第12版

上册

BRAUNWALD'S
HEART DISEASE
A TEXTBOOK OF CARDIOVASCULAR MEDICINE

BRAUNWALD
心脏病学

(影印中文导读版)

第12版

上册

BRAUNWALD'S
HEART DISEASE
A TEXTBOOK OF CARDIOVASCULAR MEDICINE

BRAUNWALD
心脏病学
(影印中文导读版)

编审委员会顾问专家　高润霖
编审委员会主任委员　吴永健　张　健　姚　焰

Edited by

PETER LIBBY, MD
Mallinckrodt Professor of Medicine
Harvard Medical School
Brigham and Women's Hospital
Boston, Massachusetts

ROBERT O. BONOW, MD
Max and Lilly Goldberg Distinguished Professor of Cardiology
Department of Medicine
Northwestern University Feinberg School of Medicine
Chicago, Illinois

DOUGLAS L. MANN, MD
Lewin Distinguished Professor of Cardiovascular Disease
Washington University School of Medicine in St. Louis
Saint Louis, Missouri

GORDON F. TOMASELLI, MD
Professor of Medicine (Cardiology)
The Marilyn and Stanley M. Katz Dean
Albert Einstein College of Medicine
Executive Vice President and Chief Academic Officer
Montefiore Medicine
Bronx, New York

DEEPAK L. BHATT, MD, MPH
Executive Director of Interventional Cardiovascular Programs
Brigham and Women's Hospital
Senior Physician
Brigham and Women's Hospital
Professor of Medicine
Harvard Medical School
Boston, Massachusetts

SCOTT D. SOLOMON, MD
The Edward D. Frohlich Distinguished Chair
Professor of Medicine
Harvard Medical School
Senior Physician
Brigham and Women's Hospital
Boston, Massachusetts

Founding Editor and Online Editor

EUGENE BRAUNWALD, MD, MD(Hon), ScD(Hon), FRCP
Distinguished Hersey Professor of Medicine
Harvard Medical School
Founding Chairman, TIMI Study Group
Brigham and Women's Hospital
Boston, Massachusetts

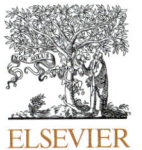

ELSEVIER

Braunwald XINZANGBINGXUE（DI 12 BAN）（YINGYIN ZHONGWEN DAODUBAN）（SHANGCE）

图书在版编目（CIP）数据

Braunwald 心脏病学：第 12 版：影印中文导读版：上下册＝Braunwald's Heart Disease：A Textbook of Cardiovascular Medicine，12th edition：英文 /（美）彼得·利贝（Peter Libby）等原著 . —北京：北京大学医学出版社，2023.3
ISBN 978-7-5659-2805-5

Ⅰ. ① B… Ⅱ. ①彼… Ⅲ. ①心脏病学－英文 Ⅳ. ① R541

中国国家版本馆 CIP 数据核字（2023）第 019315 号

北京市版权局著作权合同登记号：图字：01-2022-6707

Elsevier (Singapore) Pte Ltd.
3 Killiney Road, #08-01 Winsland House I, Singapore 239519
Tel: (65) 6349-0200; Fax: (65) 6733-1817

Braunwald's Heart Disease: A Textbook of Cardiovascular Medicine, 12th edition
Copyright © 2022 by Elsevier Inc. All rights reserved.
Previous editions copyrighted 2019, 2015, 2012, 2008, 2005, 2001, 1997, 1992, 1988, 1984, 1980 by Elsevier Inc.
ISBN-13: 9780323824682

This English Adaptation of Braunwald's Heart Disease: A Textbook of Cardiovascular Medicine, 12th edition by Peter Libby, Robert O. Bonow, Douglas L. Mann, Gordon F. Tomaselli, Deepak L. Bhatt, Scott D. Solomon was undertaken by Peking University Medical Press and is published by arrangement with Elsevier (Singapore) Pte Ltd.
Braunwald's Heart Disease: A Textbook of Cardiovascular Medicine, 12th edition by Peter Libby, Robert O. Bonow, Douglas L. Mann, Gordon F. Tomaselli, Deepak L. Bhatt, Scott D. Solomon 由北京大学医学出版社进行改编影印，并根据北京大学医学出版社与爱思唯尔（新加坡）私人有限公司的协议约定出版。

ISBN: 978-7-5659-2805-5
Copyright © 2023 by Elsevier (Singapore) Pte Ltd. and Peking University Medical Press.
All rights reserved. No part of this publication may be reproduced or transmitted in any form or by any means, electronic or mechanical, including photocopying, recording, or any information storage and retrieval system, without permission in writing from Elsevier (Singapore) Pte Ltd. and Peking University Medical Press. Online resources are not available with this adaptation. 本书不包含英文原版配套电子资源。

Notice

The adaptation has been undertaken by Peking University Medical Press at its sole responsibility. Practitioners and researchers must always rely on their own experience and knowledge in evaluating and using any information, methods, compounds or experiments described herein. Because of rapid advances in the medical sciences, in particular, independent verification of diagnoses and drug dosages should be made. To the fullest extent of the law, no responsibility is assumed by Elsevier, authors, editors or contributors in relation to the adaptation or for any injury and/or damage to persons or property as a matter of products liability, negligence or otherwise, or from any use or operation of any methods, products, instructions, or ideas contained in the material herein.

Published in China by Peking University Medical Press under special arrangement with Elsevier (Singapore) Pte Ltd. This edition is authorized for sale in the People's Republic of China only, excluding Hong Kong SAR, Macau SAR and Taiwan. Unauthorized export of this edition is a violation of the contract.

Braunwald 心脏病学（第 12 版）（影印中文导读版）（上册）

原　　著：	Peter Libby　Robert O. Bonow　Douglas L. Mann　Gordon F. Tomaselli　Deepak L. Bhatt　Scott D. Solomon
出版发行：	北京大学医学出版社
地　　址：	（100191）北京市海淀区学院路 38 号　北京大学医学部院内
电　　话：	发行部 010-82802230；图书邮购 010-82802495
网　　址：	http://www.pumpress.com.cn
E-mail：	booksale@bjmu.edu.cn
印　　刷：	北京信彩瑞禾印刷厂
经　　销：	新华书店
责任编辑：	高　瑾　　责任校对：靳新强　　责任印制：李　啸
开　　本：	889 mm×1194 mm　1/16　印张：127.75　字数：4100 千字
版　　次：	2023 年 3 月第 1 版　2023 年 3 月第 1 次印刷
书　　号：	ISBN 978-7-5659-2805-5
定　　价：	980.00 元（上下册）

版权所有，违者必究

（凡属质量问题请与本社发行部联系退换）

BRAUNWALD 心脏病学
第 12 版（影印中文导读版）
编审委员会

编审委员会顾问专家
  高润霖 中国医学科学院阜外医院

编审委员会主任委员
  吴永健 中国医学科学院阜外医院
  张　健 中国医学科学院阜外医院
  姚　焰 中国医学科学院阜外医院

编审委员会副主任委员
  蒋雄京 中国医学科学院阜外医院
  柳志红 中国医学科学院阜外医院
  唐熠达 北京大学第三医院
  杨　清 天津医科大学总医院
  程　翔 华中科技大学同济医学院附属协和医院
  陶　凌 空军军医大学西京医院
  李　悦 哈尔滨医科大学附属第一医院
  张　力 上海交通大学医学院附属新华医院

编审委员会委员
  吴永健 **中国医学科学院阜外医院**
  王　媛 首都医科大学附属北京友谊医院
  武德崴 首都医科大学宣武医院
  张丽华 中国医学科学院阜外医院
  王宇彬 首都医科大学宣武医院
  王彬成 中国医学科学院阜外医院
  王墨扬 中国医学科学院阜外医院
  牛冠男 中国医学科学院阜外医院

周　政　　中国医学科学院阜外医院
陈　阳　　中国医学科学院阜外医院
丰德京　　中国医学科学院阜外医院
张宇轩　　中国医学科学院阜外医院
张　健　　中国医学科学院阜外医院
贺春晖　　中国医学科学院阜外医院
冉　君　　中国医学科学院阜外医院
靳晓萌　　中国医学科学院阜外医院
李心晴　　中国医学科学院阜外医院
齐　晨　　中国医学科学院阜外医院
辛桉燃　　中国医学科学院阜外医院
陈安天　　中国医学科学院阜外医院
姚　焰　　中国医学科学院阜外医院
吴灵敏　　中国医学科学院阜外医院
张筑欣　　中国医学科学院阜外医院
范思洋　　首都医科大学附属北京朝阳医院
李　乐　　中国医学科学院阜外医院
杜忠鹏　　中国医学科学院阜外医院深圳医院
李晓飞　　中国医学科学院阜外医院
蒋雄京　　中国医学科学院阜外医院
董　徽　　中国医学科学院阜外医院
李弘武　　中国医学科学院阜外医院
柳志红　　中国医学科学院阜外医院
赵　青　　中国医学科学院阜外医院
胡美曦　　中国医学科学院阜外医院
罗　勤　　中国医学科学院阜外医院
高璐阳　　中国医学科学院阜外医院
张　毅　　中国医学科学院阜外医院
章思铖　　中国医学科学院阜外医院
赵智慧　　中国医学科学院阜外医院
李　欣　　中国医学科学院阜外医院
段安琪　　中国医学科学院阜外医院
黄志华　　中国医学科学院阜外医院
唐熠达　　北京大学第三医院
汪京嘉　　北京大学第三医院

温　军	北京大学第三医院
张　阔	北京大学第三医院
王远耕硕	北京大学第三医院
王旭梁	北京大学第三医院
孟祥彬	北京大学第三医院
王文尧	北京大学第三医院
李　晨	北京大学第三医院
郑一天	北京大学第三医院
杨　杰	北京大学第三医院
祁　雨	北京大学第三医院
郑济林	北京大学第三医院
曹宝山	北京大学第三医院
高　峻	北京大学第三医院
宋璟景	北京大学第三医院
任佳梦	北京大学第三医院
杨　清	**天津医科大学总医院**
周　欣	天津医科大学总医院
孙蓬飞	天津医科大学总医院
韩　旭	天津医科大学总医院
陶西西	天津医科大学总医院
孙浩楠	天津医科大学总医院
吴肇贵	天津医科大学总医院
李　晟	天津医科大学总医院
陈晓智	天津医科大学总医院
刘文楠	天津医科大学总医院
李　治	天津医科大学总医院
王卓群	天津医科大学总医院
宋习文	天津医科大学总医院
裴崇哲	天津医科大学总医院
程　翔	**华中科技大学同济医学院附属协和医院**
卢玉枝	华中科技大学同济医学院附属协和医院
苏冠华	华中科技大学同济医学院附属协和医院
王　亚	华中科技大学同济医学院附属协和医院
江　颖	华中科技大学同济医学院附属协和医院
张凌雪	华中科技大学同济医学院附属协和医院

陈　儒　　华中科技大学同济医学院附属协和医院
余刘玉　　华中科技大学同济医学院附属协和医院
杨　芬　　华中科技大学同济医学院附属协和医院
毛小香　　华中科技大学同济医学院附属协和医院
潘雅杰　　华中科技大学同济医学院附属协和医院
黄丹丹　　华中科技大学同济医学院附属协和医院

陶　凌　　空军军医大学西京医院
王汝涛　　空军军医大学西京医院

李　悦　　哈尔滨医科大学附属第一医院
曹宇开　　哈尔滨医科大学附属第一医院
洪　勇　　哈尔滨医科大学附属第一医院
高　强　　哈尔滨医科大学附属第一医院
虞　辉　　哈尔滨医科大学附属第一医院

张　力　　上海交通大学医学院附属新华医院
徐肖磊　　上海交通大学医学院附属新华医院

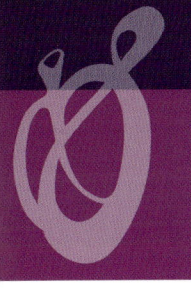

原著者名单

Keith D. Aaronson, MD, MS
Bertram Pitt MD Collegiate Professor of Cardiovascular Medicine
Professor of Internal Medicine
Division of Cardiovascular Medicine
University of Michigan
Ann Arbor, Michigan
Chapter 59. Mechanical Circulatory Support

Michael J. Ackerman, MD, PhD
Windland Smith Rice Cardiovascular Genomics Research Professor
Professor of Medicine, Pediatrics, and Pharmacology
Mayo Clinic College of Medicine and Science
Department of Cardiovascular Medicine (Division of Heart Rhythm Services and the Windland Smith Rice Genetic Heart Rhythm Clinic)
Department of Molecular Pharmacology & Experimental Therapeutics (Windland Smith Rice Sudden Death Genomics Laboratory)
Department of Pediatric and Adolescent Medicine (Division of Pediatric Cardiology)
Mayo Clinic
Rochester, Minnesota
Chapter 63. Genetics of Cardiac Arrhythmias

Philip A. Ades, MD
Endowed Professor of Medicine
Division of Cardiology
University of Vermont College of Medicine
Director, Cardiac Rehabilitation and Prevention
University of Vermont Medical Center
Burlington, Vermont
Chapter 15. Exercise Physiology and Exercise Electrocardiographic Testing

Christine M. Albert, MD
Chair and Professor of Cardiology
Smidt Heart Institute, Cedars-Sinai Medical Center
Los Angeles, California
Chapter 70. Cardiac Arrest and Sudden Cardiac Death

Michelle A. Albert, MD, MPH
Professor of Medicine
Director, Center for the Study of Adversity and Cardiovascular Disease (NURTURE Center)
University of California at San Francisco
San Francisco, California
Chapter 93. Heart Disease in Racially and Ethnically Diverse Populations

Mark J. Alberts, MD
Chief of Neurology
Hartford Hospital
Hartford, Connecticut;
Co-Physician-in-Chief
Ayer Neuroscience Institute
Hartford HealthCare
Professor of Neurology
University of Connecticut
Storrs, Connecticut
Chapter 45. Prevention and Management of Ischemic Stroke

Sadeer Al-Kindi, MD
Assistant Professor of Medicine
Case Western Reserve University
Harrington Heart and Vascular Institute
University Hospitals Cleveland Medical Center
Cleveland, Ohio
Chapter 3. Impact of the Environment on Cardiovascular Health

Nandan S. Anavekar, MBBCh
Professor of Medicine
Department of Cardiovascular Diseases
Department of Radiology
Mayo Clinic College of Medicine and Science
Rochester, Minnesota
Chapter 80. Infectious Endocarditis and Infections of Indwelling Devices

Zachi Attia, PhD
Department of Cardiovascular Medicine
Mayo Clinic College of Medicine and Science
Rochester, Minnesota
Chapter 11. Artificial Intelligence in Cardiovascular Medicine

Sonya V. Babu-Narayan, MBBS, BSc, PhD, FRCP
Adult Congenital Heart Disease
Royal Brompton Hospital
Reader, National Heart and Lung Institute
Imperial College London
London, United Kingdom
Chapter 82. Congenital Heart Disease in the Adolescent and Adult

Larry M. Baddour, MD
Professor of Medicine
Mayo Clinic College of Medicine and Science
Rochester, Minnesota
Chapter 80. Infectious Endocarditis and Infections of Indwelling Devices

Aaron L. Baggish, MD
Associate Professor of Medicine
Harvard Medical School
Director, Cardiovascular Performance Program
Massachusetts General Hospital
Boston, Massachusetts
Chapter 32. Exercise and Sports Cardiology

C. Noel Bairey Merz, MD
Women's Guild Endowed Chair in Women's Health
Director, Barbra Streisand Women's Heart Center
Erika J. Glazer Women's Heart Research Initiative Director
Director, Linda Joy Pollin Women's Heart Health Program
Barbra Streisand Women's Heart Center
Cedars-Sinai Heart Institute
Los Angeles, California
Chapter 91. Cardiovascular Disease in Women

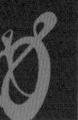

George L. Bakris, MD, MA
Professor of Medicine
Section of Endocrinology, Diabetes and Metabolism
Director, American Heart Association Comprehensive Hypertension Center
UChicago Medicine
Chicago, Illinois
Chapter 26. Systemic Hypertension: Mechanisms, Diagnosis, and Treatment

Gary J. Balady, MD
Professor of Medicine
Boston University School of Medicine
Director, Non-Invasive Cardiovascular Laboratories
Boston Medical Center
Boston, Massachusetts
Chapter 15. Exercise Physiology and Exercise Electrocardiographic Testing

David T. Balzer, MD
Professor of Pediatrics
Division of Pediatric Cardiology
Washington University School of Medicine in St. Louis
Saint Louis, Missouri
Chapter 83. Catheter-Based Treatment of Congenital Heart Disease in Adults

Joshua A. Beckman, MD
Professor of Medicine
Division of Cardiovascular Medicine
Vanderbilt University College of Medicine
Director, Section of Vascular Medicine
Vanderbilt University Medical Center
Nashville, Tennessee
Chapter 23. Anesthesia and Noncardiac Surgery in Patients with Heart Disease

Donald M. Bers, PhD
Distinguished Professor and Chair
Department of Pharmacology
University of California, Davis
Davis, California
Chapter 46. Mechanisms of Cardiac Contraction and Relaxation

Aruni Bhatnagar, PhD
Professor of Medicine
University of Louisville
Louisville, Kentucky
Chapter 28. Cardiovascular Disease Risk of Nicotine and Tobacco Products

Deepak L. Bhatt, MD, MPH
Executive Director of Interventional Cardiovascular Programs
Brigham and Women's Hospital
Senior Physician
Brigham and Women's Hospital
Professor of Medicine
Harvard Medical School
Boston, Massachusetts
Chapter 41. Percutaneous Coronary Intervention
Chapter 44. Treatment of Noncoronary Obstructive Vascular Disease

Bernadette Biondi, MD
Professor of Internal Medicine
Department of Clinical Medicine and Surgery
Federico II University
Naples, Italy
Chapter 96. Endocrine Disorders and Cardiovascular Disease

Ron Blankstein, MD
Associate Director, Cardiovascular Imaging Program
Director, Cardiac Computed Tomography
Co-Director, Cardiovascular Imaging Training Program
Brigham and Women's Hospital
Professor of Medicine and Radiology
Harvard Medical School
Boston, Massachusetts
Chapter 20. Cardiac Computed Tomography

Erin A. Bohula, MD, DPhil
TIMI Study Group and Division of Cardiology
Brigham and Women's Hospital
Harvard Medical School
Boston, Massachusetts
Chapter 38. ST-Elevation Myocardial Infarction: Management

Marc P. Bonaca, MD, MPH
Executive Director
CPC Clinical Research
Professor of Medicine
Cardiology and Vascular Medicine
University of Colorado
Aurora, Colorado
Chapter 35. Approach to the Patient with Chest Pain
Chapter 43. Peripheral Artery Diseases

Robert O. Bonow, MD
Max and Lilly Goldberg Distinguished Professor of Cardiology
Department of Medicine
Northwestern University Feinberg School of Medicine
Chicago, Illinois
Chapter 72. Aortic Valve Stenosis
Chapter 73. Aortic Regurgitation
Chapter 76. Mitral Regurgitation

Barry A. Borlaug, MD
Professor of Medicine
Mayo Medical School
Director, Circulatory Failure Research
Consultant, Cardiovascular Diseases
Mayo Clinic College of Medicine and Science
Rochester, Minnesota
Chapter 46. Mechanisms of Cardiac Contraction and Relaxation

Jason S. Bradfield, MD
Associate Professor of Medicine
Director, Specialized Program for Ventricular Tachycardia
UCLA Cardiac Arrhythmia Center
Ronald Reagan UCLA Medical Center
Los Angeles, California
Chapter 102. Cardiovascular Manifestations of Autonomic Disorders

Eugene Braunwald, MD, MD(Hon), ScD(Hon), FRCP
Distinguished Hersey Professor of Medicine
Harvard Medical School
Founding Chairman, TIMI Study Group
Brigham and Women's Hospital
Boston, Massachusetts
Chapter 1. Cardiovascular Disease: Past, Present, and Future
Chapter 39. Non-ST Elevation Acute Coronary Syndromes

Alan C. Braverman, MD
Alumni Endowed Professor in Cardiovascular Diseases
Director, Marfan Syndrome and Aortopathy Clinic
Washington University School of Medicine in St. Louis
Director, Inpatient Cardiology Firm
Barnes-Jewish Hospital
Saint Louis, Missouri
Chapter 42. Diseases of the Aorta

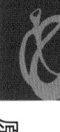

John E. Brush Jr., MD
Senior Medical Director
Sentara Health Research Center
Sentara Healthcare
Professor of Medicine
Department of Internal Medicine
Eastern Virginia Medical School
Norfolk, Virginia
Chapter 5. Clinical Decision-Making in Cardiology

Hugh Calkins, MD
Catherine Ellen Poindexter Professor of Cardiology
Professor of Medicine
Director, Cardiac Arrhythmia Service
The Johns Hopkins Medical Institutions
Baltimore, Maryland
Chapter 66. Atrial Fibrillation: Clinical Features, Mechanisms, and Management
Chapter 71. Hypotension and Syncope

John M. Canty Jr., MD
SUNY Distinguished and Albert and Elizabeth Rekate Professor of Medicine
Division of Cardiovascular Medicine
Jacobs School of Medicine and Biomedical Sciences
University at Buffalo
Buffalo, New York
Chapter 36. Coronary Blood Flow and Myocardial Ischemia

Robert M. Carney, PhD
Professor of Psychiatry
Washington University School of Medicine in St. Louis
Saint Louis, Missouri
Chapter 99. Psychiatric and Psychosocial Aspects of Cardiovascular Disease

Y.S. Chandrashekhar, MD
Professor of Medicine
Division of Cardiology
University of Minnesota
Chief of Cardiology
VA Medical Center
Minneapolis, Minnesota
Chapter 75. Mitral Stenosis

Peng-Shen Chen, MD
Cedars-Sinai Medical Center
Los Angeles, California
Chapter 71. Hypotension and Syncope

Mina K. Chung, MD
Professor of Medicine
Cardiovascular and Metabolic Sciences
Lerner Research Institute
Cleveland Clinic Lerner College of Medicine of Case Western Reserve University
Staff, Cardiovascular Medicine
Cleveland Clinic
Cleveland, Ohio
Chapter 69. Pacemakers and Implantable Cardioverter-Defibrillators

Leslie T. Cooper Jr., MD
Professor of Medicine
Chair, Department of Vascular Medicine
Mayo Clinic
Jacksonville, Florida
Chapter 55. Myocarditis

Mark A. Creager, MD
Professor of Medicine and Surgery
Geisel School of Medicine at Dartmouth
Hanover, New Hampshire;
Director, Heart and Vascular Center
Heart and Vascular Center
Dartmouth-Hitchcock Medical Center
Lebanon, New Hampshire
Chapter 43. Peripheral Artery Diseases

Paul C. Cremer, MD
Assistant Professor of Medicine
Cleveland Clinic Lerner College of Medicine of Case Western Reserve University
Associate Director of Cardiovascular Training Program
Cleveland Clinic Foundation
Cleveland Clinic
Cleveland, Ohio
Chapter 86. Pericardial Diseases

Juan A. Crestanello, MD
Professor of Surgery
Mayo Clinic College of Medicine and Science
Rochester, Minnesota
Chapter 80. Infectious Endocarditis and Infections of Indwelling Devices

Anne B. Curtis, MD
Charles and Mary Bauer Professor and Chair
SUNY Distinguished Professor
Department of Medicine
Jacobs School of Medicine and Biomedical Sciences
University at Buffalo
Buffalo, New York
Chapter 61. Approach to the Patient with Cardiac Arrhythmias

George D. Dangas, MD, PhD
Professor of Medicine (Cardiology)
Zena and Michael A Wiener Cardiovascular Institute
Icahn School of Medicine at Mount Sinai
New York, New York
Chapter 21. Coronary Angiography and Intravascular Imaging

James P. Daubert, MD
Professor of Medicine
Cardiology (Electrophysiology)
Duke University Medical Center
Durham, North Carolina
Chapter 69. Pacemakers and Implantable Cardioverter-Defibrillators

James A. de Lemos, MD
Professor of Medicine
Sweetheart Ball-Kern Wildenthal MD PhD Distinguished Chair in Cardiology
UT Southwestern Medical Center
Dallas, Texas
Chapter 40. Stable Ischemic Heart Disease

Jean-Pierre Després, PhD
Professor
Kinesiology Department
Université Laval
Scientific Director
VITAM – Centre de recherche en santé durable
Centre intégré universitaire de santé et de services sociaux de la Capitale-Nationale
Québec City, Québec, Canada
Chapter 30. Obesity: Medical and Surgical Management

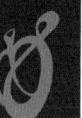

Stephen Devries, MD
Executive Director
Gaples Institute for Integrative Cardiology
Deerfield, Illinois;
Division of Cardiology
Northwestern University Feinberg School of Medicine
Chicago, Illinois
Chapter 34. Integrative Approaches to the Management of Patients with Heart Disease

Marcelo F. Di Carli, MD
Seltzer Family Professor of Radiology and Medicine
Harvard Medical School
Executive Director, Cardiovascular Imaging Program
Chief, Division of Nuclear Medicine and Molecular Imaging
Brigham and Women's Hospital
Boston, Massachusetts
Chapter 18. Nuclear Cardiology

Sharmila Dorbala, MD, MPH
Professor of Radiology
Harvard Medical School
Director, Nuclear Cardiology
Division of Nuclear Medicine and Molecular Imaging
Brigham and Women's Hospital
Boston, Massachusetts
Chapter 18. Nuclear Cardiology

Adam L. Dorfman, MD
Professor
Departments of Pediatrics and Radiology
Director, Non-Invasive Imaging, Division of Pediatric Cardiology
University of Michigan Medical School
C.S. Mott Children's Hospital
Ann Arbor, Michigan
Chapter 82. Congenital Heart Disease in the Adolescent and Adult

Dirk J. Duncker, MD, PhD
Professor of Experimental Cardiology
Department of Cardiology
Erasmus MC, University Medical Center Rotterdam
Rotterdam, The Netherlands
Chapter 36. Coronary Blood Flow and Myocardial Ischemia

Kenneth A. Ellenbogen, MD
Martha M. and Harold W. Kimmerling Professor of Cardiology
Director, Electrophysiology and Pacing
Virginia Commonwealth University School of Medicine
Richmond, Virginia
Chapter 64. Therapy for Cardiac Arrhythmias

Thomas H. Everett IV, PhD
Associate Professor of Medicine
The Krannert Institute of Cardiology and Division of Cardiology
Indiana University School of Medicine
Indianapolis, Indiana
Chapter 71. Hypotension and Syncope

James C. Fang, MD
Professor of Medicine
Division of Cardiovascular Medicine
University of Utah
Executive Director, Cardiovascular Service Line
University of Utah Health Sciences
Salt Lake City, Utah
Chapter 13. History and Physical Examination: An Evidence-Based Approach

G. Michael Felker, MD, MHS
Professor of Medicine
Vice Chief for Clinical Research
Division of Cardiology
Duke University School of Medicine
Director, Cardiovascular Research
Duke Clinical Research Institute
Durham, North Carolina
Chapter 49. Diagnosis and Management of Acute Heart Failure

Jerome L. Fleg, MD
Medical Officer
Division of Cardiovascular Sciences
National Heart, Lung, and Blood Institute
Bethesda, Maryland
Chapter 90. Cardiovascular Disease in Older Adults

Lee A. Fleisher, MD
Professor
Anesthesiology and Critical Care
Professor of Medicine
University of Pennsylvania Perelman School of Medicine
Philadelphia, Pennsylvania
Chapter 23. Anesthesia and Noncardiac Surgery in Patients with Heart Disease

Daniel E. Forman, MD
Professor of Medicine
University of Pittsburgh
Chair, Section of Geriatric Cardiology
Divisions of Geriatrics and Cardiology
University of Pittsburgh Medical Center
Director, Cardiac Rehabilitation
VA Pittsburgh Healthcare System
Pittsburgh, Pennsylvania
Chapter 90. Cardiovascular Disease in Older Adults

Kenneth E. Freedland, PhD
Professor of Psychiatry
Washington University School of Medicine in St. Louis
Saint Louis, Missouri
Chapter 99. Psychiatric and Psychosocial Aspects of Cardiovascular Disease

Paul Friedman, MD
Norman Blane & Billie Jean Harty Chair
Mayo Clinic Department of Cardiovascular Medicine Honoring Robert L. Frye, MD
Professor of Medicine
Mayo Clinic College of Medicine and Science
Rochester, Minnesota
Chapter 11. Artificial Intelligence in Cardiovascular Medicine

J. Michael Gaziano, MD, MPH
Professor of Medicine
Harvard Medical School
Chief, Division of Aging
Brigham and Women's Hospital
Director, Preventive Cardiology
VA Boston Healthcare System
Boston, Massachusetts
Chapter 2. Global Burden of Cardiovascular Disease

Thomas A. Gaziano, MD, MSc
Associate Professor
Harvard Medical School
Physician
Cardiovascular Medicine Division
Brigham & Women's Hospital
Boston, Massachusetts
Chapter 2. Global Burden of Cardiovascular Disease

Jacques Genest, MD
Professor of Medicine
Faculty of Medicine
McGill University
Research Institute of the McGill University Health Centre
Montreal, Quebec, Canada
Chapter 27. Lipoprotein Disorders and Cardiovascular Disease

Robert Gerszten, MD
Herman Dana Professor of Medicine
Harvard Medical School
Chief, Division of Cardiovascular Medicine
Beth Israel Deaconess Medical Center
Boston, Massachusetts
Chapter 8. Proteomics and Metabolomics in Cardiovascular Medicine

Linda D. Gillam, MD, MPH
Dorothy and Lloyd Huck Chair
Department of Cardiovascular Medicine
Morristown Medical Center
Morristown, New Jersey;
Professor of Medicine
Thomas Jefferson University
Philadelphia, Pennsylvania
Chapter 16. Echocardiography

John R. Giudicessi, MD, PhD
Assistant Professor of Medicine
Department of Cardiovascular Medicine (Division of Heart Rhythm Services and the Windland Smith Rice Genetic Heart Rhythm Clinic)
Mayo Clinic College of Medicine and Science
Rochester, Minnesota
Chapter 63. Genetics of Cardiac Arrhythmias

Robert P. Giugliano, MD, SM
Staff Physician
Cardiovascular Medicine
Brigham and Women's Hospital
Professor of Medicine
Harvard Medical School
Boston, Massachusetts
Chapter 39. Non-ST Elevation Acute Coronary Syndromes

Ary L. Goldberger, MD
Professor of Medicine
Harvard Medical School
Department of Medicine
Beth Israel Deaconess Medical Center
Boston, Massachusetts
Chapter 14. Electrocardiography

Jeffrey J. Goldberger, MD, MBA
Professor of Medicine
Chief, Cardiovascular Division
University of Miami Miller School of Medicine
Miami, Florida
Chapter 70. Cardiac Arrest and Sudden Cardiac Death

Samuel Z. Goldhaber, MD
Professor of Medicine
Harvard Medical School
Director, Thrombosis Research Group
Associate Chief and Clinical Director
Division of Cardiovascular Medicine
Brigham and Women's Hospital
Boston, Massachusetts
Chapter 87. Pulmonary Embolism and Deep Vein Thrombosis

William J. Groh, MD, MPH
Clinical Professor of Medicine
Medical University of South Carolina
Chief of Medicine
Ralph H. Johnson VAMC
Charleston, South Carolina
Chapter 100. Neuromuscular Disorders and Cardiovascular Disease

Martha Gulati, MD, MS
Chief of Cardiology
Professor of Medicine
University of Arizona–Phoenix
Phoenix, Arizona
Chapter 91. Cardiovascular Disease in Women

Rebecca Tung Hahn, MD
Director of Interventional Echocardiography
Center for Interventional and Vascular Therapy
Columbia University Medical Center
New York, New York
Chapter 76. Mitral Regurgitation

Gerd Hasenfuss, MD
Professor of Medicine
Chair, Department of Cardiology and Pneumology
University of Göttingen Medical Center
Göttingen, Germany
Chapter 47. Pathophysiology of Heart Failure

Howard C. Herrmann, MD
John W. Bryfogle Jr. Professor of Cardiovascular Medicine
Division of Cardiovascular Medicine
University of Pennsylvania Perelman School of Medicine
Health System Director for Interventional Cardiology
Hospital of the University of Pennsylvania
Philadelphia, Pennsylvania
Chapter 78. Transcatheter Therapies for Mitral and Tricuspid Valvular Heart Disease

Joerg Herrmann, MD
Professor of Medicine
Department of Cardiovascular Medicine
Mayo Clinic
Rochester, Minnesota
Chapter 22. Invasive Hemodynamic Diagnosis of Cardiac Disease
Chapter 57. Cardio-Oncology: Approach to the Patient

Ray E. Hershberger, MD
Professor of Internal Medicine
Director, Division of Human Genetics
Division of Cardiovascular Medicine
Section of Heart Failure and Cardiac Transplantation
Dorothy M. Davis Heart and Lung Research Institute
Wexner Medical Center at the Ohio State University
Columbus, Ohio
Chapter 52. The Dilated, Restrictive, and Infiltrative Cardiomyopathies

Carolyn Y. Ho, MD
Associate Professor of Medicine
Cardiovascular Division
Brigham and Women's Hospital
Boston, Massachusetts
Chapter 54. Hypertrophic Cardiomyopathy

Priscilla Y. Hsue, MD
Professor
Department of Medicine
University of California, San Francisco
San Francisco, California
Chapter 85. Cardiovascular Abnormalities in HIV-Infected Individuals

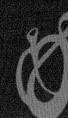

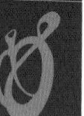

W. Gregory Hundley, MD
Professor of Medicine
Chairman, Cardiology Division
VCU School of Medicine
Director, Pauley Heart Center
Virginia Commonwealth University Health
Richmond, Virginia
Chapter 98. Tumors Affecting the Cardiovascular System

Silvio E. Inzucchi, MD
Professor, Internal Medicine (Endocrinology)
Yale University School of Medicine
Clinical Chief, Endocrinology
Director, Yale Diabetes Center
Yale-New Haven Hospital
New Haven, Connecticut
Chapter 31. Diabetes and the Cardiovascular System

Francine L. Jacobson, MD, MPH
Thoracic Radiologist
Brigham and Women's Hospital
Harvard Medical School
Boston, Massachusetts
Chapter 17. Chest Radiography in Cardiovascular Disease

James L. Januzzi Jr., MD
Physician
Cardiology Division
Massachusetts General Hospital
Hutter Family Professor of Medicine
Harvard Medical School
Boston, Massachusetts
Chapter 48. Approach to the Patient with Heart Failure

Karen E. Joynt Maddox, MD, MPH
Associate Professor of Medicine
Cardiovascular Division
Washington University School of Medicine in St. Louis
Co-Director, Center for Health Economics and Policy
Institute for Public Health at Washington University
Saint Louis, Missouri
Chapter 6. Impact of Health Care Policy on Quality, Outcomes, and Equity in Cardiovascular Disease

Jonathan M. Kalman, MBBS, PhD
Director of Cardiac Electrophysiology
Department of Cardiology
Royal Melbourne Hospital, Melbourne
Professor of Medicine
University of Melbourne
Melbourne, Victoria, Australia
Chapter 65. Supraventricular Tachycardias

Suraj Kapa, MD
Assistant Professor of Medicine
Cardiovascular Diseases
Mayo Clinic College of Medicine and Science
Rochester, Minnesota
Chapter 11. Artificial Intelligence in Cardiovascular Medicine

Morton J. Kern, MD
Professor of Medicine
University California, Irvine
Orange, California;
Chief of Medicine and Cardiology
Veterans Administration Long Beach Healthcare System
Long Beach, California
Chapter 22. Invasive Hemodynamic Diagnosis of Cardiac Disease

Scott Kinlay, MBBS, PhD
Chief, Cardiology (acting)
Director Cardiac Catheterization Laboratory and Vascular Medicine
VA Boston Healthcare System
West Roxbury, Massachusetts
Physician, Cardiovascular Division
Brigham and Women's Hospital
Associate Professor in Medicine
Harvard Medical School
Adjunct Associate Professor in Medicine
Boston University Medical School
Boston, Massachusetts
Chapter 44. Treatment of Noncoronary Obstructive Vascular Disease

Allan L. Klein, MD, FRCP(C)
Professor of Medicine
Cleveland Clinic Lerner College of Medicine of Case Western Reserve University
Director, Center for the Diagnosis and Treatment of Pericardial Diseases
Department of Cardiovascular Medicine
Heart, Vascular and Thoracic Institute
Cleveland Clinic
Cleveland, Ohio
Chapter 86. Pericardial Diseases

Robert A. Kloner, MD, PhD
Professor of Medicine (Clinical Scholar)
Cardiovascular Division
Keck School of Medicine of University of Southern California
Los Angeles, California;
Chief Science Officer
Scientific Director of Cardiovascular Research Institute
Huntington Medical Research Institutes
Pasadena, California
Chapter 84. Cardiomyopathies Induced by Drugs or Toxins

Kirk U. Knowlton, MD
Director of Cardiovascular Research
Intermountain Healthcare Heart Institute
Adjunct Professor
Department of Medicine
University of Utah
Salt Lake City, Utah;
Professor Emeritus of Medicine
University of California, San Diego
La Jolla, California
Chapter 55. Myocarditis

Eric V. Krieger, MD
Professor of Medicine
Division of Cardiology
University of Washington School of Medicine
Director, Adult Congenital Heart Service
University of Washington Medical Center
Seattle Children's Hospital
Seattle, Washington
Chapter 82. Congenital Heart Disease in the Adolescent and Adult

Harlan M. Krumholz, MD, SM
Harold H. Hines, Jr. Professor of Medicine
Section of Cardiovascular Medicine
Department of Medicine
Department of Health Policy and Management
School of Public Health
Yale School of Medicine
Center for Outcomes Research and Evaluation
Yale New Haven Hospital
New Haven, Connecticut
Chapter 5. Clinical Decision-Making in Cardiology

Dharam J. Kumbhani, MD, SM
Associate Professor of Medicine
Section Chief, Interventional Cardiology
Department of Internal Medicine
University of Texas Southwestern Medical Center
Dallas, Texas
Chapter 41. Percutaneous Coronary Intervention

Raymond Y. Kwong, MD, MPH
Professor of Medicine
Harvard Medical School
Director of Cardiac Magnetic Resonance Imaging
Cardiovascular Division
Brigham and Women's Hospital
Boston, Massachusetts
Chapter 19. Cardiovascular Magnetic Resonance Imaging

Bonnie Ky, MD, MSCE
Associate Professor of Medicine and Epidemiology
Division of Cardiovascular Medicine
Senior Scholar
Department of Biostatistics, Epidemiology and Informatics
University of Pennsylvania School of Medicine
Philadelphia, Pennsylvania
Chapter 56. Cardio-Oncology: Managing Cardiotoxic Effects of Cancer Therapies

Carolyn S.P. Lam, MBBS, PhD, MRCP, MS
Professor
Cardiovascular Academic Clinical Program
Duke–National University of Singapore
Senior Consultant Cardiologist
National Heart Centre Singapore
Singapore
Chapter 51. Heart Failure with Preserved and Mildly Reduced Ejection Fraction

Eric Larose, DVM, MD, FRCPC
Professor and Head of Cardiology Division
Department of Medicine
Chair of Research & Innovation in Cardiovascular Imaging
Université Laval
Cardiologist, Institut universitaire de cardiologie et de pneumologie de Québec – Université Laval
Quebec City, Quebec, Canada
Chapter 30. Obesity: Medical and Surgical Management

John M. Lasala, MD, PhD
Professor of Medicine
Director, Structural Heart Disease Program
Cardiology Division
Washington University School of Medicine in St. Louis
Saint Louis, Missouri
Chapter 83. Catheter-Based Treatment of Congenital Heart Disease in Adults

Daniel J. Lenihan, MD
President, International Cardio-Oncology Society
Professor of Medicine
Director, Cardio-Oncology Center of Excellence
Cardiovascular Division
Washington University School of Medicine in St. Louis
Saint Louis, Missouri
Chapter 98. Tumors Affecting the Cardiovascular System

Eric J. Lenze, MD
Professor of Psychiatry
Washington University School of Medicine in St. Louis
Saint Louis, Missouri
Chapter 99. Psychiatric and Psychosocial Aspects of Cardiovascular Disease

Martin B. Leon, MD
The Mallah Family Professor of Cardiology
Director, Center for Interventional Vascular Therapy
Columbia University Irving Medical Center
NY Presbyterian Hospital
Founder and Chairman Emeritus
Cardiovascular Research Foundation
New York, New York
Chapter 74. Transcatheter Aortic Valve Replacement

Martin M. LeWinter, MD
Professor Emeritus of Medicine and Molecular Physiology and Biophysics
Larner College of Medicine at the University of Vermont
Attending Cardiologist
University of Vermont Medical Center
Burlington, Vermont
Chapter 86. Pericardial Diseases

Peter Libby, MD
Mallinckrodt Professor of Medicine
Harvard Medical School
Brigham and Women's Hospital
Boston, Massachusetts
Chapter 10. Biomarkers and Use in Precision Medicine
Chapter 24. The Vascular Biology of Atherosclerosis
Chapter 25. Primary Prevention of Cardiovascular Disease
Chapter 27. Lipoprotein Disorders and Cardiovascular Disease
Chapter 37. ST-Elevation Myocardial Infarction: Pathophysiology and Clinical Evolution

JoAnn Lindenfeld, MD
Professor of Medicine
Samuel S Riven MD Directorship in Cardiology
Vanderbilt University Medical Center
Nashville, Tennessee
Chapter 58. Devices for Monitoring and Managing Heart Failure

Brian R. Lindman, MD, MSc
Associate Professor of Medicine
Medical Director, Structural Heart and Valve Center
Cardiovascular Division
Vanderbilt University Medical Center
Nashville, Tennessee
Chapter 72. Aortic Valve Stenosis

Michael J. Mack, MD
Chair, Cardiovascular Service Line
Baylor Scott & White Health
President, Baylor Scott & White Research Institute
Dallas, Texas
Chapter 74. Transcatheter Aortic Valve Replacement

Mohammad Madjid, MD, MS
Associate Professor of Medicine
McGovern Medical School
University of Texas Health Science Center at Houston
Interventional Cardiologist
Heart and Vascular Institute
Memorial Hermann Hospital
Houston, Texas
Chapter 94. Endemic and Pandemic Viral Illnesses and Cardiovascular Disease: Influenza and COVID-19

Douglas L. Mann, MD
Lewin Distinguished Professor of Cardiovascular Disease
Washington University School of Medicine
Saint Louis, Missouri
Chapter 47. Pathophysiology of Heart Failure
Chapter 48. Approach to the Patient With Heart Failure
Chapter 50. Management of Heart Failure Patients with Reduced Ejection Fraction

Bradley A. Maron, MD
Associate Professor of Medicine
Division of Cardiovascular Medicine
Brigham and Women's Hospital
Harvard Medical School
Department of Cardiology
Boston VA Healthcare System
Boston, Massachusetts
Chapter 88. Pulmonary Hypertension

Nikolaus Marx, MD
Professor of Medicine / Cardiology
Head of the Department of Internal Medicine I
University Hospital Aachen
Aachen, Germany
Chapter 31. Diabetes and the Cardiovascular System

Justin C. Mason, PhD, FRCP
Professor of Vascular Rheumatology
Vascular Sciences and Rheumatology
Imperial College London
London, United Kingdom
Chapter 97. Rheumatic Diseases and the Cardiovascular System

Mathew S. Maurer, MD
Arnold and Arlene Goldstein Professor of Cardiology
Professor of Medicine
Columbia University College of Physicians and Surgeons
Center for Advanced Cardiac Care
Columbia University Medical Center
Director, Clinical Cardiovascular Research Laboratory for the Elderly
New York, New York
Chapter 53. Cardiac Amyloidosis

Peter A. McCullough, MD, MPH
Consultant Cardiologist
Clinical Professor of Medicine
Department of Internal Medicine
Texas A&M College of Medicine
Dallas, Texas
Chapter 101. Interface Between Renal Disease and Cardiovascular Illness

Darren K. McGuire, MD, MHSc
Professor, Internal Medicine
Division of Cardiology
University of Texas Southwestern Medical Center
Dallas, Texas
Chapter 31. Diabetes and the Cardiovascular System

John McMurray, OBE BSc (Hons), MB ChB (Hons), MD, FRCP
Professor of Medical Cardiology
Deputy-Director (Clinical), Institute of Cardiovascular and Medical Sciences
BHF Cardiovascular Research Centre
University of Glasgow
Honorary Consultant Cardiologist
Queen Elizabeth University Hospital
Glasgow, Scotland, United Kingdom
Chapter 4. Clinical Trials in Cardiovascular Medicine

Elizabeth M. McNally, MD, PhD
Director, Center for Genetic Medicine
Northwestern University Feinberg School of Medicine
Chicago, Illinois
Chapter 100. Neuromuscular Disorders and Cardiovascular Disease

Roxana Mehran, MD
Professor of Medicine (Cardiology)
Director of Interventional Cardiovascular Research and Clinical Trials
Zena and Michael A. Wiener Cardiovascular Institute
Icahn School of Medicine at Mount Sinai
New York, New York
Chapter 21. Coronary Angiography and Intravascular Imaging

John M. Miller, MD
Professor of Medicine
Indiana University School of Medicine
Director, Cardiac Electrophysiology Services
Indiana University Health
Indianapolis, Indiana
Chapter 64. Therapy for Cardiac Arrhythmias

David M. Mirvis, MD
Professor Emeritus
Preventive Medicine
University of Tennessee College of Medicine
Memphis, Tennessee
Chapter 14. Electrocardiography

Ana Olga Mocumbi, MD, PhD
Associate Professor
Internal Medicine
Universidade Eduardo Mondlane
Head of Division
Non Communicable Diseases
Instituto Nacional de Saúde
Maputo, Mozambique
Chapter 81. Rheumatic Fever

Samia Mora, MD
Associate Professor of Medicine
Harvard Medical School
Associate Physician
Brigham and Women's Hospital
Boston, Massachusetts
Chapter 25. Primary Prevention of Cardiovascular Disease
Chapter 27. Lipoprotein Disorders and Cardiovascular Disease

Fred Morady, MD
McKay Professor of Cardiovascular Disease
Department of Medicine
University of Michigan
Ann Arbor, Michigan
Chapter 66. Atrial Fibrillation: Clinical Features, Mechanisms, and Management

Alanna A. Morris, MD, MSc
Associate Professor of Medicine
Director, Heart Failure Research
Emory University School of Medicine
Atlanta, Georgia
Chapter 93. Heart Disease in Racially and Ethnically Diverse Populations

David A. Morrow, MD, MPH
Professor of Medicine
Harvard Medical School
Boston, Massachusetts
Chapter 37. ST-Elevation Myocardial Infarction: Pathophysiology and Clinical Evolution
Chapter 38. ST-Elevation Myocardial Infarction: Management
Chapter 40. Stable Ischemic Heart Disease

Dariush Mozaffarian, MD, DrPH
Dean, Friedman School of Nutrition Science & Policy
Jean Mayer Professor of Nutrition
Tufts University School of Medicine
Boston, Massachusetts
Chapter 29. Nutrition and Cardiovascular and Metabolic Diseases

Kiran Musunuru, MD, PhD, MPH, ML
Professor of Cardiovascular Medicine and Genetics
Cardiovascular Institute
University of Pennsylvania Perelman School of Medicine
Philadelphia, Pennsylvania
Chapter 7. Applications of Genetics to Cardiovascular Medicine

Robert J. Myerburg, MD
Professor of Medicine and Physiology
Department of Medicine
University of Miami Miller School of Medicine
Miami, Florida
Chapter 70. Cardiac Arrest and Sudden Cardiac Death

Pradeep Natarajan, MD, MMSc
Director of Preventive Cardiology
Massachusetts General Hospital
Assistant Professor of Medicine
Harvard Medical School
Boston, Massachusetts;
Associate Member
Program in Medical and Population Genetics
Broad Institute of Harvard and MIT
Cambridge, Massachusetts
Chapter 7. Applications of Genetics to Cardiovascular Medicine

Stanley Nattel, MDCM
Professor
Department of Medicine
Paul-David Chair in Cardiovascular Electrophysiology
Montreal Heart Institute
University of Montreal
Montreal, Quebec, Canada
Chapter 62. Mechanisms of Cardiac Arrhythmias

Rick A. Nishimura, MD
Judd and Mary Morris Leighton Professor of Cardiovascular Diseases
Department of Cardiovascular Medicine
Mayo Clinic College of Medicine and Science
Rochester, Minnesota
Chapter 73. Aortic Regurgitation

Vuyisile T. Nkomo, MD, MPH
Cardiologist
Professor of Medicine
Department of Cardiovascular Medicine
Mayo Clinic College of Medicine and Science
Rochester, Minnesota
Chapter 77. Tricuspid, Pulmonic, and Multivalvular Disease

Peter Noseworthy, MD
Consultant
Cardiovascular Diseases
Mayo Clinic College of Medicine and Science
Rochester, Minnesota
Chapter 11. Artificial Intelligence in Cardiovascular Medicine

Patrick T. O'Gara, MD
Professor of Medicine
Harvard Medical School
Senior Physician
Cardiovascular Division
Brigham and Women's Hospital
Boston, Massachusetts
Chapter 13. History and Physical Examination: An Evidence-Based Approach
Chapter 79. Prosthetic Heart Valves

Jeffrey E. Olgin, MD
Gallo-Chatterjee Distinguished Professor
Chief, Division of Cardiology
University of California, San Francisco
San Francisco, California
Chapter 68. Bradyarrhythmias and Atrioventricular Block

Steve R. Ommen, MD
Division of Cardiovascular Diseases
Mayo Clinic College of Medicine and Science
Rochester, Minnesota
Chapter 54. Hypertrophic Cardiomyopathy

Catherine M. Otto, MD
Professor of Medicine
J. Ward Kennedy-Hamilton Endowed Chair in Cardiology
Division of Cardiology
University of Washington School of Medicine
Director, Heart Valve Clinic
Associate Director, Echocardiography
University of Washington Medical Center
Seattle, Washington
Chapter 72. Aortic Valve Stenosis

Francis D. Pagani, MD, PhD
Otto Gago MD Endowed Professor of Cardiac Surgery
Department of Cardiac Surgery
University of Michigan
Ann Arbor, Michigan
Chapter 59. Mechanical Circulatory Support

Kristen K. Patton, MD
Professor of Medicine
Division of Cardiology
University of Washington
Seattle, Washington
Chapter 68. Bradyarrhythmias and Atrioventricular Block

Patricia A. Pellikka, MD
The Betty Knight Scripps Professor of Medicine
Mayo Clinic College of Medicine and Science
Vice Chair, Academic Affairs and Faculty Development
Consultant, Department of Cardiovascular Medicine
Director, Ultrasound Research Center
Mayo Clinic
Rochester, Minnesota
Chapter 77. Tricuspid, Pulmonic, and Multivalvular Disease

Gregory Piazza, MD, MS
Staff Physician
Cardiovascular Division
Department of Medicine
Section Head, Vascular Medicine
Brigham and Women's Hospital
Boston, Massachusetts
Chapter 87. Pulmonary Embolism and Deep Vein Thrombosis

Philippe Pibarot, DVM, PhD
Professor
Department of Medicine
Québec Heart & Lung Institute
Université Laval
Québec City, Quebec, Canada
Chapter 79. Prosthetic Heart Valves

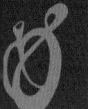

Paul Poirier, MD, PhD, FRCPC
Chief, Cardiac Prevention/Rehabilitation
Institut universitaire de cardiologie et de pneumologie de Québec – Université Laval
Professor
Faculty of Pharmacy
Université Laval
Quebec City, Quebec, Canada
Chapter 30. Obesity: Medical and Surgical Management

Dorairaj Prabhakaran, MD, DM (Cardiology), MSc, FRCP
Vice President, Research and Policy
Public Health Foundation of India
Executive Director, Centre for Chronic Disease Control
Gurgaon, Haryana, India;
Professor
Department of Epidemiology
London School of Hygiene and Tropical Medicine
London, United Kingdom
Chapter 2. Global Burden of Cardiovascular Disease

Sanjay Rajagopalan, MD
Professor of Medicine
Director, Case Cardiovascular Research Institute
Case Western Reserve University
Chief, Division of Cardiovascular Medicine
Harrington Heart and Vascular Institute
University Hospitals Cleveland Medical Center
Cleveland, Ohio
Chapter 3. Impact of the Environment on Cardiovascular Health

Michael J. Reardon, MD
Professor of Cardiothoracic Surgery
Department of Cardiovascular Surgery
Houston Methodist Hospital
Houston, Texas
Chapter 78. Transcatheter Therapies for Mitral and Tricuspid Valvular Heart Disease
Chapter 98. Tumors Affecting the Cardiovascular System

Susan Redline, MD, MPH
Peter C. Farrell Professor of Sleep Medicine
Harvard Medical School
Senior Physician
Division of Sleep and Circadian Disorders
Departments of Medicine and Neurology
Brigham and Women's Hospital
Boston, Massachusetts
Chapter 89. Sleep-Disordered Breathing and Cardiac Disease

Shereif Rezkalla, MD
Adjunct Professor of Medicine
University of Wisconsin
Madison, Wisconsin;
Department of Cardiology and Cardiovascular Research
Marshfield Clinic Health System
Marshfield, Wisconsin
Chapter 84. Cardiomyopathies Induced by Drugs or Toxins

Michael W. Rich, MD
Professor of Medicine
Division of Cardiology
Washington University School of Medicine in St. Louis
Saint Louis, Missouri
Chapter 90. Cardiovascular Disease in Older Adults
Chapter 99. Psychiatric and Psychosocial Aspects of Cardiovascular Disease

Paul M Ridker, MD, MPH
Eugene Braunwald Professor of Medicine
Harvard Medical School
Director, Center for Cardiovascular Disease Prevention
Brigham and Women's Hospital
Boston, Massachusetts
Chapter 10. Biomarkers and Use in Precision Medicine
Chapter 25. Primary Prevention of Cardiovascular Disease

Dan M. Roden, MD
Professor of Medicine, Pharmacology, and Biomedical Informatics
Senior Vice President for Personalized Medicine
Vanderbilt University School of Medicine
Nashville, Tennessee
Chapter 9. Principles of Drug Therapeutics, Pharmacogenomics, and Biologics

Frederick L. Ruberg, MD
Associate Professor of Medicine
Section of Cardiovascular Medicine
Department of Medicine and Amyloidosis Center
Boston Medical Center
Boston University School of Medicine
Boston, Massachusetts
Chapter 53. Cardiac Amyloidosis

Marc S. Sabatine, MD, MPH
Chair, TIMI Study Group
Lewis Dexter MD Distinguished Chair in Cardiovascular Medicine
Brigham and Women's Hospital
Professor of Medicine
Harvard Medical School
Boston, Massachusetts
Chapter 35. Approach to the Patient with Chest Pain

Prashanthan Sanders, MBBS, PhD
Director, Centre for Heart Rhythm Disorders
School of Medicine
University of Adelaide
Director, Cardiac Electrophysiology and Pacing
Department of Cardiology
Royal Adelaide Hospital
Director, Heart Rhythm Group
Heart Health
South Australian Health and Medical Research Institute
Adelaide, Australia
Chapter 65. Supraventricular Tachycardias

Marc Schermerhorn, MD
George H. A. Clowes Jr. Professor of Surgery
Harvard Medical School
Chief, Division of Vascular and Endovascular Surgery
Beth Israel Deaconess Medical Center
Boston, Massachusetts
Chapter 42. Diseases of the Aorta

Benjamin M. Scirica, MD, MPH
Associate Professor of Medicine
Harvard Medical School
Senior Investigator, TIMI Study Group
Associate Physician, Cardiovascular Division
Brigham and Women's Hospital
Boston, Massachusetts
Chapter 37. ST-Elevation Myocardial Infarction: Pathophysiology and Clinical Evolution

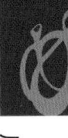

Arnold H. Seto, MD, MPA
Associate Clinical Professor
University of California, Irvine
Cardiologist
Veterans Administration Long Beach Healthcare System
Long Beach, California
Chapter 22. Invasive Hemodynamic Diagnosis of Cardiac Disease

Sanjiv J. Shah, MD
Neil Stone MD Professor of Medicine
Division of Cardiology
Northwestern University Feinberg School of Medicine
Chicago, Illinois
Chapter 51. Heart Failure with Preserved and Mildly Reduced Ejection Fraction

Shabana Shahanavaz, MBBS
Associate Professor of Pediatrics
Director, Cardiac Catheterization Laboratory
The Heart Institute
Cincinnati Children's Hospital
Cincinnati, Ohio
Chapter 83. Catheter-Based Treatment of Congenital Heart Disease in Adults

Kalyanam Shivkumar, MD, PhD
Professor of Medicine (Cardiology), Radiology, and Bioengineering
Director, UCLA Cardiac Arrhythmia Center and Electrophysiology Programs
Director, Adult Cardiac Catheterization Laboratories
Ronald Reagan UCLA Medical Center
Los Angeles, California
Chapter 102. Cardiovascular Manifestations of Autonomic Disorders

Candice K. Silversides, SM, MD
Professor of Medicine
University of Toronto Pregnancy and Heart Disease Program
Toronto, Ontario, Canada
Chapter 92. Pregnancy and Heart Disease

Samuel C. Siu, MD, SM, MBA
Professor of Medicine
Division of Cardiology
Schulich School of Medicine and Dentistry
Western University
London, Ontario, Canada
Chapter 92. Pregnancy and Heart Disease

Scott D. Solomon, MD
The Edward D. Frohlich Distinguished Chair
Professor of Medicine
Harvard Medical School
Senior Physician
Brigham and Women's Hospital
Boston, Massachusetts
Chapter 4. Clinical Trials in Cardiovascular Medicine
Chapter 16. Echocardiography
Chapter 51. Heart Failure with Preserved and Mildly Reduced Ejection Fraction
Chapter 94. Endemic and Pandemic Viral Illnesses and Cardiovascular Disease: Influenza and COVID-19

Matthew J. Sorrentino, MD
Professor of Medicine
Section of Cardiology
UChicago Medicine
Chicago, Illinois
Chapter 26. Systemic Hypertension: Mechanisms, Diagnosis, and Treatment

Randall C. Starling, MD, MPH
Professor of Medicine
Kaufman Center for Heart Failure
Heart, Thoracic and Vascular Institute
Cleveland Clinic
Cleveland, Ohio
Chapter 60. Cardiac Transplantation

William G. Stevenson, MD
Professor of Medicine
Division of Cardiology
Vanderbilt University Medical Center
Nashville, Tennessee
Chapter 67. Ventricular Arrhythmias

John R. Teerlink, MD, FRCP(UK)
Professor of Medicine
University of California School of Medicine, San Francisco,
    Director, Heart Failure
Director, Echocardiography
Section of Cardiology
San Francisco Veteran Affairs Medical Center
San Francisco, California
Chapter 49. Diagnosis and Management of Acute Heart Failure

David J. Tester, BS
Associate Professor of Medicine
Mayo Clinic College of Medicine and Science
Department of Molecular Pharmacology & Experimental Therapeutics (Windland Smith Rice Sudden Death Genomics Laboratory)
Mayo Clinic
Rochester, Minnesota
Chapter 63. Genetics of Cardiac Arrhythmias

Randal Jay Thomas, MD, MS
Professor of Medicine
Mayo Clinic Alix School of Medicine
Medical Director, Cardiac Rehabilitation Program
Division of Preventive Cardiology
Department of Cardiovascular Medicine
Mayo Clinic
Rochester, Minnesota
Chapter 33. Comprehensive Cardiac Rehabilitation

Paul D. Thompson, MD
Chief of Cardiology, Emeritus
Hartford Hospital
Hartford, Connecticut
Chapter 32. Exercise and Sports Cardiology

Gordon F. Tomaselli, MD
Professor of Medicine (Cardiology)
The Marilyn and Stanley M. Katz Dean
Albert Einstein College of Medicine
Executive Vice President and Chief Academic Officer
Montefiore Medicine
Bronx, New York
Chapter 61. Approach to the Patient with Cardiac Arrhythmias
Chapter 62. Mechanisms of Cardiac Arrhythmias
Chapter 66. Atrial Fibrillation: Clinical Features, Mechanisms, and Management
Chapter 100. Neuromuscular Disorders and Cardiovascular Disease

Mintu P. Turakhia, MD, MAS
Associate Professor of Medicine (Cardiovascular Medicine)
Executive Director, Center for Digital Health
Stanford University
Stanford, California;
Chief, Cardiac Electrophysiology
VA Palo Alto Health Care System
Palo Alto, California
Chapter 12. Wearable Devices in Cardiovascular Medicine

Anne Marie Valente, MD
Associate Professor
Pediatrics and Internal Medicine
Harvard Medical School
Director, Boston Adult Congenital Heart Program
Children's Hospital Boston
Brigham and Women's Hospital
Boston, Massachusetts
Chapter 82. Congenital Heart Disease in the Adolescent and Adult

Orly Vardeny, PharmD, MS
Associate Professor of Medicine
Center for Care Delivery and Outcomes Research
Minneapolis VA Health Care System and University of Minnesota
Minneapolis, Minnesota
Chapter 94. Endemic and Pandemic Viral Illnesses and Cardiovascular Disease: Influenza and COVID-19

David D. Waters, MD
Professor Emeritus
Department of Medicine
University of California, San Francisco
San Francisco, California
Chapter 85. Cardiovascular Abnormalities in HIV-Infected Individuals

Jeffrey I. Weitz, MD, FRCP(C)
Professor of Medicine and Biochemistry
McMaster University
Executive Director
Thrombosis and Atherosclerosis Research Institute
Hamilton, Ontario, Canada
Chapter 95. Hemostasis, Thrombosis, Fibrinolysis, and Cardiovascular Disease

Nanette Kass Wenger, MD
Professor of Medicine (Cardiology) Emeritus
Emory University School of Medicine
Consultant, Emory Heart and Vascular Center
Atlanta, Georgia
Chapter 90. Cardiovascular Disease in Older Adults

Walter R. Wilson, MD
Professor of Medicine
Mayo Clinic College of Medicine and Science
Rochester, Minnesota
Chapter 80. Infectious Endocarditis and Infections of Indwelling Devices

Justina C. Wu, MD, PhD
Assistant Professor of Medicine
Harvard Medical School
Director of Echocardiography
Brigham and Women's Hospital
Boston, Massachusetts
Chapter 16. Echocardiography

Katja Zeppenfeld, MD, PhD
Professor of Cardiology
Leiden University Medical Centre
Leiden, The Netherlands
Chapter 67. Ventricular Arrhythmias

Michael R. Zile, MD
Charles Ezra Daniels Professor of Medicine
Division of Cardiology
Medical University of South Carolina
Charleston, South Carolina
Chapter 58. Devices for Monitoring and Managing Heart Failure

To
Beryl, Oliver, and Brigitte
Pat, Rob, Sam, Laura, and Yoko
Benjamin Tan
Charlene, Sarah, Emily, and Matthew
Shanthala, Vinayak, Arjun, Ram, and Raj
Caren, Will and Lyz, Katie and Zach, and Dan

《Braunwald 心脏病学》中文导读版序言

《Braunwald 心脏病学》是培育全球心血管病医师的经典教科书，是心血管病医师的权威参考书。其内容完整、详实，既有丰富的历史沿革，又有不断更新的当代进展。从心血管病的基础研究到临床实践，用简洁明了的语言，客观生动的表述，清晰明了的图表，丰富全面的引文，充分展现了现代心血管病学的全貌。全书的每一个章节都由该领域全球最优秀的专家撰写，自出版以来，已经成为心血管病专业最具影响力和代表性的教科书和参考书，也是中国心血管病医生的必读书目。

我有幸通过参加 Braunwald 教授主持的 TIMI 全球研究等工作，直接深刻地感受到他高尚的人格和严谨的学风，科学的态度和孜孜不倦的精神。他于办公室赠送予我第 8 版《Braunwald 心脏病学》的照片作为珍贵纪念一直摆放在我的案头。陈灏珠院士曾经主持翻译了这部巨著的第 5 版，对推动我国心血管内科医师的专业教育起到了重要作用。今天非常高兴地看到由吴永健、张健、姚焰教授组织全国百位专家共同导读的《Braunwald 心脏病学》第 12 版（影印中文导读版）付梓出版，这是一种很好的、崭新的尝试。一方面凝练的导读介绍，会给读者一个相关内容的核心理念；另一方面完整保留了原文，让读者能够细致学习、品味原著的精髓；其三，之后还将根据学术进展更新电子资源中的导读内容或配上对应的中文视频讲解。多种形式、深入浅出地阐述核心内容将带给大家耳目一新的感受，有效地提高学习积极性和效果。

当代心血管病学的基础和临床研究日新月异，飞速进步。流行病学、遗传学、各种组学、影像学和生物标志物等方面的研究不断揭示和夯实了心血管病的发病机制，完善了评价体系；新药研究、新器械开发、生物工程学应用等方面的不断进展，进一步提升了心血管病治疗学的水平和能力。的确，这是一个知识爆炸的时代，也是一个充满挑战和希望的时代。我国中青年一代心血管病研究和临床工作者既要满怀热情和理想，又要踏踏实实地潜心读书，从事科学研究和临床实践。《Braunwald 心脏病学》无疑将成为我们学习心血管病学的基石，成为我们从事心血管病专业的最重要的教科书和参考书。希望此"中文导读版"对读者更好地理解原著有所裨益。

于中国医学科学院　北京协和医学院　阜外医院
国家心血管病中心
2023 年 2 月

《Braunwald 心脏病学》中文导读版前言

心血管病学是过去数十年间发展最快的学科之一，新理念、新知识、新技术层出不穷，令人目不暇接，稍有懈怠就跟不上学科发展。在浩如烟海的各种教科书和学术刊物中，《Braunwald 心脏病学》一直是经典巨著，它教育了一代又一代心血管病医生。Braunwald 本人是当代心脏病学之父。年近九旬的他依然活跃在世界心脏病领域。他主导的 TIMI 系列研究几乎代表了现代心脏病学的发展。如今在西方国家，《Braunwald 心脏病学》是心脏科医生成长的必读之书。其内容涵盖了心血管疾病的方方面面。所有参与编写的作者都是在其编写的章节领域的全世界最权威专家。该书另外一个最大的特点就是帮助年轻医生建立心脏病学的整体理念。如它会帮助您了解心脏病学发展的历史、全球心脏病的状况、环境因素和生活方式对心血管疾病的影响、心血管疾病基础和临床研究的方法和模式、医疗卫生政策与人群心血管疾病以及教您学会心血管疾病的诊治理念。

《Braunwald 心脏病学》对于中国医生同样是最好的教科书。陈灏珠教授曾经组织中国的专家将《Braunwald's HEART DISEASE》第 7 版全书翻译成中文，形成中文版的《Braunwald 心脏病学》，对于很多中国医生的成长发挥了重要的作用。随着心脏病学在各个方面的快速发展，该书反复再版，如今已是第十二版，体现了目前心脏病领域的最新进展。众多中国心脏科医生都渴望能获得此书，以作为工作中的指导和陪伴。有鉴于此，北京大学医学出版社引进出版了中文导读影印版的《Braunwald 心脏病学》，并联合玲珑医学共同组织中国的专家对每一章节进行中文导读，这样可以让阅读者快速了解该章节的大致内容，如果读者对其中的内容感兴趣，可以继续阅读原文。很多重要章节的后面配有编译者制作的中文幻灯和编译者的影像版讲解，由此提供更多、更灵活的学习形式。

受玲珑医学的委托，遵循北京大学出版社的要求，本次参与《Braunwald 心脏病学》编译的专家主要来自中国医学科学院阜外医院，同时邀请了部分兄弟医院的专家。由于这是初次尝试一种全新的编译方式，缺乏经验和参考，问题和不足在所难免，还望广大读者朋友提出批评和建议。但编译委员会相信，我国心脏科医生的英文阅读能力均有了大幅度提高，采取编译的方式也许对于我国读者来说是一种更好的尝试。我们衷心地期待这种形式能够帮助中国医生的成长，同时也希望它成为心脏科医生的好帮手。

吴永健　张健　姚焰
2023 年 1 月

Preface

The knowledge relevant to the practice of cardiology continues to grow by leaps and bounds. Scientific and clinical advances have occurred at such a rapid pace that clinicians often suffer information overload. Communications about advances in cardiovascular medicine inundate practitioners on a seemingly minute-to-minute basis through journals, mailings, text messages, newsletters, social media, webinars, advertisements, and other electronic and print media. How can a practitioner or trainee sift through this cacophony to discern reliable, durable, and important information critical for practice?

This textbook of cardiovascular medicine offers a solution to this quandary. The 12th edition of *Braunwald's Heart Disease* provides a comprehensive, carefully curated, balanced, and unbiased distillation not only of the tried and true, but especially the latest advances in our field. This volume should serve the novice and experienced practitioner alike. Trainees and those preparing for certification or recertification examinations can use this text for an overall review of contemporary cardiovascular medicine. Practitioners confronting a particular clinical problem can consult the appropriate section of the book on an as-needed basis to answer the clinical question at hand to aid on-the-spot clinical decision making. While not a basic science textbook, this volume builds on Dr. Braunwald's founding vision and reviews fundamental pathophysiologic mechanisms to furnish a foundation for informed practice where appropriate.

Cardiovascular medicine has expanded so enormously that few if any individuals can maintain mastery of the entire scope of practice. Sub-specialization and even sub-sub-specialization have increased. Yet, each of us encounters issues within these super-specialized areas when we care for and counsel our own patients. The palette of patients' problems often overlaps the fine divisions our specialty has developed. This book aims to provide a ready reference so that we can update our knowledge with recent and authoritative information in areas of cardiovascular medicine afield from our own primary areas of expertise. Indeed, with the addition of companion volumes, the *Heart Disease* family has become a living learning system and comprehensive reference.

As necessitated by evolution and progress in cardiovascular medicine, in planning this 12th edition the editors have carefully reviewed the content to reflect current knowledge. This edition has 14 totally new chapters. For example, we have added chapters on artificial intelligence in cardiology and on the use of wearables in cardiovascular medicine. These two topics will doubtless change our practices profoundly. We expect that future editions will continue to build on these and other novel areas that will provide us with innovative tools to confront our patients' problems.

We have added a new chapter, "Impact of the Environment on Cardiovascular Health," as we recognize increasingly the clinical importance of this critical interface. Another new chapter, "Cardiovascular Disease Risk of Nicotine and Tobacco Products," highlights the concerning increase in smokeless tobacco use among youth. The burgeoning field of cardio-oncology has expanded coverage in the 12th edition, with two chapters devoted to different aspects of this topic. Expanded coverage of valvular heart disease includes a new chapter on interventions for mitral and tricuspid valvulopathies, which complements an updated chapter on percutaneous interventions for the aortic valve. These additions acknowledge the growing role of structural heart disease interventions in tackling these conditions.

The period of planning and preparation of this 12th edition coincided with the pandemic caused by SARS-CoV-2. We would be remiss not to include an expanded discussion of viral heart diseases in a new chapter, as our specialty needs to prepare for likely future viral pandemics, as well as deal with the potentially long-term cardiovascular consequences of COVID-19. Of course, each and every chapter in the book has undergone extensive updating and revision to reflect advances since the last edition. To this end, a number of chapters are completely written de novo by new authors. Indeed, the 12th edition boasts almost 80 new authors, reflecting our commitment to continuous refreshment and review of the content.

Our field can take considerable pride in the rapid advances in both basic and clinical investigation that this book highlights. Yet, we face a disconnect between these advances and their application to practice. To this end we include a new chapter, "Impact of Health Care Policy on Quality and Outcomes of Cardiovascular Disease," that focuses on practical societal approaches to ensure that our patients can benefit from the clinical and basic scientific advances in our field. Moreover, closing gaps in offering progress in cardiovascular medicine to racially, ethnically, geographically diverse, or underserved populations presents a global challenge. We focus on cardiovascular conditions in particular segments of the population—women, people with diabetes, and those with HIV/AIDS—that may require specialized approaches; each of these and others have been accorded a separate chapter. The global pandemic has placed disparities and inequities in health care in stark relief, locally and globally. To address this problem, a new chapter, "Heart Disease in Racially and Ethnically Diverse Populations," deals with cardiovascular conditions that confront disadvantaged segments of our population.

Finally, the Editors were fortunate to enlist Professor Eugene Braunwald, the founder of this textbook, to contribute an opening chapter, "Cardiovascular Disease: Past, Present, and Future," which shares his vision from his uniquely broad perspective. We have striven to uphold the standards that he set for this textbook from the first five editions that he edited solo. We have aimed to emulate his editorial prowess and example of refreshing every page of this textbook in each edition to maximize its utility for all who care for patients with or at risk of developing cardiovascular disease.

Peter Libby
Robert O. Bonow
Douglas L. Mann
Gordon F. Tomaselli
Deepak L. Bhatt
Scott D. Solomon

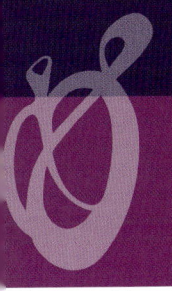

Preface to the First Edition

Cardiovascular disease is the greatest scourge affecting the industrialized nations. As with previous scourges — bubonic plague, yellow fever, and small pox — cardiovascular disease not only strikes down a significant fraction of the population without warning but also causes prolonged suffering and disability in an even larger number. In the United States alone, despite recent encouraging declines, cardiovascular disease is still responsible for almost 1 million fatalities each year and more than half of all deaths; almost 5 million persons afflicted with cardiovascular disease are hospitalized each year. The cost of these diseases in terms of human suffering and material resources is almost incalculable.

Fortunately, research focusing on the prevention, causes, diagnosis, and treatment of heart disease is moving ahead rapidly. Since the early part of the twentieth century, clinical cardiology has had a particularly strong foundation in the basic sciences of physiology and pharmacology. More recently, the disciplines of molecular biology, genetics, developmental biology, biophysics, biochemistry, experimental pathology and bioengineering have also begun to provide critically important information about cardiac function and malfunction.

In the past 25 years, in particular, we have witnessed an explosive expansion of our understanding of the structure and function of the cardiovascular system—both normal and abnormal—and of our ability to evaluate these parameters in the living patient, sometimes by means of techniques that require penetration of the skin but also with increasing accuracy, by noninvasive methods. Simultaneously, remarkable progress has been made in preventing and treating cardiovascular disease by medical and surgical means. Indeed, in the United States, a steady reduction in mortality from cardiovascular disease during the past decade suggests that the effective application of this increased knowledge is beginning to prolong human life span, the most valued resource on earth.

To provide a comprehensive, authoritative text in a field that has become as broad and deep as cardiovascular medicine, I enlisted the aid of a number of able colleagues. However, I hoped that my personal involvement in the writing of about half of the book would make it possible to minimize the fragmentation, gaps, inconsistencies, organizational difficulties, and impersonal tone that sometimes plague multiauthored texts. Although *Heart Disease: A Textbook of Cardiovascular Medicine* is primarily a clinical treatise and not a textbook of fundamental cardiovascular science, an effort has been made to explain, in some detail, the scientific bases of cardiovascular diseases.

To the extent that this book proves useful to those who wish to broaden their knowledge of cardiovascular medicine and thereby aids in the care of patients afflicted with heart disease, credit must be given to the many talented and dedicated persons involved in its preparation. I offer my deepest appreciation to my fellow contributors for their professional expertise, knowledge, and devoted scholarship, which has so enriched this book. I am deeply indebted to them for their cooperation and willingness to deal with a demanding editor.

Eugene Braunwald
1980

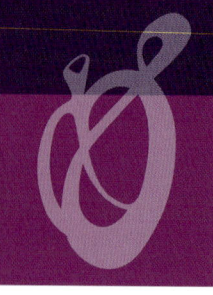

Acknowledgments

The conception and creation of this textbook of over 100 chapters and almost 2000 pages required the expertise, assistance, and skills of many dedicated individuals. We thank the contributors who have authored the chapters that comprise this textbook. We recognize the leadership of Ms. Dolores Meloni, executive content strategist at Elsevier, for her guidance and assistance at all stages of the planning and preparation of this volume. Ms. Anne Snyder, senior content development specialist, provided invaluable and detailed assistance on a daily basis. The editors owe her a great debt of gratitude. Mr. John Casey, senior project manager, cheerfully worked with the authors and the editors in executing the composition and proofing of this tome and accommodating last-minute additions and alterations to make the print edition as accurate and up to date as possible. The editors would not have been able to produce this book and ensure its quality without all of these contributions.

We also thank colleagues the world over who provided suggestions on how to improve *Braunwald's Heart Disease* and identified points that could use clarification. We welcome such input that will enable us to improve this edition in subsequent printings and plan future editions to meet our readers' needs even better.

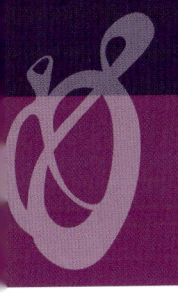

目录

第一部分　心血管医学基础
（吴永健　导读）

PART I FOUNDATIONS OF CARDIOVASCULAR MEDICINE

1　Cardiovascular Disease: Past, Present, and Future, 1
EUGENE BRAUNWALD

2　Global Burden of Cardiovascular Disease, 14
THOMAS A. GAZIANO, DORAIRAJ PRABHAKARAN, AND J. MICHAEL GAZIANO

3　Impact of the Environment on Cardiovascular Health, 31
SADEER AL-KINDI AND SANJAY RAJAGOPALAN

4　Clinical Trials in Cardiovascular Medicine, 42
SCOTT D. SOLOMON AND JOHN MCMURRAY

5　Clinical Decision-Making in Cardiology, 53
JOHN E. BRUSH JR. AND HARLAN M. KRUMHOLZ

6　Impact of Health Care Policy on Quality, Outcomes, and Equity in Cardiovascular Disease, 62
KAREN E. JOYNT MADDOX

第二部分　心血管疾病的个体化诊疗
（周欣　杨清　导读）

PART II INDIVIDUALIZING APPROACHES TO CARDIOVASCULAR DISEASE

7　Applications of Genetics to Cardiovascular Medicine, 71
PRADEEP NATARAJAN AND KIRAN MUSUNURU

8　Proteomics and Metabolomics in Cardiovascular Medicine, 87
ROBERT GERSZTEN

9　Principles of Drug Therapeutics, Pharmacogenomics, and Biologics, 92
DAN M. RODEN

10　Biomarkers and Use in Precision Medicine, 102
PETER LIBBY AND PAUL M RIDKER

11　Artificial Intelligence in Cardiovascular Medicine, 109
ZACHI ATTIA, SURAJ KAPA, PETER NOSEWORTHY, AND PAUL FRIEDMAN

12　Wearable Devices in Cardiovascular Medicine, 117
MINTU P. TURAKHIA

第三部分　患者的评估
（张力　导读）

PART III EVALUATION OF THE PATIENT

13　History and Physical Examination: An Evidence-Based Approach, 123
JAMES C. FANG AND PATRICK T. O'GARA

14　Electrocardiography, 141
DAVID M. MIRVIS AND ARY L. GOLDBERGER

15　Exercise Physiology and Exercise Electrocardiographic Testing, 175
GARY J. BALADY AND PHILIP A. ADES

16　Echocardiography, 196
JUSTINA C. WU, LINDA D. GILLAM, AND SCOTT D. SOLOMON
ILLUSTRATED BY BERNARD BULWER

17　Chest Radiography in Cardiovascular Disease, 268
FRANCINE L. JACOBSON

18　Nuclear Cardiology, 277
SHARMILA DORBALA AND MARCELO F. DI CARLI

19　Cardiovascular Magnetic Resonance Imaging, 314
RAYMOND Y. KWONG

20　Cardiac Computed Tomography, 335
RON BLANKSTEIN

21　Coronary Angiography and Intravascular Imaging, 363
GEORGE D. DANGAS AND ROXANA MEHRAN

22　Invasive Hemodynamic Diagnosis of Cardiac Disease, 385
MORTON J. KERN, ARNOLD H. SETO, AND JOERG HERRMANN

23	**Anesthesia and Noncardiac Surgery in Patients with Heart Disease, 410** LEE A. FLEISHER AND JOSHUA A. BECKMAN	36	**Coronary Blood Flow and Myocardial Ischemia, 609** DIRK J. DUNCKER AND JOHN M. CANTY JR.

第四部分　预防心脏病学
（卢玉枝　苏冠华　程翔　导读）

PART IV　PREVENTIVE CARDIOLOGY

- 24 **The Vascular Biology of Atherosclerosis, 425**
  PETER LIBBY

- 25 **Primary Prevention of Cardiovascular Disease, 442**
  SAMIA MORA, PETER LIBBY, AND PAUL M RIDKER

- 26 **Systemic Hypertension: Mechanisms, Diagnosis, and Treatment, 471**
  GEORGE L. BAKRIS AND MATTHEW J. SORRENTINO

- 27 **Lipoprotein Disorders and Cardiovascular Disease, 502**
  JACQUES GENEST, SAMIA MORA, AND PETER LIBBY

- 28 **Cardiovascular Disease Risk of Nicotine and Tobacco Products, 525**
  ARUNI BHATNAGAR

- 29 **Nutrition and Cardiovascular and Metabolic Diseases, 531**
  DARIUSH MOZAFFARIAN

- 30 **Obesity: Medical and Surgical Management, 547**
  JEAN-PIERRE DESPRÉS, ERIC LAROSE, AND PAUL POIRIER

- 31 **Diabetes and the Cardiovascular System, 556**
  NIKOLAUS MARX, SILVIO E. INZUCCHI, AND DARREN K. MCGUIRE

- 32 **Exercise and Sports Cardiology, 579**
  PAUL D. THOMPSON AND AARON L. BAGGISH

- 33 **Comprehensive Cardiac Rehabilitation, 588**
  RANDAL JAY THOMAS

- 34 **Integrative Approaches to the Management of Patients with Heart Disease, 593**
  STEPHEN DEVRIES

第五部分　动脉粥样硬化性心血管疾病
（曹宇开　李悦　导读）

PART V　ATHEROSCLEROTIC CARDIOVASCULAR DISEASE

- 35 **Approach to the Patient with Chest Pain, 599**
  MARC P. BONACA AND MARC S. SABATINE

- 37 **ST-Elevation Myocardial Infarction: Pathophysiology and Clinical Evolution, 636**
  BENJAMIN M. SCIRICA, PETER LIBBY, AND DAVID A. MORROW

- 38 **ST-Elevation Myocardial Infarction: Management, 662**
  ERIN A. BOHULA AND DAVID A. MORROW

- 39 **Non–ST Elevation Acute Coronary Syndromes, 714**
  ROBERT P. GIUGLIANO AND EUGENE BRAUNWALD

- 40 **Stable Ischemic Heart Disease, 739**
  DAVID A. MORROW AND JAMES DE LEMOS

- 41 **Percutaneous Coronary Intervention, 786**
  DHARAM J. KUMBHANI AND DEEPAK L. BHATT

- 42 **Diseases of the Aorta, 806**
  ALAN C. BRAVERMAN AND MARC SCHERMERHORN

- 43 **Peripheral Artery Diseases, 837**
  MARC P. BONACA AND MARK A. CREAGER

- 44 **Treatment of Noncoronary Obstructive Vascular Disease, 859**
  SCOTT KINLAY AND DEEPAK L. BHATT

- 45 **Prevention and Management of Ischemic Stroke, 870**
  MARK J. ALBERTS

第六部分　心力衰竭
（贺春晖　张健　导读）

PART VI　HEART FAILURE

- 46 **Mechanisms of Cardiac Contraction and Relaxation, 889**
  DONALD M. BERS AND BARRY A. BORLAUG

- 47 **Pathophysiology of Heart Failure, 913**
  GERD HASENFUSS AND DOUGLAS L. MANN

- 48 **Approach to the Patient with Heart Failure, 933**
  JAMES L. JANUZZI JR. AND DOUGLAS L. MANN

- 49 **Diagnosis and Management of Acute Heart Failure, 946**
  G. MICHAEL FELKER AND JOHN R. TEERLINK

50 **Management of Heart Failure Patients with Reduced Ejection Fraction, 975**
DOUGLAS L. MANN

51 **Heart Failure with Preserved and Mildly Reduced Ejection Fraction, 1007**
CAROLYN S.P. LAM, SANJIV J. SHAH, AND SCOTT D. SOLOMON

52 **The Dilated, Restrictive, and Infiltrative Cardiomyopathies, 1031**
RAY E. HERSHBERGER

53 **Cardiac Amyloidosis, 1052**
FREDERICK L. RUBERG AND MATHEW S. MAURER

54 **Hypertrophic Cardiomyopathy, 1062**
CAROLYN Y. HO AND STEVE R. OMMEN

55 **Myocarditis, 1077**
LESLIE T. COOPER JR. AND KIRK U. KNOWLTON

56 **Cardio-Oncology: Managing Cardiotoxic Effects of Cancer Therapies, 1091**
BONNIE KY

57 **Cardio-Oncology: Approach to the Patient, 1099**
JOERG HERRMANN

58 **Devices for Monitoring and Managing Heart Failure, 1107**
JOANN LINDENFELD AND MICHAEL R. ZILE

59 **Mechanical Circulatory Support, 1119**
KEITH D. AARONSON AND FRANCIS D. PAGANI

60 **Cardiac Transplantation, 1132**
RANDALL C. STARLING

第七部分　心律失常
（吴灵敏　姚焰　导读）

PART VII　ARRHYTHMIAS, SUDDEN DEATH, AND SYNCOPE

61 **Approach to the Patient with Cardiac Arrhythmias, 1145**
ANNE B. CURTIS AND GORDON F. TOMASELLI

62 **Mechanisms of Cardiac Arrhythmias, 1163**
STANLEY NATTEL AND GORDON F. TOMASELLI

63 **Genetics of Cardiac Arrhythmias, 1191**
JOHN R. GIUDICESSI, DAVID J. TESTER, AND MICHAEL J. ACKERMAN

64 **Therapy for Cardiac Arrhythmias, 1208**
JOHN M. MILLER AND KENNETH A. ELLENBOGEN

65 **Supraventricular Tachycardias, 1245**
JONATHAN M. KALMAN AND PRASHANTHAN SANDERS

66 **Atrial Fibrillation: Clinical Features, Mechanisms, and Management, 1272**
HUGH CALKINS, GORDON F. TOMASELLI, AND FRED MORADY

67 **Ventricular Arrhythmias, 1288**
WILLIAM G. STEVENSON AND KATJA ZEPPENFELD

68 **Bradyarrhythmias and Atrioventricular Block, 1312**
KRISTEN K. PATTON AND JEFFREY E. OLGIN

69 **Pacemakers and Implantable Cardioverter-Defibrillators, 1321**
MINA K. CHUNG AND JAMES P. DAUBERT

70 **Cardiac Arrest and Sudden Cardiac Death, 1349**
JEFFREY J. GOLDBERGER, CHRISTINE M. ALBERT, AND ROBERT J. MYERBURG

71 **Hypotension and Syncope, 1387**
HUGH CALKINS, THOMAS H. EVERETT IV, AND PENG-SHENG CHEN

第八部分　心脏瓣膜疾病
（王墨扬　吴永健　导读）

PART VIII　DISEASES OF THE HEART VALVES

72 **Aortic Valve Stenosis, 1399**
BRIAN R. LINDMAN, ROBERT O. BONOW, AND CATHERINE M. OTTO

73 **Aortic Regurgitation, 1419**
ROBERT O. BONOW AND RICK A. NISHIMURA

74 **Transcatheter Aortic Valve Replacement, 1430**
MARTIN B. LEON AND MICHAEL J. MACK

75 **Mitral Stenosis, 1441**
Y. S. CHANDRASHEKHAR

76 **Mitral Regurgitation, 1455**
REBECCA TUNG HAHN AND ROBERT O. BONOW

77 **Tricuspid, Pulmonic, and Multivalvular Disease, 1473**
PATRICIA A. PELLIKKA AND VUYISILE T. NKOMO

78 **Transcatheter Therapies for Mitral and Tricuspid Valvular Heart Disease, 1484**
HOWARD C. HERRMANN AND MICHAEL J. REARDON

79 **Prosthetic Heart Valves, 1495**
PHILIPPE PIBAROT AND PATRICK T. O'GARA

80 Infectious Endocarditis and Infections of Indwelling Devices, 1505
LARRY M. BADDOUR, NANDAN S. ANAVEKAR, JUAN A. CRESTANELLO, AND WALTER R. WILSON

81 Rheumatic Fever, 1531
ANA OLGA MOCUMBI

第九部分　心肌、心包和肺血管系统疾病
（赵青　柳志红　导读）

PART IX　DISEASES OF THE MYOCARDIUM, PERICARDIUM, AND PULMONARY VASCULATURE BED

82 Congenital Heart Disease in the Adolescent and Adult, 1541
ANNE MARIE VALENTE, ADAM L. DORFMAN, SONYA V. BABU-NARAYAN, AND ERIC V. KRIEGER

83 Catheter-Based Treatment of Congenital Heart Disease in Adults, 1587
SHABANA SHAHANAVAZ, JOHN M. LASALA, AND DAVID T. BALZER

84 Cardiomyopathies Induced by Drugs or Toxins, 1593
ROBERT A. KLONER AND SHEREIF REZKALLA

85 Cardiovascular Abnormalities in HIV-Infected Individuals, 1603
PRISCILLA Y. HSUE AND DAVID D. WATERS

86 Pericardial Diseases, 1615
MARTIN M. LEWINTER, PAUL C. CREMER, AND ALLAN L. KLEIN

87 Pulmonary Embolism and Deep Vein Thrombosis, 1635
SAMUEL Z. GOLDHABER AND GREGORY PIAZZA

88 Pulmonary Hypertension, 1656
BRADLEY A. MARON

89 Sleep-Disordered Breathing and Cardiac Disease, 1678
SUSAN REDLINE

第十部分　特定人群的心血管疾病
（王汝涛　陶凌　导读）

PART X　CARDIOVASCULAR DISEASE IN SELECT POPULATIONS

90 Cardiovascular Disease in Older Adults, 1687
DANIEL E. FORMAN, JEROME L. FLEG, NANETTE KASS WENGER, AND MICHAEL W. RICH

91 Cardiovascular Disease in Women, 1710
MARTHA GULATI AND C. NOEL BAIREY MERZ

92 Pregnancy and Heart Disease, 1723
SAMUEL C. SIU AND CANDICE K. SILVERSIDES

93 Heart Disease in Racially and Ethnically Diverse Populations, 1743
ALANNA A. MORRIS AND MICHELLE A. ALBERT

第十一部分　心血管疾病和其他器官疾病
（王文尧　唐熠达　导读）

PART XI　CARDIOVASCULAR DISEASE AND DISORDERS OF OTHER ORGANS

94 Endemic and Pandemic Viral Illnesses and Cardiovascular Disease: Influenza and COVID-19, 1751
ORLY VARDENY, MOHAMMAD MADJID, AND SCOTT D. SOLOMON

95 Hemostasis, Thrombosis, Fibrinolysis, and Cardiovascular Disease, 1766
JEFFREY I. WEITZ

96 Endocrine Disorders and Cardiovascular Disease, 1791
BERNADETTE BIONDI

97 Rheumatic Diseases and the Cardiovascular System, 1809
JUSTIN C. MASON

98 Tumors Affecting the Cardiovascular System, 1829
DANIEL J. LENIHAN, MICHAEL J. REARDON, AND W. GREGORY HUNDLEY

99 Psychiatric and Psychosocial Aspects of Cardiovascular Disease, 1841
KENNETH E. FREEDLAND, ROBERT M. CARNEY, ERIC J. LENZE, AND MICHAEL W. RICH

100 Neuromuscular Disorders and Cardiovascular Disease, 1853
WILLIAM J. GROH, ELIZABETH M. MCNALLY, AND GORDON F. TOMASELLI

101 Interface Between Renal Disease and Cardiovascular Illness, 1873
PETER A. MCCULLOUGH

102 Cardiovascular Manifestations of Autonomic Disorders, 1893
JASON S. BRADFIELD AND KALYANAM SHIVKUMAR

第一部分　心血管医学基础

吴永健　导读

心血管疾病诊疗已经经历了400余年的发展，在疾病（冠心病、心律失常、高血压、高脂血症、心脏瓣膜疾病、心力衰竭等）的诊断、评估、治疗方面，以及影像学诊断技术、介入性治疗方法、心脏外科手术治疗、疾病机制探索、急危重症辅助技术等方面迅猛发展。心血管疾病领域总体发展趋势是从解剖到功能、从宏观到微观、从有创到微创、从诊治到预防康复。但面对较高的心脏病病死率和不良事件发生率，心血管疾病领域仍存有诸多难题与挑战。（详见本部分第1章：心血管疾病：过去、现在和未来）

过去30年，心血管疾病引起的死亡占据全球总死亡人数的比例从26%增长到32%，在中低收入国家中，增长趋势尤为明显。在高收入国家，尽管心血管疾病发生率已经逐年下降，但是随着人口老龄化的加剧和寿命的延长，心血管疾病患者的总人数依然在增加。在不同的社会、文化和经济环境中，心血管疾病负担需要不同的解决方案。在高收入国家，需要关注老年患者的健康管理；而在中低收入国家，需要危险因素控制，倡导健康生活方式。中国心血管疾病患者的危险因素控制仍不理想：全国约有2.7亿烟民，其中男性吸烟率约为47.7%；中国人群的总胆固醇水平在过去30年不断升高，并主要归因于非高密度脂蛋白胆固醇水平的上升；中国人群的糖尿病负担相对欧美国家更高，中国和印度糖尿病患者的总人数在全世界占比75%；中国人群的肥胖率在近30年也显著升高，超重人口总数升高了41%，肥胖人口总数升高了97%。中国人群的心血管疾病负担仍在不断增加，未来心血管疾病给中国带来的经济卫生负担将不断加重。（详见本部分第2章：全球心血管疾病负担）

环境因素是心血管疾病的发病和预后的重要风险因素。环境污染大致分为：①空气污染；②水污染；③土壤、化学和重金属污染；④职业因素污染。据估计，环境污染导致的心血管疾病约占全部心血管疾病的20%、缺血性心脏病的25%。空气污染是导致心血管疾病最重要的环境因素，每年在全世界造成的死亡人数高达667万。空气污染可以通过多种机制来诱发或促进心血管疾病的进展。比如，PM2.5暴露可能会导致炎症、氧化应激等多种病理生理机制的激活，而增加冠心病、高血压、糖尿病、心力衰竭、心律失常等心血管系统相关疾病风险。随着对于环境因素与人体健康研究的开展，逐步认识到环境因素对心血管疾病有着至关重要的影响。（详见本部分第3章：环境对心血管健康的影响）

随机对照临床试验是现代心血管疾病医学进步的重要基础之一，为医务工作者提供最高水平的临床证据、创新有效的诊疗手段，并在实践中指导患者的治疗。研究者应当按照研究目的，选择适当的研究设计类型，如平行组设计、交叉设计等，注意随机化与盲法的应用。依据研究目的制定合理的受试者入选与排除标准，并选择恰当的变量作为研究的结局事件。医学伦理也是临床试验的关键一环。在临床研究的解读时，应注意参考临床试验网站的注册信息，关注研究主要终点与次要终点所代表的意义，以及临床试验事后分析的研究结果。（详见本部分第4章：心血管医学的临床试验）

心脏病学的临床决策包括两方面：诊断决策和治

疗决策。诊断决策的前提是充足的知识储备和临床经验，医生要凭借临床线索诊断可能的疾病，因此完善相应的检查为可能的诊断提供更有力的证据或推翻其他诊断。治疗决策首先需要权衡利弊，如何帮助患者做出理性的决定是治疗决策的难点。其次，如何根据最新的研究进展改变当前的治疗决策，需要临床医生关注新的研究。因此，临床决策是一项综合性的能力，心血管疾病临床决策应当基于以患者为中心的诊疗方式，在患者诊疗过程中对其进行依从性和疗效评估。（详见本部分第 5 章：心脏病学的临床决策）

卫生政策决定了卫生保健领域的基本规则，并从根本上决定了医疗的实施方式和医疗服务方式。平价医疗法案对医保的覆盖范围和准入政策有着深远的影响，扩大医保的覆盖与补助范围，对改善健康和福祉产生了超出财政保障的积极影响。尽管，美国每年在医疗方面投入巨大财力，但其医疗质量，尤其是心血管方面的医疗质量，却仍然存在不足，并且存在公平性的问题，突出表现为：心血管疾病患者的死亡率高，发病率、患病率以及医疗结局在不同种族、不同收入和不同区域的人群中存在着明显差异。为了提高心血管健康水平，提升优质医疗服务的公平性，政府应该以扩大保险等成功政策为基础，改进效果欠佳的政策，从而使人人享有更好、更公平的医疗。（详见本部分第 6 章：医疗政策对心血管疾病的质量、结果、公平性的影响）

PART I **FOUNDATIONS OF CARDIOVASCULAR MEDICINE**

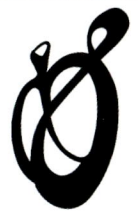

1 Cardiovascular Disease: Past, Present, and Future

EUGENE BRAUNWALD

扫描二维码阅读
第1章中文导读

THE BIRTH, 1
Early Stirrings, 1
Emergence of a Specialty, 2

CARDIAC IMAGING, 2
The Past, 2
The Present, 2

INVASIVE PROCEDURES, 2
Cardiac Catheterization, 2
Percutaneous Coronary Intervention, 3
Cardiovascular Surgery, 3
Comments, 3

HYPERTENSION, 3
The Past, 3
The Present, 4
The Future, 4

VALVULAR HEART DISEASE, 4
The Past, 4
The Present, 4

ARRHYTHMIAS, 5
The Past, 5
The Present, 5

DYSLIPIDEMIAS, 5
The Past, 5
The Present, 5
The Future, 6

ACUTE MYOCARDIAL INFARCTION, 6
Coronary Risk Factors, 6

HEART FAILURE, 7
The Past, 7
The Present, 7

ASSISTED CIRCULATION, 7
The Past, 7
The Present, 8
The Future, 8

GENOMICS AND GENETICS, 8

The Present, 8
The Future, 8
Precision Medicine, 8

PRIMORDIAL PREVENTION, 8
The Present, 8
The Future, 9

INFLAMMATION, 9
The Past, 9
The Present, 9
The Future, 9

CLONAL HEMATOPOIESIS, 9

ARTIFICIAL INTELLIGENCE, 9
The Present, 9
The Future, 11

CONCLUSIONS, 11

REFERENCES, 11

THE BIRTH

Although the heart was recognized as a vital organ in early human history, its function was not understood but was widely debated over millennia. In 1628, William Harvey, a London physician (Fig. 1.1) who had trained in the great medical school in Padua, Italy, published a monograph, *De Motu Cordis, An Anatomical Treatise on the Motion of the Heart and Blood*,[1] which concluded simply: "The blood in the animal body moves around in a circle continuously, and the function of the heart is to accomplish this by pumping." Harvey based this conclusion on detailed anatomic studies that included the valves in the veins that appeared to permit blood to flow only toward the heart. He conducted experiments in humans and rabbits and then estimated cardiac output. Importantly, Harvey's research was the first major hypothesis-driven research in biology. Although his findings were not uniformly accepted during his lifetime, they are now considered to be one of the scientific triumphs of the high Renaissance, along with the works of Isaac Newton and Galileo Galilei.

Harvey's conclusion was buttressed by two findings. The first was the description of the capillary circulation in 1661 by Marcello Malpighi,[2] who identified this last anatomic link in the circulatory chain. The other, by Richard Lower in 1668, was the role of the pulmonary circulation in changing the color of the blood as it is exposed to the air in the lungs.[3]

Early Stirrings

In 1733, Steven Hales measured arterial and venous pressures in horses and other mammals.[4] "Direct" auscultation (placing the ear on the precordium) to hear the heartbeat was used later in the 18th century. Cardiac examination accelerated after 1823, when René Laennec, a French physician, described the stethoscope.[5] In his 1775 monograph on foxglove (digitalis), William Withering described its effectiveness in the treatment of patients with "dropsy," that is, edema, presumably due to heart failure (HF).[6] William Heberden described angina in 1772[7] and 40 years later the *first* paper in the *first* issue of the *New England Journal of Medicine* by John Warren, a Boston physician, discussed this symptom.[8] However, angina does not appear to have been recognized frequently.[9] In 1879, F.A. Mahomed described hypertension not associated with renal disease, the forerunner of what is now referred to as primary or essential hypertension.[10] Several important arrhythmias were described in the mid-to-late 19th century. These included severe bradycardia by Stokes in 1854 and ventricular fibrillation (VF) by MacWilliams in 1887.[11]

By the end of the 19th century, physiologists and clinicians were aware of electrical depolarization and repolarization of the heart and could recognize some cardiac arrhythmias by cardiac auscultation and palpation of the pulse. They also knew that hypertension could occur both in the presence and absence of advanced renal disease and could be associated with ventricular hypertrophy. They

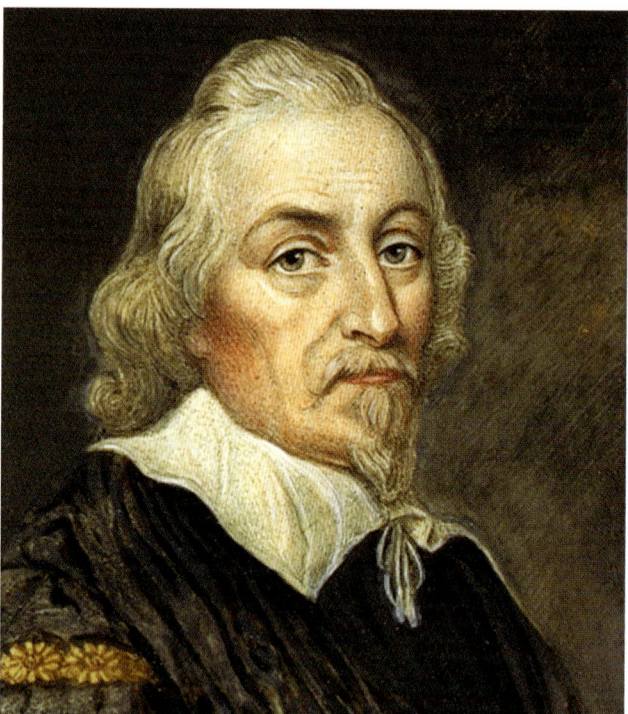

FIGURE 1.1 William Harvey (1578-1657).

recognized congenital and valvular heart disease, angina pectoris, and HF. However, cardiovascular disease was not considered to be very common; it was treated with bed rest, digitalis, nitrates, and sometimes morphine.

Emergence of a Specialty

The decade from 1895 to 1905, bridging the 19th and 20th centuries, was probably the most important in the history of cardiology because of the discovery of three critically important technologies. In 1895, Wilhelm Roentgen,[12,*] a German physicist, discovered the use of x-ray, the first technique for imaging body parts in intact humans, allowing estimation of the heart's size and shape. The noninvasive measurement of blood pressure (BP) was developed by Riva Rocci, an Italian physician, in 1896[13] and Korotkoff in Russia in 1905.[14] The first recording of the electrocardiogram using a string galvanometer by Willem Einthoven,* a Dutch clinical physiologist, was reported in 1903.[15] When added to the clinical examination, these three new technologies permitted clinical assessment of key elements of the cardiovascular system. It soon became apparent that heart disease was far more common than had been suspected. Physicians who became expert in using and interpreting these new technical wonders were dubbed "heart specialists" or "cardiologists."

Advances came rapidly in this new specialty, and it soon became necessary to develop medical journals to record them. The earliest were the *Zentrallblatt für Herz Krankenheiten* in Germany and the *Archives des Maladies du Coeur* in France, both in 1908. Subsequently, an enormous expansion of cardiac journals occurred. As of 2020, 138 cardiovascular journals are published on a regular basis.

National cardiac societies were created to bring cardiologists and their trainees from each country together to share experiences and describe advances in cardiovascular science and clinical cardiology. The first of these, the British Cardiac Club, was organized in 1922, and in 1937 it morphed into the British Cardiac Society. In addition to organizing annual meetings, these societies also publish national cardiology journals. Beginning in the last third of the 20th century, the societies have developed and promulgated clinical practice guidelines that have improved the accuracy of cardiovascular diagnosis and the quality of care. National cardiac societies have joined with their continental neighbors to form regional societies, such as the European Society of Cardiology. The development of the World Heart Federation reflects the globalization of clinical cardiology and cardiovascular research.

CARDIAC IMAGING (SEE PART III)

The Past

After the development of roentgenography, venous angiography was begun in the 1920s. Selective angiography, in which radiocontrast material is injected through an intracardiac or intravascular catheter, allowed enhanced visualization of specific sites in the heart and great vessels. In 1948, Mason Sones, a cardiologist in Cleveland, described and perfected coronary arteriography, which provided accurate anatomic assessment of the coronary arterial bed.[16]

In 1952, Edler and Herz, a Swedish cardiologist/physicist team, developed echocardiography.[17] This technique assumed growing importance for assessing cardiac structure and function, becoming the "work horse" of cardiac imaging. The devices became smaller, more portable, and even handheld. By the end of the 20th century, three-dimensional echocardiography had become a valuable clinical tool.

The development of computed tomography (CT) by Hounsfield* and Cormack* in 1973[18] and of cardiovascular magnetic resonance imaging (CMR) by Lauterbur* and Mansfield* in the same year[19] have revolutionized cardiac diagnosis. Both technologies provide precise three-dimensional displays of the cardiac chambers and great vessels. CMR is especially useful in assessing regional myocardial perfusion, tissue characteristics, systolic and diastolic function, inflammation, and scar. Although coronary calcium had been detected occasionally by fluoroscopy, the field leaped forward in 1990 when Agatston introduced calcium scoring by CT. Larger and more extensive calcium deposits in the coronary arteries were associated with a higher incidence of subsequent coronary events, thereby enhancing risk assessment (see later).[20]

The Present

Nuclear cardiology, developed in the 1930s, is now used largely to detect the presence and assess the severity of myocardial ischemia. CMR imaging is now used routinely in the diagnosis and assessment of cardiomyopathies and myocarditis and in the assessment of cardiac fibrosis and masses. CT has been shown to be particularly effective in the assessment of aortic stenosis (AS). Dobutamine stress CMR is a sensitive, accurate method of detecting and quantifying myocardial ischemia.[21] Because CMR does not require ionizing radiation, it is used repeatedly to track the progression of disease and the effects of therapeutic interventions. For CMR spectroscopy, the new 7-Tesla magnets provide higher signal-to-noise ratios and more precise quantification of myocardial high-energy phosphates.[22]

Improvements in coronary computed tomographic angiography (CCTA) with intravenous injection of contrast material provide accurate, high-quality, noninvasive visualization of the epicardial coronary arteries. This technique is now widely employed in patients with chest pain of possible cardiac ischemic origin, in whom it has reduced the need for invasive coronary arteriography.[23] Quantitative positron emission tomography has become useful in the assessment of myocardial ischemia and viability and in the evaluation of inflammatory cardiomyopathies and infective endocarditis.

INVASIVE PROCEDURES (SEE CHAPTERS 21, 22, AND 41)

Cardiac Catheterization

The first human catheterization was carried out (on himself!) by Werner Forssmann,* a German surgical resident who was forbidden to repeat the procedure, but who wisely published his experience[24] (Fig. 1.2). In the late 1940s, the technique was applied to a variety of congenital and acquired cardiac disorders by Andre Cournand*[25] and Dickinson Richards*[26] in New York. In addition to measuring pressures

---

* Names followed by an asterisk were awarded a Nobel Prize.

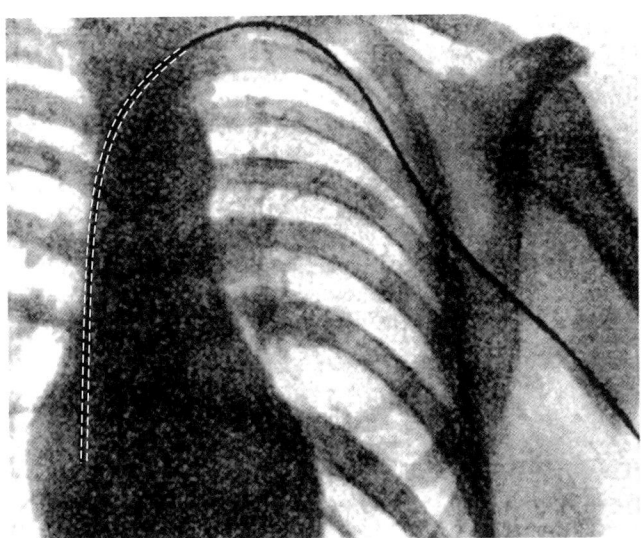

FIGURE 1.2 Cardiac catheter introduced by Werner Forssmann into his own right atrium. Forssmann W. Die Sondierung des rechten Herzens. Klin Wochenschr 1929;8:2085-2087. (Permission from Springer-Verlag, Munich, FRG.)

in the chambers of the right heart and pulmonary arteries, they also determined cardiac output at rest and during exercise. By the third quarter of the century, cardiac catheterization had become extremely important in the diagnosis of congenital and valvular heart disease.

Percutaneous Coronary Intervention

The field of invasive interventions virtually exploded in 1977 when Andreas Grüntzig, a Swiss cardiologist, described a new technique—percutaneous transluminal coronary angioplasty (PTCA), thereby ushering in a new subspecialty, interventional cardiology.[27] PTCA began with the treatment of patients with poorly controlled angina and an obstructive plaque in a proximal coronary artery. It was applied to progressively more complex lesions, and then on an emergent basis to patients with acute myocardial infarction (AMI) (see later).[28] In the late 1980s, coronary arterial stents were introduced to prevent restenosis.[29] Percutaneous coronary interventions (PCIs) expanded rapidly and began to compete with coronary artery bypass grafting (CABG). In properly selected patients it was of equivalent safety and efficacy and greatly preferred by patients who recovered in a day or two, compared with the weeks or months required after surgery.

Cardiovascular Surgery

After a number of early sporadic failures, cardiovascular surgery began in earnest in 1938 when Robert Gross of Boston successfully closed a patent ductus arteriosus.[30] Operative correction of coarctation of the aorta and of a variety of other congenital cardiac malformations soon followed. Mitral valvulotomy for stenosis was begun in 1946. A major step forward was taken by John Gibbon of Philadelphia, who developed a "heart-lung" machine in 1953, which was used for cardiopulmonary bypass[31] and led to the era of open heart surgery. This allowed repair of a large number of congenital and acquired disorders. In 1961, Albert Starr reported mitral valve replacement with a prosthetic ball valve.[32]

Beginning in the 1940s, attempts were made to treat patients with coronary artery disease (CAD) and severe angina by surgery; most were unsuccessful. In 1968, René Favaloro, a cardiac surgeon in Cleveland, Ohio described coronary artery bypass grafting,[33] which proved to be very effective in the management of severe angina pectoris and was shown in randomized clinical trials to prolong survival in patients with severe, multivessel CAD.[34]

Comments

During the last third of the 20th century, cardiology went through a major change. Before about 1970, the diagnosis of many congenital and acquired cardiac lesions were established by cardiac catheterization, often aided by selective angiography. If a mechanical therapeutic intervention was required, it was usually surgical. By the end of the century, as a consequence of the important advances in cardiac imaging, the need for diagnostic cardiac catheterization had declined. Simultaneously, catheter-based therapy advanced rapidly and expanded widely to patients with congenital and valvular heart disease. PCI became the most frequent therapy for improving coronary perfusion in ischemic heart disease and in acute myocardial infarction (AMI) (see later). Surgical therapy was reserved for patients in whom catheter-based therapy was not possible or in whom it had failed.

HYPERTENSION (SEE CHAPTER 26)

The Past

The recognition of hypertension as a critically important clinical entity was made possible by the simple noninvasive measurement of BP (see earlier) leading to the recognition of the high prevalence of the condition. The close relation between renal disease and hypertension goes back to Richard Bright, an English physician, who suggested in 1827 that patients with chronic renal disease were hypertensive.[35] In 1897, Robert Tigerstedt, a Swedish physiologist, injected an extract of rabbit kidney into a normal rabbit. He observed a prolonged elevation of arterial pressure and named the pressure-raising substance "renin."[36] In 1934, Harry Goldblatt, a Cleveland pathologist, demonstrated a rise in arterial pressure in dogs in which renal ischemia had been induced.[37] In 1940, Braun-Menendez, a physiologist in Buenos Aires, Argentina, reported that renin is an enzyme that acts on a globulin (now known as *angiotensinogen*) to produce a polypeptide with pressor properties, which he named *hypertensin* (now known as *angiotensin*), presumably produced by the ischemic kidney that had been described by Goldblatt.[38] In the first quarter of the 20th century, it became clear that in addition to renal disease, coarctation of the aorta, pheochromocytoma, and other endocrinopathies were causes of secondary hypertension. A large majority of patients with hypertension have no discernable cause; these are referred to as primary (essential) hypertension.

The clinical importance of hypertension was recognized and explicitly summarized by Soma Weiss, a Boston physician (who was a predecessor of the present author at Harvard and at the Brigham). In 1930, Weiss wrote:

> Persistently elevated arterial pressure is probably responsible for more disability and death than any other single pathological condition, including cancer and tuberculosis. Persistent hypertension combined with vascular pathology is the etiological factor in the bulk of instances of cerebral accident, myocardial failure and chronic insufficiency of the kidneys.[39]

Weiss was prescient, and today, almost a century after his paper, hypertension remains a major risk factor for stroke, AMI, HF, and renal failure. It plays a central role in cardiology and in internal medicine, neurology, and nephrology as well. However, Weiss' view was accepted very slowly until the 1950s, when systems for grading the severity of hypertension were developed, and followed by the realization of the wide spread and breadth of its serious complications.

Walter Kempner, an internist at Duke University, emphasized the use of an extremely low-salt diet (<200 mg Na^+ daily) based on rice, fruit, and juice.[40] Although this strict regimen reduced elevated BP, the diet was difficult to sustain. The most widely used antihypertensive drug in the mid-20th century was reserpine, an extract of the Indian root—*Rauwolfia serpentina*—which depresses cerebral sympathetic centers. Other early hypotensive agents included veratrum alkaloids, thought to act on the parasympathetic system, and hexamethonium derivatives, which block transmission through autonomic ganglia. The latter, while powerful, were associated with severe side effects. In patients with malignant hypertension who were not responsive to or could not tolerate potent hypotensive drugs, a splanchnic sympathectomy, championed by Reginald Smithwick, a Boston surgeon, could be considered.[41] Although it usually reduced BP, the adverse effects of this difficult operation were substantial.

Two well-designed, well-executed placebo-controlled trials in U.S. Veterans Hospitals, led by Edward D. Freis, a cardiologist in Washington, D.C., provided the first *definitive* evidence of the benefit of antihypertensive therapy. The first, conducted on patients with severe hypertension (diastolic pressures 115 to 129 mm Hg) compared treatment using the combination of hydrochlorothiazide, reserpine, and hydralazine, with placebo.[42] The second trial had a similar design and studied patients with diastolic pressures between 90 and 114 mm Hg. The risks of severe vascular events, especially HF and stroke, were markedly reduced in the treated group in both trials.[43]

The Present

By the end of the 20th century, treatment of essential hypertension had made many advances. They emphasize lifestyle changes, focusing on weight reduction, dietary salt restriction, and smoking. Of the large number of approved antihypertensive drugs, the primary agents include (1) thiazide or thiazide-like diuretics; (2) blockers of the renin-angiotensin system; and (3) calcium channel blockers. Compliance with the regimen is an important first step. Patients whose BP is not controlled with the combination of these drugs are considered to have resistant hypertension[44,45] and may require intensification of their lifestyle changes, the maximally tolerated doses of the primary agents, and/or the addition of a drug from another class, such as a mineralocorticoid receptor blocker, beta blocker, or vasodilator. The drugs for the treatment of hypertension are readily available, usually well tolerated, and inexpensive. One explanation for the inadequate control is that hypertension per se causes few if any symptoms and has been termed "the silent killer," leading to a combination of physician and patient inertia.

In the 20th century there were dozens of clinical trials, observational studies, and meta-analyses on drugs for the treatment of hypertension. The extent of clinical benefit appears to be related to five features: (1) the level of the baseline BP, (2) the event rate in the control group; (3) the extent of BP lowering by the intervention; (4) the tolerance to side effects; and (5) the duration of the trial. The higher each of these features, the greater is the clinical benefit.

The Future

Recent studies have shown a previously unrecognized primary aldosteronism in many patients with "essential" hypertension.[46] Such patients could be managed with a new nonsteroidal mineralocorticoid receptor antagonist.[47]

There have been multiple efforts to understand the genetic basis of essential hypertension, now recognized as a polygenic condition.[48] In a genome-wide association study (GWAS) in 475,000 persons, Kraja et al. identified 21 single-nucleotide polymorphisms (SNPs) and four novel loci associated with hypertension.[49] These include several candidate genes that may identify specific subgroups, with differing BP regulation and optimal therapies.

In a mendelian randomization study involving more than 600,000 subjects, triglyceride concentration, type 2 diabetes mellitus (T2DM), body mass index, alcohol dependence, insomnia, and smoking were each associated with an increased risk of hypertension, and longer sleep duration, higher high-density cholesterol concentrations, and higher education levels were each associated with a lower risk.[50] Several of these characteristics appear to be causally related, and their modification could prove to be useful in primary and/or primordial (see later) prevention. The combination of a low polygenic risk score for hypertension and adherence to a dietary approach was associated with a low BP in children.[51]

Going forward, more research on the combination of genomic and phenotypic features of hypertension is likely to provide clinically useful, actionable findings. An important goal is to identify the responders and nonresponders before the onset of therapy. In addition, there have been several observational studies suggesting that gut microbiota can influence BP. Their mechanisms are not clear but may involve levels of activation of G protein–coupled receptors.[52] Possible treatment with prebiotics, probiotics, and postbiotics to modify such microbiota may become a fertile field for future research on hypertension.

VALVULAR HEART DISEASE (SEE PART VIII)

The Past

Cardiac involvement in rheumatic fever was described by Wells in 1812.[53] Acute rheumatic fever and its sequel, rheumatic valvular disease, were common in Europe and North America until the mid-20th century and then declined with the introduction of penicillin and some relief of extreme poverty and overcrowding. However, almost simultaneously, a reciprocal increase in degenerative calcific disease of the aortic and mitral valves occurred in the rapidly growing elderly population. Acute rheumatic fever is still observed frequently in developing nations in tropical and subtropical latitudes.

The Present
Mitral Stenosis

In the mid-20th century, surgical treatment of symptomatic severe mitral stenosis (valve area <1.5 cm^2) carried out by closed mitral valvotomy was the most frequently performed cardiac operation.[54] When the valve is calcified, severely fibrotic, with subvalvular fusions, and/or accompanied by more than slight mitral regurgitation (MR), an open valvuloplasty on cardiopulmonary bypass is carried out; occasionally, mitral valve replacement is necessary. In 1983, percutaneous balloon mitral valvuloplasty (PBMV) was described by Inoue et al., a Japanese team.[55] Employing transseptal left heart catheterization[56] and echocardiographic guidance, they introduced a balloon catheter into the mitral orifice; balloon inflation opened the fused commissures. The indications for and results of PBMV are generally similar to those for closed surgical valvotomy. PBMV has gained worldwide popularity because it is relatively safe[57] and shortens the discomfort and duration of hospitalization and recovery. Favorable results have been sustained for upward of 15 years.[58]

Mitral Regurgitation (MR)

Primary MR is caused by an abnormality of the mitral valve leaflets, as in rheumatic heart disease. Secondary MR usually results from ventricular dilation caused by ischemic or nonischemic cardiomyopathy, which prevents coaptation of the normal leaflets. In 2001, Ottavio Alfieri, an Italian cardiac surgeon, treated MR by approximating the free edges of the mitral leaflets with a running suture sometimes referred to as the "Alfieri stitch."[59] In 2003, St. Goar et al. developed an endovascular "edge-to-edge" repair of the mitral valve with a valve clip in a porcine model.[60] Transcatheter mitral valve repair was extended to patients by Feldman et al.[61] Two large randomized clinical trials compared transcatheter edge-to-edge repair with guideline-directed medical therapy (GDMT) in secondary MR with HF. One of these showed superiority of the transcatheter approach,[62] whereas the other showed equivalence.[63] The 2020 American College of Cardiology/American Heart Associate (ACC/AHA) Guidelines provide a recommendation for the edge-to-edge repair in patients with moderate or severe MR with persistent symptoms despite intensive GDMT.[64] Catheter-based replacement of the mitral and tricuspid valves is under active investigation.

Transcatheter Aortic Valve Replacement

In the last third of the 20th century, symptomatic adult patients with severe AS (mean gradient >40 mm Hg) were generally treated by surgical aortic valve replacement (SAVR), and asymptomatic patients were followed closely. In 1992, Andersen et al. described the successful placement of a catheter-based bioprosthetic inflatable prosthetic aortic valve in a closed-chest porcine model.[65] This was followed a decade later by the first human percutaneous implantation of an aortic valve by Cribier et al.[66] In 2006, Webb et al. implanted a bioprosthetic valve using a catheter that was passed retrograde from the femoral artery.[67] The first large transcatheter aortic valve replacement (TAVR) trial was conducted by Leon et al. on patients whose operative risk was too high to undergo SAVR; survival was prolonged when compared with that with GDMT.[68]

Both SAVR and TAVR are effective treatments of adults with severe symptomatic AS. Both early mortality and stroke rates are somewhat lower for TAVR, but vascular complications, paravalvular regurgitation and the need for a permanent pacemaker are higher. Importantly, the length of hospital stay and recovery are much shorter for TAVR and greatly preferred by patients.[69]

TAVR was approved for high-risk patients with severe AS by the U.S. Food and Drug Administration (FDA) in 2011; the indication was extended to low-risk patients in 2019. Although TAVR is generally preferred to SAVR for patients with severe, symptomatic AS, at the time of this writing (2021), TAVR has been carried out for only 6 years and the long-term durability of the bioprosthetic valves used are not yet clear. This remains a concern when selecting TAVR for younger patients, particularly with bicuspid aortic valves.[64] Nonetheless, TAVR has transformed the management of patients with severe AS. In 2019, a total of 72,991 TAVR procedures were performed in the United States compared with 57,626 SAVR procedures.[67] In a national registry, TAVR has been shown to have a hospital mortality of 1.3%; 81% of patients reported a good quality of life after 1 year.[70]

ARRHYTHMIAS (SEE PART VII)
The Past
A "tumultuous" heartbeat was recognized in the 15th century. In 1769, Morgagni, an Italian physician, described patients with very slow heart rates and transient asystole. Although graphic tracings of irregular cardiac movements were made in the late 19th century,[71] it was the development of the string galvanometer electrocardiograph in 1903 that led Einthoven* (see earlier), Sir Thomas Lewis, and other early cardiologists to describe the majority of clinical arrhythmias.

In 1749, Senas recommended use of the bark of the cinchona tree (which contains quinine) for the treatment of palpitations. In 1918, the superiority of quinidine over quinine was recognized and subsequently a variety of other antiarrhythmic agents were developed. The mechanisms of action of these drugs were classified by Vaughan-Williams in 1970,[72] and subsequently updated.[73]

Suspicions arose in the 1970s that many of these drugs had both antiarrhythmic and proarrhythmic properties. These suspicions were proven in 1991 when the Cardiac Arrhythmia Suppression Trial (CAST) showed that several antiarrhythmic agents that markedly reduced premature ventricular contractions in post-MI patients were associated with an *increased* mortality.[74] Since then, the use of antiarrhythmic agents other than beta blockers, amiodarone, and some calcium channel blockers has been curtailed, especially in patients with structural or ischemic heart disease. Multicatheter-based invasive electrophysiologic testing, developed in the early 1970s, includes recording of electrocardiographic responses of a number of intracardiac leads to programmed electrical stimulation[75,76] before and after pharmacologic agents. This technique has proved to be extremely useful for identifying the mechanisms of arrhythmias, distinguishing between automaticity, reentry, and triggered activity and for risk stratification and selecting appropriate therapy.

In 1952, Paul Zoll, a Boston cardiologist, developed closed chest cardiac stimulation for the treatment of complete heart block and asystole.[77] In 1958, William Chardack, an American surgeon, implanted a pacemaker powered by a rechargeable battery.[78] In the same year, William Kouwenhoven, an engineer in Baltimore, described closed-chest cardiac massage.[79] In 1962, Bernard Lown, a Boston cardiologist, described direct current cardioversion of a variety of tachyarrhythmias, including atrial and VF.[80] In 1980, Michel Mirowski, a Baltimore cardiologist, described the implanted cardioverter-defibrillator. This device successfully detects and treats life-threatening arrhythmias, including ventricular tachycardia (VT) and VF.[81]

The Present
Acute supraventricular and nodal tachycardias are usually treated by vagal maneuvers, intravenous calcium channel blockers, or electrical cardioversion. To suppress chronic tachyarrhythmias, radiofrequency catheter ablation or amiodarone is frequently employed. VT is generally managed by cardioversion followed by ablation.[82] Atrial fibrillation can often be abolished early in the course by electrically disconnecting the source of arrhythmia triggers by pulmonary vein isolation sometimes using cryoballoon ablation.[83]

Sudden cardiac death (SCD) is responsible for approximately 15% of all deaths in industrialized countries. It occurs most frequently in patients with arteriosclerotic cardiovascular disease (ASCVD), especially after MI or in patients with HF, and is usually caused by VT or VF. In a minority of patients, pulseless electrical activity and asystole are responsible. SCD may also occur in children and young adults as a consequence of mutations in genes encoding ion channels (channelopathies)[84] or sarcomeric proteins (e.g., hypertrophic cardiomyopathy). Patients at high risk for SCD are managed by implantation of a ventricular defibrillator (see earlier).

DYSLIPIDEMIAS (SEE CHAPTERS 25 AND 27)
The Past
During the 20th century, CAD emerged as the most common cause of *cardiovascular* death and elevation of low-density lipoprotein cholesterol (LDL-C) as the most important cause and progression of CAD. In 1913, Nikolai Anitschkov, a pathologist in St. Petersburg, fed large quantities of cholesterol to rabbits, raising their serum concentrations to about 1000 mg/dL and producing cholesterol-containing deposits in the aorta.[85] In 1938, Carl Müller, a Norwegian physician, described families with a high incidence of both hypercholesterolemia and CAD, thus describing what we now know as heterozygous familial hypercholesterolemia.[86]

In 1954, John Gofman, a biochemist in Berkeley, California fractionated cholesterol and identified the LDL-C responsible for producing atherosclerosis.[87] In 1964, Bloch*,[88] and Lynen*,[89] separately described the multiple steps required for the biosynthesis of cholesterol. This work led to the discovery of 3-hydroxy-3methylglutaryl co-enzyme A reductase (HMGCoA reductase), the enzyme that catalyzes the synthesis of a critically important intermediary. In 1976, Akira Endo, a pharmacologist in Tokyo, Japan, identified an inhibitor of this enzyme that reduces the biosynthesis of cholesterol and lowers the concentration of circulating LDL-C.[90] In the 1970s, Michael Brown* and Joseph Goldstein* in Dallas, Texas discovered, characterized, and cloned the LDL-C receptors on cell membranes.[91] These receptors are key to the cellular uptake of LDL-C and are normally upregulated when the biosynthesis of cholesterol is lowered, thereby reducing atherogenesis.[92] Several large clinical trials showed that the administration of these inhibitors (statins) has reduced the incidence of MI and chronic CAD.[93] These agents have prolonged and improved the lives of millions of patients worldwide and along with the development of the coronary care unit (see later) represent one of the triumphs of cardiology in the 20th century.

In 2003, Marianne Abifadel, a Lebanese postdoctoral fellow working in Paris with Catherine Boileau, discovered two gain-of-function mutations in a gene that encodes proprotein convertase subtilisin/kexin type 9 (PCSK9) in patients with autosomal dominant hypercholesterolemia.[94] PCSK9 shortens the half-life of intracellular LDL-C receptors, thus reducing their recycling to the cell surface, raising circulating LDL-C and the incidence of ASCVD. In the absence or reduced concentration of PCSK9 within the hepatocyte or in the circulation, the degradation of the LDL-C receptor is lowered, raising its concentration at the cell surface, reducing circulating LDL-C and the incidence of ASCVD.[95]

The Present
Administration of monoclonal antibodies to circulating PCSK9 in two large, phase 3 clinical outcome trials, totaling more than 45,000 patients with ASCVD, lowered LDL-C by about 55% and reduced the endpoint of cardiovascular death, MI, or stroke.[96,97] Robert Giugliano, a Boston cardiologist, reported that extremely low levels of circulating LDL-C (<15 mg/dL) appear to be safe and well tolerated.[98] It now appears to be appropriate to reduce LDL-C to below 50 mg/dL on a population-wide basis, especially in patients with or at high risk for ASCVD.

siRNA-inclisiran

The need for monthly or biweekly injections of monoclonal antibodies to PCSK9 has hindered adherence to this approach for long-term therapy. In 1998, Fire,* Mello,* et al. described a small, double-stranded RNA that can interfere with gene expression.[99] This fundamental discovery is leading to a new class of drugs that include inclisiran, a small, synthetic, two-stranded interfering siRNA that inhibits hepatocellular synthesis of PCSK9, thereby reducing circulating PCSK9, upregulating LDL-C receptors on the cell surface, and lowering circulating LDL-C. In contrast to the PCSK9 monoclonal antibodies, inclisiran requires subcutaneous administration only twice yearly to reduce LDL-C by about 50% and maintain this level. This reduction has been observed in studies in healthy volunteers and patients with elevated LDL-C levels at high vascular risk, including patients with heterozygous familial hypercholesterolemia and patients receiving intensive statin therapy.[100,101] Based on the drug's biochemical efficacy, safety, and tolerance, it has been approved for lowering LDL-C. A phase 3 double-blind, placebo-controlled trial of patients with a history of ASCVD (the ORION 4 trial NCT03705234) is currently testing whether the administration of inclisiran is associated with reductions in major cardiac events. The ability to reduce LDL-C by about 50% in patients already receiving maximal LDL-C–lowering therapy and requiring only two injections annually augurs well for LDL-C control in large populations in the future.

The Future
Triglycerides

These lipids have long been known to be coronary risk factors, although not as potent as LDL-C. Genetic activation of the lipoprotein lipase gene (*LPL*) reduces serum triglycerides (TGs) and is associated with a low incidence of CAD and T2DM.[102] Angiopoietin-like 3 (ANGPTL3), a protein that is synthesized by hepatocytes, inhibits expression of *LPL*, thereby *increasing* circulating TGs. Heterozygous loss of function mutations of ANGPTL3 are associated with reductions of both LDL-C and TG,[103] lowering the risk of the development of CAD and T2DM. Three approaches to reducing ANGPTL3 are currently under investigation: (1) a hepatocyte-directed antisense oligonucleotide (vupanorsen) that reduces TG as well as apolipoproteins B and CIII[104]; (2) evinacumab, a monoclonal antibody against ANGPTL3 that reduces TG and has been approved to reduce LDL-C in patients with homozygous familial and other forms of hypercholesterolemia[105]; and (3) very preliminary studies on editing the gene encoding ANGPTL3; if the latter proves to be successful, it could provide a "one-shot long-term therapy."[103] Also, in vivo CRISPR base editing of PCSK9 has been shown to durably lower cholesterol in primates.[103a]

Lipoprotein (a)

Elevations of circulating Lp(a) are associated with four interrelated phenotypic changes, each of which increases cardiovascular risk: (1) accelerated atherogenesis; (2) intensification of vascular inflammation; (3) worsening of calcific AS;[106] and (4) enhancement of a prothrombotic state.[107] Lp(a) can be reduced with antisense oligonucleotides that target the *LPA* gene inhibiting hepatic production of Lp(a) in a dose-dependent manner.[107] Another approach is with siRNA technology. In addition, in the FOURIER-TIMI 59 trial,[96] the monoclonal PCSK9 antibody evolocumab was shown to be moderately effective in reducing elevated Lp(a).[108]

It appears likely that continued reduction of ASCVD by further population-wide suppression of LDL-C will occur, accompanied by reduction of TG and Lp(a). The maximum benefit from these measures will be obtained by starting preventive therapy early in life (see Primordial Prevention, later). The combination of these several "attacks" on the dyslipidemias, if widely carried out, could greatly reduce the incidence of ASCVD and thereby exert an enormous impact on the practice of cardiology.

ACUTE MYOCARDIAL INFARCTION (SEE CHAPTERS 37 TO 39)

In the 19th century, physiologists noted that ligation of a major coronary artery in the dog led immediately to fatal VF. It was assumed that the same occurred in patients who developed a sudden coronary occlusion. In 1910, Obraztzov and Straschenko, two Ukrainian physicians, reported that coronary occlusion in patients is associated with chest pain and AMI, but that immediate death may not occur.[109] By mid-century, AMI was regarded as the most common single cause of death in industrialized nations; many of these deaths were sudden. The introduction of the coronary care unit in 1961 by Desmond Julian, a British cardiologist,[110] was critical to the prevention of these sudden cardiac deaths and led to a reduction of mortality in AMI from about 30% to 15%. Implementation of these units spread rapidly around the world.

The major remaining risk of AMI was consequent to large infarctions that caused left ventricular failure. To reduce infarct size in patients with AMIs, it was necessary to correct the large imbalance between the oxygen supply and demand of the severely ischemic myocardium.[111] The successful restoration of perfusion of a coronary artery obstructed by a thrombus in a patient with AMI was first reported in 1976 by Yevgeny Chazov, a Soviet cardiologist, who infused a thrombolytic agent, largely streptokinase, directly into the affected coronary artery[112] (Fig. 1.3). In 1986, a large multicenter clinical trial of AMI, the GISSI trial, demonstrated a reduction in mortality with *intravenous* streptokinase.[113] GISSI was closely followed by the ISIS 2 trial led by Peter Sleight, a British cardiologist, that demonstrated that the combination of streptokinase and aspirin was even more beneficial than streptokinase alone.[114]

Ever more effective techniques of myocardial reperfusion began with the development of more potent fibrinolytic agents, such as tissue plasminogen activator,[115,116] followed by the use of percutaneous coronary angioplasty[27,28] and then coronary artery stents (see later).[117] To be effective, reperfusion has to be carried out as quickly as possible after the onset of symptoms. With successful early reperfusion, mortality fell in half again, to about 7%. Mortality was reduced further with treatment using an angiotensin-converting enzyme (ACE) inhibitor as demonstrated by Marc Pfeffer, a Boston cardiologist.[118]

Coronary Risk Factors

In 1948, U.S. President Truman established the National Heart (now Heart, Lung and Blood) Institute, which has provided substantial

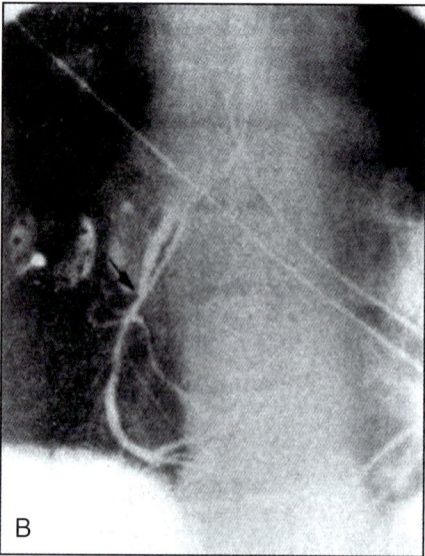

FIGURE 1.3 Acute myocardial infarction. A, Pretreatment total occlusion of right coronary artery (RCA). **B,** Post-treatment with intracoronary fibrinolytic (largely streptokinase). There is persistent nonocclusive narrowing of the RCA, with perfusion of the inferior wall of the left ventricle. (From Chazov EI, Matveeva LS, Mazaev AV, et al. Intracoronary administration of fibrinolysin in acute myocardial infarction. Ter Arkh 1976;48:8-19.)

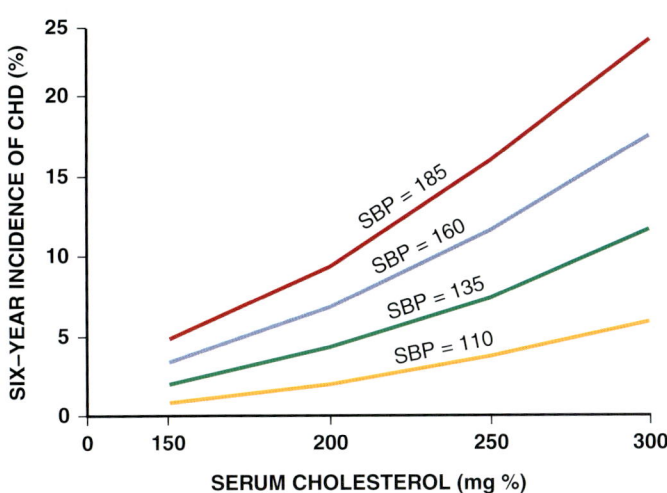

FIGURE 1.4 Synergistic effects of two coronary risk factors. Six-year incidence of coronary heart disease (CHD) according to cholesterol levels and systolic blood pressures (SBP) in men 45 to 62 years. (From Kannel WB, Dawber TR, Kagan A, et al. Factors of risk in the development of coronary heart disease: Six-year follow-up experience. The Framingham Study. Ann Int Med 1961;55:33-50.)

resources for research. One early effort of the institute was the conduct of an epidemiologic study of CAD, carried out in Framingham, near Boston, Massachusetts. The Framingham Heart Study (FHS) was the first large-scale, prospective, multigenerational observational study on a general population in the United States, established primarily to identify the determinants of CAD. In addition to the initial clinical assessments, imaging studies, biomarkers, genomics, and other "omics" technologies were included as they became available to the FHS.[119,120]

In 1961, William Kannel, an epidemiologist with the FHS, reported that the *"risk factors"* for CAD were male sex, hypertension, elevated serum cholesterol, diabetes, and electrocardiographic left ventricular hypertrophy.[121] This led to the development of the FHS risk score, a simplified version of which has been used widely in clinical practice[120] (Fig. 1.4).

HEART FAILURE (SEE PART VI)

The Past

Forty years after Harvey's publication of *De Motu Cordis*, Richard Lower, an Oxford physician-scientist, described HF as a condition "when the heart lacks the strength to preserve a constant circulation of the blood. . . . This can occur when the heart is too laden with fat or suffers from inflammation, so that it is unable to pulsate and contract."[3] In 1831, James Hope described the "backward" theory of HF, with elevation of pressures upstream of the affected ventricle or valve.[122] An opposing theory, the "forward failure" theory, was proposed about a century later by James Mackenzie,[123] who asserted that diminished cardiac output was the principal problem in HF. Irrespective of which theory was accepted, it was agreed that retention of sodium and water causes dyspnea and edema in HF. Before the 20th century, there was no effective treatment of this condition other than digitalis, and the efficacy of this drug is now in question. Mercurial diuretics became available in the 1920s and were widely used but were only moderately effective. By the 1950s, two orally active diuretics, a benzothiadiazine (chlorothiazide) and a mineralocorticoid receptor blocker, were developed and improved the care of patients with HF. More potent diuretics, the "loop" diuretics, were introduced in the 1960s.

Some members of two classes of neurohormonal blockers, beta-adrenergic blockers first described by James Black,*,[124] a British pharmacologist, as well as ACE inhibitors,[118,125] diminished the symptoms of HF, and prolonged life in patients with HF. Cardiac transplantation, introduced in 1967,[126] extended life in the small number of patients for whom a donor heart could be identified.

During the 19th and most of the 20th centuries, cardiovascular physiologists and cardiologists assumed that HF was caused by the inability of the left ventricle to eject blood during systole, and because the left ventricle dilated, its ejection fraction declined, causing HF with reduced ejection fraction (HFrEF). Other patients with HF were described in which systolic function is largely preserved, but in which ventricular filling (diastolic function) is impaired[119] because of slowed ventricular relaxation[127] and reduced ventricular compliance. This led to HF with preserved ejection fraction (HFpEF), which by the end of the century was responsible for almost half of the patients with HF.

The Present

Three types of devices introduced in the latter half of the 20th century have had beneficial effects in the treatment of HF: (1) cardiac resynchronization therapy,[128] in which multisite pacing of the ventricles enhances ventricular performance; (2) implanted cardioverter-defibrillators[81] which reduce the incidence of sudden death in patients with HF; and (3) left ventricular assist devices (LVADs, see later).[129] In the 21st century *three new* disease-modifying therapies were shown to reduce cardiovascular mortality in patients with HFrEF. The first are the mineralocorticoid receptor antagonists; spironolactone was shown by Pitt, Zannad, and colleagues to be life prolonging in patients with HFrEF (the RALES trial was published in 1999).[130] The second is sacubitril/valsartan, a first in class angiotensin neprilysin inhibitor (ARNi), which was superior to enalapril, a widely used ACE inhibitor.[131] The third are the sodium-glucose transporter 2 inhibitors (SGLT2is) that cause glucosuria and had been employed as second-tier antidiabetic agents until they were shown to reduce cardiovascular mortality and prevent HF hospitalization in patients with T2DM.[132] At the time of this writing (May 2021), three drugs in this class, dapagliflozin, empagliflozin, and sotagliflozin, have also been shown to be effective in nondiabetic patients with HFrEF.[133,134,134a] SGLT2i has been shown to be renoprotective in patients with diabetic and nondiabetic chronic kidney disease.[135]

Each of these three drug classes are relatively well tolerated, and representatives of each group can be administered together and with a beta blocker. Two trials, one with spironolactone led by Marc Pfeffer and Bertram Pitt,[136,137] and the other with sacubitril/valsartan led by Scott Solomon, a co-editor of this book,[138] have shown encouraging benefit. Innovative trials of nonpharmacologic approaches using the creation of left-to-right atrial shunting are under evaluation. Preliminary studies of an antisense oligonucleotide have reported favorable results in HF as well.[139]

ASSISTED CIRCULATION (SEE CHAPTER 58)

The Past

In 1968, the use of an intra-aortic balloon pump (IABP), was reported by Kantrowitz, a cardiac surgeon in New York.[140] This device was used in patients with cardiogenic shock, secondary to AMI or after cardiotomy. Although IABP exerted a modest favorable effect on hemodynamics, it did not improve clinical outcome with regularity and it became clear that more powerful devices were required for the treatment of severe HF. During the 1980s and 1990s, a variety of pneumatic LVADs underwent extensive animal testing and clinical trials.[129] They were used in patients in cardiogenic shock, and as a bridge to cardiac transplantation, but it was not clear whether they were superior to GDMT.

The REMATCH trial published in 2001 was the first controlled randomized trial that compared long-term LVAD support with optimal GDMT in patients with advanced (Class IV) HF who were ineligible for cardiac transplantation. This trial, led by Eric Rose, a New York cardiac surgeon, showed that 1 year after randomization, survival in the LVAD group was twice that in the medical arm.[141] This landmark trial served as a potent stimulus to the field and led the FDA to approve the LVAD employed in the trial for destination therapy, that is, for the patient's lifetime. The device, while reflecting the state of the art at the turn of the century, was bulky and noisy, with the large pulsatile pumping chamber placed in the abdomen. Although its use prolonged survival, it was associated with many adverse events, including local and systemic infections, stroke, excessive bleeding, thrombosis, and device failure.

The Present
Many refinements were made in LVADs in the last two decades. An important step was the development of an intrathoracic continuous axial flow pump, the HeartMate II,[142] which was associated with better outcomes than the pneumatic device used in REMATCH. A further development was the Heart Mate 3, a magnetically levitated centrifugal flow pump, which was even smaller, and in a trial led by Mandeep Mehra, a Boston cardiologist, it was shown to be safer as well, with elimination of pump thrombosis and lower stroke rate.[143]

Early in the 21st century, several reports appeared of a small fraction of patients on chronic LVAD support who exhibited recovery of sufficient cardiac function to allow explantation of the device.[144] Teams in London,[145] Berlin,[146] and Louisville, Kentucky[147] described the phenotypes of patients in whom recovery was possible. These patients are younger than the patients usually receiving an LVAD, have a shorter duration of HF, and are more likely to have a dilated rather than ischemic cardiomyopathy.

The Future
Although the currently available LVADs reflect striking advances when compared with their predecessors, they are still reminiscent of the Model T Ford of a century ago. With the demand for these pumps increasing steadily and the ongoing rapid strides in bioengineering and material science, it is likely that the next generation of LVADs will be smaller, easier to implant, and less likely to thrombose, with transcutaneous transmission of power without the need of a drive line, and perhaps less expensive than current versions.

Looking forward, it has been suggested that mechanical assisted circulation might also be provided by an implanted extra-aortic counterpulsation system for patients with moderately severe, chronic HF. In a preliminary feasibility trial, Abraham et al. wrapped an inflatable cuff around the ascending aorta and connected it to an external battery-powered pneumatic driver triggered by an epicardial lead.[148] This device, designed for chronic ambulatory use, would not be in contact with blood and therefore would not require anticoagulation. Possibly, it might be activated intermittently when needed. A second possible form of partial ventricular support described by Meyns et al. was implanted via a mini-thoracotomy and positioned in a subclavicular subcutaneous pocket, like a pacemaker. In a feasibility trial it showed substantial hemodynamic benefit and appeared to slow the progressive deterioration of advanced HF.[149] Although neither of these two devices is ready for clinical application, they do point to possible future directions. It is likely that further technologic advances will provide sufficient mechanical support of the circulation at an earlier stage of chronic HF and thereby reduce the need for pharmacologic inotropic support and/or the need for an LVAD of the current variety.

GENOMICS AND GENETICS (SEE CHAPTER 7)
The Present
The first decade of the 21st century was ushered in by one of the most important scientific accomplishments in the history of biology—the initial draft of the Human Genome Project (HGP), which provided an analysis of approximately 90% of the human genome.[150,151] The HGP was developed by a team at the National Institutes of Health, led by Francis Collins, and simultaneously by Celera Genomics, a private company led by Craig Venter. Each group provided maps that defined the positions of individual genes and their DNA sequences. The "finished" sequence, more than 99% complete, was published by the HGP in 2004.[152] This was soon followed by the genomes of the mouse, rat, dog, chimpanzee, and multiple bacteria and viruses and the partial genome from extinct Neanderthals.[153]

An ever-increasing number of studies have correlated specific cardiovascular disorders with single gene mutations. These include a number of dyslipidemias, a variety of arrhythmias, several cardiomyopathies, hypercoagulable and hypocoagulable states, and Marfan syndrome, among others. In many of these monogenic disorders, the diagnosis can now be established by genetic testing carried out in commercial laboratories; others require analyses in research laboratories. Screening of close relatives of patients with monogenic disorders is increasing, and many asymptomatic carriers are now being identified and counseled.

GWAS[154] have enabled discovery and mapping of DNA variants and have identified phenotypes that are controlled by multiple genes. The implications of GWAS for clinical medicine, including cardiology, are profound. For example, GWAS have been applied to CAD, T2DM, essential hypertension, and atrial fibrillation. These GWAS have identified multiple risk variants that appear to enhance the likelihood of these conditions, and they have facilitated the development of polygenic risk scores. Fortunately, the cost of GWAS is declining rapidly, and at the time of this writing the combination of GWAS and whole exome sequencing can be obtained for $230.

Direct-to-consumer (DTC) genetic testing began in 2006, and in 2017 the FDA issued its first approval of a genetic health screen. DTC is now a widely advertised, successful business. However, there is little control of the interpretation of the results and counseling of the "customers." The electronic medical record, with its description of phenotype, including clinical features, imaging, biomarkers, and responses to interventions is used increasingly to interact with genetic information, enhancing accurate diagnosis and risk of disease, that is, precision medicine.

The Future
In 2012, Emmanuelle Charpentier* a French geneticist, and Jennifer Doudna,* an American biochemist, demonstrated that CRISPR/Cas (clustered regularly interspaced short palindromic repeats with CRISPR-associated protein) can edit DNA with great precision.[155] This technique permits the identification of the specific variants that contribute to disease and will be enormously helpful in molecular diagnosis of many disorders, including those involving the cardiovascular system.[156] Initial reports of CRISPR-Cas9 editing of patients with sickle cell disease and beta-thalassemia are encouraging.[157] Gene editing in cancer, HIV, and lysosomal storage disease is ongoing.[156]

Precision Medicine
During the first two decades of the 21st century, emphasis on human variability, both inherited and acquired, increased rapidly. In many patients, important genetic differences and phenotypic features will be identified by the other so-called "omics" technologies; they need to be considered in establishing a diagnosis and developing a personalized management plan, hence the term *Personalized Medicine*.[158,159] The goal of assessing these characteristics with great precision has led to a closely related term, *Precision Medicine*,[160] which has been defined by Leopold and Loscalzo as "an integrative approach to cardiovascular disease prevention and treatment that considers an individual's genetics, lifestyle, and exposure to determinants of their cardiovascular health and disease phenotype."[161]

PRIMORDIAL PREVENTION (SEE CHAPTER 25)
The Present
The goal of *primordial* prevention is to promote health.[162] Primordial prevention is sometimes confused with primary prevention; primary prevention *reduces or eliminates established risk*, whereas primordial prevention is designed to *avoid future development of risk*. In 2010, the AHA developed a 7-item tool to promote cardiovascular health; it emphasizes a diet low in salt and cholesterol, regular physical activity, avoidance of smoking, and maintaining optimal levels of BP, body mass index, fasting blood glucose, and cholesterol.[163] Lifetime cardiovascular risk was shown to be proportional to the number of risk factors and their severity.[164,165]

Elevated BP in childhood tracks into adolescence and then adulthood and can be responsible for the development of at least two important risk factors for subsequent ASCVD: left ventricular hypertrophy and an increase in the carotid intima–medial thickness, the latter a predictor of arterial plaques.[166] Primordial prevention in children is important in preventing trends to an elevated BP, obesity, and excessive dietary salt intake while encouraging physical activity. It has become apparent that environmental influences in childhood play an important role in the subsequent trajectory of cardiovascular disease.

The Future

If GWAS is carried out in infants and neonates, it might be possible to commence primordial prevention early in life. There is increasing interest in primordial prevention even during the prenatal period. Maternal diabetes, obesity, and hypertension can be transmitted to the offspring, involving, at least in part, epigenetic mechanisms. The function of placental mitochondria may be impaired in maternal diabetes, and it has been proposed that metformin stimulates placental mitochondrial biogenesis, thereby providing protection to offspring.[167]

INFLAMMATION (SEE CHAPTER 24)

The Past

In 1858, the great German pathologist Rudolph Virchow recognized the importance of inflammation in the development and softening of arteriosclerotic plaques.[168] Sixty years later, Russell Ross, a Seattle pathologist, in a classic paper, focused on the various cell types and their DNA in atherosclerotic plaques concluded: "Atherosclerosis is clearly an inflammatory disease and does not result simply from the accumulation of lipids."[169]

Substantial research—both experimental and clinical—has provided strong, albeit circumstantial, support for the inflammatory hypothesis for atherogenesis.[170] Ridker, a Boston cardiologist, demonstrated that high-sensitivity C-reactive protein (hsCRP), an inflammatory biomarker, is as potent a predictor of cardiovascular risk as LDL-C.[171] Despite the logic and attractiveness of the inflammation hypothesis, until recently there had been no proof of its clinical relevance.

The Present

Canakinumab
In 2017, this relevance was demonstrated by the publication of the CANTOS trial, a 10,000-patient placebo-controlled trial on patients with prior MI and residual inflammation. Ridker, Libby, and colleagues used canakinumab, a humanized monoclonal antibody that blocks the interleukin (IL)-1β innate immunity pathway.[172] CANTOS validated the inflammatory hypothesis by demonstrating a statistically significant, albeit modest, reduction in lipid independent cardiovascular events.

Colchicine
Colchicine is a well-known anti-inflammatory agent that is effective in halting acute gouty arthritis, familial Mediterranean fever, and acute pericarditis. It appears to act by inhibiting tubulin polymerization and reduces activation of IL-1β. Tardif, a Canadian investigator, demonstrated that colchicine reduced major cardiovascular adverse events in post-MI patients in the COLCOT trial,[173] and Nidorf, an Australian investigator, observed a similar benefit in patients with chronic CAD in the LODOCO-2 trial.[174]

The Future

Further preclinical and clinical research on a variety of anti-inflammatory agents is being actively pursued. Attention is now directed to a proximal step in the inflammatory pathway. The activation of the NLRP3 inflammasome stimulates the formation of IL-1β and IL-18, two highly inflammatory cytokines,[175,176] which in turn activate IL-6, which enhances the production of CRP by the liver. Looking ahead, we can anticipate continued progress in the development of anti-inflammatory agents for the prevention and/or slowed progression of atherosclerosis. Just as a variety of drugs have been found to be useful in the treatment of hypertension, dyslipidemias, and HF, it is likely that a number of anti-inflammatory agents will be available as well. Their relative efficacy in patients with various manifestations and stages of atherosclerosis, their safety, tolerance, and cost will be important in selecting the right drug, at the right dose, at the right time, and for the right patient.

CLONAL HEMATOPOIESIS (SEE CHAPTER 24)

In 2014, Jaiswal et al. reported on whole exome sequencing of DNA obtained from leukocytes in the peripheral blood. They detected somatic mutations leading to expansion of hematopoietic stem cells associated with an increase in cardiovascular disease.[177] These cells acquire a progressive increase in such mutations, especially in the elderly. In an important follow-up paper[178] they referred to this condition as *clonal hematopoiesis of independent potential*, abbreviated as CHIP.

CHIP is associated with accelerated atherosclerosis, an increased risk of coronary artery calcification, MI, calcific AS, intravascular thrombosis, and T2DM (Fig. 1.5). The most commonly mutated CHIP-driver genes frequently occur in patients with severe AS and are associated with increased proinflammatory leukocytes, and an excessive mortality after successful TAVR.[179] CHIP is associated with an almost doubling in the incidence of cardiovascular disease and a 40% increase in all-cause mortality.[180]

For almost two thirds of a century, there has been broad agreement about the identity and importance of the classic risk factors for ASCVD, including elevated LDL-C, hypertension, T2DM, and smoking. During this extended period there has been some fine tuning of these factors. About 20 years ago a new risk factor—inflammation—was added (see earlier). More recently, CHIP has emerged as yet another potent risk factor independent of the classic (canonical) coronary risk factors. It is exciting to contemplate the implications of this discovery, as well as the challenges and opportunities it presents. First, the fundamental mechanisms through which the somatic mutations operate must be understood. In addition, the recognition and diagnosis of CHIP should be facilitated and therapies identified. Although no specific treatment has been described, Libby et al. have recommended aggressive control of classic risk factors.[180] It has been suggested that canakinumab, the monoclonal antibody that has been shown to block IL-1β in the CANTOS trial (see earlier) was associated with a marked reduction in the risk of major cardiovascular events in patients with CHIP.[181] This intriguing observation requires confirmation.

ARTIFICIAL INTELLIGENCE (SEE CHAPTER 11)

The Present

This is a broad field in which machines are programmed to perform a variety of complex tasks; machine learning is an important subfield. Artificial intelligence (AI) is playing a rapidly expanding role in biomedical research and in many branches of clinical medicine, especially those in which the information base is enormous, often referred to as "big data." Cardiology, with its numerous waveforms, images, genomic analyses, biomarkers, devices and their output, and detailed clinical data contained in voluminous electronic medical records, is becoming a major area to which AI can make enormous contributions.

Attia et al. at the Mayo Clinic have shown in subjects in sinus rhythm that their AI program could identify those who had previously experienced atrial fibrillation and are at risk of recurrence.[182] Similarly, they developed a program that identifies asymptomatic subjects with an abnormally low ejection fraction and subjects with normal left ventricular function at risk of future development of dysfunction.[183] Thus, with the aid of AI, a simple 12-lead ECG could become a much more powerful screening tool; it can also aid in estimating prognosis, including predicting future cardiovascular mortality in patients with

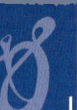

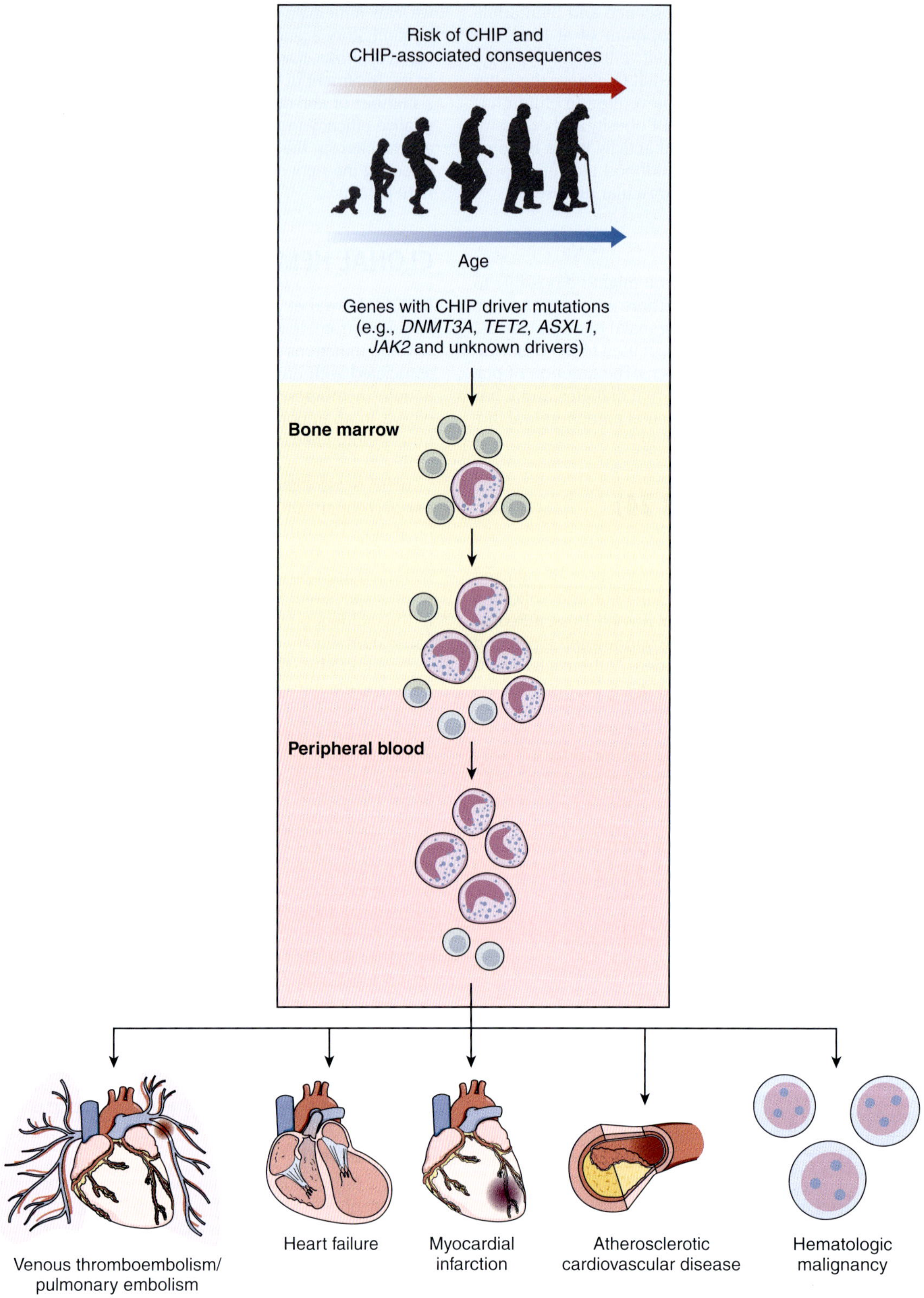

FIGURE 1.5 The progression of clonal hematopoiesis of indeterminate potential (CHIP). In ASCVD CHIP-driven expansion of myeloid cells enhances inflammation and cytokine production in the plaque. CHIP may also worsen response to pressure-induced cardiac remodeling and promotes thrombosis. (From Khetarpal SA, Qamar A, Bick AG, et al. Clonal hematopoiesis of indeterminate potential reshapes age-related CVD. J Am Coll Cardiol 2019;74[4]:578-586.)

HF.[184] AI has also been reported to use the ECG to detect hypertrophic cardiomyopathy, estimate the response to cardiac resynchronization therapy,[185] and identify patients at high risk of adverse events when undergoing TAVR.

AI appears to be useful in assessment of the rate of ventricular relaxation and in screening for diastolic dysfunction. Segar et al. have used AI to identify distinct phenotypic subgroups of patients with HFpEF. They identified three separate phenogroups with distinct clinical characteristics and outcomes.[186] Such an approach could be used to select and/or stratify patients enrolled in clinical trials of HFpEF. Given the heterogeneity of this condition, it may help in the identification of subgroups who respond to different therapies. Similar phenotyping has been reported in patients with dilated cardiomyopathy.[159] In its analysis of cardiac imaging AI can analyze both the structure and function of individual cardiac chambers and of specific regions of these chambers.[187]

The Future

The several examples of AI mentioned earlier represent pilot studies on selected patients. To determine their generalizability and to adapt this technology for routine patient care, the findings will require additional validation in specific and carefully phenotyped patient subsets. The ultimate goal of AI in clinical cardiology is to accelerate the practice of precision medicine (see earlier) and thereby to improve health care. AI could become of particular value in populations with limited access to specialists. However, concern has been raised that AI could place yet another technologic barrier between caregivers and their patients. Hopefully, it will have the opposite effect; by accomplishing complex tasks rapidly and accurately it could increase the efficiency of busy caregivers who would be freed up to provide more time for direct patient contact. Despite the initial expense of developing the necessary programs, AI could lower costs by reducing the need for expensive nonessential diagnostic procedures and shortening or avoiding hospitalizations.

CONCLUSIONS

As we approach the 400th anniversary of the publication of *De Motu Cordis*,[1] it may be of interest to consider the author of this founding document of cardiovascular science and its subsequent impact on clinical cardiology. William Harvey was a highly respected physician, the doctor to two kings of England, an admired lecturer, and, of course, an extraordinarily gifted investigator. Today he would be classified as an academic "triple threat." A majority of the investigators cited in this review were (or are) also triple threats. Eighteen have been rewarded with a Nobel Prize. Thus, cardiology is a science-based clinical specialty with a distinguished history.

Cardiovascular diseases were considered to be quite rare until the beginning of the 20th century, when over a relatively short period they became recognized as the most common causes of death in industrialized nations. Diagnosis and management of these conditions have improved immensely since 1950. It has been a unique privilege for this author to have had a ringside seat during this period and witness the enormous progress in this field. However, despite this progress, the incidence of cardiovascular morbidity and mortality remain disturbingly high.[188]

We have now reached a critical point in the history of cardiology. Going forward, it would seem wise to move in three directions: The first is to continue to apply further advances in the basic sciences to improving cardiovascular care; this has served our specialty well for almost 400 years and will continue to do so. The second, which is socioeconomic and political, is to ensure that the entire population benefits from the many advances that have been achieved.[188] This is certainly not the case today. Cardiovascular care is lagging in developing countries and in pockets of poverty and in minorities in industrialized nations. However, even when treatment and prevention are affordable they are often not employed. For example, hypertension remains a critically important risk factor for cardiac and cerebrovascular disease. Effective, well-tolerated and inexpensive antihypertensive drugs have been available for years. Yet BP is well controlled in only half of the hypertensive population in the United States. The third, and perhaps the most important direction, is to place greater emphasis, intellectual energy, and resources on prevention of cardiovascular disease and to begin this as early in life as possible.

REFERENCES

1. Harvey W. *Exercitatio anatomica de motu cordis et sanguinis in animalibus (An anatomical disquisition on the motion of the heart and blood in animals). London, 1628. Translated by Robert Willis.* Surrey, England: Barnes; 1847.
2. Malpighi M. *De Pulmonibus.* Bologna: Observationes Anatomicae; 1661.
3. Lower R. *De Corde in Gunther RT.* London: Dawnson Press; 1933.
4. Hales S. *Statical Essays Containing Haemastatics; or, an Account of Some Hydraulic and Hydrostatical Experiments Made on the Blood and Blood Vessels of Animals.* 3rd ed; 1769.
5. Laennec RTH. *Traité de l'auscultation médiate et des maladies du poumon et du Coeur.* 3rd ed; 1819.
6. Withering W. *Account of the Foxglove and Some of its Medical Uses: with Practical Remarks on Dropsy, and Other Diseases.* London: GGJ and J Robinson, Paternoster-Row; 1785.
7. Heberden W. Some accounts of a disorder of the breast. *Medical Transactions.* 1772;2:59.
8. Warren J. Remarks on angina pectoris. *N Engl J Med.* 1812;1:1–11.
9. Osler W. The Lumelian Lectures on angina pectoris *Lancet* I. 697:839.
10. Mahomed FA. Some of the clinical aspects of chronic Bright's disease. *Guys Hosp Reports.* 1879;24:363.
11. MacWilliam JA. Some applications of physiology to medicine II. Ventricular fibrillation and sudden death. *British Med J II.* 1923;215.
12. Roentgen WC. *On a New Kind of Rays.* Sitzungsberichte der Würzburger Physik.-medic. Gesellschaft; 1895.
13. Riva-Rocci S. Un Nuovo Sfigmomanometro. *Gaz Med Torino.* 1896;47:981–996.
14. Korotkoff NS. On the subject of methods of measuring blood pressure. *Bull Imp Military Med Acad.* 1905;11:365–367.
15. Einthoven W. The galvanometric registration of the human electrocardiogram, likewise a review of the use of the capillary-electrometer in physiology. *Pflüger's Arch f.d. ges Physiol.* 1903;99:472–480.
16. Sones Jr FM, Shirey EK. Cine coronary arteriography. *Mod Concepts Cardiovasc Dis.* 1962;31:735–738.
17. Edler I, Hertz CH. Use of ultrasonic reflectoscope for the continuous recording of movements of heart walls. *Kungl Fysiogr Sallsk Lund Forth.* 1954:24–40.
18. Hounsfield GN. Computerized transverse axial scanning (tomography). 1. Description of system. *Br J Radiol.* 1973;46:1016–1022.
19. Lauterbur P. Image formation by induced local interactions: examples employing nuclear magnetic resonance. *Nature.* 1973;242:190–191.
20. Agatston AS, Janowitz WR, Hildner FJ, et al. Quantification of coronary artery calcium using ultrafast computed tomography. *J Am Coll Cardiol.* 1990;15:827–832.
21. Korosoglou G, Elhmidi Y, Steen H, et al. Prognostic value of high-dose dobutamine stress magnetic resonance imaging in 1,493 consecutive patients: assessment of myocardial wall motion and perfusion. *J Am Coll Cardiol.* 2010;56:1225–1234.
22. Stoll VM, Clarke WT, Levelt E, et al. Dilated cardiomyopathy: Phosphorus 31 MR spectroscopy at 7 T. *Radiology.* 2016;281:409–417.
23. Williams MC, Hunter A, Shah ASV, et al. Use of coronary computed tomographic angiography to guide management of patients with coronary disease. *J Am Coll Cardiol.* 2016;67:1759–1768.
24. Forssmann W. Die Sondierung des rechten Herzens [Probing of the right heart]. *Klin Wochenschr.* 1929;8:2085–2207.
25. Cournand AF, Ranges HS. Catheterization of the right auricle in man. *Proc Soc Exp Biol Med.* 1941;46:462–466.
26. Richards DW. Cardiac output by the catheterization technique in various clinical conditions. *Fed Proc.* 1945;4:215–220.
27. Gruentzig AR, Senning A, Siegenthaler WE. Nonoperative dilation of coronary-artery stenosis: percutaneous transluminal coronary angioplasty. *N Engl J Med.* 1979;301:61–68.
28. Zijlstra F, de Boer MJ, Hoorntje JCA, et al. A comparison of immediate coronary angioplasty with intravenous streptokinase in acute myocardial infarction. *N Engl J Med.* 1993;328:680–684.
29. Sigwart U, Puel J, Mirkovitch V, et al. Intravascular stents to prevent occlusion and restenosis after transluminal angioplasty. *N Engl J Med.* 1987;316:701–706.
30. Gross RE, Hubbard JH. Surgical ligation of a patent ductus arteriosus: report of first successful case. *J Am Med Assoc.* 1939;112:729–733.
31. Gibbon Jr JH. Application of a mechanical heart and lung apparatus to cardiac surgery. *Minn Med.* 1954;37:171–175.
32. Starr A, Edwards ML. Mitral replacement: clinical experience with a ball-valve prosthesis. *Ann Surg.* 1961;154:726–740.
33. Favaloro RG. Saphenous vein autograft replacement of severe segmental coronary occlusion: operative technique. *Ann Thorac Surg.* 1968;5:334–339.
34. Yusuf S, Zucker D, Peduzzi P, et al. Effect of coronary artery bypass graft surgery on survival: overview of 10-year results from randomised trials by the Coronary Artery Bypass Graft Surgery Trialists Collaboration. *Lancet.* 1994;344:563–570.
35. Bright R. Tabular view of the morbid appearances in 100 cases connected with albuminurious urine. *Guy's Hosp Rep.* 1836;1:380.
36. Tigerstedt R, Bergman PG. Niere und kreislauf. *Skand. Arch. Physiol.* 1898;8:223–271.
37. Goldblatt H, Lynch J, Hanzal RF, Summerville WW. Studies on experimental hypertension: I. The production of persistent elevation of systolic blood pressure by means of renal ischemia. *J Exp Med.* 1934;59:347–379.
38. Braun-Menendez E, Fasciolo JC, Leloir LF, Munoz JM. The substance causing renal hypertension. *J Physiol.* 1940;98:283–298.
39. Weiss S. The development of the clinical concept of arterial hypertension. *N Engl J Med.* 1930;19:891–897.
40. Kempner W. Treatment of hypertensive vascular disease with rice diet. *Am J Med.* 1948;4:545–577.
41. Smithwick RH, Thompson JE. Splanchnicectomy for essential hypertension; results in 1,266 cases. *J Am Med Assoc.* 1953;152:1501–1504.
42. Veterans Administration Cooperative Study Group on Antihypertensive Agents. Effects of treatment on morbidity in hypertension I: results in patients with diastolic blood pressures averaging 115 through 129 mm Hg. *J Am Med Assoc.* 1967;202:1028–1034.
43. Veterans Administration Cooperative Study Group on Antihypertensive Agents. Effects of treatment on morbidity in hypertension II: results in patients with diastolic blood pressures averaging 90 through 114 mm Hg. *J Am Med Assoc.* 1970;213:1143–1152.
44. Whelton PK, Carey RM, Aronow WS, et al. ACC/AHA/AAPA/ABC/ACPM/AGS/APhA/ASH/ASPC/NMA/PCNA guideline for the prevention, detection, evaluation, and management of high blood pressure in adults: Executive summary: a report of the American College of Cardiology/American Heart Association Task Force on clinical practice guidelines. *Hypertension.* 2018;71:1269–1324.
45. Carey RM. Special Article - the management of resistant hypertension: a 2020 update. *Prog Cardiovasc Dis.* 2020;63:662–670.
46. Brown JM, Siddiqui M, Calhoun DA, et al. The unrecognized prevalence of primary aldosteronism: a cross-sectional study. *Ann Intern Med.* 2020;173:10–20.
47. Agarwal R, Kolkhof P, Bakris G, et al. Steroidal and non-steroidal mineralocorticoid receptor antagonists in cardiorenal medicine. *Eur Heart J.* 2021;42:152–161.
48. Morris BJ. Gene team in blood pressure genetics. *Circ Cardiovasc Genet.* 2017;10:e001776.
49. Kraja AT, Cook JP, Warren HR, et al. New blood pressure-associated loci identified in meta-analyses of 475 000 individuals. *Circ Cardiovasc Genet.* 2017;10:e001778.
50. Van Oort S, Beulens JWJ, van Ballegooijen AJ, et al. Association of cardiovascular risk factors and lifestyle behaviors with hypertension: a Mendelian randomization study. *Hypertension.* 2020;76:1971–1979.
51. Zafarmand MH, Spanjer M, Nicolaou M, et al. Influence of dietary approaches to stop hypertension-type diet, known genetic variants and their interplay on blood pressure in early childhood: ABCD study. *Hypertension.* 2020;75:59–70.
52. Muralitharan RR, Jama HA, Xie L, et al. Microbial peer pressure: the role of the gut microbiota in hypertension and its complications. *Hypertension.* 2020;76:1674–1687.
53. Wells MC. On rheumatism of the heart. *Trans Soc Improv Med and Chir Knowledge.* 1812;3:345.
54. Harken DE, Ellis LB, Ware PF, Norman LR. The surgical treatment of mitral stenosis. I. Valvuloplasty. *N Engl J Med.* 1948;239:801–809.
55. Inoue K, Owaki T, Nakamura T, et al. Clinical application of transvenous mitral commissurotomy by a new balloon catheter. *J Thorac Cardiovasc Surg.* 1984;87:394–402.
56. Ross Jr J, Braunwald E, Morrow AG. Left heart catheterization by the transseptal route. A description of the technique and its applications. *Circulation.* 1960;22:927–934.

57. Turi ZG, Reyes VP, Raju BS, et al. Percutaneous balloon versus surgical closed commissurotomy for mitral stenosis. *Circulation*. 1991;83:1179–1185.
58. Meneguz-Moreno RA, Costa Jr JR, Gomes ML, et al. Very long term follow-up after percutaneous balloon mitral valvuloplasty. *J Am Coll Cardiol Intv*. 2018;11:1945–1952.
59. Alfieri O, Maisano F, De Bonis M, et al. The double-orifice technique in mitral valve repair: a simple solution for complex problems. *J Thorac Cardiovasc Surg*. 2001;122:674–681.
60. Goar St FG, Fann JI, Komtebedde J, et al. Endovascular edge-to-edge mitral valve repair: short-term results in a porcine model. *Circulation*. 2003;108:1990–1993.
61. Feldman T, Foster E, Glower DD, et al. Percutaneous repair or surgery for mitral regurgitation. *N Engl J Med*. 2011;364:1395–1406.
62. Stone GW, Lindenfeld J, Abraham WT, et al. Transcatheter mitral-valve repair in patients with heart failure. *N Engl J Med*. 2018;379:2307–2318.
63. Obadia J-F, Messika-Zeitoun D, Leurent G, et al. Percutaneous repair or medical treatment for secondary mitral regurgitation. *N Engl J Med*. 2018;379:2297–2306.
64. Otto CM, Nishimura RA, Bonow RO, et al. 2020 ACC/AHA guideline for the management of patients with valvular heart disease: Executive summary: a report of the ACC/AHA Joint committee on clinical practice guidelines. *Circulation*. 2021;143:e35–e71.
65. Andersen HR, Knudsen LL, Hasenkam JM. Transluminal implantation of artificial heart valves. Description of a new expandable aortic valve and initial results with implantation by catheter technique in closed chest pigs. *Eur Heart J*. 1992;11:704–708.
66. Cribier A, Eltchaninoff H, Bash A, et al. Percutaneous transcatheter implantation of an aortic valve prosthesis for calcific aortic stenosis: first human case description. *Circulation*. 2002;106:3006–3008.
67. Webb JG, Chandavimol M, Thompson CR, et al. Percutaneous aortic valve implantation retrograde from the femoral artery. *Circulation*. 2006;113:842–850.
68. Leon MB, Smith CR, Mack M, et al. Transcatheter aortic-valve implantation for aortic stenosis in patients who cannot undergo surgery. *N Engl J Med*. 2010;363:1597–1607.
69. Cahill TJ, Terre J, George I. Over 15 years: the advancement of transcatheter aortic valve replacement. *Ann Cardiothorac Surg*. 2020;9:442–451.
70. Carroll JD, Mack MJ, Vemulapalli S, et al. STS-ACC TVT registry of transcatheter aortic valve replacement. *J Am Coll Cardiol*. 2020;76:2492–2516.
71. Snellen AH. *History of Cardiology*. Rotterdam: Donkor Academic Publications; 1984.
72. Vaughan-Williams EM. Classification of anti-arrhythmic drugs. In: Sandoe E, Flenstad-Jansen E, Olesen KH, eds. *Symposium on Cardiac Arrhythmias, Sotetalje, Sweden*. AB Astra; 1970:449–472.
73. Vaughan-Williams EM. A classification of antiarrhythmic actions reassessed after a decade of new drugs. *J Clin Pharmacol*. 1984;24:129–147.
74. Echt DS, Liebson PR, Mitchell LB, et al. Mortality and morbidity in patients receiving encainide flecainide, or placebo. The Cardiac Arrhythmia Suppression Trial. *N Engl J Med*. 1991;324:781–788.
75. Wellens HJJ. *Electrical Stimulation of the Heart in the Study and Treatment of Tachycardia*. Baltimore: University Park Press; 1971.
76. Haft JI. Treatment of arrhythmias by intracardiac electrical stimulation. *Prog Cardiovasc Dis*. 1974;16:539.
77. Zoll PM. Resuscitation of the heart in ventricular standstill by external electrical stimulation. *N Engl J Med*. 1952;247:768–771.
78. Chardack WM, Gage AA, Greatbatch W. A transistorized, self-contained, implantable pacemaker for the long-term correction of complete heart block. *Surgery*. 1960;48:643–654.
79. Kouwenhoven WB, Jude JR, Knickerbocker GG. Closed-chest cardiac massage. *J Am Med Assoc*. 1960;173:1064–1067.
80. Lown B, Amarasingham R, Neuman J. New method for terminating cardiac arrhythmias. Use of synchronized capacitor discharge. *J Am Med Assoc*. 1962;182. 5485-55.
81. Mirowski M, Reid PR, Mower MM, et al. Termination of malignant ventricular arrhythmias with an implanted automatic defibrillator in human beings. *N Engl J Med*. 1980;303:322–324.
82. Shivkumar K. Catheter ablation of ventricular arrhythmias. *N Engl J Med*. 2019;380:1555–1564.
83. Andrade JC, Wells GA, Deyell MW, et al. Cryoablation of drug therapy for initial treatment of atrial fibrillation. *N Engl J Med*. 2021;384:305–315.
84. Bezzina CR, Lahrouchi N, Priori SG. Genetics of sudden cardiac death. *Circ Res*. 2015;116:1919.
85. Anitschkow N, Chalatow S. Ueber experimentelle cholesterinsteatose und ihre bedeutung für die entstehung einiger pathologischer prozesse. *Zentralbl. Allg. Pathol. Anat.* 1913;24:1–9.
86. Müller C. Xanthomata, hypercholesterolemia, angina pectoris. *Acta Med Scand*. 1938;89:75–84.
87. Gofman JW, Rubin L, McGinley JP, Jones HB. Hyperlipoproteinemia. *Am J Med*. 1954;17:514–520.
88. Bloch K. The biological synthesis of cholesterol. *Science*. 1965;150:19–28.
89. Lynen F. *Der Weg von der "aktivierten Essigsaure" zu den terpenen und der Fettsäuren. Les Prix Nobel*. Stockholm: Morstedt and Sons; 1965:205–245.
90. Endo A, Kuroda M, Tanzawa K. Competitive inhibition of 3-hydroxy-3-methylglutaryl coenzyme A reductase by ML-236A and ML-236B fungal metabolites, having hypocholesterolemic activity. *FEBS Lett*. 1976;72:323–326.
91. Brown MS, Goldstein JL. A receptor-mediated pathway for cholesterol homeostasis. *Science*. 1986;232:34–47.
92. Goldstein JL, Brown MS. A century of cholesterol and coronaries: from plaques to genes to statins. *Cell*. 2015;161:161–172.
93. Collins R, Reith C, Emberson J, et al. Interpretation of the evidence for the efficacy and safety of statin therapy. *Lancet*. 2016;388:2532–2561.
94. Abifadel M, Varret M, Rabes J-P, et al. Mutations in PCSK9 cause autosomal dominant hypercholesterolemia. *Nat Genet*. 2003;34:154–156.
95. Cohen JC, Boerwinkle E, Mosley Jr TH, Hobbs HH. Sequence variations in PCSK9, low LDL, and protection against coronary heart disease. *N Engl J Med*. 2006;354:1264–1272.
96. Sabatine MS, Giugliano RP, Keech AC, et al. Evolocumab and clinical outcomes in patients with cardiovascular disease. *N Engl J Med*. 2017;376:1713–1722.
97. Schwartz GG, Steg PC, Szarek M, et al. Alirocumab and cardiovascular outcomes after acute coronary syndrome. *N Engl J Med*. 2018;379:2097–2107.
98. Giugliano RP, Pedersen TR, Park J-G, et al. Clinical efficacy and safety of achieving very low LDL-cholesterol concentrations with the PCSK9 inhibitor evolocumab: a prespecified secondary analysis of the FOURIER trial. *Lancet*. 2017;390:1962–1971.
99. Fire A, Xu S, Montgomery MK, et al. Potent and specific genetic interference by double-stranded RNA in *Caenorhabditis elegans*. *Nature*. 1998;391:806–811.
100. Ray KK, Wright RS, Kallend D, et al. Two phase 3 trials of inclisiran in patients with elevated LDL cholesterol. *N Engl J Med*. 2020;382:1507–1519.
101. Raal FJ, Kallend D, Ray KK, et al. Inclisiran for the treatment of heterozygous familial hypercholesterolemia. *N Engl J Med*. 2020;382:1520–1530.
102. Liu D, Peloso GM, Yu H, et al. Exome-wide association study of plasma lipids in >300,000 individuals. *Nature Genet*. 2017;49:1758–1766.
103. Wang X, Musunuru K. Angiopoietin-like 3. From discovery to therapeutic gene editing. *JACC (J Am Coll Cardiol): Basic Trans Sci.* 2019;4:755–762.
103a. Musunuru K, Chadwick AC, Mizoguchi T, et al. In vivo CRISPR base editing of PCSK9 durably lowers cholesterol in primates. *Nature*. 2021;593:429–434.
104. Gaudet D, Karwatowska KE, Baum SJ, et al. Vupanorsen, an N-acetyl galactosamine-conjugated antisense drug to ANGPTL3 mRNA, lowers triglycerides and atherogenic lipoproteins in patients with diabetes hepatic steatosis, and hypertriglyceridaemia. *Eur Heart J*. 2020;41:3936–3945.
105. Raal FJ, Rosenson RS, Reeskamp LF, et al. Evinacumab for homozygous familial hypercholesterolemia. *N Engl J Med*. 2020;383:711–720.
106. Thanassoulis G. Lipoprotein(a) in calcific aortic valve disease: from genomics to novel drug target for aortic stenosis. *J Lipid Res*. 2016;57:917–924.
107. Tsimikas S, Karwatowska-Prokopczuk E, Gouni-Berthold I, et al. Lipoprotein(a) reduction in persons with cardiovascular disease. *N Engl J Med*. 2020;382:244–245.
108. O'Donoghue ML, Fazio S, Giugliano RP, et al. Lipoprotein(a), PCSK9 inhibition, and cardiovascular risk. Insights from the FOURIER trial. *Circulation*. 2019;139:1483–1492.
109. Obrastzov WP, Straschenko ND. Zur Kenntniss der Thrombose der Koronartertien der Herzen. *Zeitschrift f Klin Med*. 1910;71:116.
110. Julian DG. Treatment of cardiac arrest in acute myocardial ischemia and infarction. *Lancet*. 1961;ii:840–844.
111. Maroko PR, Braunwald E. Modification of myocardial infarct size after coronary occlusion. *Ann Intern Med*. 1973;79:720–733.
112. Chazov EI, Mateeva LS, Mazaev AV. Intracoronary administration of fibrinolysin in acute myocardial infarction. *Ter Arkh*. 1976;48:8–19.
113. Gruppo Italiano per lo Studio della Streptochinasi nell'Infarto Miocardico (GISSI). Effectiveness of intravenous thrombolytic treatment in acute myocardial infarction. *Lancet*. 1986;1:397–402.
114. Second International Study of Infarct Survival Collaborative Group. Randomised trial of intravenous streptokinase, oral aspirin, both, or neither among 17,187 cases of suspected acute myocardial infarction: ISIS-2. *Lancet*. 1988;2:349–360.
115. Pennica D, Holmes WE, Kohr WJ, et al. Cloning and expression of human tissue-type plasminogen activator cDNA in E. coli. *Nature*. 1983;301:214–221.
116. TIMI Study Group. The Thrombolysis in Myocardial Infarction (TIMI) trial. Phase I findings. *N Engl J Med*. 1985;312:932–936.
117. Zhu MM, Feit A, Chadow H, et al. Primary stent implantation compared with primary balloon angioplasty for acute myocardial infarction. A meta analysis of randomized clinical trials. *Am J Cardiol*. 2001;88:297–301.
118. Pfeffer MA, Braunwald E, Moye LA, et al. Effect of captopril on mortality and morbidity in patients with left ventricular dysfunction after myocardial infarction. Results of the Survival and Ventricular Enlargement Trial. *N Engl J Med*. 1992;327:669–677.
119. Mahmood SS, Levy D, Vasan RS, Wang TJ. The Framingham Heart Study and the epidemiology of cardiovascular disease: a historical perspective. *Lancet*. 2014;383:999–1008.
120. Anderson C, Johnson AD, Benjamin EJ, et al. 70-year legacy of the Framingham heart study. *Nat Rev Cardiol*. 2019;16:687–698.
121. Kannel WB, Dawber TR, Kagan A, et al. Factors of risk in the development of coronary heart disease: six-year follow-up experience. The Framingham Study. *Ann Intern Med*. 1961;55:33–50.
122. Hope JA. *Treatise on the Diseases of the Heart and Great Vessels*. London: William-Kidd; 1832.
123. Mackenzie J. Diseases of the Heart, 3rd ed. London. Oxford University Press, 1913.
124. Black JW, Stevenson JS. Pharmacology of a new adrenergic betareceptor compound. *Lancet*. 1962;2:311–314.
125. Ondetti MA, Rubin B, Cushman DW. Design of specific inhibitors of angiotensin-converting-enzyme: new class of orally active antihypertensive agents. *Science*. 1977;196. 441–441.
126. Barnard CN. The operation. A human cardiac transplant: an interim report of a successful operation performed at Groote Schuur Hospital. *Cape Town. S. Afr Med J.* 1967;41:1271–1274.
127. Pasipoularides A, Mirsky I, Hess OM, et al. Myocardial relaxation and passive diastolic properties in man. *Circulation*. 1986;74:991–1001.
128. Abraham WT. Cardiac resynchronization therapy is important for all patients with congestive heart failure and ventricular dysynchrony. *Circulation*. 2006;114:2692–2698.
129. Holman WL, Bourge RC, McGiffin DC, Kirklin JK. Ventricular assist: experience with a pulsatile heterotopic device. *Semin Thorac Cardiovasc Surg*. 1994;6:147–153.
130. Pitt B, Zannad F, Remme WJ, et al. The effect of spironolactone on morbidity and mortality in patients with severe heart failure. *N Engl J Med*. 1999;341:709–717.
131. McMurray JJ, Packer M, Desai AS, et al. Angiotensin-neprilysin inhibition versus enalapril in heart failure. *N Engl J Med*. 2014;371:993–1004.
132. Zelniker TA, Braunwald E. Clinical benefit of cardiorenal effects of sodium-glucose cotransporter 2 inhibitors: JACC State-of-the-Art Review. *J Am Coll Cardiol*. 2020;75:435–447.
133. McMurray JJV, Solomon SD, Inzucchi SE, et al. Dapagliflozin in patients with heart failure and reduced ejection fraction. *N Engl J Med*. 2019;381:1995–2008.
134. Packer M, Anker SD, Butler J, et al. Cardiovascular and renal outcomes with empagliflozin in heart failure. *N Engl J Med*. 2020;383:1413–1424.
134a. Bhatt DL, Szarek M, Steg PG, et al. Sotagliflozin in patients with diabetes and recent worsening heart failure. *N Engl J Med*. 2020;384:117–128.
135. Heerspink HJL, Stefansson BV, Correa-Rotter R, et al. Dapagliflozin in patients with chronic kidney disease. *N Engl J Med*. 2020;383:1436–1446.
136. Pitt B, Pfeffer MA, Assmann SF, et al. Spironolactone for heart failure with preserved ejection fraction. *N Engl J Med*. 2014;370:1383–1392.
137. Braunwald E, Pfeffer MA. Treatment of heart failure with preserved ejection fraction: reflections on its treatment with an aldosterone antagonist. *JAMA Cardiol*. 2016;1:7–8.
138. Solomon SD, McMurray JJV, Anand IS, et al. Angiotensin-neprilysin inhibition in heart failure with preserved ejection fraction. *N Engl J Med*. 2019;381:1609–1620.
139. Taubel J, Hauke W, Rump S, et al. Novel antisense therapy targeting microRNA-132 in patients with heart failure: results of a first-in-human phase 1b randomized, double-blind, placebo-controlled study. *Eur Heart J*. 2021;42:178–188.
140. Kantrowitz A, Tjonneland S, Freed PS, et al. Intraaortic balloon pump. *J Am Med Assoc*. 1968;203:988.
141. Rose EA, Gelijns AC, Moskowitz AJ, et al. Long-term use of a left ventricular assist device for end-stage heart failure. *N Engl J Med*. 2001;345:1435–1443.
142. Slaughter MS, Rogers JG, Milano CA, et al. Advanced heart failure treated with continuous-flow left ventricular assist device. *N Engl J Med*. 2009;361(23):2241–2251.
143. Mehra MR, Uriel N, Naka Y. A fully magnetically levitated left ventricular assist device - Final report. *N Engl J Med*. 2019;380:1618–1627.
144. Farrar DJ, Holman WR, McBride LR, et al. Long-term follow-up of Thoratec ventricular assist device bridge-to-recovery patients successfully removed from support after recovery of ventricular function. *J Heart Lung Transplant*. 2001;21:516–521.
145. Yacoub MH. A novel strategy to maximize the efficacy of left ventricular assist devices as a bridge to recovery. *Eur Heart J*. 2001;22:534–540.
146. Dandel M, Weng Y, Siniawski H, et al. Heart failure reversal by ventricular unloading in patients with chronic cardiomyopathy: criteria for weaning from ventricular assist devices. *Eur Heart J*. 2011;32:1148–1160.
147. Birks EJ, Drakos SG, Patel SR, et al. Prospective multicenter study of myocardial recovery using left ventricular assist devices (RESTAGE-HF [Remission from Stage D Heart Failure]): Medium-Term and primary end point results. *Circulation*. 2020;142:2016–2028.
148. Abraham WT, Aggarwal S, Prabhu SD, et al. Ambulatory extra-aortic counterpulsation in patients with moderate to severe chronic heart failure. *J Am Coll Cardiol*. 2014;2:526–533.
149. Meyns B, Klotz S, Simon A, et al. Proof of concept: hemodynamic response to long-term partial ventricular support with the synergy pocket micro-pump. *J Am Coll Cardiol*. 2009;54:79–86.
150. International Human Genome Sequencing Consortium. Initial sequencing and analysis of the human genome. *Nature*. 2001;409:860–891.

151. Venter JC, Adams MD, Myers EW, et al. The sequence of the human genome. *Science*. 2001;291:1304–1351.
152. International Human Genome Sequencing Consortium. Finishing the euchromatic sequencing of the human genome. *Nature*. 2004;431:931–945.
153. Lander ES. Initial impact of the sequencing of the human genome. *Nature*. 2011;470:187–197.
154. Nikpey M, Goel A, Won H, et al. A comprehensive 1000 genomes-based genome-wide association meta-analysis of coronary artery disease. *Nat Genet*. 2015;47:1121–1130.
155. Collins FS, Doudna JA, Lander ES, Rotimi CN. Human molecular genetics and genomics - important advances and exciting possibilities. *N Engl J Med*. 2021;384:1–4.
156. Broeders JA, Herrero-Hernandez P, Ernst MPT, et al. Sharpening the molecular scissors: advances in gene-editing technology. *iScience*. 2020;23:100789.
157. Frangoul H, Altshuler D, Cappellini MD, et al. CRISPR-Cas9 gene editing for sickle cell disease and β-Thalassemia. *N Engl J Med*. 2021;384:252–260.
158. Ginsburg GS, McCarthy JJ. Personalized medicine: revolutionizing drug discovery and patient care. *Trends Biotechnol*. 2001;19:491–496.
159. Elliott PM. Personalized medicine for dilated cardiomyopathy. *Eur Heart J*. 2021;42:175–177.
160. Jameson JL, Longo DL. Precision medicine – personalized, problematic, and promising. *N Engl J Med*. 2015;372:2229–2234.
161. Leopold JA, Loscalzo J. Emerging role of precision medicine in cardiovascular disease. *Circ Res*. 2018;122:1302–1315.
162. Gaye R, Lloyd-Jones DM. Primordial prevention of cardiovascular disease: several challenges remain. *Int J Cardiol*. 2019;274:370–380.
163. Lloyd-Jones DM, Leip EP, Larson MG, et al. Prediction of lifetime risk for cardiovascular disease by risk factor burden at 50 years of age. *Circulation*. 2006;113:791–798.
164. Berry JD, Dyer A, Cai X, et al. Lifetime risks of cardiovascular disease. *N Engl J Med*. 2012;366:321–329.
165. Younus A, Aneni EC, Spatz ES, et al. A systematic review of the prevalence and outcomes of ideal cardiovascular health in US and non-US populations. *Mayo Clin Proc*. 2016;91:649–670.
166. Falkner B, Lurbe E. Primordial prevention of high blood pressure in childhood. An opportunity not to be missed. *Hypertension*. 2020;75:1142–1150.
167. Agarwal P, Morriseau TS, Kereliuk SM, et al. Maternal obesity, diabetes during pregnancy and epigenetic mechanisms that influence the developmental origins of cardiometabolic disease in the offspring. *Rit Rev Clin Lab Sci*. 2018;55:71–101.
168. Virchow R. *Cellular Pathology*. London: John Churchill; 1858.
169. Ross R. Atherosclerosis – an inflammatory disease. *N Engl J Med*. 1999;340:115.
170. Lawler PR, Bhatt DL, Godoy LC, et al. Targeting cardiovascular inflammation: next steps in clinical translation. *Eur Heart J*. 2021;42:113–131.
171. Ridker PM. From C-reactive protein to Interleukin-6 to Interleukin-1: Moving upstream to identify novel targets for atheroprotection. *Circ Res*. 2016;118:145–156.
172. Ridker PM, Everett BM, Thuren T, et al. Antiinflammatory therapy with canakinumab for atherosclerotic disease. *N Engl J Med*. 2017;377:1119–1131.
173. Tardif JC, Kouz S, Waters DD, et al. Efficacy and safety of low-dose colchicine after myocardial infarction. *N Engl J Med*. 2019;381:2497–2505.
174. Nidorf SM, Fiolet ATL, Mosterd A, et al. Colchicine in patients with chronic coronary disease. *N Engl J Med*. 2020;383:1838–1847.
175. Ridker PM. From CANTOS to CIRT to COLCOT to Clinic: will all atherosclerosis patients soon be treated with combination lipid-lowering and inflammation-inhibiting agents? *Circulation*. 2020;141:787–789.
176. Libby P. Interleukin-1 beta as a target for atherosclerosis therapy: biological basis of CANTOS and beyond. *J Am Coll Cardiol*. 2017;70:2278–2289.
177. Jaiswal S, Fontanillas P, Flannick J, et al. Age-related clonal hematopoiesis associated with adverse outcomes. *N Engl J Med*. 2014;371:2488–2498.
178. Jaiswal S, Natarajan P, Silver AJ, et al. Clonal hematopoiesis and risk of atherosclerotic cardiovascular disease. *N Engl J Med*. 2017;377:111–121.
179. Mas-Peiro S, Hoffmann J, Fichtlscherer S, et al. Clonal haematopoiesis in patients with degenerative aortic valve stenosis undergoing transcatheter aortic valve implantation. *Eur Heart J*. 2020;41:933–939.
180. Libby P, Sidlow R, Lin AE, et al. Clonal hematopoiesis. Crossroads of aging, cardiovascular disease, and cancer. *J Am Coll Cardiol*. 2019;74:567–577.
181. Svensson EC, Madar A, Campbell CD, et al. Abstract 15111: TET2-driven clonal hematopoiesis predicts enhanced response to canakinumab in the CANTOS Trial: an exploratory analysis. *Circulation*. 2018;138:A15111–A15111.
182. Attia ZI, Noseworthy PA, Lopez-Jimenez F, et al. An artificial intelligence-enabled ECG algorithm for the identification of patients with atrial fibrillation during sinus rhythm: a retrospective analysis of outcome prediction. *Lancet*. 2019;394:861–867.
183. Attia ZI, Kapa S, Yao X, et al. Prospective validation of a deep learning electrocardiogram algorithm for the detection of left ventricular systolic dysfunction. *J Cardiovasc Electrophysiol*. 2019;30:668–674.
184. Kwon J-M, Kim K-H, Jeon K-H, et al. Artificial intelligence algorithm for predicting mortality of patients with acute heart failure. *PloS One*. 2019;14:e0219302.
185. Feeny AK, Richard J, Patel D, et al. Machine learning prediction of response to cardiac resynchronization therapy. *Circ Arrhythm Electrophysiol*. 2019;12:e007316.
186. Segar MW, Patel KV, Ayers C, et al. Phenomapping of patients with heart failure with preserved ejection fraction using machine learning-based unsupervised cluster analysis. *Eur J Heart Fail*. 2020;22:148–158.
187. Zhang J, Gajjala S, Agrawal P, et al. Fully automated echocardiogram interpretation in clinical practice. *Circulation*. 2018;138:1623–1635.
188. Roth GA, Mensah GA, Johnson CO, et al. Global burden of cardiovascular diseases and risk factors, 1990-2019: Update from the GBD 2019 study. *J Am Coll Cardiol*. 2020;76:2982–3021.

2 Global Burden of Cardiovascular Disease

THOMAS A. GAZIANO, DORAIRAJ PRABHAKARAN, AND J. MICHAEL GAZIANO

SHIFTING BURDEN, 14

EPIDEMIOLOGIC TRANSITIONS, 14
Stage of Inactivity and Obesity: A Fifth Phase?, 15
Different Patterns of Epidemiologic Transition, 16

CURRENT VARIATIONS IN THE GLOBAL BURDEN, 16
High-Income Countries, 18
East Asia and Pacific, 19
Central and Eastern Europe and Central Asia, 19

Latin America and the Caribbean, 19
North Africa and Middle East, 20
South Asia, 20
Sub-Saharan Africa, 20

RISK FACTORS, 20
Tobacco, 20
Hypertension, 22
Lipids, 23
Diabetes, 23
Obesity, 23
Diet, 24
Physical Inactivity, 25

Aging Populations, 25
Fetal Influences, 26
Environmental Exposures, 26

ECONOMIC BURDEN, 26

COST-EFFECTIVE SOLUTIONS, 27
Established Cardiovascular Disease Management, 27
Risk Assessment, 27
Policy and Community Interventions, 28

SUMMARY AND CONCLUSION, 29

REFERENCES, 29

SHIFTING BURDEN

Between 1990 and 2017, deaths from cardiovascular disease (CVD) increased from 26% to 32% of all deaths globally, a reflection of the rapid epidemiologic transition, particularly in low- and middle-income countries (LMICs). Although the net percentage of deaths caused by CVD overall has increased, this reflects a rise in LMICs and a decline in high-income countries (HICs) (Fig. 2.1). CVD now causes most deaths in all low- and middle-income regions, with the exception of sub-Saharan Africa, where it is the second leading cause of death overall, and the leading cause in those 50 years and older. In absolute numbers, five times as many CVD deaths occurred in the low- and middle-income regions combined than in the High-Income region in 2017 (14.8 million to 3 million). Within the six World Bank–defined low- and middle-income regions, the CVD burden differs vastly (Fig. 2.2), with CVD deaths accounting for as much as 43.7% of all deaths in Europe and Central Asia and as little as 12.3% in sub-Saharan Africa. Cardiovascular disease accounts for 31.8% of deaths in HICs.

EPIDEMIOLOGIC TRANSITIONS

The overall increase in the global burden of CVD and the distinct regional patterns result in part from the "epidemiologic transition," which includes four basic stages (Table 2.1): Pestilence and Famine, Receding Pandemics, Degenerative and Man-Made Diseases, and Delayed Degenerative Diseases.[2,3] Movement through these stages has dramatically shifted the causes of death over the last two centuries, from infectious diseases and malnutrition in the first stage to CVD and cancer in the third and fourth stages. Although the transition through the stage of Pestilence and Famine has occurred much later in LMICs, it has also occurred more rapidly, driven largely by the transfer of low-cost agricultural technologies, the overall globalization of world economies, and public health advances.

Humans evolved during the stage of Pestilence and Famine and have lived with epidemics and hunger for most of recorded history. Before 1900, infectious diseases and malnutrition constituted the most common causes of death in virtually every part of the world, with tuberculosis, pneumonia, and diarrheal diseases accounting for a majority of deaths. These conditions, along with high infant and child mortality rates, resulted in a mean life expectancy of approximately 30 years.

Per capita income and life expectancy increased during the stage of Receding Pandemics as the emergence of public health systems, cleaner water supplies, and improved food production and distribution combined to reduce deaths from infectious disease and malnutrition. Improvements in medical education and with other public health changes, contribute to dramatic declines in infectious disease mortality rates. Rheumatic valvular disease, hypertension, and cerebrovascular accident (stroke) cause most CVD. Coronary heart disease (CHD) often occurs at a lower prevalence rate than stroke, and CVD accounts for 10% to 35% of deaths.

During the stage of Degenerative and Man-Made Diseases, continued improvements in economic circumstances, combined with urbanization and radical changes in the nature of work-related activities, led to dramatic changes in diet, activity levels, and behaviors such as smoking. For example, in the United States, deaths from infectious diseases decreased to less than 50 per 100,000 people per year, and life expectancy increased to almost 70 years. The increased availability of foods high in calories, coupled with decreased physical activity, contribute to an increase in atherosclerosis. In this stage, CHD and stroke predominate, and between 35% and 65% of all deaths are related to CVD. Typically, the ratio of CHD to stroke is 2:1 to 3:1.

In the stage of Delayed Degenerative Diseases, CVD and cancer remain the major causes of morbidity and mortality, but CVD age-adjusted mortality rates decline by almost half, accounting for 25% to 40% of all deaths. Two significant advances have contributed to the decline in CVD mortality rates: new therapeutic approaches and prevention measures targeted at people with or at risk for CVD.[4,5]

Treatments once considered advanced including the establishment of emergency medical systems, coronary care units, and the widespread use of new diagnostic and therapeutic technologies such as echocardiography, cardiac catheterization, percutaneous coronary intervention (PCI), bypass surgery, and implantation of pacemakers and defibrillators have now become the standard of care. Advances in drug development have also yielded major benefits on both acute and chronic outcomes. Efforts to improve the acute management of myocardial infarction (MI) led to the application of lifesaving interventions such as beta-adrenergic blocking agents (beta blockers), PCI, thrombolytics, statins, and angiotensin-converting enzyme (ACE) inhibitors (see Chapters 37 and 38). Advances in both heart failure and diabetes management have led to new angiotensin-receptor neprilysin inhibitors, SGLT2 inhibitors, and GLP-1 agonists which reduce cardiovascular

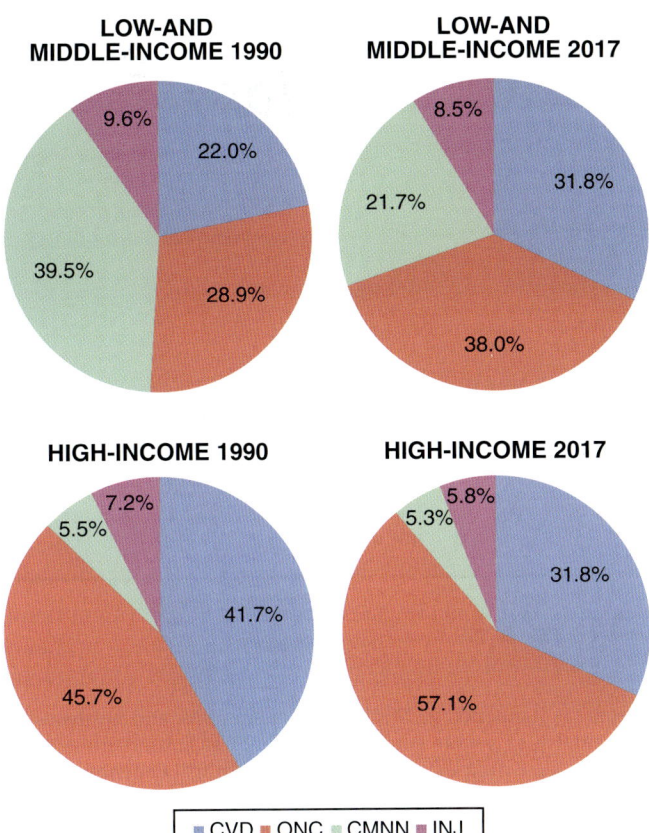

FIGURE 2.1 Changing pattern of mortality, 1990 to 2017. *CMNN*, communicable, maternal, neonatal, and nutritional diseases; *CVD*, cardiovascular disease; *INJ*, injury; *ONC*, other noncommunicable diseases. (From Global Burden of Disease Study 2017. *Age-sex Specific All-cause and Cause-specific Mortality, 1990–2017*. Seattle: Institute for Health Metrics and Evaluation; 2017.)

events. The widespread use of an "old" drug, aspirin, has also reduced the risk of dying of acute or secondary coronary events. Low-cost pharmacologic treatment for hypertension (see Chapter 26) and the development of highly effective cholesterol-lowering drugs such as statins have also made major contributions to both primary and secondary prevention by reducing CVD-related deaths (see Chapter 27).

In concert with these advances, public health campaigns have conveyed that certain behaviors increase the risk of CVD and that lifestyle modifications can reduce risk. In this regard, smoking cessation furnishes a model of success. In the United States, for example, 57% of men smoked cigarettes in 1955; in 2018, 15.6% of men smoked. The prevalence of smoking among U.S. women has fallen from 34% in 1965 to 13.7% in 2018.[6] Campaigns from the 1970s dramatically improved the detection and treatment of hypertension in the United States. This intervention likely had an immediate and profound effect on stroke rates and a subtler effect on CHD rates. Public health messages concerning saturated fat and cholesterol had a similar impact on fat consumption and cholesterol levels. Population mean cholesterol levels also declined, from 220 mg/dL in the early 1960s to 191 mg/dL by 2016,[7] with a simultaneous decrease in the prevalence of elevated low-density lipoprotein (LDL) cholesterol.

Stage of Inactivity and Obesity: A Fifth Phase?

Troubling trends in certain risk behaviors and risk factors may foreshadow a new phase of epidemiologic transition, the stage of Inactivity and Obesity (see Chapters 30 and 31).[8] In many parts of the industrialized world, physical activity continues to decline while total caloric intake increases at alarming rates, resulting in an epidemic of overweight and obesity. Consequently, the rates of type 2 diabetes, hypertension, and lipid abnormalities associated with obesity are rising, a particularly evident trend in children.[9] These changes are occurring while measurable improvements in other risk behaviors and risk factors, such as smoking, have slowed. If these trends continue, age-adjusted CVD mortality rates, which have declined over the past several decades in HICs, could plateau, as they have for young women

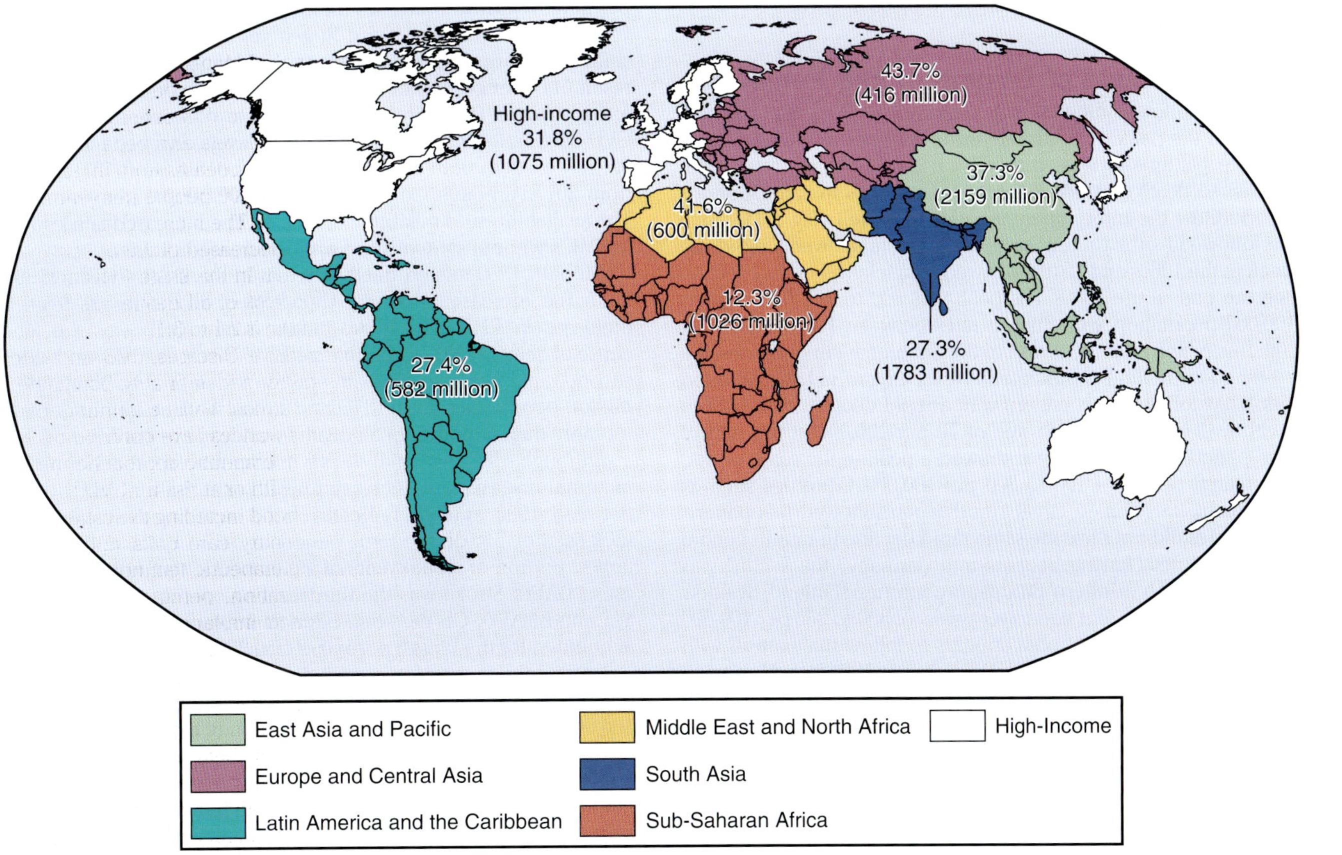

FIGURE 2.2 Cardiovascular disease deaths as a percentage of all deaths in each region and total regional population, 2017. (From Global Burden of Disease Study 2017. *Age-sex Specific All-cause and Cause-specific Mortality, 1990–2017*. Seattle: Institute for Health Metrics and Evaluation; 2017; and World Health Organization. Global Health Observatory Data Repository. Demographic and socioeconomic statistics: population data by country. http://apps.who.int/gho/data/view.main.POP2040?lang=en.)

TABLE 2.1 Five Typical Stages of Epidemiologic Transition in Cardiovascular Disease Mortality and Types

STAGE	DESCRIPTION	TYPICAL PROPORTION OF DEATHS CAUSED BY CVD (%)	PREDOMINANT TYPES OF CVD
Pestilence and famine	Predominance of malnutrition and infectious diseases as causes of death; high rates of infant and child mortality; low mean life expectancy.	<10	Rheumatic heart disease, cardiomyopathies caused by infection and malnutrition
Receding pandemics	Improvements in nutrition and public health lead to decrease in rates of deaths caused by malnutrition and infection; precipitous decline in infant and child mortality rates.	10–35	Rheumatic valvular disease, hypertension, CHD, stroke
Degenerative and man-made diseases	Increased fat and caloric intake and decreased physical activity lead to emergency of hypertension and atherosclerosis; with increased life expectancy, mortality from chronic, noncommunicable diseases exceeds mortality from malnutrition and infectious diseases.	35–65	CHD, stroke
Delayed degenerative diseases	CVDs and cancer are the major causes of morbidity and mortality; better treatment and prevention efforts help avoid deaths among those with disease and delay primary events. Age-adjusted CVD mortality declines; CVD affects older and older individuals.	40–50	CHD, stroke, congestive heart failure
Inactivity and obesity	Increasing prevalence of obesity and diabetes; some slowing of CVD mortality rates in women.	38	

CHD, Coronary heart disease; *CVD,* Cardiovascular disease.
Modified from Omran AR. The epidemiologic transition: a theory of the epidemiology of population change. *Milbank Mem Fund Q.* 1981;49:509; and Olshanksy SJ, Ault AB. The fourth stage of the epidemiologic transition: the age of delayed degenerative diseases. *Milbank Q.* 1986;64:355.

in the United States, or even increase in the coming years. This trend pertains particularly to age-adjusted stroke death rates. This concerning increase in obesity also applies to LMICs.[10]

Fortunately, recent trends in the first decade of the present century suggest a tapering in the increase in obesity rates among adults, although the rates remain alarmingly high at almost 42.4%.[11] Furthermore, continued progress in the development and application of therapeutic advances and other secular changes appear to have offset the effects from the changes in obesity and diabetes; cholesterol levels, for example, continue to decline. Overall, in this decade, age-adjusted mortality has continued to decline at about 3% per year, from a rate of 341 per 100,000 population in 2000 to 223 per 100,000 in 2013.[12]

Different Patterns of Epidemiologic Transition

The HICs have followed different patterns of the CVD transition, which differ in both the peak of death rate from CHD and the time of transition. Three patterns emerge that rely on data from countries with an established death certification system. Countries in Latin America appear to follow the three different patterns as well (Fig. 2.3).[13] One pattern, followed by the United States and Canada, showed a rapid rise and peak in the 1960s and 1970s, followed by a relatively rapid decline through the end of the 2000s. The peak was 300 to 700 CHD deaths per 100,000 population, with current rates between 100 and 200 per 100,000. This pattern also occurred in the Scandinavian countries, the United Kingdom, Ireland, Australia, and New Zealand. In Latin America, Argentina has followed this pattern with a rapid decline from 1985 to 2016 with a CHD-related death rate of 70 per 100,000 at the end of the time period. A second pattern showed a peak in the same period in CHD-related deaths of 100 to 300 per 100,000. Countries such as Portugal, Spain, Italy, France, Greece, and Japan followed this pattern. Some countries did not have the same rapid decline in rate. In central European countries (Austria, Belgium, and Germany), the decline was slower compared to northern European countries (Finland, Sweden, Denmark, and Norway), but had lower peaks of 300 to 350 per 100,000 in the 1960s and 1970s. Colombia appears to follow this pattern with relatively flat to declining levels at 150 deaths per 100,000, with a small decline from 2010 to 2015. Some countries appear to display a third pattern of continued rise (particularly many components of the former Soviet Union), and others have yet to see any significant increase, such as many countries in sub-Saharan Africa (excluding South Africa). Mexico appears to follow this pattern with rates nearly doubling from 80 to 160 per 100,000 from 1985 to 2015. Whether other LMICs will follow a "classic" pattern of significant increases then rapid declines in rates (as happened in North America, Australia, and northwestern European HICs), a more gradual rise and fall (as in southern and central European countries), or some other pattern, will depend in part on cultural differences, secular trends, and responses at the country level with regard to both public health and treatment infrastructures.

CURRENT VARIATIONS IN THE GLOBAL BURDEN

Three phenomena impact the various metrics of disease burden. First, population growth increases the overall number of deaths caused by CVD globally. Second, a trend in general aging of the population has shifted the proportion of deaths caused by CVD in most regions as a result of better control of many communicable diseases that manifest at early stages. Third, prevention of CVD and treatment for those with CVD have both improved, which reduces age-adjusted mortality rates. We rely on data from the Global Burden of Disease (GBD) study data from 2017. Although extensive, data from GBD 2017 have limitations. The availability and reliability of data on the cause of death, especially in LMICs without standardized protocols, are uncertain.

Globally, CVD-related deaths increased by 49% between 1990 and 2017. The increase in overall CVD-related deaths results from both increases in CHD and stroke-related deaths. CHD was the leading cause of death in 2017, accounting for 16% of all deaths worldwide. The second-ranking cause of death was stroke, at 11%. An estimated 15.1 million people died from CHD and stroke, which together accounted for more than a quarter of all deaths worldwide in 2017.[1]

Although still substantial, deaths from communicable, neonatal, and maternal diseases are decreasing worldwide,[1] with a 32.5% decrease between 1990 and 2017. Deaths from noncommunicable diseases increased by 53% in the same period. In 2017, CHD accounted for the largest portion of global years of life lost (YLLs) and the second highest of DALYs. Stroke was the third-ranking contributor to both global YLLs and DALYs. On the other hand, in 1990, communicable diseases accounted for the largest portion of both YLLs and DALYs.

Despite the increase in overall CVD-related deaths, the age-adjusted death rates decreased by 30.4% in the same period, from 335 to 233 per 100,000 population, suggesting significant delays in the age of occurrence and/or improvements in case-fatality rates. Unfortunately, not all countries share in the reductions. Examination of regional trends is helpful in estimating global trends in the burden of disease, particularly CVD. Because 85% of the world's population lives in LMICs, these countries largely drive global CVD rates. These estimates depend on

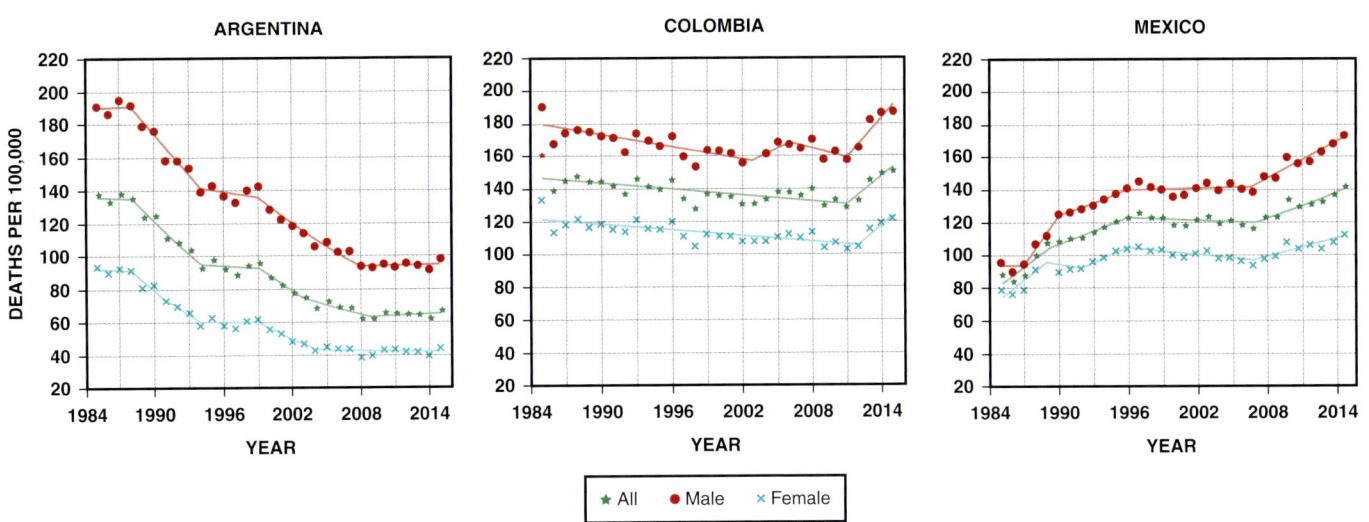

FIGURE 2.3 Trends in age-standardized mortality rates per 100,000 by sex for coronary heart disease. Argentina, Colombia, and Mexico. 1985–2015. Star: all; circle: male; cross: female. (From Arroyo-Quiroz C, Barrientos-Gutierrez T, O'Flaherty M, et al. Coronary heart disease mortality is decreasing in Argentina, and Colombia, but keeps increasing in Mexico: a time trend study. *BMC Public Health.* 2020;20(1):162. http://creativecommons.org/licenses/by/4.0/.)

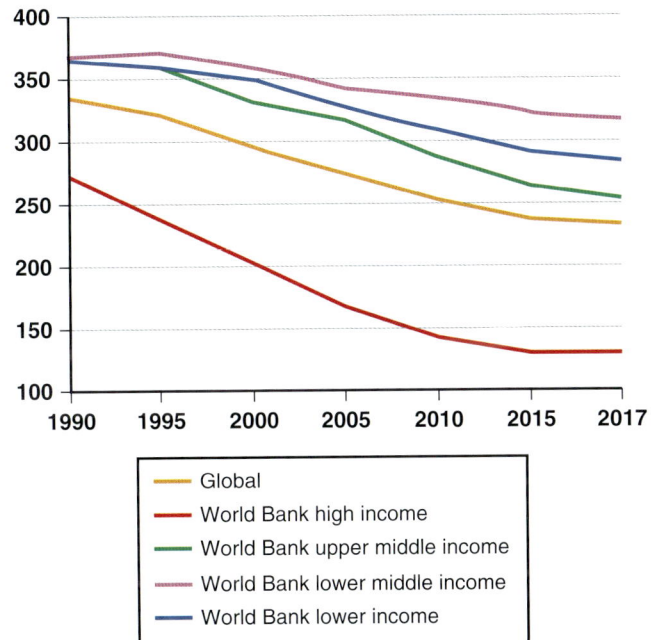

FIGURE 2.4 Cardiovascular disease death rates per 100,000 population from 1990 to 2017, by World Bank income categories. (From Global Burden of Disease Study 2017. *Age-sex Specific All-cause and Cause-specific Mortality, 1990–2017.* Seattle: Institute for Health Metrics and Evaluation; 2017.)

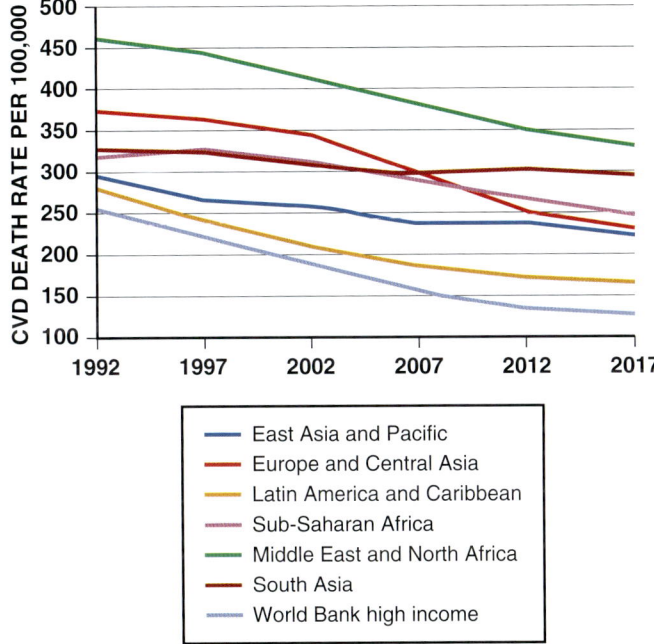

FIGURE 2.5 Cardiovascular disease death rates per 100,000 population from 1990 to 2017 in low- and middle-income countries by region, compared to World Bank high-income countries. (From Global Burden of Disease Study 2017. *Age-sex Specific All-cause and Cause-specific Mortality, 1990–2017.* Seattle: Institute for Health Metrics and Evaluation; 2017.)

modeling mortality rates in areas where established death certification–based vital registration systems do not cover the entire country. Even as age-adjusted rates have been falling globally, the pattern is different when assessed by income (Fig. 2.4) or by region (Fig. 2.5).

The magnitude of the peak of the CVD epidemic, and whether the peak has arrived at all, has a great range. Here we describe and highlight trends in the seven regions of the world as defined by the GBD project, which includes HICs as one grouping and divides the remaining LMICs into six geographic regions, further divided by sub-regions: the High-Income, East Asia and Oceania, Central and Eastern Europe and Central Asia, Latin America and Caribbean, Middle East and North Africa, and sub-Saharan Africa regions. All these regions had declines in age-adjusted CVD mortality rates from 1990 to 2017. South Asia had only a slight decrease in its age-adjusted CVD mortality rates.

Much of the variation is related to income, which is one proxy for the stages of the epidemiologic transition. Looking at age-adjusted CVD-related death rates by World Bank, the high-income regions had different trends over the last two and a half decades. In the low-income region, the death rate has decreased from 364 to 285 per 100,000 between 1990 and 2017. The Lower Middle-Income region saw a small increase (368 to 371 per 100,000) between 1990 and 1995, followed by a fall to 317 per 100,000 in 2017. The upper middle-income region saw a 30% decline, from 365 to 254 per 100,000 between 1990 and 2017. The high-income region had a 53% decline, from 272 to 128 CVD deaths per 100,000.

The LMICs have a high degree of heterogeneity with respect to the phase of the epidemiologic transition. First, LMIC sub-regions differ by age-adjusted CVD death rates (Fig. 2.6). Next, low- and middle-income sub-regions are unique, as illustrated by the different CVD disease rates by cause in each region (Fig. 2.7). Lastly, in the East Asia and Oceania region, stroke still exceeds CHD as a cause of CVD-related death.

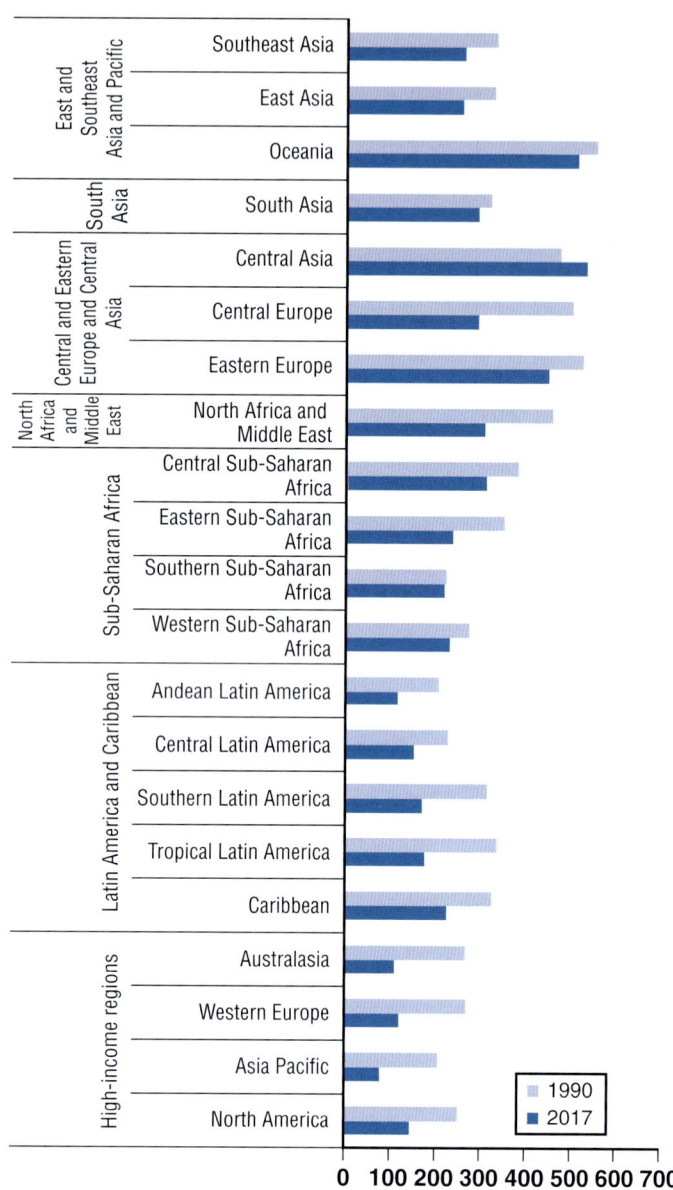

FIGURE 2.6 Age-adjusted death rates per 100,000 population for cardiovascular disease, 1990 and 2017. (From Global Burden of Disease Study 2017. *Age-sex Specific All-cause and Cause-specific Mortality, 1990–2017.* Seattle: Institute for Health Metrics and Evaluation; 2017.)

Hypertensive heart disease is the largest single contributor among remaining causes of CVD morbidity and mortality, and sub-Saharan Africa remains the region with the largest contribution from this cause.

Variability in disease prevalence among various regions likely results from multiple factors. First, the countries are in various phases of the epidemiologic transition described earlier. Second, the regions may have cultural and genetic differences that lead to varying levels of CVD risk. For example, per capita consumption of dairy products (and thus consumption of saturated fat) is much higher in India than in China, although it is rising in both countries. Third, certain additional competing pressures exist in some regions, such as war or infectious diseases (HIV/AIDS) in sub-Saharan Africa.

Because CHD affects a younger population in LMICs, the number of deaths is increased in the working population. For some LMICs, the severity of the epidemiologic transition has appeared to follow a reverse social gradient, with members of lower socioeconomic groups having the greatest rates of CHD and the highest levels of various risk factors. Unfortunately, reductions in risk factors do not follow the same trend. Compared with people in the upper and middle socioeconomic strata, those in the lowest stratum are less likely to acquire

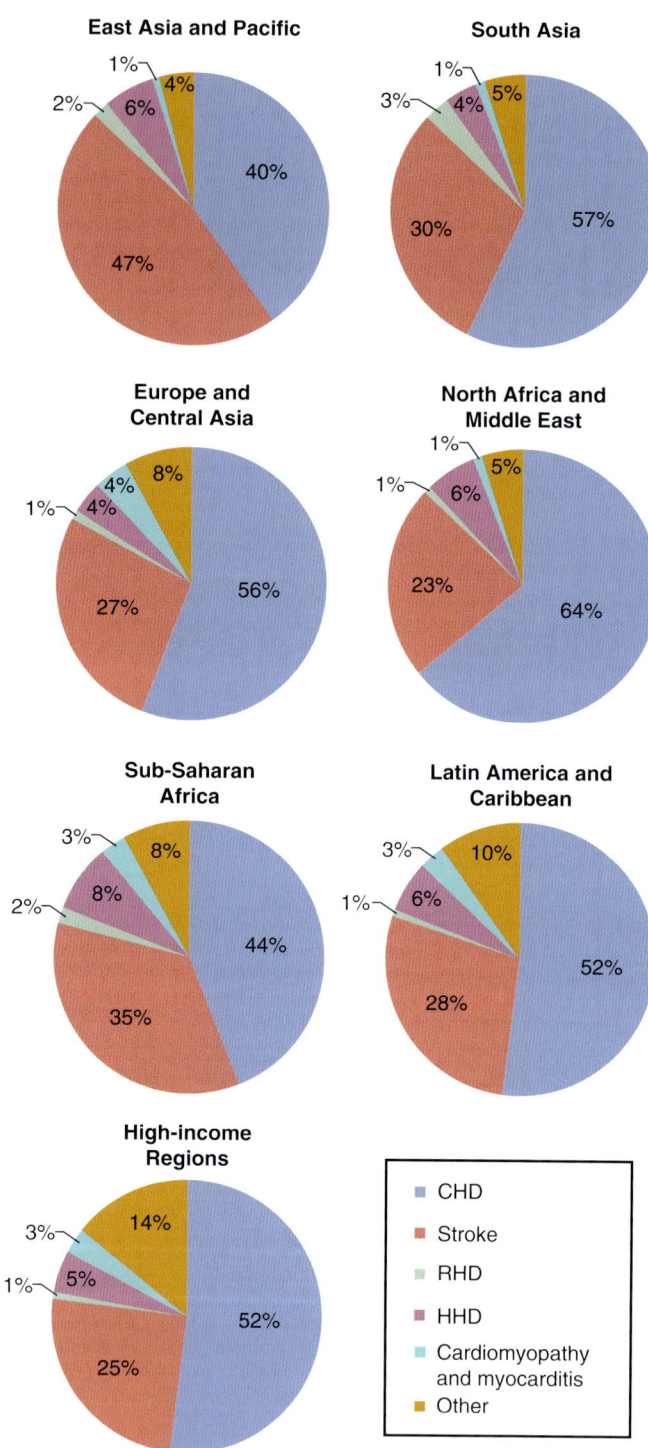

FIGURE 2.7 Cardiovascular disease death by specific cause and region. *CHD*, Coronary heart disease; *HHD*, hypertensive heart disease; *RHD*, rheumatic heart disease. (From Global Burden of Disease Study 2017. *Age-sex Specific All-cause and Cause-specific Mortality, 1990–2017.* Seattle: Institute for Health Metrics and Evaluation; 2017.)

and apply information on risk factors and behavior modifications or to have access to advanced treatment. Consequently, CVD mortality rates decline later among those of lower socioeconomic status.

High-Income Countries

In 2017, CVD accounted for almost 32% of all deaths in high-income regions, and more than half of these deaths were due to CHD (see Fig. 2.7). The movement of most HICs through the epidemiologic transition, with rising levels of risk factors and CVD death rates until the 1970s and then declines in both over the next 40 years, is similar to what occurred in the United States. CHD is the dominant form, with death rates per 100,000 twice as high as stroke rates. In Portugal however, stroke rates for women exceed CHD rates.

Age-adjusted mortality for CVD declined in all HICs. This age-adjusted decline results largely from preventive interventions that allow people to avert the disease, treatments to prevent death during an acute manifestation of the disease (particularly stroke or MI), and interventions that prolong survival once CVD manifests. Thus the average age at death from CVD continues to increase, and as a result, CVD affects a larger retired population.

Of the five sub-regions, Western Europe, with an overall CVD mortality rate of 313 per 100,000 in 2017, and Southern Latin America, with an age-standardized rate of 172 per 100,000, had the highest mortality rates, whereas Australasia and Southern Latin America tied for the lowest overall (222/100,000) rate, and high-income Asia Pacific had the lowest age-adjusted rate (80/100,000). As mentioned, high-income regions have higher mortality rates for CHD than for stroke. Japan is unique among HICs; as its communicable disease rates fell in the early 20th century, its stroke rates increased drastically. CHD rates, however, did not rise as sharply in Japan as in other industrialized nations and have remained lower than in any other industrialized country. Overall, CVD rates have dropped to 60% in Japan since the 1960s, largely because of a decrease in age-adjusted stroke rates. Japanese men and women currently have the highest life expectancy in the world: 87.3 years for women and 81.3 years for men. The difference between Japan and other industrialized countries may stem in part from genetic factors, although the traditional Japanese fish- and plant-based, low-fat diet and resultant low cholesterol levels may have also contributed. Nevertheless, as in many other countries, dietary habits in Japan are undergoing substantial changes. Since the late 1950s, cholesterol levels have progressively increased in both urban and rural populations. Although the prevalence of CVD risk factors is increasing in the Japanese population, the incidence of coronary artery disease remains low and even declined.[14] This situation could change, however, because there seems to be a long lag phase before dietary changes manifest as CHD events.

East Asia and Pacific
Demographic and Social Indices
The East Asia and Pacific (EAP) region is the most populated low- and middle-income region in the world, with 2.2 billion people; approximately 56% of the region is urban. The gross national income (GNI) per capita is $7601, ranging from $12,060 and $10,590 in Nauru and Malaysia to $1310 in Myanmar. In 2017, total health expenditure was 4.9% of total gross domestic product (GDP), or $344 per capita.[15] The region is divided into three distinct sub-regions: Southeast Asia, East Asia, and Oceania. China is by far the most populated country, representing 65% of the region. Life expectancy has risen quickly across the EAP region in past decades, up to an average of 75 years. In China the increase has been dramatic: from 37 years in the mid-1950s to 77 years in 2018.[15] This increase associates with a large rural to urban migration pattern, rapid urban modernization, aging of the population, decreased birth rates, major dietary changes, increasing tobacco use, and a transition to work requiring low levels of physical activity.

Burden of Disease
CVD caused more than 6.3 million deaths in the EAP region in 2017, accounting for 37% of all deaths in the region. Almost half of these deaths resulted from stroke, whereas 40% were caused by CHD (see Fig. 2.7). CVD death rates differ significantly between sub-regions, most notably in Southeast Asia. Age-adjusted CVD mortality rates were highest in Oceania, at 517 per 100,000 in 2017, even though the overall mortality for CVD was 253 per 100,000, suggesting that many premature deaths from CVD occurred in Oceania.

Stroke and CHD are the lead causes of death in all three sub-regions. Whereas stroke and CHD rates increased in both East Asia and Southeast Asia between 1990 and 2017, stroke rates decreased slightly in Oceania, from 87 to 83 per 100,000. China is straddling the second and third stages of a Japanese-like epidemiologic transition. Men in China age 50 to 69 have stroke death rates of 232 per 100,000, versus CHD death rates of 168 per 100,000.[1]

Central and Eastern Europe and Central Asia
Demographic and Social Indices
Of the three sub-regions that constitute this region (Central Asia, Central Europe, and Eastern Europe), Eastern Europe is the most populated. Russia alone accounts for 35% of the region's 416 million inhabitants. Sixty-seven percent of the population in the region is urban, with an average life expectancy of 73.7 years. The average GNI per capita for the region ranges from $1010 in Tajikistan to $24,500 in Slovenia. Russia has a GNI of $10,230. On average, the region spends 5.2% of its total GDP on public and private health care. Health expenditure per capita ranges from $58 per capita in Tajikistan to $1920 in Slovenia. Russia spends about $586 per capita, or 5.3% of its GDP.[15]

Burden of Disease
The highest rates of CVD mortality, both overall and age-adjusted, have occurred in this region for the entire span of the GBD project. Overall CVD mortality rates are 747 per 100,000 in Eastern Europe, 569 per 100,000 in Central Europe, and 359 per 100,000 in Central Asia. Overall rates are similar to or exceed those seen in the United States in the 1960s, when CVD peaked. CHD is generally more common than stroke, which suggests that the countries that constitute Eastern Europe and Central Asia remain largely in the third phase of the epidemiologic transition. As expected in this phase, people who develop and die of CVD have a lower average age than those in HICs. In 2017, CVD accounted for 54% of all deaths in the region, 56% of which resulted from CHD and 27% from stroke.

A country-level analysis reveals important differences in CHD profiles within the Central and Eastern Europe and Central Asia region (see Fig. 2.3). Since the dissolution of the Soviet Union, CVD rates have increased surprisingly in some of these countries, with overall rates of 956, 769, and 684 per 100,000 in Ukraine, Belarus, and Russia, respectively. Of note, deaths resulting from CHD in these countries affect not only older adults; the GBD study estimates that working-age populations (15 to 69 years) have a significant CHD burden. Almost one third of all deaths in persons age 45 to 49 years, for example, result from CVD. For people age 60 to 64 years, CVD accounts for almost half of all deaths, and 60% of CVD-related deaths are caused by CHD.[1]

Latin America and the Caribbean
Demographic and Social Indices
The Latin America and Caribbean (LAM) region comprises Andean Latin America, Central Latin America, Tropical Latin America, and the Caribbean. The region has a total population of 582 million, 80% of which is urban.[15] Brazil, the region's most populous country, represents about one third of the population (36%), with Colombia, Mexico, Peru, and Venezuela making up another 41%. The Caribbean nations account for 8% of the population in the region. Life expectancy in the LAM region is approximately 75 years but varies greatly. In 2018, for example, Haiti and Chile had life expectancies of 64 years and 80 years, respectively. Average GNI per capita in the region is about $8696 (purchasing power parity [PPP] of $15,944). The region spends an average of 8.0% of its GDP on health care. This level of spending translates into health care expenditures that range from $62 per capita in Haiti to $1772 per capita in The Bahamas.[15]

Burden of Disease
The LAM region bears a substantial CVD burden. In 2017, CVD caused 27% of all deaths in the region. As in HICs, CHD dominates among circulatory diseases (see Fig. 2.7). Mortality rates vary significantly by sub-region. The Caribbean has the highest age-standardized mortality rates for CHD and stroke: 115 deaths per 100,000 and 69 per 100,000, respectively. Andean Latin America had the lowest: 61 and 34 deaths per 100,000, respectively. As with other global trends, overall mortality for

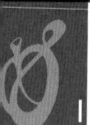

the region increased slightly between 1990 and 2017, but age-adjusted mortality declined significantly. Between 1990 and 2017, age-adjusted CVD death rates nearly halved in Tropical Latin America while decreases of 44%, 33%, and 31% occurred in Andean Latin America, Central Latin America, and the Caribbean, respectively. Together, CHD (15%), stroke (5.9%), and hypertensive heart disease (1.6%) accounted for almost one quarter of all deaths in Central Latin America in 2017. Age-adjusted overall CVD, CHD, and stroke mortality rates decreased in this sub-region between 1990 and 2017, but to a lesser extent than for global changes. The lower reductions in the LAM region may result from rapid lifestyle changes: unfavorable dietary changes, increased smoking, increased obesity, and less exercise.

North Africa and Middle East
Demographic and Social Indices
The 21 countries of the North Africa and Middle East region represent approximately 8% of the world's population (600 million people). Egypt and Iran are the two most populous countries in the region, with Egypt representing 16% of total inhabitants and Iran 14%. Approximately 65% of the population is urban, with an average life expectancy of 74 years. The average GNI per capita for the region is $7693, ranging from $1460 in Yemen to $61,150 in Qatar. Approximately 5.7% of the GDP, or approximately $459 per capita, is expended for health in the region. The per capita health expenditure ranges from $72 in Yemen to $1649 in Qatar.[15]

Burden of Disease
Thirty-nine percent of all deaths in the North Africa and Middle East region result from CVD: 26% from CHD and 10% from stroke. In 2017, the region had lower overall CVD mortality rates than global averages yet higher than global age-standardized rates. In 2017 the overall death rates per 100,000 for CHD, stroke, and overall CVD were 118, 45, and 187, respectively. The mortality rates for CHD, stroke, and overall CVD declined marginally in the region since 1990, when the rates were 130, 51, and 202 deaths per 100,000 population, respectively. However, age-adjusted mortality rates for CVD declined by 33% across the region. In 2017, CVD accounted for 26 million DALYs lost, or 16% of all DALYs lost, in the region. The DALYs lost were split differently between CHD and stroke, at 15.9 million and 6.6 million, respectively.[1]

South Asia
Demographic and Social Indices
The South Asia region (SAR), one of the world's most densely populated regions, accounts for about 23% of the world's population, with almost 1.8 billion residents. India, home to 77% of the region's inhabitants, is the largest country in the region.[16] Only 34% of the region is urban, and life expectancy is approximately 69 years. Average GNI per capita for the region is $1923, ranging from $970 in Nepal to $2970 in Bhutan. India's GNI per capita of $2020 sits near the regional average. Countries in the SAR spend an average of 3.5% of their total GDP, or $64 per capita, on health care. Bhutan spends the most per capita at $97, and India spends $70, or 3.5% of its GDP. The lowest expenditures for health care are $36 per capita in Bangladesh and $45 in Pakistan.[15]

Burden of Disease
CVD accounts for 27% of all deaths in the SAR. CHD was the lead cause of mortality in 2017, accounting for 15.5% of total reported fatalities, or 1.9 million deaths, and more than half of CVD mortality. Stroke accounted for 8.2% of all deaths and 30% of CVD deaths. The region lost almost 83.5 million DALYs from CVD in 2017, accounting for 13.5% of the total. CHD contributes 55% of the DALYs lost because of CVD, nearly twice as high as for stroke. Overall mortality rates for CVD are increasing in the region, while age-adjusted rates are slowly decreasing.[1]

CVD represents 27% of all deaths in India, the largest country in the SAR. Studies also show a higher CHD prevalence in men and in urban residents. The rise in CHD mortality contributes to the economic burden in the Indian subcontinent. Data indicate that CVD onsets at least a decade earlier in the Indian population than in comparison with those of European ancestry.[17,18]

Sub-Saharan Africa
Demographic and Social Indices
The GBD study divides sub-Saharan Africa into four sub-regions: Central, Eastern, Southern, and Western sub-Saharan Africa. Approximately one billion people live in these four regions, with Nigeria being the most populous (206 million) and Cape Verde being the least populous (545,000). Only 40% of the population in the region is urban. The average GNI per capita is $1519, ranging from $280 in Burundi to $7750 in Botswana. Overall, the region also has the lowest average life expectancy—61 years.[15] Average public and private health care expenditures for the region are 5.2% of the total GDP, or $84 per capita. The range of health care expenditures per capita for sub-Saharan Africa is similar to the GDP range for this region, from $19 in the Democratic Republic of the Congo to $499 in South Africa. Nigeria spends $74 per capita, or 3.8% of the total GDP.[15]

Burden of Disease
Communicable, neonatal, and maternal disorders still dominate causes of death in sub-Saharan Africa. HIV/AIDS and neonatal disorders are the leading causes of death, accounting for almost 19% of deaths in the region, while CHD and stroke account for 9.2%.[1] In Western sub-Saharan Africa, CVD accounts for 10.3% of all deaths. The highest portion of CVD-related deaths occurred in Southern sub-Saharan Africa, where 15.9% of all deaths were caused by CVD. Overall CVD mortality rates in the region are lower than global averages and are decreasing, while global rates have held steady. The exception is Southern sub-Saharan Africa, where rates increased from 109 to 135 per 100,000 between 1990 and 2017. Communicable, neonatal, and maternal disorders still dominate causes of death in sub-Saharan Africa.

RISK FACTORS

Worldwide, CVD is largely driven by modifiable risk factors, such as smoking, lack of physical activity, and diets high in fat and salt (see also Chapters 25 to 31). Elevated levels of blood pressure (BP) and cholesterol remain the leading causes of CHD; tobacco, obesity, and physical inactivity remain important contributors as well. The GBD project estimated that the population-attributable fraction (PAF) for individual risk factors for CHD in LMICs in 2013 were as follows: high BP, 54%; high cholesterol, 32%; overweight and obesity, 18%; dietary intake, 67%; and smoking, 18%. Because factors may contribute to similar disease mechanisms, the sum exceeds 100%. Unique features regarding some CHD risk factors in LMICs are described below.

Tobacco
By many accounts, tobacco use is the most preventable cause of death in the world. More than 1.4 billion people use tobacco worldwide, with 5.8 trillion cigarettes smoked globally in 2014.[19,20] Around 80% of the world's tobacco smokers live in LMICs, and if current trends continue unabated, tobacco will cause more than 1 billion deaths during the 21st century.

Tobacco use varies greatly across the world, as do deaths attributable to smoking in both sexes (Fig. 2.8). Although historically greatest in HICs, tobacco consumption has shifted dramatically to LMICs in recent decades; some of the highest-known tobacco use now occurs in the EAP region. Kiribati has the highest known prevalence of age-adjusted tobacco use in the world, 52.0%: 68.6% in men and 35.5% in women. For men, Indonesia, Myanmar, and Timor-Leste, all of the EAP region had similarly high tobacco use prevalence rates in 2018 (70.5%, 70.2%, and 65.8%, respectively). For women, the highest known prevalence rates in 2018 were in Serbia, Chile, and Lebanon (40.0%, 49.2%, and 49.4%, respectively).

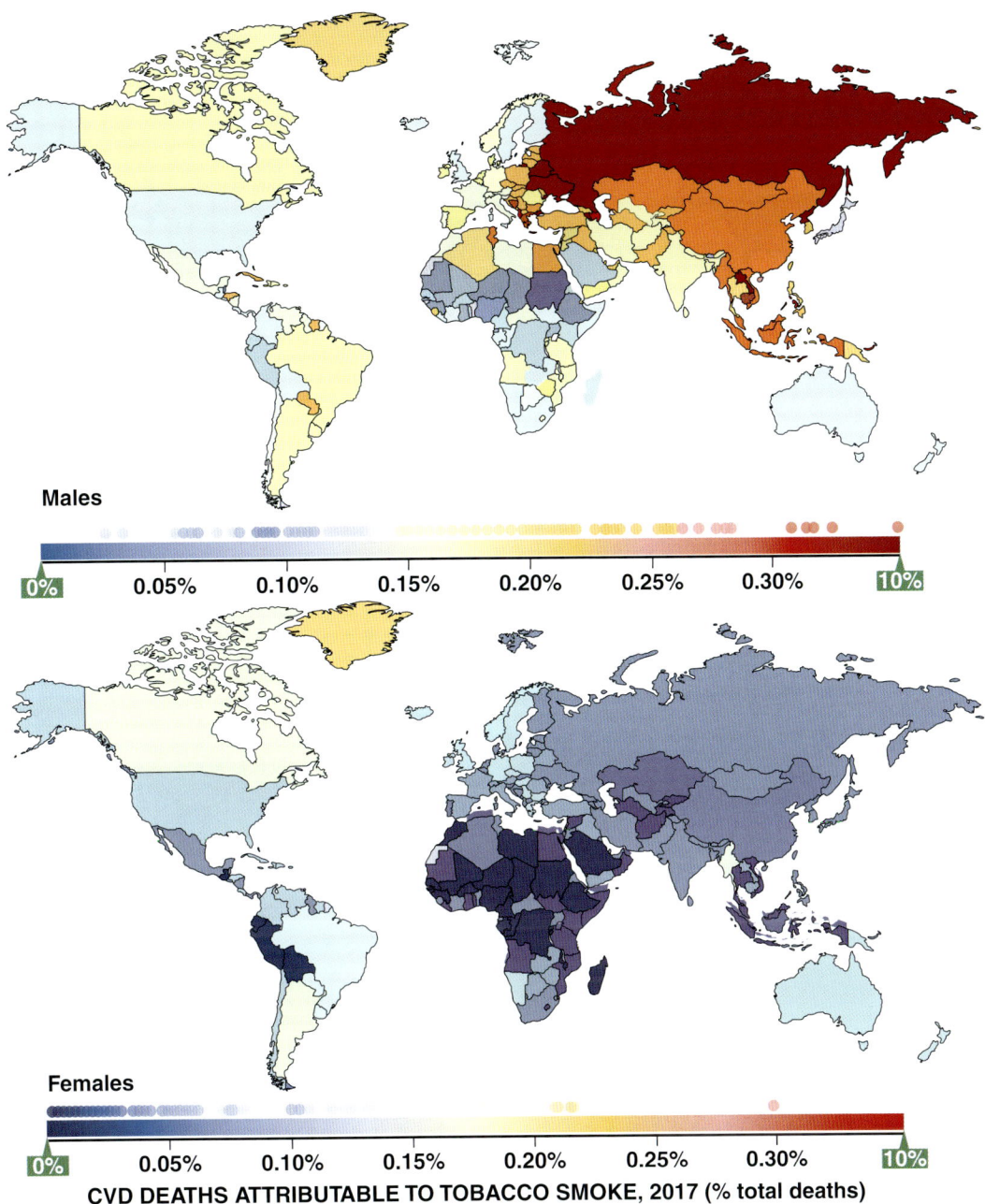

FIGURE 2.8 Cardiovascular disease mortality attributable to tobacco smoke in 2017, percentage of total deaths, males versus females. (From Institute for Health Metrics and Evaluation (IHME). *GBD Compare.* Seattle: IHME, University of Washington; 2017. http://vizhub.healthdata.org/gbd-compare.)

China is the largest consumer of tobacco in the world, with an estimated 270 million daily smokers in 2015 (40.6% prevalence in men). Daily smoking prevalence in China increased slightly from 21.4% in 1980 to 22.0% in 2015. Several countries in Central and Eastern Europe also have alarmingly high prevalence rates, including Russia (approximately 41.8% in men and 11.5% in women), Ukraine (43.7% prevalence in men), and Albania (29.1% prevalence in men). Latin America, the Middle East, and North Africa have high rates as well, although smoking is not as common among women in these regions as it is in the Pacific region. Countries in sub-Saharan Africa have some of the lowest prevalence rates; Niger and Ethiopia, for example, have less than 8% and 1% prevalence in men and women, respectively.

Women also have a high and increasing smoking prevalence in several countries, including Kiribati (22.7%), Austria (21.1%), and Greece (25.8%). In general, however, considerably more men than women smoke. Where they do occur, variations by sex can be substantial. In China, for example, tobacco use prevalence is 47.7% in men but only 1.8% in women. Indonesia has similarly diverging trends: prevalence in men is 70.5% and only 5.3% in women. Significant variations also occur in North Africa, the Middle East, and some countries in sub-Saharan Africa. Tobacco use is generally less than 4% in women in these regions but is much higher in men.

Other forms of tobacco use increase risk for CHD. Bidis (hand-rolled cigarettes common in South Asia), kreteks (clove and tobacco cigarettes), hookah pipes (water pipes used for smoking flavored tobacco), and smokeless tobacco all link to increased CHD risk (see Chapter 28). The combined use of different forms of tobacco associates with a higher risk of MI than using one type.

Secondhand smoke also contributes to CHD risk. In 2017, approximately 575,000 non-smokers died of CVD as a consequence of exposure to secondhand smoke.[1] The risk assessment analysis of 195 countries for the GBD Study 2017 found that the largest portion of secondhand smoke–related deaths in 2017 resulted from ischemic heart disease.[21] Smoking bans have both immediate and long-term effects in reducing admissions for acute coronary syndrome (ACS).[22]

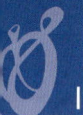

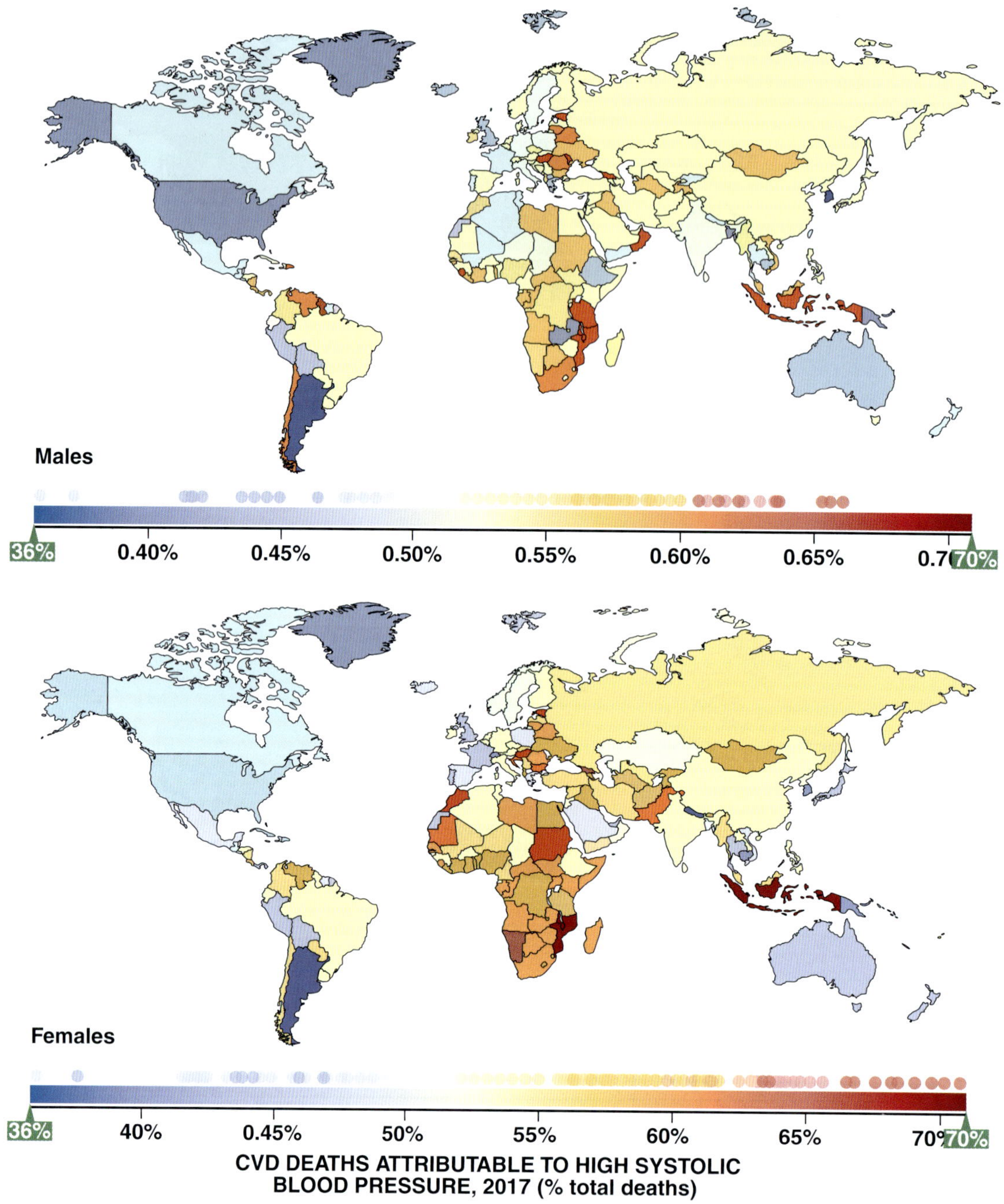

FIGURE 2.9 Cardiovascular disease mortality attributable to high systolic blood pressure in 2017, percentage of total deaths, males versus females. (From Institute for Health Metrics and Evaluation (IHME). *GBD Compare.* Seattle: IHME, University of Washington; 2017. http://vizhub.healthdata.org/gbd-compare.)

Hypertension

Elevated BP is an early indicator of an epidemiologic transition. Rising mean population BP occurs as populations industrialize and move from rural to urban settings. Worldwide, 55% of stroke-related deaths and 55% of ischemic heart disease-related deaths are attributable to sub-optimal (>115 mm Hg) systolic BP (SBP) control, accounting for 8.25 million deaths in 2017. The GBD project estimates that 19% of deaths and 9% of DALYs lost globally result from non-optimal levels of BP.[1] The high rate of undetected, and therefore untreated, hypertension presents a major concern in LMICs. The high prevalence of undetected and untreated hypertension probably drives the elevated rates of hemorrhagic stroke throughout Asia.

The most recent update of the GBD study analyzed mean SBP between 1980 and 2008 using multiple published and unpublished health surveys and epidemiologic studies. The analysis, which applied a Bayesian hierarchical model to each sex by age, country, and year, found a global decrease in mean systolic BP between 1980 and 2008 in both men and women. Worldwide, the age-standardized prevalence of uncontrolled hypertension has decreased from 33% to 29% in men and from 29% to 25% in women. However, the number of people with uncontrolled hypertension (SBP ≥140 mm Hg) has increased; in 1990, 442 million had uncontrolled hypertension, and by 2015, the number increased to 874 million.[23] The trend results largely from population growth and aging. Globally, mean SBP has decreased by 0.8 mm Hg per decade among men and by 1.0 mm Hg per decade among women. In 2008, age-standardized mean SBP values worldwide were 128.1 mm Hg in men and 124.4 mm Hg in women.

The proportion of CVD deaths attributable to BP by country in 2017 varied by sex (Fig. 2.9).

The highest mean SBP in 2015 occurred in East and West African countries, where both men and women had SBP levels that were significantly higher than global averages (men: 129.4; women: 126.2). In

Mozambique and in São Tomé and Príncipe, for example, mean SBP in women was 134.9 and 137.1 mm Hg, respectively. In men, mean SBP was as high as 138.6 mm Hg in Mozambique and 130.9 mm Hg in Niger. Men in Eastern Europe had mean SBP levels comparable to those in East and West Africa. Mean SBP was lowest in high-income regions such as Australasia (124.0 mm Hg in Australian women) and North America (122.8 mm Hg in U.S. men).

The most significant decreases occurred in the high-income Asia Pacific region, where mean SBP decreased by 2.5 mm Hg on average per decade between 1975 and 2015 in men and 3.2 mm Hg on average per decade in women. The decrease in men ranged from 0.2 to 2.5 mm Hg per decade. The decrease in mean SBP in women ranged from 1.1 mm Hg per decade in Central Asia, North Africa and the Middle East to 3.2 mm Hg per decade in High-Income Asia Pacific.

Mean SBP increased in several regions. In South Asia, SBP increased by 1.2 mm Hg on average per decade in men and 1.3 mm Hg on average per decade in women. South and East Asia saw similar increases: 1.1 mm Hg on average per decade in men and 0.8 mm Hg on average per decade in women. In Sub-Saharan Africa, mean SBP increased by 0.5 mm Hg on average per decade in men and 0.9 mm Hg on average per decade in women.

Notable sex differences occurred in Oceania and Central and Eastern Europe. In Oceania, mean SBP in women increased by 2.5 mm Hg on average per decade, the largest increase in any female cohort in the world. In men in this region, however, mean SBP increased by only 1.4 mm Hg on average per decade despite being the largest increase of all male cohorts. Data from Central and Eastern Europe show diverging trends in men and women: although mean SBP in men decreased by 0.2 mm Hg on average per decade, it decreased in women by 1.8 mm Hg.

Lipids (see Chapter 27)

Worldwide, high cholesterol causes about 42% of ischemic heart disease deaths and 9% of stroke deaths, accounting for 4.3 million deaths annually. Unfortunately, most LMICs have limited data on cholesterol levels (often only total cholesterol). In HICs, mean population cholesterol levels are generally decreasing, but in LMICs, these levels vary widely. As countries move through epidemiologic transition, mean population total plasma cholesterol levels typically rise. Changes accompanying urbanization clearly play a role, because urban residents tend to have higher plasma cholesterol levels than rural residents. This shift results largely from greater consumption of dietary fats, primarily from animal products and processed vegetable oils, and decreased physical activity. Eventually there is a decline, as seen in the last set of trend data produced by the GBD through 2009.

There has not been a systematic estimate of global trends in total cholesterol levels since 2011. More recent data also suggest that following only total cholesterol levels may be misleading. In an analysis of 438 populations from 21 Western and Asian countries totaling 82 million participants, several different patterns emerged in the lipid parameters from 1980 to 2015.[24] In Asia, for Japan and South Korea, the rise in total cholesterol was primarily due to an increase in HDL cholesterol whereas in China the risk was due primarily to non-HDL cholesterol. For most Western countries there was a decline in total cholesterol, which included the net effect of both a rise in HDL cholesterol and an even greater reduction in non-HDL, with the greatest changes occurring in New Zealand and Switzerland. Overall the total-to-HDL cholesterol ratio declined in Japan, Korea, and most Western countries.

Diabetes (see Chapter 31)

Diabetes prevalence has increased rapidly worldwide in the past 30 years. As a result, death rates of CVD attributable to diabetes have increased for many LMICs, particularly in East Asia, South Asia, and Eastern Europe and Central Asia (Fig. 2.10). According to the GBD study, an estimated 476 million people worldwide have diabetes.[25] The more expansive International Diabetes Foundation (IDF) definition which, in addition to fasting plasma glucose (FPG) as in the GBD study, includes oral glucose tolerance and hemoglobin A_{1c} tests, found that 451 million adults had diabetes in 2017.[26] Almost 50% of these cases were undiagnosed. By 2045 the number of people with diabetes is expected to increase to 693 million.[26]

Almost 80% of people with diabetes live in LMICs. The highest regional age-standardized prevalence for diabetes occurs in the Middle East and North Africa, where an estimated 8.2% of the population has diabetes. However, the top ten countries with the highest age-standardized prevalences (ranging from 14.2% to 23.5%) are all within the Southeast Asia, East Asia, and Oceania regions.[1]

Asian countries face a relatively larger burden of diabetes compared to the Europe and Central Asia or Latin America and Caribbean regions. India and China, for example, have the largest numbers of people with diabetes in the world: 67.8 million and 89.5 million, respectively.[1]

The most recent GBD study found a global increase in mean FPG. The study analyzed multiple published and unpublished health surveys and epidemiologic studies by applying a Bayesian hierarchical model for each sex by age, country, and year. Between 1980 and 2008, mean FPG increased by 0.07 mmol/L (1.26 mg/dL) per decade in men and 0.08 mmol/L (1.44 mg/dL) per decade in women. The upward trend in FPG was nearly universal.[23] In almost every region worldwide, mean FPG increased or remained unchanged; regions that displayed apparent decreases (e.g., men in the East Asia and Southeast Asia region) were not statistically different from flat trends (posterior probabilities ≤0.80).

Although some regions had unchanging mean FPG levels, other regions, including Southern and Tropical Latin America, Oceania, and High-Income regions, experienced significant increases. The most notable region is Oceania; between 1980 and 2008, mean FPG increased by 0.22 mmol/L per decade in men and 0.32 mmol/L per decade in women. By 2008, Oceania had the highest mean FPG for both sexes (6.09 mmol/L for men, 6.09 mmol/L for women) and the highest prevalence of diabetes (15.5% in men, 15.9% in women) in the world.

In addition to Oceania, the Caribbean and North Africa and the Middle East have the highest mean FPG levels worldwide: 21% to 25% of men and 21% to 32% of women in these countries have diabetes. By contrast, men in sub-Saharan Africa and women in Asia-Pacific HICs had the lowest mean FPG in 2008: 5.27 mmol/L and 5.17 mmol/L, respectively. The only significant decrease in mean FPG occurred in women in Singapore, where levels fell by 0.21 mmol/L per decade.

Trends in mean FPG also varied by sex. In sub-Saharan Africa, for example, mean FPG increased by 0.05 mmol/L per decade in men, but by 0.13 mmol/L per decade in women. The Central Asia, North Africa, and Middle East region had similar differences in sex: mean FPG increased by 0.06 mmol/L per decade in men and by 0.16 mmol/L per decade in women.

Obesity (see Chapter 30)

In 2015, an estimated 603.4 million adults and 107.7 million children were obese.[27] Global obesity prevalence was 12.0% among adults (5.0% among children) and is increasing throughout the world and particularly in LMICs, which have steeper trajectories than in HICs. Explanations for this rapid rise include changes in dietary patterns, physical activity, and urbanization. Rapid changes in the global food system have increased the availability and consumption of inexpensive, ultra-processed food and beverages rich in refined carbohydrates, fat, sugar, and salt in LMICs.[28] Physical activity declines as urbanization leads to increased use of motorized vehicles and a change to more sedentary occupations.

Unlike data from the 1980s, which showed that obesity affected predominantly the higher-income group in LMICs, a recent analysis shows a shift to the poor in the burden of overweight and obesity. Although higher-income groups still have the highest prevalence of overweight and obesity, rates are increasing faster in lower-income groups. The poor are relatively more susceptible to obesity as a developing country's GNP approaches the middle-income range. Higher GDP is also associated with faster rates of increase in the prevalence of overweight and obesity in lower-income groups.[28]

Women are more affected by obesity than men; the proportion of the world's adult women who are either overweight or obese rose from 29.8% to 38.0% between 1980 and 2013, while an increase from 28.8%

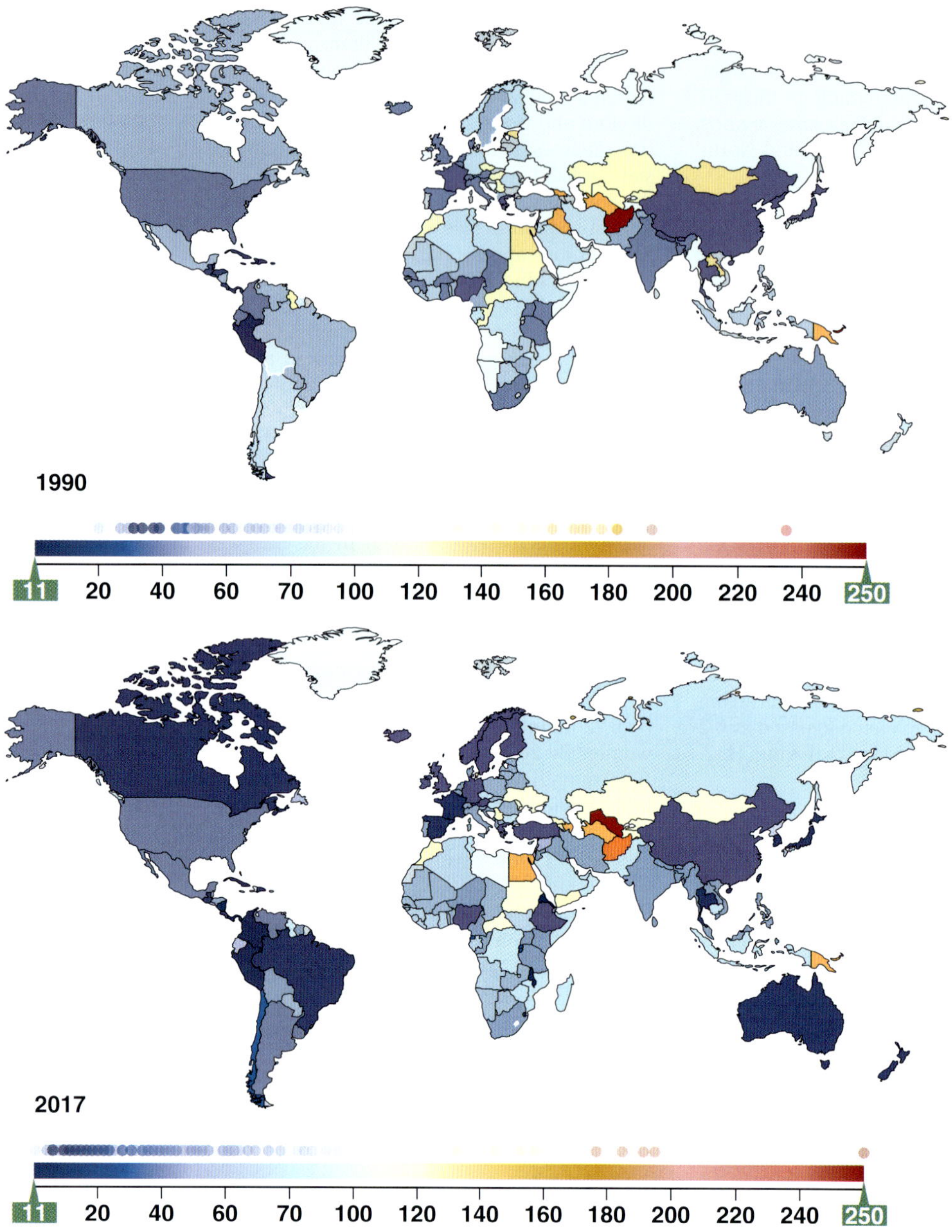

FIGURE 2.10 Cardiovascular disease mortality attributable to high fasting plasma glucose, deaths per 100,000, 1990 versus 2017. (From Institute for Health Metrics and Evaluation (IHME). *GBD Compare*. Seattle: IHME, University of Washington; 2017. http://vizhub.healthdata.org/gbd-compare.)

to 36.9% was observed for men. Adolescents are at particular risk: 18% of children and adolescents aged 5 to 19 were overweight or obese in 2016, up from 4% in 1975. The number of overweight children is increasing in countries as diverse as China, Brazil, India, Mexico, and Nigeria. The World Health Organization (WHO) estimates that in 2019, 38.2 million children younger than 5 years were overweight. In 1975 worldwide obesity prevalence was 3.2% in men and 6.4% in women. By 2014, prevalence had increased to 10.8% in men and 14.9% in women.[29]

Globally, BMI rose in both men and women. Between 1975 and 2014, global age-standardized mean BMI rose from 22.1 to 24.4 kg/m² in females and 21.7 to 24.2 kg/m² in males.[29]

BMI varies substantially between regions and by sex and over time. In more than two thirds of the countries, the contribution of obesity to attributable burden of CVD-related death rates worsened. The majority of countries that improved were from HICs, although some were from each of the LMICs that saw improvements except from South Asia (Fig. 2.11). In 2016 the age-standardized mean BMI in the United States was 29.0 kg/m² in men and 29.1 kg/m² in women. In contrast with the United States and other HICs with similarly high BMIs, the sub-Saharan Africa and Asia regions have some of the lowest mean BMIs. Men in Ethiopia, for example, have a mean BMI of 20.1 kg/m², and women in Bangladesh have a mean BMI of 22.1 kg/m².

The largest increase in BMI occurred in Oceania. Between 1980 and 2008, mean BMI rose by 1.3 kg/m² per decade in men and 1.8 kg/m² per decade in women. Of the islands in the Oceania region, Nauru had the largest BMI increase of more than 2 kg/m². BMI trends were similar in the North American high-income region (1.1 kg/m² per decade in men and 1.2 kg/m² per decade in women). In Latin America and the Caribbean, mean BMI for women increased from 0.6 to 1.4 kg/m² per decade. By contrast, mean BMI decreased in Central African men by 0.2 kg/m² per decade and remained unchanged in South Asian men. In women, mean BMI remained static, with changes less than 0.2 kg/m² per decade in Central Asia, Central Europe, and Eastern Europe.

Although regional trends generally showed concordance between sexes, some exceptions occurred. There was no change in mean BMI in South Asian men, but mean BMI in women increased at a rate close to the global average, 0.4 kg/m² per decade. The most significant discrepancy in sex trends occurred in Central Africa. BMI in men in Central Africa decreased by 0.2 kg/m² per decade, the only significant decrease in any male population in the world. In women in Central Africa, however, mean BMI increased by 0.7 kg/m² per decade, a rate greater than the world average.

Diet (see Chapter 29)

As humans have evolved, selective pressures have favored the ability to conserve and store fat as a defense against famine. This adaptive mechanism has become unfavorable in light of the larger portion sizes, processed foods, and sugary drinks that many people now regularly consume. Between 1970 and 2010, the average daily per capita caloric intake in the United States increased from 2076 to 3766 calories.[30] As per capita income increases, so does consumption of fats and simple carbohydrates, whereas intake of plant-based foods decreases. A key element of this dietary change is an increased intake of saturated animal fats and inexpensive hydrogenated vegetable fats, which contain atherogenic *trans* fatty acids. New evidence suggests that high intake of *trans* fats may also lead to abdominal obesity, another risk factor for CVD.

China provides a good example of such a "nutritional transition"—rapid shifts in diet linked to socioeconomic changes. The China Nationwide Health Survey found that between 1982 and 2002, calories from fat increased from 25% to 35% in urban areas and from 14% to 28% in rural areas, as calories from carbohydrates fell from 70% to 47%. Recently in 1980, the average BMI for Chinese adults was about 20 kg/m², and less than 1% had a BMI of 30 kg/m² or greater. From 1992 to

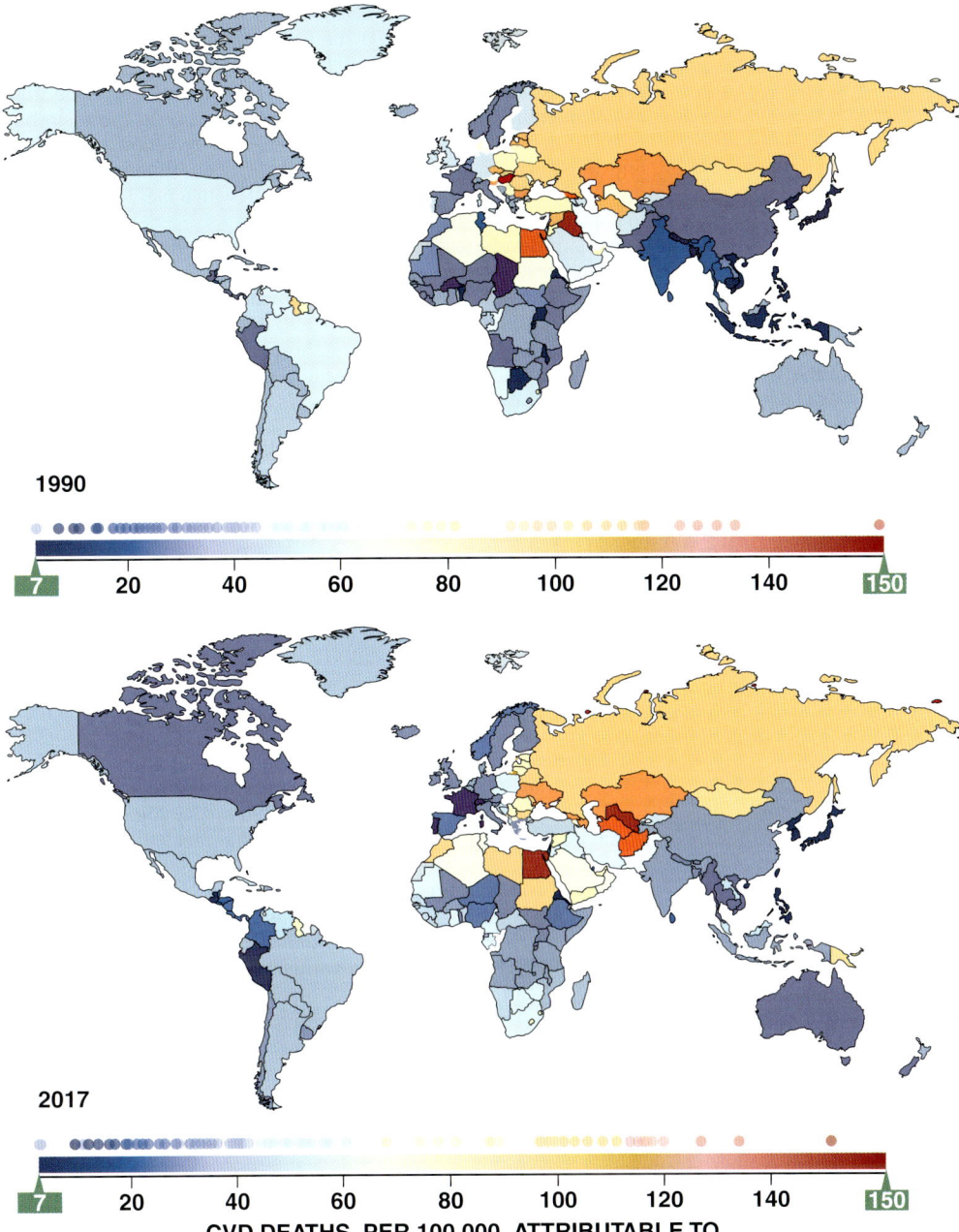

FIGURE 2.11 Cardiovascular disease mortality attributable to high body-mass index, deaths per 100,000, 1990 versus 2017. (From Institute for Health Metrics and Evaluation (IHME). *GBD Compare*. Seattle: IHME, University of Washington; 2017. http://vizhub.healthdata.org/gbd-compare.)

daily.[32] Improvements in consumption could save the United States $50 billion a year in CVD-related health costs.[31]

Physical Inactivity (see Chapters 30 and 32)

Physical inactivity is responsible for 1.3 million global deaths annually. The global age-standardized prevalence of physical inactivity has remained steady between 2001 and 2016 (28.5% to 27.5%). In HICs the widespread prevalence of physical inactivity produces a high population-attributable risk of cardiovascular consequences. Physical inactivity is also increasing in low- and middle-income regions of the world, witnessing a shift from physically demanding, agriculture-based work to largely sedentary, service industry-based and office-based work. A switch to mechanized transportation accompanies this work shift.

Current WHO recommendations call for moderate-intensity exercise for at least 150 minutes, or 75 minutes of vigorous exercise per week. In the United States, approximately one-quarter of the adult population does not participate in any leisure-time physical activity, and only 24.3% of adults reported participating in adequate leisure-time aerobic and muscle-strengthening activity to meet federal guidelines. Physical inactivity levels vary by region and by sex. The lowest levels of physical inactivity in 2016 were in men from Oceania (12.3%), East and Southeast Asia (17.6%), and sub-Saharan Africa (17.9%), while the highest levels were in women in high-income Western (42.3%), South Asia (43.0%), and Latin America and the Caribbean (43.7%). A study of adults in China using data from randomized national surveys from 2000 to 2014 found that despite increased participation in leisure-time physical activity, there were in also increases in overweight or obesity.[33]

2002, the number of overweight adults increased by 41%, and the number of obese adults increased by 97%.

China and other countries in transition have the opportunity to spare their populations from the high levels of *trans* fats that North Americans and Europeans have consumed over the past 50 years by avoiding government policies that can contribute to the CVD burden. An estimated 919 CVD-related deaths per million adults could be averted each year in the United States by eating the recommended amounts of fruits, vegetables, nuts/seeds, whole grains, polyunsaturated fats, omega-3 oils, and eliminating sugar-sweetened beverages, processed meats, and excess sodium.[31] Another facet of the nutritional transition for countries adopting a Western diet is the introduction of high-sugar beverages associated with weight gain and increased risk for type 2 diabetes. A meta-analysis suggests up to a 16% relative risk increase in CHD per unit of sugar-sweetened beverages consumed

Aging Populations (see Chapter 90)

Between 1990 to 1995 and 2015 to 2020, global life expectancy at birth increased by 7.7 years and is projected to increase by an additional 4.5 years between 2015 to 2020 and 2045 to 2050.[34] This increase is associated with a decline in overall infant mortality and fertility rates. Although older adults will constitute a greater percentage of the population in HICs, more than 53.3 million Americans were older than 65 years in 2019 and is projected to increase to 84.8 million by 2050. Low- and middle-income regions will see the population over 65 more than double from 2019 to 2050.

The time of transition to an older population is sharply shorter in LMICs. For example, whereas it took the United States and Canada more than 65 years to double their over-65 population, LMICs will do so every 25 years for the next 50 years. Such acute changes in the population structure leave less time to expand an already overburdened health infrastructure to address the chronic diseases of older adults, which prominently include cardiovascular conditions.

Genetic

A great deal of effort has recently been invested in understanding how genes impact cardiovascular health in populations. These have focused on germline genetic variants that are related to specific cardiovascular diseases as well as those that are associated with cardiovascular risk factors. In either case, every year the number of associated variants has increased meaningfully, to the point that hundreds or even thousands of variants are associated with these conditions, each explaining a small amount of the population variability in disease and risk factors. Collections of variants have been combined in polygenomic risk scores, but these too explain only a small amount of the variability of the disease in the population. More data will be available in the coming years about these associations, mechanisms that explain these associations, relationships of variants that are specific to certain tissues such as the heart or the brain, and the interactions between genetic and lifestyle factors that cause the disease. Currently, most of the data are among those with European ancestry; however, large-scale efforts are underway to understand the relationships between genes and diseases and their risk factors around the world. The early data suggest nontrivial differences among various world populations.

Fetal Influences

Adverse influences such as undernutrition during fetal life (fetal "programming") and early postnatal life appear to affect the prevalence of adult CVD and contribute to its risk factors. Barker,[35] in his "developmental origins of adult disease" hypothesis, suggested that adverse influences early in development, particularly during intrauterine life, could result in permanent changes in the physiology and metabolism of the pancreas, kidney, muscle, and vascular endothelium, resulting in adult insulin resistance, metabolic syndrome, hypertension, and CHD. Recent evidence indicates that the first thousand days of life, comprising intra-uterine life (270 days) and the first 2 years of postnatal life, is a sensitive or "critical" period of development, and any stimulus or insult during this period appears to have lasting or lifelong significance for adult-onset CVD.[36] Extensive data support these associations.[37] More recent studies tried to evaluate the role of multiple micronutrient supplementation as well, but a recent meta-analysis concluded that there is no added benefit in improving later life outcomes like childhood survival, growth, body composition, BP, respiratory or cognitive outcomes.[38] The mechanisms of increased risk appear to be both biologic (alterations in fetal tissues and postnatal epigenetic modifications) and social (cognitive impairment, low productivity, and higher prevalence of cardiovascular risk factors among those with lower birth weight and early-life adverse influences), and childhood obesity and sedentary habits aggravate this risk. Thus the prevention of adverse fetal exposures and subsequent long-term consequences require a holistic approach. An understanding of prenatal risk factors and their early childhood modifiers will provide an opportunity for interventions before the development of risk factors. Remedies include improved maternal nutrition during pregnancy and lactation, emphasis on breastfeeding through early infancy, and ensuring adequate balanced nutrition to infants. Focus on the adolescent group has shown added benefit of building maternal reserve prior to pregnancy to ensure optimal birth outcomes. On the basis of current understanding, policymakers and health care professionals should design and develop preventive strategies that effectively influence these very early determinants of CVD development.[37]

Environmental Exposures (see Chapter 3)

Environmental pollution, especially both indoor and outdoor air pollution, has emerged as a major cause of death and disease burden (see Chapter 52).[39] Exposure to particulate-matter (PM) air pollution,[40,41] heavy metals (e.g., cadmium, arsenic, lead, mercury),[42] and polyaromatic hydrocarbons[43] is associated with increased risk of mortality and morbidity from CVD. The GBD comparative risk assessment of 2017 has shown that more than 23% of all DALYs from ischemic heart disease and about 28.9% of DALYs from ischemic strokes result from environmental risk factors,[21] approximately the same as those attributable to tobacco smoke. Of these exposures, air pollution (household and ambient) is the most prominent risk factor, contributing to approximately 7 million premature deaths annually, with a majority occurring in LMICs such as India and China.

In many developing countries, populations experience a continuum of exposure to ambient air pollution (from vehicles, industry, etc.) and household air pollution (from cooking, heating, and lighting), resulting in significant contributions to the health burden, as in India, where it is the second most important risk factor for poor health. More than half of all deaths associated with air pollution exposure are through cardiovascular and cerebrovascular pathways, involving ischemic heart disease, heart failure, stroke, and hypertension.[44,45] Three pathways, listed below in order of the strength of the evidence base, may contribute to the mechanisms that link PM exposure to CVD and cerebrovascular disease:

1. Particle transport into the lungs provoking inflammatory responses and promoting systemic oxidative stress. This leads to increased risk of thrombosis, endothelial dysfunction, atherosclerosis progression, and dyslipidemia.
2. Particle transport into the lungs promoting autonomous nervous system imbalances. This leads to pathologic alterations in hypertension, endothelial dysfunction, vasoconstriction, and atherosclerosis.
3. Absorption of particles through the lungs into the bloodstream causing tissue-level interactions. This results in platelet aggregation, vasoconstriction, and endothelial dysfunction.

The epidemiologic evidence base suggests that exposure to arsenic, cadmium, and lead follows the common physiologic pathways observed with air pollution.[46] In addition, the mechanistic evidence from animal and human studies indicates that arsenic exposure is associated with carotid intima media thickness, a marker for atherosclerosis, with links to diabetes is also observed.[47]

Regardless of the primary route and the pathophysiology involved, short- or long-term exposure to various environmental pollutants is associated with an increased risk of ischemic heart disease, stroke, heart failure, and preclinical conditions such as endothelial dysfunction, thrombosis, atherosclerosis, and hypertension. Although epidemiologic evidence has been well documented for single pollutants, the synergistic impacts are understudied. From a physician's perspective, informing patients on how to avoid exposure and protect themselves should be part of primary prevention.

ECONOMIC BURDEN

Despite some overlap, at least three approaches can measure the economic burden associated with CHD. The first source of financial burden reflects the costs incurred in the health care system itself and reported in "cost-of-illness" studies. As an example, it is estimated that CVD health care costs related to poor nutrition are over $50 billion per year in the United States.[31] In these studies, the cost of CHD includes the costs of hospitalizations for angina and MI, as well as heart failure attributable to CHD. The cost of specific treatments or procedures related to CVD (e.g., thrombolytics, catheterization, PCI) and the cost associated with outpatient management and secondary prevention (e.g., office visits, pharmaceutical costs) are also included. In addition, nursing home, rehabilitation (inpatient and outpatient), and home nursing costs require consideration.

The second economic assessment is derived from microeconomic studies that assess the household impact of catastrophic health events such as MI. These studies look at out-of-pocket expenses incurred by the individual patient or family that might have other, downstream economic impacts, such as loss of savings or sale of property to cover medical costs. Many LMICs lack an extensive insurance scheme, and health care costs are almost entirely borne by individuals; over 800 million people experience financial catastrophe each year because of medical expenditures when defined by 10% of household expenditures devoted to health care expenses.[48,49] Furthermore, the limited data do not confirm the causality between chronic disease and individual or household poverty. However, expenditures for CHD or its addictive risk factors (e.g., tobacco) could lead to substantial and even impoverishing costs.

The third method of determining financial burden from CHD is based on a macroeconomic analysis. These assessments examine lost worker productivity, or the economic growth lost as a result of adults with CHD or their caregivers being partially or completely out of the workforce because of illness. The data for the impact of chronic diseases on labor supply and productivity are more robust. An additional cost usually not accounted for is the intangible loss of welfare associated with pain, disability, or suffering by the affected person. These indirect costs are often addressed by "willingness-to-pay" analyses, asking generally how much would an individual pay to avert suffering or dying prematurely from CHD. The gains are not merely improved work performance, but also enjoying activities beyond productivity. U.S. studies suggest that as much as 1% to 3% of GDP is attributable to the cost of care for CVD, with almost half of that related to CHD.[50] In China, annual direct costs of CVD are estimated at more than US$40 billion, or about 4% of GNI. In South Africa, 2% to 3% of GNI is devoted to the direct treatment of CVD, which equates to about 25% of South African health care expenditures. The indirect costs are estimated at more than double that of the direct costs. Although few cost-of-illness studies for CHD have been performed in other regions, such studies have reported on the financial burdens attributed to risk factors for CHD. For example, the direct costs caused by diabetes in the Latin American and Caribbean countries were estimated at US$10 billion. Indirect costs were estimated at more than $50 billion in 2000. The limited studies available suggest that obesity-related diseases account for 2% to 8% of all health care expenditures in HICs. In India and China, the costs for obesity are about 1.1% and 2.1% of GDP, respectively.

The costs attributable to non-optimal BP levels as mediated through stroke and MI were evaluated for all regions of the world. Globally, the healthcare costs of elevated BP represent approximately 10% of all global health care expenditures. These costs were recently confirmed in a study that showed elevated BP accounted for over $20 billion in Canada, which is 10.2% of its healthcare costs.[51] Regional variations do exist, with hypertension being responsible for up to 25% of health care costs in the Eastern Europe region (Fig. 2.12).

The high proportion of CVD burden that occurs earlier among adults of working age augments its macroeconomic impact in LMICs. Under current projections, in LMICs such as South Africa, CVD will strike 40% of adults between ages 35 and 64, compared with 10% in the United States. India and China will have death rates in the same age group that are two and three times that for most HICs. In view of the large populations in these two rapidly growing economies, this trend could have profound economic effects over the next 25 years, as workers in their prime succumb to CVD.

COST-EFFECTIVE SOLUTIONS

The large reductions in age-adjusted CVD mortality rates that have occurred in HICs result from three complementary types of interventions. One strategy targets those with acute or established CVD. A second entails risk assessment and targeting persons at high risk because of multiple risk factors for intervention before their first CVD event. The third strategy uses mass education or policy interventions directed at the entire population to reduce the overall level of risk factors. This section reviews various cost-effective interventions (see Chapter 45). Much work remains undone in LMICs to determine the best strategies given limited resources, but if implemented, these interventions could help significantly in reducing the burden. Table 2.2 lists the cost-effectiveness ratios for many high-yield interventions that could be or have been adopted in low- and middle-income regions. In 2017 the WHO published recommendations for preventing non-communicable diseases including CVD. The WHO document further divides the recommendations into 'Best buys' (interventions with cost-effectiveness analysis results less than or equal to $1000 per DALY averted in LMICs) and effective interventions (CEA >$1000/DALY averted).[52]

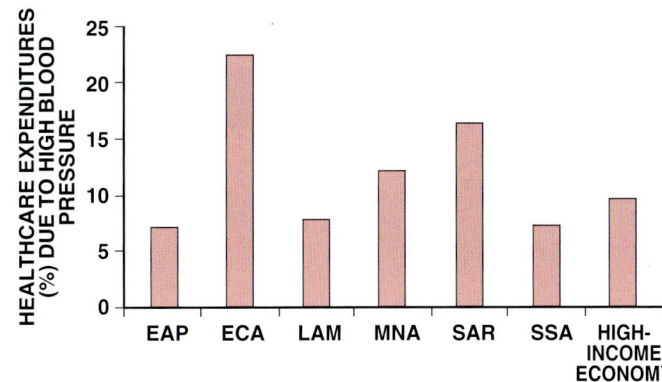

FIGURE 2.12 Percentage of health care expenditures attributed to high blood pressure. *EAP*, East Asia and Pacific; *ECA*, Europe and Central Asia; *LAM*, Latin America and the Caribbean; *MNA*, Middle East and North Africa; *SAR*, South Asia region; *SSA*, sub-Saharan Africa.

Established Cardiovascular Disease Management

People at highest risk are those having an MI or stroke; as many as half die before they ever receive medical attention. For those who do reach a hospital, many cost-effective strategies exist.[4] Four incremental strategies were evaluated for the treatment of MI and compared with a strategy of "no treatment" as a control for the six World Bank low- and middle-income regions. The four strategies compared were (1) aspirin; (2) aspirin and atenolol (beta blocker); (3) aspirin, atenolol, and streptokinase; and (4) aspirin, atenolol, and tissue plasminogen activator (t-PA). The incremental cost per quality-adjusted life-year (QALY) gained for the aspirin and beta-blocker interventions was less than $25 for all six regions. Costs per QALY gained for streptokinase were between $630 and $730 across the regions. Incremental cost-effectiveness ratios for t-PA were about $16,000/QALY gained, compared with streptokinase. Minor variations occurred between regions as a result of small differences in follow-up care based on regional costs. In some LMICs treatment with PCIs where catheterization labs are already established is now considered cost-effective.

Secondary prevention strategies have equal cost-effectiveness in LMICs. A combination of aspirin, an ACE inhibitor, a beta blocker, and a statin for secondary prevention can lead to acceptable cost-effectiveness ratios in all low- and middle-income regions. Use of currently available generic agents, even in the absence of the "polypill," could be highly cost-effective, on the order of $300 to $400 per person per QALY gained. Secondary prevention of rheumatic fever and rheumatic heart disease with prophylactic penicillin is now also recommended by the WHO. Although cost-effectiveness analyses for some therapies in most LMICs have not been conducted, the WHO recommends treatment of heart failure with beta-blockers and angiotensin-converting-enzyme inhibitors; cardiac rehabilitation post MI; and anticoagulation for medium- and high-risk non-valvular atrial fibrillation and for mitral stenosis with atrial fibrillation.

Risk Assessment

Primary prevention is paramount for the large number of people who have high risk for acquiring CVD. The WHO recommends through its 'Best buys' program drug therapy for diabetes mellitus and control of hypertension using an absolute risk approach.[52] In view of limited resources, finding low-cost prevention strategies is a top priority. Using prediction rules or risk scores to identify persons at higher risk to target specific behavioral or drug interventions is a well-established primary prevention strategy and has proved to be cost-effective.[53,54] Most such scoring systems include age, sex, hypertension, smoking status, diabetes mellitus, and lipid values; some also include family history. Other markers of risk, such as C-reactive protein, have been used that improve reclassification and discrimination. Coronary artery calcium scoring may add the most in terms of changes in C-statistic (discrimination) or

TABLE 2.2 Cost-Effectiveness for a Selection of Coronary Heart Disease Interventions in Developing Regions

INTERVENTION	COST-EFFECTIVENESS RATIO ($US/DALY)*
Drug Treatments	
Acute Myocardial Infarction	
ASA, BB (global)	11–22
ASA, BB, SK (global)	634–734
ASA, BB, t-PA (global)	15,860–18,893
Prehospital thrombolysis (Brazil)	457/LY
Secondary Treatment (CHD)	
Multidrug regimen (ASA, BB, ACEI, statin) (global)	1686–2026
Coronary artery bypass graft (global)	24,040–72,345
Primary Prevention	
Cholesterol lowering (Brazil)	441/LY
Hypertension using absolute risk approach of those with 10-year CVD risk >20% and glycemic control for those with diabetes mellitus	<100
Multidrug regimen (AR > 20%–25%) (global)	771–1195
Policy Interventions	
Tobacco	
Price increase of 33%	2–85
Nonpolicy Interventions	
(standardized packing or graphic warnings, bans on advertising and sponsorship, reduced secondhand exposure to indoor workplaces and public sites, and mass media campaigns)	33–100
Salt Reduction‡	
2–8 mm Hg reduction (via reformulation of food products to contain less sodium and setting target levels for gram of food items, mass media, and front of package labeling)	Cost-saving: 250
Fat-Related Interventions§	
Reduced saturated-fat intake	Cost-saving: 2900
Trans fat replacement: 7% reduction in CHD	50–1500
Devices	
Cardioverter-defibrillators: primary prevention (Brazil)	50,345 (US$PPP/QALY)
Physical Activity	
Community wide public education and awareness campaign and environmental programs aimed at behavioral change	<$100

*Across six World Bank regions; *DALY,* disability-adjusted life-year; *PPP,* purchasing power parity; *QALY,* quality-adjusted life-year.
‡Range includes different estimates of cost of interventions, as well as blood pressure reduction (<$0.50 to $1.00).
§Range includes estimates of cost of interventions (<$0.50 to $6.00).
ASA, Acetylsalicylic acid (aspirin); *BB,* beta blocker; *CHD,* coronary heart disease; *SK,* streptokinase; *ACEI,* angiotensin-converting enzyme inhibitor; *t-PA,* tissue plasminogen activator; *AR,* absolute risk.
Data from Gaziano TA. Cardiovascular disease in the developing world and its cost-effective management. *Circulation.* 2005;112:3547; Gaziano TA, Galea G, Reddy KS. Chronic diseases 2—scaling up interventions for chronic disease prevention: the evidence. *Lancet.* 2007;370:1939; and World Health Organization. Tackling NCDs: "Best Buys" and Other Recommended Interventions for the Prevention and Control of Noncommunicable Diseases. Geneva: World Health Organization; 2017.

the net reclassification improvement (NRI) in intermediate-risk populations, and is found to be cost-effective at least in high-income settings (see Chapter 25).[55]

More attention is now focused on developing risk scores that would be easier to use in resource-poor countries, without loss of predictive discrimination. A study based on the U.S. National Health and Nutrition Examination Survey (NHANES) follow-up cohort demonstrated that a non–laboratory-based risk tool that uses information obtained in a single encounter (age, systolic BP, BMI, diabetes status, and smoking status) can predict CVD outcomes as effectively as one that requires laboratory testing, with C-statistics of 0.79 for men and 0.83 for women that were no different from those obtained using the Framingham-based risk tool, and has been shown to correlate with other scores in other countries.[56] In LMICs with limited testing facilities, a prediction rule that requires a laboratory test may be too expensive for widespread screening, or the cost may preclude its use altogether. In response to this concern, WHO recently released risk-prediction charts for the different regions of the world, with and without cholesterol data.[57] Furthermore, community health workers can use the simple risk scores effectively, decreasing the cost of screening significantly.[58,59] The ankle-brachial index (ABI) also appears to add to risk discrimination and improve the NRI as an alternative noninvasive tool. The American Heart Association and the American College of Cardiology have recommended the use of ABI among high risk individuals while the US Preventative Services Task Force has written that there is limited information with regards to use in determining treatments in the general asymptomatic population.[60]

Policy and Community Interventions

Education and public policy interventions that have reduced smoking rates, lowered mean BP levels, and improved lipid profiles contribute to reduction in CHD rates.[4] Education and policy efforts directed at tobacco consumption have contributed substantially to the reductions in CVD. These included recommendations for reducing tobacco use, harmful effects of excessive alcohol, improved diets, and increases in physical activity.[52]

Tobacco Use

Tobacco control can be conceptualized in terms of strategies that reduce the supply of or the demand for tobacco. Most public health and clinical strategies to date focus on reducing demand through economic disincentives (taxes), health promotion (media and packaging efforts), restricted access (to advertising and tobacco), or clinical assistance for cessation. The WHO effort to catalyze the creation of a global treaty against tobacco use was a key milestone. In May 2003 the WHO World Health Assembly unanimously adopted the WHO Framework Convention in Tobacco Control (FCTC), the first global tobacco treaty. The FCTC had been ratified by 168 countries as of 2016, making it one of the most widely embraced treaties in the United Nations. The FCTC has spurred efforts for tobacco control across the globe by providing both rich and poor nations with a common framework of evidence-based legislation and implementation strategies known to reduce tobacco use.

Five "Best buys" for tobacco control include (1) increased excise taxes on tobacco, (2) standardized large graphic warnings on tobacco packaging, (3) enforce bans on advertising and promotion, (4) reduce exposure to secondhand smoke in work and public settings, and (5) implement mass media campaigns about harms of tobacco.[52]

Critically important for patients who have had a coronary event, smoking cessation saves lives at a greater rate than any individual medical treatment. Quitting smoking in the Organization to Assess Strategies in Acute Ischemic Syndromes (OASIS) 5 trial was associated with a 40% relative risk reduction for MI. Further studies suggest that varenicline leads to increased smoking cessation rates,[61] although it is unclear whether it is better than traditional NRTs.[62]

Salt, Dietary, and Lipid Reductions

The analyses on salt reduction achieved as a result of mass interventions are also quite favorable. Four WHO "Best buys" are: (1) reduce salt intake through the reformulation of food products with target levels, (2) increase options of lower sodium food options in institutions, (3) mass media campaigns for behavioral change, and (4) front of package labeling of sodium content.[52]

Elimination of trans-fat through legislation is also proven cost-effective and recommended by eh the WHO. Four other dietary recommendations that are either cost-saving or cost-effective include (1) financial incentives to those purchasing food through government food provision programs,[63] (2) taxation of sugar sweetened beverages,[64] (3) incentives to purchase healthy food items administered through government health insurance schemes,[65] and (4) menu calorie labeling regulations.[66] Simple measures such as changing prescription length for medications such as statins[67] or training community health workers to do screening for CVD can be cost-effective.[58,68]

SUMMARY AND CONCLUSION

Cardiovascular disease remains a significant global problem. The swift pace of economic and social transformation in a postindustrial world with rapid globalization presents a greater challenge for low- and middle-income economies than for high-income economies. Although CVD age-adjusted rates have declined in HICs and some of the LMICs, the number of CVD survivors continues to increase because of aging populations and improvements in case-fatality rates for acute events. From a worldwide perspective, the rate of change in the global burden of CVD is accelerating, reflecting the changes in the low- and middle-income economies, which represent 85% of the world's population. This preventable epidemic will have substantial consequences on many levels: individual mortality and morbidity, family suffering, and staggering economic costs, both the direct costs of diagnosis and treatment and the indirect costs of lost productivity.

Different regions of the world face different stages of the epidemic. In HICs, managing an ever-older population with chronic manifestations of CVD such as heart failure will strain health care budgets. Currently, the Eastern European countries and members of the former Soviet Union face enormous burdens, with more than half of all deaths attributed to CVD. Meanwhile, countries in sub-Saharan Africa are just beginning to see increases in these chronic illnesses while still grappling with HIV/AIDS. No single global solution to the rising burden of CVD exists, in view of the vast differences in social, cultural, and economic circumstances. HICs must minimize disparities, reverse unfavorable trends in CVD risk factors and behaviors, and deal with the increasing prevalence of CVD in an aging population. The most complex challenges face LMICs, with increasing access to low-cost tobacco products and ready access to less-than-favorable dietary options. Preventing the poverty-inducing effects of catastrophic CVD events will require efforts to improve access to low-cost prevention strategies at both the societal and the individual levels and must include improved financing for at least catastrophic health coverage.

A reduction in the disease burden would similarly require both policy and personal changes. In the long term, allocation of resources to lower-cost strategies will likely prove more cost-effective than dedicating resources to high-cost management of CVD. From a societal perspective, efforts to strengthen tobacco-control strategies, improve dietary choices, and increase physical activity will be paramount. At the individual level, risk assessment strategies and treatment modalities require simplification. Furthermore, alternative deployments of allied health workers such as community health workers will need evaluation, in view of the limited human resources in most LMICs. HICs must share with leading and emerging middle-income countries the burden of research and development into every aspect of prevention and treatment. Through further expansion of the knowledge base, particularly regarding the economic consequences of various treatment and prevention strategies, the efficient transfer of low-cost preventive and therapeutic strategies may alter the natural course of epidemiologic transitions in every part of the world, thereby reducing the excess global burden of preventable CVD.

REFERENCES
Epidemiology Transitions
1. *The Global Burden of Disease Study 2017 (GBD 2017)*. Institute for Health Metrics and Evaluation (IHME), University of Washington; 2017. Accessed January 2020. http://ghdx.healthdata.org/gbd-results-tool.
2. Olshansky SJ, Ault AB. The fourth stage of the epidemiologic transition: the age of delayed degenerative diseases. *Milbank Mem Fund Q*. 1986;64(3):355–391.
3. Omran AR. The epidemiologic transition: a theory of the epidemiology of population change. *Milbank Mem Fund Q*. 1971;49(4):509–538.
4. Dugani S, Gaziano TA. 25 by 25: achieving global reduction in cardiovascular mortality. *Current Cardiol Rep*. 2016;18(1):10.
5. Gaziano T, Suhrcke M, Brouwer E, et al. Costs and cost-effectiveness of interventions and policies to prevent and treat cardiovascular and respiratory diseases. In: D. Prabhakaran SA, T. Gaziano, J. Mbanya, Y. Wu, R. Nugent, ed. *Disease Control Priorities (third edition): Volume 5, Cardiovascular, Respiratory, and Related Disorders*. Washington, DC: World Bank; 2017.
6. Creamer MR, Wang TW, Babb S, et al. Tobacco product use and cessation indicators among adults — United States, 2018. *MMWR Morb Mortal Wkly Rep*. 2019;68:1013–1019.
7. National Center for Health Statistics Health, *United States*, 2018. Hyattsville, MD: Centers for Disease Control and Prevention;2019.
8. Gaziano JM. Fifth phase of the epidemiologic transition: the age of obesity and inactivity. *J Am Med Assoc*. 2010;303(3):275–276.

Variations in Global Burden
9. National Center for Health Statistics (NCHS). *Health, United States, 2015: With Special Feature on Racial and Ethnic Health Disparities*. Hyattsville, MD: NCHS; 2015. 2016.
10. Ng M, Fleming T, Robinson M, et al. Global, regional, and national prevalence of overweight and obesity in children and adults during 1980-2013: a systematic analysis for the Global Burden of Disease Study 2013. *Lancet (London, England)*. 2014;384(9945):766–781.
11. Hales C, Carroll M, Fryar C, Ogden C. *Prevalence of Obesity and Severe Obesity Among Adults: United States, 2017–2018. NCHS Data Brief, No 360*. Hyattsville, MD: National Center for Health Statistics; 2020.
12. Mozaffarian D, Benjamin EJ, Go AS, et al. Heart disease and stroke statistics-2016 update: a report from the American Heart association. *Circulation*. 2016;133(4):e38–e360.
13. Arroyo-Quiroz C, Barrientos-Gutierrez T, O'Flaherty M, et al. Coronary heart disease mortality is decreasing in Argentina, and Colombia, but keeps increasing in Mexico: a time trend study. *BMC Publ Health*. 2020;20(1):162.
14. Sekikawa A, Miyamoto Y, Miura K, et al. Continuous decline in mortality from coronary heart disease in Japan despite a continuous and marked rise in total cholesterol: Japanese experience after the Seven Countries Study. *Int J Epidemiol*. 2015;44(5):1614–1624.
15. World Development Indicators. *The World Bank*; 2018. http://data.worldbank.org. Accessed January ,2020.
16. GBD 2017 Population and Fertility Collaborators. Population and fertility by age and sex for 195 countries and territories, 1950-2017: a systematic analysis for the Global Burden of Disease Study 2017. *Lancet*. 2018;392(10159):1995–2051.
17. Prabhakaran D, Jeemon P, Roy A. Cardiovascular diseases in India: current epidemiology and future directions. *Circulation*. 2016;133(16):1605–1620.

Risk Factors
18. India State-Level Disease Burden Initiative CVD Collaborators. The changing patterns of cardiovascular diseases and their risk factors in the states of India: the Global Burden of Disease Study 1990-2016. *Lancet Glob Health*. 2018;6(12):e1339–e1351.
19. *WHO Report on the Global Tobacco Epidemic*. Geneva: World Health Organization; 2019. Licence: CC BY-NC-SA 3.0 IGO.
20. Eriksen MP, Mackay J, Schluger N, et al. *The Tobacco Atlas*. 5th ed. Atlanta, Georgia: The American Cancer Society; 2015.
21. GBD 2017 Risk Factor Collaborators. Global, regional, and national comparative risk assessment of 84 behavioural, environmental and occupational, and metabolic risks or clusters of risks for 195 countries and territories, 1990-2017: a systematic analysis for the Global Burden of Disease Study 2017. *Lancet (London, England)*. 2018;392(10159):1923–1994.
22. Frazer K, Callinan JE, McHugh J, et al. Legislative smoking bans for reducing harms from secondhand smoke exposure, smoking prevalence and tobacco consumption. *Cochrane Database Syst Rev*. 2016;2(2):Cd005992.
23. Forouzanfar MH, Liu P, Roth GA, et al. Global burden of hypertension and systolic blood pressure of at least 110 to 115 mm Hg, 1990-2015. *J Am Med Assoc*. 2017;317(2):165–182.
24. Collaboration NRF. National trends in total cholesterol obscure heterogeneous changes in HDL and non-HDL cholesterol and total-to-HDL cholesterol ratio: a pooled analysis of 458 population-based studies in Asian and Western countries. *J Epidemiol*. 2019;49(1):173–192.
25. GBD 2017 Disease and Injury Incidence and Prevalence Collaborators. Global, regional, and national incidence, prevalence, and years lived with disability for 354 diseases and injuries for 195 countries and territories, 1990-2017: a systematic analysis for the Global Burden of Disease Study 2017. *Lancet*. 2018;392(10159):1789–1858.
26. Cho NH, Shaw JE, Karuranga S, et al. IDF Diabetes Atlas: global estimates of diabetes prevalence for 2017 and projections for 2045. *Diabetes Res Clin Practice*. 2018;138:271–281.
27. The GBD 2015 Obesity Collaborators. Health effects of overweight and obesity in 195 countries over 25 years. *N Engl J Med*. 2017;377(1):13–27.
28. Popkin BM, Corvalan C, Grummer-Strawn LM. Dynamics of the double burden of malnutrition and the changing nutrition reality. *Lancet*. 2020;395(10217):65–74.
29. NCD Risk Factor Collaboration (NCD-RisC). Trends in adult body-mass index in 200 countries from 1975 to 2014: a pooled analysis of 1698 population-based measurement studies with 19.2 million participants. *Lancet (London, England)*. 2016;387(10026):1377–1396.
30. Food and Agriculture Organization of the United Nations. *New Food Balances*; 2020. http://www.fao.org/faostat/en/#data/FBS/visualize. Accessed June 14, 2020.
31. Jardim TV, Mozaffarian D, Abrahams-Gessel S, et al. Cardiometabolic disease costs associated with suboptimal diet in the United States: a cost analysis based on a microsimulation model. *PLoS Med*. 2019;16(12).
32. Huang C, Huang J, Tian Y, et al. Sugar sweetened beverages consumption and risk of coronary heart disease: a meta-analysis of prospective studies. *Atherosclerosis*. 2014;234(1):11–16.
33. Tian Y, Jiang C, Wang M, et al. BMI, leisure-time physical activity, and physical fitness in adults in China: results from a series of national surveys, 2000-14. *Lancet Diabetes Endocrinol*. 2016;4(6):487–497.
34. United Nations Department of Economic and Social Affairs Population Division. *World Population Ageing 2019*. ST/ESA/SER.A/444; 2020.
35. Barker DJ. Fetal origins of coronary heart disease. *BMJ*. 1995;311(6998):171–174.
36. Martorell R. Improved nutrition in the first 1000 days and adult human capital and health. *Am J Hum Biol*. 2017;29(2). https://doi.org/10.1002/ajhb.22952.
37. Alderman H, Behrman JR, Glewwe P, et al. Evidence of impact of interventions on growth and development during early and middle childhood. In: Bundy DAP, Silva ND, Horton S, Jamison DT, Patton GC, eds. *Child and Adolescent Health and Development*. 3rd ed. Washington (DC): The International Bank for Reconstruction and Development / The World Bank; 2017.
38. Devakumar D, Fall CHD, Sachdev HS, et al. Maternal antenatal multiple micronutrient supplementation for long-term health benefits in children: a systematic review and meta-analysis. *BMC Med*. 2016;14:90.
39. Landrigan PJ, Sly JL, Ruchirawat M, et al. Health consequences of environmental exposures: changing global patterns of exposure and disease. *Ann Glob Health*. 2016;82(1):10–19.
40. Romieu I, Gouveia N, Cifuentes LA, et al. Multicity study of air pollution and mortality in Latin America (the ESCALA study). *Res Rep*. 2012;(171):5–86.

41. Liu Z, Wang F, Li W, et al. Does utilizing WHO's interim targets further reduce the risk - meta-analysis on ambient particulate matter pollution and mortality of cardiovascular diseases? *Environmental pollution (Barking, Essex: 1987)*. 2018;242(Pt B):1299–1307.
42. Cosselman KE, Navas-Acien A, Kaufman JD. Environmental factors in cardiovascular disease. *Nat Rev Cardiol*. 2015;12(11):627–642.
43. Alshaarawy O, Elbaz HA, Andrew ME. The association of urinary polycyclic aromatic hydrocarbon biomarkers and cardiovascular disease in the US population. *Environ Int*. 2016;89–90:174–178.
44. Stafoggia M, Cesaroni G, Peters A, et al. Long-term exposure to ambient air pollution and incidence of cerebrovascular events: results from 11 European cohorts within the ESCAPE project. *Environ Health Perspect*. 2014;122(9):919–925.
45. Rajagopalan S, Al-Kindi SG, Brook RD. Air pollution and cardiovascular disease: JACC state-of-the-art review. *J Am Coll Cardiol*. 2018;72(17):2054–2070.
46. Burroughs Peña MS, Rollins A. Environmental exposures and cardiovascular disease: a challenge for health and development in low- and middle-income countries. *Cardiol Clin*. 2017;35(1):71–86.
47. Liu S, Guo X, Wu B, et al. Arsenic induces diabetic effects through beta-cell dysfunction and increased gluconeogenesis in mice. *Sci Rep*. 2014;4:6894.

Economic Burden

48. Cylus J, Thomson S, Evetovits T. Catastrophic health spending in Europe: equity and policy implications of different calculation methods. *Bull World Health Organ*. 2018;96(9):599–609.
49. Wagstaff A, Flores G, Hsu J, et al. Progress on catastrophic health spending in 133 countries: a retrospective observational study. *The Lancet Global Health*. 2018;6(2):e169–e179.
50. Mozaffarian D, Benjamin EJ, Go AS, et al. Heart disease and stroke statistics—2015 update: a report from the American Heart Association. *Circulation*. 2015;131(4):e29–e322.
51. Weaver CG, Clement FM, Campbell NRC, et al. Healthcare costs attributable to hypertension: Canadian population-based cohort study. *Hypertension*. 2015;66(3):502–508.
52. World Health Organization. *Tackling NCDs: 'best Buys' and Other Recommended Interventions for the Prevention and Control of Noncommunicable Diseases*. Geneva: World Health Organization; 2017.
53. Pandya A, Sy S, Cho S, et al. Cost-effectiveness of 10-year risk thresholds for initiation of statin therapy for primary prevention of cardiovascular disease. *J Am Med Assoc*. 2015;314(2):142–150.
54. Pandya A, Weinstein MC, Salomon JA, et al. Who needs laboratories and who needs statins?: comparative and cost-effectiveness analyses of non-laboratory-based, laboratory-based, and staged primary cardiovascular disease screening guidelines. *Circ Cardiovasc Qual Outcomes*. 2014;7(1):25–32.
55. Greenland P, Blaha MJ, Budoff MJ, et al. Coronary calcium score and cardiovascular risk. *J Am Coll Cardiol*. 2018;72(4):434–447.
56. Gaziano TA, Abrahams-Gessel S, Alam S, et al. Comparison of nonblood-based and blood-based total CV risk scores in global populations. *Glob Heart*. 2016;11(1) March:37–46.
57. Kaptoge S, Pennells L, De Bacquer D, et al. World Health Organization cardiovascular disease risk charts: revised models to estimate risk in 21 global regions. *Lancet Glob Health*. 2019;7(10):e1332–e1345.

Cost-Effective Solutions

58. Gaziano TA, Abrahams-Gessel S, Denman CA, et al. An assessment of community health workers' ability to screen for cardiovascular disease risk with a simple, non-invasive risk assessment instrument in Bangladesh, Guatemala, Mexico, and South Africa: an observational study. *Lancet Glob Health*. 2015;3(9):e556–563.
59. Abrahams-Gessel S, Denman CA, Montano CM, et al. Training and supervision of community health workers conducting population-based, noninvasive screening for CVD in LMIC: implications for scaling up. *Glob Heart*. 2015;10(1):39–44.
60. UPST F. Screening for peripheral artery disease and cardiovascular disease risk assessment with the ankle-brachial index: US preventive services Task Force recommendation statement. *J Am Med Assoc*. 2018;320(2):177–183.
61. Ebbert JO, Hughes JR, West RJ. Effect of varenicline on smoking cessation through smoking reduction: a randomized clinical trial. *J Am Med Assoc*. 2015;313.
62. Baker TB, Piper ME, Stein JH, et al. Effects of nicotine patch vs varenicline vs combination nicotine replacement therapy on smoking cessation at 26 weeks: a randomized clinical trial. *J Am Med Assoc*. 2016;315(4):371–379.
63. Mozaffarian D, Liu J, Sy S, et al. Cost-effectiveness of financial incentives and disincentives for improving food purchases and health through the US Supplemental Nutrition Assistance Program (SNAP): a microsimulation study. *PLoS Medicine*. 2018;15(10):e1002661.
64. Wilde P, Huang Y, Sy S, et al. Cost-effectiveness of a US national sugar-sweetened beverage tax with a multistakeholder approach: who pays and who benefits. *Am J Public Health*. 2018:e1–e9.
65. Lee Y, Mozaffarian D, Sy S, et al. Cost-effectiveness of financial incentives for improving diet and health through Medicare and Medicaid: a microsimulation study. *PLoS Med*. 2019;16(3):e1002761.
66. Liu J, Mozaffarian D, Lee Y, et al. Cost-effectiveness of the U.S. Federal restaurant menu calorie labeling law for improving diet and health: a microsimulation modeling study (P22-014-19). *Current Developments in Nutrition*. 2019;3(nzz042.P22-014-19).
67. Gaziano T, Cho S, Sy S, et al. Increasing prescription length could cut cardiovascular disease burden and produce savings in South Africa. *Health Aff*. 2015;34(9):1578–1585.
68. Gaziano T, Abrahams-Gessel S, Surka S, et al. Cardiovascular disease screening by community health workers can be cost-effective in low-resource countries. *Health affairs (Project Hope)*. 2015;34(9):1538–1545.

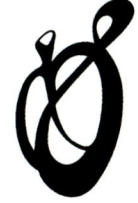

3 Impact of the Environment on Cardiovascular Health

SADEER AL-KINDI AND SANJAY RAJAGOPALAN

扫描二维码阅读
第3章中文导读

GLOBAL FOOTPRINT AND IMPACT OF POLLUTANTS ON HUMAN HEALTH, 31

AIR POLLUTION, 31
Composition and Sources of Air Pollution, 31
Assessment of Exposure, 34
Exposure-Response Function of Air Pollution, Mortality, and Cardiovascular Events, 34
Cardiovascular and Metabolic Effects of Air Pollution, 34

Mechanistic Insights Into Air-Pollution and Cardiovascular Risk, 36
Windows of Exposure, Susceptibility, and Vulnerability, 37
Air Pollution Alerts and Approaches to Communicate Risk, 37
Societal and Personal Strategies to Mitigate Cardiovascular Effects of Air Pollution, 37

CLIMATE CHANGE, 37

NOISE POLLUTION AND CARDIOVASCULAR DISEASE, 38

SYNTHETIC CHEMICALS AND CARDIOVASCULAR DISEASE, 38

METALLIC POLLUTANTS AND CARDIOVASCULAR DISEASE, 39

CHALLENGES AND OUTLOOK FOR THE FUTURE, 39

REFERENCES, 40

The Lancet Commission on pollution and health defines pollution as unwanted, often dangerous, chemical material introduced into the environment as the result of human activity, that threatens health and harms ecosystems.[1] Given the diversity of environmental exposures that an individual may encounter, the term "pollutome" is a useful encompassing term that refers to the aggregate of all exposures in the air, soil, and water (or indoor physical environment) that one is exposed to. The pollutome in turn is a subset of the exposome (i.e., the sum totality of all exposures). A framework for understanding the pollutome where zone 1 contains pollutants with well-characterized health effects; zone 2 with pollutants with emerging, but not yet definite, health effects (known and some unknowns), zone 3 including pollutants with inadequately characterized health effects (known unknowns), and finally zone 4, which may include unknown chemical exposures that are not yet recognized. The phrase "gene-environment interaction" infers that the direction and magnitude of the clinical effect that a genetic variant has on the disease phenotype can vary as the environment changes and importantly acknowledges the importance of genetic predisposition in determining the magnitude of effects. The cardiovascular system is especially vulnerable to a variety of environmental insults, including smoke, solvents, pesticides, and other inhaled or ingested pollutants, as well as extremes in noise and temperature. Our understanding of environmental factors continues to evolve with an increasing footprint attributable to pollutants than previously suspected. Thus, it is vitally important that cardiologists understand the impact of the environment on cardiovascular disease.

GLOBAL FOOTPRINT AND IMPACT OF POLLUTANTS ON HUMAN HEALTH

The global footprint of environmental pollution is very large, ranging from about 9 million deaths based on the most recent global burden of disease (GBD) estimate in 2019, to 12.6 million deaths based on a World Health Organization (WHO) estimate in 2012. These differences arise from variable definitions of the environment in the estimates. The GBD estimates are based on a more limited inventory of risk factors including air pollution: household, ambient (fine particulate matter [$PM_{2.5}$], and tropospheric ozone pollution); (2) water pollution: unsafe sanitation and unsafe water sources; (3) soil, chemical, and heavy metal pollution: lead (including contaminated sites polluted by lead from battery recycling operations), and mercury from gold mining; and (4) occupational pollution: occupational carcinogens, and occupational particulates, gases, and fumes. The WHO definition also includes noise, electromagnetic fields, occupational psychosocial risks, built environment, agricultural methods, and human-made climate and ecosystem change. It is important to emphasize that these estimates are likely a vast underestimate because all of these analyses are based on known risk factors (zone 1) for which there is convincing evidence of causal association (Fig. 3.1). Total pollution is estimated to contribute to approximately 20% of all cardiovascular disease and 25% of ischemic heart diseases (IHDs) of which air pollution is the largest contributor, responsible for over 6 million deaths annually worldwide. As such, the global impact of environmental pollution is high and is expected to worsen as population-weighted exposures increase with urbanization and increased population density.[2]

AIR POLLUTION

The GBD 2019 lists air pollution as the fourth leading risk factor for global mortality, responsible for 6.67 million deaths globally.[3] The disease burden attributable to ambient $PM_{2.5}$ estimated in disability-adjusted life-years (DALYs), increased from 70.5 (95% uncertainty interval [UI] 47.3 to 98.9) million DALYs in 1990, to 118.2 (95.9 to 138.4) million DALYs in 2019. Air pollution together with high body mass index and glucose are the only three risk factors among 87 others that account for greater than 1% of DALYs and continue in prevalence by greater than 1% per year.[3] The increase globally is almost entirely attributable to urbanization and increasing exposures in Asia, parts of the Middle East, and Africa. Although many gaseous pollutants have been linked with health effects (e.g., ozone, nitrogen oxides, sulfur oxides), fine PM (particles ≤2.5 μm, $PM_{2.5}$), principally derived from fossil fuel combustion (for the purposes of power, residential energy use, and industry) is the most extensively implicated component, and has a disproportionate impact on adverse health effects.[4–6] Over 50% of deaths attributable to air pollution is from cardiovascular causes (Fig. 3.2).[7–9]

Composition and Sources of Air Pollution

Air pollution is a complex mixture of gaseous phase and particulate constituents that varies spatially and temporally.[4] From a regulation perspective, the Environmental Protection Agency (EPA) has set National Ambient Air Quality Standards (NAAQS) for six principal pollutants, which are called "criteria" air pollutants (carbon monoxide, lead, nitrogen dioxide, ozone, particulate matter, and sulfur dioxide, Table 3.1).[10] Primary air pollutants are those that are released directly into the atmosphere, including both gaseous and particulates, whereas secondary pollutants are formed through chemical transformation through interaction with other constituents and/or in response to prevalent atmospheric conditions (sunlight, water, vapor, etc.). Many primary air pollutants such as nitrogen oxides (NO + NO_2), carbon monoxide, sulfur dioxide (SO_2), $PM_{2.5}$, as well as carbon dioxide (CO_2), originate from combustion of fuel or other anthropogenic processes. Combustion $PM_{2.5}$ is composed of many organic compounds, including organic carbon species (OC), elemental or black carbon, and trace metals (Table 3.1).[4] In addition to O_3, which is the most prevalent secondary oxidant, a number of inorganic and organic acids and volatile organic carbons (VOCs) and semivolatile organic compounds (SVOCs) formed secondarily and are found in both the gas and particle phase, are an additional large class of pollutants. Key examples are benzene, toluene, xylene, 1,3- butadiene, and polycyclic aromatic hydrocarbons (PAHs). Many VOCs contribute to the formation of O_3 and are oxidized in the atmosphere, becoming SVOCs and subsequently contribute to $PM_{2.5}$ mass. Examples of secondary pollutants include sulphates, nitrate, and ammonium which also contribute to the PM fraction of air pollution. The particulate fraction of air pollution may be broadly categorized by aerodynamic diameter: less than 10 μm (thoracic particles [PM_{10}]), less than 2.5 μm (fine particles [$PM_{2.5}$]), less than 0.1 μm (ultrafine particles [UFPs]), and between 2.5 to 10 μm (coarse [$PM_{2.5-10}$]). Although most studies have focused on one or two pollutants at a time, the reality is that pollutants coexist and vary spatially and temporally. Even though some epidemiologic studies adjust for copollutants, the significant collinearity makes it complex to separate these effects.

Particulate Air Pollutants

PM air pollution is by far the most studied and with the most evidence for health effects. The categorization of PM based on size thresholds reflects the ease of quantification and is a rough barometer of chemical composition, geographic distribution, and sources. Although regulatory thresholds exist for PM_{10} and $PM_{2.5}$ (see Table 3.1), no standards exist for UFP. PM_{10} and $PM_{2.5}$ often derive from different emissions sources and also have different chemical compositions. Emissions from combustion of gasoline, oil, diesel fuel, or wood produce much of the $PM_{2.5}$ pollution found in ambient air, as well as a significant proportion of PM_{10}. Dust from crustal material and agricultural and industrial practices contribute to the course ($PM_{10-2.5}$) or even larger particle (>PM_{10}) size ranges and may dominate composition in certain environments. PM_{10} may also include dust from road dust, tire and road wear particles, dust from construction, agricultural emissions, wildfires and brush/waste burning, industrial sources, wind-blown dust from open lands, pollen, and fragments of bacteria and lipopolysaccharide (LPS). $PM_{0.1}$ or UFPs are generated through primary combustion of fossil fuels from automobile sources, are characterized by large surface area to size ratio, and can serve as a nidus for gaseous copollutants. UFPs are short lived and are highly influenced by proximity to the sources (typically <1 km from source). The spatial and temporal colocalization of gaseous copollutants with UFPs makes it difficult to separate the health effects in epidemiologic and mechanistic research. In addition, UFP monitoring is not widely available and requires

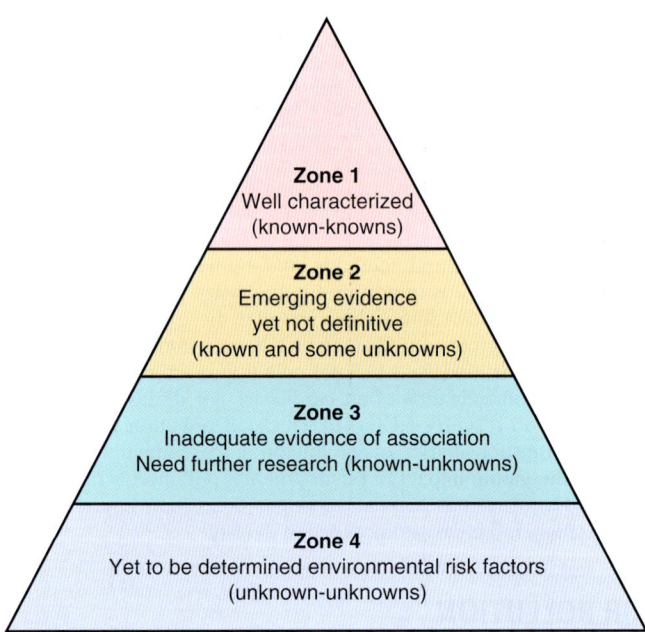

FIGURE 3.1 Zones of evidence linking environmental pollution with health effects. (Adapted from Landrigan P, Fuller R, Acosta NJ, et al. The Lancet Commission on pollution and health. *Lancet*. 2018;391:462–512.)

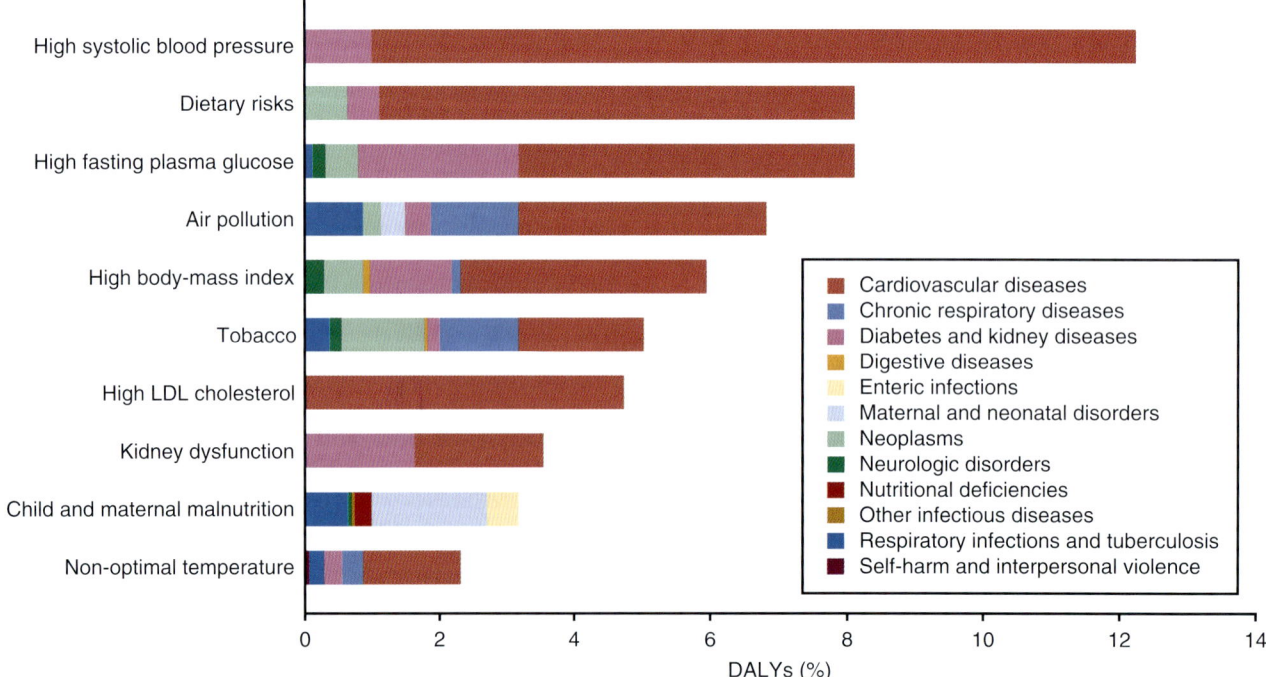

FIGURE 3.2 Estimates of global attributable deaths from various risk factors. DALYs, disability-adjusted life-years. (Adapted from GBD 2019 Risk Factors Collaborators. *Lancet*. 2020; 396:1223–1249.)

TABLE 3.1 U.S. and European Standards for Air Pollutants

Air pollution component	Size or structure	U.S. standards	European standards
PM	Coarse PM (2.5–10 μm); $PM_{2.5}$ (≤2.5 μm); PM_{10} (<10 μm)	$PM_{2.5}$: 12 μg/m³ (1 year); 35 μg/m³ (24h)	$PM_{2.5}$: 25 μg/m³ (1 year)
		PM_{10}: 150 μg/m³ (24h)	PM_{10}: 40 μg/m³ (1 year); 50 μg/m³ (24 h)
Sulfur dioxide		75 ppb (1h)	350 μg/m³ (1 h); 125 μg/m³ (24h)
Nitrogen dioxide		100 ppb (1h)	40 μg/m³ (1 year); 200 ppb (1h)
Ozone gas		0.070 ppm (8h)	120 μg/m³ (8 h)
Carbon monoxide		10 μg/m³ (8 h)	35 ppm (1h); 9 ppm (8h)
Lead		0.15 μg/m³ (3 months)	0.5 μg/m³ (1 year)

PM, particulate matter; $PM_{2.5}$, fine particulate matter; PM_{10}, coarse and fine particulate matter.

Adapted from Al-Kindi SG, Brook RD, Biswal S, et al. Environmental determinants of cardiovascular disease: lessons learned from air pollution. *Nat Rev Cardiol.* 2020;17:656–672.

specialized equipment. Recent studies have suggested heightened cardiovascular risk of UFP.[11]

Gaseous Pollutants

Ground level ozone (O_3) is the most studied gaseous pollutant with respect to health effects.[12–15] It is a secondary pollutant which is created through reaction between nitrogen oxide and volatile organic compounds, facilitated by sunlight. Although high levels of ozone clearly confer adverse health effects including increased risk of mortality and asthma, recent evidence suggests a continued relationship between ozone and health effects at levels lower than the U.S. NAAQS of 70 ppb over 8 hours.[14] The association between long-term ozone exposures and CV mortality is lower than other causes of mortality.[16] The mechanisms of ozone-related cardiovascular and mortality effects appear to be related to oxidant stress and a prothrombotic response.[5] There is paucity of data for other gaseous copollutants present in fossil fuel emissions such as VOCs and atherosclerotic cardiovascular disease (ASCVD) events, although mechanistically it is highly likely that these compounds may have important health effects. Copollutants such as NO_2 and SO_2 may not be directly toxic but function as surrogates for other copollutants and have been linked to cardiovascular events, including myocardial infarction (MI), stroke, and heart failure (HF).[17,18]

Particulate Matter Sources, Composition, and Cardiovascular Risk

Air pollution chemistry and hence health effects vary substantially by source. There is a substantial spatial and temporal variation of air pollution levels that may be important in health effects. Large urban-rural differences are found for primary combustion pollutants that originate from traffic such as nitrogen oxides (NO and NO_2), and particulate black carbon, that may drive risk. Meteorologic conditions such as atmospheric stability can significantly alter the horizontal propagation of particles and thus the size of the population exposed. Given the fact that the dynamics of air pollution chemistry and concentration may vary substantially, the detailed chemical characterization of pollution is a static time frame that in addition to being expensive may not accurately portray the chemical composition particularly for components such as ultrafine. However, speciation of common pollutants such as sulfates and nitrates or the corresponding gaseous pollutants such as NO_2 and SO_2 have been shown to be predictive of health effects.[19] A 2014 systematic review that quantified the associations between chemical components, such as sulfate, nitrate, and elemental and organic carbons, demonstrated that they were all linked to all-cause, cardiovascular, and respiratory mortality.[17] In an analysis of the American Cancer Society Cancer Prevention Study II, mortality from ischemic heart disease (IHD) associated with $PM_{2.5}$ derived from coal combustion was fivefold higher than the risk with overall $PM_{2.5}$ mass, suggesting that the source of $PM_{2.5}$ may be important in determining cardiovascular risk.[18] Examination of sources may sometimes represent a more efficient way of thinking about health effects, including regulation. For instance, traffic air pollution is perhaps the largest health threat from a source perspective in the West, with a sizeable proportion of the population living within 150 meters of a major highway and thus likely to be exposed to traffic-related ultrafine air pollution. The average Western adult spends 55 minutes a day exposed to vehicular emissions.[20] Traffic air pollution peaks during the late morning and evening rush hours, with $PM_{0.1}$ and gaseous components demonstrating substantial variation within a span of 400 m. The substantial spatial variation and reactivity of $PM_{0.1}$ fraction pose challenges for accurate quantification, and thus a simple metric such as distance from a highway has been an effective surrogate for traffic-related exposures. Fossil fuel–burning coal power plants, shipping and airplane, and agricultural emissions (e.g., crop burning) may dominate emissions in certain environments. Most individuals across the globe spend preponderant majority of time indoors and are also exposed to indoor sources. Household air pollution (HAP) encompass a range of particles from diverse sources that vary dramatically depending on geography and socioeconomic and cultural factors. For instance, with exposure to high concentrations of emissions from wood/coal-burning stoves for cooking and heat, kerosene stoves may dominate the indoor environment in developing countries reliant on solid fuels for heat and cooking. In countries with high levels of ambient air pollution, it is estimated that up to 65% of inhalation of outdoor air particles occurs when people are indoors.[21] In the West, cooking on gas stoves, burning incense and candles, use of aerosol sprays, and cleaning activities may contribute to indoor particle levels. Wood-burning communities in North America may experience high levels of UFPs during winter. The expansion of the human habitats and climate change have expanded the likelihood of exposure to air pollution from natural events such as wildfires and volcanic eruptions. Both PM and gaseous pollutants from these events can affect large populations and produce health effects in millions of people across the world.[22] For instance, crustal material from dust storms can cause dramatic increases in outdoor and indoor PM counts.[23] Mortality and respiratory morbidity have been the most frequently studied and most consistently reported outcomes of smoke exposure. Recent evidence suggests that smoke exposure from natural sources such as wildfires may be associated with cardiovascular effects with effect estimates comparable with ambient $PM_{2.5}$ from anthropogenic sources.[24]

Household Versus Ambient Air Pollution

Although the vast majority of studies on air pollution have focused on ambient air pollution owing to exposure data availability, HAP is a major contributor to global mortality, particularly in developing countries.[25,26] The burden of disease attributable to HAP has been steadily decreasing, with the most recent GBD 2019 indicating that the percentage of DALYs attributable to HAP decreasing 56%, demoting HAP as the 4th leading risk factor in 1990 to the 10th leading risk factor in 2019.[3] Although HAP is a significant cause of childhood morbidity including predisposition to respiratory tract infections and COPD, links between CVD have been recently elucidated, including association with hypertension and coronary artery disease.[27] An issue with HAP has been the estimation of reliable exposure estimates and ascertainment of mortality causes, because the predominant majority of events occur in communities with limited access to health care and standardized reporting procedures. HAP encompasses gaseous and particulate pollution generated from solid fuel use for cooking and indoor heat in developing countries.[27] In Western countries, wood-burning furnaces, indoor candle lighting, and aerosol spray use may all contribute to HAP. It is important to note that HAP and ambient air pollution also coexist, such as in developing countries and when outdoor ambient levels are very high.[25] In these environments, the indoor environment may be dominated by outdoor levels (and hence sources). The translocation of particles from ambient (outdoor) air to indoor air is determined by house insulation and the method of ventilation. Smaller particles (UFPs) have higher likelihood of translocating indoors, and this has been documented in residential areas with proximity to major highways as well as wood-burning communities in the United States.

Assessment of Exposure

Accurate assessment of exposure is of paramount importance to understand the health effects, regulate emissions, and mitigate adverse health effects. Given that studies associating exposure with health outcomes require a large number of participants who are geographically dispersed, exposure assessment needs to be pragmatic and widely available. There is a tradeoff between approaches in terms of spatial resolution (coverage), exposure assessment at the individual level, and finally temporal resolution. Satellite-based assessment approaches using aerosol optical depth of a vertical column from space, as an index of particulate air pollution, can provide ambient air annual and daily exposure assessments around the globe at spatial resolution down to 1×1 km.[28] These are frequently combined with chemical transport models, aided by statistical or machine learning–based adjustment based on ground monitors. Although these methods have been integral for GBD estimates, their accuracy for personal exposure is limited and furthermore their temporal resolution is limited.[15] Ground monitors in urban locations provide better spatial and temporal resolution, but their accuracy declines rapidly with distance, and thus some exposure models use data from multiple ground monitor sources to produce reliable estimates. It is important to emphasize that all exposure assessment approaches are only approximations of true exposure and thus can serve only as surrogates for "true personal" exposure. Personal exposure monitors (both indoor and portable) are increasingly available and promise to provide individual exposure information at a fine scale in a variety of environments, often at high temporal resolution. Such devices represent a practical way to expand the coverage of ground monitors and may facilitate real-time communication of air pollution levels and personalized assessment of environmental risk, that can be used to mitigate health risks.[15] A current challenge is their technical harmonization with current stationary approaches, especially with regards to standardization of measures and helping to resolve differential time scales.

Exposure-Response Function of Air Pollution, Mortality, and Cardiovascular Events

Understanding the relationship between continuous long-term and short-term exposure to air pollutants and health outcomes is critical for regulation, health policy, and intervention. The original integrated exposure response function (IER) used in the Global Burden of Disease 2013 study assigned estimated concentrations of $PM_{2.5}$ to inhalational exposure from a variety of sources, including secondhand smoking and active smoking, and assumed that risk is determined by the 24-hour $PM_{2.5}$ inhaled dose, regardless of the exposure source.[29] The nonlinear response curve, with steep increases at low exposure levels and flattening at higher doses, has been useful in providing a credible explanation for robust risk estimates from epidemiologic studies at low doses of air pollution, and yet reconciling studies with HAP and active smoking that are typically characterized by extremely high $PM_{2.5}$ levels. Importantly, the IER allowed derivation of credible estimates of disease events attributable to air pollution across the globe, including in areas with little to no ground level monitoring, using satellite-based assessment of $PM_{2.5}$. In GBD 2019, the inclusion of additional studies from China and India and studies of HAP allowed incorporation of a broad range of exposures and recalculation of estimates attributable to pollution from a variety of sources.[3] Importantly, the elimination of active smoking from the curves removed a significant degree of uncertainty in the estimates (Fig. 3.3). Although the epidemiology of air pollution and cardiovascular events is robust and controls for a number of factors, multiple limitations including the independent and potentially synergistic contribution by other environmental coexposures such as noise and other poorly understood socioeconomic determinants must be acknowledged.[30,31]

Cardiovascular and Metabolic Effects of Air Pollution

Both short-term and long-term exposure to $PM_{2.5}$ has been linked with the development of cardiovascular, renal, and metabolic disorders, including hypertension and type 2 diabetes. The epidemiology of the air pollution and cardiometabolic disorders involves both short-term variation typically examined in time series and case crossover analysis using referent time windows, as well as long-term exposure studies

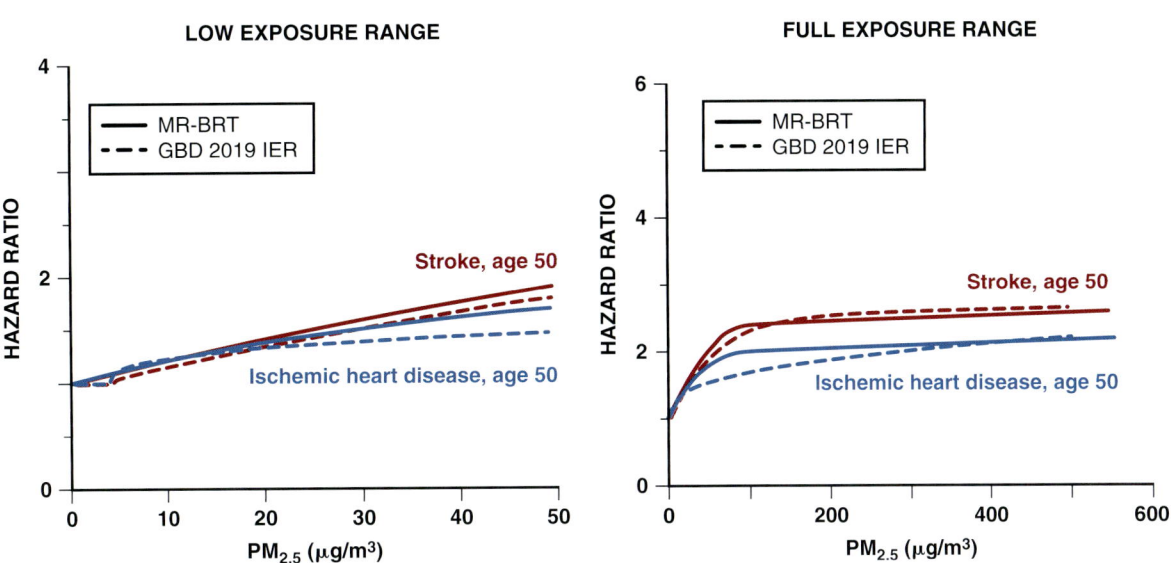

FIGURE 3.3 Ischemic heart disease (IHD) and stroke outcomes with $PM_{2.5}$. Meta-regression Bayesian, regularized, trimmed (MR-BRT). In global burden of disease (GBD) 2019, for a selected set of continuous risk factors, we modeled relative risks using MR-BRT, relaxing the log-linear assumption to allow for monotonically increasing or decreasing, but nonlinear functions using cubic splines. (Adapted from GBD 2019 Risk Factors Collaborators. *Lancet.* 2020;396 [appendix].)

involving large prospective cohorts. Together, these studies have provided a detailed portrait of the epidemiologic associations between components of air pollution and adverse cardiometabolic consequences and indeed support a strong associative link. Additional supportive mechanistic studies in animal models, short-term controlled exposure studies, interventional studies, and accountability studies have provided more or less definitive proof of air pollution as a causative environmental trigger in the genesis of cardiometabolic disease. Diabetes exposure response curves were included in GBD 2019 and suggest a steep dose response curve at lower doses with flattening at very high doses.

Ischemic Heart Disease and Cerebrovascular Events

The association between short-term $PM_{2.5}$ and cardiovascular mortality has been extensively described. Three early meta-analyses between 2012 and 2016 demonstrated that $PM_{2.5}$ was associated with cardiovascular mortality. Although some of these were at high-exposure environments, the preponderance was from low-exposure environments.[32–34] On the basis of these analyses, a short-term increase of 10 μg/m³ in $PM_{2.5}$ was associated with a 0.1% to 1.0% excess in risk of cardiovascular death. In some of these analyses, an association was also seen with other gaseous copollutants such as NO_2 and SO_2.[32] Chronic exposure studies using annual $PM_{2.5}$ concentrations have shown much higher estimates ranging from an increase of 15% to 30% per 10 μg/m³ $PM_{2.5}$ in relative risk for CV mortality at the lower range of exposures typically seen in North America.[35,36] Postinfarct mortality and quality of life are also influenced by prevailing concentrations of $PM_{2.5}$.[37] Figure 3.3 depicts the GBD 2019 IER and a meta-regression curve (meta-regression Bayesian, regularized, trimmed [MR-BRT]) that incorporates a range of cohort studies. The curves for the typical annual average exposures are depicted. In general, the incorporation of studies across the exposure range from ambient air pollution studies and some secondhand smoking studies have provided confidence across the exposure range. The GBD 2019 and meta-regression estimates are stronger than the 2017 estimates and importantly continue to demonstrate a flattening at extreme concentrations of $PM_{2.5}$ (>85 μg/m³). Given the small number of studies at such high levels and because 97% of the global population lives in countries where population-weighted outdoor exposure was less than 84 μg/m³, these results are largely relevant. An alternate Global Exposure Mortality Model (GEMM), using only ambient $PM_{2.5}$ data (excluding secondhand smoking) projected a much higher burden of disease when compared with the GBD IER estimates.[38]

There is an association between nonfatal MI and $PM_{2.5}$ levels with the evidence for ST-elevation MI being stronger than NSTEMI and unstable angina.[39–41] Men, older patients,[40] and those with risk factors for or established coronary artery disease seem to be most susceptible. Cross-sectional and prospective longitudinal cohort studies have demonstrated a positive association between estimated long-term exposure to $PM_{2.5}$, as well as distance to roadway (as a proxy for exposure), to surrogates such as endothelial function and atherosclerosis burden, when assessed by carotid intimal media thickness and coronary and abdominal aortic calcium.[42] In at least one study, an increase of 1 μg/m³ of $PM_{2.5}$ from use of CT was associated with a 62% increased incidence of "high-risk" plaque (plaque with low attenuation, spotty calcium, and positive remodeling) at follow-up.[43] The association between stroke and air pollution exposure is robust with a very consistent association between short-term exposure and stroke risk. A 2019 meta-analysis of 80 studies found a 1% increase in stroke per 10 μg/m³ increment of short-term $PM_{2.5}$ exposure. Associations were strongest for ischemic and hemorrhagic stroke.[44] Figure 3.3 demonstrates the association between long-term exposure and stroke, using GBD 2019 estimates. In general, the association between stroke and annual $PM_{2.5}$ concentrations are higher compared with that for IHD. Mechanisms underlying the association between $PM_{2.5}$ and cerebrovascular disease are likely similar to those of coronary artery disease and MI.

Blood Pressure and Hypertension

Prior meta-analyses have shown a consistent association between short-term ambient $PM_{2.5}$ levels and blood pressure (BP) levels.[5,6] Short-term (in hours to days) variation in antecedent $PM_{2.5}$, as well as controlled exposure to both fine and coarse PM, is associated with increases in BP. In large prospective cohorts, annual average $PM_{2.5}$ was associated with not only correspondingly larger increases in BP (compared with short-term elevations) but was also associated with incident hypertension. The associations between $PM_{2.5}$ and hypertension have been observed at both low levels (United States and Canada) and at high levels of $PM_{2.5}$ (China and India), with no evidence of flattening of effect estimates.[5,6] Exposure to a range of particles, including UFPs (diesel exhaust) and $PM_{2.5}$ and PM_{10} particles, has been shown to increase BP within hours in carefully performed randomized studies.[5,6] Conversely, lowering $PM_{2.5}$ using air filtration devices in randomized trials has also shown a consistent decrease in BP, suggesting a cause-and-effect relationship.[28] The mechanisms underlying BP increases in the short term in humans might involve rapid alterations in autonomic tone, redox stress, and alteration in vascular stiffness and endothelial dysfunction.[31,45] Experimental models of hypertension involving both low and high renin forms of hypertension have suggested an exacerbation of BP with $PM_{2.5}$ exposure secondary to changes in vascular redox and inflammation. Central sympathetic activation related to

Insulin Resistance and Diabetes

Studies in both low- and high-exposure environments have shown a clear association between $PM_{2.5}$ exposure incidence of diabetes and risk for diabetes-related mortality.[30,31,46] Based on exposure-response relationships derived from a cohort of veterans, ambient $PM_{2.5}$ has been suggested to contribute to approximately 3.2 million (95% UI 2.2 to 3.8) incident cases of diabetes, approximately 8.2 million (95% UI 5.8 to 11.0) DALYs and 206,105 (95% UI 153,408 to 259,119) diabetic deaths.[47] The mechanisms involve exaggeration of insulin resistance, inflammation in liver and white adipose tissue, reduced thermogenesis, and central nervous system inflammation resulting in alterations in metabolism.[46,48–50]

Heart Failure

The associations between $PM_{2.5}$ and HF are less consistent. A 2013 meta-analysis of 35 studies showed that 10 μg/m³ increments in $PM_{2.5}$ were associated with 2.12% increase in HF hospitalizations or death, with strongest associations noted on the day of exposure.[51] Based on these relationships, it was estimated that reduction of 3.9 μg/m³ of $PM_{2.5}$ in the United States would prevent approximately 8000 HF hospitalizations and save greater than 300 million U.S. dollars annually.[51] Acute increases in $PM_{2.5}$ are associated with increased right heart and filling pressures. Long-term exposure to $PM_{2.5}$ in mice leads to adverse ventricular remodeling as assessed by major histocompatibility complex isoform switch and fibrosis, alterations in flow reserve, reduced systolic function, contractile reserve, and worsening of diastolic function.[52] $PM_{2.5}$ inhalation may also lead to adverse remodeling of the right ventricle, partly due to lung inflammation and vascular remodelling.[53] The delineation of the types of HF that are most susceptible to $PM_{2.5}$ exposure need further work.

Arrhythmia

In a 2020 meta-analysis involving 572 patients with implantable cardioverter defibrillators and 1689 events, each 10 μg/m³ increment in $PM_{2.5}$ was associated with 24% increase in odds for atrial fibrillation (AF).[54] $PM_{2.5}$ has also been associated with increased stroke risk in patients with AF. In healthy individuals and in those with prior cardiovascular disease, both acute and chronic exposure to $PM_{2.5}$ has been associated with increased burden of premature ventricular contractions. The mechanisms between arrhythmic risk and $PM_{2.5}$ are unclear, although changes in autonomic tone, loading conditions, and inflammation could play a role.

Venous Thromboembolism

Various studies have shown that acute and chronic exposure to $PM_{2.5}$ leads to increase in thrombosis markers (D-dimer, fibrinogen).[5,6] Several studies have examined the association between air pollution and venous thromboembolism (VTE) events. A 2016 systematic review of 11 studies and greater than 500,000 events suggested a link between multiple $PM_{2.5}$ with VTE risk (8/11 studies).[55]

Chronic Kidney Disease

Emerging evidence has linked air pollution to chronic kidney disease (CKD). Multiple studies have suggested links between long-term $PM_{2.5}$ exposure and decline in kidney function, incident or prevalent CKD, and kidney failure in general populations.[56–58] In a study in patients with CKD and with mean glomerular filtration rate of 35 mL/min/1.73 m², each 7.5 μg/m³ (interquartile range) increase in $PM_{2.5}$ was associated with a 19% increase in risk for renal replacement therapy with evidence for a dose-response relationship. The mechanisms may involve both soluble nephrotoxic components and biologic mediators that may result in glomerular and podocyte injury.

Mechanistic Insights Into Air-Pollution and Cardiovascular Risk

Mechanistic studies have shown that a number of distinct, yet interrelated processes mediate the cardiovascular effects of $PM_{2.5}$.

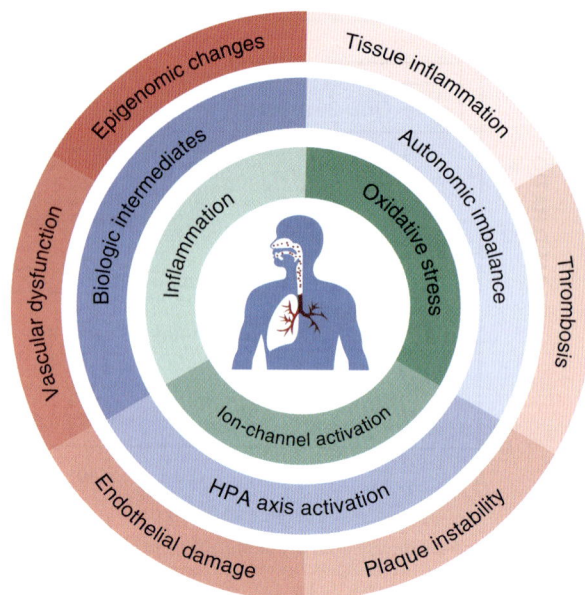

FIGURE 3.4 Mechanisms of air pollution–related cardiovascular disease. The *green circle* indicates recognition pathways. The *blue circles* indicate mechanisms of systemic transmission, and the *brown circles* indicate end-organ effector mechanisms. (Adapted from Al-Kindi S, Brook RD, Biswal S, et al. Environmental determinants of cardiovascular disease: lessons learned from air pollution. *Nat Rev Cardiol*. 2020;17:656–672.)

Importantly, these mechanisms largely overlap with conventional risk factors.[31] The mechanisms mediating cardiovascular disease in response to air pollution may be viewed as cascading responses beginning with pollutant inhalation in the lung that results in initiating responses; recognition and transmission of these responses; and finally end-organ effector mechanisms (Fig. 3.4). Initiating pathways include (a) exogenous/pollutant-mediated ion channel/receptor activation; (b) endogenous oxidative stress; and (c) pulmonary inflammation. Multiple receptors have been implicated in the initial recognition of pollutants, including families such as Toll-like receptors (TLRs) and nucleotide oligomerization domain (NOD)-like receptors (NLRs), which have been implicated in the initial sensing of particles and transduction of responses including generation of reactive oxygen species (ROS). The latter, although fundamentally important in physiology at low levels, may turn maladaptive, with generation of high levels of ROS with continued exposure over long durations and/or when antioxidant responses become inadequate.[59] Chronic oxidative stress with particulate pollution is likely facilitated through frustrated phagocytosis of particles in alveolar macrophages, depletion of antioxidant defense systems, and a failure of the inflammation to resolve not only in the lung but systemically.[60] Both innate and adaptive immune mechanisms in the lung, as well as systemically, in both human experimental animal models have been extensively implicated.[60] Transmission pathways include biologic intermediates (e.g., oxidized lipids, cytokines, microparticles, vasoconstrictors), activated immune cells, and autonomic imbalance/afferent neurologic circuits leading to sympathetic and/or hypothalamic pituitary adrenal axis activation and direct translocation of pollutants to the systemic circulation.[5,6,31,45] Nanoparticles in the ultrafine range have been shown to directly leach into the circulation and penetrate atherosclerotic plaque in humans and mice.[61] Finally, end-organ effector mechanisms responsible for cardiovascular and metabolic responses may vary in time scales from acute perturbations to chronically mediated consequences that occur with persistent exposure (see Fig. 3.4). These include: (1) endothelial barrier disruption and/or dysfunction, (2) tissue/organ inflammation, (3) heightened coagulation-thrombosis, (4) vasoconstriction/increased BP, and (5) secondary tissue damage/responses (plaque instability).[5]

Additional mechanisms can include direct disruption of the blood-brain barrier by ultrafine particulate and gaseous copollutants which may influence autonomic nervous system as well as resulting in CNS inflammation.[62–65] Acute vascular dysfunction, including arterial stiffness, conduit and microvascular alterations in flow, and alterations in thrombotic profile, that in predisposed individuals may potentiate ischemia, has been well described.[45] Chronic elevations in BP in response to exposure to $PM_{2.5}$ can result in left ventricular fibrosis and left ventricular diastolic dysfunction, progression of atherosclerosis, and multiple abnormalities associated with the insulin resistance phenotype.[66–72] Recent studies have implicated circadian rhythm alterations with $PM_{2.5}$ exposure.[73] These seem to affect both central and peripheral pathways in circadian rhythm and are similar to light at night exposure. Given the central role of circadian rhythm in organismal homeostasis including metabolic and cardiovascular responses, it is conceivable that such broad alterations may serve as common pathways that tilt the balance toward susceptibility to variety of disorders including cardiometabolic disorders and cancer. Epigenomic alterations occurring in response to pollutant exposure have been noted to occur with a number of pollutant exposures.[74] Although attractive as a facilitator of broad transcriptional reprogramming, the emerging view seems to suggest that alterations in chromatin dynamics may occur broadly, in response to any perturbation including air pollution, and may be reversible with air pollution exposure cessation at least in animal models.[73] In mice chronically exposed to $PM_{2.5}$, genome-wide reversible modifications in promoter and enhancer sequence were noted, many of which overlapped effects of high-fat diet.[73] A few studies have shown locus-specific methylation changes in CpG islands prenatally, in response to pollutants such as NO_2, that persist in the newborn, while limited human cohort studies have shown methylation changes in genes and/or within networks enriched for pathways related to inflammation, thrombosis, insulin resistance, and lipid metabolism.[75–78] These changes, although small, could be nevertheless important. The effect of air pollution exposure on genome-wide methylation status and chromatin structure in humans is not well understood.

Windows of Exposure, Susceptibility, and Vulnerability

Cohort studies involving assessment of long-term exposure consistently show higher estimates compared with short-term exposure suggestive of a cumulative effect (exposure over time).[79] Although exposure over years may promote anatomic progression of the burden of atherosclerotic plaque or other markers of cardiometabolic risk, this is ultimately not the process responsible for an acute event. However, chronic exposure may facilitate the development of "vulnerability" that may precipitate an acute coronary event including a milieu of predisposition to other triggers including acute changes in risk factors such as BP and air pollution.[43,80] The epidemiologic studies are indeed consistent with this notion, where attributable risk to $PM_{2.5}$ is related to exposures in the short and intermediate term (hours to 1 to 2 years). Larger but progressively smaller relative increases in health effects (i.e., in a less-than-additive fashion) are induced by prolonging the exposure window or follow-up period beyond 1 to 2 years.[80] Epidemiologic studies have shown that older individuals with multiple risk factors, and prior cardiovascular disease are more susceptible to $PM_{2.5}$ cardiovascular effects. Vulnerable populations include nonwhite populations in the United States living in densely populated urban environments. Nonwhites in the United States had 28% higher exposures (black individuals had 1.54 times the exposure compared with the overall population).[81] A review of 37 studies found that poorer communities often experience higher levels of air pollution in North America, Europe, Asia, Africa, and Oceania (with mixed results in Europe).[82] The interaction between susceptibility and vulnerability to $PM_{2.5}$ may identify extremely high-risk groups, for whom interventions may lead to significant improvement in health outcomes.

Air Pollution Alerts and Approaches to Communicate Risk

Currently, there is no accepted consensus on communication of air pollution levels and risk. The U.S. EPA's Air Quality Index (AQI) converts concentrations of the six regulated criteria air pollutants into levels of increasing health concern.[10] Although only a small proportion of the population follows the accompanying recommendations, those who do, can reduce exposure. Tools to communicate long-term exposure risk are needed to more accurately convey the major portion of the health risk due to air pollution. The increased access and availability of air pollution monitoring data from low-cost sensors may well have a transformative impact on understanding personal level exposures on cardiovascular health and, importantly, facilitating healthy behaviors. However, work in aligning current approaches of pollutant ascertainment with next-generation technologies is a barrier that will need to be addressed. A recent American Heart Association (AHA) statement provides a simple guide based on $PM_{2.5}$ levels and the underlying risk to help guide personal level interventions if necessary.[28]

Societal and Personal Strategies to Mitigate Cardiovascular Effects of Air Pollution

Urban strategies including land use, green belts, separation of pollution sources (industrial factories, roads), and planned residential communities that emphasize healthy living can avert not only air pollution but other concomitant exposures as well. The ultimate solution to avert air pollution exposure is its elimination. A shift to zero emissions by 2045 with near 90% elimination by 2035, a minimal requirement for averting catastrophic climate changes, should help improve air quality in the near term and produce large public health effects.[83] Two recent AHA statements reviewed policy interventions and personal-level protective measures against $PM_{2.5}$ exposure, many of which are low/no cost and logical.[28,84] Both societal (Fig. 3.5) and personal measures are necessary to protect the public living in high air-pollution environments, sus-ceptible patients, and individuals traveling to high exposure areas. Personal measures include avoiding commuting in traffic, use of car air conditioning, and closing windows while commuting in an automobile. Improvements in home and building designs that include home ventilation and air conditioning with appropriate in-duct air filters can help avert exposures while indoors. Face masks (cloth masks, surgical, N95, N99) are cheap, and widely available and have obtained widespread societal acceptance in the context of COVID-19 exposure. Cloth masks have the least filtration efficiency for $PM_{2.5}$, whereas N95 masks have the highest efficacy.[28] Multiple small randomized studies of N95 masks worn over periods of hours to days have demonstrated significant reduction in BP and improvement in markers of autonomic function (e.g., heart rate variability). Portable air cleaners (PACs) are practical and inexpensive in-home strategies suited for at-risk populations and can acutely reduce $PM_{2.5}$ exposures by as much as 30% to 60%.[85] Several small short-term human studies mostly in healthy populations but a few in susceptible patients have provided the proof of concept that reductions in $PM_{2.5}$ exposures with PACs can result in rapid, albeit small, reductions in BP and other markers of cardiometabolic risk. Ultimately, randomized controlled trials to test the efficacy of exposure mitigation on clinically relevant endpoints may be needed.

CLIMATE CHANGE

Climate change is by far the greatest existential threat confronting humanity and public health. In October 2018, the United Nations Intergovernmental Panel on Climate Change (IPCC) reported that global carbon emissions must be halved by 2030 to limit warming to 1.5°C. Greenhouse gas (GHG) emissions, primarily from fossil fuel emissions, lead to climate change but also contribute to adverse health effects, and conversely, climate change may lead to an increase in

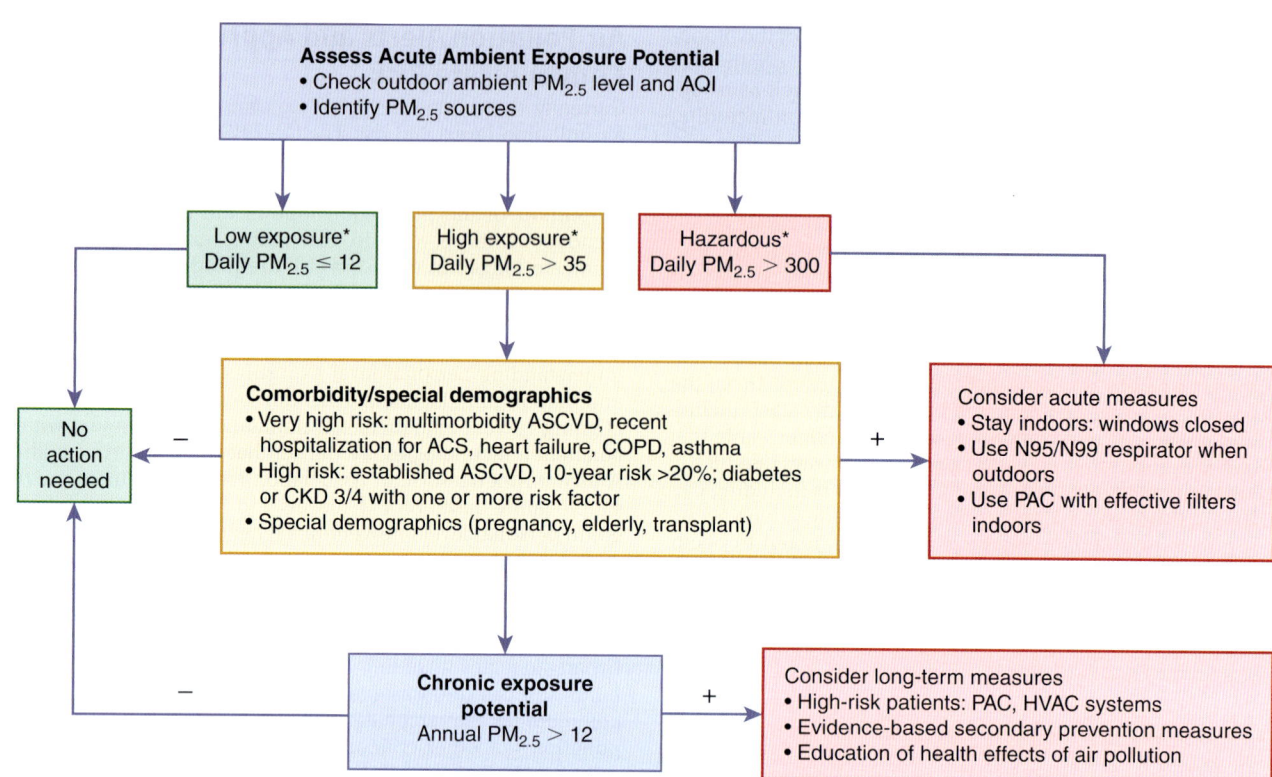

FIGURE 3.5 Public health approach based on $PM_{2.5}$ levels. (From Rajagopalan S, Brauer M, Bhatnagar A, et al. Personal-level protective actions against particulate matter air pollution exposure: a scientific statement from the American Heart Association. *Circulation*. 2010;121:2331–2378.)

PM and ground-level ozone.[19] GHGs and air pollutants are, to a large extent, emitted from the same sources. As part of climate change and global warming, extreme weather conditions, wildfires, and flooding can in turn increase both air pollution and water pollution. Rising temperature may also increase ground-level ozone that may be very difficult to eliminate. The solutions to mitigate climate change are fortunately the same that are needed to combat air pollution (see Fig. 3.5). These are structural in nature and importantly involve a total and complete shift to clean renewable energy sources. Recent data suggest that the technical and economic feasibility of achieving 90% clean (carbon-free) electricity in the United States by 2035 currently exists.[83] Not only is such a strategy imperative, but indeed strategy is critical in stimulating economic health while preserving human health.

NOISE POLLUTION AND CARDIOVASCULAR DISEASE

Emerging epidemiologic and mechanistic evidence suggests a link between noise pollution and cardiovascular disease.[30,31] The major source of chronic noise exposure is transportation (cars, trains, and airplanes) and occupational settings. Noise may result in a stress response involving the hypothalamus, the limbic system, and the autonomic nervous system with activation of the hypothalamus-pituitary-adrenal (HPA) axis with an increase in heart rate and in levels of stress hormones (cortisol, adrenalin, and noradrenaline), enhanced platelet reactivity, vascular inflammation, and oxidative stress.[86] Subconscious biologic responses may continue during nighttime in sleeping subjects, at low noise levels, and may disrupt circadian rhythm and thereby induce chronic disease. Noise is measured by decibel scale (dBA, a-weighted decibel scale adapted to human hearing frequencies). In cities in Asia, the proportion of the population reaching L_{den} levels (day-evening-night level, i.e., the average sound pressure level measured over a 24-hour period) of 60 to 64 dBA is very high.[87] For reference, an aircraft taking off is approximately 120 dBA, and a car driving is approximately 70 dBA. Several meta-analyses (including by the WHO) have shown an association between noise and CAD, with a 6% to 8% increment in incidence of coronary artery disease for each 10 dBA above 50 dBA of traffic noise.[86] These findings were consistent and persisted after adjustment for air pollution and smoking. Noise has also been linked with hypertension in multiple studies. A meta-analysis of 24 cross-sectional studies have shown that road traffic noise was associated with 3.4% increased odds of elevated BP per 5 dBA above 45 dBA.[88] The data on occupational noise are conflicting, with results from a few studies providing conflicting evidence. Noise in animal models has been shown to lead to inflammation, oxidative stress, and neurohormonal activation and is accompanied by transcriptomic changes in genes regulating vascular function, remodeling, and cell death.[89] Likewise significant endothelial dysfunction, increase in stress hormone release and BP, and a decrease in sleep quality have been noted in response to nighttime aircraft noise.[90] Studies in humans have identified amygdalar activation (using ^{18}F-FDG PET/CT imaging) in response to transportation noise and its association with arterial inflammation and major adverse cardiovascular events.[91] It is important to note that noise pollution and air pollution may coexist, especially near roadways and airports. Thus, when estimating effects of noise pollution, it is important to account for air pollutants.

SYNTHETIC CHEMICALS AND CARDIOVASCULAR DISEASE

Exposure to synthetic chemicals is ubiquitous, and humans are often exposed to low levels. These are vastly heterogenous and include synthetic chemicals, industrial solvents, pharmaceuticals, pesticides/fungicides, phytochemicals, and plastics and are present in water, soil, food, and consumer products. Many are endocrine-disrupting compounds (EDCs). Two major chemical entities include persistent organic pollutants (POPs) and plastic-associated chemicals (PACs). POPs contain a backbone of halogens (Cl, Br, or F), demonstrate resistance to degradation, and may be lipophilic or

TABLE 3.2 Sources of Metallic Pollutants and Cardiovascular Risk

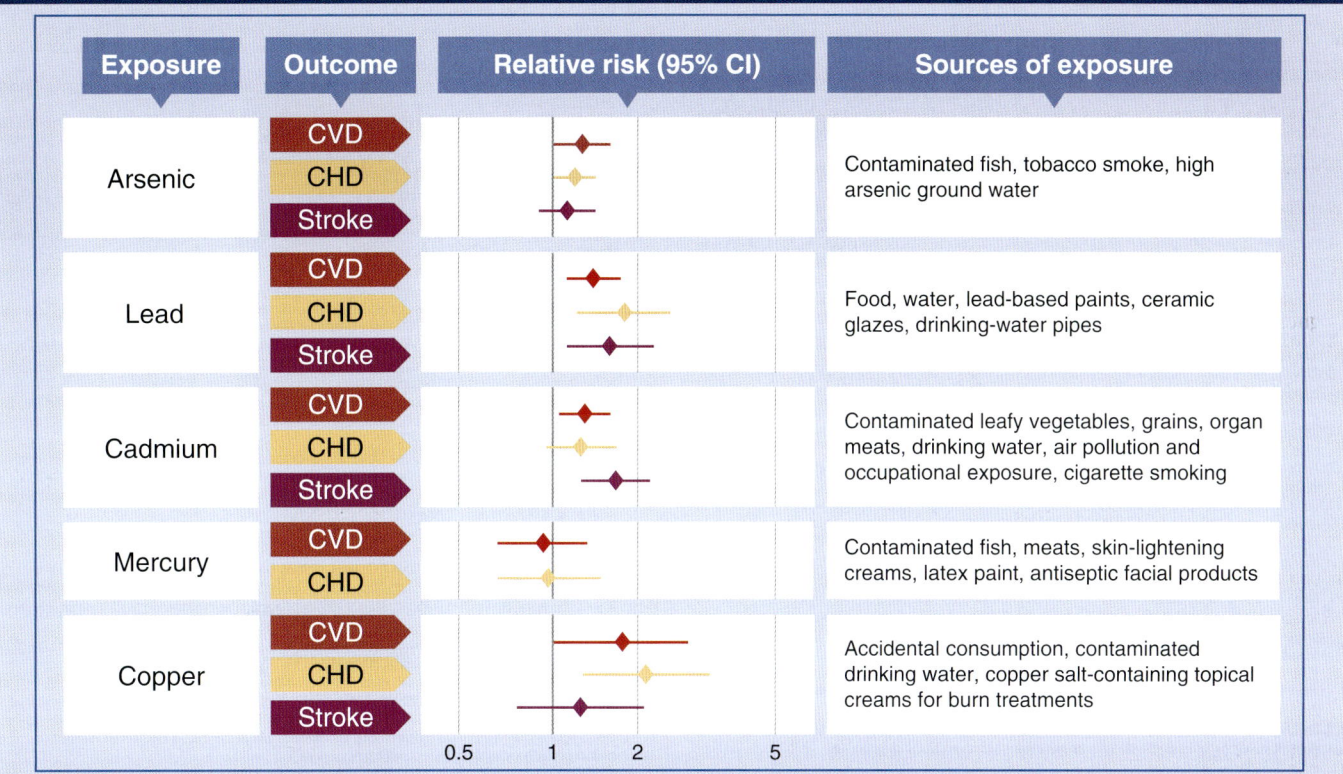

Adapted from Chowdhury R, Ramond A, O'Keeffe LM, et al. Environmental toxic metal contaminants and risk of cardiovascular disease: systematic review and meta-analysis. *BMJ*. 2018 Aug 29;362:k3310.

nonlipophilic. Lipophilic POPs include polychlorinated biphenyls (PCBs), dioxins, brominated flame retardants, and organochlorine (OC) pesticides. Nonlipophilic POPs include perfluoroalkyl substances (PFASs) encountered in water repellants and firefighting foam. Although almost all POPs and some PFASs have been banned, dietary intake from fat fish and meat from prior releases continue to be a problem. Although several cross-sectional studies link POPs with lipid abnormalities, carotid atherosclerosis, MI, and stroke, cohort studies with longitudinal data are limited. PACs are produced in high volumes for consumers and include bisphenol A (BPA), phthalates, and chemicals found in personal care products (e.g., parabens). The majority of chemicals in this group are measurable in blood routinely given their high rate of utilization in daily life. Although POPs have been associated with obesity and insulin resistance, the strongest evidence is for bisphenols and other nonpersistent chemicals.[92] A meta-analysis estimated the pooled relative risk for type 2 diabetes to be 1.45 (95% confidence interval [CI] 1.13 to 1.87) for BPA and 1.48 (95% CI 0.98 to 2.25) for phthalates.[93] Although biologic plausibility for cardiovascular disease with POPs and PACs exists, there is a need for high-quality studies to establish causation.[94]

METALLIC POLLUTANTS AND CARDIOVASCULAR DISEASE

Studies spanning greater than 50 years have linked heavy metal exposure with adverse cardiovascular health risks. The CDC's Agency for Toxic Substances and Disease Registry Priority List of Hazardous Substances provides a rank based on frequency, toxicity, and potential for human exposure. Arsenic, lead, and mercury are in the top 3 in this list, with cadmium coming in at 7. Table 3.2 provides the sources and relevant details for four major toxic metals, together with the relative risks for cardiovascular events based on a meta-analysis. Only arsenic, lead, and cadmium showed a dose-response relationship.[95] Regulations to limit lead exposure have resulted in a steep decline, and currently greater than 99% of the U.S. population have lead levels less than 10 μg/dL. However, living in older homes, occupational exposures, and atmospheric lead constitute sources of continued exposure.[96] Lead has been linked with hypertension, MI, and cardiovascular mortality.[97,98] The association between lead and BP and incident hypertension has been noted in multiple studies, with a variety of mechanisms being implicated, including kidney impairment, renin-angiotensin aldosterone system (RAAS) activation, oxidative stress, and nitric oxide dysregulation.[99-103] In the second National Health and Nutrition Examination Survey, individuals with blood lead levels of 20 to 29 μg/dL versus less than 10 μg/dL had a 46% relative increase in all-cause mortality (RR 1.46 [1.14 to 1.86]) and 39% in cardiovascular mortality (RR 1.39 [1.01 to 1.91]).[104] A meta-analysis showed that top versus bottom tertile of lead exposure was associated with an 85% risk of coronary artery disease (8 studies), 63% risk for stroke (6 studies), and 43% risk for cardiovascular disease (10 studies), with a linear dose-response relationship. Evaluation of lead exposure can be done using blood lead levels for recent exposures and x-ray fluorescence techniques for overall lead burden.

CHALLENGES AND OUTLOOK FOR THE FUTURE

Given the outsized effect of the environment on cardiovascular health, it is imperative that there be a new focus on preventable exposures.[105] The switch to green energy sources will help mitigate a number of copollutants related to air pollution but also help limit exposures to other toxic components that are released into the soil and water as well as noise. However, it is entirely conceivable that new exposures will emerge. With a high level of societal awareness facilitated through education and bold policy changes, it may be possible to eliminate almost all exposures at least to a point where their overall impact on human health is minimal.

REFERENCES

1. Landrigan PJ, Fuller R, Acosta NJ, et al. The Lancet Commission on pollution and health. *Lancet*. 2018;391:462–512.
2. Landrigan PJ, Fuller R, Acosta NJR, et al. The Lancet Commission on pollution and health. *Lancet*. 2018;391:462–512.
3. Global burden of 87 risk factors in 204 countries and territories, 1990-2019: a systematic analysis for the Global Burden of Disease Study 2019. *Lancet*. 2020;396:1223–1249.
4. Brook RD, Rajagopalan S, Pope 3rd CA, et al. Particulate matter air pollution and cardiovascular disease: an update to the scientific statement from the American Heart Association. *Circulation*. 2010;121:2331–2378.
5. Rajagopalan S, Al-Kindi SG, Brook RD. Air pollution and cardiovascular disease: JACC State-of-the-Art review. *J Am Coll Cardiol*. 2018;72:2054–2070.
6. Al-Kindi SG, Brook RD, Biswal S, Rajagopalan S. Environmental determinants of cardiovascular disease: lessons learned from air pollution. *Nat Rev Cardiol*. 2020;17:656–672.
7. Cohen AJ, Brauer M, Burnett R, et al. Estimates and 25-year trends of the global burden of disease attributable to ambient air pollution: an analysis of data from the Global Burden of Diseases Study 2015. *Lancet*. 2017;389:1907–1918.
8. Burnett R, Chen H, Szyszkowicz M, et al. Global estimates of mortality associated with long-term exposure to outdoor fine particulate matter. *Proc Nat Acad Sci*. 2018;115:9592–9597.
9. Lelieveld J, Evans JS, Fnais M, et al. The contribution of outdoor air pollution sources to premature mortality on a global scale. *Nature*. 2015;525:367–371.
10. EPA US. Air quality criteria for particulate matter (December 2016). 2016;2020.
11. Araujo JA, Barajas B, Kleinman M, et al. Ambient particulate pollutants in the ultrafine range promote early atherosclerosis and systemic oxidative stress. *Circ Res*. 2008;102:589–596.
12. Burnett RT, Smith-Doiron M, Stieb D, et al. Effects of particulate and gaseous air pollution on cardiorespiratory hospitalizations. *Arch Environ Health*. 1999;54:130–139.
13. Jerrett M, Burnett RT, Pope 3rd CA, et al. Long-term ozone exposure and mortality. *N Engl J Med*. 2009;360:1085–1095.
14. Di Q, Dai L, Wang Y, et al. Association of short-term exposure to air pollution with mortality in older adults. *J Am Med Assoc*. 2017;318.2446–2456.
15. Lim CC, Hayes RB, Ahn J, et al. Long-term exposure to ozone and cause-specific mortality risk in the United States. *Am J Respir Crit Care Med*. 2019;200:1022–1031.
16. Di Q, Wang Y, Zanobetti A, et al. Air pollution and mortality in the medicare population. *N Engl J Med*. 2017;376:2513–2522.
17. Atkinson RW, Mills IC, Walton HA, Anderson HR. Fine particle components and health—a systematic review and meta-analysis of epidemiological time series studies of daily mortality and hospital admissions. *J Expo Sci Environ Epidemiol*. 2015;25:208.
18. Thurston GD, Burnett RT, Turner MC, et al. Ischemic heart disease mortality and long-term exposure to source-related components of US fine particle air pollution. *Environ Health Perspect*. 2015;124:785–794.
19. Smith KR, Jerrett M, Anderson HR, et al. Public health benefits of strategies to reduce greenhouse-gas emissions: health implications of short-lived greenhouse pollutants. *Lancet*. 2009;374:2091–2103.
20. Transportation USD. *Bureau of Transportation Statistics, NHTS 2001 Highlights Report*; 2003.
21. Fisk WJ, Chan WR. Effectiveness and cost of reducing particle-related mortality with particle filtration. *Indoor Air*. 2017;27:909–920.
22. AghaKouchak A, Huning LS, Chiang F, et al. How do natural hazards cascade to cause disasters? *Nature*. 2018;561:458–460.
23. Kanatani KT, Okumura M, Tohno S, et al. Indoor particle counts during Asian dust events under everyday conditions at an apartment in Japan. *Environ Health Prev Med*. 2014;19:81–88.
24. DeFlorio-Barker S, Crooks J, Reyes J, Rappold AG. Cardiopulmonary effects of fine particulate matter exposure among older adults, during wildfire and non-Wildfire periods, in the United States 2008-2010. *Environ Health Perspect*. 2019;127:37006.
25. Rajagopalan S, Brook RD. The indoor-outdoor air-pollution Continuum and the burden of cardiovascular disease: an opportunity for improving global health. *Glob Heart*. 2012;7:207–213.
26. GBD 2016 Causes of Death Collaborators. Global, regional, and national age-sex specific mortality for 264 causes of death, 1980–2016: a systematic analysis for the Global Burden of Disease Study 2016. *Lancet*. 2017;390:1151–1210.
27. McCracken JP, Wellenius GA, Bloomfield GS, et al. Household air pollution from solid fuel use: evidence for links to CVD. *Glob Heart*. 2012;7:223–234.
28. Rajagopalan S, Brauer M, Bhatnagar A, et al. Personal-level protective actions against particulate matter air pollution exposure: a scientific statement from the American Heart Association. *Circulation*. 2020:CIR0000000000000931.
29. Lim SS, Vos T, Flaxman AD, et al. A comparative risk assessment of burden of disease and injury attributable to 67 risk factors and risk factor clusters in 21 regions, 1990-2010: a systematic analysis for the Global Burden of Disease Study 2010. *Lancet*. 2012;380:2224–2260.
30. Munzel T, Sorensen M, Gori T, et al. Environmental stressors and cardio-metabolic disease: part I-epidemiologic evidence supporting a role for noise and air pollution and effects of mitigation strategies. *Eur Heart J*. 2017;38:550–556.
31. Munzel T, Sorensen M, Gori T, et al. Environmental stressors and cardio-metabolic disease: part II-mechanistic insights. *Eur Heart J*. 2017;38:557–564.
32. Mustafic H, Jabre P, Caussin C, et al. Main air pollutants and myocardial infarction: a systematic review and meta-analysis. *J Am Med Assoc*. 2012;307:713–721.
33. Cai X, Li Z, Scott EM, et al. Short-term effects of atmospheric particulate matter on myocardial infarction: a cumulative meta-analysis. *Environ Sci Pollut Res Int*. 2016;23:6139–6148.
34. Lu F, Xu D, Cheng Y, et al. Systematic review and meta-analysis of the adverse health effects of ambient PM2.5 and PM10 pollution in the Chinese population. *Environ Res*. 2015;136:196–204.
35. Krewski D, Jerrett M, Burnett RT, et al. Extended follow-up and spatial analysis of the American Cancer Society study linking particulate air pollution and mortality. *Res Rep Health Eff Inst*. 2009:5–114; discussion 115-36.
36. Crouse DL, Peters PA, van Donkelaar A, et al. Risk of nonaccidental and cardiovascular mortality in relation to long-term exposure to low concentrations of fine particulate matter: a Canadian national-level cohort study. *Environ Health Perspect*. 2012;120:708–714.
37. Malik AO, Jones PG, Chan PS, et al. Association of long-term exposure to particulate matter and ozone with health status and mortality in patients after myocardial infarction. *Circ Cardiovasc Qual Outcomes*. 2019;12:e005598.
38. Burnett R, Chen H, Szyszkowicz M, et al. Global estimates of mortality associated with long-term exposure to outdoor fine particulate matter. *Proc Natl Acad Sci USA*. 2018;115:9592–9597.
39. Pope III CA, Muhlestein JB, Anderson JL, et al. Short–term exposure to fine particulate matter air pollution is preferentially associated with the risk of ST–segment elevation acute coronary events. *J Am Heart Assoc*. 2015;4:e002506.
40. Zhang Q, Qi W, Yao W, et al. Ambient particulate matter (PM(2.5)/PM(10)) exposure and emergency department visits for acute myocardial infarction in Chaoyang District, Beijing, China during 2014: a case-crossover study. *J Epidemiol*. 2016;26:538–545.
41. Gardner B, Ling F, Hopke PK, et al. Ambient fine particulate air pollution triggers ST-elevation myocardial infarction, but not non-ST elevation myocardial infarction: a case-crossover study. *Part Fibre Toxicol*. 2014;11:1.
42. Jilani MH, Simon-Friedt B, Yahya T, et al. Associations between particulate matter air pollution, presence and progression of subclinical coronary and carotid atherosclerosis: a systematic review. *Atherosclerosis*. 2020;306:22–32.
43. Yang S, Lee SP, Park JB, et al. PM2.5 concentration in the ambient air is a risk factor for the development of high-risk coronary plaques. *Eur Heart J Cardiovasc Imaging*. 2019;20:1355–1364.
44. Fu P, Guo X, Cheung FMH, Yung KKL. The association between PM2.5 exposure and neurological disorders: a systematic review and meta-analysis. *Sci Total Environ*. 2019;655:1240–1248.
45. Munzel T, Gori T, Al-Kindi S, et al. Effects of gaseous and solid constituents of air pollution on endothelial function. *Eur Heart J*. 2018;39:3543–3550.
46. Rajagopalan S, Brook RD. Air pollution and type 2 diabetes: mechanistic insights. *Diabetes*. 2012;61:3037–3045.
47. Bowe B, Xie Y, Li T, et al. The 2016 global and national burden of diabetes mellitus attributable to PM2.5 air pollution. *Lancet Planet Health*. 2018;2:e301–e312.
48. Rao X, Montresor-Lopez J, Puett R, et al. Ambient air pollution: an emerging risk factor for diabetes mellitus. *Curr Diab Rep*. 2015;15:603.
49. Chen Z, Salam MT, Toledo-Corral C, et al. Ambient air pollutants have adverse effects on insulin and glucose homeostasis in Mexican Americans. *Diabetes Care*. 2016;39:547–554.
50. Rajagopalan S, Park B, Palanivel R, et al. Metabolic effects of air pollution exposure and reversibility. *J Clin Invest*. 2020;130:6034–6040.
51. Shah AS, Langrish JP, Nair H, et al. Global association of air pollution and heart failure: a systematic review and meta-analysis. *Lancet*. 2013;382:1039–1048.
52. Wold LE, Ying Z, Hutchinson KR, et al. Cardiovascular remodeling in response to long-term exposure to fine particulate matter air pollution. *Circ Heart Fail*. 2012;5:452–461.
53. Yue W, Tong L, Liu X, et al. Short term Pm2.5 exposure caused a robust lung inflammation, vascular remodeling, and exacerbated transition from left ventricular failure to right ventricular hypertrophy. *Redox Biol*. 2019;22:101161.
54. Yue C, Yang F, Wang L, et al. Association between fine particulate matter and atrial fibrillation in implantable cardioverter defibrillator patients: a systematic review and meta-analysis. *J Intervent Cardiac Electrophysiol*. 2020:1–7.
55. Franchini M, Mengoli C, Cruciani M, et al. Association between particulate air pollution and venous thromboembolism: a systematic literature review. *Eur J Intern Med*. 2016;27:10–13.
56. Bowe B, Xie Y, Li T, et al. Particulate matter air pollution and the risk of incident CKD and progression to ESRD. *J Am Soc Nephrol*. 2018;29:218–230.
57. Chan TC, Zhang Z, Lin BC, et al. Long-term exposure to ambient fine particulate matter and chronic kidney disease: a cohort study. *Environ Health Perspect*. 2018;126:107002.
58. Yang YR, Chen YM, Chen SY, Chan CC. Associations between long-term particulate matter exposure and adult renal function in the Taipei Metropolis. *Environ Health Perspect*. 2017;125:602–607.
59. Rao X, Zhong J, Brook RD, Rajagopalan S. Effect of particulate matter air pollution on cardiovascular oxidative stress pathways. *Antioxid Redox Signal*. 2018;28:797–818.
60. Gangwar RS, Bevan GH, Palanivel R, et al. Oxidative stress pathways of air pollution mediated toxicity: recent insights. *Redox Biol*. 2020;34:101545.
61. Miller MR, Raftis JB, Langrish JP, et al. Inhaled nanoparticles accumulate at sites of vascular disease. *ACS Nano*. 2017;11:4542–4552.
62. Calderon-Garciduenas L, Solt AC, Henriquez-Roldan C, et al. Long-term air pollution exposure is associated with neuroinflammation, an altered innate immune response, disruption of the blood-brain barrier, ultrafine particulate deposition, and accumulation of amyloid beta-42 and alpha-synuclein in children and young adults. *Toxicol Pathol*. 2008;36:289–310.
63. Block ML, Elder A, Auten RL, et al. The outdoor air pollution and brain health workshop. *Neurotoxicology*. 2012;33:972–984.
64. Aragon MJ, Topper L, Tyler CR, et al. Serum-borne bioactivity caused by pulmonary multiwalled carbon nanotubes induces neuroinflammation via blood-brain barrier impairment. *Proc Natl Acad Sci USA*. 2017;114:E1968–E1976.
65. Mumaw CL, Levesque S, McGraw C, et al. Microglial priming through the lung-brain axis: the role of air pollution-induced circulating factors. *FASEB J*. 2016;30:1880–1891.
66. Wold LE, Ying Z, Hutchinson KR, et al. Cardiovascular remodeling in response to long-term exposure to fine particulate matter air pollution. *Circ Heart Fail*. 2012;5:452–461.
67. Sun Q, Wang A, Jin X, et al. Long-term air pollution exposure and acceleration of atherosclerosis and vascular inflammation in an animal model. *JAMA*. 2005;294.
68. Ying Z, Kampfrath T, Thurston G, et al. Ambient particulates alter vascular function through induction of reactive oxygen and nitrogen species. *Toxicol Sci*. 2009;111.
69. Rao X, Zhong J, Maiseyeu A, et al. CD36-dependent 7-ketocholesterol accumulation in macrophages mediates progression of atherosclerosis in response to chronic air pollution exposure. *Circ Res*. 2014;115:770–780.
70. Araujo J, Barajas B, Kleinman M, et al. Ambient particulate pollutants in the ultrafine range promote early atherosclerosis and systemic oxidative stress. *Circ Res*. 2008;102:589–596.
71. Miller MR, McLean SG, Duffin R, et al. Diesel exhaust particulate increases the size and complexity of lesions in atherosclerotic mice. *Part Fibre Toxicol*. 2013;10. 1.
72. Wold LE, Ying Z, Hutchinson KR, et al. Cardiovascular remodeling in response to long-term exposure to fine particulate matter air pollution. *Circ Heart Fail*. 2012;5.
73. Rajagopalan S, Park B, Palanivel R, et al. Metabolic effects of air pollution exposure and reversibility. *J Clin Invest*. 2020.
74. Wang T, Pehrsson EC, Purushotham D, et al. The NIEHS TaRGET II Consortium and environmental epigenomics. *Nat Biotechnol*. 2018;36.
75. Gondalia R, Baldassari A, Holliday KM, et al. Methylome-wide association study provides evidence of particulate matter air pollution-associated DNA methylation. *Environ Int*. 2019;132:104723.
76. Sayols-Baixeras S, Fernández-Sanlés A, Prats-Uribe A, et al. Association between long-term air pollution exposure and DNA methylation: the REGICOR study. *Environ Res*. 2019;176:108550.
77. Gruzieva O, Xu C-J, Breton CV, et al. Epigenome-wide meta-analysis of methylation in children related to prenatal NO2 air pollution exposure. *Environ Health Perspect*. 2016;125:104–110.
78. Breton CV, Marsit CJ, Faustman E, et al. Small-magnitude effect sizes in epigenetic end points are important in children's environmental health studies: the children's environmental health and disease prevention research center's epigenetics working group. *Environ Health Perspect*. 2017;125:511–526.
79. Al-Kindi S, Brook RD, Biswal S, Rajagopalan S. Environmental determinants of cardiovascular disease: lessons learned from air pollution. *Nat Rev Cardiol*. 2020;17.
80. Bevan GH, Al-Kindi S, Brook RD, et al. Ambient air pollution and atherosclerosis: insights into dose, time and mechanisms. *Arterioscler Thromb Vasc Biol*. 2020 Dec 17. ATVBAHA120315219.
81. Mikati I, Benson AF, Luben TJ, et al. Disparities in distribution of particulate matter emission sources by race and poverty status. *Am J Public Health*. 2018;108:480–485.
82. Hajat A, Hsia C, O'Neill MS. Socioeconomic disparities and air pollution exposure: a global review. *Curr Environ Health Rep*. 2015;2:440–450.
83. Plummeting solar, wind and battery costs can accelerate our clean electricity future. *2035 A report from the Goldman School of Public Policy, University of California, Berkeley.* http://www.2035report.com/wp-content/uploads/2020/06/2035-Report.pdf?utm_referrer=https%3A%2F%2Fwww.2035report.com%2F. Accessed October 01, 2020.
84. Kaufman JD, Elkind MSV, Bhatnagar A, et al. Guidance to reduce the cardiovascular burden of ambient air pollutants: a policy statement from the American heart association. *Circulation*. 2020:CIR0000000000000930.
85. Ravodina AM, Badgeley MA, Rajagopalan S, et al. Facile cholesterol loading with a new probe ezFlux allows for streamlined cholesterol efflux assays. *ACS Omega*. 2020;5:23289–23298.
86. Munzel T, Schmidt FP, Steven S, et al. Environmental noise and the cardiovascular system. *J Am Coll Cardiol*. 2018;71:688–697.

87. Brown AL, Lam KC, van Kamp I. Quantification of the exposure and effects of road traffic noise in a dense Asian city: a comparison with western cities. *Environ Health*. 2015;14:22.
88. van Kempen E, Babisch W. The quantitative relationship between road traffic noise and hypertension: a meta-analysis. *J Hypertens*. 2012;30:1075–1086.
89. Münzel T, Daiber A, Steven S, et al. Effects of noise on vascular function, oxidative stress, and inflammation: mechanistic insight from studies in mice. *Eur Heart J*. 2017;38:2838–2849.
90. Munzel T, Sorensen M, Gori T, et al. Environmental stressors and cardio-metabolic disease: part II-mechanistic insights. *Eur Heart J*. 2016.
91. Osborne MT, Radfar A, Hassan MZO, et al. A neurobiological mechanism linking transportation noise to cardiovascular disease in humans. *Eur Heart J*. 2020;41:772–782.
92. Kahn LG, Philippat C, Nakayama SF, et al. Endocrine-disrupting chemicals: implications for human health. *Lancet Diabetes Endocrinol*. 2020;8:703–718.
93. Song Y, Chou EL, Baecker A, et al. Endocrine–disrupting chemicals, risk of type 2 diabetes, and diabetes–related metabolic traits: a systematic review and meta-analysis. *J Diabetes*. 2016;8:516–532.
94. LaKind JS, Goodman M, Mattison DR. Bisphenol A and indicators of obesity, glucose metabolism/type 2 diabetes and cardiovascular disease: a systematic review of epidemiologic research. *Crit Rev Toxicol*. 2014;44:121–150.
95. Chowdhury R, Ramond A, O'Keeffe LM, et al. Environmental toxic metal contaminants and risk of cardiovascular disease: systematic review and meta-analysis. *BMJ*. 2018;362:k3310.
96. Leggett RW. An age-specific kinetic model of lead metabolism in humans. *Environ Health Perspect*. 1993;101:598–616.
97. Navas-Acien A, Guallar E, Silbergeld EK, Rothenberg SJ. Lead exposure and cardiovascular disease—a systematic review. *Environ Health Perspect*. 2007;115:472–482.
98. Solenkova NV, Newman JD, Berger JS, et al. Metal pollutants and cardiovascular disease: mechanisms and consequences of exposure. *Am Heart J*. 2014;168:812–822.
99. Nawrot T, Thijs L, Den Hond E, et al. An epidemiological re-appraisal of the association between blood pressure and blood lead: a meta-analysis. *J Hum Hypertens*. 2002;16:123–131.
100. Navas-Acien A, Schwartz BS, Rothenberg SJ, et al. Bone lead levels and blood pressure endpoints: a meta-analysis. *Epidemiology*. 2008:496–504.
101. Vander AJ. Chronic effects of lead on the renin-angiotensin system. *Environ Health Perspect*. 1988;78:77–83.
102. Gonick HC, Ding Y, Bondy SC, et al. Lead-induced hypertension: interplay of nitric oxide and reactive oxygen species. *Hypertension*. 1997;30:1487–1492.
103. Vaziri ND, Liang K, Ding Y. Increased nitric oxide inactivation by reactive oxygen species in lead-induced hypertension. *Kidney Int*. 1999;56:1492–1498.
104. Lustberg M, Silbergeld E. Blood lead levels and mortality. *Arch Intern Med*. 2002;162:2443–2449.
105. Münzel T, Miller MR, Sørensen M, et al. Reduction of environmental pollutants for prevention of cardiovascular disease: it's time to act. *Eur Heart J*. 2020;41:3989–3997.

4 Clinical Trials in Cardiovascular Medicine

SCOTT D. SOLOMON AND JOHN MCMURRAY

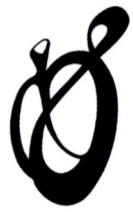

CLINICAL TRIALS VERSUS OTHER TYPES OF STUDIES, 42

COMPONENTS OF CLINICAL TRIALS, 43
Rationale and Study Background, 43
Study Design, 43
Study Execution, 44
Inclusion and Exclusion Criteria, 45
Endpoints or "Response Variables", 45

STATISTICAL CONSIDERATIONS IN TRIALS, 46
Analysis of Primary and Secondary Endpoints, 46

Power and Sample Size, 47

ETHICAL CONSIDERATIONS AND INFORMED CONSENT, 48
Equipoise in Clinical Trials, 48
Randomization to Placebo and Standard of Care, 48
Potential for Harm in Clinical Trials, 49

MONITORING OF DATA AND DATA SAFETY, 49

NOVEL APPROACHES TO CLINICAL TRIAL DESIGN AND EXECUTION, 49
Pragmatic (Large Simple) Trials, 49

Use of Electronic Medical Records in Clinical Trials, 49
Adaptive Designs, 49

INTERPRETATION OF CLINICAL TRIALS, 50
Registration and Reporting of Clinical Trials, 50
Understanding the Primary Results, 50
Secondary Endpoints, 50
Interpretation of Subgroups, 51
Post-hoc Analyses, 52

CONCLUSION, 52

REFERENCES, 52

Modern cardiovascular medicine prides itself on being evidence based. Virtually all the therapeutic advances that have informed the treatment of patients with cardiovascular disease have resulted from the findings of randomized clinical trials. Randomized trials are generally considered to provide the highest level of evidence, and this principle is reflected in the approach that all major guidelines use to support the strength of therapeutic recommendations.[1] While clinical trials are used for evidence generation in virtually all disciplines, there are few fields in which clinical trials have been so impactful as in cardiovascular medicine.

This chapter will review the basic principles of clinical trials in cardiovascular medicine, the approach to designing and executing clinical trials, and an introduction to the interpretation of clinical trials results to inform clinical practice.

CLINICAL TRIALS VERSUS OTHER TYPES OF STUDIES

Observation has always been the key to the generation of medical evidence. For centuries, astute physicians have observed patients' responses to various remedies and occasionally made insightful inferences about the benefit of new treatments. Observational studies (see also Chapter 5) can assess the natural history of disease, demonstrate relationships between risk factors and outcomes, and generate hypotheses for more definitive experimental testing. Yet observational studies are almost always biased and limited when it comes to assessing the merits of new therapies. This single-greatest inherent problem with attempting to infer effects of therapies from observational studies is termed "confounding by indication" and refers to biases, known or unknown, that influence which therapies are used for which patients and which conditions. These biases can be overcome to some extent by taking account of, or adjusting for, all the other factors that might have influenced the decision to use that medication and the outcomes in those patients. Although several novel statistical methods have been developed to attenuate indication bias in observational studies,[2] adjustment is rarely able to overcome all the potential biases because all such factors cannot be known or accounted for. Indeed, many therapies that had initially been based on observational data, such as hormone replacement therapy in postmenopausal women to reduce cardiovascular risk,[3] have been refuted by subsequent randomized trials.

In contrast to observational studies, randomized clinical trials are prospective human experiments in which an intervention (which could be a pharmacologic or device therapy or an interventional strategy) are compared with a control and in which randomization is used to eliminate the potential biases related to administration of a therapy (Fig. 4.1). In a large enough study, randomization ensures that patients in both the experimental group and the control group are similar in every respect excepting the randomly allocated therapy. While single arm studies are sometimes referred to as trials, we will in this chapter limit our discussion to multiple arm studies in which treatment allocation is randomized.

CLINICAL TRIAL PHASES

Developmental programs for drugs and devices are categorized in phases (Table 4.1). *Phase I studies* assess the safety and tolerability in the first human experience of a novel therapy typically using healthy volunteers. These studies can be open label and even single arm and collect information that can be helpful in identifying a maximally tolerated dose (dose escalation studies).

Phase II studies are designed to confirm the biologic activity of the experimental therapy in patients with the disease of interest and, in some cases, to determine the likely optimal dose for both efficacy and tolerability. The results of these studies are typically used to determine whether to proceed to a *pivotal*, or *phase III trial*, which is used for regulatory assessment. Safety and tolerability are also assessed along with other secondary and exploratory measures of efficacy that might inform further development. Phase II trials often use *surrogate endpoints* rather than clinical endpoints (see later).

Phase III, or *pivotal* studies, are designed to provide enough information on efficacy and safety for regulatory evaluation and hopefully approval. Pivotal trials require assessment of "approvable" endpoints—that is, endpoints that have been previously agreed upon by regulatory authorities such as the U.S. Food and Drug Administration (FDA) and European Medicines Agency (EMA). Approval of a new antihypertensive agent may require only demonstration of blood pressure lowering, and trials of cholesterol-lowering medication may require only demonstration of serum cholesterol lowering for approval. In contrast, other indications, such as for treatment of heart failure, may require demonstration of benefit for clinical outcomes, such as reducing death, hospitalizations for heart failure, or myocardial infarction. Phase III trials are sometimes performed for the primary purpose of determining safety for a therapy—a concern regarding cardiovascular safety for previously approved diabetes therapies prompted the FDA in 2008 to issue guidance requiring all diabetes registration programs to assess cardiovascular safety by assessing and adjudicating adverse cardiovascular events

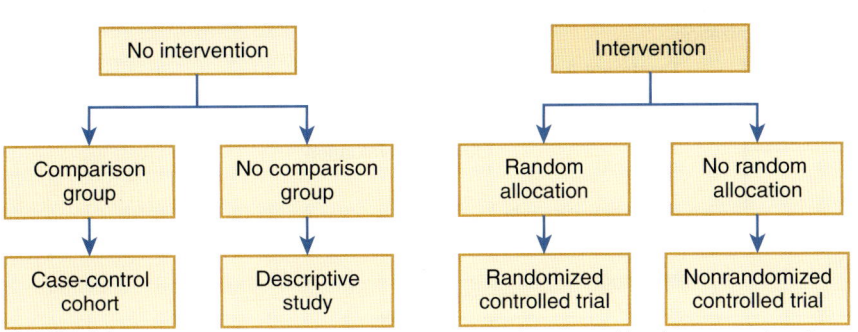

FIGURE 4.1 Types of clinical studies. Studies without intervention are considered case-control studies or descriptive studies, depending on whether or not they have a comparison group. Interventional trials can be either randomized or nonrandomized.

TABLE 4.1 Phases of Clinical Trials

PHASE	FEATURES	PURPOSE
I	First administration of new treatment	Safety and biologic plausibility
II	Early trial in patients with the disease to be studied	Efficacy—dose finding, adverse events, pathophysiologic insights
III	"Pivotal" trial large enough to test safety and efficacy	Designed to allow for regulatory approval
IV	Mechanistic, additional safety	Elucidate mechanisms, assess safety in novel populations, postmarketing surveillance

such as cardiovascular mortality, myocardial infarction, and stroke.[4] What is needed for registration is usually negotiated with regulatory authorities prior to initiation of a clinical trial. Guidance from health authorities regarding what is needed for registration has evolved over time. Recently, the FDA has indicated willingness to consider functional endpoints, such as 6-minute walk or patient-reported outcomes (PROs), for initial approval for a heart failure therapy.[5]

Phase IV trials, sometimes referred to as *post-marketing trials*, are designed to add mechanistic or other support for an indication, to extend a previous indication to a new population, or to meet a regulatory requirement such as providing additional safety information, perhaps in a specific patient population. The EVALUATE trial,[6] for example, was a phase IV trial examining the effect of sacubitril/valsartan compared with enalapril on aortic stiffness and ventricular remodeling to provide mechanistic support for the findings in PARADIGM-HF, a positive phase III outcomes trial.[7]

COMPONENTS OF CLINICAL TRIALS

Randomized clinical trials and clinical trial reports should include all the following components: *rationale, inclusion and exclusion criteria, study design, study execution, study endpoints, and analytic approach*. These components are typically codified in the study protocol, which serves as the principal documentation of the study background, objectives, design, organization, execution, and preliminary outline analysis plan.

Rationale and Study Background

Because all clinical trials are human experiments, they need to be justifiable to investigators, institutional review boards or ethics committees, and participants; a well-thought-out, clinically relevant, scientifically and ethically valid rationale is the essential first step in a clinical trial design. In short, the question should be one for which the answer is not known and for which the result would either directly inform clinical care or would provide crucial information that would inform the continued development of a particular therapy. The scientific rationale for conducting a trial can be in the form of basic research that supports a particular pathway or mechanism that may be affected by the therapy, preclinical data involving animal experiments in which a therapy was tested in a manner similar to a human trial, or early clinical or "pilot" studies that may provide some evidence that a therapy might

be efficacious. Because virtually all interventional therapies can be associated with risk, the use of a particular therapy must at least have the potential to be beneficial in a particular disease state, although early-phase trials do not necessarily need to demonstrate that benefit to be successful.

Study Design

Clinical trial designs vary, and each have distinct advantages and disadvantages. The most commonly used is a *parallel group design* (Fig. 4.2A) in which patients are randomized to two or more groups and endpoints are compared between groups. These trials can be placebo controlled or active controlled and can have multiple arms (e.g., a placebo, active comparator and study drug, or multiple doses of a study drug). In this design, patients are randomized to receive one of these therapies for the duration of the trial. This type of design can be used for either clinical outcomes trials or phase II trials in which the primary endpoint is a surrogate (e.g., cholesterol or a natriuretic peptide).

In contrast, in *crossover trials* (Fig. 4.2B), patients receive one therapy for a period of time and then are "crossed over" to receive placebo or another therapy. In this design, individual patients act as their own control, and these designs are typically used for phase II studies in which the endpoint is a measured surrogate such as a biomarker. The advantage of crossover trials is that fewer patients are needed because each patient serves as his or her own control, reducing variability. The disadvantage is that effects of a therapy from the first phase can carry over and contaminate the second phase. This issue is typically mitigated with a *washout* period, a time between therapies during which the effect of the first phase would be expected to wear off. Crossover designs are not suitable for long-acting therapies or to outcomes trials (where a clinical outcome, such as a death or hospitalization, might influence whether the patient would join the second phase).

Factorial design (Fig. 4.2C) trials are essentially parallel group studies in which there are two consecutive randomizations within the same patient population so that an individual patient would be randomized to treatment A versus B, and also to C versus D, leaving four distinct treatment groups (A+C, A+D, B+C, B+D). In a factorial design trial, each randomization is essentially treated as its own trial. Factorial trials are best when the therapies are distinct enough that there will be no "interaction" between therapies. Assuming there is no or minimal interaction between therapies, factorial designs can be executed with a modest increase in the sample size required for a single intervention. If interaction between the two therapies is suspected, sample sizes need to be increased to allow for formal interaction testing. Examples of factorial design trials include the ISIS-2 trial,[8] which randomized patients to both streptokinase or placebo and additionally randomized the same patients to aspirin or placebo, and the DREAM trial, which compared the effects of ramipril versus placebo, and rosiglitazone versus placebo on the incidence of diabetes.[7,9]

Superiority trials (Fig. 4.3) test whether therapy A is superior to therapy B, which can be either an active comparator or placebo. Superiority trials aim to reject the *null hypothesis* that there is no difference between the therapies (see statistical considerations later). In contrast, *noninferiority trials* are designed to determine whether one therapy is *noninferior* to (loosely translated to *not worse than*) another therapy. In the case of noninferiority trials, rejecting the null hypothesis requires that therapy A be *not inferior* to therapy B within a certain margin of error; this requires setting a prespecified noninferiority margin and requiring an upper 95% confidence interval to be within that margin. Noninferiority trials are typically used when it is necessary to show only that a novel therapy is "as good as" an established therapy, which may be clinically important if the novel therapy has a better side effect profile, is less expensive, or may be easier to administer. Trials can be designed to test for both noninferiority and superiority, and a particular therapy can be noninferior even if not superior (see Fig. 4.3). The VALIANT trial[10] compared the angiotensin

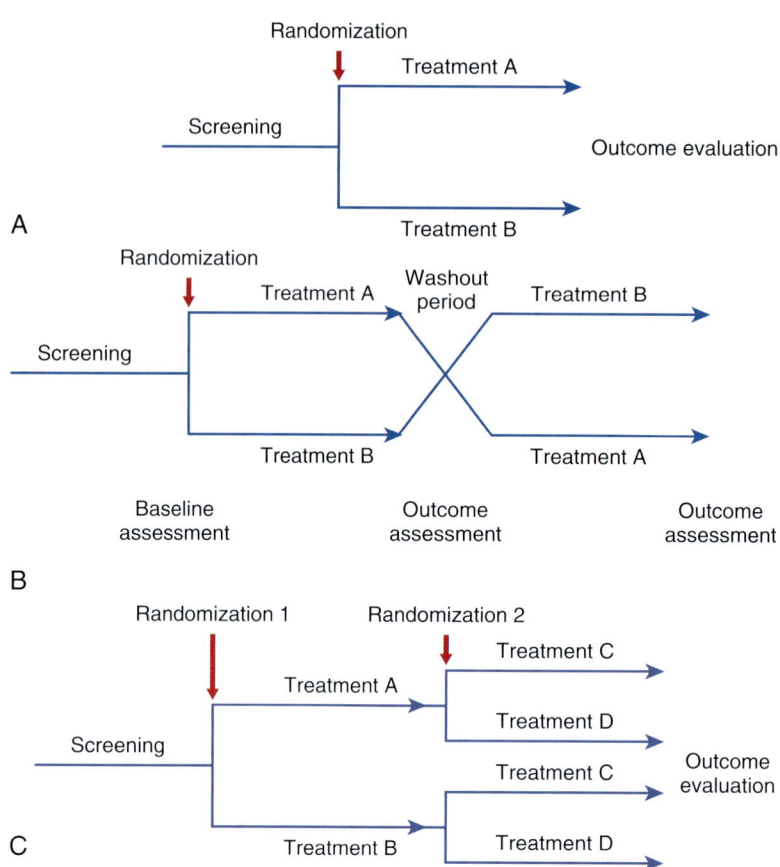

FIGURE 4.2 Clinical trial designs. Three types of clinical trial designs are illustrated. **A,** Parallel group design. **B,** Crossover design. **C,** Factorial design. Note that "treatment" can refer to an active treatment or placebo, and in factorial designs, two of four treatments could be placebo.

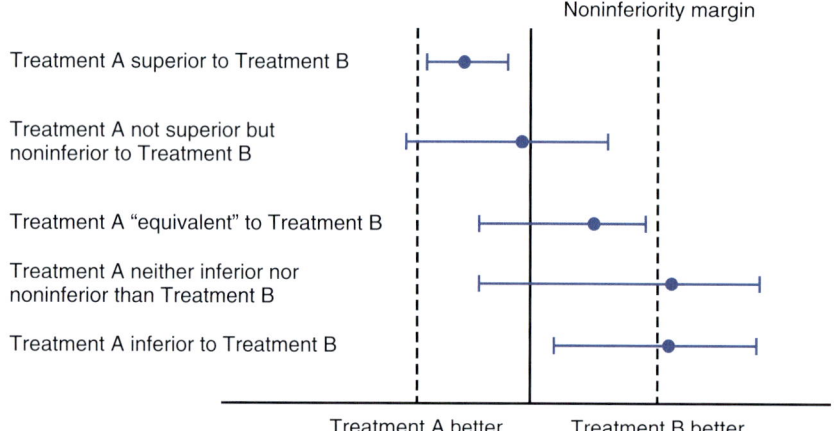

FIGURE 4.3 Superiority, noninferiority, and equivalence in clinical trials (see text).

receptor blocker (ARB) valsartan to the angiotensin-converting enzyme (ACE) inhibitor captopril (and the combination of the two) in post–myocardial infarction (MI) patients; while valsartan was not *superior* to the ACE inhibitor, it was *noninferior*, leading to an indication in post-MI patients.

Study Execution
Randomization
Randomization in a clinical trial can be as simple as a coin-toss (or the electronic equivalent) or considerably more complex, and there are a variety of approaches for randomly allocating treatment in clinical trials. Although randomization should lead to balanced groups in large trials, in smaller trials randomizing by a simple coin-toss (or random number) method can lead to imbalances at any time during the trial. For example, in a 100-patient trial, there would be a 5% risk of 60% of participants being allocated to one therapy. The commonly used *blocked* or *permuted block* randomization scheme mitigates this risk by ensuring equal number of participants assigned to each randomized group within each *block* of x, ensuring that the maximum imbalance at any given time is essentially the size of the permuted block.

While randomization in theory should lead to balanced groups in which characteristics known to be important in the disease being studied are balanced, in reality baseline imbalances are common in even relatively large trials and can influence results. For variables for which balance is especially desired, there are a variety of methods to *stratify* either at the randomization stage or the analysis stage. In stratified randomization, a participant is placed into a *stratum* (e.g., men or women) and then randomized within that stratum (ensuring balanced randomization within the stratum). This approach is more complicated than stratifying at the analysis stage, in which patients are *compared* within each stratum, an approach that is equally effective when trials are large.

Cluster randomization is a design in which groups of individuals, rather than actual individuals, are randomized. For example, trials testing specific strategies might randomly allocate clinics to one approach or another, as was done in the HOOPS trial, which randomly allocated 174 practices to pharmacist intervention or usual care to optimize use of guideline-directed therapy in patients with left ventricular dysfunction.[11] This avoids the risk of investigators applying the new strategy under investigation to "control" patients in the same clinic or practice because all patients in each practice or clinic receive one or other strategy. Cluster randomized trials require a slightly larger sample size than noncluster randomized trials.

Blinding (Masking)

Randomized trials can be blinded or unblinded, and blinded trials can be *single-blind*, *double-blind*, or *triple bind*. Blinding is designed primarily to avoid bias by allowing either participants or investigators to know which therapy a patient is on. In an open-label, or unblinded, trial, the participants and investigators will know which therapy is offered. The bias associated with this design can be mitigated using a blinded endpoint approach, often called a *prospective open-label blinded endpoint* (PROBE) design, in which the assessment is performed by individuals who are not aware of treatment assignment. An example of a PROBE design trial is one assessing cholesterol lowering where the laboratory making the cholesterol measurements was not aware of the treatment assignment and therefore could not be biased by this knowledge. It would, in contrast, be nearly impossible to eliminate bias for a patient-reported outcome in an unblinded clinical trial. Unblinded trials are less expensive and simpler to execute than blinded trials and have become an important approach to *pragmatic trial* design (see later).

A *single-blind* study is one in which the investigator, but not the participant, is aware of the study assignment, and it is also simpler to execute than fully blinded trials. If the investigator is involved, however, in collection of data and decisions about the care of the patient that might be influenced by his or her knowledge of the treatment assignment, the integrity of the trial could be compromised.

A *double-blind* study is one in which neither the participants nor the investigators are aware to which therapy a participant is assigned. Double-blind studies are considered the "gold standard" of clinical trial designs. Nevertheless, blinding can be difficult in practice, especially when investigators or patients may get "clues" about which therapy they have been assigned to (e.g., the taste of an experimental compound has unblinded participants to their therapy, and specific laboratory abnormalities, such as elevation in serum potassium, have the potential to unblind investigators). A *triple-blind* (i.e., triple-masking) study is a randomized experiment in which the treatment or intervention is unknown to (1) the research participant, (2) the individual(s) who administer the treatment or intervention, and (3) the individual(s) who assess the outcomes.

Blinding is typically accomplished by matching an experimental therapy to placebo. There are a variety of approaches used to ensure that experimental therapies are matched to placebo, including using dyes to ensure similarity in appearance of medication, overencapsulation, or various ingredients to mask taste. In device trials, there are several ways to accomplish blinding, although this is often impossible. While sham procedures can be performed, they are often impractical. Devices can be implanted but not turned on or can be programmed differently. It can even be challenging to blind the endpoints, because various diagnostic procedures (x-rays, ECGs) can unblind clinicians, investigators, and even endpoint adjudicators.

Inclusion and Exclusion Criteria

Properly defining the patient population is key to a successful clinical trial. Inclusion and exclusion criteria need to be tailored to ensure that the patients enrolled in the trial have the disease being studied and are likely to benefit from the therapy being tested if that therapy has actual benefit. For example, in a lipid-lowering therapy trial, for which the primary endpoint was degree of cholesterol lowering, patients would be required to have elevated levels of cholesterol at baseline. In a study of a similar therapy in which the primary endpoint was reduction in major adverse cardiovascular events (MACE, see later), patients enrolled need to be at risk for those events (e.g., assessment of MACEs in a primary prevention population of young adults might be impractical because of the very low event rate in that population). Often, enrichment criteria are used to ensure patients have sufficient risk—for example, in a heart failure outcomes trial, it is common to include a requirement for elevation in natriuretic peptides to ensure that patients have a high enough event rate. Exclusion criteria are based on ensuring patient safety; typical exclusions might include patients who are pregnant or may become pregnant during the course of the trial (pregnancy tests are often mandatory) if a therapy may be harmful to pregnancy or the fetus. Other exclusions might be specific to the therapy being tested. For example, a specific upper limit of serum potassium might be set when testing a drug that elevates serum potassium, such as a mineralocorticoid receptor antagonist (MRA) or renin-angiotensin system (RAS) inhibitor; alternatively, a lower blood pressure limit is typically used in heart failure trials testing drugs that tend to lower blood pressure, but this threshold may be much lower when testing an inotropic agent. Of note, specific inclusion and exclusion criteria limit the generalizability of a population—a common criticism of clinical trials, and often result in labels, guidelines, or payment decisions that reflect the specifics of those criteria.

Endpoints or "Response Variables"

Clinical trials are generally designed to evaluate both efficacy and safety. The metrics by which efficacy is assessed depend on the disease being studied, the mechanism of action of the therapy, and where the trial fits in the development lifecycle of the therapy. Measures of efficacy in cardiovascular medicine are numerous and include a variety of biomarkers including those that can be measured in the blood, such as cholesterol levels or natriuretic peptides, physical examination measures such as blood pressure or heart rate, or clinical outcomes, such as hospitalization (all cause or cause specific), or death (all cause or cause specific). Evaluation of efficacy requires a predetermined analysis plan with prespecified statistical approaches to determining whether a therapeutic benefit is met (see later). Measured endpoints—such as blood pressure—can be compared directly between treatment groups and may be measured at several time points during the course of a trial, although typically at baseline and at least once during follow-up. Usual analyses would include between-group comparisons adjusted for baseline level, although there are a variety of statistical techniques to handle multiple measures. These types of evaluation are particularly sensitive to subject drop-out leading to missing data, which can occur for a number of reasons, including subject death. For example, assessment of the effect of a drug on ejection fraction over time in a heart failure trial in which there is a high death rate, leading to many patients with missing data, can be problematic—especially if there is *differential* drop-out such that patients in one arm drop out at a greater rate, as might happen if the therapy resulted in fewer deaths, and the patients remaining alive in the placebo group were those whose ejection fraction were least likely to worsen. Such a scenario might lead to underestimation of a true treatment effect. *Surrogate endpoints* are measured endpoints that are thought to be directionally related to clinical outcomes and are often used in phase II trials. Good surrogate endpoints can usually be measured earlier than clinical outcomes, are indicative of disease progression, and are directionally related to the clinical outcome (changes in the surrogate endpoint correlate with clinical outcomes). Natriuretic peptides, for example, are often used as a surrogate in heart failure trials, and reduction in natriuretic peptides has been shown to correlate with improvement in clinical outcomes.[5] Although implanted devices have long recorded data that could be used as endpoints in trials (e.g., arrhythmia endpoints), novel endpoints from data acquired from wearable devices or smart phones are being used with greater frequency.

Clinical outcomes, such as death or hospitalization for heart failure, are typically counted and expressed as a *proportion* (i.e., percentage of patients dying over the course of the trial in each arm) or a *rate* (i.e., number of deaths per 100 patient-years). While clinical outcomes can be expressed as the proportion of patients who have an event at a certain time point (e.g., 30 days post randomization), this approach is best reserved for studies with relatively short-term outcomes. For longer outcomes trials, the *time to event* is usually incorporated by comparing the time from randomization to the event between treatment groups, thus accounting for the difference between a patient who died on the 30th day of a trial and a patient who died on the 300th day of a trial.

Clinical outcomes can be grouped into *composites* in which an "event" is said to occur if any of the several components of the composite occur, and the time to that event is based on the first occurrence of one of the component events. The designation MACE, or three-point MACE, is typically used to describe a composite of cardiovascular death, MI, or stroke. Similarly, a typical composite in heart failure trials is the combination of cardiovascular death or heart failure hospitalization[12] (or more recently, cardiovascular death or heart failure hospitalization or urgent heart failure visit[13]). Including a fatal and nonfatal component in a composite addresses the issue of *competing risk*. Patients who die in a trial are clearly not at risk for a subsequent nonfatal event; thus, assessing only nonfatal events in trials where fatal events are likely can artificially deflate the risk of the nonfatal event in the group with a higher mortality rate, because this will likely deplete higher risk individuals. The number of composite events will not simply be the sum of all the component events for a given patient because only the first event that occurs is being counted. For example, a composite event of cardiovascular death or heart failure hospitalization would not count a death event if that event occurred after a heart failure hospitalization. Similarly, a second heart failure hospitalization would not be counted in that composite either (see later for alternative approaches that incorporate multiple events).

Patient-reported outcomes have become particularly important in cardiovascular trials because they provide meaningful insight into how specific therapies truly affect how patients feel and their quality of life. PROs are assessed through instruments (or questionnaires) that have been previously validated, although the type and extent of validation can vary. Examples of specific instruments typically used in cardiovascular medicine include the Kansas City Cardiomyopathy Questionnaire (KCCQ) and the Minnesota Living with Heart Failure (MLHF) instruments commonly used in heart failure studies, and the European Quality of Life Group-5D (EQ-5D) instrument, typically used for health economic assessment. Recently, the FDA has indicated that PROs may be considered *approvable endpoints* for certain conditions.[14,15]

STATISTICAL CONSIDERATIONS IN TRIALS

Analysis of Primary and Secondary Endpoints

Clinical trials are considered *hypothesis testing*, although that initially applies only to the primary question or endpoint of the trial. The statistical methods used are designed to determine if the null hypothesis can be rejected. The null hypothesis might be that a particular blood pressure–lowering medication does not affect blood pressure or that a heart failure medication does not impact cardiovascular death or heart failure hospitalizations. The analytic methods used depend on the specific questions being asked. Assessments of measured variables (e.g., blood pressure or ejection fraction) are most often comparisons of *between-group* differences in measures at baseline and follow-up, typically adjusting for baseline values, expressed as a between-group difference in the measure (with the confidence interval). Outcome measures are typically analyzed as time to event data using Kaplan-Meier curves and Cox proportional hazards models, and results are typically expressed as a hazard ratio with a 95% confidence interval. For example, a hazard ratio of 0.80 (0.65, 0.97) for a composite of cardiovascular death or heart failure hospitalization would indicate an estimated 20% reduced hazard of this endpoint in patients treated with the experimental therapy. However, the point estimate is only an estimate of benefit (or harm), and the confidence interval provides the range of potential true treatment effects that are consistent with the data; if the experiment were repeated an infinite number of times, the confidence interval represents the range that would contain the true treatment effect in 95% of those experiments. A narrow confidence interval (CI) implies a precise effect size, while a wide CI suggests greater uncertainty about the true effect of the treatment; in an outcomes study this can be due to an insufficient number of events. Based on traditional methods of significance testing, an upper confidence bound of 1.0 would signify a *p*-value of 0.05. Additional information about the efficacy of a therapy can be gleaned from the Kaplan-Meier curves directly. For example, some therapies might not show any evidence of benefit for a period of time, which is typical of studies that look at the effect of cholesterol-lowering therapies on MACEs, but for others, the curves might diverge immediately, suggesting very rapid benefit (Fig. 4.4).

The primary endpoint of a trial represents the primary hypothesis that is being tested. Trials usually have several *secondary* endpoints to answer additional questions and can further have *exploratory* endpoints. In registration trials, all or most of the statistical power (see later) is typically allocated to the primary endpoint such that it is the only hypothesis that can be tested at the $p = 0.05$ level. Some trials use co-primary endpoints, in which the statistical power is allocated to more than one endpoint (referred to as *splitting alpha*). Secondary endpoints are tested after the primary and typically are considered only *hypothesis testing* if the primary endpoint is positive, yet might still be considered *hypothesis generating* if not. Statistical power can be allocated to secondary endpoints in a number of ways. For example, they can be assessed hierarchically, such that if a primary endpoint is positive, a first secondary endpoint is tested; if this is positive, then a second secondary endpoint is tested and so forth. Alternatively, alpha can be "split" and allocated to multiple secondary endpoints (similar splits can occur for primary endpoints). Endpoints that are considered *exploratory* do not have any alpha allocated to them and are thus always considered *hypothesis generating* rather than *hypothesis testing*.

ALTERNATIVE METHODS OF ANALYSES

There are several limitations of standard time to first event analyses of clinical outcomes. First, the outcome statistic for a time to first event analyses using Cox proportional hazards models is expressed as a hazard ratio (point estimate and 95% confidence interval). Within each group, the hazard is a measure of the instantaneous rate of an event occurring. This model assumes that these group-level hazards remain *proportional (their ratio remains constant)* during the course of the trial (proportional hazards assumption). When this is not the case, and the hazard ratio varies over the course of the trial, the proportional hazards assumptions are violated, and this method may not be accurate (and may indeed underestimate a true treatment effect). Second, time to first event analysis of a composite outcome has the limitation of counting only the first outcome of a composite, which might be a less important component than another outcome, rendering the results less clinically meaningful. Several alternative methods have been developed to assess benefit in clinical trials to mitigate some of these limitations. Finally, the concept of a reduced hazard may be difficult for both clinicians and patients to understand because this metric contains no implicit information about the absolute magnitude of benefit, or absolute risk reduction, which is dependent on the event rate in the population.

Restricted Mean Survival Time

Whereas a hazard ratio represents the reduced (or increased) hazard associated with a therapy, this method is subject to the assumption that the hazard ratio will be relatively uniform throughout the duration of the trial and is not a metric that is readily understandable. Restricted mean survival time is another approach that essentially compares the area under the curve of the two Kaplan-Meier survival curves and presents an average event-free survival for each treatment arm.[16] In this method, no assumptions are made regarding the proportionality of hazards over time. Because the mean observation time of individual trials may be relatively short compared with the residual life span of the patient, other methods using actuarial (age-based) approaches have been developed to project the lifetime benefit of therapies.[17]

Win Ratio

The win ratio is a relatively simple method in which patients in the treatment and control group are matched based on their risk profile.[18,19] A hierarchy of events is established, and the first event in the hierarchy (e.g., death) is compared between the matched patients, and a "winner" is determined. If there is no winner for that endpoint, then the approach is extended to the next component of the endpoint (e.g., heart failure hospitalization). The win ratio is calculated as the total number of winners divided by the total numbers of losers. An alternative form of this is the method described by Finkelstein and Schoenfeld in which all possible pairs are compared.[20] This method was used successfully in the ATTR-ACT trial comparing tafamidis and placebo in ATTR-amyloid heart disease.[21]

Recurrent Event Analysis

Time to first event analysis of clinical outcomes by definition ignores all outcomes that occur following the first event of a composite; a patient with a single heart failure hospitalization is counted similarly as a patient with multiple heart failure hospitalizations. Recurrent event analyses take into account not just the first event but the subsequent events and thus may more accurately assess the burden of disease in a patient in which multiple events are likely to occur. There are numerous approaches to recurrent event analyses, with a variety

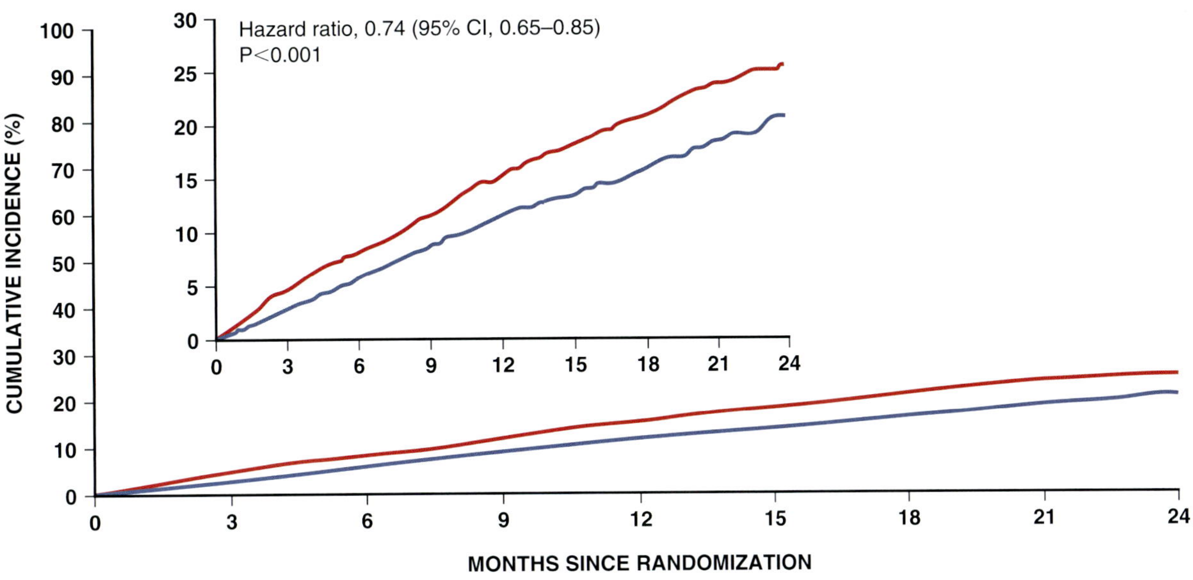

No. at risk

Placebo	2371	2258	2163	2075	1917	1478	1096	593	210
Dapagliflozin	2373	2305	2221	2147	2002	1560	1146	612	210

A

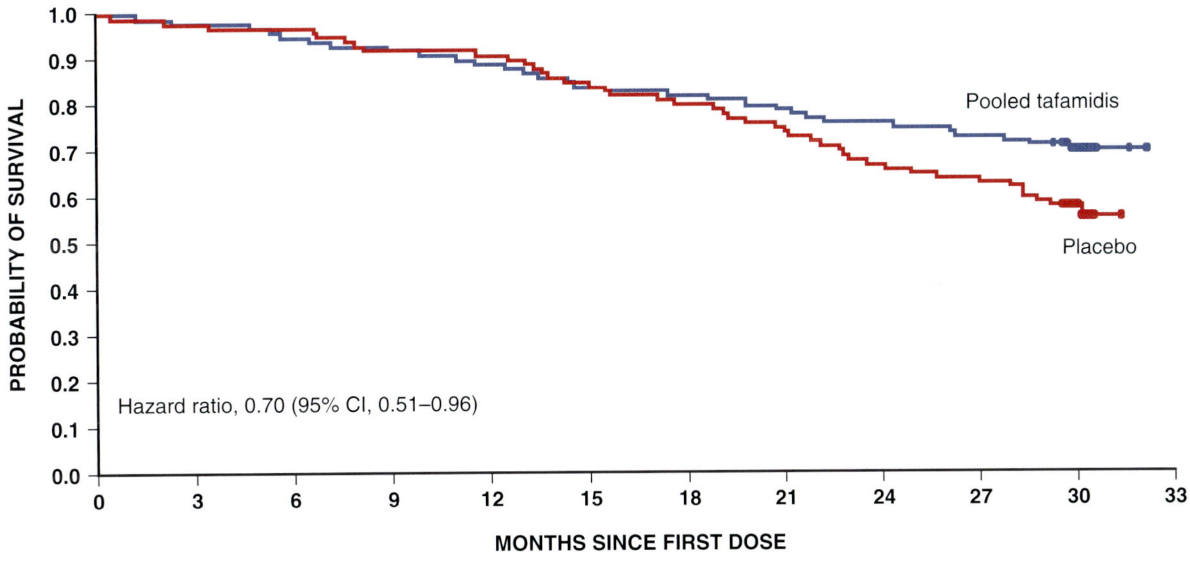

No. at risk (cumulative no. of events)

Pooled tafamidis	264 (0)	259 (5)	252 (12)	244 (20)	235 (29)	222 (42)	216 (48)	209 (55)	200 (64)	193 (71)	99 (78)	0 (78)
Placebo	177 (0)	173 (4)	171 (6)	163 (14)	161 (16)	150 (27)	141 (36)	131 (46)	118 (59)	113 (64)	51 (75)	0 (76)

B

FIGURE 4.4 Kaplan-Meier curves. **A,** The *x* axis represents time since randomization, and the *y* axis represents cumulative incidence of events. Early divergence of treatment group (dapagliflozin) and placebo. **B,** The *x* axis represents time since initial dosage, and the *y* axis represents survival probability. Late divergence in the ATTR-ACT study, likely reflecting time required for treatment to be effective. The number of participants at risk at any time point is listed on the bottom for both treatment groups. (**A** from McMurray JJV, Solomon, SD, Inzucchi SE, et al. DAPA-HF Trial Committees and Investigators. Dapagliflozin in patients with heart failure and reduced ejection fraction. *N Engl J Med.* 2019;381[21]:1995–2008. **B** from Maurer MS, Schwartz JH, Gundapaneni B, et al. ATTR-ACT Study Investigators. Tafamidis treatment for patients with transthyretin amyloid cardiomyopathy. *N Engl J Med.* 2018;379[11]:1007–1016.)

of statistical methods. Rather than simply counting the number of events, which would fail to account for the fact that individual patient events are highly correlated (i.e., patients with one event are more likely to have multiple events) as well as differences in observation time, these events use *robust variance estimation* to account for the correlation between events. Post-hoc recurrent event analyses in the CHARM-Preserved trial suggested benefit comparing candesartan to placebo in heart failure with preserved ejection fraction,[22] and the recent PARAGON-HF used a recurrent event analysis as its primary between group comparison.[23]

Power and Sample Size

Prior to embarking on a trial, investigators determine an appropriate sample size based on several assumptions. For a study assessing a "measured" endpoint, such as left ventricular ejection fraction, a sample size can be calculated from knowledge of the expected standard deviation of the endpoint, and an expected effect size. Although the former can often be estimated from prior studies, the latter needs to be assumed on the basis of biologic plausibility and clinical relevance.

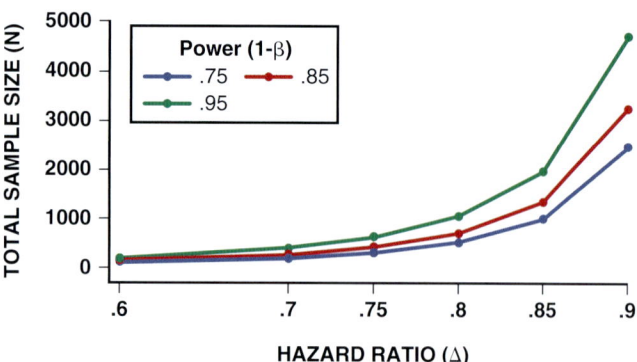

FIGURE 4.5 Relationship between hazard ratio, power, and sample size in a hypothetical clinical trial.

Parameters: $\alpha = .05$, $p_E = 1$

Another factor to consider is the desired *power*, which is defined as the probability that the test will reject a false null hypothesis—higher power increases the likelihood of success but requires greater sample size. Most cardiovascular trials are powered between 80% and 95%.

For outcomes trials, in which the primary endpoint might be time to all-cause mortality, or time to a composite of fatal and nonfatal endpoints, the analytic principles are similar regardless of the type of event or whether the event is an individual event or a composite. To determine the sample size for these types of trials, investigators need to make assumptions about the expected event rate and the expected treatment effect, as well as the desired power. The event rate can often be estimated from prior studies of similar populations. The effect size is never known beforehand, and a clinically meaningful effect size needs to be assumed. While a study can be powered to detect a very small effect size, this will require a larger sample size, which will also grow with a lower event rate (Fig. 4.5). An assumption of a large effect size (due to extreme confidence in a therapy) will lead to a small sample size but runs the risk of underpowering a trial.

Ultimately the power of an outcomes study is based not on the sample size but on the number of events. The event rates expected in outcomes trials determine the number of patients required to test a hypothesis. In diseases with very high event rates, such as advanced heart failure, effective therapies can demonstrate benefit with relatively small sample sizes; in contrast, for primary prevention, with relatively low event rates, very large sample sizes are usually required. Estimation of event rates can be difficult and is usually based on prior knowledge from previous trials or studies of similar populations. Nevertheless, these can be erroneous for a number of reasons (including due to improvement in standard of care from one trial to the next). Sample sizes can be reestimated during the course of the trial to adjust for this uncertainty (see *adaptive designs* later).

ETHICAL CONSIDERATIONS AND INFORMED CONSENT

Equipoise in Clinical Trials

There are several ethical considerations that need to be incorporated when conducting and interpreting the results of clinical trials. The primary ethical principle for conducting clinical trials is *equipoise*, which states that there is sufficient uncertainty about the value of the therapeutic interventions being tested in a trial that it is ethical to randomize a patient to any of the experimental arms.[24] Simply stated, a trial is ethical only if the trial question is worth asking and if the answer is not currently known. However, the determination about whether equipoise exists can often be quite subjective and will not always be agreed upon by individual investigators or the community at large. For example, individual clinicians may believe that one therapy is better than another although not all clinicians or even experts might agree. Many established therapies have not been subject to rigorous controlled trials, and clinicians may believe that they are nevertheless beneficial. Such therapies can be particularly difficult to test in randomized trials. When the TREAT trial was designed to assess the role of darbepoetin in reducing cardiovascular risk in patients with diabetes and chronic kidney disease, several major health authorities refused to participate because they believed that it would be unethical to deny patients this therapy, despite the fact that no rigorous assessment had been previously undertaken.[25]

Both physicians and patients have inherent biases that interfere with conduct of clinical trials. A clinician, investigator, or participant who does not believe that there is equipoise, but that one of the arms in a clinical trial is superior to the other, should not take part in a trial. This is why, in part, it can be so hard to enroll patients in trials involving surgical interventions where clinicians may believe strongly that specific procedures are beneficial. Although randomization ensures the lack of bias for the allocated treatment, it cannot remove intrinsic biases on the part of the investigators or participants which can impede the conduct of a trial by limiting the patients enrolled or the centers enrolling patients. These types of biases are particularly problematic in open-label trials, which, even when randomized, allow the investigators and participants to know which therapeutic arm they have been allocated to, which can lead to patients *crossing over* into or out of a therapeutic arm, a problem that plagued an open-label coxib safety trial in which undue concern about safety in one arm resulted in substantial crossovers.[26]

An interventional trial always has the potential to harm patients. This harm can be explicit, such as when a particular drug or therapy results in an adverse event, or implicit, such as when enrollment in a clinical trial prevents them from getting standard of care therapy that has already proven beneficial, or otherwise delays their access to care. These considerations need to be taken into account by both investigators and institutional review boards that need to approve all interventional studies.

Randomization to Placebo and Standard of Care

One common ethical question in the design of clinical trials is whether it is ethical in specific cases to randomize patients to placebo. If a condition has no proven therapy, then randomization to active therapy or placebo is usually considered ethical. If a therapy is already proven, then there are two potential approaches—to test the new therapy specifically in a head-to-head comparison with the old one, or to test the new therapy against placebo on top of *standard of care* therapy, which would typically include the old one. A head-to-head comparison requires sufficient rationale for believing the new therapy might be as good as the old one; denying those patients randomized to the new therapy from the previously accepted one does not itself present an ethical dilemma. Trials comparing ARBs to ACE inhibitors,[10,27] or sacubitril/valsartan to an ACE inhibitor in heart failure[7] are examples of active comparator trials in which a new active therapy was compared with a well-established therapy. In some cases, the goal of these trials is to prove noninferiority, which is ethically acceptable so long as there is some rationale other than commercial reasons that the second therapy may be superior in some way to the first (in the case of ARBs, there was both rationale that they would provide greater benefit than ACE inhibitors and they were known to have greater tolerability). Superiority trials comparing a novel therapy with a standard of care therapy are ethical so long as there is reasonable likelihood that the experimental therapy will be superior to, and minimal likelihood that the experimental therapy will be worse than, the standard therapy. Alternatively, studies that test novel therapies against placebo in conditions where standard of care therapies exist typically require patients to be on "optimal guideline-directed therapy." In DAPA-HF,[10] for example, which randomized patients to the sodium-glucose cotransporter-2 (SGLT-2) inhibitor dapagliflozin or placebo, participants were virtually all on ACE inhibitor/ARBs or angiotensin receptor neprilysin inhibitors (ARNIs), beta blockers, and a substantial number of patients were on MRAs—all considered standard of care background therapy in heart failure with reduced ejection fraction. Trials in which patients are not getting optimal background therapy both raise ethical dilemmas and complicate the interpretation of the results.

Potential for Harm in Clinical Trials

While there is always potential for individual benefit to participants in clinical trials, randomization ensures that some patients will not receive the experimental therapy—if it is efficacious, they will be denied the benefit. This is especially true in early-phase trials, including those with normal volunteers. This arrangement is considered ethically acceptable because of the potential benefit to the community at large, and the potential dangers of administering unproven therapies. However, the extent to which an experimental question has sufficient equipoise may change during the course of a trial due to either external evidence (e.g., information to suggest that one arm is more efficacious than another), or because of data emerging from the trial itself as assessed by unblinded individuals on the data safety monitoring committee (see later). In both cases when the equipoise calculus changes, the original rationale for the trial may become moot, or the answer sufficiently known, that the trial would no longer be ethical to continue.

MONITORING OF DATA AND DATA SAFETY

Trials are subject to several types of monitoring to ensure the integrity of the data and the safety of the participants. During the execution of the study, the data-coordinating centers typically review the incoming data to assess data accuracy and quality. These can be as simple as range checks to exclude implausible values or can be more complex to catch potential fraud. Data entered into case report forms (CRFs) which can be either on paper or, increasingly, electronic are often verified with source documentation (source verification), although more and more trials are using *risk-based monitoring* which uses statistical methods to identify data inconsistencies and discrepancies.

Virtually all clinical outcomes trials (and many phase II trials) use an independent data safety monitoring board (DSMB) or data-monitoring committee (DMC) to review the incoming unblinded data for the purpose of ensuring participant safety, maintaining trial integrity, and determining if any factors external or internal to the trial affect the equipoise that presumably existed before the trial began. They use a combination of statistical methods designed specifically to assess both safety and efficacy during the course of a trial and clinical judgment. While their principal mission is to ensure safety of participants, they are also charged with determining whether the therapy under investigation demonstrates benefit sufficient to overturn equipoise and justify discontinuation of the control group, that is, discontinuation of the trial for efficacy. Data-monitoring boards are typically completely independent of the study execution and the sponsor, should have neither financial nor intellectual conflicts of interest, and should thus be unbiased regarding the results of the trial.

DSMBs can make recommendations to alter the conduct of a trial, although these should be done in ways to avoid unblinding investigators, or can recommend stopping trials entirely. Trials can be stopped for either safety concerns or efficacy, and often DSMBs are charged with determining if proceeding with a trial is futile. DSMBs follow specific guidelines for stopping for efficacy and futility, and trials typically have built-in interim analyses in which efficacy assessments are made. The robustness of a benefit, however, typically has to be higher earlier in a trial to avoid a type 1 error. Moreover, the more times the DSMB makes this determination, the greater the chance for type I error; thus greater stringency is required when stopping a trial early, and this can be codified by various stopping boundary approaches.[28–30]

NOVEL APPROACHES TO CLINICAL TRIAL DESIGN AND EXECUTION

Over the past 25 years, clinical trials have become larger, more complex, and more expensive. Typical industry-funded trials in cardiovascular medicine cost between $10,000 and $50,000 per enrolled patient. As such, there has been growing interest in finding ways to conduct trials more efficiently and less costly. Several innovations in trial methodology and execution are being used more frequently in cardiovascular trials.[31]

Pragmatic (Large Simple) Trials

As cardiovascular therapies have shifted from the sickest patients to patients with less severe disease, and effective therapies have lowered risk, sample sizes in clinical trials have grown to ensure the event rates necessary to test hypotheses in relatively low-risk individuals. *Pragmatic trials*, also called "large, simple" trials, are designed to evaluate the effectiveness of interventions in real-life routine practice conditions, whereas traditional trials aim to test whether an intervention works under optimal situations. Pragmatic trials produce results that can be generalized and applied in routine practice settings. Since most results from traditional trials fail to be broadly generalizable, the "pragmatic design" has gained momentum. Some questions are particularly suited to these types of approaches, which include simplification of inclusion and exclusion criteria, streamlining the amount of data obtained, reducing frequency of visits, and simplifying approaches to endpoint ascertainment and adjudication. Trials in primary prevention may be particularly suited to this approach because of the large number of patients needed and the simplified logistics of outpatient trials. One approach to simplifying trials is to remove the need for blinding of therapies (e.g., providing patients with a prescription that can be filled at a local pharmacy following randomization). While simpler to administer, open-label trials are more subject to potential differential drop-out and crossover as participants' perceptions about therapies evolve.[25]

Use of Electronic Medical Records in Clinical Trials

The use of electronic medical records (EMRs) for both identifying patients who fulfill inclusion and exclusion criteria to aid recruitment and for endpoint ascertainment is becoming more commonplace in clinical trials. EMR-based approaches can be used more effectively as large health care systems consolidate medical records into single large EMR systems. Utilization of EMR platforms to identify potential participants in clinical trials can be an extremely effective approach if inclusion and exclusion criteria are captured by EMR data fields. Unfortunately, many EMRs still rely on a substantial amount of free text, and while natural language approaches have been attempted to parameterize data stored in free text, these approaches remain in early stages. Use of EMRs for endpoint ascertainment is appealing but remains problematic because endpoints are captured only when patients interact with the healthcare system and many traditional clinical trials outcomes, including death, will be incompletely captured through the EMR. It is essential to remember that EMR systems were developed primarily for clinical care, not clinical research, and are often not optimized for collecting data in the rigorous manner required by trials. Nevertheless, convergence of clinical and research data collection is happening and will greatly optimize data collection in ways that can be leveraged by trials. Several recent trials, including the SCOT trial[25] and long-term follow-up of the WOSCOPS trial,[32] have successfully used EMR-based ascertainment of events.[33]

Adaptive Designs

Traditional clinical trials are designed based on assumptions about the patient population and the efficacy of the therapy being tested, and traditionally protocols are adhered to rigorously from design to completion with minimal changes occurring along the way. *Adaptive designs* are a way of mitigating the risk associated with potential incorrect assumptions made during the design phase of trials. Simple adaptive approaches might include sample size reestimation based on observed aggregate (*blinded*) event rates during the course of a trial that deviate from the expected event rates.[34] More complex adaptive approaches involve review of *unblinded* data to make adaptations in doses used, or alterations in inclusion/exclusion criteria that might identify patients

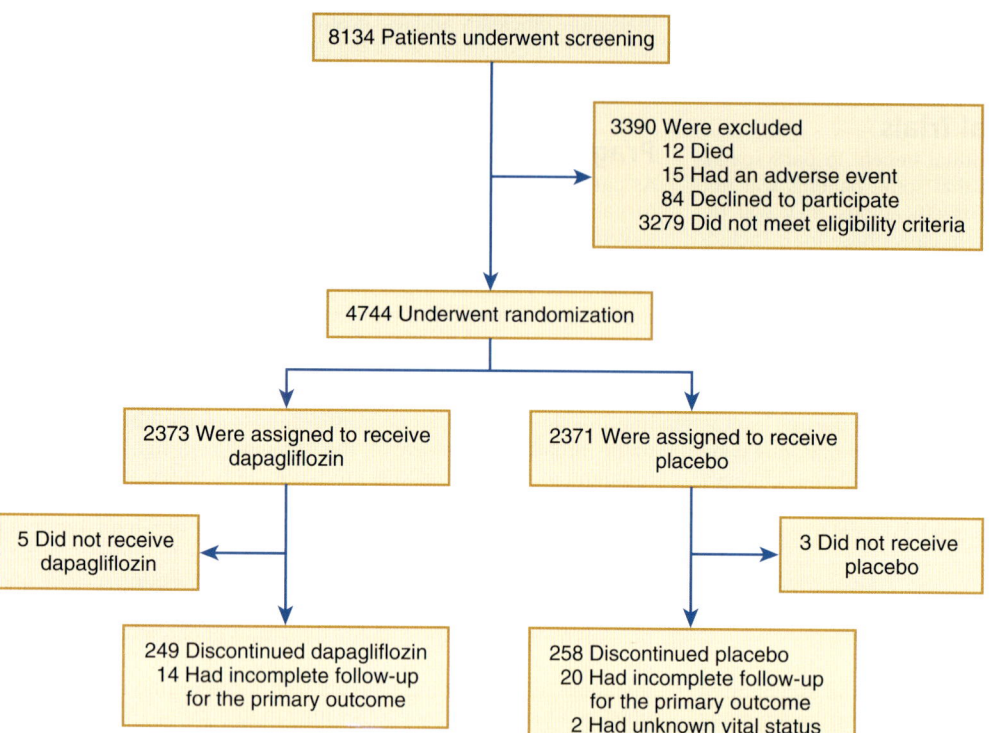

FIGURE 4.6 Typical consort diagram in a clinical trial. (From McMurray JJV, Solomon SD, Inzucchi SE, et al. Dapagliflozin in patients with heart failure and reduced ejection fraction. *N Engl J Med.* 2019;381[21]:1995–2008.)

more likely to benefit from a therapy. These approaches require appropriate safeguards to ensure that maintenance of trial integrity and not unblinding or biasing investigators—typically handled by using an unblinded group—such as a DSMB—that is firewalled from the other individuals involved in the trial, or even by computer so that no one involved in the trial conduct, is aware of the adaptations.[35]

INTERPRETATION OF CLINICAL TRIALS

Not all involved in the practice of cardiovascular medicine will design or take part in clinical trials, but every practitioner will use the results of clinical trials in their clinical decision making. Thus, understanding the statistical principles underlying the results and limitations of the analyses and reporting of trials is essential to the modern practice of medicine.

Registration and Reporting of Clinical Trials

Since 2005 there has been a requirement that all clinical trials be registered on a clinical trials registration server such as ClinicalTrials.gov prior to enrollment of the first patient, with information about the trial design, inclusion/exclusion criteria, and primary and secondary endpoints listed and publicly available. This is to ensure that trials are conducted according to the protocol and that changes to the protocol are documented, and this is to mitigate publication bias, selective reporting of results. In addition to requiring registration prior to enrollment of the first patient, high-quality journals typically require strict adherence to the protocol in reporting the primary and secondary endpoints of trials and follow and enforce the CONSORT guidelines.[36] The CONSORT statement comprises a 25-item checklist focusing on the trial design, analysis, and interpretation and also suggests a comprehensive flow diagram displaying the disposition of all trial participants (Fig. 4.6). The presentation of the primary results of a clinical trial is relatively formulaic and includes at least a description of the study population usually broken down into the randomized treatment groups (usually the first table in an article), the primary and secondary endpoint results, the primary safety results, and description of the results for prespecified subgroups. All high-quality journals also require authors to report their financial conflicts of interests.

Understanding the Primary Results

The primary results of clinical trials, whether phase II, III, or IV, are subject to the basic principles of hypothesis testing in which the primary analysis determines whether the null hypothesis has been rejected or not, and subsequent analyses are dependent on that outcome. This principle is especially sacrosanct in studies being undertaken for regulatory approval.

In phase II trials, however, where the primary goal of the studies is to decide whether to proceed to more definitive trials, this principle can be more flexible, and investigators and sponsors often use the totality of the evidence rather than simply the results of a single primary endpoint to make decisions about next steps in the investigative plan. In some cases, this is done with the help of formal statistical approaches that allow for incorporation of multiple endpoints,[37] but in other cases this is done more informally.

For clinical outcomes trials, results are typically presented as a proportion of patients within each treatment group who achieve prespecified endpoints and, in most cases, a hazard ratio with a 95% confidence interval representing the results of a Cox model, with a Kaplan-Meier curve showing either event-free survival in the treatment groups or the accumulation of events (see Fig. 4.4). A hazard ratio of 0.80 with a 95% confidence interval of 0.72, 0.91 is interpreted as a 20% reduced hazard of the primary endpoint in the treatment group compared with the control group. The confidence interval suggests that the result could be as great as 38% reduced hazard or as little as a 9% reduced hazard. When the upper bound of the 95% confidence interval crosses 1, the result is considered no longer statistically significant at the 0.05 level. The point estimate is considered a measure of the magnitude of the result and the *p*-value (or how far the upper 95% confidence interval is from 1) a measure of the robustness of the result. Thus, a hazard ratio of 0.95 with confidence interval of 0.92 to 0.98 is statistically significant, although the magnitude of the benefit might be relatively small (and possibly clinically meaningless). Conversely, a study with a primary endpoint hazard ratio of 0.70 with confidence intervals between 0.46 and 0.98 needs to be interpreted with caution because the result suggests that the benefit might be as low as a 2% difference between therapies.

Secondary Endpoints

Secondary endpoints in trials are typically considered only hypothesis testing if the primary endpoint is significant and are otherwise considered hypothesis generating. While a secondary endpoint might be significant even if a primary endpoint is not, these results need to be interpreted with caution. This is especially true for results that were not expected and for which the study may not have been powered. In the ELITE trial, which compared losartan with captopril in just over 700 heart failure patients, the primary endpoint was increase in serum creatinine, which was not different between groups. However, there was a seemingly dramatic difference in all-cause mortality (17 vs. 32 deaths, hazard ratio 0.46, 95% confidence interval 0.05, 0.69; *p* = 0.035). The trial of course was not powered for all-cause mortality, and this result was not confirmed in the properly powered and much larger ELITE II trial.

Interpretation of Subgroups

Subgroup results in clinical trials are often subject to misinterpretation.[38] All outcomes trials, and many nonoutcomes trials, prespecify certain subgroups in which the data will be assessed—typical subgroups include sex, age (often dichotomized at a particular cut point), ejection fraction (often dichotomized at a particular cut point), diabetes status, etc. (Fig. 4.7). The primary reason for identifying and analyzing subgroups is to assess for *consistency* in the treatment response, not, as many believe, to assess for differences. The primary statistical analysis of subgroups is the test for *interaction* or *heterogeneity* between the subgroups with respect to the treatment effect. This asks the question, "Does the subgroup status modify the treatment effect?" Within subgroups, there may be differences between the point estimates and even the *p*-value for a result within a subgroup may be significant, but if the *interaction p*-value is NOT significant, we cannot state that the two

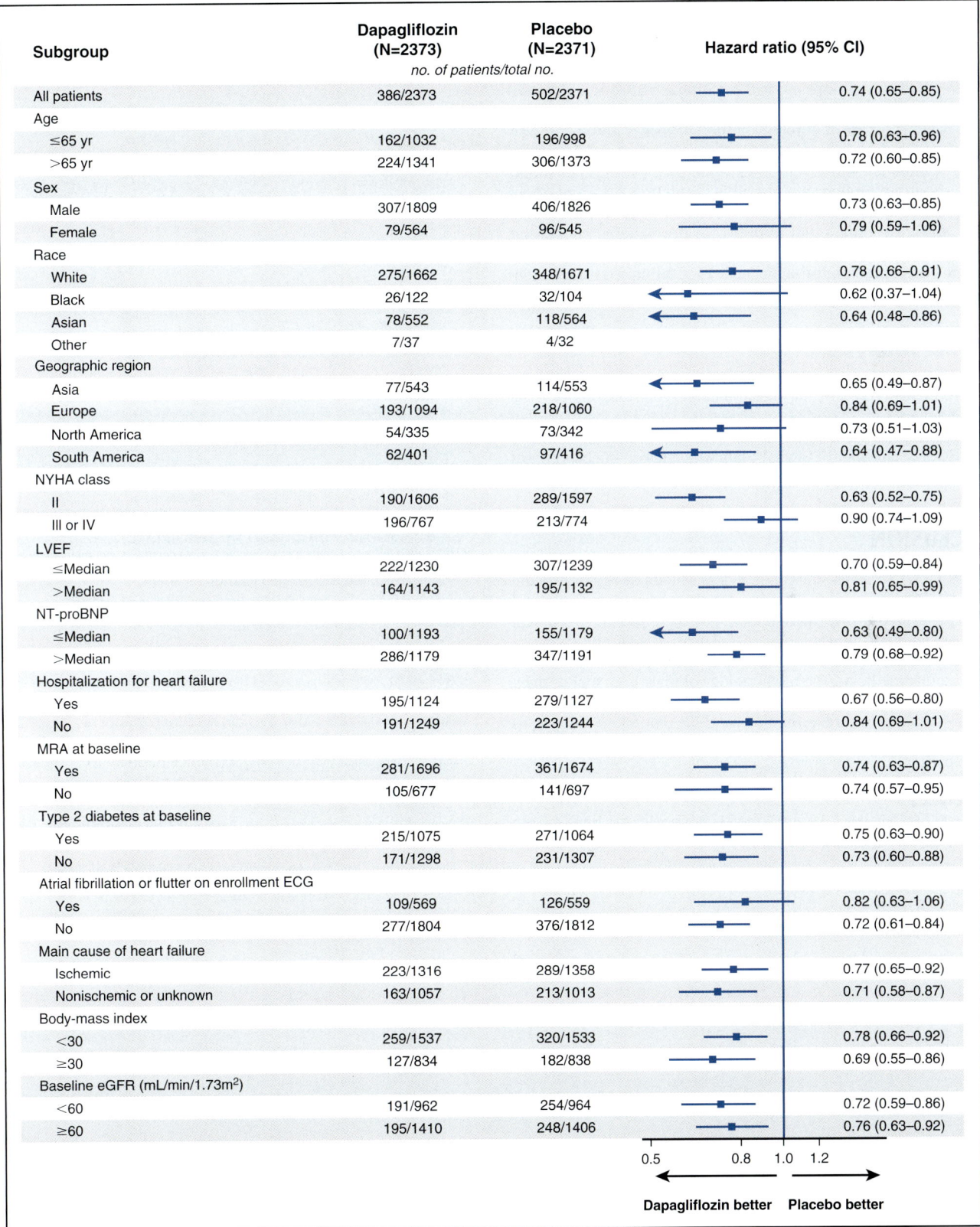

FIGURE 4.7 Subgroup "forest-plot" showing the point estimate and 95% confidence intervals within each prespecified subgroup in the DAPA-HF trial. (From McMurray JJV, Solomon SD, Inzucchi SE, et al. DAPA-HF Trial Committees and Investigators. Dapagliflozin in patients with heart failure and reduced ejection fraction. *N Engl J Med.* 2019;381[21]:1995–2008.)

subgroups are different with respect to treatment. In general, the power to assess interactions is generally lower than the power to assess main effects. Moreover, the more subgroups we assess, the more likely it is to find a significant interaction. This concept was illustrated famously in the ISIS trial in which, as an example, they showed the primary results by astrologic sign and found that patients born under Gemini or Libra had an increased risk for mortality![8]

Subgroup findings can, however, identify individuals who may respond differentially to the treatment being studied in a trial, but the bar for accepting a subgroup finding as true should be quite high. Several factors increase the plausibility of a subgroup finding. The likelihood that a subgroup finding is real is increased if a subgroup is prespecified (not post-hoc); if the subgroup is large, because smaller subgroups are less reliable and always underpowered; if the subgroup is tested for interaction and the interaction p-value is adjusted for multiplicity; if the analysis is not just univariate but multivariate (accounting for the correlation between subgroups); if there is evidence from external data (even other trials) that the subgroup findings are plausible (even from adjacent populations); and if there is biologic plausibility—the subgroup finding makes sense. The differential findings for the patients above and below the median ejection fraction of 57% in the PARAGON-HF[21] trial were considered plausible because they fulfilled the aforementioned criteria.

Post-hoc Analyses

Post-hoc analyses should always be considered hypothesis generating. Nevertheless, some of the most valuable contributions of trials have been the results of post-hoc analyses. For example, the finding of reduced atherosclerotic events in the SAVE trial provided the rationale for the HOPE, PEACE, and EUROPA trials, which tested the hypotheses generated by the post-hoc analysis.

CONCLUSION

Although most cardiovascular practitioners will not design or execute trials, virtually all will use the results of trials to care for patients, and most of the evidence presented in this book is the product of clinical trials. A rudimentary understanding of trial methodology and statistical and analytic techniques is thus essential to the modern practice of cardiovascular medicine. The methodology of trials, from trial designs, methods of recruitment, ascertainment of endpoints, and statistical analysis continues to evolve, innovate, and become more efficient as this type of evidence generation becomes essential to bring new therapies to patients.

REFERENCES

1. Gibbons RJ, Smith S, Antman E. American College of Cardiology/American heart association clinical practice guidelines: Part I. Where do they come from? Circulation. 2003;107:2979–2986.
2. Lodi S, Phillips A, Lundgren J, et al. Effect estimates in randomized trials and observational studies: comparing apples with apples. Am J Epidemiol. 2019;188(8):1569–1577.
3. Manson JE, Hsia J, Johnson KC, et al. Estrogen plus progestin and the risk of coronary heart disease. N Engl J Med. 2003;349(6):523–534.
4. Vijayakumar S, Vaduganathan M, Butler J. Glucose-lowering therapies and heart failure in type 2 diabetes mellitus: mechanistic links, clinical data, and future directions. Circulation. 2018;137(10):1060–1073.
5. Vaduganathan M, Claggett B, Packer M, et al. Natriuretic peptides as biomarkers of treatment response in clinical trials of heart failure. JACC Heart Fail. 2018;6(7):564–569.
6. Desai AS, Solomon SD, Shah AM, et al. Effect of sacubitril-valsartan vs enalapril on aortic stiffness in patients with heart failure and reduced ejection fraction: a randomized clinical trial. J Am Med Assoc. 2019;322(11):1–10.
7. DREAM (Diabetes REduction Assessment with ramipril and rosiglitazone Medication) Trial Investigators, Gerstein HC, Yusuf S, et al. Effect of rosiglitazone on the frequency of diabetes in patients with impaired glucose tolerance or impaired fasting glucose: a randomised controlled trial [published correction appears in Lancet. 2006 Nov 18;368(9549):1770]. Lancet. 2006;368(9541):1096–1105.
8. Randomised trial of intravenous streptokinase, oral aspirin, both, or neither among 17,187 cases of suspected acute myocardial infarction: ISIS-2. ISIS-2 (Second International Study of Infarct Survival) Collaborative Group. Lancet. 1988;2(8607):349–360.
9. DREAM Trial Investigators, Bosch J, Yusuf S, et al. Effect of ramipril on the incidence of diabetes. N Engl J Med. 2006;355(15):1551–1562.
10. Pfeffer MA, McMurray JJ, Velazquez EJ, et al. Valsartan, captopril, or both in myocardial infarction complicated by heart failure, left ventricular dysfunction, or both. N Engl J Med. 2003;349(20):1893–1906.
11. Lowrie R, Mair FS, Greenlaw N, et al. Pharmacist intervention in primary care to improve outcomes in patients with left ventricular systolic dysfunction. Eur Heart J. 2012;33(3):314–324.
12. McMurray JJ, Packer M, Desai AS, et al. Angiotensin-neprilysin inhibition versus enalapril in heart failure. N Engl J Med. 2014;371(11):993–1004.
13. McMurray JJV, Solomon SD, Inzucchi SE, et al. Dapagliflozin in patients with heart failure and reduced ejection fraction. N Engl J Med. 2019;381(21):1995–2008.
14. https://www.fda.gov/regulatory-information/searchfda-guidance-documents/treatment-heart-failureendpoints-drug-development-guidance-industry. Accessed August 16th, 2020.
15. https://www.fda.gov/drugs/ddt-coa-000084-kansas-city-cardiomyopathy-questionnaire-kccq.
16. Kim DH, Uno H, Wei LJ. Restricted mean survival time as a measure to interpret clinical trial results. JAMA Cardiol. 2017;2(11):1179–1180.
17. Claggett B, Packer M, McMurray JJ, et al. Estimating the long-term treatment benefits of sacubitril-valsartan. N Engl J Med. 2015;373(23):2289–2290.
18. Pocock SJ, Ariti CA, Collier TJ, Wang D. The win ratio: a new approach to the analysis of composite endpoints in clinical trials based on clinical priorities. Eur Heart J. 2012;33(2):176–182.
19. Ferreira JP, Jhund PS, Duarte K, et al. Use of the win ratio in cardiovascular trials. JACC Heart Fail. 2020;8(6):441–450.
20. Finkelstein DM, Schoenfeld DA. Combining mortality and longitudinal measures in clinical trials. Statist Med. 1999;18(11):1341–1354.
21. Maurer MS, Schwartz JH, Gundapaneni B, et al. Tafamidis treatment for patients with transthyretin amyloid cardiomyopathy. N Engl J Med. 2018;379(11):1007–1016.
22. Rogers JK, Pocock SJ, McMurray JJ, et al. Analysing recurrent hospitalizations in heart failure: a review of statistical methodology, with application to CHARM-Preserved. Eur J Heart Fail. 2014;16(1):33–40.
23. Solomon SD, McMurray JJV, Anand IS, et al. Angiotensin-neprilysin inhibition in heart failure with preserved ejection fraction. N Engl J Med. 2019;381(17):1609–1620.
24. Emanual EJ, Wendler D, Grady C. What makes clinical research ethical? J Am Med Assoc. 2000;283:2701–2711.
25. Mix TC, Brenner RM, Cooper ME, et al. Rationale–Trial to Reduce Cardiovascular Events with Aranesp Therapy (TREAT): evolving the management of cardiovascular risk in patients with chronic kidney disease. Am Heart J. 2005;149(3):408–413.
26. MacDonald TM, Hawkey CJ, Ford I, et al. Randomized trial of switching from prescribed non-selective non-steroidal anti-inflammatory drugs to prescribed celecoxib: the Standard care vs. Celecoxib Outcome Trial (SCOT). Eur Heart J. 2017;38(23):1843–1850.
27. Pitt B, Poole-Wilson PA, Segal R, et al. Effect of losartan compared with captopril on mortality in patients with symptomatic heart failure: randomised trial–the Losartan Heart Failure Survival Study ELITE II. Lancet. 2000;355(9215):1582–1587.
28. Wittes J. Stopping a trial early - and then what? Clin Trials. 2012;9(6):714–720.
29. Pocock S, Wang D, Wilhelmsen L, Hennekens CH. The data monitoring experience in the Candesartan in Heart Failure Assessment of Reduction in Mortality and morbidity (CHARM) program. Am Heart J. 2005;149(5):939–943.
30. Fleming TR, DeMets DL. Monitoring of clinical trials: issues and recommendations. Control Clin Trials. 1993;14(3):183–197.
31. Solomon SD, Pfeffer MA. The future of clinical trials in cardiovascular medicine. Circulation. 2016;133(25):2662–2670.
32. Vallejo-Vaz AJ, Robertson M, Catapano AL, et al. Low-density lipoprotein cholesterol lowering for the primary prevention of cardiovascular disease among men with primary elevations of low- density lipoprotein cholesterol levels of 190 mg/dL or above: analyses from the WOSCOPS (West of Scotland Coronary Prevention Study) 5-year randomized trial and 20-year observational follow-up. Circulation. 2017;136(20):1878–1891.
33. Barry SJ, Dinnett E, Kean S, et al. Are routinely collected NHS administrative records suitable for endpoint identification in clinical trials? Evidence from the West of Scotland Coronary Prevention Study. PloS One. 2013;8(9):e75379.
34. Packer M, Holcomb R, Abraham WT, et al. Rationale and design of the TRUE-AHF trial: the effects of ularitide on the short-term clinical course and long-term mortality of patients with acute heart failure. Eur J Heart Fail. 2017;19(5):673–681.
35. Bhatt D, Mehta C. Adaptive designs for clinical trials. N Engl J Med. 2016;375:65–74.
36. http://www.consort-statement.org.
37. Sun H, Davison BA, Cotter G, et al. Evaluating treatment efficacy by multiple end points in phase II acute heart failure clinical trials: analyzing data using a global method. Circ Heart Fail. 2012;5(6):742–749.
38. Wittes J. On looking at subgroups. Circulation. 2009;119(7):912–915.

5 Clinical Decision-Making in Cardiology

JOHN E. BRUSH JR. AND HARLAN M. KRUMHOLZ

DIAGNOSTIC DECISIONS, 53
THERAPEUTIC DECISIONS, 57
DECIDING WHEN TO CHANGE CLINICAL PRACTICE BASED ON NEW CLINICAL RESEARCH FINDINGS, 59
SHARED DECISION-MAKING, 59
MONITORING THE QUALITY OF CLINICAL DECISIONS, 60
System 1 and System 2 Thinking, 60
TEACHING CLINICAL REASONING, 60
CONCLUSION, 61
CLASSIC REFERENCES, 61
REFERENCES, 61

Medicine is an information science. Information is being produced at an unprecedented rate and is readily accessible using electronic searches and hand-held devices, making skills to parse and use the appropriate information ever more important. Memorization of medical facts is less a necessity, while processing knowledge and critical thinking remain essential for high-value medical care. Clinical decisions and recommendations are critical features of medicine and, in the midst of a rapid expansion of medical knowledge, have never been more challenging. This chapter summarizes core competencies for clinical reasoning that should be mastered by expert practicing cardiologists.

Excellent clinical decisions require a command of medical knowledge and a deep understanding of individual patients, including their preferences and goals. Good decisions take into account the limits of knowledge, uncertainty in measurements, and the play of chance.[1-3] Clinical reasoning is informed by both experiential and formal knowledge learned through years of practice and study.[4] The translation of medical knowledge into good patient-centered decisions is a key goal of clinical reasoning and is the hallmark of an expert clinician.

Clinical reasoning is often guided by simplified rules. Early in training, physicians are taught how to recognize specific clusters of signs and symptoms, place patients in diagnostic categories, and follow the rules that apply to those categories. For example, patients with particular findings might be labeled as having acute myocardial infarction (AMI), which would trigger treatment based on studies showing benefit from aspirin and beta-blocking agents. In this context, algorithmic tools are often used to direct actions. For example, guidelines recommend that a patient with a low ejection fraction should be considered for an automated implantable defibrillator, but only after considering the etiology of the systolic dysfunction and the timeframe of the disorder.

These rule-based algorithms are not intended to force actions, but to guide decisions. The best clinicians know when adherence to such algorithms is proper and when exceptions, based on the patient's particular situation or preferences, can lead to divergence from these algorithms. Divergence from guidelines may be appropriate, but requires adequate justification, documentation, and transparency.

Most of medical decision-making, however, lies outside of simple algorithms and requires judgment. There are two major settings, related to diagnosis and treatment, where clinical reasoning is critical.

First, there are decisions about classifying an individual who presents with symptoms or signs of disease into the proper diagnostic category. Book chapters and other reference materials are usually organized according to categories, such as a medical diagnosis. The chapter informs the reader about how a particular condition, such as aortic stenosis, might manifest. These labels are useful for clustering patients by common disease mechanisms, prognosis, and responses to therapeutic strategies.

But patients often do not present to medical attention fitting perfectly into pre-specified general diagnostic categories. They seek attention for symptoms, which requires the clinician to reverse the order of a typical textbook and to work inductively from a patient's signs and symptoms toward a diagnostic label before a therapeutic plan can be developed. For a patient with dyspnea on exertion and a systolic murmur, aortic stenosis is a possibility, but the diagnosis is not conclusive without further testing. In some cases, uncertainty persists. About a third of patients labeled with a principal discharge diagnosis of heart failure also receive treatments for other causes of dyspnea such as pneumonia or chronic obstructive pulmonary disease.[5] This is the reality of current practice.

Second, there are decisions about treatments. These decisions are also challenging because they involve weighing risks and benefits, speculating about estimates for these parameters, and aligning choices with the preferences of the patient. The likelihood of benefit is often probabilistic, as people are pursuing strategies to reduce risk without knowing whether they themselves will benefit. These decisions can occur in prevention, which addresses whether to intervene in the interest of preventing future health problems, based on an estimate of prognosis. In this setting, the risks and costs occur immediately while the benefit is anticipated to be in the future. These decisions can also involve treatments to address symptoms as well as reduce the immediate risk for someone with acute or chronic disease.

Risk stratification is an important application of probability and is often used to estimate patient risk and assist in decision-making. This approach generally uses the results of statistical models that have iden-tified prognostic factors and incorporated them into a tool that may assist clinicians. In recent years, many tools have been developed to assist in the rapid assessment of patients.

Recent decades have witnessed the emergence of cognitive psychology, a branch of psychology focused on how people make decisions.[6] The field demonstrated that people frequently develop useful reasoning shortcuts to circumvent the need to explicitly calculate probabilities, but these shortcuts come with biases that can lead decision-makers to deviate from the rules of logic and probability in predictable ways. Thus, a good understanding of clinical reasoning requires knowledge about logic and probability as well as cognitive psychology.

Cognitive psychologists have demonstrated how people often rely on intuition to make decisions in uncertain settings.[6,7] For cognitive psychologists, intuition is not merely guessing, but has a specialized meaning. The cognitive psychologist Herbert Simon described intuition by stating: "the situation has provided a cue; this cue has given the expert access to information stored in memory, and the information provides the answer. Intuition is nothing more and nothing less than recognition" (see Classic References). Expert clinicians learn to use intuition to recognize diagnoses and make clinical decisions. They learn to calibrate their intuitive judgments using scientific evidence and clinical experience. They may also be susceptible to cognitive biases that are associated with such decision-making.

DIAGNOSTIC DECISIONS

Patients often present with descriptions of symptoms such as chest pain. Cues are scattered, like pieces of a jigsaw puzzle. Clinicians, like all decision-makers, often use mental shortcuts called heuristics to organize cues and to turn an unstructured problem into a set of structured decisions.[3,7] They are taught to collect the cues of an unstructured clinical problem by using an organized history and physical examination.[8] When experts take a history, they use a process known as early hypothesis generation to develop a list of 3 to 5 possible diagnoses very early in the process (see Classic References). This enables the questioning to become more direct and the clinician to become more engaged in the fact-finding exercise.

Studies show that the mechanism of diagnostic hypothesis generation varies, depending on the stage of training.[8] Novice practitioners who lack clinical experience use causal reasoning, which tends to be slow and less accurate. As trainees gain experience, knowledge about diagnoses becomes encapsulated into illness scripts. An illness script is a schema or map that integrates conceptual information regarding a disease and links the concepts with case experience. As physicians gain further experience, they accrue experiential knowledge. One theory is that diagnostic experience is remembered through disease prototypes, which describe the typical features of a disease. Another theory is that experiential knowledge is remembered as specific instances called exemplars, which are memories of prior experiences that have been categorized and stored in long-term memory. With experience, a clinician accumulates exemplars that are automatically retrievable and represented in memory in a fashion that is unique to that clinician and not generalizable among clinicians. Memories of exemplars give the expert an intuitive sense of both the base rates for particular diagnostic categories and the relative frequencies of features for a diagnostic category.

Because clinicians start the diagnostic process by intuitively recognizing familiar phenotypes stored in memory as exemplars, it becomes important to study how symptoms combine in individuals as unique symptom phenotypes. A recent study showed wide variation in symptom phenotypes among patients with AMI, which may have important implications on how we teach learners to recognize a diagnosis.[9] The study also showed that women exhibited significantly more unique symptom phenotypes than men. Greater phenotypic variation could lead to more missed diagnoses and this is a promising area for further research.

After collecting, sorting, and organizing clinical data, clinicians often use a problem list as a tool to list, group, and prioritize clinical findings. With additional clinical information, a problem statement can be defined more specifically. For example, shortness of breath may be an initial problem statement that is replaced by acute systolic heart failure, as further clinical information leads to a more refined problem statement that moves from symptom to diagnosis. They then use a differential diagnosis to expand the list of possibilities to avoid premature closure of the search for the true diagnosis. This step-by-step process enables the clinician to formulate a set of hypothetical diagnostic possibilities, which can then be tested using iterative hypothesis testing. Iterative hypothesis testing allows the clinician to narrow the list of possible diagnoses and focus on the most plausible hypothesis.[1-3]

UNDERSTANDING PROBABILITY

Understanding probability is essential for good clinical decision-making.[1-3] Probability can be estimated for outcomes that are measured as continuous or categorical variables, as shown in Figure 5.1. The figure shows how probability of an outcome or event is distributed across a range of possibilities. For example, a laboratory test might be measured in a population of patients resulting in a distribution in which most patients are distributed to the middle of the range of possibilities and fewer scatter to the edges of the range, shown in the probability density curve in the left panel of Figure 5.1. The probability of categories or discrete variables can also be measured, as shown in the probability distribution graph in the right panel of Figure 5.1. If all of the diagnostic possibilities are mutually exclusive and collectively exhaustive, the probability of all of the possibilities will add up to 1, as shown by the red cumulative probability curves in Figure 5.1. Understanding cumulative probability is important for understanding sensitivity and specificity, as discussed below.

To test a diagnostic hypothesis, clinicians use conditional probability, which is the probability that something will happen, on the condition that something else happened. Conditional probability can inform the probability of a diagnosis, on the condition of some new information such as a positive test result. Bayesian reasoning is a mental process that allows clinicians to modify their perceptions by considering prior knowledge and updating that knowledge with new and evolving evidence. It enables formation of a probability estimate and revision of that estimate based on new information using conditional probability. For example, one might ask, what is the probability of coronary artery disease in a patient, given a positive stress echocardiogram? What is the probability of pulmonary embolus, given a negative D-dimer test? What is the probability of an acute coronary syndrome, given an abnormal troponin test? The post-test probability depends on a prior estimate of the probability for that particular patient, combined with the strength of the test result. Probability theory helps the clinician understand the question and calculate the answer.

Bayesian reasoning adds mathematical rigor to clinical thinking and requires both a prior estimate of probability and an estimate of the strength of a test result. Prior estimates can come from a clinician's own experience, or published data on the prevalence of a disease. A classic paper by Diamond and Forrester provides estimates of the prevalence of coronary artery disease in patients depending on age, sex and symptom features, for example (see Classic References). This type of observational research can be used to provide the prior probabilities that are needed for Bayesian reasoning.

Understanding probability is essential to interpreting laboratory tests. A laboratory test might be measured in a population of presumably normal individuals to determine a distribution and to define a normal range, shown in the probability density curve in the left panel of Figure 5.2. A normal range is commonly defined as the inner 95% cumulative probability and the abnormal range is defined as values falling outside of the normal range as shown.

Another way of defining a test result is by measuring the test result in a group of subjects who are defined as normal and abnormal by another independent "gold standard" test, as shown in the right panel of Figure 5.2. Typically, subjects with and without disease will have test results that are distributed like bell-shaped curves. A line of demarcation can be drawn to define how a new test would separate patients with positive and negative test results. Because there is overlap in subjects

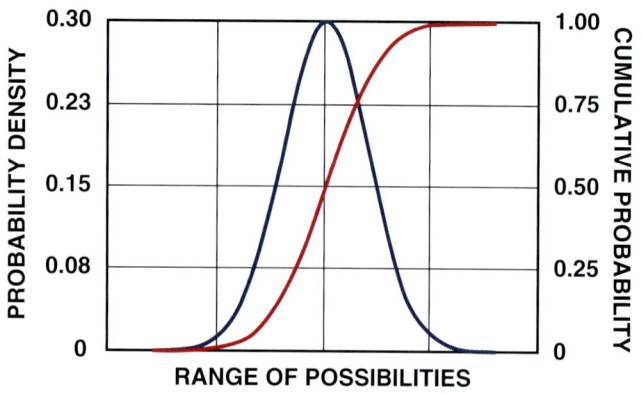
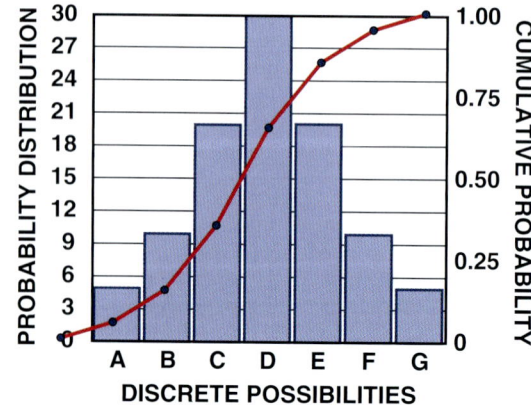

FIGURE 5.1 A probability density curve is shown in the left panel. The *blue curve* shows the probability of an event (left y-axis), across a range of possibilities (x-axis). A probability distribution is shown in the right panel. The *blue columns* show the probabilities (left y-axis) of a variety of discrete possibilities (x-axis). In both panels, the cumulative probability across the range of possibilities (x-axis) is shown by the *red curves* (right y-axis).

with and without disease, there will be false-positive and false-negative test results, as shown.

Understanding how to use clinical testing is essential to good decision-making. The utility of a test result depends, in part, on the operating characteristics of a test, namely, the sensitivity and specificity. They are rates, meaning they are proportions with different units for the numerator and denominator. The terms "true positive rate" (TPR) for sensitivity and "true negative rate" (TNR) for specificity are alternative labels. Patients with and without disease are shown separately in Figure 5.3 to show the cumulative probabilities of a true positive result (sensitivity or the TPR) on the right and of a true negative result (specificity or the TNR) on the left. Sensitivity and specificity are usually shown in a 2 × 2 table but showing the TPR and TNR in Figure 5.3 demonstrates how these rates vary, depending on the location of the line of demarcation between positive and negative test results.

The complementary probability of the TNR is the false-positive rate (FPR), as shown in the top panel of Figure 5.4. Plotting the TPR (sensitivity) of a test on the y-axis and the FPR (1-specificity) on the x-axis creates a plot called a receiver operating curve (ROC), as shown in the bottom panel of Figure 5.4. ROCs are useful for determining the optimal cutoff point for the line of demarcation of a test.

The denominators of sensitivity and specificity are patients with the disease and people without the disease, respectively. In clinical practice, when test results are reported as positive or negative, however, the results are reported using terms with different denominators. A clinician wants to know the probability that a positive test result is truly positive, or the positive predictive value (PPV), and also the probability of disease given a negative test result, which is 1 minus the negative predictive value (NPV). When changing from sensitivity and specificity to the PPV and NPV, the denominators of these rates change, making it difficult for a clinician to estimate these probabilities intuitively. In addition, the PPV and NPV depend not only on the sensitivity and specificity of the test, but also on the prevalence of the target condition in a population of test subjects.

The sensitivity and specificity are not fixed, and spectrum bias can result if the test subjects that defined the operating characteristics of the test are different from the subjects who are subsequently tested.[2,3] If the operating characteristics of the test are defined in a narrowly defined population (left panel of Fig. 5.5), but the test is used in a broadly defined population and the line of demarcation remains fixed (right panel of Fig. 5.5), the specificity, or TNR, will decrease. This commonly occurs with tests such as troponin testing, where the clinical sensitivity and specificity of the test are defined in a research setting, but the test is used indiscriminately in practice. When used as a general screening test in a broadly defined population, the width of the distribution of the subjects with no disease widens, yet the line of demarcation remains fixed, which decreases the TNR, as shown. This issue has also been shown in genetic testing.[10]

In practice, clinicians usually do not formally calculate Bayesian probabilities but, in general, use a heuristic that psychologists call "anchoring and adjusting."[3,6] Clinicians estimate a pretest probability (the anchor) and estimate the posttest probability by adjusting the anchor. For a patient with chest pain, for example, the anchor would be an estimate of the pretest probability of coronary artery disease, which would be intuitively adjusted on the basis of new information such as a stress test result to estimate a posttest probability. This is an expedient method for intuitively estimating conditional probability.

There are two potential problems when using this heuristic. One fallacy, called "anchoring," is when the decision-maker becomes too anchored on the pre-test probability estimate and does not adequately adjust in estimating the post-test probability. The second fallacy is called "base-rate neglect," when the decision maker overly responds to the new information to estimate a post-test probability, without regard for the pretest probability. For example, troponin tests may be positive because of renal failure or sepsis in patients with a low pretest probability of acute thrombotic myocardial infarction. Taking the test result at face value and initiating therapy such as antithrombotic drug therapy in such a patient would be an example of base-rate neglect.

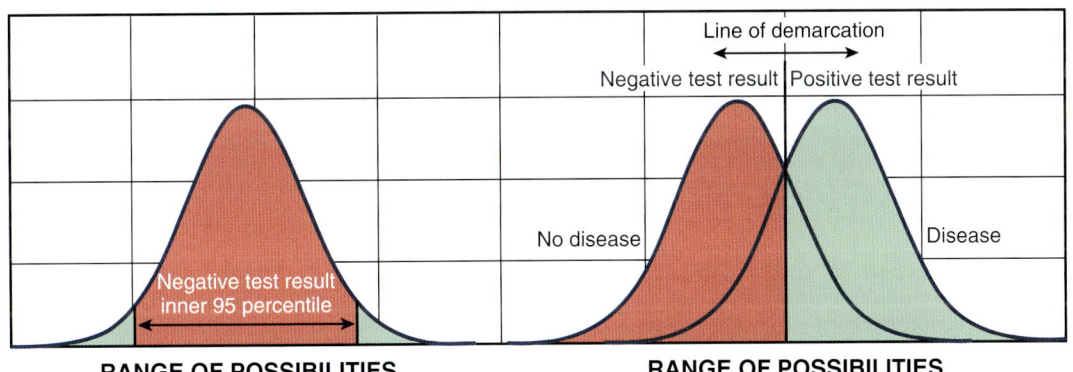

FIGURE 5.2 Left panel shows how the normal range of a test result is defined as the inner 95th percentile of a presumably normal population. Right panel shows how a normal and abnormal test result is defined by the line of demarcation between distributions of normal and abnormal test subjects, as defined by another independent "gold standard" test.

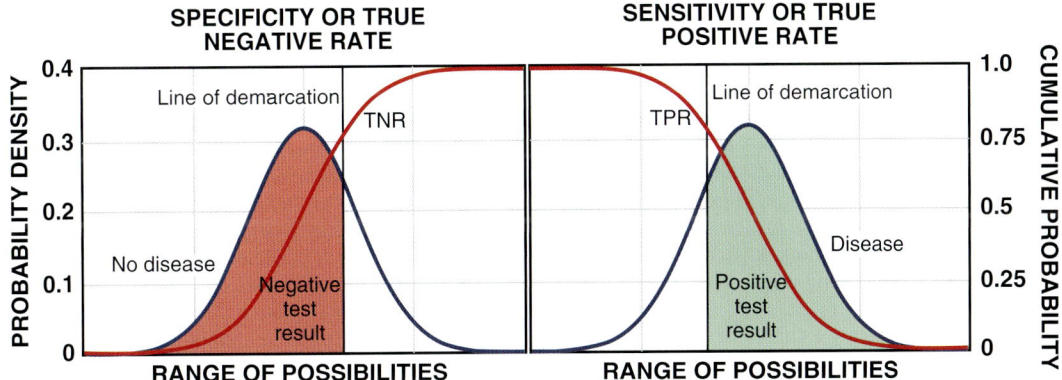

FIGURE 5.3 Distributions of normal and abnormal test subjects are shown separately to demonstrate that the true negative rate (TNR, or specificity) is the cumulative probability of a negative test result (red curve) in a distribution of subjects without disease (blue curve, left panel) and the true positive rate (TPR, or sensitivity) is the cumulative probability of a positive test result (red curve) in a distribution of subjects with disease (blue curve, right panel), depending on the location of the line of demarcation.

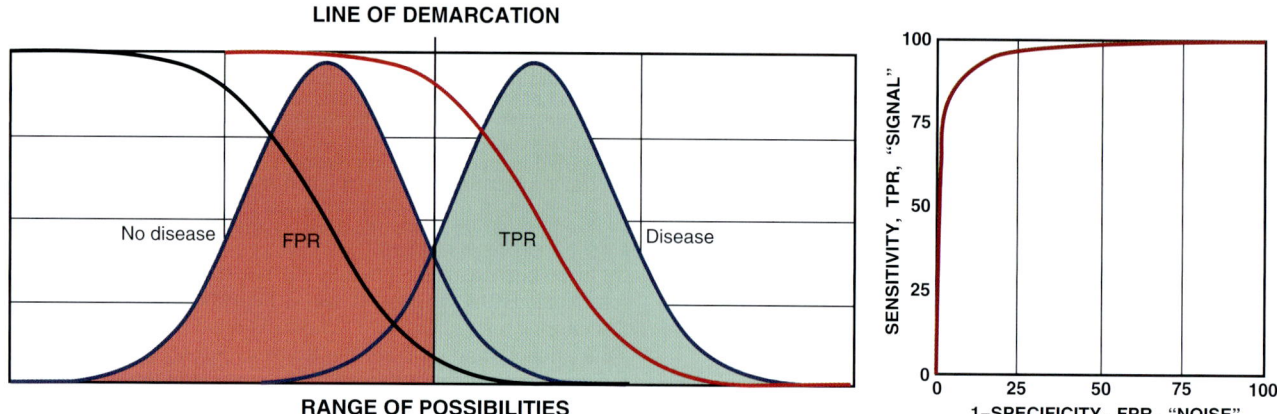

FIGURE 5.4 Distributions of patients without and with disease are shown in the left panel (*blue curves*) along with the true positive rate (TPR, or sensitivity, *red curve*) and the false-positive rate (FPR, or [1 – specificity], *black curve*). The right panel shows the TPR (sensitivity or "the signal") on the y-axis plotted against the FPR ([1 – specificity] or "the noise") on the x-axis, across the range of possibilities, depending on the location of the line of demarcation.

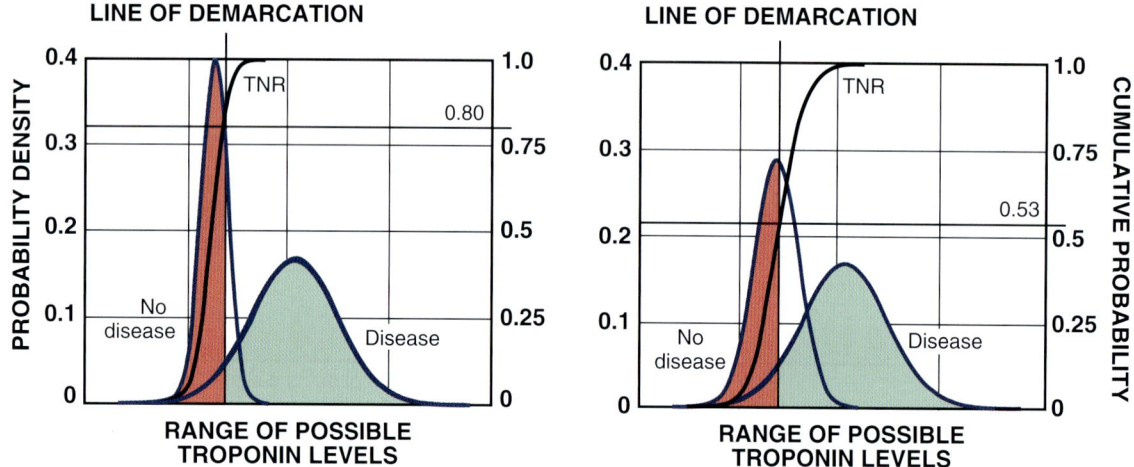

FIGURE 5.5 Distributions of patients without and with disease are shown by the *blue curves*. True negative test results are shown in *red* and true positive results are shown in *green*. The true negative rates (TNR, or specificity) are shown by the *black* cumulative probability curves. The left panel shows the results when the test is ordered on a narrowly defined population of subjects and the right panel shows the results when the test is ordered on a broadly defined population of test subjects, resulting in spectrum bias and a marked decrease in specificity of the test (80% to 53% in this example).

Likelihood ratios are useful for Bayesian reasoning. The advantage of likelihood ratios is that, unlike sensitivity and specificity, they are dimensionless numbers, so the need for keeping track of what is in the numerator and denominator is alleviated. Likelihood ratios give a measure of the persuasiveness of a positive and negative test result, and can be used intuitively, or used to actually calculate posttest odds.

A likelihood ratio is defined as the percentage of patients with a disease who have a given test result divided by the percentage of patients without disease who have that same test result. Thus, a positive likelihood ratio is the percentage of patients with disease with a *positive* test result divided by the percentage of patients without disease with a *positive* test result (TPR/FPR, or sensitivity/[1 – specificity]). A negative likelihood ratio is the percentage of patients with disease with a *negative* test result divided by the percentage of patients without disease with a *negative* test result (FNR/TNR, or [1 – sensitivity]/specificity). It is easy to calculate the positive and negative likelihood ratios from sensitivity and specificity. Once calculated, these numbers can be used to multiply the pretest odds to calculate the posttest odds of a diagnosis. They are multipliers, so a higher positive likelihood ratio, and a lower negative likelihood ratio (which is a fraction) have stronger multiplying effects. A likelihood ratio that is close to 1 is weak because it would have very little multiplying effect, meaning it has little effect on the pre-test assessment.

Figure 5.6 shows how the probability estimate of a diagnosis can shift depending on a test result. After choosing a pre-test probability estimate on the x-axis, one can trace up to either the upper curve for a positive test result or the lower curve for a negative test result, then trace over to the y-axis to read the post-test probability estimate. The diagonal line shows that there would be no change in probability for a test with a likelihood ratio of 1. A higher positive likelihood ratio or a lower negative likelihood ratio would result in positive or negative test result curves with greater deviation from the diagonal line, representing a greater shift in the post-test probability estimate based on the test result.

Some tests are asymmetrical, meaning that either their positive or negative likelihood ratio is stronger. For example, Figure 5.7, Panel A shows the probability of congestive heart failure based on congestion on a chest x-ray, which has a very strong positive likelihood ratio of 13.5 and a relatively weak negative likelihood ratio of 0.48.[3] This reflects the fact that the chest x-ray is highly specific but not very sensitive for heart failure. In other words, congestive findings on a chest x-ray are highly suggestive of heart failure, but their absence is not strong reassurance about the lack of heart failure. Tests that are highly specific are better for ruling in a diagnosis and this can be remembered using the mnemonic "SpPin." (Highly specific tests, if positive, are good for ruling in.)

On the other hand, Figure 5.7, Panel B shows that a D-dimer for pulmonary embolus has a very strong negative likelihood ratio of 0.09 and a modest positive likelihood ratio of 1.7.[3] This reflects the fact that a D-dimer is highly sensitive but not very specific for a pulmonary embolus. Tests that are highly sensitive are better for ruling out a diagnosis and this can be remembered using the mnemonic "SnNout." (Highly sensitive tests, if negative, are good for ruling out.)

The likelihood ratios, however, are only as useful as the sensitivity and specificity that are used to calculate them. They give an approximate quantitative estimate of the strength of new information that provides a mechanism for calibrating intuitive probability estimates.

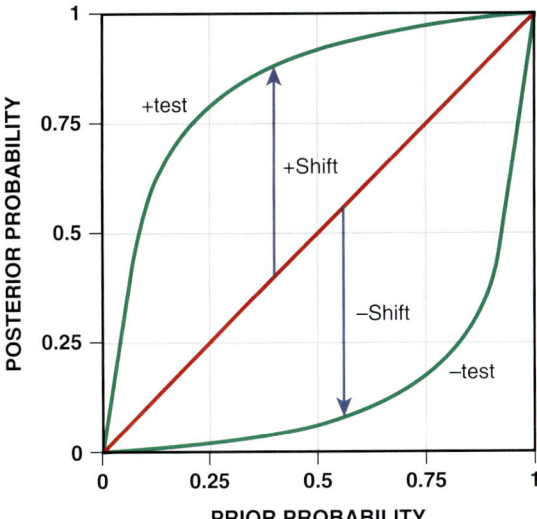

FIGURE 5.6 Leaf plot showing how the probability estimate of a diagnosis can shift depending on a test result. After choosing a pre-test probability estimate on the x-axis, one can trace up to either the upper curve for a positive test result or the lower curve for a negative test result, then trace over to the y-axis to read the post-test probability estimate.

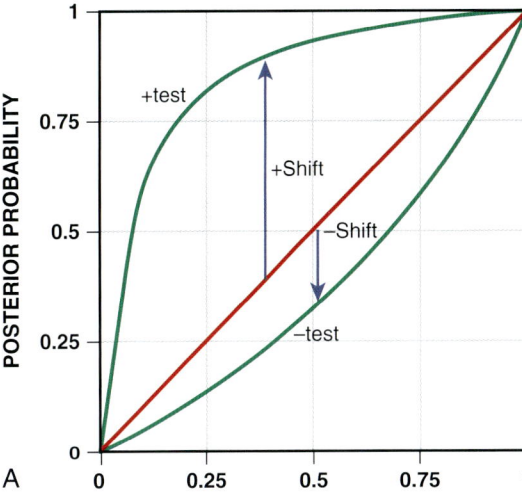

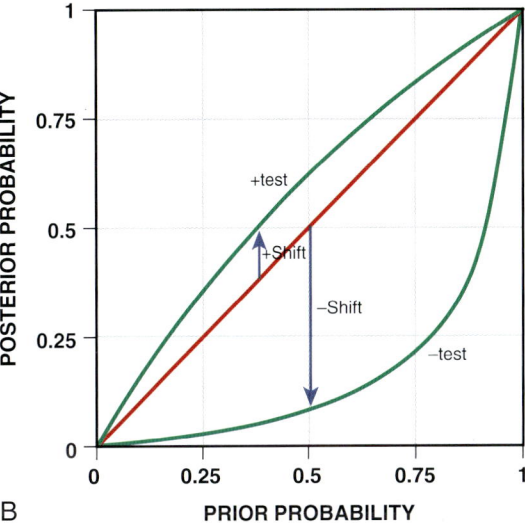

FIGURE 5.7 A, Probability estimate shift for a diagnostic test with a very strong positive likelihood ratio and a relatively weak negative likelihood ratio. **B,** Probability estimate shift for a diagnostic test with a very strong negative likelihood ratio and a modest positive likelihood ratio.

TEST ORDERING STRATEGIES

Clinical reasoning should guide not only test interpretation, but also test ordering. Tests that are ordered for good reasons are more conclusive, and tests that are ordered indiscriminately can cause clinicians to make poor judgments. Ideally, a test should be used to validate or reject an articulated hypothesis—a plausible conjecture that is generated by a patient's condition. Ideally clinicians think ahead about what they would do with test results.

To aid with test selection and avoid over-testing, the American College of Cardiology (ACC) and other organizations have developed appropriate use criteria to guide clinicians' decisions about ordering selected cardiac tests.[11] This effort is driven by both a need to avoid excessive false-positive test results and also the need to contain the costs of medical care. The goal of appropriate use guidelines is to reduce overuse errors and to maximize the value of diagnostic testing and procedures. The general principle of any test-ordering strategy is that a plausible hypothesis (a provisional diagnosis) should be formulated first, followed by testing. The appropriate use criteria are designed to avoid testing when the results are unlikely to improve patient care and outcomes.

PREDICTING RISK

Recent ACC/American Heart Association (AHA) guidelines have promoted the provision of preventive treatments according to an individual's risk of adverse outcomes.[12] The premise is that low-risk people have little to gain by preventive interventions, while high-risk individuals may have a lot to gain. These guideline recommendations emphasize the need to consider categories based on estimates of risk and prognosis, rather than merely diagnostic labels, such as hyperlipidemia. It is important for clinicians to understand the provenance of the risk scores and their performance, including in diverse populations, to know whether the tools are useful. After calculating the risk, the challenge for clinicians is communicating risk to patients in an understandable fashion. Investigators have provided infographics that can communicate risk and risk reduction in order to facilitate a discussion regarding long-term treatment options to diminish risk, and to compare the degree of risk reduction with potential side effects and costs of treatment (see Fig. 5.8). Because clinicians vary in their use of qualitative terms such as "high risk," there is a need to provide clear and understandable quantitative estimates.[13]

THERAPEUTIC DECISIONS

A preventive or therapeutic decision is a structured choice. These decisions require medical knowledge and a balanced sense of risks and benefits, as well as knowledge of patients' preferences, to make optimal therapeutic decisions.

Clinical trials report the average risk of an outcome for patients in a treatment group and in a comparison group. There may be heterogeneity of the treatment effect, in which some patients may receive a marked benefit and others receive no benefit at all. Subgroup analysis and tests for interaction can provide hints, but usually heterogeneity of treatment effect is not readily apparent, creating a challenge for clinicians trying to personalize treatment decisions. In a key example of heterogeneity, fibrinolytic therapy was effective in the treatment of suspected AMI and subgroup analyses revealed the benefit to be substantial in patients with ST-elevation but not in those without it. The challenge is that subgroup analyses introduce the possibility that associations have occurred only by chance. In the Second International Study of Infarct Survival (ISIS-2), the authors provided perspective on subgroup analyses by demonstrating that patients born under the astrological signs of Gemini or Libra were significantly less likely to benefit from fibrinolytic therapy. Thus, subgroup analysis is capable of producing important insights, but must be interpreted with caution.[14]

A weakness of relative benefit estimates is that they do not convey information about what is achieved for patients at varying levels of risk. A small relative reduction in risk may be meaningful for a high-risk patient, while a large relative reduction may be inconsequential for a very low-risk patient. Absolute risk reduction, the difference between two rates, varies with the risk of an individual patient. For example, a risk ratio of 2.0 does not distinguish between baseline risks of 80% and

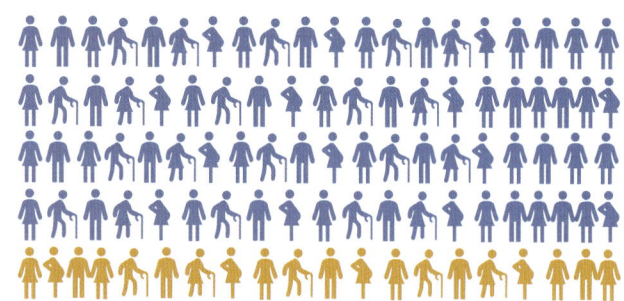
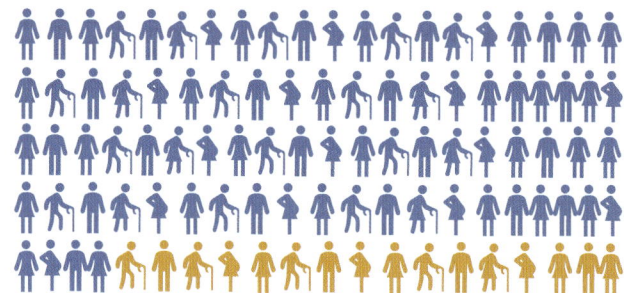

FIGURE 5.8 Infographic showing a format for demonstrating risk and benefit to patients. The infographic shows a baseline risk of a cardiovascular endpoint in patients with a baseline risk of 20%, and the 20% relative risk reduction with statin therapy.

40% and between 0.08% and 0.04%. In one case, the absolute difference is 50% (5000 per 10,000) and in the other, it is 0.05% (5 per 10,000). In one case, 1 person out of 2 benefits and in the other, 1 out of 2000 benefits. Unfortunately, absolute benefit is not emphasized adequately in many articles.[15]

Risk prediction is critically important for calculating the expected absolute risk reduction. In recent years, many tools have been developed to assist in the rapid assessment of patient risk, with variable uncertainty about their comparative performance.[15,16]

In evaluating studies of risk prediction, it is important to consider whether the approach has been validated in populations similar to the patients to whom it is applied in practice. The predictors should be collected independently of knowledge of the outcome. The outcome and timeframe should be appropriate for clinical decisions and the value of the prediction should be clear. Appropriate risk prediction can assist in calculation of absolute benefit and put the balance of risks and benefits of an intervention in proper perspective.

Several studies have shown a risk-treatment paradox in which the higher-risk patients are least likely to receive interventions that are expected to provide a benefit. This pattern is paradoxical because the high-risk patients would be expected to have the most to gain from an intervention that reduces risk, assuming that the relative reduction in risk is constant across groups defined by their baseline risk. The source of the paradox is not known, although some have suggested that it is related to an aversion to the treatment of patients with a limited functional status, or concern for greater degree of harm from the same therapy.

Cardiovascular drugs and procedures are often double-edged swords, having both benefit and harm. Also, patients may have strong preferences about potential benefit and harm. For example, a patient may have a strong fear of a side effect such as a cerebrovascular accident that may overwhelm other considerations about a treatment decision. It is important to engage patients and families in a discussion to explain the considerations that go into therapeutic decisions, particularly for nuanced decisions about treatments that have substantial risks in addition to potential benefits.

Absolute risk reduction is better than relative risk reduction for estimating a treatment effect. The inverse of the absolute risk reduction, which is a term called number needed to treat (NNT), is even more intuitive.[3]

Consider a trial with a combined event rate of 10% in the treatment group and a 15% risk in the control group, giving an absolute risk reduction of 5%. This means that 5 events are avoided for every 100 patients in the treatment group. The reciprocal of this relationship indicates that there would be 100 patients treated for every 5 events avoided. By dividing 100 by 5, which reduces the denominator to 1, there would be 20 patients treated per 1 event avoided. Thus, the NNT is 20. For NNT, the smaller the number, the better.

NNT and absolute risk reduction depend on both the relative risk reduction and the baseline risk. For conditions with a high baseline risk, the NNT can become very small (desirable). As an extreme example, for a patient with ventricular fibrillation, the baseline risk of dying without defibrillation is 100%, making the NNT for defibrillation (if always effective) equal to 1.

Primary prevention with statin drugs has a relative risk reduction of about 20% over the several-year course of a typical prevention trial.[17] The absolute risk reduction and NNT depend upon the baseline risk, which varies depending on a number of factors. At a baseline risk of 7.5%, the absolute risk reduction would be 1.5% and the NNT would be 67, a fairly high number, which suggests marginal benefit at this level of baseline risk.

NNT is a useful intuitive tool for comparing the efficacy of various treatment strategies. NNT is also a useful way to summarize the findings of a clinical trial in a single declarative sentence. For example, the PARTNER-3 trial had an NNT of 16, meaning one would need to treat 16 low-risk aortic stenosis patients with a transcatheter aortic valve replacement to prevent one composite endpoint of death, stroke, or rehospitalization over 1 year.[18] The EMPEROR-Reduced trial had an NNT of 19, meaning one would need to treat 19 patients with class II to IV heart failure and an ejection fraction of ≤40% with a sodium-glucose cotransporter 2 (SGLT-2) inhibitor for 16 months to prevent one death or hospitalization for worsening heart failure.[19] With NNT, a single sentence can provide the trial name, the magnitude of the treatment effect, the trial's entry criteria, the study drug or intervention, the duration of the trial, and the outcome measure. NNTs of 16 and 19 suggest that these treatments are strongly recommended, although some patients may not consider it worth going through the treatment if 15 of 16 people have the same outcome regardless of whether they received the intervention.

NNT is also a very personal notion of the probability of a treatment effect. Imagine bringing 19 untreated patients with congestive heart failure and an ejection fraction of ≤40% into a room and saying, "If all of you start on an SGLT-2 inhibitor, over the next 16 months, one of you will experience the benefit." Capturing the essence of a treatment effect with NNT is a useful way to intuitively convey the impact of a treatment effect. This knowledge, packaged in a way that is more intuitive, can make it easier to combine this medical knowledge with the preferences and values of individual patients to make the best therapeutic decisions.

Nevertheless, there are limitations to NNT. NNT is an index of an average treatment effect over time and does not provide information about whether the treatment effect is immediate, delayed, or highly variable. NNT does not provide information about whether there is meaningful heterogeneity in effect among different subgroups, as the NNT often is calculated based on an assumption of a uniform effect of the therapy, with the NNT just varying based on the baseline risk.

DECIDING WHEN TO CHANGE CLINICAL PRACTICE BASED ON NEW CLINICAL RESEARCH FINDINGS

Science is a quantitative discipline that uses numbers to measure, analyze, and explain nature. Evidence-based medicine has been defined by David Sackett as "the conscientious, explicit, and judicious use of current best evidence in making decisions about the care of individual patients." To practice evidence-based medicine, clinicians must remain vigilant, constantly monitoring for new research findings, accompanied by a basic knowledge of statistics to make proper inferences from clinical research.

When using statistics to compare two groups, the standard method is to assume that there is no difference between the two groups, the so-called null hypothesis. The trial results are reported, along with a p value, which is the probability of deriving the difference reported in the trial, or a more extreme difference, given the assumption that the null hypothesis is true (i.e., there is no real difference between the groups). When a trial is designed, the investigators estimate the sample sizes that are required to avoid claiming that there is a difference between treatment groups when there really is no difference (a type I error or alpha error) or claiming that there is no differences between treatment groups when there really is one (a type II error or beta error). Similar to a clinical test like a stress test that can have false-positive and false-negative test results, clinical trials can have false-positive results (alpha errors) and false-negative results (beta errors). A trial with adequate sample size and rigorous statistical methods should allow investigators to avoid these errors.

When a trial is designed, the alpha level is usually set at 0.05. If the p value of the observed data is less than 0.05, one can conclude that a very improbable event occurred, a less than 1-in-20 event, assuming the null hypothesis is valid. According to the frequentist notion of statistics, one imagines that repeating a trial many times would create a distribution of possible trial results. The p value tells us where the observed results of a particular trial would sit in that imaginary distribution of trial results.

Because the p value is so commonly used in clinical research, clinicians need to be aware of several key issues. First, the threshold of 0.05 for statistical significance is arbitrary. A p value of 0.04 implies that the data could occur 4% of the time if the null hypothesis is true and a p value of 0.06 would suggest the data would occur 6% of the time. Is the difference between 6% and 4% enough to reject the null hypothesis in one case and accept it in another? Clinicians should understand that p values are continuous values and are just one piece of information needed to assess a trial. Second, p values do not inform clinical importance. A large study sample can produce a small p value despite a clinically inconsequential difference between groups. Clinicians need to examine the size of the effects in addition to the statistical tests of whether the results could have occurred by chance.

ENDPOINTS

In evaluating evidence, clinicians should be particularly attuned to the outcomes that are assessed. Ideally, interventions are assessed for their effect on a patient's quality or quantity of life. Many studies use surrogate outcomes, measures that are more distally related to the patient experience but might be related to the likelihood that a patient's quality or quantity of life will be affected. These surrogate outcomes often reflect information about a patient's biology, and in epidemiologic studies, these outcomes may have prognostic value. However, it is not possible to know that an intervention that modifies a surrogate outcome has the expected effect on patients. There are many examples in medicine of changes in surrogate measures that did not translate into benefits for patients.

NONINFERIORITY TRIALS

Most randomized trials are designed to show the superiority of a treatment over placebo. However, some conditions already have treatments with proven benefit, making it unethical to design a trial that compares a new treatment with placebo. For example, for chronic atrial fibrillation, it was not possible to test newer oral anticoagulant drugs against a placebo arm that would have withheld the proven benefit of warfarin.

For these situations, investigators use a noninferiority trial. The premise is to show that a given treatment is at least no worse than the standard of care by more than a predefined investigator-selected margin (the treatment could be slightly worse, or even be superior for efficacy). However, because the new treatment has other ancillary advantages (e.g., fewer side effects, better costs or tolerability), it could become a reasonable alternative to the previous standard of care. This trial design requires making assumptions about the margin of decreased efficacy that would be considered acceptable before considering using a new treatment rather than an established treatment with known efficacy. Noninferiority trials are also subject to several other biases that are not seen with typical superiority trials.[20]

OBSERVATIONAL RESEARCH

There are other situations in which a randomized controlled trial is impossible, and observational studies such as case-control studies or longitudinal cohort studies are required. Randomized controlled trials have the advantage of a controlled experiment that eliminates potential biases but have the limitation of narrowly defining a study population, which may affect generalizability. Observational studies have the advantage of observing large groups of unselected subjects in the real-world setting but have the disadvantage of potentially unrecognized and unmeasured sources of bias that could produce misleading study results. There is great heterogeneity in the quality of the data and methods used in observational research and there is a need to be discerning when evaluating observational research studies.[21,22]

SHARED DECISION-MAKING

The principle of autonomy maintains that patients retain control over their bodies and must consent to undergo interventions, except in rare circumstances. Informed consent is the cornerstone of this concept.[23] Unfortunately, there is little consensus about how best to involve patients actively in decision-making. Nevertheless, given the need to align goals of therapy with the patient's preferences and values, it is important to engage them as effectively as possible. This approach is most appropriate for major decisions, those with intermediate or low certainty, and those that are not emergent.

Informed consent is a critical part of medicine, but one that has many gaps. Documentation of informed consent suggests that physicians often do not communicate in ways that address key topics necessary for informed choice.[24] It has been suggested, for example, that informed consent should be obtained with enough time before elective procedures for people to contemplate the decisions.[25] The consent about procedures should contain an easy-to-understand description of the procedure, potential benefits, potential risks, alternative strategies, out-of-pocket costs, and the experience of the health care team in performing the procedure.[26]

There are many aspects of communicating risks and benefits. First, this information takes many forms. The dimensions of risk and benefit include their identity, permanence, timing, probability, and value to an individual patient. All should be considered in decision-making. Unfortunately, there is relatively little evidence to guide physicians about how best to convey risks to patients.

It is known that patients do not always understand benefit and risk well. Many studies of patients undergoing revascularization procedures have shown that the patients can make assumptions about the survival benefits of cardiac procedures and patients often have a poor understanding of the potential for complications. There have been calls to improve medical education and medical reporting to address this problem of "risk illiteracy."[27]

The manner in which information is presented may influence patients. Like physicians, patients are also susceptible to framing effects. Patients tend to be more likely to choose a therapy that is presented as having an advantage over an alternative in relative rather than absolute terms. The relative effect is almost always much greater than the absolute change. Patients may also be influenced by the order in which information is provided.

Some techniques have been proposed to help clinicians convey risk.[28] First, clinicians should avoid descriptive terms only because they may not have a consistent meaning to patients. Terms such as "low risk" may be difficult for people to interpret. If clinicians express risk as ratios, they should use a consistent denominator (e.g., 40 out of 1000 and 5 out of 1000 instead of 1 in 25 and 1 in 200). Clinicians should offer multiple perspectives, revealing multiple ways of thinking about risk. They should use absolute numbers and natural frequencies (e.g., 1 out of 20), not relative risks or percentages. Visual aids are useful, if available, as poor numeracy or literacy skills may be a barrier for many patients. Many patients do not understand risk communication formats. In addition, clinicians should recognize that information and data are not the same, and it is incumbent on the clinician to communicate health information that is meaningful to the patient.

Figure 5.8 shows a format for demonstrating risk and benefit to patients. The infographic shows a baseline risk of a cardiovascular endpoint in patients with a baseline risk of 20%, and the 20% relative risk reduction with statin therapy.[17]

Shared decision-making can be understood as having five phases: assess, advise, agree, assist, and arrange. First, the clinician must assess the patient. Then, the clinician should advise the patient of the options, with their benefits and risks. Next, the clinician and patient should agree on a plan that is aligned with the patient's preferences and values. The clinician should then assist the patient in implementing the plan. Finally, the patient and clinician arrange follow-up.[29,30]

Clinical decision-making also involves other members of a cardiovascular team.[31,32] The model of team-based care has now become standard practice, bringing Advanced Practice Practitioners (nurse practitioners, physician assistants, and clinical pharmacists) into the decision-making process for cardiovascular care. Good communication and coordination, and the mantra of "shared goals and clear roles" are important to assure optimal team-based shared decision-making.

MONITORING THE QUALITY OF CLINICAL DECISIONS

Getting the right care to the right patient at the right time every time requires good judgment. Learning the basic competencies of good judgment and step-by-step methods of clinical reasoning can help practitioners monitor the quality of their decisions. Knowledge about clinical reasoning is a structural attribute that can lead to more reliable processes and better clinical outcomes. Awareness of the logic, probability theory, and cognitive psychology of clinical reasoning can provide a theoretical foundation for better clinical practice.

Cognitive science provides justification for many of the good habits that are part of practice, such as consistently performing a standardized history and physical examination and a conscious habit of listing a differential diagnosis. Cognitive psychologists emphasize that measurement and feedback is a crucial process for the development of expert intuition, which is so often necessary for clinical decisions.

System 1 and System 2 Thinking

Cognitive psychologists describe two general thinking modes that people use to make decisions: System 1 and System 2 thinking.[6] System 1 thinking is highly intuitive and fast, but prone to jumping to conclusions. System 2 thinking is analytical and logical, but slow, effortful, and has difficulty with uncertainty. Used together, System 2 thinking provides a double check for System 1 thinking, and System 1 thinking provides a work-around when System 2 thinking is constrained by uncertainty. Cardiology decisions require both thinking modes, and expert clinicians are able to use a balance of intuition and analytical thinking to make optimal decisions. Calibrating intuitive thinking and organizing thinking by thoughtfully monitoring clinical decisions (so called "meta-cognition") are key to good clinical practice.

Some psychologists describe three general types of fallacies: (1) hasty judgments, (2) biased judgments, and (3) distorted probability estimates.[6] Hasty judgments occur when System 1 thinking is unmonitored. For example, premature closure of a diagnostic exercise, without the use of a differential diagnosis, or becoming anchored on a diagnosis can lead to a misdiagnosis. Biased judgments occur when unconscious thoughts influence ideas, emotions, and actions. This can take the form of priming, stereotyping, overconfidence, risk aversion, or dread. Emotions can have a halo effect, influencing clinical thinking in imperceptible ways. Exaggerated fear of malpractice, financial incentives, and conflict of interest can adversely affect decisions. Decision-makers tend to overweigh the probabilities of events or propositions at the extremes. At one end, clinicians can develop an illusion of certainty, which creates certainty about something that, objectively, is not certain at all. At the other extreme is the possibility effect, which creates the impression that highly improbable events or propositions are quite probable. Knowledge of these fallacies can help clinicians develop habits that will improve the quality of their clinical reasoning.

A recent Institute of Medicine report brought attention to the high prevalence of diagnostic error.[33] Renewed interest has centered around defining diagnostic errors and measuring error rates.

A number of authors have suggested that diagnostic errors are due to cognitive biases.[33,34] To avoid cognitive biases, the cognitive psychologist Kahneman provides the following advice: "The way to block errors that originate in System 1 is simple in principle: recognize the signs that you are in a cognitive minefield and slow down, and ask for reinforcement from System 2."[6] Evans, another cognitive psychologist, counters this advice by stating, "perhaps the most persistent fallacy in the perception of dual-process theories is the idea that Type 1 processes (intuitive, heuristic) are responsible for all bad thinking and that Type 2 processes (reflective, analytic) necessarily lead to correct responses…So ingrained is this good-bad thinking idea that some dual process theories have built it into their core terminology."[35]

In fact, a number of studies show that faster response times often lead to a correct diagnosis. One study showed that when test subjects were instructed to go slow and be more analytic, there was no effect on the accuracy of diagnosis.[36]

Some investigators have advocated teaching physicians a large number of potential biases and encouraging them to routinely "debias" their thinking in practice.[34] However, studies that examined educational efforts to teach cognitive biases to medical trainees found that the instruction had no effect.[37,38] One study showed that physicians were unable to agree on what bias contributed to a diagnostic error and the study subjects were themselves affected by hindsight bias.[39]

Norman and others have argued that diagnostic error is commonly due to knowledge deficits or inability to mobilize necessary knowledge rather than flawed reasoning processes and biases.[38] Using deliberate reflection to help mobilize the necessary knowledge, as well as the use of checklists have been shown to be beneficial for reducing diagnostic error.[40] Improving diagnostic reasoning is an important goal and more research is needed to determine the most effective strategies for improvement.

Monitoring the quality of therapeutic decision-making is a broad topic and has been the focus of quality improvement efforts for decades. Explicit therapeutic decisions produce overt actions, and therefore can be easily monitored. Implicit bias, however, can have subtle effects on clinical decision-making, resulting in disparities in diagnosis, treatment, and outcomes. Implicit bias occurs when one's judgment is affected by unconscious associations between a class such as race and learned cultural prejudices and stereotypes.[41] Implicit bias related to race, sex, age, obesity, and other patient factors can unconsciously bias medical decisions. Conscious awareness of the problem through cultural competency training is helpful but may not be sufficient to alleviate implicit bias. Investigators have suggested that articulating egalitarian goals, identifying common identities with the patient, counter-stereotyping, and trying to see things from the patient's perspective are conscious mental strategies that can diminish implicit bias.[42]

TEACHING CLINICAL REASONING

Clinical reasoning can be learned through experience and continuously improved through deliberate practice and reflection. Although clinical reasoning can be learned, there are remaining questions about whether clinical reasoning can be formally taught through explicit instruction. Most teaching of clinical reasoning is through experience in the setting of clinical rotations. Formal teaching of reasoning has been promoted for centuries, but Richard Nesbit and others have posited that teaching abstract rules of reasoning fell into disfavor in the 20th century (see Classic References). The prevailing notion was that learners do not use abstract reasoning rules, but rather use domain-specific empirical rules that are better learned by experience, not instruction. There is evidence, however, that statistical heuristics, pragmatic inferential rules, and metacognitive strategies can be taught even with brief formal training.[43]

A recent study examined whether Bayesian reasoning can be taught.[44] The study showed a modest advantage for medical students randomized to receive theoretical instruction on concepts of Bayesian reasoning, suggesting that a conceptual framework can modestly improve clinical decision-making.[45]

Clinical reasoning is not a specific problem-solving skill that easily transfers from problem to problem, but rather is dependent on learned habits and a conceptual framework that enable the clinician to access, organize, and use both experiential knowledge and formal knowledge to address a clinical problem. Interleaving instruction on concepts of reasoning throughout training may strengthen the associations and provide a scaffolding for experiential knowledge to help learners make the most of their experience, calibrate their intuitive judgments, and become better at clinical reasoning.

CONCLUSION

Reliable decision-making is fundamentally important for high-quality, patient-centered medical care. Clinical decisions in cardiology are often time-sensitive, complex, and uncertain, demanding good clinical reasoning. Logic, probability theory, and cognitive science can provide a framework for good clinical reasoning. The ability to read, understand, and critique the literature is also essential. Knowledge of the components of clinical reasoning is crucial for clinical practice, for team-based care, and for shared decision-making. The ability to reason and the ability to use reasoning to stay current and monitor one's performance are the essence of professionalism. Ensuring that the patient is a participant and is part of all decisions is also essential. Integrating scientific knowledge and calibrated intuition with a patient's personal preferences and values can provide the highest quality of care.

CLASSIC REFERENCES

Simon H. Invariants of human behavior. *Annu Rev Psychol.* 1990;41:1–20.
Montgomery K. *How Doctors Think: Clinical Judgment and the Practice of Medicine.* Oxford; New York: Oxford University Press; 2006.
Elstein AS, Shulman LS, Sprafka SA. *Medical Problem Solving: An Analysis of Clinical Reasoning.* Cambridge, MA: Harvard University Press; 1978.
Diamond GA, Forrester JS. Analysis of probability as an aid in the clinical diagnosis of coronary-artery disease. *N Engl J Med.* 1979;300:1350–1358.
Nisbett RE, Fong GT, Lehman DR, Cheng PW. Teaching reasoning. *Science.* 1987;238:625–631.

REFERENCES

Access supplemental references online at Elsevier eBooks for Practicing Clinicians.

1. Kassirer JP, Wong JB, Kopelman RI. *Learning Clinical Reasoning.* Baltimore, MD: Lippincott Williams & Wilkins Health; 2010.
2. Sox HC, Higgins MC, Owens DK. *Medical Decision-Making.* 2nd ed. West Sussex, UK: Wiley-Blackwell; 2013.
3. Brush JE. *The Science of the Art of Medicine: A Guide to Medical Reasoning.* Manakin-Sabot, VA: Dementi Milestone Publishing, Inc.; 2015.
4. Norman GR, Eva KW. Diagnostic error and clinical reasoning. *Med Educ.* 2010;44:94–100.
5. Dharmarajan K, Strait KM, Tinetti ME, et al. Treatment for multiple acute cardiopulmonary conditions in older adults hospitalized with pneumonia, chronic obstructive pulmonary disease, or heart failure. *J Am Geriatr Soc.* 2016;64:1574–1582.
6. Kahneman D. *Thinking, Fast and Slow.* New York: Farrar, Straus and Giroux; 2011.
7. Gigerenzer G, Gaissmaier W. Heuristic decision making. *Ann Rev Psychol.* 2011;62:451–482.

Diagnostic Decisions

8. Brush Jr JE, Sherbino J, Norman GR. How expert clinicians intuitively recognize a medical diagnosis. *Am J Med.* 2017;130:629–634.
9. Brush Jr JE, Krumholz HM, Greene EJ, Dreyer RP. Sex differences in symptom phenotypes among patients with acute myocardial infarction. *Circ Cardiovasc Qual Outcomes.* 2020;13:e005948.
10. Manrai AK, Funke BH, Rehm HL, et al. Genetic misdiagnoses and the potential for health disparities. *N Engl J Med.* 2016;375:655–665.
11. Hendel RC, Lindsay BD, Allen JM, et al. ACC appropriate use criteria methodology: 2018 update: a report of the American College of Cardiology Appropriate use criteria task force. *J Am Coll Cardiol.* 2018;71:935–948.
12. Goff Jr DC, Lloyd-Jones DM, Bennett G, et al. 2013 ACC/AHA guideline on the assessment of cardiovascular risk: a report of the American College of Cardiology/American Heart Association task force on practice guidelines. *J Am Coll Cardiol.* 2014;63:2935–2959.
13. Spiegelhalter DJ. *The Art of Statistics: How to Learn from Data.* First US edition. New York: Basic Books; 2019.

Therapeutic Decisions

14. O'Gara PT, Kushner FG, Ascheim DD, et al. 2013 ACCF/AHA guideline for the management of ST-elevation myocardial infarction: executive summary: a report of the American College of Cardiology Foundation/American Heart Association task force on practice guidelines. *J Am Coll Cardiol.* 2013;61:485–510.
15. Damen JA, Hooft L, Schuit E, et al. Prediction models for cardiovascular disease risk in the general population: systematic review. *BMJ.* 2016;353:i2416.
16. McNamara RL, Kennedy KF, Cohen DJ, et al. Predicting in-hospital mortality in patients with acute myocardial infarction. *J Am Coll Cardiol.* 2016;68:626–635.
17. Stone NJ, Robinson JG, Lichtenstein AH, et al. 2013 ACC/AHA guideline on the treatment of blood cholesterol to reduce atherosclerotic cardiovascular risk in adults: a report of the American College of Cardiology/American Heart Association Task Force on Practice Guidelines. *J Am Coll Cardiol.* 2014;63. 2889-2834.
18. Mack MJ, Leon MB, Thourani VH, et al. Transcatheter aortic-valve replacement with a balloon-expandable valve in low-risk patients. *N Engl J Med.* 2019;380:1695–1705.
19. Packer M, Anker SD, Butler J, et al. Cardiovascular and renal outcomes with empagliflozin in heart failure. *N Engl J Med.* 2020;383:1413–1424.
20. Bikdeli B, Welsh JW, Akram Y, et al. Noninferiority designed cardiovascular trials in highest-impact journals. *Circulation.* 2019;140:379–389.
21. Califf RM, Hernandez AF, Landray M. Weighing the benefits and risks of proliferating observational treatment assessments: observational cacophony, randomized harmony. *J Am Med Assoc.* 2020. https://doi.org/10.1001/jama.2020.13319.

Shared Decision Making

22. Schuemie MJ, Ryan PB, Pratt N, et al. Principles of Large-scale Evidence Generation and Evaluation across a Network Of Databases (LEGEND). *J Am Med Inform Assoc.* 2020;27:1331–1337.
23. Spatz ES, Krumholz HM, Moulton BW. The new era of informed consent: getting to a reasonable-patient standard through shared decision making. *J Am Med Assoc.* 2016;315:2063–2064.
24. Spatz ES, Bao H, Herrin J, et al. Quality of informed consent documents among US. hospitals: a cross-sectional study. *BMJ Open.* 2020;10:e033299.
25. Spatz ES, Suter LG, George E, et al. An instrument for assessing the quality of informed consent documents for elective procedures: development and testing. *BMJ Open.* 2020;10:e033297.
26. Krumholz HM. Informed consent to promote patient-centered care. *J Am Med Assoc.* 2010;303:1190–1191.
27. Gigerenzer G, Gray JAM. *Better Doctors, Better Patients, Better Decisions: Envisioning Health Care 2020.* Cambridge, MA: MIT Press; 2011.
28. Navar AM, Wang TY, Mi X, et al. Influence of cardiovascular risk communication tools and presentation formats on patient perceptions and preferences. *JAMA Cardiol.* 2018;3:1192–1199.
29. Krumholz HM. Variations in health care, patient preferences, and high-quality decision making. *J Am Med Assoc.* 2013;310:151–152.
30. Krumholz HM, Barreto-Filho JA, Jones PG, et al. Decision-making preferences among patients with an acute myocardial infarction. *JAMA Intern Med.* 2013;173:1252–1257.
31. Brush Jr JE, Handberg EM, Biga C, et al. 2015 ACC health policy statement on cardiovascular team-based care and the role of advanced practice providers. *J Am Coll Cardiol.* 2015;65:2118–2136.
32. Rodgers GP, Linderbaum JA, Pearson DD, et al. 2020 ACC clinical competencies for nurse practitioners and physician assistants in adult cardiovascular medicine: a report of the ACC Competency Management Committee. *J Am Coll Cardiol.* 2020;75:2483–2517.

Monitoring the Quality of Clinical Decisions

33. National Academies of Sciences, Engineering, and Medicine. *Improving Diagnosis in Health Care.* Washington, DC: The National Academies Press; 2015. https://doi.org/10.17226/21794.
34. Croskerry P. From mindless to mindful practice—cognitive bias and clinical decision making. *N Engl J Med.* 2013;368:2445–2448.
35. Evans JS. Dual-processing accounts of reasoning, judgment, and social cognition. *Annu Rev Psychol.* 2008;59:255–278.
36. Sherbino J, Dore KL, Wood TJ, et al. The relationship between response time and diagnostic accuracy. *Acad Med.* 2012;87:785–791.
37. Sherbino J, Kulasegaram K, Howey E, Norman G. Ineffectiveness of cognitive forcing strategies to reduce biases in diagnostic reasoning: a controlled trial. *CJEM.* 2014;16:34–40.
38. Norman GR, Monteiro SD, Sherbino J, et al. The causes of errors in clinical reasoning: cognitive biases, knowledge deficits, and dual process thinking. *Acad Med.* 2017;92:23–30.
39. Zwaan L, Monteiro S, Sherbino J, et al. Is bias in the eye of the beholder? A vignette study to assess recognition of cognitive biases in clinical case workups. *BMJ Qual Saf.* 2017;26:104–110.
40. Schmidt HG, Mamede S. How to improve the teaching of clinical reasoning: a narrative review and a proposal. *Med Educ.* 2015;49:961–973.
41. FitzGerald C, Hurst S. Implicit bias in healthcare professionals: a systematic review. *BMC Med Ethics.* 2017;18:19.
42. Stone J, Moskowitz GB. Non-conscious bias in medical decision making: what can be done to reduce it? *Med Educ.* 2011;45:768–776.
43. Nesbitt RE. *Mindware: Tools for Smart Thinking.* New York, NY: Farrar, Straus and Giroux; 2016.
44. Brush Jr JE, Lee M, Sherbino J, et al. Effect of teaching Bayesian methods using learning by concept vs learning by example on medical students' ability to estimate probability of a diagnosis: a randomized clinical trial. *JAMA Netw Open.* 2019;2:e1918023.
45. Kulasegaram KM, Chaudhary Z, Woods N, et al. Contexts, concepts and cognition: principles for the transfer of basic science knowledge. *Med Educ.* 2017;51:184–195.

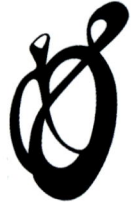

6 Impact of Health Care Policy on Quality, Outcomes, and Equity in Cardiovascular Disease

KAREN E. JOYNT MADDOX

扫描二维码阅读
第6章中文导读

WHAT IS HEALTH POLICY?, 62

INSURANCE COVERAGE AND ACCESS POLICY, 62

PAYMENT AND DELIVERY SYSTEM POLICY TO IMPROVE QUALITY AND REDUCE COSTS, 63

Public Reporting, 64
Value-Based Payment Programs: Hospitals, 65
Value-Based Purchasing: Outpatient, 65
Alternative Payment Models, 65

INEQUITIES IN CARDIOVASCULAR DISEASE RISK, CARE, AND OUTCOMES, 66

Racial and Ethnic Minorities, 66
Income, 67
Urban-Rural Geography, 67

CONCLUSIONS, 68

REFERENCES, 68

WHAT IS HEALTH POLICY?

Health policy is the collection of federal, state, and local statutes and regulations that determine the "rules of the game" in health care. Many of the major issues in health policy are driven by statute, also known as law. For example, in 1965, President Lyndon B. Johnson signed into law the Social Security Act Amendments, commonly referred to as the Medicare bill. This law established both Medicare, a health insurance program for older Americans, and Medicaid, a health insurance program for Americans living in poverty. More recently, U.S. health policy has been shaped by a number of provisions in the Affordable Care Act (ACA), signed into law by President Barack Obama in 2010.

While these laws, often hundreds or even thousands of pages in length, set specific provisions in place, they leave a great deal of detail to regulation. Regulation, in contrast to law, is not passed by Congress, but rather developed and implemented by government agencies. For example, while the ACA established a number of value-based payment (VBP) programs that will be explored in detail later in this chapter, regulatory guidance from the Centers for Medicare and Medicaid Services, commonly known as CMS, determines the annual collection of metrics, scoring systems, and payment modifications that puts them into practice.

The United States has much higher health care costs, but worse health outcomes, including cardiovascular outcomes, than other economically comparable countries. In 2018, the United States accounted for over $3.6 trillion in health care spending. Of this total, 34% was funded by private insurance, 21% by Medicare, 16% by Medicaid, 3% by public health agencies and departments, 10% by individuals in the form of "out-of-pocket" spending, and the remaining 15% by other public sources including the Veterans Health Administration, Indian Health Service, and Department of Defense (Fig. 6.1).[1] In total, this spending comprised 17.7% of the U.S. gross domestic product (GDP) in 2018, or over $11,000 per capita. Despite this spending, the United States has higher age-adjusted per-capita cardiovascular mortality and has seen fewer gains in these metrics over the past few decades than many other countries worldwide. Just as importantly, what successes the United States has had in reducing cardiovascular disease (CVD) incidence and prevalence over time have been uneven—major differences in CVD outcomes exist by race, ethnicity, income, and geography.

U.S. health policy fundamentally shapes how medicine is practiced, how care is delivered, and to some degree, the health outcomes that are achieved. A basic understanding of health policy is crucial for the practicing cardiologist as he or she works to deliver high-quality, cost-efficient care and achieve excellent outcomes for patients. Much of health policy falls into two major "buckets": coverage and access policy, and payment and delivery system policy, which will be explored in turn in this chapter. This chapter will focus primarily on public insurance (Medicaid and Medicare), because the federal and state governments largely set the norms in health policy, with private insurers often following their lead. The chapter will end with a section on health equity, since health policy also plays a major role, along with other social policies, in large and persistent cardiovascular and overall health disparities across the United States.

INSURANCE COVERAGE AND ACCESS POLICY

The primary goal of health insurance is to offer financial protection against unexpected illness or injury. Prior studies suggest that CVD is commonly associated with financial hardship. For example, almost half of patients admitted for acute myocardial infarction (AMI) report some level of financial stress.[2] Similarly, about 45% of patients with atherosclerotic CVD report financial hardship due to their medical bills, particularly among those who lack insurance or have low income.[3] Insurance coverage is therefore a key policy area in cardiovascular medicine.

However, in the United States, insurance is variable and complex. In 2018, 55% of the population had private health insurance obtained through an employer, known as employer-sponsored insurance.[4] An additional 11% of the population purchased private insurance on the individual market, meaning directly from an insurance company. Eighteen percent of the U.S. population was covered by Medicaid, a state-administered public program for people living in poverty; 18% by Medicare, a federally administered public program for people over the age of 65, with disabilities, or with end-stage renal disease or other special qualifying conditions; and 1% by other public sources. Approximately 9% of the population was uninsured. Note that since people can have more than one source of insurance coverage, these numbers add up to greater than 100%.

The ACA had profound implications for coverage and access policy. Health insurers were prevented from denying coverage based on pre-existing conditions and from dropping people's coverage when they got sick. Annual and lifetime coverage caps were prohibited. Preventative care, vaccinations, and routine medical screening were required to be exempted from co-payments or deductibles. Children were allowed to stay on their parents' insurance plans until age 26. The profit insurance companies could earn on health insurance premiums was also capped, with insurers being required to spend 80% to 85% of premiums on direct health care costs. The ACA expanded access to health insurance in two ways. First, it created insurance exchanges, which are online marketplaces that individuals and small businesses can use to compare and purchase insurance plans. States had the option to create their own state-based marketplace, but the majority rely on the federally facilitated marketplace on the healthcare.gov website. Individuals making between 100% and 400% of the federal poverty level (the FPL was $12,760 for an individual and $21,720 for a family of three in 2020)[5] and who purchase insurance through these exchanges are eligible for subsidies to lower the cost of their premiums.

The second major way that the ACA expanded coverage was via Medicaid expansion. Medicaid is a state-administered health insurance program focused on providing coverage for individuals living in poverty, and covers 76 million beneficiaries, more than half of all births, and 60% of nursing home care nationwide. Prior to the ACA, all states covered pregnant women and children in households with incomes up to 200% to 300% of FPL, but coverage for other groups varied broadly. In many states, childless adults living in poverty were not eligible for Medicaid coverage at all. The ACA provided funding for states to extend Medicaid coverage to a broader group of eligible individuals, including for parents and childless adults with incomes at or below 138% of the FPL. However, the Supreme Court's ruling in National Federation of Independent Business v. Sebelius (2012) effectively made Medicaid expansion voluntary, and as of 2020, 12 states have declined to expand (Fig. 6.2).[6]

States that have elected to expand Medicaid have seen a significant decrease in uninsurance rates, particularly among low-income populations, and a reduction in disparities in insurance coverage across major racial/ethnic categories.[7] From 2012 to 2016, the proportion of AMI admissions that were for individuals lacking insurance decreased from 18% to 8% in Medicaid expansion states, whereas it only decreased from 26% to 21% in nonexpansion states.[8]

A growing body of evidence demonstrates that health insurance coverage, and Medicaid expansion in particular, has positive effects that extend beyond financial security to improve health and well-being. Medicaid expansion has led to greater access to primary, preventative, and specialist care for low-income individuals.[9,10] Expansion states saw improvements in the identification and treatment of cardiovascular risk factors, such as diabetes, hypertension, and dyslipidemia.[11–13] Additionally, use and adherence of prescription cardiovascular medications have increased.[9,14] Medicaid expansion is also associated with better access to behavioral health services, a reduction in cigarette purchases, and an increase in smoking cessation attempts.[15]

The increase in detection and treatment of chronic disease, behavioral health conditions, and addiction associated with Medicaid expansion has had an impact on health outcomes.[9,10,16–21] Expansion is associated with fewer preventable hospitalizations,[22] although evidence on its effects on emergency department use has been mixed.[23] One study showed that even accounting for demographic, clinical, and economic differences, counties in expansion states had 4.3 fewer deaths from cardiovascular causes per 100,000 residents per year after Medicaid expansion than if they had followed the same trends as counties in nonexpansion states (roughly a 2.5% difference).[24] Studies of early Medicaid expansions suggest that gains have particularly benefited racial and ethnic minorities, with all-cause mortality reductions greatest for nonwhites (41.0% relative reduction) and residents in poorer counties (22.2% relative reduction).[16]

PAYMENT AND DELIVERY SYSTEM POLICY TO IMPROVE QUALITY AND REDUCE COSTS

Another key area of health policy refers to the group of policies that together dictate how care is reimbursed, as well as the quality metrics on which it will be measured and rewarded. Until the early 2000s, the vast majority of cardiovascular care was covered under "fee-for-service" arrangements. For the most part, such arrangements did not

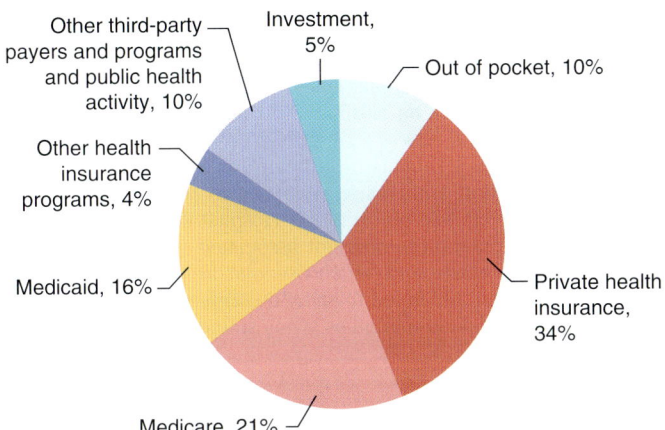

FIGURE 6.1 National health care expenditures. Pie chart of United States' national health care expenditures in 2018 broken down by payer type. Private insurance spending accounted for the largest proportion of expenditures. (Source: Centers for Medicare and Medicaid Services. NHE Fact Sheet. Available at: https://www.cms.gov/Research-Statistics-Data-and-Systems/Statistics-Trends-and-Reports/NationalHealthExpendData/NHE-Fact-Sheet. Accessed July 7, 2020.)

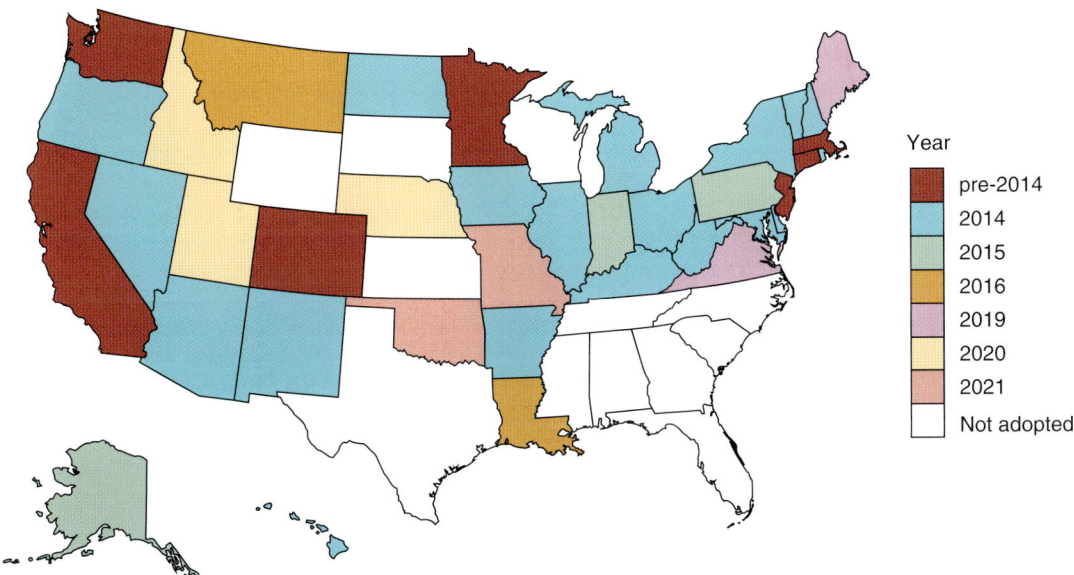

FIGURE 6.2 Map of states that have and have not expanded Medicaid. A majority of states have implemented Medicaid expansion, with only 12 states declining to expand as of 2020.

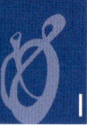

include any payment adjustments for quality or outcomes. A fixed payment was simply rendered for services provided, irrespective of the quality of care that was delivered.

However, consensus grew that cardiovascular care delivery was suboptimal. While clinical trials had made it clear which medications and procedures should be used in which situations, and guidelines began to codify those findings into statements aimed at facilitating optimal care delivery, the reality of clinical practice did not always match the guidelines. The Institute of Medicine, now known as the National Academy of Medicine, released Crossing the Quality Chasm in 2001, calling attention to the wide gap between scientific knowledge and the implementation of high-quality care.[25] A subsequent study published in 2004 demonstrated that appropriate quality of care was only being delivered 54.9% of the time, including in the acute, chronic, and preventive care domains.[26] Performance varied across cardiovascular conditions, from 68.0% guideline-concordant care for coronary artery disease, to 64.7% for hypertension, 63.9% for congestive heart failure (HF), 59.1% for cerebrovascular disease, 48.6% for hyperlipidemia, 45.4% for diabetes, and 24.7% for atrial fibrillation. A number of follow-up studies across care settings (e.g., inpatient, outpatient) and specialties (e.g., cardiovascular specialists, primary care clinicians) broadly documented suboptimal adherence to quality indicators.

As a result, several different types of health policy reform initiatives were introduced to address quality issues in cardiovascular care, many in the ACA. The majority of the changes to Medicare under the ACA were focused on moving the program away from simply paying for the volume of services rendered, and toward paying more explicitly for the quality and costs, collectively the "value," of care delivered. The sections below will outline some of these key changes and review the strength of evidence for their efficacy. Additionally, just like any evaluation of a new drug or treatment strategy in cardiovascular medicine, these policies needed to be evaluated not only in terms of their efficacy, but also in terms of their impact on patient safety. For policies, adverse "safety" events typically take the form of unintended adverse consequences, like reducing access to care, unduly penalizing clinicians for serving high-risk patients, or worsening clinical outcomes.

Public Reporting

The earliest move toward value was public reporting. In 2004, a consortium of payers and quality organizations, led by Medicare, created Hospital Compare as the first national public reporting program (Table 6.1). While participation was voluntary, hospitals that did not participate experienced a payment reduction, so nearly all hospitals joined the program within a few months of its inception. Program developers hoped that publicly posting hospitals' performance online would encourage health systems and clinicians to improve their performance through peer pressure, and allow patients the opportunity to select where to receive care based on performance. Initially, Hospital Compare only included processes of care, such as giving aspirin to patients with AMI. It later expanded to include clinical outcomes such as mortality and readmission rates for AMI and HF, added in 2008 and 2011, respectively.

Beyond these national efforts, some states implemented their own public reporting, typically focused more narrowly on mortality following cardiac procedures. In the 1990s, New York State began publicly reporting hospitals' outcomes for coronary artery bypass grafting (CABG) and percutaneous coronary intervention (PCI), as well as for individual surgeons and interventional cardiologists. Other states including Massachusetts, Pennsylvania, New Jersey, California, and Washington subsequently implemented public reporting programs as well, though some only temporarily.

Evaluations of the efficacy of public reporting programs have been underwhelming. Patients have been unlikely to utilize publicly reported information, with many preferring to rely on advice from friends or family.[27] Public reporting on Hospital Compare—either of processes or of outcomes—was not associated with improvements in mortality rates above and beyond secular trends.[28] Public reporting for PCI has similarly failed to show a consistent association with improvements in clinical outcomes. While studies have demonstrated

TABLE 6.1 Payment and Delivery System Policy Overview for Cardiovascular Conditions

POLICY	YEAR IMPLEMENTED	OVERVIEW
Public Reporting		
Hospital Compare	2004	Public reporting of clinical outcomes and processes
Value-Based Purchasing Programs		
Hospital Readmissions Reduction Program	2012	Hospitals are penalized up to 3% of their Medicare reimbursements for HF, AMI, pneumonia, COPD, joint replacement, and CABG
Hospital Value-Based Purchasing	2012	Hospitals receive bonuses or penalties based on their performance on a set of quality metrics in four core domains: safety, clinical care, efficiency and cost reduction, and patient/caregiver-centered experience
Physician Quality Reporting System	2006, 2011	Initially a public reporting program, but it transitioned into a penalty program in 2011, where physicians and group practices faced negative payment adjustments for failing to report performance data
Physician Value-Based Modifier	2015	Physicians are assigned bonuses and penalties based on performance on quality, outcome, and cost measures
Quality Payment Program	2015	Physicians must choose one of two tracks:
		Merit-Based Incentive Program, which consists of four domains: clinical quality measures, measures of electronic medical record use, measures of costs of care, and measures of practice improvement activities
		Alternative payment models, including accountable care organizations and bundled payment models
Alternative Payment Models		
Medicare Shared Savings Program	2012	Participants are paid on a fee-for-service basis, but are held accountable for their beneficiaries' quality and costs each year.
Bundled Payments for Care Improvement (and BPCI-Advanced)	2011, 2018	Quality and costs are evaluated over the course of an "episode," triggered by a hospitalization and typically 30, 60, or 90 days in length. If Medicare payments for an episode of care are less than the target, then the participant is eligible to keep a portion of the savings; however, if payments exceed the target, the participant must reimburse Medicare some of the difference.

AMI, Acute myocardial infarction; *COPD*, chronic obstructive pulmonary disease; *CABG*, coronary artery bypass grafting; *HF*, heart failure.

lower mortality among patients undergoing PCI in reporting versus nonreporting states, overall outcomes for AMI have been, if anything, worse in reporting states, suggesting that selection bias has driven the apparent improvements in procedural mortality.[29]

Public reporting for hospital processes and outcomes has not been associated with unintended consequences, but public reporting for PCI has been associated with a negative safety signal. Use of coronary angiograms and PCI for AMI are lower in reporting states compared to nonreporting states, and these differences are highest among critically ill patients, such as those in cardiogenic shock, who may benefit most from the procedure. This is likely due to risk aversion; the majority of surveyed interventional cardiologists admit to avoiding high risk but indicated PCIs due to concern that a bad outcome might negatively impact their publicly reported performance outcomes.[30] Data for CABG have been more mixed but have raised concerns about reductions in access to care for racial and ethnic minorities and clinically high-risk individuals.[29]

Concern that public reporting may lead to risk-aversive behavior and impede access to care, particularly for critically ill patients with cardiogenic shock, has prompted some states (New York, Massachusetts) to begin excluding these patients from their public reports. These policy changes have been associated with a substantial increase in the use of PCI for patients with cardiogenic shock and a reduction in associated in-hospital mortality, although PCI rates in this population still remain lower in reporting states compared with nonreporting states.[31]

Value-Based Payment Programs: Hospitals

More recently, Medicare and other payers have begun linking clinician and hospital reimbursement to performance on quality and outcome metrics through VBP programs. The premise of VBP is that paying hospitals and clinicians more if they deliver higher-quality care, or achieve better patient outcomes, will lead to quality improvement.

As part of the ACA, many hospitals across the United States were required to participate in major VBP programs. One of the first mandatory VBP programs, launched in 2012, was the Hospital Readmissions Reduction Program (HRRP). In the HRRP, hospitals are penalized up to 3% of their Medicare reimbursements based on 30-day readmission rates for HF, AMI, pneumonia, chronic obstructive pulmonary disease, joint replacement, and CABG. Hospital Value-Based Purchasing (HVBP) is another hospital VBP program that was introduced by the ACA. In this program, hospitals receive bonuses or penalties based on their performance on a set of quality metrics in four domains: safety, clinical outcomes, efficiency and cost reduction, and person and community engagement. CVD is included in each category, including specific measures for HF mortality, AMI mortality, and, most recently, condition-specific cost measures for these two conditions.

Evaluations of the HRRP and HVBP have demonstrated mixed findings in terms of their associations with improvements in care quality or patient outcomes. The HRRP has been associated with a decrease in readmission rates for Medicare beneficiaries,[32] though subsequent analyses have suggested that a significant portion of the reported improvements may have been due to changes in coding of comorbidities or regression to the mean rather than actual improvements in clinical care.[33,34] Studies have failed to find any association between the implementation of HVBP and improvement in the patient outcomes measured in the program, such as mortality for AMI and HF, or patient experience.[35–37]

In terms of potential adverse consequences, concerns have been raised that the HRRP was associated with an increase in mortality for HF patients, though findings have been mixed.[38] It is possible that the incentives put in place to reduce readmissions led to clinical interventions that ultimately did not benefit patients, such as efforts to treat and release, rather than readmit, patients from the emergency department who return within 30 days of a HF admission. However, the true underlying mechanism for these mortality patterns remains unclear.

Another unintended consequence of current VBP programs has been their disproportionate impact on hospitals that serve medically and/or socially high-risk populations. Most current claims-based risk adjustment models do not include information on frailty, cognitive function, or social determinants of health (SDOH), all of which strongly influence clinical outcomes. Consequently, models may be inequitable when used to evaluate and compare hospital performance under VBP programs. For example, the HRRP has disproportionately penalized safety-net hospitals that care for clinically and socially high-risk populations, despite data suggesting that roughly half of these hospitals' worse performance is due to the complexity of the population they serve. Similar patterns have been seen in other inpatient programs such as the Hospital-Acquired Conditions Reduction Program, as well as in VBP programs for dialysis facilities and nursing facilities.[39] Adding adjustment for social risk, and better adjustment for medical risk, to these programs could improve their ability to accurately identify high-quality and low-quality clinicians and facilities, and reduce inappropriate penalties for the safety net.

Value-Based Purchasing: Outpatient

A similar sequence of events, moving from public reporting to pay-for-performance, has occurred in clinician payment. The Physician Quality Reporting System (PQRS) was a public reporting program established in 2006. It was initially a voluntary system, but transitioned into a payment penalty program in 2011, when physicians and group practices faced negative payment adjustments for failing to report their performance data. Subsequently, a VBP program for physicians, the Physician Value-Based Modifier, created a series of bonuses and penalties that were assigned based on performance on quality, outcome, and cost measures. Building on this program, the Medicare Access and CHIP Reauthorization Act (MACRA) was passed in 2015 and created the related mandatory nationwide Quality Payment Program (QPP). The QPP consists of two "tracks" for clinicians: (1) the Merit-Based Incentive Program (MIPS) and (2) advanced Alternative Payment Models (APMs). MIPS, the default program for practicing clinicians, has four domains: clinical quality measures, measures of electronic medical record use, measures of costs of care, and measures of practice improvement activities (such as using patient portals and participating in quality improvement programs and registries). Clinicians can opt out of MIPS if they participate in a qualifying APM, which is discussed at more length later.

There has been no evidence that public reporting or VBP programs in the outpatient setting have been associated with improvements in quality or outcomes in the United States, although many of these programs were too small or short-lived to be broadly evaluated. A similar program in the UK was associated with modest improvements in quality.[40] However, early evidence suggests that MIPS has disproportionately penalized physicians and practices serving patients with high levels of social or medical risk.[41–43]

Alternative Payment Models

APMs are models that move beyond the traditional fee-for-service payment structure in order to incent high-value care delivery. The two most relevant APMs to cardiovascular care include accountable care organizations (ACOs) and episode-based or "bundled" payments.

ACOs are groups of hospitals and clinicians that assume risk for their attributed patients' quality, clinical outcomes, and total costs of care, typically on an annual basis. In Medicare's largest ACO program, the Medicare Shared Savings Program (MSSP), participants are paid on a fee-for-service basis but are held accountable for their beneficiaries' quality and costs each year. If participants' total annual spending on care for beneficiaries is below a preset target, and performance on quality is high, participants are eligible to keep a portion of the savings. A number of cardiovascular quality measures are included in the MSSP, such as preventable hospitalizations for HF, readmission rates, and the use of certain medications for patients with ischemic heart disease or HF. Thus, cardiovascular specialists can play an important role in improving quality and outcomes under this and other similar programs.

Studies examining the effectiveness of ACOs such as the MSSP have generally found that they are associated with modest savings that grow with longer participation as well as small improvements in quality or outcomes.[44,45] Specific to CVD, one study showed that participating in an ACO improved HF admission rates and all-cause unplanned admissions for patients with HF over time.[46] Another demonstrated that ACOs that included cardiologists had lower spending on beneficiaries with CVD, while achieving similar HF quality measure scores.[47] However, another found that ACOs did not improve medication adherence for patients with CVD.[48]

Another relevant APM to cardiovascular care is bundled payments, which are currently being tested by Medicare through the Bundled Payments for Care Improvement-Advanced (BPCI-A) program. Bundled payment arrangements are similar to ACOs, except that quality and costs are evaluated for an episode of care, triggered by a hospitalization for a specific condition (e.g., AMI, HF). Episodes are typically 30, 60, or 90 days in length, rather than an entire year. Similar to ACOs, if Medicare payments for an episode of care are less than a preset target, the participant can keep some of the savings; if payments exceed the target, the participant must reimburse Medicare some of the difference.

Early studies examining BPCI-A's predecessor, BPCI, have not found improvements in quality, outcomes, or costs for medical conditions including HF or AMI,[49] though longer-term follow-up has suggested that savings may begin to emerge around 2 to 3 years of participation.[50] There has been no evidence that the bundled payment programs have unintended consequences such as adverse selection or worsening patient outcomes.

Overall, there is a lack of cardiology-focused payment models. ACOs focus on primary care and population health; bundled payments focus on acute episodes. Many private health insurance plans track physician performance on cost and quality measures for 365-day episodes of care for chronic conditions such as HF, diabetes, and ischemic heart disease, but novel payment models are relatively rare in private insurance as well. There is currently no national model focused on longitudinal care for chronic CVD, such as HF, ischemic heart disease, peripheral arterial disease, or arrhythmias, all of which often require lifelong care and management by a specialist clinician. This is an area of active policy development.[51]

INEQUITIES IN CARDIOVASCULAR DISEASE RISK, CARE, AND OUTCOMES

There are clear inequities in cardiovascular risk factors, incident CVD, and cardiovascular outcomes for racial and ethnic minorities, individuals living in poverty, and those in rural areas. Yet, there is no clear evidence of a biological basis for these differences. Instead, the best evidence suggests that structural and systemic factors such as access to high-quality care, the environments and neighborhoods in which people are born, work, and live, as well as education, income, the lived experience of racism and discrimination—collectively the SDOH— drive the patterns we see. It is through this lens that these inequities are best examined, and best addressed.

Racial and Ethnic Minorities (see Chapter 93)

Black individuals have higher rates of hypertension and diabetes than their white counterparts (Fig. 6.3). Incidence rates of heart attacks, HF, stroke, and other cardiovascular events are also higher among Black people.[52] Compared to white people, Black individuals are about twice as likely to develop HF (4.6 vs. 2.4 per 1000),[53] twice as likely to experience sudden cardiac death, and have almost three times the relative risk of stroke (relative risk 2.77).[54] Black patients also have higher rates of fatal coronary heart disease compared to white patients, particularly among men (hazard ratio for Black men: 2.18, for Black women: 1.63).[54] Despite improvements in care and technology, Black patients continue to face higher rates of avoidable deaths due to heart disease, stroke, and hypertensive disease.[53] Recent evidence suggests that disparities in cardiovascular mortality for Black patients have persisted over the last two decades, and that mortality rates for some conditions (e.g., HF) are now worsening among younger Black adults.[55–57]

Latinx patients face similar inequities in cardiovascular care, although these differences are more variable and less well-studied compared to Black patients.[52] Cardiovascular risk factors are more prevalent among Latinx people. Compared to their white counterparts, Latinx individuals have a 35% higher prevalence of diabetes, and 61% of Latinx individuals report physical inactivity compared to 52% of white individuals.[53] Studies report higher rates of HF (3.5 versus 2.4 per 1000 person-years) for Latinx people compared to white and Black populations, but lower overall CVD prevalence and lower all-cause and cardiovascular-specific mortality.[58] These paradoxical findings of higher CVD risk but better CVD outcomes remain poorly understood.

Cardiovascular risk factors and outcomes are also markedly worse among Native American populations in the United States. These populations have high rates of obesity, diabetes, and hypertension, although trends vary by region and tribe.[59] In 2017, Native American individuals had the highest rate of diagnosed diabetes (14.7%) among U.S. ethnic or racial groups.[60] Additionally, Native American populations have 20% higher CVD mortality rates compared to the overall population.[59] The limited amount of available research, especially more current research, on Latinx and Native populations warrants further effort to better understand cardiovascular health in these populations.

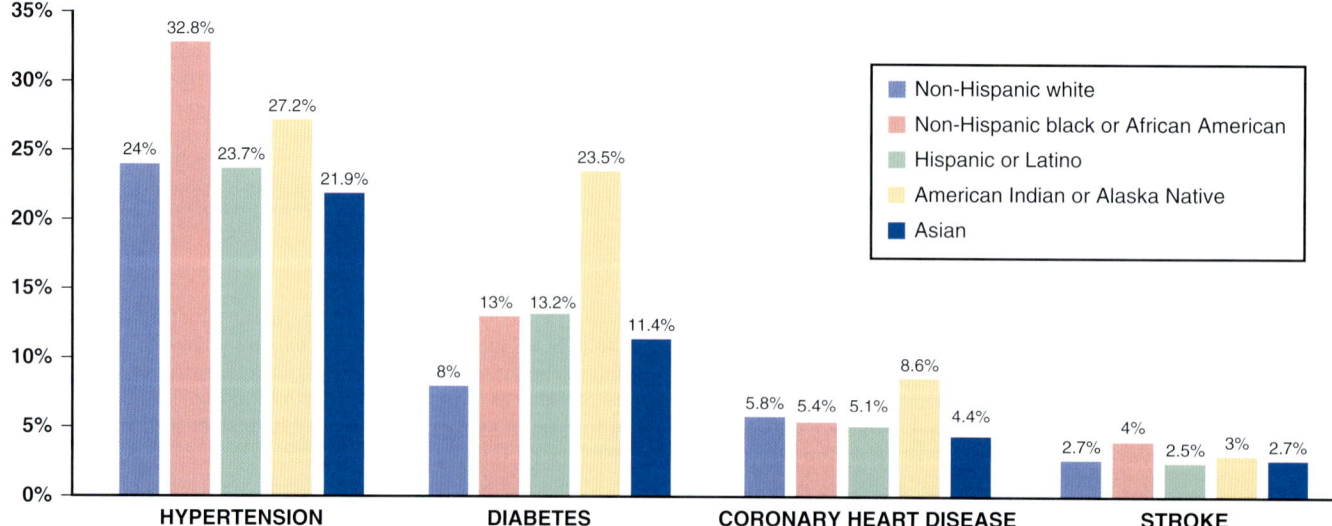

FIGURE 6.3 Racial and ethnic disparities in CVD and CVD risk factors, 2018. Minorities have higher rates of risk and incidence compared to white individuals. *CVD,* Cardiovascular disease. (Source: Centers for Disease Control and Prevention. Summary Health Statistics Tables: National Health Interview Survey. 2019. Available at: https://www.cdc.gov/nchs/nhis/shs/tables.htm. Accessed July 7, 2020.)

The reasons for these inequities are multifactorial. For example, as a result of a long history of structural and systemic racism in the United States, Black individuals are more likely to live in neighborhoods that are burdened with adverse social risk factors, and lack healthy food options, safe places to exercise, and even clean air. Long-standing discriminatory practices in housing have resulted in a disproportionate number of Black people living in areas and housing with high levels of air pollution and toxins, and this has been linked to the development of coronary artery plaque.[61]

The lived individual experience of racism and discrimination also likely play a role in the development of CVD, given the association between the experience of racism, elevated stress hormones such as cortisol and C-reactive protein, and increased blood pressure, all of which have adverse cardiovascular effects.[62] Other studies have also found associations between discrimination and preclinical atherosclerosis and coronary artery calcification for Black women and greater coronary artery obstruction for Black men.[62] Additionally, discrimination is also associated with greater risk for MI, cardiac arrest, and stroke.[62] Racial and ethnic minorities also have higher rates of adverse childhood experiences, including experiences of racism as well as other traumas, which are predictive of worse health outcomes in adulthood.[63]

Lack of access to health care, including preventive care, cardiovascular specialty care, and high-quality hospital care among Black and Latinx patients as well as Native Americans also contributes to these disparities. Racial and ethnic minority individuals are more likely to live in poverty, to be uninsured, and to face financial barriers to care.[64] Compared to white people, racial and ethnic minority patients are less likely to be treated by cardiologists versus general medicine practitioners for HF despite studies reporting lower mortality for patients treated by cardiologists.[65,66] Black patients are more likely to receive care from lower-quality surgeons for CABG procedures, and Black patients with AMI are more likely to be admitted to lower-quality hospitals that use fewer evidence-based medical treatments and have worse risk-adjusted mortality.[67]

Lack of access does not on its own explain persistent differences in care for heart transplantation, non-ST-segment-elevation myocardial infarction (NSTEMI), and other conditions.[53,68] Even within the same hospitals, where access should be similar, Black patients are less likely to receive effective cardiac procedures such as thrombolytics, PCI, CABG, cardiac resynchronization therapy, and left ventricular assist devices.[53,69] For patients with NSTEMI, Black patients are 24% less likely to receive nonaspirin antiplatelets, 29% less likely to receive angiography, and 45% less likely to receive revascularization.[68]

While most studies do not measure racial discrimination per se, it is likely that racism contributes to these differences in access and procedure use among Black, Latinx, and Native American patients. Studies have shown that some physicians perceive differences in personal characteristics based on patients' race.[70,71] And interestingly, despite overwhelming evidence to the contrary, a 2004 study found that only 34% of cardiologists believed that racial disparities in care existed.[72] Although this study may be outdated, both implicit and explicit bias have implications for clinician assessment of patients' candidacy for cardiac procedures. More work is necessary to understand and improve clinician decision-making and address the impact of racism on CVD care and outcomes.

Income

Cardiovascular and overall health outcomes are worse among individuals living in poverty compared to wealthier people. At the population level, poor counties have about 10% higher rates of hypertension, obesity, and physical inactivity compared to richer counties in the United States.[73] While the overall prevalence of these CVD risk factors has declined over time, trends vary by income: cardiovascular risk decreased from 1999 to 2014 for middle- and high-income adults, but did not change for adults with incomes at or below the FPL.[74] Adolescents show similar trends over time, with low- to middle-income adolescents showing increases in obesity rates, greater physical inactivity, and slower declines in CVD risk compared to high-income adolescents.[75]

Low income and poverty are also associated with greater CVD incidence and worse outcomes. Compared to high-income individuals, low-income individuals had higher incidence rates of coronary heart disease (6.24 versus 5.67 per 1000 person-years) and HF (10.43 vs. 6.97 per 1000 person-years).[76] Despite higher disease incidence, low-income patients are less likely to receive effective treatment for these conditions, such as left heart catheterization for MI or cardiac rehabilitation after hospitalization for a qualifying condition.[77] They are also less likely to start statin medications following AMI compared to high-income patients.[77] These disparities translate into worse outcomes even after adjusting for other sociodemographic factors. At the county level, HF mortality is strongly correlated with poverty ($r = 0.48$), and increases by 5.2 deaths per 100,000 persons for each percentage increase in county poverty.[78] Individuals living in low-income areas have a higher risk of inpatient mortality for acute stroke compared to patients living in higher-income areas (OR 1.08),[79] and higher family income is associated with a 40% to 50% decrease in all-cause and cardiovascular mortality.[80]

Income is one component of an individual's socioeconomic status, and other factors such as insurance status, employment status, and neighborhood characteristics likely contribute to low-income individuals' CVD disease risk. For example, in 2018, 84% of the uninsured population had incomes less than 400% FPL.[81] Low-income patients who lack insurance face greater financial barriers to care, which is associated with fewer annual medical exams, postponing care, and lower likelihoods of receiving preventive care.[77,81] Low-income individuals are more likely to live in food deserts, have difficulty accessing healthy food, and live in communities with fewer sidewalks and parks. This adverse environment is associated with higher rates of CVD risk factors, such as obesity and physical inactivity.[77,82] Chronic stressors driven by income and affordability barriers contribute to higher cortisol and adrenaline levels, which further increases low-income individuals' risk of chronic disease and CVD.[82]

Urban-Rural Geography

Roughly 20% of the U.S. population lives in rural areas. Rural residents tend to be older, and have higher rates of cardiovascular risk factors like diabetes, obesity, and hypertension, as well as tobacco use and physical inactivity.[83] Data from the 2018 Centers for Disease Control and Prevention (CDC) National Health Interview Survey showed a higher prevalence of heart disease among rural residents compared with their counterparts in small metropolitan and urban areas, a gap that has grown over the past decade (Fig. 6.4).[84] Rural areas have higher death rates for CVD and stroke than urban areas, and gaps are widening here too. Rural residents have a 30% higher risk for stroke mortality compared with urban residents,[85] and recent national increases in stroke mortality are steepest in the rural South.[86] Rural women face higher maternal mortality rates compared to urban women, largely driven by excess cardiovascular deaths.[87]

The reasons for these differences are again manifold. In rural areas, there are major issues in terms of access to physical facilities and medical personnel. Primary care providers (PCPs) play an important role in cardiovascular risk factor management, and rural areas have fewer PCPs per capita than urban areas. A lower supply of PCPs is associated with higher CVD mortality.[88] In addition, the average rural resident lives 10.5 miles away from a hospital, compared with 4.4 miles for urban individuals.[89] Differential outcomes related to AMI in rural regions result from lower capabilities of ambulance services, less access to timely, life-saving specialty procedures, and high reliance on transfers to definitive care.[90] Similarly, while treatment at designated stroke centers is associated with higher thrombolytic therapy rates and lower mortality, rural residents are less likely to have access to such centers than their urban counterparts.[91] As the use of endovascular therapy for stroke grows, such geographic differences have become more pronounced.[92] For less common cardiovascular conditions such as congenital heart disease, as well as procedures such as heart transplantation, left ventricular assist device implantation, and advanced mechanical circulatory support for cardiogenic shock, these issues are even more stark, as people living in rural areas may need to travel tens or even hundreds of miles to access advanced technologies.[93]

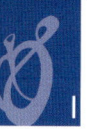

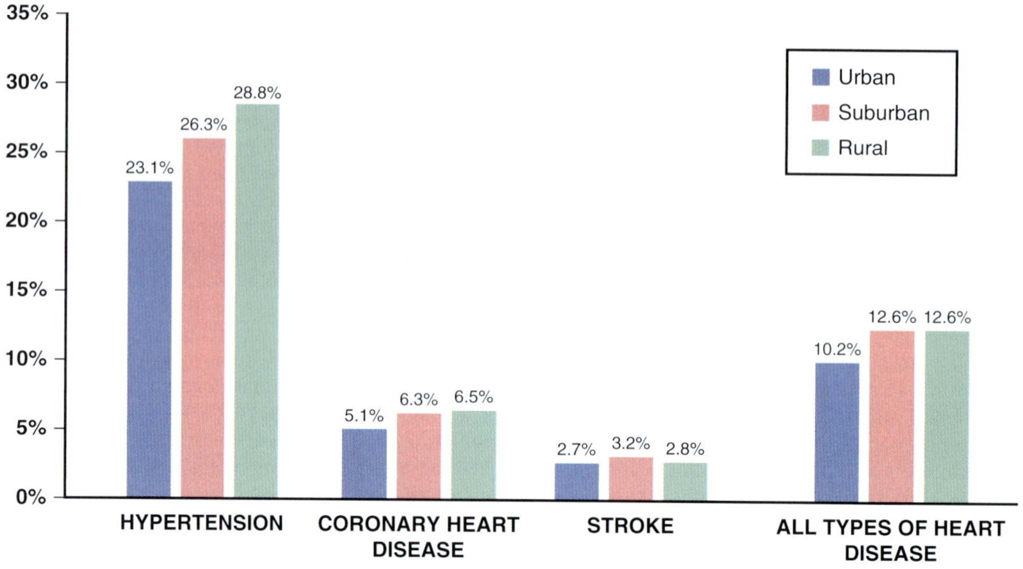

FIGURE 6.4 Urban-rural disparities in CVD, 2018. Rural areas have higher rates of CVD incidence compared to urban and suburban areas. *CVD,* Cardiovascular disease. (Source: Centers for Disease Control and Prevention. Summary Health Statistics Tables: National Health Interview Survey. 2019. Available at: https://www.cdc.gov/nchs/nhis/shs/tables.htm. Accessed July 7, 2020.)

Access continues to worsen as hospital closures have accelerated nationwide; more than 100 rural hospitals have closed since 2010,[94] and this is especially pronounced for hospitals in states which did not expand Medicaid through the ACA.[95] Studies have shown an increase in stroke and acute MI mortality associated with rural closures,[96] both in the areas with closures as well as in high-occupancy hospitals that absorb new volume; one study found that when a high-occupancy ED was exposed to a closure, 1-year mortality and 30-day readmission rates increased for acute MI, while the likelihood of receiving PCI declined.[97]

Access to high-quality care also matters for cardiovascular outcomes. Quality of care and outcomes for cardiovascular conditions in rural hospitals may be worse than urban hospitals, at least in some domains. For example, prior studies have shown higher mortality for patients with acute MI, HF, atrial fibrillation, and stroke in rural hospitals compared with urban ones.[83] Transportation challenges and long distances to services in rural areas can also result in fewer preventive or chronic care visits, which can impact cardiovascular health.[98] Rurality also poses challenges in access to, and participation in, post-acute care and rehabilitation services. For example, patients living at a distance from a cardiac or stroke rehabilitation program are less likely to participate.[99,100]

CONCLUSIONS

Health policy, while unfamiliar for many clinicians, impacts the day-to-day delivery of cardiovascular care in many ways, including access and coverage, as well as quality, costs, and reimbursement. There is also a strong relationship between health policy and equity. The evidence to date suggests that health insurance coverage is crucial for achieving optimal cardiovascular and overall health, and improvements to insurance markets as well as Medicaid expansion under the ACA have led to higher rates of coverage nationwide. The payment models introduced in the ACA have been, overall, suboptimally effective at improving outcomes or reducing costs, and may have had unintended consequences for access and equity. Major inequities in care and outcomes for racial and ethnic minorities, people living in poverty, and those in rural areas exist, despite growing recognition of their magnitude. Further research and efforts are needed to build on successful policies such as insurance expansion, improve those that have been less successful, and drive toward better and more equitable health for all.

REFERENCES

1. Centers for Medicare & Medicaid Services. *NHE Fact Sheet;* 2020. https://www.cms.gov/Research-Statistics-Data-and-Systems/Statistics-Trends-and-Reports/NationalHealthExpendData/NHE-Fact-Sheet. Accessed June 22, 2020.
2. Shah SJ, Krumholz HM, Reid KJ, et al. Financial stress and outcomes after acute myocardial infarction. *PloS One.* 2012;7:e47420.
3. Valero-Elizondo J, Khera R, Saxena A, et al. Financial hardship from medical bills among nonelderly U.S. Adults with atherosclerotic cardiovascular disease. *J Am Coll Cardiol.* 2019;73:727.
4. Berchick ER, Barnett JC, Upton RD. *Health Insurance Coverage in the United States: 2018.* Washington, DC: U.S. Government Printing Office; 2019.
5. Federal Poverty Level (FPL). Centers for Medicare & Medicaid; 2020. https://www.healthcare.gov/glossary/federal-poverty-level-fpl/. Accessed June 22, 2020.
6. Kaiser Family Foundation. *Status of State Medicaid Expansion Decisions: Interactive Map.* Kaiser Family Foundation; 2020. https://www.kff.org/medicaid/issue-brief/status-of-state-medicaid-expansion-decisions-interactive-map/. Accessed June 22, 2020.
7. Courtemanche C, Marton J, Ukert B, et al. The three-year impact of the Affordable Care Act on disparities in insurance coverage. *Health Serv Res.* 2019;54:307–316.
8. Wadhera RK, Bhatt DL, Wang TY, et al. Association of state medicaid expansion with quality of care and outcomes for low-income patients hospitalized with acute myocardial infarction. *JAMA Cardiol.* 2019;4:120–127.
9. Sommers BD, Blendon RJ, Orav EJ, et al. Changes in utilization and health among low-income adults after medicaid expansion or expanded private insurance. *JAMA Intern Med.* 2016;176:1501–1509.
10. Sommers BD, Gunja MZ, Finegold K, et al. Changes in self-reported insurance coverage, access to care, and health under the affordable care act. *J Am Med Assoc.* 2015;314:366–374.
11. Wherry LR, Miller S. Early coverage, access, utilization, and health effects associated with the affordable care act medicaid expansions: a quasi-experimental study. *Ann Intern Med.* 2016;164:795–803.
12. Kaufman HW, Chen Z, Fonseca VA, et al. Surge in newly identified diabetes among medicaid patients in 2014 within medicaid expansion States under the Affordable Care Act. *Diabetes Care.* 2015;38:833–837.
13. Cole MB, Galarraga O, Wilson IB, et al. At federally funded health centers, medicaid expansion was associated with improved quality of care. *Health Aff.* 2017;36:40–48.
14. Ghosh A, Simon K, Sommers BD. *The Effect of State Medicaid Expansions on Prescription Drug Use: Evidence from the Affordable Care Act.* Cambridge, MA: National Bureau Economic Research; 2017.
15. Cotti C, Nesson E, Tefft N. Impacts of the ACA Medicaid expansion on health behaviors: evidence from household panel data. *Health Econ.* 2019;28:219–244.
16. Sommers BD, Baicker K, Epstein AM. Mortality and access to care among adults after state Medicaid expansions. *N Engl J Med.* 2012;367:1025–1034.
17. Sommers BD, Long SK, Baicker K. Changes in mortality after Massachusetts health care reform. *Ann Intern Med.* 2015;162:668–669.
18. Baicker K, Taubman SL, Allen HL, et al. The Oregon experiment–effects of Medicaid on clinical outcomes. *N Engl J Med.* 2013;368:1713–1722.
19. Miller S, Wherry LR. Health and access to care during the first 2 years of the ACA Medicaid expansions. *N Engl J Med.* 2017;376:947–956.
20. Kaiser Family Foundation. *Health Insurance Coverage of Adults 19-64.* Kaiser Family Foundation; 2017. www.kff.org/other/state-indicator/adults-19-64/?currentTimeframe=0&sortModel=%7B%22colId%22:%22Location%22,%22sort%22:%22asc%22%7D. Accessed November 1, 2017.
21. Bhatt CB, Beck-Sagué CM. Medicaid expansion and infant mortality in the United States. *Am J Public Health.* 2018;108:565–567.
22. Wen H, Johnston KJ, Allen L, et al. Medicaid expansion associated with reductions in preventable hospitalizations. *Health Aff.* 2019;38:1845–1849.
23. Sommers BD, Blendon RJ, Orav EJ, et al. Changes in utilization and health among low-income adults after Medicaid expansion or expanded private insurance changes in access to care in low-income adults. *JAMA Intern Med.* 2016;176:1501–1509.
24. Khatana SAM, Bhatla A, Nathan AS, et al. Association of Medicaid expansion with cardiovascular mortality. *JAMA Cardiol.* 2019;4:671–679.
25. Institute of Medicine Committee on Quality of Health Care in America. In: *Crossing the Quality Chasm: A New Health System for the 21st Century.* Washington (DC): National Academies Press (US); 2001.
26. McGlynn EA, Asch SM, Adams J, et al. The quality of health care delivered to adults in the United States. *N Engl J Med.* 2003;348:2635–2645.
27. Bhandari N, Scanlon DP, Shi Y, et al. Why do so few consumers use health care quality report cards? A framework for understanding the limited consumer impact of comparative quality information. *Med Care Res Rev.* 2018;76:515–537.
28. Joynt KE, Orav EJ, Zheng J, et al. Public reporting of mortality rates for hospitalized Medicare patients and trends in mortality for reported conditions. *Ann Intern Med.* 2016;165:153–160.
29. Wasfy JH, Borden WB, Secemsky EA, et al. Public reporting in cardiovascular medicine: accountability, unintended consequences, and promise for improvement. *Circulation.* 2015;131:1518–1527.

30. Blumenthal DM, Zhao Y, Shen C, et al. *Public Reporting of PCI Outcomes and Provider Risk Aversion: The Results of a Survey of Interventional Cardiologists in Massachusetts and New York.* Anaheim, California: American Heart Association; 2017.
31. McCabe JM, Waldo SW, Kennedy KF, et al. Treatment and outcomes of acute myocardial infarction complicated by shock after public reporting policy changes in New York. *JAMA Cardiol.* 2016;1:648–654.
32. Zuckerman RB, Sheingold SH, Epstein AM. The hospital readmissions reduction program. *N Engl J Med.* 2016;375:494.
33. Ibrahim AM, Dimick JB, Sinha SS, et al. Association of coded severity with readmission reduction after the hospital readmissions reduction program. *JAMA Intern Med.* 2018;178:290–292.
34. Ody C, Msall L, Dafny LS, et al. Decreases in readmissions credited to Medicare's program to reduce hospital readmissions have been overstated. *Health Aff.* 2019;38:36–43.
35. Ryan AM, Krinsky S, Maurer KA, et al. Changes in hospital quality associated with hospital value-based purchasing. *N Engl J Med.* 2017;376:2358–2366.
36. Chee TT, Ryan AM, Wasfy JH, et al. Current state of value-based purchasing programs. *Circulation.* 2016;133:2197–2205.
37. Figueroa JF, Tsugawa Y, Zheng J, et al. Association between the value-based purchasing pay for performance program and patient mortality in US hospitals: observational study. *BMJ.* 2016;353:i2214.
38. Wadhera RK, Yeh RW, Joynt Maddox KE. The hospital readmissions reduction program - time for a reboot. *N Engl J Med.* 2019;380:2289–2291.
39. Joynt Maddox KE. Financial incentives and vulnerable populations - will alternative payment models help or hurt? *N Engl J Med.* 2018;378:977–979.
40. Navathe AS, Emanuel EJ, Bond A, et al. Association between the implementation of a population-based primary care payment system and achievement on quality measures in Hawaii. *J Am Med Assoc.* 2019;322:57–68.
41. Johnston KJ, Hockenberry JM, Wadhera RK, Joynt Maddox KE, Clinicians with high socially at-risk caseloads received reduced Merit-Based Incentive Payment System scores. *Health Aff (Millwood).* 2020;39(9):1504–1512.
42. Khullar D, Schpero WL, Bond AM, Qian Y, Casalino LP. Association between patient social risk and physician performance scores in the first year of the Merit-Based Incentive Payment System. *JAMA.* 2020;324(10):975–983.
43. Navathe AS, Dinh CT, Chen A, et al. Findings and implications from MIPS year 1 performance data. *Health Affairs Blog.* 2019. https://doi.org/10.1377/hblog20190117.305369. Accessed January 18, 2019.
44. McWilliams JM, Hatfield LA, Landon BE, et al. Medicare spending after 3 Years of the Medicare shared savings program. *N Engl J Med.* 2018;379:1139–1149.
45. McWilliams JM, Chernew ME, Landon BE. Medicare ACO program savings not tied to preventable hospitalizations or concentrated among high-risk patients. *Health Aff.* 2017;36:2085–2093.
46. Bleser WK, Saunders RS, Muhlestein DB, et al. ACO quality over time: the MSSP experience and Opportunities for system-wide improvement. *Am J ACC Care.* 2018;6:e1–e15.
47. Sukul D, Ryan AM, Yan P, et al. Cardiologist participation in accountable care organizations and changes in spending and quality for Medicare patients with cardiovascular disease. *Circ Cardiovasc Qual Outcomes.* 2019;12:e005438.
48. McWilliams JM, Najafzadeh M, Shrank WH, et al. Association of changes in medication use and adherence with accountable care organization exposure in patients with cardiovascular disease or diabetes. *JAMA Cardiol.* 2017;2:1019–1023.
49. Joynt Maddox KE, Orav EJ, Zheng J, et al. Evaluation of Medicare's bundled payments initiative for medical conditions. *N Engl J Med.* 2018;379:260–269.
50. Rolnick JA, Liao JM, Emanuel EJ, et al. Spending and quality after three years of Medicare's bundled payments for medical conditions: quasi-experimental difference-in-differences study. *BMJ.* 2020;369:m1780.
51. Maddox KJ, Bleser WK, Crook HL, et al. Advancing value-based models for heart failure. *Circ Cardiovasc Qual Outcomes.* 2020;13:e006483.
52. Graham G. Disparities in cardiovascular disease risk in the United States. *Curr Cardiol Rev.* 2015;11:238–245.
53. Youmans QR, Hastings-Spaine L, Princewill O, et al. Disparities in cardiovascular care: past, present, and solutions. *Cleve Clin J Med.* 2019;86:621–632.
54. Carnethon MR, Pu J, Howard G, et al. Cardiovascular health in African Americans: a scientific statement from the American Heart Association. *Circulation.* 2017;136:e393–e423.
55. Glynn P, Lloyd-Jones DM, Feinstein MJ, et al. Disparities in cardiovascular mortality related to heart failure in the United States. *J Am Coll Cardiol.* 2019;73:2354–2355.
56. Sidney S, Quesenberry Jr CP, Jaffe MG, et al. Recent trends in cardiovascular mortality in the United States and public health goals. *JAMA Cardiology.* 2016;1:594–599.
57. Shah NS, Lloyd-Jones DM, O'Flaherty M, et al. Trends in cardiometabolic mortality in the United States, 1999-2017. *JAMA.* 2019;322:780–782.
58. Balfour Jr PC, Ruiz JM, Talavera GA, et al. Cardiovascular disease in Hispanics/Latinos in the United States. *J Lat Psychol.* 2016;4:98–113.
59. Deen Jason F, Adams Alexandra K, Fretts A, et al. Cardiovascular disease in American Indian and Alaska native youth: unique risk factors and areas of scholarly need. *J Am Heart Assoc.* 6:e007576.
60. Centers for Disease Control and Prevention. *National Diabetes Statistics Report.* Atlanta, GA 2020.
61. Kaufman JD, Adar SD, Barr RG, et al. Association between air pollution and coronary artery calcification within six metropolitan areas in the USA (the Multi-Ethnic Study of Atherosclerosis and Air Pollution): a longitudinal cohort study. *Lancet.* 2016;388:696–704.
62. Lockwood KG, Marsland AL, Matthews KA, et al. Perceived discrimination and cardiovascular health disparities: a multisystem review and health neuroscience perspective. *Ann N Y Acad Sci.* 2018;1428:170–207.
63. Allen H, Wright Bill J, Vartanian K, et al. Examining the prevalence of adverse childhood experiences and associated cardiovascular disease risk factors among low-income uninsured adults. *Circ Cardiovasc Qual Outcomes.* 2019;12:e004391.
64. Sohn H. Racial and ethnic disparities in health insurance coverage: dynamics of gaining and losing coverage over the life-course. *Popul Res Policy Rev.* 2017;36:181–201.
65. Breathett K, Liu WG, Allen LA, et al. African Americans are less likely to receive care by a cardiologist during an intensive care unit admission for heart failure. *JACC Heart Fail.* 2018;6:413–420.
66. Eberly Lauren A, Richterman A, Beckett Anne G, et al. Identification of racial inequities in access to specialized inpatient heart failure care at an academic medical center. *Circ Heart Fail.* 2019;12:e006214.
67. Johnson A. Understanding why Black patients have worse coronary heart disease outcomes: does the answer lie in knowing where patients seek care? *J Am Heart Assoc.* 2019;8:e014706.
68. Arora S, Stouffer George A, Kucharska-Newton A, et al. Fifteen-year trends in management and outcomes of non-ST-segment-elevation myocardial infarction among Black and white patients: the ARIC community surveillance study, 2000–2014. *J Am Heart Assoc.* 2018;7:e010203.
69. Wang X, Luke AA, Vader JM, et al. Disparities and impact of medicaid expansion on left ventricular assist device implantation and outcomes. *Circ Cardiovasc Qual Outcomes.* 2020;13:e006284.
70. Schulman KA, Berlin JA, Harless W, et al. The effect of race and sex on physicians' recommendations for cardiac catheterization. *N Engl J Med.* 1999;340:618–626.
71. Kressin NR, Petersen LA. Racial differences in the use of invasive cardiovascular procedures: review of the literature and prescription for future research. *Ann Intern Med.* 2001;135:352–366.
72. Lurie N, Fremont A, Jain AK, et al. Racial and ethnic disparities in care: the perspectives of cardiologists. *Circulation.* 2005;111:1264–1269.
73. Shaw KM, Theis KA, Self-Brown S, et al. Chronic disease disparities by county economic status and metropolitan classification, behavioral risk factor surveillance system, 2013. *Prev Chronic Dis.* 2016;13:160088.
74. Odutayo A, Gill P, Shepherd S, et al. Income disparities in absolute cardiovascular risk and cardiovascular risk factors in the United States, 1999-2014. *JAMA Cardiol.* 2017;2:782–790.
75. Jackson SL, Yang EC, Zhang Z. Income disparities and cardiovascular risk factors among adolescents. *Pediatrics.* 2018;142:e20181089.
76. Fretz A, Schneider AL, McEvoy JW, et al. The association of socioeconomic status with subclinical myocardial damage, incident cardiovascular events, and mortality in the ARIC study. *Am J Epidemiol.* 2016;183:452–461.
77. Schultz WM, Kelli HM, Lisko JC, et al. Socioeconomic status and cardiovascular outcomes. *Circulation.* 2018;137:2166–2178.
78. Ahmad K, Chen Edward W, Nazir U, et al. Regional variation in the association of poverty and heart failure mortality in the 3135 counties of the United States. *J Am Heart Assoc.* 2019;8:e012422.
79. Marshall IJ, Wang Y, Crichton S, et al. The effects of socioeconomic status on stroke risk and outcomes. *Lancet Neurol.* 2015;14:1206–1218.
80. Havranek EP, Mujahid MS, Barr DA, et al. Social determinants of risk and outcomes for cardiovascular disease. *Circulation.* 2015;132:873–898.
81. Tolbert J, Orgera K, Singer N, et al. *Key Facts About the Uninsured Population.* San Francisco, CA. 2019.
82. Khullar D, Chokshi DA. *Health, Income, & Poverty: Where We Are & what Could Help.* Bethesda, MD. 2018.
83. Harrington RA, Califf RM, Balamurugan A, et al. Call to action: rural health: a presidential advisory from the American Heart Association and American Stroke Association. *Circulation.* 2020;141:e615–e644.
84. Centers for Disease Control and Prevention, National Center for Health Statistics. *Summary Health Statistics.* National Health Interview Survey; 2018, 2019.
85. Howard G, Kleindorfer DO, Cushman M, et al. Contributors to the excess stroke mortality in rural areas in the United States. *Stroke.* 2017;48:1773–1778.
86. Yang Q, Tong X, Schieb L, et al. Vital signs: recent trends in stroke death rates - United States, 2000-2015. *MMWR Morb Mortal Wkly Rep.* 2017;66:933–939.
87. Center for Disease Control and Prevention. *Pregnancy Mortality Surveillance System.* U.S. Department of Health and Human Services; 2019. https://www.cdc.gov/reproductivehealth/maternalinfanthealth/pregnancy-mortality-surveillance-system.htm. Accessed June 22, 2020.
88. Basu S, Berkowitz SA, Phillips RL, et al. Association of primary care physician supply with population mortality in the United States, 2005-2015. *JAMA Int Med.* 2019;179:506–514.
89. Lam O, Broderick B, Toor S. *How Far Americans Live from the Closest Hospital Differs by Community Type.* Pew Research Center; 2018. https://www.pewresearch.org/fact-tank/2018/12/12/how-far-americans-live-from-the-closest-hospital-differs-by-community-type/. Accessed June 22, 2020.
90. Bechtold D, Salvatierra GG, Bulley E, et al. Geographic variation in treatment and outcomes among patients with AMI: investigating urban-rural differences among hospitalized patients. *J Rural Health.* 2017;33:158–166.
91. Xian Y, Holloway RG, Chan PS, et al. Association between stroke center hospitalization for acute ischemic stroke and mortality. *J Am Med Assoc.* 2011;305:373–380.
92. Hammond G, Luke Alina A, Elson L, et al. Urban-rural inequities in acute stroke care and in-hospital mortality. *Stroke.* 2020;51:2131–2138.
93. Woo J, Anderson BR, Gruenstein D, et al. Abstract 201: travel distance among publicly insured infants with operable congenital heart disease. *Circ Cardiovasc Qual Outcomes.* 2018;11:A201-A201.
94. Cecil G. *Sheps Center for Health Services Research. 155 Rural Hospital Closures: January 2005 - Present.* The University of North Carolina at Chapel Hill; 2019. https://www.shepscenter.unc.edu/programs-projects/rural-health/rural-hospital-closures/. Accessed July 28, 2020.
95. Lindrooth RC, Perraillon MC, Hardy RY, et al. Understanding the relationship between medicaid expansions and hospital closures. *Health Aff.* 2018;37:111–120.
96. Gujral K, Basu A. *Impact of Rural and Urban Hospital Closures on Inpatient Mortality.* NBER Working Paper Series, National Bureau of Economic Research; 2019. Working Paper 26182.
97. Hsia RY, Shen YC. Emergency department closures and openings: spillover effects on patient outcomes in bystander hospitals. *Health Aff.* 2019;38:1496–1504.
98. Arcury TA, Preisser JS, Gesler WM, et al. Access to transportation and health care utilization in a rural region. *J Rural Health.* 2005;21:31–38.
99. Valencia HE, Savage PD, Ades PA. Cardiac rehabilitation participation in underserved populations. Minorities, low socioeconomic, and rural residents. *J Cardiopulm Rehabil Prev.* 2011;31:203–210.
100. Koifman J, Hall R, Li S, et al. The association between rural residence and stroke care and outcomes. *J Neurol Sci.* 2016;363:16–20.

第二部分　心血管疾病的个体化诊疗

周欣　杨清　导读

本部分内容的各个章节涉及了近年来心血管疾病个体化诊疗策略最新进展的各个环节，首先以"中心法则"为主线，概述了在基因组学/表观遗传学（第7章）和蛋白质组学/代谢组学（第8章）层面的理论基础和方法学基础；随后以此为基础，在疾病治疗学（第8章）层面介绍了药物不良反应监测、药代动力学评价和药物间相互作用的相关问题（第9章），在疾病诊断学和预后危险分层领域（第10章）介绍了基于新型组学标志物发现、评价和验证的基本策略；最后，该部分利用两个章节，阐述了近年来采用人工智能方法对多组学和表型学的高纬度数据进行深度学习并在心血管疾病诊断和危险分层中的应用原则和相关进展（第11章），以及利用可穿戴设备获取个体连续纵向健康信息的研究进展（第12章）。

第7和第8章从遗传学、蛋白质组学/代谢组学的基础理论出发，以心血管疾病发生发展过程中"marker"和"maker"是"如何被发现的"这一问题为线索，涵盖了近年来重要的基础和临床应用进展。随着近年来各种高质量大型人群研究数据向全球学者的公开，如UK-Biobank，第7章中涉及的孟德尔随机化和多基因危险评分的研究方法和策略对于致力于该领域研究的青年学者以及旨在对此领域基础理论和应用关键问题有所了解的临床医生，都具有非常高的参考价值。

从内容的连续性上，第10章的主题与第7和第8章更为紧密。在多组学marker发现的基础上，目前各种基于多变量的临床预测模型研究已经成为不同水平临床期刊发表的主流研究论文之一。然而，这些研究的质量参差不齐，尤其是缺乏统一且规范的模型构建和验证方法。结合近期发布的多变量预测模型TRIPOD（The Transparent Reporting of a multivariable prediction model for Individual Prognosis Or Diagnosis）研究规范，第10章涉及的内容从常用的统计学评价方法和经典应用范例出发，为读者提供了一个全面而系统的认识。第10章的两位作者是这个领域的资深学者（Peter Libby和Paul M. Ridker），在动脉粥样硬化炎症学说的基础和临床研究领域都有非凡的造诣。

第9章涉及的药物治疗学是临床实践和研究中涉及的经典话题。随着药物治疗学RCT研究的广泛开展和相关循证医学证据的积累，近年来各种临床指南和共识的更新频次愈发密集，广大临床医生势必面临一个新的问题，即如何在治疗策略的"add-on"模式下，优化方案、减少不必要干预、降低患者不良反应，并最终改善临床预后？第9章从临床试验中的不良反应发现入手，系统回顾了药物基因组学和时辰药动学的进展，为临床医生了解药物剂量和药物方案的优化过程提供了重要参考。

第11章概述了人工智能应用这一热点话题。首先该章节对重要的定义和常见专业名词进行了介绍，随后通过对图片以及静态和动态影像学资料（心电图和冠状动脉造影资料）人工智能研究案例的介绍、电子病历系统自然语言处理等问题的介绍，对该领域中的应用范式和范例进行了回顾。最后，该部分梳理了人工智能应用的局限性和潜在误区，对于临床医师客观解读人工智能研究、合理利用人工智能技术和手段，开拓临床大数据研究新领域提供了借鉴。

第 12 章涉及的心血管医学可穿戴设备也是当前和未来的热点话题。目前该领域的研究主要涉及心电和血压可穿戴设备，相信随着多种柔性材料、可植入材料以及微电子技术的飞速进展，其他重要的个体健康信息也会通过可穿戴设备进行连续、纵向的收集，从而对由健康向亚健康、从疾病稳定向不稳定的演变，以及相反过程转变中的关键事件和关键趋势进行高效的捕捉和获取，实现长周期、乃至全生命周期的监护。现阶段对于心电信息连续获取的应用范例当属心房颤动的识别。然而，什么是具有临床意义的心房颤动，什么是需要干预的心房颤动（比如抗凝治疗）是当前临床实践亟需解决的一个重要问题，我们既要认识到可穿戴设备的潜在巨大优势，也要避免由此产生的过度诊断和过度治疗等问题带给患者的潜在危害。

PART II INDIVIDUALIZING APPROACHES TO CARDIOVASCULAR DISEASE

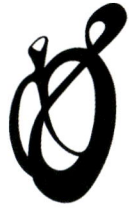

7 Applications of Genetics to Cardiovascular Medicine

PRADEEP NATARAJAN AND KIRAN MUSUNURU

扫描二维码阅读
第7章中文导读

KEY PRINCIPLES OF HUMAN GENETICS, 71
Central Dogma, 71
Heritability, 72
Genetic Architecture, 72
Genetic Variation, 72
Characterizing Human Genetic Variation, 73

GENE DISCOVERY, 75
Family-Based Studies, 75
Case-Control and Population-Based Studies, 75

CAUSAL INFERENCE OF EPIDEMIOLOGIC ASSOCIATIONS, 77

Mendelian Randomization Principles and Applications, 79

DISEASE RISK PREDICTION, 80
Pathogenicity Assessments and Monogenic Risk, 80
Polygenic Risk Scoring, 81

THERAPEUTIC RESPONSE PREDICTION, 81
Target Discovery and Clinical Trial Prediction, 81
On-Target Therapeutic Side Effect Prediction, 82
Precision Medicine, 82

NEXT-GENERATION TECHNOLOGIES AND THERAPEUTICS, 83
Somatic Genomics, 83
Epigenetics, 83
Single-Cell Ribonucleic Acid Sequencing, 84
Therapeutically Targeting the Genome, 84

FUTURE PERSPECTIVES, 85

REFERENCES, 85

Naturally occurring human genetic variation has served for decades to elucidate the root causes of disease, including cardiovascular disease. Exponential technologic advances in computation, data science, and assay development have recently enabled population-based analyses, broad clinical profiling, and direct-to-consumer genetic testing in millions of people. Because germline genetic variation is established at conception and persists for the lifetime, genetics offers a robust tool for causal inference for broader preventive and therapeutic insights.

This chapter reviews key principles in genetics, gene discovery approaches, and diverse applications of genetic association study findings toward clinical translation (Table 7.1). The molecular structure of deoxyribonucleic acid (DNA) was described approximately 70 years ago, and the Human Genome Project completed the first draft of the human genome sequence approximately 20 years ago at an estimated cost of US$2.7 billion. Over a remarkably short period of time, human genetic data have become increasingly pervasive, and their connection to disease is increasingly understood, thereby rapidly expanding their relevance to the practice of cardiovascular medicine. To highlight the diverse and emerging applications of genetics to cardiovascular medicine, we primarily focus on coronary artery disease (CAD), the leading cause of death worldwide.[1]

KEY PRINCIPLES OF HUMAN GENETICS

Central Dogma

Genes are encoded in DNA, a polymeric molecule with two intertwining strands of a deoxyribose-phosphate backbone surrounding a ladder of paired purine and pyrimidine bases in a double helical configuration. The purine nucleotides are adenine (A) and guanine (G), and the pyrimidine nucleotides are thymine (T) and cytosine (C). Purines and pyrimidines link complementarily by hydrogen bonds across opposing strands: A-T, T-A, C-G, and G-C.

The linear DNA sequence represents its primary structure, and the base-paired double helix represents its secondary structure. Geometric and steric constraints leading to differences in orientation and shape lead to the tertiary structure. Lastly, denser packing of DNA molecules around protein anchors, known as histones, into chromatin provides the quaternary structure. Further chromatin condensation and packing yields the 22 pairs of autosomal chromosomes and one pair of sex chromosomes.

The "central dogma" of molecular biology refers to the flow of information from DNA to ribonucleic acid (RNA) to proteins. Traditionally, a gene is a DNA sequence that encodes a functional protein, and roughly 20,000 genes leading to distinct proteins have been described. *Transcription* copies the information in the DNA sequence into a single-stranded coding RNA, also known as a messenger RNA (mRNA). This polymer is structurally similar to DNA but uses uracil (U) in place of thymine (T). Of the 6.4 billion base pairs in the human genome, just over 1% represent *exons*, or DNA regions that directly encode mRNA. Subsequently, *translation* copies the information in an mRNA into a sequence of amino acids that make up a protein, which can service in a variety of roles (e.g., structural elements, enzymes, hormones, gene expression regulation). Variation in DNA sequence, or *genotype*, may influence protein function or abundance directly through alteration of the amino acid sequence when occurring within exons or indirectly when occurring in noncoding regions, including effects on splicing or mRNA transcript abundance. Such effects on a protein may lead to variation in an observable characteristic, or *phenotype*.

Epigenetics refers to phenotypic changes caused by factors beyond the DNA base pair sequence that influence the process of transcription. The most common such modification is methylation of cytosine bases, typically those in CpG dinucleotides, which generally results in reduced transcription or "silencing" of a gene. Post-translational modification of histone proteins, such as acetylation of lysine residues, can influence the accessibility of DNA sequence to the transcriptional machinery. Additionally, expressed RNA molecules that do not code for proteins, termed noncoding RNAs (ncRNAs), can yield phenotypic changes. For example, long ncRNAs can regulate transcription through several mechanisms, including interactions with the cell's transcriptional machinery and with histone-modifying enzymes; this is the mechanism for X chromosome inactivation in mammals. Additionally, microRNAs, another form of ncRNA, physically bind to complementary sequences in mRNA molecules and result in either suppression of mRNA translation or degradation of the mRNAs.

TABLE 7.1 Translating Genetics to Cardiovascular Medicine

BENCH	BEDSIDE
Identify causal factors that influence disease	Biomarkers titratable to disease risk
Test epidemiologic associations for causal inference	
Penetrance estimation	Disease risk prediction
Therapeutic target prioritization	Novel therapeutic targets
Therapeutic response prediction	Maximization of therapeutic benefit
Discover and characterize the range of phenotypic consequences of therapeutic traits	Minimization of therapeutic side effects
Diverse targeting strategies	Novel medicines

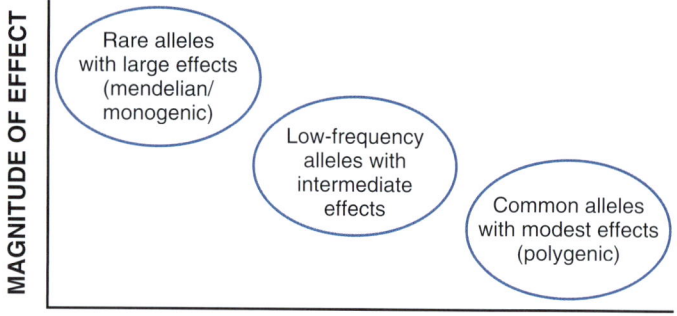

FIGURE 7.1 Relationship between allele frequency and effect magnitude of associated variants. Genome-wide assay studies, typically conducted with genome-wide genotyping arrays, typically identify common alleles with modest effects. Array coverage and imputation better enable the detection of lower frequency variants with intermediate effects. Rare alleles with larger effects are only detectable through genetic sequencing. Whole exome sequencing will detect the full allelic spectrum in coding regions, and whole genome sequencing will detect the full allelic spectrum across the genome.

Heritability

Many cardiovascular diseases, including CAD, aggregate within families. When disease occurs early, shared genetic factors may play a strong role. For example, a family history of premature CAD in a parent confers a nearly twofold risk for CAD.

Heritability refers to the fraction of interindividual variability in risk for disease attributable to additive genetic variation. Heritability is a population-based construct without clear meaning for individuals. Among individuals, 99.9% of the 6.4 billion base pairs are the same; genetic analyses leverage the 0.1% differences to understand trait or disease variation. It is estimated that CAD is 40% to 60% heritable, based on the aforementioned family-based methods or statistical genetics approaches. For common traits studied to date, heritability is typically in the 20% to 80% range. Traits with higher degrees of heritability are more suitable for gene discovery studies and genetic risk prediction. Remaining contributors to disease risk variability include environmental influences, nonadditive genetic influences (epistasis), nonadditive genotype/environment effects, errors in estimations of relatedness or disease, and random chance.

Genetic Architecture

The "genetic architecture" of a disease refers to the number and magnitude of genetic risk factors that exist in each patient and in the population, as well as their frequencies and interactions. For a given individual, diseases can result from genetic variation at a single gene (*monogenic*), few genes (*oligogenic*), or several genes (*polygenic*). In scenarios where a single gene defect is necessary to yield sufficiently large risk for disease, the condition is termed a *mendelian* disorder because it will obey classical modes of inheritance.

Typical mendelian modes of inheritance include autosomal dominant, autosomal recessive, or X-linked. In autosomal dominant disorders, a single defective copy of a gene (with most genes having two copies, one inherited from the mother and one from the father) suffices to cause the phenotype. Autosomal recessive disorders require both copies to be defective to lead to the phenotype. Familial hypercholesterolemia (FH), characterized by severely elevated blood cholesterol values and markedly increased risk for premature CAD, typically occurs due to single genetic variants in low-*LDLR*, *PCSK9*, or *APOB*. However, if both gene copies are disrupted, a more severe phenotype occurs, and thus the inheritance pattern is termed incomplete dominance. In X-linked disorders, the defective gene resides on the X chromosome. Given that men have only one X chromosome and women have two X chromosomes, men who carry the defective copy are affected with the disorder whereas women tend to be unaffected carriers, with some exceptions. Fabry disease, a lysosomal storage disease sometimes manifesting as cardiomyopathy due to disruptive mutations in *GLA* on the X chromosome, is typically more severe in hemizygous men (due to there being one X chromosome, and thus one *GLA* copy) than heterozygous women (due to there being two *GLA* copies). Thus, Fabry is not classically X-linked recessive and is generally simply termed X-linked.

Mendelian disorders imply that the presence of a pathogenic monogenic variant is deterministic for disease. However, genetic profiling in large datasets enables unbiased estimates of penetrance—the likelihood of a person with a pathogenic variant having disease—and expressivity—variation in severity of disease.[2,3]

Genetic Variation

Genetic architecture and phenotype largely dictate the diagnostic yield of genetic testing strategies (Fig. 7.1). Humans share the vast majority of DNA sequence, but variation in both coding and noncoding DNA sequences contributes to distinguishing characteristics between individuals. Due to natural selection over many generations, common genetic variation tends to link to modest phenotypic effects, whereas rarer genetic variation, arising relatively more recently in human history, can lead to larger phenotypic effects. Common genetic variation influencing phenotypes tends to occur within noncoding regulatory elements.[4] Coding sequence is less tolerant of genetic variation, and single base pair changes may lead to substantial phenotypic changes.

Current clinical cardiovascular genetics practice largely focuses on the detection of coding variants predisposing to large phenotypic changes (Fig. 7.2). DNA variation within coding sequence may not necessarily directly impact a protein's amino acid sequence. Degeneracy, or redundancy, in the genetic code refers to the observation that multiple codons (groups of three bases, the basis of the three-letter code) may yield the same amino acid. For example, variation at a G-C-A codon to G-C-G will lead to an alanine in both scenarios; such coding DNA sequence variants without impact on amino acid sequence are termed *synonymous* variants and tend to not have phenotypic consequences. Other coding variants can cause a variety of alterations in a protein—substitution of a single amino acid with another (*missense*), premature introduction of a stop codon (*nonsense*), scrambling of the amino acid sequence past the variant site (*frameshift*), or insertion or deletion of amino acids. These *nonsynonymous* variants may have a range of phenotypic effects from negligible to profound. Nonsense and frameshift variants tend to yield greater phenotypic effects than missense variants. Also, sequence variants at splice sites (the first and second bases after the end of each exon and before the beginning of each exon) can lead to a severely disrupted protein missing a domain encoded by an entire exon. Predicted loss-of-function, or protein-truncating, variants refer to nonsense, frameshift, or splice site variants; of note, such variants that occur near the downstream end of the DNA sequence may not have a significant phenotypic effect.[2,5] In silico prediction algorithms, largely weighted by assessments of evolutionary

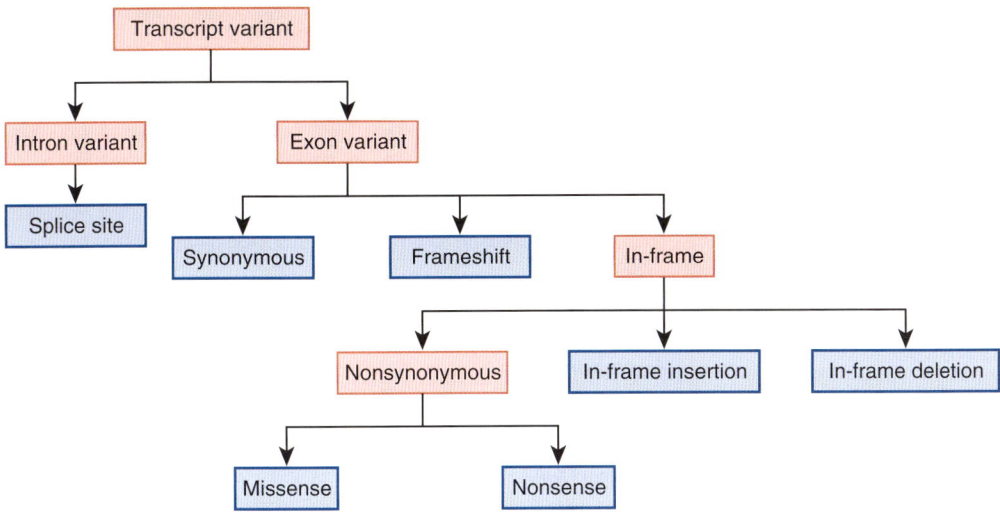

FIGURE 7.2 Protein-altering variant ontology. Key genetic variants expected to have direct impact on amino acid sequence, and therefore overall protein function, and their relationships are depicted.

conservation of DNA sequence across gene families and across species, may help to prioritize missense variants more likely to have larger phenotypic effects.[6]

Noncoding variants, although they do not directly affect the amino acid sequences of proteins, can cause phenotypic changes in other ways. A noncoding variant within regulatory elements, such as promoters or transcriptional enhancers, may result in a decreased amount of the protein product. Noncoding variants can affect the processing of RNA in other ways; for example, a noncoding variant that falls in the midst of a microRNA sequence might impair or enhance the microRNA's ability to interact with specific mRNAs. Large-scale research efforts are cross-referencing human genetic variation with diverse regulatory and intermediate effector molecule changes across tissues to help identify mechanistic links between noncoding DNA variation and phenotypes.[7]

Although most genetic variation is a single base pair change, larger DNA sequence changes may also yield phenotypic impacts. Viable aneuploidies (e.g., Down syndrome caused by trisomy 21) or chromosomal abnormalities can yield varied substantial effects. Copy number variants (CNVs) involve a variable number of repeats of a long DNA sequence (>1000 base pairs), whereas variable nucleotide tandem repeats refer to variation involving shorter nucleotide motifs. CNVs have been linked to congenital heart diseases as well as variation in atherosclerotic cardiovascular disease biomarkers, such as lipoprotein(a) [Lp(a)].

Characterizing Human Genetic Variation

In most cases, a person has two copies of each DNA sequence because of the presence of paired chromosomes, and the two copies are known as *alleles*. Exceptions are for DNA sequences on the X or Y chromosomes in men, the two sex chromosomes being quite different, and for DNA sequences in the mitochondria which are exclusively maternally inherited. For a DNA variant, the *genotype* is the identity of the two alleles at the site of the variant. The two alleles may be identical (homozygous) or different (heterozygous).

A series of genetic variants that occur together is termed a *haplotype*. After the completion of the Human Genome Project, the International HapMap Consortium performed dense sequencing of large genomic segments in hundreds of individuals and identified regions of the genome (loci) where single base pair changes, or *single nucleotide polymorphisms* (SNPs), commonly occur across individuals. Nearby common variants are often found to be inherited together and exist in a state called *linkage disequilibrium* (LD) (Table 7.2). Because the haplotype is located on a single region of the chromosome, it tends to retain the linked genotypes as it passes from parents to offspring.

TABLE 7.2 Factors Influencing Linkage Disequilibrium

FACTORS	MECHANISMS
Variable recombination rates	LD extent is inversely proportional to the recombination rate, and certain regions of the genome have higher rates of recombination than others.
Variable mutation rates	Some regions, such as CpG dinucleotides, may have high mutation rates and show little LD.
Gene conversion	During meiosis, homologous recombination between heterozygous sites may result in correction of mismatched alleles effectively copying DNA sequence.
Natural selection	Haplotypes containing favorable alleles may be quickly swept to high frequency.
Population structure	Population subdivisions promote LD patterns in humans.
Admixture	Subsequent generations after gene flow can newly establish LD between nearby markers.
Genetic drift	Random sampling of gametes in each generation can lead to allele frequency changes, more pronounced in smaller populations

DNA, Deoxyribonucleic acid; *LD*, linkage disequilibrium.

Genotyping technologies directly ascertain the genotype at prespecified variant sites. A common approach to interrogate the presence of a single variant is the polymerase chain reaction-based TaqMan assay; probes are designed to specific SNP alleles, each with a different 5′ fluorophore color that is detected during amplification. More commonly, prespecified variants are assayed in multiplex through array "chips" with the capacity to assess up to 2 million variants at once. Arrays are designed based on LD patterns detected in reference sequencing studies to ensure adequate coverage of haplotypes via "tagging" SNPs across the genome. This technology is used in conventional genome-wide assay studies and in most direct-to-consumer genetic testing services. Imputation, or statistical inference of nondirectly assayed genotypes using data from reference sequencing studies, can infer several million additional genotypes.[8] The imputed allele dosage (0 to 2 on a continuous scale) for each variant with frequency greater than 0.5% in the population is probabilistically assigned based on the combination of genotypes directly assayed on the array.

Sequencing technologies directly identify the order of base pairs in DNA (Fig. 7.3).[9] Sanger sequencing, first described in the 1970s and still in routine use, uses DNA polymerase to synthesize new DNA chains, using the DNA under study as a copy template, with trace amounts of fluorescently labeled chain-terminating nucleotides (four different colors for the four bases) to yield fragments of differing lengths that identify the base in each position by its color. Shotgun

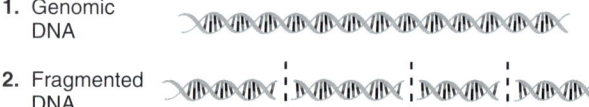
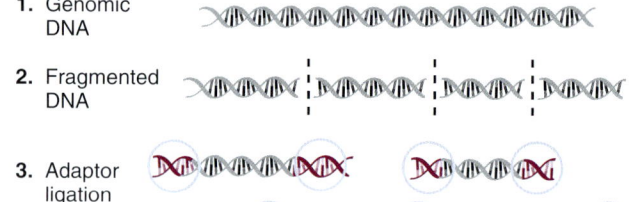
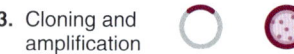
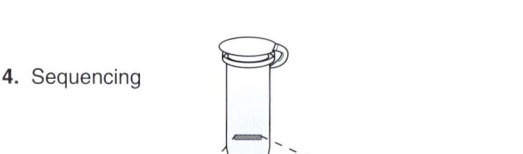
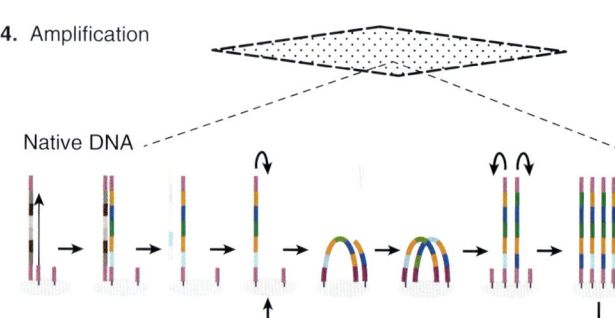
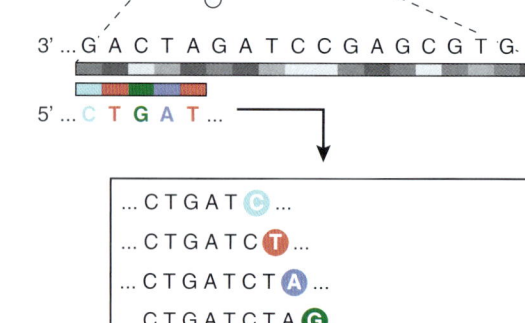
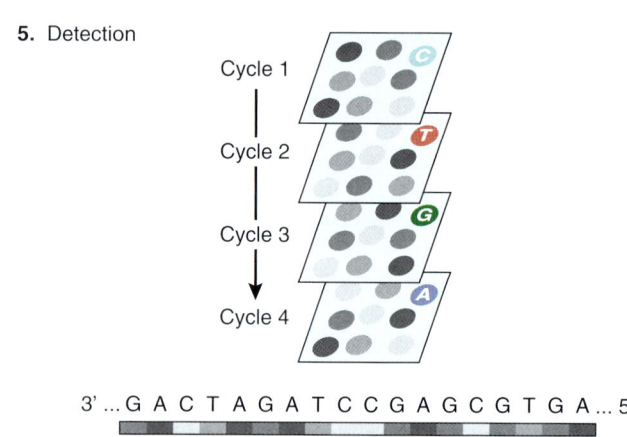
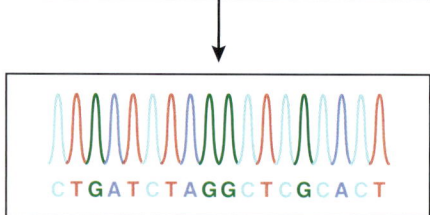
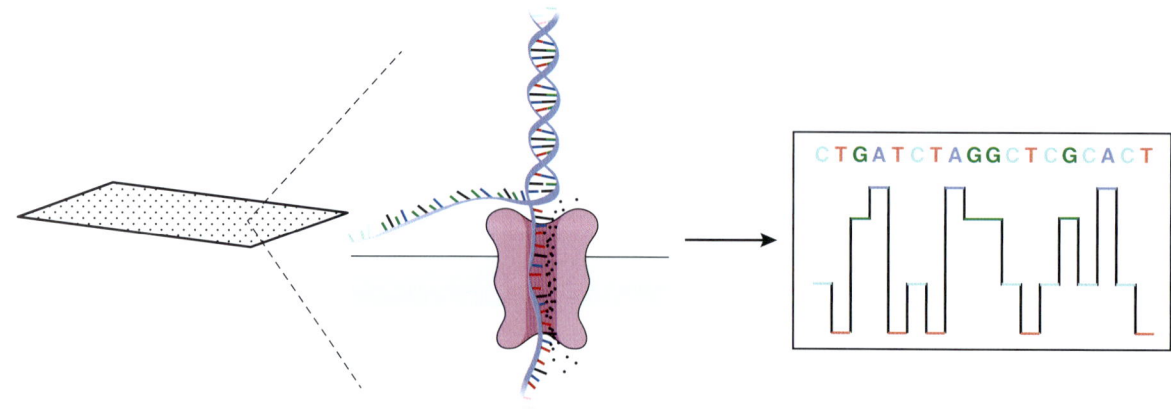

FIGURE 7.3 Schematic of DNA sequencing technologies. Second generation sequencing is also referred to as next generation sequencing. (Adapted from Shendure J, Balasubramanian S, Church GM, et al. DNA sequencing at 40: past, present and future. *Nature.* 2017;550:345–53.)

sequencing, involving the sequencing of random fragments of DNA with subsequent assembly of the sequences via overlaps between the fragments, was used for the Human Genome Project. Massively parallel "next-generation sequencing" (NGS) was developed in the late 1990s through early 2000s. In NGS, fixed DNA libraries provide templates for "sequencing-by-synthesis" in multiplex fashion. NGS can enumerate base pair changes across all 6.4 billion base pairs of the human genome (whole genome sequencing) or exclusively the protein-coding regions (whole exome sequencing). Both whole exome and whole genome sequencing are increasingly applied in population-based research analyses as well as clinical applications. To minimize biases introduced from templates (such as copying errors and sequence-dependent amplification biases) used for NGS, novel approaches such as real-time, single-molecule sequencing platforms for long-read de novo sequencing are being explored but have not yet been applied at similar scale as NGS.[10]

GENE DISCOVERY

Family-Based Studies

Conditions that occur prematurely and aggregate in families suggest important contribution from genetic variation. When classic mendelian inheritance patterns are observed for a suspected mendelian condition, genetic analyses to confirm the presence of a monogenic factor will have greater diagnostic yield than when such inheritance patterns are absent. For adult-onset conditions with strong genetic and nongenetic determinants, general familial enrichment may also result from polygenic or environmental factors. *Phenocopy* refers to a phenotype consistent with genetic predisposition but largely caused by environmental conditions for a given individual.

For novel syndromes or phenotypes without a known genetic basis or with nondiagnostic conventional genetic testing, family-based analyses may serve to discover novel implicated genes. Recruitment of multiple family members both with and without the phenotype allows for elimination of genotypes inconsistent with mendelian segregation. Both phenocopy and reduced penetrance may lead to deviation from expected inheritance patterns, and thus analyses of large extended pedigrees aid such analyses.

Previously, linkage studies were used to prioritize genomic regions that tended to cosegregate with the presence of a phenotype rather than the absence of the phenotype. Classic approaches, prior to widespread use of NGS, involved genotyping hundreds of genetic markers across the genome. Cosegregation of a marker with disease in pedigrees suggested that the causal disease mutation lay within several megabases of the marker, a region that often encompasses numerous candidate genes. Positional cloning would further narrow down the region by genotyping more markers, with subsequent sequencing used to identify the causal gene.

NGS is often now used upfront for broad gene sequencing, particularly whole exome sequencing, for family-based analyses. Variants annotated to disrupt protein function are prioritized if they are consistently observed among affected family members but not present among unaffected family members. The advent of large publicly available reference multi-ethnic whole exome and whole genome sequence databases of allele frequencies now allow for the verification of the absence of a suspected disease-causing variant among unrelated healthy individuals.[2] Once the rare genetic variant thought most likely to be the causal mutation is selected, it can be confirmed by sequencing the gene in unrelated individuals who have the same disorder. If some of these individuals have variants in the same gene (either the same or, more likely, different variants), it strongly argues that the gene is responsible for the disease.

Hypercholesterolemia and Coronary Artery Disease (see also Chapter 27)

FH afflicts approximately 1 in 300 individuals, manifesting as severely elevated blood cholesterol levels and increased risk for early-onset myocardial infarction (Fig. 7.4). Work in the 1970s and 1980s demonstrated that most cases of FH result from mutations in the *LDLR* gene, and subsequent studies implicated mutations in the gene for apolipoprotein B (*APOB*) at domains that interact with the LDL receptor.[11]

In the early 2000s, various studies identified families with apparent incompletely dominant FH but without *LDLR* or *APOB* variants. Linkage analyses and subsequent positional cloning identified *PCSK9* as the causal gene. Sequencing studies and subsequent functional work identified two different rare gain-of-function *PCSK9* variants in different families. PCSK9 increases blood cholesterol by binding to the LDL receptor and reducing the availability of the LDL receptor at the cell surface for cholesterol clearance from blood.

Also in the early 2000s, linkage and cloning analyses of families with autosomal recessive FH prioritized a large region on chromosome 1. Ultimately, homozygous mutations in *LDLRAP1* (previously known as ARH, autosomal recessive hypercholesterolemia) were implicated in several families of Sardinian origin. *LDLRAP1* encodes LDL receptor adaptor protein 1, which is required for endocytosis of the LDL receptor.

Metabolic Syndrome and Coronary Artery Disease

In 2007, linkage analysis of an extended family of Iranian ancestry with premature CAD and features of the metabolic syndrome resulted in the identification of a causal missense variant in *LRP6*. In vitro analyses indicated that the *LRP6* missense variant disrupts Wnt signaling. More recently, the same investigators used linkage analyses in three large families of Iranian ancestry with cosegregation of premature CAD and the metabolic syndrome to prioritize a region in chromosome 19.[12] Whole exome sequencing and focused analysis within the prioritized region identified a perfectly cosegregating missense variant in *DYRK1B* in all three families. Screening of morbidly obese individuals of European descent with CAD and multiple metabolic phenotypes identified a family with cosegregation of a different missense variant in *DYRK1B*. Functional analysis indicated that the variants were gain-of-function, promoting the expression of the gene encoding glucose-6-phosphatase.

Case-Control and Population-Based Studies

The technologic advances described earlier in this chapter allow unbiased assessments of the effects of genome-wide genetic variation on cardiovascular traits in large cohorts. Family-based analyses continue to be an efficient study design for families with apparently mendelian conditions with nondiagnostic genetic panel testing. However, heritability assessments for common conditions, such as CAD, indicate that naturally occurring common genetic variation may contribute to CAD risk broadly and not just in such exceptional families.

The design of studies using large cohorts focuses on maximizing power (likelihood of detecting true associations) to test hypotheses while minimizing the risk of detecting false associations. Power for genetic association analyses is determined by: (1) exposure (allele) frequency, (2) total sample size, particularly case count, (3) true effect of the exposure, and (4) threshold for statistical significance. Because there are approximately 1 million independent sites of common genetic variation in the human genome, a Bonferroni-corrected alpha threshold of 5×10^{-8} (0.05 divided by 1 million) for statistical significance is typically applied to genome-wide studies. Despite stringent thresholds for statistical significance used to mitigate false-positives in a single discovery cohort, putative novel associations should undergo independent replication in a validation cohort.[13] Both population stratification (systematic allele frequency differences between subpopulations) and cryptic relatedness (greater degree of relatedness among individuals in a cohort than is assumed) may lead to spurious associations. The use of genome-wide genotyping data to adjust for ancestry and genetic relatedness may mitigate such confounding.

Two broad analytic approaches are used—the common variant association study (CVAS) and the rare variant association study (RVAS).[14] CVAS is also termed genome-wide association study (GWAS). In a GWAS, genetic variants are sufficiently prevalent to estimate the relative difference between cases and controls or incremental change in a continuous outcome. In contrast, RVAS aims to test the collective contribution of individually rare variants to a phenotype, requiring the aggregation of rare variants into a statistical exposure unit for effect estimation.

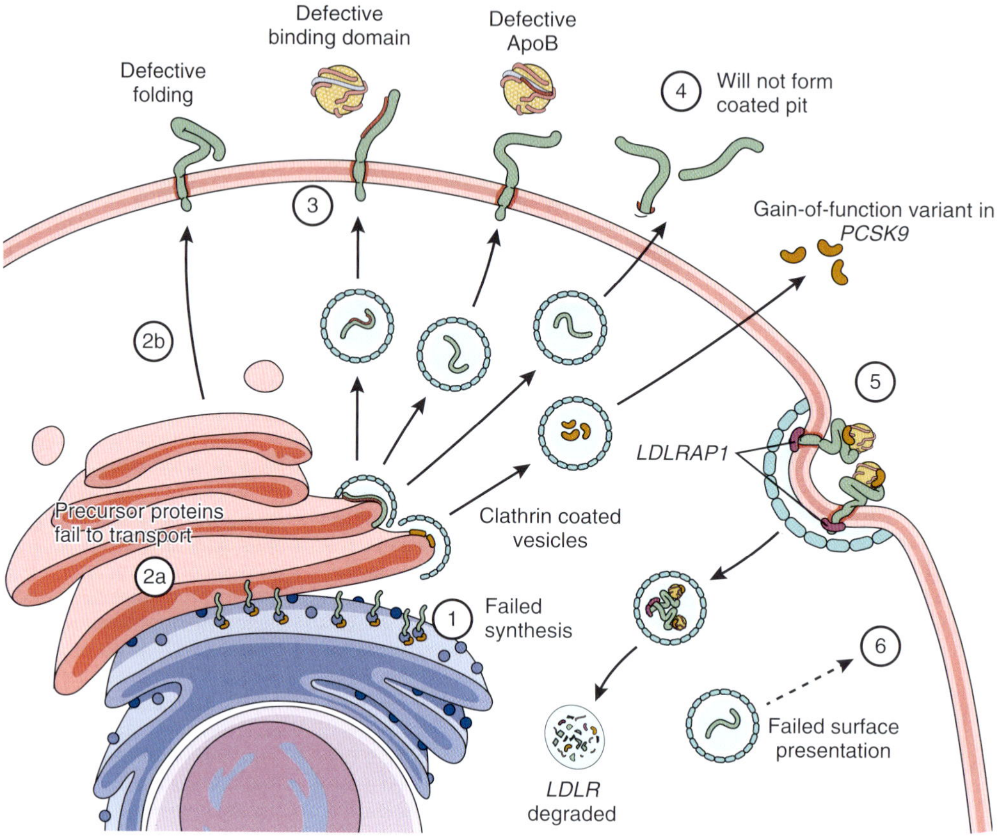

FIGURE 7.4 Mechanisms of *LDLR* dysfunction leading to familial hypercholesterolemia. Numbers refer to classes of *LDLR* variants: (1) synthesis of receptor or precursor protein is absent, (2) absent [2a] or impaired [2b] formation of receptor protein, (3) normal synthesis of receptor protein, abnormal low-density lipoprotein binding, (4) clustering in coated pits, internalization of the receptor complex does not take place, (5) receptors are not recycled and are rapidly degraded, and (6) receptors fail to be targeted in the basolateral membrane. *ApoB*, apolipoprotein B; *LDLR*, low-density lipoprotein receptor; *LDLRAP1*, low-density lipoprotein receptor associated protein 1; *PCSK9*, proprotein convertase subtilisin/kexin type 9. (Adapted from Gidding SS, Champagne MA, de Ferranti SD, et al. The Agenda for familial hypercholesterolemia: a scientific statement from the American Heart Association. *Circulation*. 2015;132:2167–92.)

GWASs use arrays comprising prespecified genetic variants, typically up to 2 million. Reference datasets may be used to impute 10 to 30 million additional variants depending on ethnicity and panel. Conventional statistical models use multivariable regression frameworks to compare each variant's allele frequency between cases or controls or with graded effect on a continuous outcome. Case-control cross-sectional study designs have a lower risk of confounding in GWAS versus in observational epidemiologic studies because putative confounders are unlikely to influence the random allocation of alleles at birth. Because case count strongly influences statistical power, case-control experimental designs are frequently used in GWASs. As broadly phenotyped mega-biobanks become increasingly available, new computationally efficient mixed model approaches to analyze unbalanced case-control phenotypes are often used.[15,16] Conventional methods ignore putative genetic interactions between loci, or epistasis; to address this omission, emerging methods aim to use multidimensional genetic architecture into genetic discovery. A novel discovery from a GWAS, typically a common noncoding SNP, represents just the first step in characterizing the biologic and clinical relevance of the genomic locus marked by the SNP, because the locus will often contain numerous candidate genes, any one of which could be causal. Follow-up efforts include comprehensive in silico and functional dissection to prioritize causal variants and genes toward understanding how the SNP genotype leads to the phenotype.

RVASs, which typically interrogate rare disruptive protein-coding variants, allow for more robust prioritization of causal genes, because any identified variants nominate the genes in which they reside. Given the infrequency of each individual variant, and the corresponding lack of statistical power, variants in the same gene are collapsed into a single statistical unit for association. Because approximately 20,000 protein-coding genes have been described in the human genome, the Bonferroni-corrected alpha threshold (i.e., corrected for multiple comparisons) for exome-wide significance is 2.5×10^{-6}. Because disruptive variants within the same gene may have bidirectional functional effects (loss-of-function variants versus gain-of-function variants), as is the case with *PCSK9* and *APOB*, specialized methods accounting for this phenomenon, such as the sequence kernel association test, are preferred.

Genome-Wide Association Studies for Lipids

Starting in 2007, GWASs have been performed on cohorts of individuals of European descent to identify SNPs associated with blood low-density lipoprotein cholesterol (LDL-C), high-density lipoprotein cholesterol (HDL-C), triglycerides, or total cholesterol. With each successive year, an increasing number of variants and loci are newly discovered due to: (1) increased sample sizes, (2) improved coverage from successive genotyping arrays, (3) incorporation of diverse ethnicities, and (4) improvements in genotype imputation. These advances also permit the characterization and association of uncommon alleles with larger effect sizes (Fig. 7.5). To date, over 350 distinct regions of the genome have been identified to be significantly associated with blood lipids.[17]

Imputation and the analysis of diverse ethnicities have enabled the detection of so-called Goldilocks alleles. Such variants represent large-effect disruptive mutations with sufficiently high allele frequencies to have statistical power in population-based studies. The analysis of founder or bottlenecked populations are well suited to identifying large-effect uncommon alleles. For example, a study of nearly 120,000 adults living in Iceland used array-derived genotypes imputed to 25.3 million variants from reference genomes from Iceland.[18] A novel rare (allele frequency 0.4%) Northern European–specific 12-base pair deletion in the fourth intron of *ASGR1* (a receptor on hepatocytes for a class of glycoproteins) was found to be associated with both reduced non–HDL-C and reduced risk for CAD. Polymerase chain reaction (PCR)-based and direct sequence analyses indicated that the intronic variant disrupted *ASGR1* mRNA splicing, leading to a truncated ASGR1 protein.

In addition to imputation, genotyping arrays enriched for exonic variant coverage ("exome chips") also identify large-effect uncommon disruptive variants. Such an approach was recently applied to lipids across diverse ethnicities, with several novel associations.[19,20] A new observation was the association of *A1CF* p.Gly398Ser with increased

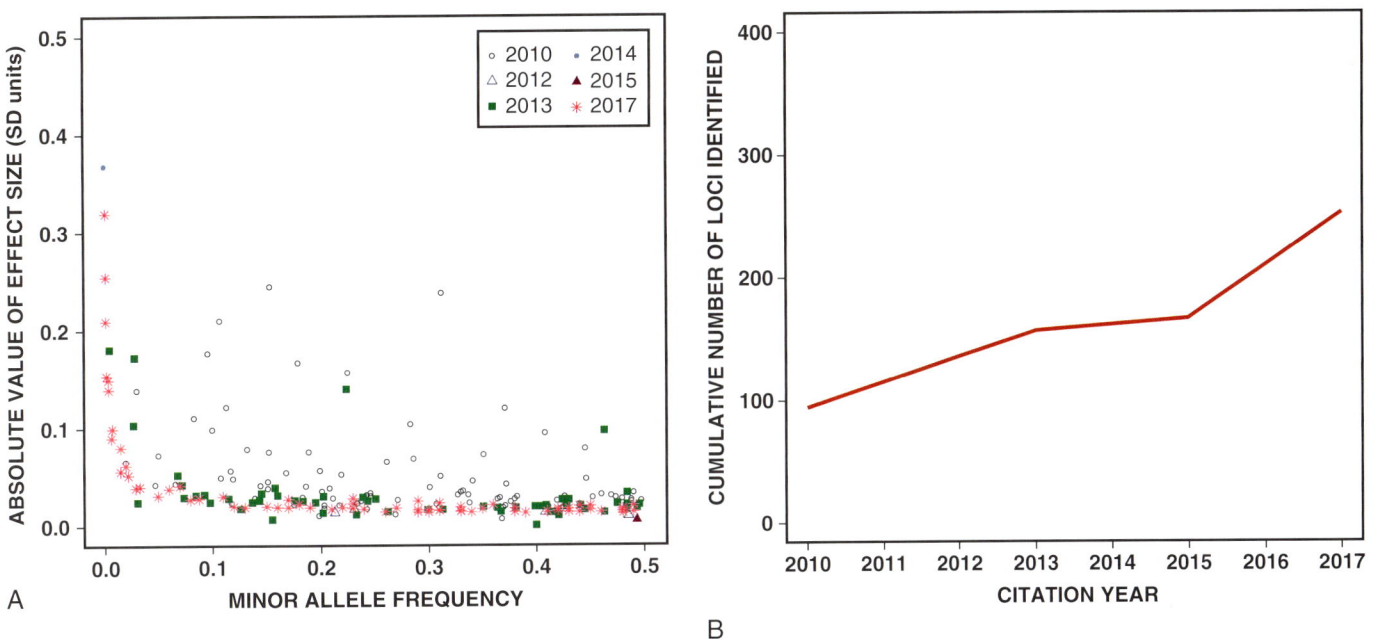

FIGURE 7.5 Identified lipid associations through genome-wide scans for plasma lipids. **A,** Compared with earlier studies, newer studies with denser arrays (including arrays enriched for coding variation), improved imputation, and larger sample sizes enable detection of variants across the allelic spectrum with more modest effects as well as lower frequency and rare variants with larger effects. **B,** Due to denser arrays, improved imputation, and larger sample sizes, genetic association studies for lipids continue to identify novel genomic loci associated with lipids. (Adapted from Peloso GM, Natarajan P. Insights from population-based analyses of plasma lipids across the allele frequency spectrum. *Curr Opin Genet Dev.* 2018;50:1–6.)

triglyceride and total cholesterol concentrations, as well as nominal association with increased risk for CAD.[19] Consistent with this observation, knock-in mice with the equivalent of the *A1CF* p.Gly398Ser mutation had increased triglycerides. A1CF is an RNA-binding protein that alters the splicing of messages that encode enzymes involved in carbohydrate metabolism.

Genome-Wide Association Studies for Coronary Artery Disease

The first GWASs for CAD were reported in 2007, all identifying a 58-kilobase interval in chromosome 9p21 not previously recognized to be relevant to CAD and not containing any protein-coding genes (a so-called gene desert). Despite intensive efforts since the discovery of this 9p21 locus, the mechanisms by which variants in the locus influence CAD risk remain unclear, highlighting how functional interrogation of disease-associated variants in genomic regions without robust pathophysiologic hypotheses remains a formidable challenge. The list of loci associated with CAD continues to expand, with 163 loci identified to date (Fig. 7.6).[21] Based on observed pleiotropy and prior biologic hypotheses, many loci may contribute to CAD risk through various established risk factors, and many other loci, including the 9p21 locus, may act through currently undiscovered pathways.

Analysis of low-frequency disruptive alleles for CAD using exome chips has also discovered newly implicated genes. *SVEP1* p.D2702G (allele frequency 3.6%) was recently found to be associated with increased risk for CAD.[22] SVEP1 encodes sushi, a cell-adhesion molecule. Interrogation of *SVEP1* p.D2702G with established CAD risk factors showed that it also led to increased blood pressure and increased risk for diabetes mellitus type 2. The CAD association appears outsized compared with the effects on blood pressure and diabetes mellitus, implicating potentially novel pathways that may contribute to CAD risk.

Evidence of association across an "allelic series"—multiple alleles with diverse frequencies (common and rare) and mechanisms (noncoding and coding) linked to the same gene—increases confidence in causal gene inference. Prior evidence strongly implicated the nitric oxide–cyclic GMP pathway in CAD risk, and CAD GWASs have detected several SNPs tagging key genes in the pathway, such as *NOS3*, *GUCY1A1* (formerly *GUCY1A3*, a guanylate cyclase subunit), *PDE5A*, *PDE3A*, and *MRVI1*. Luciferase assays for a CAD-associated noncoding variant near *GUCY1A1* show that it modulates *GUCY1A1* promoter activity.[23] Prior work linked loss-of-function mutations in *GUCY1A1* in an extended family with increased risk for premature CAD. Consistent with these findings, both common noncoding and rare coding disruptive alleles in *GUCY1A1* influence both blood pressure and CAD risk in population-based analyses.[24]

Population-Based Discovery of Rare Protein-Coding Variants Associated with Coronary Artery Disease

To date, few examples exist of aggregated rare variants significantly associated with CAD at exome-wide significance levels in RVASs. To date the only significantly associated gene to achieve exome-wide significance through this statistical procedure for CAD or myocardial infarction is *LDLR*.[25] Bolstered by strong evidence for association of *APOA5*, *APOC3*, *LPL*, *LPA*, *PCSK9*, *ANGPTL4*, *ANGPTL3*, and *NPC1L1* with atherogenic lipoproteins,[22,26-28] the observation of supportive albeit subsignificant associations of these genes with CAD at the population level supports likely causal involvement of these genes in CAD. As whole exome and whole genome datasets expand, power to detect rare variants through nonlipid pathways will improve. Focusing case-control ascertainment on extremes (early-onset cases and unaffected older control individuals) may prove to be a more efficient study design.[25]

CAUSAL INFERENCE OF EPIDEMIOLOGIC ASSOCIATIONS

Hypotheses concerning causal agents for complex diseases have often initially come from observational epidemiology. For example, seminal work in the 1960s in the Framingham Heart Study and other cohorts correlated blood cholesterol with future risk for CAD. Since then, studies have linked numerous soluble biomarkers with future risk for CAD (see also Chapter 10). How many of these biomarkers directly cause CAD, how many simply reflect other causal processes, and why is this

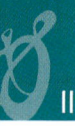

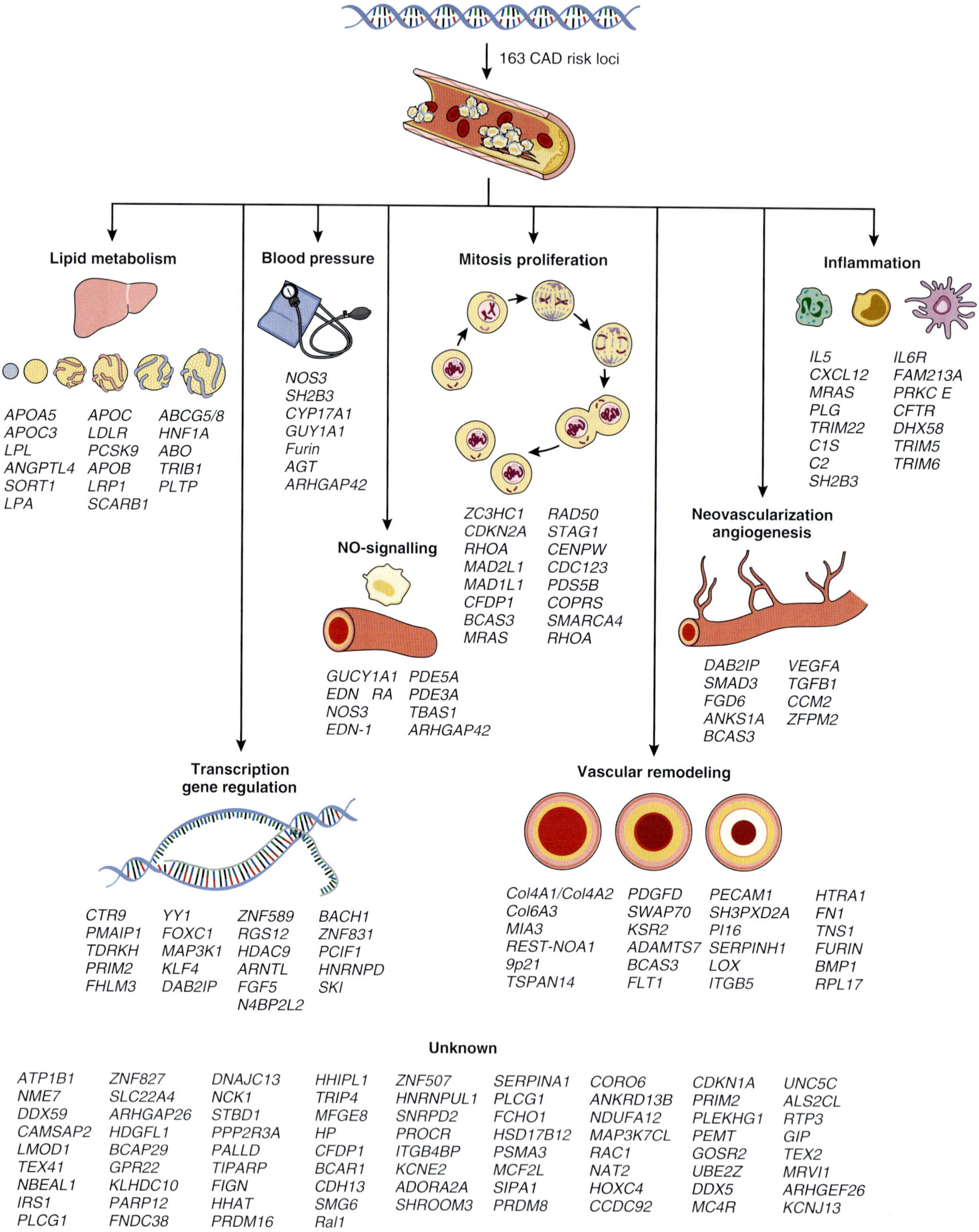

FIGURE 7.6 Genes mapped to known coronary artery disease loci from genome-wide association studies binned by atherosclerosis-related pathophysiologic pathways based on observed pleiotropy. (Adapted from Erdmann J, Kessler T, Munoz Venegas L, et al. A decade of genome-wide association studies for coronary artery disease: the challenges ahead. *Cardiovasc Res.* 2018;114:1241–57.)

question important? Both causal and noncausal biomarkers may help predict risk for future disease, but only a causal biomarker may be appropriate as a target of therapy. A randomized controlled trial (RCT) testing whether a treatment that alters the biomarker will affect risk for disease is the ultimate test for causality in humans, but RCTs are expensive and time-consuming. However, supportive human genetic evidence increases the likelihood of RCT success.[29]

Mendelian Randomization Principles and Applications

A technique termed *mendelian randomization* (MR) uses DNA sequence variants to address the question of whether an epidemiologic association between a risk factor and disease actually reflects causality (Fig. 7.7). In principle, if a DNA sequence variant directly affects an intermediate phenotype (e.g., a variant in the promoter of a gene encoding a biomarker that alters its expression) and the intermediate phenotype truly contributes to the disease, the DNA variant should be associated with the disease to the extent predicted by (1) the size of the effect of the variant on the phenotype and (2) the size of the effect of the phenotype on the disease. If the predicted association between the variant and disease does not emerge from an adequately powered study, it would argue against a causal role for the intermediate phenotype in pathogenesis of the disease.

The study design is akin to a prospective RCT in that randomization for each individual occurs at the moment of conception—genotypes of DNA variants are randomly "assigned" to gametes during meiosis, a process that avoids the typical confounders encountered in observational epidemiologic studies (Fig. 7.8). For example, a parent's disease status or socioeconomic status should not affect which of the parent's two alleles at a given SNP is passed to a child, with each allele having an equal (50%) chance of being transmitted by the gamete to the zygote. Thus, MR should mitigate confounding or reverse causation. MR has potential shortcomings, including that (1) the technique is only as reliable as the robustness of the estimates of the effect sizes of the variant on the intermediate and disease phenotypes, and (2) it assumes that the DNA variant does not influence the disease by other means (pleiotropy), which may not be true. In addition, a potential confounder of MR is that, in certain situations, a disease might cause the allele of a DNA variant passed from a parent to an offspring to be expressed in a different way (e.g., through epigenetic effects). Nevertheless, MR can prove informative for causal inference in observational human datasets.

Causal Inference for Lipoproteins (see also Chapter 27)

Numerous epidemiologic studies have positively correlated LDL-C and inversely correlated HDL-C with incident CAD risk. MR analyses support a causal relationship for LDL-C but not HDL-C. Consistently, multiple RCTs of different LDL-C–lowering medicines have demonstrated improved CAD outcomes, and multiple RCTs of different HDL-C–raising medicines have not noted any improvement in CAD outcomes. Consistent with meta-analyses implying that statins associate with an increased risk for diabetes mellitus, MR studies support a general causal inverse relationship between LDL-C and diabetes mellitus.[30] Although HDL-C is not a therapeutic target, it remains a robust biomarker for CAD risk prediction.[31]

Lp(a) is a circulating LDL-like particle covalently bound to apolipoprotein(a). Lp(a) is elevated in approximately one in five individuals and is independently associated with first and recurrent atherosclerotic cardiovascular disease events in multiple cohorts. Uniquely, Lp(a) is highly heritable across ethnicities, estimated at 85%, with associated genetic variation largely at the *LPA* locus.[32] MR studies indicate that Lp(a)-associated variants at *LPA* are also associated with CAD, supporting a causal relationship.[32,33] MR studies also extend this relationship to at least peripheral arterial disease and ischemic stroke.[34,35] Ongoing RCTs of medicines aimed at specifically lowering Lp(a) will test whether Lp(a) is causally associated with atherosclerotic cardiovascular disease. MR studies also indicate that Lp(a) is causal for aortic stenosis, for which a proven medical therapy has not yet been described.[34]

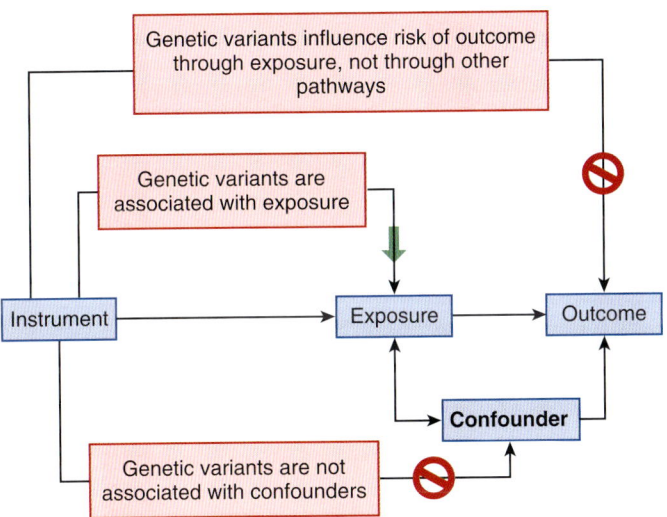

FIGURE 7.7 Mendelian randomization acyclic graph with assumptions.

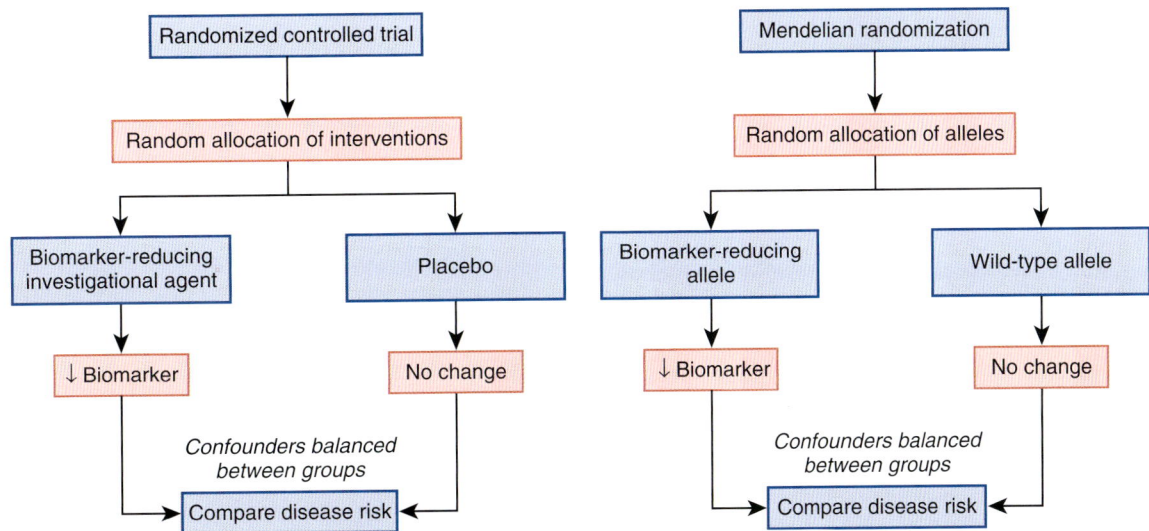

FIGURE 7.8 Parallel experimental designs between randomized controlled trials and mendelian randomization. Study randomization and the random allocation of alleles at birth facilitate the balance of putative confounders between exposure groups.

Causal Inference for Adiposity

Obesity has been correlated with diabetes mellitus type 2 and CAD risk but body fat distribution varies widely for a given body mass index (BMI). Waist-to-hip ratio (WHR) as a measure of abdominal adiposity associates independently with cardiometabolic risk in epidemiologic studies. However, reverse causation may lead to similar relationships; for example, individuals with CAD may be less prone to exercise, resulting in greater adiposity. A recent MR study, however, implied the relationship may be causal; genetic variants associated with WHR independent of BMI were strongly associated with both diabetes mellitus type 2 and CAD risks.[36] An increased WHR may occur either with increased abdominal adiposity or decreased gluteofemoral adiposity. Using dual-energy x-ray absorptiometry assessment and genotyping, MR studies indicate that abdominal adiposity and gluteofemoral adiposity may be separately deleterious and protective, respectively, for cardiometabolic disease.[37]

Mendelian Randomization Assumption Assessments

To buttress causal inferences from observational data, assumption assessments and sensitivity analyses are required. First, the hypothesis evaluated should have a strong scientific premise from observational epidemiology or experimental results from independent data sources. Second, a valid genetic instrument for the exposure of interest should be verified to mitigate weak instrument bias. After significant variants are selected and their corresponding exposure effects are tabulated from a discovery dataset, external verification of strong exposure association by examining effect estimate, model fit, and F statistic ensures validity.

After identification of a putative association, assessments of whether genetic variants influence the outcome via putative confounders correlated with the exposure of interest or independent pathways (horizontal pleiotropy) are pursued. Association of the genetic instrument with expected and measured confounders based on observational epidemiologic studies aids the assessment. The use of multiple significantly associated genetic variants in a composite score not only improves the instrument but also permits assessments of pleiotropy. For example, the more likely each variant's effect on the exposure is proportional to its effect on the outcome, the less likely pleiotropy is influencing the genetic association.[38,39] Some MR methods permit a non-zero intercept providing an estimate of unbalanced pleiotropy.[40] Novel methods now detect variant subsets that may exhibit horizontal pleiotropy to down-weight or remove outliers.[41,42]

DISEASE RISK PREDICTION

Current clinical practice focuses on the identification of monogenic variants among affected probands and asymptomatic family members. Genetic testing provides molecular confirmation for a clinical diagnosis and may inform treatments and surveillance. Because an increasing number of common genetic variants are found to be associated with cardiovascular diseases and risk factors, polygenic risk scores (PRSs) are being developed and evaluated for potential clinical application. As whole exome and genome sequencing becomes increasingly prevalent, both monogenic and polygenic factors may together improve disease risk prediction and preventive strategies.[3]

The liability threshold model of disease proposes a normal risk distribution for binary outcomes from numerous nongenetic and genetic factors, with a theoretical threshold above which a disease typically manifests. Knowledge of genotype-phenotype associations, even in the absence of identifying causal variants or genes, may inform phenotype prediction. Rare and common risk alleles as well as nongenetic risk factors, such as smoking, contribute to the overall liability of CAD risk.

Pathogenicity Assessments and Monogenic Risk

Clinical laboratories assess likelihood of disease risk on an ordinal scale using criteria put forward by the American College of Medical Genetics and Genomics (ACMG).[43] The five-tier terminology comprises: pathogenic, likely pathogenic, uncertain significance, likely benign, and benign. In addition to pathogenicity assertions, laboratories will assign inheritance patterns and associated conditions. Pathogenicity is interpreted according to: (1) scarcity in population-based datasets, (2) in silico assessments of deleteriousness, (3) functional assessments of deleteriousness, (4) cosegregation with disease in families, (5) de novo data in suitable pedigrees, (6) *trans* configuration with another pathogenic variant for autosomal recessive conditions, (7) curated reliable databases from external clinical laboratories, and (8) gene specificity for condition.[43]

The current classification system may inadvertently connote full penetrance for pathogenic variants and null risk for the remaining variants. As sequencing data are increasingly available in unselected populations, it is increasingly clear that pathogenic variants predisposing to adult-onset disease carry high disease risk but are not deterministic.[3] Approximately 1% of adults harbor a pathogenic variant for an "actionable" adult-onset condition, largely cardiovascular or oncologic. Currently, when secondarily detected in clinical testing, pathogenic variants for 59 such genes are recommended for return of results to patients according to the ACMG (Table 7.3).[44]

TABLE 7.3 American College of Medical Genetics and Genomics Cardiovascular Genes and Associated Phenotypes Recommended for Return of Secondary Findings in Clinical Sequencing

PHENOTYPE	GENE	INHERITANCE
Ehlers-Danlos syndrome, vascular type	COL3A1	AD
Marfan syndrome, Loeys-Dietz syndromes, and familial thoracic aortic aneurysms and dissections	FBN1	AD
	TGFBR1	AD
	TGFBR2	AD
	SMAD3	AD
	ACTA2	AD
	MYH11	AD
Hypertrophic cardiomyopathy, dilated cardiomyopathy	MYBPC3	AD
	MYH7	AD
	TNNT2	AD
	TNNI3	AD
	TPM1	AD
	MYL3	AD
	ACTC1	AD
	PRKAG2	AD
	GLA	XL
	MYL2	AD
	LMNA	AD
Catecholaminergic polymorphic ventricular tachycardia	RYR2	AD
Arrhythmogenic right ventricular cardiomyopathy	PKP2	AD
	DSP	AD
	DSC2	AD
	TMEM43	AD
	DSG2	AD
Romano-Ward long QT syndrome types 1, 2, and 3, Brugada syndrome	KCNQ1	AD
	KCNH2	AD
	SCN5A	AD
Familial hypercholesterolemia	LDLR	AD
	APOB	AD
	PCSK9	AD

Monogenic Coronary Artery Disease

Although FH is a well-established monogenic risk factor for CAD, the necessity of molecular confirmation after clinical diagnosis from routine lipid screening and history has been controversial.[11] Cascade testing, or screening family members of probands, has been touted as a key reason for genetic testing, but its value beyond lipid screening is less clear. Indeed, many relatives of those with FH have not had lipids assessed regardless of variant presence.[45] Two key factors have facilitated expansion of FH genetic testing in clinical practice: (1) large-scale NGS in population-based cohorts demonstrating incremental prognostic assessments[46,47] and (2) the availability of novel, expensive cholesterol-lowering medicines.

Beyond a single LDL-C value, the presence of an FH variant may yield added risk for CAD. Among individuals with severe hypercholesterolemia (LDL-C > 190 mg/dL), only 1 in 50 has an FH variant.[46,47] Among those with a clinical phenotype classified as "probable FH," 1 in 16 has an FH variant, whereas 1 in 4 with "definite" FH has an FH variant.[46] Compared with those without elevated LDL-C levels and without FH variants, severe hypercholesterolemia without an FH variant carried a 6-fold greater risk for CAD, but those with severe hypercholesterolemia and an FH variant had a 22-fold greater risk for CAD.[47] Per guidelines and current U.S. Food and Drug Administration labeling, in the primary prevention setting, more stringent LDL-C targets should be pursued in FH patients, with PCSK9 inhibitors as needed to attain those targets.[31]

Polygenic Risk Scoring

Individual common variants associated with a condition in GWASs may be leveraged for the construction of PRSs (Fig. 7.9). Early PRSs were simply a summation of uncorrelated, significantly associated risk alleles. As most genetic variants have unequal disease effects, weighting by the disease risk effect estimate improves model fit, and unweighted PRSs have largely now been abandoned for risk prediction. Because GWASs of increasing sizes detect increasing numbers of significantly associated variants, many variants not yet significantly associated with an outcome may still inform risk prediction. Novel methods focus on expanding the number of variants included in the model and reweighting to improve risk prediction, including for the creation of so-called genome-wide PRSs.

Due to their largely being informed by GWASs with individuals of European descent, the performance of contemporary PRSs continues to lag for non-European ancestries.[48] Ongoing efforts to close this gap to reduce the risk of exacerbating existing health disparities include increasingly large genetic studies in diverse ethnicities and the development of novel PRS methodologies.

Polygenic Coronary Artery Disease

Significant recent efforts have focused on polygenic risk scoring for CAD, given the prospect of facilitating earlier preventive strategies for the leading cause of death. Polygenic risk for CAD predisposes to the development of premature coronary atherosclerosis.[49,50] A CAD PRS was shown to predict future risk for CAD among individuals with or without a family history of premature CAD.[51] Recent implementation of genome-wide PRSs for CAD in the U.K. Biobank has shown improvement in the prediction of CAD beyond conventional risk factors.[52,53] Genome-wide PRSs may be particularly well suited to better identify individuals at markedly elevated risk for CAD at the distribution tails. For example, the top 5th percentile (1 in 20) carries similar odds for CAD as individuals with FH variants (1 in 300).[52] Although FH is typically readily detected by significantly elevated LDL-C concentrations, elevated CAD PRS is not readily detected by conventional risk factors. Among middle-aged adults, risk discrimination is similar to other cardiovascular disease risk factors.[54,55] A CAD PRS may be particularly helpful for middle-aged adults at intermediate cardiovascular disease risk.[56] However, a CAD PRS may prove more useful for guiding therapeutic intervention earlier in life even before the onset of conventional cardiovascular risk factors.[53,56]

THERAPEUTIC RESPONSE PREDICTION

In his 2015 State of the Union Address, President Obama launched the U.S. Precision Medicine Initiative. Although the notion of guiding preventive and treatment strategies by accounting for individual variability is not new, broad research and application are now feasible with large-scale human genetic and biologic databases, high-throughput molecular profiling, and computational advances.[57] Precision medicine aims to advance risk prediction to individualized therapies based on composite risk factors. Dense molecular and phenotyping profiling toward this goal also facilitates the discovery of broadly applicable novel therapies.

Target Discovery and Clinical Trial Prediction

Genetic variants that alter protein activity can provide robust inferences regarding the outcomes of pharmacologic manipulation before embarking on drug development. Furthermore, identification

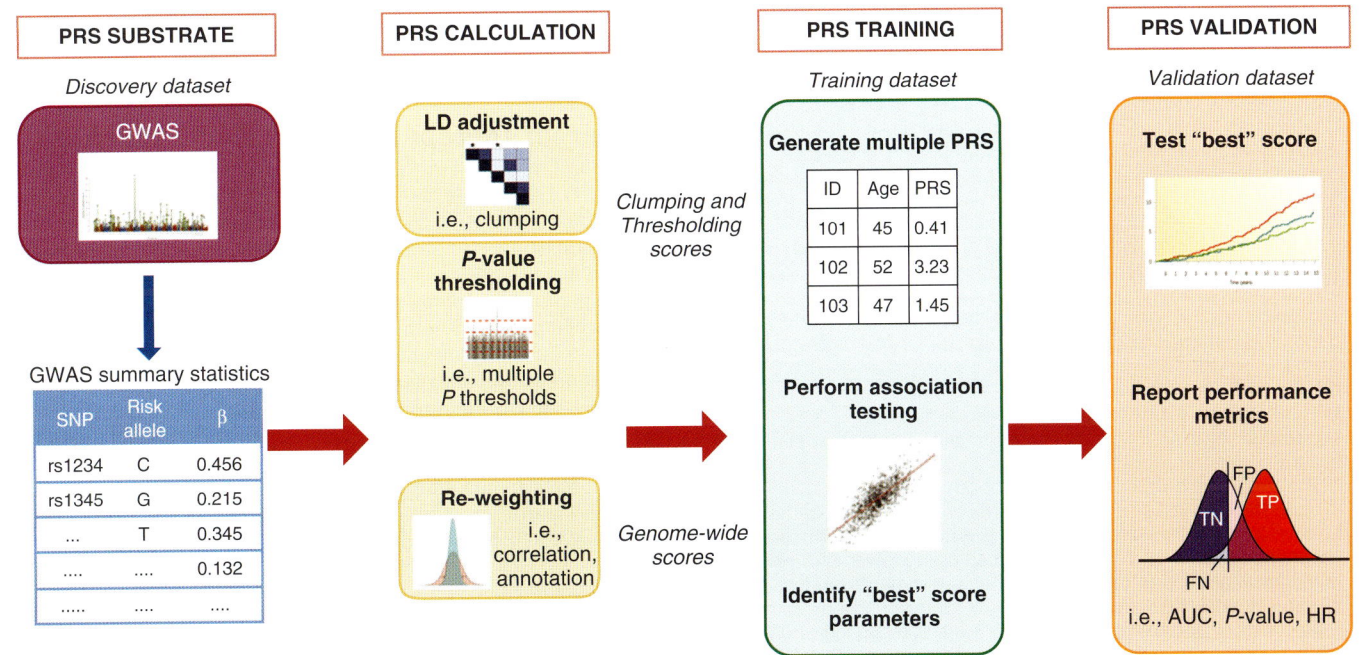

FIGURE 7.9 Development of polygenic risk scores. (Adapted from Aragam KG, Natarajan P. Polygenic scores to assess atherosclerotic cardiovascular disease risk: clinical perspectives and basic implications. *Circ Res.* 2020;126:1159–77.)

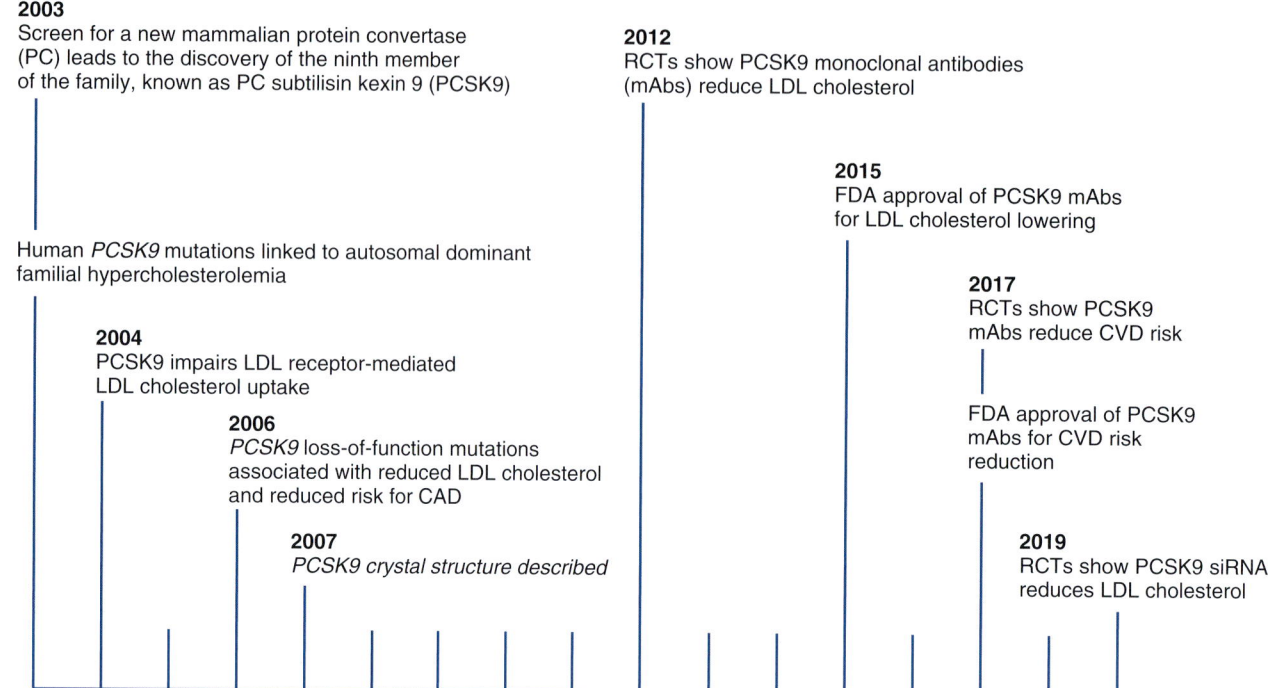

FIGURE 7.10 Timeline of PCSK9 discovery, evidence, and clinical implementation of monoclonal antibodies targeting PCSK9. (Adapted from Natarajan P, Kathiresan S. PCSK9 Inhibitors. *Cell.* 2016;165:1037.)

of putative causal biomarkers through MR with common genetic variants can also prioritize therapeutic targets. However, there are key distinctions between target modulation by genetic variation versus pharmacotherapies. First, for common diseases assessed in event-driven RCTs (often with 3 to 6 years of follow-up), reduction of events is typically assessed among individuals already with prevalent disease. In contrast, genetic variants model target modulation before the onset of disease. Second, related to the aforementioned concept, target modulation via genetic variants occurs at birth as opposed to middle age as in clinical trials. Third, target activity at the relevant tissue may be different for diverse pharmacotherapies and may not recapitulate relevant tissue-specific effects regulated by genetic alleles. Despite these caveats, a recent analysis indicated that prioritizing targets with human genetic validation may double the success rate of clinical development.[58]

PCSK9 (see also Chapter 27)

PCSK9 provides a prime example of successful therapeutic discovery from human genetics (Fig. 7.10). As discussed earlier, human genetic evidence for the relationship of *PCSK9* with blood cholesterol and CAD began with the identification of *PCSK9* gain-of-function variants in familial hypercholesterolemia families. Work described less than two decades ago identified that two nonsense *PCSK9* variants (p.Y142X and p.C679X) were particularly common (1% to 2%) specifically among individuals of African ancestry, and another disruptive missense *PCSK9* variant (p.R46L) was more common (3%) among those of European ancestry. African Americans with p.Y142X or p.C679X had 28% lower LDL-C concentration and 89% lower risk for CAD. European Americans with p.R46L had 15% lower LDL-C concentration and 50% lower risk for CAD. Additionally, rare individuals naturally carrying two nonsense *PCSK9* variants with lifelong genetic absence of PCSK9 ("human knockouts") and LDL-C levels of approximately 10 mg/dL appear to be healthy.

The aforementioned human genetic observations, as well as advances in understanding PCSK9 structure and function, spurred rapid therapeutic development. Over a relatively short period of time, PCSK9 monoclonal antibodies have come into widespread use to lower CAD risk. Two monoclonal antibodies targeting PCSK9 were shown to reduce LDL-C by approximately 50% and reduce the risk for major adverse cardiovascular events by approximately 85% over 3 years among individuals with atherosclerotic cardiovascular disease and LDL-C greater than 70 mg/dL in clinical trials.[59,60]

APOC3

Other genes, such as *APOC3*, have been similarly prioritized for CAD. Apolipoprotein C-III, encoded by *APOC3*, promotes the synthesis of and delays the clearance of triglyceride-rich lipoproteins. In 2008, genome-wide association analysis of a Lancaster Amish cohort with respect to fasting and postprandial triglycerides identified a large-effect common (5% carrier rate) noncoding variant near *APOC3*; sequencing indicated the sentinel SNP was tagging a nonsense variant in *APOC3* (p.R19X), which is now appreciated to be a founder variant in the Amish. In the Amish, presence of this variant was associated with a lower burden of subclinical coronary atherosclerosis. More recently, whole exome sequencing of European Americans and African Americans in the general population showed that *APOC3* p.R19X and other loss-of-function variants similarly reduced triglyceride concentrations and also were associated with reduced risk for CAD.[26] Among a cohort of adults living in Pakistan, where consanguinity is more common, several individuals homozygous for *APOC3* p.R19X were identified who have markedly reduced fasting and postprandial triglycerides.[5] Whether pharmacologic inhibition of apolipoprotein C-III leads to reduced CAD risk remains to be tested.

On-Target Therapeutic Side Effect Prediction

In addition to testing the association between genetic variants and primary outcomes for target efficacy assessment, one may evaluate their relationships with diverse clinical outcomes. In phenome-wide association studies (pheWASs), investigators can anticipate the beneficial and adverse consequences of modulating drug targets of interest. A systemic analysis indicates that drug side effects are more likely to occur when predicted from genetic association analyses.[61]

Among various research opportunities, contemporary densely phenotyped mega biobanks now provide the opportunity for large-scale pheWASs. The U.S. Precision Medicine Initiative led to the creation of the AllOfUs cohort, planned to comprise 1 million diverse Americans recruited through and outside of health care systems. Other cohorts of comparable size include the U.K. Biobank, Million Veterans Program, Biobank Japan, China Kadoorie Biobank, FinnGen, deCODE Genetics, and the eMERGE Network of health care system biobanks.

Precision Medicine

Pharmacogenomics refers to using genetics, in addition to clinical factors, to mitigate adverse drug reactions. Precision medicine aims to

Genetic risk	Trial	HR	95% CI	Heterogeneity
All others	JUPITER	0.68	(0.44, 1.05)	$\chi^2_2 = 0.48$, $p_{within} = 0.78$
	ASCOT-LLA	0.67	(0.46, 0.99)	
	WOSCOPS	0.76	(0.63, 0.92)	
	Summary	0.74	(0.63, 0.86)	
High	JUPITER	0.41	(0.16, 0.91)	$\chi^2_2 = 0.44$, $p_{within} = 0.80$
	ASCOT-LLA	0.54	(0.29, 0.94)	
	WOSCOPS	0.56	(0.40, 0.78)	$\chi^2_1 = 3.83$, $p_{between} = 0.05$
	Summary	0.54	(0.41, 0.71)	

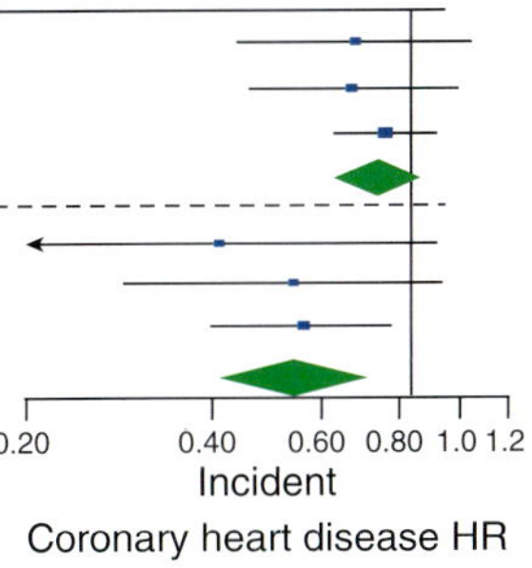

Incident Coronary heart disease HR

FIGURE 7.11 Forest plot of incident coronary artery disease risk from statin versus placebo by coronary artery disease polygenic risk group in three statin primary prevention trials. High coronary artery disease polygenic risk group refers to the top 20th percentile. For a given degree of low-density lipoprotein cholesterol lowering from statins, clinical benefit is greater among those with high coronary artery disease polygenic risk. (Adapted from Natarajan P, Young R, Stitziel NO, et al. Polygenic risk score identifies subgroup with higher burden of atherosclerosis and greater relative benefit from statin therapy in the primary prevention setting. Circulation. 2017;135[22]:2091–2101.)

extend this concept by using diverse factors, including genetics, to identify individuals more likely to benefit from preventive therapies. Currently, CAD-preventive pharmacotherapies are titrated to blood cholesterol, blood pressure, and glycemic indices, and therapies are further escalated for those with greater absolute intermediate-term risk.[31] Risk refinement from human genetics may guide therapeutic escalation. Although genetically ascertained RCTs are lacking; ongoing post-hoc analyses within completed clinical trials have led to promising hypotheses.

CYP2C19 (see also Chapter 38)
Along with the use of aspirin, inhibition of platelet P2Y purinoceptor 12 (P2Y12) receptors is standard-of-care therapy as an adjunct to percutaneous coronary intervention (PCI). Clopidogrel, the most widely prescribed P2Y12 inhibitor, is an inactive prodrug converted to its active form largely by cytochrome P-450 2C19 (CYP2C19) in the liver. Several CYP2C19 genetic polymorphisms influencing enzymatic function have been described, with two relatively common loss-of-function variants (CYP2C19*2, which disrupts splicing, and CYP2C19*3, which is a nonsense variant). The allele frequency of CYP2C19*2 is 30% in South Asians and East Asians, 17% in Europeans and Africans, and 10% in Latinos. The allele frequency of CYP2C19*3 is 6% in East Asians.

Carriers of these alleles have reduced antiplatelet effects from clopidogrel. In RCTs of clopidogrel-treated patients undergoing PCI, carriers had a greater risk of adverse outcomes, leading to a U.S. Food and Drug Administration black box warning in 2010 recommending alternative antiplatelet agents for poor metabolizers of clopidogrel. Given the lack of prospective genotype-guided RCTs when they were written, guidelines in 2016 recommended against routine CYP2C19 genotyping but noted that testing may be considered in patients at increased risk for poor clinical outcomes.[62]

More recently, a CY2C19 genotype-guided strategy was assessed in a prospective RCT among patients undergoing PCI.[63] In the genotype-guided group, carriers of CYP2C19*2 or CYP2C19*3 received ticagrelor or prasugrel, while noncarriers received clopidogrel. All participants in the standard-of-care group received ticagrelor or prasugrel. The genotype-guided group was noninferior to the standard-treatment group with respect to thrombotic events and had a 2.7% absolute risk reduction in bleeding events.

Familial Hypercholesterolemia
Retrospective observational analyses indicate a greater absolute and relative risk reduction in major adverse cardiovascular events from cholesterol lowering among those with FH variants compared with those without. Nonstatin cholesterol-lowering medicines, such as ezetimibe, PCSK9 monoclonal antibodies, and bempedoic acid, came to market with FH being the initial approved indication. In the primary prevention setting, guidelines recommend the use of additional nonstatin cholesterol-lowering medicines as needed to attain stricter LDL-C targets in patients with FH.[31]

Polygenic Coronary Artery Disease
Post hoc subgroup analyses within prospective clinical trials also indicate greater clinical cardiovascular benefit of cholesterol-lowering medicines among those with high polygenic CAD risk, even though LDL-C is typically only mildly elevated in this setting and LDL-C lowering is similar.[50,64–66] In the primary prevention setting, statin therapy versus placebo was associated with greater absolute and relative risk reduction for those with high CAD PRS versus all others (Fig. 7.11).[50,64] In the secondary prevention setting, a CAD PRS predicted recurrent events, and therapy with a PCSK9 monoclonal antibody versus placebo was associated with greater absolute and relative risk reduction for those with high CAD PRS versus all others.[65,66] A CAD PRS may help identify those more likely to clinically benefit from LDL-C-lowering therapies, which requires assessment in genotype-guided prospective clinical trials.

NEXT-GENERATION TECHNOLOGIES AND THERAPEUTICS

Human genetics, including its application to cardiovascular disease, continues to progress at a rapid rate. Novel experimental and analytic methods promise to expand our understanding of cardiovascular disease as well as develop new pharmacotherapies.

Somatic Genomics (see also Chapter 24)
Age remains the most important risk factor for CAD, but age-related factors causally contributing to CAD remain incompletely understood. Large-scale NGS of blood DNA showed that a large number of individuals (up to 1 in 10 adults older than 70 years) have clonal hematopoiesis of indeterminate potential (CHIP), an age-related phenomenon associated with the clonal selection of cancer-predisposing mutations (typically in DNMT3A, TET2, ASXL1, or JAK2) in the blood without cytopenia, dysplasia, or neoplasia. Although CHIP associates strongly with future risk of blood cancer, it has recently been linked to CAD in humans and murine models.[67–69] Inhibition of the NLRP3 inflammasome in mice with experimental atherosclerosis appears to reduce atherosclerosis burden to a greater degree in those with Tet2 loss of function versus without.[68] Applying principles of MR, investigators showed that germline genetic deficiency of IL6R, which encodes the interleukin (IL)-6 receptor in the NLRP3 inflammasome pathway, associated with a larger degree of reduced risk for CAD among those with CHIP versus without (Fig. 7.12).[69] These data indicate that modulation of this pathway may be particularly beneficial for those with CHIP.

Epigenetics
Epigenetics may contribute to CAD, because environmental factors associated with epigenetic changes such as altered histone acetylation and DNA methylation are also correlated with CAD risk and advanced atherosclerosis features.[70] For example, increased expression of histone deacetylase 3 has been observed at sites prone to atherogenesis, and increased expression of histone deacetylase 9 (HDAC9) associates with proinflammatory macrophage concentrations within atherosclerotic plaques. Common genetic variants near HDAC9 associate with vascular calcification and myocardial infarction risk, and inhibition of

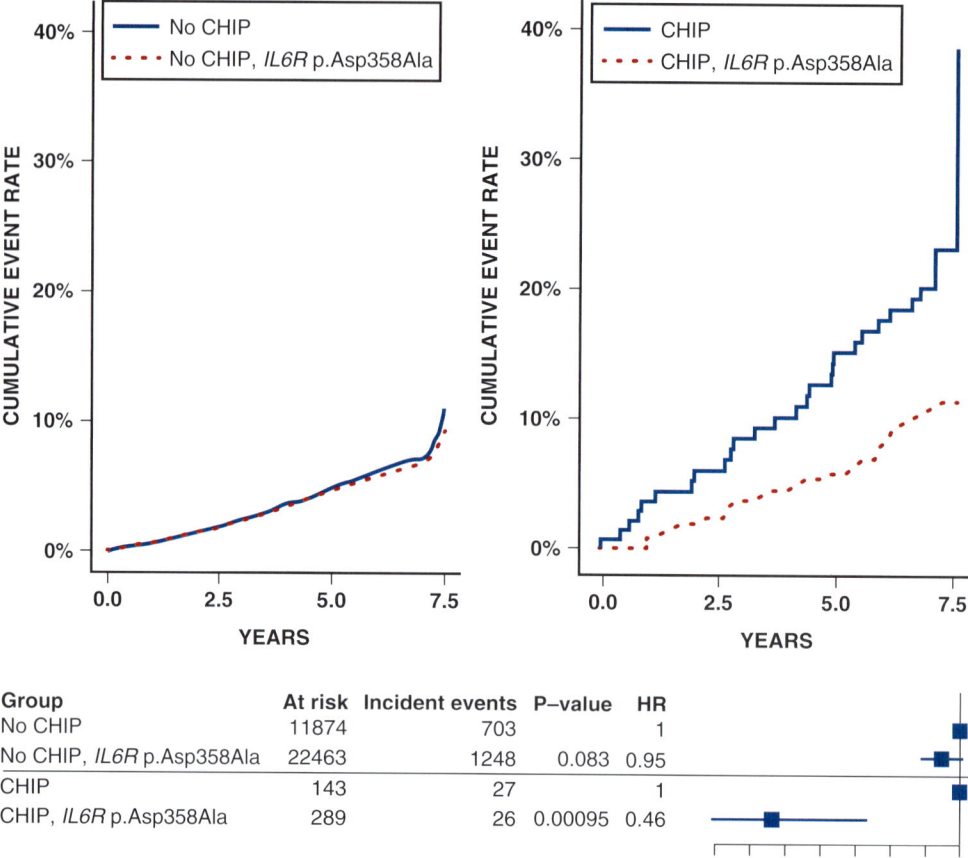

FIGURE 7.12 Cumulative incident cardiovascular risk associated with carrying *IL6R* p.Asp358Ala stratified by the presence of clonal hematopoiesis of indeterminate potential (CHIP). Cardiovascular risk reduction related to *IL6R* p.Asp358Ala is greater among those who develop CHIP with resultant cumulative risk similar to those without CHIP. (Adapted from Bick AG, Pirruccello JP, Griffin GK, et al. Genetic IL-6 signaling deficiency attenuates cardiovascular risk in clonal hematopoiesis. *Circulation*. 2019; 141[2]:124–31.)

HDAC9 in human aortic smooth muscle cells leads to reduced calcification in vitro.[71]

Methylation at specific genomic regions has been linked to CAD risk. A recent large-scale longitudinal analysis of 11,461 individuals for whom leukocyte genome-wide DNA methylation was interrogated with methylation arrays,[52] CpG methylation sites were associated with incident CAD risk.[72] MR analyses indicate that two of these CpG sites relate causally to CAD; both sites are in noncoding intergenic regions. Genetic variants associated with one of the CpG sites influence expression of *ITGA6* (which encodes integrin subunit alpha 6), and genetic variants for the other site influence expression of the long ncRNA RP4-555D20.2.

As noted in the aforementioned example, ncRNAs (microRNAs and long ncRNAs) have emerged as potential modulators of atherosclerosis. First, a high-throughput genome-wide in vitro screen for microRNAs regulating *LDLR* expression in hepatocytes prioritized miR-148a as a negative regulator.[73] In hypercholesterolemic mice, inhibition of miR-148a led to increased hepatic *LDLR* expression and a resultant decrease in LDL-C. Second, CAD risk alleles in the chromosome 9p21 GWAS locus influence the expression of the long ncRNA *ANRIL*. A linear form of *ANRIL* is enriched among those with atherosclerosis, but a circular form may control rRNA maturation in vascular smooth muscle cells and macrophages leading to apparent atheroprotection.[74]

Single-Cell Ribonucleic Acid Sequencing (see also Chapter 24)

NGS is applied to transcription profiling through RNA sequencing (RNA-seq) of tissue. Single-cell RNA sequencing (scRNA-seq) with complementary use of microfluidics may facilitate the characterization of diverse cell types in pathologic processes, discovery of novel cell populations, improved understanding of regulatory relationships between genes, and tracking of the development of specific cellular lineages. Compared with bulk RNA-seq, scRNA-seq has added technical challenges related to low starting material amount and added noise from stochastic or physiologic transcription variation. Experimental and computational tools are being developed and optimized to address these issues. Additionally, novel methods are being developed to (1) also transpose spatial information with gene expression relationships and (2) apply emerging unsupervised clustering and machine learning methods.

Immune cell profiling with atherosclerotic plaques has typically used immunostaining or fluorescence-activated cell sorting (FACS) but now frequently uses scRNA-seq technology. ScRNA-seq and single-cell proteomics analysis of carotid atherosclerotic plaques in patients with and without recent strokes identified novel activated macrophage and T cell subsets.[75] Using FACS to isolate murine vascular smooth muscle cells in atherosclerotic lesions, investigators then applied scRNA-seq to discover a new subpopulation of fibroblast-like cells termed "fibromyocytes"; scRNA-seq in human atherosclerotic lesions also identified fibromyocytes.[76] Knockout of mouse *Tcf21*, a gene prioritized from CAD GWASs, specifically in vascular smooth muscle cells led to fewer fibromyocytes.

Therapeutically Targeting the Genome

In addition to target discovery and prioritization, insights from human genetics have also led to novel approaches for therapeutic targeting. Conventional pharmacotherapies target proteins but newer classes of medicines target more proximal gene product, mRNAs. The two major RNA therapeutic approaches use (1) antisense oligonucleotides (ASOs) to inhibit mRNA translation and (2) oligonucleotides to activate RNA interference (RNAi) to inhibit mRNA translation. Even more proximally, gene therapy is used to circumvent genetically deficient gene products or augment cardioprotective genes. Lastly, emerging methods in gene editing are being explored to target genes or even correct pathogenic variants.

ASOs are synthetic single-stranded DNA sequences designed to bind and inactivate mRNAs produced by a specific gene. In addition to steric hindrance, the resultant RNA-DNA heteroduplex induces RNase H endonuclease activity that degrades in target mRNA and ultimately reduces target gene translation. ASOs are typically 20 base pairs in length and target either the initiation code or splice sites while minimizing polymorphic regions to enhance specificity. Phosphorothiolation of ASOs enables binding to plasma proteins to extend half-life, reduces renal excretion, and improve bioavailability but may lead to thrombocytopenia. Some ribose modifications to improve stability and affinity have been linked to hepatotoxicity. In 2013, the FDA approved mipomersen, an ASO targeting *APOB* mRNAs, for homozygous FH but its use is limited by hepatotoxicity. ASOs have been developed for several lipid-related targets, including *APOC3*, *ANGPTL3*, and *LPA*, and are being assessed for effects on cardiovascular outcomes. Selective targeting of RNA therapeutics to hepatocytes with oligosaccharide ligands of the asialoglycoprotein receptor can reduce the doses needed and markedly minimize unwanted actions such as injection site reactions (see also Chapter 27).

RNAi is a naturally occurring eukaryotic innate immune response of sequence-specific mRNA degradation induced by foreign long double-stranded RNAs (dsRNAs). In mammalian cells, dsRNAs induce a strong interferon response, resulting in their processing to single-stranded approximately 22-base pair small interfering RNAs (siRNAs) by Dicer. For human therapeutics, synthetic siRNAs activate RNAi by incorporating in the RNA-induced silencing complex (RISC), leading to mRNA-specific translational repression and degradation. Inclisiran, a twice-annually administered siRNA targeting *PCSK9*, reduces LDL-C safely in RCTs.[77]

Gene-editing technologies leveraging bacterial immune systems now enjoy ubiquitous use for research and have received increasing attention as a therapeutic modality. Clustered regularly interspaced short palindromic repeat (CRISPR) RNAs and CRISPR-associated proteins (Cas, particularly Cas9) can be reprogrammed to target specific genomic DNA sequences. After introducing site-specific double-stranded DNA breaks, endogenous DNA repair mechanisms are activated. Typically, error-prone nonhomologous end joining (NHEJ) is activated and can be used to produce gene knockouts. In mice, using adenovirus vectors, CRISPR-Cas9 can efficiently introduce loss-of-function mutations in *Pcsk9* in the liver, with resultant reduced cholesterol levels.[78] Alternatively, a homologous repair template can stimulate the less error-prone homology-directed repair (HDR) to facilitate desired changes; emerging methods focus on maximizing HDR efficiency versus NHEJ-mediated repair. Base editing uses fusions of Cas proteins with deaminases to facilitate transition mutations (i.e., C→T and A→G conversions). In mice, using adenovirus vectors, base editing efficiently introduced loss-of-function point mutations in *Pcsk9* and *Angptl3* in the liver.[79]

FUTURE PERSPECTIVES

Technical advances in large-scale high-throughput genomic profiling continue to yield accelerating advances for cardiovascular disease, with diverse insights and applications for the most common form—CAD. Larger-scale application of whole genome sequencing in increasingly diverse datasets will: (1) better define both lipid and nonlipid genes responsible for CAD, (2) enable interpretation of the bulk of genomic variation (rare, noncoding) which is poorly understood, and (3) improve genetic risk prediction across diverse ethnicities. Genomic interpretation for diverse clinical outcomes, including within the context of ongoing clinical trials, may facilitate therapeutic paradigms maximizing efficacy and minimizing side effects for individual patients.

Driven by public interests and scientific observations, PRSs for CAD and other diseases will likely soon become broadly available. Given the widespread availability of genetic testing and democratized interpretation, PRSs may increasingly enter clinical practice. Ethical and confidentiality issues require due considerations. Broad availability of such testing will also enable molecularly targeted RCTs to evaluate specific strategies as well as enrich for events to improve trial efficiency.

An intriguing prospect is whole genome sequencing earlier in life to inform baseline disease trajectories toward "primordial prevention."

The relationship between CHIP and cardiovascular disease implicates the prospect of novel, molecularly guided therapies. Unlike the current model of escalating therapies with the accumulation of risk factors, the presence of CHIP may prompt the orthogonal use of NLRP3/IL-1β/IL-6 inhibiting therapies.

Lastly, as the field continues to refine interpretation of the genome and prioritize therapeutic targets, advances in genome-based therapies offer the promise of durable molecular interventions to prevent and treat cardiovascular disease.

REFERENCES

1. GBD 2017 Disease and Injury Incidence and Prevalence Collaborators. Global, regional, and national incidence, prevalence, and years lived with disability for 354 diseases and injuries for 195 countries and territories, 1990-2017: a systematic analysis for the Global Burden of Disease Study 2017. *Lancet*. 2018;392:1789–1858.
2. Lek M, Karczewski KJ, Minikel EV, et al. Analysis of protein-coding genetic variation in 60,706 humans. *Nature*. 2016;536:285–291.
3. Natarajan P, Gold NB, Bick AG, et al. Aggregate penetrance of genomic variants for actionable disorders in European and African Americans. *Sci Transl Med*. 2016;8:364ra151.
4. Consortium GT, Laboratory DA, Coordinating Center -Analysis Working G, et al. Genetic effects on gene expression across human tissues. *Nature*. 2017;550:204–213.
5. Saleheen D, Natarajan P, Armean IM, et al. Human knockouts and phenotypic analysis in a cohort with a high rate of consanguinity. *Nature*. 2017;544:235–239.
6. Liu X, Wu C, Li C, Boerwinkle E. dbNSFP v3.0: a one-stop database of functional predictions and annotations for human nonsynonymous and splice-site SNVs. *Human Mutat*. 2016;37:235–241.
7. Roadmap Epigenomics Consortium, Kundaje A, Meuleman W, et al. Integrative analysis of 111 reference human epigenomes. *Nature*. 2015;518:317–330.
8. McCarthy S, Das S, Kretzschmar W, et al. A reference panel of 64,976 haplotypes for genotype imputation. *Nat Genet*. 2016;48:1279–1283.
9. Shendure J, Balasubramanian S, Church GM, et al. DNA sequencing at 40: past, present and future. *Nature*. 2017;550:345–353.
10. Jain M, Koren S, Miga KH, et al. Nanopore sequencing and assembly of a human genome with ultra-long reads. *Nature Biotechnol*. 2018;36:338–345.
11. Gidding SS, Champagne MA, de Ferranti SD, et al. The agenda for familial hypercholesterolemia: a scientific statement from the American Heart Association. *Circulation*. 2015;132:2167–2192.
12. Keramati AR, Fathzadeh M, Go GW, et al. A form of the metabolic syndrome associated with mutations in DYRK1B. *New Engl J Med*. 2014;370:1909–1919.
13. Palmer C, Pe'er I. Statistical correction of the Winner's Curse explains replication variability in quantitative trait genome-wide association studies. *PLoS Genetics*. 2017;13:e1006916.
14. Musunuru K, Kathiresan S. Genetics of common, complex coronary artery disease. *Cell*. 2019;177:132–145.
15. Loh PR, Tucker G, Bulik-Sullivan BK, et al. Efficient Bayesian mixed-model analysis increases association power in large cohorts. *Nat Genet*. 2015;47:284–290.
16. Zhou W, Nielsen JB, Fritsche LG, et al. Efficiently controlling for case-control imbalance and sample relatedness in large-scale genetic association studies. *Nat Genet*. 2018;50:1335–1341.
17. Klarin D, Damrauer SM, Cho K, et al. Genetics of blood lipids among ~300,000 multi-ethnic participants of the Million Veteran Program. *Nat Genet*. 2018;50:1514–1523.
18. Nioi P, Sigurdsson A, Thorleifsson G, et al. A Variant ASGR1 associated with a reduced risk of coronary artery disease. *New Engl J Med*. 2016;374:2131–2141.
19. Liu DJ, Peloso GM, Yu H, et al. Exome-wide association study of plasma lipids in >300,000 individuals. *Nat Genet*. 2017;49:1758–1766.
20. Lu X, Peloso GM, Liu DJ, et al. Exome chip meta-analysis identifies novel loci and East Asian-specific coding variants that contribute to lipid levels and coronary artery disease. *Nat Genet*. 2017;49:1722–1730.
21. Erdmann J, Kessler T, Munoz Venegas L, Schunkert H. A decade of genome-wide association studies for coronary artery disease: the challenges ahead. *Cardiovasc Res*. 2018;114:1241–1257.
22. Myocardial Infarction Genetics and CARDIoGRAM Exome Consortia Investigators, Stitziel NO, et al. Coding variation in ANGPTL4, LPL, and SVEP1 and the risk of coronary disease. *New Engl J Med*. 2016;374:1134–1144.
23. Kessler T, Wobst J, Wolf B, et al. Functional characterization of the GUCY1A3 coronary artery disease risk locus. *Circulation*. 2017;136:476–489.
24. Emdin CA, Khera AV, Klarin D, et al. Phenotypic consequences of a genetic predisposition to enhanced nitric oxide signaling. *Circulation*. 2018;137:222–232.
25. Do R, Stitziel NO, Won HH, et al. Exome sequencing identifies rare LDLR and APOA5 alleles conferring risk for myocardial infarction. *Nature*. 2015;518:102–106.
26. Crosby J, Peloso GM, Auer PL, et al. Loss-of-function mutations in APOC3, triglycerides, and coronary disease. *New Engl J Med*. 2014;371:22–31.
27. Myocardial Infarction Genetics Consortium Investigators, Stitziel NO, Won HH, et al. Inactivating mutations in NPC1L1 and protection from coronary heart disease. *New Engl J Med*. 2014;371:2072–2082.
28. Stitziel NO, Khera AV, Wang X, et al. ANGPTL3 deficiency and protection against coronary artery disease. *J Am Coll Cardiol*. 2017;69:2054–2063.
29. Hingorani AD, Kuan V, Finan C, et al. Improving the odds of drug development success through human genomics: modelling study. *Sci Rep*. 2019;9:18911.
30. White J, Swerdlow DI, Preiss D, et al. Association of lipid fractions with risks for coronary artery disease and diabetes. *JAMA Cardiol*. 2016;1:692–699.
31. Grundy SM, Stone NJ, Bailey AL, et al. 2018 AHA/ACC/AACVPR/AAPA/ABC/ACPM/ADA/AGS/APhA/ASPC/NLA/PCNA guideline on the management of blood cholesterol: a report of the American College of Cardiology/American Heart Association task force on clinical practice guidelines. *J Am Coll Cardiol*. 2018.
32. Zekavat SM, Ruotsalainen S, Handsaker RE, et al. Deep coverage whole genome sequences and plasma lipoprotein(a) in individuals of European and African ancestries. *Nat Commun*. 2018;9:2606.
33. Nordestgaard BG, Langsted A. Lipoprotein (a) as a cause of cardiovascular disease: insights from epidemiology, genetics, and biology. *J Lipid Res*. 2016;57:1953–1975.
34. Emdin CA, Khera AV, Natarajan P, et al. Phenotypic characterization of genetically lowered human lipoprotein(a) levels. *J Am Coll Cardiol*. 2016;68:2761–2772.
35. Klarin D, Lynch J, Aragam K, et al. Genome-wide association study of peripheral artery disease in the Million Veteran Program. *Nat Med*. 2019;25:1274–1279.
36. Emdin CA, Khera AV, Natarajan P, et al. Genetic association of waist-to-hip ratio with cardiometabolic traits, type 2 diabetes, and coronary heart disease. *J Am Med Assoc*. 2017;317:626–634.
37. Lotta LA, Wittemans LBL, Zuber V, et al. Association of genetic variants related to gluteofemoral vs abdominal fat distribution with type 2 diabetes, coronary disease, and cardiovascular risk factors. *J Am Med Assoc*. 2018;320:2553–2563.

38. Burgess S, Dudbridge F, Thompson SG. Combining information on multiple instrumental variables in Mendelian randomization: comparison of allele score and summarized data methods. *Stat Med.* 2016;35:1880–1906.
39. Greco MF, Minelli C, Sheehan NA, Thompson JR. Detecting pleiotropy in Mendelian randomisation studies with summary data and a continuous outcome. *Stat Med.* 2015;34:2926–2940.
40. Bowden J, Del Greco MF, Minelli C, et al. Assessing the suitability of summary data for two-sample Mendelian randomization analyses using MR-Egger regression: the role of the I2 statistic. *Int J Epidemiol.* 2016;45:1961–1974.
41. Verbanck M, Chen CY, Neale B, Do R. Detection of widespread horizontal pleiotropy in causal relationships inferred from Mendelian randomization between complex traits and diseases. *Nat Genet.* 2018;50:693–698.
42. Zhu Z, Zheng Z, Zhang F, et al. Causal associations between risk factors and common diseases inferred from GWAS summary data. *Nat Commun.* 2018;9:224.
43. Richards S, Aziz N, Bale S, et al. Standards and guidelines for the interpretation of sequence variants: a joint consensus recommendation of the American College of Medical Genetics and Genomics and the Association for Molecular Pathology. *Gen Med.* 2015;17(5):405–424.
44. Kalia SS, Adelman K, Bale SJ, et al. Recommendations for reporting of secondary findings in clinical exome and genome sequencing, 2016 update (ACMG SF v2.0): a policy statement of the American College of Medical Genetics and Genomics. *Gen Med.* 2017;19:249–255.
45. Alver M, Palover M, Saar A, et al. Recall by genotype and cascade screening for familial hypercholesterolemia in a population-based biobank from Estonia. *Gen Med.* 2018;21(5):1173–1180.
46. Benn M, Watts GF, Tybjaerg-Hansen A, Nordestgaard BG. Mutations causative of familial hypercholesterolaemia: screening of 98 098 individuals from the Copenhagen General Population Study estimated a prevalence of 1 in 217. *Eur Heart J.* 2016;37:1384–1394.
47. Khera AV, Won HH, Peloso GM, et al. Diagnostic yield and clinical utility of sequencing familial hypercholesterolemia genes in patients with severe hypercholesterolemia. *J Am Coll Cardiol.* 2016;67:2578–2589.
48. Martin AR, Gignoux CR, Walters RK, et al. Human demographic history impacts genetic risk prediction across diverse populations. *Am J Hum Genet.* 2017;100:635–649.
49. Khera AV, Emdin CA, Drake I, et al. Genetic risk, adherence to a healthy lifestyle, and coronary disease. *New Engl J Med.* 2016;375:2349–2358.
50. Natarajan P, Young R, Stitziel NO, et al. Polygenic risk score identifies subgroup with higher burden of atherosclerosis and greater relative benefit from statin therapy in the primary prevention setting. *Circulation.* 2017;135(22):2091–2101.
51. Tada H, Melander O, Louie JZ, et al. Risk prediction by genetic risk scores for coronary heart disease is independent of self-reported family history. *Eur Heart J.* 2016;37:561–567.
52. Khera AV, Chaffin M, Aragam KG, et al. Genome-wide polygenic scores for common diseases identify individuals with risk equivalent to monogenic mutations. *Nat Genet.* 2018;50:1219–1224.
53. Inouye M, Abraham G, Nelson CP, et al. Genomic risk prediction of coronary artery disease in 480,000 adults: Implications for primary prevention. *J Am Coll Cardiol.* 2018;72:1883–1893.
54. Elliott J, Bodinier B, Bond TA, et al. Predictive accuracy of a polygenic risk score-enhanced prediction model vs a clinical risk score for coronary artery disease. *J Am Med Assoc.* 2020;323:636–645.
55. Mosley JD, Gupta DK, Tan J, et al. Predictive accuracy of a polygenic risk score compared with a clinical risk score for incident coronary heart disease. *J Am Med Assoc.* 2020;323:627–635.
56. Aragam KG, Natarajan P. Polygenic scores to assess atherosclerotic cardiovascular disease risk: clinical perspectives and basic implications. *Circ Res.* 2020;126:1159–1177.
57. Collins FS, Varmus H. A new initiative on precision medicine. *New Engl J Med.* 2015;372:793–795.
58. Nelson MR, Tipney H, Painter JL, et al. The support of human genetic evidence for approved drug indications. *Nat Genet.* 2015;47:856–860.
59. Sabatine MS, Giugliano RP, Keech AC, et al. Evolocumab and clinical outcomes in patients with cardiovascular disease. *New Engl J Med.* 2017;376(18):1713–1722.
60. Schwartz GG, Steg PG, Szarek M, et al. Alirocumab and cardiovascular outcomes after acute coronary syndrome. *New Engl J Med.* 2018;379:2097–2107.
61. Nguyen PA, Born DA, Deaton AM, et al. Phenotypes associated with genes encoding drug targets are predictive of clinical trial side effects. *Nat Commun.* 2019;10:1579.
62. Levine GN, Bates ER, Bittl JA, et al. 2016 ACC/AHA guideline focused update on duration of dual antiplatelet therapy in patients with coronary artery disease: a report of the American College of Cardiology/American Heart Association task force on clinical practice guidelines: an update of the 2011 ACCF/AHA/SCAI guideline for percutaneous coronary intervention, 2011 ACCF/AHA guideline for coronary artery bypass graft surgery, 2012 ACC/AHA/ACP/AATS/PCNA/SCAI/STS guideline for the diagnosis and management of patients with stable ischemic heart disease, 2013 ACCF/AHA guideline for the management of ST-Elevation myocardial infarction, 2014 AHA/ACC guideline for the management of patients with non-ST-Elevation acute coronary cyndromes, and 2014 ACC/AHA guideline on perioperative cardiovascular evaluation and management of patients undergoing noncardiac surgery. *Circulation.* 2016;134:e123–e155.
63. Claassens DMF, Vos GJA, Bergmeijer TO, et al. A genotype-guided strategy for oral P2Y12 inhibitors in primary PCI. *New Engl J Med.* 2019;381:1621–1631.
64. Mega JL, Stitziel NO, Smith JG, et al. Genetic risk, coronary heart disease events, and the clinical benefit of statin therapy: an analysis of primary and secondary prevention trials. *Lancet.* 2015;385:2264–2271.
65. Damask A, Steg PG, Schwartz GG, et al. Patients with high genome-wide polygenic risk scores for coronary artery disease may receive greater clinical benefit from alirocumab treatment in the ODYSSEY OUTCOMES trial. *Circulation.* 2020;141:624–636.
66. Marston NA, Gurmu Y, Melloni GEM, et al. The effect of PCSK9 (proprotein convertase subtilisin/kexin type 9) inhibition on the risk of venous thromboembolism. *Circulation.* 2020;141:1600–1607.
67. Jaiswal S, Natarajan P, Silver AJ, et al. Clonal hematopoiesis and risk of atherosclerotic cardiovascular disease. *New Engl J Med.* 2017.
68. Fuster JJ, MacLauchlan S, Zuriaga MA, et al. Clonal hematopoiesis associated with TET2 deficiency accelerates atherosclerosis development in mice. *Science (New York, NY).* 2017;355:842–847.
69. Bick AG, Pirruccello JP, Griffin GK, et al. Genetic IL-6 signaling deficiency attenuates cardiovascular risk in clonal hematopoiesis. *Circulation.* 2019;141(2):124–131.
70. Rizzacasa B, Amati F, Romeo F, et al. Epigenetic modification in coronary atherosclerosis: JACC review topic of the week. *J Am Coll Cardiol.* 2019;74:1352–1365.
71. Malhotra R, Mauer AC, Lino Cardenas CL, et al. HDAC9 is implicated in atherosclerotic aortic calcification and affects vascular smooth muscle cell phenotype. *Nat Genet.* 2019;51:1580–1587.
72. Agha G, Mendelson MM, Ward-Caviness CK, et al. Blood leukocyte DNA methylation predicts risk of future myocardial infarction and coronary heart disease. *Circulation.* 2019;140:645–657.
73. Goedeke L, Rotllan N, Canfran-Duque A, et al. MicroRNA-148a regulates LDL receptor and ABCA1 expression to control circulating lipoprotein levels. *Nature Med.* 2015;21:1280–1289.
74. Holdt LM, Stahringer A, Sass K, et al. Circular non-coding RNA ANRIL modulates ribosomal RNA maturation and atherosclerosis in humans. *Nat Commun.* 2016;7:12429.
75. Fernandez DM, Rahman AH, Fernandez NF, et al. Single-cell immune landscape of human atherosclerotic plaques. *Nature Med.* 2019;25:1576–1588.
76. Wirka RC, Wagh D, Paik DT, et al. Atheroprotective roles of smooth muscle cell phenotypic modulation and the TCF21 disease gene as revealed by single-cell analysis. *Nat Med.* 2019;25:1280–1289.
77. Ray KK, Wright RS, Kallend D, et al. Two phase 3 trials of inclisiran in patients with elevated LDL cholesterol. *New Engl J Med.* 2020;382:1507–1519.
78. Ding Q, Strong A, Patel KM, et al. Permanent alteration of PCSK9 with in vivo CRISPR-Cas9 genome editing. *Circ Res.* 2014;115:488–492.
79. Chadwick AC, Evitt NH, Lv W, Musunuru K. Reduced blood lipid levels with in vivo CRISPR-cas9 base editing of ANGPTL3. *Circulation.* 2018;137:975–977.
80. Peloso GM, Natarajan P. Insights from population-based analyses of plasma lipids across the allele frequency spectrum. *Curr Opin Genet Dev.* 2018;50:1–6.
81. Natarajan P, Kathiresan S. PCSK9 inhibitors. *Cell.* 2016;165:1037.

8 Proteomics and Metabolomics in Cardiovascular Medicine

ROBERT GERSZTEN

NOVEL TECHNOLOGIES IN THE IDENTIFICATION OF BIOMARKERS, 87

INTRODUCTION TO PROTEOMICS AND METABOLOMICS, 87

ANALYTIC CHALLENGES FOR PROTEOMICS AND METABOLOMICS, 87

OVERVIEW OF THE DISCOVERY PROCESS, 88

APPLICATIONS OF MASS SPECTROMETRY–BASED DISCOVERY TO CARDIOMETABOLIC DISEASE, 90

FUTURE DIRECTIONS IN BIOMARKER DISCOVERY, 91

REFERENCES, 91

NOVEL TECHNOLOGIES IN THE IDENTIFICATION OF BIOMARKERS

The limitations of currently available biomarkers for screening or prognostic use underscore the importance of identifying "uncorrelated" or "orthogonal" biomarkers associated with novel disease pathways. Most current cardiovascular biomarkers have derived from extensions of targeted physiologic studies investigating known pathways such as tissue injury, inflammation, or hemostasis. By contrast, emerging technologies now enable the systematic, unbiased characterization of variation in proteins and metabolites associated with disease conditions.

INTRODUCTION TO PROTEOMICS AND METABOLOMICS

Of the emerging platforms for biomarker discovery, perhaps none have garnered more recent attention than proteomics and metabolomics. Proteomics aims to catalogue the entire protein products of the human genome. By contrast, metabolomics attempts to systemically capture smaller biochemical compounds, including simple amino acids and related amines, as well as lipids, sugars, nucleotides, and other intermediary metabolites. Although still in their infancy with respect to other approaches, proteomics and metabolomics offer insight into the full complexity of a given disease (Fig. 8.1). Because proteins and metabolites are downstream of genetic variation and transcriptional changes, they provide instantaneous "snapshots" of the state of a cell or organism. They can change rapidly in response to environmental stressors such as exercise or directly by the ingestion of foods or other compounds. Although the effects of catecholamines and natriuretic peptides on cardiovascular homeostasis are well-established, a growing body of literature suggests unanticipated roles of small proteins and metabolites in the control of biologic functions such as blood pressure and energy homeostasis.[1] Thus metabolomics and proteomics may not only identify novel biomarkers but also provide information on biology and highlight potential therapeutic targets.

The term *proteome* was coined in the 1990s with the increasing realization that, although all cells of a given organism contain an equivalent genomic content, their protein content does not represent all possible proteins that the genome can express. Selective gene expression during development and differentiation and in response to external stimuli results in each cell producing only a subset of the encoded proteins at any given time. One can speak not only of the general human proteome but also more specifically about the proteome of tissues such as the heart, of specific cells such as cardiac myocytes, and even of subproteomes that correspond to particular organelles or biologic compartments, such as mitochondria.

The proteome thus provides information beyond the messenger RNA (mRNA) expression profile of a particular genome. Studies suggest that gene expression often correlates poorly with protein levels. Protein expression depends not only on transcription but also on mRNA stability and rates of protein synthesis and degradation, so the presence or absence of mRNA may not accurately reflect levels of the corresponding protein. Following transcription and translation, proteins may undergo one or more of dozens of potential post-translational modifications (such as phosphorylation, glycosylation, acetylation, or sulfation) at multiple sites which modulate protein function. Subsequent enzymatic and nonenzymatic alterations greatly expand the number of simultaneously existing protein species.

When compared with proteomics techniques, metabolomics technologies focus on smaller compounds, generally less than 2 kDa in size. Metabolites are usually easily separated from protein constituents by simple extraction techniques and precipitation and removal of the proteins. As early as the 1970s, Arthur Robinson and Linus Pauling postulated that the quantitative and qualitative pattern of metabolites in biologic fluids reflected the functional status of the complex biologic system from which they were derived. The term "metabolic profiling" was introduced to describe data obtained from gas chromatographic analysis of a patient sample. This emerging approach to quantitative metabolic profiling of large numbers of small molecules in biofluids was ultimately termed "metabonomics" by Nicholson and colleagues and "metabolomics" by others. Recently, more focused analyses of specific metabolite families or subsets have given rise to new terms such as "lipidomics."

In terms of applications to human diagnostics, seminal studies of inborn errors of metabolism in infants have served as a key springboard. Millington and colleagues pioneered the use of mass spectrometry (MS)–based methods for monitoring fatty acid oxidation, as well as organic and selected amino acids.[2] Their work culminated in neonatal screening for metabolic disorders, thereby enabling the identification of infants with fatty acid oxidation disorders, organic acidemias, and aminoacidopathies. In certain situations, rapid identification of these disorders triggers intervention in the form of dietary modulation, conferring therapeutic benefits. A global metabolomic or proteomic analysis of more indolent, complex diseases such as atherosclerosis might similarly spotlight pathways for dietary or drug modulation.

ANALYTIC CHALLENGES FOR PROTEOMICS AND METABOLOMICS

The many classes of proteins and chemicals present analytic challenges, particularly as applied to searching for biomarkers in blood. Many different types of cells contribute to the plasma proteome and metabolome, thus increasing their complexities and presenting

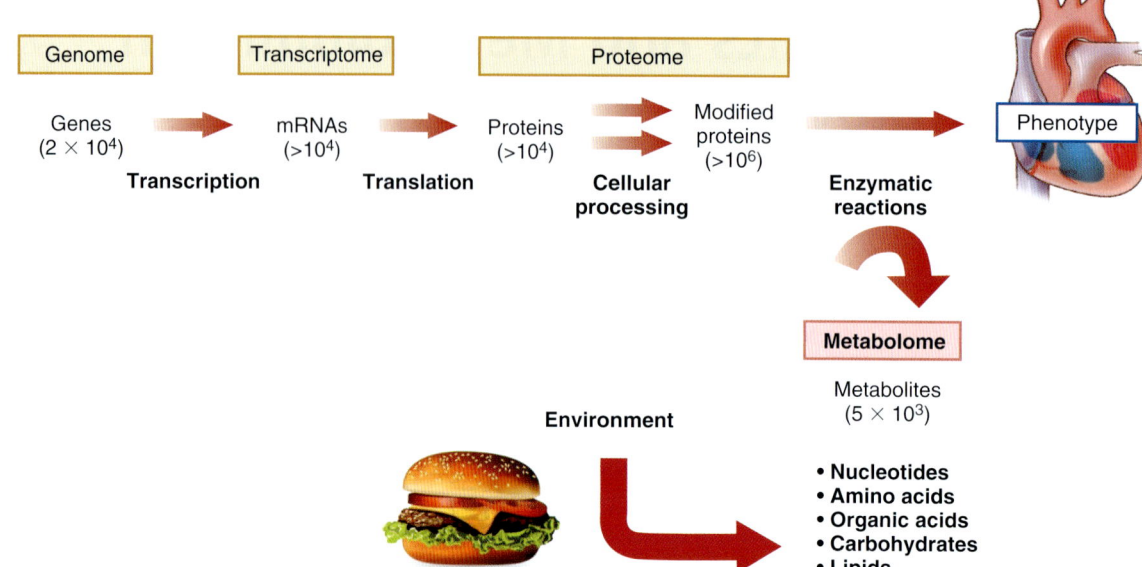

FIGURE 8.1 The conceptual relationship of the genome, transcriptome, proteome, and metabolome. Informational complexity increases from genome to transcriptome to proteome. The estimated number of entities of each type of molecule in humans is indicated in parentheses.

challenges to interpretation of the data that emerge. In the case of the blood proteome, the 22 most abundant proteins, including albumin and the immunoglobulins, account for 99% of the total proteome mass (Fig. 8.2). Many of the biologically interesting molecules relevant to human disease occur in low abundance. Cardiac markers such as troponin circulate in the nanomolar range, insulin in the picomolar range, and tumor necrosis factor in the femtomolar range. Plasma contains tens of thousands of unique protein species in concentrations spanning a range of more than 10 orders of magnitude. Indeed, some suggest that the plasma proteome might encompass the entire set of human polypeptide species resulting from splice variants and post-translational modifications because the protein content of plasma unexpectedly includes proteins of all functional classes and from apparently all cellular localizations. Many low-abundance proteins in plasma are intracellular or membrane proteins that are present in plasma as a result of cellular turnover. There is also an increasing appreciation of gut-derived small molecules and peptides (i.e., from the "microbiome") present in blood that appear to activate signaling pathways in leukocytes or metabolically active tissues.[3] Recent estimates suggest that the human metabolome consists of fewer molecular entities than the human proteome[4] and thus may be somewhat more tractable to analyze and systematize than the human proteome.

Several features contribute critically to the success of proteomic or metabolomic technologies. First, the technique must have the capability of identifying a wide breadth of proteins or metabolite analytes within complex biologic samples across a broad range of physical characteristics, including size and charge. Second, the technologies must be sensitive enough to probe the proteome or metabolome to adequate "depths"—that is, to provide resolution of biologically active compounds of the lowest abundance. Frequently, the least abundant entities play critical regulatory roles in the response to physiologic stressors. Third, tools must also work across a broad dynamic range, a notion underscored in Figure 8.2—they must be able to simultaneously identify both more abundant and less abundant proteins in the same complex mixture. Unfortunately, many analytic techniques apply well only across concentrations of several orders of magnitude. Finally, the ideal technology should be stable and reproducible, an attribute necessary for minimizing artifacts during initial discovery, validation, and testing for clinical applications.

Robust, searchable databases for validation of identified proteins or metabolites represent an increasingly crucial support for biomarker discovery. The scope of investigation addressable by these techniques has widened immeasurably since completion of the Human Genome Project. At present, the human databases are the largest and easiest to use, which will help accelerate translational investigation. Genomic databases collectively provide a catalog of all known or theoretical proteins expressed in organisms for which databases exist. Software that can search through databases for identification of candidates has proven essential to interpretation of the data; much of this software is available on the Internet. Collaborative efforts have recently begun to catalog both the human proteome and the plasma metabolome.

OVERVIEW OF THE DISCOVERY PROCESS

Figure 8.3 summarizes the essential elements of the discovery approach by using a proteomics experiment as an example. Biologic samples consist of a complex mixture containing intact and partially degraded proteins and metabolites of various molecular weights, modifications, and solubility. The chance of identifying proteins or metabolites in a mixture increases as the complexity of the mixture decreases. As suggested by Liebler, the problem of complexity and how to deal with it resembles the process of printing a book. Printing all the words on a single page could be accomplished quickly, but the resulting page would be illegibly black with ink; dividing the text into multiple pages reduces the complexity to reveal organized text. Samples can be analogously enriched for certain components through fractionation or affinity depletion columns, but all preparative procedures—including solubilization, denaturation, and reduction processes—should be compatible with the constraints of subsequent analysis steps. The quest to reduce complexity requires careful balance against the possibility that each additional step might also introduce undesired protein or metabolite modifications or loss.

Several analytic techniques can serve to identify metabolites or proteins, although MS instrumentation offers an unrivaled ability to provide several layers of complementary information, which has benefited tremendously from whole-genome analysis and the genomics revolution. MS provides accurate mass detection of peptides from proteolytic digests of complex protein mixtures or small metabolites derived from tissues or blood. The set of peptide or metabolite mass measurements can be searched in databases to obtain definitive identification of the parent proteins or metabolites of interest. Favorably compared against other proteomics and metabolomics technologies,

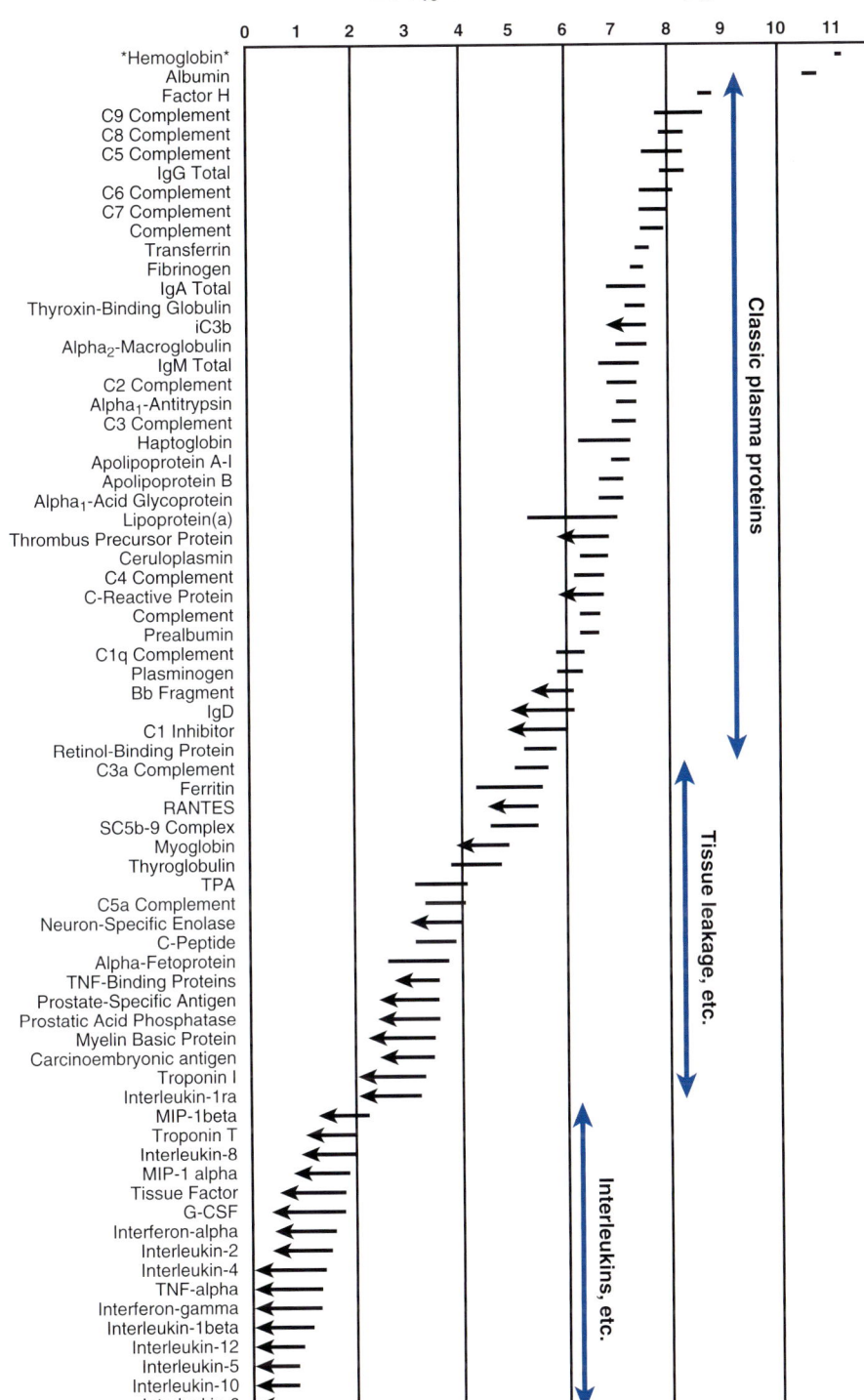

FIGURE 8.2 Reference concentration for representative protein analytes in plasma. Protein abundance is plotted on a log scale spanning 12 orders of magnitude. When only an upper limit is quoted, the lower end of the interval line shows an *arrowhead*. The classic plasma proteins are clustered to the left (high abundance), the tissue leakage markers (e.g., enzymes, troponins) are clustered in the center, and the cytokines are clustered to the right (low abundance). *G-CSF*, Granulocyte colony-stimulating factor; *MIP*, macrophage inflammatory protein; *RANTES*, regulated on activation, T cell expressed and secreted; *TNF*, tumor necrosis factor; *TPA*, tissue plasminogen activator. (From Anderson NL, Anderson NG. The human plasma proteome: history, character, and diagnostic prospects. *Mol Cell Proteomics*. 2003;2:50.)

MS offers high sensitivity and amenability to automation, thus promoting high-throughput processing. MS has a wide range of applicability and not only detects metabolites and proteins but also characterizes any post-translational modifications.

Mass spectrometers are composed of modular elements, including an ion source, mass analyzer, and a detector/recorder (Fig. 8.4). MS instruments are classified according to the ionization source and mass analyzer used, but all process samples as gas-phase ions, the movements of which are precisely measured within an electromagnetic field. An ion source generates these gas-phase ions from the analyte through a variety of available techniques, from either the solid state by matrix-assisted laser desorption/ionization (MALDI) or directly from the liquid phase by electrospray ionization (ESI). A coupled chromatographic separation step fractionates complex sample mixtures before ESI spectroscopic analysis. The gas-phase ions then enter the mass analyzer, which resolves the peptides based on their mass-to-charge (m/z) ratio. Examples of commonly used mass analyzers include the quadrupole mass filter, ion trap mass analyzer, and time-of-flight mass analyzer. Finally, the detector records the ions via an electronic multiplier and records ion intensity versus the m/z value to create the resulting MS spectra.

These technologies can be used to characterize biologic fluids either in a targeted manner or in a pattern discovery manner. In the

former, the investigator targets a predefined set of analytes to be quantitated. For example, libraries of metabolites can be purchased and their chromatographic and MS characteristics determined empirically by "spiking" reference standards into plasma. Endogenous metabolites can then be quantified based on the information ascertained from the known standards. The targeted approach now readily permits assay of several hundred metabolites in as little as tens of microliters of plasma. In the pattern discovery experiment, by contrast, the investigator confronts a complex pattern of peaks, many of which are anonymous—the molecular identities of the species that give rise to the peaks are not generally known. Although the targeted approach is more limiting, the analysis is more straightforward because the analytes yielding the signals are already known. The untargeted or "fingerprint" approach has less inherent bias, but unambiguous identification of the peaks can prove laborious and difficult. In clinical samples, considerable care must be taken to rule out spurious associations—for example, confounding related to drug treatment.

APPLICATIONS OF MASS SPECTROMETRY-BASED DISCOVERY TO CARDIOMETABOLIC DISEASE

In an initial proof-of-principle study using a targeted metabolite profiling approach, Newgard and colleagues profiled obese versus lean humans to gain a broad understanding of the metabolic and physiologic differences in these two disparate groups. Their studies identified a branched-chain amino acid signature that correlated highly with the metrics of insulin resistance while functional studies in model systems have highlighted a role for this pathway in disease pathogenesis.[5] Complementary studies in two large population-based cohorts demonstrated that branched-chain and aromatic amino acid concentrations associate significantly with incident type 2 diabetes up to 12 years before the onset of overt disease. Adjustment for established clinical risk factors did not substantially attenuate the strength of these associations. Furthermore, the branched-chain amino acid signature also predicts atherosclerosis even after adjusting for the metrics of insulin resistance and diabetes. For those in the top quartile of branched-chain amino acid levels, the odds for development of cardiometabolic disease exceeded any single-nucleotide polymorphism identified to date. Taken together, these findings have disclosed dysregulation of amino acid metabolism very early in the development of cardiometabolic diseases. Ongoing studies are examining the relative genetic versus environmental contributions to these findings. A recent report suggests that genetic variation in enzymes in branched-chain amino acid metabolism associate with both circulating amino acid levels and with diabetes in multiple large human cohorts, suggesting that this class of compounds also contributes to disease pathogenesis.[6] Such mendelian randomization analyses are now being performed for thousands of circulating proteins and metabolites in humans to assess for potential causal roles in cardiometabolic disease pathogenesis (see also Chapters 7 and 10).

In a translational study using nontargeted liquid chromatography–MS–based metabolite profiling applied to cardiovascular disease, Wang and associates first profiled the plasma of 75 individuals from a hospital-based cohort who experienced a myocardial infarction, stroke, or death in the ensuing 3 years and 75 age- and sex-matched controls who did not. Of 18 analytes that differed significantly between cases and controls, 3 demonstrated significant correlations among one another, thus suggesting a potential common biochemical pathway. Using complementary analytic methods, these metabolites were identified as betaine, choline, and trimethylamine-N-oxide, all metabolites of dietary phosphatidylcholine. Dietary supplementation of choline was sufficient to promote atherosclerosis in mice, and suppression of the intestinal bacteria responsible for the conversion of phosphatidylcholine to choline inhibited this atherogenesis. In addition to reinforcing the interaction between diet, gut bacteria, and the metabolome, this study demonstrated how metabolomic biomarker discovery can elucidate novel pathways to disease.[7]

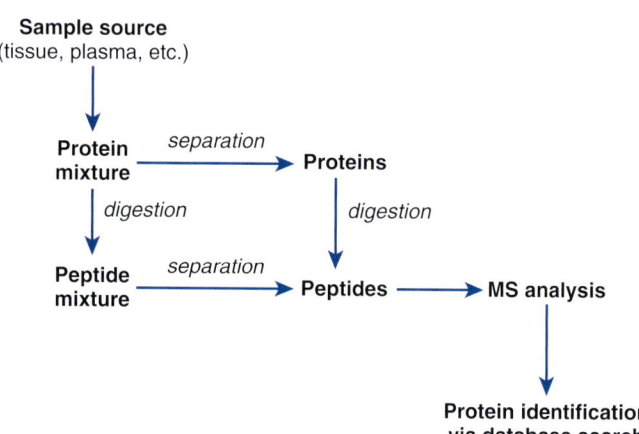

FIG. 8.3 Overview of a proteomics experiment. *MS*, mass spectrometry.

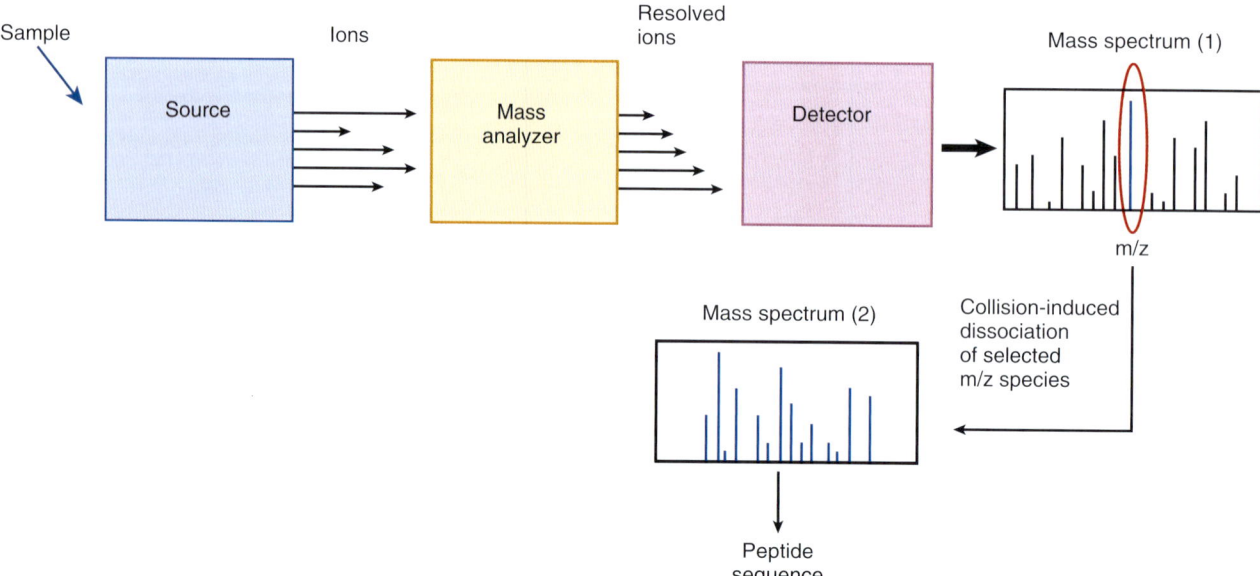

FIG. 8.4 Schematic of tandem mass spectrometry. *m/z*, mass-to-charge ratio.

FUTURE DIRECTIONS IN BIOMARKER DISCOVERY

In addition to their use in neonatal screening, MS-based assays of small molecules are increasingly used in clinical chemistry. For example, robust clinical workflows measure vitamins, sex hormones, and drug levels. By contrast, high-throughput proteomic approaches that account for the complex protein constituents of human plasma are less mature, even for research purposes. Two emerging approaches to address limitations of present tools in analyzing the blood proteome incorporate new classes of affinity (e.g., binding) reagents coupled to high-throughput readouts based on established DNA technologies. One new technique uses aptamer-based technologies to selectively probe the plasma proteome. Aptamers are small RNA or single-stranded DNA nucleic acids that can bind with great specificity to targeted proteins and related cell targets. Aptamers can be incubated with plasma and, using standard bead immobilization techniques, ultimately separated into bound and unbound fractions. Once eluted, these bound aptamers (reflecting their accompanying protein targets) are hybridized to microarrays with complementary single-stranded DNA probes to quantify the specific fluorescent tags. A second high-throughput technique conjugates antibodies with nucleotide "bar codes" which can be quantified by polymerase chain reaction (PCR) or next-generation DNA sequencing. The DNA readout mitigates interferences that severely limit the use of multiple enzyme-linked immunosorbent assays (ELISAs) performed in the same plasma sample. A recent example of the aptamer technique includes an analysis in the Heart and Soul and HUNT-3 studies that measured 1130 proteins.[8] Of these, nine proteins were identified as being predictive of vascular risk, and a risk score derived from these nine proteins was able to separate high from low risk. These new high-throughput techniques are now enabling analyses in very large, well-phenotyped, human cohorts that hold unprecedented promise to illuminate new biomarkers and cardiovascular disease pathways. Of course, the generalizability of these findings requires further work to validate clinical utility in terms or early diagnosis or reclassification and, perhaps most importantly, whether the new approaches can identify novel therapeutic targets.

Identification of new biomarkers for cardiovascular disease depends on the complementary power of genetics, transcriptional profiling, proteomics, and metabolomics. The clinical usefulness of new biomarkers will require rigorous evaluation of their ability to improve the prediction of risk or to direct and monitor management in an individual, the ultimate goal of personalized medicine (see also Chapter 10). In addition to risk biomarkers, diagnostic biomarkers could help in making challenging acute diagnoses such as reversible myocardial ischemia, pulmonary embolism, and aortic dissection. The evolution of a clinical biomarker requires a long journey and an arduous transition from the research environment to clinical practice. Emerging technologies such as those described earlier have the potential to permit systematic assessment of variation in genes, RNA, proteins, and metabolites for identification of "uncorrelated" or "orthogonal" biomarkers that probably would not emerge with a focus on candidates from well-studied pathways.

REFERENCES

1. Stanford KI, Lynes MD, Takahashi H, et al. 12,13-diHOME: an exercise-induced lipokine that increases skeletal muscle fatty acid uptake. *Cell Metab.* 2018;27:1111–1120.e3.
2. Washburn J, Millington DS. Digital microfluidics in newborn screening for mucopolysaccharidoses: a progress report. *Int J Neonatal Screen.* 2020;6:78.
3. Lavelle A, Sokol H. Gut microbiota-derived metabolites as key actors in inflammatory bowel disease. *Nature Rev Gastroenterol Hepatol.* 2020;17:223–237.
4. Chen Z-Z, Gerszten Robert E. Metabolomics and proteomics in type 2 diabetes. *Circ Res.* 2020;126:1613–1627.
5. White PJ, Newgard CB. Branched-chain amino acids in disease. *Science.* 2019;363:582.
6. Lotta LA, Scott RA, Sharp SJ, et al. Genetic Predisposition to an impaired metabolism of the branched-chain amino acids and risk of type 2 diabetes: a mendelian randomisation analysis. *PLoS.* 2016;13:e1002179.
7. Roberts A, Gu X, Buffa J, et al. Development of a gut microbe–targeted nonlethal therapeutic to inhibit thrombosis potential. *Nat Med.* 2018;24:1407–1417.
8. Ganz P, Heidecker B, Hveem K, et al. Development and validation of a protein-based risk score for cardiovascular Outcomes among patients with stable Coronary heart disease. *J Am Med Assoc.* 2016;315:2532–2541.

9 Principles of Drug Therapeutics, Pharmacogenomics, and Biologics

DAN M. RODEN

RISK VERSUS BENEFIT OF DRUG THERAPY, 92
Clinical Trials Can Define Unexpected Adverse Drug Reactions, 92
Classes of Adverse Drug Reactions, 92

PHARMACOKINETICS AND PHARMACODYNAMICS, 93

MOLECULAR AND GENETIC BASIS FOR VARIABLE DRUG RESPONSE, 96
High-Risk Pharmacokinetics, 96
Other Important Pharmacogenetic Effects, 97

OPTIMIZING DRUG DOSES, 98
Plasma Concentration Monitoring, 98
Dose Adjustments in Disease, 99

Drug Interactions, 99
Incorporating Pharmacogenetic Information into Prescribing, 100

FUTURE PERSPECTIVES, 100

REFERENCES, 101

In 2018 the total cost of health care in the United States was approximately $3.6 trillion, 17.7% of the Gross Domestic Product, and more than 10% was spent on prescription drugs.[1] Cardiovascular disease makes up the largest subcategory in this spending: in 2020 the American Heart Association estimated that the cost of care for cardiovascular disease in 2015 was $351.3 billion/year.[2]

Not every patient responds to drug therapy in the same way; efficacy varies, and adverse drug reactions (ADRs) range from minor to potentially fatal. Multiple mechanisms can result in this variability, such as poor compliance, variable impact of diverse disease mechanisms on drug actions, drug interactions, and the increasingly well-recognized role of genomic variation. Indeed, ADRs across all therapeutic categories are estimated to be the fourth to sixth most common cause of death in the United States, costing over $30 billion annually and accounting directly for 3% to 6% of all hospital admissions.[3,4]

RISK VERSUS BENEFIT OF DRUG THERAPY

The fundamental assumption underlying administration of any drug is that the real or expected benefit exceeds the anticipated risk. The benefits of drug therapy are initially defined in small clinical trials, perhaps involving several thousand patients, before a drug's marketing and approval. Ultimately, the efficacy and safety profiles of any drug are determined after the compound has been marketed and used widely in hundreds of thousands of patients. Occasionally, unexpected drug actions detected during or after a development program can result in new indications: PDE5 inhibitors for pulmonary hypertension or SGLT-2 inhibitors for heart failure are examples.

When a drug is administered for the acute correction of a life-threatening condition, the benefits are often self-evident; insulin for diabetic ketoacidosis and nitroprusside for hypertensive encephalopathy are examples. However, extrapolation of such immediately obvious benefits to other clinical situations may not be warranted.

Clinical Trials Can Define Unexpected Adverse Drug Reactions

Randomized clinical trials (RCTs) have proven invaluable both to demonstrate the efficacy of drug therapy and to identify rare but serious ADRs. One of the first examples of an RCT identifying an unexpected serious ADR was the Cardiac Arrhythmia Suppression Trial (CAST), which tested the hypothesis that suppression of ventricular ectopic activity, a recognized risk factor for sudden death after myocardial infarction (MI), would reduce mortality; this notion was highly ingrained in cardiovascular practice in the 1970s and 1980s. In CAST, sodium channel–blocking antiarrhythmic drugs did suppress ventricular ectopic beats but also unexpectedly increased mortality threefold. The use of ectopic beat suppression as a surrogate marker did not produce the desired drug action—reduction in mortality—probably because the underlying pathophysiology was incompletely understood.

Similarly, drugs with positive inotropic activity augment cardiac output in patients with heart failure but also are associated with an increase in mortality, probably because of drug-induced arrhythmias. Nevertheless, clinical trials with these agents suggest symptom relief. Thus the prescriber and the patient may elect therapy with positive inotropic drugs to realize this benefit while recognizing the risk. This complex decision making is at the heart of the broad concept of personalized medicine, which incorporates into the care of an individual patient not only genomic (or other) markers of variable drug responses, but also factors such as patients' understanding of their disease, presence of other diseases, willingness to tolerate minor or serious risks of treatment, and sociocultural factors which impact key health determinants such as exposure to pollution, ability to pay for care, and literacy and numeracy.

Classes of Adverse Drug Reactions

The risks of drug therapy may be a direct extension of the pharmacologic actions for which the drug is actually being prescribed. Hypoglycemia in a patient taking an antidiabetic agent and bleeding in a patient taking an anticoagulant are examples; sodium channel block in CAST is another. T cell activation by immune checkpoint inhibitors, with resultant myocarditis, may in this sense also be "on-target."[5]

In other cases, ADRs develop as a consequence of pharmacologic actions that were not appreciated during a drug's initial development and use in patients. Examples include rhabdomyolysis occurring with 3-hydroxy-3-methylglutaryl–coenzyme A (HMG-CoA) reductase inhibitors (statins), angioedema developing during angiotensin-converting enzyme (ACE) inhibitor therapy, and torsades de pointes during treatment with noncardiovascular drugs such as methadone or hydroxychloroquine.[6] Of importance, these rarer but serious effects generally become evident only after a drug has been marketed and extensively used. Even rare ADRs can alter the overall perception of risk versus benefit and can prompt removal of the drug from the market, particularly if alternate therapies thought to be safer are available or the benefits of drug therapy are modest or difficult to demonstrate. For example, withdrawal of the first insulin sensitizer, troglitazone, after recognition of hepatotoxicity was further spurred by the availability of other new drugs in this class.

The recognition of multiple cyclooxygenase (COX) isoforms led to the development of specific COX-2 inhibitors to retain aspirin's analgesic effects but reduce gastrointestinal side effects. However, one of these, rofecoxib, was withdrawn because of an apparent increase in cardiovascular mortality. The events surrounding the withdrawal of rofecoxib have important implications for drug development and utilization. First, specificity achieved by targeting a single molecular entity may not necessarily reduce ADRs; one possibility is that by inhibiting COX-2, the drug removes a vascular protective effect of prostacyclin. Second, drug side effects may include not only readily identifiable events such as rhabdomyolysis or torsades de pointes but also an increase—that may be difficult to detect—in events such as MI that are common in the general population.

PHARMACOKINETICS AND PHARMACODYNAMICS

Two major processes determine how the interaction between a drug and its target molecule(s) can generate variable drug actions in a patient. The first, *pharmacokinetics* (Fig. 9.1), describes drug delivery to and removal from the target molecule and includes the processes of absorption, distribution, metabolism, and excretion—collectively termed *drug disposition*. The second process, *pharmacodynamics* (Fig 9.2), describes how the interaction between a drug and its molecular target(s) generates downstream molecular, cellular, whole-organ, and whole-body effects.

Genes encoding drug-metabolizing enzymes and drug transport molecules determine pharmacokinetics. Genes encoding drug targets and the molecules modulating the biology in which the drug-target interaction occurs (including those causing the disease being treated) determine pharmacodynamics. *Pharmacogenetics* describes the concept that individual variants in the genes controlling these processes contribute to variable drug actions. *Pharmacogenomics* is often used to describe the way in which variability across multiple genes, up to whole genomes, explains differences in drug response among individuals and populations. The following overview of broad principles of pharmacokinetics, pharmacodynamics, and pharmacogenomics is followed by more detailed discussion of the specific genes, their function, and important variants influencing cardiovascular drug responses.

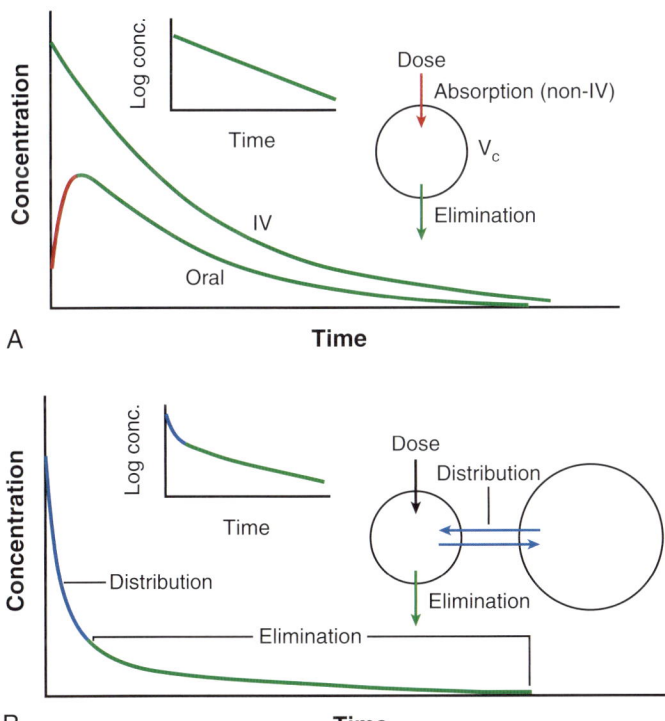

FIGURE 9.1 Models of plasma concentrations as a function of time after a single dose of a drug. **A,** The simplest situation is one in which a drug is administered as a rapid intravenous (IV) bolus into a volume (V_c), where it is instantaneously and uniformly distributed. Elimination then takes place from this volume. In this case, drug elimination is monoexponential; that is, a plot of the logarithm of concentration versus time is linear *(inset)*. When the same dose of drug is administered orally, a distinct absorption phase is required before drug entry into V_c. Most absorption (shown here in *red*) is completed before elimination (shown in *green*), although the processes overlap. In this example, the amount of drug delivered by the oral route is less than that delivered by the IV route, assessed by the total areas under the two curves, indicating reduced bioavailability. **B,** In this example, drug is delivered to the central volume, from which it is not only eliminated but also undergoes distribution to the peripheral sites. This distribution process *(blue)* is more rapid than elimination, resulting in a distinct biexponential disappearance curve *(inset)*.

PHARMACOKINETIC PRINCIPLES

Administration of an intravenous (IV) drug bolus results in maximal drug concentrations at the end of delivery of the bolus, followed by a decline in plasma drug concentrations over time (Fig. 9.1A), generally because of drug elimination. In the simplest case this decline occurs monoexponentially over time. A useful parameter to describe this decline is the half-life ($t_{1/2}$), the time in which 50% of the drug is eliminated; for example, after two half-lives, 75% of the drug has been eliminated, and after three half-lives, 87.5%. A monoexponential process can be considered almost complete in four or five half-lives. In some cases the decline of drug concentrations after administration of an IV bolus dose is multiexponential. The most common explanation is that the drug is not only eliminated (represented by terminal portion of time-concentration plot) but also undergoes more rapid distribution to peripheral tissues. Just as elimination may be usefully described by a half-life, distribution half-lives also can be derived from curves such as those shown in Figure 9.1B.

The plasma concentration measured immediately after a bolus dose can be used to derive a volume into which the drug is distributed. When the decline of plasma concentrations is multiexponential, multiple distribution compartments can be defined; these volumes of distribution can be useful in considering dose adjustments in cases of disease but rarely correspond exactly to any physical volume, such as plasma or total body water. With drugs that are highly tissue bound (e.g., some antidepressants), the volume of distribution can exceed total body volume by orders of magnitude.

Drugs are often administered by non-IV routes, such as oral, sublingual, transcutaneous, or intramuscular. Such routes of administration differ from the IV route in two ways (see Fig. 9.1A). First, concentrations in plasma demonstrate a distinct rising phase as the drug slowly enters plasma. Second, the total amount of drug that actually enters the systemic circulation may be less than that achieved by the IV route. The relative amount of drug entering by any route, compared with the same dose administered intravenously, is termed *bioavailability*, calculated as the ratio of the area under the time-concentration curves, as shown in Figure 9.1A. Some drugs undergo extensive metabolism before entry into the systemic circulation, and as a result the amount of drug required to achieve a therapeutic effect is much greater (and often more variable) than that required for the same drug administered intravenously. Thus small doses of IV propranolol (5 mg) may achieve heart rate slowing equivalent to that observed with much larger oral doses (80 to 120 mg). Propranolol is actually well absorbed but undergoes extensive metabolism in the intestine and liver before entering the systemic circulation. Another example is amiodarone; its physicochemical characteristics make it only 30% to 50% bioavailable when administered orally. Thus an IV infusion of 0.5 mg/min (720 mg/day) is equivalent to 1.5 to 2 g/day orally.

Drug elimination occurs by metabolism followed by the excretion of metabolites and unmetabolized parent drug, generally by the biliary tract or kidneys. This process can be quantified as *clearance*, the volume that is cleared of drug in any given period. Clearance may be organ specific (e.g., renal clearance, hepatic clearance) or whole-body clearance. Drug metabolism is conventionally divided into phase I oxidation and phase II conjugation, both of which enhance water solubility and, consequently, biliary or renal elimination.

The most common enzyme systems mediating phase I drug metabolism are those of the cytochrome P-450 superfamily, termed *CYPs*. Multiple CYPs are expressed in human liver and other tissues. A major source of variability in drug action is variability in CYP expression and/or genetic variants that alter CYP activity. Table 9.1 lists CYPs and other proteins important for pharmacokinetics of cardiovascular drugs. Excretion of drugs or their metabolites into the urine or bile is accomplished by glomerular filtration or specific drug transport molecules, whose level of expression and genetic variation are only now being explored. One widely studied transporter is *P-glycoprotein*, the product of expression of the *MDR1* (or *ABCB1*) gene. Originally identified as a factor mediating multiple drug resistance in patients with cancer, P-glycoprotein expression is now well recognized in normal enterocytes, hepatocytes, renal tubular cells, the endothelium of the capillaries forming the blood-brain barrier, and the testes. In each of these sites, P-glycoprotein expression is restricted to the apical aspect of polarized cells, where it acts to enhance drug efflux. In the intestine, P-glycoprotein pumps substrates back into the lumen, thereby limiting bioavailability. In the liver and kidney, it promotes drug excretion into bile or urine. In central nervous system capillary endothelium, P-glycoprotein–mediated efflux is an important mechanism limiting drug access to the brain. Transporters also play a role drug uptake into many cells. One example is OATP1B1, which is responsible for simvastatin uptake into hepatocytes; variants in *SLCO1B1*, which encodes the transporter, have been associated with an increased risk for simvastatin-induced muscle toxicity.

Pharmacodynamic Principles
Drugs can exert variable effects, even in the absence of pharmacokinetic variability. This can arise as a function of variability in the molecular targets with which drugs interact to achieve their beneficial and adverse effects, as well as variability in the broader biologic context within which the drug-target interaction takes place (see Fig. 9.2). Variability in the number or function of a drug's target molecules can arise because of genetic factors (see later) or because disease alters the number of target molecules or their state (e.g., changes in extent of phosphorylation). Simple examples of variability in the biologic context are high dietary salt, which can inhibit the antihypertensive action of beta blockers, and hypokalemia, which increases the risk for drug-induced QT prolongation. In addition, disease itself can modulate drug response. For example, the effect of lytic therapy in a patient with no clots is manifestly different from that in a patient with an acute coronary syndrome, or the vasodilating effects of nitrates, beneficial in patients with coronary disease with angina, can be catastrophic in patients with aortic stenosis. These examples highlight the requirement for precision in diagnosis to avoid situations in which risk outweighs potential benefit. One hope is that emerging genomic or other molecular approaches can add to this precision.

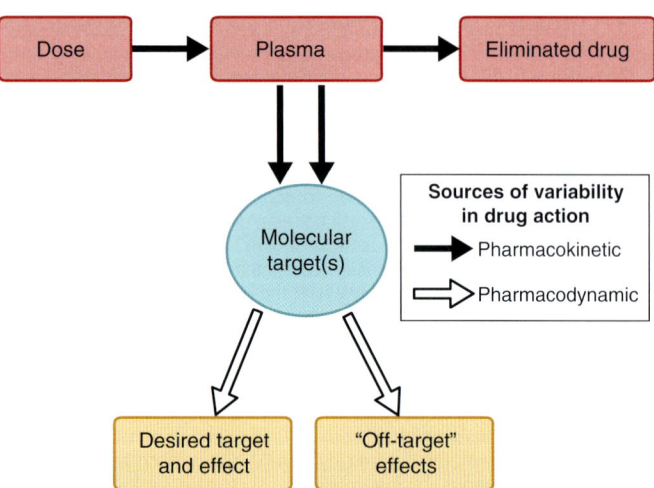

FIGURE 9.2 Pharmacokinetic and pharmacodynamic sources of variability in drug action. Pharmacokinetic processes determine drug concentration at molecular targets that through multiple mechanisms broadly termed pharmacodynamics transduce beneficial and undesirable drug effects. (From Roden DM, Van Driest SL, Wells QS, et al. Opportunities and challenges in cardiovascular pharmacogenomics: from discovery to implementation. *Circ Res*. 2018;122[9]:1176–1190.)

Drug Targets
The targets with which drugs interact to produce beneficial effects may or may not be the same as those with which drugs interact to produce ADRs. Drug targets may be in the circulation, at the cell surface, or within cells. Many drugs widely used in cardiovascular therapeutics (e.g., digoxin, amiodarone, aspirin) were developed when the technology to identify specific molecular targets was not available. Some drugs (e.g., amiodarone) have many drug targets. In other cases, however, even older drugs are found to have rather specific molecular targets. The actions of digitalis glycosides are mediated primarily by the inhibition of sodium/potassium–adenosine triphosphatase (Na^+,K^+-ATPase). Aspirin permanently acetylates a specific serine residue on the COX enzyme, an effect that is thought to mediate its analgesic effects and its gastrointestinal toxicity. Most newer drugs have been developed to interact with a specific drug target identified in the course of basic mechanistic studies; examples of such targets are HMG-CoA reductase, ACE, G protein–coupled receptors (GPCRs; e.g., alpha, beta, angiotensin II, histamine), and platelet P2Y12 receptors.

An emerging approach is to use modern genetic techniques to identify loss-of-function DNA variants that are tolerated throughout life and associated with a desired phenotype, such as greatly reduced MI risk. Inhibitors of the corresponding gene products are thus predicted to exert a beneficial effect and lack serious on-target ADRs. PCSK9 inhibitors are an excellent example (see Chapter 27), and other potential drug targets are now being identified using this approach.[7,8] Furthermore, an emerging understanding of the way in which genetic variation produces mendelian diseases such as cystic fibrosis is leading to new, mechanism-based therapies.[9] Cardiovascular diseases such as hypertrophic cardiomyopathy appear ripe for such development (see Chapter 54).[10]

Time Course of Drug Effects
With repeated doses, drug levels accumulate to a *steady state*, the condition under which the rate of drug administration is equal to the rate of drug elimination in any given period. Drug accumulation to steady state is near-complete in four to five elimination half-lives (Fig. 9.3). For many drugs, the target molecule is in plasma or readily accessible from plasma, so this time course also describes the development of pharmacologic effects. In other cases, however, although steady-state plasma concentrations are achieved in four to five elimination half-lives, steady-state drug effects take longer to achieve; there are several possible explanations for this. First, an active metabolite may need to be generated to achieve drug effects. Second, time may be required for translation of the drug effect at the molecular site to a physiologic endpoint. For example, inhibition of HMG-CoA reductase ultimately leads to a desired lowering of low-density lipoprotein (LDL) cholesterol, but the development of this desired effect may take days or weeks after the drug is started. Third, penetration of a drug into intracellular or other tissue sites of action may be required before development of a drug effect. One mechanism underlying such penetration is the variable function of the drug uptake and efflux transport proteins (discussed earlier) that control intracellular drug concentrations.

Pharmacogenomic Principles (see Chapter 7)
A range of experimental techniques have been used to establish a role for both common and rare DNA polymorphisms in pharmacokinetic and pharmacodynamic pathways as mediators of variable drug actions. Rare variants associated with mendelian diseases such as familial hypercholesterolemia and long-QT syndrome are traditionally termed *mutations*, whereas the term *polymorphism* is used more generically to describe variants that may or may not be associated with any human trait. Polymorphism frequency often varies strikingly by ancestry, and with the

TABLE 9.1 Proteins Important in Drug Metabolism and Elimination

PROTEIN	SUBSTRATES
Cytochrome P-450s (CYPs)	
CYP3A4, CYP3A5*	Erythromycin, clarithromycin; quinidine, mexiletine; many benzodiazepines; cyclosporine, tacrolimus; many antiretrovirals
	HMG-CoA reductase inhibitors: atorvastatin, simvastatin, lovastatin; not pravastatin
	Many calcium channel blockers; apixaban, rivaroxaban
CYP2D6*	Some beta blockers: propranolol, timolol, metoprolol, carvedilol
	Propafenone; desipramine and other tricyclics; codeine†; tamoxifen†; dextromethorphan
CYP2C9*	Warfarin, phenytoin, tolbutamide, losartan,† rosuvastatin
CYP2C19*	Omeprazole, clopidogrel†
Other Drug-Metabolizing Enzymes	
N-acetyltransferase*	Procainamide, hydralazine, isoniazid
Thiopurine methyltransferase*	6-Mercaptopurine, azathioprine
Pseudocholinesterase*	Succinylcholine
Serine esterase 1 (CES1)	Clopidogrel, dabigatran
Uridine diphosphate-glucuronosyltransferase*	Irinotecan,† atazanavir
Drug Transporters	
P-glycoprotein	Digoxin, dabigatran
SLCO1B1*	Simvastatin, atorvastatin; methotrexate; troglitazone; bosentan

HMG-CoA, 3-Hydroxy-3-methylglutaryl–coenzyme A.
*Clinically important genetic variants described.
†Prodrug bioactivated by drug metabolism.

advent of inexpensive sequencing, it is apparent that the vast majority of DNA polymorphisms in any individual are actually rare (minor allele frequency [MAF] < 1%) across a large population of individuals of the same ancestry. The most common type is a single nucleotide polymorphism (SNP or single nucleotide variant [SNV]); SNPs that change the encoded amino acid are termed *nonsynonymous*. Other types are short insertions or deletions (indels) or copy number variations (CNVs), in which large segments of DNA are deleted or duplicated (or more).

One of the great success stories of modern cardiovascular genetics has been the use of linkage analysis in large families to identify disease-causing rare variants (mutations) in familial syndromes with highly unusual clinical phenotypes, such as familial hypercholesterolemia (see Chapter 27), hypertrophic cardiomyopathy (see Chapter 54), and the ion channelopathies (see Chapter 63). Linkage analysis has not been widely applied to study pharmacogenomics because large kindreds with multiple individuals having clearly defined drug-response phenotypes generally are not available.

DNA variation contributes importantly to variability in common human traits, such as laboratory values or susceptibility to common disease. Methods are available to establish the extent to which that variability includes a heritable component, often by examining twins, large families, or groups of families; evidence for heritability provides strong justification for pursuing studies to identify contributing genetic variation. Indeed, this general approach has established that common phenotypes such as LDL cholesterol, blood pressure, and susceptibility to atrial fibrillation are highly heritable. The extent to which rare and common variants contribute to this variability is only now being addressed. Across populations, individual common (MAF > 5%) DNA polymorphisms rarely account for more than even 1% of variability in common traits. Variability in response to drug exposure presents a striking exception to this general rule, where even single common DNA polymorphisms may contribute substantially, 10% or more in many cases, to overall variability in drug response. It has been speculated that common variants with large effects on drug response can persist in a population because there is no evolutionary pressure against such variants because drug exposure is a recent event in human history.

One mechanism accounting for this large effect is that common SNPs in drug metabolism pathways can result in extremely large fluctuations in drug concentration and corresponding effects. Examples of specific cardiovascular phenotypes in which common SNPs have been associated with risk are presented in Table 9.2 and discussed later. Of note, rarer variants in these (or other) genes are only now being described, so their role in mediating drug response is much less well understood. In addition, virtually all studies to date have focused primarily on populations of European ancestry, and data are only now being generated on specific polymorphisms mediating variable drug actions in other ancestries.

The Candidate Gene Approach. One technique to identify associations between DNA polymorphisms and drug response (or other traits) uses an understanding of the physiology of the trait under question to identify candidate genes modulating the trait. Thus, for example, an investigator interested in variability in the PR interval might invoke

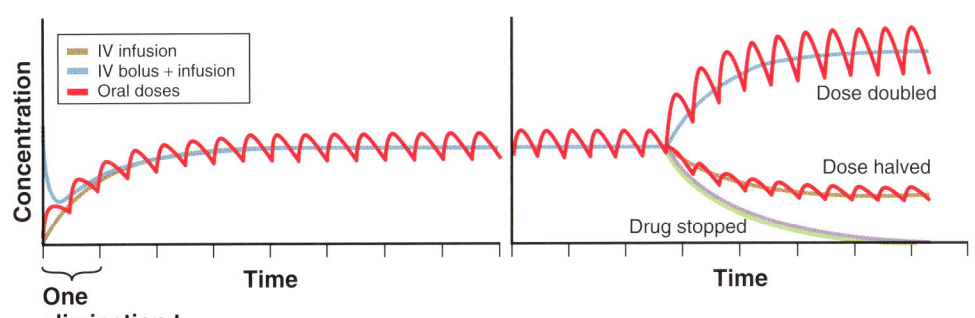

FIGURE 9.3 Time course of drug concentrations when treatment is started or dose changed. *Left,* The *hash lines* on the abscissa each indicate one elimination half-life ($t_{1/2}$). With a constant-rate intravenous (IV) infusion *(gold),* plasma concentrations accumulate to steady state in four or five elimination half-lives. When a loading bolus is administered with the maintenance infusion *(blue),* plasma concentrations are transiently higher but may dip, as shown here, before achieving the same steady state. When the same drug is administered by the oral route, the time course of drug accumulation is identical *(magenta)*; in this case the drug was administered at intervals of 50% of a $t_{1/2}$. Steady-state plasma concentrations during oral therapy fluctuate around the mean determined by IV therapy. *Right,* This plot shows that when dosages are doubled, or halved, or the drug is stopped during steady-state administration, the time required to achieve the new steady state is four or five half-lives and is independent of the route of administration.

TABLE 9.2 Examples of Common Single Nucleotide Polymorphisms Mediating Variable Drug Actions

DRUG EFFECT	PATHWAY	GENE	SNP*	DBSNP ID NUMBER	COMMENTS
Adverse outcomes during clopidogrel treatment for acute coronary syndrome	PK	CYP2C19	CYP2C19*2, CYP2C19*3: loss-of-function (LOF) variants CYP2C19*17	rs4244285	*2 and *3 result in defective clopidogrel bioactivation and decreased antiplatelet activity. About 3% of European- and 15% of Asian-ancestry individuals carry two LOF alleles. *17 increases CYP2C19 activity and has been associated with increased bleeding during clopidogrel.
Excess beta blocker effect: metoprolol, timolol	PK	CYP2D6	Many variants		
Warfarin steady-state dose	PK	CYP2C9	CYP2C9*2, *3 (European ancestry); *5, *6, *8 (African ancestry)	rs1799853 rs1057910	VKORC1 and CYP2C9 variants account for ~50% of variability in warfarin steady-state dose. VKORC1 promoter variant frequency varies by ancestry. Bleeding risk has been associated with CYP2C9*3 and variant CYP4F2.
	PD	VKORC1	Promoter variant: −1639G>A	rs9923231	
	PD	CYP4F2	V433M	rs2108622	
Statin myotoxicity	PK	SLCO1B1	SLCO1B1*5: V174A	rs4149056	Risk of simvastatin myotoxicity is increased 20-fold in homozygotes and 4-fold in heterozygotes.
Response to beta blockers for hypertension, heart failure	PD (target)	ADRB1	S49G	rs1801252	
		ADRB2	R389G	rs1801253	
Beta blocker therapy in heart failure	PD (target)	GRK5	G41L	rs17098707	
Torsades de pointes	PD	KCNE1	D85N	rs1805128	8% allele frequency in patients with torsades versus ~2% in control subjects (odds ratio ~10)

dbSNP, National Center for Biotechnology Information's SNP database; *PD,* pharmacodynamic; *PK,* pharmacokinetic; *SNP,* single nucleotide polymorphism.
*Trivial name (e.g., *2, *3) and amino acid change provided.

polymorphisms in calcium channel genes, or an investigator interested in blood pressure might invoke variation in the ACE gene. The association between polymorphisms in these candidate genes and the phenotype under study is then examined in persons with well-characterized phenotypes. The candidate gene approach is intuitively appealing because it takes advantage of what is known about underlying physiology. Despite this appeal, however, the method is now recognized to carry with it the great potential for false-positive associations, especially when small numbers of participants are studied. An important exception has been in pharmacogenomics, where the candidate gene approach has yielded important and clinically reproducible associations between single common polymorphisms and drug response. This exception probably reflects the unusually high contribution of SNPs to overall variability in drug response previously mentioned.

Unbiased Approaches, Such as Genome-Wide Association. Another approach to identifying polymorphisms contributing to variable human traits is the genome-wide association study (GWAS). Here, study participants are genotyped at hundreds of thousands or millions of sites known to harbor common SNPs across the genome. Because the GWAS platforms focus on common SNPs, effect sizes for individual SNPs are often small and difficult to identify and validate unless large numbers of participants, thousands or more, are studied. In addition, the SNPs associated with the trait usually are not themselves functional but rather serve as markers for loci that harbor truly functional variants. The great advantage of the method is that it is unbiased, in that it makes no assumptions about underlying physiology, and one of its major accomplishments has been to identify entirely new pathways underlying variability in human traits.[11] The GWAS approach has been applied to study drug response phenotypes,[12] and even in relatively small sets, it has occasionally been successful in identifying associated common variants. Sometimes these are known from candidate gene studies. In other cases, notably drug hypersensitivity reactions,[13] GWASs in relatively small numbers (tens or hundreds of patients) have identified very strong signals that have then been replicated. More recently, methods have been developed to combine multiple trait-associated SNPs into a single polygenic risk score, and these scores are showing promise in identifying patients at risk for disease and their potential to identify patients at risk for unusual drug responses is being investigated.[14,15]

The GWAS paradigm is enabled by technology to generate the dense genotype datasets. New technologies being developed to generate other types of high-dimensional data similarly hold the promise of elucidating new biologic pathways in disease and drug response. Rapid, extremely high-throughput and increasingly inexpensive sequencing technologies are detecting rare DNA sequence variants whose contribution to disease or drug response is only now being appreciated.[7] RNA sequencing ("RNA-Seq") has replaced microarray analysis as the method of choice for cataloging RNA transcript profiles and abundance by specific cellular subtype and disease, and the extension of this technique to single cells is providing important new insights into our view of common and rare diseases. Advances in mass spectrometry are similarly enabling development of catalogs (proteomic and metabolomic profiling) of all proteins or of small-molecule metabolites of cellular processes, including drug metabolites, by cell and disease. Other sources of high-dimensional data include electronic health record (EHR) systems, as discussed later, and high-density digital images. Integrating these diverse data types into a comprehensive picture of the perturbations that result in disease or variable drug responses is the goal of the evolving discipline of *systems* biology and pharmacology. It has been proposed that future drug development would be better served by a focus on pathways identified by systems approaches rather than single targets.[16]

MOLECULAR AND GENETIC BASIS FOR VARIABLE DRUG RESPONSE

Many factors contribute to variable drug responses, including the patient's age, severity of the disease being treated, presence of disease of excretory organs, drug interactions, and poor compliance. This section describes major pathways leading to variable drug responses.

High-Risk Pharmacokinetics

When a drug is metabolized and excreted by multiple pathways, absence of one of these pathways, because of genetic variants, drug interactions, or dysfunction of excretory organs, generally does not affect drug concentrations or actions. By contrast, if a single pathway plays a critical role, the drug is more likely to exhibit marked variability in plasma concentration and associated effects, a situation that has been termed *high-risk pharmacokinetics* (Fig. 9.4).

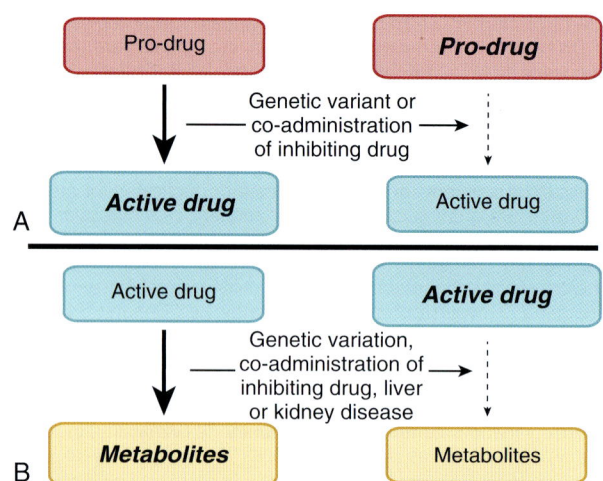

FIGURE 9.4 Two high-risk pharmacokinetic scenarios. **A,** Pro-drug activated by a single drug-metabolizing pathway. In this case, loss of function genetic variants or co-administration of a drug that inhibits the pathway will lead to failure of bioactivation and loss of drug effect. **B,** Active drug metabolized by a single pathway. In this case, loss of function genetic variants, co-administration of a drug that inhibits the pathway, or the presence of liver or kidney disease can inhibit drug elimination and thus lead to exaggerated drug action. This occurs because clinically important alternate pathways for drug elimination are absent, and increases in plasma parent drug concentrations can translate into serious drug toxicity. Note also that gain-of-function genetic variants or co-administered drugs that increase the rate of elimination will lead to decreased drug action. The overall effect is also modulated by the activity of the metabolites.

One high-risk scenario (Fig. 9.4A) involves bioactivation of a drug—that is, metabolism of the drug to active and potent metabolites that mediate pharmacologic action. Decreased function of such a pathway reduces or eliminates drug effect. Bioactivation of clopidogrel by CYP2C19 is an example; persons with reduced CYP2C19 activity (caused by genetic variants or possibly by interacting drugs; see Tables 9.1 and 9.2) have an increased incidence of cardiovascular events following coronary stent placement.[17] Similarly, the widely used analgesic codeine undergoes CYP2D6-mediated bioactivation to an active metabolite, morphine, and patients with reduced CYP2D6 activity ("poor metabolizers" [PMs]) display reduced analgesia. A small group of individuals with multiple functional copies of *CYP2D6*, and thus increased enzymatic activity ("ultrarapid metabolizers" [UMs]), has been identified; in this group, codeine may produce respiratory depression because of rapid morphine generation. In 2013 the U.S. Food and Drug Administration (FDA) label for codeine was revised to contraindicate its use in children after tonsillectomy, because deaths in UMs had been reported. A third example is the angiotensin receptor blocker losartan, which is bioactivated by CYP2C9; reduced antihypertensive effect is a risk with common genetic variants that reduce CYP2C9 activity or with co-administration of CYP2C9 inhibitors such as phenytoin.

In a second high-risk pharmacokinetic scenario (Fig. 9.4B), a drug is eliminated by only a single pathway. In this case, absence of activity of that pathway will lead to marked accumulation of drug in plasma, and for many drugs, such accumulation results in a high risk of drug toxicity. A simple example is the dependence of sotalol or dofetilide elimination on renal function; failure to decrease the dosage in a patient with renal dysfunction leads to accumulation of these drugs in plasma and an increased risk for drug-induced QT prolongation and torsades de pointes. Similarly, administration of a wide range of P-glycoprotein inhibitors will predictably elevate plasma concentration of digoxin, which is eliminated primarily by P-glycoprotein–mediated efflux into bile and urine (see Table 9.2). Propafenone is metabolized by CYP2D6 to a metabolite that has some sodium channel–blocking actions but lacks the weak beta-blocking effect of the parent drug. Administration of propafenone to PMs, or co-administration of CYP2D6 inhibitors (e.g., some SSRI antidepressants) to EMs, can lead to parent drug accumulation, bradycardia, and bronchospasm.

Other Important Pharmacogenetic Effects

Administration of CYP2D6-metabolized beta blockers, including metoprolol and carvedilol, to patients with defective enzyme activity may produce exaggerated heart rate slowing. Some antidepressants are CYP2D6 substrates; for these drugs, cardiovascular adverse effects are more common in CYP2D6 PMs, whereas therapeutic efficacy is more difficult to achieve in UMs.

The risk of aberrant drug responses caused by CYP variants is greatest in persons who are homozygous (i.e., PMs). However, for drugs with very narrow therapeutic margins (e.g., warfarin, clopidogrel), even heterozygotes may display unusual drug sensitivity. Although PMs make up a minority of persons in most populations, many drugs in common use can inhibit these enzymes and thereby "phenocopy" the PM trait. Omeprazole blocks CYP2C19 and in some studies has been associated with an increase in cardiovascular events during clopidogrel therapy; however, this effect is controversial and may not extend to other proton pump inhibitors.[18] Similarly, specific inhibitors of CYP2D6 and CYP2C9 can phenocopy the PM trait when co-administered with substrate drugs (Table 9.3).

TABLE 9.3 Drug Interactions: Mechanisms and Examples

MECHANISM	DRUG	INTERACTING DRUG	EFFECT
Decreased bioavailability	Digoxin	Antacids	Decreased digoxin effect secondary to decreased absorption
Increased bioavailability	Digoxin	Antibiotics	By eliminating gut flora that metabolize digoxin, some antibiotics may increase digoxin bioavailability. NOTE: Some antibiotics also interfere with P-glycoprotein (expressed in the intestine and elsewhere), another effect that can elevate digoxin concentration.
Induction of hepatic metabolism	CYP3A/P-glycoprotein substrates: Quinidine, Mexiletine, Verapamil, Cyclosporine, Apixaban, Rivaroxaban	Phenytoin, Rifampin, Barbiturates, St. John's wort	Loss of drug effect secondary to increased metabolism
Inhibition of hepatic metabolism	CYP2C9: Warfarin, Losartan	Amiodarone	Decreased warfarin requirement
		Phenytoin	Diminished conversion of losartan to its active metabolite, with decreased antihypertensive control
	CYP3A substrates: Quinidine, Cyclosporine, HMG-CoA reductase inhibitors: lovastatin, simvastatin, atorvastatin; not pravastatin, Apixaban, Rivaroxaban	Ketoconazole, Itraconazole, Erythromycin, Clarithromycin, Some calcium blockers, Some HIV protease inhibitors (especially ritonavir)	Increased risk for drug toxicity
	CYP2D6 substrates: Beta blockers (see Table 9.2), Propafenone, Desipramine, Codeine	Quinidine (even ultralow dose), fluoxetine, paroxetine	Increased beta blockade; Increased adverse effects; Decreased analgesia (due to failure of biotransformation to active metabolite morphine)
	CYP2C19: Clopidogrel	Omeprazole, possibly other proton pump inhibitors	Decreased clopidogrel efficacy
Inhibition of drug transport	P-glycoprotein transport: Digoxin, dabigatran	Amiodarone, quinidine, verapamil, cyclosporine, itraconazole, erythromycin, dronedarone	Increased digoxin or dabigatran plasma concentrations, with toxicity
	Renal tubular transport: Dofetilide	Verapamil	Slightly increased plasma concentration and QT effect
	Monoamine transport: Guanadrel	Tricyclic antidepressants	Blunted antihypertensive effects
Pharmacodynamic interactions	Aspirin + warfarin		Increased therapeutic antithrombotic effect; increased risk of bleeding
	Nonsteroidal anti-inflammatory drugs	Warfarin	Increased risk of gastrointestinal bleeding
	Antihypertensive drugs	Nonsteroidal anti-inflammatory drugs	Loss of blood pressure lowering
	QT-prolonging antiarrhythmics	Diuretics	Increased torsades de pointes risk secondary to diuretic-induced hypokalemia
	Supplemental potassium and/or spironolactone	ACE inhibitors	Hyperkalemia
	Sildenafil	Nitrates	Increased and persistent vasodilation; risk of myocardial ischemia

ACE, Angiotensin-converting enzyme; *HIV,* human immunodeficiency virus; *HMG-CoA,* 3-hydroxy-3-methylglutaryl–coenzyme A.

The widely used antirejection drug tacrolimus is bioinactivated by CYP3A5. A variant common in persons of European ancestry reduces enzyme activity. This variant is rare in patients of African ancestry, who therefore often require higher doses to avoid transplant rejection.[19]

A common nonsynonymous SNP in *SLCO1B1* has been associated with increased risk for simvastatin-induced myopathy by candidate studies with variability in simvastatin pharmacokinetics and by GWAS.[20]

The heart rate slowing and blood pressure effects of beta blockers and beta agonists have been associated with polymorphisms in the *drug targets*, the beta$_1$ and beta$_2$ receptors. A common variant in *ADRB1*, encoding the beta$_1$ receptor, has been implicated as a mediator of survival and prevention of atrial fibrillation[21] during therapy with the beta blocker bucindolol in heart failure. Variability in warfarin dose requirements has been clearly associated with variants in both *CYP2C9*, which mediates elimination of the active enantiomer of the drug, and *VKORC1*, part of the vitamin K complex that is the drug target. Indeed, these common variants account for up to half of the variability in warfarin dose requirement, illustrating the large impact that common SNPs can exert on drug response phenotypes. Furthermore, allele frequencies vary strikingly by ancestry, probably accounting for warfarin dose requirements being low in Asian patients and high in African patients compared with white patients.[22] Rosuvastatin plasma concentrations are higher in East Asian subjects, and variants in multiple genes have been implicated; as a result, lower doses are suggested.

Torsades de pointes during QT-prolonging drug therapy has been linked to polymorphisms not only in the ion channel that is the target for most QT-prolonging drugs (Kv11.1, encoded by *KCNH2*, also known as *HERG*) but also to other ion channel genes. A large candidate gene survey reported that a nonsynonymous SNP in *KCNE1*, a subunit for the slowly activating potassium current I_{Ks}, conferred an odds ratio of approximately 10 for torsades risk. In addition, in approximately 20% of cases, this ADR occurs in patients with clinically latent congenital long-QT syndrome, emphasizing the interrelationship among disease, genetic background, and drug therapy. Interestingly, a polygenic risk score constructed from a GWAS of baseline QT intervals was able to separate patients with drug-induced torsades de pointes and those tolerating QT-prolonging drugs.[14] Similarly, sodium channel–blocking drugs also can bring out latent Brugada syndrome. Patients with congenital long-QT syndrome or Brugada syndrome and their practitioners should be aware of websites that list potentially dangerous drugs (www.crediblemeds.org for long QT; www.brugadadrugs.org for Brugada syndrome).

The anticancer drug trastuzumab is effective only in patients with cancers that do not express the Her2/neu receptor. Because the drug also potentiates anthracycline-related cardiotoxicity, toxic therapy can be avoided in patients who are receptor negative (see also Chapters 56 and 57). More recently, rare truncating SNPs in titin, implicated in dilated cardiomyopathy, have also been associated with chemotherapy-induced cardiomyopathy.[23] Indeed, anticancer drugs and in particular newer "targeted" agents are increasingly recognized to cause diverse cardiovascular ADRs, including arterial and venous thrombosis, cardiomyopathy, myocarditis, and arrhythmias. Understanding the pathways leading to these effects could inform new approaches to prevent and treat cardiovascular disease more broadly.[24]

OPTIMIZING DRUG DOSES

The goals of drug therapy should be defined before the initiation of drug treatment. These may include acute correction of serious pathophysiology, acute or chronic symptom relief, or changes in surrogate endpoints (e.g., blood pressure, serum cholesterol, INR) that have been linked to beneficial outcomes in target patient populations. However, the lessons of CAST and of positive inotropic drugs should make prescribers skeptical about such surrogate-guided therapy in the absence of controlled clinical trials.

When the goal of drug therapy is to correct acutely a disturbance in physiology, the drug should be administered intravenously in doses designed to achieve a therapeutic effect rapidly. This approach is best justified when benefits clearly outweigh risks. Large boluses of IV drugs carry a risk of enhancing drug-related toxicity; therefore, even with the most urgent medical indication, this approach is rarely appropriate. An exception is adenosine, which must be administered as a rapidly delivered bolus because it undergoes extensive and rapid elimination from plasma by uptake into almost all cells. As a consequence, a slow bolus or infusion rarely achieves sufficiently high concentrations at the desired site of action (the coronary artery perfusing the atrioventricular node) to terminate arrhythmias. Similarly, the time course of anesthesia depends on anesthetic drug delivery to and removal from sites in the central nervous system.

The time required to achieve steady-state plasma concentrations is determined by the elimination half-life (see earlier). The administration of a loading dose may shorten this time, but only if the kinetics of distribution and elimination are known beforehand in an individual patient and the correct loading regimen is chosen. Otherwise, overshoot or undershoot during the loading phase may occur (see Fig. 9.3). Thus the initiation of drug therapy by a loading strategy should be used only when the indication is acute.

Two dose-response curves describe the relationship between drug dose and the expected cumulative incidence of a beneficial effect or an ADR (Fig. 9.5). The distance along the x axis describing the difference between these curves, often termed the *therapeutic ratio* (or index, or window), provides an index of the likelihood that a chronic dosing regimen that provides benefits without ADRs can be identified. Drugs with especially wide therapeutic indices often can be administered at infrequent intervals, even if they are rapidly eliminated (Fig. 9.5A,C).

When anticipated ADRs are serious, the most appropriate treatment strategy is to start at low doses and reevaluate the necessity for increasing drug dosages once steady-state drug effects have been achieved. This approach has the advantage of minimizing the risk of dose-related ADRs but carries with it a need to titrate doses to efficacy. Only when stable drug effects are achieved should increasing drug dosage to achieve the desired therapeutic effect be considered. An example is sotalol: because the risk of torsades de pointes increases with drug dosage, the starting dose should be low.

In other cases, anticipated toxicity is relatively mild and manageable. It may then be acceptable to start at dosages higher than the minimum required to achieve a therapeutic effect, accepting a greater-than-minimal risk of ADRs; some antihypertensives can be administered in this way. However, the principle of using the lowest dose possible to minimize toxicity, particularly toxicity that is unpredictable and unrelated to recognized pharmacologic actions, should be the rule.

Occasionally, dose escalation into the high therapeutic range results in no beneficial drug effect and no side effects. In this circumstance the prescriber should be alert to the possibility of noncompliance or drug interactions at the pharmacokinetic or pharmacodynamic level. Depending on the nature of the anticipated toxicity, dose escalation beyond the usual therapeutic range may occasionally be acceptable but only if anticipated toxicity is not serious and is readily manageable.

Plasma Concentration Monitoring

For some drugs, curves such as those shown in Figure 9.5A and B, relating drug concentration to cumulative incidence of beneficial and adverse effects, can be generated. With such drugs, monitoring plasma drug concentrations to ensure that they remain within a desired therapeutic range (i.e., greater than a minimum required for efficacy and less than a maximum likely to produce ADRs) may be a useful adjunct to therapy. Monitoring drug concentrations also may be useful to ensure compliance and to detect pharmacokinetically based drug interactions that underlie unanticipated efficacy and/or toxicity at usual dosages. Samples for measurement of plasma concentrations generally should be obtained just before the next dose, at steady state. These trough concentrations provide an index of the minimum plasma concentration expected during a dosing interval.

On the other hand, patient monitoring, whether by plasma concentration or other physiologic indices, to detect incipient toxicity is best accomplished at the time of anticipated peak drug concentrations.

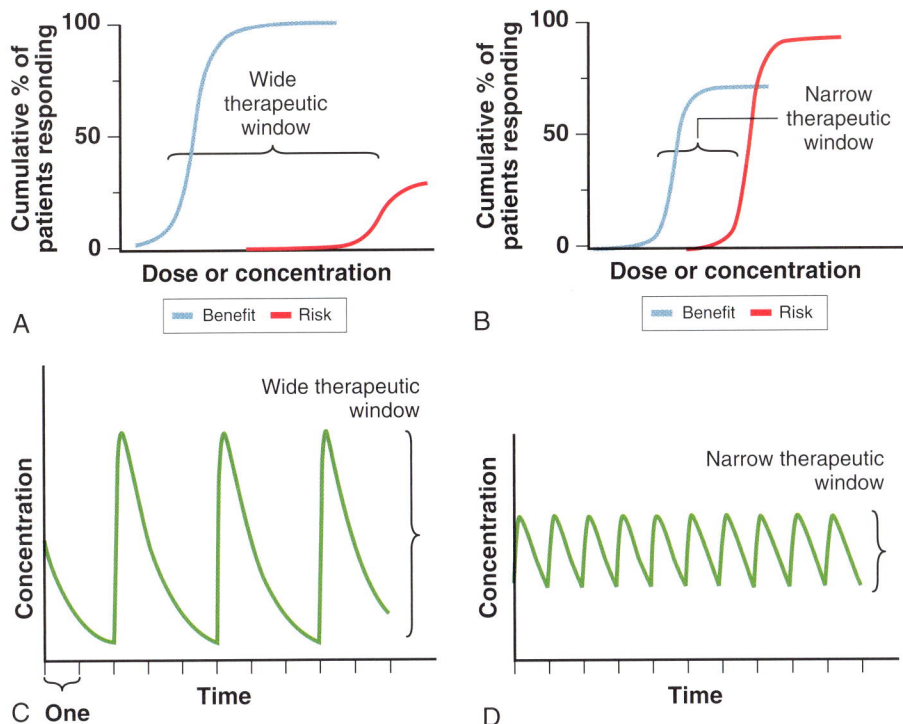

FIGURE 9.5 The concept of therapeutic ratio. **A** and **B**, Two dose-response (or concentration-response) curves. The *blue* lines describe the relationship between dose and cumulative incidence of beneficial effects, and the *magenta* lines depict the relationship between dose and dose-related adverse effects (risk). **A**, A drug with a wide therapeutic ratio displays separation between the two curves, a high degree of efficacy, and low degree of dose-related toxicity. Under these conditions, a wide therapeutic ratio can be defined. **B**, Conversely, the curves describing cumulative efficacy and cumulative incidence of adverse effects are positioned near each other, the incidence of adverse effects is higher, and the expected beneficial response is lower. These characteristics define a narrow therapeutic ratio. **C** and **D**, Steady-state plasma concentrations with oral drug administration as a function of time with wide *(left)* and narrow *(right)* therapeutic ratios. The *hash marks* on the abscissae each indicate one elimination half-life ($t_{1/2}$). **C**, When the therapeutic window is wide, drug administration every three elimination half-lives can produce plasma concentrations that are maintained above the minimum for efficacy and below the maximum beyond which toxicity is anticipated. **D**, The opposite situation is illustrated. To maintain plasma concentrations within the narrow therapeutic range, the drug must be administered more frequently.

Thus patient surveillance for QT prolongation during therapy with sotalol or dofetilide is best timed for 1 to 2 hours after the administration of a dose of drug at a steady state.

A lag between the time courses of drug in plasma and drug effects may exist (see earlier). In addition, monitoring plasma drug concentrations relies on the assumption that the concentration measured is in equilibrium with that at the target molecular site. Of note, it is only the fraction of drug not bound to plasma proteins that is available to achieve such equilibration. Variability in the extent of protein binding can therefore affect the free fraction and anticipated drug effect, even in the presence of apparently therapeutic total plasma drug concentrations.

Dose Adjustments in Disease

Polypharmacy is common in patients with varying degrees of specific organ dysfunction. Although treatment with an individual agent may be justified, the practitioner should also recognize the risk of unanticipated drug effects and interactions, particularly drug toxicity, during therapy with multiple drugs.

The presence of renal disease mandates dose reductions (or choosing alternate therapies if renal dysfunction is severe) for drugs eliminated primarily by renal excretion. Examples include dabigatran, rivaroxaban, edoxaban, digoxin, dofetilide, and sotalol. Apixaban can be used even in patients undergoing dialysis, with reduced doses in certain subgroups (e.g., older patients, those weighing <60 kg). A requirement for dose adjustment in cases of mild renal dysfunction is dictated by available clinical data and the likelihood of serious toxicity if drug accumulates in plasma because of impaired elimination. Renal failure reduces the protein binding of some drugs (e.g., phenytoin); in this case a total drug concentration value in the therapeutic range may actually represent a toxic value of unbound drug.

Advanced liver disease is characterized by decreased hepatic drug metabolism and portacaval shunts that decrease clearance, particularly first-pass clearance. Moreover, affected patients frequently have other profound disturbances of homeostasis, such as coagulopathy, severe ascites, and altered mental status. These pathophysiologic features of advanced liver disease can affect not only the dose of a drug required to achieve a potentially therapeutic effect but also the perception of risks and benefits, thereby altering the prescriber's assessment of the actual need for therapy.

Heart disease is similarly associated with several disturbances of drug elimination and drug sensitivity that may alter the therapeutic doses or the practitioner's perception of the desirability of therapy based on evaluation of risks and benefits. Patients with left ventricular hypertrophy often have baseline QT prolongation, so risks associated with use of QT-prolonging antiarrhythmics may increase; most guidelines suggest avoiding QT-prolonging antiarrhythmics in such patients (see Chapters 67 and 99).

In heart failure (see Chapter 50), hepatic congestion can lead to decreased clearance with a corresponding increased risk for toxicity with usual doses of certain drugs, including some sedatives, lidocaine, and beta blockers. On the other hand, gut congestion can lead to decreased absorption of oral drugs and decreased effects. In addition, patients with heart failure may demonstrate reduced renal perfusion and require dose adjustments on this basis. Heart failure also is characterized by a redistribution of regional blood flow, which can lead to reduced volume of distribution and enhanced risk for drug toxicity. Lidocaine probably is the best-studied example; loading doses of lidocaine should be reduced in patients with heart failure, because of altered distribution, whereas maintenance doses should be reduced in both heart failure and liver disease, because of altered clearance.

Age also is a major factor in determining drug doses, as well as sensitivity to drug effects. Doses in children generally are administered on an mg/kg body weight basis, although firm data to guide therapy are often not available. Variable postnatal maturation of drug disposition systems may present a special problem in the neonate. Older persons often have reduced creatinine clearance, even those with a normal serum creatinine level, and dosages of renally excreted drugs should be adjusted accordingly (see Chapters 90 and 101). Diastolic dysfunction with hepatic congestion is more common in older adults, and vascular disease and dementia often occur, which can lead to increased postural hypotension and risk of falling. Therapies such as sedatives, tricyclic antidepressants, or anticoagulants should be initiated only when the practitioner is convinced that the benefits of such therapies outweigh this increased risk.

Drug Interactions

As a result of therapeutic successes not only in heart disease but also in other disease areas, cardiovascular physicians are increasingly encountering patients receiving multiple medications for cardiovascular and noncardiovascular indications. Table 9.3 summarizes mechanisms that may underlie important drug interactions. Drug interactions may be based on altered absorption, distribution, metabolism, or excretion. In addition, drugs can interact at the pharmacodynamic level. A trivial example is the co-administration of two antihypertensive drugs, leading to excessive hypotension. Similarly, co-administration of platelet inhibitors and anticoagulants leads to an increased risk for bleeding, although benefits of such combinations also can be demonstrated.

The most important principle in approaching a patient receiving polypharmacy is to recognize the high potential for drug interactions. A complete medication history should be obtained from each patient at regular intervals; patients will often omit topical medications such as eye drops, health food supplements, and medications prescribed by other practitioners unless specifically prompted. Each of these, however, carries a risk of important systemic drug actions and interactions. Even high dosages of grapefruit juice, which contains CYP3A and P-glycoprotein inhibitors, can affect drug responses. Beta blocker eye drops can produce systemic beta blockade, particularly with CYP2D6 substrates (e.g., timolol) in patients with defective CYP2D6 activity. St. John's wort induces CYP3A and P-glycoprotein activity (similar to phenytoin and other drugs) and thus can greatly lower plasma concentrations of substrate drugs such as cyclosporine. As with many other interactions, this may not be a special problem provided both drugs are continued. However, if a patient stabilized on cyclosporine stops taking a concomitantly administered CYP3A inducer, plasma concentrations of the drug can rise dramatically, and toxicity can ensue. Similarly, initiation of an inducer may lead to greatly lowered cyclosporine concentrations and a risk of organ rejection. A number of natural supplements have been associated with serious drug toxicity (e.g., phenylpropanolamine-associated stroke) that has resulted in their withdrawal from the market.

Incorporating Pharmacogenetic Information into Prescribing

The identification of polymorphisms associated with variable drug responses naturally raises the question of how these data could or should be used to optimize drug doses, avoid drugs likely to be ineffective, and avoid drugs likely to produce major toxicities. Indeed, in 2007 the FDA began systematically including pharmacogenetic information in drug labels,[25] and the Clinical Pharmacogenetics Implementation Consortium (CPIC) provides in-depth reviews of the effects of specific genetic variants on drug responses.[26] Despite the intuitive appeal of a pharmacogenetically guided approach to drug therapy, however, practitioners wanting to adopt genetic testing to guide drug therapy encounter substantial practical barriers, including reimbursement and cost, varying levels of evidence supporting a role for genetics, and implementation issues such as how fast and accurately a genetic test result can be delivered. The nature of pharmacogenetic variation is that most patients will display average responses to most drugs, so systematically testing every patient in the hopes of finding the minority likely to display aberrant responses is cumbersome and seems inefficient in terms of time and cost unless the benefit for individual patients is large.[22] An example of a large benefit is that routine genotyping of all patients receiving the antiretroviral agent abacavir is now the standard of care because it avoids a potentially life-threatening skin reaction in 3% of patients. By contrast, RCTs suggest either no effect or a modest effect on time within therapeutic range when genotype information is incorporated into warfarin dosing.[22,27,28] Many of these trials were underpowered to examine bleeding risk, which has been associated with variants in *CYP4F2* or *CYP2C9* in population- or EHR-based studies.[22] Two large RCTs have compared thrombosis and bleeding risk with clopidogrel versus other platelet inhibitors (ticagrelor, prasugrel): one showed a significant benefit of using clopidogrel in patients who do not carry *CYP2C19* loss-of-function varaints,[29,30] whereas the other (not yet reported in full) trended to such a benefit but did not achieve its targeted endpoint.[31]

A difficulty with such drug-specific approaches is that the benefit of the genotype data must be large to justify the cumbersomeness and cost of testing all exposed individuals. Although the probability is small that genetic variation plays an important role in predicting the response of an individual patient to a specific drug, when many drugs are prescribed for a population of patients, each patient will display genetically determined aberrant responses to some drugs. This reasoning underlies the concept of *preemptive genotyping*, in which many genetic variants relevant to many variable drug responses are assayed in patients who have not yet been exposed to the drugs.[32,33] These data are then stored in EHR systems with advanced point-of-care decision support capabilities that deliver instantaneous advice when a drug is prescribed to a patient with known genomic variants.[34] Several technologic developments enable this vision, including advanced EHRs and multiplexed inexpensive genotyping assays or sequencing that interrogate many polymorphisms for the same cost as a handful relevant to one drug. The concept is now being tested at a few medical centers, with the goals of establishing cost and benefit, understanding how health care providers react, and optimizing decision support to integrate pharmacogenomic information seamlessly into health care.[22,34,35]

FUTURE PERSPECTIVES

The past 25 years have seen dramatic advances in the treatment of heart disease, in no small part because of the development of highly effective and well-tolerated drug therapies such as HMG-CoA reductase inhibitors, ACE inhibitors, and beta blockers. These developments, along with improved nonpharmacologic approaches, have led to dramatically enhanced survival of patients with advanced heart disease. Thus polypharmacy in an aging and chronically ill population is becoming increasingly common. In this milieu, drug effects become increasingly variable, reflecting interactions among drugs, underlying disease and disease mechanisms, and genetic backgrounds. Furthermore, despite advances in the Western world, cardiovascular disease is emerging as an increasing problem worldwide as smoking and the metabolic syndrome are increasing. Understanding how genetic background plays into disease susceptibility and responses to drug therapy, concepts largely tested in only European-ancestry populations to date, represents a major challenge in cardiovascular medicine.

More generally, genomic medicine—the application of genetic variant information in health care—is still in its infancy, so reported associations require independent confirmation and assessment of clinical importance and cost-effectiveness before they can or should enter clinical practice. Importantly, most pharmacogenomic studies reported to date have focused on common variants, and we now recognize that the vast majority of polymorphisms in any gene, including CYPs and other "pharmacogenes," are uncommon (MAF < 1%). Developing approaches to establish the clinical impact of such rare variants on drug responses, and a potential role for polygenic risk scores, is an emerging challenge.

This challenge is all the more acute because the cost of sequencing has fallen drastically since the completion of the first-draft human genome in 2000, and the less-than-$1000 whole-genome sequence is now a reality. This may be enabling for the preemptive pharmacogenomic strategy just outlined, as well as a broader vision of genome-guided health care, but presents major challenges in data storage and mining.

The relationship between the prescriber and the patient remains the centerpiece of modern therapeutics. An increasingly sophisticated molecular and genetic view of response to drug therapy should not change this view but rather complement it. Each initiation of drug therapy represents a new clinical experiment. Prescribers must always be vigilant regarding the possibility of unusual drug effects, which could provide clues about unanticipated and important mechanisms of beneficial and adverse drug effects.

REFERENCES

1. National Health Expenditure Data. 2020. https://www.cms.gov/research-statistics-data-and-systems/statistics-trends-and-reports/nationalhealthexpenddata/nationalhealthaccountshistorical.html.
2. Virani SS, Alonso A, Benjamin EJ, et al. Heart disease and stroke statistics-2020 update: a report from the American Heart Association. *Circulation*. 2020;141:e139–e596.
3. Bates DW, Slight SP. Medication errors: what is their impact? *Mayo Clin Proc*. 2014;89:1027–1029.
4. Sultana J, Cutroneo P, Trifirò G. Clinical and economic burden of adverse drug reactions. *J Pharmacol Pharmacother*. 2013;4:S73–S77.

Adverse Drug Reactions

5. Zaha VG, Meijers WC, Moslehi J. Cardio-immuno-oncology. *Circulation*. 2020;141:87–89.
6. Nguyen LS, Dolladille C, Drici MD, et al. Cardiovascular toxicities associated with hydroxychloroquine and azithromycin: an analysis of the World Health Organization Pharmacovigilance database. *Circulation*. 2020.

Pharmacogenomics

7. Stitziel NO, Kathiresan S. Leveraging human genetics to guide drug target discovery. *Trends Cardiovasc Med*. 2017;27:352–359.
8. Nelson MR, Tipney H, Painter JL, et al. The support of human genetic evidence for approved drug indications. *Nat Genet*. 2015;47:856–860.
9. Hoy SM. Elexacaftor/ivacaftor/tezacaftor: first approval. *Drugs*. 2019;79:2001–2007.
10. 2020. https://clinicaltrials.gov/ct2/show/results/NCT03442764.
11. Welter D, MacArthur J, Morales J, et al. The NHGRI GWAS Catalog, a curated resource of SNP-trait associations. *Nucleic Acids Res*. 2014;42:D1001–D1006.
12. Motsinger-Reif AA, Jorgenson E, Relling MV, et al. Genome-wide association studies in pharmacogenomics: successes and lessons. *Pharmacogenet Genomics*. 2013;23:383–394.
13. Osanlou O, Pirmohamed M, Daly AK. Pharmacogenetics of adverse drug reactions. *Adv Pharmacol*. 2018;83:155–190.
14. Strauss DG, Vicente J, Johannesen L, et al. Common genetic variant risk score is associated with drug-induced QT prolongation and torsade de Pointes risk: a pilot study. *Circulation*. 2017;135:1300–1310.
15. Lewis JP, Backman JD, Reny JL, et al. Pharmacogenomic polygenic response score predicts ischemic events and cardiovascular mortality in clopidogrel-treated patients. *Eur Heart J Cardiovas Pharmacother*. 2019;6(4):203–210.
16. MacRae CA, Roden DM, Loscalzo J. The future of cardiovascular therapeutics. *Circulation*. 2016;133:2610–2617.
17. Pereira NL, Rihal CS, So DYF, et al. Clopidogrel pharmacogenetics. *Circ Cardiovasc Interv*. 2019;12:e007811.
18. Serbin MA, Guzauskas GF, Veenstra DL. Clopidogrel-proton pump inhibitor drug-drug interaction and risk of adverse clinical outcomes among PCI-treated ACS patients: a meta-analysis. *J Manag Care Spec Pharm*. 2016;22:939–947.
19. Cascorbi I. The pharmacogenetics of immune-modulating therapy. *Adv Pharmacol*. 2018;83:275–296.
20. Bellosta S, Corsini A. Statin drug interactions and related adverse reactions: an update. *Expert Opin Drug Saf*. 2018;17:25–37.
21. Parikh KS, Piccini JP. Pharmacogenomics of bucindolol in atrial fibrillation and heart failure. *Curr Heart Fail Rep*. 2017;14:529–535.
22. Roden DM, McLeod HL, Relling MV, et al. Pharmacogenomics. *Lancet*. 2019;394:521–532.
23. Garcia-Pavia P, Kim Y, Restrepo-Cordoba MA, et al. Genetic variants associated with cancer therapy-induced cardiomyopathy. *Circulation*. 2019;140:31–41.
24. Moslehi JJ. Cardiovascular toxic effects of targeted cancer therapies. *N Engl J Med*. 2016;375:1457–1467.

Incorporating Pharmacogenetic Information into Prescribing

25. Drozda K, Pacanowski MA, Grimstein C, Zineh I. Pharmacogenetic labeling of FDA-approved drugs: a regulatory retrospective. *JACC Basic Transl Sci*. 2018;3:545–549.
26. Hoffman JM, Dunnenberger HM, Kevin Hicks J, et al. Developing knowledge resources to support precision medicine: principles from the Clinical Pharmacogenetics Implementation Consortium (CPIC). *J Am Med Inform Assoc*. 2016;23:796–801.
27. Belley-Cote EP, Hanif H, D'Aragon F, et al. Genotype-guided versus standard vitamin K antagonist dosing algorithms in patients initiating anticoagulation. A systematic review and meta-analysis. *Thromb Haemost*. 2015;114:768–777.
28. Gage BF, Bass AR, Lin H, et al. Effect of genotype-guided warfarin dosing on clinical events and anticoagulation control among patients undergoing hip or knee arthroplasty: the GIFT randomized clinical trial. *J Am Med Assoc*. 2017;318:1115–1124.
29. Claassens DMF, Vos GJA, Bergmeijer TO, et al. A genotype-guided strategy for oral P2Y12 inhibitors in primary PCI. *N Engl J Med*. 2019.
30. Roden DM. Clopidogrel pharmacogenetics—why the wait? *N Engl J Med*. 2019;381:1677–1678.
31. TAILOR-PCI: Genotype-guided Antiplatelet Therapy Post PCI Misses Mark. https://www.acc.org/latest-in-cardiology/articles/2020/03/24/16/41/sat-9am-tailor-pci-clinical-implementation-clopidogrel-pharmacogenetics-acc-2020.
32. O'Donnell PH, Danahey K, Ratain MJ. The outlier in all of us: why implementing pharmacogenomics could matter for everyone. *Clin Pharmacol Ther*. 2016;99:401–404.
33. Van Driest SL, Shi Y, Bowton EA, et al. Clinically actionable genotypes among 10,000 patients with preemptive pharmacogenomic testing. *Clin Pharmacol Ther*. 2014;95:423–431.
34. Peterson JF, Roden DM, Orlando LA, Ramirez AH, Mensah GA, Williams MS. Building evidence and measuring clinical outcomes for genomic medicine. *Lancet*. 2019;394:604–610.
35. Manolio TA, Rowley R, Williams MS, et al. Opportunities, resources, and techniques for implementing genomics in clinical care. *Lancet*. 2019;394:511–520.

10 Biomarkers and Use in Precision Medicine

PETER LIBBY AND PAUL M RIDKER

OVERVIEW OF BIOMARKERS, 102
Clinical Applications of Cardiovascular Biomarkers, 103
Novel Technologies in Biomarker Identification, 105

CLINICAL MEASURES OF BIOMARKER PERFORMANCE, 105
Sensitivity, Specificity, and Positive and Negative Predictive Value, 105
Discrimination, C-Statistics, and Receiver Operating Characteristic Curve, 106
Accuracy and Calibration, 106

Risk Reclassification, 106
External Validation and Impact Studies, 107
Practical Example: High-Sensitivity C-Reactive Protein, Lipids, and Reynolds Risk Score, 107

CONCLUSION, 107

REFERENCES, 107

Clinicians use biomarkers daily in the practice of cardiovascular medicine. Moreover, the use of biomarkers can continue to improve physicians' ability to provide clinically effective and cost-effective cardiovascular medicine in the years ahead. Appropriate risk stratification and targeting of therapies should not only help improve patient outcomes but also assist in responding to the urgent need to "bend the cost curve" of medical care. In particular, excessive use of imaging biomarkers increases the cost of medical care and can jeopardize patient outcomes (e.g., from radiation exposure or complications of administering contrast material or investigating incidental findings). Inappropriate use or interpretation of blood biomarkers (e.g., cardiac troponin levels) can lead to unnecessary hospitalization or procedures as well.

Despite the current usefulness of biomarkers, their future promise, and the critical need to use them appropriately, much misunderstanding still surrounds their current clinical application.[1] In addition, contemporary technologies can greatly expand the gamut of biomarkers relevant to cardiovascular practice. Emerging genetic, proteomic, metabolomic, and molecular imaging strategies will surely transform the landscape of cardiovascular biomarkers (see also Chapters 7, 8, and 25).

This chapter provides a primer on cardiovascular biomarkers by defining terms and discussing how the application of biomarkers can assist in clinical care. The literature abounds with descriptions of biomarkers offered to apply to various clinical situations. Advances in cardiovascular biology and the application of novel technologies have identified a plethora of novel cardiovascular biomarkers of potential clinical usefulness—begging the question of whether a novel biomarker adds value to existing and often better-validated biomarkers. Thus clinicians need tools to evaluate these emerging biomarkers, to discern which may actually elevate clinical practice and improve patient outcomes. To help the reader in this regard, we also provide a guide to the rigorous evaluation of the clinical utility of biomarkers. Chapter 8 explicates the application of proteomics and metabolomics to discover novel biomarkers.

OVERVIEW OF BIOMARKERS

For regulatory purposes, the U.S. Food and Drug Administration (FDA) first defined a *biomarker* in 1992 as "a laboratory measure or physical sign that is used in therapeutic trials as a substitute for a clinically meaningful end point that is a direct measure of how a patient feels, functions, or survives and is expected to predict the effect of the therapy." At that time the FDA considered a *surrogate endpoint* as "reasonably likely, based on epidemiologic, therapeutic, pathophysiologic, or other evidence, to predict clinical benefit." The National Institutes of Health (NIH) convened a working group in 1998 that offered some parallel operating definitions to guide the biomarker field (Table 10.1).[2] NIH defined a *biologic marker*, or biomarker, as "a characteristic that is objectively measured and evaluated as an indicator of normal biologic processes, pathogenic processes, or pharmacologic responses to a therapeutic intervention." Thus the NIH definition includes not only soluble biomarkers in circulating blood but also "bedside biomarkers," such as anthropomorphic variables obtainable with a blood pressure cuff or a tape measure at the point of care.

This broad definition encompasses measurements of biomarkers in blood (Fig. 10.1A) as well as measurements from imaging studies (Fig. 10.1B). Imaging biomarkers can include those derived from classic anatomic approaches. Imaging modalities now offer functional information, such as estimates of ventricular function and myocardial perfusion. Molecular imaging has the potential to target specific molecular processes. A functional classification of biomarkers helps sort through the plethora encountered by the clinician, in that biomarkers can reflect a variety of biologic processes or organs of origin. For example, as shown in Figure 10.1B, to a first approximation, cardiac troponin reflects myocardial injury, brain natriuretic peptide reflects cardiac chamber stretch, C-reactive protein reflects inflammation, and cystatin C and the estimated glomerular filtration rate reflect kidney function.

The NIH working group defined a *surrogate endpoint* as "a biomarker intended to substitute for a clinical endpoint. A surrogate endpoint is expected to predict clinical benefit (or harm) or lack of benefit (or harm) based on epidemiologic, therapeutic, pathophysiologic, or other scientific evidence." (Note that the NIH definitions do not include the commonly used term *surrogate marker*.) Thus a surrogate endpoint is a biomarker that has been "elevated" to surrogate status. This distinction has particular importance in the regulatory aspects of cardiovascular medicine. For example, the FDA previously accepted a certain degree of reduction in hemoglobin A_{1c} (HbA_{1c}) as a criterion for registration of a novel oral hypoglycemic agent; thus HbA_{1c} was considered a biomarker accepted as a surrogate endpoint. Current FDA guidance now requires a cardiovascular safety study for the registration of new medications that target diabetes. This policy indicates regulatory doubts about the fidelity of a decrease in HbA_{1c} as a surrogate endpoint for reduced cardiovascular risk, despite its value as a biomarker of glycemia.

The NIH working group defined a *clinical endpoint* as "a characteristic or variable that reflects how a patient feels, functions, or survives." Pivotal or phase III cardiovascular trials aspire to use clinical endpoints so defined. The distinction among biomarkers, surrogate endpoints, and clinical endpoints has crucial implications as practitioners, regulators, and payers increasingly demand evidence of improvements in actual clinical outcomes rather than mere manipulation of biomarkers as a criterion for adoption of a treatment in clinical practice.

In an effort to dispel persistent confusion regarding definitions in the biomarker arena, in 2015 a joint effort of the FDA and NIH developed an online resource denoted BEST (Biomarkers, EndpointS, and other Tools).[3] They formulated a living online resource that furnishes an extended glossary of terms to facilitate standardization (Table 10.2). The BEST definitions overlap with those of the NIH Workshop, but provide more detail of particular relevance to those interested in the regulatory aspects of biomarkers (Table 10.3).

Clinical Applications of Cardiovascular Biomarkers (see also Chapter 5)

Much of the prevailing confusion regarding biomarkers involves framing the question that the clinician wants to answer with the use of a biomarker (Fig. 10.1C). We can classify the goals of application of cardiovascular biomarkers into the following rubrics:

1. *Diagnosis.* Daily medical practice uses many biomarkers for cardiovascular diagnosis. The current universal definition of myocardial infarction, for example, requires elevation of a biomarker of myocyte injury, such as cardiac-specific isoforms of troponin.
2. *Risk stratification.* Familiar examples of biomarkers used in risk stratification in cardiovascular medicine include systolic blood pressure (SBP) and low-density lipoprotein cholesterol (LDL-C). These biomarkers reliably predict future risk for cardiovascular events on a population basis.
3. *Goals for therapy.* Contemporary guidelines often specify cutoff points for targets of treatment, for example, a specific level of a biomarker (e.g., SBP, LDL-C) in a particular group of individuals. Practitioners of cardiovascular medicine typically use the biomarker international normalized ratio (INR) to titrate the dosage of warfarin administered to an individual patient. Abundant data support the clinical benefit of maintaining the INR within a certain range in various patient groups, an example of a widely used biomarker that has proven clinical usefulness as a goal for therapy.
4. *Targeting of therapy.* In clinical practice, using biomarkers to target therapy has great usefulness and promise as we move toward a more comprehensive "personalized medicine" approach to practice. Examples of biomarkers used to target therapy include troponin measurements to triage patients with acute coronary syndromes for early invasive management and measurement of high-sensitivity C-reactive protein (hsCRP) to allocate statin treatment to individuals without elevated LDL-C.
5. *Drug development, evaluation, and registration.* Biomarkers have critical importance in the development of new pharmacologic agents. Biomarkers can provide early signals of efficacy that will help prioritize agents more likely to provide benefit on clinical endpoints in large-scale trials. Clinical trials not infrequently fail because of inappropriate dose selection. Judicious use of biomarkers can help in selecting an appropriate dose of an agent to study in a large endpoint trial. Biomarkers accepted as surrogate endpoints also prove useful to regulatory agencies in granting approval for novel therapies.

Clinical use of cardiovascular biomarkers requires a clear understanding of *how* they should be used. Many biomarkers provide

TABLE 10.1 Biomarker Definitions (NIH Working Group)

Biologic marker (biomarker) A characteristic that is objectively measured and evaluated as an indicator of normal biologic processes, pathogenic processes, or pharmacologic responses to a therapeutic intervention.

Surrogate endpoint A biomarker intended to substitute for a clinical endpoint. A surrogate endpoint is expected to predict clinical benefit (or harm) or lack of benefit (or harm) based on epidemiologic, therapeutic, pathophysiologic, or other scientific evidence.

Clinical endpoint A characteristic or variable that reflects how a patient feels, functions, or survives.

From National Institutes of Health (NIH) Biomarkers Definition Working Group, 1998.

TABLE 10.2 Biomarker Categories According to the FDA-NIH BEST Resource

Diagnostic biomarker
Monitoring biomarker
Pharmacodynamic/response biomarker
Predictive biomarker
Prognostic biomarker
Reasonably likely surrogate endpoint
Safety biomarker
Susceptibility/risk biomarker
Understanding prognostic versus predictive biomarkers
Validated surrogate endpoint

From the BEST (Biomarkers, EndpointS, and other Tools) Online Resource https://pubmed.ncbi.nlm.nih.gov/27010052/

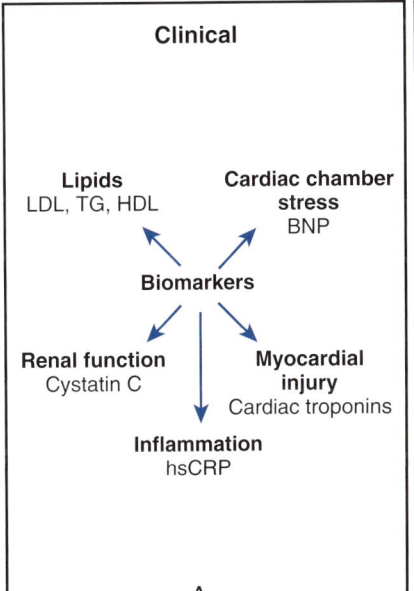
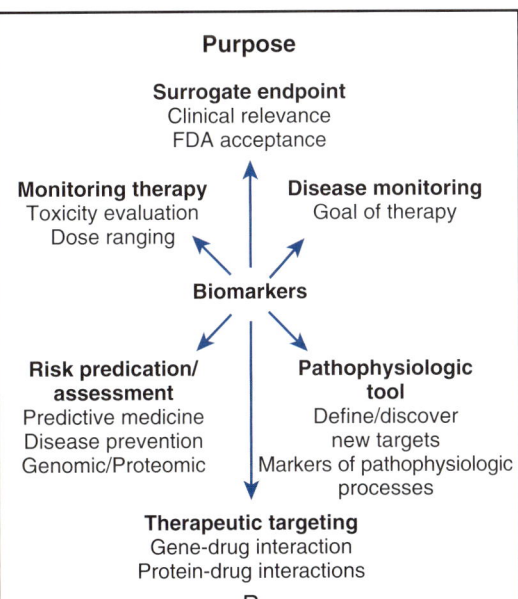
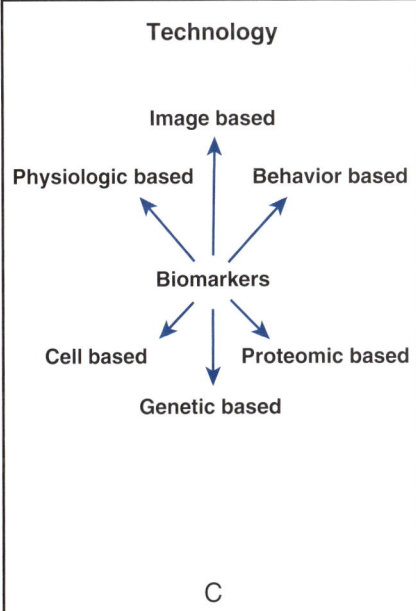

FIGURE 10.1 Examples of commonly used clinical biomarkers for cardiovascular disease **(A)**, as well as research-oriented biomarkers categorized according to purpose **(B)** and technology **(C)**. *BNP*, Brain natriuretic peptide; *hsCRP*, high-sensitivity C-reactive protein; *TG*, triglyceride.

TABLE 10.3 Selected Biomarker Definitions from the BEST Glossary

Biologic marker (biomarker): A defined characteristic that is measured as an indicator of normal biological processes, pathogenic processes, or responses to an exposure or intervention, including therapeutic interventions. Molecular, histologic, radiographic, or physiologic characteristics are types of biomarkers. A biomarker is not an assessment of how an individual feels, functions, or survives.

Surrogate endpoint: An endpoint that is used in clinical trials as a substitute for a direct measure of how a patient feels, functions, or survives. A surrogate endpoint does not measure the clinical benefit of primary interest in and of itself, but rather is expected to predict that clinical benefit or harm based on epidemiologic, therapeutic, pathophysiologic, or other scientific evidence. From a U.S. regulatory standpoint, surrogate endpoints and potential surrogate endpoints can be characterized by the level of clinical validation: validated surrogate endpoint, reasonably likely surrogate endpoint, candidate surrogate endpoint.

From the BEST (Biomarkers, EndpointS, and other Tools) Online Resource https://pubmed.ncbi.nlm.nih.gov/27010052/

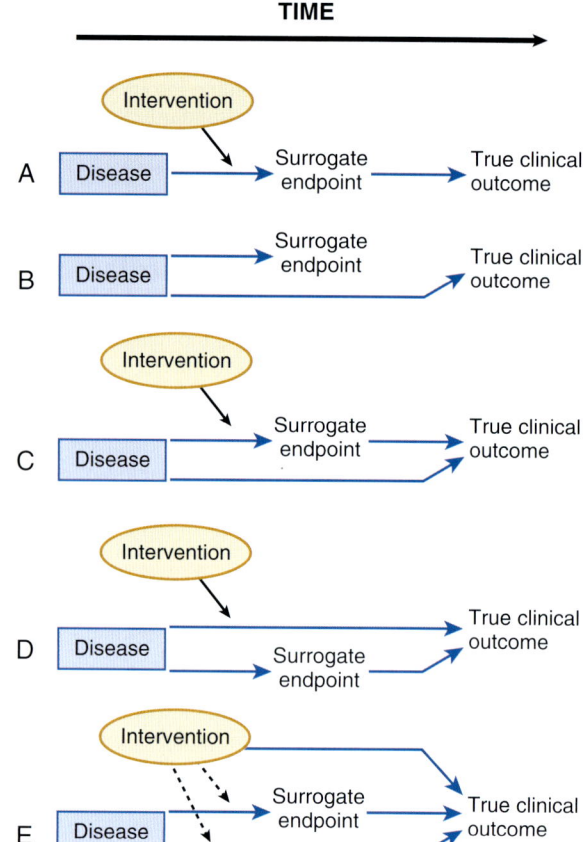

FIGURE 10.2 Biomarkers as surrogate endpoints in clinical research. **A,** The setting that provides the greatest potential for the surrogate endpoint to be valid. **B,** The surrogate is not in the causal pathway of the disease process. **C,** Of several causal pathways of disease, the intervention affects only the pathway mediated through the surrogate. **D,** The surrogate is not in the pathway of the intervention's effect or is insensitive to its effect. **E,** The intervention has mechanisms of action independent of the disease process. *Dotted lines* represent possible mechanisms of action. (Modified from Fleming TR, DeMets DL. Surrogate end points in clinical trials: are we being misled? *Ann Intern Med*. 1996;125:605.)

clinically useful information when measured once at "baseline." A baseline measurement of high-density lipoprotein cholesterol (HDL-C), for example, correlates inversely with future risk for cardiovascular events. However, serial measurement of biomarkers to document a change does not always guarantee a clinical benefit. In the case of HDL-C, recent large-scale trials that have measured clinical endpoints have cast doubt on the fidelity of a rise in HDL-C as a predictor of clinical benefit (see Chapter 27). A single measurement of coronary artery calcium score (CAC) ably predicts future events in statin naïve individuals. Yet, serial measurements of CAC may prove misleading because statin therapy increases calcification, but decreases coronary events.

Biomarkers require rigorous validation before adoption into clinical practice. In cardiovascular medicine, LDL-C has high reliability as a biomarker; it satisfies the modified Koch postulates. LDL levels prospectively predict cardiovascular risk, and decreases in LDL generally correlate with improved outcomes. Not all biomarkers, however, have proved as faithful in predicting clinical events. In the 1960s and 1970s, for example, most of the cardiovascular community considered ventricular premature depolarizations on the electrocardiogram (ECG) as important biomarkers for lethal arrhythmias. Numerous strategies have been aimed at suppressing ventricular ectopy. The Cardiac Arrhythmia Suppression Trial (CAST), however, showed that drugs capable of suppressing ventricular premature depolarizations actually worsened survival. The short-term improvements in indices of cardiac contractility produced by inotropic agents similarly led to worsened clinical outcomes, including increased mortality. These examples illustrate the necessity of rigorous validation of biomarkers before adoption into clinical practice.

Another important consideration in the use of cardiovascular biomarkers involves the question of *causality*. LDL-C exemplifies a *causal biomarker*, one that clearly participates in the pathogenesis of atherosclerosis.[4] Its levels prospectively correlate with risk for cardiovascular events and the development of atherosclerotic lesions identified by a variety of imaging modalities. A variety of independent manipulations of LDL-C levels correlate with clinical outcomes. In addition, very strong genetic evidence based on mendelian disorders (e.g., familial hypercholesterolemia) and unbiased genome-wide association scans, as well as mendelian randomization analyses, have established LDL-C as a causal risk factor in atherosclerotic cardiovascular disease and as a generally valid surrogate endpoint offering great value in clinical practice (see Chapter 27). Even a well-validated causal biomarker such as LDL-C, however, may mislead under some circumstances. For example, lowering of LDL-C with certain cholesteryl ester transfer protein inhibitors does not appear to lead to clinical benefit.[5,6] Other lipid measures such as plasma triglycerides and lipoprotein(a) predict risk, but currently lack definitive evidence that intervention reduces that risk. Ongoing trials of triglyceride reduction[7] and of lipoprotein(a) reduction[8] may move these relationships from casual to causal.

Other biomarkers, although clearly clinically useful, do not participate in the causal pathway for disease. For example, fever has served since antiquity as an important biomarker of infection. Resolution of fever correlates with successful resolution of infectious processes. However, fever does not participate causally in the pathogenesis of infection but merely serves as a biomarker of the host defenses against the infectious process. Sometimes a non-causal downstream biomarker can serve as an effective clinical surrogate for an upstream causal biomarker. For example, the use of hsCRP measurements improves the prediction of cardiovascular risk, and reductions in CRP correlate with clinical benefit in many cases. However, mendelian randomization studies do not support a causal role for CRP itself in the pathogenesis of cardiovascular disease. By contrast, intervention trials demonstrate that upstream drivers of CRP, in particular IL-1b, are indeed in the causal pathway leading to myocardial infarction, stroke, and cardiovascular events.[9]

These examples illustrate how a biomarker does not need to reside in the causal pathway of a disease to have clinical usefulness. A clear and early exposition of the uses and pitfalls in the application of biomarkers emerged from the landmark schema of Fleming and DeMets (Fig. 10.2). Biomarkers have the greatest potential for validity when there is one causal pathway and when the effect of intervention on true clinical outcomes is mediated directly through the biomarker surrogate (Fig. 10.2A). However, biomarker development can fail when the biomarker is found not to be in the causal pathway, when the biomarker is insensitive to the specific intervention's effect, or when the intervention of interest has a mechanism of action (or a toxicity) that does not involve the pathway described by the biomarker (Fig. 10.2B-E). These examples do not mean that biomarkers lack value; few if any novel biologic fields could develop without biomarker discovery and validation. Still, surrogate endpoints probably will not replace large-scale randomized trials that address whether interventions reduce actual event rates.

Novel Technologies in Biomarker Identification

The limitations of currently available biomarkers for screening or prognostic use underscore the importance of identifying "uncorrelated" or "orthogonal" biomarkers associated with novel disease pathways (see Fig. 10.1A). Most current biomarkers have been developed as an extension of targeted physiologic studies investigating known pathways such as tissue injury, inflammation, or hemostasis. By contrast, emerging technologies now enable the systematic, unbiased characterization of variation in proteins and metabolites associated with disease conditions (see Chapter 8). The rapid development of polygenic risk scores for cardiovascular disease promises to provide biomarkers that may permit the targeting of therapies particularly in primordial and primary prevention before pathological processes have progressed to the point of altering disease biomarkers (see Chapter 7.)[10-13] The applications of machine learning and artificial intelligence (see Chapter 11) will doubtless add to the development of novel candidate biomarkers that will require rigorous evaluation for clinical utility as outlined below. The burgeoning field of wearables will provide new inputs into biomarker science as well (see Chapter 12). The development of point-of-care technologies will likewise facilitate the clinical application of biomarkers by rendering their use more practical in the field and in urgent situations.[14] Digital technologies, for example, smart phone apps and implanted sensors, will also provide "real world" biomarker input outside of the confines of the traditional medical enterprise.

CLINICAL MEASURES OF BIOMARKER PERFORMANCE

When considering any biomarker in a clinical setting for risk prediction, physicians should ask two interrelated questions:
- Is there clear evidence that the biomarker of interest predicts future cardiovascular events independent of other already measured biomarkers?
- Is there clear evidence that patients identified by the biomarker of interest will benefit from a therapy that they otherwise would not have received?

Unless the answer to both these questions is a clear "yes," measurement of the biomarker will not likely have sufficient usefulness to justify its cost or unintended consequences. Such judgments require clinical expertise and will vary on a case-by-case basis.

Biomarker evaluation also typically involves repeated testing in multiple settings that include varied patient populations and that use different epidemiologic designs. *Prospective* cohort studies (in which the biomarker or exposure of interest is measured at baseline, when individuals are healthy, and then related to the future development of disease) provide a much stronger form of epidemiologic evidence than do data from *retrospective* case-control studies (in which the biomarker of interest is measured after the disease is present in the case participants).

After discovery by the technologies described earlier or identification by a candidate approach, a novel biomarker typically requires development in a translational laboratory for refinement of its assay to address issues of interassay and intra-assay variation before any clinical testing begins. Focused studies in specific patient populations typically follow and eventually broaden to encompass the population of greatest clinical interest. Beyond simple reproducibility, biomarkers under development for diagnostic, screening, or predictive purposes require further evaluation with a standard set of performance measures that include sensitivity, specificity, positive and negative predictive value (NPV), discrimination, calibration, reclassification, and tests for external validity.

Sensitivity, Specificity, and Positive and Negative Predictive Value

The validity of a screening or diagnostic test (or one used for prediction) is initially measured by its ability to categorize individuals who have preclinical disease correctly as "test positive" and those without preclinical disease as "test negative." A simple two-by-two table is typically used to summarize the results of a screening test by dividing those screened into four distinct groups (Table 10.4). In this context, sensitivity and specificity provide fundamental measures of the test's clinical validity. *Sensitivity* is the probability of testing positive when the disease is truly present and is defined mathematically as $a/(a + c)$. As sensitivity increases, the number of individuals with disease who are missed by the test decreases, so a test with perfect sensitivity will detect all individuals with disease correctly. In practice, tests with ever-higher sensitivity tend to also classify as "diseased" many individuals who are not actually affected (false positives). Thus the *specificity* of a test is the probability of screening negative if the disease is truly absent and is defined mathematically as $d/(b + d)$. A test with high specificity will rarely be positive when disease is absent and will therefore lead to a lower proportion of individuals without disease being incorrectly classified as test positive (false positives). A simple way to remember these differences is that sensitivity is "positive in disease," whereas specificity is "negative in health."

A perfect test has both very high sensitivity and specificity and thus low false-positive and false-negative classifications. Such test characteristics are rare, however, because there is a trade-off between sensitivity and specificity for almost every screening biomarker, diagnostic, or predictive test in common clinical use. For example, although high LDL-C levels usually serve as a biomarker for atherosclerotic risk, up to half of all incident cardiovascular events occur in those with LDL-C levels well within the normal range, and many events occur even when levels are low. If the diagnostic cutoff criterion for LDL-C is reduced so that more people who actually have high risk for disease will test positive (i.e., increased sensitivity), an immediate consequence of this

TABLE 10.4 Summarizing the Results of Screening, Diagnostic, or Predictive Tests

	DISEASE PRESENT	DISEASE ABSENT	
Test positive	a	b	a + b
Test negative	c	d	c + d
Total	a + c	b + d	

Sensitivity = $a/(a + c)$
Specificity = $d/(b + d)$
Positive predictive value = $a/(a + b)$
Negative predictive value = $d/(c + d)$

a = Number of individuals for whom the screening test is positive and the individual actually has the disease (true positives).
b = Number of individuals for whom the test is positive but the individual does not have the disease (false positives).
c = Number of individuals for whom the test is negative but the individual actually has the disease (false negatives).
d = Number of individuals for whom the test is negative and the individual does not have the disease (true negatives).
Modified from Biomarkers Definitions Working Group. Biomarkers and surrogate endpoints: preferred definitions and conceptual framework. *Clin Pharmacol Ther.* 2001;69:89–95.

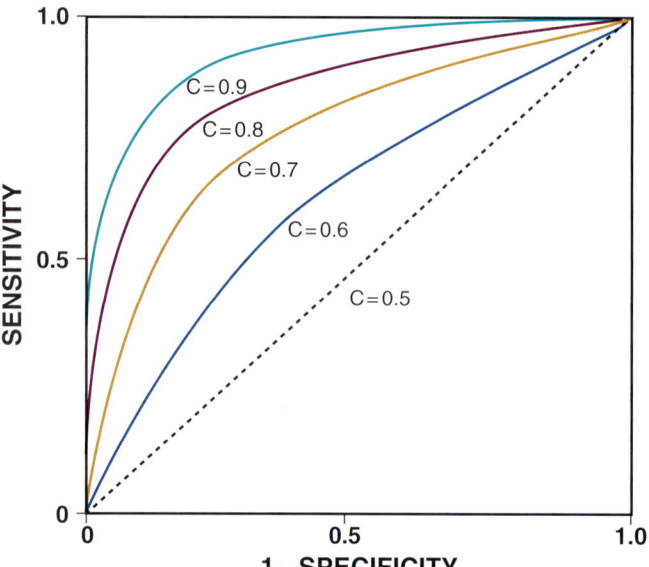

FIGURE 10.3 Receiver operating characteristic (ROC) curves for a series of biomarkers or risk prediction models with incremental improvement. The diagonal line corresponds to a random effect (C-statistic = 0.5), whereas the increasing C-statistic corresponds to improving model discrimination.

change will be an increase in the number of people without disease in whom the diagnosis is made incorrectly (i.e., reduced specificity). Conversely, if the criterion for diagnosis or prediction is made more stringent, a greater proportion of those who test negative will actually not have the disease (i.e., improved specificity), but a larger proportion of true cases will be missed (i.e., reduced sensitivity).

In addition to sensitivity and specificity, the performance or yield of a screening, diagnostic, or predictive test also varies depending on the characteristics of the population being evaluated. Positive and NPVs are terms used in epidemiology that refer to measurement of whether an individual actually has (or does not have) a disease, contingent on the result of the screening test itself.

The positive predictive value (PPV) is the probability that a person has the disease of interest, given that the individual tests positive, and is mathematically calculated as PPV = a/(a + b). High PPV can be anticipated when the disease is common in the population being tested. Conversely, the NPV is the probability that an individual is truly disease free, provided that the test has a negative result, and is mathematically calculated as NPV = d/(c + d). High NPV can be anticipated when the disease is rare in the population being tested. Although sensitivity and specificity are largely performance characteristics of the test itself (and thus tend to be fixed values), PPV and NPV depend in part on the population being tested (and thus tend to vary).

Discrimination, C-Statistics, and Receiver Operating Characteristic Curve

Discrimination is the ability of a test (or prognostic model) to separate those with disease or at high risk for disease (cases) from those without disease or at low risk for disease (controls). The most common method used to measure discrimination has been the *area under the receiver operating characteristic* (ROC) *curve* (AUC), which relates sensitivity (on the *y* axis) to (1 − specificity) (on the *x* axis) across a full range of cutoff values for the test or screening algorithm of interest (Fig. 10.3).

Given a population of individuals being evaluated, the area under the ROC curve, also called the *C-statistic*, equals the probability of correctly ranking risk for individuals by using the test or model under evaluation. A random test with no clinical usefulness would have a C-statistic (ROC AUC) of 0.5, which corresponds to the diagonal line in Figure 10.3. A perfect test that completely discriminates individuals with disease from those without disease would have a C-statistic that approaches 1.0. As the C-statistic increases from 0.5 to 1.0, model fit (or test accuracy) improves; thus the change in the C-statistic has served historically to judge whether a new biomarker can "add" significantly to those already in use. This approach permits direct comparison of the relative efficiency of multimarker panels. For example, using comparative C-statistic analyses, investigators in the Emerging Risk Factors Collaboration recently found that the incremental clinical usefulness of CRP has similar magnitude as that of total and HDL-C. Thus when change in the C-statistic can be demonstrated and the overall power to do so is adequate, this test can assist in understanding the impact of novel pathways and novel risk biomarkers on prediction and prevention.

Unfortunately, the traditional C-statistic approach is limited in that biomarkers with large associations may have minimal effect on ROC AUC. For example, a predictor (or set of predictors) would need an odds ratio (OR) as high as 16 (>2 standard deviations [SD]) to lead to a substantial increase in the C-statistic. Almost no test in common use for risk prediction or prognostication in cardiovascular medicine has an OR in this range; high cholesterol, smoking, high blood pressure, and diabetes yield an OR of less than 2 and thus have negligible individual impact on ROC AUC. Consequently, sole reliance on the C-statistic as a method for developing and evaluating new biomarkers, at least in the setting of risk prediction, is insufficient.

Accuracy and Calibration

Discrimination is only one measure of model accuracy. The other important measure is *calibration*, or the ability of a predictive model to assign risk estimates accurately compared with the actual observed risk in the population being tested. Unlike discrimination, which is based solely on relative rankings of risk, calibration compares the risk predicted from a model or test with that actually observed.

For *binary* outcomes (e.g., disease or no disease), calibration is often evaluated with the Hosmer-Lemeshow test, which places individuals within categories of estimated risk by using the test biomarker or multivariable model and compares these estimates with the proportions actually observed. These "predicted" and "observed" probabilities can be compared with standard goodness-of-fit tests across categories of risk (e.g., across estimated quintiles or estimated deciles of risk). Calibration becomes particularly important when addressing a biomarker in different populations from the population in whom it was originally developed. A biomarker may calibrate well in men but not in women, or among whites but not among blacks. This consideration also applies to multimarker panels, such as the Framingham Risk Score, which calibrates well in whites but less well in other population groups. Newer risk models such as the Reynolds Risk Score show improved calibration, as well as discrimination, compared with the traditional Framingham model.

Risk Reclassification

To address the shortcoming of biomarker validation via the C-statistic alone, contemporary biomarker development programs for risk prediction now use a series of "reclassification statistics," as initially developed by Cook and Ridker and refined by Pencina and Xanthakis and associates. Rather than addressing whether a new biomarker of interest adds to ROC AUC, reclassification addresses whether the biomarker can shift overall risk estimates upward or downward in a clinically meaningful way. Specifically, reclassification methods compare risk strata formed from prediction models with and without the new biomarker of interest and then determine which model leads to the most accurate classification of risk. Risk reclassification is particularly useful when actionable and clinically relevant risk categories already exist. For example, in primary cardiovascular prevention, 10-year estimated risk is often categorized as being less than 5%, 5% to 10%, 10% to 20%, or greater than 20%, and those above or below these cut points are frequently targeted for interventions such as aspirin and statin therapy. Thus a biomarker that reclassifies a proportion of individuals upward (or downward) might well be highly effective for targeting (or avoiding) drug therapy, even if the overall effect on discrimination is modest.

Mere reclassification of an individual by a given biomarker does not provide sufficient evidence to support clinical use. Rather, an effective biomarker should correctly reclassify risk higher or lower and thus lead to more accurate overall risk assessment. The *reclassification calibration* (RC) statistic is a tool that tests how well the average predicted risk within a given cell agrees with the observed risk of individuals who actually experience the event. Accordingly, the RC statistic addresses whether the predicted risk estimates after reclassification (using the new biomarker) are more accurate than before reclassification (without the new biomarker). Superior reclassification occurs when the new prediction model places case individuals into higher-risk categories and places control individuals into lower-risk categories, and when the net shift in these two effects is in the overall correct direction. This characteristic can be addressed by using the *net reclassification index* (NRI), analogous to a test of discrimination (the ability to separate cases from controls) in the context of a reclassification table. Broadly, the NRI does not depend as much on the actual predicted probabilities as on movement across a categorical risk border that is the result of the new probabilities predicted. When reclassification is not addressed across categories, an alternative measure is used, called the *integrated discrimination improvement* (IDI), based on the Yates slope, or the difference in predicted probabilities among case and control individuals. Despite their relatively recent introduction, reclassification statistics have rapidly become the standard for clinical evaluation of emerging biomarkers and alternative multi-biomarker prediction panels.

External Validation and Impact Studies

A final but important test for any biomarker or biomarker panel when used for prognostication, *external validation* refers to the ability of the panel to function with clinically acceptable levels of sensitivity, specificity, discrimination, and calibration in external populations, distinct from the population used for generation of the panel. As Moons and coworkers note, prognosis research and prognostic biomarkers differ from those used in diagnosis and screening.

Prognostic research involves three distinct phases in the development of multivariable prediction models. The first phase is identification of relevant predictors, assignment of weights to the model, estimation of predictive performance, and optimization of fit. The second phase involves validation or formal testing of calibration and discrimination in new patient groups, which can be similar to those used in the development stage or purposely different. The third phase involves impact studies to quantify directly whether use of a prognostic model in daily practice actually changes physician behavior and decision making, and whether this occurs in a net positive manner and is cost-effective. *Prognostic impact studies* also focus on the incremental usefulness of a given biomarker beyond simple clinical and nonclinical characteristics. Such studies tend to be less biologically driven than biomarker discovery work and recognize that prediction does not necessarily involve a causal pathway.

Practical Example: High-Sensitivity C-Reactive Protein, Lipids, and Reynolds Risk Score

The use of hsCRP in clinical practice is an example of how biomarker development programs can move from pathophysiologic principles to clinical use and onward to multinational trials evaluating novel targets for vascular risk reduction.[15] A prospective cohort of initially healthy individuals showed that hsCRP predicted future risk for a heart attack and stroke in men, an observation externally validated and quickly extended to women. Multiple commercial hsCRP assays—reproducible, internally calibrated, and externally validated to improve assay precision—then became clinically available. Multiple studies have shown that statins reduce hsCRP in a manner largely independent of reduction of LDL-C, thus suggesting that statins have both lipid-lowering and anti-inflammatory effects. The addition of hsCRP to the family history and HbA$_{1c}$ was formally incorporated into the Reynolds Risk Score in 2008.[16] This score was subsequently externally validated and shown to have superior calibration, discrimination, and reclassification over the more traditional Framingham Risk Score. Using hsCRP to define a high-risk population in need of treatment, JUPITER (Justification for the Use of Statins in Prevention: an Intervention Trial Evaluating Rosuvastatin) reported in 2008 that statin therapy (vs. placebo) in those with elevated hsCRP but low levels of LDL-C resulted in a 50% reduction in myocardial infarction and stroke and a 20% reduction in all-cause mortality. By 2010, more than 50 prospective cohort studies evaluating hsCRP were subjected to meta-analysis, which affirmed that the magnitude of vascular risk associated with a change of 1 SD in hsCRP was at least as large as that of a comparable change in cholesterol or blood pressure. An updated 2012 meta-analysis of clinical usefulness and risk prediction found that the change in C-statistic associated with hsCRP was similar to that associated with the use of total and HDL cholesterol. On this basis, several national guidelines incorporated hsCRP screening in primary and secondary prevention, and the FDA approved a labeling claim for the use of statin therapy in those with elevated hsCRP levels.

CRP itself, however, probably does not cause atherothrombosis, but rather serves as a biomarker for the underlying inflammatory process. Thus validation of the inflammatory hypothesis of atherosclerosis required measurement of clinical outcomes, not solely biomarkers. CANTOS (the Canakinumab Anti-inflammatory Thrombosis Outcomes Study), evaluated interleukin-1beta inhibition in individuals who were in a stable phase postmyocardial infarction, and were well treated with standard secondary prevention measures, but had an hsCRP greater than 2 mg/L. CANTOS demonstrated that an anti-inflammatory intervention (as gauged by lowering of hsCRP and other inflammatory biomarkers such as IL-6) that did not affect atherogenic lipoprotein levels could reduce recurrent major adverse cardiovascular events.[9,17] Trials with colchicine have validated this concept as discussed in Chapter 25,[18,19] and new trials addressing the potential role of IL-6 inhibition for atheroprotection are underway.[20] The use of hsCRP as a biomarker laid the groundwork for CANTOS, illustrating the value of biomarkers in advancing both pathophysiologic understanding and therapeutics.

Congestive heart failure is another arena where multiple biomarkers ranging for troponin to ST2 to IL-6 to GDF-15 have been proposed to have unique prognostic utility. However, other than data suggesting that interventions targeting IL-1b such as canakinumab[21] and anakinra[22,23] may reduce hospitalization for heart failure, little confirmatory evidence is available.

CONCLUSION

We use biomarkers in our daily clinical practice, and cardiovascular journals contain numerous reports regarding biomarkers, new and old, that purport to show how they may aid clinical practice. Moreover, many cardiovascular trials use biomarkers—thus the current practice of cardiovascular medicine requires a firm foundation in understanding and evaluating biomarkers. The road map to the field of biomarkers provided in this chapter, including their use, development, and methods for evaluating their usefulness for various specific applications, should give practitioners tools to sort out the various uses of biomarkers encountered in practice and in the cardiovascular literature. Informed use of biomarkers can aid in decision making in daily patient care. Biomarkers should provide a key for personalized management by directing the right therapy to the right patient at the right time. They can also shed mechanistic insight on human pathophysiology that is difficult to obtain in other ways. Rigorous and careful use of biomarkers can aid in the development of novel therapies to address the residual burden of cardiovascular risk.

REFERENCES

For citations to the older literature, see previous editions of this textbook.

Biomarkers: General Considerations

1. Libby P, King K. Biomarkers: a challenging conundrum in cardiovascular disease. *Arterioscl Thromb Vasc Biol*. 2015;35:2491–2495.
2. Biomarkers Definitions Working G. Biomarkers and surrogate endpoints: preferred definitions and conceptual framework. *Clin Pharmacol Ther*. 2001;69:89–95.
3. Robb MA, McInnes PM, Califf RM. Biomarkers and surrogate endpoints: developing common terminology and definitions. *J Am Med Assoc*. 2016;315:1107–1108.
4. Borén J, Chapman MJ, Krauss RM, et al. Low-density lipoproteins cause atherosclerotic cardiovascular disease: pathophysiological, genetic, and therapeutic insights: a consensus statement from the European Atherosclerosis Society Consensus Panel. *Eur Heart J*. 2020;41:2313–2330.

Biomarkers Versus Clinical Endpoints

5. Group HTRC. Effects of anacetrapib in patients with atherosclerotic vascular disease. *New Engl J Med*. 2017.

6. Lincoff AM, Nicholls SJ, Riesmeyer JS, et al. Evacetrapib and cardiovascular outcomes in high-risk vascular disease. *New Engl J Med.* 2017;376:1933–1942.
7. Pradhan AD, Paynter NP, Everett BM, et al. Rationale and design of the Pemafibrate to Reduce Cardiovascular Outcomes by Reducing Triglycerides in Patients with Diabetes (PROMINENT) study. *Am Heart J.* 2018;206:80–93.
8. Tsimikas S, Karwatowska-Prokopczuk E, Gouni-Berthold I, et al. Lipoprotein(a) reduction in persons with cardiovascular disease. *New Engl J Med.* 2020;382:244–255.
9. Ridker PM, Everett BM, Thuren T, et al. Antiinflammatory therapy with canakinumab for atherosclerotic disease. *New Engl J Med.* 2017;377:1119–1131.

Evolving Biomarkers

10. Khera AV, Chaffin M, Aragam KG, et al. Genome-wide polygenic scores for common diseases identify individuals with risk equivalent to monogenic mutations. *Nat Genet.* 2018;50:1219–1224.
11. Inouye M, Abraham G, Nelson CP, et al. Genomic risk prediction of coronary artery disease in 480,000 adults: implications for primary prevention. *J Am Coll Cardiol.* 2018;72:1883–1893.
12. Mosley JD, Gupta DK, Tan J, et al. Predictive accuracy of a polygenic risk score compared with a clinical risk score for incident coronary heart disease. *J Am Med Assoc.* 2020:323.
13. Aragam Krishna G, Natarajan P. Polygenic scores to assess atherosclerotic cardiovascular disease risk. *Circ Res.* 2020;126:1159–1177.
14. King KR, Grazette LP, Paltoo DN, et al. Point-of-Care technologies for precision cardiovascular care and clinical research. *JACC (J Am Coll Cardiol): Basic to Transl Sc.* 2016;1:73–86.

A Practical Application of a Biomarker

15. Ridker PM. A test in context: high-sensitivity C-reactive protein. *J Am Coll Cardiol.* 2016;67:712–723.
16. Cook NR, Paynter NP, Eaton CB, et al. Comparison of the Framingham and Reynolds Risk scores for global cardiovascular risk prediction in the multiethnic Women's Health Initiative. *Circulation.* 2012;125:1748–1756. S1-11.
17. Ridker PM, Libby P, MacFadyen JG, et al. Modulation of the interleukin-6 signalling pathway and incidence rates of atherosclerotic events and all-cause mortality: analyses from the Canakinumab Anti-Inflammatory Thrombosis Outcomes Study (CANTOS). *Eur Heart J.* 2018;39:3499–3507.
18. Tardif JC, Kouz S, Waters DD, et al. Efficacy and safety of low-dose colchicine after myocardial infarction. *New Engl J Med.* 2019;381:2497–2505.
19. Nidorf SM, Fiolet ATL, Mosterd A, et al. Colchicine in patients with chronic coronary disease. *New Engl J Med.* 2020;383:1838–1847.
20. Ridker PM, Devalaraja M, Baeres FMM et al. Effects of interleukin-6 inhibition with Ziltivekimab on biomarkers of inflammation among patients at high risk for atherosclerotic events. In press.
21. Everett BM, Cornel JH, Lainscak M, et al. Anti-inflammatory therapy with canakinumab for the prevention of hospitalization for heart failure. *Circulation.* 2019;139:1289–1299.
22. Buckley LF, Abbate A. Interleukin-1 blockade in cardiovascular diseases: from bench to bedside. *BioDrugs.* 2018;32(2):111–118.
23. Abbate A, Toldo S, Marchetti C, et al. Interleukin-1 and the inflammasome as therapeutic targets in cardiovascular disease. *Circ Res.* 2020;126:1260–1280.

11 Artificial Intelligence in Cardiovascular Medicine

ZACHI ATTIA, SURAJ KAPA, PETER NOSEWORTHY, AND PAUL FRIEDMAN

DEFINITIONS AND KEY TERMS, 109
Learning, 109
Supervised Learning, 109
Unsupervised Learning, 110
Reinforcement Learning, 110
Fully Connected and Convolutional Neural Networks, 110
Optimization and Hyperparameters, 110
Transfer Learning, 111

CLINICAL USES IN CARDIOVASCULAR MEDICINE, 111
ECG-Based Screening, Detection, and Prevention, 111
Image Interpretation and Procedural Guidance, 111
Coronary Arteriography, 113
Natural Language Processing and Structured Data Analysis, 113

Risk Scores (Deep Phenotyping), 113

IMPLEMENTING ARTIFICIAL INTELLIGENCE INTO CLINICAL PRACTICE, 113
Pitfalls and Limitations of Artificial Intelligence in Cardiovascular Medicine, 115

CONCLUSIONS, 115

REFERENCES, 115

Artificial intelligence (AI) is ubiquitous. It autocompletes the sentences we type, populates web searches before we complete our thoughts, enables our phones to understand verbal commands, permits cars to drive themselves to destinations we speak, and increasingly supports medical diagnostic tests. In medicine it has identified retinal pathology with a skill that exceeds that of a trained ophthalmologist, can tirelessly detect mammographic lesions, and identify abnormalities on a pathologic slide. Some revile it as a technology that will lead to massive unemployment, economic disruption, and serve as an existential threat to humanity; others embrace it as the tool that will liberate humanity from drudgery and elevate the most noble of human tasks.[1]

Three broad capabilities of AI apply to the field of medicine. The first is the automation of fatiguing processes that involve analysis of massive amounts of data, such as continuous ECG tracings acquired over months. In this context, AI performs human-like tasks at massive scale. AI also permits embedding technology in novel forms such as clothing and other wearables to extract physiologic information to enable continuous monitoring of health. The application of AI also, by extension, enables remote monitoring in rural locations, space exploration, and extreme conditions. The second is the ability to extract signals beyond that which a human is capable of recognizing, for example determining the presence of ventricular function from a standard 12-lead electrocardiogram or single-lead ECG acquired from a watch- or smartphone-enabled electrodes. In this context, AI brings new value to well-established medical diagnostic tests that exist in current clinical workflows and practice. Thirdly, and more broadly, the ability to specifically, richly, and uniquely characterize an individual's physiologic data allows for a new level of personalized predictive models, potentially creating a whole new category of individual "previvors" who know a disease is impending before any signs of symptoms develop, opening the doors for potential interventions, and with associated social, legal, and economic implications. This deep phenotyping may inform additional fields, such as genetics. AI in medicine is in its early stages; the promise is large, but its application requires rigorous testing, vetting, and validation, as do all tests that impact human health. Here we focus on AI and its role in cardiovascular medicine.

DEFINITIONS AND KEY TERMS

If intelligence is a cake, the bulk of the cake is unsupervised learning, the icing on the cake is supervised learning, and the cherry on the cake is reinforcement learning (RL).

Yann LeCun, 2016

AI is a lay term, referring to machine learning (ML). In his cake analogy, Dr. Yann LeCun* divides ML into its three main branches and presents one of the technology's main challenges—the amount of data required for implementation. In all three types of learning (supervised, unsupervised, and reinforcement), instead of using an explicit set of human-devised rules to interpret a signal, large volumes of data are fed to a model, which uses statistical processes to identify relationships within the data. In short, the data train the model, free from human hypothesis.

Learning

Learning is the process of improving the ability to complete a task based on experience. As the task is repeated, ML improves by getting feedback (via an error or loss function) and changing the way it performs the task (by changing with weights and biases of the mathematical functions that comprise the "neurons" in a neural network, for example), until the feedback is that the task is done correctly, or at least above a certain standard. In all three types of ML, the feedback is the loss function—the difference between a wanted outcome (how we think the task should have been performed) to the actual outcome (how the task was performed). Learning, or training, is often computationally intensive. Once trained, many networks can then operate with limited computational resources, for example on a smartphone. This makes many AI tools massively scalable.

Supervised Learning

Supervised learning is the most commonly used form of ML. Supervised learning requires labeled data (images and captions, ECGs and their rhythm description), with labels often provided by human experts. The discovery of the rules that explain the relationship between the input (a signal) to the output (a label) is called *training*. For example, if ECG samples labeled normal rhythm or atrial fibrillation (AF) are fed to a model, it will learn to differentiate between the two rhythms. The specific features of the signal used to generate model output are determined by the computer during training and are not discernible to humans (Fig. 11.1). Thus, AI is at times referred to as a "black box." In most cases, the model will be a parametric function (F) of the inputs, and it will be initialized using a set of random parameters (weights). During training, in an iterative manner, F is applied on a set of inputs with known outputs (the labels). The results of applying the function

---

*Yann LeCun, Geoffrey Hinton and Yoshua Bengio—often referred to as the "Godfathers of AI" or the founding fathers of modern AI research, have were awarded together the prestigious Turing award in 2018 for their contribution to the AI revolution.

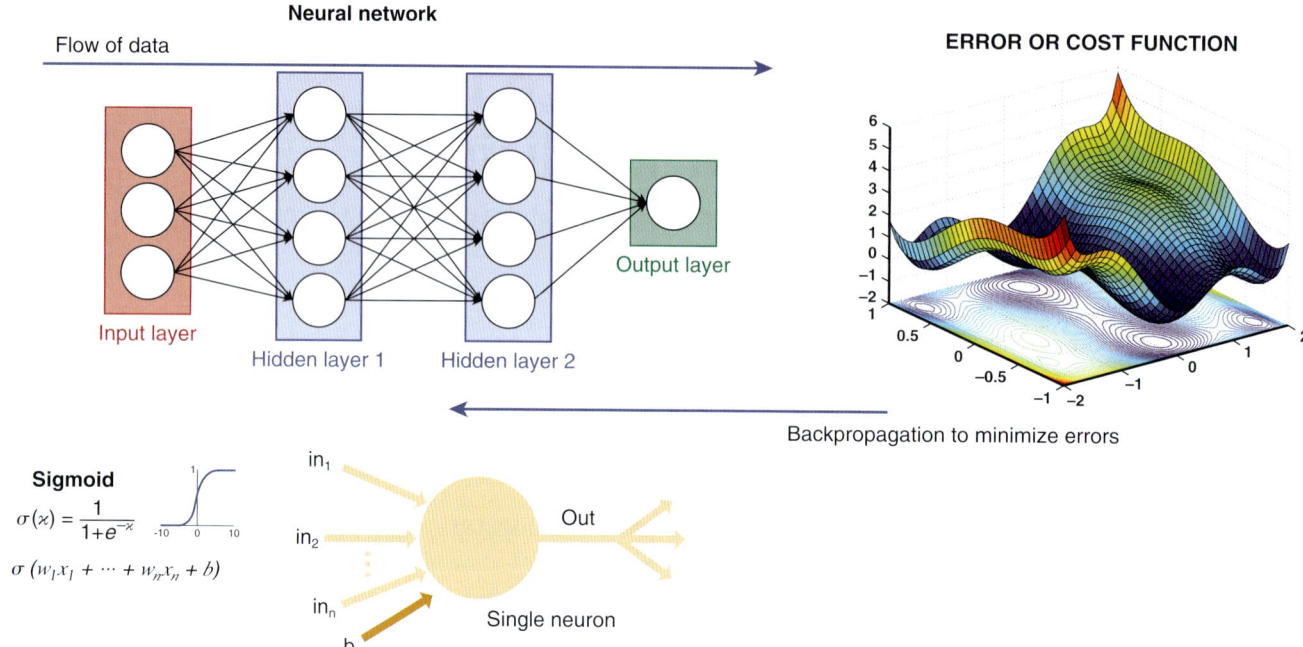

FIGURE 11.1 Graphical depiction of a neural network. **Top left:** The neural network shown contains four layers. Each layer is composed of "neurons" **(bottom panel)**. Each neuron receives multiple inputs, each multiplied by a weight (in1...inn), and a bias (offset) "b" and applies a nonlinear function to generate its output. During network training, weights and biases of each neuron are adjusted via backpropagation to minimize an error function (example error function shown **top right**).

F on the inputs yields estimated outputs (in the example, the probability of AF), and with each iteration, using the error between the estimated outputs and the real labels, model performance is assessed and the function weights are adjusted in a direction to minimize the error, improving model performance. The methods used to adjust to weights will be described in the "optimization and hyperparameters" subsection. The task can be either a classification—determination of the appropriate class for a data sample from a limited set of options (dogs versus cats, male versus female)—or a regression—a continuous value for each sample (age from an image). Because supervised learning in a neural network is an iterative process, with each step inching toward an improved solution, the biggest challenge is that large datasets are required. Because each sample in the dataset requires a label, attaching an accurate label to each element may be a limiting factor.

Unsupervised Learning

In unsupervised learning, the task revolves around the structure of the data itself. One most common form of unsupervised learning is *clustering*, in which the model clusters data based on its characteristics, instead of based on labels during the training stage. The model is fed only unlabeled data, and clusters samples based on similarity, using each sample's distance (Euclidian or other) from other samples. If the label of just a few samples in each cluster is known, the label of other samples in the cluster can be inferred because all the samples in that cluster would have similar features, but the model itself created the clusters without specific labels on the data elements. An example would be the acquisition of multiple ECG segments from a patient during a dialysis session at various potassium blood levels. The ECG segments could be clustered, and the potassium value of each cluster should be similar. Because unsupervised learning requires only the raw samples and basic assumptions regarding the data structure (such as the number of clusters), the barrier imposed by labeled data is lowered.

Reinforcement Learning

RL develops the optimal strategy for an agent in an environment with known rules and rewards. An example would be a chess player—learning chess by playing against itself, without labels or recorded human games. It uses only the rules and the game score. As RL requires known rules and rewards, its use in health care is still limited[2] and it is outside of the scope of this chapter.

Fully Connected and Convolutional Neural Networks

Inspired by the human brain, a fully connected neural network is a multi-layer parametric function that implements a nonlinear function between the inputs to the outputs (see Fig. 11.1). Each node (neuron) in each layer receives a weighted sum of all the nodes in the preceding layers and is activated using a nonlinear function. The values of the weights are defined during training, as the network learns the relationship between the input and output.

In convolutional neural networks, convolutional filters extract feature information from images in the convolutional layers, with the weights of the filters determined during training, so that the features selected are those that best define the desired network output. Both types of networks can be either used for classification tasks or for regression tasks.

Optimization and Hyperparameters

During training, the weights of the inputs to each neural in a neural network are adjusted so that the output of the function when fed samples with known labels will be the "closest" to their real labels. The difference between network output and the actual label is measured using the loss function, and a small loss value indicates network outputs close to the real labels. While weights could be randomly set to initiate a network and then randomly varied until the loss function is sufficiently small, this is clearly an inefficient and impractical way of training a network. A more efficient approach is to test a network on a set of samples, assess the effect of each of the network weights on the error function, and change the neuron weights accordingly. Mathematically, this is done by taking the derivative (actually, the gradient) of the function the network is implementing and changing the weights in the opposite direction (as the gradient points toward a higher loss). The gradient is approximated using a batch of samples, and the number of samples in the batch ("*batch size*") affects how accurate and smooth the gradient will be. While the gradient indicates the direction in which the weights should be adjusted, the magnitude of change (step size) is unknown. If a step size is too big, during training the function may step over a minimum of the error function (overcorrect), whereas if it is too small, the impact of the updated weights may be too diminutive to improve network accuracy, and the network may not converge or take a long time to train. Step size and the batch size are network "hyperparameters"—variables that affect how network parameters are changed (i.e., how the network learns during training), but which are not part of the final network function itself. Finding optimal hyperparameters requires empiric assessments of various combinations and is part of the art of network training. Assessing promising combinations of hyperparameters is typically performed on a second set of samples not used during network training called the internal validation set. Once hyperparameters and the network are finalized, the network is tested on a third set of samples not previously seen by the network referred to as the holdout testing set.

Transfer Learning

Transfer learning is a method used to apply supervised learning to problems for which the datasets available to train a network are relatively small. In this method, a network is developed to solve a problem that has enough labeled samples (the "primer"), and then it is retrained to solve a similar task with a much smaller dataset. The underlying hypothesis is that some of the patterns learned by the model are common to both tasks but can only be learned with a sufficient number of samples. This is similar to a human learning one musical instrument proficiently over years, and then requiring much less time and effort to learn a related instrument (e.g., guitar and banjo). Using transfer learning, datasets that may initially appear irrelevant can be used to solve specific tasks, and the transfer can be applied to all model parameters (basically seeding the model with weights from a trained model, instead of random weights), or to only a subset of parameters by "freezing" some model layers during training to keep the primer model values but allowing the rest to change.

CLINICAL USES IN CARDIOVASCULAR MEDICINE

ECG-Based Screening, Detection, and Prevention

Achieving human-like automated ECG interpretation has been a goal since the advent of digital ECG more than 60 years ago.[3] Early iterations of the technology were designed to identify fiducial points, make discrete measurements, and define common quantifiable abnormalities,[4–6] whereas contemporary approaches have moved beyond these rule-based approaches to recognize patterns in massive quantities of labeled ECG data.[7–9] Some early success has been achieved training deep neural networks (DNNs) on large datasets of single-lead ECGs and applying the algorithms to the 12-lead ECG,[8] sometimes outperforming expert over-readers.[7] In general, however, most algorithms lack the accuracy needed for widespread application without human oversight,[10] and it is likely that these technologies remain a tool to improve rather than replace human expertise for the foreseeable future.

For some discrete applications, these algorithms may enable rapid diagnosis on novel, patient- or consumer-facing devices. For example, algorithms have been demonstrated to be effective for AF diagnosis on a variety of single-lead ECG devices,[11–14] and there is great potential for making other important diagnoses including QT prolongation,[15] acute myocardial infarction,[16] or other arrhythmias.[17] This "democratization" of ECG technology will exponentially increase the volume of signals that demand interpretation, and this will quickly outstrip the capacity of human ECG readers. We anticipate that these models will be essential in facilitating telehealth technologies—automatic patient- and consumer-facing technologies.

By leveraging massive labeled datasets, various neural networks can be used to move beyond human-like tasks to uncover more subtle patterns in the ECG that have gone unrecognized by even expert ECG readers. In doing so, these networks can bring new diagnostic power and value to the ECG. For example, the ECG can identify low ejection fraction (EF),[18] propensity toward AF (observable during normal sinus rhythm),[19] hypertrophic cardiomyopathy,[20] left ventricular hypertrophy,[21] hyperkalemia,[22] age and sex,[23] medical comorbidity/frailty, and studies are ongoing to identity markers of valvular heart disease, amyloidosis, and many other characteristics.

The AI ECG is an example of adding AI to an existing clinical test (the 12-lead ECG), which is already embedded in clinical workflows and widely available. In that context it can readily screen for underdetected disease, for which therapies exist (Fig. 11.2A). The use of the 12-lead ECG to identify left ventricular dysfunction (present asymptomatically in 3% to 9% of people) is undergoing prospective evaluation in a large cluster-design pragmatic trial (EAGLE, discussed later); the AI ECG has also been embedded into a stethoscope form factor (i.e., a stethoscope with embedded electrodes to record the ECG during a normal examination, permitting the application of AI). Due to the potential sensitivity of AI tests to detect disease early and provide deep phenotyping, it may appear to "predict" future disease, creating a class of "previvors" who have not yet experienced a disease (Fig. 11.2B). The AI ECG may also have a role to permit inexpensive at-home follow-up of patients at risk for ventricular dysfunction, such as those receiving chemotherapy or cardiac transplants (Fig. 11.2C). Prospective studies assessing such use cases are underway (TACTIC, NCT03879629). Whether AI tests achieve a sufficient level of predictive power to warrant intervention before a disease is manifest by currently used tests requires validation (Fig. 11.3), which at present is under development. To date, AI-based tools have received FDA approval for rhythm determination (i.e., to allow scalability of human capabilities). AI to extract information beyond what humans can determine (such as ventricular dysfunction) is currently under regulatory review.

Image Interpretation and Procedural Guidance

Cardiac imaging has been a particular focus of modern AI and ML work. ML has been used to improve image acquisition, image quality, accuracy of interpretation, and enhancing insights into cardiac physiology.

Nuclear Cardiology and Stress Testing

Stress testing by ECG or by nuclear imaging can yield false-positive and false-negative results. The prognostic value of either modality depends in part effected by patient-specific pre-test likelihood of disease among other electrocardiographic, clinical, perfusion, and functional variations. The number of variables that can impact accuracy of interpretation of functional evaluations for coronary disease may lead to a wide variation in predictive accuracy of humans. One study of over 2000 patients suggested that an ML algorithm that integrated all available patient data (including clinical and electrocardiographic) along with imaging data performed better in predictive major adverse cardiac events than ML focused on imaging alone or physician interpretation. Furthermore, deep learning approaches can offer statistically significant improvements in identification of per-vessel and per-patient sensitivity for detection of obstructive coronary disease.[1,24]

Echocardiography

The clinical utility of echocardiographic images depends on several factors: (1) skill related to image acquisition; (2) image quality; and (3) accuracy and consistency of image interpretation.[25] Newer handheld devices, some of which are smartphone enabled, are inexpensive and have made bedside echocardiographic imaging available to many individuals with limited training in image acquisition and/or interpretation. Recent work has focused on using AI approaches to facilitate remote training of unskilled sonographers as well as for robot-assisted echocardiography. The latter significantly improves diagnostic process time when done in combination with telemedicine-enabled cardiac consultation. Such approaches may help scale not just the availability of tools to acquire echocardiographic images but also the capacity to acquire high-quality, interpretable images with minimal prior experience. Because embedded AI in the imaging tool recognizes images of diagnostic quality, immediate feedback is given to the bedside imager (for example, indicating an image is acceptable, or if not, suggesting specific maneuvers to acquire the desired image).

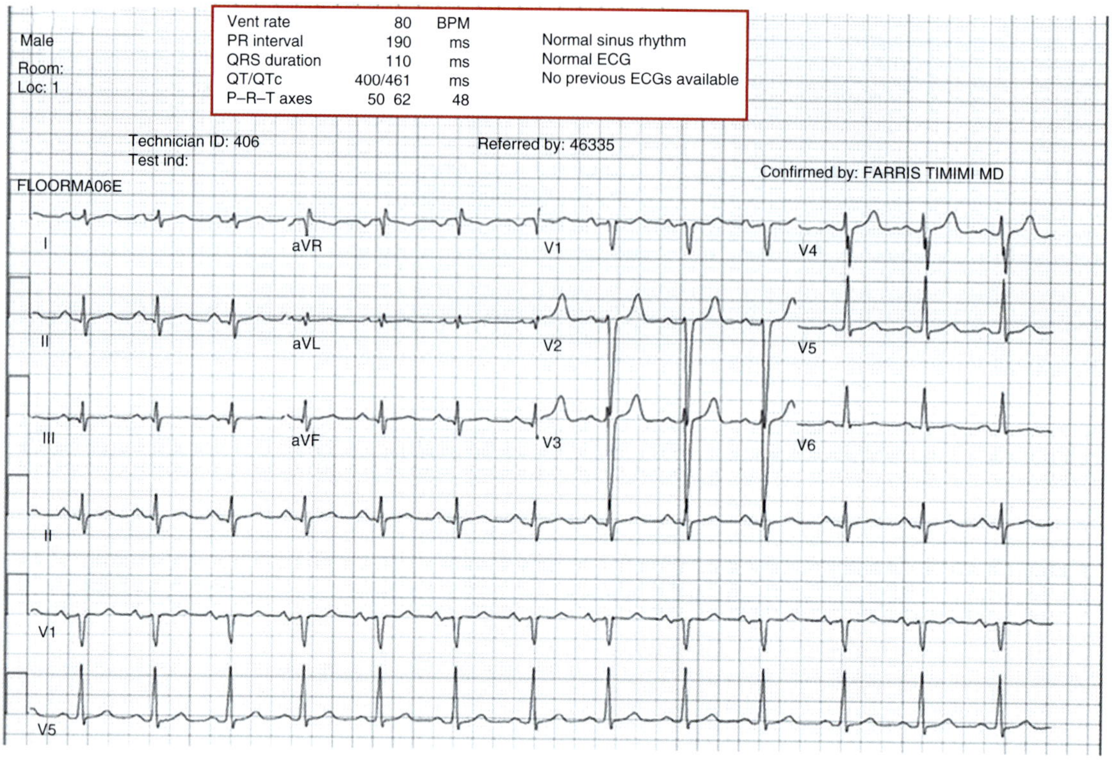

112

Vent rate	80	BPM	Normal sinus rhythm
PR interval	190	ms	Normal ECG
QRS duration	110	ms	No previous ECGs available
QT/QTc	400/461	ms	
P–R–T axes	50 62	48	

Technician ID: 406
Test ind:
Referred by: 46335
Confirmed by: FARRIS TIMIMI MD

FLOORMA06E

AI-ECG OUTPUT:
Positive for low EF (76% probability of having low EF)

Echocardiogram EF: 18%

A

Normal sinus rhythm normal ECG

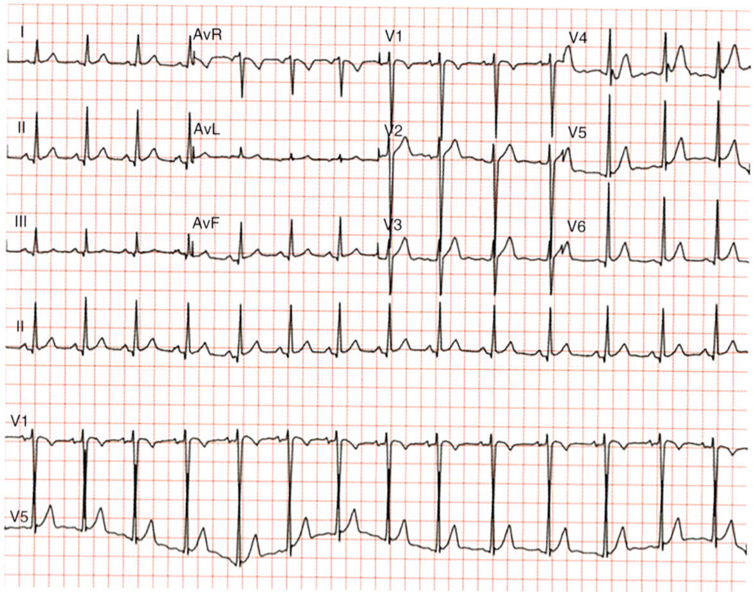

AI ECG: Positive for Low EF Echocardiographic Ejection Fraction: 50%: *False-Positive*
Ejection Fraction 5 years later at age 33: 31%

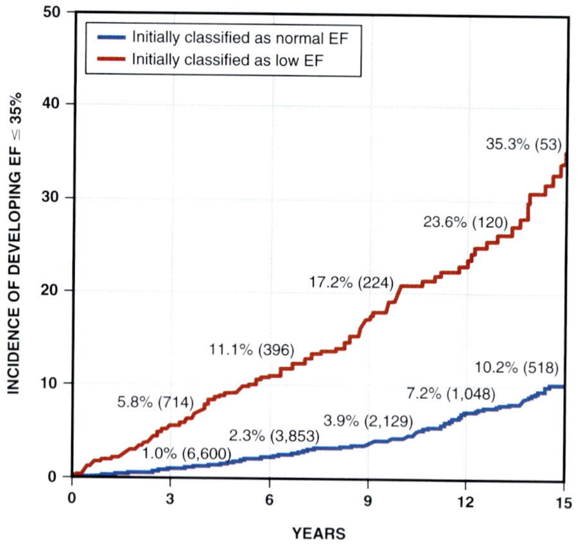

B

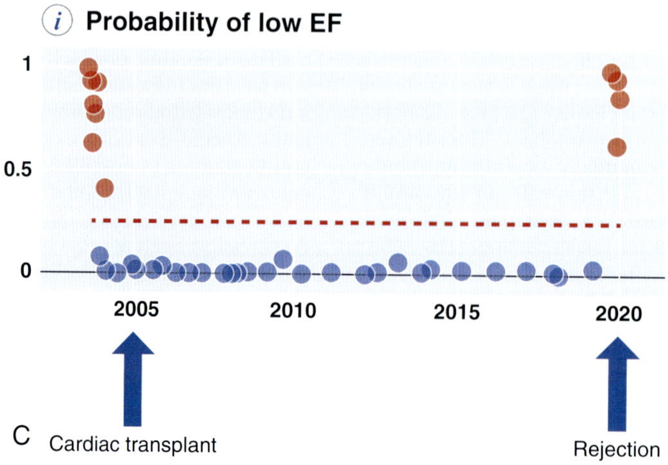

Probability of low EF

C

Cardiac transplant — Rejection

FIGURE 11.2 **A,** Electrocardiogram acquired from a 35-year-old asymptomatic man who presented after his sister died suddenly, read as normal. An AI-ECG algorithm reported a 76% probability of having a low ejection fraction. Subsequent echocardiography demonstrated an ejection fraction of 18%. He was ultimately diagnosed with familial dilated cardiomyopathy. **B,** *Left,* Electrocardiogram from a 28-year-old man, read as normal. The AI-ECG algorithm indicated a high probability of an ejection fraction less than 35% (positive test). Echocardiography at that time reported an ejection fraction (EF) of 50% suggesting a false-positive. However, the patient developed ventricular dysfunction, with an EF of 31% 5 years later. In some patients, the AI algorithm may identify subtle features that may predict future development of low EF. This situation illustrates the concept of disease "previvors," and in this case may result from pathophysiologic changes impacting ion channels and electrical impulse generation before mechanical function is affected, although the mechanism remains unproven. *Right,* The increased risk of developing left ventricular dysfunction with a positive AI-ECG screen for ventricular dysfunction. **C,** Plot of the AI-ECG outputs for all of the ECGs for an individual patient, taken from the Mayo Clinic Cardiology AI dashboard. Each point on the graph is generated by a single ECG, with the abscissa indicative of the date of the ECG, and the ordinate the probability of ventricular dysfunction. The patient had a dilated cardiomyopathy, and confirmed low ejection fraction (EF; *red points,* left of 2005 on the graph). He received a cardiac transplant, with normalization of his ejection fraction, and subsequent low probability of low EF by AI-ECG *(blue points).* In 2020 he suffered rejection and ventricular dysfunction, identified by the AI-ECG *(red points* at 2020). (**B** from Attia ZI, Kapa S, Lopez-Jimenez F, et al. Screening for cardiac contractile dysfunction using an artificial intelligence-enabled electrocardiogram. *Nat Med.* 2019;25:70–74.)

In addition to facilitating high-quality image acquisition, the scalability of echocardiographic imaging is subject to the same limitations as other imaging modalities—namely the need for expert interpretation. Several recent studies have suggested that applying ML to echocardiographic images can accurately assess several key variables (ejection fraction [heart pump strength], heart chamber size, and valve function). Such approaches, when applied broadly, may allow for rapid and accurate identification of disease, and identification of those images that warrant expert over-read.

Finally, AI approaches have the potential to address other aspects of ultrasound image acquisition, including image noise and poor image quality. In various areas of ultrasound imaging, use of ML can improve image classification, detection, and segmentation. Integrated AI algorithms may streamline methodologic tasks ranging from optimizing imaging quality through the segmentation and registration of such images.[26]

Computed Tomography and Magnetic Resonance Imaging

Similar to echocardiography and nuclear stress imaging, a key limitation of computed tomography (CT) and magnetic resonance imaging (MRI) is expert clinician interpretation. AI approaches applied to cardiac imaging may improve the consistency and accuracy of interpretation of images. Beyond interpretation, AI approaches to image acquisition may reduce the time required to acquire high-quality MRI and CT images while limiting motion or other artifact. Finally, AI can scale and improve the speed of segmentation and reconstruction of data from MRI and CT. Recent reviews have summarized this evolving area.[27]

Coronary Arteriography

A final area of modern application of AI and ML to cardiac care is in the catheterization laboratory. The accuracy of pre-procedural evaluation (reducing false-positives and false-negatives from stress testing, accurate identification of lesion severity from noninvasive CT evaluation), consistency of interpretation of images acquired in real time, to enhancement of interpretation of complex lesions, and the appropriate choices in management may be facilitated by ML and deep learning algorithms. ML approaches may extract fractional flow reserve and lesion severity from CT coronary angiography.[28] This application may improve identification of those patients appropriate for coronary intervention. In addition, AI may offer value in interventional cardiology by predicting stent size and length, likelihood of future stenosis, and complex lesion characteristics (irregular lumen shape, invasive fractional flow reserve from cinegraphic images) which would traditionally require the use of additional tools (pressure wires, intravascular ultrasound).[29]

Natural Language Processing and Structured Data Analysis

Structured data elements within the electronic health record are readily available for predictive analytics and can facilitate rapid, point-of-care decision support. However, much of the electronic health record (EHR) contains free text that requires additional processing for data abstraction. Traditional rule-based approaches to extract clinical data from free text are prone to misclassification due to the complexities of natural language structure, and more sophisticated models are emerging as more reliable alternatives. These approaches may include hybrid training of models using text vectorization and output tags that are fed into ML models or even completely unsupervised topic modeling. Because natural language processing (NLP) is not restricted by predefined diagnostic codes, an optimized NLP model has the ability to recognize even complex language patterns by comprehensively assessing all available documentation, thus improving the accuracy in capturing potentially ambiguous diagnoses.

Risk Scores (Deep Phenotyping)

The vast repositories of structured and unstructured patient data now available within EHRs offer an opportunity to generate risk scores and characterize patient phenotypes on a large scale. Such technologies promise to streamline patient care, identify individuals at risk of adverse outcome, and recognize and reinforce best practices. Often, these deep phenotyping approaches use a hybrid deep-learning model structure to distill the complicated relationships hidden in the data. This may include models that transform event structures into deep clinical-concept embedding and use a recurrent neural network (RNN) to predict outcomes over time. For example, one large-scale retrospective study using over 3 million patient records demonstrated that both traditional statistical approaches and novel ML models can predict risk of AF.[30] Similar approaches have been used to identify patients with heart failure,[31] to predict risk of hospitalization,[32] diagnose diabetes and peripheral artery disease, and generally have superior performance than relying on structured data alone.[26,33,34] Public repositories of these algorithms, such as the Phenotype KnowledgeBase (PheKB),[35] now contain algorithms for 50 to 60 medical conditions and many have demonstrated good performance when implemented across different health systems.[36-40]

IMPLEMENTING ARTIFICIAL INTELLIGENCE INTO CLINICAL PRACTICE

AI stands to increase the power of existing tests and transform many mundane accessories (e.g., stethoscopes, shirts, watches) into sources of medically diagnostic information. Several key issues need to be addressed as computational algorithms are applied to clinical cardiology practice. Standards will likely need to be set, for example, on optimal approaches to testing and validation of these algorithms. Questions such as diversity of the training and testing sets and how to ensure that an algorithm will function similarly on data acquired at centers beyond the center(s) where the initial algorithm was developed are still evolving questions. Furthermore, studies are needed to understand how best to optimize real-time, clinical implementation of AI-enabled alerts. For example, AI algorithms that streamline data acquisition, interpretation, and reporting may be more easily integrated into practice. However, as such algorithms become more integrated into systems, the potential for human oversight and correction may decrease. In turn, AI-managed alerts that allow for advanced recognition of disease (e.g., EF from a 12-lead ECG) may not have significant impact if not implemented in such a way that physicians appropriately react to the alert. Large prospective studies to assess the impact on workflow and real-world impact are needed and are

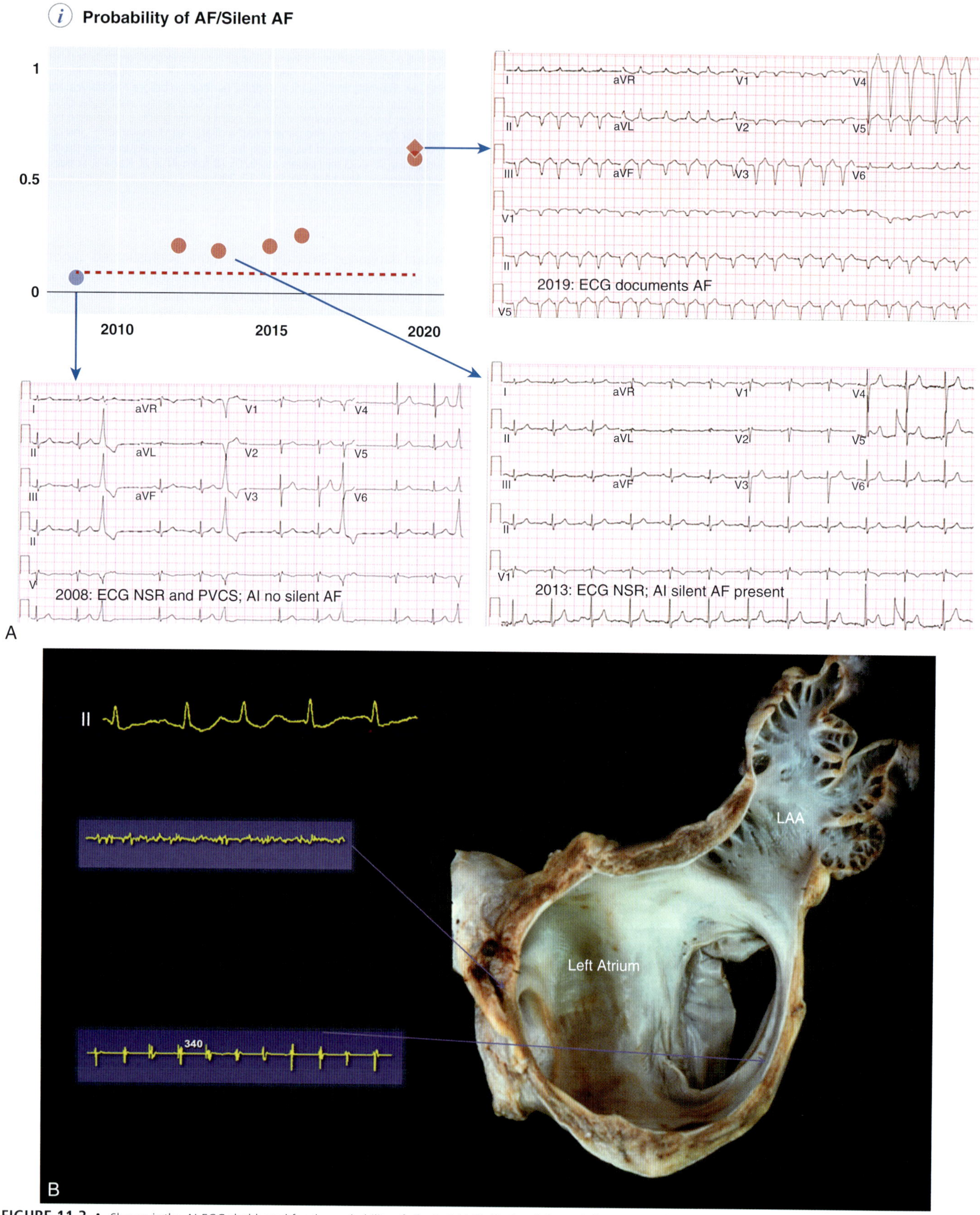

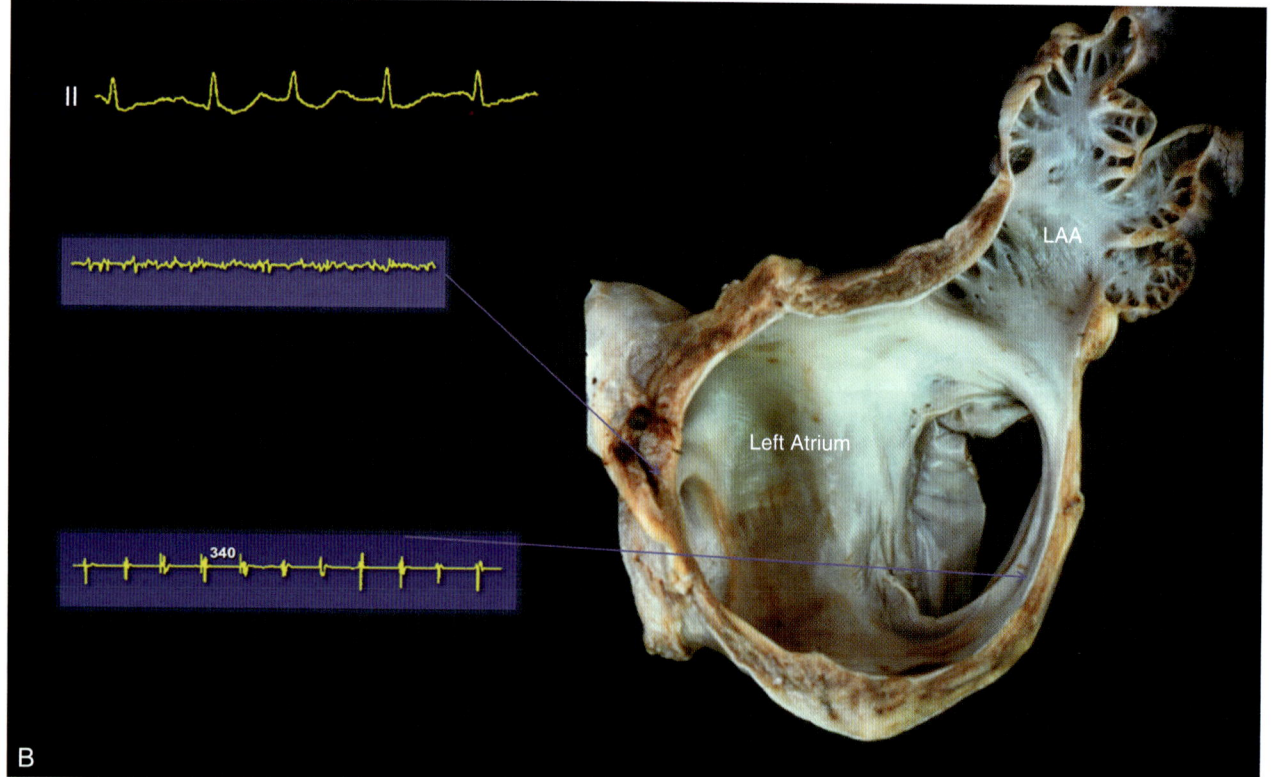

FIGURE 11.3 A, Shown is the AI-ECG dashboard for the probability of silent atrial fibrillation (AF; *top left*). In 2010, the probability of silent AF was low (representative ECG *bottom left*). From 2011 on, all ECG were recorded during sinus rhythm, but the AI ECG raised suspicion of episodic AF (*bottom right*, example from 2013), until 2019, when a tracing demonstrating AF was obtained. **B,** Surface ECG lead II (*top left*), intracardiac electrogram (EGM) acquired from interatrial septum (*left*, middle recording), and EGM acquired from the coronary sinus (*left*, bottom tracing). Note the continuous fractionated signals recorded at the septum, suggestive of fibrosis, as opposed to the discrete signals, separated by isoelectric intervals recorded simultaneously at the coronary sinus during atrial fibrillation. The structural changes and/or transient repolarization changes before or after atrial fibrillation (AF) episodes may lead to subtle changes on the ECG that are used by the AI ECG to determine episodic atrial fibrillation is present, although the mechanisms by which AI determines the presence of AF from an ECG recorded during NSR is not known. *AI*, Artificial intelligence.

underway.[41] Mayo Clinic has developed an AI dashboard accessible via the EMR that automatically ingests all ECGs available in the EMR and displays multiple AI analyses in an interactive, graphical format.

Other key areas of consideration when implementing AI and ML into clinical practice include how to allow for continuous adaptation of the algorithms to new data, associated regulatory implications, and how algorithms and data should interact. Continuous exposure to new data, which improves diversity of cases to which a clinician gets exposed thus improves clinical expertise. Ideally, systems that use AI algorithms will continue to evolve in response to their correct and incorrect interpretations, strengthening the overall model over time. However, the minimal standards to support regulatory approval of a given algorithm still require review. Furthermore, regulatory standards and approvals may vary between countries.[42] Finally, the question of how algorithms are practically deployed across institutions or countries remains to be determined. Many algorithms require such computational power as to only be operational in cloud-based systems. However, many data frameworks impose restrictions on sending data to centralized, cloud-based servers. Whether algorithms should be individually supplied to individual institutions (limiting the opportunity for continuous learning and leading to potential scalability issues due to the availability of adequate computational power at every local site) or enabled through cloud-based systems that allow data to be sent to a centralized framework (creating concerns regarding data sharing and data privacy) is an area of active discussion and will likely require policy discussions at a national and international level.

Pitfalls and Limitations of Artificial Intelligence in Cardiovascular Medicine

Despite the immense promise of ML, a number of considerations have impeded its development and require addressing. Before neural networks can be trained, data must be accessed in a usable format, and for many forms of ML, clearly labeled. This requires subject matter experts as well as technical experts. Data ownership remains an unresolved issue, particularly with patient data. Use of an individual's data in ML exposes them to risk of loss of privacy, and at the same time a third party may yield financial benefit, raising potential conflicts of interest. The training of many networks requires large quantities of data, often necessitating accumulation of data from more than a single institution, again with concerns relating to privacy and data ownership. There is currently a lack of well-established quality standards or a centralized clearinghouse for vetted technologies.

Deep learning has the capability to make deep connections within data but can only learn from data to which it was exposed. Any preexisting biases that lead to exclusion from the training set may lead to unreliable results when fed into a clinically used network. Examples have included a higher rate of misidentification of black versus white populations in facial recognition software. In medicine, false associations could lead to a prediction of increased mortality due to place of residence, socioeconomic status, and other nonmedical correlates.

Neural networks have been subject to adversarial attacks in which pixels are modified of an image with no visible effects to a human observer, yet with complete change in classification, the network output (Fig. 11.4). Such attacks could lead to misclassification and misdiagnosis and raise questions about the lack of understanding of the mechanism of network classification. This leads to the "black box issue" in that the components of a signal used by a network to make its determination are not known to humans, raising concerns about their broad spread deployment. Careful clinical testing and vetting can mitigate this concern.

Lastly, physician engagement and thoughtful assessment of workflow and implementation are essential for the adoption of AI tools in clinical practice. Technology-driven solutions (such as many EHRs) have paradoxically led to physician burnout and patient dissatisfaction and have failed to fulfill their promise. Careful attention to user interfaces, patient and physician use requirements, meticulous validation, and outcomes-based observations will be essential to permit AI to improve clinical practice.

CONCLUSIONS

In summary, the application of ML to physiologic data stands poised to transform the practice of medicine. Many AI algorithms will be integrated into devices used by clinicians (including the electronic medical record); others may be stand-alone tools. While AI is unlikely to replace physicians, physicians who use ML tools will likely supplant those who do not. Much like the electrocardiogram at the turn of the century or the echocardiogram several decades ago, ML offers new ways to probe an individual's current state and to gauge more accurately its future state, and thus work to improve the human condition. But as with any medical tool, it requires proper testing, validation, and prospective assessment, as well as a compassionate and caring clinician to deploy, apply, and interpret its findings to help the human seeking care.

REFERENCES

1. Lopez-Jimenez F, Attia Z, Arruda-Olson AM, et al. Artificial intelligence in cardiology: present and future. *Mayo Clin Proc*. 2020;95:1015–1039.
2. Shen C, Gonzalez Y, Klages P, et al. Intelligent inverse treatment planning via deep reinforcement learning, a proof-of-principle study in high dose-rate brachytherapy for cervical cancer. *Phys Med Biol*. 2019;64:115013.
3. Pipberger HV, Freis ED, Taback L, Mason HL. Preparation of electrocardiographic data for analysis by digital electronic computer. *Circulation*. 1960;21:413–418.
4. Caceres CA, Rikli AE. The digital computer as an aid in the diagnosis of cardiovascular disease. *Trans N Y Acad Sci*. 1961;23:240–245.
5. Caceres CA, Steinberg CA, Abraham S, et al. Computer extraction of electrocardiographic parameters. *Circulation*. 1962;25:356–362.
6. Rikli AE, Tolles WE, Steinberg CA, et al. Computer analysis of electrocardiographic measurements. *Circulation*. 1961;24:643–649.
7. Hannun AY, Rajpurkar P, Haghpanahi M, et al. Cardiologist-level arrhythmia detection and classification in ambulatory electrocardiograms using a deep neural network. *Nat Med*. 2019;25:65–69.
8. Ribeiro AH, Ribeiro MH, Paixao GMM, et al. Automatic diagnosis of the 12-lead ECG using a deep neural network. *Nat Commun*. 2020;11:1760.
9. Smith SW, Walsh B, Grauer K, et al. A deep neural network learning algorithm outperforms a conventional algorithm for emergency department electrocardiogram interpretation. *J Electrocardiol*. 2019;52:88–95.
10. Schlapfer J, Wellens HJ. Computer-interpreted electrocardiograms: benefits and limitations. *J Am Coll Cardiol*. 2017;70:1183–1192.
11. Halcox JPJ, Wareham K, Cardew A, et al. Assessment of remote heart rhythm sampling using the AliveCor heart monitor to screen for atrial fibrillation: the REHEARSE-AF study. *Circulation*. 2017;136:1784–1794.
12. Rajakariar K, Koshy AN, Sajeev JK, et al. Accuracy of a smartwatch based single-lead electrocardiogram device in detection of atrial fibrillation. *Heart*. 2020;106:665–670.
13. Wasserlauf J, You C, Patel R, et al. Smartwatch performance for the detection and quantification of atrial fibrillation. *Circ Arrhythm Electrophysiol*. 2019;12:e006834.
14. Perez MV, Mahaffey KW, Hedlin H, et al. Large-scale assessment of a smartwatch to identify atrial fibrillation. *N Engl J Med*. 2019;381:1909–1917.
15. Chung EH, Guise KD. QTC intervals can be assessed with the AliveCor heart monitor in patients on dofetilide for atrial fibrillation. *J Electrocardiol*. 2015;48:8–9.
16. Samol A, Bischof K, Luani B, et al. Single-Lead ECG recordings including Einthoven and Wilson Leads by a smartwatch: a new era of patient directed early ECG differential diagnosis of cardiac diseases? *Sensors*. 2019;19.
17. Ferdman DJ, Liberman L, Silver ES. A smartphone application to diagnose the mechanism of pediatric supraventricular tachycardia. *Pediatr Cardiol*. 2015;36:1452–1457.
18. Attia ZI, Kapa S, Lopez-Jimenez F, et al. Screening for cardiac contractile dysfunction using an artificial intelligence-enabled electrocardiogram. *Nat Med*. 2019;25:70–74.
19. Attia ZI, Noseworthy PA, Lopez-Jimenez F, et al. An artificial intelligence-enabled ECG algorithm for the identification of patients with atrial fibrillation during sinus rhythm: a retrospective analysis of outcome prediction. *Lancet*. 2019;394:861–867.
20. Ko WY, Siontis KC, Attia ZI, et al. Detection of hypertrophic cardiomyopathy using a convolutional neural network-enabled electrocardiogram. *J Am Coll Cardiol*. 2020;75:722–733.
21. Kwon JM, Jeon KH, Kim HM, et al. Comparing the performance of artificial intelligence and conventional diagnosis criteria for detecting left ventricular hypertrophy using electrocardiography. *Europace*. 2020;22:412–419.
22. Galloway CD, Valys AV, Shreibati JB, et al. Development and validation of a deep-learning model to screen for hyperkalemia from the electrocardiogram. *JAMA Cardiol*. 2019;4:428–436.
23. Attia ZI, Friedman PA, Noseworthy PA, et al. Age and sex estimation using artificial intelligence from standard 12-lead ECGs. *Circ Arrhythm Electrophysiol*. 2019;12:e007284.
24. Gomez J, Doukky R. Artificial intelligence in nuclear cardiology. *J Nucl Med*. 2019;60:1042–1043.
25. Seetharam K, Kagiyama N, Sengupta PP. Application of mobile health, telemedicine and artificial intelligence to echocardiography. *Echo Res Pract*. 2019;6:R41–R52.
26. Liu H, Bielinski SJ, Sohn S, et al. An information extraction framework for cohort identification using electronic health records. *AMIA Jt Summits Transl Sci Proc*. 2013;2013:149–153.
27. Dey D, Slomka PJ, Leeson P, et al. Artificial intelligence in cardiovascular imaging: JACC State-of-the-Art Review. *J Am Coll Cardiol*. 2019;73:1317–1335.
28. von Knebel Doeberitz PL, De Cecco CN, Schoepf UJ, et al. Coronary CT angiography-derived plaque quantification with artificial intelligence CT fractional flow reserve for the identification of lesion-specific ischemia. *Eur Radiol*. 2019;29:2378–2387.
29. Sardar P, Abbott JD, Kundu A, et al. Impact of artificial intelligence on interventional cardiology: from decision-making aid to advanced interventional procedure assistance. *JACC Cardiovasc Interv*. 2019;12:1293–1303.
30. Hill NR, Ayoubkhani D, McEwan P, et al. Predicting atrial fibrillation in primary care using machine learning. *PloS One*. 2019;14:e0224582.
31. Choi DJ, Park JJ, Ali T, Lee S. Artificial intelligence for the diagnosis of heart failure. *NPJ Digit Med*. 2020;3:54.
32. Xiao C, Ma T, Dieng AB, et al. Readmission prediction via deep contextual embedding of clinical concepts. *PloS One*. 2018;13:e0195024.
33. Upadhyaya SG, Murphree Jr DH, Ngufor CG, et al. Automated diabetes case identification using electronic health record data at a tertiary care facility. *Mayo Clin Proc Innov Qual Outcomes*. 2017;1:100–110.

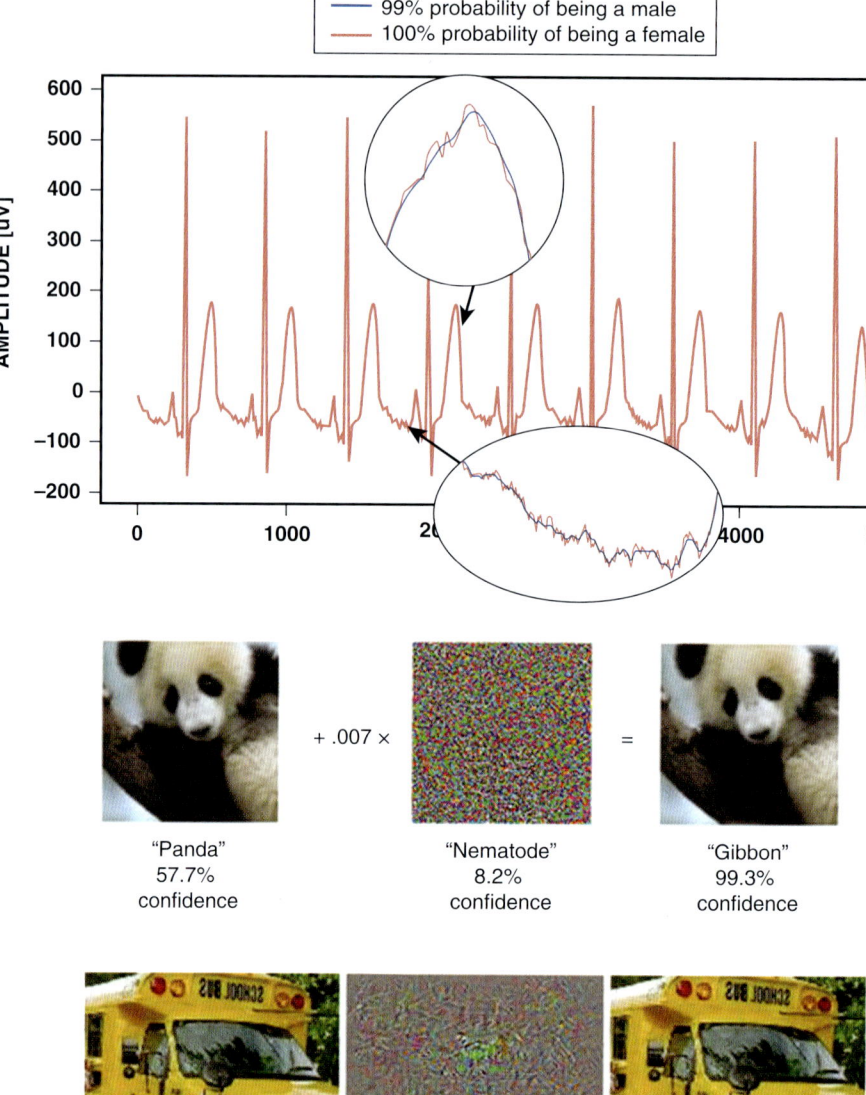

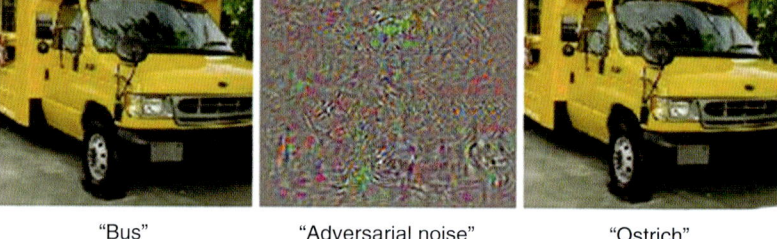

FIGURE 11.4 Examples of adversarial attacks on neural networks. An ECG *(blue tracing)* is correctly classified as being acquired from a man by a neural network. The addition of sub-clinical noise to the signal *(red tracing)* leads the network to misclassify the tracing as that belonging to a woman, despite the absence of significant change to a human observer. The images below the ECG depict similar adversarial network attacks against a network designed for image classification. The addition of apparent noise results in no visible change to a human observer, but misclassification of a panda as a gibbon by the network, as well as a similar disruption using a different image.

34. Afzal N, Sohn S, Abram S, et al. Mining peripheral arterial disease cases from narrative clinical notes using natural language processing. *J Vasc Surg*. 2017;65:1753–1761.
35. Kirby JC, Speltz P, Rasmussen LV, et al. PheKB: a catalog and workflow for creating electronic phenotype algorithms for transportability. *J Am Med Inform Assoc*. 2016;23:1046–1052.
36. Carroll RJ, Thompson WK, Eyler AE, et al. Portability of an algorithm to identify rheumatoid arthritis in electronic health records. *J Am Med Inform Assoc*. 2012;19:e162–e169.
37. Kho AN, Hayes MG, Rasmussen-Torvik L, et al. Use of diverse electronic medical record systems to identify genetic risk for type 2 diabetes within a genome-wide association study. *J Am Med Inform Assoc*. 2012;19:212–218.
38. Ritchie MD, Denny JC, Zuvich RL, et al. Genome- and phenome-wide analyses of cardiac conduction identifies markers of arrhythmia risk. *Circulation*. 2013;127:1377–1385.
39. Kawatkar A, Chu LH, Iyer R, et al. Development and validation of algorithms to identify acute diverticulitis. *Pharmacoepidemiol Drug Saf*. 2015;24:27–37.
40. Denny JC, Crawford DC, Ritchie MD, et al. Variants near FOXE1 are associated with hypothyroidism and other thyroid conditions: using electronic medical records for genome- and phenome-wide studies. *Am J Hum Genet*. 2011;89:529–542.
41. Yao X, McCoy RG, Friedman PA, et al. Clinical trial design data for electrocardiogram artificial intelligence-guided screening for low ejection fraction (EAGLE). *Data Brief*. 2020;28:104894.
42. He J, Baxter SL, Xu J, et al. The practical implementation of artificial intelligence technologies in medicine. *Nat Med*. 2019;25:30–36.

12

Wearable Devices in Cardiovascular Medicine

MINTU P. TURAKHIA

扫描二维码阅读
第12章中文导读

DEFINITIONS AND OVERVIEW, 117

ACTIVITY AND HEART RATE TRACKING FOR GENERAL CARDIOVASCULAR WELLNESS, 117

ATRIAL FIBRILLATION, 118
Photoplethysmography Detection of Irregular Rhythm, 118
Electrocardiogram, 119

HYPERTENSION, 120

CARDIAC REHABILITATION AND HEART FAILURE, 120

CARDIAC ARREST AND SUDDEN CARDIAC DEATH, 120

EVALUATION OF WEARABLE DATA AND NOTIFICATIONS, 120

Ancillary Information to the History, 120
Heart Rate and Rhythm Notifications, 120
Activity, Exercise, and Sleep, 121

LIMITATIONS, 121

THE FUTURE, 121

REFERENCES, 122

DEFINITIONS AND OVERVIEW

Wearable technology, commonly referred to as "wearables," represents a broad category of electronic, hands-free devices that are used for the measurement of physiologic signals, diagnosis of physiologic states or medical conditions, and treatment of disease. Eyeglasses, developed in 13th century, are considered to be the first wearable device. The contemporary definition refers to devices with microprocessors and connectivity to smartphones or a network. Colloquially, the term "wearables" more typically refers to technologies that can be directly acquired by the patient or consumer ("consumer-facing") and do not require interaction with the health care system for access. These devices are regarded as an example of the "Internet of Things."[1]

Wrist-worn wearables comprise almost half of the United States and international segments of the wearables market. Early wearables consisted of wristbands with dedicated functions for assessing the pulse rate and were geared toward fitness and wellness consumer markets. With advances in miniaturization, sensor technology, battery longevity, and lower manufacturing costs, these devices have become more complex and packed with a wide range of sensors. Contemporary smartwatches have the sensor capabilities to detect pulse and oxygen saturation (photoplethysmography [PPG]), movement and activity (accelerometer and gyroscope), distance and location (GPS), and sound (microphone) and record an electrocardiogram (ECG). Applications of machine learning and other forms of signal processing to streams of sensor data have enabled assessment of more complex parameters including sleep, 6-minute walk distance, irregular rhythms such as atrial fibrillation, fall detection, heart rate variability, sympathetic tone, and emotional health.

Wearable devices are part of a larger concept in medicine called, "digital health," which is a broad term that describes the application of digital information or data and communications technologies to improve patient health, population health, and care delivery. Digital health is a multidisciplinary domain that includes elements of mobile health, health information technology, wireless or connected health, big data, wearable technologies, telemedicine and remote care, precision and personalized medicine, genetics, and artificial intelligence. Digital health aims to improve all domains of medical care, including disease prevention, prediction, diagnosis, and treatment. Digital health and wearable technologies also offer solutions to improve enrollment and lower costs of clinical trials.

Cardiovascular disease has been a major focus of digital health for a variety of reasons. The sensors measure relevant physiologic parameters (heart rate, ECG), the prevalence and economic burden of disease is high, and evidence-based prevention and treatment therapies exist for a wide variety of conditions.

ACTIVITY AND HEART RATE TRACKING FOR GENERAL CARDIOVASCULAR WELLNESS

The first wearables entered the market in the consumer space for nonmedical use. In the 1970s and 1980s, calculator watches and portable music players first demonstrated the ability of placing microprocessors on compact and wearable devices. In 1987, digital hearing aids were released. In 1994, the first ECG-based smartwatches were released as physician-prescribed event recorders (Fig. 12.1). In 2009, the first major clip-on wearable devices launched and measured step counts, walking distance, and activity using an accelerometer. In the mid 2000s, the field converged to developing wrist-worn devices that embedded more sensor types, including gyroscopes and PPG.

Accelerometers can measure linear acceleration. These sensors have long been used for activity tracking including in implantable pacemakers. However, accelerometers alone are unable to differentiate type of activity. Gyroscopes sense rotation. Used together as an inertia measurement unit (IMU), the two sensors provide greater accuracy to classify gait (walking, running), exercise type, stair climbing, sleep, and even fall detection. IMUs are primarily deployed by smartwatch software for activity and exercise tracking. Built-in or smartphone-paired global positioning systems allow for more accurate estimations of distances traveled compared with pedometer calculations. Accuracy of calorie expenditure estimation is less accurate.

Most wrist-worn wearable devices have heart rate tracking. PPG is an inexpensive optical measurement technique that can estimate relative changes in blood flow. A light source is aimed at the skin, typically underneath the face of the head of the fitness band or watch. An adjacent photodetector measures the reflected light, which can estimate relative changes in blood volume. With continuous sampling, PPG can capture the cardiac cycle and estimate the pulse rate. The peak represents systole, the nadir represents diastole, and the difference approximates the relative pulse pressure. A dicrotic notch from aortic valve closure may also be detected. PPG can also measure oxygen saturation via oximetry, although most consumer watches do not provide the user this information. The core function of PPG remains

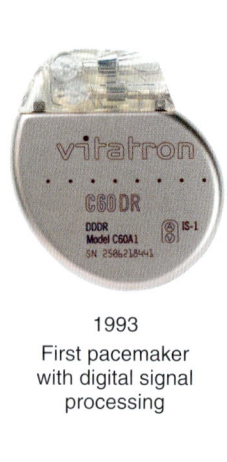
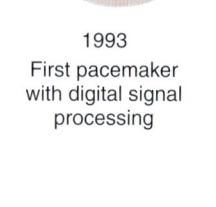
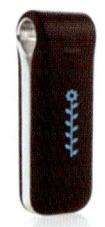
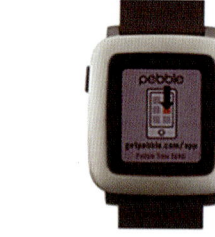
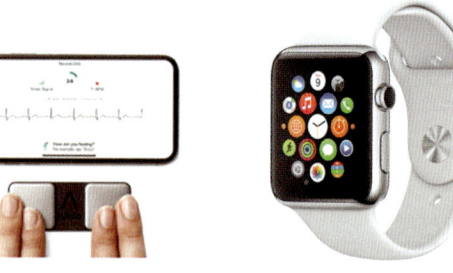
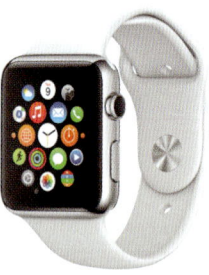
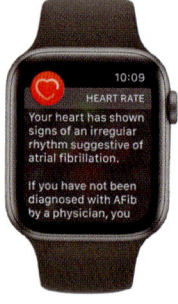
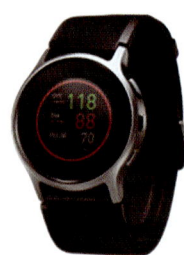

FIGURE 12.1 Timeline of wearable devices. (From Vitatron International; BioTelemetry, Inc; Google; AliveCor. Screenshots reprinted with permission from Apple Inc. Heart-Guide image courtesy of OMRON Healthcare, Inc.)

measurement of pulse rate. To preserve battery life and accuracy, heart rate sampling is typically noncontinuous and often opportunistic and will increase during exercise modes or with user-initiated measurement. On some watches, users may activate notifications for tachycardia and bradycardia during periods of inactivity (heart rate–activity discordance). The accuracy of PPG-based pulse rate may vary slightly based on the hardware, software, skin color, movement, ectopic beats, and heart rate (e.g., due to decreased ventricular filling in severe tachycardia).

ATRIAL FIBRILLATION

Photoplethysmography Detection of Irregular Rhythm

Time series analysis of PPG-derived pulse assessment can identify patterns in the pulse. Quantification of pulse rate variability or machine learning–based algorithms have been shown to successfully discriminate between sinus rhythm and atrial fibrillation using a variety of approaches.[2]

Early approaches to identify atrial fibrillation were based on a conceptual framework similar to ambulatory ECG interpretation, which is to examine a 30-second interval of pulses. This was successfully performed with transillumination of the finger from a smartphone flashlight and detection by the adjacent camera.[3] Eventually, the strategy was applied to watches. As the use cases expanded from fitness and wellness to diagnosis and disease management, these tools required greater regulatory oversight and clearance (Fig. 12.2). An early attempt using third-party software on the Apple Watch had low specificity and positive predictive value.[4] Subsequent approaches for irregular pulse identification were developed for high specificity, using a probabilistic approach of confirmatory pulse checks over hours or days. An algorithm designed for the Apple Series 1, 2, and 3 watches (Apple Inc, Cupertino, CA)[5] intermittently and passively measures pulse over 1 minute to generate a beat-to-beat pulse tachogram (Fig. 12.3). If this tachogram meets irregularity criteria, then the algorithm temporarily increases the sampling frequency. If five out of six consecutive tachograms met irregularity criteria, then the algorithm notifies the user of an irregular rhythm. Therefore, unlike the classical ECG definition of AF, which requires a consecutive duration of only 30 seconds, this PPG-based algorithm is probabilistic, requiring multiple episodes to meet criteria (see Fig. 12.3), and is therefore considered less sensitive, especially for very short AF episodes, but much more specific.

The Apple algorithm was tested at scale in a single-arm, unblinded, investigational device exemption study.[6] Inclusion criteria included age ≥22, possession of compatible Apple watches and phones, no prior history of AF, and U.S. residency. Over an 8-month period between 2017 and 2018, the study enrolled 419,297 U.S. participants. Overall 0.52% of participants received an irregular rhythm notification. Among 450 participants with notifications who received ambulatory ECG patch monitoring, AF was a detected on that patch in 34% (97.5% CI 29% to 39%). The positive predictive value for an irregular rhythm notification was 0.84 (95% CI 0.76 to 0.92). Because only notified participants received "gold standard" ECG monitoring, the study was unable to assess sensitivity or specificity.

Studies similar in design have been performed to test similar PPG-based algorithms on other smartwatch platforms. The Huawei Heart Study enrolled 246,541 participants in China to evaluate a fitness band and smartwatch and had directionally similar results, although a lower proportion receiving notifications, possibly due to a younger population or greater algorithm specificity.[7] In May 2020, Fitbit launched its own study to evaluate an algorithm on their device platform with target enrollment of 100,000 participants (https://clinicaltrials.gov/ct2/show/NCT04380415, accessed September 5, 2020).

Although these studies indicate the promise for undiagnosed AF detection in an at-risk population, the FDA views this class of algorithms as *prediagnostic* tools, rather than serving as more definitive

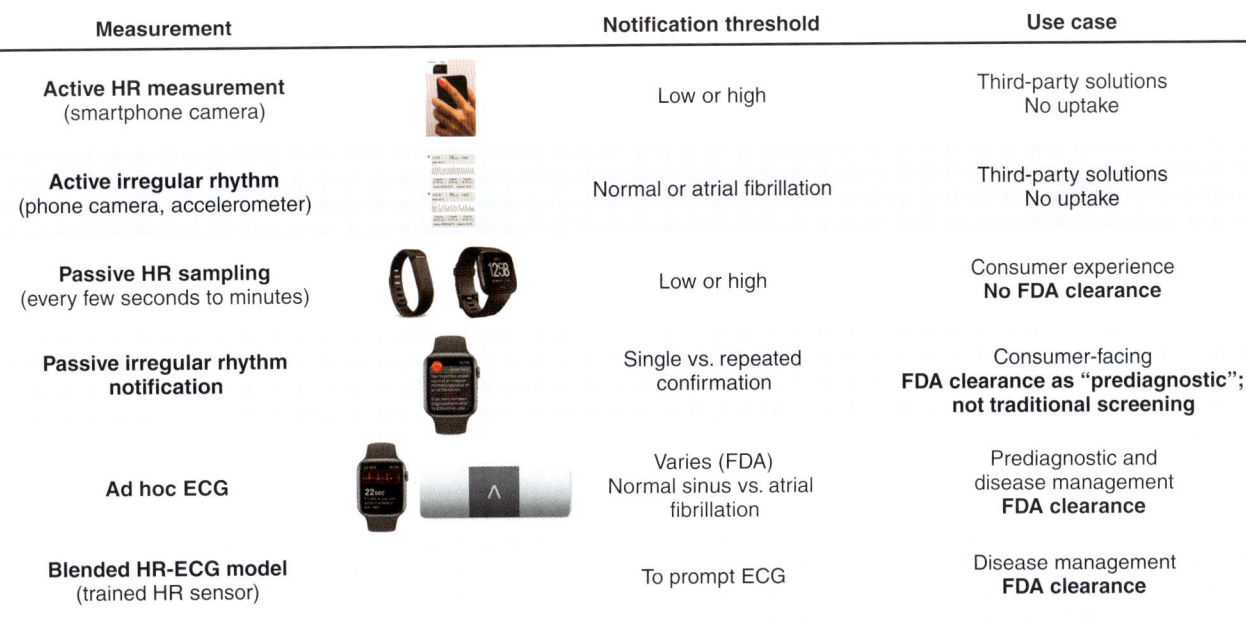

FIGURE 12.2 Evolution of consumer-facing photoplethysmography pulse measurement. (From Google, AliveCor. Screenshots reprinted with permission from Apple Inc.)

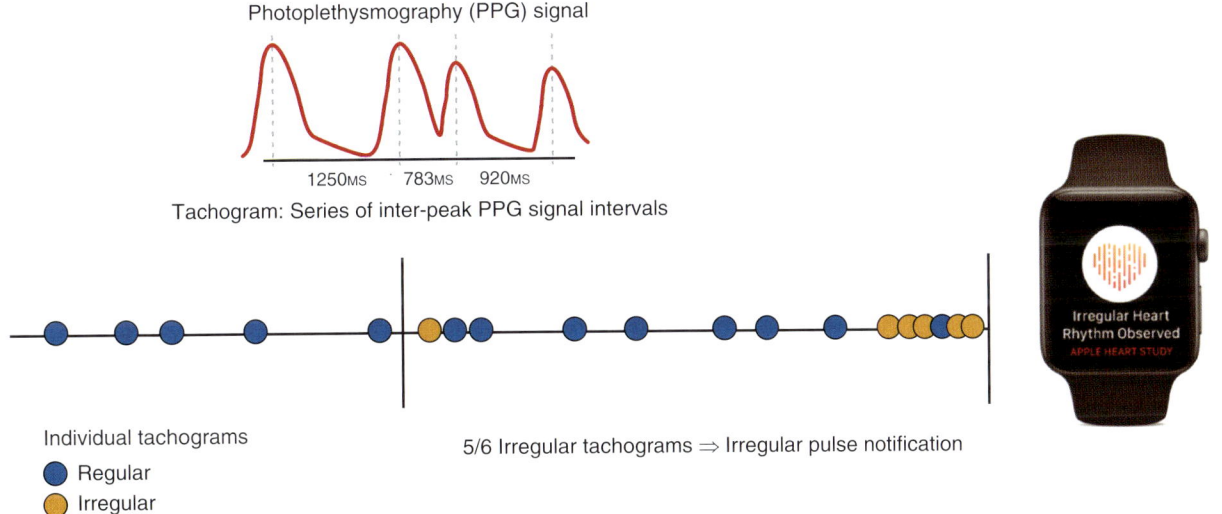

FIGURE 12.3 Irregular pulse detection algorithm. (From Perez M, Mahaffey KW, Hedlin H, et al. Large-scale assessment of a smartwatch to identify atrial fibrillation. *N Engl J Med.* 2019;381[20]:1909–1917.)

diagnostic tests. On the Apple platform, consumers must opt in to enable these features on their watches. In doing so, they receive onboarding that includes education. Because the sensitivity of these tests is not known and because they are enabled by the user rather than by a clinician as a public health intervention, these tools do not meet the classical Wilson-Jungner criteria for screening tests. Presently, there are no professional society or U.S. Preventative Services Task Force recommendations for their use for AF surveillance, screening, or diagnosis.

Electrocardiogram

More recent smartwatch models (Apple Watch Series 4 or higher, Samsung Galaxy Watch 3) have FDA-cleared single-lead ECG capability (see Fig. 12.1). The user actively records a 30-second lead I (right arm [–] to left arm [+]) ECG on the watch by pressing the crown with a finger of the hand opposite the hand with the watch body electrode. However, the first major smartphone-connected ECG was released in 2013 (AliveCor, Mountain View, CA). The Kardia device has two electrodes (one for each hand) and communicates wirelessly to a smartphone. A new six-lead consumer version (Kardia 6L) is now available that uses the right leg for additional limb and derived ECG leads.

Consumer-based ECG devices entail substantial limitations. Compared with medical 12-lead systems and patch-based ECG monitors, smartphone-connected and smartwatch ECG devices tend to have significantly more artifact. To counter this, aggressive filtering and baseline drift correction may be applied, which may obscure important ECG features. For example, a smartwatch algorithm incorrectly labeled a tracing of atrial tachycardia as atrial fibrillation (Fig. 12.4). Careful review shows that atrial tachycardia P waves have been attenuated due to filtering, which was clearly present on the medical 12-lead ECG. However, ST changes during acute coronary syndromes as measured by the Apple Watch in all 12 lead positions have shown good agreement with medical grade systems.[8]

Another major caveat is that consumer-based ECG systems also do not provide comprehensive prediagnostic information across a variety of rhythms compared with medical grade systems. Numerous examples of incorrect diagnosis, including of sustained ventricular arrhythmias, have been documented. Moreover, a ventricular rate that is out

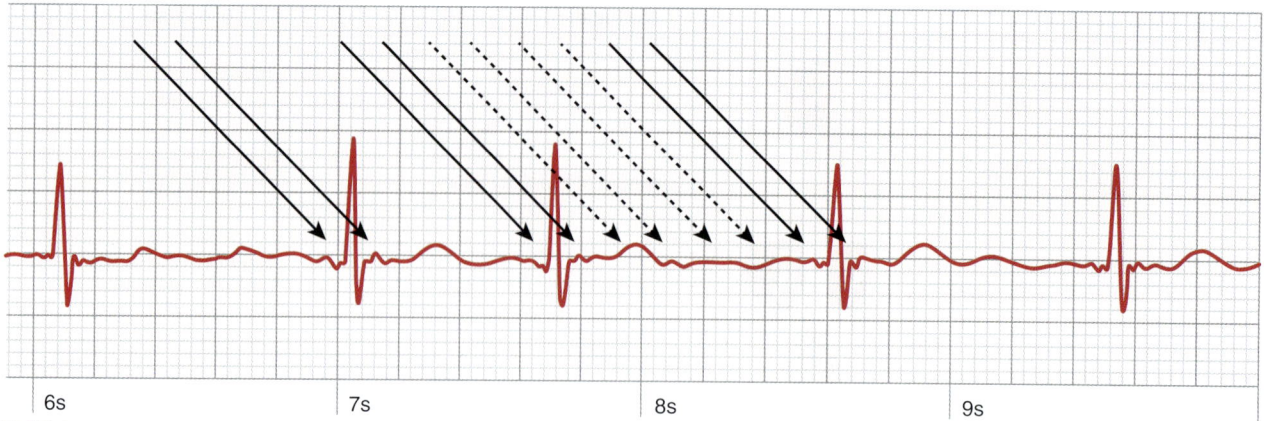

FIGURE 12.4 Atrial tachycardia misdiagnosed as atrial fibrillation due to filter attenuation. Careful observation of this Apple Watch electrocardiogram (ECG) rhythm strip identifies discrete organized atrial activity denoted by the solid arrows. The dashed arrows indicate atrial activity that appears attenuated due to filtering. A 12-lead ECG identified a macro-reentrant stable atrial tachycardia. Watch sampling was 513 Hz with 10 mm/mV gain and 25 mm/sec paper speed.

of range (<50 or >100) prevents automated ECG interpretation on the Apple Watch.

HYPERTENSION

There are hundreds of smartphone applications that allow the user to enter his or her blood pressure and track it and other vital signs over time. However, smartwatch applications and hardware that enable the device to measure blood pressure are relatively new. There are many unregulated smartphone apps that provide a blood pressure measurement based on pulse transit time derived from the PPG tracing. One such app has been found to be highly inaccurate, despite almost 150,000 paid downloads.[9] Many smartwatches available on online retail stores claim to measure blood pressure but do not have FDA clearance.

One smartwatch with FDA clearance for blood pressure uses traditional oscillometric measurement by using an inflatable cuff on the watch for blood pressure measurement (Omron Healthcare, Kyoto, Japan) (see Fig. 12.1). This watch connects to smartphones for transfer of information. A watch that uses PPG-derived pulse information to estimate blood pressure has received regulatory approval in South Korea (Samsung, South Korea) (https://news.samsung.com/global/samsung-launches-the-samsung-health-monitor-application-with-blood-pressure-measurement, accessed September 7, 2020). The device's artificial intelligence algorithm is trained and calibrated to an individual user's cuff readings. After sufficient training, the algorithm can be used to directly estimate blood pressure from the PPG data. The device is not yet approved in the United States.

CARDIAC REHABILITATION AND HEART FAILURE

Activity sensing and heart rate detection have been applied as measurement tools for heart failure and cardiac rehabilitation. Smartphone-based 6-minute walk assessments have shown high accuracy across a range of devices, applications, and disease states, including heart failure[10] and peripheral arterial disease.[11] Smart devices may have application programing interfaces to access step counts and distance traveled recorded by the watch rather than needing to access the raw data to derive these counts. Behavioral science and gamification have been incorporated into digital cardiac rehabilitation platforms. Although telehealth cardiac rehabilitation has proven at least as effective as center-based rehabilitation,[12] there remain relatively sparse randomized data on the efficacy of using mobile technology.[13]

In heart failure, mobile technology applications have focused on identifying patients at risk of heart failure and disease management (see also Chapter 11). Deep learning techniques applied to single- and multi-lead ECGs can identify systolic dysfunction with high discrimination (c-statistic 0.93),[14] although this has not been deployed in practice

at scale. A pragmatic trial is ongoing (NCT04000087). Sensor technologies to assess pulmonary congestion (thoracic impedance) and cardiac filling and emptying (ballistocardiography, seismocardiography) appear feasible but require larger trials.[15] Machine learning–based detection of obstructive hypertrophic cardiomyopathy using wearable-derived PPG has shown high discrimination.[16]

CARDIAC ARREST AND SUDDEN CARDIAC DEATH

Without reliable continuous blood pressure, ECG monitoring, or the ability to deliver therapy, treatment of cardiac arrest from a wearable sensor is challenging. Fall detection on wearable devices can be configured to call emergency medical services. Assessment of hemodynamics or circulatory arrest, if accurate, could be used to trigger medical response and bystander cardiopulmonary resuscitation.[17]

EVALUATION OF WEARABLE DATA AND NOTIFICATIONS

Ancillary Information to the History

In patients with symptoms concerning for arrhythmia, pulse rate data may be useful to correlate heart rate at time of symptoms, similar to ambulatory ECG monitoring (Fig. 12.5A). A patient can be asked by the clinician if they may view the data together on the patient's phone. It is recommended that the phone be kept by the patient and that the clinician directs him or her to access the data. This method ensures transparency and also serves to teach patients to navigate their health information on their smartphone.

If tachycardia or bradycardia is found, the activity or exercise measurement and time of day may provide useful clues as to the arrhythmia trigger and reliability of the tracing (see Fig. 12.5B). Pulse rate data may also be useful to assess ventricular response in atrial fibrillation. However, PPG may significantly and unpredictably underestimate (or overestimate) ventricular rate, especially during rapid atrial fibrillation or in the presence of structural disease such as aortic stenosis. In patients with tachycardia during AF, only 15% of earlier generation Fitbit devices and 60% of Apple Watch readings were within 10 beats of the actual ventricular rate.[18] The use of pulse rate data during syncope can be useful but must be interpreted with caution because a fall can create mechanical artifact that may create spurious readings. Patients with smart ECG devices can be counseled to immediately take an ECG if and when they have recurrent symptoms.

Heart Rate and Rhythm Notifications

Based on the positive predictive value of 0.84, a smartwatch irregular rhythm notification in a patient with no prior history of AF must

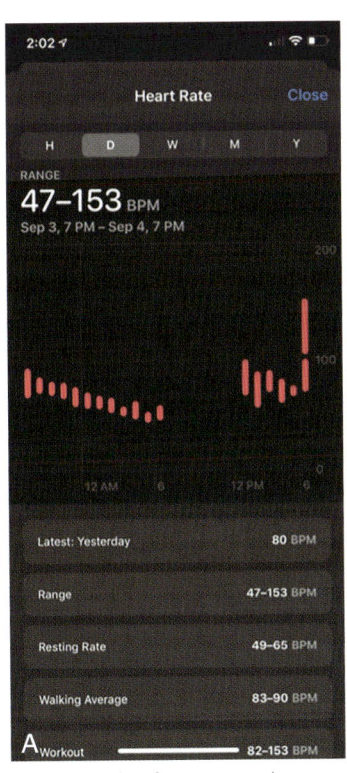 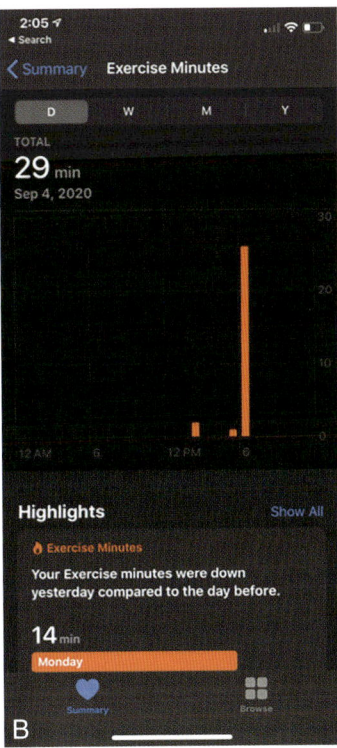 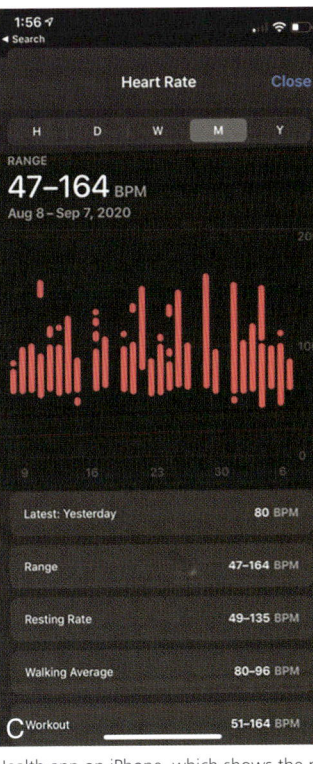

FIGURE 12.5 Pulse and activity data from a smart phone app. Data shown are pulse rate data in the Apple Health app on iPhone, which shows the pulse rate data sampled from the paired Apple Watch (Apple Inc, Cupertino, CA). **A,** Day level data show an abrupt rise in heart rate at 6 PM. **B,** Corresponding rise in activity (exercise), which is the likely cause of the tachycardia. **C,** Month level display of heart rates, which can be useful in the assessment of rate control of atrial fibrillation. (Screenshots reprinted with permission from Apple Inc.)

be taken seriously (Table 12.1). **Confirmation by an ECG is essential; the irregular rhythm notification alone is insufficient for clinical diagnosis.** The notification should prompt the clinician to ask a series of questions in the history no different than for subjective complaints: date, time, place, and context of what the patient was doing at the time of the notification. The patient should also be asked of prior notifications that were silenced or ignored. The smartphone app can also be used to collect more details and search for prior notifications.

In 25% of Apple Heart Study participants that received a notification, AF was present throughout the entire ambulatory ECG recording.[6] Therefore, an ECG taken by the patient on their watch or smart device may, with clinician verification, provide an immediate diagnosis (see Table 12.1). If AF is not present at the time of ECG, then ambulatory ECG monitoring of a minimum of 7 days and preferably 14 should be performed. If these two tests do not reveal AF, then consideration may be given for repeat ambulatory ECG monitoring or to counsel the patient to take an ECG if another notification is received. **Irregular rhythm notification alone does not suffice to make a clinical diagnosis of AF without ECG confirmation.** The feature is also not FDA cleared for use for AF disease management.

If non-AF arrhythmias are detected with ECG testing, then the clinician should inquire about symptom-arrhythmia correlation because many of ambulatory ECG findings such as infrequent atrial or ventricular ectopy could be inconsequential (see Table 12.1). Frequent or sustained non-AF rhythms could trigger irregular rhythm notifications. An appropriate work-up for these rhythms may be indicated.

Patients may also present with tachycardia or bradycardia notifications (see Table 12.1). On the Apple Watch, these are opt-in notifications where the user may set a specific threshold to be notified if the heart rate is greater than (default >120 beats/min) or less than (default <40 beats/min) specific rates while being inactive for a period of 10 minutes. Again, clinical attention should be given to the context and history. Watching sports or a movie, for example, could trigger tachycardia, and bradycardia during sleep may be normal. These features are not likely to detect exercise-induced or transient arrhythmias.

Activity, Exercise, and Sleep

The movement tracking features may be useful to provide a general sense of baseline level of activity and exercise. However, automated exercise logging, step counts, and sleep can be inaccurate, and these data are used best together with a history and patient report of activity.

LIMITATIONS

Despite the rapid innovation and incorporation of hardware and software into consumer wearables, progress has been slow to develop these tools into durable, disease management solutions. Electronic health record (EHR) integration is not robust or widely available; patients often communicate with their doctors or care team with their wearable data by electronic mail or messaging. In contrast, remote monitoring of cardiac implantable electronic devices (pacemakers, defibrillators, heart failure sensors) have tailored clinical software applications, mature workflows, stable reimbursement, clinical trials, professional society guideline recommendations, and a career path for allied health professional education.

THE FUTURE

Despite these limitations, rapid and sustained clinical adoption is likely. Large randomized trials that aim to evaluate hard outcomes are emerging. The HEARTLINE study (NCT04276441) aims to randomize 150,000 persons age ≥65 years to a smartwatch with AF detection capabilities and a study app for digital health engagement. Outcomes include clinical diagnosis of AF, anticoagulation adherence, and incidence of a composite cardiovascular outcome. Other studies are in various stages of development.

The introduction of new reimbursement codes in the United States for remote patient monitoring is expected to catalyze adoption by clinicians, practices, and health care systems. The dramatic post-pandemic shift to telehealth, including virtual visits and asynchronous care, has created new unmet needs for at-home complex cardiac diagnostics

TABLE 12.1 Management of Wearable and Smartwatch Pulse Notifications

For All Notifications

- Obtain a full detailed history for context (date, time, place, symptoms) surrounding the notification
- Ask the patient if you may view the data together on the patient's smartphone or watch; it is recommended that the patient hold the phone while the clinician directs him or her to access the data if needed
- On the phone or watch, examine the heart rate, activity, and exercise data for useful clues (time of day, whether exercising, and heart rate before and after the notification)
- Ask if this is the first notification or if there were others. The notifications can usually be found on the notification history on the connected smartphone
- Determine if the patient's watch has an ECG feature or if the patient may have other smartphone ECG devices

Tachycardia Notification	Irregular Rhythm Notification	Bradycardia Notification

• Several watch manufacturers can notify users of HR-activity discordance
• Algorithm will notify user if HR exceeds user-defined threshold (usually >100–150 beats/min) for more than 10 min while not active (based on embedded accelerometer or gyroscope)
• Assess if heart rate is appropriate (stress, anxiety, pain, dehydration, pregnancy, systemic illness, fever, deconditioning). If appropriate sinus tachycardia, then no further arrhythmia evaluation may be needed
• Examine pulse and obtain a medical-grade ECG
• Pursue appropriate diagnostic cardiac evaluation
  ○ Consider ambulatory ECG monitoring of 7–14 days or event recording of up to 30 days
	• An irregular rhythm notification alone should not be used to make the diagnosis of AF without ECG confirmation
	• The irregular rhythm notification feature is not cleared by the FDA for disease management or surveillance of established AF
	• As of January 2021, this notification is only available in the United States on the Apple watch series of products. Other hardware may access similar algorithms via the use of third-party software.
	• Determine if the patient has a history of documented arrhythmias that could explain these findings
	• Ask and look for whether a smartwatch-based ECG was taken at or near the time of notification. Counsel patient to do this when a notification is received, even in the absence of symptoms.
	• Examine pulse, and obtain a medical-grade ECG
	• If AF is not present, then perform ambulatory ECG monitoring of 7–14 days
	  ○ Consider repeat ECG monitoring based on clinical suspicion if initial test if negative
	  ○ If non-AF rhythms are identified, then inquire about symptom-arrhythmia correlation as these may be inconsequential
	• If arrhythmias are identified then pursue work-up with appropriate diagnostic evaluation
		• Algorithm will notify user if HR is less than a user-defined threshold (<40–50 beats/min) for more than 10 min
		• Examine pulse and obtain a medical-grade ECG.
		  • If there is sinus rhythm, then determine if response is normal and physiologic (high vagal tone) or secondary (medications, hypothyroidism, sleep apnea, other illnesses)
		• If rhythm is not sinus, then evaluate for structural heart disease and primary electrical disease
		• If symptoms are associated with bradycardia (presyncope, syncope, exercise intolerance), then consider ambulatory ECG monitoring and evaluation for structural heart disease
		• If there are no symptoms, then consider ambulatory ECG or diagnostic tests to look for chronotropic incompetence (exercise treadmill testing)

ECG, Electrocardiogram.

and remote monitoring. In the future, sensor technologies may move away from a wearable framework and toward contactless sensing. Sensors in the home may detect and differentiate changes in vital signs, cardiac rhythm, activity, habits, medication adherence, and psychometrics for each household member. Behavioral incentives for good health may be embedded outside of traditional health care and insurance services and on to platform technologies in computing, retail, and social media. Low-cost, minimally invasive microsensors and microimplantables may also have a role where greater sensor fidelity is needed.

REFERENCES

1. Islam SMR, Kwak D, Kabir MDH, et al. The Internet of things for health care: a comprehensive survey. *IEEE Access*. 2015;3:678–708.

Atrial Fibrillation and Other Arrythmias

2. Pereira T, Tran N, Gadhoumi K, et al. Photoplethysmography based atrial fibrillation detection: a review. *NPJ Digit Med*. 2020;3(1):3.
3. O'Sullivan JW, Grigg S, Crawford W, et al. Accuracy of smartphone camera applications for detecting atrial fibrillation. *JAMA Netw Open*. 2020;3(4):e202064.
4. Tison GH, Sanchez JM, Ballinger B, et al. Passive detection of atrial fibrillation using a commercially available smartwatch. *JAMA Cardiol*. 2018;3(5):409.
5. Turakhia MP, Desai M, Hedlin H, et al. Rationale and design of a large-scale, app-based study to identify cardiac arrhythmias using a smartwatch: the Apple Heart Study. *Am Heart J*. 2018. https://doi.org/10.1016/j.ahj.2018.09.002. Published online September.
6. Perez MV, Mahaffey KW, Hedlin H, et al. Large-scale assessment of a smartwatch to identify atrial fibrillation. *New Engl J Med*. 2019;381(20):1909–1917.
7. Guo Y, Wang H, Zhang H, et al. Mobile photoplethysmographic technology to detect atrial fibrillation. *J Am Coll Cardiol*. 2019;74(19):2365–2375.
8. Spaccarotella CAM, Polimeni A, Migliarino S, et al. Multichannel electrocardiograms obtained by a smartwatch for the diagnosis of ST-Segment changes. *JAMA Cardiol*. 2020;5(10).

Other Cardiovascular Applications

9. Plante TB, Urrea B, MacFarlane ZT, et al. Validation of the instant blood pressure smartphone app. *JAMA Intern Med*. 2016;176(5):700.
10. Brooks GC, Vittinghoff E, Iyer S, et al. Accuracy and usability of a self-administered 6-minute walk test smartphone application. *Circ Heart Fail*. 2015;8(5):905–913.
11. Ata R, Gandhi N, Rasmussen H, et al. Clinical validation of smartphone-based activity tracking in peripheral artery disease patients. *NPJ Digit Med*. 2018;1(1):66.
12. Rawstorn JC, Gant N, Direito A, et al. Telehealth exercise-based cardiac rehabilitation: a systematic review and meta-analysis. *Heart*. 2016;102(15):1183.
13. Beatty AL, Fukuoka Y, Whooley MA. Using mobile technology for cardiac rehabilitation: a review and framework for development and evaluation. *J Am Heart Assoc*. 2013;2(6):e000568.
14. Attia ZI, Kapa S, Lopez-Jimenez F, et al. Screening for cardiac contractile dysfunction using an artificial intelligence–enabled electrocardiogram. *Nat Med*. 2018;25(1):1–9.
15. DeVore AD, Wosik J, Hernandez AF. The future of wearables in heart failure patients. *JACC Heart Fail*. 2019;7(11):922–932.
16. Green EM, Mourik R van, Wolfus C, et al. Machine learning detection of obstructive hypertrophic cardiomyopathy using a wearable biosensor. *NPJ Digit Med*. 2019;2(1):57.
17. Narayan SM, Wang PJ, Daubert JP. New concepts in sudden cardiac arrest to address an intractable epidemic: JACC state-of-the-art review. *J Am Coll Cardiol*. 2019;73(1):70–88.
18. Koshy AN, Sajeev JK, Nerlekar N, et al. Smart watches for heart rate assessment in atrial arrhythmias. *Int J Cardiol*. 2018;266:124–127.

第三部分　患者的评估

张力　导读

对患者的评估是疾病诊疗的关键环节。随着医学的发展，心血管疾病的评估手段也逐渐增多，包括体格检查、心脏超声、计算机断层成像（CT）、磁共振、核素显像、冠状动脉造影以及血管内功能评估等。本部分详细阐述了目前心血管检查的主要方法及其临床应用。

体格检查始终是临床诊疗工作中的重要手段，也是心血管科医生必须掌握的基本技能。许多疾病通过体格检查发现的典型症状或体征即可基本诊断，如典型的心绞痛症状、血压升高或降低、心脏杂音、脉搏/心律不规律等。此外，详细的病史采集以及必要的全身体格检查也能提供大量线索，本部分第13章有具体论述。

心电图自1901年发明以来，迅速成为最常用、最基本的心脏血管及电生理的评估方法。第14章详细阐述了心脏电生理活动的基本特征、心电图采集的原理、正常或正常变异心电图形的特点以及异常心电图表现和诊断标准，有助于心血管科医生深入了解异常心电活动的产生机制，并提高心电图的阅读、诊断能力。

某些心血管疾病，如稳定型心绞痛，患者在静息状态下无心绞痛症状体征，且无心电图阳性发现。此时可在对患者进行安全评估后行运动负荷试验同时记录心电图变化。运动负荷试验因其设备要求低、管理操作简单、结果可靠且易解读，已在临床上广泛应用于多种心血管疾病，如冠心病、心脏瓣膜疾病、心肌病等患者的评估及预后预测。关于运动负荷试验的生理学基础（心肌氧供与氧耗平衡）、器械种类、试验流程及临床应用在第15章进行了详细论述。

超声心动图是目前最常用的、全面评估心脏功能与结构的检查方法，可获得心室舒缩功能、心腔形状及大小、瓣膜结构与运动、血流动力学等信息。其优点在于实时简便、可实现床旁快速检查以及价格低廉，但测量结果受操作者主观因素影响较大，需要经过长期专业培训以提高测量数据的准确性及可重复性。近年来，经食管超声心动图（TEE）因其较高的空间分辨率以及较少的伪影干扰，在临床上获得较大规模的普及，尤其在评估瓣膜功能、心内膜炎及心脏肿瘤方面具有独特的优势。负荷超声心动图通过评估运动状态下的心肌缺血程度以及瓣膜运动变化，实现心肌活力的测定以及瓣膜病的补充诊断。此外，3D超声心动图、组织应变成像、增强超声心动图等技术进一步拓宽了超声心动图的应用范围并提高了可视化能力（具体详见第16章）。

胸部X线检查对疾病的诊断同样能提供大量信息，并且可对重症患者行快速床旁检查，故其临床价值不可被忽视。通过胸部正侧位影像，可对多种心血管疾病进行初步诊断，如通过心影以及大血管的形态改变对结构性心脏病进行评估；通过肺水肿表现对左心衰竭严重程度进行评估等。其成像原理、解读以及临床应用详见第17章。

核心脏病学（SPECT及PET）通过静脉注射放射性核素对心血管系统进行显像，其主要优势在于功能学评估。通过与CT、MRI结合，如SPECT/CT、PET/CT/MRI，实现技术间的优势互补，从而获得高质量的影像与准确的测量结果，对心脏及血管进行更全面的评估。此外，通过定量技术，可计算整体或局部心肌血流流速。再结合负荷灌注成像，即可得出心肌血流储备，对缺血性心脏病、心肌病的诊断与评估具有重要意义，且为冠状动脉微循环障碍无创诊断的"金标准"。此外，核素显像还可评估心肌细胞活性、缺血程度等代谢性指标。但由于设备要求及检查费用较高，在一定程度上限制了其临床应用。具体成像原理、应用及解读见第18章。

心脏MRI（CMR）与CT的优势在于高时空分辨率、高质量图像以及3D重建，可对多种心血管形态、结构异常做出准确、客观的判断。CMR通过采用多种序列以及增强成像，可提供生理学相关的功能性指标以及对心肌血流灌注进行量化，对冠心病、心肌疾病、心脏瓣膜疾病以及心外膜疾病的诊断以及预后预测具有重要价值。心脏CT平扫可评估且量化冠状动脉斑块钙化情况并对患者进行危险分层，而CTA由于其高特异性，临床上多用于可疑冠心病的排除诊断。此外CTA还是经导管主动脉瓣置换术（TAVR）、经导管二尖瓣置换术（TMVR）等结构性心脏病介入术围术期的主要评估手段。近年来，人工智能（AI）飞速发展，未来将AI与CMR和CT结合，有望进一步增加检查效率、降低辐射剂量与费用、提高结果的准确性及一致性（第19、20章）。

尽管如此，冠状动脉造影依然是诊断冠心病的"金标准"，可同时提供冠状动脉解剖学与功能学信息，如狭窄程度、钙化定量、心肌桥以及冠状动脉痉挛等。而血管内成像技术，如血管内超声（IVUS）以及光学相干断层扫描（OCT），通过提供大量斑块特征（如纤维帽、脂质核等）信息并指导介入治疗，从而改善患者的长期预后，已在临床大规模使用。尽管目前造影技术相当成熟，但依然存在一定的并发症风险，故应严格掌握检查指征并遵守规范的操作流程。相关的技术要点以及图像解读于第21章详细阐述。

不同于冠状动脉造影，心导管检查可对结构性心脏病进行系统的血流动力学评估。通过测量房室压力波形、肺毛细血管楔压、瓣环面积、跨瓣流速及压差等指标，心导管检查对心脏瓣膜疾病、先天性心脏病、心肌病以及心包疾病的诊断、治疗以及危险分层具有重要指导意义。本部分第22章详细论述了心导管的检查指征、操作流程、指标解读与应用。

值得注意的是，对于患有心血管疾病或合并心血管危险因素的患者，围术期心血管并发症以及死亡风险需要得到临床医生的重视，尤其是麻醉相关的风险。术前充分评估、术后护理和疼痛治疗，以及围术期密切监测，可显著减少心血管并发症、缩短住院时长以及降低医疗费用。具体的风险评估方法以及具体的降低并发症的策略详见第23章。

总之，对患者的充分评估是日常诊疗活动的重要组成环节。心血管医生应充分掌握各项检查手段的优缺点及适应证，结合患者的具体情况进行综合评估及具体分析，进而筛选出最优检查方案，旨在通过承担最小的风险、最低的检查费用，获得准确、全面的诊断结论。

PART III EVALUATION OF THE PATIENT

13 History and Physical Examination: An Evidence-Based Approach

JAMES C. FANG AND PATRICK T. O'GARA

THE HISTORY, 123

THE GENERAL PHYSICAL EXAMINATION, 124
General Appearance, 125
Skin, 125
Head and Neck, 125
Extremities, 126
Chest and Abdomen, 126

THE CARDIOVASCULAR EXAMINATION, 126
Jugular Venous Pressure and Waveform, 126
Measuring the Blood Pressure, 128
Assessing the Pulses, 129
Inspection and Palpation of the Heart, 130
Auscultation of the Heart, 130
Cardiac Murmurs, 131
Dynamic Auscultation, 134

INTEGRATED, EVIDENCE-BASED APPROACH TO SPECIFIC CARDIAC DISORDERS, 134
Heart Failure, 134
Valvular Heart Disease, 137
Acute Coronary Syndromes, 138
Pericardial Disease, 138

FUTURE DIRECTIONS, 139

ACKNOWLEDGMENTS, 139

REFERENCES, 139

Evaluation of the patient with known or suspected cardiovascular disease begins with a directed history and targeted physical examination, the scope and duration of which depend on the clinical context of the patient encounter. Elective, ambulatory investigations allow comparatively more time for the development of a comprehensive assessment, whereas emergency department visits and urgent bedside consultations necessitate a more focused strategy. The elicitation of the history, with its emphasis on major cardiovascular symptoms and their change over time, demands a direct interaction between the clinician and patient, and should not be delegated to another nor inferred from information gleaned from a cursory chart review. The history also affords a unique opportunity to assess the patient's personal attitudes, intelligence, comprehension, acceptance or denial, motivation, fear, and prejudices. Such insights allow a more informed understanding of the patient's preferences and values regarding shared decision making. The interview also can reveal genetic or familial influences and the impact of other medical conditions on the manifesting illness. Although time constraints have limited the emphasis on careful history taking, the information gathered from the patient interview remains essential to inform the design of an efficient diagnostic and treatment plan.

Physical examination skills have declined. Only a minority of internal medicine and family practice residents recognizes classic cardiac findings in relevant diseases. Performance does not predictably improve with experience.[1] Residency work hours and health care system efficiency standards have severely restricted the time devoted to the mentored cardiovascular examination. In 2020, the SARS-CoV-2 virus pandemic drastically limited in-person interactions, catalyzed a movement to virtual visits (VV) and challenged clinicians to develop alternative means for patient assessment through real-time video observations. It is anticipated that VV will become an established feature of ambulatory patient follow-up. Less attention to bedside skills and declining confidence in the powers of observation have led to increasing use of noninvasive imaging, including the use of handheld ultrasound. Educational efforts, which utilize repetition, patient-centered teaching conferences, simulation, and visual display feedback of auscultatory and Doppler echocardiographic findings, can improve physical examination performance.[2-6]

The evidence base that links the findings from the history and physical examination to cardiovascular disease severity and prognosis is more robust for heart failure, valvular heart disease, and coronary artery disease than for other conditions. For example, vital signs and the presence of pulmonary congestion and mitral regurgitation (MR) contribute importantly to bedside risk assessment in patients with acute coronary syndromes (ACSs). The diagnosis of heart failure is fundamentally made at the bedside from symptoms and signs that reflect congestion and/or inadequate end-organ perfusion; these findings have been correlated with invasive hemodynamic measurements as well as with outcomes[7]: irregularly irregular pulse, a heart murmur suggestive of MR, a heart rate greater than 60 beats/min, and an elevated jugular venous pressure (JVP).[7] Accurate auscultation provides important insight into many valvular and congenital heart lesions. This chapter reviews the fundamentals of the cardiovascular history and physical examination and the evidence to support their utility. A diagnostic test is considered reasonably reliable if the kappa statistic is at least 0.4. A positive likelihood ratio (LR) (sensitivity/[1 − specificity]) increases the likelihood of the condition; a negative LR (1 − sensitivity)/specificity) decreases the likelihood of the condition.[8]

THE HISTORY

The major signs and symptoms associated with cardiac disease include chest discomfort (see Chapter 35), dyspnea, fatigue, edema, palpitations (see Chapter 61), and syncope (see Chapter 71). In most cases, careful attention to the specific characteristics of chest discomfort—quality, location, radiation, triggers, mode of onset, and duration—along with alleviating factors and associated symptoms can narrow the differential diagnosis (see Chapter 35). Angina pectoris can usually be differentiated from the pain associated with pulmonary embolism, pericarditis, aortic dissection, esophageal reflux, or costochondritis. Cough, hemoptysis, and cyanosis may provide additional clues as to the cause of chest pain. Claudication, limb pain, edema, and skin discoloration usually indicate a vascular disorder. The cardiovascular clinician also should be familiar with common manifestations of acute stroke and transient ischemic attack, such as sudden weakness, sensory loss, incoordination, and visual disturbance. The sudden onset of symptoms and associated diaphoresis should always elicit concern that a cardiovascular cause underlies the patient's complaints.

Typical angina should satisfy three characteristics: (1) substernal discomfort, (2) initiated by exertion or stress, and (3) relieved with rest or sublingual nitroglycerin. Chest discomfort with two of these three criteria is considered atypical angina; pain with one or none of these features is considered nonanginal. When age and sex are considered, the diagnostic accuracy for CAD using these criteria is reasonable (receiver operator curve [ROC] area under the curve [AUC] 0.713). Incorporating a history of diabetes, hypertension, smoking, and dyslipidemia improves the diagnostic accuracy (ROC AUC 0.791).[9]

Several aspects of the presenting symptom of chest pain increase or decrease the likelihood of ACS. For example, pain that is sharp (LR, 0.3; 95% CI, 0.2 to 0.5), pleuritic (LR, 0.2; 95% CI, 0.1 to 0.3), positional (LR, 0.3; 95% CI, 0.2 to 0.5), or reproducible with palpation (LR, 0.3; 95% CI, 0.2 to 0.4) usually is noncardiac, whereas discomfort that radiates to both arms or shoulders (LR, 4.1; 95% CI, 2.5 to 6.5) or is precipitated by exertion (LR, 2.4; 95% CI, 1.5 to 3.8) has a much higher likelihood of reflecting myocardial ischemia. Less classic symptoms (i.e., anginal equivalents) such as indigestion, belching, and dyspnea, also should command the clinician's attention when other features of the presentation suggest ACS, even in the absence of chest discomfort.

Women, elderly persons, and patients with diabetes more commonly present with a less typical clinical picture. A history of a prior abnormal stress test (LR, 3.1; 95% CI, 2.0 to 4.7), known CAD (LR, 2.0; 95% CI, 1.4 to 2.6) or the presence of peripheral arterial disease (PAD) (LR, 2.7; 95% CI, 1.5 to 4.8) increases the likelihood that the pain indicate an ACS.[10] However, the accuracy of traditional risk factors and symptoms for the diagnosis of ACS is weak. Clinical prediction models that incorporate aspects of the history and examination with serum biomarkers of cardiac injury (troponins) and ECG findings provide better diagnostic accuracy, especially when they have been externally validated (Table 13.1).

Dyspnea may occur with exertion or in recumbency (orthopnea) or even on standing (platypnea). Paroxysmal nocturnal dyspnea of cardiac origin usually occurs 2 to 4 hours after onset of sleep; the dyspnea is sufficiently severe to compel the patient to sit upright or stand and then subsides gradually over several minutes. The patient's partner should be questioned about any signs of sleep-disordered breathing, such as loud snoring or periods of apnea. Pulmonary embolism often associates with dyspnea of sudden onset.

Patients may use a variety of terms to describe their awareness of the heartbeat (palpitations), such as "flutters," "skips," or "pounding." The likelihood of a cardiac arrhythmia modestly increases with a known history of cardiac disease (LR, 2.03; 95% CI, 1.33 to 3.11) and decreases when symptoms resolve within 5 minutes (LR, 0.38; 95% CI, 0.22 to 0.63) or when associated with panic disorder (LR, 0.26; 95% CI, 0.07 to 1.01). A report of a regular, rapid-pounding sensation in the neck (LR, 177; 95% CI, 25 to 1251) or visible neck pulsations associated with palpitations (LR, 2.68; 95% CI, 1.25 to 5.78) increases the likelihood that atrioventricular nodal reentrant tachycardia (AVNRT) is the responsible arrhythmia. The absence of a regular, rapid-pounding sensation in the neck makes detecting AVNRT much less likely (LR, 0.07; 95% CI, 0.03 to 0.19).[11]

Cardiac syncope occurs suddenly, with rapid restoration of full consciousness thereafter. Patients with neurocardiogenic syncope may experience early warning signs (nausea, yawning), appear ashen and diaphoretic, and revive more slowly, albeit without signs of seizure or a prolonged postictal state. The complete history consists of information pertaining to traditional cardiovascular risk factors, a general medical history, occupation, social habits, activities, medications, drug allergies or intolerance, family history, and systems review. In most instances, the history, examination, and limited testing can establish the cause of syncope (Table 13.2).[12]

It is important to obtain a semiquantitative assessment of symptom severity and to document any change over time. The New York Heart Association (NYHA) and the Canadian Cardiovascular Society (CCS) functional classification systems are useful for both patient care and clinical research, despite their inherent limitations. Current technology now allows patients to self-report symptoms directly into the patient record using iterative responsive survey instruments, which can be quantified and may better reflect the patient's experience with their cardiovascular condition in contrast to the provider's interpretation of the patient's symptoms.[13]

THE GENERAL PHYSICAL EXAMINATION

The physical examination can help determine the cause of a given symptom, assess disease severity and progression, and evaluate the impact of specific therapies. It also can identify the presence of early-stage disease in patients without signs or symptoms. In general, the physical examination should be undertaken in a hypothesis-driven

TABLE 13.2 History and Exam Findings Suggestive of Cardiac Syncope

1. Known heart disease
2. Abnormal cardiovascular physical exam
3. Family history of sudden death or drowning
4. Male sex
5. Age >35 years at time of syncope
6. Two or fewer previous episodes
7. Palpitations
8. Chest pain or dyspnea

TABLE 13.1 Value of Selected History and Exam Findings For Diagnosis of Acute Coronary Syndrome

SYMPTOM	POSITIVE LR (95% CI)	PPV (%)	NEGATIVE LR (95% CI)	NPV (%)
Radiation to both arms	2.6 (1.8–3.7)	28	0.93 (0.89–0.96)	12
Radiation to left arm	1.3 (1.2–1.4)	16	0.88 (0.81–0.96)	12
Typical chest pain	1.9 (0.94–2.9)	22	0.52 (0.35–0.69)	7
Increase with exertion	1.5–1.8 (NA)	18–21	0.66–0.83 (NA)	9–11
Radiation to neck or jaw	1.5 (1.3–1.8)	18	0.91 (0.87–0.95)	12
Associated diaphoresis	1.3–1.4 (NA)	15	0.91–0.93 (NA)	12
Exam Findings				
Systolic BP <100	3.9 (0.98–15)	37	0.98 (0.95–1.0)	13
Tachypnea	1.9 (0.99–3.5)	22	0.95 (0.89–1.0)	12
Pain reproduced with palpation	0.28 (0.14–0.54)	4.0	1.2 (1.0–1.2)	15

BP, Blood pressure; *LR*, likelihood ratio; *NPV*, negative predictive value; *PPV*, positive predictive value.

manner[14] in which the pretest probability of a specific diagnosis is altered by a specific finding. Depending upon the characteristics of this finding, a post-test probability can be established to guide further testing as appropriate.

General Appearance

The examination begins with an appreciation of the general appearance of the patient, including age, posture, demeanor, and general health status. Is the patient in pain, resting quietly, or visibly diaphoretic? Does the patient choose to avoid certain positions to reduce or eliminate pain? The pain of acute pericarditis, for example, often diminishes with sitting up, leaning forward, or breathing shallowly. Pursing of the lips, a breathy quality to the voice, and an increased anteroposterior chest diameter would favor a pulmonary rather than a cardiovascular cause of dyspnea, although disorders in both etiologic categories may contribute in an individual patient. Pallor suggests anemia as a possible underlying disorder in patients with exercise intolerance or dyspnea, independent of cardiovascular disease. Cyanosis and jaundice also bear noting. Specific genetic cardiovascular disorders may be discernible from the patient's appearance. Emaciation suggests chronic heart failure or another systemic disorder (e.g., malignancy, infection).

The vital signs, including height, weight, temperature, pulse rate, blood pressure (in both arms), respiratory rate, and peripheral oxygen saturation, are used to determine the urgency of the evaluation and provide initial clues as to the presence of a cardiovascular disorder. The height and weight permit calculation of body mass index (BMI) and body surface area (BSA). Waist circumference (measured at the iliac crest) and waist-to-hip ratio (using the widest circumference around the buttocks) powerfully predict long-term cardiovascular risk. In patients with palpitations, a resting heart rate less than 60 beats/min may increase the likelihood of a clinically significant arrhythmia (LR, 3.00; 95% CI, 1.27 to 7.08).[11] Observation of the respiratory pattern may reveal signs of disordered breathing (e.g., Cheyne-Stokes respirations, obstructive sleep apnea), a finding associated with reduced survival in patients with severe systolic heart failure.[15] Mental status should be assessed and is an important gauge of adequate cerebral and systemic perfusion.

Frailty is defined as a state of decreased physiologic reserve and vulnerability to stressors. Several scales are available that incorporate quantifiable criteria such as unintentional weight loss, grip strength, gait speed, serum albumin, and hemoglobin (Table 13.3).[16] Frailty assessment, a common tool in the evaluation of patients with heart failure, is a routine feature of the preprocedural appraisal of elderly patients referred for heart valve intervention.

Skin

Central cyanosis is present with significant right-to-left shunting at the level of the heart or lungs. It also is a feature of hereditary methemoglobinemia. Peripheral cyanosis or acrocyanosis of the fingers, toes, nose, and ears is characteristic of the reduced blood flow that accompanies small-vessel constriction seen in severe heart failure, shock, or peripheral vascular disease. Differential cyanosis affecting the lower but not the upper extremities occurs with a patent ductus arteriosus (PDA) and pulmonary artery hypertension with right-to-left shunting at the great vessel level. Hereditary telangiectases on the lips, tongue, and mucous membranes (a finding in Osler-Weber-Rendu syndrome) resemble spider nevi; when present in the lungs, they can cause right-to-left shunting and central cyanosis. Telangiectasias also are seen in patients with scleroderma with or without pulmonary hypertension. Livedo reticularis, a lace-like purplish dislocation of the skin that imparts a mottled or reticulated appearance (Fig. 13.1), can occur on exposure to cold in normal individuals, but is also observed in a variety of conditions resulting in sluggish cutaneous blood flow, such as cardiogenic shock or certain autoimmune diseases. Tanned or bronze discoloration of the skin in unexposed areas can suggest iron overload and hemochromatosis. With jaundice, often first appreciated in the sclerae, the differential diagnosis is broad in scope. Ecchymoses often occur with either anticoagulant and/or antiplatelet use, whereas petechiae characterize thrombocytopenia, and purpuric skin lesions can be seen with infective endocarditis and other causes of leukocytoclastic vasculitis. Various lipid disorders can manifest with xanthomas, located subcutaneously, along tendon sheaths, or over the extensor surfaces of the extremities. Xanthomas within the palmar creases are specific for type III hyperlipoproteinemia. The leathery, cobblestone, "plucked chicken" appearance of the skin in the axillae and skinfolds of a young person is characteristic of pseudoxanthoma elasticum, a disease with multiple cardiovascular manifestations, including premature atherosclerosis. Extensive lentiginoses (freckle-like brown macules and café-au-lait spots over the trunk and neck) may be part of developmental delay–associated cardiovascular syndromes (LEOPARD, LAMB, and Carney) with multiple atrial myxomas, atrial septal defect (ASD), hypertrophic cardiomyopathy, and valvular stenoses. In a patient with heart failure or syncope, cardiovascular sarcoid should be suspected in the presence of lupus pernio, erythema nodosum, or granuloma annulare. Certain vascular disorders such as erythromelalgia, chilblains, frostbite, or lymphangitis also may be readily apparent from examination of the skin in the appropriate context.

Head and Neck

All patients should undergo assessment of the state of dentition, both as a source of infection and as an index of general health and hygiene. A high-arched palate is a feature of Marfan and other connective tissue disease syndromes. A large protruding tongue with parotid enlargement may suggest amyloidosis. Patients with Loeys-Dietz syndrome characteristically have a bifid uvula. Orange tonsils are typical of Tangier disease. Ptosis and ophthalmoplegia suggest muscular dystrophies, and congenital heart disease often is accompanied by hypertelorism,

TABLE 13.3 The Fried Criteria for Frailty

CHARACTERISTIC	METRICS
Shrinking (Unintentional weight loss)	>10 pound or >5% of total body weight in past year.
Weakness (Reduced hand grip strength)	Maximum isometric contraction in dominant hand over three attempts using hand dynamometer.
Exhaustion (Self-reported exhaustion)	Questions from the Center for Epidemiologic Studies—Depression Scale.
Slowness (Slow gait speed)	Slowest quintile according to gender/height based on time to walk 15 feet.
Inactivity (Low self-reported physical activity)	Lowest quintile of expended kcal/week using activity questionnaire.

Frail: Greater than or equal to 3 criteria present.
Intermediate/Prefrail: 1 or 2 criteria present.
From Joyce E. Frailty in advanced heart failure. *Heart Fail Clin*. 2016;12(3):363–374.

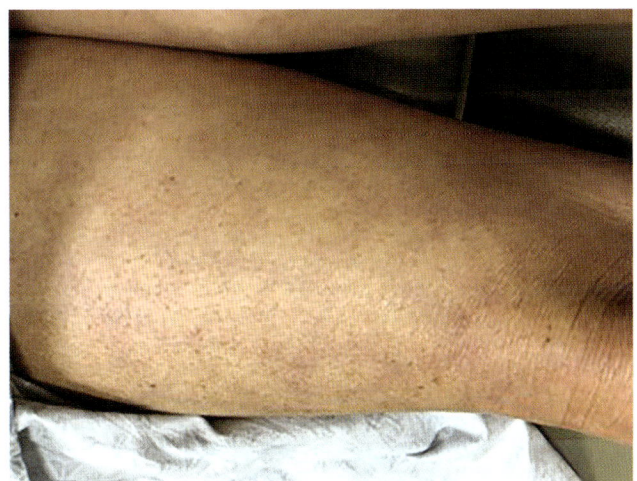

FIGURE 13.1 Appearance of livedo reticularis suggesting decreased skin perfusion.

low-set ears, micrognathia, and a webbed neck, as with Noonan, Turner, and Down syndromes. Proptosis, lid lag, and stare point to Graves hyperthyroidism. Patients with osteogenesis imperfecta may have blue sclerae, mitral or aortic regurgitation (AR), and a history of recurrent nontraumatic skeletal fractures.

Attention to the extraocular movements and the size and symmetry of the pupils may reveal a neurologic disorder. The oft-omitted funduscopic examination can aid in the evaluation of patients with hypertension, atherosclerosis, diabetes, endocarditis, neurologic signs or symptoms, or known carotid or aortic arch disease. Lacrimal gland hyperplasia is sometimes a feature of sarcoidosis. The "mitral facies" of rheumatic mitral stenosis (pink-purplish patches with telangiectasias over the malar eminences) also can accompany other disorders associated with pulmonary hypertension and reduced cardiac output. Relapsing polychondritis is suggested by inflammation of the pinnae and nasal cartilage in association with a saddle-nose deformity.

Extremities

Inspection and palpation can quickly ascertain the temperature of the extremities and the presence of clubbing, arachnodactyly, and nail changes. Clubbing implies the presence of central shunting. An unopposable "fingerized" thumb and shortened forearm bones occur in Holt-Oram syndrome. Arachnodactyly characterizes the Marfan syndrome. Janeway lesions (nontender, slightly raised areas of hemorrhage on the palms and soles), Osler's nodes (tender, raised nodules on the pads of the fingers or toes), and splinter hemorrhages (linear petechiae in the mid-nailbed) may be signs of infective endocarditis. Ulcerations and tissue loss of the fingertips may suggest thromboangiitis obliterans in the appropriate context.

Lower extremity or presacral edema with elevated JVP occurs in many volume-overloaded states, including heart failure. With a normal JVP, additional signs of venous disease, such as extensive varicosities, medial ulcers, or brownish pigmentation from hemosiderin deposition, suggest chronic venous insufficiency. A history of lower extremity vein ligation and "stripping" should be recognized. Edema also can occur with dihydropyridine calcium channel blocker therapy. Anasarca seldom occurs in heart failure, unless the condition is long standing, untreated, and accompanied by severe hypoalbuminemia. Asymmetric swelling can reflect local or unilateral venous thrombosis, the sequelae of previous vein graft harvesting, or lymphatic obstruction (lymphedema). Homan sign (calf pain elicited by forceful dorsiflexion of the foot) is neither specific nor sensitive for deep vein thrombosis. Muscular atrophy and the absence of hair in an extremity should suggest chronic arterial insufficiency or a neuromuscular disorder. Redistribution of fat from the extremities to central/abdominal stores (lipodystrophy) in some patients with HIV infection may relate to antiretroviral treatment and is associated with insulin resistance and several features of the metabolic syndrome.

Chest and Abdomen

Cutaneous venous collaterals over the anterior chest suggest chronic obstruction of the superior vena cava (SVC) or subclavian vein, especially in the presence of indwelling catheters or leads from cardiac implantable electrical devices (CIEDs). Asymmetric breast enlargement or arm swelling ipsilateral to an implanted device also may be present. Thoracic cage abnormalities, such as pectus carinatum (pigeon chest) or pectus excavatum (funnel chest), may accompany connective tissue disorders; the barrel chest of emphysema or advanced kyphoscoliosis may be associated with cor pulmonale. The severe kyphosis of ankylosing spondylitis should prompt careful auscultation for AR and scrutiny of the electrocardiogram (ECG) for first-degree atrioventricular (AV) block. The "straight back syndrome" (loss of normal kyphosis of the thoracic spine) can accompany mitral valve prolapse (MVP). A thrill may be present over well-developed intercostal artery collaterals in patients with aortic coarctation.

Patients with emphysema may exhibit prominence of the cardiac impulse in the epigastrium. The liver often is enlarged and tender in heart failure; systolic hepatic pulsations signify severe tricuspid regurgitation (TR). Patients with infective endocarditis of long duration may have splenomegaly. Ascites can develop with advanced and chronic right heart failure or constrictive pericarditis. The abdominal aorta normally may be palpated between the epigastrium and the umbilicus in thin patients and in children. The sensitivity of palpation for the detection of abdominal aortic aneurysm (AAA) disease increases as a function of aneurysm diameter and varies inversely with body size. Arterial bruits in the abdomen should be sought.

Careful chest auscultation is an essential component of the cardiovascular exam and is of prime importance when the presenting complaint is dyspnea. Technologic advances have provided important insights into often underappreciated pulmonary auscultatory phenomena (Fig. 13.2) that are commonly encountered in the evaluation of patients with cardiovascular disease.[17] Point of care ultrasound in emergency rooms and intensive care units have assumed increasing importance in the bedside evaluation of dyspnea.[18,19]

THE CARDIOVASCULAR EXAMINATION

Jugular Venous Pressure and Waveform

The JVP aids in the estimation of volume status. The external (EJV) or internal (IJV) jugular vein may be used, although the IJV is preferred because the EJV is valved and not directly in line with the SVC and right atrium. The EJV is easier to visualize when distended, and its appearance can help to discriminate between low and high central venous pressure (CVP). An elevated left EJV pressure may also signify a persistent left-sided SVC or compression of the innominate vein from an intrathoracic structure. If an elevated CVP is suspected but venous pulsations cannot be appreciated, the patient should be asked to sit upright with the feet dangling. With subsequent pooling of blood in the lower extremities, venous pulsations may be evident. SVC syndrome should be suspected if the venous pressure is elevated, pulsations are still not discernible, the face is swollen, and the skin of the head and neck appears dusky or cyanotic. When hypovolemia is suspected as a cause of hypotension, the patient may need to be lowered to a supine position to assess the waveform in the right supraclavicular fossa.

The venous waveform can sometimes be difficult to distinguish from the carotid artery pulse. The venous waveform has several characteristic features (Fig. 13.3; Table 13.4) and its individual components can usually be identified. The a and v waves, and x and y descents, are defined by their temporal relation to electrocardiographic events and heart sounds. The estimated height of the venous pressure indicates the CVP or right atrial pressure. Although observers vary widely in their estimates of the CVP, knowledge that the pressure is elevated, and not its specific value, can inform diagnosis and management.

The bedside venous pressure is usually estimated by the vertical distance between the top of the venous pulsation and the sternal inflection point, where the manubrium meets the sternum (angle of Louis). A distance of greater than 3 cm is considered abnormal. However, the distance between the angle of Louis and the mid–right atrium varies considerably as a function of body size and position. In general, use of the sternal angle as a reference leads to systematic underestimation of venous pressure. In practice, however, it is difficult to use even relatively simple thoracic landmarks. Measurements obtained by critical care nurses often will vary by several centimeters. Venous pulsations above the clavicle with the patient in the sitting position are clearly abnormal, because the distance from the right atrium is at least 10 cm. Estimated CVP correlates only modestly with direct measurement. Measurements made at the bedside, in units of centimeters of blood or water, require conversion to millimeters of mercury (1.36 cm H_2O = 1.0 mm Hg), for comparison with values measured with catheterization. Remote assessment of the JVP using video "chat" in patients with heart failure and reduced ejection fraction was demonstrated to be feasible and of comparable accuracy to bedside estimation in a pilot study using invasively measured right atrial pressure as the reference standard.[20] These findings have implications for both remote in-hospital and virtual ambulatory patient assessment (see later).

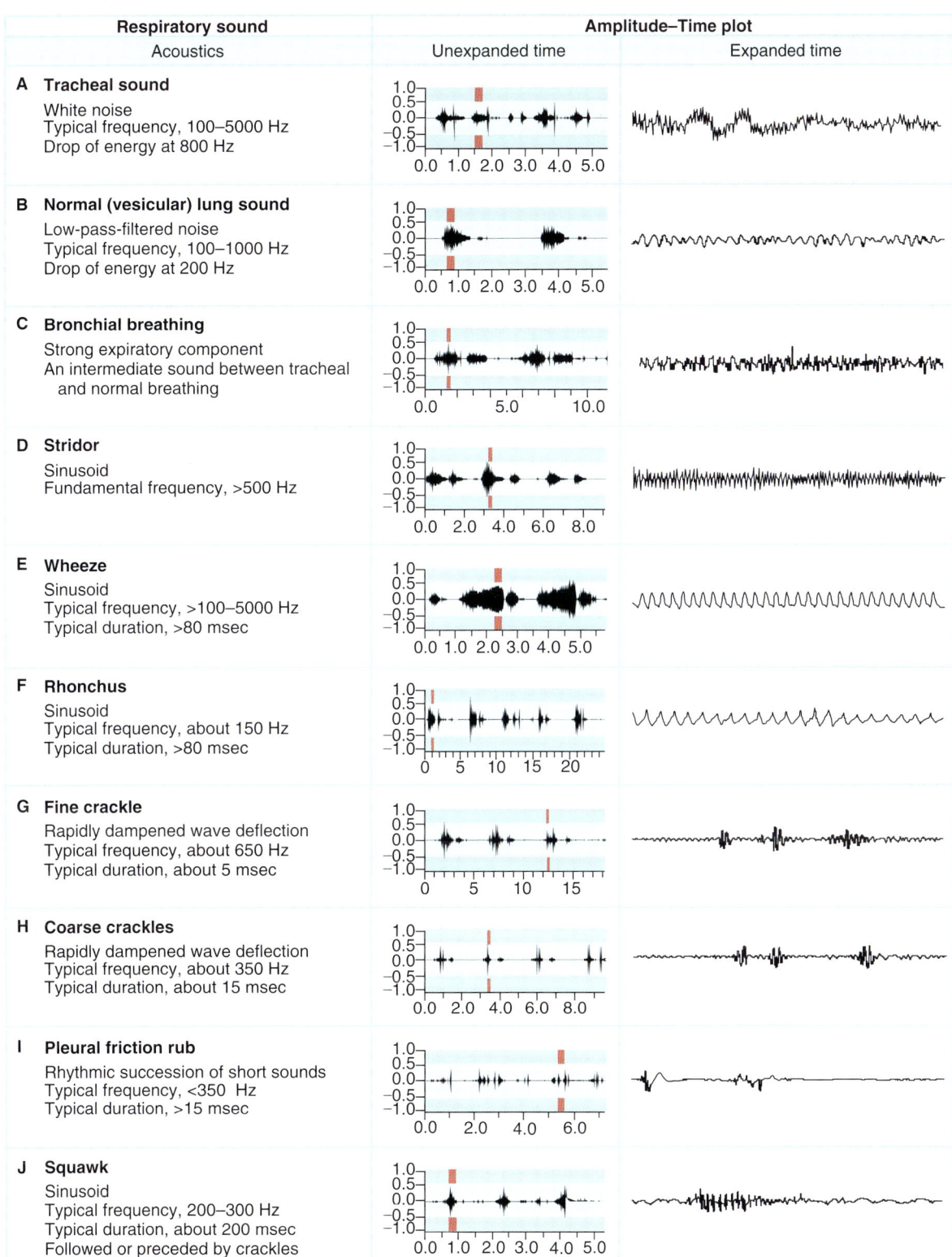

FIGURE 13.2 Respiratory sounds and the acoustic waveforms. (From Bohadana A, Izbicki G, Kraman SS. Fundamentals of lung auscultation. *N Engl J Med*. 2014;370:2053.)

The venous waveforms include several distinct peaks: *a*, *c*, and *v* (see Fig. 13.3, Table 13.4). The *a* wave reflects right atrial presystolic contraction, occurs just after the electrocardiographic P wave, and precedes the first heart sound (S_1). Patients with reduced right ventricular (RV) compliance from any cause can have a prominent *a* wave. A cannon *a* wave occurs with AV dissociation and right atrial contraction against a closed tricuspid valve. *The presence of cannon a waves in a patient with wide complex tachycardia identifies the rhythm as ventricular in origin.* The *a* wave is absent with atrial fibrillation (AF). The *x* descent reflects the fall in right atrial pressure after the *a* wave peak. The *c* wave interrupts this descent as ventricular systole pushes the closed valve into the right atrium. In the neck, the carotid pulse also may contribute to the *c* wave. As depicted in Figure 13.3, the *x* descent follows because of atrial diastolic suction created by ventricular systole pulling the tricuspid valve downward. In normal persons, the *x* descent is the predominant waveform in the jugular venous pulse. The *v* wave represents atrial filling, occurs at the end of ventricular systole, and follows just after S_2. Its height is determined

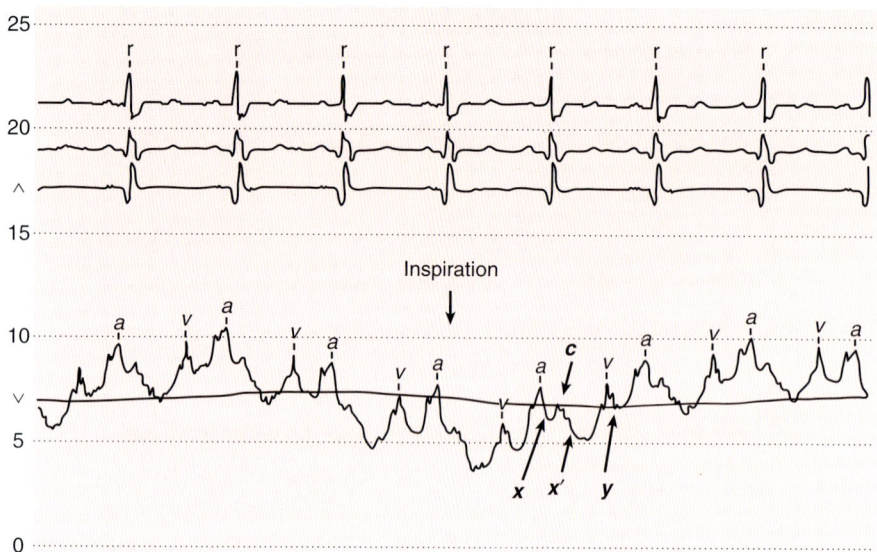

FIGURE 13.3 The normal jugular venous waveform recorded at cardiac catheterization. Note the inspiratory fall in pressure and the dominant x/x′ descent.

accommodate the enhanced volume, and the pressure rises. Increased pulmonary vascular resistance may also limit RV ejection and contribute to the Kussmaul phenomenon.

The abdominojugular reflux maneuver or passive leg elevation can elicit venous hypertension. The abdominojugular reflux maneuver requires firm and consistent pressure over the upper abdomen, preferably the right upper quadrant, for at least 10 seconds. Classically, a positive abdominojugular reflux sign has been defined as a rise of more than 3 cm in the venous pressure sustained for at least 15 seconds, although in practice a shorter time duration is usually accepted. The patient should be coached to refrain from holding their breath or performing a Valsalva-like maneuver, which can falsely elevate the venous pressure. A positive abdominojugular reflux sign can predict heart failure in patients with dyspnea, as well as a pulmonary artery wedge pressure higher than 15 mm Hg.

Measuring the Blood Pressure (see also Chapter 26)

Auscultatory measurement of blood pressure yields lower systolic and higher diastolic values than direct intra-arterial recording. Nurse or pharmacist-recorded blood pressure usually is closer to the patient's average daytime blood pressure than physician measured blood pressure. Blood pressure should be measured with the patient in the seated position, back supported, feet on the floor, with the arm at the level of the heart, using an appropriate-size cuff (Table 13.5), after 5 minutes of rest, repeated 5 minutes later, and the readings averaged. The use of an inappropriately small cuff can result in overestimation of the true blood pressure, an issue of particular relevance in obese patients.

On occasion, the Korotkoff sounds may disappear soon after the first sound, only to recur later before finally disappearing as phase 5. This auscultatory gap is more likely to occur in older, hypertensive patients with target organ damage. The systolic pressure should be recorded at the first Korotkoff sound and not when the sound reappears. This finding should be distinguished from *pulsus paradoxus* (see later). Korotkoff sounds may be heard all the way down to 0 mm Hg with the cuff completely deflated in children, in pregnant patients, in patients with chronic severe AR, or in the presence of a large arteriovenous fistula. In these cases, both the phases 4 and 5 pressures should be noted.

Blood pressure should be measured in both arms either in rapid succession or simultaneously; normally the measurements should differ by less than 10 mm Hg, independent of handedness. As many as 20% of normal subjects, however, exhibit a left-right arm blood pressure differential of more than 10 mm Hg in the absence of symptoms or other examination findings. A blood pressure differential of more than 10 mm Hg can be associated with subclavian artery disease, supravalvular aortic stenosis (SVAS), aortic coarctation, or aortic dissection. Systolic leg pressures may exceed arm pressures by as much as 20 mm Hg; greater leg-arm systolic blood pressure differences are seen in patients with severe AR (Hill sign) and patients with extensive and calcified (noncompressible) lower extremity PAD. Leg blood pressure should be measured using large thigh cuffs with auscultation at the popliteal artery or using a standard large arm cuff on the calf with simultaneous auscultation or palpation at the posterior tibial artery. Measurement of lower extremity blood pressures constitutes the basis of the ankle-brachial index (ABI) (see Chapter 43).

Consideration should be given to ambulatory blood pressure monitoring when uncertainty exists about the significance of recordings obtained in the clinic. This approach is especially useful for the patient

TABLE 13.4 Distinguishing Jugular Venous Pulse from Carotid Pulse

FEATURE	INTERNAL JUGULAR VEIN PULSE	CAROTID ARTERY PULSE
Appearance of pulse	Undulating two troughs and two peaks for every cardiac cycle (biphasic)	Single brisk upstroke (monophasic)
Response to inspiration	Height of column falls and troughs become more prominent	No respiratory change to contour
Palpability	Generally not palpable (except in severe TR)	Palpable
Effect of pressure	Can be obliterated with gentle pressure at base of vein/clavicle	Cannot be obliterated

TR, Tricuspid regurgitation.

by right atrial compliance and by the volume of blood returning to the right atrium from all sources. The *v* wave is smaller than the *a* wave because of the normally compliant right atrium. In patients with ASD, the *a* and *v* waves may be of equal height; in TR, the *v* wave is accentuated. With TR, the *v* wave will merge with the *c* wave because retrograde valve flow and antegrade right atrial filling occur simultaneously. The *y* descent follows the *v* wave peak and reflects the fall in right atrial pressure after tricuspid valve opening. Resistance to ventricular filling in early diastole blunts the *y* descent, as is the case with pericardial tamponade or tricuspid stenosis. The *y* descent will be steep when ventricular diastolic filling occurs early and rapidly, as with pericardial constriction, restrictive cardiomyopathy, or isolated, severe TR.

The normal venous pressure should fall by at least 3 mm Hg with inspiration. A rise in venous pressure (or its failure to decrease) with inspiration (Kussmaul sign) is associated with constrictive pericarditis, and with restrictive cardiomyopathy, pulmonary embolism, RV infarction, and advanced systolic heart failure. A Kussmaul sign is seen with right-sided volume overload and reduced RV compliance. Normally, the inspiratory increase in right-sided venous return is accommodated by increased RV ejection, facilitated by an increase in the capacitance of the pulmonary vascular bed. In states of RV diastolic dysfunction and volume overload, the right ventricle cannot

TABLE 13.5 Important Aspects of Blood Pressure Measurement

- Patient should be seated comfortably, with back supported and legs uncrossed and the upper arm bared.
- Upper arm should be at heart level.
- Cuff length and width should be 80% and 40% of arm circumference, respectively.
- Cuff should be deflated at <3 mm Hg/sec.
- Column or dial should be read to nearest 2 mm Hg.
- First audible Korotkoff sound is systolic pressure; last sound, diastolic pressure.
- There should be no talking between subject and observer (or other person).

From Daskalopolou SS, Rabi DM, Zarnke KB, et al. The 2015 Canadian Hypertension Education Program recommendations for blood pressure measurement, diagnosis, assessment of risk, prevention, and treatment of hypertension. *Can J Cardiol.* 2015;31:549–568; and Ringrose JS, McLean D, Ao P, et al. Effect of cuff design on auscultatory and oscillometric blood pressure measurements. *Am J Hypertens.* 2016;29(9):1063–1069.

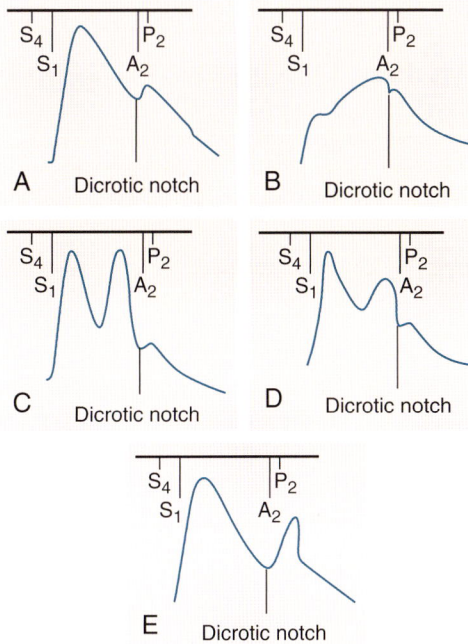

FIGURE 13.4 Carotid pulse waveforms and heart sounds. **A,** Normal. **B,** Aortic stenosis. Anacrotic pulse with slow upstroke and peak near S_2. **C,** Severe aortic regurgitation (AR): bifid pulse with two systolic peaks. **D,** Hypertrophic obstructive cardiomyopathy (HCM): bifid pulse with two systolic peaks. The second peak (tidal or reflected wave) is of lower amplitude than the initial percussion wave. **E,** Bifid pulse with systolic and diastolic peaks as may occur with sepsis or intra-aortic balloon counterpulsation. A_2, Aortic component of S_2; P_2, pulmonic component of S_2. (From Chatterjee K. Bedside evaluation of the heart: the physical examination. In: Chatterjee K, Parmley W, eds. *Cardiology: An Illustrated Text/Reference.* Philadelphia: JB Lippincott; 1991; and Braunwald E. The clinical examination. In: Braunwald E, Goldman L, eds. *Primary Cardiology.* 2nd ed. Philadelphia: WB Saunders; 2003:36.)

with suspected "white coat hypertension" (see Chapter 26).[21] Measurement of normal or even low blood pressures in the clinic with evidence of hypertensive end organ damage should suggest masked hypertension,[22] which occurs more often than clinicians appreciate and may be present in the absence of obstructive PAD that can lower extremity blood pressure.

Orthostatic hypotension (a fall in blood pressure of more than 20 mm Hg systolic and/or more than 10 mm Hg diastolic in response to moving from the supine to the standing position within 3 minutes) may be accompanied by a lack of compensatory tachycardia, a response suggestive of autonomic insufficiency, as can occur in patients with diabetes or Parkinson disease. The heart rate–blood pressure response to standing also depends on age, hydration, medications, food, conditioning, and ambient temperature and humidity. In patients with postural orthostatic tachycardia syndrome (POTS), blood pressure does not usually fall on standing.

An increase in pulse pressure can represent increased vascular stiffness, usually secondary to aging or atherosclerosis. Aortic stiffness is increased in patients with Marfan syndrome and other connective tissue disorders and may contribute to risk for dissection. Peripheral indices may not correlate well with central aortic stiffness, which is a primary determinant of ventricular-vascular coupling.

Assessing the Pulses

The carotid artery pulse wave occurs within 40 milliseconds of the ascending aortic pulse and reflects aortic valve and ascending aortic function. The temporal arteries can be easily palpated to aid in the diagnosis of temporal arteritis. One of the two pedal pulses may not be palpable in a normal subject because of unusual anatomy (posterior tibial, less than 5%; dorsal pedis, less than 10%), but each pair should be symmetric. True congenital absence of a pulse is rare, and in most cases, pulses can be detected with a handheld Doppler device when not palpable. Simultaneous palpation of the brachial or radial pulse with the femoral pulse should be performed in young patients with hypertension to screen for aortic coarctation.

The contour of the pulses depends on the stroke volume, ejection velocity, vascular capacity and compliance, and systemic resistance. The palpable pulse reflects the merging of the antegrade pulsatile flow of blood and reflection of the propagated pulse returning from the periphery. The amplitude of the arterial pulse increases with distance from the heart. Normally, the incident (percussion) wave begins with systolic ejection (just after S_1) and is the predominant monophasic pulse appreciated at the bedside (Fig. 13.4). The incisura or dicrotic notch identifies aortic valve closure. A *bounding* pulse may occur in hyperkinetic states such as fever, anemia, and thyrotoxicosis, or in pathologic states such as severe bradycardia, AR, or arteriovenous fistula. A *bifid* pulse is created by two distinct pressure peaks. This phenomenon may occur with fever or after exercise in a normal person and is consistent with increased vascular compliance. With chronic severe AR, a large stroke volume ejected rapidly into a noncompliant arterial tree produces a reflected wave of sufficient amplitude to be palpated during systole, rendering the pulse bifid. Hypertrophic cardiomyopathy (HCM) can rarely produce a bifid systolic pulse with percussion and tidal waves (see Fig. 13.4). Diastolic augmentation of pressure with an intra-aortic balloon pump also results in a bifid pulse, though with the two components separated by aortic valve closure.

A fall in systolic pressure of more than 10 mm Hg with inspiration (*pulsus paradoxus*) is considered pathologic and a sign of pericardial tamponade or severe pulmonary disease; this phenomenon also can occur in obesity and pregnancy without clinical disease. Pulsus paradoxus is detected by noting the difference between the systolic pressure at which the Korotkoff sounds are first heard (during expiration) and the systolic pressure at which the Korotkoff sounds are heard with each beat, independent of respiratory phase. Between these two pressures, the sounds will be heard only intermittently (during expiration). Appreciation of this finding requires a slow decrease of the cuff pressure. Conditions such as tachycardia, AF, and tachypnea make its assessment difficult. Pulsus paradoxus may be palpable at the brachial artery when the pressure difference exceeds 15 mm Hg (see Chapter 86). Pulsus paradoxus is not specific for pericardial tamponade and can accompany massive pulmonary embolus, hemorrhagic shock, severe obstructive lung disease, or tension pneumothorax.

Pulsus alternans is defined by the beat-to-beat variability of the pulse amplitude (Fig. 13.5). It is present when only every other phase 1 Korotkoff sound is audible as the cuff pressure is slowly lowered, in

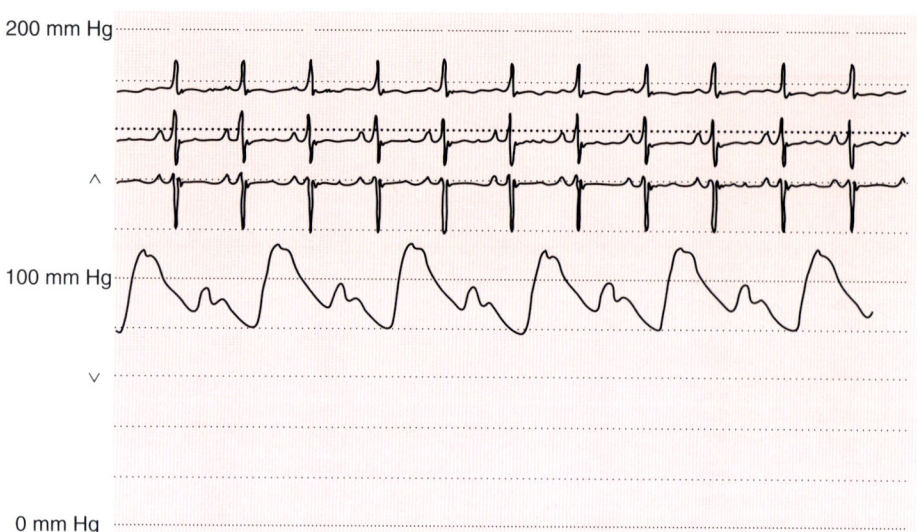

FIGURE 13.5 Pulsus alternans in a patient with severe left ventricular systolic dysfunction. The systolic pressure varies from beat to beat, independent of the respiratory cycle. The rhythm is sinus throughout.

a patient with a regular heart rhythm, independent of the respiratory cycle. Pulsus alternans generally occurs in severe heart failure, severe AR, hypertension, and hypovolemic states. It is attributed to cyclic changes in intracellular calcium and action potential duration. Association with electrocardiographic T wave alternans appears to increase arrhythmic risk.

Severe aortic stenosis may be suggested by a weak and delayed pulse (*pulsus parvus et tardus*) and is best appreciated by careful palpation of the carotid arteries (see Fig. 13.4; see Chapter 72). The delay is assessed during simultaneous auscultation of the heart sounds; the carotid upstroke should coincide with S_1. This finding is less specific in older, hypertensive patients with reduced vascular compliance and stiffer carotid arteries. An abrupt carotid upstroke with rapid fall-off characterizes the pulse of chronic AR (Corrigan or water-hammer pulse). The carotid upstroke also is rapid in older patients with isolated systolic hypertension and wide pulse pressures.

Pulsation of the abdominal aorta can be appreciated in the epigastric area. Femoral and popliteal artery aneurysms should be sought in patients with AAA disease or underlying connective tissue disease.

The history and physical examination findings can help assess the level of arterial obstruction in patients with lower extremity claudication (see Chapter 43). Auscultation for carotid, subclavian, aortic, and femoral artery bruits should be routine. The correlation between the presence of a bruit and the degree of vascular obstruction is weak. Extension of a bruit into diastole or a thrill generally indicates severe obstruction. Other causes of a bruit include arteriovenous fistulas and enhanced flow through normal arteries as, for example, in a young patient with fever.

Integrating the clinical history and presence of atherosclerotic risk factors improves the accuracy of the examination for the identification of lower extremity PAD. In an asymptomatic patient, the presence of a femoral bruit (LR, 4.8; 95% CI, 2.4 to 9.5) or any abnormality of the pulse (LR, 3.1; 95% CI, 3.1 to 6.6) increases the likelihood of PAD. The likelihood of significant PAD increases when there are lower extremity symptoms and cool skin (LR, 5.9; 95% CI, 4.1 to 8.6), pulse abnormalities (LR, 4.7; 95% CI, 2.2 to 9.9), or any bruit (LR, 5.6; 95% CI, 4.7 to 6.7). Abnormal pulse oximetry, defined by a more than 2% difference between finger and toe oxygen saturation, can also indicate lower extremity PAD and is comparable to the ABI (LR, 30.0; 95% CI, 7.6 to 121 versus LR, 24.8; 95% CI, 6.2 to 99.8).[23]

Inspection and Palpation of the Heart

The apical heartbeat may be visible in thin-chested adults. The left anterior chest wall may heave in patients with enlarged and hyperdynamic left ventricles. Right upper parasternal and sternoclavicular pulsations suggest ascending aortic aneurysm disease. A left parasternal lift indicates RV pressure or volume overload. A pulsation in the third intercostal space to the left of the sternum can indicate pulmonary artery hypertension. In very thin, tall patients, or in patients with emphysema and flattened diaphragms, the RV impulse may be visible in the epigastrium and should be distinguished from a pulsatile liver edge.

Palpation of the heart should begin with the patient in the supine position inclined at 30 degrees. If the heart is not palpable in this position, the patient should be examined either in the left lateral decubitus position with the left arm above the head or in the seated position, leaning forward. The point of maximal impulse normally is over the left ventricular (LV) apex beat and should be located in the midclavicular line at the fifth intercostal space. It is smaller than 2 cm in diameter and moves quickly away from the fingers. It is best appreciated at end-expiration, when the heart is closest to the chest wall. The normal impulse may not be palpable in obese or muscular patients or in those with thoracic cage deformities. LV cavity enlargement displaces the apex beat leftward and downward. A sustained apex beat is a sign of LV pressure overload (as in aortic stenosis or hypertension). A palpable, presystolic impulse corresponds to a fourth heart sound (S_4) and reflects the atrial contribution to ventricular diastolic filling of a noncompliant left ventricle. A prominent, rapid early filling wave in patients with advanced systolic heart failure may result in a palpable third sound (S_3), which may be present when the gallop itself is not audible. A large ventricular aneurysm may yield a palpable and visible ectopic impulse discrete from the apex beat. HOCM rarely may cause a triple cadence apex beat, with contributions from a palpable S_4 and the two components of the systolic pulse.

A parasternal lift occurs with RV pressure or volume overload. Signs of TR (jugular venous *cv* waves) and/or pulmonary artery hypertension (loud, single, or palpable P_2) should be sought. An enlarged RV can give rise to a precordial lift that can extend across the precordium and obscure left-sided findings. Rarely, patients with severe MR will have a prominent left parasternal impulse because of systolic expansion of the left atrium and forward displacement of the heart. Lateral retraction of the chest wall may be present with isolated RV enlargement secondary to posterior displacement of the systolic LV impulse. Systolic and diastolic thrills signify turbulent, high-velocity blood flow. Their locations help to identify the origins of heart murmurs.

Auscultation of the Heart
Heart Sounds
First Heart Sound (S_1)

The normal first heart sound (S_1) comprises mitral (M_1) and tricuspid (T_1) valve closure. The two components usually are best heard at the lower left sternal border in younger subjects. Normal splitting of S_1 is accentuated with complete right bundle branch block. S_1 intensity increases in the early stages of rheumatic mitral stenosis when the valve leaflets are still pliable, in hyperkinetic states, and with short P-R intervals (less than 160 milliseconds). S_1 becomes softer in the late stages of stenosis, when the leaflets are rigid and calcified, with contractile dysfunction, beta-adrenergic receptor blockers, and long P-R intervals (greater than 200 milliseconds). Other factors that can decrease the intensity of the heart sounds and murmurs include mechanical ventilation, obstructive lung disease, obesity, pendulous breasts, pneumothorax, and pericardial effusion.

Second Heart Sound (S_2)
The second heart sound (S_2) comprises aortic (A_2) and pulmonic (P_2) valve closure. With normal, or physiologic, splitting, the A_2–P_2 interval increases during inspiration and narrows with expiration. The individual components are best heard at the second left interspace with the patient in the supine position. The A_2–P_2 interval widens with complete right bundle branch block because of delayed pulmonic valve closure, and with severe MR because of premature aortic valve closure. Unusually narrow but physiologic splitting of S_2, with an increase in the intensity of P_2 relative to A_2, indicates pulmonary artery hypertension. With fixed splitting, the A_2–P_2 interval is wide and remains unchanged during the respiratory cycle, indicating ostium secundum ASD. Reverse, or paradoxical, splitting occurs as a consequence of a pathologic delay in aortic valve closure, as may occur with complete left bundle branch block, RV apical pacing, severe aortic stenosis, HCM, and myocardial ischemia. A_2 normally is louder than P_2 and can be heard at most sites across the precordium. When both components can be heard at the lower left sternal border or apex, or when P_2 can be palpated at the second left interspace, pulmonary hypertension is present. The intensity of A_2 and P_2 decreases with aortic and pulmonic stenosis, respectively. A single S_2 may result.

Systolic Sounds
An ejection sound is a high-pitched, early systolic sound that coincides in timing with the upstroke of the carotid pulse and usually is associated with congenital bicuspid aortic or pulmonic valve disease, or sometimes with aortic or pulmonic root dilation and normal semilunar valves. The ejection sound accompanying pulmonic valve disease decreases in intensity with inspiration, the only right-sided cardiac event to behave in this manner. Ejection sounds disappear as the culprit valve loses its pliability over time. They often are better heard at the lower left sternal border than at the base of the heart. Nonejection clicks, which occur after the upstroke of the carotid pulse, are related to MVP. A systolic murmur may or may not follow. With standing, ventricular preload and afterload decrease and the click and murmur move closer to S_1. With squatting, ventricular preload and afterload increase, the prolapsing mitral valve tenses later in systole, and the click and murmur move away from S_1 (Fig. 13.6).

Diastolic Sounds
The high-pitched opening snap (OS) of mitral stenosis occurs a short distance after S_2; the A_2–OS interval is inversely proportional to the height of the left atrial (LA)-LV diastolic pressure gradient. The intensity of both S_1 and OS decreases with progressive calcification and rigidity of the anterior mitral leaflet. A pericardial knock (PK) is a high-pitched early diastolic sound, which corresponds in timing to the abrupt cessation of ventricular expansion after AV valve opening and to the prominent y descent seen in the jugular venous waveform in patients with constrictive pericarditis. A tumor "plop" rarely is heard with atrial myxoma; it is a low-pitched sound sometimes only heard in certain positions that arises from the diastolic prolapse of the tumor across the mitral valve. A diastolic murmur may be present, although most myxomas cause no sound. A third heart sound (S_3) occurs during the rapid filling phase of ventricular diastole. An S_3 may be normally present in children, adolescents, and young adults, but indicates systolic heart failure in older adults and carries important prognostic weight. A left-sided S_3 is a low-pitched sound best heard over the LV apex with the patient in the left lateral decubitus position, whereas a right-sided S_3 is usually heard at the lower left sternal border or in the subxiphoid position with the patient supine

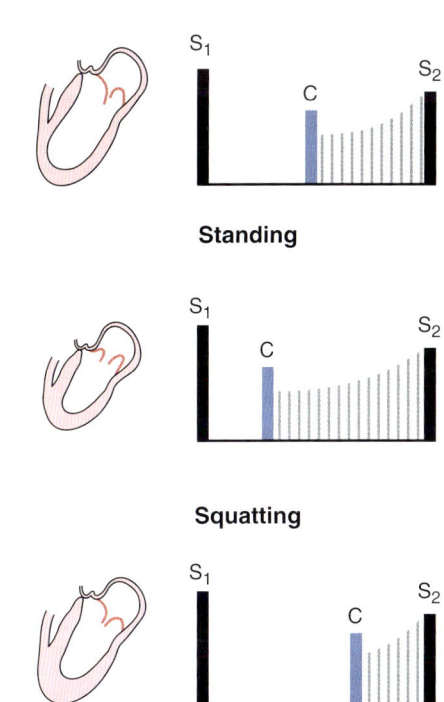

FIGURE 13.6 Behavior of the nonejection click (C) and systolic murmur of mitral valve prolapse. With standing, venous return decreases, the heart becomes smaller, and prolapse occurs earlier in systole. The click and murmur move closer to S_1. With squatting, venous return increases, causing an increase in left ventricular chamber size. The click and murmur occur later in systole and move away from S_1.

and may become louder with inspiration. A fourth heart sound (S_4) occurs during the atrial filling phase of ventricular diastole and is thought to indicate presystolic ventricular expansion. An S_4 is especially common in patients with accentuated atrial contribution to ventricular filling (e.g., LV hypertrophy).

Cardiac Murmurs
Heart murmurs result from audible vibrations caused by increased turbulence and are defined by their timing within the cardiac cycle (Tables 13.6 and 13.7; Figs. 13.7 and 13.8). Not all murmurs indicate valvular or structural heart disease. The accurate identification of a functional (benign) systolic murmur can obviate the need for echocardiography in many healthy subjects. The magnitude, dynamic change, and duration of the pressure difference between two cardiac chambers, or between the ventricles and their respective great arteries, dictate the duration, frequency, configuration, and intensity of murmurs. Intensity is graded on a scale of 1 to 6; a palpable thrill characterizes murmurs of grade 4 or higher intensity. Other important attributes that aid in identification include location, radiation, and response to bedside maneuvers, including quiet respiration.

Systolic Murmurs
Systolic murmurs are early, midsystolic, late, or holosystolic in timing. Acute severe MR results in a decrescendo, early systolic murmur because of the steep rise in pressure within the noncompliant left atrium (see Fig. 13.8). Severe MR associated with posterior mitral leaflet prolapse or flail radiates anteriorly and to the base; MR caused by anterior leaflet involvement radiates posteriorly and to the axilla. With acute TR in patients with normal pulmonary artery pressures, an early systolic murmur, which increases in intensity with inspiration, may be audible at the lower left sternal border, and regurgitant *cv* waves may be

TABLE 13.6 Principal Causes of Heart Murmurs

Systolic Murmurs

Early Systolic

Mitral—acute MR
VSD
    Muscular
    Nonrestrictive with pulmonary hypertension
Tricuspid—TR with normal pulmonary artery pressure

Midsystolic

Aortic
    Obstructive
        Supravalvular—supravalvular aortic stenosis, coarctation of the aorta
        Valvular—aortic stenosis and sclerosis
        Subvalvular—discrete, tunnel, or HCM
    Increased flow, hyperkinetic states, AR, complete heart block
    Dilation of ascending aorta, atheroma, aortitis
Pulmonary
    Obstructive
        Supravalvular—pulmonary artery stenosis
        Valvular—pulmonic valve stenosis
        Subvalvular—infundibular stenosis (dynamic)
    Increased flow, hyperkinetic states, left-to-right shunt (e.g., ASD)
    Dilation of pulmonary artery

Late Systolic

Mitral—MVP, acute myocardial ischemia
Tricuspid—tricuspid valve prolapse

Holosystolic

Atrioventricular valve regurgitation (MR, TR)
Left-to-right shunt at ventricular level (VSD)

Diastolic Murmurs

Early Diastolic

Aortic regurgitation
    Valvular—congenital (bicuspid valve), rheumatic deformity, endocarditis, prolapse, trauma, postvalvulotomy
    Dilation of valve annulus—aortic dissection, annuloaortic ectasia, cystic medial degeneration, hypertension, ankylosing spondylitis
    Widening of commissures—syphilis
Pulmonic regurgitation
    Valvular—postvalvulotomy, endocarditis, rheumatic fever, carcinoid
    Dilation of valve annulus—pulmonary hypertension; Marfan syndrome
    Congenital—isolated or associated with tetralogy of Fallot, VSD, pulmonic stenosis

Mid-diastolic

Mitral
    Mitral stenosis
    Carey Coombs murmur (mid-diastolic apical murmur in acute rheumatic fever)
    Increased flow across nonstenotic mitral valve (e.g., MR, VSD, PDA, high-output states, complete heart block)
Tricuspid
    Tricuspid stenosis
    Increased flow across nonstenotic tricuspid valve (e.g., TR, ASD, anomalous pulmonary venous return)
Left and right atrial tumors (myxoma)
Severe or eccentric AR (Austin Flint murmur)

Late Diastolic

Presystolic accentuation of mitral stenosis murmur
Austin Flint murmur of severe or eccentric AR

Continuous Murmurs

PDA
Coronary arteriovenous fistula
Ruptured sinus of Valsalva aneurysm
Aortic septal defect
Cervical venous hum
Anomalous left coronary artery
Proximal coronary artery stenosis
Mammary soufflé of pregnancy
Pulmonary artery branch stenosis
Bronchial collateral circulation
Small (restrictive) ASD with mitral stenosis
Intercostal arteriovenous fistula

AR, Aortic regurgitation; *ASD*, atrial septal defect; *HCM*, hypertrophic cardiomyopathy; *MR*, mitral regurgitation; *MVP*, mitral valve prolapse; *PDA*, patent ductus arteriosus; *TR*, tricuspid regurgitation; *VSD*, ventricular septal defect.
From Braunwald E, Perloff JK. Physical examination of the heart and circulation. In Zipes DP, et al., eds. *Braunwald's Heart Disease: A Textbook of Cardiovascular Medicine*. 7th ed. Philadelphia: Saunders; 2005:77–106; and Norton PJ, O'Rourke RA. Approach to the patient with a heart murmur. In: Braunwald E, Goldman L, eds. *Primary Cardiology*. 2nd ed. Philadelphia: Elsevier; 2003:151–168.

---

visible in the jugular venous pulse. Midsystolic murmurs begin after S_1 and end before S_2; they usually are crescendo-decrescendo in configuration. Aortic stenosis or sclerosis causes most midsystolic murmurs in adults. Accurate characterization of the severity of aortic stenosis at the bedside depends on cardiac output, stiffness of the carotid arteries, and associated findings. Other causes of a midsystolic heart murmur include HCM, pulmonic stenosis, and increased pulmonary blood flow in patients with a large ASD and a left-to-right shunt. An isolated grade 1 or 2 midsystolic murmur in the absence of symptoms or other signs of heart disease is a benign finding that does not warrant further evaluation, including echocardiography. A mid-to-late, apical systolic murmur usually indicates MVP; one or more nonejection clicks may be present. A similar murmur may be heard transiently during an episode of acute myocardial ischemia. The intensity of the murmur will vary with LV afterload, as is also the case for the murmur of chronic, secondary MR associated with ischemic or dilated cardiomyopathy. Holosystolic murmurs, which are plateau in configuration, derive from the continuous and wide pressure gradient between two cardiac chambers—the left ventricle and left atrium with chronic MR, the right ventricle and right atrium with chronic TR, and the left ventricle and right ventricle with membranous ventricular septal defect (VSD) without pulmonary hypertension. MR is best heard over the cardiac apex, TR at the lower left sternal border, and a VSD murmur at the mid-left sternal border, where a thrill is palpable in most patients. TR most commonly is secondary to annular dilation from RV enlargement with papillary muscle displacement and failure of tricuspid leaflet coaptation. Pulmonary artery hypertension also may be present.

Diastolic Murmurs

Diastolic murmurs invariably signify cardiac disease. Chronic AR causes a high-pitched decrescendo early to mid-diastolic murmur. With primary aortic valve disease, the murmur is best heard along the left sternal border, whereas with root enlargement and secondary AR, the murmur may radiate along the right sternal border. A midsystolic murmur caused by augmented and accelerated blood flow is also present with moderate to severe AR and need not signify valve or

TABLE 13.7 Interventions for Altering Intensity of Cardiac Murmurs

Respiration: Right-sided murmurs generally increase with inspiration. Left-sided murmurs usually are louder during expiration.

Valsalva maneuver: Most murmurs decrease in length and intensity. Two exceptions are the systolic murmur of HCM, which usually becomes much louder, and that of MVP, which becomes longer and often louder. After release of the Valsalva maneuver, right-sided murmurs tend to return to baseline intensity earlier than left-sided murmurs.

Exercise: Murmurs caused by blood flow across normal or obstructed valves (as in pulmonic and mitral stenosis) become louder with both isotonic and isometric (handgrip) exercise. Murmurs of MR, VSD, and AR also increase with handgrip exercise.

Positional changes: With standing, most murmurs diminish; two exceptions are the murmur of HCM, which becomes louder, and that of MVP, which lengthens and often is intensified. With squatting, most murmurs become louder, but those of HCM and MVP usually soften and may disappear. Passive leg raising usually produces the same results as squatting.

Post–ventricular premature beat or AF: Murmurs originating at normal or stenotic semilunar valves increase in intensity during the cardiac cycle after a ventricular premature beat or in the beat after a long cycle length in AF. By contrast, systolic murmurs caused by AV valve regurgitation do not change, diminish (papillary muscle dysfunction), or become shorter after a premature beat (MVP).

Pharmacologic interventions: During the initial relative hypotension after amyl nitrite inhalation, murmurs of MR, VSD, and AR decrease in intensity, whereas the murmur of AS increases in intensity because of increased stroke volume. During the later tachycardia phase, murmurs of mitral stenosis and right-sided lesions also become louder. This intervention may help distinguish the murmur of the Austin Flint phenomenon from that of mitral stenosis. The response in MVP often is biphasic (softer and then louder than control).

Transient arterial occlusion: Transient external compression of both brachial arteries by bilateral cuff inflation to 20 mm Hg greater than peak systolic pressure augments the murmurs of MR, VSD, and AR, but not murmurs from other causes.

AR, Aortic regurgitation; *HCM*, hypertrophic cardiomyopathy; *MR*, mitral regurgitation; *MVP*, mitral valve prolapse; *VSD*, ventricular septal defect.
From Bonow RO, Carabello BA, Chatterjee K, et al. ACC/AHA 2006 guidelines for the management of patients with valvular heart disease: a report of the American College of Cardiology/American Heart Association Task Force on Practice Guidelines (Writing Committee to Revise the 1998 Guidelines for the Management of Patients with Valvular Heart Disease) developed in collaboration with the Society of Cardiovascular Anesthesiologists endorsed by the Society for Cardiovascular Angiography and Interventions and the Society of Thoracic Surgeons. *J Am Coll Cardiol*. 2006;48:e18.

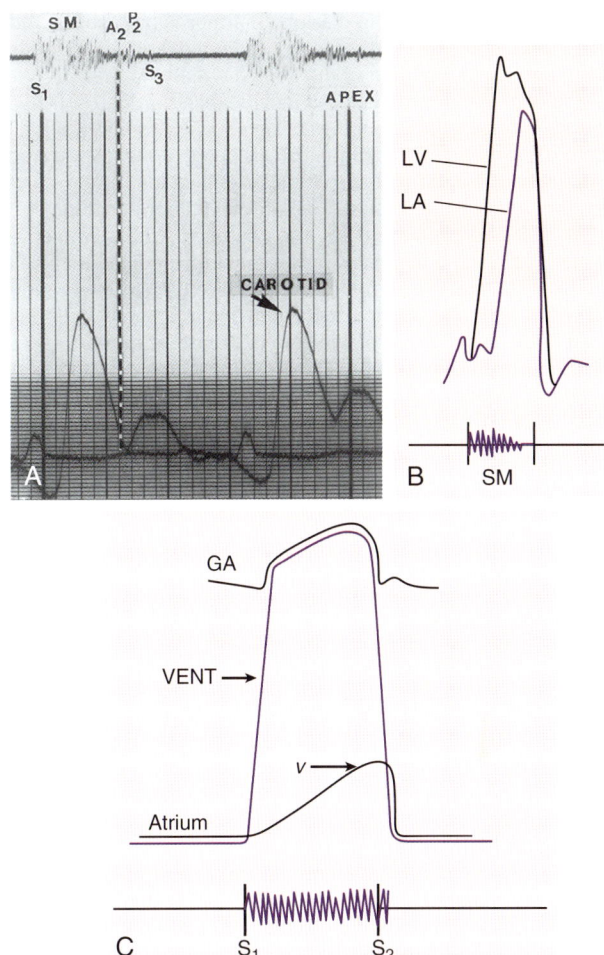

FIGURE 13.8 **A,** Phonocardiogram (*top*) obtained in a patient with acute severe mitral regurgitation (MR) showing a decrescendo early systolic murmur and diastolic filling sound (S_3). **B,** Left ventricular (LV) and left atrial (LA) pressure waveforms demonstrating the abrupt rise in LA pressure and attenuation of the LV-LA pressure gradient, resulting in the duration and configuration of the murmur. **C,** Illustration of great artery (GA) and ventricular (VENT) and atrial pressures with corresponding phonocardiogram in chronic MR or TR. Note the holosystolic timing and plateau configuration of the murmur, both of which derive from the large ventricular-atrial pressure gradient throughout systole. *SM*, Systolic murmur; *v*, v wave. (From Braunwald E, Perloff JK. Physical examination of the heart and circulation. In: Zipes D, et al. eds. *Braunwald's Heart Disease: A Textbook of Cardiovascular Medicine*. 7th ed. Philadelphia: Saunders; 2005:97.)

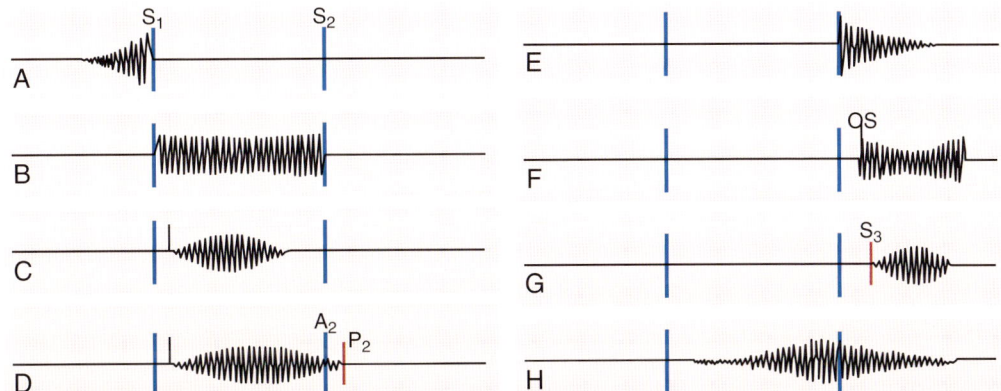

FIGURE 13.7 Diagram of principal heart murmurs. **A,** Presystolic accentuation of the murmur of mitral stenosis with sinus rhythm. **B,** Holosystolic murmur of chronic, severe mitral regurgitation or tricuspid regurgitation, or ventricular septal defect without severe pulmonary hypertension. **C,** Ejection sound and crescendo-decrescendo murmur of bicuspid aortic stenosis. **D,** Ejection sound and crescendo-decrescendo murmur that extends to P_2 in bicuspid pulmonic stenosis. **E,** Early decrescendo diastolic murmur of aortic regurgitation or pulmonic regurgitation. **F,** Opening snap (OS) and mid-diastolic rumble of mitral stenosis. **G,** Diastolic filling sound (S_3) and mid-diastolic murmur associated with severe MR, TR, or atrial septal defect with significant left-to-right shunt. **H,** Continuous murmur of patent ductus arteriosus that envelops S_2. (Modified from Wood P. *Diseases of the Heart and Circulation*. Philadelphia: Lippincott; 1968; and O'Rourke RA, Braunwald E. Physical examination of the cardiovascular system. In: Kasper D, Braunwald E, Fauci A, et al. eds. *Harrison's Principles of Internal Medicine*. 16th ed. New York: McGraw-Hill; 2005:1309.)

outflow tract obstruction. The diastolic murmur is both softer and of shorter duration in acute AR, as a result of the rapid rise in LV diastolic pressure and the diminution of the aortic-LV diastolic pressure gradient. Additional features of acute AR include tachycardia, a soft S_1, and the absence of peripheral findings of significant diastolic run-off. The murmur of pulmonic regurgitation (PR) is heard along the left sternal border and most often is due to annular enlargement from chronic pulmonary artery hypertension (Graham-Steele murmur). Signs of RV pressure overload are present. PR also can occur with a congenitally deformed valve and is invariably present after repair of tetralogy of Fallot. In these settings, the murmur is relatively softer and lower-pitched. The severity of PR after surgical repair can be underappreciated. Mitral stenosis is the classic cause of a mid- to late diastolic murmur (see Fig. 13.7). The stenosis also may be "silent"—for example, in patients with low cardiac output or large body habitus. The murmur is best heard over the apex with the patient in the left lateral decubitus position, is low-pitched (rumbling), and is introduced by an OS in the early stages of the disease. Presystolic accentuation (an increase in the intensity of the murmur in late diastole following atrial contraction) occurs in patients in sinus rhythm. Left-sided events usually obscure findings in patients with rheumatic tricuspid stenosis. Functional mitral stenosis or tricuspid stenosis refers to mid-diastolic murmurs created by increased, accelerated transvalvular flow, without valvular obstruction, in the setting of severe MR or TR, respectively, or ASD with a large left-to-right shunt. The low-pitched mid- to late apical diastolic murmur sometimes associated with AR (Austin Flint murmur) can be distinguished from mitral stenosis on the basis of its response to vasodilators and the presence of associated findings. Less common causes of a mid-diastolic murmur include atrial myxoma, complete heart block, and acute rheumatic mitral valvulitis (Carey Coombs murmur).

Continuous Murmurs

The presence of a continuous murmur implies a pressure gradient between two chambers or vessels during both systole and diastole. These murmurs begin in systole, peak near S_2, and continue into diastole. They can be difficult to distinguish from systolic and diastolic murmurs in patients with mixed aortic or pulmonic valve disease. Examples are the murmurs associated with PDA, ruptured sinus of Valsalva aneurysm, and coronary, great vessel, or hemodialysis-related arteriovenous fistulas. The cervical venous hum and mammary souffle of pregnancy are two benign variants.

Dynamic Auscultation

Simple bedside maneuvers can help identify heart murmurs and characterize their significance (see Table 13.7). Right-sided events, except for the pulmonic ejection sound, increase with inspiration and decrease with expiration; left-sided events behave oppositely (100% sensitivity, 88% specificity). The intensity of the murmurs associated with MR, VSD, and AR will increase in response to maneuvers that increase LV afterload (e.g., handgrip, vasopressor administration) and decrease after exposure to vasodilating agents (e.g., amyl nitrite). The response of the murmur associated with MVP to standing and squatting has previously been described. The murmur of HOCM behaves in a directionally similar manner, becoming softer and shorter with squatting (95% sensitivity, 85% specificity) and longer and louder on rapid standing (95% sensitivity, 84% specificity). The intensity of the murmur of HCM also increases with the Valsalva maneuver (65% sensitivity, 95% specificity). A change in the intensity of a systolic murmur in the first beat after a premature beat, or in the beat after a long cycle length in patients with AF, suggests aortic stenosis rather than MR, particularly in an older patient, in whom the murmur of aortic stenosis is well transmitted to the apex (Gallavardin effect). Systolic murmurs that are due to LV outflow obstruction, including those caused by aortic stenosis, will increase in intensity in the beat following a premature beat because of the combined effects of enhanced LV filling and post-extrasystolic potentiation of contractile function. Forward flow accelerates, causing an increase in the gradient and a louder murmur. The intensity of the murmur of MR does not change in the post-premature beat, because relatively little further increase occurs in mitral valve flow or change in the LV-LA gradient.

INTEGRATED, EVIDENCE-BASED APPROACH TO SPECIFIC CARDIAC DISORDERS

Heart Failure (see Part VI)
History

Both exertional and resting symptoms should be investigated. Common signs and symptoms include dyspnea, fatigue, exercise limitation, orthopnea, and edema. In a review of 22 studies of adult patients presenting to an emergency department with dyspnea, the probability of heart failure was best predicted by a past history of heart failure (LR, 5.8; 95% CI, 4.1 to 8.0), paroxysmal nocturnal dyspnea (LR, 2.6; 95% CI, 1.5 to 4.5), a third heart sound (LR, 11; 95% CI, 4.9 to 25), or AF (LR, 3.8; 95% CI, 1.7 to 8.8).[24] An initial clinical impression of heart failure as noted by a physician was one of the stronger clinical predictors of this diagnosis (LR, 4.4; 95% CI, 1.8 to 10.0). With the exception of paroxysmal nocturnal dyspnea, these same features also predicted heart failure when there was concomitant pulmonary disease. The addition of testing for N-terminal pro–B-type natriuretic peptide (NT-pro-BNP) increases diagnostic accuracy only modestly (C-statistic, 0.83 versus 0.86).[7]

Severe and sudden onset dyspnea indicates acute pulmonary edema, typically precipitated by ischemia, arrhythmia, sudden left-sided valvular regurgitation, and/or accelerated hypertension. It is important to exclude other causes such as pulmonary embolism and pneumothorax. The extent of limitation also should be defined because functional capacity, as assessed by NYHA classification, strongly and independently predicts the risk of death for patients with heart failure. Self-reported functional capacity and objectively measured cardiovascular performance can differ substantially. Symptoms that occur at rest may have greater predictive value for the diagnosis of heart failure than exertional symptoms. Orthopnea is not specific for heart failure and can occur in patients with asthma, ascites, or gastroesophageal reflux. Trepopnea, which is dyspnea or discomfort experienced in the lateral decubitus position, also may be present. Patients with heart failure prefer sleeping on their right side, and trepopnea probably accounts for the predominance of right-sided pleural effusions in this population. Shortness of breath may be particularly noticeable when bending forward, termed bendopnea. It is associated with higher supine right atrial and pulmonary capillary wedge pressures and is mediated by further elevations in these pressures with bending over. It is even more likely present when the resting cardiac index is low.[25] Paroxysmal nocturnal dyspnea also is common in patients with heart failure. Cheyne-Stokes respirations may be apparent when the patient is awake.[26] The prevalence of central sleep apnea or Cheyne-Stokes respirations ranges from 20% to 62% in various heart failure studies,[15] and either of these disorders is associated with an increased mortality risk.

Clinically evident edema or weight gain over days indicates volume excess but lags the clinical redistribution of intravascular volume from the splanchnic beds to the central veins. In patients with advanced right-sided heart failure, uncomfortable hepatomegaly and ascites may predominate. Patients with chronic heart failure often lack pulmonary rales or lower extremity edema. Gastrointestinal symptoms such as early satiety, nausea, vomiting, and belching are also common and are related to decreases in gastrointestinal blood flow and bowel edema, particularly in those with cardiac cachexia.[27]

Few studies have explored the predictive values of various signs and symptoms of heart failure. In a systematic review,[28] orthopnea only modestly predicted increased filling pressures. Dyspnea and edema were similarly useful but were most predictive when combined with physical examination findings (S_3, tachycardia, elevated JVP, low pulse pressure, rales, abdominojugular reflux sign). When combined with other findings, a total of three or more symptoms or signs predicted a greater than 90% likelihood of increased filling pressures if severe LV dysfunction was not known. By contrast, if one or no findings or symptoms were present, the likelihood of increased filling pressures was less than 10%. The commonly used Framingham criteria for heart failure diagnosis in patients with reduced ejection fraction have only modest specificity (63%) and sensitivity (63%).

The distinction between heart failure with reduced ejection fraction, and that with preserved ejection fraction, can be made at the bedside with modest accuracy. Systolic function is more likely to be preserved when patients are female or older and have an increased BMI, but such findings lack adequate specificity and sensitivity to guide therapy. Furthermore, diastolic dysfunction does not exclude systolic dysfunction.

Physical Examination

In most patients with heart failure who require hospitalization, the reason for admission is volume overload; failure to relieve it has negative prognostic impact. Four signs are commonly used to predict elevated filling pressures: jugular venous distention/abdominojugular reflux sign, presence of an S_3 and/or S_4, rales, and pedal edema. In general, the use of a combination of findings, rather than reliance on isolated findings, improves diagnostic accuracy. Some clinicians advocate assessment of the heart failure patient along two basic axes—volume status ("dry" or "wet") and perfusion status ("warm" or "cold")—as a useful guide to therapy. This approach has prognostic usefulness, particularly in assessing patients at discharge after admission for heart failure. For example, patients discharged with a "wet" or "cold" profile experience worse outcomes (HR, 1.5; 95% CI, 1.1 to 12.1; $P = 0.017$) compared with those discharged "warm and dry" (HR 0.9; 95% CI, 0.7 to 2.1; $P = 0.5$).[28] Advanced training may be required to achieve this level of diagnostic precision with the physical examination.

Jugular Venous Pressure

The JVP provides the readiest bedside estimate of LV filling pressure. In the Evaluation Study of Congestive Heart Failure and Pulmonary Artery Catheterization Effectiveness (ESCAPE) trial, 82% of patients whose estimated right atrial pressure was higher than 8 mm Hg (10.5 cm H_2O) had a measured right atrial pressure higher than 8 mm Hg. The same investigators also identified 9 of the 11 patients with pressures lower than 8 mm Hg.[28] Although the JVP estimates RV filling pressure, it has a predictable relationship with pulmonary artery wedge pressure. Drazner and colleagues[28] found that the right atrial pressure reliably predicted the pulmonary artery wedge pressure; the positive predictive value of a right atrial pressure higher than 10 mm Hg for a pulmonary artery wedge pressure higher than 22 mm Hg was 88%. In addition, the pulmonary artery systolic pressure could be estimated as twice the wedge pressure. In the ESCAPE trial, an estimated right atrial pressure higher than 12 mm Hg and two-pillow orthopnea were the only bedside parameters that provided incremental value to the prediction of a pulmonary artery wedge pressure higher than 22 mm Hg, and compared favorably with BNP levels.[28] Echocardiography and BNP determinations may not always provide incremental value to the clinical assessment of heart failure by experienced observers.[29]

An elevated JVP has prognostic significance. Drazner and associates[28] demonstrated that the presence of jugular vein distention signifying elevated pressures at the time of enrollment in a large clinical heart failure trial (11% of the Studies of Left Ventricular Dysfunction [SOLVD] treatment study participants), after adjustment for other markers of disease severity, predicted heart failure hospitalizations (relative risk [RR], 132; 95% CI, 1.08 to 1.62), death from pump failure (RR, 1.37; 95% CI, 107 to 1.75), and death plus heart failure hospitalization (RR, 1.30; 95%CI, 1.11 to 1.53). The investigators extended these observations to asymptomatic subjects enrolled in the SOLVD prevention study, among whom jugular vein distention was less common (1.7% of the study population).[28] In a contemporary clinical trial, physical examination evidence of congestion remained predictive of outcome and independent of symptoms, risk scores, and natriuretic peptide levels.[30] Signs of congestion have also been shown to be independently associated with cardiovascular death, heart failure hospitalization, and all-cause mortality in heart failure with preserved ejection fraction.[31]

In patients presenting with dyspnea, the abdominojugular reflux sign is useful in predicting heart failure (LR, 6.0; 95% CI, 0.8 to 51) and suggests a pulmonary artery wedge pressure higher than 15 mm Hg (LR, 6.7; 95% CI, 3.3 to 13.4). The presence of jugular vein distention, either at rest or induced, had the best combination of sensitivity (81%), specificity (80%), and predictive accuracy (81%) for elevation of the pulmonary artery wedge pressure. Ultrasound assessment of IJV dimension, both at rest and during the Valsalva maneuver, associates independently with prognosis in ambulatory heart failure patients with reduced ejection fraction.[32]

Third and Fourth Heart Sounds

The third heart sound (S_3) predicts ejection fraction poorly because it reflects primarily diastolic rather than systolic performance. In patients with heart failure, an S_3 is equally prevalent in those with and without LV systolic dysfunction. A rigorous assessment of the S_3 was conducted by Marcus and colleagues in 100 patients with various cardiovascular conditions undergoing elective cardiac catheterization. Cardiology fellows ($n = 18$; K statistic, 0.37; $P < 0.001$) and faculty ($n = 26$; K statistic, 0.29; $P = 0.003$) performed better than residents ($n = 102$; no significant agreement) in the identification of a phonocardiographically confirmed S_3.[33] Furthermore, an S_3 predicted an increase in both LV end-diastolic pressure (LVEDP) (greater than 15 mm Hg) and BNP (greater than 100 pg/mL) and depressed ventricular systolic function (ejection fraction less than 0.50), although sensitivities were low (32% to 52%).[34] An S_4 had comparable sensitivity (40% to 46%) but inferior specificity (72% to 80% for an S_4 versus 87% to 92% for an S_3). A third heart sound frequently may be heard in patients referred for cardiac transplant evaluation but is a poor predictor of elevated filling pressures. Alternatively, the lack of an S_3 cannot exclude a diagnosis of heart failure, but its presence reliably indicates ventricular dysfunction.

The prognostic value of an S_3 in chronic heart failure was established in the SOLVD treatment and prevention studies.[28] The investigators found that an S_3 predicted cardiovascular morbidity and mortality. The RR for heart failure hospitalization and death in patients with an S_3 was of comparable magnitude in the prevention and treatment cohorts. These observations remained significant after adjustment for markers of disease severity and were even more powerful when combined with the presence of an elevated JVP. An S_3 also predicts a higher risk of adverse outcomes in other settings, such as that of MI or noncardiac surgery.

Rales and Edema

In patients with chronic heart failure, approximately 75% to 80% of participants lacked rales despite elevated pulmonary artery wedge pressures, presumably because of enhanced lymphatic drainage. Recent studies have incorporated the findings from lung ultrasound (LR 7.4; 95% CI 4.2 to 12.8) in the assessment of emergency room patients with acute heart failure[35] and in ambulatory heart failure patients.[36] In the latter setting, lung ultrasound findings can identify patients with worse prognosis. When pulmonary adventitious sounds are present, specific characteristics may help elucidate a pulmonary rather than cardiac disorder (see Fig. 13.2). The chest radiograph similarly lacked sensitivity for increased filling pressures in these studies. Pedal edema is neither sensitive nor specific for the diagnosis of heart failure and has low predictive value as an isolated variable.

Valsalva Maneuver

The blood pressure response to the Valsalva maneuver can be measured noninvasively using a blood pressure cuff or commercially available devices. The Valsalva maneuver consists of four phases (Figs. 13.9 and 13.10). In a normal response, Korotkoff sounds are audible only during phases I and IV, because the systolic pressure normally rises at the onset and release of the strain phase. Two abnormal responses to the Valsalva maneuver in heart failure are recognized: (1) absence of the phase IV overshoot and (2) the square-wave response (see Fig. 13.10). The absent overshoot pattern indicates decreased systolic function; the square-wave response indicates elevated filling pressures and appears to be independent of ejection fraction. The responses can be quantified using the pulse amplitude ratio if the pulse pressure is measured during the maneuver. This ratio compares the minimum pulse pressure at the end of the strain phase against the maximum pulse pressure at the onset of the strain phase; a higher ratio is consistent with a square-wave response.

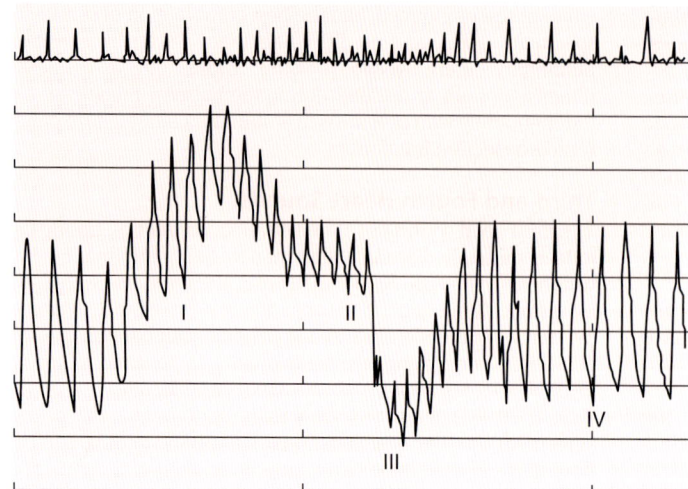

FIGURE 13.9 The normal Valsalva response. (From Nishimura RA, Tajik AJ. The Valsalva maneuver—3 centuries later. *Mayo Clin Proc.* 2004;79:577.)

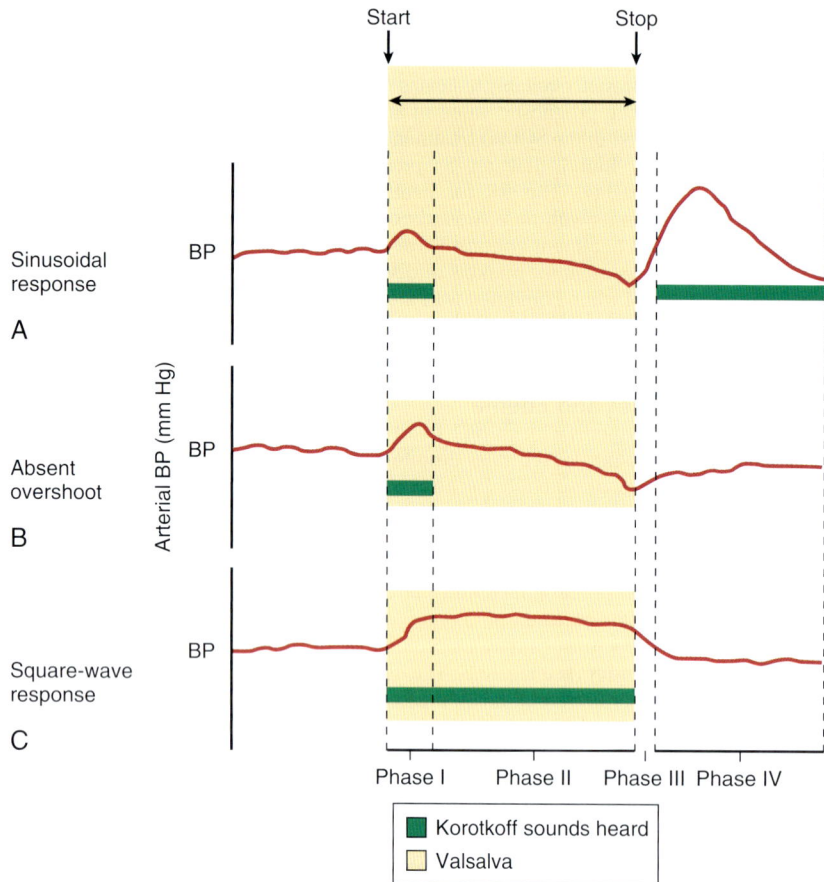

FIGURE 13.10 Abnormal Valsalva responses assessed using the pattern of Korotkoff sounds. **A,** Normal, sinusoidal response with sounds intermittent during strain and release. **B,** Briefly audible sounds during initial strain phase suggests only impaired systolic function in absence of fluid overload. **C,** Persistence of Korotkoff sounds throughout strain phase suggests elevated left ventricular filling pressures. *BP,* Blood pressure. (From Shamsham F, Mitchell J. Essentials of the diagnosis of heart failure. *Am Fam Physician.* 2000;61:1319.)

Other Findings

In the absence of hypertension, the pulse pressure is determined by the stroke volume and vascular stiffness and can be used to assess cardiac output. In a cohort of patients with chronic systolic heart failure, the proportional pulse pressure ([systolic − diastolic]/systolic) correlated well with cardiac index (correlation coefficient [r] = 0.82; $P < 0.001$), stroke volume index ($r = 0.78$; $P < 0.001$), and the inverse of systemic vascular resistance ($r = 0.65$; $P < 0.001$). Using a proportional pulse pressure of 25%, the cardiac index could be predicted: if the value was lower than 25%, the cardiac index was less than 2.2 L/min/m^2 in 91% of patients; if the value was higher than 25%, the cardiac index was higher than 2.2 L/min/m^2 in 83% of patients.[37] Circulation time has also been used to assess the cardiac output. Using oxygen as the indicator, a time from a breath hold to the nadir of finger oximetry of greater than 34 seconds has been associated with a cardiac output of less than 4 L/min.[38]

Heart rate is also a powerful indicator of prognosis in heart failure. A resting heart rate (in sinus rhythm) of greater than 70 to 75 beats/min is an independent predictor of mortality. When the heart rate is decreased by ivabradine on a background of beta-blocker therapy in patients with sinus rhythm, heart failure hospitalizations are decreased.[39] An attenuated heart rate increase with immediate standing (e.g., ≤3 beats/min) may also reflect the dysautonomia of heart failure and has been associated with death or heart failure hospitalization. A greater increase of heart rate with standing over time is associated with greater heart failure hospitalization-free survival.[40] In patients admitted with acute decompensated heart failure, a heart rate greater than the systolic blood pressure (e.g., a shock index ≥0.9) has been associated with in-hospital and 3-month mortality.[41]

Clinical experience may be the most helpful in assessing hemodynamic status. A good assessment for systemic perfusion and cardiac index appears to be overall clinical impression, the so-called "cold" profile. The gestalt of specialized heart failure clinicians performed better than proportional pulse pressure, systolic blood pressure, cool extremities, or fatigue in predicting an invasively measured cardiac index lower than 2.3 L/min/m^2.[28] This prediction rule has not been reported in other patient groups, in larger cohorts, or in more contemporary studies. Pleural effusions also are common in patients with heart failure, in whom they typically are right-sided, as noted previously. Dullness to percussion is the simplest finding to elicit in identifying a pleural effusion and is superior (LR, 8.7; 95% CI, 2.2 to 33.8) to auscultatory percussion, decreased breath sounds, asymmetric chest expansion, increased vocal resonance, crackles, or pleural friction rubs. By contrast, absence of reduced tactile vocal fremitus makes a pleural effusion less likely (negative LR, 0.21; 95% CI, 0.12 to 0.37).[42]

Patient with a Left Ventricular Assist Device
The physical examination assessment of the left ventricular assist device (LVAD) patient should be organized around the hemodynamics of durable LVAD support (e.g., volume status, presence of native aortic valve opening, mean blood pressure, end-organ perfusion) as well as the complications unique to the mechanically supported circulation (e.g., driveline infection, blood loss from either gastrointestinal bleeding or hemolysis, and neurologic complications). Jugular venous distension, lower extremity edema, and abdominal distension will indicate right heart failure, often without concomitant left heart failure. Blood pressure may be obtained with a traditional cuff but may require Doppler assessment. In general, the first Korotkoff sound obtained by Doppler will be reported interchangeably as either the systolic or mean blood pressure; a mean blood pressure of less than 90 mm Hg is optimal. The pulse should be palpated by hand at either the radial, brachial, or carotid locations; a palpable pulse should be intermittent and reflective of intermittent opening of the native aortic valve. Auscultation of the LVAD itself will elicit sounds unique to the specific LVAD device; regular changes in the LVAD hum can reflect intrinsic speed changes (a Lavare cycle) in order to provide an artificial "pulse" to the LVAD itself. Other changes to the cadence maybe indicative of LVAD dysfunction (e.g., thrombosis.)

Valvular Heart Disease (see also Part VIII)
A careful history and physical examination can reveal much regarding lesion severity, natural history, indications for intervention, and outcomes in patients with valvular heart disease. The history in patients with known or suspected valvular heart disease should rely on the use of a functional classification scheme and assessment of patient frailty when appropriate. Onset of even mild functional limitation is generally an indication for mechanical correction of the responsible valve lesion. Valvular heart disease most often is first suspected because of a heart murmur but many patients go undetected until presentation with symptoms or the discovery of a valve lesion on an echocardiogram performed for another indication.[43,44] Cardiologists can detect systolic heart murmurs with fair reliability (interobserver kappa coefficient, 0.30 to 0.48), and usually can confirm or rule out aortic stenosis, HOCM, MR, MVP, TR, and functional murmurs. The use of handheld ultrasound devices may improve detection and accuracy rates.[45]

Mitral Stenosis
In patients with mitral stenosis, survival declines following symptom onset and worsens with increasing degrees of functional limitation (NYHA class) and as pulmonary hypertension increases. Findings on physical examination vary with the chronicity of the disease, heart rate, rhythm, and cardiac output. It can be difficult to estimate the severity of the valve lesion in older patients with less pliable valves, rapid AF, or low cardiac output. Severe mitral stenosis is suggested by (1) a long or holodiastolic murmur, indicating a persistent LA-LV gradient; (2) a short A_2-OS interval, consistent with higher LA pressure; (3) a loud P_2 (or single S_2) and/or an RV lift, suggestive of pulmonary hypertension; and (4) elevated JVP with cv waves, hepatomegaly, and lower extremity edema—all signs of right heart failure with TR. Neither the intensity of the diastolic murmur nor the presence of presystolic accentuation in patients with sinus rhythm accurately reflects lesion severity.

Mitral Regurgitation
The symptoms associated with MR depend on its severity and time course of development. Acute severe MR that occurs with papillary muscle rupture or infective endocarditis usually results in sudden and profound dyspnea from pulmonary edema. Examination findings may be misleading because the LV impulse usually is neither enlarged nor displaced, and the systolic murmur is early in timing and decrescendo in configuration (see Fig. 13.10). The murmur also may be louder at the lower left sternal border or in the axilla than at the apex. A new systolic murmur developing early after an MI may not be audible in a ventilated or obese patient.

Several findings suggest chronic severe MR: (1) an enlarged, displaced, but dynamic LV apex beat; (2) an apical systolic thrill (murmur intensity of grade 4 or greater); (3) a mid-diastolic filling complex comprising an S_3 and a short, low-pitched murmur, indicative of accelerated and enhanced diastolic mitral inflow; (4) wide but physiologic splitting of S_2 caused by early aortic valve closure; and (5) a loud P_2 or RV lift. The findings in patients with MVP can vary, depending on LV loading conditions. The combination of a nonejection click and mid- to late systolic murmur predicts MVP best, as confirmed by transthoracic echocardiography criteria (LR, 2.43). Dynamic auscultation should be performed. The murmur associated with secondary MR in patients with reduced LV systolic function is often of low intensity and can be difficult to hear unless specifically sought.

Aortic Stenosis
A slowly rising carotid upstroke (*pulsus tardus*), reduced carotid pulse amplitude (*pulsus parvus*), reduced intensity of A_2, and mid- to late peaking of the systolic murmur help gauge the severity of aortic stenosis. The intensity of the murmur depends on cardiac output and body size (peak momentum transfer) and does not reliably reflect stenosis severity. In a 35-year follow-up study of 2014 apparently healthy middle-aged Norwegian men, the presence of even a low-grade systolic murmur was associated with an almost fivefold increased age-adjusted risk for aortic valve replacement.[46] No single physical examination finding has both high sensitivity and high specificity for the diagnosis of severe aortic stenosis, and only a reduced carotid upstroke amplitude may independently predict outcome. Clinical experience has established the difficulty of assessing carotid upstroke characteristics in older patients, in patients with hypertension, and in low-output states. Distinguishing the murmur of hemodynamically significant aortic stenosis from that caused by lesser degrees of stenosis is also challenging. Even with aortic sclerosis, the murmur can be of grade 2 or 3 intensity, although it peaks in midsystole. The carotid upstroke should be normal, A_2 should be preserved, and the electrocardiogram should lack evidence of LV hypertrophy. Nevertheless, TTE often is necessary to clarify this distinction, especially in older patients with hypertension. Signal analysis of digitally captured cardiovascular sounds using spectral display can distinguish the murmur of aortic sclerosis from a murmur resulting from hemodynamically significant aortic stenosis. The differential diagnosis of a systolic murmur related to LV outflow obstruction includes valvular aortic stenosis, HOCM, discrete membranous subaortic stenosis (DMSS), and SVAS. The presence of an ejection sound indicates a valvular cause. HOCM can be distinguished on the basis of the response of the murmur to the Valsalva maneuver and standing or squatting. Patients with DMSS will commonly have a diastolic murmur indicative of AR but not an ejection sound, whereas in patients with SVAS, the right arm blood pressure is more than 10 mm Hg greater than the left arm blood pressure. Assessment of fragility status in elderly patients with aortic stenosis is a routine feature of the multidisciplinary team evaluation (see Table 13.3).

Aortic Regurgitation
Patients with acute severe AR present with pulmonary edema and symptoms and signs of low forward cardiac output. Tachycardia is invariably present; systolic blood pressure is not elevated, and the pulse pressure may not be significantly widened. S_1 is soft because of premature closure of the mitral valve. The intensity and duration of the diastolic murmur are attenuated by the rapid rise in LV diastolic pressure and diminution of the aortic-LV diastolic pressure gradient. In patients with acute type A aortic dissection, the presence of a diastolic murmur (present in almost 30% of cases)

does little to change the pretest probability of dissection. Acute severe AR is poorly tolerated and mandates emergency surgery. Typical symptoms associated with chronic, severe AR include dyspnea, fatigue, chest discomfort, and palpitations. A decrescendo diastolic blowing murmur suggests chronic AR. A midsystolic murmur indicative of augmented LV outflow is invariably heard at the base. Aortic stenosis may coexist. The absence of a diastolic murmur significantly reduces the likelihood of moderate or greater AR (LR, 0.1), whereas the presence of a typical diastolic murmur increases the likelihood of moderate or greater AR (LR, 4.0 to 8.3). In addition, in patients with chronic AR, the intensity of the murmur correlates with the severity of the lesion. A grade 3 diastolic murmur has an LR of 4.5 (95% CI, 1.6 to 14.0) for distinguishing severe AR from mild or moderate AR.[47] Data conflict regarding the significance of an Austin Flint murmur. Little evidence supports the historical claims of the importance of almost all the eponymous peripheral signs of chronic AR, which number at least 12. The Hill sign (brachial-popliteal systolic blood pressure gradient higher than 20 mm Hg) may be the single exception (sensitivity of 89% for moderate to severe AR), although its supporting evidence base also is weak.

Tricuspid Valve Disease

Left-sided valve lesions often obscure the symptoms and signs of tricuspid stenosis. An elevated JVP together with a delayed *y* descent, abdominal ascites, and edema suggests severe tricuspid stenosis. Auscultatory findings are difficult to appreciate but mimic those in mitral stenosis and may be accentuated with inspiration. The symptoms of TR resemble those of tricuspid stenosis. Severe TR causes elevated JVP with prominent *cv* waves, a parasternal lift, pulsatile liver, ascites, and edema. The intensity of the holosystolic murmur of TR increases with inspiration (Carvallo sign). Murmur intensity does not accurately reflect the severity of the valve lesion. Primary and secondary causes of TR should be distinguished.

Pulmonic Valve Disease

Pulmonic stenosis may cause exertional fatigue, dyspnea, light-headedness, and chest discomfort ("right ventricular angina"). Syncope denotes severe obstruction. The midsystolic murmur of pulmonic stenosis is best heard at the second left interspace. With severe pulmonic stenosis, the interval between S_1 and the pulmonic ejection sound narrows, and the murmur peaks in late systole and may extend beyond A_2. P_2 becomes inaudible. Signs of significant RV pressure overload include a prominent jugular venous *a* wave and a parasternal lift. PR occurs most commonly as a secondary manifestation of significant pulmonary artery hypertension and annular dilation, but it may also reflect a primary valve disorder (e.g., congenital bicuspid valve) or develop as a complication of RV outflow tract surgery, in which case characteristics of the murmur and Doppler echocardiographic signs differ. Symptoms vary as a function of the severity of PA hypertension and the level of RV compensation. The diastolic murmur of secondary PR (Graham Steell) can be distinguished from that caused by AR on the basis of its increase in intensity with inspiration, its later onset (after A_2 and with P_2), and its slightly lower pitch. When a typical murmur is audible, the likelihood of PR increases (LR, 17), but the absence of a murmur does not exclude PR (LR, 0.9). With severe pulmonary artery hypertension and PR, P_2 is usually palpable and there are signs of RV pressure and volume overload on examination.

Prosthetic Heart Valves

The differential diagnosis of functional limitation after valve replacement surgery includes prosthetic valve dysfunction, prosthesis-patient mismatch, arrhythmia, and impaired ventricular function. Prosthetic valve dysfunction can occur as a result of thrombosis, pannus ingrowth, infection, or structural deterioration. Symptoms and signs mimic those of native valve disease and may arise acutely or develop gradually. The first clue that prosthetic valve dysfunction may be present often is a *change* in the quality of the heart sounds or the appearance of a new murmur. The heart sounds with a bioprosthetic valve resemble those generated by native valves. A bioprosthesis in the mitral position usually may be associated with a grade 1-2 midsystolic murmur (from turbulence created by systolic flow across the valve struts that project into the LV outflow tract) and a soft, mid-diastolic murmur that occurs with normal LV filling. The diastolic murmur usually is heard only in the left lateral decubitus position at the apex. A high-pitched or holosystolic apical murmur signifies para- or transvalvular regurgitation that requires echocardiographic verification and careful follow-up evaluation. Depending on the magnitude of the regurgitant volume, a diastolic murmur may be audible. Clinical deterioration can occur rapidly after initial manifestation of bioprosthetic failure.

A bioprosthesis in the aortic position is invariably associated with a midsystolic murmur at the base usually of grade 1-2 intensity. A diastolic murmur of AR is abnormal under any circumstance and merits additional investigation. A decrease in the intensity of either the opening or closing sounds of a mechanical prosthesis, depending on its type, is a worrisome finding. A high-pitched apical systolic murmur in patients with a mechanical mitral prosthesis, or a decrescendo diastolic murmur in patients with a mechanical aortic prosthesis, indicates paravalvular regurgitation or prosthetic dysfunction. Signs of hemolysis should be sought. Patients with prosthetic valve thrombosis may present with shock, muffled heart sounds, and soft murmurs. Pannus ingrowth is usually associated with an increase in the intensity of a systolic murmur and other signs indicative of prosthetic valve stenosis.

Acute Coronary Syndromes (see Chapters 35–39)

Risk stratification of patients with ACS informs decision making regarding the intensity and pace of management and is recommended by international guidelines.[48-50] Clinical findings indicative of high risk of short-term death or MI in patients with non-ST-elevation ACS include age greater than 75 years, tachycardia, hypotension, signs of pulmonary congestion, and/or a new or worsening murmur of MR.

Pericardial Disease (see also Chapter 86)
Pericarditis

The typical pain of acute pericarditis starts abruptly, is sharp, and varies with position. It can radiate to the trapezius ridge. Associated fever or history of a recent viral illness may provide additional clues. A pericardial friction rub is almost 100% specific for the diagnosis, although its sensitivity is not as high, because the rub may wax and wane over the course of an acute illness or may be difficult to elicit. This leathery or scratchy, typically two- or three-component sound also may be monophasic. It usually is necessary to auscultate the heart with the patient in several positions. The ECG may display concave upward ST segment elevation and P-R segment deviation (elevation in lead aVR, depression in lead II). A transthoracic ECG is routinely obtained to assess the volume and appearance of any effusion and to look for early signs of hemodynamic compromise.

Pericardial Tamponade

Pericardial tamponade occurs when intrapericardial pressure equals or exceeds right atrial pressure. The time course of its development depends on the volume of the effusion, the rate at which it accumulates, and pericardial compliance. The most common associated symptom is dyspnea (sensitivity, 87% to 88%). Hypotension (sensitivity, 26%) and muffled heart sounds (sensitivity, 28%) are relatively insensitive indicators of tamponade. A pulsus paradoxus greater than 12 mm Hg in a patient with a large pericardial effusion predicts tamponade with a sensitivity of 98%, a specificity of 83%, and a positive LR of 5.9 (95% CI, 2.4 to 14).[51] Echocardiography is indicated in all patients with suspected pericardial tamponade.

TABLE 13.8 Cardiovascular Virtual Visits: Benefits and Challenges

Benefits
- Improved access for patients
- Review in the home environment
- Medication reconciliation
- Caregiver/co-resident engagement
- Provider flexibility and engagement
- Data aspects of exam reviewable (BMI, weight, BP, HR, rhythm, urine output/quality)
- Qualitative exam possible (general appearance, neuro/mental status, skin/pallor, jugular venous distension, edema)

Challenges
- Lack of tactile and auscultatory capacity
- Reimbursement
- Change in expectations/culture
- Technology/Internet availability
- Patient and provider unfamiliarity with the technical aspects of the virtual visit
- Depersonalization of the patient-provider relationship

Constrictive Pericarditis

Constrictive pericarditis is an uncommon clinical entity that occurs with previous chest irradiation, cardiac or mediastinal surgery, chronic tuberculosis, malignancy, or a prior episode of acute pericarditis. Dyspnea, fatigue, weight gain, abdominal bloating, and leg swelling dominate the clinical presentation. The diagnosis most often is first suspected after inspection of the JVP and waveforms, with elevation and inscription of the classic M or W contour caused by prominent x and y descents and a Kussmaul sign. Evidence of pleural effusions and ascites often can be found. On rare occasion, a PK is audible. Distinction from restrictive cardiomyopathy often is not possible on the basis of the history and physical examination alone.

VIRTUAL VISITS

The COVID-19 global pandemic has accelerated the adoption of video-assisted patient encounters (VVs) into clinical practice and challenged clinicians to improve their ability to detect certain physical examination findings remotely. Despite their obvious differences from the typical in-person encounter, VVs may offer several benefits, though limitations clearly exist (Table 13.8). Evidence suggests that patients can become comfortable with VVs; in a survey of U.S. veterans, most were supportive of such encounters.

Blood pressure, HR, pulse regularity, weight, and even urine output are examples of data that can be obtained from most patients. Remote history taking may benefit from the ability to observe the patient in their home, interview other caretakers and/or home residents, and review prescription bottles. Such information is often more easily obtained during a virtual as opposed to in-person visit. These issues are particularly relevant in rural areas and urban environments when getting to in-person encounters are limited by transportation, frailty, and scheduling.

HF management may be particularly suited to the VV. Congestion can be reasonably assessed during the VV. Observations regarding JVP, peripheral edema, and weight are all possible. JVP by VV tracks closely with bedside JVP and invasively measured right atrial pressure. In a prospective study of 31 patients with 63 remote video assisted evaluations, agreement between video assisted and bedside JVP assessment was greater than 90%.[20]

FUTURE DIRECTIONS

Concerns regarding the escalating costs of medical care may reinforce the value of the traditional history and examination to guide appropriate use of imaging and invasive diagnostic modalities. Patients' perceptions of the quality of their care is often associated with the performance of the history and examination. These considerations should spur additional efforts to establish the accuracy and predictive value of bedside findings with contemporary measurement science across a spectrum of cardiovascular disorders.

The mentored patient evaluation should be revisited as a dedicated component of training programs, along with mechanisms to allow practice, repetition, and feedback. Improved teaching methods using simulation-based training aids are effective.[5] Electronic and digital stethoscopes may allow for computer automation and spectral display as means not only to enhance learning but also to improve the accuracy of diagnosis, while maintaining the physical link between the patient and provider.[6,52,53] The addition of handheld ultrasound may also improve learner performance, but whether it should replace the stethoscope is a point of contention.[54–57] Continued improvements in the technical performance characteristics and declining costs of these devices are attractive features, as is the possibility of initiating treatment at the point of care without the need for additional testing in many cases.[58,59] Insonation (e.g., ultrasound) may in fact become a pillar of the bedside exam in a way that Laennec introduced device facilitated auscultation 200 years ago.[60] Dissemination of such technology has been accelerated by the SARS-CoV-2 pandemic.[61]

Increasingly, patients will be acquiring their own digital data to review with their health care providers; how such information will be used for the patient's benefit remains to be seen.[62] Finally, the VV will become a routine part of clinical practice. Further refinements in the technology, comfort with these encounters by both patient and provider, and the decisions by payors to recognize these important care paradigms will ultimately change the delivery of cardiovascular care.

ACKNOWLEDGMENTS

The authors wish to acknowledge the previous contributions of Drs. Eugene Braunwald, Joseph Perloff, Robert O'Rourke, and James A. Shaver, which laid the foundation for this chapter.

REFERENCES

The General Physical Examination

1. Germanakis I, Petridou ET, Varlamis G, et al. Skills of primary healthcare physicians in paediatric cardiac auscultation. *Acta Paediatr*. 2013;102:e74–e78.
2. Wayne DB, Cohen ER, Singer BD, et al. Progress toward improving medical school graduates' skills via a "boot camp" curriculum. *Simul Healthc*. 2014;9:33–39.
3. Stokke TM, Ruddox V, Sarvari SI, et al. Brief group training of medical students in focused cardiac ultrasound may improve diagnostic accuracy of physical examination. *J Am Soc Echocardiogr*. 2014;27:1238–1246.
4. Kimura BJ, Shaw DJ, Amundson SA, et al. Cardiac limited ultrasound examination techniques to augment the bedside cardiac physical examination. *J Ultrasound Med*. 2015;34:1683–1690.
5. McKinney J, Cook DA, Wood D, Hatala R. Simulation-based training for cardiac auscultation skills: systematic review and meta-analysis. *J Gen Intern Med*. 2013;28:283–291.
6. Edelman ER, Weber BN. Tenuous tether. *N Engl J Med*. 2015;373:2199–2201.
7. Kelder JC, Cramer MJ, van Wijngaarden J, et al. The diagnostic value of physical examination and additional testing in primary care patients with suspected heart failure. *Circulation*. 2011;124:2865–2873.
8. McGee S. Diagnostic accuracy of physical findings. In: McGee S, ed. *Evidence-based Physical Diagnosis*. 4th ed. Philadelphia: Elsevier; 2018:13.
9. Bittencourt MS, Hulten E, Polonsky TS, et al. European Society of Cardiology-recommended coronary artery disease consortium pretest probability scores more accurately predict obstructive coronary disease and cardiovascular events than the Diamond and Forrester score: the partners registry. *Circulation*. 2016;134:201–211.
10. Fanaroff AC, Rymer JA, Goldstein SA, et al. Does this patient with chest pain have acute coronary syndrome? The rational clinical examination systematic review. *J Am Med Assoc*. 2015;314:1955–1965.
11. Thavendiranathan P, Bagai A, Khoo C, et al. Does this patient with palpitations have a cardiac arrhythmia? *J Am Med Assoc*. 2009;302(19):2135–2143.
12. Albassam OT, Redelmeier RJ, Shadowitz S, et al. Did this patient have cardiac syncope? The rational clinical examination systematic review. *J Am Med Assoc*. 2019;321:2448–2457.
13. Stehlik J, Rodriguez-Correa C, Spertus JA, et al. Implementation of real-time assessment of patient-reported outcomes in a heart failure clinic: a feasibility study. *J Card Fail*. 2017;23:813–816.
14. Garibaldi BT, Olson APJ. The hypothesis-driven physical examination. *Med Clin N Am*. 2018;102:433–442.
15. Coats AJ, Abraham WT. Central sleep apnoea in heart failure–an important issue for the modern heart failure cardiologist. *Int J Cardiol*. 2016;206(suppl):S1–S3.
16. Afilalo J, Lauck S, Kim DH, et al. Frailty in older adults undergoing aortic valve replacement: the FRAILTY-AVR study. *J Am Coll Cardiol*. 2017;70(6):689–700.
17. Bohadana A, Izbicki G, Kraman SS. Fundamentals of lung auscultation. *N Engl J Med*. 2014;370:2053.
18. Frankel HL, Kirkpatrick AW, Elbarbary M, et al. Guidelines for the appropriate use of bedside general and cardiac ultrasonography in the evaluation of critically Ill patients-Part I: general ultrasonography. *Crit Care Med*. 2015;43(11):2479–2502.
19. Levitov A, Frankel HL, Blaivas M, et al. Guidelines for the appropriate use of bedside general and cardiac ultrasonography in the evaluation of critically Ill patients-Part II: cardiac ultrasonography. *Crit Care Med*. 2016;44(6):1206–1227.

The Cardiovascular Examination

20. Kelly SA, Schesing KB, Thibodeau JT, et al. Feasibility of remote video assessment of jugular venous pressure and implications for TeleHealth. *JAMA Card.* 2020. Published online July 1, 2020. https://doi.org/10.1001/jamacardio.2020.2339.
21. Cuspidi C, Sala C, Grassi G, Mancia G. White coat hypertension: to treat or not to treat? *Curr Hypertens Rep.* 2016;18(11):80.
22. Schwartz JE, Burg MM, Shimbo D, et al. Clinic blood pressure underestimates ambulatory blood pressure in an untreated employer-based US population: results from the masked hypertension study. *Circulation.* 2016;134:1794–1807.
23. Khan NA, Rahim SA, Anand SS, et al. Does the clinical examination predict lower extremity peripheral arterial disease. *J Am Med Assoc.* 2006;295:536–546.

Integrated Evidence-Based Approach to Specific Cardiac Disorders

24. Wang CS, FitzGerald JM, Schulzer M, et al. Does this dyspneic patient in the emergency department have congestive heart failure? *J Am Med Assoc.* 2005;294:1944–1956.
25. Thibodeau JT, Turer AT, Gualano SK, et al. Characterization of a novel symptom of advanced heart failure: bendopnea. *JACC Heart Fail.* 2014;2:24–31.
26. Brack T, Thuer I, Clarenbach CF, et al. Daytime Cheyne-Stokes respiration in ambulatory patients with severe congestive heart failure is associated with increased mortality. *Chest.* 2007;132:1463–1471.
27. Sandek A, Swidsinski A, Schroedl W, et al. Intestinal blood flow in patients with chronic heart failure: a link with bacterial growth, gastrointestinal symptoms, and cachexia. *J Am Coll Cardiol.* 2014;64:1092–1102.
28. Drazner MH. Hemodynamic assessment in heart failure and cardiomyopathy: American College of Cardiology. *ACCSAP.* 2016;9.
29. From AM, Lam CS, Pitta SR, et al. Bedside assessment of cardiac hemodynamics: the impact of noninvasive testing and examiner experience. *Am J Med.* 2011;124:1051–1057.
30. Selvaraj S, et al. Prognostic implications of congestion on physical examination among contemporary patients with heart failure and reduced ejection fraction (PARADIGM-HF). *Circulation.* 2019;140:1369–1379.
31. Selvaraj S, Claggett B, Shah SJ, et al. Utility of the cardiovascular physical examination and impact of spironolactone in heart failure with preserved ejection fraction (TOPCAT). *Circ Heart Fail.* 2019;12(7):e006125.
32. Pellicori P, Kallvikbacka-Bennett A, Dierckx R, et al. Prognostic significance of ultrasound-assessed jugular vein distensibility in heart failure. *Heart.* 2015;101(14):1149–1158.
33. Marcus GM, Vessey J, Jordan MV, et al. Relationship between accurate auscultation of a clinically useful third heart sound and level of experience. *Arch Intern Med.* 2006;166:617–622.
34. Marcus GM, Gerber IL, McKeown BH, et al. Association between phonocardiographic third and fourth heart sounds and objective measures of left ventricular function. *J Am Med Assoc.* 2005;293:2238–2244.
35. Martindale JL, Wakai A, Collins SP, et al. Diagnosing acute heart failure in the emergency department: a systematic review and meta-analysis. *Acad Emerg Med.* 2016;23(3):223–242.
36. Platz E, Lewis EF, Uno H, et al. Detection and prognostic value of pulmonary congestion by lung ultrasound in ambulatory heart failure patients. *Eur Heart J.* 2016;37:1244–1251.
37. Stevenson LW, Perloff JK. The limited reliability of physical signs for estimating hemodynamics in chronic heart failure. *J Am Med Assoc.* 1989;261:884–888.
38. Kwon Y, Van't Hof J, Roy SS, et al. A novel method for assessing cardiac output with the use of oxygen circulation time. *J Card Fail.* 2016;22:921–924.
39. Swedberg K, Komajda M, Böhm M, et al. Ivabradine and outcomes in chronic heart failure (SHIFT): a randomised placebo-controlled study. *Lancet.* 2010;376(9744):875–885.
40. Maeder MT, Zurek M, Rickli H, et al. Prognostic value of the change in heart rate from the supine to the upright position in patients with chronic heart failure. *J Am Heart Assoc.* 2016;5(8):e003524.
41. El-Menyar A, Sulaiman K, Almahmeed W, et al. Shock index in patients presenting with acute heart failure: a multicenter multinational observational study. *Angiology.* 2019;70.938-846.
42. Wong CL, Holroyd-Leduc J, Straus SE. Does this patient have a pleural effusion? *J Am Med Assoc.* 2009;301:309–317.
43. Gaibazzi N, Reverberi C, Ghillani M, et al. Prevalence of undiagnosed asymptomatic aortic valve stenosis in the general population older than 65 years. A screening strategy using cardiac auscultation followed by Doppler-echocardiography. *Int J Cardiol.* 2013;168:4905–4906.
44. Chiang SJ, Daimon M, Miyazaki S, et al. When and how aortic stenosis is first diagnosed: a single-center observational study. *J Cardiol.* 2016;68:324–328.
45. Prinz C, Voigt JU. Diagnostic accuracy of a hand-held ultrasound scanner in routine patients referred for echocardiography. *J Am Soc Echocardiogr.* 2011;24:111–116.
46. Bodegard J, Skretteberg PT, Gjesdal K, et al. Low-grade systolic murmurs in healthy middle-aged individuals: innocent or clinically significant? A 35-year follow-up study of 2014 Norwegian men. *J Intern Med.* 2012;271:581–588.
47. Choudhry N, Etchells EE. The rational clinical examination. Does this patient have aortic regurgitation? *J Am Med Assoc.* 1999;281:2231–2238.
48. O'Gara PT, Kushner FG, Ascheim DD, et al. 2013 ACCF/AHA guideline for the management of ST-elevation myocardial infarction: a report of the American College of Cardiology Foundation/American Heart Association Task Force on practice guidelines. *J Am Coll Cardiol.* 2013;61:e78–e140.
49. Amsterdam EA, Wenger NK, Brindis RG, et al. 2014 AHA/ACC guideline for the management of patients with non-ST-elevation acute coronary syndromes: a report of the American College of cardiology/American heart association Task Force on practice guidelines. *J Am Coll Cardiol.* 2014;64:e139–e228.
50. Ibanez B, James S, Agewall S, et al. 2017 ESC guidelines for the management of acute myocardial infarction in patients presenting with ST-segment elevation: Task Force for the management of acute myocardial infarction in patients presenting with ST-segment elevation of the European Society of Cardiology (ESC). *Eur Heart J.* 2018;39:119–177.
51. Roy CL, Minor MA, Brookhart MA, Choudhry NK. The rational clinical examination. Does this patient with a pericardial effusion have cardiac tamponade? *J Am Med Assoc.* 2007;297:1810–1818.

Future Directions

52. Leng S, Tan RS, Chai KT, et al. The electronic stethoscope. *Biomed Eng Online.* 2015;14:66.
53. Lai LS, Redington AN, Reinisch AJ, et al. Computerized automatic diagnosis of innocent and pathologic murmurs in pediatrics: a pilot study. *Congenit Heart Dis.* 2016;11:386–395.
54. Stokke TM, Ruddox V, Sarvari SI, et al. Brief group training of medical students in focused cardiac ultrasound may improve diagnostic accuracy of physical examination. *J Am Soc Echocardiogr.* 2014;27:1238–1246.
55. Kimura BJ, Shaw DJ, Amundson SA, et al. Cardiac limited ultrasound examination techniques to augment the bedside cardiac physical examination. *J Ultrasound Med.* 2015;34:1683–1690.
56. Bank I, Vliegen HW, Bruschke AV. The 200th anniversary of the stethoscope: can this low-tech device survive in the high-tech 21st century? *Eur Heart J.* 2016;37:3536–3543.
57. Fuster V. The stethoscope's prognosis. Very much alive and very necessary. 2016;67:1118–1119.
58. Zoghbi WA. Echocardiography at the point of care: an ultra sound future. *J Am Soc Echocardiogr.* 2011;24:132–134.
59. Cardim N, Fernandez Golfin C, Ferreira D, et al. Usefulness of a new miniaturized echocardiographic system in outpatient cardiology consultations as an extension of physical examination. *J Am Soc Echocardiogr.* 2011;24:117–124.
60. Narula J, Chandrashekhar Y, Braunwald EB. Time to Add a fifth pillar to bedside physical examination: inspection, palpation, percussion, auscultation and insonation. *JAMA Cardiol.* 2018;3:346–350.
61. Khanji MY, Ricci F, Patel RS. The role of handheld ultrasound for cardiopulmonary assessment during a pandemic. *Prog Cardiovasc Dis.* 2020;63:690–695.
62. Perez MV, Mahaffey KW, Hedlin H, et al. Large scale assessment of a Smartwatch to identify atrial fibrillation. *N Engl J Med.* 2020;381:1909–1917.

14 Electrocardiography

DAVID M. MIRVIS AND ARY L. GOLDBERGER

THE NORMAL ELECTROCARDIOGRAM, 145
Atrial Activation and the P Wave, 145
Atrioventricular Node Conduction and the PR Segment, 146
Ventricular Activation and the QRS Complex, 147
Normal Variants, 149

THE ABNORMAL ELECTROCARDIOGRAM, 150
Chamber Enlargement and Hypertrophy, 150
Intraventricular Conduction Delays, 156
Myocardial Ischemia and Infarction, 160
Drug Effects, 170
Electrolyte and Metabolic Abnormalities, 170

Clinical Issues in Electrocardiographic Interpretation, 172

FUTURE PERSPECTIVES, 173

GUIDELINES, 173

REFERENCES, 174

The technology and the clinical value of the electrocardiogram (ECG or, as sometimes referred to, EKG) have continuously evolved since the invention of the string galvanometer by Einthoven in 1901. The ECG soon became the most commonly used cardiac diagnostic test, and it remains the fundamental method to assess the heart's electrical activity. This chapter provides an overview of the pathophysiology, the diagnostic criteria, and the utility of the most common ECG diagnoses in adults.

FUNDAMENTAL PRINCIPLES

The ECG is the outcome of a complex series of physiologic and technologic processes. First, transmembrane ionic currents are generated by ion fluxes across cell membranes and between adjacent cells. These currents are synchronized during cardiac activation and recovery sequences to generate a physiologically meaningful, time-varying electrical field in and around the heart.

Electrodes placed in specific locations on the extremities and torso detect the currents reaching the skin. These electrodes are configured to produce *leads*. The outputs of these leads are then amplified, filtered, digitized, and displayed to produce an ECG recording. These signals are typically analyzed by signal processing and pattern recognition software to provide a preliminary interpretation that is then subject to careful clinician review.

Genesis of Cardiac Electrical Fields
Ionic Currents and Cardiac Electrical Fields During Activation. Transmembrane ionic currents (see Chapter 62) are ultimately responsible for the potentials recorded as an ECG. As sites along a cardiac fiber are activated, the polarity of the transmembrane potential converts from negative (with the inside of the cell negative relative to the outside) to positive (with the inside of the cell positive relative to the outside of the cell), as represented in the typical cardiac action potential. Thus, sites on a cardiac fiber that have undergone excitation have positive transmembrane potentials, whereas more distal sites remaining in a resting state have negative transmembrane potentials (see Fig. 62.1).

This reversal of polarity along a fiber creates a flow of positively charged intracellular current from the already activated to the more distal, inactivated portions of the fiber. As activation of multiple adjacent fibers proceeds in synchrony, an activation *wavefront* is produced that moves in the direction of activation and that generates an electrical field characterized by positive potentials ahead and negative potentials behind it (see Fig. 62.7).

An electrode senses positive potential when an activation front is moving toward it and senses negative potentials when the activation front is moving away from it. The magnitude of the potential recorded by an electrode at any site is (1) directly proportional to the average rate of change of intracellular potential as determined by the action potential shape; (2) directly proportional to the size of the wavefront; (3) inversely proportional to the square of the distance from the activation front to the recording site; and (4) directly proportional to the cosine of the angle between the direction of activation spread and a line drawn from the site of activation to the recording site. Thus, if activation proceeds directly toward an electrode such that the angle between the direction of activation and the location of the electrode equals zero (and its cosine equals 1), the voltage sensed by the electrode will be maximal. In contrast, if activation proceeds in a direction perpendicular to that direction (cosine = 0), the sensed potential will be zero.

Cardiac Electrical Field Generation During Recovery. The cardiac electrical field during recovery differs in several important ways from that during activation. First, the gradient of intercellular potentials and thus the direction of current flow during recovery are the opposite of those described for activation. As a cell undergoes recovery, its intracellular potential becomes progressively more negative. For a cardiac fiber, the intracellular potential of the region whose recovery has progressed further (usually modelled as the region activated first) is more negative than that of the adjacent, less recovered region. Intracellular currents then flow from the less recovered toward the more recovered portion of the fiber. That is, recovery wavefronts will have an orientation opposite that of activation wavefronts.

Second, the strengths of the recovery wavefronts during recovery are lower than during activation. As noted, the strength of a wavefront is proportional to the rate of change in transmembrane potential. Rates of change in transmembrane potential during the recovery phases are considerably slower than during activation, and the strength of the resulting wavefront is lower.

Third, the rate of movement of the recovery wavefronts is much slower than that of activation fronts. Activation is rapid and occurs over only a small short length of the fiber. Recovery, by contrast, lasts 100 msec or longer and occurs simultaneously over extensive portions of the heart. Hence, the overall duration of the recovery waveforms will be longer than that of activation.

These features result in ECG differences between activation and recovery patterns. All other factors being equal (an assumption often not true, as described later), waveforms generated during recovery of a fiber with uniform recovery properties would be of opposite polarity, lower amplitude, and longer duration than those generated by activation.

Role of Transmission Factors. The activation and recovery fields are significantly perturbed by the complex three-dimensional physical environment in which they are generated. These *transmission factors* include the biophysical characteristics of the heart itself as well as those of the surrounding organs and tissues.

An important *cardiac factor* is the presence of connective tissue between cardiac fibers that disrupts efficient electrical coupling of adjacent fibers. Waveforms generated in fibers with little or no intervening connective tissue are narrow in width and smooth in contour, whereas those recorded from tissues with abnormal fibrosis are prolonged and may exhibit prominent notching.

Extracardiac factors include the effects of all the tissues and structures that lie between the activation region and the body surface, including intracardiac blood, lungs, skeletal muscle, subcutaneous fat, and skin. These tissues alter the intensity and the orientation of the wavefronts as they travel across them.

Physical factors reflect basic laws of physics. Potential magnitudes change in proportion to the square of the distance between the heart and recording electrode. In humans, the right ventricle (RV) and anteroseptal aspect of the left ventricle (LV) are closer to the anterior chest wall than are other parts of that chamber. Therefore, ECG potentials will be higher on the anterior than on the posterior chest, and the amplitudes of waveforms projected from the anterior LV to the chest wall will be greater than those generated by posterior LV regions.

An additional physical factor affecting the recording of cardiac signals is *cancellation*. When two or more wavefronts are simultaneously active, as is common during activation, the vectoral components of the wavefronts may augment (if oriented in the same directions) or cancel (if oriented in opposite directions) each other when viewed from remote electrode positions. The magnitude of this effect is substantial. During the inscription of the QRS wave, as much as 90% of cardiac activity is obscured by cancellation effects.

As a result of these factors, surface recordings have an amplitude of only 1% of the amplitude of transmembrane potentials, are smoothed in detail so that they have only a general spatial relationship to the underlying cardiac events, and preferentially reflect electrical activity in some cardiac regions over others.

Recording Electrodes and Leads Systems

Electrode Characteristics. The standard clinical ECG is recorded from electrodes placed on each of the four extremities and from six placed on the chest.[1] These electrodes are connected to form *leads* that record the potential difference between two electrodes. One electrode is designated as the positive input. The potential at the other (negative) electrode is subtracted from the potential at the positive electrode to yield the *bipolar potential*. The actual potential at either electrode is not known; only the difference between them is recorded.

In some cases, as described later, multiple electrodes are electrically connected together to form the negative member of the bipolar pair. This electrode network is commonly referred to as a *compound* or *reference electrode*. The lead then records the potential difference between a single electrode serving as the positive input (the *exploring electrode*) and the potential in the reference electrode.

The clinical ECG is performed using 12 leads: three standard *limb leads* (leads I, II, and III), six *precordial leads* (leads V_1 through V_6), and three *augmented limb leads* (leads aVR, aVL, and aVF). Specifics of electrode placement and definitions of the positive and negative inputs for each lead are presented in Table 14.1.

Standard Limb Leads. The standard limb leads record the potential differences between two limbs, as detailed in Table 14.1 and illustrated in Figure 14.1(top). Lead I registers the potential difference between the left arm (positive electrode) and right arm (negative electrode); lead II displays the potential difference between the left leg (positive electrode) and right arm (negative electrode); and lead III records the potential difference between the left leg (positive electrode) and left arm (negative electrode). The electrode on the right leg serves as an electronic reference that reduces noise and is not included in these lead configurations. Limb electrodes should be placed near the wrists and ankles or, at a minimum, distal to the shoulders and hips.

The electrical connections for each of these leads can be represented as a vector oriented from its negative toward its positive pole. These vectors form a triangle, known as the *Einthoven triangle*, in which the potential in lead II equals the sum of potentials sensed in leads I and III, that is:

$$I + III = II$$

Precordial Leads and the Wilson Central Terminal. The precordial leads register the potential at each of the six specific torso sites (see Fig. 14.1, bottom left panel) in relation to a reference potential. An exploring electrode is placed at each of six specific precordial sites and connected to the positive input of the recording system (see Fig. 14.1, bottom right). The negative input is the mean value of the potentials recorded at each of the three limb electrodes, referred to as the *Wilson central terminal* (WCT).

The potential in each V lead can be expressed as:

$$V_i = E_i - WCT$$

where

$$WCT = (LA + LL + RA)/2$$

and V_i is the potential recorded in precordial lead i, E_i is the voltage sensed at the exploring electrode for lead V_i, and WCT is the potential in the composite Wilson central terminal, and LA, LL, and RA are the potentials in the left arm, left leg, and right arm, respectively.

The potential recorded by the WCT is considered to remain relatively constant during the cardiac cycle, and the output of a precordial lead is determined predominantly by time-dependent changes in the potential recorded at that precordial site.* The potentials registered by these leads preferentially reflect activity in cardiac regions underlying the exploring electrode, with lesser although meaningful contribution by potentials generated from more distant cardiac sources.

*The precordial and the augmented limb leads are commonly referred to as "unipolar" leads. However, a true unipolar lead registers the potential at one site in relation to an absolute zero potential. Referring to these leads as unipolar is based on the assumption that the WCT represents a constant, true zero potential. In reality, the potential in the WCT is neither zero nor constant during the cardiac cycle. Hence, these leads are in reality bipolar leads with the WCT serving as the compound negative pole.

Augmented Limb Leads. The three augmented limb leads are designated aVR, aVL, and aVF. For lead aVR, the exploring electrode (Fig. 14.2) that forms the positive input is the right arm electrode, for lead aVL it is the left arm electrode, and for aVF it is the left leg electrode. The reference potential for these leads is formed by connecting the two limb electrodes not used as the exploring electrode. For lead aVL, for example, the exploring electrode is on the left arm, and the reference electrode is the combined output of the electrodes on the right arm and the left foot.

Thus,

$$aVR = RA - (LA + LL)/2$$

and

$$aVL = LA - (RA + LL)/2$$

$$aVF = LL - (RA + LA)/2$$

This modified reference system produces a signal that is larger than if the full WCT were included. When the WCT was used, the output was small, in part because the same electrode potential was included in both the exploring and the reference potential inputs. Eliminating this duplication results in a theoretical 50% increase in amplitude.

Other Lead Systems. Expanded lead systems (see Table 14.1, bottom) include recordings from additional electrodes placed on the right

TABLE 14.1 Location of Electrodes and Lead Connections for the Standard 12-Lead Electrocardiogram and Additional Leads

LEAD TYPE	POSITIVE INPUT	NEGATIVE INPUT
Standard Limb Leads*		
I	Left arm	Right arm
II	Left leg	Right arm
III	Left leg	Left arm
Augmented Limb Leads		
aVR	Right arm	Left arm plus left leg
aVL	Left arm	Right arm plus left leg
aVF	Left leg	Left arm plus right arm
Precordial Leads†		
V_1	Right sternal margin, fourth intercostal space	Wilson central terminal
V_2	Left sternal margin, fourth intercostal space	Wilson central terminal
V_3	Midway between V_2 and V_4	Wilson central terminal
V_4	Left midclavicular line, 5th intercostal space	Wilson central terminal
V_5	Left anterior axillary line at same horizontal plane as for V_4 electrode	Wilson central terminal
V_6	Left midaxillary line at same horizontal plane as for V_4 electrode	Wilson central terminal
V_7	Posterior axillary line at same horizontal plane as for V_4 electrode	Wilson central terminal
V_8	Posterior scapular line at same horizontal plane as for V_4 electrode	Wilson central terminal
V_9	Left border of spine at same horizontal plane as for V_4 electrode	Wilson central terminal

*Limb electrodes should be placed near the wrists and ankles or, at a minimum, distal to the shoulders and hips.
†The right-sided precordial leads V_3R to V_6R are placed in mirror-image positions on the right side of the chest. (See text for further details.)
From Kligfield P, Gettes LS, Bailey JJ, et al. Recommendations for the standardization and interpretation of the electrocardiogram: part I: the electrocardiogram and its technology a scientific statement from the American Heart Association Electrocardiography and Arrhythmias Committee, Council on Clinical Cardiology; the American College of Cardiology Foundation; and the Heart Rhythm Society endorsed by the International Society for Computerized Electrocardiology. *J Am Coll Cardiol.* 2007;49:1109–1127.

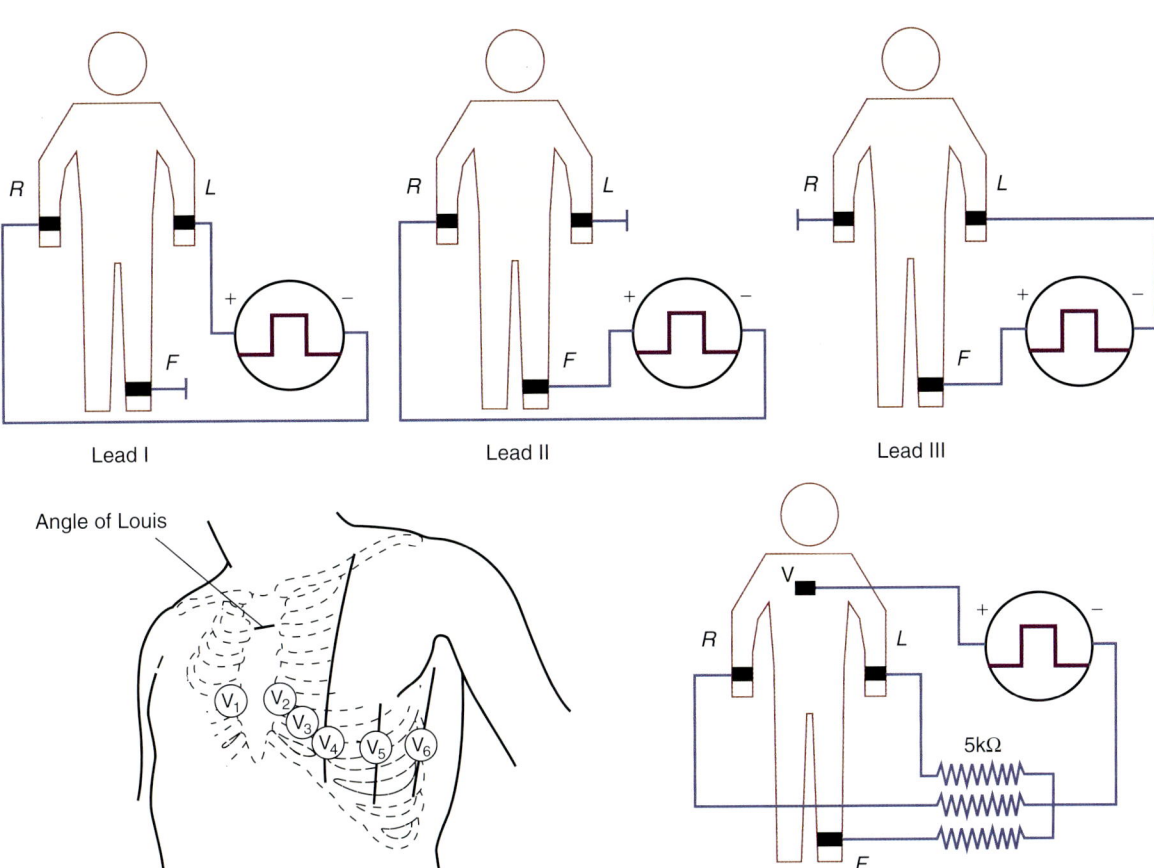

FIGURE 14.1 *Top,* Electrode connections for recording the standard limb leads I, II, and III and the augmented limb leads aVR, aVL, and aVF, with electrodes on the right arm, left arm, and left foot. *Bottom,* Electrode locations and electrical connections for recording a precordial lead. *Left,* The positions of the exploring electrode (V) for the six precordial leads. *Right,* Connections to form the Wilson central terminal for recording a precordial (V) lead. When constructing the Wilson central terminal, 5000-ohm resistors (5 kΩ) are connected to each limb electrode.

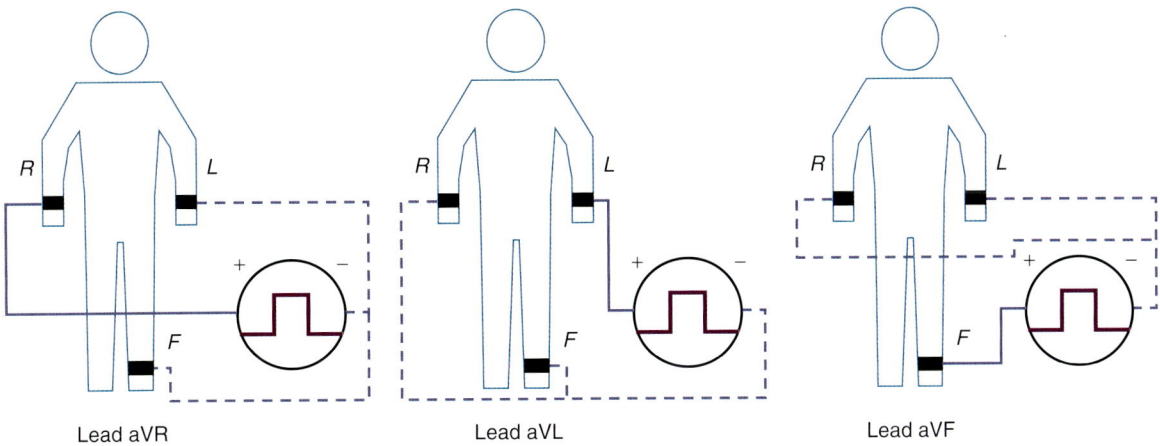

FIGURE 14.2 Electrode locations and electrical connections for recording the augmented limb leads aVR, aVL, and aVF. *Dotted lines* indicate connections to generate the reference electrode potential.

precordium to assess RV abnormalities such as RV myocardial infarction (MI). The right-sided precordial leads V_3R to V_6R are placed in mirror-image positions on the right side of the chest. Electrodes added on the left posterior torso (e.g., V_7 at the posterior axillary line at the level of V_4 and V8 at the posterior scapular line at the level of V_4) may detect acute posterolateral MI, and some placed higher on the anterior torso than normal may help detect abnormalities such as the Brugada pattern and its variants (see Chapters 63 and 70).

Other lead sets have sought to minimize movement artifacts during exercise and long-term monitoring (see Chapters 32 and 61) by placing limb electrodes on the torso rather than near the ankles and wrists. The resulting waveforms may differ substantially from those recorded from the standard ECG sites, with altered QRS and ST-T wave patterns in all 12 leads. These differences may impact the diagnostic accuracy of criteria of, for example, ventricular hypertrophy and MI.[1] Thus, these alternative lead sets should not be used to record a diagnostic ECG. Less frequently used but important lead systems include those designed to record a *vectorcardiogram* (VCG), which depicts the orientation and strength of a single cardiac vector representing overall cardiac activity throughout the cardiac cycle.

Hexaxial Reference Frame and the Electrical Axis

The three standard limb and the three augmented limb leads are aligned in the *frontal plane* of the torso. The six precordial leads are aligned in the *horizontal plane* of the chest.

Each ECG lead can be represented as a vector, the *lead vector*. The lead vectors for leads I, II, and III are directed from the negative electrode toward the positive one, e.g., from the right arm to the left arm for lead I (Fig. 14.3, *left*). For an augmented limb and for a precordial lead, the lead vector passes through the midpoint of the axis connecting

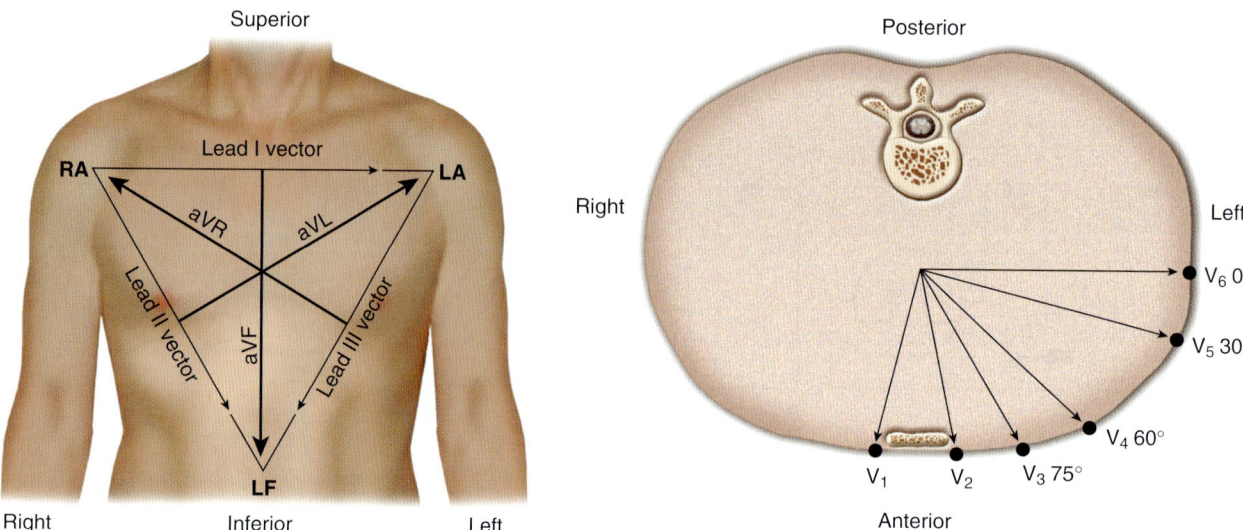

FIGURE 14.3 Lead vectors for the three standard limb leads, the three augmented limb leads (*left*), and the six unipolar precordial leads (*right*). *LA,* Left arm; *LF,* left foot; *RA,* right arm.

the electrodes that comprise the reference electrode and points to the location of the exploring electrode. That is, for lead aVL, the vector points from the midpoint of the axis connecting the right arm and left leg electrodes toward the left arm (see Fig. 14.3, *left*). For each precordial lead, the lead vector in the horizontal plane points from the center of the triangle formed by the three standard limb leads to the precordial electrode site (see Fig. 14.3, *right*).

Instantaneous cardiac activity also can be approximated as a single vector, the *heart vector,* that represents the vectoral sum of the activity of all active wavefronts. This vector's location, orientation, and intensity vary from instant to instant as cardiac activation proceeds.

The amplitude of the recorded waveform in a lead equals the length the projection of the heart vector onto the lead vector. This relation may be expressed mathematically as:

$$V_L = H \cdot \cos \theta$$

where V_L is the recorded voltage in lead L, H is the strength (length) of the heart vector, and Θ is the angle between the heart vector H and the lead vector. Thus, when the direction of activation (i.e., the direction of the heart vector) and that of the lead vector are parallel (Θ = 0 degrees and cosine Θ = 1), the recorded voltage is maximal; when the activation is perpendicular to the lead axis, the recorded potential equals zero (Θ = 90 degrees and cosine Θ = 0).

The lead axes of the six frontal plane leads can be superimposed to produce the *hexaxial reference system.* As depicted in Figure 14.4, the six lead axes divide the frontal plane into 12 segments, each subtending 30 degrees. This presentation allows calculation of the *mean electrical axis* of the heart representing the direction of activation in a theoretical "average" cardiac fiber.

The process for computing the mean electrical axis during ventricular activation in the frontal plane is illustrated in Figure 14.5. First, the mean electrical force (i.e., the heart vector) as projected onto each lead is estimated by computing the area under the QRS waveform, measured as mV-ms, in that lead. Areas above the baseline (usually the TP segment as discussed later) are assigned a positive polarity and those below the baseline are assigned a negative polarity. The overall area equals the sum of the positive and the negative areas.

Second, the area under the QRS in each lead (typically, two are chosen) is represented as a vector oriented along the appropriate lead axis in the hexaxial reference system. Third, the mean electrical axis is computed as the resultant or vector sum of the (two) vectors.

A mean electrical axis in the frontal plane directed toward the positive end of the lead axis of lead I, that is, oriented directly away from the right arm and toward the left arm, is designated as having an axis of 0 degrees. Axes oriented in a clockwise direction relative to this zero level are assigned positive values, and those oriented in a counterclockwise direction are assigned negative values (see Fig. 14.4).

The mean electrical axis in the horizontal plane can be computed in an analogous manner by using the areas under and lead axes of the six precordial leads (see Fig. 14.3, *right*). A horizontal plane axis located

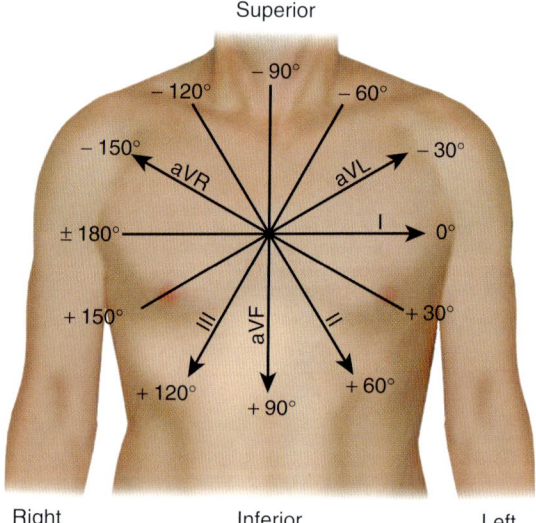

FIGURE 14.4 The hexaxial reference system constructed from the lead axes of the six frontal plane leads. The lead axes of the six frontal plane leads have been rearranged so that their centers overlie one another. Positive ends of each axis are labeled with the name of the lead.

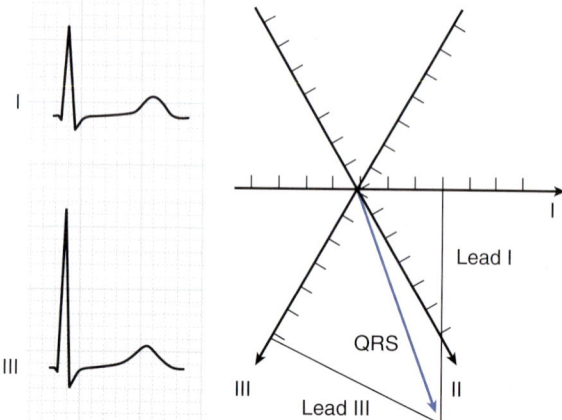

FIGURE 14.5 Calculation of the mean electrical axis during ventricular depolarization from the areas under the QRS complex in leads I and III. Magnitudes of the areas of the two leads are plotted as vectors on the appropriate lead axes, and the mean QRS axis is the sum of these two vectors. (From Mirvis DM. *Electrocardiography: A Physiologic Approach.* St Louis: Mosby–Year Book; 1993.)

along the lead axis of lead V_6 is assigned a value of 0 degrees; axes directed more anteriorly have positive values.

This approach can also be applied to compute the mean electrical axis for other phases of cardiac activity. Thus, the mean force during atrial activation is represented by the areas under the P wave and the mean force during ventricular recovery by the areas under the ST-T wave.

Electrocardiographic Processing and Display Systems
ECG recording using computerized systems includes: (1) signal acquisition, (2) data transformation, waveform recognition, and feature extraction, (3) diagnostic classification, and (4) display of the final ECG. Technical requirements for processing an ECG have been developed by various medical and engineering organizations.[1,2]

Signal Acquisition. Recorded signals are amplified, converted into digital form, and filtered to reduce noise. The standard amplifier gain for routine electrocardiography is 1000. Lower (e.g., 500, or *half-standard*) or higher (e.g., 2000, or *double-standard*) gains may be used to compensate for unusually large or small signals, respectively.

Analog signals are converted to a digital form at rates of 1000 samples per second (1000 Hz) to as high as 15,000 Hz. Too low a sampling rate may miss brief high-frequency signals such as notches in QRS complexes or pacemaker spikes. Too fast a sampling rate may introduce artifacts, including high-frequency noise, and will generate large amounts of data necessitating extensive digital storage capacity.

ECG potentials are filtered to reduce distorting signals. Low-pass filters reduce the distortions caused by high-frequency interference from, for example, muscle tremor and nearby electrical devices. High-pass filters reduce the effects of body motion or respiration. For routine electrocardiography, the standards set by professional groups require an overall bandwidth of 0.05 to 150 Hz for adults.[1] Narrower filter settings, such as 1 to 30 Hz, as typically used in rhythm monitoring, will reduce baseline wander related to motion and respiration but will distort both the QRS complex and the ST-T wave.

ECG amplifiers are *capacitor coupled*, with a capacitor stage between the input and output. The ECG may be modeled as a time-varying or alternating current (AC) signal producing the waveforms superimposed on a fixed direct current (DC) baseline. Capacitor-coupling permits the flow of AC signals, which account for the waveform shape, while blocking the nonphysiologic DC potentials such as those produced by the electrode interfaces. The elimination of the DC potential from the final product, however, means that ECG potentials are not to be calibrated against an external reference level (e.g., a ground potential). Rather, ECG potentials are measured in relation to another portion of the waveform that serves as a baseline. The *TP segment*, which begins at the end of the T wave of one cardiac cycle and ends with the onset of the P wave of the next cycle (as detailed later), is usually the most appropriate internal ECG baseline, e.g., for measuring ST-segment deviation.

Data Transformation, Waveform Identification, and Feature Extraction. The multiple cardiac cycles that are recorded for each lead and are typically overlaid electronically to form a single representative beat for each lead. This reduces the effects of minor beat-to-beat variation in the waveforms and random noise. The averaged waveforms from each lead are overlaid on each other to measure waveform intervals.[1]

Diagnostic Classification. These measurements are then compared with specific diagnostic criteria. For many diagnoses, ECG criteria are based on statistical correlations between anatomic or physiologic findings and ECG measurements in large populations (e.g., criteria for ECG diagnosis of ventricular hypertrophy). For such population-based criteria, the diagnosis is not absolute but represents a statistical probability that a structural or physiologic abnormality exists based on the presence or absence of a specified set of ECG findings. Because different populations may be studied and different ECG and structural measurements may be used as the reference standard, numerous different criteria with highly varying accuracies have been developed for common clinical conditions.

In other cases, the criteria are derived mainly from physiologic constructs and constitute the sole basis for a diagnosis, with no anatomic or functional correlation. For example, the criteria for intraventricular conduction defects are diagnostic without reference to an anatomic standard.

Display. Cardiac potentials are most often displayed as the classic *scalar* ECG, which depicts the potentials recorded from each lead as a function of time. Amplitudes are displayed on a scale of 0.1 mV/mm (for *standard gain*) on the vertical axis and time as 40 msec/mm on the horizontal scale. Leads generally are displayed in three groups—the three standard limb leads, followed by the three augmented limb leads, followed by the six precordial leads.

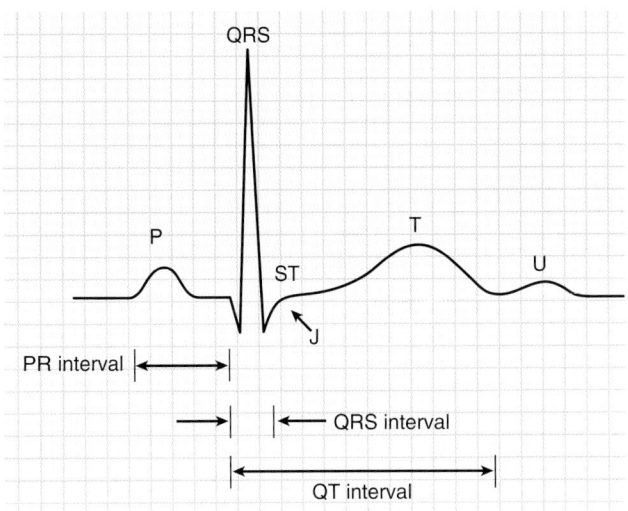

FIGURE 14.6 The waves and intervals of a normal electrocardiogram. (From Goldberger AL, Goldberger ZD, Shvilkin A. *Goldberger's Clinical Electrocardiography: A Simplified Approach*. 9th ed. Philadelphia: Elsevier; 2017.)

Alternative display formats have been proposed. One is the *Cabrera display* in which the six limb leads are displayed in the sequence of the frontal plane reference frame[3] and in which the polarity of lead aVR is inverted. In this scheme, waveforms are ordered as follows: lead aVL, lead I, inverted lead aVR, lead II, lead aVF, and lead III. Advantages of this system may include facilitating estimation of the electrical axis by presenting the leads in the order in which they appear on the frontal plane reference frame (see Fig. 14.4) and demonstrating the relevance of abnormalities in lead aVR by reversing its polarity.

THE NORMAL ELECTROCARDIOGRAM

The waveforms and intervals that make up the standard ECG are displayed schematically in Figure 14.6, and a normal 12-lead ECG is shown in Figure 14.7. The *P wave* is generated by activation of the atria, the *PR interval* corresponds to the duration of atrioventricular (AV) conduction, the *QRS complex* is produced by the activation of the two ventricles, and the *ST-T wave* reflects ventricular recovery.

Table 14.2 lists the classic normal values for the various intervals and waveforms. The range of normal values of these measurements reflects the substantial intraindividual and interindividual variability in ECG patterns. Intraindividual differences may occur between ECGs recorded days, hours, or even minutes apart because of technical issues (e.g., changes in electrode position) or the physiologic effects of changes in, for example, posture, temperature, or heart rate.

Variability between individuals may reflect differences in age, gender, race, body habitus, and physiology. For example, in the Atherosclerosis Risk in Communities (ARIC) study,[4] the upper limits for ST-segment elevation in leads V_1 and V_2 were 50 µV higher in white men than in white women and almost 100 µV higher in African American men than in white men.

Atrial Activation and the P Wave
Atrial Activation and the Normal P Wave
Atrial activation begins with impulse generation in the atrial pacemaker complex in or near the sinoatrial node (see Chapter 62). Once the impulse leaves this pacemaker site, atrial activation proceeds anteriorly and inferiorly toward the lower portion of the right atrium (RA) and the AV node.

The left atrium (LA) is normally activated after the onset of RA activation primarily by propagation across *Bachmann's bundle*, which extends from the anterior RA to the LA near the right upper pulmonary vein. Activation then continues in both atria during much of the middle

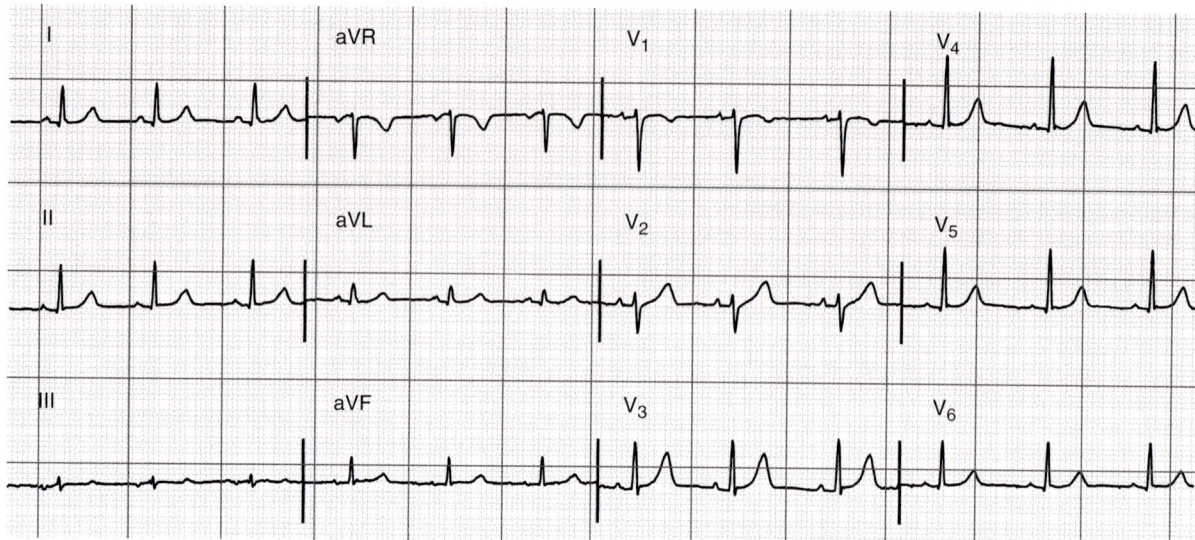

FIGURE 14.7 Normal ECG recorded from a 48-year-old woman. *Vertical lines* are spaced at 40-msec intervals. *Horizontal lines* represent voltage amplitude, with lines spaced at 0.1-mV intervals. Every fifth line on each axis is darkened. The heart rate is approximately 76 beats/min (with physiologic variations due to respiratory sinus arrhythmia); the PR interval, QRS, and QTc durations measure approximately 140, 84, and 400 msec, respectively; and the mean QRS axis is approximately +35 degrees.

TABLE 14.2 Normal Upper Limits for Durations of Electrocardiogram Waves and Intervals in Adults

WAVE OR INTERVAL	DURATION (MSEC)
P wave duration	<120
PR interval	<200
QRS duration	<110–120*
QT interval_c (corrected)	≤440–450*

*See text for further discussion.
References: Rautaharju PM, Surawicz B, Gettes LS, et al. Recommendations for the standardization and interpretation of the electrocardiogram. Part IV. The ST segment, T and U waves. *J Am Coll Cardiol.* 2009;53:982–991; and Kligfield P, Gettes LS, Bailey JJ, et al. Recommendations for the standardization and interpretation of the electrocardiogram: part I: the electrocardiogram and its technology *J Am Coll Cardiol.* 2007;49:1109–1127.

of the atrial activation period, with LA activation continuing after the end of RA activation.

The normal P wave reflects these activation patterns. P waves are positive in lead II and usually positive in leads I, aVL, and aVF, reflecting the inferior and leftward direction of normal activation. This corresponds to a mean frontal plane P wave axis of approximately 60 degrees. The pattern in leads aVL and III may be upright or downward, depending on the exact orientation of the mean P wave axis.

In the horizontal plane, early activation of the RA generates a P wave that is oriented primarily anteriorly. Later, activation shifts leftward and posteriorly as it proceeds over the LA. Thus, the P wave in the right precordial leads is typically upright. In lead V_1 and occasionally in lead V_2, the P wave may be biphasic with an initial positive deflection followed by a later, smaller negative wave. In the more lateral leads, the P wave is upright and reflects continual right-to-left spread of the activation fronts.

The upper limit for a normal P wave duration is conventionally set at 120 msec, as measured in the lead with the widest P wave. The amplitude in the limb leads normally is less than 0.25 mV, and a terminal negative deflection in the right precordial leads is normally less than 0.1 mV in depth.

Atrial Repolarization

The potentials generated by atrial repolarization are not usually seen on the surface ECG because of their low amplitude (usually <100 μV) and because they may be superimposed on the much higher-amplitude QRS complex. A repolarization wave (the T_a *wave*) may be observed as a low-amplitude wave with a polarity opposite that of the P wave during AV block, and it may be accentuated during exercise testing (see Chapter 32), with acute pericarditis (see Chapter 86), or atrial infarction (see Chapter 37).

Heart Rate Variability

Analysis of beat-to-beat changes in heart rate and related dynamics, termed *heart rate variability* (see Chapters 61 and 102), can provide insight into neuroautonomic control mechanisms and their perturbations with aging, disease, and drug effects. For example, relatively high-frequency (0.15 to 0.4 Hz) fluctuations are mediated primarily by vagus nerve traffic, such that heart rate increases during inspiration and decreases during expiration. Attenuation of this respiratory sinus arrhythmia at rest is a marker of physiologic aging and also occurs with diabetes mellitus, congestive heart failure, and a wide range of other conditions that alter autonomic tone modulation. Of note, false-positive increases in high-frequency variability, attributable to abnormal sinoatrial function and loss of vagal modulation, may occur with aging and chronic heart disease. This finding has been termed *heart rate fragmentation*.[5] Relatively lower-frequency (0.05 to 0.15 Hz) physiologic oscillations in heart rate appear to be jointly regulated by sympathetic and parasympathetic interactions. A variety of complementary signal-processing techniques have been developed to analyze heart rate variability and its interactions with other physiologic signals, including time domain statistics, frequency domain techniques based on spectral methods, and newer computational tools derived from nonlinear dynamics and complex systems theory. In addition, fluctuations in beat-to-beat QT intervals may also exhibit meaningful variability.

Atrioventricular Node Conduction and the PR Segment

The *PR segment* is the usually isoelectric region beginning with the end of the P wave and ending with the onset of the QRS complex. It forms part of the *PR interval* that extends from the onset of the P wave to the onset of the QRS complex. The normal PR interval measures 120 to 200 ms in duration in adults and is best determined from the lead with the shortest interval.

The PR segment includes atrial repolarization and slow conduction within the AV node plus the more rapid conduction through the ventricular conduction system. The segment ends when enough ventricular myocardium has been activated to initiate the QRS complex.

The potentials generated by the conduction system structures, like most atrial repolarization potentials, are too small to be detected on the body surface at amplifier gains used in clinical electrocardiography. Signals from elements of the conduction system can be recorded from intracardiac recording electrodes placed, for example, against the base of the interventricular septum (see Chapters 61 and 64).

Ventricular Activation and the QRS Complex

Normal ventricular activation is a complex process that depends on interactions between the physiology and anatomy of both the specialized ventricular conducting system and the ventricular myocardium.

Ventricular Activation. Ventricular activation is the net product of two events: endocardial activation, followed by transmural activation of the two ventricles. *Endocardial* activation is guided by the anatomic distribution and physiology of the His-Purkinje system. The rapid conduction within the broadly dispersed ramifications of this treelike (*fractal*) system results in the synchronized activation of multiple endocardial sites and the depolarization of most of the endocardial surfaces of both ventricles within several milliseconds.

The sequence of LV endocardial activation, depicted in Figure 14.8, begins at three sites on the left side of the septum: (1) the anterior paraseptal wall, (2) the posterior paraseptal wall, and (3) the center of the left side of the septum. These loci generally correspond to the sites of insertion of the fascicles of the left bundle branch (LBB). Septal activation thus begins on the left side and spreads across the septum from left to right and from apex to base.

Wavefronts then sweep from the initial sites of activation in anterior and inferior and then superior directions to activate the anterior and lateral walls of the LV. The last areas of the LV to be activated are the posterobasal regions.

Excitation of the RV endocardium begins near the insertion point of the right bundle branch (RBB) near the base of the anterior papillary muscle and spreads to the free wall. The final areas to be activated are the pulmonary conus and the posterobasal RV areas.

Thus, in both ventricles, the overall endocardial excitation pattern begins on septal surfaces, sweeps down toward the apex and then around the free walls to the basal regions, in an apex-to-base direction.

Activation then moves across the ventricular wall from endocardium to epicardium. Excitation of the endocardium begins at sites of Purkinje–ventricular muscle junctions and proceeds by muscle cell-to-muscle cell conduction toward the epicardium. Multiple regions of both ventricles are usually activated simultaneously, resulting in substantial cancellation of the electrical forces that are generated, as previously described.

Normal QRS Complex

QRS patterns are described by the sequence of waves constituting the complex. An initial negative deflection is called the *Q wave*, the first positive wave is the *R wave*, and the first negative wave after a positive wave is the *S wave*. A second upright wave following an S wave, when present, is an *R′ wave*, i.e., an *R-prime wave*. A monophasic negative complex is referred to as a *QS complex*. Tall waves are denoted by uppercase letters and smaller ones by lowercase letters. For example, the QRS complex may be described as qRS if it consists of an initial small negative wave (q) followed by a tall upright one (R) and a deep negative one (S). In an RSr′ complex, initial tall R and S waves are followed by a small positive wave (r′).

In each case, the deflection must cross the baseline to be designated a discrete wave. Changes in waveform patterns that do not cross the baseline result in *notches* or *slurs*. A notch is an abrupt change in waveform direction that does not cross the baseline. A slur exists when there is a distinct change in the slope or rate of change in waveform amplitude. The significance of these patterns is discussed later.

Early QRS Patterns. The complex pattern of activation described earlier may be simplified into two forces, the first representing septal activation and the second representing LV free wall activation (Fig. 14.9). Because RV muscle mass is considerably smaller than that of the LV, most of the electrical activity it generates is canceled by the much greater forces from the LV so that it contributes little to normal QRS complexes. Thus, the normal QRS can be represented by septal and LV activity with little meaningful oversimplification.

Initial activation forces of the interventricular septum are oriented from left to right in the frontal plane and anteriorly in the horizontal plane, corresponding to the anatomic position of the septum within the chest. These wavefronts produce initial positive wave in leads with axes directed to the right (e.g., lead aVR) or anteriorly (e.g., lead V_1). Leads with axes directed to the left (e.g., leads I, aVL, V_5, and V_6) will register initial negative waves known as *septal q waves* (discussed later). These initial forces are normally of low amplitude and are brief (<30 msec in duration).

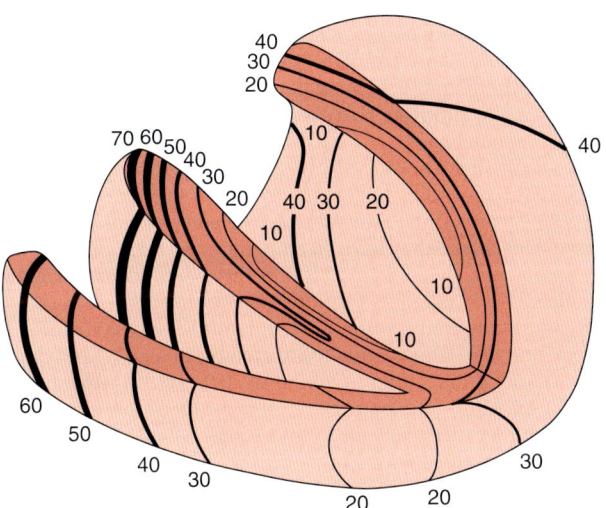

FIGURE 14.8 Activation sequence of the normal right and left ventricles. Portions of the left and right ventricles have been removed so that the endocardial surfaces of the ventricles and the interventricular septum can be seen. *Isochrone lines* connect sites that are activated at equal instants after the earliest evidence of ventricular activation. (From Durrer D. Electrical aspects of human cardiac activity: a clinical-physiological approach to excitation and stimulation. *Cardiovasc Res.* 1968;2:1–12.)

Mid- and Late QRS Patterns. Subsequent parts of the QRS complex reflect ongoing activation of, mainly, the free walls of the LV and RV. The complex interrelationships among cardiac position, conduction system function, and ventricular geometry result in a wide range of normal QRS patterns in the limb leads. The QRS pattern in leads II, III, and aVF may be predominantly upright, with qR complexes, or these leads may show rS or RS patterns. Lead I may record a qR pattern or an isoelectric RS pattern. These variations are discussed later in relation to lead axes.

Normal QRS patterns in the precordial leads follow an orderly progression from right (V_1) to left (V_6). In leads V_1 and V_2, initial r waves generated by septal activation are followed by S waves (an rS pattern), reflecting leftward and posterior activation of the LV free wall proceeding away from the precordial electrode.

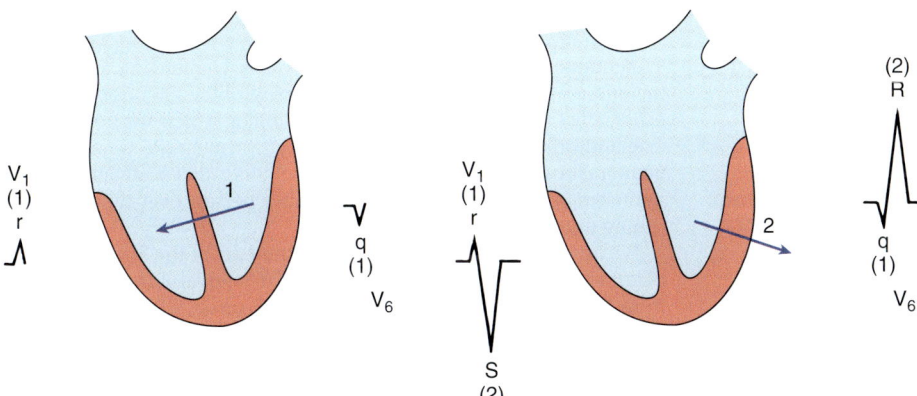

FIGURE 14.9 Ventricular depolarization shown as two sequential vectors representing septal (*left*) and left ventricular free wall (*right*) activation. QRS waveforms generated by each stage of activation in leads V_1 and V_6 are shown.

In midprecordial leads V_3 and V_4, the fronts first approach the exploring electrode and then move leftward and posteriorly, away from the exploring electrode. This sequence generates an R or r wave as it moves toward the electrode, followed by an S wave as it moves away from the electrode to produce rS or RS complexes.

As the exploring electrode moves further to the left to V_5 and V_6, the R wave becomes more dominant and the S wave becomes smaller (or totally lost by leads V_5 and V_6) because of the longer time period during which the activation front moves toward the positive end of the electrode. In the leftmost leads (i.e., leads V_5 and V_6), the normal pattern also includes the septal q wave, to produce a qR (or qRs) morphology.

Thus, in the precordial leads, the QRS complex usually is characterized by a consistent progression from an rS complex in the right precordial leads, to an RS pattern in the midprecordial leads, and to a qR pattern in the left precordial leads. The site at which the pattern changes from a dominant S wave to a dominant R wave pattern—the *transition zone*—normally occurs between lead V_3 and V_4. Transition zones that are shifted to the right (e.g., to lead V_2) are *early transitions* (previously referred to as *"counterclockwise rotation"*), and those shifted leftward (e.g., to V_5 or V_6) are *delayed transitions* (previously referred to as *"clockwise rotation"*). These patterns may have diagnostic significance in detecting, for example, ventricular hypertrophy, conduction defects, and MI, as discussed later.

Normal variability in patterns is related to demographic and physiologic factors. QRS amplitudes are greater (within the normal range) in men than in women and higher in African Americans than in those of other races. Higher-than-normal amplitudes are characteristic of chamber hypertrophy and conduction defects, as discussed later. Low-amplitude QRS complexes, that is, complexes with overall amplitudes of less than 0.5 mV in all frontal plane leads and less than 1.0 mV in the precordial leads, may occur as a normal variant or as a result of cardiac (e.g., infiltrative cardiomyopathies, myocarditis) or extracardiac (e.g., pericardial effusion, chronic obstructive pulmonary disease, pneumothorax) conditions, as discussed later in this and in other chapters.

Electrical Axis. The wide range of normal QRS patterns in the limb leads can be interpreted by referring to the hexaxial reference system in Figure 14.4. The normal mean QRS axis in adults lies between −30 degrees and +90 to 100 degrees, with physiologically vertical/inferior axes most prevalent in young adults. If the mean axis is near 90 degrees, that is, directed toward the left foot, the QRS complex in leads II, III, and aVF will be predominantly upright with qR complexes; lead I will record an isoelectric RS pattern because the heart vector lies perpendicular to its lead axis. If the mean axis is nearer 0 degrees, that is, directed toward the left arm, the patterns will be reversed; leads I and aVL will register a predominantly upright qR pattern, and leads II, III, and aVF will show rS or RS patterns. This variation largely reflects physiologic differences in the conduction system; the anatomic position of the heart within the torso has a minor role.

In adults, mean QRS axes more positive than +90 to 100 degrees (usually with an rS pattern in lead I) represent right axis deviation. Axes more negative than −30 degrees (with an rS pattern in lead II) represent left axis deviation. Mean axes lying between −90 degrees and −180 degrees (or, equivalently, between +180 and +270 degrees) are referred to as extreme axis deviations or, alternatively, as right superior axis deviations. The term indeterminate axis refers to the condition in which all six extremity leads show biphasic (QR or RS) patterns, indicating a mean electrical axis that is perpendicular to the frontal plane. This finding may occur as a normal variant or may be seen in a variety of pathologic conditions discussed later.

The Intrinsicoid Deflection. As previously described, an electrode overlying the ventricular free wall will record a rising R wave as transmural activation proceeds toward it. The peak of the R wave occurs when the activation front reaches the epicardium. After that, the full thickness of the wall under the electrode will be in an active state and the electrode will register negative potentials as activation proceeds in remote cardiac areas. This sudden reversal of potential produces a sharp downslope after the peak of the R wave, the *intrinsicoid deflection*, that approximates the timing of activation of the epicardium under the electrode. Thus, the time from the onset of the QRS to the intrinsicoid deflection (the *R-peak time*) has been interpreted as a measure of the duration of transmural spread of excitation.

Ventricular Recovery and the ST-T Wave

Genesis of Ventricular Recovery Potentials. The ST-T wave reflects activity during the plateau phase and the later repolarization phases of the cardiac action potential. ST-T wave patterns depend on the interaction of two factors: (1) the direction of intracellular current flow in cardiac fibers during repolarization, and (2) the sequence of recovery within the ventricles.

Differences in recovery times occur between regions of the LV and across the ventricular wall. In general, the repolarization sequence is the opposite of the activation sequence; that is, regions activated later have shorter action potentials than areas activated early. Thus, action potential durations are shorter in the anterobasal region than in the posteroapical region of the LV. Similarly, action potential durations are shorter in the epicardium than in the endocardium.

In each case, the shortening of recovery time is greater than the delay in onset of activation, so that repolarization ends first in areas activated last. The resulting repolarization current flow will then be directed away from the basal LV toward the apex and away from the endocardium toward the epicardium. That is, repolarization current flow will be in the same direction as during activation. The result is that normal QRS and ST-T patterns are *concordant*, with the ST-T wave having the same polarity as the QRS complex.

Evidence suggests that the regional differences in action potential duration are the major cause of ST-T wave, with lesser contribution by transmural differences.[6] In addition, some evidence suggests a role for so-called M or midmyocardial cells in the genesis of the ST-T wave.[7] These cells have longer action potentials than either endocardial or epicardial cells and repolarize last. Thus, at the end of the ST-T segment, repolarization currents flow from the epicardium toward the mid-wall, contributing to the downslope of the T wave.

The Normal ST-T Wave

The normal ST-T wave begins as a low-amplitude, slowly changing wave (the *ST segment*) that gradually evolves into a larger wave, the *T wave*. The onset of the ST-T wave, the *junction* or *J point*, is normally at or near the isoelectric baseline (typically the PR segment) of the ECG (see Fig. 14.6). The level of the ST segment generally is measured at the J point or, in some applications such as exercise testing, 40 or 80 msec after the J point (see Chapter 15).

The polarity of the normal ST-T wave generally is the same as the net polarity of the preceding QRS complex; that is, they are concordant. T waves usually are upright in leads I, II, aVL, and aVF and in the lateral precordial leads, and they have an amplitude of 1.5 mV or less. T waves are normally negative in lead aVR and variable in leads III, V_1, and V_2 (see later).

The amplitude of the normal J point and ST segment varies with race, sex, and age.[4] They typically are greatest in lead V_2, and they are higher in young men than in young women and in African Americans than in whites. Recommendations[1] for the upper limits of normal J point elevation in leads V_2 and V_3 are 0.2 mV for men age 40 or older, 0.25 mV for men younger than 40, and 0.15 mV for women. In other leads, the recommended upper limit is 0.1 mV for men and women. Higher levels, however, are common in normal persons especially among athletes. As many as 30% of athletes had ST elevation exceeding 0.2 mV in the anterior precordial leads.

The QT Interval

The QT interval extends from the onset of the QRS complex to the end of the T wave. Thus, it includes the total duration of ventricular activation and recovery and, in a general sense, corresponds to the duration of the ventricular action potential.

Accurately measuring the QT interval is challenging. Difficulties include precisely identifying the beginning of the QRS complex and especially the end of the T wave[8]; determining which lead or leads to use; and adjusting the measured interval for rate, QRS duration, and gender. These factors also make determining diagnostic thresholds and comparing QT intervals in the same person over time, such as during drug treatment, complex.

Because the onset of the QRS and the end of the T wave do not occur simultaneously in every lead, the QT interval duration will vary from lead to lead by as much as 50 to 65 msec (*QT dispersion*). In automated ECG systems, the QT interval typically is measured from a composite of all leads, beginning with the earliest onset of the QRS in any lead and terminating with the latest end of the T wave in any lead. When the interval is measured from a single lead, the lead in which the interval is the longest (most frequently lead V_2 or V_3) and in which a prominent U wave is absent (often aVR and aVL) is preferred.

Measurement of the *JT interval* (beginning at the end of the QRS complex rather than from its onset) has been proposed for patients with wide QRS complexes to adjust for the inclusion of the prolonged QRS duration in the overall QT interval.

The normal QT interval is rate dependent, decreasing as heart rate increases. This corresponds to rate-related changes in the duration of the normal ventricular action potential. Numerous formulae have been proposed to correct the measured QT interval for this rate effect.[1] The most commonly used formula is based on one proposed by Bazett in 1920. The result is the *corrected QT interval*, or *QTc*, defined by the following equation:

$$QTc = QT / \sqrt{RR}$$

where the QT and RR intervals are measured in seconds. A joint report of the American Heart Association (AHA), American College of Cardiology (ACC), and other professional organizations[1] suggested that the upper limit for QTc be set at 460 msec for women and 450 msec for men, and that the lower limit be set at 390 msec.

This formula has limited accuracy in correcting for the effects of heart rate on the QT interval. Large database studies have shown that the QTc interval based on the Bazett correction remains significantly affected by heart rate and that as many as 30% of normal ECGs may be diagnosed as having a prolonged QT interval when this formula is used.

Another commonly used correction is *Fridericia's formula* in which the adjusted QT interval is a function of the cube root of the RR interval. The AHA/ACC joint committee suggested using linear or power function regression equations.[1] One linear formula (proposed by Hodges) that has been shown to be relatively insensitive to heart rate, is:

$$QTc = QT + 1.75 (HR - 60)$$

where HR is heart rate (beats/min) and the intervals are computed as units of seconds. Other approaches include regression analyses based on the specific population studied or computing individual-specific corrections to assess serial changes such as during drug therapy.

The normal QT interval may be modified by numerous influences in addition to heart rate. These include gender (with longer intervals in women than in men), age (with increasing T intervals with increasing age), circadian rhythm (with longer intervals during sleep), and changes in autonomic tone (with decreasing intervals with increasing sympathetic tone and increasing intervals with higher parasympathetic activity). The impact of autonomic tone is demonstrated by, for example, the greater effect of increasing heart rate by exercise than with atrial pacing.

Abnormal QT prolongation occurs in numerous cardiac and noncardiac syndromes, during treatment with cardiac and noncardiac drugs, with electrolyte and metabolic abnormalities, and as a result of several gene mutations impacting ion channels (see Chapter 63). It is associated with tachyarrhythmias and sudden death (see Chapters 65–68 and 70). In the Multi-Ethnic Study of Atherosclerosis (MESA), each 10 msec increase in QT_C was associated with a 25%, 11%, and 19% increase in the development of heart failure, cardiovascular events, and stroke, respectively, during an 8-year follow-up.[9] Short QT intervals (defined by one consensus statement as <390 msec) are uncommon but identify a channelopathy with a very high risk of ventricular arrhythmias, atrial fibrillation, syncope, and sudden cardiac death (see Chapter 63).

The QRST Angle and the Ventricular Gradient

The *spatial QRST angle* is the angle, in three-dimensional space, between the vector representing the mean QRS force and the vector representing the mean ST-T force. The angle between the two vectors in the frontal plane represents a reasonable simplification and normally is less than 90 degrees for women and 107 degrees for men. If the two vectors representing mean activation and mean recovery forces are added, a third vector known as the *ventricular gradient* is created that represents the net area under the QRST complex.

These and related measures seek to quantify the level of global electrical heterogeneity in the ventricles. As described earlier, activation and repolarization forces are, in concept, concordant in direction and equal in magnitude. Thus, vectors representing the areas under the QRS complex (corresponding to the strength and orientation of overall activation forces) and under the ST-T (corresponding to overall recovery forces) should be equal and have the same orientation. That is, if the action potentials of all cells had uniform shapes and if depolarization and repolarization occurred in all regions in the same directions, the QRST angle and the ventricular gradient would equal zero.

The greater the differences in global electrical heterogeneity, the larger will be the QRST angle and the ventricular gradient. Abnormal levels of heterogeneity may occur in many conditions, including ischemia and hypertrophy, and may lead to arrhythmias, as discussed in Chapter 62. In an analysis of two large general population studies, a prediction model for sudden cardiac death demonstrated that these and related measurements were significantly and independently associated with sudden death during and after adjustment for other risk factors.[10]

Other Repolarization Waves

The U Wave

The T wave may be followed by an additional low-amplitude wave known as the *U wave*. This wave is usually less than 0.1 to 0.15 mV in amplitude, less than 160 to 200 msec in duration, and of the same polarity as the preceding T wave. Often, the U wave may merge with the end of the T wave to produce what appears to be a notched T wave, leading to what may be called a *QT(U) wave*. The U wave is generally largest in the leads V_2 and V_3 and is most often seen at slow heart rates and in patients with hypertension or hypokalemia. Its electrophysiologic basis is uncertain. Suggestions include delayed repolarization in areas of the ventricle that undergo late mechanical relaxation, late repolarization of the Purkinje fibers, and long action potentials of midmyocardial M cells. Negative U waves are uncommon and are strongly associated with adverse cardiac events.

The J Wave

A *J wave* is a dome- or hump-shaped wave or notch that appears at the end of or after the QRS complex and that has the same polarity as the preceding QRS complex. It may be prominent as a normal variant (see later), in certain pathologic conditions such as systemic hypothermia (sometimes referred to as an *Osborn wave,* described later), and in a set of conditions commonly referred to as the *J wave syndromes* that include the *Brugada patterns* (see Chapters 63 and 67) and the *early repolarization pattern* (discussed later and in Chapter 63). The origin of the J wave has been putatively associated with a prominent notch found in phase 1 of epicardial action potentials but not in those on the endocardium, creating a transmural potential gradient at the end of the QRS complex and beginning of the ST-T wave, leading to QRS notching and ST elevation.[7] A role of increased vagal tone has also been implicated in persons without structural heart disease, because benign early repolarization patterns are most apparent at slower heart rates.

Another wave occurring at the onset of repolarization is the *epsilon wave*. This uncommon wave (or set of waves) appears as a low-amplitude, high-frequency spike (or spikes) between the end of the QRS and the onset of the T wave, usually in the right precordial leads. It has been related to markedly delayed activation of islands of functional tissue interspersed among fatty or scarred tissue and, for example, is one diagnostic hallmark of arrhythmogenic right ventricular cardiomyopathy (see Chapter 52).

Normal Variants

Numerous variations in these normal ECG patterns frequently occur in persons without heart disease. The presence of such findings without coexistent cardiac pathology is particularly common among young persons and athletes (see Chapter 32). These variations are important to recognize because they may be mistaken for significant abnormalities, leading to erroneous and potentially harmful diagnoses of heart disease.

The absence of septal q waves, with QS complexes in the right precordial leads or with initial R waves in leads I, V_5, and V_6, is a common normal variant that is not generally associated with any specific cardiac disease. Recent studies using cardiac magnetic resonance (CMR)

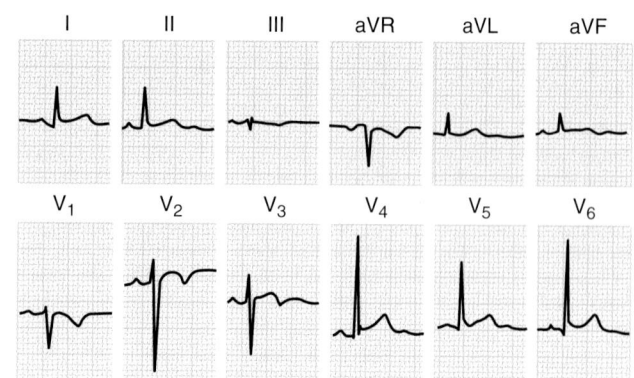

FIGURE 14.10 Normal tracing with a juvenile T wave inversion pattern in leads V_1, V_2, and V_3, as well as early repolarization pattern manifested by ST-segment elevation in leads I, II, aVF, V_4, V_5, and V_6. J point notching is also present in lead V_4. (Courtesy Dr. C. Fisch.)

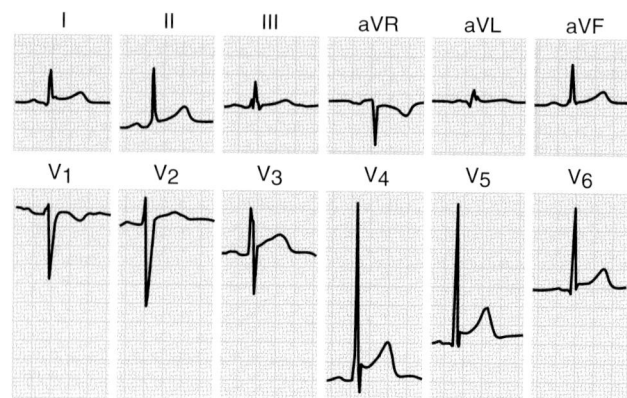

FIGURE 14.11 Normal variant with the "benign early repolarization" pattern of a J point notch and ST-segment elevation. The ST-segment elevation and a J point notch are most marked in the midprecordial lead V_4. Reciprocal ST-segment depression and PR-segment depression are absent (except in lead aVR). (From Goldberger AL, Goldberger ZD, Shvilkin A. *Goldberger's Clinical Electrocardiography: A Simplified Approach*. 9th ed. Philadelphia: Elsevier; 2017.)

imaging have, however, suggested that this finding may reflect septal scarring of ischemic or nonischemic origin.[11]

The presence of rSr′ patterns in leads V_1 and V_2 with a normal QRS duration may commonly be found in subjects without cardiac disease, including up to half of trained athletes (see Chapter 32). It may be artefactually produced by placing electrodes of leads V_1 and V_2 higher on the chest than standard. In patients with pectus excavatum, the pattern may result from changes in heart position caused by the skeletal deformity. Pathologic conditions with this pattern, discussed later, include bundle branch blocks, Brugada patterns, RV hypertrophy, preexcitation syndromes, and hyperkalemia.

T wave inversion in leads V_1 to V_3 (sometimes referred to as the *persistent juvenile pattern*) (Fig. 14.10) is common among children and adolescents and in 1% to 3% of apparently healthy adults. It is more prevalent in women than in men, in African Americans than in other racial or ethnic groups, and in as many as 30% of athletes. T wave inversion of 2 mm or greater in two leads from V_{2-6}, in leads II and aVF, or in leads I and aVL suggests underlying pathology.

Another common and important variant is the so-called *benign early repolarization pattern* (see Chapter 63). Differing diagnostic criteria have been proposed. The AHA suggested that the term be applied as an umbrella term including cases with ST-segment elevation without chest pain, with terminal QRS slurring, or with terminal QRS notching.[12]

Recent recommendations by another expert panel[7] have suggested that this ECG diagnosis may be made if (1) there is a prominent notch or J wave at the end of QRS complex or slur on the downstroke of the R wave, (2) the peak of the notch or J wave is 0.1 mV or greater in amplitude in two or more contiguous leads, excluding V_1 to V_3 (to avoid cases of Brugada pattern), and (3) the QRS duration is normal. Although commonly associated with these findings, ST-segment elevation is not required.

The elevated ST segment, when present, typically has a rapidly upsloping shape and is most prominent in the right and midprecordial leads (Fig. 14.11). Its appearance is labile, being most prominent under conditions of increased vagal tone and decreasing with exercise. This pattern occurs in as many as 30% of the general population and is most prevalent in young adults, especially African American men and in athletes.

Although most commonly a benign variant, subsets of subjects with the early repolarization phenotype have been described as tachyarrhythmias and sudden death may occur. Potentially malignant subsets of early repolarization syndrome include those with J wave patterns in multiple leads and the inferior leads, J wave amplitudes of greater than 0.2 mV, or horizontal or downsloping ST-segment elevation (see Chapters 63 and 70).[7] Specific diagnostic criteria for this syndrome, including clinical and family history criteria and genetic markers, have been proposed.[7]

Cardiac mapping studies have documented the electrophysiologic bases for these ECG findings in patients with early repolarization syndromes.[13] These include localized areas with prominent epicardial J waves followed by significantly shortened repolarization phases. The heterogeneous distribution of these regions results in large and localized repolarization potential gradients that may be arrhythmogenic.

It is important to distinguish the early repolarization pattern from other clinically important diagnoses. These include anterior MI, pericarditis, and cardiomyopathies and the Brugada patterns (see Chapter 63). QRS notches due to intraventricular conduction defects and myocardial scarring that are most common in the middle portions of the downslope of the R wave. The distinction between benign and pathologic early repolarization variants is an ongoing subject of research and some controversy.

An important set of normal variations, including benign early repolarization, are those that commonly occur in athletes (see Chapter 32). Prolonged, regular exercise can produce significant electrophysiologic changes that commonly cause variant ECG patterns. Although these changes reflect physiologic rather than pathologic effects, they may mimic the ECG patterns of various diseases and thus result in high rates of false-positive interpretations. To account for these variants, different ECG criteria separating normal from abnormal tracings have been proposed for use in atheletes.[14] These include considering increased QRS voltage, IRBBB, and right-sided T wave inversions, among other findings, to be normal variants.

THE ABNORMAL ELECTROCARDIOGRAM

The prevalence of abnormal ECGs in the general population is substantial and increases progressively with age and in certain population groups. For example, in the ARIC study of 4856 disease-free persons with normal ECGs at enrollment, 53.4% developed an abnormal ECG over the subsequent 10 years.[15] Many of these abnormalities have prognostic as well as diagnostic import. In the ARIC study, enrollees with a continuously normal ECG had a 41% lower risk of cardiovascular disease during a 13 year follow-up than did those who developed abnormal tracings.[15] Even minor ECG abnormalities (e.g., isolated ST-T wave changes) have prognostic significance; among subjects free of baseline cardiovascular disease at enrollment in the Third National Health and Nutrition Examination Survey (NHANES), each additional minor ECG abnormality was associated with a 13% increase in cardiovascular death during a 14-year follow-up.[1]

Chamber Enlargement and Hypertrophy
Atrial Abnormalities
Various pathophysiologic events can produce P wave abnormalities reflecting changes in (1) the origin of the initiating sinus node impulse, (2) conduction within the atria and from the RA to the LA, or (3) the size and shape of the atria. These may result in abnormal patterns of interatrial block, left atrial abnormalities, and right atrial abnormalities.

Abnormal Atrial Activation and Conduction. Small shifts in the site of initial activation within or near the sinoatrial node or to ectopic sites within the atria can lead to major changes in the pattern of atrial activation and in the morphology of P waves. These shifts may occur as *escape rhythms* if the normal SA nodal pacemaker fails or as *accelerated atrial rhythms* if the automaticity of an ectopic site is enhanced (see Chapter 65). Physiologic changes may also alter the P wave shapes; exercise, for example, may produce a more vertical mean P wave axis.

P wave patterns may suggest the site of impulse formation and the path of subsequent activation. A negative P wave in lead I suggests activation beginning in the LA, and an inverted P wave in the inferior leads generally corresponds to a posterior atrial activation site. However, predicting the specific location of origin from a P wave pattern is highly variable. Accordingly, these patterns, as a group, may be referred to as *atrial rhythms* rather than assigned anatomic terms inferring a specific site of origin.

Interatrial block (sometimes termed intra-atrial block [IAB]) refers to conduction delay within and between the atria that alters the duration and pattern of P waves.[16] In milder cases of delay, conduction from the RA to the LA is delayed, but the overall sequence of activation is preserved. The increased lag in LA activation relative to that of the RA increases P wave duration beyond 120 msec. P waves typically have two humps in lead II, with the first representing RA and the second reflecting LA activation.

With more advanced IAB, the normal conduction paths are blocked. The sinus node impulses reach the LA only after passing inferiorly toward the AV junction, across the mid-lower portion of the interatrial septum, and then superiorly through the LA. In these cases, P waves are wide and biphasic (an initial positive wave followed by a negative deflection) in the inferior and anterior leads. IAB may also be intermittent, varying from beat to beat.

Interatrial block is uncommon in the general population. Among over 14,000 persons in the general population enrolled in the ARIC trial, interatrial block was found in 0.5% at enrollment and an additional 1.3% developed IAB in during an average 5.9-year follow-up.[17] Rates among patients with cardiac disease or in hospitalized cohorts may, however, reach 60%. It is often, but not always, associated with ECG findings of LA enlargement, and evidence of anatomic LA remodeling and reduced atrial pump function.[18] IAB is associated with a threefold increase in the risk of developing atrial tachyarrhythmias and fibrillation (*Bayés syndrome*), and increases in the risk for ischemic strokes and cardiac death.

Left Atrial Abnormality

Anatomic abnormalities of the LA that alter the P waves include atrial dilation, atrial muscular hypertrophy, elevated intra-atrial pressures, and, as discussed earlier, conduction slowing. Because these pathophysiologic abnormalities often coexist and produce similar ECG effects, the resulting patterns are often referred to as *left atrial abnormality*.

DIAGNOSTIC CRITERIA. Abnormalities in LA structure and function produce wide and notched P waves, with prominent terminal negative deflections (P terminal forces) in the right precordial leads. The most common criteria for diagnosing left atrial abnormality are listed in Table 14.3 and illustrated in Figures 14.12 and 14.13.

Mechanisms for the Electrocardiogram Abnormalities. Prolonged activation time of the LA produces prolonged P wave duration, notching of P waves that is most prominent in inferolateral leads, and increased amplitude of the terminal negative P wave terminal force in the right precordial leads. As described earlier, the ECG changes described for LA abnormalities are very similar to those described for IAB and may reflect IAB caused by the structural changes induced by atrial hemodynamic abnormalities, sometimes referred to as "atriopathies."[18]

Diagnostic Accuracy. Studies correlating these ECG criteria with LA volumes determined by CMR[1] have demonstrated the limited accuracy of the criteria. A prolonged P wave duration has a high sensitivity (84%) but low specificity (35%). By contrast, bifid P waves and increased negative terminal P wave amplitude in lead V_1 have low sensitivities (8% and 37%, respectively) and high specificities (90% and 88%, respectively).

Clinical Significance. Because of the similarities in the ECG features of IAB and LA abnormality, the clinical significance of the two sets of abnormalities is similar. The finding of LA abnormality is associated with more severe cardiac dysfunction in patients with ischemic heart disease

TABLE 14.3 Common Diagnostic Criteria for Left and Right Atrial Abnormalities

LEFT ATRIAL ABNORMALITY	RIGHT ATRIAL ABNORMALITY*
Prolonged P wave duration to >120 msec in lead II	Peaked P waves with amplitudes in lead II to >0.25 mV
Prominent notching of P wave, usually most obvious in lead II, with interval between notches of >40 msec	Prominent initial positivity in lead V_1 or V_2 >0.15 mV
Ratio between duration of P wave in lead II and duration of PR segment >1.6	Increased area under initial positive portion of P wave in lead V_1 to >0.06 mm-sec
Increased duration and depth of terminal-negative portion of P wave in lead V_1 (P terminal force) so that the area subtended by it is >0.04 mm-sec	Rightward shift of mean P wave axis to >+75 degrees
Leftward shift of mean P wave axis to between −30 and −45 degrees	

*In addition to criteria based on P wave morphologies, right atrial abnormality is suggested by QRS changes as described in the text.
Reference: Hancock EW, Deal BJ, Mirvis DM, et al. Recommendations for the standardization and interpretation of the electrocardiogram. Part V. ECG changes associated with cardiac chamber hypertrophy. *J Am Coll Cardiol.* 2009;53:992–1002.

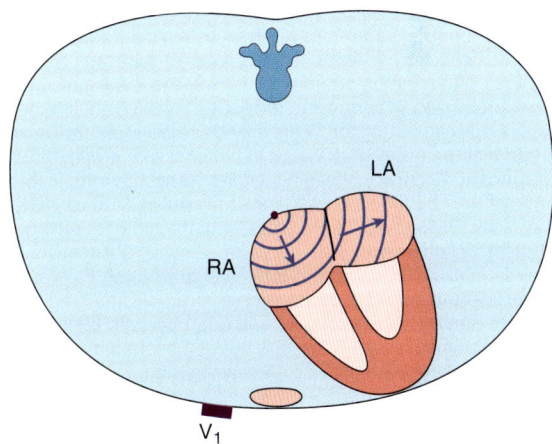

FIGURE 14.12 Top, Atrial depolarization. **Bottom,** P wave patterns associated with normal atrial activation (*left*) and with right atrial (*middle*) and left atrial (*right*) abnormalities. (Modified from Park MK, Guntheroth WG. *How to Read Pediatric ECGs.* 4th ed. St Louis: Mosby; 2006.)

(see Chapter 40) and with mitral or aortic valve disease (see Chapters 72, 73 and 75, 76). Patients with LA abnormalities also have a higher-than-normal incidence of atrial tachyarrhythmias, cerebrovascular accidents (CVAs), and all-cause and cardiovascular mortality (see Chapter 66). For example, in the ARIC study of over 14,000 persons followed for a mean of 22 years, LA abnormality defined by an abnormal P wave terminal force in V_1 was associated with an adjusted hazard rate for nonlacunar strokes of 1.49.[19]

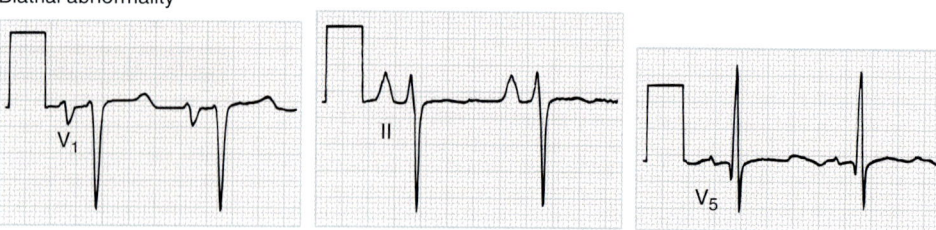

FIGURE 14.13 Biatrial abnormality, with tall P waves in lead II (right atrial abnormality) and an abnormally large terminal negative component of the P wave in lead V_1 (left atrial abnormality). The P wave is also notched in lead V_5 as part of this pattern.

Right Atrial Abnormality

The ECG features of right atrial abnormality are illustrated in Figures 14.12 and 14.13. As in the case of LA abnormality, the term *right atrial abnormality* is preferred rather than designations such as "right atrial enlargement" that suggest a particular underlying pathophysiology.

Diagnostic Criteria. P wave amplitudes in the limb and right precordial leads typically are abnormally high; P wave duration remains normal. Criteria commonly used to diagnose RA abnormality are listed in Table 14.3. In addition, RA abnormality is suggested by a qR-type pattern in the right precordial leads without evidence of MI or by low-amplitude QRS complexes in lead V_1 together with a threefold or greater increase in lead V_2.

Mechanisms for the Electrocardiogram Abnormalities. Greater RA mass and size generate greater electrical forces early during atrial activation, producing taller P waves in limb leads and increasing the initial P wave deflection in leads such as lead V_1 that face the right heart. Because RA activation occurs early during the P wave, P wave duration is not prolonged, in contrast to the pattern with LA enlargement. Downward displacement of the heart may be responsible for the increase in P-terminal force and tall P waves in patients with emphysema.

Diagnostic Accuracy. Imaging studies have shown that the ECG features of RA abnormality have limited sensitivity (7% to 10%) but high specificity (96% to 100%) for detecting anatomic RA enlargement.[1]

Clinical Significance. Patients with chronic obstructive pulmonary disease and this ECG pattern (often referred to as P pulmonale) have more severe pulmonary dysfunction and significantly reduced survival, than do others (see Chapters 87 and 88). However, comparison of ECG and hemodynamic parameters has not demonstrated a close correlation between P wave patterns and RA hypertension.

Other Atrial Abnormalities. Patients with biatrial abnormalities may have ECG patterns reflecting each defect. These include large, biphasic P waves in lead V_1 and tall, broad P waves in leads II, III, and aVF (see Fig. 14.13).

Left Ventricular Hypertrophy

Left ventricular hypertrophy (LVH) diagnosed by ECG occurs in 1% to 5% of the general population and in as many as one-third of patients with hypertension. QRS changes include greater than normal amplitudes of R waves in leads facing the LV (i.e., leads I, aVL, V_5, and V_6), and deeper than normal S waves in leads overlying the opposite side of the heart (i.e., V_1 and V_2). These changes are often associated with left axis deviation, notching or slurring of R waves, and patterns suggesting intraventricular conduction defects (Fig. 14.14). The ST segment may be normal or somewhat elevated in leads with tall R waves.

In many patients, the ST segment is depressed and followed by an inverted T wave (Fig. 14.15) in leads I, II, aVL, and V_5–V_6. The depressed ST segment is typically either flat or sloped downward from a depressed J point followed by an asymmetrically inverted T wave (the so-called *strain pattern*). These repolarization changes usually occur in patients with QRS changes but may appear alone. Additional abnormalities may include prolongation of the QT interval and evidence of LA abnormality.

These ECG features are most typical of LVH induced by pressure overload of the LV such as with hypertension (see Chapter 26). Volume overload may produce a somewhat different pattern, with tall upright T waves and narrow (<25 msec) but deep (≥0.2 mV) Q waves in leads I, aVL, and V_{4-6} (Fig. 14.16) (see Chapter 73). These distinctions have limited value in identifying hemodynamic conditions.

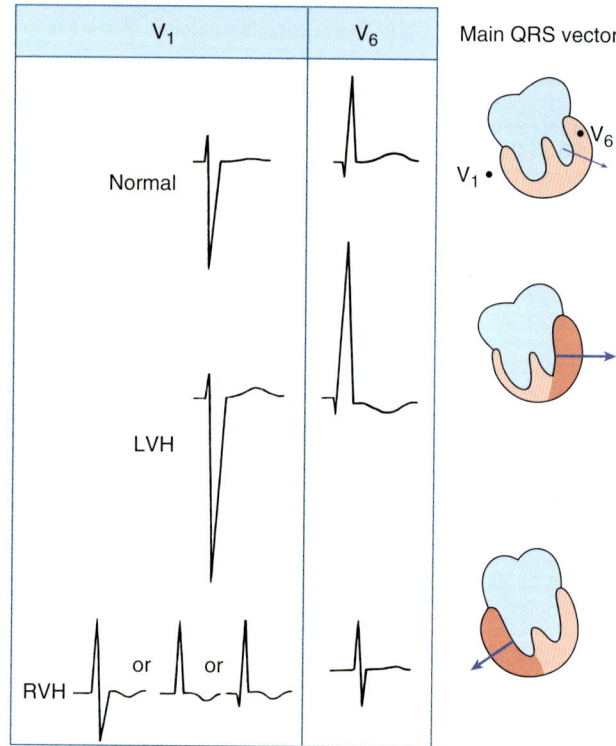

FIGURE 14.14 Left ventricular hypertrophy increases the amplitude of electrical forces directed to the left and posteriorly. In addition, repolarization abnormalities can cause ST-segment depression and T wave inversion in leads with a prominent R wave. Right ventricular hypertrophy can shift the QRS vector to the right, usually with an R, RS, or qR complex in lead V_1, especially when caused by severe pressure overload. T wave inversions may be present in the left precordial leads. (From Goldberger AL, Goldberger ZD, Shvilkin A. *Goldberger's Clinical Electrocardiography: A Simplified Approach.* 9th ed. Philadelphia: Elsevier; 2017.)

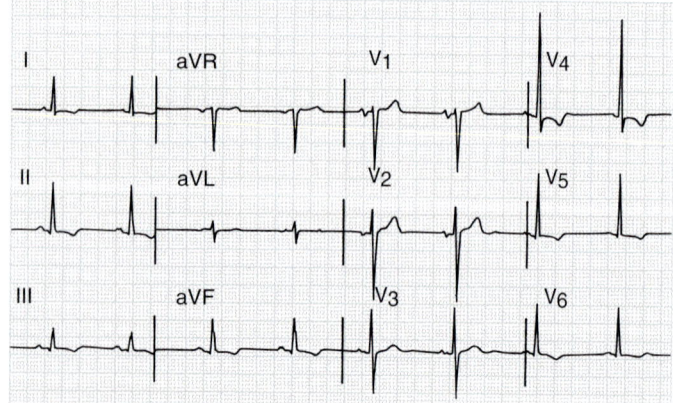

FIGURE 14.15 Marked left ventricular hypertrophy pattern with prominent precordial lead QRS voltages, ST-segment depression, and T wave inversion (compare with Fig. 14.16). Left atrial abnormality also is present.

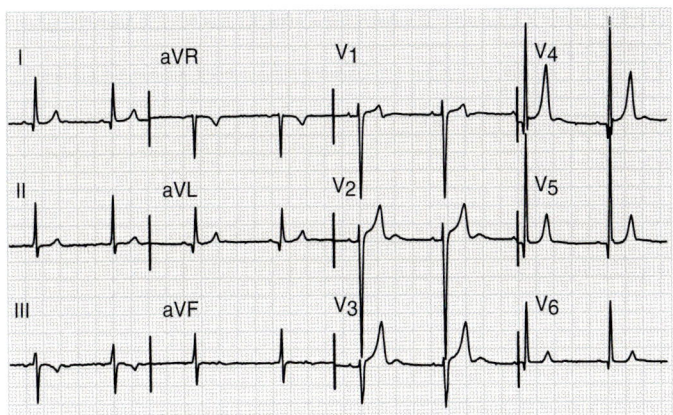

FIGURE 14.16 Left ventricular hypertrophy pattern with prominent Q waves and positive anterior T waves on an electrocardiogram from a patient with severe aortic regurgitation.

TABLE 14.4 Common Diagnostic Criteria for Left Ventricular Hypertrophy

MEASUREMENT	CRITERIA
Sokolow-Lyon voltages	$SV_1 + RV_5 > 3.5$ mV
	$RaVL > 1.1$ mV
Romhilt-Estes point score system*	Any limb lead R wave or S wave >2.0 mV (3 points)
	or SV_1 or $SV_2 \geq 3.0$ mV (3 points)
	or RV_5 to $RV_6 \geq 3.0$ mV (3 points)
	ST-T wave abnormality, no digitalis therapy (3 points)
	ST-T wave abnormality, digitalis therapy (1 point)
	Left atrial abnormality (3 points)
	Left axis deviation ≥ -30 degrees (2 points)
	QRS duration ≥ 90 msec (1 point)
	Intrinsicoid deflection in V_5 or $V_6 \geq 50$ msec (1 point)
Cornell voltage criteria	$SV_3 + RaVL > 2.8$ mV (for men)
	$SV_3 + RaVL > 2.0$ mV (for women)
Cornell regression equation	Risk of LVH = $1 / (1 + e^{-exp})$†
Cornell voltage duration measurement	QRS duration × Cornell voltage >2436 mm-sec‡
	QRS duration × sum of voltages in all leads >1742 mm-sec

LVH, Left ventricular hypertrophy; *PTF*, P terminal force; $PTFV_1$, P terminal force in lead V_1.
*Probable LVH is diagnosed with totals of 4 points, and definite LVH is diagnosed with totals of 5 or more points.
†For persons in sinus rhythm, exp = 4.558 − 0.092 (SV_3 + RaVL) − 0.306 TV_1 − 0.212 QRS − 0.278 $PTFV_1$ − 0.559 (sex). Voltages are in mV, QRS is QRS duration in milliseconds, $PTFV_1$ is the area under the P terminal force in lead V_1 (in mm-sec), and sex = 1 for men and 2 for women. LVH is diagnosed as present if exp <−1.55.
‡For women, add 8 mm.
Reference: Hancock EW, Deal BJ, Mirvis DM, et al. AHA/ACCF/HRS recommendations for the standardization and interpretation of the electrocardiogram: part V: electrocardiogram changes associated with cardiac chamber hypertrophy; a scientific statement from the American Heart Association Electrocardiography and Arrhythmias Committee, Council on Clinical Cardiology; the American College of Cardiology Foundation; and the Heart Rhythm Society. Endorsed by the International Society for Computerized Electrocardiology. *J Am Coll Cardiol.* 2009;53:992–1002.

Mechanisms for the Electrocardiogram Abnormalities. ECG changes of LVH result from interrelated structural, biochemical, and bioelectric changes.[20] Structural abnormalities include (1) an increase size of myocytes leading to an increase in mass and in the size of activation fronts moving across the thickened wall to generate higher body surface voltages, (2) thickened walls that require more time to fully activate, and (3) changes in the interstitium including fibrosis, inflammation, and degenerative changes that result in slower-than-normal and fragmented conduction across the myocardium.

Hypertrophy is also associated with cellular forms of *electrical remodeling*. This includes biochemical changes in gap junctions and ion channels that alter the intensity of current flow. In addition, changes in myocyte branching patterns alter impulse propagation. The heterogeneous distribution of these abnormalities and scattered intramural scarring associated with hypertrophy can also disrupt smooth propagation of wavefronts to produce prolongation and notching of the QRS complex. Simulation studies have demonstrated that it is the combination of the anatomic abnormalities (i.e., increased muscle mass) and slowed and disordered conduction that leads to the observed ECG changes.

ST-T abnormalities reflect several interrelated phenomena These include primary disorders of repolarization that accompany the cellular processes of hypertrophy, the mechanical consequences of hypertrophy, and myocardial ischemia-related relative inadequacy of perfusion in relation to the increased oxygen demand caused by greater muscle mass and increased wall stress.

Diagnostic Criteria

Many sets of criteria to diagnose anatomic LVH have been developed based on these ECG abnormalities. Widely used criteria are listed in Table 14.4.

Most methods predict the presence or absence of LVH as a binary function, indicating that structural LVH either does or does not exist, based on an empirically determined set of criteria. For example, the widely used Sokolow-Lyon and Cornell voltage criteria require that voltages in specific leads exceed certain values. The Cornell voltage-duration method includes measurement of QRS duration as well as amplitudes. Other methods such as the Cornell regression equation seek to quantify LV mass as a continuum, with a diagnosis of LVH based on a computed mass that exceeds an independently determined threshold.

Diagnostic Accuracy. The accuracy of these criteria depends on the ultimate outcome being predicted. This reference standard may be, as most frequently practiced, the presence or absence of structural LVH. Alternatively, the ECG criteria may be used to predict clinical outcomes, as discussed later.

The reported diagnostic accuracies of these ECG criteria to detect structural LVH are highly variable, differing with the specific criteria tested, the imaging method used to determine anatomic measurements (e.g., echocardiography or CMR) and the population studied. Most studies have reported low sensitivities and high specificities. An analysis of the MESA study which used CMR imaging to establish anatomic standards, for example, demonstrated a sensitivity and specificity of 22.4% and 95.1%, respectively, for detecting CMR-determined LVH based upon having either a positive Sokolow-Lyon or Cornell voltage criterion.[21]

Because of the limited and variable accuracy of the various criteria from one trial to another, no single criterion can be established as the preferred method. The use of combined criteria, e.g., using both the Cornell product and the Sokolow-Lyon criteria, may result in a higher sensitivity (with a modest reduction in specificity), as well as an increase in the predicted risk of future cardiovascular events, than ECG diagnoses based on only one of the criteria.[22]

Accuracy in identifying anatomic LVH also varies with sex (with women having lower QRS amplitudes than men), race (with African Americans having higher QRS amplitudes than whites), age (with lower voltages with increasing age), and body habitus (with obesity reducing QRS amplitudes).

Clinical Significance

The low sensitivities of ECG measurements limit the value of these criteria as screening tools for structural LVH in both the general population and cohorts with a higher prevalence of LVH. The significance of an ECG diagnosis of LVH may also be measured by its ability to identify patients at high risk for future cardiac clinical events.[21,23] Thus, the presence of ECG criteria for LVH may identify a subset of the general population and of those with various cardiac diseases who have a significantly increased risk for cardiovascular morbidity, independent of the presence of anatomic hypertrophy. For example, in the ALLHAT

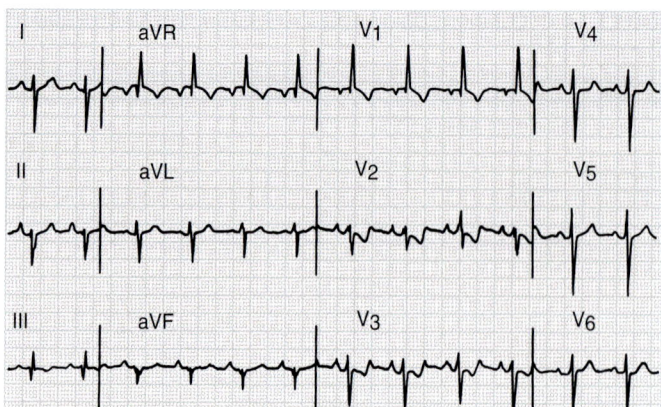

FIGURE 14.17 Right ventricular hypertrophy pattern most consistent with severe pressure overload of the right ventricle. Findings include (1) a tall R wave in V_1 (as part of the qR complex), (2) right axis deviation, (3) ST-segment depression and T wave inversion in V_1 through V_3, (4) delayed precordial transition zone (rS in V_6), (5) right atrial abnormality, and (6) an $S_1Q_3T_3$ pattern.

TABLE 14.5 Common Diagnostic Criteria for Right Ventricular Hypertrophy

Tall R in V_1 > 0.6 mV
Increased R/S in V_1 > 1
Deep S in V_5 > 1.0 mV
Deep S in V_6 > 0.3 mV
Tall R in aVR > 0.4 mV
Small S in V_1 < 0.2 mV
Small R in V_{5-6} < 0.3 mV
Reduced R/S ratio in V_5 < 0.75
Reduced R/S ratio in V_6 < 0.4
Reduced R/S in V_5 to R/S in V_1 < .04
$(R_1 + S_{III}) - (S_1 + R_{III}) < 1.5$ mV
Max R_{V1-2} + Max $S_{I,\,aVL} - S_{V1} > 0.6$ mV
$RV_1 + S_{V5-6} > 1.05$ mV
R peak V_1 > 0.035 msec
QR in V_1 present

Data from Hancock EW, et al. Deal BJ, Mirvis DM, et al. Recommendations for the standardization and interpretation of the electrocardiogram. Part V. ECG changes associated with cardiac chamber hypertrophy. *J Am Coll Cardiol.* 2009;53:992–1002.

study, baseline LVH by Cornell criteria as well as higher absolute levels of Cornell voltage were associated with 29% to 98% increases in the risks of all-cause mortality, MI, coronary heart disease events, stroke, and heart failure during a 5-year follow-up.[23]

Studies have also documented the independent predictive value of LVH diagnoses by ECG and by imaging studies. For example, the risk of cardiovascular events in patients with LVH by ECG is independent of anatomic abnormalities on echocardiography.[24] Also, the risk of cardiovascular events in patients with ECG LVH is higher than in those without these findings, whether the findings represented a true- or false-positive finding based on anatomic measurements.[21] These reports and the common discrepancies between ECG and anatomic measures of LVH may relate to the different although overlapping pathophysiologic effects of hypertrophy described earlier, i.e., structural changes assessed by imaging and electrical dysfunction and remodeling assessed by the ECG.

The clinical significance of ST-T wave changes has been demonstrated in, for example, the MESA study.[25] The presence of ST-T strain patterns was associated with an increased risk of all-cause mortality, incidence of heart failure, MI, all cardiovascular disease events during the 10-year follow-up, with hazard ratios of 1.3 to 2.8. CMR imaging in this population demonstrated that the presence of these patterns is associated with the development of abnormal cardiac remodeling, concentric hypertrophy, and LV scarring.

In addition to these clinical impacts, the ECG changes of LVH may confound or obscure ECG changes of other common conditions. The widened and notched QRS complex may mimic intraventricular conduction defects, and the ST-T wave changes may suggest myocardial ischemia or infarction. Similarly, the ECG changes of other conditions such as left anterior fascicular block (LAFB), left bundle branch block (LBBB), and right bundle branch block (RBBB) may reduce the value of ECG criteria for LVH.

Right Ventricular Hypertrophy

Right ventricular hypertrophy (RVH) changes fundamental aspects of the QRS complex, whereas an enlarged LV produces predominantly quantitative changes in underlying normal waveforms. The abnormalities associated with moderate to severe concentric RVH most often include abnormally tall R waves in anteriorly and rightward-directed leads (e.g., leads aVR, V_1, and V_2), and abnormally deep S waves and small r waves in leftward-directed leads (e.g., I, aVL, and lateral precordial leads) (Fig. 14.17). The normal R wave progression in the precordial leads is reversed, the frontal plane QRS axis is shifted to the right, and S waves in leads I, II, and III are common (the $S_I S_{II} S_{III}$ pattern).

Less severe hypertrophy, especially when limited to the outflow tract of the RV that is activated late during the QRS complex, produces less marked changes. Abnormalities may be limited to an rSr′ pattern in V_1 and persistence of s (or S) waves in the left precordial leads. This pattern is typical of RV volume overload, such as produced by an atrial septal defect and may also be seen in persons without manifest cardiac abnormalities (see later).

Diagnostic Criteria
Commonly relied-on criteria for the ECG diagnosis of RVH are listed in Table 14.5. Right axis deviation is present in most cases of significant RVH, although it is not typically included as a diagnostic criterion. Other ECG findings that are supportive although not diagnostic of RVH include an RSR′ pattern in V_1 with a QRS duration longer than 120 msec; positive S/R ratio in leads I, II and III; an S_1Q_3 pattern; negative T waves in V_{1-3}; and evidence of RA abnormality.

Diagnostic Accuracy. Common criteria typically show low sensitivities and high specificities. In the MESA study comparing ECG and CMR diagnoses of RVH in subjects without cardiac disease and normal LV morphology, most criteria had sensitivities less than 10%.[1] Although specificities were high (85% to 99%), the low prevalence of RVH resulted in a post-test positive predictive value that was similar to the pre-test probability of having RVH. Higher sensitivities have been reported with congenital heart disease and in patients with pulmonary hypertension (see Chapters 82 and 88).

Several factors contribute to the limited accuracy of standard criteria. Because the magnitude of forces generated by the RV are much lower than those generated by the LV, RVH must be severe enough to overcome the masking effects of the LV forces to be manifest on the ECG. Also, most standard criteria were developed based on autopsy studies of patients with severe disease and, hence, may have limited applicability to other populations.

Mechanisms for the Electrocardiogram Abnormalities. As in LVH, RVH increases current fluxes between hypertrophied cells and increases the size of activation fronts moving through the enlarged and thickened RV to produce higher-than-normal voltages on the body surface. In addition, the activation time of the RV is prolonged. RV activation now ends after activation of the LV is completed. As a result, cancellation of RV forces by the more powerful LV forces is reduced, so that RV forces become manifest late in the QRS complex (e.g., generation of S waves in left precordial leads). Because the RV is located anteriorly and to the right of the LV, these changes are most prominent in leads directed anteriorly and to the right, that is, in the right precordial leads.

CMR imaging has also suggested that RV enlargement may cause changes in cardiac anatomy. The RV may be shifted in a clockwise direction so that it lies under more leftward precordial electrodes than normal. Hence, leads V_4 to V_6 are more affected by RV forces than normal to show delayed transition zones with lateral S waves.[26]

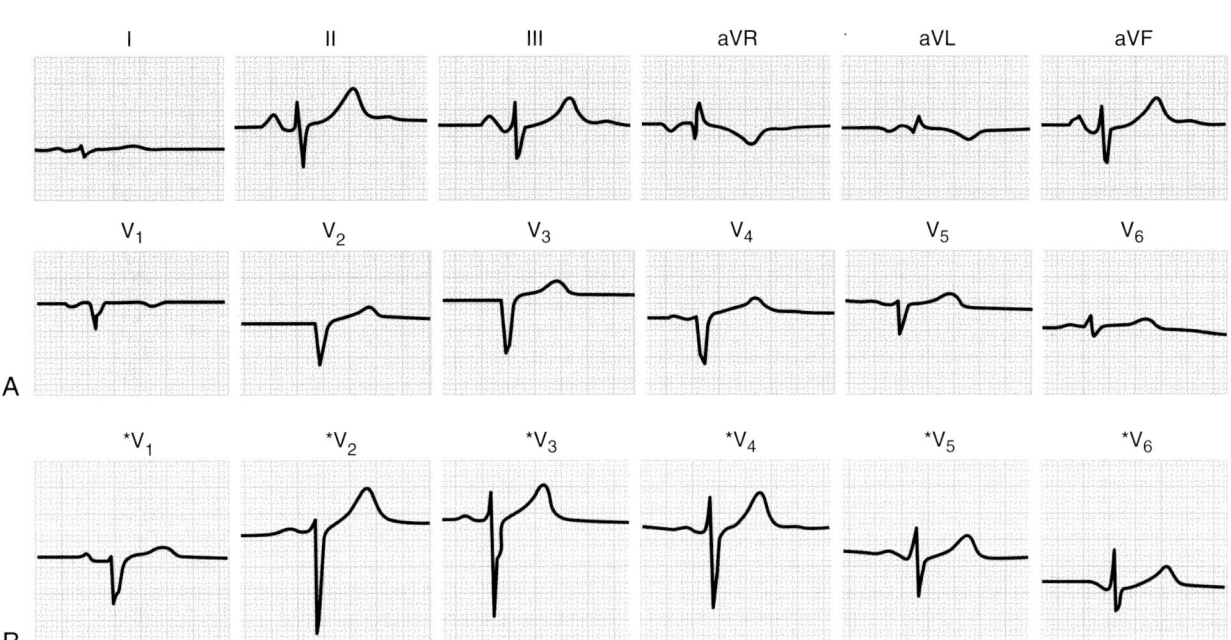

FIGURE 14.18 Pulmonary emphysema simulating anterior infarction in a 58-year-old man with no clinical evidence of coronary artery disease. **A,** Loss of anterior R waves in the precordial leads. **B,** Relative normalization of R wave progression with placement of the chest leads an interspace below their usual position (e.g., *V_1, *V_2). (Modified from Chou TC. Pseudo-infarction (noninfarction Q waves). In: Fisch C, ed. *Complex Electrocardiography.* Vol. 1. Philadelphia: FA Davis; 1973.)

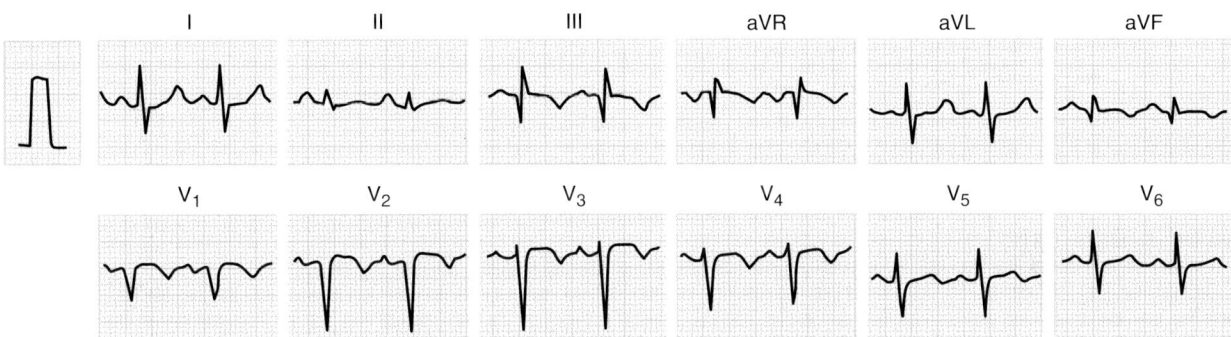

FIGURE 14.19 Acute cor pulmonale secondary to acute pulmonary embolism simulating inferior and anterior infarction. This tracing shows an $S_1Q_3T_3$ pattern, a QS in lead V_1 with slow R wave progression in the right precordial leads (clockwise rotation pattern), and right precordial to midprecordial ST elevation and T wave inversion (V_1 to V_4). (From Goldberger AL, Goldberger ZD, Shvilkin A. *Goldberger's Clinical Electrocardiography: A Simplified Approach.* 9th ed. Philadelphia: Elsevier; 2017.)

Clinical Significance

The prevalence of ECG-diagnosed RVH varies widely based on the criteria that are used. An analysis of 7857 patients in the third NHANES trial using 16 different criteria, the prevalence of diagnosed RVH varied from 0.9% to 20.7%.[27] A positive ECG diagnosis was associated with a significant increase in all-cause mortality with most criteria; mortality during the 14-year follow-up increased by 6% with each additional ECG criterion that was met.

Chronic obstructive pulmonary disease (see Chapter 88) can induce ECG changes by producing anatomic RVH, by changing the position of the heart within the chest, and by hyperinflation of the lungs (Fig. 14.18). The insulating and positional changes produced by pulmonary hyperinflation lead to reduced amplitude of the QRS complex, right axis deviation of both the P wave and QRS complex in the frontal plane, and delayed transition in the precordial leads. Evidence of true anatomic RVH includes right axis deviation, deep S waves in the lateral precordial leads, and an $S_1Q_3T_3$ pattern, with an S wave in lead I (as an RS or rS complex), an abnormal Q wave in lead III, and an inverted T wave in the inferior leads.

Pulmonary embolism causing acute RV pressure overload may generate characteristic ECG patterns (Fig. 14.19) (see Chapter 87). These include a QR or qR pattern in the right sided leads, an $S_1Q_3T_3$ pattern, ST-segment deviation and T wave inversions in leads V_1 to V_3, and incomplete or complete RBBB. Massive embolization may also cause ST-segment elevation in the right to midprecordial leads, complete RBBB, and T wave inversions in leads V_1 to V_4. In one series, the presence of the $S_1Q_3T_3$ pattern was associated with an odds ratio (OR) of 2.5 for adverse events.[28] However, the sensitivity of these findings for detecting RV dysfunction is low even with major pulmonary artery obstruction.

Biventricular Hypertrophy

Hypertrophy of both ventricles produces complex ECG patterns. In contrast to biatrial abnormality or enlargement, the result is not the simple sum of the two sets of abnormalities. The effects of enlargement of one chamber may cancel the effects of enlargement of the other. The greater LV forces generated in LVH increase the degree of RVH needed to overcome the dominance of the LV, and the anterior forces produced by RVH may cancel the enhanced posterior forces generated by LVH.

Because of these factors, specific ECG criteria for either RVH or LVH are seldom observed with biventricular enlargement. Rather, ECG patterns usually are a modification of the features of LVH, and include tall R waves in the right and left precordial leads, or evidence of LVH along with right axis deviation, deep S waves in the left precordial leads, or a shift in the precordial transition zone to the left (Fig. 14.20).

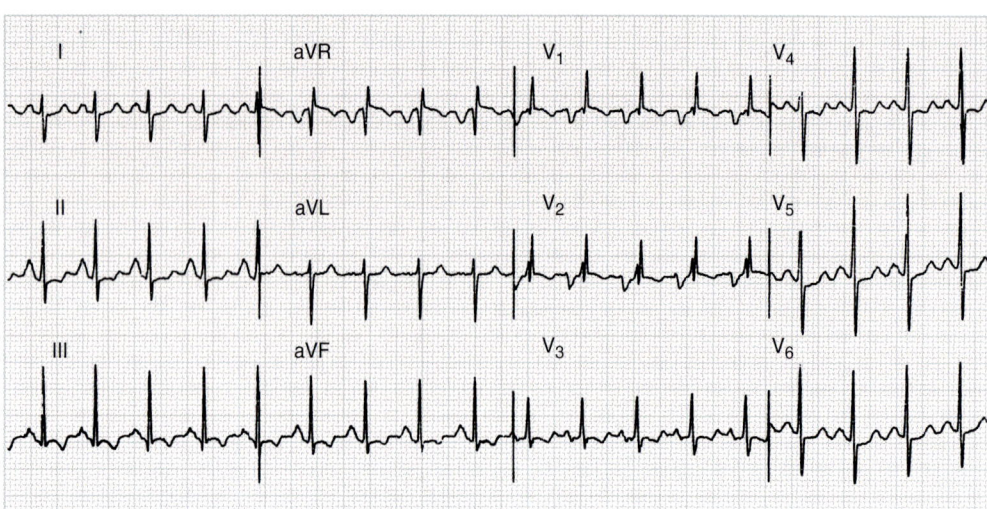

FIGURE 14.20 ECG from a 45-year-old woman with severe mitral stenosis showing right axis deviation and a tall R wave in lead V_1 consistent with right ventricular hypertrophy (RVH). The biphasic P wave in lead V_1 indicates left atrial abnormality and the tall P waves in lead II suggest concomitant right atrial abnormality. Nonspecific ST-T changes and incomplete right bundle branch block also are present. The combination of RVH and marked left or biatrial abnormality is highly suggestive of mitral stenosis. (From Goldberger AL, Goldberger ZD, Shvilkin A. *Goldberger's Clinical Electrocardiography: A Simplified Approach.* 9th ed. Philadelphia: Elsevier; 2017.)

Intraventricular Conduction Delays

Intraventricular conduction delays (IVCDs) may result from structural or functional abnormalities in the specialized conducting tissues of the LBB system, in the RBB system, or in cardiac muscle (see Chapters 65, 67, and 68). The hallmark of these disorders is significant alteration in the activation pattern of the ventricles and, hence, in the QRS complex.

Fascicular Blocks

Conduction delays in one or more of the fascicles of the LBB system result in abnormal sequences of early LV activation leading to characteristic ECG patterns of *fascicular block*. Only modest delays in conduction in one fascicle relative to that in the others are enough to alter ventricular activation sequences sufficiently to produce characteristic ECG patterns.

Left Anterior Fascicular Block

Delays in conduction through the left anterior fascicle result in delayed activation of the uppermost portion of septum, the anterosuperior portion of LV, and the left anterior papillary muscle. This results in unbalanced inferior and posterior forces early during ventricular activation (activated by the normal left posterior fascicle) followed by unopposed anterosuperior forces later during the QRS complex (the region activated late).

The diagnostic features of LAFB are listed in Table 14.6 and illustrated in Figure 14.21.[1,29] The most characteristic finding is marked left axis deviation, with a shift of the mean frontal plane QRS axis to between −45 and −90 degrees. Lower degrees of left axis deviation, with axis shifts to between −30 and −45 degrees, may be the result of less severe conduction delay or other conditions such as LVH.

> The resulting QRS pattern in the inferior leads includes initial r waves (caused by early unopposed activation of the inferoposterior LV) followed by deep S waves (caused by unopposed late activation of the anterosuperior LV). Therefore, leads II, III, and aVF show rS patterns. Leads I and aVL may show exaggerated septal q waves followed by R waves (a qR pattern).
> Precordial leads typically show the pattern of a delayed transition zone that is produced by the late activation of the anterosuperior LV. Leads V_4 through V_6 typically show deeper than normal S waves. The overall QRS duration is not prolonged; fascicular blocks alter the sequence but not the overall duration of LV activation.
> LAFB may mask or mimic ECG changes from other conditions. The larger R waves in leads I and aVL and smaller R waves but deeper S waves in leads V_5 and V_6 make LVH criteria relying on R wave amplitude less accurate. Changes that may mimic or obscure patterns of MI are discussed later.
> LAFB is common in persons without overt cardiac disease and in a variety of cardiac conditions, reflecting the delicate nature of the structure that lies in regions of turbulent blood flow near the LV outflow tract. Although generally considered to be a benign finding in the

TABLE 14.6 Common Diagnostic Criteria for Fascicular Blocks

Left Anterior Fascicular Block
Frontal plane mean QRS axis between −45 and −90 degrees
qR pattern in lead aVL
QRS duration <120 msec
Time to peak R wave in aVL ≥ 45 msec
Left Posterior Fascicular Block
Frontal plane mean QRS axis >90 degrees (or >110–120 degrees)
rS pattern in leads I and aVL with qR patterns in leads III and aVF
QRS duration <120 msec
Exclusion of other factors causing right axis deviation (e.g., normal variants, right ventricular overload patterns, lateral infarction)

Reference: Surawicz B, Childers R, Deal BJ, et al. AHA/ACCF/HRS Recommendations for the standardization and interpretation of the electrocardiogram. Part III. Intraventricular conduction disturbances. *J Am Coll Cardiol.* 2009;53:976–981.

absence of manifest cardiovascular disease, it has been associated with an increased mortality risk in patients with coronary artery or other cardiac disorders.

Left Posterior Fascicular Block

The ECG pattern of left posterior fascicular block (LPFB) is characterized by right axis deviation. Although this is traditionally defined as greater than +90 degrees, requiring an axis greater than +110 to 120 degrees may improve specificity. The QRS shows rS patterns in leads I and aVL, and qR complexes in the inferior leads (see Table 14.6 and Fig. 14.21). These changes are the result of early unopposed activation forces from the anterosuperior aspect of the LV (activated normally via the left anterior fascicle and producing the initial q and r waves) and late unopposed forces from the inferoposterior free wall (activated late via the left posterior fascicle and generating the late S and R waves). The QRS duration remains normal.

Damage to the left posterior fascicle of the LBB is less common than damage to the anterior branch because of its thicker structure and more protected location near the LV inflow tract. LPFB most often occurs with extensive cardiac disease and in association with RBBB; it is unusual in otherwise healthy persons. The specific diagnosis of LPFB, isolated or in combination with RBBB, requires first excluding other, more common causes of right axis deviation, e.g., normal variants (especially in young adults), RV overload syndromes, and extensive high or anterolateral infarction.

Other Forms of Fascicular Block

An estimated one-third of people have an anatomic third branch of the LBB system—the *left median* or *septal fascicle*—that arises most often

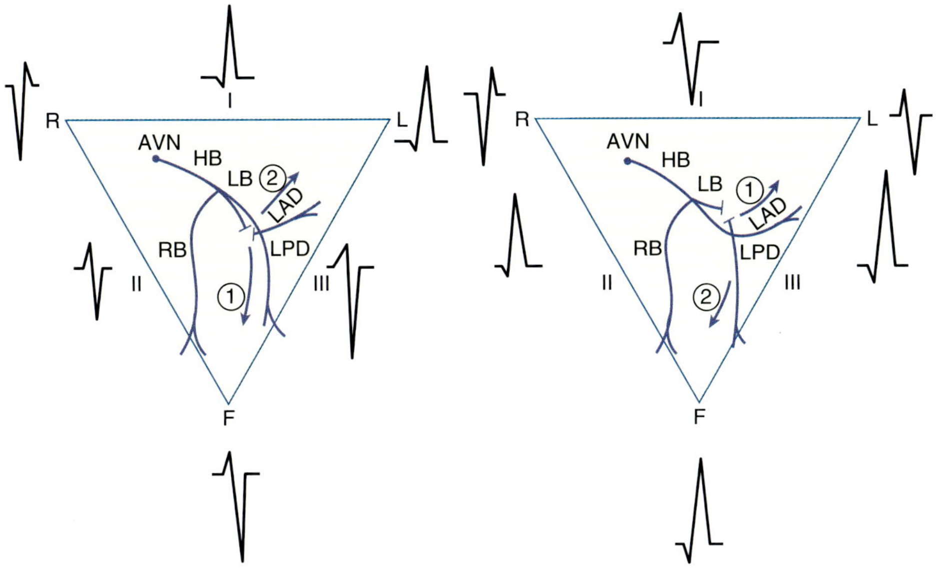

FIGURE 14.21 Diagrammatic representation of fascicular blocks in the left ventricle. **Left,** Interruption of the left anterior fascicle or division (here labeled *LAD*) results in an initial inferior (*1*) followed by a dominant superior (*2*) direction of activation. **Right,** Interruption of the left posterior fascicle or division (here labeled *LPD*) results in an initial superior (*1*) followed by a dominant inferior (*2*) direction of activation. *AVN,* Atrioventricular node; *HB,* His bundle; *LB,* left bundle; *RB,* right bundle. (Courtesy Dr. C. Fisch.)

from the left posterior fascicle and that contributes to initial left-to-right septal activation.[30] Conduction delay results in abnormal septal activation and the absence of septal q waves.

Left Bundle Branch Block

LBBB results from conduction delay or block in any of several sites in the left ventricular conduction system, including the fibers of the bundle of His that become the main LBB; the main LBB, in each of its two major fascicles; the distal conduction system of the LV, or in the ventricular myocardium. Recent mapping studies have suggested that the most common site of block may be within the bundle of His.[31] Simulation studies have also suggested that LBBB patterns may develop solely from disordered conduction within the ventricular walls even without disordered ventricular endocardial activation.[1]

Electrocardiogram Abnormalities

LBBB causes extensive reorganization of the activation and recovery patterns of the LV. The resulting ECG changes include a widened QRS complex with characteristic changes in its shape, as well as abnormalities of the ST-T wave. An example of the typical changes is shown in Figure 14.22 and the classical diagnostic criteria for LBBB are listed in Table 14.7.

Basic requirements include QRS duration of 120 msec or more; broad and, typically, notched R waves in leads I, aVL, and the left precordial leads; narrow r waves followed by broad and deep S waves in the right precordial leads; and, usually, the absence of septal q waves. The mean QRS axis may be normal, deviated to the left or, rarely, to the right.

Stricter criteria mandate a QRS duration of 140 msec or more and mid-QRS notching in left-facing leads.[1] These criteria may have better correlations with disordered endocardial activation patterns, abnormal LV mechanical function (see later), and greater benefit from resynchronization pacemaker therapy (see Chapters 58 and 69). Other criteria require a prolonged time to the peak of the R wave (≥60 msec) in the left precordial leads.

The ST segment and T wave are discordant with the QRS complex in most cases. The ST segments are depressed, and T waves are inverted in leads with positive QRS waves (e.g., leads I, aVL, V_5, and V_6). ST segments are elevated and T waves are typically upright in leads with predominantly negative QRS complexes (e.g., leads V_1 and V_2).

Incomplete LBBB (ILBBB) may result from lower degrees of conduction delay in the LBB system. Features include modest prolongation of the QRS complex (100 to 119 msec), slurring and notching of the upstroke of tall R waves, and delay in time to peak of the R wave in left precordial leads. Septal q waves may remain in many cases considered to have ILBBB. As many as one-third of patients with ILBBB develop full LBBB within 2 years.[32]

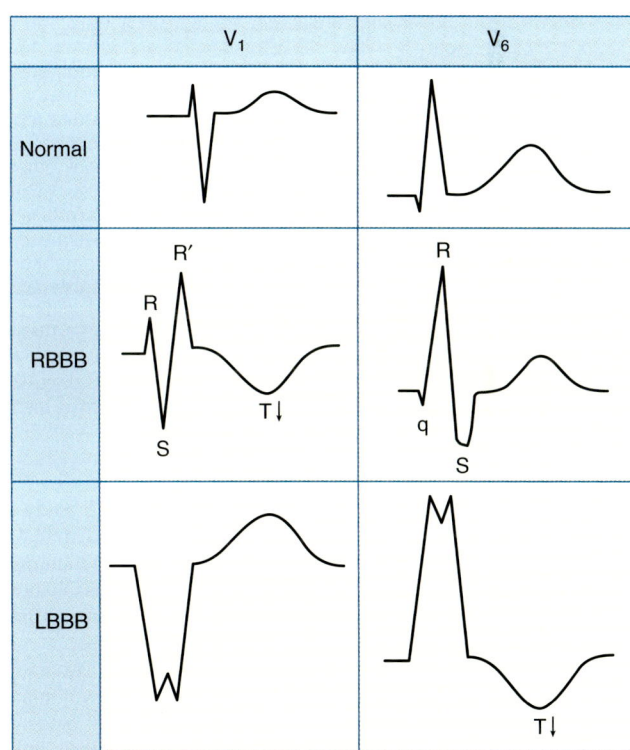

FIGURE 14.22 Comparison of typical QRS-T patterns in right bundle branch block (RBBB) (middle tracing) and left bundle branch block (LBBB) (bottom tracing) with the normal pattern (top tracing) in leads V_1 and V_6. Note the secondary T wave inversions (*arrows*) in leads with an rSR′ complex with RBBB and in leads with a wide R wave with LBBB. (From Goldberger AL, Goldberger ZD, Shvilkin A. *Goldberger's Clinical Electrocardiography: A Simplified Approach.* 9th ed. Philadelphia: Elsevier; 2017.)

Mechanisms for the Electrocardiogram Abnormalities. LBBB causes extensive reorganization of left ventricular activation. Septal activation typically begins on the right rather than on the left septal surface, leading to right-to-left (rather than normal left-to-right) activation of the septum. As a result, normal septal q waves are absent. A delay of as little as 6 msec is sufficient to produce abnormal septal activation.

In as many as one-third of cases, however, earliest septal activation occurs in the left midseptal region. This suggests initial activation of the left side of the septum by the LBB rather than by transseptal spread. In such cases, septal q waves may persist. This LBBB pattern may reflect damage to the distal LBB system, a well-developed and spared septal branch of the LBB system, or delays primarily within the ventricular myocardium.

TABLE 14.7 Common Diagnostic Criteria for Bundle Branch Blocks

Complete Left Bundle Branch Block*
QRS duration ≥120 msec
Broad, notched, or slurred R waves in leads I, aVL, V_5, and V_6
Small or absent initial r waves in leads V_1 and V_2 followed by deep S waves
Absent septal q waves in leads I, V_5, and V_6
Prolonged time to peak R wave (>60 msec) in V_5 and V_6
Complete Right Bundle Branch Block
QRS duration ≥120 msec
rsr′, rsR′, or rSR′, patterns in leads V_1 and V_2
S waves in leads I and V_6 ≥40 msec wide
Normal time to peak R wave in leads V_5 and V_6 but >50 msec in V_1

*See text for discussion of criteria.
Reference: Surawicz B, Childers R, Deal BJ, et al. AHA/ACCF/HRS Recommendations for the standardization and interpretation of the electrocardiogram. Part III. Intraventricular conduction disturbances. *J Am Coll Cardiol*. 53:976–981.

LV activation follows slow transseptal spread from the RV side of the septum and is delayed by 40 to 80 msec. The pattern of activation of the LV free wall is highly variable, depending on the type, location, and extent of the underlying cardiac disease. Spread is disrupted by regions of block, especially in patients with infarction and scarring, forcing activation wavefronts to maneuver around the block through slowly conducting myocardium. This results in a prolonged QRS complex with prominent notching and slurring. Overall activation may require more than 180 msec. In contrast, among persons with LBBB but otherwise normal hearts, activation may proceed rapidly and in a more orderly fashion.

The discordant ST-T wave pattern reflects the altered pattern of ventricular activation. With LBBB, the RV is activated and recovers earlier than the LV so that recovery currents are directed toward the right and away from the LV. Therefore, positive ST-T waves will be registered in leads over the RV that show S waves and negative ones are detected over the left sided leads showing prominent R waves. These ST-T wave changes are referred to *secondary ST-T abnormalities* because they are generated predominantly by abnormalities in conduction. As discussed later, ST-T wave changes produced by direct abnormalities of the recovery process are referred to as *primary ST-T abnormalities*.

Clinical Significance
LBBB is uncommon in the general population. In the ARIC study of over 14,000 persons free of heart disease, LBBB was observed in 0.5%.[33] However, it occurs more often in older persons and in more than one-third of patients with heart failure. As many as 70% of persons in whom LBBB develops have preceding ECG evidence of LVH, and fewer than 10% of patients have no clinically demonstrable heart disease.

In persons with or without overt heart disease, LBBB is associated with a higher-than-normal risk of mortality and morbidity from infarction, heart failure, and arrhythmias including high-grade AV block. In the ARIC study, LBBB was associated with a fourfold increase in coronary artery disease death during a 21-year follow-up.[33] In the LIFE study, among patients with hypertension, LBBB was also associated with a fourfold increase in the likelihood of developing wall motion abnormalities during 5 years of follow-up.[34]

Hemodynamic abnormalities reflect the direct effects of the abnormal ventricular activation pattern of LBBB, the ventricular remodeling that may occur with prolonged disordering of activation, and the abnormalities caused by the underlying heart disease.[35] Although normal LV contraction is highly synchronized, the contraction pattern with LBBB is less coordinated and prolonged. Early septal contraction occurs while the LV lateral wall has not yet been activated. The activated septum balloons into the LV cavity and the as yet to be activated lateral wall is stretched. Once the LV free wall is finally activated, the septum has relaxed and the LV contraction forces the septum to balloon into the RV. These forms of mechanical dysfunction can be demonstrated in approximately 60% of patients with LBBB and is more common in those with the longest QRS durations.

These abnormalities reduce the contribution of the septum and of the free wall to stroke volume by approximately 10%, increase end diastolic volume by approximately 15%, reduce cardiac efficiency, and increase myocardial work. Over time, these anomalous activation patterns likely contribute to structural remodeling, which when associated with hypertrophy of the lateral wall and thinning of the septum may cause or worsen mitral regurgitation. Such perturbations serve as a basis for resynchronization cardiac therapy (see Chapters 58 and 69).

Furthermore, the ECG changes of LBBB may obscure or simulate other ECG patterns. The diagnosis of LVH is complicated by the increased QRS amplitude intrinsic to LBBB, and the very high prevalence of anatomic LVH in patients with LBBB makes defining criteria with high specificity difficult. The diagnosis of MI may be obscured, as discussed in detail later. The impacts of the diffuse ST-T wave abnormalities related to altered activation patterns and changes in regional myocardial perfusion[1] due to disordered ventricular contraction also render unreliable the detection of ischemia on exercise ECG testing (see Chapter 15).

Right Bundle Branch Block
RBBB is a result of conduction delay in any portion of the right-sided intraventricular conduction system. The delay is most common in the distal branching portion of the bundle of His or in the main RBB; it may also occur in the more distal RV conduction system such as with damage to the RV moderator band after ventriculotomy.

Electrocardiogram Abnormalities
Major features of RBBB are illustrated in Figure 14.22, and common diagnostic criteria are listed in Table 14.7. As with LBBB, the QRS complex duration exceeds 120 msec. The right precordial leads show prominent and notched R waves with rsr′, rsR′, or rSR′ patterns, and leads I, aVL and the left precordial leads demonstrate S waves that are wider than the preceding R wave. The ST-T waves are discordant with the QRS complex; T waves are inverted in the right precordial leads and upright in the left precordial leads and in leads I and aVL. The mean QRS axis is not altered by RBBB; axis shifts can occur, however, as a result of the simultaneous occurrence of fascicular blocks along with RBBB (see later).

Incomplete RBBB may be produced by lesser delays in conduction in the RBB system or more distal damage to the RBB. It is characterized by an rSr′ pattern with a narrow r′ in lead V_1 and a QRS duration between 100 and 120 msec. These changes also may reflect underlying RVH (especially with a rightward QRS axis) without intrinsic dysfunction of the conduction system or may be a manifestation of the Brugada pattern (see Chapters 63 and 67). An rSr′ morphology in lead V_1 (and sometimes V_2) with a normal QRS duration is also a common finding in patients without cardiovascular disease, in association with pectus excavatum, and when the right precordial electrodes are placed too high in the chest.

Mechanisms for Electrocardiogram Abnormalities. With delay in the proximal RBB system, activation of the right side of the septum is initiated only after slow transseptal spread of activation from the left septal surface. The activation of the septum and RV anterior free wall are delayed, and is followed by slow activation of the remaining RV.

As a result, much or all of the RV is activated after depolarization of much of the LV has been completed. The late RV forces generated by the last areas of the RV to be activated—the right lateral wall and the outflow tract—are not cancelled by LV activation and generate increased anterior and rightward voltage observed in the latter half of the QRS in complete RBBB.

Abnormal slow and disordered LV activation patterns similar to those seen with LBBB, accompanied by LV mechanical dyssynchrony, also occurs in patients with RBBB.[1] This likely reflects the extent of the underlying cardiac disease and the associated conduction system dysfunction.

Discordant ST-T wave patterns are generated by the same mechanisms as for LBBB. With RBBB, recovery forces are directed away from the right and toward the earlier activated LV. The result is inverted T waves in the right precordial leads and positive ones in the left precordial leads.

Clinical Significance
RBBB is relatively common and is often detected as an incidental finding on routine testing. In the ARIC population-based study, RBBB was detected in 2.1% of enrollees.[33] The relatively high prevalence of RBBB

is attributable to the relative fragility of the RBB, as suggested by the development of RBBB after the minor trauma produced by right ventricular catheterization.

It is often found as an incidental finding in the absence of any demonstrable heart disease, may signal occult disease, or can develop in patients with any form of cardiovascular disorder. Although studies have reported variable effects of RBBB on prognosis, a meta-analysis of 19 studies including over 200,000 persons documented a small but significant increase in all-cause mortality (OR = 1.17) and an increase in cardiac death (OR = 1.43) in the general population.[36] Risks were similarly increased for patients with acute infarction, pulmonary embolism, and heart failure. Its frequent detection in athletes is discussed in Chapter 32.

RBBB, like LBBB, is associated with significant RV mechanical dysfunction, with higher RV end-systolic volumes and lower RV ejection fractions, especially in cases with R′ durations of over 100 msec.[37] This relation may reflect secondary damage to the RBB by mechanical stretch associated with marked RV dysfunction caused by the underlying condition. Alternatively, because of the delayed activation of the RV, peak RV contraction occurs significantly after that of the LV. These abnormalities may lead to mechanical dyssynchrony analogous to that seen with LBBB. In addition, as many as 40% of persons with RBBB (without LBBB) have abnormal LV mechanics.[38]

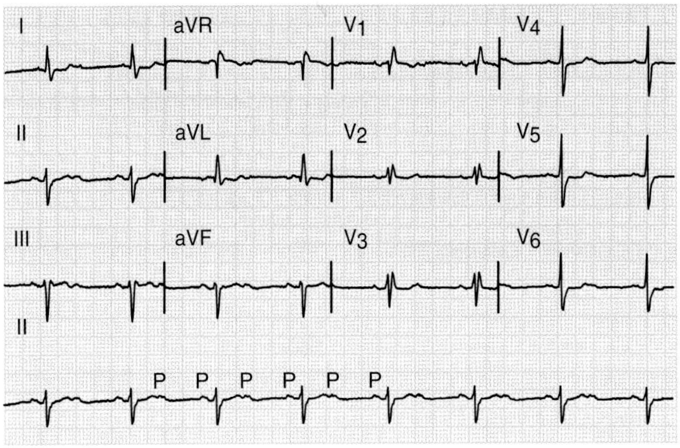

RBBB may also interfere with other ECG diagnoses. The diagnosis of RVH is more difficult to make with RBBB because of the accentuated positive potentials in lead V_1. RVH is suggested, although with limited accuracy, by the presence of an R wave in lead V_1 that exceeds 1.5 mV and a rightward shift of the mean QRS axis. An RBBB-like pattern with persistent ST-segment elevation in the right precordial leads may indicate the Brugada pattern, with susceptibility to ventricular tachyarrhythmias and sudden cardiac death (see Chapters 63 and 67).

The usual criteria for LVH have lower sensitivities than with normal conduction. RBBB reduces the amplitude of (or eliminates) the S wave in the right precordial leads and of the R waves in the left precordial leads, thus reducing the accuracy of ECG criteria for LVH. The combination of LAA or left axis deviation with RBBB does suggest underlying LVH.

FIGURE 14.23 Sinus rhythm at 95 beats/min with 2:1 atrioventricular block. Conducted ventricular beats show a pattern consistent with bifascicular block with delay or block in the right bundle and left anterior fascicle. The patient underwent pacemaker implantation for presumed infra-Hisian block.

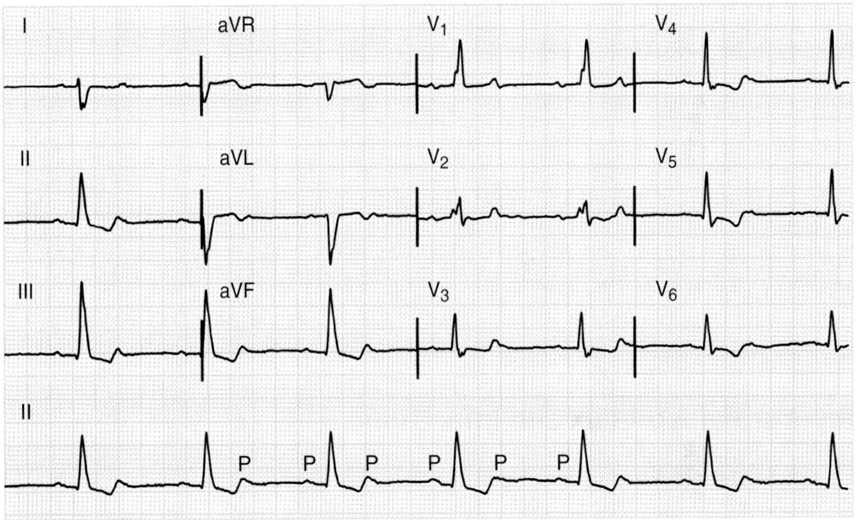

FIGURE 14.24 Sinus rhythm with 2:1 atrioventricular block. QRS morphology in the conducted beats is consistent with bifascicular block with delay or block in the right bundle and left posterior fascicle. Subsequently, complete heart block developed and the patient underwent pacemaker implantation.

Multifascicular Blocks

The term *multifascicular block* refers to conduction delay in more than one of the major structural components of the specialized conduction system. *Bifascicular block* involves delay or block in any two of these structures. It may have several forms depending on the sites of conduction delay. Delay in the RBBB and LAFB, the most common pattern, is characterized by a QRS pattern of RBBB plus left axis deviation beyond −45 degrees (Fig. 14.23). RBBB with LPFB produces a pattern of RBBB and a mean QRS axis deviation to the right of approximately +100 degrees (Fig. 14.24). LBBB alone, which may be caused by delay in both the anterior and the posterior fascicle, is also usually considered a form of bifascicular block even though the site or sites of delay are not known.

Trifascicular block involves conduction delay in the RBB plus delay in either the main LBB or in both the left anterior and the left posterior fascicle. The resulting ECG pattern depends on the relative degree of delay in the affected structures. If conduction delay exists in both the RBB and the main LBB and if the delay in the RBB is less than the delay in the LBB system, the QRS pattern will resemble that of LBBB. If the delay is greater in the RBB than in the LBB, the ECG pattern will be that of RBBB. Mixed patterns, for example, with LBBB patterns in the limb leads but RBBB patterns in the precordial leads, are also common.

A diagnosis of trifascicular block requires an ECG pattern of bifascicular block plus evidence of prolonged conduction *below* the AV node.

In bifascicular block, conduction time through the unaffected fascicle is normal and the net conduction time from the AV node to ventricular muscle is normal. In trifascicular block, however, the delay in conduction through even the least affected path is abnormally prolonged so that the minimal conduction time from the AV node to the ventricular myocardium (and the HV interval on intracardiac recordings) (see Chapter 62) also is prolonged. Only delay, not block, of conduction in at least one of the conduction pathways is required; if complete block were present in the RBB and in the LBB or in both of its fascicles, conduction would fail, and complete heart block would result.

On the surface ECG, the delay in conduction may or may not be manifested as a prolonged PR interval. The PR interval is mostly determined by the conduction time through the AV node, with a lesser contribution by the conduction time in the infranodal conduction system. Prolonged intraventricular conduction may be insufficient to extend the PR interval beyond normal limits, whereas a greatly prolonged PR interval most often reflects delay in the AV node rather than in all three intraventricular fascicles. Thus, the finding of a prolonged PR interval in the presence of an ECG pattern of bifascicular block is consistent with but is not diagnostic of trifascicular block; similarly, the presence of a normal PR interval does not exclude it.

In some cases, the path that has the longest delay can vary with the cycle length. In these cases, conduction patterns vary or alternate between two or more IVCD types to produce *alternating bundle branch block* (Fig. 14.25). This suggests severe conduction system disease and is associated with a high risk of progression to heart block.

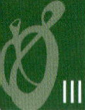

The major clinical implication of a multifascicular block is its relation to advanced conduction system as well as advanced underlying myocardial disease. It may identify patients at risk for heart block (see Fig. 14.23 and Chapter 68), although the incidence of progression appears to be low, especially with bifascicular block.[39]

Other Forms of Conduction Abnormalities

Rate-Dependent Conduction Blocks. Rate-dependent block usually occurs as a transient IVCD pattern (see Chapter 62). In *acceleration (tachycardia)-dependent block,* conduction delay occurs when the heart rate exceeds a critical value. This form of rate-related block is relatively common and can have the ECG pattern of RBBB or LBBB (Fig. 14.26). In *deceleration (bradycardia)-dependent block,* conduction delay occurs when the heart rate falls below a critical level. Deceleration-dependent block is less common than acceleration-dependent block and usually is seen only in patients with advanced conduction system disease (Fig. 14.27). The electrophysiologic bases for these patterns are discussed in Chapter 62.

Other mechanisms of ventricular aberration are discussed in Chapters 62 and 65, and Table 14.8 summarizes the major causes of a wide QRS occurring at physiologic heart rates. The more specific topic of wide complex tachycardias is discussed in Chapters 65 and 67.

Nonspecific Intraventricular Conduction Defects. This term is often used to refer to patterns with a widened QRS complex (110 to 130 msec) but without the specific pattern characteristic of RBBB or LBBB. It may represent any of a series of conditions including LBBB whose typical features are obscured by infarction, *intraventricular parietal block* (i.e., block in the distal conducting system beyond the bundle branches), or *peri-infarction block* (i.e., wide QRS complexes caused by delayed and disordered conduction around an area of infarction or scarring).[40] This term may also be applied to cases in which the limb leads have RBBB patterns but the precordial leads suggest LBBB, or vice versa.

Fragmentation of the QRS Complex. Fragmented QRS complexes represent disordered activation paths around or through areas of infarction, ischemia, or scar. They include patterns with a variety of RSR morphologies, notching in an R or S wave, or the presence of more than one r′ wave in the absence of typical LBBB or IRBB patterns. These deformities are common in patients with various cardiac disorders and are associated with an increased risk of mortality and complex arrhythmias.[41]

Myocardial Ischemia and Infarction

The ECG remains a key test for the diagnosis and management of acute and chronic coronary syndromes.[42–45] The waveform findings vary considerably depending on at least five major factors: (1) the duration of the ischemic process (acute versus evolving versus chronic), (2) its severity (ischemia with or without infarction), (3) its extent (size and degree of transmural involvement), (4) its topography (anterior versus inferior-posterior-lateral or right ventricular), and (5) the presence of other underlying abnormalities (e.g., prior infarction, LBBB, Wolff-Parkinson-White [WPW] syndrome, or pacemaker patterns) that can alter or mask the classic patterns. A critical clinical distinction is between *ST-segment elevation myocardial infarction* (or ischemia) (STEMI) and *non-STEMI infarction* (or ischemia) syndromes. With STEMI, an invasive approach aimed toward immediate reperfusion therapy with a percutaneous coronary intervention is the goal, unless contraindicated. With non-STEMI, urgent diagnostic angiography with revascularization, if feasible, is indicated by the presence of refractory angina, or hemodynamic or electrical instability (see Chapters 38 and 39).

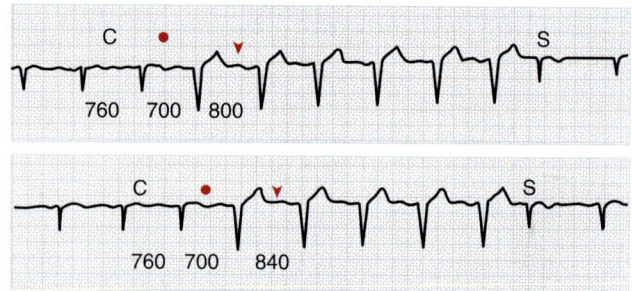

FIGURE 14.26 Acceleration-dependent QRS aberration with the persistence at a longer cycle length and normalization at a shorter cycle length than that initiating the aberration, indicating conduction hysteresis in the conduction system. The basic duration of the basic cycle (*C*) is 760 msec. LBBB appears at a cycle length of 700 msec (*dot*) and is perpetuated at cycle lengths (*arrowhead*) of 800 and 840 msec; conduction normalizes after a cycle length of 600 msec (*S*). (From Fisch C, Zipes DP, McHenry PL. Rate dependent aberrancy. *Circulation.* 1973;48:714.)

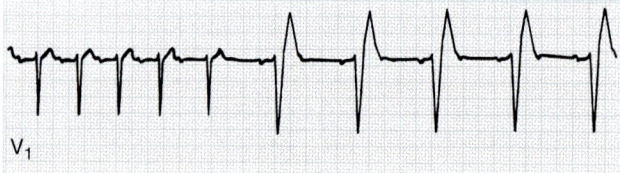

FIGURE 14.27 Deceleration-dependent aberration. The basic rhythm is sinus with a Wenckebach (type I) atrioventricular block. With 1:1 atrioventricular conduction, the QRS complexes are normal in duration; with a 2:1 atrioventricular block or after the longer pause of a Wenckebach sequence, left bundle branch block appears. (Courtesy Dr. C. Fisch.)

TABLE 14.8 Major Causes of a Wide QRS (at Physiologic Rates)

Chronic (intrinsic) intraventricular conduction delays or defects (IVCDs)
Right bundle branch block (RBBB)
Left bundle branch block (LBBB)
Nonspecific IVCDs
"Toxic" (extrinsic) conduction delays
Hyperkalemia
Drugs (especially those with class I activity)
Transient IVCDs
Rate related
Acceleration dependent
Deceleration dependent
Retrograde (transseptal) activation
Ashman type IVCD
Ventricular-originating complexes
Premature ventricular complexes (PVCs)
Ventricular escape beats
Ventricular paced beats
Ventricular preexcitation (WPW and related patterns)

WPW, Wolff-Parkinson-White syndrome.
For causes of wide-complex tachycardias, see Chapters 62 and 67.

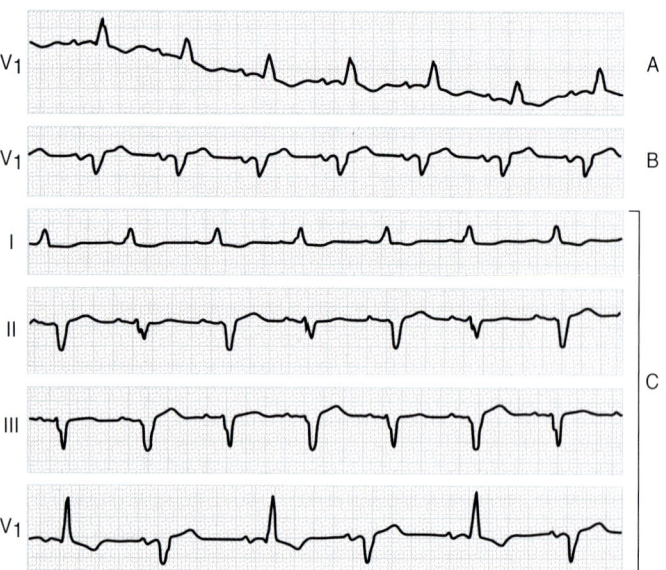

FIGURE 14.25 Multifascicular block manifested by alternating bundle branch blocks and PR intervals (sections *A–C*), recorded on separate days. *A,* Lead V$_1$ recording shows a right bundle branch block (RBBB) with a prolonged PR interval of 280 msec. *B,* Lead V$_1$ shows left bundle branch block (LBBB) with a PR of 180 msec. *C,* Leads I, II, III, and V$_1$ show alternating RBBB and LBBB patterns, along with PR alternation. The limb leads also show left anterior fascicular block (with subtle alternation of the QRS morphology). (From Fisch C. *Electrocardiography of Arrhythmias.* Philadelphia: Lea & Febiger; 1990.)

Repolarization (ST-T Wave) Abnormalities

The earliest and most consistent ECG findings during acute severe ischemia/ischemia are deviation of the ST segment occurring as a result of complicated current of injury mechanisms (see Chapter 38). Repolarization changes, including ST elevations, often precede elevation of cardiac serum biomarkers, and, therefore, the ECG plays an essential role in the emergency management of acute coronary syndromes (see Chapter 38).

Under normal conditions, the ST segment usually is nearly isoelectric, because almost all healthy myocardial cells attain approximately the same potential during the plateau phase of the ventricular action potential. Ischemia, however, produces complex time-dependent effects on the electrical properties of myocardial cells. Severe acute ischemia can reduce the resting membrane potential, shorten the duration of the action potential, and decrease the rate of rise and amplitude of phase 0 in the ischemic area (Fig. 14.28). The key concept is that these perturbations cause a *voltage gradient* between normal and ischemic zones that leads to current flow between these regions. The resulting *injury currents* are represented on the surface ECG as deviations of the ST segment.

The precise electrophysiologic mechanisms underlying injury currents and their directionality with ischemia and related conditions remain an area of active research and some controversy even after decades of study. Both "diastolic" and "systolic" injury currents have been proposed, based primarily on animal studies, to explain ischemic ST-segment elevations (Fig. 14.29). According to the "diastolic current of injury" hypothesis, ischemic ST-segment elevation is attributable to negative (downward) displacement of the electrical diastolic baseline (the TQ segment of the ECG). Ischemic cells remain relatively depolarized, probably related importantly to potassium ion leakage, during phase 4 of the ventricular action potential (i.e., lower membrane resting potential; see Fig. 14.28), and depolarized muscle carries a negative extracellular charge relative to repolarized muscle. Therefore, during electrical diastole, current (the diastolic current of injury) will flow between the partly or completely depolarized ischemic myocardium and the neighboring, normally repolarized, uninjured myocardium. The injury current vector will be directed away from the more negative ischemic zone toward the more positive normal myocardium. As a result, leads overlying the ischemic zone will record a negative deflection during electrical diastole and produce depression of the TQ segment.

TQ-segment depression appears as ST-segment elevation, because the ECG recorders in clinical practice use AC-coupled amplifiers that automatically "compensate" or adjust for any negative baseline shift, including in the TQ segment. As a result of this electronic effect, the ST segment will be proportionately elevated. Therefore, according to the diastolic current of injury theory, ST-segment elevation represents an apparent shift. The true shift, observable only with DC-coupled ECG amplifiers, is the negative displacement of the TQ baseline.

Evidence also suggests that ischemic ST-segment elevations (and hyperacute T waves) may also be related to systolic injury currents. Three pathologic factors may make acutely ischemic myocardial cells relatively positive compared with normal cells in regard to their extracellular charge during electrical systole (QT interval): (1) abbreviation of action potential duration, (2) decreased action potential upstroke velocity, and (3) decreased action potential amplitude (see Fig. 14.28). The presence of one or more of these effects will establish a voltage gradient between normal and ischemic zones during the QT interval such that the current of injury vector will be directed toward the ischemic region. This systolic current of injury mechanism, also probably related in part to potassium leakage, will result in primary ST-segment elevation, sometimes with tall positive (*hyperacute*) T waves. However, inspection of the surface ECG, with either ST elevation or ST depression ischemia, cannot differentiate between the contributions of systolic and diastolic currents of injury.

When acute ischemia is transmural (or nearly so), the overall ST vector (whether caused by diastolic or systolic injury currents, or both) usually is shifted in the direction of the outer (epicardial) layers, and ST-segment elevation and sometimes tall, positive (hyperacute) T waves are recorded over the ischemic zone (Fig. 14.30). Reciprocal ST-segment depression commonly appears in leads reflecting the contralateral surface of the heart. Occasionally, the reciprocal changes can be more apparent than the primary ST-segment elevations, leading to diagnostic confusion.

When ischemia is confined primarily to the subendocardium (approximately the inner half of the ventricular wall), the overall ST vector

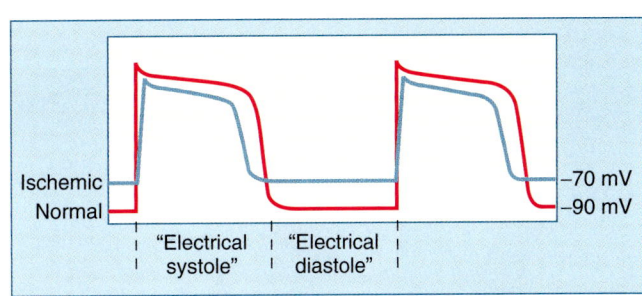

FIGURE 14.28 Acute ischemia may alter ventricular action potentials in a number of ways that result in lower resting membrane potential, decreased amplitude and velocity of phase 0, and an abbreviated action potential duration. These electrophysiologic effects, singly or in combination, create a voltage gradient between ischemic and normal cells during different phases of the cardiac electrical cycle. The resulting currents of injury are reflected on the surface ECG by deviation of the ST segment (see Fig. 14.29).

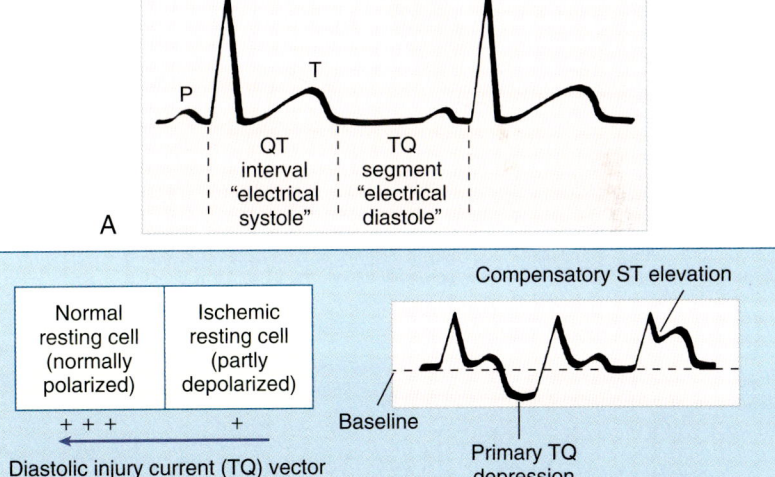

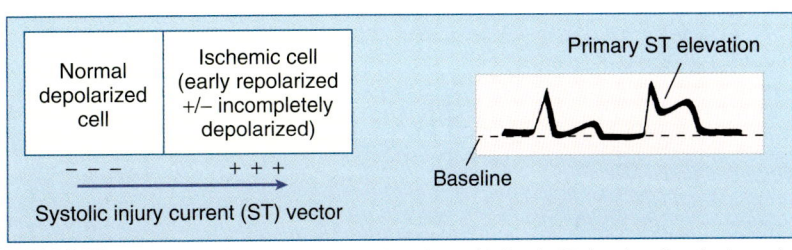

FIGURE 14.29 A simplified scheme of the pathophysiology of ischemic ST elevation. Two basic mechanisms have been advanced to explain the ST elevation seen with acute myocardial injury (**A**) based on currents of injury during ventricular electrical systole or diastole. **B,** Diastolic current of injury. In this case (first QRS-T complex), the ST vector will be directed away from the relatively negative, partly depolarized ischemic region during electrical diastole (TQ segment), and the result will be primary TQ depression. Conventional alternating current ECGs "compensate" for the baseline shift, and apparent ST-segment elevation (second QRS-T complex) results. **C,** Systolic current of injury. In this scenario, the ischemic zone will be relatively positive during electrical systole because the cells are repolarized early, and the amplitude and upstroke velocity of their action potentials may be decreased. This so-called systolic injury current vector will be oriented toward the electropositive zone, and the result will be primary ST-segment elevation. In clinical recordings, the contributions of diastolic and systolic injury currents to the observed ST-segment elevation cannot be determined (see text).

typically shifts toward the inner ventricular layer and the ventricular cavity such that the overlying (e.g., anterior precordial) leads show ST-segment depression, with ST-segment elevation in lead aVR (see Fig. 14.30). This subendocardial ischemia pattern is the typical finding during spontaneous episodes of angina pectoris or during symptomatic or asymptomatic (silent) ischemia induced by exercise or pharmacologic stress tests (see Chapter 15). Furthermore, associated alterations in myocardial conduction and action potential properties may contribute to the ST deviations observed on the ECG.[42]

Multiple factors can affect the amplitude of acute ischemic ST-segment deviations. Profound ST-segment elevation or depression in multiple leads usually indicates very severe or widespread ischemia. Conversely, prompt resolution of ST-segment elevation after reperfusion with percutaneous coronary interventions or thrombolytic therapy is a useful marker of successful reperfusion.

However, these relationships are not universal. Severe ischemia or even infarction can occur with slight or absent ST-T changes. Furthermore, a relative increase in T wave amplitude (hyperacute T waves) can accompany or precede ischemic ST-segment elevations with or without actual infarction (Fig. 14.31). Occasionally the ECG in acute coronary syndromes involving the occlusion of the left anterior descending (LAD) coronary will show a paradoxical combination of ST depressions and prominent T waves, especially in the precordial leads, sometimes now referred to as DeWinter's sign.[42] Finally, with evolving ischemia, ST-segment elevations usually become isoelectric, accompanied by T wave inversions. This evolutionary finding may lead to misclassification of an evolving ST-segment elevation MI as a non-ST elevation event.

QRS Changes

With actual infarction, depolarization (QRS) changes often accompany repolarization (ST-T) abnormalities (Fig. 14.32). Necrosis of sufficient myocardial tissue can lead to decreased R wave amplitude or frank Q waves (typically >30 to 40 msec in duration in multiple leads) a result of loss of electromotive forces in the infarcted area. Abnormal Q waves were once considered markers of transmural MI, whereas subendocardial (*nontransmural*) infarcts were thought not to produce Q waves. However, careful experimental and correlative studies based on necropsy and imaging findings have convincingly indicated that transmural infarcts can occur without Q waves and that subendocardial or other nontransmural infarcts can be associated with Q waves. Local conduction delays caused by acute ischemia also can contribute to Q wave pathogenesis in selected cases. Accordingly, evolving or chronic infarcts are more appropriately designated by ECG as *Q wave* or *non–Q wave*, rather than as "transmural" or "nontransmural."

The QRS findings may also be somewhat different with posterior or lateral infarction (Fig. 14.33). Loss of depolarization forces in these regions can reciprocally increase R wave amplitude in lead V_1 and sometimes V_2, occasionally without causing diagnostic Q waves in any of the conventional leads. The differential diagnosis for major causes of prominent right precordial R waves is presented in Table 14.9. In certain patients, fragmentation of the QRS complex, even without Q waves, may be a marker of myocardial scarring from ischemic or nonischemic causes.[41,44]

Evolution of Electrocardiogram Changes

Ischemic ST-segment elevation and hyperacute T wave changes may occur as the earliest ECG manifestations of STEMI. These are

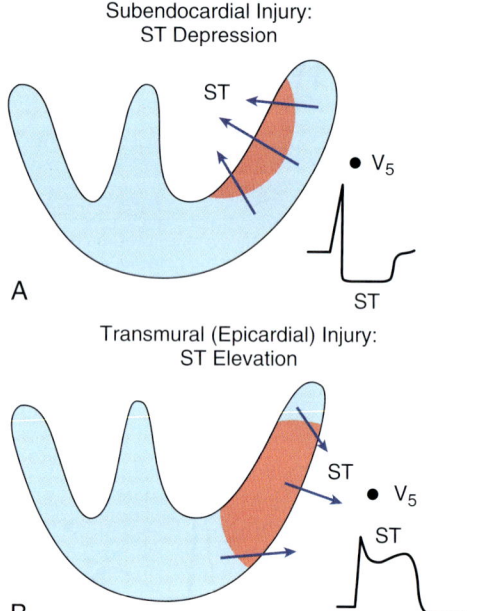

FIGURE 14.30 Directionality of current of injury patterns (ST vectors) with acute ischemia. **A,** With predominant subendocardial ischemia, the resultant ST vector is directed toward the inner layer of the affected ventricle and the ventricular cavity. Overlying leads therefore record ST depression, as may be seen during abnormal exercise stress tests or with spontaneous angina pectoris. **B,** With ischemia involving the outer ventricular layer (transmural or epicardial injury), the ST vector is directed outward. Overlying leads record ST-segment elevation.

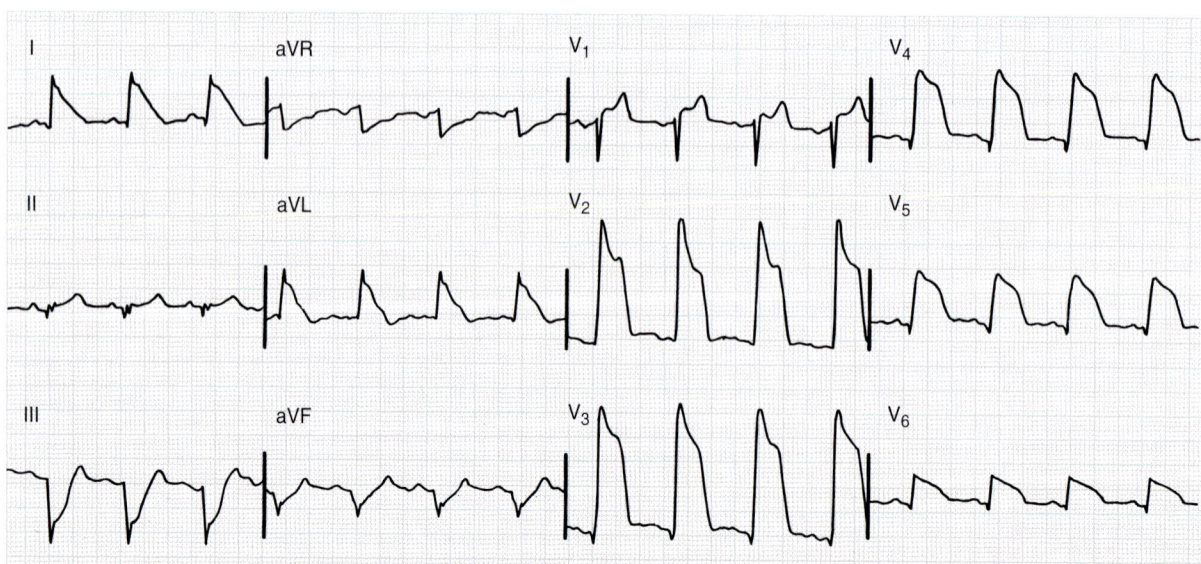

FIGURE 14.31 Hyperacute phase of extensive anterolateral myocardial infarction. Marked ST-segment elevation melding with prominent T waves is present across the precordium, as well as in leads I and aVL. ST-segment depression, consistent with a reciprocal change, is seen in leads III and aVF. Q waves are present in leads V_3 through V_6. Marked ST-segment elevations with tall T waves caused by severe ischemia are sometimes referred to as a *monophasic current of injury pattern*. A paradoxical increase in R wave amplitude (V_2 and V_3) may accompany this pattern. This tracing also shows left axis deviation with small or absent inferior R waves, possibly from a previous inferior infarct.

typically followed within hours to days by evolving T wave inversion and sometimes Q waves in the same lead distribution (see Fig. 14.32 and Chapter 38). T wave inversion from evolving or chronic ischemia correlates with increased ventricular action potential duration, and these ischemic changes are often associated with QT prolongation. The T wave inversions can resolve after days or weeks or may persist indefinitely.

In the days to weeks or longer after infarction, the QRS changes can persist or begin to resolve. Complete normalization of the ECG after Q wave infarction is uncommon but can occur, particularly with smaller infarcts, and is associated with subsequent improvement of the LV ejection fraction and regional wall motion. This development usually reflects spontaneous recanalization or good collateral circulation and is a positive prognostic sign. By contrast, persistent Q waves and ST-segment elevation seen several weeks or more after infarction correlate strongly with severe underlying wall motion disorders (akinetic or dyskinetic zone), although not necessarily a frank ventricular aneurysm. The presence of an rSr′ pattern or similar type of multiphasic complex in the mid-left chest leads or lead I is another reported marker of an LV aneurysm.[42]

Other Ischemic ST-T Patterns

Reversible transmural ischemia, such as that caused by coronary vasospasm, may result in transient ST-segment elevation (Fig. 14.34).[42] This pattern is the classic ECG marker of *Prinzmetal's variant (vasospastic) angina* (see Chapter 39). Depending on the severity and duration of such noninfarction ischemia, the ST-segment elevation either can resolve within minutes or can be followed by T wave inversions that can persist for hours or even days.

Some patients with ischemic chest pain exhibit deep coronary T wave inversions in multiple precordial leads (e.g., V_1 through V_4, I, and aVL), with or without cardiac biomarker level elevations. This finding typically is the result of severe ischemia associated with a high-grade stenosis in the proximal LAD coronary artery system (referred to as the LAD–T wave or *Wellens' pattern*).[42,45] These T wave inversions may be preceded by transient ST-segment elevations that resolve by the time

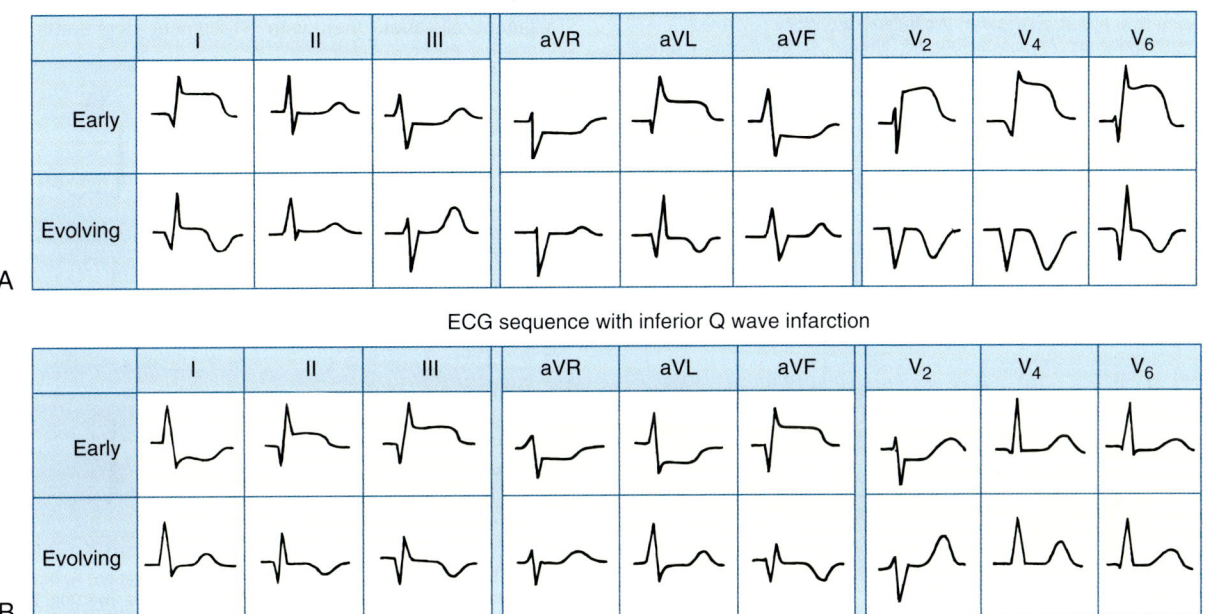

FIGURE 14.32 Sequence of depolarization and repolarization changes with acute anterior-lateral and inferior wall Q wave infarctions. **A,** With anterior-lateral infarcts, ST-segment elevation in leads I, aVL, and the precordial leads can be accompanied by reciprocal ST-segment depression in leads II, III, and aVF. **B,** Conversely, acute inferior (or posterior) infarcts can be associated with reciprocal ST-segment depression in leads V_1 to V_3. (From Goldberger AL, Goldberger ZD, Shvilkin A. *Goldberger's Clinical Electrocardiography: A Simplified Approach.* 9th ed. Philadelphia: Elsevier; 2017.)

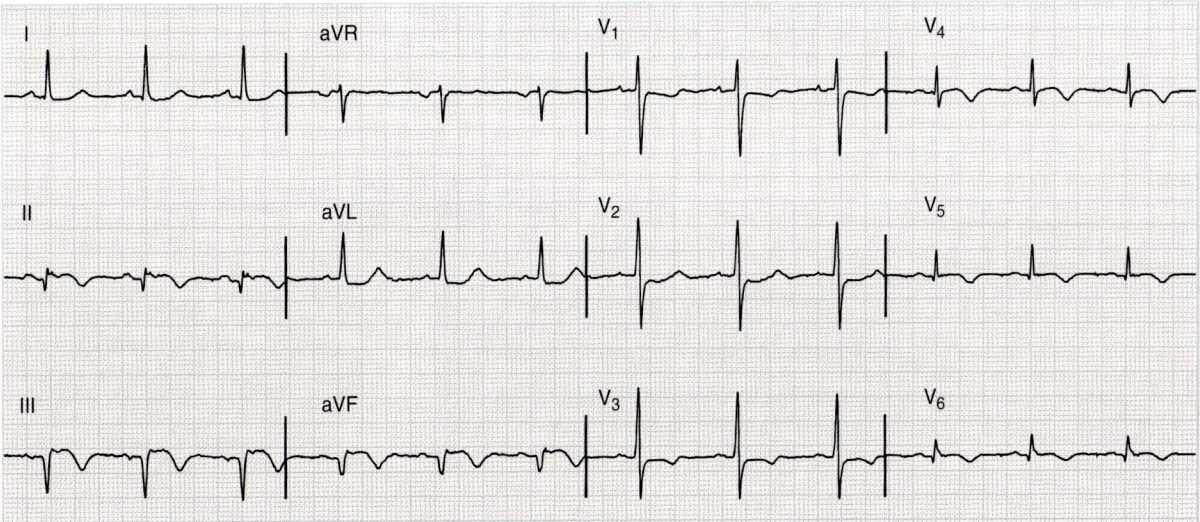

FIGURE 14.33 Evolving infero-posterolateral infarction. Note the prominent Q waves in II, III, and aVF, along with ST-segment elevation and T wave inversion in these leads, as well as V_3 through V_6. ST depression in I, aVL, V_1, and V_2 is consistent with a reciprocal change. Relatively tall R waves also are present in V_1 and V_2.

TABLE 14.9 Differential Diagnosis of Tall R Waves in Leads V_1 and V_2

Physiologic and Positional Factors
Misplacement of chest leads
Normal variants
Displacement of heart toward right side of chest (dextroversion), congenital or acquired
Myocardial Injury
Lateral or "true posterior" myocardial infarction
Duchenne muscular dystrophy (see Chapter 100)
Ventricular Enlargement
RVH (usually with right axis deviation)
Hypertrophic cardiomyopathy
Altered Ventricular Depolarization
Right ventricular conduction abnormalities
WPW patterns (caused by posterior or lateral wall preexcitation)

RVH, Right ventricular hypertrophy; *WPW,* Wolff-Parkinson-White syndrome.
Modified from Goldberger AL, Goldberger ZD, Shvilkin A. *Goldberger's Clinical Electrocardiography: A Simplified Approach.* 9th ed. Philadelphia: Elsevier; 2017.

the patient has their initial ECG. Furthermore, T wave inversions of this type, especially in the setting of an acute coronary syndrome, can correlate with segmental hypokinesis of the anterior wall and suggest a myocardial stunning syndrome (see Chapter 39). The natural history of this syndrome is unfavorable, with a high incidence of recurrent angina and MI.[42,45]

On the other hand, patients whose baseline ECG shows abnormal T wave inversion can experience paradoxical T wave normalization (*pseudonormalization*) during episodes of acute transmural ischemia (Fig. 14.35). In summary, there are four major classes of acute coronary artery syndromes in which myocardial ischemia is associated with distinct ECG findings, as shown in Figure 14.36.

Alterations in U wave amplitude or polarity have been reported with acute ischemia or infarction. For example, exercise-induced transient inversion of precordial U waves has been correlated with severe stenosis of the LAD coronary artery. Rarely, U wave inversion can be the earliest ECG sign of an acute coronary syndrome.

Electrocardiogram Localization of Myocardial Ischemia and Infarction

The ECG leads are more helpful in localizing regions associated with ST-segment elevation than with ST-segment depression. ST-segment

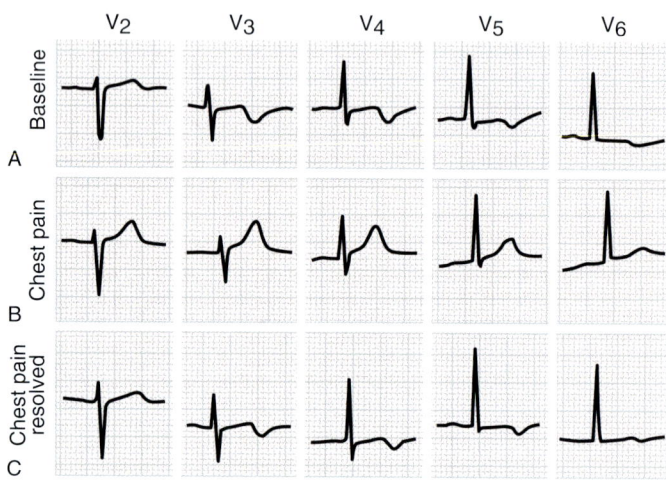

FIGURE 14.35 Pseudo- (paradoxical) T wave normalization. **A,** Baseline ECG of a patient with coronary artery disease shows ischemic T wave inversion. **B,** T wave "normalization" during an episode of ischemic chest pain. **C,** Following resolution of the chest pain, the T waves reverted to their baseline appearance. (From Goldberger AL. *Myocardial Infarction: Electrocardiographic Differential Diagnosis.* 4th ed. St Louis: Mosby–Year Book; 1991.)

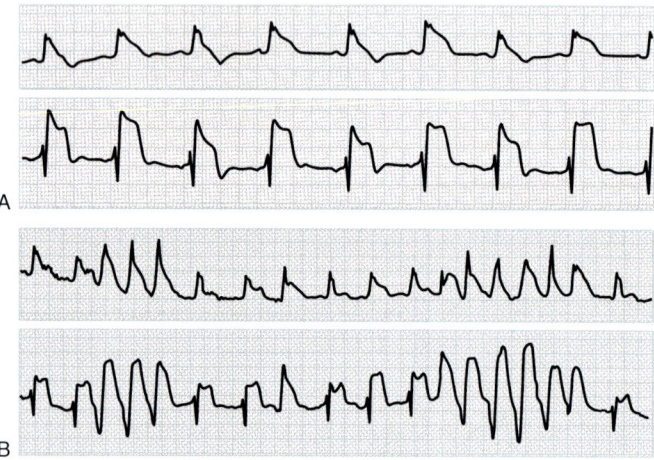

FIGURE 14.34 A, ECG tracing from a patient with Prinzmetal angina with ST-segment elevation and ST-T wave (repolarization) alternans. **B,** ECG shows ST segment elevation and T wave alternans associated with nonsustained ventricular tachycardia. (Courtesy Dr. C. Fisch.)

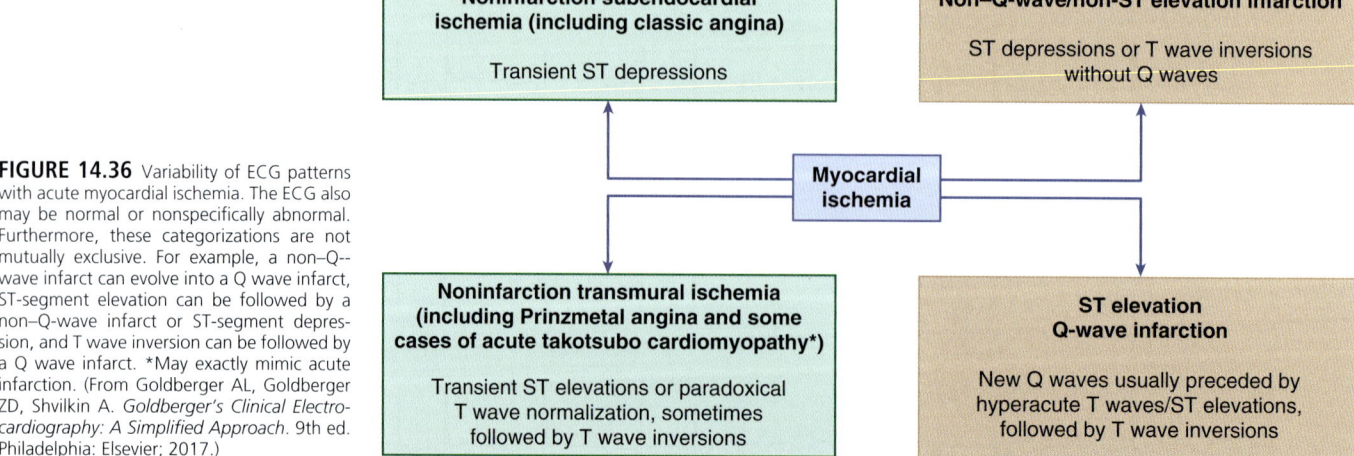

FIGURE 14.36 Variability of ECG patterns with acute myocardial ischemia. The ECG also may be normal or nonspecifically abnormal. Furthermore, these categorizations are not mutually exclusive. For example, a non–Q-wave infarct can evolve into a Q wave infarct, ST-segment elevation can be followed by a non–Q-wave infarct or ST-segment depression, and T wave inversion can be followed by a Q wave infarct. *May exactly mimic acute infarction. (From Goldberger AL, Goldberger ZD, Shvilkin A. *Goldberger's Clinical Electrocardiography: A Simplified Approach.* 9th ed. Philadelphia: Elsevier; 2017.)

elevation and hyperacute T waves are seen in the following: (1) two or more contiguous precordial leads (V_1 through V_6) and/or in leads I and aVL with acute transmural anterior or severe anterolateral wall ischemia; (2) leads V_1 to V_3 with anteroseptal or apical ischemia; (3) leads V_4 to V_6 with apical or lateral ischemia; (4) leads II, III, and aVF with inferior wall ischemia; and (5) right-sided precordial leads with RV ischemia.

In addition, posterior or posterolateral wall infarction can produce ST-segment elevation in leads placed over the back of the heart, such as leads V_7 to V_9 (see Table 14.1), associated with occlusion of the right coronary artery (RCA) or the left circumflex artery (LCA). Such blockages can produce both inferior and posterolateral injuries, which may be indirectly recognized by reciprocal ST-segment depression in leads V_1 to V_3. Similar ST changes also can be the primary ECG manifestation of anterior subendocardial ischemia.

The ECG also can also suggest more specific information about the location of an acute occlusion within the coronary system (the *culprit lesion*).[42] For example, with an acute inferior wall MI, ST-segment elevation in lead III exceeding that in lead II, particularly combined with ST-elevation in lead V_1 (and additional right-sided chest leads), is a reliable predictor of occlusion in the proximal to midportion of the RCA (Fig. 14.37). By contrast, the presence of ST-segment elevation in lead II equal to or exceeding that in lead III, especially in concert with ST-segment depressions in leads V_1 to V_3 or ST-segment elevation in leads I and aVL, suggests occlusion of the LCA or a distal occlusion of a dominant RCA.

Right-sided ST-segment elevation is indicative of acute RV injury and usually indicates occlusion of the proximal RCA. Of note is the finding that acute right ventricular infarction can project an injury current pattern in leads V_1 through V_3 or even V_4, thus simulating anterior infarction. In other cases, simultaneous ST-segment elevation in V_1 (V_2R) and ST-segment depression in V_2 (V_1R) can occur (see Fig. 14.37).

Lead aVR[46] may provide important clues to the location of artery occlusion in acute MI. Left main (or severe multivessel) coronary artery disease should be considered when leads aVR and V_1 show ST-segment elevation, especially in concert with diffuse prominent ST-segment depression in other leads.

Of note, current and future criteria to identifying the precise location of the culprit occlusion will always be subject to limitations and exceptions based on interindividual variations in coronary anatomy, the dynamic nature of acute ECG changes, the presence of multivessel involvement, collateral flow, and ventricular conduction delays. For example, in some cases, ischemia can affect more than one region of the myocardium, such as infero-posterolateral MI (see Fig. 14.33). In such cases, the ECG may show the characteristic features of involvement in each region. Sometimes, however, partial normalization can result from cancellation of opposing vectoral forces. Similarly, inferior lead ST-segment elevation accompanying acute anterior wall infarction suggests either occlusion of an LAD artery that extends onto the inferior wall of the LV (the "wraparound" vessel) or multivessel disease with jeopardized collaterals.

Clinicians should also be aware that ECG localization of the topography of infarction may not correspond to that observed with imaging studies. Distinctions between posterior, basal, and lateral regions may not map to an expected ECG designation. A noteworthy example is that the ECG label of acute anteroseptal infarction (based on changes in V_1 to V_3) may underestimate the extent of lateral or apical involvment.[42]

Electrocardiogram Diagnosis of Myocardial Infarction with Bundle Branch Blocks

The diagnosis of MI often is more difficult when the baseline ECG shows a bundle branch block pattern or when bundle branch block develops as a complication of the MI. The diagnosis of Q wave infarction usually is not impeded by the presence of RBBB, which affects primarily the terminal phase of ventricular depolarization (see earlier). The net effect is that the criteria for the diagnosis of a Q wave infarct in a patient with RBBB are the same as in patients with normal conduction (Fig. 14.38).

The diagnosis of infarction in the presence of LBBB is considerably more complicated and confusing, because LBBB alters the early and the late phases of ventricular depolarization and produces secondary ST-T changes. These changes may mask or mimic MI findings. As a result, considerable attention has been directed to the problem of diagnosing acute and chronic MI in patients with LBBB (Fig. 14.39).[47]

Infarction of the LV free (or lateral) wall ordinarily results in abnormal Q waves in the midprecordial to lateral precordial leads and in selected limb leads. However, the initial septal depolarization forces with LBBB are directed from right to left. These leftward forces produce an initial R wave in the midprecordial to lateral precordial leads, usually masking the loss of electrical potential (Q waves) caused by the MI. Therefore, acute or chronic LV free wall infarction by itself will not usually produce diagnostic Q waves in the presence of LBBB. Acute or chronic MI involving both the free wall and septum (or the septum itself) may produce abnormal Q waves (usually as part of QR-type complexes) in leads V_4 to V_6. These initial Q waves probably reflect posterior and superior forces from the spared basal portion of the septum (Fig. 14.40). Thus, a wide Q wave (>30 to 40 msec) in two or more of these leads is usually a reliable sign of underlying MI. The sequence of repolarization also is altered in LBBB, as described earlier,

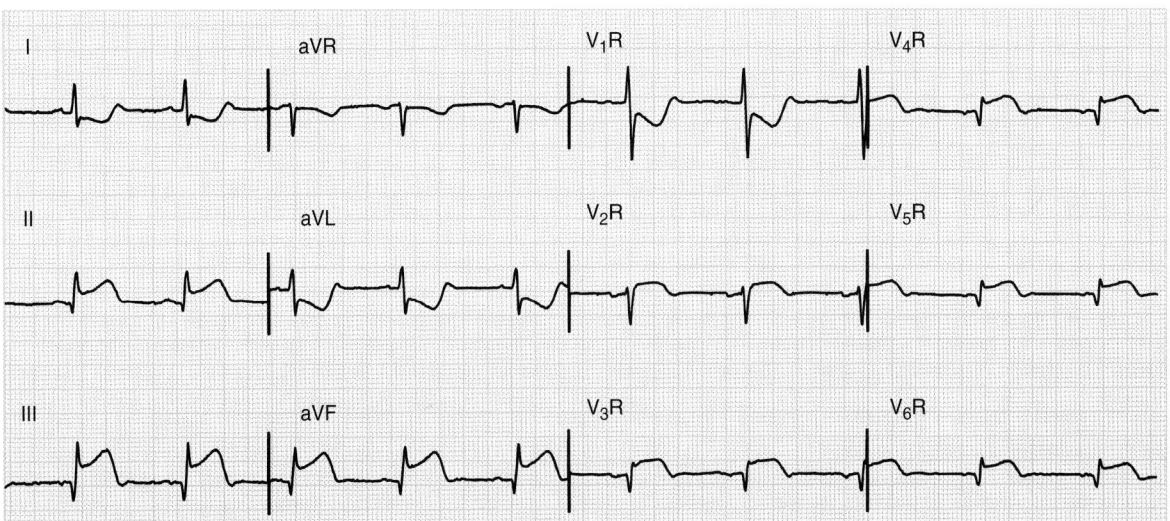

FIGURE 14.37 Acute right ventricular infarction in concert with an acute inferior wall ST-segment elevation infarction. Note the ST-segment elevation in the right precordial leads, as well as in leads II, III, and aVF, with reciprocal changes in leads I and aVL. ST-segment elevation in lead III greater than in lead II and right precordial ST-segment elevation are consistent with proximal to middle occlusion of the right coronary artery. The combination of ST-segment elevation in conventional lead V_1 (i.e., V_2R here) juxtaposed with ST-segment depression in lead V_2 (i.e., lead V_1R here) also has been reported with acute right ventricular ischemia or infarction.

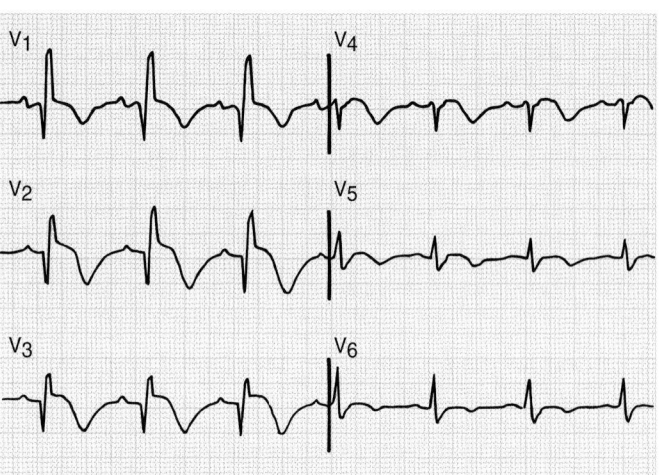

FIGURE 14.38 Right bundle branch block with acute anterior infarction. Loss of anterior depolarization forces results in QR-type complexes in the right precordial to midprecordial leads, with ST-segment elevations and evolving T wave inversions (V_1 through V_6).

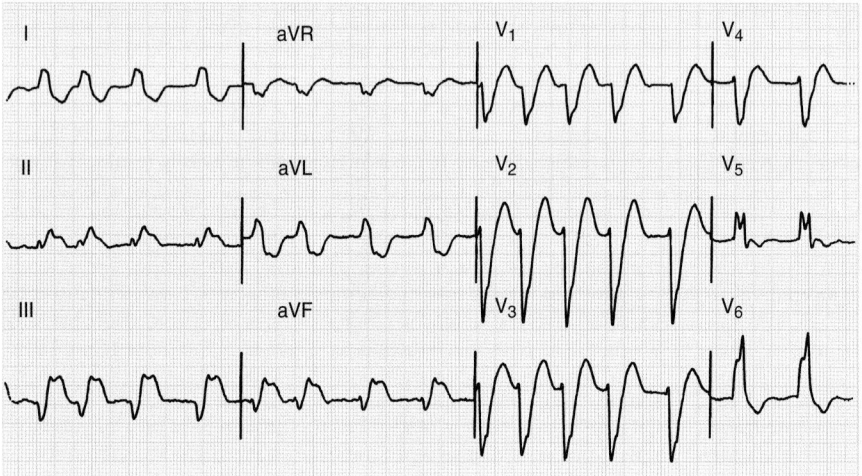

FIGURE 14.39 Complete left bundle branch block with acute inferior myocardial infarction. Note the prominent ST-segment elevation in leads II, III, and aVF, with reciprocal ST-segment depression in leads I and aVL superimposed on secondary ST-T changes. The underlying rhythm is atrial fibrillation.

and these changes can mask or simulate the ST-segment changes of actual ischemia.

The following points summarize the ECG signs of MI in LBBB:
1. ST-segment elevation with tall, positive T waves frequently is seen in the right precordial leads with uncomplicated LBBB. Secondary T wave inversions are characteristically seen in the lateral precordial leads. However, the appearance of ST-segment elevations in the lateral leads or ST-segment depressions or deep T wave inversions in leads V_1 to V_3 strongly suggests underlying ischemia. More marked ST-segment elevations (>0.5 mV) in leads with QS or rS waves also may be caused by acute ischemia, but false-positive findings occur, especially with large-amplitude negative QRS complexes. Use of the ratio of the *absolute amplitude* of the ST segment to S wave, determined in any relevant lead, of greater than 0.25 has been reported to have greater accuracy than that of the original Sgarbossa criterion.[47]
2. The presence of QR complexes in leads I, V_5, or V_6 or in II, III, and aVF with LBBB strongly suggests underlying MI.
3. Chronic MI also is suggested by notching of the ascending part of a wide S wave in the midprecordial leads or the ascending limb of a wide R wave in lead I, aVL, V_5, or V_6.

Similar principles can apply to the diagnosis of acute and chronic MI in the presence of RV pacing. Comparison between an ECG exhibiting the LBBB before the infarction and the present ECG often is helpful to show these changes.

The diagnosis of concomitant LAFB and inferior wall MI also can pose challenges. This combination can result in loss of the small r waves in the inferior leads, so leads II, III, and aVF show QS, not rS, complexes.

However, LAFB may also hide the diagnosis of inferior wall MI. The inferior orientation of the initial QRS forces caused by the fascicular block can mask inferior Q waves, with resultant rS complexes in leads II, III, and aVF. In other cases, the combination of LAFB and inferior wall MI will produce qrS complexes in the inferior limb leads, with the initial q wave the result of the infarct and the minuscule r wave the result of the fascicular block.

Atrial Infarction

A number of ECG clues to the diagnosis of atrial infarction have been suggested.[48,49] These include localized deviations of the PR segment, such as PR elevation in lead V_5 or V_6 or the inferior leads, changes in P wave morphology, and atrial arrhythmias. However, the sensitivity and specificity of these signs are limited.

Electrocardiogram Differential Diagnosis of Ischemia and Infarction

The ECG has important limitations in sensitivity and specificity in the diagnosis of coronary syndromes.[42] A normal or nondiagnostic ECG does not exclude ischemia or even acute infarction. If the initial ECG is not diagnostic, but the patient remains symptomatic, with a clinical picture strongly suggestive of acute ischemia, the ECG should be repeated at 15- to 30-minute intervals or shorter. However, a normal ECG throughout the course of an acute infarction is distinctly uncommon. As a result, prolonged chest pain without suggestive or diagnostic ECG changes on repeat ECGs should always prompt a careful search for noncoronary causes of chest pain (see Chapter 35).

Noninfarction Q Waves and Related Depolarization Changes

Q waves simulating the ECG pattern of coronary artery disease can be related to one (or a combination) of the following four factors[42] (Table 14.10): (1) physiologic or positional variants, (2) altered ventricular conduction, (3) ventricular enlargement/hypertrophy, and (4) myocardial damage or replacement. The latter category includes necrosis due to classic atherosclerotic coronary disease and nonatherosclerotic causes (see Chapter 52).

1. Prominent Q waves can be associated with a variety of positional factors that alter the orientation of the heart vis-à-vis a specific lead axis. Depending on the electrical axis, prominent Q waves (as part of QS- or QR-type complexes) can appear in the limb leads (aVL with a vertical axis and III and aVF with a horizontal axis). A QS complex can appear in lead V_1 as a normal variant but rarely in leads V_1 and V_2. Slow R wave progression, sometimes with actual QS waves, can be caused solely by improper placement of chest electrodes above their usual position. With dextrocardia (see Chapter 82), in the absence of underlying structural abnormalities, normal R wave progression can be restored by recording leads V_2 to V_6 on the right side of the chest (with lead V_1 placed in the V_2 position). A rightward mediastinal shift with left pneumothorax can contribute to the apparent loss of left precordial R waves. Other positional factors associated with slow R wave progression include pectus excavatum and congenitally corrected transposition of the great vessels.
2. An intrinsic change in the sequence of ventricular depolarization can lead to pathologic, noninfarct Q waves. The two most important conduction disturbances associated with pseudoinfarct Q waves are LBBB and the WPW preexcitation patterns (Chapter 65). With LBBB, QS complexes can appear in the right precordial to midprecordial leads and occasionally in leads II, III, and/or aVF. Depending on the location of the bypass tract, WPW preexcitation can mimic anteroseptal, lateral, or inferior-posterior infarction.

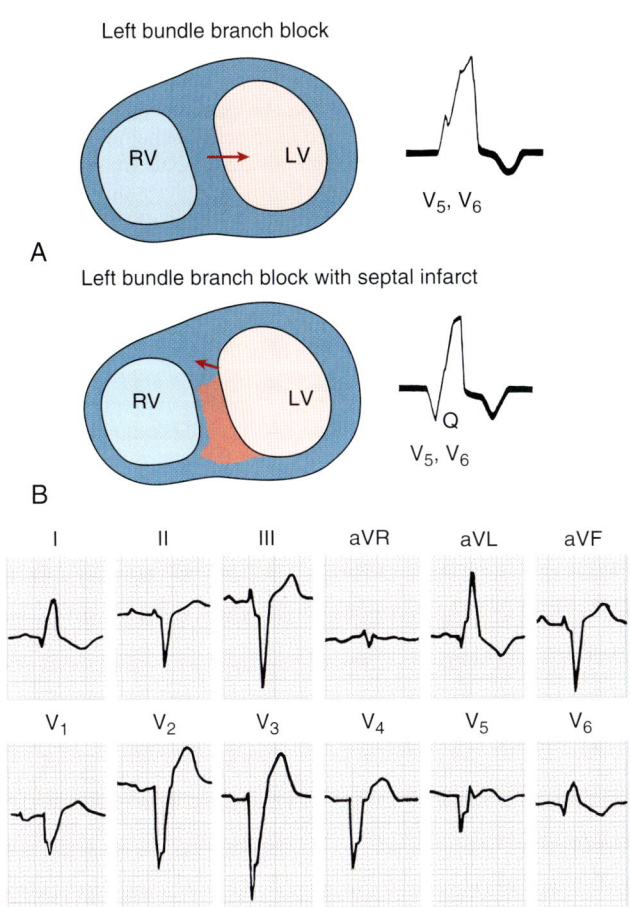

FIGURE 14.40 A, In uncomplicated (pure) left bundle branch block (LBBB), early septal forces are directed to the left (*arrow*). Therefore, no Q waves will be seen in V_5 and V_6 on the ECG tracing. **B,** With LBBB complicated by anteroseptal infarction, early septal forces can be directed posteriorly and rightward (*arrow*). Therefore, prominent Q waves may appear in leads V_5 and V_6 as a paradoxical marker of septal infarction. **C,** ECG from patient with anterior wall infarction (involving septum) with LBBB. Note the presence of QR complexes in leads I, aVL, V_5, and V_6. *LV,* Left ventricle; *RV,* right ventricle. (**A** and **B** modified from Dunn MI, Lipman BS. *Lipman-Massie Clinical Electrocardiography*. 8th ed. Chicago: Year Book; 1989.)

TABLE 14.10 Differential Diagnosis of Noninfarction Q Waves (With Select Examples)

Physiologic or Positional Factors
Normal variant "septal" Q waves
Normal variant Q waves in V_1–V_2, III, and aVF
Left pneumothorax or dextrocardia—loss of lateral R wave progression
Myocardial Injury or Infiltration
Acute processes—myocardial ischemia without infarction, takotsubo cardiomyopathy myocarditis, hyperkalemia (rare cause of transient Q waves)
Chronic myocardial processes—idiopathic cardiomyopathies, myocarditis, amyloid, tumor, sarcoid
Ventricular Hypertrophy or Enlargement
Left ventricular (slow R wave progression)*
Right ventricular (reversed R wave progression† or slow R wave progression, particularly with chronic obstructive lung disease)
Hypertrophic cardiomyopathy (can simulate anterior, inferior, posterior, or lateral infarcts
Conduction Abnormalities
LBBB (slow R wave progression*)
WPW patterns

LBBB, Left bundle branch block; *WPW,* Wolff-Parkinson-White syndrome.
*Small or absent R waves in the right precordial to midprecordial leads.
†Progressive decrease in R wave amplitude from V_1 to the midlateral precordial leads.
Modified from Goldberger AL, Goldberger ZD, Shvilkin A. *Goldberger's Clinical Electrocardiography: A Simplified Approach*. 9th ed. Philadelphia: Elsevier; 2017.

LAFB is sometimes cited as a cause of anteroseptal infarct patterns; however, LAFB usually has only minor effects on the QRS complex in horizontal plane leads. Probably the most common findings are relatively prominent S waves in leads V_5 and V_6. Slow R wave progression is not a consistent feature of LAFB, although minuscule q waves in leads V_1 to V_3 have been reported in this setting. These small (e.g., ≤20 msec duration) q waves can become more apparent if the leads are recorded one interspace above their usual position and disappear in leads that are one interspace below their usual position.

3. Slow ("poor") R wave progression is a nonspecific finding and is frequently observed with LVH, with acute or chronic RV overload (as well as in normal persons). Frank QS waves (e.g., in V_1 – V_2 /V_3) associated with ventricular overload syndromes (left, right, or biventricular) can reflect a variety of mechanisms, including a change in the balance of early ventricular depolarization forces, altered cardiac geometry and position, and electrode locations. A marked loss of R wave voltage, sometimes with frank Q waves from lead V_1 to the lateral chest leads, can be seen with severe chronic obstructive pulmonary disease (see Fig. 14.18). The presence of low limb voltage and signs of RA abnormality ("P pulmonale") can serve as additional diagnostic clues. This loss of R wave progression in part may be related to RV dilation and downward displacement of the heart in an emphysematous chest, as discussed earlier. Partial or complete normalization of R wave progression can be achieved in some of these cases by recording the chest leads an interspace lower than usual.

Other ventricular overload syndromes, acute or chronic, can also mimic ischemia and infarction. Acute cor pulmonale caused by pulmonary thromboembolism (see Chapter 87) can cause a variety of pseudoinfarct patterns. Acute RV overload in this setting can cause slow R wave progression and sometimes right precordial to midprecordial T wave inversion (sometimes still referred to as right ventricular "strain"), mimicking anterior ischemia or infarction. The classic $S_1Q_3T_3$ pattern can occur but, as noted, is neither sensitive nor specific. A prominent Q wave (usually as part of a QR complex) also can occur in lead aVF along with this pattern (see Fig. 14.19). However, acute right overload by itself does not cause a pathologic Q wave in lead II. Right-sided heart overload, acute or chronic, also may be associated with a QR complex in lead V_1, simulating anteroseptal infarction.

Pseudoinfarction patterns are also important findings in patients with hypertrophic cardiomyopathy (see Chapter 54), and the ECG changes can simulate those in anterior, inferior, posterior, or lateral infarction. The pathogenesis of depolarization abnormalities in this cardiomyopathy is not certain. Prominent inferolateral Q waves (leads II, III, aVF, and V_4 to V_6) and tall, right precordial R waves probably are related to increased depolarization forces generated by the markedly hypertrophied septum (Fig. 14.41). Abnormal septal depolarization also can contribute to bizarre QRS complexes.

4. Loss of electromotive force associated with myocardial necrosis contributes to R wave loss and Q wave formation in MI. This mechanism of Q wave pathogenesis, however, is not specific for coronary artery disease with infarction. Any process, acute or chronic, that causes sufficient loss of regional electromotive potential can result in Q waves. For example, replacement of myocardial tissue by electrically inert material such as amyloid, sarcoid, or tumor can cause noninfarction Q waves (see Chapters 52, 53, and 98). Q waves caused by myocardial injury, whether ischemic or nonischemic in origin, can appear transiently and do not necessarily signify irreversible heart muscle damage. Severe ischemia can cause regional loss of electromotive potential without actual cell death (*electrical stunning* phenomenon). Transient conduction disturbances also can cause alterations in ventricular activation and result in noninfarctional Q waves. In some cases, transient Q waves may represent unmasking of a previous Q wave infarct. New but transient

Q waves have been described in patients with severe hypotension from a variety of causes, as well as with tachyarrhythmias, acute myocarditis, Prinzmetal angina, protracted hypoglycemia, and hyperkalemia.[42]

ST-T Changes Simulating Ischemia and Infarction

The differential diagnosis of STEMI (or ischemia)[42] due to obstructive coronary disease encompasses a wide variety of clinical entities, including acute pericarditis (Fig. 14.42) (see Chapter 86), acute myocarditis (Chapter 55), normal variants (including classic "early repolarization" patterns, see Fig. 14.11), takotsubo (stress) cardiomyopathy, Brugada patterns (Chapters 63 and 67), and other conditions (Table 14.11). Acute pericarditis, unlike MI, typically induces diffuse ST-segment elevation, usually in most of the chest leads and also in leads I, aVL, II, and aVF. Reciprocal ST-segment depression is seen in lead aVR. An important clue to acute pericarditis, in addition to the diffuse nature of the ST-segment elevation, is the frequent presence of PR-segment elevation in aVR, with reciprocal PR-segment depression in other leads, caused by an atrial current of injury (see Fig. 14.42). Abnormal Q waves do not occur with acute pericarditis, and the ST-segment elevation may be followed by T wave inversion after a variable period. In addition, the J point in patients with pericarditis is typically sharp rather than slurred as in acute ischemic injury. Severe acute myocarditis can produce identical ECG patterns of acute myocardial infarction (AMI), including ST-segment elevations and Q waves. These findings can be associated with a rapidly progressive course and increased mortality. A fulminant myopericarditis-like syndrome has been reported with the COVID-19 infection, including ST elevations mimicking AMI.[50,51]

The novel SARS coronavirus may present diagnostic challenges to acute care clinicians (Chapter 94). Ischemic appearing ST-T changes may also be due to one or a combination of other pathogenetic mechanisms, including: classic "type 1" infarction precipitated by the infection (Chapter 37); takotsubo (stress) cardiomyopathy described later, Brugada pattern unmasked by fever (Chapter 63), coronary vascular injury (immune or infectious-mediated), acute right ventricular overload due to pneumonitis or pulmonary thromboembolic events (Chapter 87), and so forth.

Takotsubo cardiomyopathy (see Chapter 52), also called *transient left ventricular apical ballooning syndrome* or *stress cardiomyopathy*, is characterized by reversible wall motion abnormalities of the LV apex and midventricle.[52,53] Patients, usually postmenopausal women, may present with chest pain, ST-segment elevations, and elevated cardiac enzyme levels, mimicking AMI caused by obstructive coronary disease. The syndrome typically is reported in the setting of emotional or physiologic stress. Fixed epicardial coronary disease is absent. The exact pathophysiology is not known but may relate to coronary vasospasm or adrenergically mediated myocardial damage resulting in a variety of ST-T elevation (or

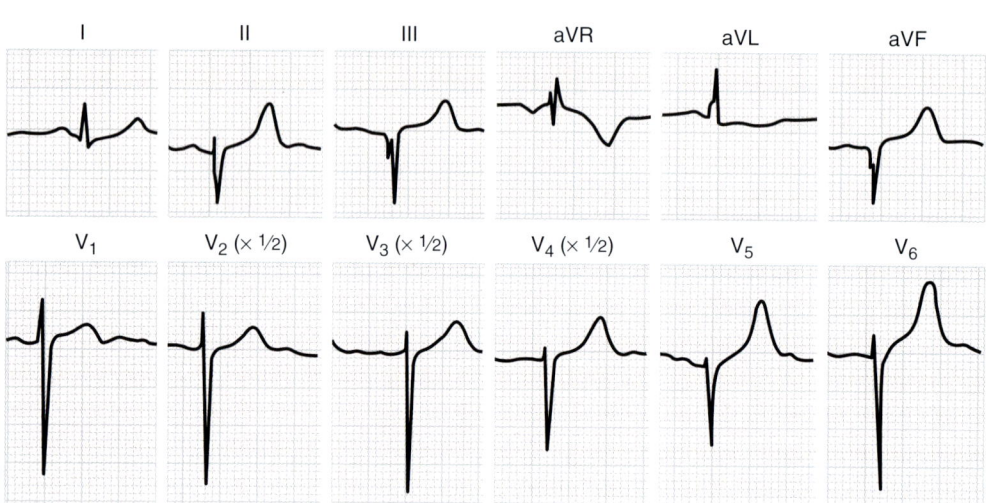

FIGURE 14.41 Hypertrophic cardiomyopathy simulating inferolateral infarction. This ECG was obtained in an 11-year-old girl who had a family history of hypertrophic cardiomyopathy. Note the W-shaped QS waves and the QRS complexes in the inferior and lateral precordial leads. (From Goldberger AL, Goldberger ZD, Shvilkin A. *Goldberger's Clinical Electrocardiography: A Simplified Approach*. 9th ed. Philadelphia: Elsevier; 2017.)

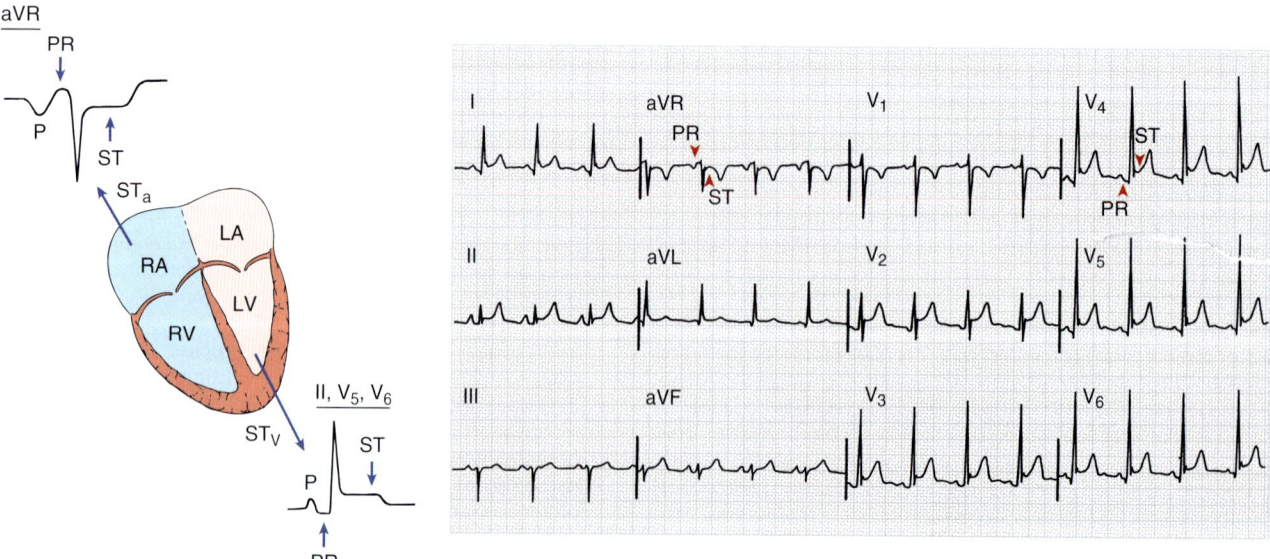

FIGURE 14.42 Acute pericarditis often is characterized by two apparent injury currents, one atrial and the other ventricular. The atrial injury current vector (ST$_a$) usually is directed upward and to the right (see diagram at *left*) and produces PR-segment elevation in aVR, with reciprocal PR depression in II, V$_5$, and V$_6$. The ventricular injury current (ST$_v$) is directed downward and to the left, associated with ST-segment elevation in leads II, V$_5$, and V$_6$. This characteristic PR-ST segment discordance is illustrated in the bottommost tracing. Note the diffuse distribution of ST-segment elevation in acute pericarditis (e.g., I, II, and V$_2$ through V$_6$, with reciprocal changes in aVR and perhaps minimally in V$_1$). *LA*, Left atrium; *LV*, left ventricle; *RA*, right atrium; *RV*, right ventricle. (From Goldberger AL. *Myocardial Infarction: Electrocardiographic Differential Diagnosis*. 4th ed. St Louis: Mosby–Year Book; 1991.)

depression) changes simulating coronary occlusion. Criteria for differentiating takotsubo syndrome from MI due to obstructive coronary disease have been proposed.[54]

A number of factors, such as digitalis, ventricular hypertrophy, hypokalemia, secondary ST-T changes, and hyperventilation, can cause *ST-segment depression* mimicking that in non–ST-segment elevation ischemic syndromes. Similarly, *tall positive T waves* do not invariably represent hyperacute ischemic changes but can reflect normal variants, hyperkalemia, cerebrovascular injury, and LV volume overloads resulting from mitral or aortic regurgitation (see Fig. 14.16), among other causes. ST-segment elevation, J point elevations, and tall positive T waves also are common chronic findings in leads V_1 and V_2 with LBBB or LVH patterns, which may simulate acute ischemia.

As noted, a variety of other factors, pathologic and sometimes physiologic, can alter repolarization, causing prominent T wave inversion, sometimes simulating ischemia or evolving MI. For example, prominent primary T wave inversions also are a well-described feature of the ECG in CVAs, particularly with subarachnoid hemorrhage. The so-called *cerebrovascular accident (CVA) T wave pattern* characteristically is seen in multiple leads, with a widely splayed appearance usually associated with marked QT prolongation (Fig. 14.43). Some studies have implicated structural damage (termed *myocytolysis*) in the hearts of patients with such T wave changes, probably induced by excessive sympathetic stimulation mediated through the hypothalamus. A role for concomitant vagal hyperactivation has also been postulated in the pathogenesis of such T wave changes, which usually are associated with bradycardia. In addition, the massive diffuse T wave inversion seen in some patients after Stokes-Adams syncope may be related to a similar neurocardiogenic mechanism. Patients with subarachnoid hemorrhage also can show transient ST-segment elevation, as well as arrhythmias including torsades de pointes. Ventricular dysfunction can even occur and may be related to takotsubo cardiomyopathy[52–54] or neurogenic stress–type syndromes (see Chapters 45 and 102).

In contrast to these primary ST-T wave abnormalities, secondary ST-T wave changes are caused by altered ventricular activation, without changes in action potential characteristics (discussed earlier). Examples include bundle branch block, WPW preexcitation, and ventricular ectopic or paced beats. In addition, transiently altered ventricular activation (associated with QRS interval prolongation) can induce T wave changes, which can persist for hours to days after normal ventricular depolarization has resumed. The term *cardiac memory T wave changes* has been used in this context to describe repolarization changes after depolarization changes caused by ventricular pacing, intermittent LBBB, intermittent WPW preexcitation, and other alterations of ventricular activation.[55,56] T wave inversions also may occur. The term *idiopathic global T wave inversion* has been applied in cases in which no identifiable cause for prominent diffuse repolarization abnormalities can be found. Some of these cases may represent unrecognized takotsubo cardiomyopathy.

When caused by physiologic variants, T wave inversion is sometimes mistaken for ischemia. T waves in the right precordial leads can be slightly inverted, particularly in leads V_1 and V_2. Some adults show persistence of the juvenile T wave pattern (see Fig. 14.10), with more prominent T wave inversion in right precordial to midprecordial leads showing an rS or RS morphology. Such patterns, especially associated with ventricular ectopy with LBBB-morphology or relevant family history, also raise strong consideration of *arrhythmogenic right ventricular cardiomyopathy* (formerly referred to as *dysplasia;* see Chapter 52).[57] The other major normal variant that can be associated with notable T wave inversion is the so-called benign *early repolarization pattern* (see Fig. 14.11). As described earlier, some persons, especially athletes, with this variant have prominent, biphasic T wave inversion in association with the ST-segment elevation. This pattern, which may simulate the initial stages of an evolving infarct, is most prevalent in young Black men and endurance athletes. These functional ST-T changes probably are the result of regional

TABLE 14.11 Differential Diagnosis of ST-Segment Elevation

Myocardial ischemia or infarction
Noninfarction, transmural ischemia (e.g., Prinzmetal angina pattern, takotsubo syndrome)
Acute myocardial infarction (caused by obstructive coronary occlusion or other causes)
Post–myocardial infarction (ventricular aneurysm pattern)
Acute pericarditis
Normal variants (including the classic "early repolarization" pattern)
LVH, LBBB (V_1, V_2 or V_3 only)
Other (rarer) causes
Acute pulmonary embolism (right to mid-chest leads)
Brugada pattern (RBBB-like pattern and ST-segment elevations in right precordial leads)*
Class IC antiarrhythmic drugs*
Hypercalcemia*
DC cardioversion (immediately after procedure)
Hyperkalemia*
Hypothermia (J or Osborn wave)
Intracranial hemorrhage
Myocardial injury (e.g., caused by trauma)
Myocarditis (may resemble myocardial infarction or pericarditis)
"Spiked-helmet" sign[†]
Tumor invading the left ventricle

DC, Direct current; *LVH*, left ventricular hypertrophy; *LBBB*, left bundle branch block; *RBBB*, right bundle branch block.
*Usually most apparent in leads V_1 to V_2.
[†]Crinion D, Abdollah H, Baranchuk A. An ominous ECG sign in critical care. *Circulation.* 2020;14:2106–2109.
Modified from Mirvis DM, Goldberger AL. Electrocardiography. In *Braunwald's Heart Disease,* 11th ed. Philadelphia: Elsevier;2019; and Goldberger AL, Goldberger ZD, Shvilkin A. *Goldberger's Clinical Electrocardiography: A Simplified Approach.* 9th ed. Philadelphia: Elsevier; 2017.

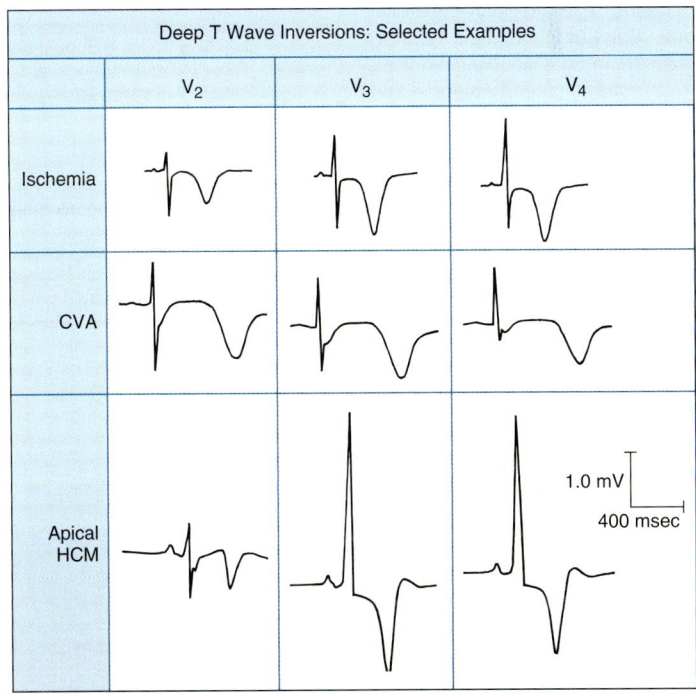

FIGURE 14.43 Deep T wave inversion can have various causes. In the *middle* tracing, note the marked QT prolongation in conjunction with the cerebrovascular accident (*CVA*) T wave pattern, caused here by subarachnoid hemorrhage. Apical hypertrophic cardiomyopathy (*HCM*), "memory T waves," and takotsubo syndrome are other causes of deep T wave inversion that can be mistaken for ischemia from acute/evolving or chronic obstructive coronary disease. (From Goldberger AL. Deep T wave inversions. *ACC Curr J Rev.* 1996;5:28–29.)

Drug Effects

Numerous drugs can affect the ECG and often are associated with nonspecific ST-T alterations.[1] More marked changes, as well as AV and intraventricular conduction disturbances, can occur with select agents (see Chapters 63 and 64).

The term *digitalis effect* refers to the relatively distinctive "scooped" appearance of the ST-T complex and shortening of the QT interval, which correlates with abbreviation of the ventricular action potential duration (Fig. 14.44). Digitalis-related ST-T changes can be accentuated by an increased heart rate during exercise, with consequent false-positive results on stress testing (see Chapter 15), and can occur with either therapeutic or toxic doses of the drug. *Digitalis toxicity* refers specifically to systemic effects (e.g., nausea, anorexia) or conduction disturbances and arrhythmias caused by drug excess or increased sensitivity.

The ECG effects and toxicities of other cardioactive agents can be anticipated in part from ion channel effects (see Chapter 62). Inactivation of sodium channels by class I agents (e.g., quinidine, procainamide, disopyramide, flecainide) can cause QRS prolongation. Class IA (e.g., quinidine) and class III (e.g., amiodarone, dronedarone, dofetilide, ibutilide, sotalol) agents can induce an *acquired long QT(U) syndrome* (see Chapters 63 and 67). Psychotropic drugs (e.g., tricyclic antidepressants, phenothiazines), which have class IA–like properties, also can lead to QRS and QT(U) prolongation (see Chapter 99). Toxicity can produce asystole or torsades de pointes. Right axis shift of the terminal 40 msec frontal plane QRS axis may be a helpful additional marker of tricyclic antidepressant overdose. QT prolongation has been reported with multiple other drugs, including methadone, and hydroxychloroquine (especially in combination with azithromycin) in some of the initial attempts to treat COVID-19.[58] Finally, cocaine (see Chapter 28) can cause a variety of ECG changes, including those of STEMI, as well as life-threatening arrhythmias.

Electrolyte and Metabolic Abnormalities

In addition to the structural and functional cardiac conditions already discussed, numerous systemic metabolic aberrations may affect the ECG, including electrolyte abnormalities and acid-base disorders, as well as systemic hypothermia.[7,42]

Calcium

Hypercalcemia and hypocalcemia predominantly alter the action potential duration. An increased extracellular calcium concentration shortens the ventricular action potential duration by shortening phase 2. By contrast, hypocalcemia prolongs phase 2. These cellular changes are reflected in abbreviation or prolongation of the ST segment portion of the QT interval with hypercalcemia or hypocalcemia, respectively (Fig. 14.45). Severe hypercalcemia (e.g., serum Ca^{2+} >15 mg/dL) also can be associated with decreased T wave amplitude, sometimes with T wave notching or

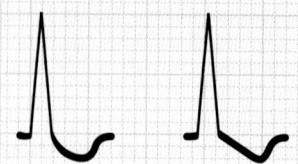

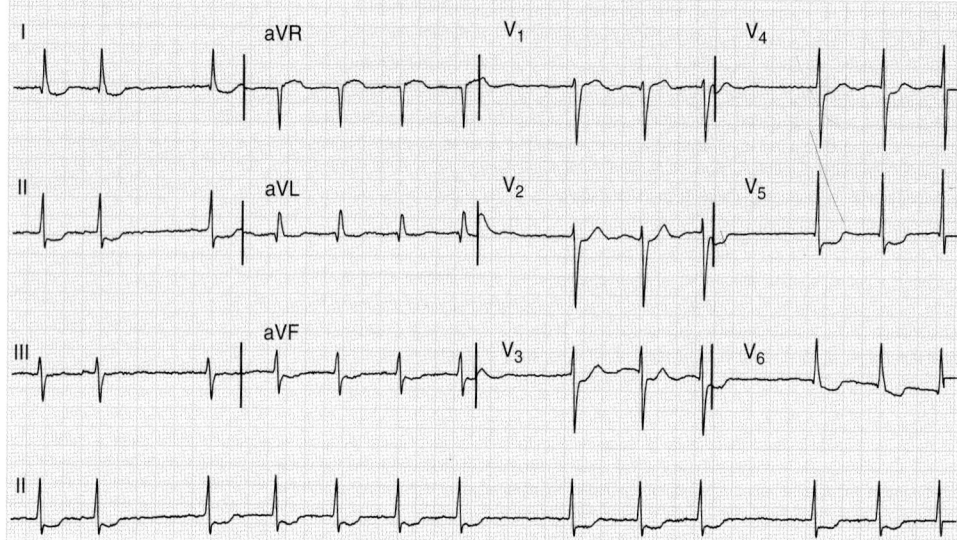

FIGURE 14.44 Top, Digitalis effect. Digitalis glycosides characteristically produce shortening of the QT interval with a scooped or downsloping ST-T complex. **Bottom,** Digitalis effect in combination with digitalis toxicity. The underlying rhythm is atrial fibrillation. A group beating pattern of QRS complexes with shortening of the R-R intervals is consistent with nonparoxysmal junctional tachycardia with probable exit block (atrioventricular Wenckebach) variant. ST-segment depression and scooping (lead V_6) are consistent with the digitalis effect, although ischemia or left ventricular hypertrophy cannot be excluded. These ECG findings are strongly suggestive of digitalis excess; the serum digoxin level was over 3 ng/mL. (**Top** from Goldberger AL, Goldberger ZD, Shvilkin A. *Goldberger's Clinical Electrocardiography: A Simplified Approach.* 9th ed. Philadelphia: Elsevier; 2017.)

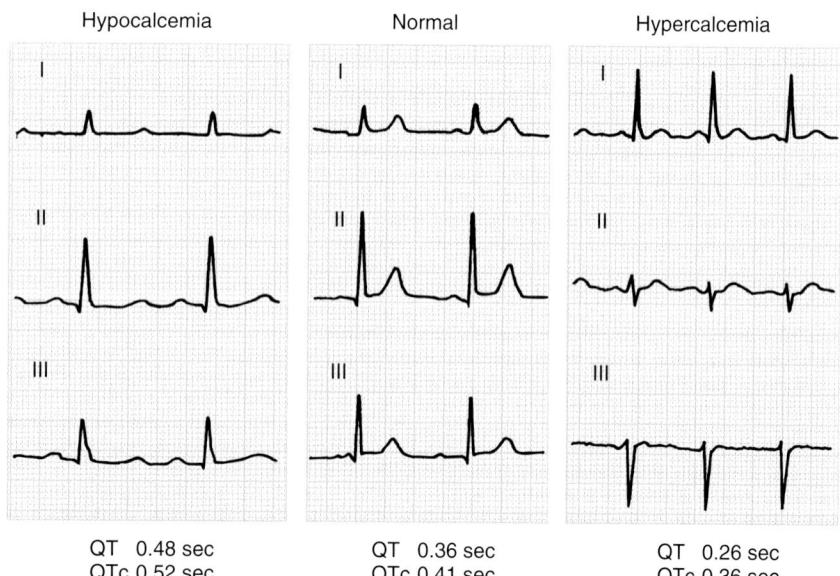

FIGURE 14.45 Prolongation of the QT interval (ST-segment portion) is typical of hypocalcemia. Hypercalcemia may cause abbreviation of the ST segment and shortening of the QT interval. (From Goldberger AL, Goldberger ZD, Shvilkin A. *Goldberger's Clinical Electrocardiography: A Simplified Approach.* 9th ed. Philadelphia: Elsevier; 2017.)

inversion. Hypercalcemia sometimes produces a high takeoff of the J point/ST segment in leads V_1 and V_2 and can thus simulate acute ischemia (see Table 14.11).

Potassium

Hyperkalemia is associated with a distinctive sequence of ECG changes (Fig. 14.46A). The earliest effect usually is narrowing and peaking (or *tenting*) of the T wave. The QT interval is shortened at this stage, reflecting a decreased action potential duration.

Progressive extracellular hyperkalemia reduces atrial and ventricular resting membrane potentials, thereby inactivating sodium channels, which decreases Vmax and conduction velocity. The QRS begins to widen, and P wave amplitude decreases. PR interval prolongation can occur, followed sometimes by second- or third-degree AV block. Complete loss of P waves may be associated with a junctional escape rhythm or putative *sinoventricular rhythm*. In the latter, sinus rhythm persists with conduction (possibly over internodal tracts or muscle bundles) between the sinoatrial and AV nodes but without producing an overt P wave.

Moderate to severe hyperkalemia occasionally induces ST elevations in the right precordial leads (V_1 and V_2), simulating an ischemic current of injury or Brugada-type patterns. Even severe hyperkalemia, however, can be associated with atypical or nondiagnostic ECG findings. Marked hyperkalemia leads to eventual asystole, sometimes preceded by a slow undulatory (or *sine wave*) ventricular flutter-like pattern. The ECG triad of peaked T waves (from hyperkalemia), QT (ST portion) prolongation (from hypocalcemia), and LVH (from hypertension) is strongly suggestive of chronic renal failure (see Chapter 101).

Electrophysiologic changes associated with hypokalemia, by contrast, include hyperpolarization of myocardial cell membranes and increased action potential duration. The major ECG manifestations are ST depression with flattened T waves and increased U wave prominence (see Fig. 14.46B). U waves can exceed the amplitude of T waves, and distinguishing T waves from U waves can be difficult or impossible from the surface ECG. Indeed, apparent U waves in hypokalemia and other pathologic settings may actually be part of T waves whose morphology is altered by the effects of voltage gradients between M, or mid-myocardial, cells and adjacent myocardial layers.[6,7] The prolongation of repolarization with hypokalemia, as part of an acquired long QT(U) syndrome, predisposes to the development of torsades de pointes (see Chapter 63) and to tachyarrhythmias during digitalis therapy.

Magnesium. Specific ECG effects of mild to moderate isolated abnormalities in magnesium ion concentration are not well characterized. Severe hypermagnesemia (e.g., serum Mg^{2+} >15 mEq/L) can cause AV and intraventricular conduction disturbances that may culminate in complete heart block and cardiac arrest. Hypomagnesemia usually is associated with hypocalcemia or hypokalemia and can potentiate certain digitalis toxic arrhythmias. The role of magnesium deficiency in the pathogenesis and treatment of the acquired long QT(U) syndrome with torsades de pointes is discussed in Chapters 63 and 67.

Other Factors. Isolated hypernatremia or hyponatremia does not produce consistent effects on the ECG. Acidemia and alkalemia are often associated with hyperkalemia and hypokalemia, respectively. Systemic hypothermia may be associated with the appearance of a distinctive convex elevation at the junction (J point) of the ST segment and QRS complex (J wave or Osborn wave) (Fig. 14.47).[7] The cellular mechanism of this type of pathologic J wave appears to be related to an epicardial-endocardial voltage gradient associated with the localized appearance of a prominent epicardial action potential notch.

Nonspecific QRS and ST-T Changes

Low QRS voltage is considered to be present when the total (positive-to-negative peak) amplitude of the QRS complexes in each of the six extremity leads is 0.5 mV or less or 1.0 mV or less in leads V_1 through V_6. Low QRS voltage, as described earlier, can be caused by a variety of mechanisms, including increased insulation of the heart by air (chronic obstructive pulmonary disease) or adipose tissue (obesity); replacement

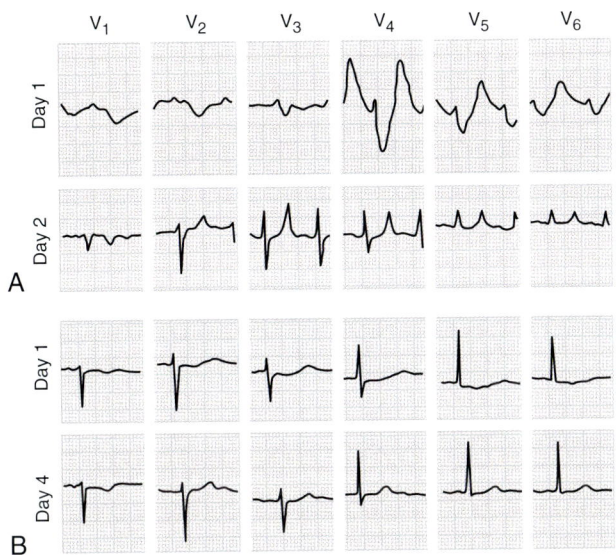

FIGURE 14.46 ECG changes in hyperkalemia (**A**) and hypokalemia (**B**). **A,** On day 1, at a K^+ level of 8.6 mEq/liter, the P wave is no longer recognizable and the QRS complex is diffusely prolonged. Initial and terminal QRS delays are characteristic of K^+-induced intraventricular conduction slowing and are best illustrated in leads V_2 and V_6. On day 2, at a K^+ level of 5.8 mEq/liter, the P wave is recognizable, with a PR interval of 0.24 second; the duration of the QRS complex is approximately 0.10 second, and the T waves are characteristically "tented." **B,** On day 1, at a K^+ level of 1.5 mEq/liter, the T and U waves are merged. The U wave is prominent and the QU interval is prolonged. On day 4, at a K^+ level of 3.7 mEq/liter, the tracing is normal. (Courtesy Dr. C. Fisch.)

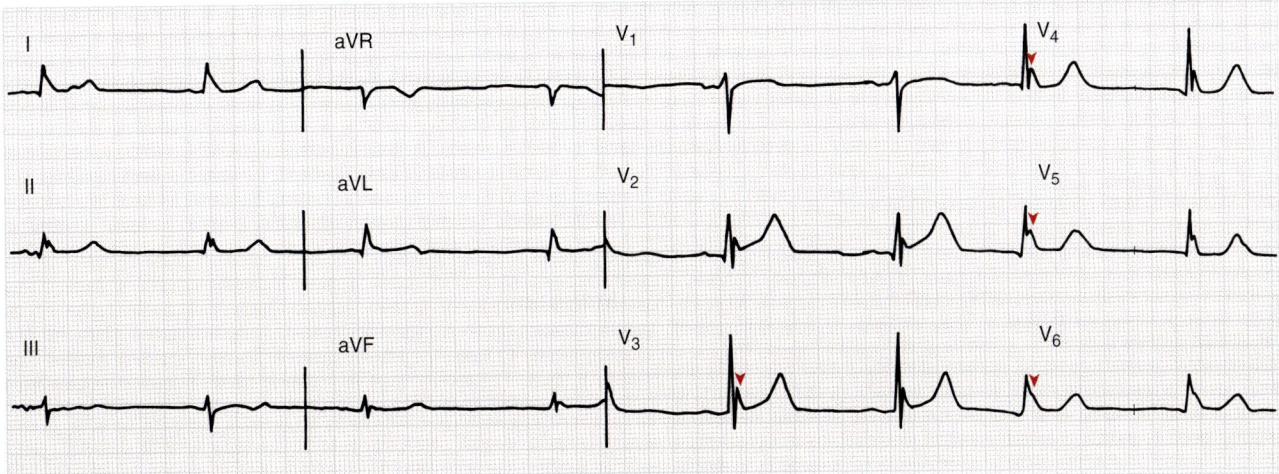

FIGURE 14.47 Systemic hypothermia. *Arrowheads* (leads V_3 through V_6) point to the characteristic convex J waves, termed *Osborn waves*. Prominent sinus bradycardia is also present, along with QT prolongation.

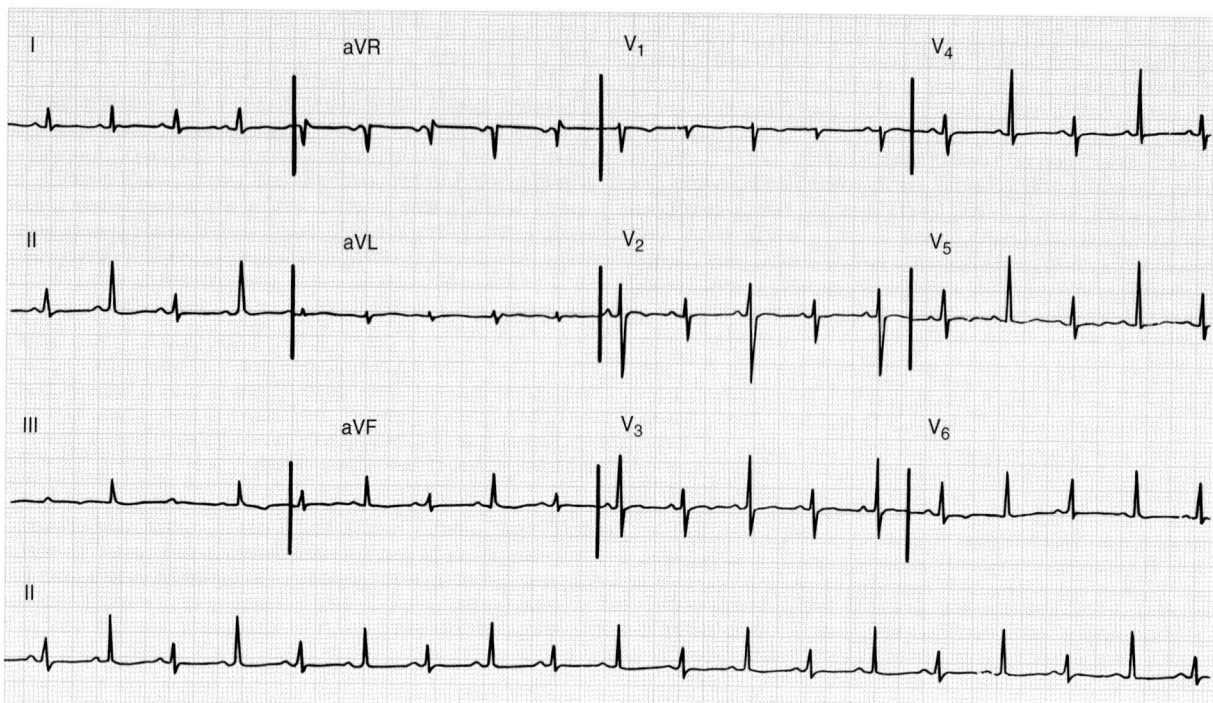

FIGURE 14.48 Total electrical alternans (P-QRS-T) caused by pericardial effusion with tamponade. This finding, particularly in concert with sinus tachycardia and relatively low voltage, is a highly specific, although not sensitive, marker of cardiac tamponade.

of myocardium by fibrous tissue (ischemic or nonischemic cardiomyopathy), amyloid, or tumor; and possibly to short-circuiting (shunting) effects resulting from low resistance of fluids (especially with pericardial or pleural effusions, or anasarca). The combination of relatively low limb voltage (QRS voltage <0.8 mV in each of the limb leads), relatively prominent QRS voltage in the chest leads (S_{V1} or S_{V2} + R_{V5} or R_{V6} >3.5 mV), and slow R wave progression (R wave < S wave amplitude in V_1 through V_4) has been reported as a relatively specific but not sensitive sign of dilated-type cardiomyopathies (initially referred to as the ECG "congestive heart failure triad").[42]

Ventricular repolarization is particularly sensitive to the effects of many factors in addition to ischemia (e.g., postural changes, meals, drugs, hypertrophy, electrolyte and metabolic disorders, central nervous system lesions, infections, pulmonary diseases) that can lead to a variety of *nonspecific ST-T changes*. The term usually is applied to slight ST-segment depression or T wave inversion or to T wave flattening without evident specific cause. Care must be taken not to over interpret such changes, especially in persons with a low prior probability of heart disease. At the same time, subtle repolarization abnormalities can be markers of coronary or hypertensive heart disease or other types of structural heart disease; these probably account for the association of relatively minor but persistent nonspecific ST-T changes with increased cardiovascular mortality in middle-aged and older men and women.

Alternans Patterns

The term *alternans* applies to conditions characterized by the sudden appearance of a periodic beat-to-beat change in some property of cardiac electrical or mechanical behavior. These abrupt changes (AAAA→ABAB pattern) are reminiscent of a generic class of patterns observed in perturbed nonlinear control systems. Many different forms of electrical alternans have been described clinically. Most familiar is total electrical alternans with sinus tachycardia, a specific but not highly sensitive marker of pericardial effusion with tamponade physiology (Fig. 14.48) (see Chapter 86). This finding is associated with an abrupt transition from a 1:1 to a 2:1 pattern in the "to-and-fro" swinging motion of the heart in the effusion.

Other alternans patterns have primary electrical rather than mechanical causes. QRS (and sometimes R-R) amplitude alternans may occur with a number of different types of supraventricular tachycardias.[1] Alternans has long been recognized as a marker of electrical instability of repolarization in cases of acute ischemia, in which it may precede ventricular tachyarrhythmia (see Fig. 14.34). Therefore, considerable interest continues to be directed at the detection of microvolt T wave (or ST-T)

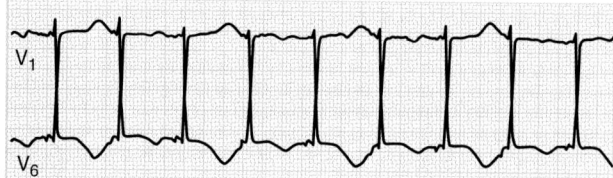

FIGURE 14.49 The QT(U) interval is prolonged (approximately 600 msec) with T-U wave alternans. The tracing was recorded in a patient with chronic renal disease shortly after dialysis. This type of repolarization alternans may be a precursor to torsades de pointes. The underlying rhythm appears to be an ectopic atrial tachycardia. (Courtesy Dr. C. Fisch.)

alternans and its variants[59] as a noninvasive marker for increased risk of ventricular tachyarrhythmias in patients with chronic heart disease (see Chapter 67). Similarly, T-U wave alternans (Fig. 14.49) may be a marker of imminent risk of torsades de pointes in hereditary or acquired long QT syndromes (see Chapter 63). Finally, with aging and advancing cardiovascular disease, fluctuations in heart rate faster than and decoupled from respiration may emerge, including sinoatrial alternans and its variants, under the proposed rubric of heart rate fragmentation.[60]

Clinical Issues in Electrocardiographic Interpretation

The clinical value of the ECG is maximized when an appropriately ordered and technically adequate recording is interpreted by a skilled professional. Key factors include reader competency, technical issues in ECG recording that impact reliability and consistency, and the appropriate application of computer technology and interpretation.

Indications

Numerous professional organizations, including the AHA, the ACC, the American College of Physicians (ACP), the U.S. Preventive Services Task Force (USPSTF), and the American College of Preventive Medicine (ACPM), have proposed appropriateness guidelines for recording an ECG[1] that have been periodically updated on their websites (Section e14.7). These include recommendations for several different populations, including persons with known or suspected heart disease, those without evidence of heart disease, and those in more specific

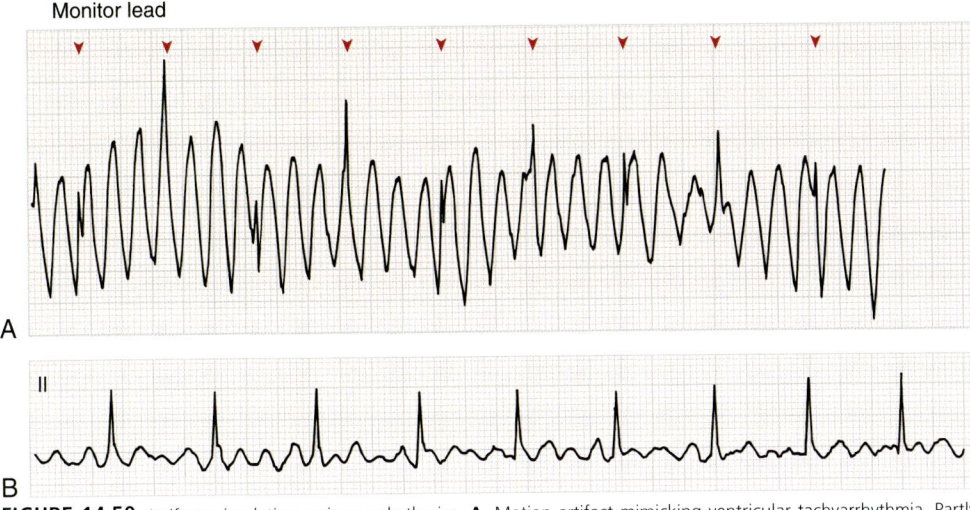

FIGURE 14.50 Artifacts simulating serious arrhythmias. **A,** Motion artifact mimicking ventricular tachyarrhythmia. Partly obscured normal QRS complexes (*arrowheads*) can be seen with a heart rate of approximately 100 beats/min. **B,** Parkinsonian tremor causing baseline oscillations mimicking atrial fibrillation. The regularity of QRS complexes may provide a clue to the source of this artifact.

groups including preoperative patients (see Chapter 23), persons with dangerous occupations, athletes (see Chapter 32), and patients taking medications with electrophysiologic effects.

Reading Competency

Developing and maintaining ECG interpretation are critical to successful clinical practice. It has been reported, however, that as many as one-third of ECG interpretations contain clinically meaningful errors and that over 10% of these lead to inappropriate management decisions.[61] Error rates are higher among noncardiologists than with cardiologists, although error rates among cardiologists as high as 40% have been reported.

A related issue is the common differences in diagnoses even among expert readers, that is, *interreader variability*. One recent study reported that, based on a test set of 20 ECGs read by 21 experts, agreement occurred in only 79% of tracings with evidence of STEMI and in only 37% of cases showing chamber hypertrophy.[1]

Professional organizations have made recommendations to aide in achieving adequate competency. The ACC recommends supervised and documented interpretation of a minimum of 3000 to 3500 ECGs covering a broad spectrum of diagnoses and clinical settings, over a 3-year training period for cardiology fellows.[62] However, the actual adequacy of training and the level of competency of trainees remain limited. In one study, cardiology fellows at an academic institution correctly interpreted only 58% of a test set of ECGs and missed 36% of potentially life-threatening abnormalities.[1] The challenge of adequate training is compounded by the number of physician specialties as well as nonphysician professionals with various levels of training performing ECG interpretation.

Technical Errors

Technical errors can lead to clinically significant diagnostic mistakes. Artifacts that interfere with interpretation can result from movement of the patient, poorly secured electrodes, electrical disturbances related to current leakage and grounding failure, and external interference from nearby electrical sources such as stimulators or cauteries. Electrical or motion (e.g., Parkinsonian tremor) artifacts can simulate life-threatening arrhythmias (Fig. 14.50). Body motion can cause excessive baseline wander that may simulate or obscure ST-segment shifts of myocardial ischemia or injury.

Misplacement of one or more electrodes is a common cause for errors. Many limb lead switches produce ECG patterns that can aid in their identification. Reversal of the two arm electrodes, for example, results in an inverted P and QRS waveforms in lead I but not in lead V_6, two leads that would normally be expected to have similar polarities.

The most common precordial electrode errors are placing V_1 and V_2 electrodes in the second or third rather than in the fourth intercostal place and the placement of the V_5 and V_6 electrodes above or below the horizontal line of V_4 or too far laterally. These misplacements may result in changes in R wave progression, accentuation of r′ waves, and ST-segment elevation in the right precordial leads simulating IVCDs or MI. In addition, variation in placement of electrodes between recordings, even small changes, may cause diagnostically confusing changes when relying on serial tracings.

As noted earlier, ECGs recorded using nonstandard electrode locations or altered filter settings such as those used for exercise testing or in intensive care settings are significantly different from those recorded using standard electrode sets. These should not be used for diagnostic purposes.[1]

Computer Interpretation

Computerized interpretation systems have the advantages of reducing analysis and reporting times, providing diagnostic prompts to clinicians to reduce overlooked abnormalities, standardizing criteria and report terminology, and increasing the ability to archive recordings to enhance serial comparisons and population studies.[63,64] The performance of these systems in identifying normal tracings is generally excellent. However, accuracy is lower for specific abnormalities including rhythm disturbances, conduction defects, and paced rhythms. Error rates as high as 30% for pattern-based diagnoses and as high as 40% for arrhythmias have been reported.

Although differences in measurements between manufacturers are clinically small, the differences increase with increasing abnormality in the ECG tracing[65] and differences may be substantial for certain diagnoses, e.g., myocardial ischemia and infarction.[66] Some of these differences may relate to differences between the information provided by analog and digital recordings and variations in methods to determine, for example, the ends of the QRS complex and T wave.[63]

An ongoing concern is common overreliance on computerized interpretations. There is a general consensus that, although computerized diagnostic algorithms have become more accurate and serve as important adjuncts to the clinical interpretation of ECGs, such systems are currently not sufficiently accurate to be relied on in critical clinical environments without expert review.

FUTURE PERSPECTIVES

Clinical electrocardiography represents a mature methodology based on extensive electrophysiologic study and clinical correlations that have evolved over more than a century of study. Several areas for expanded knowledge and clinical relevance may be suggested. These include, as examples, the application of artificial intelligence[67] and "big data"[68] approaches to interpretation and analysis, further development of clinically useful approaches to estimate epicardial potentials from body surface recordings,[69] and enhanced understanding of the genetic and cellular bases for ECG patterns (see Chapters 11 and 62).

GUIDELINES

The Guidelines for Electrocardiography are presented in the online chapter.

REFERENCES

Fundamental Principles

1. Mirvis DM, Goldberger AL. *Electrocardiography. Braunwald's Heart Disease*. 11th ed. Philadelphia, PA: Elsevier Saunders; 2019.
2. Young B, Schmidt JJ. Updates to IEC/AAMI ECG standards: a new hybrid standard. *J Electrocardiol*. 2018;51:S103–S105.
3. Lindow T, Birnbaum Y, Nikus K, et al. Why complicate an important task? An orderly display of the limb leads in the 12-lead electrocardiogram and its implications for recognition of acute coronary syndrome. *BMC Cardiovasc Dis*. 2019;19:13–20.

The Normal Electrocardiogram

4. Rautaharju PM, Zhang Z-M, Haisty WK, et al. Race- and sex-associated differences in rate-adjusted QT, QT_{peak}, ST elevation and other regional measures of repolarization: the Atherosclerosis Risk in Communities (ARIC) study. *J Electrocardiol*. 2014;47:342–350.
5. Costa MD, Davis RB, Goldberger AL. Heart rate fragmentation: a new approach to the analysis of cardiac interbeat interval dynamics. *Front Physiol*. 2017;8:255.
6. Opthof T, Janse MJ, Meijborg VM, et al. Dispersion in ventricular repolarization in human, canine and porcine heart. *Prog Biophys Mol Biol*. 2016;120:222–235.
7. Antzelevitch C, Yan GX, Ackerman MJ, et al. J-wave syndromes expert consensus conference report: emerging concepts and gaps in knowledge. *Europace*. 2017;19:665–694.
8. Vink AS, Neumann B, Lieve KVV, et al. Determination and interpretation of the QT interval. *Circulation*. 2018;138:2345–2358.
9. Beinart R, Zhang Y, Lima JC, et al. The QT interval is associated with incident cardiovascular events: the MESA study in the multi-ethnic study of atherosclerosis. *J Am Coll Cardiol*. 2014;65:2111–2119.
10. Waks JW, Sitlani CM, Soliman EZ, et al. Global electrical heterogeneity risk score for prediction of sudden cardiac death in the general population. *Circulation*. 2016;133:2222–2234.
11. Ghadban R, Alpert MA, Dohrmann ML, et al. A QS pattern in leads V_1 and V_2 is associated with septal scarring independent of etiology – a cardiac magnetic resonance imaging study. *J Electrocardiol*. 2018;51:577–582.
12. Patton K, Ellinor PT, Ezekowitz M, et al. Electrocardiographic early repolarization. A scientific statement from the American Heart Association. *Circulation*. 2016;13:1520–1529.
13. Zhang J, Hocini M, Strom M, et al. The electrophysiological substrate of early repolarization syndrome: noninvasive mapping in patients. *JACC Clin Electrophysiol*. 2017;3:894–904.
14. Sharma S, Drezner JA, Baggish A, et al. International recommendations for electrocardiographic interpretation in athletes. *J Am Coll Cardiol*. 2017;69:1057–1075.

The Abnormal Electrocardiogram

15. Soliman EZ, Zhang Z-M, Chen LY, et al. Usefulness of maintaining a normal electrocardiogram over time for predicting cardiovascular health. *Am J Cardiol*. 2017;119:249–255.
16. Bayes de Luna A, Baranchuk A, Robledo LA, et al. Diagnosis of interatrial block. *J Geriatric Cardiol*. 2017;14:161–165.
17. O'Neal WT, Zhang Z-M, Loehr LR, et al. Electrocardiographic advanced intra-atrial block and atrial fibrillation risk in the general population. *Am J Cardiol*. 216; 117:1755-1759.
18. Lacalzada-Almeida J, Izquierdo-Gomez M, Belleyo-Belkasem C, et al. Interatrial block and atrial remodeling assessed using speckled tracking echocardiography. *BMC Cardiovasc Dis*. 2018;18:38–45.
19. Kamel H, O'Neal WT, Okin PM, et al. Electrocardiographic left atrial abnormality and stroke subtype in ARIC. *Ann Neurol*. 2015;78:670–678.
20. Bacharova L. Missing link between molecular aspects of ventricular arrhythmias and QRS complex morphology in left ventricular hypertrophy. *Intern J Molec Sci*. 2019;21:48–65.
21. Bacharova L, Chen H, Estes EH, et al. Determinants of discrepancies and comparison of the prognostic significance of left ventricular hypertrophy by electrocardiographic and cardiac magnetic resonance imaging. *Am J Cardiol*. 2015;115:515–522.
22. Okin PM, Hille DA, Kjeldsen SE, Devereux RB. Combining ECG criteria for left ventricular hypertrophy improves risk prediction in patients with hypertension. *J Am Heart Assoc*. 2017;6:e007564–e007572.
23. Bang CN, Soliman EZ, Simpson LM, et al. Electrocardiographic left ventricular hypertrophy predicts cardiovascular morbidity and mortality in hypertensive patients: the ALLHAT Study. *Am J Hypertension*. 2017;30:914-822.
24. Leigh JA, O'Neal WT, Soliman EZ. Electrocardiographic left ventricular hypertrophy as a predictor of cardiovascular disease independent of left ventricular anatomy in subjects >65 years. *Am J Cardiol*. 2016;117:1831–1835.
25. Inoue YY, Soliman EZ, Yoneyama K, et al. Electrocardiographic strain pattern is associated with left ventricular concentric remodeling, scar, and mortality over 10 years: the Multi-ethnic Study of Atherosclerosis. *J Am Heart Assoc*. 2017;6:e006624–e0006632.
26. De Lazzari M, Zorzi A, Cipriani A, et al. Relationship between electrocardiographic findings and cardiac magnetic resonance phenotypes in arrhythmogenic cardiomyopathy. *J Am Heart J*. 2018;7:e009855–e009865.
27. Kowal J, Ahmad MI, Li Y, Soliman EZ. Prognostic significance of electrocardiographic right ventricular hypertrophy in the general population. *J Electrocardiol*. 2019;54:49–53.
28. Carroll BJ, Heidinger BH, Dabreo DC, et al. Multimodality assessment of right ventricular strain in patients with acute pulmonary embolism. *Am J Cardiol*. 2018;122:175–181.
29. Kusumoto FM, Schoenfeld MH, Barrett C, et al. 2018 ACC/AHA/HRS guidelines on the evaluation and management of patients with bradycardia and cardiac conduction delay. *Heart Rhythm*. 2019;16:e128–e153.
30. Elizari MV. The normal variants in the left bundle branch system. *J Electrocardiol*. 2017;50:389–399.
31. Upadhyay GA, Cherlan T, Shatz DY, et al. Intracardiac delineation of septal conduction in left bundle branch block. *Circulation*. 2019;139:1876–1888.
32. Senesael E, Calle S, Kamoen V, et al. Progression of incomplete toward complete left bundle branch block: a clinical and electrocardiographic analysis. *Ann Noninvasive Electrocardiol*. 2020;25:e12732.
33. Zhang ZM, Rautaharju PM, Prineas RJ, et al. Bundle branch blocks and the risk of mortality in the Atherosclerosis Risk in Communities study. *J Cardiovasc Med*. 2016;17:411–417.
34. Stokke IM, Li B, Cicala S, et al. Association of left bundle branch block with new onset abnormal wall motion in treated hypertensive patients with left ventricular hypertrophy: the LIFE Echo Sub-Study. *Blood Press*. 2019;28:84–92.
35. Smiseth OA, Aalen JM. Mechanism of harm from left bundle branch block. *Trends Cardiovasc Med*. 2019;29:335–342.
36. Xiong Y, Wang L, Liu W, et al. The prognostic significance of right bundle branch block: a meta-analysis of prospective cohort studies. *Clin Cardiol*. 2015;38:604–613.
37. Devarapally SR, Arora S, Ahmad S, et al. Right ventricular failure predicted from right bundle branch block: cardiac magnetic resonance imaging validation. *Cardiovasc Diagn Ther*. 2016;6:432–438.
38. Sillanmaki S, Gimelli A, Ahmad S, et al. Mechanisms of left ventricular dyssynchrony: a multinational SPECT study of patients with bundle branch block. *J Nucl Cardiol*. 2020. Feb 14. doi: 10.1007/s12350-020-02054-y. Epub ahead of print.
39. Palmisano P, Ziachhi M, Ammendola E, et al. Long-term progression of rhythm and conduction disturbances in pacemaker recipients: findings from the pacemaker expert programming study. *J Cardiovasc Med*. 2018;19:357–365.
40. Eschaller R, Ploux S, Ritter P, et al. Nonspecific intraventricular conduction delay: definitions, prognosis and implications for cardiac resynchronization therapy. *Heart Rhythm*. 2015;12:1071–1079.
41. Rattanawong P, Riangwiwat T, Kanitsoraphan C, et al. Baseline fragmented QRS increases the risk of major arrhythmic events in hypertrophic cardiomyopathy: systematic review and meta-analysis. *Ann Noninvasive Electrocardiol*. 2018;23:e12533–e12540.
42. Goldberger AL, Goldberger ZD, Shvilkin A. *Goldberger's Clinical Electrocardiography: A Simplified Approach*. 9th ed. Philadelphia: Elsevier; 2017.
43. AHA/ACC clinical performance and quality measures for adults with ST-elevation and non-ST-elevation myocardial infarction: a report of the American College of Cardiology/American Heart Association task force on performance measures. *Circulation*. 2017;10:2048–2090.
44. Chew DS, Wilton SB, Kavanagh K, et al. Fragmented QRS complexes after acute myocardial infarction are independently associated with unfavorable left ventricular remodeling. *J Electrocardiol*. 2018;51:607–612.
45. Thygesen K, Alpert JS, Jaffe AS, et al. Fourth universal definition of myocardial infarction. *J Am Coll Cardiol*. 2018;72:2231–2264.
46. Barrabés JA, Figueras J, Moure C, et al. Prognostic value of lead aVR in patients with a first non–ST-segment elevation acute myocardial infarction. *Circulation*. 2016;108:814–819.
47. Meyers HP, Limkakeng Jr AT, Jaffa EJ, et al. Validation of the modified Sgarbossa criteria for acute coronary occlusion in the setting of left bundle branch block: a retrospective case-control study. *Am Heart J*. 2015;170:1255–1264.
48. Lu ML, Nwakile C, Bhalla V, et al. Prognostic significance of abnormal P wave morphology and PR-segment displacement after ST-elevation myocardial infarction. *Int J Cardiol*. 2015;197:216–221.
49. Lu ML, De Venecia T, Patnaik S, et al. Atrial myocardial infarction: a tale of the forgotten chamber. *Int J Cardiol*. 2016;202:904–909.
50. Hendren NS, Drazner MH, Bozkurt B, Cooper Jr LT. Description and proposed management of the acute COVID-19 cardiovascular syndrome. *Circulation*. 2020;141:1903–1914.
51. Clerkin KJ, Fried JA, Raikhelkar J, et al. COVID-19 and cardiovascular disease. *Circulation*. 2020;19:1648–1655.
52. Templin C, Ghadri JR, Diekmann J, et al. Clinical features and outcomes of takotsubo (stress) cardiomyopathy. *N Engl J Med*. 2015;373:929–938.
53. de Chazal HM, Del Buono MG, Keyser-Marcus L, et al. Stress cardiomyopathy diagnosis and treatment: JACC state-of-the-art review. *J Am Coll Cardiol*. 2018;72:1955–1971.
54. Frangieh AH, Obeid S, Ghadri JR, et al. ECG criteria to differentiate between Takotsubo (stress) cardiomyopathy and myocardial infarction. *J Am Heart Assoc*. 2016;5:e003418.
55. Shvilkin A, Huang HD, Josephson ME. Cardiac memory: diagnostic tool in the making. *Circ Arrhythm Electrophysiol*. 2015;8:475–482.
56. Siontis KC, Wen S, Asirvatham SJ. Cardiac memory for the clinical electrophysiologist. *J Cardiovasc Electrophysiol*. 2019;30:2140–2143.
57. Corrado D, van Tintelen PJ, McKenna WJ, et al. Arrhythmogenic right ventricular cardiomyopathy: evaluation of the current diagnostic criteria and differential diagnosis. *Eur Heart J*. 2020;41:1414–1429.
58. Saleh M, Gabriels J, Chang D, et al. Effect of chloroquine, hydroxychloroquine and azithromycin on the corrected QT interval in patients with SARS-CoV-2 infection. *Circ Arrhythm Electrophysiol*. 2020;13:e008662.
59. Krokhaleva Y, Patel D, Shah H, et al. Increased nonalternans repolarization variability precedes ventricular tachycardia onset in patients with implantable defibrillators. *Pacing Clin Electrophysiol*. 2016;39:140–148.
60. Costa MD, Goldberger AL. Heart rate fragmentation: using cardiac pacemaker dynamics to probe the pace of biological aging. *Am J Physiol Heart Circ Physiol*. 2019;316:H1341–H1344.

Clinical Issues in Electrocardiographic Interpretation

61. Breen CJ, Kelly GP, Kernohan WC. ECG interpretation skill acquisition: a review of learning, teaching and assessment. *J Electrocardiol*. 2019;S0022–0736(18):30641–1.
62. Balady GJ, Bufalino VJ, Gulati M, et al. COCATS 4 Task Force 3: training in electrocardiography, ambulatory electrocardiography, and exercise testing. *J Am Coll Cardiol*. 65:1763–1777.
63. Macfarlane PW, Mason JW, Kligfield P, et al. Debatable issues in automated ECG reporting. *J Electrocardiol*. 2017;50:833–840.
64. Schlepfer J, Willens HJ. Computer-interpreted electrocardiograms. Benefits and limitations. *J Am Coll Cardiol*. 2017;70:1183–1192.
65. Kligfield P, Badilini F, Denjoy I, et al. Comparison of automated interval measurements by widely used algorithms in digital electrocardiography. *Am Heart J*. 2018;200:1–10.
66. Garvey JL, Zegre-Hemey J, Gregg R, Studnek JR. Electrocardiographic diagnosis of ST segment elevation myocardial infarction: an evaluation of three standard interpretation algorithms. *J Electrocardiol*. 2016;49:728–732.

Future Perspectives

67. Lyon A, Minchole A, Martinez JP, et al. Computational techniques for ECG analysis and interpretation in light of their contribution to medical advances. *J R Soc Interface*. 2018;15:20170821–21070829.
68. Estes EH. Big data and the electrocardiogram. *J Electrocardiol*. 2015;48:29–30.
69. Rudy Y. Noninvasive ECG mapping (ECGI): mapping the arrhythmic substrate of the human heart. *Int J Cardiol*. 2017;237:13–14.

15 Exercise Physiology and Exercise Electrocardiographic Testing

GARY J. BALADY AND PHILIP A. ADES

EXERCISE PHYSIOLOGY, 175
Total-Body Oxygen Uptake, 175
Myocardial Oxygen Demand and Supply Relationships During Exercise, 175

TECHNICAL COMPONENTS OF EXERCISE TESTING, 177
Patient Preparation, 177
Exercise Test Modality and Protocols, 177
Risks of Exercise Testing, 180

EXERCISE TESTING IN CORONARY ARTERY DISEASE, 180
Exercise-Induced Symptoms, 180
Functional Capacity, 181

ST-Segment Changes, 182
Pharmacologic Influences on Interpretation, 184
Diagnostic Value, 184
Assessment of Anatomic and Functional Extent of Disease, 185
Testing in Women, 185
Prognostic Value, 186
Preoperative Evaluation in Noncardiac Surgery, 189
Assessment of Therapy, 189

EXERCISE TESTING IN NONATHEROSCLEROTIC HEART DISEASE, 189
Valvular Heart Disease, 189

Hypertrophic Cardiomyopathy, 190
Adult Congenital Heart Disease, 190

ADDITIONAL USES FOR EXERCISE TESTING, 191
Chest Pain Units, 191
Physical Activity and Exercise Prescription, 192
Evaluation of Peripheral Artery Disease, 192
Patients with Diabetes, 193

SUMMARY, 194
ACKNOWLEDGMENT, 194
CLASSIC REFERENCES, 194
REFERENCES, 194

Exercise electrocardiographic testing is among the most fundamental and widely used tests for the evaluation of patients with cardiovascular disease (CVD). It is easy to administer, perform, and interpret; it is flexible and adaptable; and it is reliable, inexpensive, and readily available in hospital or practice settings. The exercise test has been used by clinicians for more than half a century, and its durability can be attributed to its evolution over time. Primarily developed to detect the presence of myocardial ischemia secondary to coronary artery disease (CAD), the exercise electrocardiogram (ECG) is now recognized for its power in predicting prognosis. Exercise test variables beyond the ST segment yield important information, particularly when used in combination with clinical information, to predict outcomes and guide therapy in a broad range of individuals, from the healthy to those disabled by heart disease. Emerging applications of exercise electrocardiography have demonstrated its usefulness in the evaluation and management of patients with a wide variety of cardiovascular conditions, including valvular heart disease, congenital heart disease, genetic cardiovascular conditions, arrhythmias, and peripheral artery disease (PAD). When used appropriately with adjunctive modalities to measure gas exchange and ventilation or with imaging techniques such as echocardiography or nuclear perfusion imaging (see Chapters 16 and 18), the power of the exercise ECG is greatly enhanced. The exercise ECG is the clinician's beacon that can guide optimal care for a great majority of patients with known or suspected CVD. This chapter provides a detailed foundation of information on the physiology of exercise testing and the exercise ECG. Other chapters address adjunctive imaging techniques and further discuss the use of exercise testing in patients with specific cardiovascular conditions.

EXERCISE PHYSIOLOGY

Total-Body Oxygen Uptake

Exercising muscles require energy to contract and relax. Most of this energy is derived from oxidative metabolism to generate adenosine triphosphate; thus, energy requirements at rest and for any given amount of physical activity (work rate) can be estimated from measurements of total-body oxygen uptake ($\dot{V}o_2$). The Fick equation (Fig. 15.1) demonstrates that $\dot{V}o_2$ is determined by the product of cardiac output and oxygen extraction at the periphery (i.e., arteriovenous oxygen difference). $\dot{V}o_2$ is easily expressed in multiples of resting oxygen requirements (metabolic equivalents [METs]), with 1 MET being resting energy expenditure and defined as approximately 3.5 mL O_2/kg body weight/min. This convenient system indexes the amount of energy used during any given physical activity against that used at rest. Accordingly, 5-MET activity requires five times the energy expenditure at rest. $\dot{V}o_2$ max is the peak oxygen uptake achieved during performance of the highest level of dynamic exercise involving large muscle groups and by definition cannot be exceeded despite increases in work rate. It is related to age, sex, heredity, exercise habits, and cardiovascular status. Cardiac output can increase as much as four to six times resting levels in the upright position. Maximum cardiac output is the result of a twofold to threefold increase in heart rate (HR) from resting levels and an increase in stroke volume. Stroke volume in healthy persons generally plateaus at 50% to 60% of $\dot{V}o_2$ max. Oxygen extraction at the periphery can increase as much as threefold, and the maximum arteriovenous O_2 difference has a physiologic limit of 15 to 17 mL O_2/100 mL blood. During clinical exercise testing, patients are prompted to exercise not until they attain $\dot{V}o_2$ max but rather to the $\dot{V}o_2$ that is attained during symptom-limited, maximum tolerated exercise; this level is termed the $\dot{V}o_2$ peak.[1]

Myocardial Oxygen Demand and Supply Relationships During Exercise

Myocardial ischemia occurs when the supply of oxygenated blood to myocardial cells is inadequate to meet demands. Many factors affect the delicate balance of supply and demand (Fig. 15.2). Exercise testing is performed to stress these relationships and observe the physiologic responses that ensue. This enables the clinician not only to assess for the development of myocardial ischemia, but also to evaluate at what level of myocardial oxygen demand and physical activity (work rate) ischemia occurs.[1]

MYOCARDIAL OXYGEN DEMAND

Myocardial oxygen demand is related to HR, blood pressure (BP), left ventricular (LV) contractility (myocardial shortening per beat), and LV wall stress. The latter is related to LV pressure, wall thickness, and cavity size. Changes in any of these interdependent factors can affect myocardial need for oxygenated blood. Of these parameters, HR and BP are the easiest to measure and monitor. The product of HR and systolic BP, termed the *rate-pressure product*, is a reliable index of myocardial oxygen demand and can be readily assessed clinically.

During acute endurance (high-repetition/low-resistance) exercise (e.g., walking or cycling), cardiac output rises in response to the

$$\text{Resting VO}_2 = \text{C.O.} \times \text{A-VO}_2 \text{ Difference}$$
$$\text{Maximal Exercise VO}_2 = \text{C.O.} \times \text{A-VO}_2 \text{ Difference}$$
$$= \text{HR (2-3x resting)} \times \text{SV (2x resting)} \times \text{A-VO}_2 \text{ Difference (3x resting)}$$

FIGURE 15.1 Fick equations at rest and during exercise. See text for details. A-VO$_2$ Difference, arteriovenous oxygen difference; C.O., cardiac output; HR, heart rate; SV, stroke volume; Vo$_2$, total body oxygen uptake.

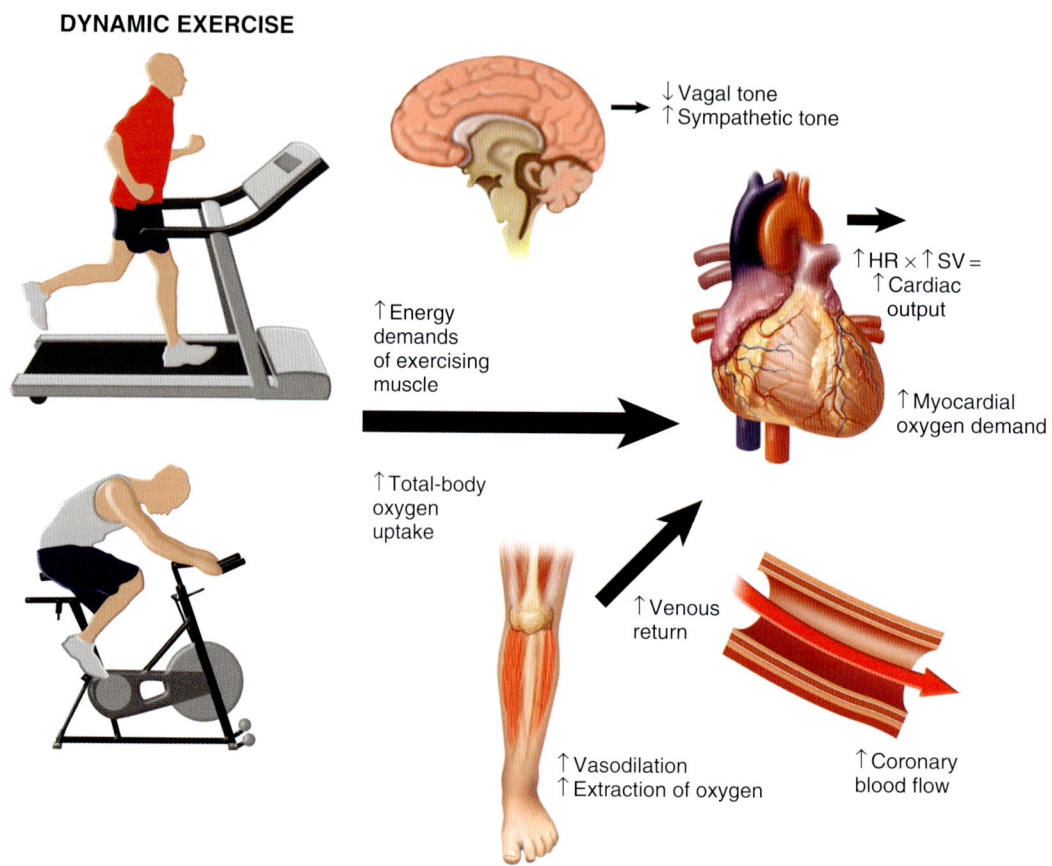

FIGURE 15.2 Physiologic responses to acute exercise. See text for details.

metabolic needs of the exercising muscles (estimated by measured $\dot{V}o_2$). Diminution of vagal tone and a rise in sympathetic tone lead to an increase in HR and LV contractility. Stroke volume also rises because of increases in venous return of blood from exercising muscles, and blood flow is redistributed from the renal, splanchnic, and cutaneous circulation to the exercising muscles. Accumulation of metabolites in the actively contracting muscles causes vasodilation of muscle arterioles, which increases skeletal muscle blood flow up to four times that of resting levels and results in a reduction in aortic outflow impedance. This in turn allows more complete systolic ejection, thereby further increasing stroke volume. Systolic BP increases mostly because of the rise in cardiac output, whereas diastolic BP either remains constant or falls as a result of the reduction in vascular resistance. The size and location of the exercising muscle groups will have different effects on the hemodynamic response to exercise. Dynamic arm exercise elicits higher HR and BP responses at any given work rate than does dynamic leg exercise. Arm work yields differences in sympathetic output, peripheral vasodilation, venous return, and metabolic requirements, which are influenced not only by the exercising muscle mass but also by the stabilizing muscles recruited during arm exercise.[1]

Resistance (low-repetition/high-load) exercise (e.g., weightlifting) is not generally used during graded exercise testing but may be used in work simulation testing or exercise training regimens. This type of exercise generates an increased sympathetic response, leading to an increase in HR; however, venous return, especially during straining, may decrease. Therefore, the rise in cardiac output is relatively small in comparison to that achieved with endurance exercise and is primarily caused by increases in HR. Muscle contraction during resistance exercise generates compressive force on muscle capillaries that leads to elevated peripheral resistance. This rise in vascular resistance coupled with an increase in cardiac output yields an increase in both systolic and diastolic BP. Elevations in systolic BP from rest to exercise are proportionally greater than the elevations in HR during resistance exercise than during endurance exercise. Therefore, both endurance exercise and resistance exercise increase myocardial oxygen demand because of variable increases in HR, BP, LV contractility, and LV wall stress (the latter caused by increases in LV pressure and/or volume during exercise).[1]

MYOCARDIAL OXYGEN SUPPLY

Coronary blood flow increases during exercise in response to neurohumoral stimulation (primarily sympathetic beta receptor stimulation) and as a result of the release of endothelial substances, including nitric oxide. In healthy persons during acute exercise, coronary arteries dilate and coronary blood flow rises in response to the increases in myocardial oxygen demand. Most often, coronary flow is compromised as a result of atherosclerotic plaque within the lumen of the coronary artery (see Chapter 36). Plaque may cause minimal stenosis or complete occlusion of the artery. Several factors influence the significance of a given luminal stenosis, including the degree of luminal obstruction, the length of the obstruction, the number and size of functioning collateral vessels, the magnitude of the muscle mass supplied, the shape and dynamic properties of the stenosis, and the autoregulatory capacity of the vascular bed. In general, a 50% to 70% reduction in luminal diameter will impair peak reactive hyperemia, whereas 90% or greater stenosis will reduce resting flow. However, exercise stimulates local changes in vasomotor tone as a result of neuromodulation, endothelial dysfunction, and local factors, and these changes can further influence the supply of oxygenated blood to the myocardium. Atherosclerotic arteries often fail to dilate and may actually constrict with exercise, thus further reducing the supply of blood in the setting of increased demand.[1]

TECHNICAL COMPONENTS OF EXERCISE TESTING

Patient Preparation

Patient Assessment

It is important to clinically assess the patient before performing the exercise test to evaluate the indications for the test, the appropriateness of the specific test that has been ordered to answer the question posed, the ability of the patient to perform exercise, and whether the patient has any contraindications to exercise testing (Table 15.1). Information from the medical history as provided by the patient, chart review, and the ordering provider and/or the patient's primary care physician or cardiologist can be most useful in this pretest evaluation. A brief physical examination that addresses the components outlined in Table 15.2 can also be helpful. A current standard resting 12-lead ECG is useful in assessing HR, rhythm, conduction abnormalities, and evidence of previous myocardial infarction (MI) and should be compared with the most recent previous ECG, if available.

Diagnostic exercise testing in patients without known CAD is best performed by withholding cardioactive medications on the day of the test to better assess for an ischemic response. On the other hand, functional testing in patients with known CAD is best performed with patients taking their usual medications to evaluate the effects of the medications on HR, BP, symptoms, and ischemia during exercise (see "Pharmacologic Influences on Interpretation").

In patients with permanent cardiac pacemakers, it is important to obtain information from the patient's cardiologist regarding the type of pacemaker (single or dual chamber), programmed mode, rate responsiveness, and pacing HR limits before the test. Similarly, in patients with implantable cardioverter-defibrillators (ICDs), information regarding ICD rhythm detection and treatment algorithms should be obtained so that the peak HR during the exercise test is maintained at least 10 beats/min below the programmed HR threshold for anti-tachycardia pacing and defibrillation.[2] Additional details of patient assessment are provided elsewhere.[1]

Symptom Rating Scales

Before exercising, patients should be made familiar with the symptom rating scales that might be used during testing. These are described further elsewhere[3] and may include the Borg Scale of Perceived Exertion.[3]

Electrocardiographic Lead Systems

As the technology of exercise electrocardiographic testing has evolved, several different types of lead systems have been developed and used. Details regarding these lead systems, along with skin preparation techniques, are provided elsewhere.[1] The importance of adequate skin preparation cannot be overstated; this is essential to optimize the quality of the exercise ECG. To obtain a high-quality 12-lead ECG during testing, electrode placement on the torso is standard for routine testing. Torso electrodes are placed under the lateral aspect of the clavicles for the arm leads and on the lower end of the rib cage or high under the rib cage for the leg leads. A standard 12-lead ECG should be performed before placement of the torso limb leads because such lead placement may alter the inferior lead complexes and result in previous Q waves being either mimicked or hidden. A standing ECG is then used as the basis for determining the presence of exercise-induced ECG changes.

Exercise Test Modality and Protocols

The testing modality and protocol should be selected in accordance with the patient's estimated functional capacity based on age, estimated physical fitness from the patient's history, and underlying disease. Several exercise test protocols are available for both treadmill and stationary cycle ergometers. Patients who have low estimated fitness levels or are deemed to be at higher risk because of underlying disease (e.g., recent MI, heart failure) should be tested with a less aggressive exercise protocol. Treadmill and cycle ergometers may use stepped or continuous ramp protocols. Work rate increments (stages) during stepped protocols can vary from 1 to 2.5 METs. Ramp protocols are designed with stages that are no longer than 1 minute and for the patient to attain peak effort within 8 to 12 minutes. Accordingly, ramp protocols must be individualized and selected to accommodate the patient's estimated exercise capacity. Because there are no widely published or standard sets of ramp protocols, individual exercise testing laboratories usually develop their own customized protocols that

TABLE 15.1 Contraindications to Exercise Testing

Absolute Contraindications
Acute myocardial infarction, within 2 days
High-risk unstable angina
Uncontrolled cardiac arrhythmia with hemodynamic compromise
Active endocarditis
Symptomatic severe aortic stenosis
Decompensated heart failure
Acute pulmonary embolism or pulmonary infarction
Acute myocarditis or pericarditis
Physical disability that precludes safe and adequate testing
Relative Contraindications
Known left main coronary artery stenosis
Moderate aortic stenosis with uncertain relation to symptoms
Tachyarrhythmias with uncontrolled ventricular rates
Acquired complete heart block
Hypertrophic cardiomyopathy with severe resting gradient
Mental impairment with limited ability to cooperate

From Fletcher GF, Ades PA, Kligfield P, et al. Exercise standards for testing and training: a scientific statement from the American Heart Association. *Circulation*. 2013;128:873–934.

TABLE 15.2 Patient Assessment for Exercise Testing

History

1. **Medical diagnoses and past medical history**—a variety of diagnoses should be reviewed, including cardiovascular disease (known existing CAD, previous myocardial infarction, or coronary revascularization); arrhythmias, syncope or pre-syncope; pulmonary disease, including asthma, emphysema, and bronchitis, or recent pulmonary embolism; cerebrovascular disease, including stroke; peripheral arterial disease; current pregnancy; musculoskeletal, neuromuscular and joint disease
2. **Symptoms**—angina; chest, jaw or arm discomfort; shortness of breath; palpitations, especially if associated with physical activity, eating a large meal, emotional upset, or exposure to cold
3. **Risk factors for atherosclerotic disease**—hypertension; diabetes; obesity; dyslipidemia; smoking
4. If patient is without known CAD, determine the pre-test probability of CAD (see Table 15.11)
5. **Recent illness, hospitalization, or surgical procedure**
6. **Medication dose and schedule**
7. **Ability to perform physical activity**

Physical Examination

1. Pulse rate and regularity
2. Resting blood pressure sitting and standing
3. Auscultation of the lungs, with specific attention to uniformity of breath sounds in all areas, particularly in patients with shortness of breath, a history of heart failure or pulmonary disease
4. Auscultation of the heart, particularly in patients with heart failure or valvular disease
5. Examination related to orthopedic, neurologic, or other medical conditions that might limit exercise

TABLE 15.3 Boston Medical Center Treadmill Ramp Protocols

STAGE*	VERY LOW RAMP			LOW RAMP			MODERATE RAMP			HIGH RAMP			ATHLETE'S RAMP		
	MPH	% GRADE	METS	MPH	% GRADE	METS	MPH	% GRADE	METS	MPH	% GRADE	METS	MPH	% GRADE	METS
1	1.0	0.0	1.8	1.0	0.0	1.8	1.5	1.5	2.5	2.1	3.0	3.5	1.8	0.0	2.4
2	1.1	0.2	1.9	1.1	0.5	1.9	1.6	2.0	2.7	2.2	4.0	3.9	2.1	0.5	2.7
3	1.2	0.4	2.0	1.2	1.0	2.1	1.7	2.5	2.9	2.3	4.5	4.2	2.4	1.0	3.2
4	1.3	0.6	2.1	1.3	1.5	2.3	1.8	3.0	3.1	2.4	5.5	4.6	2.7	1.5	3.6
5	1.4	0.8	2.2	1.4	2.0	2.5	1.9	3.5	3.4	2.5	6.0	5.0	3.3	2.0	4.1
6	1.5	1.0	2.3	1.5	2.5	2.7	2.0	4.0	3.6	2.6	7.0	5.5	3.3	2.5	4.6
7	1.6	1.2	2.5	1.6	3.0	2.9	2.1	4.5	3.9	2.7	7.5	5.8	3.6	3.0	5.2
8	1.7	1.4	2.6	1.7	3.5	3.1	2.2	5.0	4.2	2.8	8.5	6.4	3.9	3.5	6.1
9	1.8	1.6	2.8	1.8	4.0	3.4	2.3	5.5	4.5	2.9	9.0	6.8	4.2	4.0	7.3
10	1.9	1.8	2.9	1.9	4.5	3.6	2.4	6.0	4.8	3.0	10.0	7.4	4.5	4.5	8.4
11	2.0	2.0	3.1	2.0	5.0	3.9	2.5	6.5	5.1	3.1	10.5	7.8	4.8	5.0	9.5
12	2.1	2.2	3.2	2.1	5.5	4.2	2.6	7.0	5.5	3.2	11.5	8.5	5.1	5.5	10.6
13	2.2	2.4	3.4	2.2	6.0	4.5	2.7	7.5	5.8	3.3	12.0	8.9	5.4	6.0	11.5
14	2.3	2.6	3.6	2.3	6.5	4.8	2.8	8.0	6.2	3.4	13.0	9.7	5.7	6.5	12.2
15	2.4	2.8	3.8	2.4	7.0	5.1	2.9	8.5	6.6	3.5	13.5	10.1	6.0	7.0	13.0
16	2.5	3.0	3.9	2.5	7.5	5.5	3.0	9.0	7.0	3.6	14.5	10.9	6.3	7.5	13.8
17	2.6	3.2	4.1	2.6	8.0	5.8	3.1	9.5	7.4	3.7	15.0	11.4	6.6	8.0	14.7
18	2.7	3.4	4.3	2.7	8.5	6.2	3.2	10.0	7.8	3.8	16.0	12.2	6.9	8.5	15.5
19	2.8	3.6	4.5	2.8	9.0	6.6	3.3	10.5	8.3	3.9	16.5	12.6	7.2	9.0	16.4
20	2.9	3.8	4.7	2.9	9.5	7.0	3.4	11.0	8.7	4.0	17.5	13.3	7.5	9.5	17.3

METs, Metabolic equivalents.
*Stages are each 30 seconds in duration.

accommodate a wide range of fitness levels. Table 15.3 provides examples of such protocols. The American College of Sports Medicine (ACSM)[2] details a variety of treadmill and cycle ergometer testing protocols.

Exercise tests may be submaximal or maximal relative to the patient's effort. In addition to common indications for stopping the exercise test (Table 15.4), submaximal exercise testing has a predetermined endpoint, often defined as a peak HR (e.g., 120 beats/min or 70% of predicted maximum HR) or an arbitrary MET level (e.g., 5 METs). Submaximal tests are used in patients early after MI before discharge from the hospital because they can provide prognostic information to guide management. They can also be useful in the evaluation of a patient's ability to engage in daily activities after discharge and can serve as a baseline for cardiac rehabilitative exercise therapy (see "Physical Activity and Exercise Prescription"). Symptom-limited tests are designed to continue until the patient demonstrates signs and/or symptoms necessitating termination of exercise (see Table 15.4). Whatever modality or protocol is used, standard patient monitoring and measurements are made during and early after exercise (Table 15.5).

TREADMILL

Treadmill testing provides a more common form of physiologic stress (i.e., walking) in which patients are more likely to attain a higher oxygen uptake and peak HR than during stationary cycling. Cycling may be preferable when orthopedic or other specific patient characteristics limit treadmill testing or during exercise echocardiographic testing to facilitate acquisition of images at peak exercise. The most frequently used stepped treadmill protocols are the Naughton, Bruce, and modified Bruce (Table 15.6).[3]

During treadmill exercise, patients should be encouraged to walk freely and use the handrails for balance only when necessary. Excessive handrail gripping and support alter the BP response and decrease the oxygen requirement (METs) per given

TABLE 15.4 Indications for Terminating the Exercise Test

Absolute Indications

- ST elevation (>1.0 mm) in leads without Q waves due to prior MI (other than aVR, aVL, or V1)
- Drop in systolic BP of >10 mm Hg, despite an increase in workload, when accompanied by any other evidence of ischemia
- Moderate to severe angina
- Central nervous system symptoms (e.g., ataxia, dizziness, or near syncope)
- Signs of poor perfusion (cyanosis or pallor)
- Sustained ventricular tachycardia or other arrhythmia that interferes with normal maintenance of cardiac output during exercise
- Technical difficulties monitoring the ECG or systolic BP
- Patient's request to stop

Relative Indications

- Marked ST displacement (horizontal or downsloping of >2 mm) in a patient with suspected ischemia
- Drop in systolic BP of >10 mm Hg (persistently below baseline) despite an increase in workload, in the absence of other evidence of ischemia
- Increasing chest pain
- Fatigue, shortness of breath, wheezing, leg cramps, or claudication
- Arrhythmias other than sustained ventricular tachycardia, including multifocal ectopy, ventricular triplets, supraventricular tachycardia, atrioventricular heart block, or bradyarrhythmias
- Exaggerated hypertensive response (systolic blood pressure >250 mm Hg and/or diastolic blood pressure >115 mm Hg)
- Development of bundle branch block that cannot be distinguished from ventricular tachycardia

BP, Blood pressure; ECG, electrocardiogram; MI, myocardial infarction.
From Fletcher GF, Ades PA, Kligfield P, et al. Exercise standards for testing and training: a scientific statement from the American Heart Association. Circulation. 2013;128:873–934.

workload, thereby resulting in an overestimation of exercise capacity and an inaccurate HR-and BP-to-workload relationship. Exercise capacity (peak METs) can be estimated for treadmill exercise by using data provided by ACSM,[3] as long as the equipment is calibrated regularly. When precise determination of oxygen uptake is necessary, such as assessment of patients for heart transplantation (see Chapter 60), evaluation by expired gas analysis is preferred over estimation (see "Cardiopulmonary Exercise Testing"). Normal values for exercise capacity in healthy adults at different ages are available and may serve as a useful reference in the evaluation of a patient's exercise capacity.[3]

TABLE 15.5 Patient Monitoring During Exercise Testing

During the Exercise Period
- 12-lead ECG during last minute of each stage, or at least every 3 min
- Blood pressure during last minute of each stage, or at least every 3 min
- Symptom rating scales as appropriate for the test indication and lab protocol

During the Recovery Period
- Monitoring for a minimum of six minutes after exercise in sitting or supine position, or until near baseline heart rate, blood pressure, ECG and symptom measures are reached. A period of active cool-down may be included in the recovery period, particularly following high levels of exercise in order to minimize the post-exercise hypotensive effects of venous pooling in the lower extremities.
- 12-lead ECG every minute
- Heart rate and blood pressure immediately after exercise, then every one or two minutes thereafter until near-baseline measures are reached.
- Symptomatic ratings every minute as long as they persist after exercise. Patients should be observed until all symptoms have resolved or returned to baseline levels.

ECG, Electrocardiogram.

TABLE 15.6 Bruce Protocol for Treadmill Testing

STAGE	TIME	SPEED (MPH)	GRADE (%)	METS
REST	00.00	0.0	0.0	1.0
1	03.00	1.7	10.0	4.6
2	03.00	2.5	12.0	7.0
3	03.00	3.4	14.0	10.1
4	03.00	4.2	16.0	12.9
5	03.00	5.0	18.0	15.1
6	03.00	5.5	20.0	16.9
7	03.00	6.0	22.0	19.2

METS, metabolic equivalents.
Modified Bruce Protocol employs two initial low level 3–min stages at a speed of 1.7 mph and grades 0% and 5%, respectively, and then continues into the full Bruce protocol.
Data from American College of Sports Medicine Guidelines for Exercise Testing and Prescription. 10th ed. Philadelphia: Wolters Kluwer; 2018.

STATIONARY CYCLE

A cycle ergometer is smaller, quieter, and less expensive than a treadmill. Because a cycle ergometer requires less movement of the arms and thorax, quality electrocardiographic recordings and BP measurements are easier to obtain. However, stationary cycling may be unfamiliar to many patients, and its success as a testing tool is highly dependent on patient skill and motivation. Thus, the test may end before the patient reaches a true cardiopulmonary endpoint. Unlike treadmill testing, in which the work being performed involves movement of the patient's body weight at a given pace, stationary cycle work involves cycling at a given pace against an external force and is generally independent of the patient's body weight, which is supported by the seat. As shown in Table 15.7, the MET level attained at a given work rate varies with the patient's body weight. Accordingly, at the same given cycle ergometer work rate, a lighter person will attain higher METs than will a heavier person. Mechanically braked ergometers require that the patient's cycling speed be kept constant. Electronically braked cycle ergometers automatically adjust external resistance to the cycling speed to maintain a constant work rate at a given stage. Electronically braked cycle ergometers allow simple programming of ramp protocols. As with treadmill ramp protocols, customized cycle ergometer ramp protocols that accommodate a wide range of fitness levels need to be established by individual exercise testing laboratories.

ARM CYCLE ERGOMETRY

Arm ergometry is an alternative method of exercise testing for patients who cannot perform leg exercise. Although this test has diagnostic usefulness, it has been largely replaced by nonexercise pharmacologic stress techniques.

SIX-MINUTE WALK TEST

The 6-minute walk test can be used as a surrogate measure of exercise capacity when standard treadmill or cycle testing is not available. Distance walked is the primary outcome of the test. It is not useful in the objective determination of myocardial ischemia and is best used in a serial manner to evaluate changes in exercise capacity and the response to interventions that may affect exercise capacity over time. The 6-minute walk test protocol is discussed in detail elsewhere (Table 15.8).[4]

CARDIOPULMONARY EXERCISE TESTING (EXERCISE TESTING WITH GAS EXCHANGE ANALYSIS)

Because of the inaccuracies associated with estimating oxygen uptake ($\dot{V}O_2$) and METs from work rate with the treadmill or cycle ergometer, many laboratories perform cardiopulmonary exercise testing (CPX), which uses ventilatory gas exchange analysis during exercise to provide a more reliable and reproducible measure of $\dot{V}O_2$. Peak $\dot{V}O_2$ is the most accurate measure of exercise capacity and is a useful reflection of overall cardiopulmonary health. Measurement of expired gases is not necessary for all clinical exercise testing, but the additional information can provide important physiologic data that can be useful in both clinical and research applications. Measures of gas exchange primarily include $\dot{V}O_2$, carbon dioxide output ($\dot{V}CO_2$), and minute ventilation. Use of these variables in graphic form provides further information on the ventilatory threshold and ventilatory efficiency.[5]

CPX is well established as useful in the following situations:
- Evaluation of exercise capacity in selected patients with heart failure, to assist in estimation of prognosis, evaluate the response to medications and other interventions, and assess the need for cardiac transplantation.

TABLE 15.7 Approximate MET Levels During Cycle Ergometer Testing

BODY WEIGHT		EXERCISE RATE (KP • M • MIN⁻¹ AND WATTS)						
KP	LB	KPMS 300 WATTS 50	450 / 75	600 / 100	750 / 125	900 / 150	1050 / 175	1200 / 200
50	110	5.1	6.9	8.6	10.3	12.0	13.7	15.4
60	132	4.3	5.7	7.1	8.6	10.0	11.4	12.9
70	154	3.7	4.9	6.1	7.3	8.6	9.8	11.0
80	176	3.2	4.3	5.4	6.4	7.5	8.6	9.6
90	198	2.9	3.8	4.8	5.7	6.7	7.6	8.6
100	220	2.6	3.4	4.3	5.1	6.0	6.9	7.7

Kpm, kilopond-meter; *METs*, metabolic equivalents.
Data from *American College of Sports Medicine Guidelines for Exercise Testing and Prescription*. 9th ed. Philadelphia: Lippincott, Williams & Wilkins, 2013.

- Evaluation of exertional dyspnea. Such testing can provide useful information for differentiating cardiac from pulmonary limitations as a cause of exercise-induced dyspnea or impaired exercise capacity when the cause is uncertain.
- Evaluation of the patient's response to specific therapeutic interventions (e.g., medications; programmed pacing; cardiac rehabilitation) in which improvement in exercise tolerance is an important goal or endpoint.

Emerging evidence demonstrates that CPX can provide valuable clinical information in patients with hypertrophic cardiomyopathy (HCM), suspected or confirmed pulmonary hypertension, suspected myocardial ischemia, suspected mitochondrial myopathy, and confirmed chronic obstructive pulmonary disease or interstitial lung disease. More recently, utility of CPX has been demonstrated in the assessment of perioperative risk and valvular heart disease.

The technical aspects of CPX have become simplified with contemporary metabolic carts, but meticulous maintenance and calibration of these systems are required for optimal use. The personnel involved in administering and interpreting the test must be trained and proficient in this technique. The test also requires additional time, as well as patient cooperation. CPX used in combination with Doppler echocardiography can provide complementary information regarding cardiac output, myocardial contractile function, and valvular function.[5]

Exercise Test Supervision

Over the past 30 years since the American Heart Association (AHA) published its first set of *Standards for Adult Exercise Testing Laboratories*, the role of the physician in ensuring that the exercise laboratory is properly equipped and appropriately staffed with qualified personnel who adhere to a written set of policies and procedures specific to that laboratory has not changed. In subsequent iterations of their respective guidelines, the AHA, ACSM, American College of Cardiology (ACC), and American Association of Cardiovascular and Pulmonary Rehabilitation (AACVPR) have consistently addressed this issue. In 2000 the ACC/AHA/American College of Physicians/American College of Sports Medicine Competency Task Force focused its efforts on outlining the specific cognitive and training requirements for personnel involved in supervising and interpreting exercise ECGs and was the first to look beyond the specific professional type (e.g., physician, nurse, exercise physiologist) and focus on specific competencies of the individual staff member (see "Classic References"). In 2014 these recommendations were updated to define further the roles of each staff member involved with exercise testing.[6] This statement clearly defined different levels of supervision as follows: (1) "personal supervision" requires a physician's presence in the room; (2) "direct supervision" requires a physician to be in the immediate vicinity, on the premises or the floor, and available for emergencies; and (3) "general supervision" requires the physician to be available by phone or by page. Common to every guideline is the recommendation that patients be screened before exercise testing to assess their risk for an exercise-related adverse event, so that the most appropriate personnel to supervise the test can be provided. Exercise testing may be supervised by nonphysician staff members who are deemed competent according to the criteria outlined in the ACC/AHA statement.[6] In all such cases the physician should be immediately available to assist as needed (i.e., provide direct supervision). In high-risk patients the physician should personally supervise the test (i.e., provide personal supervision).

Risks of Exercise Testing

Exercise is associated with increased risk for an adverse cardiovascular event, and details regarding the safety of exercise testing and emergency preparedness in exercise laboratories are addressed in depth in guidelines from the AHA[1,5] and the ACSM.[3] Nonetheless, the safety of exercise testing is well documented, and the overall risk for adverse events is quite low. In several large series of individuals with and without known CVD, the rate of major complications (including MI and other events requiring hospitalization) was less than 1 to as high as 5 per 10,000 tests, and the rate of death was less than 0.5 per 10,000 tests. The incidence of adverse events depends on the study population. Patients with recent MI, reduced LV systolic function, exertion-induced myocardial ischemia, and serious ventricular arrhythmias are at highest risk.[1,7] A report of 5060 CPX studies performed in patients with severe functional impairment and a variety of high-risk cardiac diseases, including heart failure, HCM, pulmonary hypertension, and aortic stenosis, further supports the safety of exercise testing. The adverse event rate was 0.16%, and the most common adverse event was sustained ventricular tachycardia (VT). No fatal events were reported.[8]

Maintenance of appropriate emergency equipment, establishment of an emergency plan, and regular practice in carrying out the plan are fundamental to ensuring safety in an exercise testing laboratory (see "Classic References").

EXERCISE TESTING IN CORONARY ARTERY DISEASE

Exercise-Induced Symptoms

Any chest pain produced during the exercise test needs to be factored into the exercise test conclusion and report.

First, are the symptoms reported during the test the same or similar to the reported historical symptoms that prompted the exercise test? If the answer is yes, the provider can assess the objective test responses and discern whether they support the presence of CAD. If the answer is no, differences between the produced and historical symptoms need to be clarified. In addition, the symptoms produced need to be categorized according to whether they are consistent with angina. Distinguishing anginal from nonanginal chest pain is important at the time of occurrence of the chest pain. Angina is not well localized, pleuritic, or associated with palpable tenderness (see Chapters 13 and 35), and the only opportunity to define these qualities may be at the exercise test.

Second, exercise-induced angina is an important clinical predictor of the presence and severity of CAD, equal to or greater than ST-segment depression. Consideration of limiting versus nonlimiting chest pain, in addition to any induced angina, has been incorporated into the Duke Treadmill Score, as well as into other treadmill scores (see later). These factors will have an impact on the prognostic and diagnostic assessment of the test results, and ultimately the next step in the clinical evaluation.

Third, exercise-induced typical angina predicts an adverse prognosis and is worthy of further evaluation regardless of the ST-segment response or the exercise capacity. In a series of 3270 patients without

TABLE 15.8 Six Minute Walk Test Protocol

Testing Site

The Six Minute Walk Test Protocol should be performed indoors, along a long, flat, straight, enclosed corridor with a hard surface that is seldom traveled. The walking course must be 30 m in length. A 100-ft (30.4 m) hallway is required and its length should be marked every 3 m. The turnaround points should be marked with a cone (such as an orange traffic cone). A starting line, which marks the beginning and end of each 60-m lap, should be marked on the floor using brightly colored tape.

Measurements

Assemble all necessary equipment (lap counter, timer, clipboard, worksheet) and move to the starting point. Set the lap counter to zero and the timer to 6 min. Position the patient at the starting line. You should also stand near the starting line during the test. Do not walk with the patient. As soon as the patient starts to walk, start the timer. Do not talk to anyone during the walk. Use an even tone of voice when using the standard phrases of encouragement. Each time the patient returns to the starting line, click the lap counter once (or mark the lap on the worksheet). At the end of 6 min, tell the patient to stop walking, and measure the total distance traveled (meters). Heart rate, blood pressure and oxygen saturation should be measured at rest and at the end of exercise as well. The main outcome of this test is total distance traveled.

Patient Instructions

Standardized scripted patient instructions should be used, and are provided elsewhere

Data from American Thoracic Society: ATS statement: Guidelines for the six-minute walk test. *Am J Respir Crit Care Med.* 2002;166:111.

known coronary disease referred for exercise testing, Christman and colleagues[9] found that typical angina defined by physicians and exercise physiologists at the exercise test was a predictor of adverse events, including death, nonfatal MI, and revascularization. This was found irrespective of the presence or absence of a positive ST-segment response or good exercise capacity.

Lastly, if the patient stops exercise earlier than anticipated because of dyspnea, careful consideration should be given as to whether an anginal equivalent is present. If the presenting symptom was dyspnea with exertion, this becomes even more relevant.

Functional Capacity

Functional capacity is a strong predictor of mortality and nonfatal cardiovascular outcomes in both men and women with and without CAD.[10] Even though exercise capacity is most accurately measured by CPX, a reasonable estimate can be obtained from treadmill testing alone. The best methods for estimating predicted METs are the following simple regression equations.[1]

$$\text{Men: Predicted METs} = 18 - (0.15 \times \text{Age})$$

$$\text{Women: Predicted METs} = 14.7 - (0.13 \times \text{Age})$$

The reported exercise time can be translated into METs or METs based on the exercise test protocol. The reported METs can then be expressed as a percentage of the predicted METs. Table 15.9 provides an alternative qualitative classification of functional capacity that adjusts for age and sex.

In addition to clinical factors, functional capacity can be related to familiarity with the exercise equipment, level of training, and environmental conditions in the exercise laboratory. Patients who cannot adequately perform an exercise test or who undergo a pharmacologic stress test have a worse prognosis than do those who can perform an exercise test.[9]

Functional capacity should always be incorporated into the results, conclusions, and/or recommendations of the exercise test report. Functional capacity can be incorporated into available multivariable scores such as the Duke Treadmill Score or the Cleveland Clinic Prognostic Score to classify the prognosis as low, intermediate, or high risk (see Prognostic Value).

HEART RATE RESPONSES
Peak Heart Rate

The maximum HR with exercise is a fundamental physiologic parameter that provides the clinician relevant information concerning the intensity of exercise, the adequacy of the exercise test, the effect of medications that influence HR, the potential contribution to exercise intolerance, and the patient's prognosis.[11] The maximum achievable HR (HRmax) is unique for each patient but can be estimated by using regression equations that adjust for the patient's age. The most familiar equation, which was developed principally in middle-aged men, is:

$$\text{HRmax} = 220 - \text{Age}$$

Although easy to apply and calculate, there is considerable variability with this equation, especially in patients with CAD who are taking beta blockers. Newer equations[3] have been proposed to more accurately replace the "220 − age" rule to generate the maximum age-predicted HR (MPHR):

$$\text{Men: HRmax} = 208 - (0.7 \times \text{Age})$$

$$\text{Women: HRmax} = 206 - (0.88 \times \text{Age})$$

Chronotropic Incompetence

The inability of the heart to increase its rate to meet the demand placed on it is termed chronotropic incompetence. It is considered an independent predictor of cardiac or all-cause mortality, as well as other adverse cardiovascular outcomes.[11]

A *submaximal* study is assigned when the peak HR achieved is below the MPHR. An *inadequate* study is defined by failure to achieve a predefined goal, such as 85% of MPHR. If a patient without known CAD has an inadequate study, the term *nondiagnostic* study is often applied. As usual, this "nondiagnostic" status is relative. In the presence of any other diagnostic endpoints, such as 2-mm or greater ST-segment depression, exercise-induced hypotension, or exercise-induced anginal chest pain, the HR adequacy question becomes irrelevant.

Chronotropic incompetence typically has been defined by the adjusted HR reserve, incorporates both resting and peak HRs, as well as the age-adjusted HRmax. However, before "chronotropic incompetence" is applied, consideration should be given to the effort exerted in performing exercise, present medications, in particular beta blockers, and the reason for termination of the exercise test. Effort applied to the exercise is often defined by the symptoms produced or by indices of perceived exertion (e.g., Borg scale).[1,3] These work well in most settings but can also be defined quantitatively by using CPX parameters such as the respiratory exchange ratio. For the usual non-CPX application, the following formula defines the chronotropic index:

$$[(\text{HRmax} - \text{HRrest}) / (220 - \text{Age} - \text{HRrest})] \times 100$$

Failure to achieve a chronotropic index higher than 80% defines the presence of chronotropic incompetence and this predicts a poor prognosis.[11] Criteria for assessing chronotropic incompetence in patients with atrial fibrillation (AF) have not been established.

Heart Rate Recovery

The HR increases during exercise because of an increase in sympathetic tone and a decrease in vagal tone. At the cessation of exercise, under

TABLE 15.9 Estimated Functional Capacity Relative to Age and Sex

	ESTIMATED FUNCTIONAL CAPACITY (METS)				
AGE (YR)	POOR	FAIR	AVERAGE	GOOD	HIGH
Women					
≤29	<7.5	8–10	10–13	13–16	>16
30–39	<7	7–9	9–11	11–15	>15
40–49	<6	6–8	8–10	10–14	>14
50–59	<5	5–7	7–9	9–13	>13
≥60	<4.5	4.5–6	6–8	8–11.5	>11.5
Men					
≤29	<8	8–11	11–14	14–17	>17
30–39	<7.5	7.5–10	10–12.5	12.5–16	>16
40–49	<7	7–8.5	8.5–11.5	11.5–15	>15
50–59	<6	6–8	8–11	11–14	>14
≥60	<5.5	5.5–7	7–9.5	9.5–13	>13

METs, metabolic equivalents (1 MET = 3.5 mL/kg/min of oxygen consumption).
From Snader CE, Marwick TH, Pashkow FJ, et al. Importance of estimated functional capacity as a predictor of all-cause mortality among patients referred for exercise thallium single-photon emission computed tomography: Report of 3,400 patients from a single center. *J Am Coll Cardiol*. 1997;30:641–648.

normal circumstances, the reverse process occurs. In athletes and normal persons, there is a biexponential response, with an initial steep 30-second fall in HR followed by a shallower decline thereafter. This biexponential response disappears with the administration of atropine and becomes similar to the response in patients with heart failure. Thus, the initial steep phase is due to parasympathetic activation. Abnormal *HR recovery* (HRR) has been defined by many methods, but the most commonly accepted include less than 12 beats/min decrement after 1 minute with post-exercise slow walking cool-down, less than 18 beats/min after 1 minute with immediate cessation of movement into either the supine or sitting position, and less than 22 beats/min after 2 minutes. In healthy individuals, short-term reproducibility has been demonstrated (see "Classic References").

Abnormal HRR is associated with an increase in all-cause mortality in both asymptomatic individuals and patients with established heart disease.[12] This association is independent of the chronotropic index, beta blockade, CAD severity, LV function, Duke Treadmill Score, and ST-segment depression. HRR adds to the prognostic ability of peak $\dot{V}o_2$. When considered in a multivariable format assessing prognosis, HRR has been found to be an independent predictor of adverse outcomes even when combined with nuclear variables.[13]

BLOOD PRESSURE RESPONSES
Exercise BP responses, as with those for HR, reflect the balance between sympathetic and parasympathetic influences. Systolic BP, pulse pressure (difference between systolic and diastolic BP), HR-BP product (also called the *double product*), and double-product reserve (change in double product from peak to rest) all increase steadily as work rate increases. Diastolic BP increases only minimally or may fall. In most normal individuals, systolic BP will increase to well above 140 mm Hg and the double product to higher than 20,000.

Hypertensive Systolic Pressure Response
This response is usually defined as greater than 210 mm Hg in men and greater than 190 mm Hg in women. Even though these exercise responses are considered abnormal, they are not generally reasons to terminate exercise. Such responses may be indicative of the future development of hypertension or adverse cardiac events.[14]

Exercise-Induced Systolic Hypotension
This has been variably defined but most frequently as systolic pressure during exercise falling below resting systolic pressure.[1] Another definition is a 20 mm Hg fall after an initial rise. Either of these definitions would be an absolute reason to terminate the exercise test. The former definition is more predictive of a poor prognosis and is often related to severe multivessel CAD with LV dysfunction, especially when noted with other signs of ischemia, such as ST depression or angina at a low workload. Its positive predictive value (PPV) is higher in men than in women. Its presence usually warrants consideration of prompt invasive evaluation. Exercise-associated hypotension may also be seen in patients with cardiomyopathy, LV outflow tract obstruction, enhanced vagal tone, hypovolemia, antihypertensive medications, and arrhythmias. In addition, one study of 57,442 patients suggests that exercise-induced hypotension may be a predictor of future AF.[15]

One systolic BP response that needs to be appreciated might be called "pseudo–exercise-induced hypotension." This response occurs in patients who are anxious about the exercise study and begin exercise with a somewhat elevated systolic pressure. As exercise proceeds in the first stage, this elevated BP usually settles down or "falls" toward its customary resting level and the patient looks well. As exercise continues, continued observation reveals a gradual upward trend in BP. Considerable judgment needs to be used when interpreting this response.

Blunted Systolic Pressure Peak
A normal rise in systolic BP is approximately 10 mm Hg per MET increase. A blunted BP rise during exercise may be due to cardioactive medications, or may indicate underlying heart conditions that limit the normal increase in cardiac output during exercise (e.g., cardiomyopathy; aortic stenosis).[3]

ST-Segment Changes
For decades, the change in ST segments was the principal factor considered in the analysis of exercise ECG results (Fig. 15.3). However, the diagnostic value of ST-segment depression has been recognized to be only moderately helpful by current noninvasive test standards, with a sensitivity and specificity of 60% to 70% and 70% to 80%, respectively, based on coronary angiography. When adjusted for referral or workup bias, its sensitivity is lower (45% to 50%) and specificity higher (85% to 90%).[1] Accordingly, the overall prognostic value of ST-segment changes has been appropriately placed behind the prognostic value of non–ST-segment variables, such as functional capacity and HR responses. Despite these issues, it is still appropriate to consider ST-segment changes, but only in the context of other clinical and non–ST-segment data.

ST Depression
When considering ST-segment depression, it is important to use standards that allow application of uniform criteria. The usual criterion applied to raw data is 1 mm or greater or 0.1 mV or greater of horizontal or downsloping (i.e., <0.5 mV/sec) ST-segment depression in three consecutive beats.[3] This assumes that the PQ point (not the TP segment) is used as the isoelectric reference and that the point of ST-segment measurement is 60 to 80 milliseconds after the J point. The 60-millisecond post–J point criterion is used at HR higher than 130 beats/min. This criterion should be added to and not included with existing resting ST-segment depression. ST-segment changes in the presence of early repolarization should be measured from the isoelectric line and not the baseline ST elevation. Unlike ST-segment elevation, exercise-induced ST-segment depression does not localize ischemia to a precise region or vascular bed. The lateral precordial leads (especially lead V_5) are the best for defining positive responses. However, the inferior leads can be helpful in assessing the extent of ischemia when the lateral leads are abnormal as well. Isolated inferior ST depression is frequently falsely abnormal because of the influence of atrial repolarization in these leads.

Although raw data should always be examined, the use of signal-averaged data can be useful, especially when moderate baseline wandering or motion artifact is present. Particular care must be taken to avoid signal averaging that incorporates gross distortions as a result of motion and transient ventricular aberrations such as premature ventricular contractions and intraventricular conduction defects.

Post-exercise recovery responses are also important to assess. First, positive responses are occasionally limited to the recovery period, and these have equal significance to changes that occur at peak exercise. Second, positive changes during exercise that resolve within 1 minute of recovery are associated with a favorable prognosis and low downstream diagnostic test yield.[9] In addition, compared to ST changes longer than 1 minute, early-recovery ST changes are associated with significantly smaller summed stress scores on myocardial perfusion imaging and a lower prevalence of CAD.[16]

Upsloping ST Depression
Rapidly upsloping ST depression that resolves quickly is rarely a true-positive response and is less specific than horizontal or downsloping ST depression. However, ST-segment depression that is slowly upsloping (0.5 to 1.0 mV/sec) may be considered abnormal, especially if it occurs at low workloads. Its presence during exercise may presage horizontal or downsloping depression in recovery. HR adjustment can be applied to upsloping ST segments (see later).

Lead aVR ST Elevation
Emerging literature suggests that 1-mm or greater ST-segment elevation in lead aVR may be a significant predictor of left main CAD, proximal left anterior descending (LAD) artery disease, or at least multivessel CAD.[17] As an isolated marker, it appears to be sensitive, have moderate specificity, and a high negative predictive value (NPV). What is yet unclear is where it fits into the multivariate approach for assessing prognosis.

ST Adjustments
HR adjustments of ST segments have been proposed as an alternative way to analyze ST-segment depression.[1] However, comparative studies have not shown an increase in accuracy. Nevertheless, HR adjustments can be helpful for borderline cases in which ST depression is upsloping or barely abnormal, or traditional criteria and other clinical or exercise data suggest a false-positive result (e.g., low pretest probability or very high HR or workload achieved during exercise). HR adjustment

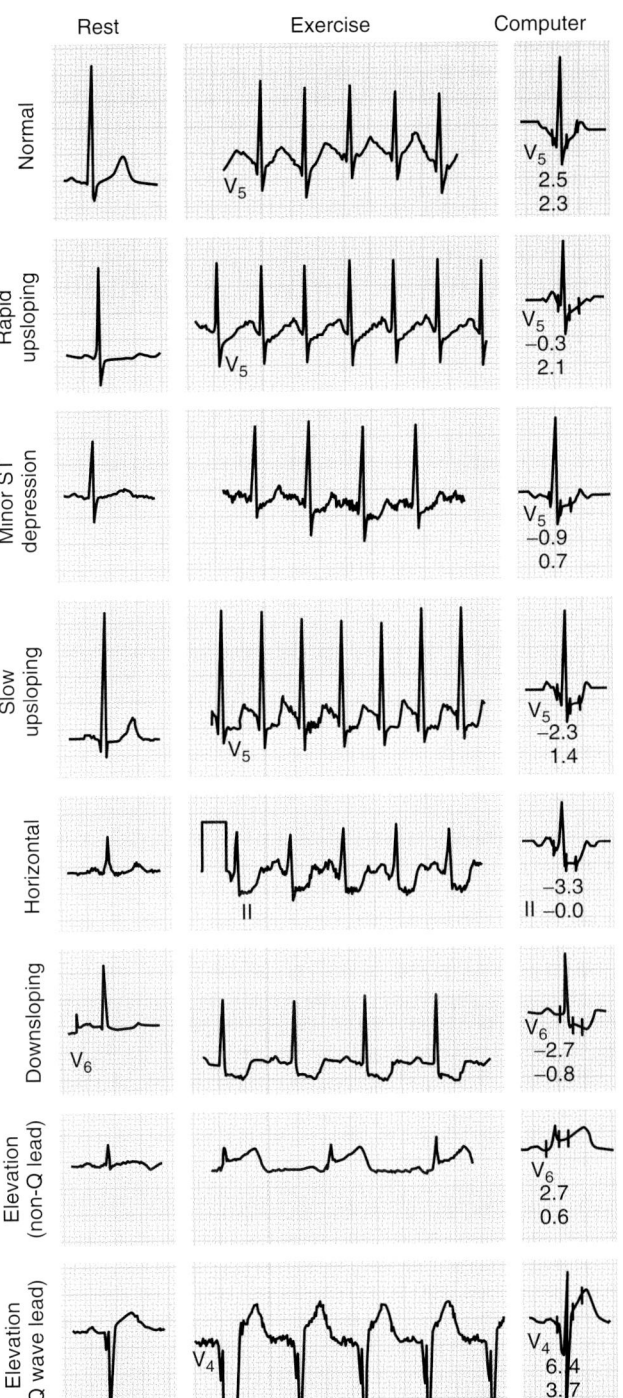

FIGURE 15.3 Eight typical exercise electrocardiographic patterns at rest and at peak exertion. The computer-processed incrementally averaged beat corresponds with the raw data taken at the same time point during exercise and is illustrated in the last column. The patterns represent worsening ECG responses during exercise. In the column of computer-averaged beats, ST80 displacement (*top number*) indicates the magnitude of ST-segment displacement 80 milliseconds after the J point relative to the PQ junction or E point. ST-segment slope measurement (*bottom number*) indicates the ST-segment slope at a fixed time point after the J point to the ST80 measurement. At least three non–computer-averaged complexes with a stable baseline should meet criteria for abnormality before the exercise ECG result can be considered abnormal. The *normal* and *rapid upsloping ST-segment* responses are normal responses to exercise. J point depression with rapid upsloping ST segments is a common response in an older, apparently healthy person. *Minor ST-segment depression* can occur occasionally at submaximal workloads in patients with coronary artery disease (CAD); in this figure, the ST segment is depressed 0.09 mV (0.9 mm) 80 milliseconds after the J point. The *slow upsloping ST-segment pattern* may suggest an ischemic response in patients with known CAD or those with a high pretest clinical risk of CAD. Criteria for slow upsloping ST-segment depression include J point and ST80 depression of 0.15 mV or more and ST-segment slope of more than 1.0 mV/sec. This pattern may also precede horizontal or downsloping ST-segment depression that will occur in recovery. *Classic criteria for myocardial ischemia* include horizontal ST-segment depression observed when both the J point and ST80 depression are 0.1 mV or more and the ST-segment slope is within the range of 1.0 mV/sec. Downsloping ST-segment depression occurs when the J point and ST80 depression are 0.1 mV or more and the ST-segment slope is –1.0 mV/sec. *ST-segment elevation in a non–Q wave noninfarct lead* occurs when the J point and ST60 are 1.0 mV or higher and represents a severe ischemic response. *ST-segment elevation in an infarct territory (Q wave lead)* indicates a severe wall motion abnormality and, in most cases, is not considered an ischemic response. (From Chaitman BR. Exercise electrocardiographic stress testing. In: Beller GA, ed. *Chronic Ischemic Heart Disease*. In: Braunwald E, series ed. *Atlas of Heart Diseases*. Vol 5. Philadelphia: Current Medicine; 1995:2.1–30.)

can be accomplished by two methods (complicated and simple). The complicated method, known as *ST/heart rate slope*, is automated and available on most stress testing machines as an option to be toggled on or off. It plots ST depression as a function of HR at numerous points during exercise and generates the terminal ST/HR slope for each lead. The criterion for abnormality is 2.4 μV/beat/min. Depending on the protocol used and the duration of exercise, the ST/HR slope will not always be calculated because of insufficient data points. The developers of the method proposed a modification of the standard Bruce protocol to increase the points available for analysis. The slightly less intensive Cornell protocol uses 2-minute rather than 3-minute stages and is useful in patients who are not anticipated to exercise beyond stage 2 of the Bruce protocol. The simple method, known as *ST/HR index*, can easily be calculated by dividing the maximum ST-segment depression in microvolts by the difference in resting and peak HR. The criterion for abnormality is 1.6 μV/beat/min.

ST Elevation

The usual criterion applied to raw data is 1 mm or greater or 0.1 mV of ST-segment elevation above the PQ point at 60 milliseconds after the J point in three consecutive beats. The J point may or may not be elevated as well. Without pathologic Q waves, exercise-induced ST elevation usually indicates either significant proximal coronary stenosis or epicardial coronary spasm. In either case the ST-segment elevation precisely localizes the transmural ischemia to a particular vascular region (e.g., anterior = LAD) and thus, coronary angiography is an appropriate next step. In most cases, coronary angiography should be performed in an expedited fashion. In contrast, when pathologic Q waves are present, ST-segment elevation is usually indicative of an LV aneurysm or significant wall motion change. Ischemia may be involved in this process, and myocardial perfusion imaging is generally required to determine this.

OTHER ELECTROCARDIOGRAM CHANGES
QRS Duration

During exercise there is a normal shortening of the QRS complex, as well as the PR and QT intervals. Exercise-induced bundle branch block (BBB) is rare and occurs at a frequency of 0.5% or less. Exercise-induced left BBB (EI-LBBB) has been reported.[1] When EI-LBBB occurs at HRs higher than 125 beats/min, this finding is not likely to reflect underlying CAD. However, the incidence of CAD does increase when EI-LBBB occurs at progressively lower HRs. One study suggested an increased association of EI-LBBB with death and major cardiac events.[18] The ST-segment changes before onset of the LBBB are still interpretable, but they become uninterpretable once the LBBB begins. Onset and offset of the LBBB usually occur at different HRs.

In contrast, exercise-induced right BBB (EI-RBBB) from one recent large Veterans Affairs series correlated with age, and was not associated with added incremental risk.[19] Limited data are available in women. EI-RBBB does not invalidate interpretation of the ST segment for the inferior (II, III, aVf) and lateral leads (V_5, V_6). However, ST-segment changes limited to V_1 to V_4 are nondiagnostic.

Exercise-Induced Rhythm Changes

Ventricular ectopic activity is noted in up to 20% of patients during exercise testing. It varies from isolated ventricular premature beats to nonsustained VT, to sustained VT. However, frequent ventricular ectopy, which is variably defined, occurs during exercise or recovery in only 2% to 3% of patients. Suppression of resting ventricular ectopic activity during exercise is essentially a normal finding that can occur with or without CAD. In clinical populations referred for testing because of symptoms, ventricular ectopic activity during exercise was predictive of mortality in most studies.[20] In addition, ventricular ectopic beats occurring during exercise or recovery increase the likelihood of future cardiac death.[1]

Exercise-induced supraventricular arrhythmias are not predictive of ischemia or any cardiovascular endpoint. However, they may be a marker for the later occurrence of AF or supraVT.

Pharmacologic Influences on Interpretation
Digitalis Glycosides

That digitalis can have an adverse effect on ST-segment interpretation is generally common knowledge. The principal issue has been false-positive results and reduced specificity. The absence of ST-segment change at rest does not eliminate the effect occurring during exercise. Sensitivity is not affected by digitalis. Therefore, a negative ST-segment response with digitalis is still reliable. For most patients taking digitalis, stress imaging is appropriate as an initial test if the goal of the test is to assess for myocardial ischemia.

Beta Adrenoreceptor Blockers

Beta blockers clearly reduce the rate-pressure product in most patients receiving adequate doses. Evidence indicates that the diagnostic sensitivity and NPV of exercise testing are adversely affected.

For those without established CAD who are undergoing a diagnostic-level exercise ECG, beta blockers should ideally be withheld to allow an adequate HR response. For those undergoing supplemental stress imaging, the issue is less critical given the availability of conversion to pharmacologic stress if the patient fails to achieve the desired HR response.

For those with established CAD, the situation is less clear and it depends on the indication for the stress test. For most patients with CAD, beta blockers are part of their standard medical therapy and have significant effects on both quality and quantity of life (i.e., their prognosis). Therefore, many laboratories do not discontinue these medications. Discontinuing beta blockers in patients with CAD creates a clinical state that is unlike their usual day-to-day existence. We are unaware of any reported studies in patients with established CAD indicating that beta blockers adversely affected the ability of exercise testing (with or without imaging) to detect prognostically important myocardial ischemia such that it would have significantly altered their clinical management. Therefore, discontinuation of beta blockers before exercise testing may be left to the discretion of the referring provider.

Diagnostic Value
Sensitivity and Specificity (see also Chapter 10)

Table 15.10 outlines the diagnostic characteristics of stress testing. Sensitivity and specificity define how effectively a test discriminates individuals with disease from those without disease. *Sensitivity* is the percentage of individuals with a disease who have abnormal test results and, in the case of CAD, is influenced by disease severity, effort level, and the use of anti-ischemic drugs. *Specificity* is the percentage of those without disease who have normal test results, and it may be affected by resting ECG patterns (e.g., LV hypertrophy, ST-T abnormalities, interventricular conduction delay) and drugs such as digoxin or flecainide. All tests have a range of inversely related sensitivities and specificities such that when sensitivity is the highest, specificity is lowest, and vice versa. These can be affected by specifying a *discriminant* or diagnostic cut point. The standard exercise test cut point of 0.1 mV

TABLE 15.10 Diagnostic Characteristics of the Exercise Electrocardiogram Test

TERM	DEFINITION
True-positive (TP)	Abnormal test result in individual with disease
False-positive (FP)	Abnormal test result in individual without disease
True-negative (TN)	Normal test result in individual without disease
False-negative (FN)	Normal test result in individual with disease
Sensitivity	Percentage of patients with CAD who have an abnormal result = TP/(TP + FN)
Specificity	Percentage of patients without CAD who have a normal result = TN/(TN + FP)
Predictive value of a positive test	Percentage of patients with an abnormal result who have CAD = TP/(TP + FP)
Predictive value of a negative test	Percentage of patients with a normal result who do not have CAD = TN/(TN + FN)
Test accuracy	Percentage of true test results = (TP + TN)/total number tests performed

Modified from Chaitman BR. Exercise stress testing. In Bonow RO, Mann DL, Zipes DP, Libby P, eds. *Braunwald's Heart Disease*. 9th ed. Philadelphia: WB Saunders: 2012.

(1 mm) of horizontal or downsloping ST-segment depression in three consecutive beats of at least a single lead has been selected as the discriminating cut point and has a sensitivity of 68% and specificity of 77% (see "Classic References").

Once a discriminant value that determines a test's specificity and sensitivity is chosen, the population tested must be considered. If the population is skewed toward individuals with a greater severity of disease, the test will have higher sensitivity. Thus the exercise test has higher sensitivity in individuals with triple-vessel disease than in those with single-vessel disease.[1] The sensitivity and specificity of stress testing are limited by the use of angiographic CAD as the diagnostic "gold standard," so most data are derived from studies in which patients underwent both exercise testing and cardiac catheterization. The data are therefore subject to workup bias, which inflates the estimated sensitivity and deflates the specificity, because patients selected for coronary arteriography are more likely to have obstructive CAD[1] and in some studies, patients with a positive test result were more likely to be referred for angiography.

The *diagnostic accuracy* of a test is the percentage of true test results (total true positives plus total true negatives) among all tests performed. Diagnostic accuracy is additionally influenced by the criteria used to determine whether an adequate level of stress has been achieved. This is currently defined as having attained 85% of the maximum age-predicted HR, with HRmax estimated as "220 – age" (see earlier, "Heart Rate Responses"). Despite many limitations in using this equation for diagnostic purposes, it remains a standard criterion for test adequacy but should not be used as a reason to terminate the test.

Positive and Negative Predictive Values

Predictive values further define the diagnostic value of a test (see Table 15.10). The predictive value of a test is heavily influenced by the prevalence of disease in the group being tested. Bayes' theorem states that the probability of a person having the disease after the test is performed is the product of the probability of the disease before testing and the probability that the test provided a true result. Thus, a test has a higher PPV and lower NPV when used in a population with a high prevalence; conversely, a higher NPV and lower PPV occur in a population with a lower prevalence. For example, an exercise ECG that demonstrates ST depression in an elderly person with typical anginal symptoms is most likely a true-positive result, whereas that in a young asymptomatic person without cardiac risk factors is most likely a false-positive result.

Pre-Test and Post-Test Probability of Disease

An important part of patient evaluation prior to exercise testing is the assessment of the pre-test probability of obstructive CAD. This can guide the clinician in deciding whether any testing is needed, and if so, what type of test might be the most helpful. This key step can affect the accuracy, yield, and cost-effectiveness of downstream diagnostic testing.[21] Table 15.11 provides a chart of the pre-test likelihood of obstructive CAD (Diamond/Forrester Score) that is contained or cited in most AHA/ACC guidelines,[22] and is widely used. It demonstrates the pretest probability of obstructive CAD based on age, sex, and symptoms. However, these data are derived from a cohort of patients who underwent diagnostic invasive coronary angiography, and as such, are subject to significant work-up bias. Hence, the probabilities listed in Table 15.11 overestimate CAD prevalence. More recently, the *CAD Consortium Clinical Score* (Fig. 15.4)[23] which is derived from data that use CT coronary angiography (≥50% stenosis) as the basis to define obstructive CAD, and take into account age, sex, type of pain, and the presence of atherosclerotic risk factors, has been shown in several studies to have significantly greater predictive accuracy regarding the likelihood of obstructive CAD than the Diamond/Forrester Score.[24] Accordingly, the CAD Consortium Clinical Score, which is now readily available (https://qxmd.com/calculate/calculator_287/pre-test-probability-of-cad-cad-consortium) can more reliably assist the clinician in pre-test patient assessment.

There are no widely used and validated calculators that assess the post-test likelihood of obstructive CAD, but several that evaluate post-test prognosis (see "Prognostic Value"). However, using exercise ST-segment criteria and knowledge of the sensitivity and specificity of the test when applied to the pre-test likelihood of disease in a given patient, the post-test likelihood of obstructive CAD can be estimated. This is further discussed in detail elsewhere.[22]

Assessment of Anatomic and Functional Extent of Disease

As discussed earlier, several factors influence the hemodynamic significance of a given coronary artery luminal stenosis, such as the length and complexity of a coronary lesion, and these factors may affect the presence and extent of myocardial ischemia relative to exercise-induced increases in myocardial oxygen demand. Furthermore, exercise-induced ST-segment depression does not provide a reliable assessment of the extent of disease or the specific coronary vessel or vessels involved. ST-segment elevation in leads without Q waves, although an uncommon response, generally reflects transmural ischemia that can be localized by the leads involved: leads V_2 to V_4 reflect LAD disease; lateral leads reflect left circumflex and diagonal vessel disease; and leads II, III, and AVF reflect right CAD (in a right-dominant circulation) (see "Classic References"). Other factors related to the probability and severity of CAD include the degree, time of appearance, duration, and number of leads with ST-segment depression or elevation. It is important to realize, however, that prognostically important CAD may be present in the absence of obstructive lesions. Therefore, the use of diagnostic ST-segment analysis alone during exercise testing is inadequate and should be done with consideration of several non–ST-segment variables, as discussed later (see "Prognostic Value").

Testing in Women

Identification of ischemic heart disease in women can be a diagnostic challenge because of several factors, including the lower prevalence of obstructive CAD in women younger than 65, more atypical manifestations of ischemic symptoms, and more frequent resting ST changes. In women with a low pre-test likelihood of CAD, exercise electrocardiographic testing results in a minimal change in assessment from pretest levels. Premenopausal women with one or fewer risk factors for CAD and with nonanginal or atypical symptoms will have a high rate of false-positive tests owing to the lower likelihood of obstructive disease in these low-risk patients. Thus, the exercise ECG in such low-risk women is of little value, except perhaps in selected cases to reassure women with atypical symptoms regarding their low likelihood of obstructive CAD when they have no exercise-induced ischemic ST changes and a low-risk Duke treadmill score.

The reported sensitivity and specificity of exercise electrocardiographic testing in symptomatic women vary greatly depending on the study characteristics and range from 31% to 71% and 66% to 86%, respectively.[25] However, exercise testing has similar diagnostic characteristics in women with an intermediate probability of CAD as it does for men. Thus, exercise testing has the greatest incremental value in intermediate-risk women, particularly when coupled with the Duke treadmill score (see "Prognostic Value"). In a series of 976 symptomatic women referred for exercise testing and coronary angiography, a low-, intermediate-, and high-risk score was associated with obstructive CAD (>75% luminal narrowing) in 19%, 35%, and 89% of women, respectively. Moreover, 2-year cardiac mortality rates in this same cohort of women with low-, moderate-, and high-risk Duke treadmill scores were 1%, 2%, and 4%, respectively. Non–ST-segment variables, including peak exercise capacity (METs), chronotropic response, HRR, and BP response, have prognostic value in women (Table 15.12),[25,26] and are most useful when incorporated into the prognostic scores discussed next. The usefulness of exercise stress testing in the assessment of ischemic heart disease in women has been reviewed and updated in detail by the AHA (Fig. 15.5).[26] The exercise ECG remains the recommended test of first choice for the assessment of symptomatic, intermediate-risk women who can exercise and have normal findings on a resting ECG. A negative and

TABLE 15.11 Pretest Likelihood of Coronary Artery Disease in Symptomatic Patients According to Age and Sex (Combined Diamond/Forrester and CASS Data)

AGE (YR)	NONANGINAL CHEST PAIN		ATYPICAL ANGINA		TYPICAL ANGINA	
	MEN	WOMEN	MEN	WOMEN	MEN	WOMEN
30–39	4	2	34	12	76	26
40–49	13	3	51	22	87	55
50–59	20	7	65	31	93	73
60–69	27	14	72	51	94	86

CASS, Coronary Artery Surgery Study.
From Fihn SD, Gardin JM, Abrams J, et al. 2012 ACCF/AHA/ACP/AATS/PCNA/SCAI/STS Guideline for the Diagnosis and Management of Patients with Stable Ischemic Heart Disease: a report of the American College of Cardiology Foundation/American Heart Association Task Force on Practice Guidelines, and the American College of Physicians, American Association for Thoracic Surgery, Preventive Cardiology Nurses Association, Society for Cardiovascular Angiography and Interventions, and Society of Thoracic Surgeons. *Circulation*. 2012;126:e354–e471.

Adapted from Diamond GA, Forrester JS. Analysis of probability as an aid in the clinical diagnosis of coronary artery disease. *N Engl J Med*. 1979;300:1350–1358; and Chaitman BR, Bourassa MG, Davis K, et al. Angiographic prevalence of high-risk coronary artery disease in patient subsets (CASS). *Circulation*. 1981;64:360–367.

Consortium prediction model to estimate presence of CAD	
Age	53
Sex (M=1, F=0)	0
Quality of chest pain (if non-specific, enter 0 for both below)	
Atypical chest pain (Yes=1, No=0)	1
Typical chest pain (Yes=1, No=0)	0
Diabetes (Yes=1, No=0)	0
HTN (Yes=1, No=0)	0
HL (Yes=1, No=0)	0
Any current or prior smoking history? (Yes=1, No=0)	0
CCS available? (Yes=1, No=0)	0
Coronary calcium score	
Probability of obstructive CAD in at least 1 vessel	Results
CAD consortium basic	5.0%
CAD consortium clinical	3.0%
Clinical + CCS	

FIGURE 15.4 CAD consortium prediction model to estimate the presence of CAD. Calculator available at https://qxmd.com/calculate/calculator_287/pre-test-probability-of-cad-cad-consortium. In this example, the calculated predicted likelihood of obstructive CAD in a 53-year-old woman with atypical chest pain, no atherosclerotic risk factors, and no available coronary artery calcium score using clinical variables is 3%. *CAD*, Coronary artery disease; *CCS*, coronary calcium score; *F*, female; *M*, male.

TABLE 15.12 Electrocardiogram and Non-Electrocardiogram Variables Associated with an Elevated Ischemic Heart Disease Risk from Exercise Testing in Women

STRESS TESTING VARIABLES	METHOD OF ASSESSMENT	HIGH-RISK VALUE
Exercise capacity	Estimated by ETT protocol (speed and grade)	<5 METs
		<100% age-predicted METs = 14.7–(0.13 × age)
HR recovery	Difference between peak HR at 1 min of recovery	≤12 bpm after 1 min recovery (upright cool-down period)
ST-segment changes	Difference in ST segment Δs (at 60 msec after the J point) between peak exercise (or recovery) and resting ECG	ST-segment depression ≥ 2 mm
		ST-segment depression ≥ 1 mm at <5 METs or >5 min into recovery
		ST-segment elevation ≥ 2 mm (not in q-wave lead or aVR)
DTS	DTS = exercise time (5× STΔ) – (4× angina index)	High-risk DTS less than or equal to –11
BP response	Assessment of BP response to exercise, change in SBP from rest to peak exercise	Decrease in SBP >10 mm Hg from rest
Ventricular arrhythmias		Persistent ventricular tachycardia/fibrillation

BP, blood pressure; *DTS*, Duke Treadmill Score; *ETT*, exercise treadmill testing; *HR*, heart rate; *METs*, metabolic equivalents; *SPB*, systolic blood pressure.
From Mieres JH, Gulati M, Bairey Merz N, et al. Role of noninvasive testing in the clinical evaluation of women with suspected ischemic heart disease: a consensus statement from the American Heart Association. *Circulation.* 2014;130:350–379.

diagnostically adequate test, particularly when associated with low risk scores, makes the likelihood of obstructive CAD very low. A positive or inconclusive test generally requires further evaluation with either a stress imaging test or coronary angiography.

Prognostic Value
Predictive Variables

The strongest predictor of prognosis derived from the exercise test is functional capacity. A weaker predictor is ST-segment depression. All other variables, such as the HR achieved, HRR, BP response, ventricular arrhythmias, and exercise-induced angina, fall between these two extremes. This prognostic hierarchy is similar in both men and women. Table 15.13 provides a summary of the available prognostic scores that use variables derived from the exercise-ECG test.

Multivariable scores are the best way to distill the relative prognostic values of many variables into a single indicator of risk that can be expressed as both continuous (e.g., 0 to 100) and ordinal variables (e.g., low, intermediate, and high). To date, three scores have been developed and validated and are worthy of consideration in analyzing exercise tests.

DUKE TREADMILL PROGNOSTIC SCORE

This score has been available since 1987 (see "Classic References") and is the most widely recognized, used, and validated score. It was cited in the 1997 and subsequent updates of the ACC/AHA exercise test guidelines. It incorporates three treadmill variables: exercise time (Bruce protocol), millimeters of any ST-segment deviation (except aVR), and angina score index (1 = nonlimiting angina and 2 = exercise-limiting angina). It is simple enough to present as the following equation:

Score = Exercise time – (5 × ST deviation) – (4 × Angina index)

ST deviation is the largest net ST-segment displacement in any lead. It is equally valid in men and women, and its prognostic value

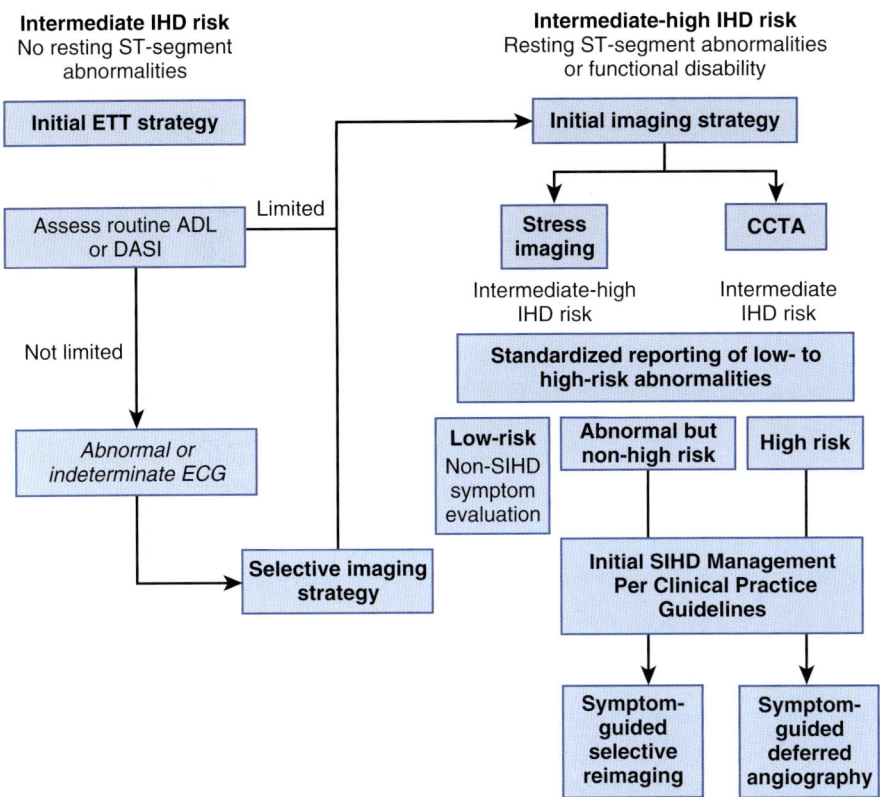

FIGURE 15.5 Diagnostic algorithm for women presenting with suspected ischemic heart disease. *ADL*, Activities of daily living; *CCTA*, coronary computed tomographic angiography; *DASI*, Duke Activity Status Index; *ETT*, exercise treadmill testing; *IHD*, ischemic heart disease; *SIHD*, stable ischemic heart disease. (From Mieres JH, Gulati M, Merz NB, et al. Role of noninvasive testing in the clinical evaluation of women with suspected ischemic heart disease: a consensus statement from the American Heart Association. *Circulation*. 2014;130:350–379.)

Investigators in Finland proposed the SCORE-exe, which included functional capacity and HR responses to exercise and recovery.[27] In a population of 1531 patients with stable CAD taking beta blockers, these three variables had significant independent prognostic value over other clinical data on cardiovascular death and heart failure admissions. This score is not yet easily applied in the clinical setting.

Park and colleagues[28] followed 898 adults without cardiac disease prospectively for up to 27 years after undergoing treadmill exercise testing. Main outcome measures were silent and overt MI. They found that ST-segment change, inability to achieve target HR, abnormal HRR, and chronotropic incompetence were independent predictors of the outcomes. An integrated scoring model using these four parameters demonstrated a stepwise increase in risk as the number of abnormal parameters increased.

Arbit and associates[13] analyzed 11,218 patients with and without CAD not receiving beta blockers and demonstrated that reduced functional capacity (<7 METs), HRR less than 22 beats after 2 minutes, and chronotropic index less than 80 added significant incremental prognostic value to myocardial perfusion imaging for cardiac death and all-cause mortality. As the number of these three abnormal treadmill variables increased, the risk of mortality increased regardless of the scan interpretation. A patient with a normal scan but two or three variables that were abnormal had the same all-cause mortality risk as a patient with a severely abnormal scan but two or three variables that were normal. This study provides a simple method to incorporate non–ST-segment variables into the interpretation of both stand-alone exercise-ECGs and myocardial perfusion studies.

is independent of clinical, coronary anatomic, and LV function data. The principal criticism of the Duke score is the absence of consideration of clinical variables, especially age, or other exercise test variables such as HR.

SEPARATE SCORES FOR MEN AND WOMEN

These scores were developed and validated in the early 2000s (see "Classic References"). Separate scores for men and women incorporate three standard exercise test variables (ST-segment depression, peak HR, exercise angina score) and several other clinical variables (Fig. 15.6). These scores are not as simple as the Duke treadmill score but lend themselves to easy clinical application.

Cleveland Clinic Prognostic Score

This score was initially reported in 2007 (see "Classic References"). It incorporates most of the important prognostic exercise test variables, as well as other important clinical variables. The originally published nomogram is more difficult to apply in routine clinical settings, but it is available in a more user-friendly, free, online software application (Fig. 15.7).

Newer Scores and Observations

Several published scores and methods for patients with and without CAD emphasize non–ST-segment variables. None of these has been validated outside the derivation institution or compared to other scores (e.g., Duke treadmill) but nevertheless demonstrate the prognostic power of the non–ST-segment variables in a variety of populations.

The Fitness Risk Score was derived using more than 58,000 adults without established heart disease (about half women) to assess for all-cause mortality.[10] Patients were followed 10 years on average. The maximum predicted HR and functional capacity were the best exercise predictors. The score equation is:

Maximum heart rate (%) + 12 (METs) − 4 (Age) + 43 (if female)

Score ranges of greater than 100, 0 to 100, −1 to −100, and less than −100 yielded mean survival at 10 years of 98%, 97%, 89%, and 62%, respectively.

Post–Myocardial Infarction Evaluation

Since 2002, when the last full set of exercise testing guidelines was updated, treatment of MI and evaluation of post-MI patients have evolved greatly. In the original guidelines, exercise testing carried class I indications before hospital discharge (submaximal, 4 to 7 days), 14 to 21 days after discharge (symptom limited if not performed before discharge), and 3 to 6 weeks after discharge (symptom limited if predischarge submaximal exercise performed). These recommendations were based largely on the existing ACC/AHA guidelines for the management of acute MI. In this setting the exercise test was found to be safe, with a reported mortality rate of 0.03% and a nonfatal event rate of 0.09%.

Since 1997, the use of coronary angiography as part of the diagnostic evaluation and treatment of MI has taken priority. This evolution has limited the role of exercise testing in the stratification of post-MI patients. The most recent guidelines for both ST-segment elevation MI (STEMI)[29] and non-STEMI[30] state that the role of the simple exercise ECG is limited to patients who did not undergo coronary angiography following thrombolytic therapy, or patients who did not receive reperfusion therapy. In addition, these patients should have a LV ejection fraction greater than 40%, no other high-risk features, should be able to exercise, and should have interpretable ECGs. This subset of patients is likely to be a small percentage of the total postinfarction group. In addition, it is highly likely that many of these patients will undergo stress imaging rather than a simple exercise test. Nevertheless, when exercise testing is performed, the variables of prognostic importance are the same as in all other settings: functional capacity, HR, systolic BP, ventricular arrhythmias and ST segment deviation.

In the present clinical environment, realistic goals of exercise testing in the post-MI setting, whenever it is performed, should be threefold: to provide (1) a functional evaluation to guide the exercise rehabilitation prescription, (2) a basis for advice concerning return to work and other physical activities, and (3) an evaluation of present therapy.

TABLE 15.13 Multivariable Prognostic Scores

PROGNOSTIC SCORE	PROGNOSTIC INFORMATION	NUMBER OF PARTICIPANTS (N)	REFERENCE
Duke treadmill	Exercise time ST-segment deviation Angina score	613	Shaw LJ et al.
Cleveland Clinic	HRR Duke treadmill score	9,454	Lauer MS et al.
Fitness risk score	Maximal HR Functional capacity Age Gender	58,000	Ahmed HM et al.
SCOREexe	Functional capacity HR response	1,531	Kiviniemi AM et al.
Rancho Bernardo	ST depression Chronotropic incompetence HRR	898	Park J-I et al.
Arbit et al.	Exercise capacity HRR Chronotropic incompetence	11,218	Arbit B et al.

HR, Heart rate; HRR, heart rate recovery.
From Shaw LJ, Peterson ED, Shaw LK, et al. Use of a prognostic treadmill score in identifying diagnostic coronary disease subgroups. *Circulation*. 1998;98:1622–1630; Lauer MS, Pothier CE, Magid DJ, et al. An Externally validated model for predicting long-term survival after exercise treadmill testing in patients with suspected coronary artery disease and a normal electrocardiogram. *Ann Intern Med*. 2007;147:821–828; Ahmed HM, Al-Mallah MH, McEvoy JW, et al. Maximal exercise testing variables and 10-year survival: fitness risk score derivation from the FIT project. *Mayo Clin Proc*. 2015;90:346–355; Kiviniemi AM, et al. Exercise capacity and heart rate responses to exercise as predictors of short-term outcome among patients with stable coronary artery disease. *Am J Cardiol*. 2015;116:1495–1501; Park J-I, Shin SY, Park SK, et al. Usefulness of the integrated scoring model of treadmill tests to predict myocardial ischemia and silent myocardial ischemia in community-dwelling adults (from the Rancho Bernardo study). *Am J Cardiol*. 2015;115:1049–1055; Arbit B, Azarbal B, Hayes SW, et al. Prognostic contribution of exercise capacity, heart rate recovery, chronotropic incompetence, and myocardial perfusion single-photon emission computerized tomography in the prediction of cardiac death and all-cause mortality. *Am J Cardiol*. 2015;116:1678–1684.

A

VARIABLE	CHOOSE RESPONSE	SUM
Maximal heart rate	Less than 100 bpm = 30	
	100 to 129 bpm = 24	
	130 to 159 bpm = 18	
	160 to 189 bpm = 12	
	190 to 220 bpm = 6	
Exercise ST depression	1 to 2 mm = 15	
	Greater than 2 mm = 25	
Age	Greater than 55 yr = 20	
	40 to 55 yr = 12	
Angina history	Definite/typical = 5	
	Probable/atypical = 3	
	Noncardiac pain = 1	
Hypercholesterolemia?	Yes = 5	
Diabetes?	Yes = 5	
Exercise test: induced angina	Occurred = 3	
	Reason for stopping = 5	
	Total score:	

Exercise test score **MEN**
Choose one per group
<40 = low probability
40-60 = intermediate probability
>60 = high probability

B

VARIABLE	CHOOSE RESPONSE	SUM
Maximal heart rate	Less than 100 bpm = 20	
	100 to 129 bpm = 16	
	130 to 159 bpm = 12	
	160 to 189 bpm = 8	
	190 to 220 bpm = 4	
Exercise ST depression	1 to 2 mm = 6	
	Greater than 2 mm = 10	
Age	Greater than 65 yr = 25	
	50 to 65 yr = 15	
Angina history	Definite/typical = 10	
	Probable/atypical = 6	
	Noncardiac pain = 2	
Smoking?	Yes = 10	
Diabetes?	Yes = 10	
Exercise test: induced angina	Occurred = 9	
	Reason for stopping = 15	
Estrogen status	Positive = –5, Negative = 5	
	Total score:	

Exercise test score **WOMEN**
Choose one per group
<40 = low probability
40-60 = intermediate probability
>60 = high probability

FIGURE 15.6 Prognostic Exercise Test Scores for Men and Women. Exercise test scores for men **(A)** and women **(B)**; *bpm*, beats per minute. To determine risk group, total points for the appropriate choice for each clinical and exercise test variable. If there is no appropriate choice for a particular variable, score points as zero for that variable. *Exercise ST depression* is only horizontal or downsloping. *Diabetes* is insulin or noninsulin requiring. *Smoking* is any current or prior cigarette smoking. *Estrogen status* positive includes women who are premenopausal, receiving hormone replacement therapy, or with intact ovaries under age 50. Otherwise, women are estrogen status negative. (From Morise AP, Jalisi F. Evaluation of pretest and exercise test scores to assess all-cause mortality in unselected patients presenting for exercise testing with symptoms of suspected coronary artery disease. *J Am Coll Cardiol*. 2003;42:842–850.)

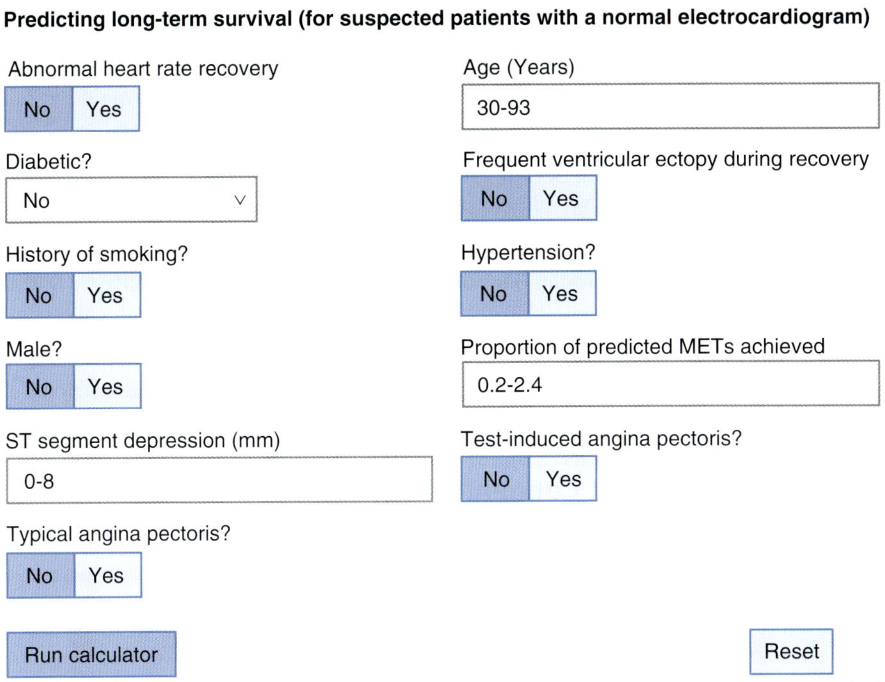

Predicting long-term survival (for suspected patients with a normal electrocardiogram)

Abnormal heart rate recovery: [No] [Yes]
Diabetic? [No ▼]
History of smoking? [No] [Yes]
Male? [No] [Yes]
ST segment depression (mm): [0-8]
Typical angina pectoris? [No] [Yes]

Age (Years): [30-93]
Frequent ventricular ectopy during recovery: [No] [Yes]
Hypertension? [No] [Yes]
Proportion of predicted METs achieved: [0.2-2.4]
Test-induced angina pectoris? [No] [Yes]

[Run calculator]   [Reset]

FIGURE 15.7 Cleveland Clinic prognostic score. Predicts 3-, 5- and 10-year survival after exercise treadmill testing. The Cleveland Clinic Risk Calculator is available at https://riskcalc.org/. Entering this URL will bring you to the site listing many scores developed at the Cleveland Clinic. Choose "Heart Disease" and then "For Patients with Suspected Coronary Artery Disease and a Normal Electrocardiogram". Definition of terms used in this calculator follow. *Typical angina*: chest discomfort that is substernal, is brought on by physical or mental exertion, and is relieved within minutes by rest or nitroglycerin. *Smoking*: regular smoking now or within the past year. *Hypertension*: resting systolic BP ≥140 mm Hg, resting diastolic BP ≥90 mm Hg, or use of medications for treatment of hypertension. *Proportion of predicted* metabolic equivalents *(METs)* (metabolic equivalents) *achieved*: in men, predicted METs = [14.7 − (0.11 × age)]; in women, [14.7 − (0.13 × age)]. *ST depression:* only count horizontal or downsloping ST depression that is at least 1 mm; otherwise record as 0. *Exercise-induced angina:* any angina is included, whether or not it is test terminating. *Abnormal heart rate recovery:* calculated as HR at the end of graded exercise minus HR 1 min later; for upright cool-down, consider abnormal if ≤12 beats/min; for supine cool-down, consider abnormal if ≤18 beats/min. *Frequent ventricular ectopy in recovery:* includes at least seven premature ventricular beats/min, frequent ventricular couplets, any ventricular triplets, nonsustained or sustained ventricular tachycardia or torsade des pointes, or ventricular fibrillation occurring in the first 5 minutes of recovery.

Preoperative Evaluation in Noncardiac Surgery (see Chapter 23)

It is estimated that noncardiac surgery has a complication rate as high as 11%, and that more than 40% of these complications are due to cardiovascular issues.[31] Cardiovascular complications are the leading cause of perioperative death within 30 days of surgery, with a rate currently estimated at 1.7% in the United States,[32] that is similar worldwide.[31] Comprehensive consideration of the type of surgery that is to be performed along with an appropriate evaluation of each specific patient aims to yield a benefit-risk assessment that guides subsequent decisions and patient management. Although stress testing is widely used in the evaluation of patients with CVD, very few randomized trials have addressed the value of preoperative stress testing. A recent comprehensive systematic review and meta-analysis of preoperative testing prior to noncardiac surgery[33] found a general lack of quality studies available. Most studies did not have a comparator group and there was a high heterogeneity among the studies. These data strongly support the current American[34] and European[31] guidelines that find no role for indiscriminate and routine preoperative stress testing. Importantly, such testing should be guided by patient history with specific signs and symptoms that suggest high risk CVD in the context of the particular type of noncardiac surgery that is to be performed. Such an assessment is integral to guide subsequent decisions regarding treatments and interventions, if any, that might mitigate postoperative adverse events.

Assessment of Therapy

The exercise ECG can be applied to assess the efficacy of therapy, whether medication, revascularization, cardiac rehabilitation, ablation, or other. Serial exercise testing can be performed to assess HR and double product at the onset of ischemia (i.e., angina or ST-segment depression). These parameters are generally chosen because of their reproducibility. Peak $\dot{V}o_2$ is the most reproducible measure, but CPX is not performed routinely.

EXERCISE TESTING IN NONATHEROSCLEROTIC HEART DISEASE

The latest iteration of ACSM guidelines on exercise testing is dominated by diagnostic and prognostic assessments of atherosclerotic CAD.[3] Less prominent are applications that pertain to certain nonatherosclerotic conditions. In each case, exercise imaging, especially with echocardiography, provides important information for evaluation of these conditions. This section emphasizes and expands on the value of the exercise-ECG test.

Valvular Heart Disease

The role of exercise ECG testing in patients with valvular heart disease is best exemplified in the current valvular heart disease guidelines from AHA/ACC, which were updated in 2020 (see Chapters 72, 73, and 75 to 77).[35] Exercise testing also has a role in patients with valvular heart disease who want to participate in competitive athletic activity.[36] Frequently, exercise testing is combined with echocardiography to assess structural and physiologic responses. This is the preferred approach in evaluating patients with mitral stenosis and disparate clinical and resting echocardiographic data, such as severe stenosis without symptoms or symptoms with mild to moderate stenosis. In patients with chronic severe mitral or aortic regurgitation, the diagnostic role of exercise testing is limited to the evaluation of functional capacity in patients with equivocal symptoms. The only valve lesion in which the simple exercise ECG still has a significant role in management is aortic stenosis. This latter topic is discussed in greater detail elsewhere.[37]

Aortic Stenosis

It is universally agreed that exercise testing is absolutely contraindicated in patients with symptomatic severe valvular aortic stenosis.[35] However, for asymptomatic patients, exercise testing has found a role in two specific scenarios (see Chapter 72).

Severe Acquired Aortic Valve Stenosis

The first scenario is asymptomatic patients with severe acquired valvular aortic stenosis, defined as a peak Doppler velocity of 4 m/sec or greater, valve area less than 1 cm^2, or a mean valve gradient greater than 40 mm Hg with associated normal LV systolic function.[38] Patients with more moderate stenosis but suspected symptoms might also be considered. When peak aortic velocity exceeds 5.5 m/sec, exercise testing should not be done even in the absence of symptoms.[39] In addition, patients with severe aortic stenosis and high-gradient and normal LV function are to be distinguished from those with low-gradient stenosis and either normal or reduced LV systolic function; this latter important issue warrants further evaluation that includes stress—echocardiography and not simple exercise—ECG testing.

Customary practice is to defer aortic valve replacement until symptoms develop (see Chapter 72). However, some patients with asymptomatic severe aortic stenosis who do not undergo early aortic valve replacement are still at increased short- and longer-term risk. The purpose of exercise testing in this setting is to induce either symptoms or an abnormal BP response, which most studies define as a lack of increase or ≤20 mm Hg increase in systolic BP (Class IIa, level of evidence B). The Class IIa indication provides a basis to recommend valve replacement in patients who do not report any of the expected symptoms of severe aortic stenosis. Exercise testing in this scenario should be performed only in those with no reported symptoms or with symptoms that are equivocal at worst, such that aortic valve surgery is not indicated on that basis. They should have no extracardiac factors that limit exercise and no contraindications to aortic valve replacement. Considering that replacement of the aortic valve can currently be performed surgically or percutaneously, absolute contraindications for replacement are evolving. Protocols less intense than the standard Bruce protocol should be used, especially in elderly or untrained individuals. A modified Bruce or other low-level protocol can be used for patients who might manifest an earlier-than-anticipated adverse response. Special emphasis should be placed on the minute-by-minute BP response, patient symptoms, and heart rhythm. Exercise should be terminated for limiting dyspnea and fatigue at a low workload, any angina or dizziness, any decrease in systolic BP, and complex ventricular ectopy. All these should be considered abnormal responses, placing the patient in a higher-risk group. Limiting dyspnea and fatigue must be interpreted carefully according to what is appropriate for age- and sex-based expectations. Isolated ST-segment depression (i.e., >2 mm of horizontal or downsloping depression) is very prevalent but is considered a nonspecific finding in severe aortic stenosis.[37] If possible, termination should include a 2-minute cool-down walk and avoidance of the supine position to obviate acute LV volume overload.

Moderate to Severe Congenital Valvular Aortic Stenosis

The second scenario consists of young or adolescent patients with congenital aortic valve stenosis that is moderate to severe, defined as a mean Doppler gradient greater than 30 mm Hg or a peak Doppler gradient greater than 50 mm Hg. Exercise testing in this specific scenario is done to provide advice for patients wanting to participate in athletic activities,[36] as well as to evaluate asymptomatic patients with severe stenosis to assess the BP response and exercise tolerance, as with acquired stenosis. The testing procedure is similar to that for acquired aortic stenosis.

Mitral Regurgitation

In asymptomatic patients with severe mitral regurgitation, exercise testing may be useful to elicit symptoms or demonstrate reduced exercise capacity, and may prompt reclassification of patients to a stage of disease that warrants structural intervention with repair, replacement or mitral clip.

Echocardiographic stress testing can provide information beyond exercise capacity and is discussed elsewhere (see Chapter 76). Alternatively, a 6-minute walk test can be used in frail or elderly patients with severe mitral regurgitation to better reflect impairments in the ability to perform activities of daily living.[40]

Hypertrophic Cardiomyopathy

Exercise testing can play an important role in the evaluation of patients with HCM (see Chapter 54). In the 2020 ACC/AHA guidelines on HCM,[41] the exercise test carries a class I recommendation (level of evidence B) for assessing dynamic outflow obstruction using exercise echocardiography and for assessing patients with nonobstructive HCM for possible cardiac transplantation using CPX. In addition, class IIa indications (level of evidence B) are provided for determination of functional capacity and for risk stratification (i.e., rhythm and BP). Several reported series have demonstrated that such testing in patients with HCM is safe with a low and acceptable incidence of fatal and nonfatal complications.

Exercise testing in patients with HCM has clinical value in three clinical situations[38]: (1) defining the presence of exercise-induced outflow tract obstruction with Doppler echocardiography in patients with no gradient at rest; (2) identifying patients with coexistent CAD; (3) detecting patients with the high-risk indicator of an abnormal BP response.

The first two questions require exercise testing with imaging since in HCM, the exercise ECG is nonspecific for the evaluation of ischemia, and Doppler echocardiography is required to assess resting and exercise induced dynamic LV outflow tract gradients. These are discussed in detail elsewhere.[38,41]

An abnormal BP response during upright treadmill exercise is a risk factor for SCD in patients with HCM (see Chapter 54). It is of greater predictive value in patients younger than 50 years. An abnormal BP response is defined as either an initial increase in systolic pressure with a subsequent fall greater than 20 mm Hg, or a continuous fall from the start of exercise greater than 20 mm Hg. The NPV for SCD is reported to be in the mid-90% range, whereas the PPV is low. Therefore, further stratification as outlined in the guidelines[41] is required beyond the abnormal BP response. It is considered reasonable to reassess the BP response after therapy to reduce the outflow tract obstruction, but no data exist on this issue.

Adult Congenital Heart Disease

The 2018 AHA/ACC Guideline for the Management of Adults with Congenital Heart Disease[42] outlines the role of the exercise test for the evaluation of patients with selected congenital defects (see Chapter 82). The guidelines provide a class IIa recommendation for CPX for baseline evaluation and serial follow-up for response to treatment. In patients unable to perform CPX, a 6-minute walk test is recommended (class IIa) as it can provide objective information regarding prognosis beyond history alone. The use of exercise testing in several specific types of adult congenital heart disease is discussed.

A 2015 scientific statement from ACC/AHA addresses the selective use of exercise testing in individuals with congenital heart disease who want to participate in competitive athletics. The specific conditions where the exercise-ECG has a role include repaired and unrepaired aortic coarctation, repaired tetralogy of Fallot, surgically and congenitally corrected transposition of the great arteries, and coronary artery anomalies. Details regarding sport-specific intensity levels and recommendations are provided.[43]

CARDIAC RHYTHM DISTURBANCES

Exercise testing can be used in the evaluation of suspected cardiac arrhythmias, premature ventricular complexes (PVCs), or nonsustained VT.[1,20] Table 15.14 summarizes indications for exercise testing in the evaluation of arrhythmias. In addition, concerning the eligibility recommendations for competitive athletes with cardiac arrhythmias, an ACC/AHA statement covers the role of exercise testing in the settings of sinus bradycardia, heart block, isolated ventricular ectopic beats, nonsustained VT, and sustained monomorphic VT.[44]

Atrial Fibrillation

The AF guidelines state that exercise testing should be performed for three specific scenarios (see Chapter 66).[45] The first indication is when myocardial ischemia is suspected and initiation of type IC antiarrhythmic drug therapy is being considered. The second indication involves assessing the adequacy of HR control across a full spectrum of activity in patients with persistent or permanent AF (class Ic). No standard method for assessment of HR control has been established to guide management in patients with AF. Criteria for HR control vary with patient age but usually involve achieving ventricular rates between 90 and 115 beats/min during moderate exercise. Lastly, exercise testing may be used to induce possible exercise-induced AF.

Ventricular Preexcitation

Exercise testing carries a class Ib recommendation in either symptomatic or asymptomatic patients with preexcitation.[46] Identifying accessory pathways that are at risk of developing rapid conduction and life-threatening ventricular arrhythmias in response to AF is an important consideration. The abrupt loss of preexcitation during exercise testing identifies a low-risk patient in this respect. Care should be taken to ensure that the delta wave is truly absent. It is noteworthy that preexcitation with conduction abnormalities is a well-known cause of false positive ST segment changes.

Ventricular Arrhythmias

The 2017 AHA/ACC/Heart Rhythm Society Guideline for the Management of Patients with Ventricular Arrhythmias and the Prevention of

TABLE 15.14 Guideline Recommendations for Exercise-Electrocardiogram Testing in Heart Rhythm Disorders

Class I

Exercise testing is useful to assess for exercise-induced ventricular arrhythmias in patients with ventricular arrhythmia symptoms associated with exertion, suspected ischemic heart disease, or catecholaminergic polymorphic ventricular tachycardia *(Level of evidence: B-NR)*.

In *asymptomatic* patients with preexcitation, the findings of abrupt loss of conduction over a manifest pathway during exercise testing in sinus rhythm is useful to identify patients at low risk of rapid conduction over the pathway *(Level of evidence B-NR)*.

In *symptomatic* patients with preexcitation, the findings of abrupt loss of conduction over the pathway during exercise testing in sinus rhythm is useful for identifying patients at low risk of developing rapid conduction over the pathway *(Level of evidence B-NR)*.

Class IIa

In patients with suspected long QT syndrome, exercise testing can be useful for establishing a diagnosis and monitoring the response to therapy *(Level of evidence B-NR)*.

Exercise testing can be useful for evaluating response to medical or ablation therapy in patients with known exercise-induced ventricular arrhythmias *(Level of evidence: B)*

In patients with suspected chronotropic incompetence, exercise electrocardiographic testing is reasonable to ascertain the diagnosis and provide information on prognosis *(Level of evidence B-NR)*.

In patients with exercise-related symptoms suspicious for bradycardia or conduction disorders, or in patients with 2:1 atrioventricular block of unknown level, exercise electrocardiographic testing is reasonable *(Level of evidence C-LD)*

In patients with exertional symptoms (e.g., chest pain, shortness of breath) who have first-degree or second-degree Mobitz type I atrioventricular block at rest, an exercise treadmill test is reasonable to determine whether they may benefit from permanent pacing *(Level of evidence C-LD)*

Atrial Fibrillation

The following are included as indications for exercise testing in atrial fibrillation, but are not given a recommendation class or level of evidence:

- If adequacy of rate control is in question.
- To reproduce exercise-induced atrial fibrillation.
- To exclude ischemia before treatment of selected patients with a class IC antiarrhythmic drug.

From Al-Khatib SM, et al. 2017 ACC/AHA/HRS guideline for management of patients with ventricular arrhythmias and the prevention of sudden cardiac death. *Circulation.* 2018;138:e210–e271; January CT, Samuel Wann L, Alpert JS, et al. 2014 AHA/ACC/HRS guideline for the management of patients with atrial fibrillation. *Circulation.* 2014;130:e199–e267; Kusumoto FM, Mark H. Schoenfeld MH, et al. ACC/AHA/HRS guideline on the evaluation and management of patients with bradycardia and cardiac conduction delay. *Circulation.* 2019;140: e382–e482; Page RL, Joglar JA, Caldwell, MA, et al. 2015 ACC/AHA/HRS guideline for the management of adult patients with supraventricular tachycardia. *Circulation.* 2016;133; e506–e574; Tracy CM, Hirsch AT, Misra S, et al. 2012 ACCF/AHA/HRS focused update of the 2008 guidelines for device -based therapy of cardiac rhythm abnormalities. *Circulation.* 2012;126:1784–1800.

Sudden Cardiac Death recommend that exercise testing be performed for known or suspected exercise-induced ventricular arrhythmias in order to provoke and diagnose the arrhythmia and determine response to the tachycardia.[20] Exercise-induced ventricular arrhythmias can be associated with CAD. Therefore, detection of ischemia with or without associated ventricular arrhythmias defines a role for the exercise test.

With respect to patients with known or suspected exercise-induced ventricular arrhythmias, it should be understood that exercise testing in this high-risk cohort is not a low-risk endeavor, and in many cases the physician should be in the room for the test. It is reasonable in these cases to have intravenous access in place.

Catecholaminergic Polymorphic Ventricular Tachycardia

This arrhythmia occurs in genetically predisposed individuals when they are subjected to intense emotional or physical stress.[38] Standard cardiac testing, including the ECG at rest, usually produces normal results. The arrhythmia is almost always inducible by a maximal exercise test and is frequently not inducible with programmed electrical stimulation. Catecholaminergic polymorphic VT generally appears in HRs above 120 to 130 beats/min and begins with polymorphic ventricular premature beats progressing to nonsustained VT and eventually to bidirectional or polymorphic VT. The purpose of the exercise test, therefore, is to achieve a diagnosis and determine the patient's response to treatment, namely, beta blockade.[20]

Long-QT Syndrome

When LQTS is suspected and the rest QTc is borderline, exercise testing can be performed safely given that arrhythmias do not usually develop in patients with LQTS during exercise (see Chapter 63). In addition, changes in the QT interval with exercise can be useful in identifying and stratifying patients with LQTS.[20] Further prolongation of (or failure to shorten) an already prolonged QT interval with exercise is typical of LQT1. LQT2 has normal shortening, whereas LQT3 has supranormal shortening of the QT interval with exercise. Beta blockade normalizes these responses. These responses can be useful in predicting and directing genetic testing in patients with LQTS.

Arrhythmogenic Right Ventricular Cardiomyopathy

Even though arrhythmias and SCD can occur during exercise in patients with arrhythmogenic right ventricular cardiomyopathy, exercise testing has no significant role in the management of these patients. Serious ventricular arrhythmias that do occur during exercise usually take the form of monomorphic VT with an LBBB pattern.[47]

ASSESSMENT OF THERAPY

Assessing the response to medical, ablative, or surgical therapy for exercise-induced ventricular arrhythmias is a class IIa, level of evidence B indication. Unlike anti-ischemic therapy, the endpoint is the presence or absence of significant ventricular arrhythmias with reasonable levels of exercise, depending on patient-specific factors.[48]

ASSESSMENT OF PACEMAKER FUNCTION

Even though earlier guidelines endorse exercise testing with rate-adaptive pacemakers to fine-tune or maximize the physiologic response, the 2012 guidelines regarding device-based treatment of cardiac arrhythmias do not even mention the use of exercise testing with implanted pacemakers.[48] This discrepancy raises a practical question. Despite the original endorsement of exercise testing in patients with rate-adaptive pacemakers, do electrophysiologists actually use exercise testing in clinical decision making for rate-adaptive pacemakers? Exercise testing could play a role with rate-adaptive pacemakers when exercise intolerance is not completely relieved by factory settings or empiric adjustments. This would be especially true in patients involved in significant physical activities or athletic participation.[38]

ADDITIONAL USES FOR EXERCISE TESTING

Chest Pain Units

Chest pain units are designed to assist in the triage and management of low-risk patients with chest pain among the millions of patients evaluated in emergency departments annually. Low-risk patients have stable hemodynamic signs, no arrhythmias, normal or near-normal findings on the ECG, and negative cardiac injury biomarkers and are appropriate for observation in a chest pain unit. Such units are designed to provide an integrated approach to further risk stratification by short-term observation, repeated ECGs, and serial cardiac injury biomarkers. In patients without further chest pain and no objective evidence of ischemia, an exercise test can be performed after 8 to 12 hours of observation. Such testing is often performed with a symptom-limited treadmill protocol. Several studies encompassing more than 3000 such patients have demonstrated that a negative test has a high NPV for subsequent cardiac events (Table 15.15). No adverse events during exercise testing have been reported. Those with a positive test are admitted for further evaluation, whereas those with a negative test can be discharged safely with outpatient follow-up. This strategy has been shown to be cost-effective compared with usual care in which such patients are admitted to the hospital.[49] Patients who are unable to exercise

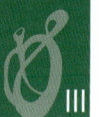

TABLE 15.15 Chest Pain Unit: Patient Selection, Testing Procedure, and End Points

Patient Selection Criteria
Able to exercise
ECG: Normal or minor ST-T changes
Hemodynamically stable, no arrhythmia
Negative cardiac injury markers
Procedure
Bruce or modified Bruce protocol
End points
Symptom-limited
Ischemia (≥0.10 mV of horizontal ST depression or elevation)
Decreased blood pressure (≥10 mm Hg systolic) during exercise test
Result
Positive: ≥0.10 mV of horizontal ST-segment depression
Negative: No exercise-induced abnormalities at 85% MPHR
Nondiagnostic: <85% MPHR with no ECG evidence of ischemia

ECG, Electrocardiogram; *MPHR*, maximum age-predicted HR.
From Amsterdam EA, Lettino M, Ahrens I, et al. Testing of low-risk patients presenting to the emergency department with chest pain: a scientific statement from the American Heart Association. *Circulation*. 2010;122:1756.

or who have baseline electrocardiographic abnormalities can undergo stress imaging tests or computed tomographic angiography. The usefulness of such tests is discussed in detail elsewhere (see Chapters 16, 18, and 20).

The advent of high-sensitivity troponin testing may re-define the role of stress testing in the emergency department or chest pain unit. A recent expert panel concludes that management algorithms that include high-sensitivity troponin testing aim to mitigate over-testing, emergency department and chest pain unit overcrowding, and the low yield of true-positive testing. In this new paradigm, stress testing plays a more limited and specific role.[50]

Physical Activity and Exercise Prescription

Data derived from the exercise test can yield valuable objective information to assist in providing physical activity recommendations for patients with CVD, specifically regarding domestic, occupational, recreational, and athletic activities (see Chapter 33). The 2011 Compendium of Physical Activities: a Second Update of Codes and MET Values (see "Classic References") and its associated web link (http://links.lww.com/MSS/A82) provide 821 codes that reflect 21 major headings, numerous specific activities and their detailed descriptions, and associated MET values that can be used to identify the energy cost associated with a given activity. By using the exercise test to measure peak exercise capacity in METs and evaluate the HR, BP, and symptomatic responses to peak and submaximal MET levels, the clinician can combine this information with that derived from the compendium to counsel patients on their ability to perform a broad spectrum of activities and tasks. Ample data for the cardiac rehabilitation literature has shown that exercise in the range of 70% to 85% of the maximal measured HR is exceedingly safe.[51] It is important to realize, however, that the exercise test does not yield information regarding the patient's ability to perform sustained tasks for long periods or take into account the environmental conditions (e.g., temperature, humidity, altitude, wind) where the activity is performed. Therefore, data from the exercise test and the compendium can serve only as a guide to prudent activity counseling. Patients must be made aware of these other factors and instructed to use subjective symptoms scales (e.g., Borg Scale of Perceived Exertion) and HR to further tailor their activity performance.

Exercise training programs are designed to maintain or improve fitness and include the prescriptive components of intensity, duration, frequency, and modality. Details regarding the exercise prescription for patients with CVD are provided elsewhere.[1,3,51] For patients with CVD, the *intensity* of dynamic aerobic exercise is usually determined from the results of a pretraining exercise test by using either of two methods: 40% to 80% of peak exercise capacity using the *HR reserve* method ([peak HR − resting HR] × [percent intensity] + [resting HR]), and in patients who have performed a CPX, the HR at 40% to 80% of the measured peak $\dot{V}O_2$. A simpler approach is to have individuals exercise at 70% to 85% of their maximal measured HR. Intensity may be modified further by using the subjective perceived exertion scale at a rating of 11 to 16 on a scale of 6 to 20. In patients with an ischemic response during exercise, the intensity should be prescribed at a HR that is at least 10 beats below the symptomatic ischemic threshold (i.e., the HR at which ischemic ST depressions and typical angina begin to occur). The goal *duration* of exercise at the prescribed intensity is generally 20 to 60 minutes per session at a *frequency* of 3 to 5 days per week. Training *modalities* should ideally incorporate exercises that include rhythmic, large muscle group activities of both the upper and the lower extremities with varying types of exercise equipment such as treadmills, cycle ergometers and elliptical trainers. A symptom limited ECG stress test can also screen for the safety of resistance training in cardiac patients as the maximal HR × BP product attained at the stress test is rarely exceeded during clinical (non-body building) strength training (see "Classic References").

Emerging data on aerobic interval training (AIT) offer promise for patients with CVD. AIT involves alternating 3- to 4-minute periods of exercise at very high intensity (90% to 95% of peak HR) with exercise at moderate intensity (60% to 70% of peak HR). When such training is performed for approximately 40 minutes, three times per week, studies demonstrate greater improvements in peak $\dot{V}O_2$, endothelial function, and metabolic parameters than with standard continuous, moderate-intensity exercise.[52] The cardiovascular risks of AIT appear to be low in a supervised cardiac rehabilitation setting. Although more studies are needed, AIT can be considered in select patients as an alternative training modality for those with CVD enrolled in cardiac rehabilitation program.

DISABILITY ASSESSMENT

The U.S. Social Security Administration defines disability as "the inability to engage in any substantial gainful activity by reason of any medically determinable physical or mental impairment(s) which can be expected to result in death or which has lasted or can be expected to last for a continuous period of not less than 12 months."[53] In several cardiovascular conditions, disability is not based solely on the diagnosis but also on the functional limitations imposed by the condition. Thus, exercise testing plays an integral role in the determination of disability for several cardiovascular conditions, including chronic heart failure, ischemic heart disease, congenital heart disease, PAD, and valvular heart disease. The Institute of Medicine (IOM) convened a panel of experts to provide recommendations for updating the Social Security listings for cardiovascular conditions. Although each of the previous conditions have specific criteria to define the condition, functional disability in almost all of them is defined by the inability to attain a directly measured peak $\dot{V}O_2$ of 15 mL/kg/min using gas exchange (or 5 estimated METs) on a symptom-limited treadmill or stationary cycle test. Table 15.16 outlines details regarding exercise test criteria for specific cardiovascular conditions as recommended by IOM.

Evaluation of Peripheral Artery Disease

Exercise testing can be performed in patients with PAD to establish further the diagnosis by noninvasive techniques, particularly in patients with calf pain and borderline ankle-brachial indices (ABIs: 0.91 to 1.0), and objectively evaluate functional limitations imposed by PAD and the subsequent response to therapies (see Chapter 43). Assessment of the time to initial claudication symptoms *(claudication onset time)* and the *peak exercise time* to maximum tolerated calf pain should be assessed by using gradual graded exercise treadmill stages, such as the Gardner protocol (Table 15.17). For functional assessment, the 6-minute walk test (see Table 15.8) can also be used; during this test, both time and distance are measured to onset and to peak calf pain.

The post-exercise ABI can provide additional diagnostic information and is done by measuring the ABI in both ankles at rest and again immediately after exercise (see Chapter 43). During leg exercise, systolic BP normally increases in the arms but decreases in the

TABLE 15.16 Exercise Test Criteria for Disability Determination in Specific Cardiovascular Conditions

CARDIOVASCULAR CONDITION	SOCIAL SECURITY CRITERIA	IOM RECOMMENDATIONS
Chronic heart failure	Inability to attain five METs due to symptoms of dyspnea, fatigue, palpitations, or chest discomfort; frequent or complex ventricular ectopy; >10 mm Hg decrease in systolic blood pressure during graded exercise; signs due to inadequate cerebral perfusion.	Exercise testing in chronic heart failure is safe; CPX testing requires less subjective endpoint interpretation, using criteria of measured peak VO_2 <15 mL/kg/min with RER >1.1; or <5 estimated METs on standard treadmill test without gas exchange; frequent exercise-induced ventricular ectopy alone should not be listed as a criterion.
Ischemic heart disease	Exercise tolerance testing that demonstrates ischemia, or ≥10 mmHg fall in systolic blood pressure at ≤5 METs	Additional specific criteria when stress imaging tests are used.
Peripheral arterial disease	≥ 50% decrease in systolic blood pressure at the ankle from resting levels that requires ≥10 minutes to recover.	
Congenital heart disease (Adults)	Intermittent right to left shunting leading to cyanosis and arterial PO_2 of ≤ 60 Torr at ≤5 METs	Intermittent right to left shunting with pulse oximetry ≤85% at ≤5 METs; Exercise capacity with peak measured VO_2 <15 mL/kg/min or <5 estimated METs
Pulmonary hypertension	No previous criteria	Exercise capacity <5 METs
Valvular heart disease	No previous criteria	Exercise capacity <5 METs

IOM, Institute of Medicine; METs, Metabolic equivalents; RER, respiratory exchange ratio; Vo_2, oxygen uptake.
Information from the Institute of Medicine of the National Academies. *Cardiovascular Disability. Updating the Social Security Listings.* Washington, DC: National Academies Press; 2010.

TABLE 15.17 Gardner Testing Protocol for Patients with Peripheral Artery Disease

STAGE*	SPEED/GRADE	METS
1	2 mph/0%	2.5
2	2 mph/2%	3.1
3	2 mph/4%	3.6
4	2 mph/6%	4.2
5	2 mph/8%	4.7
6	2 mph/10%	5.3
7	2 mph/12%	5.8
8	2 mph/14%	6.4
9	2 mph/16%	6.9
10	2 mph/18%	7.5

METs, Metabolic equivalents.
*Each stage is 2 minutes in duration.
From Gardner AW, Skinner JS, Cantwell BW, et al. Progressive vs single-stage treadmill tests for evaluation of claudication. *Med Sci Sports Exerc.* 1991;23:402–408.

TABLE 15.18 American College of Cardiology/American Heart Association Guidelines for Exercise Testing in Peripheral Artery Disease

Class I
- Patients with ABI 0.91–0.99 may possibly have PAD, and should undergo exercise ABI if the clinical suspicion of PAD is significant.
- Patients with exertional non-joint-related leg symptoms and normal or borderline resting ABI (>0.90 and ≤1.4) should undergo exercise treadmill ABI testing to evaluate for PAD.

Class IIa
- In patients with PAD and an abnormal resting ABI (≤0.90). Exercise treadmill ABI testing can be useful to objectively assess symptoms, measure change in exercise ABI in response to exercise training or revascularization, and assess functional status.
- Exercise testing can help to individualize exercise prescriptions in patients with PAD before initiation of a formal program of structured exercise training.
- Administration of a 6-minute walk test in a corridor is a reasonable alternative to treadmill ABI testing for assessment of functional status.

ABI, Ankle-brachial index; PAD, peripheral artery disease.
From Gerhard-Herman MD, Gornik HL, Barrett C, et al. 2016 AHA/ACC guideline on the management of patients with lower extremity peripheral artery disease: a report of the American College of Cardiology/American Heart Association Task Force on Clinical Practice Guidelines. *J Am Coll Cardiol.* 2017;69(11):e71–e126.

ankles because of the peripheral vasodilation that occurs in exercising leg muscles. This leads to a mild decrease in the ABI in healthy patients that returns to normal within 1 to 2 minutes of recovery. In patients with PAD, ankle pressure decreases even more, thereby leading to a further decrease in the ABI and also a prolonged recovery time. Several diagnostic criteria have been proposed and include greater than a 5% drop in post-exercise ABI from resting levels, post-exercise ABI lower than 0.9, greater than a 30 mm Hg drop in systolic BP at the ankle, and recovery time to baseline ABI longer than 3 minutes.[54] Details regarding the use of exercise testing are also discussed in the ACC/AHA guidelines for the management of patients with PAD (Table 15.18).[55]

Patients with Diabetes

CAD remains the most common cause of morbidity and mortality in patients with diabetes mellitus (see Chapter 31). In recent years, strategies for the treatment of CAD in patients with diabetes have undergone much evolution such that regardless of symptoms or documented CAD, diabetic patients are treated with preventive therapies. In this context, the ability to specifically identify diabetic patients with disease who will benefit from more aggressive and, perhaps, invasive therapies remains a challenge. Exercise electrocardiographic testing has similar diagnostic sensitivity (approximately 60%) and specificity (80%) for diabetic patients with angina as for nondiabetic patients. Considerable prognostic power of the exercise ECG test lies beyond the ST-segment response. Poor exercise capacity and slow HRR in diabetic patients are markers of an adverse outcome. The value of the Duke prognostic score in patients with diabetes has not been well studied, and unlike the Morise score and the Cleveland Clinic Foundation risk score (see "Classic References"), it did not specifically address the presence of diabetes in the original cohort study. Therefore, at present, the Morise and Cleveland Clinic scores are more appropriate to apply in patients with diabetes who have normal resting ECG findings and undergo exercise electrocardiography.

At present, evidence is inadequate for recommending routine screening of asymptomatic diabetic patients with an exercise ECG.[56] The American Diabetes Association standards of medical care conclude that in asymptomatic patients, routine screening for CAD is not recommended, even before initiation of an exercise training program, because it does not improve outcomes as long as risk factors for CVD are treated.[57] They recommend that diabetic persons who might be considered for advanced or invasive cardiac testing include those with (1) typical or atypical cardiac symptoms and (2) an abnormal resting ECG. Exercise ECG testing without or with imaging may be used initially. Pharmacologic stress echocardiography or nuclear imaging should be considered in diabetic persons in whom resting ECG abnormalities preclude exercise stress testing (e.g., LBBB or ST-T abnormalities) or in those who are not able to exercise.

SUMMARY

ECG exercise testing is a mature diagnostic testing modality with an extensive literature. It is exceedingly important as an initial diagnostic testing strategy to evaluate individuals with symptoms suggestive of coronary ischemia. It also carries invaluable prognostic information for patients in numerous clinical situations including ostensibly healthy individuals, individuals with stable CAD, individuals with chronic heart failure (aided by CPX), and individuals with valvular and other non-atherosclerotic heart diseases. Indeed, the duration of exercise performed on a standardized exercise protocol may be the simplest and best prognostic indicator in all of clinical cardiology.

ACKNOWLEDGMENT

The authors wish to acknowledge the previous contributions of Dr. Anthony Morise, which have laid the foundation for this chapter.

CLASSIC REFERENCES

Ainsworth BE, Haskell WL, Herrmann SD, et al. 2011 compendium of physical activities. *Med Sci Sports Exerc*. 2011;43:1575–1581.
Cole CR, Blackstone EH, Pashkow FJ, et al. Heart-rate recovery immediately after exercise as a predictor of mortality. *N Engl J Med*. 1999;341:1351–1357.
Gibbons RJ, Balady GJ, Timothy Bricker J, et al. ACC/AHA 2002 guideline update for exercise testing: summary article. *Circulation*. 2002;106:1883–1892.
Lauer MS, Pothier CE, Magid DJ, et al. An externally validated model for predicting long-term survival after exercise treadmill testing in patients with suspected coronary artery disease and a normal electrocardiogram. *Ann Intern Med*. 2007;147:821.
Mark DB, Hlatky MA, Harrell Jr FE, et al. Exercise treadmill score for predicting prognosis in coronary artery disease. *Ann Intern Med*. 1987;106:793–800.
Morise AP, Jalisi F. Evaluation of pretest and exercise test scores to assess all-cause mortality in unselected patients presenting for exercise testing with symptoms of suspected coronary artery disease. *J Am Coll Cardiol*. 2003;42:842–850.
Myers J, Arena R, Franklin B, et al. Recommendations for clinical exercise laboratories. *Circulation*. 2009;119:3144–3161.
Rodgers GP, Ayanian JZ, Balady G, et al. American College of Cardiology/American Heart Association clinical competence statement on stress testing. *Circulation*. 2000;102:1726–1738.
Shaw LJ, Peterson ED, Shaw LK, et al. Use of a prognostic treadmill score in identifying diagnostic coronary disease subgroups. *Circulation*. 1998;98:1622–1630.
Williams MA, Haskell WL, Ades PA, et al. Resistance exercise in individuals with and without cardiovascular disease: 2007 update: a scientific statement from the American heart association council on clinical cardiology and council on nutrition, physical activity, and metabolism. *Circulation*. 2007;116:572–584.

REFERENCES

Exercise Physiology and Technical Components of Exercise Testing

1. Fletcher GF, Ades PA, Kligfield P, et al. Exercise standards for testing and training. *Circulation*. 2013;128:873–934.
2. Pescatello LS, American College of Sports Medicine. *ACSM's Guidelines for Exercise Testing and Prescription*. 9th ed. Philadelphia: Wolters Kluwer/Lippincott Williams & Wilkins Health; 2014.
3. American College of Sports Medicine, Riebe D, Ehrman JK, Liguori G, Magal M. *ACSM's Guidelines for Exercise Testing and Prescription*. 10th ed. Philadelphia: Wolters Kluwer; 2018.
4. Holland AE, Spruit MA, Troosters T, et al. An official European Respiratory Society/American Thoracic Society technical standard: field walking tests in chronic respiratory disease. *Eur Respir J*. 2014;44:1428–1446.
5. Guazzi M, Arena R, Halle M, et al. 2016 focused update: clinical recommendations for cardiopulmonary exercise testing data assessment in specific patient populations. *Circulation*. 2016;133:e694–e711.
6. Myers J, Forman DE, Balady GJ, et al. Supervision of exercise testing by nonphysicians. *Circulation*. 2014;130:1014–1027.
7. Franklin BA, Thompson PD, Al-Zaiti SS, et al. Exercise-related acute cardiovascular events and potential deleterious adaptations following long-term exercise training: placing the risks into perspective-an update: a scientific statement from the American Heart Association. *Circulation*. 2020;141:e705–e736.
8. Skalski J, Allison TG, Miller TD. The safety of cardiopulmonary exercise testing in a population with high-risk cardiovascular diseases. *Circulation*. 2012;126:2465–2472.

Exercise Testing in Coronary Artery Disease: Diagnosis

9. Christman MP, Bittencourt MS, Hulten E, et al. Yield of downstream tests after exercise treadmill testing: a prospective cohort study. *J Am Coll Cardiol*. 2014;63:1264–1274.
10. Ahmed HM, Al-Mallah MH, McEvoy JW, et al. Maximal exercise testing variables and 10-year survival: fitness risk score derivation from the FIT Project. *Mayo Clin Proc*. 2015;90:346–355.
11. Marzlin KM, Webner C. Chronotropic incompetence. *AACN Adv Crit Care*. 2019;30:294–300.
12. Sydo N, Sydo T, Gonzalez Carta KA, et al. Prognostic performance of heart rate recovery on an exercise test in a primary prevention population. *J Am Heart Assoc*. 2018;7:e008143.
13. Arbit B, Azarbal B, Hayes SW, et al. Prognostic contribution of exercise capacity, heart rate recovery, chronotropic incompetence, and myocardial perfusion single-photon emission computerized tomography in the prediction of cardiac death and all-cause mortality. *Am J Cardiol*. 2015;116:1678–1684.
14. Schultz MG, La Gerche A, Sharman JE. Blood pressure response to exercise and cardiovascular disease. *Curr Hypertens Rep*. 2017;19:89.
15. O'Neal WT, Qureshi WT, Blaha MJ, et al. Relation of risk of atrial fibrillation with systolic blood pressure response during exercise stress testing (from the Henry Ford Exercise Testing Project). *Am J Cardiol*. 2015;116:1858–1862.
16. Chow R, Fordyce CB, Gao M, et al. The significance of early post-exercise ST segment normalization. *J Electrocardiol*. 2015;48:803–808.
17. Ghaffari S, Asadzadeh R, Tajlil A, et al. Predictive value of exercise stress test-induced ST-segment changes in leads V1 and avR in determining angiographic coronary involvement. *Ann Noninvasive Electrocardiol*. 2017;22:e12370.
18. Stein R, Ho M, Oliveira CM, et al. Exercise-induced left bundle branch block: prevalence and prognosis. *Arq Bras Cardiol*. 2011;97:26–32.
19. Stein R, Nguyen P, Abella J, et al. Prevalence and prognostic significance of exercise-induced right bundle branch block. *Am J Cardiol*. 2010;105:677–680.
20. Al-Khatib SM, Stevenson WG, Ackerman MJ, et al. 2017 AHA/ACC/HRS guideline for management of patients with ventricular arrhythmias and the prevention of sudden cardiac death: executive summary: a report of the American College of Cardiology/American Heart Association Task Force on Clinical Practice Guidelines and the Heart Rhythm Society. *Circulation*. 2018;138:e210–e271.
21. Baskaran L, Danad I, Gransar H, et al. A comparison of the updated Diamond-Forrester, CAD Consortium, and CONFIRM history-based risk scores for predicting obstructive coronary artery disease in patients with stable chest pain: the SCOT-HEART Coronary CTA Cohort. *JACC Cardiovasc Imaging*. 2019;12:1392–1400.
22. Fihn SD, Gardin JM, Abrams J, et al. 2012 ACCF/AHA/ACP/AATS/PCNA/SCAI/STS guideline for the diagnosis and management of patients with stable ischemic heart disease: a report of the American College of Cardiology Foundation/American Heart Association Task Force on Practice Guidelines, and the American College of Physicians, American Association for Thoracic Surgery, Preventive Cardiovascular Nurses Association, Society for Cardiovascular Angiography and Interventions, and Society of Thoracic Surgeons. *Circulation*. 2012;126:e354–e471.
23. Genders TS, Steyerberg EW, Hunink MG, et al. Prediction model to estimate presence of coronary artery disease: retrospective pooled analysis of existing cohorts. *BMJ*. 2012;344:e3485.
24. Bittencourt MS, Hulten E, Polonsky TS, et al. European Society of cardiology-recommended coronary artery disease consortium pretest probability scores more accurately predict obstructive coronary disease and cardiovascular events than the Diamond and Forrester score: the Partners Registry. *Circulation*. 2016;134:201–211.
25. Kohli P, Gulati M. Exercise stress testing in women. *Circulation*. 2010;122:2570–2580.
26. Mieres JH, Gulati M, Bairey Merz N, et al. Role of noninvasive testing in the clinical evaluation of women with suspected ischemic heart disease. *Circulation*. 2014;130:350–379.

Exercise Testing in Coronary Artery Disease: Prognosis

27. Kiviniemi AM, Lepojärvi S, Kenttä TV, et al. Exercise capacity and heart rate responses to exercise as predictors of short-term outcome among patients with stable coronary artery disease. *Am J Cardiol*. 2015;116:1495–1501.
28. Park J-I, Shin S-Y, Park SK, Barrett-Connor E. Usefulness of the integrated scoring model of treadmill tests to predict myocardial ischemia and silent myocardial ischemia in community-dwelling adults (from the Rancho Bernardo study). *Am J Cardiol*. 2015;115:1049–1055.
29. O'Gara PT, Kushner FG, Ascheim DD, et al. 2013 ACCF/AHA guideline for the management of ST-elevation myocardial infarction: a report of the American College of cardiology foundation/American heart association task force on practice guidelines. *Circulation*. 2013;127:e362–425.
30. Amsterdam EA, Wenger NK, Brindis RG, et al. 2014 AHA/ACC guideline for the management of patients with non-ST-elevation acute coronary syndromes: a report of the American College of Cardiology/American Heart Association Task Force on Practice Guidelines. *J Am Coll Cardiol*. 2014;64:e139–e228.
31. Kristensen SD, Knuuti J, Saraste A, et al. 2014 ESC/ESA guidelines on non-cardiac surgery: cardiovascular assessment and management: the Joint Task Force on non-cardiac surgery: cardiovascular assessment and management of the European Society of Cardiology (ESC) and the European Society of Anaesthesiology (ESA). *Eur Heart J*. 2014;35:2383–2431.
32. Smilowitz NR, Gupta N, Ramakrishna H, et al. Perioperative major adverse cardiovascular and cerebrovascular events associated with noncardiac surgery. *JAMA Cardiol*. 2017;2:181–187.
33. Kalesan B, Nicewarner H, Intwala S, et al. Pre-operative stress testing in the evaluation of patients undergoing non-cardiac surgery: a systematic review and meta-analysis. *PloS One*. 2019;14:e0219145.
34. Fleisher LA, Fleischmann KE, Auerbach AD, et al. 2014 ACC/AHA guideline on perioperative cardiovascular evaluation and management of patients undergoing noncardiac surgery: a report of the American College of Cardiology/American Heart Association Task Force on Practice Guidelines. *J Am Coll Cardiol*. 2014;64:e77–e137.

Exercise Testing in Nonatherosclerotic Heart Disease

35. Otto CM, Nishimura RA, Bonow RO, et al. 2020 AHA/ACC guideline for the management of patients with valvular heart disease: a report of the American College of Cardiology/American Heart Association Task Force on Clinical Practice Guidelines. *J Am Coll Cardiol*. 2021. https://doi.org/10.1016/j.jacc.2020.11.018.
36. Bonow RO, Nishimura RA, Thompson PD, Udelson JE. Eligibility and disqualification recommendations for competitive athletes with cardiovascular abnormalities: task Force 5: valvular Heart Disease. *J Am Coll Cardiol*. 2015;66:2385–2392.
37. Redfors B, Pibarot P, Gillam LD, et al. Stress testing in asymptomatic aortic stenosis. *Circulation*. 2017;135:1956–1976.
38. Morise AP. Exercise testing in nonatherosclerotic heart disease. *Circulation*. 2011;123:216–225.
39. Magne J, Lancellotti P, Piérard LA. Exercise testing in asymptomatic severe aortic stenosis. *JACC Cardiovasc Imaging*. 2014;7:188–199.
40. Bonow RO, O'Gara PT, Adams DH, et al. 2020 focused update of the 2017 ACC expert consensus decision pathway on the management of mitral regurgitation: a report of the American College of Cardiology Solution Set Oversight Committee. *J Am Coll Cardiol*. 2020;75:2236–2270.
41. Ommen SR, Mital S, Burke MA, et al. 2020 ACCF/AHA guideline for the diagnosis and treatment of hypertrophic cardiomyopathy: a report of the American College of cardiology foundation/American heart association task force on practice guidelines. *J Am Coll Cardiol*. 2020;76:e159–e240.
42. Stout KK, Daniels CJ, Aboulhosn JA, et al. 2018 AHA/ACC guideline for the management of adults with congenital heart disease: a report of the American College of cardiology/American heart association task force on clinical practice guidelines. *Circulation*. 2019;139:e698–e800.
43. Van Hare GF, Ackerman MJ, Evangelista JK, et al. Eligibility and disqualification recommendations for competitive athletes with cardiovascular abnormalities: task Force 4: congenital Heart Disease. *J Am Coll Cardiol*. 2015;66:2372–2384.

44. Zipes DP, Link MS, Ackerman MJ, et al. Eligibility and disqualification recommendations for competitive athletes with cardiovascular abnormalities: task Force 9: arrhythmias and conduction defects. *J Am Coll Cardiol*. 2015;66:2412–2423.
45. January CT, Wann LS, Alpert JS, et al. 2014 AHA/ACC/HRS guideline for the management of patients with atrial fibrillation: a report of the American College of cardiology/American heart association task force on practice guidelines and the heart rhythm Society. *J Am Coll Cardiol*. 2014;64:e1–e76.
46. Page RL, Joglar JA, Caldwell MA, et al. 2015 ACC/AHA/HRS guideline for the management of adult patients with supraventricular tachycardia: a report of the American College of cardiology/American heart association task force on clinical practice guidelines and the heart rhythm Society. *J Am Coll Cardiol*. 2016;67:e27–e115.
47. Massin MM. The role of exercise testing in pediatric cardiology. *Arch Cardiovasc Dis*. 2014;107:319–327.
48. Tracy CM, Epstein AE, Darbar D, et al. 2012 ACCF/AHA/HRS Focused Update of the 2008 guidelines for device-based therapy of cardiac rhythm abnormalities. *Circulation*. 2012;126:1784–1800.

Additional Uses for Exercise Testing

49. Amsterdam EA, Kirk JD, Bluemke DA, et al. Testing of low-risk patients presenting to the emergency department with chest pain: a scientific statement from the American Heart Association. *Circulation*. 2010;122:1756–1776.
50. Januzzi Jr JL, Mahler SA, Christenson RH, et al. Recommendations for institutions transitioning to high-sensitivity troponin testing: JACC Scientific Expert Panel. *J Am Coll Cardiol*. 2019;73:1059–1077.
51. American Association of Cardiovascular & Pulmonary Rehabilitation. *Guidelines for Cardiac Rehabilitation Programs*. 6th ed. Champaign, IL: Human Kinetics; 2021.
52. Quindry JC, Franklin BA, Chapman M, et al. Benefits and risks of high-intensity interval training in patients with coronary artery disease. *Am J Cardiol*. 2019;123:1370–1377.
53. Institute of Medicine (US) Committee on Social Security Cardiovascular Disability Criteria. *Cardiovascular Disability: Updating the Social Security Listings*. Washington, D.C: National Academies Press; 2010.
54. Aboyans V, Criqui MH, Abraham P, et al. Measurement and interpretation of the ankle-brachial index. *Circulation*. 2012;126:2890–2909.
55. Gerhard-Herman MD, Gornik HL, Barrett C, et al. 2016 AHA/ACC guideline on the management of patients with lower extremity peripheral artery disease: a report of the American College of Cardiology/American Heart Association Task Force on Clinical Practice Guidelines. *Circulation*. 2017;135:e726–e779.
56. Jonas DE, Reddy S, Middleton JC, et al. Screening for cardiovascular disease risk with resting or exercise electrocardiography: evidence report and systematic review for the US Preventive Services Task Force. *J Am Med Assoc*. 2018;319:2315–2328.
57. American Diabetes Association. Cardiovascular disease and risk management: standards of medical care in diabetes-2020. *Diabetes Care*. 2020;43:S111–S134.

16 Echocardiography

JUSTINA C. WU, LINDA D. GILLAM, AND SCOTT D. SOLOMON

Illustrated by Bernard Bulwer

PRINCIPLES OF ULTRASOUND AND INSTRUMENTATION, 196
Principles of Image Generation, 196
Physical Principles of Ultrasound, 197
Doppler Echocardiography in Practice, 199
Assessment of Flow and Continuity Equation, 200

THE STANDARD ADULT TRANSTHORACIC ECHOCARDIOGRAPHIC EXAMINATION, 200
M-Mode Echocardiography, 200
Assessment of Cardiac Structure and Function, 203

TRANSESOPHAGEAL ECHOCARDIOGRAPHY, 210
The Standard Transesophageal Echocardiographic Examination, 211

THREE-DIMENSIONAL ECHOCARDIOGRAPHY, 212

ULTRASOUND ENHANCING AGENTS, 212

MYOCARDIAL INFARCTION, 216
Practical Considerations in Assessment of Regional Wall Motion, 216

Echocardiographic Prognostic Indicators After Myocardial Infarction, 219

CARDIOMYOPATHIES, 220
Dilated Cardiomyopathy, 220
Hypertrophic Cardiomyopathy, 221
Other Cardiomyopathies With Regional or Global Variations in Myocardial Composition, 222
Restrictive Cardiomyopathies, 222
Heart Failure, 222
The Athlete's Heart, 224

STRESS ECHOCARDIOGRAPHY, 224

VALVULAR HEART DISEASE, 226
Mitral Valve, 226
Aortic Valve, 231
Tricuspid Valve, 234
Pulmonic Valve, 235
Prosthetic Valves, 235

PERICARDIAL DISEASE, 240
Pericardial Effusion, 240
Constrictive Pericarditis, 242

DISEASES OF THE AORTA, 244
Focal Aortopathies, 244
Aortic Emergencies, 244

PULMONARY HYPERTENSION, 248

INFECTIVE ENDOCARDITIS, 248
Role of Echocardiography in Surgery for Endocarditis, 252

CARDIAC MASSES, 253
Secondary Tumors, 253
Alternative Diagnoses, 255

ADULT CONGENITAL HEART DISEASE, 256
Atrial Septal Defect, 256
Ventricular Septal Defect, 259

TRANSCATHETER INTERVENTIONS, 260
Future Directions, 265
Handheld Echocardiography (Point of Care Ultrasound), 265

REFERENCES, 266

Echocardiography remains the most commonly used comprehensive cardiac imaging modality and is often the first test of choice for assessing cardiac structure and function. When compared with other imaging methods, echocardiography can be performed quickly at bedside, with minimal patient inconvenience or risk, and provides immediate clinically relevant information at relatively low cost. Echocardiography provides detailed data on cardiac structure, including the size and shape of cardiac chambers, as well as the morphology and function of cardiac valves. Furthermore, the real-time nature of echocardiography makes it uniquely suited to immediate non-invasive assessment of systolic and diastolic function and intracardiac hemodynamics. In most echocardiography laboratories, standard *transthoracic echocardiography* (TTE) is complemented by *transesophageal echocardiography* (TEE) imaging from within the body which offers improved resolution, and by *stress echocardiography*, which is routinely used to assess myocardial ischemia and valvular function with exercise. Technical advancements in echocardiography over the past decades have led to progressively improved diagnostic capabilities. In recent years, these included advances in three-dimensional (3D) and tissue strain imaging, expanded functionality and miniaturization of systems that can be used for point of care imaging, and contrast echocardiography for better cavity visualization, augmentation of Doppler signals and assessment of tissue perfusion.

Two-dimensional (2D) echocardiography is not a tomographic technique such as cardiac computed tomography (CT) or cardiac magnetic resonance (CMR) imaging (see Chapters 19 and 20); acquisition of ultrasound images is dependent on the operator—either a sonographer or a physician. Both acquisition and interpretation of echocardiograms require substantial training and skill. Thus, echocardiography is best described as an "examination" rather than a "test." Although cardiologists receive this training routinely, a growing number of non-cardiologists, including emergency physicians, anesthesiologists, intensivists, and in-patient hospital staff are increasingly using echocardiography in their practice, in some cases with small handheld ultrasound devices (POCUS, or point-of-care ultrasound devices). Knowledge of the basic principles, utility, and limitations of echocardiography is becoming essential for all physicians who care for patients with cardiovascular problems.

PRINCIPLES OF ULTRASOUND AND INSTRUMENTATION

Principles of Image Generation

Echocardiography is based on the standard principles of ultrasound imaging in which high-frequency sound waves in the 1 to 10 MHz range are emitted from piezoelectric crystals housed in a transducer, traverse through internal body structures, interact with tissues, reflect back to the transducer, and are then processed by microcomputers to generate an image. An understanding of the physical principles that underlie echocardiography is essential to understanding its usefulness and limitations.[1]

Ultrasound machines measure the time required for sound waves to reflect from structures and return to the transducer, and use this data to calculate the depth of reflecting structures. This information is used to generate scan lines that depict both *location* (depth of reflection) and *amplitude* (intensity of reflection). Early ultrasound equipment projected a single beam of ultrasound, which resulted in a single scan line that could be "painted" across a moving paper or screen, with depth being depicted on the vertical axis and time on the horizontal axis. This method, known as *M-mode* (for motion) echocardiography (Fig. 16.1, lower right), has largely been replaced by 2D imaging (see Fig. 16.1, lower left). However, M-mode is still used routinely and is particularly useful for characterizing high-frequency events or making linear measurements and assessments that require precise timing with respect to the cardiac cycle.

Current 2D imaging scans sectors of the heart using phased-array transducers, in which the piezoelectric crystal is precisely diced into multiple (hundreds to thousands) of elements that emit and receive sonar pulses. Phased-array transducers steer the beam electronically through an arc side-to-side to create a scan plane (Fig. 16.2). The transducer emits pulses of ultrasound in an ordered sequence and sequentially "listens" for returning echoes, referred to as the *pulse-echo principle*.

The returning sound waves are coded into electric signals, and repetition of this sequence enables reconstruction of moving images to depict the heart. The rate at which these pulses are emitted is termed the *pulse repetition frequency* (PRF). Proper interpretation of returning signals is physically limited by the speed of sound in tissues (approximately 1540 m/sec) and the depth of the tissues being interrogated, both of which dictate the time it takes for the ultrasound signal to return to the transducer. Nevertheless, improvements in processing speed have allowed "frame" rates, a major determinant of temporal resolution, to reach speeds higher than 100 image frames per second. In practice, the echo machine operator can also increase frame rate by narrowing the scan sector, imaging at shallower depths, and reducing scan line density. (On most systems, the preprocessing "zoom" feature easily narrows the sector to the region of interest to accomplish this.) 3D echocardiography extends the phased-array concept to make use of a planar waffle-like grid or matrix-array of elements (3000+), which allows both simultaneous multiplanar 2D imaging and true volumetric 3D imaging and rendering (see Three-Dimensional Echocardiography).

Physical Principles of Ultrasound

The physical characteristics of ultrasound are exploited to generate images representative of the heart. The wavelength of the ultrasound used, which is inversely related to ultrasound frequency, is the principal determinant of axial imaging resolution, which equals approximately half the wavelength. The higher the ultrasound frequency (i.e., shorter the wavelength), the higher is the spatial resolution. Imaging resolution is also dependent on the depth of the structure being interrogated. Therefore, the choice of imaging frequency involves a trade-off between image resolution and target tissue depth: higher frequencies are capable of increased resolution, but at the expense of reduced tissue penetration. Most TTE machines operate across frequencies of 2.5 to 5 MHz. Higher frequencies up to 7 to 10 MHz can be used in pediatric imaging, in TEE where the transducer is closer to the heart, or when interrogating near-field structures, such as the apex of the heart from the apical window. Current broad-bandwidth transducers allow the operator to easily modify the transmit frequency (mHz), so that one may start with higher transmit frequency for better image resolution but adjust the frequency downwards during the exam if additional tissue penetration is desired.

The speed of ultrasound through body tissues averages 1540 meters per second (m/sec), essentially the speed of sound through water, but varies minutely as ultrasound waves traverse various body constituents. These slight differences in ultrasound speed through different media (e.g., blood, muscle, fat, air) result in impedance mismatches at the tissue interfaces, which produces the *specular reflections* that mark the boundaries between different tissues. The most intense reflections occur when ultrasound strikes these interfaces perpendicularly and when the tissues differ greatly in density. When ultrasound encounters inhomogeneous tissue regions, such as myocardium, liver, or other tissues, multidirectional reflection, or *backscatter*, occurs and results in speckled-appearing images. The combination of specular reflections and backscatter, together with the unique interactions between ultrasound and tissue such as refraction, interference, and attenuation, contributes to the characteristic gray-scale appearance of ultrasound images. Ultrasound

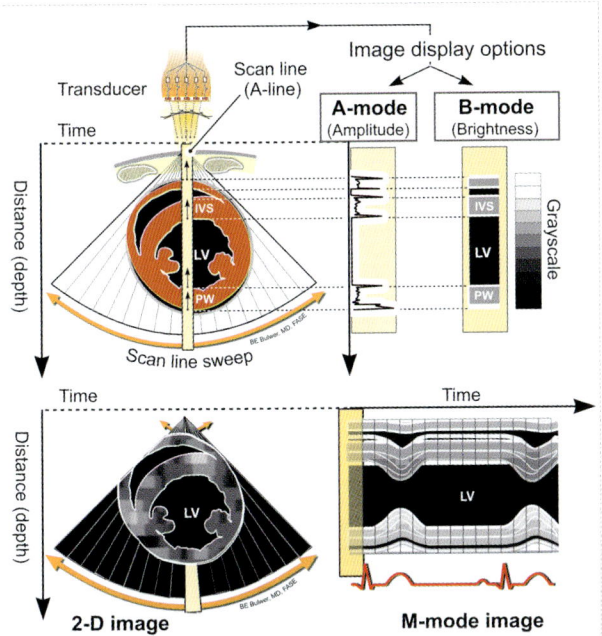

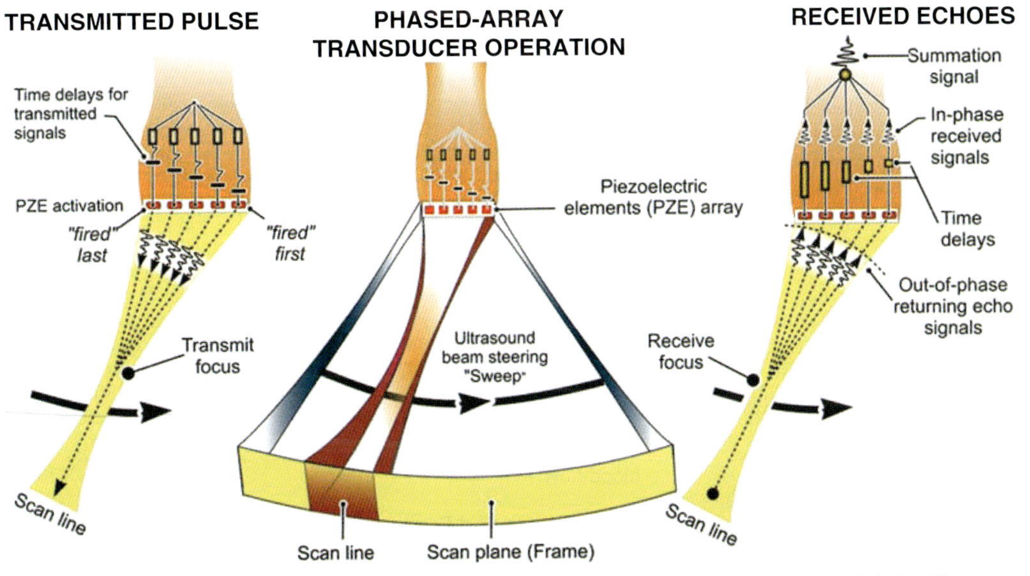

FIGURE 16.1 Generation of ultrasound images. An ultrasound pulse transmitted from piezoelectric elements housed in a transducer **(upper left)** reflects off structures and returns to the transducer. These signals are processed and displayed based on their amplitudes **(upper right)**. Echoes with the highest amplitudes emerge from tissue interfaces such as the pericardial-pleural and endocardial-blood borders. In original A-mode scans, such signals are visualized as amplitude spikes. On B-mode, the echo amplitudes are displayed via gray scale. B-mode images can then be displayed in one dimension over time, i.e., M (motion)–mode **(bottom right)**, or as a two-dimensional cross-sectional image **(bottom left)**. *IVS,* Interventricular septum; *LV,* left ventricle; *PW,* posterior wall. (Modified from Bulwer BE, Rivero JM, eds. *Echocardiography Pocket Guide: The Transthoracic Examination.* Burlington, MA: Jones & Bartlett Learning; 2011, 2013. Reprinted with permission.)

FIGURE 16.2 Phased-array transducer operation. Modern echocardiography transducers scan through a relatively wide scan sector by steering the electronic beam across the scan plane **(center)**. During transmission **(left)**, electronic time delays in firing the piezoelectric elements of the transducer cause the scan line to sweep in an arc. During reception **(right)**, the returning echo signals received by each transducer element must be time-shifted or phased before being summated and processed. (Modified from Bulwer BE, et al. Physics of echocardiography. In Savage RM, Aronson S, Shernan SK, eds. *Comprehensive Textbook of Perioperative Transesophageal Echocardiography.* Philadelphia: Wolters Kluwer; Lippincott, Williams & Wilkins; 2009:1–41.)

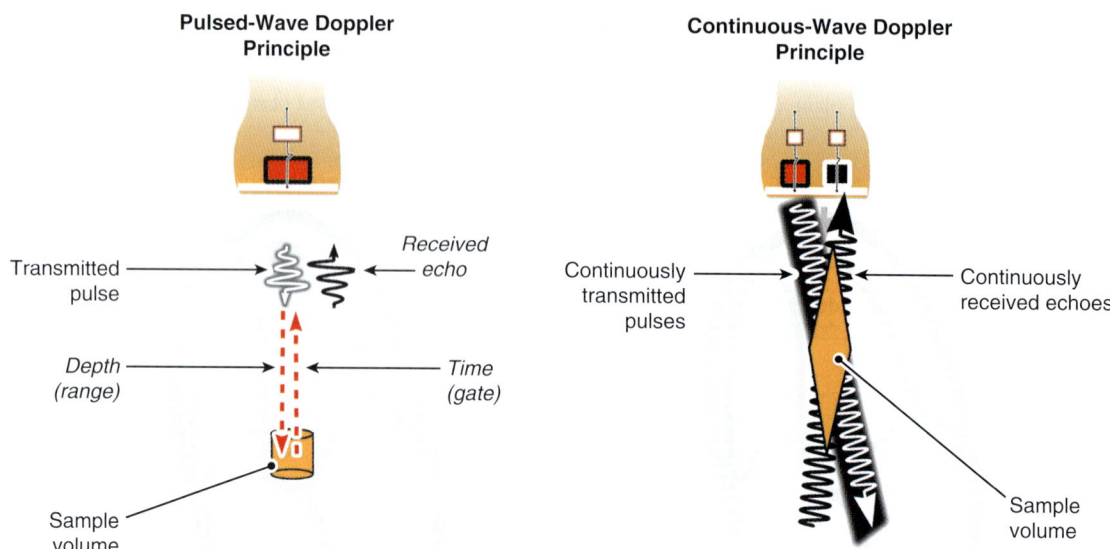

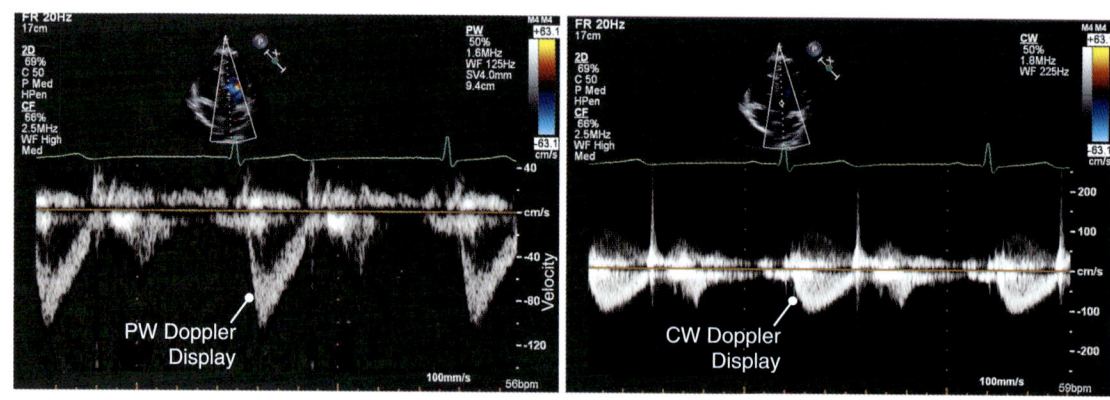

FIGURE 16.3 Pulsed-wave (PW) versus continuous-wave (CW) Doppler. **Left,** PW Doppler technique uses a single piezoelectric element that generates the pulse, interrogates a small sample volume at a specific depth, and receives the emerging echoes within the specified time window. **Right,** CW Doppler technique uses two separate transducer elements, one continuously transmitting pulses and the other receiving echoes across a large sample volume, and thus cannot localize the depth of the site with highest velocity.

penetrates poorly through air and bone, which is one of the greatest challenges to echocardiography because the heart is surrounded by the lungs and the rib cage. The ability to circumvent these limitations during image acquisition underscores the importance of the operator's skill and the advantages of a TEE approach in specific clinical situations.

Several advances in the past decade have improved the quality of ultrasonic imaging. The higher number of elements in phased-array transducers has increased the number of scan lines and thus lateral resolution. *Tissue harmonic imaging* is now the norm, in which the receiver "listens" for returning second-harmonic ultrasound signals that are twice the fundamental frequency of the emitted ultrasound. By doing so, it effectively filters out the weaker noisy and artefactual signals and has substantially improved the definition of tissue interfaces, in particular that of the endocardial borders, when compared to fundamental imaging.

PRINCIPLES OF DOPPLER IMAGING

In addition to generating images of cardiac structures, ultrasound can be used to interrogate the velocity of blood flow through the heart and to assess myocardial motion. These techniques are based on the Doppler principle, which states that the perceived frequency of a waveform bounced back from a moving object will be perceived as shifted from the emitting frequency, depending on whether the object is moving toward or away from the observer. Ultrasound that is reflected from red blood cells moving toward the emitter will appear to be at a higher frequency, whereas blood flow away from the transducer will cause the perception that a lower-frequency waveform has been reflected. This difference between the frequency emitted and that received is termed the *Doppler frequency shift* and is dependent on the speed of ultrasound through the medium and the velocity of blood flow. The basic equation for Doppler shift (f_d) is $f_d = f_t\, V/c$, where f_t is the transmitted ultrasound frequency, V is the velocity of blood flow, and c is the speed of ultrasound in the tissue. For cardiac ultrasound, multiplication by a factor of 2 occurs because the Doppler shift occurs twice (when the wave goes to and from the moving object). Notably, the velocity information obtained is most accurate when the ultrasound beam is aligned parallel to the direction of blood flow (i.e., an optimal angle of insonation is 0 degrees). When the angle of insonation (θ) cannot be physically corrected, the correction factor $\cos\theta$ may be applied. Thus the refined formula for Doppler shift is:

$$F_d = 2 f_t V (\cos\theta)$$

Ultimately, the equation above is used to solve for velocity, V, of blood flow.

Pulsed-Wave and Continuous-Wave Doppler

The two principal types of Doppler imaging are pulsed-wave (PW) and continuous-wave (CW) Doppler. In PW Doppler (Fig. 16.3, left panel), discrete pulses of ultrasound reflect off moving structures (i.e., red blood cells moving through the heart) and return to the transducer. By *gating,* or defining a specific time window during which the machine "listens" for reflected signal, this technique can be used to ascertain the velocity of blood flow at a prespecified depth within the heart. Thus, when an operator places the cursor (sample volume) on the 2D ultrasound image at a particular location, the equipment will assess the velocity at that point. Because it takes time for the pulses to reflect and return to the transducer, they cannot be transmitted too frequently, or the equipment will fail to discern whether a given pulse has returned from the defined location or some multiple of that distance from the transducer, and the velocity information obtained at that depth will be ambiguous. The PRF is essentially the sampling rate; the higher the blood flow velocity, the higher is the frequency of the Doppler shift and thus the higher the sampling rate needed to accurately sample that shift. These physical principles limit the upper range of velocities that can be interrogated with PW Doppler. The *Nyquist limit* refers to the maximum velocity that can be accurately quantified within a given sample volume and is directly related to the PRF (the numeric value equals ½ the PRF). PRF in turn is inversely related to the distance from the sample volume to the transducer. The machine is unable to assess velocities that are higher than the Nyquist limit, because the values will go off-scale and appear to "alias" (wrap around) in the generated spectrogram; adjusting the Nyquist limit setting on the machine upward effectively adjusts the PRF upward until the physical limit is reached.

With CW Doppler (see Fig. 16.3, right panel) a dedicated piezoelectric element continuously emits ultrasound, and a separate element simultaneously continuously receives the returning signals. Because the ultrasound tone is continuous rather than pulsed, depth of the target cannot be determined from the signal received. However, unlike the situation with PW Doppler, no limit is imposed on the velocities discernible with this technique. Thus *PW Doppler is primarily used to assess flow with relatively low velocity (typically ≤1.5 m/sec) present at a specific location, whereas CW Doppler is used to assess higher velocities (typically ≥1.5 m/sec) along the transducer beam, but cannot specify at what location the highest velocity occurs.* Note that PW Doppler envelopes have a linear "hollowed-out" profile because the blood within the small sample volume tends to travel at similar velocities (laminar flow), whereas CW Doppler envelopes are "filled in" because all the varying velocities along the ultrasound beam are received and recorded.

Color Flow Doppler

Color flow Doppler is a PW Doppler–based technique in which the velocities in a region of interest are encoded with colors that represent both mean velocities and directionality of the flow, which are superimposed on a 2D image in the region of interest (Fig. 16.4). By convention, flow moving away from the transducer is encoded in blue, and flow toward the transducer is encoded in red. Because color flow Doppler is a form of PW Doppler, it is subject to aliasing, such that high velocities (greater than the Nyquist limit) demonstrate "wraparound" in the color coding to the color of the opposite direction. Turbulent flow, in which a wide range of velocities exist, appears as a multicolored mosaic pattern (usually *green* and *yellow*). In some systems the variance in the velocities relative to the mean is color-coded in superimposed shades of *green*. Color flow Doppler allows direct real-time visualization of the movement of blood in the heart and is particularly useful for identifying blood flow acceleration and turbulence. Therefore, this technology is useful for delineating both regurgitant lesions, in which blood moves rapidly and opposite to the expected direction of flow, and discrete stenoses in which there is flow acceleration.

Blood Flow Profiles and Doppler Signals

Laminar Versus Turbulent Flow. Blood flow through the normal heart and great vessels is predominantly *laminar*, meaning that the direction and velocity of flow are streamlined and uniform, even across valves. Figure 16.5 shows that the spectral Doppler flow signal observed when interrogating laminar flow is characterized by a hollowed-out waveform with a narrow outline, indicating that flow velocities throughout the sample are similar. In a Doppler assessment of the left ventricular outflow tract (LVOT), for example, the Doppler profile represents the velocity of blood flow throughout systole and is usually laminar. In contrast, valvular or vessel stenoses or obstructive lesions often cause turbulent flow, in which blood moves at different velocities and in multiple directions. In these cases, if the range of velocities is still largely within the Nyquist limit, the displayed spectrum of velocities will be wider on PW Doppler, a phenomenon termed *spectral broadening*. On color Doppler, turbulent flow appears brighter with a mixture of colors.

As illustrated by the Doppler equation and discussed earlier, the velocity of blood flow determined from the Doppler shift will change with the angle of insonation (θ). If the vector of flow is not directly in line with the ultrasound beam, the velocities calculated by the Doppler

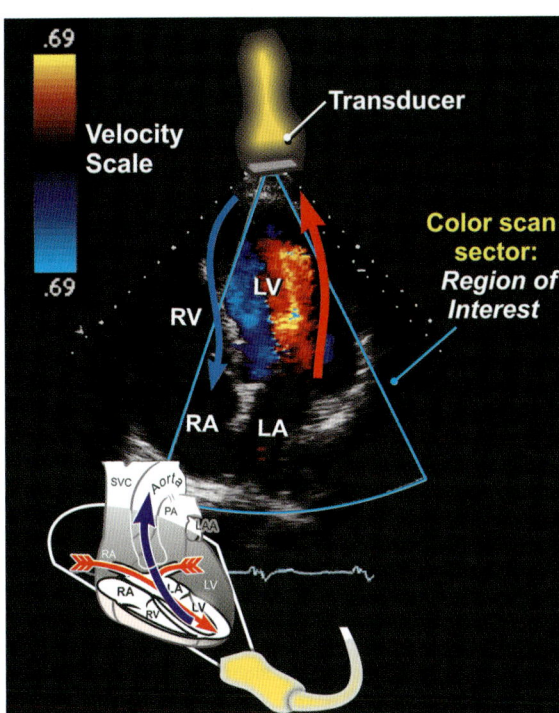

FIGURE 16.4 Color flow Doppler. By convention, blood flow moving toward the transducer is color-coded *red* and flow away from the transducer is shown in *blue*. The color velocity scale (*upper left vertical bar*) represents increasing velocities in either direction, with higher velocities depicted in progressively brighter hues. Note the Nyquist limit (69 cm/sec) displayed above and below the color scale bar. Velocities greater than the Nyquist limit cause aliasing, i.e., an apparent wraparound in the color-coding to that of the opposite direction. *LA*, Left atrium; *LV*, left ventricle; *RA*, right atrium; *RV*, right ventricle. (Modified from Bulwer BE, Rivero JM, eds. *Echocardiography Pocket Guide: The Transthoracic Examination*. Burlington, MA: Jones & Bartlett Learning; 2011, 2013:156. Reprinted with permission.)

shift will be underestimates of those of red blood cells. This problem can be corrected by applying an angle adjustment (cosθ) that is computed at the machine level. However, the further the angle of flow deviates from the angle of the beam, the greater the likelihood for error in the calculation. In practice, for cardiac ultrasound it is recommended simply to minimize the angle of insonation as much as possible by probe and patient positioning and to avoid Doppler assessments that are substantially off-angle. It is for this reason that multiple windows are used in assessing peak flow velocities of aortic stenosis (AS) and tricuspid regurgitation (TR). Ideally, the window with the lowest angle of insonation is selected to avoid underestimation. In specific cases where flow is very laminar and insonation angles are unavoidable, such as in vascular ultrasound, the angle correction factor proves to be useful.

Doppler Echocardiography in Practice

Doppler echocardiography is used primarily to assess blood flow velocity in the heart and blood vessels. Within the heart, the velocity of blood flow is itself dependent on the pressure gradient between cardiac chambers, with higher gradients resulting in higher velocities. This relationship can be described by the Bernoulli equation, which estimates the pressure gradient (ΔP) between two chambers separated by an orifice based on the velocity of flow through the orifice. The original Bernoulli equation is complex and includes variables for flow acceleration and viscous friction and a constant for fluid density. The clinical equation used in echocardiography assumes that these two factors are negligible, and that the velocity (V_1) proximal to an orifice is relatively low in comparison to that distal velocity. This leaves the vastly simplified equation for use in clinical echocardiography for ΔP:

$$P_1 - P_2 = 4V^2$$

For example, the peak flow velocity of a tricuspid regurgitant (TR) jet can be used to calculate the pressure gradient ΔP between the right

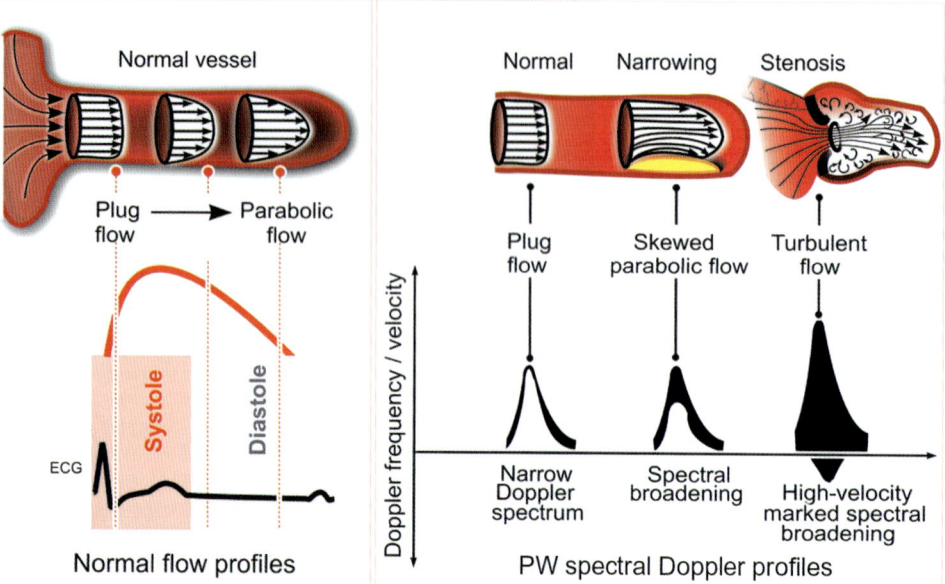

FIGURE 16.5 Flow velocity profiles on spectral Doppler. **Left,** During the cardiac cycle, most intracardiac and large arterial flows exhibit a laminar flow profile termed "plug flow" proximally that progresses distally to a more parabolic profile because of drag force and blood viscosity. **Right,** The narrowest range or spectrum of flow velocities is seen during the initial phases of systole or when valves open (plug flow). As the vessel becomes stenotic, the turbulence causes progressively wider variation in flow velocities and directions. On spectral Doppler this manifests as a splay in velocities both above and below the baseline. (Modified from Bulwer BE, et al. Physics of echocardiography. In Savage RM, Aronson S, Shernan SK, eds. *Comprehensive Textbook of Perioperative Transesophageal Echocardiography*. Philadelphia: Wolters Kluwer; Lippincott, Williams & Wilkins; 2009:23.)

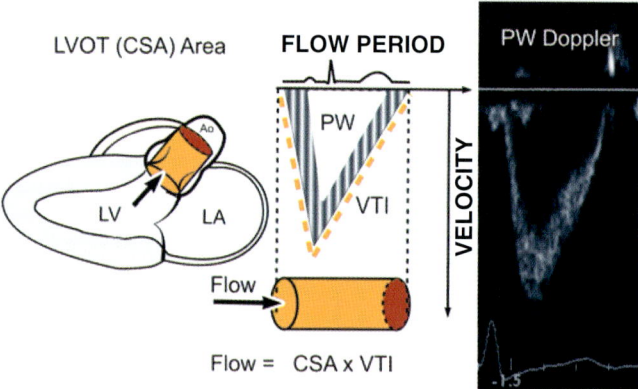

FIGURE 16.6 Volumetric flow assessments using spectral Doppler. The volume of a cylinder is cross-sectional area (CSA) multiplied by length. Using this geometric assumption and assuming constant flow during systole, stroke volume (SV) can then be derived from the CSA of the left ventricular outflow tract (LVOT) measured on the parasternal long-axis view. This is then multiplied by the Doppler velocity-time integral (VTI) measured on apical windows. *Ao,* Aorta; *LA,* left atrium; *LV,* left ventricle.

integral (VTI; i.e., integrated velocity throughout the cardiac interval) by the cross-sectional area (CSA) of the region being interrogated (Fig. 16.6). For example, stroke volume (SV) can be estimated by interrogating the LVOT region with PW Doppler and multiplying the VTI by the CSA (calculated by measuring the diameter of the LVOT and assuming a circular area = πr^2):

$$SV = VTI_{LVOT} \times Area_{LVOT}$$

The continuity principle is based on conservation of mass and states that flow in one region of the heart should be equivalent to flow in another region (assuming no intervening shunt or valve regurgitation). It can be applied to Doppler and imaging data to determine an unknown cross-sectional area, such as that of a stenotic valve. The CSA of a stenotic valve can be difficult to measure directly (i.e., by planimetry) if image quality is suboptimal. By combining the calculated CSA and measured VTI proximal to the valve with the VTI at the valve itself, the CSA of the stenosis can be calculated. Since velocities through stenotic valves are usually too high to assess with PW Doppler, CW Doppler is usually used, assuming that the highest attained velocities correspond to the narrowest region along the ultrasound beam. Because the continuity principle states that flow through the LVOT must equal flow through the aortic valve (AV);

$$VTI_{LVOT} \times Area_{LVOT} = VTI_{AV} \times Area_{AV}$$

Rearranging the equation to solve for $Area_{AV}$ will give the desired valve CSA. The accuracy of this estimate depends on the accuracy of the LVOT CSA calculation (and thus LVOT diameter measurement) and optimal positioning of the PW and CW Doppler cursors.

THE STANDARD ADULT TRANSTHORACIC ECHOCARDIOGRAPHIC EXAMINATION

The standard adult TTE examination consists of a combination of 2D, M-mode, and Doppler imaging. The recommended comprehensive examination protocol involves a series of views, each of which is described in terms of three principal components: (1) the standard transducer position or "window," (2) the orthogonal imaging planes, and (3) the anatomic region of interest (Figs. 16.7 and 16.8). At each transducer position the operator optimally acquires 2D images with M-mode images, spectral Doppler, and color flow Doppler as indicated.

M-Mode Echocardiography

M-mode echocardiography provides greater temporal resolution than standard 2D imaging and was traditionally the method of choice for certain linear measurements, particularly those that are collinear with the ultrasound beam. Standard reports continue to include measurements of septal and posterior wall thickness and left ventricular (LV) chamber dimensions on parasternal views. Figure 16.9A shows a normal M-mode at the basal left ventricle. Because M-mode echocardiography is essentially a one-dimensional imaging technique, it has several limitations that should be recognized. For accurate measurements the cursor scan line must be oriented perpendicular to the long axis of the left ventricle or left atrium, which may require operator steering or machine correction to achieve. For these reasons, convention has now shifted to using 2-dimensional measurements for standardization.[2,3] M-mode–based estimates of LV volume, mass, and function can also be inaccurate in patients with LV geometries that deviate substantially

ventricle and the right atrium, which when added to an estimate of right atrial (RA) pressure, provides an estimate of right ventricular systolic pressure (RVSP; and hence pulmonary artery systolic pressure [PASP] in most cases). Similarly, the blood flow velocity difference between the LVOT and the aorta can be used to calculate the peak instantaneous pressure gradient across a stenotic aortic valve. It is important to appreciate that Doppler echocardiography measures *velocity* but neither pressure nor flow direction. Pressure gradients are inferred from velocities based on the Bernoulli equation, but the absolute pressure within chambers cannot be directly measured as in cardiac catheterization. Similarly, the amount of flow cannot be measured directly, although there are Doppler-based methods that permit fairly accurate estimation of flow volumes (see below).

Assessment of Flow and Continuity Equation

Doppler methods are used to assess blood flow velocities, but the magnitude of flow can also be inferred by multiplying the *velocity-time*

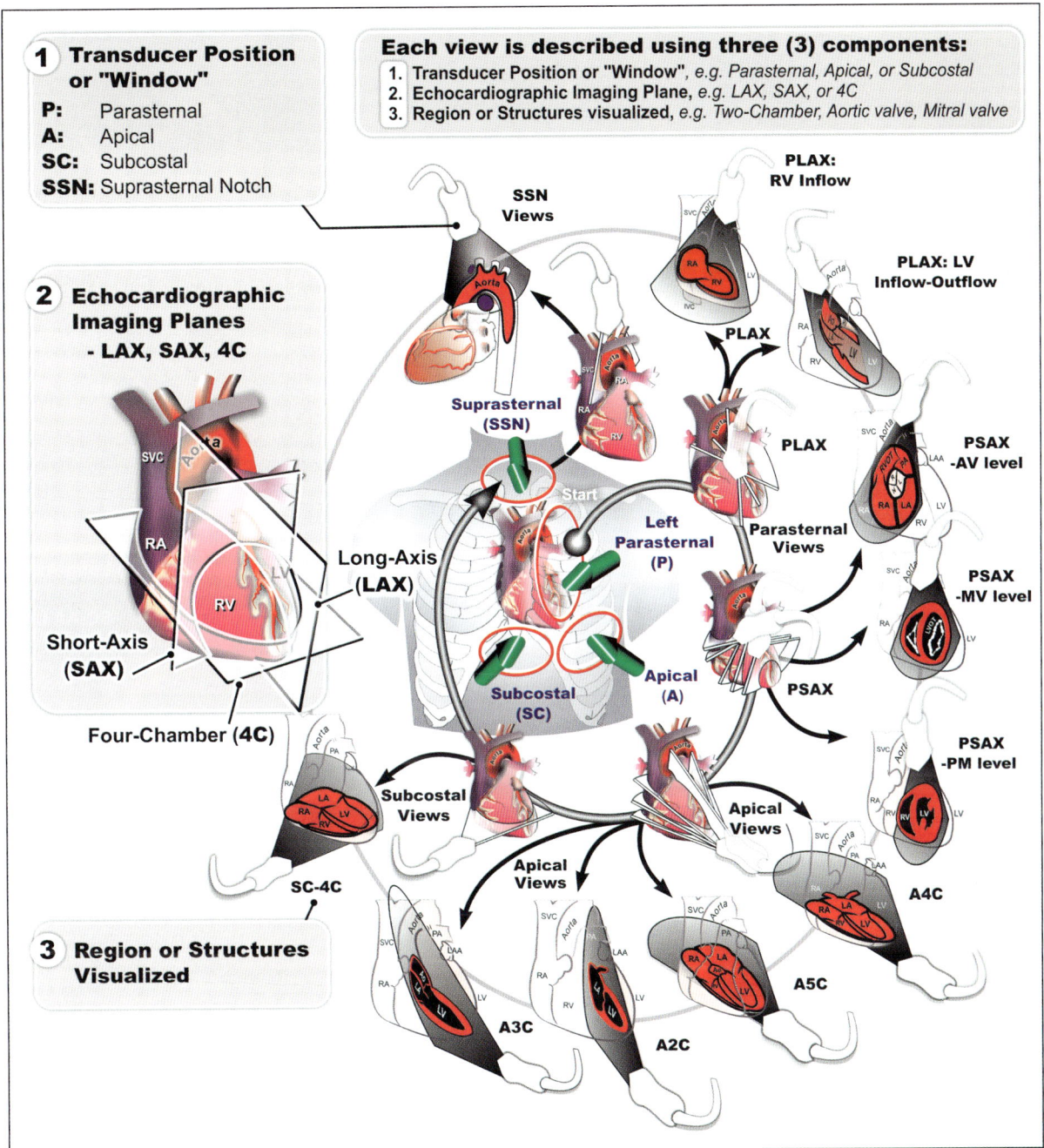

FIGURE 16.7 Standard adult transthoracic echocardiography imaging planes, protocol, and nomenclature recommended by the American Society of Echocardiography (ASE). Each echocardiographic view can be described by three parameters: window, plane, and structure visualized. See Fig. 16.8 for abbreviations. (Modified from Bulwer BE, et al. Physics of echocardiography. In Savage RM, Aronson S, Shernan SK, eds. *Comprehensive Textbook of Perioperative Transesophageal Echocardiography*. Philadelphia: Wolters Kluwer; Lippincott, Williams & Wilkins; 2009:1–41.)

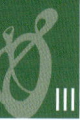

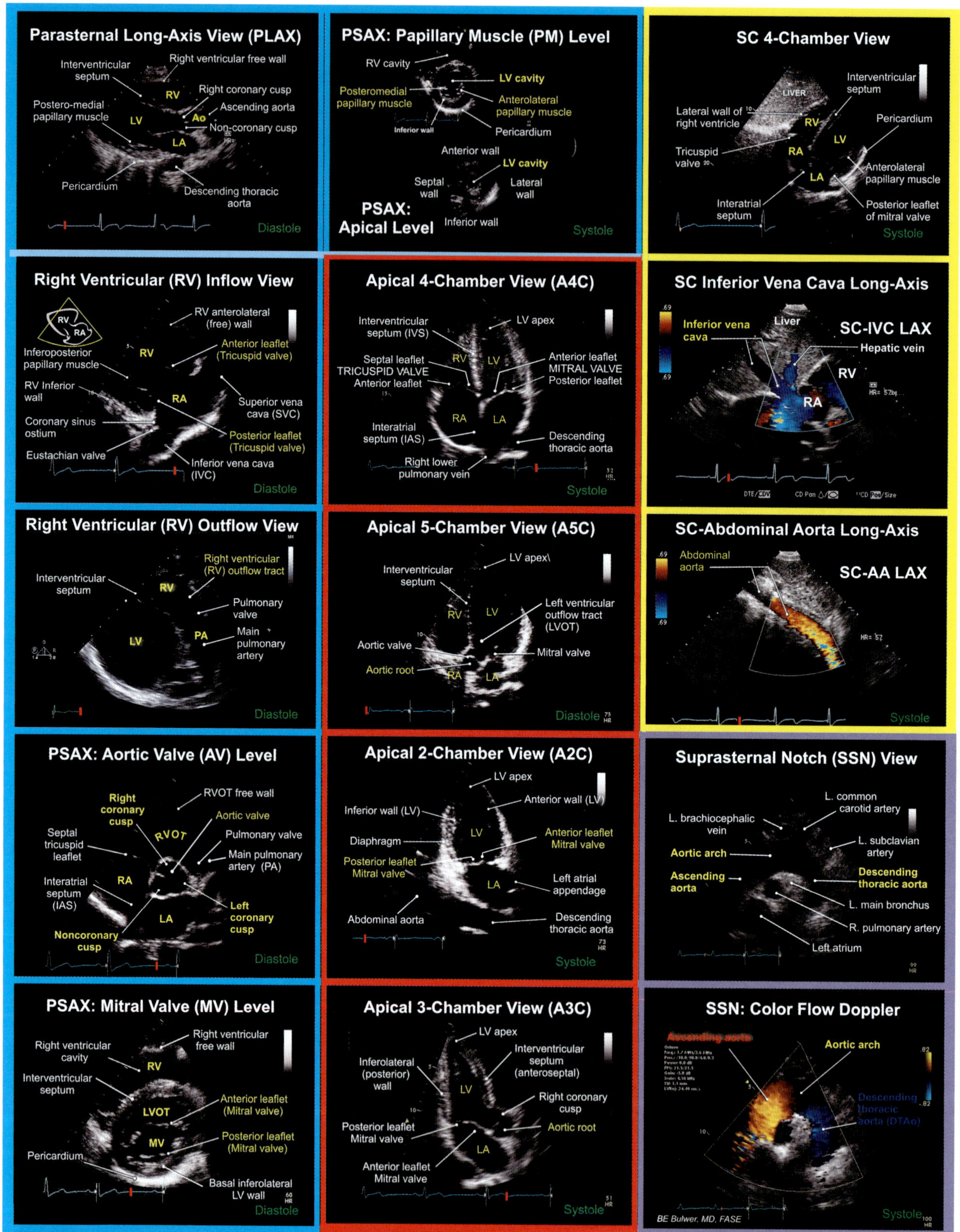

AA: abdominal aorta
Ao: aorta
Asc. Ao: ascending aorta
AV: aortic valve
BCA: brachiocephalic artery
DTAo: descending thoracic aorta
IVC: inferior vena cava
LA: left atrium
LLPV: left lower pulmonary vein
LSA: left subclavian artery
LUPV: left upper pulmonary vein
LV: left ventricle
LVOT: LV outflow tract
PA: pulmonary artery
RA: right atrium
RLPV: right lower pulmonary vein
RUPV: right upper pulmonary vein
RV: right ventricle
RVOT: RV outflow tract
SVC: superior vena cava
TV: tricuspid valve

FIGURE 16.8 Labeled still frames of standard adult TTE views. Compare with Fig. 16.7. *Ao,* Aorta; *LA,* left atrium; *RA,* right atrium; *LV,* left ventricle; *RV,* right ventricle; *PA,* pulmonary artery; *LVOT,* left ventricular outflow tract. Labeled tricuspid valve leaflets and right ventricular walls are those typically identified from these windows, although slight differences in transducer angulation can result in the display of different wall/leaflets (e.g., the inferior rather than lateral wall seen in the subcostal view).

from normal, such as those with aneurysms or focal wall motion abnormalities. M-mode of valvular leaflets is of historical importance for diagnosis and still remains useful for demonstrating abnormalities in valvular motion, including rheumatic mitral stenosis (MS), mitral valve prolapse, and systolic anterior motion of the mitral valve as occurs in obstructive hypertrophic cardiomyopathy (HCM) (Fig. 16.9).

M-mode can also be combined with 2D imaging to reveal subtle changes in interventricular septal motion and chamber wall movement in pericardial disease, particularly with respect to timing within the cardiac cycle and relative to respirophasic changes. In combination with color flow Doppler (color M-mode), accurate information about timing and direction of flow and assessment of diastolic function can also be augmented. In apical four-chamber windows, M-mode may be applied to assess RV systolic function (see Fig. 16.17).

IMAGING ARTEFACTS

Ultrasound imaging artefacts are ubiquitous in echocardiography and are incurred by the physical principles of ultrasound. Artefacts can include the semblance of structures that do not exist or can be caused by real structures, such as the ribs obscuring visualization of the heart. Most artefacts are caused by physical interactions between ultrasound and tissue (Fig. 16.10). Common artefacts include (1) *attenuation artefacts,* which result in acoustic "shadowing" typically caused by ribs or bony structures; (2) *side lobe artefacts,* which occur when lower-energy side beams (side lobes) aside from the main ultrasound beam reflect off of lateral structures and are mapped onto the central image; (3) *multiple reflection artefacts,* in which the sound waves bounce between a strong reflector—such as the pericardium, pleura, or aortic wall—and the transducer more than once, giving rise to mirror images or near-field clutter; and (4) *reverberation artefacts,* which are caused by continuing repetition of internal reflections, often seen behind mechanical valve prostheses or left ventricular assist device (LVAD) cannulae. One type of reverberation artefact, *comet-tail artefact,* can be useful diagnostically to detect interstitial fluid in the lungs, where the specific finding is known as "B-lines" (see also Heart Failure).

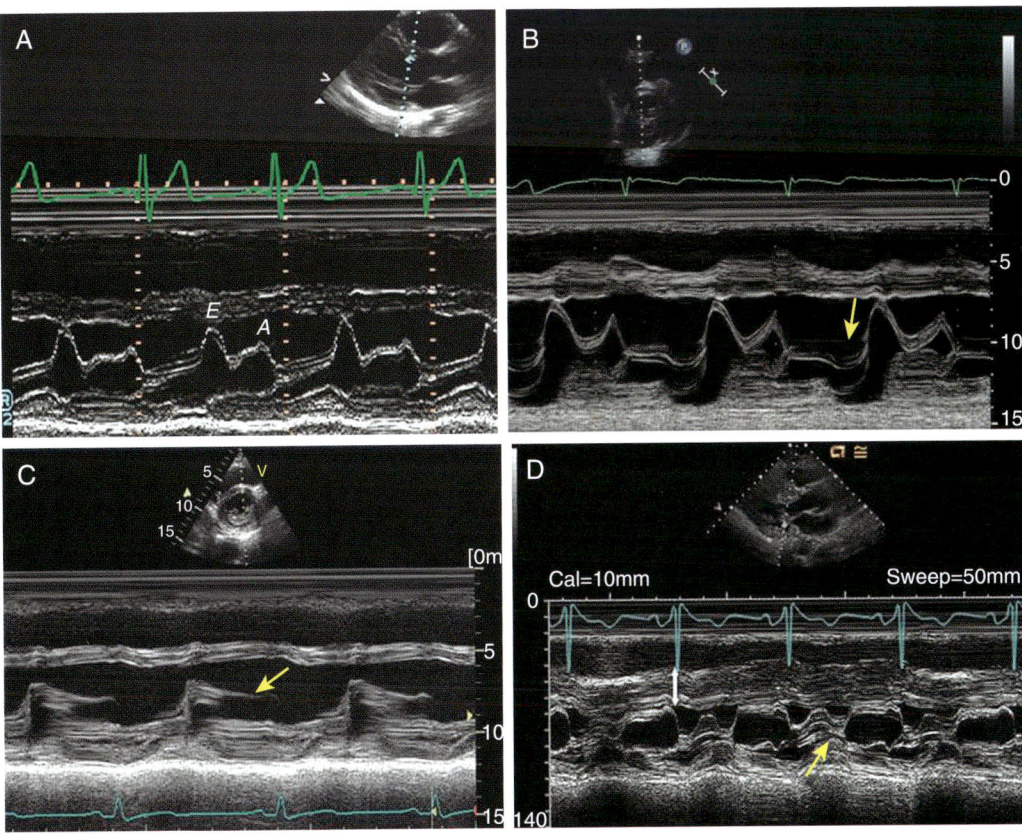

FIGURE 16.9 M-mode tracings. **A,** Normal M-mode across the base of the left ventricle at the level of the mitral leaflet tips. Note the E and A waves corresponding to the anterior mitral leaflet motion in early diastole (E) and with atrial contraction (A), respectively. Compare with **B,** which shows a patient with mitral valve prolapse, where there is late systolic posterior bowing (*arrow*) of the mitral leaflets on M-mode. **C,** Rheumatic mitral stenosis, with thickened mitral leaflets that move parallel to each other, straightening of the slope after the E wave (E-F slope), and reduced leaflet opening in diastole. **D,** Hypertrophic obstructive cardiomyopathy, displaying a very thickened interventricular septum (*white double-headed arrow*) and systolic anterior motion of the mitral valve leaflets (*yellow arrow*).

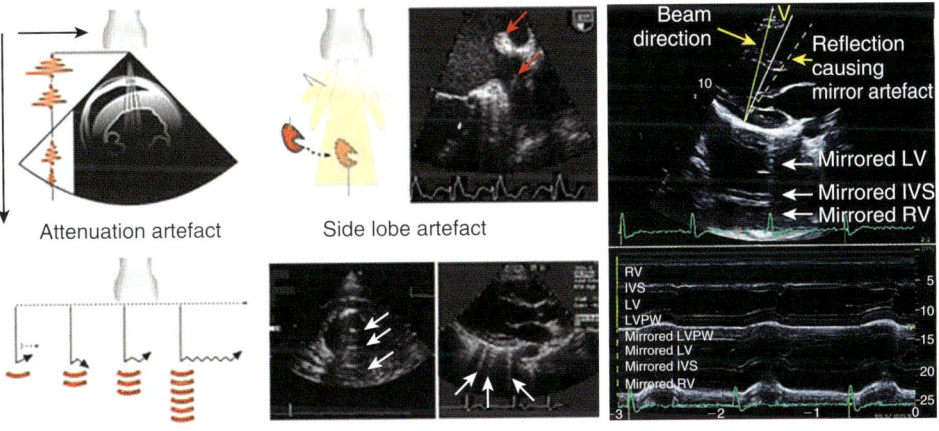

FIGURE 16.10 Common imaging artefacts seen in echocardiography. Attenuation artefacts, caused by diminution in ultrasound beam intensity with increasing depth, resulting in fading and dropout **(upper left)**. Side lobe artefacts occur when structures in the path of the side lobe beams are erroneously mapped into the image **(upper middle)**. Reverberation artefacts are common **(lower left and middle panels)**. They may be large, as in the case of reflections from the inflow tube of an LVAD (three parallel *arrows,* below center), or appear as fine comet-tail or "ring-down" artefacts because of multiple reverberations that invariably occur at the highly specular epicardial-pleural interface **(lower right)**. **Right panels,** Mirror artefact, caused by reflection between tissue interfaces and the transducer.

Assessment of Cardiac Structure and Function

The primary goal of the echocardiographic examination remains the assessment of cardiac structure and performance. Each chamber, valve, and great vessel can be assessed qualitatively and quantitatively to define any alterations in size, geometry, and function.[3] Measurements of cardiac structures are typically made in various locations throughout the heart, and linear, area, or volumetric measures can be obtained. These methods are often complementary to one another. For example, although volumetric measurements of the left ventricle (see later) are generally considered best suited to characterize LV size, many laboratories continue to record linear cavity measurements, because there is extensive literature correlating these measures with outcomes in numerous disease states. Moreover, linear measures may be subject to less variability than area- or volume-based measures and hence more reliable for assessing changes over time.

Tables 16.1 to 16.3 show established normal values on echocardiography. For LV linear dimensions and volume, Table 16.1 gives the normal ranges for the general population, but ideally one should take into account not only sex, but also body surface area (BSA) and age[2]. Current American Society of Echocardiography (ASE) consensus statements also provide partition values— that is, mild, moderate, and severely abnormal ranges—for LV size, mass, and ejection fraction (EF) and left atrial (LA) volume, but caution that the ranges were arrived at by experience-based consensus only, and that degree of abnormality does not necessarily connote a direct correlation with outcomes or prognosis (see Table 16.2). Normal values for LV parameters obtained with 3D echocardiography also exist and appear accurate and reproducible when image quality is good. In general, LV volumes calculated by 3D imaging are smaller than those generated from CMR data, but correlations with trends in sex and BSA hold true.[2]

Left Ventricular Structure: Size and Mass

Historically, LV volumes have been estimated from one of several formulas that use either linear or 2D measurements to calculate a volume based on the assumption that the left ventricle approximates a prolate ellipsoid or cylinder hemiellipsoid shape (Fig. 16.11). These approaches had the advantages of being relatively reproducible and simple to calculate. Much published research relies on M-mode data, but the estimation of LV volume is less accurate when ventricular geometry deviates from normal because of myocardial damage or remodeling. For all LV geometries, the modified biplane Simpson method of discs has been demonstrated and recommended as the most accurate method (Fig. 16.12). This method requires tracing the endocardial border in the apical four- and two-chamber views with computerized assistance to measure the diameter and height of equally distributed slices along the ventricle. With these measurements, the volume of each axial slice can be calculated, and the volume of all the slices summed to give the total chamber volume. The method is very accurate when image quality is good. However, in actual practice, suboptimal image quality can make definition of the endocardial border challenging. Moreover, foreshortening of the ventricle in one of the apical views, which can occur simply by minor changes in the transducer angle, can dramatically reduce the measured volume. The development and utilization of LV echocardiographic contrast and 3D echocardiography (see later) can

TABLE 16.1 Normal Values for Two-Dimensional Echocardiographic Parameters of Left Ventricular Size and Function According to Sex

	MALE		FEMALE	
PARAMETER	MEAN ± SD	2-SD RANGE	MEAN ± SD	2-SD RANGE
Left Ventricular (LV) Internal Dimension				
Diastolic dimension (mm)	50.2 ± 4.1	42.0–58.4	45.0 ± 3.6	37.8–52.2
Systolic dimension (mm)	32.4 ± 3.7	25.0–39.8	28.2 ± 3.3	21.6–34.8
LV Volumes (Biplane)				
LV EDV (mL)	106 ± 22	62–150	76 ± 15	46–106
LV ESV (mL)	41 ± 10	21–61	28 ± 7	14–42
LV Volumes Normalized by Body Surface Area				
LV EDV (mL/m²)	54 ± 10	34–74	45 ± 8	29–61
LV ESV (mL/m²)	21 ± 5	11–31	16 ± 4	8–24
LV EF (biplane)	62 ± 5	52–72	64 ± 5	54–74

EDV, End-diastolic volume; *EF*, ejection fraction; *ESV*, end-systolic volume; *SD*, standard deviation.
From Lang RM, Badano LP, Mor-Avi V et al. Recommendations for cardiac chamber quantification by echocardiography in adults: an update from the American Society of Echocardiography and the European Association of Cardiovascular Imaging. *J Am Soc Echocardiogr.* 2015;28:1.

TABLE 16.3 Normal Ranges for Left Ventricular (LV) Mass Indices

INDEX	WOMEN	MEN
Linear Method		
LV mass (g)	67–162	88–224
LV mass/BSA (g/m²)	*43–95*	*49–115*
Relative wall thickness (cm)	0.22–0.42	0.24–0.42
Septal thickness (cm)	*0.6–0.9*	*0.6–1.0*
Posterior wall thickness (cm)	*0.6–0.9*	*0.6–1.0*
Two-Dimensional Method		
LV mass (g)	66–150	96–200
LV mass/BSA (g/m²)	*44–88*	*50–102*

Bold/italic values: Recommended and best validated.
From Lang RM, Badano LP, Mor-Avi V, et al. Recommendations for cardiac chamber quantification by echocardiography in adults: an update from the American Society of Echocardiography and the European Association of Cardiovascular Imaging. *J Am Soc Echocardiogr.* 2015;28:1.

TABLE 16.2 Normal Ranges and Severity Partition Cutoff Values for Two-Dimensional Echocardiography–Derived Left Ventricular Ejection Fraction (LVEF) and Left Atrial (LA) Volume

	MALE				FEMALE			
	NORMAL RANGE	MILDLY ABNORMAL	MODERATELY ABNORMAL	SEVERELY ABNORMAL	NORMAL RANGE	MILDLY ABNORMAL	MODERATELY ABNORMAL	SEVERELY ABNORMAL
LVEF (%)	52–72	41–51	30–40	<30	54–74	41–53	30–40	<30
Max LA vol/BSA (mL/m²)	16–34	35–41	42–48	>48	16–34	35–41	42–48	>48

BSA, Body surface area.
From Lang RM, Badano LP, Mor-Avi V, et al. Recommendations for cardiac chamber quantification by echocardiography in adults: an update from the American Society of Echocardiography and the European Association of Cardiovascular Imaging. *J Am Soc Echocardiogr* 2015;28:1.

With all methods, care must be taken to measure the walls at end-diastole, because small errors may be exponentially multiplied depending on the calculation used; Table 16.3 shows currently accepted normal values. An LV mass index (derived from 2D echocardiographic measurements) of greater than 95 g/m² for women or more than 115 g/m² for men is considered abnormally high. Pathologically, LV *hypertrophy* is defined as increased overall LV mass and is distinct from wall thickness per se. However, in general, if LV diameter is not decreased, wall thicknesses of 12 mm or more correlate with LV hypertrophy. Alterations in LV size and mass can be categorized based on the ratio of relative wall thickness to the total LV mass index (Fig. 16.13). The specific pattern of ventricular remodeling has been related to prognosis in a variety of diseases, of both myocardial and valvular etiology.[5]

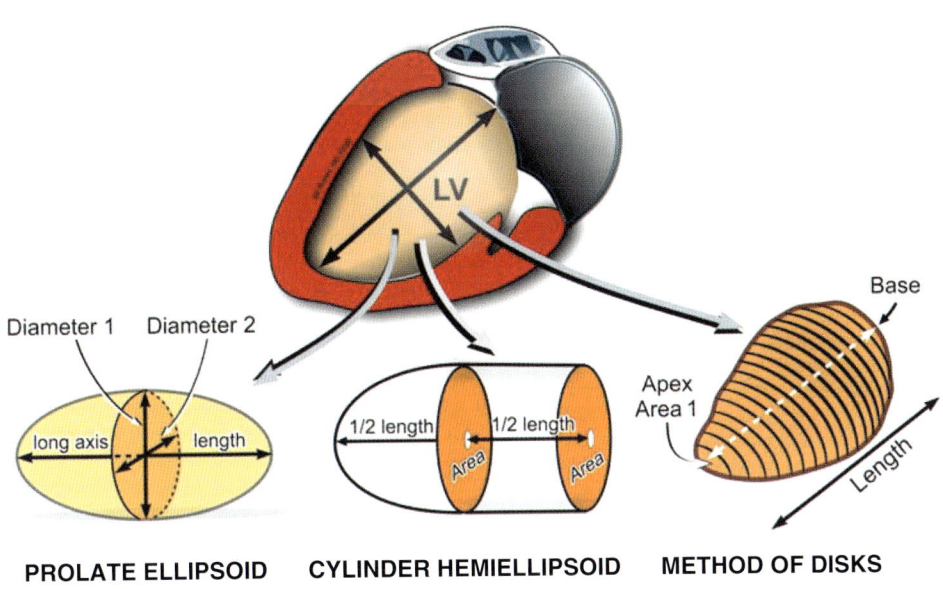

FIGURE 16.11 Geometric models and assumptions used in quantification of volumes of the left ventricle (*LV*) in two-dimensional echocardiography. (Modified from Bulwer BE, et al. Basic principles of echocardiography and tomographic anatomy. In Solomon SD, ed. *Atlas of Echocardiography*. 2nd ed. Philadelphia: Current Science/Springer Science; 2009:1–24.)

3D datasets, in which wall thicknesses are measured at a multitude of points and mass is calculated without assumptions about cavity geometry, ultimately appear more accurate but again depend on image quality. Normal values for LV mass index based on 3D data, validated against cardiac MRI, have emerged over the last several years. With less interobserver variability and automated calculations, these more sophisticated calculated values may have incremental value for outcome prediction in comparison to older 2D methods.[6]

Left Ventricular Systolic Function

Echocardiography offers several methods for assessment of systolic function. The most common remains left ventricular ejection fraction (LVEF), calculated as the difference between end-diastolic volume and end-systolic volume divided by end-diastolic volume (see Fig. 16.12). LVEF is one of the best-studied measures in cardiovascular medicine for diagnosis and risk stratification. In echocardiography the volumes are preferably calculated by the modified Simpson formula (see earlier), and normal values are 52% to 72% for men and 54%

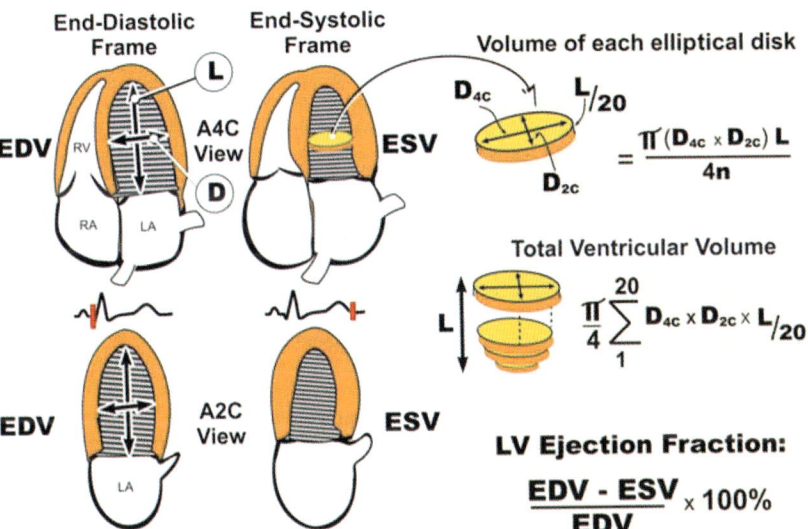

FIGURE 16.12 Simpson method of discs for quantification of left ventricular (*LV*) volumes and LV ejection fraction on two-dimensional (2D) echocardiography. *A2C,* Apical two-chamber view; *A4C,* apical four-chamber view; *D,* LV diameter; *EDV,* end-diastolic volume; *ESV,* end-systolic volume; *L,* LV length; *n,* number of discs. (Modified from Bulwer BE, et al. Basic principles of echocardiography and tomographic anatomy. In Solomon SD, ed. *Atlas of Echocardiography*. 2nd ed. Philadelphia: Current Science/Springer Science; 2009:1–24.)

mitigate the impact of these limitations and appear to permit greater accuracy and reproducibility.

LV mass may be calculated by using one of several formulas that take into account both wall thickness and chamber size,[2] typically using either linear (M-mode) or 2D measurements together with geometric modeling of the shape of the LV myocardial "shell". These formulas have been validated in normal ventricles; however, as in volume calculations, accuracy suffers when applied to those that are abnormally shaped.

to 74% for women.[2] Most echocardiography machines have basic analysis packages for automatically estimating the LVEF based on linear measurements at the base of the heart (e.g., Teicholz and Quinones formulas), which are helpful for a quick approximation but are less accurate in remodeled ventricles. In reality, the accuracy of all methods is affected by image quality, endocardial border definition, ventricular geometry, and imaging plane. When one or more of these factors are suboptimal, a visual "eyeball" estimation

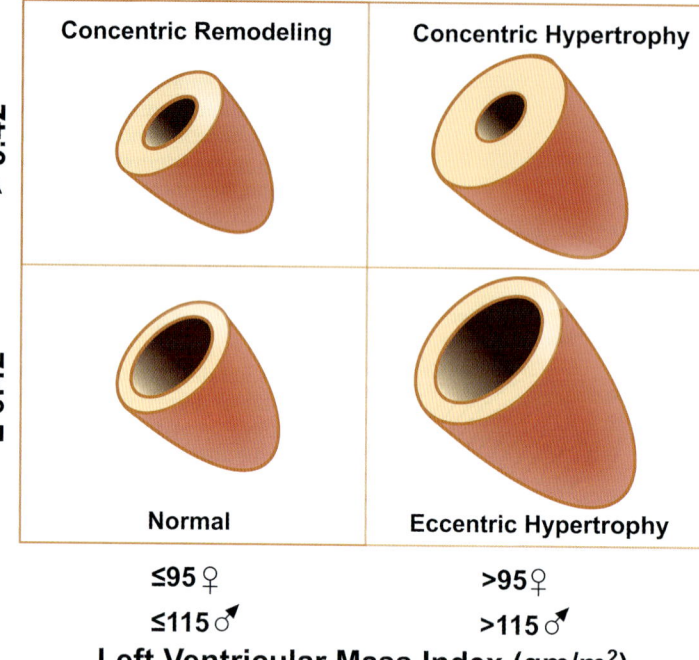

FIGURE 16.13 Patterns of left ventricular (LV) remodeling. Three patterns of adverse LV remodeling can be defined based on measurement of left ventricular mass index (LVMI) and relative wall thickness (RWT): concentric remodeling (normal LVMI and increased RWT), eccentric hypertrophy (increased LVMI and normal RWT), and concentric hypertrophy (both LVMI and RWT are increased). (Modified from Konstam MA, Kramer DG, Patel AR, et al. Left ventricular remodeling in heart failure. current concepts in clinical significance and assessment. *J Am Coll Cardiol Imaging.* 2011;4:98.)

by experienced echocardiographers can be reliable and sufficient for most clinical scenarios. Although this is common practice and can actually be more accurate than mathematical computation in many cases, the presence of intra- and interobserver variability needs to be acknowledged, and reproducibility should be monitored.[7] Current echocardiography systems can now automatically calculate the LVEF using the Simpson's method of discs from 2D or 3D datasets, which are accurate and reproducible, but only in patients with good image quality. 3D volumes can also be used to calculate LVEF.[2]

Other approaches are commonly used in addition to LVEF to assess systolic function. Stroke volume can be determined from 2D or 3D images by subtracting end-systolic volume from end-diastolic volume. An alternative method is to use Doppler data (discussed earlier), in which the VTI within the LVOT is multiplied by the LVOT CSA to calculate SV (see Fig. 16.6). Multiplication of SV by the heart rate gives the cardiac output.

Several other methods have been proposed for assessment of both LV and RV function. The *myocardial performance index* (MPI), also known as the Tei index, is defined as the sum of isovolumic relaxation time (IVRT) and isovolumic contraction time divided by ejection time, and this method takes into account both systolic and diastolic performance. A higher index is associated with worse function.[2] In adults, values of LV MPI greater than 0.40 and RV MPI greater than 0.43 are considered abnormal. This measure has been related to outcomes in a variety of conditions, including heart failure and following myocardial infarction (MI). *Doppler tissue imaging* (DTI) can be used to assess myocardial contraction velocity, or S', although this technique is also frequently used in assessment of diastolic function (see later).

Myocardial Strain Imaging

Myocardial deformation, or strain imaging, has evolved to become a sensitive method for assessment of cardiac function. *Strain* refers to the percent deformation between two regions, such as shortening of myocardial muscle in systole or lengthening in diastole.[2] It was initially measured by Doppler of the myocardial tissues to derive the change in distance between points, but an alternate method, 2D speckle-tracking has been found to be more robust and reliable and has proven its utility in clinical applications. The technique has been validated by sonomicrometry and takes advantage of the coherent speckle within the myocardial tissue digital signature to determine regions that are contracting versus those that are moving passively. Strain can be estimated in the longitudinal, circumferential, and radial directions by using the appropriate imaging plane (Fig. 16.14). Normal values for longitudinal and circumferential strain are negative whereas for radial strain, values are normally positive reflecting the normal change in the relative positions of myocardial targets in each of these directions.

Current equipment can assess regional strain and then calculate global longitudinal strain (GLS) either by averaging regional strain values or by determining the percent difference in the endocardial perimeter between systole and diastole (Fig. 16.15). Longitudinal deformation reflects function of the subendocardial myocardial fiber bands primarily, whereas circumferential deformation, best assessed on short-axis views, may reflect the function of more epicardial layers.

Global strain, particularly *global longitudinal strain* (GLS, or the maximal deformation of the LV myocardium at peak systole averaged over the entire ventricle), has emerged as an important measure of cardiac performance that adds incremental predictive value to standard measures such as the LVEF.[8] GLS is expressed as a percentage, and since the overall deformation is towards compression (negative), values closer to zero represent worse function. Several diseases have been associated with a reduction in GLS, including hypertension, diabetes mellitus, renal insufficiency, infiltrative cardiomyopathies, HCM, and valvular heart disease. This measure also appears to predict survival or the development of heart failure in patients following MI. Global strain measurements are also useful in assessing the effect of cardiotoxic chemotherapies on individual patients over time, and may be useful in identifying acute subclinical rejection in cardiac transplant patients.

Myocardial deformation imaging has been used for the evaluation of cardiac synchrony by assessing the time to peak strain (maximal contraction) across many cardiac regions. Both regional timing, reflecting synchrony, and myocardial peak strain, reflecting contractile function, have prognostic significance in patients undergoing cardiac resynchronization therapy (CRT) (see Chapters 50 and 69). The identification of patients who will benefit most from CRT has been a challenge. No single echocardiographic parameter has been found to date that can unequivocally predict response, although radial strain appears to more accurate than other parameters. Ultimately, utilizing regional strain data during CRT placement to help guide optimal lead position may be a more effective approach.[8]

In addition to assessment of global function, strain imaging can be used to assess and quantify regional function. Regional strain correlates with the degree of myocardial scar in patients with ischemic heart disease (see Chapter 36) and in HCM[8,9] (Chapter 54). These measures can also be used to assess ischemia during stress echocardiography. Moreover, a pattern in which strain is preserved apically relative to that at the midventricular and basal levels is suggestive of amyloid cardiomyopathy.[8] An offshoot of myocardial strain imaging has been the quantitative assessment of ventricular twist and torsion, or the wringing motion of the heart during contraction and relaxation.[10]

There are several limitations of strain imaging based on 2D echocardiography. First, myocardial deformation occurs in three dimensions, and out-of-imaging plane movement is lost. Second, these measures are subject to the same limitations as conventional ultrasound images, including frame rate and image quality, with limited temporal resolution at high heart rates. Third, the technique, data acquisition and calculations, and normal values were initially not standardized among the many vendors, making it difficult to compare data in individual cases. The industry has now converged to provide consensus on standardization as well as automated strain measurements, which has amplified the utility of this tool in routine clinical practice.[9]

Left Ventricular Regional Function

Although measures of global LV function provide quantification of overall cardiac performance and carry prognostic value, regional

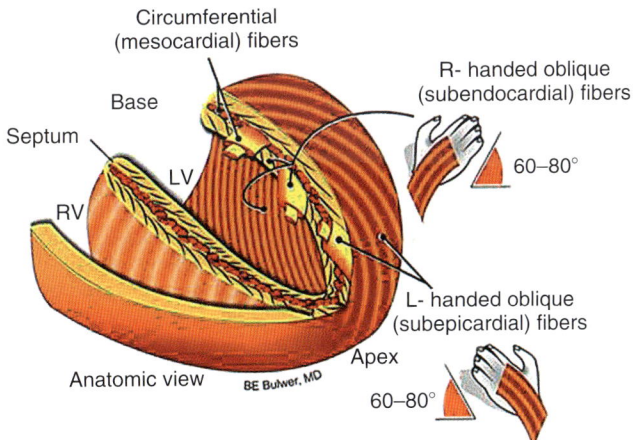

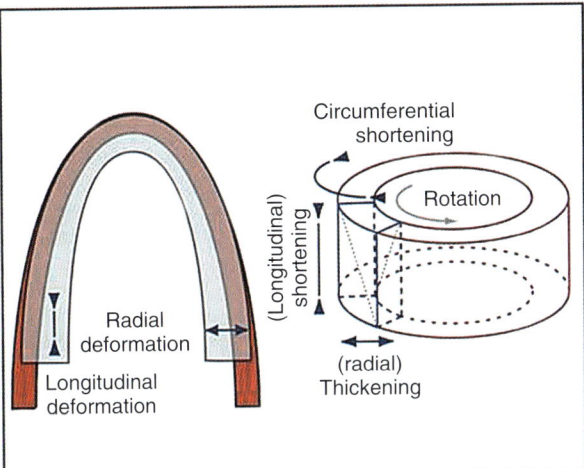
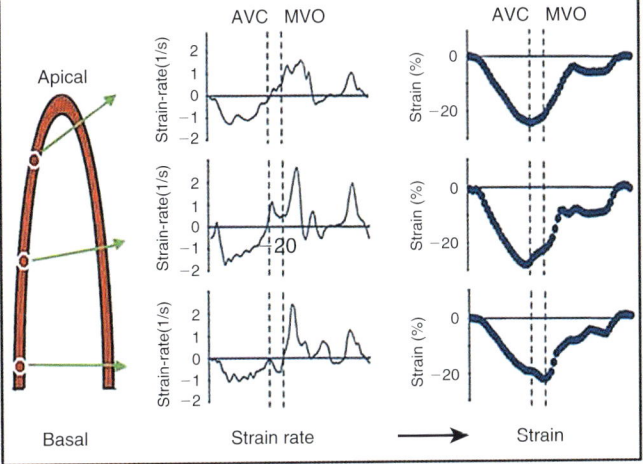

FIGURE 16.14 Normal myocardial fiber orientation, deformation planes, and typical longitudinal strain rate and strain traces. **Upper panel,** Left ventricular endo- and epicardial longitudinal fibers and their opposing oblique directions, midmyocardial circumferential fibers. **Lower panel: Left,** The three planes of myocardial motion and deformation at systole: longitudinal shortening, radial thickening, and circumferential shortening. **Right,** Typical traces of longitudinal strain rate and strain from a healthy adult. *AVC,* Aortic valve closure; *MVO,* mitral valve opening. (From Cikes M, Solomon SD. Beyond ejection fraction: an integrative approach for assessment of cardiac structure and function in heart failure. *Eur Heart J.* 2016;37:1642.)

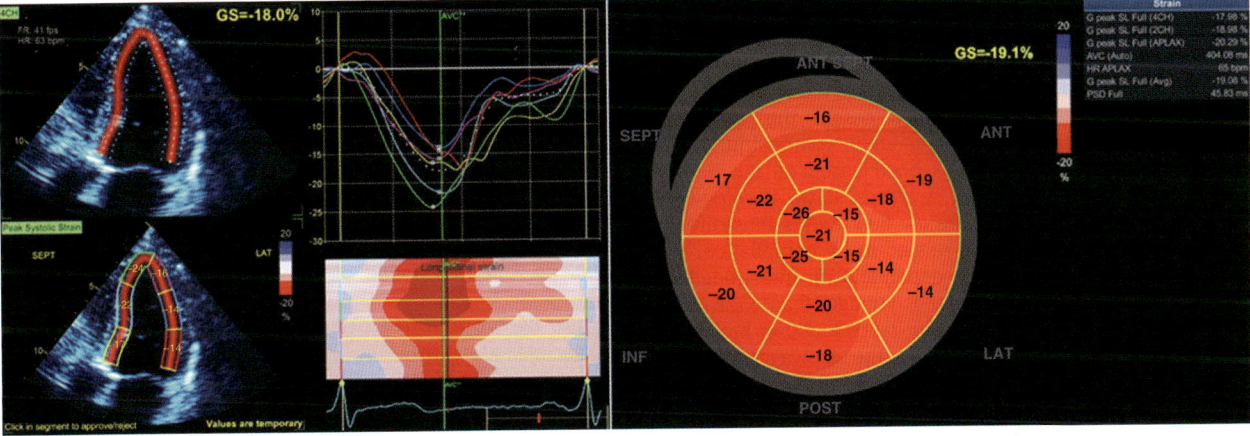

FIGURE 16.15 Global longitudinal strain (GLS) GLS is measured in the three apical planes, mapped onto a bulls-eye plot, and averaged.

function can vary substantially, particularly when affected by ischemic heart disease or other focal processes. Acute MI can cause segmental wall motion abnormalities, that is, altered contractility—visualized on echocardiography as an inwards centripedal segmental motion or wall thickening—of a focal segment of the myocardium. Although there is variability, each specific myocardial region has a typical coronary artery blood supply (see later, Myocardial Infarction). Regional wall motion may be assessed qualitatively or semiquantitatively with a scoring system. The most popular current scoring system is based on a 17-segment model advocated by the ASE in which each segment is scored as normal (1 point), hypokinetic (2 points), akinetic (3 points), or dyskinetic (4 points). The *wall motion score index* (WMSI) is equal to the sum of these grades divided by the number of segments visualized, so a normally contracting ventricle should have a score of 1.0. A WMSI of 1.7 or higher is usually associated with the physical examination findings of heart failure. A higher score is also an independent predictor of mortality and morbidity, including increased hospitalization for heart failure following MI.

One main goal of detecting regional myocardial dysfunction is to identify patients with coronary artery disease (CAD). The hallmark of a significant MI is the appearance of discrete regions of severe hypokinesis (decreased systolic thickening), akinesis (no thickening), or even dyskinesis (bulging outwards in systole). Hypokinesis as a focal wall motion abnormality can be apparent even within the first few minutes of acute MI, thus making echocardiography particularly suited for diagnosis in the acute setting, for example, in patients with acute chest pain and equivocal abnormalities on the electrocardiogram (ECG) in whom a new discrete wall motion abnormality might argue for early intervention (see Chapters 38 and 39). Ultrasound cannot easily distinguish between old and new wall motion abnormalities, although local myocardial thinning and increased echo-brightness would be suggestive of chronic infarction and scar tissue. Although MI, either acute or old, is the most prevalent reason for regional wall motion abnormalities, other conditions such as myocarditis, stress cardiomyopathy (Takotsubo syndrome) or sarcoidosis can affect the myocardium regionally, but these generally will not present in a clear coronary distribution. The LV dysfunction that can accompany valvular or hypertensive heart disease may also have some minor regional variability.

Assessment of regional wall motion is particularly important in stress echocardiography, in which induced focal wall motion abnormalities in the setting of exercise-induced or pharmacologic stress indicate myocardial ischemia. For stress echocardiography, regions are compared before and after stress in a side-by-side fashion, and wall segments with unchanged or worsening systolic function are compared qualitatively and scored (see later).

Left Ventricular Diastolic Function

Diastolic dysfunction is extremely prevalent in patients with hypertension and in older adults (see Chapter 26 and 51). It is described mechanistically as impaired LV relaxation and increased LV stiffness. The historical "gold standard" for assessment of diastolic function has been the invasively obtained pressure-volume loop, in which diastolic function is assessed as the instantaneous relationship between pressure and volume. By echocardiography, assessment of, left atrial pressure, left ventricular end-diastolic pressure (LVEDP) and diastolic dysfunction is multifaceted and can be nuanced.[11] Analysis of diastolic dysfunction must be carried out with acknowledgment that (1) there are no absolute cutoffs for echo values that define the presence and degree of diastolic dysfunction at any LVEF; (2) the age, hemodynamics, and presence of other cardiac disease (particularly mitral disease) may affect many values; and (3) no single index is accurate in isolation.

Mitral Inflow Patterns

Mitral inflow Doppler can be used to assess flow from the left atrium to the left ventricle during diastole. The transmitral inflow velocity at a given point in time correlates with the pressure gradient between the chambers. The E wave occurs during early diastole when the ventricle is filling passively. The A wave represents the velocity of blood flow during late diastole during atrial contraction. Initial classification of diastolic function has been based on the pattern (i.e., relative heights) of the E and A waves. E wave velocity is dependent on the transmitral pressure gradient and is thus directly related to LA pressure and inversely related to LV compliance. The height of the A wave is additionally dependent on the strength of atrial contraction. Normally in individuals younger than 65, E wave height is greater than A wave height, with ratios of 1.0 or higher. LV compliance declines with age, and so the E wave generally diminishes. Simultaneously, the A wave typically increases as atrial contraction augments to compensate for the reduced LV compliance. Moreover, the deceleration time (DT) of the E wave increases as compliance worsens initially. However, as diastolic function continues to worsen and LA pressures rises, the E wave will heighten again, and the size of the A wave declines as LV pressure rises and LA function begins to worsen, so the E/A ratio may revert to relatively normal (*pseudonormalization*). Because pseudonormal patterns can appear similar to normal patterns, E and A measures alone can be misleading. Further worsening of diastolic function leads to the so-called restrictive pattern, in which the descending slope of the E wave becomes very steep (rapid DT) because of abrupt cessation of mitral inflow. Thus, both the pattern of the E and the A waves and the mitral DT follow a biphasic course as diastolic function worsens, which limits the usefulness of these measures alone in assessment of diastolic function.

Doppler Tissue Imaging

DTI applies Doppler imaging principles to the assessment of myocardial contraction and relaxation. Rather than assessing signals from rapidly moving red blood cells, DTI uses filters to optimize reception of the higher-amplitude signals that arise from the much slower-moving myocardium. When applied to assess myocardial motion at the mitral annulus (typically at both medial and lateral sampling points), the Doppler velocities are recorded over the cardiac cycle. Three distinct waveforms are seen: systolic contraction (the S′ wave) toward the relatively fixed apex, followed by early (e′) and late relaxation (a′) signals in diastole. The timing of the e′ and a′ waves is coincident and analogous in many ways to standard Doppler of mitral inflow, but the movement is in the opposite direction to blood flow and of much lower velocity. The e′ peak value is inversely related to tau (τ), the time constant of ventricular relaxation. The e′ velocity ranges up to greater than 20 cm/sec in children and young adults but declines rapidly in early adulthood and beyond. Values less than 5 cm/sec are seen in patients with severe diastolic dysfunction (e.g., amyloidosis).

Because E velocity reflects the atrial-to-ventricular pressure gradient, it is dependent on both LV compliance and LA pressure (i.e., preload dependent). In contrast, DTI e′ in principle is a measure of LV compliance alone. Therefore, dividing E by e′ yields a measure that reflects LA pressure, which usually approximates LVEDP. An E/e′ ratio greater than 14 is considered abnormally high at any age and is usually indicative of elevated LVEDP. However, this ratio may be insensitive to acute changes and thus may not be suitable for monitoring patients during therapy.[11]

Pulmonary Venous Doppler Flow Patterns

Pulmonary flow patterns are complementary to mitral inflow Doppler patterns for assessment of diastolic function. Pulmonary vein flow has three components: (1) the S wave, which consists of forward flow from the pulmonary veins to the left atrium during ventricular systole; (2) the D wave, which consists of passive flow during ventricular diastole; and (3) the AR wave, which is the slight flow reversal into the pulmonary veins during atrial contraction. Patients with impaired LV relaxation will demonstrate blunting of the S wave relative to the D wave. Reduced LV compliance may also result in greater flow into the pulmonary veins during atrial contraction (broader A wave).

A number of other Doppler parameters change with declining diastolic function. The *isovolumic relaxation time* represents the period between closure of the aortic valve and the start of ventricular filling (i.e., end of LVOT flow and beginning of mitral inflow E wave). Prolongation of the IVRT is associated with abnormal relaxation, and shortening of the IVRT can occur in patients with restrictive LV filling. Mitral E wave DT is the interval from peak to no mitral inflow in early diastole. In early diastolic dysfunction, DT can actually increase. However, in patients with severe restrictive physiology where the stiff ventricle reaches its volume limit suddenly, the DT will be very rapid (<140 ms). This has been associated with an adverse prognosis in patients with heart failure and after MI (i.e., in patients with both systolic and advanced diastolic dysfunction).

Color M-Mode and Flow Propagation

Color M-Mode can be used to assess transmitral flow propagation velocity (Vp). While performing color flow Doppler through the mitral valve in apical windows, one can initiate the M-mode function to superimpose the color flow information onto the M-mode image. The slope of the E wave flow (Vp) represents flow propagation, which correlates inversely with tau, the time constant of relaxation. Patients with impaired active relaxation will have a reduced "suction" action of the left ventricle, with abrupt slowing of blood once it enters the ventricle. On color M-mode, this manifests as a more shallow slope of Vp (abnormal is considered <0.45 in middle-aged adults, and <0.55 in younger adults). In practice, despite refinements in calculation of parameters based on flow propagation, Vp measures have lower reproducibility and appear reliable only in patients with depressed LVEF.[11]

Assessing Diastolic Function in Clinical Practice

In clinical practice, assessment of diastolic function requires an integrated approach. Main parameters and rough cutoffs for initial

TABLE 16.4 Expected Findings for Left Ventricular (LV) Relaxation, Filling Pressures, and Two-Dimensional and Doppler Findings According to LV Diastolic Function

PARAMETER	NORMAL	GRADE I	GRADE II	GRADE III
LV relaxation	Normal	Impaired	Impaired	Impaired
LA pressure	Normal	Low or normal	Elevated	Elevated
Mitral E/A ratio	≥0.8	≤0.8	>0.8 to <2	>2
Average E/e′ ratio	<10	<10	10–14	>14
Peak TR velocity (m/sec)	<2.8	<2.8	>2.8	>2.8
LA volume index	Normal	Normal or increased (>34 ml/m²)	Increased	Increased

LA, Left atrial; *TR,* tricuspid regurgitation.
From Nagueh SF, Smiseth OA, Appleton CP, et al. Recommendations for the evaluation of left ventricular diastolic function by echocardiography: an update from the American Society of Echocardiography and the European Association of Cardiovascular Imaging. *J Am Soc Echocardiogr.* 2016;29:277.

TABLE 16.5 Normal Values for Right Ventricular (RV) Chamber Size

PARAMETER	MEAN ± SD	NORMAL RANGE
RV basal diameter (mm)	33 ± 4	25–41
RV mid diameter (mm)	27 ± 4	19–35
RV longitudinal diameter (mm)	71 ± 6	59–83
RVOT PLAX diameter (mm)	25 ± 2.5	20–30
RVOT proximal diameter (mm)	28 ± 3.5	21–35
RVOT distal diameter (mm)	22 ± 2.5	17–27
RV wall thickness (mm)	3 ± 1	1–5
RVOT EDA (cm²)		
Men	17 ± 3.5	10–24
Women	14 ± 3	8–20
RV EDA indexed to BSA (cm²/m²)		
Men	8.8 ± 1.9	5–12.6
Women	8.0 ± 1.75	4.5–11.5
RV ESA (cm²)		
Men	9 ± 3	3–15
Women	7 ± 2	3–11
RV ESA indexed to BSA (cm²/m²)		
Men	4.7 ± 1.35	2.0–7.4
Women	4.0 ± 1.2	1.6–6.4
RV SEDV indexed to BSA (mL/m²)		
Men	61 ± 13	35–87
Women	53 ± 10.5	32–74
RV ESV indexed to BSA (mL/m²)		
Men	27 ± 8.5	10–44
Women	22 ± 7	8–36

BSA, Body surface area; *EDA,* end-diastolic area; *ESA,* end-systolic area; *PLAX,* parasternal long-axis view; *RVOT,* RV outflow tract.
From Lang RM, Badano LP, Mor-Avi V, et al. Recommendations for cardiac chamber quantification by echocardiography in adults: an update from the American Society of Echocardiography and the European Association of Cardiovascular Imaging. *J Am Soc Echocardiogr.* 2015;28:1.

assessment include mitral inflow Doppler (particularly E/A ratio) and tissue Doppler (é and E/é′ ratio) criteria, but also estimates of PASP and LA volume (Table 16.4). A majority of evidence (initially at least two of four) of these abnormal parameters is required to parse diastolic dysfunction, with use of additional parameters as needed for corroboration.[11] Several schemes have been developed to grade diastolic function based on these parameters (Table 16.4). Their application, particularly for assessing LV filling pressures, should also take into consideration LV systolic function and the presence of underlying cardiomyopathies. Although these schemes allow for some standardization in description of diastolic dysfunction, data on the relationship between specific grades, resting hemodynamics, and clinical outcomes remain limited. Abnormalities in diastole are extremely prevalent in patients with hypertension and in elderly patients but are not necessarily associated with clinical symptoms or overt heart failure.[11,12] Assessment of diastolic function during exercise, termed the "diastolic stress test," may help unmask abnormalities that contribute to symptoms only during exertion.[12]

Right Ventricular Structure and Function

Assessment of the right ventricle has proved especially challenging for 2D echocardiography. Whereas the left ventricle is relatively easily characterized as a prolate ellipsoid, the odd crescentic shape of the right ventricle makes modeling of volumes considerably more complex. Moreover, because visualization of the entire right ventricle is not encompassed by any single 2D plane, multiple measurements from multiple views are necessary to fully assess this chamber. Normal linear RV measurements are shown in Table 16.5. Under normal conditions, the right ventricle is accustomed to low pulmonary vascular resistance (PVR) and is thus extremely sensitive to changes in afterload. Conditions that increase PVR acutely, such as pulmonary embolism (see Chapter 87), will cause marked RV dilation and dysfunction. Conditions that cause a chronic increase in PVR will lead to RV hypertrophy and dilation, but RV function is usually maintained until the late stages of disease (see Chapter 88).

Several methods are commonly used to assess global RV function initially on conventional echocardiography (Table 16.6).[2] RV fractional area change (FAC) (Fig. 16.16) is easily determined by calculating the RV area in diastole (RVAd) and systole (RVAs) on the apical four-chamber view:

$$FAC = (RVAd - RVAs)/RVAd$$

Assessment of RV function by FAC has been shown to provide incremental prognostic value in patients with heart failure and following MI.[13] *Tricuspid annular plane systolic excursion* (TAPSE) is a measure of RV contractility that is readily measured with M-mode imaging in the apical four-chamber view (Fig. 16.17). This longitudinal motion of the tricuspid annulus can similarly be assessed with pulsed or tissue Doppler as the peak velocity of the systolic wave, S′ (see Fig. 16.17, right). Also exactly analogous to the left ventricle, an RV Tei index and RV GLS values can similarly be obtained. RV regional, as opposed to global, dysfunction has particular importance in conditions in which RV afterload increases abruptly, such as pulmonary embolism (see later), in which regional RV function is often preserved in the apical and basal free wall segments but dyskinetic or akinetic in the midregion. Both global and segmental RV wall motion abnormalities also notably occur in RCA infarcts and RV cardiomyopathies.

3D imaging of the right ventricle is now available, and reconstructed views beautifully illustrate its geometric complexity (Fig. 16.18). 3D imaging allows for calculation of volumes that are not as angle dependent as all the measures previously discussed. Image acquisition still relies on an experienced sonographer, and the volume measurements require additional training, are only semiautomatic, and must be done off-line. However, normal reference values for RV volumes and RV ejection fractions now exist (see Tables 16.5 and 16.6).[2] Similar to LV volume data, the accuracy appears comparable with that of CMR imaging, although volumes tend to be lower on echocardiography.

Left and Right Atria

LA enlargement has been associated with adverse cardiovascular outcomes. The left atrium enlarges under several pathologic conditions, including LV systolic and diastolic dysfunction and atrial fibrillation (AF). Other frequent causes of LA enlargement include hypertension and mitral valve regurgitation or stenosis. LA size is thought to reflect LV filling pressure and thus has been considered a useful indicator of diastolic function over time. Indeed, left atrial volume (corrected for BSA) is a key element of the assessment of diastolic function in the ASE guidelines. Several methods can be used to quantify LA size. A linear measurement of the left atrium is traditionally obtained on the parasternal long axis view and in the early days of echocardiography was the initial screen of LA size. A longstanding reference standard for parasternal long-axis LA dimension has been 3.8 cm as the upper limit of normal in women and 4.0 cm in men (or 2.3 cm/m² BSA for both). Other axes in the apical windows may also be measured. However, any single linear measurement is inadequate, and LA area is more fully assessed from orthogonal apical views, with volume subsequently calculated by applying the Simpson biplane method.

Volumes are typically indexed to BSA (see Table 16.2). LA function contributes to overall cardiac performance and is itself also affected by LV compliance.

Assessment of the right atrium is best performed from the apical and subcostal views. RA size is a reflection of right-sided filling pressure and volume. The most frequent causes of RA enlargement are AF and TR. Isolated right heart enlargement should always raise the question of whether interatrial (left-to-right) shunting is occurring, and a search for an atrial septal defect should be undertaken with intravenous (IV) saline contrast if necessary. Biatrial enlargement can occur with AF or with restrictive cardiomyopathy.

Indexed RA volumes based on volumetric assessment are similar to LA volumes in healthy men and are slightly smaller in healthy women. Assessment of both the right atrium and the inferior vena cava (IVC) is important in the estimation of RA pressure, which is essential for calculating PASP from TR velocity. Qualitative evidence of elevated RA pressure includes a dilated right atrium, dilation of the IVC, or attenuation of IVC collapse during inspiration. Several methods have been used to estimate RA pressure by echocardiography, but most involve a combination of IVC size and the amount that the IVC collapses with inspiration. A rough scale of RA pressure has been developed that combines assessment of IVC size using a cutoff of 2.1 cm and respirophasic collapse (Table 16.7) using a cutoff of 50%. Notably, the IVC is occasionally dilated in healthy young individuals and in athletes, particularly when imaged completely supine. It does not provide a consistent measure of RA pressure in mechanically ventilated patients due to positive end-expiratory pressure.[14]

TRANSESOPHAGEAL ECHOCARDIOGRAPHY

TEE is an alternative method to obtain ultrasound images of the heart in which a smaller ultrasound transducer is introduced into the patient's esophagus through a manipulable flexible probe. Similar to transthoracic scanning, multiplane 2D and 3D, color flow, and spectral Doppler imaging can be performed at the bedside, but with a higher-frequency transducer and from a position that is posterior and closer to the heart than can be achieved with TTE. The result is superior image quality and spatial resolution with less artefact, particularly when assessing the left atrium and left-sided valves, which are directly adjacent to the esophagus. Because it is semi-invasive, TEE is generally used as an adjunctive or follow-up test to an initial TTE if additional information is sought or the TTE images are inconclusive. Table 16.8 summarizes the advantages and disadvantages of TTE versus TEE.

TEE is particularly useful in the evaluation of valve dysfunction, diagnosis or follow-up of endocarditis (see Chapter 80), searching for potential causes of stroke, and for better characterization of cardiac masses and congenital heart disease.[15,16] In some circumstances, TEE is appropriately the first test of choice, such as evaluation of aortic pathology and assessment for LA appendage thrombi (see Diseases of the Aorta and Cardiac Masses).[17] TEE can be used to determine the presence of thrombus in patients in whom rapid cardioversion of AF is necessary (see Chapter 66) or when elective atrial arrhythmia ablation/cardioversion is planned, particularly in the patient found to be underanticoagulated or at high risk for stroke. In addition, TEE has a major role in optimizing and evaluating cardiac surgical and percutaneous procedures, particularly with respect to valvular procedures, closure of intracardiac shunts, implantation of LVADs, and left atrial appendage occlusion.

TABLE 16.6 Normal Values for Parameters of Right Ventricular (RV) Function

PARAMETER	MEAN ± SD	ABNORMALITY THRESHOLD
TAPSE (mm)	24 ± 3.5	<17
Pulsed Doppler S wave (cm/sec)	14.1 ± 2.3	<9.5
Color Doppler S wave (cm/sec)	9.7 ± 1.85	<6.0
RV fractional area change (%)	49 ± 7	<35
RV free wall 2D strain* (%)	−29 ± 4.5	>−20[†]
RV 3D EF (%)	58 ± 6.5	<45
Pulsed Doppler MPI	0.26 ± 0.085	>0.43
Tissue Doppler MPI	0.38 ± 0.08	>0.54
E wave deceleration time (msec)	180 ± 31	<119 or >242
E/A	1.4 ± 0.3	<0.8 or >2.0
e′/a′	1.18 ± 0.33	<0.52
e′	14.0 ± 3.1	<7.8
E/e′	4.0 ± 1.0	>6.0

*Limited data; values may vary depending on vendor and software version.
[†]<20 in magnitude with the negative sign.
MPI, Myocardial performance (Tei) index; TAPSE, tricuspid annular plane systolic excursion.
From Lang RM, Badano LP, Mor-Avi V, et al. Recommendations for cardiac chamber quantification by echocardiography in adults: an update from the American Society of Echocardiography and the European Association of Cardiovascular Imaging. J Am Soc Echocardiogr. 2015;28:1.

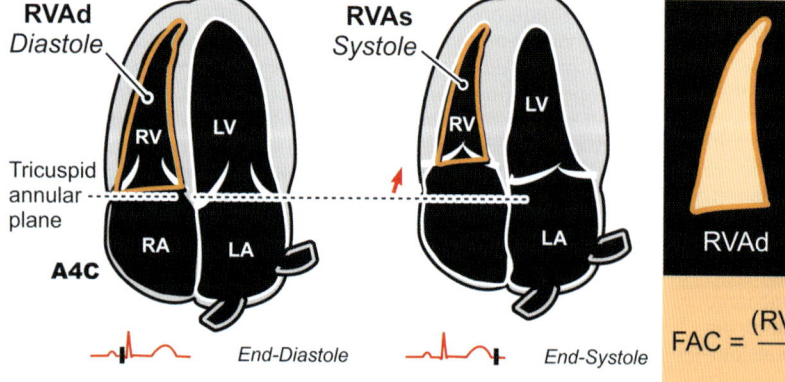

FIGURE 16.16 Right ventricular area (RVA) measurement and fractional area change (FAC) used to assess RV function with the apical four-chamber view (A4C). LA, Left atrium; LV, left ventricle; RA, right atrium; RV, right ventricle.

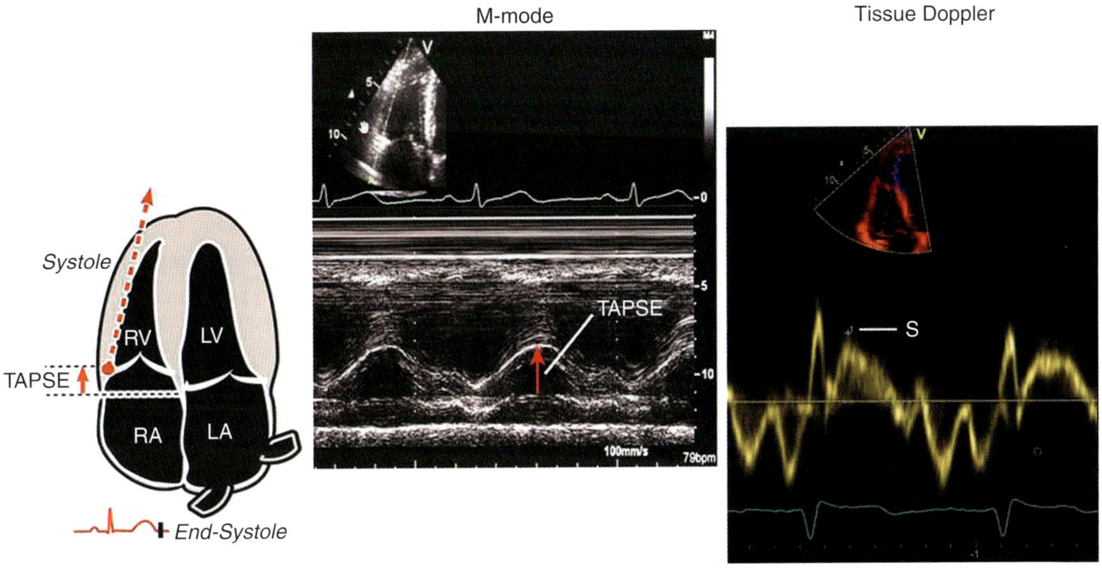

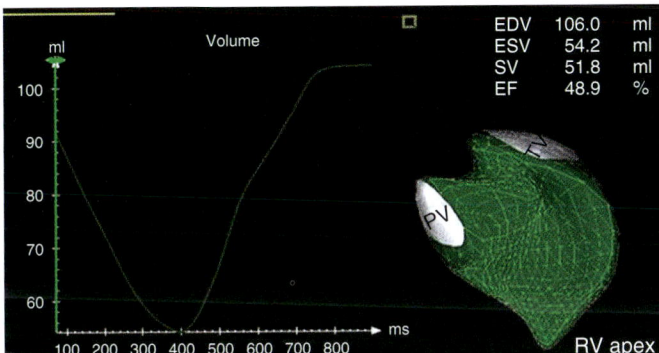

FIGURE 16.17 M-mode and Doppler tissue imaging (DTI) measurements of RV systolic function. **Left and middle panels,** On M-mode, the tissue annular plane systolic excursion (TAPSE) can be measured. **Right,** DTI is used to map tricuspid annular motion, where *S* is the analogous measurement to TAPSE.

FIGURE 16.18 Three-dimensional measurements of right ventricular (RV) volume and function. A 3D echocardiographic reconstruction of the RV shape and volume, as viewed from the septal surface. The graph at *left* shows RV volumes plotted against time over the cardiac cycle, with data obtained from RV-focused apical four-chamber windows. RV stroke volume (SV) = EDV − ESV. RV ejection fraction (EF) = SV/EDV. *EDV,* end-diastolic volume; *ESV,* end-systolic volume; *PV,* pulmonic valve; *TV,* tricuspid valve.

TABLE 16.7 Estimation of Right Atrial Pressure Based on Inferior Vena Cava (IVC) Diameter and Collapse

VARIABLE	NORMAL (0–5 [3] mm Hg)		INTERMEDIATE (5–10 [8] mm Hg)	HIGH (15 mm Hg)
IVC diameter	≤2.1 cm	≤2.1 cm	>2.1 cm	>2.1 cm
Collapse with sniff	>50%	>50%	<50%	<50%
Secondary indices				Restrictive filling by tricuspid valve inflow
				Tricuspid E/e′ >6
				Diastolic flow predominance in hepatic veins (systolic filling <55%)

Ranges are provided for low and intermediate categories, but for simplicity, midrange values of 3 mm Hg for normal and 8 mm Hg for intermediate are suggested. Intermediate (8 mm Hg) RA pressures may be downgraded to normal if no secondary indices of elevated RA pressure are present, upgraded to high if minimal collapse with nasal inhalation (<35%) and secondary indices of elevated RA pressure are present, or left at 8 mm Hg if uncertain.

From Rudski LG, Lai WW, Afilalo J, et al. Guidelines for the Echocardiographic Assessment of the Right Heart in Adults: A Report from the American Society of Echocardiography. *J Am Soc Echocardiogr.* 2010:23:685.

TEE may be performed on an inpatient or outpatient basis, and most patients require topical anesthesia and/or IV conscious sedation for comfort. This is usually achieved with IV midazolam and fentanyl or alternatively with propofol if issues with respiratory or hemodynamic stability or patient comfort are anticipated. Risks are relatively low but include trauma to the oropharynx and esophagus, aspiration, bronchospasm or laryngospasm, accidental tracheal intubation, and arrhythmia, as well as risks associated with sedation (transient hypotension) and theoretically with neck manipulation. General anesthesia is used for patients in the operating room and during some transcatheter procedures and, in this context, TEE may be associated with higher complication rates (as high as 1.2% for major complications), particularly during prolonged procedures.[17,18] The most serious complication is upper gastrointestinal perforation, which typically occurs in the esophagus or hypopharynx. Patients with esophageal diverticula or strictures, significant thoracic radiation-induced fibrosis, distorted anatomy of the mediastinal organs, or difficult probe placement are at higher risk. TEE may also cause bleeding (0.02% to 1.0%) from direct abrasion or laceration of the mucosa, esophageal varices, or tumor. The overall risk for major adverse events with TEE is 0.2% to 0.5% in the nonsurgical setting, and the overall mortality rate is exceedingly low (0.0004%). These risks may be minimized by screening patients for potential contraindications; if one is found, TEE is best deferred until the situation can be better assessed or ameliorated. Alternatively, another imaging modality (e.g., intravascular ultrasound [IVUS] or epiaortic scanning, CT or CMR) or management strategy could be considered if an underlying risk factor cannot be mitigated.

The Standard Transesophageal Echocardiographic Examination

Figure 16.19 shows a standard TEE examination. It is usually prudent to address the main indication first in the event that the examination must be aborted because of clinical instability. If the patient remains stable, a comprehensive examination is performed, with the majority of the images at the midesophageal level (probe tip approximately 35 cm from the incisors). For a frame of reference with respect to the imaging planes, at midesophageal level with the transducer angle set at 0 to 30 degrees and the probe flexed, the imaging plane cuts the heart in

TABLE 16.8 Advantages and Disadvantages of Transesophageal Echocardiography (TEE) Relative to Transthoracic Echocardiography (TTE)

ADVANTAGES	DISADVANTAGES
Useful in percutaneous and surgical procedures, as well as at the bedside	Semi-invasive—usually requires sedation, hence associated risks with probe intubation (gastrointestinal and pulmonary implications) and sedation effects (hypotension). Long procedures may necessitate general anesthesia.
	Generally a minimum of two staff members required: one operator and one person to monitor the sedation needed.
	Aerosol-generating procedure (risk of transmission of airborne pathogens)
Higher resolution: better to definitively detect vegetations, thrombi, masses, and intracardiac shunts. Superior imaging of valves, especially the mitral and aortic, left atrium and appendage, left ventricle, thoracic aorta and arch, and interatrial septum, as well as the pulmonary veins	May not view the LV apex or right-sided structures well (structures that are further from probe, particularly in large patients)
"Continuous" acoustic window when compared with TTE (no ribs to cause acoustic shadowing)	"Blind spot" of acoustic shadowing where the trachea is interposed between the esophagus and heart
	Much of the abdominal aorta is out of range
Superior imaging of the mitral valve and mitral prostheses in general, with the ability to precisely localize valvular and paravalvular defects	Mechanical aortic prostheses can cause excessive shadowing
	May be technically difficult to achieve the best angle of insonation (i.e., less reproducible and accurate) for assessing aortic stenosis gradients
	Maneuvers to increase or decrease preload may be more difficult (e.g., Valsalva maneuver), although most patients can cooperate
	Real-time 3D imaging and reconstruction dependent on a slow regular heart rate and "stable" window (i.e., still patient)

a short-axis (transverse) plane. A TEE transducer angle of 90 to 120 degrees corresponds to a long-axis (longitudinal, or sagittal) plane.

Most transesophageal examinations start with the standard four-chamber view of the heart, similar to the transthoracic apical four-chamber view. At midesophageal level, 0 degrees, this is achieved by slight retroflexion of the probe to tilt the imaging plane in order to include the cardiac apex. At this level the multiplane "omni" controller is used to rotate the scanning plane counterclockwise to slice the left ventricle into two-chamber (approximately 90-degree) and then three-chamber (long-axis or 120-degree) views. These views are optimal for assessing the left ventricle, left atrium, and mitral valve structure and function. If desired, the LA appendage may be thoroughly examined by withdrawing the probe slightly cephalad, centering the image sector on the appendage, and scanning from 30 to 150 degrees. To examine the aortic valve, the operator retracts the probe slightly, and the aortic valve should be imaged just superior to the mitral valve, at approximately 30 degrees for short-axis images and 120 degrees for long-axis views. The tricuspid valve may be examined at approximately 45 degrees, with subsequent views of the right ventricular outflow tract (RVOT), pulmonary artery and valve, and pulmonary bifurcation sought by gradually increasing the omni angle up toward 120 degrees. The tricuspid valve may be best seen by advancing the probe to about 40 cm from the incisors which typically is in the vicinity of the gastroesophageal junction. Minor additional manipulations of the TEE probe and transducer angle will provide views of the pulmonary veins, right atrium, interatrial septum, superior vena cava (SVC), IVC, coronary sinus, and abdominal aorta. For transgastric windows, the TEE probe is advanced gently past the gastroesophageal sphincter with the transducer plane reset back to 0 degrees and the probe in a neutral position (unflexed). One can view the left ventricle and mitral valve in the short axis and also obtain transaortic gradients from an apical five- or three-chamber view if needed. By increasing the omni angle up to 90 degrees and rotating the transducer plane to the right, more detailed views of the tricuspid valve and right side of the heart are attainable. Lastly, the thoracic aorta is usually examined in cross-sectional and longitudinal views as the probe is withdrawn, to document any significant atherosclerosis or other pathology.

THREE-DIMENSIONAL ECHOCARDIOGRAPHY

Acquisition and display of 3D images have been a long-term goal of echocardiography. Although 3D datasets can be obtained by reconstruction from transthoracic or transesophageal rotational 2D acquisition, true 3D echocardiography is accomplished by using a matrix-array transducer that emits and receives stacked beams of ultrasound which allows the real-time acquisition of a pyramidal dataset in three dimensions (Fig. 16.20). Matrix-array probes for both transthoracic and transesophageal use are available. The 3D datasets can be used to display simultaneous orthogonal 2D images (e.g., four- and two-chamber apical views) or a 3D-rendered image. 3D echocardiography offers the potential to better orient valvular structures (see Valvular Heart Disease) or congenital abnormalities and can be particularly useful in planning surgical and percutaneous interventions. As discussed earlier, 3D echocardiography can also improve the accuracy of quantification of LV and RV volume and function. Useful 3D imaging depends heavily on good 2D images, and in fact there is some loss of spatial and temporal resolution in comparison. However, 3D echocardiography has become extremely useful as a way to delineate complex structures that extend beyond one plane or to find and localize measurements and abnormalities that are difficult to encompass using 2D images. Examples include finding clefts and localizing prolapsed segments in the mitral valve, delineating paravalvular leaks, measuring the distance of the coronary artery origins from the aortic valve, and providing comprehensive quantitative analysis of the valve leaflets and annuli (Fig. 16.21), as well as guiding percutaneous device implantation (see Transcatheter Interventions). 3D acquisition is now becoming standard in echocardiography and in the operating room.

ULTRASOUND ENHANCING AGENTS

Contemporary echocardiographic enhancing agents, also called ultrasound "contrast" agents, are stabilized gas microspheres of 1.1 to 4.5 μm, similar in size to red blood cells, and can move through the circulatory system accordingly after IV injection. Currently approved agents consist of high-molecular weight gases, chosen because of their resistance to diffusion into the blood, which are enclosed within either albumin or phospholipid shells. Unlike the larger bubbles created by agitating saline, commercial contrast bubbles are uniform in size and small enough to transit the pulmonary vascular bed and are therefore capable of opacifying the left side of the heart.

Because their shells are somewhat resilient, contrast bubbles will contract in response to the peak acoustic pressure of the sinusoidal ultrasound wave and expand when acoustic pressure is lowest. Optimal

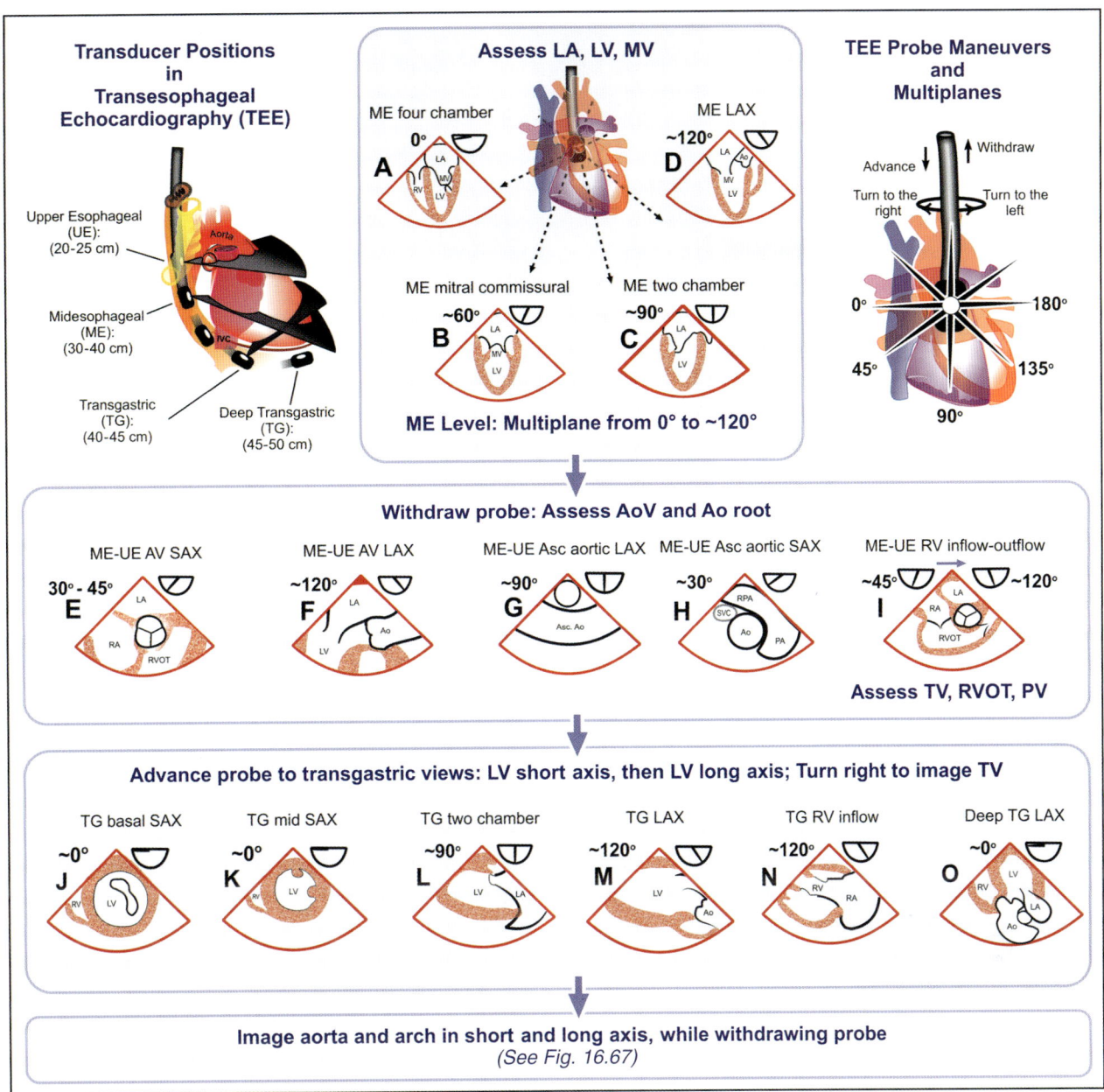

FIGURE 16.19 A suggested standard TEE examination, showing basic probe positioning, manipulations, and views. The sequence illustrated allows a basic survey of all the cardiac chambers and valves. Additional views are obtained as required for the specific indication. *Ao,* Aorta; *AoV,* aortic valve; *Asc,* ascending; *AV,* aortic valve; *Desc,* descending; *LAX,* long axis; *ME,* midesophageal; *PV,* pulmonic valve; *SAX,* short axis; *TG,* transgastric; *TV,* tricuspid valve; *UE,* upper esophageal.

imaging of contrast agents capitalizes on the way in which this oscillation in size varies with ultrasound system transmit power (mechanical index). When exposed to sound waves at lower mechanical indices, the bubbles will undergo resonant oscillation in a linear fashion and reflect sound at the same fundamental frequency. With higher transmit frequencies, the bubbles will resonate in a nonlinear fashion and reflect sound at both fundamental and harmonic frequencies, multiples of the fundamental frequency. At even higher transmit powers, the bubbles will be destroyed, thereby generating very strong nonlinear backscatter of extremely short duration. Therefore, to distinguish bubbles from surrounding tissue, ultrasound systems are set at low mechanical indices (0.15 to 0.3) that will generate nonlinear resonance without bubble destruction and then selectively "listen" only at harmonic frequencies, thereby improving the strength of the bubble signal relative to that of tissue.

By opacifying the blood pool, ultrasound enhancing agents improve detection of the endocardial–blood pool interface and thus facilitate assessment of ventricular volume, as well as global and regional ventricular function (Fig. 16.22).[20] It has been demonstrated that enhancing agents can convert nondiagnostic (defined as inadequate visualization of two or more of six LV segments seen on apical views) to diagnostic studies in up to 90% of patients. This can be particularly helpful in the intensive care unit (ICU), as well as with stress echocardiography, in which obtaining adequate images in the immediate postexercise period may be challenging. By better delineating the cardiac anatomy, enhancing agents facilitate the discovery of aneurysms and diverticula, mechanical complications of MI such as free wall rupture and pseudoaneurysms, apical hypertrophy, transient apical ballooning, endomyocardial fibrosis, and the spongelike trabeculations of noncompaction cardiomyopathy. Contrast is also helpful in

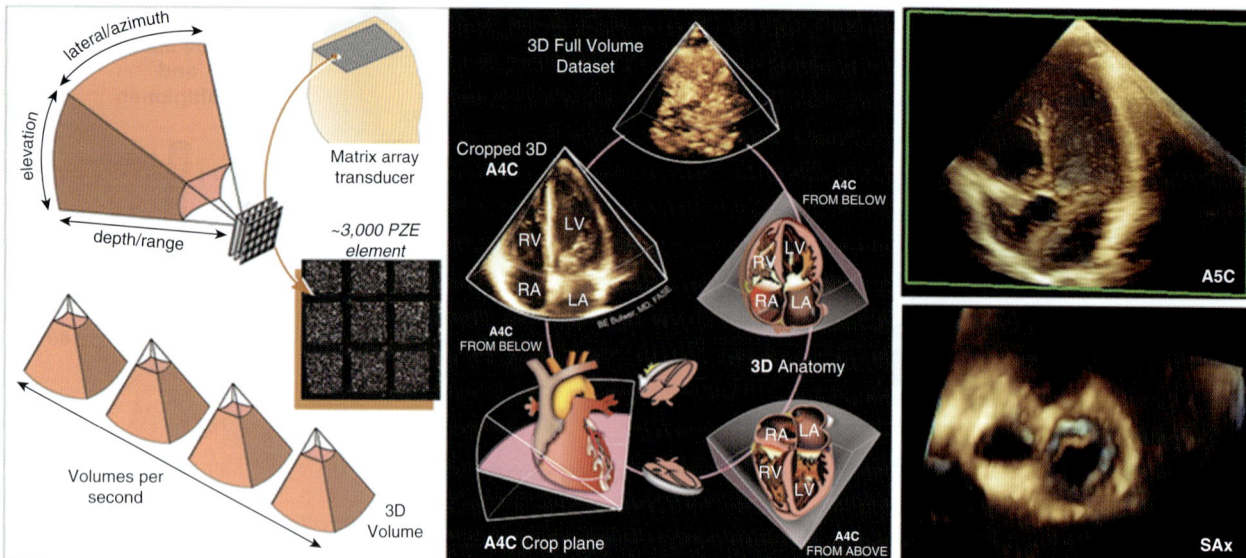

FIGURE 16.20 Three-dimensional echocardiography using a matrix-array transducer. A waffle-like matrix array **(left panel)** is used to obtain pyramidal "volumes" for real-time 3D data sets that can be cropped **(middle panel)** and rendered in three dimensions. Alternatively, two-dimensional planes can be "cut" through any part of the 3D data set (**right panels**, showing apical 5 chamber cut plane on top and short-axis cuts across the mitral and tricuspid valves on bottom). *A4C*, Apical four-chamber view; *A5C*, Apical five-chamber view, *SAx*, short-axis view. (Modified from Bulwer BE, Rivero JM, eds. *Echocardiography Pocket Guide: The Transthoracic Examination*. Burlington, MA: Jones & Bartlett Learning, 2011, 2013:208. Reprinted with permission.)

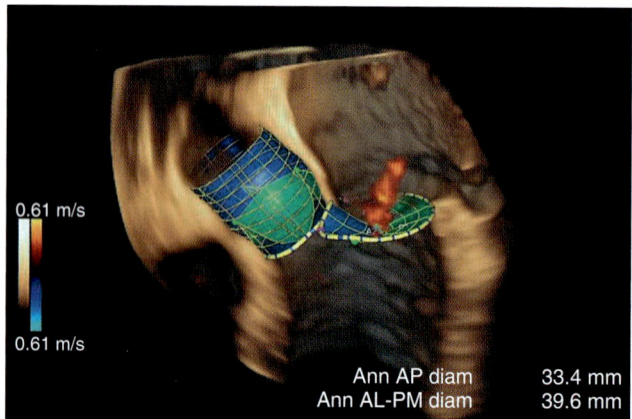

FIGURE 16.21 Three-dimensional TEE reconstructed view of the heart, showing the aortic and mitral valve geometry with mitral regurgitant jet (*red*) originating between the midscallops of the mitral valve.

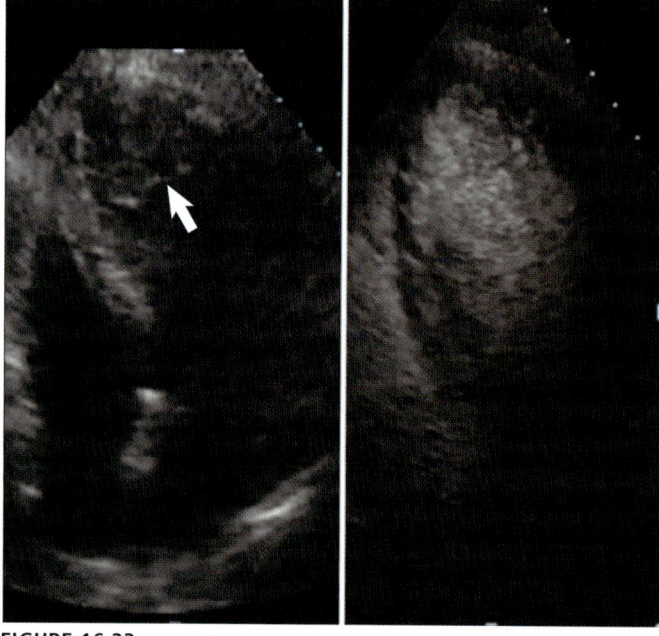

FIGURE 16.23 Apical four-chamber unenhanced **(left)** and contrast-enhanced **(right)** images. In the unenhanced image a thrombus-like structure is visualized in the apical region (*arrow*). The enhanced version shows that there is no filling defect, thus suggesting that this was an acoustic artefact and not a true thrombus.

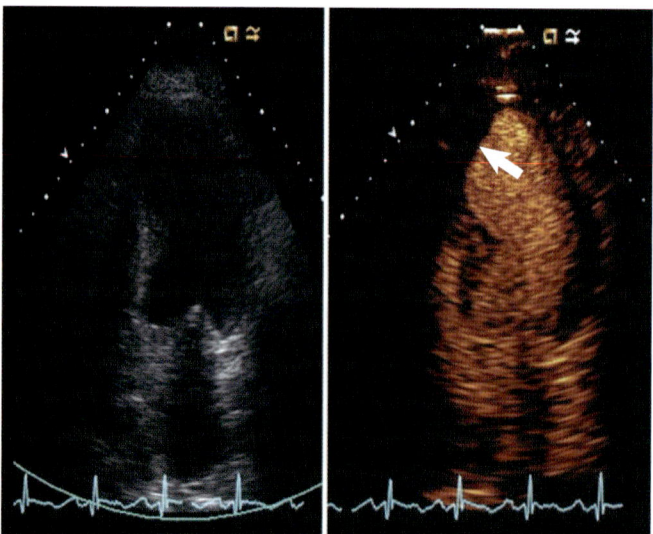

FIGURE 16.22 Unenhanced **(left)** and contrast-enhanced **(right)** apical four-chamber systolic images. In the unenhanced image it is impossible to define the endocardium, whereas with contrast enhancement the endocardium is clearly delineated and the straight margin characteristic of a sessile apical thrombus (*arrow*) is appreciated.

detecting intracardiac masses such as thrombi and tumors and assessing their vascularity. In addition, these agents may help distinguish imaging artefact from pathology (Fig. 16.23). Ultrasound enhancing agents may also be used (off-label) to intensify spectral Doppler signals, which may be particularly helpful in defining TR signals and gradients in AS, and can delineate extracardiac pathology such as vascular dissection. Finally, in patients undergoing alcohol septal ablation for obstructive HCM (see Chapter 54), contrast agents are used to delineate the perfusion bed of target septal perforators.

Myocardial perfusion contrast-enhanced echocardiography is another application that is based on the ability of ultrasound to detect contrast bubbles within the myocardial vasculature. Approaches depend on the fact that a burst of ultrasound with a high mechanical index "flash" will predictably destroy all microbubbles in the sector,

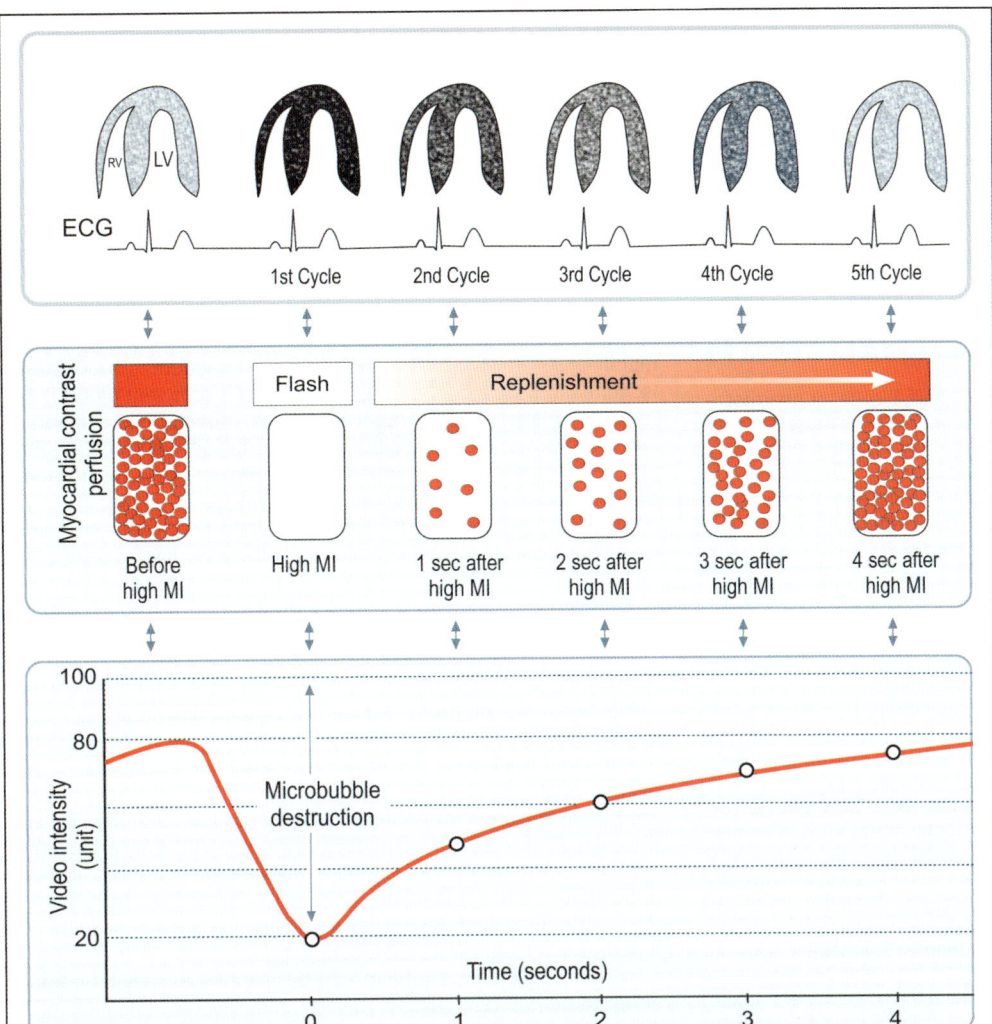

FIGURE 16.24 Myocardial contrast-enhanced echocardiography: schematic demonstrating the approach to myocardial perfusion imaging during steady-state infusion of a contrast agent. A high–mechanical index impulse (MI) destroys all the intramyocardial bubbles to yield an unenhanced image that will serve as the reference baseline. Subsequently, bubbles will return by coronary perfusion and progressively enhance the myocardium until a steady-state concentration is reached. This may be monitored by either a triggered approach in which imaging is performed on end-systolic images at increasing numbers of beats after the flash (1, 2, 3, 4, etc.) or by using low-MI continuous imaging. Enhancement will increase until a steady-state level is achieved (in this hypothetical example, at a five-beat pulsing interval or after 4 seconds of low-MI imaging). The rate at which replenishment occurs and the degree of enhancement under steady-state conditions, as quantitated by video intensity, reflect myocardial perfusion. (Modified from Wei K, Jayaweera AR, Firoozan A, et al. Quantification of myocardial blood flow with ultrasound-induced destruction of microbubbles administered as a constant venous infusion. *Circulation.* 1998;97:473.)

and the rate at which myocardial contrast will subsequently be replenished depends on myocardial blood flow (Fig. 16.24). There are two options for imaging protocols following the high–mechanical index flash: continuous low–mechanical index real-time imaging, which preserves the ability simultaneously to see wall motion in the segment, versus a higher–mechanical index approach with progressively longer intervals between ultrasound frames, which enhances the perfusion signal but at the expense of attaining wall motion information. Although myocardial perfusion imaging has been shown to be of value in both rest and stress imaging for detecting ischemia and identifying viable but stunned or hibernating myocardium,[21] contrast perfusion imaging requires expertise and special machine capabilities, which currently limits its mainstream use.

ECHOCARDIOGRAPHY IN THE CONTEXT OF CARDIAC IMAGING

The arsenal of noninvasive cardiovascular imaging modalities includes nuclear imaging (single-photon emission computed tomography [SPECT] and positron emission tomography [PET]), cardiac CT, and CMR (see Chapters 18 to 20) and will undoubtedly continue to expand. Of these choices, echocardiography continues to hold the major advantage of being the most rapid, portable, and real-time imaging modality available today. Therefore, TTE or TEE is often the first tool used in emergency situations such as cardiac tamponade, aortic dissection, peri-infarct or postoperative complication, and shock, in which rapid assessment of a very unstable patient may be carried out at the bedside. When a large number of patients need to be screened or patients need to be monitored long term with serial examinations, the fact that ultrasound imaging involves no ionizing radiation or potentially toxic contrast is a particularly important consideration. It is thus ideal for monitoring valvular dysfunction, cardiotoxic chemotherapy, and cardiomyopathies. Although the spatial resolution of other modalities such as CMR or CT may be greater than that of echocardiography, the superior temporal resolution of TTE and TEE render these techniques ideal for detection of small mobile vegetations, thrombi, and fibrinous strands in the heart, which move too rapidly to be easily visualized by techniques with slower frame rates. Echocardiography also allows the simultaneous assessment of the impact of these lesions on valvular function, i.e., extent of regurgitation.

On the other hand, PET with ^{18}F-fluorodeoxyglucose (FDG) has emerged as a sensitive method for detecting inflammation and abscesses (see Chapter 80) when suspicion of endocarditis and intracardiac abscess is high but TEE is nondiagnostic.[16,22] Use of contrast-enhanced CT for diagnosis of aortic dissections has increased over the past two decades, largely because of the increasing accessibility of high-speed scanners and their ability to scan the entire aorta expeditiously. More recently, CT angiography has emerged as a feasible alternative for detecting left atrial and prosthetic valve thrombus, as well as for device surveillance after endovascular left atrial appendage closure.[23] These radiologic modalities serve as a useful alternative or adjunct, particularly if the patient has contraindications to TEE, or if risk of aspiration or aerosolization of contagious pathogens are a large concern (as in the recent Covid-19 pandemic).

In addition to diagnosing structural abnormalities of the myocardium, pericardium, valves, and vessels, echocardiography can directly demonstrate the consequent physiologic and hemodynamic derangements. This is particularly true for pericardial effusions (see Chapter 86), in which echocardiography can demonstrate evidence of impending or actual tamponade in real time within seconds. For more refined tissue characterization, CMR often offers higher resolution and specificity in defining tumor characteristics such as tissue density and vascularity, infiltrative/inflammatory processes, and nontransmural fibrosis. CT is particularly useful in defining calcified cardiac structures, and CT angiography is capable of imaging the coronary arteries along their full extent much more reliably than echocardiography (provided that the patient has a relatively slow and regular heart rate). Defining the thickness of the pericardium is also another "Achilles heel" of echocardiography; CT and CMR provide a more sensitive and comprehensive method of evaluation. However, echocardiography remains the first-line modality for detecting the characteristic respirophasic septal bounce and respiratory variation in cardiac output caused by constriction and continues to be the mainstay of follow-up regardless of treatment.[24]

Acoustic shadowing from prosthetic valves, ventricular assist devices (VADs), calcification, or air between the transducer and the far-field portions of the heart can preclude adequate visualization of portions of the heart by echocardiography. In these cases, fluoroscopy and CT are useful alternative or adjunctive modalities. A common example would be the dysfunctional mechanical aortic prosthesis, which can be difficult to visualize directly on TEE because of acoustic shadowing. However, the valve discs and disc excursion are easily visible on fluoroscopy or CT angiography. Similarly, because the sternum and ribs impede transthoracic ultrasound imaging and the air-filled trachea produces a "blind spot" on TEE, echocardiographic evaluation of the aorta is limited to the proximal root, arch, and segments of the thoracic and abdominal aorta. However, for unstable patients (e.g., after a motor vehicle accident or those in profound shock), TTE or TEE is often the only suitable bedside tool and is sufficient to diagnose or rule out most type A dissections (see Chapter 42). With TEE one can also expeditiously determine whether the proximal coronary arteries and arch vessels are patent without the use of nephrotoxic contrast material.

Stress echocardiography using either treadmill, bicycle, or pharmacologic (dobutamine or vasodilator) stress has proved to be more accurate than the exercise ECG alone for diagnosing flow-limiting CAD, particularly in women and patients with LV hypertrophy.[25] When compared with nuclear imaging, stress echocardiography is equally sensitive and specific. It also has the advantage of allowing simultaneous assessment of hemodynamics, valvular disease (particularly aortic and MS), and estimation of PASPs in the same examination. However, the presence of previously infarcted segments, known multivessel CAD, and a left bundle branch block (LBBB) may decrease the sensitivity and specificity of stress echocardiography because of difficulty interpreting wall thickening in the presence of resting regional dysfunction and translational motion.

It should be emphasized that in many cases the use of two or more modalities is appropriate and complementary to diagnose more definitively the nature and extent of a pathology and plan appropriate treatment.[15] This is particularly true in cases of ischemic and nonischemic cardiomyopathy for which CMR, SPECT and FDG PET methods can more clearly define the locations of hypertrophy, fibrosis, or inflammation. Extensive aortic dissections in which one needs to define precisely the extent to which major coronary, head, and systemic arteries are involved also often calls for multimodality imaging.[26] Nuclear molecular imaging is also useful for confirming or refuting suspected diagnoses of sarcoidosis and ATTR amyloidosis (see Chapter 53) made initially on clinical and echocardiographic grounds.

Significant valvular pathology may necessitate the use of other modalities after initial echocardiographic assessment (see Multimodality Imaging, later): CT calcium scores have been found useful to risk-stratify calcific AS that may benefit from aortic valve replacement.[27] In patients with valvular regurgitation, where the degree of regurgitation appears significant but unclear, CMR is indicated to determine the regurgitant volume.[16] Fusion imaging, in which images from different modalities (e.g., TEE and fluoroscopy, or FDG-PET and CT angiography) are hybridized, has been shown to be feasible for real-time images and may more accurately guide the deployment of devices in transcatheter structural heart disease interventions.[28,29]

Echocardiography can unfortunately render a variety of artefacts that mimic masses, thrombi, tumors, or related tissue flaps. Although most can be discerned as false findings by experienced echocardiographers, a minority may require additional tailored echocardiographic views in varying tissue planes to put the question to rest. The adjunctive use of 3D echocardiography and echocardiographic enhancing agents can often reveal the true nature of these artefacts without the nephrotoxic effects of the iodinated and gadolinium agents used in radiologic imaging.

Currently, the newer techniques for assessing tissue strain, dyssynchrony, and diastolic function have evolved in almost parallel fashion in echocardiography and CMR.[30] These techniques have been used extensively in research and are being validated in a clinical setting with larger populations. In summary, although ultrasound and radiology continue to advance, familiarity with the relative advantages and limitations of each imaging modality greatly assists in determining which tool is best suited to answer the clinical question at hand.

MYOCARDIAL INFARCTION

Echocardiography plays an essential diagnostic and prognostic role in assessing patients during and after acute MI. Normal wall contractility (normokinesis) is seen as wall thickening caused by the contraction of individual myocardial fibers during systole. On echocardiography the radial distance between the epicardial and endocardial borders normally increases by at least 20% during systole. Global LVEF, as calculated by 2D echocardiography and preferably by the 2D biplane method of discs, provides an indication of overall infarct size and its impact on function. It has remained the single measure with the greatest prognostic and clinical significance during and after MI.[31]

Myocardial ischemia affects LV systolic function both focally and globally. Focal hypokinesis—decreased systolic thickening—occurs within seconds of the onset of myocardial ischemia, before chest pain and changes on the ECG. This pathognomonic finding will occur in the region of the left and/or right ventricle supplied by the compromised artery (at least 70% stenosis) and give the appearance of a hinge point compared with adjacent perfused segments. Ischemia may also manifest as delayed contraction of a segment (tardokinesis). Ischemia may be a dynamic condition, and if sufficient blood flow is restored in time, either through a decrease in metabolic demand (as when a stress test ends) or through reperfusion, contractility of the affected segment can recover rapidly. However, after reperfusion, a marked reduction in LVEF during the initial few days after MI can be secondary to myocardial stunning rather than permanent myocardial dysfunction and can improve substantially over days to weeks (see Chapter 36).

Persistence or increasing severity of the wall motion abnormality after the initial insult implies that the tissue is becoming nonfunctional (i.e., not metabolically active or hibernating) or nonviable (infarcted). Akinetic myocardial segments do not thicken at all, and dyskinetic segments bulge paradoxically outward in systole, thus implying that no functioning myocardium is present. Thinning of the walls to less than 6 mm, echo brightness, and dyskinesis usually indicate scar. Sudden dilation of the left ventricle and a decrease in the LVEF are predictive signs of larger areas of ischemia (more proximal and/or multivessel disease). More refined techniques, including IV echocardiographic contrast enhancement to examine myocardial perfusion, low-dose dobutamine echocardiography, or regional strain analysis, may be useful in demonstrating whether segments that are still akinetic after reperfusion remain viable but hibernating.[31]

Specific regions in the heart can be mapped to specific coronary artery territories (Fig. 16.25), thereby allowing determination of the infarct-related vessel in patients with MI or detection of ischemic territory during stress echocardiography (see later, Stress Echocardiography). Very proximal CAD can actually be detected by examining the ostia of the coronary arteries with TEE. A proximal coronary artery stenosis will cause wall motion abnormality in a large territory (i.e., an entire wall from base to apex), whereas more distal blockage will affect only more apical segments. An acute left main occlusion will result in such extensive dysfunction (anterior septum, anterior and lateral walls) that if untreated, it is usually lethal. Proximal right coronary artery (RCA) lesions can additionally cause RV dysfunction and infarction. The presence of previously existing CAD can modify the extent of new wall motion abnormalities seen during acute MI. Collateral vessels from other unobstructed coronary arteries can develop and perfuse the peripheral territory of affected vessels, thus diminishing the dysfunctional region. Wall motion scoring can be used as a complementary tool to the EF for quantifying the extent and severity of LV systolic function.

Practical Considerations in Assessment of Regional Wall Motion

It is important to distinguish carefully between wall thickening as opposed to just epicardial or endocardial border movement during systole. The many pitfalls in diagnosing wall motion abnormalities include false-positives because of poor visualization of the endocardium, superior angulation of the probe such that the membranous nonmuscular portion of the upper interventricular septum is misinterpreted as an akinetic myocardial segment, extracardiac compression of the inferior wall by ascites or abdominal contents ("pseudodyskinesis"), and paradoxical or dyssynchronous septal motion as a result of bundle branch block or the postsurgical state. False-negatives, such as missing a wall motion abnormality that is present, can also occur

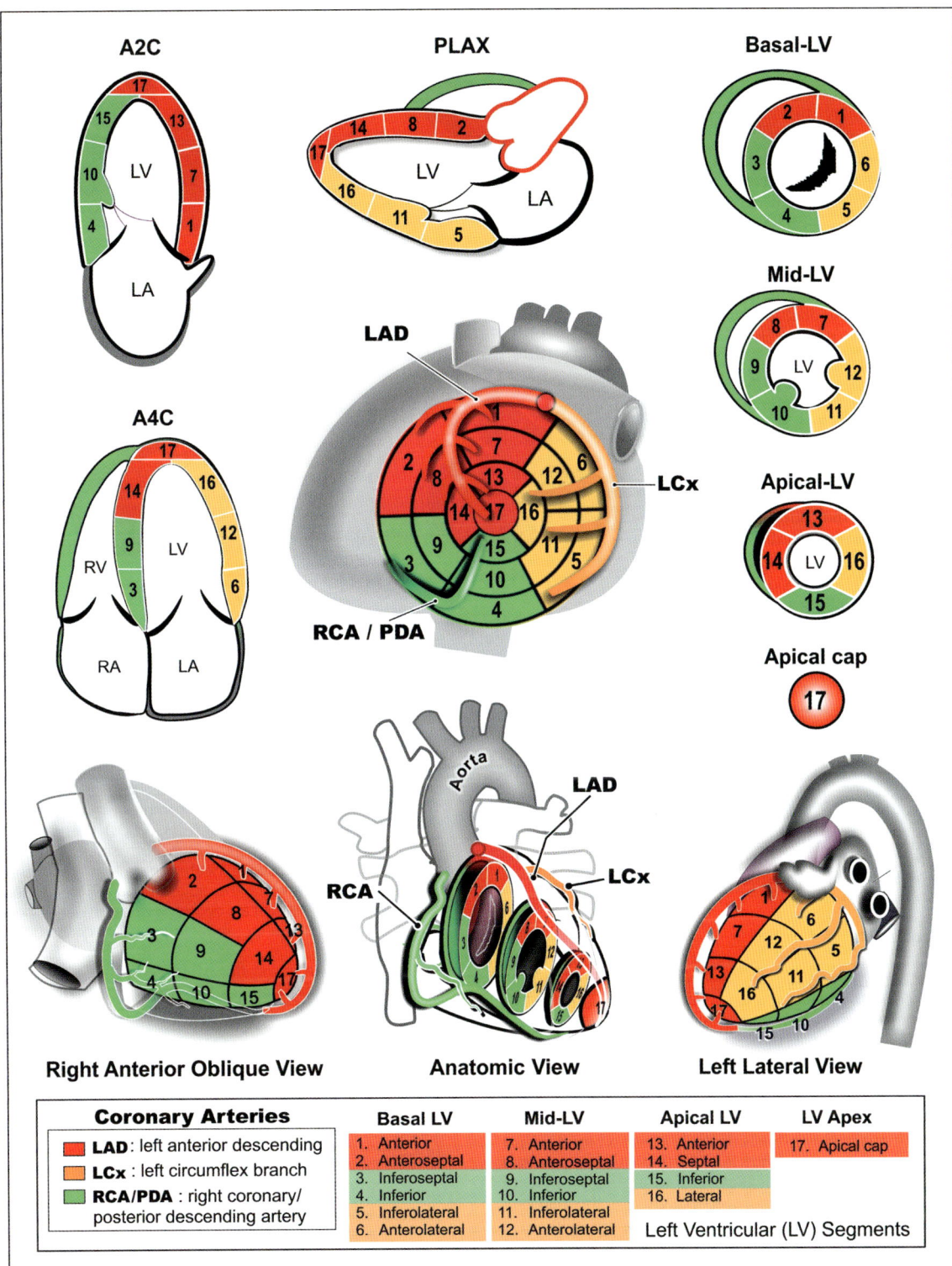

FIGURE 16.25 Coronary artery territories. The main epicardial coronary arteries each supply distinct myocardial territories, which may be mapped and evaluated during the ultrasound examination. For standardization, the left ventricle (LV) is divided along the long axis into anterior, inferior, septal, and lateral quadrants. At the basal and midventricular levels, the septal and lateral walls are further subdivided into anterior and inferior segments. Each wall is further sectioned in short-axis planes into basal, middle, and apical thirds, with the distal apex beyond the LV cavity forming a cap segment, to yield a total of 17 wall segments. Most of the blood supply to the heart is from the left main coronary artery, which divides into the left anterior descending (LAD) and left circumflex (LCx) arteries. The LAD supplies most of the anterior ventricular wall, and its septal branches supply the anterior two thirds of the septum. In addition, diagonal branches of the LAD supply the anterolateral wall. Large LADs may wrap around the apex of the heart and supply the distal-most portion of the inferior wall. The LCx runs in the atrioventricular groove, and its obtuse marginal branches supply the inferolateral wall. The right coronary artery (RCA) supplies blood to the inferior third of the septum and the inferior wall. The RCA also supplies the right ventricle. *A2C,* apical two-chamber view; *A4C,* apical four-chamber view; *LA,* left atrium; *PDA,* posterior descending artery; *PLAX,* parasternal long axis; *RA,* right atrium; *RV,* right ventricle. (Modified from Bulwer BE, Rivero JM, eds. *Echocardiography Pocket Guide: The Transthoracic Examination.* Burlington, MA: Jones & Bartlett Learning; 2011, 2013:131. Reprinted with permission.)

because of poor image quality or off-axis imaging. Injection of an IV ultrasound enhancing agent can often help delineate the endocardial borders.

Notably, echocardiography in a patient who is free of chest pain at the time of imaging may not reveal a resting wall motion abnormality (because of decreased demand or reperfusion at that point in time). Furthermore, this technique is relatively insensitive for small areas of subendocardial or microvascular ischemia. Nevertheless, when a patient has ongoing acute chest pain but echocardiography does not reveal new wall motion abnormalities, a broader differential diagnosis than epicardial coronary artery occlusion must be entertained. Possible nonischemic cardiac causes of chest pain that can be also diagnosed by cardiac ultrasound include aortic or coronary aneurysm or dissection, myocarditis, cardiac contusion, and ruptured mitral chordae. Taken in context, the presence of a pericardial effusion may support a diagnosis of pericarditis. Noncardiac causes include pulmonary emboli (which can cause acute right-sided heart dysfunction in a distinctive pattern), as well as gastroenterologic processes (reflux, peptic ulcer disease, esophageal spasm), pleuritis, and costochondritis.

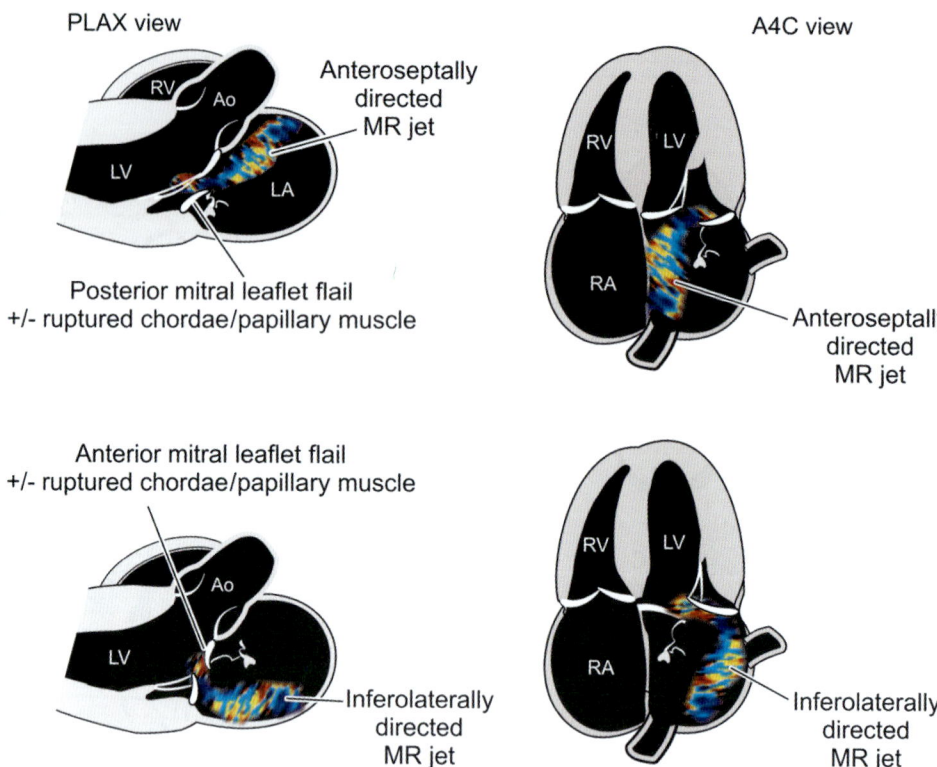

FIGURE 16.26 Acute structural mitral regurgitation (MR). The consequences of rupture of the posterior papillary muscle and chordae **(upper figure)** versus the anterior papillary muscle and chordae **(lower figure)** are shown with respect to the direction of the MR jet. Posterior mitral leaflet flail will cause a very eccentric jet to be directed anteroseptally, and this can occasionally cause clinicians to erroneously detect a "new aortic stenosis" murmur. Anterior mitral leaflet flail will cause the MR jet to be directed inferolaterally, and this murmur may be missed unless one auscultates the back. *A4C,* Apical four-chamber; *Ao,* aorta; *LA,* left atrium; *LV,* left ventricle; *PLAX,* parasternal long axis; *RA,* right atrium; *RV,* right ventricle.

MECHANICAL COMPLICATIONS AFTER MYOCARDIAL INFARCTION

MI can cause serious collateral damage from tissue necrosis and bleeding, which is often heralded by cardiogenic shock (see Chapter 38). These events may appear within days of the initial infarct or may be delayed by years. All cardiologists should be familiar with causes of infarct-related shock and their appearance on echocardiography.[14,32]

Mitral Regurgitation

Acute severe mitral regurgitation (MR) is most often caused by infarction and consequent rupture of a papillary muscle. It results in "flail" of the associated mitral leaflet into the left atrium during systole with valve incompetence. The anterolateral papillary muscle receives dual blood supply from both the left anterior descending (LAD) coronary artery and its diagonals and the left circumflex artery (see Chapter 21); thus a very large infarct would be required to disrupt this papillary muscle, which supports more of the anterior mitral leaflet. In contrast, the posterior descending artery, which arises from the RCA in right-dominant individuals, is the sole blood supply of the posteromedial papillary muscle. For this reason, papillary muscle rupture and flail posterior leaflet occur more frequently with inferior infarcts. There is, however, overlap between the papillary muscle support of the leaflets, and only one head or a tip of a papillary muscle may be disrupted rather than the entire trunk. Thus, in small infarcts there may be a focally flail segment or just the tip of an opposing mitral leaflet affected. The jet of MR is eccentric and directed *away* from the affected mitral leaflet; that is, posterior leaflet flail directs the MR jet anteroseptally, whereas anterior leaflet flail directs the regurgitant jet posterolaterally (Fig. 16.26). If clinical suspicion for acute infarct-related MR is high and TTE is not definitive, proceeding expeditiously to surgical consultation and TEE is recommended.

Ventricular Septal Defect

Defects in the ventricular septum may appear as discrete areas of echo dropout with interventricular flow coursing through, as demonstrated by color Doppler). Echocardiography should define the location, type (simple or complex), and size of the defect. Anterior ventricular septal defects (VSDs) tend to be simple (i.e., direct slitlike perforations through both sides of the septum at the same level) and are usually located more apically. In contrast, inferior infarctions often involve the adjacent basal inferior septum or even the right ventricle and can be complex (with serpiginous or multiple fissures). Unless the defect is very large, 2D echocardiographic images alone may only be suggestive of thinned or focally absent myocardium, but color flow Doppler can definitively demonstrate both location and extent of the shunt at the "break" area. A small (restrictive) VSD will have a high interventricular pressure gradient, whereas a large (unrestrictive) VSD will have lower gradients and is more likely to be associated with further tissue damage, including even papillary muscle rupture or free wall rupture in catastrophic cases. By applying the Bernoulli equation, the pressure gradient across a restrictive VSD can be calculated. RV systolic pressure should be equal to systolic blood pressure minus the interventricular pressure gradient. Significant and prolonged shunting across the VSD can lead to biventricular failure and eventually cause right-sided pressures to increase and the amount of left-to-right shunting paradoxically to decrease over time.

Pseudoaneurysm

A pseudoaneurysm is a ventricular free wall perforation that is locally contained by adjacent pericardium and adhesions. Pseudoaneurysms appear more often after inferior MI, although they may arise in the lateral and apical regions. On echocardiography, pseudoaneurysms appear as echo-free spaces or extra chambers adjacent to and continuous with the LV cavity. The appearance can be similar to that of a true LV aneurysm or diverticulum, but unlike these two pathologies, the definitive feature of a pseudoaneurysm is disruption of all three layers: endocardium, myocardium, and epicardium. Thus a pseudoaneurysm is more likely to have distinguishing traits such as a narrower neck with more ragged edges and turbulent bidirectional flow (as opposed to the smoother margins and flow pattern typically seen with true aneurysms). However, no single echocardiographic criterion is specific enough to distinguish false from true LV aneurysms definitively. IV ultrasound enhancing agents can be very helpful in delineating the area of the perforation and extravasation into the pericardial space if the patient is sufficiently stable. Although pseudoaneurysms are typically subacute complications of MI and may hemorrhage suddenly, a fair percentage of pseudoaneurysms are surprisingly stable and go undetected for months and even years. In stable patients, historically LV angiography was used to confirm pseudoaneurysm, but contemporary use of CMR or CT angiography can noninvasively render higher resolution anatomy and also assess for regional myocardial viability.

Free Wall Rupture
Free wall rupture is usually so acutely lethal that it is rarely imaged, but findings consist of a sudden new pericardial effusion in a patient with marked thinning and akinesis at the terminal myocardial territory of the occluded artery. Echocardiographic features of tamponade are usually present. The pericardial effusion may contain spontaneous echocardiographic contrast or organized clot (*hemopericardium*) Demonstration of low-velocity color Doppler flow or extravasation of IV echocardiographic contrast from the LV cavity into the effusion (ewould confirm wall rupture, but care must be taken not to confuse rupture with the low-velocity color signal generated within pericardial fluid by the adjacent moving heart.

Tamponade
Mechanical causes of tamponade related to infarcts include pseudoaneurysm and free wall rupture, as previously described, but also aortic dissection (in some cases caused iatrogenically by percutaneous intervention). All cause frank bleeding into the pericardial sac. Hemopericardium is associated with a distinctive gel-like appearance of pericardial fluid on echocardiography. Fully organized thrombus found in otherwise echolucent pericardial effusions may be indicative of past wall rupture that has been sealed off in the interim (i.e., intermittent bleeding).

Other Causes of Cardiogenic Shock in Myocardial Infarction
In addition to the mechanical complications described earlier, there are other potential explanations for hypotension in the setting of acute MI.[32] Simple loss of pump function in large infarcts is probably the most common reason. RV infarction can occur concomitantly with inferoposterior injury or as isolated RV injury in a patient with occlusion of a nondominant RCA (see Chapter 38). It may reveal itself when nitroglycerin is administered and decreases preload. The most reliable echocardiographic sign of RV infarction is new dilation and hypokinesis of the right ventricle. Typically, the lateral, diaphragmatic or posterior RV walls are most affected (the posterior wall represents the distal most RCA territory), with sparing of the apex (which is also supplied by the distal LAD). Depressed RV function can often be illustrated by a low tissue Doppler peak systolic velocity of the tricuspid annulus (S′ wave) or by a slow upstroke to the TR Doppler envelope (low dP/dT), and can be quantified by a low RV ejection fraction or FAC.[13] Annular dilation may cause associated TR and RA dilation with relatively low or normal peak TR flow velocity (because of low or normal RV systolic pressure). Because RV walls are thinner than those of the left ventricle, the right ventricle can recover relatively quickly from ischemic insults and return to normal function after revascularization. Other potential causes of hypotension and cardiogenic shock include reocclusion of coronary arteries with infarct expansion, related effusive pericarditis (Dressler syndrome), and acute dynamic LVOT obstruction with mitral systolic anterior motion, when the basal portion of the heart becomes hypercontractile as compensation for more apical wall motion abnormalities in patients with upper septal hypertrophy.

LATE COMPLICATIONS OF MYOCARDIAL INFARCTION
Even after an MI is completed, ongoing changes in heart structure and function can cause negative sequelae that can be clinically silent. *Left ventricular aneurysms* are discrete dyskinetic outpouchings of the left ventricle with preservation of the integrity of the three heart layers (endocardium, myocardium, and epicardium). The most common locations of LV aneurysms are the basal inferior wall and the apex, where they may grow to a size that rivals the other cardiac chambers.

Spontaneous echocardiographic contrast within the aneurysms signifies local stasis of blood flow.

In the absence of anticoagulation, ongoing stagnant flow within an LV aneurysm may lead to the formation of *left ventricular thrombus* (Fig. 16.27A). Patients with large aneurysms, anterior MIs, or LVEF less than 40% are at particular risk for LV thrombus. Intracavitary thrombi may be detected within the first 1 to 2 weeks after MI and appear as discrete, homogeneously echogenic, deformable masses abutting the endocardial border of an akinetic or dyskinetic wall segment. Earlier studies indicated that the sensitivity and positive predictive value (PPV) of echocardiography for LV thrombus were decently high, compared with surgical/pathologic or radionuclide imaging. However, compared with CMR, the sensitivity and PPV appear to be significantly less than originally assumed.[33] Accuracy is undoubtedly affected by pretest probability, image quality, and the size and type of thrombus (the mural type being more difficult to detect). The use of IV ultrasound enhancing agents can double the detection rate of intracavitary thrombi (sensitivity up to 60%, and PPV increases to 93%) and is highly recommended (see Fig. 16.22). Thrombi may appear mural (i.e., fixed, flattened, and adherent to the endocardial wall, as in Fig. 16.27A) or may have independently mobile and protuberant portions. Larger and more mobile thrombi, as well as those residing adjacent to hyperkinetic myocardial segments, are more likely to embolize. As the thrombi age, they tend to become less mobile, more compact, and echobright in appearance. With anticoagulation, LV thrombi have been observed to resolve in almost 50% of patients by 1 year and in approximately 75% by 2 years of follow-up.

The left ventricle can continue to expand in size and mass and display hypokinesis in noninfarcted areas, even after the initial insult has ended, a process termed *left ventricular remodeling*. In the broadest context, remodeling is defined as an increase in LV volume, but concomitant changes in the geometry of the ventricle are also frequently observed. An increase in the globular shape of the heart is quantified by the *sphericity index*. On 2D echocardiography, this is the ratio of the long-axis dimension to the short-axis dimension. Sphericity index is 1.5 or higher in normal hearts but approaches 1.0 in globular hearts (see later, Dilated Cardiomyopathy).

Ischemic MR refers to mitral incompetence in the setting of ischemic LV dysfunction and in the absence of structural abnormalities, such as prolapse, thickening, calcification, or papillary muscle rupture that would otherwise cause regurgitation (see Chapter 76). It is a subset of secondary (functional) MR. This process has been intensively studied, and there appears to be interplay between the LV, mitral, and subvalvular components, as well as the left atrium, all of which contribute to the pathophysiology of MR and an imbalance between the closing and tethering forces that normally maintain valve competence.[34] Displacement of the papillary muscle positions inferiorly and toward the apex contributes to tethering of the mitral leaflets at abnormal angles that restrict leaflet closure. Impaired LV systolic function reduces closing forces. Mitral annular and LA dilation and decreased LV basal myocardial rotation all appear to play a role in enhancing ischemic MR as well (Fig. 16.27B). The imaging hallmark of ischemic MR is pathologic systolic leaflet tethering which may be associated with a hockey-stick appearance. Dysfunction of the papillary muscles per se does not cause ischemic MR and may, in fact, mitigate leaflet tethering. Quantitation of ischemic MR may be challenging but the *effective regurgitant orifice area* (EROA) derived from color and spectral Doppler measurements has a direct correlation with overall mortality (see later, Mitral Regurgitation).

Echocardiographic Prognostic Indicators After Myocardial Infarction
After acute MI, echocardiography can assist in assessing (1) the prognosis for patients at risk for recurrent ischemia and heart failure and (2) overall risk for morbidity and mortality. LVEF is one of the most important predictors of overall morbidity and mortality after acute MI and is used as a surrogate endpoint in most major clinical trials of medical and procedural interventions. As LVEF declines, the rate of sudden cardiac death (SCD) increases. Based on current evidence, an LVEF of ≤30% to 40% (cutoff varies depending on other clinical characteristics) is a Class I indication for implantation of an implantable cardioverter-defibrillator (ICD)

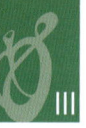

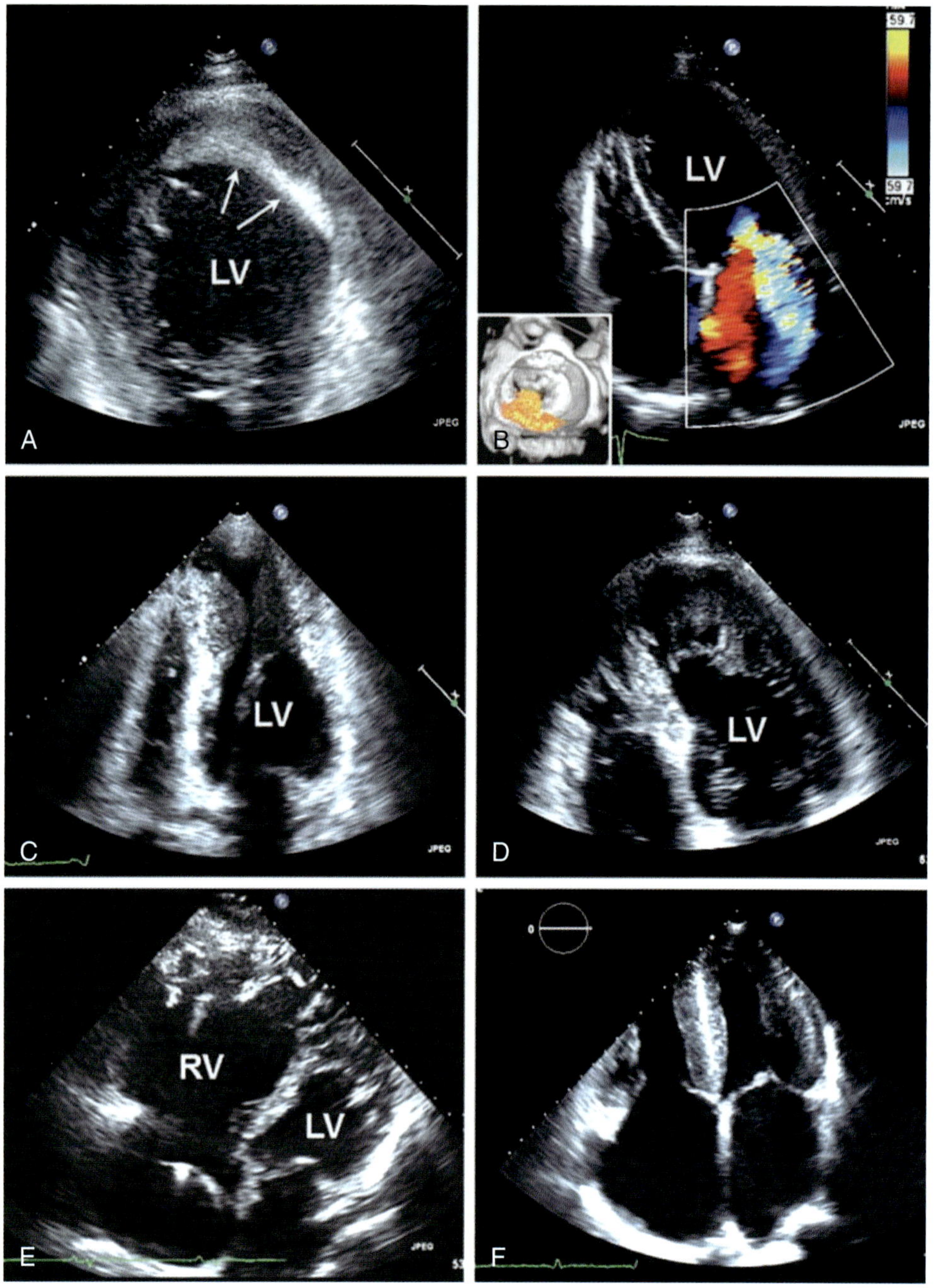

independently predictive of heart failure in patients with stable CAD include increasing LV mass index (LVMI >90 g/m^2), a restrictive pattern of diastolic dysfunction (E/é' ratio >15, DT <130 msec), an LVOT VTI less than 22 mm, an LA volume index greater than 32 mL/m^2, and estimated PASP greater than 35 mm Hg. The presence of at least moderate MR (especially if EROA ≥20 mm^2 or regurgitant volume ≥30 mL) is now well established as an independent predictor of cardiac mortality as well as heart failure. RV systolic function, in particular an RV GLS ≤−22%, also appears to be associated with increased risk.[31]

The WMSI may be a more discriminatory measure than LVEF (as measured by echocardiography or nuclear methods) in predicting cardiac events, in particular, rehospitalization for heart failure. On resting echocardiography, WMSI higher than 1.5 that persists after treatment of MI suggests a substantial (>20%) perfusion defect and increased risk for complications. In stress echocardiography, WMSI higher than 1.7 at peak stress and LVEF of 45% or less are independent markers of patients at high risk for recurrent MI or cardiac death. When there is a question of whether revascularization will improve akinetic but viable areas, dobutamine or contrast-enhanced echocardiography may delineate the extent of myocardium that is hibernating (hypocontractile yet viable and still perfused)[25] (see later, Stress Echocardiography).

Finally, it should be noted that wall motion abnormalities are indicative of focal myocardial dysfunction but are not entirely specific for atherosclerosis-related MI. Vasospasm, inflammation, or fibrosis secondary to myocarditis; swelling from intramural hematoma or edema; Takotsubo cardiomyopathy (see Chapter 52); and any focal myocardial insult are also causes of wall motion abnormality. A comprehensive synthesis of the history, clinical and physical examination findings, and ECG together with appropriate cardiac imaging will allow the clinician to narrow down the differential diagnoses and pursue appropriate therapy.

FIGURE 16.27 Cardiomyopathies. **A,** Ischemic cardiomyopathy illustrating an apical aneurysm and thrombus (*arrows*). **B,** Ischemic cardiomyopathy illustrating severe functional MR. **C,** Apical hypertrophic cardiomyopathy with midcavity systolic obliteration and an apical aneurysm. **D,** LV noncompaction. **E,** Arrhythmogenic RV dysplasia. **F,** Amyloid heart disease. *LV,* Left ventricle; *RV,* right ventricle.

for primary prevention in selected patients, with an increasing proportion receiving biventricular pacing (CRT) as well (see Chapters 50, 58, and 69).[35] As mentioned previously, after reperfusion, stunned or hibernating myocardium may recover function days to weeks later, so it is generally recommended that one wait at least 40 days after acute MI, or as long as 3 months after coronary artery bypass graft (CABG) or percutaneous revascularization, to reevaluate LVEF before making a decision on ICD implantation for primary prevention. Reduced global longitudinal (GLS <−14%) and circumferential strain have emerged as important risk indicators for death or heart failure after MI. A high degree of dyssynchrony, quantitated by the same technique, is also a risk factor.[2,5,31,35] In addition to LVEF, overall LV size (as assessed by LV end-diastolic diameter and volume) and sphericity are important prognostic indicators. Other measures

CARDIOMYOPATHIES

Dilated Cardiomyopathy

Dilated cardiomyopathies share the common characteristics of an enlarged LV and/or RV cavity with systolic dysfunction (see Chapter 52). Left ventricular end-diastolic (LVED) and end-systolic volumes, as well as LVED dimensions and overall LV mass, are increased (with normal or thinned walls), and the overall LVEF is subnormal. With persistence of the underlying condition, the left ventricle becomes less ellipsoid and more globular in shape, and the sphericity index

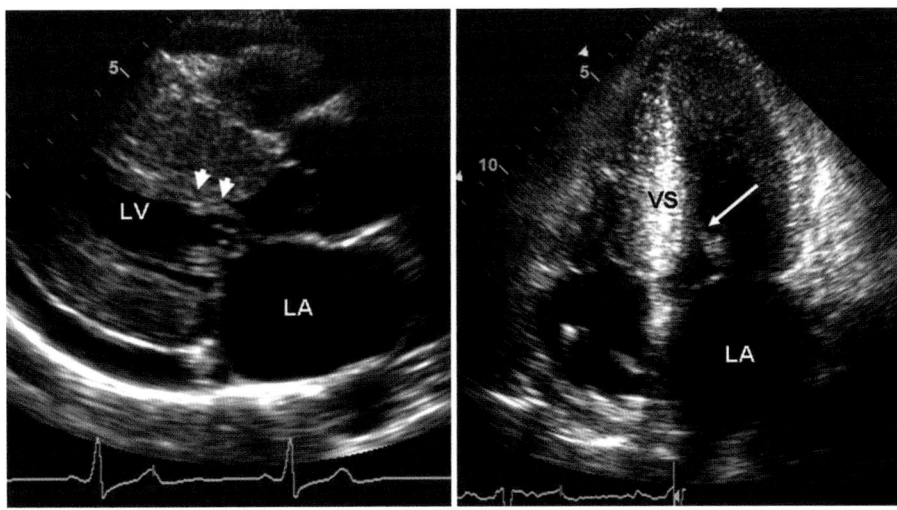

FIGURE 16.28 Hypertrophic cardiomyopathy. A parasternal long-axis view **(left)** shows markedly increased septal wall thickness and systolic anterior motion of the mitral valve (*arrows*), also visualized in the apical four-chamber view **(right)**. Note the sigmoid, banana-shaped septum. *LA*, Left atrium; *LV*, left ventricle; *VS*, interventricular septum.

less confers a worse prognosis in patients with dilated cardiomyopathy.

Functional (secondary) MR with incomplete leaflet coaptation, caused by multiple processes similar to that seen with ischemic cardiomyopathy, often accompanies and exacerbates dilated cardiomyopathy (see Fig. 16.27B).[34] If the patient begins to experience right-sided heart failure because of left-sided heart failure (i.e., elevated LVED pressure), the pulmonary venous inflow patterns will show diminution of systolic inflow (the S wave) because of elevated atrial pressure, and this may precede a rise in estimated PASP (as reflected by TR velocity).

Regardless of cause, a worse prognosis is associated with declining LVEF and elevated end-diastolic and end-systolic volume, increasing LV mass, the development of restrictive physiology by Doppler indices, and the presence of right-sided heart failure, pulmonary hypertension, and severe TR.[11,39] If the LVEF is 35% or lower and the patient has an intraventricular conduction delay and clinical heart failure, CRT (see Chapters 58 and 69) may improve pump cardiac output, reverse the LV remodeling, and improve functional MR[40] (see later, Echocardiography in Heart Failure). Whereas chamber enlargement and systolic dysfunction are the prominent features in dilated cardiomyopathies, in *hypertrophic* and *restrictive cardiomyopathies* the ventricles are not dilated, but diastolic filling of the ventricle is impaired. Declining systolic function and chamber enlargement typically appears only very late in the process. Both cardiomyopathies typically have thickened LV walls, caused by infiltration, myocyte hypertrophy, or both. Biatrial enlargement is frequent because the atria become the low-compliance reservoirs for cardiac inflow, particularly if AF is present.

Hypertrophic Cardiomyopathy

HCM is a primary, genetic disease of the sarcomere in which the ventricular walls are inappropriately hypertrophied and frequently asymmetrically thickened (see Chapter 54). HCM should be distinguished from the more common *focal upper septal hypertrophy*, a discrete septal bulge frequently observed in older adults, not usually associated with significant LVOT obstruction, and with a benign prognosis. In contrast, the most common forms of HCM of the obstructive type show these echocardiographic features (Fig. 16.28): a small, hyperdynamic left ventricle with a thick sigmoid septum and/or banana-shaped cavity, asymmetric septal hypertrophy (septal thickness ≥ 1.6 times the thickness of the posterior wall), a relatively small LVOT, elevated flow velocity in the LVOT that peaks in late systole (when the LVOT is smallest), systolic anterior motion of the mitral valve, and often a significant amount of posteriorly directed MR. The LVOT gradient (ΔP) is calculated from PW Doppler LVOT peak velocity by the Bernoulli equation $\Delta P = 4(V_{LVOT})^2$. It reflects the degree of outflow obstruction caused by altered LV and mitral valve geometry. The combination of small LVOT area and motion of a relatively large, anteriorly positioned, slack mitral apparatus causes the mitral leaflets to be pushed into the LVOT in early systole by flow drag forces and, to a lesser extent, by suctioning via the LVOT gradient and Venturi effect. A maximum wall thickness greater than 30 mm or a resting LVOT gradient greater than 30 mm Hg is associated with increased risk for SCD and progression to New York Heart Association (NYHA) Functional Class III heart failure. The LVOT obstruction is highly dynamic: in some individuals the LVOT obstruction and gradient can be significantly augmented by conditions that decrease preload and consequently also diminish LVOT size. Such movements include the Valsalva maneuver, sudden standing, and exercise, all of which may be performed during echocardiographic evaluation of these patients.

decreases toward 1. The actual SV and cardiac output may remain preserved because of increased overall ventricular volumes, as well as increased heart rate.

Dilated cardiomyopathies due to viral, postpartum, genetic, chemotherapeutic, tachycardia-mediated, and toxic-metabolic causes typically display diffuse LV hypokinesis; those caused by more focal processes such as sarcoidosis are more likely to have discrete areas of hypokinesis or akinesis. Ischemic heart disease is often accompanied by focal wall motion abnormalities in a coronary distribution, as well as visible atherosclerotic plaque in the aortic root and other portions of the aorta. One clue to the presence of focal inflammatory processes is wall motion abnormalities that do not follow a coronary distribution and associated thickening secondary to edema. Approximately half of symptomatic patients with Chagas disease classically have segmental abnormalities such as an apical or inferobasal aneurysm, but more advanced cases feature global hypokinesis and RV dysfunction.[37] *Takotsubo cardiomyopathy*, which appears to be a stress- or neuroendocrine-mediated process, is unique in displaying a distinctive pattern of apical ballooning and basal hyperkinesis in the majority (>80%) of patients.[38] Although the degree of dysfunction can be impressive in stress cardiomyopathy, remarkable and complete resolution often occurs within days to weeks. Rarer "reverse" or alternate patterns of stress cardiomyopathy have also been encountered, in which basal or midventricular wall motion abnormalities occur with preservation of apical function. With sustained left-sided heart failure (and thus secondary pulmonary hypertension) or systemic causes of myocardial dysfunction, the right ventricle may also become dilated and hypokinetic, and enlargement of both atria—and thus four-chamber enlargement—is also common.

The degree of impairment in LV contractility is quantifiable by several means (see earlier, Assessment of Cardiac Structure and Function). Historically, M-mode findings such as increased separation of the mitral E point from the interventricular septum, decreased mitral leaflet opening, and early closure of the aortic valve are known to correlate with poor cardiac output. A universally used measure of systolic function is LVEF, which is considered subnormal if less than 50%. The total SV of the ventricle (reflected by VTI_{LVOT}) may be diminished, and tissue Doppler S′ (systolic) excursion is diminished. RV size and contractility may be assessed by parallel means (see Tables 16.5 and 16.6), although it is more difficult to assess RV volume without the use of 3D echocardi-ography. One easily obtainable measure of RV function is TAPSE, which reflects shortening in the long-axis dimension of RV myocardial fibers; a TAPSE of less than 17 mm is considered abnormal, and 14 mm or

Other forms of HCM may easily be recognized by echocardiography and facilitated with the use of an ultrasound enhancing agent. In *apical* HCM, basal wall thickness may be normal, but the midventricular and apical portions are unusually thickened, and a midcavity gradient may exist; in more advanced cases, a distal apical aneurysmal area may develop (see Fig. 16.27C) and may be associated with a higher incidence of arrhythmias, stroke, and SCD.[41] In a minority (10% to 15%) of patients with HCM, systolic dysfunction ultimately develops, and the heart becomes progressively more dilated and globally hypokinetic. For screening purposes, it is important to keep in mind that some patients with HCM by genotype may have normal or only slightly increased wall thickness or may not manifest hypertrophy until late in adulthood.[42,43]

Other Cardiomyopathies With Regional or Global Variations in Myocardial Composition

Left Ventricular Noncompaction

LV noncompaction is a myocardial phenotype that is thought in many cases to be genetically determined. It is characterized by abundant trabeculations and deep endothelial-lined recesses extending into the myocardial layer that have failed to compact. On echocardiography this confers a double-layered architecture to the myocardium: there is a "spongy" appearance to the inner layer, whereas the outer layer closer to the epicardium has the normal "compacted" morphology (see Fig. 16.27D). Using color flow Doppler and/or echocardiographic contrast enhancement, blood extending between the intratrabecular recesses and the LV cavity can be demonstrated. With noncompaction there is a spectrum of expression: the condition may affect the entire mid- and apical ventricle or merely a portion of the apicolateral wall in less affected individuals, and the severity of trabeculation may vary. There is rising awareness of the condition, but to complicate the issue there is also a high prevalence of trabeculations that appear to be acquired in patients with chronically increased LV preload and afterload, and even in athletes. Hence, the appearance may resemble or overlap that of genetic or sporadically occurring noncompaction and may represent a common end-pathway. Accordingly, the definitive imaging and clinical criteria for noncompaction continue to be debated. There is general agreement that on echocardiography, a ratio of trabeculated/compacted layer thickness of greater than 2 as measured on short-axis views at the mid- and apical levels, is likely to be consistent with noncompaction.[44] More specific sets of criteria are listed in Chapter 52.

Arrhythmogenic Cardiomyopathy

Arrhythmogenic cardiomyopathy (ACM) appears in many cases to be caused by autosomal dominant mutations in a gene encoding desmosomal proteins. It is distinct from the other nonischemic cardiomyopathies in that the right ventricle is usually primarily affected (see Chapter 52), hence the older term arrhythmogenic right ventricular dysplasia (ARVD). However, as use of CMR and familial screening has increased, we now know that biventricular or even LV-predominant expressivity also occurs in up to 76% of patients. In the most classic form, RV dilation (RVOT long-axis dimension ≥ 32 mm or short-axis dimension ≥ 36 mm) is the most commonly associated abnormality, and RV global hypokinesis (FAC ≤ 33%) is present in most (see Fig. 16.27E). Segmental wall motion abnormalities, including thinning, akinetic areas, and aneurysms, may be present and are caused by fibrofatty infiltration. The inferoposterior wall of the RV inflow tract is the most frequent segment affected. RV trabecular derangement and subsequent TR secondary to annular dilation is common. Echocardiography alone is insufficiently sensitive or specific for the diagnosis of ACM, and other causes of right-sided heart dilation and arrhythmia need to be considered.[44,45]

Restrictive Cardiomyopathies

Systemic diseases that can infiltrate the heart may lead to restrictive cardiomyopathies (see Chapters 52 and 53); the most common is *amyloidosis*. Deposition of amyloid proteins in the heart causes a very distinct appearance on echocardiography, including increased LV and RV wall thickness in association with a very finely granular or "scintillating" echobright appearance of the myocardium and initially a preserved LVEF (see Fig. 16.27F). Advanced diastolic dysfunction is manifested both by Doppler indices and by worsening longitudinal strain measured by speckle tracking. Features that distinguish infiltrative cardiomyopathy from true LV hypertrophy include the concomitant presence of diffusely thickened valves, biatrial enlargement ("owl eyes" pattern), RV hypertrophy, pericardial effusion, and low voltage on the ECG. Although LVEF can appear to be normal even in clinically affected individuals, there is often marked systolic dysfunction in the longitudinal axis, as detected by both tissue Doppler and strain imaging. Amyloidosis in particular has a characteristic regional pattern of severely reduced longitudinal strain at the base of the left ventricle, but relatively preserved apical strain ("apical sparing") (see Chapter 53).[46] The classic echocardiographic features of amyloid are not specific enough to distinguish between the types of amyloidosis (i.e., light chain from transthyretin amyloidosis), and clinical features and additional MRI or radionuclide imaging often need to be incorporated into a diagnostic and treatment plan.

Apart from amyloid heart disease, echocardiography is frequently used to screen for cardiac involvement by other infiltrative diseases.[47] It may reveal abnormalities ranging from dilated to restrictive phenotypes, but no specific pattern is pathognomonic of any single cause. Heart failure develops in more than one third of patients with idiopathic or hereditary *hemochromatosis*, and their echocardiograms reveal LV and LA dilation and global hypokinesis with normal LV wall thickness. A restrictive filling pattern may occur earlier than the manifestations of systolic heart failure. All these parameters of function have been shown to improve with iron removal therapy. *Fabry disease* is associated with accumulation of glycosphingolipid in the heart and a high incidence of cardiovascular signs and symptoms in addition to renal, dermatologic, and neurologic abnormalities. More than 80% of individuals with Fabry disease will display concentric LV hypertrophy (men earlier and more prominently than women), although concentric remodeling and asymmetric hypertrophy, as well as RV hypertrophy occur in a smaller proportion. The presence of LV hypertrophy is associated with lower alpha-galactosidase activity and more cardiovascular symptoms. Longitudinal strain reduction in one or more segments has been shown to correlate with regions of fibrosis on MRI in patients with Fabry disease. Mitral leaflet thickening and significant MR are common, and focal or global LV systolic dysfunction occurs in a minority of patients. Fabry disease may mimic the findings of HCM.

Endomyocardial fibrosis, also termed *Loeffler endocarditis*, is a rare restrictive cardiomyopathy frequently accompanied by peripheral eosinophilia, which may be idiopathic or associated with helminthic infection in the tropics. Eosinophilic endocarditis and infiltration of the myocardium lead to changes that can be striking on echocardiography. LV size and systolic function may be preserved, but a hallmark of this condition is the formation of prominent diffuse thrombi along the endocardium in one or both LV apices that may embolize and can grow large enough to actually obliterate the cavities. The ventricular cavities themselves are small with restrictive physiology because of the fibrotic process. Patients may display retracted and incompetent atrioventricular valves and marked biatrial enlargement. Because most patients are identified relatively late in the disease, the time course of development of these changes is unclear.

Heart Failure

Echocardiography is key in the diagnosis and management of patients with heart failure (see Chapters 50 and 51). Determination of LVEF is the primary method to distinguish heart failure with reduced ejection fraction (HFrEF) from heart failure with preserved ejection fraction (HFpEF), with the former generally being considered when the LVEF is 40% or less. The exact EF cutoff for HFpEF has been subject to debate, and recent guidelines have used the term heart failure with mid-range ejection fraction (HFmrEF) to denote patients in the LVEF range of 40% to 49%.[48] Echocardiography can help distinguish among the different types and narrow down the potential causes of heart failure.

Abnormalities in diastolic function are common in patients with heart failure and either reduced or preserved LVEF and may have prognostic implications. MR can occur in heart failure patients secondary to apical displacement of the papillary muscles, annular dilation, or both, and progressive ventricular dilation can develop in patients with primary valvular MR (see Chapter 76). Increasing degrees of MR are associated with a poor outcome in patients with heart failure.

Assessment of Ventricular Synchrony

CRT is used to reduce heart failure and death in patients with reduced LV function and a wide QRS complex (see Chapters 58 and 69). Use of CRT can reverse ventricular remodeling and improve pump performance; in numerous studies it has also been associated with marked improvement in LV end-diastolic and end-systolic volume, EF, RV function, and LA size. While the benefit of CRT is seen most often in patients with LVEF ≤30% to 35%, QRS greater than 130 msec on ECG, and heart failure symptoms, 30% to 35% of those treated turn out to be nonresponders. Although echocardiography has been used to identify patients for CRT placement, no single parameter reliably predicts a positive clinical or echocardiographic response to CRT in the referred population.[48]

Nevertheless, echocardiography is useful in quantifying dyssynchrony and cardiac function before and after CRT. In patients with LBBB, significant dyssynchrony can be grossly visualized as an early systolic movement of the interventricular septum towards the center of the LV, followed immediately by movement in the opposite direction (a paradoxic motion). Because this affects only the basal and midportion, as the apex continues to move inwards throughout systole it may appear to rock relative to the proximal septum translating outwards; a key distinction is that the septum will still thicken overall in systole if myocardium is viable and functional, unlike a true wall motion abnormality. Also, in the normal LV, all segments contract and thicken simultaneously, but with LBBB, the time to activate the more lateral segments increases and these will thicken later than the septal segments, contributing to the rocking appearance. Because these abnormal motion patterns are subtle, visual assessment alone is only qualitative and subjective. However, longitudinal and radial strain measured by speckle-tracking has been shown to be quantitative and reproducible in assessing baseline dyssynchrony and demonstrating improvement due to CRT. Prior to or during device implantation, echocardiography may be used in select patients to discriminate appropriately paceable regions from scar and thereby optimize placement of the LV and coronary venous leads. Post-CRT implant, echocardiography is sometimes used to quantify both LVOT stroke volume and degree of MR at bedside, so that atrioventricular intervals and interventricular intervals may be tailored to produce the best forward cardiac output. In summary, LVEF remains a cornerstone for CRT patient selection, and echocardiography and myocardial deformation imaging may be useful on a case-by-case basis for optimizing CRT and quantifying the effects on heart mechanics and remodeling.[49]

Assessment After Orthotopic Heart Transplantation

Echocardiography is used both to certify that cardiac structure and function are normal in potential heart donors and to monitor for rejection in cardiac transplant recipients (see Chapter 60).[50] After uncomplicated orthotopic heart transplantation, the "normal" transplanted heart should display normal LV size and systolic function, although mild LV hypertrophy is common. GLS is often slightly lower than normal reference values. The RV is usually mildly enlarged with reduced measures of RV systolic function and free wall strain, although some recovery is often seen within a year after transplant. In patients who have undergone the standard Shumway-Lower technique of transplantation, the resultant atria are very enlarged and deformed because of the retained upper portion of the dilated native heart. In these patients the anastomosis between the donor and recipient heart may be visible as a thickened ridge of plicated tissue that encircles the atria. The ridge may be mistaken for thrombus by inexperienced observers. Newer surgical methods retain no recipient myocardium (i.e., total atrioventricular transplantation) or retain only a limited cuff of LA wall with pulmonary vein ostia (in the bicaval technique) and thus preserve more normal atrial architecture with less obvious suture lines. A "normal" transplanted heart often has slight paradoxical septal motion—anterior motion of the septum in systole and a slight decrease in septal systolic thickening—that persists in the postoperative state. Over time, in part because of distortions in atrial geometry, supraventricular arrhythmias, and repeated endomyocardial biopsies causing incidental damage to the tricuspid valve, significant TR and MR, as well as atrial thrombi, may develop in the allograft heart.

Cardiac allograft dysfunction may result from acute rejection, coronary artery vasculopathy, myocardial fibrosis, acute myocarditis from opportunistic infections, or tachycardia-mediated cardiomyopathy. Cardiac ultrasound may detect the "downstream" effects of these pathologic mechanisms. Acute cellular rejection, which results in edema and interstitial infiltrates in the myocardium, has been shown to cause detectable increases in LV wall thickness and mass, systolic dysfunction, and Doppler indices of elevated LA pressure and restrictive physiology (increased E wave velocity, decreased IVRT and mitral DT), but these changes are of insufficient sensitivity and specificity to rely on for routine clinical screening. Speckle tracking has shown that that in addition to EF, GLS is generally lower in patients with rejection, but the differences in a given individual are not significant enough to detect biopsy-proven rejection.[51] For now the gold standard for detecting acute rejection remains endomyocardial biopsy, although echocardiography and GLS evaluation have an appropriate supplementary role in monitoring for graft dysfunction and other complications after transplantation.

For detecting cardiac allograft vasculopathy, coronary angiography is the standard of care, with coronary IVUS as the ultimate gold standard at experienced centers, if more specific imaging is needed. Among noninvasive imaging techniques, echocardiography is the most widely investigated and used.[52] The presence of depressed LVEF or focal wall motion abnormalities on a *resting* echocardiogram is relatively specific (>80% in multiple studies) for allograft vasculopathy but has poor (<50%) sensitivity. Some centers use dobutamine stress echocardiography (DSE), which is preferred over exercise stress echocardiography because denervation of the allografted heart blunts the heart rate response to exercise. Meta-analysis of the published data on the accuracy of DSE indicates a pooled mean sensitivity between 60% and 70% and a specificity of 86%.[53,54] The use of longitudinal strain rate imaging or myocardial echocardiographic contrast enhancement with DSE may increase the sensitivity. For prognostic purposes, however, normal findings on DSE have been shown to have a high negative predictive value for adverse cardiac events (0.6% incidence) over short-term follow-up. Conversely, worsening findings on serial DSE confer increased risk in comparison to stable findings. Currently, therefore, DSE (as well as SPECT) is considered by the International Society of Heart and Lung Transplantation as possibly being useful (class IIa, level of evidence B) in transplant recipients who are unable to undergo invasive evaluation. Some centers use DSE to minimize exposure of transplant patients to coronary angiography, although currently no noninvasive imaging modality is sufficiently accurate to supplant it.

Assessment of Left Ventricular Assist Devices

The advent and increasing use of a variety of VADs for both bridge and destination therapy (see Chapter 59) have mandated that echocardiography play an integral role in assisting in the optimal selection of patients for left and right VADs, implantation, optimization, and troubleshooting. Here we address the principles for the more widely used HeartMate devices, which are now continuous-flow pumps with the latest models using centrifugal design.

All LVADs work by unloading the ventricle (i.e., removing some or all of the inflow and pumping it to the aorta). Echocardiography is useful for evaluation of the patient preoperatively for VAD implantation and for evaluating LV as well as RV function.[55] If RV failure is too severe, as may be indicated by a number of parameters such as RV FAC, TAPSE, and the RV Tei index (see earlier), there will be insufficient preload to fill the VAD and left ventricle. The incidence of right-sided heart failure is 20% to 30% in patients implanted with an isolated LVAD, and a preoperative RV FAC less than 20% is associated with RV failure on activation of the LVAD. In addition, echocardiography (TTE and/or TEE) can identify aortic insufficiency, intracardiac shunting, thrombi in the LV or LA appendage, or structural problems with inflow and outflow site cannulation such as excessive necrosis or atherosclerotic plaque, which are detrimental to proper LVAD function. *Intraoperatively*, TEE is used to ensure proper LV apical coring, de-airing, and cannula position and to reassess RV function on initial start-up of the LVAD. Extreme RV failure may mandate placement of an RV assist device (RVAD) as well.

Postoperatively the echocardiogram may be used to identify causes of LVAD dysfunction and fine-tune its operation[56]. When the LVAD is working properly, the ventricle should be "decompressed," that is, smaller than its original dilated size with the interventricular septum in a neutral position. The aortic valve in a completely decompressed heart stays completely closed throughout the cardiac cycle. Thickening and fusion of the aortic valve often occurs over time with nonpulsatile LVADs; it is desirable to adjust flow settings to permit at least occasional opening of the aortic valve (i.e., on a 1:3 or smaller cyclic ratio) to avoid this valvulopathy and associated aortic regurgitation (AR, which develops in approximately 25% of patients). This is ideally assessed with both M-mode and 2D imaging of the aortic valve over multiple beats. Enlargement of the left ventricle, distention of the interventricular septum rightward, and rising estimated PASP are signals of a relatively underfunctioning device that may be caused by an inadequate pump rate, worsening ventricular function, AR, volume overload, or systemic factors (e.g., sepsis). If the left ventricle appears small with a left-shifted interventricular septum, this indicates inadequate preload to the ventricle, and factors such as RV failure, pulmonary embolus, tamponade, hypovolemia (e.g., bleeding) should be sought. Obstruction of the inflow cannula is another important complication and may be caused by LV thrombus, a papillary muscle or chorda, or bending or slippage of the cannula or outlet graft. Such abnormalities may be demonstrated by 2D imaging or by increased velocities and turbulence seen with Doppler evaluation at the cannula/graft orifices. The LVAD inflow cannula should be visible at the apex, and the outflow graft/cannula can occasionally be detected by angling into the ascending aorta with a right parasternal view. Occasionally, positional kinks in the LVAD cannulae or the aortic outflow graft, which tend to occur in smaller patients, can be demonstrated by scanning the patient in the supine, sitting, and standing positions. In some patients, echocardiography "ramp" studies are performed for continuous-flow LVADs, in which the aforementioned parameters (LV and RV dimensions, septal position, aortic valve opening, valvular insufficiency, and calculated PASP) are tracked at incrementally varying pump rpm settings, with the aim of optimizing LV unloading and diagnosing malfunction, in particular thrombosis.[55,56] Assessing the IVC as a surrogate for RA filling pressure may also be useful. In the latest centrifugal pump (HeartMate 3), much narrower speed ranges are needed to optimize hemodynamics, leading to a decreased need to perform routine ramp tests in these patients.

Percutaneously implanted ventricular assist devices (PVADs) are often used to provide temporary or partial support for the left ventricle. These are increasingly replacing intra-aortic balloon pumps for short-term LV support. Echocardiography is useful for confirming that the cannulas are positioned appropriately across the interatrial septum (in the case of the TandemHeart PVAD, CardiacAssist, Pittsburgh, PA) or the aortic valve/LVOT (for the Impella), with vigilance for either obstruction or prolapse. The Impella is placed retrograde across the aortic valve into the LVOT, where it takes blood from the left ventricle and pumps it into the ascending aorta just distal to the valve. Echocardiographic imaging and color Doppler are frequently used to optimize device placement. As imaged in the parasternal long axis view, the inflow portion (a teardrop-shaped cage) of the Impella should be in the LV approximately 3.5 cm from the aortic annulus and color mosaic flow generated from the outlet portion of the cannula should be seen above the aortic valve.

Extracorporeal membrane oxygenation (ECMO) uses a pump to circulate blood through an oxygenator in order to provide short-term support for the lungs and heart in patients with acute severe respiratory failure (e.g., ARDS) or refractory cardiogenic shock (e.g., post MI or cardiac arrest, or failure to wean from cardiopulmonary bypass). There are two types of ECMO, venovenous (VV, in which a cannula takes blood from the femoral vein and returns oxygenated blood to the right atrium via the IVC or SVC) and venoarterial (VA, in which the return catheter is placed into the femoral artery to bypass a failing right ventricle). Catheters may also be placed more centrally, directly into the right atrium and ascending aorta, if a sternotomy is being performed. Transthoracic or TEE is used to evaluate left and RV function and ensure no significant valvular regurgitation is present in candidates for ECMO. Echocardiography is also used to select and confirm cannula positioning sites, assess RV function, and rule out cannula obstruction or thrombus.

Lung Ultrasound in Heart Failure

Lung ultrasound is a technique that can provide semiquantitative assessment of lung fluid in patients with heart failure. *B-lines* are vertical echogenic reverberation artefacts that arise from the pleural line and extend raylike to the far field of the imaging window with respirophasic movement. They are caused by reverberations at the interface between interstitial/alveolar fluid and air, and hence are markers of increased extravascular lung water. B-lines are most frequently seen in pulmonary edema but also in other processes such as acute respiratory distress syndrome and pulmonary fibrosis.[57] In patients with heart failure, the presence of B-lines appears more sensitive for lung congestion than even lung auscultation and chest x-ray, and correlates with N-terminal pro-brain natriuretic peptide (NT-proBNP) levels. B-lines within prespecified thoracic segments also clear contemporaneously with treatment. In patients admitted with acute heart failure, an increased number of B lines found early in admission is a prognostic marker for in-hospital adverse events. The number present at discharge is associated incrementally with increased short-term hospital readmission for heart failure and death.

The simplicity and availability of this ultrasound technique make it attractive for early diagnosis and monitoring of therapy, particularly in limited-resource environments. During the COVID-19 pandemic, lung ultrasound performed with portable ultrasound units was helpful in qualitatively assessing the burden of lung pathology, and had the added advantage of reducing the potential for viral transmission throughout hospitals. B-lines alone did not clearly distinguish between congestive heart failure and ARDS in patients with COVID respiratory distress. However, the concomitant presence of pleural thickening and irregularity and subpleural consolidations together with preserved LV systolic function seen on POCUS was indicative of significant interstitial-alveolar damage and correlated with lung CT findings of ground-glass opacities and COVID pneumonia. Lung ultrasound is also a very effective tool for rapid diagnosis of pneumothorax, an occasional complication of the positive-pressure ventilation frequently needed to treat patients with severe heart failure or COVID-19 pneumonia.[32]

The Athlete's Heart

Physiologic changes, including enlargement of the heart and bradycardia, can be induced in the heart through intensive athletic training. Echocardiography, along with ECG and ECG exercise testing, is often used to distinguish the athlete's beneficial cardiac adaptive changes from pathologic entities such as hypertrophic, arrhythmogenic, or other cardiomyopathies that are associated with SCD. Different forms of exercise are hypothesized to favor different remodeling patterns: endurance athletes have been well documented to develop LV (and actually four chamber) dilation together with a balanced increase in wall thickening (eccentric hypertrophy), whereas strength/isometric training is predisposed towards concentric hypertrophy (LV walls thickened relative to LV diameter, or RWT >0.42).[58] Although strict cutoff values for normal LVED diameter are not advocated for distinguishing physiologic from pathologic remodeling (a variable percentage of athletes have diameters >60 mm), absolute wall thicknesses greater than 15 mm in men or 12 mm in women are unusual even in elite athletes and should trigger further investigation for HCM, particularly if the hypertrophy is asymmetric. Typically, the resting LVEF is in the low-normal (approximately 50%) range in trained athletes. The standard flow and tissue Doppler metrics of diastolic dysfunction are normal or even supranormal (higher E' velocities and transmitral E/A >2) in athletes compared with HCM patients, and speckle-based local and GLS parameters are generally higher as well. Further CMR testing, exercise testing (to confirm LV augmentation and document high exercise capacity), and in "gray-zone" cases even a period of detraining (to see if LV hypertrophy regresses) may be necessary to distinguish the athlete's heart from a true cardiomyopathy.[59]

STRESS ECHOCARDIOGRAPHY

Stress echocardiography is a well-validated tool for the evaluation of ischemia. In particular, it is an appropriate first-line test in patients who have baseline abnormalities on the ECG that preclude interpretation of exercise ECGs, and it is both time- and cost-efficient. The accuracy of stress echocardiography is similar to that of stress radionuclide perfusion imaging (see Chapter 18). From meta-analyses, as well as from comparisons of the accuracy of stress echocardiography and nuclear imaging in the same patient population, the sensitivity of stress echocardiography for significant CAD (generally defined as >50% coronary artery stenosis by angiography) averages approximately 88% and its specificity is 83%.[60] The specificity of stress echocardiography appears to be higher than that of nuclear imaging for left main and triple-vessel CAD. As with other tests, stress echocardiography is best used for diagnosis or to identify the extent, severity, and location of ischemia in patients with an intermediate pretest probability of disease.

The Stress Echocardiographic Protocol

In the standard stress protocol, baseline images are obtained at rest, before the patient exercises on either a treadmill or stationary bicycle. The same Bruce protocol used for routine (ECG only) exercise stress tests is standard (see Chapter 15), with echocardiographic imaging performed at rest and during immediate recovery as close to the peak exercise time as possible. If a stationary (upright or supine) bicycle is used, the workload is increased by 25 W every 2 or 3 minutes, and echocardiographic images can be monitored continuously and captured precisely at the time of peak stress. The test endpoint is exercise-limiting symptoms or completion of the protocol (reaching at least 85% of the age-predicted maximal heart rate). Absolute indications to terminate the test early include moderate to severe angina, ST-segment elevation, sustained ventricular tachycardia, near-syncope or signs of poor perfusion, a drop in systolic blood pressure of more than 10 mm Hg from baseline when accompanied by any other evidence of ischemia, and patient request to stop (intolerable symptoms). Relative indications to stop early include a hypertensive response (systolic blood pressure >220 mm Hg and/or diastolic blood pressure >120 mm Hg).[60]

Patients who cannot exercise can undergo pharmacologic stress with a graded dobutamine infusion of up to 40 μg/kg/min (and added atropine, if necessary, to achieve the target heart rate), which increases the heart rate and myocardial contractility. This method, although less physiologic than exercise, produces a smaller rise in blood pressure and also allows imaging exactly at the time of peak stress. Vasodilator stress with dipyridamole and pacing stress—via a preexisting permanent pacemaker or a transesophageal pacing catheter—are also possible but less widely used. If not combined with myocardial contrast perfusion techniques, vasodilator stress echocardiography relies on ischemia-associated wall motion abnormality to define a positive test unlike nuclear vasodilator stress test which addresses flow redistribution.

The risks associated with exercise echocardiography or DSE are very low. In the largest survey to date, the overall rate of life-threatening events was 1 per 1000 examinations (0.015% for exercise and 0.18% for dobutamine).[25] The most frequent complications were acute MI or ventricular tachycardia or fibrillation.

If a previous echocardiogram has not been performed, a brief survey of the ventricular chambers, valves, and aortic root should be performed to screen for significant pathology or contraindications to stress and to ensure adequate image quality (usually obtainable in at least 90% of patients with harmonic imaging). If endocardial resolution is poor in two or more segments, IV echocardiographic contrast enhancement should be used to improve accuracy. Images of the left ventricle are then obtained in the parasternal long, parasternal short, and apical windows at rest and then with stress. Side-by-side comparison of the baseline versus stress digitized images, which are gated by the ECG and synchronized in systole, allows quantification of overall LV size and systolic function, as well as identification of regional wall motion abnormalities. The standard 17-segment ASE model is used as the guide for grading function in each segment as normal, hyperkinetic, hypokinetic, akinetic, or dyskinetic at rest and with exercise or increasing doses of dobutamine. A normal ventricle has normal size and wall thickness and an EF of 50% or higher with no focal wall motion abnormalities (WMSI = 1.0); with stress the ventricle should become hypercontractile and the cavity size should shrink. The presence of baseline wall motion abnormalities that remain "fixed" (unchanged) with stress is indicative of a previous infarct. The development of a new or worsening wall motion abnormality indicates a flow-limiting stenosis in the coronary artery supplying the abnormal segment or segments (Fig. 16.29). A large ischemic territory—such as left main or multivessel disease—will manifest as diminished global LVEF and chamber dilation with stress (i.e., transient ischemic LV dilatation).

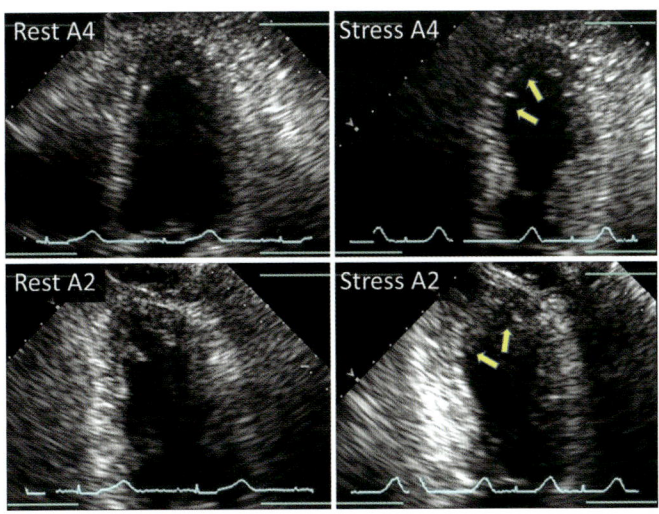

FIGURE 16.29 Stress echocardiography showing evidence of ischemia in the left anterior descending (LAD) distribution. Resting and stress echocardiograms in the apical four-chamber (*A4*) and apical two-chamber (*A2*) views reveal new severe mid to distal septal, apical, and distal inferior LV hypokinesis (*arrows*). This patient was found to have greater than 90% mid-LAD stenosis on cardiac catheterization.

Limitations of Stress Echocardiography

When compared with the gold standard of coronary angiography, the results of stress echocardiography can be discrepant. The primary causes of a false-negative result include suboptimal level of stress (from inadequate exercise capacity or beta-blocker use), limited image quality, a small area of ischemia (particularly for single-vessel or left circumflex disease), or preexisting conditions such as marked LV hypertrophy or a hyperdynamic state. False-positive results may also occur, particularly when the pretest probability is low. Diagnosis of wall motion abnormalities is particularly challenging in patients with LBBB or septal dyssynchrony (e.g., as a result of pacing or the postoperative state). In these patients, because exercise can exaggerate the abnormal septal motion and thereby obfuscate interpretation, DSE is recommended. A focus on wall thickening rather than on endocardial excursion may also be helpful in such situations. Other conditions that can cause nonspecific or nondiagnostic findings include the presence of preexisting wall motion abnormalities that tether adjacent segments, severe hypertension, HCM, and other cardiomyopathies in which myocardial perfusion reserve is diminished as a result of microvascular disease.[60]

Risk Stratification with Stress Echocardiography

Numerous studies have demonstrated that in patients who complete normal exercise or pharmacologic stress echocardiograms (demonstrating good exercise capacity and/or reaching target heart rate), the risk for cardiac events is very low and at or close to that of a "normal" population (<1% per year for exercise and <2% per year for pharmacologic tests). In patients with suspected or known CAD, both the extent of resting wall motion abnormalities and the extent of ischemia—specifically quantified by an increase in WMSI, four or more LV wall segments affected, and/or no change or decrease in exercise LVEF—correlate with a fourfold or greater increased risk for cardiac death or MI.[60]

Assessment of Myocardial Viability

DSE can also be used to quantify viability (contractile reserve) and thus functional recovery after reperfusion.[60] Although its overall sensitivity appears to be slightly lower than that of nuclear and CMR studies, DSE has better specificity for predicting recovery of systolic function of viable segments. A biphasic response, in which improvement in wall thickening occurs at low-dose dobutamine but then deteriorates with high-dose dobutamine, is the most specific sign. However, any improvement in wall motion abnormality by at least one grade in two or more segments during stress is likely to signify viability (either stunned or hibernating myocardium).

Coronary Flow Reserve and Perfusion

To provide additional prognostic information, it is feasible to assess coronary flow and flow reserve (see Chapter 36), most reliably in the LAD territory, by using Doppler TTE and vasodilators (adenosine or dipyridamole). Coronary flow reserve reduced to less than 1.9 to 2.0 in the LAD territory correlates with greater than 70% angiographic stenosis and is a predictor of future adverse cardiac events. Microperfusion of the myocardium at rest and with stress echocardiography may also be demonstrated with the use of ultrasound enhancing agents on 2D and 3D images (see Ultrasound Enhancing Agents and Fig. 16.24). In laboratories with expertise, both techniques of assessing myocardial perfusion appear to have acceptable agreement compared with angiography and nuclear stress tests. However, technical challenges and a learning curve presently exist, which has currently limited widespread adoption of these methods.[25,60]

Stress echocardiography is also used to assess factors beyond LV systolic function, particularly in patients who are dyspneic for unclear reasons. Valvular disease, diastolic function, pulmonary hypertension, and hemodynamics may all be assessed under stress conditions.[60,61]

Stress Echocardiography in Valvular Heart Disease

Resting echocardiography may lead to conflicting interpretations of the degree of AS in patients with very calcified valves and low LVEF, because leaflet excursion and both the LVOT and the aortic velocities are diminished simply by low forward flow (see Chapter 72). In patients with "low-gradient, low-output aortic stenosis" and LV dysfunction (defined classically as a calculated aortic valve area (AVA) by Doppler ≤1.0 cm^2 [0.6 cm^2/m^2]), mean transaortic gradient <40 mm Hg, and reduced LVEF, variably defined as <45% or 50%, DSE can be used to assess both the true severity of AS and the amount of LV contractile reserve (see later, Aortic Stenosis). In this test, dobutamine is infused in graded doses from 5 to 20 µg/kg/min, typically for longer stages than used for ischemia testing, to allow for steady-state measurements of PW Doppler of the LVOT and CW Doppler across the aortic valve. SV is calculated from VTI_{LVOT}. An increase of 20% or higher in SV is indicative of significant contractile reserve. The test is indeterminate if little or no augmentation of LV function takes place (no contractile reserve, or ΔSV <20%). AVA is calculated at both baseline and with dobutamine; in true AS, the transvalvular gradients increase and the valve area remains in the severe AS range, whereas in "pseudosevere" or "functional" AS, the aortic gradients change relatively little while the LVOT VTI increases, and the calculated valve area increases as the leaflets open more. Patients with true severe AS generally benefit from aortic valve replacement, but if contractile reserve is absent or concomitant CAD is present, surgical mortality is high.[61,62] TAVR may provide a valuable option in this patients.

A subset of patients with advanced AS have been described who have "paradoxical" low-gradient/low-flow states despite preserved LVEF (see Chapter 72).[62] These are defined as having AVA ≤1.0 cm^2 (0.6 cm^2/m^2), mean transaortic gradient <40 mm Hg, LVEF ≥50% and BSA-corrected forward SV <35 cc/m, measured when the systolic BP is <140. While there are many causes of low flow despite preserved LVEF including MR or stenosis, AF and constriction, these patients are often women with small ventricles and hypertension. DSE has limited utility for these patients as it may be difficult to augment SV but where there is a response, those with true AS tend to maintain low AVAs and demonstrate modest gradient augmentation. These patients have a poor prognosis, which is improved by aortic valve replacement. The explanation appears to be pronounced LV concentric remodeling and myocardial fibrosis that results in severe restrictive physiology and low SV. Optimizing antihypertensive therapy is important as higher gradients may emerge with better BP control. Given its limited utility, DSE has largely been replaced by CT with calcium scoring or hybrid CT-Doppler imaging in evaluating these patients.[63]

Patients with rheumatic or calcific MS may have severe exertional symptoms despite relatively modest gradients on the resting echocardiogram. Conversely, sedentary patients with severe MS may be relatively asymptomatic because they are inactive. Valve gradients are notoriously dependent on the flow rate and heart rate. Stress

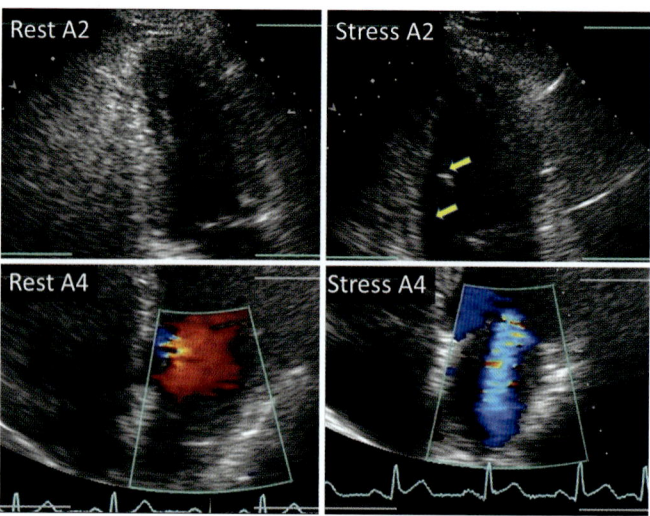

FIGURE 16.30 Stress echocardiography with evidence of ischemia in the right coronary artery (RCA) territory and acute ischemic MR. Resting and stress echocardiograms in the apical two-chamber (*A2*) and apical four-chamber (*A4*) views with color Doppler reveal new stress-induced inferior hypokinesis (*arrows*) in the area containing the posteromedial papillary muscle and increased MR. This patient was found to have 90% stenoses of the RCA and left circumflex artery on cardiac catheterization.

echocardiography can define the true exercise capacity and quantitate the degree of valvular stenosis and regurgitation. A rise in the mean transmitral pressure gradient greater than 15 mm Hg or an increase in calculated PASP to greater than 60 mm Hg is correlated with significant MS, and such patients should be considered for valvotomy (if the cause is rheumatic and there is no more than mild MR) or mitral valve replacement (see Chapter 75).[61,64] Mitral valve surgery might also be considered if severe MR is elicited with stress. If symptoms and PASP increase markedly while transmitral gradients remain low, however, a pulmonary cause should be sought.

In patients with MR, stress echocardiography may be instrumental in revealing worsening ischemic MR caused by inferior wall ischemia (Fig. 16.30). This would characteristically be associated with stress-induced inferior wall motion abnormalities and improvement in both abnormalities during recovery. In chronic severe primary MR, stress echocardiography may unmask exercise induced LV dysfunction as well as assess exercise capacity. An exercise induced PASP of ≥ 60 mm Hg has been proposed for risk stratification but does not appear in current guidelines for intervention.[64]

Stress echocardiography may be refined or tailored in other conditions. In patients with HCM, exercise can bring out latent gradients and is also used to monitor response to therapy and assess symptoms such as syncope (see Chapter 54). In patients or family members of those with known or suspected pulmonary hypertension, stress echocardiography may also be helpful and should include calculation of PVR as well as PA pressure. In conjunction with cardiopulmonary testing, stress echocardiography may aid in identifying other causes of dyspnea and fatigue, such as diastolic dysfunction. Delayed diastolic relaxation, as measured by strain and strain rate imaging, may also be a more sensitive and persistent indicator of exercise-induced ischemia than wall thickening. With the advent of real-time 3D and four-dimensional (4D) imaging, automatic endocardial border tracking, and volumetric imaging, there is now the capability to capture images of LV systolic and diastolic function simultaneously at peak exercise, thereby potentially improving the sensitivity, accuracy, and reproducibility of this test for ischemia.

VALVULAR HEART DISEASE (SEE PART VIII)

Mitral Valve (see Chapters 75 and 76)

Mitral Valve Anatomy

The mitral valve apparatus is a complex structure consisting of two leaflets attached to the left atrium by the mitral annulus and to the left

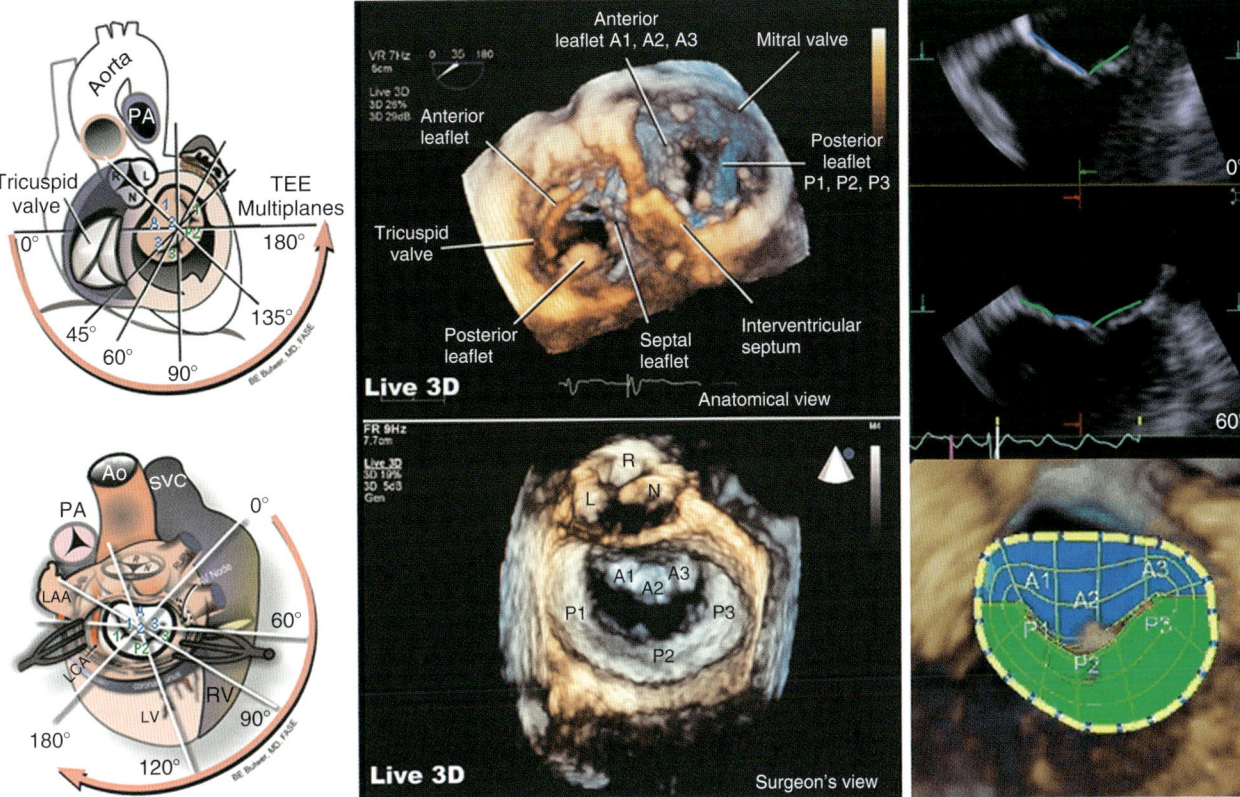

FIGURE 16.31 Mitral valve anatomy from TEE. **Left,** Two-dimensional (2D) TEE approach involving adjustment of probe position and omni orientation (degrees), sweeping to image all scallops. **Middle,** Three-dimensional (3D) appearance of the valve from the TEE view **(upper)** and surgeon's view **(lower)** with the mitral leaflet scallops labeled. **Right,** 3D TEE images delineating the mitral valve scallops at 0 degrees (four-chamber) and 60 degrees (two-chamber) planes, and below superimposed 3D analysis of leaflet areas from the left atrial aspect. *Ao,* Aorta; *PA,* pulmonary artery, *LAA,* left atrial appendage. The aortic valve right (*R*), left (*L*), and non- (*N*) coronary cusps are also shown. (See Video 16.34.)

ventricle through the mitral chordae and papillary muscles. The posterior leaflet is divided naturally into three scallops termed P1, P2, and P3 (using the Carpentier nomenclature), with P1 being lateral and P3 being medial. Opposing scallops of the anterior leaflet are termed A1, A2, and A3. Localization of pathology to specific scallops is important, particularly in surgical decision making for primary degenerative MR. The annulus is a nonplanar saddle-shaped structure, with its highest points seen on the parasternal long-axis view and its nadir seen in the apical four-chamber view (see Fig. 16.21). The chordae consist of a complex arcade of primary (first-order) and secondary (second-order) chordae radiating from both papillary muscles, with the former being inserted along the free margin of both leaflets and the latter serving as strut supports to the leaflet undersurfaces. Tertiary (third-order) chordae arise from the ventricular wall and insert into the base of the posterior leaflet only (Fig. 16.31).

Although it is possible to identify each of the scallops with 2D TTE on the parasternal short-axis view at the level of the mitral valve, it may be challenging to identify the scallops in the other views. Consequently, TEE plays a particularly important role in assessment of the mitral valve. 3D TEE has rapidly become an essential tool because of its ability to provide images that replicate the surgeon's view of the valve (see Fig. 16.31), as well as improved methods for assessing mitral pathophysiology in a variety of disease states. Leaflet morphology, focal disruptions, and detailed measurements can now be made virtually real-time. Congenital anomalies of the mitral valve are unusual, but those that might be newly diagnosed in adulthood include double-orifice and parachute mitral valve, as well as isolated clefts.

Mitral Stenosis

Echocardiographic Features

Commissural fusion, chordal thickening and fusion, as well as leaflet thickening and calcification that develop in patients with rheumatic MS result in narrowing of the mitral orifice, classically with a fish-mouth configuration (Fig. 16.32). Other pathognomonic echocardiographic features of rheumatic mitral disease are best appreciated on the parasternal long- and short-axis views and apical views. Commissural fusion results in restricted diastolic excursion of the tips of the

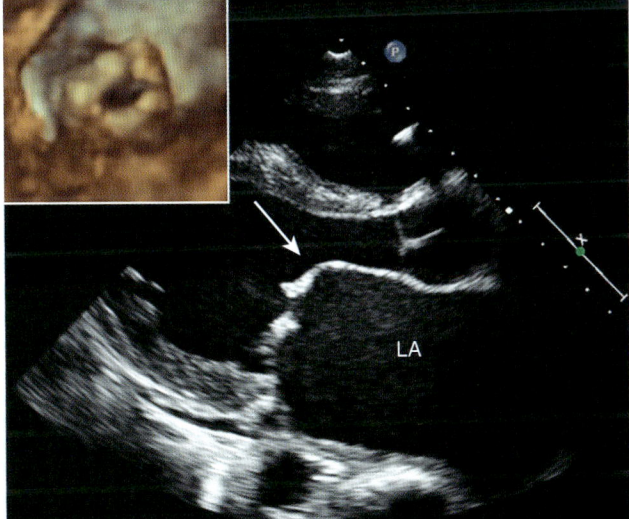

FIGURE 16.32 Rheumatic mitral stenosis. Parasternal long-axis view (diastolic frame) of a rheumatic mitral valve. Diastolic doming of the anterior mitral leaflet (*arrow*) is present, as well as a fixed posterior leaflet. *Inset,* Doming and fish-mouth appearance of the valve, as seen by 3D TTE from the LV aspect. *LA,* Left atrium.

leaflets, with relatively preserved mobility of the belly of the leaflet, particularly in early or milder forms of the disease. The result is a pattern of opening in which excursion of the midsection of the leaflet exceeds that of the leaflet tips, termed *doming*. Doming is also seen in rheumatic tricuspid stenosis and congenital anomalies of the aortic valve (discussed later). In rheumatic mitral disease, anterior leaflet doming is more readily appreciated because the posterior leaflet is shorter and tends to become immobilized early in the rheumatic process. Leaflet and chordal thick-ening with or without calcification is also seen. Despite the fact that degenerative mitral annular calcification is a very common anomaly that occurs with aging and renal disease, it infrequently causes significant MS unless very severe.

Quantification of Severity

The normal mitral valve area (MVA) is 4 to 5 cm^2, and severe MS usually correlates with MVA ≤1.0 to 1.5 cm^2.[65] Direct planimetry of the orifice area from a parasternal short-axis view was first validated in the pre-Doppler era. It relies on meticulous positioning of the imaging plane at the level of the flow-limiting orifice; misleadingly larger-appearing "orifices" will be captured if the plane used is at the level of more mobile leaflet segments. It is equally important for the gain to be set at the lowest possible setting that will provide a complete orifice. Overgained images will underestimate the true MVA. 3D echocardiography has proved to be a valuable tool because it provides a robust means of precisely identifying the valve orifice (Fig. 16.33).

Determination of the mean gradient is the simplest Doppler method for assessing the severity of MS. Given the degree to which gradients are influenced by flow rate, it is important to report the heart rate at which the gradient was determined and to be cognizant of the impact of concomitant MR, which can increase overall transmitral flow (and hence the inflow gradients, leading to overestimation of MS). Conversely, abnormalities that increase LV diastolic pressure independent of transmitral flow, such as reduced LV compliance and AR, can attenuate the transmitral gradient and result in underestimation of the severity of MS.

Doppler echocardiography also provides alternative methods to planimetry for determining MVA. The most widely used approach is the pressure half-time (PHT) method, which relies on the rate at which LA and LV pressures equalize. Using a simplified derivation of a catheterization laboratory–validated method, MVA is calculated as 220 divided by PHT, with 220 being an empirically derived constant. PHT is the time that it takes the initial transvalvular gradient to fall to half its initial value. This calculation can rapidly be done online with the basic analysis packages available on echocardiographic machines (Fig. 16.34). There are caveats: the PHT method should not be used in the immediate postvalvuloplasty setting because acute changes in both the LA-LV compliance relationship and in the initial transmitral gradient may have occurred. As discussed, it may also be invalid in the setting of significant AR and reduced LV compliance, each of which will result in overestimation of MVA. Additionally, the PHT may be indeterminate when the mitral inflow Doppler spectrum has a biphasic contour. Finally, this method has not been validated for other causes of MS, such as mitral annular calcification, or for prosthetic valves.

An alternative method is the *proximal isovelocity surface area* (PISA) approach (Fig. 16.35), in which MVA = $2(\pi r^2)(V_{aliasing})/(\text{Peak } V_{mitral}) \times \alpha/180$, where α is the angle formed by the doming cusps, or a simplification of this equation in which α is assumed to be 100 degrees. A 2D/Doppler-based method based on the principle of flow continuity may also be used, which calculates MVA = $\pi(D_{LVOT}/2)^2(VTI_{LVOT}/VTI_{MV})$, where D is the diameter of the LVOT measured on the parasternal long-axis view. As with other forms of valvular heart disease, an approach that integrates imaging and Doppler findings will optimize assessment of mitral stenotic severity.

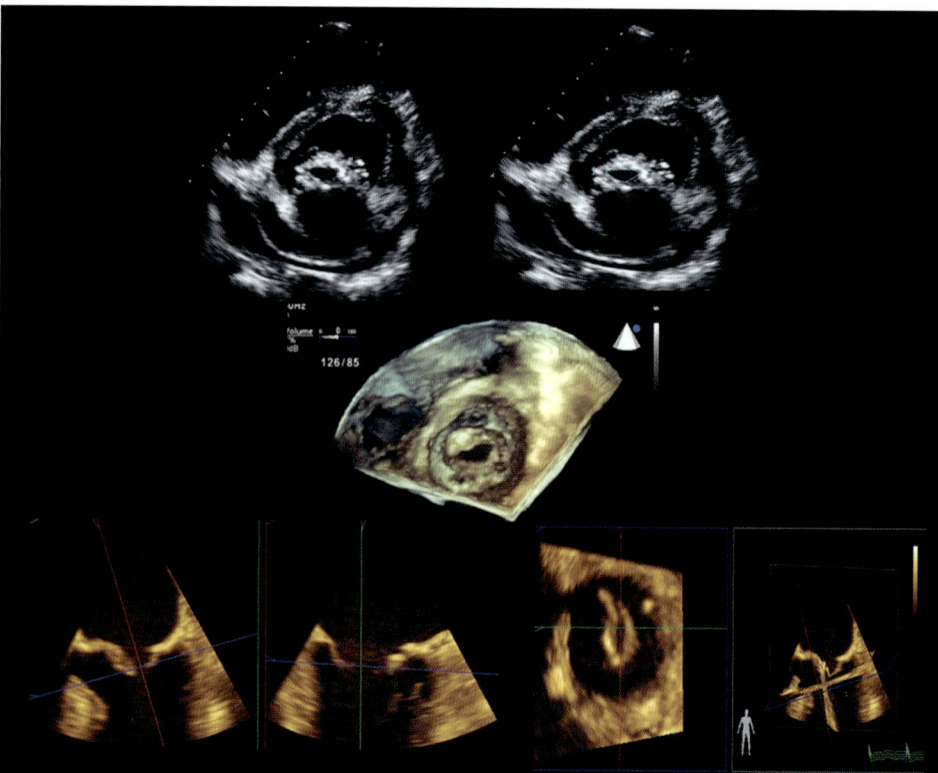

FIGURE 16.33 Approaches to planimetry of the mitral valve area (MVA) in rheumatic mitral stenosis. **Top,** Planimetry of 2D parasternal short-axis images. **Middle,** 3D TEE view of the stenotic orifice from the perspective of the left ventricle, which can be directly planimetered. **Bottom,** Multiplanar reconstruction of 3D TEE volumes can ensure that a short-axis view precisely at the level of the limiting orifice is selected for planimetry.

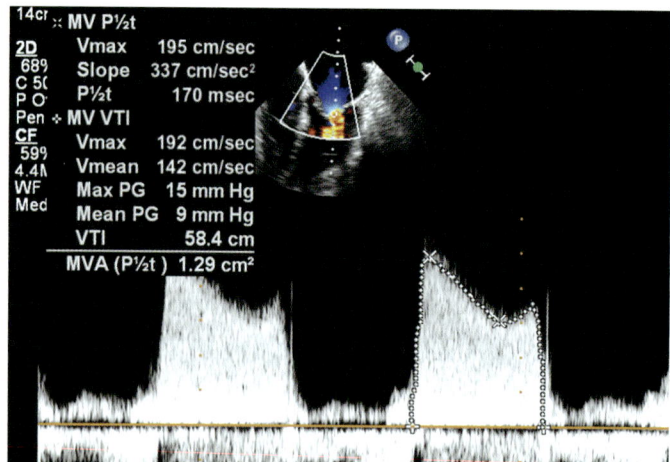

FIGURE 16.34 Tracing the CW mitral stenotic spectrum (*dotted line*) for VTI provides the mean transvalvular gradient, whereas assessment of the rate at which the gradient between the left atrium and left ventricle falls (marked by the two Xs) can be used to calculate valve area from the pressure half-time method ($P\frac{1}{2}t$). *MV,* Mitral valve; *MVA,* MV area; *PG,* pressure gradient.

Patient Selection for Balloon Valvuloplasty

In patients with severe MS in whom transcatheter intervention is planned, the Wilkins echocardiographic scoring system is useful in determining the likelihood of overall procedural success (Table 16.9); the less widely used Padial scoring system is useful in predicting freedom from severe MR. A Wilkins score greater than 8 or Padial score of 10 or more are predictors of poorer outcomes. It is also important to determine the amount of associated MR on echocardiography, because percutaneous balloon mitral valvotomy will increase the severity of regurgitation by at least one grade; thus the presence of moderate or greater MR should deter one from pursuing

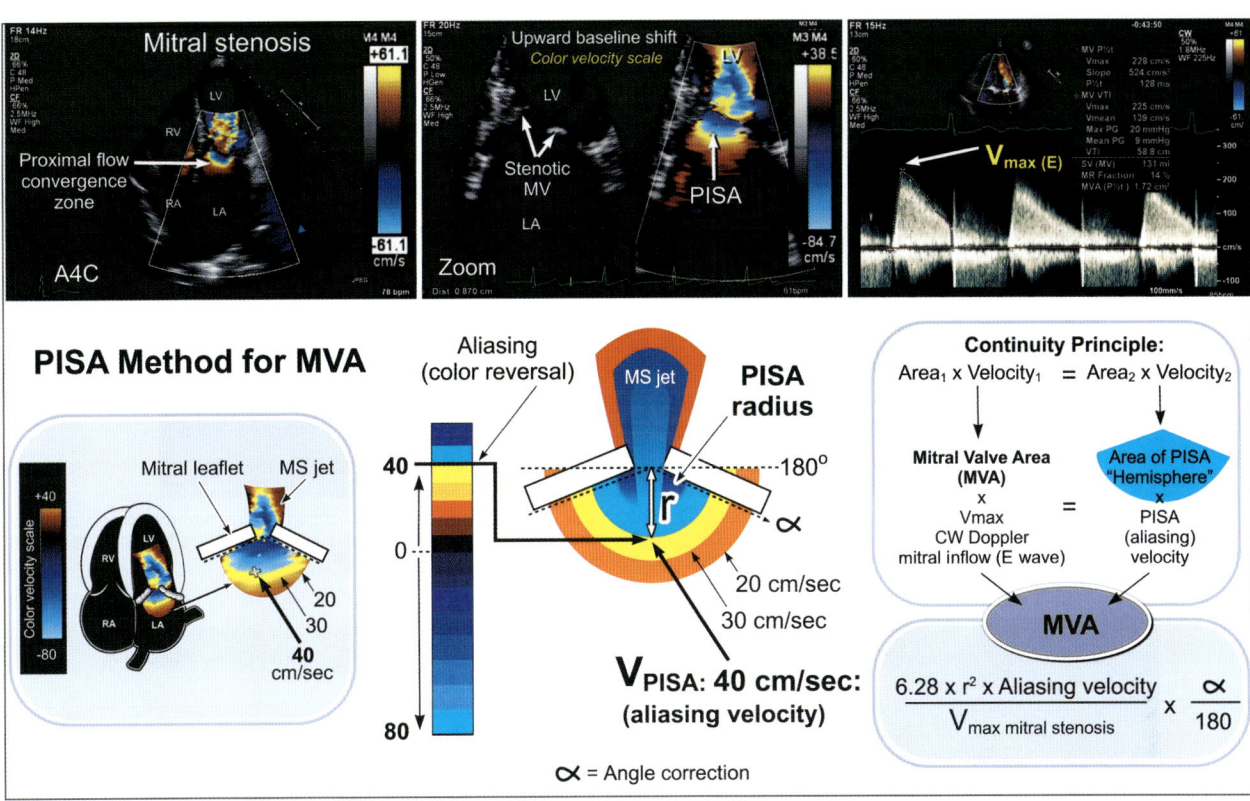

FIGURE 16.35 Proximal isovelocity surface area (PISA) method for calculation of MVA. In patients with mitral stenosis (MS), flow acceleration proximal to the stenotic orifice will result in a flow convergence zone that is characterized by color aliasing and a PISA shell **(upper left)**. The definition of the PISA shell and thus accuracy of the PISA radius measurement can be improved by shifting the baseline Nyquist limit in the direction of flow **(upper middle)**. In the **lower left** and **middle panels,** the aliasing velocity is 40 cm/sec. Application of the continuity equation allows MVA to be calculated as MVA = $[2(\pi r^2)(V_{aliasing})/(Peak\ V_{mitral})] \times \alpha/180$. The angle correction is used to correct for deviation of the shell from hemisphericity. *A4C,* Apical four-chamber view.

TABLE 16.9 Wilkins Scoring System for Mitral Valvuloplasty

GRADE	LEAFLET MOBILITY	VALVE THICKENING	CALCIFICATION	SUBVALVULAR THICKENING
1	Highly mobile	Minimal thickening	Single area of brightness	Minimal chordal thickening
2	Reduced mobility	Thickened tips	Scattered areas at leaflet margins	Chordal thickening up to one-third
3	Basal leaflet motion only	Entire leaflet thickened	Brightness extends to mid leaflets	Distal third of chordae thickened
4	Minimal motion	Marked leaflet thickening	Extensive leaflet brightness	Extensive thickening to papillary muscles

A desirable score is 8 or lower.

a percutaneous approach. The presence of LA appendage thrombus, which must be ruled out by TEE, is also a contraindication to percutaneous intervention because of the risk of embolization from guidewires and catheters.

Mitral Regurgitation

Causes of Mitral Regurgitation

Minor leakage of the mitral valve is a common physiologic finding. There are many causes of pathologic regurgitation, and echocardiography should be used not only to diagnose and quantify MR, but also to determine the underlying functional disturbance and, when possible, to identify the disease causing the disturbance (see Chapter 76). Carpentier proposed a useful classification system based on the pathophysiology of MR that lends itself to an echocardiographic approach. In type I, leaflet motion is normal, and the most common abnormalities are leaflet perforation, alteration in coaptation because of bulky vegetation, or annular dilation secondary to chronic AF. In type II, at least one leaflet overrides the most superior plane of the annulus, that is, mitral prolapse or flail on the basis of either intrinsic valvular abnormality or rupture of either the chordae or papillary muscles. In type IIIA, leaflet motion is restricted during both systole and diastole, usually because of rheumatic disease, whereas in type IIIB, motion is limited in systole because of pathologic tethering on the basis of LV systolic dysfunction and remodeling. This is the most common scenario in secondary or functional MR.

Primary (Degenerative) Mitral Regurgitation

Mitral prolapse or flail that is attributable to primary leaflet and/or chordal pathology is termed *degenerative* MR. Echocardiography is the gold standard for the diagnosis of mitral prolapse or flail, distinguished as follows: in mitral flail, the unsupported free edge of the mitral leaflet falls back into the left atrium because of loss of chordal support, whereas in mitral prolapse, the free edge remains tethered by chordae, and the body of the leaflet billows pathologically into the left atrium. The diagnosis of prolapse is made from the parasternal long-axis view when any part of the leaflet extends 2 mm above a line drawn from the insertion of the anterior and posterior leaflets (Fig. 16.36). This line represents the most superior aspect of the saddle-shaped annulus (see Fig. 16.21 for 3D mitral valve shape). In the apical four- and two-chamber views, some extension of leaflet tissue above the annular boundaries is a normal variant. Hence these views should not be used to diagnose or define prolapse, although they may demonstrate the classic billowing motion of a truly prolapsing mitral valve. It may be difficult to differentiate between mitral prolapse and flail with TTE alone, but TEE can assist in making the correct diagnosis.

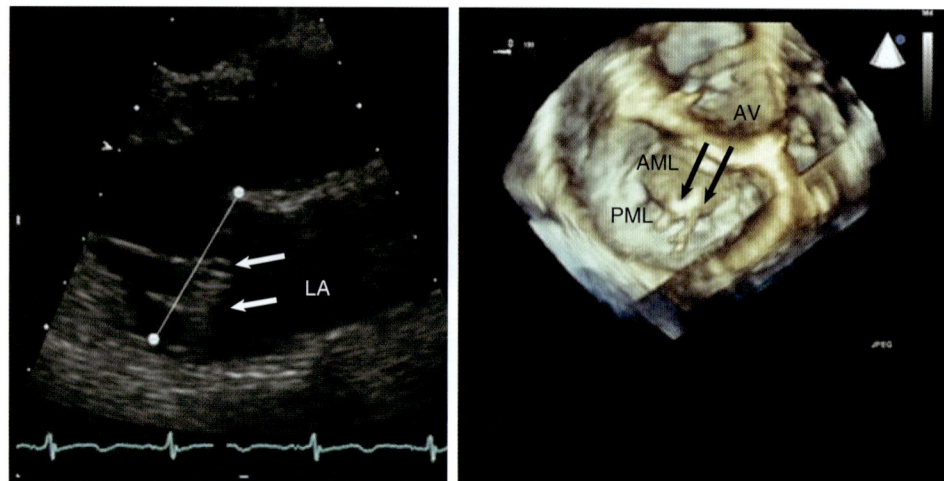

FIGURE 16.36 Degenerative MR. **Left,** Parasternal long-axis view showing bileaflet prolapse, as evidenced by billowing of both leaflets (*arrows*) above the annular plane, defined by the insertion of the anterior and posterior leaflets (*line*). **Right,** 3D TEE image of the mitral valve from the left atrial perspective. There is a large flail segment of the anterior mitral leaflet (*AML*). Arrows point to ruptured chordae. *AV,* Aortic valve; *LA,* left atrium; *PML,* posterior mitral leaflet.

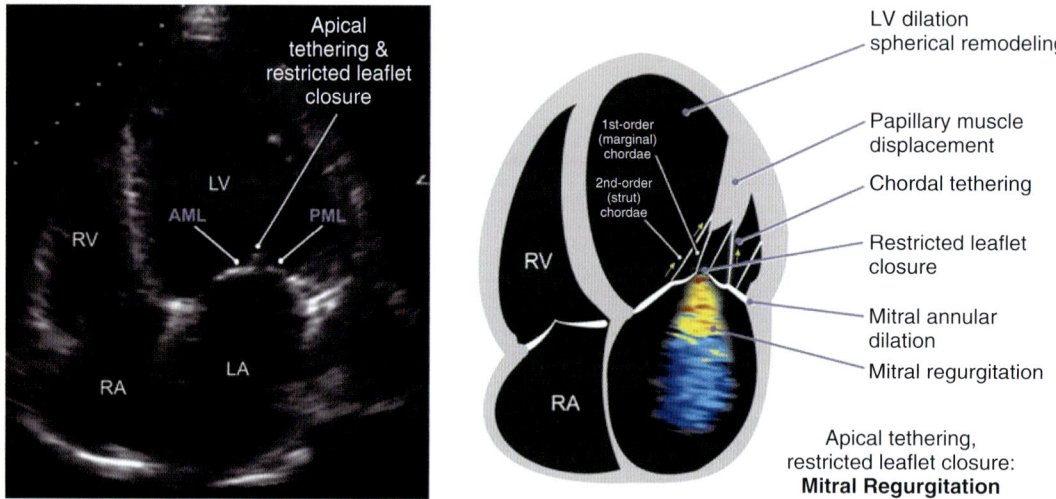

FIGURE 16.37 Functional/ischemic MR. Mitral tethering forces are increased because of both annular dilation and papillary muscle traction, which occur as a result of LV remodeling. Closing forces are reduced because of impaired LV systolic function. The end result is apical displacement of leaflet coaptation, as shown in the apical four-chamber view on the left. *AML,* Anterior mitral leaflet; *LA,* left atrium; *LV,* left ventricle; *PML,* posterior mitral leaflet; *RA,* right atrium; *RV,* right ventricle.

The anatomic substrate for degenerative MR spans the spectrum from diffuse myxomatous change (Barlow) to localized abnormalities characterized as fibroelastic deficiency. Mitral valve prolapse is more prevalent in patients with Marfan syndrome, Ehlers-Danlos syndrome, osteogenesis imperfecta, and other connective tissue disorders. 3D echocardiographic assessment of the extent of billowing has been reported to be useful in characterizing the nature of the pathology but, more importantly, has assumed a key role in determining precisely which scallop(s) are prolapsing or flail. This information is essential in predicting the likelihood of successful repair, whether surgical or with transcatheter approaches. Isolated P2 pathology is the most common pattern, and successful repair is highly probable. Next in frequency and ease of repair is A2 disease, followed by abnormalities in the medial and lateral scallops. 3D TEE is also helpful in identifying involvement of multiple scallops or unexpected associated anomalies such as localized mitral valve clefts. The latter are particularly important in mitral clip repair as they may impact effective leaflet grasping. In the absence of 3D capability, a systematic approach to assessment of all three scallops via 2D TEE can be used (see Fig. 16.31). Complete assessment of the mitral scallops is difficult with TTE, although when achievable, high-quality 3D TTE images may be used for this purpose.

Secondary (Functional) Mitral Regurgitation

The term *secondary or functional* MR is used when the leaflets, chords and papillary muscles are structurally normal. Most commonly, the root cause of functional MR is LV systolic dysfunction and remodeling (Carpentier Type IIIB). When the dysfunction is on the basis of CAD, the term *ischemic MR* is used. Recently, functional MR that occurs with preserved ventricular function has been recognized when the primary abnormality is annular dilation, typically due to AF (Carpentier Type I), termed "atrial functional MR." 3D echocardiography has shown that functional MR reflects an imbalance between the forces that close versus those that tether the mitral leaflets (Fig. 16.37).[33] The end result is pathologic tethering seen as apical displacement of leaflet coaptation. This pattern, which is appreciable on parasternal long-axis or apical views, is the echocardiographic hallmark of functional MR. Reduced closing forces are attributable to impaired LV systolic function, whereas pathologic tethering forces can occur because of traction on the mitral leaflets from either their annular insertion (as a result of annular dilation and/or reduced annular contraction) or from their chordal connection to the papillary muscles. The latter has been shown to result from geometric displacement of the papillary muscles either apically (in the case of global remodeling) or inferiorly (due to regional remodeling from focal infarct). It has been shown convincingly that papillary muscle contractile dysfunction per se does not cause functional/ischemic MR.

Quantitation of Mitral Regurgitation

The ASE recommends an integrated approach to the quantitation of MR[66] that incorporates semiquantitative measures such as assessment of jet area (ratio of jet area to LA area), the size of the peak mitral E

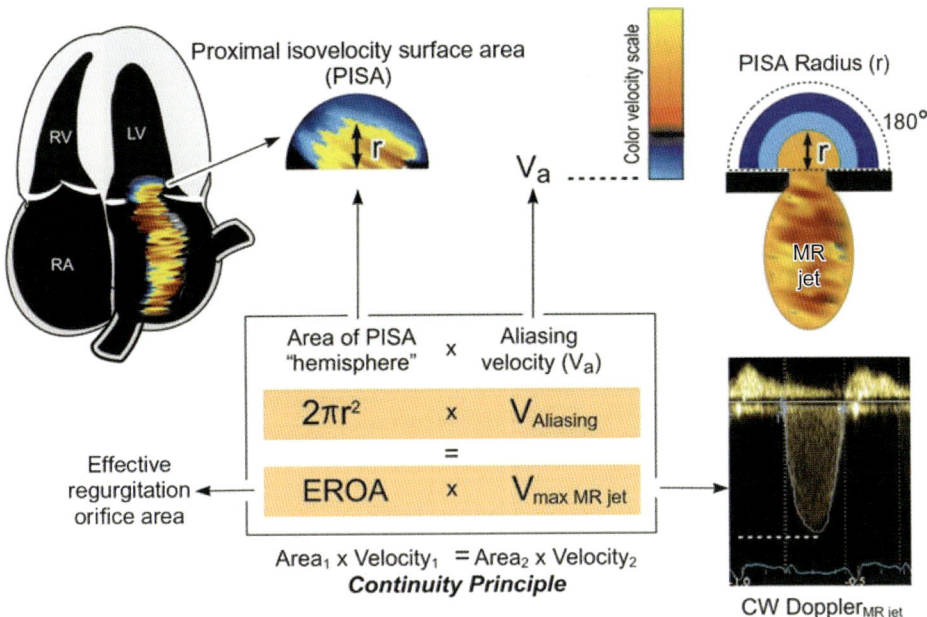

FIGURE 16.38 PISA approach to quantitating the effective regurgitant orifice area (EROA) for MR. To optimize the PISA shell, the baseline is shifted in the direction of the jet. EROA is computed as EROA = $2(\pi r^2)(V_{aliasing})/(V_{MaxMR})$. Regurgitant volume can be calculated as EROA × VTI_{MR}, where VTI_{MR} is the velocity-time integral of the MR spectrum.

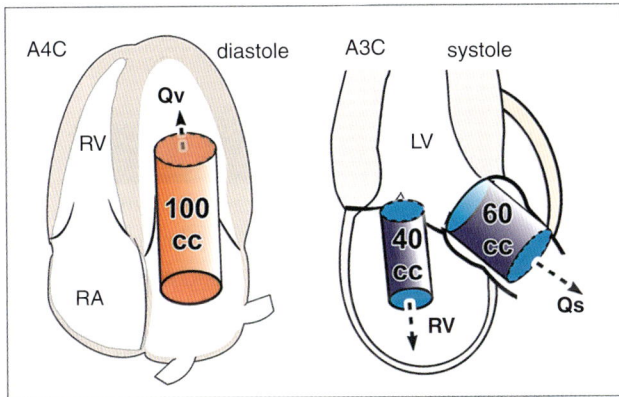

FIGURE 16.39 Quantitative Doppler approach to assessing the severity of MR. Regurgitant volume (RV) is calculated as the difference between total transmitral flow (Qv) and antegrade flow across the LVOT (Qs). Qv and Qs are calculated via the continuity method approach (CSA × VTI). Alternatively, Qv, which is identical to LV SV in the absence of a ventricular shunt or aortic regurgitation, may be calculated as LVEDV − LVESV, where LVEDV and LVESV are the LV end-diastolic and end-systolic volumes, respectively. *A4C*, Apical four-chamber view; *RA*, right atrium.

wave, vena contracta diameter, and pulmonary venous flow patterns in addition to the imaging appearance of the mitral valve, left atrium and left ventricle. The peak E velocity reflects the initial diastolic gradient between the left atrium and left ventricle and will be elevated when MR has resulted in elevation of LA pressure. The vena contracta is the narrowest region of a jet and is best assessed in zoom mode on the parasternal long-axis view. Pulmonary venous flow patterns reflect the impact of the MR jet on flow into the left atrium with, in some cases, severe regurgitant systolic flow reversal. Quantitation of regurgitant volume and the EROA is possible with the PISA approach, which is based on the concept of acceleration of flow proximal to the regurgitant orifice (Fig. 16.38). The quantitative Doppler approach that uses the continuity equation provides a means of calculating regurgitant volume and fraction by comparing the total antegrade flow across the mitral valve with that across a nonstenotic nonregurgitant reference valve, typically the aortic valve (Fig. 16.39). In general, an EROA of ≥ 0.4 cm^2 and RV volume of ≥ 60 mL is indicative of severe MR.

Even though the color jet size approach is easy and widely utilized, it is influenced by machine settings and many other factors.[66] It underestimates MR severity with eccentric jets and overestimates severity with non-holosystolic MR. It should not be the only tool used to quantitate more than mild MR. The PISA method is limited in situations where the assumption of a hemispheric PISA shell and circular regurgitant orifice is invalid; this is often true for eccentric jets caused by degenerative MR, as well as for functional MR cases where the PISA shell is flatter and hemi-elliptical. In fact, for functional ischemic MR, the PISA values that correlate with poor clinical outcome are lower than those used for primary MR. This is in part because studies have consistently shown that any degree of ischemic MR is prognostically important, but also because the regurgitant orifice is elliptical rather than circular, causing 2D PISA measures to commonly underestimate ischemic MR severity. 3D planimetry may provide a superior method of determining the EROA.[65] Conversely, in nonholosystolic MR (e.g., late systolic MR that frequently occurs in MV prolapse), the EROA calculated with the PISA approach will overestimate severity because it reflects the maximum EROA rather than the EROA averaged over all of systole. The major limitation of the quantitative Doppler technique lies in the assumption of circular or oval mitral orifice geometry in calculating transmitral flow. The use of LV SV calculated from echocardiographically measured LV volume versus aortic outflow has been suggested as an alternative approach. The advent of 3D echocardiography has provided methods for direct planimetry of regurgitant orifices, an approach that is increasingly used but that typically requires the spatial resolution of TEE. 3D techniques for optimizing assessment of nonhemispheric PISA shells have also been reported but are not yet widely used clinically.

It is important to recognize that secondary, and to a lesser degree primary, MR is afterload dependent, and thus determination of severity must take into account LV systolic pressure. Clinical decision making based on echo parameters made under general anesthesia is to be avoided, because anesthesia is associated with a predictable fall in systemic vascular resistance which may dramatically reduce the degree of regurgitation.

Aortic Valve (see Chapters 72 to 74)

Aortic Valve Anatomy

The normal aortic valve consists of three symmetric cusps that are supported by the aortic annulus and extend into the aortic root. The right and left coronary cusps lie within the sinuses of Valsalva that give rise to the corresponding coronary arteries, and the remaining cusp is termed the *noncoronary* cusp. The ideal views for assessing aortic valvular anatomy are the parasternal short- and long-axis views (see Fig. 16.8) and their comparable views on TEE (see Fig. 16.19E,F). The short-axis view shows all three cusps, which when open create a triangular-shaped orifice and when closed have a Y-shaped appearance. The long axis typically displays the right and noncoronary cusps, which when normally open will flatten against the walls of the aortic root and with normal closure will meet centrally without prolapse below the plane of the aortic annulus.

The most common congenital abnormalities of the aortic valve result from failure of cusp development and include, in order of decreasing frequency, bicuspid, unicuspid, and quadricuspid valves (Fig. 16.40). There are several approaches to the classification of congenitally abnormal valves. The most widely used is the Sievers classification based on the number of raphes (vestigial commissures) and their orientation. Type 0 is the classic bicuspid valve with no raphe, Type 1 (one raphe) is the most common with left-right fusion the most prevalent orientation. Type 2 is least common and corresponds to a functionally unicuspid valve. Quadricuspid valves are not included in this classification. Because of the inability of bicuspid valves to open fully, the systolic orifice of a bicuspid aortic valve is oval when seen in short axis, whereas the long-axis view demonstrates convex bulging of the leaflet midportions into the aortic lumen

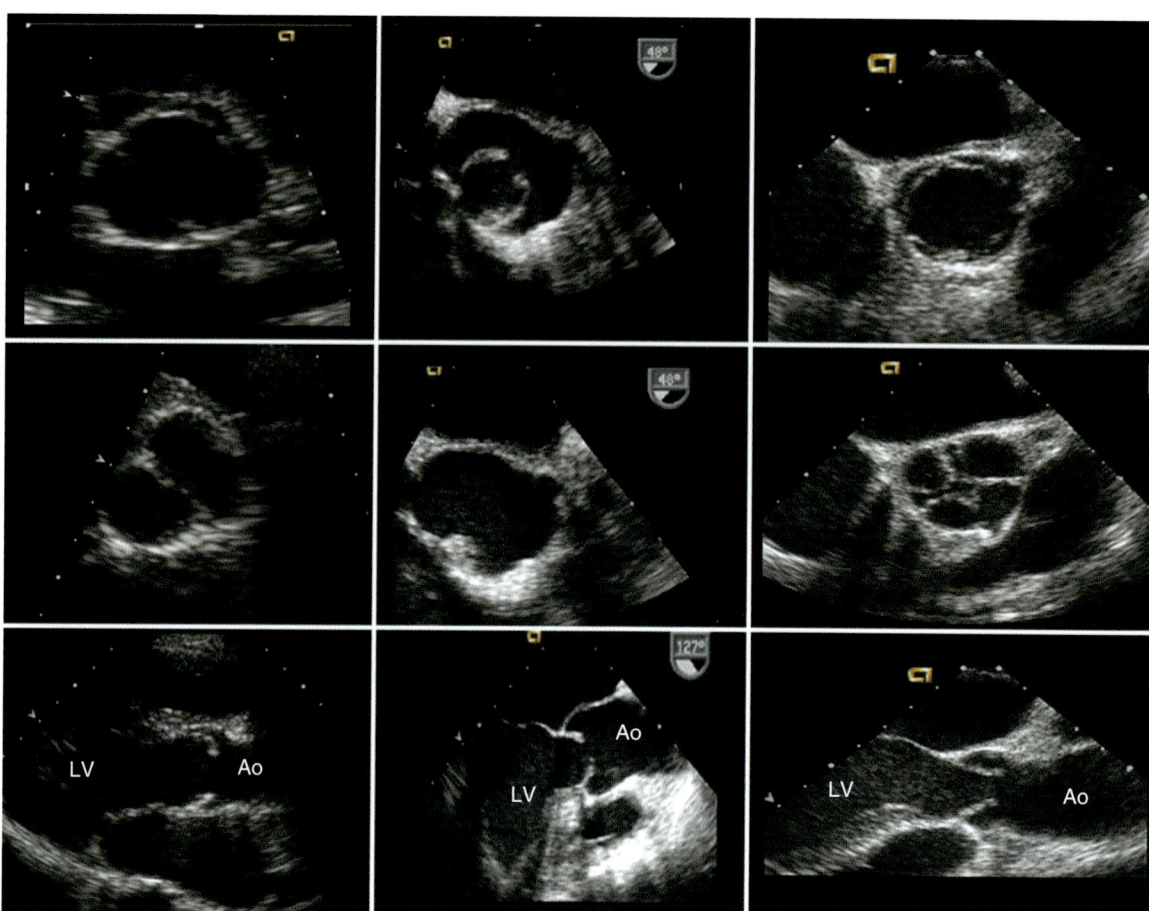

FIGURE 16.40 Congenital abnormalities of the aortic valve with (top to bottom) systolic short-axis, diastolic short-axis, and systolic long-axis views. **Left panels,** Bicuspid aortic valve. **Middle panels,** Unicuspid unicommissural aortic valve. **Right panels,** Quadricuspid aortic valve. *Ao,* Aorta; *LV,* left ventricle.

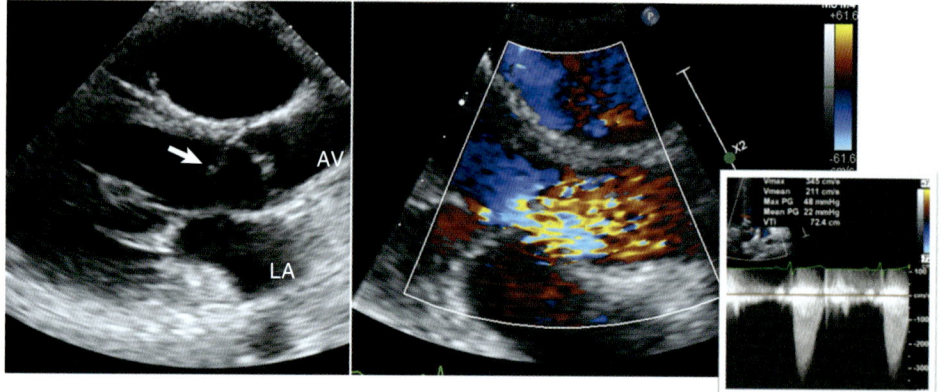

FIGURE 16.41 Parasternal long-axis view demonstrating **Left,** a subaortic membrane (*arrow*) extending from the anterior mitral leaflet to the septum. The aortic valve (*AV*) is about to open. *LA,* Left atrium. **Right,** color Doppler showing turbulent brisk flow across the membrane. Right inset, CW Doppler showing a peak gradient across the LVOT of 48 mm Hg.

LVOT for evidence of obstruction. Associated valvular AR is seen frequently and results from valve trauma caused by the subaortic stenotic jet. Supravalvular AS is a rare phenomenon that consists of localized or diffuse narrowing of the ascending aorta distal to the sinuses of Valsalva.

Aortic Stenosis

Although the impeded cusp excursion of a congenitally bicuspid or unicuspid aortic valve is the most frequent cause of AS in young patients, calcium deposition on a previously structurally normal tricuspid aortic valve is a common cause of AS in elderly adults. The echocardiographic appearance is restricted cusp excursion with irregular nodular cusp thickening (Fig. 16.42).

(doming). Although bicuspid aortic valves classi-cally have a single line of closure and no raphe (type 0), these account for only 7% of cases. The majority (88%) have an echogenic ridge or raphe that represents a vestigial commissure between two "would-be" cusps on a trileaflet valve. The closed appearance of such valves may be echocardiographically indistinguishable from a tricuspid valve. Thus, bicuspid aortic valve is a systolic diagnosis. Unicuspid valves (Type 2) typically have circular openings that may be central or asymmetrically positioned, and quadricuspid valves have a square appearance in systole and a crosslike appearance in diastole.

Congenital abnormalities of the LVOT include subaortic membranes, characterized by linear echoes extending from the anterior mitral leaflet to the septum or fibromuscular tunnels in which there is an echogenic ridge extending into the LVOT (Fig. 16.41). The presence of subaortic systolic turbulence on color Doppler should prompt close inspection of the

Quantitation of Severity

The normal AVA is 3 to 4 cm². In adults, severe AS usually occurs with an AVA less than 1.0 cm². Indexing of the AVA for BSA (<0.6 cm²/m² for severe AS) is important in children and small adults.[67] Application of the Bernoulli equation to CW Doppler interrogation of transvalvular flow provides accurate measures of the mean and peak instantaneous gradients in AS. Typically, the simplified form of the equation ($\Delta P = 4V^2$) may be used, but when LVOT velocity significantly exceeds 1 m/sec, the expanded version, $\Delta P = 4(V_2^2 - V_1^2)$, where V_2 is transaortic velocity and V_1 is LVOT velocity, should be used.

In recognition of the importance of recording Doppler signals parallel to flow, aortic gradients are best recorded from the apical five- or three-chamber, suprasternal notch, and right parasternal windows;

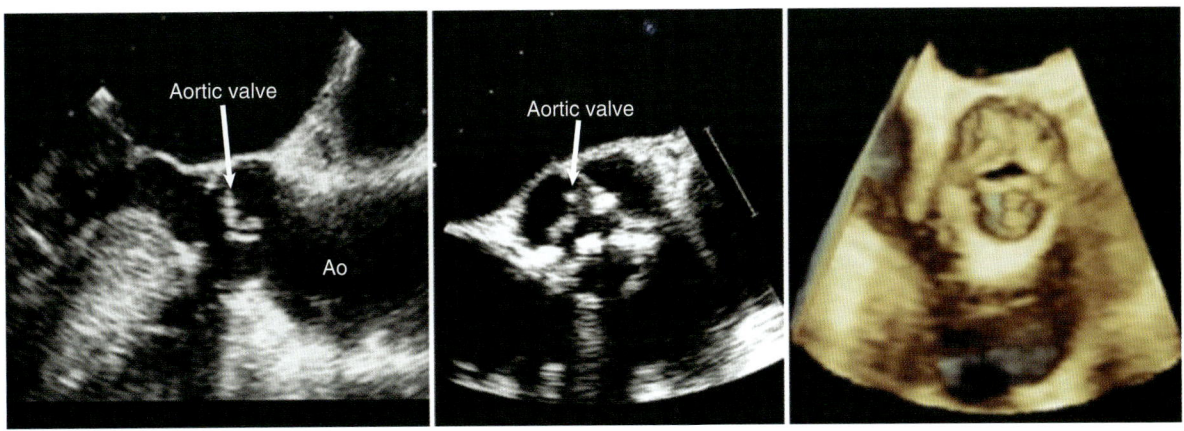

FIGURE 16.42 Systolic TEE images of calcific aortic stenosis in a patient with a tricuspid valve. **Left,** Two-dimensional long axis. There is minimal opening of the valve. *Ao,* Aorta. **Middle,** Short axis. **Right,** Three-dimensional image. The latter two views better demonstrate the distribution of calcium.

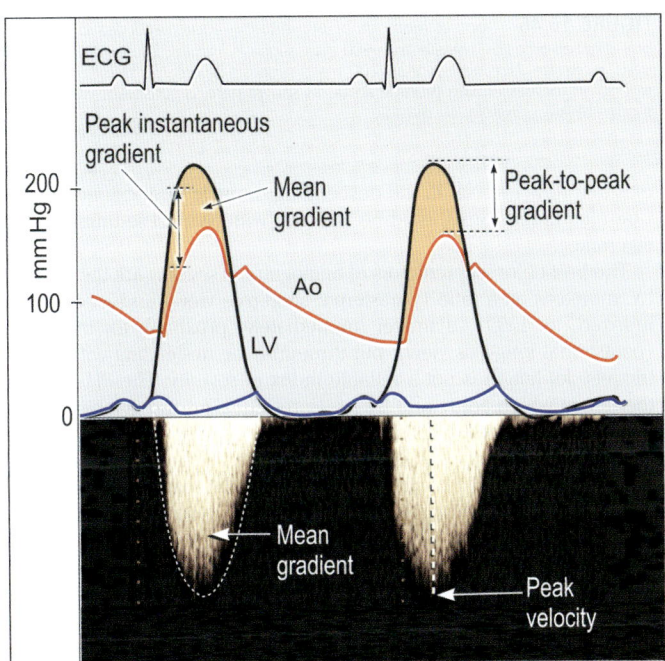

FIGURE 16.43 Doppler methods provide peak instantaneous and mean gradients. The peak instantaneous gradient is typically higher than the peak-to-peak gradient calculated from invasively measured peak left ventricular (*LV*) and aortic (*Ao*) pressure, which is not instantaneous, although mean gradients measured with both techniques are identical.

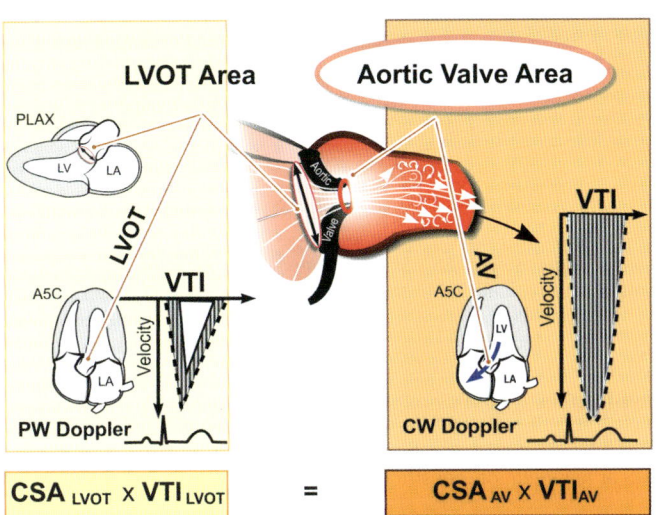

FIGURE 16.44 Continuity equation approach to calculating aortic valve area. The cross-sectional area (CSA) of the aortic valve (CSA_{AV}) is calculated as ($CSA_{LVOT} \times VTI_{LVOT}$)/$VTI_{AV}$). LVOT CSA is calculated as $\pi(D/2)^2$, where *D* is LVOT diameter. LVOT VTI should be measured from the modal rather than the maximal velocity (see Fig. 16.45).

typically, the highest velocities are found on the right parasternal view. The nonimaging Pedoff probe has a small footprint, making it essential for optimal assessment of patients with AS. When TEE is used, velocities are recorded from the deep transgastric views (see Fig. 16.19, position O). It should be noted that although echocardiographically derived mean gradients are generally identical to those obtained invasively, the echocardiographically derived peak *instantaneous* gradient is typically higher than the *peak-to-peak* gradient calculated in the catheterization laboratory (see Chapter 22). The latter is the arithmetic difference between peak LV and aortic pressure (Fig. 16.43), which may not be coincident in time.

Although gradients alone provide a reasonable assessment of the severity of AS when transaortic flow is normal, they may underestimate severity in the setting of low-flow states and overestimate severity when flow is elevated (e.g., high-output states such as those caused by sepsis and anemia). For this reason it is important to determine AVA. Direct planimetry of TEE images may be used for this purpose, but TTE planimetry is not sufficiently accurate. The most common approach is therefore by application of the continuity equation (Fig. 16.44). AVA is calculated as follows:

$$AVA = (CSA_{LVOT} \times VTI_{LVOT})/VTI_{AV}$$

Less desirable is the simplified version:

$$AVA = (CSA_{LVOT} \times V_{LVOT})/V_{AV}$$

where V represents peak velocity. The CSA of the LVOT is typically calculated by assuming circular geometry with the formula $CSA = \pi(D/2)^2$, where D is the systolic LVOT diameter measured on the parasternal or TEE-equivalent long-axis view. According to the ASE convention, the diameter is measured just proximal to the aortic annulus. It is cautioned that because the LVOT velocity incorporated into the calculation is the *modal* velocity, displayed as the densest part of the pulsed Doppler envelope, the VTI should not be traced by using the outer edge of the spectrum, which represents the maximal (not modal) velocity at each time point (Fig. 16.45). Optimal sample volume placement for pulse wave Doppler is in the LVOT immediately proximal to the site of subvalvular flow acceleration, typically 1 to 2 mm proximal to the valve on the apical five- or three-chamber (TTE) or deep transgastric (TEE) views.

Low-Gradient Severe Aortic Stenosis

In the setting of reduced SV because of LV systolic dysfunction, leaflet excursion may appear reduced and calculated effective orifice area may be small despite low gradients, and it becomes important to

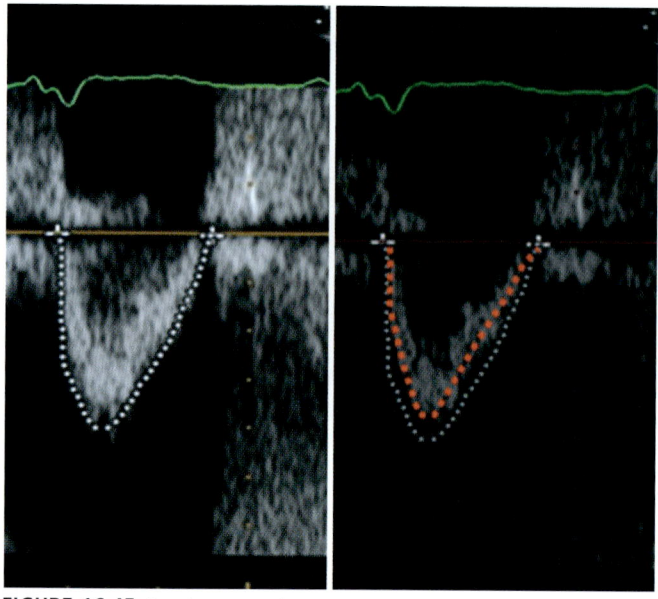

FIGURE 16.45 Doppler spectra demonstrating the error that may be introduced if the maximal (*white dotted line*) rather than the modal (*red dotted line*) velocity is measured. The modal velocity (the most commonly occurring velocity) corresponds to the brightest portion of the Doppler spectrum.

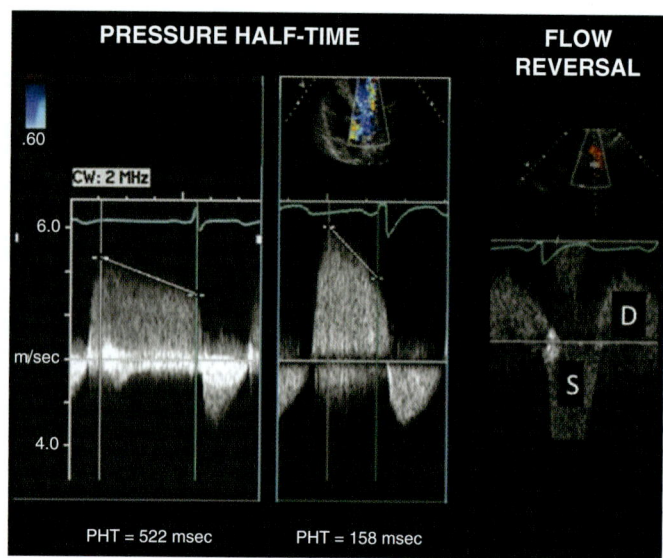

FIGURE 16.46 Doppler methods of quantitating aortic regurgitation (AR). A pressure half-time (PHT) greater than 500 msec suggests mild AR, 200 to 500 msec suggests moderate AR, and less than 200 msec suggests severe AR. Holodiastolic flow reversal in the descending thoracic aorta, as shown here, is consistent with at least moderate AR. *S*, Systole; *D*, diastole.

determine whether the valve obstruction is fixed (true severe AS) or the valve is intrinsically capable of opening more fully at higher flow rates (pseudosevere AS). As noted previously, DSE is routinely used in this setting, typically with close physician supervision to determine the true AVA as well as LV contractile reserve (i.e., augmentation of segmental and global contractility). The effective orifice area may also be severely reduced despite low gradients when the LVEF is within the normal range but SV is impaired, so-called paradoxical low-gradient, preserved–EF, severe AS (discussed earlier) that can occur with small restrictive ventricles or other causes of reduced forward flow including MS or regurgitation, constrictive physiology, or poorly controlled AF.[62,64]

Subvalvular or Supravalvular Aortic Stenosis

CW Doppler echocardiographic assessment of peak and mean gradients is the cornerstone in evaluating patients with LVOT obstruction below or above the valve (see Fig. 16.41). However, by demonstrating the site of flow acceleration relative to the 2D images, color Doppler may provide a clue that the obstruction is not at the level of the valve and prompt more detailed imaging investigation of the pathophysiology. In some patients, evaluation is complicated by the presence of obstruction at multiple levels, such as the presence of both subaortic and valvular AS. In such cases, because of the trade-off between range resolution and the inability to measure accurately high velocities that is inherent in the PW Nyquist limit, it may be impossible to precisely quantitate the gradients created at each level of obstruction.

Aortic Regurgitation (see Chapter 73)

AR may result from abnormalities in the valve cusps, normal cusps whose coaptation is altered by enlargement of the annulus and/or sinuses, or rarely, prolapse of an aortic dissection flap through the valve (see Diseases of the Aorta). Echocardiographic imaging (TTE and TEE) will establish a causative diagnosis and typically demonstrates LVED enlargement if the regurgitation is hemodynamically significant. High-frequency fluttering of the anterior mitral leaflet caused by the impact of the regurgitant jet may be evident on M-mode, and in cases of acute severe regurgitation, the mitral valve may close prematurely before ventricular systole because of a rise in LV pressure exceeding the LA pressure before ventricular contraction.

The diagnosis of AR is most easily made when a diastolic color Doppler jet is seen in the LVOT. Small transient jets can be normal variants. Again, an integrated approach is best for determining the severity of AR, with elements including evidence of LV enlargement, color jet dimensions, spectral Doppler signal intensity, PHT, vena contracta, and diastolic flow reversal in the descending thoracic or abdominal aorta. Color jet dimensions should be assessed with Nyquist settings of 50 to 60 cm/sec.

The best color jet predictors of angiographic severity are the jet area/LV short-axis area ratio (parasternal short-axis view) and jet diameter indexed to LVOT diameter immediately proximal to the valve (parasternal long-axis view), but these may be misleading with eccentric jets. Jet length is not a reliable index of severity. The PHT reflects the rate at which aortic and LV pressures equalize and is most reliable in the setting of acute AR, as long as care is taken to ensure that the early diastolic velocity is captured accurately (Fig. 16.46). The vena contracta is the waist (smallest diameter) of the regurgitant flow jet at the level of the valve measured in zoom mode on a parasternal long-axis or TEE-equivalent view. A measurement > 6 mm generally correlates with severe AR. Holodiastolic flow reversal in the descending thoracic aorta as detected with the pulsed Doppler is a marker of at least moderate AR (see Fig. 16.46). Reversal of comparable duration as measured in the abdominal aorta generally reflects severe AR. Regurgitant volume and fraction can be calculated using a continuity-based 2D/Doppler approach. This approach calculates regurgitant volume by comparing flow through the LVOT with that across a competent nonstenotic valve; it is most robust when the pulmonic valve is used as the reference for normal flow (image quality permitting). The mitral valve can theoretically be used as the reference but is more geometrically complex and thus more prone to error. Alternatively, both measures and EROA may be calculated with the PISA approach similar to the principles used in MR. A regurgitant volume of $\geq$ 60 mL and EROA of $\geq$ 0.30 cm^2 are consistent with severe AR.[64,65]

Tricuspid Valve (see Chapter 77)

Tricuspid Valve Anatomy

The tricuspid valve is the largest cardiac valve and is anatomically complex, with anterior, posterior, and septal leaflets extending from a saddle-shaped tricuspid annulus to chordae and variable papillary muscle/trabecular attachments. Even though the anterior and septal leaflets are well seen on multiple echocardiographic views, the posterior leaflet is visualized only on the RV inflow tract view and on short-axis views of the right ventricle (which can display all three leaflets). Because of its importance in imaging the tricuspid valve, on TTE the RV inflow tract view must be acquired in a manner that displays the inferior (diaphragmatic) wall but avoids the interventricular septum and septal leaflet of

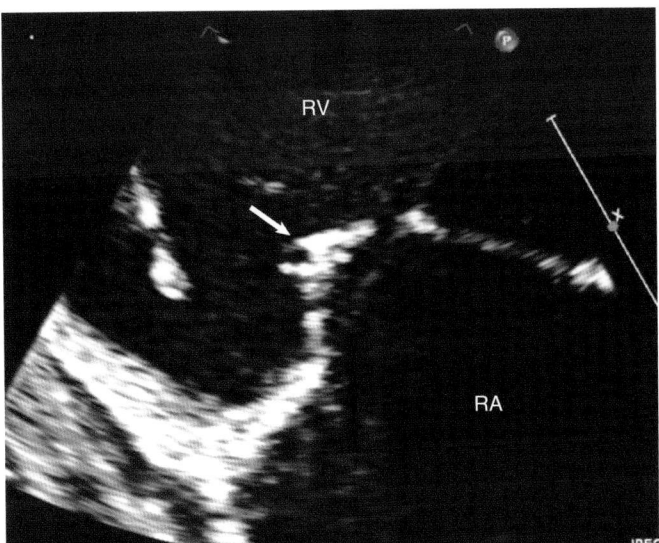

FIGURE 16.47 Right ventricular inflow tract view demonstrating diastolic doming of the posterior leaflet (arrow) characteristic of rheumatic tricuspid valve disease. RA, Right atrium; RV, right ventricle.

Quantitation of Tricuspid Regurgitation

Quantitation of TR is similar to that for MR and consists of an integrated parametric approach,[66] including measures of jet size, vena contracta, and PISA-derived regurgitant volume and EROA. Systolic flow reversal into the hepatic veins is specific for severe TR and may be appreciated with color and PW Doppler or with saline contrast.

Pulmonic Valve (see Chapter 77)

Pulmonic Valve Anatomy

The normal pulmonic valve is tricuspid with a structure that is similar to that of the aortic valve. The cusps are named right, left, and anterior, although it is unusual to be able to see all three cusps simultaneously with 2D imaging. The pulmonic valve can be seen on parasternal and subcostal views, as well as on anteriorly oriented apical views. TEE windows include the midesophageal, deep transgastric, and high esophageal (at the level of the aortic arch). The most common congenital anomaly is valvular stenosis, based on developmental abnormalities that mimic those of a bicuspid aortic valve. It is characterized by systolic doming and a jump rope–like appearance of the valve. Congenital pulmonic stenosis may be isolated or may occur as a feature of more complex congenital anomalies. Acquired pulmonic disease is rare with causes that include carcinoid and endocarditis, as well as iatrogenic regurgitation due to disruption of the valve from balloon or surgical valvuloplasty for congenital stenosis.

Quantitation of Valve Dysfunction

Pulmonic stenosis is most reliably quantitated with mean and peak gradients, although the continuity equation provides a means of calculating valve area. Pulmonic regurgitation is usually graded on the basis of jet dimensions, with the caveat that there may be little turbulence in the setting of severe regurgitation with normal pulmonary pressure, which can lead to inadvertent underestimation of the true severity. Using Doppler, a wide color jet origin width plus laminar regurgitant flow and rapid diastolic flow deceleration on spectral Doppler are clues to severe regurgitation. (Figs. 16.49E and 16.50). Mild-to-moderate degrees of pulmonic regurgitation may be seen in patients with dilatation of the pulmonary artery and pulmonary hypertension.

Prosthetic Valves (see Chapter 79)

Echocardiographic assessment of prosthetic valves requires an understanding of valve design, normal functional characteristics, and the imaging artefacts introduced by valve elements.

The most commonly encountered mechanical valves are bileaflet or single, tilting disc valves. Ball-and-cage valves, which are no longer implanted, are now quite rare. Most bioprosthetic valves are stented porcine or bovine pericardial valves, although freestyle (stentless) xenograft, cadaveric homograft, autograft (Ross procedure), and transcatheter and sutureless surgical valves are also available. Prosthetic annular rings are also often used for mitral and tricuspid repair. The sewing rings of all valves, as well as the occluders of mechanical valves, may cause acoustic shadowing that limits imaging and Doppler assessment; the exceptions to this are the stentless, homograft, and autograft valves, which may be indistinguishable from native valves. Additionally, the material of the ball in ball-and-cage valves transmits sound more slowly than human tissue does, with the result that the ball appears much larger than its actual size when imaged echocardiographically.

Even normally functioning prostheses tend to be intrinsically stenotic, with the degree of stenosis inversely related to valve size. Additionally, trivial degrees of valvular regurgitation are normal findings, and although not normal, trivial paravalvular regurgitation is not uncommon. Intraventricular microcavitations (apparent "microbubbles," thought to be caused by transient localized pressure drop at the site of prosthetic valve closure vaporizing blood) are often seen in the left heart in the presence of mechanical valves and are considered normal. Figures 16.51 to 16.53 demonstrate the normal echocardiographic appearance of the most common

the tricuspid valve (see Fig. 16.8). Although all 3 leaflets can often be seen in transgastric TEE views, 3D echocardiography more reliably permits visualization of all the leaflets in an en-face view from the atrial or RV side.

Acquired Disorders of the Tricuspid Valve

Tricuspid stenosis occurs in approximately 11% of patients with rheumatic mitral disease and is characterized by diastolic leaflet doming, as well as by leaflet and chordal thickening (Fig. 16.47). Severity is best assessed by Doppler-derived mean gradients. Methods for calculating valve area, including the PHT approach, have not been validated for tricuspid stenosis (see Chapter 77).

Pathologic TR most frequently occurs on a functional basis, that is, attributable to RV (and RA) enlargement or dysfunction. RV pathology, in turn, may be due to pulmonary hypertension and left-sided cardiac abnormalities. Isolated RA and tricuspid annular enlargement may be the consequence of AF. The echocardiographic hallmark of functional TR is apical tethering, which when severe may result in a visible regurgitant orifice (noncoaptation of the leaflets) (Fig. 16.48). Under these conditions the regurgitant jet could be laminar (nonturbulent) and relatively low velocity because of the almost complete equalization of pressures between the right ventricle and the right atrium and could lead to underestimation of the severity of the TR. Similarly, estimation of PASP from TR jet velocity will be inaccurate in this situation.

Myxomatous tricuspid valve disease, the most common cause of primary TR, has been less well studied than mitral disease. It accompanies MVP in 20% of patients. Because there is great variability in the mobility and size of the three tricuspid leaflets, there are less clear-cut criteria for the diagnosis in the TV. Unlike the mitral valve, spontaneous flail of the tricuspid valve virtually never occurs. Less common acquired causes of primary TR include carcinoid, rheumatic disease, endocarditis, trauma (including iatrogenic injury to the valve during RV biopsy as well as blunt trauma), and deformation or damage by pacemaker and defibrillator wires. The characteristic echocardiographic appearance of carcinoid heart disease is drumstick-like, rigid, and shortened leaflets with at times a visible regurgitant orifice (Fig. 16.49). Carcinoid involvement of the tricuspid valve may be associated with mixed tricuspid stenosis and regurgitation; the pulmonic valve may be similarly involved. Carcinoid involvement of the mitral valve is rare and suggests either pulmonary metastases or a right to left shunt. Absence of concomitant mitral involvement may help distinguish carcinoid from rheumatic tricuspid disease.

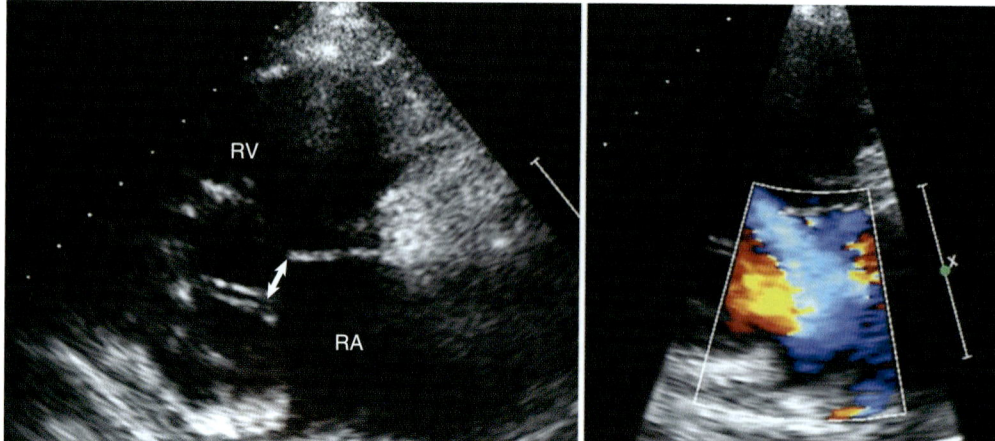

FIGURE 16.48 Left, Right ventricular inflow tract view showing failure of coaptation of the anterior and posterior leaflets (*arrow*) in a patient with severe functional tricuspid regurgitation. *RA,* Right atrium; *RV,* right ventricle. **Right,** Severity may be underestimated because of its low velocity and monochromatic appearance.

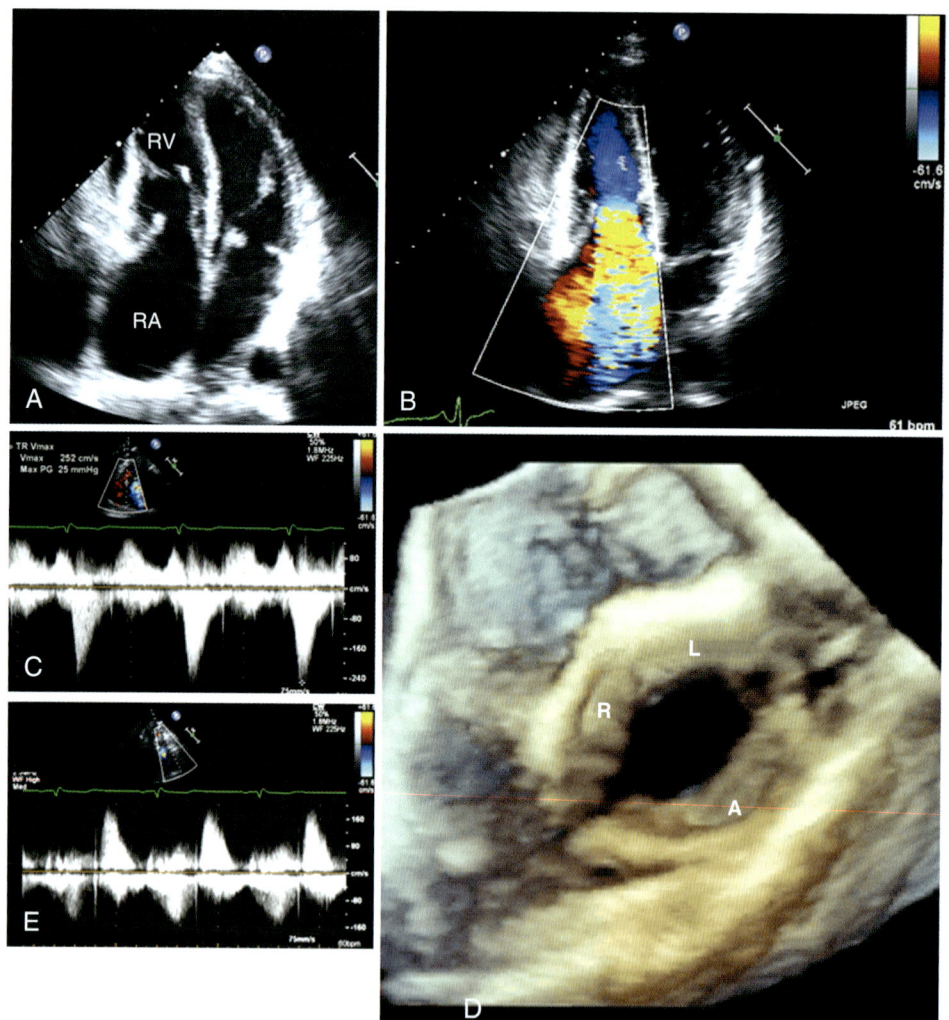

FIGURE 16.49 Carcinoid heart disease. **A,** Apical 4-chamber view, demonstrating the thickened and retracted tricuspid valve, characteristic drumstick-like appearance, frozen in the half-open, half-closed position. The interventricular septum is distended leftwards and the right atrium is severely enlarged. *RA,* Right atrium; *RV,* right ventricle. **B,** Severe tricuspid regurgitation through the wide-open valve. **C,** CW Doppler of the tricuspid antegrade and regurgitant flow, illustrating a mildly stenotic valve but severe tricuspid regurgitation. The remarkably rapid slope of deceleration of the tricuspid regurgitant jet is indicative of severely elevated right atrial pressure. **D,** 3D live TEE view from the pulmonary arterial aspect of the similarly thickened and retracted pulmonic valve (*R,* right; *L,* left; *A,* anterior leaflet). **E,** CW Doppler of the pulmonic antegrade and regurgitant flow (from transthoracic echocardiogram), illustrating only a mildly stenotic pulmonic valve but severe pulmonic regurgitation, as evidenced by the dense jet with a very rapid deceleration time.

prostheses. More current data, including recently introduced prostheses, are collated from the literature and valve manufacturers at www.valveguide.ch.[68] A helpful rule of thumb when valve size is unknown is that for common-size prostheses in patients with physiologic heart rates and SV, the peak transaortic velocity should be less than 3 m/sec and the mean transmitral gradient 5 to 6 mmHg or lower.[68,69] Stentless bioprosthetic valves, which have little or no acoustic shadowing due to lack of a rigid annulus, are designed to have lower hemodynamic profiles (i.e., lower gradients) than their equivalently sized first-generation predecessors and appear useful for implantation in patients with a small annulus or severely reduced LV function.

The echocardiographic approach to prosthetic valves is similar to but often more challenging than that of native valves. Peak and mean gradients are calculated by using the conventional application of the Bernoulli equation, and effective orifice area may be calculated with the continuity equation. Additionally, the Doppler velocity or "dimensionless" index, defined as the ratio of the VTI (or peak velocity) proximal to the valve to that distal to the valve, provides an alternative metric of aortic prosthetic function that is useful when LVOT diameter cannot be measured. A value less than 0.25 is highly suggestive of valvular obstruction. As for native valves, it is critical that LVOT sampling be proximal to the site of flow acceleration; in the case of transcatheter or sutureless valves, the sampling volume should be proximal to the inlet of the metal frame because in these valves there is acceleration of flow at the inlet, as well as at the level of the cusps. For mitral prostheses, the comparable measure is the ratio of mitral to aortic VTI with values less than 2.2 considered normal. In the patient with AF, matching of cycle lengths for beats used for LVOT and valvular VTIs is preferred to averaging over multiple beats. Beats corresponding to physiologic heart rates should be used if available. Although the PHT may be useful in a relative sense in patients with mitral prostheses (with PHT ≥ 130 ms considered suggestive of obstruction),[69] it does not provide a valid measure of effective orifice area.

In many centers, intraoperative TEE is performed routinely during valve procedures, and these studies can both alert the surgeon to remediable complications before chest closure and serve as reference studies for follow-up evaluation. It is also recommended that TTE be performed soon—either before hospital discharge or within 3 months—after implantation to define the baseline appearance and structure with this modality and under more physiologic conditions than those present in the immediate postpump period (see Chapter 79). For all studies, chamber dimensions and function and estimated PASP, as well as heart rate, blood pressure, and BSA, should be included in the report. For postoperative echocardiographic evaluation, it is important to obtain information on valve type and size and details of the valve implantation when possible.

Abnormalities in Valve Appearance

Abnormalities in valve appearance include evidence of an unusual implantation position or valvular dehiscence, which when extensive is characterized by pathologic valve rocking. Although extensive bioprosthetic cusp thickening is typically associated with functional disturbance (see later), mild abnormalities may not affect valve function. Similarly, valve vegetation and thrombus may be functionally silent. Therefore, echocardiographic evaluation must focus on structure even when function is normal, with ensuing TEE planned if TTE images are nondiagnostic.

Approach to Assessing Elevated Prosthetic Gradients

The diagnosis of prosthetic stenosis is suggested when gradients are elevated and the effective orifice area is reduced relative to published norms. Comprehensive guidelines from national echocardiography societies have been published (and more recently reviewed)[69]. For aortic prostheses, a Doppler velocity index less than 0.25 or a ratio of acceleration to ejection times greater than 0.4 supports the diagnosis. For mitral prostheses per ASE guidelines, a PHT >200 msec, peak E wave ≥ 2.5 m/sec, or VTI_{MV}/VTI_{LVOT} of ≥ 2.5 suggests severe stenosis vs normal values of less than 130 msec, less than 1.9 and less than 2.2 m/sec respectively. As with native valves, gradients must be interpreted in the context of heart rate. Causes of prosthetic stenosis include restricted leaflet/disc motion because of thrombus (Fig. 16.54), pannus ingrowth (Fig. 16.55), vegetation, or in the case of bioprostheses, cusp calcification and degeneration (Fig. 16.56). Differentiation between pannus and thrombus may be challenging, although thrombi tend to have a softer echotexture than pannus and may be larger with extension beyond the sewing ring. Clinical factors suggesting thrombus include the acuity of symptom onset and a history of inadequate anticoagulation. Because the restricted motion may be intermittent, it is important to capture multiple beats if prosthetic dysfunction is clinically suspected. TEE is frequently required to image valves optimally, and fluoroscopy or CTA may be helpful when abnormal occluder motion is suspected in mechanical valves.

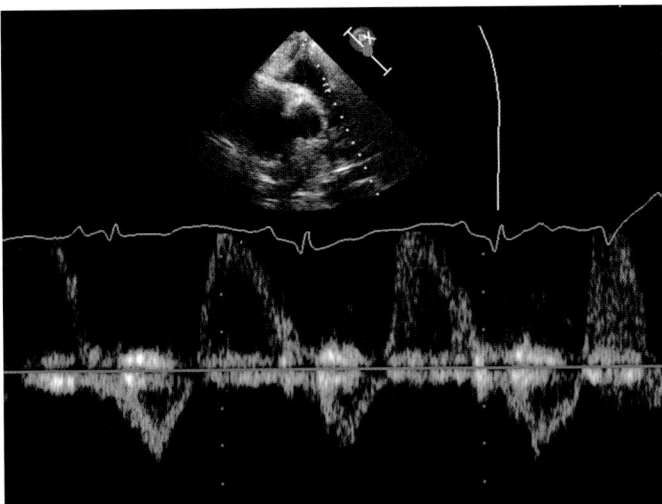

FIGURE 16.50 PW Doppler interrogation of the RVOT in a patient who has undergone pulmonary valvotomy. There is severe pulmonic regurgitation resulting in a laminar regurgitant signal.

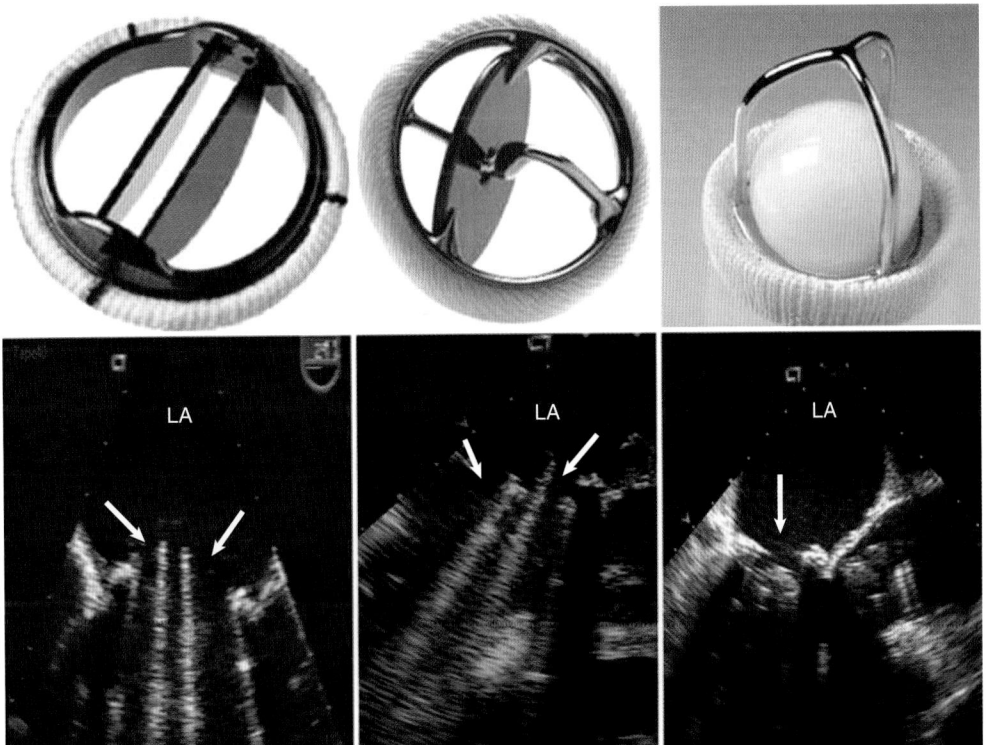

FIGURE 16.51 Mechanical prostheses and their transesophageal echocardiographic (TEE) appearance when implanted in the mitral position. **Left panels**, St. Jude bileaflet valve. *Arrows* indicate discs in the open position. **Middle panels**, Medtronic-Hall tilting single disc valve. The *right arrow* indicates the disc in the open position, and the *left arrow* indicates reverberation from the central pivot. **Right panels**, Starr Edwards ball-and-cage valve. The *arrow* points to the valve in the open position. *LA,* Left atrium.

Notably, elevated gradients do not always reflect prosthetic stenosis. *Patient-prosthesis mismatch* (PPM) refers to the situation in which the implanted valve, although functioning normally, has elevated gradients (see Chapter 79). This occurs when patient anatomy necessitates the implantation of a smaller-than-ideal valve. The diagnosis is made by confirming that the calculated effective orifice area is consistent with normal function, but the *indexed* orifice area is ≤0.85 cm^2/m^2 for aortic prostheses and less than 1.2 cm^2/m^2 for mitral prostheses. For aortic prostheses an indexed effective orifice area less than 0.65 cm^2/m^2 is considered severe PPM, a phenomenon encountered in 2% to 11% of patients. PPM is best studied for the aortic valve and is reportedly associated with poorer outcomes, although in obese patients it is unclear whether the indexed effective orifice area should be calculated on the basis of lean rather than actual body mass.

Elevated gradients may also be a consequence of significant regurgitation, which when paravalvular in origin may be underappreciated on initial evaluation. A final important cause of elevated gradients in aortic prostheses, *pressure recovery*, refers to the tendency for Doppler-derived gradients to overestimate those registered invasively.

This occurs because Doppler measures the largest gradient, typically encountered at the vena contracta, whereas invasive measurements reflect pressure distal to the valve where there has been recovery either because blood has moved from the narrow valve orifice into the wider aorta (i.e., a flask-shaped aortic root, which is a significant factor only in the setting of aortas measuring <3 cm) or, in the case of bileaflet mechanical valves, because the lower pressure encountered in the central orifice is augmented by higher pressure caused by eddies at the lateral orifices. Pressure recovery is most important clinically in the setting of small (≤ 21 mm) bileaflet valves in the aortic position. As demonstrated, the measurements most representative of invasive gradients is obtained by carefully interrogating the lateral orifices, but this generally requires TEE. Alternatively, it has been suggested that gradients recorded through the central orifice may be corrected by applying the pressure loss coefficient of 0.64.

Prosthetic Regurgitation

Trivial degrees of valvular regurgitation are normal findings, although the location of normal jets varies depending on the valve type. Pathologic regurgitation which is termed *central* (*trans*valvular) originates from within the sewing ring (central, transvalvular origin), which should be distinguished from *para*valvular regurgitation which arises external to the annulus. Valvular regurgitation in mechanical valves typically reflects occluder malfunction as a result of pannus, thrombus, vegetation, or rarely, retained mitral valve apparatus preventing full leaflet closure, whereas in bioprostheses, this is typically a result of cusp degeneration or disruption from endocarditis. Paravalvular regurgitation may be a residual finding resulting from suboptimal implantation or may develop de novo from endocarditis or spontaneous valve dehiscence. Some degree of paravalvular regurgitation is a common finding after transcatheter aortic valve implantation (see Chapter 72), but moderate or greater degrees appear to be associated with a worse prognosis (Fig. 16.57).

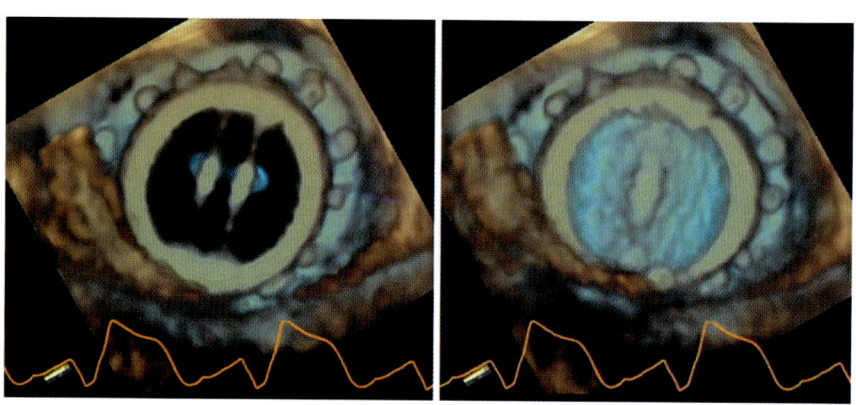

FIGURE 16.52 Three-dimensional TEE views of a bileaflet mechanical prosthesis as viewed from the left atrial aspect in diastole (**left**, with discs open) and systole (**right**, with discs closed).

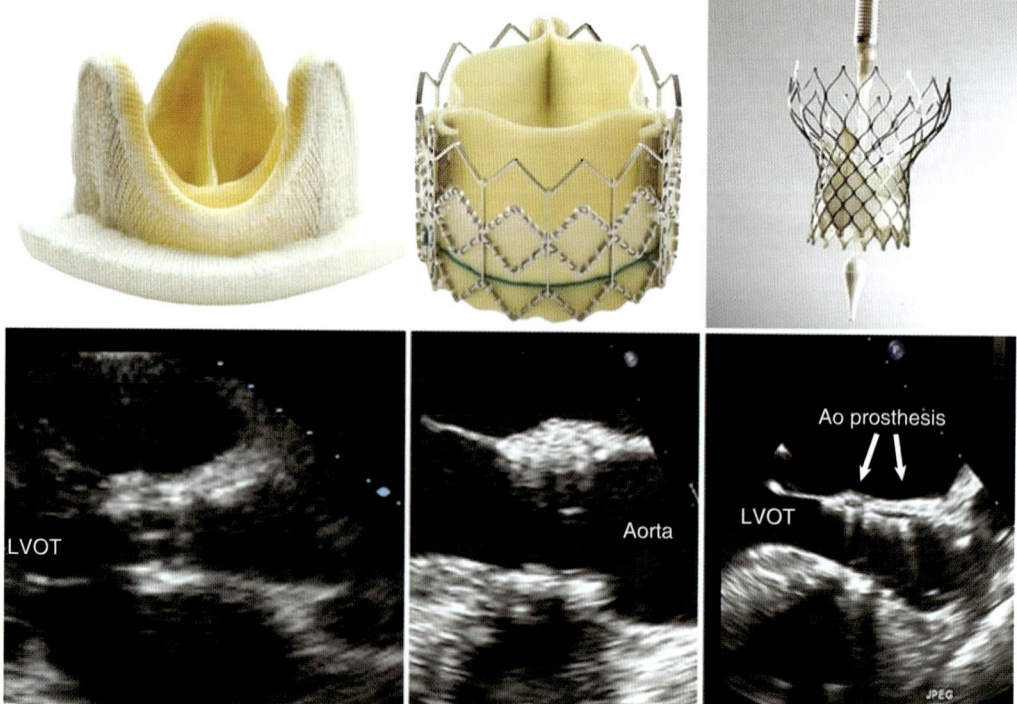

FIGURE 16.53 Bioprostheses and their echocardiographic long-axis appearance when implanted in the aortic (*Ao*) position. **Left panels,** Heterograft stented bioprosthesis. **Middle panels,** Sapien balloon expandable transcatheter aortic valve. **Right panels,** CoreValve self-expanding transcatheter aortic valve. *LVOT,* Left ventricular outflow tract.

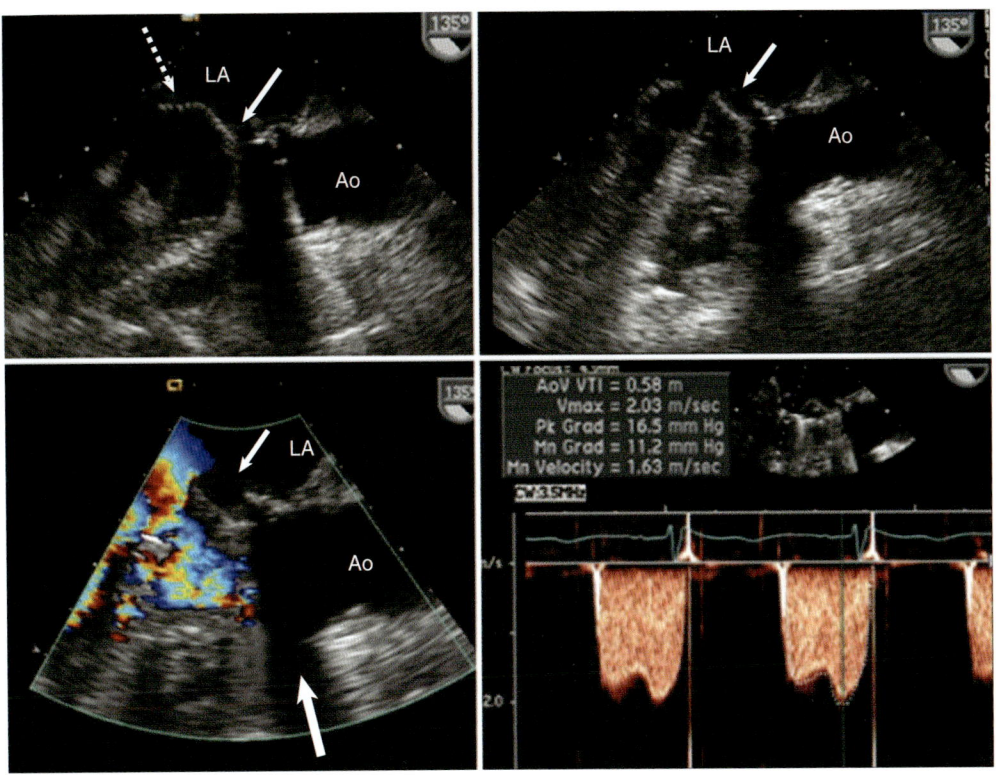

FIGURE 16.54 TEE showing a bileaflet mechanical mitral prosthesis in which one disc is immobilized because of thrombus. **Upper left,** Systolic frame showing that neither disc (*arrows*) closes completely. **Upper right,** While the left disc opens fully, the right disc is immobile. **Lower left,** Color flow Doppler demonstrating high-velocity flow through a single orifice. The *large arrow* indicates acoustic shadowing because of the mitral sewing ring. **Lower right,** Doppler demonstrating an elevated transmitral gradient (11 mm Hg at a heart rate of 65 beats/min). *Ao,* Aorta; *LA,* left atrium.

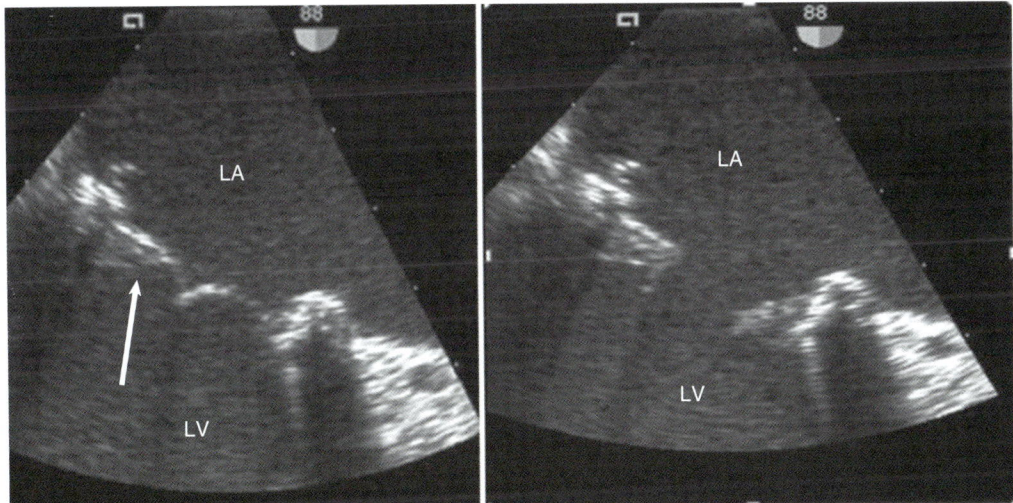

FIGURE 16.55 TEE appearance of pannus ingrowth (*arrow*) in a mitral bioprosthesis. **Left,** Systole. **Right,** Diastole. The pannus has immobilized the base of the left-sided cusp and created a hinge point midway along the cusp and an narrow orifice. *LA,* Left atrium; *LV,* left ventricle.

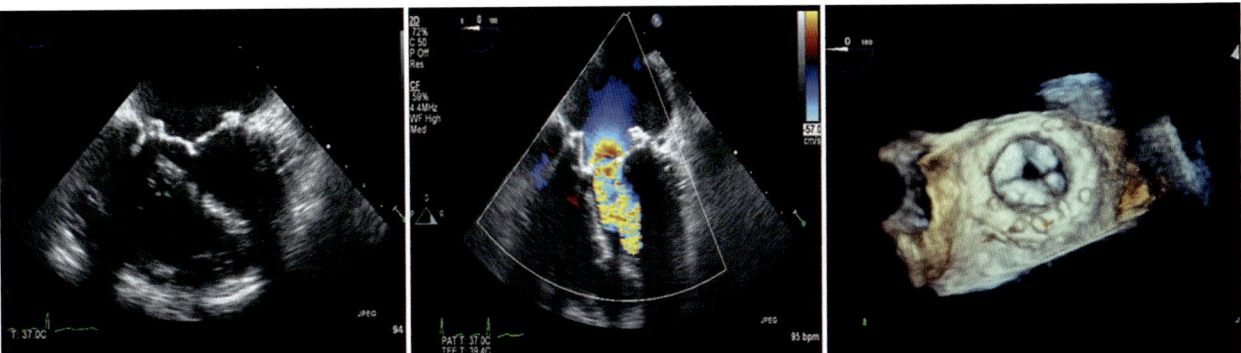

FIGURE 16.56 TEE demonstrating a degenerated bioprosthesis. **Left,** Diastolic frame showing grossly restricted cusp motion. **Middle,** Color Doppler demonstrating turbulent transmitral flow and an easily identifiable proximal isovelocity hemispheric surface area shell. **Right,** 3D TEE view of the prosthesis from the left atrial perspective. The mitral orifice is greatly restricted.

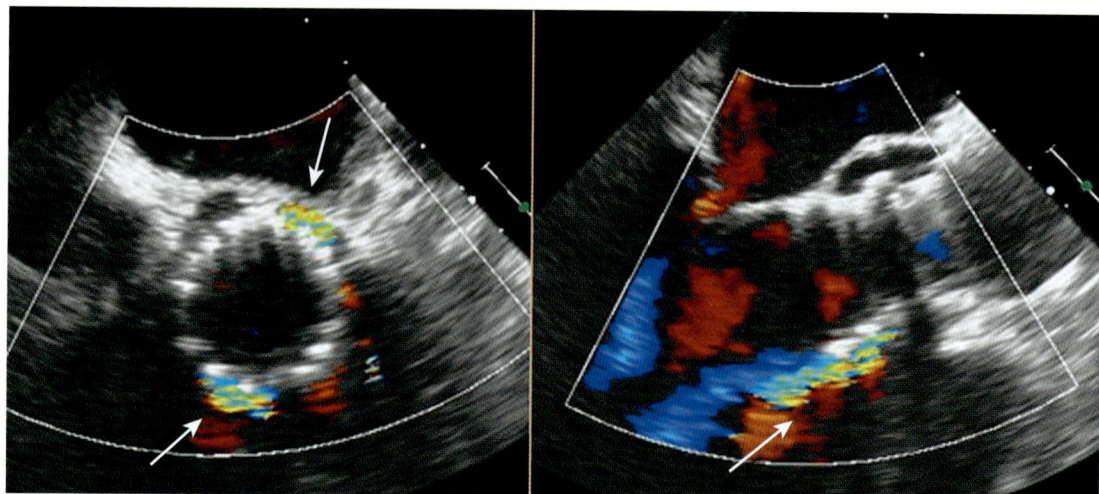

FIGURE 16.57 Orthogonal TEE views of a balloon-expandable aortic prosthesis (TAVI, CoreValve) with at least two sites of significant paravalvular regurgitation (*arrows*), seen as turbulent diastolic flow on **left panel** (45 degrees) and **right panel** (120 degrees).

Detection of prosthetic regurgitation may require nonstandard views. Quantitation of prosthetic regurgitation may be challenging because jets frequently are highly eccentric and may be multiple, thus limiting the value of approaches based on jet dimensions. For mechanical valves the acoustic shadowing cast by mitral prostheses can greatly limit detection of MR, because the shadowing predictably falls directly over the left atrium in TTE views. The use of TEE is extremely advantageous in this respect since it insonifies the valve from an aspect posterior and directly adjacent to the left atrium. Assessment of paravalvular regurgitation in transcatheter or sutureless valves is particularly difficult because multiple pinhole jets may be present and the stents may obscure portions of the color flow jet.[70] As in native AR, the presence of a shortened PHT (<200 msec) and holodiastolic flow reversal in the descending thoracic or abdominal aorta are clues to significant regurgitation. For mitral prostheses, VTI_{MV}/VTI_{LVOT} of ≥2.8 (as seen in stenotic valves as well), but in particular an elevated E wave (i.e., peak gradient elevated out of proportion to the mean gradient) and pulmonary venous flow reversal in systole, should raise suspicion for significant regurgitation. The quantitative Doppler approach using the pulmonic valve as the reference may also be helpful for aortic prostheses. As in native valvular regurgitation, regurgitant volume values less than 30 mL, 30 to 59 mL, and ≥60 mL and regurgitant fraction values less than 30%, 30% to 50%, and greater than 50% are consistent with mild, moderate, and severe prosthetic AR, respectively. For mitral valves the presence of well-defined flow convergence suggests significant regurgitation, and the PISA approach may be used to quantitate central valvular or well-defined single paravalvular jets. 3D TEE approaches that allow direct planimetry of regurgitant orifices and better localization of paravalvular leaks facilitate these tasks and may be more accurate.

Prosthetic tricuspid and pulmonic valves are much less common than their left-sided counterparts. In general, methods developed for assessment of the mitral and aortic valves are extrapolated to the tricuspid and pulmonic valves, although the evidence base for their use is less robust.

PERICARDIAL DISEASE (SEE CHAPTER 86)

Echocardiography is the imaging modality of choice for the identification of pericardial effusion and is an important tool in the diagnosis of tamponade and pericardial constriction (see Chapter 86).

Pericardial Effusion

Identification of pericardial effusion was one of the earliest applications of echocardiography.[71,72] The diagnosis is made when an echo-free space separates the visceral and parietal pericardial echoes throughout the cardiac cycle, including diastole (Fig. 16.58). Systolic separation alone may be a normal finding reflecting normal

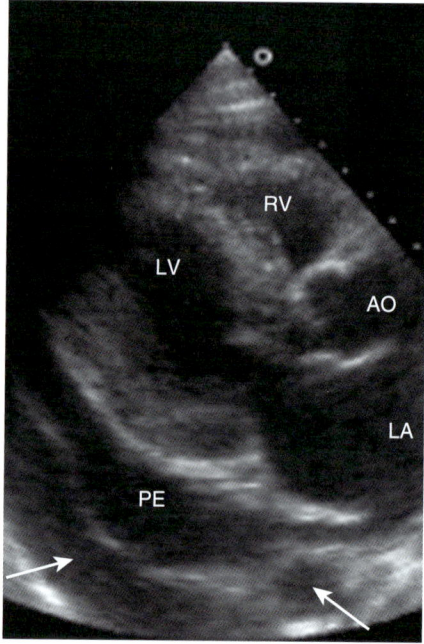

FIGURE 16.58 Pericardial effusion. A parasternal long-axis view shows both pericardial effusion (*PE*) and pleural effusion (*left arrow*). Note that the descending thoracic aorta (*right arrow*) is displaced from the heart by the pericardial effusion. With isolated pleural effusion, the descending aorta (*Ao*) remains immediately posterior to the heart. In this case the pericardial effusion extends posterior to the left atrium (*LA*), although this is not always the case. *LV*, Left ventricle; *RV*, right ventricle.

lubricating pericardial fluid. In most cases the diagnosis of pericardial effusion is straightforward because the parietal pericardium is a strong echo reflector and the visceral pericardium is adherent to the epicardial surface of the heart. "Echo free" is defined as having an echotexture that is equivalent to that of the intracardiac blood pool. Although it is typically black, in some cases suboptimal image quality results in both blood pool and pericardial effusion with a grayish or intermediate echotexture. In such cases it may be difficult to differentiate a small pericardial effusion from epicardial fat, although the latter typically has a more reticulated inhomogeneous appearance than a fluid effusion.

Another source of confusion may be left pleural effusion. Differentiating features include displacement of the aorta from the heart by pericardial (but not pleural) fluid and extension of pleural (but not pericardial) fluid behind the left atrium (see Fig. 16.58). Of the two features, the relative position of the aorta is the most definitive: pericardial effusions may extend cephalad beyond the atrioventricular groove but will be anterior to the aorta, whereas fluid posterior to the aorta is pleural in nature. It is therefore essential that sonographers routinely provide views that demonstrate the descending thoracic aorta and its position relative to the heart. Multiple windows—particularly the subcostal view, because fluid is gravity dependent and thus tends to collect inferiorly—are essential to rule out localized effusions.

Sizing of pericardial effusions is typically somewhat subjective, with the terms *trace, small, medium,* and *large* being used. For reporting the size of effusions when longitudinal comparison will be important, it is helpful to report the maximal diameter of the effusion while noting the view(s) and time of the cardiac cycle (systole versus diastole) when the measurement is taken. Earlier estimates of the volume of the effusion, calculated using linear measures of pericardial and epicardial diameter, relied on a symmetric distribution of fluid and assumptions on the shape of the pericardial sac and heart. Semiquantitatively, systolic separation alone is consistent with a trace (physiologic) collection. Effusions with linear dimensions of less than 1 cm (small) correspond with less than 300 mL of fluid, whereas 1 to 2 cm (moderate) corresponds with 500 mL, and a dimension greater than 2 cm (large) is usually associated with greater than 700 mL of pericardial fluid.[72]

Pericardial Hematoma

Pericardial hematoma results from bleeding into the pericardial space and may be caused by bleeding along suture lines after open heart surgery, trauma, myocardial rupture, or aortic dissection. It may occur as a complication of catheter-based or surgical intervention. Hematomas typically have an echotexture that is more coalescent and echodense than that of free fluid. They may be unevenly distributed and localized to the bleeding site, such as the anterior mediastinum post-CABG. When images are obtained in the acute setting, there may be evidence of both clot and free fluid (Fig. 16.59).

Echocardiographic Markers of Tamponade

Echocardiographic markers of cardiac tamponade fall into two categories: (1) cardiac chamber invagination reflecting *elevated intrapericardial pressure* and the resultant pressure gradients across the chamber walls and (2) echocardiographic markers of pulsus paradoxus, which reflect exaggerated respiratory variation in left-sided heart filling and ejection relative to that of the right side of the heart (*ventricular interdependence*).

Right atrial inversion is a dynamic phenomenon with onset when RA volume and pressure are lowest: in late ventricular diastole immediately after atrial contraction (Fig. 16.60, left panel). Inversion continues through a variable portion of ventricular systole and resolves as the right atrium fills and RA pressure rises. This sign can be detected in any view where the RA wall and adjacent effusion are well seen, typically the parasternal short-axis view at the level of the great vessels and the apical and subcostal four-chamber views. This sign is highly sensitive (100%) but may be present when hemodynamic disturbances are invasively detectable but fall below the threshold for the clinical diagnosis of tamponade, resulting in a specificity for clinical tamponade of 82%. Empirically, an RA inversion time index (readily calculated as number of frames during which the right atrium is inverted divided by number of frames per cardiac cycle) of at least 0.33 is associated with clinically evident tamponade (100% specificity, 95% sensitivity). *Left atrial inversion* as a marker of tamponade is rare and typically occurs in the setting of loculated effusions or those in which the pericardial reflection is relatively high and the left atrium is exposed to the effects of intrapericardial pressure.

Right ventricular inversion has its onset when RV volume and pressure are lowest: during isovolumic relaxation (Fig. 16.60, right panel). It continues through a variable portion of ventricular diastole, with the RV contour normalizing as the ventricle fills and RV pressure rises. This sign is most easily detected on the parasternal long-axis view, which displays

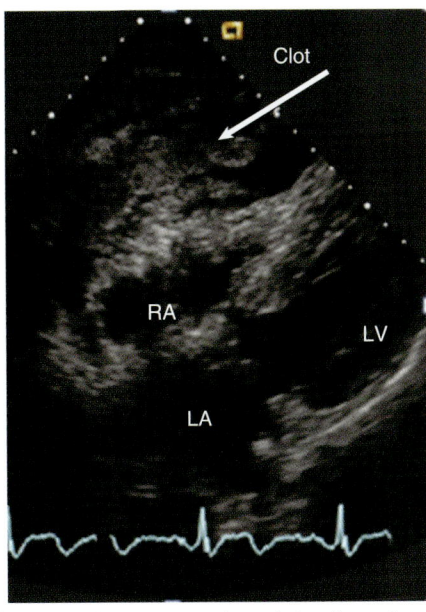

FIGURE 16.59 Pericardial hematoma. A subcostal view shows clotted (*arrow*) and free blood (black echotexture) within the pericardial space. In this patient the cause was acute aortic dissection. *LA,* Left atrium; *LV,* left ventricle; *RA,* right atrium.

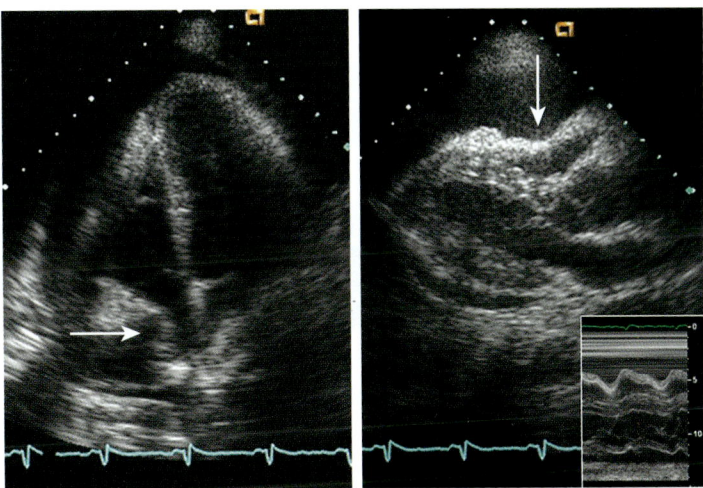

FIGURE 16.60 Signs of cardiac tamponade. **Left,** Apical four-chamber view showing RA inversion (*arrow*), a marker of tamponade. In this case, inversion, which is initiated in late ventricular diastole, has persisted well into ventricular systole. **Right,** Parasternal long-axis view showing RV collapse in diastole (*arrow*). *Inset,* An M-mode cursor placed down the RVOT shows diastolic inversion of the RV wall (note timing with respect to the ECG, closed aortic valve, and open mitral valve).

the RVOT. Its reported sensitivity is 82% to 94%, with a specificity of 88% to 100%.

It is important to note that RA inversion and RV inversion are defined by actual wall invagination rather than by the normal flattening that may occur with respective chamber systole. RA or RV inversion may also be absent (i.e., false-negative) in the setting of underlying right-sided heart dysfunction associated with elevated intracavitary pressure. With pericardial hematoma in which no free blood is present, dynamic inversion of the chambers will not be observed, but the presence of fixed compression and underfilling of the cardiac chambers may be clues to the presence of tamponade physiology.

There are echocardiographic correlates to the clinical phenomenon of pulsus paradoxus. In the normal state, a slight increase (up to 17%) in flow velocities through the right heart occurs on inspiration, with a reciprocal but smaller decrease (up to 10%) in flow velocities through the left heart in systole. These tendencies are exaggerated

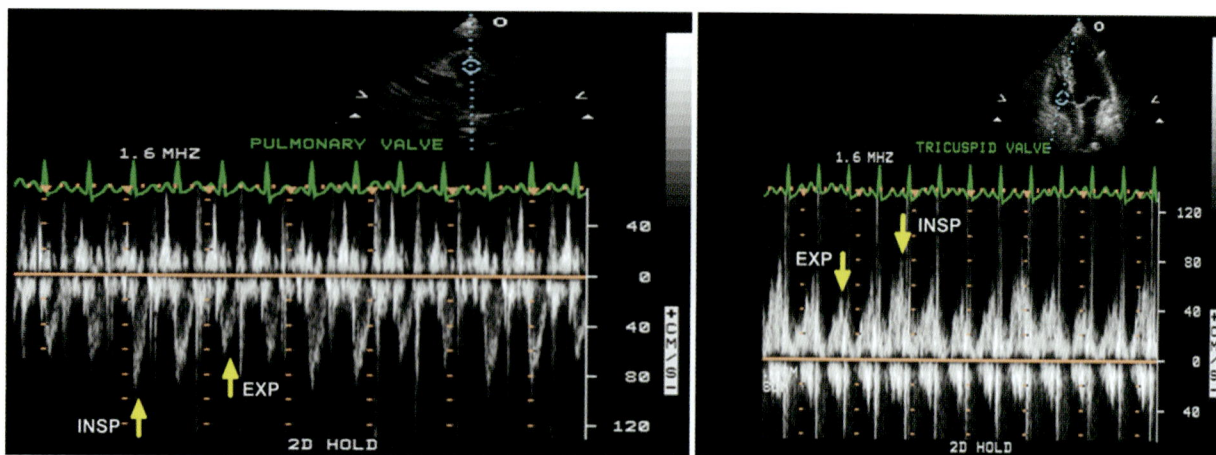

FIGURE 16.61 Doppler spectra showing the characteristic exaggerated respiratory variation in right-sided pulmonary valve outflow **(left panel)** and tricuspid valve inflow **(right panel)** peak flow velocities. On inspiration, right-sided flow increases. In the left heart, PW tracings of LVOT outflow and mitral valve inflow (not shown) would demonstrate reciprocal reductions in left-sided flow on inspiration. *EXP,* Expiration; *INSP,* inspiration.

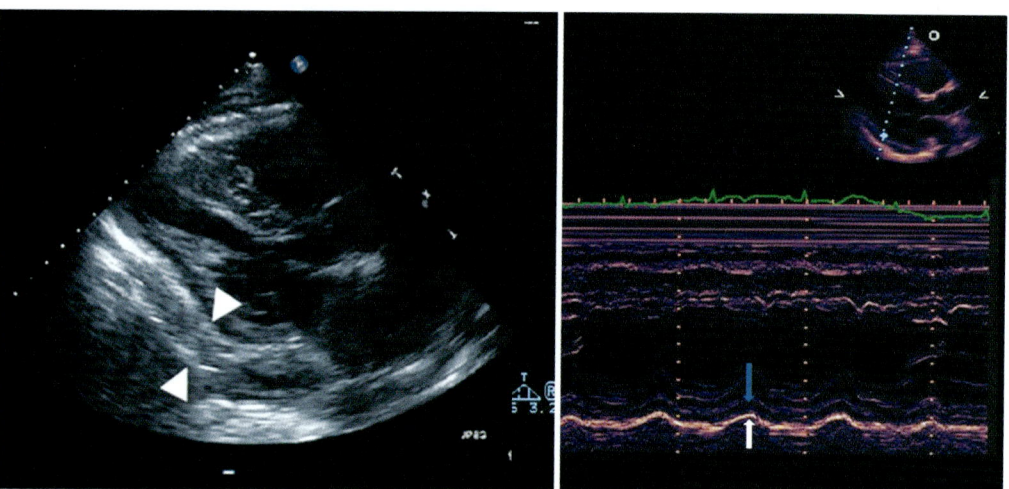

FIGURE 16.62 Left, Parasternal long-axis view demonstrating thickened pericardium (between *arrows*). **Right,** M-mode echocardiogram. The bright posterior echo (*white arrow*) representing the parietal pericardium moves in parallel with the visceral pericardial/epicardial echoes (*blue arrow*), a finding indicative of adhesion between the two layers. If the pericardial space were expanded by free fluid (pericardial effusion), the parietal pericardial echo would be relatively stationary (compare with the M-mode *inset* of Fig. 16.60).

when a tense, fluid-filled pericardium constrains the overall heart size and increases interdependence between the right and left ventricles. The most widely used signs are an exaggerated (>25%, and often >60% in frank tamponade) inspiratory increase in the tricuspid inflow Doppler E wave peak velocities with a reciprocal decrease (of >30%) in the mitral E wave velocities (Fig. 16.61), as well as corresponding changes in the pulmonic and aortic (or LVOT) systolic Doppler spectra. Additional signs of tamponade include the characteristic appearance of the heart oscillating or "swimming" in the pericardial fluid, which has its counterpart in electrical alternans on ECG, and a dilated IVC consistent with elevated RA pressures.

Pericardiocentesis

Echocardiography may also be useful in guiding needle pericardiocentesis, particularly in the setting of loculated effusions. Imaging may help identify the best puncture site and angle of needle introduction, then confirm that the needle has entered the pericardial space. The latter is accomplished by the injection of a small amount of agitated saline, which will opacify the pericardial effusion with proper needle placement but will result in intracardiac contrast bubbles if the needle inadvertently penetrates the heart. Echocardiography is used to document the reduction in effusion size that should occur with successful drainage.

Constrictive Pericarditis

Pericardial constriction occurs when there is thickening, with or without calcification, of the pericardium that results in impaired cardiac diastolic filling, particularly during inspiration (Fig. 16.62). The clinical features mimic those of biventricular heart failure, although the presence of a pericardial knock and Kussmaul sign (inspiratory increase in jugular venous pressure) should raise suspicion for constriction. Frequently, when the patient is referred for echocardiographic evaluation, the clinical differential diagnosis is "restrictive cardiomyopathy" versus pericardial constriction, since EF is generally preserved in both. Pericardial thickening is a hallmark of constriction but is a relatively insensitive finding; furthermore, echocardiography is relatively insensitive for detecting pericardial thickening compared with CT and CMR. When the pericardial space is expanded because of adhesions and fibrous tissue, the visceral and parietal pericardia are separated by tissue of variable echogenicity, unlike the echolucent appearance of pericardial effusion. Also, with effusion the parietal pericardial echo will be relatively stationary, whereas with pericardial thickening, visceral and parietal pericardial echoes will move in tandem. Calcification will result in acoustic shadowing.

Restrictive and constrictive physiology share a mitral diastolic filling pattern characterized by a prominent E wave (E/A ratio >2) and shortened DT caused by rapid early filling, biatrial enlargement, and a fixed dilated IVC that does not change size with a sniff. However, the two may be distinguished by tissue and color Doppler diastolic indices, as well as respirophasic effects on septal motion (ventricular interdependence and septal bounce) that are not seen with restriction. Mitral annular DTI waves generally have normal or increased amplitude in constriction (peak e′ ≥8 cm/sec is reported to be 89% sensitive and 100% specific for constriction), reflecting compensatory exaggerated longitudinal motion of the heart, in contrast to the reduced e′ seen with restriction. Notably, the peak e′ of the lateral site may be smaller than that of the medial annulus, which is the opposite of the normal pattern; this phenomenon is termed *annulus reversus* and is believed to result from calcification and tethering effects of the pericardium on the lateral heart wall. Color M-mode propagation velocity is typically normal or even increased in constriction but reduced in restriction. In addition, PASP rarely exceeds 50 mm Hg in constriction.

In constriction the rigid pericardium abruptly limits filling to a fixed volume. When inspiration causes increased venous return to the right side of the heart, there is a sudden leftward septal shift and thus obligatory reduction in the amount of blood that the left ventricle can accommodate. The leftward septal shift may be seen on echocardiography during inspi-ration (Fig. 16.63), and often a transient left-right septal "bounce" occurs in both early and late diastole, giving the appearance of a double bounce. This ventricular interdependence occurs in tamponade, but pericardial encase-ment has the additional effect of isolating the heart chambers (but not pulmonary veins) from swings in intrathoracic pressure. This affects blood flow into the heart:

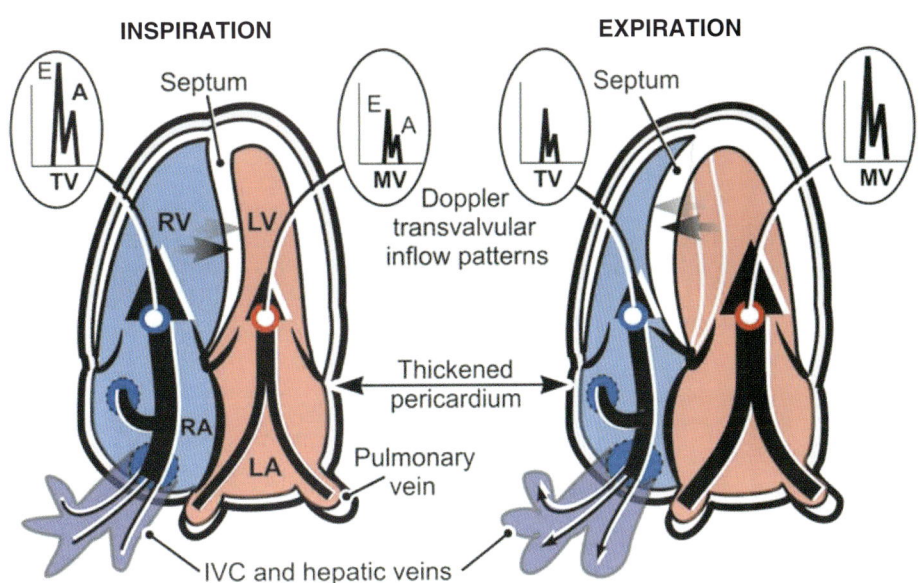

FIGURE 16.63 Schematic representing the echocardiographic manifestations of constriction that may be appreciated on the apical four-chamber view and PW Doppler. Mitral (*MV*) and tricuspid (*TV*) valve Doppler spectra are characterized by an increased E/A ratio and shortened deceleration time. With inspiration there is increased venous return to the right side of the heart, which can be accommodated within the rigid pericardium only by displacement of the interventricular septum to the left and reduced left-sided filling. On expiration, left-sided filling increases, the septum moves to the right, and there is flow reversal in the hepatic veins (see Fig. 16.64). *IVC*, Inferior vena cava; *LA*, left atrium; *LV*, left ventricle; *RA*, right atrium; *RV*, right ventricle. (Modified from Bulwer BE, Rivero JM, eds. *Echocardiography Pocket Guide: The Transthoracic Examination*. Burlington, MA: Jones & Bartlett Learning; 2011, 2013:141. Reprinted with permission.)

with inspiration there is a decrease in intrathoracic pressure and hence a reduction in pulmonary venous pressures driving flow into the left heart, and with expiration there is a rise in intrathoracic (and therefore pulmonary venous) pressures, augmenting flow into the left heart but diminishing RV filling due to septal rightwards motion. There are also exaggerated respirophasic changes in the magnitude of the mitral and tricuspid E-waves (in opposing directions, similar to the patterns in tamponade). Additional markers of constriction include premature opening of the pulmonic valve, which is most pronounced with inspiration (reflecting a rapid rise in end-diastolic RV pressure that exceeds pulmonary artery pressure), diastolic MR, and expiratory diastolic hepatic vein flow reversal consistent with venous congestion (Fig. 16.64). In digital echocardiography laboratories where acquisitions are frequently limited to one to three beat clips, it is essential that longer captures with respiratory gating be obtained to assess the impact of respiration.

Parasternal views can be helpful with M-mode echocardiography over multiple cycles to parse the leftward (posterior) motion of the septum on inspiration and the diastolic septal bounce. In addition, diastolic flattening of the posterior myocardial endocardium rather than the normal continued posterior motion during diastole may be present and reflects abrupt ventricular filling. One may also demonstrate two thickened adhered pericardial layers moving in parallel throughout the cardiac cycle (see Fig. 16.62). Strain analysis shows that GLS is often preserved, but regional analysis demonstrates that there is decreased LV lateral wall and RV free wall strain with preserved septal strain ("strain reversus"), which is theorized to be due to myocardial tethering to the pericardium (analogous to the annulus reversus of mitral annular TDI).[71]

Differentiation between constriction and restriction can be further complicated by coexisting pathologies in the patient. Fibrotic involvement extending from the pericardium into the myocardium may result in mixed constrictive-restrictive physiology. Echocardiographic reassessment after removal of the pericardial fluid causing tamponade may unmask underlying constriction (i.e., effusive-constrictive physiology while the effusion was present).

MALIGNANT INVOLVEMENT OF THE PERICARDIUM

Malignant pericardial disease typically occurs on the basis of local spread or distal metastases, with lung and breast cancer being the most

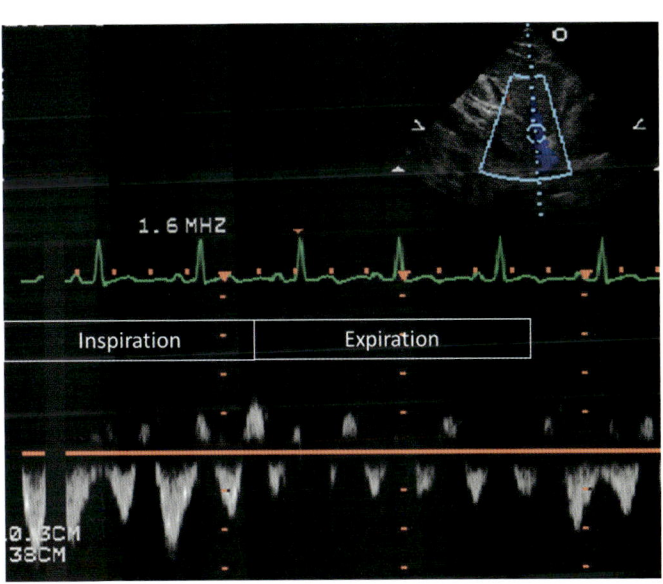

FIGURE 16.64 Hepatic venous flow recordings demonstrate expiratory diastolic flow reversal, seen in constriction.

common primaries. Primary pericardial tumors are uncommon. The echocardiographic appearance may be that of pericardial effusion and/or solid tumor, which frequently invades locally into the myocardium (Fig. 16.65).

OTHER PERICARDIAL PATHOLOGY

Congenital absence of the pericardium is a rare abnormality that usually involves the left pericardium and is associated with a leftward shift in the position of the heart, as well as exaggerated translation. The net result is an echocardiographic pattern that mimics RV volume overload. A *pericardial cyst* is a benign abnormality that is typically detected as an incidental finding of an echo-free mass adjacent to the heart.

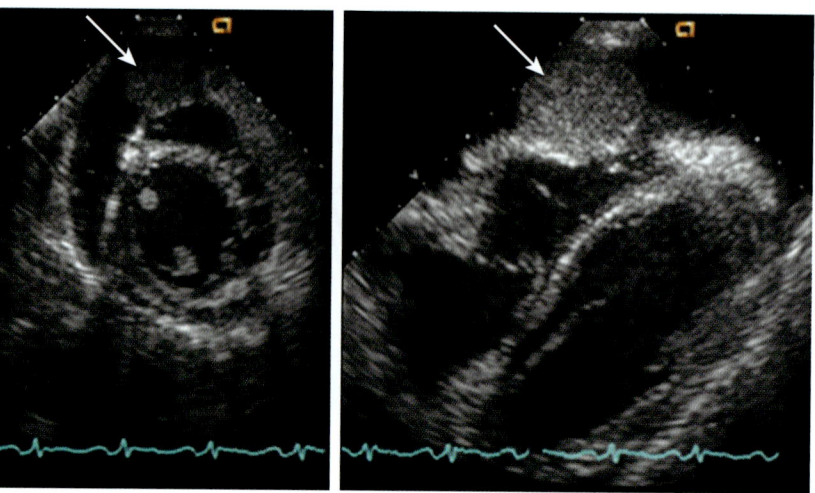

FIGURE 16.65 Subcostal echocardiograms showing a tumor metastasis *(arrows)* within the pericardial space and invading the right ventricular myocardium. The tumor is surrounded by pericardial effusion.

DISEASES OF THE AORTA (SEE CHAPTER 42)

TTE is a first-line tool to assess the thoracic aorta for pathologic processes (see Chapter 42).[15,27] TTE can visualize the aortic root and proximal ascending aorta, aortic arch up to the isthmus (takeoff of the left subclavian artery), and limited portions of the descending thoracic and proximal abdominal aorta (Fig. 16.66). TEE can be used to more comprehensively examine the entire thoracic aorta (Fig. 16.67), with the exception of a small area of distal ascending aorta (which is obscured by shadowing from the air-filled trachea interposed between the esophagus and the heart), the so-called echo blindspot. Therefore, for screening purposes and for serially monitoring a known aortic abnormality for stability, TTE may be sufficient. Higher degrees of suspicion for an acute aortic process or for disease extending beyond the TTE windows require TEE evaluation (or alternatively, CT or magnetic resonance angiography [MRA]).[26]

During the standard echocardiographic examination, the normal diameter of the aorta should be assessed at the aortic annulus, sinuses of Valsalva and sinotubular junction (aortic root), and ascending aorta. The upper limit of normal varies with age, sex, and BSA (Table 16.10). More of the ascending aorta can be viewed by moving the transthoracic probe up one interspace, angling the probe more cephalad, or utilizing right parasternal windows.

Focal Aortopathies

Atherosclerotic plaque can be visualized as irregular, heterogeneous, or echobright calcified foci adherent to the endothelial side of the lumen. These plaques often accumulate at the sinotubular junction and aortic arch. Plaque that is thicker than 5 mm or that has mobile or protruding elements appears to be at higher risk of being associated with stroke (Fig. 16.68A). *Ulcerated aortic plaque* is thought to be a potential precursor to intramural hematomas (see later). In patients with bicuspid valves, the descending aorta should always be evaluated carefully for narrowing and blood flow acceleration at the isthmus, to rule out *aortic coarctation*.

Aortic Emergencies

Aortic aneurysms, technically defined as vessel dilation greater than 50% above the normal diameter of the aorta, may occur anywhere along the course of the aorta (Fig. 16.68B), although they are more common in the abdominal location. Patients with connective tissue syndromes (e.g., Marfan, Loeys-Dietz, Ehlers-Danlos type IV) and patients with bicuspid aortic valves are thought to have defects in the elastic and smooth muscle composition of the aorta which render them prone to the development of ascending aneurysms (generally defined as ascending aortic diameter >4.0 cm). Marfan syndrome in particular often affects only the sinuses of Valsalva symmetrically, whereas diameters at the sinotubular junction and ascending aorta are relatively preserved. The portion of the aortic wall proximal to the coronary orifices is often elongated, giving the root an "onion-bulb" appearance. If the aneurysm involves the ascending aorta and the proximal root up to and including the annulus (termed *aortoannular ectasia*), the resulting incomplete cusp coaptation may cause aortic insufficiency and necessitate valve repair as well. Isolated *sinus of Valsalva aneurysms* are focal dilations that asymmetrically affect only one sinus (most often the right, as shown in Fig. 16.69). They are usually discovered incidentally, and their cause is uncertain. Although not considered an acute aortic emergency, there have been case reports of rupture of these aneurysms into the right ventricle, right atrium, and other locations. In contrast to *ascending* aneurysms, most *descending* aortic aneurysms are associated with atherosclerosis. Whereas ascending aneurysms are typically fusiform, abdominal aneurysms may be more irregular, focal, and saccular in shape.

The most common emergency indication for echocardiography in patients with aortic diseases is to detect *aortic dissection*, a tear in the aortic intima that enables blood to force its way between the other layers of the vessel wall. Although it can arise de novo, aortic dissection and rupture are the most feared sequelae of aortic aneurysms and thus share the same causative associations and risk factors, including connective tissue disorders, aortic valve disease (personal or family history), hypertension, smoking, and atherosclerosis. Figures 16.66 and 16.67 show examples of aortic dissection and their location and appearance. Recent aortic manipulation, such as cardiac catheterization, cardiac surgical bypass, placement of intra-aortic balloon pumps, and intravascular stenting, is also considered a high-risk condition.[26] Serious morbidity from compromised blood flow to the coronary arteries, central nervous system, renal arteries, and other organs may occur, and if the dissection ruptures through all three layers, massive bleeding and death can rapidly ensue. Dissection tends to propagate in antegrade fashion (i.e., from the proximal toward the distal aorta), although retrograde extension may also occur all the way back to the sinuses, causing aortic insufficiency or occluding coronary artery ostia. The mortality rate is high, and surgical treatment has been shown to be the most effective therapy for patients with ascending (DeBakey types I and II or Stanford type A) dissections. *Blunt chest trauma*, in particular rapid-deceleration injuries such as in motor vehicle accidents, may cause tears at the ligamentum arteriosum (near the aortic isthmus, just distal to the left subclavian artery), which demarcates a hinge point between the relatively tethered descending thoracic aorta and the more mobile arch and ascending aorta. Tertiary syphilis, now a rare disease in the developed world, can cause *aortitis*, that is, inflammation of the aortic adventitia, weakening of the walls, and subsequent development of descending aortic aneurysms and dissections. Rarely, other systemic arteritides, such as giant cell arteritis, can also cause aneurysm formation in the ascending aorta.

TTE has somewhat limited sensitivity for aortic dissection (70% to 80% for all locations with higher sensitivity in type A dissections) and specificity (63% to 93%) because of limited views of the abdominal aorta. TEE has been shown to have a sensitivity reaching 99% and specificity of 89%, particularly with ascending dissections.[26] An aortic dissection flap on echocardiography appears as a linear or thin serpiginous tissue plane extending parallel (in the long-axis plane) (Fig. 16.70A; see also Fig. 16.66A,C) or semicircumferentially (in the short-axis plane) (see Fig. 16.67I) to the aortic walls. It represents the intima that has split from the other layers of the aorta. An acute, unthrombosed flap will undulate independently and usually bulge outward from the true lumen in pulsatile fashion during systole. These characteristics can be demonstrated by M-mode and can be used to distinguish true disease from reverberation artefact. If color Doppler is used to sweep

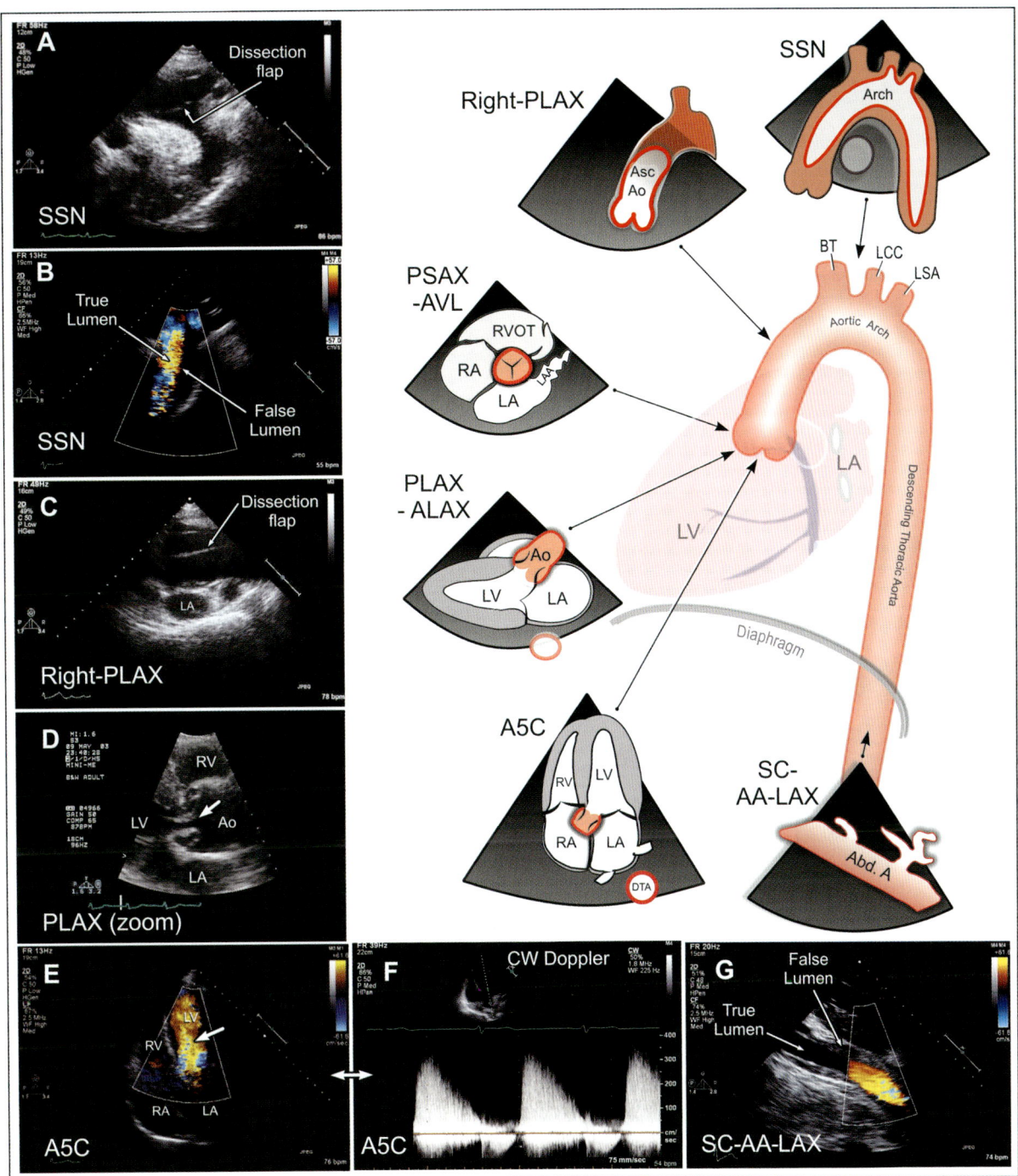

FIGURE 16.66 Transthoracic views of the aorta and examples of acute aortic pathologies from each window. The composite illustrates **(A, B)** suprasternal notch 2D and color Doppler views of a type A dissection flap that is seen extending into the brachiocephalic artery; **(C, D)** a type A dissection flap that originates at the level of the aortic sinuses, prolapses through the aortic valve, and also extends into the ascending aorta in the parasternal long-axis view; **(E, F)** color and spectral Doppler apical five-chamber views illustrating the resultant severe aortic insufficiency; and **(G)** an abdominal aortic type B dissection with a small central true lumen and chronic thrombus in the circumferential false lumen in the subcostal long-axis view. *ALAX,* Apical long axis; *PLAX,* parasternal long axis; *PSAX,* parasternal short axis; *SSN,* suprasternal notch; *SC,* subcostal; *Ao,* aorta; *AVL,* aortic valve level; *BT,* brachiocephalic trunk; *DTA,* descending thoracic aorta; *LCC,* left common carotid artery; *LSA,* left subclavian artery; *TL,* true lumen; *FL,* falselumen.

along the flap, one may occasionally be able to identify the site of the primary tear as a communication between the false and true lumen. The false lumen may be seen to contain more spontaneous echocardiographic contrast or even formed thrombus. By color and spectral Doppler, forward flow in systole can also help identify the true lumen (Fig. 16.70B,E). Complications arising from aortic dissection that may be directly imaged by ultrasound include: (1) extension of the flap into the coronary arteries with loss of the diastolic-dominant coronary flow by spectral and color Doppler and wall motion abnormality signaling MI; (2) AR (see Fig. 16.66E,F) which may be caused by interference with leaflet coaptation due to diastolic prolapse of the flap across the aortic valve, enlargement of the annulus or root, and/or displacement of the cusps relative to one another; (3) extension of the flap into the carotid arteries (causing stroke) or the innominate or subclavian arteries (see Fig. 16.66A); (4) pericardial effusion, which is frequently frank hemopericardium; (5) pleural effusion, which is more common on the left than on the right side; and (6) periaortic hematoma, signifying a leak into the adventitia and impending complete rupture.

Other aortic emergencies are less common but equally life threatening. *Aortic transection* occurs as a result of severe deceleration injury and consists of complete shearing of the aorta at the isthmus, with the

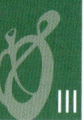

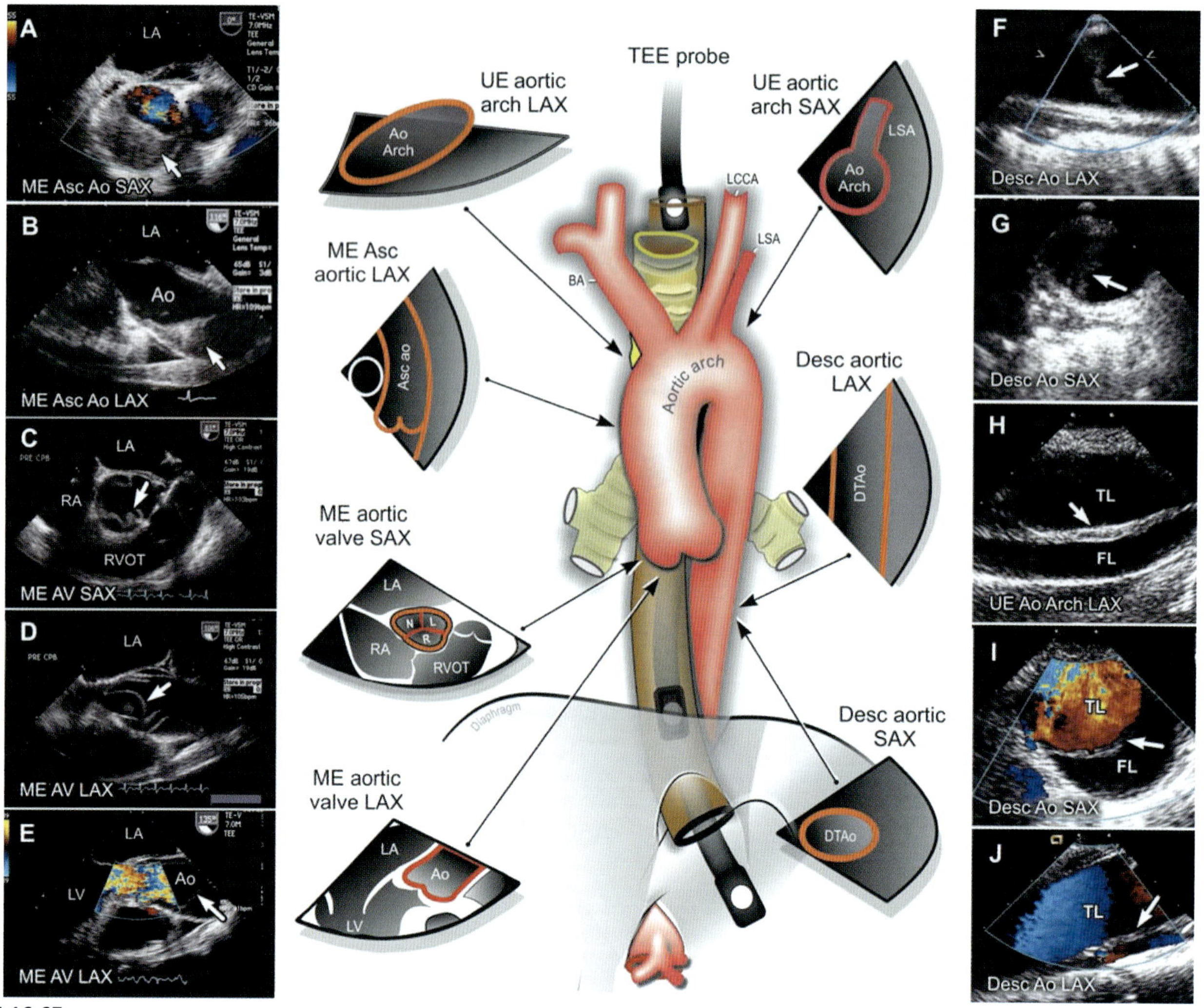

FIGURE 16.67 This TEE composite illustrates **(A, B)** short- and long-axis views of an intramural hematoma in the ascending aorta (*arrow*); **(C, D)** a type A dissection flap that originates at the level of the aortic sinuses, prolapses through the aortic valve, and also extends into the ascending aorta; **(E)** severe aortic insufficiency resulting from dissection in the same patient; **(F, G)** long- and short-axis views of partial aortic transection occurring in the descending thoracic aorta just distal to the origin of the left subclavian artery as a result of sudden deceleration during a motor vehicle accident; and **(H-J)** long- and short-axis views of a type B aortic dissection flap A (*arrow*) visualized in the distal descending thoracic aorta. *FL*, False lumen; *TL*, true lumen; *ME*, midesophageal; *ME*, midesophageal; *UE*, upper esophageal.

TABLE 16.10 Normal Values for Aortic Size in Adults

AORTIC ROOT	ABSOLUTE VALUES (cm)		INDEXED VALUES (cm/m²)	
	MEN	WOMEN	MEN	WOMEN
Annulus	2.6 ± 0.3	2.3 ± 0.2	1.3 ± 0.1	1.3 ± 0.1
Sinuses of Valsalva	3.4 ± 0.3	3.0 ± 0.3	1.7 ± 0.2	1.8 ± 0.2
Sinotubular junction	2.9 ± 0.3	2.6 ± 0.3	1.5 ± 0.2	1.5 ± 0.2
Proximal ascending aorta	3.0 ± 0.4	2.7 ± 0.4	1.5 ± 0.2	1.6 ± 0.3

From Lang RM, Badano LP, Mor-Avi V, et al. Recommendations for cardiac chamber quantification by echocardiography in adults: an update from the American Society of Echocardiography and the European Association of Cardiovascular Imaging. *J Am Soc Echocardiogr* 2015;28:1.

severed ends of the aorta floating freely within hematoma. This is so lethal that examples are rarely captured on TEE during emergency surgery or endovascular repair, although local containment of blood within the mediastinum can permit a very brief window of survival.

A partial transection is shown in Fig. 16.67F,G. *Aortic intramural hematoma* is an accumulation of blood that remains contained within the aortic media; it accounts for approximately 5% to 20% of acute aortic syndromes (see Fig. 16.67A, B). On echocardiography, intramural hematoma appears as a smooth, homogeneously echogenic bulge within the medial layer of aortic wall. It is hypothesized to arise from rupture of a penetrating atherosclerotic ulcer, spontaneous rupture of the vasa vasorum, or more frequently, blunt trauma. Intramural hematomas are distinguished from atherosclerotic plaque (which is typically focal, echobright, and irregular), in that they lie within the aortic wall and extend smoothly and longitudinally along the aorta. On cross-sectional views the hematoma appears as a crescentic or circular area of homogeneous thickening around the central aortic lumen. Unlike dissection, the intimal layer is still intact and is not mobilized, so there is no detectable intimal tear and no blood flow communication with the aortic lumen. If the intramural hematoma is relatively small, additional imaging with CT or MRA may be required to identify the hematoma definitively and distinguish it from the differential diagnoses of plaque or periaortic fat. Intramural hematomas can arise in either ascending or descending aortic locations and may enlarge or progress to frank aortic dissection and may have similar mortality rates. Thus the principles of medical and surgical management are essentially the same as for typical aortic dissections.[26]

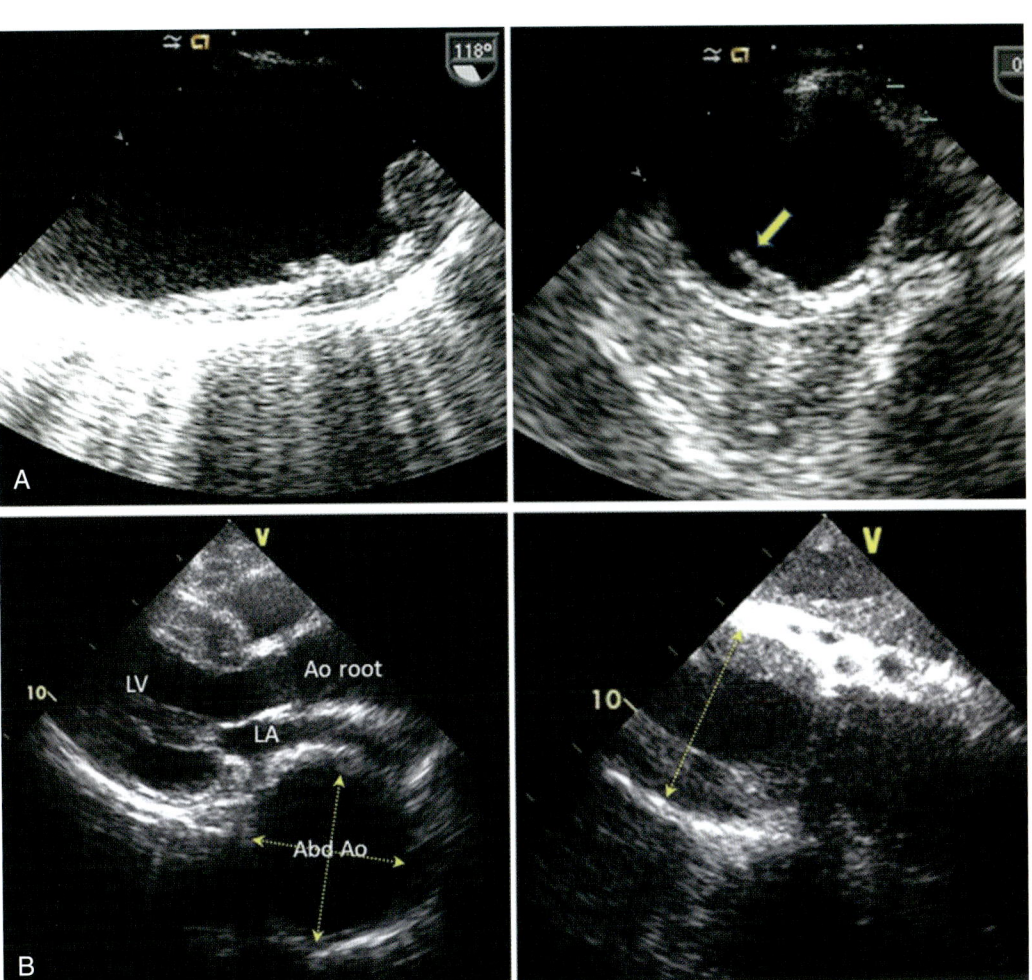

FIGURE 16.68 Aortic atheroma and aneurysm. **A,** TEE views of complex aortic atheroma in the ascending aorta. In the long-axis view **(left),** the atheroma is seen to be irregular and measures up to 1.0 cm in thickness. In the short-axis view **(right),** a protuberant finger-like atheroma is seen and is independently mobile. **B,** Transthoracic parasternal long-axis **(left)** and subcostal **(right)** views of a large 7-cm-diameter descending thoracoabdominal aortic aneurysm (dotted arrows spanning the diameter) compressing the posterior aspect of the left atrium (LA), within which diffuse circumferential thick mural thrombus is layered. Ao, Aortic; LV, left ventricle.

PULMONARY EMBOLISM (SEE CHAPTER 87)

Echocardiography can be extremely useful in the diagnosis and management of acute pulmonary embolism. Indeed, in the acutely unstable patient with known risk factors for hypercoagulability, echocardiographic evidence of RV dysfunction can prompt consideration for immediate reperfusion therapy without further testing.[73] For patients who are hemodynamically stable, however, CT pulmonary angiography is preferred for the definitive diagnosis of pulmonary embolism because of its higher accuracy. Echocardiography provides supplemental information, has prognostic value, and may inform or monitor therapy (particularly if CT angiography is not feasible). Echocardiography performed for other indications, including dyspnea, chest pain, and hypotension, also occasionally leads to the incidental discovery of pulmonary embolus as certain echocardiographic findings can be virtually pathognomonic.

The thrombi of pulmonary embolism generally arise from the deep venous system in the legs. Thus they may have a pathognomonic appearance of sausage-link like casts of the veins from which they have originated. Echocardiography may be used to directly visualize thrombus anywhere from the IVC to the mainstem pulmonary arteries (Fig. 16.71). Those in the pulmonary arteries generally can be visualized to just past the bifurcation with TTE; when found, they are associated with RV dysfunction and high early mortality. Although TEE can image slightly farther into the main pulmonary artery branches, it is not sensitive enough to be relied upon as a primary diagnostic modality for pulmonary embolism. The pulmonary artery bifurcation should be carefully assessed from the short-axis views in patients with suspected pulmonary embolism, and it is not uncommon for so-called saddle emboli to become lodged at the bifurcation (Fig. 16.71, right). Putative thrombi must be distinguished from other cardiac masses, including myxomas, fibroelastomas, and vegetations (see later, Cardiac Masses).

The characteristic echocardiographic findings in pulmonary embolism result in part from the unique physiology of the right ventricle and are summarized in Figure 16.72. The normal right ventricle is generally accustomed to low PVR and thus extremely low afterload, and RV systolic pressure normally is low. In acute pulmonary embolism, PVR rises substantially and abruptly, which results in RV dilation and, in severe cases, failure. Thus, RV dilation is the echocardiographic hallmark of pulmonary embolism, and is found in ≥ 25% of patients with pulmonary embolus. It is best visualized on the apical four-chamber view, where classic findings include RV diameter greater than LV diameter (ratio >1.0) and a small, underfilled, but normally functioning left ventricle. A distinctive regional wall motion abnormality has been recognized in acute pulmonary embolism in which the free RV midwall becomes dyskinetic, with relative sparing of the apex and base. This pattern, known as the *McConnell sign,* is highly specific for conditions in which PVR increases abruptly[74] but cannot be relied on to distinguish pulmonary embolus from other causes of respiratory decompensation. RV TAPSE may also be decreased in patients with acute pulmonary embolus. Both RV dilation and RV regional dysfunction will be less apparent in patients in whom PVR has been elevated for a longer period, resulting in RV hypertrophy. In these patients, pulmonary pressure will ultimately rise, and the right ventricle may not show evidence of acute dilation or dysfunction in acute pulmonary embolism. Thus the classic echocardiographic RV patterns are of lower sensitivity and have low negative predictive value in patients with longstanding pulmonary hypertension, such as those with chronic obstructive pulmonary disease (COPD) or chronic thromboembolic disease.

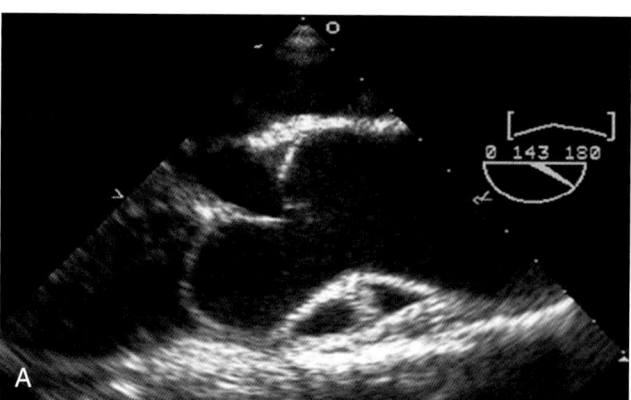
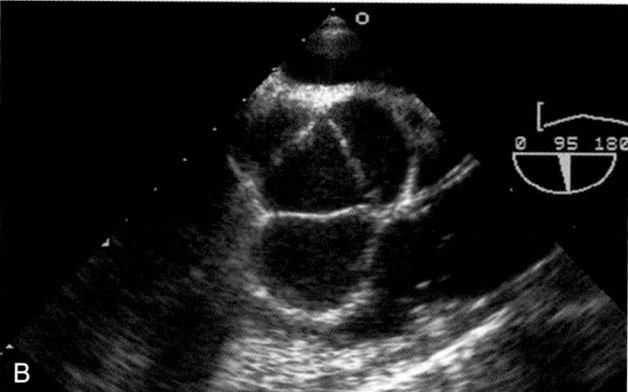

FIGURE 16.69 Sinus of Valsalva aneurysm. **A,** TEE long-axis view of a right sinus of Valsalva aneurysm (measuring 2.5 × 2.8 cm). **B,** TEE short-axis view of the trileaflet aortic valve in the open position showing the right sinus aneurysm in cross section. The patient had mild aortic insufficiency.

In patients without a previous history of pulmonary hypertension, even in the setting of acute pulmonary embolus, the TR velocity will remain relatively normal, rarely exceeding 3 m/sec. Patients with pre-existing pulmonary vascular disease, however, may have increased TR velocity consistent with elevated pulmonary systolic pressure. Assessment of RV dilation and dysfunction has now been incorporated into treatment algorithms and is particularly useful in triaging highly unstable and intermediate-risk patients.[73] Their presence is an independent predictor of adverse outcomes and short-term mortality, even in hemodynamically stable patients. In terms of response to therapy, improvement in RV function can be seen on echocardiography within several days of successful treatment—reperfusion by either embolectomy or thrombolysis—of pulmonary embolism.

PULMONARY HYPERTENSION (SEE CHAPTER 88)

Echocardiography can noninvasively assess for pulmonary hypertension and causative conditions. Pulmonary hypertension is defined by a mean pulmonary artery pressure of at least 20 to 25 mm Hg. It is classified as Group 1: pulmonary arterial hypertension; Group 2: due to left heart disease; Group 3: due to lung disease and/or chronic hypoxia; Group 4: due to pulmonary emboli and Group 5: due to blood and other disorders including sickle cell disease, in which pulmonary hypertension is an important cause of morbidity and mortality.

With the exception of some Group 2 cases, the common echocardiographic appearance is an enlarged right side with an intrinsically normal left ventricle but septal flattening in systole and diastole (Fig. 16.73). Echocardiography is well suited to identify underlying left heart pathology as well as other causes of pulmonary hypertension including congenital shunts (VSDs, PDAs or less commonly ASDs). In general, most of the indices of pulmonary artery pressure and right-sided heart failure (e.g., TAPSE, FAC) have been shown to be predictors of mortality in patients with diverse causes of pulmonary hypertension.[75]

2D echocardiographic findings in patients with pulmonary hypertension include flattening of the interventricular septum (predominantly in systole but often, due to concomitant RV dilation, in diastole as well), dilation of the pulmonary artery, RV hypertrophy, RV dilation, and ultimately RV dysfunction. Other signs are enlargement of the right atrium, dilation of the IVC and hepatic veins, loss of respirophasic size variation in the IVC and systolic notching of the pulmonic valve (dubbed the "flying W" sign). Typical Doppler findings include elevated TR velocity (≥3.0 m/sec), which is used to calculate the RVSP (See example in Fig. 16.73D). The calculation is based on the Bernoulli-derived pressure gradient between the right ventricle and right atrium and estimated RA pressure derived from the size and inspiratory collapsibility of the IVC. The equation for estimating PASP is:

$$PASP = 4\ (TRpeak\ velocity)^2 + RA\ pressure$$

where TRpeak velocity is measured in m/sec and RA pressure in mm Hg. In the absence of right ventricular outflow obstruction, the RVSP equals the PA systolic pressure (PASP). The normal IVC diameter measured 1 to 2 cm from the IVC-RA junction is less than 2.1 cm and normal collapsibility, elicited with a sniff, is at least 50%. If size and collapsibility are normal, the RA pressure is assumed to be 3 mm; if one is abnormal, 8 mm Hg; and if both are abnormal, 15 mm Hg (see Table 16.7).

If TR is not present or the TR jet is acquired off-axis, this measurement will be impossible to make or will underestimate the severity of pulmonary hypertension. Additionally in severe TR, the RA pressure is grossly elevated and the standard approach will underestimate PASP. A shortened PA acceleration time has also been reported as a Doppler marker of pulmonary hypertension but is limited by its reproducibility.

If there is pulmonic regurgitation, PA diastolic pressure can be calculated as the diastolic gradient between the PA and RV plus the RA pressure. Mean PA pressure can be calculated in one of several ways, most commonly by integration of the TR jet to determine mean RV to RA pressure gradient and adding RA pressure. In addition to PA pressure assessment, the PVR in Woods units (PVR) can be calculated non-invasively by using the formula:

$$PASP = 10\ (TRpeak\ velocity/VTI_{RVOT}) + 0.1$$

where TR peak velocity is measured in m/sec and VTI_{RVOT} in cm. This approach may have utility in distinguishing high PASP caused by increased pulmonary blood flow (as occurs in high-output states such as hyperthyroidism, anemia, and obesity) from that caused by elevated PVR.

Assessment of RV size and function is essential in pulmonary hypertension. RV FAC, TAPSE, RV Tei index, and tricuspid annular systolic velocity (S′) are typical quantitative measures to assess RV function in patients with pulmonary hypertension (see Table 16.6). RV longitudinal and free wall strain, as well as RV EF and increased RV indexed volumes as determined by 3D echocardiography are newer echocardiographic indices that have been shown to predict poor outcome in pulmonary hypertension.[75]

There are several features that may assist in distinguishing between pulmonary hypertension and acute pulmonary embolism on echocardiography. Acute pulmonary embolism is not usually associated with RV hypertrophy, elevation in PAP, or flattening of the interventricular septum in systole, unless there is pre-existing disease (e.g., longstanding thromboembolic disease with resultant pulmonary hypertension). In addition, the regional RV dysfunction in acute pulmonary embolism may spare the apex, whereas there is global RV hypokinesis in pulmonary hypertension.

INFECTIVE ENDOCARDITIS (SEE CHAPTER 80)

Echocardiography is the first-line modality in the diagnosis, evaluation, and management of endocarditis. The American College of Cardiology/American Heart Association guidelines regard echocardiography as a Class I indication in the following settings: (1) in patients with suspected endocarditis to characterize the hemodynamic severity of valvular lesions, assess ventricular function and pulmonary pressures, and detect complications; (2) TTE and/or TEE are recommended for

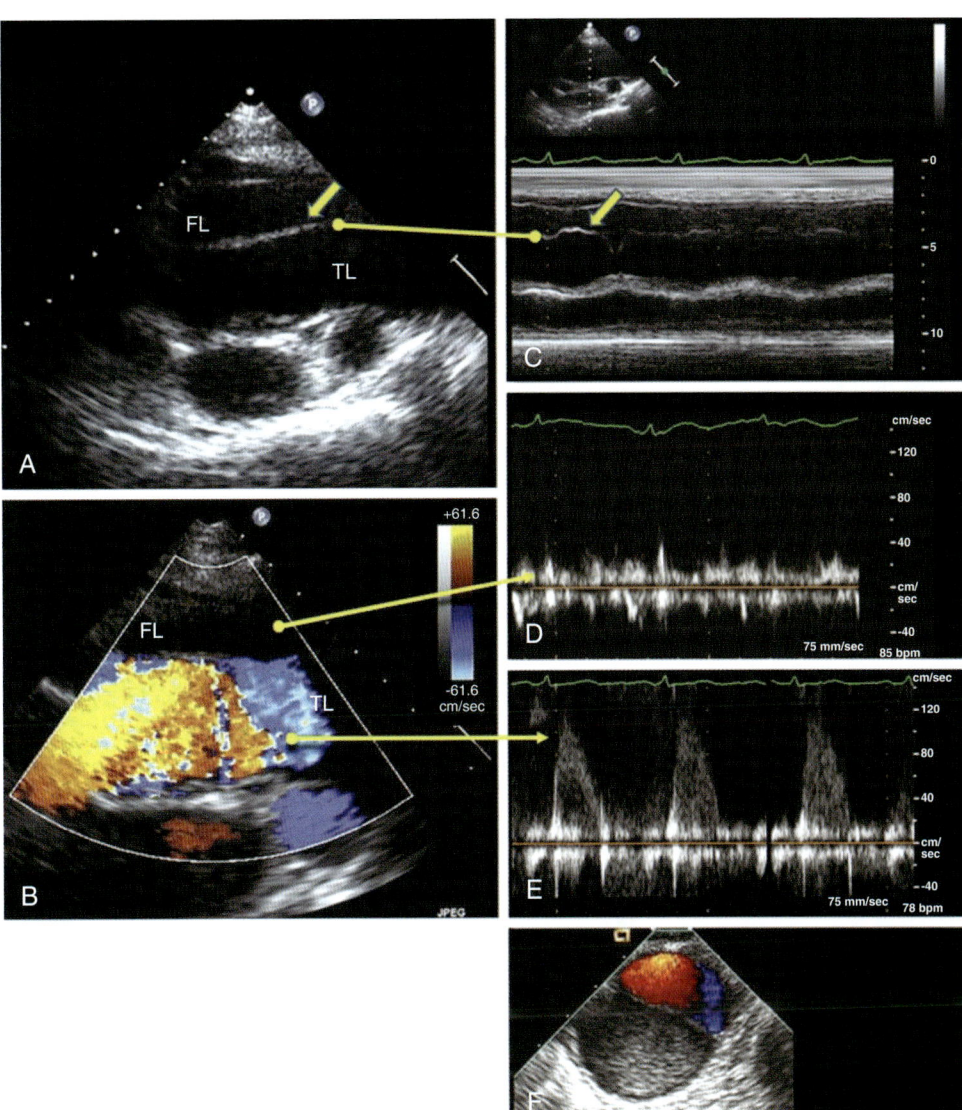

FIGURE 16.70 Aortic dissection demonstrating true and false lumens. **A,** TTE high parasternal long-axis view of a type A aortic dissection. The linear dissection flap is indicated by the *arrow*. *FL,* False lumen; *TL,* true lumen. **B,** TTE view at the same level with color flow Doppler illustrating brisk and turbulent color flow within the true lumen. **C,** M-mode illustrating systolic pulsation of the dissection flap *(arrow)* outward from the true aortic lumen. **D,** Low-velocity spectral Doppler flow without clear cyclic variation in the false lumen. **E,** Systolic forward high-velocity spectral Doppler flow in the true lumen. **F,** TEE short-axis view of the ascending aorta in a different type A dissection case demonstrating spontaneous echocardiographic contrast in the false (larger) lumen and brisk systolic flow in the true (smaller) lumen by color Doppler.

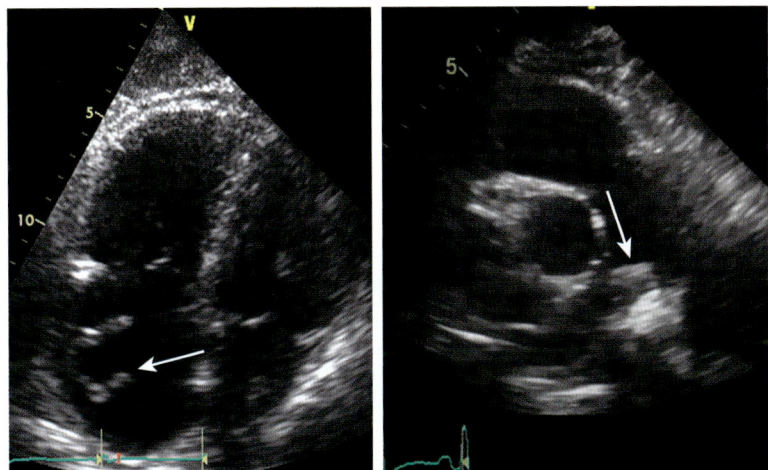

FIGURE 16.71 Left, Thromboembolus in the right atrium (*RA*). The *arrow* indicates a serpentine mass that is a thrombotic "cast" of a deep vein of the lower extremities that has embolized to the RA. Note the right-sided heart dilation and hypokinesis, clues indicating that a significant acute pulmonary embolus has also occurred. **Right,** Saddle embolus at the bifurcation of the pulmonary artery *(arrow)*.

re-evaluation of patients with endocarditis who have a change in clinical signs or symptoms (e.g., new murmur, embolism, persistent fever, HF, abscess, or atrioventricular heart block) and in patients at high risk of complications (e.g., extensive infected tissue/large vegetation on initial echocardiogram or staphylococcal, enterococcal, fungal infections); (3) in patients with known or suspected endocarditis, TEE is recommended when TTE is nondiagnostic, when complications have developed or are clinically suspected, or when intracardiac device leads are present; and (4) Intraoperative TEE should be performed for patients undergoing valve surgery for IE.[65,76] Following completion of antibiotic therapy, TTE is also recommended to re-evaluate cardiac and valve structure and function.

Infective endocarditis is definitively diagnosed by culture or pathologic examination of a vegetation (in situ or embolized) or intracardiac abscess. However, many cases are diagnosed on clinical grounds by using the modified Duke criteria as a guideline. The first criterion is positive blood cultures consistent with infective endocarditis. The second major criterion is an echocardiogram demonstrating (1) a vegetation (Fig. 16.74AB) (an oscillating intracardiac mass on a valve, in the path of a regurgitant jet, or on implanted material) in the absence of an alternative anatomic explanation, (2) an abscess or pseudoaneurysm (Fig. 16.74C), or (3) new partial dehiscence of a prosthetic valve (Fig. 16.74D).[76] Variations on the extent and location of destroyed endocardial tissue can lead to distinct associated pathologies such as pseudoaneurysms, leaflet aneurysms or perforations, and fistulas between neighboring cavities.

The sensitivity of TTE ranges up to 63% (up to 71% in patients without prosthetic valves), with a specificity close to 100%. Endocarditis of the mitral and aortic valves are unlikely without evidence of regurgitation. The suboptimal sensitivity often results from physical imaging factors causing poor image quality and acoustic shadowing and also depends on the size of the vegetation. Because of its higher 2D resolution and different windows, TEE has much higher sensitivity (94% to 100%) and is especially advantageous in assessing prosthetic valves and diagnosing paravalvular extension of infection with abscess. Thus, a reasonable diagnostic approach is to use TTE as the first-line screening tool; if this is nondiagnostic, one may turn to TEE if clinical suspicion for endocarditis is

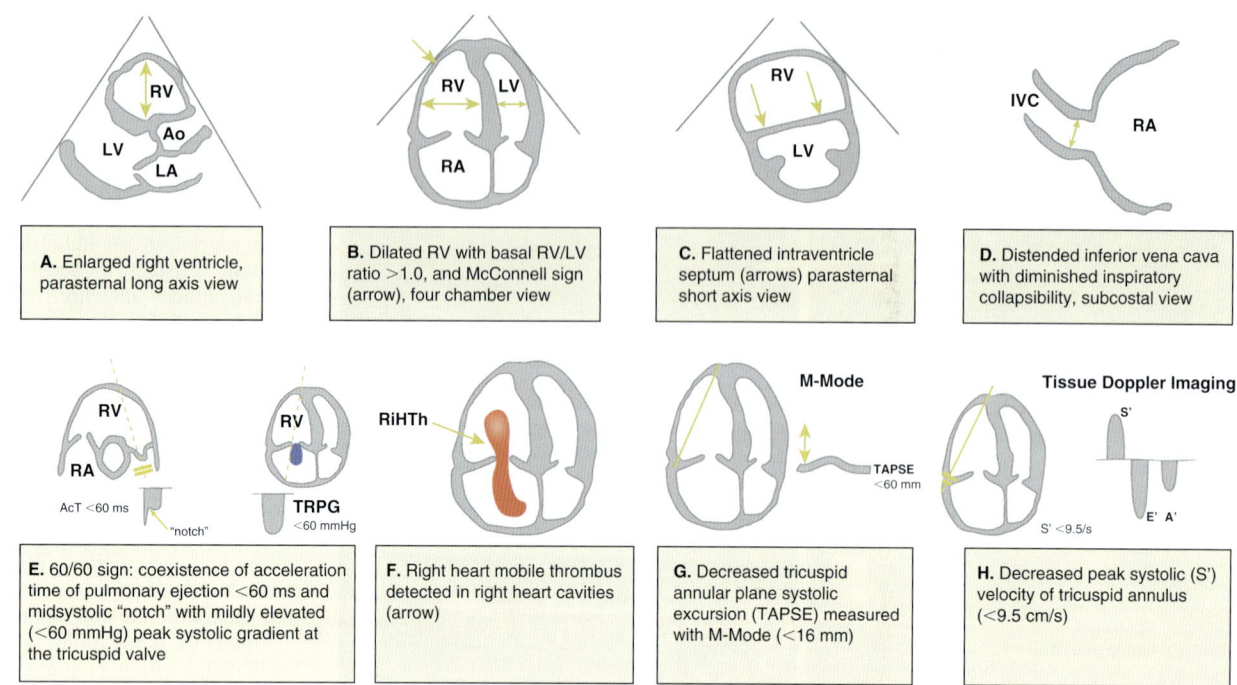

FIGURE 16.72 Echocardiographic signs of RV pressure overload that may be associated with pulmonary embolus. *A′*, peak late diastolic (during atrial contraction) velocity of tricuspid annulus by tissue Doppler imaging; *AcT*, right ventricular outflow Doppler acceleration time; *Ao*, aorta; *E′*, peak early diastolic velocity of tricuspid annulus by tissue Doppler imaging; *IVC*, inferior vena cava; *LA*, left atrium; *LV*, left ventricle; *RA*, right atrium; *RiHTh*, right heart thrombus (or thrombi); *RV*, right ventricle/ventricular; *S′*, peak systolic velocity of tricuspid annulus by tissue Doppler imaging; *TAPSE*, tricuspid annular plane systolic excursion; *TRPG*, tricuspid valve peak systolic gradient. (From Konstantinides SV, Meyer G, Becattini C, et al. 2019 ESC guidelines on the diagnosis and management of acute pulmonary embolism developed in collaboration with the European Respiratory Society (ERS): The Task Force for the diagnosis and management of acute pulmonary embolism of the European Society of Cardiology (ESC). *Eur Heart J.* 2020;41:543.)

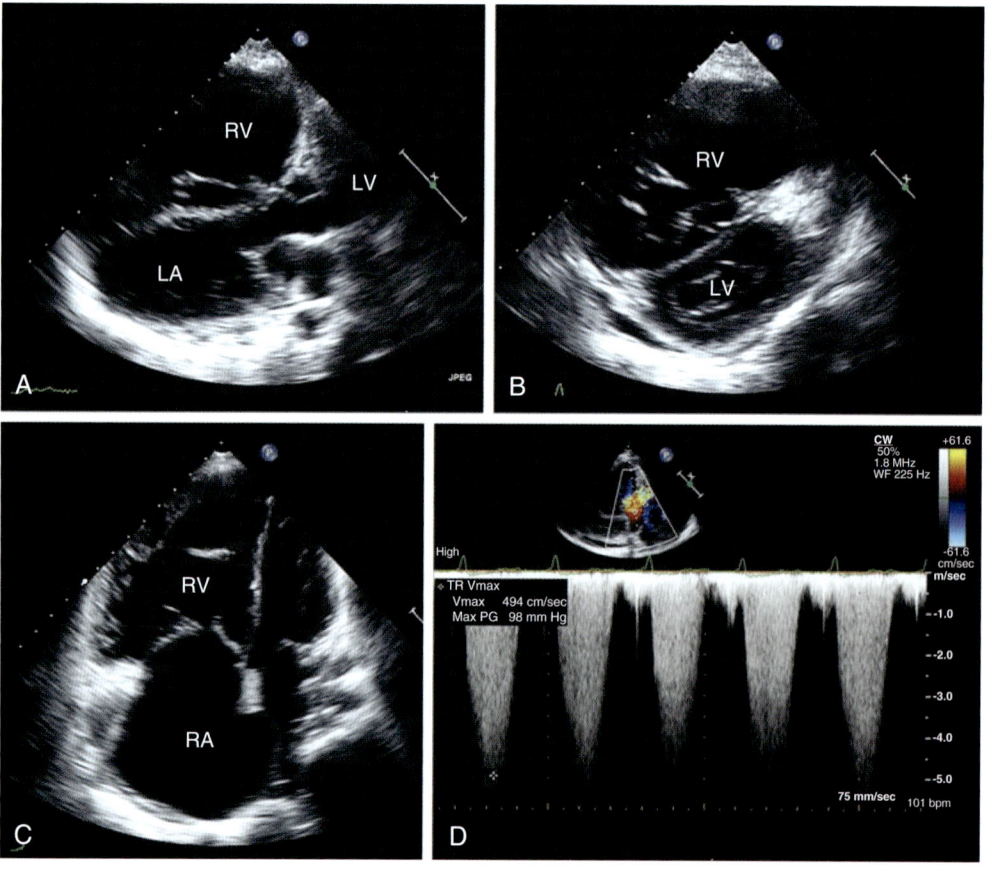

FIGURE 16.73 Pulmonary hypertension secondary to chronic thromboembolic disease. **A,** Parasternal long-axis view illustrating a small left ventricular cavity and enlarged right ventricular outflow tract. **B,** Parasternal short-axis view demonstrating the D-shaped left ventricular cavity caused by systolic and diastolic septal flattening, i.e., pancyclic elevated right ventricular pressure. **C,** Apical four-chamber view. Note the dilated right atrium and tricuspid annulus with incomplete closure of the tricuspid valve, as well as leftward distention of the interatrial septum. **D,** Severe tricuspid regurgitation (TR) with an elevated TR velocity corresponding to a calculated right ventricular systolic pressure of 98 mm Hg plus right atrial pressure. The upslope of the tricuspid regurgitant jet is slow, indicative of poor right ventricular contractility. *LA,* Left atrium; *LV,* left ventricle; *RA,* right atrium; *RV,* right ventricle.

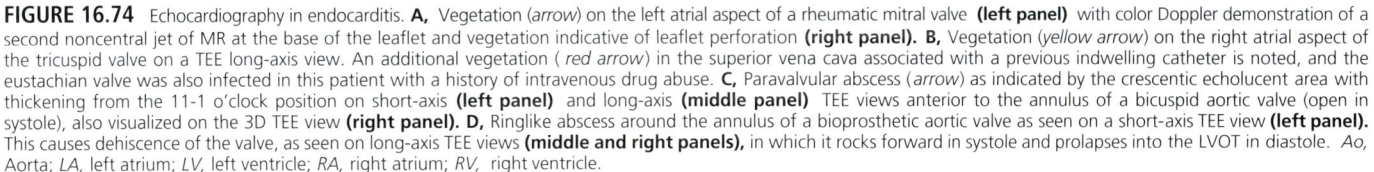

FIGURE 16.74 Echocardiography in endocarditis. **A,** Vegetation (*arrow*) on the left atrial aspect of a rheumatic mitral valve **(left panel)** with color Doppler demonstration of a second noncentral jet of MR at the base of the leaflet and vegetation indicative of leaflet perforation **(right panel)**. **B,** Vegetation (*yellow arrow*) on the right atrial aspect of the tricuspid valve on a TEE long-axis view. An additional vegetation (*red arrow*) in the superior vena cava associated with a previous indwelling catheter is noted, and the eustachian valve was also infected in this patient with a history of intravenous drug abuse. **C,** Paravalvular abscess (*arrow*) as indicated by the crescentic echolucent area with thickening from the 11-1 o'clock position on short-axis **(left panel)** and long-axis **(middle panel)** TEE views anterior to the annulus of a bicuspid aortic valve (open in systole), also visualized on the 3D TEE view **(right panel)**. **D,** Ringlike abscess around the annulus of a bioprosthetic aortic valve as seen on a short-axis TEE view **(left panel)**. This causes dehiscence of the valve, as seen on long-axis TEE views **(middle and right panels)**, in which it rocks forward in systole and prolapses into the LVOT in diastole. *Ao*, Aorta; *LA*, left atrium; *LV*, left ventricle; *RA*, right atrium; *RV*, right ventricle.

high, as in the patient with a prosthetic valve or predisposing condition, clinical features suspicious for a complicated endocarditis, or a potential indication for cardiac surgery.[78] Selected patients with suspected endocarditis—often those with obscured areas or acoustic shadowing on echocardiography, degenerative changes that are difficult to distinguish from infectious processes, vascular grafts, or those at high risk of complications during TEE—will benefit from additional imaging with other techniques such as CT angiography, CMR, or metabolic imaging modalities such as FDG PET or white blood cell imaging. These complementary modalities are particularly helpful in the setting of prosthetic valves (see Multimodality Imaging and Future Directions).

Vegetations appear as discrete echogenic masses that are adherent to but have motion that is distinct from that of valve itself. A typical mitral vegetation is shown in Fig. 16.74A. Characteristics of vegetations that aid in distinguishing them from other masses include localization, texture, motion, shape, and associated abnormalities. Vegetations are typically located on the upstream, or low-pressure, sides of valves (i.e., the atrial aspect of atrioventricular valves or the ventricular aspect of semilunar valves); less often, they are attached to the periphery of septal defects (on the low-pressure side), to chordae, or to the mural endocardium. The *echodensity* of a vegetation is usually similar to that of myocardium, although advanced vegetations can be inhomogeneous, with findings indicative of liquefaction (which is echolucent) or fibrosis/calcification (which is echodense or bright). Independent *motion* of vegetations is often described as oscillating or erratic. Large vegetations can create a "ball-and-chain" effect that causes leaflet prolapse and flail into the upstream chamber and consequent regurgitation. Vegetations vary tremendously in *shape* but often appear as compact multilobulated or pedunculated, amorphous, and friable agglomerations compared with tumor tissue or thrombus. The vegetation can extend some distance from the valve to which it is tethered and may occur in multiples on the same or different valves. *Associated abnormalities* such as regurgitation, abscesses, leaflet perforation, and intracardiac fistulas can accompany advanced endocarditis. 3D TEE appears to provide more accurate assessment of overall vegetation size, and in some cases can better visualize and define the extent of complications involving valves and surrounding anatomic structures.[78] There are no distinguishing characteristics that are organism specific, although staphylococcal infections (particularly methicillin-resistant *Staphylococcus aureus* and *S. lugdunensis*) tend to be more destructive and form abscesses, and fungal infections are often impressively large and dendritic in appearance.

Vegetations devoid of microorganisms are the hallmark of *noninfectious endocarditis*, also called "nonbacterial thrombotic" or "nonbacterial marantic" endocarditis (see Chapter 80). The typical lesions are small (1 to 5 mm), verrucous, nondestructive nodules that adhere to the upstream side of the valve (typically mitral or aortic) along the line of closure and contain only cellular and fibrin elements. These aseptic lesions are seen in up to 43% of patients with systemic lupus erythematosus (SLE) and 29% of those with antiphospholipid syndrome (APS), in whom they can cause cerebral embolization. These also occur in patients with advanced neoplasms, sepsis, and prothrombotic tendencies in association with clinical features indistinguishable from those of typical infective endocarditis (see later, Systemic Diseases and Echocardiography).[77]

It is important to note that the presence of preexisting thickening and degenerative changes in leaflets can render the diagnosis challenging. On occasion, myxomatous leaflets, ruptured chordae, calcified structures, and fibrin strands can either mask or mimic a vegetation. Papillary fibroelastomas and thrombi can resemble valvular vegetations. In these circumstances, clinical correlation with other Duke diagnostic criteria is important. Comparison with previous echocardiograms should also be undertaken; a stable finding over years is unlikely to represent a vegetation. Use of TEE for higher-resolution images is often indicated, particularly if a cardiac device is involved, a complication (e.g., embolization, valve destruction, abscess) is suspected or an aggressive organism such as *S. aureus* is involved.[78,79]

Among patients with endocarditis, 66% to 75% have risk factors for infection, and echocardiography should be used to scrutinize the relevant structures at risk particularly carefully. Patients with any type of prosthetic valve or closure device, complex cyanotic congenital heart disease, and surgical systemic-pulmonary shunts are at relatively high risk. Previous endocarditis and IV drug abuse are strong predisposing factors for tricuspid and pulmonic valve endocarditis. Those with bicuspid aortic valves, rheumatic heart disease, or mitral valve prolapse are predisposed but at lower risk. Other intracardiac structures that are prone to infection, usually at the time of placement or access, include defibrillator/pacemaker wires and chronic indwelling IV catheters, particularly when used for total parenteral nutrition or hemodialysis in immunocompromised patients. Echocardiographic characteristics associated with a poorer prognosis and/or embolization include vegetation size greater than 1.0 cm on 2D images (which confers a 2.5-fold higher risk for embolization, especially if on the mitral valve), increasing size of the vegetation over time despite therapy, very mobile vegetation, and paravalvular abscess. The latter is more common with prosthetic valves and increases mortality twofold. Other findings such as severe left-sided regurgitation or prosthetic valve dysfunction, low LVEF, pulmonary hypertension, and premature mitral valve closure or other signs of elevated diastolic pressures also portend poor outcome.[76,79]

The natural history of vegetations after medical therapy is of interest because most will still be apparent on follow-up echocardiography in 1 to 2 months, even after successful medical treatment. Approximately half will become more echodense over time. These observations probably reflect the varied components of the vegetation, which include not only bacteria but also inflammatory cells, fibroblasts, and extracellular matrix. Growth of a vegetation over time and increasing valvular regurgitation are additional poor prognostic signs. However, the mere persistence of vegetations in the absence of symptoms or positive blood cultures is not associated with increased clinical complications. Thus, treatment of endocarditis should not be guided by the echocardiographic morphology of the vegetation over time but by clinical response to therapy.

Role of Echocardiography in Surgery for Endocarditis

If left untreated, infective vegetations are destructive via pathways that are apparent on echocardiograms and ECGs and by clinical sequelae. If present, these sequelae are indications for surgery, particularly if recalcitrant to medical therapy. Indications include (1) embolism to the coronary arteries, brain, lungs, spleen, kidney, or extremities; (2) severe valvular regurgitation and heart failure secondary to leaflet malcoaptation, perforations, or flail; (3) abscess, which may invade the cardiac conduction system; (4) mycotic aneurysms of vessels and valves; (5) pseudoaneurysms or fistulas of the heart; and (6) suppurative or hemorrhagic pericarditis.

Typical paravalvular extension patterns can be detected on echocardiograms (and ECGs). At the *aortic valve*, involvement of the right cusp can lead to necrosis of the membranous interventricular septum, aneurysm of the right sinus of Valsalva, and, prosthetic valve dehiscence. Embolization into the RCA can also occur and cause MI. Involvement of the left cusp can affect the intervalvular fibrosa and extend to infect the base of the anterior mitral valve leaflet. There is also the potential to form an aortic-to-LVOT fistula, or prosthetic paravalvular leak. Involvement of the noncoronary cusp can extend to the posterior interventricular septum, where the His conduction fibers are located, which can lead to the development of an intra- or infra-hisian block (third-degree atrioventricular block) or bundle branch block.

Severe infection of the *mitral valve* less frequently leads to conduction disturbances. Although first- or second-degree atrioventricular block can occur, supraventricular tachycardias are more common. *Tricuspid valve* infection can extend to involve the tricuspid annulus and eustachian valves (Fig. 16.74B), seed the pulmonic valve, and cause septic pulmonary emboli in 25% to 80% of cases.

SYSTEMIC DISEASES AND ECHOCARDIOGRAPHY

Aside from conditions that directly affect the heart itself, many systemic diseases with cardiac manifestations are detectable on echocardiography. Uncontrolled hypertension causes symmetrically increased wall thickness and LV hypertrophy in association with LA enlargement and diastolic dysfunction. Renal disease causes early calcification of the valves and potentially uremic pericardial effusions. Hypothyroidism can be associated with a myxedematous pericardial effusion. COPD can cause conspicuous right-sided heart enlargement, RV hypertrophy, elevated TR velocity, and a prominent pericardial fat pad secondary to corticosteroid treatment.

There are diseases that affect all tissue layers of the heart. Amyloidosis is notorious for causing restrictive cardiomyopathy (see earlier and Fig. 16.27F), but also frequently causes valvular thickening and pericardial effusions. Infiltration of amyloid into the atrial walls leads to poor atrial contractility and a high prevalence of atrial thrombi, even when sinus rhythm is still present.[47] Granulomatous diseases such as sarcoidosis can cause a focal myocarditis with granulomas, which results in very localized areas of akinesis in a noncoronary distribution. Pericarditis, valvulitis, and also coronary and aortic arteritis have been reported with Wegener granulomatosis. Although scleroderma is known to cause direct myocardial fibrosis histologically, on echocardiography this becomes apparent in only a minority of patients, usually late in the course of disease. Instead, the most common echocardiographic abnormalities in scleroderma are elevated RV systolic pressure, RV dilation, and pericardial effusion, as well as LA enlargement and diastolic dysfunction.

Other diseases that have echocardiographic manifestations include human immunodeficiency virus (HIV) infection (see Chapter 85), in which the most common abnormalities are dilated cardiomyopathy, pericardial effusion (seen in 12% to 25% of cases), and also HIV-related pulmonary hypertension and cardiac lymphomas. The prolonged duration of HIV infection and combination antiretroviral therapy regimens may contribute directly and indirectly (via lipodystrophic effects and chronic inflammation) to both cardiomyopathy and the excess risk of CAD in this population. Overall however, with increasing access to combination antiretroviral therapy, the prevalence of clinically significant HIV-associated cardiomyopathy and pericardial effusions appears to be decreasing.[80]

Similarly, even when cancers spare the heart by way of direct involvement, the radiation and chemotherapy regimens used to attack the neoplasms can have cardiac effects (see Chapters 56 and 57). Ideally, the early detection of cardiomyopathy in patients who receive chemotherapy, particularly with anthracyclines (as well as tyrosine kinase inhibitors and immunomodulators), allows modification of the protocol before irreversible damage occurs. Screening for LVEF is the most widely used strategy (with a suggested cutoff of decline in LVEF ≥10% to an absolute value < 53% as a sign of LV dysfunction), but a decrease in peak systolic GLS (>15% change from baseline) is a more sensitive and earlier predictor of cardiotoxicity.[81,82] Baseline and serial determination of GLS is becoming more widely accepted as reproducibility improves and vendors converge to standardize measurements. It is not yet known if decrements in GLS during chemotherapy will predict chronic irreversible heart failure, and thus it remains to be seen if cancer treatment should be altered based on a new reduction in GLS alone. Aside from chemotherapy damage, survivors of Hodgkin disease also frequently have early thickening and stenosis of the aortic and less commonly mitral valves, as well as accelerated CAD from radiotherapy. Hence, screening echocardiograms for even asymptomatic patients who have had radiation therapy are recommended at 10 years post-radiation and every 5 years thereafter. For symptomatic patients with valvular disease, echocardiography is suggested annually.

Several other conditions predispose to valvular abnormalities (see earlier, Valvular Heart Disease). Rheumatic carditis and its sequelae are well-known historical examples and are still a significant cause of heart disease in developing nations (see Chapter 81). Up to 60% of patients with carcinoid tumors have cardiac involvement in which plaquelike deposits build up on the right- sided heart valves (typically the ventricular aspect of the tricuspid valve and the arterial aspect of the pulmonic valve). This causes a characteristic retracted fixed, "half-open" appearance of the tricuspid and pulmonary leaflets and a combination of valvular stenosis and regurgitation (see Fig. 16.49). Cardiac involvement confers a worse median survival time for carcinoid. The hematologic malignancies and any thrombophilic state (e.g., sepsis, disseminated intravascular coagulation, SLE, APS) can cause nonbacterial marantic endocarditis in which the sterile vegetations and fibrin strands undergo frequent cycles of growth and subsequent fragmentation and embolization, with associated valvulitis and leaflet destruction. The systemic vasculitides such as Takayasu arteritis and Behçet disease are notable causes of AR and aortic root dilatation, particularly in younger patients.[83]

CARDIAC MASSES (SEE CHAPTER 98)

Cardiac tumors are relatively rare, ranging from an incidence of 1% to 2% in general autopsy series but up to 4% to 8% in cancer patient autopsies, so routine screening is not recommended. Among primary tumors of the heart, up to 90% or more are detected incidentally and three quarters are benign. It is the location of an intracardiac or extracardiac mass—in the context of the patient's age, clinical findings, and comorbidities—that is often the best indicator of the type of tumor; morphologic features of the mass play a secondary role in identification (Table 16.11).[84]

Nonetheless, the overall appearance of the mass (with respect to size, solid versus cystic, shape, degree of independent mobility, and fragility), its attachments, and the extent of myocardial, endocardial, or pericardial invasion can offer clues to its nature. Calcified or fibrotic areas appear echobright, whereas cystic degeneration causes echolucent foci on echocardiography. Obstruction to caval or valvular inflow will cause increases in peak spectral Doppler velocities, often with a mosaic color Doppler pattern signifying turbulent flow. MS and MR caused by an LA myxoma prolapsing across the mitral valve is a classic example (Fig. 16.75). When myxomas present this way, the echocardiographic appearance of this entity may be so pathognomonic that no further workup is required before surgical resection. Although 70% of myxomas originate from the left side of the fossa ovalis, they may arise in other locations and may be multiple, so that complete echocardiographic evaluation of the heart is indicated. Similarly, papillary fibroelastomas occur so characteristically on the aortic and mitral valves and are so commonly seen as filamentous or amorphous growths that shimmer, undulate, and prolapse, that further assessment may not be required before surgery (Fig. 16.76). However, the smaller lesions may be difficult to differentiate from highly mobile Lambl excrescences or even vegetation.

In select patients, to refine the diagnostic possibilities, IV echocardiographic contrast material may be used to determine whether a tumor hyperenhances. Hyperenhancement indicates that the mass is neovascularized and thus more likely to be malignant than a benign stromal tumor or thrombus.[21] One can also use 3D echocardiography to better illustrate the overall size, location, and attachments of intracavitary masses. Following diagnosis, echocardiography is a convenient way to monitor for recurrence, growth, or adverse sequelae after excision or treatment.[85]

COMMON PRIMARY TUMORS

Myxoma accounts for more than 50% of primary cardiac tumors in adults, followed by papillary fibroelastomas and lipomas. Myxoma is a primary benign tumor believed to arise from mesenchymal (endocardial) cells. It typically arises in the left atrium (75% of cases, with the other 20% occurring in the right atrium and 5% in the ventricles) and is attached to the interatrial septum near the fossa ovalis by a stalklike pedicle. Attachments to the mitral valve have been described in a small percentage of cases. Grossly and on echocardiography, myxoma frequently appears as a gelatinous, compact mass, but there is a spectrum of morphologies. Smaller tumors tend to be more papillary or villous and are friable and thus prone to embolize. Larger myxomas have a smoother, globular, or grape cluster–like appearance and can grow large enough to fill the left atrium and cause both MS and a renowned tumor "plop" on auscultation as the mass prolapses into the left ventricle in diastole (see Fig. 16.75). Approximately 7% of cases result from an autosomal dominant mutation and are part of the "Carney complex" syndrome, associated with skin lentiginosis and endocrine disorders.[85]

In adults, *papillary fibroelastomas* are the next most common cardiac benign tumors and the most common valvular tumor. Most (>80%) are found on left-sided (aortic or mitral) valves, although any valve may be affected, and 9% occur as multiple lesions. Pathologists usually classify fibroelastomas as an advanced or more florid form of *Lambl excrescences*, which are degenerative changes in the valves. Fibroelastomas tend to appear on either side of the aortic valve or on the atrial side of the mitral valve. Less frequently, they have also been known to arise on mitral chordae or papillary muscles. On echocardiography, papillary fibroelastomas appear round, oval, or irregular in shape and homogeneous in texture (see Fig. 16.76). Almost half have a short stalk, which confers more mobility. Fibroelastomas are found most frequently in older adults as solitary lesions. Shedding of the threadlike elements and associated clot accounts for their frequent manifestation as embolization (transient ischemic attack or stroke, angina, or sudden death).[84,85]

Lipomas are encapsulated collections of benign fat cells that tend to occur in subepicardial or subendocardial locations and may grow into the pericardial space. Although benign, usually discovered incidentally, and easily distinguished by CMR characteristics (see Chapter 19), these tumors tend to increase progressively and can cause mass effect, heart block, or tachyarrhythmias. *Lipomatous hypertrophy of the interatrial septum* is a generally benign finding, particularly in elderly or obese patients and is technically hyperplasia of epicardial adipocytes within the groove between the LA and RA walls and inferior pyramidal space, which spares the fossa ovalis and produces a characteristic dumbbell-shaped mass. Although lipomatous hypertrophy is unencapsulated and may reach an impressive thickness (1 to 2 cm or more), if the location is typical and no associated atrial arrhythmias or caval obstruction are present, no treatment is indicated.[86]

Pericardial cysts are benign fluid-filled tumors of the parietal pericardium and are thought to be a congenital abnormality.[72,87] They may be solitary or multilocular, and some have been documented to grow to massive (>20 cm) size. They account for approximately 20% of benign primary cardiac masses (overall incidence of 1 in 10,000) and usually occur near the cardiophrenic borders (right more often than the left). This gives the appearance of cardiomegaly on chest radiographs and an encapsulated echolucent mass on echocardiography. Among known cases, 75% are asymptomatic. If large, however, pericardial cysts may cause atypical chest pain, breathlessness, AF, persistent cough, or compressive problems such as RVOT obstruction. Rare cases of cardiac tamponade secondary to intrapericardial rupture and hemorrhage have been reported.

Rhabdomyomas are the most common primary cardiac neoplasm in children and are usually found during the first year of life. They tend to be solid intramyocardial lesions containing striated myocyte fibers, and 90% occur as multiple tumors. Although most patients are asymptomatic, larger tumors have been known to cause arrhythmias, LVOT obstruction, and heart failure. Half the cases are associated with tuberous sclerosis. Most regress spontaneously, and overall these tumors are rare in young adults.[84,85]

Fibromas are the second most common pediatric cardiac neoplasm. They arise in the ventricular myocardial layer, are five times more common in the left ventricle, and consist of solid tumors containing fibroblasts. These tumors often occur in the LV septum or free wall, where they appear broad-based and can become quite large and develop calcific foci. Unlike rhabdomyomas, fibromas do not spontaneously regress and may grow to a size that obliterates the heart chamber, interferes with valvular function, or causes arrhythmia and thus necessitates surgical resection.[85]

Secondary Tumors

Secondary cardiac tumors outnumber primary ones by 20 to 40 to 1. In principle, any malignant tumor may metastasize to the heart. The most

TABLE 16.11 Site-Specific Differential Diagnosis of Cardiac Tumors

SITE	ONCOLOGIC	ALSO CONSIDER NON-NEOPLASTIC MASSES	NORMAL OR VARIANT STRUCTURES
Left atrium	Myxoma Lipoma Bronchogenic carcinoma Sarcoma (involving the wall/pericardium) Hemangioma Paraganglioma	Thrombus Endocardial blood cyst	Lipomatous hypertrophy of interatrial septum External compression (by hernia, thoracic aorta, bezoar) Echocardiographic artefact: left upper pulmonary vein limbus ("Coumadin ridge") Appendage pectinate muscles Atrial suture anastomosis after heart transplantation Inverted LA appendage (postoperative) Aberrant LA chorda
Right atrium	Myxoma Nephroblastoma, renal cell cancer Hepatocellular carcinoma Sarcoma (angiosarcoma) Paraganglioma Adrenal tumors	Thrombus (deep venous or in situ) or fibrin casts (of previous indwelling catheter/wire) Vegetation (on pacer/ICD wires) Lipomatous hypertrophy of interatrial septum	Eustachian valve Chiari network Crista terminalis Interatrial septal aneurysm Pectus excavatum
Left ventricle	Rhabdomyoma (often multiple) Fibroma Hamartomas Purkinje cell tumors (usually infants)	Thrombus Apical hypertrophic cardiomyopathy Subaortic membrane	Calcified or multilobed papillary muscles Redundant or severed mitral chordae Trabeculations, false tendons Focal upper septal hypertrophy Swirling from inhomogeneous intravenous echocardiographic contrast distribution
Right ventricle	Rhabdomyoma Fibroma	Thrombus	Redundant tricuspid chordae Tricuspid papillary muscle Moderator band
Valves/annuli	Papillary fibroelastoma Myxoma Hamartoma Lipomas	Lambl excrescences Focal or caseous mitral annular calcification Vegetation Marantic endocarditis Thrombus (especially on prosthetics) Pannus (especially on prosthetics) Abscess Blood cyst Rheumatoid nodule	Nodules of Arantius Myxomatous/degenerative changes Pannus; loose suture; bioglue or pledgets around prosthetic valves
Pericardium	Malignant involvement from lung, breast, lymphoma/leukemia, or gastrointestinal tract melanoma Mesothelioma Primary: spindle cell tumor, fibrous tumors, lipoma, liposarcoma, teratoma Paraganglioma	Pericardial or bronchogenic cyst Rheumatoid nodule Thrombus Hydatid cyst (*Echinococcus*)	Epicardial or mediastinal fat Pectus excavatum Atelectatic lung or fibrin in pleural/peritoneal spaces Vascular pseudoaneurysm Thymus (in infants)

ICD, Implantable cardioverter-defibrillator; *LA*, left atrial.
Modified from Wu J. Cardiac tumors and masses. In: Stergiopoulos K, Brown DL, eds. *Evidence-Based Cardiology Consult*. New York: Springer Science + Business Media; 2014.

common site of involvement is the pericardium, with invasion of the myocardium seen next in frequency.[84]

Pericardial involvement in cancers may arise from direct invasion of tumor from adjacent lung or mediastinum (e.g., mesothelioma, lymphoma), or there may be more diffuse involvement and effusive/constrictive changes. The most frequent sources of malignant pericardial disease are lung cancer, lymphoma/leukemia, and breast cancer because of their relatively high prevalence, and proximity to the heart. Metastatic pericardial disease may invade the myocardium as well. Of all malignancies, *melanoma* has the highest predilection to metastasize to the heart and pericardium. Cardiac metastases from any source typically are small and multiple or cause effusion or diffuse thickening of the pericardium. However, bulky large solitary tumor lesions may also occur and, unlike benign tumors, may extend from the blood pool into the myocardium or pericardium (see Fig. 16.65).

Secondary tumors may also invade the heart by direct extension[85]: renal cell carcinoma, Wilms tumor, uterine leiomyosarcoma, hepatomas, angiosarcomas, and adrenal tumors can be detected extending into the right atrium via the IVC on echocardiography. Bronchogenic carcinomas can invade the left atrium through the pulmonary veins. An important teaching point is that all four pulmonary veins should be comprehensively evaluated when a left atrial mass is identified.

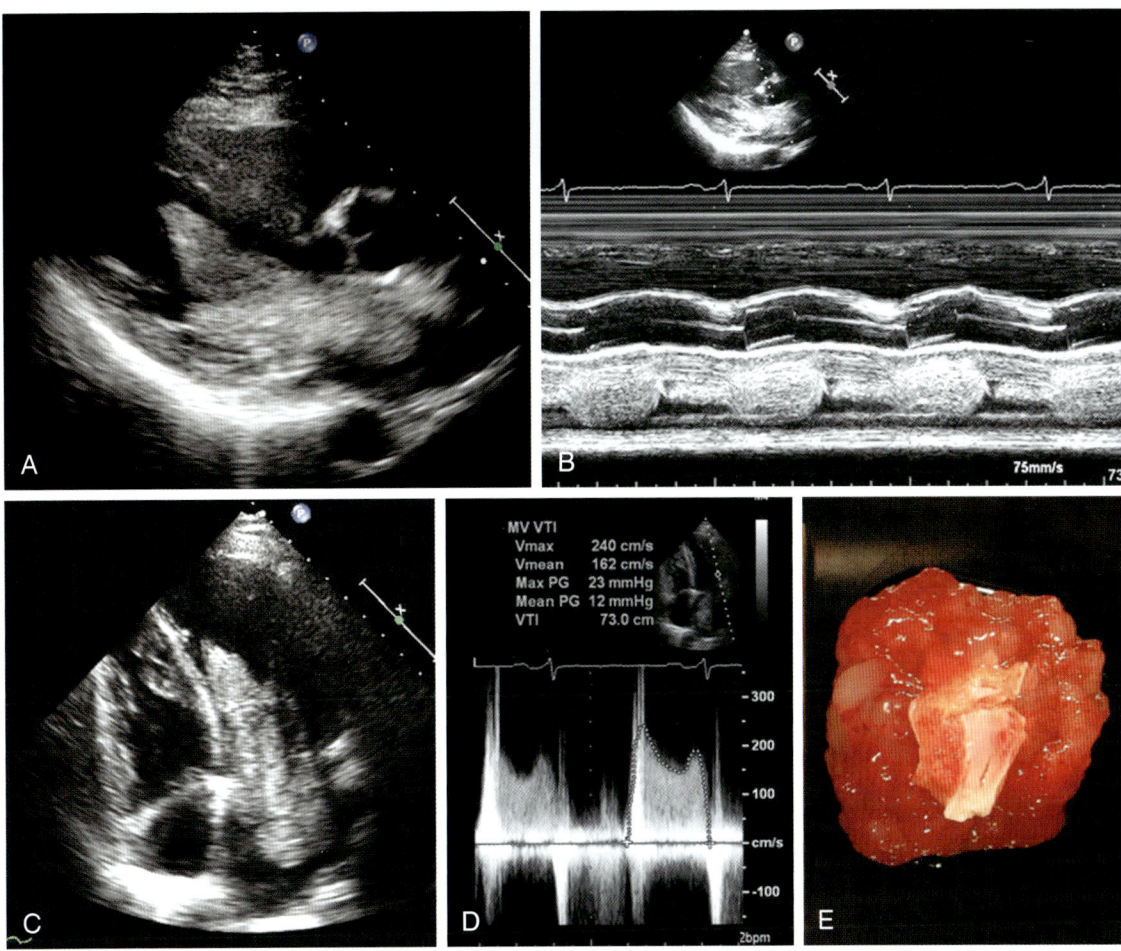

FIGURE 16.75 Left atrial myxoma. **A,** Parasternal long-axis view. **B,** M-mode view showing the mass prolapsing through the mitral valve into the left ventricle in diastole. **C,** Apical 4-chamber view. **D,** Transmitral gradients (mitral stenosis) as shown by CW Doppler, with peak and mean gradients of 23 and 12 mm Hg. **E,** Gross pathological specimen. (Modified from Wu J. Cardiac tumors and masses. In Stergiopoulos K, Brown DL, eds. *Evidence-Based Cardiology Consult*. New York: Springer Science + Business Media; 2014.)

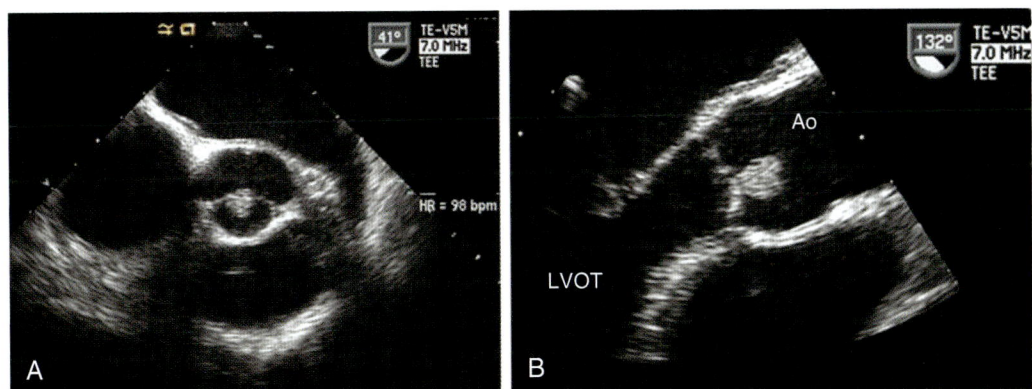

FIGURE 16.76 Papillary fibroelastoma on the aortic valve. **A,** TEE short-axis view showing the mass on the aortic aspect of the noncoronary cusp. **B,** TEE long-axis view. *Ao,* Aorta; *LVOT,* left ventricular outflow tract. (Modified from Wu J: Cardiac tumors and masses. In: Stergiopoulos K, Brown DL, eds. *Evidence-Based Cardiology Consult*. Springer Science + Business Media, Inc., 2014.)

Evidence of pulmonary venous involvement is pathognomonic of a malignant process. Lymphatic and hematogenous routes are also pathways to the heart. The location and mass effect of the metastases, rather than type of primary, tend to determine the patient's symptomatology.

Alternative Diagnoses
Pseudoneoplasms
With the abundance of cardiac imaging being performed by various modalities, it is inevitable that normal or slight variants of normal structures, degenerative or benign acquired lesions, and nonneoplastic masses may be detected. The onus is on the cardiologist or radiologist to distinguish between the following entities (listed in Table 16.11) and a true neoplasm.

Intracardiac Thrombus
Masses such as thrombi and vegetations have obvious clinical implications. On echocardiography, formed thrombi appear relatively homogeneous in echodensity and have a gel-like or deformable appearance (Fig. 16.77B). Old thrombi may have more echobright regions and a compact immobile or laminated appearance (see Fig. 16.27A). Clues that a mass is actually a thrombus include residence in areas of stasis (e.g., tip of LA appendage or within LV aneurysm), "wisps" of spontaneous echocardiographic contrast associated with the surface (Fig. 16.77A), and associated predisposing cardiac conditions, including MS, prosthetic valves, cardiomyopathy, aneurysms of any chamber, or AF. Ropelike vacillating masses in the right side of the heart often represent thromboemboli from the deep venous system (see Fig. 16.71, left). If one is found, then the IVC, as well as the pulmonary arteries, should be inspected for

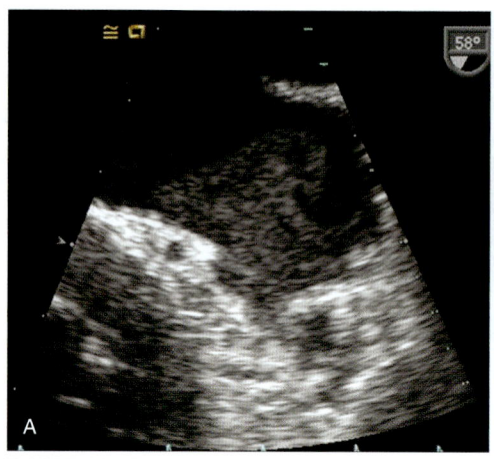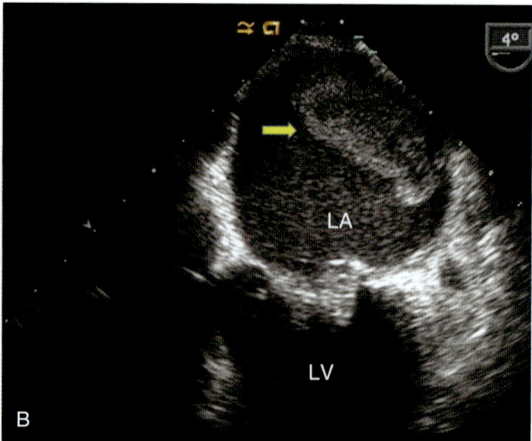

FIGURE 16.77 Spontaneous echocardiographic contrast and left atrial appendage thrombus. **A,** Zoomed TEE view of spontaneous echocardiographic contrast in the left atrial appendage in a patient with a bileaflet mechanical mitral prosthesis who was subtherapeutic with warfarin treatment. **B,** TEE view of organized thrombus (*arrow*) in the left atrial appendage in a patient following mitral annuloplasty. *LA,* Left atrium; *LV,* left ventricle.

portions of the same clot. With anticoagulation, intracardiac thrombi frequently regress or remain stable.

The presence of LV aneurysms or severe dilated cardiomyopathy should always prompt vigilance for thrombi. Conversely, it would be highly unusual for a thrombus to form in an area with normal wall motion. Use of a high-frequency (7 to 8 MHz) probe to focus on the cardiac apex, angling it at unconventional views and sweeping across the field as needed, can better distinguish thrombus versus myocardium or trabeculations and will also decrease noise and reverberation artefact. Ultrasound enhancing agents are often the key, particularly when endocardial border or thrombus definition is poor.

With its higher resolution and proximity to the base of the heart, TEE plays a major role in ruling out intracardiac thrombi (or other sources of emboli, such as atheroma or vegetation) when no identifiable source is found after TTE and after imaging the head and neck arteries. An embolic stroke or unusually high transvalvular gradients in a patient with a mechanical (or even bioprosthetic) valve should prompt referral for TEE, contingent on the assumption that the findings on TTE were nondiagnostic and that they would alter management. TEE is also frequently used to facilitate the decision to anticoagulate, cardiovert, or perform radiofrequency ablation of a tachyarrhythmia, particularly in high-risk patients (i.e., those with the predisposing cardiac conditions mentioned earlier or those found to be underanticoagulated before a planned procedure). TEE should be performed before percutaneous mitral valvuloplasty for rheumatic MS to rule out LA thrombus (as well as to better define the mitral anatomy and degree of regurgitation) and thus avert potentially catastrophic embolic complications.[15,26,77]

Vegetations and Pannus
Vegetations tend to arise on the lower pressure (regurgitant) side of valves or at areas of flow turbulence. Valves with degenerative changes, prosthetic valves, and indwelling catheters or pacemaker/defibrillator wires are well-recognized nidi for infection. Thick, immobile, heaped-up irregular masses affixed to the annuli of older prosthetic valves may represent pannus (fibrovascular granulation tissue) (see Fig. 16.55). For both thrombi and vegetations, the larger and/or highly mobile masses that threaten the pulmonary, systemic, or cerebral circulation with embolization or cause severe valvular dysfunction may compel emergency surgical resection (see earlier, Infective Endocarditis).

Normal Variants and Artefacts
Normal or mild variants of normal structures have also been mistaken for neoplasms on echocardiography (see Table 16.11). The most common are lipomatous hypertrophy, upper septal hypertrophy, redundant and/or calcified mitral chordae, prominent/multilobed papillary muscle, interatrial septal aneurysm, or pericardial fat. Degenerative changes such as valvular calcification or external compression of chambers of the heart by adjacent structures (e.g., from esophageal hernia indenting the posterior wall of left atrium) can give the appearance of a large mass when viewed in only one plane. In the case of a hiatal hernia, having the patient ingest a carbonated beverage to create "contrast" in the hernia can be diagnostic. Knowledge of the typical appearance of these abnormalities, use of echocardiographic enhancing agents, and either careful tilting and sweeping of the transducer plane or use of 3D echocardiography to track the boundaries and attachments of these entities can reveal their true nature.

ADULT CONGENITAL HEART DISEASE (SEE CHAPTER 82)

Echocardiography plays a critical role in the evaluation and management of both children and adults with congenital heart disease. Consequently, this section focuses on the role of echocardiography in diagnosing common shunts (ASDs and VSDs), as well as transposition of the great arteries (TGA) and tetralogy of Fallot, complex lesions that may be seen by cardiologists caring for adults. The use of echocardiography for the selection and implantation of ASD closure devices is also covered.

Atrial Septal Defect
ASDs account for approximately 10% of all congenital heart disease and 20% to 40% of congenital heart disease occurring in adulthood. The initial diagnosis of ASD is often made during echocardiography for nonspecific symptoms or for a heart murmur in an asymptomatic individual.

General Imaging Principles
Figure 16.78 provides the anatomic classification of ASDs. Although secundum defects are often isolated anomalies, ASDs of other types are frequently associated with other structural anomalies. Multiple ASDs may be encountered in the same patient. Secundum and primum ASDs can generally be diagnosed with 2D TTE, but TEE is typically required to detect sinus venosus and coronary sinus defects. On TTE, although parasternal and apical views are useful, the subcostal view is particularly important because it optimizes the Doppler detection of shunts and minimizes the chance that normal thinning of the fossa will be mistaken for a secundum defect. In the absence of significant pulmonary hypertension, ASD flow is typically left to right, reflecting normal intracardiac pressures. However, agitated saline injections may demonstrate the transient right-to-left shunts that can occur in patients with ASDs or show negative contrast enhancement ("ghosting") when the shunt flow from the left atrium meets the contrast-enhanced RA blood pool.

Regardless of location, hemodynamically significant ASDs will be associated with evidence of RV volume overload, characterized by RV enlargement and diastolic flattening of the interventricular septum. Pulmonary hypertension, which may complicate large defects, will result in flattening that persists through systole. This 2D appearance of RV volume overload and right-sided heart enlargement is considered evidence of a hemodynamically significant shunt ($Q_p/Q_s \geq 1.5:1$). For ASDs, Q_p/Q_s, or the ratio of pulmonic to systemic flow is the ratio of RV output (RV SV) to LV output (LV SV) and may be calculated directly by applying the principles of the continuity equation:

$$Q_p/Q_s = \left(\pi[D_{RVOT}/2]^2 \times VTI_{RVOT}\right)/\left(\pi[D_{LVOT}/2]^2 \times VTI_{LVOT}\right)$$

where D indicates the diameter of the RVOT and LVOT, respectively (Fig. 16.79). Additionally, PVR can be calculated in Wood units (see earlier, Pulmonary Hypertension); normal PVR is 0.5 to 1.5 Wood units.[75]

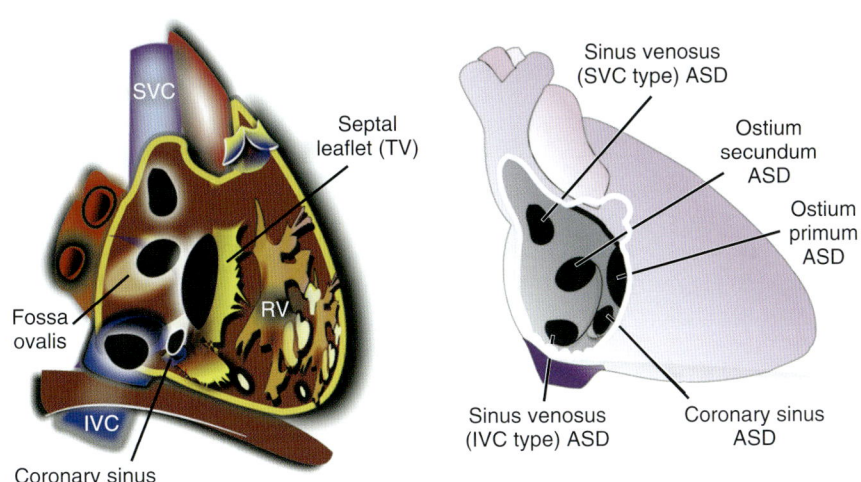

FIGURE 16.78 Classification of atrial septal defects (ASDs). *IVC, SVC,* Inferior, superior vena cava; *RV,* right ventricle; *TV,* tricuspid valve.

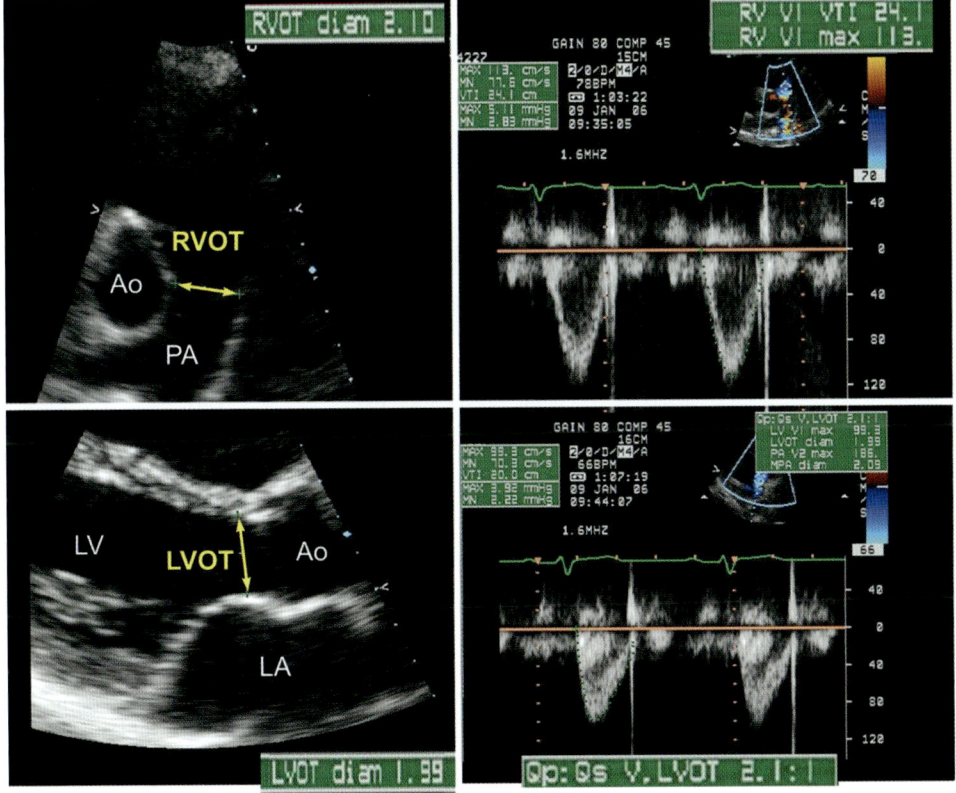

FIGURE 16.79 Q_p/Q_s calculation. For ASDs, Q_p is equivalent to RV stroke volume (SV), which equals $CSA_{RVOT} \times VTI_{RVOT}$, in which $CSA_{RVOT} = \pi(D/2)^2$. Q_s is equivalent to LV SV calculated as $CSA_{LVOT} \times VTI_{LVOT}$, where $CSA_{LVOT} = \pi(D/2)^2$. The **upper and lower panels** illustrate the derivation of RV and LV SV, respectively, from echo data. *Ao,* Aorta; *LA,* left atrium; *PA,* pulmonary artery.

Secundum Atrial Septal Defect

Secundum ASDs account for 75% of all ASDs and 30% to 40% of congenital disease seen in patients older than 40 (see Chapter 82). Figures 16.80 and 16.81 show the 2D TTE and TEE echocardiographic appearance of these defects. They are the only ASDs that are eligible for catheter-based closure. In planning transcatheter closure, TEE is used to (1) ensure that only one (or more) secundum ASDs is present, excluding other interatrial shunts that cannot be closed percutaneously, (2) size the defect, and (3) ensure that there is enough adjacent tissue rim to anchor the device. 3D TEE is especially advantageous for displaying en face displays of the septum before and during implantation.[77,88] Of the two devices currently approved by the U.S. Food and Drug Administration, the Amplatzer may be used for defects up to 38 mm, whereas the Cardioform device may be used only for defects up to 17 to 18 mm, although it may be placed successfully in patients with deficient anterior rims.

With 2D TEE, orthogonal diameters are recorded during ventricular systole, and a screen for presence of fenestrations is performed. 3D echocardiography allows en face displays of the entire defect in relation to the surrounding landmarks; measurements can be performed online with less risk of undersizing the defect compared to standard 2D imaging, particularly in those of irregular shape (see Fig. 16.81). Acceptable rim margins are at least 3 mm for the anterior rim and 5 mm for all other rims. Deficiency of the anterior rim is the most common (Fig. 16.81, right, and Fig.16.82).

Device closure is guided by either TEE or intracardiac echocardiography (ICE). In sequential order, the key steps are placement of the guidewire across the defect (avoiding any smaller secondary fenestrations), balloon sizing of the defect, occluder placement followed by a tug to ensure optimal seating, assessment for residual shunt by color Doppler, and a survey for any complications such as pericardial effusion. Small residual shunts may be present immediately following deployment but often resolve after endothelialization of the device. Fig. 16.83 illustrates the 2D and 3D TEE appearance of a successfully deployed Amplatzer device. The occluder halves should appear well-apposed and aligned on both sides of the interatrial septum, without unusual tilting or prolapse of any portion through the defect, and ideally with no significant shunting by color Doppler or saline contrast. If there is misalignment of the device, particularly causing it to impinge upon the aortic root, there is a risk of erosion through the tissue.[88]

A *patent foramen ovale* (PFO) is a related condition characterized by incomplete fusion of the septum primum and septum secundum following birth. It may be detected by saline contrast demonstration of a right-to-left interatrial shunt, typically with maneuvers that raise RA pressure (cough, Valsalva or Müller maneuver). PFO is a very common condition that occurs in 20% to 35% of the normal population. It is also frequently associated with aneurysm of the interatrial septum. Echocardiography with saline contrast injection is often used to elucidate a PFO that could allow a paradoxical embolism to occur in patients without a clear source of left-sided embolic events, i.e., cryptogenic stroke. Evaluation for a PFO is one reason for performing TTE and TEE in patients with transient ischemic attacks, embolic stroke, or other embolic events.[79]

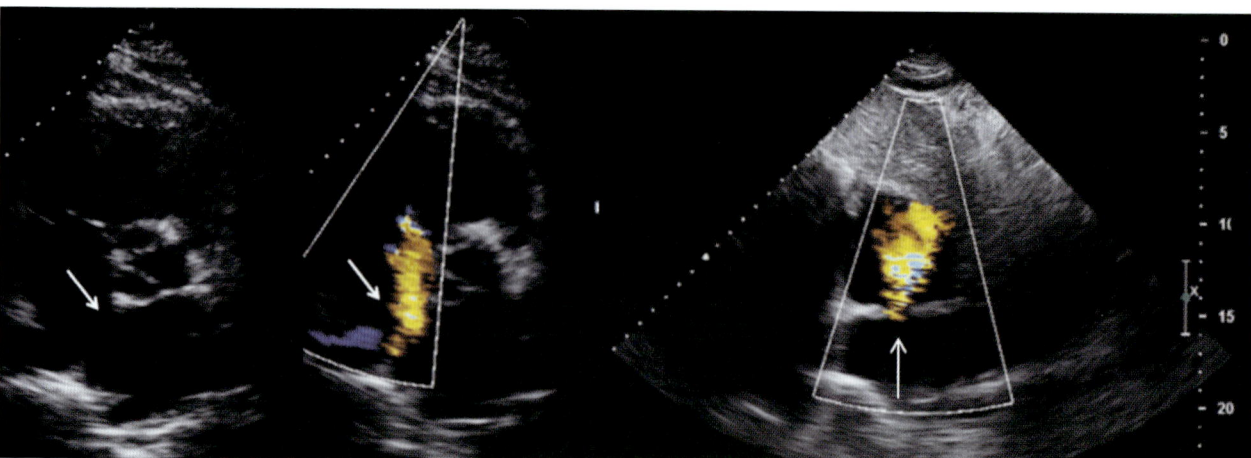

FIGURE 16.80 Parasternal (**left and middle panels**) and subcostal (**right panel**) images of a secundum ASD and its associated left-to-right shunt (*arrows*).

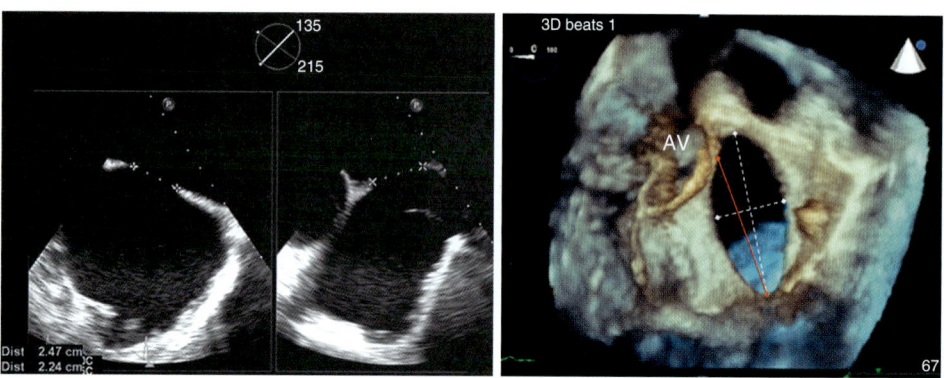

FIGURE 16.81 Biplane two- and three-dimensional TEE measurement of ASD dimensions. **Left**, Biplane 2D TEE measurement of ASD dimensions. The 0 to 45-degree midesophageal view can be used to measure the anterior (toward aorta) and posterior (toward pulmonary veins) rims, whereas the 90- to 120-degree view images the superior (toward SVC) and inferior (toward IVC) rims. **Right**, Large secundum ASD viewed by 3D TEE from the left atrial perspective. Note that the 2D TEE–measured diameter (*red line*) is typically smaller than that measured by 3D TEE (*white dotted lines*). Also note that there is a deficient anterior rim, i.e., no separation between the defect and the aortic valve (*AV*).

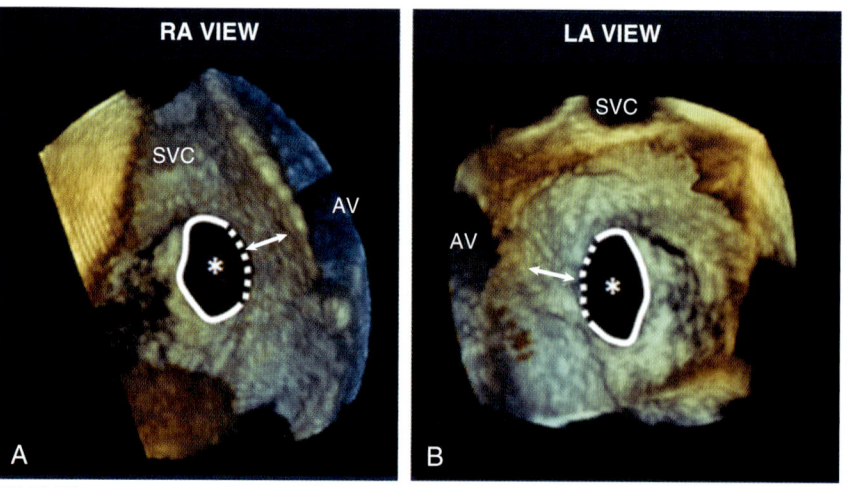

FIGURE 16.82 Assessment of ASD rims with 3D TEE in **A**, right atrial (RA) and **B**, left atrial (LA) views. The anterior rim is represented as the distance between the *dotted line* and the aorta (*arrow*). *Asterisk*, secundum ASD. *AV*, Aortic valve. (From Saric M, et al. Imaging atrial septal defects by real-time three-dimensional transesophageal echocardiography: step-by-step approach. *J Am Soc Echocardiogr.* 2010;23:1128.)

Primum Atrial Septal Defect
Primum ASDs account for 15% to 20% of ASDs and occur as part of the spectrum of atrioventricular canal defects. They may occur as isolated defects (partial atrioventricular canal defect) or may be accompanied by inlet VSDs (complete atrioventricular canal defect). Partial atrioventricular canal defects typically have an associated cleft mitral valve. In complete atrioventricular canal defects there is a common single atrioventricular valve. atrioventricular canal defects are the most common congenital heart abnormality in Down syndrome. Primum defects can be seen on apical or subcostal views if posterior angulation is ensured to demonstrate the inlet portion of the ventricular septum (Fig. 16.84). These defects must be closed surgically.

Sinus Venosus Atrial Septal Defect
Sinus venosus ASDs account for 2% to 10% of ASDs and occur in two locations. The SVC type creates a confluence among the left atrium, right atrium, and SVC as it enters the right atrium. It is frequently accompanied by partial anomalous drainage of the right upper pulmonary vein, which is created when this vein enters the confluence. Partial anomalous drainage contributes to the left-to-right shunt. IVC-type defects are less common and create a confluence among the left atrium, right atrium, and IVC as it enters the right atrium. They may be accompanied by partial anomalous drainage of the right lower pulmonary vein. These defects should be suspected in patients with markers of RV volume overload without apparent cause. Typically, TEE is required to make the diagnosis, although SVC-type defects may be demonstrated with subcostal TTE. Figure 16.85 shows the TEE appearance of a sinus venosus ASD with partial anomalous pulmonary venous drainage. Sinus venosus ASDs must be closed surgically.

Coronary Sinus Atrial Septal Defect
Coronary sinus ASDs are rare and may be associated with fenestrations or complete unroofing of the coronary sinus into the left atrium. They are frequently associated with a persistent left SVC, a more frequent

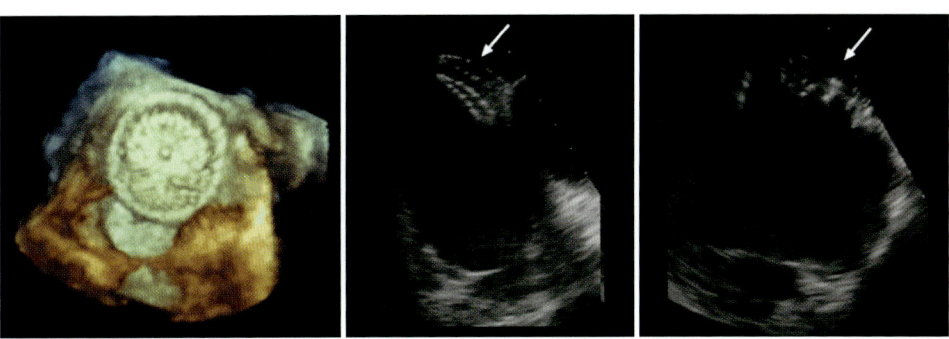

FIGURE 16.83 Postimplantation appearance of an Amplatzer ASD closure device. **Left panel,** 3D left atrial perspective. **Middle and right panels,** Orthogonal 2D TEE views. The *arrow* points to the left atrial disc.

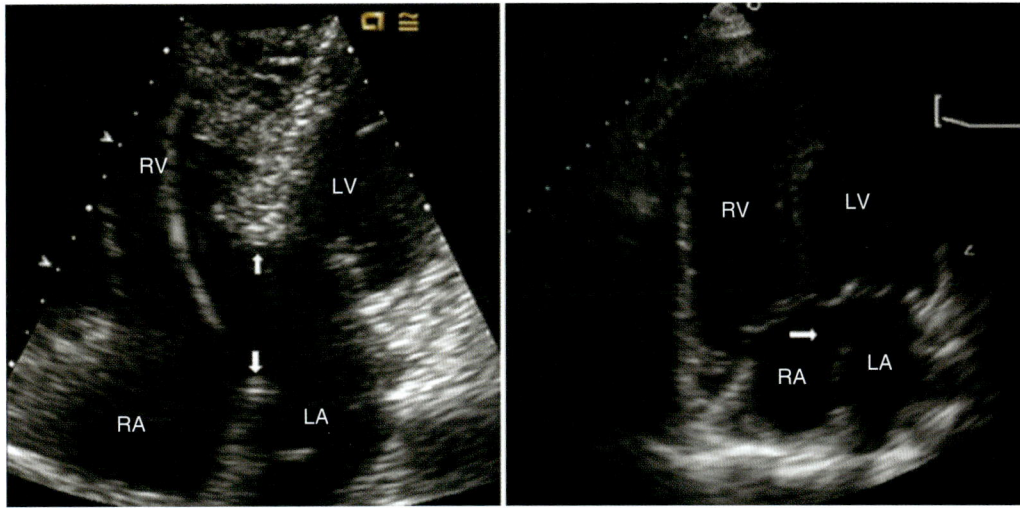

FIGURE 16.84 Apical four-chamber views showing complete **(left)** and partial **(right)** atrioventricular canal defects. In the **left panel,** *arrows* outline a large defect with atrial and ventricular components. In the **right panel** there is a primum ASD (*arrow*) with an intact ventricular septum. *LA,* Left atrium; *LV,* left ventricle; *RA,* right atrium; *RV,* right ventricle.

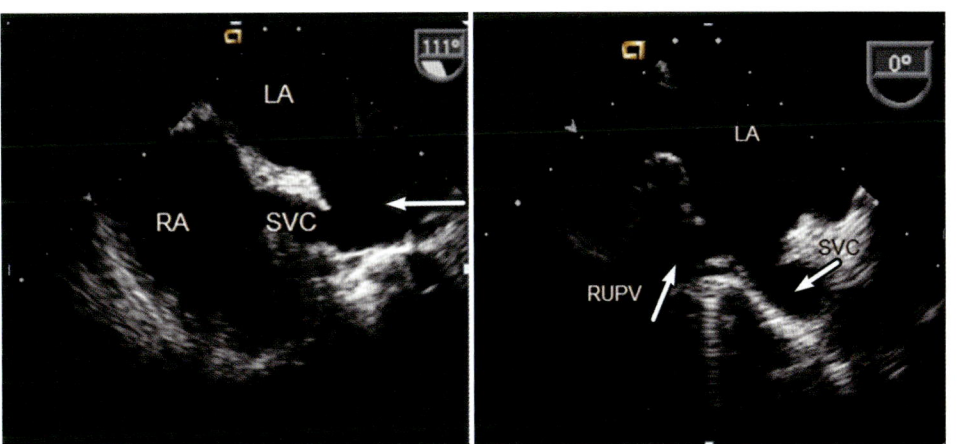

FIGURE 16.85 TEE images of a sinus venosus ASD (SVC type) with anomalous drainage of the right upper pulmonary vein (*RUPV*). A confluence is created between the superior vena cava (*SVC*), RUPV, and adjoining atria. *LA,* Left atrium; *RA,* right atrium.

finding (0.3% of the general population) and the most common cause of a dilated coronary sinus in general. The diagnosis is facilitated with TEE. Isolated persistent left SVC can be easily confirmed by TTE by injecting agitated saline contrast into a left cubital vein and demonstrating opaci-fication of the coronary sinus first, followed by contrast within the right atrium. It is usually an incidental finding that is generally not clinically important, but it can complicate transvenous placement of catheters or pacemaker/AICD leads if not recognized.

Ventricular Septal Defect

There are a number of classifications for VSDs. Figure 16.86 shows one anatomic classification, and Figure 16.87 outlines the division of the interventricular septum into its membranous, inlet, outlet, and trabecular portions along with the echocardiographic views that may be used to identify defects in each of these locations. VSDs vary in size and are considered to be small (restrictive) when less than half the size of the aortic root and when the LV-RV pressure gradient is greater than 64 mm Hg. Moderately restrictive VSDs are approximately half the size of the root, with gradients of approximately 36 mm Hg. With larger nonrestrictive defects, LV and RV systolic pressures are equalized. These latter defects are those that most often result in irreversible pulmonary vascular changes (Eisenmenger syndrome). Echocardiography may be used to size defects and LV-RV gradients. Shunting may be assessed by both color flow mapping and Q_p/Q_s calculated with the continuity equation. Although chamber size may be normal in the setting of small defects, LV and LA enlargement is expected in those that are hemodynamically significant.

Membranous (Paramembranous) and Outlet Ventricular Septal Defects

Eighty percent of VSDs involve the membranous septum. They vary in size, but even small defects can generally be detected on the parasternal long-axis view, as revealed by a high-velocity color Doppler jet. Membranous defects may be associated with wind-sock aneurysms that reflect varying degrees of spontaneous closure (Fig. 16.88). Even though the jets of membranous and outlet (supracristal) defects appear similar on the parasternal long-axis view, these defects may be distinguished from one another on short-axis views at the level of the great vessels. Membranous defects will be directed toward the septal leaflet of the tricuspid valve (10 to 11 o'clock position on the short-axis clock face), whereas outlet defects will be associated with jets that are directed toward the pulmonic valve (at 2 to 3 o'clock on the short axis clock face) (Fig. 16.87 and 16.89). Either defect may be accompanied by aortic cusp prolapse and consequent AR.

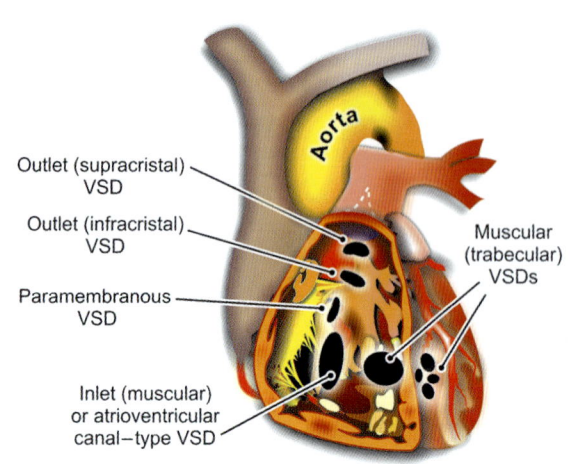

FIGURE 16.86 Anatomic classification system for ventricular septal defects (VSDs).

Inlet Ventricular Septal Defects
Inlet defects have been addressed in the preceding discussion of complete atrioventricular canal defects. Although often easily detected (see Fig. 16.84, left panel), inlet VSDs may be partially closed by adjacent atrioventricular valve tissue. In such situations, nonstandard views and TEE may be required to detect the ventricular component of the atrioventricular canal defect.

Muscular Ventricular Septal Defects
Muscular defects vary considerably in size and location and may be multiple. When small and serpiginous, they may easily be missed with conventional echocardiographic views. Because these small defects are associated with loud murmurs with or without a thrill, a detailed evaluation using nonstandard views, such as sliding/tilting the transducer systematically down the barrel of the left ventricle with color Doppler sweeps, is warranted in any patient with these clinical manifestations (Fig. 16.90).

TRANSPOSITION OF THE GREAT ARTERIES
TGA arises from failure of the aorticopulmonary septum to take its normal spiraling course (see Chapter 82). In dextro (D)–TGA the aorta lies anterior and to the right of the pulmonary artery and arises from the right ventricle, with the pulmonary artery arising from the left ventricle. D-TGA accounts for 5% to 7% of all congenital heart disease and, in the absence of shunting (VSD, ASD, patent ductus arteriosus) or surgery, D-TGA would be fatal. The most common associated anomalies are VSD (30% to 45%), pulmonary outflow tract obstruction (25%), and coarctation. Patients seen by cardiologists treating adults with congenital heart disease will have undergone corrective surgery consisting of either an atrial baffle/switch (Mustard or Senning) procedure in the past (up until ~1985), or more recently an arterial switch procedure.[89]

With baffle procedures the systemic venous baffle directs deoxygenated blood across the mitral valve into the left ventricle, from which it is ejected into the pulmonary artery. The pulmonary venous baffle directs oxygenated blood returning from the lungs to the tricuspid valve and into the right ventricle, from which it is pumped into the aorta. The end result is a "physiologic" circulation. Although short- and mid-term results are good, the right ventricle ultimately fails because of its inability to sustain its role as the systemic ventricle. Other complications detectable by echocardiography include baffle obstruction, baffle leaks, and pulmonary hypertension (the cause of which is incompletely understood).

The echocardiographic hallmark of transposition is parallel orienta-tion of the great vessels, best appreciated on parasternal long-axis or apical views (Fig. 16.91). The diagnosis can be confirmed by demonstrating that the posterior great vessel (the pulmonary artery) bifurcates and the anterior aorta gives off arch vessels. In patients with D-TGA who have undergone atrial switch surgery, the baffles can be traced as they crisscross the atrium, with color flow mapping and spectral Doppler identifying areas of obstruction and baffle leak. The hypertrophied right ventricle has the rounded contour typically associated with the left ventricle, whereas the left ventricle is crescentic, a result of reversal of the normal septal curvature because of systemic RV pressures. RV systolic function may be reduced with accompanying functional TR.

Levo (L)–TGA, also termed *congenitally corrected transposition*, is rare and accounts for less than 1% of all congenital heart disease. In L-TGA, transposition, with the aorta anterior and typically to the left of the pulmonary artery, is also accompanied by ventricular inversion. Thus, systemic venous blood returning to the right atrium drains into the morphologic left ventricle and is pumped into the pulmonary artery. Pulmonary venous blood returning to the left atrium crosses the tricuspid valve into the morphologic right ventricle, from which it is ejected into the aorta. Therefore the circulation is "normalized". Associated abnormalities are common and include VSD (70% of patients), pulmonary outflow tract obstruction that is typically subvalvular (40%), and abnormalities of the tricuspid (systemic atrioventricular) valve (90%). Patients, particularly those without associated anomalies, may remain undiagnosed until adulthood, but eventually the morphologic right ventricle will fail because it cannot meet the pressure demands of the systemic circulation.

Echocardiographic features of L-TGA again include parallel orientation of the great vessels as with all cases of transposition, but on apical views, ventricular inversion becomes apparent. Ventricular morphology may be determined by the structure of its atrioventricular valve and the pattern of trabeculation. The morphologic right ventricle is associated with a tricuspid atrioventricular valve, which is identified by the presence of three leaflets and leaflet insertion that is apical to that of the mitral valve. The morphologic right ventricle is coarsely trabeculated with a moderator band, whereas the morphologic left ventricle is smooth walled and has two discrete papillary muscles. In assessing ventricular morphology by the four-chamber view, it is essential to maintain standard transducer orientation and avoid rotating the transducer so that an image is created in which the right and left ventricles occupy their expected positions. Figure 16.92 illustrates ventricular inversion in a patient with L-TGA. As with D-TGA, the morphologic right ventricle is hypertrophied with a round contour, and the morphologic left ventricle is crescentic. The septal curvature is reversed, consistent with the systemic pressure in the morphologic right ventricle.[89]

TETRALOGY OF FALLOT
Tetralogy of Fallot is the most common form of cyanotic congenital heart disease and accounts for 10% of all congenital heart cases. The tetralogy of abnormalities consists of an overriding aorta, nonrestrictive subaortic VSD, RVOT obstruction (typically infundibular with variable valvular abnormalities), and secondary RV hypertrophy. Each of these features is readily identifiable with echocardiography (Fig. 16.93). *Pentalogy of Fallot* refers to the condition in which an ASD is also present.

Surgery for tetralogy consists of patching the VSD and a tailored approach to relieving the RVOT obstruction. Pulmonic regurgitation, sometimes severe, is a frequent finding after surgery for tetralogy of Fallot and may drive the need for repeated surgery. Other problems to remain vigilant for in the years after surgery include residual infundibular (subvalvular) and supravalvular pulmonic stenosis, as well as aneurysmal degeneration of the patch used to open up the infundibulum and/or pulmonary artery.[90]

TRANSCATHETER INTERVENTIONS (SEE CHAPTERS 74 AND 78)

Transcatheter intervention for the treatment of structural heart disease has been a rapidly evolving field with an expanding number of devices and applications.[70] Throughout every phase in the development and clinical application of these procedures, echocardiography has remained indispensable in selecting candidates with suitable anatomy and pathophysiology, guiding device selection, and providing both intra-procedural guidance and post-procedure assessment. This has held true for older devices (plugs and occluders) used to treat paravalvular leaks and shunts as well as ever-expanding options for valvular disease that have emerged in recent decades, including transcatheter aortic valve replacement (TAVR), mitral and tricuspid repair/replacement, and atrial appendage occlusion.

Currently, TAVR using either balloon-expandable or self-expanding valves is widely available for symptomatic AS. Since 2017, TAVR has surpassed the number of standard surgical aortic valve replacements for AS in Europe and North America. Much less commonly, it is used for bioprosthetic or native valve aortic insufficiency. While TAVR is typically a percutaneous transfemoral procedure, more invasive alternative access sites, including trans-axillary and trans-aortic, may be used.

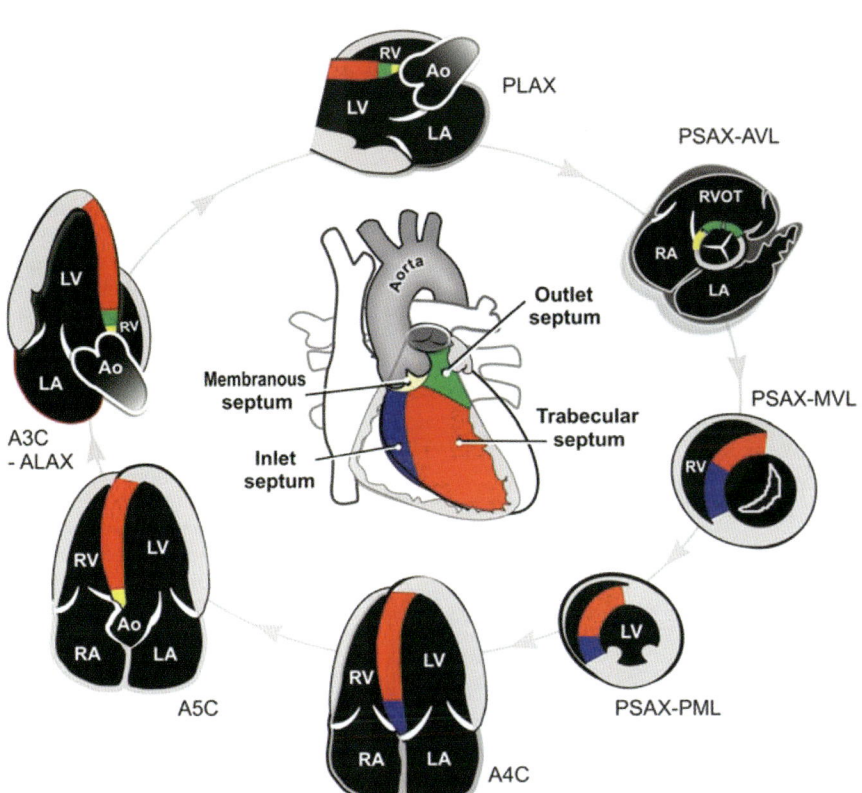

FIGURE 16.87 Echocardiographic views used in imaging the interventricular septum. *A3C*, Apical three-chamber view; *Ao*, aorta; *AVL*, aortic valve level; *LA*, left atrium; *LV*, left ventricle; *MVL*, mitral valve leaflet; *PLAX*, parasternal long-axis view; *PML*, papillary muscle level; *RA*, right atrium; *RV*, right ventricle. (Modified from Bulwer BE, Rivero JM, eds. *Echocardiography Pocket Guide: The Transthoracic Examination*. Burlington, MA: Jones & Bartlett Learning; 2011, 2013:142. Reprinted with permission.)

The latter have largely replaced the trans-apical approach used in early TAVR experience. Pre-procedural assessment routinely includes TTE to verify AS severity, provide input into device selection (type and size) and identify features that would constitute a hostile landing zone for the valve, such as extensive annular or LVOT calcification. Pre-procedural CTA is routinely used to assess vascular access and aortic annular and root size, but in cases where there are contraindications to CT, 3D TEE may be used. 3D capability is important to accurately size the annulus given its non-circularity and is uniquely able to determine the height of the coronary arteries relative to the annulus based on reconstructed views. The latter is important since low coronary ostia pose a risk of occlusion by displaced native leaflets at the time of implantation. Analytic enhancements incorporating artificial intelligence permit detailed online and offline measurements throughout the cardiac cycle (4D TEE) and volume reconstruction at the bedside.

Intraprocedural TEE may be used to ensure that the stented valve is properly seated across the aortic annulus and to immediately assess for complications. Many experienced structural heart programs have transitioned from routine intra-procedural TEE to intraprocedural fluoroscopy alone with immediate post-procedural TTE, reserving planned intra-procedural TEE for patients at higher risk for complications but having TEE on standby should a complication occur.

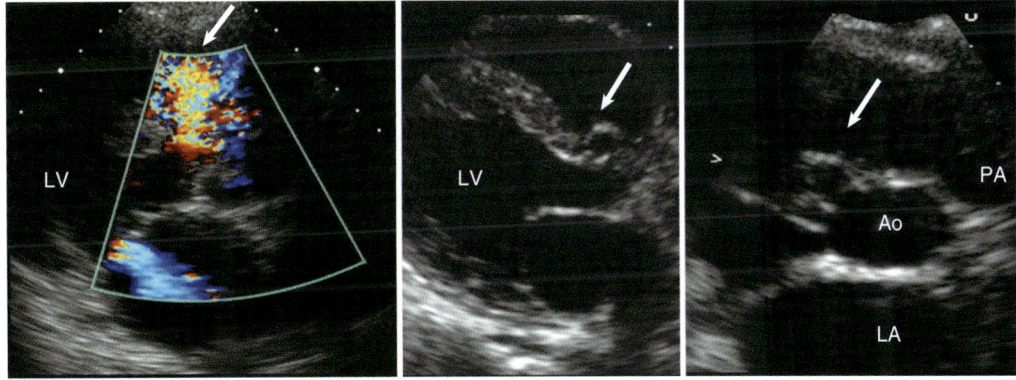

FIGURE 16.88 Parasternal views of a membranous VSD partially closed with a wind-sock aneurysm. **Left,** A systolic left-to-right jet is identified. **Middle,** With slight angulation, a wind-sock aneurysm representing partial spontaneous closure of the defect is identified. *LV*, Left ventricle. **Right,** In the short-axis view, the wind sock helps localize the VSD to the 11 o'clock position, as opposed to outlet defects, which are seen in the 12 to 2 o'clock position (compare with Fig. 16.89). *Ao*, Aorta; *LA*, left atrium; *PA*, pulmonary artery.

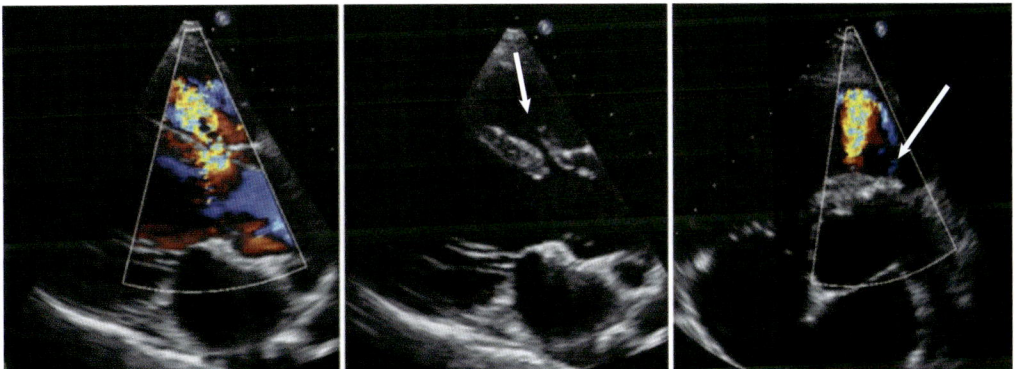

FIGURE 16.89 Parasternal images illustrating an outlet VSD. In the parasternal long-axis view **(left** and **middle panels)**, the VSD jet and the defect (*arrow*) may be indistinguishable from those of a membranous defect. However, in the short axis **(right panel)**, the jet is seen at the 12 o'clock position immediately next to the pulmonic valve (*arrow*). (Compare with Fig. 16.89.)

Post-deployment paravalvular aortic insufficiency is not uncommon, though seen less frequently with newer generation valves (see Fig. 16.57); if the degree is significant, further re-expansion of the stented valve or even implantation of a second valve within the first one may solve the problem. Intra- or post-procedural echocardiography also serves to survey for iatrogenic complications such as acute infarcts caused by coronary ostial inclusion, annular rupture, MR, and pericardial effusion.[70] As experience has grown, TAVR is now used successfully in some patients with bicuspid valves although associated aortopathy can preclude its use in some patients.

Post-procedure follow-up is similar to that for surgical bioprostheses with the exception that TAVR valve design results in acceleration of flow at two levels—the first at the level of the stent frame inlet and the second at the level of the valve cusps. For this reason, care must be taken to record LVOT velocity proximal to the valve inlet. LVOT diameter is typically measured as the outer to outer edge diameter of the lower end of the valve frame. The identification of paravalvular regurgitation also requires some attention to detail; jets may be seen on color Doppler short axis images outside the perimeter of the frame that are trapped within the device skirt and do not actually reach the left ventricle. To be considered paravalvular regurgitation, jets must be demonstrated to reach the LV. Quantitation based on color jet dimensions may be challenging due to the frequent jet eccentricity.

Additionally, valve in valve procedures (TAVR implanted into another TAVR or surgical bioprosthetic AVR) may be performed for initially failed TAVR attempts or subsequent TAVR or surgical valve degeneration. Along the same lines, valves designed for aortic implantation may be used to address mitral bioprosthetic dysfunction (typically MR) or, rarely, mitral

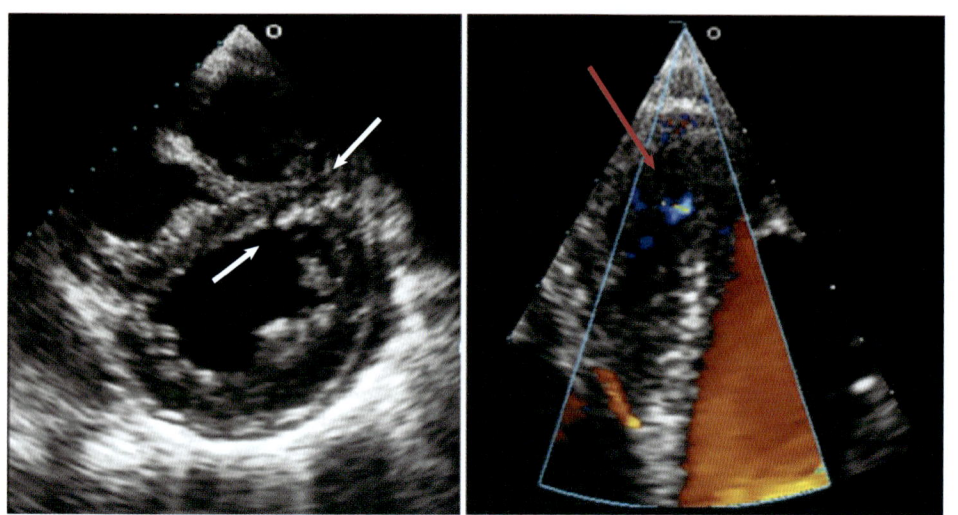

FIGURE 16.90 Parasternal short-axis **(left)** and off-axis apical **(right)** views demonstrating a serpiginous muscular VSD. The *white arrows* point to LV and RV entry points. The *red arrow* identifies a small left-to-right shunt.

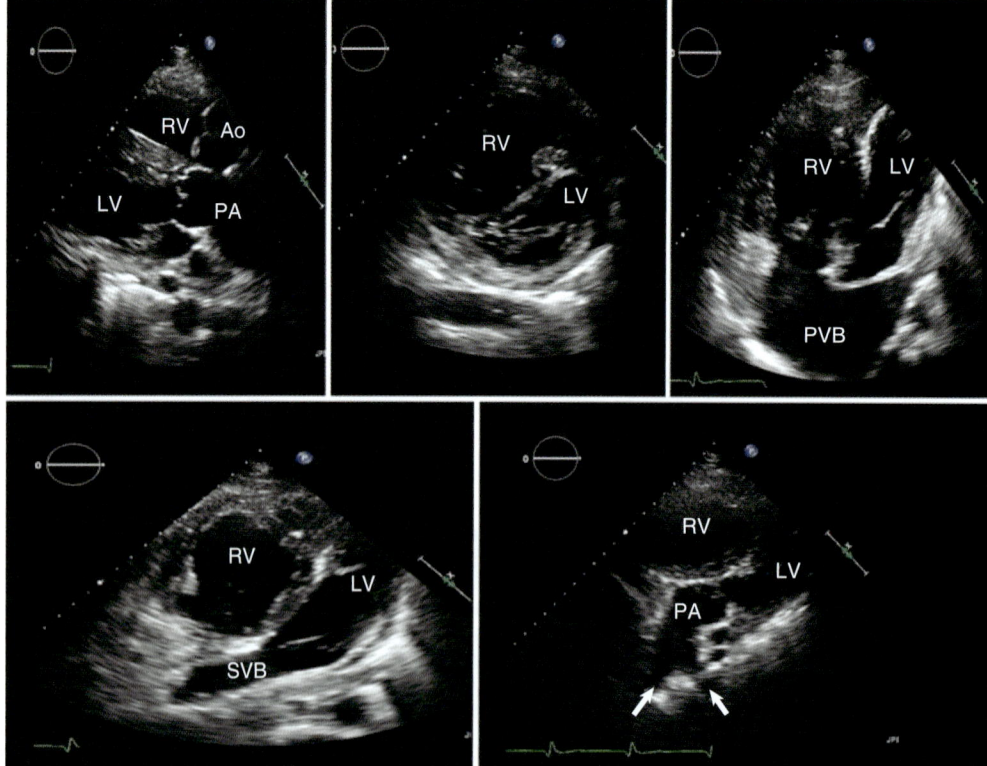

FIGURE 16.91 D-Transposition of the great arteries after Mustard baffle surgery. **Top left,** Parasternal long-axis view showing parallel orientation of the aorta (*Ao*) and pulmonary artery (*PA*). The aorta is anterior. **Top middle,** Parasternal short-axis view showing septal inversion reflecting the fact that the right ventricle (*RV*) is the systemic ventricle. **Top right,** Apical four-chamber view showing the pulmonary venous baffle (*PVB*), which directs pulmonary venous flow across the tricuspid valve into the RV. **Bottom left,** The four-chamber view has been angulated to demonstrate the systemic venous baffle (*SVB*), which directs systemic venous return across the mitral valve into the left ventricle (*LV*). Note the right ventricular hypertrophy and enlargement. **Bottom right,** The four-chamber view is angulated anteriorly to demonstrate the connection between the LV and PA. *Arrows* point to the PA bifurcation.

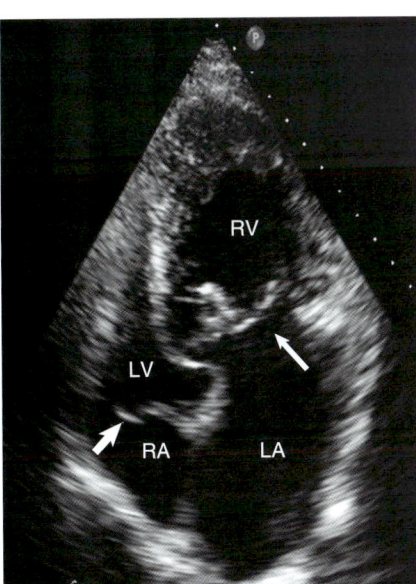

FIGURE 16.92 Apical four-chamber view in patient with L-transposition of the great arteries. The ventricles are inverted with the right ventricle (*RV*) to the right, identified on the basis of its heavy trabeculation and tricuspid atrioventricular valve (*thin arrow*). Although the insertion of the tricuspid valve is always apical to that of the mitral valve, in this case the offset is accentuated, consistent with the Ebstein anomaly. Unlike isolated Ebstein anomaly, that seen with L-TGA does not have a sail-like leaflet or adherence of the septal leaflet to the septum. The *thick arrow* points to the mitral valve. *LA,* Left atrium; *LV,* left ventricle; *RA,* right atrium.

annular calcification. *Transcatheter pulmonary valve implantation* with balloon expandable valves is now routine in pediatric centers experienced in congenital heart disease.

Balloon valvuloplasty for MS is a relatively common procedure in parts of the world where rheumatic disease is still prevalent. As previously discussed (see Mitral Stenosis), echocardiographic scoring systems may help with patient selection and TEE is used to exclude intra-atrial thrombus.[65] Intra-procedural guidance includes fluoroscopy and TEE, the latter preferentially performed with 3D or intracardiac ultrasound. Measures of success include a decrease in mean gradient without an increase in degree of MR. Of note, the PHT is invalid for calculating MVA in the early post-valvuloplasty period, due to acute changes in left atrial and ventricular compliance.

Interventions for MR can be divided into repair and replacement with options for repair further divided into those procedures that directly alter the leaflets or their chordal support and annuloplasty (direct or indirect). To date, these approaches have been modeled on established surgical techniques. Currently, the only FDA-approved device is the mitral clip edge-to-edge repair system (MitraClip) although others are at varying stages of investigation. An array of devices for transcatheter mitral valve replacement are being evaluated.

The mitral clip (MitraClip) is modeled on the surgical Alfieri procedure and joins the anterior and posterior leaflets, typically at their mid portion, to create a double orifice valve. It may be used for both degenerative and secondary MR and echocardiography plays a critical role in patient selection. Implantation is done under fluoroscopic and TEE guidance ideally with 3D. Key steps are transseptal puncture, orienting the device so that it is aligned with the target jet (ideally P2-A2), advancing the device into the left ventricle, grasping the leaflets with

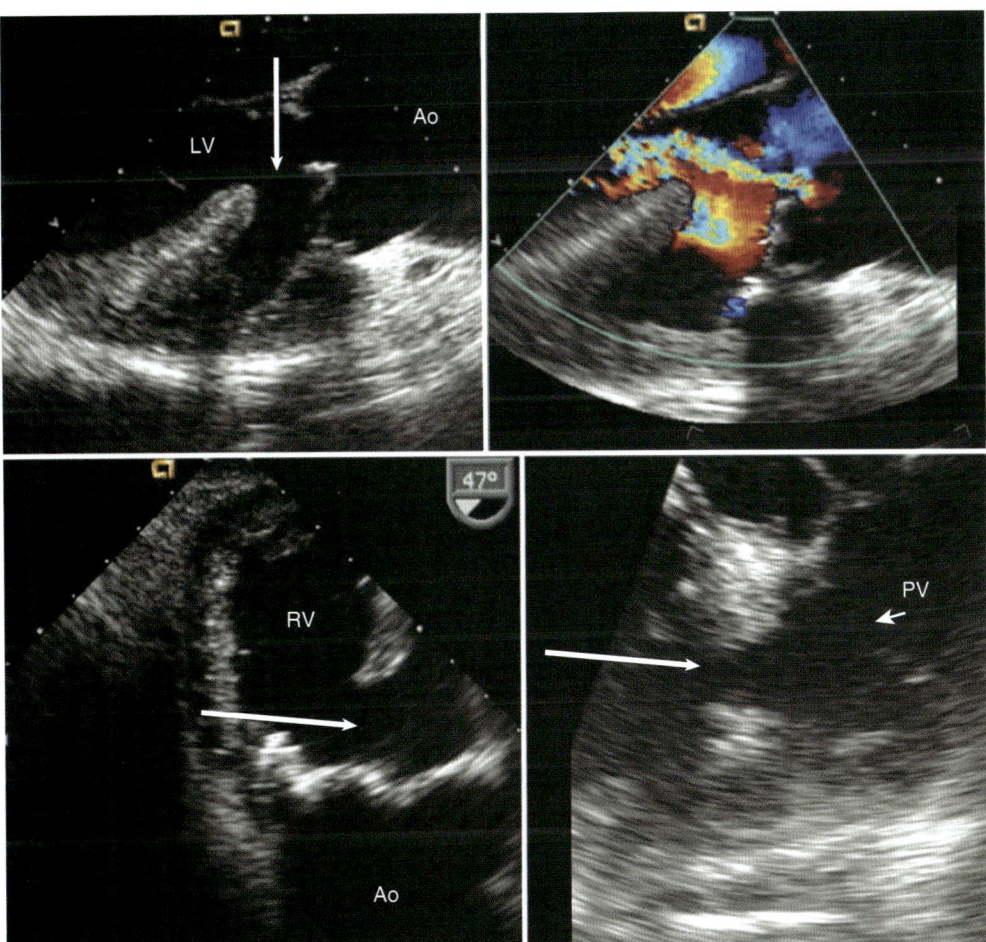

FIGURE 16.93 TEE images of a patient with tetralogy of Fallot. **Upper left,** Midesophageal image showing the aorta (*Ao*) overriding a large (nonrestrictive) VSD (*arrow*). **Upper right,** There is mild aortic regurgitation. **Lower left,** From a deep transgastric view, severe right ventricular hypertrophy is seen. The *arrow* points to the VSD. **Lower right,** In this midesophageal view, focal infundibular narrowing is seen (*arrow*). The pulmonic valve (*PV*) is not well seen but, in other views, was shown to be normal. *LV,* Left ventricle; *RV,* right ventricle.

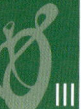

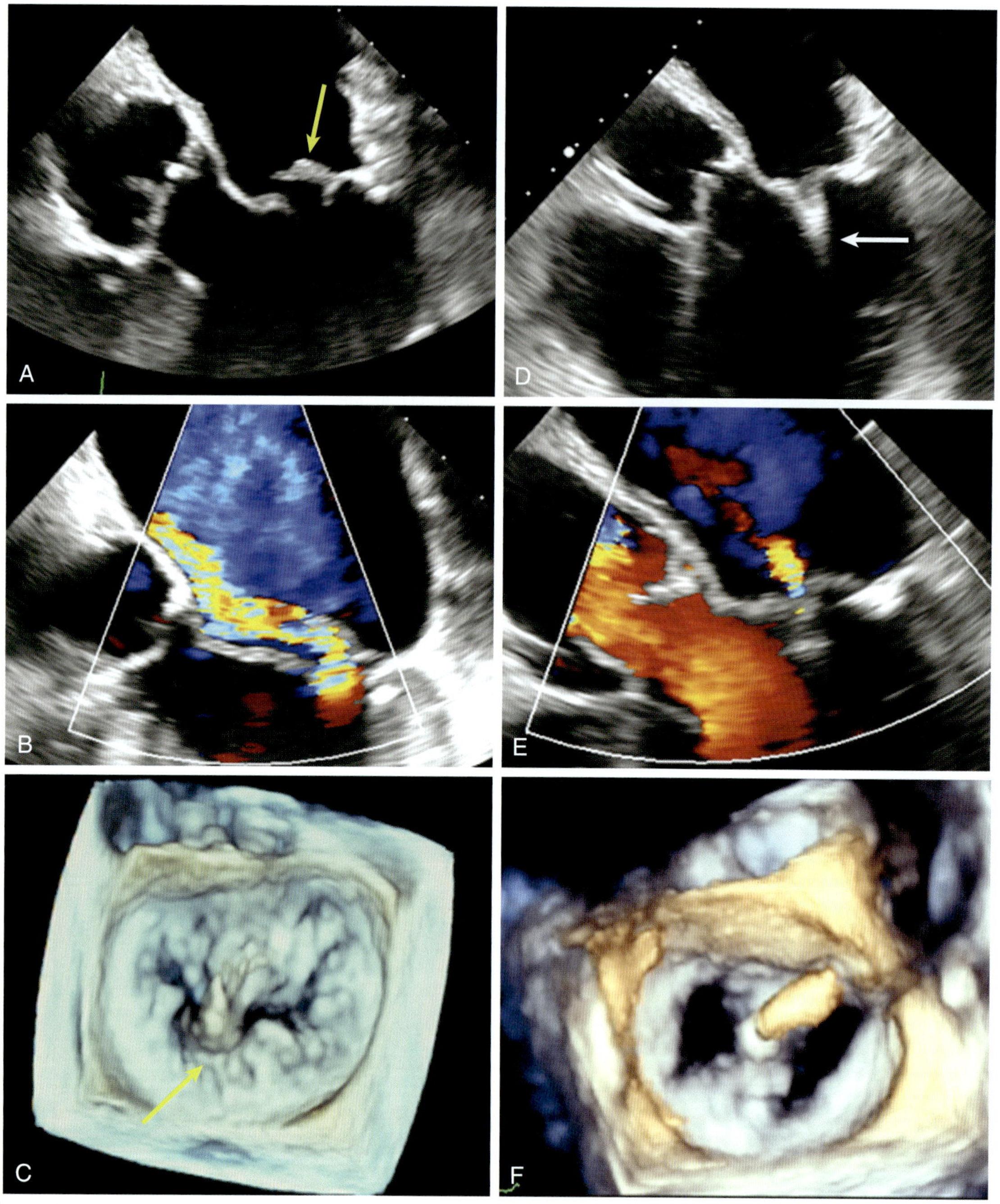

FIGURE 16.94 MitraClip repair of posterior mitral valve leaflet flail. 2- and 3-D TEE images in a patient with posterior mitral leaflet flail (**Left panels, yellow arrows**) followed by MitraClip placement (**Right panels, white arrow**). **A,** Posterior leaflet flail segment with ruptured chordae. **B,** Corresponding eccentric severe MR. **C,** 3D TEE view as viewed from the left atrial aspect; **D,** MitraClip is seen attached to both leaflets in the LV. **E,** with reduced MR on color Doppler. **F,** 3D TEE view of the double orifice created by the MitraClip (note the delivery catheter is still attached on the left atrial side.

device grippers and subsequently device arms, assessing residual MR and degree of MS and excluding complications including pericardial effusion. Intra-procedure assessment of MR relies on color jet dimensions, pulmonary venous flow, 3D planimetered EROA and pulmonary artery pressure. Real-time multiplanar reconstruction, a recent advance in 3D technology is particularly helpful during these procedures[70] (Fig. 16.94). Multiple MitraClips may be placed in a valve with a large orifice as needed to reduce MR, but antegrade mitral gradients and estimated PASP must be followed to prevent iatrogenic MS.

Transcatheter tricuspid valve interventions have emerged more recently, with strategies of leaflet approximation, annuloplasty, or total valve replacement. These are all in clinical trials currently. Procedural success will likely be heavily dependent upon pre-procedural evaluation of the tricuspid valve, TR, and the right heart.[92]

In the subspecialty of electrophysiology, occlusion of the LA appendage is possible with a variety of devices and is targeted toward patients at high risk for recurrent strokes (despite anticoagulation or unable to take anticoagulants). TEE is performed before the procedure primarily to size the LA appendage and ensure that it can receive an appropriately sized device, as well as to exclude appendage thrombus. For the Watchman device, the ostia of the appendage diameters are measured at several angles, and the appendage must be longer than its width to properly select and seat the occluder. ICE may alternatively be used for transseptal puncture and to guide device delivery.[93] Post-procedure surveillance is performed by TEE in the 1 to 2 months following implantation to assess for any residual flow between the appendage and left atrial body.

There is a small cautionary note to the exponential increase in transcatheter interventions: While generally safe and absolutely essential to deployment of many of these devices, recently there has been increasing recognition that the constant probe manipulation during TEE-guided procedures engenders a potential for esophageal injury. This is particularly true with mitral clip placement, long procedure times, and in patients with risk factors such as prior GI bleed, low body weight, and chronic immunosuppressive medications such as steroids.[19,91] These risks underscore the importance of pre-screening patients, giving appropriate informed consent, and strategizing TEE mechanics. The risks may potentially be mitigated by the use of real time 3D-TEE and fusion imaging (see next), which allows for faster and more intuitive display of the device with respect to cardiac structures.

Future Directions
Multimodality and Fusion Imaging

Simultaneous advances in nuclear medicine and radiology have occurred hand-in-hand with the clinical implementation of the above transcatheter devices. Although TTE and TEE give real-time information particularly on the dynamic function of the heart chambers and valves, there are specific areas that may not be accessible for ultrasound imaging due to acoustic shadowing (e.g., portions of the aorta, mechanical valve or VAD artefacts, extracardiac structures). Furthermore, TEE is semi-invasive, usually requires at least IV conscious sedation with its inherent risks, and is an aerosol-generating procedure with the potential for airborne transmission of respiratory pathogens. The latter was of particular concern with the COVID-19 pandemic, and prompted an appropriate shift to alternative modalities such as CT angiography, MRI, and nuclear/PET scanning in selected cases.

Common clinical indications in which alternative or adjunct modalities to echocardiography are helpful follow: For aortic disease such as aneurysm and dissection, it is recommended the imaging modality able to visualize the affected segments with the lowest iatrogenic risk be used. Hence TTE and TEE are useful for first-line screening and following chronic disease in the aortic root and proximal ascending aorta. For acute aortic syndromes, CT angiography is often used due to the ability to image the complete aorta, speed, and sensitivity. If there is renal insufficiency, pregnancy, or an allergy to iodinated contrast, the modality with the least radiation exposure is recommended except in the case of emergency. For long-term follow-up, the same modality should be used in order to compare similar measurements, but repetitive radiation exposure in younger adults is to be avoided.[15,94]

TTE followed by TEE remains the mainstay for diagnosing endocarditis. However, in carefully selected cases, particularly those involving prosthetic valves or other implanted devices, CT angiography, metabolic imaging (with ^{18}F-FDG-PET scanning), and radionuclide-labeled white blood cell imaging which detects areas of inflammation are useful ancillary diagnostic tools that can be used to circumvent some of the limitations of echocardiography (see Infective Endocarditis). These radiologic modalities should also be considered in conditions where TEE is impractical or risky for either the patient or the provider. Cardiac PET and CTA images may be fused to confirm which cardiac structures are infected, which is particularly useful if vascular grafts are involved or there is extensive degenerated tissue. Although echocardiography permits high resolution 2D and moving 3D images of highly mobile or tiny structures in the heart, CMR has the advantage of more detailed tissue characterization and less angle dependence than ultrasound. Hence it is very useful for characterizing masses and discerning between myocardial damage, edema, and fibrosis. In many cases of endocarditis, it is very appropriate to use two or more modalities to examine the heart.[15,76,95]

Handheld Echocardiography (Point of Care Ultrasound)

The era of miniaturization has ushered in increasingly smaller and capable portable ultrasound machines, which were introduced commercially in 2004. Current laptop-size devices are a lightweight alternative to the traditional 400-lb full-size machines and have virtually all the same capabilities, including Doppler and strain imaging, stress and TEE studies, automatic quantification of LVEF, and 4D imaging. They can operate wirelessly. Many systems allow the performance of vascular, abdominal, and obstetric ultrasound on the same machine and can accommodate a wide range of transducers, including pediatric ones. There are miniaturized disposable TEE probes, designed to stay in patients for up to 72 hours, which may prove useful in the care of ICU patients after cardiac surgery.

The Covid-19 pandemic ignited a rocketing demand for handheld ultrasound devices to perform studies at the bedside (point-of-care ultrasound, or POCUS; see Chapter 94). These devices, developed over the last 20 years, are similar in size to a cellphone and can fit in the physician's coat pocket. Some models consist of a standalone transducer (which may be interchangeably cardiac, vascular, abdominal, or obstetric) which is plugged into a smartphone or tablet that serves as the display. One model uses a silicon chip that produces a 2D array of microsensors in lieu of piezocrystals, giving it the unique capability to act as multiple transducers in a single unit. In the hands of experienced sonographers, the current devices offer 2D and color Doppler imaging with adequate image quality and accuracy compared with conventional machines.[96] Currently, none of the handhelds support spectral Doppler and thus cannot perform quantification of valve stenosis or assess intracardiac pressures. Additionally, without the specialized presets of full-featured systems, echocardiographic enhancing agents (contrast) are less effective. Features of various models include wireless data transmission (in some cases to the cloud), as well as the ability to connect and share real-time images at the bedside for interpretation, teleguidance, and even remote control of settings by an expert consultant. At least one system has piloted an artificial intelligence feature to help the user correctly capture heart images and automatically computes an LVEF.

In COVID-19, SARS-CoV-2 primarily affects the lungs but also causes right and left heart failure, thrombosis, and acute kidney injury, a single streamlined instrument that could rapidly assess the heart, lungs, and blood vessels suddenly became ideal. POCUS units, being easier to carry, use, and disinfect, enabled frequent serial exams at the bedside while reducing the risk of viral transmission and conserving resources. A single focused exam can help distinguish between pneumonia and heart failure, as well as crudely estimate RA filling pressures. Apart from its unique utility in epidemics, handheld ultrasound clearly has the potential to extend the physical exam, educate others, and obtain quantitative serial data at the bedside. From a more global aspect, the affordability and portability of these POCUS units also renders echocardiography more accessible for health care outside the hospital and in underdeveloped regions.

Despite these remarkable developments in handheld units, POCUS is operator-dependent and, like conventional echocardiography, requires an understanding of cardiac anatomy and physiology as well as training in image interpretation for optimal use by noncardiologists.[97] With sufficient user experience and continual improvements in design and function, these instruments will likely become a bedside tool as familiar as the stethoscope in clinical settings. At present, however, they do not supplant a complete formal echocardiographic study with a high-end machine and experienced sonographer.

Recent Echocardiography Techniques

Echocardiography has evolved over five decades to become a cornerstone in cardiac imaging. Although its fundamentals are based on the immutable physics of ultrasound, revolutionary advances in the processing and application of data continue to not only improve imaging, but also to provide more functional cardiac evaluation and applicability to clinical treatment. 4D imaging and speckle-based strain measurements have moved into the clinical realm. The potential utility of these techniques is being explored in avenues such as valvular, ischemic, and oncologic heart disease.[98] Strain and strain rate measurements in the right ventricle and left atrium may be more discerning indicators of function and filling pressures than our current parameters. 3D strain, the analysis of myocardial deformation in all vectors, is a recent development that may prove useful in cardio-oncology and heart failure. These measurements are currently hampered by limits in temporal and spatial resolution, and need validation and standardization, but research into their clinical and prognostic potential is ongoing. With regard specifically to valvular disease, the high prevalence of TR that persists or worsens after interventions on the left heart, has spurred a new interest in evaluating patients for TV surgical or transcatheter intervention.

Fusion imaging, in which two or more imaging modalities are combined to form one image (see Echocardiography in the Context of Cardiac Imaging), has already demonstrated utility in endocarditis cases where areas of inflammation (by FDG-PET) can be localized to infected valves or tissue (seen on CT angiography). Using software, it is also possible to overlay 3D echo images with cardiac CT to demonstrate the functional abnormalities (in LV wall motion or strain) that correlate with coronary artery stenoses as well as structural abnormalities such as shunts and defects. 3D TEE images may also be integrated with fluoroscopic markers to more accurately guide transcatheter interventions such as ASD closure, LAA occlusion, and potentially valvular interventions.[99]

Artificial Intelligence (see Chapter 11)

Artificial intelligence (AI), in the sense of automating tedious or complicated tasks, is already in use in echocardiography: automated endocardial border detection and EF calculation, 2- and 3D strain analysis and calculation of GLS, and automatic calculations of EROAs and volumes on 3D echos are some examples. For handheld ultrasounds, AI can be used to assist a novice in scanning, by combining real-time image assessment with adaptive anatomic guidance. Machine learning algorithms can be automated to expedite the analyses of ventricular size, mass, and global/regional function, but also could demonstrably automate complex assessments of valvular stenoses and regurgitation and diastolic function (by grouping relevant images together, and quantitatively assessing the multiple quantitative and semi-quantitative parameters). One could envision that the integrated data may populate reporting templates and trigger corresponding statements and conclusions.

However, in the context of actual machine learning, the full potential of AI is yet to be realized. AI can theoretically be used for largescale screening of diseases such as dilated or HCM, amyloidosis, or pulmonary hypertension. Using cluster analysis and additional clinical data, it appears that computers can be tasked, unsupervised, to parse complex echocardiographic phenotypes or subtle characteristics—perhaps too indistinct for the human eye to easily discern, as in the case of strain—in order to identify subgroups of patients with propensity to poor outcomes (e.g., male diabetics with LV hypertrophy and systolic dysfunction). Given the human skills, training, and nuances currently required to perform and interpret echocardiograms, there are obviously limitations to AI. AI presently cannot substitute for an echocardiologist's experience and ability to integrate clinical data in a specific patient, but is undoubtedly poised to enhance the accuracy, efficiency, and utility of echocardiography in clinical practice, education, and research.[100,101]

REFERENCES

Principles of Ultrasound Imaging

1. Cikes M, D'hooge J, Solomon SD. Physical principles of ultrasound and generation of images. In: Solomon SD, ed. *Essential Echocardiography*. Philadelphia, PA: Elsevier, Inc; 2019.
2. Lang RM, Badano LP, Mor-Avi V, et al. Recommendations for cardiac chamber quantification by echocardiography in adults: an update from the American Society of Echocardiography and the European Association of Cardiovascular Imaging. *J Am Soc Echocardiogr*. 2015;28:1.
3. Mitchell M, Rahko PS, Blauwet LA, et al. Guidelines for performing a comprehensive transthoracic echocardiographic examination in adults: recommendations from the American Society of Echocardiography. *J Am Soc Echocardiogr*. 2019;32:1.
4. Mizukoshi K, Takeuchi M, Nagata Y, et al. Normal values of left ventricular mass index assessed by transthoracic three-dimensional echocardiography. *J Am Soc Echocardiogr*. 2016;29:51.
5. Stewart MH, Lavie CJ, Shah S, et al. Prognostic implications of left ventricular hypertrophy. *Progress in Cardiovasc Dis*. 2018;61:446.
6. Guta AC, Badano LP, Ochoa-Jimenez RC, et al. Three-dimensional echocardiography to assess left ventricular geometry and function. *Expet Rev Cardiovasc Ther*. 2019;17:11.
7. Cole GD, Dhutia NM, Shun-Shin JG, et al. Defining the real-world reproducibility of visual grading of left ventricular function and visual estimation of left ventricular ejection fraction: impact of image quality, experience and accreditation. *Int J Cardiovasc Imaging*. 2015;31:1303.
8. Hernandez-Suarez DF. Strain imaging echocardiography: what imaging cardiologists should know. *Curr Cardiol Rev*. 2017;13(2):118–129.
9. Tops LF, Delgado V, Marsan NA, et al. Myocardial strain to detect subtle left ventricular systolic dysfunction. *Eur J Heart Fail*. 2017;19:307.
10. Stöhr EJ, Shave RE, Baggish AL. Left ventricular twist mechanics in the context of normal physiology and cardiovascular disease: a review of studies using speckle tracking echocardiography. *Am J Physiology-Heart Circulatory Physiol*. 2015;311:H633.
11. Nagueh SF, Smiseth OA, Appleton CP, et al. Recommendations for the evaluation of left ventricular diastolic function by echocardiography: an update from the American Society of Echocardiography and the European Association of Cardiovascular Imaging. *J Am Soc Echocardiogr*. 2016;29:277.
12. Nagueh SF. Left ventricular diastolic function: understanding pathophysiology, diagnosis, and prognosis with echocardiography. *J Am Coll Cardiol Img*. 2020;13:228.
13. Rallidi LS, Makavos G, Nihoyannopoulos P. Right ventricular involvement in coronary artery disease: role of echocardiography for diagnosis and prognosis. *J Am Soc Echocardiogr*. 2014;27:223.
14. Porter TR, Shillcutt SK, Adams MS, et al. Guidelines for the use of echocardiography as a monitor for therapeutic intervention in adults: a report from the American Society of Echocardiography. *J Am Soc Echocardiogr*. 2015;28:40.
15. Doherty JU, Kort S, Mehran R, et al. ACC/AATS/ AHA/ASE/ASNC/HRS/SCAI/SCCT/SCMR/STS 2019 appropriate use criteria for multimodality imaging in the assessment of cardiac structure and function in nonvalvular heart disease: a report of the American College of Cardiology appropriate use criteria task force, American Association for Thoracic Surgery, American Heart Association, American Society of Echocardiography, American Society of Nuclear Cardiology, Heart Rhythm Society, Society for Cardiovascular Angiography and Interventions, Society of Cardiovascular Computed Tomography, Society for Cardiovascular Magnetic Resonance, and Society of Thoracic Surgeons. *J Am Coll Cardiol*. 2019;73:488.
16. Doherty JU, Kort S, Mehran R, Schoenhagen P, et al. ACC/AATS/ AHA/ASE/ASNC/HRS/SCAI/SCCT/SCMR/STS 2017 appropriate use criteria for multimodality imaging in valvular heart disease: a report of the American College of Cardiology appropriate use criteria task force, American Association for Thoracic Surgery, American Heart Association, American Society of Echocardiography, American Society of Nuclear Cardiology, Heart Rhythm Society, Society for Cardiovascular Angiography and Interventions, Society of Cardiovascular Computed Tomography, Society for Cardiovascular Magnetic Resonance, and Society of Thoracic Surgeons. *J Am Soc Echocardiog*. 2018;31:381.
17. Thaden JJ, Malouf JF, Rehfeldt KH, et al. Adult intraoperative echocardiography: a comprehensive review of current practice. *J Am Soc Echocardiogr*. 2020;33:735.
18. Purza R, Ghosh S, Walker C, et al. Transesophageal echocardiography complications in adult cardiac surgery: a retrospective cohort study. *Annals Thoracic Surg*. 2017;103:795.
19. Freitas-Ferraz AB, Rodés-Cabau J, Junquera V, et al. Transesophageal echocardiography complications associated with interventional cardiology procedures. *Am Heart J*. 2020;221:19.
20. Porter TR, Mulvagh SL, Abdelmoneim SS, et al. Clinical applications of ultrasonic enhancing agents in echocardiography: 2018 American Society of Echocardiography guidelines update. *J Am Soc Echocardiog*. 2018;31:241.
21. Seol SH, Lindner JR. A primer on the methods and applications for contrast echocardiography in clinical imaging. *J Cardiovasc Ultrasound*. 2014;22:101.
22. Bruun NE, Habib G, Thuny F, et al. Cardiac imaging in infectious endocarditis. *Eur Heart J*. 2014;10:624.
23. Saw J, Lopes JP, Reisman M, McLaughlin P, et al. Cardiac computed tomography angiography for left atrial appendage closure. *Can J Cardiol*. 2016;32:1033.
24. Klein AL, Abbara S, Agler DA, et al. American Society of Echocardiography clinical recommendations for multimodality cardiovascular imaging of patients with pericardial disease. *J Am Soc Echocardiogr*. 2013;26:965.
25. Sicari R, Cortigiani L. The clinical use of stress echocardiography in ischemic heart disease. *Cardiovasc Ultrasound*. 2017;15:7.
26. Erbel R, Aboyans V, Boileau C, et al. 2014 ESC Guidelines on the diagnosis and treatment of aortic diseases: document covering acute and chronic aortic diseases of the thoracic and abdominal aorta of the adult. The Task Force for the Diagnosis and Treatment of Aortic Diseases of the European Society of Cardiology (ESC). *Eur Heart J*. 2014;35:2873.
27. Clavel MA, Pibarot P, Messika-Zeitoun D, et al. Impact of aortic valve calcification, as measured by MDCT, on survival in patients with aortic stenosis: results of an international registry study. *J Am Coll Cardiol*. 2014;64:1202.
28. Balzer J, Zeus T, Veulemans V, et al. Hybrid imaging in the catheter laboratory: real-time fusion of echocardiography and fluoroscopy during percutaneous structural heart disease interventions. *Interv Cardiol*. 2016;11:59.
29. Afzal S, Piayda K, Maier O, et al. Current and future aspects of multimodal imaging, diagnostic, and treatment strategies in bicuspid aortic valve and associated aortopathies. *J Clin Med*. 2020;9:662.
30. Amzulescu MS, De Craene M, Langet H, et al. Myocardial strain imaging: review of general principles, validation, and sources of discrepancies. *Eur Heart J - Cardiovasc Imaging*. 2019;20:605.

Myocardial Infarction

31. Prastaro M, Pirozzi E, Gaibazzi N, et al. Expert review on the prognostic role of echocardiography after acute myocardial infarction. *J Am Soc Echocardiog*. 2017;30:431.
32. Lancellotti P, Price S, Edvardsen T, et al. The use of echocardiography in acute cardiovascular care: recommendations of the European Association of Cardiovascular Imaging and the acute cardiovascular care association. *Eur Heart J*. 2015;16:119.
33. Roifman I, Connelly KA, Wright GA, et al. Echocardiography vs. Cardiac magnetic resonance imaging for the diagnosis of left ventricular thrombus: a systematic review. *Can J Cardiol*. 2015;31:785.
34. Dudzinski DM, Hung J. Echocardiographic assessment of ischemic mitral regurgitation. *Cardiovasc Ultrasound*. 2014;12:46.
35. Malhotra S, Canty JM. Structural and physiological imaging to predict the risk of lethal ventricular arrhythmias and sudden death. *JACC Cardiovasc Imaging*. 2019;12:2049.
36. Cikes M, Solomon SD. Beyond ejection fraction: an integrative approach for assessment of cardiac structure and function in heart failure. *Eur Heart J*. 2016;37:1642.

Cardiomyopathies

37. Nunes MCP, Badan LP, Marin-Neto JA, et al. Multimodality imaging evaluation of Chagas disease: an expert consensus of Brazilian Cardiovascular Imaging Department (DIC) and the European Association of Cardiovascular Imaging (EACVI). *Eur Heart J Cardiovasc Imaging*. 2018;19:459.
38. Citro R, Lyon AR, Meimoun P, et al. Standard and advanced echocardiography in takotsubo (stress) cardiomyopathy: clinical and prognostic implications. *J Am Soc Echocardiogr*. 2015;28:57.
39. Omar AM, Bansal M, Sengupta PP. Advances in echocardiographic imaging in heart failure with reduced and preserved ejection fraction. *Circ Res*. 2016;119:357.
40. Katbeh A, Van Camp G, Barbato E, et al. Cardiac resynchronization therapy optimization: a comprehensive approach. *Cardiology*. 2019;142:116.
41. Parato VM, Antoncecchi V, Sozzi F, et al. Echocardiographic diagnosis of the different phenotypes of hypertrophic cardiomyopathy. *Cardiovasc Ultrasound*. 2016;14:30.
42. Maron BJ. Clinical course and management of hypertrophic cardiomyopathy. *N Engl J Med*. 2018;379:655.
43. Asatryan B, Marcus FI. The ever-expanding landscape of cardiomyopathies. *J Am Coll Cardiol Case Rep*. 2020;2:361.
44. Oechslin E, Jenni R. Left ventricular noncompaction: from physiologic remodeling to noncompaction cardiomyopathy. *J Am Coll Cardiol*. 2018;71:723.

45. Towbin JA, McKenna WJ, Abrams DJ, et al. 2019 HRS expert consensus statement on evaluation, risk stratification, and management of arrhythmogenic cardiomyopathy: executive summary. *Heart Rhythm*. 2019;16:e373.
46. Dorbala SD, Cuddy S, Falk RH. How to image cardiac amyloidosis: a practical approach. *J Am Coll Cardiol: Cardiovasc Imaging*. 2019;13:1368.
47. Perry R, Selvanayagam JB. Echocardiography in infiltrative cardiomyopathy. *Heart Lung Circ*. 2019;28:1365.
48. Gorscan J, Bhupendar T. Newer echocardiographic techniques in cardiac resynchronization therapy. *Heart Fail Clin*. 2017;13:53.
49. Ponikowski P, Voors AA, Anker SD, et al. 2016 ESC Guidelines for the diagnosis and treatment of acute and chronic heart failure: the Task Force for the diagnosis and treatment of acute and chronic heart failure of the European Society of Cardiology (ESC) Developed with the special contribution of the Heart Failure Association (HFA) of the ESC. *Eur Heart J*. 2016;37:2129.
50. Ingvarsson A, Werther Evaldsson A, Waktare J, et al. Normal reference ranges for transthoracic echocardiography following heart transplantation. *J Am Soc Echocardiog*. 2018;31:349.
51. Clemmensen TS, Løgstrup BB, Eiskjær H, et al. Changes in longitudinal myocardial deformation during acute cardiac rejection: the clinical role of two-dimensional speckle-tracking echocardiography. *J Am Soc Echocardiogr*. 2015;28:330.
52. Badan LP, Miglioranza MH, Edvardsen T, et al. European Association of Cardiovascular Imaging/Cardiovascular Imaging Department of the Brazilian Society of Cardiology recommendations for the use of cardiac imaging to assess and follow patients after heart transplantation. *Eur Heart J Cardiovasc Imaging*. 2015;16:919.
53. Olymbios M, Kwiecinski J, Berman DS, et al. Imaging in heart transplant patients. *J Am Coll Cardiol Cardiovasc Imaging*. 2018;11:1514.
54. Elkaryoni A, Abu-Sheasha G, Altibi AM, et al. Diagnostic accuracy of dobutamine stress echocardiography in the detection of cardiac allograft vasculopathy in heart transplant recipients: a systematic review and meta-analysis study. *Echocardiography*. 2019;36:528.
55. Stainback RF, Estep JD, Agler DA, et al. Echocardiography in the management of patients with left ventricular assist devices: recommendations from the American Society of Echocardiography. *J Am Soc Echocardiogr*. 2015;28:853.
56. Bouchez S, Van Belleghem Y, De Somer F, et al. Haemodynamic management of patients with left ventricular assist devices using echocardiography: the essentials. *Eur H J Cardiovasc Imaging*. 2019;20:373.
57. Platz E, Campbell RT, Claggett B, et al. Lung ultrasound in acute heart failure. *J Am Coll Cardiol Heart Failure*. 2019;7:849.
58. Baggish AL, Battle RW, Beaver TA, et al. Recommendations on the use of multimodality cardiovascular imaging in young adult competitive athletes: a report from the American Society of Echocardiography in collaboration with the society of cardiovascular computed tomography and the society for cardiovascular magnetic resonance. *J Am Soc Echocardiog*. 2020;33:523.
59. Wasfy MM, Weiner RB. Differentiating the athlete's heart from hypertrophic cardiomyopathy. *Curr Opin Cardiol*. 2015;30:500.

Stress Echocardiography

60. Pellikka P, Arruda-Olson A, Chaudhry FA, et al. Guidelines for performance, interpretation, and application of stress echocardiography in ischemic heart disease: from the American Society of Echocardiography. *J Am Soc Echocardiog*. 2020;33:1.
61. Garbi M, Chambers J, Vannan MA, et al. Valve stress echocardiography: a practical guide for referral, procedure, reporting, and clinical implementation of results from the HAVEC Group. *JACC Cardiovasc Imaging*. 2015;8:724.
62. Clavel MA, Burwash IG, Pibarot P. Cardiac imaging for assessing low-gradient severe aortic stenosis. *J Am Coll Cardiol Cardiovasc Imag*. 2017;10:185.
63. Delgado V, Clavel MA, Hahn RT, et al. How do we reconcile echocardiography, computed tomography, and hybrid imaging in assessing discordant grading of aortic stenosis severity? *J Am Coll Cardiol Cardiovasc Imaging*. 2019;12:267.
64. Lancellotti P, Pellikka PA, Budts W, et al. The clinical use of stress echocardiography in non-ischaemic heart disease: recommendations from the European Association of Cardiovascular Imaging and the American Society of Echocardiography. *J Am Soc Echocardiogr*. 2017;30:101.

Valvular Heart Disease

65. Otto CM, Nishimura RA, Bonow RO, et al. 2020 ACC/AHA Guideline for the management of patients with valvular heart disease. A Report of the American College of Cardiology/American Heart Association Joint Committee on Clinical Practice Guidelines. *Circulation*. 2021;143(5):e35–e71.
66. Zoghbi WA, Adams D, Bonow RO, et al. Recommendations for noninvasive evaluation of native valvular regurgitation: a report from the American Society of Echocardiography developed in collaboration with the society for cardiovascular magnetic resonance. *J Am Soc Echocardiogr*. 2017;30:303.
67. Baumgartner H, Hung J, Bermejo J, et al. Recommendations on the echocardiographic assessment of aortic valve stenosis: a focused update from the European Association of Cardiovascular Imaging and the American Society of Echocardiography. *J Am Soc Echocardiogr*. 2017;30:372.
68. Frank M, Ganzoni G, Starck C, et al. Lack of accessible data on prosthetic heart valves. *Int J Cardiovasc Imaging*. 2016;32:439.
69. Blauwet LA, Miller Jr FA. Echocardiographic assessment of prosthetic heart valves. *Prog Cardiovasc Dis*. 2014;57:100.
70. Zamorano J, Goncalves A, Lancellotti P, et al. The use of imaging in new transcatheter interventions: an EACVI review paper. *Eur Heart J Cardiovasc Imag*. 2016;17:835.

Pericardial Disease

71. Chetrit M, Xu B, Verma BR, et al. Multimodality imaging for the assessment of pericardial diseases. *Curr Cardiol Rep*. 2019;21:41.
72. Cosyns B, Plein S, Nihoyanopoulos P, et al. European Association of Cardiovascular Imaging (EACVI) position paper: multimodality imaging in pericardial disease. *Eur Heart J Cardiovasc Imaging*. 2015;16:12.

Pulmonary Embolism

73. Konstantinides SV, Meyer G, Becattini C, et al. 2019 ESC guidelines on the diagnosis and management of acute pulmonary embolism developed in collaboration with the European Respiratory Society (ERS): the Task Force for the diagnosis and management of acute pulmonary embolism of the European Society of Cardiology (ESC). *Eur Heart J*. 2020;41:543.
74. Mediratta A, Addetia K, Medvedofsky D, et al. Echocardiographic diagnosis of acute pulmonary embolism in patients with McConnell's sign. *Echocardiography*. 2016;33:696.

Pulmonary Hypertension

75. Cordina RL, Playford D, Lang I, Celermajer DS. State-of-the-Art review: echocardiography in pulmonary hypertension. *Heart Lung Circ*. 2019;28:1351.

Infective Endocarditis

76. Habib G, Lancellotti P, Antunes MJ, et al. 2015 ESC guidelines for the management of infective endocarditis. The task force for the management of infective endocarditis of the European Society of Cardiology (ESC). Endorsed by the European Association for Cardio-Thoracic Surgery (EACTS) and the European Association of Nuclear Medicine (EANM). *Eur Heart J*. 2015;36:3075.
77. Flachskampf FA, Wouters PF, Edvardsen T, et al. Recommendations for transoesophageal echocardiography: EACVI update 2014. *Eur Heart J Cardiovasc Imaging*. 2014;15:353.
78. Sedgwick JF, Scalia GM. Advanced Echocardiography for the Diagnosis and Management of Infective Endocarditis. Firstenberg MS (ed). Contemporary Challenges in Endocarditis. 2016 In Tech.
79. Saric M, Armour AC, Anaout MS, et al. Guidelines for the use of echocardiography in the evaluation of a cardiac source of embolism. *J Am Soc Echocardiogr*. 2016;29.

Systemic Disease and Echocardiography

80. Manga P, McCutcheon K, Tsabede N, et al. HIV and nonischemic heart disease. *J Am Coll Cardiol*. 2017;69:83.
81. Plana JC, Galderisi M, Barac A, et al. Expert consensus for multimodality imaging evaluation of adult patients during and after cancer therapy: a report from the American Society of Echocardiography and the European Association of Cardiovascular Imaging. *J Am Soc Echocardiogr*. 2014;27:911.
82. Kang Y, Scherrer-Crosbie M. Echocardiography imaging of cardiotoxicity. *Cardiol Clinics*. 2019;37:419.
83. Bois J, Anand V, Anavekar N. Detection of inflammatory aortopathies using multimodality imaging. *Circ: Cardiovasc Imaging*. 2019;12:e008471.

Cardiac Masses

84. Wu JC. Cardiac tumors and masses. In: Stergiopoulos K, Brown DL, eds. *Evidence-Based Cardiology Consult*. New York: Springer Science+Business Media; 2014.
85. Palaskas N, Thompson K, Gladish G, et al. Evaluation and management of cardiac tumors. *Curr Treatment Options Cardiovasc Med*. 2018;20:29.
86. Laura DM, Donnino R, Kim EE, et al. Silbiger JJ, Bazaz R, Trost B. Lipomatous atrial septal hypertrophy: a review of its anatomy, pathophysiology, multimodality imaging, and relevance to percutaneous interventions. *J Am Soc Echocardiog*. 2016;29:717.
87. Tower-Rader A, Kwon D. Pericardial masses, cysts and diverticula: a comprehensive review using multimodality imaging. *Prog Cardiovasc Dis*. 2017;59:389.

Congenital Heart Disease in Adults

88. Akagi T. Current concept of transcatheter closure of atrial septal defect in adults. *J Cardiol*. 2015;65:17.
89. Cohen MS, Eidem BW, Cetta F, et al. Multimodality imaging guidelines of patients with transposition of the great arteries: a report from the American Society of Echocardiography developed in collaboration with the society for cardiovascular magnetic resonance and the society of cardiovascular computed tomography. *J Am Soc Echocardiogr*. 2016;29:571.
90. Valente AM, Cook S, Festa P, et al. Multimodality imaging guidelines for patients with repaired tetralogy of Fallot: a report from the American Society of Echocardiography developed in collaboration with the society for cardiovascular magnetic resonance and the society for pediatric radiology. *J Am Soc Echocardiogr*. 2014;27:111.

Transcatheter Interventions

91. Freitas-Ferraz AB, Bernier M, Vaillancourt, et al. Safety of transesophageal echocardiography to guide structural cardiac interventions. *J Am Coll Cardiol*. 2020;75:3174.
92. Hahn RT, Nabauer M, Zuber M, et al. Intraprocedural imaging of transcatheter tricuspid valve interventions. *J Am Coll Cardiol Cardiovasc Imaging*. 2019;12:532.
93. Vainrib AF, Harb SC, Jaber W, et al. Left atrial appendage occlusion/exclusion: procedural image guidance with transesophageal echocardiography. *J Am Soc Echocardiogr*. 2018;31:454.

Future Directions

Multimodality Imaging

94. Rozado J, Martin M, Pascual I, et al. Comparing American, European and Asian practice guidelines for aortic diseases. *J Thorac Dis*. 2017;9:S551.
95. Afonso L, Kottam A, Reddy V, et al. Echocardiography in infective endocarditis: state of the art. *Echocardiogr*. 2017;19:127.

Handheld Echocardiography (Point of Care Ultrasound)

96. Cahmsi-Pasha MA, Sengupta PP, Zoghbi WA. Handheld echocardiography: current state and future perspectives. *Circulation*. 2017;136:2178.
97. Cardim N, Dalen H, Voigt J-U, et al. The use of handheld ultrasound devices: a position statement of the European Association of Cardiovascular Imaging (2018 update). *Eur Heart J Cardiovasc Imag*. 2019;20:245.

Newer Techniques

98. Voigt J-U, Cvijic M. 2- and 3-dimensional myocardial strain in cardiac health and disease. *J Am Coll Cardiol Cardiovasc Imaging*. 2019;12:1849.
99. Takaya Y, Ito H. New horizon of fusion imaging using echocardiography: its progress in the diagnosis and treatment of cardiovascular disease. *J Echocardiog*. 2020;18:9.

Artificial Intelligence

100. Dey D, Slomka PJ, Leeson P, et al. Artificial intelligence in cardiovascular imaging: JACC state-of-the-art review. *J Am Coll Cardiol*. 2019;73:1317.
101. Narang A, Lang RM. Artificial Intelligence and Echocardiography. Expert Analysis. https://www.acc.org/latest-in-cardiology/articles/2019/06/18/07/43/artificial-intelligence-and-echocardiography.

17 Chest Radiography in Cardiovascular Disease

FRANCINE L. JACOBSON

OVERVIEW, 268
PA and Lateral CXR, 268

APPROACH TO CXR EVALUATION, 269
Radiographic Densities, 270
CXR Anatomy, 270

Common Anatomic Variants, 270
Localization Within Cardiac Silhouette, 271

SPECIFIC CARDIOVASCULAR CONDITIONS, 273
Congenital Heart Disease, 273

Acquired Heart Disease, 274
Advanced Imaging in ICU, 275

REFERENCES, 276

The chest radiograph (CXR) has endured, despite all advances in technology, due to its instantaneous capture of patient health as a snapshot in time. Like photographic snapshots, CXRs can also be collected over time to tell the story of disease in a particular patient and provide valuable information at the bedside when a patient is critically ill. The CXR is the first medical imaging for a wide variety of medical conditions, including suspected cardiovascular disease (Table 17.1).[1,2]

OVERVIEW

Understanding how CXRs are made will provide an appreciation for how the best radiographs can be obtained under the most difficult of situations. Understanding the imaging process increases the value of CXRs at the bedside in the intensive care unit (ICU) where there may not be availability of immediate consultation from a radiologist. The American College of Radiology maintains evidence-based guidelines that are reviewed and updated annually by leaders in radiology and other specialties.[2-5]

Though partnership between clinicians and radiologists supports high-quality patient care while conserving patient exposure to ionizing radiation, keeping the dose "as low as reasonably achievable (ALARA)" is the principle that guides the creation of every CXR.[6]

The appearance of the heart and lungs on CXRs can be very specific for some disease processes, including congenital and acquired heart diseases, based on anatomy. Chest radiography is frequently the first imaging study ordered and may be available before the first visit with a cardiologist. Anatomic structure identification is enhanced by common calcifications and radiopaque devices that supply additional landmarks within regions of radiographically undifferentiated tissue. Fully utilizing the lateral view along with the frontal posteroanterior (PA) view, when available, maximizes the information available from CXR. Approach to the evaluation of the CXR and uses for CXR in patient care will be the central components of this chapter. The first principles presented will provide a foundation for approaching CXRs in patients with diseases beyond the examples in this chapter.

PA and Lateral CXR

Magnification of structures follows the inverse square law by which magnification increases as the square of distance. With distance, sharp edges become less sharp. These two directly related principles guide the making of the standard CXR examination including PA and lateral views, made in the erect position for adults able to stand. For the PA radiograph, the anterior chest wall is placed as close as possible to the detector, thereby minimizing magnification of the heart. Despite this, the left lung is less well imaged than the right lung due to the presence of the heart primarily in the left hemithorax. This is balanced by providing a slight advantage to the left lung on lateral radiograph by placing the receptor against the left side of the patient, providing the sharpest depiction of vessels and other structures in the left lung. The inverse square law thus results in magnification of the right hemithorax and right ribs compared with the left hemithorax and left ribs, as shown in Figures 17.1 and 17.2. Thus, when a normal CXR is made, the left lung and ribs will be projected within the right hemithorax. This is an important means by which pathology is localized. The patient's arms are positioned for both views to minimize the overlap of scapula with lungs. The lungs are positioned where sensors will best account for the difference in tissue density, thereby making an image that is correctly exposed for both heart and lungs.

The CXR is obtained at relatively high 120 to 140 kV to deliberately decrease obscuration of structures by the ribs and other bones encasing the thorax. It is for this reason that CXR may not identify calcifications, particularly larger calcifications. The radiation dose from one standard adult CXR is approximately 0.1 mSV. This is equivalent to 10 days of natural background radiation. These figures are convenient for comparing radiation dose from other imaging studies such as computed tomography (CT). The radiation exposure while on a plane flying at 40,000 feet is approximately 30% higher than our background radiation at sea level. This can be used to reassure a patient who becomes distressed about radiation exposure when many serial CXRs are required. Radiology department professional staffs include radiation physicists who can also assist with calculating patient-specific doses of ionizing radiation.[6]

Portable Chest Radiographs

The ICU is a much more complex environment in which to perform chest radiography. Safety of ICU personnel and logistics for making the best possible images benefit from partnership between radiology technologists, nurses, and respiratory therapists to secure support lines away from regions of interest. The portable CXR machine provides a lower maximum dose of radiation and may lose capability if it is battery powered as battery level decreases toward a level at which it must be recharged. This type of unit can be most desirable when ICU outlets are in short supply.[5,6]

Beyond Standard Radiographs

A hybrid type of exam is frequently performed for patients in the emergency department and for patients on stretchers. The frontal radiograph is made in the anteroposterior (AP) projection like a portable CXR while using the standard radiography equipment. If the patient can sit straight up on the stretcher, a lateral view can be made. Using the radiography room in the radiology department results in a near-standard CXR. This can be especially valuable for obese patients for whom portable CXR may be inadequate due to tube limitations regarding radiation dose. When a patient needs to be flat, the standard radiography cross-table lateral will be superior to the same examination performed at the bedside in the ICU. This can be important when a lateral view is required for localization of malpositioned support line. While it takes more effort to organize the trip to the radiology department, considered use of this strategy can improve patient care, decrease cumulative radiation dose, and decrease delay in optimizing patient care.

Inspiration-Expiration CXR
Inspiration-expiration CXR is infrequently ordered, although it can demonstrate diaphragmatic excursion and the range in apparent size of a particular patient's heart. This CXR can be obtained as PA or AP views. The expiration CXR alone can be used to increase visibility of a pneumothorax, although this is infrequently performed in academic medical centers where thoracic radiologists read all CXRs using PACS (picture archive and communication system) workstation display and tools.

Frontal CXR Variations
Oblique, lordotic, and reverse lordotic views are useful for problem solving. Forty-five-degree oblique views of the chest are familiar to cardiologists as a standard plane for evaluation of the aorta. The hallmark of the 45-degree obliquity used to image the aorta is a projection of the trachea to the right of the spine. Shallow 15-degree oblique views do not shift structures significantly, just enough to differentiate between nodules, vessels, and bone findings. Shallow oblique views are superior to lordotic and reverse lordotic views for assessment of lung nodules, especially in the lung apices. Shallow obliques are also useful for differentiating between breast nipples from lung nodules. A four view CXR refers to PA, lateral, and bilateral oblique views that can often substitute for chest fluoroscopy when used to determine whether a nodule is present. This and chest fluoroscopy have largely given way to CT for these differentiations, although CT carries more significant risk of additional findings leading to additional CT scans and anxiety for the patient. They are presented here because the equivalent information and views are frequently available in the cardiac catheterization laboratory, sparing the patient additional procedures.

Chest Fluoroscopy
Chest fluoroscopy is performed at lower kV than CXRs and is capable of detecting benign patterns of calcification in lung nodules. This function has been largely replaced by CT with chest fluoroscopy now used almost exclusively for functional evaluation of the diaphragm, referred to commonly as a "sniff" test. This is best performed as an outpatient procedure and contraindicated for patients requiring mechanical ventilation. It is best at detecting unilateral diaphragmatic paralysis and limited in value for detecting bilateral diaphragmatic paralysis because it depends on the asymmetry between the normal and abnormal hemidiaphragm. The exam begins in the erect position and is repeated in the supine position, especially when normal in the erect position, in order to decrease the effectiveness of accessory muscles or respiration. Abdominal muscles in particular are unable to adequately move the hemidiaphragms in the supine position. Deep inspiration and deep expiration demonstrate the overall diaphragmatic excursion. The sniff maneuver, breathing sharply through the nose while the mouth is closed, will provoke paradoxical motion, whereby the paralyzed hemidiaphragm will rise during the special sniff maneuver. A patient report of sleep position is often revealing as sleeping on a paralyzed hemidiaphragm will tend to awaken the patient. This is because the lung that is down does the primary work of breathing. This positional difference can also be exploited with radiography.

Decubitus Views
Although decubitus position in adults is most often used for evaluation of pleural effusion size and mobility, the decubitus position in an adult will also result in the upper lung being held in inspiration. Restoration of a sharp costophrenic sulcus can confirm mobility of the pleural effusion when it shifts into the mediastinum. Paired right and left lateral decubitus views are not always needed for diagnostic purposes, but the paired images will provide inspiratory examination of both lungs in a patient who is unable to stand or cooperate in taking a deep breath.

TABLE 17.1 American College of Radiology (ACR) Appropriateness Criteria for Cardiac Diseases Algorithms for Disease Group Specific Workup Using Multiple Imaging Modalities and Appropriate Use for Specific Imaging Modalities

PRESENTATION OF SYMPTOMS AND INITIAL IMAGING	SPECIFIC APPROPRIATENESS CRITERIA
Asymptomatic Patient	At Risk for Coronary Artery Disease (CAD)
Acute chest pain	Possible acute coronary syndrome (ACS)
	High probability of CAD
	Low probability of CAD
	Suspected aortic dissection
	Suspected pulmonary embolism
Blunt chest trauma	Suspect cardiac injury
Chronic chest pain	High probability of CAD
	Low to intermediate probability of CAD
Heart failure	New-onset and chronic heart failure
Adult congenital heart disease	Known or suspected congenital heart disease
Use of chest radiograph (CXR)	Routine CXR
	Portable CXR

From American College of Radiology. Appropriateness criteria table, for cardiac diseases. (https://acsearch.acr.org/list). Accessed 3/11/2021.

APPROACH TO CXR EVALUATION

A systematic approach to the evaluation of the PA-lateral CXR is greatly facilitated by placing the two views side by side. When looking at PA and lateral views together, levels are matched based on readily visible anatomy. The top of the aortic arch, the carina (at approximately the same level as the bottom of an ectatic aorta), and pulmonary venous confluence are accessible for basic orientation on the lateral view. This provides a check on any hypothesis about localization based on any frontal view. Discordance requires a new hypothesis. This strategy, combined with imaging physics and a few basic radiographic signs, derives maximum information from every CXR.[7]

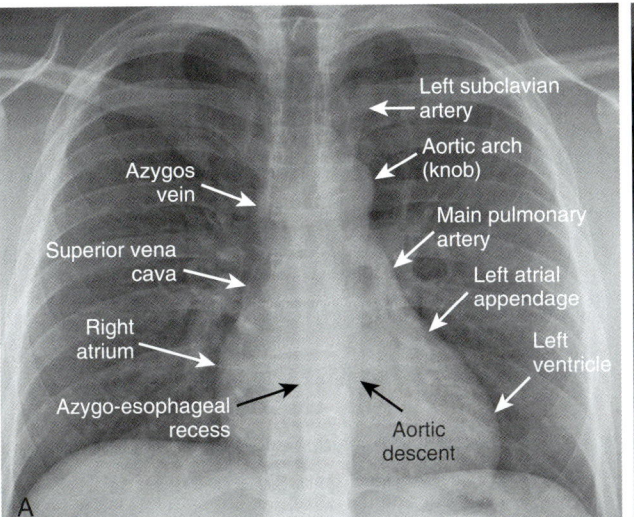 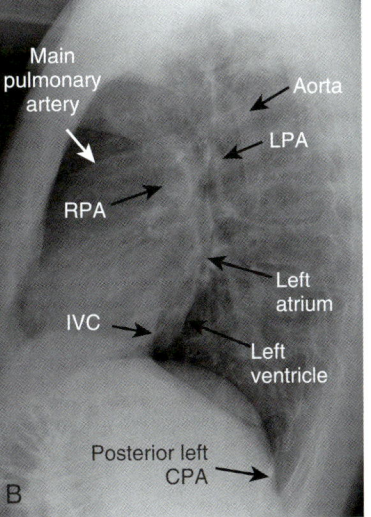

FIGURE 17.1 Normal standard two-view chest radiograph. PA **(A)** and lateral **(B)** views of the chest depict various normal cardiovascular structures. *CPA,* costophrenic angle; *IVC,* inferior vena cava; *LPA,* left pulmonary artery; *RPA,* right pulmonary artery. (From Javidan-Nejad C, Balla S. The chest radiograph in cardiovascular disease. In Zipes DP, et al. (editors): Braunwald's Heart Disease: A Textbook of Cardiovascular Medicine. 11th ed. Philadelphia: Elsevier; 2019, pp 252-260.)

Radiographic Densities

Radiographic densities are air, fat, water, calcification, and metal. Water density is the density of a wide variety of soft tissues including fluid, muscle, and solid organs. The differentiation of fat in regions of air can also result in water attenuation for pleural and pericardial fat. Calcifications provide delineation of anatomic structures for which we do not have a radiographic difference in density. These, and an ever-increasing variety of radiopaque devices, help to provide internal anatomic landmarks in the heart on CXRs. Some, such as the intra-aortic balloon pump and with luck some replacement valves, can also reveal the phase of the cardiac cycle in which a radiograph has been obtained.

The limited differentiation of tissues requires a lexicon for CXR in order to communicate accurately the findings and the significance of the findings. The most basic of terms, cardiac silhouette must be understood to include more than just the heart. The cardiac silhouette may become enlarged by one or more chamber enlargements. A pericardial effusion surrounding the heart can also enlarge the cardiac silhouette. We expand this to cardiovascular silhouette to include the aorta, great vessels, pulmonary artery, and vascular pedicle. To this we add the entire mediastinum when we refer to the cardiomediastinal contour. Pulmonary vascular redistribution is an important term from the point of view of cardiology practice.

Interpreting CXR Pearl
The most valuable advice about looking at CXRs in medical school came to me from an elderly radiologist who said, "The answer is in the jacket." When caring for a patient who has had many CXRs, you can often find the same findings on a prior CXR and read the radiologist's report to support your own reading of a new CXR that has not yet been interpreted by a radiologist. It is even more valuable to expand this concept to include looking at other modalities in the now-virtual radiology jacket. The information that might be gained from ordering a CT scan may already be available from a prior examination, saving money, time, and radiation exposure.

CXR Anatomy
PA Radiograph

The heart border is composed of a series of landmarks, right heart border being the normal heart landmark that extends to the right of the spine. The interface with the lung is provided by the right atrium. A minimally dilated aorta is often seen just above the right ventricle in adult patients, especially those with hypertension and heart disease (Fig. 17.3). A small double density is often created by this divergence that is also coincidentally at the same level as the junction of the superior vena cava and the right atrium, frequently referred simply as the cavo-atrial junction, an important landmark for vascular support line placements. The superior vena cava can be followed to the right paratracheal region above the level of the azygous arch (see Fig. 17.1). The azygous vein drains into the superior vena cava at the level of the carina, allowing it to appear as an almond-shaped structure along the right side of the tracheobronchial angle. The upper limit of the normal size range for this structure is 11 mm, a useful guide for determining pulmonary vascular engorgement. The aortic arch will cross over the trachea with variable visibility depending on patient age and disease. The side of the aortic arch is fundamental for determination of situs. In infants and children, this may need to be inferred by the side on which it creates an impression on the trachea. With age and disease, the aorta becomes a major landmark by which one can imagine picking up the mediastinum. The normal left-sided aorta will descend to the left of the spine. As it enlarges and elongates, it will become a tortuous retrocardiac structure. Great vessels emanating from the aorta course upward and may be seen at and above the clavicles. Coming down the left side of the cardiovascular silhouette brings the eye to the main pulmonary and left pulmonary artery. The pulmonary arteries introduce subtle asymmetry due to the difference in arterial position relative to airways. The left hilum is 1 to 2 cm higher than the right hilum, creating what is referred to as the hilar angle. Alterations in hilar angle indicate volume loss in one or both lungs. The AP window is at the point where the direction of the contours changes from aorta to left pulmonary artery. This space may be enlarged by invagination of lung only in the case of absence of the pericardium that binds the aorta and pulmonary artery together. The upper portion of the left heart border is created by the left atrium and most prominent when the left atrial appendage is enlarged as in mitral valve disease. The lower left heart border is created by the left ventricle. Midline structures include posterior and anterior junction lines, and the azygo-esophageal line that defines the azygo-esophageal recess behind the heart. Additional midline structures that are also frequently visible include the manubrium and hiatal hernia. After completing the tour of the heart border, the right ventricle will not have been border forming, only seen if enlarged and creating a double density sign.

Lateral Radiograph

The first heart border encountered on the lateral chest radiographic is the right ventricle in continuity with the main pulmonary artery with the aorta seen more posteriorly and extending higher (see Fig. 17.1). The upper posterior heart border is created by the left atrium. Left atrial enlargement can elevate the left mainstem bronchus on the frontal radiograph. The lower posterior border of the heart is created by the left ventricle. The inferior vena cava creates an interface extending up from the diaphragm. In a well-positioned lateral radiograph of a 70 kg man with a normal size heart, the left ventricle would extend less than 1.7 cm posterior to the IVC and 2 cm above the diaphragm. A handy rule of thumb is to use up 2 cm and back 2 cm for a more forgiving reference relative to the position and size of the patient. Left ventricular enlargement can create the appearance of right ventricular enlargement on the lateral radiograph due to mass effect elevating the right ventricle. The right pulmonary artery is seen with the heart more anteriorly while the left pulmonary artery is higher and more posterior. The aortic-pulmonary window lies between the aorta and left pulmonary artery. The right paratracheal region will be projected with and just anterior to the trachea.

Common Anatomic Variants

Understanding anatomic variants in anatomy on chest x-rays is facilitated by an understanding of embryology. The heart itself arises from mesoderm within the trilaminar embryonic disc. It begins as a pair of tubes within the pericardial cavity and folds under the direction of cilia. In absence of cilia, folding will be random, with equal probability for each fold in the development of normal situs. Aortic arches are formed sequentially from paired pharyngeal arches (previously referred to as branchial arches). A sequence of remodeling leads to the normal asymmetric arrangement of great vessels. The paired system provides opportunities to recover

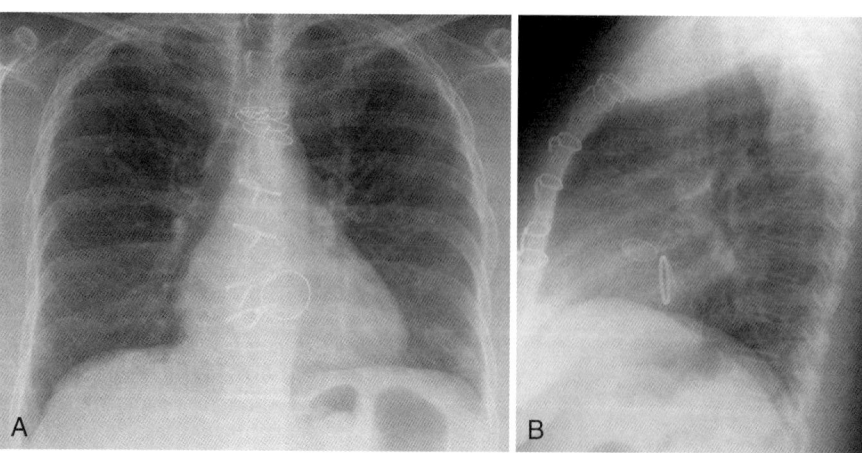

FIGURE 17.2 PA and lateral chest x-ray in a patient with bioprosthetic aortic and mitral valves. A, PA view reveals mitral valve ring and linear appearance of aortic valve ring that is in center of heart. The mitral valve is located inferior to the aortic valve. **B,** Lateral view shows typical magnification of the right hemithorax and right ribs compared with the left hemithorax and left ribs. Mitral valve annulus is posterior to the aortic valve.

from missed steps in sequence. The variations in arch anatomy are well known. Variations also occur beyond the aortic arch, using vessels that connect between right and left circulation to overcome small errors in development. Resulting tortuosity of the aorta may become more apparent as vessels enlarge over the life cycle.

Azygous Lobe Variant

Incomplete migration of the azygous vein during embryologic development can result in the azygous vein being variably placed or mobile within an azygous fissure. Although not strictly speaking a lobe, it is often referred to as the azygous lobe variant. It is extremely rare for the azygous vein to leave the fissure even in the setting of a large pneumothorax. The normal almond-shaped azygous vein normally measuring up to 11 mm in transverse diameter will not be seen abutting the carina. It is important to recognize this variant as dilation of the azygous vein contributes to widening of the vascular pedicle that can be valuable observation in the setting of pulmonary vascular engorgement.

Aortic Arch Variants

Anatomic arch anomalies arise from developmental differences in embryology, often as compensation for slight differences or "mistakes" in development as the paired aortic arches are joined.

Localization Within Cardiac Silhouette

Chest radiography is not able to differentiate between fluid and muscle, resulting in a very homogeneous density of the heart. The fluid density of the heart can be separated from three different distinct radiographic densities: fat, calcification, and metal.

Fat

In a normal heart, epicardial fat immediately adjacent to the heart and pericardial fat outside the pericardium are seen without separation, if visible at all on CXRs. The fat in these locations can be separated by a pericardial effusion. This is most frequently seen on the lateral CXR immediately behind the anterior chest wall. This is sometimes referred to as the "Oreo cookie" sign and can be sensitive for small pericardial effusion. On the frontal view of the chest, globular enlargement of the heart is more likely to raise concern for pericardial effusion with the heart appearing to be in a "water bottle" (Fig. 17.4). Large pericardial effusions can cause the edge of the heart to be differentiated from the effusion going around the heart on either or both frontal and lateral views.

Calcifications

Calcifications are powerful definers for intracardiac anatomy with localization based primarily on anatomy.[8] Coronary artery calcifications are frequently visible on CT although infrequently reported on chest radiography. Thoracic aortic calcification is a common finding and in extreme cases deserves the term "porcelain aorta" (Fig. 17.5). Mitral annulus calcification with characteristic "C" shape and location on both frontal and lateral CXRs is very easily identified (Fig. 17.6). This C-shaped fibrocalcification is frequently found in older patients (see Chapter 75) and provides a good reference for internal cardiac anatomy. If very exuberant, it can obstruct inflow to left ventricle and be associated with ischemic and, rarely, embolic stroke. Aortic valve calcification is infrequently seen by comparison, but the fact that these two valves share a common attachment can be helpful to identify smaller amounts of calcification in the aortic valve.

Differentiating calcified muscle from pericardial calcification is facilitated by the anatomy itself (Figs. 17.7 and 17.8). Pericardial calcification can extend over boundaries between cardiac chambers. It will be best seen on the view in which it is most closely perpendicular to the direction of the x-ray beam and may be completely inapparent on the opposite orthogonal view. Calcific pericarditis completely encasing the heart can be diagnosed by chest radiography alone. Pericardial calcifications can be caused by infection, most commonly tuberculosis, and intrapericardial hemorrhage (see Chapter 86).

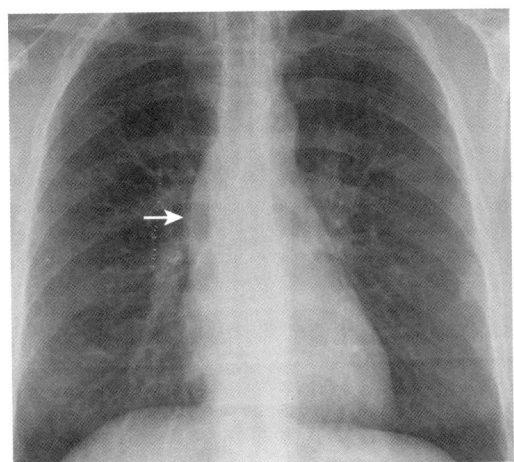

FIGURE 17.3 Ectatic ascending aorta *(arrow)* in a patient with aortic stenosis.

Pulmonary Vasculature

Pulmonary edema can occur through both increased pressure and increased permeability of vessels and these may be seen in combination (Fig. 17.9). Permeability edema can occur with or without diffuse alveolar damage. Distension of pulmonary veins most typically appears as cephalization on supine radiographs. The distribution of pulmonary edema follows the course of least resistance within any given patient position. Cephalization, dependent on the presence of upper lobe vessels, may be absent in the setting of significant emphysema. A patient position preference may introduce lateralization.[9]

Slowly evolving pulmonary edema is more likely to produce pulmonary interlobular septal thickening due to veins and lymphatics. This process produces what are usually referred to as Kerley B lines along with small pleural effusion(s) (Fig. 17.10). Kerley B lines are most apparent at the right lung base on the frontal chest x-ray. Visualization of Kerley B lines can become permanent due to hemosiderin deposition following repeated episodes of interstitial pulmonary

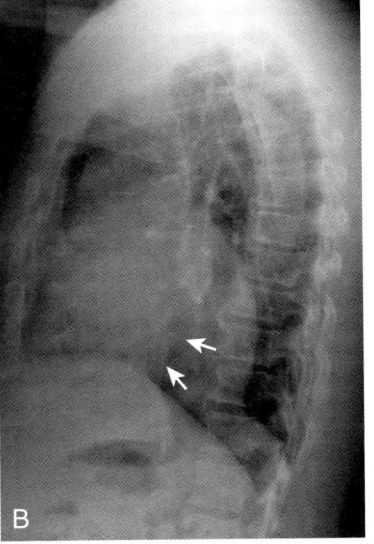

FIGURE 17.4 PA **(A)** and lateral **(B)** chest radiographs in a patient with a large pericardial effusion. The PA view reveals marked enlargement of heart with a hot water bottle shape. This can also have shape of an Erlenmeyer flask. The lateral view reveals the normal size heart *(arrows)* inside the pericardial effusion. Separation of epicardial from pericardial fat may be most apparent anteriorly.

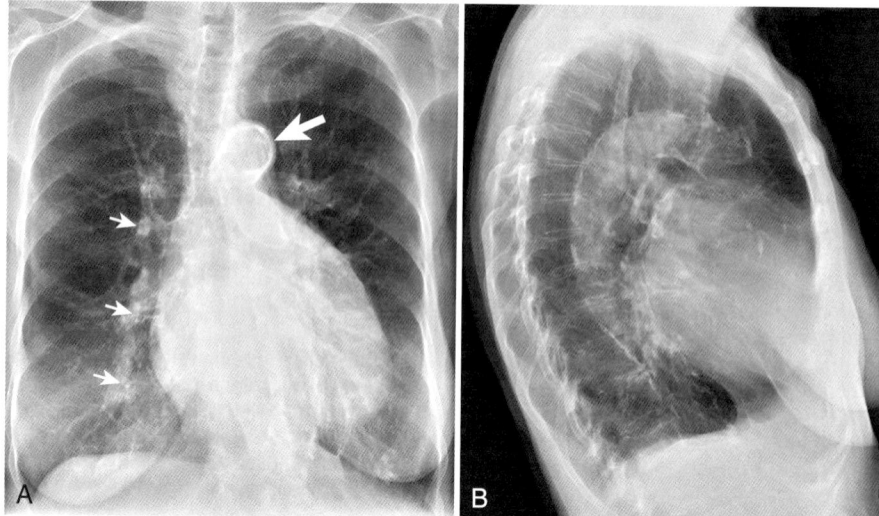

FIGURE 17.5 PA **(A)** and lateral **(B)** chest radiographs in a patient with aortic calcification. This is best seen on the PA view with long summation shadow-gram of aortic arch *(large arrow)*. The PA view also shows calcification of tracheobronchial tree *(small arrows)*, which is occasionally encountered in patients receiving warfarin. The lateral view reveals extensive calcification of aorta as well as origins of great vessels and coronary arteries.

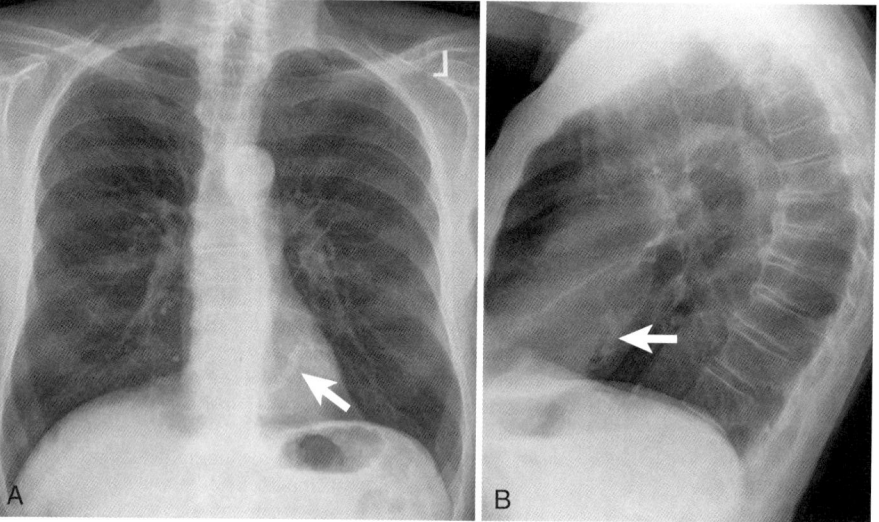

FIGURE 17.6 PA **(A)** and lateral **(B)** chest radiographs in a patient with mitral annular calcification *(arrows)*.

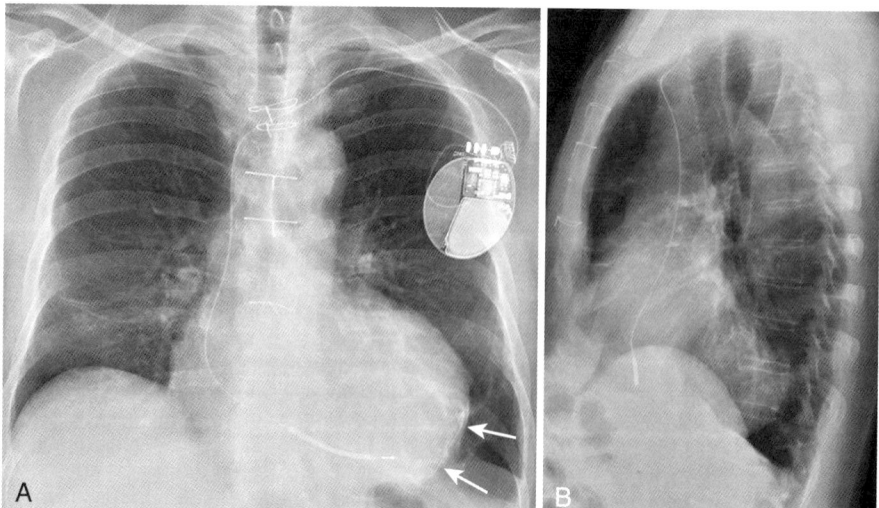

FIGURE 17.7 PA **(A)** and lateral **(B)** chest radiographs in a patient with a calcified left ventricular pseudoaneurysm *(arrows)*. The lateral view reveals posterior extension of the pseudoaneurysm.

edema or hemorrhage. Kerley B lines are also associated with viral pneumonia and lymphangitis carcinomatosis. Dilatation of pulmonary veins, blurring of pulmonary vascular margins, and fissures are subtle signs of congestive heart failure.

Pulmonary hypertension causes characteristic features involving the pulmonary vasculature. Idiopathic pulmonary hypertension causes marked enlargement of main pulmonary artery. Central pulmonary artery branches are enlarged with peripheral pruning (Fig. 17.11). Extremely large central artery branch pruning may result in normal-appearing peripheral branches despite marked decrease in size.

Support Lines and Devices

Intravascular support lines demonstrate individual anatomy extremely well. Malpositioned intravascular catheters are frequently found following the course of smaller vessels and anomalous vessels, many of which are derived from the embryologic development of the heart. The suitability of line placements in structures such as persistent left superior vena cava can be addressed by comparison with historical chest CT scan in addition to bedside assessment. Common vascular line malposition locations also include azygous vein and arch and superior intercostal vein (responsible for aortic nipple).

Radiopaque intracardiac devices include devices placed by both cardiologists and cardiac surgeons. Normal positions of the four intracardiac valve replacements and valve repair rings are readily identified on radiographs (see Fig. 17.2). Right ventricular pacemaker leads (see Fig. 17.6) characteristically rise to go through the tricuspid valve. Right atrial leads are directed anteriorly and superiorly toward the sinoatrial node. Use of a third lead to the coronary sinus has become common (see Chapter 58) with additional recent alternative placement to the atrioventricular node, seen on radiographs projected within the region of tricuspid valve. The atrial appendage occlusion device, to prevent thromboembolic events due to atrial fibrillation, is placed in the left atrial appendage as an alternative to atrial ablation and surgical maze procedures (see Chapter 66).

Pearls for Evaluating Portable CXR

The radiologist will approach the individual CXR beginning with placement of support lines, tubes, and devices. The position of the endotracheal tube terminating in the right mainstem bronchus can markedly narrow the differential diagnosis for opacification of the left hemithorax to left lung collapse. The sudden onset of a new lung parenchymal abnormality may be tied to an event such as aspiration, hemorrhage, or flash pulmonary edema. The distribution of abnormality is a powerful differentiator between these possibilities. Central distribution is characteristic of perihilar "bat wing" pulmonary edema. Hemorrhage is likely to produce asymmetric bilateral consolidation. Aspiration in the ICU setting is most often seen in left lower lobe due to the posterior angulation of the left mainstem bronchus. Sterile aspiration, also known as Mendelson syndrome, can simulate acute pulmonary edema and is frequently associated

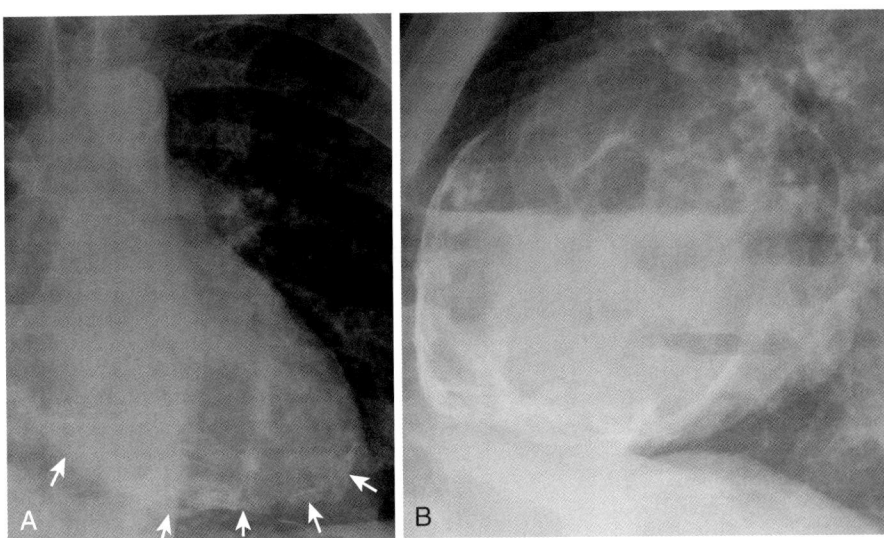

FIGURE 17.8 PA **(A)** and lateral **(B)** coned down views in a patient with constrictive pericarditis *(arrows)*. The PA view reveals pericardial calcification extending across expected cardiac chamber boundaries and extending through the atrial-ventricular groove, resulting in severe constrictive pericarditis, while the lateral view shows extensive anterior, apical, and inferior calcification.

with a side hole of the enteric tube left in the esophagus, setting up a route for reflux from the stomach to the esophagus. Portable CXRs are routinely used following procedures and placement of devices to rule out hemorrhage, pneumothorax, and pneumomediastinum (Fig. 17.12).

Serial CXRs provide more information over time. Pulmonary edema will clear over 24 hours. Hemorrhage will clear more slowly with the shift from consolidation to coarse interstitial pattern, with the periphery of the lung developing sharply defined sparing with complete resolution after about 3 days. Aspiration may be transient or lead to pneumonia that will clear slowly over a longer period. Physiologic changes such as increasing and decreasing pulmonary edema can be helpful for the management of patients with heart disease.

Viewing multiple images as a group also provides compensation between individually limited nonstandard images. An opacity due to a healed rib fracture may be more obvious on one image and avoid consideration of a pulmonary nodule in another image. The patient's progress in recovering from cardiac surgery may be followed through the succession of support line removals with an ability to point out the time and duration of a setback in recovery allowing more thoughtful consideration of potential complication that required the extended use of a particular support line or device.

Clinical ICU care has historically over-relied on routine daily portable CXRs. Harmonizing clinical care routines can increase the value of each radiograph for managing support lines, tubes, and devices and decrease the total number of images required for optimum care in the ICU. The American College of Radiology Appropriateness Criteria for CXRs in ICU patients and for routine chest radiography are maintained by periodic interdisciplinary panel review.[10]

Value of Baseline CXR. The most valuable CXRs for any patient with heart disease are baseline PA and lateral views of the chest. New baseline CXRs are generally acquired 4 to 6 weeks following cardiac surgery in order to allow time for perioperative findings to resolve. The same is not always followed for patients with medically managed heart disease, limiting evaluation for subtle changes.

SPECIFIC CARDIOVASCULAR CONDITIONS

Congenital Heart Disease

The range of congenital heart disease is very broad, ranging from a single embryologic error that can go undetected throughout life to very complex abnormalities that become apparent even before birth.[11-14] Early-life diagnosed and treated congenital heart disease may have increasing physiologic consequences in adulthood for which the individual patient history will be paramount (see Chapter 82). In the context of adult heart disease, it is most valuable to focus on initial diagnosis of congenital heart disease in adults.

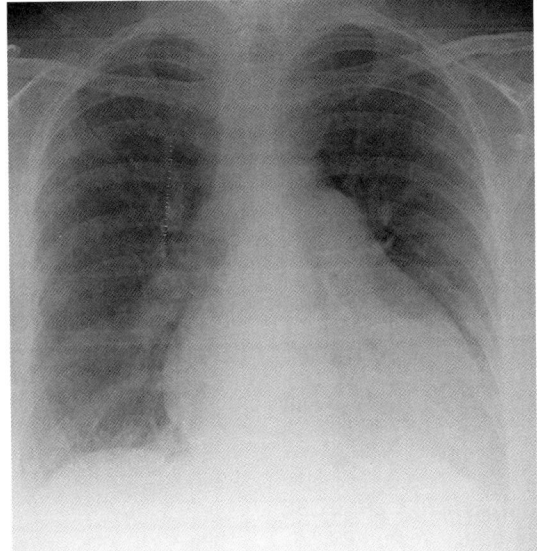

FIGURE 17.9 PA chest radiograph in a patient with congestive heart failure. There is enlargement of the left ventricle, left atrium, and main pulmonary artery, with pulmonary venous congestion.

The most common congenital heart disease is bicuspid aortic valve. This may go undetected until a patient becomes symptomatic due to critical aortic stenosis (see Chapter 72). Dilatation of the aorta, resulting in greater ectasia of the ascending aorta, is often the primary radiologic finding (see Fig. 17.3), followed by left ventricular enlargement should the aortic valve become regurgitant.

Aortic arch anomalies reflect disordered embryogenesis during the folding of the primitive tube that becomes the heart and the integration between the dual embryonic right and left main arteries and veins. If the right and left aorta persist, a doubled aortic arch will result.

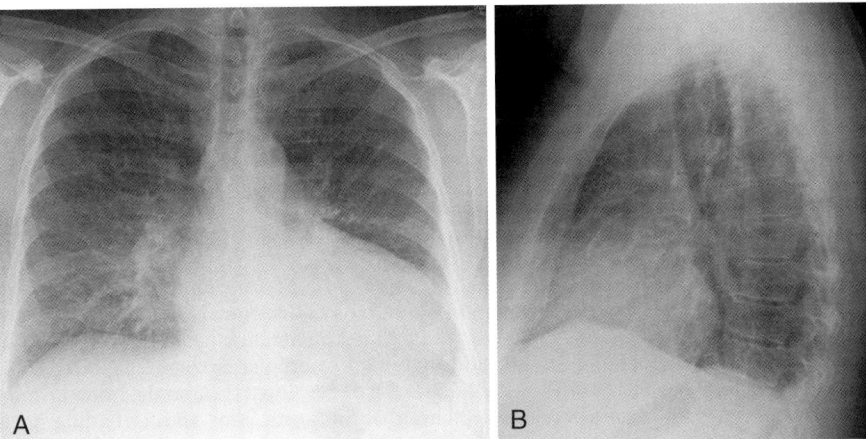

FIGURE 17.10 PA **(A)** and lateral **(B)** chest radiographs in a patient with left ventricular dilation and pulmonary edema. PA view shows venous cephalization, blurring of pulmonary vascular margins, and fissures and Kerley B lines. Lateral view shows pleural effusions.

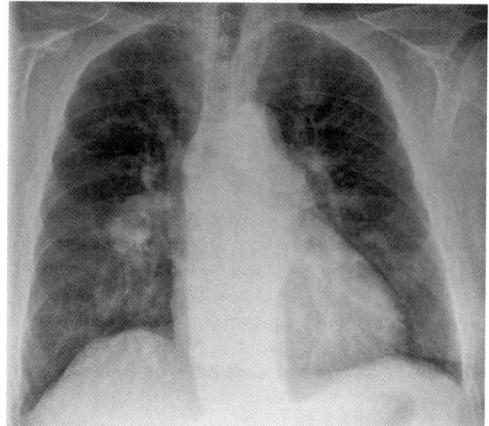

FIGURE 17.11 PA chest radiograph in a patient with idiopathic pulmonary hypertension. Idiopathic pulmonary hypertension causes marked enlargement of main pulmonary artery. Central pulmonary artery branches are enlarged with peripheral pruning. Extremely large central artery branch pruning may result in normal-appearing peripheral branches despite marked decrease in size.

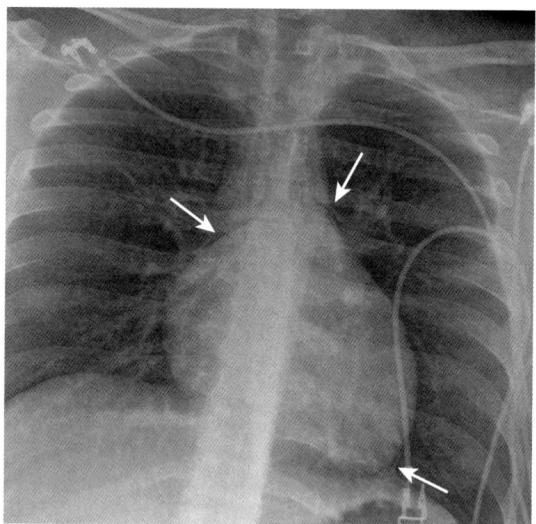

FIGURE 17.12 Portable chest x-ray demonstrating gas along central pulmonary arteries as well as around the cardiac apex (arrows). Pericardial insertion is along underside of aorta, limiting gas going around the aorta within the intact pericardium.

The right arch is generally higher than the left arch with both impressing on the aorta.

Cilia direct the normal development of cardiac chambers to normally produce *situs solitus* with left-sided aortic arch, left-sided cardiac apex, and left-sided stomach on CXRs. Anomalous branching of the great vessels is not frequently evident on adult CXRs. One common great vessel branching anomaly can become visible on CXRs and lead to both gastrointestinal dysmotility and false identification of significant lung nodule in later life. The right subclavian artery is normally the first great vessel leaving the aortic ring. This small embryologic error can be an isolated event with the right subclavian artery arising last and coursing behind the esophagus, resulting in an aberrant subclavian artery. The artery is subject to the processes of atherosclerosis with enlargement and calcification possible in later life. When enlarged, the vessel is well seen focally displacing the trachea on the lateral view simulating a dominant upper lobe lung nodule. The vessel has a more subtle diagonal course on frontal view when enlarged that is helpful for a radiologist to avoid overcalling a lung nodule. The aberrant subclavian artery is *always* contralateral to the aortic arch. Thus a patient with a right-sided aortic arch would have a left-sided aberrant subclavian artery and lower probability of complex congenital heart disease than the alternative of mirror image branching of the aorta.

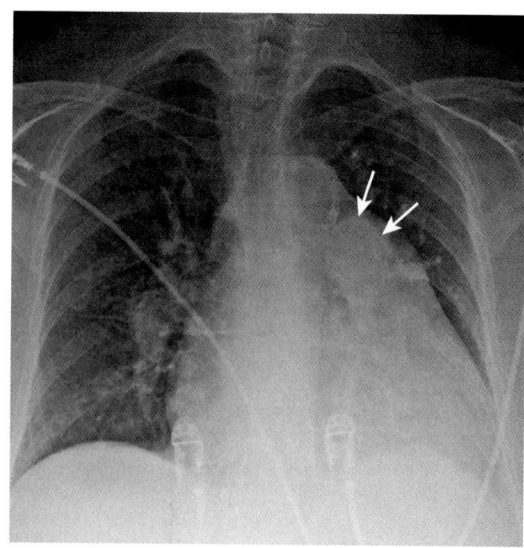

FIGURE 17.13 PA chest radiograph in a patient with congenital heart disease with pulmonary arterial hypertension. The calcified pulmonary artery (arrows) indicates that it has carried systemic pressure. The patient is now presenting with Eisenmenger's physiology and mild interstitial pulmonary edema. Note Kerley B lines in the base of the right lung.

Coarctation of the aorta can also be identified on CXRs. The characteristic notching of the posterior third to eight ribs that occurs in 75% of cases may be more apparent than the narrowing of the aortic arch (see Chapter 42). The rib notching occurs due to pulsatile collateral blood flow through the intercostal arteries. This feature would not be expected in pseudocoarctation due to the dilation and elongation of the aorta causing a folding of the proximal descending thoracic aorta.

In adult patients with complex forms of congenital heart disease, echocardiography, CT, and cardiac magnetic resonance imaging (MRI) are most helpful in determining cardiac chamber location, size, and function, as well as the anatomy of the great vessels (see Chapters 16, 19, and 20). However, CXRs often provide important clues for clinical diagnosis and management, including evidence of pulmonary hypertension and pulmonary edema (Figs. 17.13 to 17.16).

Acquired Heart Disease

In addition to cardiomyopathies, valvular heart disease, and coronary artery disease (CAD),[15,16] additional types of acquired heart disease include cardiac tumors, such as benign atrial myxoma and malignant sarcomas, which may be primary or secondary to prior radiation therapy, and pericardial disease.[17-19] Pericardial effusion may decrease visibility of pulmonary edema and result in long-term restriction associated with calcific pericarditis. Cardiovascular diseases are increasingly viewed in a unified fashion throughout the body, connecting stroke syndromes, aortic aneurysms, dissections, and transections.

Valvular Heart Disease

Echocardiography is the primary method for diagnosing and following valvular heart disease whether congenital, rheumatic, or degenerative (see Chapter 16). The radiographic findings of critical importance include evidence of ventricular or atrial dilation, valvular calcification, dilations of the aorta or pulmonary arteries, and evidence of pulmonary venous congestion. Most common causes of aortic valve disease include congenital bicuspid valves, acquired calcific disease, and rheumatic heart disease (see Chapters 72 and 73). Aortic regurgitation also develops commonly from primary diseases causing dilation of the aortic root and ascending aorta. Mitral valve disease primarily results from myxomatous disease and rheumatic heart disease, but mitral regurgitation can also occur as a secondary phenomenon due to left ventricular remodeling from

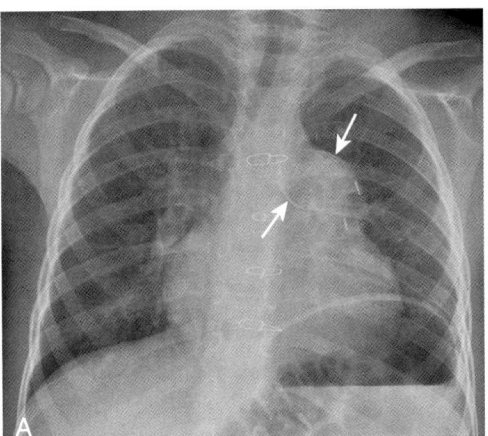 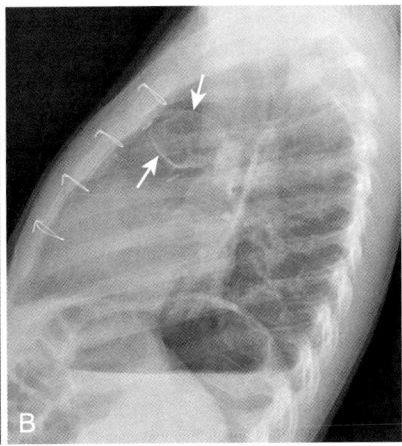

FIGURE 17.14 PA (A) and lateral (B) chest radiographs in a patient with truncus arteriosus. There is dilation of the main pulmonary artery, which is calcified (arrows) as a marker of chronic pulmonary arterial hypertension.

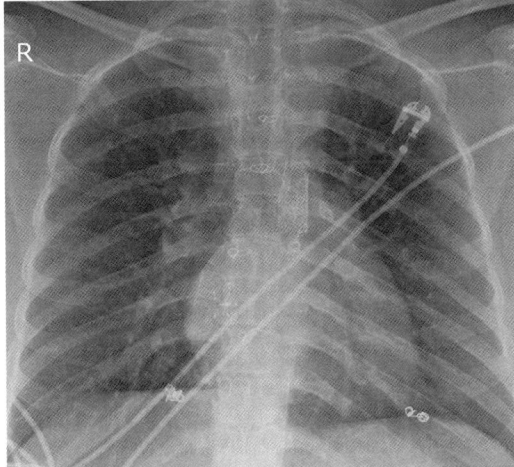

FIGURE 17.15 PA chest radiograph in a 22-year-old patient with hypoplastic left heart and a left aortic arch, initially treated with Blalock-Tausig shunt, subsequently replaced by a Glenn procedure and Fontan procedure with creation of an atrial septal defect (ASD). The ASD has been closed percutaneously, and a stent has been placed to revise the Fontan baffle to the pulmonary artery.

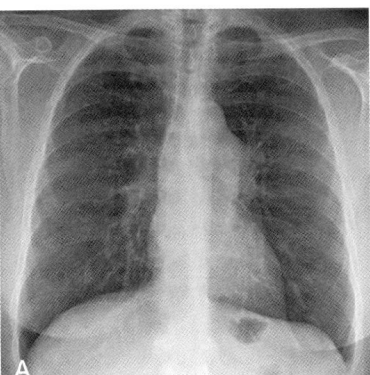 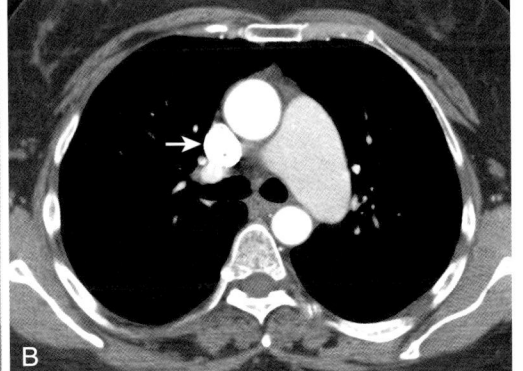

FIGURE 17.16 Congenital pulmonic stenosis. A, PA chest radiograph shows poststenotic dilation of the left pulmonary artery. Right pulmonary artery is normal. B, Axial CT image confirms enlargement of left pulmonary artery (arrow).

dilated cardiomyopathy or ischemic left ventricular dysfunction (see Chapter 76).

Coronary Artery Disease

Chest radiography is not a primary diagnostic modality for CAD but is central to the evaluation of chest pain[20] and postinfarction left ventricular dysfunction.

Heart Failure

CXRs are invaluable in managing patients with heart failure, including initial diagnosis and serial imaging to assess worsening signs and symptoms of heart failure (Fig. 17.17) or improvement following therapy. CXR assists in establishing baseline chamber dilation and status of the pulmonary vascular markings and also in identifying potential undiagnosed valve disease and cardiomyopathy, coexisting lung diseases such as emphysema that also alter the capillary bed capacity of lung parenchyma, and common changes to the cardiovascular silhouette related to sustained hypertension: The increased systemic pressure causes enlargement and elongation of the aorta causing it to assume an uncoiled configuration.[21]

In the outpatient setting, standard PA and lateral CXR views provide the proper snapshot for following the ongoing variations in patient physiology. The size of the heart, the appearance of lung parenchyma, and ancillary findings including lymphadenopathy and pleural effusions provide central information for medical management on an ongoing basis.

Patients with acute heart failure symptoms are seen more frequently in the emergency room and cardiac ICU where basic imaging is performed at the bedside with portable CXRs.[22]

Heart Failure CXR Pearls. Patients with symptomatic heart failure have generally had multiple episodes of pulmonary edema, leaving hemosiderin deposition along interlobular septae in lungs, which contribute to Kerley B lines. In compensated heart failure, little or no pulmonary vascular engorgement will be evident. The vascular pedicle will be normal and the central hilar vessels will be sharp. The lack of pulmonary vascular redistribution, most commonly seen as cephalization, is a very useful sign of equilibrium for a patient receiving medical management of congestive heart failure.

Cardiogenic pulmonary edema arising from rapid elevation hydrostatic pressure causes airspace filling around the pulmonary hila, resulting in bat wing pulmonary edema, sometimes referred to as flash pulmonary edema. This may occur very suddenly in the ICU whether or not it is related to myocardial infarction. As noted previously, when the onset of pulmonary edema occurs very gradually, the lymphatics provide drainage, resulting in Kerley B lines that are particularly easy to identify in the base of the right lung and typically accompanied by small pleural effusions (see Figs. 17.10 and 17.13). In the ICU setting, injury pulmonary edema may be seen in setting of sepsis and multiple organ system failure. Decreased pulmonary compliance and stiffening of lung parenchyma can lead to diffuse alveolar damage and clinical adult respiratory distress syndrome (ARDS).

Advanced Imaging in ICU

A series of portable CXRs can be thought of as a filmstrip or time lapse photography allowing a series of images to provide greater physiologic information than might be obtained from a CT scan, which is limited to a single point in time. Prior outpatient CT scans can provide valuable insight and clarification in the interpretation of portable CXR. Many emergency departments have dedicated CT scanners. A patient presenting with chest pain and shortness of breath may undergo CT angiography to detect pulmonary emboli. It also provides information about lungs, pleural effusions, and cardiovascular anatomy. CT and MRI examinations performed for inpatients are often limited by symptoms, limiting patient cooperation and breath-holding ability. For these reasons, as well as likely presence of acute confounding abnormalities, CT scan for follow-up of small lung nodules should not be performed during hospitalization. The

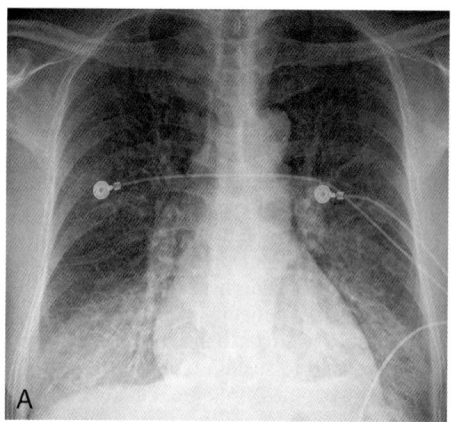
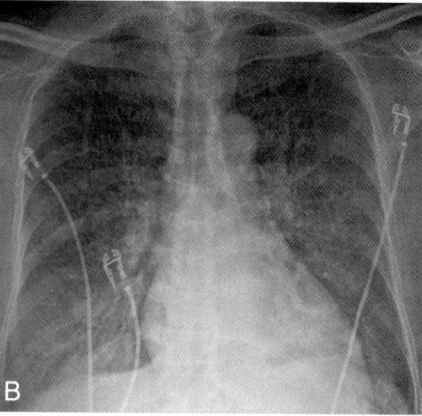

FIGURE 17.17 PA chest radiographs in a patient with chronic heart failure after several myocardial infarctions. **A,** CXR shows chronic interstitial pulmonary edema. **B,** CXR in the same patient following a new myocardial infarction, showing acute on chronic pulmonary edema.

American College of Radiology website provides detailed appropriateness criteria for ordering of advanced imaging including within the inpatient acute care setting.[2-6]

REFERENCES

Overview

1. Goldschlager R, Roth H, Solomon J, et al. Validation of a clinical decision rule: chest X-ray in patients with chest pain and possible acute coronary syndrome. *Emerg Radiol.* 2014;21:367–372.
2. *ACR Appropriateness Criteria Table for Cardiac Diseases.* https://acsearch.acr.org/list. Accessed on 3/11/2021.
3. *ACR-SPR-STR Practice Parameters for the Performance of Portable (mobile Unit) Chest Radiography.* https://www.acr.org/-/media/ACR/Files/Practice-Parameters/Port-Chest-Rad.pdf. Accessed 3/11/2021.
4. *ACR Appropriateness Criteria for Routine Chest Radiography, Last Review Date 2015.* https://acsearch.acr.org/docs/69451/Narrative/. Accessed on 3/11/2021.
5. *ACR Appropriateness Criteria for Portable Chest X-ray in Intensive Care Unit Patients, Revised 2020.* https://acsearch.acr.org/docs/69452/Narrative/. Accessed on 3/11/2021.
6. *ACR-AAPM-SIIM-SPR Practice Parameter for Digital Radiography.* https://www.acr.org/-/media/ACR/Files/Practice-Parameters/Rad-Digital.pdf. Accessed on 3/11/2021.

Approach to CXR Evaluation

7. Arndt H, Busse A, Meinel FG. Heart and lung in x-ray images: lost art? *Radiologe.* 2020;60:1122–1130.
8. Ahmed T, Ahmad M, Mungee S. *Cardiac Calcifications in: StatPearls [Internet].* Treasure Island (FL): StatPearls Publishing; 2021. https://pubmed.ncbi.nlm.nih.gov/32491621/. Accessed on 3/11/2021.
9. Handagala R, Ralapanawa U, Jayalath T. Unilateral pulmonary edema: a case report and review of the literature. *J Med Case Rep.* 2018;12:219.
10. Amorosa JK, Bramwit MP, Mohammed T-LH, et al. ACR appropriateness criteria routine chest radiographs in intensive care unit patients. *J Am Coll Radiol.* 2013;10:170–174.

Congenital Heart Disease

11. Lindsey SE, Butcher JT, Yalcin HC. Mechanical regulation of cardiac development. *Front Physiol.* 2014;5:318.
12. Bhat V, Belaval V, Gaddananahalli K, et al. Illustrated imaging essay on congenital heart diseases: multimodality approach part I: clinical perspective, anatomy and imaging techniques. *J Clin Diagn Res.* 2016;10:TE01–TE06.
13. Bhat V, Belaval V, Gaddananahalli K, et al. Illustrated imaging essay on congenital heart diseases: multimodality approach part II: acyanotic congenital heart disease and extracardiac abnormalities. *J Clin Diagn Res.* 2016;10:TE01–TE06.
14. Bhat V, Belaval V, Gaddananahalli K, et al. Illustrated imaging essay on congenital heart diseases: multimodality approach part III: cyanotic heart diseases and complex congenital abnormalities. *J Clin Diagn Res.* 2016;10:TE01–TE10.

Acquired Heart Disease

15. Basu J, Sharma S. Early recognition vital in acute coronary syndrome. *Practitioner.* 2016;260:19–23.
16. Lempel JK, Bolen MA, Renapurkar RD, et al. Radiographic evaluation of valvular heart disease with computed tomography and magnetic resonance correlation. *J Thorac Imaging.* 2016;31:273–284.
17. Khayata M, Alkharabsheh S, Shah NP, Klein AL. Pericardial cysts: a contemporary comprehensive review. *Curr Cardiol Rep.* 2019;21:64.
18. Chang SA, Oh JK. Constrictive pericarditis: a medical or surgical disease? *J Cardiovasc Imaging.* 2019;27:178–186.
19. Avondo S, Andreis A, Casula M, Imazio M. Update on diagnosis and management of neoplastic pericardial disease. *Expert Rev Cardiovasc Ther.* 2020;18:615–623.
20. Hunter BR, Martindale J, Abdel-Hafez O, Pang PS. Approach to acute heart failure in the emergency department. *Prog Cardiovasc Dis.* 2017;60:178–186.
21. Inamdar AA, Inamdar AC. Heart failure: diagnosis, management and utilization. *J Clin Med.* 2016;5:62–90.
22. Bentz MR, Primack SL. Intensive care unit imaging. *Clin Chest Med.* 2015;36:219–234.

18 Nuclear Cardiology

SHARMILA DORBALA AND MARCELO F. DI CARLI

PRINCIPLES OF IMAGING, 277
Single Photon Emission Computed Tomography, 277
Positron Emission Tomography, 278
Hybrid SPECT/CT, PET/CT, and PET/MR, 279
Radiotracers and Protocols, 280

SYSTEMATIC INTERPRETATION OF IMAGES, 287
Image Quality, 287

Image Display, 287
Image Review and Interpretation, 287
Photon Attenuation and Attenuation Correction, 288

REDUCING RADIATION DOSE, 288

PATIENT-CENTERED CLINICAL APPLICATIONS, 290
Ischemic Heart Disease, 290
Heart Failure and Cardiomyopathies, 298

Infective Endocarditis, 307
Cardio-Oncology, 310

MACHINE LEARNING AND ARTIFICIAL INTELLIGENCE, 311

TRANSLATIONAL MOLECULAR IMAGING, 311
Aortic Valve Disease, 312

REFERENCES, 312

Nuclear cardiology encompasses multiple quantitative imaging techniques with established clinical applications in ischemic heart disease, heart failure, cardiac and vascular inflammation and infection, with emerging applications in valvular heart disease and peripheral arterial disease (PAD). Extensive literature over the last 50 years supports a role for nuclear cardiology imaging to diagnose cardiovascular disease, stratify risk, and guide management. Over the past two decades, novel radiotracers, software improvements, instrumentation advances, and personalized low radiation dose protocols have transformed nuclear cardiology. This chapter reviews the principles of single photon emission computed tomography (SPECT) and positron emission tomography (PET) imaging, stress testing protocols, imaging protocols, and systematic scan interpretation, and methods to reduce radiation dose. We will discuss the diagnostic and prognostic value of nuclear cardiology in the context of case-based patient-centered clinical applications. We conclude with a brief overview of the emerging role of machine learning in nuclear cardiology and summarize some emerging clinical applications.

PRINCIPLES OF IMAGING

The primary nuclear cardiology techniques are SPECT and PET.

Single Photon Emission Computed Tomography
Conventional SPECT
Conventional SPECT scanners consist of one or more (most commonly, two) detector heads mounted on a rotating gantry, thereby allowing three-dimensional (3D) SPECT in addition to two-dimensional (2D) planar imaging. Each camera head contains a radiation detector, consisting of a large scintillation crystal coupled to photomultiplier tubes and associated electronics, and a collimator (Fig. 18.1). The scintillation crystal converts energy from each gamma ray (high-energy photon) into many low-energy photons (light), which are converted to an electronic signal using a light sensor and subsequently amplified by an array of photomultiplier tubes. Gamma rays emitted from radiotracers in the patient spread out in all directions such that a 2D image formed on a bare detector would be inevitably blurred. Collimators are sheets of lead or other highly absorbent material mounted on the surface of the detector with a pattern of holes that restricts acceptance of high-energy photons that have traveled a path with a narrow range of angles (most other photons are absorbed) and help provide a clear 2D view. The most commonly used collimator has parallel holes. Although collimators are needed to localize the photons, most are absorbed and only 0.1% of the counts emitted from the patient reach the detector.[1] Conventional SPECT scanners collect planar images at multiple angles around the patient (called projection images) using two heads in a 90- or 180-degree configuration for cardiac imaging. The American Society of Nuclear Cardiology (ASNC) recommends a 180-degree angular image acquisition, with two heads in a 90-degree configuration, and 60 projection images (30 per detector), 3-degree rotation per stop, 25 to 30 seconds of imaging per stop (13- to 16-minute scan duration), and gated imaging. The images are then reconstructed using a computer algorithm before review.

Because images are derived from multiple planar projections over the scan duration (step and shoot or continuous mode), that is, at any given time data are acquired at only two angular projections, dynamic imaging to quantify absolute radiotracer activity is challenging. In obese patients who cannot fit on the scanner table and for certain imaging applications (such as gated blood pool imaging), images can be acquired in a 2D planar mode (only left anterior oblique, left lateral, and anterior projections). Finally, the quality of SPECT images is determined by the number of counts collected. Some of the photons are attenuated by tissue, with more photon attenuation in obese persons, and they do not reach the detector and contribute to the image. The next two sections discuss novel image reconstruction software and scanner designs that have enhanced image quality.

Novel Image Reconstruction Software
Compared with conventional SPECT reconstruction methods, newer SPECT reconstruction algorithms have substantially enhanced image quality, making possible reduced radiation dose and/or rapid imaging protocols. Previously, analytical reconstruction approaches such as filtered back projection (FBP) were used; these images were often smoothed to reduce statistical noise, resulting in degradation of spatial resolution and image quality. Most current SPECT and PET scanners use iterative approaches such as ordered subset expectation maximization (OSEM). The advantages of these algorithms over FBP are better handling of noise and improved accuracy due to the ability to model the physics of photon attenuation and scatter, and to restore spatial resolution. The resolution of nuclear cardiology images is spatially variant, depending on the distance of the heart from the detector and the collimator geometry. With iterative reconstruction, this distance-dependent image blur can be estimated and corrected in a process called resolution recovery. These novel reconstruction algorithms lead to better spatial resolution and improved accuracy. In addition, improved noise compensation allows for reduced dose and/or scan duration with improved image quality. A significant practical advantage of these novel reconstruction methods is that they can be easily incorporated into older systems, as only software modifications are needed.

Novel SPECT Scanners
Modern SPECT scanners include innovative gantry designs with cardiofocal or 360-degree detector geometry, semiconductor detectors and, in some cases, the potential for quantitative imaging.

Solid-state detectors convert photon energy directly to electrons, eliminating the need for bulky photomultiplier tubes. Importantly, the cardiocentric design allows for an approximately fivefold higher count sensitivity and improved spatial resolution, by nearly twofold. Protocols can thus be personalized into rapid protocols or low radiation dose protocols. Rapid protocols improve test tolerability, minimize patient motion, allow for multiposition imaging, and can provide early and rapid poststress ejection fraction (EF) measurements. With low radiation dose protocols, stress images can be performed first with a <2 mSv dose. Some dedicated cardiac scanners allow imaging in a seated position, further improving test tolerability. Novel detector geometries provide for simultaneous angular sampling over 180 degrees (cardiac scanners) or 360 degrees (novel whole-body scanners). Because all detectors acquire images simultaneously, patient motion can be challenging to detect. On the other hand, if the scan is prematurely terminated for any reason, tomographic SPECT images can still be reconstructed with the acquired data; this is not possible with conventional SPECT. A major advantage of the 360-degree geometry scanners and some dedicated cardiac scanners, compared with rotating conventional SPECT scanners, is that complete tomographic data are acquired simultaneously, making dynamic imaging and quantification of myocardial blood flow possible. These novel scanners have greatly expanded the range of cardiac SPECT applications.

Positron Emission Tomography

The fundamental principle of positron tomography is that positron emitting radionuclides (e.g., ^{11}carbon, ^{13}nitrogen, ^{15}oxygen, ^{18}fluorine) decay by emitting "positively" charged electrons (positrons). Once released from the nucleus, these positrons travel short distances in tissue and annihilate when they encounter a nearby electron. This annihilation releases energy in the form of two high-energy gamma rays or photons that are emitted at 180 degrees from each other. These opposite high-energy photons (511 keV) are captured externally by an array of radiation detector elements (scintillators) in the PET gantry (Fig. 18.2). The most common PET detector materials are bismuth germanate (BGO), gadolinium oxyorthosilicate (GSO), lutetium oxyorthosilicate (LSO), and lutetium yttrium orthosilicate (LYSO).[2] The electronics of the PET system are arranged to facilitate detection of 511-keV photons arriving at opposite detectors within a narrow temporal window, and rejection of scattered photons arriving outside the preset temporal window (so-called electronic collimation), thereby enhancing the spatial and contrast resolution. Because there is no need for a physical collimator, as in SPECT, the sensitivity of PET is much higher. If one of the two photons is attenuated by tissue and does not reach a detector, the entire event is rejected by the system, amplifying the adverse effects of attenuation on image quality.[2] Attenuation correction is, therefore, necessary for PET. A radionuclide transmission image or, most commonly, a computed tomography (CT)-based transmission image provides soft tissue densities from which photon attenuation maps are generated and used to correct the inhomogeneities caused by soft tissue attenuation on the PET emission images. Older generation PET scanners operate in a 2D mode using lead septa to separate detector rings; this improves image quality by minimizing detection of cross-slice scattered counts. However, these septa also

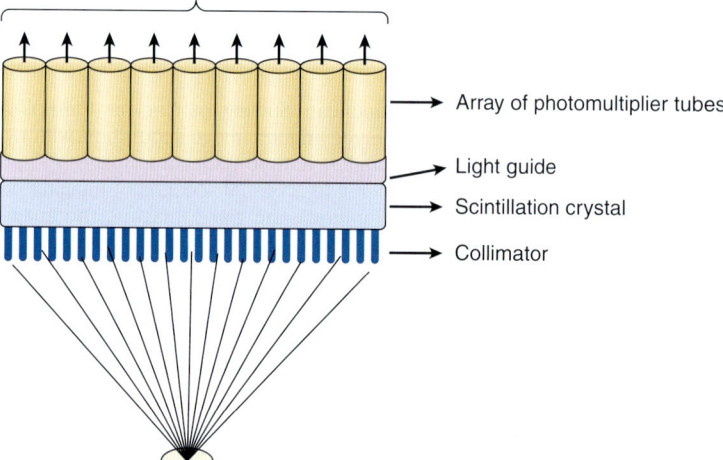

FIGURE 18.1 Principles of conventional SPECT. Conventional SPECT scanners include a collimator (blocks scattered photons and provides a clear view of the imaged object), a scintillation crystal (typically sodium iodide), light sensor (conversion of light into an electronic signal), and an array of photomultiplier tubes (amplification of the electronic signal).

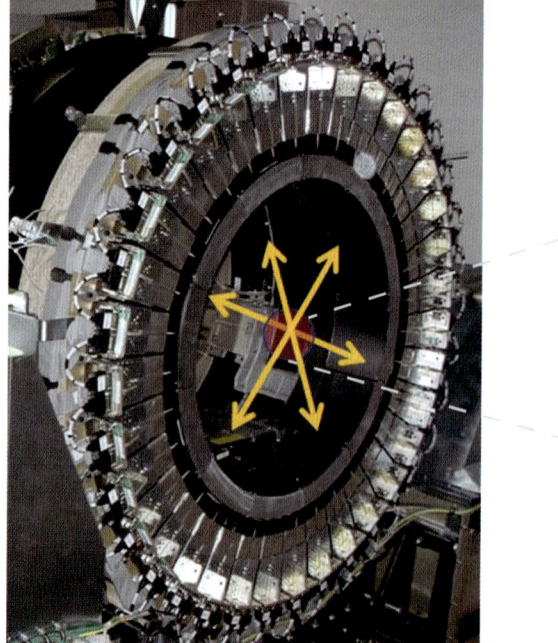

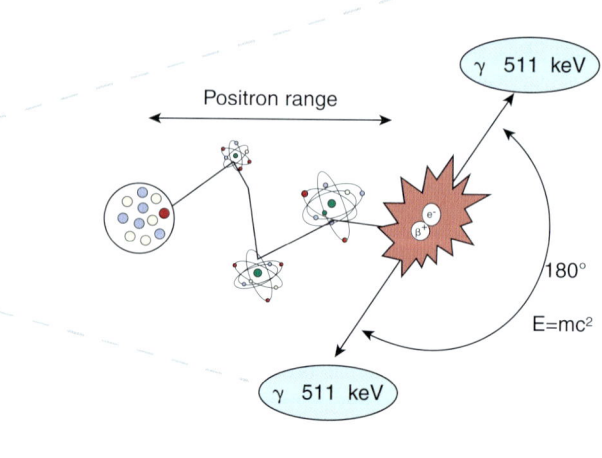

FIGURE 18.2 Principles of PET. The PET scanner consists of a series of rings of detector blocks that are typically integrated with a computed tomography (CT) scanner in the PET/CT gantry. The collision of a positron with a nearby electron produces an annihilation reaction that typically releases two high-energy photons (511 keV) that are emitted at 180 degrees from each other and captured by opposite detectors to form a coincidence line.

reduce true count rates, because they limit detection of photon pairs that are coincident to those detected in the same or adjacent rings. Current generation PET scanners are manufactured as 3D scanners without lead septa. Although the lack of collimation increases scatter and reduces effective spatial resolution, the 3D scanner design leads to substantially increased count rates, allowing rapid imaging and low radiotracer dose imaging.[2] Newer digital PET scanners include solid-state detectors with silicon photomultipliers with very high count rate capabilities that reduce radiotracer dose even more and allow for very rapid imaging. However, PET scanners are not widely available, and perfusion tracers and expertise with PET imaging remains limited. PET offers several advantages as listed in Table 18.1.

Indications for cardiac PET myocardial perfusion imaging (MPI) and myocardial blood flow measurement with PET are listed in Table 18.2.

TABLE 18.1 Advantages of Positron Emission Tomography

High spatial and contrast resolution
Capability for tomographic dynamic imaging with high temporal resolution
Accurate and depth-independent attenuation correction
High count sensitivity, making possible rapid protocols
Low radiation dose protocols (due to short half-life of the PET tracers)
Quantitation of absolute radiotracer concentration in tissue, including myocardial blood flow
CT hybrid imaging for quantification of atherosclerotic burden and localizing hot spot imaging tracers
Availability of a wide array of molecularly targeted clinical and research radiotracers that can image molecular processes in the pico and nano molar concentrations

TABLE 18.2 Indications for Cardiac Positron Emission Tomography Myocardial Perfusion Imaging and Myocardial Blood Flow Measurements

Rest-stress myocardial perfusion PET is a first-line preferred test for patients with known or suspected CAD who meet appropriate criteria for a stress imaging test and are unable to complete a diagnostic-level exercise stress imaging study
Rest-stress myocardial perfusion PET is recommended for patients with suspected active CAD, who meet appropriate use criteria for a stress imaging test, and who also meet one or more of the following criteria: • Prior stress imaging study that is of poor quality, equivocal or inconclusive, affected by attenuation artifact, or discordant with clinical impressions or other diagnostic test results including findings at coronary angiography   • Body characteristics that commonly affect image quality such as large breasts, breast implants, obesity, etc.   • High-risk patients in whom diagnostic error carries even greater clinical implications, such as chronic kidney disease stages 3, 4, or 5; diabetes mellitus; and high-risk CAD   • Young patients with established CAD who are expected to need repeated exposures to radiation associated cardiac procedures   • Patients in whom myocardial blood flow quantitation is needed   • Patients without known CAD who present with symptoms suspicious for myocardial ischemia   • Increased suspicion of multivessel CAD   • Suspected heart transplant vasculopathy   • Patients with known CAD in whom more specific physiologic assessment is desired

CAD, coronary artery disease.
From Bateman TM, et al. American Society of Nuclear Cardiology and Society of Nuclear Medicine and Molecular Imaging Joint Position Statement on the Clinical Indications for Myocardial Perfusion PET. J Nucl Cardiol 2016;23:1227-1231.

Hybrid SPECT/CT, PET/CT, and PET/MR

Hybrid SPECT/CT and PET/CT scanners, in which the gantry integrates a CT scanner with a PET or SPECT scanner, are available. Depending on the type of CT scanner, CT images can be used for attenuation correction, quantification of coronary artery calcium, and/or CT coronary angiography (see Chapter 20). Attenuation correction CT is a low-dose, noncontrast, ungated free tidal breathing scan of the chest. A calcium score CT scan is a noncontrast, prospectively gated CT scan for dose reduction, acquired during an inspiratory breath-hold. With hybrid scanners, coronary artery calcification can be assessed either on the attenuation correction CT scan or using a dedicated calcium score CT scan. Calcium score, in conjunction with SPECT and PET MPI, plays a major diagnostic role, particularly in the evaluation of patients without prior known coronary artery disease (CAD) and with normal MPI (see section Patient-Centered Clinical Applications).

A coronary CT angiogram (CTA) is a prospectively electrocardiogram (ECG)-gated CT, with iodinated contrast, acquired during an inspiratory breath-hold (see Chapter 20). Unlike calcium score imaging, PET or SPECT MPI combined with coronary CTA is associated with a high radiation burden; therefore it is not recommended routinely. Sequential imaging (CTA followed by MPI or vice versa) can be helpful in complex cases. Radionuclide imaging has limited anatomic resolution and hybrid CT imaging (without or with iodinated CT contrast) provides localization of the tracer uptake, which is helpful in hot spot imaging (e.g., ^{99m}Tc-pyrophosphate for amyloidosis or 2-deoxy-2-[^{18}F] fluoro-D-glucose [^{18}F-FDG] for sarcoidosis or infection imaging).

PET/MR (magnetic resonance) scanners are currently used primarily for research. Attenuation correction is challenging in these scanners, but PET/MR offers the advantages of respiratory motion compensation and simultaneous imaging of dual physiologic processes. Details of PET/MR imaging are beyond the scope of this chapter, and readers are referred to more comprehensive reviews on this topic (see Chapter 19).

SPECT and PET Image Acquisition

There are four common modes of image acquisition with SPECT or PET: list mode, static, ECG gated, or dynamic. PET scanners and certain advanced SPECT scanners can acquire data in list mode (i.e., information is stored for every detected event). The list mode data can be summed into a single frame and reconstructed as a static image, binned into 8 to 16 cardiac cycle frames to evaluate cardiac function, or binned into time frames and reconstructed into dynamic image series for absolute quantification of radiotracer concentration in tissue (e.g., myocardial blood flow).

ECG-gated images allow assessment of regional wall motion and quantification of left ventricular (LV) volumes and EF [(LV end-diastolic volume − LV end-systolic volume/LV end-diastolic volume)×100]. Compared with echocardiography, gated SPECT or PET provides tomographic information and measurement of LVEF. Ventricular dyssynchrony can also be assessed using specialized software. Typically, a 8- or 16-frame gating is used with MPI (a higher frame gating of 24 or 32 frames is used for gated blood pool imaging).

Dynamic imaging allows tracking of radiotracer transit through the blood vessels and the heart starting with the time of radiotracer injection. These images can be analyzed using compartmental analysis, with an image-derived input function from arterial blood and tissue time activity curves from the myocardium. Myocardial blood flow estimates can be derived by this approach, incorporating corrections for radiotracer extraction characteristics, radiotracer decay, and the effects of limited spatial resolution. This can be performed at rest and during peak pharmacologic stress to compute rest and stress myocardial blood flow, respectively. The ratio of stress to rest myocardial blood flow is termed myocardial flow reserve (MFR). Dynamic imaging for myocardial blood flow quantitation requires pharmacologic stress testing with vasodilators (preferred) or dobutamine. During treadmill exercise stress, radiotracer injection occurs outside the PET gantry. Postexercise myocardial blood flow quantification is not feasible because of the lack of an arterial input function.

Radiotracers and Protocols

Nuclear cardiology uses radionuclide tracers with distinct molecular structures to probe various physiologic processes in the heart and vasculature. This section will mainly focus on clinically recommended radiotracers and standard stress and imaging protocols recommended by the ASNC.

Radiotracers

A wide array of radiotracers has been validated for the evaluation of myocardial blood flow, metabolism, innervation, amyloidosis, and microcalcification (Table 18.3), and several other radiotracers are currently under development.

Myocardial Perfusion Imaging Tracers. An ideal radiotracer for MPI should be extracted by the myocardium at a rate that is linearly related to myocardial blood flow. As shown in Fig. 18.3, most SPECT and PET perfusion radiotracers demonstrate linear extraction at relatively low blood flow rates, as in the resting state, or when there is significant obstructive CAD with a reduction in stress myocardial blood flow. As myocardial blood flow increases with exercise or pharmacologic stress, radiotracer extraction falls off and, consequently, myocardial blood flow is underestimated. Accuracy can be increased by using radiotracers with greater extraction at high flow rates; this is particularly important for the evaluation of nonobstructive CAD, diffuse CAD, or microvascular dysfunction. ^{15}O-water is close to an ideal tracer, as it is freely diffusible and the relationship between radiotracer extraction and blood flow remains linear at high flow rates. However, because it is freely diffusible, myocardial perfusion images are difficult to interpret, requiring special corrections or the use of parametric flow maps. Most software programs for myocardial blood flow quantitation correct for the expected roll off phenomenon at high flow rates; therefore ^{82}rubidium, ^{13}N-ammonia, and ^{15}O-water can all be used to quantify myocardial blood flow; the first two are approved by the U.S. Food and Drug Administration (FDA) in the United States.

SPECT MPI Tracers. ^{99m}Tc-sestamibi, ^{99m}Tc-tetrofosmin, and ^{201}thallium are FDA-approved SPECT myocardial perfusion tracers. ^{99m}Tc is produced by a ^{99m}molybdenum generator and then compounded into ^{99m}Tc-sestamibi or ^{99m}Tc-tetrofosmin. ^{99m}Tc emits 140-keV gamma rays and have a half-life of 6 hours. After intravenous (IV) injection, ^{99m}Tc perfusion tracers passively diffuse into cardiomyocytes at rates proportional to blood flow and bind to the mitochondria within the first 60 to 90 seconds after injection. There is no significant redistribution of ^{99m}Tc perfusion tracers and imaging can be delayed for up to several hours. Because of the 6-hour half-life of ^{99m}Tc, these SPECT perfusion tracers are commercially available as unit doses, increasing their accessibility. They are also suitable for exercise or pharmacologic stress testing.

In contrast, ^{201}thallium is produced by a cyclotron, emits lower energy photons (80 keV), and has a half-life of 73 hours. ^{201}Thallium circulates to the heart at a rate proportional to blood flow and enters the cardiomyocytes via the Na$^+$/K$^+$ ATPase pump. ^{201}Thallium washes out of normally perfused and hypoperfused regions at different rates. Early perfusion defects on ^{201}thallium images represent reduced blood flow from ischemia or scar. Perfusion defects may resolve over time because of redistribution of ^{201}thallium in ischemic and hibernating regions; therefore poststress ^{201}thallium images are obtained within 10 to 15 minutes after injection. Because of its long half-life and relatively low photon energy, ^{201}thallium imaging is associated with a higher radiation dose. For this reason, it is currently not recommended for perfusion imaging; instead, it is used for viability assessment at sites without access to other viability tests (e.g., PET or cardiac magnetic resonance [CMR] imaging). Because of the high radiation dose, injected doses are low, leading to high levels of statistical noise and limited image quality. The newer solid-state scanners with high sensitivity provide much higher quality ^{201}thallium images and provide good quality gated images.

PET MPI Tracers. ^{82}Rubidium and ^{13}N-ammonia are FDA-approved PET perfusion tracers, whereas ^{15}O-water and ^{18}F-flurpiridaz are novel tracers that are currently under development.

^{82}Rubidium is a monovalent cation that enters the cardiomyocyte via the Na$^+$/K$^+$ ATPase pump. Because it has a very short half-life (76 seconds), (1) it is produced from a ^{82}strontium/^{82}rubidium generator housed in an infusion cart next to the PET scanner, (2) exercise stress imaging is not feasible, and (3) rapid sequential imaging is possible.

^{13}N-ammonia enters the cardiomyocytes passively where it is converted into ^{13}N-glutamine and trapped in the glutamate pool. Compared with ^{82}rubidium, it has a higher extraction fraction and a shorter positron range and is produced by a cyclotron. Because of its short (9.96 minutes) half-life, (1) an on-site cyclotron is required, (2) exercise PET is feasible, and (3) lower injected doses are administered compared with ^{82}rubidium. Exercise PET with ^{13}N-ammonia can be logistically challenging. Close coordination is required with the cyclotron for delivery of the tracer, and exercise stress protocols may have to be modified to minimize radiotracer decay during the exercise period. Also, as mentioned earlier, exercise PET does not allow for quantitation of myocardial blood flow, which is an important advantage of PET MPI.

The superior extraction characteristics of PET tracers, compared with SPECT perfusion tracers, makes them more suitable for quantifying myocardial blood flow (see Fig. 18.3). ^{82}Rubidium and ^{13}N-ammonia have shorter half-lives compared with SPECT perfusion radiotracers, leading to a lower radiation dose for patients and rapid clinic throughput. However, unlike SPECT tracers, these PET perfusion tracers cannot be transported as single unit doses because of the short half-lives. ^{18}F-flurpiridaz is a novel PET perfusion tracer with a half-life of 109 minutes. This will make unit dose radiotracer delivery possible, which will greatly improve access to PET MPI. The extraction characteristics of ^{18}F-flurpiridaz are superior to those of ^{13}N-ammonia and ^{82}rubidium and image resolution is superior to that of ^{99m}Tc-SPECT MPI (see section Translational Molecular Imaging).

Myocardial Metabolic Imaging Tracers. A number of SPECT and PET radiotracers have been developed to study myocardial metabolism.[3] SPECT tracers of fatty acid metabolism (^{123}I-IPPA, phenylpentadecanoic acid, ^{123}I-BMIPP, 15-(p-iodophenyl)-3-(R,S)-methyl-pentadecanoic acid) are not approved by the FDA in the United States; therefore

TABLE 18.3 Characteristics of Clinically Used Radiotracers

	MECHANISM OF UPTAKE	EXTRACTION FRACTION	ENERGY	SOURCE
SPECT				
^{201}Thallium	Na$^+$/K$^+$ ATPase pump	85%	69-81 keV	Cyclotron
^{99m}Tc-sestamibi	Mitochondrial uptake	65%	140 keV	Generator
^{99m}Tc-tetrofosmin	Mitochondrial uptake	60%	140 keV	Generator
^{99m}Tc-PYP, DPD, MDP	Unknown	N/A	140 keV	Generator
^{123}I-meta iodobenzylguanidine (MIBG)	Active uptake via norepinephrine transporter	N/A	159 keV	
PET				
^{13}N-ammonia	Passive diffusion and incorporation into the glutamate pool	75%	511 keV	Cyclotron
^{82}Rubidium(^{82}Rb)	Na$^+$/K$^+$ ATPase pump	55%	511 keV	Generator
^{15}Oxygen-water*	Diffusion	100%	511 keV	Cyclotron
^{18}F-flurpiridaz*†	Mitochondrial complex 1 inhibitor	94%	511 keV	Cyclotron
2-deoxy-2-[^{18}F]fluoro-D-glucose (FDG)†	Active uptake via glucose transporters	N/A	511 keV	Cyclotron
^{18}F-sodium fluoride (NaF)	Microcalcification	N/A	511 keV	Cyclotron

*Not approved by the U.S. Food and Drug Administration for use in the United States.
†Shipped as unit doses.
DPD, 3,3-diphosphono-1,2-propanodicarboxylic acid; *HMDP*, hydroxymethylene diphosphonate; *PYP*, pyrophosphate; ^{99m}Tc, 99m technetium.

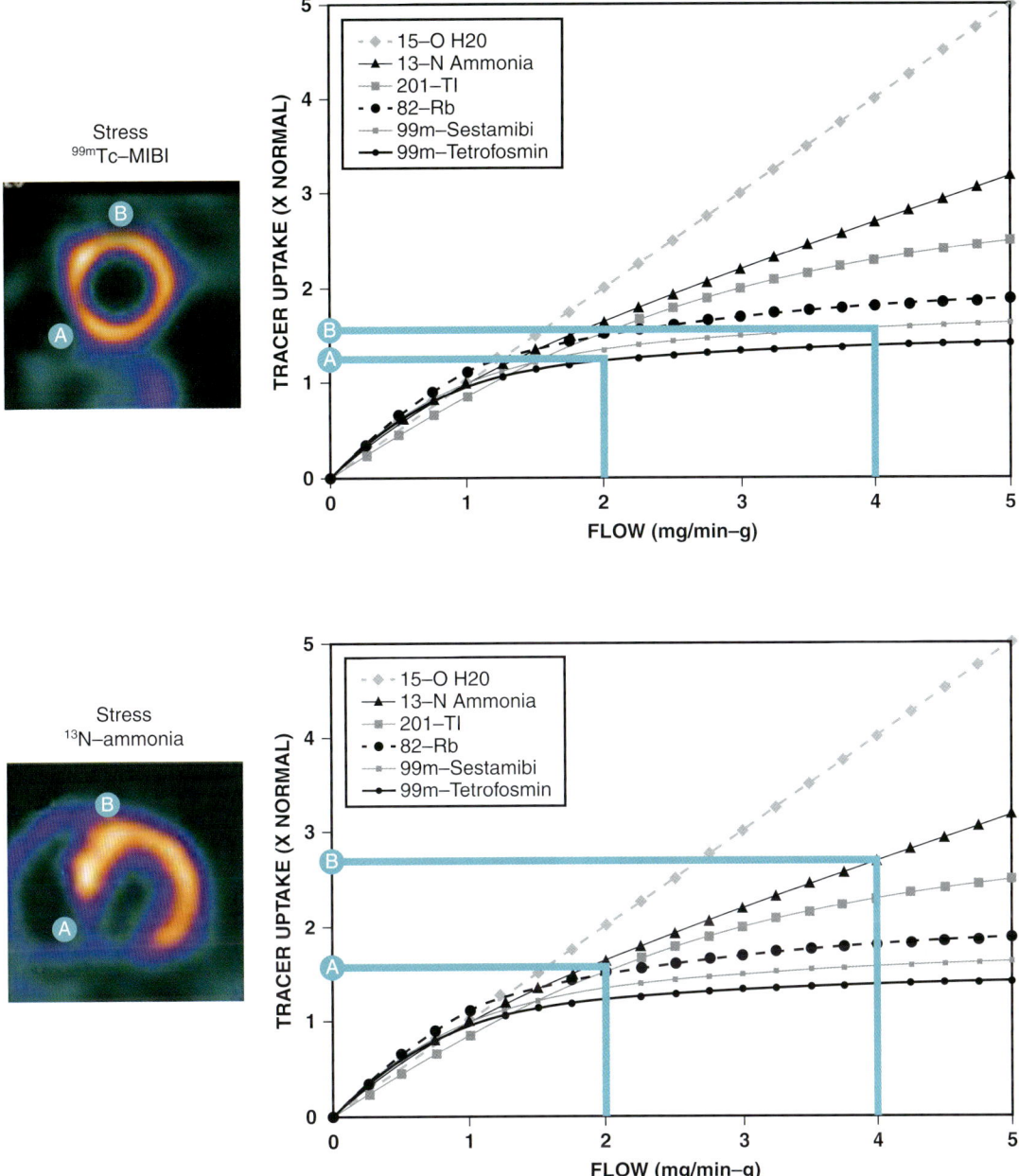

FIGURE 18.3 Relationship between myocardial blood flow, radiotracer uptake, and perfusion defect contrast. The linear scatter plot shows the characteristic roll-off in myocardial retention with increasing myocardial blood flow, which in turn determines perfusion defect contrast, for different radiotracers used in single photon emission computed tomography and positron emission tomography imaging. *Top:* Patient with an approximately 50% coronary stenosis imaged with ^{99m}Tc-sestamibi. The marked roll-off of sestamibi uptake at high flow rates leads to minimal contrast between tracer retention in the diseased coronary territory (*point A*) and the normal coronary artery (*point B*) and a relatively normal image. *Bottom:* Improved defect contrast when the same patient is imaged with ^{13}N ammonia, which has a less marked roll-off in tracer retention at high flow rates. (Adapted from Salerno M, Beller GA. Noninvasive assessment of myocardial perfusion. Circ Cardiovasc Imaging 2009;2:412-424.)

they are not used in clinical practice. PET tracers have been developed to image glucose metabolism (^{18}F-FDG, ^{11}C-glucose), oxidative metabolism (^{11}C-palmitate, ^{15}O$_2$), fatty acid metabolism (^{11}C-palmitate, ^{18}F-FTHA[14(R,S)-[F-18]Fluoro-6-thia-heptadecanoic acid], FTP[4-thia palmitate], FCPHA[trans-9-F-18-fluoro-3,4-methyleneheptadecanoic acid]), lactic acid metabolism (^{11}C-lactate),[3] and myocardial innervation (^{11}C-hydroxyephedrine[HED], ^{18}F-N-[3-bromo-4-(3-fluoro-propoxy)-benzyl]-guanidine [(18)F-LMI1195]). The only clinically available FDA-approved tracer to image myocardial metabolism is ^{18}F-FDG.

^{18}F-FDG is a glucose analog used to image myocardial glucose metabolism. The primary clinical applications of cardiac ^{18}F-FDG PET are for imaging myocardial viability, myocardial and vascular inflammation, and infective endocarditis.[2] ^{18}F-FDG enters the cardiomyocytes through glucose transporters (GLUT 1 and 4), where it is phosphorylated by the enzyme hexokinase and trapped as ^{18}F-FDG-6-phosphate. Unlike glucose-6-phosphate, ^{18}F-FDG-6-phosphate cannot be metabolized. Normal myocytes are metabolic omnivores that can use glucose, fatty acids, or lactic acid based on substrate availability, neurohormonal milieu, and cardiac work.[3] Insulin, ischemia, and hypoxia induce translocation of glucose transporters to the plasma membrane and increase myocyte glucose uptake. Ischemic and hypoxic cells overexpress GLUTs and preferentially use glucose for their metabolic needs, independent of the substrate or insulin availability. Malignant cells and inflammatory cells are also characterized by significantly increased glucose uptake by an insulin-independent mechanism.[4] Myocardial metabolism can be forced to switch to using glucose or fatty acids by dietary manipulation. Dietary preparation to switch myocardial metabolism to glucose or fatty acids forms the basis for the use ^{18}F-FDG to image myocardial viability (glucose load with IV insulin) and cardiovascular inflammatory conditions (low-carbohydrate, high-fat diet followed by prolonged fasting) such as sarcoidosis, infective endocarditis, and vasculitis.

Physiologic Basis for Stress Testing

The heart extracts oxygen nearly maximally at rest (60% to 80%).[5] With exercise stress (or dobutamine infusion) there is a severalfold increase

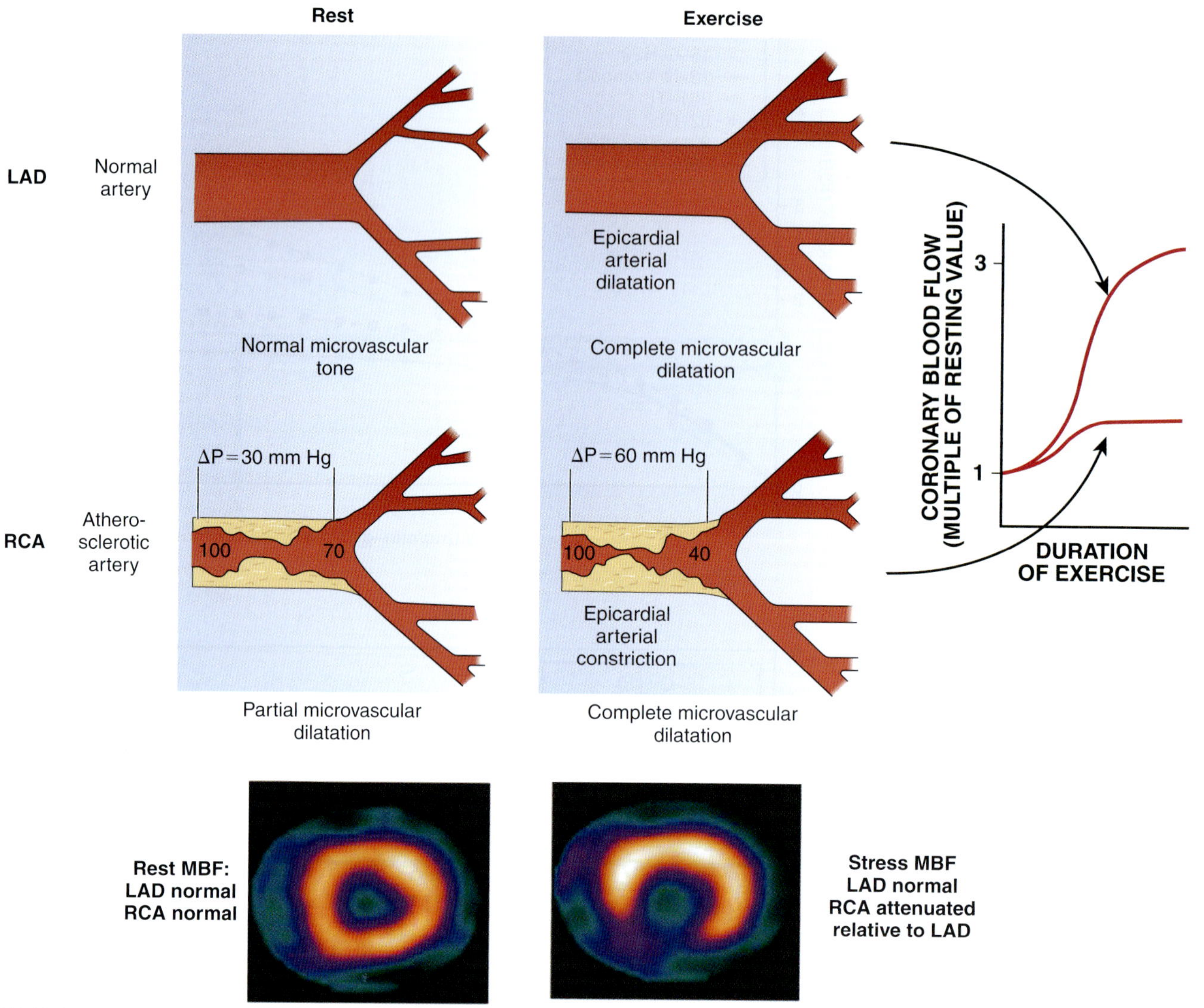

FIGURE 18.4 Physiologic basis of myocardial perfusion imaging. Schematic of two coronary arteries (left anterior descending [LAD], nondiseased, and right coronary artery [RCA], diseased). In the normal LAD artery, exercise stress causes vasodilation of the epicardial and microvascular bed increasing myocardial blood flow two- to fourfold compared to rest. However, the diseased RCA shows blunted coronary vasodilation in response to exercise. This difference in myocardial perfusion between diseased and nondiseased coronary arteries forms the basis for stress perfusion imaging. (Adapted from Wilson RF. Assessing the severity of coronary-artery stenoses. N Engl J Med 1996;334:1735-1737.)

in oxygen demand from high heart rate, contractility, and ventricular work that is met physiologically by increased blood supply from metabolic vasodilation. If the myocardial oxygen demand with exercise exceeds supply in any coronary territory, exercise-induced ischemia is provoked.

Normal coronary arteries have a coronary blood flow at rest of 0.7 to 1 mL/min, which can increase three- to fivefold during maximal vasodilation.[5] Coronary blood flow remains constant over a wide range of coronary perfusion pressures through dynamic changes in tone in arterioles and other resistance vessels,[5] and it only falls in the presence of very severe upstream coronary stenosis (>90% luminal narrowing; see Chapter 36). However, augmentation of myocardial blood flow in response to exercise/vasodilator stress is progressively blunted with increasing severity of upstream coronary stenosis (Fig. 18.4) and forms the basis for the use of stress radionuclide MPI for detection of obstructive CAD. These changes in myocardial perfusion represent the earliest event in the ischemic cascade, which ultimately leads to changes in myocardial metabolism, mechanical function, ischemic ECG changes, and angina (Fig. 18.5).

In contrast to exercise stress, vasodilator stress does not increase oxygen demand; the diseased and nondiseased territories manifest differential hyperemic responses due to differences in resting microvascular dilation. In myocardial territories supplied by coronary arteries with critical stenosis (>90%), where the microvasculature is maximally vasodilated at rest, vasodilation of the epicardial coronaries by vasodilator stress agents can redistribute flow away from the subendocardium causing coronary steal,[5] which can often manifest as ischemic ST depression during vasodilator stress testing. Finally, if there is severe multivessel obstructive CAD and coronary blood flow is reduced in all vascular territories, this can result in an apparently normal appearing relative myocardial perfusion image with no perfusion defects, also known as balanced ischemia. As discussed later in the chapter, integration of data from myocardial perfusion images with clinical, ECG, and hemodynamic response to exercise stress, and calcium score (when available), or myocardial blood flow (with quantitative PET MPI) may raise the suspicion of balanced ischemia. If balanced ischemia is suspected, further testing with coronary angiography (invasive for patients with high-risk stress features or symptoms, or coronary CTA for patients without high-risk features).

Stress Testing Protocols

Exercise stress, vasodilator stress, and dobutamine stress have been shown to have equally high diagnostic accuracy to identify obstructive epicardial CAD. Exercise is most commonly used. If not feasible or contraindicated, vasodilator agents are used. If they are not feasible or contraindicated, dobutamine/atropine stress is used with radionuclide MPI.

Exercise Stress

Stress testing using exercise stress with treadmill or bicycle is safe and is the preferred mode of stress in conjunction with radionuclide MPI.

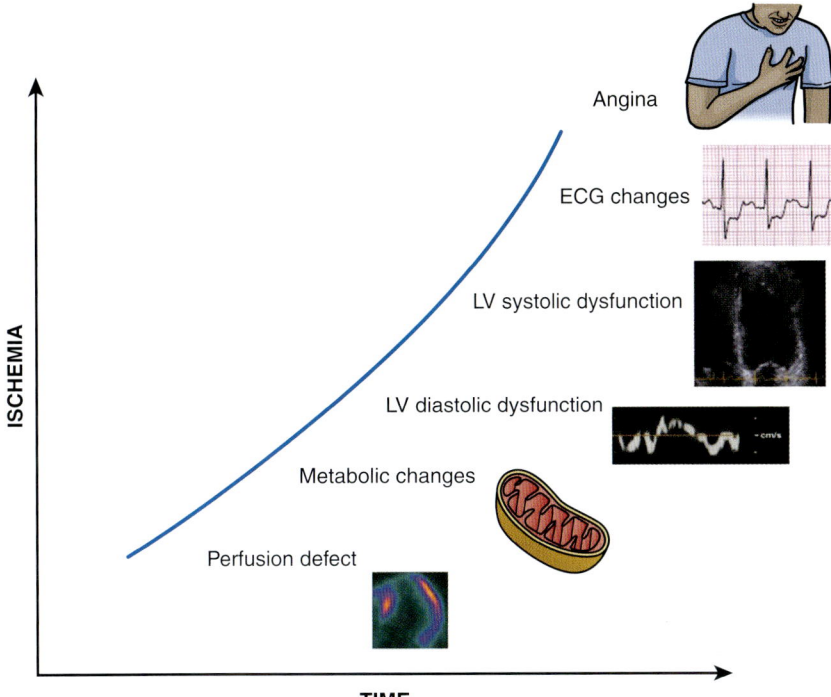

FIGURE 18.5 Ischemic cascade. Reduced regional myocardial perfusion is the initial stage in myocardial ischemia, setting the stage for mismatch between oxygen supply and demand. This leads to cellular metabolic changes, left ventricular diastolic dysfunction, systolic dysfunction, electrocardiogram (ECG) changes, and finally, angina. Typically, stress tests coupled with imaging myocardial perfusion are more sensitive than those that rely on detection of abnormalities in regional wall motion or ECG changes. (The image depicting metabolic changes is from Huss JM, Kelly DP. Mitochondrial energy metabolism in heart failure: a question of balance. J Clin Invest 2005;547-555.)

A standard Bruce treadmill exercise is the most widely used protocol. See Chapter 15 for more details on contraindications, protocols, indications for premature termination of exercise, and treatment of complications. Exercise stress is preferred as it is physiologic, providing information on symptoms, functional capacity, and hemodynamic and ECG changes with stress. However, submaximal exercise decreases test sensitivity to detect ischemia and should be avoided. Pharmacologic stress testing provides an excellent alternative if exercise stress is not feasible (orthopedic or other limitations), contraindicated (recent acute coronary syndrome [ACS], or recent deep vein thrombosis, very large aortic aneurysm, etc.), or if patients are unable to exercise maximally. Maximal exercise is defined as ability to achieve an exercise heart rate of at least 85% of age-predicted maximal heart rate (220-age). To evaluate anginal symptoms on maximal medical therapy in patients with known prior CAD, a symptom-limited stress test irrespective of heart rate is often adequate if a reasonable workload of at least 5 metabolic equivalents (METS) is achieved. To evaluate anginal symptoms in patients without documented prior CAD, maximal heart rate response is desirable with exercise stress. If not, the radiotracer is not administered, and stress test is converted to a vasodilator stress. In those instances, regadenoson, a non–weight-based fixed dose stress agent is well suited for administration on the treadmill or soon after termination of exercise.

Pharmacologic Stress

Pharmacologic stress testing is the preferred stress modality for radionuclide MPI (SPECT and PET) in patients who are unable to exercise adequately, and for evaluation of residual ischemia in patients with recent ACS/myocardial infarction (MI) (see section Patient-Centered Clinical Applications).

Adenosine, dipyridamole, and regadenoson are the three most commonly used vasodilator stress agents. Adenosine binds to four types of adenosine receptors. Binding to A_{2A} receptors causes coronary vasodilation, whereas binding to the A1, A_{2B}, and A3 receptors causes side effects of heart block, wheezing, and peripheral vasodilation, respectively.[6] Dipyridamole causes coronary vasodilation by increasing endogenous adenosine levels. Regadenoson is a specific A_{2A} receptor agonist that was developed to avoid the side effects of the nonspecific vasodilators. Vasodilator agents are contraindicated in patients with active wheezing, high-grade atrioventricular (AV) block without a functioning pacemaker, systolic blood pressure (BP) <90 mm Hg, and any contraindications for stress testing (acute MI, unstable angina, aortic dissection, acute pulmonary embolism). A few reports indicated that regadenoson stress testing is associated with seizures; thus it is contraindicated in patients with a history of seizures that are not well controlled or in those with structural brain injury (ischemic or hemorrhagic stroke or brain tumors). In those patients, a short-acting vasodilator like adenosine or dobutamine can be used.

Vasodilator agents provoke maximal hyperemia and thus are well suited for tests relying on perfusion imaging. As shown in Fig. 18.6, adenosine (140 mcg/kg/min) and dipyridamole (0.56 mg/kg) are weight-based infusions administered over 4 minutes, whereas regadenoson is a fixed-dose rapid IV bolus over 10 seconds (0.4 mg/5 mL prefilled solution administered as a rapid bolus over 10 seconds).[6] Vasodilator stress agents often cause symptoms of hyperemia in about 50% of patients including an urge to breathe deeply, chest tightness, headache, flushing, a 10 to 20 beat increase in heart rate, and a 10-mm Hg decrease in systolic BP. These side effects occur acutely with adenosine but are typically short-lived (due to the 3-second half-life of adenosine) and terminate when the infusion is completed. Exercise, including swinging the legs on the side of the bed, hand grip exercise, or low-level treadmill exercise, improves symptoms and reduces heart block, which is common during adenosine infusion. Unlike exercise, which shunts blood to the exercising muscles, vasodilator agents cause splanchnic hyperemia and intense radiotracer uptake in the liver that may scatter into the inferior wall of the left ventricle; addition of low-level treadmill exercise has been shown to improve heart to liver ratio.[6] Methylxanthines are competitive agonists of the adenosine receptors and can reverse the vasodilatory effects of adenosine, dipyridamole, and regadenoson. For this reason, they need to be held for at least 12 hours before vasodilator stress (see section Imaging Protocols). IV aminophylline (1 to 2 mg/kg slow push over 1 to 2 minutes) is used as an antidote for side effects of vasodilator stress agents. Vasodilator stress has been shown to be safe for evaluation of myocardial ischemia within 24 to 48 hours after presentation with ACS or uncomplicated MI. When vasodilators are contraindicated or cannot be used because of caffeine intake, dobutamine stress testing is used.

Dobutamine is administered as a weight-based graded infusion starting at 10 mcg/kg/min and escalating every 3 minutes by 10 mcg/kg/min to a maximum of 40 mcg/kg/min. The infusion is terminated 1 minute after injection of the radiotracer. If target heart rate is not achieved, atropine is administered as 0.5 mg IV followed by increments of 0.25 mg IV to a maximum of 2 mg IV (see Chapter 16). Dobutamine-atropine testing is less well tolerated compared with vasodilator agents and nearly 80% of the patients experience side effects from dobutamine. Dobutamine plus atropine stress testing with maximal heart rate response has been shown to increase myocardial blood flow equivalently to vasodilator stress. Atropine is contraindicated in patients with angle closure glaucoma and prostatism. For more details about indications and contraindications for stress agents, readers are referred to the ASNC stress protocols and tracers document.[6]

Imaging Protocols
General Principles

Given the number of scanners, software, and radiotracer choices, and clinical questions, many possible protocols can be used for nuclear

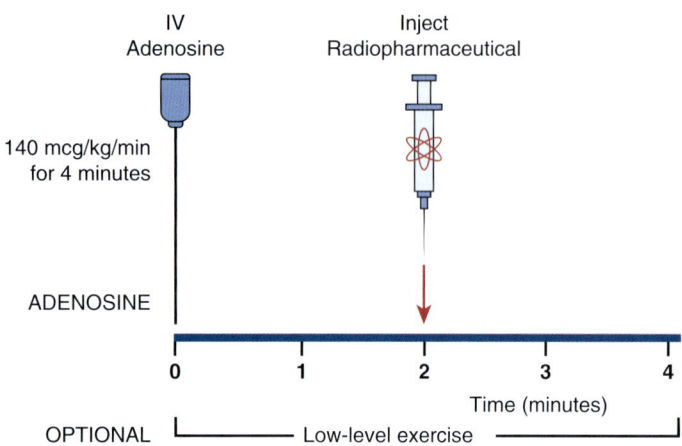

A. Adenosine protocol

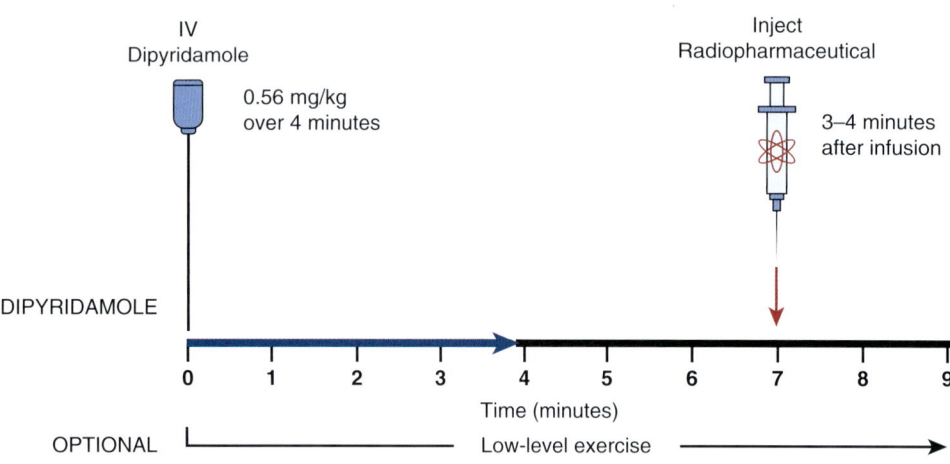

B. Dipyridamole protocol

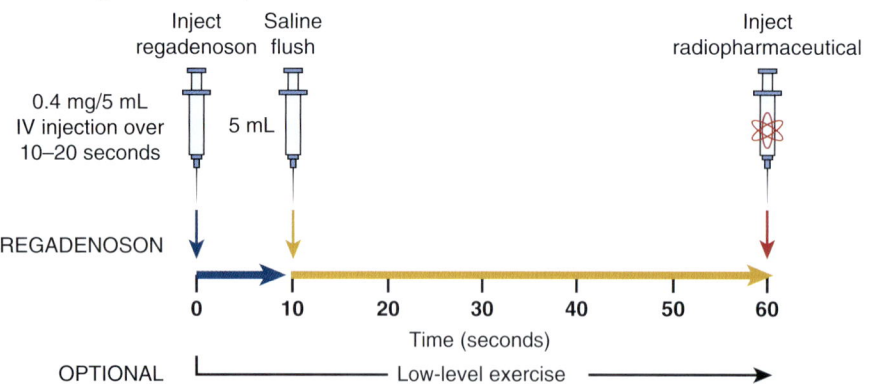

C. Regadenoson protocol

FIGURE 18.6 Pharmacologic stress protocols. Adenosine **(A)** and dipyridamole **(B)** are weight-based infusions administered over 4 minutes, whereas regadenoson **(C)** is a non–weight-based slow bolus injection administered over 10 to 20 seconds. Each of these pharmacologic stressors can be combined with low-level exercise.

PREPARATION FOR NUCLEAR CARDIOLOGY TESTING
Stress Testing
Patients are typically prepared with a 4 to 6 hour fast before a stress test and asked to abstain from smoking for 6 hours prior. Caffeine intake (including caffeine-containing medications) should be withheld for 12 hours, and theophylline-containing medications and oral dipyridamole are withheld for 48 hours before vasodilator testing. Patients with known CAD are generally tested on their anti-ischemic therapy. Patients without known CAD are ideally tested by withholding their beta blockers and antianginal medications for 12 hours before testing when feasible. Patients on dialysis are typically scheduled for their test on the day after dialysis. For more details of preparation readers are referred to ASNC/Society of Nuclear Medicine and Molecular Imaging (SNMMI) SPECT MPI guidelines.[1]

^{18}F-FDG for Viability Testing
Patients are prepared by a 6-hour fast. On arrival, fingerstick glucose level is checked and they are given an oral glucose drink. Forty-five minutes later fingerstick glucose is checked again and IV regular insulin is administered to drive down the blood glucose level to <150 mg/dL before administration of ^{18}F-FDG. For more details of preparation readers are referred to ASNC imaging guidelines/SNMMI procedure standard for PET nuclear cardiology procedures.[2]

^{18}F-FDG for Inflammation/Infection
Patients are prepared by using a high-fat, low to zero carbohydrate diet for at least two large meals 24 hours before the test followed by overnight fast (8 to 12 hour fast). For more details of preparation readers are referred to ASNC/SNMMI expert consensus recommendations.[7]

Amyloidosis Imaging and Gated Blood Pool Scans
No specific dietary preparation is necessary for gated blood pool scanning[8] or for amyloidosis imaging with ^{99m}Tc-pyrophosphate, 3,3-diphosphono-1,2-propanodicarboxylic acid (DPD), or hydroxymethylene diphosphonate (HMDP) imaging.

SPECT Protocols
Myocardial Perfusion Imaging
With SPECT MPI the imaging protocol can be personalized to the patient and the clinical question. ^{99m}Tc-radiotracers with gated SPECT imaging is recommended. When available, advanced hardware (cadmium zinc telluride [CZT] SPECT scanners, novel collimators, attenuation correction) and advanced reconstruction methods (advanced iterative reconstruction and resolution recovery with noise reduction) should be used.[1] Stress first and single-day rest followed by stress MPI are the mostly widely used protocols (Fig. 18.7A–B). Two-day protocols with stress first followed by rest on another day if stress MPI is abnormal are used in patients with large body habitus (see Fig. 18.7C).

cardiology studies. Imaging protocols are optimally planned before the patient arrives for the test.[1] The optimal protocol is one that provides the best image quality with the lowest radiation dose and in the most expeditious manner.

A. Stress-first single-day protocol

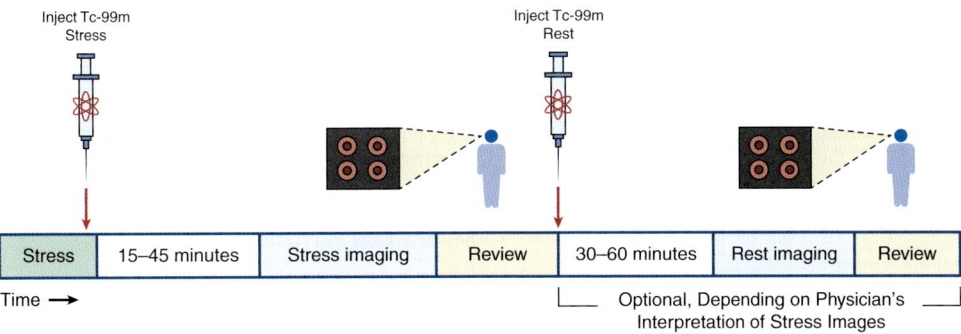

B. Rest-first single-day protocol

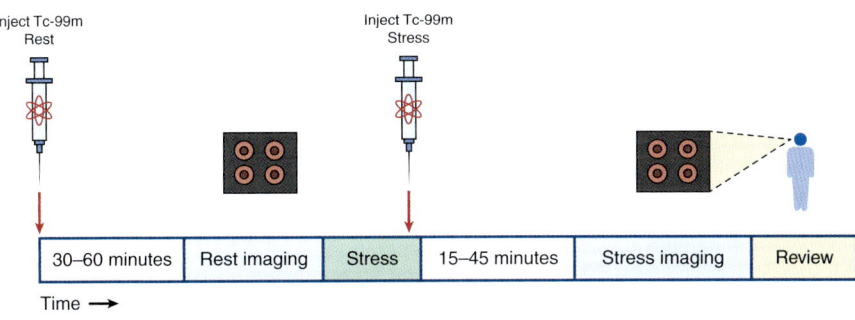

C. Stress-first two-day protocol

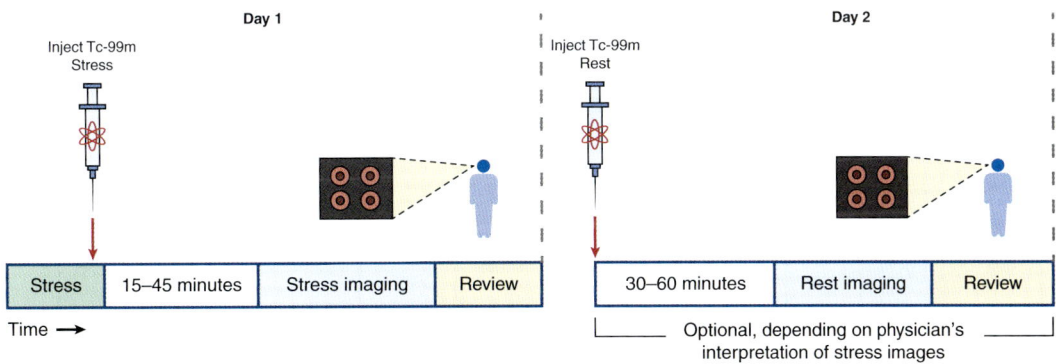

D. ⁹⁹ᵐTc-PYP/DPD/HMDP SPECT/CT protocol

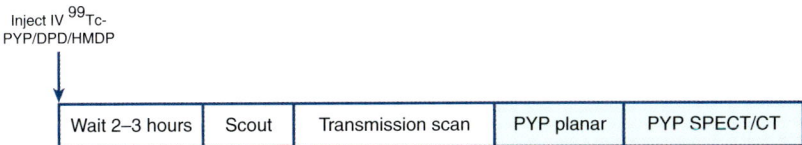

FIGURE 18.7 SPECT imaging protocols. A–C, Recommended protocols for myocardial perfusion imaging. Two-day protocol is typically used for large patients or for young patients for low radiation dose studies. **D,** Recommended protocol for imaging cardiac amyloidosis. A dose of 15 to 20 mCi of ^{99m}Tc-PYP/DPD/HMDP is administered; after a 2- to 3-hour delay, planar and SPECT images are obtained. If available, SPECT/CT imaging is recommended to better delineate blood pool from myocardial retention.

In a stress-first protocol, stress MPI is performed first and only followed by rest imaging when stress images are abnormal. This protocol is preferred for patients without prior CAD because it is most efficient and associated with the lowest radiation dose to the patient. Stress-first MPI requires careful patient selection, review of the stress images as soon as they are completed, and a definitive scan interpretation as normal. Advances in machine learning algorithms will soon guide the imaging teams on which patients to safely avoid rest imaging and improve the workflow for stress-first MPI. Also, this protocol is most effective with attenuation correction and advanced scanners. If stress-first MPI is performed using conventional scanners, multiposition imaging (supine/prone or upright/supine) and/or novel reconstruction

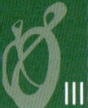

methods may help mitigate artifacts and minimize the need for additional rest MPI.[1] Most patients referred for SPECT MPI are candidates for stress-first imaging, except for patients with documented prior MI, those needing viability assessment, or those presenting with ACS who may benefit from rest and stress imaging. A normal stress-first imaging has been proven to have excellent prognostic value and portends very low likelihood of major adverse cardiac events (MACE).[1]

For single-day ^{99m}Tc-rest-first MPI, the low rest radiotracer dose (4 to 8 mCi) is typically followed by a larger stress radiotracer dose (12 to 25 mCi, approximately three times the initial dose) to overcome the shine through of the first injection.[1] This is not necessary for two-day protocols where an equal amount of radioactivity is used, with stress imaging performed first, so that rest is only performed if needed (i.e., stress is not normal). Two-day protocols provide the lowest possible radiation dose and optimal image quality because there is no shine through of rest radiotracer activity.

SPECT and PET perfusion tracers are administered intravenously and extracted by cardiomyocytes within 60 to 90 seconds after injection. The images reflect myocardial perfusion at the time of radiotracer injection (rest or peak stress). Therefore it is important to maintain maximal stress (exercise or vasodilator) for at least 1 minute after injection of the radiotracer. In contrast, the ECG-gated images reflect myocardial function, EF, and volumes at the time of the scan acquisition. SPECT MPI scans are typically acquired 15 to 45 minutes after stress radiotracer injection. Hence, most patients with reversible perfusion defects do not demonstrate regional wall motion abnormalities on the gated SPECT studies, unless ischemia is severe leading to postischemic stunning. In contrast, PET MPI-gated images are obtained immediately after completion of vasodilator stress and during peak dobutamine infusion. A lack of increase in LVEF with vasodilator stress or a decrease in LVEF post vasodilator stress with ^{82}rubidium PET has been shown to be a marker of significant obstructive multivessel CAD (see section Patient-Centered Clinical Applications).[2]

Transthyretin Cardiac Amyloidosis Imaging

Transthyretin cardiac amyloidosis (ATTR-CA) can be imaged using 10 to 20 mCi ^{99m}Tc-PYP, ^{99m}TcDPD, ^{99m}Tc-HMDP (see section Infiltrative Cardiomyopathy: Amyloidosis), and planar and SPECT (SPECT/CT if available) imaging 2 to 3 hours after injection of the radiotracer (see Fig. 18.7D).[8]

PET Protocols
Myocardial Perfusion Imaging

For PET,[2] a single-day rest and stress MPI is performed with ^{82}rubidium or ^{13}N-ammonia (Fig. 18.8A). With most advanced scanners, images are acquired in a list mode and reconstructed into static, gated, and dynamic images. With hybrid PET/CT MPI a dedicated noncontrast gated cardiac CT can be obtained for calculation of a coronary artery calcium score. The low-dose free-breathing CT obtained for attenuation correction can also be reviewed to assess semiquantitatively the presence and extent of coronary calcification. Although this is specific, it may be insensitive for detection of milder degrees of coronary artery calcification.

^{18}F-FDG Metabolic Imaging Protocols

For viability imaging, glucose/insulin preparation is necessary. Then, ^{18}F-FDG (5 to 10 mCi) is administered intravenously and cardiac PET/CT images are acquired 60 minutes later (see Fig. 18.8B).[2] For cardiac sarcoidosis (see Fig. 18.8C), infection, or vasculitis imaging (see Fig. 18.8D), patients undergo the high-fat/low-carbohydrate dietary preparation. Cardiac and partial or full-body PET/CT images are acquired 90 minutes after IV injection of ^{18}F-FDG. For viability imaging and for sarcoidosis imaging rest MPI is performed before

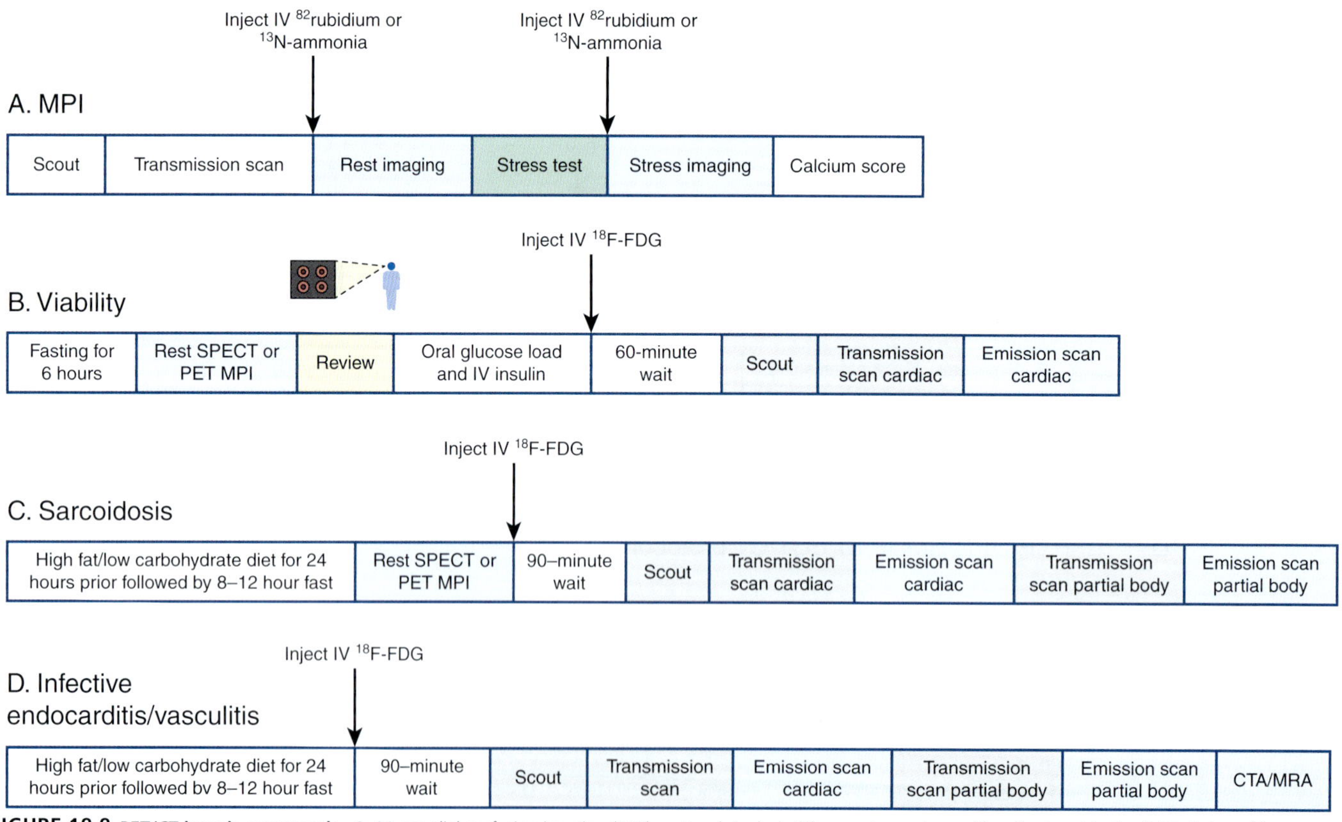

FIGURE 18.8 PET/CT imaging protocols. A, Myocardial perfusion imaging (MPI) protocols include (1) a scout scan to position the heart in the field of view; (2) nongated, low-dose CT transmission scan for attenuation correction; and (3) emission scan. MPI is typically performed in association with pharmacologic stress. However, exercise PET MPI is possible with ^{13}N ammonia because of its longer physical half-life. In patients without known coronary artery disease, a gated CT scan to measure coronary artery calcium score can be added. **B–D,** ^{18}F-FDG PET/CT protocols for myocardial viability, sarcoidosis, and infective endocarditis/vasculitis assessment. Specific dietary preparation is required for each of these ^{18}F-FDG protocols as discussed in the text and in American Society of Nuclear Cardiology guidelines. Myocardial perfusion imaging is required for the evaluation of myocardial viability and cardiac sarcoidosis. Limited whole-body (chest, abdomen, and pelvis) ^{18}F-FDG imaging is recommended for sarcoidosis, whereas whole-body (scalp to toes) imaging is recommended for infective endocarditis and vasculitis. *CTA,* CT angiography useful in cases of infective endocarditis; *IV,* intravenous; *MRA,* magnetic resonance angiography useful in cases of aortitis and vasculitis.

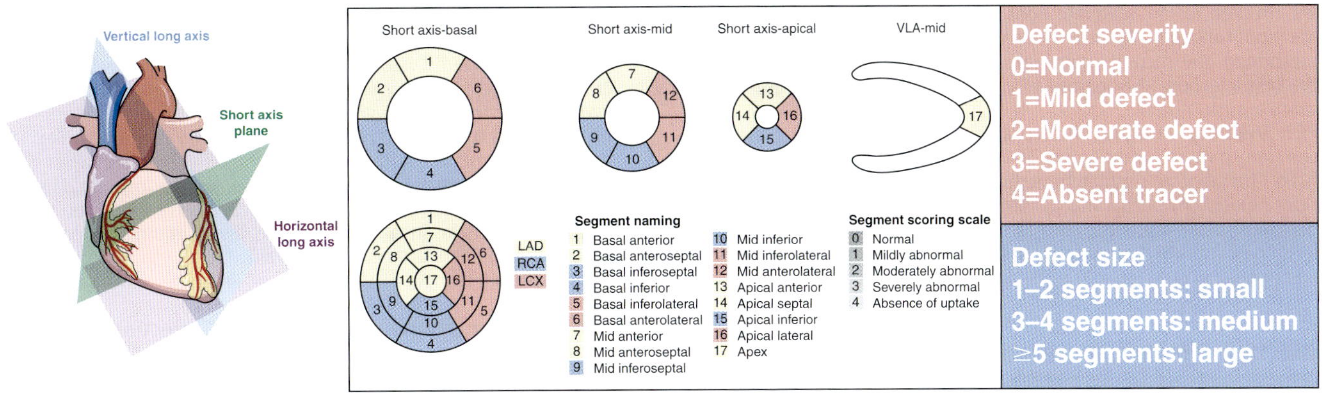

FIGURE 18.9 Myocardial segmentation model. A 17-segment heart model is recommended for segmental evaluation of myocardial perfusion and metabolic imaging. For semiquantitative scan interpretation, myocardial perfusion in each segment is scored from normal to absent tracer uptake and defect size estimated from small to large, as shown in the figure. Short-axis, vertical long-axis, and horizontal long-axis images are in a plane parallel to the mitral valve, the septum, and the inferior wall, respectively. (From Dorbala S, et al. Single photon emission computed tomography (SPECT) myocardial perfusion imaging guidelines: instrumentation, acquisition, processing, and interpretation. J Nucl Cardiol 2018;25:1784-1846.)

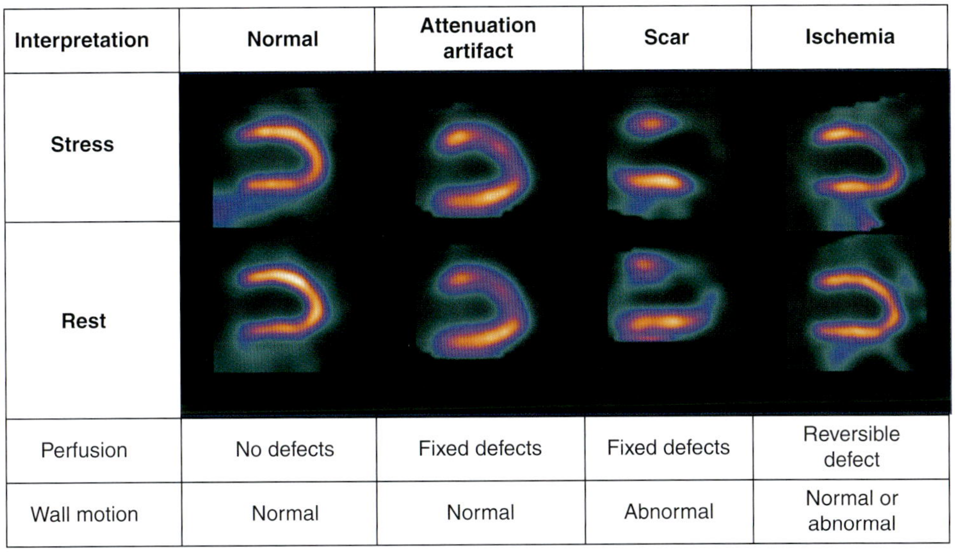

Interpretation	Normal	Attenuation artifact	Scar	Ischemia
Stress				
Rest				
Perfusion	No defects	Fixed defects	Fixed defects	Reversible defect
Wall motion	Normal	Normal	Abnormal	Normal or abnormal

FIGURE 18.10 Interpretation of myocardial perfusion images. Patterns of regional myocardial perfusion and corresponding regional wall motion associated with scans showing normal myocardial perfusion, attenuation artifact, scar, and ischemia.

the ^{18}F-FDG scan. A coronary CTA, and a vascular CTA or MR angiogram (MRA), is also added for endocarditis and vasculitis protocols, respectively. Please review ASNC guidelines for more protocol details.[2,7]

SYSTEMATIC INTERPRETATION OF IMAGES

A systematic review of images will improve diagnostic accuracy of scan interpretation and intra/interreader variability.[1]

Image Quality

Following image acquisition, each image is checked for quality and appropriate measures taken to mitigate any artifacts before the patient leaves. The projection images are viewed sequentially in a cine loop format to identify patient motion on conventional SPECT. Vertical motion is easier to identify on the rotating projection images and the sinogram may provide a clue to horizontal motion. Motion is more challenging to identify on novel multidetector SPECT (semiconductor detector scanners) and PET scanners because of simultaneous acquisition of projection images. Identification of distortion or blurriness on reconstructed images may provide some clues to motion artifact. Identification of motion on cardiac PET images is also possible by a review of the cine loop display of the multiframe dynamic images. Misregistration of the transmission and emission images is checked in a fusion screen.

Image Display

The perfusion images are interpreted using cardiac projection images of short-axis, vertical-long axis, and horizontal-long axis images. The rest and stress images are viewed simultaneously in alternate rows. Adequate alignment of rest and stress slices is required.

Image Review and Interpretation

Scan interpretation starts with a visual evaluation of rest, stress images for LV size, right ventricular (RV) size, and tracer uptake. Any transient changes in size of the left ventricle or RV tracer uptake from rest to stress are noted.

Perfusion Imaging Interpretation. The perfusion images are reviewed visually and semiquantitatively. Interpretation is performed in a segmental fashion using a 17-segment heart model (Fig. 18.9) and a 0 to 4 scale (where each of the 17 segments are scored using 0 = normal, 1 = mild, 2 = moderate, 3 = severe, and 4 = absent tracer uptake). The sum of the stress scores, rest scores, and their difference is termed summed stress score (SSS), summed rest score (SRS), and summed difference score (SDS), respectively. These visual scores are often converted into percentage myocardium abnormal [(SSS/68) x 100], ischemic [(SDS/68) x 100] or scarred [(SRS/68) x 100] Well-validated commercially available software programs provide semiautomatic estimates of perfusion defect size, extent, and severity (in terms of percentage myocardium abnormal, ischemic, or scarred).

Fig. 18.10 illustrates the common patterns of stress and rest myocardial perfusion images including normal, fixed defect, and reversible defect. Common normal variants in MPI include apical thinning (a fixed perfusion defect in the apical inferior wall or septum with normal wall motion) on SPECT or PET/MPI and a fixed basal lateral perfusion defect with normal wall motion on ^{13}N-ammonia PET/CT. The differential diagnosis of a fixed perfusion defect includes artifact (if wall motion is normal) or real defect (if wall motion is abnormal). Real fixed perfusion defects can be further evaluated for myocardial viability using radionuclide methods, CMR, or low-dose dobutamine echocardiography (see Chapters 16 and 19). High-risk features of MPI are listed in Table 18.4.

ECG-Gated Image Interpretation. The gated images are reviewed for regional wall motion, wall thickening, and calculation of LV volumes and EF. Dyssynchrony can also be evaluated using specialized software.

PET/SPECT Dynamic Image Interpretation[9]. For cardiac PET MPI, absolute myocardial blood flow images are checked for quality and motion. Motion correction is applied if necessary. An image-derived input function is placed in the left atrium or ascending aorta and positioned to capture the peak blood pool activity. The time activity curves are checked for an adequate tight bolus of radiotracer (sharp peak of the input function). When low-dose/high-dose ¹³N-ammonia studies are performed, the second images are corrected for residual activity from the first injection.[9] Myocardial blood flow is displayed in segmental or vascular distribution.

PET Viability Imaging Interpretation. Fig. 18.11 illustrates the common patterns of MPI and ¹⁸F-FDG viability imaging including perfusion-metabolism mismatch, perfusion-metabolism match, and perfusion-metabolism partial match. Segmental radiotracer uptake on rest perfusion polar maps can also be used to guide viability assessment. Resting counts are normalized to peak counts and expressed as percentage of peak activity (counts in the pixels with highest uptake considered 100%, and all other pixel values compared relative to that maximal uptake). Myocardial segments with >60% peak activity of perfusion tracer are considered viable, those with <40% peak activity are considered nonviable, and those with 40% to 60% of peak activity are further evaluated for myocardial viability.

PET Imaging of Infiltrative and Inflammatory Processes. Fig. 18.12 shows the common patterns of MPI and ¹⁸F-FDG imaging in cardiac sarcoidosis. Hot-spot images (sarcoidosis, amyloidosis, and infective endocarditis) are quantified using target to background ratio (myocardium to rib uptake in amyloidosis and myocardium to blood activity in sarcoidosis), standardized uptake value (SUV), volume of myocardial pixel above a threshold SUV mean value, and other advanced metrics.

Photon Attenuation and Attenuation Correction

In patients with excess soft tissue, the photons emitted by the heart may be attenuated (stopped by soft tissue) or scattered before they reach the detectors and cause artifactual perfusion defects. Attenuation artifacts are more prominent in obese patients, in patients with large chest size, and in those who are unable to raise their left arm for MPI. Anterior wall attenuation in women from overlying breast tissue (Fig. 18.13A) and inferior wall attenuation in men from diaphragmatic muscle are common sources of attenuation artifacts.

Attenuation artifacts are mitigated by multiposition imaging, ECG-gated SPECT imaging, or radionuclide or CT-based transmission imaging for attenuation correction.[1] Multiposition SPECT imaging (supine/prone and upright/supine) may improve attenuation artifacts, particularly inferior wall artifacts, while true defects remain unchanged. ECG-gated SPECT imaging showing normal wall motion despite a fixed perfusion defect is another way to discern attenuation artifacts. Attenuation- and scatter-corrected SPECT improves the specificity and normalcy of MPI.[1] Most attenuation artifacts typically result in fixed defects, but variable attenuation may result in pseudo-reversible perfusion defects, which can be challenging to detect and attenuation correction is optimal in those instances.

Measurement of photon attenuation and correction using radionuclide or CT transmission imaging is the most direct way to correct for attenuation artifacts. Attenuation correction is depth independent and more robust with PET compared with SPECT imaging (see Fig. 18.13B).[1]

Older generation SPECT and PET scanners used a transmission scan based on a rotating line source of a radionuclide such as Gd-153 (gamma rays with energies of 97 and 103 keV). This image takes about 3 to 4 minutes or longer based on the life of the line source. Current generation SPECT and PET scanners most commonly use a CT-based transmission imaging (a low-dose, free tidal breathing, noncontrast CT) for attenuation correction.[10] High-resolution chest CT images are transformed into a low-resolution attenuation map of the chest based on density of bone, soft tissue, or air. The transmission images are obtained sequentially before or after the emission images; hence accurate alignment of the transmission and emission images is important for accurate attenuation correction. It is particularly important to ensure adequate coregistration of the emission and CT to avoid misregistration artifacts that typically result in regional perfusion defects from incorrect attenuation correction of the myocardial counts caused by overlap with lung tissue (Fig. 18.14).[2] If the emission image overlies a metallic object, such as implantable cardiac defibrillator (ICD) leads, the emission image is overcorrected resulting in artifactual hot spots that can interfere with interpretation of inflammation or infection images (see section Patient-Centered Clinical Applications).

REDUCING RADIATION DOSE

Radiation risks from diagnostic nuclear cardiology imaging are small and challenging to estimate as the effects are stochastic with a potential unknown risk of cancer several decades after exposure (extrapolated from atom-bomb survivor studies).[11] A large body of evidence accumulating over the last 50 years strongly supports the power

TABLE 18.4 High-Risk Features

Myocardial Perfusion Imaging
Large single or multiterritorial fixed and/or reversible myocardial perfusion defects involving >15% of the LV mass
Transient ischemic dilation of the left ventricle
Stress-induced myocardial stunning with a drop in LVEF poststress
Transient RV tracer uptake
Increased pulmonary tracer uptake
Stress Test
Significant (>3 mm) ST-segment depression
Prolonged ST-segment depression
ST depression at low workload
Multilead ST depression
ST-segment elevation (>1 mm)
Hypotension (>10 mm Hg) with exercise
Sustained ventricular tachycardia

LVEF, Left ventricular ejection fraction; *RV*, right ventricular.

Interpretation	Hibernation	Scar	Nontransmural scar
Perfusion	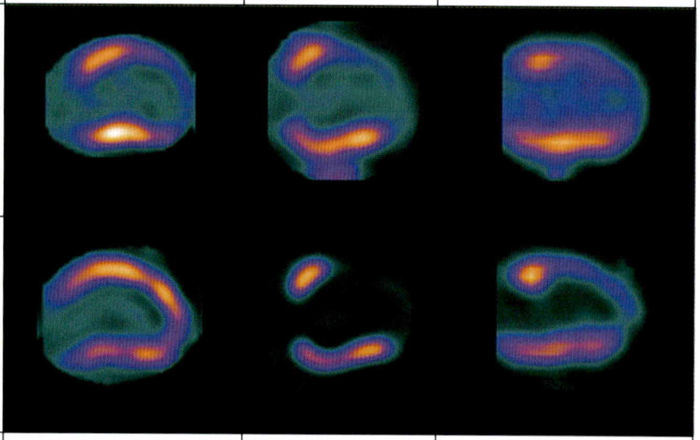		
Glucose metabolism			
Perfusion	Defect	Defect	Defect
Wall motion	Abnormal	Abnormal	Normal/Abnormal
¹⁸F-FDG uptake	Increased	Absent	Partial uptake
Pattern	Mismatch	Match	Partial mismatch

FIGURE 18.11 Patterns of myocardial perfusion and ¹⁸F-FDG in viability imaging. Patterns of regional myocardial perfusion, metabolism, and corresponding regional wall motion associated with scans showing viable and nonviable myocardium. The most common perfusion-metabolism patterns are mismatch (perfusion defect with preserved ¹⁸F-FDG uptake, representing hibernating myocardium), match (perfusion defect with concordantly reduced ¹⁸F-FDG uptake, representing myocardial scar), and partial match (nontransmural perfusion defect with concordantly reduced ¹⁸F-FDG uptake, representing nontransmural scar). Occasionally, a reversed mismatch (normal perfusion but reduced ¹⁸F-FDG uptake) can be seen in association with myocardial stunning, left bundle branch block, or both.

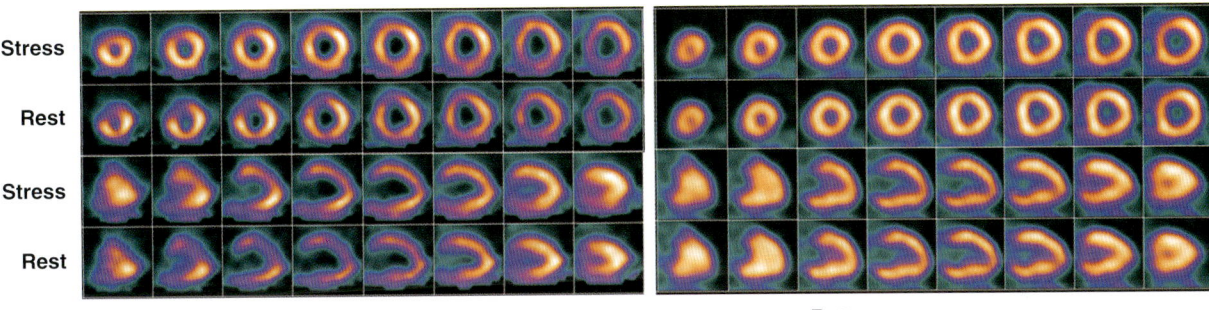

FIGURE 18.12 Patterns of myocardial perfusion and ^{18}F-FDG images in cardiac sarcoidosis. In patients undergoing evaluation for cardiac sarcoidosis, ^{18}F-FDG images are typically interpreted in conjunction with perfusion images. Normal perfusion with no myocardial ^{18}F-FDG uptake is normal and diffuse ^{18}F-FDG uptake is nonspecific. Normal or abnormal perfusion with focal ^{18}F-FDG uptake is abnormal and indicates focal myocardial inflammation. Myocardial perfusion defect with no myocardial ^{18}F-FDG uptake indicates myocardial fibrosis (*last panel* shows intense blood pool activity without myocardial ^{18}F-FDG uptake).

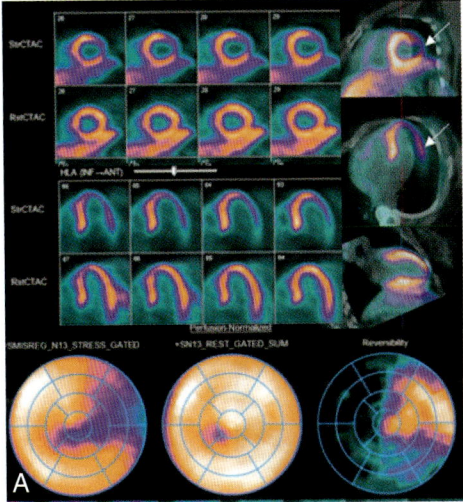
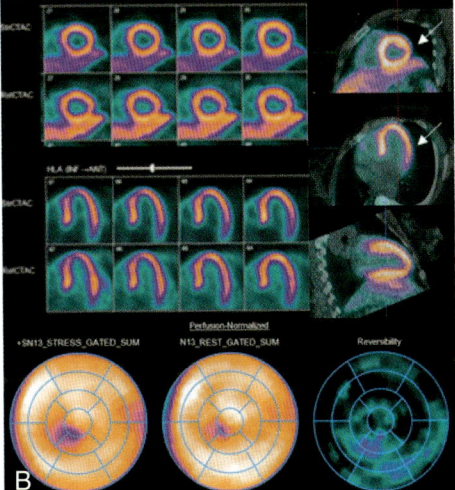

FIGURE 18.13 Breast attenuation artifact. ^{99m}Tc-sestamibi SPECT MPI **(A)** and ^{82}rubidium positron emission tomography (PET)/computed tomography (CT) MPI **(B)** of a 59-year-old woman with a body mass index of 31 kg/m² are shown. SPECT images show a medium-sized perfusion defect of moderate intensity in the mid and apical anterior wall that was fixed. Gated SPECT images (not shown) demonstrated diffuse global left ventricular hypokinesis and an ejection fraction of 35%. A cardiac PET was ordered because of concern for anterior wall attenuation artifact versus nontransmural scar. ^{82}Rubidium PET MPI was normal confirming attenuation artifact on SPECT MPI. In this and subsequent figures, short-axis images (*rows 1 and 2*) are shown from apex to base (left to right). Vertical long-axis images (*rows 3 and 4*) are shown from the septum to the lateral wall and horizontal long-axis images (not shown in this figure) are shown from inferior to anterior walls. *MPI,* Myocardial perfusion imaging.

FIGURE 18.14 Misregistration artifact on hybrid PET/CT imaging. A, Stress and rest ^{13}N-ammonia PET/CT images and corresponding polar maps show a medium-sized and severe perfusion defect in the anterolateral wall that is reversible. A review of the stress transmission and emission fused images show misalignment of the CT and perfusion images with the lateral wall on the PET images overlying the lung field on the CT (*white arrows*). **B,** Proper realignment of the perfusion and CT images and new reconstruction of the PET images resulted in a normal study.

of nuclear cardiology testing in the diagnosis, management, and risk assessment of patients with heart diseases. Hence any theoretical long-term effects of radiation from the use of radiotracers must be carefully weighed against the established short-term benefits from this test. There are several strategies for dose reduction. These include ensuring appropriate use of the test, use of weight-based radiotracer dosing, avoiding dual isotope and thallium protocols for MPI, and employing stress-first protocols, novel scanners, and processing software to allow for lower injected dose, and cardiac PET, particularly with 3D PET. Novel scanner technologies (CZT SPECT) and weight-based tracer dosing have cut radiation dose by more than half while maintaining or even improving image quality. PET MPI is associated with a substantially lower radiation dose compared with SPECT MPI. But a recent worldwide survey[12] has identified marked variability in the use of these radiation dose reduction practices across countries. Effective radiation dose reduction efforts must begin before the test (by ensuring the test is appropriate for the clinical question), continue during the test (by use of advanced protocols, technology, and lowest possible radiation dose for high-quality imaging), and after the test (clear reporting of test results will minimize layered testing and reduce radiation dose).[11] Following the principles of justification of the test and optimization of imaging will ensure that the risks of ionizing radiation, if any, will far outweigh its benefits. Indeed, stress-only imaging can be performed with <1.7 mSv for CZT SPECT and <1 mSv for PET.[11] Radiation dose for common nuclear cardiology studies can be calculated using the SNMMI radiation dose tool (see http://www.snmmi.org/clinicalpractice/dosetool.aspx?itemnumber=1).

PATIENT-CENTERED CLINICAL APPLICATIONS

Ischemic Heart Disease
Principles of Perfusion Imaging
The basic principle of radionuclide MPI for detecting CAD is based on the ability of a radiotracer to identify a transient regional perfusion deficit in a myocardial region subtended by a coronary artery with a flow-limiting stenosis. A reversible myocardial perfusion defect is indicative of ischemia, whereas a fixed perfusion defect generally reflects scarred myocardium from prior MI (see Fig. 18.10). Generally, myocardial perfusion defects during stress develop downstream to a epicardial stenosis with ≥50% to 70% luminal narrowing and become progressively more severe with increasing degree of stenosis. It is noteworthy that coronary stenosis of intermediate severity (e.g., 50% to 90%) is associated with significant variability in the resulting maximal myocardial blood flow, which in turns affects the presence and/or severity of regional perfusion defects. For any degree of intermediate luminal stenosis, the observed physiologic variability is multifactorial and includes geometric factors of coronary lesions not accounted for by a simple measure of minimal luminal diameter or percentage of stenosis (see Chapter 36). These factors include shape, eccentricity, and length, which are known to modulate coronary resistance; collateral blood flow; and the presence of diffuse coronary atherosclerosis and microvascular dysfunction. All these factors account for the frequent disagreements between angiographically defined CAD and its associated physiologic severity by radionuclide perfusion imaging.

Suspected Stable Coronary Artery Disease
Patients with New-Onset Chest Pain
Radionuclide MPI is appropriate in symptomatic patients with suspected CAD (Fig. 18.15). Although in younger patients coronary CT angiography may be an excellent choice to screen for CAD, it is probably not ideal in older patients who are more likely to show coronary artery calcifications, especially in patients with cardiometabolic risk factors. The diagnostic accuracy of SPECT MPI for detecting obstructive CAD as defined by invasive coronary angiography was examined in a recent large meta-analysis including 86 studies (10,870 patients).[13] The pooled sensitivity was 87% and the specificity was 78% with similar accuracy for exercise and pharmacologic stress. However, one needs to keep in mind that the reported accuracies of noninvasive testing for radionuclide MPI (and other modalities) are limited by the referral biases intrinsic to the design of most studies in this area, especially partial verification bias that refers to selective referral to the reference standard (catheterization) based on the results of the test being studied. That is, very few patients with normal noninvasive tests will be

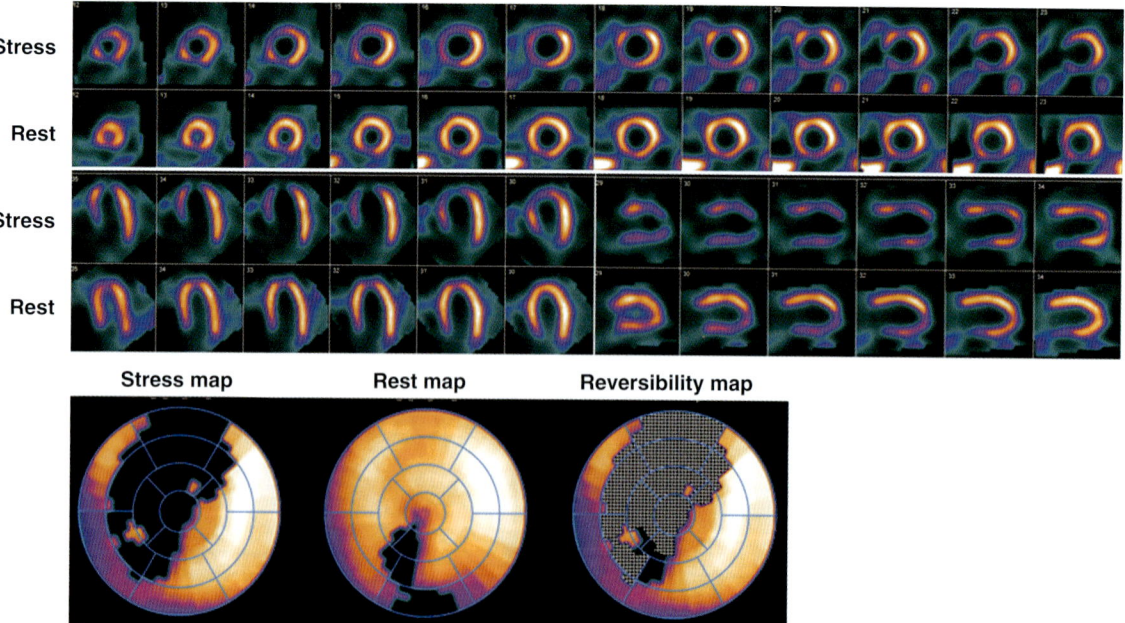

FIGURE 18.15 High-risk myocardial perfusion SPECT study. Exercise-stress and rest ^{99m}Tc-MIBI myocardial perfusion imaging of an 80-year-old man presenting with atypical chest pain and dyspnea. Exercise was terminated because of chest pain, with associated decrease in blood pressure and 3-mm downsloping ST-segment depression in the inferolateral leads. Images demonstrate transient left ventricular (LV) dilatation and a large and severe perfusion defect throughout the anterior, anteroseptal, and apical LV segments and the LV apex, showing complete reversibility. In addition, there was a medium-sized perfusion defect of severe intensity in the mid and basal inferior and inferoseptal walls, showing moderate reversibility. Polar maps confirmed these findings. There was also a decrease in LV ejection fraction after exercise. These findings are highly predictive of high-risk coronary artery disease, which was confirmed on coronary angiography.

referred to catheterization, whereas many more with abnormal tests will be referred for coronary angiography, resulting in relatively fewer true or false-negatives and more true- or false-positives, yielding an increase in sensitivity and a marked reduction in specificity.

Fig. 18.16 underscores that despite its widespread use and acceptance, a recognized limitation of semiquantitative visual assessment of radionuclide myocardial perfusion images with SPECT and PET often uncovers only coronary territories supplied by coronary arteries with the most severe stenosis. Consequently, it is relatively insensitive to accurately delineate the extent of obstructive angiographic CAD, especially in the setting of multivessel CAD. As illustrated in this example, quantification of myocardial blood flow (in mL/min/g) and MFR (calculated as the ratio of maximum hyperemic myocardial blood flow over that at rest) showed that myocardial ischemia was far more extensive than predicted by the visual extent of perfusion abnormalities. The severely reduced MFR corresponded with the high-risk angiographic findings.

A number of studies have demonstrated a relationship between myocardial blood flow and flow reserve and percentage diameter stenosis on angiography; that is, there is a progressive reduction in myocardial blood flow and flow reserve with increasing severity of angiographic stenosis. These observations have served as the basis for the clinical use of quantitative myocardial blood flow to improve identification of obstructive CAD and, especially, to exclude the presence of severe angiographic multivessel CAD.

Recent meta-analyses,[14,15] a prospective European multicenter study (Evaluation of Integrated CAD Imaging in Ischemic Heart Disease [EVINCI]),[16] and a prospective comparative effectiveness study (Prospective Comparison of Cardiac PET/CT, SPECT/CT Perfusion Imaging and CT Coronary Angiography With Invasive Coronary Angiography [PACIFIC])[17] support the notion that PET MPI is one of the most accurate noninvasive techniques for detecting flow-limiting CAD.[17] As discussed earlier, one unique advantage of PET over SPECT is that it allows routine quantification of myocardial blood flow and MFR. These quantitative measures of myocardial perfusion improve the sensitivity and negative predictive value of PET for ruling out high-risk angiographic CAD. Indeed, an MFR >2.0 is associated with a >97% negative predictive value for ruling out high-risk angiographic CAD.

Risk Stratification with Radionuclide Myocardial Perfusion Imaging

Radionuclide MPI provides robust prognostic assessments of patients with suspected stable CAD, which has been documented for over four decades and forms the basis of its widespread use and clinical utility. The power of radionuclide MPI (including SPECT and PET) for risk stratification is based on the fact that major determinants of prognosis in patients with CAD are readily available from gated MPI. These include the amount of myocardial scar, the extent and severity of stress-induced ischemia, degree of LV dilatation, and reduced LVEF. Optimal risk stratification is based on the concept that the risk associated with a normal study is sufficiently low that referral to revascularization will not further improve patient outcomes; hence catheterization is an unlikely option after testing. Conversely, patients with abnormal stress imaging results are at greater risk of adverse events and, thus, are potential candidates for intervention, and the magnitude of their risk is related to the extent and severity of the imaging abnormalities.

A normal or low-risk rest/stress radionuclide MPI with SPECT or PET was associated with an annual risk of MACE of 0.85% and 0.4%, respectively.[18] The low risk associated with normal SPECT MPI has recently been extended to the radiation-sparing, stress-only radionuclide MPI protocols and to PET MPI as well.[10,18,19] However, the risk associated with a normal radionuclide MPI has not necessarily been low (<1%) in higher risk cohorts (e.g., diabetes, chronic kidney impairment, elderly). The reasons for the observed increased adverse event rate in higher risk cohorts despite a visually normal radionuclide MPI are likely multifactorial. On one hand, coexisting comorbidities including hypertension, obesity, and others increase clinical risk even in the absence of obstructive CAD. On the other hand, and notwithstanding the clinical utility of SPECT MPI, it is a somewhat insensitive test to uncover diffuse obstructive and nonobstructive atherosclerosis and/or coronary microvascular dysfunction (CMD) associated with myocardial ischemia and increased risk of adverse events. Consequently, absolute quantification of myocardial blood flow and flow reserve by PET (an integrated marker of epicardial stenosis, diffuse atherosclerosis, and microvascular dysfunction) is a definite advantage in higher-risk patients. In such patients, a relatively preserved MFR identifies truly low-risk individuals among high-risk patients.[20] For example, patients with diabetes without known CAD but abnormal MFR had a cardiac mortality risk similar to that in nondiabetics with known

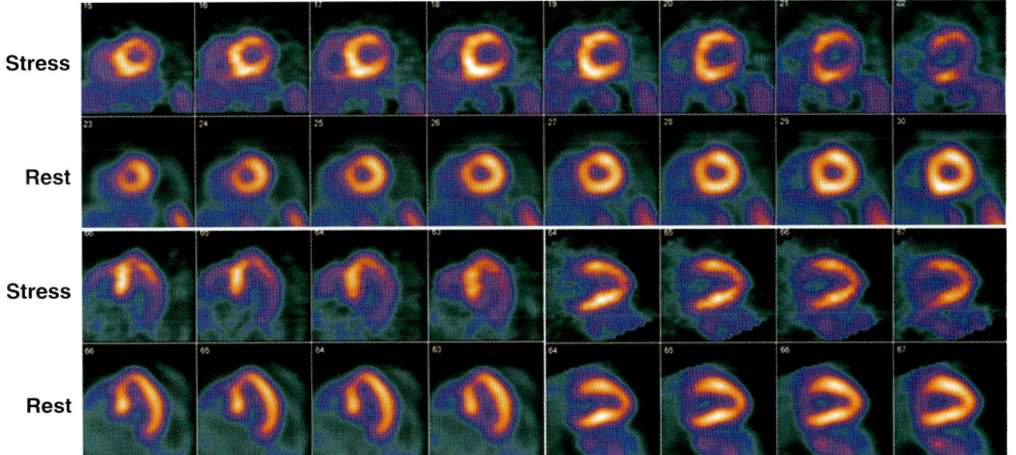

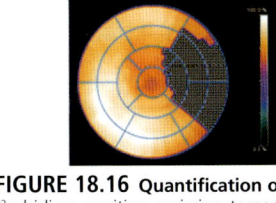

Quantitative myocardial blood flow and MFR

	Rest	Stress	MFR
LAD	1.21	1.19	0.99
LCX	1.16	0.82	0.71
RCA	1.30	1.73	1.33
Global LV	1.22	1.22	1.00

FIGURE 18.16 Quantification of myocardial blood flow and multivessel obstructive CAD. Rest and vasodilator-stress [82]rubidium position emission tomography scan of an 85-year-old woman presenting with exertional dyspnea. Stress images demonstrate a medium-sized perfusion defect of severe intensity throughout the lateral wall showing complete reversibility, consistent with single-vessel left circumflex (LCX) ischemia. However, the quantitative myocardial blood flow and myocardial flow reserve data show a severely blunted hyperemic flow response to vasodilator stress and reduced flow reserve in all coronary territories. The noncontrast computed tomography scan showed severe coronary artery calcification of the left main, left anterior descending (LAD), and LCX arteries (images not shown). Follow-up coronary angiography showed severe left main and LCX disease. *LV*, left ventricle; *RCA*, right coronary artery.

CAD. Conversely, diabetic individuals without overt CAD with relatively preserved MFR had an annual risk of <1% that was comparable to subjects without diabetes or CAD. Similar findings have been shown in patients with chronic kidney disease.[21]

The risk associated with an abnormal radionuclide MPI study is not only greater than that after a normal MPI but increases as a function of the extent and severity of perfusion abnormalities (Fig. 18.17). This concept is applicable to both SPECT and PET MPI, vasodilator and exercise stress testing, and virtually all patient groups. The prognostic information provided by the results of radionuclide MPI is incremental to that provided by demographics and medical history data and that from exercise stress testing. Most importantly, the postscan risk increases with the degree of perfusion and LV functional abnormalities present on the radionuclide MPI. Importantly, the presence of LV dilatation and/or reduced LVEF further increases clinical risk across all levels of myocardial perfusion abnormalities. Finally, fixed perfusion defects (and the presence of often associated LV dilatation and reduced LV function) are associated with a greater risk of cardiac death, whereas reversible or ischemic defects are more closely associated with the occurrence of nonfatal MI. The constellation of extensive myocardial scar (fixed defects), LV remodeling, and reduced EF represents the highest risk subgroup.

As discussed previously, the quantitative regional and global myocardial blood flow and MFR information obtained with PET MPI provide incremental information that is useful in risk stratification. Indeed, for any amount of ischemic and/or scarred myocardium, a severely reduced global MFR is associated with a higher risk of death than in the setting of relatively preserved MFR (Fig. 18.18). The increased risk of adverse events in patients with reduced MFR (<2.0) also applies to patients with visually normal radionuclide MPI. In the majority of these patients, the reduced MFR reflects a combination of diffuse nonobstructive atherosclerosis and CMD and is found frequently in symptomatic men and women without overt obstructive CAD (51% and 54%, respectively). Importantly, the noninvasive PET measure of MFR improves risk reclassification, especially among high-risk cohorts (e.g., patients with diabetes, non-ST elevation MI [NSTEMI], chronic renal impairment, and high coronary calcium scores). Thus the ability to quantify MFR allows a level of risk assessment well beyond that achieved thus far using semiquantitative analysis of regional perfusion defects, with the potential to incorporate measures of endothelial function and vascular health status into routine patient evaluations.

Symptomatic Patients Without Angiographic Obstructive Coronary Artery Disease

CMD is quite common in symptomatic patients with risk factors (Fig. 18.19) and the relative frequency and severity of CMD is similar in women and men, but numerically there is a larger number of women with CMD than men. When present, symptomatic patients with CMD have a worse prognosis than asymptomatic patients. Because it is a diffuse process, conventional exercise stress testing and stress imaging tests, such as with echocardiography or SPECT imaging, lack sensitivity and specificity for detecting CMD and thus have a relatively limited role in its diagnosis. Because the coronary microcirculation is beyond the resolution of invasive or noninvasive coronary angiography, direct interrogation of coronary microvascular function is necessary to establish the diagnosis of CMD. There are several noninvasive and invasive approaches for this evaluation, each with advantages and limitations, and quantitative PET imaging is considered the most accurate and reproducible noninvasive technique. Reduction of stress myocardial blood flow and MFR reflects the combined effects of altered coronary fluid dynamics caused by diffuse atherosclerosis and microcirculatory dysfunction. Diffuse nonobstructive atherosclerosis in the epicardial coronary arteries is a common finding in symptomatic patients with CMD and can be identified using coronary artery calcium scoring (Fig. 18.19). The combined effects of extensive nonobstructive atherosclerosis and CMD increases the clinical risk compared to the risks associated with either one alone.[22] This consideration highlights the important complementary role of delineating atherosclerotic burden with a noncontrast coronary artery calcium score or contrast CTA in addition to MPI.

Evaluation Before Organ Transplantation

Pretransplant patients are part of a special population and optimal strategies for detection of CAD in these patients are yet to be defined. However, there is general agreement that it may be reasonable to consider noninvasive testing in patients with multiple risk factors for CAD. The choice of the ideal test remains controversial and there is high

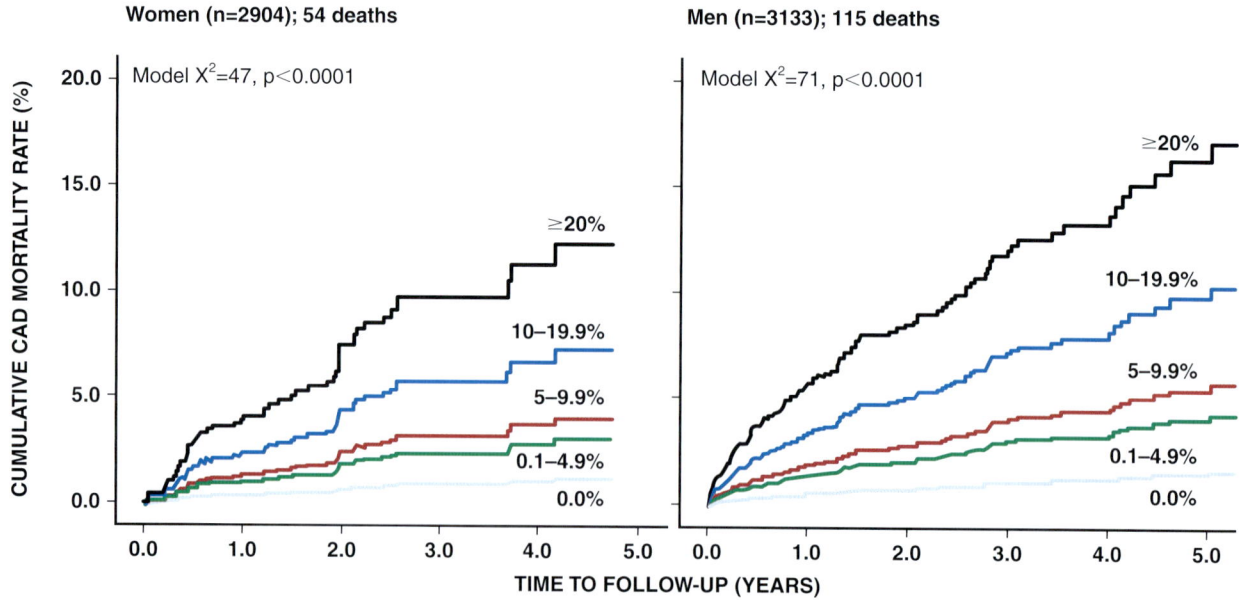

FIGURE 18.17 **Annualized coronary artery disease mortality stratified by magnitude of perfusion abnormality.** Multicenter data in 7061 patients at four institutions show a progressive increase in cardiac mortality with increasing extent of perfusion abnormality on position emission tomography, based on percentage of left ventricular myocardium, in both women (*left*) and men (*right*). (From Kay J, et al. Influence of sex on risk stratification with stress myocardial perfusion Rb-82 positron emission tomography: Results from the PET (Positron Emission Tomography) Prognosis Multicenter Registry. J Am Coll Cardiol 2013;62:1866-1876.)

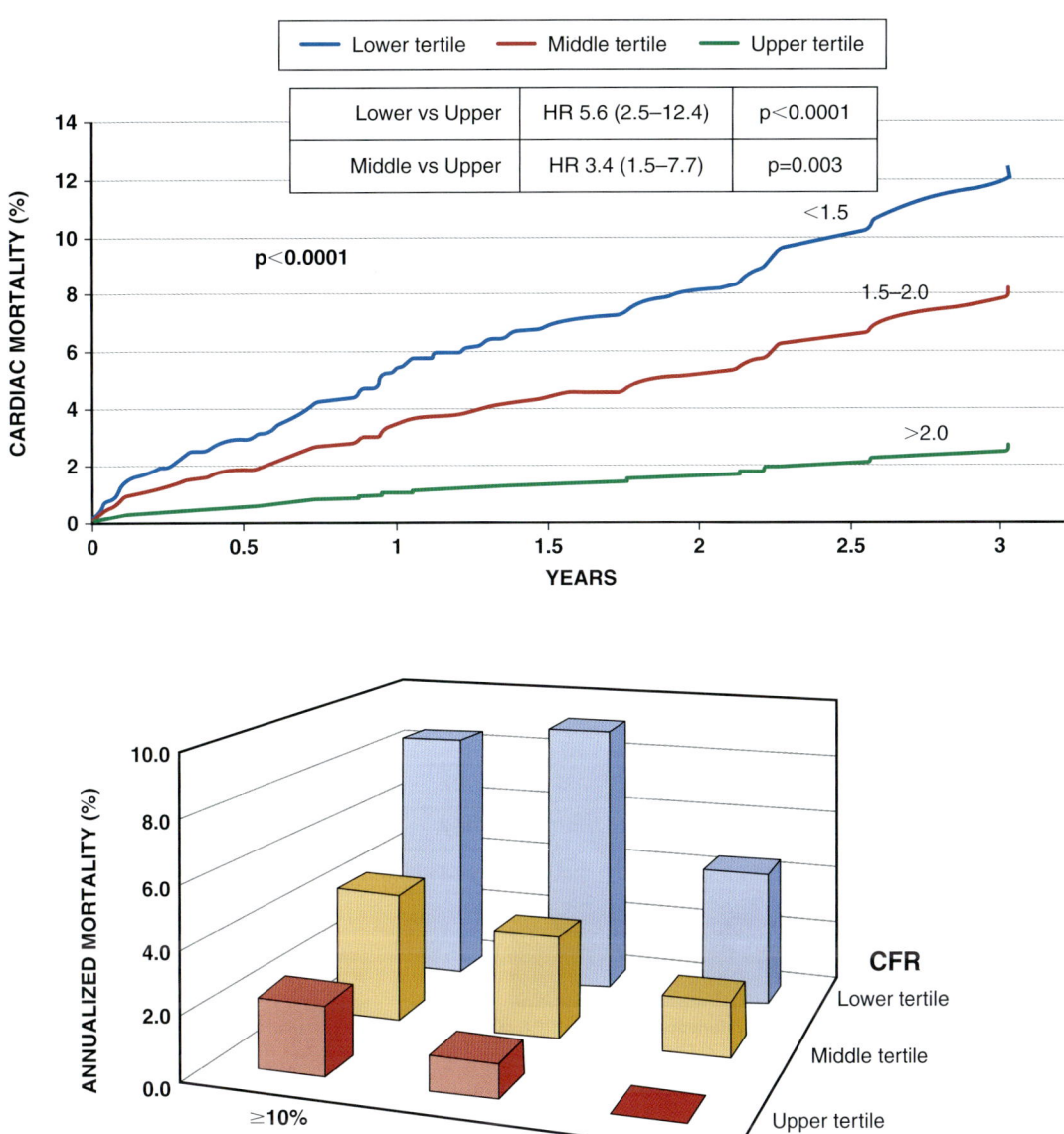

FIGURE 18.18 Risk stratification with myocardial flow reserve by PET MPI. *Top*, Probability of cardiac mortality in 2783 patients by tertiles of coronary flow reserve (CFR) with the highest risk corresponding to patients with the lowest tertile of CFR (<1.5). *Bottom*, Bar graph shows that annualized cardiac mortality is consistently higher for patients in the lowest CFR tertile across all levels of myocardial perfusion abnormalities. (From Murthy VL, et al. Improved cardiac risk assessment with noninvasive measures of coronary flow reserve. Circulation 2011;124:2215-2224.)

regional variability depending on availability and local expertise. Coronary CTA may be reasonable in young patients undergoing evaluation for organ transplantation because they are unlikely to show extensive coronary calcifications. However, noninvasive stress imaging may be more appropriate for patients over the age of 55, especially those with chronic kidney disease who are more likely to show coronary calcifications. Although exercise stress testing is preferred if the patient is likely to achieve an adequate cardiac workload, many patients require pharmacologic stress testing because of reduced functional capacity. There is a wealth of data on the diagnostic and prognostic utility of radionuclide MPI in renal transplant patients. A number of studies have shown that abnormal MPI is associated with both short- and long-term adverse cardiac events in patients with chronic kidney disease including renal transplant patients, and that a normal MPI study has a high negative predictive value. PET perfusion imaging offers the advantage of flow quantification, which provides incremental prognostic information beyond that of conventional perfusion imaging in patients on hemodialysis evaluated for renal transplantation.[23] Similar data have been reported for patients undergoing evaluation for liver transplantation. In summary, given the limited number of organs available for transplantation, surgeons and transplant teams are generally inclined to ensure that transplant recipients are free of severe CAD and have the best chance of meaningful event-free survival after transplantation.

Suspected Acute Coronary Syndrome
Patients with Nondiagnostic Electrocardiogram and Troponin Elevation

Normal radionuclide perfusion imaging in patients with low-level cardiac troponin elevation without typical symptoms or ECG changes and intermediate risk (TIMI risk score <5) is associated with very low short-term cardiac mortality. Conversely, an abnormal perfusion study identifies patients at significantly higher clinical risk. In such patients, the magnitude of stress-induced ischemia quantified by perfusion imaging helps guide the subsequent need of referral to cardiac catheterization and revascularization (see Chapter 39). In a prior large study of patients with ST-segment elevation MI (STEMI) and NSTEMI undergoing adenosine SPECT MPI, patients with low-risk scans (small defects with no or mild ischemia) had significantly lower risk than those with high-risk scans (large defects with significant residual ischemia) (rate

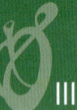

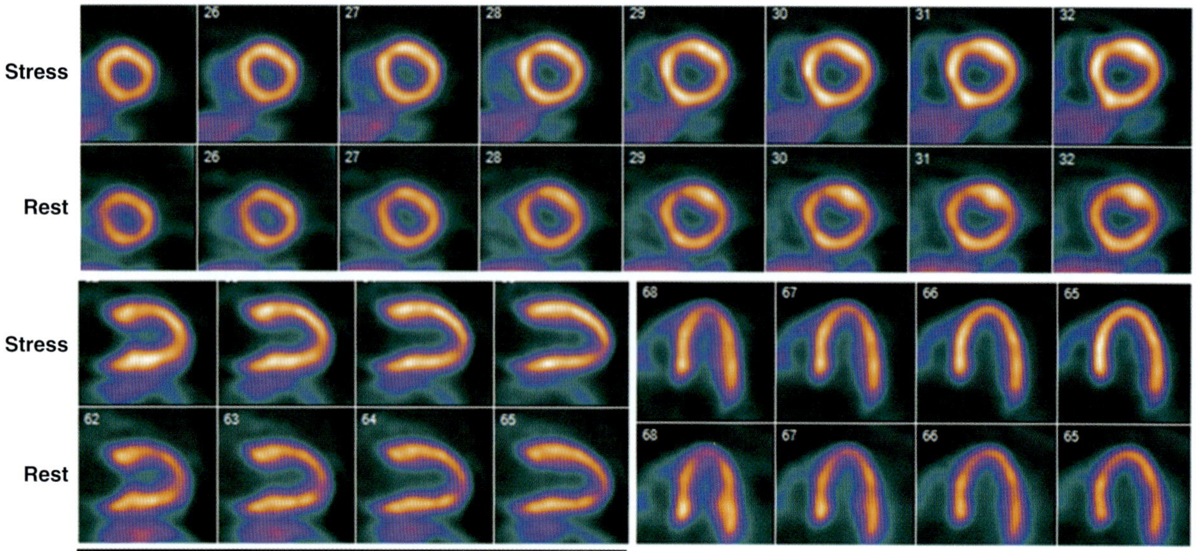

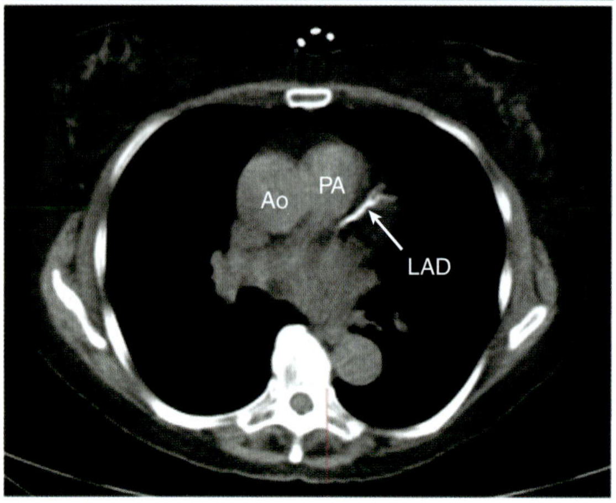

Quantitative myocardial blood flow (mL/min/g) and MFR

	Rest	Stress	MFR
LAD	0.91	1.57	1.73
LCX	0.92	1.53	1.66
RCA	0.83	1.46	1.76
Global LV	0.88	1.50	1.70

FIGURE 18.19 Evaluation of coronary microvascular dysfunction. Cardiac PET/CT images of a 76-year-old woman with dyslipidemia, hypertension, and nonobstructive angiographic coronary artery disease who presented with atypical chest pain and dyspnea. Vasodilator-stress and rest ^{13}N ammonia PET images demonstrate visually normal myocardial perfusion. The ECG gated images demonstrated a rest left ventricular (LV) ejection fraction of 71% that increased to 73% during stress with normal LV volumes (not shown). The CT transmission scan showed severe coronary artery calcification (*lower left*). Quantitative stress myocardial blood flow and myocardial flow reserve was moderately reduced in all coronary territories and globally. The abnormal quantitative findings are consistent with myocardial ischemia from nonobstructive atherosclerosis and coronary microvascular dysfunction. *Ao,* Aorta; *LAD,* left anterior descending artery; *LCX,* left circumflex artery; *PA,* pulmonary artery; *RCA,* right coronary artery.

of death 5.4%, 14%, and 18.6% and rate of MI 1.8%, 9.2%, and 11.6% for low-risk, intermediate-risk, and high-risk findings, respectively).[24]

The pathophysiology of minimally elevated levels of serum cardiac troponin in the absence of an ACS is heterogeneous. In one study, impaired global MFR in the absence of obstructive CAD as measured by PET was independently associated with troponin elevation, suggesting an association between chronic microvascular ischemia and myocardial injury, especially among patients with diffuse atherosclerosis.[25] More importantly, this quantitative imaging marker provides prognostic information incremental to other clinical markers of risk (Fig. 18.20).[25] Therefore, in intermediate-high risk patients with low-level elevation of cardiac troponin, quantitative stress PET perfusion imaging may offer an advantage compared with SPECT and may be preferable if available.

Patients with Known Stable Coronary Artery Disease

Radionuclide MPI is commonly used to facilitate diagnosis and management in patients with known CAD, including those with prior MI and revascularization with recurrent symptoms, worsening LV function, and/or arrhythmias. In these patients, diagnosis and quantification of myocardial ischemia is important for risk stratification and, especially, for guiding the potential need of revascularization (see Chapter 40).

Patients with Prior PCI and Recurrent Symptoms

Radionuclide MPI is appropriate for diagnosis of ischemia and risk stratification among patients with prior revascularization presenting with new-onset or worsening symptoms of angina or anginal equivalents such as dyspnea. In patients with prior percutaneous coronary intervention (PCI) or coronary artery bypass surgery (CABG), radionuclide MPI provides localization and quantification of myocardial ischemia that helps with risk prediction and management decisions regarding the potential need for targeted revascularization (Fig. 18.21). In these patients, exercise stress is ideal and should be performed when feasible because it provides important prognostic information and helps reproduce exertional symptoms. However, it is important to avoid submaximal exercise as this reduces the sensitivity of the test for detection of myocardial ischemia. In such cases, conversion to vasodilator stress helps avoid nondiagnostic tests. Among patients with known CAD, both PET and SPECT MPI offer high sensitivity. However, PET has higher specificity compared with SPECT, and consequently higher diagnostic accuracy. The addition of quantitative myocardial blood flow information is useful in patients with prior PCI but less so in those with prior CABG, as they have extensive disease in the native vessels, which can lead to a blunted flow response to vasodilator-stress despite patent grafts.

Patients with Recent Myocardial Infarction Evaluated for Potential Staged PCI

Stress radionuclide imaging is appropriate and commonly used to quantify the magnitude of residual stress-induced ischemia after MI, which aids in diagnosis, localization of ischemia, and risk stratification as discussed previously. The assessment of functional significance of

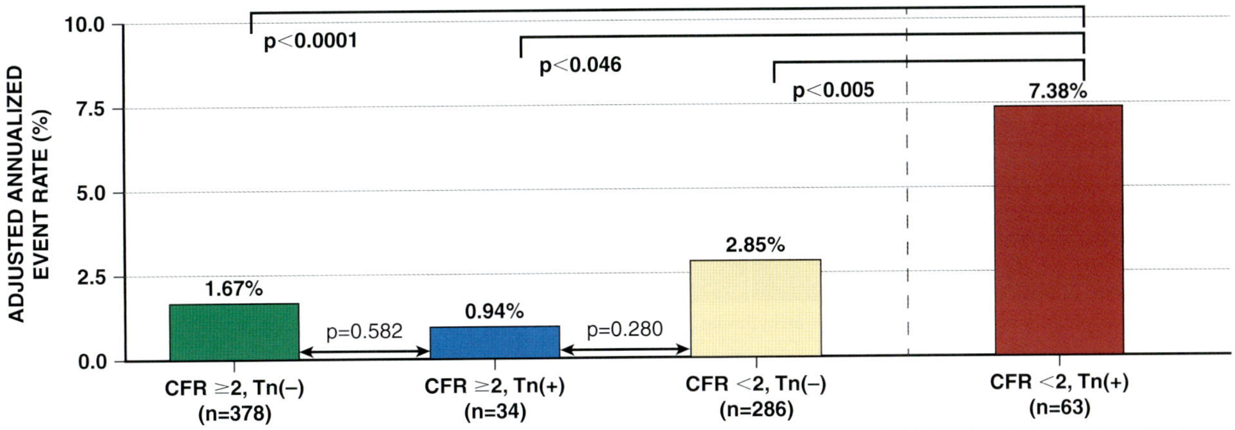

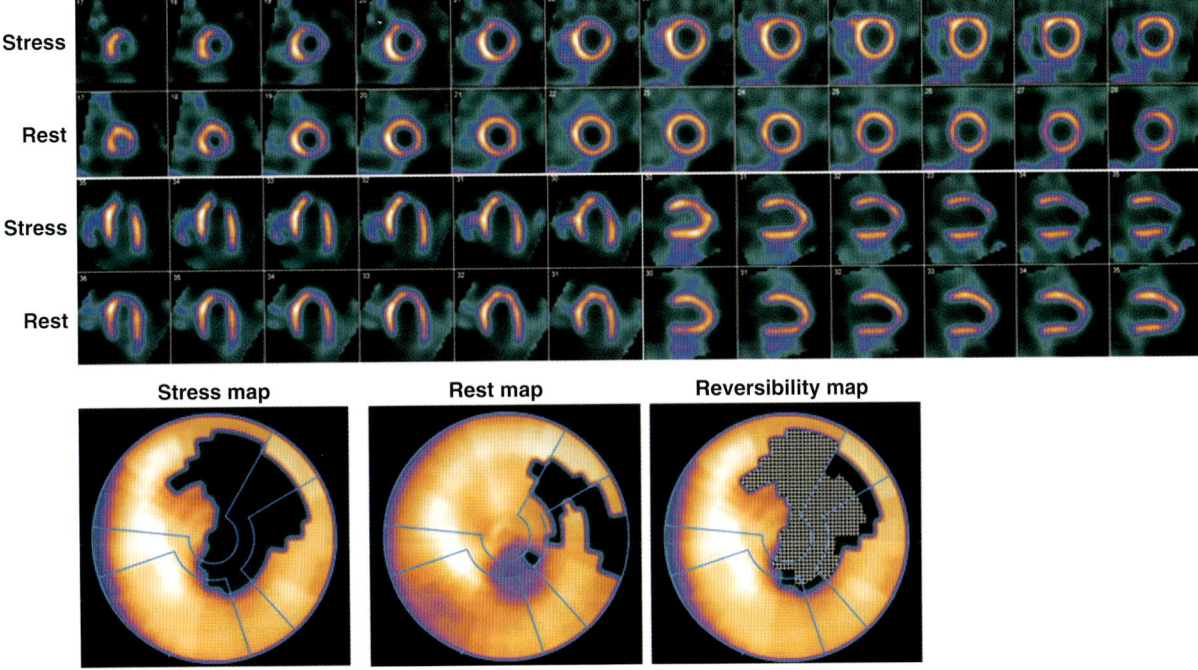

FIGURE 18.20 Incremental risk stratification by quantitative PET in patients with non-ST elevation myocardial infarction. Patients with positive troponin (Tn+) and impaired coronary flow reserve (CFR) (*red bar*) have a higher annualized event rate compared with those with a positive Tn but preserved CFR (*blue bar*). (From Taqueti VR, et al. Interaction of impaired coronary flow reserve and cardiomyocyte injury on adverse cardiovascular outcomes in patients without overt coronary artery disease. Circulation 2015;131:528-535.)

FIGURE 18.21 SPECT MPI in a patient with prior PCI and recurrent symptoms. Vasodilator-stress and rest ^{99m}Tc-sestamibi SPECT MPI of a 58-year-old woman who underwent PCI of the left circumflex (LCX) and left anterior descending (LAD) coronary arteries 3 years ago, now presenting with atypical angina and dyspnea. During vasodilator stress, there was 1-mm downsloping ST-segment depression in the inferolateral leads, which resolved 5 minutes into recovery. Myocardial perfusion images and associated polar maps demonstrate a large perfusion defect of severe intensity in the mid and apical anterior and anterolateral walls with significant but not complete reversibility. Follow-up coronary angiography demonstrated a long segment of severe diffuse disease in the mid-distal LAD including a diagonal branch, and a 50% proximal LCX lesion with total occlusion of the first marginal branch.

residual stenosis requires a maximal stress test. As maximal exercise testing is relatively contraindicated in the immediate post MI setting, a vasodilator stress is commonly used.

Patients with Prior Myocardial Infarction and Ventricular Arrhythmias

Myocardial ischemia is a cause of sustained ventricular arrhythmias/ventricular fibrillation and observational studies have shown that revascularization in addition to arrhythmia management afforded improved survival compared with arrhythmia management alone.[26] Consequently, investigation of stress-induced ischemia is common in these patients (Fig. 18.22). In addition to ischemia assessment, either SPECT or PET imaging can effectively quantify the extent of myocardial scar and provide effective arrhythmic risk stratification in patients with ischemic and nonischemic cardiomyopathy. For example, in a study of 439 patients with LVEF ≤35% (65% ischemic cardiomyopathy, 35% nonischemic) undergoing rest/stress PET MPI, patients without myocardial scar demonstrated a significantly lower annualized rate of major arrhythmic events (i.e., sudden cardiac arrest [SCA], resuscitated SCA, or appropriate ICD therapy for ventricular tachyarrhythmia) compared with those with any scar (2.1% vs 8.4% per year).[27] Importantly, myocardial scar was an independent predictor of major arrhythmic events, whereas other perfusion PET variables including ischemic burden, the presence of nontransmural scar/hibernation, peri-infarct ischemia, and MFR were not. These studies highlight the excellent prognostic value conferred by low scar burden detected by standard radionuclide perfusion imaging, and its ability to further identify a low-risk subgroup, among patients traditionally perceived to be at a high risk of lethal arrhythmic events.

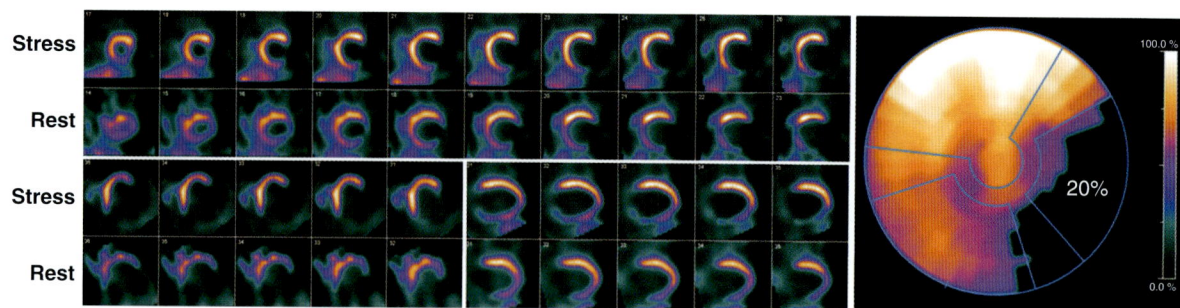

FIGURE 18.22 SPECT MPI in a patient with ventricular arrhythmias. Vasodilator-stress and rest ^{99m}Tc-sestamibi SPECT MPI of a 60-year-old woman with sustained monomorphic ventricular tachycardia 3 years following a large lateral wall myocardial infarction complicated by papillary muscle rupture with cardiogenic shock and need for mitral valve replacement. The myocardial perfusion images demonstrate a mildly dilated left ventricle and a large perfusion defect of severe intensity throughout the inferior and inferolateral and basal anterolateral walls, which was irreversible. Her ECG-gated images demonstrated a left ventricular ejection fraction of 40%.

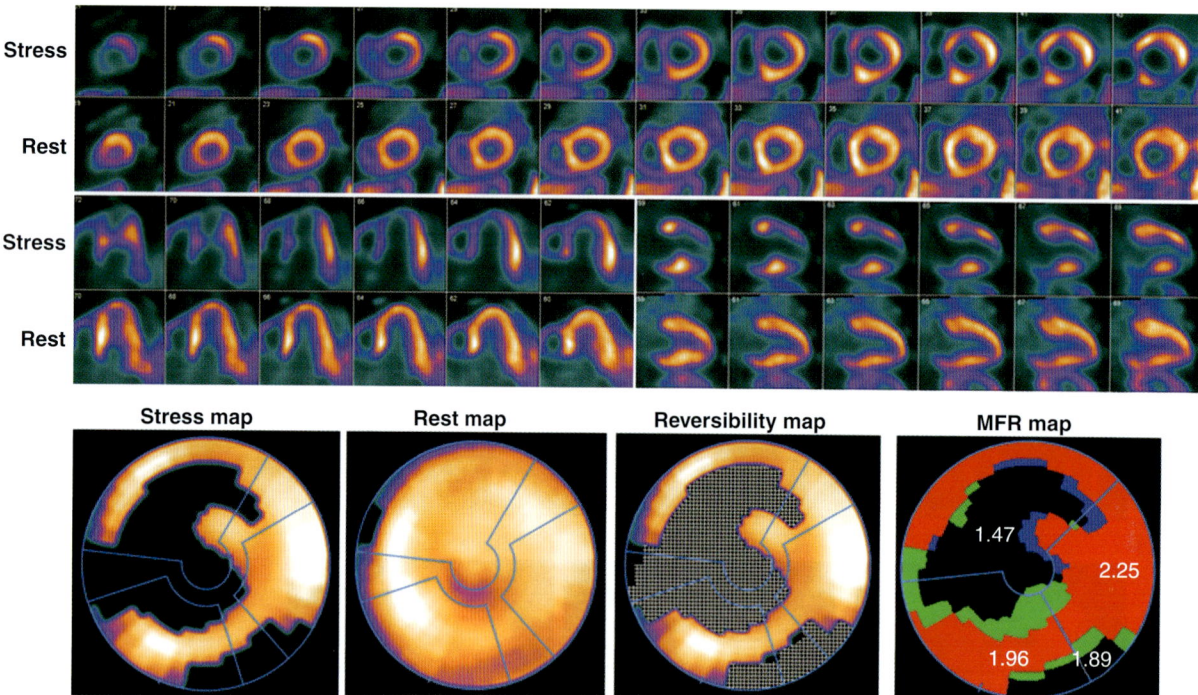

FIGURE 18.23 Quantitative PET in a patient with chronic total coronary occlusion. Vasodilator-stress and rest ^{13}N ammonia PET MPI of a 64-year-old man with known chronic total occlusion (CTO) of the LAD coronary artery who presented with nonanginal chest pain and exertional dyspnea. PET images demonstrate transient left ventricular (LV) dilatation with stress and a large perfusion defect of severe intensity throughout the anteroseptal and anterior walls and LV apex, showing complete reversibility. There is a small but severe perfusion defect involving the basal inferolateral wall, also showing complete reversibility. The ECG-gated images demonstrated a transient increase in the LV end-systolic volume during stress with a decrease in LV ejection fraction from 58% at rest to 51% during stress associated with severe hypokinesis of the anterior and anteroseptal walls, apical LV segments, and LV apex, all consistent with postischemic stunning. The study shows complete viability of the LAD territory with evidence of severe stress-induced ischemia, and a small area of moderate stress-induced ischemia in the inferolateral wall. Myocardial flow reserve is severely reduced in the territory of LAD CTO and relatively preserved in the right coronary artery and left circumflex territories. The patient underwent successful percutaneous coronary intervention of the LAD CTO.

Patients with Chronic Total Coronary Artery Occlusion

Coronary chronic total occlusions (CTOs) are quite common among patients undergoing coronary angiography with a prevalence rate estimated between 18% and 52%. The rapid expansion of dedicated equipment and techniques along with improved operator experience has led to a rapid growth in the number of patients with refractory symptoms despite optimal guideline-directed medical therapy (GDMT) being considered for CTO PCI, in addition to more traditional referral to CABG (see Chapter 41). In experienced centers, CTO PCI may substantially reduce myocardial ischemia and improve quality of life. In such patients, demonstration of significant myocardial ischemia and viability within the territory supplied by a coronary vessel with a CTO is generally accepted as a useful approach to help inform the risk versus benefit of CTO PCI. Radionuclide perfusion imaging is well suited for this task as it is able to provide more detailed quantitative assessments of ischemia than other noninvasive techniques (e.g., stress echocardiography). One additional advantage of PET imaging is its ability to provide quantitative blood flow and flow reserve data, which helps refine the interrogation of physiologic significance in non-CTO vessels and inform the extent of revascularization (Fig. 18.23).

Patients with Cardiac Allograft Vasculopathy. Cardiac allograft transplantation has transformed the lives of patients with advanced heart failure. However, cardiac allograft vasculopathy remains a leading cause of mortality and retransplantation in these individuals (see Chapter 60). Because of myocardial denervation, silent ischemia is common. Annual surveillance with invasive angiography, endomyocardial biopsy, and imaging is routine in these patients. Transplant vasculopathy develops as diffuse disease that may not result in discrete perfusion defects on MPI (Fig. 18.24). Emerging data from multiple centers have provided evidence that cardiac PET-measured myocardial blood flow is a sensitive tool with high diagnostic value to identify cardiac allograft vasculopathy (Fig. 18.25A). Moreover, patients with PET-defined vasculopathy are at significantly higher risk of mortality (see Fig. 18.25B). Indeed, in patients with serial PET assessments, patients with a decline in myocardial blood flow had worse prognosis.

Patients with Coronary Artery Disease Associated with Complex Congenital Heart Disease. Highly successful surgical

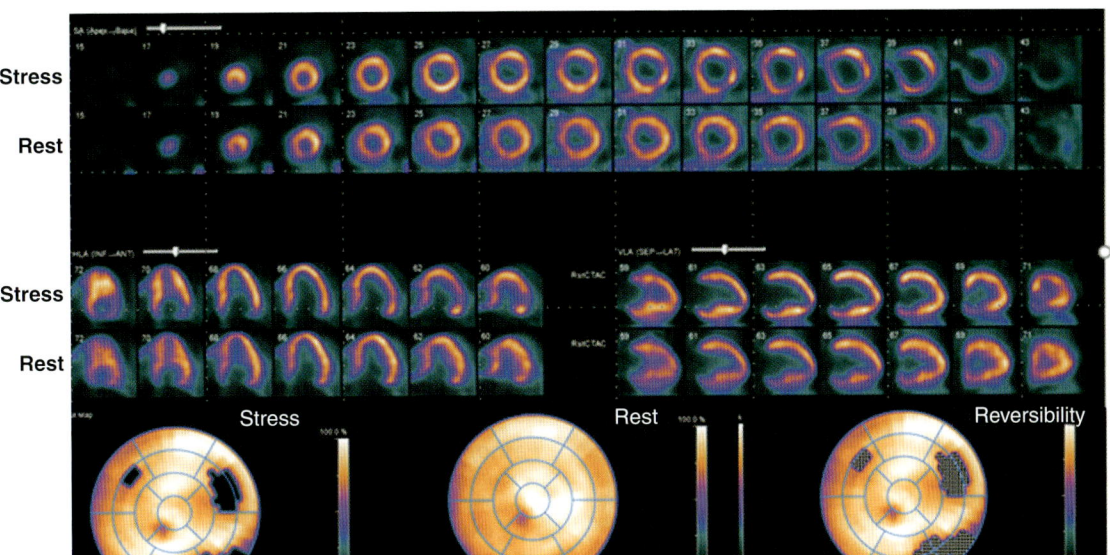

FIGURE 18.24 Quantitative PET imaging in a patient with prior cardiac transplantation. Vasodilator stress and rest ^{13}N-ammonia PET images of a 54-year-old woman with cardiac transplantation 3 years earlier who presented with syncope. Myocardial perfusion images show a dilated left ventricle with a medium-sized region of moderate stress-induced ischemia in the mid to basal inferolateral and anterolateral walls. Her left ventricular ejection fraction (LVEF) was 44%. Myocardial blood flow was elevated at rest (>1.0 mL/min/g) in all three vascular territories (common in patients with cardiac transplant) and her stress myocardial blood flow and flow reserve were reduced in all three coronary territories but worse in the left circumflex distribution. The reduced LVEF and abnormal quantitative blood flow are consistent with severe coronary allograft vasculopathy. She underwent a percutaneous coronary intervention to the left circumflex and right coronary arteries, but unfortunately, died 8 weeks later. Autopsy confirmed severe cardiac allograft vasculopathy (bottom right).

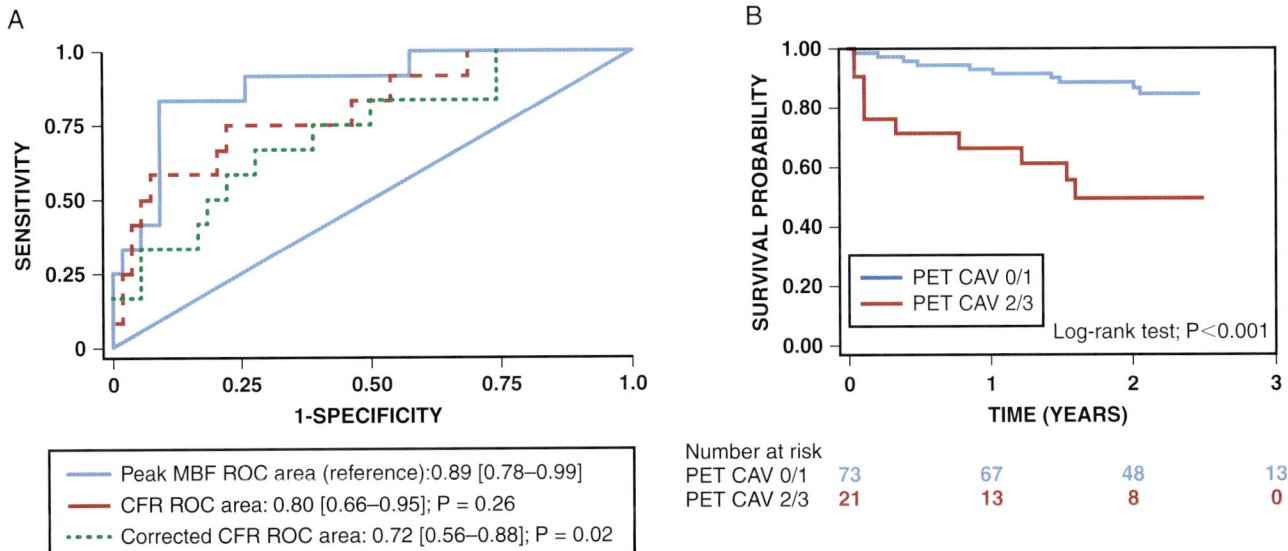

FIGURE 18.25 Diagnostic and prognostic value of quantitative PET after cardiac transplantation. **A,** In a study of 94 patients with prior cardiac transplantation and cardiac PET myocardial perfusion imaging, peak stress myocardial blood flow (MBF) showed the highest accuracy in identifying grade 2 or 3 cardiac allograft vasculopathy (CAV) as defined by the International Society for Heart and Lung Transplantation classification. **B,** In the same study, PET CAV grade 2/3 predicted worse event-free survival. (*PET CAV grade 2/3* is defined as multivessel perfusion defects or single-vessel perfusion defect with peak stress MBF <1.7 mL/min/g, or no perfusion defects but peak stress MBF <1.7 and ejection fraction ≤45%.) (From Bravo PE, et al. Diagnostic and prognostic value of myocardial blood flow quantification as non-invasive indicator of cardiac allograft vasculopathy. Eur Heart J 2018;39:316-323.)

interventions and advances in medical therapy have substantially increased the life expectancy of patients with complex congenital heart disease (see Chapter 82). Atherogenic risk factors increase the risk for ischemic heart disease in adult survivors with complex congenital heart disease. Additionally, these patients are at risk of ischemia due to congenital coronary abnormalities, surgical reimplantation of coronary arteries, mechanical obstruction of coronary arteries caused by compression from abnormal cardiac structures or implanted devices, and atherosclerosis. Finally, device and prosthetic material infections are increasing in this population and ^{18}F-FDG PET/CT may play a role.

Echocardiography is the usual first test for the evaluation of ischemia in these patients. However, stress echocardiography can be challenging to interpret particularly in those with complex congenital heart disease. CMR is also often used to study anatomy, but stress CMR is limited to pharmacologic stress, which is not suitable to provoke ischemia in compressive physiologies. Radionuclide MPI, particularly SPECT with novel scanners or PET, is performed with very low radiation doses. Exercise stress is preferable in these patients and is feasible with SPECT and with ^{13}N-ammonia PET (Fig. 18.26). Pharmacologic PET with flow quantitation can play a role in the evaluation of patients with atherosclerotic coronary artery stenosis including familial hypercholesterolemia and Kawasaki disease. Patients with transposition of great arteries (arterial switch and systemic right ventricle), anomalous left coronary artery from pulmonary artery, Fontan surgery, cyanotic heart disease, and Kawasaki disease have been shown to have significantly reduced peak stress myocardial blood flow and flow reserve. Radionuclide imaging is also playing an increasing role in the evaluation of device and prosthetic material infection in these complex patients.

Interpretation of the images can be challenging as the current software is not optimized for review of MPI in complex anatomies. When evaluating complex congenital heart disease patients with radionuclide imaging it is important to evaluate perfusion to the systemic ventricle. Knowledge of prior surgical repairs and patches improves specificity of interpretation, and hybrid SPECT/CT and PET/CT help in the interpretation. Because of the high burden of lifetime procedures and related radiation dose, protocols should be personalized to minimize radiation dose.[28] Stress-first imaging, novel scanners, two-day protocols, and cardiac PET are some methods used to reduce radiation dose.

Heart Failure and Cardiomyopathies
Patients with Newly Diagnosed Left Ventricular Systolic Dysfunction

An important question in patients presenting with newly diagnosed LV systolic dysfunction is whether significant obstructive CAD is present and likely represents the underlying cause of heart failure. This question can be addressed by invasive coronary angiography or noninvasive imaging including coronary CTA or radionuclide MPI. Both the American and European practice guidelines recommend a diagnostic strategy largely based on symptoms and clinical presentation, patient history, and the likelihood that revascularization may be necessary. There is general agreement that patients with heart failure, severe LV dysfunction, and severe angina should be referred to coronary angiography provided the patient is otherwise suitable for revascularization. However, the initial diagnostic approach for patients without angina or history of MI, or those with prior MI but no angina, is less clear. The latter two categories of patients probably make up the majority of heart failure patients. In patients without angina or a prior history of MI, coronary CTA may be an attractive option, especially in younger patients who are less likely to show coronary calcifications. Another reasonable option includes radionuclide MPI, which may be preferred in older patients with chronic kidney disease. Previous studies have shown that a completely normal radionuclide MPI study is associated with a very high negative predictive value to rule out significant CAD as the likely etiology of heart failure. If available, PET MPI may be preferred as it allows quantification of myocardial blood flow and MFR. The absence of perfusion defects involving a typical coronary artery territory and normal MFR would support a diagnosis of nonischemic cardiomyopathy (Fig. 18.27). In patients without angina but a history of MI, radionuclide MPI helps define the extent of scarred and viable myocardium and the magnitude of residual stress-induced ischemia, which in turn helps inform patient management (Fig. 18.28).

Patients with Ischemic Cardiomyopathy and Heart Failure

LVEF is a well-established and powerful predictor of poor outcome after MI, especially when associated with heart failure. In selected patients, high-risk revascularization appears to afford long-term survival benefit.[29] However, selection of patients with severe LV dysfunction for high-risk revascularization remains controversial. Noninvasive imaging can help determine the presence and severity of myocardial ischemia and viability and, consequently, can help identify patients who may benefit from revascularization.

Pathophysiology of Ischemic Left Ventricular Dysfunction

For many years, chronic LV dysfunction at rest in patients with CAD was thought to represent previous MI and, thus, irreversible damage. However, it is now clear that myocardium that has been subjected to acute or chronic ischemia may remain viable and demonstrate regional and global LV dysfunction that can be improved with revascularization. Such reversible contractile dysfunction may be caused by myocardial stunning or hibernation (see Chapter 36).

Myocardial stunning is a reversible state of regional contractile dysfunction that can occur after restoration of coronary blood flow following a brief episode of ischemia despite the absence of myocardial necrosis. In humans, stunned myocardium can be demonstrated in patients undergoing reperfusion therapy for acute MI, following attacks of unstable angina, and in some patients with exercise-induced ischemia. Although commonly regarded as an acute phenomenon, stunned myocardium may also occur in patients with chronic coronary stenoses who experience recurrent episodes of ischemia (symptomatic or asymptomatic) in the same territory. The latter mechanism is probably the most common form of stunning in patients with chronic LV dysfunction caused by CAD. Myocardial stunning is considered a form of reperfusion injury, in which reintroduction of oxygen after a period of ischemia induces a transient calcium overload that damages the contractile apparatus. The postischemic contractile abnormality is fully reversible provided that recurrent ischemia (followed by stunning) does not occur and sufficient time is allowed for the myocardium to recover.

Myocardial hibernation refers to a state of persistent LV dysfunction associated with chronically reduced blood flow but preserved viability. This chronic downregulation in contractile function at rest is thought to represent a protective mechanism in which the heart reduces its oxygen requirements to ensure myocyte survival. However, this protective mechanism can result in a considerable amount of myocardium that is rendered hypocontractile, thus, it may contribute to overall LV dysfunction.

It is generally accepted that stunning and hibernation represent a continuum of severity that depends on the critical interplay between the severity of angiographic CAD, associated reduction in MFR, and severity of myocardial ischemia. Initially, the presence of a flow-limiting coronary artery stenosis leads to a reduction in coronary vasodilator reserve with preserved resting coronary blood flow. The reduced flow reserve in turn results in episodes of ischemia during periods of increased oxygen demand. Ultimately, these transient, recurrent episodes of ischemia lead to a state of persistent LV dysfunction (so-called repetitive stunning). As the severity of coronary stenosis increases, coronary vasodilator reserve becomes critically reduced and resting coronary blood flow eventually falls. The presence of resting hypoperfusion marks the transition from "repetitive" stunning to hibernation. The varying degree of flow deficit underlying these two conditions likely explains the distinct morphologic changes present in stunned and hibernating myocytes. This precarious balance between perfusion and viability in hibernating myocardium cannot be maintained indefinitely, and myocardial necrosis ultimately occurs if blood flow is not restored.

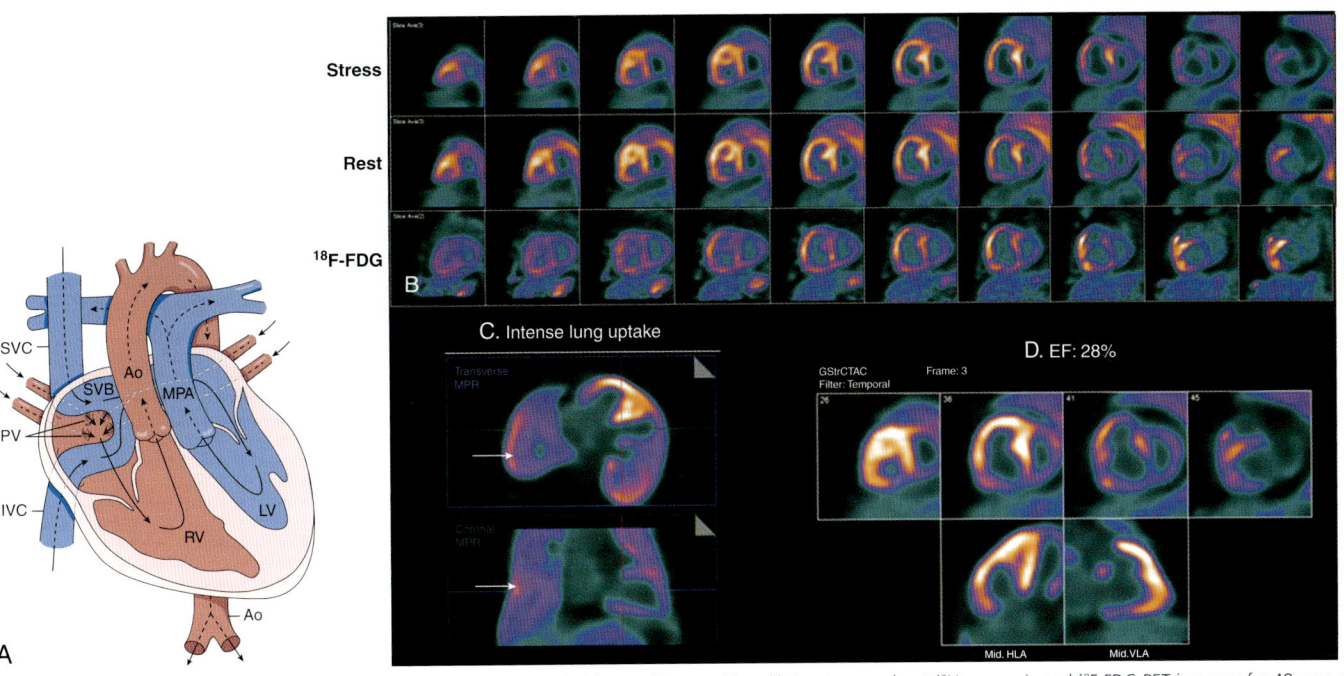

FIGURE 18.26 Cardiac PET scan in an adult patient with congenital heart disease. Vasodilator stress and rest ^{13}N-ammonia and ^{18}F-FDG PET images of a 48-year-old man with D-transposition of great arteries with prior atrial switch operation (Mustard repair) **(A)**, with prior inferior myocardial infarction and residual systemic right ventricular systolic dysfunction, presenting with dyspnea and progressive heart failure. **B,** PET images demonstrate an anteriorly positioned and dilated systemic right ventricle associated with moderately increased lung uptake **(C)** (*arrows*). The subpulmonic left ventricle showed little radiotracer uptake, as expected. There was a medium-sized and severe perfusion defect in the inferior wall of the systemic right ventricle with a partial mismatch on the ^{18}F-FDG images. **D,** The gated images showed global hypokinesis of the systemic right ventricle with akinesis of the inferior segments. These findings were consistent with a small area of viable but hibernating myocardium in the right coronary artery (RCA) territory. He underwent a repeat coronary angiography, which demonstrated a patent RCA. *PV,* pulmonary veins; *Ao,* aorta; *MPA,* main pulmonary artery; *SVC,* superior venacava; *IVC,* inferior vena cava; *RV,* right ventricle; *LV,* left ventricle; *SVB,* systemic venous baffle.

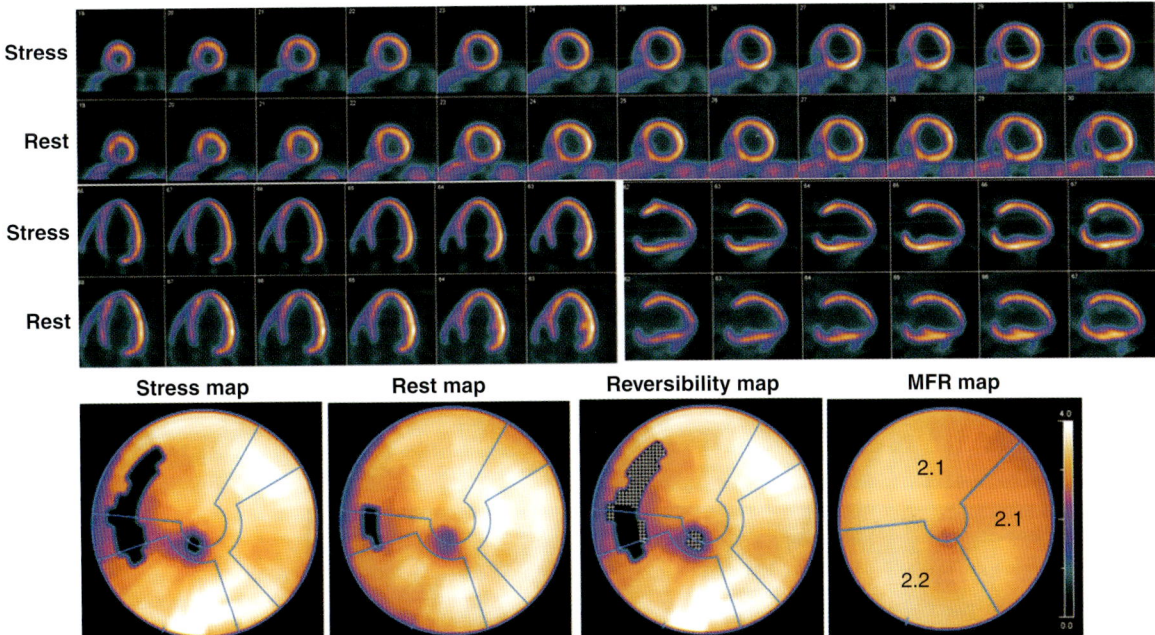

FIGURE 18.27 Myocardial perfusion imaging in a patient with cardiomyopathy. Vasodilator stress and rest ^{13}N-ammonia PET images of a 74-year-old woman with hypertension, diabetes, and chronic kidney dysfunction who presented with new-onset exertional dyspnea. The ECG showed left bundle branch block (LBBB). PET MPI shows a severely dilated left ventricle and a small septal perfusion defect showing apparent reversibility, likely secondary to LBBB. The ECG-gated images demonstrated an ejection fraction of 15% that rose to 20% during peak stress, and evidence of septal dyssynchrony. Myocardial flow reserve was preserved in all coronary territories. These findings are consistent with a nonischemic cardiomyopathy, which was subsequently confirmed on coronary angiography *LBBB,* left bundle branch block.

Radionuclide Imaging Approaches to Assess Myocardial Ischemia and Viability

The evaluation of patients with severe LV dysfunction and angiographic CAD often requires the combination of stress testing to quantify the extent of myocardium at risk and metabolic imaging to distinguish viable from nonviable myocardium (Fig. 18.29).

SPECT MPI can be used to assess the extent and severity of myocardial ischemia using exercise or pharmacologic stress in combination with ^{99m}Tc-labeled radiotracers or ^{201}thallium, as described earlier in this chapter. For viability assessment, attenuation-corrected SPECT MPI is preferable. One advantage of ^{201}thallium is that it provides a more accurate assessment of viable myocardium, especially in the setting

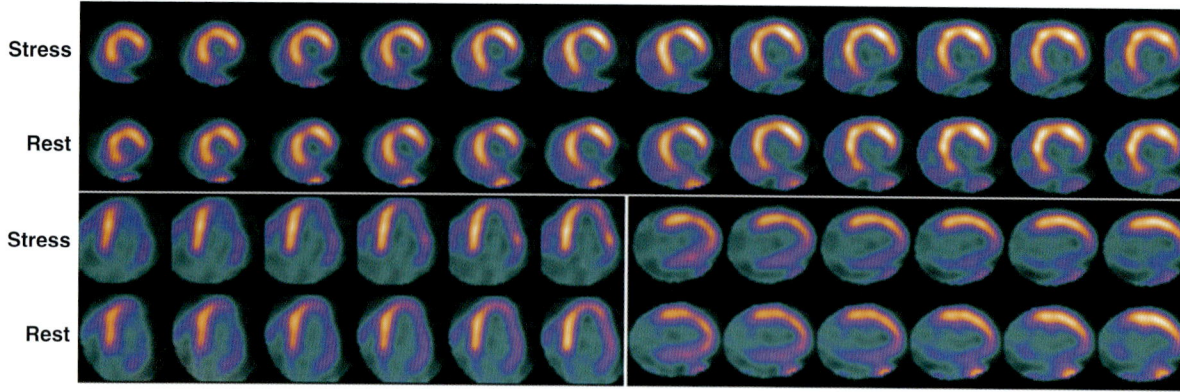

Quantitative myocardial blood flow and MFR

Coronary territory	Rest (mL/min/g)	Stress (mL/min/g)	MFR
LAD	0.83	0.89	1.07
LCX	0.86	1.01	1.17
RCA	0.64	0.66	1.03

FIGURE 18.28 Quantitative myocardial perfusion imaging in a patient with ischemic cardiomyopathy. Vasodilator-stress and rest ^{13}N-ammonia PET images of a patient with prior myocardial infarction (MI) who presented with worsening heart failure. His left ventricular ejection fraction was estimated at 30%. Myocardial perfusion images MPI demonstrate a large and severe perfusion defect throughout the inferior and inferolateral walls, which was irreversible and consistent with prior MI. However, the quantitative myocardial blood flow and flow reserve (MFR) data show blunted augmentation of flow during stress, resulting in a severe reduction in MFR in all three vascular territories. Coronary angiography demonstrated severe multivessel obstructive coronary artery disease. *LAD*, left anterior descending artery; *LCX*, left circumflex artery; *RCA*, right coronary artery.

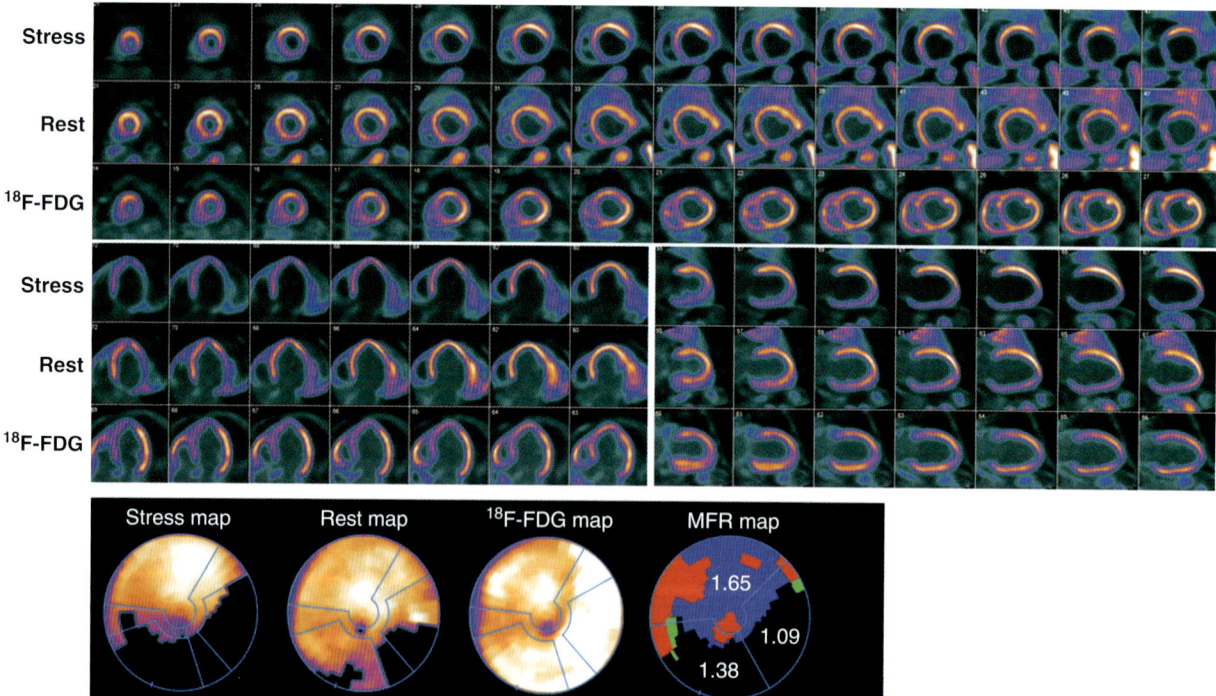

FIGURE 18.29 Assessment of myocardial ischemia and viability in a patient with ischemic cardiomyopathy. Vasodilator stress and rest ^{13}N-ammonia and ^{18}F-FDG PET images of a 70-year-old man with progressive dyspnea, hypotension, and new severe biventricular systolic dysfunction with elevated natriuretic peptides. Coronary angiography demonstrated multivessel coronary artery disease with left circumflex (LCX) chronic total occlusion (filled by left-to-left collaterals), serial severe right coronary artery (RCA) lesions (80% to 90%), and moderate left anterior descending (LAD) stenosis (40% to 50%) in the proximal mid segments. PET images demonstrate severe left ventricular (LV) dilatation and mild right ventricular (RV) dilatation with increased RV uptake of ^{18}F-FDG, consistent with pulmonary hypertension. Stress perfusion images show a large and severe perfusion defect throughout the inferoseptal, inferior, and inferolateral walls, with moderate reversibility. The ^{18}F-FDG images demonstrate normal glucose uptake in all hypoperfused LV segments (perfusion-^{18}F metabolism mismatch). Quantitative PET confirmed severely reduced flow reserve (MFR) in the LCX and RCA territories, consistent with the severe stress perfusion defects. In addition, MFR was also moderately reduced in the LAD territory. The ECG-gated images demonstrated a rest LV ejection fraction (LVEF) of 14% and end-systolic volume index (ESVI) of 158 mL/m^2. Poststress LVEF was 17% with ESVI 155 mL/m^2. The findings are consistent with extensive areas of mixed stress-induced ischemia and hibernating myocardium throughout the LCX and RCA territories, and a flow-limiting stenosis in the LAD territory. The patient underwent successful three-vessel coronary artery bypass graft surgery.

of severe resting hypoperfusion. A common approach to improve detection of hibernating myocardium is the use of nitrates to improve collateral flow at rest and enhance radiotracer uptake in areas of severe hypoperfusion.

PET imaging provides a more comprehensive approach for the evaluation of patients with ischemic cardiomyopathy and its use for this application is growing worldwide. As was discussed earlier, the advantages of PET include its more accurate quantitative assessment of ischemia and the use of ^{18}F-FDG to assess myocardial metabolism and myocardial viability. The use of metabolic ^{18}F-FDG imaging for viability assessment requires careful patient preparation before imaging. For a detailed step-by-step description of the available methods for patient preparation before ^{18}F-FDG imaging, the reader should review the Guidelines for PET Imaging published by the ASNC.[2]

Myocardial Viability Imaging to Guide Revascularization in Patients with Ischemic Heart Failure

Several studies using different PET approaches have shown that the gain in global LVEF after revascularization is related to the magnitude of ischemic and/or viable myocardium assessed preoperatively. These data demonstrate that clinically meaningful changes in global LV function can be expected after revascularization only in patients with relatively large areas of hibernating and/or stunned myocardium (~20% of the LV mass). Similar to other noninvasive imaging modalities, the extent of nonviable or scarred myocardium by ^{18}F-FDG PET correlates inversely with changes in LVEF after revascularization.

Consistent data from single-center, observational studies demonstrate that the presence of ischemic, viable myocardium among patients with severe LV dysfunction identifies patients at higher clinical risk, and that prompt revascularization in selected patients is associated with improved LV function, symptoms, and survival compared with medical therapy alone. The PARR-2 clinical trial, in which patients were randomized to PET-guided management versus standard clinical care, however, did not demonstrate an overall benefit of PET; it did show in a post hoc analysis that image-guided decisions regarding revascularization were associated with improved clinical outcomes following revascularization if treatment decisions adhere to imaging recommendations[30] (Fig. 18.30).

Nonetheless, the main criticism of those older studies is that they were retrospective and medical therapy did not reflect current accepted management of heart failure nor was it standardized in any way. The results of the Surgical Treatment of Ischemic Heart Failure (STICH) trial, especially its ancillary viability substudy, have challenged all prior data as they failed to demonstrate a significant interaction between ischemia or viability information, revascularization, and improved survival compared with optimal medical therapy[29] (Fig. 18.31). This casts significant uncertainty whether noninvasive characterization of ischemia, viability, and scar can actually provide useful information to guide management decisions. This issue is currently undergoing intense debate in the medical community. As we begin to incorporate the results of the STICH trial into clinical practice, it is important to consider the strengths and weaknesses of the STICH substudies.

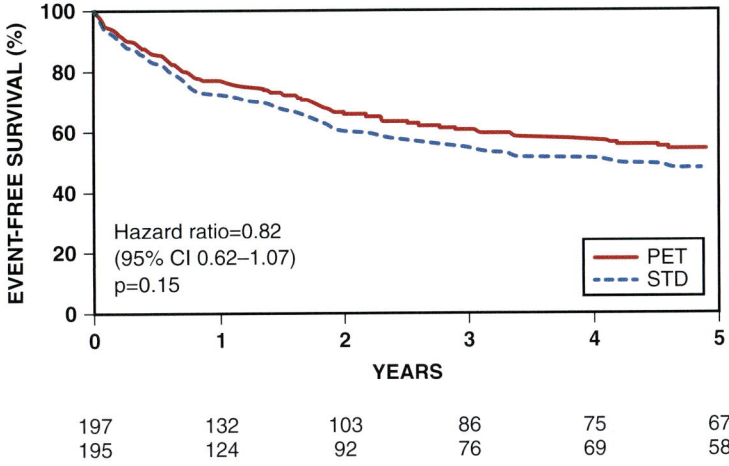
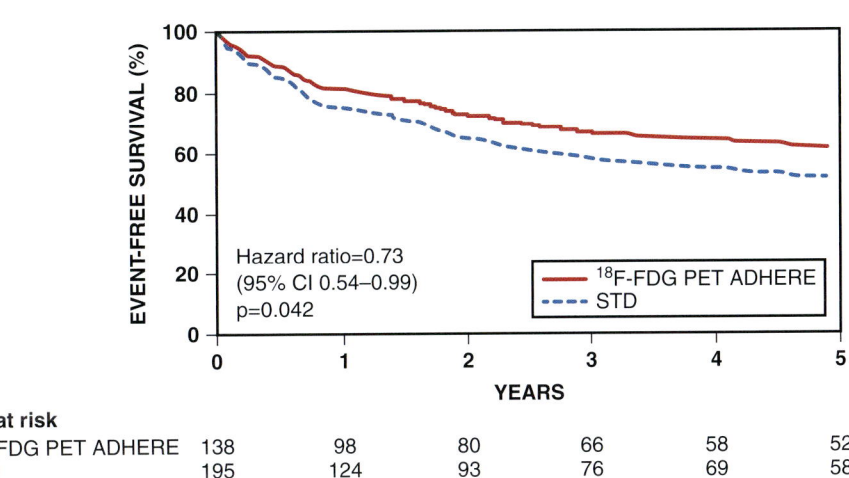

FIGURE 18.30 PET-guided revascularization in ischemic cardiomyopathy. *Top,* Event-free survival in patients randomized to a PET-guided approach versus standard care (STD) in the PARR-2 study. There was no difference in survival between the standard arm and the PET-guided arm. *Bottom,* In post hoc analysis, PET-guided management showed improved survival compared with standard care among patients in whom management decisions adhered to the PET recommendation (i.e., revascularization for hibernating myocardium; medical therapy alone for scar). (From McArdle B, et al. Long-term follow-up of outcomes with F-18-fluorodeoxyglucose positron emission tomography imaging-assisted management of patients with severe left ventricular dysfunction secondary to coronary disease. Circ Cardiovasc Imaging 2016;9:e004331.)

The STICH viability[31] and ischemia substudies are the largest reports to date relating myocardial viability and ischemia to clinical outcomes of patients with CAD and LV dysfunction associated with heart failure. They are also the first to assess these relationships prospectively among patients who were all eligible for CABG as well as optimal medical management alone. As mentioned previously, medical therapy in the STICH trial was standardized and followed published guidelines that were current during the course of the trial (angiotensin converting enzyme inhibitors or angiotensin receptor blockers, beta blockers, statins, and aspirin). However, these studies also have important limitations. First, viability data were only available in half of the STICH population, which is likely to introduce some selection bias. In fact, patients in the STICH viability study had higher prevalence of prior MI, lower frequency of limiting angina symptoms, lower LVEF, and more advanced LV remodeling compared with those who did not receive viability imaging before randomization. Second, the definition of viability in the STICH substudy was quite broad resulting in 81% of the total study population considered as having "viability" by study criteria. This number is a great deal higher than that seen in other studies using similar methodologies for viability assessment. Third, neither PET nor CMR was used to evaluate ischemia or viability. On the other hand, medical therapy did not include newer agents that might further improve outcome of medically treated patients, such as sacubitril-valsartan and sodium-glucose cotransporter-2 inhibitors (see Chapter 50). An important additional consideration to

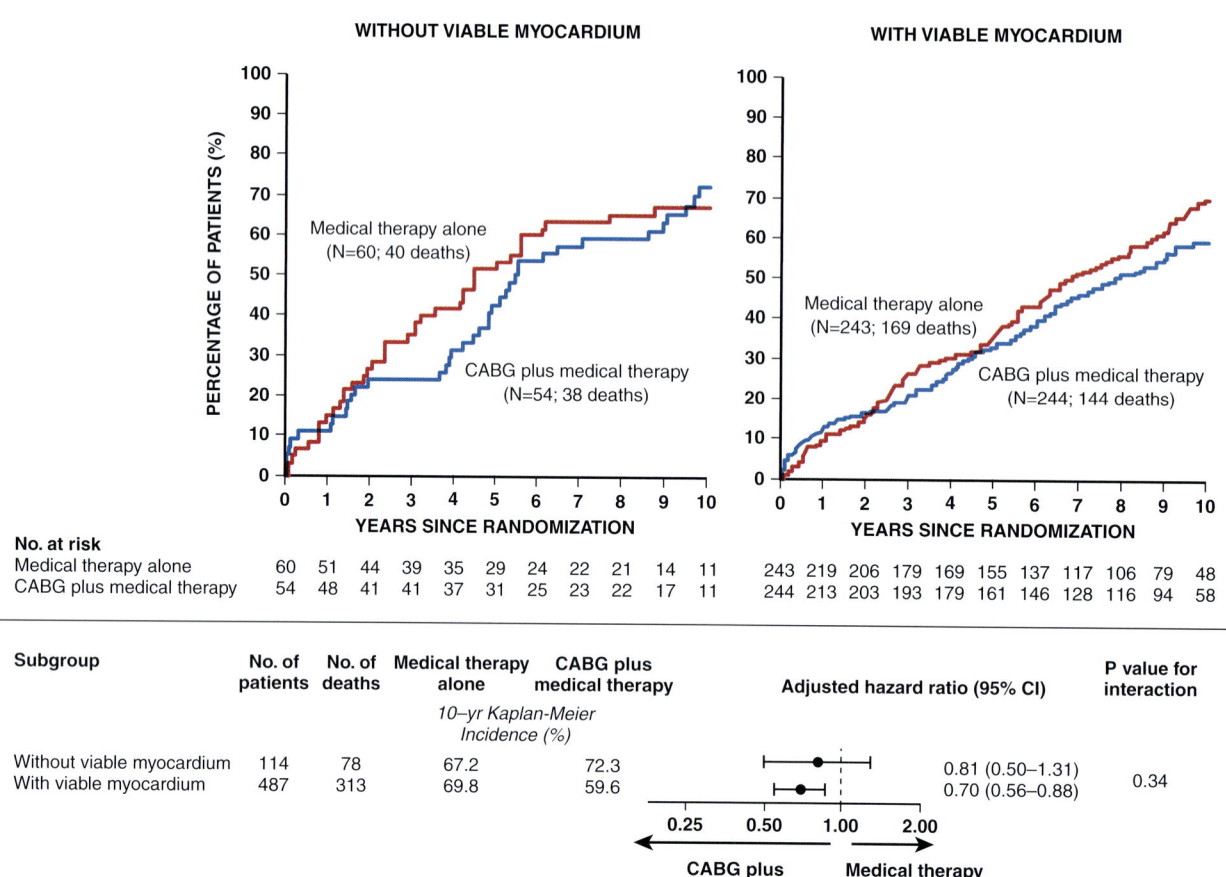

FIGURE 18.31 Role of viability imaging in the STICH study. Survival probability in patients without (*left*) and with (*right*) myocardial viability by treatment assignment in the long-term follow-up of the STICH patients included in the viability substudy. *Bottom*, Results of a Cox proportional-hazards model that tested for the interaction between myocardial viability and treatment with adjustment for baseline covariates, which was not significant. *CABG*, Coronary artery bypass graft surgery. (From Panza JA, et al. Myocardial viability and long-term outcomes in ischemic cardiomyopathy. N Engl J Med 2019;381:739-748.)

understand the generalizability of the STICH substudies is that patients in the main trial in general, and those in the viability and ischemia studies in particular, had end-stage LV remodeling. Indeed, the mean LV end-diastolic volume index was >120 mL/m², and LV end-systolic volume index approached 100 mL/m². This degree of advanced LV remodeling has generally been associated with poor outcomes regardless of the presence of ischemia or viability and treatment applied. In summary, the STICH trial and its imaging substudies suggest that among patients with *heart failure* and *end-stage LV remodeling*, identification of moderate ischemia or viability is not associated with a significant survival advantage from revascularization. Although the benefits of optimal medical therapy in patients with ischemic cardiomyopathy are undeniable, we cannot and should not generalize the STICH findings to all patients with heart failure and severe systolic dysfunction, especially those with a lesser degree of LV remodeling, as these patients were not studied in the STICH trial. As data from randomized clinical trials in such patients are limited, careful integration of clinical, anatomic, and functional information regarding ischemia and viability from noninvasive imaging is necessary to individualize difficult management decisions based on the best available evidence and sound clinical judgment.

Neuronal Imaging to Identify Patients at Risk for Sudden Cardiac Death.

There is experimental and clinical evidence supporting the concept that sympathetic activation plays an important role as a potential trigger of ventricular arrhythmias after MI. Indeed, MI and ischemia can lead to sympathetic denervation in both the infarct and peri-infarct zone. Viable but denervated myocardial regions show supersensitive shortening of effective refractory period in response to the infusion of norepinephrine and are more vulnerable to ventricular arrhythmias. This suggests that direct imaging of cardiac sympathetic innervation may have an important clinical role in risk stratification of patients after MI.

For radionuclide imaging, tracer analogues to the sympathetic neurotransmitter norepinephrine (NE), the parasympathetic mediator acetylcholine (ACh), and postsynaptic adrenergic receptors have been used to visualize and quantify autonomic innervation and receptor density and function. Most of the clinical evidence regarding the potential applications of neuronal imaging in heart failure has been obtained with NE analogue ^{123}I-meta-iodobenzylguanidine (MIBG), currently the only FDA-approved imaging tracer for this application. PET radiotracers have also been used including ^{11}C-meta-hydroxyephedrine (^{11}C-HED).

AdreView Myocardial Imaging for Risk Evaluation in Heart Failure (ADMIRE-HF), the largest study to date, included 961 patients with class II–III heart failure and LVEF ≤ 35% who were initially followed over a median of 17 months for the occurrence of worsening HF class, cardiac death, and life-threatening ventricular arrhythmias defined as a spontaneous sustained (>30 seconds) ventricular tachyarrhythmia, a resuscitated cardiac arrest, or an appropriate ICD discharge (anti-tachycardic pacing or defibrillation).[32] The principal finding of this study was that patients with a quantitative heart to mediastinum ratio (HMR) of ^{123}I-MIBG <1.6 had a higher rate of adverse events than those with HMR ≥ 1.6 (37% vs. 15%) (Figs. 18.32 and 18.33).[32] Importantly, patients with an HMR ≥ 1.6 had a mortality rate below 1%.

The Prediction of ARrhythmic Events with Positron Emission Tomography (PAREPET) study tested the hypothesis that the extent of inhomogeneity in myocardial sympathetic innervation and/or hibernating myocardium increased the risk of arrhythmic death independent of LV function in patients with ischemic cardiomyopathy (LVEF ≤ 35%).[33] The study included 204 patients who were eligible for primary prevention ICDs. Myocardial sympathetic denervation was quantified with ^{11}C-HED and PET imaging. The primary endpoint was SCA defined as arrhythmic death or ICD discharge for ventricular fibrillation or ventricular tachycardia > 240 beats/min. Compared with patients in the lowest tertile of cardiac sympathetic denervation assessed by HED PET, those in the highest tertile showed a greater than six-fold increase in the risk of SCA.[33] In multivariable analysis, the extent of PET-defined sympathetic denervation, LV end-diastolic volume index, and creatinine were significantly associated with the risk of SCA.[33]

In summary, the available evidence suggests that cardiac neuronal imaging with NE analogues including ^{123}I-MIBG and ^{11}C-HED are clinically useful tools for risk stratification of patients with heart failure.

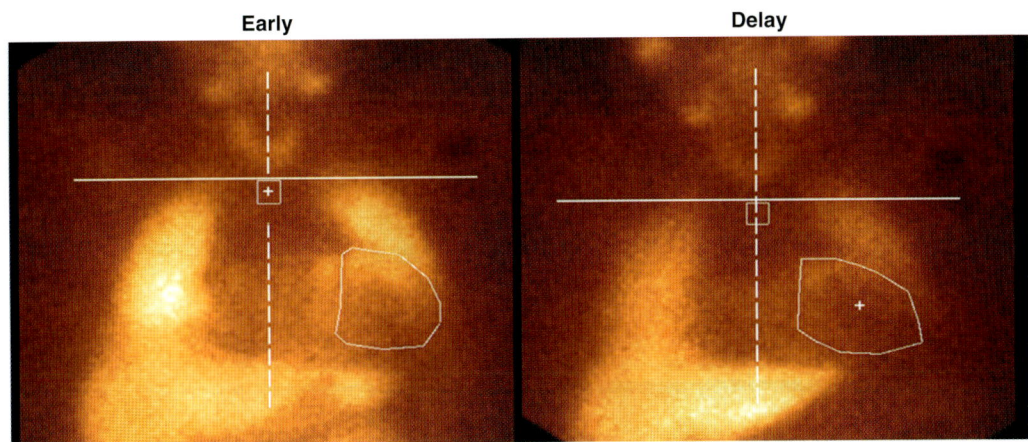

FIGURE 18.32 Assessment of heart to mediastinum ratio (HMR) with ^{123}I-MIBG. These planar chest images illustrate the calculation of HMR with MIBG imaging. Regions of interest are drawn over the heart and upper mediastinum on the early (15-minute) and delayed (4-hour) images, and corresponding mean counts used to calculate the HMR. (Images courtesy Dr. Mark Travin, Montefiore Medical Center, Bronx, NY.)

	Early			Late		
	Counts	Pixels	Mean	Counts	Pixels	Mean
Heart	188855	601	314.2	100370	548	183.2
Mediastinum	10715	49	218.7	7630	49	155.7
HMR			1.44			1.18

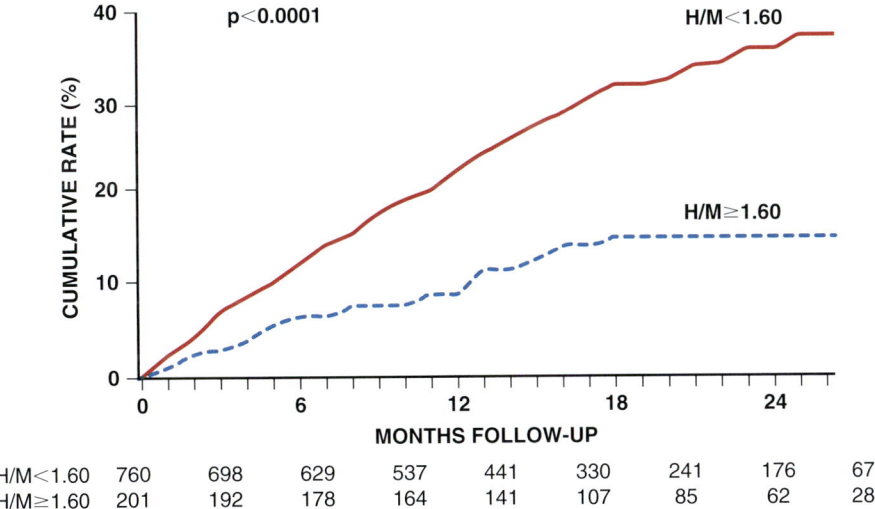

| n: H/M<1.60 | 760 | 698 | 629 | 537 | 441 | 330 | 241 | 176 | 67 |
| n: H/M≥1.60 | 201 | 192 | 178 | 164 | 141 | 107 | 85 | 62 | 28 |

FIGURE 18.33 Prognostic value of ^{123}I-MIBG in heart failure. In the ADMIRE-HF study, 961 subjects with heart failure (New York Heart Association [NYHA] class II/III) and left ventricular ejection fraction (LVEF) of ≤35% underwent ^{123}I-MIBG imaging. The cumulative rate of events (time to first NYHA class progression, potentially life-threatening arrhythmia, or cardiac death) was significantly higher in patients with a heart to mediastinum ratio (H/M) <1.6 than in those with H/M ≥1.6. (From Jacobson AF, et al. Myocardial iodine-123-meta-iodobenzylguanidine imaging and cardiac events in heart failure. Results of the prospective ADMIRE-HF (AdreView Myocardial Imaging for Risk Evaluation in Heart Failure) study. J Am Coll Cardiol 2010;55:2212-2221.)

However, it is still uncertain if such evidence is sufficient to guide selection of heart failure patients for primary prevention ICD implantation beyond LVEF and conventional clinical risk stratification parameters as recommended by practice guidelines.

Infiltrative Cardiomyopathy: Amyloidosis

Cardiac amyloidosis is a protein misfolding disorder in which misfolded proteins deposit in various organs as fibrils causing a diffuse infiltrative cardiomyopathy (see Chapter 53). The two common forms of amyloidosis that affect the heart are immunoglobulin light chain amyloidosis (AL amyloidosis, a plasma cell dyscrasia) and transthyretin amyloidosis (wild-type ATTR or hereditary ATTR).[34] Both AL and ATTR-CA present as heart failure with preserved EF (HFpEF), and a multitude of clinical symptoms that cannot distinguish AL from ATTR-CA. AL amyloidosis is treated with chemotherapy. Wild-type TTR-CA is treated by TTR stabilization (tafamidis) and for hereditary TTR neuropathy is treated by silencing TTR gene products (patisiran and inotersen). Hence once a diagnosis of ATTR-CA is confirmed, genetic testing is indicated to exclude TTR gene mutation.

The diagnosis of cardiac amyloidosis is often delayed because of its perceived rarity and multifaceted clinical presentation (Fig. 18.34; see Fig. 72.13). An evaluation for cardiac amyloidosis includes clinical history and examination, cardiac biomarkers, evaluation for light chain amyloidosis, cardiac imaging, endomyocardial or organ biopsy, and genetic testing in patients with ATTR-CA.[34] Echocardiography and CMR (see Fig. 19.13) are important first tests that raise the suspicion of cardiac amyloidosis (see Chapters 16 and 19). Radionuclide scintigraphy (SPECT bone-avid radiotracers or amyloid PET radiotracers)[34] is emerging as a key diagnostic study for ATTR-CA.

Although myocardial uptake of bone-avid radiotracers in cardiac amyloidosis has been recognized for almost 40 years, it is now established that such increased uptake is more consistently seen in ATTR-CA. Multiple studies have established the high accuracy of bone scintigraphy to diagnose ATTR-CA. About 20% to 25% of patients with AL cardiac amyloidosis also manifest significant myocardial uptake of bone-avid radiotracers. Exclusion of AL amyloidosis using serum free light chain assay, serum, and urine immunofixation electrophoresis is thus critical to maintain the high specificity of ^{99m}Tc-PYP/DPD/HMDP scan for ATTR-CA and to ensure timely consideration of chemotherapy if AL amyloidosis is diagnosed. A multicenter study of 1498 patients revealed that a grade 2 or 3 positive ^{99m}Tc-PYP/DPD/HMDP scan can identify cardiac ATTR amyloidosis with nearly 100% specificity and 71% sensitivity, if AL amyloidosis is excluded, avoiding an endomyocardial biopsy.[35] Furthermore, there is growing evidence that nearly 13% to 18% of older adults with HFpEF, and nearly 25% to 30% of those with severe aortic stenosis have underlying ATTR-CA by bone-avid tracer cardiac scintigraphy (see Chapters 51 and 72). These findings are particularly important now as ATTR-CA is a treatable cause of HFpEF.

A multisocietal expert consensus document recommends multimodality imaging in cardiac amyloidosis, including the key role of bone scintigraphy for identification of ATTR amyloidosis.[36] As per these recommendations, cardiac AL amyloidosis can be diagnosed by biopsy or clinical measures (Table 18.5) and cardiac ATTR amyloidosis can be diagnosed by biopsy or by imaging. Indications for ^{99m}Tc-PYP/DPD/HMDP imaging include Black patients age >60 with HFpEF or LV thickening; non-Black patients age >60 with HFpEF and LV thickening;

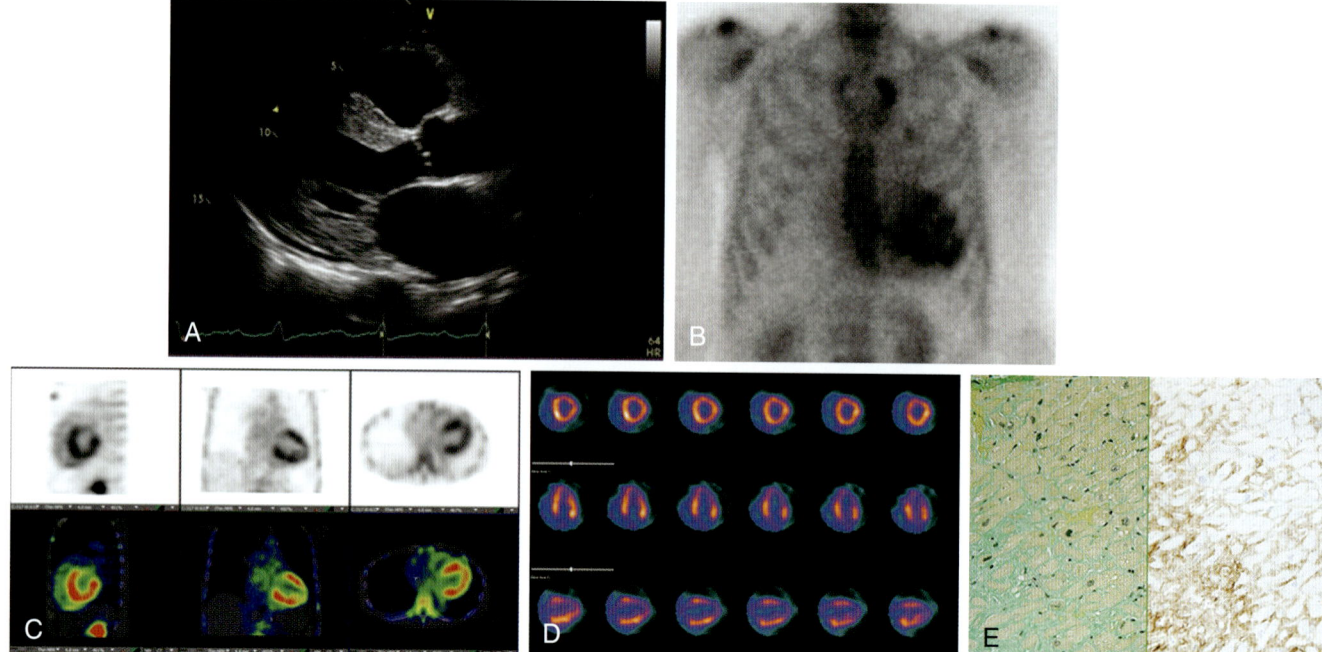

FIGURE 18.34 Role of bone scintigraphy in the diagnosis of cardiac amyloidosis. **A,** Echocardiogram in a 78-year-old man with heart failure and recently diagnosed cardiac amyloidosis showed severe concentric left ventricular (LV) thickening (18 mm) and moderately reduced LV ejection fraction (35%). **B,** The ^{99m}Tc-PYP SPECT/CT scan showed intense myocardial PYP uptake (grade 3) on the planar and **(C and D)** SPECT/CT images. **E,** Endomyocardial biopsy with sulfated Alcian blue staining and immunohistochemistry-confirmed transthyretin (TTR) cardiac amyloidosis. Serum free light chain assay and serum and urine immunofixation were normal and excluded light chain amyloidosis. A genetic test excluded TTR mutations and confirmed wild-type A TTR amyloidosis.

TABLE 18.5 Diagnostic Criteria for Cardiac Amyloidosis

Endomyocardial biopsy: documenting amyloid deposits with Congo red positivity and immunohistochemistry or mass spectrometry typing of fibril

Extracardiac biopsy: documenting amyloid deposits with Congo red positivity and immunohistochemistry or mass spectrometry typing of fibril AND

Cardiac AL or ATTR amyloidosis can be diagnosed by typical imaging features* (echo wall thickness >12 mm, late gadolinium enhancement, or expanded extracellular volume >0.40) OR Cardiac AL amyloidosis can be diagnosed by elevated cardiac biomarkers* (age-adjusted NT proBNP or troponin T)

Clinical diagnosis: cardiac ATTR amyloidosis can be diagnosed by endomyocardial biopsy or a strongly positive bone-avid cardiac scintigraphy (PYP/DPD/HMDP) in patients with typical imaging features* and without a plasma cell dyscrasia (normal serum free light chain assay as well as serum and urine immunofixation electrophoresis).

*When all other causes of imaging features or cardiac biomarker release are excluded. From Dorbala S, et al. ASNC/AHA/ASE/EANM/HFSA/ISA/SCMR/SNMMI expert consensus recommendations for multimodality imaging in cardiac amyloidosis: Part 2 of 2-Diagnostic criteria and appropriate utilization. J Nucl Cardiol 2019;26:2065-2123.

heart failure with unexplained peripheral sensory neuropathy; known or suspected hereditary ATTR-CA; and follow-up of progressive symptoms in known AL amyloidosis or ATTR-CA. Once a diagnosis of ATTR-CA is made, the next step is to evaluate for TTR gene mutations as that may identify need for different therapies, a different prognosis, and implications for family members.[34]

The typical imaging protocol for ^{99m}Tc bone scintigraphy includes the use of SPECT imaging (preferably SPECT/CT if available) 2 to 3 hours after the IV administration of the bone-avid radiotracer. Planar imaging with measurement of heart to contralateral lung ratio has been used and it can be helpful when negative. However, when positive planar imaging is limited it is difficult to distinguish blood pool from myocardial retention. ^{99m}Tc-PYP/DPD/HMDP images are typically interpreted visually comparing radiotracer uptake in myocardium in relation to that in the ribs using the following grading system: grade 0 = absent myocardial uptake, grade 1 = rib uptake, grade 2 = rib uptake, and grade 3 = rib uptake (Fig. 18.35). Quantitative imaging of bone-avid scintigraphy with SPECT/CT is emerging as a novel technique,[37] which may allow detection of early disease, assessment of response to therapy, and determination of prognosis. Bone-avid scintigraphy can detect early amyloid deposition in the heart before increase in myocardial wall thickening,[34] but emerging data indicate that bone scintigraphy may be negative in certain hereditary forms of cardiac amyloidosis. Consequently, if hereditary ATTR-CA is suspected and the bone scintigram is negative, further evaluation including endomyocardial biopsy should be considered. Also, ^{99m}Tc-MDP, a common bone scanning tracer in the United States, has low sensitivity and is not recommended for evaluation of ATTR-CA.[34] The presence of ATTR-CA by bone scintigraphy has been associated with worse outcome.[38]

Amyloid imaging using targeted PET radiotracers approved for diagnosis of Alzheimer disease is emerging as a novel method to accurately diagnose cardiac AL and ATTR amyloidosis.[39] Amyloid-targeted PET tracers are quantitative and provide a measure of whole-heart and whole-body amyloid load and can be repeated, making it a potentially promising tool to evaluate response to therapy. Notably, these tracers are the only clinically available tracers to image AL cardiac amyloidosis. ^{123}I-serum amyloid P-component SPECT is used in the United Kingdom for systemic AL amyloidosis imaging, but it does not image cardiac AL amyloidosis and is not available in the United States. Limited whole-body images (^{18}F-florbetapir,[40] and other tracers) have identified AL amyloid deposits in various organs before clinical suspicion of organ involvement. Importantly, recent data indicate that early cardiac AL amyloid deposits can be identified using ^{18}F-florbetapir[41] and ^{11}C-Pittsburgh-B-Compound imaging[39] before clinically evident changes in cardiac structure (increased LV thickness) or cardiac biomarker release.

Inflammatory Cardiomyopathy: Sarcoidosis

Sarcoidosis is a granulomatous disorder of unknown etiology that effects multiple organs and cardiac involvement is present in approximately 20% to 25% of patients (see Chapter 52).[7] Women and Black patients are specially predisposed to sarcoidosis.[7] Sarcoidosis is characterized by focal noncaseating granulomas with multinucleated giant cells and macrophages formed as a result T cell-mediated immune response to an unknown trigger. The granulomas may remain

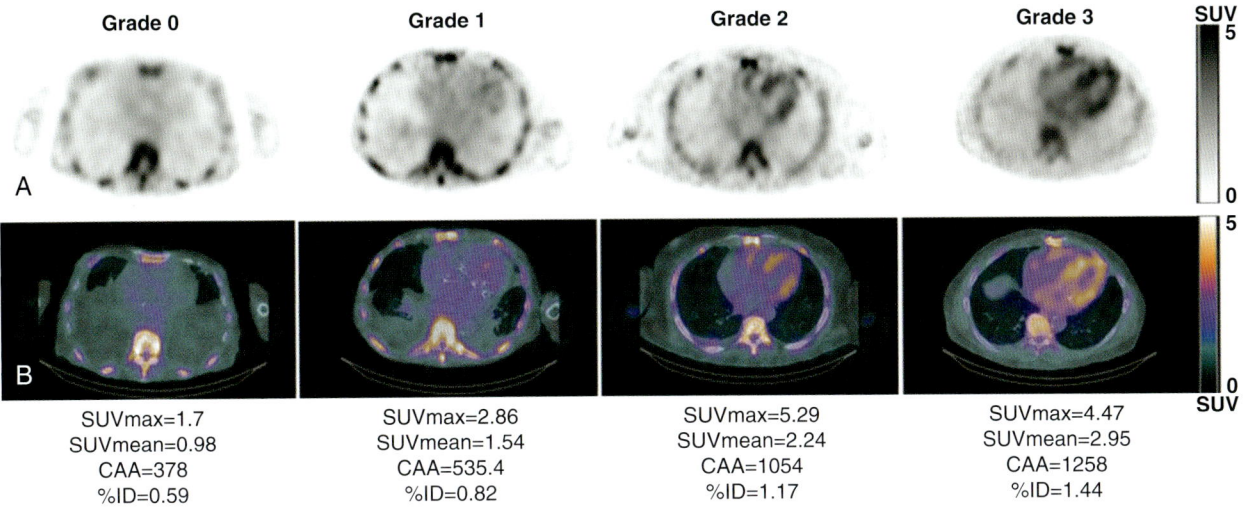

FIGURE 18.35 Quantification of 99mTc-PYP uptake. Selected cross-sectional 99mTc-PYP SPECT **(A)** and fused SPECT/CT **(B)** images of the chest illustrating visual grades of PYP uptake and their corresponding absolute quantitative metrics including standardized uptake value (*SUV*), cardiac amyloid activity (*CAA*), and percentage injected dose (*%ID*). (From Dorbala S, et al. Absolute quantitation of cardiac (99m)Tc-pyrophosphate using cadmium zinc telluride-based SPECT/CT. J Nucl Med 2020;62:716-722.)

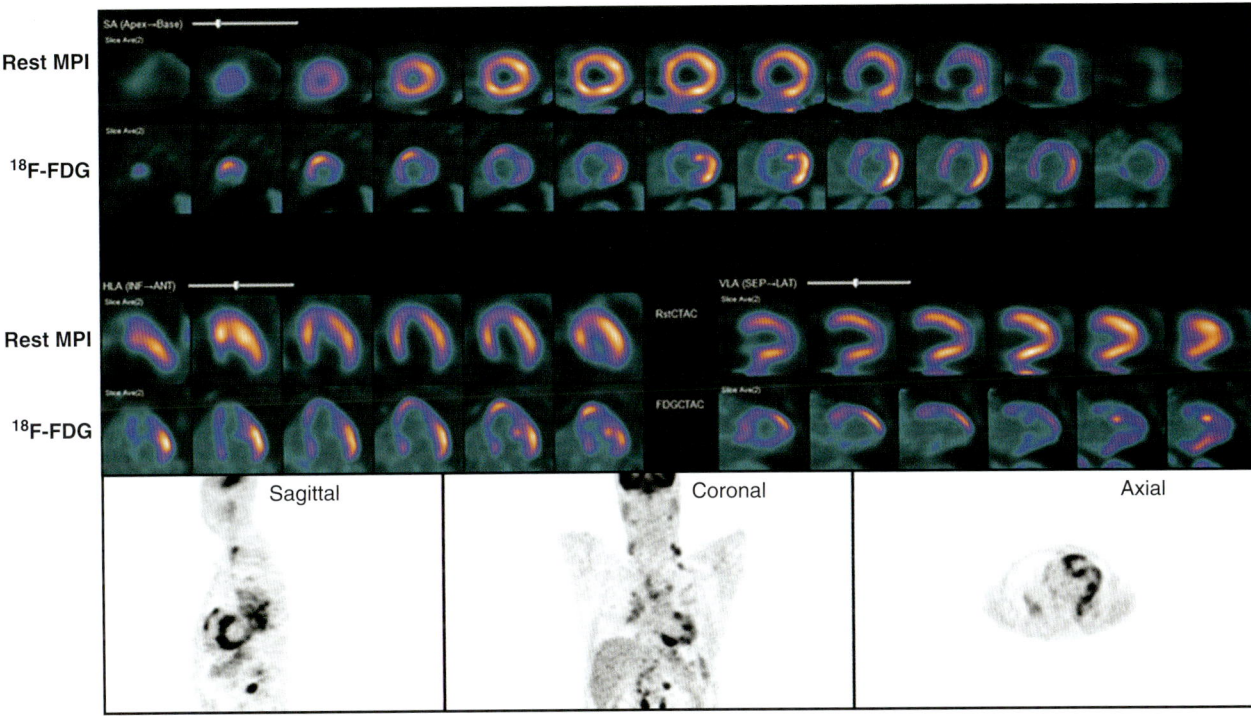

FIGURE 18.36 **18F-FDG PET/CT in a patient with suspected cardiac sarcoidosis.** Rest 99mTc-sestamibi SPECT/CT and 18F-FDG PET/CT scan of a 43-year-old man with progressive dyspnea, prominent hilar lymphadenopathy on chest CT scan, and patchy subepicardial regions of late gadolinium enhancement involving the mid to basal inferoseptal wall of the left ventricle and the right ventricular (RV) free wall in the region of the RV outflow tract on cardiac magnetic resonance imaging (not shown). PET scan demonstrates multiple focal regions of intense myocardial uptake including the apical anteroseptal and mid and basal lateral walls (maximum standardized uptake value [SUVmax]: 7.3). There is also moderate RV uptake. In addition, there are multiple intensely 18F-FDG-avid supraclavicular, mediastinal, and right-sided internal mammary lymph nodes (SUV max: 11.2). The perfusion images show a small perfusion defect in the basal inferoseptal wall without corresponding 18F-FDG uptake (matched reduction in perfusion and metabolism 18F-) consistent with myocardial scar. His left ventricular ejection fraction was 60%. The volume of inflamed myocardium (using an SUV threshold of 2.7) was 77 cc. Endomyocardial biopsy confirmed nonnecrotizing granulomas with focal granulomas consistent with sarcoidosis.

actively inflamed, resolve spontaneously, or progress to a fibrotic phase. Patients can be asymptomatic or present with syncope, sudden death, heart block, atrial or ventricular tachyarrhythmias, and heart failure (Fig. 18.36). RV endomyocardial biopsy has a low yield because of frequent sampling errors given the focal nature of the cardiac sarcoidosis most frequently affecting the left ventricle. Most importantly, any given patient may harbor active granulomas, healing granulomas, or scar and a biopsy with blind sampling may underestimate the burden and variety of pathologies in cardiac sarcoidosis. CMR and PET imaging play a critical role in the clinical diagnosis of cardiac sarcoidosis (Figs. 18.36 and 18.37; see Fig. 19.12).[7] The diagnostic criteria for cardiac sarcoidosis are shown in Table 18.6.

18F-FDG PET imaging has a significant advantage over endomyocardial biopsy in identifying cardiac and systemic involvement, identifying extracardiac sites for biopsy, and facilitating the evaluation of response to anti-inflammatory therapy. CMR is typically the first test when cardiac sarcoidosis is suspected with specific features that may suggest sarcoidosis (see Chapter 19). However, the presence of late gadolinium enhancement does not differentiate fibrosis from active inflammation, and T2-weighted edema signal is insensitive to diagnose active cardiac sarcoidosis. Currently, the only clinical test to image myocardial inflammation is 18F-FDG PET, which is used when CMR is positive, unavailable, contraindicated, or inconclusive. 18F-FDG PET is necessary, even when CMR is positive, to guide the potential need of anti-inflammatory therapy (Fig. 18.38).

TABLE 18.6 Criteria to Diagnose Cardiac Sarcoidosis

JAPANESE MINISTRY OF HEALTH AND WELFARE (JMHW)	HEART RHYTHM SOCIETY (HRS)
Histologic Diagnosis Group	**Histologic Diagnosis From Myocardial Tissue**
CS confirmed by EMB, and histologic or clinical diagnosis of extracardiac sarcoidosis	Noncaseating granulomas on EMB with no alternative cause identified
Clinical Diagnosis Group	**Clinical Diagnosis**
Histologic or clinical diagnosis of extracardiac sarcoidosis AND	Probable diagnosis of CS exists IF
Two or more major criteria OR	There is histologic diagnosis of extracardiac sarcoidosis* AND
One major criterion and two or more minor criteria	One or more of the following is present
Major Criteria	**Major Criteria**
Advanced atrioventricular block	Cardiomyopathy or atrioventricular block responsive to immunosuppressive treatment*
	Unexplained reduced LVEF (<40%)
Basal thinning of intraventricular septum	Unexplained ventricular tachycardia
67-Ga uptake in heart	Mobitz II second- or third-degree heart block
Depressed LVEF (<50%)	^{18}F-FDG uptake on cardiac PET consistent
	Patchy with CS*
Minor Criteria	**Minor Criteria**
Electrocardiography: ventricular tachycardia, PVCs, RBBB, abnormal axis, abnormal Q wave	Late gadolinium enhancement on cardiac MRI consistent with CS
Echocardiography: structural or wall motion abnormality	Cardiac 67-Ga uptake AND
Nuclear medicine: perfusion defect, 201Tl, 99mTc*	Exclusion of other causes of cardiac manifestations
Cardiac MRI: late gadolinium enhancement	
EMB: moderate fibrosis or monocyte infiltration	

*Significant difference between Japanese Ministry Health Welfare and Heart Rhythm Society criteria.
FDG, Fluorodeoxyglucose; *LVEF*, left ventricular ejection fraction; *MRI*, magnetic resonance imaging; *PVC*, premature ventricular contractions; *RBBB*, right bundle branch block; *CS*, cardiac sarcoidosis; *EMB*, endomyocardial biopsy; *Ga*, gallium; *Tl*, thallium; *Tc*, technetium.
From Chareonthaitawee P, et al. Joint SNMMI-ASNC expert consensus document on the role of (18)F-FDG PET/CT in cardiac sarcoid detection and therapy monitoring. J Nucl Cardiol 2017;24:1741-1758.

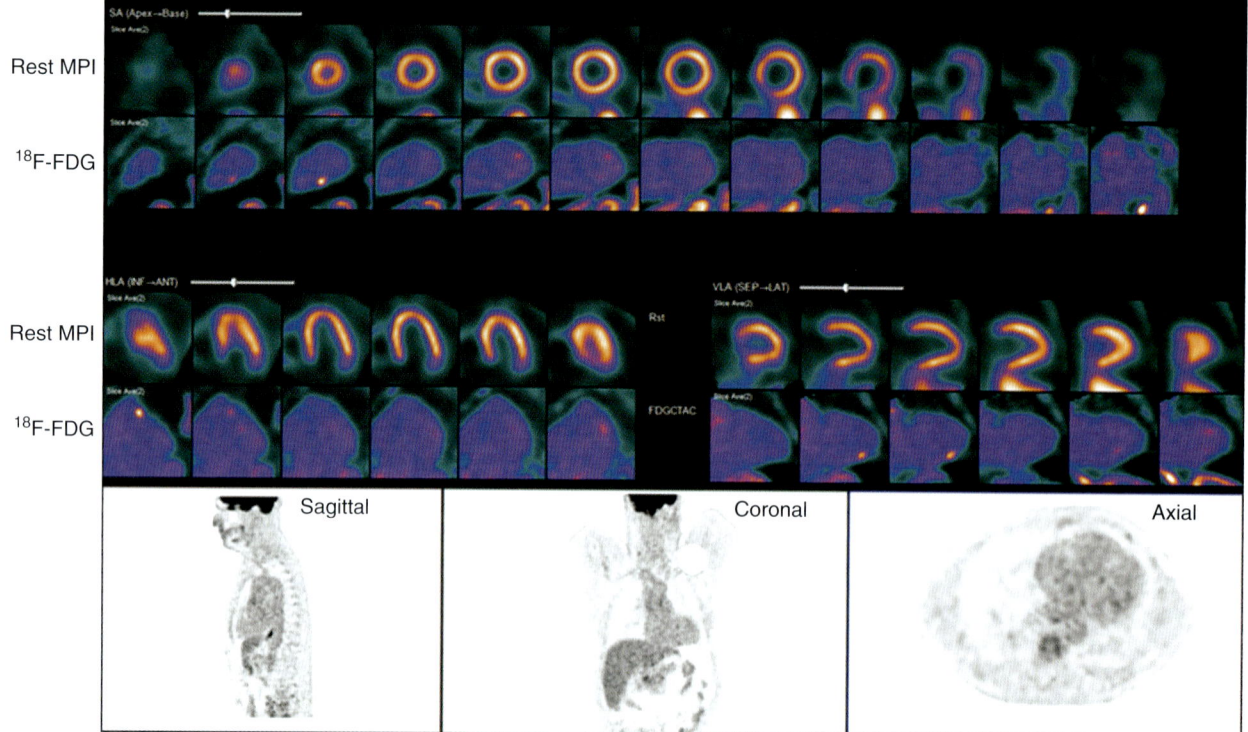

FIGURE 18.37 ^{18}**F-FDG PET/CT to assess treatment response in cardiac sarcoidosis.** Follow-up PET images of the patient described in Fig. 18.36 after 6 months of antiinflammatory therapy showed complete resolution of myocardial and extracardiac ^{18}F-FDG uptake. The severe perfusion defect in the basal inferoseptal wall remained unchanged and consistent with focal myocardial scarring.

^{18}F-FDG PET uptake in the heart, however, is not specific for sarcoidosis and can represent normal myocardium, inflamed myocardium, malignancy, or hibernating myocardium. Hence the ^{18}F-FDG PET scan is performed with a special diet of low-carbohydrate and high-fat meals for 24 hours before the test followed by prolonged fasting of at least 12 hours.[7] A myocardial perfusion scan is performed in conjunction with the ^{18}F-FDG PET study to identify areas of myocardial scar or burned out cardiac sarcoidosis. In patients with intracardiac devices, both attenuation-corrected, and non–attenuation-corrected images are interpreted to avoid artifactual focal uptake of ^{18}F-FDG in the regions with the metallic leads. Fig. 18.12 summarizes the typical patterns of myocardial perfusion and ^{18}F-FDG imaging in cardiac sarcoidosis.

^{18}F-FDG PET plays an important role in the evaluation and management of cardiac sarcoidosis. In relation to the Japanese Ministry of Health and Welfare criteria or Japanese Heart Rhythm Society criteria, ^{18}F-FDG PET is highly sensitive and specific to diagnose cardiac sarcoidosis. In a meta-analysis, pooled sensitivity was 89% and pooled specificity was 78%. As ^{18}F-FDG PET may be more sensitive than the Japanese ministry criteria, the reference used in these meta-analyses, these estimates may be biased.[7] Also, ^{18}F-FDG PET provides significant prognostic value. Among patients with known or suspected sarcoidosis, the presence of myocardial perfusion defects and focally increased ^{18}F-FDG uptake in the left and/or right ventricles are high-risk markers (Fig. 18.39).[42] ^{18}F-FDG is performed at baseline before initiation of immunosuppressive therapy and to monitor response to therapy (see Fig. 18.37).[43] Quantitative ^{18}F-FDG PET imaging using SUV, volume of inflamed myocardium using an SUV threshold, and target to background ratio (myocardium to left atrium or blood pool ratio) are usually included in the evaluation of the response to therapy.[43,44]

Infective Endocarditis

Infective endocarditis is a multisystem acute inflammatory/infectious disease that is increasing in prevalence and is associated with a very high mortality (see Chapter 80). Echocardiography, particularly transesophageal echocardiography (TEE), plays a central role in the evaluation and management of patients with infective endocarditis. However, as echocardiography is not tomographic and does not image the whole body, it is limited in evaluating complications of endocarditis. It is also limited in prosthetic valve/device/implanted prosthetic material infection caused by artifact from the prosthetic material.

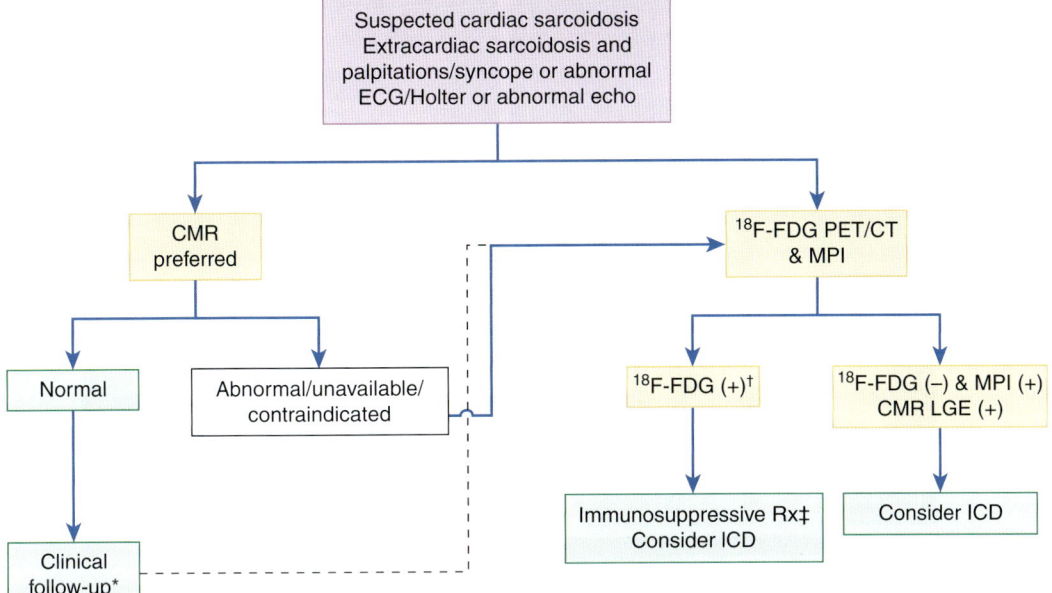

FIGURE 18.38 Role of ^{18}F-FDG PET/CT in sarcoidosis. This flowchart illustrates the role of ^{18}F-FDG PET in the evaluation of patients with suspected cardiac sarcoidosis. *High clinical suspicion. †Identifies coexistent inflammation. Immunosuppressive Rx may be considered, taking into account the amount of inflammation. *CMR*, Cardiac magnetic resonance imaging; *ICD*, implantable cardioverter defibrillator; *MPI*, myocardial perfusion imaging.

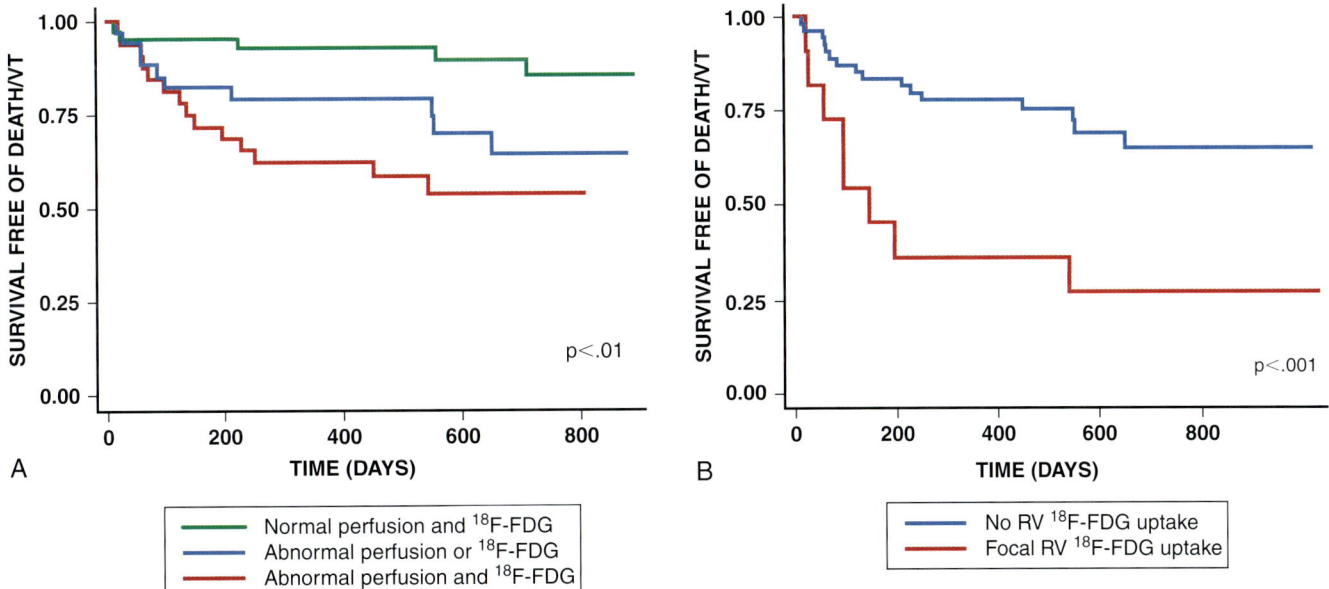

FIGURE 18.39 Prognostic value of ^{18}F-FDG PET/CT in cardiac sarcoidosis. Event-free survival of different patterns of ^{18}F-FDG uptake in the left ventricular **(A)** and right ventricular **(B)** myocardium in patients with known or suspected sarcoidosis referred for ^{18}F-FDG PET/CT. *VT*, Ventricular tachycardia. (From Blankstein R, et al. Cardiac positron emission tomography enhances prognostic assessments of patients with suspected cardiac sarcoidosis. J Am Coll Cardiol 2014;63:329-336.)

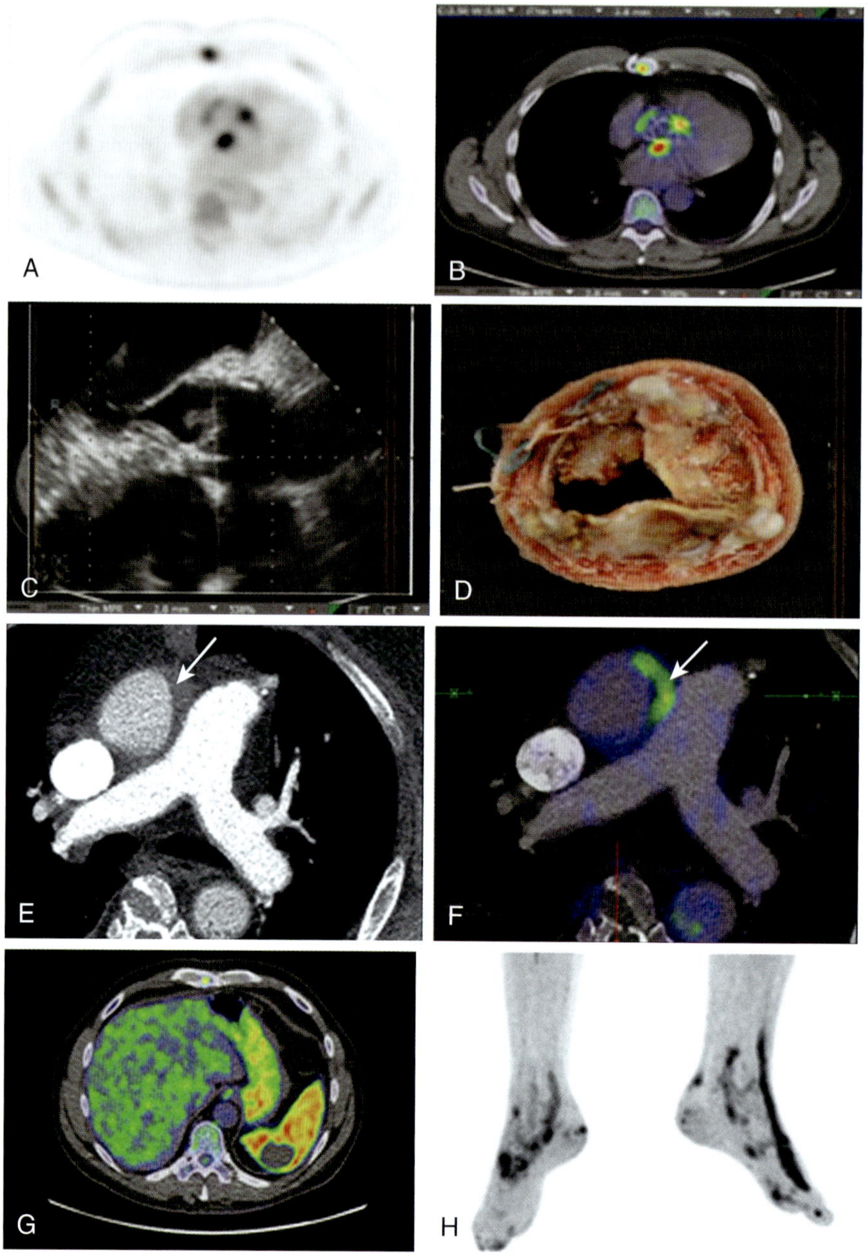

FIGURE 18.40 **^{18}F-FDG PET/CT and multimodality imaging of infective endocarditis.** Images of a 54-year-old man with a history of bioprosthetic aortic valve and aortic root replacement who presented with multiple episodes of transient vision loss and bacteremia with *Cardiobacterium valvarum*. **A** and **B,** Selected axial ^{18}F-FDG PET and fused PET/CT images showing focal FDG uptake in the aortic valve annulus. **C,** Transesophageal echocardiogram (*TEE*) (120-degree long axis) shows a 1.25 × 1 cm vegetation on the bioprosthetic aortic valve and a thickened aortic root that could represent abscess. **D,** Explanted aortic valve showing valve destruction from endocarditis. **E** and **F,** Selected axial view of a CT angiogram and its corresponding ^{18}F-FDG image at the level of the pulmonary artery bifurcation shows increased soft tissue density around the aortic root (*arrow*) with increased metabolic activity suspicious for abscess. **G,** Selected axial whole-body ^{18}F-FDG PET image shows a focal region with absent ^{18}F-FDG uptake in the spleen consistent with a splenic infarct, likely embolic. **H,** ^{18}F-FDG images of the feet demonstrate multiple focal areas of uptake consistent with septic emboli.

^{18}F-FDG PET and cardiac CTA are emerging as important adjuncts to echocardiography to identify complications of endocarditis, prosthetic valve/device infection, and systemic embolization (Fig. 18.40). Contrast-enhanced CT along with ^{18}F-FDG PET enhances the evaluation of complications from infective endocarditis. In a recent study, the combination of ^{18}F-FDG PET and cardiac CTA yielded higher diagnostic performance compared with ^{18}F-FDG PET/CT alone (Fig. 18.41).[45] ^{18}F-FDG PET is also a useful method to image response to therapy in patients in whom removal of the infected prosthetic material is not feasible (e.g., conduits or descending aortic stents). As with sarcoidosis imaging, patients must be adequately prepared with a high-fat/low-carbohydrate diet and undergo dedicated cardiac imaging followed by whole-body imaging to delineate possible sites of septic embolization. Nonspecific ^{18}F-FDG uptake can be seen after surgery. The presence of focal (as opposed to diffuse) and intense radiotracer uptake is consistent with infection. Images are reconstructed with and without attenuation correction. As with sarcoidosis, non–attenuation-corrected ^{18}F-FDG emission images are also reviewed in patients with mechanical heart valves and metallic cardiovascular implantable electronic devices to ensure that any focal uptake seen on the attenuation-corrected images does not represent an artifact from overcorrection of attenuation from a metallic object.

The incremental diagnostic value of ^{18}F-FDG PET for prosthetic valve and native valve endocarditis, intracardiac device infection, and LV-assist device infection was studied by several investigators[46] and summarized in a recent systematic review.[47] In addition, a recent study demonstrated the prognostic value of ^{18}F-FDG PET/CT. In this study, 173 patients with native ($n = 64$) or prosthetic valve ($n = 109$) endocarditis were followed for a mean of 225 days for major cardiac events (in hospital and 1-year death, recurrent infective endocarditis, unscheduled cardiovascular hospitalization, and new embolic events on antibiotics). MACE occurred in 94 patients, and on multivariable analysis, C-reactive protein level ≥100 mg/L, a positive 18F-FDG PET/CT, and a moderate to intense 18F-FDG PET/CT valvular uptake remained independently associated with MACE. This study showed that moderate to severe 18F-FDG uptake associated with predictive of new embolic events within the first year after diagnosis of infective endocarditis (hazard ratio [HR] 7.5; 95% confidence interval [CI]: 1.2 to 45.2; P = 0.03).[48] The 2015 European Society of Cardiology (ESC) guidelines on infective endocarditis[49] included an abnormal 18F-FDG PET/CT (abnormal 18F-FDG activity around the site of the prosthetic valve implantation detected by PET/CT only if prosthesis was implanted >3 months prior), or radiolabeled leukocyte SPECT/CT, or cardiac CT showing a definite paravalvular lesion as major criterion for infective endocarditis. In the ESC guidelines,[49] 18F-FDG PET or leukocyte-labeled SPECT/CT was also indicated for cases with possible/rejected infective endocarditis with high clinical suspicion for prosthetic valve endocarditis. A recent algorithmic approach to the evaluation of infective endocarditis proposes using 18F-FDG PET/CT after a positive or nondiagnostic TEE study, a positive cardiac CTA study, and a positive white blood cell scintigraphy study.[47]

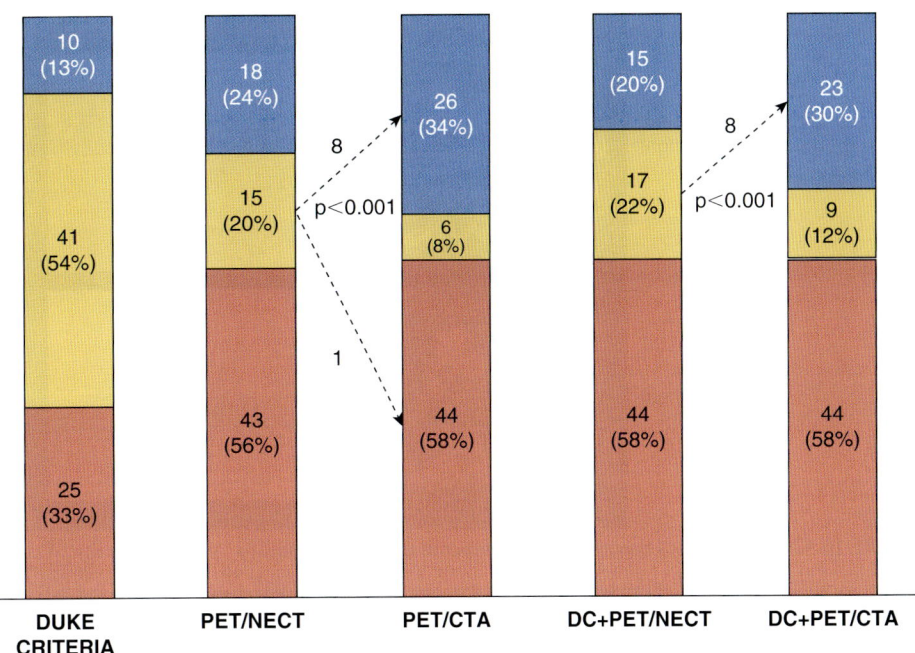

FIGURE 18.41 **Value of 18F-FDG PET/CTA in diagnosis of infective endocarditis.** This stacked bar graph demonstrates the incremental value of 18F-FDG PET/CTA over modified Duke criteria to enhance diagnostic certainty in patients with suspected prosthetic valve or cardiac device infection. (From Pizzi MN, et al. Improving the diagnosis of infective endocarditis in prosthetic valves and intracardiac devices with 18F-fluorodeoxyglucose positron emission tomography/computed tomography angiography: initial results at an infective endocarditis referral center. Circulation 2015;132:1113-1126.)

Radionuclide Imaging in Vasculitis

Vasculitis can be challenging to diagnose. The initial evaluation in patients with suspected vasculitis typically includes clinical history and serum biomarkers, followed by anatomic assessment of vascular involvement by ultrasound, MRA, CTA or invasive angiography, and 18F-FDG PET/CT imaging (see Chapters 43 and 97). The clinical manifestations of vasculitis and serum biomarker changes are usually nonspecific. A positive vascular biopsy is usually confirmatory but limited by false-negatives. Imaging plays a central role in the diagnosis and management of vasculitis. Anatomic imaging methods identify wall thickening, thrombus, luminal stenosis, and aneurysms, which typically represent advanced disease manifestations that may not be reversible. [67]Gallium-SPECT and radiolabeled white blood cell scans are obsolete because of poor sensitivity. 18F-FDG PET/CT is the test of choice to ascertain the presence of inflammation in large-vessel vasculitis (Fig. 18.42).[50] Moreover, 18F-FDG PET/CT can guide the most appropriate site of biopsy, identify disease at an inflammatory stage where it may be more amenable to therapy, and can quantify the extent and severity of inflammation that is useful in the evaluation of response to anti-inflammatory therapy. Typically, 18F-FDG PET/CT is used in conjunction with MRA or CTA to evaluate the anatomic abnormalities from the vasculitis.

As with cardiac sarcoidosis, 18F-FDG PET/CT for vasculitis is often performed after a high-fat, low-carbohydrate diet for 24 hours, especially for evaluation of the aortic root. Whole-body images are obtained a minimum of 90 minutes after injection of radiotracer. 18F-FDG is interpreted visually in relation to liver uptake as grade 0 = no vascular uptake (≤ mediastinum), grade 1 = low-grade uptake (< liver), grade 2 = vascular uptake = liver, and grade 3 = vascular uptake > liver uptake.[50] Grade 0 (no uptake) or grade 1 (low-grade uptake) are considered negative for vasculitis, grade 2 (intermediate-grade uptake) is possible vasculitis, and grade 3 (high-grade uptake) is considered positive for vasculitis. In conjunction with magnetic resonance imaging (MRI) images, the vasculitis patterns can be classified as normal (both MRI and PET normal), inflammatory (PET uptake > liver uptake and abnormal MRI), and fibrous (abnormal MRI, but PET uptake ≤ liver uptake). Target to background SUV ratios (vessel to blood pool ratio) are used for quantitative evaluation.[50]

18F-FDG PET/CT has a pooled sensitivity and specificity of 90% and 98% for diagnosis of giant cell arteritis, and a pooled sensitivity and specificity of 80% and 89%, respectively, for the diagnosis of Takayasu arteritis.[50] Sensitivity of 18F-FDG PET/CT to detect inflammation may be

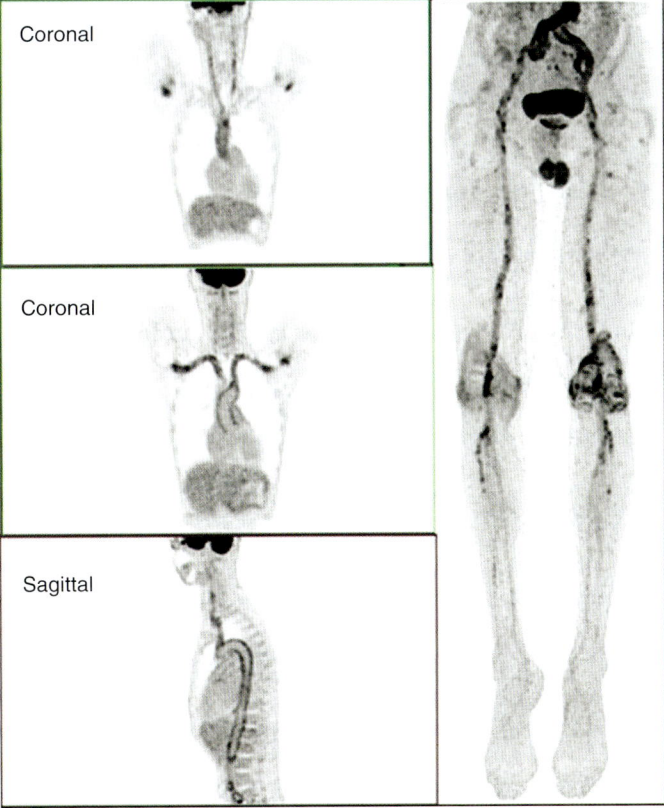

FIGURE 18.42 **18F-FDG PET/CT imaging in large-vessel vasculitis.** Selected 18F-FDG PET images of a 69-year-old man with a history of ulcerative colitis and polymyalgia rheumatica presenting with night sweats and weight loss. CT angiography showed diffuse circumferential wall thickening of the aorta and main branches (images not shown). The PET images show intense 18F-FDG uptake in the thoracic and abdominal aorta and subclavian, carotid, and femoral arteries bilaterally, consistent with large-vessel vasculitis. Giant cell arteritis was excluded and he was started on oral prednisone 60 mg/day with a reduction in C-reactive protein and erythrocyte sedimentation rate.

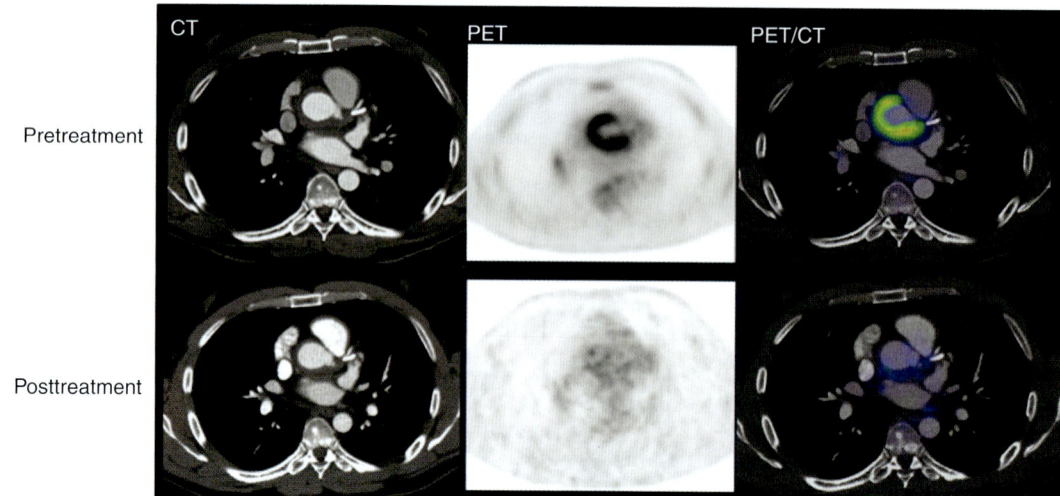

FIGURE 18.43 ¹⁸F-FDG PET/CT imaging to assess response to therapy in aortitis. Selected axial chest CT angiograms (CTAs) (*left*), ¹⁸F-FDG PET (*middle*), and fused CTA and ¹⁸F-FDG PET images (*right*) of a patient with Behçet disease. Pretreatment images (*top row*) show peri-aortic thickening on the CT images with near circumferential intense ¹⁸F-FDG uptake consistent with inflammation. Posttreatment scans (*bottom row*) demonstrate persistent wall thickening on the CT images, but near complete resolution of ¹⁸F-FDG uptake indicating excellent response to therapy.

reduced after more than 3 days of glucocorticoid therapy.[50] ¹⁸F-FDG offers the advantage to demonstrate change after successful immunosuppressive therapy (Fig. 18.43), whereas anatomic imaging methods may be limited as they may continue to demonstrate vessel wall abnormalities even in the fibrotic phase of vasculitis. However, the definitive role of ¹⁸F-FDG to evaluate longitudinal disease course and response to therapy remains unclear, with some studies indicating decreased ¹⁸F-FDG uptake after therapy and other studies finding no difference in relapsing and nonrelapsing patients.[50] In addition to large-vessel vasculitis, comprising giant cell arteritis and Takayasu arteritis, ¹⁸F-FDG PET/CT can also be helpful in diagnosing and monitoring response to therapy in aortitis, Behçet disease, and IgG4-related disease.

Cardio-Oncology

Radionuclide imaging can be used to evaluate possible cardiovascular complications from chemotherapy and radiotherapy in patients with cancer (see Chapters 56 and 57). The incidence and prognosis of cardiotoxicity from cancer therapy can vary depending on the age at treatment, sex, agent(s) used, cumulative dose, concomitant treatment with other cardiotoxic therapies, and other factors, including underlying cardiovascular risk factors. There are several other forms of cardiotoxicity associated with cancer therapy including ventricular dysfunction, CAD, hypertension, myocarditis, valvular heart disease, pericardial disease, venous thromboembolic disease, arrhythmias, and conduction system abnormalities. Additionally, neoplasms can involve the heart as primary cardiac tumors, or as a site of metastases. The following is a brief description of the most common applications of radionuclide imaging in patients undergoing cancer treatment or in cancer survivors.

Assessment of Ventricular Function

The American Society of Clinical Oncology recommends assessment of LVEF at baseline in all patients who meet criteria for increased risk with reassessment within 1 year of completing anthracycline therapy. Patients at increased risk for ventricular dysfunction and heart failure include those receiving high-dose anthracycline therapy (e.g., doxorubicin ≥ 250 mg/m^2); those receiving concomitant high-dose radiation therapy (≥30 Gy) with the heart is in the treatment field; those receiving lower-dose anthracycline therapy in combination with lower-dose radiation therapy where the heart is in the field; those receiving lower-dose anthracycline or trastuzumab therapy alone and have any of the following risk factors including ≥2 cardiovascular risk factors, age ≥60, or known cardiovascular disease; and those receiving treatment with lower-dose anthracycline followed by trasutuzmab.[51] The guideline recommends discontinuation of doxorubicin if there is an absolute decrease in LVEF of ≥10% from baseline to ≤50%.

Although echocardiography is currently the modality of choice for baseline and serial assessment of LV function in patients with cancer, gated blood pool scanning (also known as equilibrium radionuclide angiography can also be used to determine regional and global LV function. The technique consists of radiolabeling the patient's own red blood cells, which are then re-injected for imaging. For a full description of the technique, please refer to the SNMMI Procedure Standard.[52] Briefly, there are two methods for labeling the red blood cells: (1) in vivo or modified in vivo/in vitro methods (e.g., using 2 to 3 mg stannous pyrophosphate 15 minutes before injection of ^{99m}Tc) and (2) commercial in vitro kit, which is the most commonly used. Radiolabeled blood cells are then re-injected and, after 1 to 2 minutes, ECG-gated equilibrium blood pool imaging is obtained with planar or SPECT imaging. End-diastolic and end-systolic volumes are then measured to calculate LVEF.

Evaluation of Coronary Artery Disease

CAD, a frequent comorbid illness in patients diagnosed with cancer, has increased in prevalence in cancer survivors as this population continues to live longer, and is a known form of cardiotoxicity of several cancer therapies.[53] Radiation therapy in particular has been associated with an increased risk of obstructive CAD. Because of this, guidelines recommend functional stress testing for the evaluation of obstructive CAD 5 to 10 years after exposure in high-risk patients, even if they are asymptomatic (e.g., lymphoma). Radiation therapy with the heart in the treatment field remains the cancer therapy associated with the highest risk for development of CAD. The risk of radiation-associated CAD increases linearly with mean radiation dose to the heart, with no apparent threshold. MPI with SPECT or PET is commonly used for this application similar to that described previously for noncancer patients. An advantage of PET is its ability to quantify myocardial blood flow and flow reserve, which increases the sensitivity for detection of myocardial ischemia.

Evaluation of Primary or Metastatic Cardiac Neoplasms

Cardiac neoplasms are rare and multimodality imaging plays a critical role in the evaluation and management of these patients. Although CMR is the modality of choice for the evaluation of cardiac masses, ¹⁸F-FDG PET/CT can be helpful in the evaluation of both primary malignancies and metastatic disease to the heart. Imaging with ¹⁸F-FDG PET to identify metabolically active tissue and integrated anatomic assessment with CT can provide useful diagnostic information and help plan therapeutic interventions such as surgical resection.

MACHINE LEARNING AND ARTIFICIAL INTELLIGENCE

Machine learning and artificial intelligence applications are transforming several aspects of cardiology and cardiovascular imaging (see Chapter 11). The use of artificial intelligence in nuclear cardiology can be applied to image processing, enhancement of image quality, image interpretation, and risk assessment. Machine learning approaches integrating imaging data with the vast amounts of clinical and stress data have been shown to improve diagnosis, risk assessment, and management of ischemic heart disease. The REFINE SPECT registry included high-efficiency solid-state CZT SPECT scanner MPI data with follow-up data for prognosis from 5 medical centers on 20,418 patients, and diagnostic data (patients without known CAD, MI, or coronary revascularization and with invasive coronary angiography) on 2079 patients from 9 centers. In one study from this registry, deep learning improved the identification of obstructive CAD[54] compared with conventional semiquantitative visual interpretation. In another analysis from this registry, a score developed from machine learning methods accurately predicted in which patients a rest MPI could be safely canceled.[55] Machine learning including clinical and imaging data demonstrated high accuracy for predicting 3-year risk of MACE and was superior to machine learning–based evaluation of imaging or conventional measures of stress or ischemic perfusion defects alone.[56]

TRANSLATIONAL MOLECULAR IMAGING

Cardiovascular molecular imaging is a cutting-edge field with several exciting translational research applications, some of which are discussed in the following section.

Peripheral Arterial Disease

PAD is prevalent and associated with high morbidity and mortality. (see Chapter 43). Conventional approaches to diagnosis of PAD including the ankle-brachial index (ABI) and angiography (invasive and noninvasive) can only assess the extent and severity of macrovascular atherosclerosis. There is growing recognition that microvascular abnormalities in PAD contribute to patient symptoms and portend adverse clinical outcomes including wound healing, infection, and limb amputation. However, microvascular abnormalities and associated skeletal muscle remodeling are poorly captured by standard diagnostic modalities. Radionuclide imaging with SPECT and PET provide accurate, quantitative assessments of the integrated effects of macrovascular and microvascular abnormalities on skeletal muscle perfusion, thereby complementing angiographic information.[57] Beyond skeletal muscle perfusion, radionuclide molecular imaging techniques are emerging as promising tools to evaluate the effects of novel cell–based and gene-based therapies.[57]

Atherosclerosis

By integrating the detailed anatomic information from CT with the high sensitivity of radionuclide imaging to evaluate targeted molecular and cellular abnormalities in the myocardium and vasculature, hybrid imaging may play a key role in shaping the future of molecular diagnostics and therapeutics. One of the areas of greatest research interest has been centered on the evaluation of inflammation within atheroma (see Chapter 24). Because there is marked heterogeneity in the composition of human atherosclerotic plaques, targeted molecular imaging has been used to characterize the composition of such plaques, thereby allowing the determination of their risk for complications (e.g., erosion and rupture). Such imaging tools provide mechanistic insights into atherothrombotic processes, better risk stratification, optimal selection of therapeutic targets, and the means for monitoring therapeutic responses.

PET/CT is a powerful technique because it is highly sensitive in detecting low quantities of molecularly targeted radiotracers to assess biologic processes involved in atherosclerosis (e.g., inflammation, microcalcification). Although the use of radionuclide imaging in atherosclerosis remains a research tool at the moment, it is an area of very active investigation.

For example, ^{18}F-FDG PET has been the most commonly applied imaging marker of vascular inflammation. In patients with carotid disease, ^{18}F-FDG uptake has been shown to accurately differentiate culprit and high-risk from lower-risk carotid atherosclerotic plaques. A meta-analysis of data from 539 patients in 14 studies showed that ^{18}F-FDG uptake was significantly higher in culprit carotid arteries than in nonculprit arteries in patients with transient ischemic attack or stroke.[58] ^{18}F-FDG is of limited value for imaging atherosclerotic disease activity in the coronary vasculature because under most physiologic conditions the tracer is avidly taken up by the myocardium.

Focus is beginning to shift toward other more specifically targeted PET ligands because of the limitations of plaque imaging using ^{18}F-FDG.[59] For example, ^{18}F-sodium fluoride (NaF) enables the study of vascular calcification resulting from intense plaque inflammation. Because it is not taken up by normal cardiomyocytes, ^{18}F-NaF has demonstrated superior ability to differentiate high-risk coronary lesions compared with ^{18}F-FDG.[60,61] The mitochondrial membrane translocator protein (TSPO) receptor involved in cholesterol transport, immunomodulation, and apoptosis is widely expressed in the body, it is abundant in macrophages, and it has been evaluated in experimental and human atherosclerosis. ^{68}Ga-Pentixafor binds to C-X-C chemokine receptor 4 (CXCR4) and is the receptor for CXCL12 and the chemokine macrophage migration inhibitory factor that is expressed in endothelial cells, smooth muscle cells, monocytes, and other leukocytes. In patients with recent MI, ^{68}Ga-pentixafor retention was higher in culprit than nonculprit coronary lesions.[62] Finally, the ^{68}Ga-dotatate has also been used to evaluate plaque inflammation. It targets the somatostatin receptor subtype-2 (SSTR2), which is overexpressed in activated macrophages and other inflammatory cells. Binding of ^{68}Ga-dotatate was demonstrated in CD68-positive macrophage-rich carotid plaque regions and there was a strong correlation between its in vivo retention signals and SSTR2 and CD68 gene expression.[63]

Novel PET Perfusion Tracers

^{18}F-flurpiridaz is a novel ^{18}F-labeled PET perfusion tracer that binds to mitochondrial complex I, demonstrates rapid myocardial uptake, and has higher extraction than ^{13}N-ammonia even at high myocardial blood flow rates.[64] It is produced by a cyclotron, but because of its long half-life (110 minutes) it can be transported as unit doses to various sites, vastly enhancing access to PET MPI globally. Data from a phase III study demonstrate its superior accuracy in relation to SPECT MPI. In the study, 795 patients (mean age 62.3 ± 9.5 years, 31% women, 55% obese, 71% pharmacologic stress) from 92 sites in the United States and Canada underwent ^{99m}Tc-SPECT, ^{18}F-flurpiridaz PET, and invasive coronary angiography.[64] ^{18}F-flurpiridaz PET MPI was more sensitive to ^{99m}Tc-SPECT MPI in diagnosing ≥50% obstructive CAD (sensitivity 71.9 [95% CI 67.0% to 76.3%] vs. 53.7% [95% CI 48.5% to 58.8%], $p < 0.001$). But its specificity did not meet prespecified criteria of noninferiority (76.2% [95% CI, 71.8% to 80.1%] vs. 86.6% [95% CI, 83.2% to 89.8%], p = nonsignificant [NS]). Perfusion defect size, image quality, and radiation dose were better delineated by ^{18}F-flurpiridaz PET compared with ^{99m}Tc-SPECT MPI. ^{18}F-flurpiridaz PET was superior to SPECT in subgroups of women, obese individuals, patients undergoing pharmacologic stress, and in patients with small LV volumes.[64] Because of its long half-life, exercise PET is feasible and nearly 30% of the patients in the study underwent exercise PET.[64] A second phase III study is currently underway.

Whole-Body PET Imaging

PET using targeted radiotracers is the most sensitive method for imaging biologic processes. A novel PET scanner that is 194 cm long has been recently developed. This scanner provides high spatial and temporal resolution imaging, rapid imaging of the whole body (<2 minutes), very low radiation dose imaging (<1 mCi), delayed imaging of physiologic processes (10-hour imaging for ^{18}F-FDG), and whole-body dynamic imaging.[65] Whole-body coverage allows for real-time tracking of blood flow to the heart and various organs opening novel clinical research applications. Atherosclerosis and several cardiovascular diseases are systemic diseases, and this system offers unprecedented opportunities to study cardiovascular pathophysiology including heart and brain connections. High temporal resolution allows for imaging tracers with short half-lives. The rapid imaging minimizes patient motion and freezes respiratory and cardiac motion further improving spatial resolution of the images. The high-count sensitivity allows for detection of radiotracer for several hours after injection and can provide novel applications to track metabolic processes over a long duration of several hours.[65] The whole-body PET scanner has transformed cardiovascular molecular imaging with several ongoing research studies.

Aortic Valve Disease

Calcific aortic valve stenosis is one of the most common valvular disease of aging (see Chapter 72). Currently, the only effective therapy is aortic valve replacement, which is most effective when applied before onset of irreversible interstitial myocardial fibrosis. Echocardiography is usually the first imaging test in the evaluation of valvular heart disease and aortic disease and provides information of EF, mass, and global longitudinal strain (see Chapter 16). CMR additionally provides evidence of extracellular volume expansion (see Chapter 19). Radionuclide imaging is playing an emerging role in imaging inflammation, microvascular calcification, ATTR amyloidosis (see Fig. 72.13), infection, and microvascular dysfunction in patients with aortic valve disease.

Patients with severe aortic stenosis may remain asymptomatic and accurate prediction of disease progression remains challenging. Inflammation and microcalcification have been proposed as potential mechanisms that lead to progressive aortic stenosis. In one study 30 patients with aortic stenosis underwent ^{18}F-NaF and ^{18}F-FDG PET/CT.[66] In 12 of these patients the excised valves after surgery were evaluated for inflammation (CD68 staining) and microcalcification (alkaline phosphatase and osteocalcin) and 18 patients underwent aortic valve calcium scoring at baseline and after 1 year (see Fig. 72.12). ^{18}F-FDG imaging did not correlate with CD68 staining.[66] Baseline ^{18}F-NaF, but not ^{18}F-FDG, correlated closely with increase in aortic valve calcification on CT ($r = 0.66$; $P < 0.01$).[66] Ongoing studies will inform us whether ^{18}F-NaF-guided management of aortic stenosis is superior to current clinical management.

Severe aortic stenosis increases LV wall thickness, wall stress, and afterload, each of which decreases coronary microvascular function. Advanced phenotyping of patients with severe asymptomatic aortic stenosis using myocardial perfusion reserve is identifying an advanced disease phenotype that may benefit from valve replacement before advanced irreversible LV remodeling. In a study of 43 patients with aortic stenosis or sclerosis and a matched cohort of 43 patients without aortic valve disease, global MFR decreased with increasing aortic valve stenosis.[67] Reduced MFR was associated with worse function (global longitudinal strain) and survival free of MACE after a median follow-up of 7 years. Adjusted annualized MACE rates were determined by MFR and global longitudinal strain, and they were highest in patients with both abnormal values and lowest in those with both normal values (30.99% vs. 1.86%, $P = 0.002$).[67]

Wild-type ATTR-CA and aortic stenosis are both diseases of aging and a prevalent cause of heart failure in the elderly. Transcatheter aortic valve replacement (TAVR) has revolutionized the treatment of aortic stenosis making it accessible to patients with severe comorbidities precluding surgery (see Chapter 74). In aortic stenosis the left ventricle is thickened because of myocyte hypertrophy, whereas in amyloidosis the left ventricle is thickened because of infiltration by amyloid fibrils. Both conditions are characterized by high intraventricular pressures, high wall stress, high filling pressures, subendocardial and microvascular ischemia, heart failure, arrhythmia, contractile dysfunction, angina, syncope, and death (see Chapters 53 and 72). Patients with very advanced aortic stenosis may manifest features of myocardial disease, reduced cardiac output, and poor prognosis. Both diseases can potentiate heart failure and small initial reports suggested that patients with dual pathology of ATTR-CA and aortic stenosis were at higher risk of post-TAVR mortality.[68] More recent studies refute those initial reports and suggest no differences in post-TAVR mortality. A recent two-center study of 204 patients undergoing TAVR for severe aortic stenosis showed that after a mean follow-up of 2 years, post-TAVR survival was similar in aortic stenosis patients with and without ATTR-CA.[69] However, 1-year heart failure hospitalization rate was higher in those with dual aortic stenosis and ATTR-CA.[69]

REFERENCES

Principles of Imaging, Interpretation of Images, and Radiation Dose

1. Dorbala S, Ananthasubramaniam K, Armstrong IS, et al. Single Photon Emission Computed Tomography (SPECT) myocardial perfusion imaging guidelines: instrumentation, acquisition, processing, and interpretation. *J Nucl Cardiol*. 2018;25:1784–1846.
2. Dilsizian V, Bacharach SL, Beanlands RS, et al. ASNC imaging guidelines/SNMMI procedure standard for Positron Emission Tomography (PET) nuclear cardiology procedures. *J Nucl Cardiol*. 2016;23:1187–1226.
3. Taegtmeyer H, Young ME, Lopaschuk GD, et al. Assessing cardiac metabolism: a scientific statement from the American Heart Association. *Circ Res*. 2016;118:1659–1701.
4. Viola A, Munari F, Sanchez-Rodriguez R, et al. The metabolic signature of macrophage responses. *Front Immunol*. 2019;10:1462.
5. Duncker DJ, Koller A, Merkus D, Canty Jr JM. Regulation of coronary blood flow in health and ischemic heart disease. *Prog Cardiovasc Dis*. 2015;57:409–422.
6. Henzlova MJ, Duvall WL, Einstein AJ, et al. ASNC imaging guidelines for SPECT nuclear cardiology procedures: stress, protocols, and tracers. *J Nucl Cardiol*. 2016;23:606–639.
7. Chareonthaitawee P, Beanlands RS, Chen W, et al. Joint SNMMI-ASNC expert consensus document on the role of (18)F-FDG PET/CT in cardiac sarcoid detection and therapy monitoring. *J Nucl Cardiol*. 2017;24:1741–1758.
8. Dorbala S, Ando Y, Bokhari S, et al. ASNC/AHA/ASE/EANM/HFSA/ISA/SCMR/SNMMI expert consensus recommendations for multimodality imaging in cardiac amyloidosis: Part 1 of 2-evidence base and standardized methods of imaging. *J Nucl Cardiol*. 2019;26:2065–2123.
9. Murthy VL, Bateman TM, Beanlands RS, et al. Clinical quantification of myocardial blood flow using PET: joint position paper of the SNMMI cardiovascular council and the ASNC. *J Nucl Cardiol*. 2018;25:269–297.
10. Dorbala S, Di Carli MF, Beanlands RS, et al. Prognostic value of stress myocardial perfusion positron emission tomography: results from a multicenter observational registry. *J Am Coll Cardiol*. 2013;61:176–184.
11. Dorbala S, Blankstein R, Skali H, et al. Approaches to reduce radiation dose from radionuclide myocardial perfusion imaging. *J Nucl Med*. 2015;56:592–599.
12. Einstein AJ, Pascual TN, Mercuri M, et al. Current worldwide nuclear cardiology practices and radiation exposure: results from the 65 country IAEA Nuclear Cardiology Protocols Cross-Sectional Study (INCAPS). *Eur Heart J*. 2015;36:1689–1696.

Clinical Applications–Ischemic Heart Disease

13. Medical Advisory S. Single photon emission computed tomography for the diagnosis of coronary artery disease: an evidence-based analysis. *Ont Health Technol Assess Ser*. 2010;10:1–64.
14. Takx RA, Blomberg BA, El Aidi H, et al. Diagnostic accuracy of stress myocardial perfusion imaging compared to invasive coronary angiography with fractional flow reserve meta-analysis. *Circ Cardiovasc Imaging*. 2015;8:e002666.
15. Driessen RS, Danad I, Stuijfzand WJ, et al. Comparison of coronary computed tomography angiography, fractional flow reserve, and perfusion imaging for ischemia diagnosis. *J Am Coll Cardiol*. 2019;73:161–173.
16. Neglia D, Rovai D, Caselli C, et al. Detection of significant coronary artery disease by noninvasive anatomical and functional imaging. *Circ Cardiovasc Imaging*. 2015;8:e002179.
17. Danad I, Raijmakers PG, Driessen RS, et al. Comparison of coronary CT angiography, SPECT, PET, and hybrid imaging for diagnosis of ischemic heart disease determined by fractional flow reserve. *JAMA Cardiol*. 2017;2:1100–1107.
18. Shaw LJ, Hage FG, Berman DS, Hachamovitch R, Iskandrian A. Prognosis in the era of comparative effectiveness research: where is nuclear cardiology now and where should it be? *J Nucl Cardiol*. 2012;19:1026–1043.
19. Patel KK, Spertus JA, Chan PS, et al. Extent of myocardial ischemia on positron emission tomography and survival benefit with early revascularization. *J Am Coll Cardiol*. 2019;74:1645–1654.
20. Murthy VL, Naya M, Foster CR, et al. Improved cardiac risk assessment with noninvasive measures of coronary flow reserve. *Circulation*. 2011;124:2215–2224.
21. Charytan DM, Skali H, Shah NR, et al. Coronary flow reserve is predictive of the risk of cardiovascular death regardless of chronic kidney disease stage. *Kidney Int*. 2018;93:501–509.
22. Naya M, Murthy VL, Foster CR, et al. Prognostic interplay of coronary artery calcification and underlying vascular dysfunction in patients with suspected coronary artery disease. *J Am Coll Cardiol*. 2013;61:2098–2106.
23. Shah NR, Charytan DM, Murthy VL, et al. Prognostic value of coronary flow reserve in patients with dialysis-dependent ESRD. *J Am Soc Nephrol*. 2016;27:1823–1829.
24. Mahmarian JJ, Shaw LJ, Filipchuk NG, et al. A multinational study to establish the value of early adenosine technetium-99m sestamibi myocardial perfusion imaging in identifying a low-risk group for early hospital discharge after acute myocardial infarction. *J Am Coll Cardiol*. 2006;48:2448–2457.
25. Taqueti VR, Everett BM, Murthy VL, et al. Interaction of impaired coronary flow reserve and cardiomyocyte injury on adverse cardiovascular outcomes in patients without overt coronary artery disease. *Circulation*. 2015;131:528–535.
26. Al-Khatib SM, Stevenson WG, Ackerman MJ, et al. 2017 AHA/ACC/HRS guideline for management of patients with ventricular arrhythmias and the prevention of sudden cardiac death: a report of the American College of Cardiology/American Heart Association task force on clinical practice guidelines and the Heart Rhythm Society. *Circulation*. 2018;138:e272–e391.
27. Gupta A, Harrington M, Albert CM, et al. Myocardial scar but not ischemia is associated with defibrillator shocks and sudden cardiac death in stable patients with reduced left ventricular ejection fraction. *JACC Clin Electrophysiol*. 2018;4:1200–1210.
28. Partington SL, Valente AM, Bruyere Jr J, et al. Reducing radiation dose from myocardial perfusion imaging in subjects with complex congenital heart disease. *J Nucl Cardiol*. 2019. https://doi.org/10.1007/s12350-019-01811-y.

Clinical Applications–Heart Failure and Cardiomyopathies

29. Panza JA, Ellis AM, Al-Khalidi HR, et al. Myocardial viability and long-term outcomes in ischemic cardiomyopathy. *N Engl J Med*. 2019;381:739–748.
30. Mc Ardle B, Shukla T, Nichol G, et al. Long-term follow-up of outcomes with F-18-Fluorodeoxyglucose positron emission tomography imaging-assisted management of patients with severe left ventricular dysfunction secondary to coronary disease. *Circ Cardiovasc Imaging*. 2016;9:e004331.
31. Bonow RO, Maurer G, Lee KL, et al. Myocardial viability and survival in ischemic left ventricular dysfunction. *N Engl J Med*. 2011;364:1617–1625.
32. Jacobson AF, Senior R, Cerqueira MD, et al. Myocardial iodine-123 meta-iodobenzylguanidine imaging and cardiac events in heart failure. Results of the prospective ADMIRE-HF (AdreView Myocardial Imaging for Risk Evaluation in Heart Failure) study. *J Am Coll Cardiol*. 2010;55:2212–2221.
33. Fallavollita JA, Heavey BM, Luisi Jr AJ, et al. Regional myocardial sympathetic denervation predicts the risk of sudden cardiac arrest in ischemic cardiomyopathy. *J Am Coll Cardiol*. 2014;63:141–149.
34. Dorbala S, Cuddy S, Falk RH. How to image cardiac amyloidosis: a practical approach. *JACC Cardiovasc Imaging*. 2020;13:1368–1383.
35. Gillmore JD, Maurer MS, Falk RH, et al. Nonbiopsy diagnosis of cardiac transthyretin amyloidosis. *Circulation*. 2016;133:2404–2412.
36. Dorbala S, Ando Y, Bokhari S, et al. ASNC/AHA/ASE/EANM/HFSA/ISA/SCMR/SNMMI expert consensus recommendations for multimodality imaging in cardiac amyloidosis: Part 2 of 2-Diagnostic criteria and appropriate utilization. *J Nucl Cardiol*. 2019;26:2065–2123.
37. Dorbala S, Park MA, Cuddy S, et al. Absolute quantitation of cardiac (99m)Tc-pyrophosphate using cadmium zinc telluride-based SPECT/CT. *J Nucl Med*. 2020. https://doi.org/10.2967/jnumed.120.247312.
38. Singh V, Falk R, Di Carli MF, et al. State-of-the-art radionuclide imaging in cardiac transthyretin amyloidosis. *J Nucl Cardiol*. 2019;26:158–173.

39. Rosengren S, Skibsted Clemmensen T, Tolbod L, et al. Diagnostic accuracy of [(11)C]PIB positron emission tomography for detection of cardiac amyloidosis. *JACC Cardiovasc Imaging.* 2020;13:1337–1347.
40. Ehman EC, El-Sady MS, Kijewski MF, et al. Early detection of multiorgan light-chain amyloidosis by whole-body (18)F-florbetapir PET/CT. *J Nucl Med.* 2019;60:1234–1239.
41. Cuddy SAM, Bravo PE, Falk RH, et al. Improved quantification of cardiac amyloid burden in systemic light chain amyloidosis: redefining early disease? *JACC Cardiovasc Imaging.* 2020;13:1325–1336.
42. Blankstein R, Osborne M, Naya M, et al. Cardiac positron emission tomography enhances prognostic assessments of patients with suspected cardiac sarcoidosis. *J Am Coll Cardiol.* 2014;63:329–336.
43. Slart R, Glaudemans A, Lancellotti P, et al. A joint procedural position statement on imaging in cardiac sarcoidosis: from the cardiovascular and inflammation & infection Committees of the European Association of Nuclear Medicine, the European Association of Cardiovascular Imaging, and the American Society of Nuclear Cardiology. *J Nucl Cardiol.* 2018;25:298–319.

Clinical Applications–Endocarditis, Vasculitis, Cardio-Oncology

44. Miller RJH, Cadet S, Pournazari P, et al. Quantitative assessment of cardiac hypermetabolism and perfusion for diagnosis of cardiac sarcoidosis. *J Nucl Cardiol.* 2020. https://doi.org/10.1007/s12350-020-02201-5.
45. Pizzi MN, Roque A, Fernandez-Hidalgo N, et al. Improving the diagnosis of infective endocarditis in prosthetic valves and intracardiac devices with 18F-fluordeoxyglucose positron emission tomography/computed tomography angiography: initial results at an infective endocarditis referral center. *Circulation.* 2015;132:1113–1126.
46. Swart LE, Gomes A, Scholtens AM, et al. Improving the diagnostic performance of (18)F-fluorodeoxyglucose positron-emission tomography/computed tomography in prosthetic heart valve endocarditis. *Circulation.* 2018;138:1412–1427.
47. Gomes A, Glaudemans A, Touw DJ, et al. Diagnostic value of imaging in infective endocarditis: a systematic review. *Lancet Infect Dis.* 2017;17:e1–e14.
48. San S, Ravis E, Tessonier L, et al. Prognostic value of (18)F-fluorodeoxyglucose positron emission tomography/computed tomography in infective endocarditis. *J Am Coll Cardiol.* 2019;74:1031–1040.
49. Habib G, Lancellotti P, Antunes MJ, et al. 2015 ESC guidelines for the management of infective endocarditis: the task force for the management of infective endocarditis of the European Society of Cardiology (ESC). Endorsed by: European Association for Cardio-Thoracic Surgery (EACTS), the European Association of Nuclear Medicine (EANM). *Eur Heart J.* 2015;36:3075–3128.
50. Slart R. FDG-PET/CT(A) imaging in large vessel vasculitis and polymyalgia rheumatica: joint procedural recommendation of the EANM, SNMMI, and the PET Interest Group (PIG), and endorsed by the ASNC. *Eur J Nucl Med Mol Imaging.* 2018;45:1250–1269.
51. Armenian SH, Lacchetti C, Barac A, et al. Prevention and monitoring of cardiac dysfunction in survivors of adult cancers: American Society of Clinical Oncology clinical practice guideline. *J Clin Oncol.* 2017;35:893–911.
52. Farrell MB, Galt JR, Georgoulias P, et al. SNMMI procedure standard/EANM guideline for gated equilibrium radionuclide angiography. *J Nucl Technol.* 2020;48:126–135.
53. Lancellotti P, Nkomo VT, Badano LP, et al. Expert consensus for multi-modality imaging evaluation of cardiovascular complications of radiotherapy in adults: a report from the European Association of Cardiovascular Imaging and the American Society of Echocardiography. *Eur Heart J Cardiovasc Imaging.* 2013;14:721–740.

Artificial Intelligence and Translational Molecular Imaging

54. Betancur J, Commandeur F, Motlagh M, et al. Deep learning for prediction of obstructive disease from fast myocardial perfusion SPECT: a multicenter study. *JACC Cardiovasc Imaging.* 2018;11:1654–1663.
55. Hu LH, Miller RJH, Sharir T, et al. Prognostically safe stress-only single-photon emission computed tomography myocardial perfusion imaging guided by machine learning: report from REFINE SPECT. *Eur Heart J Cardiovasc Imaging.* 2020. https://doi.org/10.1093/ehjci/jeaa134.
56. Betancur J, Otaki Y, Motwani M, et al. Prognostic value of combined clinical and myocardial perfusion imaging data using machine learning. *JACC Cardiovasc Imaging.* 2018;11:1000–1009.
57. Stacy MR, Paeng JC, Sinusas AJ. The role of molecular imaging in the evaluation of myocardial and peripheral angiogenesis. *Ann Nucl Med.* 2015;29:217–223.
58. Chowdhury MM, Tarkin JM, Evans NR, et al. (18)F-FDG uptake on PET/CT in symptomatic versus asymptomatic carotid disease: a meta-analysis. *Eur J Vasc Endovasc Surg.* 2018;56:172–179.
59. Tarkin JM, Joshi FR, Rudd JH. PET imaging of inflammation in atherosclerosis. *Nat Rev Cardiol.* 2014;11:443–457.
60. Dweck MR, Chow MW, Joshi NV, et al. Coronary arterial 18F-sodium fluoride uptake: a novel marker of plaque biology. *J Am Coll Cardiol.* 2012;59:1539–1548.
61. Joshi NV, Vesey AT, Williams MC, et al. 18F-fluoride positron emission tomography for identification of ruptured and high-risk coronary atherosclerotic plaques: a prospective clinical trial. *Lancet.* 2014;383:705–713.
62. Derlin T, Sedding DG, Dutzmann J, et al. Imaging of chemokine receptor CXCR4 expression in culprit and nonculprit coronary atherosclerotic plaque using motion-corrected [(68)Ga]pentixafor PET/CT. *Eur J Nucl Med Mol Imaging.* 2018;45:1934–1944.
63. Tarkin JM, Joshi FR, Evans NR, et al. Detection of atherosclerotic inflammation by (68)Ga-DOTATATE PET compared to [(18)F]FDG PET imaging. *J Am Coll Cardiol.* 2017;69:1774–1791.
64. Maddahi J, Lazewatsky J, Udelson JE, et al. Phase-III clinical trial of fluorine-18 flurpiridaz positron emission tomography for evaluation of coronary artery disease. *J Am Coll Cardiol.* 2020;76:391–401.
65. Badawi RD, Shi H, Hu P, et al. First human imaging studies with the EXPLORER total-body PET scanner. *J Nucl Med.* 2019;60:299–303.
66. Dweck MR, Jenkins WS, Vesey AT, et al. 18F-sodium fluoride uptake is a marker of active calcification and disease progression in patients with aortic stenosis. *Circ Cardiovasc Imaging.* 2014;7:371–378.
67. Zhou W, Bajaj N, Gupta A, et al. Coronary microvascular dysfunction, left ventricular remodeling, and clinical outcomes in aortic stenosis. *J Nucl Cardiol.* 2019. https://doi.org/10.1007/s12350-019-01706-y.
68. Falk RH, Dorbala S. Transthyretin cardiac amyloidosis in patients with severe aortic stenosis. *Eur Heart J.* 2020;41:2768–2770.
69. Rosenblum H, Masri A, Narotsky DL, et al. Unveiling outcomes in coexisting severe aortic stenosis and transthyretin cardiac amyloidosis. *Eur J Heart Fail.* 2020. https://doi.org/10.1002/ejhf.1974.

19 Cardiovascular Magnetic Resonance Imaging

RAYMOND Y. KWONG

PRINCIPLES OF MAGNETIC RESONANCE IMAGING, 314
Basic Physics of Magnetic Resonance Imaging, 314

CLINICAL APPLICATIONS OF CMR, 320
Coronary Artery Disease, 320
Cardiomyopathies, 322
Idiopathic Dilated Cardiomyopathy, 326
Other Cardiomyopathies, 327

Valvular Heart Disease, 328
Pericardial Disease, 329

NOVEL CMR IMAGING TECHNIQUES AND FUTURE PERSPECTIVES, 333

REFERENCES, 333

The multicomponent capability of cardiovascular magnetic resonance (CMR) provides morphologic, structural, and physiologic information relevant to a broad array of cardiovascular diseases. CMR offers technical advantages of unrestricted tomographic imaging in arbitrary scan planes, various types of tissue characterization, and a lack of need for ionizing radiation. In this chapter, we will review the current cardiac clinical applications of CMR.

PRINCIPLES OF MAGNETIC RESONANCE IMAGING

Basic Physics of Magnetic Resonance Imaging

Clinical magnetic resonance imaging (MRI) is based on generating signal from the abundant hydrogen nuclei in the human body. When placed inside the magnetic field (called B_0), the ^1H nuclei in a patient's body align with B_0, either with or against the direction of the B_0 field (known as the z-axis). The summed magnetic effect from all the ^1H nuclei is referred to as the equilibrium magnetization, which is excitable by a radiofrequency pulse to generate an MRI signal. The ^1H nuclei in different tissue environments (fat, complex protein, simple fluids, etc.) have characteristic frequencies. A radiofrequency pulse is designed so that it has a specific frequency that can activate the ^1H nuclei to generate a measurable MRI signal specific to the tissue. The spatial location of a ^1H nuclei is organized by three-dimensional (3D) magnetic field gradients inside the scanner. After delivery of a radiofrequency pulse, the electromagnetic energy absorbed by the ^1H nuclei will be released back to the environment by two coexisting mechanisms, longitudinal magnetization recovery and transverse magnetization decay. The rates of longitudinal magnetization recovery and transverse magnetization decay are measured by T1 and T2 (or T2*) values, respectively. They are important because MRI can use different pulse sequence designs to capture patterns of change in these rates to generate signal differences (contrast) on an image to identify tissue types, differentiate normal versus pathologic states, and quantify severity of pathophysiology at the tissue level. The choice of signal contrast weighting of the imaging method is partly dictated by the physiologic characteristics of the tissue being studied. For qualitative interpretation, signal enhancement (from T1 effects) is in general preferred in CMR, thus most pulse sequences used in CMR are T1-weighted techniques. Current common T1-weighted CMR techniques include gradient echo cine, myocardial perfusion, late gadolinium enhancement (LGE), and phase contrast blood flow imaging. T2-weighted and T2*-weighted CMR are primarily for imaging of myocardial edema and iron content, respectively. Cine steady-state free precession (SSFP), the standard pulse sequence for quantifying cardiac volumes and functions, employs a mixed T2/T1 weighting.

CONTRAST AGENTS IN CMR

Gadolinium-based contrast agents (GBCAs) are most commonly used in clinical CMR. When injected as an intravenous bolus, a GBCA transits through cardiac chambers and coronary arteries over 15 to 30 seconds (first-pass phase) before it diffuses into the extracellular space. At approximately 10 to 15 minutes after injection, a transient equilibrium between contrast washing-in into the extracellular space and washing-out to the blood pool is reached. At present, myocardial perfusion CMR and most magnetic resonance angiograms (MRAs) are performed during the first-pass phase, whereas LGE images are obtained during the equilibrium phase. All GBCAs are chelated to render them nontoxic and to facilitate renal excretion. GCBA use is associated with mild reactions (nausea, mild skin rash) in ~1% and severe reactions are extremely rare. In patients with severe renal dysfunction, GBCA use may expose the patient to the toxic nonchelated free gadolinium (Gd^{3+}), which can lead to nephrogenic systemic fibrosis (NSF), an interstitial inflammatory reaction that can lead to severe skin induration, contracture of the extremities, fibrosis of internal organs, and death. Risk factors to developing NSF include estimated glomerular filtration rate (eGFR) <30 mL/min/1.73 m^2, need for hemodialysis, acute renal failure, and presence of concurrent proinflammatory events. With implementation of routine screening of those at risk with creatinine clearance, weight-based dosing, avoidance of GBCA use in patients with eGFR <30 mL/min/1.73 m^2, and the use of a macrocyclic form (group II) of GBCA, NSF from GBCA had a near-zero incidence globally over the past decade. In April 2020, the American College of Radiology considered the risk of NSF from group II GBCA as sufficiently low or possibly nonexistent such that questionnaire screening and eGFR testing are no longer mandatory.

CMR IMAGING METHODS

To overcome blurring from cardiac motion, data acquisition is synchronized to the electrocardiogram (ECG) signal (cardiac gating), which is either prospective (ECG triggering follows imaging data acquisition in each cardiac cycle) or retrospective (continuous data acquisition with subsequent reconstruction based on ECG timing). For cine imaging, retrospective gating is preferred because it covers the entire cardiac cycle. Many CMR pulse sequences fractionate the data acquisition of an image to occur within a narrow window of the cardiac cycle over several heartbeats (segmented approach). To overcome blurring from respiratory motion, patient breath-holding, tracking of diaphragmatic position and motion (navigator methods), averaging of respiratory motion, and combinations can be used. In patients who cannot breath-hold or have irregular heart rhythms, static single-shot and real-time cine imaging (both involve rapid acquisition of whole images within a cardiac cycle) can achieve diagnostic studies at reduced temporal and spatial resolutions. Table 19.1 shows a summary of the most common clinical CMR pulse sequence techniques at our center. CMR uses bright-blood cine SSFP imaging or dark-blood fast spin-echo (FSE) imaging to assess cardiac morphology and structure. Cine SSFP can image the heart in motion at a high temporal resolution of 30 to 45 msec during a breath-hold of <10 seconds. For dark-blood techniques, T1-weighted FSE is used for morphology of cardiac chambers, vascular structures, pericardium, and imaging of fat. T2-weighted FSE with fat suppressed can image for myocardial edema. Myocardial tagging has been extensively validated to assess myocardial strain by marking the myocardium with dark lines or a grid to quantify the deformational change across the cardiac cycle. This type of intrinsic myocardial performance can be quantified global and regional in circumferential, longitudinal, and radial directions. However, the detection and tracking of tagged grids requires significant postprocessing effort and time, limiting clinical efficiency. Feature

TABLE 19.1 Summary of Common Clinical Cardiac Magnetic Resonance (CMR) Pulse Sequence Techniques at Brigham and Women's Hospital

CMR TECHNIQUES	PULSE SEQUENCE OPTIONS	DARK/BRIGHT BLOOD	CONTRAST WEIGHTING	TYPICAL IN-PLANE SPATIAL/TEMP. RESOLUTIONS AND OTHER IMAGING PARAMETERS	BREATH-HOLD REQUIRED	GADOLINIUM CONTRAST REQUIRED	RELATIVE MERITS OF THE PULSE SEQUENCE OPTIONS	IMAGE EXAMPLE
Cine cardiac structure and ventricular function	• Cine SSFP* • Cine FGRE • Real-time cine SSFP	Bright	T2/T1W for cine SSFP and real-time cine SSFP; T1W for FGRE	• 1.5–2.5 mm/~45 msec per phase • Adjust number of lines of K-space per cardiac cycle (segments) to balance temporal resolution and duration of patient breath-holds • 2.3–3.2mm/~60ms for real-time cine	Yes for ECG-gated cine SSFP and FGRE. Optional for real-time cine	No	Cine SSFP has higher SNR and CNR (between endomyocardium and blood) than FGRE but is sensitive to field inhomogeneity (especially at 3T), giving rise to banding artifact FGRE has weaker endocardial definition than cine SSFP, but it is an alternative when severe artifact exists in cine SSFP Good shimming or frequency scout would be needed at 3T to eliminate banding artifact Real-time cine SSFP: Use in patients with significant arrhythmia or difficulty breath-holding. It has the lowest spatial and temporal resolutions	Cine SSFP
Quantitative regional myocardial strain	Myocardial tagging (newer but less widely available techniques for regional strain exist, see text)	Bright	T1W	• Tag spacing 5–10 mm • Temporal resolution ~45 msec • Low flip angle, on order of 10° to limit tag fading	Yes	No	Tissue-tracking quantitation of intramyocardial motion Disadvantages: Tag lines fade near end of cardiac cycle and time-consuming strain analysis (postprocessing)	
Structure, morphology, and fat imaging	• Standard FSE* • SS FSE (or HASTE)	Dark	T1W ± fat suppression	• 0.8–1.5 mm/every cardiac cycle	Yes for standard fast SE. No for SS FSE	No	• Standard FSE has better image quality but relatively long scan time • Fat suppression can be achieved by fat saturation pulse (more specific) or by suppressing tissues with short T1 (a technique known as STIR, which is less specific for fat, in particular post Gd contrast). • SS FSE covers the whole heart quickly and is useful in patients with arrhythmia or limited breath-holding	

Continued

TABLE 19.1 Summary of Common Clinical Cardiac Magnetic Resonance (CMR) Pulse Sequence Techniques at Brigham and Women's Hospital—cont'd

CMR TECHNIQUES	PULSE SEQUENCE OPTIONS	DARK/ BRIGHT BLOOD	CONTRAST WEIGHTING	TYPICAL IN-PLANE SPATIAL/ TEMP. RESOLUTIONS AND OTHER IMAGING PARAMETERS	BREATH-HOLD REQUIRED	GADOLINIUM CONTRAST REQUIRED	RELATIVE MERITS OF THE PULSE SEQUENCE OPTIONS	IMAGE EXAMPLE
Myocardial scar by LGE imaging	• Standard 2D segmented FGRE* • 2D SS SSFP technique • 3D whole-heart techniques (breath-hold or navigator-guided) • Segmented or SS PSIR (phase sensitive image reconstruction)	Bright or Dark (if "black-blood" LGE is used)	T1W (10-30 minutes after 0.1-0.2 mmol/ kg GBCA injection)	• 1.5-2.0 mm/150-200 msec (for standard 2D) • Adjust inversion time and time delay after ECG detection to null "normal" myocardium and to image in diastole, respectively	Yes for standard 2D technique. No for SS technique	Yes	• Standard 2D technique has higher spatial and temporal resolutions than the SS technique • 2D SS technique covers the whole heart quickly and is useful in patients with arrhythmia or difficulty breath-holding • PSIR is less inversion time-sensitive and gives improved contrast when normal myocardium is not perfectly nulled • New 3D application using navigator-guidance yields higher SNR than 2D and can achieve spatial resolution of <1 mm without the need for breath-holding • Black-blood LGE imaging helps better identify small subendocardial scar	2D segmented LGE
Myocardial perfusion imaging	Saturation prepared gradient-echo based 2D techniques: - FGRE* - Hybrid GE-echoplanar (EPI) - SSFP	Bright	T1W	• 2.0-3.0 mm • 130-180 msec per slice • 3-4 locations every cardiac cycle or 6-8 locations every two cardiac cycles during vasodilator stress and rest • 0.05-0.1 mmol/kg IV GBCA injected at 4 or 5 mL/ sec (qualitative assessment only)	No, but breath-hold is preferable	Yes	• Breath-holding useful to track contrast-enhancement in specific segments • Parallel-imaging acceleration and sparse sampling to reduce acquisition time per slice and extend slice coverage of the heart, but carries signal-to-noise penalty	

Myocardial edema imaging	• T2W FSE* • STIR FSE • T1W EGE$_r$ • T2 prep SSFP • T2 map	Dark (FSE-based), Bright (SSFP-based)	• T2W + fat suppression (for T2W techniques) • T1W (for EGE technique)	• In-plane spatial and temporal resolutions similar to standard FSE • Slice thickness 7-10 mm to improve SNR • For qualitative assessment, algorithm needed to correct for the distance of the heart from the receiver surface coils is required • T2 map for quantification (insensitive to signal non-uniformity)	Yes	No/Yes for early gadolinium enhancement (EGE)$_r$	• Myocardial edema appears as a transmural area of high SI on T2W images • In FSE techniques, beware of artifacts from slow flow especially adjacent to regional wall motion abnormality or the LV apex, which may mimic edema • Regional myocardial signal variation from phase array coils may mimic edema • In absence of LGE, T2W edema reflects reversible myocardial injury • Using T2W FSE techniques, an SI ratio of myocardium over skeletal muscle >1.9 has been reported to be abnormal in myocarditis • An EGE, between myocardium and skeletal muscle of ≥4 or an absolute myocardial SI increase of 45% after contrast are considered abnormal in myocarditis • The bright-blood SSFP-based technique has improved CNR and is less susceptible to slow flow artifact • T2 map is insensitive to surface coil related signal inhomogeneity and slow flowing blood-related artifact
Myocardial iron content imaging	T2*W multiple echo times FGRE	Bright	T2*W	• 2.0-3.0 mm/ ~100-150 msec • One short-axis mid-ventricular location • A series of images with 6-8 echoes that goes from ~2 to 35 msec • Axial ungated acquisition of the liver for comparison	Yes	No	• Measurement is most accurate and reproducible in the mid septum • T2* value describes the exponential decay of myocardial SI as the echo time increases • At 1.5T, T2* value of <20 msec with LV dysfunction (without other obvious cause) indicates iron-overload cardiomyopathy

Continued

EVALUATION OF THE PATIENT

TABLE 19.1 Summary of Common Clinical Cardiac Magnetic Resonance (CMR) Pulse Sequence Techniques at Brigham and Women's Hospital—cont'd

CMR TECHNIQUES	PULSE SEQUENCE OPTIONS	DARK/ BRIGHT BLOOD	CONTRAST WEIGHTING	TYPICAL IN-PLANE SPATIAL/ TEMP. RESOLUTIONS AND OTHER IMAGING PARAMETERS	BREATH-HOLD REQUIRED	GADOLINIUM CONTRAST REQUIRED	RELATIVE MERITS OF THE PULSE SEQUENCE OPTIONS	IMAGE EXAMPLE
Cardiac thrombus	• LGE with long inversion time • EGE imaging	Bright	T1W	• In-plane spatial and temporal resolutions similar to LGE imaging • EGE is acquired within the first 5 min after gadolinium injection	Yes	Yes	• LGE imaging with inversion time set at 600 msec or longer or EGE imaging can detect thrombus indicated by an intense "black" regions • Look for thrombus in locations of stagnant flows	H
Cardiac blood flow	Phase contrast imaging cine GE	Bright	Velocity-related signal phase shift	• 1.5–2.5 mm/50 msec per phase • Keep number of lines of K space (segments) low to improve temporal resolution during free breathing studies	No (multiple signal averages used)	No	• Multiple averages can reduce ghosting artifacts from respiratory motion during free breathing • Should keep velocity encoding strength slightly > the highest expected flow velocity to avoid velocity aliasing while maximizing accuracy • Background phase correction may be needed for accurate results	I
Coronary MRA	• 3D whole heart volume using SSFP or FGRE* • Target-vessel approach	Bright	T2 prepared 3D SSFP or FGRE technique	• ~0.6–1.0 mm in-plane • Free-breathing navigator-guided 3D technique is currently most widely used	No, but yes for target-vessel approach	Yes at 3T or optional at 1.5T (no need for contrast with SSFP-based technique)	• Compared with the target-vessel approach, 3D coronary MRA has higher SNR and provides volumetric whole-heart coverage • T2-prepared SSFP sequence with suppression of the adjacent epicardial fat provides the strong blood vessel contrast • Contrast-enhanced FGRE-based technique is used in 3T	J

Anatomy for electrophysiologic mapping of the pulmonary vein	• 3D FGRE MRA of the left atrial volume and pulmonary veins	Bright	T1W FGRE	• 1.5-2.5 mm isotropic volume • Timing bolus is required to achieve proper timing of imaging during first-pass transit of the contrast bolus • Gating is optional but may improve border definition at the expense of prolonging breath-hold • Free-breathing navigator-guided 3D technique is being increasingly used	Yes	Yes	• Subtraction mask scan is necessary to enhance the MRA images • Coronal (more common) or axial 3D MRA of the entire left atrium and the pulmonary vein is generated for electrophysiologic mapping • Use same parameters as in the subtraction mask scan
T1 mapping for assessment of extracellular volume expansion and diffuse fibrosis	• Look-Locker (LL), or modified LL 2D gradient echo	Varying (depending on T1)	GRE LL or SS SSFP (MOLLI)	• 1.5-2.0 mm in-plane resolution • LL requires complete relaxation between repetitions • MOLLI has lower T1 resolution	Yes	Yes (measurements pre- and postcontrast required)	• MOLLI acquires all images during single cardiac phase to allow calculation of T1 maps • MOLLI requires SSFP read-outs • LL can provide high T1 resolution for short T1s

*More commonly used option.

Note: Dark-blood techniques and myocardial iron content by T2* imaging should be performed before administration of gadolinium contrast.

CNR, Contrast-to-noise ratio; *EGE*, early gadolinium enhancement ratio; *FGRE*, fast gradient-recalled echo; *FSE*, fast spin-echo; *LGE*, late gadolinium enhancement; *SI*, signal intensity; *SNR*, signal-to-noise ratio; *SS*, single-shot; *SSFP*, steady-state free precession; *T1W*, T1-weighted.

tracking detects and tracks the pattern of a patch of pixel of the myocardium ("feature") at blood pool-myocardial border across successive time frames. Given the feature tracking can be applied onto routine cine SSFP imaging, this application has gained increasing clinical adaptation. LGE is a T1-weighted imaging that detects accumulation of GBCA in the myocardium due to infarction, infiltration, or fibrosis. LGE is detected 5 to 15 minutes after an intravenous injection of GBCA (0.1 to 0.2 mmol/kg) (hence the term "late"). LGE data can be captured in 2D or 3D. Phase-sensitive inversion recovery (PSIR) reconstruction is routinely used in LGE imaging to enhance myocardial tissue contrast. In patients who cannot perform breath-holding, LGE imaging can be acquired using either the single-shot method or navigator guidance. CMR perfusion imaging examines the first-pass transit of an intravenous bolus of GBCA as it travels through the coronary circulation. Several perfusion techniques are available; fast bright-blood gradient-echo imaging acquires three to five short-axis slices of the heart every cardiac cycle during the injection of a GBCA bolus. Gadolinium provides strong signal enhancement in well-perfused region compared with hypoenhancement (dark regions) in poorly perfused myocardium. At a spatial resolution of approximately 2 mm in-plane, CMR perfusion can provide information of myocardial blood flow at the endocardial/epicardial or at a segmental level. T2-weighted imaging detects myocardial edema from ischemic injury or inflammation, and it has been shown to have high correlation to the area-at-risk after acute myocardial infarction (MI). It also complements LGE in determining the chronicity of an MI and allowing for accurate measurement of *salvageable myocardium*. The pulse sequence options for T2-weighted imaging include black-blood short T1 inversion recovery (STIR) FSE and the newer SSFP-type methods and their merits are listed in Table 19.1. T2* is a transverse relaxation parameter well-validated method for measuring tissue iron content. A T2* of <20 msec (normal myocardium ~40 to 50 msec) is diagnostic of myocardial iron overload and a T2* of <10 msec is evidence of severe iron overload. Despite challenges from small luminal sizes and cardiac and respiratory motions, technical advances in coronary MRA imaging have favored the use of whole-heart 3D acquisition (with or without navigator guidance). Phase contrast imaging allows quantitation of velocities of blood flow and myocardial motion and intravascular flow rates. Data acquisition in MRI is slow as it acquires lines of raw data and takes approximately 200 msec to construct a single image. Parallel imaging are techniques that speed this up, using knowledge of the spatial coverage of the phased-array surface coils, to reduce the number of lines of raw data needed to be acquired by two- to threefold. It is routinely used in all commercial MRI systems to reduce acquisition time and/or improve temporal resolution. Similarly, by taking advantage of the correlation between images at different times (either within or between cardiac cycles), methods that reconstruct images at a higher efficiency using a reduced number of data (known as k-t accelerated imaging) have been in routine clinical use.

T1 and T2 Mapping
T1 mapping estimate in quantitative terms the expansion of the extracellular space in the myocardium where GBCA distribute. This method has demonstrated good correlation with collagen content of the interstitial space in conditions where diffuse fibrosis or infiltration occurs and can serve as a noninvasive method in monitoring disease progression or treatment response. Using both pre- and postcontrast T1 measurements, one determines the change of R1 (=1/T1) between pre- and postcontrast states in myocardium relative to the change of R1 in blood. This ratio estimates the tissue volume fraction filled by extracellular GBCA. Compare to T1-weighted imaging such as LGE, T1 mapping provides quantitation of the spectrum of extracellular volume (ECV) expansion from fibrosis or infiltration. T1 mapping techniques characterized myocardial pathology not visible by LGE imaging. Myocardial T2 mapping, which involves acquisition of a series of images with different T2 weighting, provides a quantitative measurement of regional fraction of free water in the myocardium. Compared to T2-weighted imaging, T2 mapping renders the detection of myocardial edema more reliable and is less prone to artifacts due to either motion or arrhythmia.

Patient Safety in CMR
U.S. Food and Drug Administration (FDA)-approved MRI-conditional pacemakers and implantable cardioverter defibrillators (ICDs), that allow patients to safely undergo a MRI under specific imaging settings, are now widely available. With a standard procedure of device interrogation before and after the MRI scanning established, patients with pacemakers and ICDs that are not MRI-conditional ("legacy" devices) are now routinely undergoing CMR in many experienced centers. In a series of 1509 patients with a legacy device who underwent 2103 MRI studies, device reset was noted in 0.4%, with only one case of post-MRI device dysfunction needing replacement.[1] Sternal wires, mechanical heart valves, annuloplasty rings, coronary stents, non-metallic catheters, and orthopedic or dental implants are also safe under usual clinical CMR scanning. Common hazardous implants include cochlear implants, neurostimulators, hydrocephalus shunts, metal-containing ocular implants, most breast tissue expanders, or metallic cerebral aneurysm clips. Claustrophobia has become uncommon with the use of wide-bore scanners (~2% of patients) and most can be managed with oral sedation administered before scanning.

CLINICAL APPLICATIONS OF CMR

Coronary Artery Disease
Assessing Stable Chest Pain Syndromes
Collective evidence from the past decade demonstrated that vasodilating stress CMR perfusion imaging is accurate in diagnosing and risk stratifying for CAD in patients with stable chest pain syndromes. Stress CMR perfusion has fewer artifacts, is free from ionizing radiation, and has threefold higher spatial resolution than single-photon emission computed tomography (SPECT) (see Chapter 18). Several studies had reported that stress CMR perfusion has excellent accuracy in detecting single or multivessel coronary disease, which is higher than SPECT[2] (Fig. 19.1). The physiologic significance of stress CMR complements sensitive assessment of coronary atherosclerosis by calcium scoring (see Chapter 20).[3] Annualized cardiac event rates in patients with stable chest pain syndromes who had a negative stress CMR are consistently low across numerous single and multicenter studies.[4] In a recent multicenter registry study of 2349 patients, patients with a negative stress CMR experienced cardiac events in 0.6% annually during 5 years of follow-up[5] (Fig. 19.2). The use of stress CMR in this setting had been found to be cost-effective.[6] Quantitative stress CMR perfusion using automated algorithms is becoming the standard of care in some experienced CMR centers, with its potential advantages over qualitative methods in minimizing reader's bias, assessing microvascular coronary disease (Fig. 19.3), and improving diagnostic accuracy especially in cases of possible multivessel coronary artery disease (CAD)[7] (Fig. 19.4) and prognosticating of adverse cardiac events.[8] Multiple clinical studies and a meta-analysis had demonstrated excellent correlation of stress CMR perfusion against invasive measurement of fractional flow reserve (FFR), showcasing its high accuracy in determining the physiologic significance of coronary stenosis. In a recent randomized trial of patients with stable angina, a stress CMR strategy led to a lower incidence of coronary revascularization than invasive FFR but was noninferior in cardiac outcomes.[9] Dobutamine stress CMR captures change in both regional cine function and perfusion. It is less often used than vasodilating stress CMR perfusion imaging as it is often reserved for patients who have a contraindication to receiving vasodilating stress infusion but nonetheless demonstrated excellent sensitivity and specificity in detecting CAD regardless of the presence of underlying resting wall motion abnormality. Multiple clinical studies have shown that dobutamine cine CMR provides strong prognostic value in risk assessment of patients. In a few specialized centers, stress CMR with exercise treadmill stress has shown promising results.[10]

CMR Assessment of Myocardial Viability and Benefit from Coronary Revascularization
CMR offers multicomponent assessment of structure and physiology to inform about myocardial viability (see Chapter 36). A combined criteria of end-diastolic wall thickness of >5.5 mm and cine systolic wall thickening of >2 mm has sensitivity and specificity between 85% and 90% in the prediction of segmental contractile recovery after revascularization. In addition, the transmural extent of myocardial scar detected by LGE imaging accurately depicts a progressive stepwise decrease in functional recovery despite successful coronary revascularization, especially robust in myocardial regions of akinesia or dyskinesia. LGE is easy to perform and interpret, and a 50% transmurality cutoff is sensitive in detecting segmental contractile recovery. On the other hand, low-dose dobutamine cine imaging can provide a physiologic assessment of the mid-myocardial and subepicardial contractile

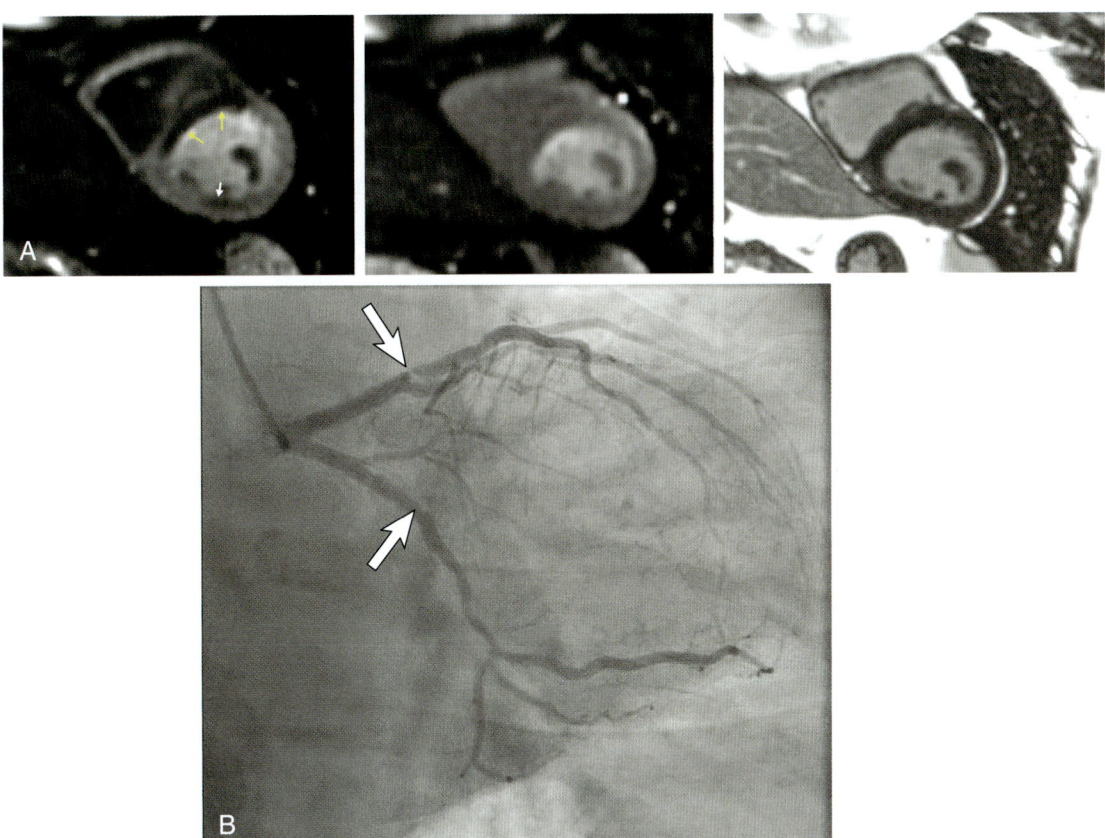

FIGURE 19.1 Stress CMR assessment of myocardial ischemia. **A,** Stress CMR perfusion (**left**) in a patient with intermittent chest pain shows severe hypoperfusion in the basal to mid septum *(yellow arrows)* and the inferolateral wall *(white arrow)*. These defects appear reversible as no significant perfusion defect is seen at rest (**middle**), and the myocardium appears viable without LGE (**right**). **B,** Coronary angiography demonstrates severe proximal left anterior descending stenosis and moderate left circumflex stenosis.

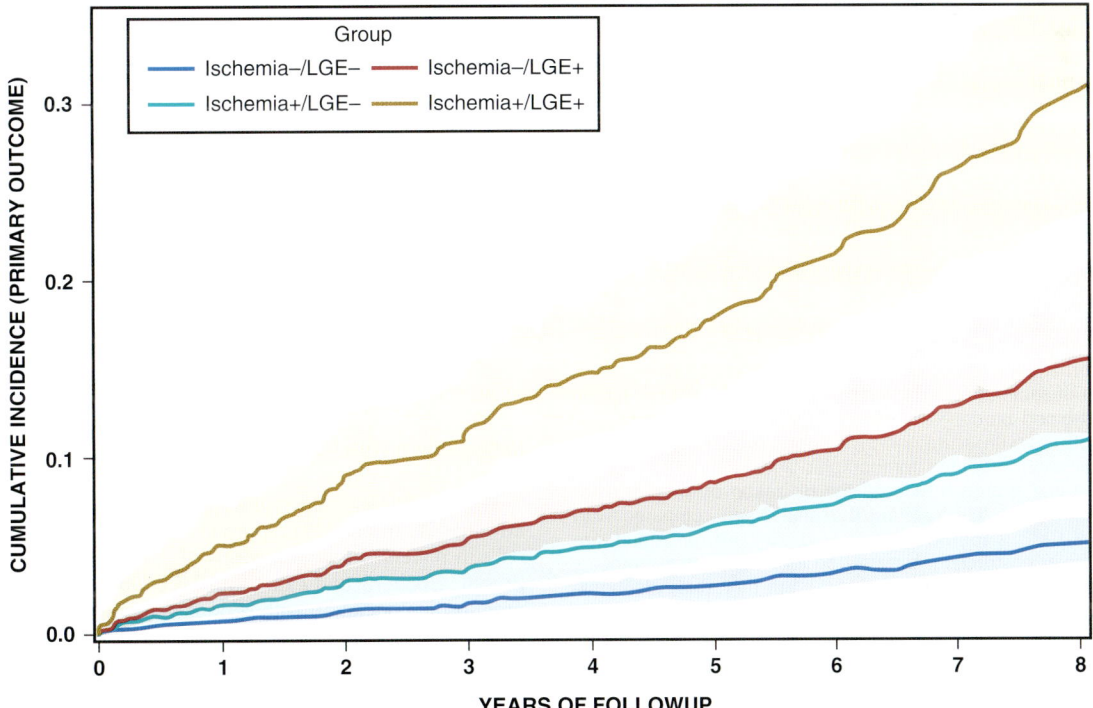

FIGURE 19.2 Stress CMR and cardiac outcome. Cumulative incidence function for the primary outcome of cardiac death or nonfatal MI in a multicenter cohort of 2349 patients presenting with stable chest pain syndromes. Patients with no ischemia (by qualitative CMR perfusion analysis) and no LGE evidence of infarction had very low incidence of primary outcome during study follow-up. (From Kwong RY, et al. Cardiac magnetic resonance stress perfusion imaging for evaluation of patients with chest pain. J Am Coll Cardiol 2019;74:1741-1755.)

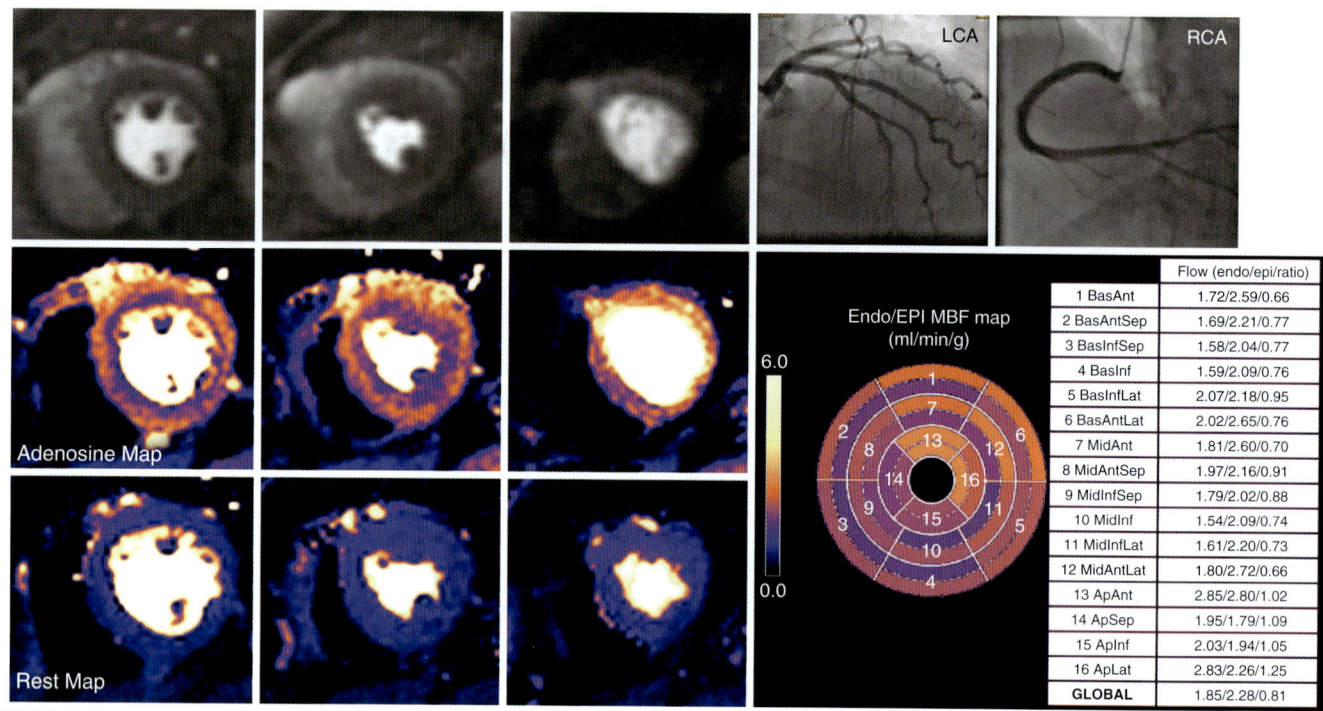

FIGURE 19.3 Microvascular coronary disease. Adenosine CMR perfusion exam in a woman with diabetes mellitus, hypertension, exertional chest discomfort, and normal coronary arteriogram reveals a diffuse subendocardial defect, prominent at the basal and mid-levels, best seen on quantitative perfusion maps. Myocardial blood flow quantification demonstrates a gradient across the myocardial wall with flow values lower in the subendocardium than the epicardium, consistent with small vessel ischemia. (Images courtesy Peter Kellman, PhD; W. Patricia Bandettini, MD.)

reserve and may be useful when tissue edema is prominent (e.g., early after an acute coronary syndrome), making infarct transmurality assessment challenging.

Assessing Acute Coronary Syndromes

In a single session, MR assesses the spectrum of myocardial changes from an acute coronary syndrome using cine cardiac structure and function, myocardial perfusion, LGE imaging of infarction, and T1- or T2-weighted or mapping of myocardial edema or other tissue characteristics. At a spatial resolution of 1.5 to 2 mm and a high contrast-to-noise ratio, CMR LGE imaging is at present the most sensitive and accurate imaging method in detecting subendocardial infarction and quantifying infarct size, respectively. CMR is not indicated as a routine first-line imaging after an acute MI, but it is useful in assessing the most common issues after an acute MI, including addressing the perfusion status of MI or the extent of noninfarct salvageable myocardium, or complications such as formation of aneurysm, intracavitary thrombus, microvascular obstruction (Fig. 19.5), pericarditis, or ventricular septal defect (Fig. 19.6). In patients with an acute reperfused MI, regions of ischemic area-at-risk, microvascular obstruction (no-reflow), and intramyocardial hemorrhage can be quantified by T1 or T2 mapping, LGE, and T2* mapping, respectively. Dark-blood LGE imaging improves the detection of subendocardial infarction by enhanced discrimination of the infarct-blood border[11] (Fig. 19.7). In a small randomized clinical trial of patients with acute non-ST elevation MI, CMR in conjunction with coronary computed tomographic angiography (CTA) as a combined first-line approach reduced the utilization of invasive angiography without adversely affecting outcome when compared with routine care.[12] CMR is the noninvasive gold standard for infarct size and microvascular obstruction. Not only do these CMR measurements contribute to long-term prognosis after MI,[12] but they allow identification of potential benefits associated with new cardioprotective strategies both in experimental and clinical trials.[13] In patients presenting with a ST-segment elevation myocardial infarction (STEMI) after a primary percutaneous coronary intervention (PCI), CMR has also shown moderate-good agreement with invasive FFR assessment of the significance of nonculprit coronary lesions.[14]

CMR is effective in diagnosing and guiding the management of acute chest pain syndromes. In a randomized study of acute chest pain patients with elevated troponins, a combined CMR and coronary CTA strategy imaging for infarction, myocardial salvage, and coronary stenosis resulted in more efficient utilization of invasive coronary angiography.[15]

In a cohort of 388 patients with acute elevation of serum troponins but with nonobstructive coronary arteries, CMR identified the causes for abnormal troponins in approximately three-fourths of patients as myocarditis, acute MI, or other cardiomyopathies. The remaining one-fourth with no abnormality on CMR had a favorable prognosis.[16] In a recent study of 229 patients with elevated troponins and nonobstructed coronary arteries, the use of a new 3D free-breathing (navigator-prepped) LGE imaging method enabled an in-plane resolution of 1.3 mm in infarct detection and reduced inconclusive diagnosis by 29%[17] (Fig. 19.8).

Cardiomyopathies

Overall Approach to Undiagnosed Cardiomyopathy

CMR is an invaluable tool for assessing various cardiomyopathies given its multifaceted interrogation of ventricular structure and myocardial physiology in matching arbitrary scan planes. CMR assessment of rest and stress myocardial perfusion, regional function, LGE, and T2-weighted imaging is useful in differentiating causes of cardiomyopathies and providing guidance for management. In the past few years, T1, ECV fraction, and other tissue mapping methods have provided novel diagnostic insights and validated noninvasive estimates of severity of fibrosis or infiltration from various causes of cardiomyopathy.[18] Inclusion of a stress CMR component is complementary to LGE imaging of infarction in ruling out ischemia as a factor in cardiomyopathy. Multiple multinational registries now exist with CMR incorporated to advance the understanding of the interacting roles of genotypes and risks in patients in various forms of genetic cardiomyopathies.[19] The presence, pattern, and extent of LGE continue to demonstrate strong prognostic association with serious ventricular arrhythmias and sudden cardiac death in various types of cardiomyopathies, although specific guidance of ICD therapies is a matter of ongoing research.[20]

Hypertrophic Cardiomyopathy

Compared with echocardiography, CMR provides a more complete 3D morphologic pattern of left ventricular (LV) hypertrophy and tissue characteristics in patients with hypertrophic cardiomyopathy (HCM) and can monitor the progression of disease at a higher precision than echocardiography (see Chapter 16).[21] CMR has higher sensitivity than

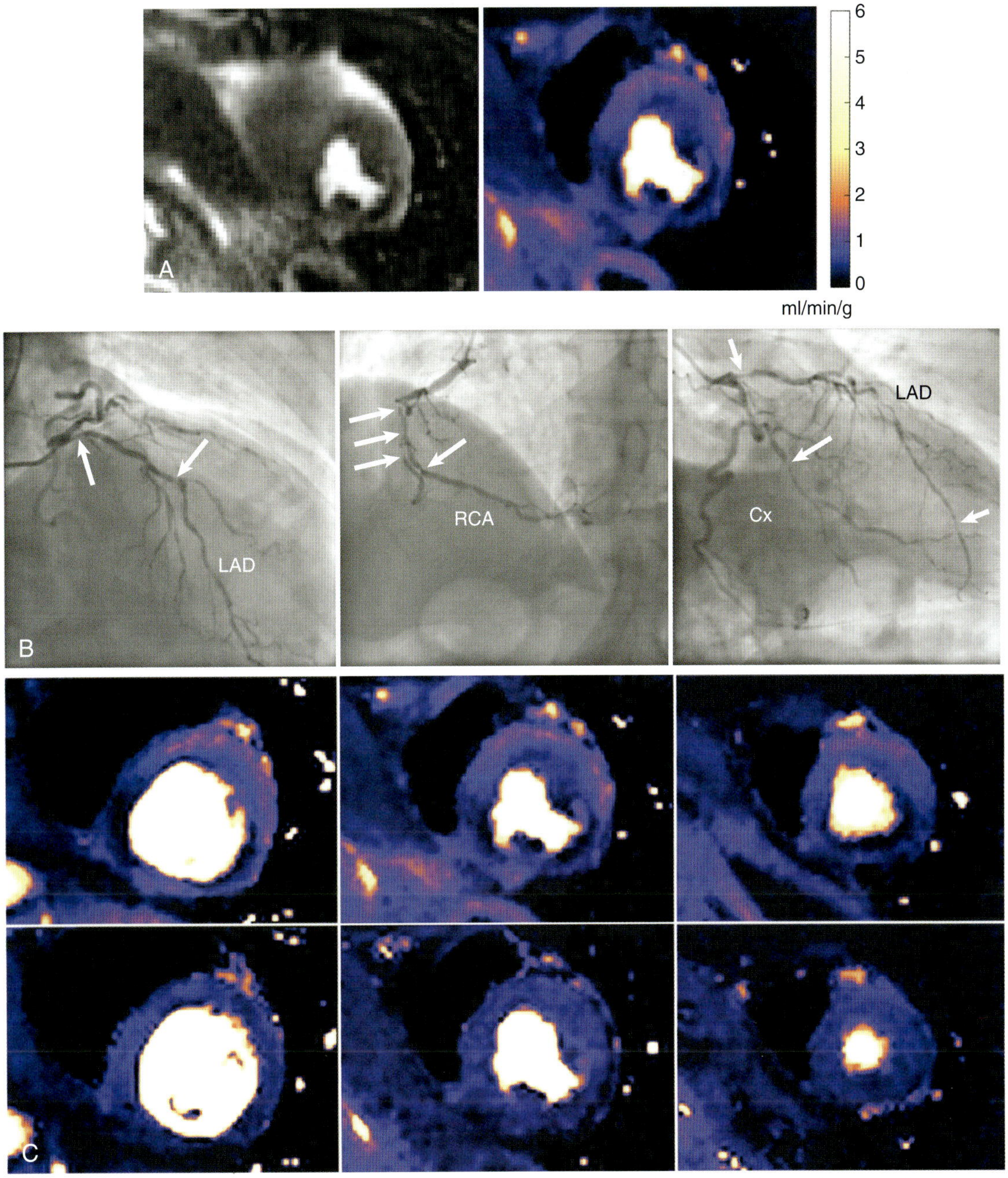

FIGURE 19.4 Quantitative CMR perfusion mapping in multivessel CAD. **A,** First-pass adenosine stress perfusion image **(left)** and corresponding quantitative myocardial perfusion map **(right)** in a patient with angiographically confirmed unbalanced three-vessel CAD **(B).** Visual analysis suggested discrete stress perfusion defects whereas perfusion maps show more extensive global ischemia consistent with three vessel disease **(C).** (Images courtesy Peter Kellman, PhD, NIH, Bethesda, MD, USA and Drs. Tushar Kotecha and Marianna Fontana, Royal Free Hospital, London, UK.)

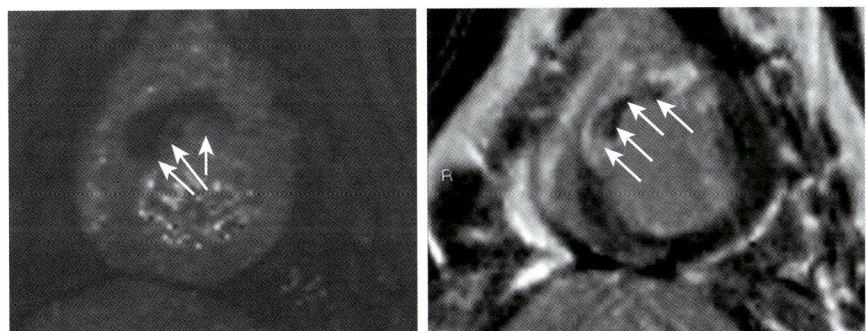

FIGURE 19.5 Microvascular obstruction. **Left,** Short-axis T2*-weighted image from a porcine model of reperfused MI demonstrating intramyocardial hemorrhage in the anteroseptum. **Right,** Short-axis phase-sensitive inversion recovery LGE image in the same animal demonstrating transmural LGE with a mid-wall region of intramyocardial hemorrhage. (Courtesy Christopher Kramer, MD and Michael Salerno, MD, PhD, University of Virginia Health System.)

echocardiography for diagnosing HCM by capturing hypertrophy of the basal anterior wall or apical aneurysm, which are occasionally missed by echocardiography (Fig. 19.9 and 19.5). LV mass index varies widely with maximal LV wall thickness due to heterogeneity of the HCM phenotype (see Chapter 54). Markedly elevated LV mass index (men >91 g/m² and women >69 g/m²) and maximal wall thickness of >30 mm have been shown to be sensitive and specific markers of risk of cardiac death, respectively. In a large series, the extent of LGE was indicative of heterogeneous fibrosis and was associated with ventricular arrhythmias, progressive LV dilation, and cardiac events, regardless of presence of outflow obstruction or prior septal myectomy.[22] The

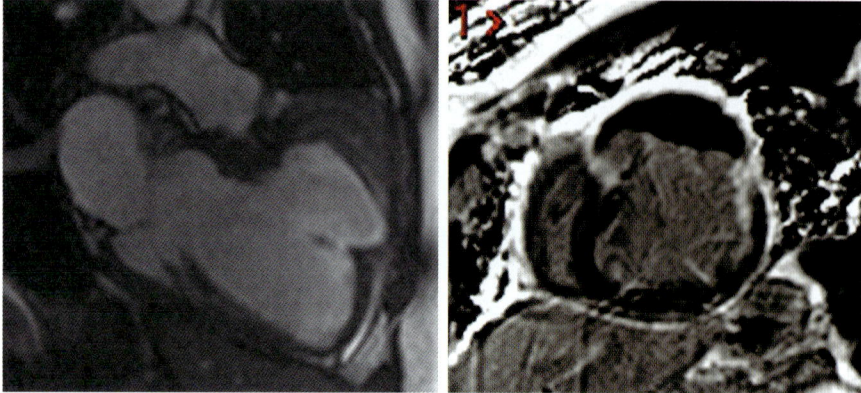

FIGURE 19.6 Ventricular pseudoaneurysm. **Left,** A two-chamber long-axis SSFP cine image at end-diastole in a patient 5 years after anterior MI demonstrating a chronic anterior pseudoaneurysm. Note the narrowed neck of the pseudoaneurysm. **Right,** Short-axis phase-sensitive inversion recovery LGE image from the same patient demonstrating enhancement of the fibrous outer layer of the pseudoaneurysm, which is lined with thrombus, which appears black. (Courtesy Christopher Kramer, MD and Michael Salerno, MD, PhD, University of Virginia Health System.)

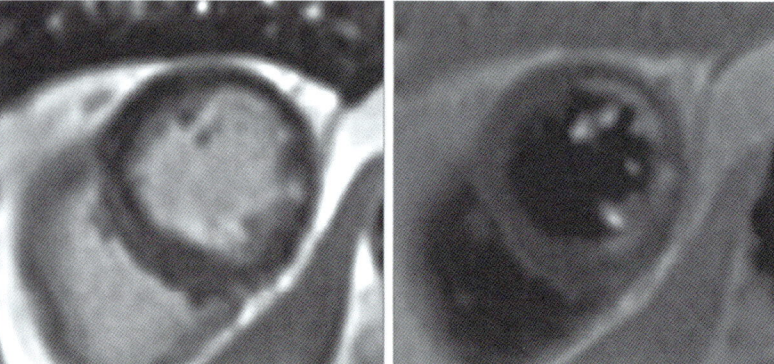

FIGURE 19.7 Dark-blood LGE. Dark-blood LGE imaging increases the contrast between endocardial infarction and blood pool, which allows better delineation of the subendocardial infarct border and increased sensitivity in infarct detection. (Courtesy Peter Kellman, PhD, NIH, Bethesda, MD, USA.)

multifaceted approach by CMR allows an individualized characterization of abnormal myocardial pathophysiology secondary to coronary microvascular dysfunction, fibrosis, and hypertrophy. Quantifying left atrial remodeling by cine CMR, LGE, and regional strain imaging estimates the risk of atrial fibrillation in HCM patients.[23] Recent work from specialized centers demonstrated that in vivo myocardial disarray could be imaged by diffusion tensor CMR. The directionality of myocardial disarray (known as fractional anisotropy) was shown to have strong association with ventricular arrhythmia independent of presence of fibrosis.[24] A National, Heart, Lung, and Blood Institute (NHLBI)-funded prospective multinational registry (HCMR) has recently completed enrollment of 2755 HCM patients incorporating CMR, genetic data, biomarker data, and clinical outcomes.[25] On the other hand, CMR has also been included in the large international Sarcomeric Human Cardiomyopathy Registry (SHaRe) describing long-term national history of HCM patients with LV dysfunction.[26]

Arrhythmogenic Cardiomyopathy

Arrhythmogenic cardiomyopathy distinguishes itself from other cardiomyopathies by (1) a predisposition toward ventricular arrhythmia that precede overt morphologic abnormalities and even histologic substrate and (2) diverse phenotypic manifestations including LV or biventricular involvement (see Chapter 52). CMR offers advantages over echocardiography by its quantitative and volumetric assessment of right ventricular (RV) function and its fibrofatty tissue characterization of myocardium. The 2010 Task Force Criteria affirmed CMR as an integral and a standardized component in the workup of arrhythmogenic cardiomyopathy, in which it described a combination of regional RV akinesia/dyskinesia/dyssynchronous contraction and significant RV dilation or dysfunction as constituting major diagnostic criteria. These abnormalities are typically observed in predilection

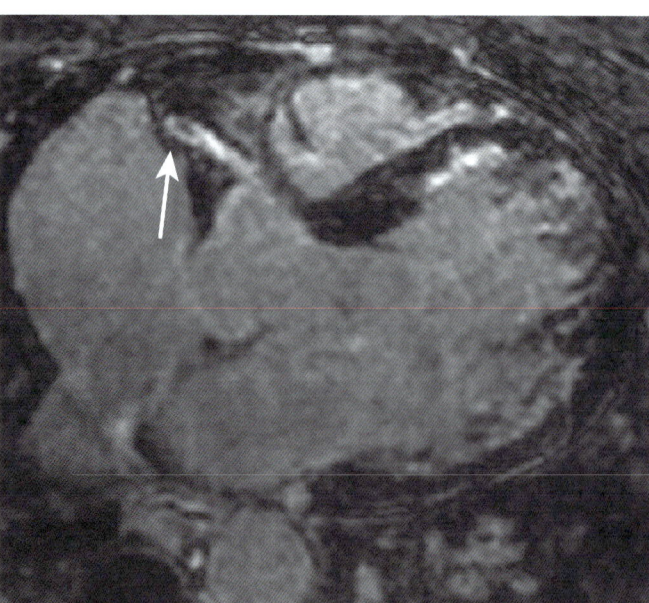

FIGURE 19.8 High resolution 3D late gadolinium enhancement. A free-breathing 3D CMR dataset that captures both coronary anatomy (arrow) and an anteroseptal and apical myocardial infarction. Compressed sensing data acquisition and reconstruction were used to shorten the scan time. (Courtesy Reza Nezafat, PhD, Beth Israel Deaconess Medical Center.)

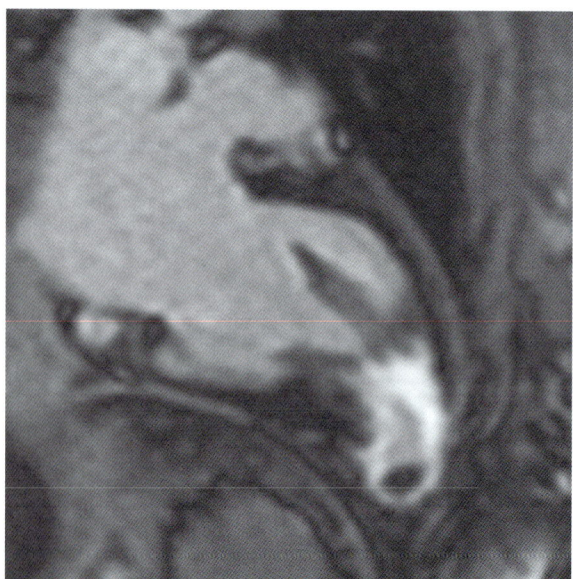

FIGURE 19.9 Apical hypertrophic cardiomyopathy with apical thrombus. CMR in a 36-year-old man with syncope demonstrates "burnt out" apical HCM with evidence of an apical LV thrombus on LGE imaging and cine functional four- and two-chamber imaging. The apical thrombus resolved with anti-coagulation and an ICD was implanted. (Courtesy Naeem Merchant, MD and Bobak Heydari, MD, MPH. Stephenson Cardiac Imaging Center, University of Calgary, Calgary, Canada.)

areas, including the subtricuspid region, basal RV free wall, and LV posterolateral wall.[21] Evidence of RV fat by CMR as an isolated finding is of limited diagnostic specificity, but fat-suppressed LGE imaging of the RV fibrosis has shown a high correlation with endomyocardial biopsy and the inducibility of ventricular arrhythmias. In a recent cohort of 140 patients with a definite diagnosis of arrhythmogenic cardiomyopathy who were followed for 5 years, biventricular, isolated LV and isolated RV involvement were reported in 37%, 12%, and 41%, respectively. Patients with LV involvement experienced substantially higher risk of sudden death or arrhythmic events than those with solitary RV involvement, and no events were observed in those with a negative CMR[27] (Fig. 19.10).

Myocarditis

CMR targets the three main pathophysiologic components of myocarditis (see Chapter 55): myocardial edema by T2-weighted imaging, regional hyperemia and capillary leak by early gadolinium enhancement ratio (EGE_r), and myocardial necrosis or fibrosis by LGE imaging. From the Lake Louise Criteria Guideline using pooled data of the single-center studies, T2-weighted imaging, EGE_r, and LGE have individual sensitivities and specificities of 70% and 71%, 74% and 83%, and 59% and 86%, respectively. A combined approach using T2-weighted images and LGE provides high diagnostic accuracy for acute myocarditis. However, two recent meta-analyses found that T1 or T2 mapping increased diagnostic accuracies over the conventional Lake Louise diagnostic criteria.[28,29] The subepicardium and midmyocardium of the inferolateral walls have been described in parvovirus-related cases, whereas septal involvement has been associated with human herpesvirus 6 with potentially more serious sequelae. T2 mapping has been shown to differentiate acute versus healed stages of myocarditis in cases where chronicity of myocarditis is uncertain.[30] Several large single-center studies have indicated LGE pattern to be a strong prognostic marker,[31,32] and monitoring of LGE changes may identify a higher risk cohort than captured by serum troponins or inflammatory biomarkers[33,34] (Fig. 19.11).

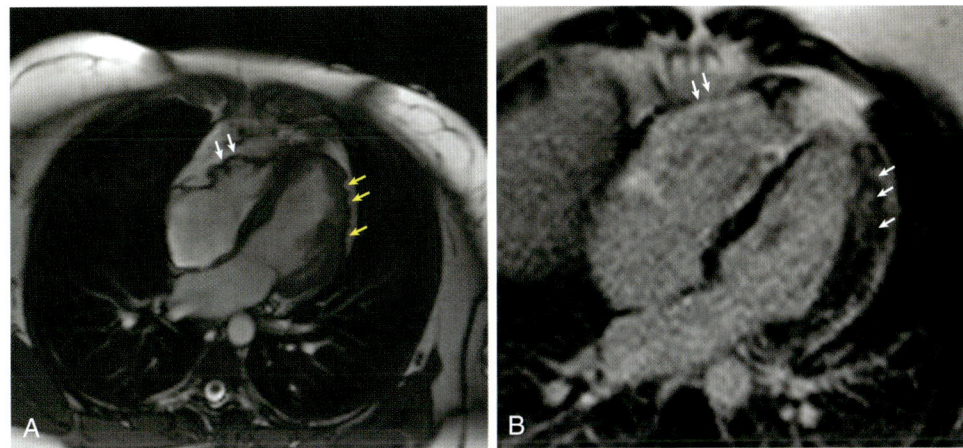

FIGURE 19.10 Arrhythmogenic cardiomyopathy. CMR images in a woman who developed heart failure following birth of her second child. The ECG showed left anterior fascicular block and frequent ventricular couplets. Echocardiography demonstrated mild LV and RV dysfunction, with hyperdynamic function of the RV apex relative to the rest of the right ventricle (McConnell's sign). The differential diagnosis included peripartum cardiomyopathy, pulmonary embolism, myocarditis, arrhythmogenic cardiomyopathy, and cardiac sarcoidosis. **A**, End-systolic frame from cine CMR shows "crinkling" or "accordion sign" of the RV base *(white arrows)* and notching of the LV epicardium due to fatty infiltration *(yellow arrows)*. **B**, Post-contrast T1-weighted inversion recovery image shows LGE of the RV free wall and LV epicardium *(arrows)*. These findings are highly suggestive of arrhythmogenic cardiomyopathy. Subsequent genetic testing revealed pathogenic mutations in PKP2 and Asn557Asp, confirming this diagnosis. (Courtesy Amit Patel, MD, University of Chicago Medicine.)

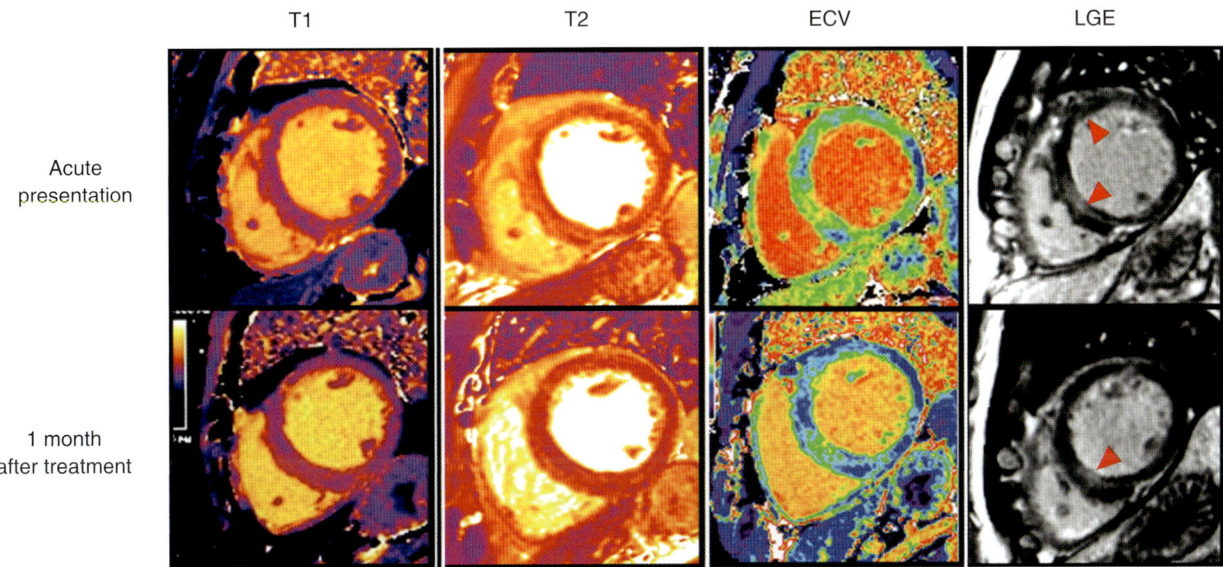

FIGURE 19.11 Serial assessment of myocarditis. **Top**, CMR at 1.5T in a 54-year-old man with fever, chills, rash, and elevated troponin, sedimentation rate, and C-reactive protein revealed dilated cardiomyopathy with a LV ejection fraction of 28%. There were diffuse inflammatory abnormalities with T1 >1300 msec, T2 >70 msec, ECV ~50%, and patchy mid-wall enhancement on LGE imaging, consistent with acute myocarditis. He was treated with intravenous immunoglobulin, methylprednisolone, tofacitinib, and tocilizumab. **Bottom**, Serial CMR aided in monitoring response to therapy, demonstrating reduction in T1 to 1100 ms, T2 to 55 ms, ECV to ~40%, and extent of LGE, as well as improvement, but not normalization, in LV volume and ejection fraction (39%). (Courtesy Drs. W. Patricia Bandettini and Alessandra Brofferio, National Heart, Lung, and Blood Institute, Bethesda, Maryland.)

Cardiac Sarcoidosis

CMR may enhance disease detection through the successive histologic stages of disease: tissue edema, noncaseating granulomatous infiltration, and patchy myocardial fibrosis (see Chapter 52). LGE imaging has been reported to identify myocardial abnormalities due to sarcoidosis at a higher sensitivity than the modified Japanese Ministry of Health guidelines. Most commonly, cardiac infiltration based on LGE imaging is seen in multiple locations involving the septum and basal anterior part of the right ventricle. Typical cases demonstrate expansion of the wall thickness matched with LGE infiltration and occasionally high signal on T2-weighted imaging indicative of edema (Fig. 19.12). In cases where septal LGE is seen, CMR may also guide sampling during endomyocardial biopsy and increase tissue yield. In a recent cohort of 321 patients with biopsy-proven systemic sarcoidosis, CMR had higher sensitivity in screening for cardiac involvement than echocardiography. During follow-up, LGE presence portended a near sixfold increased risk of adverse cardiac outcomes, whereas echocardiographic parameters were not predictive.[35] In patients with known cardiac sarcoidosis, current evidence suggests that presence, multiple foci, extent of LGE, RV systolic dysfunction, and RV LGE are the strongest risk markers for mortality or significant ventricular arrhythmias.[36,37] Per current American College of Cardiology (ACC)/American Heart Association (AHA) guideline, patients with cardiac sarcoidosis, the presence of LGE is a Class IIa indication for ICD therapy in patients with an expected meaningful survival >1 year.[38]

Cardiac Amyloidosis

In patients with cardiac amyloidosis (see Chapter 53), CMR typically demonstrates morphologic changes of a restrictive cardiomyopathy, circumferential and diffuse LGE in the LV with possible RV subendocardial involvement, and in some cases microvascular dysfunction on first-pass perfusion matching the LGE regions. Its diagnostic accuracy is excellent in published series and may obviate the need for endomyocardial biopsy (Fig. 19.13; see also Fig. 72.13F, G). Cardiac amyloidosis from ATTR appears to show more ventricular remodeling of increased myocardial mass, transmural LGE, and RV involvement than the AL subtype, although these patterns overlap in a minority of patients. Myocardial T2 consistent with edema is highest in untreated cases and appears to reflect response to chemotherapy.[39] Both native myocardial T1 and ECV are increased from amyloid protein of either AL or ATTR subtypes. The transmurality and extent of LGE represent advanced cardiac amyloidosis, and these findings are associated with patient mortality incremental to common risk markers including systolic and diastolic function. However, myocardial ECV quantitation has become a part of the standard diagnostic algorithm because it offers a more complete quantitation of the regional and global severity of amyloid infiltration as well as in monitoring treatment response. Multiple studies and a recent meta-analysis demonstrated that ECV provided incremental diagnostic and prognostic values over LGE and native T1.[40] Patients with the uncommon cardiomyopathy secondary to hypereosinophilic syndromes may mimic amyloidosis on echocardiography but have characteristic features on CMR including diffuse endocardial fibrosis and mural thrombi (Fig. 19.14).

Idiopathic Dilated Cardiomyopathy

CMR in idiopathic dilated cardiomyopathy (see Chapter 52) can rule out ischemic or myocardial infiltration as cause of cardiomyopathy, detect patterns of LGE (which have diagnostic and prognostic values), and monitor treatment response and disease progression. Current

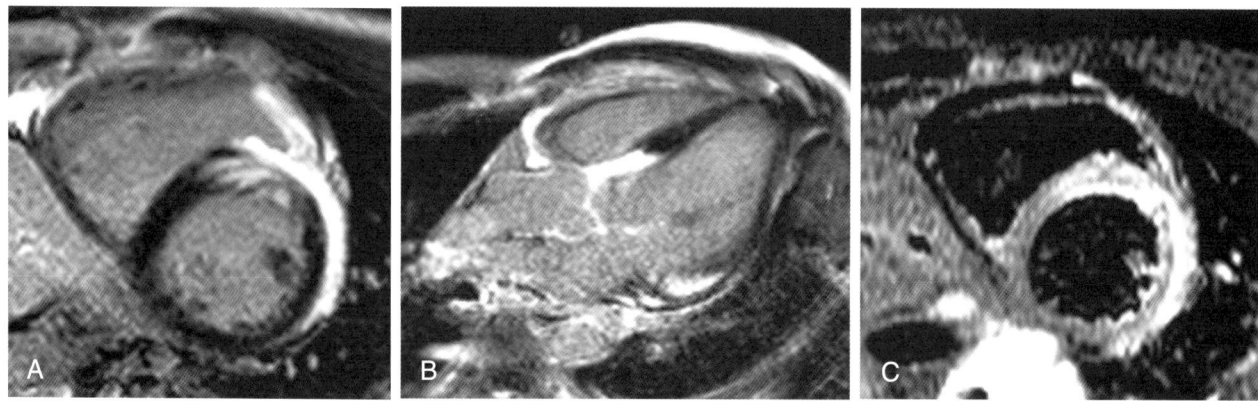

FIGURE 19.12 Cardiac sarcoidosis. CMR in a 48-year-old woman with new-onset complete heart block and history of pulmonary sarcoidosis demonstrated extensive LV subepicardial late gadolinium enhancement in short axis **(A)** and long axis **(B)** images, consistent with cardiac involvement, and myocardial edema on T2-weighted imaging suggesting active inflammation **(C)**. Intravenous pulse steroids resulting in resolution of the heart block. (Courtesy Naeem Merchant, MD and Bobak Heydari, MD, MPH. Stephenson Cardiac Imaging Center, University of Calgary, Calgary, Canada.)

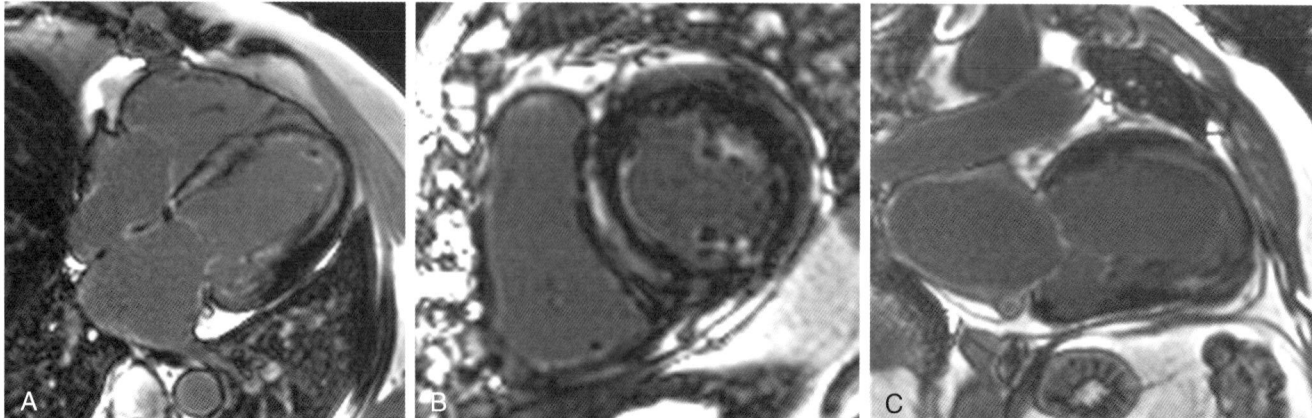

FIGURE 19.13 Cardiac amyloidosis. CMR in a 75-year-old man with worsening heart failure with persevered ejection fraction demonstrated extensive mid-wall LV **(A** and **B)** and left atrial **(C)** LGE consistent with cardiac amyloidosis. Subsequent RV biopsy confirmed the diagnosis of transthyretin (ATTR) amyloidosis. (Courtesy Naeem Merchant, MD and Bobak Heydari, MD, MPH. Stephenson Cardiac Imaging Center, University of Calgary, Calgary, Canada.)

evidence indicates that in absence of infarct LGE or perfusion abnormality, ischemic causes of LV dysfunction can be excluded (Fig. 19.15). This gatekeeper approach has been robust in most experienced CMR centers, where many patients can be spared the procedural risk, efforts, and costs of an invasive angiography. In about 30% of patients with idiopathic dilated cardiomyopathy, a patch or linear mid-wall striae septal LGE has been reported and its extent is associated with a lack of response to medical therapy, sudden death, and inducible ventricular tachycardia, independent of LV size and function.[41] ECV mapping has been validated histologically, and it has been shown that a diffuse extent of fibrosis is a stronger marker for heart failure outcomes than LGE.[18] Currently in investigation, the use of feature tracking and myofiber orientation appear promising to better understand of cardiac mechanics toward heart failure outcome,[42,43] whereas novel tissue characterization may allow better understanding of arrhythmic risks in this condition.[44]

Other Cardiomyopathies

Iron-overload cardiomyopathy is either inherited or acquired (see Chapter 52). In patients with transfusion-dependent thalassemia major, cardiac death as a result of myocardial iron toxicity occurs in 50% of patients. Global systolic LV function is usually preserved, especially in anemic thalassemic patients, until severe cardiac toxicity has developed, and thus provides little if any guidance to chelation therapy. Quantitative T2* was extensively validated and demonstrated an inverse exponential relationship with myocardial iron content. The use of T2* in guiding the use of iron-chelation therapy had led to a substantial reduction of mortality in patients with thalassemia major. In patients with reduced ventricular function, a T2* <20 msec (at 1.5T) is consistent with iron overload, whereas a myocardial T2* <10 msec indicates a high risk of clinical heart failure, despite normal LV function, within 1 year. T2* imaging on a 3T scanner provides similar clinical guidance as 1.5T, although measurements have higher reproducibility at 1.5T for iron-overload cases.[45] On the other hand, recent data indicates that T1 has high concordance with T2* in characterizing myocardial iron; indeed using a cutoff value of 800 msec (at 1.5T) is more sensitive in detecting mild iron overload than T2*. Transient LV apical ballooning syndrome (or Takotsubo cardiomyopathy), precipitated by elevated catecholamines from severe emotional or physical stress, is characterized by a transient circumferential contractile dysfunction of the apex, which is in stark contrast to basal hyperkinesia. A variant of mid-LV akinesia sparing the apex has been reported affecting as many as 40% of patients. Myocardial edema by T2-weighted imaging and perfusion defects consistent with microvascular dysfunction, matching the segments with severe systolic dysfunction, are common. LGE imaging in most cases are negative

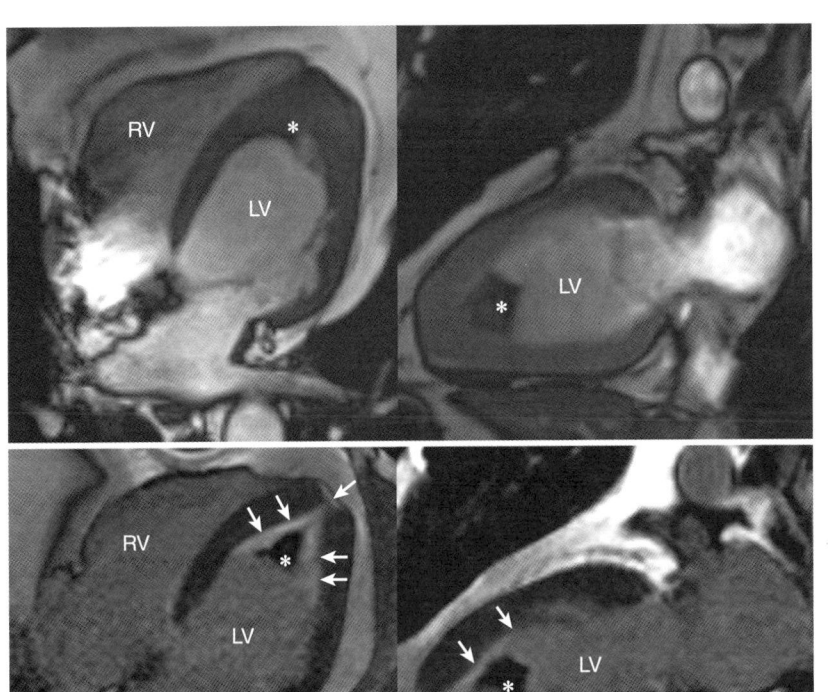

FIGURE 19.14 Loffler's cardiomyopathy. **Top,** CMR in a 63-year-old man with fatigue, elevated eosinophil count, and echocardiogram suggestive of LV apical thrombus revealed normal LV and RV systolic function with obliteration of the LV apex on SSFP cine sequences in four-chamber and two-chamber projections. **Bottom,** LGE imaging with phase-sensitive inversion recovery revealed subendocardial LGE at the LV apex (arrows) with overlying apical thrombus (asterisk). Collectively these findings are consistent with endomyocardial fibrosis (Loeffler's endocarditis). (Courtesy Aldo Schenone, MD, Brigham and Women's Hospital, Boston.)

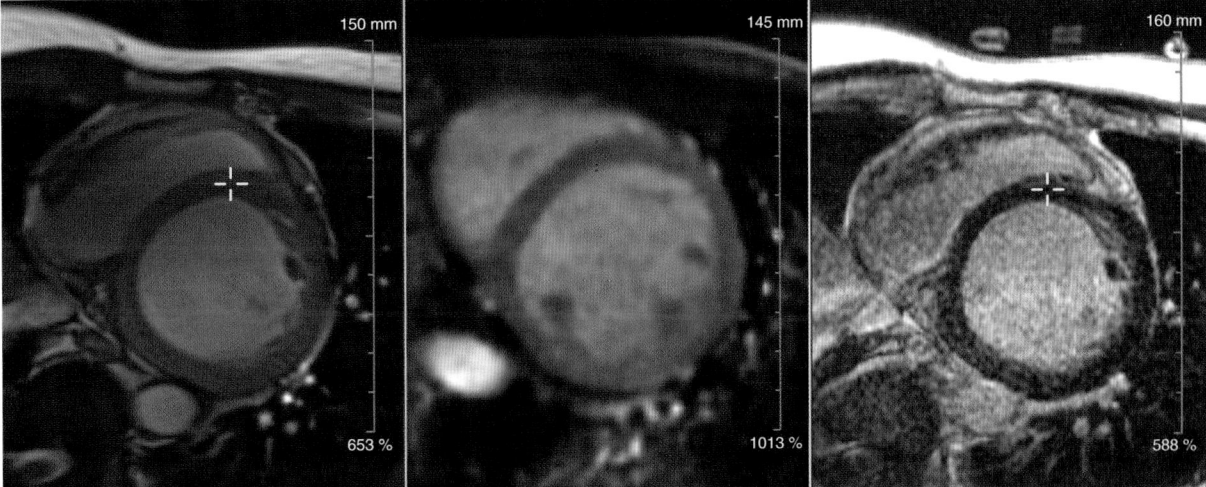

FIGURE 19.15 Idiopathic dilated cardiomyopathy. CMR diagnosis of nonischemic dilated cardiomyopathy relies on demonstration of LV dilation and systolic dysfunction **(left)** and ruling out other causes of cardiomyopathy. In this case, there was absence of both stress perfusion defect **(middle)** and LGE **(right)** so that infarction and infiltration were ruled out. In approximately 30% of patients with idiopathic cardiomyopathy, there is a characteristic mid-wall striate of LGE.

or showing only a low-intensity diffuse enhancement (<5 SD above remote myocardium) in the dysfunctional segments. Indeed, significant LGE should raise the suspicion for an alternative diagnosis of an acute coronary event. A recent study of ultrasmall superparamagnetic iron-oxide enhanced CMR demonstrated that macrophage-mediated inflammation may last for several months and is associated with clinical heart failure in patients with Takotsubo cardiomyopathy.[46]

At an investigational level, tissue mapping and feature-tracking strain analysis have expanding applications. CMR tissue mapping has remarkably high negative predictive value for clinically significant cardiac allograft rejection for obviation of routine invasive endomyocardial biopsy and capability of monitoring treatment.[47,48] For patients with pulmonary hypertension, CMR feature tracking RV strain correlates well with invasive RV-pulmonary arterial uncoupling and RV end-diastolic stiffness.[49] In patients who received anthracyclic chemotherapy, T1, T2, and ECV mapping appears to have higher sensitivity than global longitudinal strain in detecting subclinical cardiotoxicity and may help in dose titration.[50]

Valvular Heart Disease (see Part VIII)

With capability to quantify cardiac volumes, valvular and great vessel flow hemodynamics, 3D angiography, and the lack of acoustic window limitation, CMR is complementary to echocardiography in quantifying valvular dysfunction and its associated cardiac consequences.

Aortic Stenosis

For aortic stenosis (see Chapter 72), aortic valve area, by planimetry or estimates from pressure gradients, is reliable and can be measured in most native aortic valves without severe calcifications.[51] As myocardial consequences are the most common in severe valvular disease if not timely managed, some argue that CMR methods can better time intervention than an isolated assessment of valvular severity. Diffuse (patchy LGE) or replacement (endocardial) myocardial fibrosis often coexist in the pressure-loaded LV myocardium in patients with severe aortic stenosis. (see Figs. 72.6 and 72.7) In one study, presence of LGE scar, seen in 57% of the cohort, was associated with severe adverse LV remodeling, a doubling of mortality risk over 3.6 years.[52] Another study observed that ECV fraction by CMR before transcatheter aortic valve replacement (TAVR) provided strong association with mortality adjusted to LV ejection fraction and LGE (see Fig. 72.8A).[53] Using CMR spectroscopy, it has been reported that a de-energized myocardial state already developed in most moderate grade aortic stenosis.[54] These studies in combination challenges the notion if an earlier CMR-guided TAVR intervention should be implemented to improve patient outcomes. In elderly patients, coexistence of amyloidosis was noted by CMR in 8% of patients manifesting a low-flow low-gradient pattern, and it has poor prognosis.[55] CMR is a useful tool in assessing patients before or after TAVR (see Chapter 74). Compared with transthoracic echocardiography, CMR is more accurate in sizing the aortic annulus before the procedure, which predicts the severity of aortic regurgitation after TAVR. It has also been shown to be more sensitive in detecting significant paravalvular aortic regurgitation after TAVR. Metallic artifacts from prosthetic aortic valve may limit CMR assessment of aortic valvular dysfunction.

Aortic Regurgitation

For aortic regurgitation (see Chapter 73), CMR phase contrast imaging quantifies regurgitant volume without the need for geometric assumption, thus has higher reproducibility than echocardiography and is more suitable for serial monitoring (Fig. 19.16

see also Fig. 73.6). A recent study of 232 patients with chronic aortic regurgitation, CMR and echocardiography were discordant by two or more grades in 41% of patients, the majority of whom were considered to have severe aortic regurgitation by echocardiography. At a 3-year follow-up, only N-terminal pro-BNP and severe aortic regurgitation by CMR were significant predictors for heart failure and death.[56] The ability of CMR to provide high quality imaging of structure and physiology of the great vessels may complement the assessment of valvular

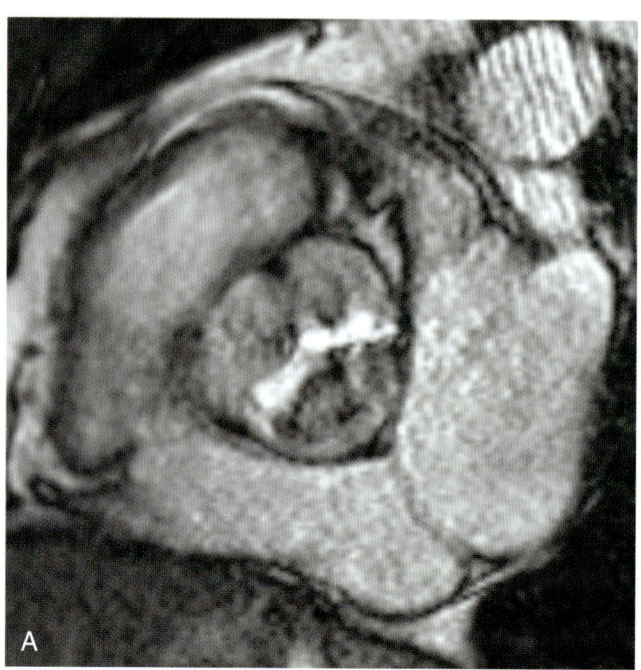

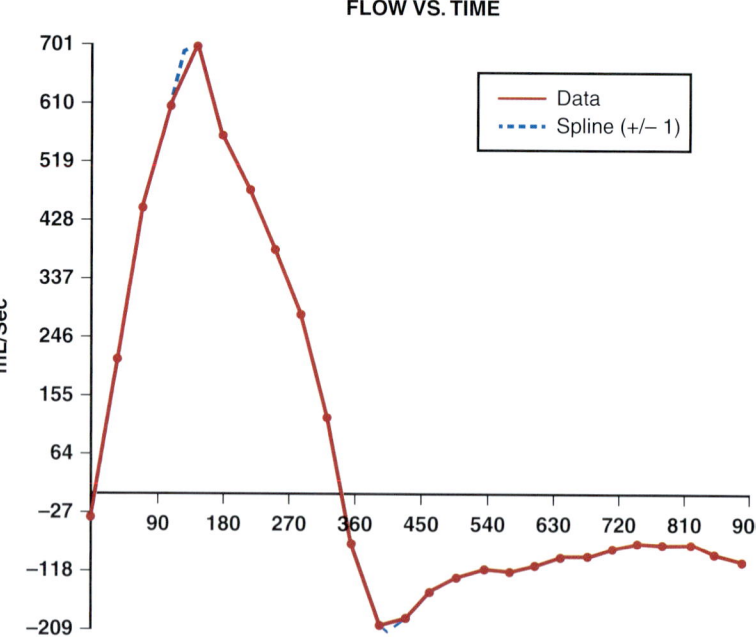

FIGURE 19.16 Bicuspid aortic valve with aortic regurgitation and ascending aortic aneurysm. **A,** CMR of a patient with bicuspid aortic valve with significant calcific degenerative changes. **B,** Severe aortic regurgitation (regurgitant volume 60 mL on velocity flow mapping). Serial imaging revealed severe aortic regurgitation (regurgitant volume 60 mL on velocity flow mapping), moderate LV dilation, normal ejection fraction (58%), and ascending aortic aneurysm. He developed symptoms and underwent aneurysm repair and valve replacement with a bioprosthesis, which is well seated without regurgitation, with associated reverse remodeling with LV end-diastolic volume decreasing from 279 mL to 137 mL.

dysfunction. 4D flow imaging can identify vortical blood flow pattern in the pulmonary artery and estimate mean pulmonary arterial pressures noninvasively. In addition, in patients with bicuspid aortic valve, visualization of vascular "vector" flow can determine vascular wall shear stress and systolic flow eccentricity, potentially predicting development of bicuspid aortic valvular aortopathy.

Mitral Regurgitation

Echocardiography is highly available and clinically adapted in assessment of mitral regurgitation as the principal technique, but it has significant interpretive variability due to characteristics of the regurgitant jet and requires major assumptions in its quantitative methods. Similar to echocardiography, CMR can visualize mitral leaflet and regurgitant jet morphology in multiple views (see Chapters 16 and 76). However, CMR can quantify mitral regurgitation without major assumption, as the difference between LV stroke volume and forward stroke volume using cine SSFP and phase-contrast imaging, respectively. CMR also provides highly accurate and reproducible assessment of LV and left atrial function and volumes. Cine CMR and phase-contrast are most often acquired in 2D currently; thus some efforts and experience are needed to ensure precise placement of imaging scan planes and elimination of base phase offset errors.[57] Significant discordance had been reported between echocardiography and CMR, where an agreement of severe regurgitant status achieved in less than 70% was reported in most studies. When echocardiographic flow convergence and Doppler-based methods or 3D echocardiography were used to quantify regurgitant volume, the agreement with CMR slightly increased. In general, 2D echocardiography diagnoses severe mitral regurgitation substantially more frequently and reports higher regurgitant volume than CMR. CMR has the advantage of accounting for flows in the entire cardiac cycle rather than reliance on a single point in time by some echocardiographic Doppler methods. CMR may provide more robust prediction of subsequent development of an indication for mitral valve surgery or heart failure mortality than echocardiography.[58] In patients who had severe mitral regurgitation by echocardiography and underwent mitral valve surgery, CMR regurgitant volume demonstrated stronger correlation to postsurgery reversal of LV remodeling than echocardiography. Adding tissue characterization to CMR scanning of mitral regurgitation may help with patient risk assessment. A single-center study demonstrated that LGE evidence of fibrosis was prevalent in patients with mitral regurgitation secondary to leaflet prolapse, and it was associated with ventricular arrhythmic events or sudden death.[59] In patients with CAD, LGE infarct size and ischemic mitral regurgitation severity by CMR were additive in patient risk assessment[60] (Fig. 19.17).

Tricuspid Regurgitation

CMR quantifies tricuspid regurgitant volume by the difference of RV stroke volume and pulmonary arterial forward volume. In small studies, moderate to high agreement was reported between echocardiography and CMR grading of tricuspid regurgitation severity.[61]

Pericardial Disease (see Chapter 86)

Echocardiography in most cases should be performed first-line as it offers a rapid assessment of the pericardial structures and physiologic significance from pericardial constriction or cardiac tamponade, but a

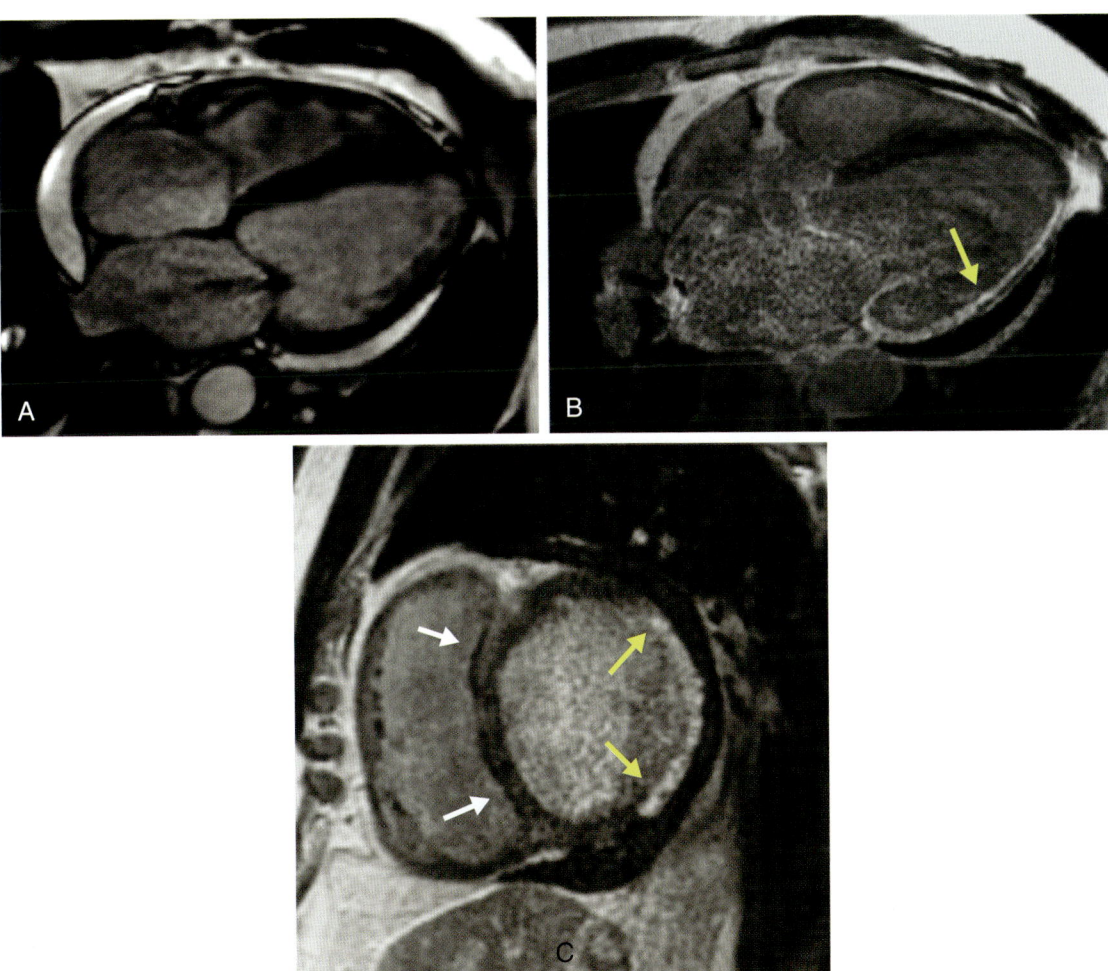

FIGURE 19.17 Ischemic mitral regurgitation. **A,** CMR in a 70-year-old man with new-onset heart failure in the setting of ischemic cardiomyopathy revealed severe biventricular dysfunction, akinesia of the lateral wall, and severe mitral and tricuspid regurgitation. Volumetric analysis confirmed marked LV dilation and dysfunction (LVEDV 185 mL and ejection fraction 21%). Flow velocity mapping across the aortic valve showed a stroke volume of 20 mL, with a regurgitant fraction of 48%, confirming severe mitral regurgitation. **B** and **C,** LGE images showed a lateral wall transmural myocardial infarction (*yellow arrows*) together with tethering of the posterior mitral leaflet. In addition, midwall septal fibrosis (*white arrows*) suggested mixed ischemic and nonischemic cardiomyopathy.

CMR offers a comprehensive assessment complementary to echocardiography in hemodynamically stable patients. A typical CMR protocol for pericardial diseases includes cine SSFP (pericardial structures), T1- and T2-weighted black-blood FSE (structures and T2-STIR imaging for edema), and LGE imaging (pericardial inflammation). In patients with suspected constriction, real-time cine SSFP (with or without Valsalva) may detect respirophasic septal shift due to ventricular interdependence. First-pass perfusion and contrast T1-weighted imaging may determine vascularity of a pericardial mass (e.g., differentiate tumor versus thrombus). Myocardial tagging (dark lines or grids) may identify regional concordance from pericardial adhesions. Pericardial thickness can be shown on either black-blood FSE or cine imaging, where up to 2 mm is considered normal; however, minimal but diffuse increased thickness is observed in 20% of patients with significant pericardial constriction. Pericardial LGE after the administration of GBCA indicates active pericardial inflammation and has been shown to complement C-reactive protein levels in diagnosing active pericarditis and predicting reversibility of pericardial inflammation and even constrictive physiology in response to anti-inflammatory medical therapies (Fig. 19.18). A recent study demonstrated quantitative pericardial LGE extent could predict the likelihood of clinical recurrence of pericarditis, incremental to clinical and inflammatory biomarkers.[62] Simple pericardial cysts usually have thin smooth walls without internal septa and their transudative contents appear homogeneous dark on T1-weighted images and bright on T2-weighted images, with no enhancement after contrast. Proteinaceous cysts are bright on T1 but dark on T2-weighted images. Exudative pericardial fluid has medium intensity on T1-weight images. Hemorrhagic effusion is bright on both T1- and T2-weighted images but darkens as hemosiderin deposition occurs as it develops into a hematoma with variable intensity. All of the previously mentioned interpretations of signal intensities on T1- and T2-weighted images need to consider the effects of through-plane flow in black-blood imaging with time-of-flight effects. Pericardial metastases are far more common (from lung, breast, and lymphomas) than primary pericardial tumors. Malignant invasion of the pericardium often shows focal obliteration of the pericardial line and a pericardial effusion. Most neoplasms appear dark or gray on noncontrast T1-weighted images except metastatic melanoma owing to its paramagnetic metals bound by melanin. Similar to CMR, computed tomography (CT) also accurately assesses the pericardial and cardiac structures, but it offers less tissue characterization or physiologic information than CMR.

APPLICATIONS IN CARDIAC ELECTROPHYSIOLOGY

CMR is helpful in planning electrophysiologic procedures given its ability to identify potential sites of ablation or scar and provide a 3D volume mapping of the atria or ventricles. For patients with paroxysmal atrial fibrillation (AF) undergoing pulmonary venous isolation (see Chapters 64 and 66), left atrial emptying function and LGE evidence of fibrosis are strong markers of AF recurrence. For those with postablation AF recurrence, atrial LGE from prior ablation can improve the success rate of a repeat pulmonary venous isolation by localizing ablation gaps and reduce procedural duration and radiofrequency application time. Although still early in development, CMR offers promise in characterizing mechanical dyssynchrony in heart failure patients and information relevant to placement of the LV pacing lead, such as coronary venous anatomy and LV scan location.

Risk Stratifying Patients at Risk of Sudden Death

CMR contributes to assessment of patients at risk of sudden death (SD) by quantitation of LV ejection fraction, RV pathology, detection of myocardial scar using LGE, anomalous coronary arteries, and less commonly T2* mapping for iron overload.[38] LV structures and LGE pattern in combination differentiate most patients in this setting as ischemic, nonischemic, and infiltrative, which provides clinical guidance and patient risk profile (see Chapter 70). In SD survivors, LGE identified unexpected myocardial scar and a potential arrhythmic substrate in more than 70% of patients. For patients with CAD, multiple single-center studies have

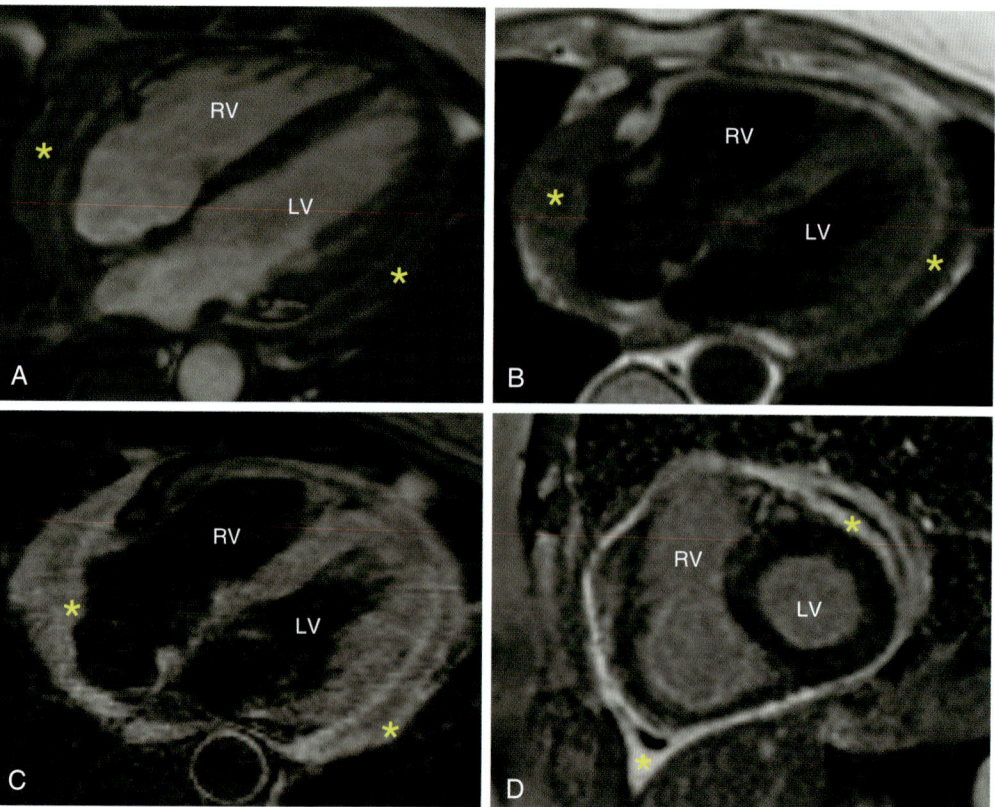

FIGURE 19.18 Constrictive pericarditis. CMR in a 66-year-old woman with recent acute pericarditis and worsening pain and dyspnea despite anti-inflammatory therapy revealing normal LV and RV systolic function. Both SSFP cine **(A)** and T1-weighted fat suppressed **(B)** sequences revealed diffuse pericardial thickening *(asterisks)*. **C,** Both pericardial layers exhibited diffuse hyperintensity on T2-weighted images consistent with pericardial edema *(asterisks)*. **D,** The pericardium enhanced on first-pass perfusion images and demonstrated severe concentric LGE *(asterisks)* signaling pericardial inflammation. There was no respirophasic shift of the interventricular septum on real-time cine acquisition with Valsalva to support a diagnosis of transient constriction. With evidence of acute pericarditis without constriction, the patient was treated with prednisone in addition to nonsteroidal anti-inflammatory agents and colchicine with eventual symptomatic improvement. (Courtesy Aldo Schenone, MD, Brigham and Women's Hospital, Boston, MA.)

reported LGE size as robust risk marker for SD independent of left ven-tricular ejection fraction (LVEF). Larger than 5% of LV mass has been reported to be a risk marker in both ischemic and nonischemic cardiomyopathies. Scar texture and scar heterogeneity might carry additional information. A multicenter long-term follow-up outcome study of heart failure patients with implanted ICD equipped with cardiac resynchronization therapy showed that a lack of LGE fibrosis was protective but greater presence of border zone channel heterogeneity identified life-threatening ventricular arrhythmias incrementally, thus raising the possibility for better triage of ICD candidates.[63] For patients with non-ischemic cardiomyopathy, a mid-wall septal LGE pattern has a noted in many patients with dilated cardiomyopathy and its size has been reported to be associated with inducibility of ventricular arrhythmias and SDs. LV LGE in patients with systemic sarcoidosis has a high risk of SD. More research is needed to define how the LGE extent can improve the current practice guidelines specifically toward ICD therapy.

ADULT CONGENITAL HEART DISEASE

CMR can complement other imaging for adult congenital heart disease (see Chapter 82) based on several factors: lack of radiation exposure to young patients, 3D tomographic imaging of thoracic structures and anatomy (compared with the more limited echocardiographic windows with body growth), and correlation of complex anatomy with blood flow and physiology.

Atrial and Ventricular Septal Defects

CMR offers a less invasive alternative to transesophageal echocardiography and even diagnostic catheterization for patients presenting with right-sided volume overload from a suspected left-to-right shunt. A CMR study can detect the presence of an atrial septal defect (ASD), assess suitability for transcatheter ASD closure (Fig. 19.19), quantify right heart size and function by cine SSFP, determine pulmonary-to-systemic shunt ratio (Qp/Qs) using velocity-encoded phase-contrast, and identify any coexisting anomalous pulmonary venous return using 3D contrast-enhanced MRA. Phase-contrast imaging positioned in a plane parallel to the atrial septum and set at a low velocity range (100 cm/sec) can visualize the ASD *en face* with good correlation with defect size measured invasively. Phase-contrast imaging of the tricuspid regurgitation can estimate the pulmonary arterial systolic pressure. Because most closure devices are MRI compatible, CMR can be used to assess for residual shunt and proper device deployment. Patients with a ventricular septal defect (VSD) can be assessed using similar CMR techniques. In addition, LGE imaging may help to determine if a VSD has developed as a complication from an MI.

Anomalous Pulmonary Venous Connection

Using a large field of view, 3D MRA can capture abnormal intra-thoracic structures and vascular dynamics in anomalous pulmonary venous return (Fig. 19.20). Near-isotropic in-plane resolution can be achieved allowing reformatting in any plane to detect anomalous venous structures as small as 1 mm. The magnitude of any left-to-right shunt can be assessed by either direct blood flow measurement in the anomalous pulmonary vein or Qp/Qs ratio described previously, which is in general more accurate than invasive oximetry measurements due to the errors from mixed venous return in the right atrium.

Coarctation of the Aorta

Gadolinium-enhanced 3D MRA is sufficient in defining the site of aortic narrowing in most cases of aortic coarctation. Cine SSFP in a long-axis "candy-cane" view can further delineate the aortic anatomy, the degree of obstruction, and aortic valvular dysfunction. Cine SSFP is the gold standard for LV size, LV function, and myocardial mass. Black-blood FSE is useful to evaluate the entire aorta because it is less affected by metallic artifacts from implanted endovascular stent than gradient-echo techniques. Phase-contrast imaging can characterize the descending-to-ascending aorta flow ratio and estimate pressure gradient across the coarctation and collaterals formation (Fig. 19.21).

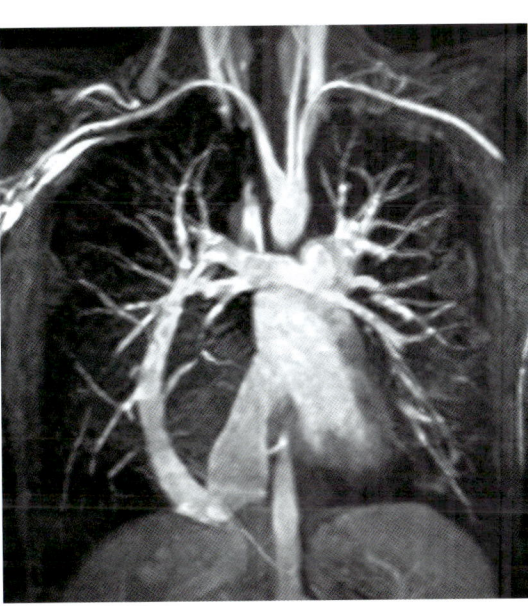

FIGURE 19.20 Scimitar syndrome. Gadolinium-enhanced 3D MRA (oblique coronal subvolume maximal intensity projection) in an adult with scimitar syndrome. (Courtesy Drs. Andrew J. Powell and Rahul H. Rathod, Boston Children's Hospital.)

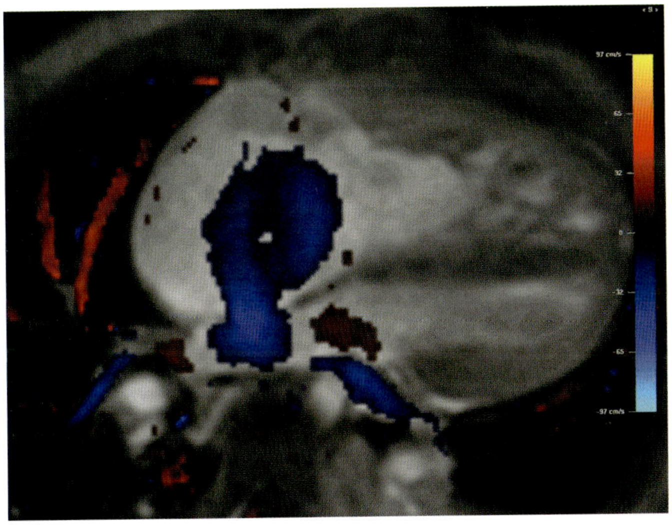

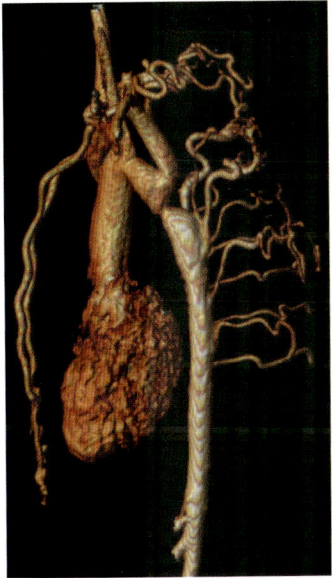

FIGURE 19.19 Secundum atrial septal defect. Color-coded phase contrast imaging demonstrated large left atrial to right atrial flow with resultant right atrial and ventricular dilation. (Courtesy Drs. Andrew J. Powell and Rahul H. Rathod, Boston Children's Hospital.)

FIGURE 19.21 Aortic coarctation. Volume rendered gadolinium-enhanced 3D MRA in a patient with aortic coarctation reveals several tortuous collateral vessels and dilated internal mammary arteries. (Courtesy Drs. Andrew J. Powell, MD, and Rahul H. Rathod, MD, Boston Children's Hospital.)

Conotruncal Anomalies

Tetralogy of Fallot (TOF) is an increasingly common referral. In patients being planned for surgical repair, key elements provided by CMR include depiction of all sources of pulmonary blood flow (including pulmonary arterial, aortopulmonary collateral, and ductus-arterial sources) in presence of RV outflow obstruction, quantitation of the severity of infundibular or pulmonary stenosis, assessment of RV function, and ruling out a coexisting anomalous coronary artery. In patients who have undergone surgery for TOF, CMR provides relevant assessment for any RV outflow aneurysm, pulmonary regurgitation fraction (patients who underwent patching of the pulmonary valve with postoperative pulmonary regurgitation), biventricular size and function, and any residual shunt. LGE imaging has been proposed for detection of myocardial fibrosis, which is associated with ventricular dysfunction, exercise intolerance, and arrhythmias. The principle physiologic abnormality in D-loop transposition of the great arteries (TGA, D-loop being the most common type of TGA) is profound hypoxemia due to ventriculoarterial discordant connection where systemic venous blood goes to the aortic and oxygenated pulmonary venous blood returns to the lung. Survival is dependent on systemic-pulmonary circulatory mixing via a ductus arteriosus, an ASD, or a VSD. An arterial switch operation is now the most common corrective surgery, but many adult patients have undergone an atrial switch procedure. CMR is useful in monitoring these patients after surgical correction by serially assessing ventricular size and function, flow across the postoperative LV and RV outflow tracts, and aortopulmonary collaterals. Systemic RV LGE is strongly associated with adverse clinical outcome especially arrhythmia in transposition of the great arteries; thus LGE CMR should be incorporated in risk stratification of these patients.

CARDIAC THROMBUS AND MASS

The differential diagnoses of an intracardiac mass includes a thrombus, tumor, or vegetation (see Chapter 98). LGE imaging can detect thrombus at a higher sensitivity than echocardiography by depicting high contrast between the dark thrombus and its adjacent structures and by imaging in 3D. Mural thrombus does not enhance on first-pass perfusion and often has a characteristic "etched" appearance on LGE imaging, thus providing higher diagnostic specificity than anatomical information alone. Multiple pulse sequences can be used to detect vascularity of tumor after contrast injection and allow differentiation from thrombus (Fig. 19.22). A pattern of hyperintensity/isointensity (compared with normal myocardium) with short TI and hypointensity with long TI was very frequent in thrombi (94%), rare in tumors (2%), and the highest accuracy (95%) for the differentiation of both entities. Common benign cardiac tumors include atrial myxoma, rhabdomyoma, fibroma, and endocardial fibroelastoma. Atrial myxomas are often seen as a round or multilobar mass in the left atrium (75%), right atrium (20%), and ventricles or mixed chambers (5%) (Fig. 19.23). They typically have inhomogeneous brightness in the center on cine SSFP imaging due to gelatinous contents and may have a pedunculated attachment to the fossa ovalis. Metastatic cardiac malignancy is much more common than primary cardiac malignancy; malignant lesions include cardiac involvement from direct invasion (lung and breast), lymphatic spread (lymphomas and melanomas), and hematogenous spread (renal cell carcinoma). Primary cardiac malignancies occur more often in children or young adults. They include angiosarcoma, fibrosarcoma, rhabdomyosarcoma, and liposarcoma. CMR in a multicenter trial correctly diagnosed 97% of these cases although a differential diagnosis was necessary in 42%.

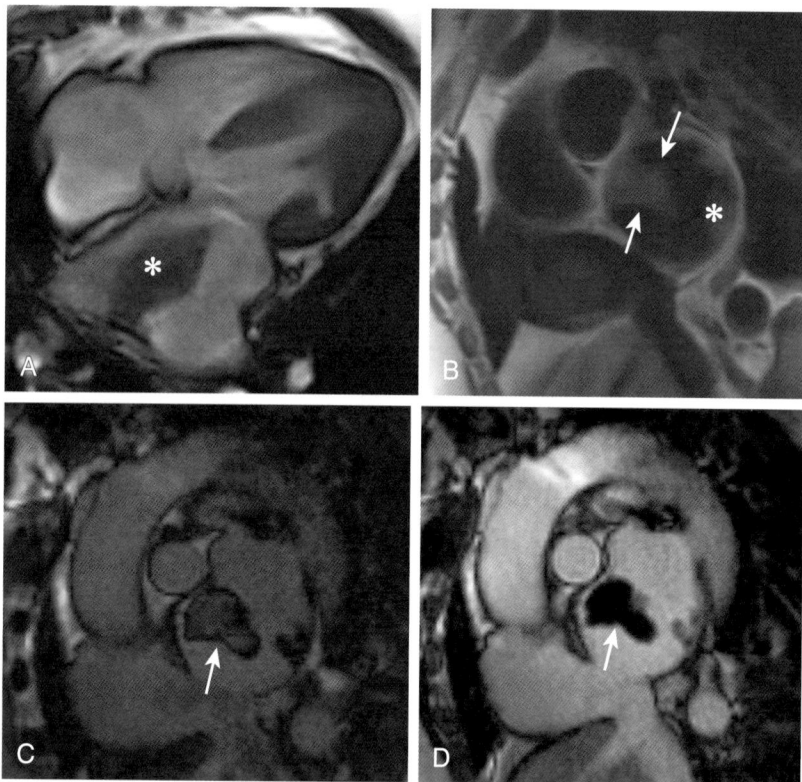

FIGURE 19.22 Cardiac thrombus. CMR in a 66-year-old woman with factor V Leiden mutation and antiphospholipid syndrome and finding of a mass on echocardiography. **(A)** Steady-state free precession image, four-chamber view demonstrates an isointense mass in the left atrium posterior wall *(asterisk)*. **(B)** T1-weighted black-blood image, short-axis view demonstrates an isointense mass attached to the left atrial wall *(arrows)*. There is another small mass in the posterior wall of the atrium *(asterisk)*, which suggests presence of multiple thrombi. **(C)** On LGE image, short-axis view, the mass appears to be heterogeneously hyperintense, while **(D)** on LGE, long inversion time (T1) image (T1 = 600 ms), short-axis view, the mass was nulled completely suggesting lack of enhancement. These findings are consistent with multiple intracardiac thrombi.

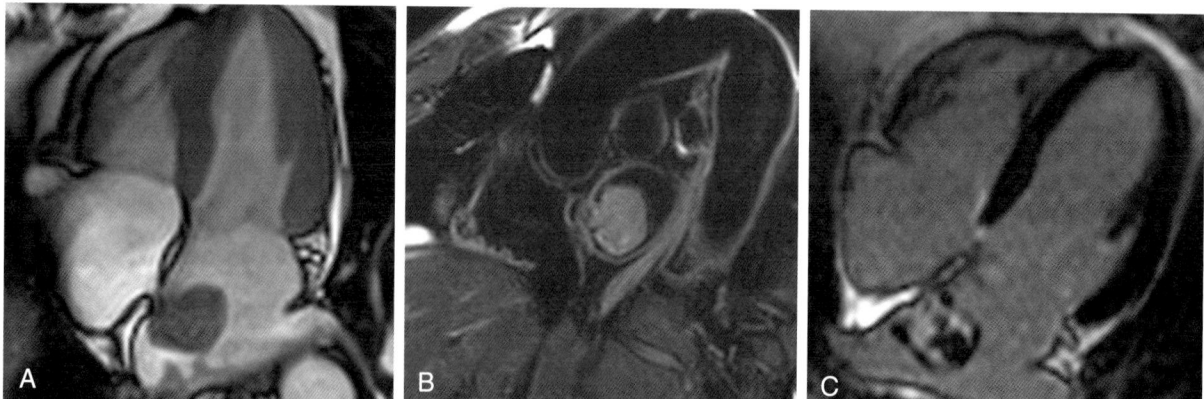

FIGURE 19.23 Cardiac myxoma. **A,** CMR in a 24-year-old woman with and suspicion of a left atrial mass on echocardiography revealed evidence of a left atrial myxoma adherent to the interatrial septum on cine functional four-chamber and basal short-axis. **B,** Tissue characterization revealed hyperintense signal on T2-weighted sequence suggestive of tissue edema. **C,** There was heterogenous signal intensity on LGE imaging. Subsequent histopathology confirmed the diagnosis after surgical resection resulting in symptom resolution. (Courtesy Naeem Merchant, MD, and Bobak Heydari, MD, MPH. Stephenson Cardiac Imaging Center, University of Calgary, Calgary,Canada.)

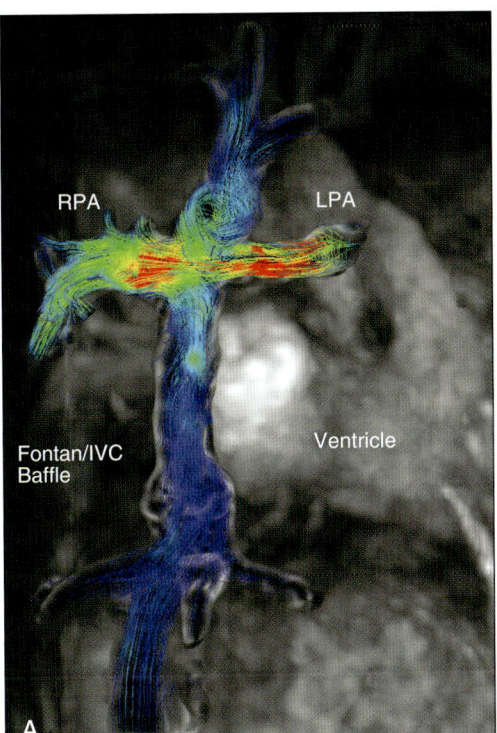 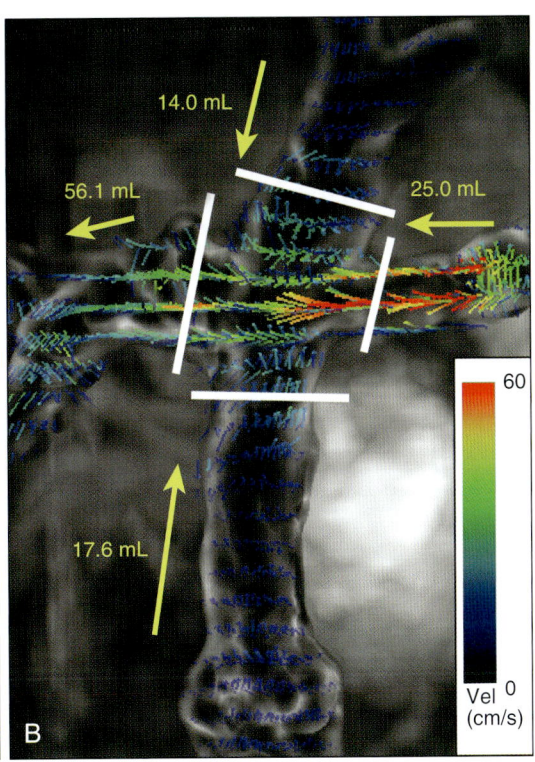

FIGURE 19.24 Four-dimensional flow imaging in a 12-year-old girl with congenital heart disease, including right dominant atrioventricular defect and previous Fontan operation. Routine clinical MRA showed a hypoplastic left pulmonary artery (LPA) without stenosis and a moderately dilated right pulmonary artery (RPA). **A,** 4D flow visualization using time-resolved pathlines and vector representations demonstrated the unique case that all caval flow was directed to the RPA, and there was complete retrograde flow in the LPA due to an extensive aortopulmonary collateral burden to the left lung. These observations were confirmed by comprehensive flow quantification in the Fontan connection: 2D planes were retrospectively placed in the 4D flow MRI to quantify flow in the superior vena cava and inferior vena cava baffle (SVC, IVC), as well as the RPA and LPA. **B,** For flow quantification accuracy assurance, 4D flow MRI could be used to check flow conservation: Using the net flow values depicted in **(B)** net flows (|LPA|+|SVC|+|IVC|) = 56.6 mL/cycle, which was equal to RPA net flow. **A,** Depicts 3D streamlines in mid diastole released from the Fontan anastomoses. **B,** A zoomed-in view depicts vectorized representation of flow velocities, with large yellow arrows indicating the primary direction of flow. White lines indicate retrospective placement of 2D orthogonal analysis planes for 4D flow quantification, with associated numbers representing net flow through each plane (mL/cycle). (Courtesy Liliana Ma, Cynthia Rigsby, Matthew Cornicelli, and Michael Markl, Departments of Medical Imaging and Radiology, Northwestern University.)

NOVEL CMR IMAGING TECHNIQUES AND FUTURE PERSPECTIVES

Technologic advance of CMR in the next years will likely focus on improving the study throughput, protocol consistency, and patient tolerability. Compressed sensing was a signal processing breakthrough in 2004, which discovered that digital images can be reconstructed with data sample rates even lower than Nyquist's Law because information content of CMR images is compressible. Compressed sensing has shown promise in substantially improving the efficiency of CMR cine, perfusion, 4D flow (Fig. 19.24), and coronary MRA.[64] It allows increasing clinical use of high quality real-time imaging of cardiac function without any need for cardiac gating or breath holding or acquisition of the whole-heart cine at high resolution in a single breath-hold. Pulse sequences that acquire a 3D dataset achieve a whole cardiac coverage at higher consistency than 2D and have shown clinical promise in perfusion imaging and LGE imaging. Automated motion correction reduces blurring from cardiac motions and has become standard in many pulse sequences because it not only improves qualitative visual displays but also facilitates quantitative measurements. Artificial intelligence-guided cardiac localization and scanning algorithms have been developed and are now commercially available to increase scanning consistency and may reduce scan time by 40% to 60%. Although MRI technology in general moves in the direction of higher field strength owing to the benefits of improved signal-to-noise ratio, low field CMR (field strength <1.0T) is a focus of active investigations and is promising in enhancing the clinical adaptation of CMR. Compared with current routine of 1.5 or 3T, low field CMR has potential benefits unique to cardiac patients: lower scanner and site construction cost, fewer artifacts and easier performance, and less heat deposition and thus safer for patients with metallic devices.[65] It appears that the loss in signal-to-noise ratio can be gained back by the use of SSFP methods or appropriate revision of pulse sequence settings (e.g., increasing flip angle) without significant risk of tissue heating.[66]

REFERENCES

Principles of Magnetic Resonance Imaging

1. Nazarian S, Hansford R, Rahsepar AA, et al. Safety of magnetic resonance imaging in patients with cardiac devices. *N Engl J Med*. 2017;377:2555–2564.

Coronary Artery Disease

2. Foley JRJ, Kidambi A, Biglands JD, et al. A comparison of cardiovascular magnetic resonance and single photon emission computed tomography (SPECT) perfusion imaging in left main stem or equivalent coronary artery disease: a CE-MARC substudy. *J Cardiovasc Magn Reson*. 2017;19:84.
3. Rijlaarsdam-Hermsen D, Lo-Kioeng-Shioe M, van Domburg RT, et al. Stress-only adenosine CMR improves diagnostic yield in stable symptomatic patients with coronary artery calcium. *JACC Cardiovasc Imaging*. 2020;13:1152–1160.
4. Vincenti G, Masci PG, Monney P, et al. Stress perfusion CMR in patients with known and suspected CAD: prognostic value and optimal ischemic threshold for revascularization. *JACC Cardiovasc Imaging*. 2017;10:526–537.
5. Kwong RY, Ge Y, Steel K, et al. Cardiac magnetic resonance stress perfusion imaging for evaluation of patients with chest pain. *J Am Coll Cardiol*. 2019;74:1741–1755.
6. Ge Y, Pandya A, Steel K, et al. Cost-effectiveness analysis of stress cardiovascular magnetic resonance imaging for stable chest pain syndromes. *JACC Cardiovasc Imaging*. 2020;13:1505–1517.
7. Biglands JD, Ibraheem M, Magee DR, et al. Quantitative myocardial perfusion imaging versus visual analysis in diagnosing myocardial ischemia: a CE-MARC substudy. *JACC Cardiovasc Imaging*. 2018;11:711–718.
8. Knott KD, Seraphim A, Augusto JB, et al. The prognostic significance of quantitative myocardial perfusion: an artificial intelligence based approach using perfusion mapping. *Circulation*. 2020;141:1282–1291.
9. Nagel E, Greenwood JP, McCann GP, et al. Magnetic resonance perfusion or fractional flow reserve in coronary disease. *N Engl J Med*. 2019;380:2418–2428.
10. Le TT, Bryant JA, Ting AE, et al. Assessing exercise cardiac reserve using real-time cardiovascular magnetic resonance. *J Cardiovasc Magn Reson*. 2017;19:7.
11. Kim HW, Rehwald WG, Jenista ER, et al. Dark-blood delayed enhancement cardiac magnetic resonance of myocardial infarction. *JACC Cardiovasc Imaging*. 2018;11:1758–1769.
12. Symons R, Pontone G, Schwitter J, et al. Long-term incremental prognostic value of cardiovascular magnetic resonance after ST-segment elevation myocardial infarction: a study of the collaborative registry on CMR in STEMI. *JACC Cardiovasc Imaging*. 2018;11:813–825.

13. Ibanez B, Aletras AH, Arai AE, et al. Cardiac MRI endpoints in myocardial infarction experimental and clinical trials: JACC scientific expert panel. *J Am Coll Cardiol*. 2019;74:238–256.
14. Everaars H, van der Hoeven NW, Janssens GN, et al. Cardiac magnetic resonance for evaluating nonculprit lesions after myocardial infarction: comparison with fractional flow reserve. *JACC Cardiovasc Imaging*. 2020;13:715–728.
15. Smulders MW, Kietselaer B, Wildberger JE, et al. Initial imaging-guided strategy versus routine care in patients with non-ST-segment elevation myocardial infarction. *J Am Coll Cardiol*. 2019;74:2466–2477.
16. Dastidar AG, Baritussio A, De Garate E, et al. Prognostic role of CMR and conventional risk factors in myocardial infarction with nonobstructed coronary arteries. *JACC Cardiovasc Imaging*. 2019;12:1973–1982.
17. Lintingre PF, Nivet H, Clement-Guinaudeau S, et al. High-resolution late gadolinium enhancement magnetic resonance for the diagnosis of myocardial infarction with nonobstructed coronary arteries. *JACC Cardiovasc Imaging*. 2020;13:1135–1148.

Cardiomyopathies

18. Vita T, Grani C, Abbasi SA, et al. Comparing CMR mapping methods and myocardial patterns toward heart failure outcomes in nonischemic dilated cardiomyopathy. *JACC Cardiovasc Imaging*. 2019;12:1659–1669.
19. Charron P, Elliott PM, Gimeno JR, et al. The Cardiomyopathy Registry of the EURObservational Research Programme of the European Society of Cardiology: baseline data and contemporary management of adult patients with cardiomyopathies. *Eur Heart J*. 2018;39:1784–1793.
20. Di Marco A, Anguera I, Schmitt M, et al. Late gadolinium enhancement and the risk for ventricular arrhythmias or sudden death in dilated cardiomyopathy: systematic review and meta-analysis. *JACC Heart Fail*. 2017;5:28–38.
21. Hindieh W, Weissler-Snir A, Hammer H, et al. Discrepant measurements of maximal left ventricular wall thickness between cardiac magnetic resonance imaging and echocardiography in patients with hypertrophic cardiomyopathy. *Circ Cardiovasc Imaging*. 2017;10:e006309.
22. Mentias A, Raeisi-Giglou P, Smedira NG, et al. Late gadolinium enhancement in patients with hypertrophic cardiomyopathy and preserved systolic function. *J Am Coll Cardiol*. 2018;72:857–870.
23. Sivalokanathan S, Zghaib T, Greenland GV, et al. Hypertrophic cardiomyopathy patients with paroxysmal atrial fibrillation have a high burden of left atrial fibrosis by cardiac magnetic resonance imaging. *JACC Clin Electrophysiol*. 2019;5:364–375.
24. Ariga R, Tunnicliffe EM, Manohar SG, et al. Identification of myocardial disarray in patients with hypertrophic cardiomyopathy and ventricular arrhythmias. *J Am Coll Cardiol*. 2019;73:2493–2502.
25. Neubauer S, Kolm P, Ho CY, et al. Distinct subgroups in hypertrophic cardiomyopathy in the NHLBI HCM registry. *J Am Coll Cardiol*. 2019;74:2333–2345.
26. Marstrand P, Han L, Day SM, et al. Hypertrophic cardiomyopathy with left ventricular systolic dysfunction: insights from the SHaRe registry. *Circulation*. 2020;141:1371–1383.
27. Aquaro GD, De Luca A, Cappelletto C, et al. Prognostic value of magnetic resonance phenotype in patients with arrhythmogenic right ventricular cardiomyopathy. *J Am Coll Cardiol*. 2020;75:2753–2765.
28. Kotanidis CP, Bazmpani MA, Haidich AB, et al. Diagnostic accuracy of cardiovascular magnetic resonance in acute myocarditis: a systematic review and meta-analysis. *JACC Cardiovasc Imaging*. 2018;11:1583–1594.
29. Oka E, Iwasaki YK, Maru Y, et al. Prevalence and significance of an early repolarization electrocardiographic pattern and its mechanistic insight based on cardiac magnetic resonance imaging in patients with acute myocarditis. *Circ Arrhythm Electrophysiol*. 2019;12:e006969.
30. von Knobelsdorff-Brenkenhoff F, Schuler J, Doganguzel S, et al. Detection and monitoring of acute myocarditis applying quantitative cardiovascular magnetic resonance. *Circ Cardiovasc Imaging*. 2017;10.
31. Grani C, Eichhorn C, Biere L, et al. Prognostic value of cardiac magnetic resonance tissue characterization in risk stratifying patients with suspected myocarditis. *J Am Coll Cardiol*. 2017;70:1964–1976.
32. Aquaro GD, Perfetti M, Camastra G, et al. Cardiac MR with late gadolinium enhancement in acute myocarditis with preserved systolic function: ITAMY study. *J Am Coll Cardiol*. 2017;70:1977–1987.
33. Aquaro GD, Ghebru Habtemicael Y, Camastra G, et al. Prognostic value of repeating cardiac magnetic resonance in patients with acute myocarditis. *J Am Coll Cardiol*. 2019;74:2439–2448.
34. Berg J, Kottwitz J, Baltensperger N, et al. Cardiac magnetic resonance imaging in myocarditis reveals persistent disease activity despite normalization of cardiac enzymes and inflammatory parameters at 3-month follow-up. *Circ Heart Fail*. 2017;10:e004262.
35. Kouranos V, Tzelepis GE, Rapti A, et al. Complementary role of CMR to conventional screening in the diagnosis and prognosis of cardiac sarcoidosis. *JACC Cardiovasc Imaging*. 2017;10:1437–1447.
36. Velangi PS, Chen KA, Kazmirczak F, et al. Right ventricular abnormalities on cardiovascular magnetic resonance imaging in patients with sarcoidosis. *JACC Cardiovasc Imaging*. 2020;13:1395–1405.
37. Coleman GC, Shaw PW, Balfour Jr PC, et al. Prognostic value of myocardial scarring on CMR in patients with cardiac sarcoidosis. *JACC Cardiovasc Imaging*. 2017;10:411–420.
38. Al-Khatib SM, Stevenson WG, Ackerman MJ, et al. 2017 AHA/ACC/HRS guideline for management of patients with ventricular arrhythmias and the prevention of sudden cardiac death: a report of the American College of Cardiology/American Heart Association Task Force on clinical practice guidelines and the heart rhythm society. *Circulation*. 2018;138:e272–e391.
39. Kotecha T, Martinez-Naharro A, Treibel TA, et al. Myocardial edema and prognosis in amyloidosis. *J Am Coll Cardiol*. 2018;71:2919–2931.
40. Pan JA, Kerwin MJ, Salerno M. Native T1 mapping, extracellular volume mapping, and late gadolinium enhancement in cardiac amyloidosis: a meta-analysis. *JACC Cardiovasc Imaging*. 2020;13:1299–1310.
41. Halliday BP, Cleland JGF, Goldberger JJ, Prasad SK. Personalizing risk stratification for sudden death in dilated cardiomyopathy: the past, present, and future. *Circulation*. 2017;136:215–231.
42. von Deuster C, Sammut E, Asner L, et al. Studying dynamic myofiber aggregate reorientation in dilated cardiomyopathy using in vivo magnetic resonance diffusion tensor imaging. *Circ Cardiovasc Imaging*. 2016;9:e005018.
43. Romano S, Judd RM, Kim RJ, et al. Feature-tracking global longitudinal strain predicts death in a multicenter population of patients with ischemic and nonischemic dilated cardiomyopathy incremental to ejection fraction and late gadolinium enhancement. *JACC Cardiovasc Imaging*. 2018;11:1419–1429.
44. Muthalaly RG, Kwong RY, John RM, et al. Left ventricular entropy is a novel predictor of arrhythmic events in patients with dilated cardiomyopathy receiving defibrillators for primary prevention. *JACC Cardiovasc Imaging*. 2019;12:1177–1184.
45. Alam MH, Auger D, McGill LA, et al. Comparison of 3 T and 1.5 T for T2* magnetic resonance of tissue iron. *J Cardiovasc Magn Reson*. 2016;18:40.
46. Scally C, Rudd A, Mezincescu A, et al. Persistent long-term structural, functional, and metabolic changes after stress-induced (Takotsubo) cardiomyopathy. *Circulation*. 2018;137:1039–1048.
47. Imran M, Wang L, McCrohon J, et al. Native T1 mapping in the diagnosis of cardiac allograft rejection: a prospective histologically validated study. *JACC Cardiovasc Imaging*. 2019;12:1618–1628.
48. Dolan RS, Rahsepar AA, Blaisdell J, et al. Multiparametric cardiac magnetic resonance imaging can detect acute cardiac allograft rejection after heart transplantation. *JACC Cardiovasc Imaging*. 2019;12:1632–1641.
49. Tello K, Dalmer A, Vanderpool R, et al. Cardiac magnetic resonance imaging-based right ventricular strain analysis for assessment of coupling and diastolic function in pulmonary hypertension. *JACC Cardiovasc Imaging*. 2019;12:2155–2164.
50. Galan-Arriola C, Lobo M, Vilchez-Tschischke JP, et al. Serial magnetic resonance imaging to identify early stages of anthracycline-induced cardiotoxicity. *J Am Coll Cardiol*. 2019;73:779–791.

Valvular Heart Disease

51. Woldendorp K, Bannon PG, Grieve SM. Evaluation of aortic stenosis using cardiovascular magnetic resonance: a systematic review & meta-analysis. *J Cardiovasc Magn Reson*. 2020;22:45.
52. Musa TA, Treibel TA, Vassiliou VS, et al. Myocardial scar and mortality in severe aortic stenosis. *Circulation*. 2018;138:1935–1947.
53. Everett RJ, Treibel TA, Fukui M, et al. Extracellular myocardial volume in patients with aortic stenosis. *J Am Coll Cardiol*. 2020;75:304–316.
54. Peterzan MA, Clarke WT, Lygate CA, et al. Cardiac energetics in patients with aortic stenosis and preserved versus reduced ejection fraction. *Circulation*. 2020;141:1971–1985.
55. Cavalcante JL, Rijal S, Abdelkarim I, et al. Cardiac amyloidosis is prevalent in older patients with aortic stenosis and carries worse prognosis. *J Cardiovasc Magn Reson*. 2017;19:98.
56. Kammerlander AA, Wiesinger M, Duca F, et al. Diagnostic and prognostic utility of cardiac magnetic resonance imaging in aortic regurgitation. *JACC Cardiovasc Imaging*. 2019;12:1474–1483.
57. Uretsky S, Argulian E, Narula J, Wolff SD. Use of cardiac magnetic resonance imaging in assessing mitral regurgitation: current evidence. *J Am Coll Cardiol*. 2018;71:547–563.
58. Penicka M, Vecera J, Mirica DC, et al. Prognostic Implications of magnetic resonance-derived quantification in asymptomatic patients with organic mitral regurgitation: comparison with Doppler echocardiography-derived integrative approach. *Circulation*. 2018;137:1349–1360.
59. Kitkungvan D, Nabi F, Kim RJ, et al. Myocardial fibrosis in patients with primary mitral regurgitation with and without prolapse. *J Am Coll Cardiol*. 2018;72:823–834.
60. Cavalcante JL, Kusunose K, Obuchowski NA, et al. Prognostic Impact of ischemic mitral regurgitation severity and myocardial infarct quantification by cardiovascular magnetic resonance. *JACC Cardiovasc Imaging*. 2020;13:1489–1501.
61. Zhan Y, Senapati A, Vejpongsa P, et al. Comparison of echocardiographic assessment of tricuspid regurgitation against cardiovascular magnetic resonance. *JACC Cardiovasc Imaging*. 2020;13:1461–1471.

Pericardial Disease; Cardiac Electrophysiology; Novel Techniques

62. Kumar A, Sato K, Yzeiraj E, et al. Quantitative pericardial delayed hyperenhancement informs clinical course in recurrent pericarditis. *JACC Cardiovasc Imaging*. 2017;10:1337–1346.
63. Acosta J, Fernandez-Armenta J, Borras R, et al. Scar characterization to predict life-threatening arrhythmic events and sudden cardiac death in patients with cardiac resynchronization therapy: the GAUDI-CRT study. *JACC Cardiovasc Imaging*. 2018;11:561–572.
64. Hirai K, Kido T, Kido T, et al. Feasibility of contrast-enhanced coronary artery magnetic resonance angiography using compressed sensing. *J Cardiovasc Magn Reson*. 2020;22:15.
65. Schukro C, Puchner SB. Safety and efficiency of low-field magnetic resonance imaging in patients with cardiac rhythm management devices. *Eur J Radiol*. 2019;118:96–100.
66. Simonetti OP, Ahmad R. Low-field cardiac magnetic resonance imaging: a compelling case for cardiac magnetic resonance's future. *Circ Cardiovasc Imaging*. 2017;10:e005446.

20 Cardiac Computed Tomography

RON BLANKSTEIN

BASICS OF CARDIAC COMPUTED TOMOGRAPHY, 335
Different Types of Cardiac Computed Tomography Exams, 335

CORONARY ARTERY CALCIUM TESTING, 337
Test Performance and Acquisition, 337
Clinical Data, 337
Special Populations, 337
Clinical Indications and Management Recommendations, 338
Limitations of Coronary Artery Calcium Testing, 340

CORONARY COMPUTED TOMOGRAPHY ANGIOGRAPHY, 340
Diagnostic Accuracy, 340
Prognostic Implications, 341
Coronary Computed Tomography Angiography in Acute Chest Pain, 341
Coronary Computed Tomography Angiography in Stable Chest Pain, 342
Coronary Computed Tomography Angiography Plaque Characteristics, 344
Plaque Characteristics and Incident Risk, 345
Physiologic Evaluation of Coronary Artery Disease, 347

Implications of the ISCHEMIA Trial for Coronary Computed Tomography Angiography, 349
Patient Management Considerations, 350
Special Populations, 352
Guidelines, 353

ASSESSMENT OF CARDIOVASCULAR STRUCTURE AND FUNCTION, 354
Pericardial and Myocardial Disease, 354
Valvular Heart Disease, 354
Evaluation of Cardiac Masses, 361

FUTURE DIRECTIONS, 361

REFERENCES, 361

Over the last 15 years, cardiac computed tomography (CT) has evolved considerably and is now an essential noninvasive tool for evaluating various forms of heart disease. The technical advances that have permitted this evolution include the development of scanner systems with improved spatial and temporal resolution, thereby allowing the acquisition of high-resolution images with virtually no motion artifacts. At the same time, improvements in scan acquisition techniques, such as axial acquisition using prospective electrocardiogram (ECG) gating, have resulted in a substantial reduction in radiation dose.[1]

Although there are currently several different types of cardiac CT, the most common clinical use is for coronary CT angiography (CCTA) where information on the amount and type of coronary plaque, as well as the severity of stenosis, is provided. The increased use of this technique is because of data demonstrating diagnostic accuracy, prognostic value, and clinical effectiveness in patients with stable or acute chest pain. Nevertheless, there have been advances in several multimodality imaging techniques, and selecting appropriate candidates for cardiac CT, and understanding which indications are most and least useful, remains fundamental for ensuring that the potential benefits of this test are fully realized. This chapter provides an overview of the various clinical applications of cardiac CT for multiple different clinical indications.

BASICS OF CARDIAC COMPUTED TOMOGRAPHY

Different Types of Cardiac Computed Tomography Exams

Cardiac CT, with or without contrast, uses x-rays to obtain high resolution three-dimensional (3D) datasets. There are various different type of cardiac CT.

- *Coronary artery calcium (CAC) scan:* Non–contrast-enhanced ECG gated study during a single cardiac phase used to identify the presence and amount of calcified coronary plaque.
- *CCTA:* Contrast-enhanced ECG gated study performed to identify the presence and amount of both calcified and noncalcified plaque, and to estimate the severity of luminal stenosis.
- *Cardiac CT to evaluate noncoronary structures:* Contrast-enhanced ECG gated images to evaluate various pathologies ranging from valvular heart disease and cardiac function to cardiac masses and pulmonary venous anatomy. Depending on the indication, certain types of cardiac CT acquire data throughout the cardiac cycle to display cine imaging. The ability to view the heart throughout the cardiac cycle can be used to determine left or right ventricular systolic function, visualize cardiac masses that are mobile, or assess for valvular heart disease.

TECHNICAL CONSIDERATIONS/IMAGE ACQUISITION

CT scanners require an x-ray source that directs photons past a collimator and through the part of the body being imaged (Fig. 20.1). As photons pass through various parts of the body they become attenuated based on the x-ray absorption characteristics of the objects through which they pass. Those that pass through the patient reach the detectors that are located on the opposite side of the patient from the x-ray source. These x-rays are recorded by the detector electronics as a string of binary numbers that can be reconstructed to two-dimensional (2D) and 3D images.

Multidetector CT scanners have multiple parallel rows of detector elements that can acquire data more rapidly and more uniformly because of improved coverage along the z-axis (i.e., longitudinal axis of patient). The detector width is an important determinant of spatial resolution (i.e., the ability to differentiate small structures from each other). The gantry rotation speed is an important determinant of temporal resolution, or the ability to freeze the motion of the heart. The temporal resolution is also based on whether a scanner utilizes a single x-ray source and detector array or two x-ray sources and detector arrays. With a single source system, ~180 degrees of rotation of the gantry (plus the "fan angle" related to the width of the detector array) is required to acquire an image, whereas a dual source system allows data acquisition to be reduced to an approximately 90-degree rotation. Thus if a scanner has gantry rotation speed of 280 msec and uses a single x-ray source, the temporal resolution would be approximately 140 msec, versus 70 msec with a dual source system.

During a cardiac CT, a patient is placed on the scanner bed and is connected to ECG leads. Image acquisition, with or without contrast, is then performed during predetermined "phases" of the cardiac cycle. The combination of fast image acquisition, and ECG gating (i.e., obtaining data during specific portions of the cardiac cycle) enable "freezing" of the motion of the heart. Data acquisition requires the operator to select various parameters (Table 20.1). Higher tube voltage (kilovolt

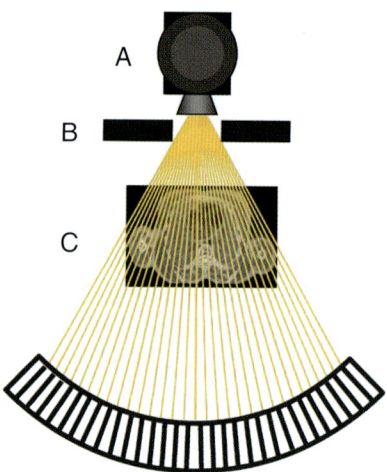

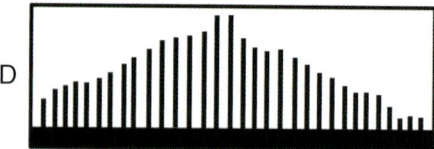

FIGURE 20.1 Computed tomography imaging requires an x-ray source *(A)* that directs photons past a collimator *(B)*. Photons are attenuated by organs in a differential pattern related to their material densities. Photons not attenuated reach multiple detectors *(C)* at which a scintillation reaction occurs. At each detector, a photon flux is generated that is a product of the number of photons emitted from the x-ray tube (milliamperes, mA), the photon energy (kilovolts, kV), and the organ tissue properties. These are calculated for every detector element *(D)*.

[kV]) allows for greater tissue penetration, but it decreases the brightness of administered intravenous (IV) contrast.

Higher tube current (milliamperes [mA]) increases the total number of photons that ultimately reach the detector elements. Both higher kV and higher mA increase the radiation dose associated with cardiac CT imaging.

RADIATION PRINCIPLES/PATIENT SAFETY

The radiation dose of cardiac CT is dependent on several parameters (see Table 20.1) determined during scan acquisition. The CT tube voltage, measured in kV, determines the energy of the emitted photons, whereas the tube current, measured in mA or milliamperes second (mAs), determine the number of photons emitted. Higher tube voltage (kV) allows for greater tissue penetration, whereas higher photon count (mA) increases the total number of photons that ultimately reach the detector elements. Both higher kV and higher mA increase the radiation dose associated with cardiac CT imaging, yet an insufficiently low setting can result in excess image noise and reduced image quality. Thus scan settings must be selected based on body habitus and the desired image quality. For instance, in obese patients, where a high degree of noise and photon attenuation is expected, higher kV is usually preferable. A higher kV may also be beneficial in cases where coronary stents or dense coronary calcifications are present. Although it is essential for imagers to understand how to select these parameters, many modern scanner systems have algorithms that may assist in selecting certain scan acquisition parameters based on the image noise that is present on the scout images.

A prospective multicenter registry study has shown that over the last decade, the estimated radiation dose associated with cardiac CT has decreased by ~78%. Specifically the median dose-length product (DLP) of CCTA decreased from 885 mGy × cm (in 2007) to 195 mGy × cm (in 2017). This DLP results in an estimated effective dose of 2.7 mSv when applying the conversion factor of k = 0.014.[1] This reduction has been

TABLE 20.1 Image Acquisition Parameters During Cardiac Computed Tomography Acquisition

		TYPICAL SETTING	EXPLANATION OF PARAMETER	IMPLICATIONS ON RADIATION DOSE OR IMAGE QUALITY	ADDITIONAL CONSIDERATIONS
Contrast	Amount of contrast	60-75 cc		Neutral	Faster scanners require less contrast; evaluation of right heart structures or a larger field of view may require more contrast
	Injection rate	5-7 cc/s	Faster injection rate increases contrast opacification of the coronary vessels	Neutral	Use of lower kV allows for improved contrast and may enable use of lower injection rate
Scan range (in z-axis)	Coverage	12-16 cm	Determined when setting the acquisition field of view based on localizer images	Linear association with radiation dose	Larger coverage necessary when evaluating bypass grafts or other vascular pathology
Photon energy/amount	Tube voltage (kV)	80, 100, 120	Can be selected based on anticipated image noise versus desired radiation	Logarithmic association with radiation dose	In the presence of stents or metallic objects, higher kV may be beneficial
	Tube current (mA or mAs)	Scanner dependent (e.g., 100-400)		Linear association with radiation dose	Noncoronary studies (e.g., calcium scan) can be performed with lower mA
Acquisition mode	Axial versus helical	Axial preferred	Image acquisition during predefined portions of the cardiac cycle	Use of axial acquisition associated with ~70% lower dose (versus helical acquisition)	Axial acquisition requires regular heart rate to avoid misregistration artifacts
	ECG triggering	Prospective	When using axial acquisition, prospective ECG triggering is used		
	Phases	65%-75%	A wider phase acquisition window enables reconstruction of images from multiple portions of the cardia cycle	A wider phase acquisition window will results in higher dose	Acquisition of more phases may be beneficial when heart rate is elevated or irregular
	Tube current modulation	Turn "on" if helical acquisition performed	A technique to lower tube current across certain portions of the cardiac cycle	Used to lower radiation dose when helical acquisition is performed	The percentage reduction in tube current may be selected, depending on scanner used

ECG, Electrocardiogram; *kV*, kilovolt; *mA*, milliamperes; *mAs*, milliamperes second.

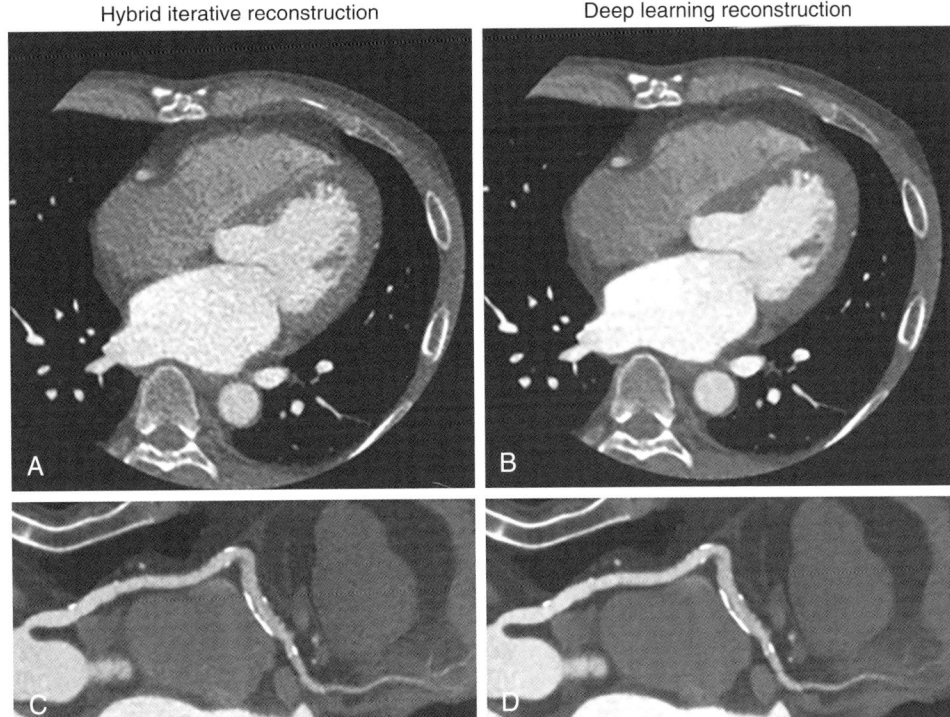

FIGURE 20.2 Reconstruction techniques for radiation reduction and coronary computed tomography angiography (CCTA) image quality. CCTA radiation dose can be reduced while maintaining high image quality by using deep learning reconstruction techniques, which provide superior image quality compared with hybrid iterative reconstruction techniques. Axial CCTA sections reconstructed by using **(A)** hybrid iterative and **(B)** deep learning techniques are shown, as is multiplanar reformatting of the right coronary artery using **(C)** hybrid iterative reconstruction and **(D)** deep learning reconstruction. (From Abdelrahman KM, et al. Coronary computed tomography angiography from clinical uses to emerging technologies. J Am Coll Cardiol 2020;76:1226-1243.)

achieved because of wider adoption of dose-saving techniques, including axial acquisition using prospective ECG triggering, low tube voltage, iterative image reconstruction (which reduces image noise, thereby allowing for image acquisition using lower kV and mA), and high-pitch helical scanning modes. Novel image reconstruction techniques using convolution neural networks and artificial intelligence are expected to further improve image quality, thus allowing for a lower radiation dose[2] (Fig. 20.2).

CORONARY ARTERY CALCIUM TESTING

Test Performance and Acquisition

CAC testing uses a noncontrast ECG gated scan to measure the amount of calcified coronary plaque. The test can be performed during a single breath-hold and does not require an IV, premedications, or any special patient preparation. When contemporary techniques are employed, the radiation dose is approximately 1 to 1.5 mSv, which is similar to the dose of a mammogram. Following image acquisition, the overall amount of calcifications can be quantified using commercially available programs, most commonly using the Agatston technique,[3] where the total calcium score is based on the amount and density of calcified plaque (Fig. 20.3).

The overall amount of coronary plaque can then be categorized as absent (CAC = 0), minimal (1 to 9), mild (10 to 99), moderate (100 to 299), severe (300 to 999), or extreme (≥1000). A CAC scan may also provide information regarding pericardial calcifications or thickness, aortic calcifications, valvular calcification, and in some cases the presence of fatty liver disease. In addition to providing information on the overall calcified plaque (i.e., total Agatston score), a CAC study should also report the CAC score of each coronary vessel, and the age-, sex-, and race-based percentiles.[4] It may also be useful to report the MESA (Multi-Ethnic Study of Atherosclerosis) coronary heart disease (CHD) score (https://www.mesa-nhlbi.org/MESACHDRisk/MesaRiskScore/RiskScore.aspx), which allows for calculation of the 10-year risk of CHD events, with and without CAC data.[5] In the near future, a MESA calculator, which will allow for the calculation of the 10-year atherosclerotic cardiovascular disease (ASCVD) risk based on the CAC test results, will allow clinicians to determine how the 10-year ASCVD risk is affected by having information on the overall amount of calcified plaque.

Clinical Data

Calcifications in the coronary arteries indicate the presence of coronary atherosclerosis, and there is a direct association between the amount of coronary calcifications and long-term risk of future cardiovascular events in both men and women, and across different races.[6] Importantly, information on CAC has been shown to provide incremental data beyond risk factors,[7-9] and results in a significant improvement in risk reclassification and discrimination.[10-12] Although the absolute CAC score is the strongest predictor of future risk, the age- and sex-based percentile is useful for determining relative risk, and it may be especially important among younger (e.g., <50) or older (e.g., >70) patients.

Although many studies have focused on the use of CAC to identify high-risk individuals, the absence of coronary calcifications (i.e., CAC score of zero) has been shown to be associated with a very low 10-year event rate, especially among individuals with a 10-year ASCVD risk that is <20%.[6,13,14] In fact, among borderline- and intermediate-risk patients, as defined by the 2018 multisociety cholesterol guideline, ~50% of individuals may have a CAC score of zero, a finding associated with a 10-year ASCVD risk that is <7.5%.[13] In such individuals it is reasonable to defer statin therapy and focus instead on lifestyle interventions, if there is a strong preference to avoid lipid-lowering therapy.

In addition to being a strong predictor of CHD events, increased CAC can also be used to predict other forms of cardiovascular disease (CVD), including atrial fibrillation, stroke, and congestive heart failure.[15-17] In addition, high CAC is associated with a higher rate of cancer and noncardiovascular death.[18,19]

Special Populations

Although CAC testing is generally only recommended for adults over the age of 40, there are studies that suggest that CAC scoring may be used selectively in adults <40 years of age. The Coronary Artery Risk Development in Young Adults (CARDIA) study included community-based participants who were 32 to 46 years old at the time of CAC testing.[20] In this unselected population, only 10% of young adults had coronary artery calcifications, yet with the use of a risk score, a subgroup of individuals with 45% prevalence of CAC could be identified.[20] The CAC Consortium is a large multicenter registry that included patients who were referred for testing and found that 34% of adults aged 30 to 49 had CAC, including 21.8% of those 30 to 39 years of age. In both of these studies, the presence of any CAC was associated with a significantly higher risk of incident CVD. Collectively, these findings

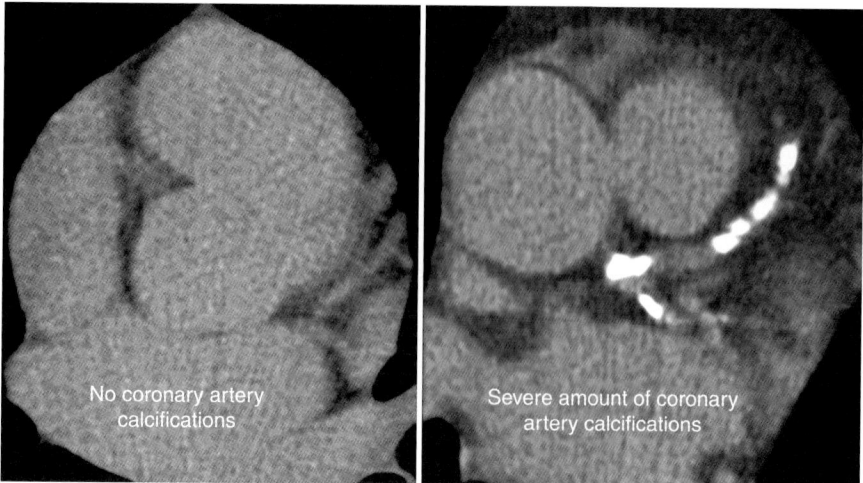

FIGURE 20.3 Examples of images from coronary artery calcium (CAC) testing. *Left:* example of patient with no evidence of calcified coronary plaque and an Agatston CAC score of zero. *Right:* example of patient with severe amount of calcified coronary plaque.

suggest that selective use of CAC in certain high-risk individuals who are 30 to 40 years of age may be reasonable, but the absence of CAC in this age group should not be reassuring and should not be used as a basis to defer any therapies. Because women, on average, develop CAC later than men, the role of CAC testing in women under the age of 40 may be even more limited.

Several studies have shown that the absence of CAC can be used to identify lower risk older adults in whom statin therapy can be deferred. Among a study evaluating 5805 BioImage participants with a mean age of 70, the presence of CAC ≤10 was found in 38% and was associated with a negative likelihood ratio of 0.2 for CHD, implying an 80% lower risk than would be expected based on traditional risk factor asssesment.[21] The use of CAC as a "negative risk marker" among older adults was also established in the CAC Consortium study, in which among 2474 asymptomatic patients with a mean age of 79, those with CAC of 0 to 9 or less than the 25th percentile had a lower risk of cardiovascular and all-cause mortality.[22]

Although at any given age, women have less CAC than men, CAC has been found to predict risk in a similar manner for both men and women.[6,23] Moreover, a meta-analysis of 5 large population cohorts of women with an ASCVD risk <7.5% found that CAC was present in 36%, and that the presence of any CAC was associated with a twofold increase in incident ASCVD events.[24]

Clinical Indications and Management Recommendations
Clinical Indications

Potential uses of CAC testing in cardiovascular medicine are listed in Table 20.2. The current 2018 AHA/ACC multisociety cholesterol guideline states that in intermediate-risk or selected borderline-risk adults (i.e., 10-year ASCVD risk of 5%–20%), if the decision about statin use remains uncertain, it is reasonable to use CAC testing in the decision to withhold, postpone, or initiate statin therapy (Fig. 20.4). When CAC testing is used in this context, if the CAC score is zero, it is reasonable to withhold statin therapy and reassess in 5 to 10 years, as long as higher risk conditions are absent (diabetes mellitus, family history of premature CHD, cigarette smoking). The AHA/ACC guidelines indicate that if the CAC score is 1 to 99, it is reasonable to initiate statin therapy, especially in those ≥55 years of age. If the CAC score is 100 or higher or in the 75th percentile or higher, it is recommended to initiate statin therapy (Fig. 20.5). However, it is noteworthy that the finding of any CAC (i.e., CAC >0) in individuals with borderline or intermediate (5% to <20%) risk should generally favor statin therapy, as also suggested by the National Lipid Association recommendations.[13,25,26]

Management Recommendations

Because patients with elevated CAC scores have a higher risk of CVD, management recommendations focus on treatment of all underlying risk factors using lifestyle and pharmacologic therapies (see Chapters 25 and 27). The vast majority of patients with coronary artery calcifications and a baseline 10-year risk of ASCVD events >5% have a sufficiently high risk of future ASCVD events (i.e., >7.5% 10-year risk) and would benefit from lipid-lowering therapies. However, there is a linear increase with risk as the burden of calcified plaque increases. Accordingly, individuals with moderate to severe CAC should be considered for high-intensity statins.[26]

Although there are no clinical trials that have assessed the efficacy of aspirin therapy among patients with CAC, prior modeling studies from the MESA study[27,28] have suggested that individuals with a CAC score >100, and especially those with a CAC >400, may be more likely to benefit from aspirin therapy. These studies applied the estimated relative risk reduction associated with aspirin therapy to the observed event rate in individuals who have coronary artery calcifications. Accordingly, among individuals with CAC >100, the estimated number needed to treat over 5 years to reduce a cardiovascular event was lower than the number needed to harm. Based on this data, it may be reasonable to consider aspirin therapy in patients with CAC >100 who do not have bleeding-related contraindications.[29]

Individuals who have evidence of severe CAC (>300), and especially those with extreme CAC (>1000), have an annual cardiovascular event rate that is similar to the event rate observed in high-risk secondary prevention trials.[30] Accordingly, it is reasonable to consider such patients for advanced therapies that are usually reserved for secondary prevention. Although CAC measurements have not been used in prior clinical trials, several recent clinical cardiovascular outcome trials are now including the presence of underlying CAC as a potential inclusion criteria.

A common question is whether individuals with severe CAC require further testing. Because coronary revascularization has not been shown to improve outcomes among various high-risk subgroups,[31-33] individuals who are asymptomatic should be treated with aggressive preventive therapies but are unlikely to benefit from additional testing. When there is uncertainty regarding patient symptoms or exercise capacity, exercise testing may be reasonable. Even in the setting of CAC >1000, significant ischemia is only detected in ~15% of patients.[34] When further testing is considered, positron emission tomography myocardial perfusion imaging (PET MPI) may be particularly beneficial as normal myocardial blood flow reserve can be used to exclude high-risk anatomy and inform prognosis.[35,36] Invasive angiography should not be performed in asymptomatic individuals with severe CAC.

A valid concern is that CAC testing can lead to unnecessary downstream noninvasive and invasive testing. In the EISNER (Early Identification of Subclinical Atherosclerosis by Noninvasive Imaging Research) study of 2137 volunteers randomized to CAC scoring versus no CAC scoring, those receiving CAC scoring achieved lower systolic blood pressure, low-density lipoprotein (LDL) cholesterol levels, abdominal girth, and weight.[37] In this study, individuals with CAC ≥1000 had a marked increase in medical costs but constituted only 2.2% of the study population. In an economic analysis, the CAC group experienced costs and medical testing similar to those not undergoing CAC scanning.[37,38] A subsequent meta-analysis evaluating the impact of CAC testing on subsequent preventive therapies has also shown that the identification of calcified plaque is associated with increased use of lipid-lowering therapies, blood pressure–lowering therapies, use of aspirin, and dietary changes.[39]

TABLE 20.2 Potential Uses of Coronary Artery Calcium Testing

POPULATION	PURPOSE	CLINICAL INDICATIONS/DETAILS
Asymptomatic persons without established ASCVD	Screening among *select* low- and borderline-risk patients	• CAC testing may be useful for risk assessment, particularly if this will impact the use of preventive therapies • Individuals who may benefit from such testing include those with strong family history of premature CAD or systemic inflammatory disease
	Shared decision making among *selected* borderline- and intermediate-risk adults in whom the decision regarding statin use is uncertain	• In intermediate-risk or selected borderline-risk adults (i.e., 10-year ASCVD risk of 5%-20%), if the decision about statin use remains uncertain, it is reasonable to use a CAC score in the decision to withhold, postpone, or initiate statin therapy (see Fig. 20.4)
	Shared decision making among *select* high-risk adults who are unable to tolerate statin therapy	• In select high-risk adults who do not have known ASCVD and are unable to tolerate statin therapy, CAC testing may be reasonable for further risk stratification if this could impact the use of additional therapies (e.g., PCSK9 inhibitors)
Symptomatic persons with no known CAD	Low-risk patients with suspected CAD	• CAC testing may be useful to identify low-risk patients who have a low likelihood of obstructive CAD versus those with CAC >0 who may benefit from additional testing
Symptomatic persons with no known CAD	As add-on to other functional testing techniques	• Among individuals who do not have known CAD, who are referred for an ischemic evaluation, add-on CAC testing may be useful to determine the presence and severity of coronary plaque (see Chapter 18 for details)

ASCVD, Atherosclerotic cardiovascular disease; *CAC*, coronary artery calcium; *CAD*, coronary artery disease.

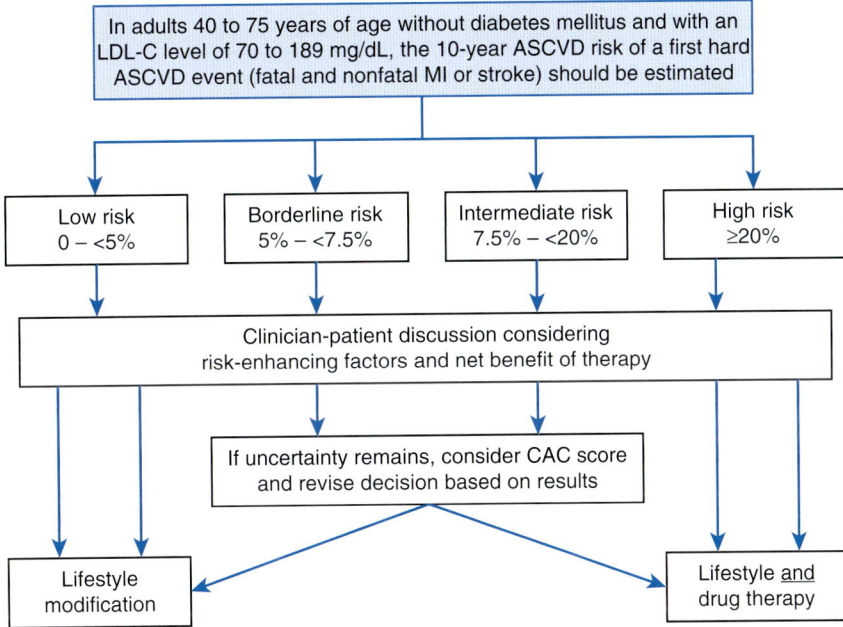

FIGURE 20.4 Overview of role of coronary artery calcium testing in deciding on therapy for the primary prevention of atherosclerotic cardiovascular disease. (From Lloyd-Jones DM, et al. RS. Use of risk assessment tools to guide decision-making in the primary prevention of atherosclerotic cardiovascular disease: a special report from the American Heart Association and American College of Cardiology. J Am Coll Cardiol 2019;73:3153-3167.)

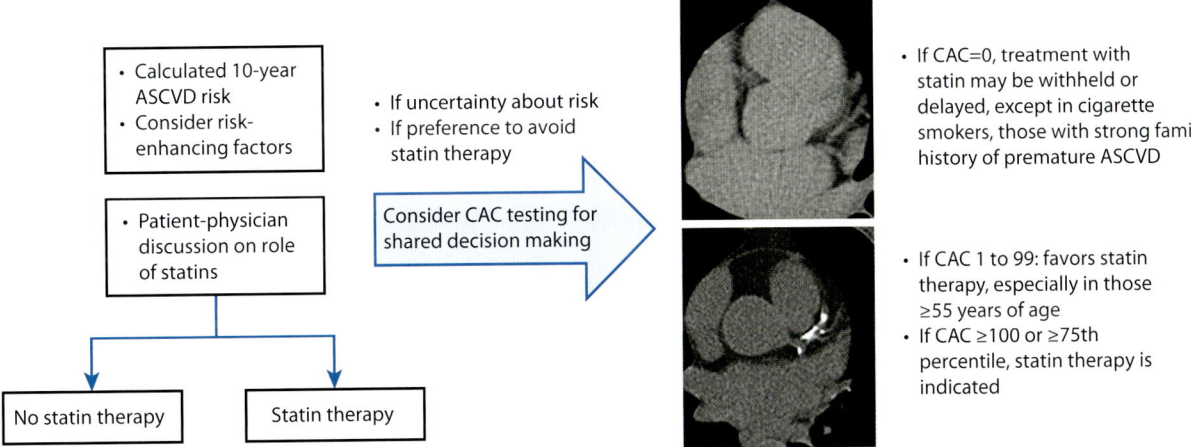

FIGURE 20.5 Overview of how to use coronary artery calcium (CAC) testing for shared decision making among borderline- and intermediate-risk individuals for whom CAC may be used to guide the decision to withhold, postpone or initiate statin therapy. (Based on Stone NJ, Bailey AL, et al. 2018 AHA/ACC/AACVPR/AAPA/ABC/ACPM/ADA/AGS/APhA/ASPC/NLA/PCNA Guideline on the Management of Blood Cholesterol. J Am Coll Cardiol 2019;73:e285-e350.[116])

Limitations of Coronary Artery Calcium Testing

The amount of CAC cannot be reduced with therapy, in fact, some studies have shown that statin therapy may be associated with a mild increase in CAC progression. Nevertheless, the strong association of CAC with future cardiovascular events is robust in patients who are on lipid-lowering therapies. Because the amount of CAC cannot be lowered, repeat CAC testing is not useful to assess response to therapy. Although there is substantial data on the use of CAC testing in various registries and clinical trials, there have been no large-scale clinical trials demonstrating the efficacy of CAC testing for lowering cardiovascular events.

Clinical Trials Using Coronary Artery Calcium

In the St. Francis Heart Study, 1005 patients with CAC greater than the 80th percentile were randomized to atorvastatin (20 mg) versus placebo.[40] At a 4.3-year follow-up, no differences were observed in the composite CVD endpoint (6.9% vs. 9.9%; $P = 0.08$). However, this was an underpowered study, and in a post hoc analysis, participants with a baseline CAC >400 did have a lower event rate (8.7% vs. 15.0%; $P = 0.046$) with statin therapy. Although several trials have been proposed to further investigate the potential efficacy of CAC testing, no trials have been completed to date.

Given ethical issues inherent to withholding therapy in individuals who have CAC and the increased adoption of statin therapy in primary prevention, as now promoted in various guidelines, it is unlikely that there will be a large-scale randomized trial that will randomize patients to treatment based on CAC results. A trial design only including individuals who do not currently have an indication for statin therapy will have a low event rate, thus requiring a very large sample size or a long follow-up period. As a result, such a trial would likely be prohibitively expensive.

When evaluating various future potential trial designs, it is important to recognize that the role of CAC testing has shifted form a "screening test" to a "shared decision-making test," where testing is now most commonly performed among individuals who already have an indication for statin therapy (see previous section on Clinical Indications). Recognizing these challenges, a recent National Heart Lung and Blood Institute (NHLBI) workshop proposed several possible trials using CAC testing in primary prevention. The potential opportunities identified included (1) studies evaluating the efficacy of shared decision tools using CAC, (2) studies using artificial intelligence to identify CAC on noncardiac CT and subsequently notify clinicians, (3) studies using CAC testing to enhance prevention in young adults (i.e., <45 years), and (4) studies using CAC testing in low-risk older adults to identify "healthy vascular agers" in whom treatment can be avoided.[41]

CORONARY COMPUTED TOMOGRAPHY ANGIOGRAPHY

How Is the Test Performed?

Image acquisition for cardiac CT was described previously (see Technical Considerations/Image Acquisition; see Table 20.1). Prior to contrast-enhanced cardiac CT exams, an 18-gauge IV is inserted to allow for rapid injection (e.g., 5 to 7 cc/s) of contrast during the scan; in some cases a 20-gauge IV may be sufficient in smaller patients. When CCTA is performed, patients are often administered nitroglycerin to dilate the coronary arteries and beta blockers (oral, or in some cases IV) to achieve a sufficiently low heart rate, in part depending on the type of scanner being used. Thus it is important to screen patients for any contraindications for these medications.

Image acquisition is performed approximately 15 to 25 seconds after starting the contrast injection to allow for maximal contrast enhancement in the coronary arteries. This can be achieved by using either a bolus tracking technique, whereby the attenuation in the ascending or descending aorta is monitored during contrast injection, or by first performing a test bolus and measuring the amount of time from injection of 10 to 15 cc of contrast until peak contrast enhancement in the ascending aorta. The scan is performed during a single breath-hold, usually lasting 5 to 10 seconds. Subsequently, the raw data obtained from the CT scanner is used to reconstruct high-resolution images that are then transferred to a dedicated workstation for interpretation.

Contraindications to CCTA include inability to tolerate contrast because of renal dysfunction (glomerular filtration rate [GFR] <30), severe contrast allergy, or uncontrolled tachycardia. Relative contraindications include the presence of atrial fibrillation, morbid obesity (e.g., body mass index [BMI] >40 kg/m^2), extensive coronary calcifications, or the presence of small stents. All of these conditions will degrade CT image quality and CT should generally be avoided unless there is a high likelihood of obtaining diagnostic image quality. For instance, some scanners have algorithms that allow for successful scanning of patients in atrial fibrillation who have controlled heart rates.[42,43] With respect to obesity, the upper weight limit for most scanners is around 450 pounds, and some scanners have certain acquisition modes that may enhance image quality in these scenarios. Although most contemporary scanners can achieve good image quality with BMI <40 kg/m^2, individuals with obesity are more likely to have reduced image quality and may have nondiagnostic scans even when maximal scanner output is used.

The presence of extensive coronary calcifications can be problematic because of calcium blooming artifacts, which may interfere with the ability to visualize the lumen and estimate the severity of stenosis. Blooming artifacts occur because of limited spatial resolution and are caused by partial volume averaging of different densities within a single voxel. As a result, the actual size of the calcium is exaggerated making the lumen smaller. Although the amount of calcium blooming has reduced considerably with new-generation scanners that have better spatial resolution, the inability to fully exclude stenosis remains an important limitation when there are dense focal calcifications. The amount of calcium "blooming" can be reduced by using higher resolution scanners,[44] reconstructing the thinnest possible slices, using a sharper reconstruction kernel, and optimizing display settings (e.g., wider grayscale window with a higher center). In addition, there are vendor-specific algorithms that are being developed to help mitigate these artifacts.[45]

Diagnostic Accuracy

The diagnostic accuracy of CCTA compared with invasive angiography has been evaluated in multiple multicenter and single-center trials. A meta-analysis[46] across 9 studies has identified a sensitivity of 97% (93 to 99) with a specificity of 78% (67 to 86) for detecting >50% stenosis. The same analysis showed that CCTA has the highest sensitivity of any noninvasive imaging technique to detect the presence of anatomic stenosis. When evaluating the diagnostic accuracy of CCTA to detect functionally significant coronary artery disease (CAD), as defined by an invasive fractional flow reserve (FFR) ≤0.80, the sensitivity of CCTA was 93% (89 to 96) with a specificity of 53% (37 to 68). The lower specificity of CTA versus invasive FFR in this meta-analysis may have been influenced by the fact that several studies excluded, by design, patients with nonobstructive CAD.

An important challenge in comparing the diagnostic accuracy of different tests is that each study is usually performed on a different group of patients. To address this challenge, two prospective studies were designed to allow for a better head-to-head comparison by having each patient undergo multiple tests.

The EVINCI (Evaluation of Integrated Cardiac Imaging for the Detection and Characterization of Ischemic Heart Disease) study was a multicenter prospective study designed to compare the diagnostic accuracy of noninvasive anatomic and functional imaging in identifying patients with significant CAD defined by invasive angiography.[47] Among 475 patients who each underwent multiple imaging tests including CCTA, single-photon emission computed tomography (SPECT), or PET MPI, and either cardiac magnetic resonance (CMR) or stress echocardiography, CCTA had the highest diagnostic accuracy to detect significant CAD, defined by invasive angiography as >50% stenosis of the left main stem, >70% stenosis in a major coronary vessel, or 30% to 70% stenosis with FFR ≤0.8. The sensitivity of CCTA was 91% (86 to 95), whereas the specificity was 92% (89% to 95%).

The PACIFIC trial (Prospective Comparison of Cardiac PET/CT, SPECT/CT Perfusion Imaging and CT Coronary Angiography With Invasive Coronary Angiography) provided a head-to-head comparison of different techniques against invasively measured FFR ≤0.80 as the reference standard.[48] In this study, CCTA (90%) and PET (87%) had the highest sensitivity, whereas PET and SPECT had the highest specificity. The overall diagnostic accuracy to detect lesion-specific ischemia was highest for PET.

Collectively, the available data (see side insert) support CCTA as a highly sensitive test for detecting coronary stenosis, and accordingly a high negative predictive value (NPV) to rule out CAD, especially in populations that have a lower prevalence of disease. However, the specificity of CCTA to identify ischemia is limited, as is also the case for invasive angiography (see the section Physiologic Evaluation of Coronary Artery Disease).

Prognostic Implications

Multiple studies have evaluated the prognostic capabilities of CCTA to identify high-risk patients. The Coronary CT Angiography Evaluation for Clinical Outcomes: an International Multicenter Registry (CONFIRM) study evaluated a cohort of 24,775 patients without known CAD who underwent CCCTA between 2005 and 2009.[49] Over a mean follow-up of 2.3 years, nonobstructive and obstructive CAD were associated with higher risk of mortality, including a 2.6-fold increased risk of death for patients with >70% stenosis, and a 1.6-fold increased risk of death for those with <50% stenosis. Increasing risk of mortality was observed for patients with a greater number of vessels with stenosis. Importantly, incident rates of all-cause death were very low in the absence of CAD by CCTA, with an annualized rate of 0.28%.[49]

The prognostic value of CCTA has subsequently been evaluated across multiple cohorts, registries, and prospective studies, all showing an increase in events among patients who have a greater extent or severity of plaque or stenosis.[50] In the Partners registry, 3242 patients who underwent CCTA were followed over a median of 3.6 years. The presence of nonobstructive plaque was associated with a higher rate of cardiovascular death or myocardial infarction (MI). Moreover, patients who had greater than four segments with plaque (i.e., segment involvement score [SIS] >4) had the same risk of incident cardiovascular death or MI as those who had one-vessel obstructive CAD.[51] Similar increase in mortality among patients with nonobstructive plaque (SIS >4 or involving 3 vessels) was also observed in a prospective 2 center study.[52]

The prognostic value of CCTA and functional testing were compared in the PROMISE trial, where 4500 patients were randomly assigned to CCTA and 4602 were randomly assigned to functional testing.[53] The prevalence of obstructive CAD and myocardial ischemia was low (11.9% vs. 12.7%, respectively), and both finding had similar prognostic value over a median follow-up of 26.1 months. However, the overall discriminatory ability of CCTA in predicting events was significantly better than functional testing (c-index, 0.72; 95% confidence interval [CI], 0.68–0.76 vs. 0.64; 95% CI, 0.59–0.69; $P = 0.04$), a finding that was driven by the fact that CCTA identified nonobstructive CAD, a prognostically relevant finding, especially when the overall burden of ischemia and obstructive CAD are low.[53]

As suggested by the previous studies, an important aspect of CCTA is the ability to further stratify risk beyond just the presence or absence of anatomic stenosis. Indeed, emerging data have suggested that the overall amount of plaque, and various high-risk plaque (HRP) features (see the next section), may provide incremental prognostic information.

Plaque Burden and Prognosis

The Western Denmark Heart Registry[54] evaluated the prognostic value of CCTA among 23,759 symptomatic patients who underwent CCTA and were followed for the primary endpoint of major CVD (MI, stroke, and all-cause death). The overall risk of major CVD events increased in a stepwise manner with both atherosclerotic disease burden (determined by the total CAC score) and number of vessels with ≥50% stenosis. When stratified by groups of increasing CAC, patients with nonobstructive CAD had a risk of CVD events similar to those with obstructive CAD, suggesting that plaque burden, not stenosis, was the main predictor of future CVD events.[54] These findings reinforce the importance of assessing overall plaque burden, rather than just stenosis, in deciding on the role of secondary prevention therapies. As has also been shown in the PROMISE trial (see later), the vast majority (~65%) of events occurred among patients who did not have obstructive CAD.

Coronary Computed Tomography Angiography in Acute Chest Pain

To date there have been several randomized trials evaluating the safety and efficacy of using CCTA to evaluate patients with acute chest pain. Collectively, these studies have shown that the use of CCTA can reduce the time to diagnosis, hospital length of stay, and emergency department cost compared with a standard evaluation.[55] The improved efficiency of CCTA was due, in part, to the fact that this test does not require patients to be "ruled out" for MI, and can be performed after one set of negative cardiac enzymes. However, in the era of high-sensitivity troponin testing (hsTn), other testing options (including deciding on deferral of any testing) can now be pursued without a prolonged delay and patients can be more rapidly discharged from the emergency department.

Evaluating the comparative effectiveness of testing in the current era of hsTn, the Better Evaluation of Acute Chest Pain by Computed Tomography Angiography (BEACON) trial was a prospective multicenter randomized trial that compared the diagnostic strategy of early CCTA with the use of hsTn among 500 patients with suspected acute coronary syndrome (ACS).[56] In contrast to earlier trials, this study did not shorten hospital length of stay in the emergency department. In addition, there was no significant difference in the rate of revascularization within 30 days and incidence of major adverse cardiovascular events (MACE) at 30 days. However, the CCTA approach allowed for significantly reduced downstream outpatient testing and a reduction in direct medical cost.[56]

Although most studies evaluating the use of CCTA only evaluated short-term outcomes, the CATCH trial evaluated whether postdischarge CCTA-guided care in patients with normal ECG and troponin values improved long-term outcomes. The primary endpoint was a composite of cardiac death, MI, hospitalization for unstable angina, late symptom-driven revascularizations, and readmission for chest pain. Over a median follow-up of 18 months, patients randomized to CCTA-guided treatment strategy experienced fewer events compared with those evaluated using a standard of care strategy (11% vs. 16%; $P = 0.04$; hazard ratio [HR] 0.62).

With respect to long-term outcomes, one potential advantage of using CCTA is that it can detect nonobstructive CAD, and thus be used to initiate preventive therapies. Although the implementation of such therapies following CCTA have been shown to occur among patients with stable chest pain who are treated in the outpatient setting, one challenge to the use of CCTA in the acute setting is that nonurgent findings are less likely to impact future medical therapy.[57] Accordingly, better systems are needed to use information from CCTA (and other tests obtained in the emergency department) to improve long-term preventive treatments.

When considering the prospective clinical trials of CCTA for acute chest pain, it is important to recognize that most of them were performed in low-risk patients, where ultimately <10% were found to have an ACS, and of those only a small proportion represented patients with MI.

Coronary Computed Tomography Angiography in Non–ST Elevation Myocardial Infarction

Although initial trials using CCTA for the evaluation of patients with acute chest pain excluded individuals with elevated troponin levels, recent data have suggested that CCTA can be effective at excluding obstructive CAD in low- and intermediate-risk non–ST-segment elevation MI (NSTEMI) patients. A subanalysis of the Very EaRly vs Deferred Invasive evaluation using Computerized Tomography (VERDICT) trial, which included non-ST elevation ACS patients who underwent a CCTA and invasive angiography showed that the NPV of CCTA to exclude ≥50% stenosis was 91%.[58] A small randomized trial of 207 patients with elevated hsTn and inconclusive enzymes found that the use of CCTA resulted in ~33% reduction in invasive angiography while achieving similar outcomes.[59] Accordingly the 2020 European Society of Cardiology (ESC) recommends CCTA as an alternative to invasive angiography to exclude ACS when there is low-to-intermediate likelihood of CAD and when cardiac troponin and/or ECG are normal or inconclusive.[60] The selective use of CCTA to evaluate patients with elevated cardiac enzymes with potential ACS has also been used throughout the COVID-19 pandemic and has been suggested as a useful testing option by several international expert guidance documents.[61]

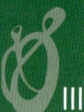

Age (years)	Chest pain		Dyspnea	
	Men	Women	Men	Women
30–39	≤4	≤5	0	3
40–49	≤22	≤10	12	3
50–59	≤32	≤13	20	9
60–69	≤44	≤16	27	14
70+	≤52	≤27	32	12

Pretest probability based on age, sex and symptoms	Low ≤15%	Intermediate-high >15%		
Pretest probability based on CAC Score*	≤15%	>15%–50%		>50%
	CAC=0	CAC 1–99	CAC≥100–999	CAC≥1000

FIGURE 20.6 Pretest probability (PTP) of obstructive coronary artery disease (CAD) in symptomatic patients. The PTP shown is for patients with anginal symptoms. Patients with lower risk symptoms would be expected to have lower PTP. The *dark green shaded regions* denote the groups in which noninvasive testing is most beneficial (PTP >15%). The *light green shaded regions* denote the groups with PTP of CAD ≤15% in which the testing for diagnosis may be considered based on clinical judgment. If information on coronary artery calcium testing is available, it can also be used to further define the pretest probability estimate. The vast majority of symptomatic patients have a PTP of obstructive CAD <50%. (Data from Juarez-Orozco LE, et al. Impact of a decreasing pre-test probability on the performance of diagnostic tests for coronary artery disease. Eur Heart J Cardiovasc Imag 2019;20:1198-1207; and Winther S, et al. Incorporating coronary calcification into pre-test assessment of the likelihood of coronary artery disease. J Am Coll Cardiol 2020;76:2421-2432; Gulati M, Levy PD, Mukherjee D, et al. 2021 AHA/ACC/ASE/CHEST/SAEM/SCCT/SCMR guideline for the evaluation and diagnosis of chest pain: a report of the American College of Cardiology/American Heart Association Joint Committee on Clinical Practice Guidelines. J Am Coll Cardiol. 2021.)

Coronary Computed Tomography Angiography in Stable Chest Pain

The most common use of CCTA is to evaluate patients with symptoms that raise suspicion for CHD. When symptoms are chronic and associated with consistent precipitants, such as exertion or emotional stress, they are often categorized as "stable." The use of CCTA in this setting has been shown to accurately diagnose both nonobstructive and obstructive CAD, improve diagnostic certainty, and improve patient outcomes. Appropriate patient selection and management based on CCTA results is essential for maximizing the value of CCTA.

Selecting Appropriate Candidates for Coronary Computed Tomography Angiography

Although CCTA has robust capabilities to estimate the amount and severity of CAD, like other imaging tests, the accuracy and effectiveness of this test are dependent on selecting appropriate patients in whom high-quality images can be achieved. Use of contemporary scanners, which along with other advances offer improved spatial and temporal resolution, is also helpful for achieving optimal image quality. For instance, scanners that have dual source capabilities will allow imaging at higher heart rates because of improved temporal resolution. Scanners that have better spatial resolution will have less calcium blooming–related artifacts. Patients who are ideal candidates for CCTA have no known CAD, can achieve a low heart rate (e.g., <70 beats/min with medications), can hold their breath during image acquisition, and can tolerate the administration of IV contrast.

Pretest Probability of Obstructive Coronary Artery Disease

Although older guidelines have suggested that CCTA may be most effective in patients who have a low to intermediate pretest probability (PTP) of having obstructive CAD, it is noteworthy that most algorithms overestimate the likelihood of having obstructive CAD.[62-64] The latest ESC Chronic Coronary Syndrome guideline and the 2021 AHA/ACC chest pain guideline provide a useful PTP tool that was derived from 15,815 symptomatic patients according to age, sex, and type of symptoms. When evaluating this PTP tool (Fig. 20.6), the only group of patients with a PTP >50% is men over the age of 70 with chest pain, but even in this group the PTP was 52% or lower. Other recent PTPs have shown an even lower likelihood of obstructive CAD,[65] further reinforcing that risk scores alone may not be sufficient in identifying patients who truly have a high PTP of obstructive CAD.

The 2021 AHA/ACC chest pain guideline indicates that patients with stable chest pain who have a low PTP of obstructive CAD (e.g., PTP <15%) may not require further testing, whereas patients with intermediate and high PTP are most likely to benefit from further testing with either CCTA or functional testing. The severity of underlying coronary artery calcifications may be important in identifying patients with a high PTP of obstructive CAD.[65] Accordingly, when available, prior CT images should be reviewed for the presence of extensive coronary calcifications. The absence of extensive coronary calcifications may favor CCTA, whereas the presence of such findings may favor stress testing.

Patient Outcomes Following Coronary Computed Tomography Angiography

There have been several randomized controlled trials comparing CCTA with functional testing among patients with stable symptoms (these trials evaluated the impact of CCTA on diagnosis, symptoms, risk stratification, clinical management, and patient outcomes).

The SCOT-HEART (Scottish Computed Tomography of the HEART) trial was a prospective multicenter trial that randomized 4146 participants to standard care plus CCTA or standard care alone. The addition of CCTA led to a lower frequency of diagnosing angina caused by CHD, and a higher diagnostic certainty.

The CAPP (Cardiac CT for the Assessment of Patients With Pain and Plaque) and CRESCENT trials[66,67] were designed to assess the impact of CCTA on angina symptoms compared with a functional testing strategy. The use of CCTA was associated with lower levels of angina after 12 months of follow-up. Similar improvements in symptoms were seen in the SCOT-HEART trial, especially in those demonstrated to have normal coronary arteries or those with obstructive disease who underwent coronary revascularization.[50]

Hard Clinical Outcomes

The SCOT-HEART and PROMISE trials are the largest trials to date to examine the impact of CCTA on clinical outcomes. The SCOT-HEART was a prospective multicenter trial of 4146 patients with stable chest pain who were recruited across 12 centers across Scotland and

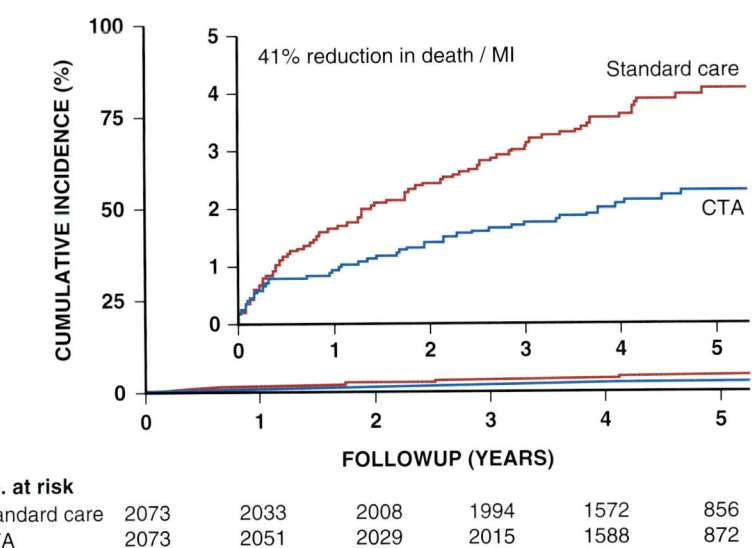

FIGURE 20.7 Cumulative incidence of death from coronary heart disease or nonfatal myocardial infarction in the SCOT-HEART trial. The figure shows cumulative event curves for the primary endpoint of death from coronary heart disease or nonfatal myocardial infarction among patients assigned to computed tomography angiography in addition to standard care and those assigned to standard care alone. (From Newby DE, et al. Coronary CT angiography and 5-year risk of myocardial infarction. N Engl J Med 2018;379:924-933.)

randomized to standard care plus CCTA or to standard care alone. In both groups, standard of care included the use of exercise treadmill testing in 85% of patients, while stress imaging was infrequent (9%). Over a median follow-up of 4.8 years, the addition of CCTA to standard of care resulted in a 41% reduction in the combined endpoint of CHD death or nonfatal MI (2.3% vs. 3.9%; HR 0.59; $P = 0.004$; Fig. 20.7).

The PROMISE trial compared a strategy of CCTA versus functional testing (67% nuclear stress testing, 27% stress echocardiography, 10% exercise electrocardiography). The composite primary endpoint was death, MI, hospitalization for unstable angina, or major procedural complication. Over a median follow-up of 25 months, 164 patients (3.3%) in the CCTA group and 151 (3.0%) in the functional-testing group experienced the primary outcome (HR 1.04; $P = 0.75$). Although there was no difference in this primary outcome, the use of CCTA was associated with a lower rate of death or MI at 12 months (HR 0.66; $P = 0.049$). The use of CCTA was associated with a lower incidence of invasive angiography showing no obstructive CAD during the 90 days after randomization, which was a prespecified secondary endpoint. However, more patients in the CCTA group underwent invasive angiography within 90 days of randomization (12.2% vs. 8.1%) and more patients in the CCTA group underwent coronary revascularization (6.2% vs. 3.2%). Limitations of the PROMISE study included a low event rate, as there was a total of 315 events while 800 events were anticipated to achieve 90% power to detect a 20% reduction in events. The PROMISE trial used a pragmatic design to enhance the generalizability of the results, thus patient care decisions were determined by local sites, and at a time when there was little guidance for clinicians on how to act on various CCTA findings.

A prespecified post hoc analysis from the PROMISE study was to examine cardiovascular outcomes in 2144 patients with diabetes. Patients with diabetes who underwent CCTA had a lower risk of cardiovascular death or MI compared with those who were randomized to functional stress testing (CCTA 1.1% vs. 2.6%; HR 0.39; $P = 0.01$).[68]

There are several additional nonrandomized studies suggesting that the use of CCTA may be associated with a lower event rate. A meta-analysis evaluating hard outcomes following CCTA versus usual care included the results of the PROMISE trial, the SCOT-HEART initial findings over a median follow-up of 1.7 years, and the CAPP trial. In this study, using CCTA was associated with a 30% reduction in incident MI (HR 0.69 [95% CI, 0.49–0.98]).[69] Similar reductions in MI have also been reported in a large (n = 86,705) observational Danish registry (HR 0.71 [95% CI, 0.61–0.82]).[70] The lower risk of MI was similar when comparing with patients who underwent exercise treadmill testing or those who underwent SPECT MPI.

Mechanisms Underlying Improved Patient Outcomes. A key question related to the aforementioned studies is regarding the mechanism for the reduction in event rates following CCTA. In the PROMISE and SCOT-HEART trials, and the Danish registry, when compared with functional testing approaches, the use of CCTA was associated with greater use of preventive therapies such as statins and aspirin. Further supporting these findings, other registries have also showed a stepwise increase in the use and intensity of preventive therapies when more severe stenosis is identified by CCTA.[71] The 5-year results from the SCOT-HEART trial showed that higher use of statin and antiplatelet therapies was sustained over the entire trial period. Furthermore, the observed reduction in events observed in this trial was explained by modeling, which accounted for the benefits of medical therapy.[72] Reinforcing the importance of preventive therapies, the PROMISE investigators reported that the majority of events in patients randomized the functional testing group occurred in those who did not have any abnormalities.[53] Although some have suggested that the higher use of coronary revascularization following CCTA may have contributed to a reduction in events, there are no data that such procedures are associated with improved outcomes (see the section Implications of the ISCHEMIA Trial for Coronary Computed Tomography Angiography).

Use of Invasive Angiography Following Coronary Computed Tomography Angiography

An appropriate criticism of CCTA has been that it can lead to a higher use of invasive angiography and coronary revascularization. In the PROMISE study, there was an ~50% higher use of invasive angiography and twofold increase in coronary revascularization in the CCTA arm compared with the functional testing arm. There were no significant differences in the SCOT-HEART trial, although the absolute rate of coronary revascularization was higher in the SCOT-HEART trial when compared with PROMISE (10.5% vs. 4.7%). In the SCOT-HEART trial, although the initial rates of invasive coronary angiography and coronary revascularization were higher in the CCTA group, the overall rates were similar at 5 years. In fact, when examining the utilization of such procedures beyond 12 months, the rates of invasive coronary angiography and coronary revascularization were higher in the standard-care group. These findings suggest that although CCTA may lead to a higher initial rate of invasive angiography and coronary revascularization, over longer-term follow-up these initial differences may no longer be present.

When considering the differences in revascularization following CCTA versus functional testing between SCOT-HEART and PROMISE, it is possible that geographic differences in practice patterns may play a role. In addition, in the SCOT-HEART trial CCTA was performed in addition to functional testing, most often exercise treadmill testing. It is plausible that reassuring results from functional testing may have been helpful in avoiding invasive angiography. Another factor that may account for the higher use of invasive testing following CCTA in these studies is that the PROMISE study was a pragmatic trial that started enrollment over a decade ago. Yet, this was at a time when there was a paucity of guidance to clinicians on how to manage patients based on the CCTA results (see section Patient Management Following CCTA).

Cost-Effectiveness Data

Several cost-effectiveness studies comparing CCTA with functional testing have been reported collectively showing that the costs of CCTA are similar to those that occur following stress testing. An economic analysis using hospital bills to estimate hospital-based costs in the PROMISE study showed that CCTA had costs similar to the stress testing approaches.[31] Although patients in the CCTA arm had less follow-up noninvasive testing, they had higher costs related to downstream invasive angiography and revascularization. Similarly, results from the SCOT-HEART trial revealed slightly higher costs associated with randomization to CTA, although the cost difference of $462 was mostly attributable to the additional cost of undergoing CCTA. In the CRESCENT trial,[67] referral to exercise electrocardiography was associated with a higher rate of additional diagnostic testing and a 16% higher cost of care. Nearly half of patients in the stress testing arm had induced diagnostic testing procedures compared with only 1 in 4 in the CCTA arm ($p < 0.0001$). The cost savings achieved in the CTA arm of the CRESCENT trial were also related to the fact that 42% of this arm had a CAC score of zero and did not undergo follow-up CCTA.

A comprehensive cost analysis comparing CCTA to functional testing was also conducted by the NICE guidelines.[50] This analysis determined that CCTA has the lowest cost per correct diagnosis, and was projected to save the National Health Service approximately £16 million each year by excluding CAD with a high NPV. Based on these projections, an initial testing approach with CCTA was recommended to allow for selective use of higher cost stress testing in a smaller proportion of patients with stable chest pain.

One potential advantage of using CCTA in stable chest pain patients is the identification and treatment of nonobstructive plaque, yet the benefits of such preventive therapies are often not realized in the short term. A cost-effectiveness analysis based on patient data from the PROMISE trial that modeled the impact of preventive therapies when nonobstructive plaque was detected showed that CCTA was cost-effective, while the addition of FFRCT further lowered cost and resulted in a dominant strategy. Moreover, over a lifetime, the use of CCTA resulted in a gain of 6 months in perfect health compared with functional testing. In probabilistic sensitivity analyses, anatomic approaches were cost-effective in more than 65% of scenarios, assuming a willingness-to-pay threshold of $100,000/quality-adjusted life year (QALY). Although this study was limited by various assumptions used in the Markov model, the results suggested that anatomic strategies may present a more favorable initial diagnostic option in the evaluation of low-risk stable chest pain.[73]

Coronary Computed Tomography Angiography Plaque Characteristics

There are several CCTA-based adverse plaque characteristics (APCs) associated with a higher risk of future events (Table 20.3). An important but unknown question is whether the increased risk conferred by such plaque is caused by identification of plaque that is more likely to rupture (i.e., "vulnerable plaques"), plaque that is more likely to rapidly progress, or plaque that is more likely to result in ischemia. Regardless, it is important to recognize HRP characteristics, the presence of which could prompt intensification of preventive medical therapies, or in selected cases, referral for further testing.

High-Risk Plaque Characteristics
Low-Attenuation Plaque

Low-attenuation plaque on CCTA (Hounsfield units [HU] <30; Fig. 20.8) corresponds to lipid-rich plaque whereas noncalcified plaque with higher CT attenuation correlates with fibrous tissues. However, it is important to recognize that there is variability in CT values within plaque types that prevents the reliable subclassification of noncalcified plaques. Furthermore, CT measurements of coronary plaques can be influenced by several factors: concentration of adjacent intraluminal iodinated contrast agent, image noise, tube voltage, and the reconstruction filter.

Low-attenuation plaque is more often seen in patients with ACS,[74] and has been found to be associated with ruptured fibrous caps,[75] lesion-specific ischemia,[76] and a future risk of MI.[77] In the SCOT-HEART trial, low-attenuation plaque burden was a strong independent predictor of incident fatal or nonfatal MI (HR 1.60, 95% CI, 1.10–2.34 per doubling) beyond the CAC score or stenosis severity. Patients with low-attenuation plaque burden greater than 4% were nearly 5 times more likely to have subsequent MI[77].

Positive Remodeling

Positive remodeling describes compensatory enlargement of the vessel wall as plaque size increases outward to preserve the luminal area. This feature is associated with a larger burden of plaque, a larger necrotic core, and also higher likelihood of thin-cap fibroatheroma (TCFA) by intravascular ultrasound (IVUS).

The remodeling index is calculated as the vessel cross-sectional area at the site of maximal stenosis divided by the average of the proximal and distal reference segments' crosssectional areas. A remodeling index threshold of ≥ 1.1 is typically used to define positive remodeling by CCTA (Fig.20.9).

TABLE 20.3 CCTA-Based Measurements Associated With Increased Risk

CATEGORY	MEASURE	EXPLANATION
Stenosis	Stenosis	• Luminal narrowing estimated as minimal (1%-24%), mild (25%-49%), moderate (50%-69%), severe (70%-99%), or occluded (100%)
Plaque burden	CAC scores	• Overall burden of calcified plaque, which serves as an effective surrogate for overall plaque burden, and provides strong prognostic data
	Segment involvement score	• Number of coronary segments with plaque, which can provide an estimate of the overall extent of plaque, which can provide incremental prognostic value
	Plaque volume	• Quantitative assessment of the overall amount of plaque. Higher plaque volume is associated with higher risk of adverse events and a higher likelihood of flow-limiting CAD
Adverse plaque characteristics (see Fig. 20.11)	Positive remodeling	• Compensatory enlargement of the vessel wall that occurs at the site of the atherosclerotic lesion as the plaque size increases, resulting in the preservation of luminal area
	Low-attenuation plaque	• Correspond to lipid rich plaques (HU <30)
	Spotty calcifications	• Small, dense (>130 HU) plaque component surrounded by noncalcified plaque tissue
	Napkin-ring sign	• A central area of low CT attenuation in contact with the lumen that has a ring-like higher attenuation plaque surrounding this central area
Hemodynamics	FFR_{CT}	• Measure of lesion-specific hemodynamic significance that estimates FFR by applying computational fluid dynamics to rest CCTA data (see Fig. 20.12)
	ESS	• ESS is the tangential force generated by the friction of flowing blood on the endothelial surface of the arterial wall
		• Low ESS triggers an endothelial cell gene expression resulting in reduced nitric oxide production, increased LDL uptake, and local oxidative stress and inflammation. These processes may lead to the development of high-risk lesions
Inflammation	Pericoronary fat attenuation index (FAI)	• Reflects inflammation in the perivascular adipose tissue resulting from nearby coronary inflammation (see Fig. 20.14 for details.)

CAC, Coronary artery calcium; *CAD*, coronary artery disease; *CCTA*, coronary computed tomography angiography; *ESS*, endothelial shear stress; *FFR*, fractional flow reserve; *FFRCT*, fraction flow research computed tomography; *HU*, Hounsfield units; *LDL*, low-density lipoprotein.

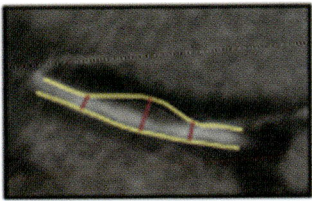
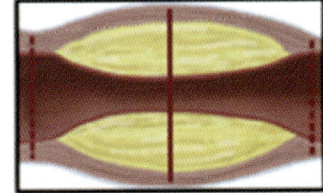

Positive remodeling

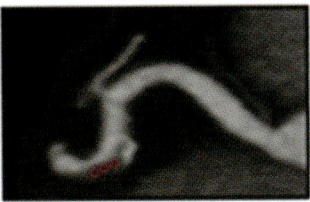
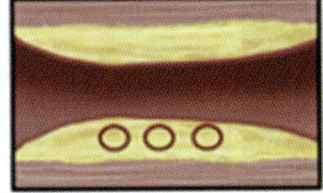

Low HU

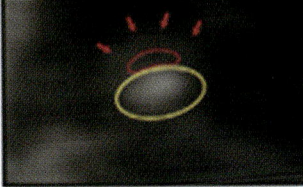
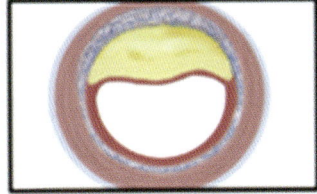

Napkin ring sign

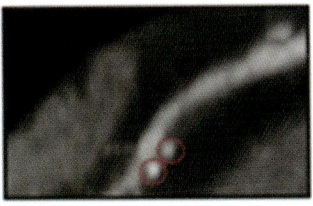
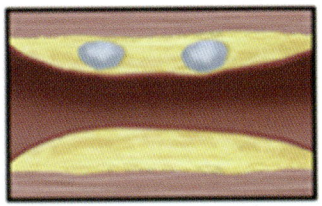

Spotty calcium

FIGURE 20.8 High-risk coronary plaque features. Positive remodeling: noncalcified plaque with positive remodeling. The two *dotted red lines* demonstrate the vessel diameters at the proximal and distal references (both 1.8 mm), and the *solid red line* demonstrates the maximal vessel diameter in the midportion of the plaque (2.7 mm). The remodeling index is 1.5. Low Hounsfield units (HU) plaque: partially calcified plaque in the mid right coronary artery with low <30 HU plaque. The *red circles* demonstrate the three regions of interest, with mean computed tomography (CT) numbers of 22, 19, and 20 HU. Napkin-ring sign: napkin-ring sign plaque in the mid left anterior descending coronary artery. Schematic cross-sectional view of the napkin-ring sign. The *red line* demonstrates the central low HU area of the plaque adjacent to the lumen (*yellow ellipse*) surrounded by a peripheral rim of the higher CT attenuation (*red arrows*). Spotty calcium: partially calcified plaque in the mid right coronary artery with spotty calcification (diameter <3 mm in all directions; *red circles*). (Adapted from Puchner SB, et al. High-risk plaque detected on coronary CT angiography predicts acute coronary syndromes independent of significant stenosis in acute chest pain: results from the ROMICAT-II Trial. J Am Coll Cardiol 2014;64:684-692.)

Napkin-Ring Sign

Napkin-ring sign (NRS) describes plaques that on cross-section have a ring-like peripheral enhancement surrounding low CT attenuation in the center (Fig. 20.10). The central area of low attenuation represents, based on pathologic correlation, a large necrotic core, and the higher surrounding ring-like attenuation may be caused by fibrous plaque. However, the peripheral enhancement may also be caused by the vasa vasorum.[78] NRS has been shown to have a high specificity to identify TCFA on optical coherence tomography (OCT), or culprit ACS lesions, and future risk of ACS.[78] Plaques with the NRS contain large necrotic cores and, although infrequent, they have a higher association with future events than other APCs.

Spotty Calcifications

Spotty calcifications are defined as small, dense (>130 HU) plaque components surrounded by noncalcified plaque tissue. Compared with intermediate (1 to 3 mm) calcifications, small (<1 mm) spotty calcification have the strongest association with HRP features defined by virtual histology IVUS, and may represent plaques that are more likely to accelerate.[78] However, the impact of spotty calcifications on plaque stability is controversial, and this feature is a weaker marker of future risk compared with other APCs, such as low-attenuation plaque and positive remodeling.

Plaque Characteristics and Incident Risk

When interpreting CCTA results, it is useful to identify the presence of potential HRP, or APCs. However, such findings are common and have a low specificity for predicting future events. In the SCOT-HEART study, 34% of participants had at least one APC (low-attenuation plaque, positive remodeling, NRS, or spotty calcifications), including 40% of those with nonobstructive plaque and 75% of those with obstructive plaque.[79] As expected, the frequency was higher among individuals who were older or had more risk factors. Although participants who experienced CHD death or MI were 3 times as likely to have at least one APC, the positive predictive value of these findings was low (4.1% when APCs present vs. 1.4% if APCs absent). Notably, APCs were not associated with increased risk once accounting for overall plaque burden, as measured by CAC.[79] In the PROMISE study,[80] HRP characteristics (which only included positive remodeling, low CT attenuation, and NRS) occurred in 15% of patients and were associated with a higher risk of future events (HR 2.7). However, the predictive value was stronger among women, young individuals, and those with nonobstructive plaque.

Recognizing the limited specificity of APCs for identifying high-risk patients, plaque features should not just be thought of as binary (i.e., present or absent). For instance, the larger the low-attenuation plaque volume and the more expansive the positive remodeling, the greater is the risk of plaque rupture.[50] Also plaques that have multiple APCs have higher risk. For instance, patients with plaques that have both low-attenuation and positive remodeling (so-called two-feature positive plaque) have been shown to have a higher risk of future events. When evaluating patient risk, the abovementioned factors should always be interpreted in the context of other risk factors and the overall amount of plaque and severity of coronary stenosis.[50,71]

Plaque Features and Myocardial Ischemia

Because it is well recognized that anatomic stenosis, whether by CCTA or invasive angiography, is often inadequate for identifying ischemia,[81,82] a common question is what plaque characteristics are more likely to cause myocardial ischemia. Although the aforementioned HRP features that predict a higher risk of adverse events have also been associated with lesion-specific ischemia,[50] these features have not consistently been found to add incremental data to the evaluation of stenosis.[83] Furthermore, it is unclear if the predictive value of HRP is caused by the identification of specific types of plaque, or if these features are simply markers of having larger plaque burden. A prospective multicenter study of 252 patients from 17 centers evaluated the role of APCs, including positive remodeling, low-attenuation plaque, and spotty calcifications for identification of ischemia-causing coronary artery lesions.[76] A dose-response relationship was noted for increasing numbers of APCs and ischemia, with two or more APCs associated with a 12-fold increase in the rate of ischemia. This improvement for identification of ischemia existed only for positive remodeling (odds ratio [OR] 5.3) and low-attenuation plaque (OR 2.1), with no improvement noted for spotty calcifications. Importantly, arteries exhibiting positive remodeling were useful for diagnosis of lesion-specific ischemia for stenoses of 50% or greater and 50% or less, the latter present in almost 17% of ischemic lesions.[76]

One of the most robust markers of ischemia by CCTA is the percentage aggregate plaque volume (%APV), which is the sum of the entire plaque volume within a vessel divided by the sum of the vessel volume from the artery ostium to the distal end of the coronary lesion. In a study of 58 lesions, %APV demonstrated high discriminatory capacity to identify vessel ischemia beyond traditional diameter stenosis alone (0.85 vs. 0.68).[84]

The CREDENCE trial provided further data that the overall amount and type of plaque is a strong determinant of ischemia. This was a multicenter trial of 612 patients designed to compare the diagnostic accuracy of comprehensive anatomic versus functional imaging measures

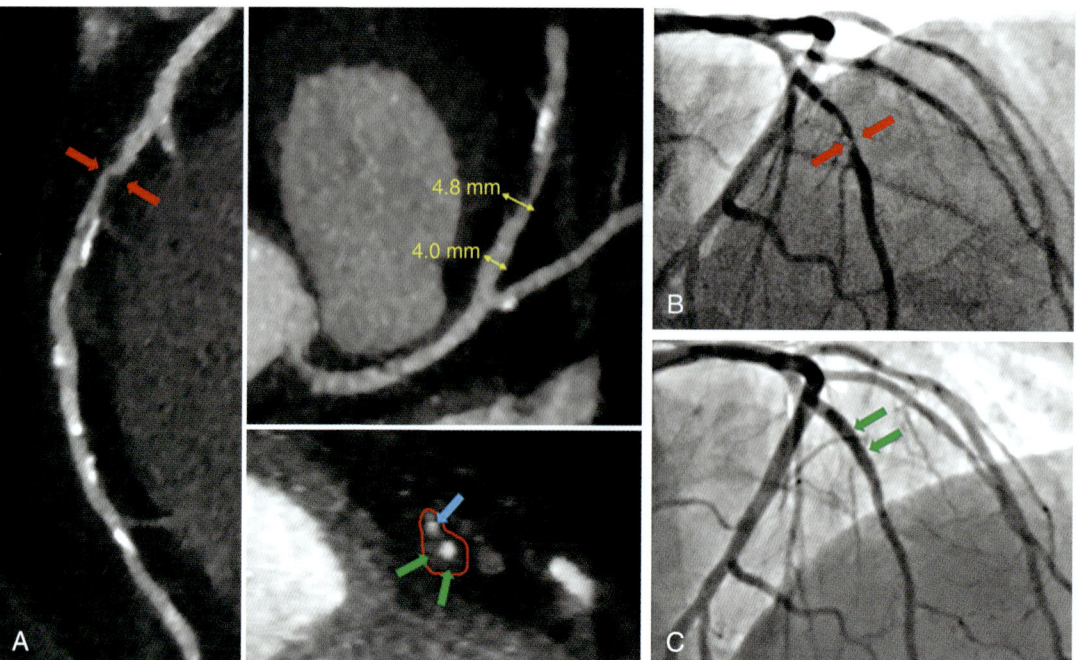

FIGURE 20.9 Example of severe stenosis associated with high-risk plaque features. A 74-year-old man with hypertension and hyperlipidemia presented with several months of intermittent chest pain. Electrocardiogram and echocardiogram were unremarkable. Coronary computed tomography angiography showed **(A)** large amount of predominantly noncalcified plaque in the mid left anterior descending (LAD) artery resulting in severe stenosis (70%–99%) (*red arrows*). High-risk plaque features included (1) positive remodeling: *two yellow double-headed arrows* demonstrate the maximal vessel diameters at the proximal (4.0 mm) and the mid portion of the plaque (4.8 mm); remodeling index is 1.2; (2) low Hounsfield units plaque (<30 HU) (*green arrows*); and (3) spotty calcification (*blue arrow*). **B,** Invasive angiography showed severe stenosis of the mid LAD (*red arrows*). **C,** Status post successful percutaneous coronary intervention of the mid LAD (*green arrows*).

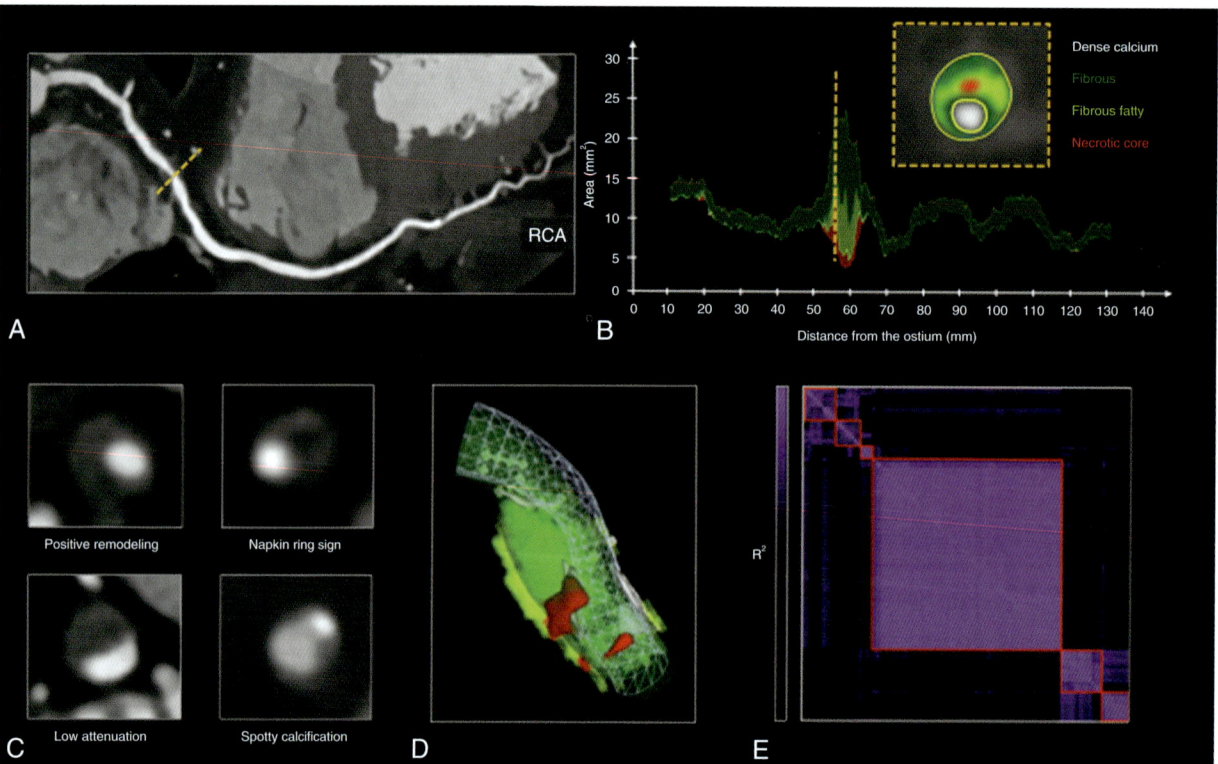

FIGURE 20.10 Identification of high-risk plaque features using radiomics. **A,** Curved multiplanar reconstruction of the right coronary artery with a noncalcified plaque showing positive remodeling *(dashed line)*. **B,** Volumetric plaque quantification. Contribution of different plaque components at each cross-sectional area along the vessel. A representative cross section is shown in the boxed inset. **C,** Qualitative high-risk plaque features. **D,** Volume-rendered image of the plaque in which the different plaque components are shown using different colors. **E,** Heat map showing the regression R^2 value between each pair of radiomic features. The information can be used for clustering analysis to show unique structural components. (Courtesy Drs. M. Kolossvary and P. Maurovich-Horvat, Semmelweis University, Budapest, Hungary.)

for estimating vessel-specific invasive FFR.[85] Overall, an invasive FFR ≤ 0.80 was present in 26.5% of 1727 vessels. The comprehensive com-posite of anatomic variables (stenosis severity, percentage of noncalcified atheroma volume, lumen volume, the number of lesions with HRP, and the number of lesions with stenosis greater than 30%) had superior discrimination to detect abnormal invasive FFR than MPI (area under the curve [AUC] for CCTA of 0.81 vs. 0.67 for MPI; $P < 0.001$). Of note, FFRCT was not additive to the comprehensive anatomic model, supporting the concept that plaque burden and plaque characteristics are important determinants of pressure decrement across a vessel. Although the extensive quantitative plaque characterization that was performed in this study is currently not used in clinical practice, it is likely that future software will enable greater adoption of such measures.

PLAQUE PROGRESSION AND MEDICAL THERAPY

There have been several studies evaluating the impact of various medical and lifestyle therapies on coronary plaque, as assessed by CCTA. The PARADIGM (Progression of AtheRosclerotic PlAque DetermIned by Computed TomoGraphic Angiography Imaging) study was a multicenter registry that included 1255 patients who underwent serial CCTA. In this study, statin use was associated with slower progression of overall coronary plaque volume, with increased calcified plaque and reduction of HRP features.[86] The EVAPORATE trial (Effect of Vascepa on Improving Coronary Atherosclerosis in People With High Triglycerides Taking Statin Therapy) used serial CCTA to evaluate the impact of adding 4 g/day of icosapent ethyl to statin and diet therapy. The study included 80 patients and showed significant regression of low-attenuation plaque and noncalcified plaque over 18 months.[87]

Perivascular Fat Attenuation

An emerging novel marker of risk on CCTA is the perivascular fat attenuation index[88] (FAI) and perivascular fat radiomic profile[89] (FRP) (Fig. 20.11). Coronary inflammation drives phenotypic changes in perivascular adipose tissue (PVAT) that can be captured by measuring a CT-derived perivascular FAI. Persistence of vascular inflammation leads to further changes in PVAT composition, characterized by increased extracellular fibrosis and local angiogenesis. These changes may be detected by radiomic phenotyping of PVAT using the signature FRP. FAI and FRP provide incremental prognostic value for future fatal or nonfatal cardiac events.[88,89]

Physiologic Evaluation of Coronary Artery Disease

A known limitation of CCTA, and invasive angiography, is that anatomy alone is often insufficient for determining whether there is myocardial- or lesion-specific ischemia. Cardiac CT techniques that can be used to determine this include CT FFR and CT perfusion.

Computed Tomography Fractional Flow Reserve

FFR derived from CCTA (CT FFR) is a method for deriving three-vessel FFR values using typically acquired CCTA (Fig. 20.12; see Fig. 36.17). Because CT FFR is determined from the CCTA dataset, it requires no additional testing and no additional radiation. The advantage of CT FFR is that it provides lesion-specific ischemia, and thus may help inform revascularization decisions.

FFRCT calculations are based on the application of computational fluid dynamics to CCTA to determine coronary fluid pressure, velocity, and flow. To calculate FFRCT, coronary arteries and left ventricular myocardium are segmented with subvoxel resolution. Rest coronary flow for each artery is calculated as a function of the myocardial mass it subtends and a calculation of distal intramyocardial microcirculatory resistance. Hyperemia is then modeled by estimating the response of the coronary arteries to adenosine. The final step in the calculation of FFRCT is the distribution of tetrahedral meshes through each artery and its branch, then solving the fluid dynamic equations to estimate FFR values at every point along the coronary artery bed.

Diagnostic Accuracy (see Fig. 36.17)

The diagnostic performance of FFRCT has been evaluated in multiple prospective multicenter trials, with more recent trials representing improvement in FFRCT technology related to improved image segmentation and flow modeling. The Analysis of Coronary Blood Flow Using CT Angiography: Next Steps (NXT) was a prospective multicenter trial that included 254 patients referred for clinically indicated invasive angiography. CCTA and FFRCT were performed, with 484 vessels directly interrogated by invasive FFR. The area under the receiver operating characteristic (ROC) curve for FFRCT was 0.90 and 0.93 on a per-patient and per-vessel basis, respectively, which corresponded to an overall per-vessel diagnostic accuracy of 86%.[90]

A post hoc analysis from the PACIFIC trial[91] evaluated the diagnostic accuracy of FFRCT among the 208 patients included in this trial, with FFRCT evaluable in 505 (83%) vessels that were thus included in the primary per-vessel analysis. When evaluating this population, the AUC for FFRCT was 0.94 (95% CI, 0.92–0.96), and significantly higher than CCTA alone (0.83; 95% CI, 0.80–0.86; $P < 0.001$), SPECT (0.70; 95% CI, 0.65–0.74; $P < 0.001$), and PET (0.87; 95% CI, 0.83–0.90; $P < 0.001$). The sensitivity of FFRCT (90%) was higher than any of the other modalities, whereas the specificity of FFRCT (86%) was comparable to CCTA and PET. A notable limitation of this substudy was that 17% of vessels were nonevaluable by FFRCT and were excluded from the primary analysis.

Although the specificity of FFRCT is comparable to other functional techniques, it is notable that it is a lesion-specific measure, which is fundamentally different from measuring abnormalities in myocardial flow (see Chapter 18).

Clinical Effectiveness

FFRCT has been assessed for its ability to alter the clinical management of patients undergoing noninvasive and invasive testing. In the crossover-design Prospective Longitudinal Trial of FFRCT Outcome and Resource Impacts (PLATFORM), 584 symptomatic patients with suspected CAD were assigned to either usual care or a CCTA-FFR$_{CT}$-based evaluation to determine the rates of nonobstructive CAD (<50%) at invasive coronary angiography (ICA). Two separate cohorts were studied, referred for invasive assessment and for noninvasive stress testing. Among patients intended to undergo invasive angiography, a CCTA-FFRCT approach resulted in a significantly higher rate of obstructive CAD at ICA (73% vs. 12%) and also resulted in 61% of ICAs being canceled after CCTA-FFRCT findings were known. These cancellations were associated with 32% lower costs and similar quality-of-life measures by a CCTA-FFRCT algorithm compared with usual care, a finding that extended to the 1-year follow-up. In contrast, among patients referred to noninvasive imaging, the rates of nonobstructive CAD at ICA were not statistically different (13% vs. 6%). For these patients undergoing noninvasive imaging, quality-of-life measures were higher with a CCTA-FFRCT-based strategy than with usual care, although with higher costs ($2766 vs. $2137).

The Assessing Diagnostic Value of Non-invasive FFRCT in Coronary Care (ADVANCE) registry was a prospective multicenter registry that included 5083 patients from 38 sites who were referred for CCTA with FFRCT.[92] This study found that the addition of FFRCT to CCTA results in a modification to the anticipated treatment plan in two-thirds of patients. However, the true magnitude of how often FFRCT may impact care was likely overestimated as anticipated treatment plans were made by a core lab reviewing angiographic findings alone. The ADVANCE registry also evaluated the safety of deferring revascularization when FFRCT is greater than 0.8. Over a 90-day follow-up, none of the 1952 subjects with negative FFRCT experienced death, MI, or unplanned hospitalization for ACS and urgent revascularization. In contrast, there were 19 adverse events (10 deaths, 4 MIs, and 5 hospitalizations for urgent revascularization) in patients with positive FFRCT (HR 19.75; $P < 0.001$).[92] At 1 year, there was a trend toward lower MACE ($P = 0.062$) and significantly lower cardiovascular death or MI ($P = 0.01$) in patients with a negative FFRct compared with patients with abnormal FFRCT.[93]

The utility of FFRCT following CCTA was also evaluated in a large single-center registry of 3674 consecutive patients with stable chest pain who were evaluated with CCTA followed by selective FFRCT for those with intermediate stenosis (30% to 70%).[94] FFRCT was performed for 697 patients (18% of the cohort), reflecting the fact that this test is only needed for a minority of CCTA cases, when there is stenosis of uncertain hemodynamic significance. Notably, patients

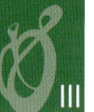

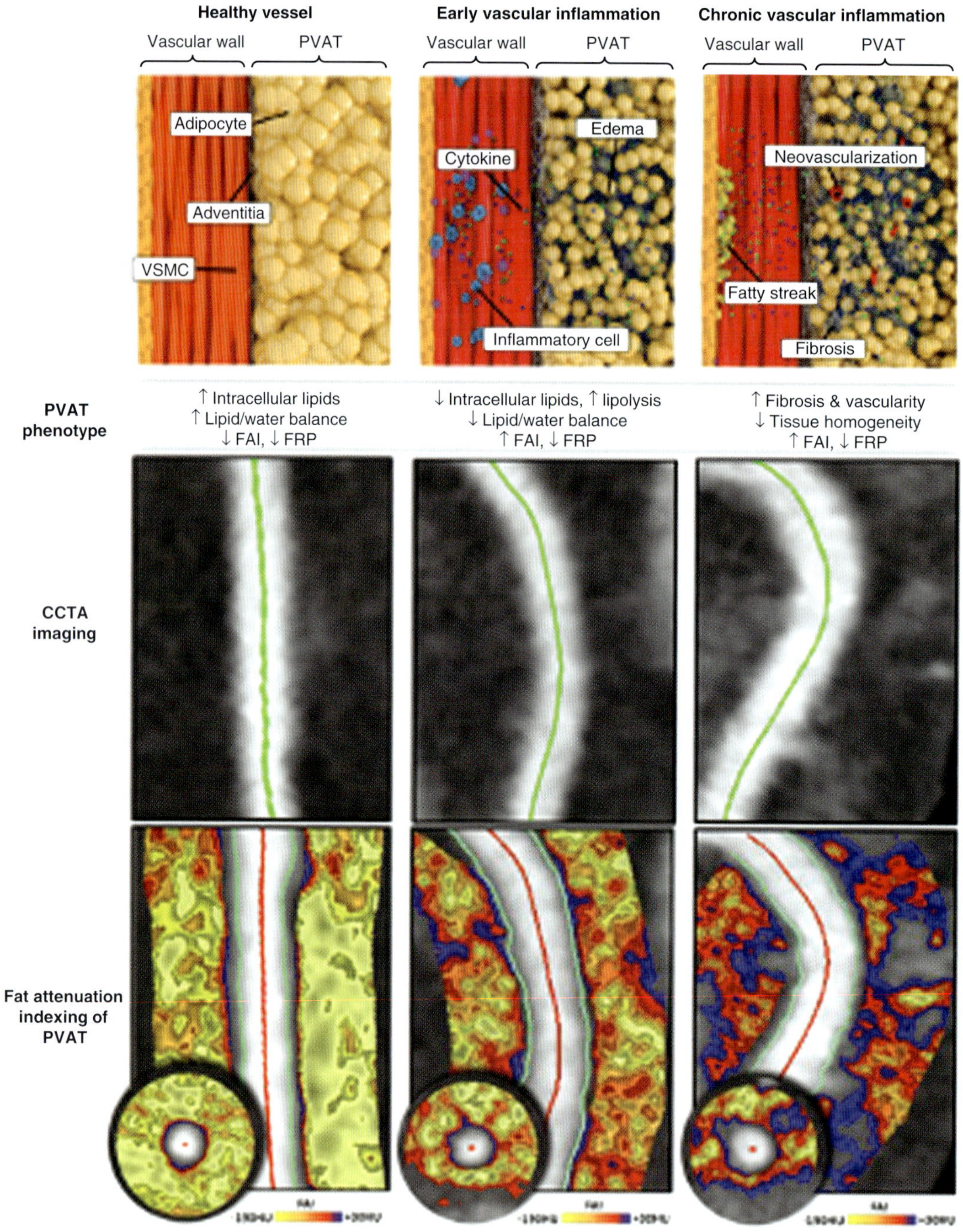

FIGURE 20.11 Schematic representation of the biology underlying fat attenuation index (FAI) and fat radiomic profile (FRP). Early coronary inflammation drives lipolysis and inhibits adipogenesis in perivascular adipocytes, shifting the composition of perivascular adipose tissue (PVAT) toward the aqueous phase, at the expense of the lipid phase (*top middle panel*). Persistent chronic vascular inflammation may lead to further changes of the perivascular space, such as fibrosis and angiogenesis (*top right panel*). These changes may not be visible on coronary computed tomography angiography, as they may precede plaque formation (*middle panels*). Perivascular fat attenuation indexing identifies arteries with low inflammation (*bottom left panel*), early vascular inflammation (*bottom middle panel*), or chronic vascular inflammation (*bottom right panel*). Early vascular inflammation is quantified by the perivascular FAI and chronic vascular inflammation by the perivascular FRP. (Courtesy Charalambos Antoniades, MD, PhD, University of Oxford.)

with intermediate stenosis who had a negative FFRCT (>0.80) had similar long-term outcomes when compared with patients with no to minimal stenosis (0% to 30%) by CCTA. On the other hand, adverse events were higher among patients with an abnormal FFRCT who were not referred for invasive angiography. Although the latter findings may be influenced by selection bias (i.e., patients who were not treated could have been higher risk), the overall findings from this trial support the safety of using CT-FFR to defer coronary revascularization in patients who have intermediate lesions that are deemed non–flow limiting.[94]

When integrating data from FFRCT into clinical management decisions, there are several important factors to consider. FFRCT may aid decision making in lesions that have intermediate stenosis (i.e., 40% to 70%) in the proximal or mid-coronary vessel (see Table 20.4 for guideline-based recommendations). Because FFRCT declines along the length of the vessel with serial focal lesions or areas of diffuse disease, it is important to correlate the pressure loss to specific lesions, which can only be established by direct comparison between the CCTA lesion location and the FFRct 3D model.[95] When doing so, FFRCT >0.80 indicates that a lesion is unlikely to be hemodynamically significant and revascularization can be safely deferred. Although most studies have used a dichotomous interpretation strategy, FFRCT values (similar to invasive FFR) have a continuous relationship, and the lower the FFRct values, the higher the likelihood of hemodynamic significance and the risk of adverse events.[95] When FFRCT is between 0.76 and 0.80, additional information may be useful for deciding on

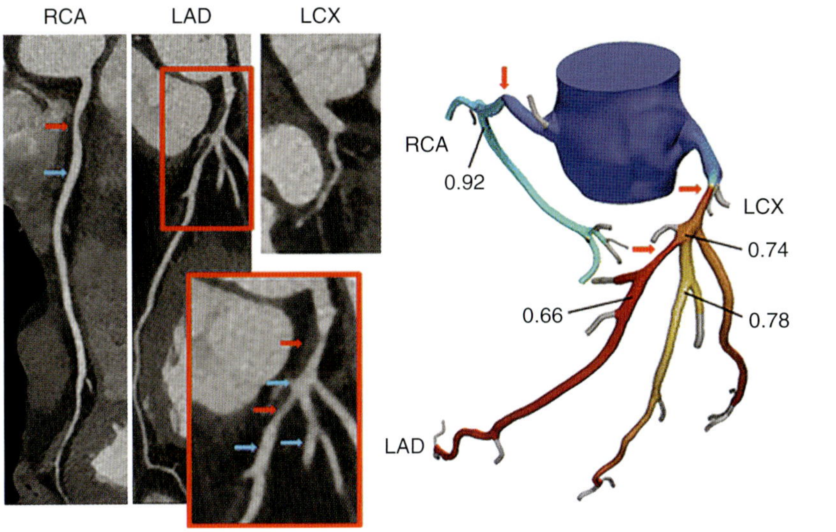

FIGURE 20.12 FFR$_{CT}$ assessment in vessels with serial lesions in a 53-year-old man with typical angina. *Left:* Coronary computed tomography angiography curved multiplanar reconstructions demonstrate a proximal 60% right coronary artery (RCA) stenosis (*red arrow*) and two serial stenoses in the left anterior descending artery (LAD) (one lesion in the proximal segment with 70% or greater diameter stenosis, and a 50% to 69% diameter stenosis lesion distal to the takeoff of the second diagonal [*red arrows*]). *Blue arrows* indicate where the FFR$_{CT}$ values were assessed. *Right:* in the FFR$_{CT}$ three-dimensional model, the FFR$_{CT}$ value 10 mm distal to the proximal LAD stenosis was 0.74 and thus had hemodynamic significance, whereas FFR$_{CT}$ 15 mm distal to the second LAD stenosis was 0.66. FFR$_{CT}$ 10 mm distal to the lower border of the proximal RCA stenosis was 0.92, thus this lesion had low likelihood of being hemodynamically significant. Of note, pressure recovery was observed in the proximal part of the second diagonal with a step-up in FFR$_{CT}$ from 0.74 in the LAD to 0.78 when moving downstream the diagonal branch. LCX = left circumflex coronary artery. (From Nørgaard BL, et al. Coronary CT angiography-derived fractional flow reserve testing in patients with stable coronary artery disease: recommendations on interpretation and reporting. Radiol Cardiothorac Imaging 2019;1:e190050.)

the potential role of revascularization, including lesion location, presence of HRP features, patient symptoms, or the translesional FFRCT gradient.[95]

There are several noteworthy limitations of FFRCT. At present, this technique is performed by a single vendor and is associated with additional cost, although this has been shown to be cost-effective because of the avoidance of invasive angiography and coronary revascularization in a subgroup of patients.[73] FFRCT requires excellent CCTA image quality, and artifacts, such as motion, misalignment, low contrast, or blooming from coronary calcification, may impair the diagnostic reliability of this technique. FFRCT is not recommended in vessels with prior stents or in patients who have undergone bypass surgery.

Coronary Tomography Perfusion

CT perfusion is a technique in which the myocardium can be visualized on CT datasets to determine whether there is a stress-induced or rest myocardial perfusion defects. On rest CCTA images, a resting perfusion defect (i.e., subendocardial hypoenhancement of the myocardium) can be used to identify areas of prior infarction or high-grade stenosis. Other features of a prior infarction on CCTA include areas of fatty metaplasia, intramyocardial calcifications, wall thinning, and wall motion abnormalities, in cases where multiphase data were acquired. Several small studies have shown the incremental data of resting myocardial perfusion defects beyond CCTA alone, especially for the detection of ACSs among patients with acute chest pain.

Stress Computed Tomography Perfusion

CT stress perfusion imaging can performed when images are acquired during vasodilator stress.[96] Typically, two separate acquisitions are performed: (1) a rest CCTA, which is used for evaluation of the coronary arteries and resting MPI, and (2) a stress CT, which is used for the evaluation of stress-induced perfusion defects. The sequence of imaging depends on the clinical scenario. In patients with known CAD in which stress perfusion is desired, there are advantages to acquiring this data first, and then obtaining the CCTA dataset 15 to 20 minutes later. Another approach is to first obtain the rest CCTA dataset, especially if the absence of significant CAD may be used to avoid the stress component of the exam.

Multiple single-center studies and two multicenter studies have evaluated the diagnostic accuracy of various stress CT perfusion protocols against both invasive and noninvasive techniques, showing good accuracy for detecting anatomic stenosis or myocardial ischemia.[96] The value of stress CT perfusion is greatest when added to the CCTA data, where CT perfusion can increase the specificity of anatomic stenosis measures to detect myocardial ischemia.

Stress CT perfusion can provide simultaneous data on both CCTA and myocardial perfusion. Furthermore, it can be performed on-site, and at the same time as the CCTA exam. CT perfusion can also be performed in patients who have significant coronary calcification and stents, and it is generally less dependent on high image quality than CCTA, as it does not require high spatial resolution. However, when compared with nuclear and CMR myocardial perfusing imaging, CT has lower contrast resolution. In addition, there are certain artifacts that may impact the diagnostic accuracy of CT perfusion including beam-hardening artifacts and motion-related artifacts. CT perfusion also requires a higher amount of contrast and higher radiation dose than routine CCTA studies. Despite robust data on the diagnostic accuracy of this technique, there is currently a paucity of clinical effectiveness data, insufficient insurance coverage, and limited clinical expertise; thus this technique has not been widely adopted and remains mostly investigational.

Comparing and Integrating Different Techniques

A single-center study of 147 consecutive patients scheduled for invasive angiography with invasive FFR who underwent both FFR-CT and stress CT perfusion showed that both FFRCT and stress CT perfusion improved specificity and positive predictive values compared with CCTA alone. Although this study suggests that both techniques may be comparable for evaluating the functional significance of CAD lesions,[97] there is a paucity of data comparing these techniques, and overall significantly more data supporting the accuracy and safety of CT-FFR.

Implications of the ISCHEMIA Trial for Coronary Computed Tomography Angiography

The ISCHEMIA trial[31] found that among stable patients who had evidence of moderate to severe ischemia on stress testing, an initial invasive strategy, when compared with an initial conservative strategy, was not associated with a reduction in the primary outcome of cardiovascular death, MI, hospitalization for unstable angina, hospitalization for heart failure, or resuscitated cardiac arrest over a median follow-up of 3.3 years. Similar results were also observed for the prespecified secondary endpoint of cardiovascular death or MI, and across multiple other prespecified subgroup analyses. However, an initial invasive strategy was associated with a reduction in angina and improved quality of life, but only in those who had frequent symptoms of angina. In this trial, CCTA was useful for excluding left main disease (~5%) or nonobstructive CAD (~14%). Thus, in the presence of significant ischemia, if a decision is made to pursue medical management alone, CCTA should be considered for excluding high-risk anatomy.

The ISCHEMIA trial did not evaluate the effectiveness of any single imaging strategy; instead it reinforced the concept that contemporary medical therapy is highly effective in reducing the risk of cardiovascular outcomes. In fact, over a median follow-up of 3.3 years, the primary composite endpoint occurred in only 15.5% of patients in the conservative arm and 13.8% of patients in the invasive arm ($P = 0.34$).[31] The are several notable implications of this trial when considering the role of CCTA in evaluating patients with stable CAD.

TABLE 20.4 Select U.S. and European Guideline Recommendations

GUIDELINES	CLINICAL SCENARIO	RECOMMENDATION
U.S. Multisociety Cholesterol Guidelines[116]	CAC testing in prevention	• In intermediate-risk or selected borderline-risk adults, if the decision about statin use remains uncertain, it is reasonable to use a CAC score in the decision to withhold, postpone, or initiate statin therapy (COR 2a; LOE: B-NR)
2019 ESC Guidelines for the diagnosis and management of chronic coronary syndromes[117]	Initial diagnostic management of symptomatic patients with suspected coronary artery disease	• Noninvasive functional imaging for myocardial ischemia* or CCTA is recommended as the initial test to diagnose CAD in symptomatic patients in whom obstructive CAD cannot be excluded by clinical assessment alone (Class 1, Level B) Additional guidance: "Coronary CTA is the preferred test in patients with a lower range of clinical likelihood of CAD, no previous diagnosis of CAD, and characteristics associated with a high likelihood of good image quality" • CCTA should be considered as an alternative to invasive angiography if another noninvasive test is equivocal or nondiagnostic (Class 2a, Level C) • CCTA is not recommended when extensive coronary calcification, irregular heart rate, significant obesity, inability to cooperate with breath-hold commands, or any other conditions make obtaining good image quality unlikely (Class 3, Level C)
	Recommendations for investigations in patients with suspected vasospastic angina	• Invasive angiography or CCTA is recommended in patients with characteristic episodic resting angina and ST-segment changes, which resolve with nitrates and/or calcium antagonists, to determine the extent of underlying coronary disease (Class 1, Level C)
	Recommendations for valvular disease in chronic coronary syndromes	• CCTA should be considered as an alternative to coronary angiography before valve intervention in patients with severe valvular heart disease and low probability of CAD (Class 2a, Level C)
2020 ESC Guidelines for management of ACS[60]	Patients presenting without persistent ST-segment elevations	• CCTA is recommended as an alternative to invasive angiography to exclude ACS when there is a low-to-intermediate likelihood of CAD and when cardiac troponin and/or ECG are normal or inconclusive (Class 1, Level A) • In patients with no recurrence of chest pain, normal ECG findings, and normal levels of cardiac troponin (preferably high sensitivity), but still with a suspected ACS, a noninvasive stress test (preferably with imaging) for inducible ischemia or CCTA is recommended before deciding on an invasive approach (Class 1, Level B)
2021 AHA/ACC and others: Guideline for the Evaluation and Diagnosis of Chest Pain[118]	Patients with acute chest pain	• For intermediate-risk patients with acute chest pain and no known coronary artery disease eligible for diagnostic testing following a negative or inconclusive evaluation for acute coronary syndrome, CCTA is useful for exclusion of atherosclerotic plaque and obstructive coronary artery disease (Class 1, Level A)
	Patients with stable chest pain	• For intermediate–high risk patients with stable chest pain and no known coronary artery disease, CCTA is effective for diagnosis of CAD, for risk stratification, and for guiding treatment decisions. (Class 1, Level A) • For intermediate–high risk patients with stable chest pain and known coronary stenosis of 40% to 90% in a proximal or middle coronary segment on CCTA, FFRCT can be useful for diagnosis of vessel-specific ischemia and to guide decision-making regarding the use of coronary revascularization (Class 2a, Level B)
	Patients with prior bypass surgery	• In patients with prior CABG surgery presenting with acute chest pain who do not have ACS, performing stress imaging is effective to evaluate for myocardial ischemia or CCTA for graft stenosis or occlusion. (Class 1, Level C) • In patients who have had prior coronary artery bypass surgery presenting with stable chest pain who are suspected to have myocardial ischemia, it is reasonable to perform stress imaging or CCTA to evaluate for myocardial ischemia or graft stenosis or occlusion. (Class 2a, Level C)
	Patients with stable chest pain and known nonobstructive plaque	• For symptomatic patients with known nonobstructive CAD who have stable chest pain, CCTA is reasonable for determining atherosclerotic plaque burden and progression to obstructive CAD, and guiding therapeutic decision making (Class 2a, Level B-NR)

*Stress echocardiography, stress cardiac magnetic resonance, single-photon emission CT, or positron emission tomography
ACC, American College of Cardiology; *ACS*, acute coronary syndrome; *AHA*, American Heart Association; *CAC*, coronary artery calcium; *CAD*, coronary artery disease; *CCTA*, coronary computed tomographic angiography; *ECG*, electrocardiogram; *ESC*, European Society of Cardiology; *FFR*, fractional flow reserve.

Patient Management Considerations

Among patients who do not have known CAD, CCTA can identify the need and intensity of medical therapy (Fig. 20.13) and identify patients who may benefit from additional noninvasive or invasive testing to determine the need for coronary revascularization. Pertinent to the ISCHEMIA trial results, CCTA may be useful to rule out underlying high-risk coronary anatomy, particularly when symptoms are infrequent and conservative management is being considered. Indeed, one of the strengths of CCTA lies in its ability to identify a wide spectrum of CAD, ranging from nonobstructive plaque to extensive multivessel disease. Another advantage of using CCTA as a front-line test has to do with its diagnostic efficiency: the majority of individuals with no history of CAD who are evaluated with CCTA will have no CAD, or nonobstructive CAD, and will not need further testing. For example, in the PROMISE study only 14% of patients had ≥50% stenosis,[98] and in the CRESCENT I and II trials only 14% had ≥50% stenosis.[99] In the absence of significant CAD, CCTA can also identify various other alternative explanations for a patient's symptoms ranging from aortic or pulmonary disease to pericardial and esophageal pathologies (Fig. 20.14).

The finding that most patients with stable symptoms can be effectively treated with medical therapy has implications for how CCTA results should be used in patient management (see Fig. 20.13). Specifically, most patients only require preventive therapies following CCTA, and invasive angiography should be reserved for patients that have

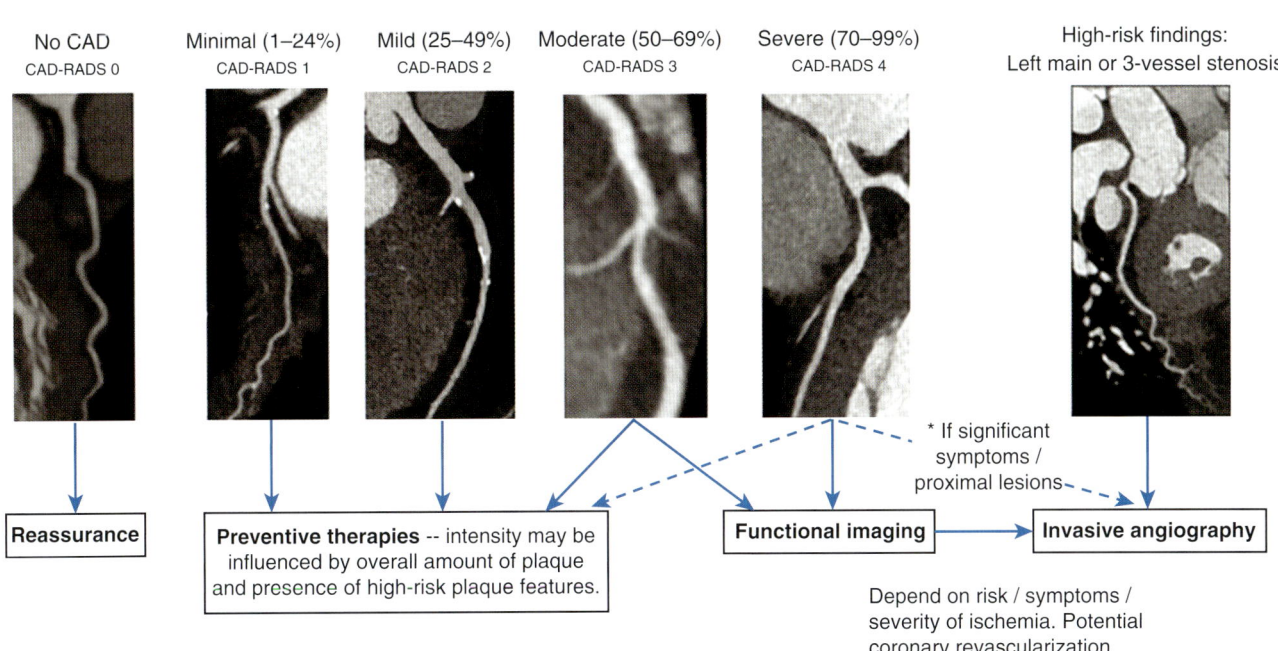

FIGURE 20.13 Patient management recommendation following coronary computed tomography angiography in stable chest pain.

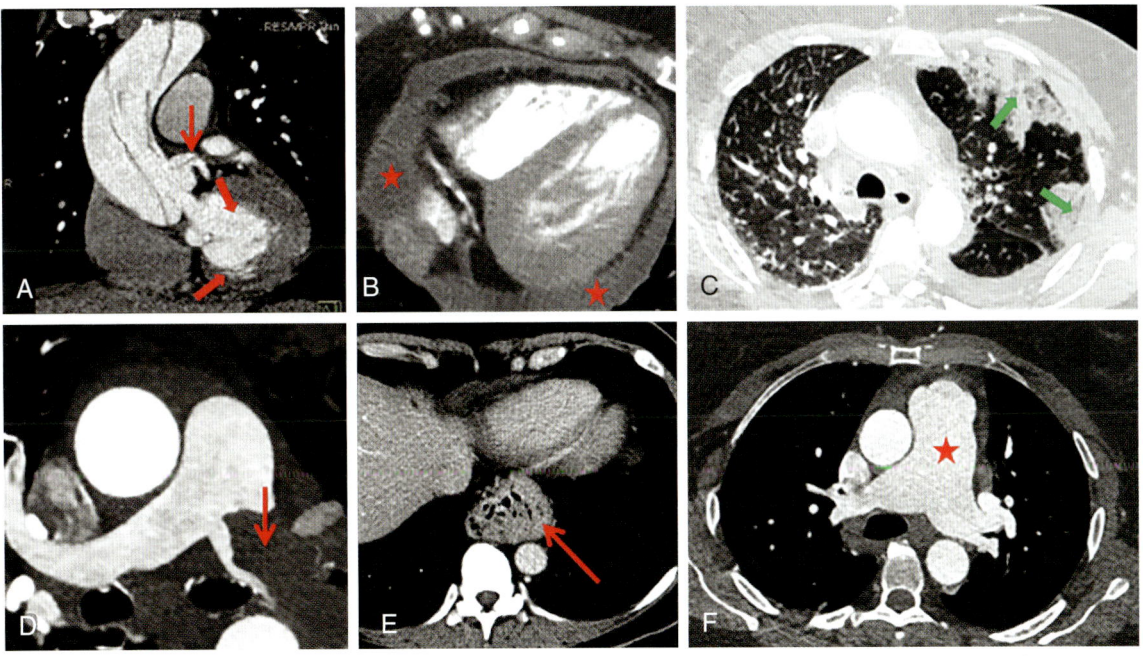

FIGURE 20.14 Examples of various etiologies of chest pain or dyspnea diagnosed on cardiac computed tomography. **A,** Aortic dissection extending into the left main coronary artery. **B,** Pericardial effusion. **C,** Pulmonary infarction. **D,** Pulmonary embolus. **E,** Hiatal hernia. **F,** Dilated pulmonary artery in a patient with pulmonary hypertension.

high-risk anatomy (e.g., left main stenosis or three-vessel obstructive CAD), or those with obstructive CAD with frequent or unstable symptoms. Nevertheless, in some patients it may be unclear if their symptoms are related to their underlying CAD, and in such cases functional testing, including exercise testing alone, may be helpful for establishing the potential benefit of coronary revascularization (see Chapter 15).

Patient Management Recommendations

Patient management recommendations are summarized in Fig. 20.13, and they are based on an expert consensus document (CAD-RADS),[100] recent guidelines, and implications of the ISCHEMIA trial discussed previously.

Normal CCTA (CAD-RADS 0): Patients who have no plaque or stenosis should be reassured that they have an excellent prognosis, and a nonatherosclerotic cause of symptoms should be considered.

Preventive lifestyle therapies should be the main focus for reducing the risk of future events, as should be the case in all adults, and for all the following groups.

Nonobstructive plaque (CAD-RADS 1 or 2): Patients with minimal (1% to 24%) or mid (25% to 49%) stenosis should also be evaluated for potential nonatherosclerotic causes of their symptoms, as it is unlikely that their plaque is flow limiting. In select cases of mild (25% to 49%) stenosis in which there is a large amount of diffuse plaque or HRP features, a noninvasive evaluation for ischemia can be considered, if there are frequent symptoms and a high suspicion for ongoing ischemia. Patient management should focus on lifestyle and pharmacologic preventive therapies, as per prevention guidelines (see Chapter 25). However, for patients who are not on such therapies, the identification of plaque, especially if extensive, should prompt the initiation or intensification of pharmacotherapy. When

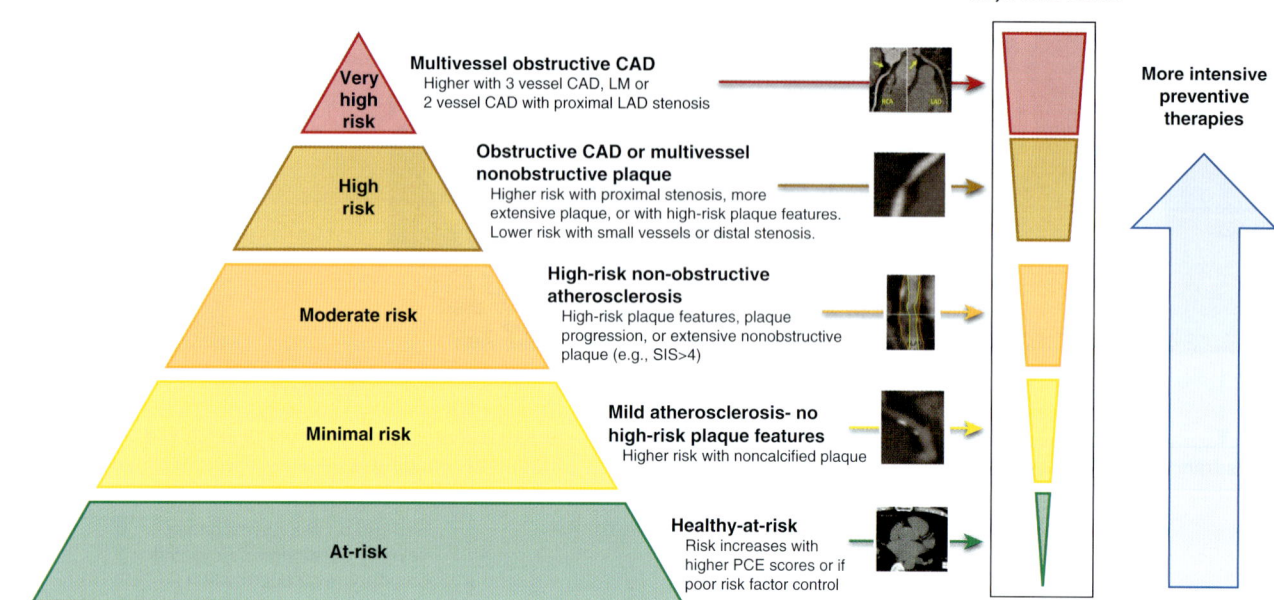

FIGURE 20.15 Stages of atherosclerosis. Patients with more extensive, multivessel coronary artery disease are at highest risk, whereas those without any plaque or stenosis comprise those at lowest risk. (From Shaw LJ, et al. Society of Cardiovascular Computed Tomography/North American Society of Cardiovascular Imaging—Expert Consensus Document on Coronary CT Imaging of Atherosclerotic Plaque. J Cardiovasc Comput Tomogr 2021;15:93-109.)

deciding on the intensity of preventive therapies, it is important to consider the level of risk by integrating data on clinical risk factors and the level of risk associated with the CCTA findings. Fig. 20.15 provides an overview of various stages of atherosclerosis detected by CCTA. Risk level can be determined based on the amount or extent of plaque (e.g., number of segments or vessels that have coronary plaque and CAC score, if available), the presence of HRP features (see section Coronary Computed Tomography Angiography Plaque Characteristics), plaque progression, lesion location, and extent of obstructive CAD. Patients who have moderate to high risk have an event rate that is similar to secondary prevention cohorts and are more likely to benefit from high-intensity lipid-lowering therapy and antiplatelet therapy, if there are no contraindications.

Moderate stenosis (50% to 69%; CAD-RADS 3). In addition to the previous recommendation regarding preventive therapies, functional assessment may be considered if there are frequent symptoms. Routine invasive angiography should be avoided unless there are frequent or unstable symptoms.

Severe stenosis (70% to 99%; CAD-RADS 3). In addition to the previous recommendation regarding preventive therapies, either functional assessment or invasive angiography may be considered if there are frequent symptoms. In the presence of left main disease or three-vessel obstructive (≥70%) CAD, invasive angiography is recommended.

Total occlusion (100%; CAD-RADS 4). In addition to the previous recommendation regarding preventive therapies, invasive angiography and/or viability assessment should be considered. In such cases it is important to consider CCTA factors that can predict the likelihood of successful revascularization, including amount of coronary calcifications and the length of the occluded segment.

Special Populations

Diabetes (see also Chapter 31): While routine CCTA in asymptomatic individuals who are on baseline preventive therapies has not been shown to improve patient outcomes, subgroup analyses from both the PROMISE and SCOT-HEART studies suggested that the use of CCTA among symptomatic patients with diabetes may be associated with improved outcomes (see the previous section Hard Clinical Outcomes) when compared with functional testing approaches.[101] Given that individuals with diabetes are more likely to have diffuse plaque, have faster plaque progression, and have a higher rate of adverse cardiovascular events, it is plausible that CCTA may have unique advantages in identifying patients who may benefit from more aggressive interventions. Integration of plaque volume, HRP features, and luminal stenosis may provide the most robust long-term risk prediction.[102]

Women (see also Chapter 91): Although women are less likely to have obstructive CAD than men, CCTA allows for the accurate detection of nonobstructive plaque, including overall plaque extent, and HRP features. CCTA has similar accuracy and prognostic value in men and women, although in the PROMISE study the prognostic value of HRP was stronger in women than in men.[80] In the multicenter ROMICAT II trial, women with acute chest pain had a greater reduction in length of stay than men when CCTA was compared with standard of care, a finding which likely reflects the lower prevalence and severity of CAD in women (58% of women had a normal CCTA vs. 37% of men; $P < 0.001$).[23] CCTA is also the only noninvasive test that can be used to detect spontaneous coronary artery dissection (SCAD; see Fig. 20.16, for example), although this diagnosis requires excellent CCTA image quality, and is limited in evaluating small distal vessels.[103]

Anomalous coronary arteries: CCTA is a useful noninvasive test used to evaluate patients with known or suspected anomalous origin of the coronary arteries (Fig. 20.17). When such abnormalities are identified, CCTA can describe the type of abnormality and various features that may help inform patient management (Fig. 20.18).[104,105] In general, vessels with a retroaortic or prepulmonic course are considered benign, whereas the highest risk of sudden death is attributed when there is an anomalous left main coronary artery arising from the right cusp with an interarterial course; this is an infrequent variant. Patients who have a right coronary artery arising from the left cusp with an interarterial course, or those with a subpulmonic (also known as transseptal) left main arising from the right cusp have a variable level of risk and require a careful assessment that integrates clinical and imaging findings. Among 5991 consecutive patients evaluated by CCTA in the PARTNERS registry, the prevalence of an anomalous coronary artery originating from the opposite sinus of Valsalva (ACAOS) was 1.7%, and the vast majority were benign variants. CCTA-derived features that were associated with subsequent revascularization included slit-like narrowing of the origin, interarterial course, intramural course, and narrowing of proximal anomalous vessel of >5.4 mm in length.[104] (Fig. 20.18 shows examples of various features.)

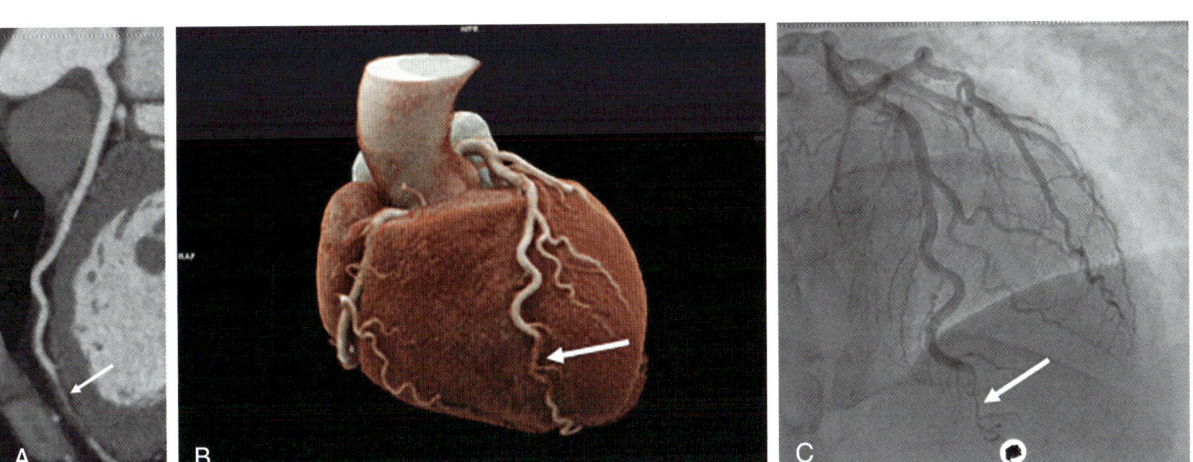

FIGURE 20.16 Example of spontaneous coronary artery dissection diagnosed by coronary computed tomography angiography. Images show dissection of distal left anterior descending artery (*white arrow*) on curved multiplanar reformatting image **(A)**, three-dimensional cinematic volume-rendered image **(B)**, and invasive angiography **(C)**. (Courtesy of Dr. Sumit Gupta, Brigham and Women's Hospital, Boston.)

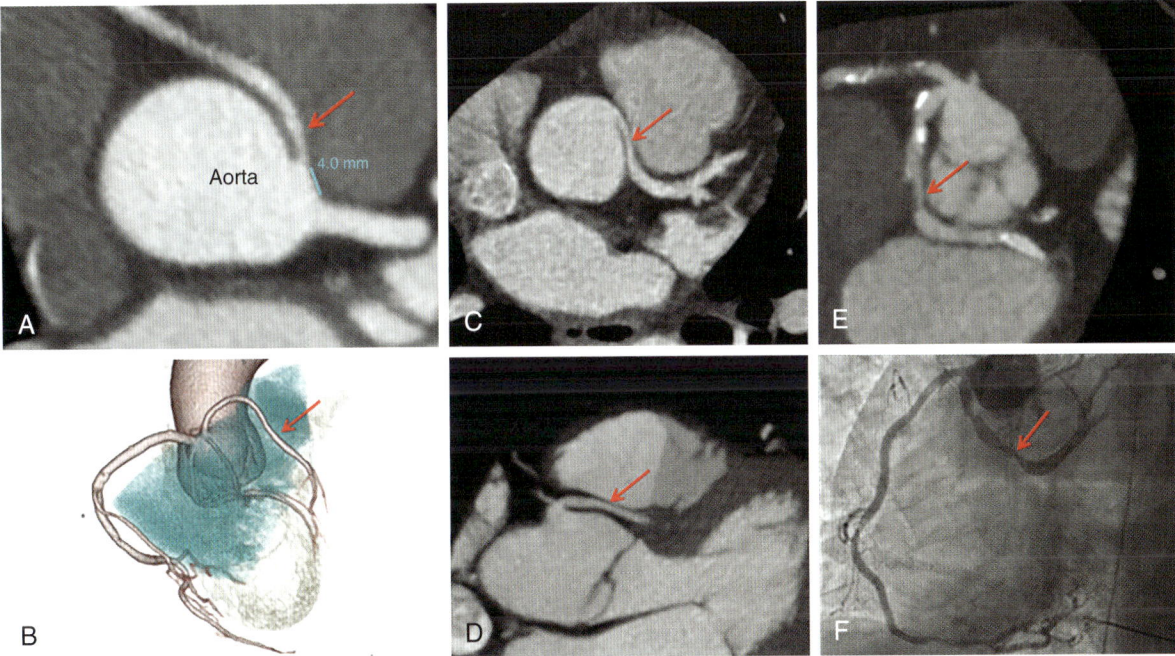

FIGURE 20.17 Examples of anomalous aortic origin of the coronary arteries from the opposite cusp. **A**, Right coronary artery arising from the left coronary cusp with an interarterial course between the aorta and the pulmonary artery. **B**, Three-dimensional volume-rendered image showing the left anterior descending (LAD) artery arising from the right coronary artery with a prepulmonic LAD (i.e., anterior to the pulmonary artery) The *translucent blue volume* is used to show the right ventricular outflow tract and pulmonary artery. **C**, Left main arising from the right coronary cusp with an interarterial course. **D**, Left main arising from the right coronary cusp below the pulmonic valve traveling in a transeptal course. **E**, Left circumflex (LCX) arising from the right coronary cusp and traveling in a retroaortic course posterior to the aorta. The LCX has a large amount of plaque and moderate stenosis (*red arrow*). **F**, Invasive angiography images corresponding to **(E)** illustrating the retroaortic LCX.

Coronary Artery Bypass Grafts: CCTA has been shown to be highly accurate for detecting stenosis in arterial or venous bypass grafts. However, the evaluation of native coronary arteries in patients with prior coronary artery bypass grafting can be challenging, because of the common occurrence of underlying severe coronary calcifications of the native vessels. Therefore, CCTA may be better suited if the main clinical question pertains to patency of the bypass grafts.[50]

Prior heart transplantation: CCTA has been used as a surrogate for invasive angiography to diagnose coronary allograft vasculopathy (CAV) following cardiac transplantation. The use of CCTA in this setting requires expertise, and it may be challenging in patients who have elevated heart rate. A meta-analysis of 13 studies evaluating the diagnostic performance of CCTA compared with invasive angiography found that on a per-patient basis, CCTA detected any CAV (any luminal irregularities) or significant CAV (≥50% stenosis) with a sensitivity of 97% and 94%, and specificity of 81% and 92%, respectively.[50] FFRct may further improve the identification of hemodynamically significant CAD.

Guidelines

Table 20.4 provides an overview of key CCTA recommendations from the most recent ESC and AHA/ACC guidelines. Both guidelines provide a class I recommendation for use of CCTA as an initial testing option in stable and acute chest pain. Nevertheless, there are multiple available testing options across these clinical scenarios. Although guideline-based recommendations are often lacking in this regard, clinicians are required to select the best initial testing option for each patient. This requires a careful consideration of various factors, including clinical data (e.g., the anticipated impact of the test on patient management), the results of prior tests (when available), the likelihood of having high image quality, and local availability and expertise.

The 2019 ESC guidelines stated that CCTA is the preferred test in patients with a lower range of clinical likelihood of CAD, no previous diagnosis of CAD, and characteristics associated with a high likelihood of good image quality. The 2021 AHA/ACC guidelines stated that CCTA may be preferred among patients less than 65 years of age and those

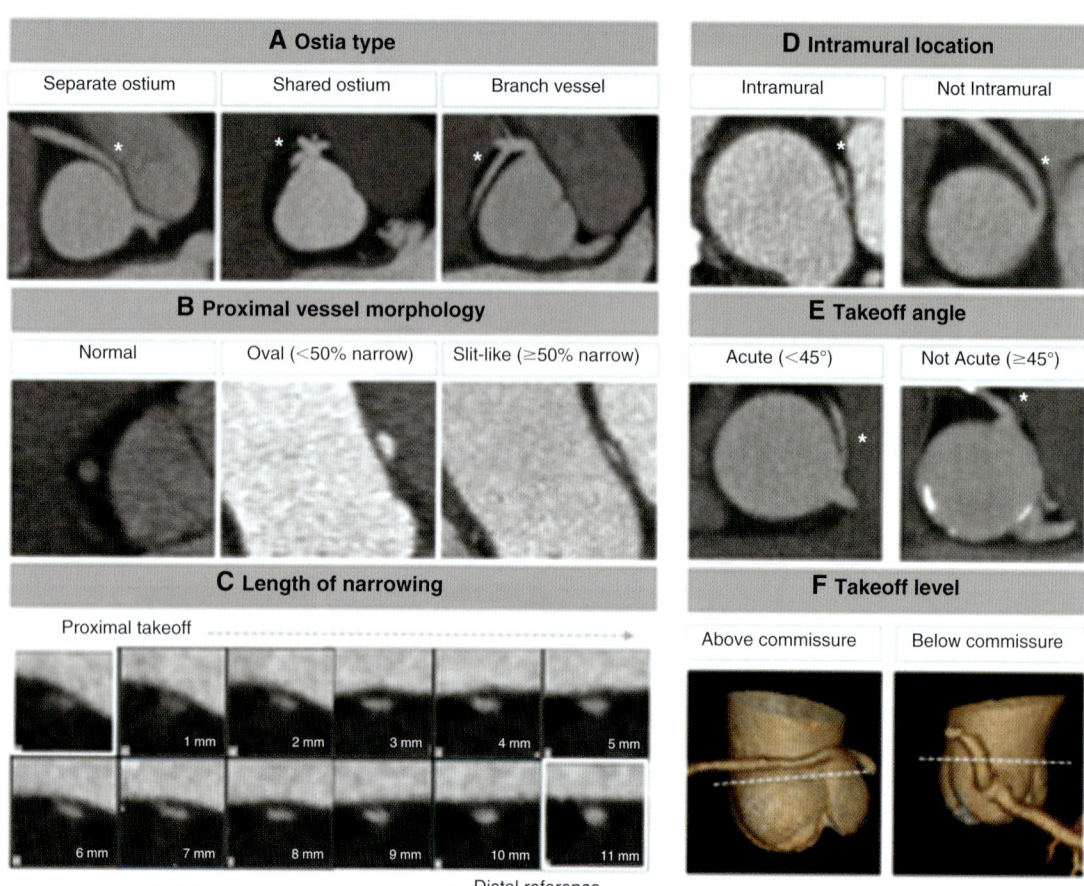

FIGURE 20.18 Coronary computed tomography (CT) angiography features for evaluating patients with anomalous aortic origin of the coronary arteries (AAOCA). **A,** Multiplanar axial CT reconstruction at the level of the coronary artery takeoff demonstrating AAOCA ostia types (separate ostium, shared ostium, and branch vessel). **B,** Proximal vessel morphology in double oblique view using the percentage of lumen diameter narrowing compared with normal distal reference (not shown), stratified by normal, oval shape (<50% narrowing), and slit-like narrowing (≥50% narrowing). **C,** Centerline length of vessel narrowing shown in double oblique view extending from the AAOCA vessel takeoff to the normal caliber distal reference. **D,** Multiplanar axial reformation demonstrating AAOCA vessels with and without an intramural takeoff (proximal course within the aortic wall). **E,** AAOCA takeoff angle obtained in the multiplanar axial reconstruction at the level of the AAOCA ostium. **F,** AAOCA vessel takeoff level (above/below aortic valve commissure) shown in three-dimensional reformatted images. Asterisk denotes anomalous coronary artery. (From Cheezum MK, et al. Anomalous aortic origin of a coronary artery from the inappropriate sinus of Valsalva. J Am Coll Cardiol 2017;69:1592-1608.)

not on optimal preventive therapies (see the sections Pretest Probability of Obstructive Coronary Artery Disease and Selecting Appropriate Candidates for Coronary Computed Tomography Angiography).

Table 20.5 provides a summary of the Society of Cardiovascular Computed Tomography (SCCT) CCTA expert consensus recommendations,[50] which address the use of CCTA and cardiac CT for various cardiovascular conditions.

ASSESSMENT OF CARDIOVASCULAR STRUCTURE AND FUNCTION

Beyond coronary artery stenosis and plaque, cardiac CT can be used to visualize various cardiac pathologies including pericardial, myocardial, and valvular heart disease.

Pericardial and Myocardial Disease

Pericardial thickening and calcifications visualized on cardiac CT can be useful in assessing patients with suspected pericardial constriction, and the use of multiphase imaging can also be used to identify individuals who have pericardial adhesions. Other pericardial pathologies that can be detected on cardiac CT include pericardial cysts, pericardial effusions, and pericardial masses (see Chapter 86).

There are various forms of myocardial and infiltrative heart disease that can be identified on routine cardiac CT (Fig. 20.19). Images at end diastole can be used to measure left and right ventricular wall thickness, and left and right ventricular size. When a multiphase dataset is obtained during image acquisition, a qualitative or quantitative assessment of left and right ventricular systolic function can be obtained,[106] and images can be evaluated for regional wall motion abnormalities. Since the acquisition of multiphase data is associated with a higher radiation dose (because of the use of a helical acquisition, or when using either a helical or axial acquisition mode from opening of the phase acquisition window to include data throughout the cardiac cycle), most CCTA studies should be performed in diastole only. However, a multiphase acquisition may be helpful when data regarding left or right ventricular function are desired, in selected cases with congenital heart disease, when evaluating right ventricular morphology in suspected arrhythmogenic right ventricular cardiomyopathy (ARVC), or when evaluating for scar prior to ablation procedures.

Late enhancement imaging on CT refers to the acquisition of images ~8 minutes after contrast administration. Similar to late gadolinium enhancement imaging on CMR, iodinated contrast is an extracellular contrast agent that has delayed washout from areas of abnormal myocardium. In individuals who are unable to undergo CMR, late enchantment imaging on CT may be used to detect myocardial scar. Recent studies have also shown that CT can identify individuals with cardiac amyloidosis by quantifying the extracellular volume (ECV), a technique that may have a potential future role when evaluating patients prior to transcatheter aortic valve replacement (TAVR).[107]

Valvular Heart Disease (see Part VIII)

Cardiac CT has emerged as a useful test to evaluate various forms of valvular heart disease. Although all four cardiac valves can be assessed when a multiphase acquisition is performed (Fig. 20.20), imaging of the tricuspid valve is more challenging, but is now used to guide various emerging percutaneous repair options. The severity of aortic stenosis can be determined by calculating the Agatston calcium score of the

TABLE 20.5 Summary of Society of Cardiovascular Computed Tomography Coronary Computed Tomography Angiography Expert Consensus Recommendations

Evaluation of Stable CAD: CCTA in Native Vessels

- It is appropriate to perform CCTA as the first-line test for evaluating patients with no known CAD who present with stable typical or atypical chest pain, or other symptoms that are thought to represent a possible anginal equivalent (e.g., dyspnea on exertion, jaw pain)
- It is appropriate to perform CCTA as a first-line test for evaluating patients with known CAD who present with stable typical or atypical chest pain, or other symptoms that are thought to represent a possible anginal equivalent (e.g., dyspnea on exertion, jaw pain)
- It is appropriate to perform CCTA following a nonconclusive functional test to obtain more precision regarding diagnosis and prognosis, if such information will influence subsequent patient management
- It is recommended to perform CCTA as the first-line test when considering evaluation for revascularization strategies using the ISCHEMIA Trial
- It may be appropriate to perform CCTA in selected asymptomatic high-risk individuals, especially in those who have a higher likelihood of having a large amount of noncalcified plaque
- It is rarely appropriate to perform CCTA in very low-risk symptomatic patients, e.g., <40 years of age with noncardiac symptoms (chest wall pain, pleuritic chest pain)
- It is rarely appropriate to perform CCTA in low- and intermediate-risk asymptomatic patients

Evaluation of Stable CAD: CCTA Post-Revascularization

- It is appropriate to perform CCTA in symptomatic patients with intracoronary stent diameter ≥3.0 mm. Measures to improve accuracy of stent imaging should be used to include strict heart rate control (goal <60 beats/min), iterative reconstruction, sharp kernel reconstruction, and mono-energetic reconstructions (when available). Protocols to optimize stent imaging should be developed and followed
- It may be appropriate to perform CCTA in symptomatic patients with stents <3.0 mm, especially those known to have thin stent struts (<100 mm) in proximal, nonbifurcation locations
- It is appropriate to perform CCTA for evaluation of patients with prior CABG, particularly if graft patency is the primary objective
- It is appropriate to perform CCT to visualize grafts and other structures prior to re-do cardiac surgery

Evaluation of Stable CAD: CCTA with FFR or CTP

- It may be appropriate to perform CT-derived FFR and CT myocardial perfusion imaging to evaluate the functional significance of intermediate stenoses on CCTA (30%-90% diameter stenosis) particularly in the setting of multivessel disease to help guide ICA referral and revascularization treatment planning. LM stenosis ≥50% and severe triple vessel disease should undergo invasive coronary angiography
- Adding FFRCT and stress-CTP to CCTA increases specificity, positive predictive value, and diagnostic accuracy over regular CCTA
- FFRCT and stress-CTP may be largely comparable in diagnostic utility. CTP is a potentially valuable alternative particularly when CT-FFR is technically difficult (e.g., suboptimal CCTA quality, prior revascularization)

Evaluation of Stable CAD: CCTA and CCT in Other Conditions

- It is appropriate to perform CCTA for coronary artery evaluation prior to noncoronary cardiac surgery as an equivalent alternative to invasive angiography in selected patients, e.g., low-intermediate probability of CAD, younger patients with primarily nondegenerative valvular conditions
- CCTA may be considered an appropriate alternative to other noninvasive tests for evaluation of selected patients prior to noncardiac surgery
- It is appropriate to perform CCTA to exclude CAD in patients with suspected nonischemic cardiomyopathy
- It may be appropriate to perform late-enhancement CT imaging to detect infiltrative heart disease or scar in selected patients who have nonischemic or ischemic cardiomyopathy and who cannot undergo cardiac MRI. Such imaging may be performed if it has the potential to impact the diagnosis and/or treatment (e.g., planning for ablation therapy)
- It may be appropriate to perform CCTA as an alternative to invasive coronary angiography for the screening of patients for coronary allograft vasculopathy in selected clinical practice settings
- It is appropriate to perform CCTA for the evaluation of coronary anomalies
- It is appropriate to ECG gate aortic dissection and aneurysm CTA, as well as pulmonary embolus studies in men >45 years and women >55 years, and analyze and report the coronary arteries
- CCT with a limited delayed image (60 s) is an appropriate alternative to TEE when the primary aim is to exclude LA/LAA thrombus and in patients where the risks associated with TEE outweigh the benefits. In all situations, CCT and TEE should be discussed with the patient in the setting of shared decision making
- It may be appropriate to perform late enhancement CT imaging for the evaluation of myocardial viability in selected patients who cannot undergo cardiac MRI. Such imaging may be performed if it has the potential to impact the diagnosis and/or treatment (e.g., planning for revascularization)

Reporting on CCT Coronary and Noncoronary Information

- CAD-RADs reporting is recommended
- It is appropriate to report prior myocardial infarction when its features are evident on CCT
- It is appropriate to report remote myocardial infarction when fatty metaplasia or calcification within an area of infarction are present

CABG, Coronary artery bypass grafting; *CAD*, coronary artery disease; *CAD-RADs*, Coronary Artery Disease-Reporting and Data System; *CCTA*, coronary computed tomography angiography; *CTP*, computed tomography perfusion; *FFRCT*, computed tomography–derived FFR; *ICA*, invasive coronary angiography; *LA*, left atrium; *LAA*, left atrial appendage; *LM*, left main coronary; *MRI*, magnetic resonance imaging; *TEE*, transesophageal echocardiogram.
Adapted from Narula J, et al. SCCT 2021 Expert Consensus Document on Coronary Computed Tomographic Angiography: a report of the Society of Cardiovascular Computed Tomography. J Cardiovasc Comput Tomogr. 2020;S1934-5925(20)30473-1.

aortic valve (see Figs. 72.3 and 72.11), in which a measure >2065 in men and >1274 in women has been found to provide good discriminatory value for diagnosing severe aortic stenosis, and identifying patients with adverse prognosis.[108] In addition, direct planimetry at the level of the aortic valve leaflet tips can be performed to measure the aortic valve area. Similarly, the presence of aortic regurgitation can be accurately evaluated by assessing for aortic valve closure during diastole. Several studies have shown that direct planimetry of the regurgitant orifice can be used to estimate the severity of aortic regurgitation.

One particular advantage of cardiac CT is the ability to evaluate patients with mechanical valves, as such valves often have significant artifacts on echocardiography. When there is suspicion for valve dysfunction, cardiac CT can evaluate for valvular thrombosis and pannus (Fig. 20.21; see Fig. 79.5C). When endocarditis is suspected,

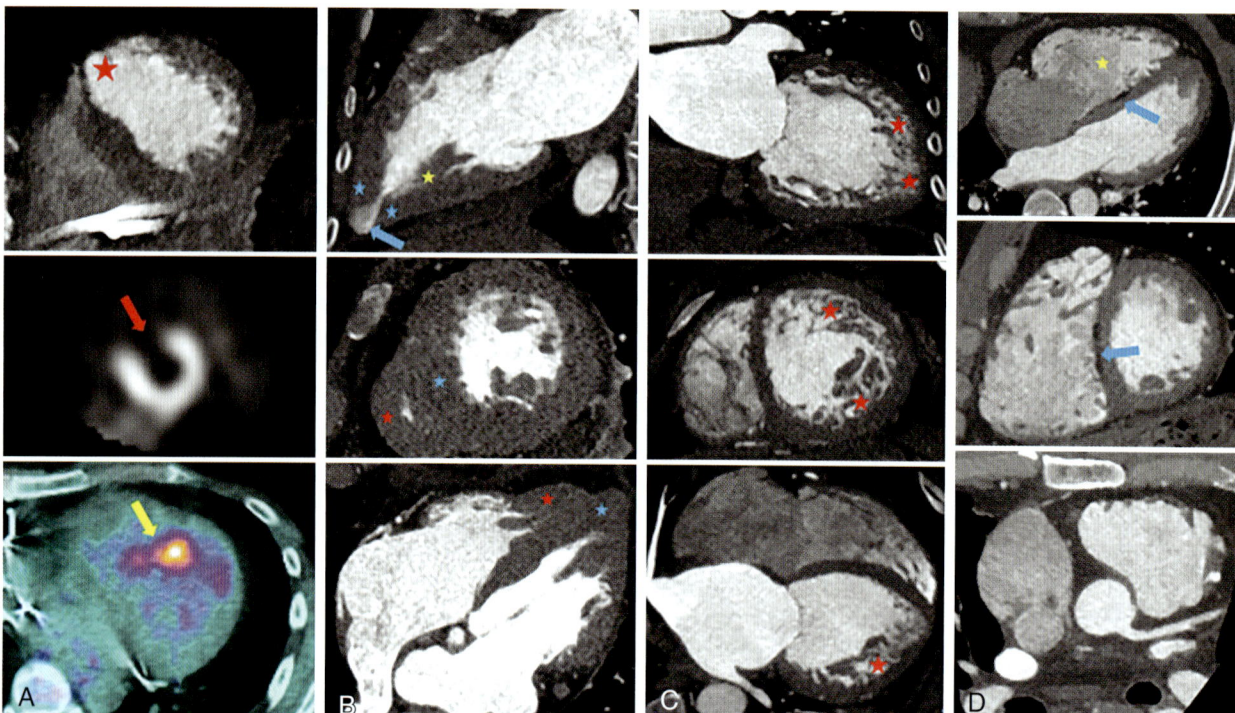

FIGURE 20.19 Examples of various cardiomyopathies on cardiac computed tomography (CT). A, Cardiac sarcoidosis. *Top panel:* Cardiac CT showing a large aneurysm of the mid anterior and anteroseptal segments associated with myocardial thinning and akinesis (*red star*). *Middle panel*: Resting technetium-99m perfusion scan showing a severe perfusion defect in the mid anterior and anteroseptal segments (*red arrow*). *Bottom panel*: F18-fluorodeoxyglucose (FDG) positron emission tomography (PET)/CT scan demonstrating a small region of intense FDG uptake in the same region (*yellow arrow*). **B,** Apical hypertrophic cardiomyopathy. Increased left ventricular (LV) apical wall thickness (*blue stars*) and apical displacement of the papillary muscle (*yellow star*). There is an LV apical aneurysm (*blue arrow*) without LV cavity thrombus. In addition, there is hypertrophy of the right ventricular apex (*red stars*). **C,** LV noncompaction cardiomyopathy. There are prominent LV trabeculations along the anterior, inferior, and lateral walls, and the LV apical segments (*red stars*). Gated CT images also showed a reduced LV ejection fraction of 20% with global hypokinesis. The end-diastolic ratio of noncompacted to compacted myocardium was 3.8 (normal <2.3). **D,** Arrhythmogenic cardiomyopathy. Cardiac CT images showing a dilated right atrium and right ventricle (*yellow star*). There is also fatty infiltration of the interventricular septum (*blue arrow*). Coronary CT angiography showed no evidence of plaque or stenosis. (Courtesy Dr. Vasvi Singh, Brigham and Women's Hospital, Boston.)

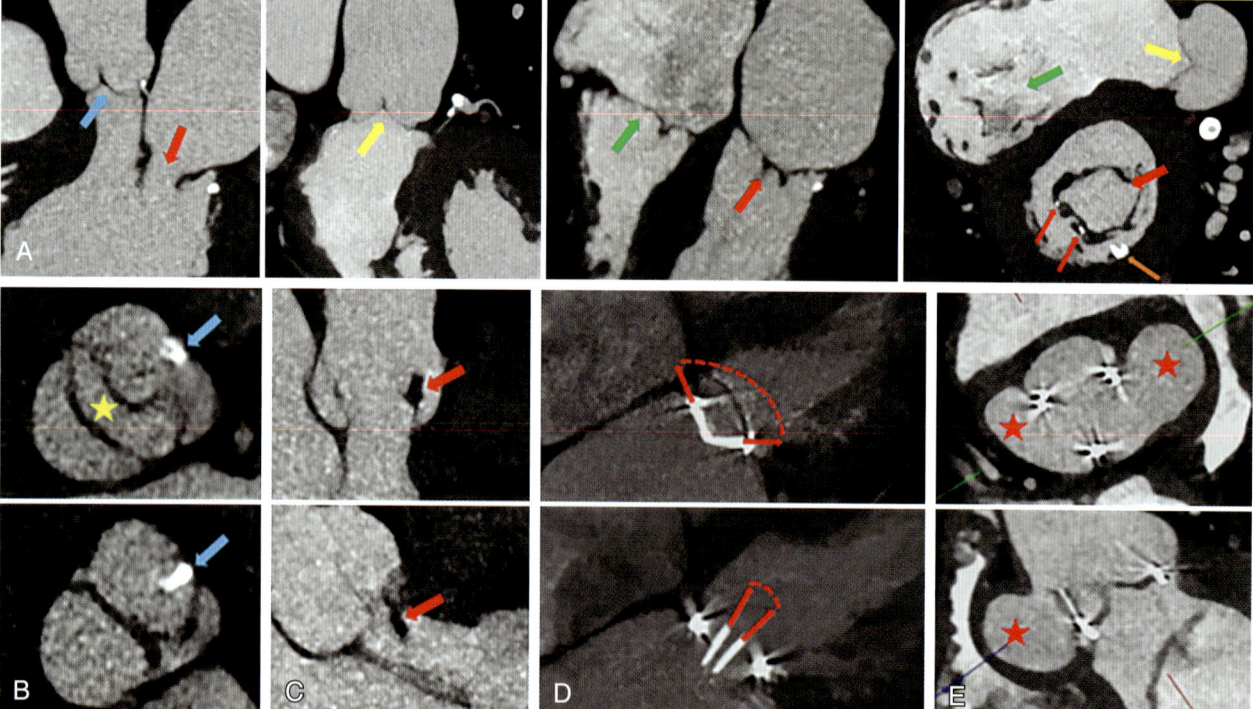

FIGURE 20.20 Examples of assessing valvular heart disease on cardiac computed tomography. A, Normal appearances of aortic valve (*blue arrow*), pulmonic valve (*yellow arrows*), and tricuspid valve (*green arrows*) in different phases of the cardiac cycle. Mitral valve (*red arrows*) in different phases of the cardiac cycle; the mitral valve leaflets are mildly thickened with calcifications (*small red arrow*), and there is mild posterior mitral annular calcification (*small orange arrow*). **B,** Bicuspid aortic valve during systole and diastole. There is fusion of the right and left coronary cusps with calcification of the fusion raphe (*blue arrows*). The bicuspid valve has an elliptical opening (*yellow star*) visualized during systole. **C,** Mobile aortic valve vegetation (*red arrows*) visualized during systole and diastole (prolapses into the left ventricular outflow tract) in a patient with gram-positive bacteremia and sepsis. **D,** Normal functioning St. Jude's mechanical bileaflet mitral valve prosthesis during ventricular systole and diastole. The prosthetic leaflets have normal closing and opening angles (*red arrows*). **E,** Pseudoaneurysms (*red stars*) developed as a complication of bioprosthetic aortic valve infective endocarditis, visualized during systole and diastole. (Courtesy Dr. Vasvi Singh, Brigham and Women's Hospital, Boston.)

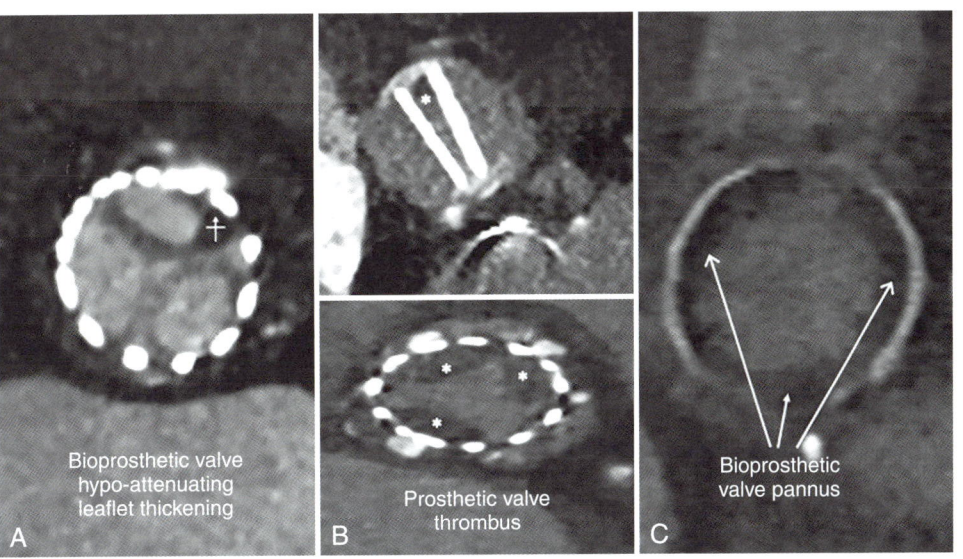

FIGURE 20.21 Examples of valve thrombosis versus pannus. **A**, Bioprosthetic valve demonstrating hypoattenuation leaflet thickening consistent with subclinical thrombosis. **B**, Mechanical (*top*) and bioprosthetic (*bottom*) valves with thrombus. **C**, Bioprosthetic valve with pannus.

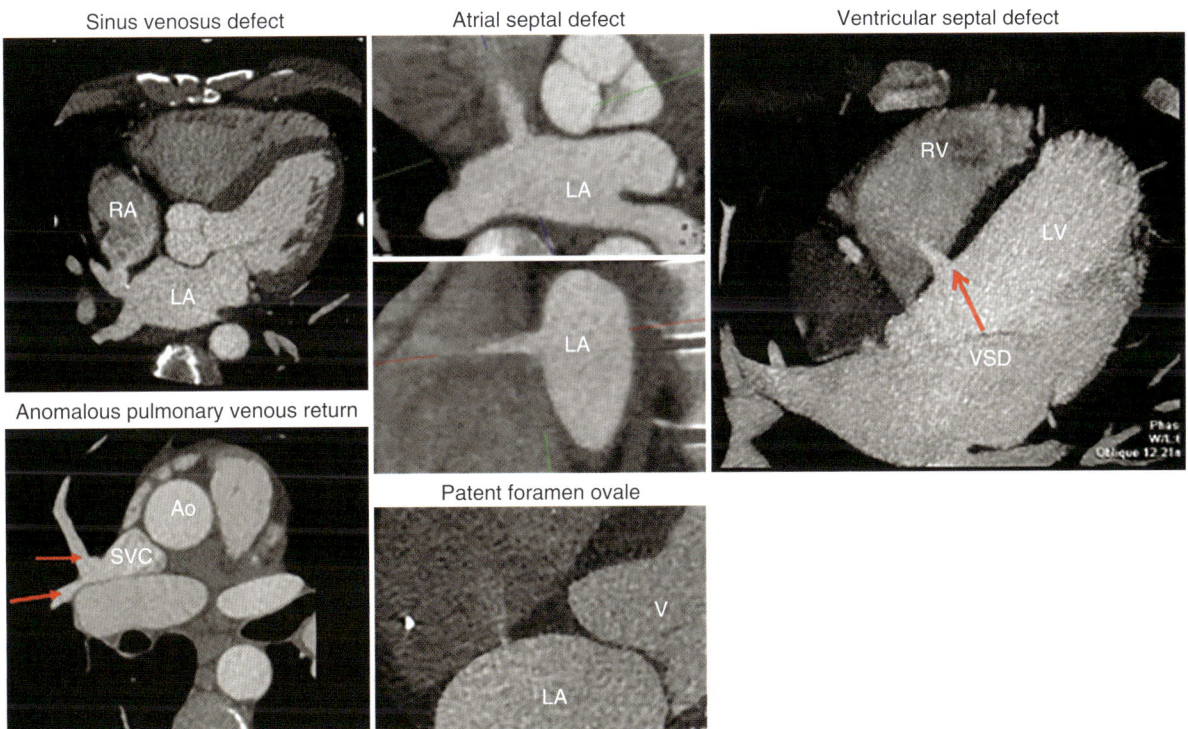

FIGURE 20.22 Examples of various intracardiac shunts on cardiac computed tomography. *Ao*, Aorta; *LA*, left atrium; *RA*, right atrium; *SVC*, superior vena cava, *VSD*, ventricular septal defect.

cardiac CT can be useful for the evaluation of both native and prosthetic valves. In native valves, cardiac CT can detect vegetations with a high diagnostic accuracy, although very small vegetations can be challenging to detect. In prosthetic valves, cardiac CT can identify paravalvular lesions, such as a pseudoaneurysm, abscess, or fistula. The 2015 ESC Guidelines for Management of Infective Endocarditis categorize paravalvular lesions by CCT as a major criteria for diagnosing endocarditis as part of the modified criteria for the diagnosis of infective endocarditis.[109]

Shunts

Cardiac CT can be useful for assessing for various intracardiac defects including atrial septal defects, ventricular septal defects, and anomalous pulmonary venous drainage (Fig. 20.22). In addition, CCT can detect patent foreman ovale, sinus venous defects, and unroofed coronary sinus. When such defects are identified, cardiac CT may be helpful in assessing the feasibility of percutaneous versus surgical closure techniques.

Use of Cardiac Computed Tomography for Structural Heart Disease Interventions

Cardiac CT has evolved to become an important imaging modality for preprocedural guidance and postprocedural follow-up for many of structural heart disease interventions. These include imaging for transcatheter heart valve replacement, left atrial appendage occlusion, and arrhythmia ablation.

Pre-Transcatheter Aortic Valve Replacement

Cardiac CT is an essential imaging test prior to TAVR, and it has been shown to improve procedural outcomes and prevent complications (Fig. 20.23).[110] CT imaging prior to TAVR generally includes two scans using a single contrast injection: (1) cardiac ECG gated dataset of the aortic root and heart followed by (2) nongated vascular CTA of the chest, abdomen, and pelvis. An alternative option is to acquire an ECG gated dataset of the entire chest and then to acquire a nongated

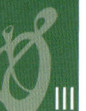

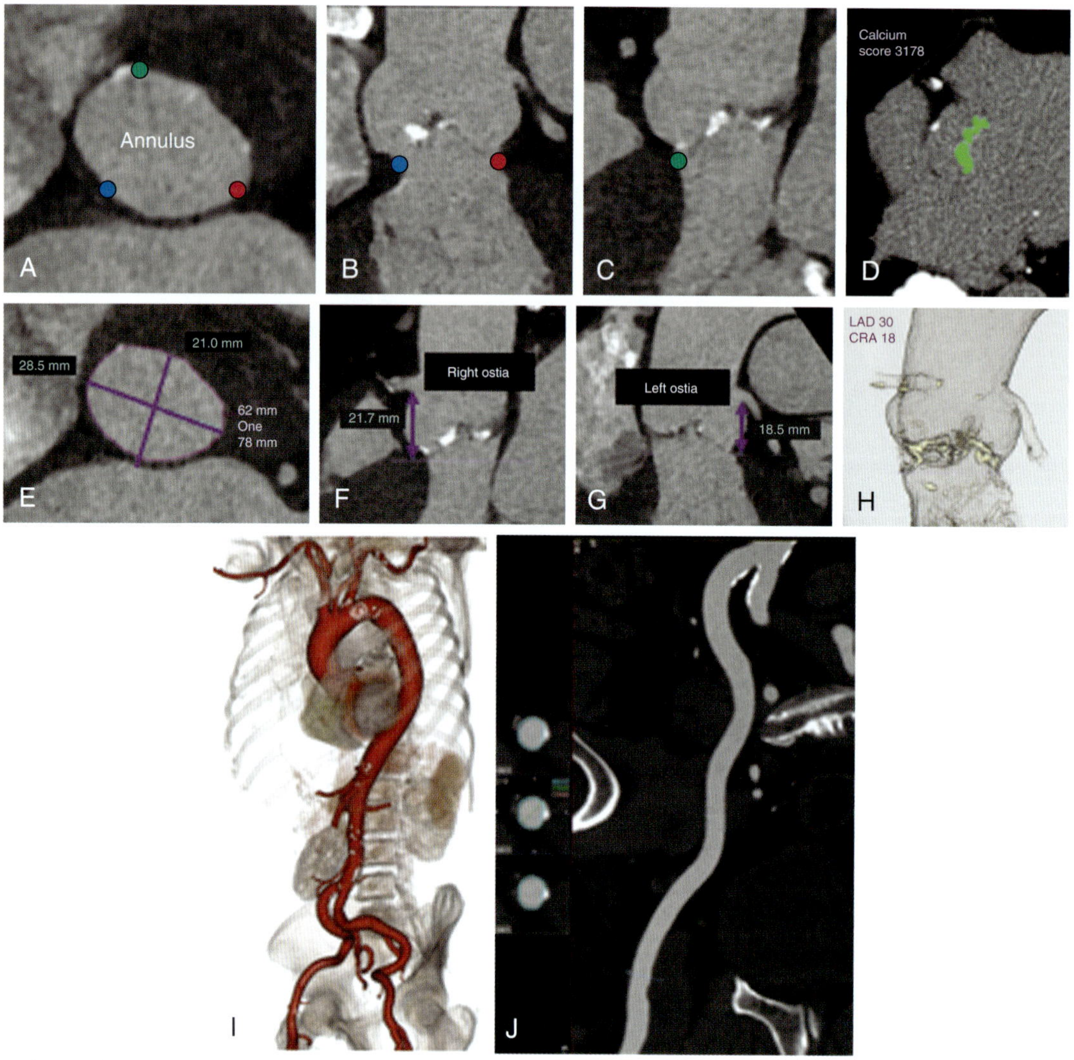

FIGURE 20.23 Cardiovascular computed tomography for preprocedural planning of transcatheter aortic valve replacement (TAVR). **A,** Short-axis view of the aortic annulus to mark the nadir of each cusp (*green, right cusp; red, left cusp; blue, noncoronary cusp*). **B** and **C,** Corresponding long-axis views of the aortic root showing the correct placement of the markers on the nadirs. **D,** Aortic valve calcium score for stenosis severity. **E,** Annulus view for major and minor axis diameters, area, and perimeter. **F** and **G,** Coronary ostia height measurements. **H,** Three-dimensional virtual reality (3DVR) showing the en face annular plane for TAVR deployment planning. **I,** 3DVR for access vessel tortuosity and calcification. **J,** Curved multiplanar reformat for access vessel diameters. (Courtesy Michael Steigner, Brigham and Women's Hospital, Boston, MA.)

vascular CTA of the abdomen and pelvis. Because the aortic root dimensions are usually larger in systole, systolic imaging is required (if only one portion of the cardiac cycle is acquired); however, coverage during the entire cardiac cycle may be beneficial. In addition, if there is uncertainty regarding whether severe aortic stenosis is present, a noncontrast ECG gated scan covering the aortic root may be added, as the aortic valve calcium score may be helpful in assessing aortic stenosis severity. (see section Valvular Heart Disease). The previously mentioned protocol uses a contrast volume ranging from 50 to 100 mL using a flow rate of 4 to 6 ms/s. A slower flow rate may be helpful when trying to minimize the amount of contrast, together with using lower tube voltage (e.g., 80 kV). Prospective high-pitch imaging is an alternative option that can help lower the contrast dose while maintaining a high image quality. Table 20.6 summarizes the recommendations on aortic root data that should be evaluated and reported prior to potential TAVR.[110]

Post-Transcatheter Aortic Valve Replacement (see Chapter 74)

Following TAVR, cardiac CT may be considered if there is clinical concern for valve thrombosis, infective endocarditis, or structural valve degeneration. Concern for thrombosis may exist if there is an increase in aortic valve gradients on echocardiography, especially if these also occur in the presence of any signs or symptoms of aortic stenosis. Features of leaflet thrombosis on cardiac CT include hypoattenuated leaflet thickening (HALT) (Fig. 20.24) and reduced leaflet motion, also referred to as hypoattenuation affecting motion (HAM). Leaflet thickening appears meniscal-shaped on the long axis, with greater thickness at the base than toward the center of the leaflet. Such thickening should be described based on location, extent in length, and overall thickness. Restricted motion should be reported as present or absent. Most cases of HALT with reduced leaflet motion are likely subclinical. Oral anticoagulation is associated with a lower rate of developing HALT or HAM. When such abnormalities are identified, initiation of oral anticoagulation is associated with a subsequent reduction in leaflet thickening. Nevertheless, it is unclear if treatment of subclinical leaflet thrombosis is beneficial or if it can lead to a lower rate of valve degeneration.

Evaluation Pre-Transcatheter Mitral Valve Replacement (see Chapter 78)

Cardiac CT has an essential role in selecting potential candidates for transcatheter mitral valve replacement (TMVR) by measuring the mitral valve dimensions and area and also estimating the risk of paravalvular regurgitation or left ventricular outflow track (LVOT) obstruction. The latter is achieved by using 3D visualization software to simulate the position of the implanted mitral valve and measuring the resulting "neo-LVOT" and thus the potential risk of LVOT obstruction (Fig. 20.25). Cardiac CT can also be used for 3D geometry of the mitral valve, which has a complex D-shaped structure with a saddle-shaped morphology. A single-center retrospective study has estimated that ~50% of patients evaluated for TMVR have a contraindication for the procedure based on cardiac CT such as high

TABLE 20.6 Aortic Root Assessment During Transcatheter Aortic Valve Replacement

	DETAILS TO REPORT	TIPS/RATIONALE
Aortic annulus	• Annular area, dimensions (long- and short-axis), perimeter	• Select phase with largest annular dimensions
Landing zone calcium (landing zone includes the valve cusps, annulus, and the LVOT)	• None, mild, moderate, severe • Annular and subannular calcifications should be described as crescent/flat/adherent or protruding and its relation to the aortic cusps	• Severe subannular calcification may indicate a higher risk of heart block/need for a pacemaker, especially if preexisting RBBB • Large protruding nodules of calcification, particularly below the noncoronary cusp, may increase the risk of annular rupture/paravalvular regurgitation

Valve morphology	• BAV morphology:
	  • Number of commissures
	  • Presence of absence of a raphe
	  • Presence and degree of raphe calcification (mild, moderate, severe)
		• BAV and severe raphe calcification associated with higher likelihood of paravalvular regurgitation

Coronary ostial height and sinus of Valsalva assessment	• Low coronary ostial height from the annulus • Sinus of Valsalva mean diameter	• Low coronary height (<12 mm) and sinus of Valsalva mean diameter <30 mm associated with higher risk of coronary occlusion • Coronary height and sinus of Valsalva width should be interpreted in the context of annular dimensions, overall root dimensions, and the anticipated THV size
Aortic root measurements	• STJ diameter and height • Ascending aorta dimensions	• When using balloon-expandable devices in low STJ height, STJ diameter should be compared with the anticipated THV size
Optimal fluoroscopic angles	• Reported as degrees LAO or RAO with the corresponding values for cranial or caudal angulation	• Only valid if patient positioned supine in the CT scanner

BAV, Bicuspid aortic valve; *CT*, computed tomography; *LVOT*, left ventricular outflow track; *RBB*, right bundle branch block; *STJ*, sinotubular junction; *THV*, transcatheter heart valve.

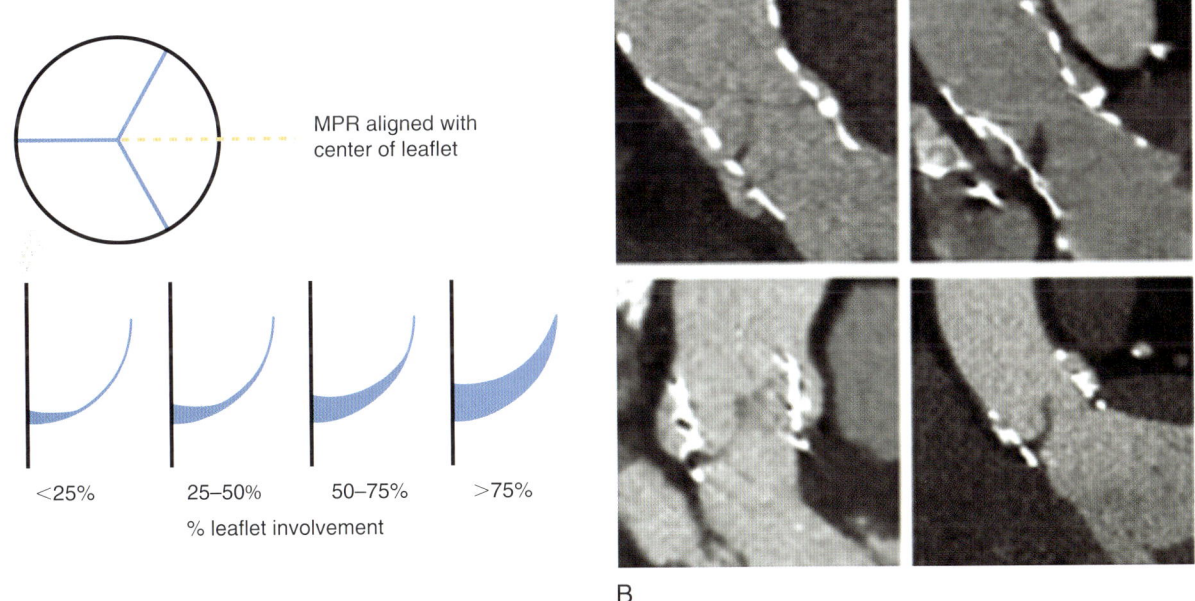

FIGURE 20.24 Post transcatheter aortic valve replacement assessment. **A,** How to use multiplanar (MPR) alignment for semiquantitative grading of hypoattenuated leaflet thickening. The *dashed yellow line* indicates the orientation of the long-axis views in the lower row, aligned with the center of the cusps. The extent of leaflet thickening can be graded on a subjective four-tier grading scale along the curvilinear orientation of the leaflet. Typically, hypoattenuated leaflet thickening appears meniscal shaped on long-axis reformats, with greater thickness at the base than toward the center of the leaflet. **B,** Examples of hypoattenuated leaflet thickening in both self-expandable (*upper row*) and balloon-expandable devices (*lower row*) with varying degree of thickening. Limited to base, i.e., <25% leaflet involvement (*left column*) and near complete leaflet involvement, i.e., >75% (*right column*). (From Blanke P, et al. Computed tomography imaging in the context of transcatheter aortic valve implantation (TAVI)/transcatheter aortic valve replacement (TAVR): an expert consensus document of the Society of Cardiovascular Computed Tomography. J Cardiovasc Comput Tomogr 2019;13:1-20.)

risk of LVOT obstruction, a large annular size, or an insufficient amount of mitral annular calcifications.[110a] As future generations of transcatheter mitral valves will expand the feasibility of TMVR procedures, cardiac CT will continue to play an integral role in patient and device selection.

Evaluation of Left Atrial Appendage (for Thrombus, Pre–Left Atrial Appendage Occlusion Devices)

Cardiac CT can be used to image the left atrial appendage (LAA) morphology and size and exclude the presence of an LAA clot.[50] Notably, a filling defect in the LAA can represent slow flow, and thus postcontrast delayed imaging may be necessary to confirm the presence of a clot (Fig. 20.26). A meta-analysis that included 19 studies identified a sensitivity and specificity of cardiac CT of 96% and 92%; however, when only studies (n = 7) that included delayed imaging were evaluated, the sensitivity and specificity increased to 100% and 99%.[111] A large single-center study that used a combination of transesophageal echocardiogram (TEE) and intracardiac echocardiography as the reference standard also demonstrated a sensitivity and NPV of 100% when using cardiac CT with delayed imaging. In this study, the specificity of cardiac CT when combining positive and equivocal CCT results was 98%.[112]

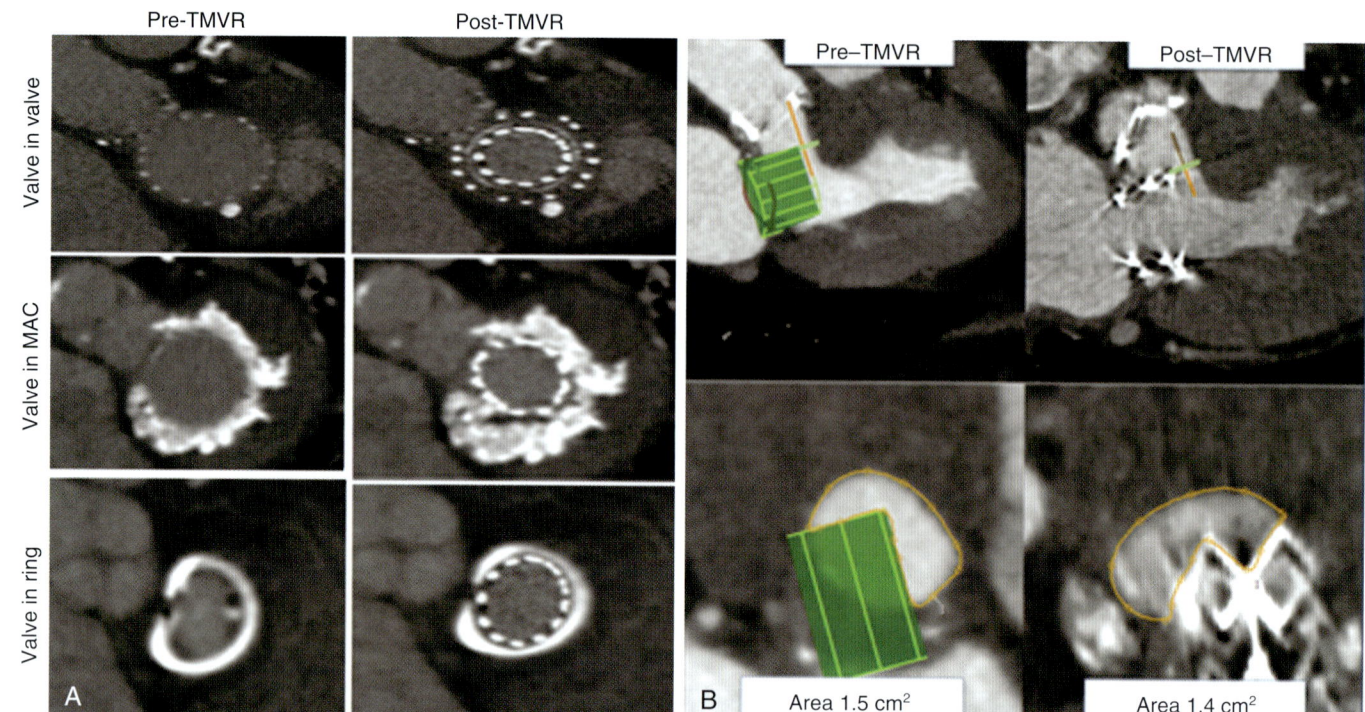

FIGURE 20.25 **A,** Pre- and post-transcatheter mitral valve replacement (TMVR) evaluation using cardiac computed tomography (CCT) for a valve-in-valve, valve-in-mitral angular calcification, and valve-in-ring scenarios. **B,** Pre-TMVR CCT in a valve-in-valve case projected a neo-left ventricular outflow tract (LVOT) area of 1.5 m². Post-TMVR CCT demonstrated a neo-LVOT area of 1.4 cm². (A, From Ge Y, et al. Role of cardiac CT in pre-procedure planning for transcatheter mitral valve replacement. JACC Cardiovasc Imaging 2021 [online ahead of print]. doi:10.1016/j.jcmg.2020.12.018)

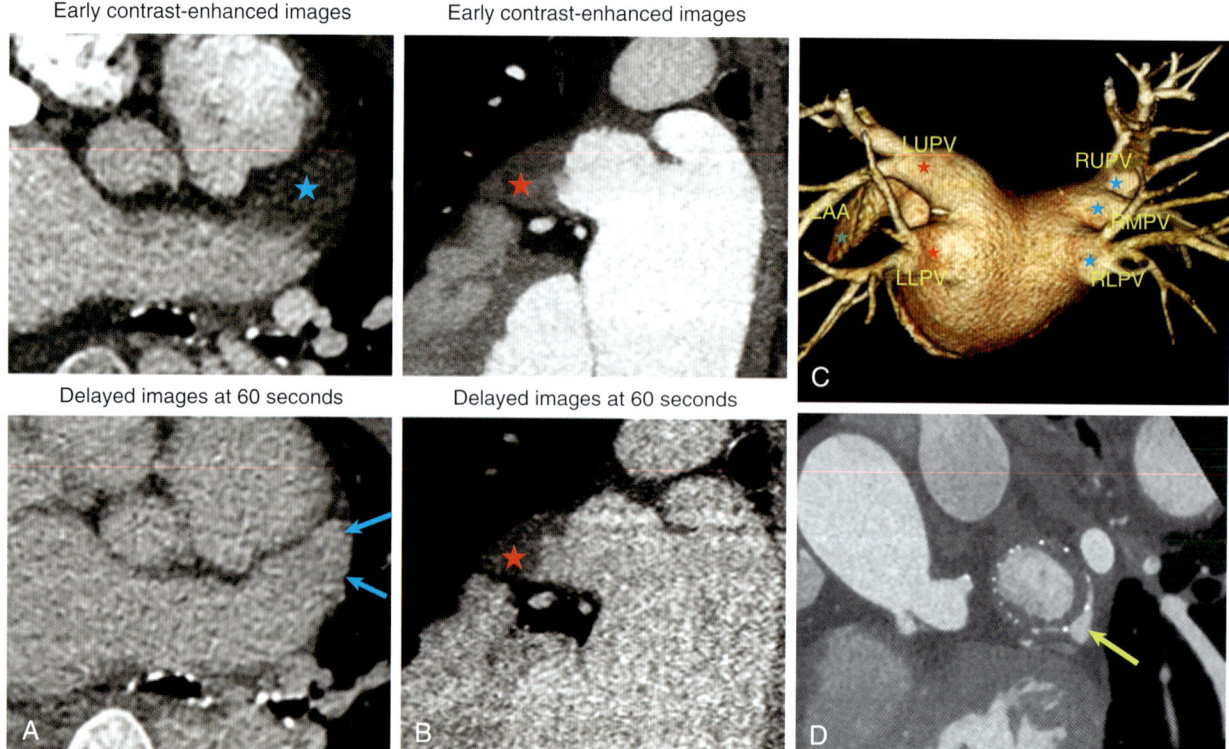

FIGURE 20.26 Evaluation of left atrial appendage and pulmonary venous anatomy. **A,** *Top:* Early contrast-enhanced images showing a filling defect in the left atrial appendage (LAA), which can represent low-flow state or a thrombus (*blue star*). *Bottom:* Delayed images acquired after 60 seconds demonstrates complete contrast opacification of the LAA (*blue arrows*) confirming the absence of a LAA thrombus. **B,** *Top panel:* Early contrast-enhanced images showing a filling defect in the LAA. *Bottom panel:* Delayed images acquired after 60 seconds demonstrate a persistent filling defect, thereby confirming the presence of a LAA thrombus (*red star*). **C,** Three-dimensional volume-rendered reconstruction of pulmonary vein anatomy. There are two pulmonary veins (PVs) on the left (*red stars*) (left upper [LUPV] and left lower [LLPV]), and three PVs on the right (*blue stars*) (right upper [RUPV], right middle [RMPV], and right lower [RLPV]). The LAA (*green star*) is adjacent to the LUPV. **D,** Incomplete contrast opacification following LAA occlusion device, including a gap (*yellow arrow*) at the ostium of the appendage.

Although TEE and CCT have overlapping capabilities in evaluating the LAA, selecting the best test may depend on the specific clinical situation. When it is important to also evaluate for underlying valvular disease, TEE is the preferred modality. In patients who are being evaluated for a pulmonary vein isolation (PVI) or LAA occlusion device placement, cardiac CT may be preferred if this test is already being performed for evaluating pulmonary vein or LAA anatomy.

Cardiac CT is increasingly being used to evaluate patients prior to LAA occlusion device implantation and in selected cases as follow-up to assess procedure success (see Fig. 20.26).

Evaluation of Cardiac Masses

Cardiac CT can provide useful information when evaluating patients with cardiac masses.[113] Although echocardiography and CMR are often the preferred initial testing options for such patients, cardiac CT may be helpful for masses that may involve the coronary arteries, for instance, when there is uncertainty whether a mass encases the coronary arteries, or when determining whether the coronary arteries provide blood supply to the mass. In addition, cardiac CT can be helpful for evaluating pseudoaneurysms of the heart (where high spatial resolution may be helpful in differentiating an aneurysm from a pseudoaneurysm), especially if these involve bypass grafts or the coronary arteries.[114]

FUTURE DIRECTIONS

CAC and CCTA are likely to have an increasing role in allocating preventive therapies in primary prevention.[41] With respect to CAC testing, future scan acquisition and image processing techniques will further lower the radiation dose of this exam, enhancing the prognostic value. Current ongoing research, including the SCOT-HEART 2 trial (https://clinicaltrials.gov/ct2/show/NCT03920176), will assess the potential efficacy and cost-effectiveness of CCTA in primary prevention. Ultimately, the distinction between primary and secondary prevention may lessen, as the amount of underlying plaque, and thereby risk level, may be incorporated in clinical trials and guidelines.

As CCTA becomes increasingly used in the evaluation of symptomatic patients with suspected CAD, future studies will be required to demonstrate how it is being used in clinical care, and the impact of this test on subsequent medical therapies, downstream procedures, and patient outcomes. Ultimately, findings on CCTA, including the overall amount and type of plaque, will be used to determine patient risk and guide the intensity of medical therapy. To achieve this paradigm, future clinical trials will be required to assess the efficacy of various treatments based on CCTA or CAC inclusion criteria. Because the clinical effectiveness of CCTA relies on obtaining high image quality and ensuring that the test results are used appropriately, continued technologic advances that promote high quality imaging and educational efforts to ensure the test in interpreted and used correctly remain essential.[115] Ultimately, the acquisition and interpretation of CCTA findings may be enhanced by artificial intelligence, making this technology easier to disseminate across different practice environments.

REFERENCES

1. Stocker TJ, Deseive S, Leipsic J, et al. Reduction in radiation exposure in cardiovascular computed tomography imaging: results from the PROspective multicenter registry on radiaTion dose Estimates of cardiac CT anglOgraphy iN daily practice in 2017 (PROTECTION VI). *Eur Heart J*. 2018;39:3715–3723.
2. Abdelrahman KM, Chen MY, Dey AK, et al. Coronary computed tomography angiography from clinical uses to emerging technologies. *J Am Coll Cardiol*. 2020;76:1226–1243.
3. Agatston AS, Janowitz WR, Hildner FJ, et al. Quantification of coronary artery calcium using ultrafast computed tomography. *J Am Coll Cardiol*. 1990;15:827–832.
4. McClelland RL, Chung H, Detrano R, et al. Distribution of coronary artery calcium by race, gender, and age: results from the Multi-Ethnic Study of Atherosclerosis (MESA). *Circulation*. 2006;113:30–37.
5. McClelland RL, Jorgensen NW, Budoff M, et al. 10-Year coronary heart disease risk prediction using coronary artery calcium and traditional risk factors: derivation in the MESA (Multi-Ethnic Study of Atherosclerosis) with validation in the HNR (Heinz Nixdorf Recall) study and the DHS (Dallas Heart Study). *J Am Coll Cardiol*. 2015;66:1643–1653.
6. Budoff MJ, Young R, Burke G, et al. Ten-year association of coronary artery calcium with atherosclerotic cardiovascular disease (ASCVD) events: the multi-ethnic study of atherosclerosis (MESA). *Eur Heart J*. 2018;39:2401–2408.
7. Nasir K, Rubin J, Blaha MJ, et al. Interplay of coronary artery calcification and traditional risk factors for the prediction of all-cause mortality in asymptomatic individuals. *Circ Cardiovasc Imaging*. 2012;5:467–473.
8. Silverman MG, Blaha MJ, Krumholz HM, et al. Impact of coronary artery calcium on coronary heart disease events in individuals at the extremes of traditional risk factor burden: the Multi-Ethnic Study of Atherosclerosis. *Eur Heart J*. 2014;35:2232–2241.
9. Blankstein R, Budoff MJ, Shaw LJ, et al. Predictors of coronary heart disease events among asymptomatic persons with low low-density lipoprotein cholesterol MESA (Multi-Ethnic Study of Atherosclerosis). *J Am Coll Cardiol*. 2011;58:364–374.
10. Erbel R, Mohlenkamp S, Moebus S, et al. Coronary risk stratification, discrimination, and reclassification improvement based on quantification of subclinical coronary atherosclerosis: the Heinz Nixdorf Recall study. *J Am Coll Cardiol*. 2010;56:1397–1406.
11. Polonsky TS, McClelland RL, Jorgensen NW, et al. Coronary artery calcium score and risk classification for coronary heart disease prediction. *J Am Med Assoc*. 2010;303:1610–1616.
12. Mahabadi AA, Möhlenkamp S, Lehmann N, et al. CAC score improves coronary and CV risk assessment above statin indication by ESC and AHA/ACC primary prevention guidelines. *JACC (J Am Coll Cardiol): Cardiovasc Imaging*. 2017;10:143–153.
13. Nasir K, Bittencourt MS, Blaha MJ, et al. Implications of coronary artery calcium testing among statin candidates according to American College of Cardiology/American Heart Association cholesterol management guidelines: MESA (Multi-Ethnic study of atherosclerosis). *J Am Coll Cardiol*. 2015;66:1657–1668.
14. Sarwar A, Shaw LJ, Shapiro MD, et al. Diagnostic and prognostic value of absence of coronary artery calcification. *JACC Cardiovasc Imaging*. 2009;2:675–688.
15. Bakhshi H, Ambale–Venkatesh B, Yang X, et al. Progression of coronary artery calcium and incident heart failure: the multi–ethnic study of atherosclerosis. *J Am Heart Assoc*. 2017;6:e005253.
16. Gibson AO, Blaha MJ, Arnan MK, et al. Coronary artery calcium and incident cerebrovascular events in an asymptomatic cohort. The MESA Study. *JACC Cardiovasc Imaging*. 2014;7:1108–1115.
17. O'Neal WT, Efird JT, Dawood FZ, et al. Coronary artery calcium and risk of atrial fibrillation (from the multi-ethnic study of atherosclerosis). *Am J Cardiol*. 2014;114:1707–1712.
18. Handy CE, Desai CS, Dardari ZA, et al. The association of coronary artery calcium with noncardiovascular disease: the multi-ethnic study of atherosclerosis. *JACC Cardiovasc Imaging*. 2016.
19. Dzaye O, Al Rifai M, Dardari Z, et al. Coronary artery calcium as a synergistic tool for the age- and sex-specific risk of cardiovascular and cancer mortality: the coronary artery calcium Consortium. *J Am Heart Assoc*. 2020;9:e015306.
20. Carr J, Jacobs Jr DR, Terry JG, et al. Association of coronary artery calcium in adults aged 32 to 46 years with incident coronary heart disease and death. *JAMA Cardiol*. 2017.
21. Mortensen MB, Fuster V, Muntendam P, et al. Negative risk markers for cardiovascular events in the elderly. *J Am Coll Cardiol*. 2019;74:1–11.
22. Wang FM, Rozanski A, Arnson Y, et al. Cardiovascular and all-cause mortality risk by coronary artery calcium scores and percentiles among older adult males and females. *Am J Med*.
23. Truong QA, Rinehart S, Abbara S, et al. Coronary computed tomographic imaging in women: an expert consensus statement from the Society of Cardiovascular Computed Tomography. *J Cardiovasc Comput Tomogr*. 2018;12:451–466.
24. Kavousi M, Desai CS, Ayers C, et al. Prevalence and prognostic implications of coronary artery calcification in low-risk women: a meta-analysis. *J Am Med Assoc*. 2016;316:2126–2134.
25. Orringer CE, Blaha MJ, Blankstein R, et al. The National Lipid Association scientific statement on coronary artery calcium scoring to guide preventive strategies for ASCVD risk reduction. *J Clin Lipidol*. 2021;15(1):33–60.
26. Hecht H, Blaha MJ, Berman DS, et al. Clinical indications for coronary artery calcium scoring in asymptomatic patients: expert consensus statement from the Society of Cardiovascular Computed Tomography. *J Cardiovasc Comput Tomogr*. 2017;11:157–168.
27. Cainzos-Achirica M, Miedema MD, McEvoy JW, et al. Coronary artery calcium for personalized allocation of aspirin in primary prevention of cardiovascular disease in 2019: the MESA study (Multi-Ethnic study of atherosclerosis). *Circulation*. 2020;141:1541–1553.
28. Miedema MD, Duprez DA, Misialek JR, et al. Use of coronary artery calcium testing to guide aspirin utilization for primary prevention: estimates from the multi-ethnic study of atherosclerosis. *Circ Cardiovasc Qual Outcomes*. 2014;7:453–460.
29. Arnett DK, Blumenthal RS, Albert MA, et al. 2019 ACC/AHA guideline on the primary prevention of cardiovascular disease: a report of the American College of Cardiology/American Heart Association task force on clinical practice guidelines. *Circulation*. 2019;140:e596–e646.
30. Peng AW, Mirbolouk M, Orimoloye OA, et al. Long-term all-cause and cause-specific mortality in asymptomatic patients with CAC >/=1,000: results from the CAC Consortium. *JACC Cardiovasc Imag*. 2020;13:83–93.
31. Maron DJ, Hochman JS, Reynolds HR, et al. Initial invasive or conservative strategy for stable coronary disease. *N Engl J Med*. 2020;382:1395–1407.
32. Muhlestein JB, Lappe DL, Lima JA, et al. Effect of screening for coronary artery disease using CT angiography on mortality and cardiac events in high-risk patients with diabetes: the FACTOR-64 randomized clinical trial. *J Am Med Assoc*. 2014;312:2234–2243.
33. Young LH, Wackers FJ, Chyun DA, et al. Cardiac outcomes after screening for asymptomatic coronary artery disease in patients with type 2 diabetes: the DIAD study: a randomized controlled trial. *J Am Med Assoc*. 2009;301:1547–1555.
34. Berman DS, Wong ND, Gransar H, et al. Relationship between stress-induced myocardial ischemia and atherosclerosis measured by coronary calcium tomography. *J Am Coll Cardiol*. 2004;44:923–930.
35. Naya M, Murthy VL, Taqueti VR, et al. Preserved coronary flow reserve effectively excludes high-risk coronary artery disease on angiography. *J Nucl Med*. 2014;55:248–255.
36. Naya M, Murthy VL, Foster CR, et al. Prognostic interplay of coronary artery calcification and underlying vascular dysfunction in patients with suspected coronary artery disease. *J Am Coll Cardiol*. 2013;61:2098–2106.
37. Rozanski A, Gransar H, Shaw LJ, et al. Impact of coronary artery calcium scanning on coronary risk factors and downstream testing the EISNER (Early Identification of Subclinical Atherosclerosis by Noninvasive Imaging Research) prospective randomized trial. *J Am Coll Cardiol*. 2011;57:1622–1632.
38. Shaw LJ, Min JK, Budoff M, et al. Induced cardiovascular procedural costs and resource consumption patterns after coronary artery calcium screening results from the EISNER (early identification of subclinical atherosclerosis by noninvasive imaging research) study. *J Am Coll Cardiol*. 2009;54:1258–1267.
39. Gupta A, Lau E, Varshney R, et al. The identification of calcified coronary plaque is associated with initiation and continuation of pharmacological and lifestyle preventive therapies: a systematic review and meta-analysis. *JACC Cardiovasc Imaging*. 2017;10:833–842.
40. Arad Y, Spadaro LA, Roth M, et al. Treatment of asymptomatic adults with elevated coronary calcium scores with atorvastatin, vitamin C, and vitamin E: the St. Francis Heart Study randomized clinical trial. *J Am Coll Cardiol*. 2005;46:166–172.
41. Greenland P, Michos ED, Redmond N, et al. Primary prevention trial designs using coronary imaging. *JACC Cardiovasc Imaging*. 2020.
42. Andreini D, Pontone G, Mushtaq S, et al. Atrial fibrillation: diagnostic accuracy of coronary CT angiography performed with a whole-heart 230-μm spatial resolution CT scanner. *Radiology*. 2017;284:676–684.
43. Yang L, Zhang Z, Fan Z, et al. 64-MDCT coronary angiography of patients with atrial fibrillation: influence of heart rate on image quality and efficacy in evaluation of coronary artery disease. *Am J Roentgenol*. 2009;193:795–801.
44. Pontone G, Bertella E, Mushtaq S, et al. Coronary artery disease: diagnostic accuracy of CT coronary angiography—a comparison of high and standard spatial resolution scanning. *Radiology*. 2014;271:688–694.
45. Li P, Xu L, Yang L, et al. Blooming artifact reduction in coronary artery calcification by A new de-blooming algorithm: initial study. *Sci Rep*. 2018;8:6945–6945.
46. Knuuti J, Ballo H, Juarez-Orozco LE, et al. The performance of non-invasive tests to rule-in and rule-out significant coronary artery stenosis in patients with stable angina: a meta-analysis [illegible]

47. Neglia D, Rovai D, Caselli C, et al. Detection of significant coronary artery disease by noninvasive anatomical and functional imaging. *Circ Cardiovasc Imaging*. 2015;8:e002179–e002179.
48. Danad I, Raijmakers PG, Driessen RS, et al. Comparison of coronary CT angiography, SPECT, PET, and hybrid imaging for diagnosis of ischemic heart disease determined by fractional flow reserve. *JAMA Cardiol*. 2017;2:1100–1107.
49. Min JK, Dunning A, Lin FY, et al. Age- and sex-related differences in all-cause mortality risk based on coronary computed tomography angiography findings results from the International Multicenter CONFIRM (Coronary CT Angiography Evaluation for Clinical Outcomes: an International Multicenter Registry) of 23,854 patients without known coronary artery disease. *J Am Coll Cardiol*. 2011;58:849–860.
50. Narula J, Chandrashekhar Y, Ahmadi A, et al. SCCT 2021 expert consensus document on coronary computed tomographic angiography: a report of the society of Cardiovascular Computed Tomography. *J Cardiovasc Comput Tomogr*. 2020 Nov 20;S1934–5925(20)30473-1.
51. Bittencourt MS, Hulten E, Ghoshhajra B, et al. Prognostic value of nonobstructive and obstructive coronary artery disease detected by coronary computed tomography angiography to identify cardiovascular events. *Circ Cardiovasc Imaging*. 2014;7:282–291.
52. Lin FY, Shaw LJ, Dunning AM, et al. Mortality risk in symptomatic patients with nonobstructive coronary artery disease. A prospective 2-center study of 2,583 patients undergoing 64-detector row coronary computed tomographic angiography. 2011;58:510–519.
53. Hoffmann U, Ferencik M, Udelson JE, et al. Prognostic value of noninvasive cardiovascular testing in patients with stable chest pain. *Circulation*. 2017;135:2320–2332.
54. Mortensen MB, Dzaye O, Steffensen FH, et al. Impact of plaque burden versus stenosis on ischemic events in patients with coronary atherosclerosis. *J Am Coll Cardiol*. 2020;76:2803–2813.
55. Hulten E, Pickett C, Bittencourt MS, et al. Outcomes after coronary computed tomography angiography in the emergency department: a systematic review and meta-analysis of randomized, controlled trials. *J Am Coll Cardiol*. 2013;61:880–892.
56. Dedic A, Lubbers MM, Schaap J, et al. Coronary CT angiography for suspected ACS in the era of high-sensitivity troponins: randomized multicenter study. *J Am Coll Cardiol*. 2016;67:16–26.
57. Chang AM, Litt HI, Snyder BS, et al. Impact of coronary computed tomography angiography findings on initiation of cardioprotective medications. *Circulation*. 2017;136:2195–2197.
58. Linde JJ, Kelbæk H, Hansen TF, et al. Coronary CT angiography in patients with non-ST-segment elevation acute coronary syndrome. *J Am Coll Cardiol*. 2020;75:453–463.
59. Smulders MW, Kietselaer BLJH, Wildberger JE, et al. Initial imaging-guided strategy versus routine care in patients with non–ST-segment elevation myocardial infarction. *J Am Coll Cardiol*. 2019;74:2466–2477.
60. Collet J-P, Thiele H, Barbato E, et al. ESC Guidelines for the management of acute coronary syndromes in patients presenting without persistent ST-segment elevation: the Task Force for the management of acute coronary syndromes in patients presenting without persistent ST-segment elevation of the European Society of Cardiology (ESC). *Eur Heart J*. 2020;42:1289–1367. 2021.
61. Choi AD, Abbara S, Branch KR, et al. Society of cardiovascular computed tomography guidance for use of cardiac computed tomography amidst the COVID-19 pandemic endorsed by the American College of Cardiology. *J Cardiovasc Comput Tomogr*. 2020.
62. Foldyna B, Udelson JE, Karády J, et al. Pretest probability for patients with suspected obstructive coronary artery disease: re-evaluating Diamond–Forrester for the contemporary era and clinical implications: insights from the PROMISE trial. *Eur Heart J Cardiovasc Imaging*. 2018;20:574–581.
63. Juarez-Orozco LE, Saraste A, Capodanno D, et al. Impact of a decreasing pre-test probability on the performance of diagnostic tests for coronary artery disease. *Eur Heart J Cardiovasc Imaging*. 2019;20:1198–1207.
64. Bittencourt MS, Hulten E, Polonsky TS, et al. European society of cardiology-recommended coronary artery disease Consortium pretest probability scores more accurately predict obstructive coronary disease and cardiovascular events than the diamond and forrester score: the Partners registry. *Circulation*. 2016;134:201–211.
65. Winther S, Schmidt SE, Mayrhofer T, et al. Incorporating coronary calcification into pre-test assessment of the likelihood of coronary artery disease. *J Am Coll Cardiol*. 2020;76:2421–2432.
66. McKavanagh P, Lusk L, Ball PA, et al. A comparison of cardiac computerized tomography and exercise stress electrocardiogram test for the investigation of stable chest pain: the clinical results of the CAPP randomized prospective trial. *Eur Heart J Cardiovasc Imaging*. 2015;16:441–448.
67. Lubbers M, Dedic A, Coenen A, et al. Calcium imaging and selective computed tomography angiography in comparison to functional testing for suspected coronary artery disease: the multicentre, randomized CRESCENT trial. *Eur Heart J*. 2016;37:1232–1243.
68. Sharma A, Coles A, Sekaran NK, et al. Stress testing versus CT angiography in patients with diabetes and suspected coronary artery disease. *J Am Coll Cardiol*. 2019;73:893–902.
69. Bittencourt MS, Hulten EA, Murthy VL, et al. Clinical outcomes after evaluation of stable chest pain by coronary computed tomographic angiography versus usual care: a meta-analysis. *Circ Cardiovasc Imaging*. 2016;9:e004419.
70. Jorgensen ME, Andersson C, Norgaard BL, et al. Functional testing or coronary computed tomography angiography in patients with stable coronary artery disease. *J Am Coll Cardiol*. 2017;69:1761–1770.
71. Shaw LJ, Blankstein R, Bax JJ, et al. Society of Cardiovascular Computed Tomography / North American Society of Cardiovascular Imaging – expert consensus document on coronary CT imaging of atherosclerotic plaque. *J Cardiovasc Comput Tomogr*. 2021;15(2):93–109.
72. Adamson PD, Williams MC, Dweck MR, et al. Guiding therapy by coronary CT angiography improves outcomes in patients with stable chest pain. *J Am Coll Cardiol*. 2019;74:2058–2070.
73. Karády J, Mayrhofer T, Ivanov A, et al. Cost-effectiveness analysis of anatomic vs functional index testing in patients with low-risk stable chest pain. *JAMA Network Open*. 2020;3:e2028312–e2028312.
74. Motoyama S, Kondo T, Sarai M, et al. Multislice computed tomographic characteristics of coronary lesions in acute coronary syndromes. *J Am Coll Cardiol*. 2007;50:319–326.
75. Ozaki Y, Okumura M, Ismail TF, et al. Coronary CT angiographic characteristics of culprit lesions in acute coronary syndromes not related to plaque rupture as defined by optical coherence tomography and angioscopy. *Eur Heart J*. 2011;32:2814–2823.
76. Park HB, Heo R, OHartaigh B, et al. Atherosclerotic plaque characteristics by CT angiography identify coronary lesions that cause ischemia: a direct comparison to fractional flow reserve. *JACC Cardiovasc Imaging*. 2015;8:1–10.
77. Williams MC, Kwiecinski J, Doris M, et al. Low-attenuation noncalcified plaque on coronary computed tomography angiography predicts myocardial infarction. *Circulation*. 2020;141:1452–1462.
78. Maurovich-Horvat P, Ferencik M, Voros S, et al. Comprehensive plaque assessment by coronary CT angiography. *Nat Rev Cardiol*. 2014;11:390–402.
79. Williams MC, Moss AJ, Dweck M, et al. Coronary artery plaque characteristics associated with adverse outcomes in the SCOT-heart study. *J Am Coll Cardiol*. 2019;73:291–301.
80. Ferencik M, Mayrhofer T, Bittner DO, et al. Use of high-risk coronary atherosclerotic plaque detection for risk stratification of patients with stable chest pain: a secondary analysis of the PROMISE randomized clinical trial. *JAMA Cardiol*. 2018;3:144–152.
81. Tonino PA, Fearon WF, De Bruyne B, et al. Angiographic versus functional severity of coronary artery stenoses in the FAME study fractional flow reserve versus angiography in multivessel evaluation. *J Am Coll Cardiol*. 2010;55:2816–2821.
82. Blankstein R, Di Carli MF. Integration of coronary anatomy and myocardial perfusion imaging. *Nat Rev Cardiol*. 2010;7:226–236.
83. Bakhshi H, Meyghani Z, Kishi S, et al. Comparative effectiveness of CT-derived atherosclerotic plaque metrics for predicting myocardial ischemia. *JACC Cardiovasc Imaging*. 2019;12:1367–1376.
84. Nakazato R, Shalev A, Doh JH, et al. Aggregate plaque volume by coronary computed tomography angiography is superior and incremental to luminal narrowing for diagnosis of ischemic lesions of intermediate stenosis severity. *J Am Coll Cardiol*. 2013;62:460–467.
85. Stuijfzand WJ, Van Rosendael AR, Lin FY, et al. Stress myocardial perfusion imaging vs coronary computed tomographic angiography for diagnosis of invasive vessel-specific coronary physiology. *JAMA Cardiol*. 2020.
86. Lee S-E, Chang H-J, Sung JM, et al. Effects of statins on coronary atherosclerotic plaques. *JACC Cardiovascular Imag*. 2018;11:1475–1484.
87. Budoff MJ, Bhatt DL, Kinninger A, et al. Effect of icosapent ethyl on progression of coronary atherosclerosis in patients with elevated triglycerides on statin therapy: final results of the EVAPORATE trial. *Eur Heart J*. 2020;41:3925–3932.
88. Oikonomou EK, Marwan M, Desai MY, et al. Non-invasive detection of coronary inflammation using computed tomography and prediction of residual cardiovascular risk (the CRISP CT study): a post-hoc analysis of prospective outcome data. *Lancet*. 2018;392:929–939.
89. Oikonomou EK, Williams MC, Kotanidis CP, et al. A novel machine learning-derived radiotranscriptomic signature of perivascular fat improves cardiac risk prediction using coronary CT angiography. *Euro Heart J*. 2019;40:3529–3543.
90. Nørgaard BL, Leipsic J, Gaur S, et al. Diagnostic performance of noninvasive fractional flow reserve derived from coronary computed tomography angiography in suspected coronary artery disease: the NXT trial (Analysis of Coronary Blood Flow Using CT Angiography: next Steps). *J Am Coll Cardiol*. 2014;63:1145–1155.
91. Driessen RS, Danad I, Stuijfzand WJ, et al. Comparison of coronary computed tomography angiography, fractional flow reserve, and perfusion imaging for ischemia diagnosis. *J Am Coll Cardiol*. 2019;73:161–173.
92. Fairbairn TA, Nieman K, Akasaka T, et al. Real-world clinical utility and impact on clinical decision-making of coronary computed tomography angiography-derived fractional flow reserve: lessons from the ADVANCE Registry. *Eur Heart J*. 2018.
93. Patel MR, Nørgaard BL, Fairbairn TA, et al. Bax JJ and Leipsic J. 1-Year impact on medical practice and clinical outcomes of FFR(CT): the ADVANCE registry. *JACC Cardiovasc Imaging*. 2020;13:97–105.
94. Norgaard BL, Terkelsen CJ, Mathiassen ON, et al. Clinical outcomes using coronary CT angiography and FFRCT-guided management of stable chest pain patients. *J Am Coll Cardiol*. 2018.
95. Nørgaard BL, Fairbairn TA, Safian RD, et al. Coronary CT angiography-derived fractional flow reserve testing in patients with stable coronary artery disease: recommendations on interpretation and reporting. *Radiol Cardiothoracic Imaging*. 2019;1:e190050.
96. Patel AR, Bamberg F, Branch K, et al. Society of cardiovascular computed tomography expert consensus document on myocardial computed tomography perfusion imaging. *J Cardiovasc Comput Tomogr*. 2020;14:87–100.
97. Pontone G, Baggiano A, Andreini D, et al. Stress computed tomography perfusion versus fractional flow reserve CT derived in suspected coronary artery disease: the PERFECTION study. *JACC Cardiovasc Imaging*. 2019;12:1487–1497.
98. Park H-B, Heo R, ó Hartaigh B, et al. Atherosclerotic plaque characteristics by CT angiography identify coronary lesions that cause ischemia: a direct comparison to fractional flow reserve. *JACC Cardiovascular Imag*. 2015;8:1–10.
99. Nous FMA, Budde RPJ, Lubbers MM, et al. Impact of machine-learning CT-derived fractional flow reserve for the diagnosis and management of coronary artery disease in the randomized CRESCENT trials. *Eur Radiol*. 2020;30:3692–3701.
100. Cury RC, Abbara S, Achenbach S, et al. CAD-RADS(TM) coronary artery disease - reporting and data system. An expert consensus document of the Society of Cardiovascular Computed Tomography (SCCT), the American College of Radiology (ACR) and the North American Society for Cardiovascular Imaging (NASCI). Endorsed by the American College of Cardiology. *J Cardiovasc Comput Tomogr*. 2016;10:269–281.
101. Cardoso R, Dudum R, Ferraro RA, et al. Cardiac computed tomography for personalized management of patients with type 2 diabetes mellitus. *Circ Cardiovasc Imag*. 2020;13:e011365.
102. Halon DA, Lavi I, Barnett-Griness O, et al. Plaque morphology as predictor of late plaque events in patients with asymptomatic type 2 diabetes. *JACC Cardiovasc Imaging*. 2019;12:1353–1363.
103. Gupta S, Meyersohn NM, Wood MJ, et al. Role of coronary CT angiography in spontaneous coronary artery dissection. *Radiol Cardiothorac Imaging*. 2020;2:e200364.
104. Cheezum MK, Ghoshhajra B, Bittencourt MS, et al. Anomalous origin of the coronary artery arising from the opposite sinus: prevalence and outcomes in patients undergoing coronary CTA. *Eur Heart J Cardiovasc Imaging*. 2017;18:224–235.
105. Cheezum MK, Liberthson RR, Shah NR, et al. Anomalous aortic origin of a coronary artery from the inappropriate sinus of Valsalva. *J Am Coll Cardiol*. 2017;69:1592–1608.
106. Rizvi A, Deaño RC, Bachman DP, et al. Analysis of ventricular function by CT. *J Cardiovasc Comput Tomogr*. 2015;9:1–12.
107. Oda S, Kidoh M, Takashio S, et al. Quantification of myocardial extracellular volume with planning computed tomography for transcatheter aortic valve replacement to identify occult cardiac amyloidosis in patients with severe aortic stenosis. *Circ Cardiovasc Imaging*. 2020;13:e010358.
108. Pawade T, Clavel M-A, Tribouilloy C, et al. Computed tomography aortic valve calcium scoring in patients with aortic stenosis. *Circ Cardiovasc Imaging*. 2018;11:e007146.
109. Habib G, Lancellotti P, Antunes MJ, et al. 2015 ESC guidelines for the management of infective endocarditis: the task force for the management of infective endocarditis of the European Society of Cardiology (ESC)Endorsed by: European Association for Cardio-Thoracic Surgery (EACTS), the European Association of Nuclear Medicine (EANM). *Eur Heart J*. 2015;36:3075–3128.
110. Blanke P, Weir-McCall JR, Achenbach S, et al. Computed tomography imaging in the context of transcatheter aortic valve implantation (TAVI) / transcatheter aortic valve replacement (TAVR): an expert consensus document of the Society of Cardiovascular Computed Tomography. *J Cardiovasc Comput Tomogr*. 2019;13:1–20.
110a. Ge Y, Gupta S, Fentanes E, et al. Role of cardiac CT in pre-procedure planning for transcatheter mitral valve replacement. *JACC Cardiovasc Imaging*. 2021 Apr 7:S1936-878X(20)31110-4. https://doi.org/10.1016/j.jcmg.2020.12.018. Epub ahead of print.
111. Romero J, Husain SA, Kelesidis I, et al. Detection of left atrial appendage thrombus by cardiac computed tomography in patients with atrial fibrillation. *Circ Cardiovasc Imaging*. 2013;6:185–194.
112. Bilchick KC, Mealor A, Gonzalez J, et al. Effectiveness of integrating delayed computed tomography angiography imaging for left atrial appendage thrombus exclusion into the care of patients undergoing ablation of atrial fibrillation. *Heart Rhythm*. 2016;13:12–19.
113. Kassop D, Donovan MS, Cheezum MK, et al. Cardiac masses on cardiac CT: a review. *Curr Cardiovasc Image Rep*. 2014;7:9281.
114. Hulten EA, Blankstein R. Pseudoaneurysms of the heart. *Circulation*. 2012;125:1920–1925.
115. Choi AD, Thomas DM, Lee J, et al. 2020 SCCT guideline for training Cardiology and radiology trainees as independent practitioners (level II) and advanced practitioners (level III) in cardiovascular computed tomography: a statement from the society of cardiovascular computed tomography. *JACC Cardiovasc Imaging*. 2021;14:272–287.
116. Grundy SM, Stone NJ, Bailey AL, et al. 2018 AHA/ACC/AACVPR/AAPA/ABC/ACPM/ADA/AGS/APhA/ASPC/NLA/PCNA guideline on the management of blood cholesterol. *J Am Coll Cardiol*. 2019;73:e285–e350.
117. Knuuti J, Wijns W, Saraste A, et al. 2019 ESC Guidelines for the diagnosis and management of chronic coronary syndromes. *Eur Heart J*. 2020;41:407–477
118. Gulati M, Levy PD, Mukherjee D, et al. 2021 AHA/ACC/ASE/ CHEST/SAEM/SCCT/SCMR guideline for the evaluation and diagnosis of chest pain: a report of the American College of Cardiology/American Heart Association Joint Committee on Clinical Practice Guidelines. J Am Coll Cardiol. 2021.

21 Coronary Angiography and Intravascular Imaging

GEORGE D. DANGAS AND ROXANA MEHRAN

INDICATIONS FOR CORONARY ANGIOGRAPHY, 363
Appropriate Use Criteria, 364

CORONARY ARTERIOGRAPHY TECHNIQUE, 366
Patient Preparation, 366
Access Sites, 366
Basic Technique, 367
Catheters for Diagnostic Procedures, 367
Ventriculography, 369
Selection of Contrast Media, 371
Automatic and Manual Injection of Contrast Media, 371

ANGIOGRAPHIC PROJECTIONS, 371
CORONARY ANATOMY, 372
CORONARY ARTERY ANOMALIES, 373
PITFALLS OF CORONARY ANGIOGRAPHY, 374
Myocardial Bridging, 374
Coronary Artery Spasm, 374
ANGIOGRAM EVALUATION, 375
SYNTAX SCORE, 375
Quantification of the Stenosis, 376
Evaluation of Microvascular Blood Flow, 376

SPECIAL LESION CONSIDERATIONS, 377
Chronic Total Occlusion, 377
Calcific Lesions, 377
Thrombotic Lesions, 377
Bifurcation Lesions, 378
Coronary Dissections, 378

CORONARY INTRAVASCULAR IMAGING, 378
Intravascular Ultrasound, 378
Optical Coherence Tomography, 380

ACKNOWLEDGMENTS, 383
REFERENCES, 383

Coronary angiography consists of the visualization of the coronary anatomy under fluoroscopy, facilitated by direct injection of contrast media into the epicardial coronary arteries through a catheter advanced from a peripheral artery to the aortic root and into the coronary ostia.

The history of coronary angiography starts in the 19th century with the discovery of x-rays by Roentgen in 1895. One month later, Haschek and Lindenthal injected a mixture of calcium carbonate in the blood vessels of an amputated hand and were able to visualize the vascular bed using a roentgenogram. Meanwhile, Andre Cournand and Dickinson Richards at Columbia University performed the first experiments on cardiac catheterization in animals, which led to the description of heart hemodynamics and the application to humans of crucial techniques and principles, such as the Fick method to measure cardiac output and pressure manometry (see Chapter 22). Forssmann performed the first human cardiac catheterization on himself in 1928, advancing a catheter through an antecubital vein into his right atrium, and acquired roentgenograms to document it.

Selective coronary angiography was first attempted in 1958 by Mason Sones, who cannulated a right coronary artery with a catheter inserted through a brachial artery.[1] In the 1960s, angiographic studies for the determination of coronary artery disease (CAD) were performed in extremely ill patients in the few tertiary care centers in the United States with the necessary resources. Coronary angiography remained a purely diagnostic technique until 1977, when Gruentzig performed the first percutaneous transcatheter coronary angioplasty (see Classic References, Ryan). In the early 1990s the field of coronary angiography entered a period of explosive growth, such that by 2010, an estimated 1,029,000 inpatient diagnostic cardiac catheterization procedures and 954,000 inpatient percutaneous coronary intervention (PCI) procedures (see Chapter 41) were performed per year in the United States alone.[2] Recent years have seen rapid development and maturation of the field, with continuous introduction of new materials, techniques, and innovations for coronary angiography and intracoronary interventions.

Despite the availability of noninvasive imaging techniques such as computed tomographic coronary angiography (CTCA) and magnetic resonance coronary angiography (MRCA) that allow visualization of the coronary anatomy without the risks related to an invasive percutaneous procedure (see Chapters 19 and 20), selective coronary angiography remains the gold standard to determine the extent of CAD because it is the only technique that can simultaneously provide both functional and anatomic information for the estimation of ischemic burden of CAD. Although coronary angiography technique is well established, it is important to keep in mind that it is an invasive procedure with potential complications. Therefore, indications for coronary angiography are clearly defined in the current American Heart Association and American College of Cardiology (AHA/ACC) clinical practice guidelines.[3,4] This chapter reviews the indications for coronary angiography, the basic technique, and interpretation of angiographic images, with an overview of the available intravascular imaging techniques.

INDICATIONS FOR CORONARY ANGIOGRAPHY

Selection of candidates for invasive coronary angiography is based on the pretest probability of CAD, which is estimated on the basis of the clinical evaluation of the patient, the patient's clinical presentation, and the results of noninvasive diagnostic testing such as electrocardiography, echocardiography, blood tests, stress test, and CTCA or MRCA if performed[5,6] (see Chapters 15, 16, and 18 to 20). Current guidelines and indications for coronary angiography by clinical presentation are summarized in Chapters 37 to 40.[37]

In patients with low pretest probability of CAD, first-line noninvasive assessment of cardiovascular risk is necessary to decide whether to proceed to coronary angiography. Traditionally, stress test findings can be defined as low, intermediate, or high risk, which are associated with a cardiac mortality of less than 1%, 1% to 3%, and greater than 3% per year, respectively. For patients with intermediate-risk pretest probability, coronary angiography may be considered, whereas for patients with high-risk pretest probability, angiography should be performed without delay and with no need for further testing. Patients presenting with acute coronary syndrome (ACS), unstable angina (UA), or non–ST-segment elevation myocardial infarction (NSTEMI) with hemodynamic instability or who are at high clinical risk should undergo early invasive evaluation. For hemodynamically stable UA/NSTEMI patients without high clinical risk, a delayed invasive strategy may be justified, although an initially noninvasive risk stratification may be practiced outside the United States. Patients presenting with ST-segment elevation myocardial infarction (STEMI) should generally undergo urgent invasive intervention as soon as possible after symptom onset.[7] Patients with delayed cases may be treated conservatively, as described in other chapters.

Appropriate Use Criteria

In 2012 the appropriate use criteria (AUC) for diagnostic coronary angiography were released.[4] This and a more recent focused update document provide a classification schema for procedures into *appropriate*, *may be appropriate*, and *rarely appropriate* care based on specific criteria. The proportion of "inappropriate" nonacute PCI has been reduced overall.[8] Clinical indications for PCI are beyond the scope of this chapter, but the AUC for diagnostic catheterization are mentioned here to highlight the appropriate selection of patients referred for coronary angiography for diagnostic purposes, since coronary angiography itself may be an unnecessary invasive procedure that could trigger an inappropriate coronary intervention in some cases.[9] The rate of angiographically normal or minimally diseased coronary arteries in patients undergoing elective procedures is approximately 39%.[10] In particular, the use of coronary angiography and PCI in asymptomatic patients is uncertain. A recent study showed that among a sample of 300,000 patients receiving coronary angiography in the United States, 25% were asymptomatic at the time of the elective coronary angiography. Furthermore, the rate of angiographic procedures in asymptomatic patients directly correlated with the number of inappropriate PCI procedures performed.[9] Therefore, strategies to verify the correct referral of patients for diagnostic coronary angiography are required to avoid unnecessary procedures, reduce health care costs, and prevent the therapeutic cascade that may lead from diagnostic angiography to inappropriate PCI.

Contraindications to Coronary Angiography

There are no absolute contraindications to coronary angiography listed in the clinical practice guidelines. However, specific conditions should be taken into account when weighing risks and benefits of the procedure. Based on the patient's cardiovascular risk and the clinical presentation, a decision should be made whether to avoid or postpone the procedure or proceed with coronary angiography using prophylactic measures to reduce the probability of periprocedural complications. Relative contraindications that should be taken into account are known anaphylactoid reaction to contrast media, moderate to severe kidney impairment, decompensated heart failure and pulmonary edema that prevent the patient from lying down during the procedure, uncontrolled hypertension, active infection, coagulopathy, and gastrointestinal bleeding.[11] In addition, coronary angiography requires the use of radiation to visualize the wires and catheters advanced through the blood vessels and to obtain images of the coronary arteries. Therefore, pregnant women should not undergo angiography unless strictly necessary and on exhaustive explanation of the risks related to radiation exposure, medications, and contrast media for both the mother and the fetus.[12] The presence of comorbidities that can increase the risk of complications should be critically considered before referring patients for coronary angiography.[13]

Complications of Coronary Angiography

Complications during coronary angiography are rare, occurring in approximately 2% of patients, with serious complications such as cerebrovascular accident (CVA), or stroke, or myocardial infarction (MI) accounting for less than 1% of all patients. Mortality rate is lower than 0.1%.[13] Complications during PCI are more common (see Chapter 41). Table 21.1 lists complications that may be encountered during coronary angiography.

Although rare, the most common complications are allergic reactions to contrast, vascular complications, and worsening of kidney function (see next section). Vascular complications at the access site include hematoma, pseudoaneurysm, aneurysm, and dissection. The risk of a vascular complication increases with the diameter of the sheath used, age of the patient, and degree of local calcifications. Iatrogenic coronary dissection or perforation occurs infrequently but is potentially life-threatening and could require urgent coronary stenting[14] (Fig. 21.1). Ventricular and atrial arrhythmias are relatively common. Intracoronary injection of contrast media itself can induce arrhythmias. In particular, during injection of contrast media into the right coronary artery (RCA), one should take care to avoid deep cannulation of the RCA and injection of contrast media directly into the conus branch because this can result in ventricular fibrillation (VF).[15] In addition, when performing ventriculography, the mechanical stress of the catheter on the ventricular walls can trigger ventricular arrhythmias ranging from isolated premature ventricular complexes (PVCs) to runs of ventricular tachycardia (VT). Usually, these arrhythmias are self-resolving with catheter relocation and do not require medical intervention. Embolic events are rare but can occur and may involve the coronary arteries, central nervous system, or peripheral arteries.[16] Highly calcific axillary or subclavian arteries can increase the likelihood of embolization.

In addition, advanced age, diabetes mellitus, emergency coronary angiography, prior stroke, renal failure, and congestive heart failure (CHF) have been reported as risk factors for periprocedural stroke.[16] Infections are exceptionally rare in immunocompetent patients, and prophylactic antibiotic therapy is not usually required. Bleeding is usually minor, except when precipitated by vascular complications. In general, the use of anticoagulation during diagnostic angiography should be dosed based on the length of the procedure, weight of the patient, and presence of comorbidities such as kidney impairment to avoid the risk of bleeding when the sheath is removed from the access site. Use of radial access rather than femoral access has significantly reduced the rate of vascular and bleeding complications[17] (see Chapter 41).

Contrast-Induced Acute Kidney Injury. Contrast-induced acute kidney injury (CI-AKI) is defined as an acute deterioration of renal function, defined as an increase in creatinine of 0.5 mg/dL or more or 25% or greater compared with baseline.[18] It generally develops 24 to 72 hours after administration of an intravascular contrast agent in the absence of other identifiable causes (see Classic References, Goldenberg and Matetzky). This complication significantly impacts the duration of hospital stay and related health care costs. CI-AKI also has marked repercussions on short- and long-term morbidity and mortality.[19] In particular, studies in patients with moderate to severe renal dysfunction (estimated glomerular filtration rate [eGFR] <60 mL/min/1.73 m^2) undergoing coronary angiography or angioplasty show that the development of CI-AKI in such patients is a negative prognostic factor of clinical outcome both short and long term.[20] The incidence of CI-AKI ranges from 2% in low-risk patients to 12% to 50% in patients with diabetes and known chronic kidney disease (CKD) (see Chapters 31 and 101). The mechanisms of CI-AKI are only partially understood. Certainly, toxic damage caused by the passage of iodine molecules in the interstitial kidney is one of the causes. Another mechanism is related to the redistribution of flow in the kidney tissue secondary to contrast administration. In particular, after injection of contrast media, blood flow increases in the cortex and decreases in the medulla. Unfortunately, the medulla is particularly vulnerable to ischemic injury for the basal hypoxic condition (P_{O_2} = 20 mm Hg) because of high metabolic activity (e.g., sodium transporter channels). Therefore, blood flow reduction in the medulla after contrast injection further decreases oxygen tension, leading to endothelial dysfunction. Other important elements affecting kidney function are the physical and chemical characteristics of the contrast agents, in particular osmolality and viscosity. Contrast agents with a high osmolality and viscosity significantly increase hypoxemia and tubular stress. The downstream effect consists of an increase of free radicals, a reduction of nitric oxide (NO) bioavailability, and an increase in cellular death.[19,20]

The risk of CI-AKI depends largely on baseline renal function. The eGFR is a valid index to describe the level of renal function. Patients with an eGFR value below 60 mL/min are at high risk of CI-AKI. However, eGFR is not able to identify subclinical or latent forms of renal dysfunction. Therefore, a careful assessment of CI-AKI risk is essential, particularly before interventional procedures that may require high contrast medium volume (Fig. 21.2) (see Classic References, Mehran et al.).

TABLE 21.1 Risks Associated with Coronary Angiography

COMPLICATION	RISK (%)
Mortality	0.11
Myocardial infarction	0.05
Cerebrovascular accident	0.07
Arrhythmias	0.38
Vascular complications	0.43
Contrast agent reaction	0.37
Hemodynamic complications	0.26
Perforation of heart chamber	0.03
Other complications	0.28
Total of major complications	1.70

Modified from Scanlon P, et al. ACC/AHA guidelines for coronary angiography. J Am Coll Cardiol 1999;33:1756.

Risk of CI-AKI can be stratified using a risk score model that includes patients' baseline and procedural characteristics.[21]

In high-risk patients, prevention is crucial and consists of pharmacologic and nonpharmacologic measures. Individual risk-benefit ratios should be carefully estimated for each patient, and the utility of an alternative noninvasive diagnostic test should be evaluated. If the use of contrast medium is necessary for diagnostic purposes, the volume used should be minimized, and the use of monomeric low- or iso-osmolality contrast agents is recommended. Hydration plays a pivotal role in reducing the incidence of CI-AKI. Depending on the clinical condition (e.g., CHF), the Contrast-Induced Nephropathy (CIN) Consensus Working Panel recommendations state that an infusion of 1.0 to 1.5 mL/kg/hr of isotonic saline solution, from 3 to 12 hours before until 6 to 24 hours after the procedure, is suitable to minimize the incidence of CIN.[22] Recently, a clinical trial specifically investigated the efficacy and safety of a left ventricular (LV) end-diastolic pressure–guided hydration protocol with good results; thus filling pressure–guided fast hydration may be employed in the catheterization laboratory.[23] Moreover, to obtain effective hydration, devices have been developed that balance the volume of infusion and fluids lost through diuresis.[24] N-Acetylcysteine has been considered for the prevention of CI-AKI for years. In animal models of ischemia-reperfusion injury, the use of N-acetylcysteine significantly limited kidney damage mainly through its antioxidant properties.[25] However, the efficacy of N-acetylcysteine in humans in clinical studies remains unclear, given the high heterogeneity in study protocols and populations.[26] Similarly, some studies report that the use of isotonic sodium bicarbonate is associated with a higher reduction in the incidence of CI-AKI than saline solution. These findings were attributed to a potential reduction in the production of reactive oxygen species in the renal parenchyma. However, recent meta-analyses did not show superiority of sodium bicarbonate over saline solution.[27,28] For this reason, both N-acetylcysteine and sodium bicarbonate have minimal roles in the latest guidelines on prevention (i.e., no benefit) and the routine prevention of CIN in patients undergoing percutaneous coronary angiography and interventions.

Risks Related to Radiation Exposure

Coronary catheterization may result in radiation-related injury, which although infrequent, may be potentially serious. Radiation injury may be *deterministic* (i.e., dose-dependent), which can present weeks after exposure, or *stochastic*, which is genetically determined and not dose-dependent. Stochastic injury can result in cancer, pregnancy complications, and inheritable diseases. Deterministic injury may result in skin injury, hair loss, and lens injury. However, the

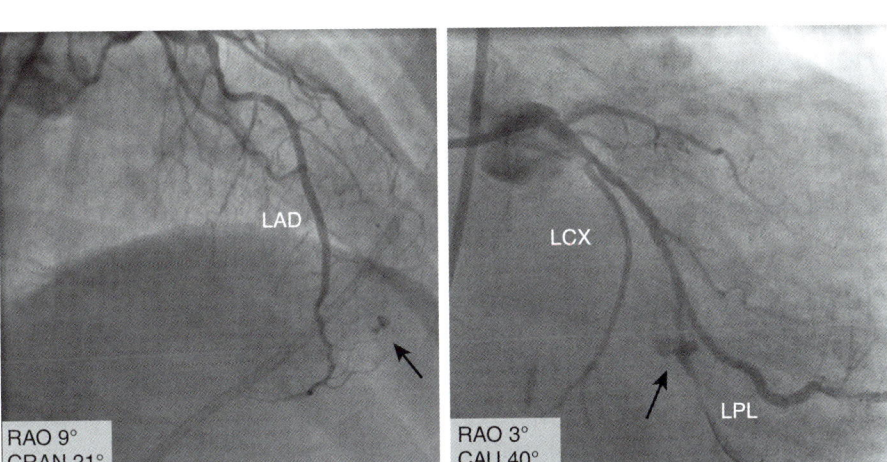

FIGURE 21.1 Iatrogenic coronary perforations. Left, Wire perforation of distal left anterior descending artery (*LAD*). **Right,** Perforation of a left posterolateral branch (*LPL*) after rotational atherectomy. *Black arrows* indicate contrast media extravasation. *CAU*, Caudal; *CRAN*, cranial; *LCX*, left circumflex artery; *RAO*, right anterior oblique. (Angiographic images courtesy Dr. Annapoorna Kini, Icahn School of Medicine at Mount Sinai, New York, NY.)

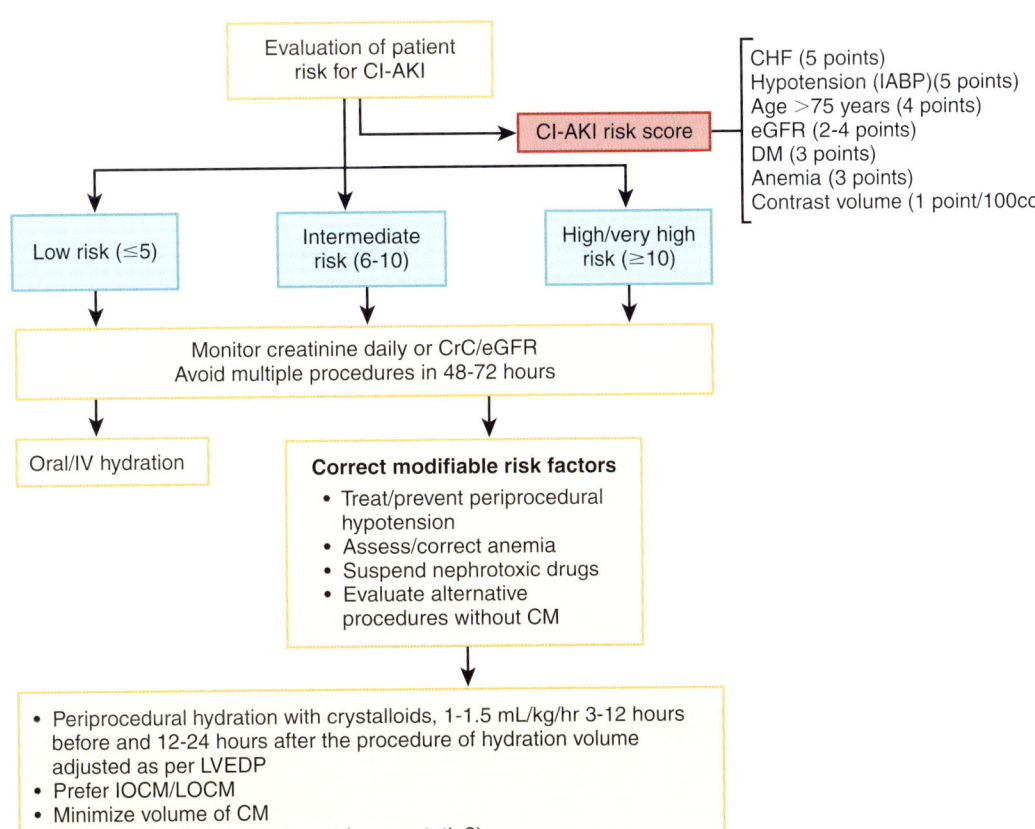

FIGURE 21.2 Risk score to determine the probability of contrast-induced acute kidney injury. *BID*, Twice daily; *CHF*, congestive heart failure; *CI-AKI*, contrast-induced acute kidney injury; *CM*, contrast media; *CrC*, creatinine clearance; *DM*, diabetes mellitus; *eGFR*, estimated glomerular filtration rate; *IOCM*, iso-osmolar contrast media; *IV*, intravenous; *LOCM*, low-osmolar contrast media; *LVEDP*, left ventricular end-diastolic pressure. See also Chapter 101 and Figure 101.7 for a management strategy for CI-AKI.

most common location of radiation-induced lesions in cardiac catheterization is the skin of the back, and common patterns include erythema, telangiectasia, and plaques.[29] The sensitivity of the skin to radiation exposure is differentiated by site; areas at risk in decreasing order of sensitivity include anterior neck, antecubital and popliteal areas, flexor extremities, chest and abdomen, face, back, extensors, nape of the neck, scalp, palms, and soles.[30] Although uncommon in contemporary practice, early reports from coronary catheterization indicate deep and extensive skin rashes and burns at the site of radiation exposure, some requiring skin grafting.

PCI procedures may result in 10-fold higher radiation exposure compared with diagnostic catheterization (see Chapter 41). An average PCI results in 150 times more exposure than a chest radiograph and five times the annual radiation exposure received as environmental background radiation.[31] Measures used to assess patient dose include dose-area product (DAP; the absorbed dose multiplied by the area irradiated), air kerma (AK; *kinetic energy released per unit mass* of air), and fluoroscopy time (FT), which are routinely measured and documented.[32] All procedures should be performed using the ALARA (as low as reasonably achievable) principle.[33] Exposure can be minimized in several ways: reduced FT and acquisition time, use of multiple angles rather than a single working camera position, reduced fluoroscopy dose, avoidance of high magnification, use of collimator beams and filters, avoidance of high angulation, and reduction in the flat-panel image detector as much as possible. For exposures of absorbed radiation greater than 5 Gy, patients should be advised to watch for areas of erythema; for those greater than 10 Gy, a medical physicist should be consulted to calculate the peak dose in 2 to 4 weeks; greater than 15 Gy is regarded as a hospital risk management event. Similarly, in the event that FT exceeds 60 minutes, physicians must be vigilant for late radiation effects.

From the perspective of occupational radiation exposure, operators should be cognizant of the need to wear protective personal equipment during catheterization procedures, including a lead apron, thyroid drape, lead eyeglasses, and dosimeters.[33] Table height and distance from the x-ray source are important, and radiation risk decreases as the inverse square of distance from the source. Operators should also optimally position lead shields and skirts and should be compliant with use of radiation dosimeters for monitoring exposure to the whole body (chest) and eye. Novel dosimeters providing real-time monitoring and alerts can serve to decrease operator radiation exposure.[34] Monitoring, reporting, and audit of radiation exposure can promote improved awareness and practice in the operator and catheterization laboratory staff. Systematic tracking of FT and radiation exposure is expanding through inclusion in the procedure report as well as in quality assurance databases (national/statewide).

CORONARY ARTERIOGRAPHY TECHNIQUE
Patient Preparation

Patients should receive a comprehensive explanation of the diagnostic angiographic procedure and of the coronary intervention potentially required. Risks of angiography should be discussed in-depth and weighed against both the clinical benefit and the risks related to refusal of the procedure. Patients are required to provide written informed consent before coronary angiography. Women of childbearing age should be questioned on their pregnancy status and advised on the additional risks of radiation exposure for pregnant women. A thorough medical history, including comorbidities, current medications, and allergies, needs to be obtained before the procedure. In the event of an emergency procedure, as with a STEMI presentation, a brief evaluation of the patient history with particular attention to known CKD and known allergies to contrast media should be obtained if possible. In patients with prior coronary artery bypass graft (CABG) procedure, a report stating the type, arterial or venous graft(s), and position of the graft(s) should be attained if available to facilitate the cannulation and subsequent imaging of the grafts. Patients may receive mild sedation with a benzodiazepine before the procedure according to the hospital standard practice.[35] In case of hemodynamic instability or respiratory distress, anesthesiologist support might be necessary. In most patients, however, general anesthesia and deep sedation are unnecessary for coronary angiography. Conscious sedation with short-term agents such as midazolam or fentanyl is most common. Constant monitoring of the patient's ECG, heart rate, blood pressure, respiratory rate, and oxygen saturation is required periprocedurally. A venous access line should be readily available for the infusion of fluids or medications. Local anesthesia with topical anesthetic cream or subcutaneous injection of 1% lidocaine or mepivacaine (0.5 to 1 mL for radial access and 2 to 5 mL for femoral access) should be performed in all patients before puncturing the peripheral artery and introducing the sheath.[36] An adequate local anesthetic will not only make the patient more comfortable but, by reducing the pain during the arterial cannulation, also reduce the risk of peripheral artery spasm.

Access Sites (see Chapter 41)

Possible access sites for coronary angiography are the femoral artery and the radial artery. Although the radial access approach is associated with fewer vascular and bleeding complications, femoral access is still commonly used in the United States. Femoral access allows for larger-diameter equipment that could be necessary in case of PCI. In addition, accessing from the femoral artery usually grants an easier advancement of the catheter to the aortic root due to the lack of tortuosity in the descending aorta. After disinfection and appropriate local anesthesia at the access site, the common femoral artery (CFA) is punctured with a base-metal needle approximately 1 cm below the inguinal line with a 45- to 60-degree angulation.[35] In obese patients, the ideal puncture site is sometimes difficult to determine. The head of the femur, visualized under fluoroscopy, can be used as a landmark. Ultrasound can localize the common femoral artery and its bifurcation. Puncture should be performed with the needle leveled at half the head of the femur. Multiple punctures should be avoided to reduce the risk of bleeding and vascular damage. A J-tip flexible guide is inserted through the needle into the CFA. The needle is then removed and a sheath advanced around the wire into the artery. Once the sheath is fully advanced in the artery, the dilator and wire are removed, and the sheath is flushed with saline.[37] Usually, a 6 French (6F) sheath (French units: F = 0.33 mm) is used for coronary angiography and coronary interventions. Verification of the correct position of the sheath in the vessel can be ascertained simply by drawing blood from the sheath.

Radial access should always be considered first, before resorting to the femoral approach, especially for diagnostic coronary angiography.[38] The procedure for the sheath insertion is similar to that described for the femoral artery. The modified Allen test is performed by applying pressure on both the ulnar and the radial artery of one wrist to occlude them while the patient keeps the hand elevated with the fist clenched for approximately 30 seconds. Once opened, the hand appears pale. The compression on the ulnar artery is then removed while pressure is maintained on the radial artery. If the ulnar artery supply to the hand is adequate, the color quickly returns to the hand and the test is normal. Conversely, if color does not return, the ulnar artery supply is insufficient, meaning that the radial artery supports the entire circulation of the hand. In this case the radial artery should not be punctured, because this may compromise the blood flow to the hand. This rule may be bypassed if an oximeter is placed in the thumb during radial artery occlusion, and resurgence of pulsation and oxygenation is documented after its initial disappearance ("Barbeau method").

When both radial arteries are acceptable access sites, the patient's right, closer to the operator, is preferred for technical reasons. However, the left subclavian artery may be less tortuous than the innominate artery. The ideal puncture site is 1 to 2 cm proximal to the radial styloid with the wrist slightly hyperextended. After local anesthesia, usually 0.5 to 1 mL of 1% lidocaine, the needle is advanced angled 30 to 45 degrees to the skin until a flashback of blood is visualized. A straight-tip wire is gently inserted through the needle. After removing the needle, a 5F or 6F sheath is inserted in the radial artery over the wire. A small incision 1 mm long can be made on the skin to facilitate advancement of the sheath. Because the radial artery is extremely vasoactive, the risk of spasm is high, especially in women; therefore, as soon as access is obtained, an intra-arterial spasmolytic agent such as nitroglycerin (100 to 200 μg) or verapamil (2.5 mg) diluted into 10 mL of saline should be administered.[35] A hydrophilic-coated sheath can further reduce the likelihood of spasm and regional pain. To prevent thromboembolic events and radial artery occlusion, weight-adjusted unfractionated heparin (UFH), 40 to 70 U/kg up to 5000 U, is administered either intravenously or intra-arterially.[39]

Radial access appears associated with fewer periprocedural events and should be preferred whenever possible. It should be noted, however, that the axillary-subclavian axis can be tortuous and calcific, particularly in elderly patients, and it can therefore be technically difficult to advance the catheter to the aortic root. Brachial access is very uncommon, but unlike radial access, it avoids the small-caliber arteries in the forearm and therefore may be required in the event that radial access is not available or fails. Brachial access can be obtained with a percutaneous or cutdown approach. On the other hand, there is no alternative blood supply to the forearm in case of closure.

Basic Technique

Coronary angiography is an invasive procedure based on the intravascular advancement of angiographic guidewires and catheters from a percutaneous access using the Seldinger technique. After a valved sheath is inserted into the access site artery (see Access Sites), a flexible metallic J-tipped guidewire is inserted through the sheath and advanced slowly under fluoroscopic imaging through the arterial axis until the aortic root is reached. A fluid-filled catheter is then advanced over the angiographic guidewire, while the wire itself is maintained in place. Once the catheter is in the aortic root, the wire is fully extracted from the sheath, and the catheter is flushed and connected to the contrast media injection apparatus. Under fluoroscopic imaging, and with the help of small injections of contrast, the coronary ostium is engaged with the tip of the catheter.[40] At this point, the x-ray tube is positioned appropriately (see Projection), and angiographic images are obtained while injecting contrast directly into the cannulated coronary artery.

Catheters for Diagnostic Procedures

There are several types of diagnostic catheters, characterized by differing lengths, diameters, and shapes. In general, catheters are composed of an external layer, which is not thrombogenic or lubricious, and by a lubricious inner layer. These two layers include a fine metallic core required to confer stability, improve maneuverability, and reduce the risks of kinking. Lengthwise, the catheter is divided into three parts: hub, body, and tip. Through a female Luer-Lok, the *hub* connects the catheter to the contrast injection system and facilitates the catheter grip and rotation with winged tips. The *body*, mostly strong and rigid, transmits to the tip the movements impressed on the hub by the operator. The *tip* can be divided, starting from the distal end, into three curves: primary, secondary, and tertiary, which allows the best possible fit to the aortic root curvature. The size of the catheter is another important characteristic. Compared with guiding catheters used for PCI (see Chapter 41), diagnostic catheters have a thicker wall, which considerably reduces their internal lumen. The 5F catheter allows an optimal balancing between contrast flow and satisfactory catheter manipulation, particularly for the radial approach. Catheter length can vary from 80 to 110 cm (32 to 44 inches), depending on the anatomic characteristics and the access site (radial, brachial, or femoral). However, the standard length for adult left-heart catheterization by both the radial and the femoral approach is 100 cm (40 inches), while 80 cm is suitable for brachial access.

Among the diagnostic catheters, the most commonly used are the Judkins and the Amplatz catheters. *Judkins catheters* can be used both for the femoral and for the right/left radial approach. A preformed left Judkins (JL) presents a primary curve of 90 degrees and a secondary curve of 180 degrees, whereas the right Judkins (JR) presents a primary curve of 90 degrees and secondary curve of 30 degrees (Fig. 21.3). Since the JL is preformed, after removing the angiographic guide, it automatically engages the ostium of the left coronary artery (LCA). The JR, in contrast, once positioned in the right coronary sinus, requires a clockwise rotation to engage the ostium of the RCA from any vascular approach. In both JL and JR catheters, the distance between the primary and secondary curves (termed *arm*) is variable; for example, JL4 has a 4.2-cm length arm, and JL5 and JL6 have 5.2- and 6.2-cm-long

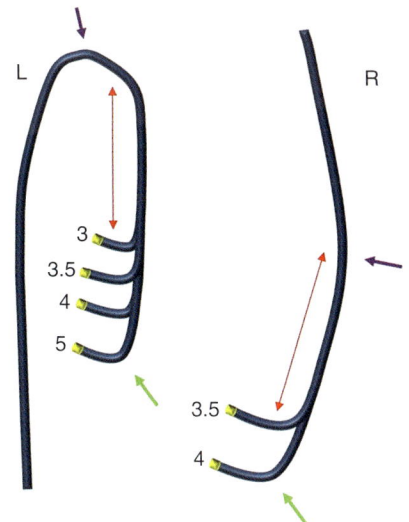

FIGURE 21.3 Judkins catheters. *Left* (L), for left coronary artery. *Right* (R), for right coronary artery. *Green arrows* indicate the primary curve. *Purple arrows* show the secondary curve. *Red arrows* indicate the distance between the primary and the secondary curve. To determine the correct catheter's tip, the operator should evaluate the approach (femoral or radial), the patient's height, and diameter of the aortic root. In particular, it would be helpful to add 0.5 cm for a femoral approach and for a dilated or horizontal aorta.

arms, respectively (see Fig. 21.3). Catheter selection depends on the approach (radial or femoral), the height of the patient, and the aortic diameter and curvature. For example, when using a femoral access, the JL4 is the most adaptable catheter for the LCA, whereas for the radial access, the JL3.5 catheter may be more suitable. Moreover, the presence of a dilated aortic root or the anatomy of particularly tall patients (>180 cm [72 inches]) may increase the length required between the primary and secondary curves and might require the selection of a catheter with a longer arm. In addition to their conventional use, JR catheters may be used for saphenous vein graft (SVG) and left internal mammary artery graft study through femoral and left radial approach.

Amplatz catheters for the LCA (AL) and RCA (AR) represent a valid alternative to Judkins catheters (Fig. 21.4). The available lengths and sizes are the same as for the Judkins catheters, but the tip morphology of the left Amplatz (AL) catheter differs, allowing for easier coronary engagement in specific settings, such as short left main ostium, separate ostium of circumflex (Cx)–left anterior descending (LAD) artery branches, and RCA with anterior-high origin. Conversely, the right Amplatz (AR) catheter allows engagement of RCAs with inferior orientation. Amplatz catheters may also be used with confidence for the study of SVGs. *Multipurpose* (MP) *catheters* present a single bend (MPA 1 and 2 have a 45- to 60-degree primary curve, while MPB 1 and 2 have approximately an 80-degree primary curve) and may be used for the cannulation of coronary ostia that are difficult to reach with other catheters, as well as for engagement of SVGs. *Internal mammary artery* (IMA) *catheters* have a high angulated primary curve tip (80 degrees) to facilitate the engagement of the IMA through either the femoral or the radial approach. These catheters can also be used to engage the upward-pointing RCA (see Fig. 21.4). It should be specified that the catheters just described are the ones most frequently used to perform diagnostic coronary angiography. Additional catheter types are available, although less frequently used, in case of specific coronary anatomic variables.

Selective Coronary Artery Cannulation

Left Coronary Artery. The JL4.0 coronary catheter is used most often to engage the LCA (Fig. 21.5). The catheter is advanced over the guidewire until it reaches the aortic root. There, the catheter is rotated clockwise to direct it toward the left sinus of Valsalva. Once in position, the wire is removed, and the catheter regains its primary bent and should engage the ostium of the LCA. When the ascending aorta is dilated or the aortic arch is unfolded, advancement of the JL4.0 or JL5.0 might be necessary. If the tip of the JL catheter advances beyond the ostium of the LCA without engaging the ostium, the catheter can be advanced

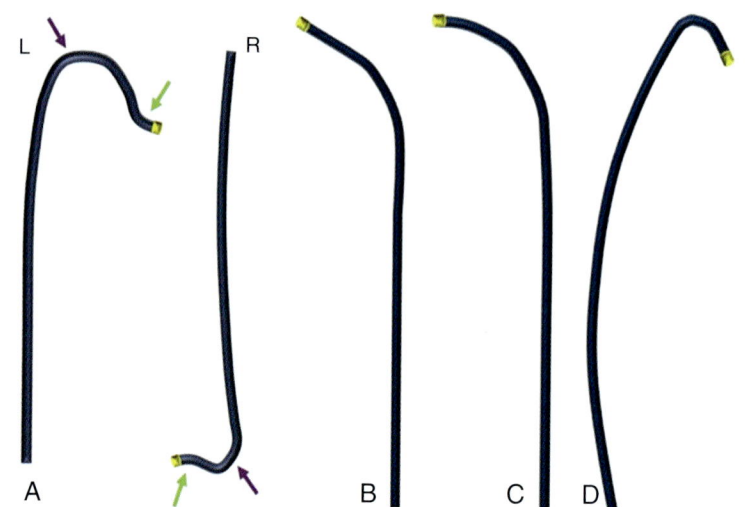

FIGURE 21.4 A, Amplatz catheters, left (L), for left coronary artery; right (R), for right coronary artery. *Green arrows* indicate the primary curve. *Purple arrows* show the secondary curve. **B,** Multipurpose A catheter. **C,** Multipurpose B catheter. **D,** Internal mammary artery catheter.

clockwise to engage the vessel. The height of the catheter during the rotation may need to be adjusted by gently withdrawing the catheter to engage the ostium.

In patients with prior CABG, cannulation might be challenging because the locations of graft ostia are more variable, even when surgical clips or ostia markers are used. Whenever possible, the number, type, and course of the bypass grafts should be obtained before the procedure.

Saphenous Vein Grafts

SVGs from the aorta to the distal RCA or posterior descending artery (PDA) originate from the right anterolateral aspect of the aorta approximately 5 cm (2 inches) superior to the sinotubular ridge. SVGs to the LAD artery (or diagonal branches) originate from the anterior portion of the aorta approximately 7 cm superior to the sinotubular ridge (Fig. 21.6). SVGs to the obtuse marginal branches arise from the left anterolateral aspect of the aorta 9 to 10 cm superior to the sinotubular ridge. In most patients, all SVGs can be engaged with a single catheter, such as a JR4.0 or a modified Amplatz right 1 or 2.

Viewed in the LAO projection, the catheter should be rotated anteriorly from the leftward position as it is rotated in a clockwise direction. This movement should be repeated with the catheter at various heights in the ascending aorta, 5 to 10 cm above the sinotubular ridge, and with various degrees of rotation. Small test injections of contrast media can be used to verify that the catheter is in the SVG. If the graft is occluded, usually it is possible to visualize a "stump" during contrast injection. The surgical clips can be used to verify that all the grafts have been visualized. If one or more SVGs cannot be visualized, it can be useful to perform an ascending aortogram (preferably in biplane) to visualize all SVGs and their course to the coronary arteries. When visualizing an SVG, it is important to evaluate the ostium and the anastomotic site for irregularities or stenosis. It is also important to evaluate the flow distal to the anastomosis. *Sequential grafts* are those that supply two different epicardial branches in a side-to-side fashion (for the more proximal epicardial artery) and terminate in an end-to-side anastomosis (for the more distal epicardial artery). A Y graft is characterized by a proximal anastomosis in an end-to-side fashion to another saphenous vein or arterial graft, with two distal end-to-side anastomoses to the two epicardial grafts from these two grafts. It should be noted that with severe calcifications of the ascending aorta, the SVG could depart from the descending aorta to reach lateral wall branches.

Internal Mammary Artery Grafts. The left IMA (LIMA) can be cannulated with a specially designed J-tip IMA catheter. The catheter is advanced into the aortic arch distal to the origin of the left subclavian artery, then rotated counterclockwise and gently withdrawn with the tip pointing in a cranial direction, allowing entry into the left subclavian artery. The right anterior oblique (RAO) or anteroposterior (AP) projections can be used to visualize the IMA (Fig. 21.7). For the right IMA (RIMA), first the innominate artery is entered with the guidewire in the LAO projection, then the IMA catheter is advanced to a point distal to the expected origin of the RIMA. The catheter is withdrawn slowly in the LAO view and rotated to cannulate the RIMA. Small injections of contrast are used to assess the position and the cannulation of the IMA. If the IMA cannot be selectively engaged and arteriography of the subclavian artery can be used, this usually allows for the opacification of all or most of the IMA, although weak. The IMA can also be visualized with semiselective contrast injection; to avoid injury of the ostium, the catheter can simply be oriented toward the IMA without cannulating it. The correct orientation can be obtained by advancing a guidewire in the IMA to stabilize the position of the catheter during injection.

Radial Grafts

Radial artery (RA) grafts represent the most popular arterial grafts after the LIMA and RIMA. Similar to SVGs, radial grafts require a double anastomosis, one on the aorta and one on the coronary vessel. Because of potential early spasm, RA grafts were abandoned in the 1970s and 1980s. In the 1990s, however, this procedure was rediscovered, and with specific surgical techniques and pharmacologic prophylaxis, it has safely been used with good short- and long-term results.

Gastroepiploic Artery. Rarely the right gastroepiploic artery (GEA) can be used for CABGs. To cannulate the GEA, first a special catheter called the "cobra" is inserted into the common hepatic artery. Next, a hydrophilic-coated guidewire is advanced to the gastroduodenal artery and then to the right GEA. The cobra catheter is then exchanged for an MP or JR catheter, which is used for the selective cannulation of the GEA (Fig. 21.8).

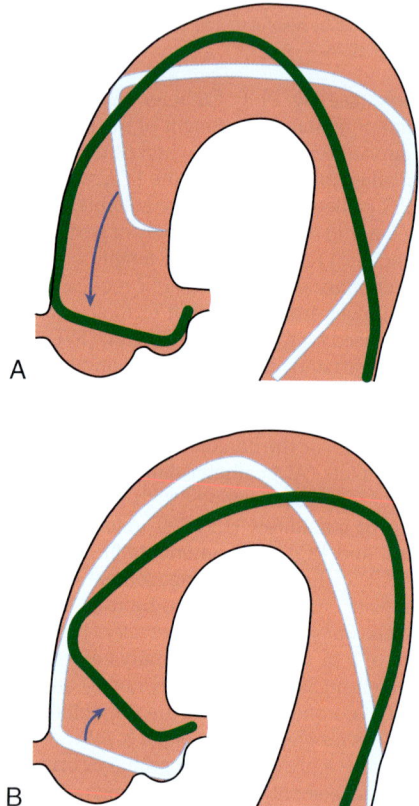

FIGURE 21.5 A, Push-pull technique for catheterization of the left coronary artery (LCA) with the Judkins left catheter. In the LAO view, the coronary catheter is positioned in the ascending aorta over a guidewire, and the guidewire is removed. The catheter is advanced so that the tip enters the left sinus of Valsalva. **B,** If the catheter does not selectively engage the ostium of the LCA, further slow advancement into the left sinus of Valsalva creates a temporary acute angle at the catheter. Prompt withdrawal of the catheter allows easy entry into the artery. (From Popma JJ, et al. Coronary angiography and intracoronary imaging. In Mann D, et al, editors: Braunwald's Heart Disease: A Textbook of Cardiovascular Medicine. 10th ed. Philadelphia: Elsevier; 2014.)

farther until the tip enters the left sinus and the catheter body assumes an acute angle. At that point, prompt withdrawal of the catheter should allow the tip to "pop" into the ostium of the LCA.

Right Coronary Artery. The RCA is cannulated in the left anterior oblique (LAO) position (see later, Angiographic Projections). Once the JR or modified Amplatz catheter reaches the aortic root, it must be rotated

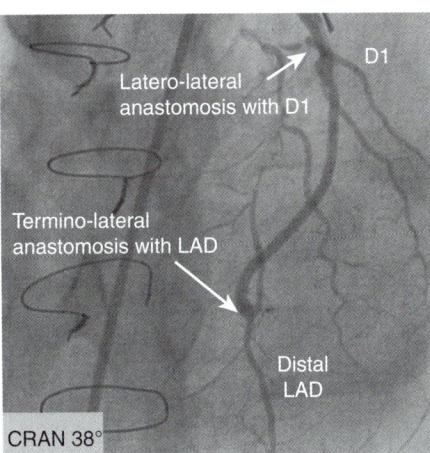

FIGURE 21.6 Sequential saphenous vein graft to the first diagonal branch (*D1*) and left anterior descending artery (*LAD*) with latero-lateral anastomosis to D1 and termino-lateral anastomosis to the distal LAD. *CRAN,* Cranial. (Courtesy Dr. Annapoorna Kini, Icahn School of Medicine at Mount Sinai, New York.)

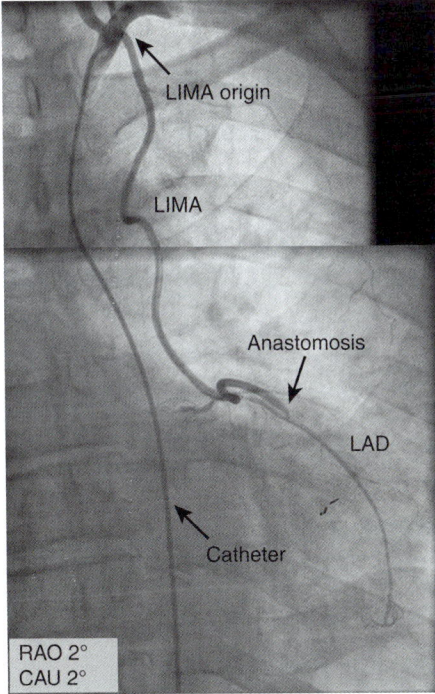

FIGURE 21.7 Arterial graft of left internal mammary artery (*LIMA*) to the left anterior descending artery (*LAD*). RAO, Right anterior oblique; CAU, caudal. (Courtesy Dr. Annapoorna Kini, Icahn School of Medicine at Mount Sinai, New York, NY.)

Ventriculography
Left Ventriculography

Left ventriculography provides important information about volumes, global and segmental function, and anatomic abnormalities such as ventricular septal defect, ventricular thrombus, and valvular dysfunction. However, it is not routinely performed in the current era given the continuous evolution of noninvasive technologies such as echocardiography, CT, or MRI and concerns for complications and contrast volume. Incomplete ventricular opacification with hand-injection of up to 10 cc of contrast through a JR catheter has been become popular as a method to verify an already known normal LV function based on earlier noninvasive studies.

Since the physiologic high pressure developed during each cycle in the left ventricle, the operator should inject a rather high volume of contrast agent in a rather short time for an effective opacification. Accordingly, 6F to 8F catheters with multiple lateral holes are the best option since the single end-hole catheter could be unstable during the

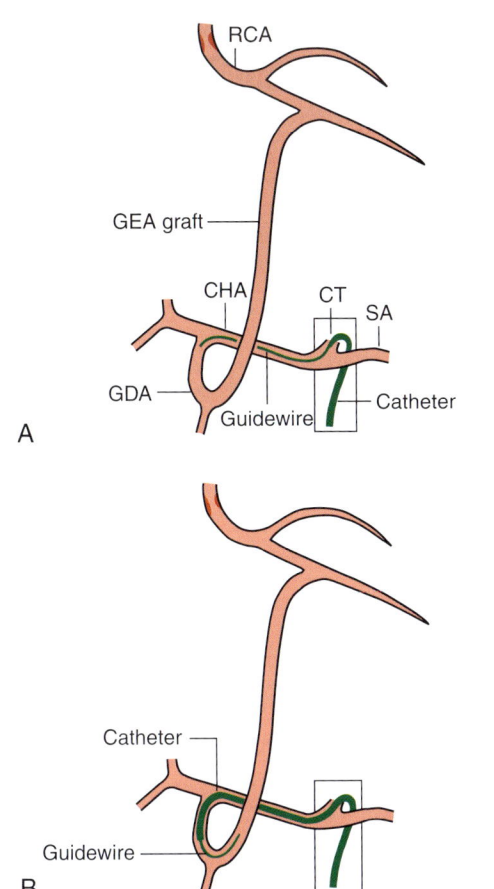

FIGURE 21.8 Catheterization of right gastroepiploic artery (*GEA*) graft. **A,** The celiac trunk (*CT*) is selectively engaged with a cobra catheter, and a guidewire is gently advanced to the gastroduodenal artery (*GDA*) and the GEA. **B,** The catheter is advanced over the guidewire for selective arteriography of the GEA graft. *CHA,* Common hepatic artery; *SA,* splenic artery. (From Popma JJ, et al. Coronary angiography and intracoronary imaging. In Mann D et al, editors. Braunwald's Heart Disease: A Textbook of Cardiovascular Medicine. 10th ed. Philadelphia: Elsevier; 2014.)

high-pressure injection, thus increasing the risk of arrhythmias or inadequate ventricle opacification. The pigtail catheter, including multiple side holes and a "pigtail-like" end-configuration, is frequently used for several reasons. First, usually, the pigtail catheter easily crosses the aortic valve, either directly or by prolapsing across the valve leaflets. Second, the loop shape keeps the end-hole of the catheter away from the cardiac wall, thus decreasing the risk of endocardium trauma, intramyocardial ventricular staining, and arrhythmias. Third, the simultaneous delivery of the contrast agent along the numerous side holes allows a correct opacification of the left ventricle and a further stabilization of the catheter. The pigtail catheter is available with a preformed straight shaft or with a 145- to 155-degree angled shaft, allowing a central position also for that ventricle having an accentuate angle between the aortic root and long axis of the chamber. Crossing the aortic valve requires careful movements, despite the safety profile of the pigtail catheter, and watchful rhythm observation since VT occurrence may require immediate wire/catheter manipulations and even retraction. A common approach is advancing the pigtail close to the aortic valve with a 0.035-inch J-tip guidewire up to the end of the straight catheter section and rotate the catheter to achieve a "6" shape on a RAO projection. Then the catheter should be pushed against the aortic plane to obtain a U-shape curve, and following a deep inspiration or under pullback and clockwise rotation, the tip of the catheter usually falls into the left ventricle. An alternative to the pigtail could be the Halo-type catheters, constituted by a perpendicular helix, inwardly and upwardly directed, and a single end-hole, thus decreasing the risk of ectopic beats and allowing a superior pressure measurement when necessary (e.g., hypertrophic cardiomyopathy). Other catheters can be used to better suit the anatomic variability and facilitate the crossing through the aortic valve. The Judkins catheter for the RCA may be more appropriate for the small aortic roots, whereas

TABLE 21.2 Settings, Suggested Projection and Structure Observed in Patients Undergoing Left or Right Ventriculography

	SETTINGS	SUGGESTED PROJECTION	STRUCTURES OBSERVED
Left Ventricle	Flow rate 10-15 mL/sec Total contrast volume 30-45 mL Pressure limit 750-1200 psi 0- to 0.5-second rise	30-degree right anterior oblique and 0-degree cranial angulation	• Global ventricular function • Segmental wall motion (anterobasal, anterolateral, apical, diaphragmatic, and inferobasal) • Mitral valve
		60-degree left anterior oblique and 25-degree cranial angulation	• Segmental wall motion (lateral, posterolateral, apical septal, and basal septal) • Interventricular septum integrity • Aortic valve
Right Ventricle	Flow rate 8-10 mL/sec Total contrast volume 20-30 mL Pressure limit 750 psi	30-degree right anterior oblique and 0-degree cranial angulation	• Global ventricular function • Segmental wall motion (right ventricle dysplasia)
		Anteroposterior view	• Congenital heart disease evaluation

PSI, Pounds per square inch.

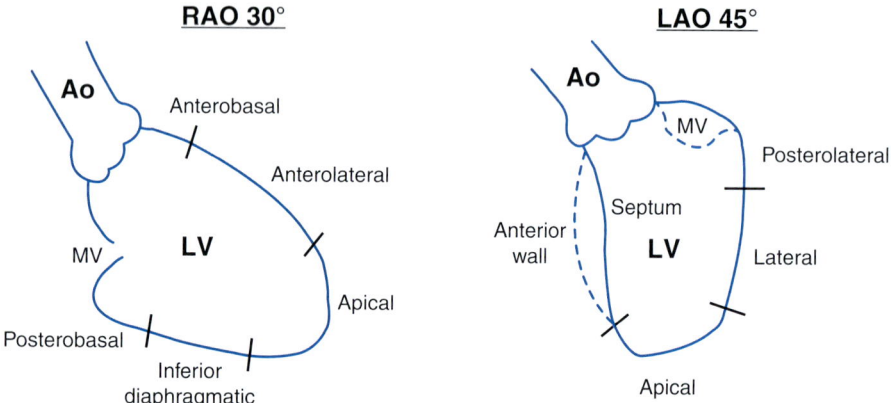

FIGURE 21.9 Projections for left ventriculography. *Ao*, Aorta; *LAO*, left anterior oblique; *LV*, left ventricle; *MV*, mitral valve; *RAO*, right anterior oblique.

the AL or multipurpose catheters might be used to cross bicuspid valves or stenotic aortas. In severe aortic valve stenosis, straight rather than J-tipped guidewires are used, including the straight Glidewire, which may afford faster crossing but also requires greater care to avoid microperforations.[41] Of note, regardless of the type of catheter used to cross the valve, it may need to be exchanged over a 0.035-inch J-tip guidewire with a Pigtail catheter for the following indications: (1) the complete ventriculography via power-injector, (2) detailed hemodynamic assessment of stenosis (dual-lumen pigtail) particularly with excessive femoral pressure amplification of any significant aortoiliac arterial stenosis, (3) if an end-hole catheter is specifically required (e.g., Halo or multipurpose) for slow pull-back hemodynamic measurements, and (4) for advancement of the stiff pigtail-end guidewires to the ventricular apex, as necessary for aortic valve interventions. For optimal ventriculography technique, the catheter should be in midcavity and the RAO projection selected. Table 21.2 and Fig. 21.9 summarize settings and other structures that can be evaluated. Both qualitative and quantitative assessment requires at least two free extra-beats periods since the evaluation of ectopic or post ectopic beats will over- or underestimate the ventricular function and regurgitation entities as well.

Complications related to left ventriculography are as follows: (1) cardiac arrhythmias (both supraventricular and ventricular) often requiring dynamic repositioning, (2) microembolization, (3) intramyocardial contrast staining, (4) contrast associated issues, including nephropathy or high volume load in end-stage heart failure or dialysis patients.

The wall motion pattern is graded from normokinesis, hypokinesis, akinesis, and dyskinesis. Anterobasal, anterolateral, apical, diaphragmatic, and inferobasal segments can be evaluated in RAO projection; lateral, posterolateral, apical septal, and basal septal are viewed in LAO projection. Ejection fraction can be determined qualitatively with a visual estimation or quantitatively assessing end-diastolic and end-systolic contours (centerline method).

The degree of mitral regurgitation can be scored by Sellers classification (see Classic References, Sellers et al.).

Trivial (+1): A minimal jet with a brief and incomplete atrial opacification during systole, rapidly clearing during each cycle without atrial enlargement.

Mild (+2): A moderate opacification of the left atrium with each cycle, clearing with the subsequent beats. The atrium is less opacified than the left ventricle, usually with preserved dimensions.

Moderate (+3): A complete opacification of the left atrium, equal intensity to ventricular opacification. There is delayed atrial clearing over several cycles and a significant enlargement of the left atrium.

Severe (+4): A complete and immediate opacification of the left atrium, even denser than the ventricle. The left atrium is typically severely enlarged and opacification of pulmonary veins may be visible.

Aortography

Dos Santos first described aortography in 1929 by a direct abdominal aorta puncture. Ascending aortography, as practiced by Sones, is indicated to assess the following: (1) aortic valve regurgitation, (2) dimensions, (3) aortic coarctation, (4) sub- or supravalve aortic stenosis, (5) shunts, and (6) identification of bypass grafts.

The standard approach of LAO 30-degree projection allows the best view of ascending aorta, aortic arch, the innominate artery, and the left subclavian and carotid arteries; RAO is preferred for aortic valve evaluation and related interventions. The typical set up for aortic injection is flow rate 15 to 20 mL/sec, volume of the contrast agent 30 to 45 mL, rate of rising 0 to 0.5 s, and pressure limit 750 to 1000 psi.

The less traumatic side-hole pigtail catheter should be preferred for complete opacification. After tight connection of the catheter to the power injector with high-pressure tubing, the operator should ensure any air bubbles are removed from the injector system. The loop of the pigtail catheter must *not* be in Valsalva sinus and the operator should avoid iatrogenic regurgitation minimizing catheter-valve contact.

Aortic regurgitation may be trivial, mild, moderate, or severe depending on ventricular opacification after the third cycle following contrast injection.

Trivial or grade 1 (1+): minimal regurgitation jet with a brief and incomplete left ventricle opacification during diastole and fast clearance of the contrast agent.

Mild or grade 2 (+2): regurgitation jet causing a moderate ventricular opacification, which less dense than in the ascending aorta and is cleared within one to two cardiac cycles.

Moderate or grade 3 (+3): regurgitation jet causing complete ventricular opacification within two cycles, as dense as in the ascending aorta and with delayed clearing from the ventricle over several cycles, often associated with dilated left ventricle.

Severe or grade 4 (+4): complete and immediate opacification of the left ventricle, denser than observed in the ascending aorta.

Right Ventriculography

The optimal position is the midcavity that allows only few ventricular premature beats. Right ventriculography is indicated to assess right-to-left ventricular shunts, right ventricle dimensions or dysplasia, abnormalities of the RV outflow tract (RVOT), and pulmonary stenosis or global and segmental ventricular function. However, it is not valuable for assessing tricuspid regurgitation due to the presence of the catheter across that valve. A multiple-hole pigtail might be used. The 7F Berman balloon-directed multiple-sidehole catheter is frequently used. The septum and RVOT can be evaluated using an AP cranial or AP lateral projections. Typically, 20 to 30 mL of contrast material is injected at 8 to 10 mL/sec (but if the ventricle is severely dilated, the volume could be increased up to 40 to 50 mL at 12 to 18 mL/sec).

Selection of Contrast Media

Since the introduction of intravascular contrast agents (ICAs) in the 1950s, clinical practice has become increasingly dependent on their use, particularly as the use of computed tomography (CT) and cardiac catheterization procedures has expanded markedly in recent years. All currently used ICAs are classified on the basis of their physical and chemical structure, specifically osmolality, iodine content, ionization in solution, and viscosity. The most useful classification in clinical practice divides available ICAs into high-osmolar contrast agents (HOCAs), low-osmolar contrast agents (LOCAs), and iso-osmolar contrast agents (IOCAs). The HOCAs have an osmolality four to five times higher than blood (300 Osm). LOCAs have an osmolality twice as high as blood. The latest-generation IOCAs have the same osmolality as blood. Ionic high-osmolality ICAs were the first class of ICA used. However, the high-osmolality and calcium-chelating proprieties often resulted in heart rhythm disorders (sinus bradycardia, atrioventricular blocks, QRS prolongation, long QT, ST-T, giant T-wave inversion, and extremely rarely, VT and VF) and altered LV contractility. Therefore, in recent decades, new-generation ICAs have been developed with low osmolality and neutral chemical characteristics that allow a significant reduction of adverse events.[42] In large cohort studies, the incidence of all types of adverse reactions to contrast was approximately 12% with a high-osmolality agent, compared with only 3% with a low-osmolality ICA (see Classic References, Katayama et al.). For this reason, LOCAs and IOCAs are now considered the safest ICAs to use for vascular diagnostic procedures.

Automatic and Manual Injection of Contrast Media

Manual contrast injection with a manifold permits a constant modulation of the pressure of the injection and allows the operator to feel the resistance of the vessel to the injection. However, careful evaluation of the line should be performed before the injection to ensure the absence of air bubbles in the system. Manual injection was the only technique used to deliver contrast media until 10 years ago, when power injections were introduced. These automatic systems can detect air bubbles in the tubes and stop the injection accordingly. The maximum volume of contrast delivered, as well as the maximum pressure, can be preset to reduce the risk of iatrogenic artery dissection. Current systems also allow for operator touch-sensitive, variable-volume, and pressure injections. For the RCA, 4 to 6 mL/sec is usually injected to optimally visualize the entire vessel, with a maximal pressure of 450 psi. For the LCA, a volume of 6 to 8 mL/sec is injected at a pressure of 450 to 600 psi.

The use of automatic injection systems is now preferred in most catheterization laboratories in Europe, whereas in the United States, 50% of sites still use manual injection. Automatic injections can significantly reduce the volume of contrast used for coronary procedures, and some studies report that they might reduce the risk of CI-AKI.[43;44]

Adverse Reactions to Contrast Media and Prophylactic Therapy

Adverse reactions after injection of ICA may be acute or delayed and can further be classified as allergic or allergic-like (physiologic). *Allergic reactions* can present with a variety of clinical symptoms, ranging from itching to skin rash, local edema, asthma, and full-blown anaphylactoid reaction. The pathophysiologic mechanisms hinge on the activation of different components of the immune system. *Allergic-like reactions* have a similar clinical presentation as the classic allergic response but are independent of immune system activation. Allergic-like reactions revolve around a physiologic response to contrast (e.g., nausea, vomiting, vasovagal reaction, hypertension, flushing).[45] The incidence of acute adverse reactions is related to the chemical and physical characteristics of ICAs. In particular, as previously described, high-osmolar ICAs have approximately a 12% rate of acute adverse events, whereas that of low- or iso-osmolality ICAs is significantly lower (see Classic References, Katayama et al.). In a cohort of 545 patients undergoing CT, the use of nonionic ICAs led to an allergic reaction rate of only 0.6%, of which only 23% were graded moderate to severe.[46]

Temporally, acute reactions occur within seconds or minutes of contact with the ICA. Delayed reactions, on the other hand, may develop from 30 minutes up to 1 week after injection of ICA and usually present with cutaneous manifestations. A prospective study of 539 patients by Loh and colleagues demonstrated that the percentage of delayed adverse events with the use of the dimeric low-molecular group (iohexol) is 14.3% compared with 2.5% observed in the no-contrast group.[47] Moreover, among the different types of ICA, nonionic dimeric agents show a higher percentage of delayed events than nonionic monomer agents. Because the rate of true allergic reaction to contrast is so low, prophylactic therapy is indicated only in patients with a history of allergic adverse events. In elective patients at risk for allergic reactions, in particular those with a history of anaphylactoid reaction, prophylactic treatment must include prednisone, 50 mg by mouth (PO), or hydrocortisone, 200 mg intravenous (IV) at 13 hours, 7 hours, and 1 hour before ICA injection, plus diphenhydramine, 50 mg IV, intramuscularly (IM), or PO, 1 hour before ICA administration (see Classic References, Lasser et al.). Methylprednisolone, 32 mg PO, 12 hours and 2 hours before ICA injection, plus an antihistamine can also be used. In addition, careful selection of ICA in addition to prophylactic therapy can help to further reduce the risk of adverse reactions, which are very uncommon (0.2% to 1.6%). Reactions to contrast agents may be more difficult to manage in patients receiving beta-blocker therapy. Recurrence rates may approach 50% on repeat exposure to contrast agents, and prophylactic use of H_1 and H_2 histamine receptor–blocking agents and aspirin therapy has been recommended.

ANGIOGRAPHIC PROJECTIONS

To identify and interpret the severity of coronary lesions, proper visualization of every segment of the main epicardial vessels and their branches is crucial. Although the coronary anatomy has a certain degree of variability, specific angulations of the x-ray tube are typically used during coronary angiography to ensure that vessel segments are not foreshortened or overlapping. The projections depend on the position of the x-ray tube and image intensifier. The AP view is obtained with the image intensifier in perpendicular position above the patient, with the x-ray beam traveling back to front. The intensifier can then be angled toward the patient's left or right side to obtain LAO and RAO views. The beam can be angulated cranially if the intensifier is tilted toward the head of the patient and caudally if it is moved toward the patient's feet. The degree of angulation can be changed to prevent overlapping of vessels or obstruction of vessel segments caused by superimposition of implantable devices or other structures, such as spine, bone, or diaphragm. As a general rule, in LAO views, the LAD is visible on the right side of the spinal column. Conversely, in RAO projections, the LAD is on the left side of the spinal column. Cranial and caudal tilting is used to "open" overlapped segments. Caudal views are mostly used for the proximal segment of the LCA, whereas cranial views avoid foreshortening and allow for the evaluation of the mid- and distal portion of the vessel and its bifurcations. Table 21.3 lists common projections for every coronary artery, and Figs. 21.10 and 21.11 provide examples for the LCA and RCA, respectively.

CORONARY ANATOMY

The heart vasculature comprises three main epicardial arteries that divide into smaller, thinner branches that eventually form the arterioles. The arterioles have a muscular wall and are the main site of vascular resistance that can modulate the blood pressure reaching the capillary net downstream (see Chapter 36). This section reviews the coronary anatomy of the main epicardial vessels that can be visualized with coronary angiography.

The main epicardial vessels are the left main coronary artery (LMCA) and the RCA. The LMCA originates from the left sinus of Valsalva and divides into the LAD and the Cx arteries. Occasionally, a third branch can originate from the LMCA, the ramus intermedius (RI), usually attributed to the Cx artery.

The LAD artery runs along the anterior interventricular sulcus and provides circulation for the anterior and anterolateral wall of the left ventricle with diagonal vessels and the anterior two-thirds of the interventricular septum with the septal branches. The number of diagonal and septal branches may vary greatly, and for the purpose of coronary description, they are simply numbered sequentially (D1, D2 ... S1, S2, S3). Based on the length of the vessel, the LAD can be classified into type 1 if it does not reach the LV apex, type 2 if it reaches the LV apex, and type 3 if it reaches and wraps around the LV apex, supplying also the posterior apex. The Cx artery courses along the left atrioventricular (AV) groove and provides branches for the left atrium, occasionally giving rise to the sinoatrial (SA) branch (40% of cases). The Cx also supplies the LV lateral and posterior walls with branches called *obtuse marginal* (OM) branches, which are numbered sequentially similar to the diagonal branches (see Fig. 21.10). There is high anatomic variability in the number of diagonal, septal, and OM branches present in the LCA.

The RCA originates from the right sinus of Valsalva and courses across the right AV groove. The proximal branches provided by the RCA are atrial branches for the right atrium, the SA node in 60% of cases, and the branch to the conus that supplies the right ventricular outflow tract. Once it reaches the acute margin of the ventricle, the RCA provides the acute margin branch. The RCA then continues to the crux cordis (where the AV groove intersects the posterior interventricular sulcus), where it branches into the PDA and the posterolateral (PL) branches (see Fig. 21.11). This anatomy is the most common and is termed *right coronary dominance*. Dominance can also be left or balanced, based on the origin of the PDA and the PL branches. Approximately 80% of the population displays a right dominance, meaning both the PDA and the PL branches are supplied by the RCA, while 10% of the population has a *left coronary dominance*, with PDA and PL branches deriving from the Cx artery. The remaining 10% display *codominance*, or *balanced coronary dominance*, with the PDA arising from the RCA and the PL branches arising from the Cx.

The subdivision of the coronary arteries into segments is crucial to describe the localization of lesions during angiography.

TABLE 21.3 Standard Angiographic Projections

PROJECTION/DEGREES	ANATOMIC DESCRIPTION
Right Coronary Artery	
LAO 45	Vessel engagement projection
	Ostium and RCA along AV sulcus
LAO 10-30, CRAN 30	PDA, PL branches, and RCA after crux
RAO 30	PDA ostium, PDA septal branches, right ventricular branches, acute margin branches
Left Coronary Artery	
Anteroposterior, CAUD 10	LMCA engagement projection
LAO 20-45, CAUD 30-45	"Spider projection": LMCA and proximal segment of LAD, Cx, and ramus (if present)
LAO 20-45, CRAN 30-60	Mid- and distal LAD and its branches, Cx PDA, and Cx PL branches if present
RAO 15-30, CAUD 10-30	All LAD and branches, Cx and OM branches
RAO 15-30, CRAN 10-30	Mid- and distal LAD and branches, mid-Cx and branches

AV, Atrioventricular; *CAUD*, caudal; *CRAN*, cranial; *Cx*, circumflex artery; *LAO*, left anterior oblique; *LMCA*, left main coronary artery; *OM*, obtuse marginal; *PDA*, posterior descending artery; *PL*, posterolateral; *RAO*, right anterior oblique; *RCA*, right coronary artery.

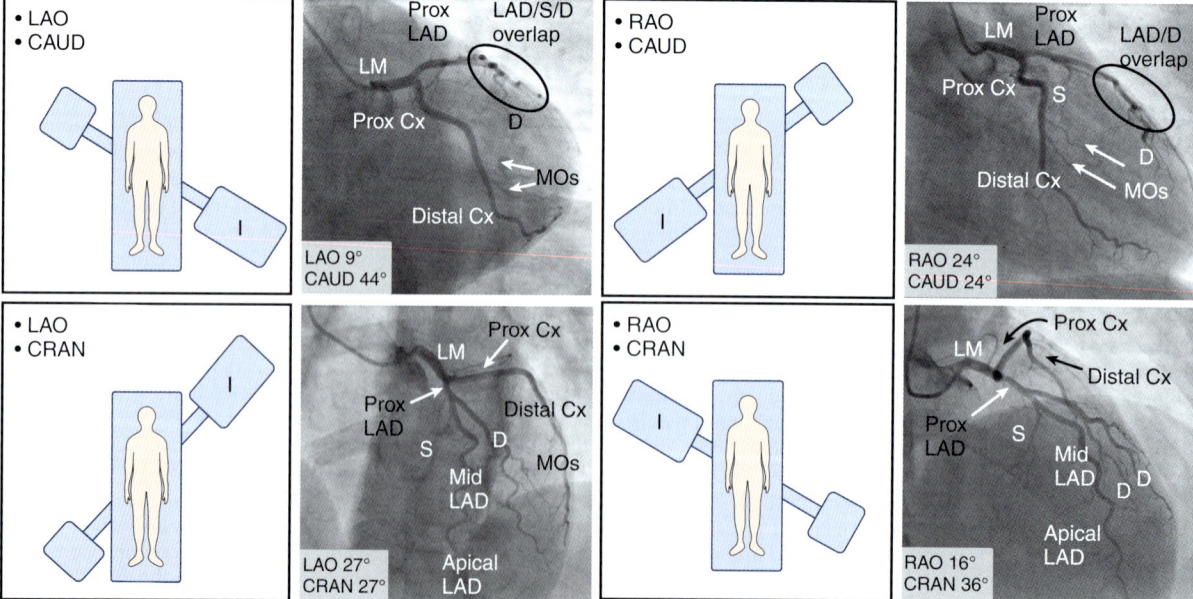

FIGURE 21.10 Angiographic projection for the left coronary artery and anatomic evaluation. *CAUD*, Caudal; *CRAN*, cranial; *Cx*, circumflex artery; *D*, diagonal branch(es); *I*, intensifier; *LAD*, left anterior descending artery; *LAO*, left anterior oblique; *LM*, left main coronary artery; *MOs*, obtuse marginal branch(es); *Prox*, proximal; *RAO*, right anterior oblique; *S*, septal branch(es). (Angiographic images courtesy Dr. Annapoorna Kini, Icahn School of Medicine at Mount Sinai, New York, NY.)

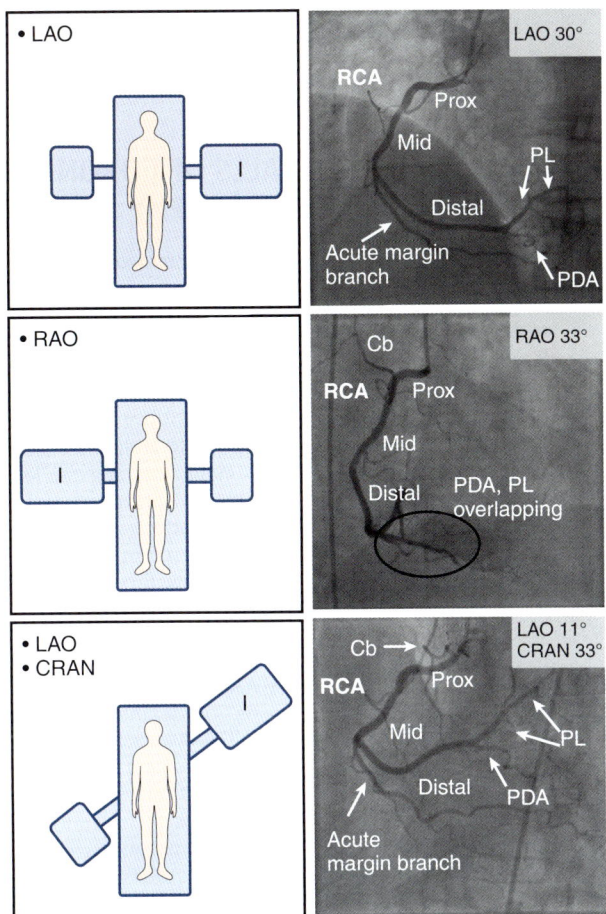

FIGURE 21.11 Angiographic projection for the right coronary artery (*RCA*) and anatomic evaluation. *Cb*, Conus branch; *CRAN*, cranial; *I*, intensifier; *LAO*, left anterior oblique; *PDA*, posterior descending artery; *PL*, posterolateral branches; *prox*, proximal; *RAO*, right anterior oblique. (Angiographic images courtesy Dr. Annapoorna Kini, Icahn School of Medicine at Mount Sinai, New York, NY.)

TABLE 21.4 Incidence of Coronary Anomalies in 1950 Angiograms

VARIABLE	NUMBER	FREQUENCY (%)
Coronary anomalies	110	5.64
Split RCA	24	1.23
Ectopic RCA (right cusp)	22	1.13
Ectopic RCA (left cusp)	18	0.92
Fistulas	17	0.87
Absent left main coronary artery	13	0.67
LCx arising from right cusp	13	0.67
LCA arising from right cusp	3	0.15
Low origin of RCA	2	0.1
Other anomalies	3	0.15

LCA, Left coronary artery; *LCx*, left circumflex artery; *RCA*, right coronary artery. From Angelini P, editor. Coronary Artery Anomalies: A Comprehensive Approach. Philadelphia: Lippincott Williams & Wilkins; 1999, p 42.

TABLE 21.5 Classification of Coronary Anomalies Based on Ischemia

ISCHEMIA	CLASSIFICATION
Absence of ischemia	Most anomalies (split RCA, ectopic RCA from right cusp; ectopic RCA from left cusp)
Episodic ischemia	Anomalous origin of a coronary artery from the opposite sinus (ACAOS); coronary artery fistulas; myocardial bridge
Typical ischemia	Anomalous left coronary artery from the pulmonary artery (ALCAPA); coronary ostial atresia or severe stenosis

CORONARY ARTERY ANOMALIES

The prevalence of coronary artery anomalies (CAAs) in patients undergoing coronary angiography averages 1% to 5%[48] (Table 21.4). Despite being rare in the general population, CAAs are the second most common cause of sudden cardiac death (SCD) among young athletes.[49]

There are many ways to classify CAAs. From a clinical standpoint, CAAs can be divided based on the presence of myocardial ischemia, into anomalies without ischemia, anomalies with episodic ischemia, and anomalies with obligatory ischemia (Table 21.5). Despite this important functional assessment, physicians often categorize CAAs based on anatomic characteristics. Use of CTCA and MRCA have increased the capability to detect and characterize anatomic abnormalities and help to determine optimal management of patients with a CAA. The most common anatomic classification of CAAs includes anomalies of ostium, anomalous origin of coronary artery, anomalous termination, congenital absence, and hypoplasia.[49]

Congenital Atresia of Coronary Ostium

Coronary ostial hypoplasia or atresia can occur as an isolated lesion or as a concomitant anomaly with other CAAs. The life expectancy of patients with coronary ostial hypoplasia or atresia depends on the presence of collateral circulation from other vessels that can supply the distal coronary bed.

Anomalous Origin of Coronary Artery

Anomalous origin of coronary arteries is a common type of CAA. Coronary arteries with ectopic origin can arise either from the wrong sinus of Valsalva (e.g., the Cx artery arising from the right coronary sinus) or from a different structure, including the pulmonary artery (PA), a branch of another coronary artery, or even a ventricular chamber.[49] The course of the anomalous coronary arteries can be assessed by angiography in the RAO view. The LCA arising from the right aortic sinus usually follows one of these four courses: prepulmonic, retroaortic, interarterial, or transseptal (Fig. 21.12). The interarterial course of an anomalous LCA from the right sinus is associated with SCD during or shortly after exercise in young individuals. The hemodynamic mechanism underlying the risk of SCD remains unclear. Some authors hypothesize that distention of the aortic root and the pulmonary trunk during exercise or stress might exacerbate the preexisting angulation of the anomalous coronary artery, resulting in compression of the coronary artery lumen. In other cases the vessel might have an aberrant course within the aortic wall that favors compression of the coronary artery. Similarly, origin of the RCA from the left aortic sinus with an interarterial course is associated with myocardial ischemia and SCD. Once this anomaly is diagnosed, CABG is recommended, although a stenting strategy has also been reported. A benign variation of the RCA origin is represented by the high anterior origin. This variation has no hemodynamic significance but might result in a challenging cannulation.

Anomalous pulmonary origin of any coronary artery (APOCA) is a very rare occurrence. If all three coronary arteries arise from the PA, prognosis is poor; patients with this anomaly usually die within the first month of life (see Classic References, Yamanaka and Hobbs). Anomalous origin of the LCA from PA (ALCAPA), also known as Bland-White-Garland syndrome, was reported for the first time in 1956 and represents the most common APOCA. Almost 90% of patients with this CAA die during the first year of life. Only very few, with extensive collateral circulation from the RCA, survive into adulthood. If diagnosed in time, the preferred treatment for APOCA is CABG or unroofing and re-implantation (with or without a patch). Partial ALCAPA (e.g., only of the LAD) has also been reported.[50]

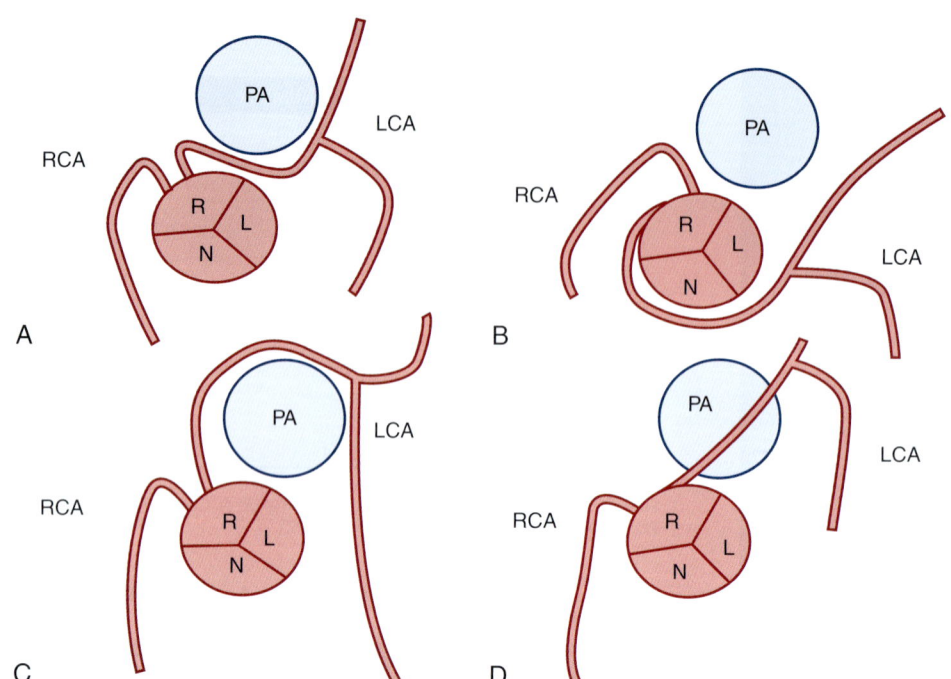

FIGURE 21.12 Four possible courses of the anomalous left coronary artery (*LCA*) arising from the right coronary sinus: **A,** Interarterial. **B,** Retroaortic. **C,** Prepulmonic. **D,** Transseptal. *L,* Left sinus of Valsalva; *N,* noncoronary sinus; *PA,* pulmonary artery; *R,* right sinus of Valsalva; *RCA,* right coronary artery.

Congenital Absence

Lack of an LMCA is the most common form of congenital coronary absence, with a rate of 0.41% to 0.67% in the general population. In the absence of LMCA, the LAD and Cx arteries simply arise directly from the left sinus of Valsalva with separate origins. This anomaly is considered a benign condition and is an occasional finding during coronary angiography. The congenital absence of either the Cx or the RCA has been reported and associated with a benign prognosis.[51]

Hypoplasia

Hypoplasia of a coronary artery is defined as the maldevelopment of at least one of the major epicardial arteries or its branches. One, two, or all three coronary territories can be involved. Hypoplastic coronary arteries usually have a small diameter and a shortened course. A luminal diameter of less than 1.5 mm in a major epicardial vessel, with no nearby compensatory branches, has been proposed as the threshold for diagnosis. The prognosis of single-vessel hypoplasia of the Cx or RCA is relatively good, but SCD can occur in two-vessel hypoplasia.

Anomalous Termination

Congenital coronary artery fistulas (CAFs) are rare anomalies, with an estimated incidence in the general population of approximately 0.002%. As an incidental finding, CAFs are reported in 0.3% to 0.8% of patients undergoing coronary angiography for any indication. CAFs are defined as abnormal direct communication between one or more coronary arteries with another major vessel or a chamber, such as the vena cava, left or right ventricle, pulmonary vein, or PA (Fig. 21.13).

CAFs can originate from any of the major epicardial vessels and involve the RCA in 33% to 55%, the LAD in 35% to 49%, and the Cx in 17% to 18% of cases. Simultaneous involvement of both the left and the right coronary system exists in about 4% to 18% of CAFs.[52,53] Most of the fistulas drain into low-pressure structures, such as the right ventricle (40%), right atrium (26%), PA (17%), coronary sinus (7%), and superior vena cava (1%). Although possible, drainage of CAFs into left-sided chambers is less frequent (left atrium 5%, left ventricle 3%).[52,54]

Coronary angiography is the gold standard for the diagnosis of CAFs. However, in clinical practice, most CAFs are incidental findings during CTCA in low-risk patients. The clinical presentation of patients with CAF depends on size and volume of the shunt, location of the shunt, and concomitance with other cardiac disease. Approximately 50% of patients with CAF are asymptomatic. When present, common symptoms are dyspnea, fatigue, palpitation, and chest pain. The first manifestation of CAF can also include CHF, arrhythmias, SCD, and infective endocarditis. Symptomatic patients with large fistulas should be treated with surgical closure or interventional closure.

PITFALLS OF CORONARY ANGIOGRAPHY

Improper interpretation of angiographic images can result from the use of inadequate projection views, CAAs, vessel foreshortening or superimposition of branches, and deep engagement of the catheter into the vessel, potentially resulting in oversight of ostial lesions. In addition, obesity or instrument malfunctioning can lead to low image quality and erroneous image interpretation. Inadequate vessel opacification because of enhanced blood flow or competitive flow from a bypass graft might result in oversight of stenosis in collateral branches or in overestimation of the degree of thrombosis in a vessel. Also, when reading coronary angiograms, borderline lesions may require multiple views and potentially intracoronary imaging or evaluation of the fractional flow reserve (FFR) to adequately assess the severity of the lesion. Moreover, a myocardial bridge or a coronary spasm can result in a minus defect in the coronary artery that can be misinterpreted as atherosclerotic disease, leading to unnecessary treatment (see next section). In the case of ostial occlusion of a vessel, especially for primary or secondary branches of main epicardial vessels, it can be challenging to notice the missing vessel unless a collateral perfusion is present that allows for partial visualization of the downstream portion of the occluded vessel.[55]

Myocardial Bridging

Myocardial bridging is not a coronary lesion per se, although in the long term it can lead to local coronary damage. It can also be mistaken for a coronary stenosis because bridging might cause filling defects. Myocardial bridging consists of a segment of an epicardial artery that descends into the myocardium for a variable distance (Fig. 21.14). It occurs in approximately 5% to 10% of patients and usually involves the LAD. As it runs in the myocardium, during systole the arterial segment is constricted by the muscle fibers and appears as a narrowing on the angiogram. However, these segments are usually easily identifiable because the narrowing disappears during diastole. Although bridging is not thought to be of any hemodynamic significance in most cases, myocardial bridging has been associated with angina, arrhythmia, depressed LV function, myocardial stunning, early death after cardiac transplantation, and SCD.[56] Treatment with beta blockers can be considered. Alternatively, surgical treatment can be attempted in selected cases.

Coronary Artery Spasm

Coronary spasm is a dynamic reversible focal restriction or occlusion of a coronary artery caused by the constriction of the smooth muscle cells in the vessel wall (Fig. 21.15) (see Chapter 36). Coronary spasm, when prolonged, can cause Prinzmetal angina and lead to transitory ECG changes. Cigarette smoking, cocaine use, alcohol, intracoronary irradiation, and administration of catecholamines can promote

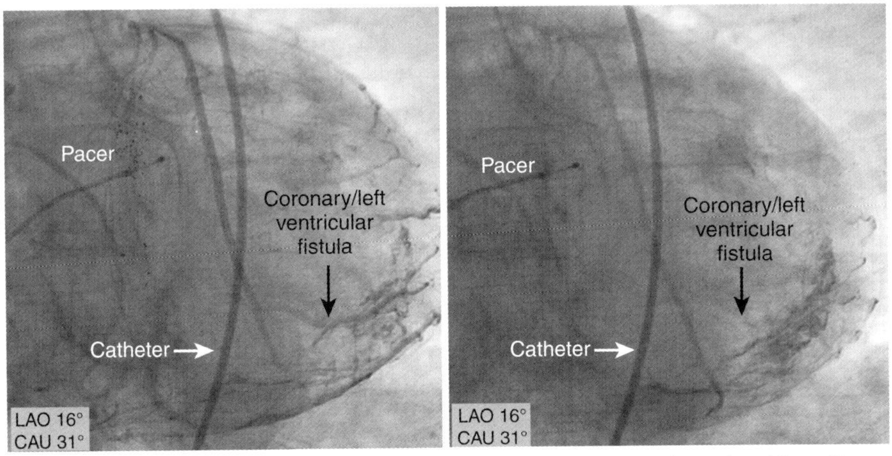

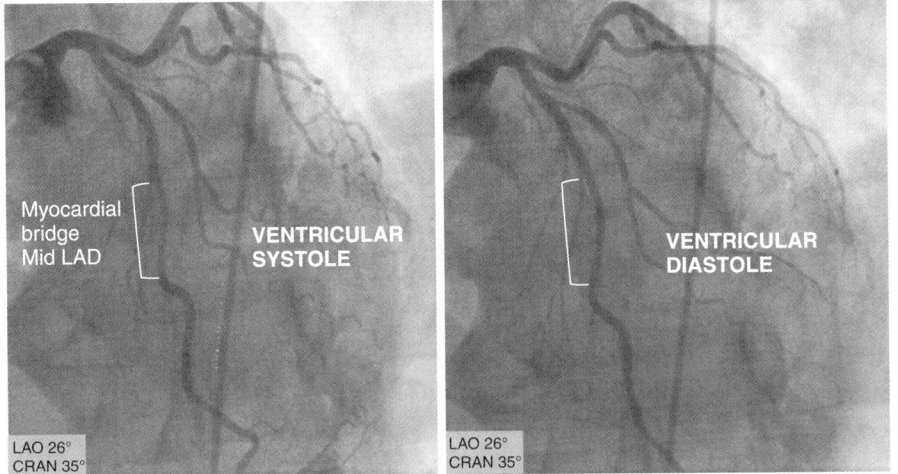

FIGURE 21.13 Coronary fistula with the left ventricle. *CAU*, Caudal; *LAO*, Left anterior oblique. (Courtesy Dr. Annapoorna Kini, Icahn School of Medicine at Mount Sinai, New York, NY.)

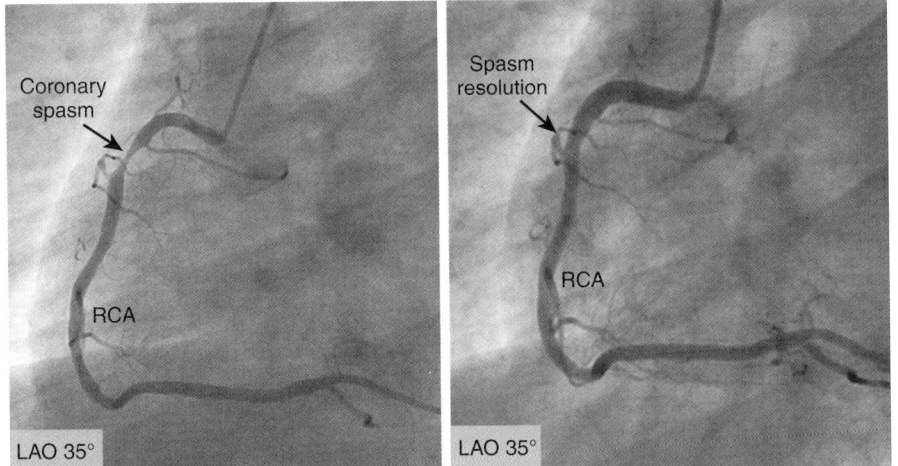

FIGURE 21.14 Myocardial bridge. Left, Narrowing of the middle left anterior descending artery (*LAD*) can be observed during the ventricular systolic phase. **Right,** The vessel diameter returns to normal during the ventricular diastolic phase. *CRAN*, Cranial; *LAO*, left anterior oblique. (Courtesy Dr. Annapoorna Kini, Icahn School of Medicine at Mount Sinai, New York, NY.)

FIGURE 21.15 Left, Coronary spasm in the proximal segment of the right coronary artery (*RCA*). **Right,** Resolution of the spasm. *LAO*, Left anterior oblique. (Courtesy Dr. Annapoorna Kini, Icahn School of Medicine at Mount Sinai, New York, NY.)

coronary artery spasm. If a coronary spasm is suspected, a diagnosis can be made with several provocative tests, most often IV ergonovine maleate, IV acetylcholine, and hyperventilation. The physiologic response to ergonovine is a diffuse coronary vasoconstriction in all epicardial vessels. In patients with coronary spasm, however, ergonovine can induce focal coronary spasm often associated with chest pain and ECG changes. Intracoronary nitroglycerin is used to relieve the spasm. Acetylcholine (ACh) is a vasodilator acting on the muscarinic receptors of the vascular smooth muscle cells. Incremental doses of ACh (20, 30, and 50 μg) are injected directly into the coronary artery. In the presence of endothelial dysfunction, cells cannot produce NO in response to ACh, resulting in local vasoconstriction. Adverse reactions to ACh include hypotension, bradycardia, dyspnea, and flushing. Also, hyperventilation during coronary angiography can elicit spasm, although it is a much less sensitive test compared with the others. If no spasm can be documented, the diagnosis relies instead on clinical features and the response to treatment with nitrates and calcium channel blockers.

ANGIOGRAM EVALUATION

When reading coronary angiograms, the entire extension of every coronary artery and its branches should be carefully evaluated in all the acquired views. First, the coronary dominance can be assessed. Next, the presence of abnormalities in the course of the coronary arteries should be investigated. The following elements should be part of the evaluation of diseased coronary vessels: (1) extension and localization of the lesion, (2) severity of the stenosis, (3) morphologic characteristics of the lesion, (4) evaluation of the downstream flow, (5) presence of collateral blood vessel circles, and (6) changes compared with previous angiograms, if available.

SYNTAX SCORE

The SYNTAX score is a valuable tool for the assessment of CAD severity. Developed in the context of the eponymous trial, this algorithm integrates several historical anatomical scores including the ACC/AHA, Medina bifurcation, and CTO classifications, as well as the AHA categorization of the three coronary segments and finally the modified Leaman score.[57,58] Although the primary purpose of this score was not to assess prognosis, several trials and prospective registries have shown a significant correlation between the high score tertiles and worse outcomes, irrespective of clinical presentation and follow-up length. Therefore, in patients with LM or multivessel disease, current guidelines recommend SYNTAX score to assess the anatomical complexity of CAD, as well as the long-term risk of mortality and morbidity after PCI. Accordingly, higher tertiles move indication for surgery, while low score tertile for PCI.

Even the residual SYNTAX score has been found strongly related to long-term adverse events. In particular, a post-hoc analysis from the SYNTAX trial has shown that a residual SYNTAX score >8 was an independent predictor of 5-year mortality; observation corroborated in different clinical contexts including patients with ACS.[59,60] This finding has important clinical implications. In patients with multivessel disease in which

Quantification of the Stenosis

A coronary stenosis is a reduction of the caliber of the vessel that is not caused by the progressive thinning of the vessel along its course but rather by pathologic local conditions. The degree of the stenosis can be evaluated by comparing the minimum diameter of the vessel at the level of the lesion to the diameter of the adjacent segment upstream of the stenosis. The degree of stenosis is usually underestimated compared with postmortem evaluation or intravascular ultrasound (IVUS) because the adjacent healthy lumen to which the stenosis is compared might present with vasospasm or diffuse atherosclerosis despite appearing normal on the angiogram. This often leads to underestimation of the stenosis. In addition, it is particularly difficult to evaluate long lesions since the arteries physiologically narrow during their course, and there might be a marked mismatch between the diameters of the normal segment upstream and downstream of a long stenosis.

Stenoses are defined as *minimal* if the narrowing is visually less than 50%, *moderate* between 50% and 70%, and *severe* with diameter reduction 70% or more.[55] Evaluation of stenosis severity can be estimated visually by the interventional cardiologist reading the angiogram, or it can be measured with quantitative coronary angiography (QCA) methodologies based on the selection of the area of interest and vessel diameter measurements, which can be automatic, semiautomatic, or manual. Most programs can be calibrated using the diameter of the catheter and can automatically detect the edge of the vessel across its length and measure the minimum diameter of the stenosis and the length of the stenosis. Alternatively, rather than edge detection, densitometric methodology can be used. This technique avoids the errors of edge detection caused by geometric assumptions required for software calculations. Densitometry measures the stenosis based on the area containing ICA when the vessel is fully opaque. There is usually good agreement between edge detection and densitometry techniques. QCA reduces interoperator variability of reading, which is estimated around 20%, and usually results in 10% to 20% lower values than visual stenosis estimation.[61]

When evaluating a coronary lesion, the diameter and length of the stenosis are only two of many characteristics to consider. Also important are morphologic characteristics of the lesion, including the presence of thrombus, extent of calcification, and tortuosity of the vessel involved. The AHA has classified coronary artery lesions into three main types based on easily identifiable characteristics on the angiogram. This classification has predictive value for the success of a PCI procedure (see Chapter 41). Type A lesions have a procedural success rate of 92% and a low complication rate, type B lesions have a 72% success rate with a 10% rate of complications, and type C lesions have only a 61% success rate and a 21% rate of complications (Table 21.6). Additional classifications of lesion severity are the Society for Cardiovascular Angiography and Interventions (SCAI) and the Ellis systems.[62]

Evaluation of Microvascular Blood Flow

Evaluation of the downstream flow provides additional information not only on the severity of the stenosis but also on the status of the microcirculation in the affected territory. It has been proven that often the microcirculation is impaired in the territory affected by epicardial vessel lesions. Prognostic information can be obtained from the degree of blood flow through the lesion. The most common classification is the Thrombolysis in Myocardial Ischemia/Infarction (TIMI) flow grade[35] (Table 21.7). In the presence of good blood flow in the coronary artery (TIMI 3) after PCI, patients can additionally be stratified using the TIMI frame count (TFC) score based on the number of angiographic frames necessary for the contrast to reach a standardized distal point in the vessel. The angiographic film should be acquired at 30 frames per second and contrast injection performed with a 6F catheter to measure TFC. The first frame is where the origin of the vessel appears fully opacified. The last frame is predefined for each coronary vessel: For the LAD and Cx arteries, it is the most distal bifurcation, whereas for the RCA, it is the emergence of the first PL branch. For the LAD, the apical segment is the milestone for the TFC. Because the LAD is usually longer than the other vessels, a correction factor needs to be used when calculating this score in the LAD by dividing TFC in the LAD by 1.7. Normal TFCs are 36 ± 3 (or 21 ± 2 if corrected) for the LAD, 22 ± 4 for the Cx, and 20 ± 3 for the RCA.[37] This score provides quantitative information on the status of the microcirculation in the infarcted areas and is a predictor of functional recovery and clinical outcomes after primary PCI. In fact, while most primary PCIs obtain patency of the epicardial flow and a TIMI flow grade 3, the tissue-level perfusion will determine the extent of the myocardial damage or the muscle recovery. Similarly, the *myocardial blush* score provides a semiquantitative measure of peripheral perfusion (Table 21.8). It represents the arrival of the contrast in the capillaries and therefore can be appreciated only with angiographic acquisitions prolonged after the contrast has washed out of the main epicardial vessel. The myocardial blush grade is superior to TIMI flow grade for predicting postprocedural cardiac death and major adverse cardiovascular event (MACE).[63]

TABLE 21.6 AHA/ACC Lesion Classification

Type A	• Length <10 mm • Discrete • Concentric readily accessible • <45-degree angle • Smooth contour	• Little or no calcification • Less than totally occluded • Not ostial • No major side branch involvement • Absence of thrombus
Type B B1 if only one characteristic is present B2 if two or more characteristics are present	• Length 10-20 mm • Eccentric • Moderate tortuosity of proximal segment • 45- to 90-degree angle • Irregular contour • Presence of any thrombus grade	• Moderate or heavy calcification • Total occlusion <3 months old • Ostial lesion • Bifurcation lesion requiring two guidewires
Type C	• Length >20 mm • Diffuse • Excessive tortuosity of proximal segment • >90-degree angle • Total occlusion >3 months old and/or bridging collaterals inability to protect major side branches • Degenerated vein graft with friable lesions	

TABLE 21.7 Thrombolysis in Myocardial Ischemia/Infarction (TIMI) Flow Rate

TIMI 0 Flow	No penetration of contrast beyond the stenosis (100% stenosis, occlusion)
TIMI 1 Flow	Penetration of contrast beyond the stenosis but no perfusion of the distal vessel (99% stenosis, subtotal occlusion)
TIMI 2 Flow	Contrast reaches the distal vessel but at reduced rate of filling or clearing compared with other coronary arteries (partial perfusion)
TIMI 3 Flow	Contrast reached the distal vessel and clear at the same rate as the other coronary arteries

Collateral Vessel Circulation

The coronary arteries represent the end circulation of the heart, and thus there is very little redundancy in the vascularization of each myocardial territory. However, collateral vessels can form under specific circumstances. Collateral blood vessels are anastomotic connections between two segments of the same artery or between different native coronary arteries. They function as natural bypasses and represent an alternative source of blood supply for a coronary territory. Clearly, collateral circulation becomes very important in the event that the main vessel serving the territory becomes occluded. There are two main mechanisms by which collateral vessels can be formed: arteriogenesis and angiogenesis. *Arteriogenesis* is the growth of preexisting arterioles that transform into functional collateral arteries, as a muscular layer forms and viscoelastic and vasomotor properties are acquired. Arteriogenesis is promoted by the pressure gradient across the stenosis that favors the blood flow through the small, preexisting anastomotic vessels upstream of the stenosis. *Angiogenesis,* on the other hand, involves the de novo formation of vessels starting from primitive postcapillary venules. The process is favored by hypoxic stimuli such as local production of vascular endothelial growth factor (VEGF) and hypoxia-inducible factors (HIFs)[64] (see Chapter 36). The collateral vessel net can be intracoronary if it connects different segments of the same coronary artery or the two LCAs and intercoronary if it connects the RCA with one or both of the LCAs.

When evaluating coronary stenosis, it is important to take into account the presence of collateral vessels that may have formed over time. Collateral flow can allow visualization of an occluded vessel by retrograde opacification of the vessel downstream of the occlusion. Based on the presence of contrast in the collateral vessels and the degree of retrograde opacification of the epicardial vessel, collateral circulation can be classified with the Rentrop grade[65] (see Classic References) (Fig. 21.16).

SPECIAL LESION CONSIDERATIONS

Chronic Total Occlusion

A chronic total occlusion (CTO) is the complete or almost-complete blockage of a coronary artery for 30 or more days. It can be an incidental finding in patients referred for diagnostic angiography. To visualize the vessel downstream to the CTO, a retrograde technique can be used by injecting the patent coronary artery; if collateral vessels are present between the two arteries, the vessel downstream of the CTO can be visualized (see Rentrop classification for collateral vessels previously described). CTOs are considered very complex lesions and contribute greatly to the SYNTAX score (see Chapters 40 and 41); less than 50% of CTO lesions in the SYNTAX trial were successfully treated by PCI. A specific score, the J-CTO, has been developed to predict the probability of successful guidewire CTO crossing within 30 minutes; independent predictors were previously failed lesion, blunt stump type, vessel bending, presence of calcification, and occlusion length of 20 mm or more. For the purpose of CTO angioplasty, another way to visualize the vessel distal to the CTO is the preprocedural use of CTCA. Using co-registration software, the vessel portion that is "missing" in the coronary angiogram is integrated with the CT image, thus providing guidance for the advancement of the intracoronary guidewire.

Calcific Lesions

Atherosclerotic calcifications are an important predictor of successful PCI. Although invasive coronary angiography can detect calcific coronary lesions, it has a low sensitivity for calcium and can only detect moderate to severe calcifications[66]. The gold standard for the evaluation of calcific lesions is CTCA (see Chapter 20). The extent of CAC correlates with the plaque burden, and because of the high sensitivity of CT scan for calcium, this imaging modality can detect plaque burden at a very early stage. As an alternative to CTCA, IVUS has been shown to have significantly higher sensitivity to detect coronary calcification than standard angiography, especially for milder calcifications.[66] Presence of a calcific arc greater than 180 degrees by IVUS is considered a severe calcification.[67]

The correct assessment of the calcium burden of a coronary lesion is important to determine the most appropriate treatment strategy. Highly calcific lesions are not compliant, and despite dilation before stent deployment, the risk of suboptimal stent apposition is high. Vessel dissection and distal embolization with aggressive vessel dilation before or after stent deployment are also possible complications. CABG might not be a valid alternative to PCI with extensive calcifications that do not allow for graft insertion on the native coronary artery, particularly in multivessel calcific disease. Atherectomy (rotational or orbital) may specifically treat calcific lesions during PCI (see Chapter 41).

Thrombotic Lesions

Presence of thrombus is usually associated with plaque rupture observed during ACSs (see Chapters 24 and 37 to 39). However, patients with generalized prothrombotic states can develop thrombus in the absence of plaque rupture. Thrombi are associated with higher rates of periprocedural complications. Thrombus load has been graded with the TIMI score as follows:

Grade 0, no cineangiographic characteristics of thrombus present;
Grade 1, images suggestive but not diagnostic for thrombus: reduced contrast density, haziness, and irregular lesion contour;
Grade 2, small thrombus present that is one-half or less the vessel diameter;
Grade 3, moderate-size thrombus present with greatest linear dimension more than one-half the vessel diameter but less than two vessel diameters (Fig. 21.17);
Grade 4, large thrombus present with a dimension that is two vessel diameters or greater;
Grade 5, recent total occlusion, which can involve some collateralization but usually does not involve extensive collateralization and tends to have a "beak" shape and a hazy edge or appearance of distinct thrombus; and
Grade 6, CTO, which usually involves extensive collateralization, tends to have a distinct, blunt cutoff or edge and will generally clot to the nearest proximal side branch.

TABLE 21.8 Myocardial Blush Score

Grade 0	No myocardial blush or contrast density
Grade 1	Minimal myocardial blush or contrast density
Grade 2	Moderate myocardial blush but less than that obtained from the ipsilateral non–infarct-related coronary artery
Grade 3	Normal myocardial blush or contrast density comparable to that obtained during angiography of a contralateral or ipsilateral non–infarct-related artery

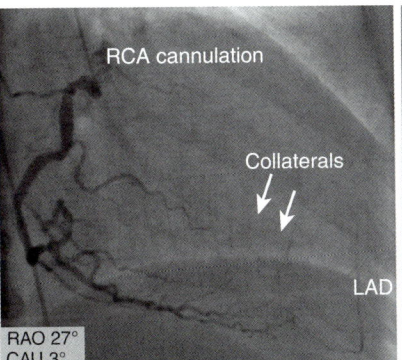 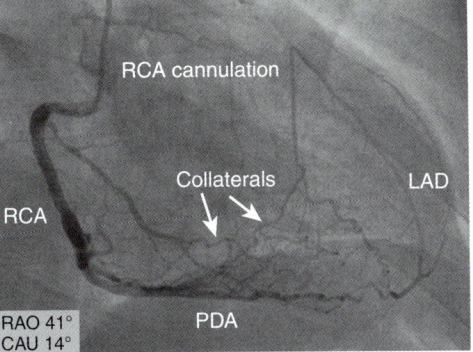

FIGURE 21.16 Collateral circulation from the right coronary artery to the left coronary artery. **Left,** Rentrop 2. **Right,** Rentrop 3. *CAU,* Caudal; *LAD,* left anterior descending coronary artery; *PDA,* posterior descending artery; *RAO,* right anterior oblique; *RCA,* right coronary artery. (Courtesy Dr. Annapoorna Kini, Icahn School of Medicine at Mount Sinai, New York, NY.)

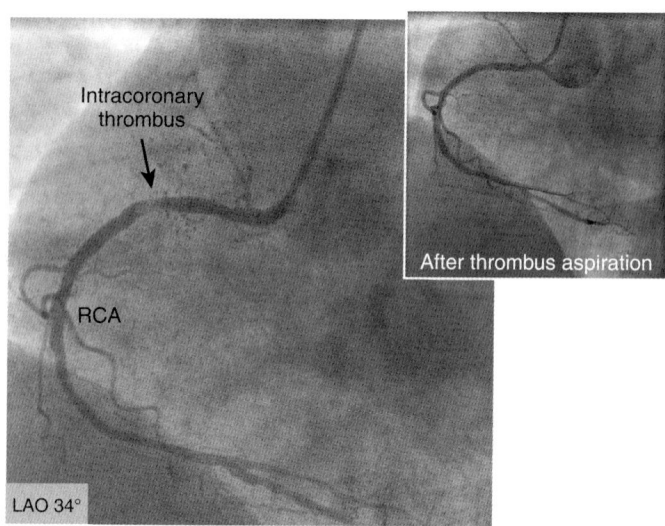

FIGURE 21.17 Grade 3 intracoronary thrombus in the proximal segment of the right coronary artery (*RCA*). **Right inset,** Absence of visible thrombus after aspiration. *LAO,* Left anterior oblique. (Courtesy Dr. Annapoorna Kini, Icahn School of Medicine at Mount Sinai, New York, NY.)

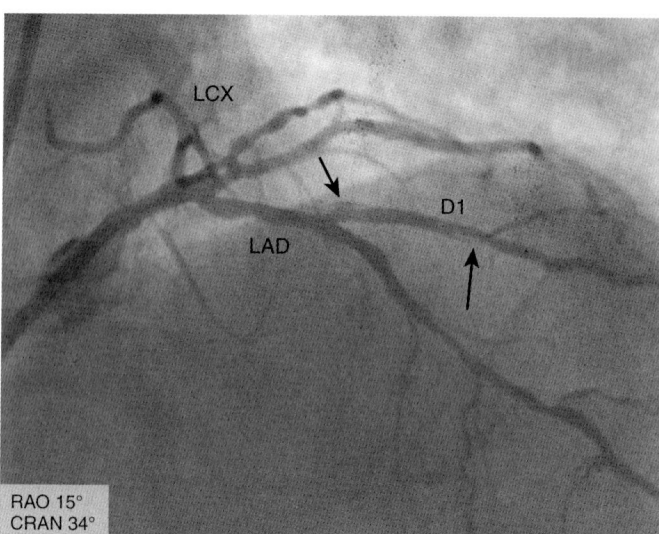

FIGURE 21.18 Type B coronary dissection. The *arrows* show two dissection sites in the diagonal branch. *CRAN,* Cranial; *RAO,* right anterior oblique. (Courtesy Dr. Annapoorna Kini, Icahn School of Medicine at Mount Sinai, New York, NY.)

Bifurcation Lesions

Bifurcation lesions account for approximately 15% of lesions requiring PCI. Bifurcation lesions are difficult to assess and treat because they may require intervention not only on the main vessel but also on the side branch as well. Thus, these lesions are associated with increased complications during and after PCI. During coronary angiography, bifurcations are evaluated according to the Medina classification, a three-digit system based on the evaluation of three distinct vessel segments in the following order: main artery in the segment proximal to the bifurcation, main artery in the segment distal to the bifurcation, and the side branch. To each segment, the operator can assign 0 if no significant CAD or 1 if a significant stenosis is present.

Coronary Dissections

Coronary artery dissection can be a life-threatening complication during PCI or a spontaneous event. Iatrogenic dissections can be caused by the advancement of the guidewire into the coronary artery or by plaque fracture after intracoronary balloon inflation. Based on their angiographic appearance, dissections can be classified (Fig. 21.18). Not all dissections require treatment. Type A and B dissections are usually considered benign and might not require intervention, whereas types C and F are often major dissections associated with morbidity and mortality. Whenever necessary, the management of coronary dissection is stent deployment.

Spontaneous coronary artery dissections (SCADs) are rare. Their pathophysiology is not clear, but since they are more common in young women age 40 to 50 without any other cardiovascular risk factors, the etiology of SCAD has been associated with steroid hormones (see Chapter 91). In accordance with this theory, SCADs are more common within 2 weeks postpartum, when marked changes in hormonal levels are usually observed. Another possible explanation is the presence of undetected fibromuscular dysplasia (FMD), an arteriopathy that can involve different vascular districts, including renal arteries and coronary arteries (see Chapter 43). FMD can cause intramural hematomas that may result in SCADs. For example, in a study of 50 patients with SCAD, 86% were found to have FMD.[68]

CORONARY INTRAVASCULAR IMAGING

The diffusion of techniques for intravascular imaging has advanced the understanding of coronary atherosclerotic disease and has provided additional information to angiography for the guidance of intracoronary stenting. IVUS and OCT are the main imaging modalities currently available in the catheterization laboratory for intravascular imaging.

Intravascular Ultrasound

An invasive coronary angiogram is a luminogram with poor specificity. Intravascular imaging such as IVUS and OCT can facilitate detailed assessment and characterization of CAD and aid optimization of revascularization with stent implantation. OCT provides better definition of the vascular endothelium and fibrous cap of atheromas,[69] while IVUS has higher vessel wall penetration that ensures a more detailed characterization of the atheroma core.

Principles. IVUS employs an intracoronary catheter with a transducer at the tip, which generates sound waves by converting electrical energy into acoustic energy.[70] The waves are reflected off arterial vessel walls, returned to the transducer, and subsequently converted into a working image for qualitative and quantitative evaluation. Contemporary IVUS catheters include transducers emitting sound waves at frequencies of 20 to 60 MHz, which provide high penetration (5 to 10 mm) for accurate assessment of vessel size and plaque burden. However, the low resolution (70 to 200 μ; 100-μ micron axial resolution parallel to radius and 200-μ lateral resolution perpendicular to radius) of gray-scale IVUS results in imperfect plaque characterization.[71] Virtual histology IVUS (VH-IVUS) overcomes the drawback of gray-scale IVUS and allows detailed interpretation of plaque morphology in the different stages of phenotypic plaque evolution, namely, pathologic intimal thickening, fibrotic plaque, thick- and thin-cap fibroatheroma, and fibrocalcific plaque.[72] VH-IVUS also clearly demonstrates necrotic core, dense calcium, and areas of plaque rupture. Comparatively, OCT using light wave technology permits a higher resolution of 5 to 10 μ, although with low penetration for optimal assessment of plaque morphology, as well as differentiation between thrombus and plaque.[73] Finally, near-infrared spectroscopy (NIRS) technology promotes understanding of coronary plaque lipid burden and may be used in conjunction with IVUS or OCT.[74]

Technology. There are two types of IVUS systems: single-element transducers and phased array transducers with multiple crystals arranged around the end of the delivery catheter.[70] A single-element transducer uses one element that generates and receives sound waves; a phased array system uses multiple transducers, which can be pulsed separately. The single-element type of catheter is commercially available with a transducer frequency of 40 to 60 MHz and a crossing profile of 2.9F to 3.2F compatible with 5F and 6F guides. Two such catheters are the Revolution (Volcano, California) and the Opticross (Boston Scientific). In contrast, the Eagle Eye Platinum catheter (Volcano) employs a phased array transducer with 20-MHz frequency and 2.9F crossing profile compatible with 5F guides. This catheter combines gray-scale and radiofrequency VH-IVUS assessment. The working length of the catheter is 150 cm (60 inches), and the proximal end is connected to the IVUS console for image reconstruction, which may be operated within the catheterization laboratory by radiation scientists. A console connected to the angiography table permits the operator to obtain measurements online during the procedure.

Indications for Use. Intracoronary imaging is used in the vast majority of PCI procedures in Japan. Current guidelines on the use of IVUS[75] are summarized. ACC/AHA recommends IVUS use for assessment of indeterminate lesions in the LMCA (class IIa, level of evidence B) and non-LMCA (IIb, B) coronary arteries to determine the need for revascularization. IVUS is also recommended for optimization of stent implantation, particularly in the LMCA (IIa, B). Indeed, the use of IVUS in observational data has been associated with implantation of larger and longer stents and higher pressures for postprocedural dilation.[76] After PCI, IVUS is recommended for the investigation of stent failure to determine the mechanism of both in-stent restenosis (IIa, C) and stent thrombosis (IIb, C). Some investigators have also advocated IVUS use for the assessment and diagnosis of SCAD to visualize the tissue flap, true and false lumens, and intramural hematoma, thereby facilitating more accurate diagnoses.[77]

The European guidelines recommend use of IVUS to assess lesion severity and optimize the treatment for unprotected left main coronary lesions (Class IIa, level of evidence B). Furthermore, IVUS should be considered to detect stent-related mechanical problems leading to restenosis (Class IIa, level of evidence C) and to optimize stent implantation in selected patients (Class IIa, level of evidence B).[78]

Procedure

Similar to a standard PCI procedure, IVUS examination is performed through a coronary guide catheter system over a 0.0014-inch guidewire using standard techniques. The crossing profile of the IVUS catheter varies from 2.9F to 3.2F, which is compatible with a 5F to 6F guide catheter. It is conventional an adequate dose of anticoagulation for thrombus prevention and a bolus dose of intracoronary nitroglycerin to prevent arterial spasm and allow better imaging assessment.[62] Onceat the desired location distal to the lesion, pullback of the catheter is initiated, which may be automated or manual, with a typical pullback rate of 0.5 mm/sec. IVUS-related complications are rare and usually self-resolving. The risk of coronary dissection or perforation with IVUS use is estimated at 1.6%.[79] Complications with IVUS catheter use may be related to size of the vessel and force used to advance the catheter.

Interpretation

IVUS identifies three layers in normal vessel architecture, including the intima, media, and adventitia (Fig. 21.19). The *intima* is an echogenic, bright inner layer. The *media* is a hypoechoic, homogeneous area between the intima and adventitia composed of smooth muscle cells, collagen, elastic tissue, and proteoglycans. The *adventitia* is the outer reflective layer.[70] In the presence of atherosclerosis, there is evidence of medial thinning and deposition of plaque in the intima. This is typically noted to be heterogeneous due to variable impedance of the different plaque components (Fig. 21.20). Thrombus in the lumen may appear similar to plaque and cannot be clearly differentiated on gray-scale IVUS in the absence of a distinct interface between thrombus and plaque. Occasionally, IVUS may indicate the presence of blood flow through luminal thrombus. VH-IVUS identifies different plaque morphologies in a color-coded manner, and necrotic core, dense calcification, and fibrous and fibrofatty areas are all clearly noted.[72]

A coronary dissection may be diagnosed on IVUS with documentation of tissue flap, true and false lumens, and intramural hematoma.[80] Implanted coronary stents can be assessed using IVUS for both expansion and apposition. A gap between the stent struts and the vessel wall indicates malapposition; the greater the distance between the stent strut and the vessel wall, the worse the malapposition. Stent underexpansion and malapposition are correlated with long-term adverse outcomes, including stent thrombosis. Real-time assessment of stent apposition and the need for post-dilation can be made online to allow specific management during PCI. Post-PCI neointimal hyperplasia caused by in-stent restenosis can be assessed using IVUS and appears as a hypoechoic area within the stent.[70]

In addition to immediate qualitative assessment of images for nature and extent of CAD, automated software analysis is available for both online and offline quantitative measurement of plaque burden and vessel size. Several validated measurements may be taken for evaluation of minimum lumen area, minimum lumen diameter, external elastic membrane (EEM) area, EEM diameter, plaque and media area (EEM area–lumen area), and plaque burden (plaque and media area/EEM area)[71] (Fig. 21.21). General criteria for significant obstructive disease include minimum lumen area less than 6 mm^2 in the LMCA or less than 4 mm^2 in the proximal LAD and other major vessels.[81]

For VH-IVUS, the gray-scale IVUS images recorded during pullback are combined with raw radiofrequency data captured on top of the R wave and reconstructed in a color-coded map by the IVUS-VH data recorder. The color-coded map identifies necrotic core (red), dense calcium (white), fibrofatty tissue (light green), and fibrous tissue (dark green). Thin-cap fibroatheroma on VH-IVUS is diagnosed in the presence of a greater than 30-degree arc of necrotic core abutting the lumen in three consecutive slices.[71]

Clinical Data

Several observational and randomized trial have shown long-term benefit from IVUS use for PCI attributed to greater minimum stent area and lower MACE. In the Assessment of Dual Antiplatelet Therapy with Drug-Eluting Stents (ADAPT-DES) study, IVUS was used in 39% of cases and was associated with longer stents, larger stent diameters, and higher inflation pressures in 74% of IVUS-guided cases.[76] The MATRIX (Comprehensive Assessment of Sirolimus-Eluting Stents in Complex

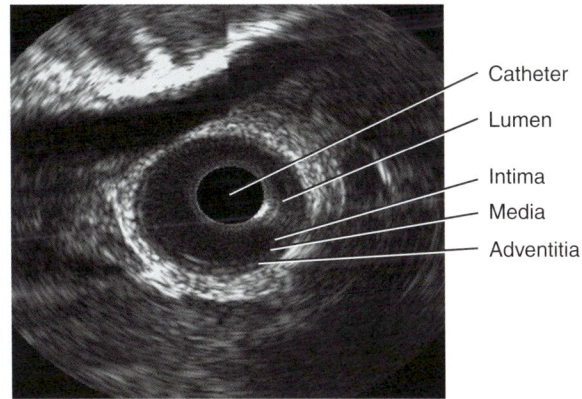

FIGURE 21.19 Normal vessel architecture on intravascular ultrasound (IVUS) demonstrating three layers: intima, media, and adventitia. (Courtesy Dr. Annapoorna Kini, Icahn School of Medicine at Mount Sinai, New York, NY.)

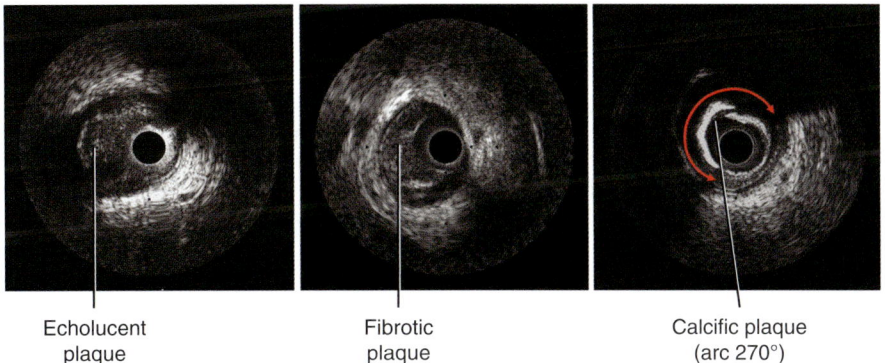

Echolucent plaque — Fibrotic plaque — Calcific plaque (arc 270°)

FIGURE 21.20 Heterogeneous nature of different plaque components caused by variable impedance on IVUS. (Courtesy Dr. Annapoorna Kini, Icahn School of Medicine at Mount Sinai, New York, NY.)

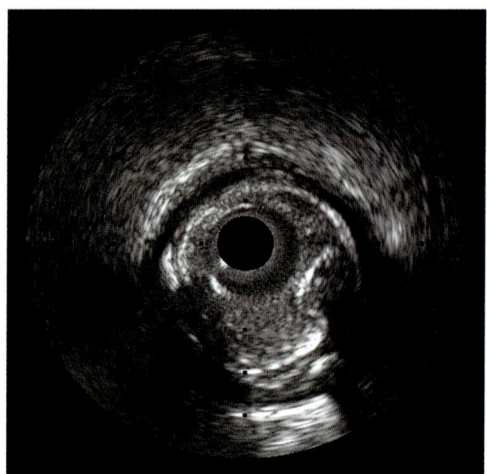
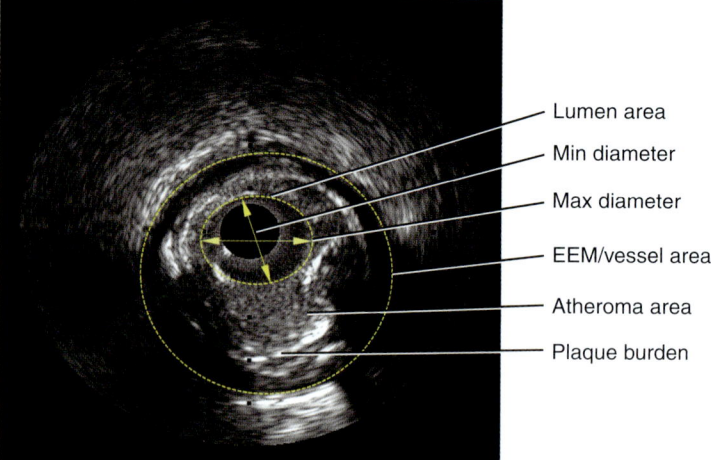

FIGURE 21.21 IVUS quantitative measurements for evaluation of lumen diameter and lumen area, external elastic membrane (EEM) area, and plaque burden. (Courtesy Dr. Annapoorna Kini, Icahn School of Medicine at Mount Sinai, New York, NY.)

Lesions) registry compared patients undergoing IVUS-guided versus non-IVUS-guided PCI. Both short- and long-term outcomes were significantly reduced with IVUS use.[82]

Furthermore, several randomized clinical trials have compared IVUS-guided with angiography-guided PCI. A meta-analysis summarizing those evidences confirmed benefits of IVUS guided PCI compared with PCI alone with a reduction in major adverse events, including cardiovascular death, MI, and target lesion revascularization.[83] Results confirmed in the following published Intravascular Ultrasound Guided Drug Eluting Stents Implantation in "All-comers" Coronary Lesions (ULTIMATE) trial, randomized a total of 1448 all-comer patients undergoing PCI to IVUS-guided PCI or angiography-guided PCI. At 12-month follow-up, this study showed that IVUS-guided DES implantation was associated with reduction in target vessel failure (0.530 [0.312 to 0.901]; $P = 0.019$).

The greater the complexity or lesion burden, the higher should be the use of intravascular imaging. For example, the EXCEL trial comparing 1905 patients with left main disease to PCI with cobalt-chromium everolimus-eluting stents versus CABG has shown an extensive use of intravascular imaging, pre- and post-stent implantation. In particular, IVUS guidance was performed in 722 of 935 (77.2%) patients who underwent PCI. Furthermore, in the Providing Regional Observations to Study Predictors of Events in the Coronary Tree (PROSPECT) study, almost 700 patients presenting with ACS underwent three-vessel coronary angiography and IVUS after PCI. The study showed that nonculprit lesion–related MACE (composite of all-cause death, cardiac arrest, MI, or rehospitalization due to unstable or progressive angina) was associated with plaque burden of 70% or more, minimum lumen area of 4 mm² or less, and thin-cap fibroatheroma less than 65 µ.[79] However, at 3 years, MACE was equally related to culprit and nonculprit vessel lesions. Use of intracoronary imaging may facilitate early detection and treatment of vulnerable plaque in nonculprit lesions and decrease long-term MACE.

An important limitation of IVUS interpretation is the need for coaxial catheter position during image acquisition.[84] However, dedicated software that allows real-time co-registration between angiogram and intravascular images has significantly improved this technique limitation (see paragraph Co-registration of Intravascular Imaging and X-Ray Angiography for Patients Undergoing PCI). The low resolution prevents clear differentiation between thrombus and plaque burden. In regard to applicability to the workflow of a busy catheterization laboratory, routine IVUS use is perceived to be expensive, time-consuming, and limited by operator skill. Further, IVUS does not allow visualization of the plaque lipid content, which might have important prognostic repercussions. To overcome this limitation, NIRS can be used.

Plaque Lipid Core Detection
The NIRS catheter emits near-infrared waves with a wavelength of 0.8 to 2.5 µ. Based on differences in absorption pattern of the light, different components of plaque and lipid are demonstrated in a map or chemogram of lipid deposition along the coronary artery.[85] The TVC Insight Catheter (Infraredx, Massachusetts) combines NIRS and IVUS (40 MHz), with a crossing profile of 3.2F compatible with 6F guide catheter systems. The TVC composite system allows superimposed imaging from NIRS-IVUS, which can provide information on vessel size, plaque burden, and areas of lipid-rich plaque.[86]

Hybrid catheters are also available, combining FFR-IVUS and IVUS-OCT to provide complementary data from these dual technologies. NIRS can be used before PCI to identify lipid-rich plaques that might be at risk of periprocedural myonecrosis and distal embolization, to evaluate the necessity of distal protection filters.[87] The Coronary Assessment by Near-infrared of Atherosclerotic Rupture-prone Yellow (CANARY) Trial was a randomized clinical study on 57 patients undergoing coronary angiography and NIRS-IVUS imaging. Patients were randomized to angioplasty with or without a distal embolic protection device. The results showed that lipid-rich plaques identified by NIRS are associated with higher rates of periprocedural MI. However, the use of a distal protection filter did not prevent myonecrosis after PCI at lipid-rich plaques.[88]

Optical Coherence Tomography
Cardiovascular OCT is a catheter-based imaging technique that uses light and its reflection to create images of the coronary wall. Initially developed to perform imaging of the retina, OCT technology rapidly expanded to various biomedical and clinical applications.

Principles. OCT is based on a fiberoptic wire with a rotating lens that emits near-infrared light (approximately 1300 nm) and records the light reflected from the analyzed tissue. One of the most valuable properties of OCT is its high resolution, up to 10 µ for axial resolution and 20 µ for lateral resolution (i.e., superior to IVUS). Although resolution is high, tissue penetration ranges from 1.0 to 3.5 mm (i.e., inferior to IVUS).

The images created by OCT are derived from the delay that results from the light traveling to the target tissue and back to the lens. Images are generated by measuring the echo time delay and the intensity of reflected light. The speed of light does not allow direct measurement of the echo time delay, so a technique known as *interferometry* has been developed to analyze the reflected light signal. With this technique the light reflected from target tissue is measured by correlating it with light that has traveled a known reference distance. Cross-sectional images of the vessel are created by obtaining multiple axial scans as the fiberoptic wire is simultaneously rotating and pulled back rapidly along the vessel.

Two types of OCT imaging systems have been developed: *time-domain* OCT (TD-OCT) and Fourier-domain OCT, also known as *frequency-domain* OCT (FD-OCT). Using a novel wavelength-swept laser as a light source, FD-OCT imaging systems provide superior signal-to-noise ratio and allow significantly faster imaging speed compared with the earlier time-domain technology. Recent FD-OCT imaging systems are capable of acquiring images at a rate of 180 frames/second at a pullback speed of up to 36 mm/sec. One single pullback allows imaging of up to 75 mm of the vessel.

Early OCT technology required a complete displacement of blood from the viewing field to generate high-quality images. An over-the-wire low-pressure occlusion balloon catheter with distal flush ports to infuse saline or Ringer lactate can be used to remove erythrocytes from the viewing field. However, the accelerated pullback speed provided by FD-OCT no longer requires occlusion of the vessel, with a shift toward a nonocclusive approach with flushing of contrast.

Clinical Applications

OCT can be used to guide diagnosis during coronary angiography as well as procedure planning and assessment of PCI, as indicated in an initial clinical study.[89]

Normal Vessel Wall

In a healthy vessel, OCT visualizes the coronary artery wall as a three layered structure (Fig. 21.22). The intima appears as a thin, highly reflective, and signal-rich layer. Although not able to visualize the "healthy" intima layer since that is beyond its resolution, OCT can identify intimal thickening: an early stage of atherosclerosis that appears as a signal-rich, homogeneous, thin rim of tissue. The media layer appears as a dark, low-reflective band with a mean media thickness of 200 μm delimited by the internal elastic lamina, an adluminal signal-rich line, and the external elastic lamina, an abluminal signal-rich line. With its limited tissue penetration (1 to 1.5 mm), OCT is not able to characterize vessel remodeling. Finally, the adventitia appears as a signal-rich, heterogeneously textured outer layer.

Stable Coronary Artery Disease

In patients with stable CAD, OCT imaging is used for quantitative assessment of the lesion by measuring the minimal lumen area (MLA). For the identification of hemodynamically severe coronary stenosis, OCT was shown to have only moderate diagnostic efficiency, when using the gold standard FFR as a reference, and similar accuracy compared with IVUS.[90]

Plaque Morphology

High-risk features of plaques, including a large lipid core, thin fibrous cap, and increased macrophage infiltration, can be detected by OCT.[91]

First, OCT provides the possibility to distinguish between fibrotic, lipid-rich, and calcified lesions. Lipids are signal-poor regions with diffuse borders, while fibrous tissue appears as a signal-rich homogenous region, and fibrocalcific or calcific tissue appear as well-delineated, signalpoor regions with sharp borders.

Second, OCT is the only imaging technique that in vivo allows an accurate evaluation of the fibrous cap and macrophage content. Smooth muscle cells organized in a collagenous-proteoglycan matrix, with varying degrees of infiltration by macrophages and lymphocytes, compose the fibrous cap of the plaque. Thin fibrous cap, lower collagen density, thinner collagen fibers, or low number of smooth muscle cells (SMCs) are highly related to plaque rupture. OCT has shown high accuracy in detecting thin fibrous cap, with a specificity of 79% and sensitivity of 90%.[92] The implemented polarization-sensitive OCT (PS-OCT) technology is able to assess collagen density and its polarization as well as quantify the presence of the SMCs. In particular, PS-OCT allows measurement of birefringence, a property that is elevated in tissues containing proteins with an ordered structure such as collagen and SMCs actin/myosin. Accordingly, a high positive correlation between PS-OCT with thick collagen fiber content and SMC density has been demonstrated.

Finally, OCT may allow visualization of plaque's macrophages that appear as a signal-rich punctate dots, distinct or confluent, which exceed the intensity of background speckle noise. Macrophages may often be distributing at the boundary between the bottom of the cap and the top of a necrotic core. Also for the evaluation of macrophages, dedicated software has been developed that provides a higher accuracy than simple visual inspection.

Acute Coronary Syndrome

In patients with ACS, OCT has not only high sensitivity to detect intraluminal thrombus but also the capability of discriminating between red and white thrombus (Fig. 21.23). Furthermore, OCT has higher sensitivity in detecting fibrous cap rupture (Fig. 21.24) and fibrous cap erosion compared with IVUS.[89] The capability of OCT to discriminate the underlying mechanism of ACS has direct impact on further treatment

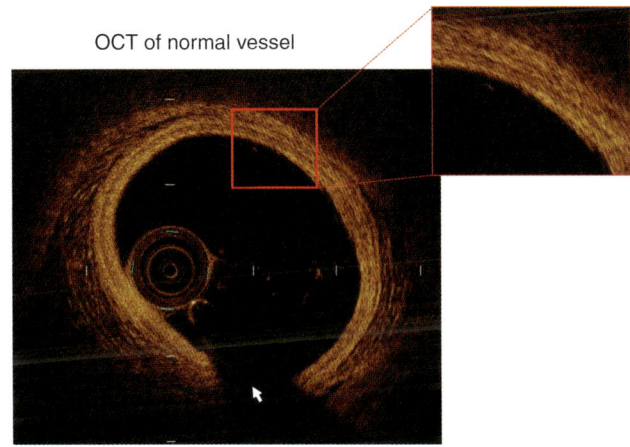

FIGURE 21.22 Optical coherence tomography (OCT) of a healthy vessel: The coronary artery wall is visualized as a layered structure. (Courtesy Dr. Annapoorna Kini, Icahn School of Medicine at Mount Sinai, New York, NY.)

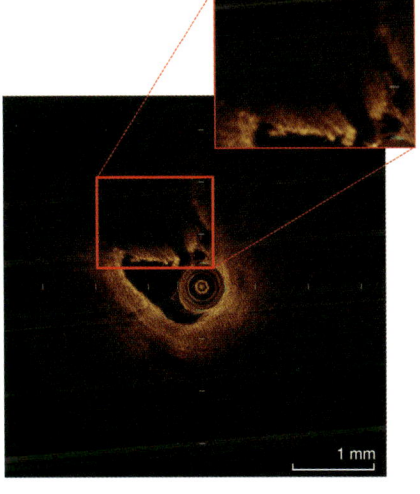 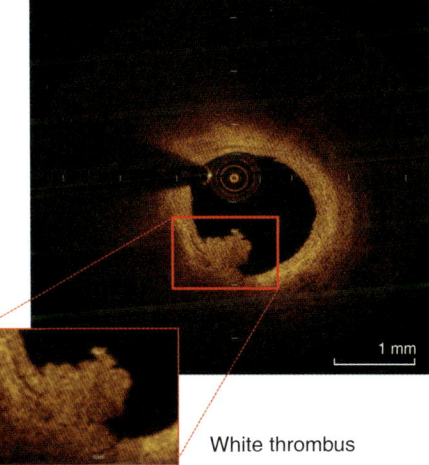

FIGURE 21.23 OCT is capable of discriminating between red **(left)** and white **(right)** thrombus. (Courtesy Dr. Annapoorna Kini, Icahn School of Medicine at Mount Sinai, New York, NY.)

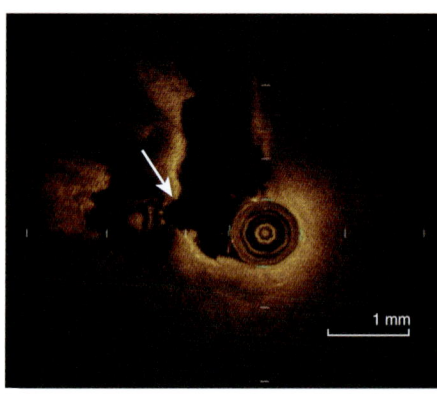

FIGURE 21.24 OCT of a ruptured fibrous cap. *Arrow* indicates the rupture site. (Courtesy Dr. Annapoorna Kini, Icahn School of Medicine at Mount Sinai, New York, NY.)

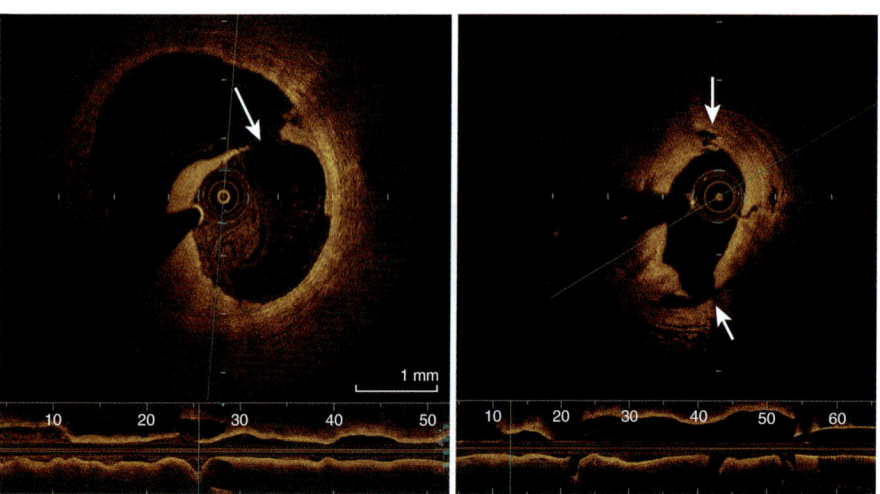

FIGURE 21.25 OCT of a dissected vessel. **Left,** Spontaneous coronary artery dissection (SCAD). **Right,** Dissection after balloon pre-dilation. *Arrows* indicate the sites of rupture. (Courtesy Dr. Annapoorna Kini, Icahn School of Medicine at Mount Sinai, New York, NY.)

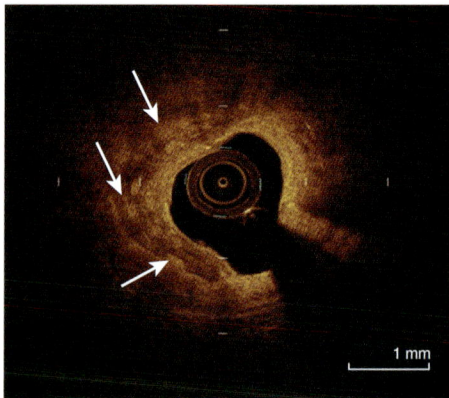

FIGURE 21.26 OCT of a severely calcified lesion. *Arrows* indicate some of the calcifications. (Courtesy Dr. Annapoorna Kini, Icahn School of Medicine at Mount Sinai, New York, NY.)

Concentric but thin calcium allows the use of regular or scoring balloons, whereas thicker concentric calcium may require atherectomy[93] (Fig. 21.26). OCT imaging can guide adequate lesion preparation, which is crucial for optimal stent deployment, but it can also be helpful for stent selection. Stent diameter, as well as length, can be chosen according to measurements of the reference vessel diameter both proximal and distal to the target lesion, as well as the lesion length. The fast-pullback acquisition of images makes FD-OCT less susceptible to artifacts resulting from heart motion, and therefore an optimal tool for accurate measurement of lesion length.

Assessment After Percutaneous Coronary Intervention

Post-PCI OCT offers the possibility to detect postprocedural complications and to provide information on the potential need for further procedural steps. OCT is used for ensuring appropriate stent expansion and evaluating apposition of the stent with the vessel wall (Fig. 21.27). Stent underexpansion, associated with small minimal stent area measured by OCT, was shown to be an independent predictor of device-oriented clinical endpoints, including cardiac death, target vessel–related MI, target lesion revascularization, and stent thrombosis.[94] By allowing the determination of the distance of each stent strut from the vessel wall, OCT is capable of detecting the percentage of malapposed stent struts, which were shown to be associated with delayed neointimal coverage.[95] The presence of uncovered stent struts detected by OCT was proposed as an independent predictor of late stent thrombosis in drug-eluting stents.[96] In particular, for bioresorbable scaffolds, the rate of stent thrombosis seems to increase significantly in malapposition. Therefore, use of OCT is strongly recommended after deployment of such a stent. *Stent edge dissection* (SED) is another post-PCI complication that is detectable by OCT that has been shown to be associated with adverse clinical outcomes.[97] However, the vast majority of SEDs diagnosed by OCT heal without further treatment, and additional stenting should be reserved for the presence of intramural hematoma, as recently suggested.[93] Deployment of stent edges within the normal vessel wall and appropriate selection of stent diameter may help to avoid SED.[97] Compared with SED, tissue protrusion is a less investigated post-PCI complication. Irregular tissue protrusion was shown to be associated with device-related clinical endpoints, which were primarily driven by target lesion revascularization.[94] However, the further management of tissue protrusion detected by OCT is not yet clear.

CO-REGISTRATION OF INTRAVASCULAR IMAGING AND X-RAY ANGIOGRAPHY FOR PATIENTS UNDERGOING PERCUTANEOUS CORONARY INTERVENTION. During coronary invasive procedures, it may be difficult to identify corresponding segments between intracoronary imaging and angiography. To overcome this limitation, several tools have been recently developed, providing a real-time point-to-point co-registration that allow a precise integration of angiographic and intravascular imaging. Co-registration tools are available for both IVUS and OCT. These technologies offer more precise localization and characterization of the lesions and support an optimal stent implantation. To understand the impact of co-registration on the angiographic results, several studies have been conducted. The prospective single-arm DOCTOR (Does Optical Coherence Tomography Optimize Revascularization) study, including patients admitted for elective PCI, assessed the relevance of co-registration for a correct stent implantation. Without access to co-registered data, the segment of the target lesion indicated by OCT was left uncovered by the stent in approximately 70% of the stented population.[98]

strategy. Furthermore, the possibility to detect vulnerable plaques among the nonculprit lesions is also extremely important to prevent recurrence of ischemic events. In SCAD (Fig. 21.25), one of the non-CAD-related causes that can be detected by OCT, unnecessary stent implantation, can be avoided.

Procedure Planning and Lesion Preparation

In procedural planning for PCI, OCT is a valuable tool for assessing the landing zone and especially for measuring calcium thickness.

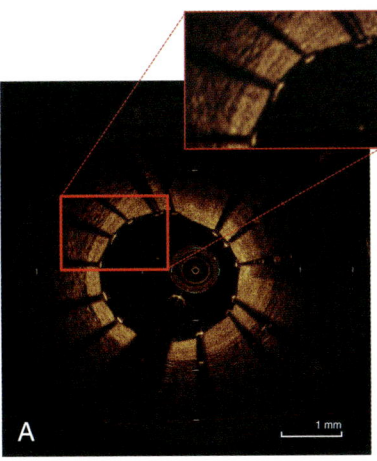
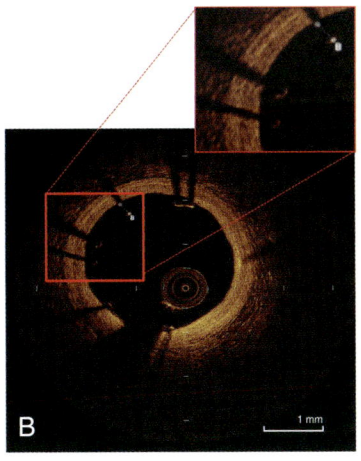

FIGURE 21.27 OCT is capable of evaluating apposition of a stent. **Left,** Good stent apposition. **Right,** Stent malapposition. (Courtesy Dr. Annapoorna Kini, Icahn School of Medicine at Mount Sinai, New York, NY.)

ACKNOWLEDGMENTS
The authors thank Dr. Sabato Sorrentino for editorial assistance.

CLASSIC REFERENCES

Goldenberg I, Matetzky S. Nephropathy induced by contrast media: pathogenesis, risk factors and preventive strategies. *Can Med Assoc J.* 2005;172:1461–1471.

Katayama H, Yamaguchi K, Kozuka T, et al. Adverse reactions to ionic and nonionic contrast media: a report from the Japanese Committee on the Safety of Contrast Media. *Radiology.* 1990;175:621–628.

Lasser EC, Berry CC, Talner LB, et al. Pretreatment with corticosteroids to alleviate reactions to intravenous contrast material. *N Engl J Med.* 1987;317:845–849.

Mehran R, Aymong ED, Nikolsky E, et al. A simple risk score for prediction of contrast-induced nephropathy after percutaneous coronary intervention: development and initial validation. *J Am Coll Cardiol.* 2004;44:1393–1399.

Rentrop KP, Cohen M, Blanke H, Phillips RA. Changes in collateral channel filling immediately after controlled coronary artery occlusion by an angioplasty balloon in human subjects. *J Am Coll Cardiol.* 1985;5:587–592.

Ryan TJ. The coronary angiogram and its seminal contributions to cardiovascular medicine over five decades. *Circulation.* 2002;106:752–756.

Sellers RD, Levy MJ, Amplatz K, et al. Left retrograde cardioangiography in acquired cardiac disease: technique, indications and interpretation in 700 cases. *Am J Cardiol.* 1964;14:437.

Yamanaka O, Hobbs RE. Coronary artery anomalies in 126,595 patients undergoing coronary arteriography. *Cathet Cardiovasc Diagn.* 1990;21:28–40.

REFERENCES

Indications, Appropriate Use, and Risks

1. Oudkerk M, ed. *Coronary Radiology.* 1st ed. 2013.
2. Writing Group M, Mozaffarian D, Benjamin EJ, et al. Executive summary: heart disease and stroke Statistics-2016 update: a report from the American Heart Association. *Circulation.* 2016;133(4):447–454.
3. Amsterdam EA, Wenger NK, Brindis RG, et al. 2014 AHA/ACC guideline for the management of patients with non-ST-elevation acute coronary syndromes: a report of the American College of Cardiology/American Heart Association Task Force on Practice Guidelines. *J Am Coll Cardiol.* 2014;64(24):e139–228.
4. Patel MR, Bailey SR, Bonow RO, et al. ACCF/SCAI/AATS/AHA/ASE/ASNC/HFSA/HRS/SCCM/SCCT/SCMR/STS 2012 appropriate use criteria for diagnostic catheterization: a report of the American College of Cardiology Foundation Appropriate Use Criteria Task Force, Society for Cardiovascular Angiography and Interventions, American Association for Thoracic Surgery, American Heart Association, American Society of Echocardiography, American Society of Nuclear Cardiology, Heart Failure Society of America, Heart Rhythm Society, Society of Critical Care Medicine, Society of Cardiovascular Computed Tomography, Society for Cardiovascular Magnetic Resonance, and Society of Thoracic Surgeons. *J Am Coll Cardiol.* 2012;59(22):1995–2027.
5. Kumamaru KK, Arai T, Morita H, et al. Overestimation of pretest probability of coronary artery disease by Duke clinical score in patients undergoing coronary CT angiography in a Japanese population. *J Cardiovasc Comput Tomogr.* 2014;8(3):198–204.
6. Arbab-Zadeh A. Stress testing and non-invasive coronary angiography in patients with suspected coronary artery disease: time for a new paradigm. *Heart Int.* 2012;7(1):e2.
7. O'Gara PT, Kushner FG, Ascheim DD, et al. 2013 ACCF/AHA guideline for the management of ST-elevation myocardial infarction: executive summary: a report of the American College of Cardiology Foundation/American Heart Association Task Force on Practice Guidelines: developed in collaboration with the American College of Emergency Physicians and Society for Cardiovascular Angiography and Interventions. *Catheter Cardiovasc Interv.* 2013;82(1):E1–E27.
8. Desai NR, Bradley SM, Parzynski CS, et al. Appropriate use criteria for coronary revascularization and trends in utilization, patient selection, and appropriateness of percutaneous coronary intervention. *J Am Med Assoc.* 2015;314(19):2045–2053.
9. Bradley SM, Spertus JA, Kennedy KF, et al. Patient selection for diagnostic coronary angiography and hospital-level percutaneous coronary intervention appropriateness: insights from the National Cardiovascular Data Registry. *JAMA Intern Med.* 2014;174(10):1630–1639.
10. Bradley SM, Maddox TM, Stanislawski MA, et al. Normal coronary rates for elective angiography in the Veterans Affairs Healthcare System: insights from the VA CART program (Veterans Affairs Clinical Assessment Reporting and Tracking). *J Am Coll Cardiol.* 2014;63(5):417–426.
11. Bjerking LH, Hansen KW, Madsen M, et al. Use of diagnostic coronary angiography in women and men presenting with acute myocardial infarction: a matched cohort study. *BMC Cardiovasc Discord.* 2016;16:120.
12. Pradhan AD, Visweswaran GK, Gilchrist IC. Coronary angiography and percutaneous interventions in pregnancy. *Minerva Ginecol.* 2012;64(5):345–359.
13. Tavakol M, Ashraf S, Brener SJ. Risks and complications of coronary angiography: a comprehensive review. *Global J Health Sci.* 2012;4(1):65–93.
14. Eshtehardi P, Adorjan P, Togni M, et al. Iatrogenic left main coronary artery dissection: incidence, classification, management, and long-term follow-up. *Am Heart J.* 2010;159(6):1147–1153.
15. Chen J, Gao L, Yao M, Chen J. Ventricular arrhythmia onset during diagnostic coronary angiography with a 5F or 4F universal catheter. *Rev Esp Cardiol.* 2008;61(10):1092–1095.
16. Werner N, Zahn R, Zeymer U. Stroke in patients undergoing coronary angiography and percutaneous coronary intervention: incidence, predictors, outcome and therapeutic options. *Expert Rev Cardiovasc Ther.* 2012;10(10):1297–1305.
17. Baker NC, O'Connell EW, Htun WW, et al. Safety of coronary angiography and percutaneous coronary intervention via the radial versus femoral route in patients on uninterrupted oral anticoagulation with warfarin. *Am Heart J.* 2014;168(4):537–544.
18. Mehran R, Dangas GD, Weisbord SD. Contrast-associated acute kidney injury. *N Engl J Med.* 2019;380(22):2146–2155.
19. James MT, Ghali WA, Knudtson ML, et al. Associations between acute kidney injury and cardiovascular and renal outcomes after coronary angiography. *Circulation.* 2011;123(4):409–416.
20. James MT, Ghali WA, Tonelli M, et al. Acute kidney injury following coronary angiography is associated with a long-term decline in kidney function. *Kidney Int.* 2010;78(8):803–809.
21. Rudnick MR, Goldfarb S, Wexler L, et al. Nephrotoxicity of ionic and nonionic contrast media in 1196 patients: a randomized trial. The Iohexol Cooperative Study. *Kidney Int.* 1995;47(1):254–261.
22. McCullough PA, Stacul F, Becker CR, et al. Contrast-Induced Nephropathy (CIN) consensus working panel: executive summary. *Rev Cardiovasc Med.* 2006;7(4):177–197.
23. Brar SS, Aharonian V, Mansukhani P, et al. Haemodynamic-guided fluid administration for the prevention of contrast-induced acute kidney injury: the POSEIDON randomised controlled trial. *Lancet.* 2014;383(9931):1814–1823.
24. Briguori C, Visconti G, Focaccio A, et al. Renal Insufficiency After Contrast Media Administration Trial II (REMEDIAL II): RenalGuard system in high-risk patients for contrast-induced acute kidney injury. *Circulation.* 2011;124(11):1260–1269.
25. Koc F, Ozdemir K, Kaya MG, et al. Intravenous N-acetylcysteine plus high-dose hydration versus high-dose hydration and standard hydration for the prevention of contrast-induced nephropathy: CASIS—a multicenter prospective controlled trial. *Int J Cardiol.* 2012;155(3):418–423.
26. Sun Z, Fu Q, Cao L, et al. Intravenous N-acetylcysteine for prevention of contrast-induced nephropathy: a meta-analysis of randomized, controlled trials. *PloS One.* 2013;8(1):e55124.
27. Brar SS, Hiremath S, Dangas G, et al. Sodium bicarbonate for the prevention of contrast induced-acute kidney injury: a systematic review and meta-analysis. *Clin J Am Soc Nephrol.* 2009;4(10):1584–1592.
28. Zoungas S, Ninomiya T, Huxley R, et al. Systematic review: sodium bicarbonate treatment regimens for the prevention of contrast-induced nephropathy. *Ann Intern Med.* 2009;151(9):631–638.
29. Mann DL, Zipes DP, Libby P, Bonow RO. In: *Braunwald's Heart Disease: A Textbook of Cardiovascular Medicine.* 10th ed. 2014.
30. Brown KR, Rzucidlo E. Acute and chronic radiation injury. *J Vasc Surg.* 2011;53(suppl 1):15S–21S.
31. Chambers CE, Fetterly KA, Holzer R, et al. Radiation safety program for the cardiac catheterization laboratory. *Catheter Cardiovasc Interv.* 2011;77(4):546–556.
32. Christopoulos G, Makke L, Christakopoulos G, et al. Optimizing radiation safety in the cardiac catheterization laboratory: a practical approach. *Catheter Cardiovasc Interv.* 2016;87(2):291–301.
33. Naidu SS, Aronow HD, Box LC, et al. SCAI expert consensus statement: 2016 best practices in the cardiac catheterization laboratory (endorsed by the Cardiological Society of India, and Sociedad Latino Americana de Cardiologia Intervencionista; Affirmation of value by the Canadian Association of Interventional Cardiology-Association Canadienne de cardiologie d'intervention). *Catheter Cardiovasc Interv.* 2016;88(3):407–423.
34. Christopoulos G, Papayannis AC, Alomar M, et al. Effect of a real-time radiation monitoring device on operator radiation exposure during cardiac catheterization: the radiation reduction during cardiac catheterization using real-time monitoring study. *Circ Cardiovasc Interv.* 2014;7(6):744–750.

Technique

35. Kern MS, P.Lim MJ. *Cardiac Catheterization Handbook.* 6th ed. 2015.
36. Hamid A. Anesthesia for cardiac catheterization procedures. *Heart Lung Vessel.* 2014;6(4):225–231.
37. Moscucci M. *Grossman & Baim's Cardiac Catheterization, Angiography, and Intervention.* 8th ed. 2013.

38. Valgimigli M, Gagnor A, Calabro P, et al. Radial versus femoral access in patients with acute coronary syndromes undergoing invasive management: a randomised multicentre trial. *Lancet*. 2015;385(9986):2465–2476.
39. Ho HH, Jafary FH, Ong PJ. Radial artery spasm during transradial cardiac catheterization and percutaneous coronary intervention: incidence, predisposing factors, prevention, and management. *Cardiovasc Revasc Med*. 2012;13(3):193–195.
40. Topol EJ, TPS. *Textbook of Interventional Cardiology*. 7th ed. 2015.
41. Sharma SK, Dangas G, Israel D, et al. Prospective evaluation of a stiff shaft glide wire compared with the standard straight wire in crossing severely stenotic aortic valves. *Am J Cardiol*. 1997;80(1):103–105.
42. Dickinson MC, Kam PC. Intravascular iodinated contrast media and the anaesthetist. *Anaesthesia*. 2008;63(6):626–634.
43. Godley 2nd RW, Joshi K, Breall JA. A comparison of the use of traditional hand injection versus automated contrast injectors during cardiac catheterization. *J Invasive Cardiol*. 2012;24(12):628–630.
44. Minsinger KD, Kassis HM, Block CA, et al. Meta-analysis of the effect of automated contrast injection devices versus manual injection and contrast volume on risk of contrast-induced nephropathy. *Am J Cardiol*. 2014;113(1):49–53.
45. Manual on Contrast Media of the American College of Radiology (ACR) Committee on Drugs and Contrast Media. Version 10.2. 2016.
46. Wang CL, Cohan RH, Ellis JH, et al. Frequency, outcome, and appropriateness of treatment of nonionic iodinated contrast media reactions. *AJR Am J Roentgenol*. 2008;191(2):409–415.
47. Loh S, Bagheri S, Katzberg RW, et al. Delayed adverse reaction to contrast-enhanced CT: a prospective single-center study comparison to control group without enhancement. *Radiology*. 2010;255(3):764–771.

Coronary Anatomy

48. Ouali S, Neffeti E, Sendid K, et al. Congenital anomalous aortic origins of the coronary arteries in adults: a Tunisian coronary arteriography study. *Arch Cardiovasc Dis*. 2009;102(3):201–208.
49. Villa AD, Sammut E, Nair A, et al. Coronary artery anomalies overview: the normal and the abnormal. *World J Radiol*. 2016;8(6):537–555.
50. Alexi-Meskishvili V, Nasseri BA, Nordmeyer S, et al. Repair of anomalous origin of the left coronary artery from the pulmonary artery in infants and children. *J Thorac Cardiovasc Surg*. 2011;142(4):868–874.
51. Yurtdas M, Gulen O. Anomalous origin of the right coronary artery from the left anterior descending artery: review of the literature. *Cardiol J*. 2012;19(2):122–129.
52. Ata Y, Turk T, Bicer M, et al. Coronary arteriovenous fistulas in the adults: natural history and management strategies. *J Cardiothorac Surg*. 2009;4:62.
53. Saboo SS, Juan YH, Khandelwal A, et al. MDCT of congenital coronary artery fistulas. *AJR Am J Roentgenol*. 2014;203(3):W244–W252.
54. Sohn J, Song JM, Jang JY, et al. Coronary artery fistula draining into the left ventricle. *J Cardiovasc Ultrasound*. 2014;22(1):28–31.
55. Bhatt DL. *Cardiovascular Intervention: A Companion to Braunwald's Heart Disease*. 1st ed. 2015.
56. Ishikawa Y, Akasaka Y, Suzuki K, et al. Anatomic properties of myocardial bridge predisposing to myocardial infarction. *Circulation*. 2009;120(5):376–383.
57. Serruys PW, Morice MC, Kappetein AP, et al. Percutaneous coronary intervention versus coronary-artery bypass grafting for severe coronary artery disease. *N Engl J Med*. 2009;360(10):961–972.
58. Medina A, Suarez de Lezo J, Pan M. A new classification of coronary bifurcation lesions. *Rev Esp Cardiol*. 2006;59(2):183.
59. Farooq V, Serruys PW, Bourantas CV, et al. Quantification of incomplete revascularization and its association with five-year mortality in the synergy between percutaneous coronary intervention with taxus and cardiac surgery (SYNTAX) trial validation of the residual SYNTAX score. *Circulation*. 2013;128(2):141–151.
60. Kobayashi Y, Lonborg J, Jong A, et al. Prognostic value of the residual SYNTAX score after functionally complete revascularization in ACS. *J Am Coll Cardiol*. 2018;72(12):1321–1329.
61. Nallamothu BK, Spertus JA, Lansky AJ, et al. Comparison of clinical interpretation with visual assessment and quantitative coronary angiography in patients undergoing percutaneous coronary intervention in contemporary practice: the Assessing Angiography (A2) project. *Circulation*. 2013;127(17):1793–1800.
62. Popma JJK S, Bhatt DL. *Coronary Arteriography and Intracoronary Imaging. Braunwald's Heart Disease: A Textbook of Cardiovascular Medicine*. 10th ed. Elsevier; 2015.
63. Kaya MG, Arslan F, Abaci A, et al. Myocardial blush grade: a predictor for major adverse cardiac events after primary PTCA with stent implantation for acute myocardial infarction. *Acta Cardiol*. 2007;62(5):445–451.
64. Rosendorff. *Essential Cardiology: Principles and Practice*. 3rd ed. 2013.
65. Rentrop KP, Cohen M, Blanke H, Phillips RA. Changes in collateral channel filling immediately after controlled coronary artery occlusion by an angioplasty balloon in human subjects. *J Am Coll Cardiol*. 1985;5(3):587–592.
66. Madhavan MV, Tarigopula M, Mintz GS, et al. Coronary artery calcification: pathogenesis and prognostic implications. *J Am Coll Cardiol*. 2014;63(17):1703–1714.
67. Chirumamilla AP, Maehara A, Mintz GS, et al. High platelet reactivity on clopidogrel therapy correlates with increased coronary atherosclerosis and calcification: a volumetric intravascular ultrasound study. *JACC Cardiovasc Imaging*. 2012;5(5):540–549.
68. Michelis KC, Olin JW, Kadian-Dodov D, et al. Coronary artery manifestations of fibromuscular dysplasia. *J Am Coll Cardiol*. 2014;64(10):1033–1046.

Intravascular Imaging

69. Kini AS, Vengrenyuk Y, Yoshimura T, et al. Fibrous cap thickness by optical coherence tomography in vivo. *J Am Coll Cardiol*. 2017;69(6):644–657.
70. Caixeta A, Maehara A, Mintz GS. *Intravascular Ultrasound: Principles, Image Interpretation, and Clinical Applications Interventional Cardiology: Principles and Practice*; 2011.
71. Maehara A, Cristea E, Mintz GS, et al. Definitions and methodology for the grayscale and radiofrequency intravascular ultrasound and coronary angiographic analyses. *JACC Cardiovasc Imaging*. 2012;5(suppl 3):S1–S9.
72. Garcia-Garcia HM, Mintz GS, Lerman A, et al. Tissue characterisation using intravascular radiofrequency data analysis: recommendations for acquisition, analysis, interpretation and reporting. *EuroIntervention*. 2009;5(2):177–189.
73. Sinclair H, Bourantas C, Bagnall A, et al. OCT for the identification of vulnerable plaque in acute coronary syndrome. *JACC Cardiovasc Imaging*. 2015;8(2):198–209.
74. Roleder T, Kovacic JC, Ali Z, et al. Combined NIRS and IVUS imaging detects vulnerable plaque using a single catheter system: a head-to-head comparison with OCT. *EuroIntervention*. 2014;10(3):303–311.
75. Levine GN, Bates ER, Blankenship JC, et al. 2011 ACCF/AHA/SCAI guideline for percutaneous coronary intervention: a report of the American College of Cardiology Foundation/American Heart Association Task Force on Practice Guidelines and the Society for Cardiovascular Angiography and Interventions. *Catheter Cardiovasc Interv*. 2013;82(4):E266–E355.
76. Witzenbichler B, Maehara A, Weisz G, et al. Relationship between intravascular ultrasound guidance and clinical outcomes after drug-eluting stents: the assessment of dual antiplatelet therapy with drug-eluting stents (ADAPT-DES) study. *Circulation*. 2014;129(4):463–470.
77. Saw J, Ricci D, Starovoytov A, et al. Spontaneous coronary artery dissection: prevalence of predisposing conditions including fibromuscular dysplasia in a tertiary center cohort. *JACC Cardiovasc Interv*. 2013;6(1):44–52.
78. Neumann FJ, Sousa-Uva M, Ahlsson A, et al. 2018 ESC/EACTS Guidelines on myocardial revascularization. *Eur Heart J*. 2019;40(2):87–165.
79. Stone GW, Maehara A, Lansky AJ, et al. A prospective natural-history study of coronary atherosclerosis. *N Engl J Med*. 2011;364(3):226–235.
80. Saw J, Mancini GB, Humphries KH. Contemporary review on spontaneous coronary artery dissection. *J Am Coll Cardiol*. 2016;68(3):297–312.
81. de la Torre Hernandez JM, Hernandez Hernandez F, Alfonso F, et al. Prospective application of pre-defined intravascular ultrasound criteria for assessment of intermediate left main coronary artery lesions results from the multicenter LITRO study. *J Am Coll Cardiol*. 2011;58(4):351–358.
82. Claessen BE, Mehran R, Mintz GS, et al. Impact of intravascular ultrasound imaging on early and late clinical outcomes following percutaneous coronary intervention with drug-eluting stents. *JACC Cardiovasc Interv*. 2011;4(9):974–981.
83. Raber L, Mintz GS, Koskinas KC, et al. Clinical use of intracoronary imaging. Part 1: guidance and optimization of coronary interventions. An expert consensus document of the European Association of Percutaneous Cardiovascular Interventions. *EuroIntervention*. 2018;14(6):656–677.
84. Lotfi A, Jeremias A, Fearon WF, et al. Expert consensus statement on the use of fractional flow reserve, intravascular ultrasound, and optical coherence tomography: a consensus statement of the Society of Cardiovascular Angiography and Interventions. *Catheter Cardiovasc Interv*. 2014;83(4):509–518.
85. Brugaletta S, Garcia-Garcia HM, Serruys PW, et al. NIRS and IVUS for characterization of atherosclerosis in patients undergoing coronary angiography. *JACC Cardiovasc Imaging*. 2011;4(6):647–655.
86. Sanon S, Dao T, Sanon VP, Chilton R. Imaging of vulnerable plaques using near-infrared spectroscopy for risk stratification of atherosclerosis. *Curr Atheroscler Rep*. 2013;15(2):304.
87. Kini AS, Baber U, Kovacic JC, et al. Changes in plaque lipid content after short-term intensive versus standard statin therapy: the YELLOW trial (reduction in yellow plaque by aggressive lipid-lowering therapy). *J Am Coll Cardiol*. 2013;62(1):21–29.
88. Stone GW, Maehara A, Muller JE, et al. Plaque characterization to inform the prediction and prevention of periprocedural myocardial infarction during percutaneous coronary intervention: the CANARY trial (Coronary Assessment by Near-Infrared of Atherosclerotic Rupture-Prone Yellow). *JACC Cardiovasc Interv*. 2015;8(7):927–936.
89. Kubo T, Imanishi T, Takarada S, et al. Assessment of culprit lesion morphology in acute myocardial infarction: ability of optical coherence tomography compared with intravascular ultrasound and coronary angioscopy. *J Am Coll Cardiol*. 2007;50(10):933–939.
90. Gonzalo N, Escaned J, Alfonso F, et al. Morphometric assessment of coronary stenosis relevance with optical coherence tomography: a comparison with fractional flow reserve and intravascular ultrasound. *J Am Coll Cardiol*. 2012;59(12):1080–1089.
91. Akasaka T, Kubo T, Mizukoshi M, et al. Pathophysiology of acute coronary syndrome assessed by optical coherence tomography. *J Cardiol*. 2010;56(1):8–14.
92. Kume T, Okura H, Yamada R, et al. Frequency and spatial distribution of thin-cap fibroatheroma assessed by 3-vessel intravascular ultrasound and optical coherence tomography: an ex vivo validation and an initial in vivo feasibility study. *Circ J*. 2009;73(6):1086–1091.
93. Roleder T, Jakala J, Kaluza GL, et al. The basics of intravascular optical coherence tomography. *Postepy Kardiol Interwencyjnej*. 2015;11(2):74–83.
94. Soeda T, Uemura S, Park SJ, et al. Incidence and clinical significance of poststent optical coherence tomography findings: one-year follow-up study from a multicenter registry. *Circulation*. 2015;132(11):1020–1029.
95. Gutierrez-Chico JL, Regar E, Nuesch E, et al. Delayed coverage in malapposed and side-branch struts with respect to well-apposed struts in drug-eluting stents: in vivo assessment with optical coherence tomography. *Circulation*. 2011;124(5):612–623.
96. Guagliumi G, Sirbu V, Musumeci G, et al. Examination of the in vivo mechanisms of late drug-eluting stent thrombosis: findings from optical coherence tomography and intravascular ultrasound imaging. *JACC Cardiovasc Interv*. 2012;5(1):12–20.
97. Chamie D, Bezerra HG, Attizzani GF, et al. Incidence, predictors, morphological characteristics, and clinical outcomes of stent edge dissections detected by optical coherence tomography. *JACC Cardiovasc Interv*. 2013;6(8):800–813.
98. Hebsgaard L, Nielsen TM, Tu S, et al. Co-registration of optical coherence tomography and X-ray angiography in percutaneous coronary intervention. The Does Optical Coherence Tomography Optimize Revascularization (DOCTOR) fusion study. *Int J Cardiol*. 2015;182:272–278.

22 Invasive Hemodynamic Diagnosis of Cardiac Disease

MORTON J. KERN, ARNOLD H. SETO, AND JOERG HERRMANN

INTRODUCTION TO INVASIVE HEMODYNAMIC DIAGNOSIS OF CARDIAC DISEASE, 385
Indications for Cardiac Catheterization and Hemodynamic Assessment, 385
Vascular Access, 386
Left-Heart Catheterization, 390
Right-Heart Catheterization, 391
Technical Aspects and Artifacts of Pressure Measurements, 391
Computations for Hemodynamic Measurements, 392
Cardiac Output Measurements, 393

NORMAL RIGHT AND LEFT HEART WAVEFORMS AND VALVULAR HEMODYNAMICS INCLUDING HOCM (LVOT GRADIENTS), 394

The Cardiac Cycle and Generation of Pressure Waves, 394
Normal Pressure Waveforms, 395
Evaluation of Valvular Heart Disease, 398
Calculation of Stenotic Valve Orifice Areas, 398
Aortic Valve Stenosis, 399
Low-Flow, Low-Gradient Aortic Stenosis, 400
Hypertrophic Obstructive Cardiomyopathy, 400
Mitral Valve Stenosis, 401
Pulmonary and Tricuspid Valve Stenosis, 401
Aortic Regurgitation, 401
Mitral Regurgitation, 402
Pulmonary and Tricuspid Valve Regurgitation, 402

SEPTAL DEFECTS AND LEFT-TO-RIGHT/ RIGHT-TO-LEFT SHUNTS, 403
Pericardial Disease and Restrictive Cardiomyopathy, 404
Normal Pericardial Function and Pathophysiology of Constriction, 404
Cardiac Tamponade, 405

PHYSIOLOGIC AND PHARMACOLOGIC MANEUVERS AND PV LOOPS, 405
Exercise Provocation, 406
Dynamic Exercise, 406
Static Exercise, 406
Pacing Tachycardia, 406
Pharmacologic Challenges, 407
Pressure-Volume (PV) Relationships, 408

ACKNOWLEDGMENT, 409

REFERENCES, 409

INTRODUCTION TO INVASIVE HEMODYNAMIC DIAGNOSIS OF CARDIAC DISEASE

The cardiac catheterization laboratory serves multiples roles, which include not only angiography and vascular interventions but also, structural interventions. The latter are directed to percutaneously correct valve diseases, atrial and ventricular septal defects, and septal ablation for hypertrophic cardiomyopathy. Six to seven decades ago the cardiac catheterization laboratory was essential for the hemodynamic assessment and understanding of various disease entities and provided the diagnostic foundation for the application of surgical structural interventions as they arose in those days. At the end of the 1970s the pendulum started to shift with the advancing development of two-dimensional and Doppler echocardiography, which allowed for an alternative assessment of both cardiac anatomy and hemodynamics in patients with structural heart disease. Coupled with the excitement of being able to perform percutaneous coronary interventions (PCIs), the focus of many cardiac catheterization laboratories shifted to coronary artery disease, leading to dwindling interest and expertise in invasive hemodynamic assessment of cardiac diseases. This loss, however, had to be regained with the advent of transcatheter aortic valve replacement (TAVR) in the 21st century, especially as contemporary studies indicate that the correlation between noninvasively (echocardiography) and invasively (cardiac catheterization) measured aortic valve area and gradient is imperfect. This is critically important when decisions on valve procedures are made as well as when gauging the success of these interventions instantly in the catheterization laboratory. With the renaissance of hemodynamic assessment of cardiac diseases, cardiologists of today, especially those engaged in the catheterization laboratory, must have a proper understanding of the principles and nuances of invasive hemodynamic assessment as well as their limitations for proper interpretation and patient management decisions. This chapter will address these concepts and the technical aspects of the cardiac catheterization. As with most diagnostic tools in medicine, hemodynamics cannot be used in a vacuum and must be coupled with the clinical presentation, physical examination, and adjunctive imaging modalities to arrive at accurate results.

Indications for Cardiac Catheterization and Hemodynamic Assessment

The scope of indications for cardiac catheterization are summarized.[1] As outlined, the cardiac catheterization laboratory enables invasive testing for cardiac disease and includes the acquisition of tissue samples (biopsies), imaging of vasculatures and heart chambers (intravascular and intracardiac ultrasound, optical coherence tomography, angiograms, and ventriculograms), and hemodynamic assessments (fractional flow reserve, vascular resistance, cardiac output, pressure gradients, etc.). Clinical history, physical examination, and additional (noninvasive) diagnostic studies guide the invasive hemodynamic evaluation. The ACC/AHA valvular heart disease guidelines, for instance, make it clear (class III recommendation) that the invasive assessment is not the default first-step diagnostic modality in the evaluation of patients with structural heart diseases. Hemodynamics are to be used, however, in case of discrepancies in the results of noninvasive evaluations (in particular the echocardiogram but also additional imaging and stress studies) with the clinical presentation and examination.

Contraindications to cardiac catheterization include fever, anemia, coagulopathy, electrolyte imbalance (especially hypokalemia predisposing to arrhythmias), and other systemic illnesses or conditions needing stabilization. The clinical necessity of cardiac catheterization should also be carefully considered when the diagnostic information or therapeutic intervention will not meaningfully impact patient management and outcomes. Furthermore, the procedure is to be done only with full explanation of its benefits and risks and informed consent of the patient. Most catheterization laboratories will also mandate that "do not resuscitate/do not intubate" orders will be suspended during the procedure.

Complications and Risks

For diagnostic catheterization, an analysis of the complications in more than 200,000 patients indicated the incidences of risks were death, ~0.2%; myocardial infarction, ~0.05%; stroke, ~0.07%; serious ventricular arrhythmia, ~0.5%; and major vascular complications (thrombosis, bleeding requiring transfusion, or pseudoaneurysm), ~1%. Compared with femoral or radial artery access, vascular complications occurred more often when the brachial artery approach was used and least when the radial approach was used.

Vascular Access
Arterial Access
Percutaneous Radial Artery Technique

Radial artery access has become the default approach for many labs (Fig. 22.1).[2] Compared with femoral artery access, transradial procedures have a lower risk of bleeding and vascular complications, superior patient comfort, and improved efficiency in post-procedural care. Documentation of adequate dual blood supply to the hand by either the Allen or the Barbeau test is no longer required in most patients.

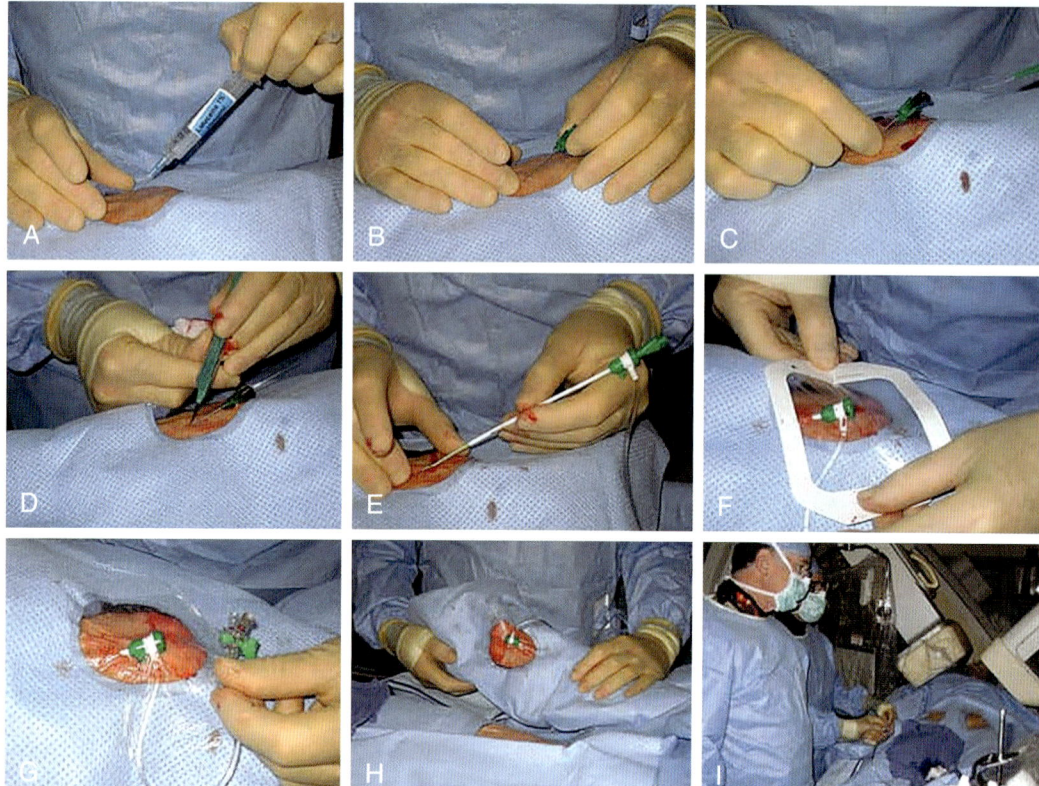

FIGURE 22.1 Radial artery access and sheath introduction. Once draped, the radial pulse is palpated. The point of puncture should be 1 to 2 cm cranial to the bony prominence of the distal radius. **A,** Administer a small amount of lidocaine into the skin. **B,** Use the needle (micropuncture needle shown here) at a 30- to 45-degree angulation. Slowly advance until blood pulsates out of needle. It will not be a strong pulsation because of the small bore of the needle. **C,** Fix needle position and carefully introduce a 0.018-inch guidewire with twirling motion. There should be little or no resistance to wire introduction. Remove needle. **D,** Make a small incision over the wire in preparation for sheath introduction (this step is optional). **E,** Advance the sheath over the wire into the artery. If sheath moves easily, advance to hub. If resistance is felt with sheath halfway in artery, remove wire and administer vasodilator cocktail. Reinsert wire and continue to advance the sheath. **F** and **G,** After the sheath is positioned and flushed, secure sheath with clear plastic dressing or suture (also optional). **H** and **I,** The arm can now be moved to the patient's side for catheter introduction. (From Sorraja P, et al. Kern's Cardiac Catheterization Handbook. 2020, p 104.)

In preparation for radial access, the arm should be placed on an appropriate board, abducted at a 30- to 45-degree angle, and the wrist should be hyperextended over a gauze roll. Unless prompted by anatomy or demand (e.g., left internal mammary artery injection), the right radial artery is used. Its distal course can be mapped by palpation or ultrasound; the latter reduces the difficulty of access and can be used to screen for small radial arteries or anatomical challenges before radial sheath insertion.[3] Only a small amount of 1% lidocaine (up to 1 mL) is injected at the skin entry site, which should be 1 to 2 cm cranial to the bony prominence of the distal radius. The radial artery is accessed by either a micropuncture needle (anterior wall technique) or a 20-gauge angiocatheter needle (posterior wall technique) at a 30- to 45-degree angle. With pulsatile blood return, a 0.018-inch guidewire is advanced into the artery, and there should be little or no resistance to wire advancement. If this were to be noted, access should be reexamined before proceeding. Otherwise, the needle is removed and the sheath is advanced over the wire into the artery. Once the sheath is in place, typically, 5000 units of unfractionated heparin are given as a bolus, or weight-adjusted (50 units per kg), to prevent postprocedural radial artery occlusion. Practices differ but one should consider smaller sizes for women (4 to 5F) yet larger sizes (6F, maximum 7F in men) if coronary intervention is likely. Overstretching of the artery is to be avoided as it leads to higher postprocedural occlusion rates. A longer sheath (up to 16 cm) has been considered to protect more against vasospasm at the level of the forearm. However, other studies suggest that it is the hydrophilic coating rather than the length of the sheath that reduces spasms. Arterial vasospasm is a complicating factor and prevented by adequate sedation, avoidance of limb cooling, and administration of vasodilators. Most commonly, nitroglycerin (100 to 200 mcg) and verapamil (2.5 mg) are given. Other approaches are sublingual nitroglycerin, and/or intra-arterial (local) administration of diltiazem or nicardipine. With these preparations, coronary angiographic catheters are advanced over a 0.035-inch floppy or small J-tipped guidewire into the ascending aorta and then manipulated to engage the coronary artery ostia. Some operators note catheter instability or poor coronary ostial engagement from the radial approach. Larger (>7F) sheath sizes that may be required for complex PCI also present a challenge for radial access.

After the procedure is completed, arterial puncture hemostasis is most often obtained with air-bladder compression bands or other similar closure devices (Fig. 22.2). In addition to adequate initial anticoagulation, the use of "patent hemostasis" (occlusion to the point of bleeding control but not complete vessel occlusion) minimizes the risk of radial artery occlusion. Hematomas, while uncommon, can lead to pseudoaneurysms and very rarely compartment syndrome. Other risks include radial artery vasospasm, dissections, transient hand dysfunction, and potentially a higher risk of future coronary artery bypass graft (CABG) radial graft dysfunction.

Percutaneous Femoral Artery Technique

Femoral artery access was the standard access over the last four decades.[4] Femoral artery access uses the Seldinger needle puncture technique with the insertion of a valved sheath (6 to 8F or larger) and use of preshaped "Judkins" catheters. The optimal puncture location is the common femoral artery (CFA). Familiarity with the anatomy will

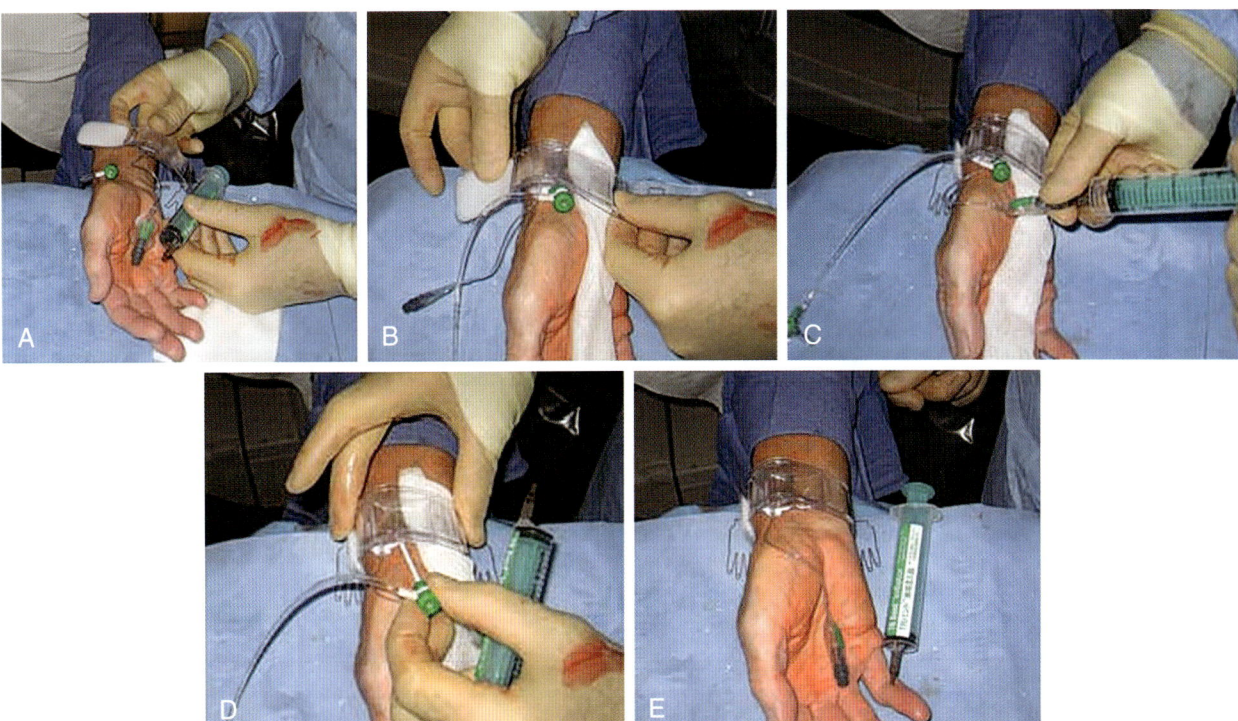

FIGURE 22.2 **A,** Radial sheath removal with Terumo band, which has an inflatable compression pad for hemostasis. **B,** Band is applied around the wrist with green dot over the arterial (not skin) puncture. A thin gauze wick is placed beneath the band to absorb blood when pressure is released to assess proper compression pressure in pad. **C,** Compression pad inflated. **D,** Sheath removed. **E,** Final result. (From Sorraja P, et al. Kern's Cardiac Catheterization Handbook. 7th ed. Elsevier; 2020, p 109.)

assist in identifying the point of needle entry, usually 1 to 3 cm below the inguinal ligament, in line with the palpable course of the CFA (Figs. 22.3 and 22.4). Superficial anatomic landmarks such as the inguinal crease can be misleading in obese as well as very thin individuals. Identifying the inferior edge of the femoral head by fluoroscopy using a hemostatic clamp is used to begin the puncture. Ultrasound imaging provides the best visualization and definition of the vascular location (Fig. 22.5) and has been shown to improve first-pass success rates and reduce vascular complications in general.[5] Correct placement of the sheath in the CFA will reduce the chance of retroperitoneal hematoma (as occurs with puncture that are above the inferior epigastric artery) or pseudoaneurysm and arteriovenous fistula formation (as occurs with punctures below the profunda and superficial femoral artery bifurcation). Accidental cannulation of the superficial or profunda femoral artery may result in limb ischemia or inability to accommodate vascular closure devices.

Once localization of the vessel is completed, local anesthesia with 1% lidocaine is given and a small incision is performed followed by insertion of an 18- to 21-gauge needle into the CFA in a modified Seldinger technique (Fig. 22.6). Upon pulsatile blood return, a 0.038-inch guidewire is advanced and should pass freely through the vessel. Symptoms of pain or excessive resistance on wire advancement may indicate vascular trauma, such as dissections or perforations, and should be recognized immediately. The advantages of the Judkins technique are the relative ease, speed, and reliability, and yet vigilance is still required to ensure quality and safety.

After the procedure, femoral hemostasis can be achieved with a vascular closure device or with manual compression. Despite their perceived benefit, vascular closure devices are not superior to manual compression in general and may in fact be inferior in patients who have had multiple vascular access needle attempts. Vascular closure devices do play an important role in cases of large-bore (>10F) access which are now common in the era of TAVR with sheath sizes of 18F to 24F. Femoral sheaths should not be removed until the activated clotting time (ACT) is less than 160 to 180 seconds unless a vascular closure device is being used.

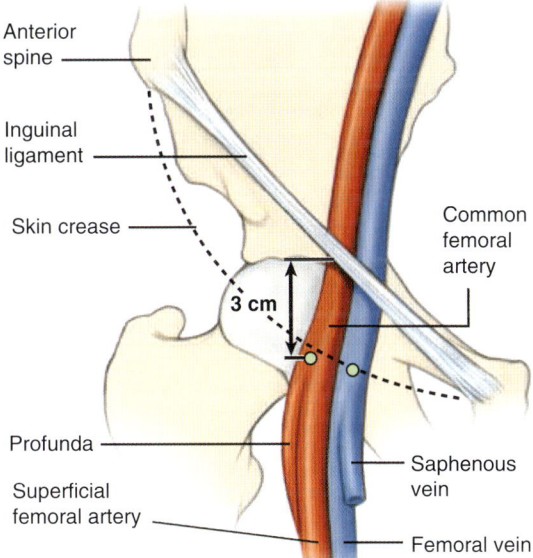

FIGURE 22.3 Regional anatomy relevant to percutaneous femoral arterial and venous catheterization. Diagram showing the right femoral artery and vein coursing underneath the inguinal ligament, which runs from the anterior superior iliac spine to the pubic tubercle. The arterial skin nick should be placed approximately 3 cm below the ligament and directly over the femoral arterial pulsation; the venous skin nick should be placed at the same level but approximately one fingerbreadth more medially. Although this level corresponds roughly to the skin crease in most patients, anatomic localization relative to the inguinal ligament provides a more constant landmark. (From Baim DS, Grossman W: Percutaneous approach, including transseptal and apical puncture. In Baim DS, Grossman W, editors: Cardiac Catheterization, Angiography, and Intervention. 7th ed. Philadelphia: Lea & Febiger; 2006, p 81.)

Patients with a history of peripheral arterial disease (PAD) require particular attention. Before the procedure, one should carefully review what types of interventions were performed in the past (e.g., balloon

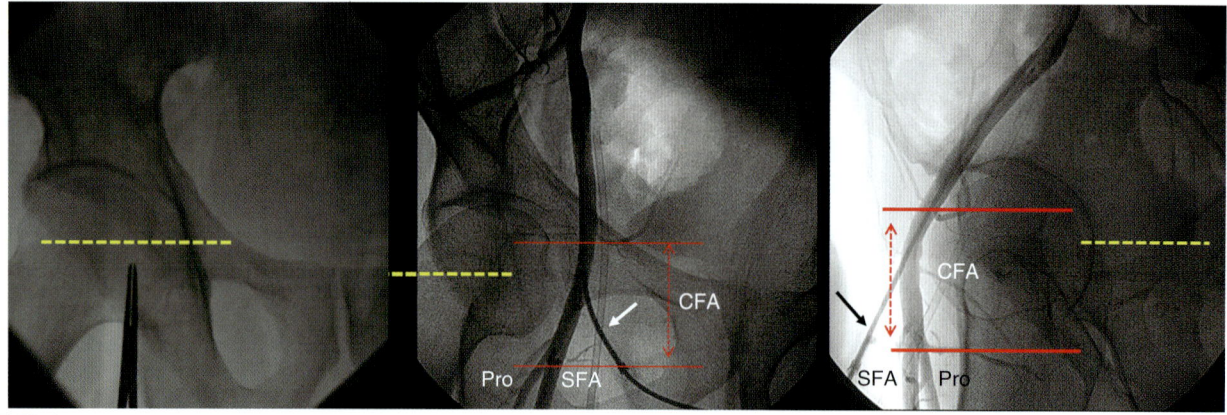

FIGURE 22.4 Left, Fluoroscopic localization of the skin nick (marked by the tip of the clamp). The middle of the femoral head is marked by the dashed yellow line. **Middle,** Angiogram of sheath in the femoral artery with a catheter (*arrow*) inserted in the common femoral artery. CFA is bounded by lower red line of the bifurcation of the superficial femoral artery (SFA) and profunda (Pro) branches and the upper red line of the inferior epigastric artery. **Right,** Lateral view of CFA (bounded by red lines) showing the relationship between the CFA and the bony femoral head, making manual compression effective.

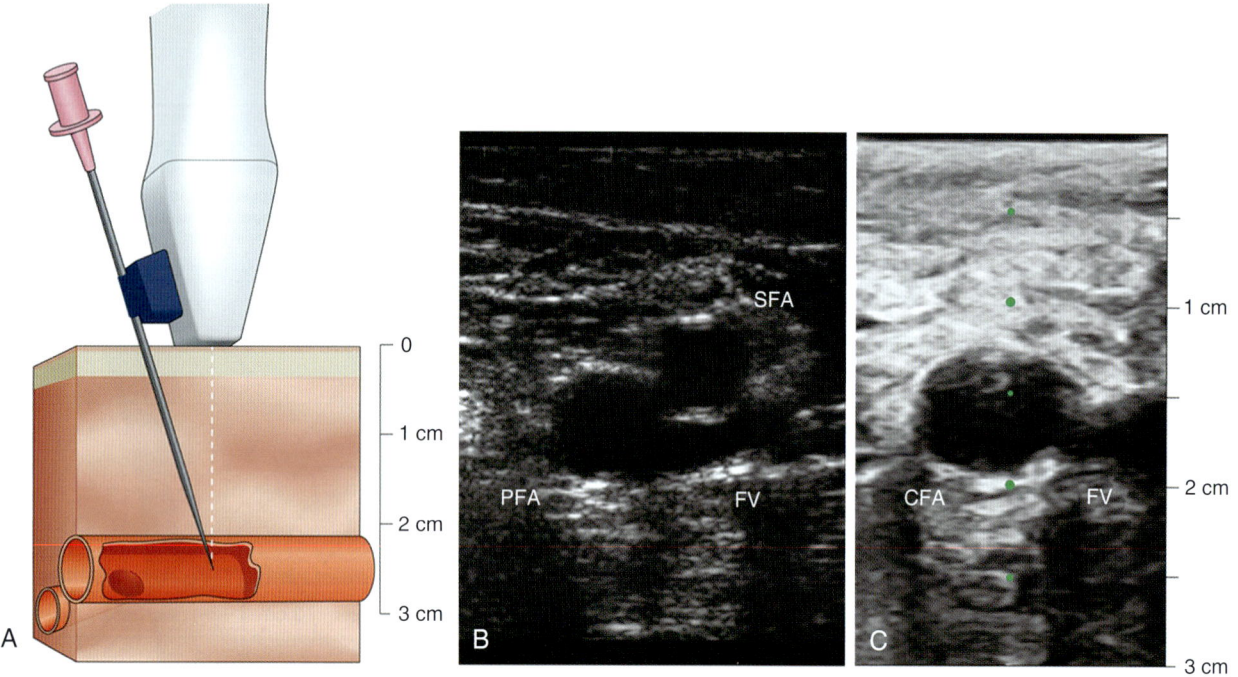

FIGURE 22.5 Ultrasound-guided femoral artery access. A, The attached needle guide fixes the needle's angle of entry to intersect the vessel at the imaging plane 1.5 cm, 2.5 cm, or 3.5 cm below the skin, depending upon the guide chosen. The vessel bifurcation is kept inferior to the probe at the time of insertion. **B,** The right femoral artery bifurcation is imaged in the axial plane, identifying the separation of the profunda femoral artery (PFA) and superficial femoral artery (SFA). Compression is used to differentiate arteries from the femoral vein (FV). **C,** The probe is moved superiorly until the common femoral artery (CFA) is visualized. During needle advancement, the anterior wall of the vessel is kept under the central target line (*green dots*), which indicates the path of the needle. (From Seto A, et al. Real-time ultrasound guidance facilitates femoral arterial access and reduces vascular complications: FAUST (Femoral Artery Access with Ultrasound Trial). JACC Cardiovasc Interv 2010;3:751.)

angioplasty, patch endarterectomy, arterial conduits, and prosthetic grafts). The vascular anatomy should be defined for location and size such that large devices may be accommodated. Prosthetic peripheral vascular grafts are the most problematic vascular challenges, not because they cannot be cannulated but rather because of the lack of adequate closure and potential for thrombotic occlusion. For these reasons, these grafts are usually avoided.

Venous Access

Right-heart hemodynamic assessment is critical to accurately provide a set of differential diagnoses for the causes of dyspnea, the severity and types of pulmonary hypertension, and the determination of cardiac output, among others. Many patients may require simultaneous right- and left-heart pressure measurements. Venous access may use femoral, brachial, or internal jugular approaches.

Percutaneous Femoral Vein Access

Using the femoral arterial pulse as a landmark, the femoral vein sits approximately 1 cm medial to the femoral artery. If a combined arterial and venous access is needed, the entry skin area is infiltrated by lidocaine sufficient to cover both puncture sites. The venous puncture site is 0.5 to 1 cm medial and 0.5 to 1 cm caudal to the planned arterial entry site. Because venous pressure is low, a 10- or 20-mL syringe is attached to the Seldinger needle and gently aspirated during needle advancement. The operator inserts the needle through the skin at a 30- to 45-degree angle to the horizontal plane while palpating the femoral arterial pulse with light pressure so as to not occlude the vein. If arterial pulsations are felt at the tip of the needle, the needle is withdrawn and redirected at a slightly more medial angle. Ultrasound imaging guidance can improve successful cannulation and reduce accidental arterial puncture. Upon entry of the vein, venous (nonpulsatile) dark blood should flow easily into the syringe. If the vein has not been entered, the needle is withdrawn,

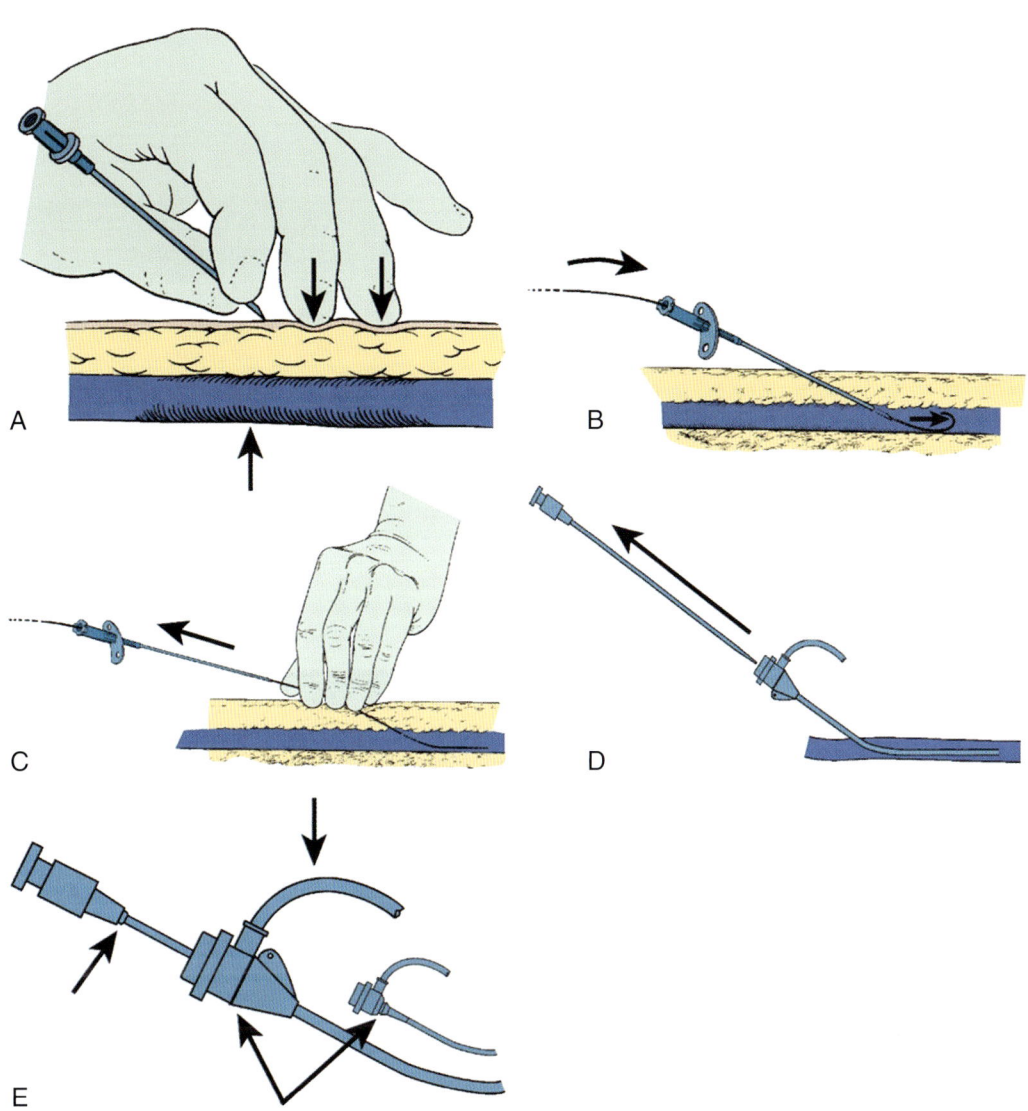

FIGURE 22.6 A, Femoral artery has been entered by a large-bore needle with backflow of blood. Note the operator's finger positions. As soon as the needle passes into the vessel through the anterior wall, brisk pulsatile flow occurs. This technique is called the "front wall stick." It prevents occult bleeding through the posterior wall. **B,** The flexible tip of the guidewire is passed through the needle into the vessel. **C,** Introducing a valve sheath into the artery. The needle is withdrawn, the artery is compressed, and the wire is pinched and fixed. **D,** The valve sheath is advanced over a guidewire, and the dilator and guidewire are removed. **E,** *Arrows* indicate position of sewing rings to attach valve to skin should prolonged insertion be required. (**A, B, C,** and **E** from Uretsky B, editor. Cardiac Catheterization: Concepts, Techniques, and Applications. Walden, Mass: Blackwell Science; 1997; **D** and **E** courtesy of Cordis Corporation, Miami, FL.)

flushed, and reintroduced in a slightly more lateral or medial direction. The remainder of the venous sheath placement is completed in the same fashion as described for the femoral arterial sheath insertion.

A vein that has been entered mistakenly during a femoral artery puncture attempt should be used only if the needle tip did not puncture both walls of the artery and go into the vein behind it. Placing a sheath through the artery into the vein may create an arteriovenous (AV) fistula or cause uncontrolled bleeding from a large hole in the posterior wall of the femoral artery.

After the procedure is completed, venous hemostasis can be achieved with light finger pressure applied over the vein as described for femoral artery sheath removal. Usually only 5 to 10 minutes of compression is needed to obtain adequate hemostasis.

Percutaneous Brachial Vein Access
In conjunction with radial artery catheterization, the brachial or antecubital vein may be considered for venous access for right-heart catheterization. Access to the antecubital vein can be obtained using a 20-gauge IV or ultrasound-guided needle puncture. Application of a tourniquet above the elbow will facilitate the identification of a suitable vein. A medial antecubital vein is preferable over a lateral antecubital vein to avoid the acute angulation of the cephalic vein system as it joins with the axillary vein in the shoulder. Before sheath insertion, administration of 1% lidocaine over the puncture site will reduce discomfort. The arm vein sheath size is usually 5F sheath but can be as large as 7F with a suitably sized balloon-tipped pulmonary artery (PA) catheter. Advancing the PA catheter is often straightforward, but if venous tortuosity or valve obstruction is present, the operator can facilitate advancement with an angioplasty guidewire or use an injection of saline to straighten and stiffen the catheter and expand the vein. The balloon should not be expanded until the catheter is in the subclavian system.

Percutaneous Internal Jugular Vein Access
The internal jugular (IJ) vein, especially the right IJ, is the preferred venous access given the anatomic ease and for prolonged placement of sheath or PA catheter. The IJ approach allows for greater patient comfort and lower infectious risk than a femoral approach, and is preferred over the subclavian approach because of reduced risk of pneumothorax. Use of a micropuncture kit with a 21-gauge needle and introducer will minimize inadvertent puncture of the carotid artery or

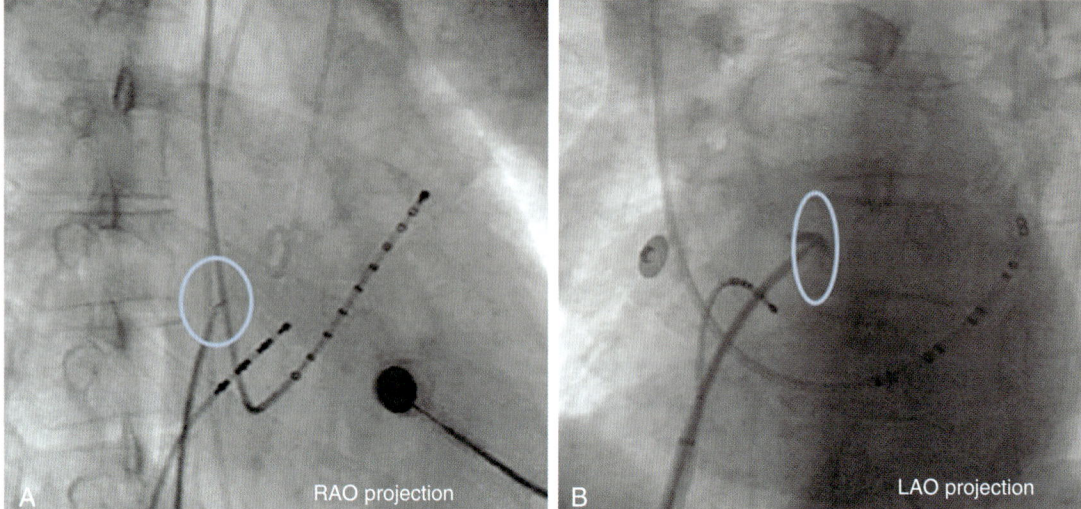

FIGURE 22.7 Septum crossing in fluoroscopy-guided transseptal puncture engaging the fossa ovalis in the right anterior oblique (RAO) **(A)** and left anterior oblique (LAO) **(B)** projections. Blue circle/oval indicate the fossa ovalis. Note the staining of the fossa ovalis in the LAO view. A pigtail is present in the RAO projection to mark the anterior location of the aorta.

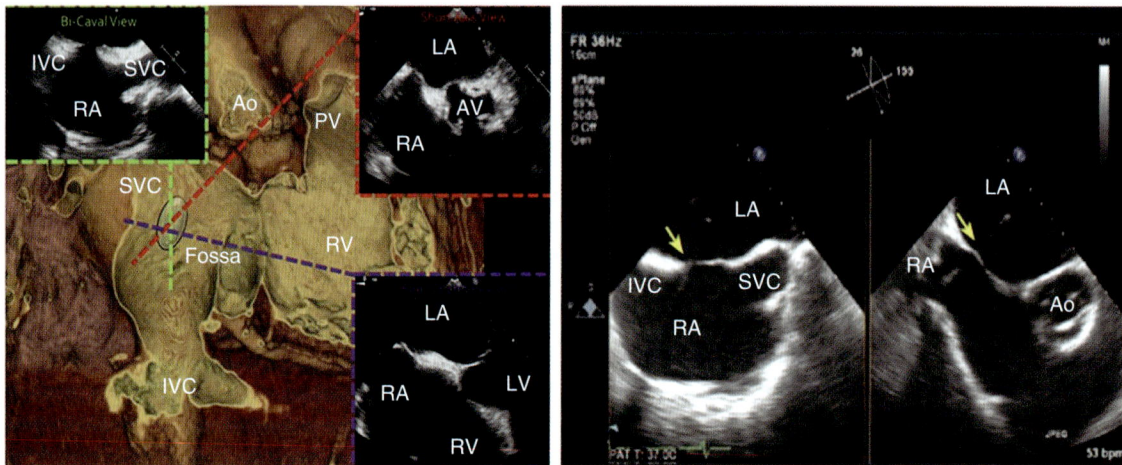

FIGURE 22.8 Biplane transesophageal echocardiography for transseptal puncture. *AV,* Aortic valve; *PV,* pulmonary vein; *SVC,* superior vena cava; other abbreviations as in Figure 22.2. (From Alkhouli M, et al. JACC Cardiovasc Interv 2016;9:2465-2480.)

lung. After entering the jugular vein, the micropuncture assembly can be exchanged for any larger sheath (e.g., 7F) for right-heart catheterization or right ventricular biopsy.

The internal jugular vein is located lateral to the carotid artery in the anatomic triangle of the two heads of the sternocleidomastoid muscle and the clavicle. For access, the patient is instructed to lie supine with the head turned 30 degrees to the contralateral side. Patients with low venous pressure may require leg elevation to increase venous filling volume. Routine use of ultrasound imaging facilitates localization of the IJ and can verify its patency. The use of ultrasound is recommended by national guidelines and reduces the overall risk of complications (carotid artery puncture, in particular) by 70%.[6]

Transseptal Catheterization

With increasing demands for certain structural heart disease evaluations and interventions (e.g., mitral valve disease) and some arrhythmia mapping procedures, transseptal catheterization has become an essential technique. In brief, the technique uses a right femoral venous access, through which a 0.032-inch guidewire and transseptal needle and catheter assembly is advanced into the right atrium and on into the superior vena cava (SVC). This catheter assembly is then brought back into the fossa ovalis using angiographic landmarks. Transesophageal or intracardiac echocardiography are also typically utilized, especially in difficult cases (e.g., large right atrium, postsurgical condition, anatomic variant) (Figs. 22.7 and 22.8). Once confident in its correct position, the needle and catheter are advanced through the fossa ovalis and into the left atrium. Transseptal catheterization of the left atrium is described in detail elsewhere.[7]

Left-Heart Catheterization

Retrograde access to the left ventricle is commonly performed using a straight or angled pigtail-shaped catheter, initially advanced over a 0.035-inch J-tip guidewire and initially positioned at the level of the AV. (Fig. 22.9). A common approach to crossing the AV is to position the pigtail catheter into the anterior sinus of Valsalva taking a "figure 6" configuration in the right anterior oblique (RAO) projection. The catheter is then pushed against the AV to form a U-shape. With deep inspiration, slight pullback and clockwise rotation, the tip loop usually falls across the valve into the left ventricle. Once inside the left ventricle, the catheter resumes a "figure 6" configuration with the loop directed toward the apex. Alternatively, the catheter can be positioned in front of the mitral valve, but not so deep as to interfere with its function or become entangled in the chordae. Repeated catheter repositioning may be required to eliminate ventricular ectopy.

With dilated aortic roots or horizontally oriented hearts, an angled pigtail catheter is preferable, whereas small aortic roots may require a right coronary Judkins for initial wiring and subsequent exchange for

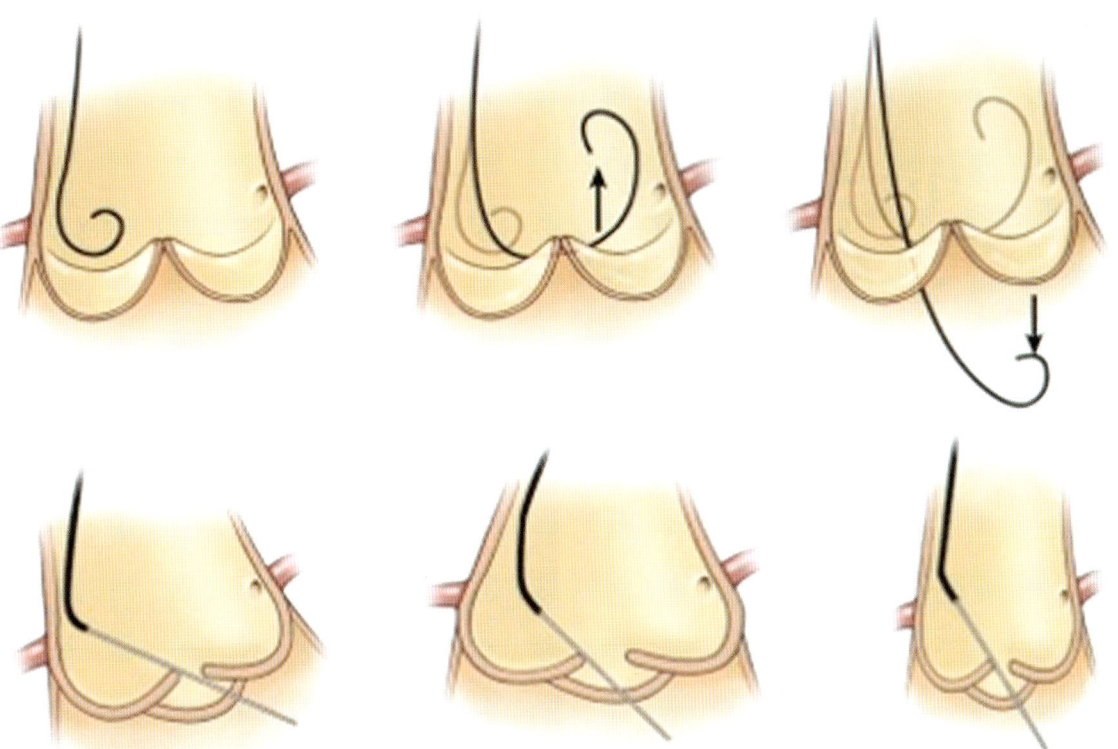

FIGURE 22.9 Technique for retrograde crossing of an aortic valve by a pigtail catheter. **Top row,** Technique for crossing a normal aortic valve. **Bottom row:** *Left,* Use of a straight guidewire and pigtail catheter in combination. Increasing the length of the protruding guidewire straightens the curve of the catheter and causes the wire to point more toward the right coronary ostium; reducing the length of the protruding wire restores the pigtail contour and deflects the tip of the guidewire toward the left coronary artery. When the correct length of wire and the correct rotational orientation of the catheter have been determined, repeated advancement and withdrawal of the catheter and guidewire together allow retrograde passage across the valve. *Middle,* In a dilated aortic root, an angled pigtail catheter is preferable. *Right,* In a small aortic root, a right coronary Judkins catheter may have advantages. In patients with bicuspid valves an Amplatz left catheter is often used because it directs the wire more superiorly. (From Baim DS, Grossman W. Percutaneous approach including transseptal and apical puncture. In Baim DS, Grossman W, editors. Cardiac Catheterization, Angiography, and Intervention. 6th ed. Philadelphia: Lea & Febiger; 2006, p 93.)

a pigtail catheter. In patients with bicuspid valves, a left Amplatz catheter directs the wire tip more superiorly and is also useful for placement of a guidewire into the left ventricle. A left Amplatz is also useful in patients with aortic stenosis, or a multipurpose catheter, depending on the angulation of the AV (more horizontal or more vertical). For sclerotic or stenotic AVs, straight rather than J-tipped guidewires facilitate probing of the AV orifice but also have greater potential for dislodging material from the AV or aorta with the risk of embolic ischemic events (including myocardial infarction and stroke).

For pressure measurements and contrast injections in the left ventricle, a pigtail catheter is preferred because of the high safety profile and inability to entrap the catheter tip in the LV musculature. Catheter tip entrapment leading to erroneous pressure signal readings is a problem for hypertrophic obstructive cardiomyopathy (HOCM) studies when end-hole catheters are used.

Aortic stenosis hemodynamics are best measured with simultaneous aortic and left ventricular (LV) pressures from a dual lumen catheter or use of a multipurpose catheter through which a 0.014-inch high-fidelity pressure sensor guidewire is advanced into the left ventricle while the catheter remains in the aorta. For gradients across the mitral valve, LV and pulmonary capillary wedge (PCW) or left atrial pressures are recorded simultaneously with two transducers. LV measurements include systolic, diastolic, and end-diastolic pressure; dP/dt can also be calculated. Details of obtaining and interpreting pressure measurements are discussed later in this chapter.

Right-Heart Catheterization

Right-heart catheterization is one of the central elements in the hemodynamic evaluation in the catheterization laboratory. The choice of venous access and catheter depends on the clinical presentation and patient-specific characteristics. The most commonly used right heart catheters are pulmonary balloon-tipped flotation (e.g., Swan-Ganz) catheters with multiple lumens for pressure recording and a thermistor sensor for thermodilution-based cardiac output measurement (Fig. 22.10). Single-lumen balloon wedge catheters have similar rigidity, larger caliber, less catheter whip artifact, and thus higher fidelity for pressure measurement but lack the capacity to determine cardiac output by thermodilution.

A standard pulmonary balloon-tipped catheter is relatively easy to advance into the right atrium, the right ventricle, and on to the pulmonary artery and PCW position (Fig. 22.11). Although catheter location can be noted from pressure tracings alone, fluoroscopy is advisable, especially if any structural and functional difficulties (e.g., severe right atrial enlargement, severe TR, severe right ventricular [RV] dilation) are encountered or pacing/defibrillator leads are present. Even more so under the latter circumstances, fluoroscopy should be considered for a left IJ approach. Some maneuvering of the catheter may require guidewire assistance.

Technical Aspects and Artifacts of Pressure Measurements

Before addressing the normal and abnormal pressure waveforms used in the hemodynamic diagnosis of cardiac disease, a basic understanding of factors and artifacts affecting the accurate recording of pressure waveforms is required. A correct interpretation of the pressure waveforms requires confidence in the data. A *pressure wave* is the cyclic force generated by cardiac muscle contraction, and its amplitude and duration are influenced by various mechanical and physiologic parameters. The pressure waveform is influenced by the force of the contracting chamber. The waveform is also a function of chamber compliance, both intrinsic and extrinsic (i.e., the surrounding structures, including the contiguous chambers of the heart, pericardium, lungs, and vasculature). Physiologic variables of heart rate, respiratory cycle, and vascular resistance all influence the pressure waveform.

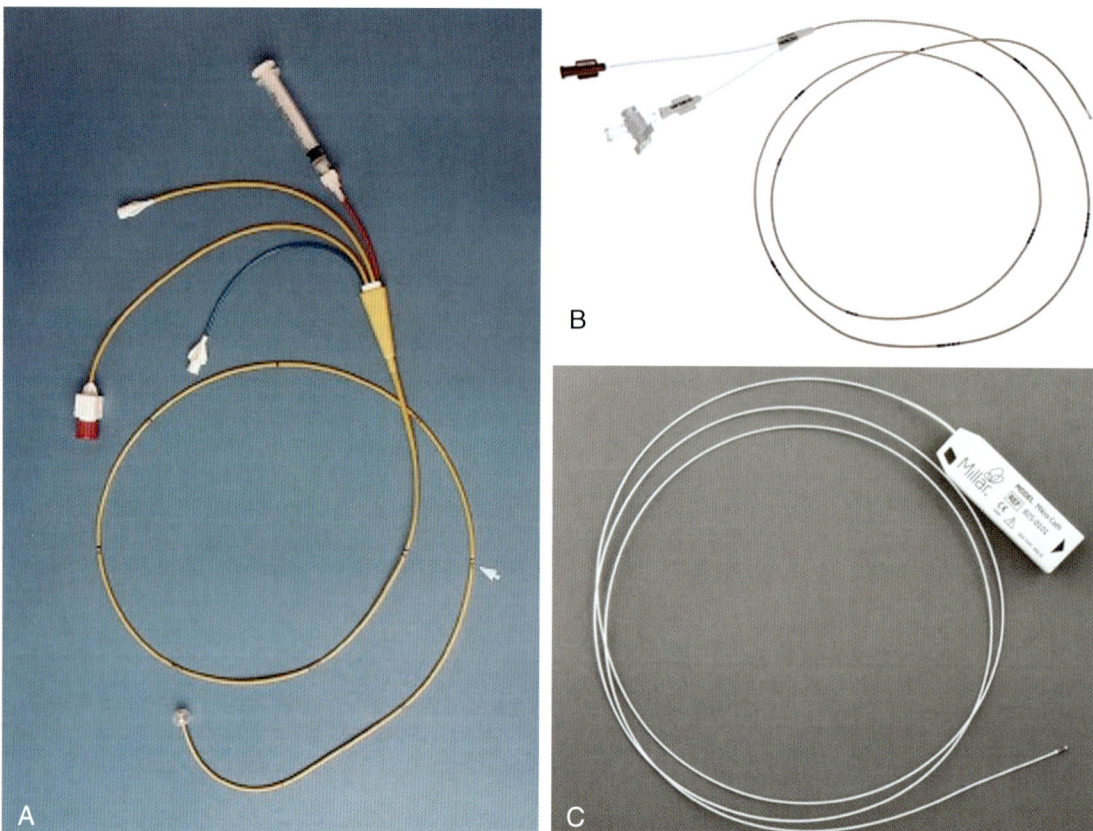

FIGURE 22.10 A, Typical Swan-Ganz catheter. The proximal ports, left to right, are the proximal injection hub, thermistor connector, distal lumen hub, and balloon inflation valve with syringe. The distal end of the catheter has a balloon and a distal end hole. The proximal injectate port exits 30 cm from the distal end of the lumen (*arrow*). The thermistor lies just proximal to the balloon. **B,** Example of a balloon wedge catheter, which has only one port besides the balloon inflation valve. **C,** Example of a diagnostic pressure catheter. (**A** from Davidson CJ, Bonow RO. Cardiac catheterization. In Mann DL, et al., editors: Braunwald's Heart Disease: A Textbook of Cardiovascular Medicine. 10th ed. Philadelphia: Elsevier; 2012, p 364; **B** from Arrow, Teleflex, Morrisville, NC; **C,** from Mikro-Cath, Millar, Houston, TX.)

Fluid-Filled Pressure Systems

Catheter-based pressure recording is accomplished by converting the force of the pressure wave from the catheter tip into an electrical signal by a transducer. A fluid-filled system (catheter plus tubing and connectors) transmits the pressure wave to the transducer in which the distortion of a diaphragm is converted into an electrical analog or digital signal to be visualized on the hemodynamic display monitor/recorder.

Various factors influence the pressure signal, which can impact signal accuracy. In such cases, the output amplitude would not be a true representation of the physiologic input amplitude. The most common technical artifacts of fluid filled systems are underdamping (also known as excessive resonant artifact or ringing) (Fig. 22.12), over-dampening (e.g., blunted waveforms), and improper calibrations or setting (i.e., zeroing) the transducer to atmospheric pressure. An output-to-input ratio less than 1 represents *damping* (dissipation of energy), as may be caused by friction. This cause of error can be reduced by using a short, wide-bore, noncompliant tubing system that is directly connected to the transducer. Damped signals are frequently associated with air bubbles, blood, or contrast in the tubing. Aspiration and catheter flushing with saline will produce more accurate measurements. The higher the density of the liquid (e.g., contrast media) within the catheter, the greater is the damping effect. Furthermore, any luminal compromise ("kink") of the catheter-tubing system is also a source of damping and needs to be considered with any unexpected or unexplained pressure drop (e.g., during extensive catheter torquing or manipulation). Another explanation for a damped signal may be catheter tip obstruction by small vessel orifices or by engagement against vessel walls or thrombus within a catheter. Other sources of error are related to catheter motion artifact or impacts on the catheter (internal) or tubing (external). An impact artifact (a brief, very high-frequency signal) can be noted when the catheter is struck by the walls or valves of the cardiac chambers.

Critical for all measurements is correct positioning (heart level) and calibration of the pressure transducer against atmospheric pressure, a function known as *zeroing*. This is performed by placing the fluid-filled tubing to the transducer open to air at the level of the atria, which corresponds to the mid-axillary line. Because fluid-filled transducer signals may fluctuate over time, the signal may "drift" from its initial zero calibration. To address signal drift, all transducers should be zeroed immediately before any simultaneous recordings.

Micromanometer Catheters and Pressure Sensor Guidewires

Micromanometer pressure catheters and sensor guidewires allow for superior pressure recording because they have a miniaturized high-fidelity solid-state pressure transducer mounted at the tip, which eliminates the interposing fluid column and its damping effect as well as the 30- to 40-millisecond delay in wave transmission (see later). The pressure wave-form is less distorted and the whip (motion) artifact is greatly reduced. High-fidelity catheters can assess the rate of rise in ventricular pressure (dP/dt), wall stress, rate of decay in ventricular pressure (−dP/dt), and time constant of relaxation (τ), and when coupled to impedance catheters can provide ventricular pressure-volume relationships. Catheters with two transducers separated by a short distance allow for accurate determination of gradients within chambers (e.g., intraventricular gradient in HCM) and across structures (e.g., stenotic AV). Some high-fidelity micromanometer systems allow for over-the-wire insertion and angiography.

Computations for Hemodynamic Measurements

When the pressure waveform data have been obtained, computations are made to quantify various cardiac and vascular functions. The most common computations and standard formulas are provided in Table 22.1. These computations provide metrics to determine cardiac work,

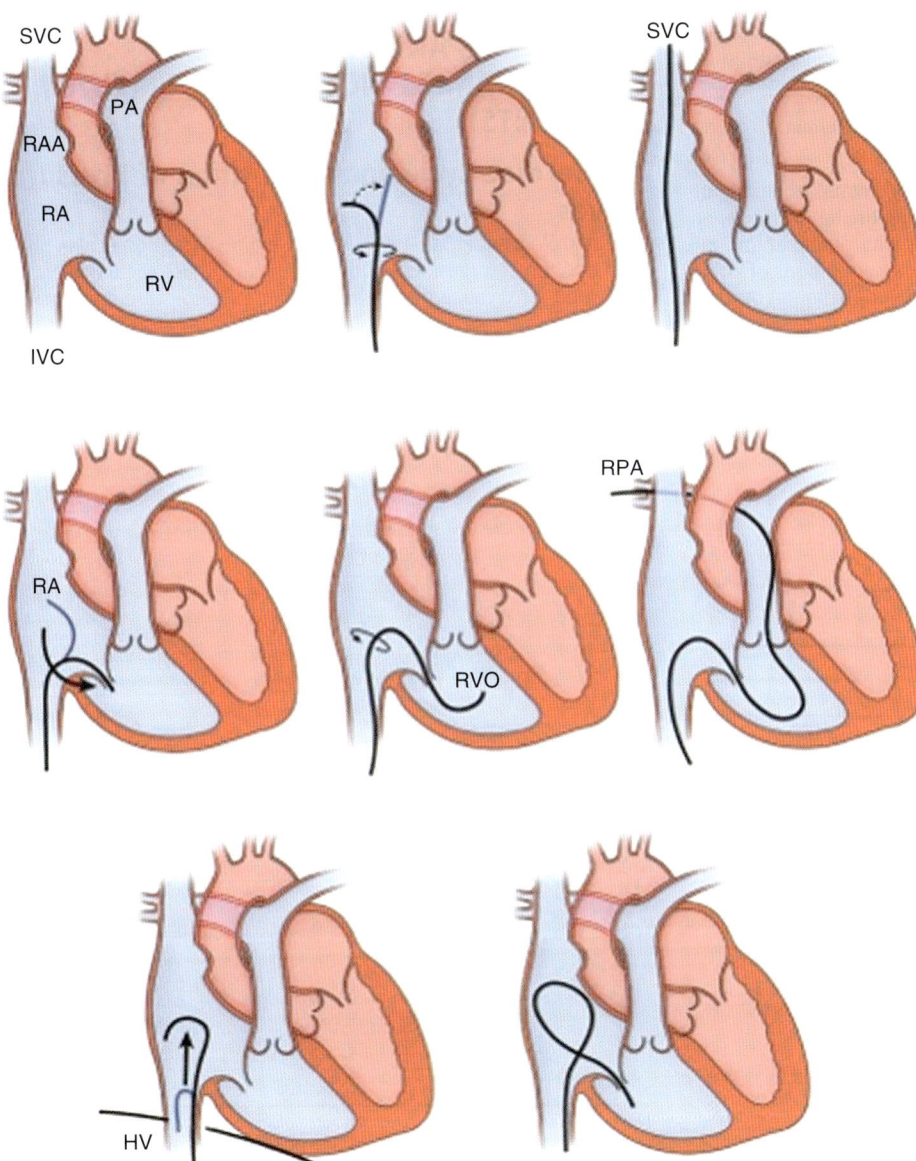

FIGURE 22.11 Right-heart catheterization via the femoral venous approach. Top row, The right-heart catheter is initially placed in the right atrium (RA) aiming at the lateral atrial wall. Counterclockwise rotation then directs the catheter posteriorly and allows advancement into the superior vena cava (SVC). Although it is not evident in the figure, clockwise catheter rotation into an anterior orientation would lead to advancement into the right atrial appendage (RAA) and thereby preclude SVC catheterization. *IVC,* Inferior vena cava; *PA,* pulmonary artery; *RA,* right atrium; *RV,* right ventricle. **Center row,** The catheter is withdrawn back into the RA and aimed laterally. Clockwise rotation causes the tip of the catheter to sweep anteromedially and cross the tricuspid valve. With the catheter tip in a horizontal orientation just beyond the spine, it is positioned below the RV outflow (RVO) tract. Additional clockwise rotation causes the catheter to point straight up and allows advancement into the main PA and from there into the right PA (RPA). **Bottom row,** Two maneuvers useful in catheterization of a dilated right heart. A larger loop with a downward-directed tip may be required to reach the tricuspid valve and can be formed by catching the tip of the catheter in the hepatic vein (HV) and advancing the catheter quickly into the RA. The reverse-loop technique (right) gives the tip of the catheter an upward direction, aimed toward the outflow tract. (From Baim DS, Grossman W. Percutaneous approach, including transseptal and apical puncture. In Baim DS, Grossman W, editors. Cardiac Catheterization, Angiography, and Intervention. 7th ed. Philadelphia: Lea & Febiger; 2006, p 86.)

flow resistance, valve areas, and shunts. Specific derivations and applications of these formulas can be found elsewhere.[8]

Cardiac Output Measurements

Catheterization-derived cardiac output measurements represent only estimates of the true cardiac output. The most common methods used in the catheterization laboratory are thermodilution and the Fick method.

Thermodilution Method

Thermodilution utilizes the indicator-dilution method for flow assessment with the indicator being temperature change after injection of a saline bolus cooler than blood temperature. The faster the circulation or flow (i.e., cardiac output), the quicker the neutralization of the temperature change. A distal thermistor records the temperature change in the blood that is induced by injection of a set amount (10 cc) of room temperature (25°C) saline at the proximal injection port. The change in temperature over time is displayed as a curve function, and the cardiac output correlates inversely with the area under the curve. The cardiac output can be calculated provided that the temperature and volume of the injectate along with a computation constant from each pulmonary artery catheter are known (Fig. 22.13).

The advantage of this method is the relative ease of use and results. However, thermodilution is less accurate in patients with significant tricuspid or pulmonic regurgitation, intracardiac shunts, low cardiac output, or irregular rhythms.

Fick Method

As blood circulates, oxygen is extracted by the tissues at the capillary level. The degree of oxygen extraction is inversely proportional to the rate of oxygen delivery. The Fick method relies on this principle that blood flow (cardiac output) is inversely proportional to the extent of oxygen extraction, that is, the difference in the concentration of oxygen between arterial and venous blood and the rate of oxygen uptake in the lungs (Fig. 22.14). It further assumes that pulmonary blood flow (PBF) is equal to systemic blood flow (SBF) in the absence of an intracardiac shunt. In other words, the same number of red blood cells (RBCs) that enter the lung must leave the lung in the absence of an intracardiac shunt. Therefore, knowing the number of oxygen molecules attached to RBCs entering the lung, the number of oxygen molecules attached to RBCs leaving the lung, and the number of oxygen molecules added during travel through the lung, the rate of RBC flow through the lung can be determined. This can be expressed in the following terms:

$$CO = \frac{O_2 \ consumption \left(\frac{mL}{min}\right)}{A-Vo_2 \ difference \left(\frac{mLO_2}{100 \ mL \ blood}\right) \times 10}$$

where $A-Vo_2$ is the arterial-venous oxygen saturation difference. Oxygen consumption is best measured from a metabolic hood or cart. Because of limited metabolic cart availability, the oxygen consumption is more commonly estimated as 3 mL O_2/kg or 125 mL/min/m² (generating an "assumed Fick" measurement). These estimated values may differ as much as 40% compared with the measured oxygen consumption. The arteriovenous oxygen difference is calculated from arterial–mixed venous (PA) O_2 content, where O_2 content = saturation × 1.36 × hemoglobin. For example, if the arterial saturation is 95%, then the O_2 content = 0.95 × 1.36 × 13.0 g = 16.7 mL, PA saturation is 65%, and O_2 consumption is 210 mL/min (i.e., 70 kg × 3 mL/kg) or a measured value. CO would be determined as follows:

$$\frac{210}{(0.95 - 0.65) \times 1.36 \times 13.0 \times 10} = \frac{210}{53} = 3.96 \text{ L/min}$$

In contrast to thermodilution, the Fick method retains accuracy in patients with low cardiac output and tricuspid regurgitation. However, the Fick method should not be used in patients with significant mitral regurgitation (MR) or AR and is not suitable under conditions of rapid changes in flow. Also, patients should not be on supplemental oxygen during the measurement period.

NORMAL RIGHT AND LEFT HEART WAVEFORMS AND VALVULAR HEMODYNAMICS INCLUDING HOCM (LVOT GRADIENTS)

The Cardiac Cycle and Generation of Pressure Waves

Dr. Carl J. Wiggers (1883–1963) was an eminent cardiovascular physiologist and the 21st president of the American Physiological Society. He is renowned for creating the classic diagram of cardiovascular physiology

TABLE 22.1 Common Hemodynamic Calculations

The cardiac index (CI, L/min/m²) is calculated as follows:

$$CI = \frac{CO \text{ (ml/beat)}}{BSA \text{ (m}^2\text{)}}, \text{ where BSA is body surface area.}$$

The stroke volume (SV, mL/beat) is calculated as follows:

$$SV = \frac{CO \text{ (ml/min)}}{HR \text{ (bpm)}}, \text{ where HR is heart rate.}$$

The stroke volume index (SI, mL/beat/m²) is calculated as follows:

$$SI = \frac{SV \text{ (ml/beat)}}{BSA \text{ (m}^2\text{)}}, \text{ where BSA is body surface area.}$$

The pulmonary vascular resistance (PVR, Wood units) is calculated as follows:

$$PVR = \frac{\text{mean pulmonary arterial pressure} - \text{mean LA pressure (or mean PCW)}}{CO}$$

The total pulmonary resistance (TPR, Wood units) is calculated as follows:

$$TPR = \frac{\text{mean pulmonary arterial pressure}}{CO}$$

The systemic vascular resistance (SVR, Wood units) is calculated as follows:

$$SVR = \frac{\text{mean systemic arterial pressure} - \text{mean right atrial pressure}}{CO}$$

Note: Resistance calculations follow the form of the Ohm law, $R = \Delta p/\dot{Q}$, where R is resistance; Δp is mean pressure differential across the vascular bed; and $\dot{Q}$ is blood flow. Resistance units (mm Hg/L/min) are also called hybrid resistance units or Wood units. To convert Wood units to metric resistance (dynes × s × cm⁻⁵), multiply by 80.

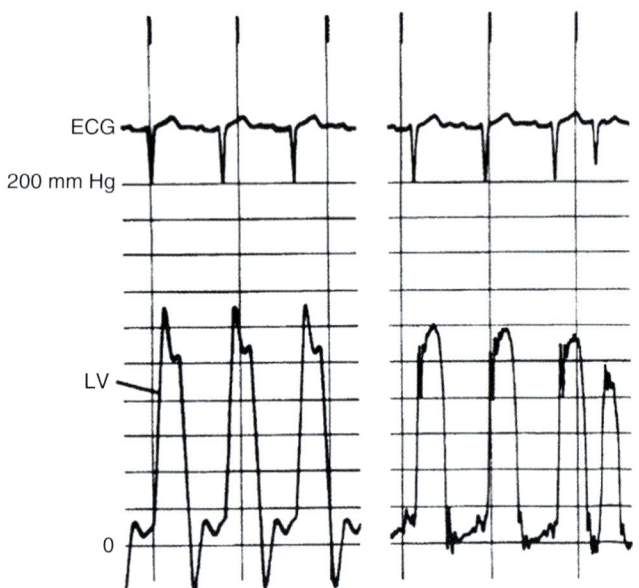

FIGURE 22.12 Left ventricular (LV) pressure with a 7F pigtail catheter using fluid-filled transducers. Left panel demonstrates "ringing" artifact with overshoot of the pressure signal during ejection and an exaggerated negative response during relaxation. On the right, a correctly damped LV pressure signal with minimal ringing during diastasis and no overshoot during systole. (From Kern MJ, et al. Hemodynamic Rounds. 4th ed. Elsevier; 2019.)

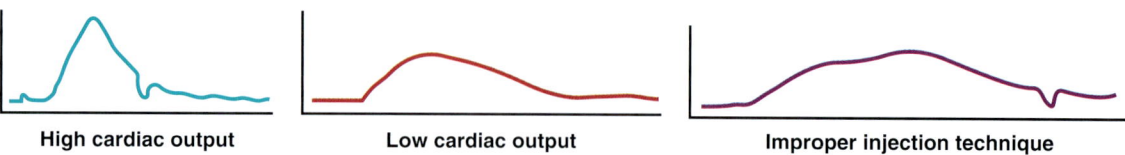

$$Q = \frac{V \times (Tb - Ti) K1 \times K2}{Tb(t) \, dt}$$

Q = cardiac output
V = injected volume
Tb + blood temperature
Ti = injectate temperature
K1 and K2 = corrections for specific heat and density of the onjectate and for blood and dead space volume
Tb(t) dt = change in blood temperature as a function of time

FIGURE 22.13 Display of a normal cardiac output reading by the thermodilution method (*top*), which plots temperature change over time; the area under the curve is converted into flow L/min by the Stewart-Hamilton formula. *Bottom*, Configurations of thermodilution curves in high and low cardiac output states and with improper injection technique. (Modified from Davidson CJ, Bonow RO. Cardiac catheterization. In Mann DL, et al., editors. Braunwald's Heart Disease: A Textbook of Cardiovascular Medicine. 10th ed. Philadelphia: Elsevier; 2012, p 364.)

that summarizes the cardiac cycle. By reviewing the electrical and mechanical activity of the heart as shown on the Wigger's diagram (Fig. 22.15), one can understand each of the pressure waves of the cardiac cycle.

The timing of mechanical events such as myocardial contraction and relaxation can be matched with an electrical stimulus as marked by the electrocardiogram (ECG). Each electrical event (e.g., P wave, QRS, T wave) is followed normally by a corresponding mechanical function resulting in a specific pressure wave. The ECG P wave is responsible for atrial contraction. The QRS complex triggers ventricular activation beginning the generation of ventricular (LV or RV) pressure rise and ejection. The T wave is the signal for ventricular repolarization and muscular relaxation. This normal chronology of electrical-mechanical activity is disturbed by arrhythmias and conduction defects, while principally anatomic pathologies (valvular disease, cardiomyopathy, pericardial disease) will affect the characteristics of pressure waveforms but less often their sequence of activation.

Rate of indicator out = rate in + rate added

$$Q \times C_{out} = Q \times C_{in} + \dot{V}$$

$$Q = \frac{\dot{V}}{(C_{out} - C_{in})}$$

When O_2 is used as indicator:

$$Q = \frac{\dot{V}o_2}{Cao_2 - C\bar{v}o_2}$$

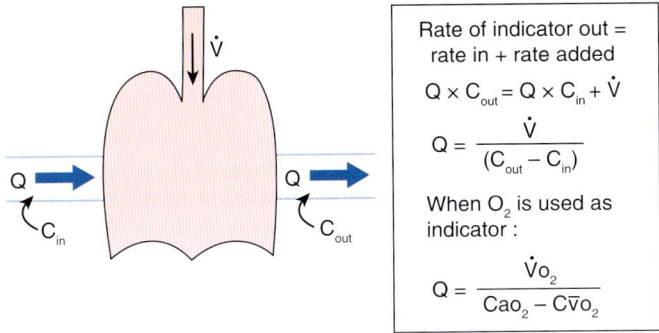

FIGURE 22.14 Schematic illustration showing measurement of flow by the Fick principle. Fluid containing a known concentration of an indicator enters a system at flow rate (C in). As the fluid passes through the system, indicator is continuously added at rate, thereby raising the concentration in the outflow (C out). In a steady state the rate of indicator leaving the system must equal the rate at which it enters plus the rate at which it is added. When oxygen is used as the indicator, cardiac output can be determined by measuring oxygen consumption, arterial oxygen content, and mixed venous oxygen content. (From Winniford MD, et al. Blood flow measurement. In Pepine CJ, et al., editors. Diagnostic and Therapeutic Cardiac Catheterization. 3rd ed. Baltimore: Williams & Wilkins; 1998, p 400.)

Normal Pressure Waveforms

The cardiac cycle starts with the electrocardiographic P wave, which initiates atrial contraction. The pressure waves of atrial systole and diastole are denoted as the *a* wave (see Fig. 22.15) and *x* descent, respectively. The P wave is followed by the QRS, triggering depolarization of the ventricles. The LV pressure at the end of the *a* wave is called the end-diastolic pressure (also known as LVEDP). The LVEDP corresponds to the ECG R wave. About 15 to 30 msec after the QRS, the ventricles contract, the LV (and RV) pressure increases rapidly before blood is ejected. This phase is called the isovolumetric contraction period. When the LV pressure rises above the aortic pressure, the AV opens. Systolic ejection with matching increases in LV and aortic pressures continues until repolarization, signaled by the T wave, ends contraction and starts LV muscular relaxation with a corresponding fall in the LV and aortic pressures. When the LV pressure falls below the aortic pressure, the AV closes, forming the dicrotic notch on the aortic

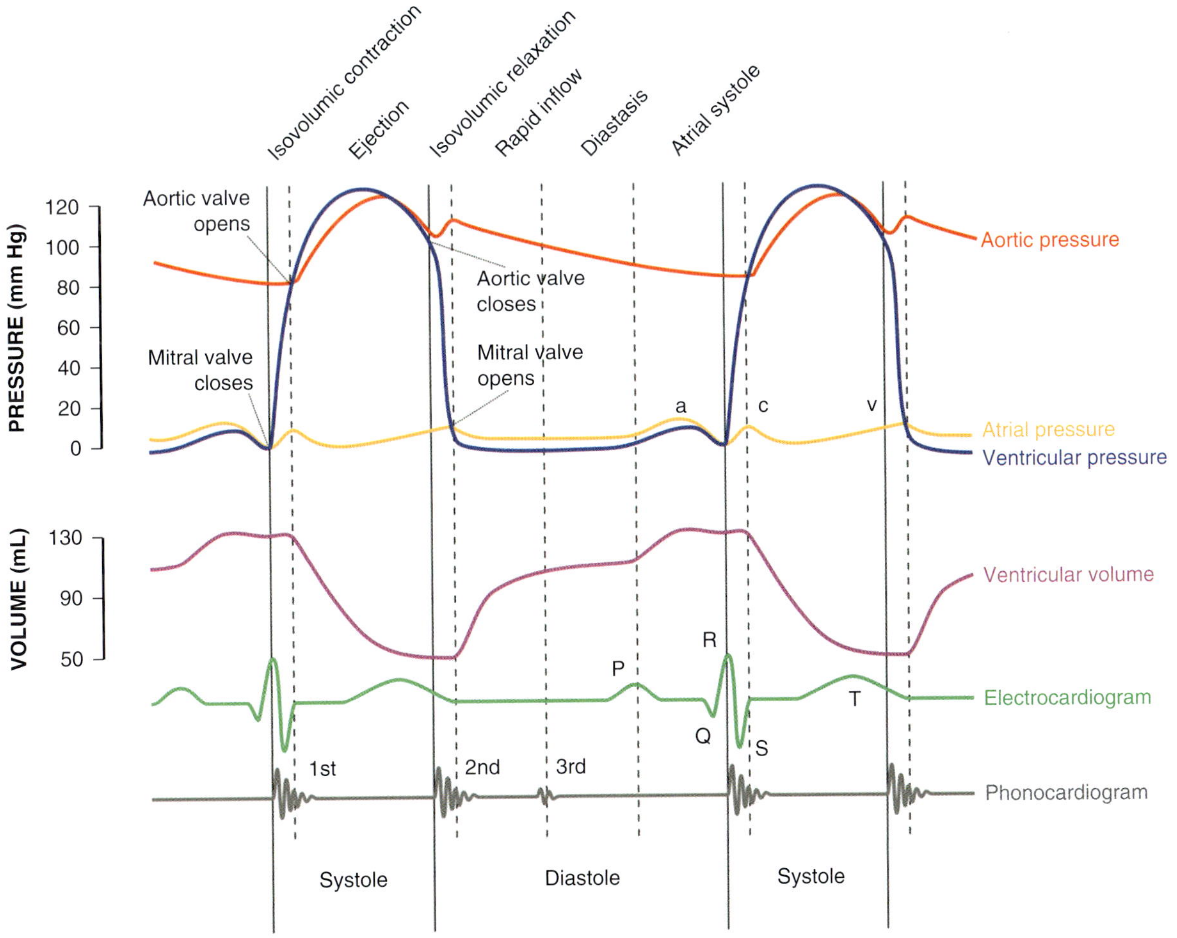

FIGURE 22.15 Wigger's diagram. Pressure curves of the left atrium and left ventricle are superimposed with the corresponding portions of the electrocardiogram at bottom. In the atrial pressure plot: wave *a* corresponds to atrial contraction, wave *c* corresponds to an increase in pressure from the mitral valve bulging into the atrium after closure, and wave *v* corresponds to passive atrial filling. In the electrocardiogram: wave *P* corresponds to atrial depolarization, waves *QRS* correspond to ventricular depolarization, and wave *T* corresponds to ventricular repolarization. In the phonocardiogram: The sound labeled first contributes to the S1 heart sound and is the reverberation of blood from the sudden closure of the mitral valve (left A-V valve) and the sound labeled "second" contributes to the S2 heart sound and is the reverberation of blood from the sudden closure of the aortic valve. (From https://commons.wikimedia.org/wiki/File:Wiggers_Diagram_2.svg.)

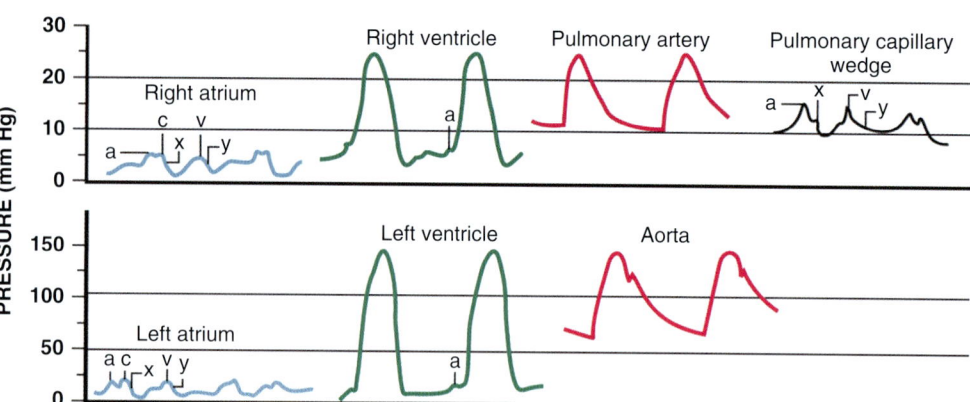

FIGURE 22.16 Normal pressure waveforms. From Normal right- and left-heart pressures recorded from fluid-filled catheter systems in a human. (In Zipes. Braunwald's Heart Disease: A Textbook of Cardiovascular Medicine. 7th ed.)

TABLE 22.2 Normal Pressure and Vascular Resistance Values

PRESSURE	MEAN (mm Hg)	RANGE (mm Hg)
Right Atrium		
a wave	6	2-7
v wave	5	2-7
Mean	3	1-5
Right Ventricle		
Peak systolic	25	15-30
End-diastolic	4	1-7
Pulmonary Artery		
Peak systolic	25	15-30
End-diastolic	9	4-12
Mean	15	9-19
Pulmonary Capillary Wedge		
Mean	9	4-12
Left Atrium		
a wave	10	4-16
v wave	12	6-21
Mean	8	2-12
Left Ventricle		
Peak systolic	130	90-140
End-diastolic	8	5-12
Central Aorta		
Peak systolic	130	90-140
End-diastolic	70	60-90
Mean	85	70-105

VASCULAR RESISTANCE	MEAN (DYNE-SEC · CM^{-5})	RANGE (DYNE-SEC · CM^{-5})
Systemic vascular resistance	1100	700-1600
Total pulmonary resistance	200	100-300
Pulmonary vascular resistance	70	20-130

waveform. The ventricular pressure continues to fall without a change in volume, a phase called isovolumic relaxation. When the LV pressure falls below the left atrial (LA) pressure, the mitral valve opens and the LA empties into the LV. The slope of the fall is LV pressure during the isovolumic period and is one of several indicators of normal or abnormal diastolic function.

Normal cardiac pressure waveforms are shown on Figure 22.16 and reference values are defined for all hemodynamic parameters in Table 22.2. Intrathoracic pressure and respiration influence these values, particularly for the right-sided chambers. Inhalation leads to a drop in intrathoracic and right atrial pressure, and exhalation has the opposite effect. The reverse is true for patients on mechanical ventilation. Pressure measurements should be obtained at end-expiration for consistency and averaged over several respiratory cycles.

Atrial Pressures

Focusing on atrial physiology, the atrial waveform has three positive deflections or waves (*a*, *c*, and *v*) and two negative deflections or descents (*x* and *y*) (Fig. 22.17). The *a* wave follows the P wave on the ECG and reflects atrial contraction, and atrial contractility and downstream resistance determine its height. Following the *a*, the *x* descent represents atrial relaxation and downward pulling of the tricuspid annulus as the right ventricle contracts. The *x* descent is interrupted by a second peak, the *c* wave, due to the atrioventricular (tricuspid or mitral) valve bulging into the atria during isovolumic ventricular contraction (early systole). Over the remainder of ventricular systole, atrial pressure slowly rises with atrial filling reaching its maximum at the end of ventricular isovolumetric relaxation, producing a peaked ventricular filling wave, the *v* wave. As ventricular pressure continues to drop below atrial pressure and the atrioventricular valve opens and ventricular filling begins, atrial pressure drops, called the *y* descent.

The pressure waveforms are strongly influenced by the specific pressure-volume relationship (also known as compliance) of the chamber in which the pressure is measured. The *a* wave is usually smaller than the *v* wave in the right atrium while the reverse tends to be true for the left atrium because the right atrium can easily decompress through the SVC and inferior vena cava (IVC), whereas the left atrium is constrained posteriorly by the pulmonary veins. While valvular regurgitation is often cited as one cause for large *v* waves, a highly compliant atrium may accommodate a large amount of volume from acute valvular regurgitation and produce only small *v* waves. Conversely, stiff, poorly compliant chambers can produce exaggerated pressure waves with normal filling volumes.

Pulmonary Capillary Wedge Pressure

The pulmonary capillary wedge pressure (PCWP) derived its name from advancing an end-hole catheter to the most distal part of the pulmonary artery and wedging it in place to register the pressure reflected through the pulmonary veins from the left atrium. A balloon-tipped (Swan-Ganz) catheter floated through the right heart to the pulmonary artery made this technique safer and more efficient. The PCWP is an indirect measure of the LA pressure transmitted through the pulmonary vein and pulmonary capillaries.

There are two common methods to confirm an accurate PCWP that closely agrees with LA pressure. The operator should confirm that PCWP wave is not a damped PA pressure by identifying clear *a* and *v* waveforms timed against the ECG or LV pressure. Fidelity is higher with the use of an end-hole catheter that is connected to the pressure transducer with stiff, short pressure tubing thoroughly flushed and bubble free. The operator should note the time delay (i.e., phase shift) of the PCW *v* wave to match the LV down stroke. The PCW position can also be confirmed by obtaining an oxygen saturation > 95% reflecting oxygenated pulmonary venous blood.

The PCWP waveform represents a slightly damped and delayed reflection of the left atrial pressure waveform, and *c* waves may not be seen (Fig. 22.18). With the normally low resistance of the pulmonary circulation, pulmonary artery diastolic pressure matches mean PCWP. This is not the case under circumstances of elevated pulmonary vascular resistance (hypoxemia, pulmonary embolism, chronic pulmonary hypertension). Also, PCWP may not reflect left atrial pressure as accurately as needed for mitral valve assessment. In general, "over wedging" of the balloon catheter causes an excessively damping signal leading to falsely low values, whereas "under wedging" with a signal contaminated in part by higher PA pressure leads to falsely high pressure readings. These two scenarios can be recognized by the pressure waveform lacking its desired atrial waveform configuration: noticeably flat with over wedging and appearing as a dampened pulmonary artery pressure (PAP) tracing with under wedging. For optimal left atrial pressure measurements, a transseptal puncture and direct chamber access should be used.

Aortic and Pulmonary Artery Pressure Waveforms

During systole, ventricular ejection transmits pressure to the great vessels (aorta and pulmonary artery) through the semilunar aortic and pulmonary valves. Normally, the upstroke of aortic pressure matches that of the LV pressure. As diastole begins, peak aortic and ventricular pressures decline together until LV pressure falls below aortic pressure at which time the AV closes producing an abrupt cessation of the pressure signal, the dicrotic notch. Aortic pressure slowly dissipates as blood is distributed into the peripheral vascular circulation. An identical but lower amplitude set of waveforms is observed for the right ventricle and pulmonary artery. The shape and magnitude of the aortic pressure is also the result of systemic wave reflections and summation. In the normal subject,

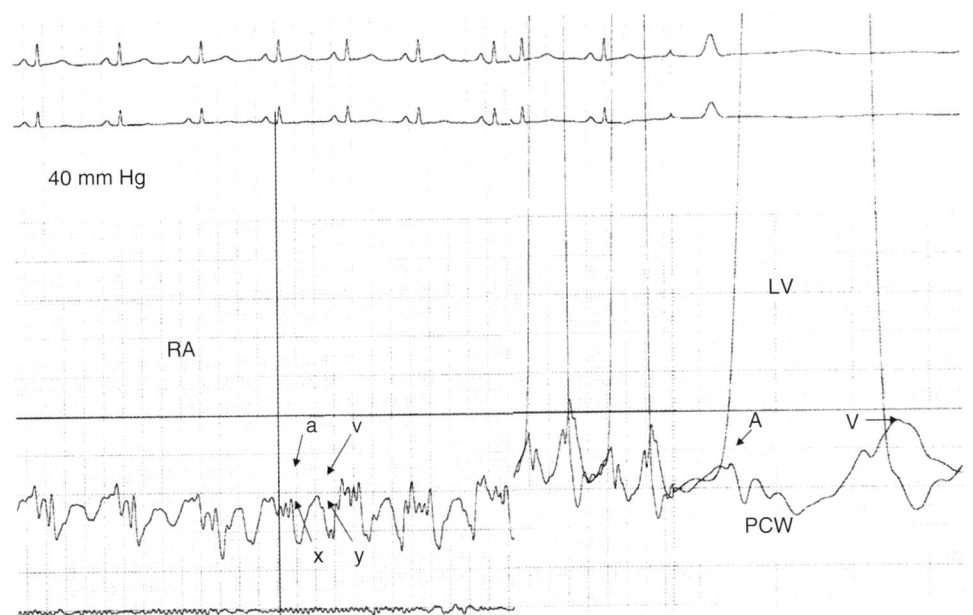

FIGURE 22.17 Left, Normal right atrial (RA) pressure with *a* and *v* waves and their associated *x* and *y* descents. The timing of any individual wave can be established from the ECG (vertical line from the R wave); in this case denotes atrial contraction. **Right,** Left ventricular (LV) and pulmonary capillary wedge (PCW) waveforms. The LA is usually higher than the RA and left-sided *v* waves are usually larger than right-sided *v* wave due to atrial chamber compliance and pressure.

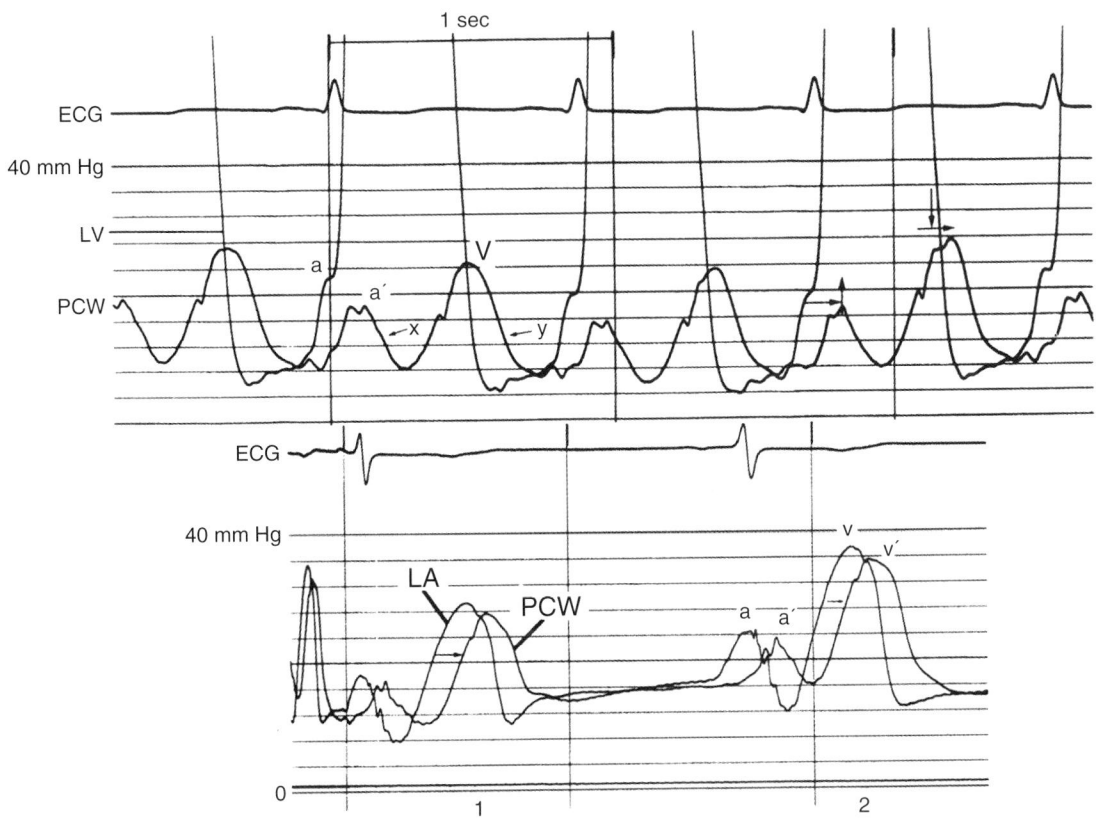

FIGURE 22.18 Top, Simultaneous left ventricular and pulmonary capillary wedge pressures (PCWPs) measured with fluid-filled catheters. Note the delay in pressure waves in the PCW compared with the LV, particularly the *a* and *a'* waves. The *v* wave from the PCW is also delayed on or after the LV downstroke. **Bottom,** Simultaneous LA and PCW tracings showing time delay in the PCW relative to the LA pressure waves.

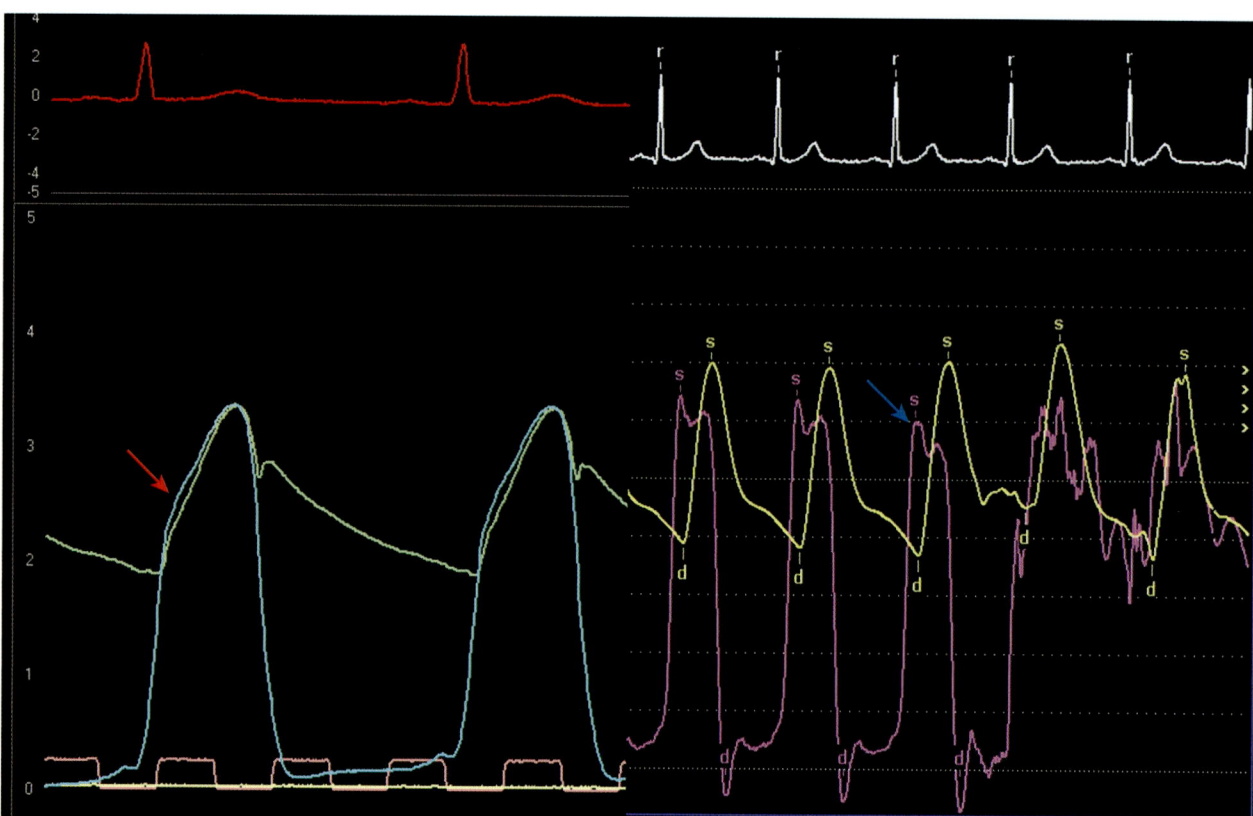

FIGURE 22.19 Normal LV and aortic pressures. **Left,** Micromanometer dual transducer pressure catheter with near ideal waveforms of aortic and left ventricular pressure. *Red arrow* denotes anacrotic shoulder and small normal impulse LV outflow tract gradient. **Right,** Pressures measured with fluid-filled transducer systems using 5F pigtail catheter through a 6F femoral artery sheath side arm. Note the resonant artifact (fling or ringing, *blue arrow*).

the backward-traveling wave arrives at end-systole and contributes to the closing of the AV and to increasing diastolic perfusion pressure. In the hypertensive subject, the backward-traveling wave reaches the proximal aorta in early systole and contributes to the late systolic peak in pressure. The magnitude of the reflected wave (and the late systolic pressure) has a well-validated and independent prognostic significance.[9]

Ventricular Pressure Waveforms

The LV pressure reflects the ejection force of blood into the higher resistance circuit of the systemic circulation while the RV ejects into the lower resistance pulmonary circuit. Although similar in morphology, the right and LV pressure differ in magnitude, timing of activation, and force of contraction. Under normal conditions, the magnitude of the LV waveform is significantly higher than that of the RV waveform. The duration of LV systole, isovolumic contraction, and relaxation are longer, and the ejection period is shorter than that for the right ventricle. In the early rapid-filling phase of diastole, ventricular pressures initially drop quickly below atrial pressures (often producing suction, i.e., a LA-LV gradient promoting rapid ventricular filling). Across diastole, as the LV fills, ventricular pressure rises, reaching a plateau (diastasis) ending in a more rapid upward deflection due to atrial contraction (the ventricular *a* wave). The end diastolic pressure after the *a* is taken at the onset of isovolumic contraction usually corresponding to the R wave on the simultaneous ECG (Fig. 22.19).

Normally, the LVEDP is only marginally higher than the PCWP but in certain states, such as hypertrophy or other causes of low ventricular compliance, it can be significantly higher. Although this post-*a* LVEDP value represents the true preload exerted on the ventricle, the PCWP correlates better with a pre-*a* LVEDP, which reflects the mean LV filling pressure.

Evaluation of Valvular Heart Disease

Cardiac catheterization and hemodynamic evaluation plays an important part in the diagnosis of patients with valvular pathology, particularly if there is discordance in the estimated degree of severity by physical examination and noninvasive tests such as echocardiography. The need for hemodynamic evaluation depends on the accuracy of the echocardiographic data, invasive assessment being most valuable in borderline or low-flow clinical states.

Calculation of Stenotic Valve Orifice Areas

The orifice area of a valve can be calculated from hydraulic principles. The volume of flow (F) across an orifice equals the area of the orifice (A) times the velocity of flow (V): $F = A \times V$, and accordingly, the orifice area can be calculated as $A = F/V$. F equals the cardiac output, and V can be calculated from the transvalvular gradient based on a special case of the Bernoulli principle called Torricelli's law:

$$V = \sqrt{2gh}$$

where g is the effect of gravity and h the pressure gradient (derived from the height of a water column).

Gorlin and Gorlin refined this equation in 1951, which has become known as the "Gorlin formula" for the calculation of valve areas[10]:

$$A = F / \left(C_c \times C_v \sqrt{2gh} \right)$$

C_c is the coefficient of orifice contraction, which accounts for the fact that fluids tend to move through the center of an orifice, generating a physiologic orifice that is smaller than the anatomic orifice. C_v is the velocity coefficient, which allows for the pressure gradient not being fully converted to flow because some of the velocity is lost to friction. Neither of these two coefficients has ever been determined. Instead, an empiric value has been used to align the calculated area with the actual area on autopsy or surgery in 11 patients with mitral valve disease. The maximal discrepancy between the actual mitral valve area and calculated values was just 0.2 cm² for a constant C of 0.85. Importantly, such direct comparison data have never been obtained for any of the other three valves, and not even empiric constants were developed for these. Rather, a constant of 1.0 has been assumed for any valve other than the mitral valve, which points out that the derived areas are best estimates only.

To derive a more accurate AV area, because flow across the AV occurs only during systole, the cardiac output is divided by the actual systolic ejection period (SEP), the period from opening to closure of the AV, times the heart rate (HR). In agreement with the Gorlin formula and factoring in a combined constant of 44.3 for C_c and C_v, the AV area (AVA) can be calculated as follows:

$$\text{AVA (cm}^2\text{)} = \frac{[\text{Cardiac output (mL/min)} \div (\text{SEP} \times \text{HR})]}{\left[44.3 \times \sqrt{\text{Mean gradient}}\right]}$$

The normal AVA is 2.6 to 3.5 cm² in adults. Valve areas <1.0 cm² represent severe aortic stenosis.

The calculation is similar for the mitral valve area (MVA). Because mitral flow occurs only during diastole, cardiac output is corrected for the diastolic filling period (DFP), the period of opening to closure of the mitral valve, yielding the following formula:

$$\text{MVA (cm}^2\text{)} = \frac{[\text{Cardiac output (mL/min)} \div (\text{DFP} \times \text{HR})]}{\left[37.7 \sqrt{\text{Mean gradient}}\right]}$$

The normal MVA is 4 to 6 cm², and severe mitral stenosis is present with valve areas smaller than 1.0 cm².

A simplified formula has been proposed by Hakki and colleagues.[11] The effects of SEP and DFP are relatively constant at normal heart rates, which leads to the following equation:

$$\text{AVA (cm}^2\text{)} = \frac{\text{Cardiac output (L/min)}}{\sqrt{\text{PeakLV} - \text{peak Ao or Mean gradient}}}$$

Of note, mean aortic transvalvular gradient and peak-to-peak gradient yield similar correlation with the Gorlin formula and thus can be used in this formula. For the MVA, only the mean gradient was validated:

$$\text{MVA (cm}^2\text{)} = \text{Cardiac output (L/min)} \div \sqrt{\text{Mean gradient}}$$

The valve area estimated by using the Hakki formula can differ by almost 20% from the valve area using the Gorlin formula in patients with bradycardia or tachycardia. As readily evident from the formulas, the accuracy of the measurements of pressure gradient and cardiac output is critical for obtaining the correct valve values, which are a major determinant for management decisions.

There are several sources of errors in the valve area calculations. Because the square root of the mean gradient is used, miscalculation of the cardiac output leads to more erroneous valve areas than miscalculation of the gradient. The imprecision in calculating the cardiac output is greatest in patients with a low cardiac output, in whom the pressure gradient is often inappropriately low and the severity of stenosis relies even more on accurate valve area determinations. In these patients, as well as in those with tricuspid regurgitation (TR), the Fick method should be used. Both the thermodilution and the Fick method overestimates stenosis severity in patients with mixed valvular disease (stenosis and regurgitation) of the same valve. If both AR and MR are present, accurate assessment of either the aortic or the MVA is not possible.

Inherent to the Gorlin formula area calculation is the dependence on transvalvular flow. Although greater flow could lead to greater opening pressure and thus greater valve area, correlation studies with planimetry by transesophageal echocardiography (TEE) argue against this occurring. Accordingly, even under increasing flow conditions, the AVA by planimetry remains unchanged, whereas it increases with use of the Gorlin formula, suggesting that at high flow states the Gorlin equation may overestimate true valve area.

Aortic Valve Stenosis

Aortic stenosis is one the most common valvular stenosis encountered in practice. For optimal hemodynamic assessment of the AV, simultaneous aortic and LV pressures are required. A single pressure pullback recording from the left ventricle into the aorta should only be used as a screening technique given the risk that premature contractions

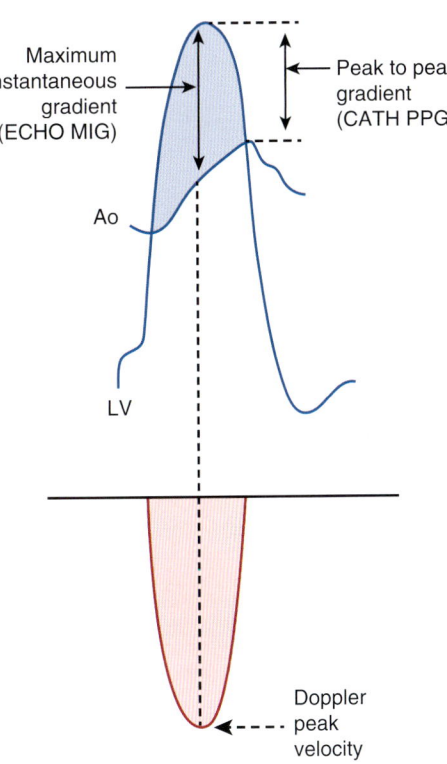

FIGURE 22.20 Top, Simultaneous left ventricular (LV) and central aortic (Ao) pressures in a patient with aortic stenosis. The optimal way to measure the gradient in a patient with aortic stenosis is to use these simultaneous pressures. The peak-to-peak gradient is the difference between the peak left ventricular and peak aortic pressures, which is a nonphysiological measurement because the peak pressures occur at different points in time. The mean pressure gradient (the integrated gradient between the left ventricular and aortic pressure throughout the entire systolic ejection period) should be used to determine the severity of the aortic stenosis. **Bottom,** ECHO vs. CATH gradients: ECHO maximum instantaneous gradient (MIG), CATH peak-to-peak gradient (PPG), CATH mean gradient (ΔP mean) (dotted area), and ECHO Δp mean (shaded area). ECHO MIG is the gradient between the peak LV pressure and the aortic pressure at the same point in time. CATH PPG is the gradient between the peak LV pressure and the peak aortic pressure at two different points in time. ECHO MIG is inherently higher than PPG. However, ECHO and CATH ΔP mean are closer in value in the absence of significant pressure recovery. (From Abbas AE, Pibarot P. Hemodynamic characterization of aortic stenosis states. Catheter Cardiovasc Interv 2019;93:1002-1023.)

or respiration changes the relative values. In the past, femoral artery (FA) pressure measured from the sheath side arm was compared with LV pressure that was obtained from a smaller size catheter placed through the sheath to the LV. FA pressure approximates but mostly overestimates central aortic pressure due to resonance and peripheral amplification of pressure. Using a dual-lumen catheter or micromanometers eliminates any difference in pressure transmission time or effect of peripheral amplification. Figure 22.19 shows the LV-aortic pressure measured from a high-fidelity catheter with micromanometer pressure transducers above and below the AV compared with a fluid-filled LV catheter with the fluidfilled FA sheath pressure.

The mean integrated gradient between the left ventricle and aortic pressure waves over the systolic ejection period is the best measure of the stenosis severity. The AV area is calculated as detailed above, and as alluded to, the Hakki formula should only be used as an estimate of AV area as it does not correlate with Doppler maximal velocity (a true measure of peak instantaneous gradient)[11] (Fig. 22.20).

Abbas and Pibarot[12] reviewed the detailed pathophysiology of the stenosed AV. The ejection of blood from the LV is forced through the fixed reduced aortic orifice area (i.e., the anatomic orifice area [AOA]). Energy is lost due to valvular resistance, resulting in a pressure drop and acceleration of flow. After crossing the AV, (i.e., the effective orifice area [EOA]), part of the kinetic energy is reconverted back to potential energy, and the pressure increases (also called the "pressure recovery"). Doppler echocardiography

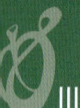

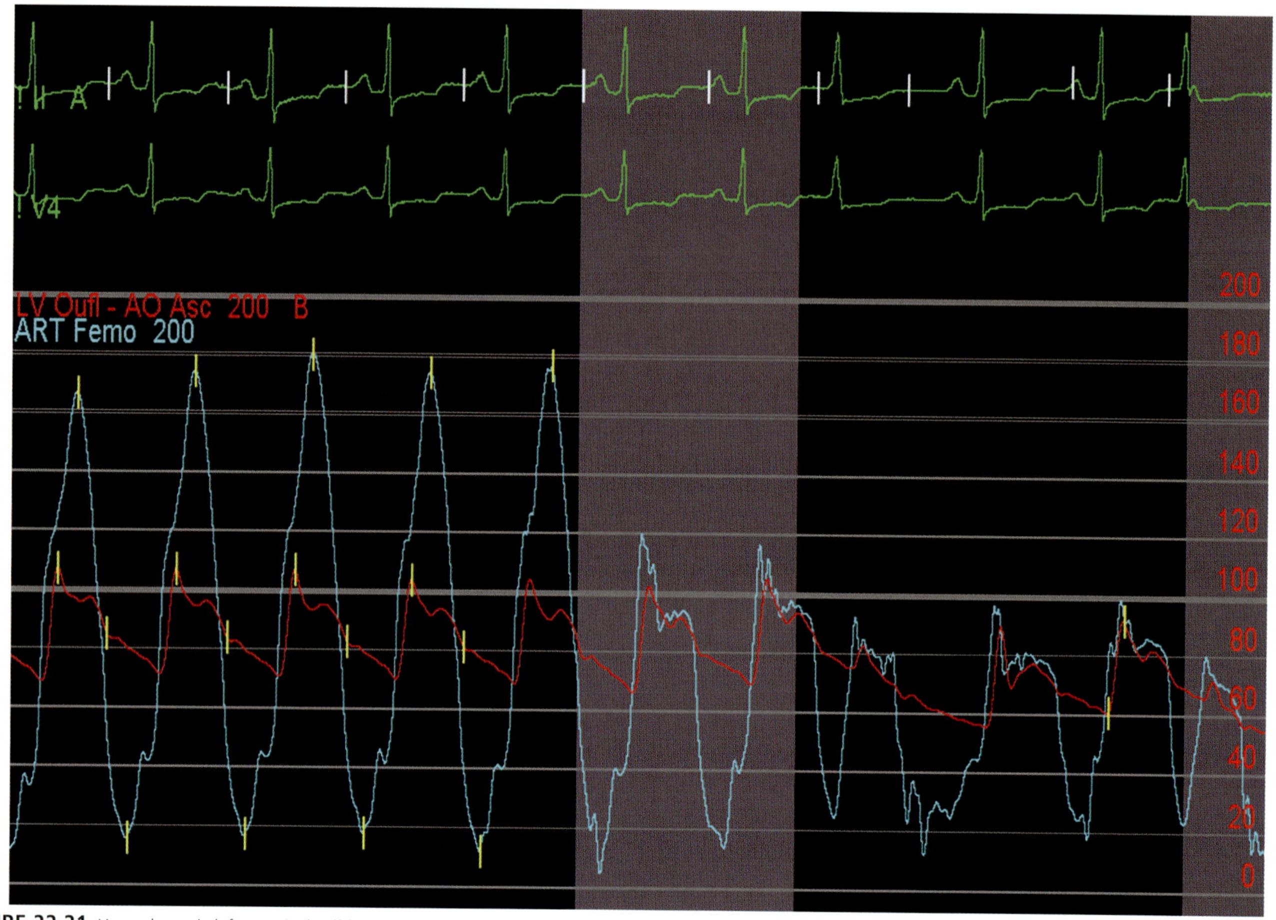

FIGURE 22.21 Hemodynamic left ventricular (*blue*) and aortic (*red*) pressure tracings in patient with hypertrophic cardiomyopathy. The LV catheter is pulledback from distal LV (*left side*) to subaortic position (*right side*). Not the reduction in LV-Ao pressure gradient while still recording LV pressure. In addition, one can appreciate the configuration of the aortic pressure matching the LV upstroke with a typical "spike-and-dome" appearance.

measures the peak instantaneous gradient across the entire outflow tract and aorta and is thus able to capture this phenomenon of pressure recovery. Because catheter-based measurement of aortic pressure is typically acquired several centimeters distal in the aorta after pressure recovery has already occurred, it is less affected by pressure recovery.

Low-Flow, Low-Gradient Aortic Stenosis

In patients with low-flow, low-gradient (LF/LG) severe aortic stenosis (AS) (i.e., valve area <1 cm^2 but mean gradient <40 mm Hg), pharmacologic maneuvers can help to establish the true anatomic severity of the stenosis for decisions regarding valve replacement. In patients with low-gradient severe AS with a preserved ejection fraction (paradoxical LF/LG AS), cardiac output is limited by relaxation abnormalities, low stroke volume, and impaired ventriculovascular coupling rather than systolic function. For such paradoxical LF/LG severe AS, lowering of the peripheral resistance with nitroprusside should lead to an increase in the AV gradient without a change in the valve area.[13]

In patients with LG/LF AS with a reduced ejection fraction, a dobutamine challenge will increase cardiac output and permit reassessment of the valve gradient and area in the setting of an improved cardiac performance. In patients with mild or minimal AS, in response to low-dose dobutamine, the valve area should increase by >0.2 cm^2 with minimal or no change in the transvalvular gradient. In patients with true anatomic stenosis, the valve gradient should increase with a higher cardiac output while the AV area will remain small. Dobutamine also provides prognostic information, as patients without an adequate contractile reserve (e.g., stroke volume increase <20%) have poor outcomes irrespective of valve intervention.

Hypertrophic Obstructive Cardiomyopathy

An LV outflow gradient can be present not only at the AV but also at the subvalvular level within the ventricle. Whereas valvular AS is structural in nature and the gradient is usually constant in daily life, the LVOT-aortic gradient caused by HOCM is dynamic and sensitive to ventricular loading conditions and changes in contractility.[14,15] A low LVOT gradient at rest should be challenged with dynamic and provocative maneuvers (e.g., variation with respiration, post-PVC accentuation, isometric exercise) to identify the true obstructive nature of the disease and suitability for septal myectomy or percutaneous alcohol septal ablation.

Confirmation of the subvalvular location of the intracavitary gradient is obtained by pressure pullback from the LV apex to a position just beneath the AV. The location of the intraventricular gradient is defined by the resolution point of the aortic-LV gradient while still registering LV pressure. A standard pigtail catheter has shaft side holes and is not suitable for gradient location assessment because some or all of the holes may be positioned above the intracavitary obstruction producing an erroneously small LVOT gradient. Alternative methods for the invasive assessment of intracavitary gradients include the use of a dual-lumen catheter, a double-sensor micromanometer catheter, or an end-hole catheter in the LV outflow tract and a second catheter in the left ventricle placed by transseptal puncture.

Compared with fixed AV obstruction, in dynamic subaortic outflow tract obstruction the aortic and LV waveforms display distinctly different characteristics (Fig. 22.21). Patients with valvular AS have a slow and delayed upstroke (*parvus et tardus*) in the aortic waveform. In contrast, HOCM patients have a rapid rise of the aortic pressure corresponding to the LV pressure at the onset of AV opening. The rapid rise is followed by a blunted and rounded wave in late systole, leading to a "spike-and-dome contour", which is characteristic of a dynamic LV outflow obstruction. While both AS and HOCM have increased post-PVC

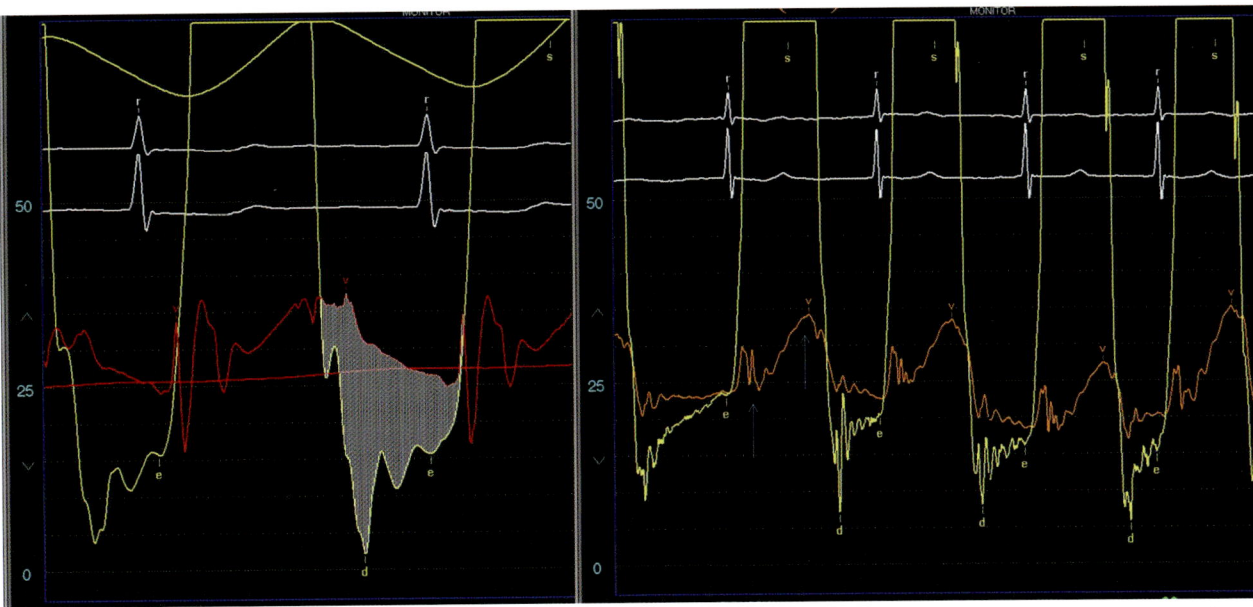

FIGURE 22.22 Hemodynamic tracings in a patient with mitral stenosis. *Left,* LV and PCW tracings show a large mitral valve gradient of approximately 20 mm Hg (pressure scale is 0 to 50 mm Hg). *Right,* LV and directly measured LA pressures (via transseptal approach) show higher fidelity pressure waveforms and marked reduction in the mitral pressure gradient (6 mm Hg). On the LA pressure, the c notch and v wave are distinct compared with the waveforms on the PCW.

LVOT gradients, HOCM tracings show a smaller post-PVC aortic pulse pressure. The diminished aortic pulse pressure following a PVC is the pathognomonic hemodynamic pattern of HOCM, named the Braunwald-Brockenbrough-Morrow sign.

Other provocative maneuvers used in the hemodynamic evaluation of HOCM include alteration of loading conditions with Valsalva maneuver, inhalation of amyl nitrate, or increasing contractility by a dobutamine or isoproterenol infusion. Each of these has the potential to exacerbate the LVOT gradient and reveal the underlying physiology, just as physical examination maneuvers can increase (Valsalva, standing up) or reduce (squatting, leg raise) the murmur of HOCM.

Symptomatic patients, refractory to medical therapy with appropriate morphologic abnormalities of HOCM, may benefit from myectomy or percutaneous alcohol septal ablation. The specific details of the alcohol septal ablation are described elsewhere.[16]

Mitral Valve Stenosis

The hemodynamic assessment of the stenotic mitral valve is performed initially with combined left and right heart hemodynamics examining the LV-PCW (LA) pressure gradient at rest. In patients with borderline normal/abnormal findings, measurements should be made during exercise (e.g., arm lifting with weights or bicycle ergometer). Important to recall is the fact that the PCWP often overestimates LA pressure in patients with mitral stenosis or prosthetic mitral valves due to delayed and poor-quality pressure transmission.

For patients with elevated PCWP and suspected mitral valve abnormalities, direct measurement of the LA pressure by transseptal puncture is the most accurate method for decisions regarding mitral valvuloplasty or replacement. Figure 22.22 shows a PCWP (red) and a LA pressure (orange) demonstrating different timing of V waves and higher mean for PCWP which falsely increased the mitral valve gradient measurement. However, if the PCW/LV pressure tracings show no significant gradients, transseptal catheterization is often unnecessary. A simplified formula for the estimation of the mean mitral valve gradient (MVG = mean left atrial pressure − LVEDP/2) has been proposed.[17] MVA can be calculated as outlined above.

The classic hemodynamic sign of mitral stenosis on left atrial pressure tracing is a markedly elevated *a* wave. Further, due to the stenosis of the mitral valve, the pressure only gradually decreases after opening and the *y* descent is gradual. The LV pressure waveform may show a lower end-diastolic pressure due to the impaired filling and a reduced atrial kick (i.e., *a* wave amplitude).

Pulmonary and Tricuspid Valve Stenosis

The same principles and techniques outlined above apply to right-sided valvular heart diseases. For the pulmonic valve, the transvalvular gradient is not infrequently obtained on catheter pullback from the pulmonary artery into the right ventricle, although ideally it should be measured simultaneously using multi-lumen catheters or two separate catheters. Invasive hemodynamic measurements are performed when the severity of pulmonary stenosis is unclear, when an infundibular stenosis is suspected, and when balloon valvotomy is considered.

With tricuspid stenosis, the obstruction of blood flow from the right atrium into the right ventricle, the volume of blood in the right atrium and the mean right atrial pressure are increased in diastole, generating a diastolic pressure gradient between these two chambers. This translates into a markedly elevated *a* wave. Opening of the stenotic tricuspid valve leads to a slow decrease in right atrial pressure and gradual *y* descent. Right ventricular pressure tracings show a reduced end-diastolic *a* wave amplitude secondary to the reduced atrial filling.

Aortic Regurgitation

Aortic regurgitation (AR) occurs when there is inadequate closure or malcoaptation of the AV leaflets, allowing blood to enter the LV cavity from the aorta during diastole. Common causes of aortic regurgitation include aortic root dilation, bicuspid AV, and endocarditis. An aortogram can be used to visualize and semi-quantitatively measure the degree of aortic regurgitation by the extent the regurgitation of contrast volume injected into the aortic root is opacifying the left ventricle.

It is important to be cognizant that the results are influenced by catheter position, volume of contrast, and chamber size and contractility, not just regurgitant volume alone. Nevertheless, the semi-quantitative classification scheme by Sellers and colleagues remains the reporting standard:

1+ Minimal regurgitant jet seen.
    Clears rapidly from the proximal chamber with each beat.
2+ Moderate opacification of the proximal chamber and clearing with subsequent beats.
3+ Intense opacification of the proximal chamber that becomes equal to that of the distal chamber.
4+ Intense opacification of the proximal chamber that becomes denser than that of the distal chamber. Opacification often persists over the entire series of images obtained.

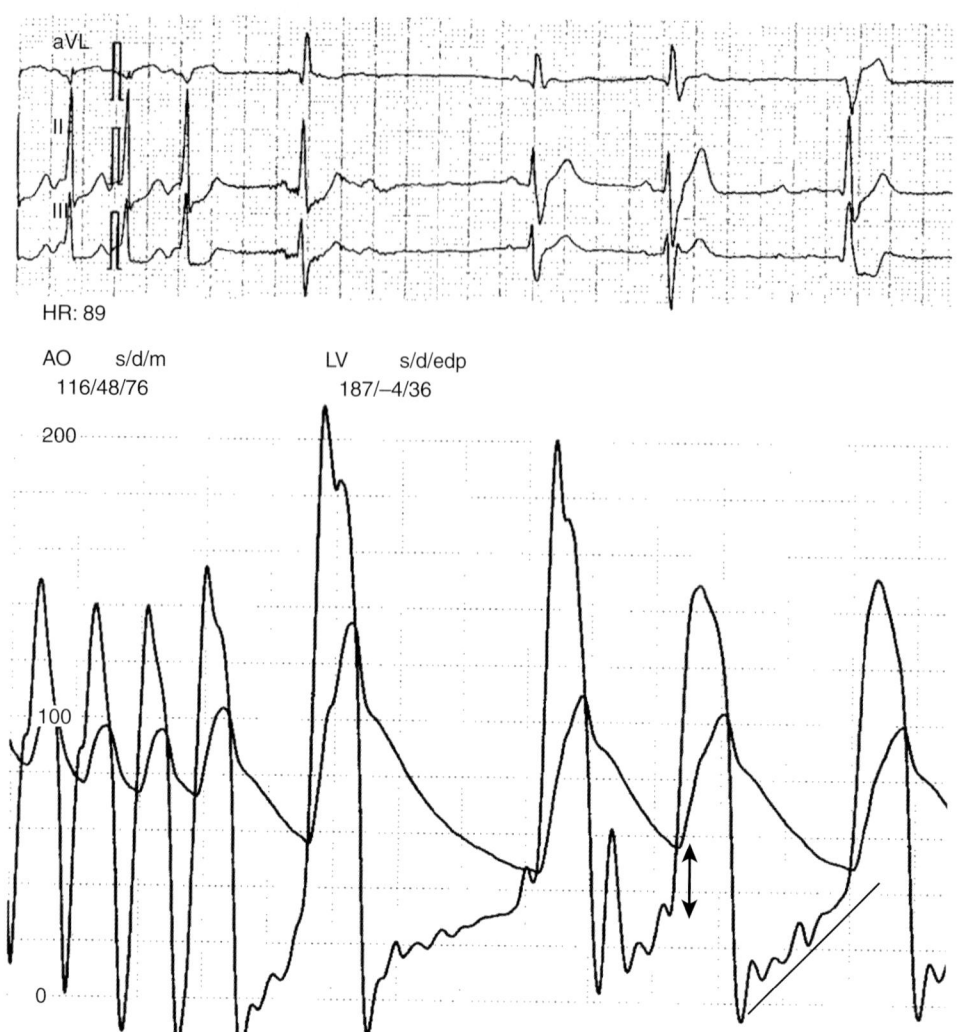

FIGURE 22.23 Hemodynamics of combined mixed AS and AI with LV-Ao systolic gradient and rapidly increasing diastolic LV filling pressure (*diagonal line*), wide pulse pressure, and close approximation of aortic diastolic pressure with LVEDP (*double arrowhead*).

Occasionally, measurements made with a stiff exchange wire across a severely calcific stenotic valve may prop the leaflet open and produce an artifactual hemodynamic picture of severe AR.

Mitral Regurgitation

Mitral regurgitation (MR) is typically the result of the mitral apparatus failing to maintain the coaptation of the mitral leaflets during systole. The mitral apparatus consists of four components: the annulus, the anterior and posterior leaflets, the chordae tendineae, and the papillary muscles. Failure of any of these structures can result in leaflet malcoaptation with valvular regurgitation. Semi-quantitative assessment of MR with left ventriculography remains a useful screening tool during coronary angiography.

In particular, pulmonary artery pressure (PAP) and PCWP at rest and with exercise are important parameters for clinical assessment of MR. With severe MR, a prominent v wave is characteristic and the hemodynamic consequence is postcapillary pulmonary hypertension, especially under conditions of increased workload. It is a class I ACC/AHA guideline recommendation to perform a hemodynamic evaluation of either aortic or mitral regurgitant lesions when PAPs are disproportionate to the severity of regurgitation on noninvasive testing or when clinical and noninvasive findings are inconsistent.

Acute MR produced by stretching or tearing of leaflets is characterized by a large v wave (Fig. 22.24). However, as with all hemodynamic waveforms, atrial and ventricular compliance determine the waveform and thus a large v wave, may be present due to low compliance of the LA rather than MR (Fig. 22.25). A new large v wave after mitral balloon valvuloplasty, however, is usually a valid demonstration of acute MR. Freihage et al.[18] reported that the ratio of the area under the v wave to the LV systolic area, that is Va/LVa, correlates best with the degree of MR.

By cardiac catheterization the regurgitant volume can be calculated as the fraction of the stroke volume that does not contribute to net cardiac output, that is,

Regurgitant stroke volume = angiographic stroke volume − forward stroke volume.

The regurgitant stroke volume can also be used to produce a regurgitant fraction, that is

Regurgitant fraction (RF) = regurgitant stroke volume / angiographic stroke volume

The angiographic stroke volume is calculated by the cardiac output measurement on the left ventriculogram, the forward stroke volume by Fick or thermodilution cardiac output measurement; either value is then divided by the heart rate. Prerequisites for this calculation are similar heart rates for both output measurements, stable hemodynamic states between measurements, and the presence of only a single regurgitant valve. Considering these limitations, volumetric approaches by echocardiography and MRI provide easier and more precise quantitative measurements.

The three typical hemodynamic findings of AR are widened aortic pulse pressure, rapid upstroke of LV diastolic filling pressure, and near equilibration of end-diastolic aortic and LV pressure. Figure 22.23 shows a patient with mixed AS and regurgitation. Note the wide pulse pressure and rapid LV diastolic filling slope up to the LVEDP.

Pulmonary and Tricuspid Valve Regurgitation

Invasive hemodynamic assessment of patients with pulmonary regurgitation serves primarily the purpose of determining pulmonary arterial pressures and pulmonary vascular resistance, especially as part of comprehensive assessment when other structural cardiac abnormalities are present and/or pulmonary valve intervention is considered. The hemodynamic characteristics of severe pulmonary regurgitation include low pulmonary artery end-diastolic pressure, wide pulmonary pulse pressure, and increased RV end-diastolic pressure. With severe degrees of regurgitation, PAP tracings may take on the appearance of an RV pressure tracing ("ventricularization").

In patients with tricuspid regurgitation (TR), measurement of pulmonary pressures and pulmonary vascular resistance will assist in determining secondary causes of regurgitation, for example pre- or postcapillary pulmonary hypertension and septal defects. The characteristic hemodynamic finding is an elevated v wave generated by the open communication between the two chambers and the volume ejection from the right ventricle into the right atrium with the onset of systole. The magnitude of the v wave pressure elevation is determined

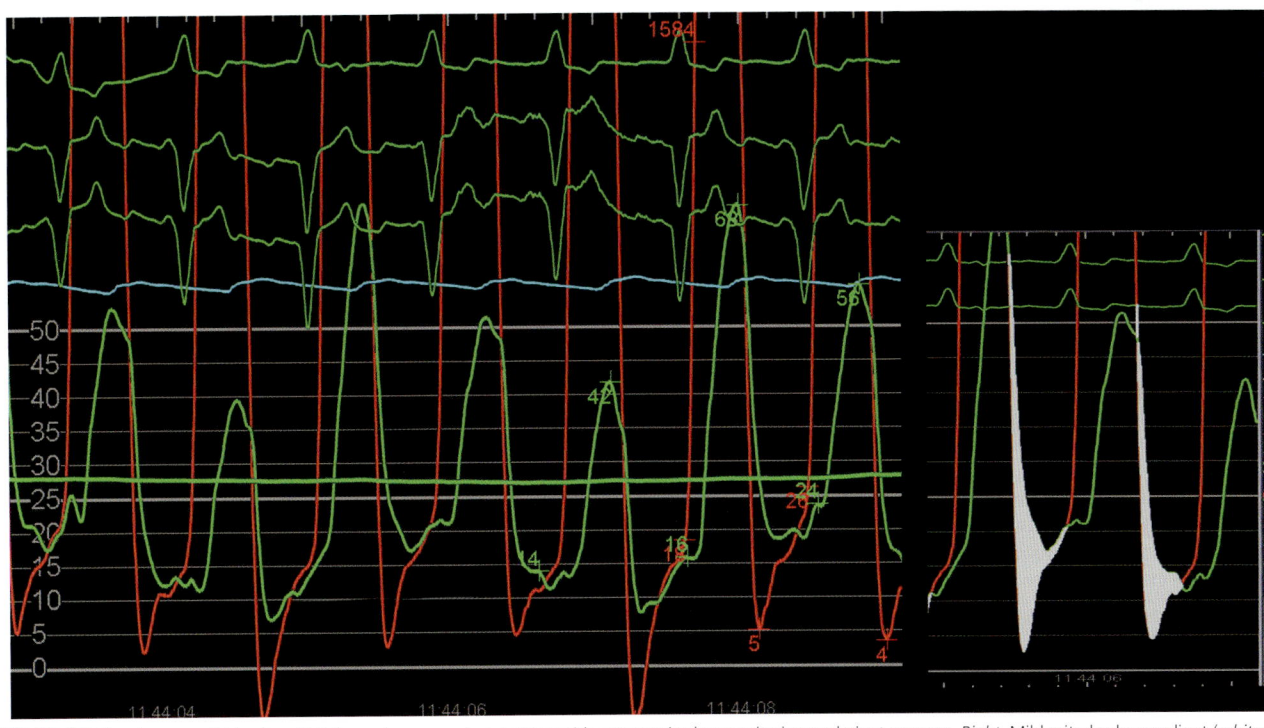

FIGURE 22.24 Simultaneous LV (*red*) and LA (*green*) pressure in a patient with severe mitral regurgitation and giant *v* waves. *Right,* Mild mitral valve gradient (*white shaded area*) with large *v* waves. Scale is 0 to 50 mm Hg.

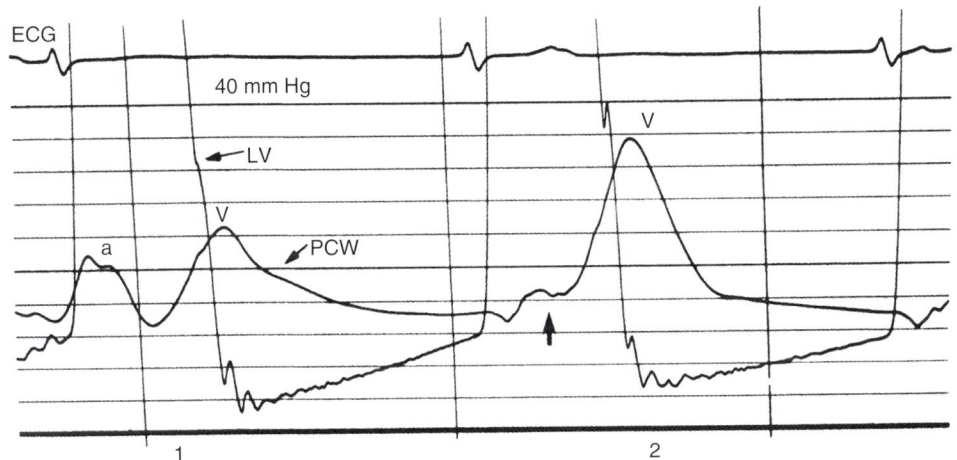

FIGURE 22.25 Left ventricular (LV) and pulmonary capillary wedge pressure in patient with mitral stenosis without evidence of mitral regurgitation. Beat 1 demonstrates large *a* with prominent *v* wave, an 12 mm Hg mitral gradient. Beat 2 shows a junction beat with a retrograde P wave (*arrow*) producing a significantly large *v* wave and larger gradient in the absence of regurgitation due to low compliance of the diseased left atrium.

not only by the regurgitant volume but also by the compliance of the right atrial chamber. Accordingly, *v* wave amplitude and mean right atrial pressure may be very minimally elevated in relation to the chronicity of TR. Furthermore, right atrial distension due to chronic volume expansion with evolving reduction in contractility also leads to a reduction in the *a* wave.

SEPTAL DEFECTS AND LEFT-TO-RIGHT/RIGHT-TO-LEFT SHUNTS

As with valvular heart disease, echocardiography takes the leading role in the initial diagnosis of atrial or ventricular defects and pulmonary arteriovenous malformations. Hemodynamic assessment is used in the determination and quantification of the extent and consequences of shunts. Hemodynamics provide information on the status of PAP, resistance, and their reversibility in case of elevation.

The systemic and pulmonary circulations operate in series, and thus normally their output is the same. Any abnormal communication between them then generates a short circuit or shunt. This can be from the systemic circulation to the pulmonary circulation (left-to-right shunt), from the pulmonary circulation to the systemic circulation (right-to-left shunt), or in both directions (bidirectional shunt). Most shunt assessments in the cardiac catheterization laboratory are made by determination of the oxygen content in the blood at different levels of the circuit given the normally very well defined and distinct oxygenation values in the systemic and pulmonary circulation.

As a general rule, pulmonary artery oxygen saturations exceeding 80% should raise the suspicion for a left-to-right shunt. On the contrary, systemic, arterial oxygen saturations <93% that persist after several deep breaths to counteract alveolar hypoventilation (as seen with over sedation or pulmonary venous congestion) should raise suspicion for a right-to-left shunt.

In addition to pulmonary artery oxygen sampling, a screening oxygen saturation should also be obtained from the SVC routinely with right-heart catheterization to possibly detect even small left-to-right shunts. If the difference in oxygen saturation between these two samples is ≥8%, a left-to-right shunt may be present, and the oximetry run should be extended to also include samples from the IVC, right atrium, and right ventricle. In fact, if an inter-atrial shunt is suspected, samples should be obtained at the level of the low, mid, and high right atrium, and for an inter-ventricular shunt from the RV inflow tract, apex, and outflow tract. An absolute increase in oxygen saturation by 5% or more defines a significant step-up and the location of the shunt.

A small left-to-right shunt might be missed if the right atrium is used for screening purposes because of incomplete mixing of blood in the right atrium from the SVC, IVC, and coronary sinus. When taking blood samples in the right atrium, the catheter should always be directed away from the coronary sinus, which has one of the lowest oxygen saturations in the human body. Further to note oxygen saturation in the IVC is higher than in the SVC as oxygen extraction of the internal organs and lower extremity muscles is lower in a fasting and resting state than that of the brain. The best method for determination of the mixed venous saturation is by Flamm's formula, which is based on IVC and SVC samples (see later).

A full saturation run entails samples from the high and low IVC; high and low SVC; high, middle, and low right atrium; RV inflow, midcavity, and outflow tract; main pulmonary artery; left or right pulmonary artery; pulmonary vein and left atrium, if possible; left ventricle; and distal aorta. Right-to-left shunt assessments require samples from the pulmonary veins, left atrium, left ventricle, and aorta. A decrease (stepdown) in oxygen saturation is expected in such cases.

To quantify the extent of a shunt, PBF and SBF need to be calculated, which is, in essence, oxygen consumption divided by the difference in oxygen content across the pulmonary or systemic bed. The effective blood flow (EBF) is the fraction of mixed venous return received by the lungs without contamination by shunt flow. Under normal conditions, PBF, SBF, and EBF are equal.

These equations are as follows:

$$PBF = VO_2 \div [(PvO_2 - PaO_2) \times Hb \times 1.36 \times 10]$$

$$SBF = VO_2 \div [(SaO_2 - MvO_2) \times Hb \times 1.36 \times 10]$$

$$EBF = VO_2 \div [(PvO_2 - MvO_2) \times Hb \times 1.36 \times 10]$$

VO_2 (oxygen content) is determined as outlined in the section on Fick cardiac output. PvO_2, PaO_2, SaO_2, MvO_2 are oxygen saturation of pulmonary venous, pulmonary arterial, systemic arterial, and mixed venous blood, respectively.

MvO_2 is calculated by Flamm's formula:

$$[MvO_2 = (3 \times SVC\,O_2 + 1 \times IVC\,O_2)/4]$$

Systemic arterial oxygen saturation may be substituted for pulmonary venous sampling, if at least 95%. Otherwise, in the absence of a right-to-left shunt, systemic arterial oxygen content is used. If a right-to-left shunt is present, pulmonary venous oxygen content is calculated as 98% of the oxygen capacity.

The size of an isolated left-to-right shunt is

$$L \rightarrow R\ shunt = PBF - SBF$$

If an additional right-to-left shunt is present (bidirectional shunt), the approximate size of the left-to-right shunt is

$$L \rightarrow R\ shunt = PBF - EBF$$

and the approximate size of the right-to-left shunt is

$$R \rightarrow L\ shunt = SBF - EBF$$

Clinically, the ratio of PBF to SBF (or Qp/Qs) is often used to express shunt significance. A ratio <1.5 indicates a small left-to-right shunt, a ratio of 1.5 to 2.0 a moderate-sized shunt, and a ratio of >2.0 a large left-to-right shunt. A flow ratio <1.0 indicates a net right-to-left shunt.

If oxygen consumption is not measured, the PBF/SBF ratio may be calculated as follows:

$$PBF/SBF\ ratio = (SaO_2 - MvO_2) \div (PvO_2 - PaO_2)$$

where SaO_2, MvO_2, PvO_2, and PaO_2 are systemic arterial, mixed venous, pulmonary venous, and pulmonary arterial blood oxygen saturation, respectively.

Pericardial Disease and Restrictive Cardiomyopathy

Impairment of ventricular filling or diastolic dysfunction can be caused by a number of intrinsic and extrinsic pathologies. Intrinsic causes of diastolic dysfunction include hypertrophic cardiomyopathies, infiltrative diseases such as amyloid, sarcoid, or hemochromatosis, scarring after radiation or chemotherapy, and other restrictive myopathic conditions. Extrinsic impairment of diastolic filling is most commonly due to pericardial constraint from pericarditis, cancer with metastases to the pericardial space, or pericardial effusion with tamponade physiology from a number of causes. Rarely, very large pleural effusions can limit cardiac filling and masquerade as pericardial constriction, though more frequently pleural effusions are the result rather than the cause of the abnormal physiology.

Normal Pericardial Function and Pathophysiology of Constriction

While not critical to maintenance of normal cardiovascular function, the pericardium has important subsidiary functions including stabilization of intrathoracic cardiac motion, balancing right and LV cardiac output through diastolic and systolic interactions, limiting acute cardiac dilation, minimizing friction between cardiac chambers and surrounding thoracic structures, and providing an anatomic barrier to infection from the lung and other contiguous structures. The diseased pericardium becomes stiffer, thicker, and less compliant (from progressive inflammation). Ultimately the pericardium can become adherent to the myocardium and limit cardiac filling through its constrictive effect on the global cardiac volume.

Differentiating between constrictive and restrictive causes for impaired cardiac filling may occur through the patient history, as the causes of intrinsic myocardial restriction are often distinct from constrictive pericardial diseases. From a hemodynamic standpoint, both constrictive and restrictive diseases produce elevation and equalization of right and LV diastolic pressures. Both demonstrate abrupt cessation of early ventricular filling (Fig. 22.26), classically described as a "dip and plateau" waveform of the ventricular pressures.

Unique to restrictive cardiomyopathy is the decreased ventricular chamber compliance due to increased myocardial stiffness. The steep compliance curve results in an abnormal increase in impedance throughout the entire diastolic period and a reduced atrial filling component at end-diastole (often associated with biatrial enlargement). In contrast, in constrictive pericarditis, the ventricular chamber compliance is normal in early diastole, allowing for normal or rapid early filling. In mid-diastole, ventricular filling is abruptly decelerated as the intracardiac volume approaches the fixed limit of the constricting pericardium. The limitation in global cardiac volume results in an increase in ventricular interdependence or ventricular coupling; that is, the right and left ventricles are unable to fill independently of each other. The intraventricular septum shifts over the course of the respiratory cycle such that the filling of one ventricle impairs the filling of the other ventricle. These dynamic respiratory changes of ventricular interdependence allow for accurate discrimination of constrictive pericarditis from restrictive cardiomyopathy.

In addition, the constricting pericardium dissociates the intrathoracic from the intracardiac pressures such that intrathoracic pressure is not fully transmitted through the diseased pericardium to the intracardiac structures. Normally, decreased intrathoracic and intracardiac pressures increases systemic venous return as the SVC and IVC are mostly extrathoracic and flow can proceed to the lower-pressure right heart structures. This causes right-sided cardiac output and murmurs to increase during inspiration (Carvallo sign). LV filling is mostly unchanged with respiration as the pulmonary veins are intrathoracic and any changes to thoracic pressure are transmitted to the LA/LV, though a small decrease in LV filling occurs with increased pulmonary pooling of blood volume with inspiration.

In contrast, in the setting of constriction, inspiration leads to decreased pulmonary venous pressure (as these are intrathoracic and extrapericardial) without a decrease in intracardiac pressures, resulting in significantly reduced left-sided preload and stroke volume during inspiration. At the same time, right-sided filling is augmented by increased IVC flow and paradoxically increasing jugular venous pressure with inspiration, termed Kussmaul's sign. Kussmaul's sign is only occasionally seen in patients with cardiac tamponade wherein the increase in negative intrathoracic pressure is generally still transmitted

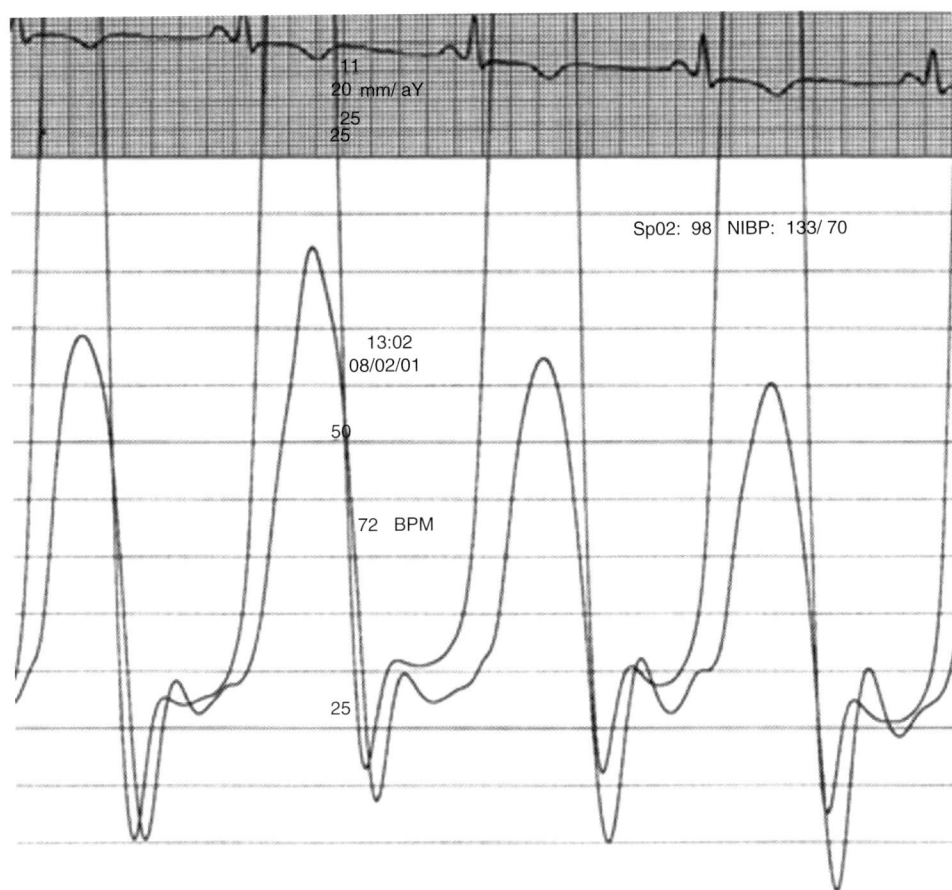

FIGURE 22.26 LV and RV hemodynamic pressure pattern of constrictive/restrictive physiology demonstrating an abrupt cessation of early diastolic filling with a "dip and plateau" configuration. While common, this pattern is not diagnostic of constrictive pericarditis (scale 0 to 40 mm Hg).

be positive in constriction but not in restriction (1.4 ± 0.2 versus 0.92 ± 0.019; $P < 0.0001$). A systolic area index ≥1.1 has a sensitivity of 97% and predicted accuracy of 100% for identifying constriction.[20] In real time, ventricular interdependence (indicative of constriction) is often assessed in the catheterization laboratory by observing discordance in the movement of peak RV and LV systolic pressures over the respiratory cycle.

Cardiac Tamponade

Cardiac tamponade is a clinical syndrome associated with extrinsic compression of the heart by elevated pericardial pressures, usually due to accumulation of pericardial fluid, bleeding, or masses. Increased intrapericardial pressure results in an inability to fill the heart, leading to reduced stroke volumes, cardiac output, arterial pressure, and ultimately death. The classic signs in cardiac tamponade (Beck's triad) include hypotension, jugular venous distension, and muffled heart sounds. Elevated pericardial pressures have characteristic hemodynamic and echocardiographic findings even before full clinical signs manifest. The magnitude of pericardial pressure increase depends on the rate of fluid accumulation and the compliance of the pericardium.

One of the classically associated clinical signs is pulsus paradoxus, the exaggerated decline (>10 mm Hg) in systemic arterial pressure during inspiration. Although characteristic of cardiac tamponade, it can also be seen with restrictive and constrictive physiology, but to a lesser degree. When fluid accumulates in the pericardial space, intrapericardial pressure increases, leading to compression of the RA and RV, increasing their diastolic pressures. Right-heart filling becomes more heavily reliant on decreased intrathoracic pressures during inspiration to fill, exaggerating the left-sided cardiac output and arterial blood pressure change over each respiratory cycle. The interventricular septum shifts to the left during inspiration and encroaches on the left ventricle, leading to a further reduction in stroke volume of the left ventricle and enhancing the pulsus paradoxus.

Cardiac tamponade produces elevation and near equalization of diastolic chamber pressures matching intrapericardial pressures. As described above, there is also inspiratory increase in right-sided volumes and reduction in left-sided volumes that are responsible for pulsus paradoxus (Fig. 22.27A). Incomplete resolution of elevated right atrial pressure and RV filling after pericardiocentesis can indicate the presence of both constrictive and tamponade physiologies, termed effusive-constrictive physiology (Fig. 22.27B). This phenomenon may occur in as many as 16% of cases in recent series and not necessarily require pericardiectomy as previously believed.[21]

PHYSIOLOGIC AND PHARMACOLOGIC MANEUVERS AND PV LOOPS

It is important to be aware of the fact that even clinically significant cardiac disease states can be diagnostically silent until revealed by physiological or provocation maneuvers such as exercise, strain or Valsalva, Mueller maneuvers, pharmacologic stimulation, or cardiac pacing. Every case should be thoroughly reviewed for the clinical question

to the right side of the heart in the absence of a constrictive component to the physiology (effusive-constrictive, see later).

The traditional hemodynamic criteria for the diagnosis of constrictive pericarditis include (1) end-diastolic pressure equalization (LV end-diastolic pressure minus RV end-diastolic pressure >5 mm Hg), (2) PAP <55 mm Hg, (3) RV end-diastolic pressure divided by RV systolic pressure >1/3, (4) dip and plateau diastolic pressure morphology as reflected by the height of the LV rapid filling wave (>7 mm Hg), (5) and Kussmaul's sign (lack of an inspiratory fall in mean right atrial pressure) (Table 22.3). Unfortunately, these criteria are neither highly specific nor sensitive to differentiate constrictive from restrictive physiology.

Dynamic ventricular interdependence (correspondence of LV-RV systolic pressures) exhibited during respiration, on the other hand, is the most sensitive and specific hemodynamic finding differentiating constrictive pericarditis from restrictive physiology. Hurrell et al.[19] examined dynamic respiratory changes in LV and RV pressures in 36 patients: 15 with surgically proven constrictive pericarditis and 21 with congestive heart failure. The dissociation of the intrathoracic and intracardiac pressures was assessed at end inspiration and end expiration. The exaggerated respiratory variation was significantly greater in those with constrictive pericarditis than restrictive diseases. During peak inspiration, there was discordance between RV and LV function with an increase in RV systolic pressure and simultaneous decrease in LV systolic pressure. In contrast, patients with congestive heart failure (and other restrictive cardiomyopathies) usually demonstrate concordant changes in right and LV systolic pressures during peak respiration. Dynamic respiratory variation in this study was 100% sensitive and 95% specific for the diagnosis of constrictive pericarditis.

Recently, the ratio of the RV to the LV systolic pressure–time area in inspiration versus expiration, the *systolic area index,* was noted to

TABLE 22.3 Comparison of Traditional and Dynamic Respiratory Criteria for Diagnosis of Constrictive Pericarditis

	CRITERIA	SENSITIVITY (%)	SPECIFICITY (%)	PPV	NPV
Traditional	LVEDP versus RVEDP <5	60	38	4	57
	RVEDP versus RVSP >1/3	93	38	52	89
	PASP <55	93	24	47	25
	Right ventricular free wall >7 mm	93	57	61	92
	Respiratory: Change of right atrial pressure <3 mm Hg	93	48	58	92
Dynamic Respiratory Factors	Pulmonary capillary wedge versus LV >5 mm Hg	93	81	78	94
	LV/RV interdependence	100	95	94	100

LVEDP–RVEDP, Left and right ventricular end-diastolic pressure; *RVSP,* right ventricular systolic pressure; *PASP,* pulmonary artery systolic pressure; *PPV,* positive predictive value; *NPV,* negative predictive value; *RFW,* rapid filling wave; *RAP,* right atrial pressure; *PCWP,* pulmonary capillary wedge pressure; *RV,* right ventricular.
From Hurrell DG, et al. Value of dynamic respiratory changes in left and right ventricular pressures for the diagnosis of constrictive pericarditis. Circulation 1996;93:2007-2013.

to be addressed and the cardiac catheterization protocol should be planned accordingly. Poor planning of critical measurements may lead to inconclusive results or, even worse, false conclusions.

Exercise Provocation

Exercise is a commonly used and valid provocation method, aiming to recapitulate what patients are experiencing in daily life. An adequate response to exercise entails a normal ventilatory response (i.e., oxygen consumption), a normal chronotropic response (i.e., HR increases in response to an increase in demand), a normal blood pressure response (i.e., systolic BP increases as a consequence of increased CO), normal ventricular volume responses (i.e., decrease in cardiac filling pressures due to higher CO and increase in diastolic relaxation), and adequate metabolic substrate use (i.e., appropriate use of glucose as an energy source without generating lactic acid). Right-heart (and left-heart as needed) catheterization pressures are measured before, during every phase or stage of exercise, and after exercise. Two forms of exercise are to be distinguished in this context: dynamic and static.

Dynamic Exercise

Dynamic exercise is still the most physiologic way of challenging the heart to unmask cardiac pathology. In the catheterization laboratory, this can be performed by arm exercise with weights or by leg exercise with supine bicycle ergometry. Using a pulmonary artery balloon flotation catheter (inserted from the arm or internal jugular vein), upright bicycle and treadmill exercise can also be performed with hemodynamic monitoring outside the catheterization laboratory.

Supine exercise differs from normal upright exercise in several ways: (1) Ventricular volumes are larger when the patient is supine rather than upright, (2) HR and diastolic arterial pressure are higher when the patient is upright rather than supine, (3) pulmonary and intracardiac filling pressures are lower when the patient is upright, (4) SV increases by 100% with maximal exercise when the patient is upright and only 20% to 50% when the patient is supine, and (5) both upright and supine exercise is normally associated with increases in LV end-diastolic volume (EDV) and decreases in end-systolic volume (ESV), with a concomitant increase in LV ejection fraction. In patients with coronary artery disease (CAD), these findings may either be absent or limited due to exercise limitation.

Under normal conditions, the increased oxygen demand induced by exercise is met by an increase in cardiac output and peripheral oxygen extraction. Cardiac dysfunction impairs the increase in cardiac output, and the demands of exercise can only be met by increased peripheral oxygen extraction, leading to often profound drops in mixed venous oxygen saturation and thus marked increases in arteriovenous oxygen difference. The fact that cardiac output and oxygen consumption are linearly correlated allows for a prediction of the cardiac index (CI) at a given level of oxygen consumption. This linear relationship forms the basis to calculate the exercise index (also known as the Dexter index), the ratio of the observed to the predicted CI. The predicted CI with exercise is equal to $2.99 \times 0.0059 \times$ measured O_2 consumption index with exercise. The measured CI is the CO divided by body surface area (BSA). The normal Dexter index equals the measured CI with exercise divided by the predicted CI. A value of ≥ 0.8 reflects a normal cardiac output response to exercise.

Another way of expressing the same relationship is the *exercise factor,* defined as the increase in cardiac output divided by the increase in oxygen consumption. An exercise factor of ≥ 6 is normal; that is, for every 100 mL/min increase in oxygen consumption, cardiac output should increase by at least 600 mL/min with exercise.

There are important nuances to supine exercise as performed in the cardiac catheterization lab. In the early phase of exertion, there is increased venous return, augmenting LVEDV and stroke volume. However, at progressively higher levels of exercise, LVESV and LVEDV decrease, minimizing stroke volume increase. The augmentation in cardiac output with this form of stress testing is primarily due to an increase in heart rate. Exercise-induced cardiac output may be limited in patients with chronotropic incompetence in the absence of other cardiac disease.

Despite these caveats, invasive hemodynamics during exercise are very useful for the diagnostic evaluation of patients with suspected heart failure with preserved ejection fraction (HFpEF) or valvular heart disease, particularly as many patients have only mild hemodynamic abnormalities at rest.[22] Exercise increases LVEDP, PCWP, and PAP in patients with HFpEF. It increases transvalvular mitral gradient and PAP in mitral stenosis. In patients with clinically relevant valvular regurgitation, exercise increases LVEDP, PCWP, PAP, and SVR in conjunction with a reduced exercise index (<0.8) and abnormal exercise factor (<6). Simultaneous echocardiographic evaluation of valvular regurgitation and invasive hemodynamic assessment is also useful in equivocal cases.

Static Exercise

Isometric exercise consists of skeletal muscle contraction without shortening. In the cardiac catheterization laboratory, isometric exercise commonly is performed using a handgrip with a graded hand dynamometer. Measurements of hemodynamics and ventricular function are obtained during sustained handgrip at a predetermined range (15% to 50% of the maximal handgrip contraction) for a period of 3 to 4 minutes. The size of the involved muscle group is unimportant, provided that maximal voluntary contraction is maintained to increase oxygen demand during the isometric exercise period. Isometric exercise is easy to perform (repeatedly) and requires only minimal (inexpensive) equipment. It does not involve body motion that may interfere with hemodynamic measurements. An involuntary Valsalva maneuver may occur during unsupervised isometric exercise. Careful monitoring, patient cooperation, and practice with the use of the handgrip dynamometer will minimize false hemodynamic information. In patients with CAD, isometric exercise rarely precipitates ischemia but may induce new LV wall motion abnormalities, a decrease in LV ejection fraction, and an increase in ESV with no change in diastolic volume. SV and CO may decline during isometric exercise. In patients with CHF, HR and systemic pressure may rise appropriately with a fall in SV and CO, resulting in an increase in LVEDV and PA pressure.

Pacing Tachycardia

Although rarely used, rapid atrial or RV pacing increases myocardial oxygen consumption and myocardial blood flow, LVEDV decreases

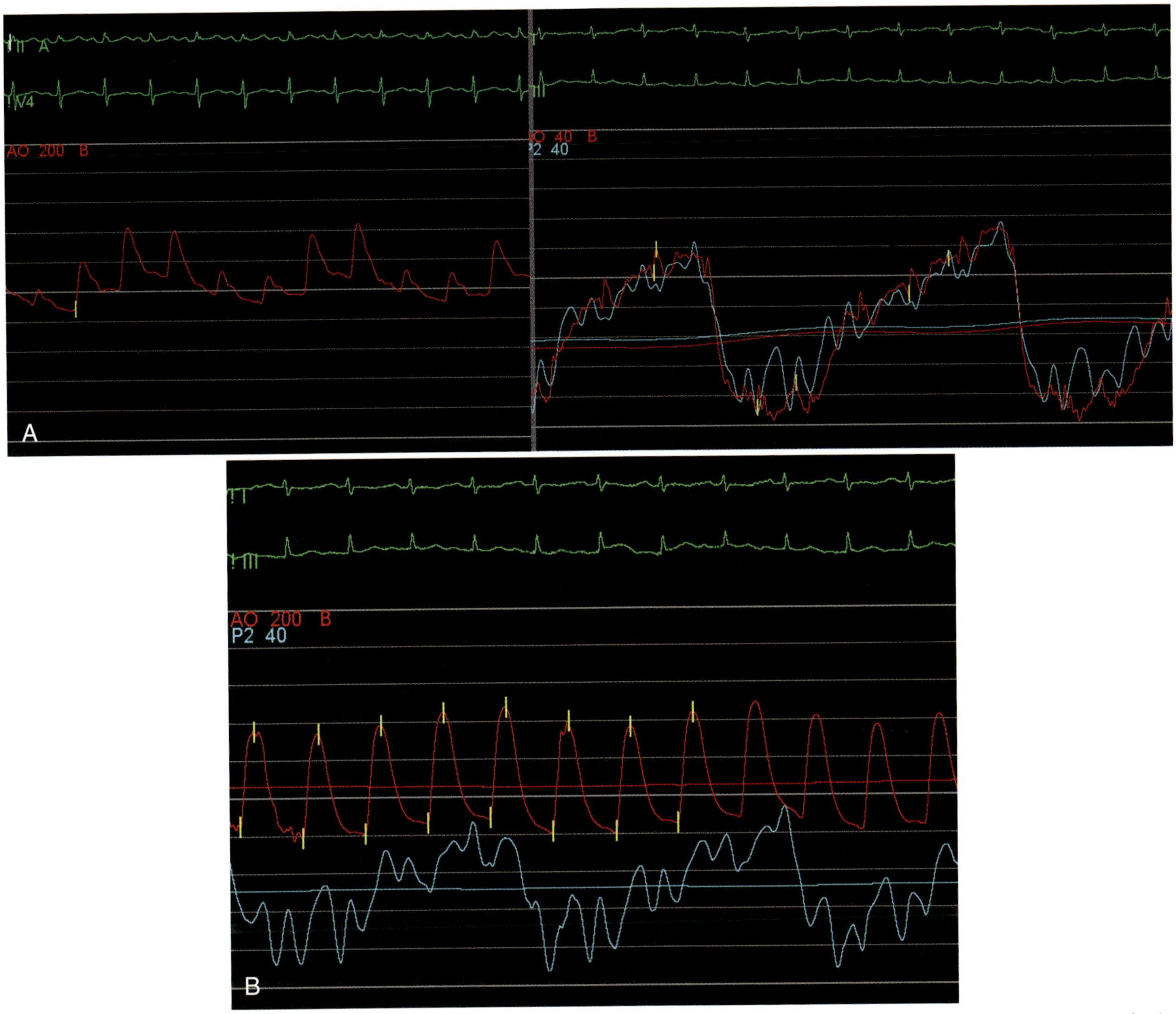

FIGURE 22.27 A, *Left,* Arterial pressure in patient with cardiac tamponade (scale 0 to 200 mm Hg). Note the large respiratory decrease in systolic pressure of pulsus paradoxus. *Right,* Left atrial (*red*) and pericardial pressure at the beginning of the pericardiocentesis. Atrial waveforms are blunted without distinct *a* or *v* waves. (scale 0 to 40 mm Hg). **B,** Arterial (*red*) and LA pressure (*blue*) after withdrawal of pericardial fluid. Note the return of normal arterial waveform and response to respiration.

with little change in cardiac output. It can be a useful method to define the severity of mitral valve stenosis and is safe with the ability to immediately terminate pacing if needed.

Physiologic Maneuvers and Volume Challenge

Various physiologic maneuvers can be used to alter the filling conditions of the heart. For example, the Valsalva maneuver in the strain phase decreases venous return and thus LV preload, which increases the systolic LV outflow tract pressure gradient in patients with HCM. In these patients, induction of a premature ventricular beat paradoxically decreases the pulse pressure (Brockenbrough-Braunwald-Morrow sign) and accentuates the spike-and-dome configuration on the aortic pressure waveform of the subsequent ventricular beat as the LV outflow gradient increases.

Another very useful physiologic challenge is rapid volume loading, which may distinguish pericardial constriction from myocardial restriction. Both conditions share hemodynamic patterns of early rapid filling dynamics and equalization of LV and RV pressure at end-expiration. Since pericardial restraint does not allow any overall volume expansion of the cardiac chambers, any volume expansion of the right ventricle will be at the cost of volume contraction of the left ventricle and vice versa, so-called exaggerated ventricular interdependence. Volume loading can cause equalized diastolic pressures between the two ventricles to differ in the setting of constriction.

Pharmacologic Challenges

Drugs that enhance contractility or vasodilate are useful for the hemodynamic diagnosis of various conditions and are readily available in the cardiac catheterization laboratory. Several of these have been previously discussed.

Dobutamine

Up to one-third of patients with LF/LG AS may be incorrectly defined as having severe AS by the Gorlin formula. To differentiate true from pseudo–severe AS, dobutamine can be infused at 5 μg/kg/min and increased by 3 to 10 μg/kg/min every 5 minutes. The test is ended once a maximum dose of 40 μg/kg/min is reached, the heart rate is >140 beats/min and/or cardiac output is increased by 50%, or the mean gradient increased to >40 mm Hg. Patients with a final AVA <1.2 cm² and mean gradient >30 mm Hg are considered to have severe AS. Excluding ischemia during the dobutamine infusion is important and a coronary angiogram is advised before dobutamine infusion in those patients. For patients with systemic hypertension and severe AS, afterload reduction with sodium nitroprusside can be useful to define the degree of AS.

Isoproterenol

In patients with HCM, various physical and pharmacologic manipulations can be performed to confirm the dynamic nature of the LV outflow tract gradient. The LVOT gradient is increased by isoproterenol due to increased inotropy and chronotropy and by nitroglycerin or amyl nitrate due to decreased preload and afterload. The dynamic LVOT outflow tract gradient can be reduced by administering phenylephrine thus increasing afterload (SVR).

Pulmonary Vasodilators

In patients with pulmonary hypertension, the response to pulmonary vasodilators can dictate future therapies. Vasodilator testing with epoprostenol, adenosine, nitroprusside, or nitric oxide is used to identify potential responders to therapy with calcium channel blockers and to establish prognosis.[23] In these cases, right-heart catheterization is required for the diagnosis of pulmonary arterial hypertension, which is defined by a mean PAP (mPAP) >25 mm Hg, a PCWP or LVEDP <15, and a pressure-volume relationship (PVR) >3 Wood units.

Vasodilator hemodynamic testing is also an important part of the evaluation for patients with advanced systolic heart failure who are being considered for orthotopic heart transplantation (OHTx). Relative contraindications to OHTx include a PVR ≥5, a pulmonary vascular resistance index (PVRI) ≥6, and a transpulmonary gradient (TPG) ≥16. A PA systolic pressure ≥60 mm Hg and any of the aforementioned elevations in pulmonary pressures are associated with increased mortality after OHTx. For these reasons, RHC is required in all OHTx candidates and should be repeated annually until transplantation or every 3 to 6 months if the patient has documented pulmonary hypertension.

Vasodilator testing is recommended in potential OHTx candidates with a pulmonary artery systolic pressure (PASP) ≥50, TPG ≥15, or PVR ≥3. Ideally, patients should have a PCWP <25 before testing to limit contribution from ongoing pulmonary venous congestion. Agents (e.g., nitroglycerine, nitroprusside, inhaled nitric oxide, epoprostenol, or milrinone) are also used to assess pulmonary pressures in patients with advanced heart failure. If acute vasodilator testing fails, patients are often admitted for 48 to 72 hours of continuous infusion therapy with milrinone and diuretics to optimize pulmonary pressures.

Nitric Oxide

Nitric oxide is an endothelium-derived vasodilator administered by inhalation and rapidly inactivated, making it safe to use without causing sustained systemic hypotension. It produces a pulmonary vasodilator response, the magnitude of which is a fairly accurate predictor of the response to oral vasodilator medical therapy and of overall prognosis. The pulmonary and systemic hemodynamic effects can be observed during escalating doses (doubling) in 2- to 5-minute intervals from 10 to 80 ppm. Cardiac output, PAP, and PCWP are the key study parameters, allowing for the calculation of PVR. A positive vasodilator response (i.e., reversibility) is defined as a decrease in mean PAP of ≥10 mm Hg to an absolute mean PAP of ≤40 mm Hg without a decrease in cardiac output.

A cautionary note for patients with elevated PCWP at baseline: Inhaled nitric oxide can reduce PVR leading to pulmonary edema. The mechanism is increased forward flow through the pulmonary vasculature with increased filling of left-sided heart chambers that have already reached their maximum compliance, precipitating further increase in PCWP and pulmonary congestion.

Nitroprusside

In patients with an elevated PCWP, sodium nitroprusside is preferred to document if reduction in afterload and LV filling pressure also lowers PAP and improves cardiac output. This holds true in cases of MR, dilated cardiomyopathy, and HFpEF. A typical protocol is to commence the infusion at 0.25 to 0.5 μg/kg/min following acquisition of baseline hemodynamic data and to up-titrate at the same dose range in 2- to 5-minute intervals until PCWP is <18 mm Hg, systemic blood pressure <90 mm Hg, or development of symptoms (e.g., lightheadedness).[24,25] On reaching those hemodynamic endpoints, a positive response is usually defined as a drop in PVR of at least 20%.

Pressure-Volume (PV) Relationships

The ejection fraction is the most commonly used parameter to reflect on cardiac function, but it remains sensitive to afterload as well as preload and heart size. A widely used invasive parameter is the maximal rate of pressure rise during isovolumic contraction (dP/dtmax); however, this parameter is also influenced by preload and heart rate as well as cardiac dyssynchrony. Relating cardiac pressure to cardiac volume has come the closest to providing the ideal parameter of cardiac contractility, one that is independent of preload, afterload, heart rate, and remodeling. A series of pressure-volume (PV) loops can be obtained to describe contractile function, relaxation properties, stroke volume, cardiac work, and myocardial oxygen consumption. Hemodynamic alterations and interventions change the PV relationship in predictable ways, and comparisons of various hemodynamic interventions can be made more precisely by examining the PV loop (Fig. 22.28). For example, increasing peripheral resistance decreases stroke volume while raising blood pressure, whereas reducing afterload has the opposite effect. Positive and negative inotropes increase and decrease stroke volume and stroke work by increasing or decreasing the slope of the end-systolic elastance (Ees).

A PV loop plots the changes of these variables over a cardiac cycle.[26-28] Each PV loop (see Fig. 22.28) represents one cardiac cycle. Beginning at end-diastole (point a), LV volume has received the atrial contribution and is maximal. Isovolumic contraction (a to b) increases LV pressure with no change in volume. At the end of isovolumic contraction, LV pressure exceeds aortic pressure, the aortic valve opens, and blood is ejected from the LV into the aorta (point b). Over the systolic ejection phase, LV volume decreases, and as ventricular repolarization occurs, LV ejection ceases and relaxation begins. When LV pressure falls below aortic pressure, the aortic valve closes, a point also known as the end-systolic pressure-volume point (ESPV) (point c). Isovolumic relaxation occurs until LV pressure decreases below the atrial pressure, opening the mitral valve (point d).

The stroke volume (SV) is represented by the width of the PV loop, the difference between end-systolic and end-diastolic volumes. The area within the loop represents stroke work. Load-independent LV contractility, also known as Emax, is defined as the maximal slope of the ESPV points under various loading conditions, the line of these points is the ESPV relationship (ESPVR). Effective arterial elastance (Ea), a measure of LV afterload, is defined as the ratio of end-systolic pressure to stroke volume. Maximal LV performance as measured as stroke work occurs when Ea = Emax. LV performance is more efficient when, for a given stroke work, myocardial oxygen consumption is lower, which occurs when Ea = 0.5 Emax.

Acute changes in cardiac function, for example, in the setting of an acute myocardial infarction (AMI), are also easily demonstrated. In AMI, LV contractility (Emax) is reduced; LV pressure, SV, and LV stroke work may be unchanged or reduced; and LVEDP is increased. In more severe cases of myocardial infarction, which evolve into cardiogenic shock, LV contractile function (Emax) is more severely reduced with associated significant increases in end-diastolic volume (LVEDV) and pressure (LVEDP). The LV impairment results in a markedly reduced stroke volume, acute diastolic dysfunction, and increased myocardial oxygen demand.

Most reports using PV loops characterize only LV hemodynamics. For research into RV function or extra-cardiac problems, the standard PV loops become complex and affected by additional factors altering the PV loop configuration and interpretation.[29]

Last but not least, it should be mentioned that careful assessment of the hemodynamics in the catheterization laboratory not only helps to diagnose and define the patient's cardiac disease status but also aids in its dynamic management. Examples include guidance for preload and afterload and optimization of cardiac filling pressures, initiation of inotropic therapy, and mechanical circulatory support. These elements integrate into the management of heart failure. Likewise, the invasive measurement of pulmonary arterial pressures and resistance and their modulation by pulmonary vasodilator therapy plays a central element in the management of patients with pulmonary arterial hypertension. This is further outlined in the corresponding disease chapters.

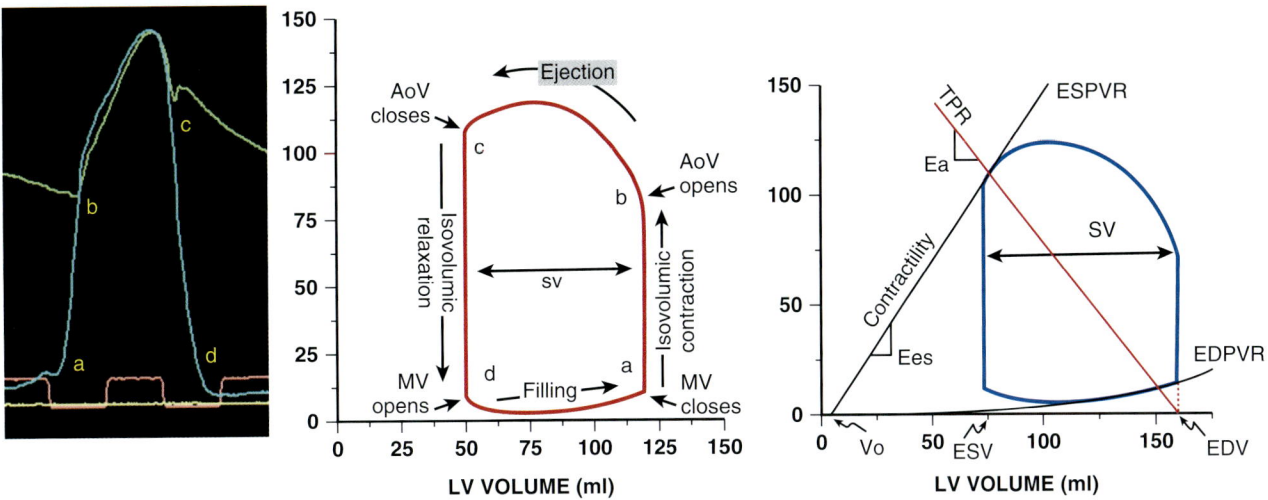

FIGURE 22.28 Origin of the pressure-volume loop relationship. **Left,** LV aortic pressure curves are used to generate the PV loop. Point a is LVEDP and the initiation of isovolumetric contraction. Point b is aortic valve opening as LV pressure exceeds aortic pressure. Systolic ejection continues until repolarization causes LV pressure to fall, crossing aortic pressure, point c, with the aortic pressure dicrotic notch beginning isovolumetric relaxation. The width of the PV loop is the stroke volume (SV). The width of the loop represents the difference between EDV and ESV, which is by definition the SV. The area within the loop is the ventricular stroke work. **Right,** Ventricular filling occurs along the end-diastolic pressure-volume relationship (EDPVR), or passive filling curve for the ventricle. The slope of the EDPVR is the reciprocal of ventricular compliance. Changes in ventricular compliance alter the slope of the passive filling curve. The maximal pressure that can be developed by the ventricle at any given left ventricular volume is defined by the end-systolic pressure-volume relationship (ESPVR), which represents the inotropic state of the ventricle.

ACKNOWLEDGMENT

This section extends the corresponding chapter of prior editions of *Braunwald's Heart Disease*, which was authored by Drs. Charles J. Davidson and Robert O. Bonow.

REFERENCES

1. Bashore TM, Balter S, Barac A, et al. 2012 American College of Cardiology Foundation/Society for Cardiovascular Angiography and Interventions expert consensus document on cardiac catheterization laboratory standards update: a report of the American College of cardiology foundation task force on expert consensus documents developed in collaboration with the Society of Thoracic Surgeons and Society for Vascular Medicine. *J Am Coll Cardiol*. 2012;59:2221–2305.
2. Mason PJ, Shah B, Tamis-Holland JE, et al. An update on radial artery access and best practices for transradial coronary angiography and intervention in acute coronary syndrome: a scientific statement from the American Heart Association. *Circulation: Cardiovasc Interv*. 2018;11(9):e000035.
3. Seto AH, Roberts JS, Abu-Fadel MS, et al. Real-time ultrasound guidance facilitates transradial access: RAUST (Radial Artery access with Ultrasound Trial). *JACC Cardiovasc Interv*. 2015;8:283–291.
4. Skelding KA, Tremmel JA. Arterial and venous access. In: Kern M, Lim M, Sorajja P, eds. *The Cardiac Catheterization Handbook*. 6th ed. Philadelphia: Elsevier; 2016:55–98.
5. Sobolev M, Slovut DP, Lee Chang A, et al. Ultrasound-guided catheterization of the femoral artery: a systematic review and meta-analysis of randomized controlled trials. *J Invasive Cardiol*. 2015;27:318–323.
6. Brass P, Hellmich M, Kolodziej L, et al. Ultrasound guidance versus anatomical landmarks for internal jugular vein catheterization. *Cochrane Database Syst Rev*. 2015;1:CD006962.5.
7. Alkhouli M, Rihal CS, Holmes Jr DR. Transseptal techniques for emerging structural heart interventions. *JACC Cardiovasc Interv*. 2016 Dec 26;9(24):2465–2480. https://doi.org/10.1016/j.jcin.2016.10.035.
8. Sorajja P, Lim MJ, Kern MJ, eds. *Kern's Cardiac Catheterization Handbook*. 7th ed. Philadelphia: Elsevier; 2020.
9. Nagueh SF, Smiseth OA, Appleton CP, et al. Recommendations for evaluation of left ventricular diastolic function by echocardiography: an update from the American society of Echocardiography and the European Association of Cardiovascular Imaging. *J Am Soc Echocardiogr*. 2016;29:277–314.
10. Gorlin R, Gorlin SG. Hydraulic formula for calculation of stenotic mitral valve, other cardiac valves, and central circulatory shunts. *Am Heart J*. 1951;41:1–29.
11. Hakki AH, Iskandrian AS, Bemis CE, et al. A simplified valve formula for the calculation of stenotic cardiac valve areas. *Circulation*. 1981;63:1050.
12. Abbas AE, Pibarot P. Hemodynamic characterization of aortic stenosis states. *Catheter Cardiovasc Interv*. 2019;93:1002–1023.
13. Lloyd JW, Nishimura RA, Borlaug BA, Eleid MF. Hemodynamic response to nitroprusside in patients with low-gradient severe aortic stenosis and preserved ejection fraction. *J Am Coll Cardiol*. 2017;70(11):1339–1348.
14. Maron BJ. Clinical course and management of hypertrophic cardiomyopathy. *N Engl J Med*. 2018;379:655–668. https://doi.org/10.1056/NEJMra1710575.
15. Geske JB, Ommen SR, Gersh BJ. Hypertrophic cardiomyopathy - clinical update. *JACC (J Am Coll Cardiol): Heart Fail*. 2018;6(5). https://doi.org/10.1016/j.jchf.2018.02.010.
16. Spaziano M, Sawaya FJ, Lefèvre T. Alcohol septal ablation for hypertrophic obstructive cardiomyopathy: indications, technical aspects, and clinical outcomes. *J Invasive Cardiol*. 2017;29(12):404–410.
17. Cui W, Dai R, Zhang G. A new simplified method for calculating mean mitral pressure gradient. *Catheter Cardiovasc Interv*. 2007;70:754–757.
18. Freihage JH, Joyal D, Arab D, et al. Invasive assessment of mitral regurgitation: comparison of hemodynamic parameters. *Catheter Cardiovasc Interv*. 2007;69:303–312.
19. Hurrell DG, Nishimura RA, Higano ST, et al. Value of dynamic respiratory changes in left and right ventricular pressures for the diagnosis of constrictive pericarditis. *Circulation*. 1996;93:2007–2013.
20. Talreja DR, Nishimura RA, Oh JK, Holmes DR. Constrictive pericarditis in the modern era: novel criteria for diagnosis in the cardiac catheterization laboratory. *J Am Coll Cardiol*. 2008;51:315–319.19 (constrict v restrict).
21. Kim KH, Miranda WR, Sinak LJ, et al. Effusive-constrictive pericarditis after pericardiocentesis: incidence, associated findings, and natural history. *JACC Cardiovasc Imaging*. 2018;11(4):534–541. https://doi.org/10.1016/j.jcmg.2017.06.017.
22. Borlaug BA, Nishimura RA, Sorajja P, et al. Exercise hemodynamics enhance diagnosis of early heart failure with preserved ejection fraction. *Circ Heart Fail*. 2010;3:588–595.
23. Galiè N, Humbert M, Vachiery JL, et al. 2015 ESC/ERS guidelines for the diagnosis and treatment of pulmonary hypertension: the joint task force for the diagnosis and treatment of pulmonary hypertension of the European Society of Cardiology (ESC) and the European Respiratory Society (ERS): Endorsed by: Association for European Paediatric and Congenital Cardiology (AEPC), International Society for Heart and Lung Transplantation (ISHLT). *Eur Heart J*. 2016;37:67–119.
24. Schwartzenberg S, Redfield MM, From AM, et al. Effects of vasodilation in heart failure with preserved or reduced ejection fraction implications of distinct pathophysiologies on response to therapy. *J Am Coll Cardiol*. 2012;59:442–451.
25. Yancy CW, Jessup M, Bozkurt B, et al. 2017 ACC/AHA/HFSA focused update of the 2013 ACCF/AHA guideline for the management of heart failure: a report of the American College of Cardiology/American Heart Association task force on clinical practice guidelines and the Heart Failure Society of America. *J Am Coll Cardiol*. 2017;70(6):776–803.
26. Burkhoff D, Mirsky I, Suga H. Assessment of systolic and diastolic ventricular properties via pressure-volume analysis: a guide for clinical, translational, and basic researchers. *Am J Physiol Heart Circ Physiol*. 2005;289(2):H501–H512.
27. Borlaug BA, Kass DA. Invasive hemodynamic assessment in heart failure. *Heart Fail Clin*. 2009;5(2):217–228.
28. Seemann F, Arvidsson P, Nordlund D, et al. Noninvasive quantification of pressure-volume loops from brachial pressure and cardiovascular magnetic resonance. *Circ Cardiovasc Imaging*. 2019;12(1):e008493.
29. Kapur NK, Esposito ML, Bader Y, et al. Mechanical circulatory support devices for acute right ventricular failure. *Circulation*. 2017;136:314–326.

23 Anesthesia and Noncardiac Surgery in Patients with Heart Disease

LEE A. FLEISHER AND JOSHUA A. BECKMAN

ASSESSMENT OF RISK, 410
Ischemic Heart Disease, 410
Hypertension, 411
Heart Failure, 411

THE DECISION TO UNDERGO DIAGNOSTIC TESTING, 412
Risk Calculators, 415

TESTS TO IMPROVE IDENTIFICATION AND DEFINITION OF CARDIOVASCULAR DISEASE, 416

OVERVIEW OF ANESTHESIA FOR CARDIAC PATIENTS UNDERGOING NONCARDIAC SURGERY, 417
Regional Anesthesia, 418
Monitored Anesthesia Care, 418
Intraoperative Hemodynamics and Myocardial Ischemia, 418

POSTOPERATIVE MANAGEMENT, 418
Postoperative Response to Surgery, 418

SURVEILLANCE AND IMPLICATIONS OF PERIOPERATIVE CARDIAC COMPLICATIONS, 419

STRATEGIES TO REDUCE THE RISK ASSOCIATED WITH NONCARDIAC SURGERY, 420
Coronary Artery Revascularization, 420
Pharmacologic Interventions, 421

CONCLUSION, 423

CLASSIC REFERENCES, 423

REFERENCES, 424

Cardiovascular morbidity and mortality represent a special concern in patients with known (or with risk factors for) cardiovascular disease who undergo noncardiac surgery. The cost of perioperative myocardial injury adds substantially to the total health care expenditure, with an average increased length of stay (LOS) of 6.8 days for patients with perioperative myocardial ischemic injury. Perioperative cardiovascular complications not only affect the immediate period but may also influence the outcome over subsequent years with an increased risk of readmission and death. The evidence base for managing patients with cardiovascular disease in the context of noncardiac surgery has grown in recent decades, beginning with identification of those at greatest risk and progressing to randomized trials to identify strategies for reducing perioperative cardiovascular complications. Guidelines provide information for the management of high-risk patients and disseminate best practices published by three major groups. Indeed, over the last decade, mortality rates for all major surgeries have decreased in parallel with implementation of these practices. This chapter distills this information by incorporating guidelines available from the American College of Cardiology and American Heart Association (ACC/AHA),[1] the European Society of Cardiology (ESC),[2] and the Canadian Cardiovascular Society (CCS).[3] The ACC/AHA Guideline was updated in 2014 with a focused update on dual antiplatelet therapy in 2016.[4]

ASSESSMENT OF RISK

Numerous points of entry lead to evaluation of patients before they undergo noncardiac surgery. Primary physicians or cardiologists may encounter such patients. History and physical examination represent the cornerstone of surgical risk evaluation, but risk assessment testing is rarely performed unless changes in management will result. Many patients undergo evaluation just before surgery by the surgeon or anesthesiologist. Importantly, several cardiovascular conditions require assessment independent of the time before surgery.

Ischemic Heart Disease

The stress related to noncardiac surgery increases metabolic requirements and activates the sympathetic nervous system and may raise the heart rate (HR) preoperatively, which is associated with a high incidence of symptomatic and asymptomatic myocardial ischemia. Preoperative clinical evaluation of patients may therefore identify stable or unstable coronary artery disease (CAD). Patients with acute manifestations of CAD such as unstable angina or other cardiac disease like decompensated heart failure (HF) have a high risk for the development of further decompensation, myocardial infarction (MI), and death during the perioperative period. Such patients clearly warrant further evaluation and medical stabilization prior to surgery. If the noncardiac surgery is truly an emergency, several small older case series have shown that intra-aortic balloon pump counterpulsation can provide short-term myocardial protection beyond that afforded by maximal medical therapy, although this measure is seldom used today.

If the patient is clinically stable, identification of known asymptomatic or symptomatic stable CAD or risk factors for CAD can foster the implementation of guideline-based risk reduction therapies. There is currently no significant adjunctive therapy that ameliorates cardiovascular surgical risk. In determining the extent of preoperative evaluation, it is important not to perform testing unless the results will affect perioperative management. In addition, the use of medications or interventions should mirror those that would be implemented in the absence of surgery. Infrequently, these changes in management may include cancellation of surgery (if the risk-benefit ratio is prohibitive) and consideration of palliative therapy, delay of surgery for further medical management, coronary investigation and interventions before surgery, use of an intensive care unit (ICU), and changes in monitoring. As discussed later, few evidence-based therapies are available independent of treating the underlying atherosclerotic risk, and except in the case of left main coronary artery stenosis, current data challenge the benefit of preoperative coronary revascularization. Thus, the primary reason to perform risk assessment is to determine clinical cardiovascular instability and suitability for surgery.

Over the last two decades, there has been a secular decrease in the rates of perioperative type 1 MI and mortality. Finks and colleagues reported a 36% decrease in death after open abdominal aortic aneurysm repair from 2000 to 2008, to a risk-adjusted mortality of 2.8%.[1] More recent data substantiate a decreasing frequency of type 1 MI and increasing rate of type 2 MI, indicating a predominance of subendocardial ischemic events resulting from hemodynamic challenge and more sensitive biomarker testing.[1] Although these events are characterized by increases in troponin and are strongly associated with death, the interval between troponin elevation and adverse events and the higher rate of nonvascular than cardiovascular mortality suggest that this is a marker of illness rather than a mechanism of mortality.

Traditionally, assessment of the coronary risk associated with noncardiac surgery in patients with previous MI was based on the time between the MI and surgery. Multiple older studies have demonstrated an increased incidence of reinfarction after noncardiac surgery if the previous MI had occurred within 6 months of the operation. Improvements in MI management and perioperative care have shortened this interval. Although in some patients after a recent MI the myocardium may still be at risk for subsequent ischemia and infarction, most patients in the United States will have had critical coronary stenoses identified and revascularized when appropriate and should already be receiving maximal medical therapy. The AHA/ACC Task Force on Perioperative Evaluation of the Cardiac Patient Undergoing Noncardiac Surgery has suggested that the highest-risk patients are those within 30 days of MI, during which time plaque and myocardial healing occur. After this period, risk stratification is based on the features of the disease (i.e., those with active ischemia are at highest risk). It should be noted that a study using administrative data from California demonstrated that the rate of perioperative cardiac morbidity and mortality remained elevated for at least 60 days after an MI, and the current iteration of the guidelines supports such a time frame.[1]

Hypertension

In the 1970s a series of case studies changed the prevailing thought that the use of antihypertensive agents should be discontinued before surgery. The reports suggested that poorly controlled hypertension was associated with untoward hemodynamic responses and that antihypertensives should be continued perioperatively. However, several large prospective studies were unable to establish mild to moderate hypertension as an independent predictor of postoperative cardiac complications including cardiac death, postoperative MI, HF, or arrhythmias. The approach to patients with hypertension therefore relies mostly on management strategies from the nonsurgical literature.

Blood pressure (BP) excursions in the operative and postoperative period portend worsening outcome. A hypertensive crisis in the postoperative period—defined as diastolic BP higher than 120 mm Hg and clinical evidence of impending or actual end-organ damage—poses a definite risk for MI and cerebrovascular accident (CVA, stroke). Iatrogenic precipitants of hypertensive crises include abrupt withdrawal of clonidine or beta blocker therapy before surgery, chronic use of monoamine oxidase inhibitors with or without sympathomimetic drugs, and inadvertent discontinuation of antihypertensive therapy. Similarly, intraoperative hypotension is associated with both type 2 MI and increases in postoperative mortality.[5]

Although postulated to predict an increased rate of myocardial ischemia, none of the recent large clinical trials has shown that chronic hypertension predisposes patients to perioperative cardiovascular events.[1] This finding likely reflects, in part, the excellent perioperative management of hypertension in the current era. The pharmacologic management of patients with hypertension should be continued perioperatively, and BP should be maintained near preoperative levels to reduce the risk for myocardial ischemia. In patients with more severe hypertension, such as a diastolic BP higher than 110 mm Hg, little evidence suggests a benefit of delaying surgery to optimize antihypertensive medications in the absence of a hypertensive urgency or emergency. Currently, debate surrounds the optimal decision on withholding angiotensin-converting enzyme inhibitors and angiotensin receptor blockers on the day of surgery to avoid intraoperative hypotension. Studies support both continuation and withholding, although continuation may require treatment with vasopressin for intractable hypotension. It is important to restart these agents as soon as possible postoperatively.

The importance of perioperative BP management was studied in the Intraoperative Norepinephrine to Control Arterial Pressure (INPRESS) study, a multicenter, randomized, clinical trial of an individualized management strategy aimed at achieving a systolic BP within 10% of the reference value (i.e., patient's resting systolic BP) or standard management strategy of treating systolic BP less than 80 mm Hg or lower than 40% from the reference value during and for 4 hours following surgery. Among 292 patients who completed the trial, management targeting an individualized systolic BP, compared with standard management, reduced the risk of postoperative organ dysfunction.[6]

Heart Failure

HF is associated with perioperative cardiac morbidity after noncardiac surgery in virtually all studies. Since the early work of Goldman and colleagues, who identified signs of HF as a significant risk of adverse perioperative events, HF has become more common with more varied presentations, including the presence or absence of ischemia and of reduced left ventricular ejection fraction. The underlying causes in patients with signs or symptoms of HF who are scheduled for noncardiac surgery require characterization. HF may eclipse CAD as a cause of postoperative adverse events. The 30-day postoperative mortality rate was significantly higher in patients with both nonischemic (9.3%) and ischemic (9.2%) HF compared to those with CAD (2.9%) in a population-based data analysis of 38,047 consecutive patients.[1]

The preoperative evaluation should aim to identify the underlying coronary, myocardial, and valvular heart disease and assess the severity of the systolic and diastolic dysfunction. Hammill and associates used Medicare claims data to evaluate short-term outcomes in patients with HF, CAD, or neither who underwent major noncardiac surgery. Elderly patients with HF who underwent major surgical procedures had substantially higher risk for operative mortality and hospital readmission than other patients, including those with CAD, admitted for the same procedures. A study using the American College of Surgeons (ACS) National Surgical Quality Improvement Program (NSQIP) database demonstrated that worsening preoperative HF is associated with a significant increase in postoperative morbidity and mortality when controlling for other comorbidities.[7] In the absence of a surgical emergency, patients with decompensated HF should be treated to achieve a euvolemic, stable state before operation. Ischemic cardiomyopathy is of greatest concern because the patient has the additional substantial risk for the development of further ischemia, which can lead to myocardial necrosis and potentially induce a downward spiral.

Hypertrophic Cardiomyopathy

Treatment of decompensated hypertrophic cardiomyopathy differs from that of dilated cardiomyopathy, and thus the preoperative evaluation can influence perioperative management in this setting (see Chapter 54). In particular, this assessment may influence perioperative fluid and vasopressor management. Obstructive hypertrophic cardiomyopathy was formerly regarded as a high-risk condition associated with high perioperative morbidity. A retrospective review of perioperative care in 35 patients, however, suggested low risk related to general anesthesia and major noncardiac surgery in such patients. This study also suggested that spinal anesthesia was a relative contraindication in view of the sensitivity of cardiac output to preload in this condition. Haering and colleagues studied 77 patients with asymmetric septal hypertrophy identified retrospectively from a large database; 40% had one or more adverse perioperative cardiac events, including one patient with MI and ventricular tachycardia who required emergency cardioversion. Most of the events consisted of perioperative congestive HF, and no perioperative deaths occurred. Unlike the finding in the original cohort of patients, the type of anesthesia was not an independent risk factor. Important independent risk factors for an adverse outcome (as seen generally) included major surgery and increasing duration of surgery.

VALVULAR HEART DISEASE

Aortic stenosis places patients at increased risk. Critical stenosis is associated with the highest risk for cardiac decompensation in patients undergoing elective noncardiac surgery (see Chapter 72). Thus, the presence of any of the classic triad of angina, syncope, and HF in a patient with aortic stenosis should prompt further evaluation and potential interventions (usually valve replacement). Preoperative patients with aortic systolic murmurs warrant a careful history and physical examination—and often further evaluation. Several recent case series of patients with critical aortic stenosis have demonstrated that when necessary, noncardiac surgery can be performed with acceptable risk. In a matched-sample study using the Danish Health Care System, Andersson and colleagues demonstrated that patients with asymptomatic aortic stenosis did not experience a higher rate of major adverse cardiovascular events (MACE) or mortality in elective surgery.[8] Emergency surgery type and symptomatic aortic stenosis increased both MACE and mortality. Aortic valvuloplasty is a bridging option for selected patients who cannot undergo valve replacement or percutaneous intervention in the short term. The substantial risk for procedure-related morbidity and mortality and little evidence to demonstrate a perioperative risk reduction mandate careful consideration before recommending this strategy.[1,9]

Mitral valve disease is associated with a lower risk for perioperative complications than aortic stenosis, although occult rheumatic mitral stenosis can sometimes lead to severe left-sided HF in patients with tachycardia (e.g., uncontrolled atrial fibrillation [AF]) and volume loading (see Chapter 75). In contrast to aortic valvuloplasty, mitral valve balloon valvuloplasty often yields both short- and long-term benefit, especially in younger patients with predominant mitral stenosis but without severe mitral valve leaflet thickening or significant subvalvular fibrosis and calcification.

In perioperative patients with a functioning prosthetic heart valve, antibiotic prophylaxis and anticoagulation require management (see Chapter 79). All patients with prosthetic valves who undergo procedures that can cause transient bacteremia should receive prophylaxis. In patients with prosthetic valves, the risk for increased bleeding during a procedure while receiving antithrombotic therapy must be weighed against the increased risk for thromboembolism caused by stopping the therapy. Common practice in patients undergoing noncardiac surgery with a mechanical prosthetic valve in place is cessation of warfarin 3 days before surgery. This allows the international normalized ratio (INR) to fall to less than 1.5 times normal; oral anticoagulants can then be resumed on postoperative day 1. A multicenter, single-arm cohort study of 224 high-risk patients (prosthetic valves, AF, and a major risk factor) investigated the use of low-molecular-weight heparin (LMWH) as a preoperative bridge to warfarin anticoagulation in which warfarin was withheld for 5 days and LMWH was given 3 days preoperatively and at least 4 days postoperatively. The overall rate of thromboembolism was 3.6% and of cardioembolism 0.9%. Major bleeding was seen in 6.7% of patients, although only 8 of 15 episodes occurred during the administration of LMWH. LMWH is cost-effective because it helps reduce the duration of the hospital stay, but two studies have shown a residual anticoagulation effect in as many as two thirds of patients.[10]

Many current prosthetic valves have a lower risk for valve thrombosis than the older designs, so the risk associated with heparin may outweigh its benefit in the perioperative setting. According to the 2020 AHA/ACC guidelines on management of valvular heart disease,[9] heparin can usually be reserved for high-risk patients. *High risk* is defined by the presence of a mechanical mitral or tricuspid valve or a mechanical aortic valve in the presence of certain risk factors, including AF, previous thromboembolism, hypercoagulable condition, older-generation mechanical valves, an ejection fraction lower than 30%, or more than one mechanical valve. Bridging anticoagulation therapy with heparin during the preoperative time interval when the INR is subtherapeutic should be made on an individualized basis, with the risks of bleeding weighed against the benefits of thromboembolism prevention. Subcutaneous LMWH or unfractionated heparin offers an alternative outpatient approach but has received only a tentative recommendation. Discussion between the surgeon and cardiologist regarding optimal perioperative management is critical. The 2020 ACC/AHA guidelines also note that it is reasonable to consider the need for bridging anticoagulant therapy around the time of invasive procedures in patients with bioprosthetic heart valves or annuloplasty rings who are receiving anticoagulation for AF on the basis of the CHA2DS2-VASc score weighed against the risk of bleeding.[9]

CONGENITAL HEART DISEASE IN ADULTS (SEE ALSO CHAPTER 82)

Congenital heart disease afflicts 500,000 to 1 million adults in the United States. The nature of both the underlying anatomy and any anatomic correction affects the perioperative plan and incidence of complications, which include infection, bleeding, hypoxemia, hypotension, and paradoxical embolization. In a study using the NSQIP database, prior cardiac surgery in a population age 19 to 39 years significantly increased the risk of death, MI, stroke, reoperation, and LOS.[11] Pulmonary hypertension and Eisenmenger syndrome present a major concern in patients with congenital heart disease. Regional anesthesia has traditionally been avoided in these patients because of the potential for sympathetic blockade and worsening of the right-to-left shunt. However, a review of 103 cases found that overall perioperative mortality was 14%; patients receiving regional anesthesia had a mortality of 5%, whereas those receiving general anesthesia had a mortality of 18%. The authors concluded that most deaths probably resulted from the surgical procedure and the disease rather than from anesthesia. Although perioperative and peripartum mortality was high, many anesthetic agents and techniques have been used with success. Patients with congenital heart disease are at risk for infective endocarditis and should receive antibiotic prophylaxis (see Chapter 82).

ARRHYTHMIAS

Cardiac arrhythmias frequently occur in the perioperative period, particularly in older adults or patients undergoing thoracic surgery.[12] Predisposing factors include previous arrhythmias, underlying heart disease, hypertension, perioperative pain (e.g., hip fractures), severe anxiety, and other situations that heighten adrenergic tone. In a prospective study of 4181 patients 50 years or older, supraventricular arrhythmia occurred in 2% during surgery and in 6.1% after surgery. Perioperative AF raises several concerns, including the incidence of stroke (see Chapters 45 and 66). In a study of 317 patients without AF undergoing major vascular surgery reported by Winkle et al. (see "Classic References"), the incidence of new-onset AF was 4.7% and was associated with more than a sixfold increase in cardiovascular death, MI, unstable angina, and stroke in the first 30 days and a fourfold increase over the next 12 months. Early treatment to restore sinus rhythm or control the ventricular response and initiate anticoagulation may be indicated. Prophylactic use of intravenous (IV) diltiazem and esmolol in randomized, placebo-controlled trials of patients undergoing high-risk thoracic surgery reduced the incidence of clinically significant atrial arrhythmias.[12]

Although older studies identified ventricular arrhythmias as a risk factor for perioperative morbidity, recent studies have not confirmed this finding. Current guidelines cite studies of patients undergoing major noncardiac surgical procedures reporting that preoperative arrhythmias are associated with intraoperative and postoperative arrhythmias, but not with nonfatal MI and cardiac death. However, this remains controversial as a population-based study by van Diepen et al. reported that the risk of mortality at 30 days was 6.4% in patients with preoperative AF compared with 2.9% for patients with CAD (see "Classic References").[1] These findings suggest that a preoperative arrhythmia should provoke a search for underlying cardiopulmonary disease, ongoing myocardial ischemia or infarction, drug toxicity, or electrolyte or metabolic derangements as suggested by other clinical circumstances.

Conduction abnormalities can increase perioperative risk and may require placement of a temporary or permanent pacemaker. On the other hand, patients with intraventricular conduction delays, even in the presence of a left or right bundle branch block but without a history of advanced heart block or symptoms, rarely progress to complete heart block perioperatively. The availability of transthoracic pacing units has decreased the need for temporary transvenous pacemakers.

THE DECISION TO UNDERGO DIAGNOSTIC TESTING

The ACC/AHA and ESC proposed algorithms for CAD evaluation based on the available evidence and incorporated the class of recommendations and level of evidence into each step (Figs. 23.1 and 23.2). Current algorithms use a stepwise Bayesian strategy that relies on assessment of clinical markers, previous coronary evaluation and treatment, functional capacity, and surgery-specific risk. Successful use of the ACC/AHA algorithm requires an appreciation of the different levels of risk attributable to the combination of clinical circumstances and type of surgery, levels of functional capacity, and how the information from any diagnostic testing will influence perioperative management.

Multiple studies have attempted to identify clinical risk markers for perioperative cardiovascular morbidity and mortality. As described earlier, patients with unstable coronary syndromes and severe valvular disease have active cardiac conditions. Risk can be divided into low (<1%) and elevated clinical risk. The 2014 ACC/AHA guidelines advocate using a risk index.[1] This includes either the ACS NSQIP risk calculator or myocardial infarction and cardiac arrest (MICA) risk calculator, which incorporates both surgical and clinical risk. Alternatively, the clinician can incorporate the revised cardiac risk index (RCRI) with the estimated surgical risk to differentiate low from elevated risk (Table 23.1). Cardiovascular disease also has clinical risk markers classified as "low-risk factors," each of which is associated with variable levels of perioperative risk. Recent investigation of more than 3 million patients using the United States National Surgical Quality Improvement Program shows patients without hypertension, diabetes mellitus, or current smoking have a postoperative MI and death rate of 0.1% and 0.47%, respectively.[13] The previous classification of perioperative, active clinical risk markers to assess the need for further testing includes issues beyond ischemic heart disease (Table 23.2).

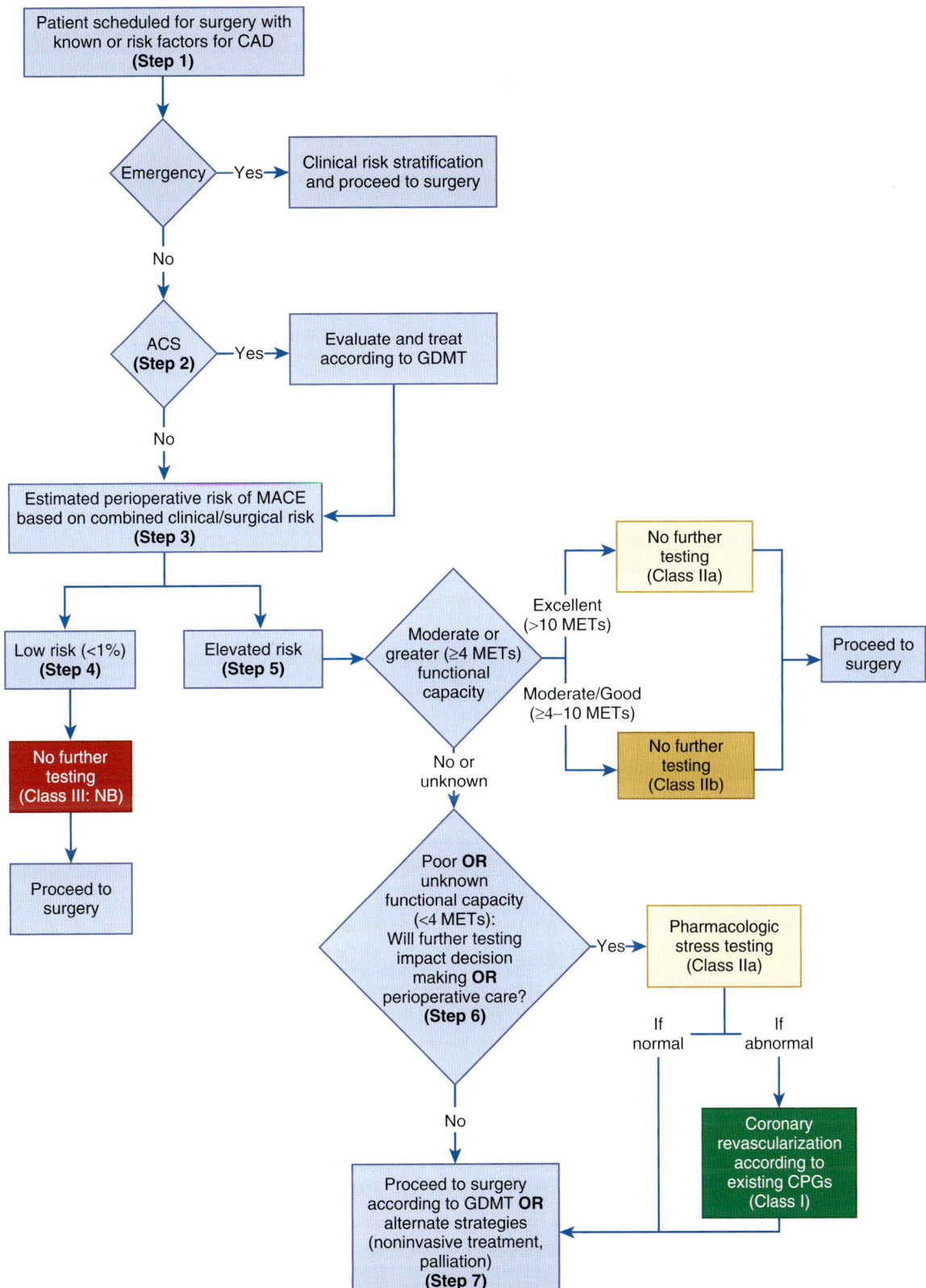

FIGURE 23.1 The 2014 ACC/AHA guideline algorithm depicting the stepwise approach to perioperative cardiac assessment for CAD. *ACS*, Acute coronary syndrome; *CAD*, coronary artery disease; *CPG*, clinical practice guideline; *GDMT*, guideline-directed medical therapy; *MACE*, major adverse cardiac event; *MET*, metabolic equivalent; *NB*, no benefit; *PCI*, percutaneous coronary intervention. (From Fleisher LA, Fleischmann KE, Auerbach AD, et al. 2014 ACC/AHA guideline on perioperative cardiovascular evaluation and management of patients undergoing noncardiac surgery: a report of the American College of Cardiology/American Heart Association Task Force on Practice Guidelines. *J Am Coll Cardiol*. 2014;64:e77–e137.)

Exercise tolerance is one of the strongest determinants of perioperative risk and the need for invasive monitoring. Several scales based on activities of daily living have been proposed to assess exercise tolerance; current guidelines advocate the Duke Activity Scale Index (Table 23.3).

The type of surgical procedure significantly impacts perioperative risk and the amount of preparation required to perform anesthesia safely. For surgical procedures not associated with significant stress or a high incidence of perioperative myocardial ischemia or morbidity, the cost and procedural delay of the evaluation often exceed any

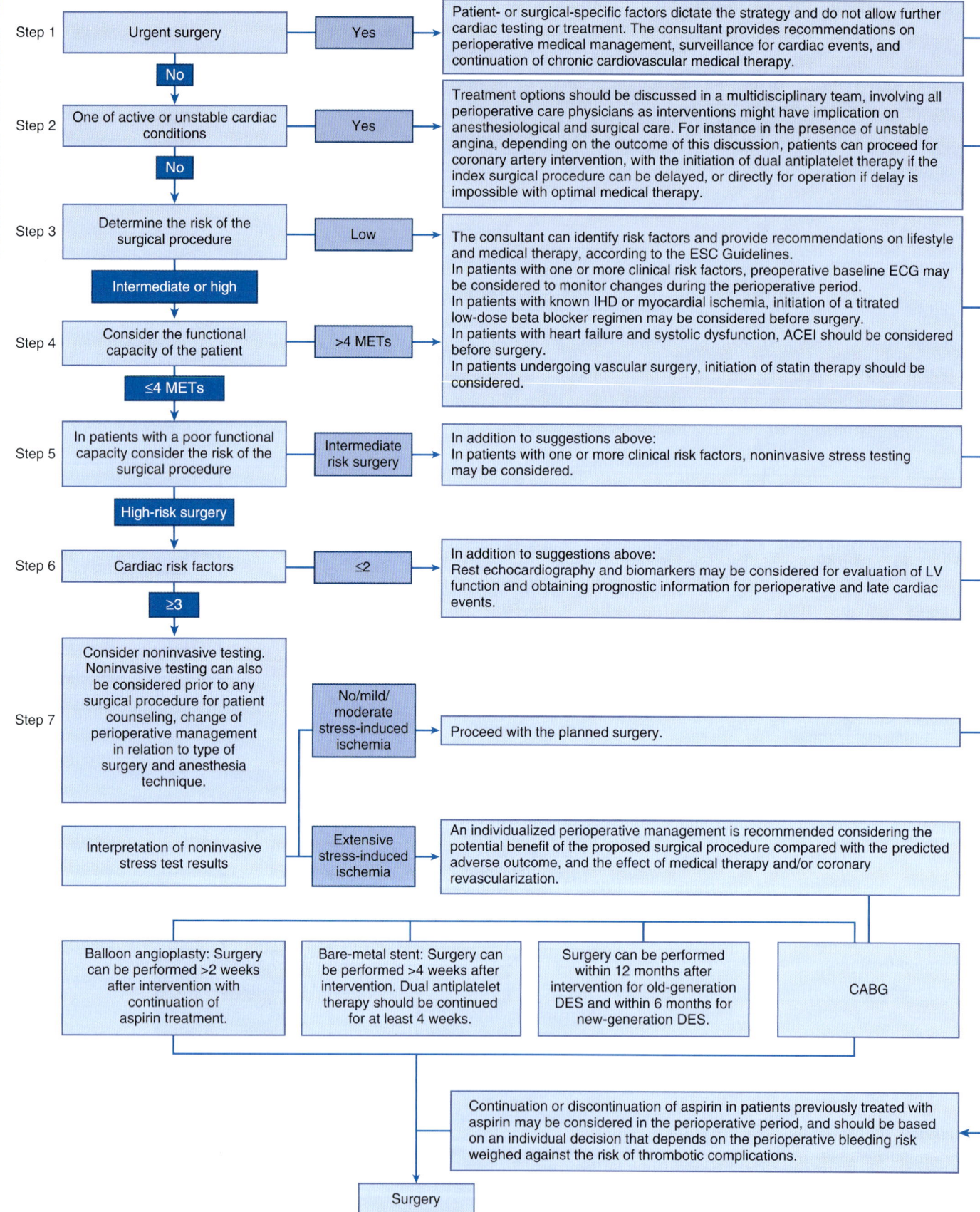

FIGURE 23.2 Summary of preoperative cardiac risk evaluation and perioperative management. *ACEI*, Angiotensin-converting enzyme inhibitors; *CABG*, coronary artery bypass graft; *DES*, drug-eluting stents; *IHD*, ischemic heart disease; *LV*, left ventricular; *METs*, metabolic equivalents. (From Kristensen SD, Knuuti J, Saraste A, et al. 2014 ESC/ESA guidelines on non-cardiac surgery: cardiovascular assessment and management: The Joint Task Force on Non-Cardiac Surgery: Cardiovascular Assessment and Management of the European Society of Cardiology (ESC) and the European Society of Anaesthesiology (ESA). *Eur Heart J*. 2014;35:2383–2431.)

TABLE 23.1 Cardiac Risk* Stratification for Noncardiac Surgical Procedures

RISK STRATIFICATION	EXAMPLES OF PROCEDURES
High (reported cardiac risk often >5%)	Aortic and other major vascular surgery Peripheral vascular surgery
Intermediate (reported cardiac risk generally 1%–5%)	Intraperitoneal and intrathoracic surgery Carotid endarterectomy Head and neck surgery Orthopedic surgery Prostate surgery
Low† (reported cardiac risk generally <1%)	Endoscopic procedures Superficial procedure Cataract surgery Breast surgery Ambulatory surgery

*Combined incidence of cardiac death and nonfatal myocardial infarction.
†These procedures do not generally require further preoperative cardiac testing.
From Fleisher LA, Beckman JA, Brown KA, et al. 2009 ACCF/AHA focused update on perioperative beta blockade incorporated into the ACC/AHA 2007 guidelines on perioperative cardiovascular evaluation and care for noncardiac surgery: a report of the American College of Cardiology Foundation/American Heart Association Task Force on Practice Guidelines. *J Am Coll Cardiol.* 2009;54:e77–e137.

TABLE 23.2 Active Cardiac Conditions for Which Patients Should Undergo Evaluation and Treatment Before Noncardiac Surgery (Class I; Level of Evidence: B)

CONDITION	EXAMPLES
Unstable coronary syndromes	Unstable or severe angina* (CCS class III or IV)† Recent myocardial infarction (MI)‡
Decompensated HF (NYHA functional class IV; worsening or new-onset HF)	
Significant arrhythmias	High-grade atrioventricular block Mobitz II atrioventricular block Third-degree atrioventricular heart block Symptomatic ventricular arrhythmias Supraventricular arrhythmias (including atrial fibrillation) with an uncontrolled ventricular rate (heart rate >100 beats/min at rest) Symptomatic bradycardia Newly recognized ventricular tachycardia
Severe valvular disease	Severe aortic stenosis (mean pressure gradient >40 mm Hg, aortic valve area <1.0 cm², or symptomatic) Symptomatic mitral stenosis (progressive dyspnea on exertion, exertional presyncope, or HF)

*According to Campeau L, Enjalbert M, Lespérance J, et al. Atherosclerosis and late closure of aortocoronary saphenous vein grafts: sequential angiographic studies at 2 weeks, 1 year, 5 to 7 years, and 10 to 12 years after surgery. *Circulation.* 1983;68(Suppl II):1–7.
†May include "stable" angina in patients who are unusually sedentary.
‡The American College of Cardiology National Database Library defines "recent" MI as more than 7 days but 1 month or less (within 30 days) although the 2014 guidelines suggest 60 days.
CCS, Canadian Cardiovascular Society; *HF,* heart failure; *NYHA,* New York Heart Association.
From Fleisher LA, Beckman JA, Brown KA, et al. 2009 ACCF/AHA focused update on perioperative beta blockade incorporated into the ACC/AHA 2007 guidelines on perioperative cardiovascular evaluation and care for noncardiac surgery: a report of the American College of Cardiology Foundation/American Heart Association Task Force on Practice Guidelines. *J Am Coll Cardiol.* 2009;54(22):e77–e137.

TABLE 23.3 Estimated Energy Requirements for Various Activities

	CAN YOU …
1 MET	Take care of yourself? Eat, dress, or use the toilet? Walk indoors around the house? Walk a block or two on level ground at 2–3 mph (3.2–4.8 kph)?
4 METs	Do light work around the house such as dusting or washing dishes? Climb a flight of stairs or walk up a hill? Walk on level ground at 4 mph (6.4 kph)? Run a short distance? Do heavy work around the house such as scrubbing floors or lifting or moving heavy furniture? Participate in moderate recreational activities such as golf, bowling, dancing, doubles tennis, or throwing a baseball or football?
>10 METs	Participate in strenuous sports such as swimming, singles tennis, football, basketball, or skiing?

MET, Metabolic equivalent; *mph,* miles per hour; *kph,* kilometers per hour.
Modified from Hlatky MA, Boineau RE, Higginbotham MB, et al. A brief self-administered questionnaire to determine functional capacity (the Duke Activity Status Index). *Am J Cardiol.* 1989;64:651–654; and Fleisher LA, Beckman JA, Brown KA, et al. 2009 ACCF/AHA focused update on perioperative beta blockade incorporated into the ACC/AHA 2007 guidelines on perioperative cardiovascular evaluation and care for noncardiac surgery: a report of the American College of Cardiology Foundation/American Heart Association Task Force on Practice Guidelines. *J Am Coll Cardiol.* 2009;54:e77–e137.

benefit from the information gained by preoperative assessment. Outpatient procedures, for example, cause minimal morbidity and mortality; in such patients, cardiovascular status rarely changes perioperative management unless the patient has unstable angina or overt HF. In fact, 30-day mortality after outpatient surgery may actually be lower than that expected if the patient did not undergo surgery. In contrast, open surgery for vascular disease entails a high risk for morbidity and the potential for ischemia. Intra-abdominal, thoracic, and orthopedic procedures are associated with elevated risk, which, when combined with clinical risk factors, determine overall perioperative risk. Endovascular procedures fall into this intermediate-risk category because of their associated perioperative morbidity and mortality, although long-term survival appears to be similar to that in patients who undergo open procedures.

In addition to the risk related to the surgical procedure itself, risk is also correlated with the surgical volume in a given center. Several studies have demonstrated differential mortality rates in both cancer and vascular surgery, with higher mortality occurring in low-volume centers, although recent studies have demonstrated that low-volume centers may also have low mortality rates if proper care systems are in place. Surgical mortality rates may therefore be institution specific, which may influence the decision to perform further perioperative evaluations and interventions.

Risk Calculators

Much of the contemporary study of perioperative cardiac risk has focused on the development of clinical risk indices. The most widely used index was developed in a study of 4315 patients age 50 or older undergoing elective major noncardiac procedures in a tertiary care teaching hospital. The index includes six independent predictors of complications in a *revised cardiac risk index*: high-risk type of surgery, history of ischemic heart disease, history of congestive HF, history of cerebrovascular disease, preoperative treatment with insulin, and preoperative serum creatinine concentration greater than 2.0 mg/dL. Cardiac complication rates rise with an increasing number of these risk factors. Patients are stratified into low, intermediate, or high cardiovascular risk on the basis of having 0, 1 or 2, or 3 or more factors included in the RCRI, respectively. The RCRI has become a standard tool for assessing the probability of perioperative cardiac risk in a given individual and serves to direct the decision to perform cardiovascular testing and implement perioperative management protocols. The RCRI has undergone validation in vascular surgery populations and serves to predict long-term outcome and quality of life, although one group has advocated inclusion of age as a risk factor and its outcomes are derived from data a quarter century old.

Additional risk indices were developed from the ACS-NSQIP database. Gupta and colleagues developed a risk calculator for predicting perioperative *myocardial infarction and cardiac arrest* (see "Classic References") in a study of 211,410 patients, of whom perioperative MI or cardiac arrest developed in 1371 (0.65%).[1] Multivariate logistic regression analysis identified five predictors of perioperative MI or cardiac arrest: type of surgery, dependent functional status, abnormal creatinine level, American Society of Anesthesiologists class, and increasing age.

A universal risk calculator developed to predict multiple outcomes was based on 1,414,006 patients encompassing 1557 unique surgical procedure codes, which had excellent performance for mortality (C-statistic = 0.944) and morbidity (C-statistic = 0.816). Morbidity is defined as any of the following intraoperative or postoperative events: surgical site infection, wound disruption, pneumonia, unplanned intubation, pulmonary embolism, on ventilator greater than 48 hours, progressive renal insufficiency, acute renal failure, urinary tract infection, stroke/CVA, cardiac arrest, MI, deep venous thrombosis, (systemic sepsis), pneumonia, cardiac event (cardiac arrest or MI), SSI, UTI, VTE, and renal failure (progressive renal insufficiency or acute renal failure) (http://riskcalculator.facs.org).[1] The risk calculator incorporates 21 preoperative risk factors and therefore has more discriminative ability than the MICA-specific risk calculator. Glance and colleagues demonstrated variability in the predicted risk of cardiac complications using different risk-prediction tools, also suggesting that the ACS-NSQIP risk calculator is the best option.[14]

In 2019 American University of Beirut-Pre-Operative Cardiovascular Evaluation Study (AUB-POCES) prospectively derived and validated a new preoperative cardiovascular risk index (CVRI).[15] It was subsequently renamed the AUB-HAS2 based on the six predictors of risk identified by multivariate logistic regression analysis in the derivation cohort: history of **H**eart disease, **H**eart symptoms of angina or dyspnea, **A**ge ≥75 years, **A**nemia with hemoglobin less than 12 mg/dL, vascular **S**urgery, and emergency **S**urgery. Patients were assigned a score of 0, 1, 2, 3, and greater than 3 based on the number of predictors. The incidence of the primary outcome of death, MI, or stroke at 30 days increased steadily across the increasing scores. A subsequent analysis of the performance of AUB-HAS2 in 9 surgical specialty groups and 8 site-specific surgeries using 1,167,278 noncardiac surgeries from the NSQIP database demonstrated superior discriminatory power compared with the RCRI. The performance of the AUB-HAS2 index was superior to that of the RCRI in all surgical subgroups ($P < 0.001$) but needs further evaluation.[15]

THE GUIDELINES APPROACH

The ACC/AHA Task Force for Guidelines for Perioperative Cardiovascular Evaluation and Management for Noncardiac Surgery presented their recommendations in algorithmic form as a framework for determining which patients are candidates for cardiac testing (see Fig. 23.1). Given the availability of the evidence, the writing committee included the level of the recommendations and strength of evidence for each of the pathways. The current algorithm focuses exclusively on the evaluation for CAD. Valvular or other forms of heart disease are not included in the current algorithm.

Step 1: The consultant should determine the urgency of performing noncardiac surgery. In many cases, patient- or surgery-specific factors dictate an obvious strategy (e.g., emergency surgery) that may not allow further cardiac assessment or treatment.

Step 2: Does the patient have an acute coronary syndrome? Acute coronary syndromes include previous MI with evidence of substantial ischemic risk as determined by clinical symptoms or noninvasive study, unstable or severe angina, and new or poorly controlled ischemia-mediated HF. Depending on the results of tests or interventions and the risk inherent in delaying surgery, it may be appropriate to proceed to the planned surgery with maximal medical therapy.

Step 3: What is the estimated perioperative risk of a MACE based on the combined clinical and surgical risk? The use of a validated risk index is advocated, either of the ACS-NSQIP risk indices or combining the RCRI with the estimated surgical risk.

Step 4: Does the patient have low perioperative risk (<1%)? In such cases, no further testing is required.

Step 5: Does the patient have elevated risk? Such circumstances merit assessment of functional capacity. If the patient has at least moderate exercise capacity (≥4 metabolic equivalents), management rarely changes on the basis of the results of any further cardiovascular testing, and it is therefore appropriate to proceed with the planned surgery. The strength of the evidence and the recommendation depends on the degree of exercise capacity, with excellent capacity having stronger evidence and recommendation. In the recently published METS study, subjectively assessed functional capacity should not be used for preoperative risk evaluation. The authors suggested that clinicians could instead consider a standardized measure such as Duke Activity Status Index (DASI) for cardiac risk assessment.

Step 6: In patients with poor (<4 METs) or unknown functional capacity, the physicians and patient should jointly determine if further testing will impact decision making or perioperative care. If not, proceeding to surgery with goal-directed medical therapy is appropriate. In the current guidelines, the identification of elevated risk with poor functional capacity may also lead to the decision to proceed with alternative strategies, such as noninvasive treatment or palliation.

The CCS Guidelines use an entirely different approach and include the RCRI combined with the Brain Natriuretic Peptide (BNP) or NT-proBNP for risk assessment for more extensive postoperative monitoring as opposed to advocating preoperative cardiovascular testing.[3] There is no management strategy to mitigate risk discussed after testing.

TESTS TO IMPROVE IDENTIFICATION AND DEFINITION OF CARDIOVASCULAR DISEASE

The use of testing to identify patients at high cardiovascular risk requires the acknowledgement of several secular outcome changes over time. First, overall results from surgery are excellent, with mortality rates for all patients hovering around 1% in all comers and continual improvement in higher-risk surgery.[1] Second, type 1 MI requiring postoperative revascularization is uncommon. In a recent large, randomized trial of patients at high risk on the basis of an elevated troponin postoperatively requirement for study entry, fewer than 4% of this group underwent coronary revascularization.[16] Indeed, mortality in recent trials is driven more by non-vascular events than vascular ones.[17] From these data, we recommend the focus of testing remain actionable management changes, either providing a target for risk remediation or cancelling of surgery.

Several noninvasive diagnostic methods can diagnose and indicate the extent of CAD before noncardiac surgery. The exercise electrocardiogram (ECG) has traditionally served as an initial evaluation for the presence of CAD. As noted earlier, patients with excellent exercise tolerance in daily life will rarely benefit from further testing. Patients with poor exercise capacity, in contrast, may not achieve an adequate HR and BP for diagnostic purposes on electrocardiographic stress tests. Such patients often require concomitant imaging. Recent work demonstrates the common inappropriate use and lack of predictive value of stress testing in patients undergoing low risk surgery. Among more than 800,000 patients undergoing total hip or knee arthroplasty, half had a low-risk RCRI score of 0 and stress test acquisition resulted in no difference in the primary outcome of MI or cardiac arrest among patients with an RCRI score of ≥1.[18]

Many high-risk patients either cannot exercise or have limitations to exercise (e.g., patients with intermittent claudication or knee arthritis). Pharmacologic stress testing, therefore, has become popular, particularly as a preoperative test in patients undergoing vascular surgery. Several studies have shown that the presence of a redistribution defect on dipyridamole or adenosine thallium or sestamibi imaging in patients undergoing peripheral vascular surgery predicts an increased risk for postoperative cardiac events (see Chapter 18). Pharmacologic stress imaging is best used in patients at moderate clinical risk. Several strategies may increase the predictive value of such tests. The redistribution defect can be quantitated, with larger areas of defect associated with increased risk. Additionally, either increased lung uptake or dilation of the left ventricular cavity indicate ventricular dysfunction with ischemia. Several investigative groups have demonstrated that delineation of low-risk and high-risk myocardial perfusion scans (larger area of defect, increased lung uptake, and dilation of the left ventricular cavity) greatly improves the test's predictive value. Patients with high-risk scans have a particularly increased risk for perioperative morbidity and long-term mortality.

Stress echocardiography has also been used widely as a preoperative test (see Chapter 16). One advantage of this test is that it dynamically assesses myocardial ischemia in response to increased inotropy and HR, stimuli relevant to the perioperative period. The presence of new wall motion abnormalities occurring at a low HR is the best predictor of increased perioperative risk, with large areas of contractile dysfunction having secondary importance. As part of the DECREASE studies, Boersma and colleagues (as cited in the guidelines) assessed the value of dobutamine stress echocardiography with respect to the extent of wall motion abnormalities and the ability of preoperative treatment with beta blockers to attenuate risk in patients undergoing major aortic surgery. They assigned 1 point for each of the following characteristics: age older than 70 years, current angina, MI, congestive HF, previous cerebrovascular disease, diabetes mellitus, and renal failure. As the total number of clinical risk factors increases, perioperative cardiac event rates also increase. Furthermore, with a high-risk score, abnormal findings on an echocardiogram predict higher risk.

Several groups have published meta-analyses examining various preoperative diagnostic tests. Such studies report good predictive values for ambulatory electrocardiographic monitoring, radionuclide angiography, dipyridamole-thallium imaging, and dobutamine stress echocardiography. Shaw and colleagues also demonstrated excellent predictive values for dipyridamole thallium imaging and dobutamine stress echocardiography.[2] Beattie and colleagues performed a meta-analysis of 25 stress echocardiography studies and 50 thallium imaging studies.[1] The likelihood ratio for stress echocardiography was more indicative of a postoperative cardiac event than that for thallium imaging (likelihood ratio), 4.09; (95% confidence interval (CI), 3.21 to 6.56; versus LR, 1.83; 95% CI, 1.59 to 2.10; $P < 0.001$). The difference was attributable to fewer false-negative stress echocardiograms. A moderate to large abnormality found by either test predicted a greater risk of postoperative MI and death.

Institutional expertise should guide the choice of preoperative testing. The relevant clinical questions also influence the choice of test. For example, if valve function or ventricular wall thickness is of interest, echocardiography has advantages over perfusion imaging. Stress nuclear imaging may have slightly higher sensitivity, but stress echocardiography may have fewer false-positive results. The role of newer imaging modalities such as magnetic resonance imaging, multislice computed tomography, coronary calcium scores, and positron emission tomography in preoperative risk assessment is rapidly evolving.

Over the past decade, cardiopulmonary exercise testing (CPET) has been used as a preoperative test (see Chapter 15), particularly in Great Britain. A consistent finding of the studies was that a low anaerobic threshold was predictive of perioperative cardiovascular complications, postoperative death, or midterm and late death after surgery. An anaerobic threshold of approximately 10 mL O_2/kg/min was proposed as the optimal discrimination point, with a range in these studies of 9.9 to 11 mL O_2/kg/min. The METS study was designed to address the value of subjective assessment of exercise capacity, the objective Duke Activity Specific Index (DASI) questionnaire and a biomarker N-terminal pro-B-type natriuretic peptide (NT-pro-BNP) to predict death or complications after major elective non-cardiac surgery.[19] The investigators documented the poor discriminative ability of anesthesiologists to subjectively predict functional capacity; however, the DASI was predictive of myocardial injury and death. Although CPET did not have increased predictive ability for cardiac events, some of the measured variables were predictive of complications after surgery. CPET is therefore currently under evaluation as a means of determining both the need for and value of "prehabilitation," in which a strategy of exercise is initiated to increase aerobic capacity before surgery.[20] Several groups are studying the value of CPET to inform shared decision making in determining the appropriateness of surgery given the intermediate- and long-term outcomes in high-risk patients.

The use of biomarkers in risk stratification before surgery has also been investigated. A meta-analysis of 18 studies demonstrated that preoperative BNP measurement independently predicted perioperative cardiovascular events in studies that considered only the outcomes of death, or nonfatal MI (odds ratio [OR], 1.9; 95% CI, 1.38 to 2.58).[1] In a large substudy of the Vascular Events in Noncardiac Surgery Cohort Evaluation (VISION) trial of more than 10,400 patients, higher preoperative levels of NT-proBNP associated directly with higher levels of cardiovascular events.[21] In a stepwise pattern, the 30-day risk of vascular mortality increased from 0.2% in subjects with a NT-proBNP of less than 100 g/mL and increased directly with increasing NT-proBNP to 2.1% in patients with NT-proBNP ≥ 1500 pg/mL (HR 6.8 compared to referent). Thirty-day all-cause mortality increased with the previous thresholds from 0.3% to 3.4% (HR 8.4 compared to referent).[21] Similar to exercise and imaging testing above, the lack of a management algorithm after abnormal measurement limits the ability of the clinician to modify surgical risk based on this test. Maile and coworkers reviewed 6030 patients with troponin measured in the 30 days before nonemergent noncardiac surgery and found a 30-day mortality of 4.7% in the group without detectable troponin levels, but a 12.7% mortality in the group with the highest tercile of troponin elevation.[22] The closer in time that an elevated troponin was drawn to the date of surgery, the higher the risk.

OVERVIEW OF ANESTHESIA FOR CARDIAC PATIENTS UNDERGOING NONCARDIAC SURGERY

Three classes of anesthetics exist: general, regional, and local/sedation or monitored anesthesia care (MAC). General anesthesia can be defined best as a state that includes unconsciousness, amnesia, analgesia, immobility, and attenuation of autonomic responses to noxious stimulation, and it can be achieved with inhalational agents, IV agents, or a combination of these (frequently called a "balanced technique"). Contemporary general anesthesia does not always require an endotracheal tube. Laryngoscopy and intubation were traditionally considered the time of greatest stress and risk for myocardial ischemia, but extubation may actually engender even greater risk. Alternative methods for delivering general anesthesia include the use of a mask or a laryngeal mask airway—a device that fits above the epiglottis and does not require laryngoscopy or intubation.

> Five inhalational anesthetic agents (in addition to nitrous oxide) are currently approved in the United States, although enflurane and halothane are rarely used today. All inhalational agents have reversible myocardial depressant effects and lead to decreases in myocardial oxygen demand. The degree to which they depress cardiac output depends on their concentration, their effects on systemic vascular resistance, and their effects on baroreceptor responsiveness; agents therefore differ in their specific effects on HR and BP. Isoflurane causes negative inotropic effects and potent vascular smooth muscle relaxation and has minimal effects on baroreceptor function. Desflurane has the fastest onset and is commonly used in the outpatient setting. The onset and offset of action of sevoflurane are intermediate to those of isoflurane and desflurane; the major advantage of sevoflurane is an extremely pleasant smell, which makes it the agent of choice in children.
>
> Issues have arisen regarding the safety of inhalational agents in patients with CAD. Several large-scale, randomized and nonrandomized studies of patients undergoing coronary artery bypass grafting (CABG), however, demonstrated no increased incidence of myocardial ischemia or infarction in patients receiving inhalational agents versus narcotic-based techniques. The use of inhalational anesthetics in patients with CAD also has theoretical advantages. Several investigative groups demonstrated in vitro and in animals that inhalational agents have protective effects on myocardium similar to ischemic preconditioning, although the clinical relevance of this remains unclear.
>
> High-dose narcotic techniques offer the advantages of hemodynamic stability and lack of myocardial depression. Narcotic-based anesthetics were frequently considered the "cardiac anesthesia" and were

advocated for use in all high-risk patients, including those undergoing noncardiac surgery. The disadvantage of these traditional high-dose narcotic techniques is the requirement for postoperative ventilation. The ultrashort-acting narcotic remifentanil obviates the need for prolonged ventilation but provides hemodynamic stability. This agent can assist in early extubation of patients undergoing cardiac surgery and may aid in managing short periods of intense intraoperative stress in high-risk patients.

Despite the theoretical advantages of a high-dose narcotic technique, large-scale trials in patients undergoing CABG showed no difference in survival or major morbidity compared to the inhalation-based technique. This observation has contributed to the abandonment of high-dose narcotics in much of cardiac surgery and to an emphasis on early extubation. Most anesthesiologists use a balanced technique involving the administration of lower doses of narcotics with an inhalational agent. This approach allows the anesthesiologist to derive the benefits of each of these agents while minimizing side effects.

The IV agent propofol is an alternative mode of delivering general anesthesia. An alkyl phenol that can be used for both induction and maintenance of general anesthesia, propofol can cause profound hypotension because of reduced arterial tone with no change in HR. Its major advantage is rapid clearance with few residual effects on awakening, but because it is expensive, its current use tends to be limited to operations of brief duration. Despite its hemodynamic effects, propofol has been used extensively to assist in early extubation after CABG.

Current evidence indicates that there is no single "best" general anesthetic technique for patients with CAD who are undergoing noncardiac surgery, which has led to abandonment of the concept of a cardiac anesthetic.

Regional Anesthesia

Regional anesthesia includes spinal, epidural, and peripheral nerve blocks, and each technique has advantages and risks. Peripheral techniques, such as brachial plexus, femoral nerve, or Bier blocks, offer the advantage of causing minimal or no hemodynamic effects. These techniques are frequently used for orthopedic surgery. In contrast to peripheral nerve blocks, spinal or epidural techniques can produce sympathetic blockade, which can reduce BP and slow the HR. Spinal anesthesia and lumbar or low thoracic epidural anesthesia can also evoke reflex sympathetic activation mediated above the level of blockade, which might lead to myocardial ischemia.

The primary clinical difference between epidural and spinal anesthesia is the ability to provide continuous anesthesia or analgesia with placement of an epidural catheter, as opposed to a single dose with spinal anesthesia, although some clinicians will place a catheter in the intrathecal space. Even though the speed of onset depends on the local anesthetic agent used, spinal anesthesia and its associated autonomic effects occur sooner than when the same agent is administered epidurally. A catheter, usually left in place for epidural anesthesia, permits titration of the agent. Epidural catheters can also be used postoperatively to provide analgesia.

Extensive research has compared regional with general anesthesia for patients with CAD, particularly in those undergoing infrainguinal bypass surgery. In one meta-analysis, overall mortality was reduced by approximately one third in patients allocated to neuraxial blockade, although the findings were controversial because most of the benefit was observed in older studies. Reductions in MI and renal failure also occurred. A large-scale study of regional versus general anesthesia in noncardiac surgery patients did not demonstrate a difference in outcome.

Regional anesthesia has become very common with recent advances in ultrasound-guided administration and development of *enhanced recovery after surgery* (ERAS) protocols. Regional anesthesia offers the opportunity to provide excellent pain relief after surgery, which has proved advantageous and reduces perioperative cardiac stress.[24]

Monitored Anesthesia Care

MAC encompasses local anesthesia administered by the surgeon, with or without sedation. In a large-scale cohort study, MAC was associated with increased 30-day mortality compared with general anesthesia in a univariate analysis, although it did not remain significant in multivariate analysis once patient comorbidity was taken into account. The major issue with MAC is the ability to block the stress response adequately because the tachycardia associated with inadequate analgesia may be worse than the potential hemodynamic effects of general or regional anesthesia. Since the introduction of newer, short-acting IV agents, general anesthesia can now be administered essentially without an endotracheal tube. This approach allows the anesthesiologist to provide intense anesthesia for short or peripheral procedures without the potential effects of endotracheal intubation and extubation and therefore blurs the distinction between general anesthesia and MAC. An analysis of closed insurance claims demonstrated a high incidence of respiratory complications with MAC.

Intraoperative Hemodynamics and Myocardial Ischemia

Over the last two decades, numerous studies have explored the relationship between hemodynamics and perioperative ischemia and MI. Tachycardia is the strongest predictor of perioperative ischemia. Although traditionally an HR greater than 100 beats/min defines tachycardia, slower HRs may result in myocardial ischemia. As described later, control of HR with beta blockers decreases the incidence of myocardial ischemia and infarction. In the DECREASE studies, HR control reduced the incidence of perioperative MI, with the greatest benefit achieved if HR was controlled to less than 70 beats/min. Although some are concerned about beta blockers causing intraoperative hypotension in patients with CAD, no evidence supports this contention. However, the Perioperative Ischemic Evaluation (POISE) trial demonstrated that an acute high-dose beta blockade protocol in patients naïve to beta adrenergic blockade therapy was associated with hypotension and a higher rate of stroke in the metoprolol arm.[25] During CABG, the vast majority of episodes of intraoperative ischemia are not correlated with hemodynamic changes. In the absence of tachycardia, hypotension is not associated with myocardial ischemia.

POSTOPERATIVE MANAGEMENT

Postoperative Response to Surgery

Understanding the pathophysiology of perioperative cardiac events helps in determining the best approach to preoperative testing. A full discussion of the pathophysiology of perioperative MI has been published.[26] All surgical procedures cause a stress response, although the extent of the response depends on the extent of the surgery and the use of anesthetics and analgesics to reduce the response. The stress response can increase HR and BP, which can precipitate episodes of myocardial ischemia in areas distal to coronary artery stenoses. Prolonged myocardial ischemia (either prolonged individual episodes or prolonged cumulative duration of shorter episodes) can cause myocardial necrosis and perioperative MI and death. Identification of patients at high risk for coronary artery stenosis, through either the history or cardiovascular testing, can lead to the implementation of strategies to reduce morbidity as a result of supply-demand mismatches. Recent work with highly sensitive markers of myocardial damage has shown a high rate of cardiac injury even in the absence of frank infarction. In the POISE trial, 8.3% of the patients had an elevated cardiac biomarker without other evidence of infarction, whereas 5% also had a second confirmatory marker of MI.[25]

A major mechanism of MI in the nonoperative setting is plaque rupture with subsequent coronary thrombosis (see Chapters 24 and 37). Inasmuch as the perioperative period is marked by tachycardia and a hypercoagulable state, plaque disruption and thrombosis may occur more often than appreciated. Several observations support this contention. Because noncritical stenosis can furnish the nidus for coronary artery thrombosis, preoperative cardiac evaluation may fail to identify patients at risk before surgery. The areas distal to the noncritical stenosis might not have developed collateral coronary flow, and therefore any acute thrombosis may have a greater detrimental effect than it would in a previously severely narrowed vessel. If a prolonged increase in myocardial oxygen demand in a patient with one or more critical fixed stenoses provoked postoperative MI, preoperative testing would probably identify such a patient.

Evidence from several autopsy and postinfarction angiography studies after surgery supports both mechanisms. Ellis and colleagues demonstrated that one third of all patients sustained events in areas distal to noncritical stenoses. Dawood and associates, as cited in the guidelines, demonstrated that fatal perioperative MI occurs predominantly in patients with multivessel coronary disease, especially left main and three-vessel disease, but the severity of preexisting stenosis did not predict the infarct territory. This analysis suggested that fatal events occurred primarily in patients with advanced fixed stenoses, but that the infarct may result from plaque rupture in a mild or only moderately stenotic segment of the diseased vessel. Duvall and colleagues reviewed hospital records and coronary angiograms from patients who underwent noncardiac surgery complicated by perioperative MI from 1998 to 2006. The distribution of demand, thrombotic, and nonobstructive MI was 55%, 26%, and 19%, respectively. In contrast, Gualandro and colleagues found that almost 50% of patients with perioperative acute coronary syndromes have evidence of ruptured coronary plaque. The evidence therefore shows that several mechanisms may cause perioperative MI. That said, the incidence of type-1, plaque-rupture MI is likely much lower than feared. Wilcox and colleagues reported an all-comers risk of MI of 0.36% in more than 3 million surgeries.[13] Similarly, in the POISE trial of higher cardiovascular risk patients, only 0.04% of patients underwent coronary revascularization in the postoperative period.[25]

POSTOPERATIVE INTENSIVE CARE

Provision of intensive care by intensivists has now become a patient safety goal. Pronovost and coworkers performed a systematic review of the literature on physician staffing patterns and clinical outcomes in critically ill patients (see "Classic References"). They grouped ICU physician staffing into low-intensity (no intensivist or elective intensivist consultation) and high-intensity (mandatory intensivist consultation or closed ICU [all care directed by an intensivist]) groups. High-intensity staffing was associated with lower hospital mortality in 16 of 17 studies (94%) and with a pooled estimate of the relative risk for hospital mortality of 0.71 (95% CI, 0.62 to 0.82). High-intensity staffing was associated with lower ICU mortality in 14 of 15 studies (93%) and with a pooled estimate of the relative risk for ICU mortality of 0.61 (95% CI, 0.50 to 0.75). High-intensity staffing reduced hospital LOS in 10 of 13 studies and reduced ICU LOS in 14 of 18 studies without case-mix adjustment. High-intensity staffing was associated with reduced hospital LOS in two of four studies and lowered ICU LOS in both studies that adjusted for case mix. No study found increased LOS with high-intensity staffing after case-mix adjustment. High-intensity versus low-intensity ICU physician staffing was associated with reduced hospital and ICU mortality and LOS.

POSTOPERATIVE PAIN MANAGEMENT

Postoperative analgesia may reduce perioperative cardiac morbidity. Because postoperative tachycardia and catecholamine surges probably promote myocardial ischemia and/or rupture of coronary plaque, and because postoperative pain can produce tachycardia and increase catecholamines, effective postoperative analgesia may reduce cardiac complications. Postoperative analgesia may also reduce the hypercoagulable state. Epidural anesthesia may decrease platelet aggregability compared with general anesthesia. Whether this decrease relates to intraoperative or postoperative management is unclear. In an analysis of Medicare claims data, the use of epidural analgesia (as determined by billing codes for postoperative epidural pain management) was associated with decreased risk for death at 7 days. As previously noted, regional anesthesia may be advantageous for postoperative pain relief. Future research will focus on how best to deliver postoperative analgesia to maximize the potential benefits and reduce complications.[14]

SURVEILLANCE AND IMPLICATIONS OF PERIOPERATIVE CARDIAC COMPLICATIONS

The optimal and most cost-effective strategy for monitoring high-risk patients for major morbidity after noncardiac surgery is unknown. Myocardial ischemia and infarctions that occur postoperatively are usually silent, most likely because of the confounding effects of analgesics, postoperative surgical pain, and their hemodynamic demand mismatch origin. Intraoperative hypotension confers a fourfold increase in the risk of troponin elevation.[6] Most perioperative MIs do not cause ST-segment elevation, and less specific ST-T wave changes are common after surgery with or without MI. These considerations therefore render the diagnosis of perioperative MI particularly difficult to make.

A marked elevation in mortality associated with postoperative MI provides continuing impetus for improved methods of detection and management. Biomarkers may help identify myocardial necrosis. Lee and colleagues found that troponin T had similar efficacy as creatine kinase (CK) MB in diagnosing perioperative MI but significantly better correlation with major cardiac complications developing after acute MI. Mohler and colleagues evaluated troponin I (cTnI) and CK-MB in 784 high-risk vascular surgery patients on the day of surgery and at 24, 72, and 120 hours postoperatively. They reported a sensitivity of 51% and a specificity of 91% for the defined cardiovascular event by using a receiver operating characteristic (ROC)–defined cutoff point for CK-MB of 3.1 ng/mL.[1]

In the VISION study, 15,133 participants undergoing noncardiac surgery had troponin T measurements performed between 6 and 12 hours postoperatively and on postoperative days 1, 2, and 3.[17] Troponin T levels above the baseline level of 0.01 ng/mL or lower were associated with increased rates of 30-day mortality. Indeed, a troponin T level of 0.02 ng/mL was associated with more than a twofold risk for death. With a troponin T level of 0.3 ng/mL or higher, the hazard ratio (HR) for death increased to more than 10-fold above that in patients without any elevation in troponin. Mortality was 16.9% with a troponin T level of 0.3 ng/mL or higher, versus 1% in the group without troponin elevation. Although troponin T levels stratified the rate of mortality across a low spectrum of positive levels, it could not predict the cause of death. Both vascular and nonvascular death increased similarly with increasing troponin T levels, and more than half of all deaths were from nonvascular causes. An elevated troponin T level thus provides adverse prognostication without direction for appropriate therapy.

Three important points can be made from these data. First, noncardiovascular causes of mortality now outnumber cardiovascular causes, indicating important new areas for research. Second, even if there is evidence of troponin elevation, death is remote from the event, suggesting that troponin elevation is not causally related to an immediate event but is a marker of illness and clinical instability. Third, true type 1 MI is rare. In the POISE trial, 7521 participants were screened to find 697 (9.2%) with troponin elevations, but only two individuals of the total cohort were referred for coronary revascularization.[1] In our opinion, troponin measurement should be avoided in the asymptomatic patient without hemodynamic embarrassment or ischemic ECG change. Troponin elevations in this setting provide neither diagnostic direction nor specific management to implement. Should future trials identify management strategies for troponin elevations, we would reconsider routine troponin measurement in high-risk patients.

Evidence for the first step toward a management plan for elevations in troponin after operation is provided by the MANAGE trial[27] which randomly assigned 1754 postoperative noncardiac surgery patients with an elevated troponin level to dabigatran 110 mg BID or placebo. The dabigatran-treated patients had fewer of the primary composite outcome events (vascular mortality and non-fatal MI, non-hemorrhagic stroke, peripheral arterial thrombosis, amputation, and symptomatic venous thromboembolism). The study enrolled slowly, so the investigators reduced the sample size by 45% and expanded the primary outcome. Nearly half the patients discontinued the study drug. Moreover, there was a significant increase in important bleeding, even if criteria for major bleeding (>4 g/dL decline in hemoglobin or ≥3 units of red blood cell transfusion) weren't met. The study raises the possibility of benefit for treatment of patients identified by postoperative troponin elevations, but additional investigation is required before a recommendation can be made.[27]

Several studies have evaluated BNP in the postoperative period showing the impact of markers of increased volume. A meta-analysis showed that the addition of postoperative BNP measurements to a risk prediction model of 30-day death and MI had a net reclassification

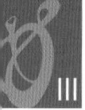

index of 20%.[28] Moreover, elevated postoperative BNP increased the rate of death and MI by 3.7-fold.

Traditionally, perioperative MI has been associated with 30% to 50% short-term mortality, but recent series have reported a fatality rate of less than 20% for perioperative MI. Studies from the 1980s suggested a peak incidence on the second and third postoperative days. Puelacher and colleagues, using troponin T as a marker for MI in high-cardiac-risk patients, suggested that the highest incidence occurred during the immediate postoperative days,[29] as confirmed in other studies. The finding that tachycardia, hypotension, and hypertension in the operative suite predicted release of troponin suggests a hemodynamic consequence rather than plaque rupture event (type 2 vs. type 1 MI).[16] Further, acute surgical anemia, expressed as a greater than 35% drop on preoperative hemoglobin, increases major acute coronary morbidity.[1] Thus the change is probably related to more robust surveillance methods, not to a fundamental shift in how or when myocardial ischemia or infarction occurs.

Increasing evidence has associated perioperative MI or biomarker elevation with worse long-term outcome. Oberweis and colleagues[30] studied 3050 patients who underwent orthopedic surgery. Of the 179 in whom myocardial necrosis occurred, mortality was 16.8% in patients with biomarker elevation at a mean follow-up of 3 years compared to 5.8% in patients without elevation. Landesberg and coworkers, as cited in the guidelines, demonstrated that postoperative CK-MB and troponin, even at low cutoff levels, are independent and complementary predictors of long-term mortality after major vascular surgery. Mahla and colleagues have also shown that elevations in BNP are associated with a fivefold increased long-term risk for cardiac events. The appropriate use of screening biomarkers in current preoperative risk assessment algorithms remains unstudied because there is no evidence-based intervention to apply in response to a biomarker elevation.

STRATEGIES TO REDUCE THE RISK ASSOCIATED WITH NONCARDIAC SURGERY

Coronary Artery Revascularization

The treatment of patients before noncardiac surgery should follow the same trajectory as in the absence of impending surgery. As such, it should be noted that the recently completed International Study of Comparative Health Effectiveness with Medical and Invasive Approaches (ISCHEMIA) trial showed that coronary revascularization in patients with moderate or severe stable CAD neither reduces MI nor death in patients with or without advanced kidney disease.[31] Indeed, over optimum medical treatment, coronary revascularization in stable patients has limited value.[1] Despite this evidence and recent data that the postoperative incidence of type 1 MI requiring revascularization is 0.3% to 0.5%, some have suggested coronary revascularization as a means of reducing the perioperative risk related to noncardiac surgery.[32] This view is derived from retrospective evidence of patients who survived initial surgery in the Coronary Artery Surgery Study (CASS) registry, which enrolled patients from 1978 to 1981, an era that antedates almost all the current therapies shown to be effective for reducing coronary events. This observational analysis did not randomly assign patients, however, and reflects a different era in preventive strategies and higher rates of adverse outcomes after noncardiac surgery.

Several cohort studies have examined the benefit of percutaneous coronary intervention (PCI) before noncardiac surgery. Posner and colleagues, as cited in the guidelines, used an administrative dataset of patients who underwent PCI and noncardiac surgery.[1] They matched patients with coronary disease undergoing noncardiac surgery with and without previous PCI and examined cardiac complications. In this nonrandomized analysis, they noted a significantly lower rate of 30-day cardiac complications in patients who underwent PCI at least 90 days before the noncardiac surgery. PCI within 90 days of noncardiac surgery did not improve outcomes. The advent of drug-eluting stents requiring prolonged antiplatelet therapy may promote operative bleeding complications or increase subacute stent thrombosis if antiplatelet treatment is stopped perioperatively.

Several randomized trials have now addressed the value of both CABG and PCI in a subset of patients. McFalls and coauthors reported the results of a multicenter randomized trial in the Veterans Affairs Health System in which patients with documented CAD on coronary angiography, excluding those with left main CAD or a severely depressed ejection fraction (≤20%), were randomly assigned before elective major vascular surgery to CABG (59%) or PCI (41%) versus routine medical therapy.[1] At 2.7 years after randomization, mortality in the revascularization group did not differ significantly (22%) from that in the no-revascularization group (23%). Within 30 days after the vascular operation, postoperative MI, defined as elevated troponin levels, occurred in 12% of the revascularization group and in 14% of the no-revascularization group ($P = 0.37$). The authors suggested that coronary revascularization is not indicated in patients with stable CAD and that PCI or CABG for one- or two-vessel disease before noncardiac surgery does not prevent perioperative MI. A reanalysis of the data found that the completeness of revascularization affects the rate of perioperative MI, with CABG being more effective than PCI. Similarly, Garcia and colleagues analyzed both randomly and nonrandomly assigned patients who underwent coronary angiography before vascular surgery in the CARP trial registry; 4.6% of these patients had unprotected left main CAD. Only this subset of patients showed a benefit of preoperative coronary artery revascularization.

Monaco and associates studied 208 patients at moderate clinical risk who underwent major vascular surgery and were randomly allocated to either a "selective strategy" group, in whom coronary angiography was performed on the basis of noninvasive test results, or to a "systematic strategy" group, in whom preoperative coronary angiography was systematically performed. The strategy of routine coronary angiography had no effect on the short-term outcome, but the long-term outcome was improved in surgical patients with peripheral arterial disease at medium to high risk.

One issue in interpreting the results is that the length of time between coronary revascularization and noncardiac surgery most likely affects its protective effect and potential risks. Back and colleagues studied 425 consecutive patients undergoing 481 elective major vascular operations at an academic Veterans Affairs Medical Center. Coronary revascularization was classified as "recent" (CABG, <1 year; percutaneous transluminal coronary angioplasty [PTCA], <6 months) in 35 cases, as "previous" (CABG, 1 to 5 years; PTCA, 6 months to 2 years) in 45 cases, and as "remote" (CABG, >5 years; PTCA, >2 years) in 48 cases. Patients with previous PTCA had similar outcomes as those after CABG. Significant differences in adverse cardiac events and mortality were found between patients with CABG performed within 5 years or PTCA within 2 years (6.3% and 1.3%, respectively), individuals with remote revascularization (10.4% and 6.3%, respectively), and nonrevascularized patients stratified at high risk (13.3% and 3.3%, respectively) or intermediate to low risk (2.8% and 0.9%, respectively). The authors concluded that previous coronary revascularization (CABG, <5 years; PTCA, <2 years) provides only modest protection against adverse cardiac events and mortality following major arterial reconstruction.

In our opinion, the randomized controlled trials provide strong evidence of limited to no benefit of preoperative coronary artery revascularization to reduce cardiovascular risk. In the absence of unusual circumstances, percutaneous and surgical revascularization should not be pursued before noncardiac surgery.

Percutaneous Coronary Intervention and Noncardiac Surgery

PCI using coronary stenting poses several special issues (see Chapter 41).[4] Kaluza and colleagues reported the outcome of 40 patients who underwent prophylactic coronary stent placement less than 6 weeks before major noncardiac surgery requiring general anesthesia. They reported seven MIs, 11 major bleeding episodes, and eight deaths. All the deaths and MIs, as well as 8 of the 11 bleeding episodes, occurred in patients subjected to surgery less than 14 days after stenting. Four patients died after undergoing surgery 1 day after stenting. Wilson and colleagues, as cited in the guidelines, reported on 207 patients in whom noncardiac surgery was performed within 2 months of stent placement. Eight patients died or had an MI, and all of them were among the 168 patients who underwent surgery 6 weeks after stent placement. Vincenzi and coworkers studied 103 patients and reported that the risk for a perioperative cardiac event was 2.11-fold greater in patients with recent stents (<35 days before surgery) than in those undergoing PCI more than 90 days before surgery. These data point to the importance of delaying surgery after stenting, even though the investigators either continued antiplatelet drug therapy or only briefly interrupted it, and all patients received heparin.

Drug-eluting stents may represent an even greater problem during the perioperative period. Emerging data from a series of recent analyses in the nonoperative setting and several perioperative case reports suggest that the risk for thrombosis continues for at least 1 year after insertion. Several reports suggest that drug-eluting stents may represent an additional risk over a prolonged period (up to 12 months), particularly if the use of antiplatelet agents is discontinued.

Schouten retrospectively evaluated 192 patients who underwent noncardiac surgery after successful PCI for unstable CAD within 2 years of the procedure. Drug-eluting stents accounted for 52% of the stents placed. Of the 192 patients, 30 underwent surgery before the recommended discontinuation of dual-antiplatelet therapy for the particular stent (30 days for bare-metal stents and up to 6 months for sirolimus-eluting stents). In patients in whom antiplatelet therapy was stopped before the required time for use of clopidogrel (early-surgery group), the incidence of death or nonfatal MI was 30.7% compared with 0% in patients who continued antiplatelet therapy. The elevated risk for stent thrombosis and cardiovascular events, however, seems to abate over time. In the Evaluation of Drug-Eluting Stents and Ischemic Events (EVENT) registry of 4637 consecutive patients, 4.4% underwent major noncardiac surgery in the ensuing year. A relative 27-fold increased rate of cardiovascular events occurred in the week after surgery versus any other week after stent implantation, but the absolute rate was only 1.9%.

Wijeysundera and colleagues evaluated 8116 patients who underwent noncardiac surgery in Ontario, Canada, and found that 34% had a coronary stent implanted within the 2 years before surgery.[1] Drug-eluting stents represented one third of the stents placed. Patients with bare-metal stents implanted less than 45 days before surgery had a 6.7% cardiovascular event rate, which dropped to 2.6% with a stent implanted 45 to 180 days before surgery. Patients with a drug-eluting stent had a 20.2% cardiovascular event rate in the first 45 days after stent implantation, and the rate became similar to that in patients without stenting when the stent was implanted more than 180 days before surgery. Bangalore and colleagues studied the impact of drug-eluting stents compared with bare-metal stents placed preoperatively in 8415 patients in Massachusetts.[33] In this cohort the death, MI, and bleeding event rate was 8.6% in the first 30 days after PCI, dropping to 5.2% when surgery was performed more than 90 days after coronary revascularization. Using propensity matching to compare the bare-metal stent and drug-eluting stent populations, the death and MI rate was higher in the bare-metal stent cohort.

In a Scotland-wide retrospective cohort analysis, perioperative death and ischemic cardiac events were much more common within the first 6 weeks after stent implantation than after 6 weeks, 42.4% versus 12.8%, respectively.[1] Forty-five percent of the revascularizations in this cohort were performed for an acute coronary syndrome, increasing the baseline risk of the cohort. The event rate was higher in patients who underwent revascularization because of acute coronary syndromes within 6 weeks, in whom it reached 65%. In contrast to other reports, no temporal differences were noted between the bare-metal and drug-eluting stent groups.

Data from more recent large observational studies suggest that the time frame of increased risk of stent thrombosis is on the order of 6 months, regardless of stent type (bare metal or drug eluting). In a large cohort of patients from the Veterans Health Administration hospitals, the increased risk of surgery for the 6 months after stent placement was most pronounced in patients in whom the indication for PCI was an MI.[1]

In 2016, ACC/AHA published a focused update on duration of dual-antiplatelet therapy in CAD patients, including revising the perioperative guidelines.[4] The current recommendations for delay after coronary stent placement include 30 days for bare-metal stent implantation and 6 months after drug-eluting stent placement (Fig. 23.3). The guidelines writing committee noted that elective noncardiac surgery may be considered more than 180 days after drug-eluting stent implantation if the risk of delay is thought to be greater than the risk of stent thrombosis. The guideline committee gave a class IIb recommendation that elective surgery may be considered after 3 months for patients in whom the P2Y12 inhibitor needs to be discontinued if further delay of surgery is greater than the risk of stent thrombosis. In patients with illness requiring more timely surgery, strategies for bridging the cessation of antiplatelet therapy until the procedure include the use of IV eptifibatide and tirofiban, but these strategies lack outcomes data.

Pharmacologic Interventions
Beta-Adrenergic Blocking Agents

Beta-adrenergic blocking agents have undergone extensive study in perioperative risk management. As noted earlier, some of the trial data used to support recent recommendations on the titrated use of beta blockers from Poldermans and colleagues have become uncertain. A recent meta-analysis of all the beta blocker trials demonstrates that beta blockers decrease nonfatal MI but increase stroke and death.[34] As a result, ACC/AHA guidelines[1] suggest that perioperative beta blockers can be considered on a case-by-case basis in patients with significant myocardial ischemia, three or more RCRI risk factors, or a compelling long-term indication for beta blockers. Aggregate impact of beta blockers seems to be low. Of the more than 10,000 participants in the trials, 75 nonfatal MIs were prevented and 19 strokes and 35 deaths instigated (Table 23.4).

Most of these trials did not titrate beta blockers in the same manner as they are used in other conditions, such as HF or hypertension. For example, in the POISE trial, Devereaux and colleagues randomly assigned 8351 high-risk patients undergoing noncardiac surgery to metoprolol succinate, 200 mg daily, or matching placebo.[25] The use of high-dose, long-acting medications may have worsened outcomes by limiting the physician's flexibility to modify treatment on the basis of the rapidly shifting perioperative environment. Other trials used lower doses without titration to hemodynamic parameters as well. Administration of beta blockers as performed in the clinical trials clearly does not provide a benefit sufficient for their routine use.

Current guidelines suggest that beta blockade may be reasonable in patients with intermediate- or high-risk myocardial ischemia reported in preoperative noninvasive testing or patients with three or more RCRI risk factors, although there is no direct evidence to support routine use even in this higher-risk population.[1] If beta blockers are to be used, it is recommended that initiation begin 1 day or more before surgery. Initiation on the day of surgery has been associated with an increase in stroke and mortality.[1] In hospital, short-acting oral or IV beta blockers should be used to permit titration to hemodynamics. No specific BP or HR targets have been validated, although BP control to less than 140/90 mm Hg and HRs of 60 to 80 beats/min may be reasonable when beta blockers are used.

Statin Therapy

Statins are routinely recommended for patients with atherosclerosis and diabetes (see Chapters 25 and 27). Their role in patients undergoing noncardiac surgery is less well defined. In a retrospective analysis of 750 patients, 10% of whom had the composite outcome (30-day death, MI, and AF), statin use was associated with a 45% reduction in adverse events, including a 5% absolute reduction in 30-day mortality. In addition to their cholesterol-lowering properties, statins have anti-inflammatory actions that may provide benefit as well. In an NSQIP study of 7777 patients undergoing various surgeries, statin use was associated with reductions in noncardiac events, including a 47% reduction in respiratory complications, 59% reduction in VTE, and 35% reduction in infectious complications.[35] The evidence suggests that statin therapy should be continued during the perioperative period. Le Manach and associates evaluated the effect of statin discontinuation in a vascular surgery population. When compared with a control population, discontinuation of statins was associated with more than a twofold increase

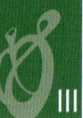

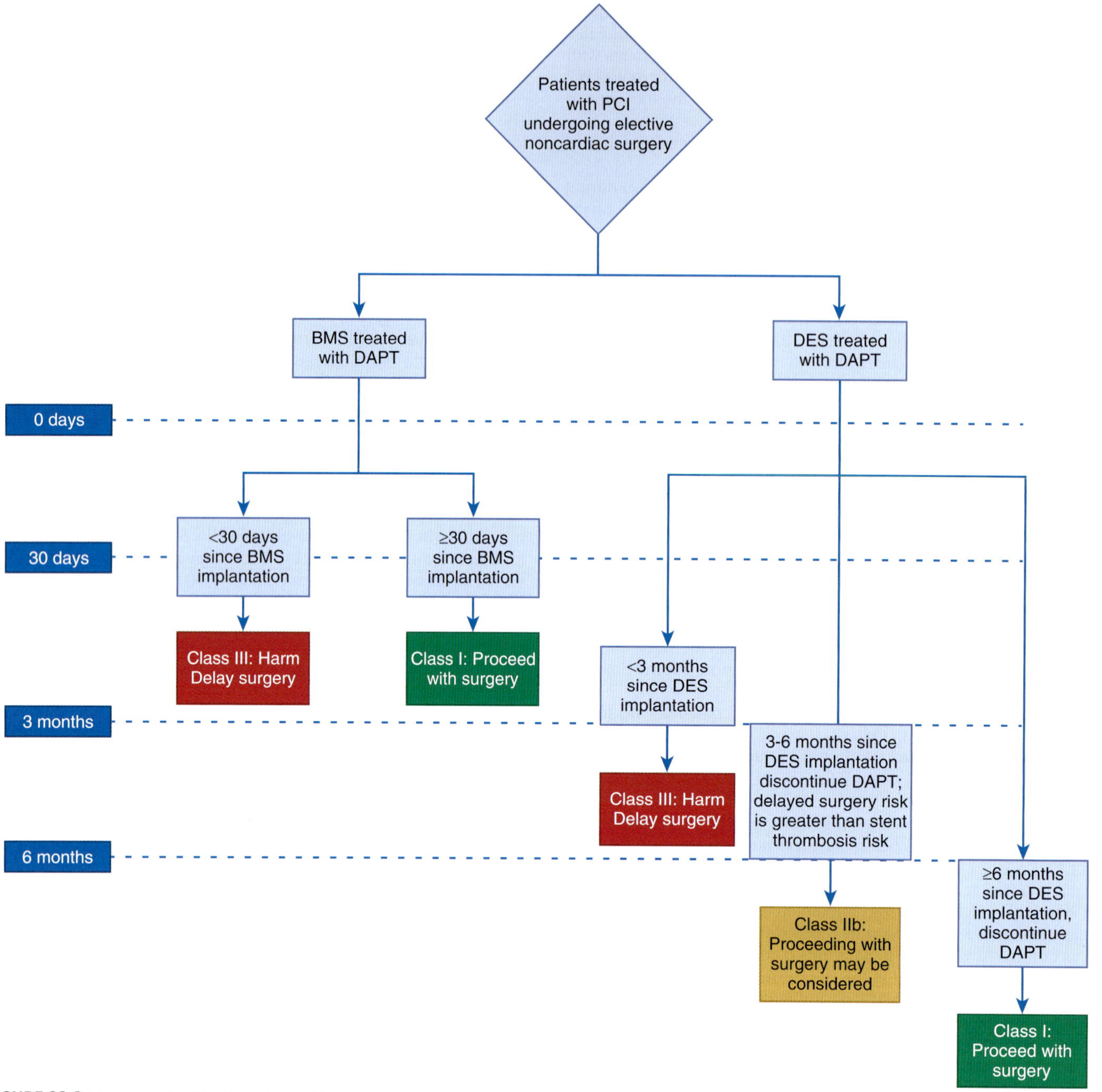

FIGURE 23.3 Treatment algorithm for patients with coronary stents undergoing noncardiac surgery. *BMS*, Bare metal stent; *DAPT*, dual-antiplatelet therapy; *DES*, drug-eluting stent; *PCI*, percutaneous coronary intervention. (From Levine GN, Bates ER, Bittl JA, et al. 2016 ACC/AHA guideline focused update on duration of dual antiplatelet therapy in patients with coronary artery disease: a report of the American College of Cardiology/American Heart Association Task Force on Clinical Practice Guidelines. *J Am Coll Cardiol.* 2016;68:1082–1115.)

in troponin elevation, whereas continuation reduced the rate of troponin release by more than 40%. In patients already receiving statins, a prospective randomized trial of 500 patients with stable CAD about to undergo emergency surgery randomly received placebo or atorvastatin (80 mg) 2 hours before surgery. In the group who received the statin, cardiac death, MI, or unplanned revascularization occurred in 2.4% of patients compared with 8% in the placebo arm.[36] Indeed, starting statin therapy should be considered in patients who meet ACC/AHA lipid guideline recommendations and in cardiovascular high-risk patients, because they merit this treatment even without surgery.

Other Therapies

POISE 2, a blind randomized trial with a 2 × 2 factorial design, allowed separate evaluation of low-dose clonidine versus placebo and low-dose aspirin versus placebo in 10,010 patients with, or at risk for, atherosclerotic disease who were undergoing noncardiac surgery.[37] Low-dose clonidine did not reduce the rate of death or nonfatal MI but was associated with an increased risk of clinically important hypotension and nonfatal cardiac arrest. Administration of aspirin was not associated with any difference in the rate of death or nonfatal MI but increased the risk of major bleeding.[38]

Two small, randomized trials have evaluated the potential protective effect of prophylactic nitroglycerin in reducing perioperative cardiac complications after noncardiac surgery. Neither established a benefit for the prophylactic use of nitroglycerin. Because prophylactic nitroglycerin has considerable hemodynamic effects and is not known to prevent MI or cardiac death, the data do not support its routine use.

As described above, the MANAGE trial has a 2 × 2 factorial design testing the efficacy of dabigatran and omeprazole in patients undergoing noncardiac surgery who develop an elevated troponin or

TABLE 23.4 Recommendations for Perioperative Therapy with Beta Blockers

Class I
- Continue beta blockers in patients who are receiving beta blockers chronically.

Class IIa
- Guide management of beta blockers after surgery by clinical circumstances.

Class IIb
- In patients with intermediate- or high-risk preoperative tests, it may be reasonable to begin beta blockers.
- In patients with ≥3 Revised Cardiac Risk Index (RCRI) factors, it may be reasonable to begin beta blockers before surgery.
- Initiating beta blockers in the perioperative setting as an approach to reduce perioperative risk is of uncertain benefit in those with a long-term indication but no other RCRI risk factors.*
- It may be reasonable to begin perioperative beta blockers long enough in advance to assess safety and tolerability, preferably >1 day before surgery.

Class III
- Beta blocker therapy should not be started on the day of surgery.

*Clinical risk factors include a history of ischemic heart disease, history of compensated or previous heart failure, history of cerebrovascular disease, diabetes mellitus, and renal insufficiency (defined in the RCRI as a preoperative serum creatinine level of 2 mg/dL).
From Fleisher LA, Beckman JA, Brown KA, et al. 2014 ACC/AHA guideline on perioperative cardiovascular evaluation and management of patients undergoing noncardiac surgery: a report of the American College of Cardiology/American Heart Association Task Force on Practice Guidelines. J Am Coll Cardiol. 2014;64:e77–e137.

CK-MB level with evidence of an ischemic event or no alternative explanation for biomarker elevation.[27] Although a benefit was noted with therapy, the incomplete follow up, change in endpoint, and high discontinuation rate render recommendation of dabigatran in this setting difficult.

NONPHARMACOLOGIC INTERVENTIONS

Temperature
Frank and colleagues, as cited in the guidelines, completed a randomized trial of regional versus general anesthesia for lower extremity vascular bypass procedures and noted an association between hypothermia (temperature <35°C) and myocardial ischemia. They subsequently performed a trial in 300 high-risk patients undergoing a diverse range of intermediate- and high-risk procedures and randomly assigned to maintenance of normothermia or routine care. They observed a significantly reduced incidence of perioperative cardiac morbidity and mortality within 24 hours of surgery in the normothermic group.

Electrocardiographic, Hemodynamic, and Echocardiographic Monitoring
Multiple studies have demonstrated the predictive value of correlating perioperative ST-segment changes and major cardiac events, as described earlier. Furthermore, the duration (cumulative or continuous) of perioperative ST changes strongly predicts poor outcomes. ST-segment monitoring has therefore become standard during the intraoperative and ICU periods for high-risk patients. However, ST-segment changes may also develop in patients at low to moderate risk. These changes may not reflect true myocardial ischemia, as suggested in a recent series.

Postoperative patients may have the greatest risk for a cardiac event when on the ward and unmonitored. Few studies have tested the efficacy of ST-segment telemetric monitoring during the perioperative period. The issue of whether early treatment of prolonged ST-segment changes improves outcomes in this situation remains unresolved.

Much controversy surrounds the value of pulmonary artery (PA) catheterization for noncardiac surgery. Several small, randomized trials did not demonstrate a significant reduction in major cardiac morbidity and mortality in patients so monitored during aortic surgery. In a large-scale cohort study, Polanczyk and colleagues found that patients with PA catheters who were matched to those without catheters by a propensity score also failed to demonstrate significant benefit (see "Classic References"). In fact, they observed an increased incidence of congestive HF and untoward noncardiac outcomes in the catheter group. A total of 1994 patients were randomly allocated to goal-directed therapy guided by a PA catheter or to standard care without the use of a PA catheter in patients undergoing urgent or elective major surgery. No difference in survival occurred, but pulmonary embolism developed at a higher rate in the catheter group than in the standard-care group. Current evidence therefore does not support the routine use of PA catheterization for high-risk patients undergoing major noncardiac surgery. Determining whether these results apply to the high-risk vascular surgical population and whether use of a PA catheter provides benefit in specific clinical situations will require further work.

Transesophageal echocardiography (TEE) represents another means of assessing intraoperative cardiac function (see Chapter 16). This tool sensitively monitors intraoperative wall motion abnormalities and fluid status. In patients undergoing aortic cross-clamping, TEE showed significantly better sensitivity in detecting intraoperative ischemia than electrocardiographic monitoring. For noncardiac surgery, a study of TEE, 2-lead electrocardiography, and 12-lead electrocardiography demonstrated minimal additive value of TEE over 2-lead electrocardiography. TEE monitoring may nonetheless prove valuable in guiding treatment in patients with unstable hemodynamics who have uncertain fluid status and myocardial function.

Transfusion Threshold
Much controversy surrounds the optimal hemoglobin level at which transfusion is indicated in high-risk noncardiac surgical patients. No randomized trials have evaluated the optimal transfusion threshold, although much anecdotal evidence exists. A large-scale trial of transfusion triggers in the ICU did not document increased morbidity or mortality when a hemoglobin concentration lower than 7 g/dL was used as a transfusion threshold, but trends toward increased morbidity emerged in the subset of patients with ischemic heart disease. In the FOCUS (Transfusion Trigger Trial for Functional Outcomes in Cardiovascular Patients Undergoing Surgical Hip Fracture Repair) trial, Carson and colleagues randomly assigned hip fracture patients to a liberal transfusion strategy (hemoglobin threshold of 10 g/dL) or a restrictive transfusion strategy (symptoms of anemia or at physician's discretion for hemoglobin level <8 g/dL).[1] A liberal transfusion strategy, compared with a restrictive strategy, did not reduce rates of death or inability to walk independently on 60-day follow-up and did not reduce in-hospital morbidity in elderly patients at high cardiovascular risk. The impact of transfusion may depend on the severity of the precipitating anemia. Smilowitz and coworkers followed 3050 patients after orthopedic surgery.[39] In this cohort the presence of anemia, hemorrhage, and transfusion were independently associated with long-term mortality. Interestingly, the effect of transfusion was attenuated by the severity of anemia. For patients with no anemia, transfusion increased the HR 4.4-fold; for those with mild anemia, HR was only 2.3-fold; and for those with moderate/severe anemia (hemoglobin <11 g/dL), there was benefit, with HR of 0.81. These data suggest a restrictive policy of transfusion may be the most beneficial for patients undergoing noncardiac surgery.

CONCLUSION

Three trends are notable in the perioperative management of patients undergoing noncardiac surgery: (1) the rate of MI and cardiovascular death are declining; (2) noncardiovascular death now accounts for the majority of perioperative mortality; and (3) the evidence base supporting current management practices continues to grow rapidly. As overall mortality risk declines over time, the future goal of preoperative assessment will be to identify patients at clinically inapparent increased risk and devise and test interventions to reduce this risk. Additionally, preoperative risk assessment will increasingly serve to determine if the long-term benefits of surgery outweigh the perioperative risks. The predictive value of biomarkers and treatment of biomarker elevations, novel medications, and presurgical rehabilitation (prehabilitation) are currently under investigation and may represent the next frontier in perioperative management.

CLASSIC REFERENCES
Gupta PK, Gupta H, Sundaram A, et al. Development and validation of a risk calculator for prediction of cardiac risk after surgery. Circulation. 2011;124:381–387.

Pronovost PJ, Jenckes MW, Dorman T, et al. Organizational characteristics of intensive care units related to outcomes of abdominal aortic surgery. JAMA. 1999;281:1310–1317.

Polanczyk CA, Rohde LE, Goldman L, et al. Right heart catheterization and cardiac complications in patients undergoing noncardiac surgery: an observational study. *JAMA*. 2001;286:309–314.

van Diepen S, Bakal JA, McAlister FA, Ezekowitz JA. Mortality and readmission of patients with heart failure, atrial fibrillation, or coronary artery disease undergoing noncardiac surgery: an analysis of 38 047 patients. *Circulation*. 2011;124:289–296.

Winkel TA, Schouten O, Hoeks SE, et al. Prognosis of transient new-onset atrial fibrillation during vascular surgery. *Eur J Vasc Endovasc Surg*. 2009;38:683–688.

REFERENCES

Assessment of Risk

1. Fleisher LA, Fleischmann KE, Auerbach AD, et al. 2014 ACC/AHA guideline on perioperative cardiovascular evaluation and management of patients undergoing noncardiac surgery: a report of the American College of Cardiology/American Heart Association Task Force on practice guidelines. *J Am Coll Cardiol*. 2014;64:e77–137.
2. Kristensen SD, Knuuti J, Saraste A, et al. 2014 ESC/ESA Guidelines on non-cardiac surgery: cardiovascular assessment and management: The Joint Task Force on non-cardiac surgery: cardiovascular assessment and management of the European Society of Cardiology (ESC) and the European Society of Anaesthesiology (ESA). *Eur Heart J*. 2014;35:2383–2431.
3. Duceppe E, Parlow J, MacDonald P, et al. Canadian Cardiovascular Society guidelines on perioperative cardiac risk assessment and management for patients who undergo noncardiac surgery. *Can J Cardiol*. 2017;33:17–32.
4. Levine GN, Bates ER, Bittl JA, et al. 2016 ACC/AHA guideline focused update on duration of dual antiplatelet therapy in patients with coronary artery disease: a report of the American College of Cardiology/American Heart Association Task Force on clinical practice guidelines. *J Am Coll Cardiol*. 2016;68:1082–1115.
5. Hallqvist L, Martensson J, Granath F, et al. Intraoperative hypotension is associated with myocardial damage in noncardiac surgery: an observational study. *Eur J Anaesthesiol*. 2016;33:450–456.
6. Futier E, Lefrant JY, Guinot PG, et al. Effect of individualized vs standard blood pressure management strategies on postoperative organ dysfunction among high-risk patients undergoing major surgery: a randomized clinical trial. *J Am Med Assoc*. 2017;318:1346–1357.
7. Maile MD, Engoren MC, Tremper KK, et al. Worsening preoperative heart failure is associated with mortality and noncardiac complications, but not myocardial infarction after noncardiac surgery: a retrospective cohort study. *Anesth Analg*. 2014;119:522–532.
8. Andersson C, Jorgensen ME, Martinsson A, et al. Noncardiac surgery in patients with aortic stenosis: a contemporary study on outcomes in a matched sample from the Danish Health Care System. *Clin Cardiol*. 2014;37:680–686.
9. Otto CM, Nishimura RA, Bonow RO, et al. 2020 Guideline for the management of patients with valvular heart disease: a report of the American College of Cardiology/American Heart Association Task Force on clinical practice guidelines. *J Am Coll Cardiol*. 2021. https://doi.org/10.1016/j.jacc.2020.11.018.
10. Douketis JD, Spyropoulos AC, Kaatz S, et al. Perioperative bridging anticoagulation in patients with atrial fibrillation. *N Engl J Med*. 2015;373:823–833.
11. Maxwell BG, Wong JK, Lobato RL. Perioperative morbidity and mortality after noncardiac surgery in young adults with congenital or early acquired heart disease: a retrospective cohort analysis of the National Surgical Quality Improvement Program database. *Am Surg*. 2014;80:321–326.
12. Rohatgi N, Smilowitz NR, Lansberg MG. Perioperative stroke risk reduction in patients with patent foramen ovale. *JAMA Neurol*. 2020. https://doi.org/10.1001/jamaneurol.2020.2619.

The Decision to Undergo Diagnostic Testing

13. Wilcox T, Smilowitz NR, Xia Y, et al. Cardiovascular risk factors and perioperative myocardial infarction after noncardiac surgery. *Can J Cardiol*. 2020. https://doi.org/10.1016/j.cjca.2020.04.034.
14. Glance LG, Faden E, Dutton RP, et al. Impact of the choice of risk model for identifying low-risk patients using the 2014 American College of Cardiology/American Heart Association perioperative guidelines. *Anesthesiology*. 2018;129:889–900.
15. Dakik HA, Sbaity E, Msheik A, et al. AUB-HAS2 cardiovascular risk index: performance in surgical subpopulations and comparison to the revised cardiac risk index. *J Am Heart Assoc*. 2020;9:e016228.
16. Abbott TEF, Pearse RM, Archbold RA, et al. A prospective international multicentre cohort study of intraoperative heart rate and systolic blood pressure and myocardial injury after noncardiac surgery: results of the VISION study. *Anesth Analg*. 2018;126:1936–1945.
17. Vascular Events in Noncardiac Surgery Patients Cohort Evaluation Study Investigators; Devereaux PJ, Chan MT, et al. Association between postoperative troponin levels and 30-day mortality among patients undergoing noncardiac surgery. *JAMA*. 2012;307:2295–2304.
18. Rubin DS, Hughey R, Gerlach RM, et al. Frequency and outcomes of preoperative stress testing in total hip and knee arthroplasty from 2004 to 2017. *JAMA Cardiol*. 2020. https://doi.org/10.1001/jamacardio.2020.4311.
19. Wijeysundera DN, Pearse RM, Shulman MA, et al. Assessment of functional capacity before major non-cardiac surgery: an international, prospective cohort study. *Lancet*. 2018;391:2631–2640.
20. Levett DZ, Grocott MP. Cardiopulmonary exercise testing, prehabilitation, and Enhanced Recovery After Surgery (ERAS). *Can J Anaesth*. 2015;62:131–142.
21. Duceppe E, Patel A, Chan MTV, et al. Preoperative N-terminal pro-B-type natriuretic peptide and cardiovascular events after noncardiac surgery: a cohort study. *Ann Intern Med*. 2020;172:96–104.
22. Maile MD, Jewell ES, Engoren MC. Timing of preoperative troponin elevations and postoperative mortality after noncardiac surgery. *Anesth Analg*. 2016;123:135–140.

Overview of Anesthesia for Cardiac Patients Undergoing Noncardiac Surgery

23. Kunst G, Klein AA. Peri-operative anaesthetic myocardial preconditioning and protection - cellular mechanisms and clinical relevance in cardiac anaesthesia. *Anaesthesia*. 2015;70:467–482.
24. Tan M, Law LS, Gan TJ. Optimizing pain management to facilitate Enhanced Recovery after Surgery pathways. *Can J Anaesth*. 2015;62:203–218.
25. POISE Study Group, Devereaux PJ, Yang H, et al. Effects of extended-release metoprolol succinate in patients undergoing non-cardiac surgery (POISE trial): a randomised controlled trial. *Lancet*. 2008;371:1839–1847.

Postoperative Management

26. Devereaux PJ, Sessler DI. Cardiac complications and major noncardiac surgery. *N Engl J Med*. 2016;374:1394–1395.
27. Devereaux PJ, Duceppe E, Guyatt G, et al. Dabigatran in patients with myocardial injury after non-cardiac surgery (MANAGE): an international, randomised, placebo-controlled trial. *Lancet*. 2018;391:2325–2334.
28. Rodseth RN, Biccard BM, Le Manach Y, et al. The prognostic value of pre-operative and postoperative B-type natriuretic peptides in patients undergoing noncardiac surgery: B-type natriuretic peptide and N-terminal fragment of pro-B-type natriuretic peptide: a systematic review and individual patient data meta-analysis. *J Am Coll Cardiol*. 2014;63:170–180.
29. Puelacher C, Lurati Buse G, Seeberger D, et al. Perioperative myocardial injury after noncardiac surgery: incidence, mortality, and characterization. *Circulation*. 2018;137:1221–1232.
30. Oberweis BS, Smilowitz NR, Nukala S, et al. Relation of perioperative elevation of troponin to long-term mortality after orthopedic surgery. *Am J Cardiol*. 2015;115:1643–1648.

Strategies to Reduce the Cardiac Risk Associated With Noncardiac Surgery

31. Bangalore S, Maron DJ, O'Brien SM, et al. Management of coronary disease in patients with advanced kidney disease. *N Engl J Med*. 2020;382:1608–1618.
32. Smilowitz NR, Berger JS. Perioperative cardiovascular risk assessment and management for non-cardiac surgery: a review. *J Am Med Assoc*. 2020;324:279–290.
33. Bangalore S, Silbaugh TS, Normand S-LT, et al. Drug-eluting stents versus bare metal stents prior to noncardiac surgery. *Catheter Cardiovasc Interv*. 2015;85:533–541.
34. Wijeysundera DN, Duncan D, Nkonde-Price C, et al. Perioperative beta blockade in noncardiac surgery: a systematic review for the 2014 ACC/AHA guideline on perioperative cardiovascular evaluation and management of patients undergoing noncardiac surgery: a report of the American College of Cardiology/American Heart Association Task Force on practice guidelines. *J Am Coll Cardiol*. 2014;64:2406–2425.
35. Iannuzzi JC, Rickles AS, Kelly KN, et al. Perioperative pleiotropic statin effects in general surgery. *Surgery*. 2014;155(3):398–407.
36. Xia J, Qu Y, Shen H, Liu X. Patients with stable coronary artery disease receiving chronic statin treatment who are undergoing noncardiac emergency surgery benefit from acute atorvastatin reload. *Cardiology*. 2014;128:285–292.
37. Devereaux PJ, Sessler DI, Leslie K, et al. Clonidine in patients undergoing noncardiac surgery. *N Engl J Med*. 2014;370:1504–1513.
38. Devereaux PJ, Mrkobrada M, Sessler DI, et al. Aspirin in patients undergoing noncardiac surgery. *N Engl J Med*. 2014;370:1494–1503.
39. Smilowitz NR, Oberweis BS, Nukala S, et al. Association between anemia, bleeding, and transfusion with long-term mortality following noncardiac surgery. *Am J Med*. 2016;129:315–323.e312.

第四部分 预防心脏病学

卢玉枝 苏冠华 程翔 导读

流行病学数据显示，心血管疾病是当前世界疾病负担的主要原因，心血管疾病的总患病人数和死亡人数均在全球范围内高居榜首。干预心血管疾病的传统危险因素（如高血压、高血脂、吸烟）可以显著降低心血管疾病的发病率及死亡率，显示了预防心脏病学的重要性。预防心脏病学旨在通过饮食行为干预、药物治疗、心脏康复等综合手段控制危险因素，做到早发现、早诊断、早治疗，减少心血管疾病的发病率、复发率及死亡率，改善患者预后。

动脉粥样硬化是诸多心血管疾病的共同病理生理学机制，第24、25章基于正常血管结构，介绍了动脉粥样硬化的发病机制、并发症以及特殊类型的动脉粥样硬化，阐述了心血管疾病相关的危险因素和生物标志物的检测及意义，为后续章节内容的展开打下基础。

高血压和脂蛋白紊乱是心血管疾病常见且重要的危险因素。近年来随着多项临床试验结果的公布，高血压及血脂异常的诊断及治疗理念发生了一些变化。2017年美国心脏病学会/美国心脏协会（ACC/AHA）高血压指南将诊室血压≥130/80 mmHg定义为1期高血压，并建议对10年动脉粥样硬化性心血管疾病（ASCVD）风险≥10%的1期高血压患者进行药物治疗。该指南支持强化降压以获得最大心血管获益，但其带来的负面作用也需考虑。目前心血管疾病强化降压相关的临床试验正在进行中，这可能会影响我们未来的临床决策。总胆固醇和低密度脂蛋白胆固醇（LDL-C）升高、高密度脂蛋白胆固醇降低被证实与冠心病发病相关，高甘油三酯也参与其中。生活方式和药物干预调节脂质代谢是治疗和预防急性冠脉综合征最有效的手段。最新的ACC/AHA指南推荐根据LDL-C绝对值、是否合并糖尿病或动脉粥样硬化性疾病和10年ASCVD风险等级决定何时启用饮食控制或药物治疗，并指导他汀治疗强度的选择。PCSK9抑制剂显示出良好的降脂效果，尤其适用于他汀不耐受或最大剂量他汀联合其他降脂药物后血脂仍不达标的患者。PCSK9反义RNA药物正在临床试验阶段，其3~6个月给药一次，将明显增加患者依从性，其临床结果值得期待。同时我们也应关注n-3脂肪酸可能的心血管保护作用。该部分内容在第26、27章详细讲述。

心血管疾病是吸烟者主要死亡原因。尽管全球吸烟率逐年下降，但烟草消费量却在不断增加，二手烟暴露严重。尼古丁和烟草产品影响血管内皮细胞功能，导致血压升高、交感兴奋、冠脉痉挛、动脉粥样硬化、血栓形成等。基于此，本部分新增了第28章《尼古丁和烟草制品的心血管疾病风险》，旨在强调及早戒烟对心血管疾病防治的有益作用。

饮食习惯、肥胖及糖尿病均与心血管疾病相关，三者相互影响，且可影响血压、血脂等心血管代谢，是心血管疾病防治的重要内容。随着营养学的发展，目前强调饮食模式而非独立营养素在心血管疾病防治中的作用。建议减少精制谷物、淀粉、添加糖、加工肉类等的摄入，取代以全谷物、水果、蔬菜、坚果、鱼贝、适量奶制品、不饱和脂肪酸的摄入，均衡营养，以达到最佳心血管保护作用。超重/肥胖越来越引起人们的重视。内脏脂肪堆积被认为可增加心血管疾病风险，与脂肪重量相比我们更应关注脂肪的质量及功能。对肥胖者需强调生活方式改变（包括饮食、运动、睡眠及压力管理等）的作用。现阶段减肥药物缺乏心血管获益证据，既有减重又具有心血管保护作用的降糖药物可能是一个较好的选择，而对于严重肥胖患者减重手术可获得心血管益处。与非糖尿病患者相比，糖尿病患者心血管疾病风险及死亡率明显升高。随着新的临床研究结果揭晓，临床医生对糖尿病患者的治疗理念逐渐发生了转变。现阶段不应只追求药物的降糖效果，而更应关注降糖药物的心血管安全性及疗效。多种钠-葡萄糖协同转运蛋白2（SGLT2）抑制剂和胰高血糖素样肽1（GLP-1）受体激动剂被证实具有心血管保护作用，指南也推荐这两类药物作为糖尿病合并心血管疾病高风险人群的优先选择。第29、30、31章详细讲述了饮食、肥胖及糖尿病在心血管疾病中的作用及可采取的控制手段。

除控制上述危险因素外我们也应关注心血管疾病特殊人群。长期运动人群或运动员可能出现一些心血管症状（如胸痛、晕厥），存在一定的运动相关风险。第32章描述了心血管系统对运动训练的适应及体育活动的心血管风险，介绍了运动人群的心血管疾病特征，有助于临床医生评估其是否为正常变异，平衡运动的风险和获益，制订正确的管理和指导方案。

对心脏病患者的综合管理是预防心脏病学的重要组成部分。随着科技进步和生物医学发展，基于人工智能、组学测序、基因编辑等的应用将进一步推动预防心脏病学的发展。心血管疾病防治过程应强调个人、家庭、社会共同参与，同时需要心血管、内分泌、营养学、运动学、康复学、护理等多学科协作。第33、34章聚焦心脏康复和心脏病患者的综合管理，建议关注心血管疾病患者的营养和生活方式干预，调动患者主观能动性，积极进行心脏康复，同时强调家庭社会共同参与。我国预防心脏病学起步较晚，心血管疾病患者人口基数大、社会负担重，亟需各方的共同努力来改变这一局面，促进人民健康福祉。

PART IV PREVENTIVE CARDIOLOGY

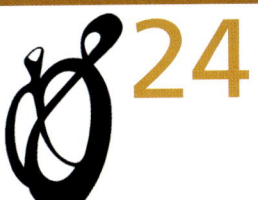

24 The Vascular Biology of Atherosclerosis

PETER LIBBY

扫描二维码阅读
第24章中文导读

OVERVIEW AND BACKGROUND, 425
STRUCTURE OF THE NORMAL ARTERY, 425
Cell Types Composing the Normal Artery, 425
Layers of the Normal Artery, 427

ATHEROSCLEROSIS INITIATION, 428
Extracellular Lipid Accumulation, 428
Leukocyte Recruitment and Retention, 430
Focality of Lesion Formation, 431
Intracellular Lipid Accumulation: Foam Cell Formation, 432

EVOLUTION OF ATHEROMA, 432
Innate and Adaptive Immunity: Mechanisms of Inflammation in Atherogenesis, 432

Smooth Muscle Cell Migration and Proliferation, 432
Smooth Muscle Cell Death During Atherogenesis, 433
Arterial Extracellular Matrix, 433
Angiogenesis in Plaques, 434
Plaque Mineralization, 435

COMPLICATION OF ATHEROSCLEROSIS, 435
Arterial Stenoses and Clinical Implications, 435
Thrombosis and Atheroma Complication, 435
Plaque Rupture and Thrombosis, 435
Thrombosis Caused by Superficial Erosion of Plaques, 437

Thrombosis and Healing in Progression of Atheroma, 437
Diffuse and Systemic Nature of Plaque Susceptibility to Rupture and Inflammation in Atherogenesis, 437

SPECIAL CASES OF ARTERIOSCLEROSIS, 438
Restenosis After Arterial Intervention, 438
Accelerated Arteriosclerosis After Transplantation, 438
Aneurysmal Disease, 439
Infection, the Microbiome, and Atherosclerosis, 440

REFERENCES, 440

OVERVIEW AND BACKGROUND

The 20th century witnessed a remarkable evolution in concepts concerning the pathogenesis of atherosclerosis. This disease has a venerable history, having left traces in the arteries of mummies.[1,2] Atherosclerosis became epidemic as populations increasingly survived early mortality associated with communicable diseases and malnutrition. Economic development and urbanization promoted poor diet (e.g., a surfeit of saturated fats) and diminished physical activity, which can favor atherogenesis. These environmental factors have spread steadily, such that we face an epidemic of atherosclerosis that reaches far beyond Western societies.[3]

Views of the pathogenesis of atherosclerosis have evolved considerably over time (Fig. 24.1).[4] In the mid-19th century, Rudolf Virchow recognized the participation of cells in atherogenesis. A controversy raged between Virchow, who viewed atherosclerosis as a proliferative disease, and Carl von Rokitansky, who believed that atheroma derived from healing and resorption of thrombi. Experiments were performed in the early part of the 20th century using dietary modulation to produce fatty lesions in the arteries of rabbits and ultimately identified cholesterol as the culprit. These observations, followed by the characterization of human lipoprotein particles in the mid-20th century, found that lipids are a cause for atherosclerosis. Elements of all these mechanisms indeed contribute to atherogenesis. This chapter summarizes evidence from human studies, animal experimentation, and in vitro work and presents a synoptic view of atherogenesis from the biologic perspective.[4]

Acquaintance with the vascular biology of atherosclerosis should prove useful to the practitioner. Our daily contact with this common disease lulls us into a complacent belief that we understand it better than we actually do. For example, we have begun to understand why atherosclerosis affects certain regions of the arterial tree preferentially and why its clinical manifestations occur only at certain times. Despite systemic exposure to risk factors such as dyslipidemia and hypertension and smoking, atherosclerosis preferentially produces focal stenoses in certain locations.

Atherosclerosis also displays dispersion in time; this disease has both chronic and acute manifestations. Few human diseases have a longer "incubation" period than atherosclerosis, which begins to affect the arteries of many Americans in the second and third decades of life. Indeed, many young Americans often have abnormal thickening of the coronary arterial intima; yet typically, symptoms of atherosclerosis emerge only after several decades of delay, characteristically appearing even later in women. Despite this indolent time course and prolonged period of clinical inactivity, the dreaded complications of atheroma—myocardial infarction (MI) and stroke—often occur suddenly and without warning.

Another poorly understood aspect of atherogenesis is its role in the narrowing, or stenosis, of some vessels and in the dilation or ectasia of others. Traditionally, cardiologists have focused on stenoses in coronary arteries, but atherosclerosis can also commonly manifest as aneurysms, as in the aorta. Even in the life history of a single atherosclerotic lesion, a phase of ectasia known as *positive remodeling*, or *compensatory enlargement*, precedes the formation of stenotic lesions. Contemporary vascular biology has begun to shed light on some of these puzzling aspects of atherosclerosis.

STRUCTURE OF THE NORMAL ARTERY

Cell Types Composing the Normal Artery

Endothelial Cells

The endothelial cell (EC) of the arterial intima constitutes the crucial contact surface with blood. Arterial ECs possess many highly regulated mechanisms of capital importance in vascular homeostasis that often go awry during the pathogenesis of arterial diseases. For example, the EC provides one of the only surfaces, either natural or synthetic, that can maintain blood in a liquid state during protracted contact (Fig. 24.2). This remarkable blood compatibility derives in part from the expression of heparan sulfate proteoglycan molecules on the surface of the EC. Like heparin, these molecules, can serve as a cofactor for antithrombin III, causing a conformational change that allows this inhibitor to bind to and inactivate thrombin. The surface of the EC also contains *thrombomodulin*, which binds thrombin molecules and can exert antithrombotic properties by activating proteins S and C. Should a thrombus begin to form, the normal EC possesses potent fibrinolytic mechanisms associated with its surface. The EC can produce both tissue-plasminogen activator (t-PA) and urokinase-type plasminogen activator (u-PA). These

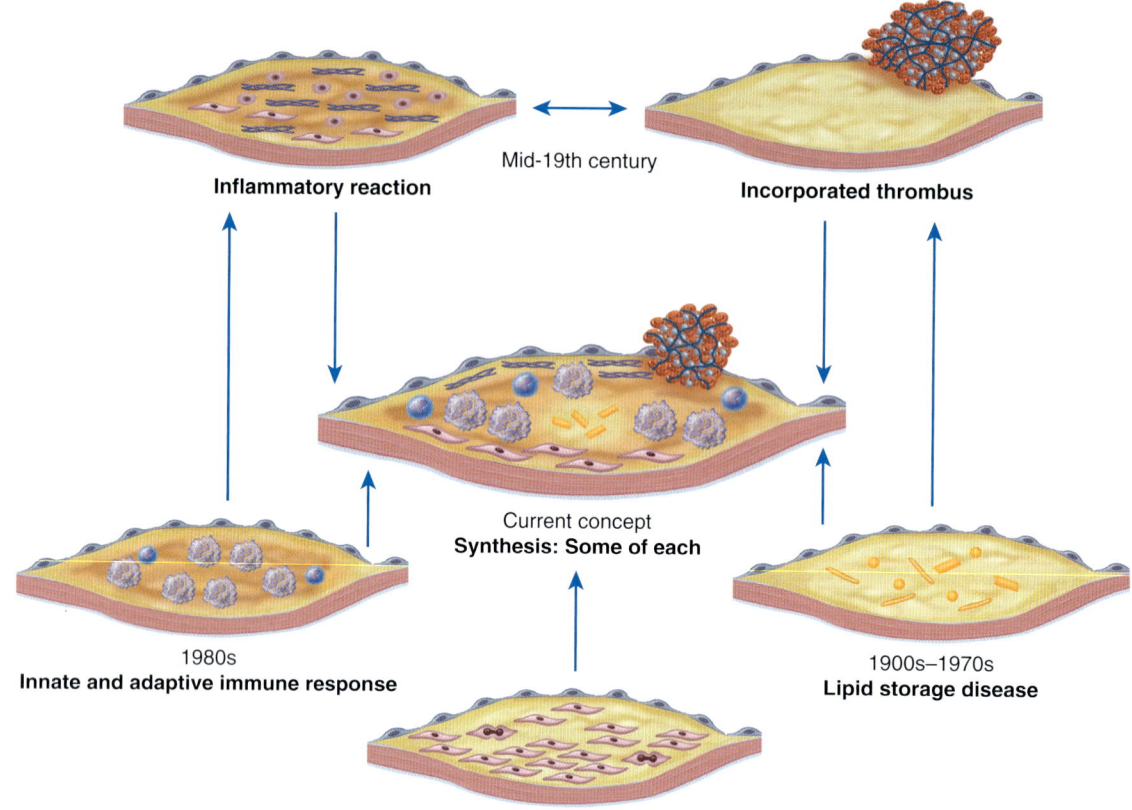

FIGURE 24.1 Evolution of concepts of the pathogenesis of atherosclerosis. The diagrams represent the dominant formulation of mechanisms of atherogenesis as they emerged over time (clockwise). In the mid-19th century, Virchow and von Rokitansky fueled a heated controversy regarding the role of incorporated thrombus in atherosclerosis (top pair of diagrams). The experiments of an Anichkov and many others lead to a predominant view of atherosclerosis as primarily a lipid storage disease. This concept prevailed for much of the 20th century. The pioneering work of Ross and of Benditt in the 1970s emphasized the role of smooth muscle proliferation in lesion formation. The initial formulation of the "response to injury" hypothesis accorded an initiating role to endothelial denudation and did not invoke a role for inflammatory cells. Work in the 1980s and beyond used the evolving tools of immunology to define operation of both innate and adaptive immunity in atherogenesis, coming full circle to Virchow's older observations implicating inflammation pathways in atherogenesis. Our current synthetic view of atherogenesis (center) encompasses elements of each of these pathogenic processes unraveled through the years. (From Libby P, Hansson GK. From focal lipid storage to systemic inflammation. *J Am Coll Cardiol.* 2019;74:1594–1607.)

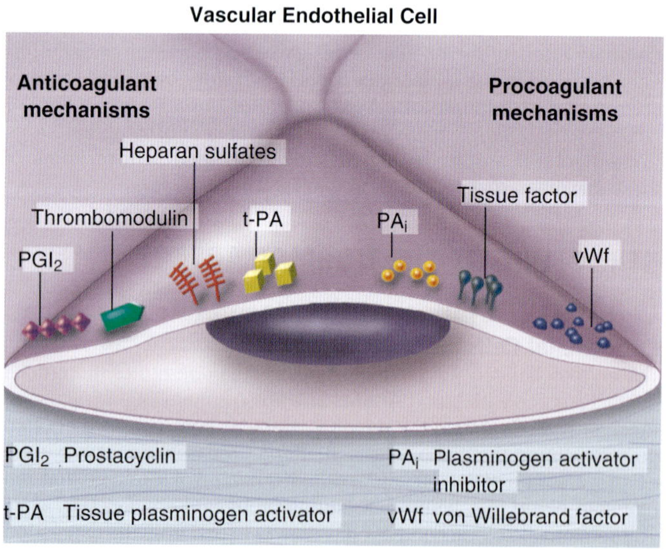

FIGURE 24.2 The endothelial thrombotic balance. This diagram depicts the anticoagulant profibrinolytic functions of the endothelial cell (*left*) and certain procoagulant and antifibrinolytic functions (*right*).

enzymes—t-PA and u-PA—catalyze the activation of plasminogen into *plasmin*, a fibrinolytic enzyme. (See Chapter 95 for a complete discussion on the role of the endothelium in hemostasis and fibrinolysis.)

ECs have a common origin but are considerably heterogeneous. The use of single cell analyses has increased appreciation of the functional attributes and anatomic distribution of three to four distinct EC populations.[5–8] An example from mouse atheroma shows EC populations expressing genes implicated in lipid handling, angiogenesis, and lymph functions (Fig. 24.3).

Arterial Smooth Muscle Cells

The second major cell type of the normal artery wall, the smooth muscle cell (SMC), has many important functions in normal vascular homeostasis, as a target of therapies in cardiovascular medicine and in the pathogenesis of arterial diseases.[9] These cells contract and relax and thus control blood flow through the various arterial beds, generally at the level of the muscular arterioles. However, in larger arteries involved in atherosclerosis, abnormal smooth muscle contraction may cause *vasospasm,* a complication of atherosclerosis that may impede blood flow. SMCs synthesize the bulk of the complex arterial extracellular matrix (ECM) that plays a key role in normal vascular homeostasis and in the formation and complication of atherosclerotic lesions. These cells also can migrate and proliferate, contributing to the formation of intimal hyperplastic lesions, including atherosclerosis and restenosis; stent stenosis after percutaneous intervention; or anastomotic hyperplasia, complicating vein grafts. Death of SMCs may promote destabilization of atheromatous plaques or may favor ectatic remodeling and ultimately aneurysm formation.

In contrast with ECs, which are thought to come from a common precursor, SMCs can arise from many sources. After ECs form tubes, the rudimentary precursor of blood vessels, they recruit the cells that will become SMCs or *pericytes* (smooth muscle–like cells associated with microvessels). In the descending aorta and arteries of the lower body, the regional mesoderm serves as the source of smooth muscle

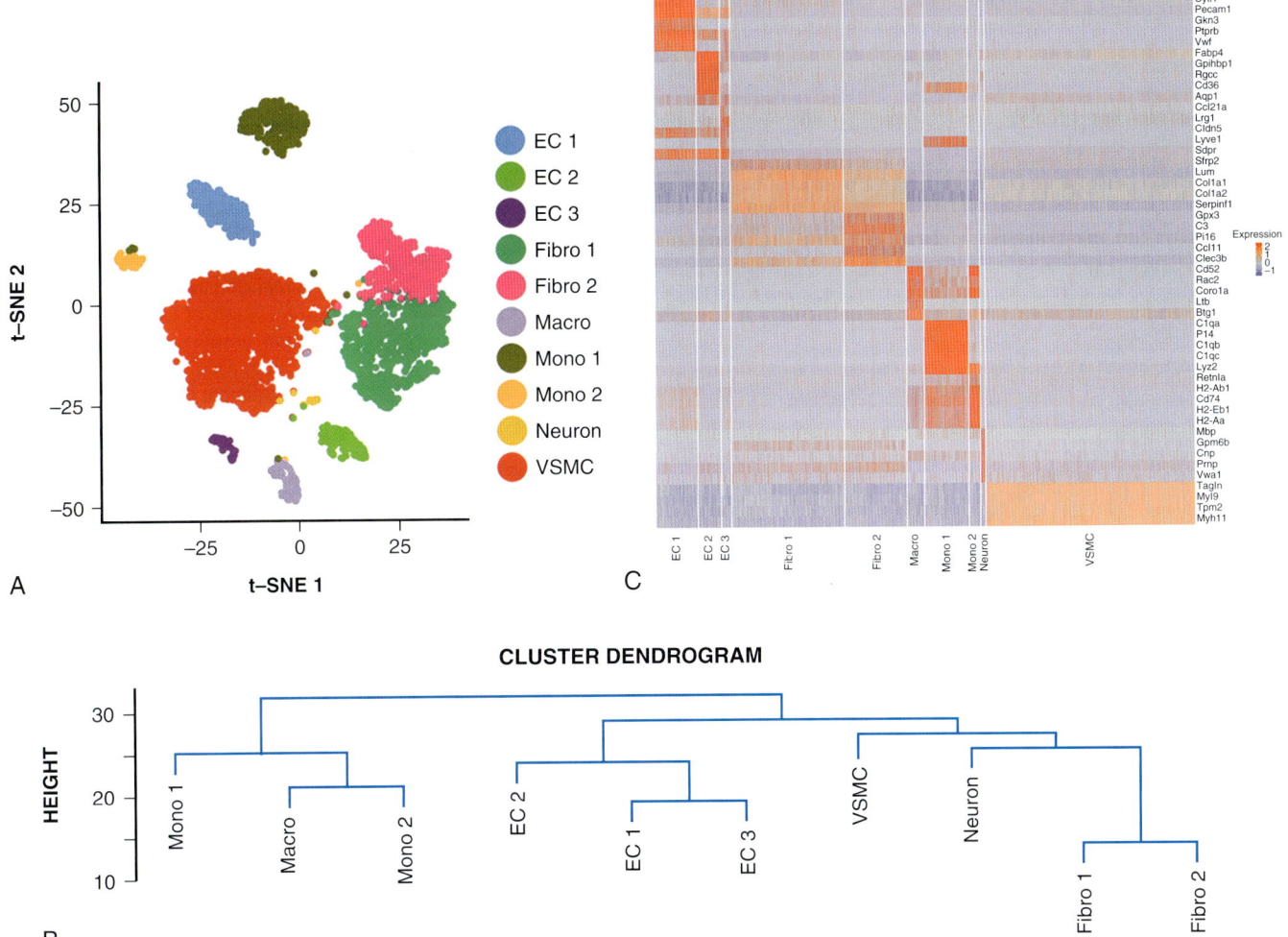

FIGURE 24.3 Subpopulations within cell types identified from single-cell RNA-sequencing. **A,** T-Distributed Stochastic Neighbor Embedding (t-SNE) demonstrating 10 clusters identified as comprising the aorta. **B,** Dendrogram summarizing similarity between aortic cell subpopulations. **C,** Heat map identifying markers of each cellular subpopulation. *EC,* endothelial cells; *Fibro,* fibroblasts; *Macro,* macrophages; *Mono,* monocytes; and *VSMC,* vascular smooth muscle cells. (From Kalluri AS, Vellarikkal SK, Edelman ER, et al. Single-cell analysis of the normal mouse aorta reveals functionally distinct endothelial cell populations. *Circulation.* 2019;140:147–163.)

precursors. The mesodermal cells in somites give rise to the SMCs that make up much of the distal aorta and its branches. However, in arteries of the upper body, SMCs can derive from a completely different germ layer—the neuroectoderm, rather than mesoderm. Also, the precursors of coronary artery SMCs arise from another embryologic source, a structure known as the *proepicardial* organ.

The heterogeneity of SMCs may have direct clinical implications to help understand several common observations, such as the propensity of certain arteries or regions of arteries to develop atherosclerosis or heightened responses to injury (e.g., proximal left anterior descending coronary artery), and medial degeneration (e.g., proximal aorta in Marfan syndrome). Differential responses of SMCs to regulators of ECM production help explain why the clinical manifestations of systemic defects in fibrillin and elastin characteristically occur locally in the ascending aorta. The plasticity of SMCs may even give rise to cells with characteristics and functions of mononuclear phagocytes in murine atherosclerotic plaques.[9,10] SMCs can expand clonally in atheromata, exert proinflammatory functions, and contribute to formation of the plaques' necrotic core,[11] as discussed below.[12]

Layers of the Normal Artery

Intima
An understanding of the pathogenesis of atherosclerosis first requires knowledge on the structure and biology of the normal artery and its indigenous cell types. Normal arteries have a well-developed trilaminar structure (Fig. 24.4). The innermost layer, the tunica intima, is generally thin at birth in humans and in many nonhuman species. Although it is often depicted as a monolayer of ECs abutting directly on a basal lamina, the adult human intima actually has a much more complex and heterogeneous structure. The endothelial monolayer resides on a basement membrane containing nonfibrillar collagen types, such as type IV collagen, laminin, fibronectin, and other ECM molecules. With aging, human arteries develop a more developed intima containing arterial SMCs and fibrillar forms of interstitial collagen (types I and III). SMCs produce these ECM constituents of the arterial intima. Most adult human arteries have a more complex intima, known by pathologists as "diffuse intimal thickening." Some locales in the arterial tree tend to develop a thicker intima than other regions, even in the absence of atherosclerosis (Fig. 24.5).[13] For example, the proximal left anterior descending coronary artery often contains a more fully developed diffuse intimal thickening or an intimal cushion of SMCs than that in typical arteries. The diffuse intimal thickening process does not necessarily go hand in hand with lipid accumulation and may occur in persons without a substantial burden of atheroma. The internal elastic membrane binds the tunica intima abluminally and serves as the border between the intimal layer and the underlying tunia media.

Tunica Media
The tunica media lies under the intima and internal elastic lamina. Like in the aorta, the media of elastic arteries has well-developed concentric layers of SMCs, interleaved with layers of elastin-rich ECM (see Fig. 24.4). This structure appears well adapted to the storage of the kinetic energy of left ventricular systole by the walls of great arteries.

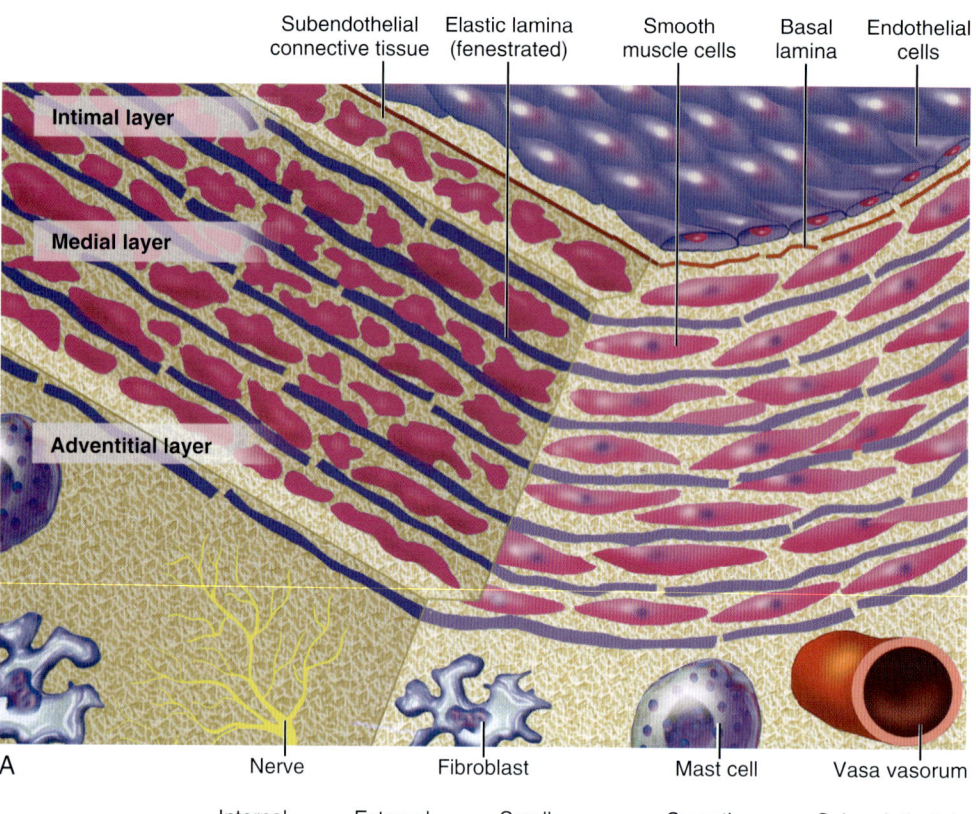

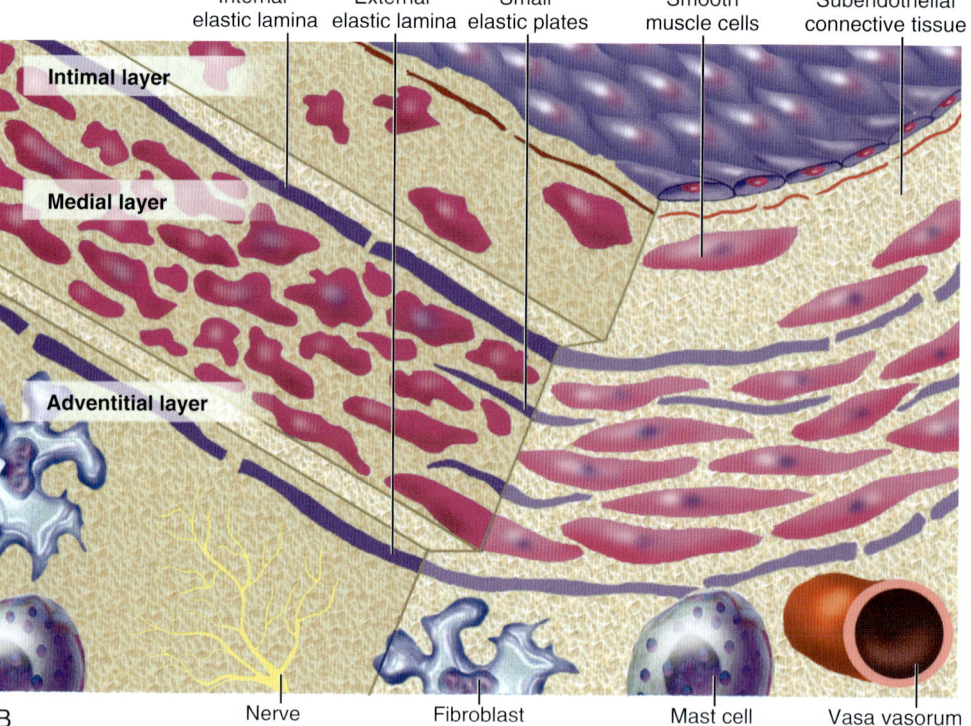

FIGURE 24.4 The structures of normal arteries. **A,** Elastic artery. Note the concentric laminae of elastic tissue that form sandwiches with successive layers of smooth muscle cells (SMCs). Each level of the elastic arterial tree has a characteristic number of elastic laminae. **B,** Muscular artery. In the muscular artery, a collagenous matrix surrounds the SMCs, but the architecture lacks the concentric rings of the well-organized elastic tissue characteristic of larger arteries.

are low. In the normal artery, a state of ECM homeostasis also typically prevails: rates of arterial matrix synthesis and dissolution usually balance each other. The external elastic lamina bounds the tunica media abluminally, forming the border with the adventitial layer.

Adventitia

The adventitia of arteries typically has received little attention, although appreciation of its potential roles in arterial homeostasis and pathology has increased. The adventitia contains collagen fibrils in a looser array than that usually encountered in the intima. Vasa vasorum and nerve endings localize in this outermost layer of the arterial wall. The cellular population in the adventitia is sparser than in other arterial layers. Cells found in this layer include fibroblasts and mast cells (see Fig. 24.4). Emerging evidence suggests a role for mast cells in atheroma and aneurysm formation in animal models, but their importance in humans remains speculative.[14] The adventitia also contains aggregates of lymphocytes known as tertiary lymphoid organs that may contribute to local periarterial immune responses.[15]

ATHEROSCLEROSIS INITIATION

Extracellular Lipid Accumulation

The first steps in human atherogenesis remain largely conjectural, but the integration of observations of tissues obtained from young humans with the results of experimental studies of atherogenesis in animals provides hints in this regard. On initiation of an atherogenic diet, typically rich in cholesterol and saturated fat, small lipoprotein particles accumulate in the intima (Fig. 24.6, steps 1 and 2).[16] These lipoprotein particles appear to decorate the proteoglycan of the arterial intima and tend to coalesce into aggregates (Fig. 24.7). Detailed kinetic studies of labeled lipoprotein particles indicate that a prolonged residence time characterizes sites of early lesion formation in rabbits. The binding of lipoproteins to proteoglycan in the intima leads to their capture and retention, accounting for their prolonged residence time. Lipoprotein particles bound to proteoglycan have increased susceptibility to oxidative or other chemical modifications, considered by many to contribute to the pathogenesis of early atherosclerosis (step 2 in Fig. 24.6). Other studies suggest that permeability of the endothelial monolayer increases at sites of lesion predilection to low-density lipoprotein (LDL). Contributors to oxidative

The lamellar structure also certainly contributes to the structural integrity of the arterial trunks. The media of smaller muscular arteries usually has a less stereotypic organization. SMCs in these smaller arteries generally embed in the surrounding matrix in a more continuous than lamellar array. The SMCs in normal arteries seldom proliferate. Indeed, under usual circumstances, the rates of cell division and cell death

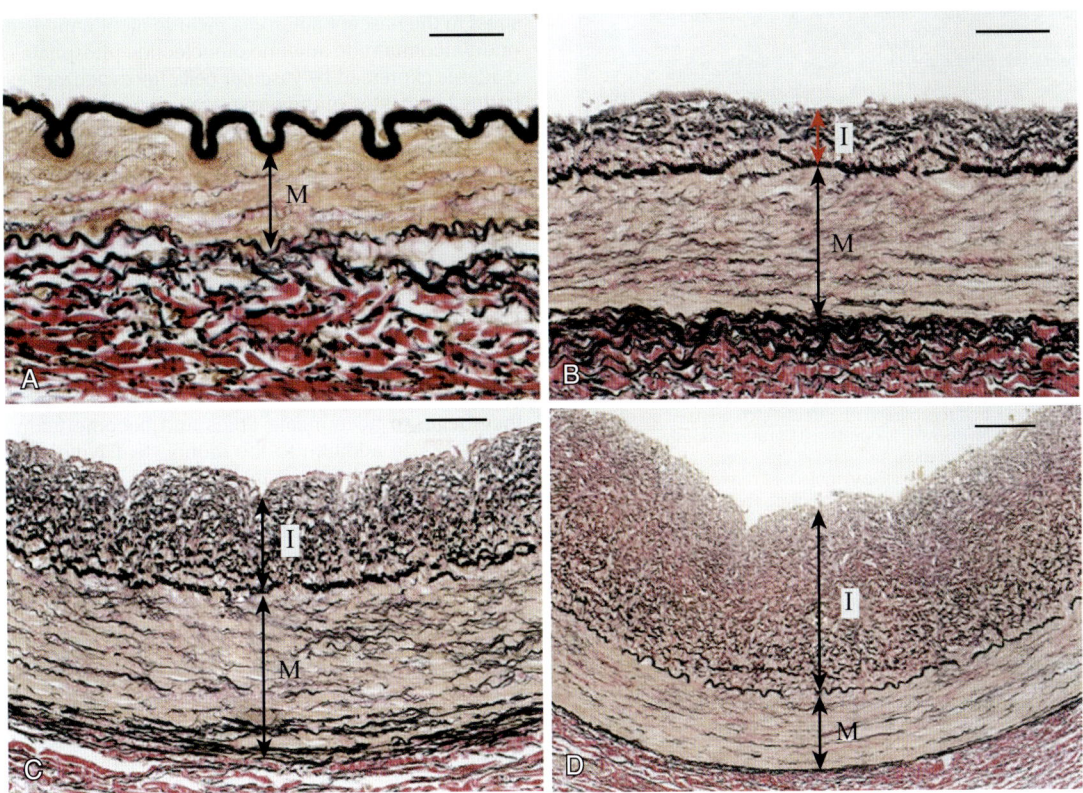

FIGURE 24.5 Diffuse intimal thickening (DIT) in proximal coronary arteries. **A,** Right coronary artery (RCA) of a 7-day-old girl. **B,** Left anterior descending artery (LAD) of a 5-year-old girl. **C,** LAD of a 15-year-old girl. **D,** LAD of a 29-year-old woman. Bars in parts **A, B, C,** and **D** represent 25, 50, 50, 100 µm, respectively. *I,* intima; *M* media. (From Nakashima Y, Chen Y-X, Kinukawa N, et al . Distributions of diffuse intimal thickening in human arteries: preferential expression in atherosclerosis-prone arteries from an early age. *Virchows Arch.* 2002;441:279–288.)

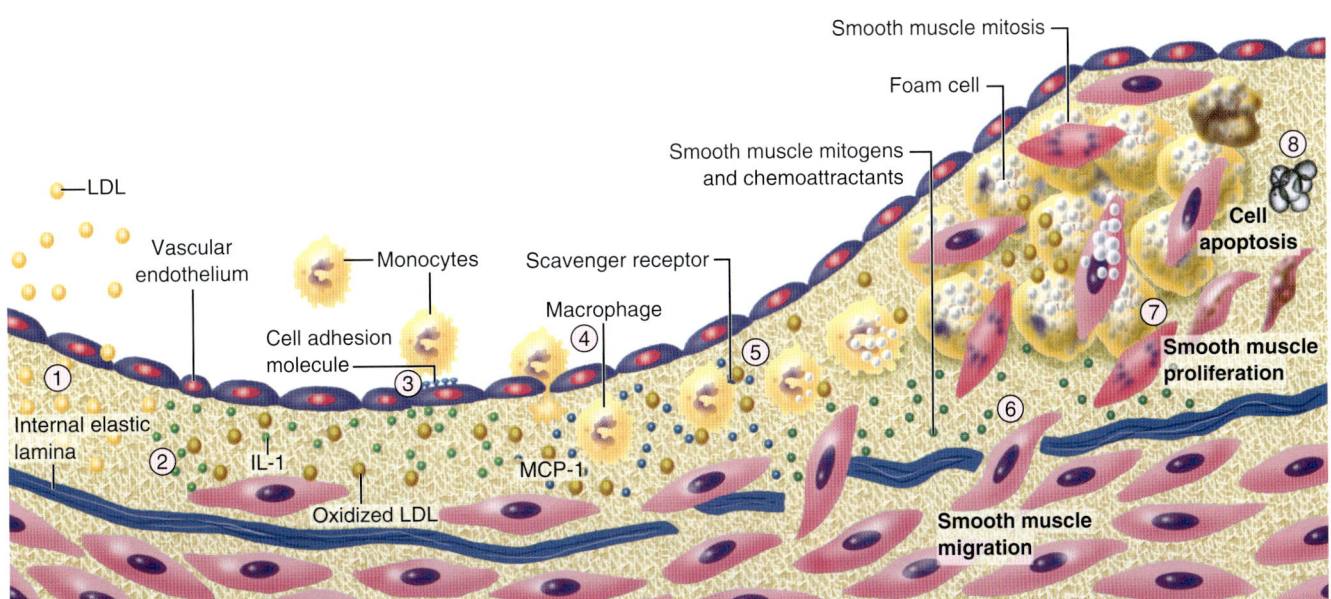

FIGURE 24.6 Schematic of the evolution of the atherosclerotic plaque. *1,* Accumulation of lipoprotein particles in the intima (*yellow spheres*). The modification of these lipoproteins is depicted by the *darker color.* Modifications include oxidation, glycation, and aggregation. *2,* Oxidative stressors, including products found in modified lipoproteins, can induce local cytokine elaboration (*green spheres*). *3,* The cytokines thus induced increased expression of adhesion molecules (*blue stalks on endothelial surface*) for leukocytes that cause their attachment and chemoattractant molecules that direct their migration into the intima. *4,* Blood monocytes, on entering the artery wall in response to chemoattractant cytokines such as monocyte chemoattractant protein 1 (*MCP-1*), encounter stimuli such as macrophage colony-stimulating factor that can augment their expression of scavenger receptors. *5,* Scavenger receptors mediate the uptake of modified lipoprotein particles and promote the development of foam cells. Macrophage foam cells produce mediators, such as additional cytokines and effector molecules such as hypochlorous acid, superoxide anion (O_2^-), and matrix metalloproteinases. *6,* Smooth muscle cells (SMCs) migrate into the intima from the media. *7,* SMCs can then divide and elaborate the extracellular matrix, promoting ECM accumulation in the growing atherosclerotic plaque. In this manner, the fatty streak can evolve into a fibrofatty lesion. *8,* In later stages, calcification can occur (*not depicted*) and fibrosis continues, sometimes accompanied by SMC death (including programmed cell death or apoptosis), yielding a relatively acellular fibrous capsule surrounding a lipid-rich core that also may contain dying or dead cells and their detritus. *IL,* Interleukin; *LDL,* low-density lipoprotein.

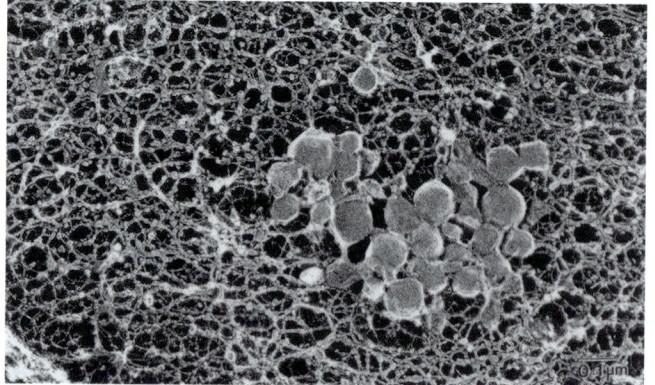

FIGURE 24.7 Scanning electron micrograph of a freeze-etch preparation of rabbit aorta after injection of human low-density lipoprotein (LDL) intravenously. Round LDL particles decorate the strands of proteoglycan found in the subendothelial region of the intima. By binding LDL particles, proteoglycan molecules can retard their traversal of the intima and promote their accumulation. Proteoglycan-associated LDL appears particularly susceptible to oxidative modification. Accumulation of extracellular lipoprotein particles is one of the first morphologic changes noted after initiation of an atherogenic diet in experimental animals. (From Nievelstein PF, Fogelman AM, Mottino G, Frank JS. Lipid accumulation in rabbit aortic intima 2 hours after bolus infusion of low density lipoprotein: a deep-etch and immunolocalization study of ultrarapidly frozen tissue. *Arterioscler Thromb.* 1991;11:1795.)

stress in the nascent atheroma include nicotinamide adenine dinucleotide/nicotinamide adenine dinucleotide phosphate (NADH/NADPH) oxidases expressed by vascular cells, lipoxygenases expressed by infiltrating leukocytes, or the enzyme myeloperoxidase.

Leukocyte Recruitment and Retention

Another hallmark of atherogenesis is leukocyte recruitment and accumulation (step 4 in Fig. 24.6), also occurs early in lesion generation (Fig. 24.8).[17] The normal EC generally resists adhesive interactions with leukocytes. Even in inflamed tissues, most recruitment and trafficking of leukocytes occurs in postcapillary venules and not in arteries. However, very soon after initiation of hypercholesterolemia, leukocytes adhere to the endothelium and move between EC junctions, or even penetrate through ECs (transcytosis) to enter the intima, where they begin to accumulate lipids and become foam cells (step 5 in Fig. 24.6).[18] In addition to the monocyte, T lymphocytes also tend to accumulate in early human and animal atherosclerotic lesions. The expression of certain leukocyte adhesion molecules on the surface of the EC regulates the adherence of monocytes and T cells to the endothelium.[17] Several categories of leukocyte adhesion molecules exist. Members of the *immunoglobulin* (Ig) superfamily include vascular cell adhesion molecule-1 (VCAM-1), or cluster of differentiation (CD)106. This adhesion molecule is of particular interest in the context of early

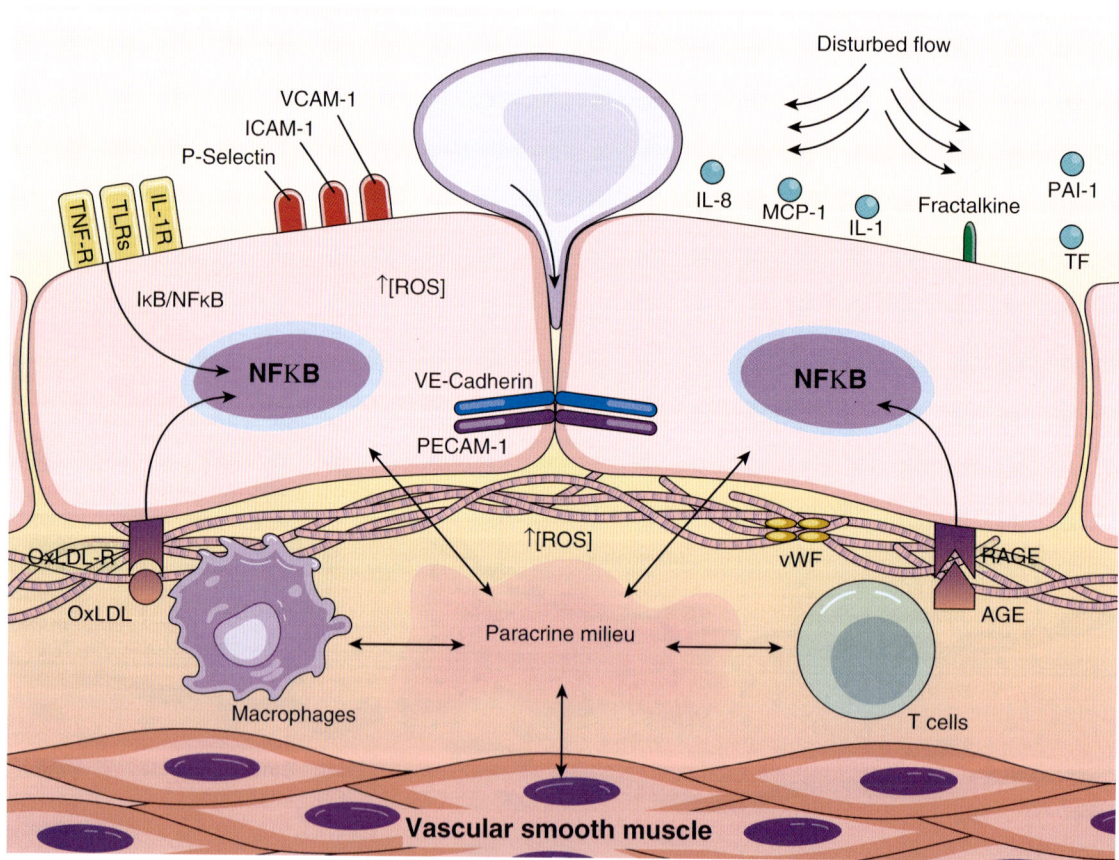

FIGURE 24.8 Endothelial proinflammatory activation. In lesion-prone regions of the arterial vasculature, the actions of proinflammatory agonists (e.g., interleukin [IL]-1, tumor necrosis factor [TNF], and endotoxin), oxidized lipoproteins (Ox-LDL) and advanced glycation end products (AGE), and biomechanical stimulation by disturbed blood flow, leads to endothelial activation. These biochemical and biomechanical stimuli signal predominantly via the pleiotropic transcription factor nuclear factor-κB (NF-κB), resulting in a coordinated program of genetic regulation within the endothelial cell. This includes the cell surface expression of adhesion molecules (e.g., vascular cell adhesion molecule-1 [VCAM-1]), secreted and membrane-associated chemokines (e.g., monocyte chemoattractant protein [MCP]-1 and fractalkine), and prothrombotic mediators (e.g., tissue factor [TF], von Willebrand Factor [vWF], and the inhibitor of fibrinolysis plasminogen activator inhibitor [PAI]-1). These events foster the selective recruitment of monocytes and various types of T lymphocytes, which become resident in the subendothelial space. The concerted actions of activated endothelial cells, smooth muscle cells, monocyte/macrophages, and lymphocytes result in the production of a complex paracrine milieu of cytokines, growth factors, and reactive oxygen species (ROS) within the vessel wall, which perpetuates a chronic proinflammatory state and fosters atherosclerotic lesion progression. IL-R, TNF-R indicates receptor(s) for IL-1, TNF; *Ox-LDL-R,* receptor for oxidized LDL; *RAGE,* receptor for AGE; *TLRs,* Toll-like receptors. (Illustration Credit: Ben Smith; From Gimbrone MA, García-Cardeña G. Endothelial cell dysfunction and the pathobiology of atherosclerosis. *Circ Res.* 2016;118:620–636.)

atherogenesis because it interacts with an integrin, very late antigen-4 (VLA-4), characteristically expressed by only those classes of leukocytes that accumulate in nascent atheroma—monocytes and T cells. Moreover, experimental studies have shown expression of VCAM-1 on ECs overlying very early atheromatous lesions. Other members of the Ig superfamily of leukocyte adhesion molecules include intercellular adhesion molecule-1 (ICAM-1). This molecule is more promiscuous in the types of leukocytes it binds and in its wide and constitutive expression at low levels by ECs in many parts of the circulation.

Selectins constitute the other broad category of leukocyte adhesion molecules. The prototypic selectin, E-selectin or CD62E (E stands for "endothelial," the cell type that selectively expresses this particular family member), probably has little to do with early atherogenesis. E-selectin preferentially recruits polymorphonuclear leukocytes, a cell type seldom found in early atheromata (but an essential protagonist in acute inflammation and host defenses against bacterial pathogens). Moreover, ECs overlying atheroma do not express high levels of this adhesion molecule. Other members of this family, including P-selectin, or CD62P (P stands for "platelet," the original source of this adhesion molecule), may play a greater role in leukocyte recruitment in atheroma, because ECs overlying human atheroma express this adhesion molecule. Selectins tend to promote saltatory or rolling locomotion of leukocytes over the endothelium. Adhesion molecules belonging to the immunoglobulin superfamily tend to promote tighter adhesive interactions and immobilization of leukocytes. Studies in genetically altered mice have proven roles for VCAM-1 and P-selectin (including both platelet-derived and endothelium-derived P-selectin) in experimental atherosclerosis. Increasing evidence supports the accumulation in atheromas of distinct subtypes of mononuclear phagocytes.[19] The functional consequences of this heterogeneity of macrophage populations in plaques require further study, especially in humans.[20,21] In mice, a particularly proinflammatory subset of monocytes accumulates in the spleen and peripheral blood in response to hypercholesterolemia and preferentially populates nascent atheroma.[22]

Once adherent to the endothelium, leukocytes must receive a signal to penetrate the endothelial monolayer and enter the arterial wall (step 4 in Fig. 24.6). The current concept of directed migration of leukocytes involves the action of protein molecules known as chemoattractant cytokines, or *chemokines*. Observations on human atheroma and functional studies in vitro and in genetically altered mice point to causal roles of various chemokines in atherogenesis.[23] In addition to recruitment, the accumulation of leukocytes in the arterial wall depends on factors that cause their retention in the intimal lesions. Retention factors include netrin-1 interacting with its receptor UNC5b (both induced by hypoxia), a protein that impairs macrophages from exiting plaques.[24]

Focality of Lesion Formation

The spatial heterogeneity of atherosclerosis is challenging to explain in mechanistic terms. Equal concentrations of blood-borne risk factors such as lipoproteins bathe the endothelium throughout the vasculature. It is difficult to envisage how injury resulting from inhalation of cigarette smoke could produce any local rather than global effect on arteries, yet stenoses caused by atheromas typically form focally. Some researchers have evoked a multicentric origin hypothesis of atherogenesis, proposing that atheromas arise as benign leiomyomas of the artery wall. The monotypia of various molecular markers in individual atheromas supports this monoclonal hypothesis of atherogenesis. Contemporary lineage mapping studies support clonal expansion of SMCs as noted earlier.[12]

The location of the lesion predilection at proximal portions of arteries after branch points or bifurcations at flow dividers, suggests a hydrodynamic basis for early lesion development. Arteries without many branches (e.g., the internal mammary and radial arteries) tend not to develop atherosclerosis.[25] Two concepts can aid in understanding how local flow disturbances might render certain foci sites of lesion predilection. Locally disturbed flow could induce alterations that promote the steps of early atherogenesis. Alternatively, the laminar flow that usually prevails at sites that do not tend to develop early lesions may elicit antiatherogenic homeostatic mechanisms (atheroprotective functions).[17] The EC experiences the laminar shear stress of normal flow and the disturbed flow (usually yielding decreased shear stress) at sites of predilection. Multiple transduction mechanisms operate to signal the local shear stress environment to ECs.[26] For example, these cells have cilia on their luminal surface and adhesion receptors in their lateral cell membrane that can sense tension, transmit forces to the cortical cytoskeleton, and potentially regulate ion channels or G protein–coupled receptors that signal changes in gene expression (Fig. 24.9). In vitro data suggest that laminar shear stress can augment the expression of genes that may protect against atherosclerosis, including forms of the enzymes superoxide dismutase (SOD) and nitric oxide synthase (NOS). SOD can reduce oxidative stress by catabolizing the reactive and injurious superoxide anion. Endothelial NOS produces the well-known endogenous vasodilator nitric oxide (NO). Beyond its vasodilating actions, NO can resist inflammatory activation of endothelial functions, including the expression of VCAM-1. NO appears to exert this anti-inflammatory action at the level of gene expression by interfering with the transcriptional regulator nuclear factor kappa B (NF-κB). NO increases the production of IκBα, an intracellular inhibitor of this important transcription factor. NF-κB regulates numerous genes involved in inflammatory responses in general and in atherogenesis in particular.

Studies also implicate transcription factors, notably Krüppel-like factor 2 (KLF2), as important regulators of endothelial anti-inflammatory properties. KLF2 can induce endothelial NOS expression and also inhibits NF-κB function by sequestering cofactors needed to boost NF-κB transcriptional activity, resulting in inhibition of the expression of the cassette of NF-κB–dependent genes involved in the inflammatory pathways that operate during atherogenesis. Thus, several atheroprotective mechanisms operate such that under usual conditions of laminar shear

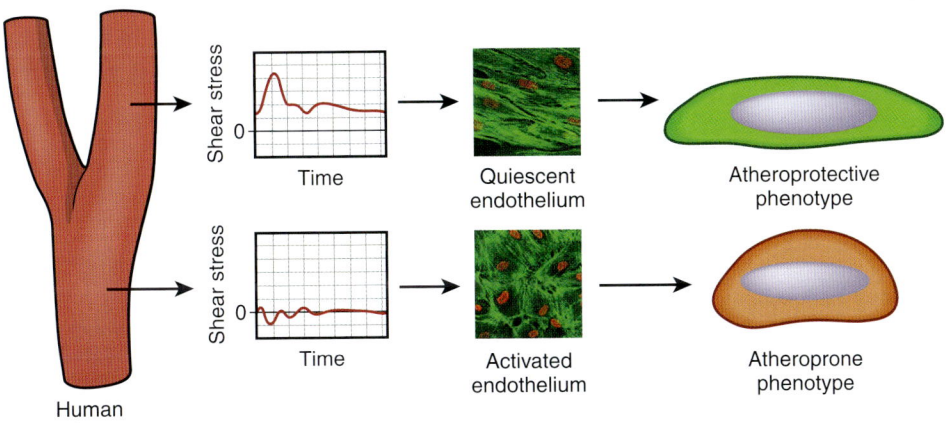

FIGURE 24.9 Hemodynamics determine endothelial functions. Computational analyses of blood flow patterns in vivo in the normal human carotid artery bifurcation provided representative near-wall shear stress waveforms from two hydrodynamically distinct locations known to have distinct predilection to atherogenesis: the distal internal carotid (a region that generally resists lesion formation) and the carotid sinus (a common location for plaque formation). The exposure of monolayers of human endothelial cell in culture to these different biomechanical environments yielded substantially different cell morphologies (depicted by cytoskeletal actin staining) and functions. Pulsatile (unidirectional) laminar flow induced the pivotal transcription factors (Krüppel-like factor [KLF]-2, KLF4, and nuclear factor erythroid 2–related factor [Nrf]-2), which coordinately elicit a palette of atheroprotective functions. In contrast, disturbed (oscillatory) flow enhanced expression of NF-κB, a central transcription factor that governs a number of proinflammatory and proatherogenic functions. (From Gimbrone MA, García-Cardeña G. Endothelial cell dysfunction and the pathobiology of atherosclerosis. *Circ Res.* 2016;118:620–636.)

stress in normal arteries, the endothelium tonically expresses locally acting anti-inflammatory function.[17] Studies in intact pigs and humans show that sites of low shear stress in coronary arteries are associated with the development of plaque characteristics associated with rupture and thrombosis.[27]

Intracellular Lipid Accumulation: Foam Cell Formation

The monocyte, once recruited to the arterial intima, can imbibe lipid and become a foam cell or lipid-laden macrophage (step 5 in Fig. 24.6). Although most cells can express the classic cell surface receptor for LDL, that receptor does not mediate foam cell accumulation (see Chapter 27). This assertion agrees with the clinical finding of tendinous xanthomas filled with foamy macrophages that develop in patients lacking functional LDL receptors (familial hypercholesterolemia homozygotes). The LDL receptor does not mediate foam cell formation, because of its exquisite regulation by cholesterol. As soon as a cell collects enough cholesterol for its metabolic needs from LDL capture, an elegant transcriptional control mechanism quenches expression of the receptor.[28]

Instead of the classic LDL receptor, various *scavenger* receptors appear to mediate the excessive lipid uptake characteristic of foam cell formation. These surface molecules, belonging to several families, bind modified rather than native lipoproteins and participate in their internalization.[29] Because scavenger receptors have functions such as recognition of apoptotic cells and modified lipoproteins, they likely have complex roles during different stages of atherosclerosis (see Chapter 27).

Once macrophages have taken up residence in the intima and become foam cells, they can replicate. In experimental atherosclerosis in mice, monocyte recruitment from blood initially populates the nascent lesion with mononuclear phagocytes, but local proliferation predominates in the established lesion.[22] The factors that trigger macrophage cell division in the atherosclerotic plaque probably include hematopoietic growth factors such as macrophage colony-stimulating factor (M-CSF), granulocyte-macrophage colony-stimulating factor (GM-CSF), and interleukin-3 (IL-3). These co-mitogens and survival factors for mononuclear phagocytes exist in human and experimental atheromatous lesions.

Up to this point, the lesion consists primarily of lipid-engorged macrophages. Complex features such as fibrosis, thrombosis, and calcification do not characterize the *fatty streak*, which is the precursor lesion of the complex atheroma. Several lines of evidence suggest that such fatty streaks can regress, at least to some extent. The relative contributions of reduced recruitment, death of cells within lesions, and egress of cells to reduce the accumulation on mononuclear phagocytes in atheromata under conditions of lipid lowering remain controversial.

EVOLUTION OF ATHEROMA

Innate and Adaptive Immunity: Mechanisms of Inflammation in Atherogenesis

During the past decade, the convergence of basic and clinical evidence has demonstrated a fundamental role for inflammation and immunity in atherogenesis (see Chapter 25).[4,30–34] The macrophage foam cells recruited to the artery wall early in this process serve as a reservoir for excess lipid, and in the established atherosclerotic lesion also furnish many proinflammatory mediators, including proteins (e.g., cytokines, chemokines), various eicosanoids, and other lipid mediators. These phagocytic cells also can elaborate large quantities of oxidant species, such as superoxide anion or hypochlorous acid, in the milieu of the atherosclerotic plaque. This ensemble of inflammatory mediators can promote inflammation in the plaque and thereby contribute to the progression of lesions. The term *innate immunity* describes this type of amplification of the inflammatory response that does not depend on antigenic stimulation (Fig. 24.10).

In addition to innate immunity, mounting evidence supports a prominent role for antigen-specific or *adaptive immunity* in plaque progression.[30] In addition to the mononuclear phagocytes, dendritic cells in atherosclerotic lesions can present antigens to the T cells that constitute an important minority of the leukocytes in atherosclerotic lesions. Candidate antigens that stimulate this adaptive immune response include modified or native lipoproteins, heat shock proteins, beta$_2$-glycoprotein Ib, and infectious agents.[30] The antigen-presenting cells (macrophages, dendritic cells, or ECs) allow the antigen to interact with T cells in a manner that triggers their activation. The activated T cells can then secrete copious quantities of cytokines that modulate atherogenesis.

The helper T cells (bearing CD4) fall into two general categories (see Fig. 24.10). Cells of the T helper 1 (Th1) subtype elaborate proinflammatory cytokines such as interferon (IFN)-γ, lymphotoxin, CD40 ligand, and tumor necrosis factor (TNF)-α. This panel of Th1 cytokines can in turn activate vascular wall cells and orchestrate alterations in plaque biology that can lead to plaque destabilization and heightened thrombogenicity. On the other hand, helper T cells slanted toward the production of Th2 cytokines, such as IL-10, can inhibit inflammation in the context of atherogenesis. Cytolytic T cells (bearing CD8) can express Fas ligand and other cytotoxic factors that can promote cytolysis and apoptosis of target cells, including SMCs, ECs, and macrophages. The death of all these cell types can occur in the atherosclerotic lesion and may contribute to plaque progression and complication.[16] Regulatory T cells (Tregs) can elaborate transforming growth factor (TGF)-β and IL-10. Treg lymphocytes bear the markers CD4 and CD25. Both TGF-β and IL-10 can exert anti-inflammatory effects. Several experimental preparations suggest an antiatherosclerotic function of Tregs in vivo.[35] Distinct from such anti-inflammatory mechanisms, the operation mediators of resolution may provide another avenue to dampening the inflammatory response during atherogenesis.[36]

The role of B cells and antibody in atherosclerosis remains incompletely explored. Humoral immunity may have either atheroprotective or atherogenic properties, depending on the circumstances.[30,31,33] B1 cells that produce natural antibodies, many of which recognize oxidatively modified LDL, can protect against experimental atherosclerosis.[37,38] B2 cells generally aggravate atherosclerosis in mice by promoting proinflammatory cytokine production, which created interest in immunotherapy to mitigate atherosclerosis.[39,40]

Smooth Muscle Cell Migration and Proliferation

Whereas the early events in atheroma initiation involve primarily altered endothelial function and recruitment and accumulation of leukocytes, the subsequent evolution of atheroma into more complex plaques also involves SMCs (steps 6 and 7 in Fig. 24.6). SMCs in the normal arterial tunica media differ considerably from those in the intima of an evolving atheroma. Some SMCs probably arrive in the arterial intima early in life; others accumulate in advancing atheroma after recruitment from the underlying media into the intima or arise from blood-borne precursors. Some cells bearing macrophage markers in mouse atheromata appear to derive from SMCs.[9,41,42]

SMCs in the atherosclerotic intima appear to exhibit a less mature phenotype than that for the quiescent SMCs in the normal arterial medial layer. Instead of expressing primarily isoforms of smooth muscle myosin characteristic of adult SMCs, those in the intima have higher levels of the embryonic isoform of smooth muscle myosin. Thus, SMCs in the intima seem to recapitulate an embryonic phenotype. These intimal SMCs in atheroma appear to be morphologically distinct; they contain more rough endoplasmic reticulum and fewer contractile fibers than do normal medial SMCs.

Although replication of SMCs in the steady state appears uncommon in mature human atheroma, clonal expansion likely occurs over time, and bursts of SMC replication may occur during the life history of a given atheromatous lesion.[9,11,12] For example, as discussed later, episodes of plaque disruption with thrombosis may expose SMCs to potent mitogens, including the coagulation factor thrombin itself. Thus, accumulation of SMCs during atherosclerosis and growth of the intima

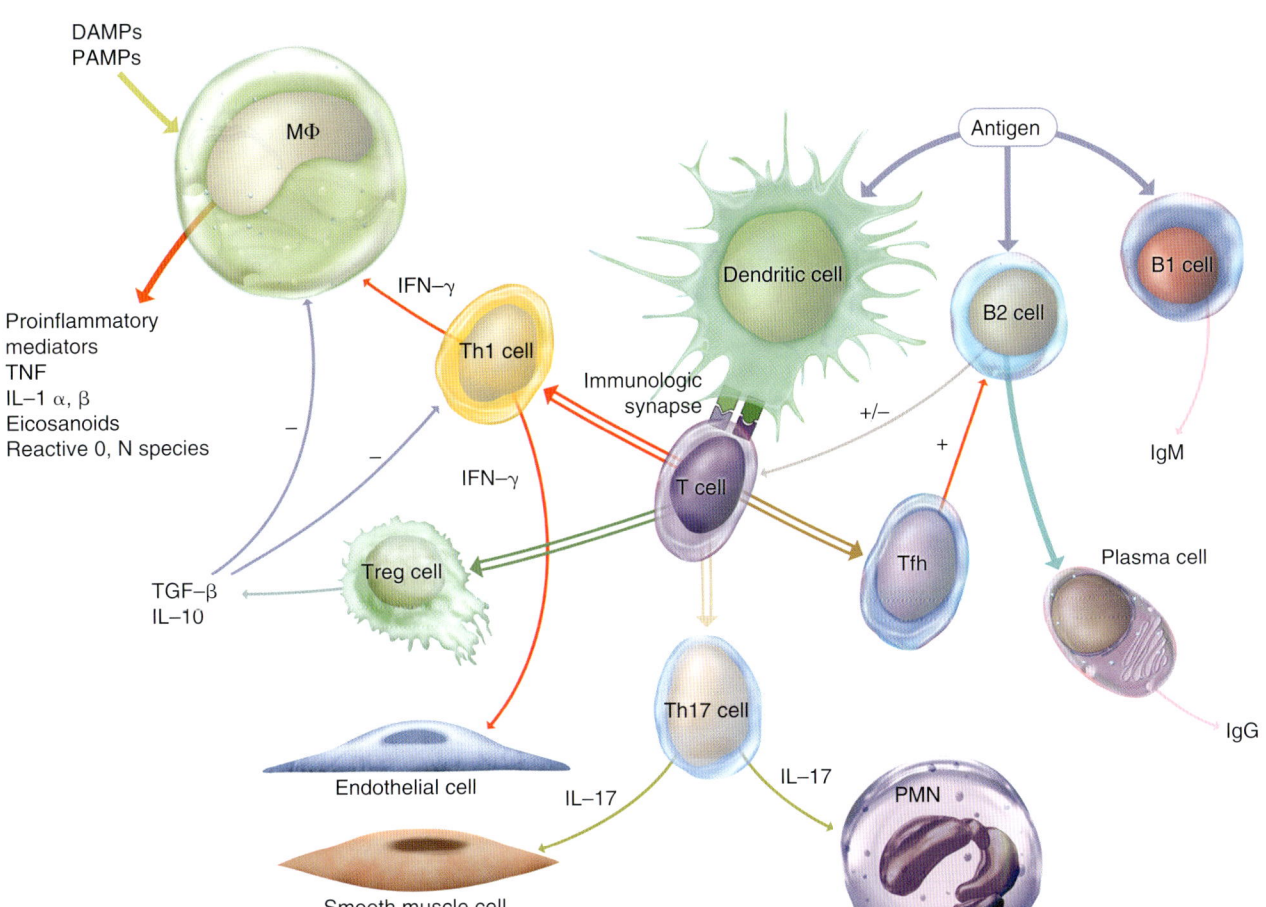

FIGURE 24.10 A simplified view of the operation of innate and adaptive immunity as thought to operate in atherogenesis. Innate immunity initiates when macrophages (MΦ) recognize pathogen-associated molecular patterns (PAMPs) and damage-associated molecular patterns (DAMPs) binding to their pattern recognition receptors. This interaction leads to production of a host of proinflammatory molecules including cytokines (e.g., interleukin [IL]-1-α and IL-β and tumor necrosis factor [TNF]) and small molecules such as eicosanoids. Adaptive immune responses follow the processing of antigens (foreign or autologous) by dendritic cells (DCs). Proteolytic cleavage of protein antigens into peptides within the DC prepares the antigen for presentation on the DC surface bound to major histocompatibility complex (MHC) molecules (human leukocyte antigens in humans). Antigen-specific immune cells recognize the nominal antigen in the context of self MHC (immunologic synapse). T cells can recognize peptide-human leukocyte antigens complexes via specific antigen receptors. Antigen recognition in combination with signals produced by the DC prompts the T cell to activate and differentiate. Activated CD4β T cells may differentiate into several cell types with different functions. Among them, Th1 cells produce interferon (IFN)-g and TNF, are highly proinflammatory, and strongly stimulate macrophage activation and vascular inflammation. Regulatory T cells (Treg), on the other hand, make 2 anti-inflammatory and immunoregulatory cytokines, namely transforming growth factor (TGF)-β and IL-10. IL-17 produced by Th17 cells activates granulocytes and stimulates collagen production, as does TGF-β B cells recognize antigens that ligate their surface-bound immunoglobulins. The most prevalent type of B cell, the B2 cell, receives help from T follicular helper (Tfh) cells and can develop into plasma cells specialized in production of immunoglobulin G (IgG) antibodies. In addition, B2 cells produce cytokines that can modulate inflammation. Another B cell subset, the B1 cell, produces immunoglobulin M (IgM) antibodies and does not require Tfh cell help. B1 cells largely produce "natural" antibodies encoded by the germline, while the genes that encode IgG antibodies generally undergo somatic mutations to achieve greater affinity for the particular antigen with time. *Single-line arrows* indicate signaling molecules; *double-line* and *thick arrows* show cell development. *PMN,* polymorphonuclear leukocytes. (From Libby P, Hansson GK. From focal lipid storage to systemic inflammation. *J Am Coll Cardiol.* 2019;74:1594–1607.)

may not occur in a continuous and linear manner. Rather, "crises" may punctuate the history of an atheroma, during which bursts of smooth muscle activity may occur (Fig. 24.11).

Smooth Muscle Cell Death During Atherogenesis

In addition to SMC replication, death of these cells also may participate in the complication of the atherosclerotic plaque (step 8 in Fig. 24.6).[9,16] Some examples of programmed cell death or apoptosis SMCs in advanced human atheroma exhibit fragmentation of their nuclear DNA. Apoptosis may occur in response to inflammatory cytokines present in the evolving atheroma. In addition to soluble cytokines that may trigger programmed cell death, T cells in atheroma may participate in eliminating some SMCs. In particular, certain T cell populations known to accumulate in plaques can express Fas ligand on their surface. Fas ligand can engage Fas on the surface of SMCs and, in conjunction with soluble proinflammatory cytokines, lead to SMC death.

Thus, SMC accumulation in the growing atherosclerotic plaque probably results from a tug-of-war between cell replication and cell death. Contemporary cell and molecular biologic research has identified candidates for mediation of both the replication and the attrition of SMCs, a concept that originated from Virchow's careful morphologic observations made in the mid-19th century.[4] Referring to the SMCs in the intima, Virchow noted that early atherogenesis involves a "multiplication of their nuclei" but also noted that cells in lesions can "hurry on to their own destruction."

Arterial Extracellular Matrix

Rather than cells themselves, ECM makes up much of the volume of an advanced atherosclerotic plaque. Accordingly, extracellular constituents of plaque also require consideration. The major ECM macromolecules that accumulate in atheroma include interstitial collagens (types I and III) and proteoglycans such as versican, biglycan, aggrecan, and decorin. Elastin fibers also may accumulate in atherosclerotic plaques. Arterial SMCs produce these ECM molecules in disease, just as they do during development and maintenance of the normal artery (step 7 in Fig. 24.6). Stimuli for excessive collagen production by SMCs include platelet-derived growth factor (PDGF) and TGF-β, a constituent of platelet granules, and a product of many cell types found in lesions, including Treg lymphocytes.

As with accumulation of SMCs, ECM secretion also depends on a balance, as noted earlier. In this case, the counterpoise to biosynthesis of the ECM molecules is breakdown catalyzed in part by catabolic enzymes, notably the matrix metalloproteinases (MMPs). Dissolution of ECM macromolecules undoubtedly contributes to the migration of SMCs as they penetrate into the intima from the media through a dense ECM, traversing the elastin-rich internal elastic lamina.

ECM breakdown also likely plays a role in arterial remodeling that accompanies lesion growth. During the early life of an atheromatous lesion, plaques grow outwardly, in an abluminal direction, rather than inwardly, in a way that would lead to luminal stenosis. This outward growth of the intima leads to an increase in the caliber of the entire artery. This so-called positive remodeling or compensatory enlargement must involve turnover of ECM molecules to accommodate the circumferential growth of the artery. Luminal stenosis tends to occur only after the plaque burden exceeds approximately 40% of the cross-sectional area of the artery.

Angiogenesis in Plaques

Due to endothelial migration and replication, atherosclerotic plaques develop their own microcirculation as they grow. Histologic examination with appropriate markers for ECs reveals a rich neovascularization in evolving plaques. These microvessels probably form in response to angiogenic peptides overexpressed in atheroma. These angiogenesis factors include vascular endothelial growth factor (VEGF) forms of fibroblast growth factors, placental growth factor (PlGF), and oncostatin M.

These microvessels within plaques probably have considerable functional significance. For example, the abundant microvessels in plaques provide a relatively large surface area for the trafficking of leukocytes, which could include both entry and exit of leukocytes. Indeed, in the advanced human atherosclerotic plaque, the microvascular endothelium displays mononuclear cell–selective adhesion molecules such as VCAM-1 much more prominently than does the macrovascular endothelium overlying the plaque. The microvascularization of plaques may allow growth of the plaque, overcoming diffusion limitations on oxygen and nutrient supply, analogous to the concept of tumor angiogenic factors and growth of malignant lesions. Consistent with this view, administration of inhibitors of angiogenesis to mice with experimentally induced atherosclerosis limits lesion expansion. Further, the plaque microvessels may be friable and prone to rupture, as with the neovessels in the diabetic retina. Hemorrhage and thrombosis in situ could promote a local round of SMC proliferation and matrix accumulation in the area immediately adjacent to the microvascular disruption (Fig. 24.12). This scenario illustrates a special case of the crises described earlier in the evolution of the atheromatous plaque (see Fig. 24.11). Attempts to augment myocardial perfusion by enhancing new vessel growth through the transfer of angiogenic proteins or their genes may have

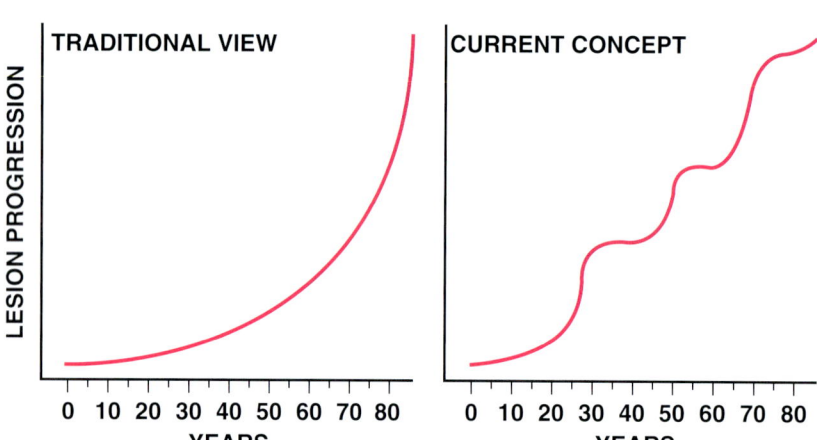

FIGURE 24.11 The time course of atherosclerosis. **Left,** Traditional teaching held that atheroma formation followed an inexorably progressive course with age, as depicted by the smooth upward curve. **Right,** Current thinking suggests an alternative model, a step function rather than a monotonically upward course of lesion evolution in time, as depicted by the serpentine curve. According to this latter model, "crises" can punctuate periods of relative quiescence during the life history of a lesion. Such crises might follow an episode of plaque disruption, with mural thrombosis and healing, yielding a spurt in smooth muscle proliferation and matrix deposition. Intraplaque hemorrhage from rupture of a friable microvessel might produce a similar scenario. Such episodes usually are clinically inapparent. Extravascular events, such as an intercurrent infection with systemic cytokinemia or endotoxemia, could elicit an "echo" at the level of the artery wall, evoking a round of local cytokine gene expression by "professional" inflammatory leukocytes resident in the lesion. The episodic model of plaque progression fits better with human angiographic data than does the traditional model of continuous function.

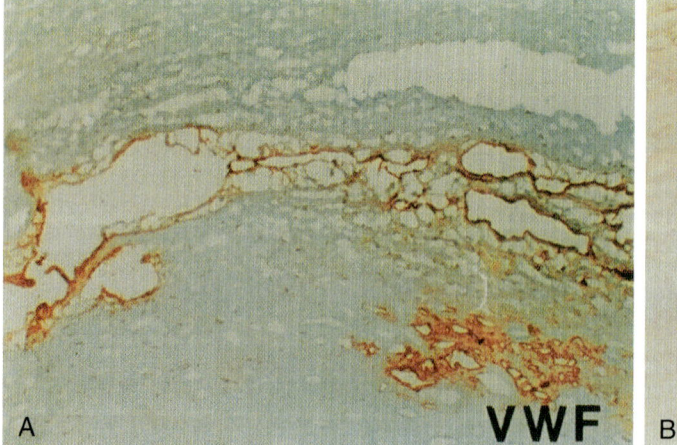 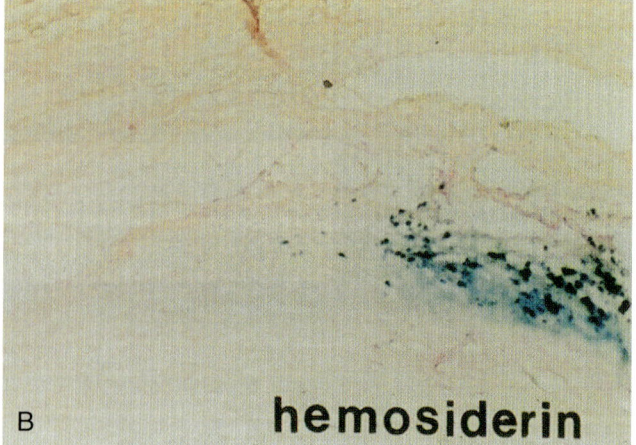

FIGURE 24.12 Intraplaque hemorrhage surrounding neovessels in an atheroma. Typical human atherosclerotic plaque, stained for von Willebrand factor (VWF) **(A)** and for iron by Prussian blue **(B).** The VWF stains the endothelial cells that line the microvascular channels and lakes. Note the extravasated VWF, which colocalizes with iron deposition, indicating hemosiderin deposition consistent with an intraplaque hemorrhage. (After Brogi E, Winkles JA, Underwood R, et al. Distinct patterns of expression of fibroblast growth factors and their receptors in human atheroma and non-atherosclerotic arteries: association of acidic FGF with plaque microvessels and macrophages. *J Clin Invest.* 1993;92:2408.)

adverse effects on lesion growth or may induce clinical complications of atheroma by these mechanisms.

Plaque Mineralization

Plaques often develop areas of calcification as they evolve. Indeed, Virchow recognized morphologic features of bone formation in atherosclerotic plaques in early microscopic descriptions of atherosclerosis. Understanding of mineralization mechanism during the evolution of atherosclerotic plaques has advanced considerably.[43] Some subpopulations of SMCs may foster calcification by enhanced secretion of cytokines such as bone morphogenetic proteins, homologues of TGF-β. Atheroma calcification shares many mechanisms with bone formation. Receptor activator of NF-κB ligand (RANKL), a member of the TNF family, appears to promote SMC mineral formation through a bone morphogenetic protein-4–dependent pathway. *Osteoprotegerin* can antagonize plaque mineralization by inhibiting RANKL signaling. Genetic absence of osteoprotegerin augments calcification of mouse atheromas, and administration of exogenous osteoprotegerin limits it. The transcription factor Runx-2, activated by inflammatory mediators and oxidative stress among other stimuli, can promote SMC mineral formation by activating AKT (i.e., protein kinase B). Markers of inflammation colocalize with foci of mineralization in nascent mouse atheromata. Microparticles elaborated by macrophages may provide nidi for plaque calcification, yielding another link between inflammatory cells and cardiovascular calcification.[44] Sortilin (Sort-1), a genome-wide association study (GWAS) "hit" on atherosclerosis, regulates the loading of alkaline phosphatase into extracellular vesicles, thereby promoting calcification.[45]

COMPLICATION OF ATHEROSCLEROSIS

Arterial Stenoses and Clinical Implications

The phases of the atherosclerotic process generally last many years, during which the affected person often has no symptoms. After the plaque burden exceeds the capacity of the artery to remodel outward, encroachment on the arterial lumen begins. During the chronic asymptomatic or stable phase of lesion evolution, growth probably occurs discontinuously, with periods of relative quiescence punctuated by episodes of rapid progression (see Fig. 24.11). Human angiographic studies support this discontinuous growth of coronary artery stenoses. Eventually, the stenoses may progress to a degree that impedes blood flow through the artery. Lesions that produce stenoses of greater than 60% can cause flow limitations under conditions of increased demand. This type of athero-occlusive disease commonly produces chronic stable angina pectoris or intermittent claudication on increased demand. Thus, the symptomatic phase of atherosclerosis usually begins many decades after lesion initiation.

In many cases of MI, however, no history of previous stable angina precedes the acute event. Acute coronary syndromes may result from thrombi that form as a consequence of disruption of plaques that do not produce a critical stenosis.[46] These findings do not imply that small atheromas cause most MIs. Indeed, culprit lesions of acute MI may be sizable but may not produce a critical luminal narrowing because of compensatory enlargement. Critical stenoses do cause MIs, however, and high-grade stenoses more likely cause acute MI than do nonocclusive lesions. Because the noncritical stenoses by far outnumber the tight focal lesions in a given coronary tree, however, the lesser stenoses cause more MIs, even though high-grade stenoses have a greater individual likelihood of causing infarction.

Thrombosis and Atheroma Complication

Several major modes of plaque disruption provoke most coronary thrombi.[46] The first mechanism, accounting for about two thirds of acute MIs, involves a fracture of the plaque's fibrous cap (Fig. 24.13, *left*). Another mode involves a superficial erosion of the intima (Figs. 24.13, *right*, and 24.14), accounting for a quarter to a third of acute MIs.

Plaque Rupture and Thrombosis

The rupture of the plaque's fibrous cap probably reflects an imbalance between the forces that impinge on the cap and the mechanical strength of the cap. Interstitial forms of collagen provide most of

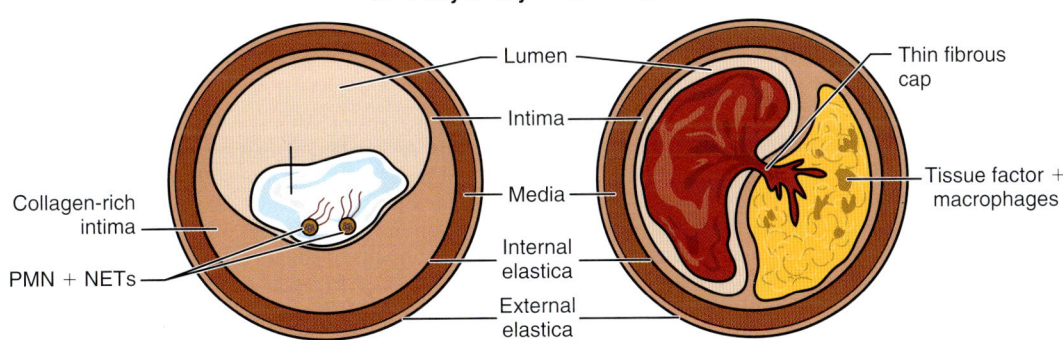

FIGURE 24.13 Distinct mechanisms may cause coronary thrombosis resulting from superficial erosion versus fibrous cap rupture. **Left,** Thrombosis caused by erosion, associated with a sessile, "white" thrombus superimposed on a lesion with abundant extracellular matrix and limited expansive remodeling. Endothelial cell desquamation or death can uncover collagen within the plaque that can trigger such platelet-rich thrombi. Polymorphonuclear leukocytes (PMN) that arrive on the scene can then contribute to a second wave of amplification and propagation of thrombosis resulting from their elaboration of neutrophil extracellular traps (NETs). Erosion may also more frequently cause non–ST-segment elevation myocardial infarction (non-STEMI) than STEMI. **Right,** Thrombosis resulting from rupture, usually associated with lesions with a thin fibrous cap. Such thrombi have more of the character of a "red" fibrin-rich clot. Tissue factor produced by the numerous macrophages in ruptured plaques promote thrombosis. The lesions that rupture and cause thrombi may more often have undergone outward remodeling and are more likely to cause STEMI than non-STEMI.

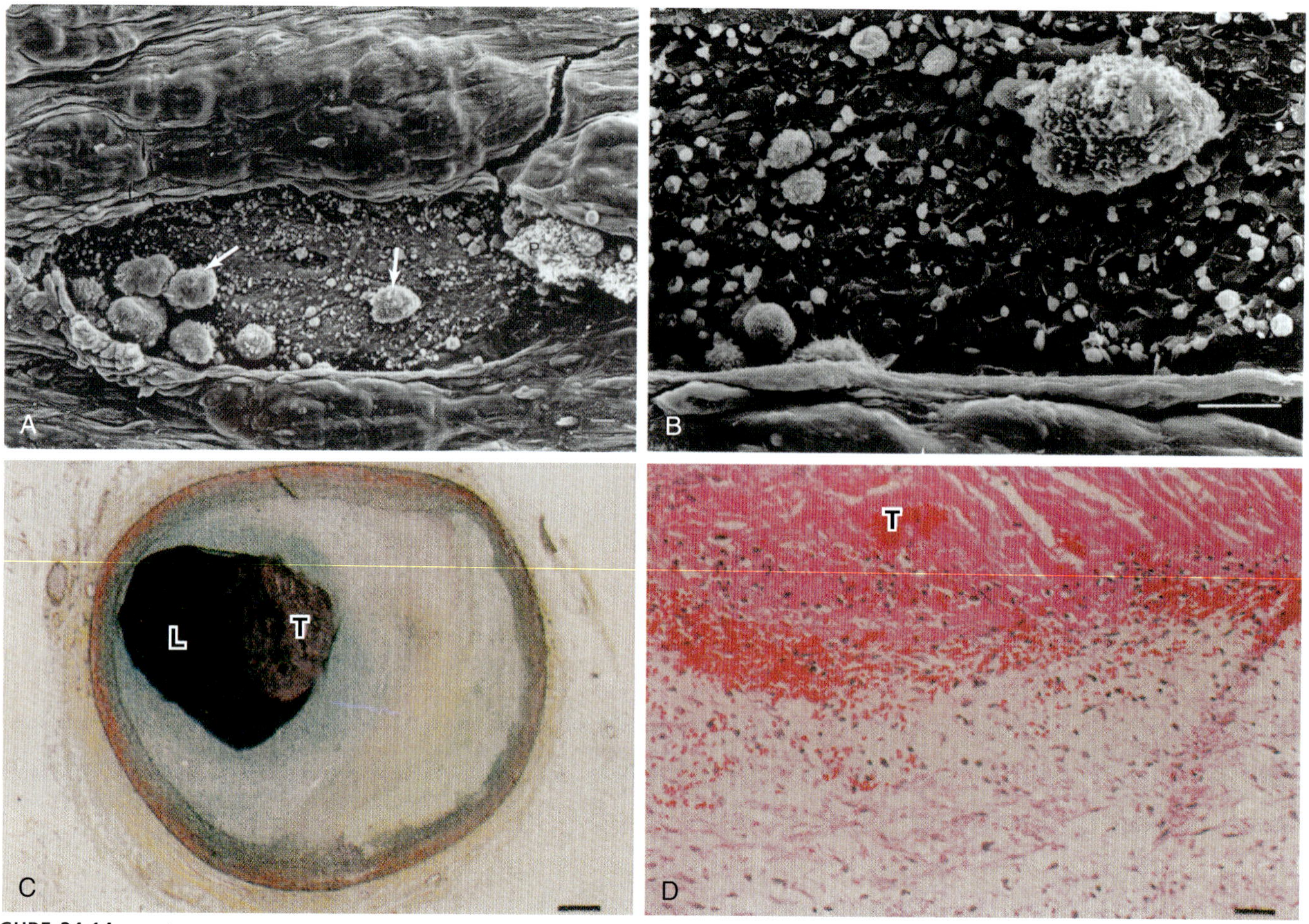

FIGURE 24.14 Superficial erosion of experimental atherosclerotic lesions on scanning electron microscopy. Advanced atherosclerotic plaques can promote thrombosis by superficial erosion of the endothelial layer, exposing the blood and platelets to the subendothelial basement membrane containing collagen, which promotes platelet activation and thrombosis. **A,** Low-power view shows a rent in endothelium. Leukocytes (*arrows*) have adhered to the subendothelium, which is beginning to be covered with a carpet of platelets. **B,** High-power view is a field selected from the center of **A** that shows the leukocytes and platelets adherent to the subendothelium. **C,** Low-power histologic section through a coronary artery, thrombosed as a result of superficial erosion. **D,** High-power histologic section through a coronary artery, also thrombosed as a result of superficial erosion. *L,* Lumen; *T,* thrombus. (**A** and **B** from Faggiotto A, Ross R, Harker L. Studies of hypercholesterolemia in the nonhuman primate. I. Changes that lead to fatty streak formation. *Arteriosclerosis* 1984;4:323-340. **C** and **D** from Farb A, Burke AP, Tang AL, et al. Coronary plaque erosion without rupture into a lipid core: a frequent cause of coronary thrombosis in sudden coronary death. *Circulation.* 1996;93:1354.)

the biomechanical resistance to disruption of the fibrous cap. Thus, the metabolism of collagen probably participates in regulating the propensity of a plaque to rupture (Fig. 24.15). Factors that decrease collagen synthesis by SMCs can impair their ability to repair and to maintain the plaque's fibrous cap. For example, the T cell–derived cytokine IFN-γ potently inhibits SMC collagen synthesis. On the other hand, as already noted, certain mediators released from platelet granules during activation (e.g., TGF-β, PDGF) can increase SMC collagen synthesis, tending to reinforce the plaque's fibrous structure.

In addition to reduced de novo collagen synthesis by SMCs, increased catabolism of the ECM macromolecules that comprise the fibrous cap also can contribute to weakening of this structure, rendering it susceptible to rupture and thus thrombosis. The same matrix-degrading enzymes thought to contribute to smooth muscle migration and arterial remodeling also may contribute to weakening of the fibrous cap (see Fig. 24.15).[46,47] Macrophages in advanced human atheroma overexpress MMPs and elastolytic cathepsins, which can break down the collagen and elastin of the arterial ECM. Therefore, the strength of the plaque's fibrous cap undergoes dynamic regulation, linking the inflammatory response in the intima with the molecular determinants of plaque stability and thus thrombotic complications of atheroma. Thin fibrous caps associate with plaque rupture, probably resulting from reduced collagen synthesis and increased degradation.

A relative lack of SMCs also characterizes plaques that have caused fatal MIs. As explained earlier, inflammatory mediators, both soluble and associated with the surface of T lymphocytes, can provoke programmed death of SMCs. Dropout of SMCs from regions of local inflammation within plaques probably contributes to the relative lack of SMCs at points of plaque rupture. Because these cells produce new collagen needed to repair and to maintain the matrix of the fibrous cap, the lack of SMCs may contribute to weakening of the fibrous cap and the propensity of that plaque to rupture.[46,47]

Plaques that have fatally ruptured exhibit another microanatomic feature: prominent accumulation of macrophages with a large lipid pool. From a strictly biomechanical viewpoint, a large lipid pool can serve to concentrate biomechanical forces on the shoulder regions of plaques, where they frequently fracture. From a metabolic standpoint, the activated macrophage characteristic of the plaque's core region produces the cytokines and the matrix-degrading enzymes thought to regulate aspects of matrix catabolism and SMC apoptosis in turn. Apoptotic macrophages and SMCs can generate particulate tissue factor, a potential instigator of microvascular thrombosis after spontaneous or iatrogenic plaque disruption. The success of lipid-lowering therapy in reducing the incidence of acute MI or unstable angina in patients at risk may result from a reduced accumulation of lipid and a decrease in inflammation and plaque thrombogenicity. Animal studies and accumulated data from monitoring peripheral markers of inflammation in humans support this concept.[46–48]

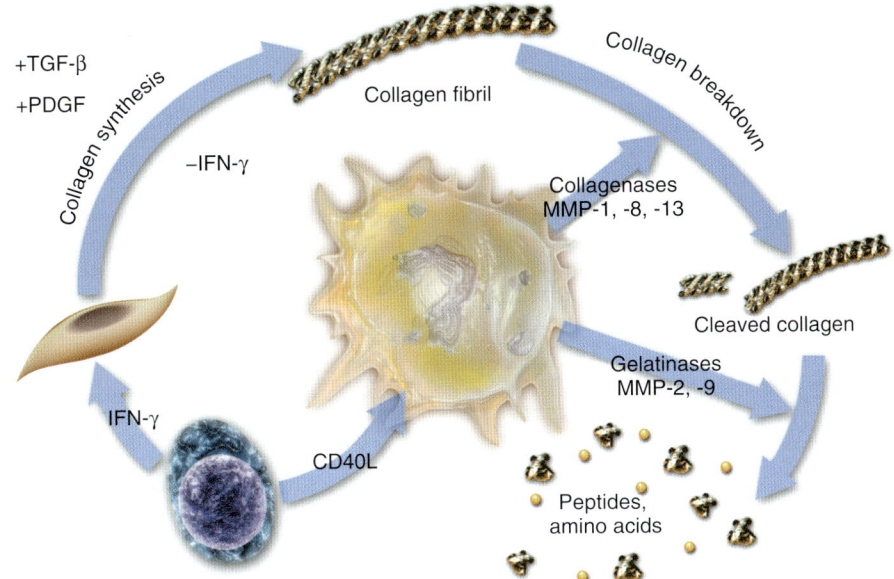

FIGURE 24.15 Inflammation regulates metabolism of fibrillar collagen, which may influence atherosclerotic plaque disruption. The T lymphocyte releases proinflammatory cytokines such as interferon (IFN)-γ (*lower left*) that inhibit smooth muscle cells from producing the new collagen required to lay down the collagenous matrix of the plaque's fibrous cap, which protects the plaque from rupture. The T cell–derived cytokine CD40L stimulates mononuclear phagocytes (*center*) to elaborate interstitial collagenases including matrix metalloproteinase (MMP)-1, MMP-8, and MMP-13, which catalyze the initial proteolytic cleavage of the intact collagen fibril. The cleaved collagen can then undergo additional degradation by gelatinases such as MMP-9. In this way, inflammation can threaten the stability of atherosclerotic plaques and increase their tendency to rupture, thereby causing thromboses, which trigger most acute coronary syndromes. *PDGF*, Platelet-derived growth factor; *TGF*, transforming growth factor. (From Libby P. The molecular mechanisms of the thrombotic complications of atherosclerosis. *J Intern Med*. 2008;263:517.)

Thrombosis Caused by Superficial Erosion of Plaques

The underlying molecular and cellular mechanisms of superficial erosion have received much less attention than those involved in plaque rupture (Fig. 24.13, *left*).[49–51] In experimental atherosclerosis in the nonhuman primate, areas of endothelial loss and platelet deposition occur in more advanced plaques (see Fig. 24.14). Apoptosis of ECs could contribute to desquamation of ECs in areas of superficial erosion. Likewise, MMPs, such as certain gelatinases specialized in degrading the nonfibrillar collagen found in the basement membrane (e.g., collagen type IV), also may sever the tetherings of the EC to the subjacent basal lamina and promote their desquamation. Vasospasm of atherosclerotic coronary arteries in rabbits can promote endothelial damage, thrombosis, and MI.[46]

The lesions that provoke superficial erosion appear quite distinct from those that cause plaque rupture (see Fig. 24.13). Lesions associated with superficial erosion contain abundant proteoglycan and glycosaminoglycan, as opposed to the collagen-depleted fibrous cap characteristic of ruptured plaques. Eroded lesions have few macrophages, whereas these chronic inflammatory cells abound in ruptured plaques. In contrast, plaques complicated by superficial erosion have thrombi that contain many granulocytes, acute inflammatory cells. Activated granulocytes release many pro-oxidant and proinflammatory mediators, and when they die, they extrude their nuclear DNA to form neutrophil extracellular traps (NETs). These strands of DNA bind many of the released neutrophil products and provide a "solid-state reactor" that can aggravate the local pro-oxidant, proinflammatory, and prothrombotic environment (Fig. 24.16).[52–54]

Recent work has implicated the innate immune receptor Toll-like receptor 2 (TLR2) in signaling endothelial alterations that may predispose to superficial erosion. ECs subjected to disturbed flow in vitro or those overlying atheroma-prone regions of arteries in hyperlipidemic mice overexpress TLR2. Hyaluronic acid in eroded-type plaques may serve as an endogenous ligand for TLR2, causing chronic smoldering endothelial activation that predisposes to sloughing of these cells. Experimentally, neutrophil depletion preserves the endothelial barrier function and limits desquamation of intimal ECs in regions of disturbed flow in arteries with fibrous intimal hyperplasia, reminiscent of plaques that undergo erosion in humans.[55,56] Macrophage accumulation in eroded plaques link to worsened outcomes, indicating participation of these chronic innate immune cells in this process.[57] Adaptive immunity may also contribute to erosion. Coronary artery sampling from patients with ACS due to erosion shows a predominance of CD8+ T cells, capable of hastening EC death and hence desquamation.[58]

Thrombosis and Healing in Progression of Atheroma

Most plaque disruptions do not give rise to clinically apparent coronary events. Careful pathoanatomic examination of hearts obtained from patients who have succumbed to noncardiac death has shown a surprisingly high incidence of focal plaque disruptions with limited mural thrombi. Moreover, hearts fixed immediately after explantation from persons with severe but chronic stable coronary atherosclerosis who had undergone transplantation for ischemic cardiomyopathy show similar evidence for ongoing but asymptomatic plaque disruption. Experimentally, in atherosclerotic nonhuman primates, mural platelet thrombi can complicate plaque erosions without causing arterial occlusion. Therefore, repetitive cycles of plaque disruption, thrombosis in situ, and healing probably contribute to lesion evolution and plaque growth.[59] Such episodes of thrombosis and healing constitute one type of crisis in the history of a plaque that may cause a burst of SMC proliferation, migration, and matrix synthesis (see Fig. 24.11). TGF-β and PDGF released from platelet granules may promote healing at the site of thrombosis by stimulating migration and collagen synthesis by SMCs, as noted earlier. Thrombin, generated at sites of mural thrombosis, potently stimulates SMC proliferation. The "burned-out" fibrous and calcific atheroma may represent a late stage of a plaque that previously was lipid rich with characteristics associated with rupture, but that has become fibrous and hypocellular because of a wound-healing response mediated by the products of thrombosis and calcification seeded by cell death.[59–61]

Diffuse and Systemic Nature of Plaque Susceptibility to Rupture and Inflammation in Atherogenesis

Studies at autopsy of atherosclerotic plaques that caused fatal thrombosis brought out the notion of "vulnerable" or "high-risk" plaque. This observation stimulated many investigators to seek ways of identifying and treating such high-risk atherosclerotic lesions. Current evidence, however, suggests that more than one such high-risk plaque often resides in a given coronary tree, and that plaques with these characteristics actually rupture rather infrequently.[62] Moreover, the inflammation thought to characterize the so-called vulnerable plaque is widespread. The application of various imaging modalities generally has found an association of lesions that cause acute manifestations ("culprit lesions") with positive remodeling or compensatory enlargement of arteries, radiolucency, and spotty calcification.

Multiple studies have shown that systemic markers of inflammation, such as C-reactive protein, increase in patients at risk for ACS (see Chapter 25). Inflammation often precedes ACS, as revealed by profiling

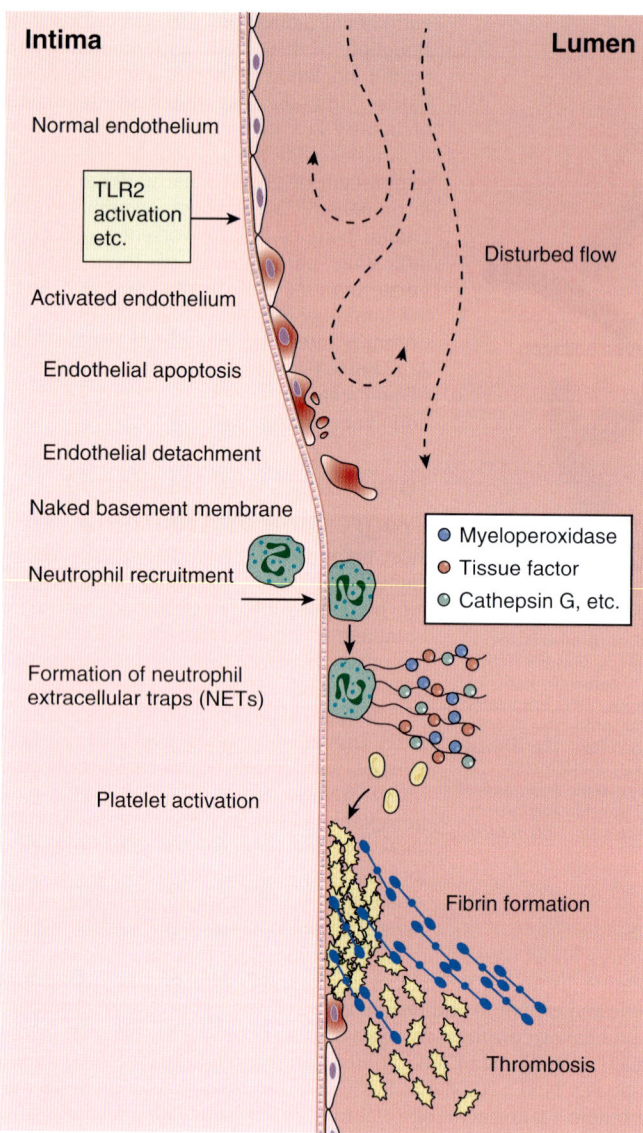

FIGURE 24.16 Pathways implicated in arterial thrombosis caused by superficial erosion. Stimuli such as disturbed flow or engagement of innate immune receptors such as Toll-like receptor-2 (TLR2) can activate the endothelial cells that line the arterial intima. These cells can undergo cell death, e.g., by apoptosis, depicted by the cell with the interrupted membrane and pyknotic nucleus. Injured or dying endothelial cells can desquamate, uncovering the basement membrane. Neutrophils attracted by chemokines produced by activated endothelial cells can congregate on the denuded intima and can in turn degranulate and die, releasing neutrophil extracellular traps (NETs). These strands of extruded DNA can bind the contents of the neutrophil granules and other proteins, e.g., myeloperoxidase or tissue factor. The NETs can constitute a solid-state reactor that generates oxidants such as hypochlorous acid and stimulates coagulation locally. Platelets interacting with the basement membrane can activate, release their granular contents, including chemokines that can recruit further leukocytes, and form the nidus of a white thrombus. (From Crea F, Libby P. Acute coronary syndromes. *Circulation.* 2017;136:1155–1166.)

of the platelet transcriptome, providing a window on gene transcription many days before the acute event.[46] Thus a combination of imaging studies and investigations using inflammatory markers supports the diffuse and systemic nature of instability of atheromas in individuals with or at risk for ACS. This recognition has important therapeutic implications. In addition to appropriately deployed local revascularization strategies, affected patients also should receive systemic therapy aimed at stabilizing the usually multiple high-risk lesions that may cause recurrent events (see Chapters 25, 38–40).

Thrombosis depends not only on the "solid state" of the plaque that may rupture or erode to trigger thrombosis, but also on the "fluid phase" of blood that determines the consequences of a given plaque disruption (Fig. 24.17).[63] The amount of tissue factor in the lipid core of a plaque (the solid state) can control the degree of clot formation that will ensue after disruption. The level of fibrinogen in the fluid phase of blood can influence whether a plaque disruption will cause an occlusive thrombus that can precipitate an acute ST-segment elevation myocardial infarction (STEMI) or yield merely a small asymptomatic mural thrombus. Likewise, elevated levels of inhibitors of fibrinolysis, such as plasminogen activator inhibitor-1 (PAI-1), will impede the ability of endogenous thrombolytic enzymes to limit thrombus growth or persistence. Inflammation regulates both the fluid-phase and the solid-state factors delineated earlier, including tissue factor, fibrinogen, and PAI-1. These considerations help to explain the links between inflammation and thrombotic complications of atherosclerosis that have emerged from laboratory and clinical investigations.

SPECIAL CASES OF ARTERIOSCLEROSIS

Restenosis After Arterial Intervention

The problems of restenosis and in-stent stenosis after percutaneous arterial intervention are special cases of arterial hyperplastic disease (see Chapter 41). Work on the pathophysiology of restenosis after angioplasty initially focused on smooth muscle proliferation. Much of the thinking regarding the pathobiology of restenosis or in-stent stenosis depended on the extension to the human situation of the results of withdrawal of an overinflated balloon or overexpanded stents in previously normal animal arteries. Studies on balloon-injured rat carotid arteries led to a precise understanding of the kinetics of intimal thickening after this type of injury, but the attempts to transfer this information to human restenosis ended with considerable frustration. This disparity between experimental injury of animal arteries and human restenosis should not be surprising. The substrate of the animal studies was usually a normal artery rather than an atherosclerotic one, with all the attendant cellular and molecular differences.[64] These animal studies, however, did reveal evidence for sustained inflammation in injured arteries.

The widespread use of stents refocused the restenosis problem. The process of in-stent stenosis, in contrast with restenosis after balloon angioplasty, depends primarily on intimal thickening as opposed to negative remodeling. The stent provides a firm scaffold that prevents constriction from the adventitia. The use of drug-eluting stents (DES) that release agents with anti-inflammatory and antiproliferative properties has greatly reduced in-stent stenosis, and newer-generation DES appear to have a limited potential for augmenting late stent thrombosis associated with earlier DES. The risk of late thrombosis after radiation brachytherapy or with stents that contain antiproliferative agents may relate to impaired endothelial healing, with attendant loss of the anticoagulant and profibrinolytic properties of the normal intimal lining (see Fig. 24.2).

Accelerated Arteriosclerosis After Transplantation

Since the advent of effective immunosuppressive therapy including calcineurin inhibitors, the major limitation to long-term survival of cardiac allografts is the development of an accelerated form of arterial hyperplastic disease (see Chapter 60).[65] The term *arteriosclerosis* (hardening of the arteries) rather than atherosclerosis (gruel-hardening) is preferable in describing this process because of the inconstant association with lipids (the "gruel" in atherosclerosis). This form of arterial disease often presents a diagnostic challenge. The patient may not experience typical anginal symptoms because of post-transplantation cardiac denervation. In addition, graft coronary disease is concentric and diffuse, not only affecting the proximal epicardial coronary vessels but also penetrating smaller intramyocardial branches (Fig. 24.18). For this reason, the angiogram, well suited to visualize focal and eccentric stenoses, consistently underestimates the degree of transplantation arteriosclerosis. Computed tomographic angiography is a newer avenue to diagnose this condition but still has limitations, although it avoids invasive contrast arteriography.[66,67]

In most centers, most patients undergoing transplantation have atherosclerotic disease and ischemic cardiomyopathy, but a sizable

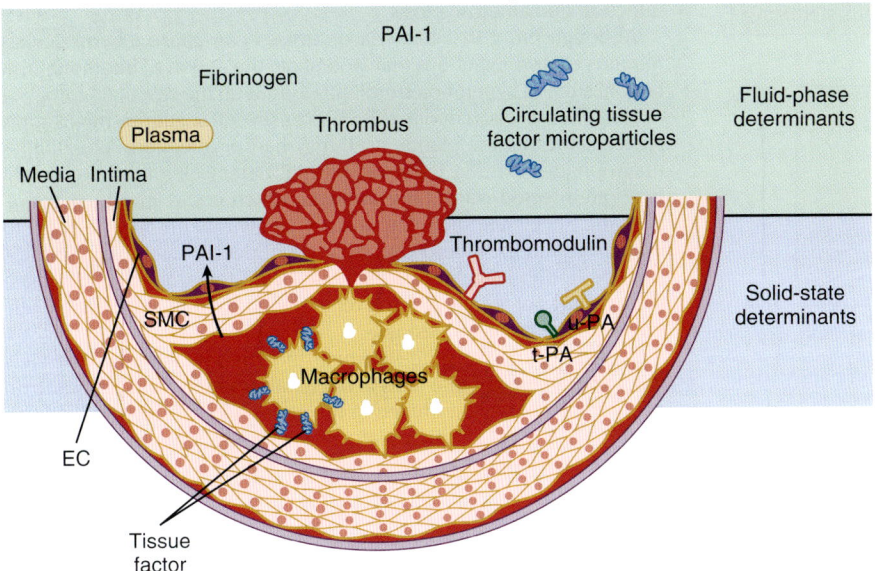

FIGURE 24.17 A two-state concept of atherothrombosis. The high-risk atheroma has a thin fibrous cap overlying a large lipid core that contains tissue factor–bearing macrophages. When the fibrous cap fractures, coagulation proteins in the fluid phase of blood gain access to tissue factor–associated macrophages and tissue factor–bearing microparticles derived from apoptotic cells in the solid state of the plaque. These events trigger thrombus formation on the ruptured plaque. The clinical consequences depend on the amount of tissue factor and apoptosis in the plaque's core and on the levels of fibrinogen and plasminogen activator inhibitor (PAI)-1 in the fluid phase of blood. The interaction of the fluid phase with the solid state determines whether a given plaque disruption provokes a partial or transient coronary artery occlusion (that can be clinically silent or less often cause an episode of unstable angina) or a devastating persistent and occlusive thrombus that can precipitate an acute myocardial infarction. Inflammation regulates the thrombotic/fibrinolytic balance in both the solid state and the fluid phase, because PAI-1 and fibrinogen both are acute-phase reactants and because the inflammatory mediator CD40 ligand (CD154) induces tissue factor expression. *EC*, Endothelial cell; *SMC*, smooth muscle cell; *t-PA*, tissue plasminogen activator; *u-PA*, urokinase-type plasminogen activator. (From Libby P, Theroux P. Pathophysiology of coronary artery disease. *Circulation.* 2005;111:3481.)

Considerable evidence from both human and experimental studies currently supports this viewpoint.[69] ECs in the transplanted coronary arteries express histocompatibility antigens that can engender an allogeneic immune response from host T cells. The activated T cells can secrete cytokines (e.g., IFN-γ) that can augment histocompatibility gene expression, recruit leukocytes by induction of adhesion molecules, and activate macrophages to produce SMC chemoattractants and growth factors. Interruption of IFN-γ signaling can prevent experimental graft coronary disease in mice.

Therefore, graft arteriosclerosis represents an extreme case of immunologically driven arterial hyperplasia (Fig. 24.19) that can occur in the absence of other risk factors. At the other extreme, patients with homozygous familial hypercholesterolemia can develop fatal atherosclerosis in the first decade of life solely from an elevation in LDL. Atherosclerosis in most patients falls somewhere between these two extremes. Analysis of usual atherosclerotic lesions shows evidence for a chronic immune response and lipid accumulation. The study of the extreme cases, such as transplantation arteriopathy and familial hypercholesterolemia, provided insight into elements of the pathophysiology that contribute to the multifactorial form of atherosclerosis that affects most patients.

Aneurysmal Disease

Atherosclerosis also produces aneurysmal disease (see Chapter 42). Why is a single disease process manifested in directionally opposite ways, for example, most often producing stenoses in the coronary arteries but then causing ectasia of the abdominal aorta? In particular, aneurysmal disease characteristically affects the infrarenal abdominal aorta. This region is highly prone to the development of atherosclerosis. Data from the Pathobiological Determinants of Atherosclerosis in Youth (PDAY) study show that the dorsal surface of the infrarenal abdominal aorta has a particular predilection for the development of fatty streaks and raised lesions in Americans younger than 35 years who died of noncardiac reasons.[70] Because of the absence of vasa vasorum, the relative lack of blood supply to the tunica media in this portion of the abdominal aorta might explain the regional susceptibility of this part of the arterial tree to aneurysm formation. In addition, the lumbar lordosis of the biped human may alter the hydrodynamics of blood flow in the distal aorta, causing flow disturbances that may promote lesion formation.

Histologic examination shows considerable distinction between occlusive atherosclerotic disease and aneurysmal disease. In typical coronary artery atherosclerosis, expansion of the intimal lesion produces stenotic lesions. The tunica media underlying the expanded intima often is thinned, but its general structure remains relatively well preserved. By contrast, transmural destruction of the arterial architecture occurs in aneurysmal disease. In particular, the usually well-defined laminar structure of the normal tunica media disappears with obliteration of the elastic laminae. The tunica media of advanced aortic aneurysms have few SMCs, which are often prominent in typical stenotic lesions.

Study of the pathophysiology that underlies these anatomic-pathologic findings has proved frustrating. Experimental aneurysm formation in animals has uncertain relevance to the clinical disease.[64] The human specimens obtainable for analysis generally represent the late stages of this disease. Nonetheless, recent work has identified several mechanisms that may underlie the peculiar pathology of aneurysmal disease. Widespread destruction of the elastic laminae suggests a degradation of elastin, collagen, and other constituents by

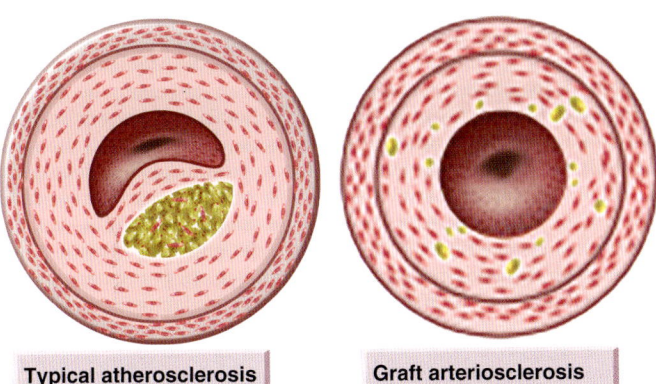

FIGURE 24.18 Comparison of typical and transplantation arteriosclerosis. **Left,** Typical atherosclerosis characteristically forms an eccentric lesion with a lipid core and fibrous cap. **Right,** By contrast, the lesion of transplantation-associated accelerated arteriosclerosis characteristically exhibits a concentric intimal expansion without a clear, central lipid core.

minority undergo heart transplantation for idiopathic dilated cardiomyopathy and may have few (if any) risk factors for atherosclerosis. Even in the absence of traditional risk factors, this latter patient group can develop arteriosclerosis.

The selective involvement of the engrafted vessels, with sparing of the host's native arteries, suggests that accelerated arteriopathy does not merely result from immunosuppressive therapy or other systemic factors in the transplantation recipient. Rather, these observations suggest that the immunologic differences between the host and recipient vessels might contribute to the pathogenesis of this disease.[68]

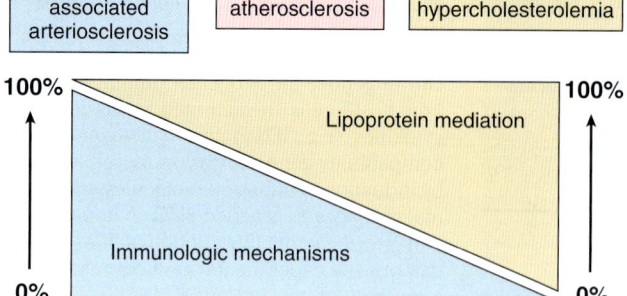

FIGURE 24.19 Multifactorial view of pathogenesis of atherosclerosis, depicting relative contributions of main pathogenic mechanisms in two extreme cases of atherosclerosis. In transplantation-associated disease (*left*), accelerated arteriosclerosis can occur in the transplanted heart in the absence of traditional coronary risk factors. This disease probably represents primarily immune-mediated arterial intimal disease. At the other extreme (*right*), familial hypercholesterolemia, the patient may succumb to rampant atherosclerosis in the first decade of life solely because of an elevated low-density lipoprotein (LDL) level caused by a mutation in the LDL receptor (homozygous familial hypercholesterolemia). Between these two extremes lie most cases of atherosclerosis, probably involving various mixtures of immune and inflammatory or lipoprotein-mediated disease. One can further consider that this diagram extends to a third dimension that would involve other candidate risk factors, such as hypertension lipoprotein(a), infection, and tobacco abuse.

the arterial ECM. Many studies have documented overexpression of matrix-degrading proteinases, including MMPs, in human aortic aneurysm specimens. Clinical trials have tested the hypothesis that MMP inhibitors can reduce the expansion of aneurysms. In atherosclerotic mice, angiotensin II potentiates aneurysm formation. Mutations that alter TGF-β signaling, among a number of other genetic determinants, can predispose to aneurysm formation.[71]

Thus, heightened elastolysis may explain the breakdown of the usually ordered structure of the tunica media in this disease.[72,73] A slant toward Th2 cell populations in aneurysmal versus occlusive disease may contribute to the overexpression of certain elastolytic enzymes. In addition, aortic aneurysms show evidence for considerable inflammation, particularly in the adventitia. The lymphocytes that characteristically abound on the adventitial side of aneurysmal tissue suggest that apoptosis of SMCs triggered by inflammatory mediators (e.g., soluble cytokines, Fas ligand) elaborated by these inflammatory cells may contribute to SMC destruction and promote aneurysm formation. Although ECM degradation and SMC death also occur in sites where atherosclerosis causes stenosis, these processes appear to predominate in regions of aneurysm formation and to affect the tunica media much more extensively, for reasons that remain obscure.

Infection, the Microbiome, and Atherosclerosis

Interest persists in the proposition that infections may cause atherosclerosis.[74] A considerable body of seroepidemiologic evidence supported a role for certain bacteria, notably *Chlamydia pneumoniae*, and certain viruses, notably cytomegalovirus (CMV), in the etiology of atherosclerosis. These studies spurred a number of in vivo and in vitro experiments that have lent various degrees of support to this concept. Indeed, multiple clinical trials have not shown benefit of antibiotic therapy in secondary prevention of atherosclerotic events.[75]

Several caveats apply in the evaluation of the seroepidemiologic evidence. First, confounding factors should be carefully considered. For example, smokers may have a higher incidence of bronchitis caused by *C. pneumoniae*. Therefore, evidence for infection with *C. pneumoniae* may merely serve as a marker for tobacco use, a known risk factor for atherosclerotic events. In addition, a strong bias favors the publication of positive rather than negative studies. Thus, meta-analyses of seroepidemiologic studies may be slanted toward the positive merely because of underreporting of negative studies. Also, atherosclerosis is a common and virtually ubiquitous disease in developed countries. Many adults have serologic evidence of previous infections with members of the Herpesviridae (e.g., CMV) and respiratory pathogens (e.g., *C. pneumoniae*). Sorting out coincidence from causality is difficult when a majority of the population studied exhibit evidence of both infection and atherosclerosis.

Although proof that bacteria or viruses can cause atherosclerosis remains elusive, infections may potentiate the action of traditional risk factors, such as hypercholesterolemia. Based on the vascular biology of atherosclerosis discussed in this chapter, several scenarios might apply. First, cells within the plaque itself may harbor infection. For example, macrophages existing in an established atherosclerotic lesion might become infected with *C. pneumoniae*, which could spur their activation and accelerate the inflammatory pathways currently believed to operate within the atherosclerotic intima. Specific microbial products, such as lipopolysaccharides, heat shock proteins, or other virulence factors, may act locally at the level of the artery wall to potentiate atherosclerosis in infected lesions.

Increased focus on the intestinal microbiome supports the view that exposure of vascular cells to bacterial products such as endotoxin applies in vivo. A slight breach in the integrity of the intestinal epithelium, with release of microbial danger signals, could have a direct effect on vascular cells or could alter systemic risk factors by activating inflammation in visceral adipose tissues, contributing to insulin resistance and other features of the "metabolic syndrome" cluster.[76] Moreover, metabolites produced by gut microflora from dietary constituents may augment atherogenesis.[77]

Extravascular infection also may potentially influence the development of atheromatous lesions and cause complications. For example, circulating endotoxin or cytokines produced in response to a remote infection can act locally at the level of the artery wall to promote the activation of vascular cells and of leukocytes in preexisting lesions, producing an "echo" at the level of the artery wall of a remote infection.[78] The acute-phase response to an infection in a nonvascular site also may affect the incidence of thrombotic complications of atherosclerosis by increasing fibrinogen or PAI or by otherwise altering the balance between coagulation and fibrinolysis. Such disturbance in the prevailing prothrombotic, fibrinolytic balance may critically influence whether a given plaque disruption will produce a clinically inapparent, transient or nonocclusive thrombus or sustained and occlusive thrombus that could cause an acute coronary event (see Fig. 24.17).

Acute infections also can produce hemodynamic alterations that could trigger coronary events. For example, the tachycardia and increased metabolic demands of fever can augment the oxygen requirements of the heart, precipitating ischemia in an otherwise compensated individual.[74] Such mechanisms may contribute to the myocardial injury commonly encountered in hospitalized patients with COVID-19,[79,80] and explain the association of cardiovascular events in individuals with influenza or other acute infections.[81,82] These various scenarios illustrate how infectious processes, either local in the atheroma or extravascular, may aggravate atherogenesis, particularly in preexisting lesions or in concert with traditional risk factors.

REFERENCES

The Structure of Arteries and Their Cellular Components

1. Allam AH, Mandour Ali MA, Wann LS, et al. Atherosclerosis in ancient and modern Egyptians: the Horus study. *Glob Heart*. 2014;9:197–202.
2. Hajar R. Coronary heart disease: from mummies to 21(st) century. *Heart Views*. 2017;18:68–74.
3. Herrington W, Lacey B, Sherliker P, et al. Epidemiology of atherosclerosis and the potential to reduce the global burden of atherothrombotic disease. *Circ Res*. 2016;118:535–546.
4. Libby P, Hansson GK. From focal lipid storage to systemic inflammation. *J Am Coll Cardiol*. 2019;74:1594–1607.
5. Kalluri AS, Vellarikkal SK, Edelman ER, et al. Single-cell analysis of the normal mouse aorta reveals functionally distinct endothelial cell populations. *Circulation*. 2019;140:147–163.
6. Vanlandewijck M, He L, Mäe MA, et al. A molecular atlas of cell types and zonation in the brain vasculature. *Nature*. 2018;554:475–480.
7. Fernandez DM, Rahman AH, Fernandez NF, et al. Single-cell immune landscape of human atherosclerotic plaques. *Nat Med*. 2019.
8. Williams JW, Winkels H, Durant CP, et al. Single cell RNA sequencing in atherosclerosis research. *Circ Res*. 2020;126:1112–1126.
9. Bennett MR, Sinha S, Owens GK. Vascular smooth muscle cells in atherosclerosis. *Circ Res*. 2016;118:692–702.
10. Dobnikar L, Taylor AL, Chappell J, et al. Disease-relevant transcriptional signatures identified in individual smooth muscle cells from healthy mouse vessels. *Nature Commun*. 2018;9:4567.
11. Schwartz S, Virmani R, Majesky M. An update on clonality: what smooth muscle cell type makes up the atherosclerotic plaque? *F1000Res*. 2018;7:1969.
12. Wang Y, Nanda V, Direnzo D, et al. Clonally expanding smooth muscle cells promote atherosclerosis by escaping efferocytosis and activating the complement cascade. *Proc Nat Acad Sci*. 2020;117:15818.
13. Nakashima Y, Chen Y-X, Kinukawa N, Sueishi K. Distributions of diffuse intimal thickening in human arteries: preferential expression in atherosclerosis-prone arteries from an early age. *Virchows Arch*. 2002;441:279–288.

14. Kovanen PT, Bot I. Mast cells in atherosclerotic cardiovascular disease – activators and actions. *Eur J Pharmacol.* 2017;816:37–46.
15. Akhavanpoor M, Gleissner CA, Akhavanpoor H, et al. Adventitial tertiary lymphoid organ classification in human atherosclerosis. *Cardiovasc Pathol.* 2018;32:8–14.
16. Libby P, Buring JE, Badimon L, et al. Atherosclerosis. *Nat Rev Dis Primers.* 2019;5.
17. Gimbrone MA, García-Cardeña G. Endothelial cell dysfunction and the pathobiology of atherosclerosis. *Circ Res.* 2016;118:620–636.
18. Cybulsky MI, Cheong C, Robbins CS. Macrophages and dendritic cells: partners in atherogenesis. *Cir Res.* 2016;118:637–652.
19. Zernecke A, Winkels H, Cochain C, et al. Meta-analysis of leukocyte diversity in atherosclerotic mouse aortas. *Circ Res.* 2020;127:402–426.
20. Thomas GD, Hamers AAJ, Nakao C, et al. Human blood monocyte subsets. *Arterioscler Thromb Vasc Biol.* 2017;37:1548–1558.
21. Hamers Anouk AJ, Dinh Huy Q, Thomas Graham D, et al. Human monocyte heterogeneity as revealed by high-dimensional mass cytometry. *Arterioscler Thromb Vasc Biol.* 2019;39:25–36.
22. Fayad ZA, Swirski FK, Calcagno C, et al. Monocyte and macrophage dynamics in the cardiovascular system: JACC macrophage in CVD series (Part 3). *J Am Coll Cardiol.* 2018;72:2198–2212.
23. Noels H, Weber C, Koenen RR. Chemokines as therapeutic targets in cardiovascular disease. *Arterioscler Thromb Vasc Biol.* 2019;39(4):583–592.
24. Schlegel M, Moore KJ. A heritable netrin-1 mutation increases atherogenic immune responses. *Atherosclerosis.* 2020;301:82–83.
25. Kraler. The internal mammary artery and its resilience to atherogenesis: the key to combat residual cardiovascular risk? *Nat Rev Cardiol.* 2020.
26. Baeyens N, Bandyopadhyay C, et al. Endothelial fluid shear stress sensing in vascular health and disease. *J Clin Invest.* 2016;126:821–828.
27. Bajraktari A, Bytyçi I, Henein MY. The relationship between coronary artery wall shear strain and plaque morphology: a systematic review and meta-analysis. *Diagnostics (Basel).* 2020 Feb 8;10(2):91.

Mechanisms and Mediators of Risk Factor Enhancement of Atherosclerosis

28. Goldstein JL, Brown MS. A century of cholesterol and coronaries: from plaques to genes to statins. *Cell.* 2015;161:161–172.
29. PrabhuDas MR, Baldwin CL, Bollyky PL, et al. A consensus definitive classification of scavenger receptors and their roles in health and disease. *J Immunol.* 2017;198:3775.
30. Ketelhuth DFJ, Hansson GK. Adaptive response of T and B cells in atherosclerosis. *Circ Res.* 2016;118:668–678.
31. Srikakulapu P, McNamara CA. B cells and atherosclerosis. *Am J Physiol Heart Circ Physiol.* 2017;312(5):H1060–H1067.
32. Zhao TX, Mallat Z. Targeting the immune system in atherosclerosis: JACC state-of-the-art review. *J Am Coll Cardiol.* 2019;73:1691–1706.
33. Sage AP, Tsiantoulas D, Binder CJ, Mallat Z. The role of B cells in atherosclerosis. *Nat Rev Cardiol.* 2018.
34. Ley K. Role of the adaptive immune system in atherosclerosis. *Biochem Soc Trans.* 2020.
35. Saigusa R, Winkels H, Ley K. T cell subsets and functions in atherosclerosis. *Nature Rev Cardiol.* 2020;17(7):387–401.
36. Fredman G, Tabas I. Boosting inflammation resolution in atherosclerosis: the next frontier for therapy. *Am J Pathol.* 2017;187:1211–1221.
37. Binder CJ, Papac-Milicevic N, Witztum JL. Innate sensing of oxidation-specific epitopes in health and disease. *Nat Rev Immunol.* 2016;16:485–497.
38. Que Y, Hung M-Y, Yeang C, et al. Oxidized phospholipids are proinflammatory and proatherogenic in hypercholesterolaemic mice. *Nature.* 2018;558:301–306.
39. Chyu K-Y, Dimayuga PC, Shah PK. Vaccine against arteriosclerosis: an update. *Ther Adv Vaccines.* 2017;5(2):39–47.
40. Nilsson J, Hansson Göran K. Vaccination strategies and immune modulation of atherosclerosis. *Circ Res.* 2020;126:1281–1296.
41. Wang Y, Dubland JA, Allahverdian S, et al. Smooth muscle cells contribute the majority of foam cells in ApoE (Apolipoprotein E)-deficient mouse atherosclerosis. *Arterioscl Thromb Vasc Biol.* 2019;39:876–887.
42. Allahverdian S, Alencar GF, Owens GK. Revealing the origins of foam cells in atherosclerotic lesions. *Arterioscler Thromb Vasc Biol.* 2019;39:836–838.
43. Rogers MA, Aikawa E. Cardiovascular calcification: artificial intelligence and big data accelerate mechanistic discovery. *Nat Rev Cardiol.* 2019;16:261–274.
44. Ruiz JL, Hutcheson JD, Aikawa E. Cardiovascular calcification: current controversies and novel concepts. *Cardiovasc Pathol.* 2015;24:207–212.
45. Goettsch C, Hutcheson JD, Aikawa M, et al. Sortilin mediates vascular calcification via its recruitment into extracellular vesicles. *J Clin Invest.* 2016;126:1323–1336.
46. Crea F, Libby P. Acute coronary syndromes. *Circulation.* 2017;136:1155–1166.
47. Libby P. Mechanisms of acute coronary syndromes and their implications for therapy. *N Engl J Med.* 2013;369:2004–2013.

Mechanisms of the Thrombotic Complications of Atherosclerosis

48. Libby P. How does lipid lowering prevent coronary events? New insights from human imaging trials. *Eur Heart J.* 2015;36:472–474.
49. Luscher TF. Substrates of acute coronary syndromes: new insights into plaque rupture and erosion. *Eur Heart J.* 2015;36:1347–1349.
50. Partida RA, Libby P, Crea F, Jang IK. Plaque erosion: a new in vivo diagnosis and a potential major shift in the management of patients with acute coronary syndromes. *Eur Heart J.* 2018;39:2070–2076.
51. Libby P, Pasterkamp G, Crea F, Jang IK. Reassessing the mechanisms of acute coronary syndromes. *Circ Res.* 2019;124:150–160.
52. Martinod K, Wagner DD. Thrombosis: tangled up in NETs. *Blood.* 2014;123:2768–2776.
53. Quillard T, Franck G, Mawson T, et al. Mechanisms of erosion of atherosclerotic plaques. *Curr Opin Lipidol.* 2017.
54. Döring Y, Libby P, Soehnlein O. Neutrophil extracellular traps participate in cardiovascular diseases. *Circ Res.* 2020;126:1228–1241.
55. Quillard T, Araujo HA, Franck G, et al. TLR2 and neutrophils potentiate endothelial stress, apoptosis and detachment: implications for superficial erosion. *Eur Heart J.* 2015;36:1394–1404.
56. Franck G, Mawson T, Sausen G, et al. Flow perturbation mediates neutrophil recruitment and potentiates endothelial injury via TLR2 in mice - implications for superficial erosion. *Circ Res.* 2017;121:31–42.
57. Montone RA, Vetrugno V, Camilli M, et al. Macrophage infiltrates in coronary plaque erosion and cardiovascular outcome in patients with acute coronary syndrome. *Atherosclerosis.* 2020;311:158–166.
58. Leistner DM, Kränkel N, Meteva D, et al. Differential immunological signature at the culprit site distinguishes acute coronary syndrome with intact from acute coronary syndrome with ruptured fibrous cap: results from the prospective translational OPTICO-ACS study. *Eur Heart J.* 2020;41:3549–3560.
59. Vergallo R, Crea F. Atherosclerotic plaque healing. *N Engl J Med.* 2020;383:846–857.
60. Fracassi F, Crea F, Sugiyama T, et al. Healed culprit plaques in patients with acute coronary syndromes. *J Am Coll Cardiol.* 2019;73:2253–2263.
61. Russo M, Fracassi F, Kurihara O, et al. Healed plaques in patients with stable angina pectoris. *Arterioscl Thromb Vasc Biol.* 2020;40:1587–1597.
62. Libby P, Pasterkamp G. Requiem for the 'vulnerable plaque'. *Eur Heart J.* 2015;36:2984–2987.
63. Wang Y, Fang C, Gao H, et al. Platelet-derived S100 family member myeloid-related protein-14 regulates thrombosis. *J Clin Invest.* 2014;124:2160–2171.
64. Libby P. Murine "model" monotheism: an iconoclast at the altar of mouse. *Circ Res.* 2015;117:921–925.

Special Forms of Atherosclerosis

65. Libby P, Hasan AA, Nohria A. Drugs targeting inflammation. In: Bhatt DL, ed. *Opie's Cardiovascular Drugs: A Companion to Braunwald's Heart Disease.* Elsevier; 2020.
66. Patel B, Ahuja A, Kassab G, Labarrere C. Diagnosis of cardiac allograft vasculopathy: challenges and opportunities. *Front Biosci (Elite Ed).* 2017;9:161–161.
67. Olymbios M, Kwiecinski J, Berman DS, Kobashigawa JA. Imaging in heart transplant patients. *JACC (J Am Coll Cardiol): Cardiovasc Imaging.* 2018;11:1514–1530.
68. Libby P. Inflammation in atherosclerosis. *Arterioscler Thromb Vasc Biol.* 2012;32(9):2045–2051.
69. Merola J, Jane-Wit DD, Pober JS. Recent advances in allograft vasculopathy. *Curr Opinion Organ Transplant.* 2017;22:1–7.
70. Head T, Henn L, Andreev VP, et al. Accelerated coronary atherosclerosis not explained by traditional risk factors in 13% of young individuals. *Am Heart J.* 2019;208:47–54.
71. Pinard A, Jones Gregory T, Milewicz D M. Genetics of thoracic and abdominal aortic diseases. *Circ Res.* 2019;124:588–606.
72. Liu CL, Guo J, Zhang X, et al. Cysteine protease cathepsins in cardiovascular disease: from basic research to clinical trials. *Nat Rev Cardiol.* 2018;15:351–370.
73. Libby P, Sukhova GK, Ozaki CK, Shi GP. Tilting at the tilted protease balance in arterial aneurysmal disease. *Cardiovasc Res.* 2017;113(11):1279–1281.
74. Libby P, Loscalzo J, Ridker PM, et al. Inflammation, immunity, and infection in atherothrombosis: JACC review topic of the week. *J Am Coll Cardiol.* 2018;72:2071–2081.
75. Campbell LA, Rosenfeld ME. Persistent C. pneumoniae infection in atherosclerotic lesions: rethinking the clinical trials. *Front Cell Infect Microbiol.* 2014;4:34.
76. Aron-Wisnewsky J, Clement K. The gut microbiome, diet, and links to cardiometabolic and chronic disorders. *Nat Rev Nephrol.* 2016;12:169–181.
77. Tang WHW, Backhed F, Landmesser U, Hazen SL. Intestinal microbiota in cardiovascular health and disease: JACC state-of-the-art review. *J Am Coll Cardiol.* 2019;73:2089–2105.
78. Libby P, Nahrendorf M, Swirski FK. Leukocytes link local and systemic inflammation in ischemic cardiovascular disease. *J Am Coll Cardiol.* 2016;67:1091–1103.
79. Libby P. The heart in COVID-19: primary target or secondary bystander? *JACC Basic to Transl Sci.* 2020;5:537–542.
80. Libby P, Lüscher T. COVID-19 is, in the end, an endothelial disease. *Eur Heart J.* 2020;41:3038–3044.
81. Musher DM, Abers MS, Corrales-Medina VF. Acute infection and myocardial infarction. *N Engl J Med.* 2019;380:171–176.
82. Kwong JC, Schwartz KL, Campitelli MA, et al. Acute myocardial infarction after laboratory-confirmed influenza infection. *N Engl J Med.* 2018;378:345–353.

25 Primary Prevention of Cardiovascular Disease

SAMIA MORA, PETER LIBBY, AND PAUL M RIDKER

OVERVIEW, 442
Trends in Cardiovascular Disease and Risk Factors, 442
Types of Prevention: Primordial, Primary, and Secondary, 442

CARDIOVASCULAR DISEASE RISK ASSESSMENT, 443
Cardiovascular Health and Life's Simple 7, 443
Global Risk, 444
Lifetime Risk, 445
Vascular Imaging in Preventive Practice: Coronary Artery Calcium and Coronary Computed Tomographic Angiography, 445
Society Guidelines for Cardiovascular Risk Assessment and Statin Therapy, 445

RISK FACTORS FOR CARDIOVASCULAR DISEASE, 446
Traditional Risk Factors, 446
Risk-Enhancing Factors, 451
Biomarkers, 453

CARDIOVASCULAR PREVENTION IN WOMEN, 457
Premature Menopause and Pregnancy-Associated Conditions, 457
Menopause and Postmenopausal Hormone Therapy, 458

LIFESTYLE FACTORS AND INTERVENTIONS, 458
Nutrition and Diet, 458
Physical Activity, 461

PHARMACOLOGIC THERAPIES, 462
Shared Decision-Making, 462
Aspirin, 463
N-3 Fatty Acids, 464

NOVEL APPROACHES TO PREVENTIVE CARDIOLOGY, 465
The Polypill in Current Practice, 465
Precision Medicine Versus Preventive Care, 466
Community Interventions, 467
Mobile Health, Remote Monitoring, and Wearables, 467

GAPS IN THE EVIDENCE AND FUTURE PERSPECTIVES, 467
Regional and International Perspectives, 468

REFERENCES, 468

OVERVIEW

Trends in Cardiovascular Disease and Risk Factors

Global Trends

Cardiovascular disease remains the leading cause of death worldwide, accounting for approximately 18 million deaths in 2017, with most deaths (approximately 70%) now occurring in low- and middle-income countries (see Chapter 2).[1] During the past decade, total cardiovascular disease deaths have increased globally by approximately 20%, at the same time that the age-adjusted cardiovascular deaths have decreased by approximately 10%. Total death rates are based on the total number of cardiovascular deaths divided by the population, while age-adjusted rates remove variations from differences in age structures in populations. Despite the decline in age-adjusted cardiovascular death rates, the total number of cardiovascular deaths have increased due to both population growth and aging, and in some countries also due to increases in age-specific cardiovascular mortality rates which may relate to rising obesity and diabetes rates.[1]

The age-adjusted decline in deaths from ischemic heart disease and stroke in high-income countries since the mid-1970s results from advances in both prevention (improvement in risk factors) and treatment (improvement in medical and surgical interventions), with each of prevention and treatment accounting for approximately half the decline. The age-adjusted rate of cardiovascular disease disability-adjusted life-years (DALYs) has also improved over the past several decades, but significant variations by country result from differences in risk factor prevalence and control. The largest contributors to the age-adjusted decline in cardiovascular death are lower cholesterol and blood pressure and smoking cessation.[2] On the other hand, increases in ischemic heart disease mortality in China may relate to increases in smoking and cholesterol, while rates have increased in Mexico due to increases in obesity and diabetes.[2] These observations underscore the importance of preventing and treating cardiovascular risk factors to reduce disparities in mortality. Recent global increases in obesity and diabetes and their long-term consequences on cardiovascular mortality currently present enormous challenges in cardiovascular prevention and controlling cardiovascular mortality. The decline in age-adjusted cardiovascular disease burden over the past several decades has recently slowed, requiring new global preventive measures.

Trends in the United States

Over the past 50 years, age-adjusted cardiovascular and ischemic heart disease death rates in the United States have declined by half. The annual incidence of coronary heart disease hospitalizations in the United States is estimated at 720,000 for new events and 335,000 for recurrent events per year, and for stroke the estimates are 610,000 new and 185,000 recurrent strokes per year.[1] Incidence of myocardial infarction has declined, with the greatest decrease in pre-hospital fatal events. The US age-adjusted rate of cardiovascular disease DALYs has also improved over the past few decades. Yet substantial disparities across the key demographic categories persist, including geographic, socioeconomic, education, sex, race, and ethnicity variation, and in some cases the disparities have increased with growing economic inequality (see Chapters 6 and 93). The greatest cardiovascular disease burden is in the stroke belt of the southeastern United States along the Mississippi River, and worse in blacks regardless of age.[2] These disparities link closely to differences in the prevalence of major cardiovascular risk factors, highlighting the importance of prevention in reducing cardiovascular disparities and mortality.

Furthermore, cardiovascular disease accounts for 14% of US health expenditures and is projected to increase substantially over the next decade.[1] Precision medicine approaches, such as the National Institutes of Health All of Us program that is collecting cardiovascular risk factor and event data over time in ≥ 1 million US participants will contribute to understanding future trends and more precise strategies for the prevention and treatment of cardiovascular disease.[2]

Types of Prevention: Primordial, Primary, and Secondary

Primordial prevention is the prevention of the development of risk factors, while primary prevention aims to prevent the clinical manifestation of cardiovascular disease in individuals without clinical cardiovascular disease (Fig. 25.1).[3] Primordial prevention focuses on social determinants of health and health inequities (e.g., poverty and

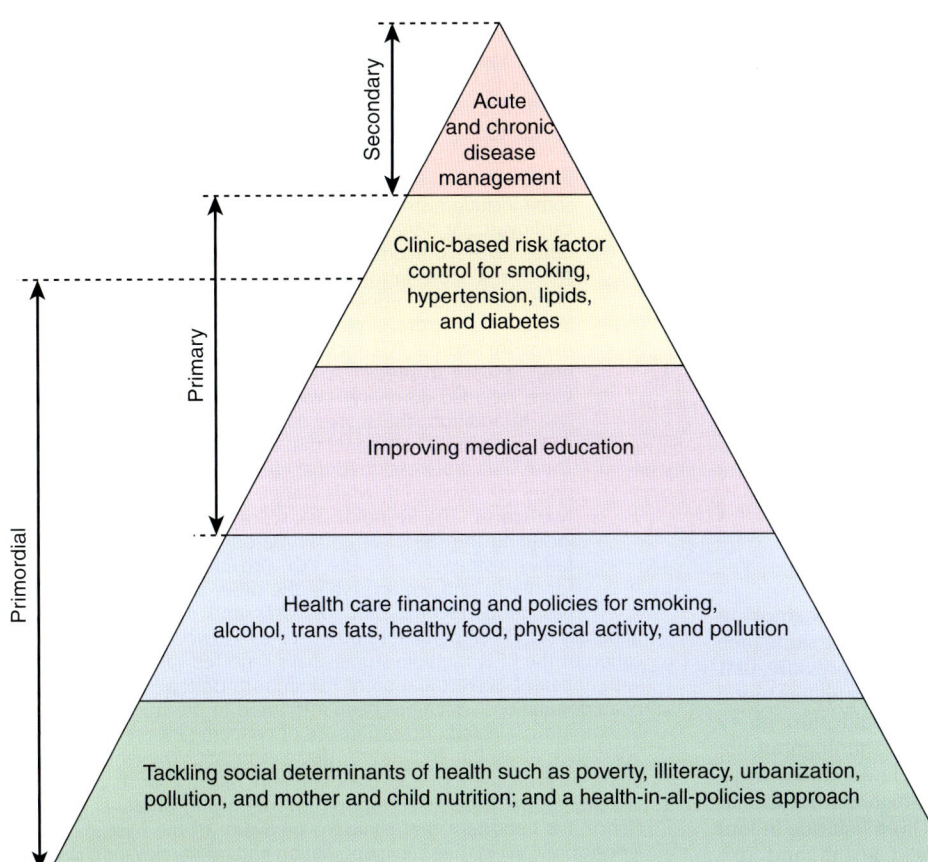

FIGURE 25.1 Types of prevention. Primordial prevention is the prevention of the development of risk factors. Primary prevention is the prevention of the first clinical manifestation of cardiovascular disease. Secondary prevention is the prevention of recurrent cardiovascular events in patients with established disease. (From Gupta R, Wood DA. Primary prevention of ischaemic heart disease: populations, individuals, and health professionals. *Lancet.* 2019;394:685–696.)

living conditions, urbanization, air pollution, education, sedentary behavior, psychosocial stress), while primary prevention focuses on controlling cardiovascular risk factors among high-risk individuals through lifestyle approaches and treatment of established risk factors. On the other hand, secondary prevention targets patients with established disease to reduce risk of recurrent cardiovascular events and mortality.

Lifetime cardiovascular risk estimates suggest that lowering the burden of cardiovascular disease requires all three types of prevention. The American Heart Association (AHA) guidelines emphasize the importance of primordial prevention by addressing the impact of social determinants of health. The World Health Organization also recommends this approach to achieve its noncommunicable disease goals (United Nations Sustainable Development Goals), in particular for improving daily living conditions and distribution of power, money, and resources. This model of "health-in-all-policies" includes universal health care, better health care financing, and improvements in agriculture, transportation, and employment, in addition to reducing poverty, illiteracy, smoking, alcohol abuse, and poor diet. Scandinavian countries which now have the lowest ischemic heart disease prevalence in Europe have demonstrated the success of this approach.[3]

Primordial and primary prevention can eliminate most cardiovascular events.[4] In the Prospective Urban Rural Epidemiology (PURE) study of 155,722 participants (mean age 50 years) from 21 countries followed for nearly a decade, greater than 70% of cardiovascular disease and myocardial infarction cases could be attributed to a small number of modifiable risk factors, consistent with prior results from the Global Burden of Disease and other studies. The largest contribution to cardiovascular risk was from metabolic risk factors (41% of the population attributable fraction) of which 22% were attributed to hypertension followed by non-HDL cholesterol (8%), while the biggest contribution to all-cause deaths was from behavioral risk factors (26%) and low education (12.5%).[5] For myocardial infarction, the largest risk factor was high non-HDL cholesterol, followed by hypertension, smoking, abdominal obesity, and diabetes.[5] Population-based interventions that aim to improve nationwide health include bans on trans fats and smoking, reducing salt, sugar, and alcohol intake, and improving diet and physical activity. Disparities in cardiovascular disease could be reduced with multi-factorial programs for the entire population, plus more targeted interventions for specific high-risk communities and individuals. Healthy People 2020 and 2030 are national initiatives in the United States designed to improve health for all population groups and eliminate disparities by emphasizing key cardiovascular health goals and tracking them.[6]

CARDIOVASCULAR DISEASE RISK ASSESSMENT

Cardiovascular Health and Life's Simple 7

Maintaining cardiovascular health across the lifespan is critical for primary prevention and depends on health-promoting activities that occur both within and outside of the health care system.[6] The AHA introduced Life's Simple 7 cardiovascular health metrics in 2010 to shift the focus from disease toward cardiovascular and overall health and well-being. The seven health metrics are smoking status, body mass index (BMI), physical activity, diet, cholesterol, blood pressure, and glucose. Levels of poor, intermediate, and ideal health are defined for each metric, with ideal cardiovascular health defined as the absence of clinical cardiovascular disease together with ideal levels of all seven components in the absence of medication treatment (Fig. 25.2).[1] For US and non-US populations, the prevalence of 6 to 7 ideal metrics is low (approximately 0.5% to 15%), worse for diet and physical activity, differs by demographics (e.g., worse for African Americans and those with lower education), and associates with higher risk of cardiovascular disease, mortality, and other outcomes (cancer, depression, and cognitive impairment).[7] By 2020, some of

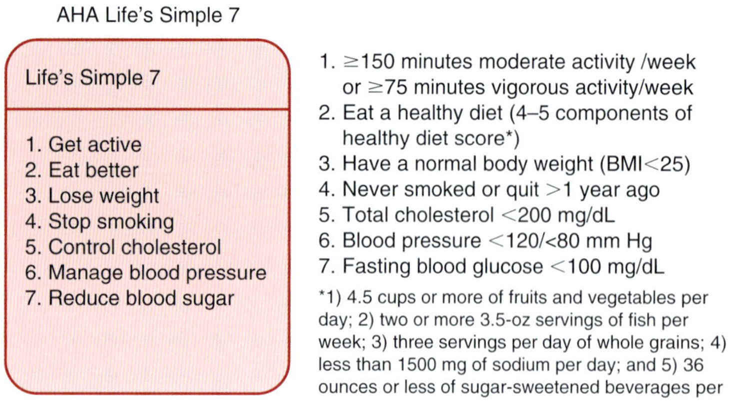

FIGURE 25.2 The American Heart Association (AHA) Life's Simple 7 cardiovascular health metrics. (Adapted from Lloyd-Jones DM, Hong Y, Labarthe D, et al. Defining and setting national goals for cardiovascular health promotion and disease reduction: the American Heart Association's strategic Impact Goal through 2020 and beyond. *Circulation*. 2010;121:586–613.)

these metrics improved in the United States, with overall less smoking, more physical activity, and lower cholesterol, yet during the same time other metrics have worsened with increases in blood pressure, BMI, and diabetes mellitus, and in youth, lower activity and higher blood glucose.[1,6] While achieving ideal cardiovascular health throughout the lifetime confers most benefit when maintained throughout life, tracking with less subclinical atherosclerosis and fewer cardiovascular events, benefit also derived from starting at high cardiovascular health levels even if they decreased over time. Given that one in four children start with less-than-ideal cardiovascular health, and 70% experience decline in cardiovascular health by early adulthood,[8] it is more important than ever to promote ideal cardiovascular health early in life in particular for children, adolescents, and young adults. Recognizing that behavior influences overall health and well-being, the 2030 AHA goals emphasize an even broader vision of health and well-being that includes health equity, with the goal to increase health-adjusted life expectancy (HALE), that is, the number of years that a population can anticipate living in good health (commonly known also as healthy life expectancy) from 66 years to at least 68 years of age in the United States and from 64 years of age to at least 67 years of age globally.[6] This new focus on healthy life expectancy incorporates overall health, disease conditions, quality and longevity of life, and well-being, with an emphasis on equity and improvements for all.[6]

Global Risk

Current guidelines recommend targeting the intensity of preventive cardiovascular interventions (e.g., blood pressure lowering, cholesterol lowering, and aspirin when appropriate) to the level of the individual's absolute risk. For almost half a century, interventions to reduce the risk of heart attack and stroke among adults without known cardiovascular disease have largely used a two-step process based on absolute risk. First, using a global risk–estimating algorithm for primary prevention in individuals ages 20 to 79 years old, 10-year risk is usually calculated and categorized into low, intermediate, and high. Then, based on shared decision-making, guidelines have traditionally targeted lifestyle interventions to those individuals at low risk while limiting pharmacologic interventions (such as statin therapy) to those with high-risk profiles, while sometimes recommending further laboratory or imaging assessments for refinement of risk among those at intermediate risk. In the United States, cardiovascular risk assessment used a global risk score such as that used in the third report of the Adult Treatment Panel of the National Cholesterol Education Program (ATP-III), a subsequent score that added family history of premature myocardial infarction and high-sensitivity C-reactive protein (hsCRP) to the traditional risk factors (the Reynolds risk score),[9] or the most recent 2013 American College of Cardiology (ACC)/AHA atherosclerotic cardiovascular disease (ASCVD) risk assessment algorithm which is based on the Pooled Cohorts Equations (PCE).[10,11]

All of these scores predict absolute risk of an event over the subsequent 10 years using sex-specific equations that take into account age, blood pressure, antihypertensive medication use, smoking status, and cholesterol measurements, and some include history of diabetes either as a risk factor or as a cardiovascular disease risk equivalent. These global risk scores differ in the outcomes that they predict. For example, the ATP-III risk score (also known as the Framingham risk score) predicted hard coronary heart disease events (myocardial infarction and coronary death). By comparison, the Reynolds risk score and the PCE included stroke in addition to coronary heart disease to predict ASCVD, but while the Reynolds risk score included coronary revascularization, the PCE score did not. In addition, the scores differ somewhat in the variables and associated coefficients that are included in the equations. The ATP-III score excluded diabetes as it was considered a coronary risk equivalent, while diabetes was included in the other two scores. The Reynolds risk score is distinct in additionally including the use of an inflammatory biomarker (hsCRP) and family history. Finally, the PCE provides different equations for blacks and whites, while the other two do not. The PCE has good discrimination of cases and noncases (C-statistic generally >0.7) comparable to other scores. However, since the publication of the PCE, multiple studies have reported variable calibration, with apparent overestimation of risk in both United States and European populations which has been attributed to the study populations being highly selected, increasing use of concomitant preventive therapies such as aspirin and statins, decreasing ASCVD event rates, and under-ascertainment of event rates in more recent cohorts which usually rely on participant self-reports for identifying potential events.[12] Hence it is important that clinicians be aware of the baseline prevalence of ASCVD in their clinic population and other relevant characteristics that may influence the pretest probability (e.g., socioeconomic status, lifestyle, comorbidities). Overprediction of risk may be more pronounced in income strata such as individuals with higher socioeconomic status, while underprediction of risk may pertain to those with lower socioeconomic status or high-risk ethnic groups.

The cut points for low, intermediate, and high risk also have changed over the past few decades. The 2013 AHA/ACC guidelines recommended that the intermediate-risk category be expanded to include individuals with a 10-year absolute risk of a hard event of greater than 5% to 20%, with the argument that this lower 5% cut point for intermediate risk identifies a group of individuals, especially women or younger individuals, who may benefit more from more aggressive lipid-lowering and lifestyle modification as compared to those with a 10-year absolute risk less than 5%.[10] The 2018 and 2019 guidelines recommended to further divide the intermediate risk category into "borderline" (5% to <7.5%) and "intermediate" subgroups (7.5% to <20%).[4,11]

Several variations of the US scores have been developed in Europe, such as the European Society of Cardiology (ESC) recommended SCORE (Systematic Coronary Risk Evaluation, predicting fatal cardiovascular events) and the UK's QRISK (which incorporates family history and social deprivation to predict cardiovascular events).[13,14] Estimating 10-year cardiovascular risk in low- and middle-income countries has expanded with the World Health Organization CVD risk chart that estimates 10-year risk of fatal and nonfatal cardiovascular disease in 21 world regions from greater than 1 million individuals, finding substantial variation in risk across regions.[15]

While robust evidence exists that changing some of the modifiable risk factors that comprise the global risk scores (e.g., blood pressure management, cholesterol lowering, smoking cessation) decreases cardiovascular risk, it is unclear if providing global risk information to patients or clinicians results in better outcomes. In a Cochrane review of 41 randomized trials from 6422 reports involving 194,035 participants without cardiovascular disease, providing risk score information slightly improved cardiovascular risk factors and resulted in greater preventive medication use without evidence of harm, but there was substantial heterogeneity across the studies and the evidence was rated as low quality.[16] This result agreed with an overview of systematic reviews that included both trials and observational studies.[17]

Lifetime Risk

Lifetime risk assessment was developed to address limitations of 10-year risk assessments and has been highlighted in recent guidelines.[11,13] Since age is the predominant determinant of cardiovascular risk, risk may be underestimated by relying on short-term (10-year) risk in younger individuals with multiple risk factors in whom cumulative exposure to these risk factors may be substantial over a lifetime, whereas older individuals with optimal levels of risk factors may have their risk overestimated as they are deemed high risk based on their age alone. Within the low- and intermediate-risk groups, there is variation in lifetime risk. To address this limitation, lifetime risk assessments (e.g., QRISK-Lifetime, Million Hearts longitudinal ASCVD risk assessment tool, LIFE-CVD) estimate risk over longer periods, yet such scores may not be accurate given that they may be derived from older cohorts, may not account for change in risk factors over time, or may be limited by disease ascertainment. Future risk scores should also address cumulative exposure and change in risk factors over time as well as comorbidities or factors that may modify risk. Finally, while risk estimates (short- or long-term) may inform shared decision-making discussions between clinicians and patients regarding initiation and maintenance of therapies, as well as quality assessments when risks and benefits of interventions are in question, it is important to remember that all risk estimates are probabilities of future clinical disease, and do not provide diagnostic or prognostic certainty.

Vascular Imaging in Preventive Practice: Coronary Artery Calcium and Coronary Computed Tomographic Angiography

In contrast to biologic factors that predispose to disease and are included in global risk scores, direct imaging of preclinical atherosclerosis provides an alternative method to detect high-risk individuals who might benefit from early preventive interventions. Of several imaging techniques developed over the past decade, computed tomography to detect coronary artery calcification (CAC) has emerged as a leading imaging tool for the preventive cardiology community.[18]

The advantages of CAC include wide availability, consistency across epidemiologic cohorts, and reproducible findings with regard to car-diovascular risk. CAC augments risk prediction across the full spectrum of primary prevention patients using either contemporary ESC or AHA/ACC guidelines.[19] The AHA/ACC guidelines suggest use of CAC among those with estimated 10-year risk between 5% and 20% in the context of shared decision-making when either the physician or patient is otherwise uncertain about use of specific preventive therapies, in particular statins.[4,11] CAC may also identify high-risk patients who would benefit from diet, exercise, smoking cessation, and other behavioral intervention, yet who have lacked motivation to do so. Some preventive cardiologists employ CAC scanning in lower-risk patients when there is a family history of premature coronary artery disease (see also Family History).

However, CAC scanning even with modern technology entails radiation exposure and results in increased downstream testing consequent to unanticipated false-positive findings particularly when tomography includes the full pulmonary bed. Further, therapeutic trials based on CAC are lacking (in contrast for example to LDL cholesterol or high-sensitivity C-reactive protein [hs CRP]) and evidence is inconsistent as to whether knowledge of CAC changes patient behaviors. In addition, CAC only detects calcified plaques (which are less likely to rupture) and does not detect the noncalcified thin-capped lesions that underlie many clinical events; as such, even CAC scores of zero do not eliminate atherosclerotic risk, particularly over long-term follow-up, and repeat testing after 5 years may be needed.[11] Finally, as statins increase rather than reduce coronary calcification, scanning those already taking these agents has little utility, and repeat testing has no role once a decision to start lipid-lowering has been made. Patterns of CAC use thus vary widely in the preventive cardiology community; among those favoring imaging, utilization of CAC has clearly increased while measures of carotid intimal medial thickness have waned.

The second imaging modality gaining broader acceptance in the prevention community is coronary computed tomographic angiography (CCTA; see Chapter 20). In the open-label, parallel-group SCOT-HEART trial of 4146 patients with stable chest pain, participants randomized to CCTA as compared to usual care had a lower rate of nonfatal myocardial infarction or coronary death at 5 years, an effect due to earlier use of coronary revascularization and more aggressive use of preventive and anti-anginal therapies.[20] Further, while obstructive coronary disease was more prevalent among those with prior coronary disease events than among those with possible angina or those with non-anginal symptoms, the benefits of CCTA seen at 5 years were present among all three of these groups. Moreover, among patients with stable chest pain, lowattenuation noncalcified plaque burden most strongly predicted fatal or nonfatal myocardial infarction, irrespective of risk score, CAC, or coronary artery area stenosis, and nearly half of all incident infarctions occurred among those without clear obstructive disease. These emerging data suggest that use of CCTA in high-risk secondary prevention can improve certainty of the diagnosis of obstructive coronary disease, better target angiography and revascularization, and results in higher levels of prescription and adherence to preventive therapies. Given recent trial evidence that those with moderate ischemia do not preferentially benefit from an initial invasive as compared to conservative strategy, use of CCTA may increase in the future though its superiority over functional testing using exercise electrocardiography, nuclear stress testing, or stress echocardiography remains uncertain (see Chapters 15, 16, and 18).

Society Guidelines for Cardiovascular Risk Assessment and Statin Therapy (see Chapter 27)

The 2018 and 2019 AHA/ACC cholesterol and prevention guidelines are summarized in Fig. 25.3 and Table 25.1,[4,11] and the European guidelines are summarized in Table 25.2.[14] The US and European guidelines share many recommendations, but European guidelines additionally recommend treatment goals for lipids. A healthy lifestyle remains the foundation for cardiovascular risk reduction across the life span. Class I recommendations for statin therapy include three subgroups of patients: (1) patients from secondary prevention with clinical ASCVD (history of acute coronary syndrome, myocardial infarction, stable or unstable angina, coronary or arterial revascularization, stroke, transient ischemic attack, or peripheral arterial disease) should be treated with maximally tolerated statin and nonstatin therapy to achieve LDL cholesterol reduction of 50% or more, (2) individuals from primary prevention with LDL cholesterol greater than or equal to 190 mg/dL, as this indicates primary hypercholesterolemia and should be treated with high-intensity statin or the highest intensity tolerated, aiming for LDL cholesterol reduction of 50% or more which can be achieved with addition of non-statin medication, and (3) patients from primary prevention with diabetes, age 40 to 75 years old, and LDL cholesterol 70 to 189 with no clinical ASCVD, should be treated with moderate-intensity therapy, or high intensity if multiple ASCVD risk factors present in addition to diabetes. The guidelines recommend assessing 10-year ASCVD risk every 5 years in all asymptomatic adults age 40 to 75 years old, using the sex- and race-specific PCE. In individuals with borderline (5% to <7.5%) or intermediate (7.5% to <20%) risk, the guidelines recommend refining risk by assessing lifetime risk, use of clinical risk enhancers (see Table 25.1), or if there is still uncertainty about the risk estimate, then using CAC to evaluate for subclinical coronary atherosclerosis and reclassify risk. These factors should enter into the clinician-patient discussion to guide shared decision-making regarding starting statin therapy, in addition to considerations of adverse drug effects, drug-drug interactions, cost, and patient preferences.

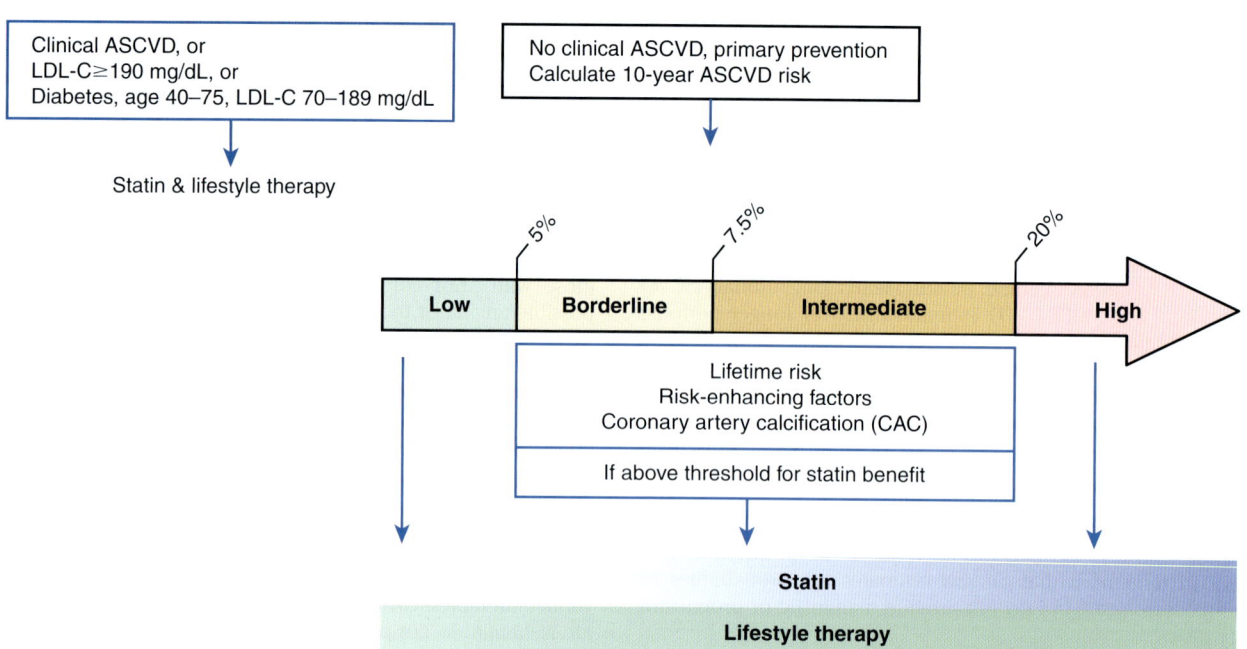

FIGURE 25.3 The 2018/2019 American College of Cardiology (ACC)/American Heart Association (AHA) assessment for risk of atherosclerotic cardiovascular disease (ASCVD) uses the Pooled Cohorts Equations for adults aged 40 to 79 years to calculate the 10-year absolute risk of ASCVD to guide discussions regarding lifestyle and statin treatment. *LDL-C*, LDL cholesterol. (Adapted from Grundy SM, Stone NJ, Bailey AL, et al. 2018 AHA/ACC/AACVPR/AAPA/ABC/ACPM/ADA/AGS/APHA/ASPC/NLA/PCNA guideline on the management of blood cholesterol: A report of the American College of Cardiology/American Heart Association Task Force on Clinical Practice Guidelines. *J Am Coll Cardiol*. 2019;73:e285–e350; and Arnett DK, Blumenthal RS, Albert MA, et al. 2019 ACC/AHA guideline on the primary prevention of cardiovascular disease: a report of the American College of Cardiology/American Heart Association Task Force on Clinical Practice Guidelines. *J Am Coll Cardiol*. 2019;74:e177–e232.)

TABLE 25.1 ACC/AHA Atherosclerotic Cardiovascular Disease Risk Enhancers Used in the ACC/AHA Guidelines

Family history of premature ASCVD (men <55 years, women <65 years)
Primary hypercholesterolemia (LDL-C ≥160 mg/dL [4.1 mmol/L]; non-HDL-C ≥190 mg/dL [4.9 mmol/L])
Chronic kidney disease (eGFR 15–59 mL/min/1.73 m², not on dialysis or kidney transplant)
Metabolic syndrome
Conditions specific to women (e.g., preeclampsia, premature menopause)
Chronic inflammatory conditions (especially rheumatoid arthritis, lupus, psoriasis, HIV)
High-risk race/ethnicity (e.g., South Asian ancestry)
Lipids/Biomarkers
Persistently elevated triglycerides (≥175 mg/dL [2 mmol/L], fasting or nonfasting)
In selected individuals if measured:
hsCRP ≥2 mg/L
Lipoprotein(a) ≥50 mg/dL or ≥125 nmol/L
Apolipoprotein B ≥130 mg/dL
Ankle-brachial index <0.9

ACC, American College of Cardiology; *AHA*, American Heart Association; *ASCVD*, atherosclerotic cardiovascular disease.

TABLE 25.2 Summary of the European Dyslipidemia Guidelines

CVD risk estimation
• Risk estimation (e.g., SCORE) is recommended for asymptomatic adults aged >40 years without evidence of CVD, DM, CKD, FH, or LDL-C >4.9 mmol/L (>190 mg/dL). IC
• High- and very high-risk individuals (CVD, DM, moderate-to-severe renal disease, very high-risk factors, FH, or a high SCORE risk) are a priority for advice and management of all risk factors. IC
Lipid analyses for CVD risk estimation
• **Total cholesterol** for estimation of total risk of CVD. IC
• **HDL-C** for further refining risk estimation. IC
• **LDL-C** is the primary lipid analysis method for screening, diagnosis, and management. IC
• **TGs** are recommended in routine lipid analysis. IC
• **Non-HDL-C** is recommended for risk assessment, particularly if high TGs, DM, obesity, or very low LDL-C. IC
• **Apolipoprotein B** is recommended for risk assessment, particularly in people with high TGs, DM, obesity, MetS, or very low LDL-C. Can be used as an alternative to LDL-C, if available, as the primary measurement for screening, diagnosis, and management, and may be preferred over non-HDL-C in people with high TGs, DM, obesity, or very low LDL-C. IC
Treatment goals for LDL-C in primary prevention
In individuals at very high risk, LDL-C reduction ≥50% and an LDL-C goal of <1.4 mmol/L (<55 mg/dL). IC
In individuals at high risk, LDL-C reduction ≥ 50% and LDL-C goal of <1.8 mmol/L (<70 mg/dL). IA

CKD, chronic kidney disease; *CVD*, cardiovascular disease; *FH*, familial hypercholesterolemia; *SCORE*, Systematic Coronary Risk Evaluation, predicting fatal cardiovascular events

RISK FACTORS FOR CARDIOVASCULAR DISEASE

Traditional Risk Factors

Smoking and e-Cigarettes (see Chapter 28)

As described in the 2020 Surgeon General's report on smoking,[21] tobacco use remains the single most important preventable cause of death and disability in the United States. Approximately 34 million American adults smoke cigarettes, most on a daily basis, resulting in excess health care spending of $170 billion annually.

Cigarette consumption contributes causally to one of every five deaths in the United States; the majority due to complications of coronary disease, lung cancer, and chronic obstructive pulmonary disease. From a cardiovascular perspective alone, smoking doubles the incidence of coronary disease and increases coronary deaths by more than 50%, with risks increasing with age and the number of cigarettes consumed. Smoking further is associated with increased rates of recurrent myocardial infarction, sudden cardiac death, aortic aneurysm rupture, symptomatic peripheral arterial disease, ischemic stroke, hemorrhagic stroke, coronary bypass surgery, and percutaneous coronary interventions. In women, smoking acts synergistically with oral contraceptives, placing younger women at additionally elevated risks for venous thromboembolism. Smokers lose at least one decade of life expectancy compared with never-smokers. Mechanisms underlying these multiple adverse effects include smoking-induced elevations of blood pressure and vascular tone, coronary spasm, lowered arrhythmia thresholds, impaired endothelium-dependent vasodilation, systemic pro-inflammatory effects, spontaneous platelet aggregation, reduced fibrinolytic function, and augmented insulin resistance.

Largely as a result of aggressive public health campaigns, between 1965 and 2017, the prevalence of current smoking in the United States declined from 52% to 16% in men and from 34% to 12% in women.[21] Smoking prevalence, however, is greater today among the young than among the elderly and there remain large disparities in tobacco use across strata defined by education, socioeconomic status, and ethnic background with the highest rates observed among adults living below the federal poverty level. By contrast to gains seen in North America, smoking prevalence is increasing in most developing economies worldwide. Today, more than 80% of the world's 1 billion smokers live in low- and middle-income countries.

The Surgeon General's 2020 report appropriately focuses on smoking cessation with an intent of helping all current smokers quit.[21] US government-related interventions include the full funding of comprehensive statewide tobacco control programs, enforcing higher retail pricing of cigarettes to at least $10 per pack; complete protection of the US population from second-hand smoke; public funding of high-impact media campaigns; more aggressive product warnings; and ensuring barrier-free cessation insurance coverage. With regard to global health, the WHO EMPOWER program seeks on an international basis to increase pricing of tobacco products; promote anti-tobacco media campaigns; implement smoke-free laws for workplaces and public spaces; and most importantly place strong restrictions on the advertising and promotion of tobacco products.

At an individual level, multiple approaches to smoking cessation exist and can be effective. First and foremost, smokers need to understand that quitting will reduce the excess risk of a coronary event by 50% within the first 2 years after cessation, with much of this benefit seen within the first few months. Risk further falls within the first 1 to 2 years of cessation with the risk in former smokers approaching that of never smokers after 3 to 5 years. Moreover, the beneficial effects on cardiovascular disease and all-cause mortality accrue even in the elderly, supporting the idea that it is never too late to quit smoking for the purpose of reducing cardiovascular risk. The magnitude of benefit conferred by smoking cessation equals or exceeds that of alternative secondary prevention efforts that typically receive greater attention from physicians and the pharmaceutical industry, including the use of lipid-lowering drugs. Unfortunately, though the elevated cardiovascular risks associated with smoking diminish significantly after cessation, the risks for development of cancers of the lungs, pancreas, and stomach persist for more than a decade.

Three of five US adults who have ever smoked have quit, and roughly two of every three current smokers want to quit. Many insurers now cover behavioral approaches and pharmacotherapy for smoking cessation. As of 2019, the US Food and Drug Administration has approved five nicotine replacement therapies and two non-nicotine oral medications that target smoking cessation, agents considered cost-effective. Implementation programs have shown effectiveness across multiple settings, including among low-income populations. Recent evidence suggests that combinations of short- and long-term nicotine replacement therapies may increase smoking cessation efficacy, as do text messaging services and web-based interventions that can serve as positive reminders and incorporate behavioral change techniques. A 2019 Cochrane review of 51 trials inclusive of 22,000 people found no overall difference in effectiveness between abrupt quitting and reduction-to-quit interventions, although with use of varenicline as a reduction aid the reduction-to-quit approach did appear somewhat better. Reduction aided by fast-acting nicotine replacement or varenicline was modestly better than reduction without pharmacologic aid, but this was not seen with nicotine patch or bupropion pharmacologic therapies.[22] A previous Cochrane review found that nicotine replacement could be effective both with and without counseling and found no evidence that nicotine replacement increased short-term vascular risk.

Whether or not nicotine exposure from e-cigarettes reduces long-term risks of heart disease and lung cancer when compared to traditional smoking remains controversial, as is the premise that e-cigarettes in general lead to smoking cessation; the Surgeon General's 2020 report explicitly found evidence supporting this hoped-for benefit inadequate (see Chapter 28).[21] Initial promotion of e-cigarettes falsely presumed that vaping would not lead to new smokers nor impact upon the young. Quite to the contrary, while the prevalence of adult smoking has declined, the prevalence of e-cigarette use (vaping) has dramatically increased among youth. In a recent cross-sectional survey conducted in North America, e-cigarette use was 27.5% among high school students and 10.5% among middle school students.[23] Much of this increase is due to flavored products specifically intended for a youth market, as less than 5% of adults report current e-cigarette use.

E-cigarettes certainly can cause a severe and life-threatening form of toxic inhalation pneumonitis known as e-cigarette or vaping associated lung injury (EVALI). EVALI represents an industry-induced health epidemic that could have been avoided had these products not entered the market in the first place. In response to these concerns, the Centers for Disease Control and Prevention has recommended that e-cigarette and related vaping products never be used by youths, young adults, or pregnant women. The above issues notwithstanding, preventing smoking in the first place must receive greater emphasis. School-, community-, and physician-based primary prevention remain the most important components of any smoking reduction strategy.

Hypertension

Elevated blood pressure is a major risk factor for cardiovascular diseases including coronary disease, heart failure, cerebrovascular disease, sudden cardiac death, peripheral arterial disease, renal failure, atrial fibrillation, and total mortality, as well as loss of cognitive function and increased incidence of dementia (see Chapter 26).[24] Globally, hypertension affects an estimated 1 billion people, while systolic blood pressure ≥ 110 to 115 mm Hg affects 3.5 billion adults and accounts for approximately one in five total deaths (>10 million deaths) and more than half of cardiovascular deaths.[25] Based on surveys from 154 countries with 8.69 million participants, the Global Burden of Disease study estimated that over the past 25 years the rates of annual deaths associated with systolic blood pressure ≥ 110 to 115 mm Hg increased from 135.6 to 145.2 per 100,000 adults, and annual deaths associated with systolic blood pressure ≥ 140 mm Hg increased from 97.9 to 106.3 per 100,000 adults.[25] DALYs from cardiovascular and other diseases increased concomitantly (by 40%), with the greatest burden seen in five countries (China, India, Russia, Indonesia, United States).[25] In 2015, elevated systolic blood pressure was the third-leading risk factor for global DALYs in both men and women, and the second-leading risk factor for DALYs from cardiovascular disease (dietary risks ranked #1).[26]

In the United States, 46% of Americans have hypertension (defined as systolic ≥130 or diastolic ≥80 mm Hg), with an estimated lifetime risk ranging from approximately 70% for white women to greater than 85% for black men and women, yet the prevalence of hypertension is increasing across all race/ethnicity and age groups.[1] Hypertension contributes to more cardiovascular deaths in the United States than any of the other major modifiable cardiovascular risk factors and is one of the most common reasons for clinic visits.[1] Strong socioeconomic, racial/ethnic, and sex disparities persist in the prevalence of elevated blood pressure and in the timing of blood pressure transition in the life course (see Chapter 93). The prevalence of hypertension in blacks in the United States is among the highest in the world, and is increasing.[1] The predominant drivers of elevated blood pressure are behavioral, specifically diet (high salt, low fruits, and vegetables), physical inactivity, and overweight/obesity, highlighting opportunities for prevention of cardiovascular disease and reducing mortality.[26]

Prospective studies indicate that death from both coronary disease and stroke increases progressively from blood pressure levels as low as 115 mm Hg systolic and 75 mm Hg diastolic.[24] Regardless of the definition of hypertension (≥130/80 or ≥ 140/90 mm Hg) both systolic and diastolic blood pressure are associated with risk as demonstrated in a study of 1.3 million US adults using electronic health care records, with systolic blood pressure having stronger association than diastolic blood pressure with cardiovascular outcomes.[27]

Guideline Recommendations (See Chapter 26)

INTERVENTIONS TO REDUCE BLOOD PRESSURE. The risk factors and markers for development of hypertension include increasing age, ethnicity, family history of hypertension, genetic factors, lower education and socioeconomic status, greater weight, lower physical activity, tobacco use, psychosocial stressors, sleep apnea, dietary factors (including increased dietary fats, higher sodium intake, lower potassium intake, tobacco, and excessive alcohol intake), and changes in the gut microbiome. The core strategies to prevent and treat high blood pressure are lifestyle (weight loss, sodium reduction, potassium supplementation, healthy diet, increased activity, and moderation of alcohol intake) and drug therapy. Controlling dietary and lifestyle risk factors can prevent much hypertension.

Diet is one of the main drivers for hypertension, and the benefits of healthy dietary interventions can lower blood pressure.[24] A meta-analysis of 24 randomized controlled trials including greater than 23,000 individuals found that dietary modifications lowered blood pressure, with the Dietary Approaches to Stop Hypertension (DASH) intervention (low sodium combined with high fruits, vegetables, low-fat dairy, and naturally high potassium) having the largest mean effect on lowering blood pressure (up to −7.6 mm Hg reduction in systolic blood pressure, and −4.2 mm Hg reduction in diastolic blood pressure), with clinically meaningful blood pressure-lowering benefits also seen for low-sodium, high-potassium, low-calorie, or Mediterranean diets.[28] Notably, blood pressure lowering by these dietary interventions resembles in magnitude drug monotherapy.

Physical activity protects against hypertension. In a meta-analysis of 29 studies of greater than 330,000 individuals, the risk of incident hypertension was lower by 6% for each 10 metabolic equivalents (MET hour/week) increment in leisure-time physical activity, with more benefit with higher activity (e.g., up to 33% lower risk of hypertension with 60 MET hour/week).[29] In overweight or obese adults with elevated blood pressure or hypertension, weight loss through a combination of reduced intake and increased activity is a key recommendation to reduce blood pressure.[24] Weight loss of 1 kilogram achieved through lifestyle/diet is associated with approximately 1 mm Hg systolic blood pressure reduction in a dose-response manner, with greater reductions in patients with higher blood pressures.[24,30]

DRUG THERAPY (SEE CHAPTER 26). Initiation of drug therapy depends on blood pressure and the absolute level of cardiovascular risk. Multiple randomized trials in patients with hypertension have demonstrated that blood pressure reductions as small as 3 to 5 mm Hg result in large and clinically significant reductions in risk for stroke, cardiovascular mortality, congestive heart failure, and coronary disease in middle-aged subjects, elderly persons, and specified high-risk patients such as those with diabetes and peripheral arterial disease.[24]

Metabolic Syndrome, Insulin Resistance, and Diabetes

Insulin resistance and diabetes rank among the major cardiovascular risk factors; the presence of diabetes confers an equivalent risk to aging 15 years, an impact comparable with if not greater than that of smoking (see Chapter 31). More than one third of US adults (88 million people) have some degree of abnormal glucose tolerance or prediabetes, a condition along with obesity that markedly increases the risk for type 2 diabetes and premature atherothrombosis.[4] Approximately 13% of US adults (34.1 million) have diabetes (most of which is type 2 diabetes), with significant heterogeneity by age, sex, race/ethnicity, and socioeconomic status, and it is estimated that by 2050 one in three US adults will have diabetes if current trends continue. A particular area of concern is the role of childhood adiposity as a future determinant of adult diabetes and cardiovascular risk. Overweight or obese children who become obese adults suffer concomitant increases in risks for development of type 2 diabetes, hypertension, dyslipidemia, and early-onset atherosclerosis, whereas obese children who avoid adult obesity avoid many of these complications.

Patients with diabetes have twofold to eightfold higher rates of future cardiovascular events as compared with age- and ethnically matched nondiabetic subjects, and 75% of all deaths in diabetic patients result from coronary disease. Compared with unaffected persons, patients with diabetes have a greater atherosclerotic burden in the major arteries, as well as of microvascular disease. Insulin resistance alone confers an elevated risk of congestive heart failure. Moreover, the risk of cardiovascular disease starts to increase long before the onset of clinical diabetes. These effects loom even larger in ethnic minority populations and in patients with other concomitant risk factors.

Although hyperglycemia associates with microvascular disease, insulin resistance itself promotes atherosclerosis even before it produces frank diabetes, and available data corroborate the role of insulin resistance as an independent risk factor for atherothrombosis. This finding has prompted recommendations for increased surveillance for the *metabolic syndrome*, a cluster of glucose intolerance and hyperinsulinemia accompanied by hypertriglyceridemia (both fasting and postprandial), low-HDL cholesterol levels, a predominance of small dense LDL particles and elevation of LDL particles and apolipoprotein B (apoB) levels, central obesity, hypofibrinolysis, hypertension, microalbuminuria, and elevated inflammatory biomarkers such as hsCRP. (See Chapters 27, 30, and 31.) ApoB or non-HDL cholesterol may be elevated in the absence of abnormal LDL cholesterol due to the excess of small dense LDL particles.[14,31] Controversy continues regarding insulin resistance as a unifying pathophysiologic pathway that accounts for all of the features of metabolic syndrome, and whether coalescence of risk factors incorporated in the concept of the metabolic syndrome augment risk over and above the sum of risk attributable to the individual components. Nonetheless, multiple studies document that individuals with the metabolic syndrome have elevated cardiovascular event rates. Increases in fasting glucose also associate with increased rates of cardiovascular deaths, cancer deaths, and nonvascular, noncancer mortality. Inflammation also provides a unifying concept that links elements of metabolic syndrome, and levels of hsCRP both predict incident diabetes and increase the specificity of metabolic syndrome definitions.

Despite ongoing controversies, many clinicians find the concept of metabolic syndrome useful because it fits the profile of many patients presenting in primary care in contemporary practice. Some argue that the concept of metabolic syndrome can encourage physicians to engage in tighter control of risk factors and lifestyle modification and to encourage patients to adhere to lifestyle modification or therapy designed to address the individual components of metabolic syndrome as mandated by prevailing guidelines. Skeptics, however, note the lack of evidence that the construct of metabolic syndrome can influence physicians or the public to adopt or maintain a healthy lifestyle or preventive therapies. The 2018 and 2019 AHA/ACC guidelines now consider the metabolic syndrome as a risk-enhancing factor to consider in shared decision making regarding statin initiation or intensification decisions (see Table 25.1), in particular among individuals who are borderline or intermediate risk based on their 10-year risk score.[4,10] Further, the guidelines provide diabetes-specific cardiovascular risk enhancers that are independent of other risk factors in diabetes, and these include long duration of diabetes, nephropathy (eGFR <60 mL/min/1.73 m^2 or albuminuria ≥ 30 μg albumin/mg creatinine), retinopathy, neuropathy, and ankle-brachial index (ABI) less than 0.9.[4,10] In addition to systemic metabolic abnormalities, hyperglycemia causes accumulation of advanced glycation end products associated with vascular damage. Diabetic and prediabetic patients also commonly have abnormalities of endogenous fibrinolysis and impaired endothelium-dependent (nitric oxide–mediated) vasodilation.

Interventions to Reduce Cardiovascular Risk among Patients with Diabetes

Therapeutic interventions for patients with diabetes are reviewed elsewhere (see Chapters 30 and 31). Beyond diet, exercise, and other lifestyle interventions, multiple randomized trials now demonstrate cardiovascular risk reduction among those with diabetes using new classes of glucose-lowering agents, in particular for glucagon-like peptide-1 receptor agonists (GLP-1RA) and for sodium-glucose cotransporter 2 (SGLT-2) inhibitors, which both reduce cardiovascular events and improve glycemic control.[4,32] Almost all patients with diabetes should be considered for statin therapy (Fig. 25.3), and the presence of diabetes-specific risk enhancers could be used in shared decision-making discussions about statin intensification. Statins plus fibrate or niacin combinations have not been shown to improve cardiovascular outcomes. However, the pharmaceutical grade preparation of the n-3 fatty acid eicosapentaenoic acid (EPA, icosapent ethyl) administered in high dose (2 g twice daily) to patients who met the entrance criteria for REDUCE-IT did benefit (see Chapter 27). Low-dose aspirin may be considered for primary prevention of cardiovascular disease in patients with diabetes and increased cardiovascular risk who are not at increased risk of bleeding given the recent ASCEND trial showing 12% risk reduction in the primary cardiovascular endpoint, although at the cost of 30% increased risk of major bleeding, while aspirin should be used in those with diabetes and cardiovascular disease unless there is a contraindication (see section on Aspirin). Surgical approaches to diabetes and diabetes prevention can prove effective and in selected patients, metabolic surgery can provide long-term glycemic control, reductions in event rates, and increased longevity (see Chapter 30).

Regrettably, though lifestyle recommendations remain a core concern for obesity and diabetes prevention, interventions to improve fitness and lose weight have had limited long-term success even among highly motivated patients. These findings suggest the need for novel approaches to diabetes prevention that better integrate social supports and issues of poverty and food quality along with medical and surgical interventions.

Obesity (see Chapter 30)

Across all ethnic and race groups, across genders, and across all socioeconomic levels, obesity is a major risk factor for premature death, elevated morbidity, lost productivity, and increased medical costs of care. Unfortunately, obesity is very difficult to treat after it has developed, and thus prevention of unhealthy weight gain is easier and more effective than reversing it afterward.

An assessment of weight, height, and a calculation of BMI should be part of every cardiovascular prevention visit. BMI is calculated as weight in kilograms divided by height in meters squared; using this metric, a BMI of ≥25 kg/m^2 is considered "overweight," a BMI ≥30 kg/m^2 is used to define "obesity," and a BMI ≥35mkg/m^2 is used to define "severe obesity." In turn, patients with a calculated BMI of 30 kg/m^2 or greater should be considered for intensive, multi-component behavior interventions and in some cases for drug and surgical therapy.[33] Support for this recommendation comes, in part, from a recent meta-analysis inclusive of 122 randomized trials; compared to controls, participants in behavior-based interventions had greater weight loss (−2.4 kg) at 12 months and less weight regain (−1.6 kg) at 18 months.[34] In the same meta-analysis, studies of medical interventions also improved outcomes modestly when added to a successful behavioral program, while both intervention strategies lowered the risk of developing diabetes among prediabetic patients. Weight-loss medications, but not behavioral interventions, associated with increased rates of harm, though these were of low absolute magnitude.

In the United States, obesity prevalence has increased in a stable and predictable manner over the past 30 years. Using state-level longitudinal BMI data from over 6 million adults participating in the Behavioral Risk Factor Surveillance Systems Survey which were corrected for self-reporting bias using direct obesity measures from the National Health and Nutrition Examination Survey, alarming trends in obesity can be projected forward on a regional basis (Fig. 25.4).[35] Specifically, by 2030, nearly one in every two American adults is projected to be obese, with a prevalence higher than 50% in 29 states and not below 35% in any state.[35] Moreover, if national trends do not change, nearly 25% of the United States will have "severe obesity" (BMI >35 kg/m^2), a category not even ascertained two decades ago. Reflecting the social determinants of health, all of these findings are more extreme among women, minorities, and those with low annual household incomes. Similar disturbing rates of increasing childhood obesity affect the entire United States.

Obesity also has major adverse effects on global health. The worldwide prevalence of obesity is estimated to be 108 million children and 604 million adults, and the rate of increase in childhood obesity over the past 30 years has increased faster than the rate of adult obesity. Elevated BMI accounts for 4 million deaths globally with more than two-thirds related to cardiovascular disease.[36]

Adult obesity strongly predicts incident cardiovascular and coronary diseases as well as hypertension, dyslipidemia, type 2 diabetes, osteoarthritis, sleep apnea, some cancers, low quality of life, depression, and anxiety, with risk increasing as BMI levels rise. Obese children have a risk for short-term health consequences including dramatic increases in insulin resistance, diabetes, breathing difficulties, and fractures. Obese children also have long-term risks for cardiovascular disease and diabetes as childhood obesity tracks closely with adult obesity. Nonobese adults who were overweight or obese during childhood have risks of these outcomes similar to those who were never obese.

Whether obesity is a "risk factor" or a "risk marker" is an area of long-term controversy in the epidemiologic community and helps to explain why BMI is not part of the traditional global risk scores. On the one hand, obesity tracks with diabetes, hyperlipidemia, and hypertension, all components of traditional risk scores. On the other hand, obesity tracks with prediabetic insulin resistance, low-grade systemic inflammation as measured by hsCRP, none of which usual preventive risk scores capture. An exception to this rule is the Reynolds Risk Score which also includes measures of inflammation and family history. The distribution of body fat also is a factor in the development of coronary disease, with abdominal obesity posing a substantial risk in both men and women. The waist-to-hip ratio, a surrogate for centripetal or abdominal obesity, independently predicts cardiovascular risk in women and older men. Chapter 30 discusses the mechanisms that link these anthropometric measures and cardiovascular risk.

Regardless of causal pathways, obesity challenges practitioners. Treatment strategies targeting obesity involve a multifaceted approach, including dietary counseling, behavioral modification, increased physical activity, psychosocial support, and potential pharmacologic and surgical interventions. Critical diet-related priorities to reduce adiposity include reductions in refined grains, starches, sugars, and processed meats and increasing intake of fruits, vegetables, nuts, fish, vegetable oils, and whole grains, in the context of regular physical activity. Data from numerous observational studies and short-term randomized trials support the substantial health benefits that accrue with weight loss. Even modest weight reductions of 5% to 10% confer significant improvement in blood pressure, improved lipoprotein profiles yielding lower levels of serum triglyceride-rich lipoproteins and LDL cholesterol while raising HDL cholesterol, and improvement in glucose tolerance and insulin resistance. However, behavioral weight loss trials have not definitively demonstrated reductions in incident cardiovascular events and mortality due primarily to participant inability to maintain weight loss on a long-term basis. Among motivated individuals, little convincing evidence establishes the superiority of any specific diet or dietary pattern in sustained weight reduction. Intermittent fasting displays diverse clinical benefits even in the absence of substantive weight loss.[37] Dietary strategies relevant to cardiovascular disease prevention are discussed below.

By contrast to medical intervention trials, randomized trials indicate that metabolic surgery improves diabetes control, hypertension, lipid levels, sleep apnea, and osteoarthritis and show a trend toward improved mortality.[38] (See Chapter 30 for details regarding operative approaches to obesity management.)

On a population basis, an increased intake of energy-dense foods and sugar-sweetened beverages, a decrease in physical activity, and an increase in sedentary behaviors because of changes in work, transportation, and urbanization all contribute to the obesity

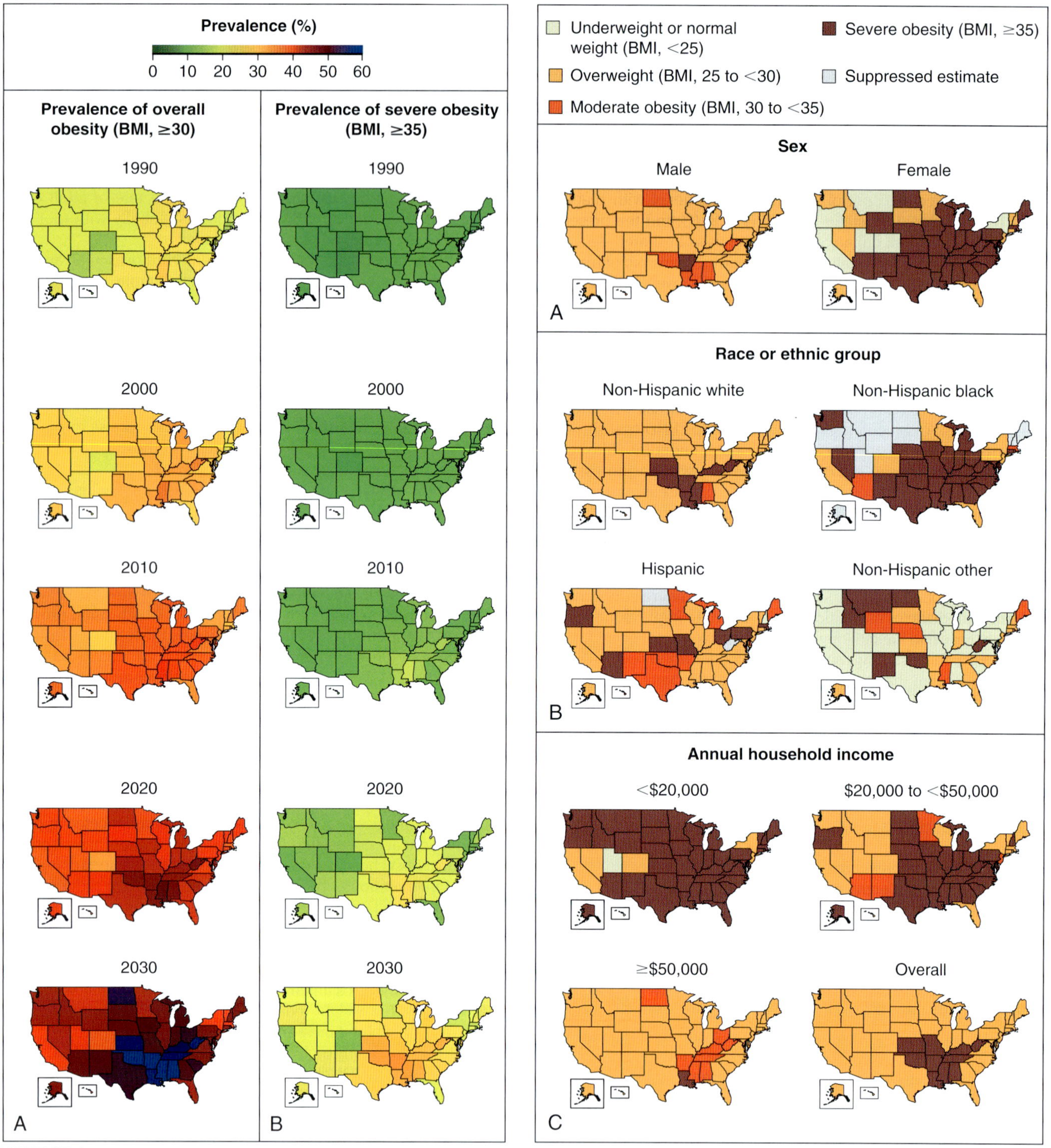

FIGURE 25.4 Estimated prevalence of obesity (body-mass index [BMI] >30 kg/m²) in the United States, from 1990 to 2030 *(left)* and the most common projected BMI category in 2030 (underweight or normal weight, overweight, moderate obesity, or severe obesity), according to sex, race/ethnicity, and annual income *(right)*. (Ward ZJ, Bleich SN, Cradock AL, et al. Projected U.S. state-level prevalence of adult obesity and severe obesity. *N Engl J Med.* 2019;381:2440–2450.)

epidemic. Interventions to reduce obesity prevalence must therefore go beyond behavioral changes and medical prescriptions to include substantive societal change and government coordination. These concerns extend beyond the emerging economies; in the United States, three interventions can reduce childhood obesity and save more money than they cost to implement: the introduction of a sugar-sweetened beverage excise tax, elimination of the existing tax subsidy for advertising unhealthy food to children, and the provision of nutrition standards for food and beverages sold in schools outside of school meals.[39] Critical examination should address how the built environment influences physical activity, diet, and weight change, and how government programs designed to oversee nationwide food production can inadvertently promote obesity both at home and abroad. Because a substantial burden of obesity and poor dietary intake exists among poor and less-educated groups, community-based efforts to make healthy choices an easier and more economic part of people's lives is essential. Novel approaches can move beyond traditional environmental-focused policy measures, such as collaboration with the food and restaurant industry to achieve responsible marketing especially to children, expand available health food choices, and reduce fat, sugar, and salt content of processed foods. None of these interventions, however, can occur without broad

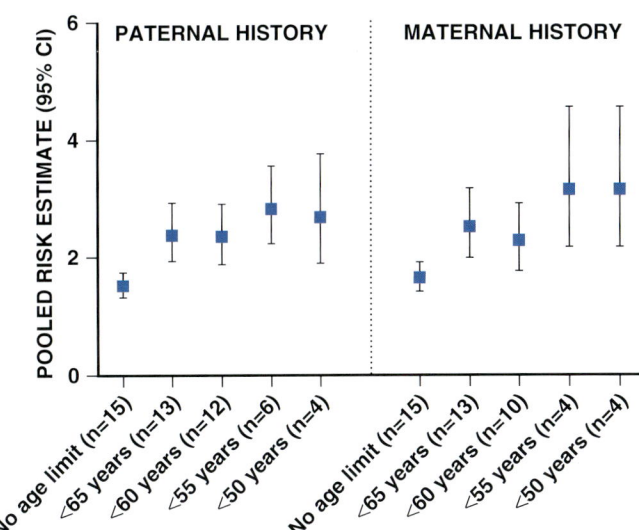

FIGURE 25.5 Age- and sex-adjusted pooled risk estimates of offspring risk for cardiovascular disease by parental age of onset in a systematic review of 26 studies. n, number of studies. (From Weijmans M, van der Graaf Y, Reitsma JB, et al. Paternal or maternal history of CVD and risk of CVD in offspring. Systematic review and meta-analysis. *Int J Cardiol.* 2015 Jan 20;179:409–416.)

political support, an effort that can and should involve the preventive cardiology community.

Family History

Premature cardiovascular disease generally refers to clinical cardiovascular disease occurring before age 65 years in women or before age 55 years in men, to distinguish it from conventional disease which occurs at older ages. Since cardiovascular disease drives much premature mortality, identifying individuals at risk of premature cardiovascular disease events is crucial. World leaders committed to reducing premature deaths from non-communicable diseases when the World Health Assembly and later the World Heart Federation adopted "25×25" to reduce these premature deaths by 25% by the year 2025 by improving 6 preventable factors (tobacco and alcohol use, salt intake, obesity, blood pressure, and glucose), and the United Nations Sustainable Development Goals aimed to reduce them by one-third by the year 2030 through prevention and treatment.[40] At the global level, the increased burden of premature myocardial infarction has affected several countries including United Kingdom, Australia, Canada, and the United States, where the rates of myocardial infarction incidence and/or mortality among younger adults have decreased to a lesser extent and are possibly increasing, with worse outlooks for women than men.[1]

Routine preventive practice should include evaluation of family history, and the 2018 and 2019 AHA/ACC guidelines now include family history of premature cardiovascular disease as a risk-enhancing factor that could be useful for initiating or intensifying statin therapy in adults with borderline or intermediate risk (see Table 25.1).[4,11] The guidelines now consider family history of premature ASCVD or genetic dyslipidemias an indication for assessing lipids and other risk factors, as well as a relative indication for measuring lipoprotein(a).[11] A systematic review of 26 studies showed that a positive maternal or paternal history of cardiovascular disease conferred a similar degree of increased risk in the offspring by about 1.5- to 2-fold, with the highest risks observed for maternal history less than 50 years or paternal history less than 55 years (Fig. 25.5).[41] These effects compare in magnitude with those of smoking, hypertension, and hyperlipidemia. The Justification for the Use of Statins in Prevention: An Intervention Trial Evaluating Rosuvastatin (JUPITER) trial affirmed the importance of family history as a clinical marker of risk. Within JUPITER, those subjects with a family history of premature atherosclerosis experienced a 62% reduction in first vascular events associated with statin therapy as compared with a 39% reduction among those without a family history, with even greater statin-related risk reductions seen in women with family history versus men, which has led recent US guidelines to emphasize family history as a risk-enhancing factor when considering statin treatment.[11] Even among individuals with coronary artery calcium (CAC) scores of 0, family history is associated with increased cardiovascular risk.[42] Hence, family history could be considered a coronary disease risk equivalent for purposes of statin prescription in primary prevention. Several widely used global cardiovascular risk scores (e.g., Reynolds Risk Score and the PROCAM score) have incorporated family history of myocardial infarction at less than 60 years,[9] highlighting the importance of family history as a variable that reflects both shared genetics and environment.

Risk-Enhancing Factors

Social Determinants of Health (see Chapters 6 and 93)

Non-medical health-related social needs affect not only individual health outcomes but also health care utilization and costs, yet clinical assessments and interventions addressing these needs have lagged the evidence base. Recognizing their importance, the 2019 AHA/ACC prevention guidelines gave a class I recommendation that patient-centered approaches to cardiovascular prevention should be informed by social determinants of health.[4] Social determinants include factors related to the environment over which an individual has little control (e.g., health inequities, lack of resources, public and environmental safety), and factors related to the individual and social factors seen in the clinical setting (e.g., disability status, race, ethnicity, insurance, ZIP code, income inequality) (Fig. 25.6).[43]

To aid clinicians, communities, and systems of care in assessing these social determinants to identify unmet needs and reduce barriers to health care, the Centers for Medicare & Medicaid Services Accountable Health Communities developed an evidence-based simple 10-item standardized screening tool on five core domains (housing instability, food insecurity, transportation difficulties, utility assistance needs, and interpersonal safety). Another tool that may be more useful for health care programs rather than clinical practice is the Social Deprivation Index, which was developed to calculate disadvantage levels and to address health inequities. The strengths and limitations of these and other tools for cardiovascular care are reviewed elsewhere.[43]

In a systematic review of 18 studies, neighborhood environment characteristics (e.g., residential density, traffic volume, recreation facilities, fast food restaurants, grocery stores) were significantly associated with cardiovascular risk factors (e.g., physical activity, obesity, blood pressure, diabetes) and major cardiovascular outcomes.[44] For example, neighborhood green space has been found to be associated with approximately 20% lower risk of coronary events, heart failure, and atrial fibrillation, which is partly mediated by cardiometabolic risk factors, and several studies showed lower cardiovascular and all-cause mortality with more greenness.[45] Importantly, environments are modifiable and amenable to community-level and policy interventions, but they require a systems-level approach. For clinicians, better routine assessment and attention to societal determinants could help alert clinicians that these factors may impact patient care and help them to address these patient needs as part of a team-based approach, since these are complex issues that require multiple team members with varying expertise (e.g., patient navigators, public health workers, community partners).

Psychosocial Factors (see Chapter 99)

Psychosocial factors such as depression, stress and anxiety, hostility and anger, social isolation, and perceived lack of social support have consistently been linked with cardiovascular risk factors (e.g., tobacco use, diet, physical activity, obesity, diabetes, and blood pressure) and with the risk of cardiovascular disease and mortality outcomes, and often cluster together in individuals or groups. They may impede treatment adherence or lifestyle changes.[46] Low socioeconomic status (e.g., low education, low income) is associated with 30% to twofold increased risk of cardiovascular disease and mortality.[13] In the PURE study of 154,169 participants from 20 countries, lower educational level associated strongly with 1.5- to 2-fold increased risk of cardiovascular events and mortality independent of household wealth and other risk factors, with the strongest association noted in low- and middle-income

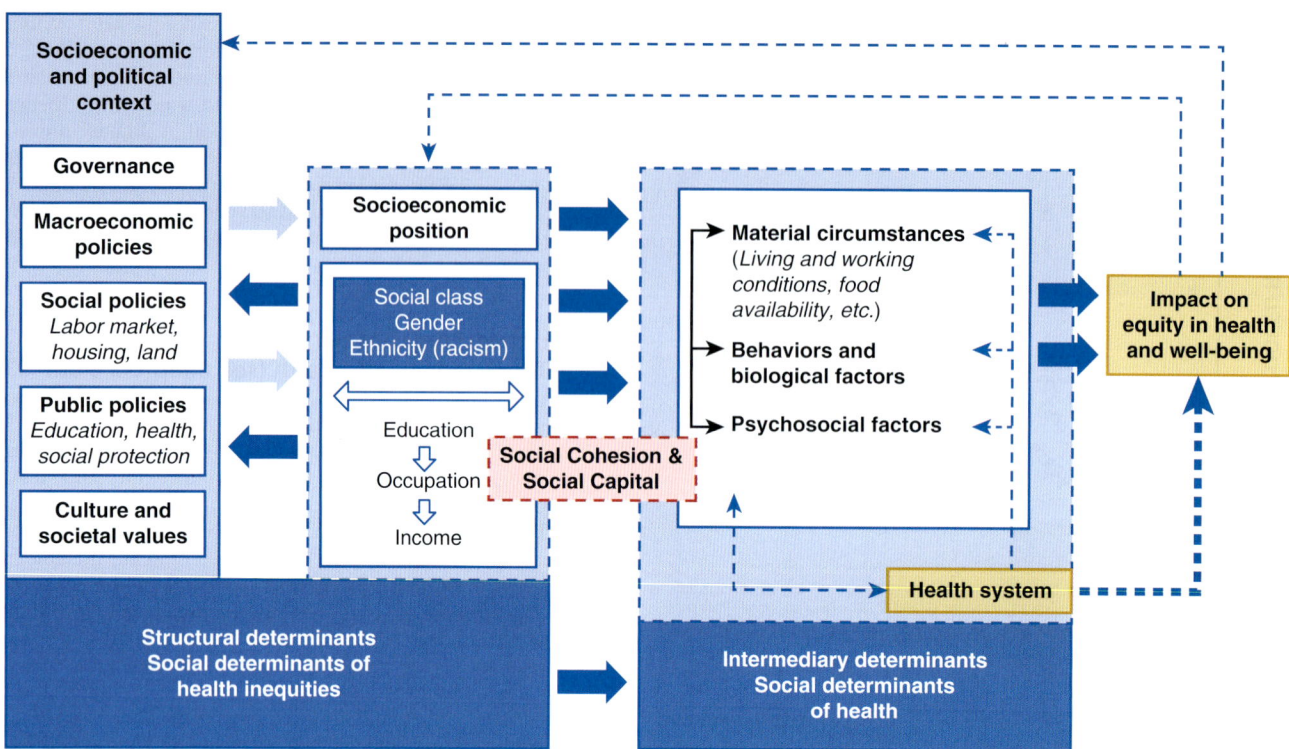

FIGURE 25.6 World Health Organization social determinants of health framework. (Reprinted from Solar O, Irwin A. A Conceptual Framework for Action on the Social Determinants of Health: Social Determinants of Health Discussion Paper 2 (Policy and Practice). Geneva, Switzerland: World Health Organization; 2010; From White-Williams C, Rossi LP, Bittner VA, et al. Addressing social determinants of health in the care of patients with heart failure: a scientific statement from the American Heart Association. Circulation. 2020;141[22]:e841–e863.)

countries and to a lesser degree in high-income countries.[47] Notably, in the PURE study, out of 14 potentially modifiable cardiovascular risk factors, the largest contributor to death was low education which accounted for 16% of deaths, exceeding that of smoking or hypertension (11% each), household pollution, diet, or grip strength (8% each).[5] Negative emotions, particularly depression, consistently and independently are associated with the development of cardiovascular morbidity and mortality in patients without known cardiovascular disease; moreover, patients with known cardiovascular disease have higher prevalence of depression. Depression in otherwise healthy persons almost doubles the risk of developing coronary heart disease.[48] Major depression is associated with worse prognosis in patients with coronary heart disease and constitutes a risk factor for poor prognosis in patients with acute coronary syndromes and stroke including adverse health outcomes, disability, mortality, and health care costs.[48,49]

Mental stress has gained recognition as a source of cardiovascular risk with meta-analyses demonstrating stress as a risk factor for incident cardiovascular disease in asymptomatic individuals and for cardiovascular events in patients with established cardiovascular disease, with stronger stress-cardiovascular associations seen for patients at higher cardiovascular risk or those with established disease.[50] Both work stress and private-life stress correlate with up to 60% higher risk of cardiovascular events, with twofold or greater increased risk among patients at high cardiovascular risk.[50] Work stress has two components—job strain, which combines high work demands and low job control, and effort-reward imbalance, which more closely reflects economic factors in the workplace. Both components are associated with increased risk for coronary events and stroke, with a multicohort consortium of 90,164 individuals finding approximately 15% increased risk of incident coronary events for effort-reward imbalance independent of the job strain experienced.[51] Other psychological metrics, including anger and hostility scales as well as negative social interactions, also are associated with elevated cardiovascular risk.[52] Lifetime exposure to traumatic psychological stress increases risk for morbidity and mortality in patients with cardiovascular disease. In addition to the effects of these chronic stressors, a body of observational evidence implicates acute emotional and stress triggers in precipitating an acute coronary syndrome or stroke via stress-induced ischemia, increased sympathetic activity and hemodynamic responses, and a variety of other potential mechanisms including proinflammatory and prothrombotic processes that contribute to plaque rupture or disruption.

Psychosocial risk factors have gained recognition as risk factors for cardiovascular disease and several clinical guidelines or expert statements now recommend assessment and treatment. A few small-scale randomized trials have shown efficacy in reducing major cardiovascular events, while other trials have shown benefits on surrogate outcomes, mood scales, and quality of life.[50] Effective treatment options for depression include shared decision making and collaborative care interventions, cognitive behavioral therapy, pharmacologic interventions, and physical activity. A systematic review of 14 randomized controlled trials found that shared decision-making interventions, in particular those using decision tools or collaborative care interventions, improved patient satisfaction and engagement and were feasible in the clinical management of depression and mood disorders, while the trials that used collaborative care (i.e., including patients' families and other health professionals) plus shared decision making additionally improved depression outcomes or medication adherence.[53] In one clinical trial of 119 patients with 8-year follow-up, collaborative care for depression reduced by half the future risk of cardiovascular disease among older, depressed patients.[54] In an observational study from the Translational Research Investigating Underlying Disparities in Acute Myocardial Infarction Patients' Health Status acute myocardial infarction registry, untreated depression is associated with about twofold increase in 1-year mortality, while treated depression did not associate with risk in post-myocardial infarction patients.[55] Recognizing the scarce clinical trial data and gaps in evidence, European prevention guidelines nonetheless recommended assessment of psychosocial factors and their consideration as risk modifiers in cardiovascular risk prediction, especially for intermediate- or borderline-risk individuals when treatment decisions are unclear.[13] They gave a class I recommendation for treating psychosocial factors with specialized multimodal behavioral interventions that integrate health education, physical exercise, and psychological therapy for patients with established cardiovascular disease and psychosocial symptoms, and gave a grade IIa recommendation for treating psychosocial risk factors for the prevention of cardiovascular disease.[13] The most recent AHA Scientific Statement on depression and coronary heart disease recommends screening of patients with coronary heart disease for depression,[48] and the AHA/American Stroke Association Scientific Statement on depression and stroke recommends timely screening and prompt evidence-based management of depression in stroke patients while calling for further research on the best treatment strategies.[49] A better understanding of psychosocial factors and the risk of adverse cardiovascular events may provide additional opportunities for cardiovascular prevention and management and for broader population-wide public health and policy programs, especially for older adults or those with lower socioeconomic status and greater health inequities. Cardiovascular practice often omits this important aspect of patient care.

Ankle-Brachial Index (see Chapter 43)

Atherosclerosis, a systemic disease, affects not only the coronary and cerebrovascular beds but other vascular beds including the aorta and the peripheral arteries, and each affected vascular bed is considered a marker of cardiovascular risk.[56,57] Patients with peripheral arterial disease are at highly increased risk of cardiovascular events and mortality, and are considered for secondary (not primary) prevention therapies addressing not only symptoms of peripheral arterial disease but more importantly comprehensive risk factor management (smoking cessation, heart-healthy diet, weight loss, regular exercise, and appropriate pharmacologic therapies).[14,57] The ABI for lower extremities is obtained noninvasively and calculated by dividing each of the ankle pressures by the higher of the brachial artery pressures. For cardiovascular risk assessment, the lowest ABI between the two legs is used. A normal resting ABI is greater than 0.9 to 1.3 (borderline abnormal is ABI 0.91 to 0.99). An ABI ≤0.9 is abnormal (low), diagnostic for lower extremity arterial disease, and is associated with more than doubling of the 10-year cardiovascular risk, while ABI ≥1.4 is also abnormal (high) as it represents arterial stiffening, vascular calcification, and noncompressibility, and is also associated with higher cardiovascular risk.[57] ABI is useful for diagnosing and preventing progression of lower extremity arterial disease and events, but also for general cardiovascular risk assessment as an adjunct to the global risk score. Guidelines differ in their recommendations for screening ABI.[58] The AHA/ACC and ESC guidelines support screening ABI measurements particularly among individuals at increased risk of peripheral arterial disease,[4,11,14] while the US Preventive Services Task Force concluded there was insufficient evidence for screening.[59] Factors that increase the risk of peripheral arterial disease are an age greater than 65 years old, the presence of other cardiovascular risk factors (e.g., diabetes, history of smoking, hyperlipidemia, hypertension), family history of peripheral arterial disease, or known atherosclerosis in another vascular bed (coronary or non-coronary).[56] The European guidelines recommended targeting men and women aged greater than 65 years, in particular those classified at high cardiovascular risk and with a family history of lower extremity arterial disease.[14] The AHA/ACC guidelines consider ABI less than 0.9 as a risk-enhancing factor that can be useful for further risk stratification and statin decisions among individuals with borderline or intermediate risk based on the PCE equations (see Table 25.1).[4,11]

Biomarkers (see Chapter 10)
Lipids/Lipoproteins
Standard Lipid Testing (see Chapter 27)

The burden of risk for cardiovascular disease begins early. Cholesterol levels measured early in life influence long-term cardiovascular risk, and the burden of risk factors for atherosclerosis, including hypercholesterolemia, correlate with autopsy-proven fatty streak and raised lesion formation in the arterial tree and future cardiovascular outcomes. Cholesterol screening for children with a nonfasting sample should start early (age 10 years) and be repeated every 5 years.[60] If there is a family history of hypercholesterolemia or premature cardiovascular disease, cholesterol screening should start earlier at age 2 and repeated every 3 to 5 years for early identification of familial hypercholesterolemia and hereditary dyslipoproteinemias, even if the initial profile is normal. Adults should have the traditional cardiovascular risk factors assessed at least every 5 years starting at age 20, and by age 40 all adults should undergo a cardiovascular risk assessment with a global risk score to estimate the absolute 10-year risk of ASCVD to guide discussions and decisions about preventive therapies.[4,11,14] However, absolute risk alone should not solely guide decisions regarding prevention, and risk calculators may underestimate or overestimate risk for a particular individual.[4] For younger adults, lifetime risk assessment is better than 10-year risk, since age is the predominant driver of risk and early interventions could prove most effective. Risk assessment requires measurement of total and HDL cholesterol, while LDL cholesterol and non-HDL cholesterol (total minus HDL cholesterol) are used for guiding statin initiation, response, and intensification.

Standard lipid testing, assessed by total, LDL, HDL cholesterol, and triglycerides, is well-established laboratory testing for cardiovascular risk prediction and management. In general, the higher the cholesterol (especially the LDL or non-HDL cholesterol), the higher the short- and long-term risk of cardiovascular disease. Premenopausal women tend to have higher HDL cholesterol levels than men, and hence their total cholesterol level may be higher due to the elevated HDL cholesterol. Yet, a large proportion of patients with cardiovascular disease have average or even low levels of total or LDL cholesterol. Usually these individuals have other predisposing factors that promote atherosclerosis, such as atherogenic dyslipoproteinemia (increased levels of small dense LDL particles despite normal or low LDL cholesterol, increased triglycerides and remnants, and low HDL cholesterol), obesity (particularly abdominal obesity), metabolic syndrome/insulin resistance, diabetes, physical inactivity, unhealthy diet, chronic inflammatory conditions, or genetic susceptibility (commonly polygenic or less commonly, monogenic variants).

FASTING VERSUS NONFASTING. The rationale behind using nonfasting testing is appealing physiologically. We live most of our lives in the nonfasting state, which is the most representative of our physiology. Nonetheless, fasting samples have been the standard for measurement of lipid profiles, which traditionally have been measured after an 8- to 12-hour overnight fast. Over the past several decades, numerous large prospective studies have verified the adequacy of nonfasting lipids for general screening of cardiovascular risk. An evidence-based review of the published literature from greater than 300,000 individuals found no attenuation of lipid relationships with predicting incident cardiovascular events for nonfasting lipids, including for triglycerides.[61] At least three large statin clinical trials (involving nearly 43,000 patients) have used nonfasting lipids as entry criteria.

Concern that population-level risk associations would not capture individual variability based on fasting status has been raised as a critique against adopting widespread nonfasting testing. Recent data published on 8270 participants from the Anglo-Scandinavian Cardiac Outcomes Trial-Lipid Lowering Arm (ASCOT-LLA) trial with prospective follow-up provided robust evidence addressing this concern.[62] Both fasting and nonfasting lipids in the same individuals were measured 4 weeks apart with no intervention or advice given between the two visits. The association of baseline lipids with cardiovascular events was similar irrespective of fasting status, and importantly, results were similar by randomized allocation to statin versus placebo. Risk algorithms use total and HDL cholesterol (not triglycerides or LDL cholesterol), hence there is little impact of nonfasting on risk estimates using these methods. The ASCOT-LLA study found no significant misclassification that would adversely affect the decision for initiation of statin therapy, with high concordance (95%) between fasting and nonfasting lipids measured from the same individuals for classification into risk categories.[62]

Further, genetic studies using mendelian randomization have linked nonfasting triglycerides and remnant cholesterol to increased risk of cardiovascular disease and mortality. In certain patients, including those with metabolic syndrome, diabetes mellitus, or specific genetic abnormalities, fasting can mask abnormalities in triglyceride metabolism which is captured by nonfasting measurements. One of the major reasons for slow adoption of nonfasting measurements has been clinician concern regarding misclassification of individuals into a lower risk category when evaluating LDL cholesterol in nonfasting panels due to variability in triglycerides affecting LDL cholesterol calculation by the Friedewald equation. However, differences in routine lipids according to fasting status are clinically small: HDL cholesterol change is negligible; slightly lower levels are seen (up to −8 mg/dL) for nonfasting total cholesterol, LDL cholesterol, and non-HDL cholesterol compared with fasting, and modest changes (up to 26 mg/dL higher) for triglycerides. Given the independent risk conferred by elevated triglycerides and triglyceride-rich lipoproteins, the question of what constitutes high-risk nonfasting triglycerides has also been studied. Most guidelines, including the latest US and European guidelines, define elevated nonfasting triglycerides as ≥175 mg/dL (≥2 mmol/L) based on a cut point that has been prospectively validated.[63] The 2018 and 2019 AHA/ACC guidelines also consider fasting or nonfasting triglycerides ≥175 mg/dL as a risk-enhancing factor that could prompt consideration for initiating or intensifying statin therapy.[4,11] 2016 marked the approval of several international recommendations for nonfasting lipid testing. The European Atherosclerosis Society, European Federation of Laboratory Medicine, and ESC all allowed for use of nonfasting lipid testing as the standard of care for patients.[61,64] The Canadian Hypertension Education Program guidelines removed fasting as a requirement in 2016 and that same year the Canadian Cardiovascular Society dyslipidemia guidelines designated nonfasting lipid testing as a suitable alternative to fasting.[65] In 2017 the American Association of Clinical Endocrinologists and American Association of Endocrinology allowed for nonfasting testing. Finally, in 2018 and 2019 the AHA/ACC cholesterol and prevention guidelines modified previous 2013 recommendations for fasting tests and allowed for the use of nonfasting testing for routine screening.[4,11]

LDL Cholesterol

Extensive epidemiologic, genetic, and clinical trial studies demonstrate that LDL cholesterol is a causal risk factor for cardiovascular disease.[66] In addition to the magnitude of elevation of LDL cholesterol, the cumulative lifelong exposure to high LDL is a key determinant of LDL-related cardiovascular risk, as it reflects the exposure of the arterial tissues to LDL particles.[66] While treating to a pre-specified LDL cholesterol target is no longer as rigorously advocated as before, most guidelines use LDL cholesterol levels or percentage reduction in LDL cholesterol for guiding decisions to initiate or intensify statin and other lipid-lowering therapies, tailoring the level of LDL cholesterol reduction to the individual's level of cardiovascular risk.

Clinical trials of LDL-lowering therapies across the spectrum of LDL cholesterol have shown a significant relationship between on-treatment LDL cholesterol levels and the reduction in risk of ASCVD events, supporting the principle that "lower is better."[11] On average, the lowering of LDL cholesterol by 1% corresponds to approximately a 1% lower risk of cardiovascular events.[11] Most of these trials have evaluated the effects of statin versus placebo or high- versus low-intensity statin on cardiovascular outcomes. In the Cholesterol Treatment Trialists meta-analysis of 27 randomized statin trials ($N = 174{,}149$ individuals, 27% women), every 1 mmol/L (39 mg/dL) in LDL cholesterol with statin versus placebo (22 trials) or more- versus less-intensive statin (5 trials) was associated with 21% reduction in major vascular events over median follow-up of 4.9 years, with significant risk reductions in all-cause mortality (10%) driven by reduction in vascular mortality (12%), major coronary events (23%), coronary revascularization (24%), and stroke (15%), with no effect on incident cancer or cancer mortality.[67] The relative risk reductions were similar for primary or secondary prevention populations, although individuals from primary prevention had lower absolute risks and hence lower absolute benefits. Similar results were obtained from a Cochrane meta-analysis of 18 randomized trials of statin versus placebo on 56,934 individuals from primary prevention, with 14% relative risk reduction in all-cause mortality and 25% reduction in vascular events.

Some have expressed concern that low LDL cholesterol could impair health. However, the meta-analysis of more than 170,000 patients treated with statins has shown long-term treatment with statins to be safe with low risk of clinically relevant adverse effects and no increase in cancer incidence or non-cardiovascular mortality in patients treated to very low LDL cholesterol with statins or non-statins.[67]

HDL Cholesterol

Prospective epidemiologic data demonstrate a strong inverse relationship between HDL cholesterol and cardiovascular risk. In general, observational data suggest that each 1 mg/dL higher increment in HDL cholesterol is associated with approximately 2% to 3% lower risk of total cardiovascular disease, in particular for coronary events. Some recent studies suggest that very high HDL cholesterol may paradoxically associate with increased risk, although whether this is related to HDL or due to confounding by comorbidities such as alcohol or other factors remains unclear and more evidence is needed. HDL cholesterol (along with total cholesterol) is included in global risk prediction algorithms, and the ratio of total to HDL cholesterol as well as non-HDL cholesterol (total minus HDL cholesterol) are among the most potent lipid-based predictors of cardiovascular risk. Most observational and clinical trials studies have measured HDL cholesterol based on the reference method of ultracentrifugation/precipitation, with HDL defined as the lipoprotein fraction in the density range of 1.063 to 1.21 g/mL. Like LDL cholesterol, this is an "operational" definition for HDL cholesterol.[31] Currently, most clinical laboratories measure HDL cholesterol using direct assays which can have substantial error depending on the type of assay, especially in dyslipidemic samples.[31]

While HDL cholesterol strongly and inversely indicates cardiovascular risk, this has not translated into clinical benefit. Mendelian randomization studies suggest that HDL cholesterol *per se* is not causally associated with cardiovascular disease, but this is complicated by the strong inverse correlations between HDL cholesterol and atherogenic particles, in particular the triglyceride-rich lipoproteins.[14] Large-scale clinical trials have found no evidence that increasing HDL cholesterol reduces clinical events and in some cases have carried a suggestion of harm.[14] In the Randomized Evaluation of the Effects of Anacetrapib Through Lipid Modification (REVEAL) trial, cholesteryl ester transfer inhibition with anacetrapib increased HDL cholesterol by twofold, but the modest clinical benefit (9% relative risk reduction) may have been due to the concomitant modest reduction in atherogenic particles.[68]

Given the extreme heterogeneity of HDL structure and function, measuring only the cholesterol content of HDL will, at best, only partially reflect the potential role of HDL in cardiovascular risk assessment and therapeutic drug development. This has led to interest in developing HDL metrics and targets that might better indicate the atheroprotective functions of HDL. Proposed measurements include HDL particle number (HDL-p), average size, subclasses, functional assays (efflux, anti-inflammatory function, anti-glycemic, etc.), and the HDL lipidome or proteome. Of the alternate HDL metrics, the concentration of HDL particles (HDL-p) and efflux function have shown the most promise to date in cardiovascular prevention. Data from the Multi-Ethnic Study of Atherosclerosis and the placebo arm of JUPITER showed that HDL cholesterol is no longer predictive of cardiovascular disease after adjusting for HDL-p; on the other hand, HDL-p remained inversely associated with cardiovascular disease after adjusting for HDL cholesterol or efflux function.[69] More research is needed to better understand the impact of therapies that alter HDL function or structure beyond HDL cholesterol.

Triglycerides

Plasma triglycerides are primarily produced in the intestines (where dietary triglycerides rapidly enter the circulation within circulating chylomicrons) and within the liver (where triglycerides assembled from de novo synthesized fatty acids are secreted in VLDL) (see Chapter 27). Elevated triglyceride concentrations associate with increased risk of cardiovascular disease, and serve as a marker of the triglyceride-rich lipoproteins (e.g., remnant/VLDL cholesterol). While some studies found independent associations for triglycerides with cardiovascular disease risk, a meta-analysis of 68 prospective studies (>300,000 individuals) found that the association of triglycerides with cardiovascular risk was lost after adjusting for non-HDL cholesterol or apoB. Genetic studies support the causality of the association between plasma triglycerides and cardiovascular risk, but many genetic variants are pleiotropic, and often also associate with differences in VLDL/remnant cholesterol, apoB, or HDL cholesterol, making it challenging to identify the causal atherogenic component. In a meta-analysis of recent trials ($N = 374{,}358$ from 25 statin trials and 24 nonstatin trials), triglyceride lowering is associated with lower cardiovascular risk (approximately 15% lower risk per 1 mmol/L reduction in triglycerides), which was somewhat lower than for LDL cholesterol (approximately 20% lower risk per 1 mmol/L reduction in LDL cholesterol).[70]

Hypertriglyceridemia is multifactorial arising from the interaction of genetic and nongenetic factors. Plasma triglycerides are usually mildly to moderately elevated in patients with insulin resistance, metabolic syndrome, or diabetes, who often have abdominal obesity and poor lifestyle. Severe elevation in triglycerides often reflects the combination of lifestyle (unhealthful diet, inadequate physical activity) on a background susceptibility of multiple genetic defects.[71] Therefore, treatment is based first on lifestyle modifications, including weight reduction in overweight individuals, limiting alcohol intake, reducing caloric intake, increasing exercise, and withdrawal of hormones (estrogens and progesterone or anabolic steroids). Primary causes of hypertriglyceridemia (see Table 27.5) include the rare monogenic syndromes in several genes related to the regulation of lipoprotein lipase activity, and the much more common polygenic or multifactorial cases, which could include contributions from rare heterozygote variants in these genes and/or other common variants associated with elevated triglycerides. Genetic screening of siblings of patients with monogenic disorders is mandated.[71]

Recent guidelines have shifted to measuring nonfasting or fasting lipids for general risk screening or assessment.[11,14,31,61] Nonfasting triglycerides are associated equally or more strongly with cardiovascular endpoints than fasting levels.[61] Guidelines consider nonfasting triglycerides ≥ 2 mmol/L (175 mg/dL) as abnormal, while for fasting triglycerides the corresponding level is ≥ 1.7 mmol/L (150 mg/dL).[11,14,61] The 2018 and 2019 AHA/ACC guidelines consider fasting or nonfasting triglycerides greater than 175 mg/dL as a risk-enhancing factor that could prompt consideration for initiating or intensifying statin therapy.[4,11] There are some differences in the guideline cut points for severe hypertriglyceridemia, defined as fasting triglycerides ≥ 500 mg/dL (5.7 mmol/L) in US guidelines[11] and greater than 10 mmol/L (885 mg/dL) in European guidelines.[14] Guidelines recommend using non-HDL cholesterol or apoB instead of calculated LDL cholesterol in patients with hypertriglyceridemia, as direct LDL cholesterol assays may also be inaccurate.[31]

Current guidelines do not establish a target value for triglycerides, and pharmacologic triglyceride reduction is not broadly recommended other than for patients at high risk for pancreatitis. Dietary measures (in particular reducing saturated fats and refined carbohydrates), exercise, and weight reduction are recommended for lowering triglycerides, together with avoidance of estrogens or other medications that raise triglycerides. Agents for reducing triglycerides include n-3 fatty acid supplements (see section on n-3 fatty acids) and fibrates, which moderately reduce triglycerides. Fibrates are weak peroxisome proliferator-activated receptor (PPAR)-α agonists and reduce triglycerides by approximately 25% to 50% depending on baseline levels, but in 2016 the US Food and Drug Administration withdrew its earlier approval for fenofibric acid with statins to treat dyslipidemia, citing the lack of efficacy in randomized trials (e.g., the Fenofibrate Intervention and Event Lowering in Diabetes [FIELD] and the Action to Control Cardiovascular Risk in Diabetes [ACCORD trials]). Meta-analysis of these trials also found no cardiovascular or mortality benefit overall.[72] Subgroup analyses suggested cardiovascular benefit among patients with high triglycerides and low HDL cholesterol, an issue not yet addressed prospectively in a large endpoint-driven trial. Nicotinic acid (niacin) is no longer approved in Europe or the United States after two large, randomized trials showed no benefit and an increase in adverse events.

Novel biological agents for triglyceride lowering are being evaluated (see Chapter 27) and include therapies that target genes critical in the regulation of triglyceride-rich lipoproteins, such as apoCIII, lipoprotein lipase, angiopoietin-like protein 3 (ANGPTL3), or selective peroxisome proliferator-activated receptor modulators (SPPARMs). No short-term safety signals have been noted with these agents, but long-term safety and efficacy assessment is ongoing. Volanesorsen is an apoCIII inhibitor used for familial hyperchylomicronemia syndrome as an adjunct to diet and reduces triglycerides by 70%. Evinacumab is a monoclonal anti-ANGPTL3 antibody that binds circulating ANGPTL3 to form immune complexes. This augments plasma lipase activity, reducing triglycerides (approximately 50% to 75%).[73] Pemafibrate is a novel potent SPPARM that reduces triglycerides by up to 45% in patients with diabetes and hypertriglyceridemia, in addition to reducing non-HDL cholesterol and remnant cholesterol, apoB and apoCIII, and increasing HDL cholesterol, without significant effect on LDL cholesterol. In short-term studies, it appears well tolerated with a safety profile similar to fenofibrate. PROMINENT (Pemafibrate to Reduce Cardiovascular Outcomes by Reducing Triglycerides in Patients With Diabetes) is an international phase 3 randomized placebo-controlled trial in approximately 10,000 patients (two thirds with prior cardiovascular disease) with type 2 diabetes and mild to moderate hypertriglyceridemia (2.26 to 5.64 mmol/L, or 200 to 499 mg/dL) and low HDL cholesterol (≤1.03 mmol/L or 40 mg/dL) that is evaluating efficacy of pemafibrate on a background of statin therapy in reducing cardiovascular events.[74]

Alternative Lipid Measures

LIPOPROTEIN(a). Lipoprotein(a) [Lp(a)] comprises a class of circulating lipoprotein particles composed of a single copy of apoB covalently linked to an apolipoprotein(a) molecule that varies in length due to genetically mediated kringle-IV type 2 copy number variation. Individuals with higher numbers of kringle IV type 2 repeats have lower circulating lipoprotein(a) levels. Lp(a) likely contributes to cardiovascular disease through multiple mechanisms including pro-atherogenic, pro-inflammatory, and pro-thrombotic effects. Abundant prospective epidemiologic data link elevated Lp(a) levels to increased risk of myocardial infarction, stroke, and aortic valve calcification and stenosis, but not consistently with venous thromboembolism.[75] Both mendelian randomization and genome-wide association studies have made a strong argument that lipoprotein(a), largely mediated through polymorphism in the *LPA* gene, plays a causal role in these disorders.

HOMOCYSTEINE. Homocysteine is a sulfhydryl-containing amino acid derived from the demethylation of dietary methionine. In patients with rare inherited defects of methionine metabolism, severe hyperhomocysteinemia (plasma levels >100 mmol/L) can develop; such patients have greatly elevated risk for premature atherothrombosis as well as venous thromboembolism. Mechanisms that may account for these effects include endothelial dysfunction, accelerated oxidation of LDL cholesterol, impairment of flow-mediated endothelium-derived relaxing factor with subsequent reduction in arterial vasodilation, platelet activation, and oxidative stress. By contrast, mild to moderate hyperhomocysteinemia (plasma levels >15 mmol/L) is common, primarily due to insufficient dietary intake of folic acid.

Polymorphism in the methylene tetrahydrofolate reductase gene (*MTHFR*) that encodes a thermolabile protein is also linked to homocysteine metabolism. The *MTHFR* polymorphism, however, appears to have marginal clinical importance as heterozygous persons display little evidence of elevated homocysteine levels and only a modest increase in atherosclerotic risk. Because folate supplementation is crucial in the general population to reduce the risk of neural tube defects, screening for *MTHFR* has little utility in settings where fortification exists, such as in North America. Fortification of the food supply has also reduced the frequency of low folate and elevated homocysteine levels. Finally, a series of randomized trials of homocysteine lowering have failed to show reduction in myocardial infarction or mortality, including in a trial of patients with advanced kidney disease, with a Cochrane meta-analysis finding at most a potentially small reduction in stroke.[76] For all of these reasons, screening for homocysteine has greatly decreased in preventive cardiology practice.

High-Sensitivity C-Reactive Protein and Other Biomarkers of Inflammation (see Chapter 10)

Inflammation characterizes all phases of the atherothrombotic process and provides a critical pathophysiologic link between plaque formation and acute rupture, leading to occlusion and infarction. Inflammatory cytokines such as interleukin (IL)-1 implicated in atherogenesis and activated by the NLRP3 inflammasome, elicit the expression of the messenger cytokine IL-6, which can travel from local sites of inflammation to the liver and change the program of protein synthesis to produce the acute-phase response.[77]

In clinical practice, the best-studied and most easily applied biomarker of this inflammatory process is the downstream acute-phase reactant CRP. More than 80 prospective cohorts in primary prevention, secondary prevention, and post-acute coronary syndrome indicate that CRP, when measured with high-sensitivity assays (hsCRP), independently predicts risk of myocardial infarction, stroke, peripheral artery disease, and sudden cardiac death, even when LDL cholesterol levels are low.[78] In comprehensive meta-analyses, the multivariable hazard associated with hsCRP resembles in magnitude of risk to blood pressure or hyperlipidemia, and hsCRP yields an incremental increase in C-statistic virtually identical in magnitude to that of total and HDL cholesterol.

Based on JUPITER and other studies, current US guidelines consider hsCRP ≥2 mg/L as a risk-enhancing factor that could be used in global risk evaluation, in particular when statin decision making is otherwise uncertain (borderline- or intermediate-risk individuals),[4,11] while hsCRP levels of less than 1 mg/L are lower risk. Values of hsCRP in excess of 8 mg/L may represent an acute-phase response caused by an underlying inflammatory disease or intercurrent infection and should lead to repeat testing in approximately 2 to 3 weeks. Because hsCRP levels are otherwise stable over long periods of time, exhibit minimal circadian variation, and do not depend on prandial state, outpatients can undergo screening at the cholesterol evaluation.

Levels of hsCRP correlate only modestly with underlying atherosclerotic disease as measured by carotid intima media thickness or by coronary calcification. This observation suggests that hsCRP does not simply reflect the presence of subclinical disease but indicates an increased propensity for plaque disruption and/or thrombosis. Autopsy data support this hypothesis: elevated hsCRP levels are more common in patients with frankly ruptured plaques than in those with erosive disease or those who died of nonvascular causes. Elevated levels of hsCRP predict not only cardiovascular events but also the onset of type 2 diabetes, perhaps because hsCRP levels correlate with several components of the metabolic syndrome, including those not easily measured in clinical practice such as insulin sensitivity, endothelial dysfunction, and impaired fibrinolysis.

In primary prevention, diet, exercise, and smoking cessation are the first-line interventions for those with elevated hsCRP, as with elevated LDL cholesterol or other risk factors. At a minimum, an elevated hsCRP should provide considerable motivation to improve lifestyle, particularly for those previously told that they were not at risk because of an absence of hyperlipidemia.

The large-scale multinational JUPITER trial demonstrated that statin therapy, previously shown to lower hsCRP levels independent of LDL cholesterol lowering, markedly reduces vascular event rates among apparently healthy men and women with hsCRP ≥2 mg/L and LDL cholesterol less than 130 mg/dL. In JUPITER, random allocation to rosuvastatin 20 mg daily as compared to placebo resulted in a 44% lower risk of the trial primary endpoint of all vascular events, a 54% reduction in myocardial infarction, a 48% reduction in stroke, a 46% reduction in need for arterial revascularization, and a 20% reduction in all-cause mortality. All prespecified subgroups within JUPITER significantly benefited from statin therapy, including women, nonsmokers, those without metabolic syndrome, and those with low global risk scores. In an additional prespecified analysis, rosuvastatin reduced incident venous thromboembolism by 43%, a result with clinical relevance and an important observation regarding pleiotropic effects of statin therapy. The JUPITER trial also demonstrated that achieving low levels of both LDL cholesterol and hsCRP after the initiation of statin therapy greatly maximizes clinical benefits, an observation corroborated in the IMPROVE-IT trial of ezetimibe combined with simvastatin.

In demonstrating that individuals with elevated levels of hsCRP but low levels of LDL cholesterol markedly benefit from statins, JUPITER influenced clinical guidelines and resulted in much wider use of statin therapy. However, by using a statin—an LDL-lowering drug with concomitant anti-inflammatory effects—JUPITER was not a formal test of the inflammation hypothesis of atherothrombosis. That evidence arose from the Canakinumab Anti-inflammatory Thrombosis Outcomes Study (CANTOS) which provided direct proof-of-principle that inflammation inhibition in the absence of lipid lowering can significantly reduce cardiovascular event rates.[79] Among 10,061 stable atherosclerosis patients with residual inflammatory risk who were already on statin therapy, those allocated to higher doses of canakinumab—a monoclonal antibody that binds IL-1β—experienced a 15% reduction in major adverse cardiovascular events when compared to a placebo. CANTOS helped to define the inflammatory pathway from IL-1 to IL-6 to CRP as a target for atheroprotection, with the magnitude of clinical benefit for individual patients tracking with the degree of inflammation inhibition as assessed by on-treatment levels of both IL-6 and CRP. CANTOS also implicated the IL-18 pathway and by proxy the upstream NLRP3 inflammasome as therapeutic targets in atherosclerosis.[80] Canakinumab treatment in CANTOS is associated with a small but significant risk in infections, including fatal infections, counterbalanced by a decrease in cancer mortality.

In contrast, the Cardiovascular Inflammation Reduction Trial (CIRT) of 4786 stable atherosclerosis patients with diabetes or metabolic syndrome reported that low-dose methotrexate did not reduce major adverse cardiovascular events.[81] Yet, low-dose methotrexate also failed to reduce plasma levels of IL-1β, IL-6, or CRP. As such, in the context of CANTOS, CIRT can be viewed as providing informative neutral data supporting the concept that adequate inhibition of the IL-1β to IL-6 pathway of innate immunity is necessary to secure long-term cardiovascular benefits.

Subsequently, the Colchicine Cardiovascular Outcomes Trial (COLCOT) and the Low Dose Colchicine 2 trial (LoDoCo2) provided independent affirmation of the inflammation hypothesis of atherosclerosis using the anti-inflammatory agent colchicine in patients post myocardial infarction.[82,83] Colchicine is an anti-mitotic agent that inhibits tubulin polymerization and microtubule generation. As a consequence, part of colchicine's anti-inflammatory effect may derive in part from its ability to inhibit NLRP3 inflammasome assembly and thus indirectly reduce IL-1β activation leading to downstream reductions in both IL-6 and CRP. Colchicine has shown efficacy to treat and prevent classical inflammasome/IL-1β activation disorders including gout and familial Mediterranean fever. In COLCOT, treatment with colchicine 0.5 mg daily as compared to placebo over a 2-year period among 4745 post-myocardial infarction patients resulted in a 23% relative reduction in the primary trial endpoint inclusive of myocardial infarction, stroke, resuscitated cardiac arrest, urgent hospitalization for angina leading to revascularization, and cardiovascular death. While the benefit of colchicine was significant only for the coronary revascularization and stroke components of this primary endpoint, all cardiovascular outcomes were directionally consistent, providing reassurance. Further, effects in COLCOT were of greater magnitude in analyses including all post-randomization cardiovascular events as well as first events. These benefits came with modest risk as colchicine was associated with increases in pneumonia and nausea. In LoDoCo2, colchicine 0.5 mg as compared to placebo among 5522 patients with stable coronary disease resulted in a similar 28% relative reduction in major recurrent adverse cardiovascular events. Rates of coronary revascularization and coronary death were also reduced although no reduction in all-cause mortality was observed. Subsequent analyses of LoDoCo2 have shown anticipated reductions in both hsCRP and IL-6, as previously shown in CANTOS.

By contrast to canakinumab, colchicine is widely available and relatively inexpensive. Thus, if benefit is confirmed in other ongoing trials such as the Clear Synergy trials, colchicine could provide an important adjunctive therapy for high-risk atherosclerosis patients. Due to renal excretion, chronic use of colchicine may be contraindicated for those with advanced kidney dysfunction. At high doses or in the setting of inadvertent overdose, colchicine toxicity can be a "fatal masquerader."

CANTOS, CIRT, COLCOT, and LoCoCo2 have stimulated considerable interest in several novel anti-inflammatory and anti-cytokine agents that also target the NLRP3 to IL-1 to IL-6 to CRP pathway (Fig. 25.7).[84] These will likely include direct upstream inhibitors of the NLRP3 inflammasome (which would additionally lower IL-18 activation) as well as inhibitors of IL-6 signaling. IL-6 is widely seen as the central mediator of the pro-inflammatory atherosclerotic response and a probable causal target based upon mendelian randomization analyses. At least one anti-IL-6 monoclonal antibody, ziltivekimab, is being developed specifically for atherothrombotic applications.[84a] At this time, the use of any targeted anti-inflammatory agent (including colchicine) should be considered only as an adjunct to statin therapy in high-risk, secondary prevention patients.

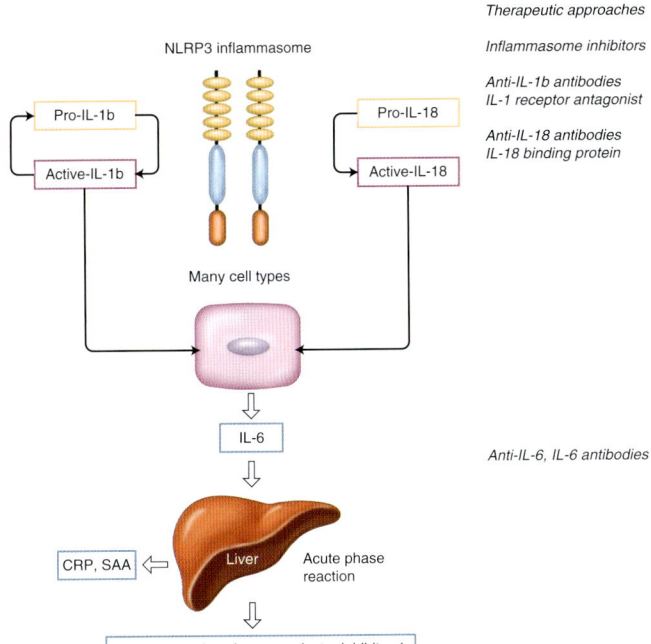

FIGURE 25.7 Potential therapeutic targets in the NLRP3 inflammasome to interleukin-1 to interleukin-6 to C-reactive protein (CRP) signaling pathway. In response to various pro-inflammatory stimuli and crystalline structures (including cholesterol crystals), the proteinase caspase-1 contained in the NLRP3 inflammasome cleaves pro-interleukin-18 and pro-interleukin-1β into activated interleukin-18 and interleukin1β, triggering robust pro-inflammatory signaling through interleukin-6. Interleukin-18, interleukin-1β, and interleukin-6 have direct vascular effects while interleukin-6 also induces the acute phase response and concomitant hepatic production of CRP. CRP, when measured with high-sensitivity assays (hsCRP), is used in clinical practice as a biomarker to detect inflammatory risk. Yellow boxes indicate targets of this signaling pathway and, where available, approved agents that potentially could be repurposed as vascular therapeutics. NLRP3 inflammasome, NOD-like receptor family pyrin domain containing 3 inflammasome; IL-18, interleukin-18; IL-6, interleukin-6; IL-1β, interleukin-1β; IL-1βmAB, interleukin-1β monoclonal antibody; IL-1 TRAP, dimeric fusion protein of an interleukin-1 receptor component and an IL-1 receptor accessory protein; IL-1Ra, interleukin-1 receptor antagonist. (From Libby P, et al. Drugs targeting inflammation. In Bhatt DL, ed. *Opie's Cardiovascular Drugs: A Companion to Braunwald's Heart Disease*. 9th ed. Elsevier; 2021.)

Beyond hsCRP, other inflammatory biomarkers may have a role in the future of preventive cardiology. During chronic inflammation, inflammatory proteins not only experience changes in circulatory concentrations but also in their glycan structure, leading to modifications in the interaction with receptors and changes in their function, and glycans serve in various essential cellular mechanisms and molecular pathways, including cytokines and inflammatory pathways.[85] Post-translational modifications of proteins via enzymatic regulation of glycans have been explored to identify new biomarkers of cardiovascular development and progression. GlycA as well as IgG glycan signatures have shown promising results, with risk associations that were additive or independent of hsCRP.[86,87] Studies have shown that IgG galactosylation and sialylation are strongly associated with hsCRP levels and poor metabolic health.[88] In addition, IL-6 provides additive information on vascular risk after adjustment for hsCRP. By contrast, in another contemporary study, hsCRP remained significantly associated with risk regardless of atherogenic lipids level or pooled cohort risk. Considerable promise has also been reported for the neutrophil-to-lymphocyte ratio. Other inflammatory biomarkers, such as the IL-1 family member ST2, myeloperoxidase, sICAM-1, sCD40, fibrinogen, and Lp-PLA2 have generally not shown additional benefits beyond hsCRP and are not recommended in current guidelines. Trials of targeted phospholipase inhibitors failed to reduce vascular event rates.

In cardiovascular practice, three times as many patients have "residual inflammatory risk" defined as a post-statin LDL cholesterol less than 70 mg/dL but an hsCRP greater than 2 mg/L than have "residual cholesterol risk" defined as a post-statin LDL cholesterol greater than 70 mg/dL and an hsCRP less than 2 mg/L. In the setting of suspected acute coronary syndrome, a recent analysis of over 100,000 patients continues to demonstrate that hsCRP predicts mortality beyond that of troponin.[89] The movement of "residual inflammatory risk" into clinical practice as a distinct concept beyond "residual cholesterol risk" has helped to open cardiovascular disease prevention to several novel pathways with the potential for atheroprotection.

CARDIOVASCULAR PREVENTION IN WOMEN (SEE CHAPTER 91)

Although cardiovascular disease mortality has declined in the United States and other high-income countries over the past several decades, cardiovascular disease remains the leading cause of death in women and men in the United States, with greater than 1 in 4 women dying of cardiovascular disease, similar to cardiovascular mortality in men.[1] The age-adjusted rate of cardiovascular disease DALYs has improved over the past three decades but the improvement has lagged in women compared with men in all 50 US states. Women also suffer from a disproportionate rate of death from stroke, in particular after age 65 years.[1] As a result of increasing longevity and large population sizes, cardiovascular mortality rates for older women in low- and middle-income countries are twice as high compared with women in high-income countries, and account for more than 80% of cardiovascular deaths in women.

Sex (biological) and gender (sociocultural) differences in cardiovascular risk are multifactorial and arise from differences in the pathophysiology, incidence, and clinical manifestations of cardiovascular disease, prevalence and sequelae of cardiovascular risk factors, response to treatments, adverse reactions, and risk factor control.[90] Many cardiovascular risk factors are associated differentially with sex and gender. Current cardiovascular risk scores, including the PCE equations, are sex-specific, with separate equations for women and men and for African Americans and whites. These risk scores, and many others, do not incorporate female-specific risk factors. To address this limitation, recent guidelines in the United States have added two female-specific factors (premature menopause and preeclampsia) as risk-enhancing factors that could guide treatment decisions regarding statin initiation or intensification for primary prevention of cardiovascular disease.[4,11] Additional risk-enhancing factors include systemic inflammatory conditions, such as autoimmune collagen-vascular disease (lupus, rheumatoid arthritis), which predominate in women.

Compared with men, women have a steeper rise in blood pressure that starts in young adulthood, and a greater lifetime burden of hypertension, which becomes more common in women than men after age 65 years. The adverse long-term sequelae of hypertension (e.g., left ventricular hypertrophy, concentric remodeling, reduced longitudinal strain, heart failure with preserved ejection fraction) are also more common in women than men, yet women are undertreated to goal, in particular for African Americans, Asian Americans, and Hispanic Americans. Diabetes carries greater cardiovascular risk for women compared with men, yet women are often undertreated for diabetes compared with men. Smoking, obesity, and psychosocial factors also carry greater cardiovascular risk in women than men. Furthermore, obesity, physical inactivity, and depression are more common in women than men. Lifestyle interventions and evidence-based preventive therapies including statins, antihypertensive medications, and glucose-modifying medications, benefit women and men to a similar degree. Yet women are less likely to be treated (e.g., statins, aspirin) or achieve goals (e.g., antihypertensive therapy) or receive referral to cardiac rehabilitation programs.[90]

Premature Menopause and Pregnancy-Associated Conditions (see Chapters 91 and 92)

A comprehensive pregnancy history should be obtained as part of the cardiovascular risk assessment for women, as pregnancy-related risk factors are early indicators of a woman's future cardiovascular risk. This is particularly relevant for younger women in whom global risk scores based on traditional risk factors are often low risk. The two recently added two risk-enhancing factors specific for women, specifically premature menopause (<40 years old) and preeclampsia (elevated blood pressure and proteinuria after 20 weeks of gestation), increase cardiovascular risk to a similar extent as standard risk factors.[4,11]

While the guidelines emphasize premature menopause and preeclampsia as risk-enhancing factors, other pregnancy-related cardiovascular risk factors include hypertensive disorders of pregnancy (gestational hypertension [blood pressure >140/90 mm Hg on two separate occasions after 20 weeks of gestation]), HELLP syndrome (hemolysis, elevated liver function tests, low platelets), gestational diabetes, preterm delivery, and having a small for gestational age infant. Hypertensive disorders of pregnancy also increase the risk for peripartum cardiomyopathy and future risk of hypertension, heart failure, and valvular disease.[91] Other conditions that carry increased risk of subclinical atherosclerosis and cardiovascular disease include premature menarche (≤10 years), polycystic ovarian syndrome (excess androgens, ovulatory dysfunction, and polycystic ovaries), or recurrent (2 or more) spontaneous pregnancy loss.[90,91]

Menopause and Postmenopausal Hormone Therapy

Age-specific coronary heart disease death rates in women lag approximately 10 years behind those of men, and this risk increases after either natural or surgical menopause. Premature menopause (<40 years old) is now considered a risk-enhancing factor. This increased risk after menopause may be related to adverse changes in lipids (increases in LDL cholesterol and triglycerides, and a decrease in HDL cholesterol), glucose metabolism (an increase in glucose intolerance), and changes in hemostatic factors and vascular function.

Although non-randomized observational studies among women who began hormone therapy around the time of menopause consistently suggested coronary heart disease benefits of hormone replacement therapy, the randomized trial data demonstrated that estrogen and progestin replacement does not confer cardiovascular protection, especially among older women. In the Women's Health Initiative (WHI) trial, one arm included 16,608 postmenopausal women, 50 to 79 years of age, with an intact uterus and evaluated the combined hormone therapy of conjugated estrogen plus medroxyprogesterone acetate versus placebo.[92] The active hormone arm had significantly increased risk of coronary heart disease, stroke, venous thromboembolism, and breast cancer, exceeding the benefits on reductions of fracture and colon cancer. Two years later, the unopposed estrogen versus placebo arm of the WHI, which included 10,739 generally healthy postmenopausal women 50 to 79 years of age without a uterus, also was halted early because of an increased risk of stroke, particularly in subjects 60 years of age or older, in the absence of net health benefits. Subgroup analyses of the WHI trial data raised a number of unanswered questions about the role of estrogens and other hormones in the biology and etiology of cardiovascular disease and suggested that age, the presence of cardiovascular risk factors, and time since menopause may modulate the effect of estrogen on cardiovascular risk. The WHI provided clear evidence that postmenopausal hormone therapy did not prevent coronary disease in women who started treatment distant from menopause onset (>10 years). Long-term observational follow-up of the WHI participants found no increase in mortality from either intervention during a follow-up of 18 years.[92] The question remains as to whether estrogen therapy initiated close to menopause onset may reduce coronary heart disease risk (see Chapter 91). Because of its risks, many professional organizations have recommended against (class III) the use of hormone therapy at any age to prevent coronary heart disease and other chronic diseases.

LIFESTYLE FACTORS AND INTERVENTIONS

Nutrition and Diet (see Chapters 29 and 30)

Dietary factors have an important impact on risk of coronary heart disease, stroke, neurocognitive health, hypertensive disorders, diabetes, lipids, obesity, and many types of cancer. Poor diet is a major challenge for prevention of cardiovascular disease. Overall, dietary quality has improved over the past three decades, but diet quality varies substantially across the world, with better diet quality in Mediterranean countries and worse quality in Eastern and Northern Europe, Central Asia, and the South Pacific.[93] Diet was the leading risk factor for causes of death in the United States.[94] Diet accounted for more than half a million US deaths in 2016 alone, with the vast majority (84%) of these deaths due to cardiovascular disease.[94] Compared with other risk factors, diet was the leading contributor to worse cardiovascular disease DALYs and the third leading contributor to overall DALYs. The majority of the US population eats a diet that is low in fruits, vegetables, whole grains, and unsaturated oils, and high in sugar, refined grains, red meat, and processed meat.

The 2015 and the 2020 Dietary Guidelines Committees[95] emphasize healthful dietary patterns (e.g., a healthy Mediterranean-style pattern, a healthy US-style pattern, and a healthy vegetarian pattern). The Dietary Guidelines, along with the companion website (Choose My Plate), offer evidence-based nutrition education and practical tutorials for patients and clinicians. Common to these three recommended dietary patterns is the emphasis on greater intake of fruits, vegetables, other plant foods such as beans and nuts, and in many patterns, whole grains and fish; with more limited or occasional dairy products; and limiting red meats or processed meats and fewer refined carbohydrates and other processed foods. These patterns conform to the food-based priorities for cardiovascular health that include foods that are higher in dietary fiber, healthy fatty acids, vitamins, antioxidants, potassium, other minerals, and phytochemicals, and lower in refined carbohydrates, sugars, salt, saturated fatty acids, dietary cholesterol, and trans fats. A dietary approach that uses single foods or nutrients as dietary supplements in the prevention of disease neglects the complexity of overall diet and its relationship with risk. In contrast, the dietary pattern approach overcomes these limitations by capturing individual and combined effects among a variety of foods that comprise the dietary pattern.

In addition, data from meta-analysis of small randomized trials, supported by prospective observational studies, show that replacing dietary saturated fat with unsaturated fat (mostly polyunsaturated fat from soybean oil) reduced cardiovascular events by approximately 30%.[96,97] These trials included both primary prevention and patients post myocardial infarction and were conducted mostly before the statin era when cholesterol levels were higher, but the trials did show reductions in LDL cholesterol that could explain the concomitant reduction in cardiovascular events. In contrast, replacing saturated fat with carbohydrates (in particular refined carbohydrates) does not reduce cardiovascular events. Reducing *total* dietary fat however is not recommended by current guidelines.[96]

The AHA's Life's Simple 7 includes healthy diet as one of the simple 7 cardiovascular health metrics, with an ideal diet defined as 4 to 5 components (and poor diet one or less) of the following five diet elements: (1) 4.5 cups or more of fruits and vegetables per day, (2) two or more 3.5-oz servings of fish per week, (3) three servings per day of whole grains, (4) less than 1500 mg of sodium per day, and (5) 36 ounces or less of sugar-sweetened beverages per week. Yet despite some studies showing modest improvement recently in the consumption of sugar-sweetened beverages, poor diet remains the most prevalent risk behavior, compared with other cardiovascular health metrics.

Low-Risk Populations

The US Preventive Services Task Force conducted a systematic review among adults without known cardiovascular disease and not at high cardiovascular risk (without traditional risk factors) and identified four trials (total *N* = 51,356) of high-intensity diet interventions in relation to all-cause or cardiovascular mortality.[98] Compared with controls, healthful diet interventions resulted in favorable outcomes in several intermediate risk factors over a period of 6 months or more, with dose-response effects for blood pressure (−1.3 mm Hg mean reduction in systolic blood pressure, 22 trials), LDL cholesterol (−2.6 mg/dL mean reduction in LDL cholesterol, 13 trials), and adiposity (−0.4 BMI mean reduction, −1.2 cm waist circumference mean reduction, 20 trials) with no reductions noted in pooled analyses for HDL cholesterol, triglycerides, or fasting glucose.[98] Very few trials reported longer-term

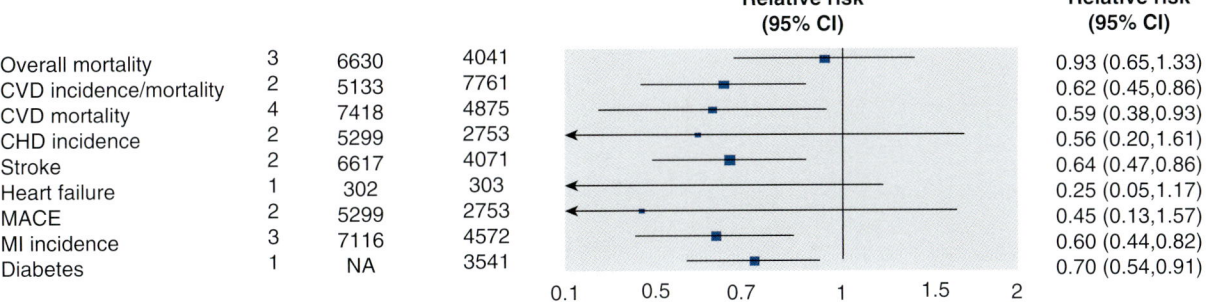

FIGURE 25.8 Umbrella review of meta-analyses on greater than 12.8 million individuals demonstrating that greater adherence to a Mediterranean dietary pattern is associated with risk reductions in cardiovascular mortality and incident cardiovascular events including myocardial infarction and stroke. *CHD,* Coronary heart disease; *CVD,* cardiovascular disease; *MACE,* major adverse cardiovascular events; *MI,* myocardial infarction. (From Dinu M, Pagliai G, Casini A, et al. Mediterranean diet and multiple health outcomes: an umbrella review of meta-analyses of observational studies and randomised trials. *Eur J Clin Nutr.* 2018;72[1]:30–43.)

effects on intermediate outcomes. Over a range of study follow-up periods (3 to 15 years), there were few all-cause deaths in these low-risk populations, and no significant differences between intervention and control groups. These trials included the WHI dietary modification trial (n = 48,835 postmenopausal women, evaluated low-fat diet) and the Trials of Hypertension Prevention Collaborative Research Group (TOHP, N = 2415, evaluated sodium reduction). The TOHP intervention follow-up period was only 18 months and showed reduction in blood pressure with sodium reduction. But long-term (10 to 15 years) observational post-intervention follow-up found significant treatment-related reduction in cardiovascular events (30% relative risk reduction). The WHI dietary modification trial, which examined a low-fat diet (reducing fat intake from baseline of approximately 35% to 20% of total energy, together with increasing intake of fruits and vegetables [to 5 servings/day] and grains [to 6 servings/day]) versus usual care, also found no significant reduction in major cardiovascular events over the trial intervention period of 8.1 years. However, after longer-term observational follow-up of nearly 20 years, in a subgroup analysis of 23,000 women without baseline hypertension or prior cardiovascular disease, there was 15% to 30% treatment-related reduction in coronary events, and a similar reduction in new-onset insulin-dependent diabetes.[99]

High-Risk Populations and Randomized Trials of the Mediterranean Diet

In two randomized controlled trials conducted among higher-risk individuals, Mediterranean dietary pattern interventions significantly lowered risk of cardiovascular events. The Lyon Heart Study was a secondary prevention trial in central, non-Mediterranean France comparing a low-fat diet with a Mediterranean diet which included a margarine high in alpha-linolenic-acid. There were significantly fewer primary cardiovascular events in the Mediterranean diet group (8/302) compared with the control group (33/303). The Mediterranean group changed their entire dietary pattern, specifically increasing intake of fruits, vegetables, legumes, breads, and margarine, and less meat, processed meat, butter, and cream. Limitations of this trial included a very small number of events and early stopping of the trial for benefit but apparently without an *a priori* rule, and a study population of only men post myocardial infarction.

More recently, the Prevención con Dieta Mediterránea (PREDIMED) study was a large-scale primary prevention parallel-group randomized trial conducted in 7447 Spanish men and women at high cardiovascular risk recruited based on cardiovascular risk factors. The study was originally published in 2013, but because of some trial irregularities in the randomization procedures, the study was retracted and republished in 2018.[100] Over a follow-up period of 4.8 years, this trial found that a Mediterranean dietary intervention supplemented either with nuts or extra virgin olive oil compared with a low-fat dietary pattern significantly reduced the primary endpoint of major cardiovascular events by 30% and favorable reduction in other outcomes. PREDIMED was not just a supplementation trial with extra virgin olive oil or nuts, as there was comprehensive dietary modification in the two Mediterranean diet groups with both group and individual participant diet modification training targeting increased intake of fruits, legumes, fish or seafood, and decreased meat or meat products and sweets during the trial. In post-hoc analysis of PREDIMED, higher intake of fruits, vegetables, legumes, fiber, and whole grains and lower intake of red meat and processed meats were associated with lower risk of cardiovascular disease. In an umbrella review of meta-analyses including observational studies and randomized trials (N > 12.8 million individuals), greater adherence to the Mediterranean diet associated with reduced risk of cardiovascular diseases (including myocardial infarction and stroke), cardiovascular mortality, diabetes, and other chronic conditions (Fig. 25.8).[101]

Mechanistic evidence from small-scale clinical studies and from PREDIMED biomarker analyses found that the Mediterranean diet favorably affects multiple cardiovascular risk factors including improving inflammation, insulin resistance and glucose metabolism, hypertension, atherogenic dyslipidemia, and may also have antiarrhythmic properties shown by reductions in sudden cardiac death and atrial fibrillation. The Mediterranean diet supplies abundant polyphenols from extra virgin olive oil, fresh fruit, vegetables, nuts, and legumes which have beneficial effects on blood lipids, oxidative stress, platelet aggregation, and endothelial cell adhesion molecules. Nuts have unsaturated fatty acids, tocopherols, and polyphenols and are associated with lower risk of cardiovascular disease. Whole grains contain vitamins, trace minerals, and phenolic acids, which have beneficial antioxidant and antithrombotic properties. The combined effects from these foods contribute to the effectiveness of the Mediterranean diet pattern in reducing cardiovascular risk.

In the 2019 EAT-Lancet Commission, a leading panel of nutritional experts and scientists proposed a healthy diet from a sustainable food system. The proposed diet shares many foods with the Mediterranean diet and emphasizes vegetables, fruits, whole grains, legumes, nuts, and unsaturated oils, with low to moderate amounts of seafood and poultry, and low or no red meat, processed meat, added sugar, refined grains, and starchy vegetables. They estimated 15% to 30% reductions in cardiovascular risk and approximately 10% reductions in mortality if red meat (1 serving/day) is replaced with other protein sources.[102] The authors estimated that moving the global population to this diet would provide healthy foods for the estimated global population of 10 billion people by 2050, in addition to concomitant large reductions in food losses and waste consistent with the US Sustainable Development Goals.

Alcohol Consumption

The relationships between alcohol consumption, cardiovascular events, and all-cause mortality are complex and recent epidemiologic and genetic data challenge long-held views that low-dose alcohol consumption (≈ 1 drink per day) confers cardioprotection. In view of disparate international guidelines regarding alcohol consumption, it is important to understand the implications of evolving evidence.

Though cultural norms vary widely, mild to moderate alcohol consumption is typically defined as roughly one drink-equivalent per day using as a reference a 12-ounce regular beer (5% alcohol), 5 fluid

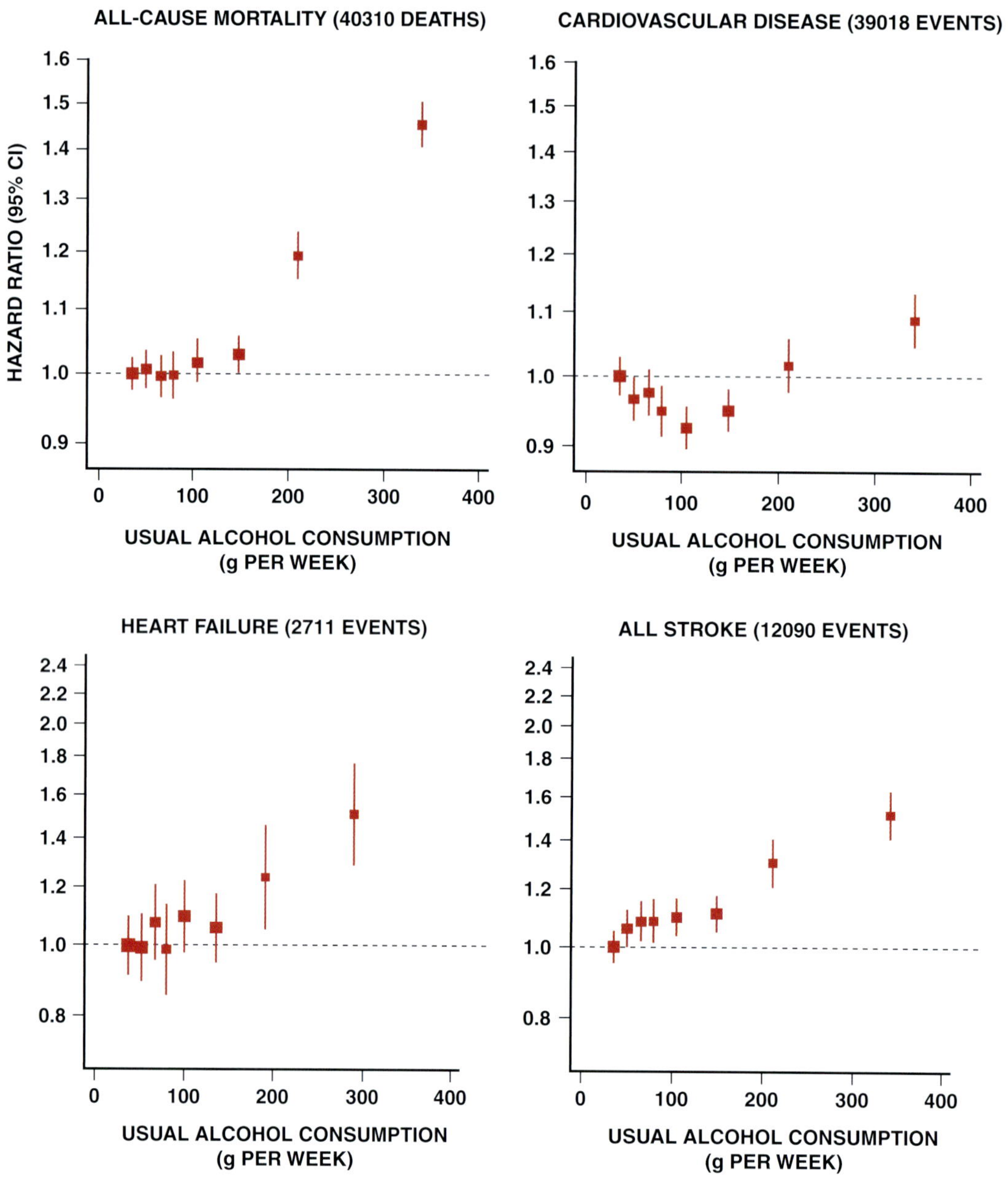

FIGURE 25.9 Relationships of alcohol consumption with all-cause mortality *(upper left)*, cardiovascular disease *(upper right)*, heart failure *(lower left)*, and stroke *(lower right)* among nearly 600,000 participants in 83 prospective studies. (From Wood AM, Kaptoge S, Butterworth AS, et al. Risk thresholds for alcohol consumption: combined analysis of individual-participant data for 599 912 current drinkers in 83 prospective studies. *Lancet.* 2018;391:1513–1523.)

ounces of wine (12% alcohol), or 1.5 fluid ounce of 80-proof distilled spirit (40% alcohol) for an approximate 12 to 14 g of alcohol per beverage. Habitual heavy alcohol consumption, defined as 8 or more drinks per week for women, 15 or more drinks per week for men, or binge drinking for either gender, is a major cause of preventable death. Levels of alcohol consumption at or above these thresholds increase risks of total mortality, cardiovascular mortality, coronary disease, and stroke; fatal traffic accidents; liver damage; harm in pregnancy; risk of developing breast cancer and other tumors in both women and men; and depression and violence. There is no controversy that consumption at these levels is hazardous for health and for all-cause mortality (Fig. 25.9).[103] Binge drinking in particular carries multiple health hazards.

What is newly controversial is whether a biologically informative J-shaped curve exists in the relationship between alcohol consumption and cardiovascular events, and if so, at what level that threshold is. For total cardiovascular disease, most studies show a J-shaped relationship such that risks appear lowest at roughly one alcohol beverage daily.[103] However, some recent work suggests that this overall J-shaped curve for total cardiovascular disease reflects a more complex set of curves that suggest benefit for myocardial infarction, but net hazard for other endpoints such as stroke, heart failure, and cardiovascular deaths. These subtleties may reflect directionally divergent effects of alcohol on specific vascular risk factors, such as an increase in systolic blood pressure (and thus a potential increase in stroke) and a concomitant increase in HDL cholesterol (and thus a potential reduction in myocardial infarction). Recent mendelian randomization studies, themselves disputed, have added to this controversy by challenging the causality of observed relationships.[104]

Given these uncertainties, recommendations related to alcohol consumption as a potential preventive method for overall cardiovascular disease remain complicated. Any individual or public health recommendation must consider the complexity of alcohol's metabolic, physiologic, and psychological effects. Because of the health hazards of alcohol associated with higher intake, moderate alcohol use does not offer a population-based strategy to reduce cardiovascular risk, even for myocardial infarction where epidemiologic data remain consistent. Discussions of alcohol consumption require individual consideration and should take into account other medical problems, coronary risk factors, comorbid conditions, concurrent medications, pregnancy, and family history of alcoholism. Patients who are heavy drinkers should be

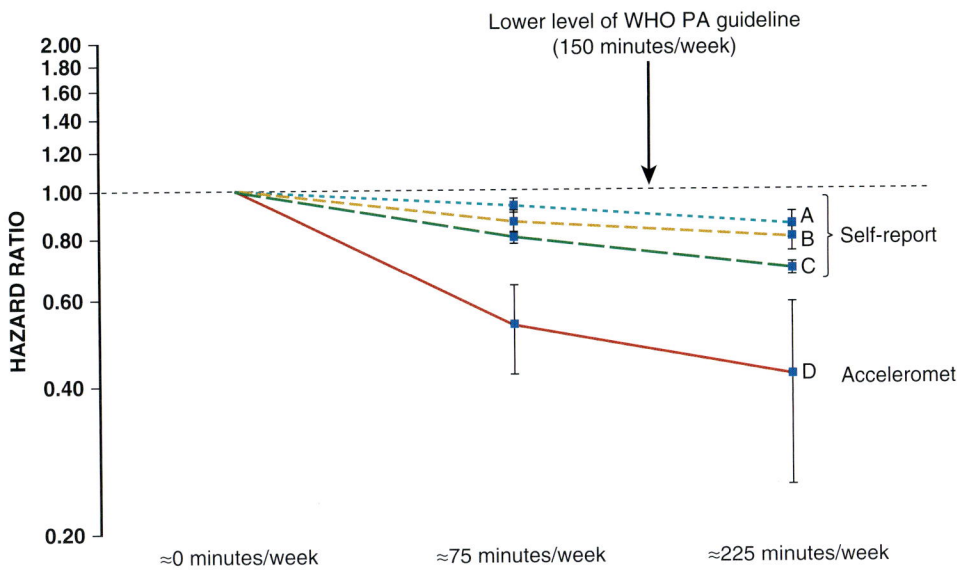

FIGURE 25.10 Physical activity has a curvilinear relation with all-cause mortality as shown by self-reported (*dashed lines*) and accelerometer-assessed (*solid line*) moderate-to-vigorous physical activity. Risk reduction was substantially greater in magnitude when using accelerometer compared with self-reported data, with risk reductions seen at much lower levels of moderate-vigorous physical activity than the recommended minimum of 150 minutes/week. (From Ekelund U, Dalene KE, Tarp J, et al. Physical activity and mortality: what is the dose response and how big is the effect? *Br J Sports Med.* 2020;54[19]:1125–1126.)

counseled to limit intake. The initiation of moderate alcohol consumption is not recommended, especially in view of other known preventive measures, such as dietary discretion, physical activity, lipid and blood pressure control, and smoking cessation.

Physical Activity (see Chapters 32 and 33)

The large body of epidemiologic evidence that has accumulated since the 1950s demonstrates that physical activity unequivocally is associated with health benefits including reduced rates of cardiovascular morbidity and mortality, all-cause and premature mortality, and multiple non-communicable diseases including hypertension, diabetes, depression, dementia, and at least 8 cancers including breast and colorectal cancer. Physical inactivity is a major risk factor for cardiovascular disease, peripheral arterial disease, and heart failure, and meeting guideline-recommended activity levels is one of the AHA LS7 components.[1] Currently there is a global pandemic of physical inactivity. Worldwide, more than 1.4 billion adults have insufficient activity levels, with higher age-standardized prevalence of insufficient activity in women than men (31.7% vs. 23.4%) and high- versus low-income countries (36.8% vs. 16.2%).[105] In the United States, the prevalence of self-reported physical inactivity in adults has decreased over the past decade from 40.2% to 25.9%, but ethnic/racial, socioeconomic, and gender disparities continue, with greater activity levels among educated non-Hispanic white men.[1] At least 10% of deaths could be avoided if guideline-recommended activity levels were met.

The US federal government issued its first-ever physical activity guidelines in 2008 and updated them in 2018, asking adults to do at least 150 to 300 minutes (2.5 to 5 hours) per week of moderate-intensity aerobic physical activity (e.g., brisk walking), or 75 to 150 minutes per week of vigorous aerobic activity (e.g., jogging), or a combination of activities of both intensities that expends an equivalent amount of energy, preferably spread throughout the week.[106,107] In addition, the guidelines recommended muscle-strengthening activities (e.g., push-ups) on 2 or more days per week, as these activities provide additional benefits. New since 2008 is that the updated guidelines no longer require activities to occur for periods of at least 10 minutes' duration, promoting even small increases that do not take 10 minutes. For those persons who do not meet the recommended minimum, the guidelines state encouragingly that *some physical activity is better than none*. Although the guidelines stipulate a total amount of physical activity, spacing of episodes throughout the week may minimize the risk of musculoskeletal injuries. Furthermore, the new guidelines also incorporated growing evidence about the relationship between activity and sedentary behavior, underscoring the dual importance of being more active and sitting less throughout the day.[107–109]

Notable advances in recent years include elucidation of the curvilinear dose-response relation (i.e., what percent risk reduction is associated with different levels of physical activity), as well as research showing that sedentary behavior may constitute an independent risk factor, even among persons who engage in sufficient physical activity to meet the current guidelines. Compared with those engaging in no leisure time activity, individuals meeting the recommended activity minimum had 31% lower risk of mortality with lesser but significant 20% lower mortality even among those performing less than the recommended minimum.[110] Risks continued to decline at higher levels of energy expenditure albeit with more modest magnitudes of additional mortality benefit, with maximum mortality benefit (39% lower risk) for those performing 3 to 5 times the recommended minimum, with no evidence of harm at 10 times or more the recommended minimum. A similar curvilinear dose-response curve pertains for mortality from cardiovascular disease and cancer, and for moderate- and vigorous-intensity activities (1 minute of vigorous intensity activity approximates 2 minutes of moderate-intensity activity based on energy expenditure). Among older women (mean age 72 years), as few as 4400 steps/day was associated with 40% risk reduction in mortality compared with 2700 steps/day, with greater benefit for more steps taken per day until approximately 7500 steps/day.[111] Risk reductions for moderate-to-vigorous activity with mortality is substantially greater in magnitude when using an accelerometer compared with self-reported data (Fig. 25.10).[112] Therefore, different intensities of activity can be combined in a variety of ways to achieve health benefits.

For people who consume a usual American diet, the level of physical activity recommended by the federal guidelines may not suffice to prevent the weight gain that occurs with age. Weight control is complex and depends on energy expenditure and energy intake, and a significant relationship exists between greater activity and attenuated weight gain in adults.[106,107] Nonetheless, the available data clearly indicate that physical activity lowers cardiovascular risk among not only individuals with normal BMI but also those who are overweight or obese, those with other cardiovascular risk factors, and patients with clinical cardiovascular disease and other chronic conditions.[107] Because of the difficulty in maintaining sustained weight loss among overweight and obese persons, the importance of physical activity—even without weight loss—for cardioprotection should be emphasized to patients.

Finally, physical activity can be associated with adverse events which can be minimized by wearing protective equipment, choosing safe environments, and making sensible choices, including the types and amounts of activity that are appropriate for an individual's fitness level, and increasing activity levels gradually over time, in particular for those with chronic conditions ("start low and go slow").[107] The most common adverse events are musculoskeletal injuries, and risks relate directly to the amount and intensity of physical activity undertaken. At the level recommended by the federal guidelines, risk is low. One of the most severe adverse events related to physical activity is the risk of a sudden cardiac event (e.g., sudden death) during or shortly after exercise, but these events are extremely rare. *Vigorous intensity* activities can precipitate such events, particularly when unaccustomed. Adding a small amount of light to moderate intensity activity (e.g., walking, 5 to 15 minutes per session, two or three times a week) carries no known risk for sudden severe cardiac events, compared with periods of less intense activity or at rest. Compared with inactive people, active people are at lower overall risk for cardiovascular disease, because when averaged over the whole day, the risk during activity and during all other periods in active people yields a lower average risk than in inactive people. The benefits of regular physical activity clearly outweigh the inherent risk of adverse events.

Sedentary Behavior

The 2018 guidelines highlight the complex interaction between physical inactivity and sedentary behavior, but does not specify quantitative parameters for sitting time or sitting patterns.[106,107] One expert statement recommended reducing work time sitting for up to 4 hours per day, but this advice was not evidence based.[113] Recently, interest has burgeoned in understanding the role of sedentary behaviors on health, independent of physical activity level, because one can be both sedentary and physically active (e.g., an office worker who sits during most of the workday but who also jogs regularly). In a meta-analysis of 34 studies (1.3 million individuals), there was a non-linear relationship after adjusting for physical activity levels between sedentary behavior, all-cause and cardiovascular mortality, with increased risk seen above a threshold of 6 to 8 hours per day of total sitting and 3 to 4 hours per day of television viewing.[114] The authors estimated that for every 1 hour of sitting time, there was 1% to 2% increased risk of mortality that was independent of activity levels, and that television viewing (which was worse than sitting) accounted for approximately 5% of cardiovascular mortality, 8% of all-cause mortality, and 29% of type 2 diabetes, suggesting an important burden of deaths that could be avoided with decreasing television viewing.[114] Higher physical activity levels, however, modify the association between sedentary behavior and cardiovascular death, such that increased risks for sitting time with cardiovascular mortality were most pronounced in the inactive group who had a clear dose-response association between sitting and cardiovascular death; there was no association between sedentary behavior and cardiovascular mortality in the most active group (≥60 minutes of moderate intensity activity per day), while less active groups had significantly increased risk of cardiovascular sitting only for those who sat greater than 8 hours/day.[114] Similar effect modification was also noted for all-cause mortality, whereby associations with increased mortality for sedentary behavior were eliminated in the most active group.[114] These studies underscore the synergy between activity levels and sedentary time, whereby individuals who cannot avoid large amounts of sitting could increase their physical activity levels to counteract the detrimental effects of sedentary behavior. It is unknown if sedentary breaks (without increasing physical activity) could result in benefit.

Interventions to Increase Physical Activity

Evidence-based strategies to increase physical activity include those that focus on individuals or small groups as well as more upstream approaches that target community-level programs and policies.[106,107] Individual approaches toward increasing physical activity levels, although important, have limited impact, because they focus only on a single patient. A comprehensive public health approach would involve health agencies; schools; businesses; policy, advocacy, nutrition, recreation, planning, and transport agencies; and health care organizations. In addition to the important role that health care professionals and health care systems play in assessing, counseling, advising, and promoting activity programs, the National Physical Activity Plan outlines multiple societal sectors that should be involved in promoting activity, including businesses, community recreation/parks, educational settings, faith-based settings, mass media outlets and messages, public health departments and organizations, the sports sector (in particular for youth sports), and the transportation/public transit sector.[115] Wearable devices and step counters can be useful to provide feedback to individuals and for remote monitoring and behavioral interventions. A recent meta-analysis of activity monitors used in 14 studies found a trend in benefit for increasing activity levels in adults with overweight or obesity compared to interventions that did not use an activity monitor.[116] Based on a comprehensive review of the literature, the World Health Organization and the Lancet physical activity series have advocated prioritizing environmental over individual approaches for physical activity promotion.[117] Future studies should work across disciplines and sectors to scale up the impact and make translation of research into evidence-based interventions a priority. Until then, a simple message of "sit less, move more and more often" is the key take-home message.[112]

PHARMACOLOGIC THERAPIES

Shared Decision-Making

Patients play a central role in shared decision-making as they ultimately make decisions regarding how to lead their lives. These choices impact their health, the effectiveness of recommended treatments, and their use of medical resources. Therefore, to improve the health of patients, the role of health care professionals extends beyond practicing evidence-based medicine and should include providing patients with easy-to-understand dual assessments of both the risks and benefits of various treatments. Support tools can be easily incorporated into the electronic health record to facilitate the appropriate preventive and therapeutic approaches by health care providers. Such tools could provide personalized estimates for the potential for absolute risk reduction (number needed to treat, NNT) with a medication or intervention weighed against the potential for adverse events (number needed to harm, NNH), with net clinical benefit calculated as NNT minus NNH. Shared decision-making is particularly important for primary prevention of cardiovascular disease, where patients are asymptomatic and there is a long latency period before the clinical onset of disease. The 2019 ACC/AHA prevention guidelines gave a class I (LOE B-R [moderate quality evidence]) for shared decision-making in cardiovascular disease prevention based on data supporting that patient input and collaboration with clinicians decreases potential barriers to treatments.[4,118] Health care providers and patients together could make more informed choices regarding the risks and benefits of various preventive treatments including lifestyle and medical therapies.[4,10,11,14]

Statins (see Chapter 27)

Statins inhibit cholesterol synthesis by inhibiting the enzyme hydroxymethylglutaryl coenzyme A (HMG-CoA) reductase and preventing the formation of mevalonate, the rate-limiting step of sterol synthesis. Statins also have anti-inflammatory effects independent of LDL cholesterol lowering. Statins lower LDL cholesterol in a non-linear dose-response manner. Statins vary in intensity from high-intensity (average lowering of LDL cholesterol by ≥50%) to moderate-intensity (30% to 49%) and low-intensity (<30%). Statins reduce LDL cholesterol and non-HDL cholesterol more than reducing apoB and triglycerides, and effects on HDL cholesterol are variable. Statins do not reduce Lp(a).[31] Concomitant drugs that interfere with the metabolism of statins by inhibiting the cytochrome P-450 3A4 (which metabolizes lovastatin, simvastatin, and atorvastatin) and 2C9 can increase plasma concentrations of statins.[11] The starting dose selected depends on the patient's cardiovascular risk, age, polypharmacy, and other clinical characteristics (renal function, liver function, hypothyroidism, prior history or family history of previous statin intolerance or muscle disorders, history of hemorrhagic stroke, Asian ancestry).[10] Statin side effects include adverse effects on muscle, glucose metabolism, and hemorrhagic stroke.[119] The major side effects of statins are muscle symptoms (statin-associated muscle symptoms [SAMS]) ranging from diffuse myalgias (normal creatine kinase without functional loss), seen in up to 10% to 15% of statin users, to myositis, defined as diffuse muscle pain with evidence of muscle inflammation and elevated creatine kinase levels, which necessitate discontinuation of use of the drug in less than 1% of patients. Rarely, statin use is associated with rhabdomyolysis, which is often associated with predisposing factors (advanced age, frailty, renal failure, shock, concomitant use of antifungal agents, antibiotics, the fibric acid derivative gemfibrozil, and hypothyroidism).[11] The use of statins is associated with a small but significant dose-dependent increase in new-onset diabetes of approximately 1 per 1000 person-years, in particular among adults with other diabetes risk factors.[119] The overwhelming benefits of statins in subjects at high risk for or in the secondary prevention of cardiovascular disease exceeds the small risk for development of diabetes. The cumulative evidence from large-scale clinical outcomes data supports the concept that reaching a low total cholesterol and LDL cholesterol state is related directly to lower cardiovascular risk. In the Cholesterol Treatment Trialists meta-analysis of 27 randomized statin trials ($N = 174,149$ individuals, 27% women), every 1 mmol/L (39 mg/dL) in LDL cholesterol with statin versus placebo (22 trials) or more versus less intensive statin (5 trials) was associated with 21% reduction in major vascular events over median follow-up of 4.9 years, with significant risk reductions in all-cause mortality (10%) driven by reduction in vascular mortality (12%), major coronary events (23%), coronary revascularization (24%), and stroke (15%), with no effect on incident cancer or cancer mortality.[67] The relative risk reductions were similar for primary or secondary prevention populations. Similar results were obtained from a Cochrane meta-analysis on 18 randomized trials of statin versus placebo on 56,934 individuals from primary prevention, with 14% relative risk reduction in all-cause mortality and 25% reduction in vascular events. Not all agents that lower LDL cholesterol lower vascular event rates, so physicians should exercise caution when using agents that have not been evaluated in randomized clinical outcomes trials.

Monitoring of Therapy

Before initiation of statin therapy, either a fasting or nonfasting lipid panel should be obtained along with baseline transaminase levels (alanine aminotransferase) and creatine kinase.[10] After initiation of statin therapy, the response should be checked with a repeat lipid panel (fasting or nonfasting) within the first 1 to 3 months to determine the patient's adherence and response. Thereafter, clinical judgment should dictate the interval between follow-up visits. Although frequent visits are probably not useful for the detection of serious side effects, they serve to encourage compliance and adherence to diet and lifestyle changes. Nevertheless, statin and other lipid modifying therapy should accompany a diet and exercise program aimed at achieving a healthy diet and ideal body weight, and glucose should be monitored in statin-treated individuals with risk factors for diabetes. While treating to a pre-specified LDL cholesterol target is no longer as rigorously advocated, recent guidelines specify the importance of percentage reduction in LDL cholesterol in assessing LDL lowering therapies. Controversy persists about whether the smaller differences between apoB (or LDL particle concentration) and non-HDL (or LDL cholesterol) for cardiovascular risk prediction are sufficient to offset the potentially higher health care costs from additional testing. European guidelines suggest that although LDL cholesterol is the primary target of lipid-lowering therapy, non-HDL cholesterol or apoB are secondary treatment targets, in particular for patients who also have cardiometabolic risk factors (e.g., triglycerides >175 mg/dL, obesity, metabolic syndrome, or diabetes) or low LDL cholesterol.[14]

Aspirin

Low-dose aspirin provides proven clinical benefit in the secondary prevention of cardiovascular disease. Among patients with previous myocardial infarction, stroke, bypass surgery, angioplasty, peripheral arterial disease, or angina, aspirin use as compared to placebo is associated with a 19% reduction in any serious cardiovascular events, a 31% reduction in nonfatal myocardial infarction, a 20% reduction in major coronary heart disease, and a 19% reduction in total stroke. In absolute terms, this represents an annual benefit of aspirin versus control for serious vascular events of 6.7% versus 8.2% per year; in total stroke, 2.08% versus 2.54%; and in coronary events, 4.3% versus 5.3%. In this secondary prevention setting, reductions are of similar magnitude for men and women, but come with a small though nonsignificant increase in hemorrhagic stroke and with increased risk of gastrointestinal bleeding. For high-risk secondary prevention individuals, aspirin use is associated with cardioprotective effects on top of optimal medical therapy such as achieving LDL cholesterol levels below 70 mg/dL with high-intensity statin therapy. Thus, in secondary prevention, low-dose aspirin remains of major importance.

In primary prevention, however, the role of aspirin is not straightforward, particularly in the post-statin era where the absolute risk of a cardiovascular event is lower and the risk of major adverse effects including bleeding remain the same. Given the complex matrix of benefits and risks, the use of aspirin in primary prevention requires individualized shared decision-making.[120,121] Earlier aspirin trials in primary prevention provided evidence of cardiovascular benefits, albeit with an increased risk of bleeding. The 2016 US Preventive Services Task Force recommended individualized use of aspirin based on factors including age, 10-year risk of cardiovascular disease, and bleeding risk.[122] These recommendations were based on their systematic review of 11 major aspirin primary prevention trials ($n = 118,445$). Overall, aspirin associated with a 22% significant relative risk reduction in nonfatal MI, 6% significant reduction in all-cause mortality, 5% to 6% nonsignificant reductions in cardiovascular mortality and nonfatal stroke, and in the seven trials that evaluated aspirin ≤100 mg/day, there was a significant 14% relative risk reduction in nonfatal stroke.[122] Yet many of the early aspirin prevention trials were conducted when smoking was common, blood pressure control suboptimal, and aggressive lipid lowering rare. Thus, until recently, the risks and benefits of prophylactic aspirin in contemporary preventive practice remained uncertain.

In 2018, three contemporary primary prevention trials of aspirin were reported: ASCEND (a trial of patients with diabetes),[123] ARRIVE (a trial intended to evaluate high-risk patients without diabetes),[124] and ASPREE (a trial of older individuals).[125] Of these three trials, only ASCEND was statistically powered for cardiovascular events, while ARRIVE and ASPREE were underpowered. ASCEND randomly allocated 15,480 patients with diabetes (estimated absolute 10-year risk of cardiovascular disease 10%, i.e., intermediate risk) to aspirin 100mg daily or matching placebo. During a mean follow-up of 7.4 years, aspirin was associated with a 12% reduction in cardiovascular events, yet at a cost of a 29% increase in major bleeds. In ASCEND, all-cause mortality was neutral.

ARRIVE was intended to investigate the role of 100 mg aspirin daily or placebo among higher-risk primary prevention patients without diabetes. During 5 years of follow-up among 12,456 participants, however, observed risk estimates were substantially lower than predicted and the trial was underpowered. Thus, ARRIVE should be interpreted as a trial of borderline to intermediate risk primary prevention (estimated 10-year risk of cardiovascular disease 7%). In this context, aspirin conferred no vascular benefit but resulted in a significant twofold increase in gastrointestinal bleeding. In ARRIVE, all-cause mortality was again neutral.

ASPREE included 19,114 participants 70 years of age and older (estimated 10-year risk of cardiovascular disease 8%) who were free of cardiovascular disease, dementia, or disability at trial entry and who were randomly allocated to 100 mg enteric coated aspirin or placebo for up to 5 years. In ASPREE, aspirin as compared to placebo conferred no benefit on the primary endpoint of survival without dementia or persistent physical disability. The trial halted early due to likely futility for the primary outcome (life free of dementia and physical disability). ASPREE was underpowered for cardiovascular events, and there was no evidence of cardiovascular benefit for the total cardiovascular endpoint that included heart failure events, while major bleeds increased. By contrast with all prior primary prevention aspirin trials and with ASCEND and ARRIVE, ASPREE reported a small increase in the secondary endpoint of all-cause mortality (HR 1.14, 95% CI 1.01 to 1.29).

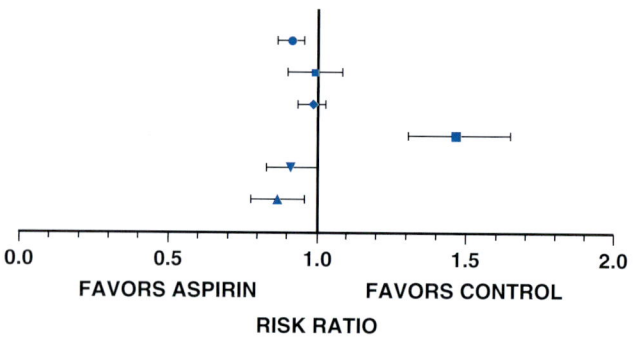

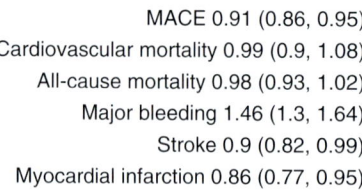

FIGURE 25.11 Meta–analysis of 13 randomized controlled trials involving 164,225 participants comparing the effects of aspirin versus control for primary prevention of cardiovascular disease. *MACE*, Major adverse cardiovascular events. (From Gelbenegger G, Postula M, Pecen L, et al. Aspirin for primary prevention of cardiovascular disease: a meta-analysis with a particular focus on subgroups. *BMC Med.* 2019;17:198.)

Several meta-analyses conducted since then that include all the primary prevention trials agree with prior meta-analyses. For example, a 2019 systematic review and meta-analysis of 13 trials and 164,225 participants (estimated 10-year risk of cardiovascular disease 10%) showed significant 11% reduction in cardiovascular events (NNT 241, with absolute benefit depending on absolute risk), with a concomitant increased risk of major bleeding of 43% (NNH 210).[126] Hence, in adults with 10-year risk of 10% or more, the number of cardiovascular events prevented is similar to the number of bleeding events. Similar results were obtained in another meta-analysis (Fig. 25.11), which additionally found that aspirin was associated with potentially greater benefit in statin-treated compared with non-statin-treated patients.[127] Statins in primary prevention are associated with a 25% reduction in cardiovascular events for every 1 mmol/L reduction in LDL cholesterol, without the bleeding complications associated with aspirin. In the International Polycap Study-3 (TIPS-3) trial, a daily fixed-dose combination polypill (simvastatin, ramipril, atenolol, and hydrochlorothiazide) plus low-dose aspirin (75 mg) as compared to placebo among 5713 intermediate risk individuals (mostly Asian) resulted in a 31% relative risk reduction in the primary cardiovascular endpoint, with increases in dizziness and hypotension in the polypill arm.[128] Notably, the combination of the polypill (which included a statin) with aspirin was more effective than the polypill alone (31% vs. 21% relative risk reductions).[128]

Various clinical societies provide recommendations on the use of aspirin for primary prevention. European guidelines recommend against aspirin for primary prevention.[14] For adults with diabetes, the American Diabetes Association suggests low-dose aspirin may be considered for those who are at increased cardiovascular risk, after a comprehensive discussion with the patient regarding the risks and benefits.[32] The 2019 AHA/ACC guidelines recommend low-dose aspirin might be considered for the primary prevention of cardiovascular disease among adults 40 to 70 years who have increased cardiovascular risk but not increased bleeding risk, and recommend against aspirin among adults who have increased risk of bleeding.[4] While clinical practice guidelines are essential, it is often challenging to integrate the benefit and risk profile into clinical decision making regarding whether or not to initiate aspirin therapy for a particular patient, and shared decision-making support tools have been developed that calculate the dual bleeding and cardiovascular risks.[120,121] Some clinicians will continue to prescribe aspirin in primary prevention for individuals at very high risk for atherosclerosis, particularly among those where concomitant bleeding risks are low. Major risk factors for gastrointestinal bleeding include male sex, history of upper gastrointestinal disorder, older age (doubling with each decade, and particularly increased for age >70 years), hepatic or renal disease, multiple cardiovascular risk factors, and use of other medicines (e.g., non-steroidal anti-inflammatory drugs, corticosteroids, antiplatelets, antithrombotics, and selective serotonin reuptake inhibitors). Thus, the best strategy for aspirin in the primary prevention of cardiovascular disease is an individualized precision-medicine approach that balances the individual's estimated risk and benefit in a shared decision-making approach.

N-3 Fatty Acids

Omega-3 (n-3) fatty acids are polyunsaturated fatty acids with pleiotropic physiologic actions, including favorable changes in the lipidome (reducing plasma triglycerides, ceramides, and diacylglycerols), and as precursors to bioactive lipid mediators pivotal to resolving inflammation. n-3 fatty acids include (EPA, 20:5) and docosahexaenoic acid (DHA, 22:6). EPA and DHA are converted by cyclooxygenases (COX) or lipoxygenases (LOX) to generate potent specialized pro-resolving mediators and bioactive lipids including prostaglandins, prostacyclins, resolvins, and thromboxanes. n-3 fatty acids may have other beneficial cardiovascular effects through other mechanisms including molecular and gene-regulatory effects such as favorable effects on insulin signaling and energy use; lowering blood pressure and heart rate; reducing susceptibility to ventricular arrhythmias; and regulating inflammation, thrombosis, platelet function, vascular tone, and endothelial function.[129]

Many randomized clinical trials have evaluated n-3 fatty acid interventions and cardiovascular clinical outcomes.[129] These trials differed in their study populations (low or high risk), the specific formulation for the interventions, dose, presence or absence of a placebo arm, type of placebo oil used, and clinical outcomes. With the exception of the *VIT*amin D and Omeg*A*-3 Tria*L* (VITAL) that was conducted in a general primary prevention American population at usual risk, the rest of the trials were conducted in patients from secondary prevention or at high cardiovascular risk. Before 2019, most meta-analyses of n-3 fatty acid supplementation found no benefit or at most modest benefit for coronary death but not for stroke or major cardiovascular events. For example, a 2018 meta-analysis from the Omega-3 Treatment Trialists' Collaboration examined aggregate study-level data from 10 randomized trials (EPA dose ranged from 226 to 1800 mg/day; 9 trials tested combined EPA+DHA) conducted in high-risk populations ($n = 77,917$ individuals; 12,001 cardiovascular events) and found no significant reduction in major cardiovascular or coronary events, with a trend toward 7% relative risk reduction in coronary deaths.[130] Several landmark n-3 fatty acid supplementation trials were published in 2018 or later, and these as well as meta-analyses that included them are discussed in more detail in the next section.

Primary Prevention

The VITAL trial is the only primary prevention trial of n-3 fatty acid supplementation in a general usual-risk population selected only on age and not selected on high cardiovascular risk. VITAL was a randomized, double-blind, placebo-controlled trial of marine n-3 fatty acids (1 g/day Omacor fish-oil capsule with 840 mg of n-3 FAs, including EPA+DHA (1.3:1 ratio) versus placebo (olive oil), and in a 2×2 factorial design also tested vitamin D_3 (2000 IU/day) versus placebo in the primary prevention of cardiovascular disease and cancer among 25,871 US men aged ≥ 50 and women ≥ 55 with no prior cardiovascular disease.[131] Compared with placebo, n-3 fatty acids did not significantly reduce the primary endpoint of major cardiovascular events (a composite of myocardial infarction, stroke, and cardiovascular mortality; hazard ratio (HR)=0.92 [95% confidence interval 0.80 to 1.06]) but significantly reduced myocardial infarction (a prespecified secondary endpoint) by 28% and total coronary heart disease events by 17%. While there was significant reduction in myocardial infarction and coronary heart disease, there was no significant reduction in stroke, which resulted in no significant reduction in major cardiovascular disease, the primary endpoint of the trial. However, two VITAL study subgroup analyses deserve further investigation in future trials. First, in the subgroup of individuals with low baseline fish intake (below the study median of 1½ servings/week), n-3 supplementation was associated with a significant 19% reduction in the trial primary endpoint of major cardiovascular events, including a 40% reduction in myocardial infarction, while no benefit was found for n-3 supplementation in those with greater than 1½ fish servings/week. Second, in the 5106 African American participants, n-3 supplementation resulted in a significant 77% reduction in myocardial infarction irrespective of baseline fish intake, and nearly 40% reduction in coronary heart disease, while other racial/ethnic groups had smaller reductions. Whether the racial/ethnic difference in benefit relates to genetic variation, cardiovascular risk, environmental or other factors remains to be determined. Observational studies suggest that genetic variation in fatty acid enzymes such as the fatty acid desaturase genes (*FADS1*, *FADS2*) or genes in LOX or COX pathways could interact with diet to influence cardiovascular outcomes. Overall, the n-3 fatty acid intervention of 1 g/day in VITAL was well tolerated, with no treatment-associated increase in bleeding or gastrointestinal symptoms.[131]

High-Risk Primary Prevention

In 2018, A Study of Cardiovascular Events in Diabetes (ASCEND) trial reported results of supplementation with 1g/day fish oil capsule (840 mg EPA+DHA, same ratio and formulation as used in the VITAL trial) versus placebo (olive oil), and in a 2×2 factorial design, which also tested low dose aspirin versus placebo in 15,480 UK patients with diabetes but without clinical evidence of cardiovascular disease. There was no n-3 treatment-related reduction in composite vascular events over a 7.4-year follow-up period.[132] In ASCEND, there was a significant reduction in vascular death (19%), driven by coronary death, with no reduction in stroke or stroke death.

Subsequently, in a higher-risk patient population than ASCEND, The Reduction of Cardiovascular Events with Icosapent Ethyl–Intervention Trial (REDUCE-IT) trial examined a high-risk patient population of statin-treated patients ($N = 8179$; 90% white), with elevated triglycerides (median baseline triglycerides 216 mg/dL, LDL cholesterol 75 mg/dL) and with either known cardiovascular disease (70.7% of the study population) or high-risk patients with diabetes and one or more additional cardiovascular risk factors.[133] The trial tested a high-dose purified synthetic EPA (icosapent ethyl, 4 g/day) versus placebo (mineral oil). Over a 5-year follow-up, there was a significant 26% reduction in major cardiovascular events, including significant reductions of 31%, 28%, and 20% in total myocardial infarction, total stroke, and cardiovascular death, respectively.[133] The n-3 intervention arm had more atrial fibrillation (5.3% vs. 3.9%) and a trend toward increased bleeding. In the primary prevention cohort of high-risk patients with diabetes, there was 12% nonsignificant relative risk reduction in the primary endpoint (vs. 27% in the secondary prevention cohort), p for interaction 0.14.

Updated Meta-Analyses and Summary

A 2019 meta-analysis of 30 trials of n-3 supplementation ($N > 130,000$) that included VITAL and ASCEND, but not REDUCE-IT, reported modest (7%) significant relative risk reductions for myocardial infarction and total coronary events with nonsignificant reduction in cardiovascular mortality and no reduction in stroke.[134] A subsequent meta-analysis of 13 marine n-3 trials ($N = 127,477$) included the three trials (VITAL, ASCEND, and REDUCET-IT) (Fig. 25.12). Analyses that excluded REDUCE-IT found significant relative risk reductions (5% to 8%) in myocardial infarction, coronary heart disease, and coronary deaths, and % significant reductions (3% to 5%) in total cardiovascular events and death from cardiovascular disease. After including REDUCE-IT the reduction in myocardial infarction was greater (12% risk reduction), but with evidence of significant heterogeneity. Additional analyses suggested a linear dose-response association with cardiovascular events. Every 1 g/day of marine n-3 supplementation corresponded to a 9% lower risk of myocardial infarction and 7% lower risk of total coronary events. There was no significant reduction in stroke risk.

The Statin Residual Risk Reduction With EpaNova in HiGh CV Risk PatienTs With Hypertriglyceridemia (STRENGTH) trial tested a different high-dose purified formulation of n-3 carboxylic acids (Epanova 4 g/day, EPA+DHA, ratio 2.75:1) versus placebo (corn oil).[135] The trial was stopped early in 2020 for futility to reduce major cardiovascular events in 13,086 patients with hypertriglyceridemia and low HDL cholesterol on maximally tolerated statins and with established atherosclerotic disease or at high cardiovascular risk. It is uncertain if the differences in outcome results for STRENGTH vs REDUCE-IT relate to differences in the n-3 formulations, placebo, or the study populations.

In the United States, there are currently five prescription n-3 treatments approved for treating hypertriglyceridemia, with various amounts, ratios, and bioavailability of EPA and DHA.[129] For over the counter n-3 fatty acid supplements, the typical pill content is 180 mg for EPA and 120 mg for DHA, and the analytical content of EPA and DHA was found to be mostly consistent with the labeled amounts.[129] Absorption of n-3 fatty acids (in particular for ethyl esters which have lower bioavailability compared with free fatty acid supplements[129]) is improved by dietary fat. The dose-response curve for many favorable n-3 fatty acid cardiovascular effects appears to plateau at doses of 0.5 to 1 g/day, including lowering heart rate, blood pressure, and arrhythmias, while other clinical effects such as triglyceride lowering or anti-thrombotic effects may require higher doses.[129] In 2017, the AHA published a scientific statement that did not address primary prevention (since the VITAL trial at the time was ongoing) but suggested that treatment is reasonable for secondary prevention of coronary events and sudden cardiac death among patients with prevalent coronary disease, or for secondary prevention in patients with heart failure.[129] Based on the VITAL study results and previous studies, a reasonable approach would be to consider using n-3 fatty acid supplements among primary prevention adults with low fish consumption or among African Americans. For secondary prevention or high-risk primary prevention patients, high-dose EPA provides additional cardiovascular benefit among maximally statin-treated patients with high triglycerides and other risk factors. Fish intake ≥2 servings/week should be encouraged for both primary and secondary prevention, in particular as part of an overall healthful diet such as the Mediterranean diet to replace less healthful foods.

NOVEL APPROACHES TO PREVENTIVE CARDIOLOGY

The Polypill in Current Practice

Although much of cardiovascular disease prevention is conducted on a risk-based model, alternative population-based approaches have merit when the prevalence of absolute risk is high and in settings where the resources required for individualized care are limited.

In secondary prevention, fixed-dose "polypill" preparations which might include a statin, aspirin, and various blood pressure lowering agents in a single capsule have theoretical advantages particularly in the developing world where a single inexpensive intervention might provide improved delivery at reduced cost, and perhaps through the use of trained non-physician health care workers. Beyond the simplicity of using a daily pill to improve adherence to therapy, the polypill approach can minimize or even eliminate dose adjustments, a relevant issue for blood pressure lowering where multiple low-dose agents are commonly given and known to be safe. Several studies conducted predominantly in low- to middle-income countries demonstrate that combined agents significantly reduce blood pressure and lipids levels, improve overall medication compliance, and in some studies lower vascular event rates.[136]

In primary prevention where risk is considerably lower, effects of different therapies have not always proved to be additive as assumed. In the HOPE-3 trial, the benefit observed compared to placebo when two anti-hypertensive agents were added to a statin were not significantly greater to that with the statin alone, except in a subgroup analysis of patients with baseline systolic blood pressure greater than 143 mm Hg. However, in the TIPS-3 trial of intermediate risk individuals (mostly Asian), a fixed-dose combination polypill plus aspirin versus double placebo resulted in 31% relative risk reduction in cardiovascular events, with greater benefit seen when aspirin was added to the polypill versus polypill alone.[128]

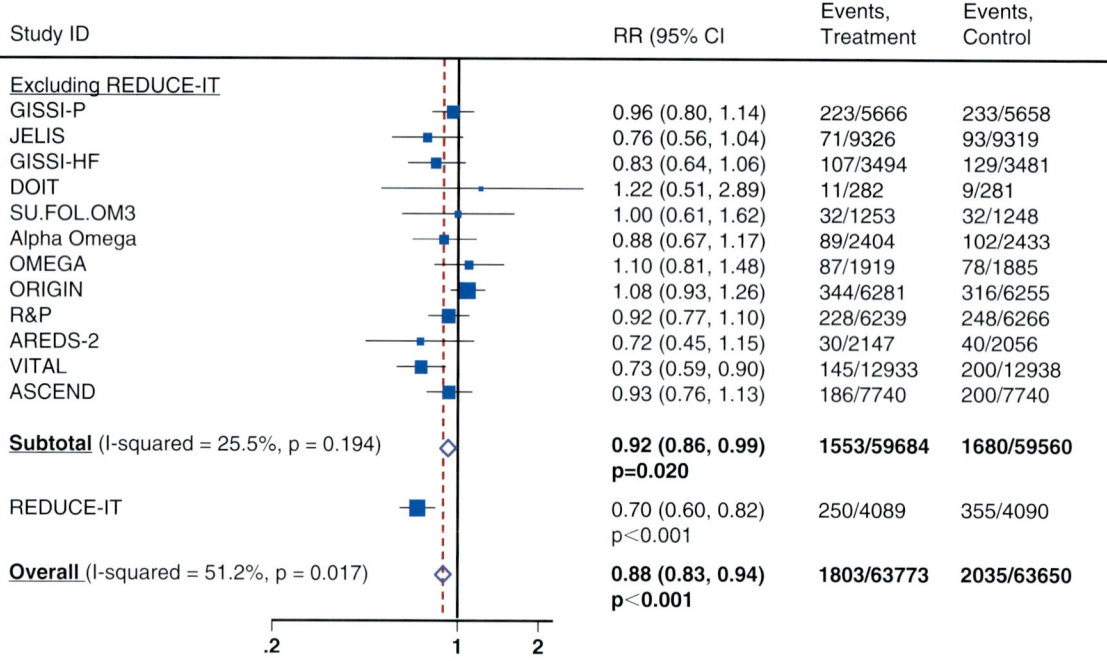

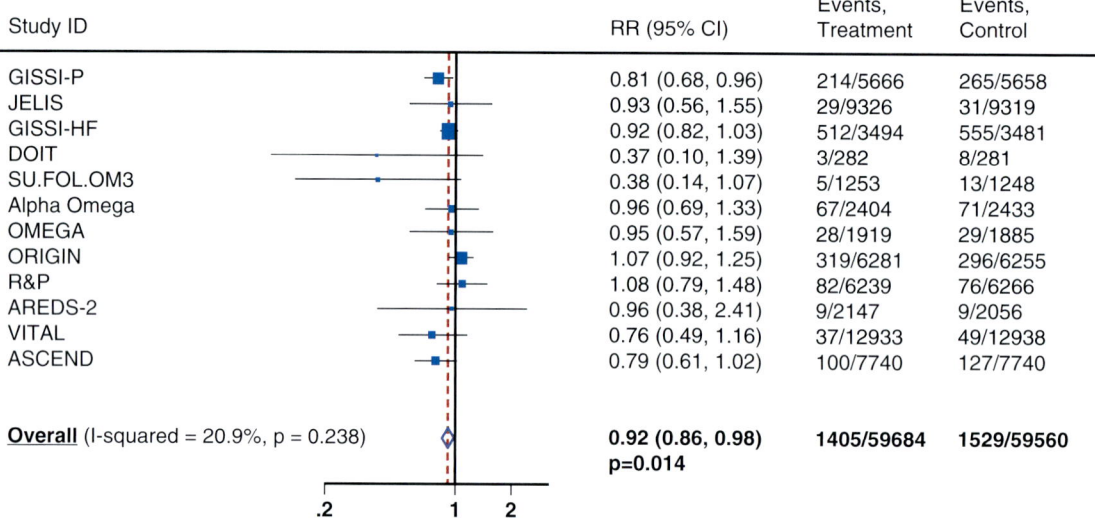

FIGURE 25.12 Meta-analysis of 13 randomized controlled trials involving 127,477 participants evaluating omega-3 (n-3) treatment versus control. Each 1 g/day of n-3 was associated with 9% lower risk of myocardial infarction and 7% lower risk of coronary heart disease (CHD) death. (Adapted from Hu Y, Hu FB, Manson JE. Marine omega–3 supplementation and cardiovascular disease: an updated meta-analysis of 13 randomized controlled trials involving 127477 participants. *J Am Heart Assoc.* 2019;8[(19]:e013543.)

The polypill approach may prove attractive for primary prevention in resource-limited settings, including in North America, where fewer than half of those with hypertension and only a third of those with hyperlipidemia are successfully treated.[24] In a recent trial conducted in the Southern US region, African American participants with very low annual incomes achieved greater reductions in systolic blood pressure and LDL cholesterol when an inexpensive polypill was provided rather than usual care.[137]

Precision Medicine Versus Preventive Care

Getting the right drug to the right patient at the right time is a central mantra of precision medicine. Formally, precision medicine in cardiovascular settings has been described as an integrative approach that considers an individual's genetics, lifestyle, and exposures as determinants of their overall cardiovascular health and disease phenotypes.[138]

In contrast to the polypill approach, a precision medicine focus explicitly pushes back against general assumptions that all patients with the same signs and symptoms of a disease share common characteristics and thus a common treatment strategy. The precision medicine approach incorporates the belief that technologic advances in data portability and analysis, combined with advances in systems biology and network analyses, will ultimately improve health outcomes.

Evidence is accumulating that the practice of preventive cardiology can benefit from a precision medicine approach. For example, interindividual variability in statin response has repeatedly been shown to influence outcomes; in waterfall plots of LDL reduction achieved in statin trials, individual variation is broad and a major determinant of clinical event reduction, even among fully compliant patients. Similarly, in recent inflammation inhibition trials, the magnitude of cardiovascular benefit was directly related to the magnitude of individual-level response as ascertained by treatment levels of IL-6 and hsCRP.

In a third example of precision medicine, cluster analytic techniques have been used to differentiate between five pathophenotypic subtypes of adult-onset diabetes, each with different rates of progression to differential outcomes such as the time to develop chronic kidney disease, microalbuminuria, end stage renal failure, retinopathy, and coronary artery disease.[139]

If linked to a specific targeted therapy, such phenotypic "subprofiling" has the potential to markedly alter strategies for cardiovascular disease prevention. For inexpensive agents with broad application, such precision medicine approaches are more controversial, particularly when tied to genetics. Polygenic risk scores, for example, can define populations with greater or lesser benefit from statin therapy, yet opinion varies widely as to whether such approaches should be implemented in practice (see Chapter 7).[140,141]

"Precision Public Health" is an emerging novel approach which seeks to identify, perhaps through biologic or genetic testing, segments of the population for whom targeted prevention strategies might be provided.[142] Those prone to metabolize alcohol more slowly or nicotine more quickly might be targeted for differential alcohol and smoking cessation programs, while national screening programs for familial hypercholesterolemia might provide a targeted way to treat those with the very highest lipid levels. Implementation science trials will be needed to ensure that such approaches better predict risk and improve treatment response.

Community Interventions

A major initiative in the preventive cardiology community must be to move prevention and wellness out of hospital settings and into the communities where our patients live, work, and play. Daily decisions related to physical activity, dietary choices, smoking, and individual wellness all take place outside the traditional health care system yet are major determinants of long-term health.

Community-based prevention strategies can also be reframed in terms of health rather than in terms of disease (e.g., the AHA's Life's Simple 7). These preventive cardiology concepts have also been expressed as "50 × 50 × 50" to represent maintaining the prevalence of ideal cardiovascular health at a level of 50% or greater, at ages 50 years and younger, by the target date of 2050 or sooner.[143]

Achieving these goals requires a societal transformation that addresses health care inequities in both access and literacy. As simple examples, school-based and community center-based programs will need to replace hospital-based programs if we are to reach patients long before cardiovascular interventions are required but when prevention must begin. Some early successes, such as blood pressure management in barbershops,[144] suggest that health care delivery can in fact be restructured. Other interventions that are known to improve health and save money will require political will similar to that used to implement bans on smoking advertisements 40 years ago. For example, three interventions to reduce childhood obesity that save more than they cost to implement include the introduction of a sugar-sweetened beverage excise tax, the elimination of existing tax subsidies for advertising unhealthy food to children, and the provision of nutrition standards for food and beverages sold in schools.[39]

Appropriate messaging free from industry-bias, such as the healthy foods pyramid (Fig. 25.13) developed by researchers at the Harvard T.H. Chan School of Public Health), provides simple and pragmatic application of these concepts for school, community, and home-based settings.

Mobile Health, Remote Monitoring, and Wearables (see Chapter 12)

Mobile health involves the application of social media, health related apps, location-tracking devices, artificial intelligence, and a variety of biologic sensors to obtain and analyze data related to diagnosis and disease management. With smartphone technology becoming almost

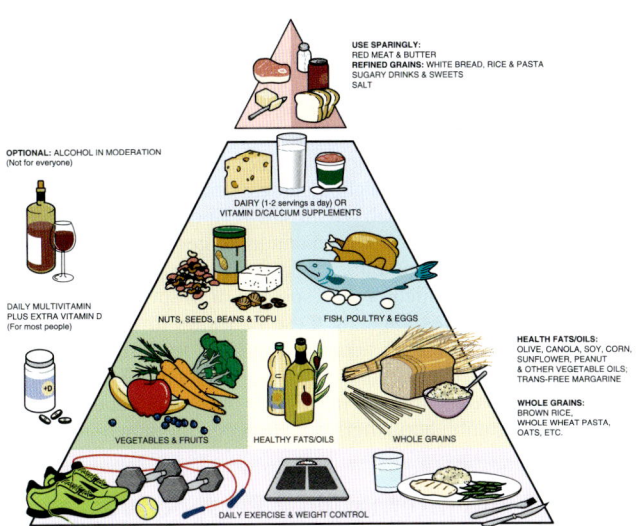

FIGURE 25.13 Appropriate messaging free from industry-bias, such as the healthy foods pyramid developed by researchers at the Harvard School of Public Health, provides simple and pragmatic application of these concepts for school, community, and home-based settings). (Sources: https://www.hsph.harvard.edu/nutritionsource/healthy-eating-pyramid; Copyright © 2008. For more information about The Healthy Eating Pyramid, please see The Nutrition Source, Department of Nutrition, Harvard T.H. Chan School of Public Health, www.thenutritionsource.org.)

universally available in the developed world, the potential utility of mobile health in cardiovascular disease prevention and chronic cardiovascular disease management is exceptionally broad.

Beyond camera capabilities, most current smartphones can passively measure acceleration and geographic position as well as atmospheric and touchscreen pressure, attributes that have been used creatively for diverse medical purposes such as the estimation of heart rate and rhythm, pulmonary function, seizure activity, sleep apnea, and gait stability. When remote monitoring is combined with active sensing (which should greatly reduce recall bias) and repeated functional assessments (such as a smartphone-based 6-minute walk test), a future can be imagined where symptom management is done on an as needed basis rather than only after annual or bi-annual office visits. Delivery of behavioral therapy through targeted text messaging and chat features are under evaluation for patients with hypertension, diabetes, and congestive heart failure.

Legal, ethical, privacy, regulatory, and logistic barriers remain that will slow the introduction of wearables and remote sensing devices into clinical care. High drop-out rates even among motivated individuals electing to purchase activity tracking devices for step-counting suggests that greatly improved engagement strategies are needed. Perhaps most important, and largely missing to date, is clear evidence that resources used for eHealth purposes will result in net clinical gain for patients. For example, while pragmatic studies have shown that remote monitoring may be useful to identify atrial fibrillation,[145] outcome data based on this information is not available. By contrast, at least among inpatients with type 2 diabetes, automated closed loop insulin-delivery systems have resulted in better glycemic control compared to usual care without increasing risk of hypoglycemia.[146]

System-wide implementation of remote management based upon clinical algorithms, computerized case screening, and participant engagement through non-physician "navigators" can also be an effective and potentially transformational way to provide optimal lipid and blood pressure management. Similar programs to address whether remote management can be applied for more complicated patients with heart failure and diabetes are under evaluation.

GAPS IN THE EVIDENCE AND FUTURE PERSPECTIVES

The future of cardiovascular care will need to address not only hyperlipidemia and hypertension, but additionally the innate pro-inflammatory response. More intensive LDL cholesterol lowering agents will be coupled with antiinflammatory therapies to maximize vascular benefit. Bempedoic acid, an agent that provides concomitant LDL cholesterol and hsCRP lowering, is currently being evaluated in outcome trials. Ezetimibe monotherapy (which lowers LDL cholesterol but not hsCRP) augments CRP reduction when combined with statin therapy. More potent combinations might include, as examples, a PCSK9 inhibitor (evolocumab, alirocumab) or an siRNA (inclisiran) given in combination with an IL-1 inhibitor (canakinumab, gevokizumab, anakinra, rilonacept) or an IL-6 inhibitor (tocilizumab, sarilumab, sirukumab, olokizumab). The production of bi-specific or tri-specific therapeutic monoclonal antibodies targeting these pathways in a single chemical entity could provide an additional method for industry to move forward. Given well-described interactions between lipids and innate immunity, it is possible that the magnitude of clinical benefit deriving from intensive combination therapy will exceed the sum of the parts.[84]

Regional and International Perspectives (see Chapters 2 and 93)

In the United States, while heart disease mortality has generally declined over the past 40 years, the absolute number of deaths from ischemic heart disease has increased reflecting both an aging society and persistent racial and ethnic disparities.[2] Disparities are a local as well as regional phenomena; as immediately apparent from neighborhood-by-neighborhood maps of obesity prevalence in local communities, the social determinants of health must be addressed for effective preventive cardiovascular care.[35]

Worldwide, cardiovascular disease and atherothrombotic stroke remain the leading causes of death, accounting for close to 18 million deaths or 32% of all-cause mortality.[147] The highest prevalence of cardiovascular disease is now seen in low- and middle-income countries where resources to address prevention are limited and nearly three-quarters of all cardiovascular morbidity exists.[148] Many of these countries are in the midst of a transition from classic infectious risks in younger individuals to non-communicable disease risks in middle-aged and older individuals. Regrettably, many of these countries are also experiencing adverse population trends in the prevalence of smoking, diabetes, and obesity with concomitant declines in physical activity and a movement away from natural food products. Physicians concerned with cardiovascular disease prevention in the developing world will need to move beyond traditional treatment paradigms and embrace prevention programs that address societal and economic factors.

REFERENCES

Trends in Cardiovascular Disease and Risk Factors

1. Virani SS, Alonso A, Benjamin EJ, et al. Heart disease and stroke statistics-2020 update: a report from the American Heart Association. *Circulation*. 2020;141:e139–e596.
2. Mensah GA, Wei GS, Sorlie PD, et al. Decline in cardiovascular mortality: possible causes and implications. *Circ Res*. 2017;120:366–380.
3. Gupta R, Wood DA. Primary prevention of ischaemic heart disease: populations, individuals, and health professionals. *Lancet*. 2019;394:685–696.
4. Arnett DK, Blumenthal RS, Albert MA, et al. 2019 ACC/AHA guideline on the primary prevention of cardiovascular disease: a report of the American College of Cardiology/American Heart Association task force on clinical practice guidelines. *J Am Coll Cardiol*. 2019;74:e177–e232.
5. Yusuf S, Joseph P, Rangarajan S, et al. Modifiable risk factors, cardiovascular disease, and mortality in 155 722 individuals from 21 high-income, middle-income, and low-income countries (PUREe): a prospective cohort study. *Lancet*. 2020;395:795–808.
6. Angell SY, McConnell MV, Anderson CAM, et al. The American Heart Association 2030 impact goal: a presidential advisory from the American Heart Association. *Circulation*. 2020;141:e120–e138.
7. Younus A, Aneni EC, Spatz ES, et al. A systematic review of the prevalence and outcomes of ideal cardiovascular health in US and non-US populations. *Mayo Clin Proc*. 2016;91:649–670.
8. Allen NB, Krefman AE, Labarthe D, et al. Cardiovascular health trajectories from childhood through middle age and their association with subclinical atherosclerosis. *JAMA Cardiol*. 2020;5:1–10.

Cardiovascular Disease Risk Assessment

9. Cook NR, Ridker PM. Calibration of the pooled cohort equations for atherosclerotic cardiovascular disease: an update. *Ann Intern Med*. 2016;165:786–794.
10. Stone NJ, Robinson JG, Lichtenstein AH, et al. 2013 ACC/AHA guideline on the treatment of blood cholesterol to reduce atherosclerotic cardiovascular risk in adults: a report of the American College of Cardiology/American Heart Association task force on practice guidelines. *Circulation*. 2014;129:S1–S45.
11. Grundy SM, Stone NJ, Bailey AL, et al. 2018 AHA/ACC/AACVPR/AAPA/ABC/ACPM/ADA/AGS/APHA/ASPC/NLA/PCNA guideline on the management of blood cholesterol: a report of the American College of Cardiology/American Heart Association task force on clinical practice guidelines. *J Am Coll Cardiol*. 2019;73:e285–e350.
12. Mora S, Wenger NK, Cook NR, et al. Evaluation of the pooled cohort risk equations for cardiovascular risk prediction in a multiethnic cohort from the women's health initiative. *JAMA Intern Med*. 2018;178:1231–1240.
13. Piepoli MF, Hoes AW, Agewall S, et al. 2016 european guidelines on cardiovascular disease prevention in clinical practice: the sixth joint task force of the European Society of Cardiology and other societies on cardiovascular disease prevention in clinical practice (constituted by representatives of 10 societies and by invited experts)developed with the special contribution of the European Association for Cardiovascular Prevention & Rehabilitation (EACPR). *Eur Heart J*. 2016;37:2315–2381.
14. Mach F, Baigent C, Catapano AL, et al. 2019 ESC/EAS guidelines for the management of dyslipidaemias: lipid modification to reduce cardiovascular risk. *Eur Heart J*. 2020;41:111–188.
15. World Health Organization. World Health Organization cardiovascular disease risk charts: revised models to estimate risk in 21 global regions. *Lancet Glob Health*. 2019;7:e1332–e1345.
16. Karmali KN, Persell SD, Perel P, et al. Risk scoring for the primary prevention of cardiovascular disease. *Cochrane Database Syst Rev*. 2017;3:Cd006887.
17. Studziński K, Tomasik T, Krzysztoń J, et al. Effect of using cardiovascular risk scoring in routine risk assessment in primary prevention of cardiovascular disease: an overview of systematic reviews. *BMC Cardiovasc Disord*. 2019;19:11.
18. Greenland P, Blaha MJ, Budoff MJ, et al. Coronary calcium score and cardiovascular risk. *J Am Coll Cardiol*. 2018;72:434–447.
19. Mahabadi AA, Möhlenkamp S, Lehmann N, et al. CAC score improves coronary and CV risk assessment above statin indication by ESC and AHA/ACC primary prevention guidelines. *JACC Cardiovasc Imaging*. 2017;10:143–153.
20. Newby DE, Adamson PD, Berry C, et al. Coronary CT angiography and 5-year risk of myocardial infarction. *N Engl J Med*. 2018;379:924–933.

Risk Factors for Cardiovascular Disease

21. U.S. Department of Health and Human Services. *Smoking Cessation: A Report of the Surgeon General*. Atlanta, GA: Department of Health and Human Services, Centers for Disease Control and Prevention, National Center for Chronic Disease Prevention and Health Promotion, Office on Smoking and Health; 2020.
22. Lindson N, Klemperer E, Hong B, et al. Smoking reduction interventions for smoking cessation. *Cochrane Database Syst Rev*. 2019;9:Cd013183.
23. Cullen KA, Gentzke AS, Sawdey MD, et al. E-cigarette use among youth in the United States, 2019. *J Am Med Assoc*. 2019;322:2095–2103.
24. Whelton PK, Carey RM, Aronow WS, et al. 2017 ACC/AHA/AAPA/ABC/ACPM/AGS/APHA/ASH/ASPC/NMA/PCNA guideline for the prevention, detection, evaluation, and management of high blood pressure in adults: a report of the American College of Cardiology/American Heart Association task force on clinical practice guidelines. *J Am Coll Cardiol*. 2018;71:e127–e248.
25. Forouzanfar MH, Liu P, Roth GA, et al. Global burden of hypertension and systolic blood pressure of at least 110 to 115 mm Hg, 1990-2015. *J Am Med Assoc*. 2017;317:165–182.
26. Global, regional, and national comparative risk assessment of 79 behavioural, environmental and occupational, and metabolic risks or clusters of risks, 1990-2015: a systematic analysis for the global burden of disease study 2015. *Lancet*. 2016;388:1659–1724.
27. Flint AC, Conell C, Ren X, et al. Effect of systolic and diastolic blood pressure on cardiovascular outcomes. *N Engl J Med*. 2019;381:243–251.
28. Gay HC, Rao SG, Vaccarino V, et al. Effects of different dietary interventions on blood pressure: systematic review and meta-analysis of randomized controlled trials. *Hypertension*. 2016;67:733–739.
29. Liu X, Zhang D, Liu Y, et al. Dose-response association between physical activity and incident hypertension: a systematic review and meta-analysis of cohort studies. *Hypertension*. 2017;69:813–820.
30. Semlitsch T, Jeitler K, Berghold A, et al. Long-term effects of weight-reducing diets in people with hypertension. *Cochrane Database Syst Rev*. 2016;3:Cd008274.
31. Langlois MR, Chapman MJ, Cobbaert C, et al. Quantifying atherogenic lipoproteins: current and future challenges in the era of personalized medicine and very low concentrations of LDL cholesterol. A consensus statement from EAS and EFLM. *Clin Chem*. 2018;64:1006–1033.
32. American Diabetes Association. Addendum. 10. Cardiovascular disease and risk management: standards of medical care in diabetes-2020. *Diabetes Care*. 2020;43(suppl 1):S111–s134.
33. Curry SJ, Krist AH, Owens DK, et al. Behavioral weight loss interventions to prevent obesity-related morbidity and mortality in adults: us preventive services task force recommendation statement. *J Am Med Assoc*. 2018;320:1163–1171.
34. LeBlanc ES, Patnode CD, Webber EM, et al. Behavioral and pharmacotherapy weight loss interventions to prevent obesity-related morbidity and mortality in adults: updated evidence report and systematic review for the us preventive services task force. *J Am Med Assoc*. 2018;320:1172–1191.
35. Ward ZJ, Bleich SN, Cradock AL, et al. Projected U.S. State-level prevalence of adult obesity and severe obesity. *N Engl J Med*. 2019;381:2440–2450.
36. Afshin A, Forouzanfar MH, Reitsma MB, et al. Health effects of overweight and obesity in 195 countries over 25 years. *N Engl J Med*. 2017;377:13–27.
37. de Cabo R, Mattson MP. Effects of intermittent fasting on health, aging, and disease. *N Engl J Med*. 2019;381:2541–2551.
38. Schauer PR, Bhatt DL, Kirwan JP, et al. Bariatric surgery versus intensive medical therapy for diabetes - 5-year outcomes. *N Engl J Med*. 2017;376:641–651.
39. Gortmaker SL, Wang YC, Long MW, et al. Three interventions that reduce childhood obesity are projected to save more than they cost to implement. *Health Aff*. 2015;34:1932–1939.
40. UN Division for Sustainable Development Group. *Sustainable Development Goals: 17 Goals to Transform Our World; United Nations Sustainable Development Knowledge Platform [online Platform]*. United Nations; 2015.
41. Weijmans M, van der Graaf Y, Reitsma JB, et al. Paternal or maternal history of cardiovascular disease and the risk of cardiovascular disease in offspring. A systematic review and meta-analysis. *Int J Cardiol*. 2015;179:409–416.
42. Cohen R, Budoff M, McClelland RL, et al. Significance of a positive family history for coronary heart disease in patients with a zero coronary artery calcium score (from the multi-ethnic study of atherosclerosis). *Am J Cardiol*. 2014;114:1210–1214.
43. White-Williams C, Rossi LP, Bittner VA, et al. Addressing social determinants of health in the care of patients with heart failure: a scientific statement from the American Heart Association. *Circulation*. 2020;141:e841–e863.
44. Malambo P, Kengne AP, De Villiers A, et al. Built environment, selected risk factors and major cardiovascular disease outcomes: a systematic review. *PloS One*. 2016;11:e0166846.
45. Rojas-Rueda D, Nieuwenhuijsen MJ, Gascon M, et al. Green spaces and mortality: a systematic review and meta-analysis of cohort studies. *Lancet Planet Health*. 2019;3:e469–e477.
46. Doyle F, Rohde D, Rutkowska A, et al. Systematic review and meta-analysis of the impact of depression on subsequent smoking cessation in patients with coronary heart disease: 1990 to 2013. *Psychosom Med*. 2014;76:44–57.
47. Rosengren A, Smyth A, Rangarajan S, et al. Socioeconomic status and risk of cardiovascular disease in 20 low-income, middle-income, and high-income countries: the prospective urban rural epidemiologic (PURE) study. *Lancet Glob Health*. 2019;7:e748–e760.
48. Lichtman JH, Froelicher ES, Blumenthal JA, et al. Depression as a risk factor for poor prognosis among patients with acute coronary syndrome: systematic review and recommendations: a scientific statement from the American Heart Association. *Circulation*. 2014;129:1350–1369.

49. Towfighi A, Ovbiagele B, El Husseini N, et al. Poststroke depression: a scientific statement for healthcare professionals from the American Heart Association/American Stroke Association. *Stroke.* 2017;48:e30–e43.
50. Kivimäki M, Steptoe A. Effects of stress on the development and progression of cardiovascular disease. *Nat Rev Cardiol.* 2018;15:215–229.
51. Dragano N, Siegrist J, Nyberg ST, et al. Effort-reward imbalance at work and incident coronary heart disease: a multicohort study of 90,164 individuals. *Epidemiology.* 2017;28:619–626.
52. Mostofsky E, Penner EA, Mittleman MA. Outbursts of anger as a trigger of acute cardiovascular events: a systematic review and meta-analysis. *Eur Heart J.* 2014;35:1404–1410.
53. Samalin L, Genty JB, Boyer L, et al. Shared decision-making: a systematic review focusing on mood disorders. *Curr Psychiatry Rep.* 2018;20:23.
54. Stewart JC, Perkins AJ, Callahan CM. Effect of collaborative care for depression on risk of cardiovascular events: data from the impact randomized controlled trial. *Psychosom Med.* 2014;76:29–37.
55. Smolderen KG, Buchanan DM, Gosch K, et al. Depression treatment and 1-year mortality after acute myocardial infarction: insights from the triumph registry (translational research investigating underlying disparities in acute myocardial infarction patients' health status). *Circulation.* 2017;135:1681–1689.
56. Gerhard-Herman MD, Gornik HL, Barrett C, et al. 2016 AHA/ACC guideline on the management of patients with lower extremity peripheral artery disease: executive summary: a report of the American College of Cardiology/American Heart Association task force on clinical practice guidelines. *Circulation.* 2017;135:e686–e725.
57. Aboyans V, Ricco JB, Bartelink MEL, et al. 2017 ESC guidelines on the diagnosis and treatment of peripheral arterial diseases, in collaboration with the European Society for Vascular Surgery (ESVS): document covering atherosclerotic disease of extracranial carotid and vertebral, mesenteric, renal, upper and lower extremity arteriesendorsed by: the European Stroke Organization (ESO)the task force for the diagnosis and treatment of peripheral arterial diseases of the European Society of Cardiology (ESC) and of the European Society for Vascular Surgery (ESVS). *Eur Heart J.* 2018;39:763–816.
58. Chen Q, Li L, Chen Q, et al. Critical appraisal of international guidelines for the screening and treatment of asymptomatic peripheral artery disease: a systematic review. *BMC Cardiovasc Disord.* 2019;19:17.
59. Curry SJ, Krist AH, Owens DK, et al. Screening for peripheral artery disease and cardiovascular disease risk assessment with the Ankle-Brachial Index: US preventive services task force recommendation statement. *J Am Med Assoc.* 2018;320:177–183.
60. de Ferranti SD, Steinberger J, Ameduri R, et al. Cardiovascular risk reduction in high-risk pediatric patients: a scientific statement from the American Heart Association. *Circulation.* 2019;139:e603–e634.
61. Nordestgaard BG, Langsted A, Mora S, et al. Fasting is not routinely required for determination of a lipid profile: clinical and laboratory implications including flagging at desirable concentration cutpoints-a joint consensus statement from the European Atherosclerosis Society and European Federation of Clinical Chemistry and Laboratory Medicine. *Eur Heart J.* 2016;37:1944–1958.
62. Mora S, Chang CL, Moorthy MV, et al. Association of nonfasting vs fasting lipid levels with risk of major coronary events in the anglo-scandinavian cardiac outcomes trial-lipid lowering arm. *JAMA Intern Med.* 2019;179:898–905.
63. White KT, Moorthy MV, Akinkuolie AO, et al. Identifying an optimal cutpoint for the diagnosis of hypertriglyceridemia in the nonfasting state. *Clin Chem.* 2015;61:1156–1163.

Management of Cardiovascular Risk

64. Catapano AL, Graham I, De Backer G, et al. 2016 ESC/EAS guidelines for the management of dyslipidaemias. *Eur Heart J.* 2016;37:2999–3058.
65. Anderson TJ, Grégoire J, Pearson GJ, et al. 2016 Canadian Cardiovascular Society guidelines for the management of dyslipidemia for the prevention of cardiovascular disease in the adult. *Can J Cardiol.* 2016;32:1263–1282.
66. Borén J, Chapman MJ, Krauss RM, et al. Low-density lipoproteins cause atherosclerotic cardiovascular disease: pathophysiological, genetic, and therapeutic insights: a consensus statement from the European Atherosclerosis Society Consensus Panel. *Eur Heart J.* 2020;41:2313–2330.
67. Fulcher J, O'Connell R, Voysey M, et al. Efficacy and safety of LDL-lowering therapy among men and women: meta-analysis of individual data from 174,000 participants in 27 randomised trials. *Lancet.* 2015;385:1397–1405.
68. Bowman L, Hopewell JC, Chen F, et al. Effects of anacetrapib in patients with atherosclerotic vascular disease. *N Engl J Med.* 2017;377:1217–1227.
69. Khera AV, Demler OV, Adelman SJ, et al. Cholesterol efflux capacity, high-density lipoprotein particle number, and incident cardiovascular events: an analysis from the JUPITER trial (justification for the use of statins in prevention: an intervention trial evaluating rosuvastatin). *Circulation.* 2017;135:2494–2504.
70. Marston NA, Giugliano RP, Im K, et al. Association between triglyceride lowering and reduction of cardiovascular risk across multiple lipid-lowering therapeutic classes: a systematic review and meta-regression analysis of randomized controlled trials. *Circulation.* 2019;140:1308–1317.
71. Hegele RA, Borén J, Ginsberg HN, et al. Rare dyslipidaemias, from phenotype to genotype to management: a European Atherosclerosis Society Task Force consensus statement. *Lancet Diabetes Endocrinol.* 2020;8:50–67.
72. Keene D, Price C, Shun-Shin MJ, et al. Effect on cardiovascular risk of high density lipoprotein targeted drug treatments niacin, fibrates, and cetp inhibitors: meta-analysis of randomised controlled trials including 117,411 patients. *BMJ.* 2014;349:g4379.
73. Hegele RA, Tsimikas S. Lipid-lowering agents. *Circ Res.* 2019;124:386–404.
74. Pradhan AD, Paynter NP, Everett BM, et al. Rationale and design of the pemafibrate to reduce cardiovascular outcomes by reducing triglycerides in patients with diabetes (PROMINENT) study. *Am Heart J.* 2018;206:80–93.
75. Nordestgaard BG, Langsted A. Lipoprotein (a) as a cause of cardiovascular disease: insights from epidemiology, genetics, and biology. *J Lipid Res.* 2016;57:1953–1975.
76. Martí-Carvajal AJ, Solà I, Lathyris D, et al. Homocysteine-lowering interventions for preventing cardiovascular events. *Cochrane Database Syst Rev.* 2017;8:Cd006612.
77. Libby P, Rocha VZ. All roads lead to IL-6: a central hub of cardiometabolic signaling. *Int J Cardiol.* 2018;259:213–215.
78. Ridker PM. Clinician's guide to reducing inflammation to reduce atherothrombotic risk: JACC review topic of the week. *J Am Coll Cardiol.* 2018;72:3320–3331.
79. Ridker PM, Everett BM, Thuren T, et al. Antiinflammatory therapy with canakinumab for atherosclerotic disease. *N Engl J Med.* 2017;377:1119–1131.
80. Ridker PM, MacFadyen JG, Thuren T, et al. Residual inflammatory risk associated with interleukin-18 and interleukin-6 after successful interleukin-1β inhibition with canakinumab: further rationale for the development of targeted anti-cytokine therapies for the treatment of atherothrombosis. *Eur Heart J.* 2020;41:2153–2163.
81. Ridker PM, Everett BM, Pradhan A, et al. Low-dose methotrexate for the prevention of atherosclerotic events. *N Engl J Med.* 2019;380:752–762.
82. Tardif JC, Kouz S, Waters DD, et al. Efficacy and safety of low-dose colchicine after myocardial infarction. *N Engl J Med.* 2019;381:2497–2505.
83. Nidorf SM, Fiolet ATL, Mosterd A, et al. Colchicine in patients with chronic coronary disease. *N Engl J Med.* 2020;383:1838–1847.
84. Ridker PM. From cantos to cirt to colcot to clinic: will all atherosclerosis patients soon be treated with combination lipid-lowering and inflammation-inhibiting agents? *Circulation.* 2020;141:787–789.
84a. Ridker PM, Devalaraja M, Baeres FMM, et al. IL-6 inhibition with ziltivekimab in patients at high atherosclerotic risk (RESCUE): a double-blind, randomised, placebo-controlled, phase 2 trial. *Lancet* 2021;May 17, 2021.
85. Lawler PR, Mora S. Glycosylation signatures of inflammation identify cardiovascular risk: some glyc it hot. *Circ Res.* 2016;119:1154–1156.
86. Akinkuolie AO, Buring JE, Ridker PM, et al. A novel protein glycan biomarker and future cardiovascular disease events. *J Am Heart Assoc.* 2014;3:e001221.
87. Lawler PR, Akinkuolie AO, Chandler PD, et al. Circulating n-linked glycoprotein acetyls and longitudinal mortality risk. *Circ Res.* 2016;118:1106–1115.
88. Gudelj I, Lauc G, Pezer M. Immunoglobulin G glycosylation in aging and diseases. *Cell Immunol.* 2018;333:65–79.
89. Kaura A, Panoulas V, Glampson B, et al. Association of troponin level and age with mortality in 250 000 patients: cohort study across five UK acute care centres. *BMJ.* 2019;367:l6055.
90. Cho L, Davis M, Elgendy I, et al. Summary of updated recommendations for primary prevention of cardiovascular disease in women: JACC State-of-the-art review. *J Am Coll Cardiol.* 2020;75:2602–2618.
91. Agarwala A, Michos ED, Samad Z, et al. The use of sex-specific factors in the assessment of women's cardiovascular risk. *Circulation.* 2020;141:592–599.
92. Manson JE, Aragaki AK, Rossouw JE, et al. Menopausal hormone therapy and long-term all-cause and cause-specific mortality: the women's health initiative randomized trials. *J Am Med Assoc.* 2017;318:927–938.
93. Wang DD, Li Y, Afshin A, et al. Global improvement in dietary quality could lead to substantial reduction in premature death. *J Nutr.* 2019;149:1065–1074.
94. Mokdad AH, Ballestros K, Echko M, et al. The state of us health, 1990-2016: burden of diseases, injuries, and risk factors among US states. *J Am Med Assoc.* 2018;319:1444–1472.
95. Dietary Guidelines Advisory Committee. *Scientific Report of the 2020 Dietary Guidelines Advisory Committee: Advisory Report to the Secretary of Agriculture and Secretary of Health and Human Services*. Washington, DC: U.S. Department of Agriculture; 2020.
96. Sacks FM, Lichtenstein AH, Wu JHY, et al. Dietary fats and cardiovascular disease: a presidential advisory from the American Heart Association. *Circulation.* 2017;136:e1–e23.
97. Hooper L, Martin N, Jimoh OF, et al. Reduction in saturated fat intake for cardiovascular disease. *Cochrane Database Syst Rev.* 2020;5:Cd011737.
98. Patnode CD, Evans CV, Senger CA, et al. Behavioral counseling to promote a healthful diet and physical activity for cardiovascular disease prevention in adults without known cardiovascular disease risk factors: updated evidence report and systematic review for the US Preventive Services Task Force. *J Am Med Assoc.* 2017;318:175–193.
99. Prentice RL, Aragaki AK, Howard BV, et al. Low-fat dietary pattern among postmenopausal women influences long-term cancer, cardiovascular disease, and diabetes outcomes. *J Nutr.* 2019;149:1565–1574.
100. Estruch R, Ros E, Salas-Salvadó J, et al. Primary prevention of cardiovascular disease with a mediterranean diet supplemented with extra-virgin olive oil or nuts. *N Engl J Med.* 2018;378:e34.
101. Dinu M, Pagliai G, Casini A, et al. Mediterranean diet and multiple health outcomes: an umbrella review of meta-analyses of observational studies and randomised trials. *Eur J Clin Nutr.* 2018;72:30–43.
102. Willett W, Rockström J, Loken B, et al. Food in the anthropocene: the EAT-Lancet Commission on healthy diets from sustainable food systems. *Lancet.* 2019;393:447–492.
103. Wood AM, Kaptoge S, Butterworth AS, et al. Risk thresholds for alcohol consumption: combined analysis of individual-participant data for 599 912 current drinkers in 83 prospective studies. *Lancet.* 2018;391:1513–1523.
104. Mukamal KJ, Stampfer MJ, Rimm EB. Genetic instrumental variable analysis: time to call mendelian randomization what it is. The example of alcohol and cardiovascular disease. *Eur J Epidemiol.* 2020;35:93–97.
105. Guthold R, Stevens GA, Riley LM, et al. Worldwide trends in insufficient physical activity from 2001 to 2016: a pooled analysis of 358 population-based surveys with 1.9 million participants. *Lancet Glob Health.* 2018;6:e1077–e1086.
106. U.S. Department of Health and Human Services. *Physical Activity Guidelines for Americans*. 2nd ed. Washington, DC: U.S. Department of Health and Human Services; 2018.
107. Piercy KL, Troiano RP, Ballard RM, et al. The physical activity guidelines for Americans. *J Am Med Assoc.* 2018;320:2020–2028.
108. Ekelund U, Steene-Johannessen J, Brown WJ, et al. Does physical activity attenuate, or even eliminate, the detrimental association of sitting time with mortality? A harmonised meta-analysis of data from more than 1 million men and women. *Lancet.* 2016;388:1302–1310.
109. Ekelund U, Tarp J, Steene-Johannessen J, et al. Dose-response associations between accelerometry measured physical activity and sedentary time and all cause mortality: systematic review and harmonised meta-analysis. *BMJ.* 2019;366:l4570.
110. Arem H, Moore SC, Patel A, et al. Leisure time physical activity and mortality: a detailed pooled analysis of the dose-response relationship. *JAMA Intern Med.* 2015;175:959–967.
111. Lee IM, Shiroma EJ, Kamada M, et al. Association of step volume and intensity with all-cause mortality in older women. *JAMA Intern Med.* 2019;179:1105–1112.
112. Ekelund U, Dalene KE, Tarp J, et al. Physical activity and mortality: what is the dose response and how big is the effect? *Br J Sports Med.* 2020;54(19):1125–1126.
113. Buckley JP, Hedge A, Yates T, et al. The sedentary office: an expert statement on the growing case for change towards better health and productivity. *Br J Sports Med.* 2015;49:1357–1362.
114. Patterson R, McNamara E, Tainio M, et al. Sedentary behaviour and risk of all-cause, cardiovascular and cancer mortality, and incident type 2 diabetes: a systematic review and dose response meta-analysis. *Eur J Epidemiol.* 2018;33:811–829.
115. National Physical Activity Plan Alliance. *U.S. National Physical Activity Plan*. Columbia, SC: NPAP; 2016.
116. de Vries HJ, Kooiman TJ, van Ittersum MW, et al. Do activity monitors increase physical activity in adults with overweight or obesity? A systematic review and meta-analysis. *Obesity (Silver Spring).* 2016;24:2078–2091.
117. World Health Organization. *Global Action Plan on Physical Activity 2018-2030: More Active People for a Healthier World: At-A-Glance*. World Health Organization; 2018.
118. Buhse S, Kuniss N, Liethmann K, et al. Informed shared decision-making programme for patients with type 2 diabetes in primary care: cluster randomised controlled trial. *BMJ Open.* 2018;8:e024004.
119. Mach F, Ray KK, Wiklund O, et al. Adverse effects of statin therapy: perception vs. The evidence - focus on glucose homeostasis, cognitive, renal and hepatic function, haemorrhagic stroke and cataract. *Eur Heart J.* 2018;39:2526–2539.
120. Mora S, Ames JM, Manson JE. Low-dose aspirin in the primary prevention of cardiovascular disease: shared decision making in clinical practice. *J Am Med Assoc.* 2016;316:709–710.
121. Mora S, Manson JE. Aspirin for primary prevention of atherosclerotic cardiovascular disease: advances in diagnosis and treatment. *JAMA Intern Med.* 2016;176:1195–1204.
122. Bibbins-Domingo K. Aspirin use for the primary prevention of cardiovascular disease and colorectal cancer: U.S. Preventive Services Task Force recommendation statement. *Ann Intern Med.* 2016;164:836–845.
123. Bowman L, Mafham M, Wallendszus K, et al. Effects of aspirin for primary prevention in persons with diabetes mellitus. *N Engl J Med.* 2018;379:1529–1539.
124. Gaziano JM, Brotons C, Coppolecchia R, et al. Use of aspirin to reduce risk of initial vascular events in patients at moderate risk of cardiovascular disease (ARRIVE): a randomised, double-blind, placebo-controlled trial. *Lancet.* 2018;392:1036–1046.

125. McNeil JJ, Wolfe R, Woods RL, et al. Effect of aspirin on cardiovascular events and bleeding in the healthy elderly. *N Engl J Med.* 2018;379:1509–1518.
126. Zheng SL, Roddick AJ. Association of aspirin use for primary prevention with cardiovascular events and bleeding events: a systematic review and meta-analysis. *J Am Med Assoc.* 2019;321:277–287.
127. Gelbenegger G, Postula M, Pecen L, et al. Aspirin for primary prevention of cardiovascular disease: a meta-analysis with a particular focus on subgroups. *BMC Med.* 2019;17:198.
128. Yusuf S, Joseph P, Dans A, et al. Polypill with or without aspirin in persons without cardiovascular disease. *N Engl J Med.* 2020.
129. Siscovick DS, Barringer TA, Fretts AM, et al. Omega-3 polyunsaturated fatty acid (fish oil) supplementation and the prevention of clinical cardiovascular disease: a science advisory from the American Heart Association. *Circulation.* 2017;135:e867–e884.
130. Aung T, Halsey J, Kromhout D, et al. Associations of omega-3 fatty acid supplement use with cardiovascular disease risks: meta-analysis of 10 trials involving 77 917 individuals. *JAMA Cardiol.* 2018;3:225–234.
131. Manson JE, Cook NR, Lee IM, et al. Marine n-3 fatty acids and prevention of cardiovascular disease and cancer. *N Engl J Med.* 2019;380:23–32.
132. Bowman L, Mafham M, Wallendszus K, et al. Effects of n-3 fatty acid supplements in diabetes mellitus. *N Engl J Med.* 2018;379:1540–1550.
133. Bhatt DL, Steg PG, Miller M, et al. Cardiovascular risk reduction with icosapent ethyl for hypertriglyceridemia. *N Engl J Med.* 2019;380:11–22.
134. Khan SU, Khan MU, Riaz H, et al. Effects of nutritional supplements and dietary interventions on cardiovascular outcomes: an umbrella review and evidence map. *Ann Intern Med.* 2019;171:190–198.
135. Nicholls SJ, Lincoff AM, Garcia M, et al. Effect of high-dose omega-3 fatty acids vs corn oil on major adverse cardiovascular events in patients at high cardiovascular risk: the strength randomized clinical trial. *J Am Med Assoc.* 2020;324:2268–2280.
136. Roshandel G, Khoshnia M, Poustchi H, et al. Effectiveness of polypill for primary and secondary prevention of cardiovascular diseases (polyiran): a pragmatic, cluster-randomised trial. *Lancet.* 2019;394:672–683.
137. Muñoz D, Uzoije P, Reynolds C, et al. Polypill for cardiovascular disease prevention in an underserved population. *N Engl J Med.* 2019;381:1114–1123.
138. Leopold JA, Loscalzo J. Emerging role of precision medicine in cardiovascular disease. *Circ Res.* 2018;122:1302–1315.
139. Ahlqvist E, Storm P, Käräjämäki A, et al. Novel subgroups of adult-onset diabetes and their association with outcomes: a data-driven cluster analysis of six variables. *Lancet Diabetes Endocrinol.* 2018;6:361–369.
140. Levin MG, Rader DJ. Polygenic risk scores and coronary artery disease: ready for prime time? *Circulation.* 2020;141:637–640.
141. Khan SS, Cooper R, Greenland P. Do polygenic risk scores improve patient selection for prevention of coronary artery disease? *J Am Med Assoc.* 2020;323:614–615.
142. Bilkey GA, Burns BL, Coles EP, et al. Optimizing precision medicine for public health. *Front Public Health.* 2019;7:42.
143. Labarthe D, Lloyd-Jones DM. 50×50×50: cardiovascular health and the cardiovascular disease endgame. *Circulation.* 2018;138:968–970.
144. Victor RG, Lynch K, Li N, et al. A cluster-randomized trial of blood-pressure reduction in black barbershops. *N Engl J Med.* 2018;378:1291–1301.
145. Perez MV, Mahaffey KW, Hedlin H, et al. Large-scale assessment of a smartwatch to identify atrial fibrillation. *N Engl J Med.* 2019;381:1909–1917.
146. Bally L, Thabit H, Hartnell S, et al. Closed-loop insulin delivery for glycemic control in noncritical care. *N Engl J Med.* 2018;379:547–556.
147. GBD-2017 Causes of Death Collaborators. Global, regional, and national age-sex-specific mortality for 282 causes of death in 195 countries and territories, 1980-2017: a systematic analysis for the global burden of disease study 2017. *Lancet.* 2018Vol.392:1736–1788.
148. GBD 2017 Disease and Injury Incidence and Prevalence Collaborators. Global, regional, and national incidence, prevalence, and years lived with disability for 354 diseases and injuries for 195 countries and territories, 1990-2017: a systematic analysis for the global burden of disease study 2017. *Lancet.* 2018;392:1789–1858.

26 Systemic Hypertension: Mechanisms, Diagnosis, and Treatment

GEORGE L. BAKRIS AND MATTHEW J. SORRENTINO

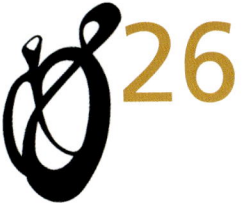

DEFINITIONS OF HYPERTENSION, 471

EPIDEMIOLOGY, 471

PATHOPHYSIOLOGY, 473
Pressure Natriuresis and Salt Sensitivity, 473
Renin-Angiotensin-Aldosterone System, 474
Sympathetic Nervous System, 476
Natriuretic Peptides, 477
Endothelium, 477
Arterial Stiffness in Hypertension, 478

FACTORS INVOLVED IN PREDISPOSITION TO HYPERTENSION, 478
Genetics, 478
Obesity, 478

A DIAGNOSTIC APPROACH TO PRIMARY HYPERTENSION, 480
History and Physical Examination, 480
Blood Pressure Measurement, 481

Integrating Home Blood Pressure Into Clinical Practice, 483
Laboratory and Other Complementary Tests, 483

DIAGNOSTIC APPROACH FOR SECONDARY HYPERTENSION, 484
Endocrine Causes, 484
Nonendocrine Causes, 487
Nonlifestyle, Nonendocrine Causes, 488

THERAPEUTIC OPTIONS AND APPROACHES FOR PRIMARY HYPERTENSION, 490
Goals of Therapy, 490
Effect of Lifestyle Intervention in the Older People (>65 years), 490

BLOOD PRESSURE–LOWERING MEDICATIONS, 490

THERAPEUTIC OPTIONS AND APPROACHES FOR SUBGROUPS OF HYPERTENSION, 490
Pharmacologic Intervention in the Older People (>65 years), 490

MANAGEMENT OF HYPERTENSION IN CHRONIC KIDNEY DISEASE, 492
Blood Pressure Management in Patients Undergoing Dialysis, 492

HEART FAILURE, 493

RESISTANT HYPERTENSION, 494
Renal Denervation, 495
Baroreceptor-Activation, 496

HYPERTENSIVE URGENCY AND EMERGENCY, 497

REFERENCES, 498

Primary hypertension is a key contributor to premature morbidity and mortality in the United States[1] and consistently ranks among the top two risk factors worldwide for global disease burden in 2015.[2] After tobacco use and diabetes, uncontrolled primary hypertension is the most important risk factor for peripheral vascular disease (the second leading cause of loss of limbs in the United States).[3]

Uncontrolled primary hypertension is the most important modifiable risk factor for stroke, the leading contributor to all common forms of heart failure, the second most common cause of end-stage kidney disease, and also contributes to memory loss.[4]

DEFINITIONS OF HYPERTENSION

Blood pressure (BP) is the phenotypic expression of the genetically predisposed disease hypertension and is a continuous variable. As more data became available, the guideline-based definition of hypertension has evolved over the past 40 years. The traditional "threshold BP value" to secure a diagnosis of hypertension comes from large epidemiologic studies demonstrating a higher mortality at levels above 140/90 mm Hg.[4] More recent guidelines, however, define the level at which one is considered hypertensive based on level of cardiovascular (CV) risk rather than just the BP number. This is true of the most recent US guidelines that define hypertension as ≥130/80 mm Hg and the European Guidelines which use a slightly different approach to risk and define hypertension as ≥140/90 mm Hg (Table 26.1).[5–7] Thus, in most people up to age 80 years and those with comorbidities, a BP ≥130/80 mm Hg is considered hypertension requiring treatment in the United States. However, medical treatment is not accepted in everyone with low risk and around the world for BP 130 to 140/80 to 90 mm Hg (Table 26.1).[6,7]

EPIDEMIOLOGY

The global burden of hypertension is estimated at approximately 1.4 billion individuals, and by 2025 at the current rate will exceed 1.6 billion.[8] CV risk attributable to elevated BP dates back to 1948 and the origin of the Framingham Heart Study.[2,9–11] The continuous relationship between BP level and risk of events in the brain, heart, and kidney are well documented.[9–12] A natural history study involving almost 12,000 veterans, followed over 15 years, noted that BP level correlated with risk for end-stage kidney disease (Fig. 26.1).[13] Note that, in this study, the highest risk for end-stage kidney disease was found at levels above the renal autoregulatory range (i.e., a systolic BP >180 mm Hg). A natural history study of over a million people demonstrates that CV risk becomes most pronounced above levels of 140/90 mm Hg (Fig. 26.2).[4]

Increasing age is a major risk factor for developing hypertension, as well as a very strong confounder of its independent influence on CV and renal events due to increased arterial stiffness and reduced nitric oxide (NO) release (see Fig. 26.2).[14] In an analysis of 61 epidemiologic studies followed for an average of 13.3 years, those with BP levels in the highest decile had approximately the same risk for death from either ischemic heart disease or stroke as people who were 20 years older but had BP levels in the lowest decile.[4] In the Framingham study the lifetime risk of 55- to 65-year-old men or women for developing hypertension was above 90%.[15] In this study, those who survived to ages 65 to 89 years, systolic BP (SBP) elevations were found in 87% of the hypertensive men and 93% of the hypertensive women. In an analysis of the Framingham data set, classification of people with hypertension older than age 60 years into the appropriate BP stages was done correctly in 99% of the cases using SBP rather than diastolic BP (DBP).[16]

These data highlight the public health importance of SBP, particularly among people older than 50 years of age. In such individuals, SBP is a much better predictor of hypertensive target-organ damage and future CV and renal events than is DBP.[4,17,18] Overall, each 20-mm Hg increase in SBP doubled the risk for CV death.[4] Although uncontrolled hypertension in the United States in 2014 was noted in nearly 54% of people 60 years of age and older,[19] antihypertensive drug therapy reduces CV events with its greatest absolute benefit in older people, including individuals older than 80 years of age.[20–22] Moreover, data clearly show that people with sustained BP control have fewer CV events than others; however, in spite of multiple international guidelines including US guidance for initial *dual therapy* to help achieve BP control, initial dual therapy fails to be adopted to achieve this benefit (Fig. 26.3).[23,24]

TABLE 26.1 Guidelines Comparison: US and European

GUIDELINE DIFFERENCES	AMERICAN COLLEGE OF CARDIOLOGY/AMERICAN HEART ASSOCIATION (ACC/AHA)		EUROPEAN SOCIETY OF CARDIOLOGY/EUROPEAN SOCIETY OF HYPERTENSION (ESC/ESH)	
Level of Blood Pressure (BP) Defining Hypertension	Systolic and/or Diastolic		Systolic and/or Diastolic	
	(mm Hg)	(mm Hg)	(mm Hg)	(mm Hg)
Office/clinic BP	≥130	≥80	≥140	≥90
Daytime mean	≥130	≥80	≥135	≥85
Nighttime mean	≥110	≥65	≥120	≥70
24-hr mean	≥125	≥75	≥130	≥80
Home BP mean	≥130	≥80	≥135	≥85
BP targets for treatment	<130/80		Systolic targets	<140 and close to 130
Initial combination therapy	Initial single-pill combination therapy		Initial single-pill combination in patients >20/10 mm Hg above BP goal therapy in patients ≥ 140/90 mm Hg	
Hypertensive requiring	>130/80 mm Hg		≥140/90 mm Hg intervention	
Guidelines Similarities				
Importance of home	Take BP at home, twice in the morning and twice in the evening, in the week before clinic BP monitoring		Bring the BP machine in annually for validation	
Therapy	Restrict beta blockers to patients with comorbidities or other indications		Initial single-pill combination as initial therapy	
Follow-up	Detect poor adherence and focus on improvement		BP telemonitoring and digital health solutions recommended	

From Bakris G, Ali W, Parati G. ACC/AHA versus ESC/ESH on hypertension guidelines: JACC guideline comparison. *J Am Coll Cardiol.* 2019;73:3018–3026.

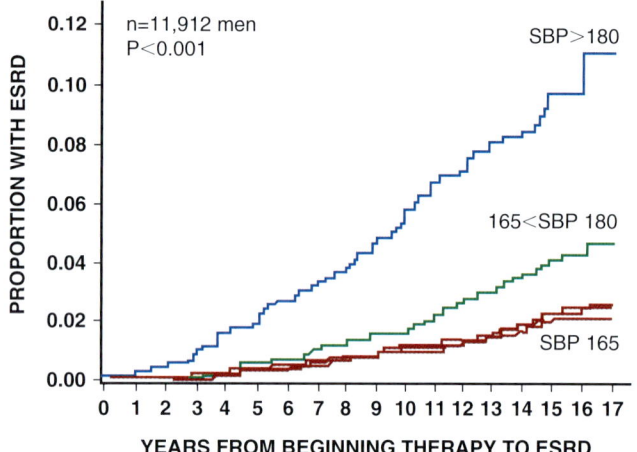

FIGURE 26.1 Natural history of untreated hypertension in 12,000 people followed over 15 years. (From Perry HM, Jr., Miller JP, Fornoff JR, et al. Early predictors of 15-year end-stage renal disease in hypertensive patients. *Hypertension.* 1995;25:587–594.)

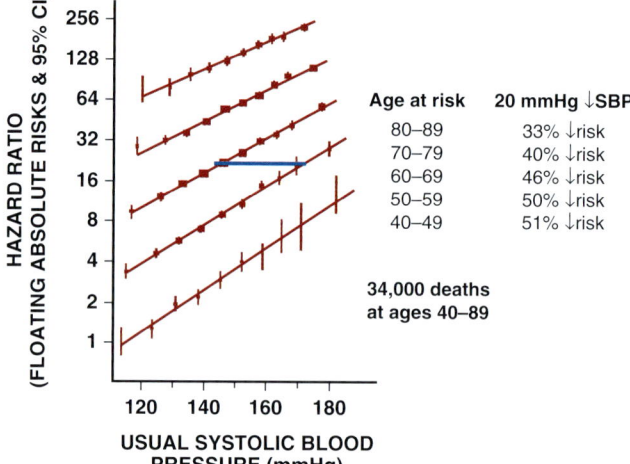

FIGURE 26.2 Natural history of over a million people demonstrates that CV risk becomes most pronounced above levels of 140/90 mm Hg.[4] Note also the line signifying the difference in risk at a given age and level of blood pressure.

Currently there are more than 125 different medications, almost all of which are generically available, from eight different antihypertensive drug classes to help lower BP (Fig. 26.4). Moreover, there are more than 15 fixed-dose single-pill combination agents (Table 26.2).[25] Note that all clinical trials over the past 30 years have used more than one medication for BP control (Fig. 26.5). In spite of this, BP control remains suboptimal in many parts of the world.[2,10,19,26-28] What is missing is a focus on obesity reduction and wide availability of single-pill two-drug combinations to control BP as is strongly advocated by the European hypertension guidelines (see Table 26.1).[6]

The diagnosis of hypertension in children and adolescents is becoming more important, due to the epidemic of obesity in young Americans.[29] Current US guidelines recommend BP measurement in children at least annually, but "normative values" depend on sex, age, and height of the child.[30] As a result, interpretation of BP levels in children and adolescents usually involves comparison of a child's average BP (from three visits) to a comprehensive table that provides threshold values for "elevated" (traditionally, BP between the 90th and 95th percentiles), "hypertension" (BP between the 95th and 99th percentiles), and "severe hypertension" (99th percentile or higher).

Non-Hispanic Blacks have approximately a 50% higher prevalence of hypertension than non-Hispanic Whites, even after age adjustment (41.2% versus 28.0%) (see Chapter 93).[19] The prevalence of hypertension is geographically heterogeneous, with the highest prevalence in both Blacks and Whites in the southeastern United States. However, non-Hispanic Blacks had the highest awareness (at 85.7%) and treatment (at 77.4%) of hypertension in National Health and Nutrition Examination Survey (NHANES) 2011 to 2012, but their BP control rate in 2011 to 2014 lagged that of non-Hispanic Whites (48.5% to 55.7%, age adjusted). This pattern has been consistent over the past decade.[31]

The prevalence of hypertension has increased since 1988, with the greatest increase for non-Hispanic Blacks, compared with either Mexican Americans or non-Hispanic Whites. In contrast to non-Hispanic Whites and Mexican Americans, a slightly higher prevalence of hypertension was observed in NHANES 2011 to 2014 for non-Hispanic Black women, compared with men (41.5% versus 40.8%).[32] In all three racial/

JNC 7 (2003)
ASH Initial Combo Report (2010)
ACC/AHA BP Guidelines (2017)
%
40.6
40.4
40.2
40
39.8
39.6
39.4
39.2
30
TOTAL (2005–2008)
TOTAL (2009–2012)
TOTAL (2013–2016)

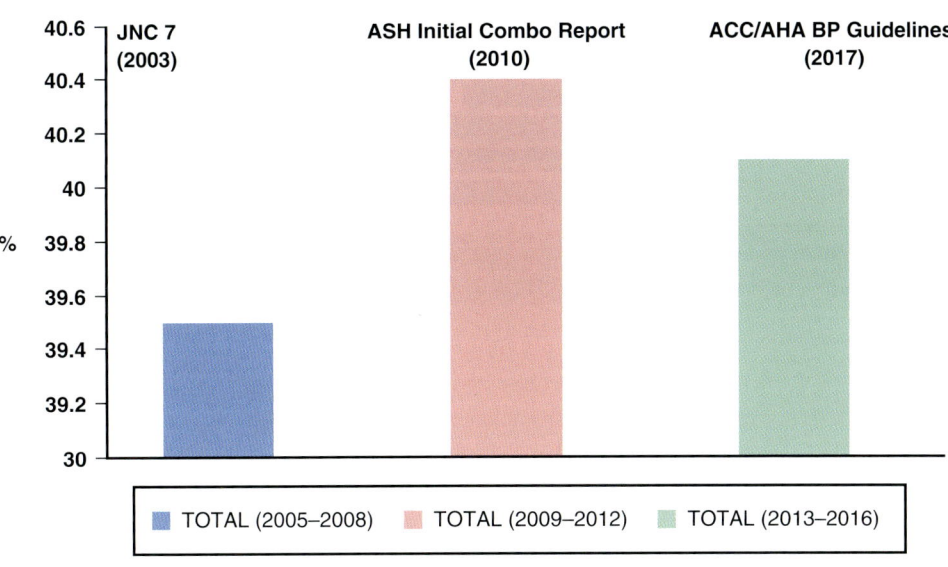

FIGURE 26.3 Data over the past 15 years evaluating combination therapy use and guideline recommendations.

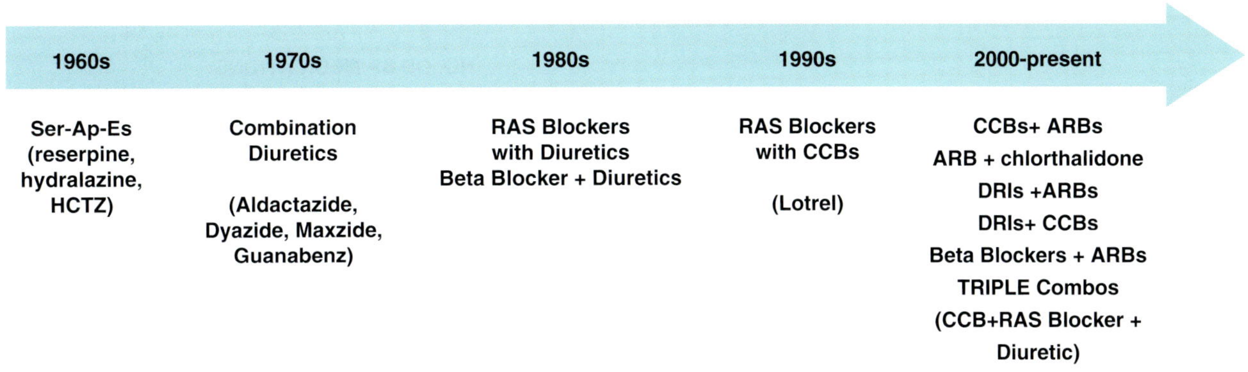

1960s
1970s
1980s
1990s
2000-present
Ser-Ap-Es (reserpine, hydralazine, HCTZ)
Combination Diuretics
(Aldactazide, Dyazide, Maxzide, Guanabenz)
RAS Blockers with Diuretics
Beta Blocker + Diuretics
RAS Blockers with CCBs
(Lotrel)
CCBs+ ARBs
ARB + chlorthalidone
DRIs +ARBs
DRIs+ CCBs
Beta Blockers + ARBs
TRIPLE Combos
(CCB+RAS Blocker + Diuretic)

FIGURE 26.4 Evolution of different antihypertensive drug classes over time.

TABLE 26.2 Drug Combinations in Hypertension: Recommendations from the American Society of Hypertension

Preferred
ACE inhibitor/diuretic*
ARB/diuretic*
ACE inhibitor/CCB*
ARB/CCB*Acceptable
Beta blocker/diuretic*
CCB (dihydropyridine)/beta blocker
CCB/diuretic
Renin inhibitor/diuretic*
Thiazide diuretics/K^+-sparing diuretics*Less effective
ACE inhibitor/ARB
ACE inhibitor/beta blocker
ARB/beta blocker
CCB (nondihydropyridine)/beta blocker
Centrally acting agent/beta blocker

*Single-pill combinations approved in the United States.

ACE, Angiotensin-converting enzyme; *ARB*, angiotensin receptor blocker; *CCB*, calcium channel blocker.

Adapted from Gradman AH, Basile JN, Carter BL, et al. Combination therapy in hypertension. *J Clin Hypertens (Greenwich)*. 2011;13:146–154.

ethnic groups, women had higher rates of awareness, treatment, and control of BP than men in NHANES 2011 to 2014.

In 2014, the age-adjusted death rate from heart disease was 24% higher in Blacks, as was stroke (by 41%) and hypertension or hypertensive renal disease (by 111%).[33] Incident end-stage renal disease (ESRD) was 3.1 or 1.2 times more common in 2014 in Blacks or Native Americans, compared with whites.[34]

Although the prevalence of hypertension in Hispanics is lower than in non-Hispanic Blacks and whites, hypertension is a concern. Mexican Americans continue to have the lowest age-adjusted prevalence of controlled hypertension in both men and women (25.6% and 31.9%, respectively, in NHANES 1999 to 2006, compared with 37.0% and 49.2% in NHANES 2007 to 2014).[1]

BP control rates (to <140/90 mm Hg) have improved substantially in the United States since 1974 and have stabilized at just over 50% in the last four biennial NHANES reports.[1] Successful national efforts to increase hypertension treatment and control rates have been associated with significant reductions in CV hospitalizations or death in both Canada[28] and the United Kingdom.[35] With new hypertension goals, those with apparent treatment-resistant hypertension and the prevalence of uncontrolled hypertension are greater for undiagnosed, untreated, or older individuals and for SBP (rather than DBP).[36]

PATHOPHYSIOLOGY

The factors that generate BP comprise the integration of cardiac output (CO) and systemic vascular resistance (SVR): BP = CO × SVR. Note that CO = heart rate × stroke volume; SVR = 80 × (mean arterial pressure – central venous pressure)/CO.

Pressure Natriuresis and Salt Sensitivity

To fully understand BP regulation, one has to appreciate that the kidney is a regulatory organ that tries to maintain a homeostatic

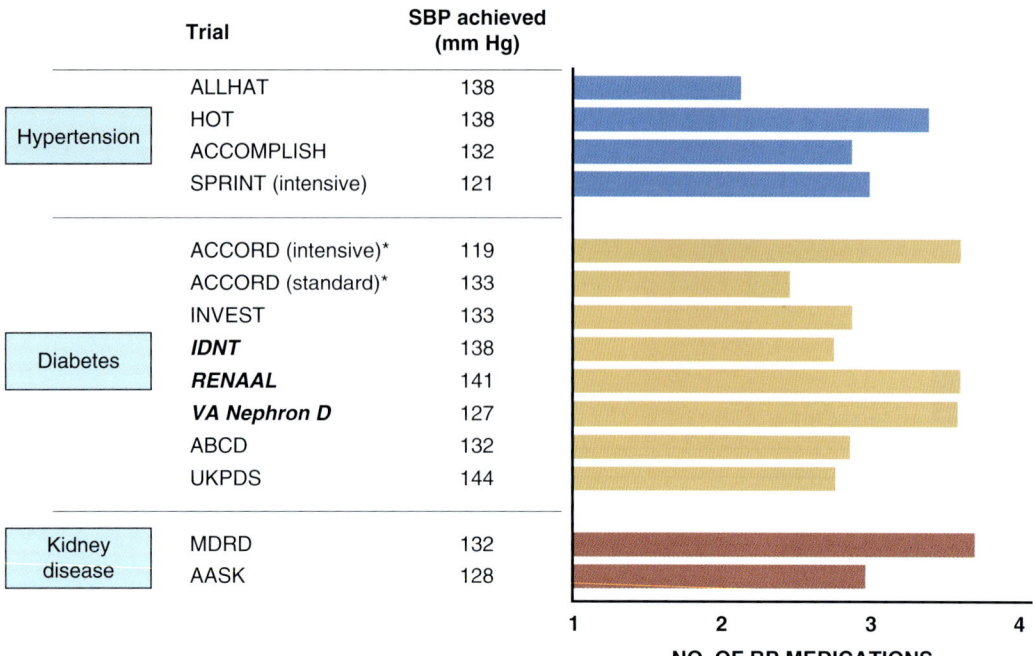

FIGURE 26.5 Summary of clinical trials with blood pressure (BP) heart or kidney endpoints and average number of medications used to attain BP level <140 mm Hg.

environment under a variety of changes not only in BP but electrolytes and acid-base balance. Hence, because sodium conservation is one of its principle jobs, any large increase in pressure will lead to pressure natriuesis.[37]

Pressure natriuresis is defined as the increase in renal sodium excretion due to mild increases in BP, typically because of extracellular fluid volume expansion, allowing BP to remain in the normal range.[37–39] This concept is essential to the understanding of the sustainability of hypertension. If one understands the "set-point BP" as the BP at the point when extracellular volume and pressure natriuresis are in equilibrium, it necessarily follows that an increase in BP can be sustained only if pressure natriuresis is abnormal. Pressure natriuresis occurs over hours to days and is modulated by both biophysical and humoral factors.

In the normal state, increased sodium intake causes an increase in extracellular volume and BP. Because of the steep relationship between volume and pressure, small increases in BP produce natriuresis that restores sodium balance and returns BP to normal (Fig. 26.6A). Expansion of extracellular fluid volume and increased BP result in a rise in blood flow through the vasa recta, which stimulates the production of paracrine factors such as NO and ATP, which can inhibit tubular sodium reabsorption at multiple sites of the nephron.[40] NO blunts the myogenic response of arteriolar autoregulation, thus allowing increased blood flow that is necessary to increase renal blood flow and interstitial pressure (Fig. 26.6B).[37,40]

The kidneys adapt to sodium loading quickly, adapting to fluctuations in sodium intake as high as 50-fold,[39] but this response is markedly blunted in the setting of chronic hypertension, resulting in a need for much higher BP levels to promote natriuresis. These states of abnormal sodium handling lead to sodium-sensitive hypertension, such as in conditions of reduced glomerular filtration rate (GFR) or high levels of angiotensin II. In such situations the change in extracellular fluid volume is relatively small (3% to 5%), but a state of chronic high BP develops resulting from increased SVR. The mechanisms responsible for this vascular effect are not completely understood but likely involve increased activity of the renin-angiotensin-aldosterone system (RAAS) (high angiotensin II levels) and several other vasoconstricting substances.[37] Because abnormalities in pressure-sodium relationships are essential to maintaining chronic elevations in BP, they represent a fundamental step in the pathogenesis of any type of hypertension, not only primary, but also in the maintenance phase of most secondary causes, such as renal and renovascular hypertension, hyperaldosteronism, glucocorticoid excess, coarctation of the aorta, and pheochromocytoma.

The interplay between renal sodium retention and hypertension involves changes in sodium handling throughout the nephron. A theory with substantial experimental support proposes that increased renal vasoconstriction due to a variety of possible mechanisms (e.g., increased levels of angiotensin II, catecholamines, uric acid, or progressive aging) induces a preglomerular (afferent) arteriolopathy that results in impaired sodium filtration.[41,42] In addition, renal vasoconstriction results in tubular ischemia, another mediator of increased sodium avidity.

Renin-Angiotensin-Aldosterone System

The RAAS has wide-ranging effects on BP regulation. Figure 26.7 summarizes the most relevant elements of the RAAS and its role in the pathogenesis of hypertension and its complications. The different elements of the RAAS have key roles in mediating sodium retention, pressure natriuresis, salt sensitivity, vasoconstriction, endothelium dysfunction, and vascular injury; and use of RAAS blockers is an effective means of treating hypertension.[37] Taken together, the RAAS has an important role in the pathogenesis of hypertension. However, there are a number of unanswered issues about this relationship. A very large genome-wide association study (GWAS) of 2.5 million genotyped or imputed single-nucleotide polymorphisms (SNPs) in 69,395 individuals of European ancestry from 29 studies[43] showed that the majority of SNPs associated with BP involved issues with natriuretic peptides. Thus natriuretic peptides play a prominent role in the pathogenesis of hypertension and may be more important than the RAAS system, which did not have prominent SNPs associated with hypertension in this analysis. Another meta-analysis evaluating the relationship between polymorphisms in key RAAS genes (angiotensin-converting enzyme [ACE], angiotensinogen gene [AGT], and CYP11B2) and salt sensitivity also found no significant role of RAAS polymorphisms.[44]

Despite these genetic inconsistencies, a wealth of experimental evidence links the RAAS to hypertension. Tissue expression of different elements of the RAAS is also important, including in the protection of animals from the development of hypertension after targeted elimination of renal ACE activity.[45] Paradoxically the same experiments indicate that the absence of ACE in other tissues may also be protective from hypertension caused by triggers that do not involve the RAAS (such as NO inhibition), therefore raising the possibility that other (extrarenal) sites may also be relevant.[46]

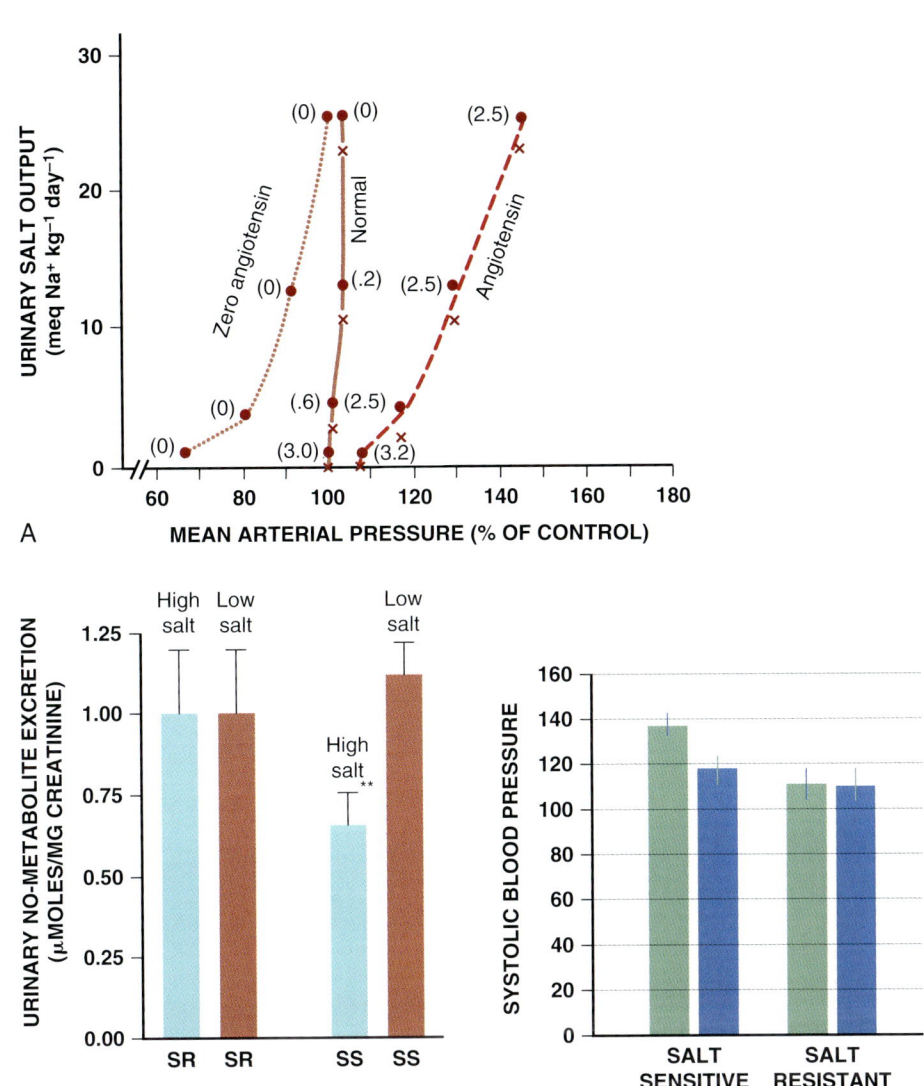

FIGURE 26.6 A, Relationship between volume and pressure, where small increases in blood pressure (BP) produce natriuresis that restores sodium balance and returns BP to normal. **B,** Evidence that nitric oxide (NO) blunts the myogenic response of arteriolar autoregulation, thus allowing increased blood flow to increase renal blood flow and interstitial pressure.

receptor (AT_1R), angiotensin II is a potent vasoconstrictor of vascular smooth muscle, causing systemic vasoconstriction as well as increased renovascular resistance and decreased medullary flow, which is a mediator of salt sensitivity. Angiotensin II produces increased sodium reabsorption in the proximal tubule by increasing the activity of the sodium:hydrogen exchanger (NHE3), the sodium-bicarbonate exchanger, and Na^+-K^+-ATPase and by inducing aldosterone synthesis and release from the adrenal zona glomerulosa. Angiotensin II is associated with endothelial cell dysfunction and produces extensive fibrotic and inflammatory changes, largely mediated by increased oxidative stress, resulting in renal, cardiac, and vascular injury, thus giving angiotensin II a tight link to target-organ injury in hypertension. In contrast, stimulation of the angiotensin II type 2 receptor (AT_2R) is associated with opposite effects, resulting in vasodilation, natriuresis, and antiproliferative effects.

The relative importance of the renal and vascular effects of angiotensin II was evaluated in classic cross-transplantation studies using both wild-type mice and mice lacking the AT_1R.[49,50] By cross-transplanting the kidneys of wild-type mice into AT_1R knockout mice and vice versa, investigators were able to generate animals that were selective renal AT_1R knockouts or selective systemic (nonrenal) AT_1R knockouts. In physiologic conditions, renal, systemic, and total knockout animals had lower BP than wild-type animals, indicating a role of both renal and extrarenal AT_1R in BP regulation.[50] The systemic AT_1R absence was associated with approximately 50% lower aldosterone levels, but the lower BP observed in this group was independent of this lower aldosterone production, as BP remained low despite aldosterone infusions to supraphysiologic levels following adrenalectomy in the systemic knockout animals. In addition, the BP reduction in kidney knockout animals occurred despite normal aldosterone excretion, again confirming the importance of aldosterone-independent renal angiotensin II effects.

When hypertension is present, the presence of renal AT_1R mediates both hypertension and organ injury.[50] When animals were infused with angiotensin II for 4 weeks, animals lacking renal AT_1R did not develop sustained hypertension, whereas wild-type and systemic knockout mice had a significant increase in BP. In addition, only animals with elevated BP developed cardiac hypertrophy and fibrosis. This indicates that cardiac injury is largely dependent on hypertension and not on the presence of AT_1R in the heart, because the (hypertensive) systemic knockout animals developed significant cardiac abnormalities despite the absence of AT_1R in the heart.[49] In summary, these experiments indicate that both systemic and renal actions of angiotensin II are relevant to physiologic BP regulation, but in hypertension, the detrimental effects of angiotensin II are mediated via its renal effects.

The enzyme renin and prorenin are synthesized and stored in the juxtaglomerular cell apparatus located in the kidney adjacent to the afferent arteriole and distal tubule. Renin is released in response to decreased renal afferent perfusion pressure, decreased sodium delivery to the macula densa, and activation of renal nerves (via $β_1$-adrenergic receptor stimulation) and by a variety of metabolic products, including prostaglandin E_2 and several others. The main function of renin is to cleave angiotensinogen into angiotensin I.[37]

Prorenin, previously viewed as an inactive substrate for renin production, is known to stimulate the (pro)renin receptor (PRR). This receptor leads to more efficient cleavage of angiotensinogen and activates downstream intracellular signaling through the mitogen-activated protein (MAP) kinases extracellular signal–regulated kinases 1 and 2 (ERK1/2) pathways that have been associated with profibrotic effects in some, but not all, experimental models.[47,48] It is still uncertain if the PRR is involved in the genesis or complications of hypertension in a manner that is independent of the effects of angiotensin II (see Fig. 26.7).[47]

Angiotensin II, formed by the cleavage of angiotensin I by ACE, is at the center of the pathogenetic role of the RAAS in hypertension. Primarily through its actions mediated by the angiotensin II type 1

Aldosterone, the adrenocortical hormone synthesized in the zona glomerulosa, plays a critical role in hypertension through its effects on sodium reabsorption largely mediated by transcriptional effects, via activation of the mineralocorticoid receptor, leading to increased expression of the epithelial sodium channel (ENaC). An extensive body of literature has identified other genomic and nongenomic effects of aldosterone with relevance to hypertension. Extensive nonepithelial effects include vascular smooth muscle cell proliferation, vascular

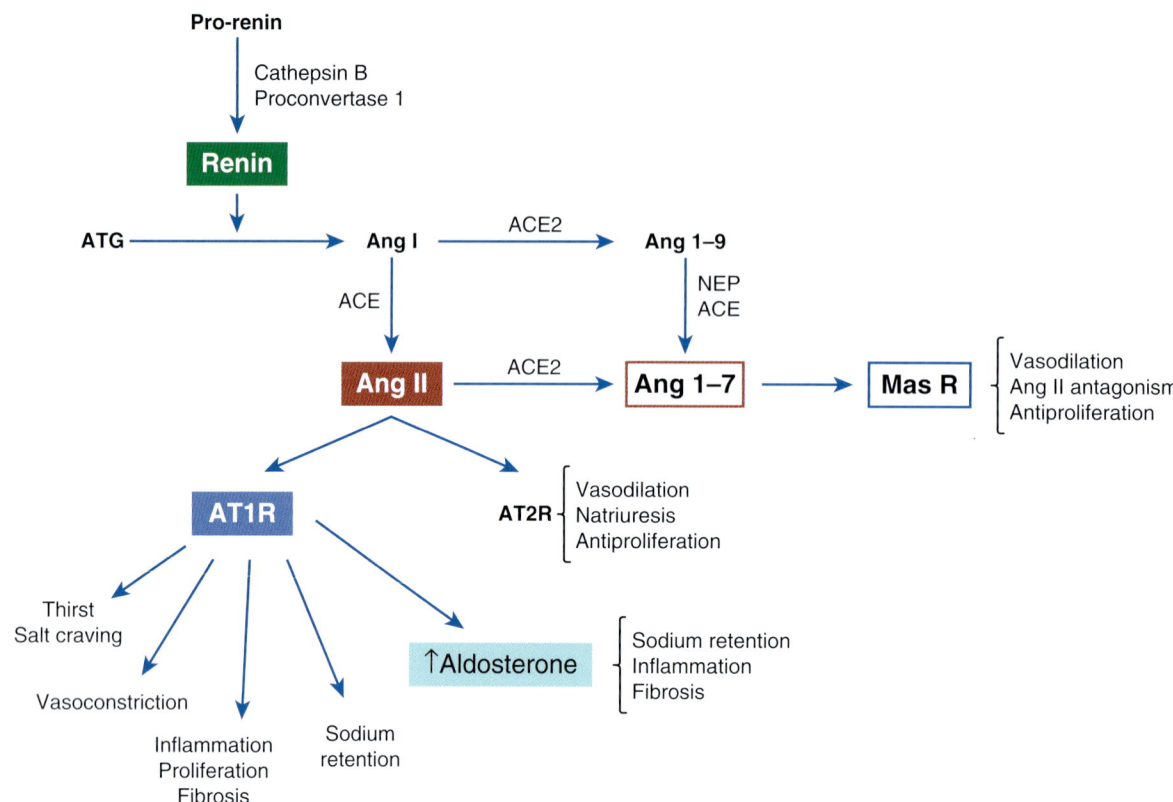

FIGURE 26.7 Factors involved in the renin-angiotensin-aldosterone system.

extracellular matrix deposition, vascular remodeling and fibrosis, and increased oxidative stress leading to endothelial dysfunction and vasoconstriction.[51]

Several other elements of the RAAS have potentially important roles in hypertension. The importance of ACE2 and angiotensin (1 to 7) to BP regulation and angiotensin II–associated target-organ injury has become apparent. ACE2 is expressed largely in the heart, kidney, and endothelium; it has partial homology to ACE and is unaffected directly by ACE inhibitors (ACEIs).[52] It has a variety of substrates, but its most important action is the conversion of angiotensin II to angiotensin (1 to 7). Angiotensin (1 to 7) is formed primarily though the hydrolysis of angiotensin II by ACE2, and its actions are opposite to those of angiotensin II, including vasodilatory and antiproliferative properties that are mediated by the Mas receptor, a G protein–coupled receptor that, upon activation, forms complexes with the AT_1R, thus antagonizing the effects of angiotensin II.

The vasodilatory effects are mediated by increased cyclic guanosine monophosphate, decreased norepinephrine release, and amplification of bradykinin effects. Studies have identified ACE2 and angiotensin (1 to 7) as protective factors in the development of atherosclerosis and cardiac and renal injury,[52,53] and administration of recombinant ACE2 or its activator, xanthenone, has resulted in improved endothelial function, decreased BP, and improved renal, cardiac, and perivascular fibrosis in hypertensive animals.[54-56] However, a phase 1 study of recombinant ACE2 in healthy humans did not show any BP-lowering effects despite appropriate modulation of the RAAS, including sustained increase in angiotensin (1 to 7) levels.[57] Therefore, the clinical value of the manipulation of any of the elements of this vasodepressor component of the RAAS remains to be determined.[58]

Sympathetic Nervous System

The sympathetic nervous system (SNS) is consistently activated in patients with hypertension compared with normotensive individuals, particularly in the obese. Many patients with hypertension are in a state of autonomic imbalance that encompasses increased sympathetic and decreased parasympathetic activity.[59,60] SNS hyperactivity is relevant to both the generation and maintenance of hypertension and is observed in human hypertension from the very earliest stages. Studies in humans have identified markers of sympathetic overactivity in normotensive individuals with a family history of hypertension.[59] Among patients with hypertension, increasing severity of hypertension is associated with increasing levels of sympathetic activity measured by microneurography.[61,62] In human hypertension, plasma catecholamine levels, microneurographic recordings, and systemic catecholamine spillover studies have consistently found elevation of these markers in obesity, the metabolic syndrome, and hypertension complicated by heart failure or kidney disease.[59] In addition, SNS hyperactivity is observed in most hypertensive subgroups, although it appears more pronounced in men than in women, and in younger than in older patients.[63]

Several experimental models have outlined the importance of the SNS in generating hypertension. Different models of obesity-related hypertension indicate that the SNS is activated early in the development of increased adiposity,[60] and the key factor in the maintenance of sustained hypertension is increased renal sympathetic nerve activity and its attendant sodium avidity.[63]

SNS-mediated induction of salt sensitivity is a key element to sustaining high BP in other models of hypertension as well. For instance, rats receiving daily infusions of phenylephrine for 8 weeks developed hypertension during the infusions, but BP normalized under a low-salt diet after discontinuation of phenylephrine.[64] However, once exposed to a high-salt diet, the animals again became hypertensive. The degree of BP elevation on a high-salt diet was directly related to the degree of renal tubulointerstitial fibrosis and decrement of GFR. These findings can be interpreted within the paradigm that catecholamine-induced hypertension causes renal interstitial injury that associates with a salt-sensitive phenotype even after sympathetic overactivity is no longer present.[63] In addition, enhanced SNS activity results in α_1-receptor–mediated endothelial dysfunction, vasoconstriction, vascular smooth muscle proliferation, and arterial stiffness, all of which contribute to the development of hypertension. Finally, evidence indicates that sympathetic overactivity results in salt sensitivity due to a reduction in the activity of serine/threonine-protein kinase WNK4. This results in increased sodium avidity through the thiazide-sensitive sodium

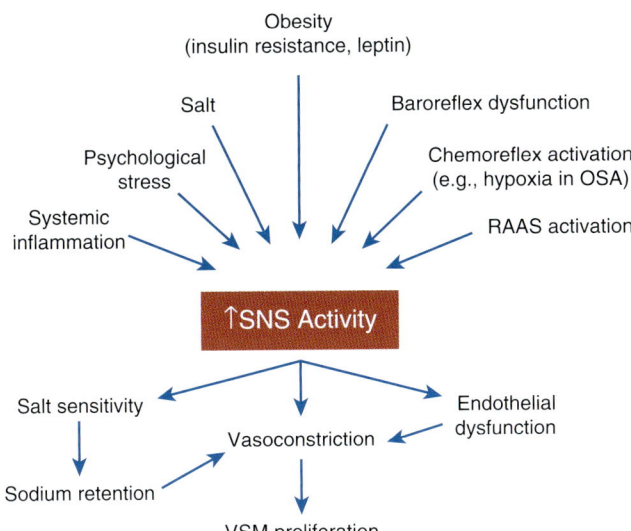

FIGURE 26.8 Demonstration of sympathetic overactivity leading to salt sensitivity due to a reduction in the activity of serine/threonine-protein kinase WNK4.

chloride symporter NCC.[65] Figure 26.8 summarizes the causes and consequences of SNS activation in the genesis of hypertension.

In a meta-analysis of hypertension trials, heart rate reduction during treatment with beta blockers was paradoxically associated with increased risk for death and CV events in patients with hypertension.[66] In contrast, in a very large ($n = 10,000$) patient outcome trial, a post hoc analysis of heart rate at baseline demonstrated that those with a resting heart rate above 80 beats/min even with a BP below 140/90 mm Hg had a higher mortality rate.[67] Therefore, although apparent that SNS activation is deleterious to patients with CV disease, and presumably with hypertension, a cause for the overactivity should be sought and an attempt made to affect that mechanism.

Natriuretic Peptides

Natriuretic peptides (atrial [ANP], brain [BNP], and urodilatin) play an important role in salt sensitivity, heart failure, and hypertension.[68] These peptides have important natriuretic and vasodilatory properties that allow maintenance of sodium balance and BP during sodium loading. Upon administration of a sodium load, atrial and ventricular stretch leads to release of ANP and BNP, respectively, which result in immediate BP lowering due to systemic vasodilation and decreased plasma volume, the latter caused by fluid shifts from the intravascular to the interstitial compartment.[69] All natriuretic peptides directly increase GFR, which in volume-expanded states is mediated by an increase in efferent arteriolar tone and increased filtration coefficient (K_f). Natriuretic peptides also inhibit renal sodium reabsorption through both direct and indirect effects. Direct effects include decreased activity of Na$^+$-ATPase and the sodium-glucose cotransporter in the proximal tubule and inhibition of the ENaC in the distal nephron.[68] The inhibitory effects of natriuretic peptides on renin and aldosterone release mediate indirect effects. Unfortunately, understanding the contribution of natriuretic peptides to the development of hypertension in humans is complicated by the elevation of their levels in association with increased BP (due to increased afterload) and hypertensive heart disease.

Some studies have tested whether polymorphisms in ANP or BNP genes resulting in higher levels of these peptides would be associated with lower BP; results of these studies have been inconsistent, and effects have been small.[70-72] There are no published studies evaluating sequential changes in natriuretic peptides and risk for incident hypertension.

Endothelium

The endothelium is a major regulator of vascular tone and thus plays a key role in BP regulation. Endothelial cells produce a host of vasoactive substances, of which NO is the most important to BP regulation. NO is continuously released by endothelial cells, especially in response to flow-induced shear stress in arteries and arterioles, leading to vascular smooth muscle relaxation through activation of guanylate cyclase and generation of intracellular cyclic guanosine monophosphate.[73,74] Interruption of NO production via inhibition of the constitutively expressed nitric oxide synthase 3 (eNOS) causes BP elevation and development of hypertension in both animals and humans. Using brachial artery flow-mediated vasodilation and measurement of urinary excretion of NO metabolites as methods to evaluate NO activity in humans, several studies have demonstrated decreased whole-body production of NO in patients with hypertension compared with normotensive controls.

Several elements are responsible for endothelial dysfunction in hypertension. Normotensive offspring of patients with hypertension have impaired endothelium-dependent vasodilation despite normal endothelium-independent responses, thus suggesting a genetic component to the development of endothelial dysfunction.[75] In addition to direct pressure-induced injury in the setting of chronically elevated BP, a mechanism of major importance is increased oxidative stress. Reactive oxygen species are generated from enhanced activity of several enzyme systems, reduced nicotinamide adenine dinucleotide phosphate-oxidase (NADPH-oxidase), xanthine oxidase, and cyclooxygenase in particular, and decreased activity of the oxygen free radical detoxifying enzyme superoxide dismutase.[76,77]

Angiotensin II is a major enhancer of vascular NADPH-oxidase activity and plays a central role in the generation of oxidative stress in hypertension, although several other factors are also involved, including cyclic vascular stretch, endothelin-1 (ET-1), uric acid, systemic inflammation, norepinephrine, free fatty acids, and tobacco smoking.[78]

ET-1 is the endothelial cell product that counteracts NO to maintain balance between vasodilation and vasoconstriction. ET-1 expression is increased by shear stress, catecholamines, angiotensin II, hypoxia, and several proinflammatory cytokines such as tumor necrosis factor-α, interleukins 1 and 2, and transforming growth factor-β.[76] ET-1 is a potent vasoconstrictor through stimulation of ET-A receptors in vascular smooth muscle.[79] In hypertension, increased ET-1 levels are not consistently found. However, there is a trend of increased sensitivity to the vasoconstrictor effects of ET-1. ET-1 therefore is considered a relevant mediator of BP elevation because ET-A and ET-B receptor antagonists attenuate or abolish hypertension in several experimental models of hypertension (angiotensin II–mediated models, deoxycorticosterone acetate–salt hypertension, and Dahl salt-sensitive rats) and are effective in lowering BP in humans.[80]

NO is not the only gas relevant to vascular biology. Hydrogen sulfide (H_2S) has received recent attention due to potential treatment relevance.[81] H_2S is a vasodilating gas produced from sulfated amino acids by action of one of two key enzymes, cystathione gamma-lyase (CSE) and cystathione beta-synthase. CSE homozygous knockout mice have approximately 80% decreased H_2S expression in heart and aorta and approximately 60% reduction in serum, and both homozygous and heterozygous animals demonstrate impaired endothelial function and develop age-dependent hypertension.[82] The mechanisms underlying the BP effects of H_2S are multiple, including enhanced NO-mediated vasodilation, activation of potassium-ATP channels, activation of protein kinase G1α, inhibition of phosphodiesterase type 5, and inhibition of SNS activity.[81] Modulation of H_2S levels with the administration of gaseous H_2S or H_2S donors (sodium hydrosulfide or sodium thiosulfate) results in lower BP and decreased CV and renal injury in several experimental models.[81] If delivery systems permit and successful oral use of these agents are developed, it is possible that H_2S may become a therapeutic target in hypertension and vascular disease.

Taken together, the net result observed in patients with hypertension is one of endothelial dysfunction. In cross-sectional analyses, the greater the extent of endothelial dysfunction as measured by the lower the degree of forearm flow-mediated vasodilation, the greater the prevalence of hypertension.[77,83] Prospective cohort studies have used flow-mediated vasodilation as a measure of endothelial dysfunction (regardless of specific mechanism) to evaluate its relationship with hypertension and test whether endothelial dysfunction is cause or consequence of hypertension, or both.[84] These studies have shown conflicting results, but the larger of them was unable to demonstrate an association between endothelial dysfunction and incident hypertension among 3500 patients followed for 4.8 years.[84] Furthermore, endothelial dysfunction carries a genetic predisposition that is independent of BP and may be improved by agents that have little or no impact on BP (e.g., some antioxidants).[85] Therefore, as it stands, the evidence is stronger for endothelial dysfunction as a consequence, not a cause, of hypertension.[83,85]

Arterial Stiffness in Hypertension

Arterial stiffness is an important factor in the pathogenesis of hypertension, particularly the syndrome of isolated systolic hypertension with aging, because it is a common accompaniment of elevated SBP and pulse pressure. High-sodium/lower-potassium diets over time predispose to increased arterial stiffness.[86] Cullin-3 mutations in vascular smooth muscle appear to be responsible for arterial aging.[87] Arterial stiffness develops as a result of structural changes in large arteries, particularly elastic arteries.[87,88] These include loss of elastic fibers and substitution with less distensible collagen fibers. Factors strongly associated with arterial stiffening include aging, hypertension, diabetes mellitus, chronic kidney disease (CKD), smoking, and high-sodium intake.[89]

A commonly used measure to assess arterial stiffness in humans is carotid-femoral pulse wave velocity (cf-PWV). The traditional view linking arterial stiffness (measured as increased cf-PWV) to hypertension invoked that faster PWV produced faster reflection of the incident pulse wave, which resulted in an earlier reflected wave that returned to the central circulation before the end of systole, resulting in increased SBP.[90]

What is the clinical importance of arterial stiffness? Increased arterial stiffness predicts the onset of ESRD in adults with polycystic kidney disease.[91] Basically, increased arterial stiffness should be interpreted as a poorer and reduced response of NO to any vasoconstricting stimuli, resulting in more labile hypertension and increased BP variability.

Evidence from several studies indicates that arterial stiffness may precede and predispose to hypertension.[90] For example, in the Framingham Heart Study, markers of arterial stiffness (cf-PWV and amplitude of the forward pressure wave) were associated with a 30% to 60% increased risk for incident hypertension (per standard deviation of each variable) during 7 years of follow-up in a cohort with a baseline mean age of 60 years.[92] Conversely, baseline BP levels did not associate with future changes in arterial stiffness. Certain studies corroborate these findings, but other studies suggest a bidirectional relationship such that arterial stiffness is also a consequence of chronic hypertension.[90] In contraposition, a recent cohort study of younger adults (baseline age 36 years) indicated that higher BP was associated with higher large artery stiffness, not the opposite.[93] These differences in results between younger and older adult populations may indicate that earlier in life, hypertension is mediated by factors that are largely independent of large vessel stiffness, whereas later in life, arterial stiffness has a more important causal role in the development of hypertension.

Arterial stiffening is relevant to target-organ damage in hypertension. Increased PWV is associated with increased mortality and CV events[94] as well as with a variety of subclinical CV injury markers, such as coronary calcification, cerebral white matter lesions, abnormal ankle-brachial index, and albuminuria. A relationship with cardiac complications has been suggested: increased impedance to left ventricular ejection results in left ventricular hypertrophy (LVH), diastolic dysfunction, and subendocardial myocardial ischemia.

Immune System in Hypertension

Immune responses, both innate and adaptive, participate in several of the mechanisms discussed earlier, including the generation of reactive oxygen species, mediation of the afferent arteriolopathy thought important to maintain salt sensitivity, and participation in the inflammatory changes noted in the kidneys, vessels, and brain in hypertension.[95,96] Innate responses, especially those mediated by macrophages, have been linked to hypertension induced by angiotensin II, aldosterone, and NO antagonism. Reductions in macrophage infiltration of the kidney or the periadventitial space of the aorta and medium-sized vessels lead to improvements in BP and salt sensitivity in several experimental models (Fig. 26.9).[96–98] Adaptive responses via T cells have been linked to the genesis and complications of hypertension. T cells express AT_1R and mediate angiotensin II–dependent hypertension, as demonstrated by the observations that adoptive transfer of T cells restored the hypertensive phenotype in response to angiotensin II infusion that was absent in mice without lymphocytes.[97] Abnormalities in both proinflammatory T cells and regulatory T cells alike are implicated in complications of hypertension, because they appear to regulate vascular and renal inflammation that underlies target-organ injury.

Suppression of these inflammatory responses can improve BP control.[95,96,99] B lymphocytes may also play a causative role in hypertension as suggested by reports of several autoantibodies, including agonistic antibodies against adrenergic receptors, vascular calcium channels, and AT_1R, and antibodies against endothelial cells causing endothelial dysfunction, or heat shock proteins (hsp70) causing salt-sensitive hypertension. Further research will determine if manipulation of immune targets is of value in the prevention and treatment of hypertension.

FACTORS INVOLVED IN PREDISPOSITION TO HYPERTENSION

Genetics (see Chapter 7)

Hypertension clusters in families; an individual with a family history of hypertension has a fourfold greater chance of developing hypertension,[100] and it is estimated that the heritability of hypertension ranges from 31% to 68%. GWASs in several multinational cohorts have identified a large number of SNPs associated with hypertension.[101] However, these individual SNPs are responsible for only minor BP effects (0.5 to 1 mm Hg), and the overall impact of these identified SNPs on the overall BP variance is only approximately 1% to 2%.[100] Among these genes, *FOS* (fos protooncogene) and *PTGS2* (COX-2) have been replicated in a number of studies. The shortcomings of the use of GWAS and other large population approaches are multiple and discussed elsewhere.[102] To advance progress toward personalized medicine in hypertension, a GWAS based on the large United Kingdom Biobank Study cohort performed functional and transcript expression analyses of candidate genes in target tissues in vitro (vascular smooth muscle cells, aortic fibroblasts, and endothelial cells) with the goal of identifying potential therapeutic targets.[101] The study developed and validated an unbiased genetic risk score that included clinical and genotype information including data on a total of 107 independent risk loci to generate estimates of risk of hypertension and risk of specific hypertension-related outcomes (stroke, coronary disease, and any CV outcome). These analyses showed a sex-adjusted SBP difference of 9.3 mm Hg between the lowest and highest risk quintile (higher in the high-risk group, which also had 2.3-fold greater odds of hypertension and a 1.35-fold increase in the odds of any CV outcome).[101] These results indicate the potential value for genetic risk-based clinical scoring.

With the improvement in techniques that allow expeditious, cheaper whole-exome or whole-genome analyses and the expansion of precision medicine, it is possible that greater mechanistic insights on the genetics of hypertension will become available. Unfortunately, compared with other clinical phenotypes, the heavy influence of lifestyle and environmental factors in hypertension makes it unlikely that the simple analysis of genome sequence will have a great impact in hypertension.[103] Further in-depth discussion is beyond this chapter, and the reader is referred elsewhere.[104]

Monogenic causes of hypertension, although quite rare, have provided substantial insight into the pathogenesis of hypertension. Of the monogenic forms of hypertension with well-described molecular mechanisms, all have one thing in common: a defect in renal sodium handling. Table 26.3 summarizes the well-recognized syndromes of familial hypertension.

Obesity

Obesity-related hypertension is characterized primarily by impaired sodium excretion and endothelial dysfunction, both of which are

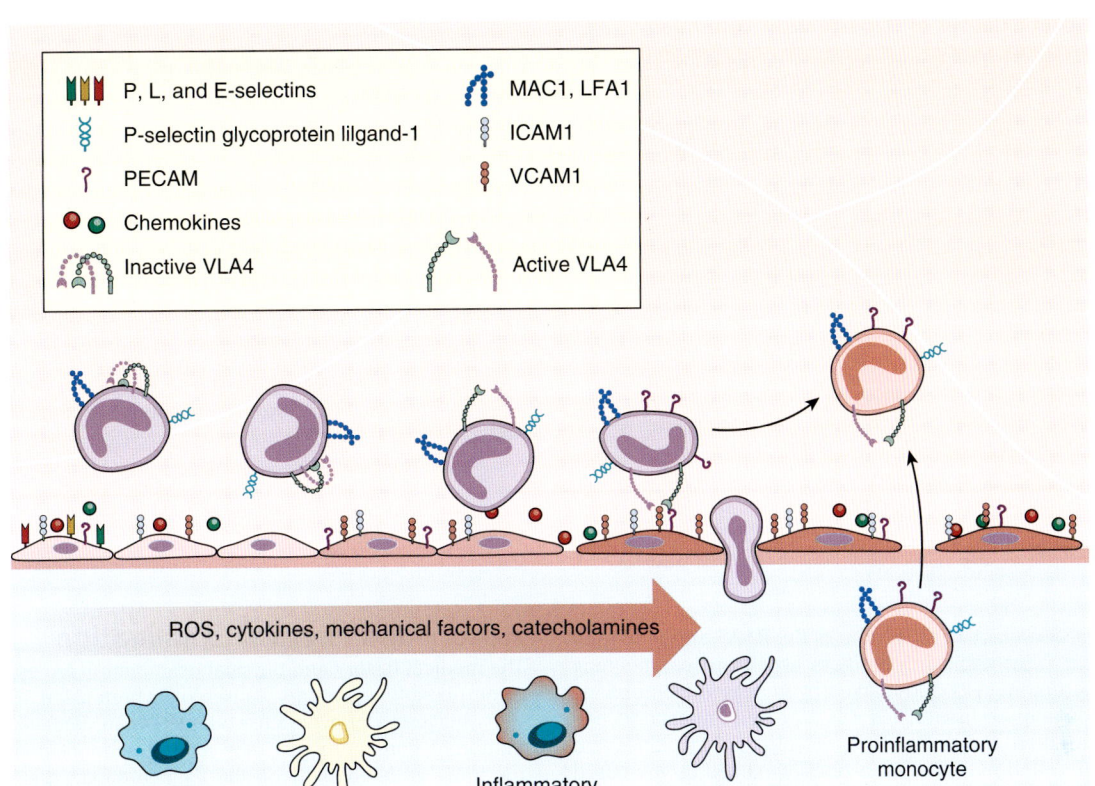

FIGURE 26.9 Overview of how the immune system modulates blood pressure levels through changes in the inflammatory response.

TABLE 26.3 Genetic Causes of Hypertension

SPECIFIC CONDITIONS	POSSIBLE CAUSES OF FAMILIAL HYPERTENSION	CLINICAL CLUES
Catecholamine-Producing Tumors		
Pheochromocytoma, paraganglioma	Familial cases are responsible for approximately 30% of cases, including MEN2A and MEN2B, von Hippel-Lindau disease, neurofibromatosis, and familial paraganglioma syndromes (SDH complex mutations)	Paroxysmal palpitations, headaches, diaphoresis, pale flushing; syndromic features of any of the associated disorders
Neuroblastomas (adrenal); aortic or renovascular lesions	1%–2% of neuroblastomas are familial	
Coarctation of the aorta	Overrepresented in families but no familial distribution	Asymmetry between upper- and lower-extremity BP, radial-formal pulse delay; associated with Turner syndrome, Williams syndrome, and bicuspid aortic valve
Renal artery stenosis caused by fibromuscular dysplasia or inherited arterial wall lesions	<10% familial with AD pattern	Abnormal renal vascular imaging results; vascular disease in the carotid territory at an early age; common in neurofibromatosis and Williams syndrome; also present in tuberous sclerosis, Ehlers-Danlos syndrome, and Marfan syndrome
Parenchymal kidney disease GN	Alport disease (X-linked, AR, or AD), familial IgA nephropathy (AD with incomplete penetrance)	Proteinuria, hematuria, low eGFR
PKD	AD PKD type 1 or 2, AR PKD	Multiple renal cysts (as few as three in patients <30 years)
Adrenocortical disease; glucocorticoid-remediable aldosteronism (familial hyperaldosteronism type I)	AD chimeric fusion of the 11β-hydroxylase and aldosterone synthase genes	Cerebral hemorrhages at young age, cerebral aneurysms; mild hypokalemia; high plasma aldosterone, low renin
Familial hyperaldosteronism II	AD; unknown defect	Severe type 2 hypertension in early adulthood; high plasma aldosterone, low renin; no response to glucocorticoid treatment
Familial hyperaldosteronism type III	AD; unknown defect	Severe hypertension in childhood with extensive target organ damage; high plasma aldosterone, low renin; marked bilateral adrenal enlargement
Congenital adrenal hyperplasia	AR mutations in 11β-hydroxylase or 21-hydroxylase	Hirsutism, virilization; hypokalemia and metabolic alkalosis; low plasma aldosterone and renin

continued

TABLE 26.3 Genetic Causes of Hypertension continued

SPECIFIC CONDITIONS	POSSIBLE CAUSES OF FAMILIAL HYPERTENSION	CLINICAL CLUES
Monogenic Primary Renal Tubular Defects		
Gordon syndrome	AD mutations of *KLHL3*, *CUL3*, *WNK1*, and *WNK4*; AR mutations of *KLHL3*	Hyperkalemia and metabolic acidosis with normal renal function
Liddle syndrome	AD mutations of the epithelial sodium channel	Hypokalemia and metabolic alkalosis; low plasma aldosterone and renin
Apparent mineralocorticoid excess	AD mutation in 11β-hydroxysteroid dehydrogenase type 2	Hypokalemia and metabolic alkalosis; low plasma aldosterone and renin
Geller syndrome; hypertension-brachydactyly syndrome	AD mutation in the mineralocorticoid receptor AD mutations in the phosphodiesterase E3A enzyme	Hypokalemia and metabolic alkalosis; low plasma aldosterone and renin; increased BP during pregnancy or exposure to spironolactone; short fingers (small phalanges) and short stature; brain stem compression from vascular tortuosity in the posterior fossa
Essential hypertension	Polygenic	When obesity or metabolic syndrome is present, likelihood of essential hypertension is higher

AD, Autosomal dominant; *ADPKD*, autosomal dominant polycystic kidney disease; *AR*, autosomal recessive; *ARPKD*, autosomal recessive polycystic kidney disease; *BP*, blood pressure; *eGFR*, estimated glomerular filtration rate; *GN*, glomerulonephritis; *IgA*, immunoglobulin A; *MEN*, multiple endocrine neoplasia; *PKD*, polycystic kidney disease; *SDH*, succinate dehydrogenase.

dependent on SNS overactivity, activation of the RAAS, and increased oxidative stress.[59,105] Fat tissue in obesity is hypertrophied, meaning larger cells versus more cells, and marked by increased macrophage infiltration in the adipose tissue.[106] As it is now well understood, adipose tissue is not inert and secretes a wide variety of cytokines and chemokines with abnormal profiles in obesity, marked by increased levels of leptin, resistin, interleukin-6, and tumor necrosis factor-α secretion, elevated free fatty acid release, and reduced adiponectin level. Decreased adiponectin levels results in insulin resistance, decreased induction of eNOS, and possibly increased sympathetic activity.

Resistin impairs NO synthesis (eNOS inhibition) and enhances ET-1 production, shifting the vasodilation/vasoconstriction balance toward vasoconstriction. Hyperleptinemia directly stimulates the SNS through complex mechanisms that involve central leptin receptors as well as activation of the pro-opiomelanocortin system (via the melanocortin 4 receptor).[105]

Lastly, visceral adipocyte mass is directly correlated with aldosterone secretion by the zona glomerulosa, a process mediated by angiotensinogen production by adipocytes as well as increased secretion of Wnt signaling molecules that modulate steroidogenesis.[107–109] In addition, despite yet unclear mechanisms, there is consistent evidence that obese individuals tend to have lower natriuretic peptides than lean individuals,[105] and this relative deficiency is amplified in obese hypertensives.[110] All of these factors compound the tendency toward sodium retention and shifting the pressure-natriuresis curve to the right. Activation of these systems leads to a proinflammatory state related to increased reactive oxygen species, factors directly associated with endothelial dysfunction and vascular proliferation. Therefore, multiple mechanisms contribute to the development and maintenance of hypertension in obese individuals.

A DIAGNOSTIC APPROACH TO PRIMARY HYPERTENSION

The evaluation of patients with hypertension focuses on six key components: (1) the confirmation that the patient is indeed hypertensive through careful measurements of BP; (2) an assessment of clinical features that might suggest specific remediable causes of hypertension; (3) the identification of comorbid conditions that confer additional CV risk, or that may impact treatment decisions; (4) the discussion of patient-related lifestyle factors and preferences that will affect management; (5) the systematic evaluation of hypertensive target-organ damage; and (6) shared decision making about the treatment plan. To accomplish this, the clinician often needs multiple visits, a targeted clinical examination, and selected laboratory and imaging tests.

History and Physical Examination

The medical history and physical examination are essential to uncovering possible secondary causes of hypertension, identifying symptoms suggestive of hypertensive target-organ damage, and diagnosing comorbid conditions that may affect treatment decisions. Although the focus is traditionally on the CV, neurologic, and renal systems, a complete review of systems is recommended when the patient is first evaluated, to identify comorbid conditions that may influence the BP. Some patients will present with hypertension because of sleep apnea (snoring, witnessed apneas/gasping), hyperthyroidism or hypothyroidism (each with their litany of possible symptoms), hyperparathyroidism (symptoms of hypercalcemia), Cushing syndrome (symptoms of cortisol excess), pheochromocytoma or paraganglioma (symptoms of catecholamine excess), or acromegaly with its distinctive physical findings. These conditions are discussed in detail later in this chapter.

High BP is typically asymptomatic, but some symptoms are common among patients with very high BP levels, such as headaches, epistaxis, dyspnea, chest pain, and faintness, all of which were present in more than 10% of patients presenting with DBP levels above 120 mm Hg.[111] Other common symptoms include nocturia and unsteady gait, whereas treated patients often complain of fatigue in addition to symptoms related to specific side effects of medications. In patients with lower BP levels, the occurrence of symptoms is often difficult to tie to observed BP, as demonstrated in a study evaluating the relationship between headaches and BP levels, where the frequently observed headaches in patients with hypertension did not correlate well with office or ambulatory BP levels.[112]

When evaluating for target-organ damage, symptoms are elicited that may suggest a previous stroke or transient ischemic attack, previous or ongoing coronary ischemia, heart failure, peripheral arterial disease, or a past history of kidney disease or current symptoms such as hematuria or flank pain.

Obtaining a detailed family history as it pertains to hypertension is essential. Focus should be on the development of hypertension at a young age or clustering of endocrine (pheochromocytoma, multiple endocrine neoplasia [MEN], primary aldosteronism) or renal problems (polycystic kidney disease or any inherited form of kidney disease). The young patient with hypertension and a family history of hypertension poses a particular challenge and should be evaluated in detail. Table 26.3 provides a guide to possible familial causes to be considered.[113]

Knowledge of several conditions with potential relevance to treatment is important. For example, issues related to CV risk management such as diabetes mellitus, hypercholesterolemia, inflammation (C-reactive protein), obesity, and tobacco smoking need to be evaluated. Patients with established CV disease will need treatment for both their hypertension and their underlying disorder (e.g., beta blockers for angina pectoris), so knowledge of specific CV diagnoses is essential. Lastly, some non-CV conditions may have an impact on treatment options. For example, patients with reactive airways disease (asthma) probably should not receive nonspecific beta blockers, patients with prostatic hyperplasia may benefit from a regimen that includes an alpha blocker, and patients with attention-deficit/hyperactivity disorder or anxiety may benefit from a central sympatholytic (e.g., guanfacine), whereas those with major depression should probably not be treated with this drug class.

When obtaining the history, the clinician should explore issues related to lifestyle, cultural beliefs, and patient preferences that will be essential in designing an effective treatment plan. It is important to define dietary and physical activity patterns and, when problems are identified, to determine if the patient is willing and/or able to modify them. Cultural beliefs related to the treatment of hypertension, health illiteracy, and mistrust in physicians and the pharmaceutical industry are several items that can affect the relationship with the patient and that should be openly raised. This is critical for patients to participate in shared decision making about their treatment, an essential tenet of patient-centered care.

The physical examination is designed to complement the items discussed in the history. One should pay attention to syndromic features of cortisol excess (moon face, central obesity, frontal balding, cervical and supraclavicular fat deposits, skin thinning, abdominal striae), hyperthyroidism (tachycardia, anxiety, lid lag/proptosis, hypertelorism, pretibial myxedema), hypothyroidism (bradycardia, coarse facial features, macroglossia, myxedema, hyporeflexia), acromegaly (frontal bossing, widened nose, enlarged jaw, dental separation, acral enlargement, carpal tunnel syndrome), neurofibromatosis (neurofibromas, café au lait spots, as neurofibromatosis is associated with pheochromocytoma and renal artery stenosis), or tuberous sclerosis (hypopigmented ash leaf patches, facial angiofibromas, as tuberous sclerosis is associated with renal hypertension, usually related to angiomyolipomas). Many other even rarer associations exist but fall beyond the scope of this chapter.

A coarctation of the aorta should be considered in younger patients with unexplained, difficult-to-treat hypertension and is evaluated by measurement of BP in both arms and in one thigh. If present, there will be a significantly lower BP in the thigh (typically by more than 30 mm Hg). Sometimes, in case of a lesion proximal to the left subclavian, there may be a significant interarm BP difference, lower on the left. In addition, there is significant decrease in intensity of the femoral pulses and a palpable radial-femoral pulse delay.

A funduscopic examination is recommended to evaluate for vascular changes associated with hypertension, especially if present for a long period of time (i.e., greater than 5 to 10 years). The retinal changes are associated with severity of both acute and chronic BP elevation. Acute changes can happen quite abruptly (hours to days) and range from arteriolar spasm in most patients with uncontrolled BP to retinal infarcts (exudates) and microvascular rupture (flame hemorrhages), to papilledema once the protection afforded by vasoconstriction is overcome. Chronic changes take much longer to develop and include vascular tortuosity (arteriovenous nicking) due to perivascular fibrosis, followed by progressive arteriolar wall thickening that prevents visualization of the blood column, thus leading to the appearance of copper wiring, then silver wiring. Several studies have demonstrated a relationship between severity of hypertensive retinopathy and risk for LVH and stroke.

Although bedside ophthalmoscopy is not commonly performed, it can provide a valuable insight into the vasculature. An important recent development is the availability of smartphone-based technology that allows use of a condensing lens coupled with the smartphone's camera for video and photography of the retina in place of a conventional ophthalmoscope.[114] In a study of hypertensive patients seen in the emergency room, use of this technology resulted in improved identification of abnormal retinal findings (exudates, hemorrhages, and papilledema) by an observer with very little clinical experience compared with conventional bedside ophthalmoscopy, while requiring about half the time to complete the exam (74 versus 130 seconds).[115] However, one has to purchase this device.

The CV examination focuses on the identification of volume overload (jugular venous distension, lung crackles, edema), cardiac enlargement (deviated cardiac impulse), and the presence of a third or fourth heart sound as markers of impaired left ventricular compliance. Subclinical atherosclerosis can be identified by the presence of bruits over the carotid arteries, as the prevalence of carotid atherosclerosis is increased in patients with hypertension, as well in the abdomen, primarily looking for renal arterial bruits heard over the epigastrium and/or flanks. These bruits are of greater significance if occurring on both systole and diastole. Finally, the detailed palpation of the peripheral pulses of the arms and legs is important to look for signs of peripheral arterial disease.

To wrap up the examination, a focused neurologic examination looks for obvious cranial nerve abnormalities, motor deficits, or speech or gait abnormalities. Any further testing is based on specific symptoms or on focal findings on the screening examination.

Blood Pressure Measurement

Because treatment decisions are based largely on BP levels, accurate BP measurement is essential. Cuff-based brachial BP is the most used method to measure BP, typically in the office setting. Table 26.4 lists the proper method for measuring BP. However, a rapidly growing body of evidence points to the value of out-of-office BP methods, such as 24-hour ambulatory BP monitoring (ABPM) and home BP monitoring, as superior methods to evaluate BP burden and evaluate BP-related risk in patients with hypertension.[116,117] Additionally, the most recent guidelines point to much more careful assessment of BP in the office setting.[5,7]

Office Blood Pressure Measurement

Office BP measurement is the time-honored method for the diagnosis and management of hypertension. It is strongly associated with hypertension-related outcomes based on more than 50 years of observational and clinical trial data. Accordingly, guidance provided to clinicians for the diagnosis and treatment of hypertension by most major guidelines is based on office BP values.[11] The most recent American College of Cardiology (ACC)/American Heart Association (AHA) guidelines on hypertension assessment strongly recommend the following approach for BP assessment in the office setting (see Table 26.4).[7]

Because attention to measurement technique is essential, it is important to follow the techniques outlined in Table 26.4 when checking BP. Most patients should have their BP measured in the arm while in the seated position. Once an arm is selected it should always be used for subsequent BP readings. In selected situations, such as malformations, injuries, or extensive vascular disease of the upper extremities, or when comparing BP levels in the upper and lower extremities, it may be necessary to use thigh measurements with an appropriately sized thigh cuff, which should be obtained in the prone position to allow the cuff to be at the level of the heart. Mercury sphygmomanometers are

TABLE 26.4 Key Steps for Proper Blood Pressure Measurement

1. Properly prepare the patient (e.g., quiet area, seated in chair, back firmly supported and feet flat on the ground, arm supported with appropriately size cuff placed). Wait 5 min, then check BP three times 1 min apart. Eliminate the first reading and average the next two readings.
2. Provide BP readings to patient.
3. Selection of proper cuff size as a function of arm circumference:

Arm circumference (cm)	Usual cuff size
22–26	Small adult
27–34	Adult
35–44	Large adult
45–52	Adult thigh

BP, Blood pressure.
Adapted from Whelton PK, Carey RM, Aronow WS, et al. 2017 ACC/AHA/AAPA/ABC/ACPM/AGS/APhA/ASH/ASPC/NMA/PCNA guideline for the prevention, detection, evaluation, and management of high blood pressure in adults: executive summary: a report of the American College of Cardiology/American Heart Association Task Force on Clinical Practice Guidelines. *J Am Coll Cardiol* 2018;71(19):2199–2269.

now seldomly available in clinical practice because of environmental concerns. Aneroid and electronic oscillometric manometers are accurate but should have periodic maintenance (every 12 months) to ensure that they are properly calibrated, as well as any time poor function is suspected.

The phenomenon of masked hypertension is defined as a clinical condition in which a patient's office BP level is normal but ambulatory or home BP readings are in the hypertensive range. This phenomenon, the opposite of white-coat hypertension (WCH), would suggest the necessity for measuring out-of-office BP in persons with apparently normal or well-controlled office BP.

When assessing BP on the initial visit, orthostatic BP should be obtained, especially among older patients, in whom it occurs in 8% to 34% of patients.[118] Additionally, people with neurologic disorders such as Parkinson disease and other neurologic disorders such as baroreceptor dysfunction have orthostatic hypotension as a common problem. Some guidelines now provide specific recommendations for measurement of standing BP to screen for orthostatic hypotension in older patients with hypertension, as well as in patients at increased risk for autonomic dysfunction, such as those with diabetes and kidney disease.[119,120]

Orthostatic vital signs (heart rate and BP) are best obtained after at least 5 minutes in the supine position followed by immediate assumption of the standing position, when sequential measurements are taken for up to 3 minutes. The difficulties of following this protocol in a busy clinical practice are recognized, so it is acceptable to compare values in the seated position with those after standing for 1 minute; this approach results in decreased sensitivity for the detection of orthostatic hypotension but is better than no measurement at all.[121] To account for this fact, a fall of 15/7 mm Hg may be used for the definition of orthostatic hypotension when the test is performed using the seated BP as baseline as compared with the generally accepted definition of orthostatic hypotension as a drop in BP of more than 20/10 mm Hg that occurs after 3 minutes of standing.[36]

Office Versus Home Blood Pressure

Office BP measurement is the time-honored method to evaluate hypertension. It is easy to perform and is widely available at low cost. Home BP is also widely available, although accessibility to low-income patients is still a problem despite the availability of low-cost devices. ABPM, on the other hand, is less widely available due to costs and limited reimbursement by third-party payers in the United States. Both home BP monitoring protocols and ABPM include larger numbers of readings, thus decreasing variability and improving reproducibility.[122]

In the past 30 years, ABPM and home BP have become accepted as better markers of hypertensive target-organ damage and adverse clinical outcomes. ABPM has stronger associations with LVH, albuminuria, kidney dysfunction, retinal damage, carotid atherosclerosis, and aortic stiffness than office BP, although this is not consistent among studies.[123] Likewise, home BP is a better marker than office BP for LVH and proteinuria, though it is not consistently superior for other measures of target-organ damage.

In the assessment of hard CV endpoints, out-of-office BP has consistently outperformed office BP in studies that account for the values observed in the office; in other words, no matter what the office BP, it is the out-of-office BP that decisively drives outcomes. In a systematic review by the National Institute for Health and Care Excellence (NICE) clinical guidelines group in the United Kingdom of nine cohort studies comparing ABPM with office BP, ABPM was superior in eight and equal to office BP in one of the studies.[124] For home BP, three studies compared similarly with office BP; home BP was superior in two and equal in one. Lastly, two studies compared ABPM, home BP, and office BP; of these, one showed superiority of both ABPM and home BP, while the other study did not show differences among any of the three methods. In meta-analyses of studies that evaluated both office and ABPM on outcomes, only ABPM values retained significance and was useful in masked hypertension.[125,126] Likewise, in the largest home BP cohort study that included simultaneous use of office and home BP to predict CV events and mortality, only home BP remained significantly associated with adverse outcomes.[127] Similar observations of the superior prognostic performance of out-of-office methods exist for patients with resistant hypertension, CKD, hemodialysis, and the general population.

In summary, evidence from prospective cohort studies convincingly demonstrates the superiority of out-of-office BP measurements as predictors of hypertension outcomes. Treated patients with hypertension who retain a white coat effect have the same overall risk as treated patients whose BP was controlled both in the office and at home. Moreover, an updated meta-analysis of 14 observational ABPM studies revealed an increase in risk of CV events and CV mortality among WCH patients compared with normotensive controls, but no statistically significant increase in stroke or all-cause death. As in previous analyses, sustained normotension was associated with lower risk.[128,129]

Because WCH and masked hypertension afflict a substantial number of patients and have diametrically different impact on outcomes, their identification improves the outcome prediction in patients with hypertension.

The ability to evaluate BP during sleep was a characteristic until now restricted to ABPM, although newer home BP monitors can be programmed for activation during sleep. In some, but not all studies, nighttime BP is a better marker of CV disease than daytime or 24-hour-average BP.[130–132] The importance of nighttime BP (compared with daytime levels) appears greater among treated patients, perhaps because antihypertensive treatment, often taken in the morning, might result in better BP control during the day than during the night.[133]

The pattern of BP fluctuation between day and night also associates with prognosis. The normal circadian BP pattern includes a fall in BP of approximately 15% to 20% during sleep. Patients who lack this normal BP dip during sleep are called "nondippers" (arbitrarily defined as a sleep BP that falls by less than 10% compared with awake levels) and have increased target-organ damage and overall CV risk. In large observational studies, patients whose SBP falls by 20% or more during the night have lower fatal and nonfatal CV event rates than those whose BP decreases by less than 20%, whereas those whose BP does not fall at all during the night have significantly worse CV outcomes than all other patients.[134]

ABPM also provides information on BP variability throughout the day. This may add further prognostic information. Increased BP variability (measured as the standard deviation of BP) has been associated with increased event rates, although these findings are of small magnitude when taken independently from BP values.[135]

Despite these observations, objective evidence demonstrating that outcomes are better when patients are managed using an out-of-office method is lacking. Three randomized clinical trials have compared management of hypertension with office or out-of-office BP, one using 24-hour ABPM[136] and two using home BP.[137–139] All of these studies showed that more patients managed with out-of-office methods could have treatment stopped or de-escalated, thus resulting in marginal cost savings. However, none of them could demonstrate the superiority of ABPM or home BP in achieving better BP control (the primary outcome of all three trials) or less LVH (evaluated in all studies as a secondary outcome).

Clinical Use of Ambulatory and Home Blood Pressure Monitoring

ABPM has been in clinical use for almost 50 years. In the United States, problems related to limited reimbursement have significantly limited its expansion compared with other parts of the world. Despite this limitation, there is general agreement on its value in several clinical circumstances.[140,141]

Although not feasible in many clinical settings, 24-hour ABPM is recommended for all newly diagnosed individuals with hypertension to eliminate the diagnosis of WCH or masked hypertension and to evaluate dipping status while sleeping.[142,143]

ABPM is performed, typically, over a period of 24 hours, although it can be extended for longer periods (e.g., 48 hours) to provide information covering more than one wake/sleep cycle, or to cover a specific period in detail, such as a 2-day interdialytic period for a patient undergoing hemodialysis. Clinicians should use an independently validated monitor (for a list, refer to www.dableducational.org). A typical measurement interval is every 20 minutes during the daytime (7 AM to 11 PM) and every 30 minutes at night (11 PM to 7 AM), although the frequency and time windows can be adjusted based on clinical needs, such as the need to identify frequent BP swings, atypical sleep patterns, etc. Patients should keep a log of activities during the day, the time of retiring to bed and waking up, and time of taking vasoactive medications (if applicable). It is preferred that the periods designated as "night" and "day" reflect the actual periods of sleep and wakefulness obtained from the patient's diary. Most patients tolerate the procedure well, although sometimes sleep is compromised (<10% of cases), and, rarely, patients have excessive bruising or discomfort from the frequent cuff inflations. Instructions on how to perform and interpret ABPM studies are available in guideline format from the European Society of Hypertension[6] and the ACC/AHA Blood Pressure Guidelines.[5,7]

Home BP is performed by the patient in the home (or sometimes work) environment. It is used commonly in clinical practice and is associated with improved adherence to therapy. It has been used successfully for self-titration of BP medications and is amenable to telemedicine approaches, in which the patient can upload BP values via telephone or direct entry to a Web server so that clinicians can inspect the BP logs and make treatment decisions remotely.

Just as with office BP, it is important that the equipment fits the patient's arm well and that measurements are obtained using the same technique as outlined earlier for office BP. Independently validated devices are listed at www.dableducational.org; unfortunately, many of the marketed devices have not been independently validated. The preferred devices use arm cuffs.[144] **Finger cuffs are inaccurate and should not be used.** Wrist cuffs often provide incorrect readings because of inappropriate technique but, if used correctly, can be convenient and accurate, and particularly useful in obese patients.

Smartphone applications are often marketed to obtain biologic information from users, including BP, and it is likely that in the near future their use will become important in the care of hypertensive patients. However, currently, none of the available technologies has been adequately validated, and a clinical validation study of the best sold BP application ("Instant Blood Pressure" [IBP]) showed wildly unreliable performance, leading to immediate removal of the application from the market upon publication of the article.[145]

To allow management decisions, home BP monitoring is best performed using specific periods of monitoring. For most patients, a BP log obtained over 7 days before each office visit suffices because it retains excellent reproducibility.[144] We recommend that the patient obtain readings in duplicate (approximately 1 minute apart), twice daily (in the morning before taking medications and in the evening before dinner). In selected situations, more frequent or more prolonged monitoring may be needed. For example, patients with hypotensive symptoms may benefit from BP measurements during peak action of medications, such as in the mid-to late morning or late evening, depending on the time when medications are taken. Likewise, patients with labile BP can be monitored more often to capture the overall BP variability, although ABPM is preferred in such patients. As for ABPM, detailed home BP guidelines are available from the European Society of Hypertension[117] and the ACC/AHA.[5]

Normative values for the interpretation of ABPM and home BP results are available based on observed outcomes in longitudinal studies.[127] For ease of use, these thresholds were matched to specific office BP levels at which the observed rate of CV events was the same, thus allowing clinicians to relate to office values that have historically driven clinical decisions. For ABPM, other measures such as the nocturnal dip, early morning surge (magnitude of BP rise during the first hours post awakening), BP load (percentage of time BP remains above a certain threshold, such as 140/90 mm Hg during the day and 120/80 mm Hg during the night), and overall BP variability (standard deviation of the 24-hour BP or awake BP), were not studied in relationship to hard outcomes for precise normative results.

Integrating Home Blood Pressure Into Clinical Practice

All current hypertension guidelines recognize the value of out-of-office BP in the diagnosis of hypertension, while the UK NICE guidelines, the US Preventive Services Taskforce, and the ACC/AHA guidelines formally recommend its use to confirm the diagnosis of hypertension in patients with elevated office BP prior to initiating treatment.

The ACC/AHA guidelines recommend the use of out-of-office BP to evaluate patients who are receiving treatment for hypertension but remain above goal in the office, with the explicit caveat that the recommendation is based on expert opinion. The high prevalence (approximately 40% to 51%) of a white coat effect in patients with resistant hypertension supports this recommendation. Patients with office BP above 160/100 mm Hg do not need further confirmation of hypertension and should be treated.

Laboratory and Other Complementary Tests

Similar to the history and physical examination, laboratory tests, imaging, and other complementary tests focus on the evaluation of comorbid conditions, established target-organ damage, and possible secondary causes. In the absence of worrisome signs or symptoms during the initial evaluation, a basic set of tests include renal function; electrolytes, calcium, glucose, and hemoglobin; a lipid profile; urinalysis; and an electrocardiogram.[5]

Further testing may be required if any of these initial test results are abnormal or if specific symptoms or physical findings suggest a diagnosis (see Secondary Hypertension section). Patients who are resistant to treatment during follow-up have higher rates of secondary causes of hypertension, in particular sleep apnea, hyperaldosteronism, and renovascular disease, thus deserving a more dedicated search for secondary causes in their evaluation.

Echocardiography

LVH is the most common target-organ damage in hypertension and is independently associated with worse prognosis, marked by increased risk for CV events (coronary, cerebrovascular), heart failure, and death.[146] The electrocardiogram is very specific but insensitive for the detection of LVH. The prevalence of LVH among patients with hypertension is approximately 18% based on electrocardiographic criteria, whereas this number increases to approximately 40% when more sensitive echocardiographic criteria are used. The echocardiogram provides information on left ventricular diastolic function, which is often impaired early in the course of hypertensive heart disease even in the absence of LVH. Echocardiography allows identification of left ventricular systolic dysfunction, which is uncommonly present in hypertension (approximately 4%) but is associated with worse prognosis. Even though echocardiography is not recommended as a routine test in patients with hypertension, it often provides important information to help guide treatment, such as defining the need to initiate or escalate treatment in patients with borderline office or ambulatory BP levels.

Evaluation of Sodium and Potassium Intake

Because of the importance of sodium and potassium as dietary interventions in hypertension, it is often useful to quantify intake objectively. A 24-hour urine collection for electrolytes can be performed on a patient on a stable dose of a diuretic. It is important to not allow hypokalemia, because that will increase BP.

Renin Profiling

The evaluation of plasma renin activity has been proposed as an empiric method for the evaluation and treatment of hypertension.[147] The premise for this approach is mechanistic: patients with high plasma renin activity levels (>0.65 ng/mL/hr, and particularly >6.5 ng/mL/hr) have vasoconstriction mediated by the RAAS as the primary operative mechanism of hypertension, whereas those with suppressed plasma renin activity levels (<0.65 ng/mL/hr) are volume overloaded. Accordingly, patients with high levels of plasma renin activity are treated with blockers of the RAAS (ACEIs, angiotensin receptor antagonists, renin inhibitors, beta blockers), and those with low levels of renin are treated with diuretics (including aldosterone antagonists), calcium channel blockers (CCBs), or alpha blockers. The approach not only includes using drugs that directly address the underlying pathophysiology but also proposes removal of drugs from the opposite group because there are reports of paradoxical BP elevations in such cases.[148] A case

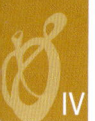

series using renin guidance reported streamlined drug regimens and improved BP control in patients with resistant hypertension, and a small randomized trial of renin-guided therapy versus conventional therapy yielded greater SBP lowering with the renin-guided system (−29 versus −19 mm Hg, $P = 0.03$).[149] Renin profiling is rarely used, and a good history and physical are as reliable as renin profiling; however, it is reasonable to entertain renin profiling, especially in patients who do not respond to initial therapy.

DIAGNOSTIC APPROACH FOR SECONDARY HYPERTENSION

Secondary (or remediable) hypertension is elevated BP due to a specific cause.[116,142] It should always be considered in every newly diagnosed or referred patient with hypertension, especially those with a history of hypokalemia. Secondary causes of hypertension are most commonly associated with endocrine abnormalities which are generally benign with a few exceptions. The most common cause of secondary hypertension is primary hyperaldosteronism, accounting for approximately 20% to 25% of all secondary hypertension cases.[150,151] Coarctation of the aorta and renovascular disease are two common nonendocrine causes of resistant hypertension. Additional factors contributing to resistance include dietary issues around sodium and potassium as well as commonly used over-the-counter medications.

Endocrine Causes (see Chapter 96)
Primary Hyperaldosteronism

Primary hyperaldosteronism as a form of secondary hypertension has been increasing in prevalence worldwide over the past 25 years[152,153] and is generally due to one of six subtypes: (1) an aldosterone-producing ("Conn") adenoma, nearly always in one adrenal gland (approximately 35% of cases); (2) bilateral adrenal hyperplasia (also known as "idiopathic primary hyperaldosteronism," approximately 60% of cases); (3) primary (or unilateral) adrenal hyperplasia (approximately 2% of cases); (4) aldosterone-producing adrenal carcinoma (approximately 35 cases in the world's literature); (5) familial hyperaldosteronism, which takes one of two forms: glucocorticoid-suppressible hyperaldosteronism, due to a chimeric chromosome 8, in which the 5′-regulatory sequence for corticotropin responsiveness of 11β-hydroxylase is fused to the enzyme-coding sequence for aldosterone synthase (<1% of cases), or familial occurrences of either an aldosterone-producing adenoma or bilateral adrenal hyperplasia (<2% of cases); or (6) ectopic production of aldosterone by an adenoma or carcinoma outside the adrenal gland (<0.1% of cases). In addition, obstructive sleep apnea (OSA) and sleep-disordered breathing also cause hyperaldosteronism. This is classically described as secondary hyperaldosteronism, but its evaluation and medical treatment are often quite similar to that of bilateral adrenal hyperplasia.

The prevalence of primary hyperaldosteronism depends on where and how one looks and is controversial. Some referral centers report a prevalence of hyperaldosteronism related to sleep apnea at approximately 20%, similar to the original prevalence of aldosterone-secreting adenomas estimated by Conn in the 1950s. In large population-based studies the prevalence of primary hyperaldosteronism has been estimated at approximately 10% to 11.2% of hypertensives. The condition appears to be more common in people with higher levels of BP (2% for BP levels 140 to 159/90 to 99 mm Hg, 8% for BP levels 160 to 179/100 to 109 mm Hg, and 13% for BP levels >180/110 mm Hg), treatment-resistant hypertension (17% to 23% in several series), patients with hypertension with either spontaneous or diuretic-associated hypokalemia, and hypertension with a serendipitously discovered adrenal mass (1% to 10%).[154,155]

In the last millennium, hypokalemia was thought to be very common (if not nearly universal) among patients with primary hyperaldosteronism, particularly if provoked by diuretic therapy. Today, however, more afflicted patients have eukalemia than hypokalemia, although sometimes more severe cases have weakness, muscle cramps, and even periodic paralysis. Patients with primary hyperaldosteronism experience higher CV morbidity and mortality than age-, gender-, and BP-matched patients with primary hypertension.[156]

Screening for primary hyperaldosteronism is most efficiently performed in potassium-repleted patients, using the ratio of plasma aldosterone concentration to plasma renin activity (ARR). The ARR can be affected by many factors, including antihypertensive drug therapy, dietary sodium restriction, posture, time of day, and sample handling, as well as a number of agents that can confound the diagnosis of true hypertension (Table 26.5). Most authorities recommend sustained-release verapamil, hydralazine, and peripheral α_1-adrenoceptor antagonists as medications that have little, if any, effect on the ARR. The likelihood of a false-positive ARR is increased by a low plasma renin activity (e.g., <0.5 ng of angiotensin II per milliliter per hour), so some investigators require the plasma aldosterone concentration to be above a given threshold (e.g., >15 ng/dL), for the screening to be considered positive, but levels between 12 and 15 ng/dL need to be considered individually, as some patients with proven aldosteronism have values in this range. Confirmation of primary aldosteronism in patients with aldosterone levels below 10 ng/dL, on the other hand, is rare. The most common cutoff value for an ARR that usually leads to further investigation is 30 (when aldosterone level is measured in nanograms per deciliter and plasma renin activity in nanograms of angiotensin II per milliliter per hour), but higher thresholds lead to more falsely negative tests.

Clinical practice guidelines from the Endocrine Society recommend one of four confirmatory tests before proceeding to an imaging study, because of the expense and radiation involved in the latter. There are only a few comparative studies of these four tests; they seem to have similar performance characteristics (75% to 90% sensitivity, 80% to 100% specificity). Cost, patient preference, local experience, local laboratory methods, and insurance reimbursement all factor into which confirmatory test is chosen.

The traditional "saline-loading test" (2 L infused over 4 hours) is confirmatory if the postinfusion plasma aldosterone concentration

TABLE 26.5 Drug-Induced Hypertension

Drugs or substances associated with apparent mineralocorticoid excess or activation of the renin-angiotensin system
1. Glucocorticoids and their derivatives
2. Glycyrrhizin acid (licorice)
3. Ketoconazole, itraconazole
4. Abiraterone acetate
5. Synthetic estrogens combined with progestin
Drugs or substances with direct vasopressor properties
1. Alcohol
2. Immunosuppressive agents (cyclosporine, tacrolimus, and calcineurin inhibitors)
3. Recombinant human erythropoietin
4. Drugs targeting the vascular endothelial growth factor (VEGF) pathway, including monoclonal antibodies and small-molecule receptor tyrosine kinase inhibitors
Drugs or substances activating the sympathetic nervous system
1. Illicit drugs of abuse, such as cocaine and amphetamines
2. Epinephrine or phenylephrine derivatives present in over-the-counter oral, nasal, or ophthalmic decongestants
3. Ephedrine alkaloids (*Ephedra* or herbal ma-huang)
4. Antidepressants, including venlafaxine, bupropion, monoamine oxidase inhibitors, and tricyclic agents
5. Appetite suppressants for weight loss
6. Modafinil
Drugs or substances with diverse mechanisms of action
1. Antiretroviral drugs (lopinavir and ritonavir)
2. Nonselective nonsteroidal antiinflammatory drugs (NSAIDs) and selective cyclooxygenase 2 inhibitors

is greater than 10 ng/mL. Patients with aldosterone concentrations between 5 and 10 ng/mL are considered indeterminate and should be retested. Note, intravenous saline is not often recommended for patients with heart failure, CKD, or uncontrolled hypertension.

Many centers have reported success with an oral sodium-loading protocol, which involves liberalizing sodium intake to approximately 6 g/day for 3 to 5 days and then assaying 24-hour urine collections for sodium (to ensure loading) and aldosterone content. The test is considered positive if the urinary aldosterone excretion is greater than 12 to 14 µg/day, but oral sodium loading can be as problematic in some patients as intravenous saline.

The fludrocortisone suppression test involves giving 0.1 mg of fludrocortisone every 6 hours for 4 days, and then assaying the plasma aldosterone concentration when the patient is standing upright. It is considered confirmatory if the concentration is greater than 6 ng/dL and plasma renin activity and serum cortisol levels are low. Execution of the test may be difficult for patients who have a long journey to the office or who are nonadherent.

Lastly, the captopril challenge test is performed by assaying the plasma aldosterone concentration before and 1 and 2 hours after administration of 25 to 50 mg of oral captopril. It is considered confirmatory if the plasma aldosterone concentration remains elevated (and unchanged from baseline), but many false-negative and equivocal captopril challenge test results have been reported.

After the diagnosis of primary aldosteronism is confirmed, a computed tomography (CT) scan of the adrenals is undertaken, which is useful in detecting large masses that might be adrenal carcinomas. Adrenal carcinomas typically have larger size (>4-cm diameter), an inhomogeneous character (often with internal hemorrhage), internal calcifications (in approximately 40%), and irregular borders (often due to micrometastases) and show enhancement after intravenous contrast medium is administered compared with adenomas. Aldosterone-producing adenomas are most commonly small (<2-cm diameter), hypodense, unilateral nodules. Idiopathic hyperaldosteronism usually has normal-appearing adrenal glands, but sometimes nodular changes and/or general enlargement are visible in one or both adrenals. Magnetic resonance imaging (MRI) is no better at detecting these abnormalities than CT, which is usually less expensive. Both techniques often detect nonfunctioning nodules, especially in older patients. At some centers, patients with hypertension with proven primary hyperaldosteronism who are younger than 40 years of age with a single typical hypodense nodule in one adrenal gland are directly offered an adrenalectomy.

Because CT scans identify unilateral adrenal disease with a sensitivity of only 78% and specificity of only 75%, the Endocrine Society recommends adrenal venous sampling for most surgical candidates.[157] Despite being invasive, expensive, technically challenging, and potentially dangerous and requiring an experienced and well-coordinated team, it has a sensitivity and specificity of 95% and 100%, respectively, for detecting unilateral aldosterone production. It is commonly performed at 8 AM, with continuous cosyntropin administration, and simultaneous adrenal vein cortisol level measurement. Most centers use a 4:1 cutoff value of the cortisol-corrected aldosterone ratio (i.e., the ratio between the aldosterone/cortisol ratios on each side) to define a positive lateralization.

Genetic testing for familial forms of primary hyperaldosteronism is recommended for those who are younger than 20 years of age at diagnosis and in those with a family history of primary aldosteronism or stroke at an early age (typically <30 years of age). This strategy was successful in approximately half of large, qualifying, unrelated cohorts. Genetic testing by either Southern blot or long polymerase chain reaction techniques is both sensitive and specific for glucocorticoid-remediable hyperaldosteronism (familial hyperaldosteronism, type I, the most common monogenetic cause of hypertension). Such testing is expensive, so many managed care organizations will not pay for the test unless an appropriate response (in both BP and plasma aldosterone concentration) is seen after weeks of empirical glucocorticoid administration. Familial hyperaldosteronism type II is genetically heterogeneous, despite being autosomal dominant in most affected cases. Genetic testing is not yet available for this more common type of familial hyperaldosteronism, so the diagnosis is primarily clinical, based on the biochemical findings and the pedigree.

Laparoscopic procedures for unilateral adrenalectomy have improved to the point that most patients with adrenal venous sampling–proven hyperaldosteronism have shorter hospital stays, fewer complications, and lower costs than open procedures. Although nearly all return to eukalemia, hypertension is "cured" (i.e., follow-up BP levels of less than 140/90 mm Hg without antihypertensive drug therapy) in only approximately 50%. "Cure" is more likely in younger people, those with a short duration of hypertension, prior BP control with only one or two agents, and a pedigree that includes fewer than two first-degree relatives with hypertension. Typically, plasma aldosterone concentration and plasma renin activity are measured shortly after successful surgery, and potassium supplementation and aldosterone antagonists are discontinued. Intravenous saline is often required because the remaining adrenal gland needs to recover its normal function, which may take a few weeks. The nonsurgical option for patients with idiopathic hyperaldosteronism is the aldosterone antagonist spironolactone, which has significantly better efficacy than its successor, eplerenone. Most physicians use dexamethasone or prednisone at bedtime (over twice-daily hydrocortisone) for glucocorticoid-remediable hyperaldosteronism, but the doses are kept low to avoid iatrogenic Cushing syndrome.

Apparent Mineralocorticoid Excess States

There are a number of conditions associated with elevated aldosterone that are secondary. These include obesity, sleep-disordered breathing, heart failure, liver disease, and other causes. Sleep-disordered breathing is relevant to hypertension and briefly discussed.

Hyperaldosteronism Associated with Sleep-Disordered Breathing (see Chapter 89)

The association of sleep-disordered breathing and hyperaldosteronism is thought to account for approximately 20% of resistant hypertension and typically responds well to selective aldosterone antagonists such as spironolactone.[158] Polysomnography is the "gold standard" test for OSA diagnosis but requires overnight evaluation and is expensive. The Berlin questionnaire, which includes questions about snoring, daytime somnolence, body mass index, and hypertension, is a brief validated screening tool that identifies persons in the community who are at high risk for OSA. The ratio of serum aldosterone to plasma renin activity is most often used to diagnose the condition. A therapeutic trial of spironolactone may be warranted, especially if the Berlin questionnaire or the sleep study is sufficiently suggestive.

Pheochromocytoma

A pheochromocytoma is a rare catecholamine-secreting tumor that arises from the chromaffin cells of the adrenal medulla. Occasionally, extra-adrenal pheochromocytomas may occur (referred to as catecholamine-secreting paragangliomas), most often in the abdomen. Pheochromocytomas are very uncommon, compromising only approximately 0.2% of patients with hypertension, although many remain undiagnosed through life. Rarely a pheochromocytoma occurs as a part of a familial disorder such as MEN type 2.[159] Approximately 90% of pheochromocytomas arise in the adrenal gland, 10% of patients have more than one tumor, and 10% are malignant. Patients typically present in their 40s or 50s with exaggerated adrenergic symptoms including headaches, palpitations, tachycardia, diaphoresis, and labile BP. Alternatively, a pheochromocytoma may be suspected from an abdominal imaging study showing an adrenal mass that may suggest a cause of adrenergic symptoms. Although labile hypertension is a typical finding in patients with a pheochromocytoma, many patients may have a BP pattern suggesting essential or resistant hypertension. A pheochromocytoma may cause a nonischemic cardiomyopathy secondary to the impact of the catecholamines on the heart.

Pheochromocytomas play important parts in the MEN syndromes, especially MEN2A (pheochromocytoma in approximately 50%—usually bilateral, medullary carcinoma of the thyroid, parathyroid adenomas, and cutaneous lichen amyloidosis, associated with the *RET* proto-oncogene), and MEN2B (usually bilateral pheochromocytomas, medullary carcinoma of the thyroid, submucosal neuromas, hyperplastic corneal nerves, joint laxity, Hirschsprung disease, and sometimes marfanoid body habitus). Pheochromocytomas are also found in patients with phakomatoses.

Approximately 20% of patients with von Hippel-Lindau disease type 2 (retinal and/or cerebellar hemangioblastomas, occasionally with clear cell renal carcinoma, pancreatic neuroendocrine tumors, retinal angiomas or hemangioblastomas, mediated by the *VHL* tumor suppressor gene, located on chromosome 3p25-26) will have pheochromocytomas or paragangliomas. Approximately 2% of patients with neurofibromatosis type 1 (autosomal dominant von Recklinghausen disease: neurofibromas, with café au lait spots, axillary and/or inguinal freckling, hamartomas of the iris—Lisch nodules, bony abnormalities, central nervous system gliomas, and sometimes macrocephaly, or cognitive deficits, mediated by the *NF1* tumor-suppressor gene on chromosome 17q11.2) will develop a catecholamine-secreting tumor, usually an adrenal pheochromocytoma. Both of these conditions can be diagnosed using genetic screening, although this is often more fruitful for screening family members after an index case has been identified.

Neither the prevalence nor the genetics of pheochromocytoma in Sturge-Weber syndrome (choroidal and leptomeningeal angiomas, port-wine stain in the trigeminal distribution) or tuberous sclerosis (sometimes called Bourneville or Pringle disease: adenoma sebaceum, subungual fibromas, and occasionally mental retardation) is as well understood. Familial paraganglioma is an autosomal dominant syndrome with paragangliomas in the skull base and neck, thorax, abdomen, pelvis, or urinary bladder wall; much work in the past 2 decades has characterized mutations in one of several genes that code for components of the mitochondrial succinate dehydrogenase complex: *SDHD*, located on chromosome 11q23, or *SDHB*, located on chromosome 1p35–36. Availability of genetic testing for these mutations has made disease surveillance for those who carry these genes (typically relatives of index cases) much simpler.

A pheochromocytoma can be suspected in patients with exaggerated adrenergic symptoms, although symptoms of headache, palpitations, and diaphoresis are very common and usually not caused by a pheochromocytoma. Suspicion for a pheochromocytoma can also be raised in patients with adrenal adenomas and hypertension, patients who have an exaggerated pressor response to anesthesia, patients with an unexplained cardiomyopathy, and familial disorders known to be associated with the tumor. The diagnosis of a pheochromocytoma must be made with biochemical evidence for catecholamine excess. Imaging of the adrenal gland alone is not sufficient to make the diagnosis because most adrenal adenomas do not release hormone and are benign findings.

A pheochromocytoma is suspected if there is a twofold or greater elevation above the upper limit of normal of a 24-hour urine collection of catecholamines and metanephrines or a significant elevation in plasma metanephrines. The diagnostic sensitivity of a 24-hour urine or plasma measurement of metanephrines is approximately the same. The sensitivity of plasma catecholamines for making the diagnosis of a pheochromocytoma is poor and not recommended as a screening test. The specificity of plasma metanephrines, however, may be poor, and most patients with elevated metanephrines will not be found to have a pheochromocytoma. Certain drugs may cause an elevation in catecholamines and metanephrines including withdrawal from clonidine, tricyclic antidepressants, certain decongestants, levodopa, buspirone, and other psychoactive agents. Withdrawal of these agents before diagnostic evaluation is usually needed to make a biochemical diagnosis of a pheochromocytoma.

Once a biochemical diagnosis of a pheochromocytoma is established, imaging studies are needed to localize the tumor. Because nearly 90% of the tumors arise from the adrenal gland, an abdominal CT or MRI is recommended as an initial imaging test. Because benign adrenal adenomas are very common, imaging studies for a pheochromocytoma are recommended only after a biochemical diagnosis is suggested. CT scans with contrast are safe and do not precipitate a hypertensive crisis. MRI may have some advantage over CT because T2-weighted images may be able to distinguish a more hyperintense pheochromocytoma from a benign adenoma.

Metaiodobenzylguanidine (MIBG) scintigraphy can be performed to detect extra-adrenal tumors or multiple tumors. MIBG resembles norepinephrine and is taken up by adrenergic tissue (including normal adrenal tissue). Prior to performing this scan, certain antihypertensive medications should be discontinued if possible for at least 7 to 10 days before the test. These classes include: calcium antagonists (i.e., amlodipine), alpha/beta blockers (i.e., labetalol), and many other non–BP-lowering agents.[160] When a MIBG scan localizes a potential tumor, the findings need to be corroborated with standard imaging studies before surgical removal. Fluorodeoxyglucose positron emission tomography (FDG-PET) is used for detection of metastatic disease. These imaging tests are recommended when there is a high index of suspicion for an extra-adrenal pheochromocytoma.

The role of genetic testing in routine care of patients with pheochromocytoma is evolving; current guidelines recommend a shared decision-making process, often involving more family members than just the index patient.[161] Eight studies have shown a high prevalence of germline mutations in patients with presumed sporadic pheochromocytoma/ganglioma, so some authorities recommend genetic screening for all afflicted patients; others base the decision on the pedigree, syndromic features, or extent of disease (multifocal, bilateral, or metastatic tumors at diagnosis).

Pheochromocytomas need to be surgically removed to adequately treat the labile BP and because of their malignant potential. Removal of a pheochromocytoma can be difficult because of the potential of causing a hypertensive crisis when the tumor is surgically manipulated. Adequate alpha- and beta-adrenergic blockade is required before surgical removal. Alpha blockade is essential before beta blockade to reduce the risk for a hypertensive crisis. The irreversible long-acting alpha blocker phenoxybenzamine is started 7 to 10 days prior to surgery at 10 mg once or twice daily and increased as needed to control the BP and prevent sudden spikes in BP. Beta blockade, for example with metoprolol, is begun after adequate alpha blockade is achieved. Most pheochromocytomas can be removed laparoscopically.

Hypercortisolism (Cushing disease)

Chronic exposure to excess glucocorticoids can lead to the signs and symptoms of Cushing syndrome. Causes of Cushing syndrome include iatrogenic glucocorticoid use, Cushing disease (corticotropin [ACTH] dependent), ectopic ACTH syndrome, adrenal tumors, and other rare conditions such as adrenal hyperplasia. Most cases of Cushing syndrome today are iatrogenic (due to prescribed oral corticosteroids), but occasional sporadic cases are still seen and were found in 0.5% to 1.0% of hypertensive subjects in two large series. The pathophysiology of hypertension in Cushing syndrome overlaps somewhat with mineralocorticoid excess states, because excess cortisol often overwhelms the capacity of 11β-hydroxysteroid dehydrogenase type 2 to selectively degrade cortisol to cortisone in the aldosterone-producing cells of the adrenal cortex and can increase circulating levels of deoxycorticosterone, which has only mineralocorticoid activity.

The full-blown Cushing syndrome of hypertension, dyslipidemia, truncal obesity with striae, diabetes, hirsutism, acne, hyperglycemia, hypokalemia, and muscular weakness is less common today than in Cushing's era. After an appropriate screening test (urinary-free cortisol, late-night salivary cortisol, or overnight dexamethasone suppression test) has positive results, an endocrine referral for a second test is recommended before imaging studies are ordered. In some centers, plasma corticotropin levels are used to discriminate between corticotropin (ACTH)-dependent Cushing syndrome (>15 pg/mL, probably 85% to 90% of cases) and corticotropin-independent Cushing syndrome (<5 pg/mL). In the majority of cases, dynamic testing of the hypothalamic-pituitary-adrenal axis is performed next, with either a corticotropin-releasing hormone test (which assays plasma cortisol and corticotropin levels before and after intravenous releasing hormone) or a high-dose dexamethasone (2 mg every 6 hours) suppression test (which assays serum cortisol level).

This evaluation can localize a tumor to the pituitary gland in 60% to 75% of the cases, a single adrenal gland in approximately 20% (split approximately 60:40 between adenomas and carcinomas), or ectopic production of corticotropin (10% to 12%, most often by small cell lung cancers), with less than 1% due to ectopic production of corticotropin-releasing hormone (typically by bronchial carcinoid tumors). Petrosal venous sinus sampling is not needed very often today. The anatomic site of hormonal overproduction is then usually approached surgically, although other modalities (e.g., radiation of the sella turcica) can be used in special circumstances. Medical therapy is also possible in some cases, especially those in which surgery is not feasible.

Thyroid Dysfunction

The literature about thyroid dysfunction being associated with hypertension is inconsistent. Many patients with hyperthyroidism have wide pulse pressures (and therefore elevated SBP levels) and high pulse rates, but this is seldom missed, especially in younger patients. The ultrasensitive serum thyroid-stimulating hormone (TSH) level is widely available and most commonly used for screening. After diagnosis, a nonselective beta blocker such as propranolol may be specifically useful because it treats the tachycardia and hypertension and may inhibit peripheral conversion of thyroxine to triiodothyronine.

The role of hypothyroidism as a potential cause of hypertension (especially isolated diastolic) is less clear. The hypertension in hypothyroidism is predominantly diastolic and usually less than 99 mm Hg. In children and adolescents, especially in areas of iodide deficiency, a positive association between serum TSH and BP has been seen. It is likely that targeted screening of patients with hypertension for hypothyroidism with determination of serum TSH level may be useful, but routine screening for all newly diagnosed patients with hypertension for thyroid disease is not currently recommended by any national or international guidelines.[162]

Acromegaly

Hypertension occurs in more than 40% of patients with excessive growth hormone release causing acromegaly, and it can be exacerbated by concomitant sleep apnea.[163] Most of such patients are easily identified by symptoms or signs of acral bony overgrowth, particularly in children or adolescents before epiphyseal closure, although some patients ignore or tolerate these changes for a decade or more. The vast majority (98%) of cases are caused by a pituitary adenoma; serum insulin-like growth factor-1 is the most useful initial laboratory screening test, although other tests (including the response of plasma growth hormone levels to an oral 75-g glucose load and prolactin levels) are often performed.

Successful treatment of acromegaly usually lowers BP, but hypertension often persists, especially in older and overweight patients.[164] No specific antihypertensive drug therapy seems to be more effective than others, but considering that acromegaly is a very unusual cause of resistant hypertension, standard antihypertensive drug therapy is usually effective.

Nonendocrine Causes
Lifestyle Factors

Although generally not considered in most discussions of secondary (or remediable) hypertension, BP can be influenced by prescription or nonprescription medications or both,[152] excessive dietary sodium intake,[165] body weight/obesity, and excessive alcohol intake.[142] The health care provider or the patient may not immediately appreciate some of these factors. Appropriate attention to these issues can result in improved BP profiles and a better prognosis.[166]

Modification of these factors is the cornerstone of therapy for primary hypertension and can mimic secondary hypertension. Of these factors, the most common issues relate to excessive sodium intake, poor sleep hygiene (i.e., getting less than 6 hours of uninterrupted sleep a night),[167] excessive caffeine or other stimulants, and use of nonsteroidal antiinflammatory drugs (NSAIDs).

Drug-Induced Hypertension

Patients presenting with hypertension should be questioned about exposure to substances that can raise BP (see Table 26.5). These include drugs of abuse and over-the-counter and prescription medications. Oral contraceptive pills (OCPs) can cause hypertension, although modern low-estrogen pills have rates much lower than older preparations. Stopping the OCP can cure the hypertension after several weeks to months in most, but not all, women. NSAIDs result in a modest average hypertensive effect (up to approximately 5 mm Hg), but some patients can have larger, clinically significant BP elevation. NSAID-induced hypertension may also present as loss of BP control in patients taking a diuretic or a blocker of the renin-angiotensin system, whereas CCBs tend to be less affected in NSAID users.

Sympathomimetic amines (legal or illegal) usually cause hypertension acutely following ingestion. Alcohol has an acute hypotensive effect, but chronic use in large amounts (>4 to 5 drink-equivalents per day) is associated with increased BP. Glucocorticoids and mineralocorticoids can produce a dose-dependent rise in BP. Glucocorticoids with low mineralocorticoid activity (dexamethasone, budesonide) induce lesser pressor responses.

Selective serotonin reuptake inhibitors (SSRIs) and serotonin-norepinephrine reuptake inhibitors (SNRIs) can increase BP modestly, but some patients receiving SNRIs may have a severe hypertensive response. Interestingly, when these medications are used for hypertensive patients with depression, BP often improves as depressive symptoms improve. Angiogenesis inhibitors, such as anti-vascular endothelial growth factor (VEGF) antibodies (bevacizumab, ramucirumab) and tyrosine kinase inhibitors (sorafenib, sunitinib) can produce hypertension that often persists despite discontinuation. Because hypertension during the use of these drugs correlates with better oncologic outcomes (likely a reflection of successful antiangiogenic effect), treatment is usually continued unless reasonable BP control is not achievable or if severe kidney injury develops.[168]

Sleep Deprivation and Sleep-Disordered Breathing (see Chapter 89)

Poor sleep quality, if chronic, can cause paroxysmal hypertension and consistently elevated BP, especially during the afternoon and evening hours. Poor sleep quality can be the result of OSA and a host of other sleep disorders including restless leg syndrome and insomnia of a various causes.[169] Many times, these different sleep disorders coexist and prevent the patient from achieving proper restful sleep.

Poor sleep quality (i.e., getting fewer than 6 hours of sleep nightly over a period of weeks) can lead to increase BP and increased BP variability. Moreover, data from the Nurses' Health study show increases of 60% to 70% over 10 years in mortality in people with this problem.[170,171] There is also increased risk of hypertension and BP variability in these patients. Correcting the sleep problem without antihypertensive medications alleviated both the hypertension and the variability.[172]

The mechanism of poor sleep quality contributing to elevated BP and paroxysmal bouts of very high BP relates to activation of both the sympathetic and RAAS.[173,174] Sympathetic activity is also increased in sleep deprivation, restless leg syndrome, and OSA.[173,174]

Patients without OSA who suffer from sleep deprivation, defined as less than a minimum of 6 hours of uninterrupted sleep, also have increased sympathetic activity. In this case, it is a consequence of reduced time in non–rapid eye movement (NREM) or slow wave sleep that also affects the nocturnal dip in BP.[174] This supports the hypothesis that disturbed NREM sleep quantity or quality is a mechanism by which sleep deprivation or restless leg syndrome leads to an increase in sympathetic tone. Prolonged periods (i.e., months without adequate sleep time, that is, >7 hours) can generate hypertension and increase BP variability and irritability. Correcting sleep independent of adding BP medications in many cases not only reduces BP but also reduces the number of medications for hypertension.[172]

Rapid eye movement (REM) sleep is generally associated with a greater propensity for upper airway closure because of inhibition of muscle tone during this stage of sleep. As a result, the likelihood of OSA or worsening of OSA in REM sleep is increased. In addition, REM sleep is also associated with increased sympathetic activity which can contribute to a rise in BP.

OSA should be suspected in patients (men more so than women) who report severe snoring, daytime somnolence, and witnessed nocturnal choking or gasping and have a "crowded oropharynx" (limited or no visualization of the soft palate) on physical examination.

Formal diagnosis is based on an ambulatory sleep study or in-center polysomnography.[175]

In contrast to reduced sleep time and quality, the increase in sympathetic activity associated with OSA is a function of intermittent hypoxia as the acute rise in BP parallels the severity of oxygen desaturation at night.[176] Indeed, increased sympathetic activity is seen in animal models subjected exclusively to intermittent hypoxia.[177] It is also important to note that OSA-associated hypertension is only slightly reduced by continuous positive airway pressure (CPAP) treatment.[178] However, patients who have more severe hypertension, more severe OSA, higher daytime sleepiness scores, and greater adherence to CPAP (average use >4 hours per night) tend to have greater responses.[179] Despite modest benefits, addressing sleep disorders or sleep habits is relevant when considering the risk of either developing or controlling preexistent hypertension.

Nonlifestyle, Nonendocrine Causes
Intrinsic Kidney Disease
Hypertension can be both a cause and a consequence of CKD (i.e., estimated GFR [eGFR] <60 mL/min/1.73 m^2). In 2020, after diabetes, poorly controlled hypertension remains the second-most common cause of kidney failure worldwide resulting in renal replacement therapy (Fig. 26.10).[180] It is often difficult to discern which occurred first when a patient presents initially with both hypertension and CKD, but the screening and diagnostic processes are identical to those used for each individually. CKD is currently diagnosed and staged using the 2012 Kidney Disease: Improving Global Outcomes (KDIGO) criteria from the National Kidney Foundation: persistent (≥3 months) evidence of kidney damage (e.g., proteinuria, abnormal urinary sediment, abnormal blood or urine chemistry levels, imaging studies, or biopsy) (Fig. 26.11).[181,182] Although it is clear both urine albumin and eGFR are needed to properly stage CKD, in most cases only eGFR is used. Note, it is possible to have CKD with eGFR greater than 60 mL/min/1.73 m^2 if you have more than 300 mg/g albuminuria. Most authorities recommend this threshold for common use. Management strategies for hypertension due to CKD are also identical to those used in primary hypertension except that doses and frequency of antihypertensive (and other) medications normally cleared by the kidney are decreased inversely to the eGFR. Although most antihypertensive drugs do not need dose adjustments in stage 3b or higher CKD, some agents that affect the RAAS mechanistically should theoretically be reduced. Renally excreted beta blockers (e.g., atenolol, metoprolol, bisoprolol, nadolol, and acebutolol), and all ACE inhibitors, except fosinopril and trandolapril, are reduced in dose or dosing frequency, but no serious adverse effects (other than possibly hyperkalemia) have been reported, if no adjustment of dosing is performed. Also note that losartan and valsartan, normally twice-daily agents from the angiotensin receptor blocker (ARB) class when kidney function is normal, should be dosed once daily among those with an eGFR less than 60 mL/min/1.73 m^2.

Restriction of dietary protein intake had been recommended in the past, based on several small trials, but had marginal success in the Modification of Diet in Renal Disease trial[183] and is usually challenging to carry out effectively, even in tertiary centers with a dedicated renal nutritionist. Dietary sodium restriction, although somewhat a lesser challenge, has benefits in patients with CKD and hypertension, not only to lower BP but also to reduce urinary protein (and albumin) excretion.[184]

Renovascular Hypertension
It is estimated that approximately 1% to 5% of people have renovascular disease as an underlying cause of hypertension. Renovascular hypertension is most commonly due to atherosclerotic disease. Fibromuscular dysplasia is a less frequent cause. Atherosclerotic renal artery disease occurs commonly in association with peripheral arterial disease and coronary artery disease. The prevalence is higher in individuals older than 65 years of age. In contrast, fibromuscular dysplasia tends to affect women between the age of 15 to 50 years, although some patients are not identified until older. Hemodynamically significant renal artery disease can cause refractory hypertension and lead to ESRD. Patients with atherosclerotic renal artery disease are at significantly increased risk for other vascular events, including coronary and cerebrovascular complications.

Fibromuscular dysplasia is a nonatherosclerotic noninflammatory disease of unknown cause. There may be genetic factors involved, because it is more commonly found in first-degree relatives of affected patients. Smoking may be associated with the disease as well. Fibromuscular disease can also involve the internal carotid artery and rarely additional vascular beds. In the renal arteries, fibromuscular lesions tend to involve the mid- or distal renal arteries and can lead to severe stenosis and aneurysms. In contrast, atherosclerotic renal artery disease more commonly involves the proximal portion of the renal arteries. Over one-third of patients with fibromuscular dysplasia will have progression of the disease.

Renal artery disease can be suspected in individuals with resistant hypertension defined as BP above target despite optimal treatment with

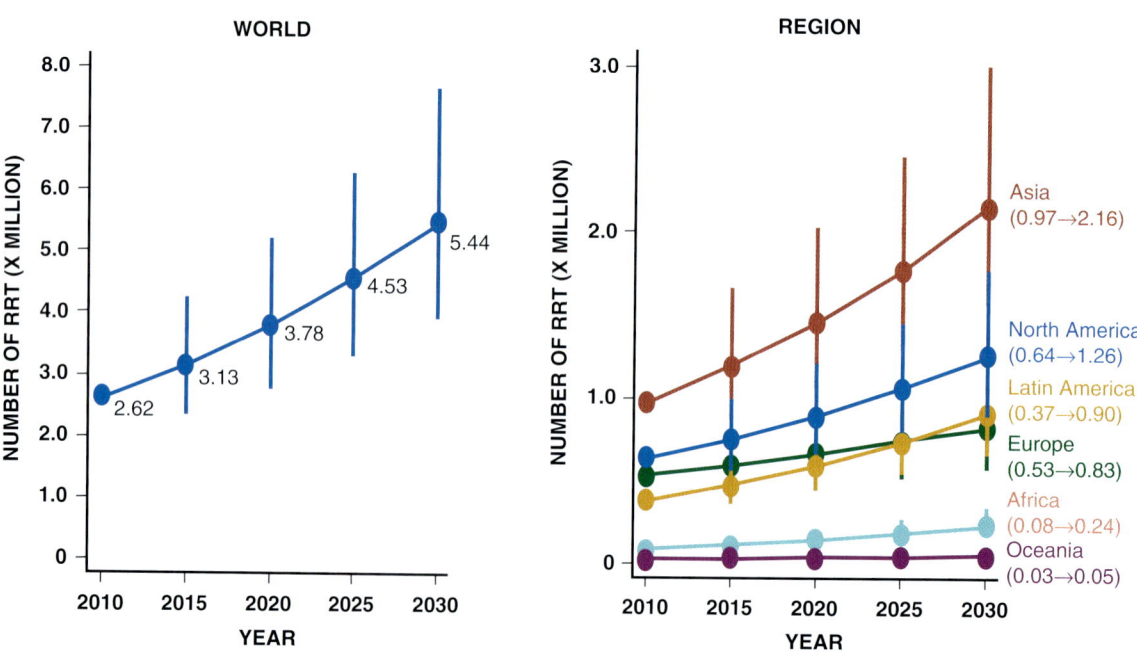

FIGURE 26.10 Trends in end-stage kidney disease development around the world. RRT, renal replacement therapy.

three antihypertensive agents with one of the medications being a thiazide diuretic. Fibromuscular disease should be considered in younger women with hypertension or presenting with carotid artery disease or stroke. Atherosclerotic disease can be considered in older patients with known atherosclerotic disease, hypertension associated with renal insufficiency, and hypertension associated with episodes of heart failure. Renal artery stenosis, by decreasing perfusion to the kidneys, tends to cause overstimulation of the RAAS. In some patients, treatment with a RAAS blocker can cause a marked worsening of renal function, suggesting dependence of kidney perfusion on renin. A greater-than-expected reduction in renal function with an ACEI or an ARB suggests the presence of hemodynamically significant bilateral renal artery stenosis.

Hemodynamically significant renal artery stenosis can be diagnosed by duplex ultrasound in the majority of individuals. A high-velocity signal correlates with a significant pressure difference across the stenosis. A clear Doppler signal may be difficult to obtain in patients with significant obesity or be obscured by bowel gas. MRA or CTA imaging can effectively diagnose renal artery stenosis, but the use of these imaging modalities may be limited in patients with renal insufficiency, due to increased risk for toxicity due to the contrast medium. Digital-subtraction angiography or selective renal angiography can be performed with minimal amounts of contrast to reduce the risk of contrast nephropathy.

Medications that block the RAAS are agents of first choice to treat renovascular hypertension due to overactivation of this hormonal system. Serum creatinine will usually increase with the introduction of an ACEI or ARB, although the increase is generally less than 30% from baseline. A significantly greater increase in creatinine suggests hemodynamically significant bilateral renal artery stenosis. In individuals with significant bilateral disease, balloon angioplasty and stenting can effectively increase renal perfusion, reduce BP or the number of antihypertensive medications, and preserve renal function. Balloon angioplasty and stenting is usually the treatment of choice for fibromuscular dysplasia of the renal arteries because this disease is frequently bilateral. In patients with fibromuscular disease, predictors of success of angioplasty include age less than 40 years at diagnosis, hypertension duration of less than 5 years, and SBP less than 160 mm Hg.[185] Angioplasty and stenting are not recommended for unilateral renal artery stenosis because no outcome advantage with respect to clinical events was seen when angioplasty was added to optimal medical therapy using a RAAS blocker in patients with atherosclerotic renal artery disease.[186] In general, renal artery revascularization is considered in patients with new-onset severe hypertension, failure or intolerance of optimal medical therapy, recurrent flash pulmonary edema, or unexplained progression of renal insufficiency.

Coarctation of the Aorta

A coarctation of the aorta is a narrowing of the descending aorta typically located just distal to the left subclavian artery at the insertion of the ductus arteriosus. BP is significantly increased proximal to the coarctation and can lead to pressure overload of the heart. Although most discrete constrictions of the aorta occur in or near the ductus arteriosus, there is growing awareness that this fifth-most common form of congenital CV disorders constitutes a spectrum of aortic and vasculopathic disorders and is not always "cured" by surgical procedures that relieve the obstruction. A bicuspid aortic valve, ventricular septal defect, and cerebral aneurysms are associated with coarctation of the aorta. There is a higher incidence of a coarctation in patients with Turner syndrome. Most patients with the condition are hypertensive[187,188] and are diagnosed in infancy or childhood, but some escape detection until adulthood. Many cases are identified by suggestive physical findings (e.g., murmur, BP lower in the legs than the arms, radial-femoral pulse delay), some after imaging studies done for other reasons (e.g., rib notching or a "3" sign on chest radiograph, the latter of which results from indentation of the aorta, with prestenotic and poststenotic dilation), and others during investigation of associated abnormalities (e.g., bicuspid aortic valve).

Echocardiography can accurately diagnosis and localize the coarctation, although some patients (especially adults and those with associated anomalies) may require angiography. Most patients can be treated with percutaneous catheter balloon dilation with aortic stent placement; this can be followed by definitive surgical correction later, if needed. Unfortunately, 25% to 68% of patients with a coarctation have

Prognosis of CKD by GFR and Albuminuria Categories: KDIGO				Persistent albuminuria categories Description and range		
				A1	A2	A3
				Normal to mildly increased	Moderately increased	Severely increased
				<30 mg/g <3 mg/mmol	30–300 mg/g 3–30 mg/mmol	>300 mg/g >30 mg/mmol
GFR categories (mL/min/1.73 m²) Description and range	G1	Normal or high	≥90			
	G2	Mildly decreased	60–89			
	G3a	Mildly to moderately decreased	45–59			
	G3b	Moderately to severely decreased	30–44			
	G4	Severely decreased	15–29			
	G5	Kidney failure	<15			

Green: low risk (if no other markers of kidney disease, no CKD); Yellow: moderately increased risk; Orange: high risk; Red: very high risk.

FIGURE 26.11 The "heat map" staging system for chronic kidney disease developed by the International Guideline committee for Kidney Disease (KDIGO). *GFR*, glomerular filtration rate.

persistent hypertension despite satisfactory procedure results, with age at the time of surgery, age at follow-up, and the type of intervention being strong predictors of persistent hypertension.[189] Standard hypertension management of elevated BP due to coarctation of the aorta, including the use of beta blockers, can successfully lower the BP in many patients.

THERAPEUTIC OPTIONS AND APPROACHES FOR PRIMARY HYPERTENSION

Goals of Therapy

Antihypertensive therapy should be started when (1) the patient has a confirmed diagnosis of hypertension, meaning more than two separate readings at separate times with BP levels consistently above 130/80 mm Hg and (2) dietary and lifestyle intervention has been tried for a brief period. If BP is greater than 20/10 mm Hg above the goal, then both lifestyle and antihypertensive therapy should be started concomitantly.[5,25]

Blood Pressure Guidelines

There are numerous guidelines published every few years that document goals and approaches to BP control to reduce risk of cardiorenal events and death. The most recent guidelines were published in 2017 in the United States and 2018 in Europe. Although these two guidelines are very similar in many aspects, there are differences. These are summarized in Table 26.1. One of the key factors emphasized in all guidelines is proper measurement of BP (see Table 26.4). This methodology allows for almost total exclusion of WCH, a very common problem with mortality similar to partially treated hypertension.[190]

Hundreds of clinical trials have evaluated the efficacy and safety of the eight different classes of antihypertensive medications. All BP-lowering agents need to have at least two appropriately powered, placebo-controlled studies to meet specific US Food and Drug Administration (FDA) criteria for approval as antihypertensive agents. This section will not focus on the details of these studies but rather on data supporting BP reductions with certain BP-lowering classes and the impact on CKD progression, as well as trials evaluating CV outcomes in patients with kidney disease.

Meta-analyses of all commonly used antihypertensive drug classes demonstrate that, regardless of the agent used, reduction in BP corresponds to reduction in CV events if BP reduction is achieved.[191–193] This reduction in CV risk, however, is predominantly seen in people with stage 2 hypertension (≥140/90 mm Hg) with much less outcome data to support risk reduction in stage 1 hypertension (systolic 130 to 139 mm Hg or diastolic 80 to 89 mm Hg).

Events that drive CV risk reduction are derived predominantly from reduced incidence of stroke, myocardial infarction, and heart failure. In all trials to date the group with the best overall BP control has the best outcomes. An exception to this generalization is Avoiding Cardiovascular Events Through Combination Therapy in Patients Living with Systolic Hypertension (ACCOMPLISH), a CV outcome trial in over 11,000 people.[194] In this trial, both groups had similar BP control, and both were randomized to the same ACEI (benazepril), yet the group initially randomized to a single-pill combination of benazepril with a calcium antagonist had a 20% CV risk reduction compared with the ACEI plus diuretic group. The observed benefit for the benazepril-amlodipine combination also extended to slowing CKD progression.[195]

Almost all people with an eGFR of less than 60 mL/min/1.73 m² and hypertension will require two or more medications to achieve a BP goal of less than 140/90 mm Hg. Single-pill combinations, including the combination of a RAAS blocker with either a calcium antagonist or diuretic, are preferred agents.[25,116] These combinations when given, generally in an additive fashion, reduce CV events and CKD progression. Other combinations that are efficacious for reducing BP but not tested in clinical trials include beta blockers with a dihydropyridine (DHP) calcium antagonist and DHP calcium antagonists with diuretics.[25]

There have been a number of trials assessing both CV outcome and changes in CKD progression. All these trials assume adherence with antihypertensive medications. However, according to one report, only 71% of subjects with hypertension in the United States are on treatment, and only 48% have their BP under adequate (<140/90 mm Hg) control. Moreover, two separate studies, one in the United Kingdom and the other in Germany, evaluating medication adherence, showed that only approximately 45% of patients who claimed to be taking BP-lowering medication actually were, as assessed by urine analysis of drug metabolites.[196,197] Although there has been significant reduction in the age-adjusted death rate for stroke and coronary artery disease since the early 1980s as a result of better BP control (and better treatment of other risk factors such as hyperlipidemia), heart disease and stroke remain the first and third leading causes of death in Western countries. This emphasizes the importance of identifying and treating patients with hypertension.

Dietary Approaches

All guidelines regardless of origin place emphasis on lifestyle modifications with emphasis on sodium restriction. Many studies document the effects of both sodium and potassium intake on BP. Table 26.6 summarizes the key lifestyle changes clearly shown to reduce BP levels and are adapted from the ACC/AHA Hypertension Guidelines of 2017.[7] It is very important to properly educate patients on the importance of a low-sodium diet. If a patient does not adhere to a low-sodium diet, the renin-angiotensin system will be suppressed reducing the efficacy or RAAS blockers.

Effect of Lifestyle Intervention in the Older People (>65 years)

In the Trial of Nonpharmacologic Interventions in the Elderly (TONE),[198] the combination of weight loss and sodium restriction showed a drop of 5.3 ± 1.2 mm Hg in the SBP and 3.4 ± 0.8 mm Hg DBP in obese, older patients with hypertension. The goal of sodium restriction was 1.8 g/24 hr, and the goal for weight reduction was 10 lb. Other lifestyle changes recommended in the older patient include watching potassium intake to keep the level of serum potassium in a safe range. Patient education about high-potassium foods is important. Intake of NSAIDs should be decreased to a minimum, because older patients are more likely to take NSAIDs for arthritis and pain. These drugs are known to cause elevations in BP by inhibiting the production of vasodilatory prostaglandins and may increase BP by as much as 6 mm Hg.[199,200] NSAIDs' BP-raising effects can be blunted by both calcium antagonists and, to less extent, diuretics.[201]

BLOOD PRESSURE–LOWERING MEDICATIONS

The American Society of Hypertension published a compendium summarizing more than 120 antihypertensive medications in eight drug classes.[202] There has been no newly approved antihypertensive medications since 2007. The following will briefly comment on these classes and make some specific observations regarding treatment.

Although both US and European guidelines focus on assessing CV risk before pursuing management, both agree that either a RAAS blocker, CCB, or thiazide-type diuretic be the initial treatment started in patients. Moreover, the European guidelines mandate initial therapy be a combination of a RAAS blocker with either a diuretic or calcium blocker, while US guidelines recommend single-pill combinations for those who are 20/10 mm Hg above the goal BP or higher. Only the US guidelines define hypertension as ≥130/80 mm Hg. The next closest group with this goal is the Canadian guidelines, but they reserve 130/80 mm Hg for those with higher CV risk only. All other international guidelines define hypertension as ≥140/90 mm Hg with a goal to get to 130/80 mm Hg.[7]

THERAPEUTIC OPTIONS AND APPROACHES FOR SUBGROUPS OF HYPERTENSION

Pharmacologic Intervention in the Older People (>65 years)

The primary agents used in the treatment of hypertension in older people with the greatest efficacy are thiazide-type diuretics and CCBs. ACEI

TABLE 26.6 Best Proven Nonpharmacologic Interventions for Prevention and Treatment of Hypertension

	NONPHARMACOLOGIC INTERVENTION	DOSE	APPROXIMATE IMPACT ON SBP HYPERTENSION	NORMOTENSION
Physical activity	Aerobic	• 90–150 min/wk • 65%–75% heart rate reserve	−5/8 mm Hg	−2/4 mm Hg
	Dynamic resistance	• 90–150 min/wk • 50%–80% 1 rep maximum • 6 exercises, 3 sets/exercise, 10 repetitions/set	−4 mm Hg	−2 mm Hg
	Isometric resistance	• 4× 2 min (hand grip), 1 min rest between exercises, 30%–40% maximum voluntary contraction, 3 sessions/wk • 8–10 wk	−5 mm Hg	−4 mm Hg
Healthy diet	DASH dietary pattern	Diet rich in fruits, vegetables, whole grains, and low-fat dairy products with reduced content of saturated and total fat	−11 mm Hg	−3 mm Hg
Weight loss	Weight/body fat	Ideal body weight is best goal but at least 1 kg reduction in body weight for most adults who are overweight	−5 mm Hg	−2/3 mm Hg
Reduced intake of dietary sodium	Dietary sodium	<1500 mg/day is optimal goal but at least 1000 mg/day reduction in most adults	−5/6 mm Hg	−2/3 mm Hg
Enhanced intake of dietary potassium	Dietary potassium	3500–5000 mg/day, preferably by consumption of a diet rich in potassium	−4/5 mm Hg	−2 mm Hg
Moderation in alcohol intake	Alcohol consumption	In individuals who drink alcohol, reduce alcohol to: • Men: <2 drinks daily • Women: <1 drink daily	−4 mm Hg	−3 mm Hg

SBP, Systolic blood pressure.

and ARBs are effective adjuncts but because of the lower renin status in older people they are not as successful in lowering BP. This is also true for younger African Americans patients.[203] Although other drug classes are available, confirmation that these agents decrease clinical outcomes to a similar extent as the primary agents is either lacking or safety and tolerability may relegate their role to use as secondary agents.[25] Specifically, there is inadequate evidence to support the initial use of beta blockers for hypertension in the absence of specific CV comorbidities. In considering the initial drug treatment of high BP, several different strategies may be contemplated. Many patients can be started on a single agent, but consideration should be given to starting with a single-pill two-drug combination for those greater than 20/10 mm Hg above the goal of 130/80 mm Hg.[204] Many patients started on a single agent will subsequently require two or more drugs from different pharmacologic classes to reach their BP goals (Fig. 26.5).

Knowledge of the pharmacologic mechanisms of action of each agent is important. Drug regimens with complementary activity, where a second antihypertensive is used to block compensatory responses to the initial agent or affect a different pressor mechanism, can result in a more than additive or synergistic lowering of BP. The use of combination therapy may also allow for treatment with lower doses of individual agents, which serves to minimize adverse effects and improve adherence. Several two- and three-drug single-pill fixed combinations of antihypertensive therapy are available in generic form with complementary mechanisms of action among the components (see Fig 26.4).[25]

Thiazide diuretics such as hydrochlorothiazide, chlorthalidone, indapamide, and bendrofluazide, as well as calcium antagonists, are recommended for initiating therapy in the older patient.[8,12] Diuretics cause an initial reduction of intravascular volume, peripheral vascular resistance, and BP in more than 50% of patients and are well tolerated and inexpensive.[205,206] However, they can cause hypokalemia, hypomagnesemia, and hyponatremia and are therefore not recommended in patients with baseline electrolyte abnormalities or those with a history of hyponatremia. Serum potassium level should be monitored, and supplementation should be given if needed.

In the Systolic Blood Pressure Intervention Trial (SPRINT), the older group of patients randomized to a lower level of BP less than 120 mm Hg did well and in many cases better than those at BPs targeted to less than 140 mm Hg, leading to the assertion that older patients should be treated to lower levels of BP. Other trials, however, in which people with much stiffer vessels were evaluated (i.e., pulse pressure >90 mm Hg), do not support this assertion. Thus, each patient's BP should be lowered to a level of tolerability where they can function and not be at risk of complications such as falls.[22,207,208]

Calcium antagonists are well suited for older patients whose hypertensive profile is based on increasing arterial dysfunction secondary to decreased atrial and ventricular compliance. This class of drugs dilates coronary and peripheral arteries in doses that do not severely affect myocardial contractility.[209,210] Most adverse effects relate to vasodilation, causing ankle edema, headache, or postural hypotension. Ankle edema is not secondary to sodium retention, because calcium antagonists are natriuretic when given initially, but the profound vasodilation with poor venous return in older people is the major contributor. First-generation immediate-release drugs, such as nifedipine, verapamil, and diltiazem, should be avoided in patients with left ventricular dysfunction. Non-DHPs can precipitate heart blocks in older adults with underlying conduction defects.

RAAS blockers, such as ACEIs, ARBs, and direct renin inhibitors, may be used in older adults.[211] Theoretically, as aging occurs, there is a reduction in angiotensin levels; thus, ACEIs may not be as effective in older adults. The use of ACEIs is beneficial in the reduction of morbidity and mortality in patients with myocardial infarction, reduced systolic function, heart failure, and reduction in the progression of diabetic renal disease and hypertensive nephrosclerosis.[212] RAAS blockers may provide greater benefit for CV and renal risk reduction than diuretics, based on data from the ACCOMPLISH trial. ACCOMPLISH suggested that a CCB-ACEI combination led to fewer people going on dialysis than a diuretic-ACEI combination; an outcome not explained by the BP difference of 1.2 mm Hg systolic between the two arms.[212,213]

It must be noted that individuals older than 70 years of age tend to

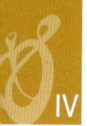

drink small amounts of fluid, and hence this makes them more vulnerable to decline in kidney function by RAAS blockade. Thus it is recommended that elderly patients increase their fluid intake to prevent volume depletion.

The clinical benefits of beta blockers as monotherapy in uncomplicated older patients are poorly documented. They may have a role in combination therapy, especially with diuretics. Beta blockers have established roles in patients with hypertension complicated by certain arrhythmias, migraine headaches, senile tremors, coronary artery disease, or heart failure.[214,215] Nebivolol, a selective beta$_1$ blocker with NO properties, does not show associated symptoms of depression, sexual dysfunction, dyslipidemia, and hyperglycemia in older adults, unlike earlier generations of beta blockers.[216]

Potassium-sparing diuretics are useful when combined with other agents only in people with an eGFR greater than 45 mL/min otherwise the rise of hyperkalemia is increased.[217] Aldosterone-blocking agents like spironolactone and eplerenone reduce vascular stiffness and SBP.[218,219] They are very helpful for patients with hypertension with heart failure or primary hyperaldosteronism. Gynecomastia and sexual dysfunction are the limiting adverse reactions that may occur in men using spironolactone but are less frequent with eplerenone. The epithelial sodium transport antagonists (amiloride, triamterene) are most useful when combined with another diuretic.

Other agents, such as alpha blockers, centrally acting drugs (e.g., clonidine), and nonspecific vasodilators (e.g., minoxidil), should not be used as first- or second-line agents in an older adult with hypertension. Instead, they are reserved as part of a combination regimen to maximize BP control after other agents have been deployed.

MANAGEMENT OF HYPERTENSION IN CHRONIC KIDNEY DISEASE

Both the Kidney Disease Outcomes Quality Initiative (KDOQI) and the KDIGO guidelines focus on the evidence for certain BP levels and classes of medication in patients with CKD. The strongest level of evidence to support slowing of CKD progression argues for BP levels below 140/90 mm Hg and the use of RAAS-blocking agents in people with stage 3 or higher CKD who have very high albuminuria. There is weaker evidence to support RAAS-blocker use in people with CKD without proteinuria, and very weak evidence supporting a BP of less than 130/80 mm Hg even for those who have a urine albumin level of 1 g or more and an eGFR of less than 60 mL/min/1.73 m^2.[220,221] BP levels and recommendations for RAAS blockers are focused on the primary outcome of slowing CKD progression.

The SPRINT included a cohort of patients with nondiabetic kidney disease but failed to reach a convincing endpoint of slowing CKD progression. Nevertheless, guidelines were put out arguing for a BP goal of less than 120/80 mm Hg for everyone with CKD. Unfortunately, this is not supported by the totality of the data and hence, the prior guidelines that recommended the BP goal of 130/80 mm Hg should be adhered to despite no further renal benefit, although there is CV risk reduction at this level.[222]

The ACC/AHA BP guidelines focus on CV risk reduction rather than a focus on renal preservation, because the BP range of 125 to 130 mm Hg has not been shown to harm the kidneys yet can further reduce CV events.[223]

Nuances in the management of BP in the patient with CKD are necessary because these patients have problems not seen in the general population. First, hyperkalemia is a risk in certain subgroups of patients. A review of clinical trials where hyperkalemia developed when managing hypertension in CKD found three risk predictors: (1) eGFR of less than 45 mL/min/1.73 m^2, (2) serum potassium level above 4.5 mEq/L, and (3) body mass index of less than 25.[217] Hyperkalemia limits the ability to assess whether RAAS blockers are effective in slowing CKD progression in stage 3b and higher CKD. Newer agents to manage hyperkalemia will allow safer management of CKD and expanded use of RAAS blockers for this population.[224,225] The use of the potassium-binding agent patiromer was applied to achieve BP control in resistant hypertension in the AMBER trial. In this phase 2 multicenter, randomized, double-blind, parallel-group, placebo-controlled study, 295 participants were stratified by serum potassium measurement (4.3 to <4.7 mmol/L versus 4.7 to 5.1 mmol/L) and history of diabetes and CKD with the focus to enable participants with resistant hypertension to achieve BP goals by using spironolactone. The results of the trial demonstrated a significantly higher number of participants on patiromer remained on spironolactone therapy.[226,227]

Further, critically important nuances in BP management in CKD patients are sodium restriction to less than 2400 mg/day, reduced alcohol consumption, and aerobic but not isometric exercise.[228] To demonstrate the importance of exercise, 296 dialysis patients were randomized to normal physical activity (control; n = 145) or walking exercise (n = 151) over a 6-month period. Those in the active group using a simple, personalized, home-based, low-intensity exercise program managed by dialysis staff improved physical performance and quality of life.[228]

Studies evaluating the effect of sodium intake on BP control in people with stage 4 CKD show that approximately every 400 mg above a sodium intake base of 3000 mg/day requires an additional BP medication to maintain BP control.[229] Moreover, failure to reduce sodium intake suppresses the RAAS system and hence reduces efficacy of RAAS blockers. Thus failure to reduce sodium intake is a cause of resistant hypertension.

The role for initial combination therapy in patients with CKD with a BP that is 20/10 mm Hg above the goal has been championed to enhance adherence and efficacy.[25,142] Studies evaluating initial monotherapy versus single-pill combination among those with an eGFR greater than 60 mL/min/1.73m^2 uniformly show an advantage of achieving BP goal more quickly and with better tolerability with single-pill combination therapy.[230,231]

The Action to Control Cardiovascular Risk in Diabetes (ACCORD) trial is a seminal trial to evaluate level of glycemic control and BP control on CV outcomes in people with diabetes. The results of the BP arm of the ACCORD trial failed to show a reduction in major CV events from more aggressive BP control.[232,233] Although the primary data from the ACCORD trial for BP control were underwhelming, two important studies using ACCORD data emerged that have changed the treatment landscape in diabetes. The first study used SPRINT inclusion criteria applied to the ACCORD database and compared CV outcomes showing a significant reduction in the intensive BP group in the primary endpoint.[234] Two further studies evaluated the change in serum creatinine and CV outcomes in ACCORD and demonstrated that up to a 30% increase in serum creatinine during the trial was associated with reduced CV outcomes.[235,236] This was not seen among those with a greater than 30% increase in serum creatinine.

The United Kingdom Prospective Diabetes Study (UKPDS) like ACCORD did not show a benefit from the lower BP group, which averaged well above 140/90 mm Hg.[237] Additional findings from post hoc analyses of diabetes subgroups of other trials also failed to show CV outcome benefit of BP levels below 130/80 mm Hg.

A number of studies demonstrate that some classes of antihypertensive drugs should be used preferentially in patients with diabetes who have nephropathy. The effect of RAAS blockers in diabetic nephropathy to retard hard kidney endpoints such as ESRD has been well documented in multiple studies.[5,238] However, this class of agents does not possess any specific advantages over other antihypertensive classes in people with diabetes who do not have nephropathy or albuminuria with levels at or above 300 mg/day.[239,240] Moreover, there is no evidence that RAAS blockers benefit people with normotension with or without microalbuminuria from developing declines in kidney function.[120,240,241]

Blood Pressure Management in Patients Undergoing Dialysis

Elevations in BP in dialysis patients are almost exclusively due to excessive volume. Hypertension control related directly to volume management is a more common problem in hemodialysis than in peritoneal dialysis. There are no large multicenter randomized trials in patients undergoing dialysis to evaluate different levels of BP on CV outcomes. A prospective, randomized trial evaluated the effects of an

ACEI versus a beta blocker on LVH, and CV mortality was performed in patients undergoing dialysis.[242] Subjects were randomly assigned to either open-label lisinopril ($n = 100$) or atenolol ($n = 100$), each administered three times per week after dialysis. Monthly monitored home BP was controlled to less than 140/90 mm Hg with medications, dry weight adjustment, and sodium restriction. The results demonstrated no between-group difference in 44-hour ambulatory BP; however, monthly measured home BP was consistently higher in the lisinopril group despite the need for both a greater number of antihypertensive agents and a greater reduction in dry weight. An independent data safety monitoring board recommended termination because of CV safety. Serious CV events were more prominent in the lisinopril group (20 events, atenolol versus 43 events, lisinopril; $P = 0.001$). Combined serious adverse events of myocardial infarction, stroke, and hospitalization for heart failure or CV death were much lower in the atenolol group ($P = 0.021$). Thus, it appears that beta blocker therapy is superior to RAAS blockade in patients undergoing hemodialysis to reduce CV morbidity and all-cause hospitalizations.

Retrospective analysis of patients on hemodialysis supports other beta blockers such as carvedilol for lowering CV events in hypertensive patients undergoing hemodialysis. The effect of beta blocker use on mortality among a cohort of patients undergoing hemodialysis was evaluated in a database analysis from the Dialysis Outcomes and Practice Patterns Study phase II of 2286 randomly selected patients on hemodialysis in Japan.[243] The main outcome measure was all-cause mortality. The authors found beta blocker use was low (i.e., only 247 patients [10.8%] were administered beta blockers, and 1828 patients [80%] were not). A Kaplan-Meier analysis revealed that all-cause mortality rates were significantly ($P < 0.007$) decreased in patients treated with beta blockers compared with the group not on beta blockers. In multivariable, fully adjusted models, treatment with beta blockers was also independently associated with reduced all-cause mortality (HR, $0.48; P = 0.02$).[241]

Data from the United States Renal Data System demonstrate a U-shaped relationship between SBP goals in patients undergoing dialysis and CV outcomes, suggesting that BP should be consistently above 120 mm Hg and below 150 mm Hg.[244] A meta-analysis of antihypertensive medications in patients undergoing dialysis demonstrates that regardless of class, reducing BP reduces CV events.[245] Data from epidemiologic studies consistently show that in patients undergoing maintenance dialysis, low BP values are associated with higher death rates when compared with normal to moderately high values.

An international consensus report provides guidance on appropriate management in dialysis patients, stating that in patients with ESRD treated with hemodialysis or peritoneal dialysis, hypertension is quite common and often poorly controlled.[233,246] BP recordings obtained before or after hemodialysis display a J-shaped or U-shaped association with CV events and survival, but this most likely reflects the low accuracy of these measurements and the peculiar hemodynamic setting related with dialysis treatment. Elevated BP by home or ABPM is clearly associated with shorter survival. Sodium and volume excess is the prominent mechanism of hypertension in dialysis patients, but other pathways, such as arterial stiffness, activation of the RAAS and SNSs, endothelial dysfunction, sleep apnea, and the use of erythropoietin-stimulating agents may also be involved. Nonpharmacologic interventions targeting sodium and volume excess are fundamental for hypertension control in this population.

If BP remains elevated after appropriate treatment of sodium-volume excess, the use of antihypertensive agents is necessary. Drug treatment in the dialysis population should take into consideration the patient's comorbidities and specific characteristics of each agent, such as dialyzability (i.e., metoprolol and atenolol are both 50% dialyzable, so effect dose is reduced).[233]

Although there is no generalizable approach to manage BP in dialysis, the following points are vital to have an accurate assessment of BP: (1) the most representative BP is the one taken the morning after dialysis, and (2) there should be a minimum of two and ideally three readings obtained 1 to 2 minutes apart during those morning readings and then averaged.[245] Given that heart failure and sudden death are the most common causes of death in dialysis patients, beta blockers have an important role in the BP-lowering armamentarium, unlike the general population. However, ensuring euvolemia is the key to controlling BP. The clinical examination is fundamental in determining volume status, but newer techniques of bioimpedance, blood volume monitoring, and inferior vena cava ultrasound are effective in improving the definition of dry weight and could be considered, particularly in patients with uncontrolled BP despite conventional dry weight assessment using the clinical examination.[247,248]

HEART FAILURE (SEE PART VI)

Hypertension has traditionally been associated with heart failure, and it has been relatively easy to infer empirically a cause-and-effect relationship. However, although the evidence is irrefutable that hypertension is a *risk factor* for heart failure, it has been less clear that hypertension is a *causal factor* for heart failure. Further, it is important to recognize the unique contribution of hypertension to HFpEF, a phenotype of heart failure which is now the predominant clinical syndrome recognized in hospital settings and responsible for more than 50% of all acute heart failure admissions.[249] Unlike HFrEF, in which clarity of the pathophysiology exists, the cellular and molecular aspects of the pathophysiology of HFpEF remain elusive. Prevailing considerations implicate fibrosis, ventricular noncompliance, hypertrophy, and ischemia; all of which can be impacted by hypertension.[250] Likely, there is no overarching maladaptive pathway that is the root cause of this important condition, but hypertension, when aligned with coronary artery disease, obesity, diabetes, and atrial fibrillation, explains the majority of concomitant comorbidities associated with clinical HFpEF.

Therapeutic considerations are clear for HFrEF but less certain for HFpEF. Management of HFpEF is hindered by the absence of a clear mechanism of left ventricular dysfunction and by the heterogeneity of persons with HFpEF. There are reasonable but not definitive data suggesting a potential benefit of mineralocorticoid receptor antagonists[251] and early signals that neprilysin inhibition in combination with renin-angiotensin-aldosterone blockade may be helpful.[246] The best guidance continues to prompt a unique focus on concomitant comorbidities, including hypertension, for which evidence-based clinical practice guidelines exist.

For HFrEF, defined treatment algorithms are available and are populated with evidence-based therapies proven to improve outcomes. ACC/AHA/Heart Failure Society of America (HFSA) clinical practice guidelines make clear the importance of both prevailing standard bearers of therapy: ACEI, ARBs, evidence-based beta-blockers, mineralocorticoid receptor antagonists, hydralazine and isosorbide dinitrate (ISDN), and implantable cardioverter-defibrillator/cardiac resynchronization therapy (ICD/CRT); and newer therapies: valsartan/sacubitril and ivabradine.[252] The expected outcomes of optimal therapy for HFrEF are now substantially better than historical expectations. Yet, whether the condition of heart failure is HFrEF, HFpEF, or even HF with improved or borderline ejection fraction, it remains clear that prevention is the more preferable intervention.

The American College of Cardiology Foundation (ACCF)/AHA guideline for the management of heart failure has adopted a stepwise progression to characterize the natural history of heart failure.[250] This framework organizes treatment strategies for preventing and controlling risk factors like hypertension (stage A), treating subclinical structural and functional changes like LVH and mechanical dysfunction (stage B), and reducing morbidity and mortality in symptomatic heart failure (stages C and D). This framework emphasizes the importance of intervening early in the progression of heart failure during stages A and B before the development of symptoms.[253]

Of all potential strategies that might reduce the incidence of heart failure, none appears to have higher yield than the treatment of hypertension. There are significant data to suggest that the incidence of heart failure may be favorably modified through optimal management of hypertension, especially in those with a higher burden of CV risk.[250] The earliest clinical trials testing antihypertensive drugs from the Veterans Administration Cooperative Study Groups reported reductions in heart failure events, but sample size was small and events were few.[254,255]

BP control and reduction are especially useful in older people to prevent heart failure. The Systolic Hypertension in Elderly Program (SHEP) was one of the first hypertension trials to include a prespecified endpoint examining the efficacy of antihypertensive therapy (chlorthalidone 12.5 to 25 mg plus atenolol 25 to 50 mg, if needed) in the prevention of heart failure.[207] Participants randomized to diuretic-based stepped care had a 49% reduction in fatal and nonfatal heart failure events during an average follow-up of 4.5 years.[256]

Similarly, in the Hypertension in the Very Elderly Trial (HYVET), patients randomized to the indapamide plus perindopril (as needed to achieve a target BP of 150/80 mm Hg) group achieved a 64% reduction in heart failure events compared with placebo at 2 years.[21]

Trials such as the Heart Outcomes Prevention Evaluation (HOPE) study demonstrated that ACEIs could also reduce heart failure events in high-risk participants.[257] In the HOPE study, among participants with diabetes mellitus or established vascular disease, ramipril treatment was associated with a 23% reduction in heart failure events after a mean of 4.5 years of follow-up.

The Antihypertensive and Lipid-Lowering Treatment to Prevent Heart Attack Trial (ALLHAT) was one of the largest clinical trials in hypertension management that tested the efficacy of chlorthalidone compared with lisinopril, amlodipine, and doxazosin in 42,418 participants with hypertension and at least one other CV risk factor.[258] Among the other comparisons, chlorthalidone was associated with a 38% reduction in heart failure compared with amlodipine and was associated with a 19% reduction in heart failure compared with lisinopril at a mean follow-up of 4.9 years. It is notable that ALLHAT included a significant proportion of African-American subjects in whom reduced responsiveness to ACEI therapy was observed.[258] A recent network meta-analysis confirmed the relative efficacy of thiazide diuretics, especially chlorthalidone, compared with other antihypertensive drug classes for heart failure prevention 10 years later.[259] In the 26 trials identified, the three most effective antihypertensive drug classes for reducing heart failure were thiazide diuretics, ACEIs, and ARBs. In direct and indirect comparisons, thiazide diuretics were marginally superior to ACEIs and ARBs; CCBs, beta blockers, and alpha blockers were the least effective agents for heart failure prevention.

Other meta-analyses have also focused on the magnitude of BP lowering as a key driver of heart failure prevention. In a recent high-quality meta-analysis of 123 BP-lowering trials, including 613,815 total participants, meta-regression demonstrated that for every 10–mm Hg reduction in SBP the risk of heart failure was reduced by 27%.[193] However, in this meta-analysis as well, investigators noted the *greater efficacy of thiazide diuretics* and *inferiority of CCBs for heart failure prevention*. In summary, hypertension treatment and control with thiazide diuretics plus ACEIs or ARBs are essential parts of a heart failure prevention strategy.

Because many of the same neurohormonal abnormalities that lead to HFrEF have been implicated in the pathogenesis of HFpEF, therapeutic trials for HFpEF have tested similar agents.[260,261] However, unlike with HFrEF, clinical trials testing beta blockers, nitrates, ACEIs, and especially ARBs and mineralocorticoid receptor antagonists have had largely disappointing results (see Chapter 51).

The role of ARBs in HFpEF has been studied in the Candesartan in Heart Failure: Assessment of Reduction in Mortality and Morbidity (CHARM)-Preserved and Irbesartan in Heart Failure with Preserved Ejection Fraction Study (I-PRESERVE).[262,263] Both trials failed to meet their primary outcome that included composite endpoints consisting of all-cause mortality, CV death, heart failure hospitalization, and/or hospitalization for a CV cause. Although candesartan therapy reduced heart failure hospitalizations in CHARM-Preserved in secondary analyses, this signal was not seen for I-PRESERVE.

The Randomized Aldosterone Antagonism in Heart Failure with Preserved Ejection Fraction (RAAM-PEF) study and the Aldosterone Receptor Blockade in Diastolic Heart Failure (Aldo-DHF) both tested the effects of mineralocorticoid receptor antagonists in patients with HFpEF.[264,265] Both trials demonstrated improvements in diastolic function in patients treated with mineralocorticoid receptor antagonists, but this did not translate to improvements in exercise capacity. The Treatment of Preserved Cardiac Function Heart Failure with an Aldosterone Antagonist (TOPCAT) was the largest trial to test the effects of mineralocorticoid receptor antagonists in patients with HFpEF.[266] After a mean follow-up of 3.3 years, spironolactone did not reduce the primary outcome of composite CV events, but it did reduce heart failure hospitalizations by 17%. Subsequent secondary and post hoc analyses suggested that clinical benefits primarily occurred in patients with higher BNP levels and those enrolled in the Americas.

A meta-analysis on the current state of evidence for mineralocorticoid receptor antagonists in HFpEF[267] identified 14 trials and found that mineralocorticoid receptor antagonists reduced the risk of heart failure hospitalization by 17%, improved quality of life, and improved multiple diastolic parameters on the echocardiogram. There was, however, no observed effect on all-cause mortality.

ACCF/AHA guidelines reflect the uncertainty from HFpEF trials by not recommending any specific agents with class I indications for HFpEF. Instead, guidelines recommend following hypertension guidelines for BP management and treating with diuretics for volume control.[252]

A meta-analysis using individual participant data from 51,917 participants included in 11 trials from the Blood Pressure Lowering Treatment Trialists' Collaboration provides empiric support for using risk assessment to guide BP-lowering treatment decisions.[268] These analyses demonstrated that the relative risk reduction for major CV events from active or more intensive BP-lowering therapy was similar across four risk strata; and consequently, absolute benefits from BP-lowering therapy were progressively greater as baseline risk increased. Importantly, these findings were consistent for all cause-specific CV outcomes but were qualitatively greatest for heart failure endpoints (Fig. 26.12).

These findings are even more relevant in the context of the SPRINT, in which participants at high risk for CV disease (e.g., 10-year cardiovascular disease [CVD] risk ≥15%, age ≥75 years, CKD or established vascular disease) were randomized to standard BP lowering (target SBP <140 mm Hg) versus intensive BP lowering (target SBP <120 mm Hg).[269] After a median follow-up of 3.3 years, intensive treatment was associated with a 25% reduction in major CV events, inclusive of heart failure, compared with standard treatment. However, the beneficial effect was primarily driven by a 38% reduction in heart failure and a 43% reduction in CV death. These studies establish the imperative to treat BP intensively in high-risk individuals to prevent heart failure.

RESISTANT HYPERTENSION

Resistant hypertension is defined as the failure to achieve a goal BP of less than 140/90 mm Hg in patients who are adherent with maximal tolerated doses of three antihypertensive drugs, one of which must be a diuretic appropriate for kidney function.[152] The increasing prevalence of obesity and hypertension in the general population has resulted in a higher incidence of resistant hypertension. Large-scale population-based studies such as the NHANES have specifically examined the prevalence and incidence of resistant hypertension and associated risk factors. The findings suggest the prevalence of resistant hypertension is approximately 8% to 12% of adult patients with hypertension (6 to 9 million people).[270] The increasing prevalence of resistant hypertension contrasts with the improvement in BP control rates during the same period. Studies also show that patients with resistant hypertension who are older than 55 years, of Black ethnicity, with high body mass index, diabetes, or CKD have an increased risk for CV events compared with patients with nonresistant hypertension. The effects of WCH and pseudoresistant hypertension have not been factored into many of the prevalence studies, and hence the true prevalence is not known. The white coat effect contributes greatly to the high-perceived incidence of resistant hypertension, as was evidenced by the over 60% screen failure in the Renal Denervation in Patients with Uncontrolled Hypertension (SYMPLICITY HTN-3) trial of renal denervation (RDN) due to WCH.[241,271]

Common causes of resistant hypertension include nonadherence with medication and volume overload secondary to poor kidney function and nonadherence with a low-sodium diet. Once a diagnosis of resistant hypertension is made, a fourth drug is needed after use of a calcium antagonist, diuretic, and RAAS blocker. A mineralocorticoid

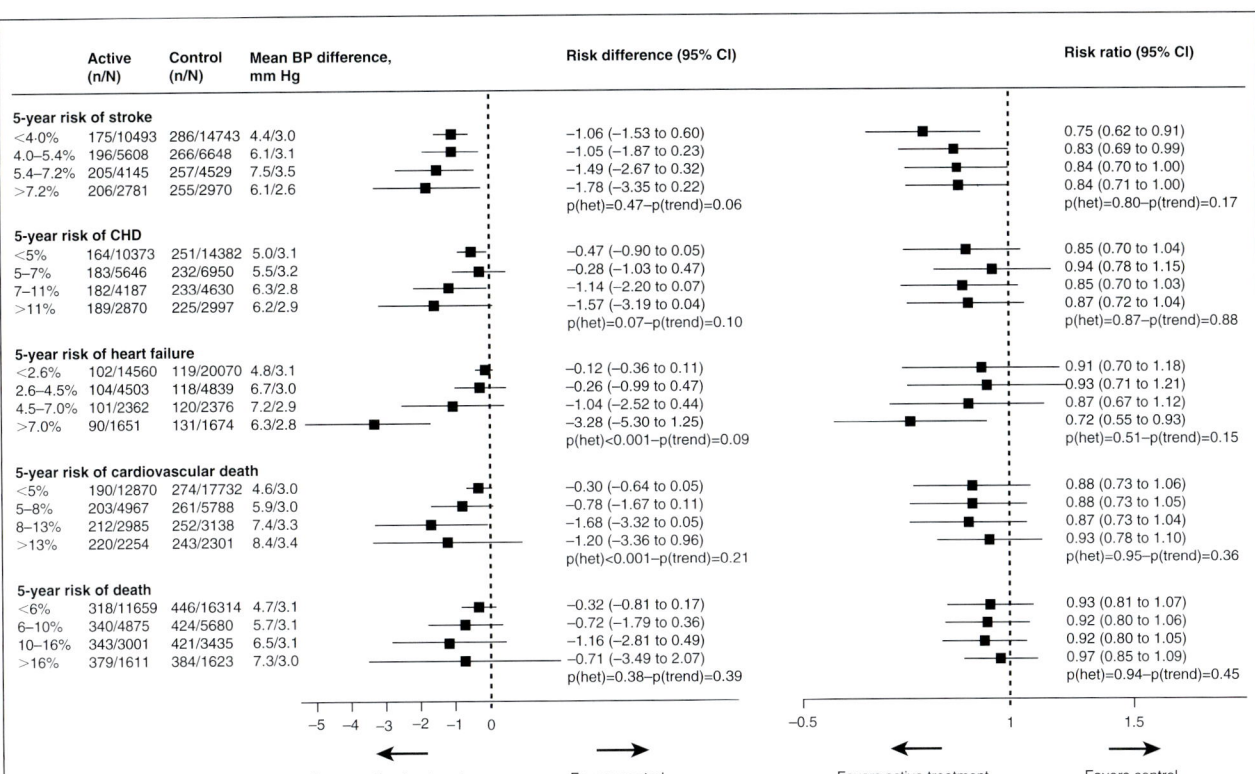

FIGURE 26.12 Meta-analysis of clinical trials demonstrating 5-year risk of heart failure and other cardiovascular events.

inhibitor such as spironolactone has demonstrated significant benefit in controlling BP in these patients.[272–274]

Nondrug Therapy for Resistant Hypertension Device Therapy

There are multiple different nondrug therapy approaches involving different devices for treatment of resistant hypertension. None of these are currently approved in the United States; however, most show great promise in reducing BP in people with resistant hypertension. Device approaches to resistant hypertension involve disruption of either the renal sympathetic nerves or stimulation of the carotid body baroreceptors. A comprehensive review that discusses the clinical studies and the basic science studies surrounding these technologies to better understand the effects of these treatments is referenced.[275]

Renal Denervation

The renal nerves enter the kidney at the hilum and branch out into segmental arteries throughout the kidney. They contain sympathetic efferent and sensory afferent fibers and are recognized as important controllers of kidney function and BP.[276] Additionally, sympathetic efferent fibers innervate the renal arteries, arterioles, renin-secreting juxtaglomerular cells, veins, and most tubular segments.[276,277] Stimulation of renal sympathetic nerves increases renal vascular resistance, tubular reabsorption of NaCl, and renin release depending on stimulation frequency.

Two initial clinical studies evaluated RDN in a multicenter study that enrolled 45 patients with SBP greater than 160 mm Hg on three or more antihypertensive drugs including a diuretic but did not include a sham control. Reductions in office SBP/DBP after RDN were impressive, averaging −22/−11 and −27/−17 mm Hg after 6 and 12 months, respectively. In 10 patients, renal norepinephrine spillover, measured using an isotope dilution method, was reduced by an average of 47%, demonstrating that the RDN procedure was moderately effective in ablating the renal nerves.[276] In a more recent study, doing a proper denervation involving branched nerves within the kidney reduced norepinephrine by 92%.[277]

These data generated the first definitive randomized, sham-controlled trial, SYMPLICITY HTN-3. A total of 533 patients with resistant hypertension taking at least three different BP medications were randomly assigned in a 2:1 ratio to undergo denervation or a sham procedure. The average decreases in SBP at 6 months were −14.1 and −11.7 mm Hg in RDN and sham groups, respectively, with no significant differences in 24-hour ambulatory SBP. After 12 months, the reductions in office BP were similar in the RDN and sham groups.[271]

The main reasons for the poor outcome revolved around procedural adequacy of denervation and location of denervation. In a retrospective analysis of angiographic and procedural records, 74% of patients did not have even one fully circumferential application of radiofrequency energy to the renal arteries, suggesting that effective denervation was not achieved in many patients.[277,278] Additionally, the location of the denervation was not adequate because there were very few nerves in that area, as was later discovered.[277] Also, there were medication changes in 38% of patients in the RDN group and 40% in the sham-control group despite the protocol mandating constant antihypertensive medication regimens. These limitations led some to conclude that, although the design of SYMPLICITY HTN-3 had many strengths compared with earlier studies, including a blinded sham-control design and relatively large patient enrollment, execution of the trial was flawed and therefore it cannot be considered definitive.[241]

Learning from all the mistaken assumptions and other trial issues as well as discussions with the FDA, a new catheter was invented (SPYRAL), and the SPYRAL HTN-OFF MED and SPYRAL HTN-ON MED trials ensued (Fig. 26.13).[279] These prospective, randomized, double-blind, sham-controlled studies were designed to assess the impact of RDN in patients with uncontrolled BP and who were medication naive or had discontinued medication and in patients being treated with one to three commonly prescribed antihypertensive medications. Both studies used a new multielectrode catheter designed to permit reliable circumferential four-quadrant renal nerve ablation. Also, RDN was performed in the main renal arteries and branches, an approach that likely produces more complete renal nerve ablation. Both studies showed significant reductions in BP through 3 months, compared with

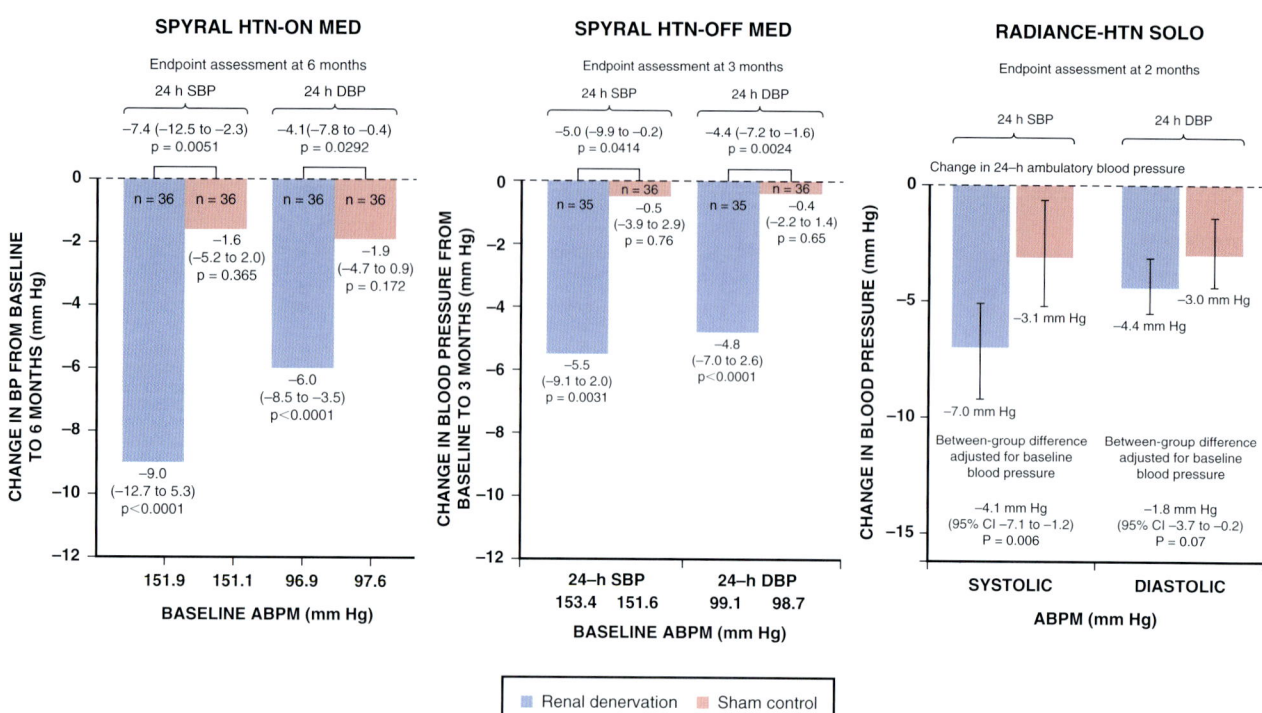

FIGURE 26.13 Summary of three randomized trials of renal denervation demonstrating the differences from placebo in blood pressure reduction. *ABPM,* Ambulatory blood pressure monitoring; *DPB,* diastolic blood pressure; *MED,* medication; *SBP,* systolic blood pressure.

sham controls, with no major adverse events. The primary results from the SPYRAL HTN-OFF MED trial confirmed earlier results demonstrating a clear 6.6/4.4–mm Hg reduction in office systolic pressure.[280] In contrast to SYMPLICITY HTN-3 in which participants received an average of greater than 5 antihypertensive agents, the effect of the sham procedure was negligible with changes in ambulatory SBP/DBP from baseline of only –0.5/–0.4 mm Hg.[271]

In the SPYRAL HTN-ON MED trial, medication adherence was approximately 60% in RDN and control groups and varied for individual patients throughout the study. Eligible patients ($n = 467$) had an office SBP between 150 and 180 mm Hg, a DBP of ≥90 mm Hg, and a 24-hour ambulatory SBP between 140 and 170 mm Hg; were on one to three antihypertensive drugs (thiazide diuretic, DHP CCB, beta blocker, and an ACEI or ARB with stable doses for at least 6 weeks); and were randomly assigned to RDN or sham control (see Fig. 26.12).[281] Office and 24-hour ambulatory BP decreased significantly from baseline to 6 months in the RDN group but not in controls, and baseline-adjusted treatment differences in 24-hour SBP/DBP averaged –7.0/–4.2 mm Hg. The BP reductions with RDN increased during 6 months of follow-up, and there were no procedural or intermediate-term adverse safety events reported. Like previous studies, nonadherence to antihypertensive drugs was common in patients with hypertension (see reference for comprehensive review of all trials).[279,282]

Baroreceptor-Activation

There are four trials involving baroreceptor activation by various procedures.

DEBuT-HT

The DEBuT-HT European trial (Device Based Therapy in Hypertension Trial) evaluated 45 patients with resistant hypertension, SBP ≥160/DBP ≥90 mm Hg. Medications were kept constant before and over the 3 months of the trial, but medication adherence was not critically assessed.[283] At each visit, the device was temporarily turned off to assess BP without activation. At that time, BP increased rapidly toward baseline levels, confirming the sustained antihypertensive effects of baroreceptor-activation (BA) therapy, and demonstrating the rapid off transient response to deactivation.

Rheos Pivotal Trial

In the Rheos Pivotal Trial, subjects were implanted with the Rheos system, and 265 patients were randomized 2:1 1 month after surgery to receive BA the first 6 months (immediate BA) or to delay BA for the first 6 months of the trial (delayed BA). For the immediate BA group, SBP was reduced by 16 mm Hg at 6 months and 27 mm Hg at 12 months when compared with the 1-month postimplant values before activation. For the delayed BA group, reductions in SBP were 9 and 25 mm Hg at 6 and 12 months, respectively. The trial was successful in meeting the prespecified sustained 12-month efficacy endpoint; however, the acute 6-month primary efficacy endpoint was missed.[284] The failure to meet the prespecified acute efficacy endpoint was apparently due primarily to a larger and more variable reduction than expected in SBP at 6 months in the group with the inactive implants and likely reflected the less-than-optimal trial design.[284] Beyond efficacy considerations, the prespecified endpoint for procedural safety was not met, with 9% of patients developing transient or permanent nerve injury and 5% having general surgical complications.

After completion of the DEBut-HT and Rheos Pivotal studies, trial participants were enrolled in separate open-label, observational follow-up studies. Follow-up findings were reported after patients had completed 2 to 4 and 5 to 6 years of therapy.[285,286] In both follow-up studies, the pressure reductions reported in the initial trials were sustained or even enhanced. Although all patients in the Rheos trial received bilateral implants, the majority of subjects had their devices programmed for unilateral activation. During regular office visits, the decision to activate either unilaterally or bilaterally was based on acute dose-response tests for BP lowering while adjusting stimulation parameters.

To optimize battery longevity, unilateral stimulation was chosen in 75% of the subjects because the acute fall in BP was not greater with bilateral stimulation. Most importantly, the Rheos-HT study (Rheos-Hypertension) showed that unilateral carotid sinus stimulation was sufficient to produce appreciable and sustained reductions in BP in patients with resistant hypertension.[285]

Barostim Neo Trial

The Barostim Neo trial was a single-arm, open-label study that evaluated efficacy and safety of the second-generation system for BA in 30 patients with resistant hypertension. The implant procedure was minimally invasive and required only unilateral suturing of a miniaturized electrode on to the surface of the carotid sinus. The primary efficacy objective of this trial was to describe reductions in office BP through 6 months of BA.[287] Compared with the Rheos-HT trial, the number of patients who suffered from procedural complications decreased from 25% to 3%. Of particular interest, 6 of the 30 patients enrolled in the Barostim Neo trial underwent previous RDN, which was unsuccessful in lowering BP. After 6 months of BA, reductions in SBP and HR were comparable in these patients when compared with the subjects with intact renal innervation.

MobiusHD Device for Baroreflex Amplification

An alternate approach for chronically activating the carotid baroreflex is being evaluated in clinical trials. Rather than increasing baroreceptor afferent activity by electrically stimulating the carotid sinus, the concept behind the MobiusHD system (Vascular Dynamics, Inc) is amplification of the signal sensed by carotid baroreceptors during distortion of their nerve endings by vascular stretch during systole. Signal amplification is achieved by a passive, flexible, self-expanding endovascular implant that reshapes the carotid sinus during systole, increasing the radius while preserving pulsatility. In so doing, this increases wall strain and, thus, baroreceptor activation during spontaneous changes in systolic pressure.

Support for this approach comes from an acute study in dogs, but long-term mechanistic studies have not been conducted. The device has received CE marking for treatment of resistant hypertension in the European Economic Area and in an open-label, uncontrolled study in 30 patients with resistant hypertension, BP was reduced substantially after 6 months of unilateral endovascular baroreceptor amplification.[288] An uncontrolled open-label study evaluating the safety and efficacy of the MobiusHD implant in patients with resistant hypertension is currently in progress in the United States (http://www.clinicaltrials.gov/ct/show/NCT01831895).

HYPERTENSIVE URGENCY AND EMERGENCY

A hypertensive emergency is the combination of elevated BP levels (with no specific diagnostic BP level) and signs or symptoms of acute, ongoing target-organ damage. Such patients are traditionally admitted to an intensive care unit and given parenteral infusions of short-acting antihypertensive agents to restore autoregulation in vascular beds. This is done because historical data from the early 1900s (antedating effective antihypertensive drug therapy) showed a very poor prognosis, similar to that of many cancers. Traditionally, patients who presented with significantly elevated BP levels usually above an SBP of 180 mm Hg, but no acute, ongoing target-organ damage, were diagnosed with a "hypertensive urgency." They were observed for a few hours after treatment with one or more oral antihypertensive agents and then discharged to a site of ongoing care for their hypertension.[289] This practice is considered safe because two retrospective studies, one involving 1016 patients seen in an emergency department[290] and another involving 58,535 outpatients, demonstrated very low rates of morbidity/mortality, and no significant difference in prognosis for those treated acutely, compared with those who were discharged with rapid follow-up.[291]

The initial evaluation of a severely hypertensive patient includes a thorough inspection of the optic fundi (looking for acute hemorrhages, exudates, or papilledema); a mental status assessment; a careful cardiac, pulmonary, and neurologic examination; a quick search for clues that might indicate secondary hypertension (e.g., abdominal bruit, striae, radial-femoral delay); and laboratory studies to assess renal function (dipstick and microscopic urinalysis, determination of serum creatinine level).

Several options for intravenous drug treatment exist, but nitroprusside is the least expensive and most widely available. It must be kept in the dark and is metabolized to cyanide and/or thiocyanate, particularly during long-term infusions. Fenoldopam mesylate, a dopamine-1 agonist, is very effective and acutely improves several parameters of renal function. Clevidipine is a DHP calcium antagonist that is hydrolyzed within minutes by ubiquitous serum esterases; it is administered in an emulsion containing soy and egg proteins (either of which can cause immunologic reactions in allergic patients). Its elimination is not importantly affected by hepatic or renal functional impairment. Clevidipine and its older, longer-acting cousin, nicardipine, are often used for patients with coronary disease, because the reflex tachycardia is usually offset by coronary vasodilation. Nimodipine is typically used only for subarachnoid hemorrhage. Labetalol can be given as an intravenous infusion and easily converted to an ongoing oral dose.

The quickest therapeutic response to a hypertensive emergency is recommended for an acute aortic dissection (see Chapter 42). In this condition the BP should be lowered *within 20 minutes* to an SBP below 120 mm Hg (neither of which is supported by a strong evidence base), typically with a beta blocker (to reduce shear stress on the dissection) and a vasodilator. Controversy exists about if, and when, BP lowering should be attempted in the setting of an acute ischemic stroke. If the patient is a candidate for acute thrombolytic therapy and the BP is higher than 180/110 mm Hg, acute BP lowering is recommended. Most US authorities suggest attempting slow and gradual BP lowering only if the BP is "very high" (e.g., ≥180/110 mm Hg) with a short-acting, rapidly titratable drug. However, two large, randomized trials done outside the United States have suggested that BP lowering in this setting is safe but does not produce significant outcome benefits in either ischemic[268] or hemorrhagic stroke.[292] All other types of hypertensive emergencies can be handled with a gradual lowering of BP (typically 10% to 15% during the first hour and a further 10% to 20% during the next hour, for a total of approximately 25%).

Frequent monitoring of the patient's clinical status is important because not all patients can reestablish the normal autoregulatory capacity of the circulation in important vascular beds during the same short time period. Because hypertensive encephalopathy is a diagnosis of exclusion, it is often very rewarding to monitor these patients closely because their mental status improves markedly (and usually rather quickly) as the BP is carefully lowered.

Patients who present with hypertensive crises involving cardiac ischemia/infarction or pulmonary edema can be managed with nitroglycerin, clevidipine, nicardipine, or nitroprusside, although typically a combination of drugs (including an ACEI for heart failure or left ventricular dysfunction) is used in these settings. Efforts to preserve myocardium and open the obstructed coronary artery (by thrombolysis, angioplasty, or surgery) also are indicated.

Hypertensive emergency involving the kidney commonly is followed by a further deterioration in renal function even when BP is lowered properly. The most important predictor of the need for acute dialysis is not the BP level but instead the degree of renal dysfunction (both eGFR and degree of albuminuria). Some physicians prefer fenoldopam to nicardipine or nitroprusside in this setting because of its lack of toxic metabolites and specific renal vasodilating effects. The need for acute dialysis often is precipitated by BP reduction in patients with preexisting stage 3 to 5 CKD, but many patients are able to avoid dialysis (and a remarkable few even discontinue it) in the long term if BP is carefully and well controlled during follow-up.

Hypertensive emergency resulting from catecholamine excess states (e.g., pheochromocytoma, monoamine oxidase inhibitor crisis, cocaine intoxication) are most appropriately managed with an intravenous alpha blocker (e.g., phentolamine), with a beta blocker added later, if needed. Many patients with severe hypertension caused by sudden withdrawal of antihypertensive agents (e.g., clonidine) are easily managed by giving one acute dose of the missed drug.

Hypertensive emergency during pregnancy must be managed in a more careful and conservative manner because of the presence of the fetus (see Chapter 92). Magnesium sulfate, methyldopa, and hydralazine are the drugs of choice, with oral labetalol and nifedipine being drugs of second choice in the United States; nitroprusside, ACEIs, and ARBs are contraindicated.[293] Delivery of the infant is often hastened by the obstetrician to assist in management of hypertension in pregnancy.

Whether hypertensive urgencies (elevated BP, but without acute ongoing target-organ damage) ought to be treated acutely is controversial because there is no evidence that such treatment improves prognosis. The BP in many such patients spontaneously falls during a 30-minute period of quiet rest. Conversely, immediate-release nifedipine capsules can cause precipitous hypotension, stroke, myocardial infarction, and death. According to the FDA, they "should be used with great caution, if at all." In such instances, true "hypotension" (e.g., SBP <90 mm Hg) may not be observed, yet the BP may fall below the autoregulatory threshold (which is likely different for every patient, and unknown to the treating physician until it is surpassed), precipitating ischemia.

Clonidine, captopril, labetalol, several other short-acting antihypertensive drugs, and even amlodipine have been used in this setting, but none has a clear advantage over the others, and each is usually effective in most patients. The most important aspect of managing a hypertensive urgency is to refer the patient to a good source of ongoing care for hypertension, where adherence to antihypertensive therapy during long-term follow-up will be more likely.

In short, patients presenting with a hypertensive emergency should be diagnosed quickly and started promptly on effective parenteral therapy (often nitroprusside 0.5 µg/kg/min) in an intensive care unit. BP should be reduced by approximately 25%, gradually over 2 to 3 hours. Oral antihypertensive therapy should be instituted, usually after approximately 8 to 24 hours of parenteral therapy; evaluation for secondary causes of hypertension may be considered after transfer from the intensive care unit. Because of advances in antihypertensive therapy and management, "malignant hypertension" is a term that should be eliminated because the prognosis of patients with this condition has improved greatly since the term was introduced in 1927.

REFERENCES
Epidemiology
1. Benjamin EJ, Blaha MJ, Chiuve SE, et al. Heart disease and stroke statistics-2017 update: a report from the American Heart Association. *Circulation*. 2017;135:e146–e603.
2. Lim SS, Vos T, Flaxman AD, et al. A comparative risk assessment of burden of disease and injury attributable to 67 risk factors and risk factor clusters in 21 regions, 1990-2010: a systematic analysis for the Global Burden of Disease Study 2010. *Lancet*. 2012;380:2224–2260.
3. Barnes JA, Eid MA, Creager MA, Goodney PP. Epidemiology and risk of amputation in patients with diabetes mellitus and peripheral artery disease. *Arterioscler Thromb Vasc Biol*. 2020: ATVBAHA120314595.
4. Lewington S, Clarke R, Qizilbash N, et al. Age-specific relevance of usual blood pressure to vascular mortality: a meta-analysis of individual data for one million adults in 61 prospective studies. *Lancet*. 2002;360:1903–1913.
5. Whelton PK, Carey RM, Aronow WS, et al. 2017 ACC/AHA/AAPA/ABC/ACPM/AGS/APhA/ASH/ASPC/NMA/PCNA guideline for the prevention, detection, evaluation, and management of high blood pressure in adults: executive summary: a report of the American College of Cardiology/American Heart Association Task Force on clinical practice guidelines. *Hypertension*. 2018;71:1269–1324.
6. Williams B, Mancia G, Spiering W, et al. 2018 ESC/ESH Guidelines for the management of arterial hypertension. *Eur Heart J*. 2018;39:3021–3104.
7. Bakris G, Ali W, Parati G. ACC/AHA versus ESC/ESH on hypertension guidelines: JACC guideline comparison. *J Am Coll Cardiol*. 2019;73:3018–3026.
8. Egan BM. Hypertension in military veterans is associated with combat exposure and combat injury. *J Hypertens*. 2020;38:1255–1256.
9. Franklin SS, Jacobs MJ, Wong ND, et al. Predominance of isolated systolic hypertension among middle-aged and elderly US hypertensives: analysis based on National Health and Nutrition Examination Survey (NHANES) III. *Hypertension*. 2001;37:869–874.
10. Forouzanfar MH, Liu P, Roth GA, et al. Global burden of hypertension and systolic blood pressure of at least 110 to 115 mm Hg, 1990-2015. *J Am Med Assoc*. 2017;317:165–182.
11. Joffres M, Falaschetti E, Gillespie C, et al. Hypertension prevalence, awareness, treatment and control in national surveys from England, the USA and Canada, and correlation with stroke and ischaemic heart disease mortality: a cross-sectional study. *BMJ Open*. 2013;3:e003423.
12. Franklin SS, Gustin W, Wong ND, et al. Hemodynamic patterns of age-related changes in blood pressure. The Framingham Heart Study. *Circulation*. 1997;96:308–315.
13. Perry Jr HM, Miller JP, Fornoff JR, et al. Early predictors of 15-year end-stage renal disease in hypertensive patients. *Hypertension*. 1995;25:587–594.
14. Golshiri K, Ataei Ataabadi E, Portilla Fernandez EC, et al. The importance of the nitric oxide-cGMP pathway in age-related cardiovascular disease: focus on phosphodiesterase-1 and soluble guanylate cyclase. *Basic Clin Pharmacol Toxicol*. 2019.
15. Vasan RS, Beiser A, Seshadri S, et al. Residual lifetime risk for developing hypertension in middle-aged women and men: the Framingham Heart Study. *J Am Med Assoc*. 2002;287:1003–1010.
16. Lloyd-Jones DM, Evans JC, Larson MG, et al. Differential impact of systolic and diastolic blood pressure level on JNC-VI staging. Joint national committee on prevention, detection, evaluation, and treatment of high blood pressure. *Hypertension*. 1999;34:381–385.
17. Haider AW, Larson MG, Franklin SS, et al. Systolic blood pressure, diastolic blood pressure, and pulse pressure as predictors of risk for congestive heart failure in the Framingham Heart Study. *Ann Intern Med*. 2003;138:10–16.
18. Jafar TH, Stark PC, Schmid CH, et al. Progression of chronic kidney disease: the role of blood pressure control, proteinuria, and angiotensin-converting enzyme inhibition: a patient-level meta-analysis. *Ann Intern Med*. 2003;139:244–252.
19. Yoon SS, Carroll MD, Fryar CD. *Hypertension Prevalence and Control Among Adults: United States, 2011-2014*. NCHS Data Brief; 2015:1–8.
20. Elliott WJ. Management of hypertension in the very elderly patient. *Hypertension*. 2004;44:800–804.
21. Beckett NS, Peters R, Fletcher AE, et al. Treatment of hypertension in patients 80 years of age or older. *N Engl J Med*. 2008;358:1887–1898.
22. Williamson JD, Supiano MA, Applegate WB, et al. Intensive vs standard blood pressure control and cardiovascular disease outcomes in adults aged >/=75 Years: a randomized clinical trial. *J Am Med Assoc*. 2016;315:2673–2682.
23. Bowling CB, Davis BR, Luciano A, et al. Sustained blood pressure control and coronary heart disease, stroke, heart failure, and mortality: an observational analysis of ALLHAT. *J Clin Hypertens*. 2019;21:451–459.
24. Derington CG, King JB, Herrick JS, et al. Trends in antihypertensive medication monotherapy and combination use among US adults, national health and nutrition examination Survey 2005-2016. *Hypertension*. 2020;75:973–981.
25. Gradman AH, Basile JN, Carter BL, Bakris GL. American society of hypertension writing G. Combination therapy in hypertension. *J Clin Hypertens*. 2011;13:146–154.
26. Chow CK, Teo KK, Rangarajan S, et al. Prevalence, awareness, treatment, and control of hypertension in rural and urban communities in high-, middle-, and low-income countries. *J Am Med Assoc*. 2013;310:959–968.
27. Kearney PM, Whelton M, Reynolds K, et al. Global burden of hypertension: analysis of worldwide data. *Lancet*. 2005;365:217–223.
28. Campbell NR, Brant R, Johansen H, et al. Increases in antihypertensive prescriptions and reductions in cardiovascular events in Canada. *Hypertension*. 2009;53:128–134.
29. Ogden CL, Carroll MD, Lawman HG, et al. Trends in obesity prevalence among children and adolescents in the United States, 1988-1994 through 2013-2014. *J Am Med Assoc*. 2016;315: 2292–2299.
30. Flynn JT, Kaelber DC, Baker-Smith CM, et al. Clinical practice guideline for screening and management of high blood pressure in children and adolescents. *Pediatrics*. 2017;140.
31. Ostchega Y, Fryar CD, Nwankwo T, Nguyen DT. *Hypertension Prevalence among adults aged 18 and over: United States, 2017-2018*. NCHS Data Brief; 2020:1–8.
32. Samanic CM, Barbour KE, Liu Y, et al. Prevalence of self-reported hypertension and antihypertensive medication use by county and rural-urban classification - United States, 2017. *MMWR Morb Mortal Wkly Rep*. 2020;69:533–539.
33. Kochanek KD, Murphy SL, Xu J, Tejada-Vera B. Deaths: final data for 2014. *Natl Vital Stat Rep*. 2016;65:1–122.
34. System USRD. *USRDS 2016 Annual Data Report: Atlas of Chronic Kidney Disease and End-Stage Renal Disease in the United States*; 2016.
35. Falaschetti E, Mindell J, Knott C, Poulter N. Hypertension management in England: a serial cross-sectional study from 1994 to 2011. *Lancet*. 2014;383:1912–1919.
36. Patel KV, Li X, Kondamudi N, et al. Prevalence of apparent treatment-resistant hypertension in the United States according to the 2017 high blood pressure guideline. *Mayo Clin Proc*. 2019;94:776–782.

Pathophysiology
37. Hall MHJ. Pathogenesis of hypertension. In: Bakris GS, MJ, ed. *Hypertension: A Companion to Braunwald's Heart Disease*. 3rd ed. Philadelphia, PA: Elsevier; 2018:33–51.
38. Guyton AC. Kidneys and fluids in pressure regulation. Small volume but large pressure changes. *Hypertension*. 1992;19:I2–I8.
39. Guyton AC. Blood pressure control–special role of the kidneys and body fluids. *Science*. 1991;252:1813–1816.
40. Ivy JR, Bailey MA. Pressure natriuresis and the renal control of arterial blood pressure. *J Physiol*. 2014;592:3955–3967.
41. Johnson RJ, Herrera-Acosta J, Schreiner GF, Rodriguez-Iturbe B. Subtle acquired renal injury as a mechanism of salt-sensitive hypertension. *N Engl J Med*. 2002;346:913–923.
42. Rodriguez-Iturbe B, Romero F, Johnson RJ. Pathophysiological mechanisms of salt-dependent hypertension. *Am J Kidney Dis*. 2007;50:655–672.
43. International Consortium for Blood Pressure Genome-Wide Association S, Ehret GB, Munroe PB, et al. Genetic variants in novel pathways influence blood pressure and cardiovascular disease risk. *Nature*. 2011;478:103–109.
44. Sun J, Zhao M, Miao S, Xi B. Polymorphisms of three genes (ACE, AGT and CYP11B2) in the renin-angiotensin-aldosterone system are not associated with blood pressure salt sensitivity: a systematic meta-analysis. *Blood Press*. 2016;25:117–122.
45. Gonzalez-Villalobos RA, Janjoulia T, Fletcher NK, et al. The absence of intrarenal ACE protects against hypertension. *J Clin Invest*. 2013;123:2011–2023.
46. Reudelhuber TL. Where hypertension happens. *J Clin Invest*. 2013;123:1934–1936.
47. Danser AH. The role of the (Pro)renin receptor in hypertensive disease. *Am J Hypertens*. 2015;28:1187–1196.
48. Rosendahl A, Niemann G, Lange S, et al. Increased expression of (pro)renin receptor does not cause hypertension or cardiac and renal fibrosis in mice. *Lab Invest*. 2014;94:863–872.
49. Crowley SD, Gurley SB, Herrera MJ, et al. Angiotensin II causes hypertension and cardiac hypertrophy through its receptors in the kidney. *Proc Natl Acad Sci U S A*. 2006;103:17985–17990.
50. Crowley SD, Gurley SB, Oliverio MI, et al. Distinct roles for the kidney and systemic tissues in blood pressure regulation by the renin-angiotensin system. *J Clin Invest*. 2005;115:1092–1099.
51. McCurley A, Jaffe IZ. Mineralocorticoid receptors in vascular function and disease. *Mol Cell Endocrinol*. 2012;350:256–265.
52. Tikellis C, Bernardi S, Burns WC. Angiotensin-converting enzyme 2 is a key modulator of the renin-angiotensin system in cardiovascular and renal disease. *Curr Opin Nephrol Hypertens*. 2011;20:62–68.
53. Ferrario CM. ACE2: more of Ang-(1-7) or less Ang II? *Curr Opin Nephrol Hypertens*. 2011;20:1–6.
54. Fraga-Silva RA, Costa-Fraga FP, Murca TM, et al. Angiotensin-converting enzyme 2 activation improves endothelial function. *Hypertension*. 2013;61:1233–1238.
55. Hernandez Prada JA, Ferreira AJ, Katovich MJ, et al. Structure-based identification of small-molecule angiotensin-converting enzyme 2 activators as novel antihypertensive agents. *Hypertension*. 2008;51:1312–1317.
56. Wysocki J, Ye M, Rodriguez E, et al. Targeting the degradation of angiotensin II with recombinant angiotensin-converting enzyme 2: prevention of angiotensin II-dependent hypertension. *Hypertension*. 2010;55:90–98.
57. Haschke M, Schuster M, Poglitsch M, et al. Pharmacokinetics and pharmacodynamics of recombinant human angiotensin-converting enzyme 2 in healthy human subjects. *Clin Pharmacokinet*. 2013;52:783–792.
58. Li XC, Zhang J, Zhuo JL. The vasoprotective axes of the renin-angiotensin system: physiological relevance and therapeutic implications in cardiovascular, hypertensive and kidney diseases. *Pharmacol Res*. 2017.
59. Mancia G, Grassi G. The autonomic nervous system and hypertension. *Circ Res*. 2014;114:1804–1814.
60. DiBona GF. Sympathetic nervous system and hypertension. *Hypertension*. 2013;61:556–560.
61. Grassi G, Cattaneo BM, Seravalle G, et al. Baroreflex control of sympathetic nerve activity in essential and secondary hypertension. *Hypertension*. 1998;31:68–72.
62. Smith PA, Graham LN, Mackintosh AF, et al. Relationship between central sympathetic activity and stages of human hypertension. *Am J Hypertens*. 2004;17:217–222.
63. DeLalio LJ, Sved AF, Stocker SD. Sympathetic nervous system contributions to hypertension: updates and therapeutic relevance. *Can J Cardiol*. 2020;36:712–720.
64. Johnson RJ, Gordon KL, Suga S, et al. Renal injury and salt-sensitive hypertension after exposure to catecholamines. *Hypertension*. 1999;34:151–159.
65. Mu S, Shimosawa T, Ogura S, et al. Epigenetic modulation of the renal beta-adrenergic-WNK4 pathway in salt-sensitive hypertension. *Nat Med*. 2011;17:573–580.
66. Bangalore S, Sawhney S, Messerli FH. Relation of beta-blocker-induced heart rate lowering and cardioprotection in hypertension. *J Am Coll Cardiol*. 2008;52:1482–1489.
67. Julius S, Palatini P, Kjeldsen SE, et al. Usefulness of heart rate to predict cardiac events in treated patients with high-risk systemic hypertension. *Am J Cardiol*. 2012;109:685–692.
68. Ichiki T, Burnett Jr JC. Atrial natriuretic peptide- old but new therapeutic in cardiovascular diseases. *Circ J*. 2017;81:913–919.

69. Curry FR. Atrial natriuretic peptide: an essential physiological regulator of transvascular fluid, protein transport, and plasma volume. *J Clin Invest*. 2005;115:1458–1461.
70. Hu BC, Li Y, Liu M, et al. Blood pressure and urinary sodium excretion in relation to 16 genetic polymorphisms in the natriuretic peptide system in Chinese. *Endocr J*. 2014;61:861–874.
71. Newton-Cheh C, Larson MG, Vasan RS, et al. Association of common variants in NPPA and NPPB with circulating natriuretic peptides and blood pressure. *Nat Genet*. 2009;41:348–353.
72. Maimaitiming S, Roussel R, Hadjadj S, et al. Association of common variants in NPPA and NPPB with blood pressure does not translate into kidney damage in a general population study. *J Hypertens*. 2010;28:1230–1233.
73. Robles-Vera I, Toral M, Duarte J. Microbiota and hypertension: role of the sympathetic nervous system and the immune system. *Am J Hypertens*. 2020.
74. Sartori C, Lepori M, Scherrer U. Interaction between nitric oxide and the cholinergic and sympathetic nervous system in cardiovascular control in humans. *Pharmacol Ther*. 2005;106:209–220.
75. Taddei S, Virdis A, Mattei P, et al. Endothelium-dependent forearm vasodilation is reduced in normotensive subjects with familial history of hypertension. *J Cardiovasc Pharmacol*. 1992;20(suppl 12):S193–S195.
76. Spieker LE, Flammer AJ, Luscher TF. The vascular endothelium in hypertension. *Handb Exp Pharmacol*. 2006;249–283.
77. Dharmashankar K, Widlansky ME. Vascular endothelial function and hypertension: insights and directions. *Curr Hypertens Rep*. 2010;12:448–455.
78. Popolo A, Autore G, Pinto A, Marzocco S. Oxidative stress in patients with cardiovascular disease and chronic renal failure. *Free Radical Research*. 2013;47:346–356.
79. Kohan DE, Barton M. Endothelin and endothelin antagonists in chronic kidney disease. *Kidney Int*. 2014;86:896–904.
80. Lazich I, Bakris G. Initial combination antihypertensives: let's ACCELERATE. *Lancet*. 2011;377:278–279.
81. van Goor H, van den Born JC, Hillebrands JL, Joles JA. Hydrogen sulfide in hypertension. *Curr Opin Nephrol Hypertens*. 2016;25:107–113.
82. Yang G, Wu L, Jiang B, et al. H2S as a physiologic vasorelaxant: hypertension in mice with deletion of cystathionine gamma-lyase. *Science*. 2008;322:587–590.
83. Quyyumi AA, Patel RS. Endothelial dysfunction and hypertension: cause or effect? *Hypertension*. 2010;55:1092–1094.
84. Shimbo D, Muntner P, Mann D, et al. Endothelial dysfunction and the risk of hypertension: the multi-ethnic study of atherosclerosis. *Hypertension*. 2010;55:1210–1216.
85. Taddei S, Bruno RM. Endothelial dysfunction in hypertension: achievements and open questions. *J Hypertens*. 2016;34:1492–1493.
86. Baldo MP, Brant LCC, Cunha RS, et al. The association between salt intake and arterial stiffness is influenced by a sex-specific mediating effect through blood pressure in normotensive adults: the ELSA-Brasil study. *J Clin Hypertens*. 2019;21:1771–1779.
87. Agbor LN, Ibeawuchi SC, Hu C, et al. Cullin-3 mutation causes arterial stiffness and hypertension through a vascular smooth muscle mechanism. *JCI Insight*. 2016;1:e91015.
88. Quinn U, Tomlinson LA, Cockcroft JR. Arterial stiffness. *JRSM Cardiovasc Dis*. 2012;1.
89. Zieman SJ, Melenovsky V, Kass DA. Mechanisms, pathophysiology, and therapy of arterial stiffness. *Arterioscler Thromb Vasc Biol*. 2005;25:932–943.
90. Mitchell GF. Arterial stiffness: insights from Framingham and Iceland. *Curr Opin Nephrol Hypertens*. 2015;24:1–7.
91. Sagi B, Kesoi I, Kesoi B, et al. Arterial stiffness may predict renal and cardiovascular prognosis in autosomal-dominant polycystic kidney disease. *Physiol Int*. 2018;105:145–156.
92. Kaess BM, Rong J, Larson MG, et al. Aortic stiffness, blood pressure progression, and incident hypertension. *J Am Med Assoc*. 2012;308:875–881.
93. Chen W, Li S, Fernandez C, et al. Temporal relationship between elevated blood pressure and arterial stiffening among middle-aged Black and white adults: the bogalusa heart study. *Am J Epidemiol*. 2016;183:599–608.
94. Ben-Shlomo Y, Spears M, Boustred C, et al. Aortic pulse wave velocity improves cardiovascular event prediction: an individual participant meta-analysis of prospective observational data from 17,635 subjects. *J Am Coll Cardiol*. 2014;63:636–646.
95. Rodriguez-Iturbe B, Pons H, Quiroz Y, Johnson RJ. The immunological basis of hypertension. *Am J Hypertens*. 2014;27:1327–1337.
96. Harrison DG. Inflammation and immunity in hypertension. In: Bakris GS, MJ, ed. *Hypertension: A Companion to Braunwald's Heart Disease*. 3rd ed. Philadelphia, PA: Elsevier; 2018:60–69.
97. Guzik TJ, Hoch NE, Brown KA, et al. Role of the T cell in the genesis of angiotensin II induced hypertension and vascular dysfunction. *J Exp Med*. 2007;204:2449–2460.
98. Xiao L, Harrison DG. Inflammation in hypertension. *Can J Cardiol*. 2020;36:635–647.
99. Herrera J, Ferrebuz A, MacGregor EG, Rodriguez-Iturbe B. Mycophenolate mofetil treatment improves hypertension in patients with psoriasis and rheumatoid arthritis. *J Am Soc Nephrol*. 2006;17:S218–S225.
100. Ehret GB, Caulfield MJ. Genes for blood pressure: an opportunity to understand hypertension. *Eur Heart J*. 2013;34:951–961.
101. Warren HR, Evangelou E, Cabrera CP, et al. Genome-wide association analysis identifies novel blood pressure loci and offers biological insights into cardiovascular risk. *Nat Genet*. 2017;49:403–415.
102. Lander E, Kruglyak L. Genetic dissection of complex traits: guidelines for interpreting and reporting linkage results. *Nat Genet*. 1995;11:241–247.
103. Kotchen TA, Cowley Jr AW, Liang M. Ushering hypertension into a new era of precision medicine. *J Am Med Assoc*. 2016;315:343–344.
104. Vasudeva K, Balyan R, Munshi A. ACE-triggered hypertension incites stroke: genetic, molecular, and therapeutic aspects. *NeuroMolecular Med*. 2020;22:194–209.
105. Hall JE, do Carmo JM, da Silva AA, et al. Obesity-induced hypertension: interaction of neurohumoral and renal mechanisms. *Circ Res*. 2015;116:991–1006.
106. Dorresteijn JA, Visseren FL, Spiering W. Mechanisms linking obesity to hypertension. *Obes Rev*. 2012;13:17–26.
107. Flynn C. Increased aldosterone: mechanism of hypertension in obesity. *Semin Nephrol*. 2014;34:340–348.
108. Schinner S, Willenberg HS, Krause D, et al. Adipocyte-derived products induce the transcription of the StAR promoter and stimulate aldosterone and cortisol secretion from adrenocortical cells through the Wnt-signaling pathway. *Int J Obes*. 2007;31:864–870.
109. Ehrhart-Bornstein M, Lamounier-Zepter V, Schraven A, et al. Human adipocytes secrete mineralocorticoid-releasing factors. *Proc Natl Acad Sci U S A*. 2003;100:14211–14216.
110. Asferg CL, Nielsen SJ, Andersen UB, et al. Relative atrial natriuretic peptide deficiency and inadequate renin and angiotensin II suppression in obese hypertensive men. *Hypertension*. 2013;62:147–153.

Clinical Assessment

111. Zampaglione B, Pascale C, Marchisio M, Cavallo-Perin P. Hypertensive urgencies and emergencies. Prevalence and clinical presentation. *Hypertension*. 1996;27:144–147.
112. Gus M, Fuchs FD, Pimentel M, et al. Behavior of ambulatory blood pressure surrounding episodes of headache in mildly hypertensive patients. *Arch Intern Med*. 2001;161:252–255.
113. Peixoto AJ. A young patient with a family history of hypertension. *Clin J Am Soc Nephrol*. 2014;9:2164–2172.
114. Muiesan ML, Salvetti M, Paini A, et al. Ocular fundus photography with a smartphone device in acute hypertension. *J Hypertens*. 2017;35:1660–1665.
115. Muiesan ML, Padovani A, Salvetti M, et al. Headache: prevalence and relationship with office or ambulatory blood pressure in a general population sample (the Vobarno Study). *Blood Press*. 2006;15:14–19.
116. Weber MA, Schiffrin EL, White WB, et al. Clinical practice guidelines for the management of hypertension in the community a statement by the American Society of Hypertension and the International Society of Hypertension. *J Hypertens*. 2014;32:3–15.
117. Parati G, Stergiou G, O'Brien E, et al. European Society of Hypertension practice guidelines for ambulatory blood pressure monitoring. *J Hypertens*. 2014;32:1359–1366.
118. Shibao C, Lipsitz LA, Biaggioni I, American Society of Hypertension Writing G. Evaluation and treatment of orthostatic hypotension. *J Am Soc Hypertens*. 2013;7:317–324.
119. Wheeler DC, Becker GJ. Summary of KDIGO guideline. What do we really know about management of blood pressure in patients with chronic kidney disease? *Kidney Int*. 2013;83:377–383.
120. de Boer I, Bangalore S, Benetos A, et al. Diabetes and hypertension: a position statement by the American Diabetes Association. *Diabetes Care*. 2017.
121. Freeman R, Wieling W, Axelrod FB, et al. Consensus statement on the definition of orthostatic hypotension, neurally mediated syncope and the postural tachycardia syndrome. *Clin Auton Res*. 2011;21:69–72.
122. Stergiou GS, Baibas NM, Gantzarou AP, et al. Reproducibility of home, ambulatory, and clinic blood pressure: implications for the design of trials for the assessment of antihypertensive drug efficacy. *Am J Hypertens*. 2002;15:101–104.
123. Bliziotis IA, Destounis A, Stergiou GS. Home versus ambulatory and office blood pressure in predicting target organ damage in hypertension: a systematic review and meta-analysis. *J Hypertens*. 2012;30:1289–1299.
124. McManus RJ, Caulfield M, Williams B, National Institute for H, Clinical E. NICE hypertension guideline 2011: evidence based evolution. *BMJ*. 2012;344:e181.
125. Conen D, Bamberg F. Noninvasive 24-h ambulatory blood pressure and cardiovascular disease: a systematic review and meta-analysis. *J Hypertens*. 2008;26:1290–1299.
126. Palla M, Saber H, Konda S, Briasoulis A. Masked hypertension and cardiovascular outcomes: an updated systematic review and meta-analysis. *Integr Blood Press Control*. 2018;11:11–24.
127. Niiranen TJ, Hanninen MR, Johansson J, et al. Home-measured blood pressure is a stronger predictor of cardiovascular risk than office blood pressure: the Finn-Home study. *Hypertension*. 2010;55:1346–1351.
128. Briasoulis A, Bakris GL. Current status of renal denervation in hypertension. *Curr Cardiol Rep*. 2016;18:107.
129. Briasoulis A, Androulakis E, Palla M, et al. White-coat hypertension and cardiovascular events: a meta-analysis. *J Hypertens*. 2016;34:593–599.
130. Fagard RH, Celis H, Thijs L, et al. Daytime and nighttime blood pressure as predictors of death and cause-specific cardiovascular events in hypertension. *Hypertension*. 2008;51:55–61.
131. Salles GF, Reboldi G, Fagard RH, et al. Prognostic effect of the nocturnal blood pressure fall in hypertensive patients: the ambulatory blood pressure collaboration in patients with hypertension (ABC-H) meta-analysis. *Hypertension*. 2016;67:693–700.
132. Kasai T, Bradley TD, Friedman O, Logan AG. Effect of intensified diuretic therapy on overnight rostral fluid shift and obstructive sleep apnoea in patients with uncontrolled hypertension. *J Hypertens*. 2014;32:673–680.
133. Boggia J, Li Y, Thijs L, et al. Prognostic accuracy of day versus night ambulatory blood pressure: a cohort study. *Lancet*. 2007;370:1219–1229.
134. Fagard RH, Thijs L, Staessen JA, et al. Night-day blood pressure ratio and dipping pattern as predictors of death and cardiovascular events in hypertension. *J Hum Hypertens*. 2009;23:645–653.
135. Hansen TW, Thijs L, Li Y, et al. Prognostic value of reading-to-reading blood pressure variability over 24 hours in 8938 subjects from 11 populations. *Hypertension*. 2010;55:1049–1057.
136. Staessen JA, Byttebier G, Buntinx F, et al. Antihypertensive treatment based on conventional or ambulatory blood pressure measurement: a randomized controlled trial. Ambulatory Blood Pressure Monitoring and Treatment of Hypertension Investigators. *J Am Med Assoc*. 1997;278:1065–1072.
137. Verberk WJ, Kroon AA, Lenders JW, et al. Self-measurement of blood pressure at home reduces the need for antihypertensive drugs: a randomized, controlled trial. *Hypertension*. 2007;50:1019–1025.
138. Verberk WJ, Kessels AG, Thien T. Telecare is a valuable tool for hypertension management, a systematic review and meta-analysis. *Blood Press Monit*. 2011;16:149–155.
139. Staessen JA, Den Hond E, Celis H, et al. Antihypertensive treatment based on blood pressure measurement at home or in the physician's office: a randomized controlled trial. *J Am Med Assoc*. 2004;291:955–964.
140. Boonyasai RT, McCannon EL, Landavaso JE. Automated office-based blood pressure measurement: an overview and guidance for implementation in primary care. *Curr Hypertens Rep*. 2019;21:29.
141. Kario K, Shin J, Chen CH, et al. Expert panel consensus recommendations for ambulatory blood pressure monitoring in Asia: the HOPE Asia Network. *J Clin Hypertens*. 2019;21:1250–1283.
142. Chobanian AV. The seventh report of the joint national committee on prevention, detection, evaluation, and treatment of high blood pressure: The JNC 7 Report. *J Am Med Assoc*. 2003;289:2560.
143. Pickering TG. Why don't we use nitrates to treat older hypertensive patients? *J Clin Hypertens*. 2005;7:685–687.90.
144. Parati G, Omboni S. Role of home blood pressure telemonitoring in hypertension management: an update. *Blood Press Monit*. 2010;15:285–295.
145. Bakris GL, Molitch ME. Should restrictions Be relaxed for metformin use in chronic kidney disease? Yes, they should Be relaxed! What's the fuss? *Diabetes Care*. 2016;39:1287–1291.
146. Santos M, Shah AM. Alterations in cardiac structure and function in hypertension. *Curr Hypertens Rep*. 2014;16:428.
147. Laragh JH. Renin profiling for diagnosis, risk assessment, and treatment of hypertension. *Kidney Int*. 1993;44:1163–1175.
148. Blumenfeld JD, Laragh JH. Renin system analysis: a rational method for the diagnosis and treatment of the individual patient with hypertension. *Am J Hypertens*. 1998;11:894–896.
149. Egan BM, Basile JN, Rehman SU, et al. Plasma Renin test-guided drug treatment algorithm for correcting patients with treated but uncontrolled hypertension: a randomized controlled trial. *Am J Hypertens*. 2009;22:792–801.
150. Tapolyai MB, Petho A, Fulop T. Whole-body imaging procedures in resistant hypertension: evaluating for secondary causes or to define end-organ damages? *J Clin Hypertens*. 2017;19:23–25.
151. Noilhan C, Barigou M, Bieler L, et al. Causes of secondary hypertension in the young population: a monocentric study. *Ann Cardiol Angeiol*. 2016;65:159–164.
152. Elliott WJ. Drug interactions and drugs that affect blood pressure. *J Clin Hypertens*. 2006;8:731–737.
153. Karashima S, Kometani M, Tsujiguchi H, et al. Prevalence of primary aldosteronism without hypertension in the general population: results in Shika study. *Clin Exp Hypertens*. 2018;40:118–125.
154. Kayser SC, Deinum J, de Grauw WJ, et al. Prevalence of primary aldosteronism in primary care: a cross-sectional study. *Br J Gen Pract*. 2018;68:e114–e122.
155. Young WJ. Primary hyperaldosteronism. In: Bakris G, Sorrentino MJ, eds. *Hypertension: A Companion to Braunwald's Heart Disease*. 3rd ed. Philadelphia: Elsevier; 2018:126–135.
156. Milliez P, Girerd X, Plouin PF, et al. Evidence for an increased rate of cardiovascular events in patients with primary aldosteronism. *J Am Coll Cardiol*. 2005;45:1243–1248.

157. Denimal D, Duvillard L. 2016 Endocrine Society guidelines update for the diagnosis of primary aldosteronism: are the proposed aldosterone-to-renin ratio cut-off values relevant in the era of fully automated immunoassays? *Ann Clin Biochem*. 2016;53:714–715.
158. Carey RMCD, Bakris G, Brook RD, et al. Resistant hypertension: diagnosis, evaluation, and treatment: a scientific statement from the American Heart Association professional education committee of the council for high blood pressure research. *Hypertension*. 2018;72(5):e53–e90.
159. Cohen DF L. Pheochromocytoma and paraganglioma. In: Bakris G, Sorrentino MJ, eds. *Hypertension : A Companion to Braunwald's Heart Disease*. 3rd ed. Philadelphia: Elsevier; 2018:136–143.
160. Stefanelli A, Treglia G, Bruno I, et al. Pharmacological interference with 123I-metaiodobenzylguanidine: a limitation to developing cardiac innervation imaging in clinical practice? *Eur Rev Med Pharmacol Sci*. 2013;17:1326–1333.
161. Lenders JW, Duh QY, Eisenhofer G, et al. Pheochromocytoma and paraganglioma: an endocrine society clinical practice guideline. *J Clin Endocrinol Metab*. 2014;99:1915–1942.
162. Berta E, Lengyel I, Halmi S, et al. Hypertension in thyroid disorders. *Front Endocrinol*. 2019;10:482.
163. Melmed S, Casanueva FF, Klibanski A, et al. A consensus on the diagnosis and treatment of acromegaly complications. *Pituitary*. 2013;16:294–302.
164. Sardella C, Urbani C, Lombardi M, et al. The beneficial effect of acromegaly control on blood pressure values in normotensive patients. *Clin Endocrinol*. 2014;81:573–581.
165. Poggio R, Gutierrez L, Matta MG, et al. Daily sodium consumption and CVD mortality in the general population: systematic review and meta-analysis of prospective studies. *Public Health Nutr*. 2015;18:695–704.
166. Cook NR, Appel LJ, Whelton PK. Lower levels of sodium intake and reduced cardiovascular risk. *Circulation*. 2014;129:981–989.
167. Bruno RM, Palagini L, Gemignani A, et al. Poor sleep quality and resistant hypertension. *Sleep Med*. 2013;14:1157–1163.
168. Carey RM, Calhoun DA, Bakris GL, et al. Resistant hypertension: detection, evaluation, and management: a scientific statement from the American Heart Association. *Hypertension*. 2018;72:e53–e90.
169. Pepin JL, Borel AL, Tamisier R, et al. Hypertension and sleep: overview of a tight relationship. *Sleep Med Rev*. 2014;18:509–519.
170. Ayas NT, White DP, Manson JE, et al. A prospective study of sleep duration and coronary heart disease in women. *Arch Intern Med*. 2003;163:205–209.
171. Patel SR, Ayas NT, Malhotra MR, et al. A prospective study of sleep duration and mortality risk in women. *Sleep*. 2004;27:440–444.
172. Ali W, Gao G, Bakris GL. Improved sleep quality improves blood pressure control among patients with chronic kidney disease: a pilot study. *Am J Nephrol*. 2020;51:249–254.
173. Gangwisch JE, Heymsfield SB, Boden-Albala B, et al. Short sleep duration as a risk factor for hypertension: analyses of the first National Health and Nutrition Examination Survey. *Hypertension*. 2006;47:833–839.
174. Sayk F, Teckentrup C, Becker C, et al. Effects of selective slow-wave sleep deprivation on nocturnal blood pressure dipping and daytime blood pressure regulation. *Am J Physiol Regul Integr Comp Physiol*. 2010;298:R191–R197.
175. Cano-Pumarega I, Duran-Cantolla J, Aizpuru F, et al. Obstructive sleep apnea and systemic hypertension: longitudinal study in the general population: the Vitoria Sleep Cohort. *Am J Respir Crit Care Med*. 2011;184:1299–1304.
176. Itani O, Jike M, Watanabe N, Kaneita Y. Short sleep duration and health outcomes: a systematic review, meta-analysis, and meta-regression. *Sleep Med*. 2017;32:246–256.
177. Dematteis M, Julien C, Guillermet C, et al. Intermittent hypoxia induces early functional cardiovascular remodeling in mice. *Am J Respir Crit Care Med*. 2008;177:227–235.
178. Gottlieb DJ, Punjabi NM, Mehra R, et al. CPAP versus oxygen in obstructive sleep apnea. *N Engl J Med*. 2014;370:2276–2285.
179. Iftikhar IH, Kline CE, Youngstedt SD. Effects of exercise training on sleep apnea: a meta-analysis. *Lung*. 2014;192:175–184.

Management

180. Liyanage T, Ninomiya T, Jha V, et al. Worldwide access to treatment for end-stage kidney disease: a systematic review. *Lancet*. 2015;385:1975–1982.
181. Van der Niepen P, Rossignol P, Lengele JP, et al. Renal artery stenosis in patients with resistant hypertension: stent it or not? *Curr Hypertens Rep*. 2017;19:5.
182. Levey AS, de Jong PE, Coresh J, et al. The definition, classification, and prognosis of chronic kidney disease: a KDIGO Controversies Conference report. *Kidney Int*. 2011;80:17–28.
183. Klahr S, Levey AS, Beck GJ, et al. The effects of dietary protein restriction and blood-pressure control on the progression of chronic renal disease. Modification of Diet in Renal Disease Study Group. *N Engl J Med*. 1994;330:877–884.
184. D'Elia L, Rossi G, Schiano di Cola M, et al. Meta-analysis of the effect of dietary sodium restriction with or without concomitant renin-angiotensin-aldosterone system-inhibiting treatment on albuminuria. *Clin J Am Soc Nephrol*. 2015;10:1542–1552.
185. Dworkin LD, Cooper CJ. Clinical practice. Renal-artery stenosis. *N Engl J Med*. 2009;361:1972–1978.
186. Cooper CJ, Murphy TP, Cutlip DE, et al. Stenting and medical therapy for atherosclerotic renal-artery stenosis. *N Engl J Med*. 2014;370:13–22.
187. Hager A. Hypertension in aortic coarctation. *Minerva Cardioangiol*. 2009;57:733–742.
188. Aronow WS, Fleg JL, Pepine CJ, et al. ACCF/AHA 2011 expert consensus document on hypertension in the elderly: a report of the American College of Cardiology foundation Task Force on clinical expert consensus documents developed in collaboration with the American Academy of Neurology, American Geriatrics Society, American Society for Preventive Cardiology, American Society of Hypertension, American Society of Nephrology, Association of Black Cardiologists, and European Society of Hypertension. *J Am Coll Cardiol*. 2011;57:2037–2114.
189. Canniffe C, Ou P, Walsh K, et al. Hypertension after repair of aortic coarctation–a systematic review. *Int J Cardiol*. 2013;167:2456–2461.
190. Cohen JB, Lotito MJ, Trivedi UK, et al. Cardiovascular events and mortality in white coat hypertension: a systematic review and meta-analysis. *Ann Intern Med*. 2019;170:853–862.
191. Emdin CA, Rahimi K, Neal B, et al. Blood pressure lowering in type 2 diabetes: a systematic review and meta-analysis. *J Am Med Assoc*. 2015;313:603–615.
192. Thomopoulos C, Parati G, Zanchetti A. Effects of blood pressure lowering on outcome incidence in hypertension: 7. Effects of more vs. less intensive blood pressure lowering and different achieved blood pressure levels - updated overview and meta-analyses of randomized trials. *J Hypertens*. 2016;34:613–622.
193. Ettehad D, Emdin CA, Kiran A, et al. Blood pressure lowering for prevention of cardiovascular disease and death: a systematic review and meta-analysis. *Lancet*. 2016;387:957–967.
194. Jamerson K, Weber MA, Bakris GL, et al. Benazepril plus amlodipine or hydrochlorothiazide for hypertension in high-risk patients. *N Engl J Med*. 2008;359:2417–2428.
195. Bakris G, Vassalotti J, Ritz E, et al. National Kidney Foundation consensus conference on cardiovascular and kidney diseases and diabetes risk: an integrated therapeutic approach to reduce events. *Kidney Int*. 2010;78:726–736.
196. Jung O, Gechter JL, Wunder C, et al. Resistant hypertension? Assessment of adherence by toxicological urine analysis. *J Hypertens*. 2013;31:766–774.
197. Tomaszewski M, White C, Patel P, et al. High rates of non-adherence to antihypertensive treatment revealed by high-performance liquid chromatography-tandem mass spectrometry (HP LC-MS/MS) urine analysis. *Heart*. 2014;100:855–861.
198. Whelton PK, Appel LJ, Espeland MA, et al. Sodium reduction and weight loss in the treatment of hypertension in older persons: a randomized controlled trial of nonpharmacologic interventions in the elderly (TONE). TONE Collaborative Research Group. *J Am Med Assoc*. 1998;279:839–846.
199. Johnson AG, Nguyen TV, Owe-Young R, et al. Potential mechanisms by which nonsteroidal anti-inflammatory drugs elevate blood pressure: the role of endothelin-1. *J Hum Hypertens*. 1996;10:257–261.
200. Izhar M, Alausa T, Folker A, et al. Effects of COX inhibition on blood pressure and kidney function in ACE inhibitor-treated blacks and hispanics. *Hypertension*. 2004;43:573–577.
201. Ishiguro C, Fujita T, Omori T, et al. Assessing the effects of non-steroidal anti-inflammatory drugs on antihypertensive drug therapy using post-marketing surveillance database. *J Epidemiol*. 2008;18:119–124.
202. Ferdinand KC. A compendium of antihypertensive therapy. *J Clin Hypertens*. 2011;13:636–638.
203. The AO, Coordinators for the ACRG. Major outcomes in high-risk hypertensive patients randomized to angiotensin-converting enzyme inhibitor or calcium channel blocker vs diuretic: the Antihypertensive and Lipid-Lowering Treatment to Prevent Heart Attack Trial (ALLHAT). *J Am Med Assoc*. 2002;288:2981–2997.
204. Whelton PK, Carey RM, Aronow WS, et al. 2017 ACC/AHA/AAPA/ABC/ACPM/AGS/APhA/ASH/ASPC/NMA/PCNA guideline for the prevention, detection, evaluation, and management of high blood pressure in adults: a report of the American College of Cardiology/American Heart Association Task Force on clinical practice guidelines. *Hypertension*. 2018;71:e13–e115.
205. Birkenhager WH. Diuretics and blood pressure reduction: physiologic aspects. *J Hypertens Suppl*. 1990;8:S3–S7.
206. Bakris GL. Recognition, pathogenesis, and treatment of different stages of nephropathy in patients with type 2 diabetes mellitus. *Mayo Clin Proc*. 2011;86:444–456.
207. Prevention of stroke by antihypertensive drug treatment in older persons with isolated systolic hypertension. Final results of the Systolic Hypertension in the Elderly Program (SHEP). SHEP Cooperative Research Group. *J Am Med Assoc*. 1991;265:3255–3264.
208. Bulpitt CJ, Beckett NS, Peters R, et al. Blood pressure control in the Hypertension In The Very Elderly Trial (HYVET). *J Hum Hypertens*. 2012;26:157–163.
209. Frishman WH. Comparative pharmacokinetic and clinical profiles of angiotensin-converting enzyme inhibitors and calcium antagonists in systemic hypertension. *Am J Cardiol*. 1992;69:17C–25C.
210. Chen N, Zhou M, Yang M, et al. Calcium channel blockers versus other classes of drugs for hypertension. *Cochrane Database Syst Rev*. 2010:CD003654.
211. Pappoe LS, Winkelmayer WC. ACE inhibitor and angiotensin II type 1 receptor antagonist therapies in elderly patients with diabetes mellitus: are they underutilized? *Drugs Aging*. 2010;27:87–94.
212. Xie J, Sert Kuniyoshi FH, Covassin N, et al. Nocturnal hypoxemia due to obstructive sleep apnea is an independent predictor of poor prognosis after myocardial infarction. *J Am Heart Assoc*. 2016;5.
213. Ahmed MI, Ekundayo OJ, Mujib M, et al. Mild hyperkalemia and outcomes in chronic heart failure: a propensity matched study. *Int J Cardiol*. 2010;144:383–388.
214. Moser M, Menard J. Clinical significance of the metabolic effects of antihypertensive drugs. *J Hum Hypertens*. 1993;7(suppl 1):S50–S55.
215. Moen MD, Wagstaff AJ. Nebivolol: a review of its use in the management of hypertension and chronic heart failure. *Drugs*. 2006;66:1389–1409; discussion 410.
216. Ladage D, Reidenbach C, Rieckeheer E, et al. Nebivolol lowers blood pressure and increases weight loss in patients with hypertension and diabetes in regard to age. *J Cardiovasc Pharmacol*. 2010;56:275–281.
217. Lazich I, Bakris GL. Prediction and management of hyperkalemia across the spectrum of chronic kidney disease. *Semin Nephrol*. 2014;34:333–339.
218. Liu Y, Dai S, Liu L, et al. Spironolactone is superior to hydrochlorothiazide for blood pressure control and arterial stiffness improvement: a prospective study. *Medicine (Baltim)*. 2018;97:e0500.
219. Currie G, Taylor AH, Fujita T, et al. Effect of mineralocorticoid receptor antagonists on proteinuria and progression of chronic kidney disease: a systematic review and meta-analysis. *BMC Nephrol*. 2016;17:127.
220. Taler SJ, Agarwal R, Bakris GL, et al. KDOQI US commentary on the 2012 KDIGO clinical practice guideline for management of blood pressure in CKD. *Am J Kidney Dis*. 2013;62:201–213.
221. Upadhyay A, Uhlig K. Is the lower blood pressure target for patients with chronic kidney disease supported by evidence? *Curr Opin Cardiol*. 2012;27:370–373.
222. Oparil S, Acelajado MC, Bakris GL, et al. Hypertension. *Nat Rev Dis Primers*. 2018;4:18014.
223. Cheung AK, Rahman M, Reboussin DM, et al. Effects of intensive BP control in CKD. *J Am Soc Nephrol*. 2017.
224. Bakris GL, Pitt B, Weir MR, et al. Effect of patiromer on serum potassium level in patients with hyperkalemia and diabetic kidney disease: the AMETHYST-DN randomized clinical trial. *J Am Med Assoc*. 2015;314:151–161.
225. Packham DK, Rasmussen HS, Lavin PT, et al. Sodium zirconium cyclosilicate in hyperkalemia. *N Engl J Med*. 2015;372:222–231.
226. Agarwal R, Rossignol P, Romero A, et al. Patiromer versus placebo to enable spironolactone use in patients with resistant hypertension and chronic kidney disease (AMBER): a phase 2, randomised, double-blind, placebo-controlled trial. *Lancet*. 2019;394:1540–1550.
227. Agarwal R, Rossignol P, Garza D, et al. Patiromer to enable spironolactone use in the treatment of patients with resistant hypertension and chronic kidney disease: rationale and design of the AMBER study. *Am J Nephrol*. 2018;48:172–180.
228. Manfredini F, Mallamaci F, D'Arrigo G, et al. Exercise in patients on dialysis: a multicenter, randomized clinical trial. *J Am Soc Nephrol*. 2017;28:1259–1268.
229. Boudville N, Ward S, Benaroia M, House AA. Increased sodium intake correlates with greater use of antihypertensive agents by subjects with chronic kidney disease. *Am J Hypertens*. 2005;18:1300–1305.
230. Feldman RD, Zou GY, Vandervoort MK, et al. A simplified approach to the treatment of uncomplicated hypertension: a cluster randomized, controlled trial. *Hypertension*. 2009;53:646–653.
231. YHaBG. Use of combination therapy. In: BGaSM, ed. *Hypertension-Companion to Braunwald's the HEART*. 3rd ed. Philadelphia: Elsevier; 2018:261–267.
232. Group AS, Cushman WC, Evans GW, et al. Effects of intensive blood-pressure control in type 2 diabetes mellitus. *N Engl J Med*. 2010;362:1575–1585.
233. Sarafidis PA, Persu A, Agarwal R, et al. Hypertension in dialysis patients: a consensus document by the European Renal and Cardiovascular Medicine (EURECA-m) working group of the European Renal Association - European Dialysis and Transplant Association (ERA-EDTA) and the hypertension and the kidney working group of the European Society of Hypertension (ESH). *J Hypertens*. 2017;35:657–676.
234. Buckley LF, Dixon DL, Wohlford 4th GF, et al. Effect of intensive blood pressure control in patients with type 2 diabetes mellitus over 9 years of follow-up: a subgroup analysis of high-risk ACCORDION trial participants. *Diabetes Obes Metab*. 2018;20:1499–1502.
235. Collard D, Brouwer TF, Olde Engberink RHG, et al. Initial estimated glomerular filtration rate decline and long-term renal function during intensive antihypertensive therapy: a post hoc analysis of the SPRINT and ACCORD-BP randomized controlled trials. *Hypertension*. 2020;75:1205–1212.

236. Collard D, Brouwer TF, Peters RJG, et al. Creatinine rise during blood pressure therapy and the risk of adverse clinical outcomes in patients with type 2 diabetes mellitus. *Hypertension*. 2018;72:1337–1344.
237. UK Prospective Diabetes Study Group. Tight blood pressure control and risk of macrovascular and microvascular complications in type 2 diabetes: UKPDS 38. UK Prospective Diabetes Study Group. *BMJ*. 1998;317:703–713.
238. Lv J, Perkovic V, Foote CV, et al. Antihypertensive agents for preventing diabetic kidney disease. *Cochrane Database Syst Rev*. 2012;12:CD004136.
239. Chavers BM, Bilous RW, Ellis EN, et al. Glomerular lesions and urinary albumin excretion in type I diabetes without overt proteinuria. *N Engl J Med*. 1989;320:966–970.
240. Mauer M, Zinman B, Gardiner R, et al. Renal and retinal effects of enalapril and losartan in type 1 diabetes. *N Engl J Med*. 2009;361:40–51.
241. Bakris GL, Townsend RR, Liu M, et al. Impact of renal denervation on 24-hour ambulatory blood pressure: results from SYMPLICITY HTN-3. *J Am Coll Cardiol*. 2014;64:1071–1078.
242. Agarwal R, Sinha AD, Pappas MK, et al. Hypertension in hemodialysis patients treated with atenolol or lisinopril: a randomized controlled trial. *Nephrol Dial Transplant*. 2014;29:672–681.
243. Nakao K, Makino H, Morita S, et al. Beta-blocker prescription and outcomes in hemodialysis patients from the Japan dialysis outcomes and practice patterns study. *Nephron Clin Pract*. 2009;113:c132–c139.
244. Port FK, Hulbert-Shearon TE, Wolfe RA, et al. Predialysis blood pressure and mortality risk in a national sample of maintenance hemodialysis patients. *Am J Kidney Dis*. 1999;33:507–517.
245. Agarwal R, Peixoto AJ, Santos SF, Zoccali C. Out-of-office blood pressure monitoring in chronic kidney disease. *Blood Press Monit*. 2009;14:2–11.
246. McMurray JJ, Packer M, Desai AS, et al. Angiotensin-neprilysin inhibition versus enalapril in heart failure. *N Engl J Med*. 2014;371:993–1004.
247. Taler SJ, Textor SC, Augustine JE. Resistant hypertension: comparing hemodynamic management to specialist care. *Hypertension*. 2002;39:982–988.
248. Khan YH, Sarriff A, Adnan AS, et al. Diuretics prescribing in chronic kidney disease patients: physician assessment versus bioimpedence spectroscopy. *Clin Exp Nephrol*. 2017;21:488–496.
249. Gerber Y, Weston SA, Redfield MM, et al. A contemporary appraisal of the heart failure epidemic in Olmsted County, Minnesota, 2000 to 2010. *JAMA Intern Med*. 2015;175:996–1004.
250. Writing Committee M, Yancy CW, Jessup M, et al. 2013 ACCF/AHA guideline for the management of heart failure: a report of the American College of Cardiology Foundation/American Heart Association Task Force on practice guidelines. *Circulation*. 2013;128:e240–e327.
251. Pfeffer MA, Braunwald E. Treatment of heart failure with preserved ejection fraction: reflections on its treatment with an aldosterone antagonist. *JAMA Cardiol*. 2016;1:7–8.
252. Writing Committee M, Yancy CW, Jessup M, et al. 2016 ACC/AHA/HFSA focused update on new pharmacological therapy for heart failure: an update of the 2013 ACCF/AHA guideline for the management of heart failure: a report of the American College of Cardiology/American Heart Association Task Force on clinical practice guidelines and the Heart Failure Society of America. *Circulation*. 2016;134:e282–e293.
253. Yancy CW, Januzzi Jr JL, Allen LA, et al. 2017 ACC expert consensus decision pathway for optimization of heart failure treatment: answers to 10 pivotal issues about heart failure with reduced ejection fraction: a report of the American College of Cardiology Task Force on expert consensus decision pathways. *J Am Coll Cardiol*. 2018;71:201–230.
254. Effects of treatment on morbidity in hypertension. Results in patients with diastolic blood pressures averaging 115 through 129 mm Hg. *J Am Med Assoc*. 1967;202:1028–1034.
255. Effects of treatment on morbidity in hypertension. II. Results in patients with diastolic blood pressure averaging 90 through 114 mm Hg. *J Am Med Assoc*. 1970;213:1143–1152.
256. Kostis JB, Davis BR, Cutler J, et al. Prevention of heart failure by antihypertensive drug treatment in older persons with isolated systolic hypertension. SHEP Cooperative Research Group. *J Am Med Assoc*. 1997;278:212–216.
257. Heart Outcomes Prevention Evaluation Study I, Yusuf S, Sleight P, et al. Effects of an angiotensin-converting-enzyme inhibitor, ramipril, on cardiovascular events in high-risk patients. *N Engl J Med*. 2000;342:145–153.
258. ALLHAT Officers and Coordinators for the ACRG. Major outcomes in high-risk hypertensive patients randomized to angiotensin-converting enzyme inhibitor or calcium channel blocker vs diuretic: the Antihypertensive and Lipid-Lowering Treatment to Prevent Heart Attack Trial (ALLHAT). *J Am Med Assoc*. 2002;288:2981–2997.
259. Sciarretta S, Palano F, Tocci G, et al. Antihypertensive treatment and development of heart failure in hypertension: a Bayesian network meta-analysis of studies in patients with hypertension and high cardiovascular risk. *Arch Intern Med*. 2011;171:384–394.
260. Edelmann F, Tomaschitz A, Wachter R, et al. Serum aldosterone and its relationship to left ventricular structure and geometry in patients with preserved left ventricular ejection fraction. *Eur Heart J*. 2012;33:203–212.
261. Leenen FHH, Wang HW, Hamlyn JM. Sodium pumps, ouabain and aldosterone in the brain: a neuromodulatory pathway underlying salt-sensitive hypertension and heart failure. *Cell Calcium*. 2020;86:102151.
262. Yusuf S, Pfeffer MA, Swedberg K, et al. Effects of candesartan in patients with chronic heart failure and preserved left-ventricular ejection fraction: the CHARM-Preserved Trial. *Lancet*. 2003;362:777–781.
263. Massie BM, Carson PE, McMurray JJ, et al. Irbesartan in patients with heart failure and preserved ejection fraction. *N Engl J Med*. 2008;359:2456–2467.
264. Edelmann F, Wachter R, Schmidt AG, et al. Effect of spironolactone on diastolic function and exercise capacity in patients with heart failure with preserved ejection fraction: the Aldo-DHF randomized controlled trial. *J Am Med Assoc*. 2013;309:781–791.
265. Deswal A, Richardson P, Bozkurt B, Mann DL. Results of the Randomized Aldosterone Antagonism In Heart Failure With Preserved Ejection Fraction trial (RAAM-PEF). *J Card Fail*. 2011;17:634–642.
266. Pitt B, Pfeffer MA, Assmann SF, et al. Spironolactone for heart failure with preserved ejection fraction. *N Engl J Med*. 2014;370:1383–1392.
267. Frankenstein L, Seide S, Tager T, et al. Relative Efficacy of Spironolactone, Eplerenone, and cAn-Renone in patients with Chronic Heart failure (RESEARCH): a systematic review and network meta-analysis of randomized controlled trials. *Heart Fail Rev*. 2020;25:161–171.
268. Blood Pressure Lowering Treatment Trialists' Collaboration. Blood pressure-lowering treatment based on cardiovascular risk: a meta-analysis of individual patient data. *Lancet*. 2014;384:591–598.
269. Group SR, Wright Jr JT, Williamson JD, et al. A randomized trial of intensive versus standard blood-pressure control. *N Engl J Med*. 2015;373:2103–2116.
270. Sarafidis PA, Georgianos P, Bakris GL. Resistant hypertension–its identification and epidemiology. *Nat Rev Nephrol*. 2013;9:51–58.
271. Bhatt DL, Bakris GL. Renal denervation for resistant hypertension. *N Engl J Med*. 2014;371:184.
272. Azizi M, Sapoval M, Gosse P, et al. Optimum and stepped care standardised antihypertensive treatment with or without renal denervation for resistant hypertension (DENERHTN): a multicentre, open-label, randomised controlled trial. *Lancet*. 2015;385:1957–1965.
273. Williams B, MacDonald TM, Morant S, et al. Spironolactone versus placebo, bisoprolol, and doxazosin to determine the optimal treatment for drug-resistant hypertension (PATHWAY-2): a randomised, double-blind, crossover trial. *Lancet*. 2015;386:2059–2068.
274. Rosa J, Widimsky P, Tousek P, et al. Randomized comparison of renal denervation versus intensified pharmacotherapy including spironolactone in true-resistant hypertension: six-month results from the Prague-15 study. *Hypertension*. 2015;65:407–413.
275. Lohmeier TE, Hall JE. Device-based neuromodulation for resistant hypertension therapy. *Circ Res*. 2019;124:1071–1093.
276. Iliescu R, Lohmeier TE, Tudorancea I, et al. Renal denervation for the treatment of resistant hypertension: review and clinical perspective. *Am J Physiol Renal Physiol*. 2015;309:F583–F594.
277. Mahfoud F, Tunev S, Ewen S, et al. Impact of lesion placement on efficacy and safety of catheter-based radiofrequency renal denervation. *J Am Coll Cardiol*. 2015;66:1766–1775.
278. Kandzari DE, Bhatt DL, Brar S, et al. Predictors of blood pressure response in the SYMPLICITY HTN-3 trial. *Eur Heart J*. 2015;36:219–227.
279. Kiuchi MG, Esler MD, Fink GD, et al. Renal denervation update from the international sympathetic nervous system summit: JACC state-of-the-art review. *J Am Coll Cardiol*. 2019;73:3006–3017.
280. Bohm M, Kario K, Kandzari DE, et al. Efficacy of catheter-based renal denervation in the absence of antihypertensive medications (SPYRAL HTN-OFF MED Pivotal): a multicentre, randomised, sham-controlled trial. *Lancet*. 2020;395:1444–1451.
281. Kandzari DE, Bohm M, Mahfoud F, et al. Effect of renal denervation on blood pressure in the presence of antihypertensive drugs: 6-month efficacy and safety results from the SPYRAL HTN-ON MED proof-of-concept randomised trial. *Lancet*. 2018;391:2346–2355.
282. Cheng X, Zhang D, Luo S, Qin S. Effect of catheter-based renal denervation on uncontrolled hypertension: a systematic review and meta-analysis. *Mayo Clin Proc*. 2019;94:1695–1706.
283. Wustmann K, Kucera JP, Scheffers I, et al. Effects of chronic baroreceptor stimulation on the autonomic cardiovascular regulation in patients with drug-resistant arterial hypertension. *Hypertension*. 2009;54:530–536.
284. Bisognano JD, Bakris G, Nadim MK, et al. Baroreflex activation therapy lowers blood pressure in patients with resistant hypertension: results from the double-blind, randomized, placebo-controlled rheos pivotal trial. *J Am Coll Cardiol*. 2011;58:765–773.
285. de Leeuw PW, Bisognano JD, Bakris GL, et al. Sustained reduction of blood pressure with baroreceptor activation therapy: results of the 6-year open follow-up. *Hypertension*. 2017;69:836–843.
286. Bakris GL, Nadim MK, Haller H, et al. Baroreflex activation therapy provides durable benefit in patients with resistant hypertension: results of long-term follow-up in the Rheos Pivotal Trial. *J Am Soc Hypertens*. 2012;6:152–158.
287. Yoruk A, Bisognano JD, Gassler JP. Baroreceptor stimulation for resistant hypertension. *Am J Hypertens*. 2016;29:1319–1324.
288. Spiering W, Williams B, Van der Heyden J, et al. Endovascular baroreflex amplification for resistant hypertension: a safety and proof-of-principle clinical study. *Lancet*. 2017;390:2655–2661.
289. Levy PD, Mahn JJ, Miller J, et al. Blood pressure treatment and outcomes in hypertensive patients without acute target organ damage: a retrospective cohort. *Am J Emerg Med*. 2015;33:1219–1224.
290. Patel KK, Young L, Howell EH, et al. Characteristics and outcomes of patients presenting with hypertensive urgency in the office setting. *JAMA Intern Med*. 2016;176:981–988.
291. Anderson CS, Heeley E, Huang Y, et al. Rapid blood-pressure lowering in patients with acute intracerebral hemorrhage. *N Engl J Med*. 2013;368:2355–2365.
292. Steiner T, Al-Shahi Salman R, Beer R, et al. European Stroke Organisation (ESO) guidelines for the management of spontaneous intracerebral hemorrhage. *Int J Stroke*. 2014;9:840–855.
293. Podymow T, August P. Antihypertensive drugs in pregnancy. *Semin Nephrol*. 2011;31:70–85.

27 Lipoprotein Disorders and Cardiovascular Disease

JACQUES GENEST, SAMIA MORA, AND PETER LIBBY

LIPOPROTEIN TRANSPORT SYSTEM, 502
Biochemistry of Lipids, 502
Lipoproteins, Apolipoproteins, Receptors, and Processing Enzymes, 504
Lipoprotein Metabolism and Transport, 505

LIPOPROTEIN DISORDERS, 509
Definitions, 509
Genetic Lipoprotein Disorders, 509
Triglyceride-Rich Lipoproteins, 510
High-Density Lipoproteins, 513

PHARMACOLOGIC MANAGEMENT OF LIPID RISK, 515
Hydroxymethylglutaryl–Coenzyme A Reductase Inhibitors (Statins), 515
Pro-Protein Convertase Subtilisin/Kexin Type 9 Inhibitors, 517
Ezetimibe, 518
Fibric Acid Derivatives (Fibrates), 518
Nicotinic Acid (Niacin), 518
Bile Acid–Binding Resins, 519
Fish Oils and Pure Eicosapentaenoic Acid, 519
Phytosterols, 520
Novel Medications[78,] 520

CLINICAL APPROACH TO THE TREATMENT OF LIPOPROTEIN DISORDERS, 521
Lifestyle Changes: Diet, 521
Treatment of Combined Lipoprotein Disorders, 521
Residual Cardiovascular Risk, 522

FUTURE PERSPECTIVES, 522
Gene Therapy, 522
Societal Changes, 522

GUIDELINES, 523

REFERENCES, 523

Atherosclerotic cardiovascular diseases (ASCVDs) represent a major burden to society and on national health care systems.[1-3] Despite public health measures aimed at decreasing saturated fat consumption and cigarette smoking and targeted pharmacologic therapies that can modify cardiovascular risk, an aging population with increased comorbidities, such as obesity, diabetes, and high blood pressure, continues to pose a considerable challenge (see also Chapters 2 and 25).[4]

Lipoprotein disorders, especially those that increase exposure of the arterial wall to cholesterol, constitute a major modifiable cardiovascular risk factor. Modulation of plasma cholesterol levels by lifestyle or, when required, pharmacologic therapy (statins), has proven to be one of the most effective interventions for the prevention and treatment of ASCVD.

The lipid transport system in animals has evolved to serve two main purposes: first, to bring ingested fats (mostly in the form of triglycerides) to muscle; when dietary fat is unavailable, the liver and adipose tissue deliver a constant supply of triglycerides. The second transport system is the delivery of cholesterol to tissues that require it for membrane synthesis, for the synthesis of steroidal hormones and bile acids. The remarkable redundancy in the ability of cells and tissues to synthetize, import, and export cholesterol attests to its critical importance in life processes.

Lipids constitute approximately 70% (by mass) of the dry weight of plasma.[5] Approximately half of circulating lipids are sterols, the other major components include glycerophospholipids (phospholipids) and glycerolipids (triglycerides), which circulate in lipoproteins. Thus, circulating lipoproteins continuously bathe vascular endothelial cells, and the interaction between lipoproteins and cells of the arterial wall contribute causally to the pathogenesis of human atherosclerosis (see also Chapter 24).

The "cholesterol hypothesis" states that "decreasing blood cholesterol significantly reduces coronary heart disease." Decades of research in basic research, epidemiology, animal experiments, and mendelian randomization studies have shown strong support for a causal role of cholesterol in the pathogenesis of atherosclerosis.[6] Observational data show a strong and consistent association across populations between elevated blood cholesterol and low-density lipoprotein cholesterol (LDL-C) with ASCVD, especially coronary artery disease (CAD). Experimental data in animals show that the development of atherosclerosis requires cholesterol. Human genetic studies provide strong support of causality for genes related to LDL-C levels, to atherogenic lipoprotein particles, and to cholesterol associated with triglyceride-rich lipoproteins (TRLs) (see also Chapter 7).[7] Most important, however, a large body of clinical trials have shown that reducing LDL-C with statins prevents ASCVD, cardiovascular deaths, and total mortality. Thus, LDL meets the modified Koch postulates as a causal risk factor for ASCVD.[8]

The terms *dyslipidemia* or *dyslipoproteinemia* reflect disorders of the lipid and lipoprotein transport pathways associated with arterial disease more appropriately than *hyperlipidemia*. *Dyslipidemia* encompasses patterns often encountered in clinical practice, such as low high-density lipoprotein cholesterol (HDL-C) and elevated triglyceride concentrations but average total plasma cholesterol or LDL-C levels. *Dyslipidemia* also includes elevated lipoprotein(a) (Lp[a]) and uncommon genetic or acquired disorders of lipoprotein metabolism. Certain rare lipoprotein disorders can cause overt clinical manifestations, but most common dyslipoproteinemias themselves seldom cause symptoms or clinical signs. Rather, they require laboratory tests for detection. Proper recognition and management of dyslipoproteinemias can reduce cardiovascular and total mortality rates. The fundamentals of lipidology presented here have importance for the daily practice of cardiovascular medicine.

LIPOPROTEIN TRANSPORT SYSTEM

Biochemistry of Lipids

Life requires fats. The biochemistry of lipids and lipoproteins is complex. The clinically relevant lipoproteins (Table 27.1), apolipoproteins (Table 27.2), receptors and processing enzymes (Table 27.3), and current (and potential) drug targets are shown. Biologic lipids usually refer to a broad grouping of naturally occurring molecules that include fatty acids, waxes, eicosanoids, monoglycerides, diglycerides, triglycerides, phospholipids, sphingolipids, sterols, terpenes, prenols, and fat-soluble vitamins (A, D, E, and K), in contrast to the other major groupings of biologic molecules, namely, nucleic acids, proteins, amino acids, and carbohydrates. The major biologic functions of lipids include critical contributions to biologic membranes, energy storage, and the backbones or modifiers of many signaling molecules. Certain lipids, especially fatty acids, readily undergo oxidation and can generate substances highly toxic to cells. Fatty acids can be metabolized in the mitochondrion by beta-oxidation, whereas the sterol nucleus resists enzymatic degradation. Elimination of cholesterol therefore requires excretion as bile acids or conversion into steroidal hormones.

Lipids generally do not dissolve in water. The lipid transport system has evolved in animals to carry hydrophobic molecules (fat) from sites of origin (the intestines and the liver) to sites of use (muscles and rapidly dividing tissues) through the aqueous (water) environment of

TABLE 27.1 Plasma Lipoprotein Composition and Apolipoproteins

	ORIGIN	DENSITY (G/ML)	SIZE (NM)	% PROTEIN	[CHOLESTEROL] IN PLASMA MG/DL (MMOL/L)*	[TRIGLYCERIDE] IN FASTING PLASMA (MMOL/L)†	MAJOR APO	OTHER APO
Chylomicrons‡	Intestine	<0.95	100–1000	1–2	0.0	0	B48	A-I, Cs
Chylomicron remnants‡	Chylomicron metabolism	0.95–1.006	30–80	3–5	0.0	0.0	B48, E	A-I, A-IV, Cs
VLDL	Liver	<1.006	40–50	10	4–15 mg% (0.1–0.4)	15–100 mg% (0.2–1.2)	B100	A-I, Cs
IDL	VLDL	1.006–1.019	25–30	18	4–12 mg% 0.1–0.3	10–25 mg% (0.1–0.3)	B100, E	
LDL	IDL	1.019–1.063	20–25	25	50–130 mg% (1.5–3.5)	15–35 mg% (0.2–0.4)	B100	
HDL	Liver, intestine	1.063–1.210	6–10	40–55	35–62 mg% (0.9–1.6)	10–15 mg% (0.1–0.2)	A-I, A-II	A-IV
Lp(a)	Liver	1.051–1.082	25	30–50			B100, (a)	

Indirect effect.
Apo, Apolipoprotein; *HDL*, high-density lipoprotein; *IDL*, intermediate-density lipoprotein; *LDL*, Low-density lipoprotein; *Lp(a)*, lipoprotein(a); *VLDL*, very-low-density lipoprotein.
*In mmol/L; for mg/dL, multiply by 38.67.
†In mmol/L; for mg/dL, multiply by 88.5.
‡In the fasted state, serum (or plasma) should not contain chylomicrons or their remnants.

TABLE 27.2 Apolipoproteins (Clinically Relevant)

NAME	PREDOMINANT LIPOPROTEIN	MWT (KDA)	ROLE	PLASMA CONCENTRATION (MG/DL)	HUMAN DISEASE	DRUG TARGET
Apo (a)	Lp(a)	250-800	Unknown	0.2-200	Lp(a) excess	AKCEA-APO(a)-LRx
Apo A-I	HDL	28.3	ACAT activation, structural	90-160	HDL deficiency	
Apo A-IV	HDL	45	Structural, absorption	10-20		
Apo A-V	VLDL, HDL		TRL metabolism		Hypertriglyceridemia	
Apo B100	LDL, VLDL	512	Structural, LDL-R binding	50-150	Hypobetalipoproteinemia	Mipomersen
Apo B48	Chylomicrons	241	Structural	0-100	abetalipoproteinemia	
Apo C-II	Chylomicrons, VLDL	8.84	LPL activation	3-5	Hyperchylomicronemia	
Apo C-III	Chylomicrons, VLDL	8.76	LPL inhibition	10-14	Hypertriglyceridemia	Volanesorsen
Apo E	Chylomicrons remnant, IDL	34	LDL-R, apo E receptor binding	2-8	Type III hyperlipoproteinemia	
Apo H	Chylomicrons, VLDL, LDL, HDL	38-50	Beta$_2$-glycoprotein / Platelet aggregation	1.4 -1.6	Cardiolipin-binding defect	

See Tables 27.1 and 27.3 for abbreviations. *TRL*, Triglyceride-rich lipoprotein

plasma. Proteins highly conserved through evolution, termed *apolipoproteins* (apo), mediate this process. Most apolipoproteins derive from an ancestral gene and contain both hydrophilic and hydrophobic domains. This amphipathic structure enables these proteins to bridge the interface between the aqueous environment of plasma and the phospholipid constituents of lipoprotein. The major types of lipids that circulate in plasma include cholesterol and cholesteryl esters, glycerophospholipids, sphingolipids, and glycerolipids (triglycerides) (Fig. 27.1). The LIPID maps (Lipid Metabolites and Pathways Strategy) consortium has provided standardized nomenclature for lipids, although this area is rapidly evolving with advanced lipidomics technologies.[9]

The membranes of mammalian cells and their subcellular organelles require *cholesterol*. This lipid gives rise to steroid hormones and bile acids and contributes to the integrity of the epidermis. Many cell functions depend critically on membrane cholesterol, and cells regulate tightly their cholesterol content. Importantly, all mammalian cells have retained the ability to synthetize cholesterol de novo from acetyl coenzyme A (CoA). Most of the cholesterol in plasma circulates as *cholesteryl esters* in the core of lipoprotein particles. The enzyme lecithin-cholesterol acyltransferase (LCAT) forms cholesteryl esters in the blood compartment by transferring a fatty acyl chain from phosphatidylcholine to cholesterol.

Glycerolipids (*triglycerides*) consist of a three-carbon glycerol backbone covalently linked to three fatty acid chains ($R_{1–3}$). The fatty acid composition varies in terms of chain length and the presence of double bonds (degree of saturation). The highly hydrophobic triglyceride molecules circulate in the core of the lipoprotein. Hydrolysis of triglycerides by lipases generates the free fatty acids (FFAs) used for energy.

Glycerophospholipids, found in all cellular membranes, consist of a glycerol molecule linked to two fatty acids (designated R; see Fig. 27.1). Fatty acids differ in length and in the number of double bonds. The third carbon of the glycerol backbone carries a phosphate group linked to one of four molecules: choline (phosphatidylcholine, also called lecithin), ethanolamine (phosphatidylethanolamine), serine (phosphatidylserine), or inositol (phosphatidylinositol). More complex phospholipids include phosphatidylglycerol (cardiolipin is formed by the fusion of two phosphatidylglycerol molecules -antibodies against cardiolipin often occur in systemic lupus), and plasmalogens, an important constituent of eukaryotic membranes. Another phospholipid, *sphingomyelin*, has special functions in the plasma membrane in the formation of membrane microdomains such as rafts and caveolae. The structure of sphingomyelin resembles that of phosphatidylcholine. The backbone of sphingolipids uses the amino acid serine rather than glycerol. Phospholipids are polar molecules, more water soluble than triglycerides or cholesterol or its esters. Phospholipids participate in signal transduction pathways: hydrolysis by membrane-associated phospholipases generates second messengers, including diacylglycerols, lysophospholipids, phosphatidic acids, and FFAs such as arachidonate, that regulate many cell functions. The phosphorylation of phosphatidylinositol contributes critically to membrane and cell organelle signaling and transport.

Fish oils and eicosapentaenoic acid (EPA) n-3 fatty acids are essential polyunsaturated fatty acids (PUFAs) that are commonly found in plants and marine life. Beyond their triglyceride lowering effects, they have pleiotropic actions with beneficial cardiovascular effects that are key to resolving inflammation and regulating adaptive immunity.[10] n-3

TABLE 27.3 Lipoprotein Processing Enzymes, Receptors, Modulating Proteins

ABBREVIATION	NAME	ROLE	GENE	HUMAN DISEASE	DRUG TARGET
ABCA1	ATP-binding cassette A1	Cellular phospholipid efflux	ABCA1	Tangier disease	
ABCG5/G8	ATP-binding cassette G5 and G8	Intestinal sitosterol transporter	ABCG5 ABCG8	Sitosterolemia	
ACLY	ATP citrate lyase	Cholesterol and fatty acid synthesis	ACLY		Bempedoic acid
ANGPTL3	Angiopoietin-like protein 3	Inhibit LDL and EL	ANGPTL3	Familial hypolipoproteinemia 2	Evinacumab, vupanorsen
CETP	Cholesteryl ester transfer protein	Lipid exchange in plasma	CETP	Elevated HDL-C	
Cyp27A1	Cytochrome	Sterols hydroxylation	CYP27A1	Cerebrotendinous xanthomatosis	
DGAT1	Acyl CoA:Diacylglycerol acyltransferase 1	Triglyceride synthesis	DGAT1	Elevated triglycerides	Pradigastat
EL	Endothelial lipase	Phospholipid hydrolysis	LIPG		
HL	Hepatic lipase	Triglyceride hydrolysis	LIPC	Remnant accumulation	
HMGCR	HMG CoA Reductase	Cholesterol synthesis	HMGCR		Statins
LCAT	Lecithin-cholesterol acyltransferase	Cholesterol esterification (plasma)	LCAT	LCAT deficiency, low HDL	
LDL-R	Low-density lipoprotein receptor	LDL uptake	LDLR	Familial hypercholesterolemia	PCSK9 inh. (statins) (bempedoic acid) AAV8.TBG.hLDLR
LDL-R AP1	LDL-R adapter protein	LDL uptake	LDLRAP1	Recessive FH	
LAL	Lysosomal Acid Lipase	Cholesteryl ester storage	LIPA	Wollman disease, CESD	
MTTP	Microsomal triglyceride transfer protein	Apo B assembly	MTTP	Abetalipoproteinemia	Lomitapide
NPC1	Niemann-Pick C gene product	Cellular cholesterol transport	NPC1	Niemann-Pick type C	
NPC1L1	Niemann-Pick C1-like 1 protein	Intestinal cholesterol absorption	NPC1L1		Ezetimibe
PCSK9	Proprotein convertase, subtilisin/kexin-9	Protein cleavage	PCSK9	Hypercholesterolemia	Alirocumab, Evolocumab, Inclisiran
SMPD1	Sphingomyelinase phosphodiesterase	Sphingomyelin hydrolysis	SMPD1	Niemann-Pick types A and B	

fatty acids derive their name from the first double, which is located on the n-3 position (between the third and fourth carbons from the terminal methyl [omega] end). n-3 metabolites serve as precursors of potent lipid mediators (eicosanoids), and have effects on other lipids (ceramides, lysophosphatidylcholines, diacylglycerols) and amino acids (leucine, glutamine). Moreover, n-3 derived eicosanoids form downstream potent oxylipins which play a critical role in regulating inflammation, vascular tone, and endothelial function.[10] n-3 fatty acids may have favorable antiarrhythmic effects by stabilizing the plasma membrane, metabolic effects through insulin signaling and energy use, and at high doses may also block coagulation. These pleiotropic effects have given rise to the hypothesis that dietary n-3 treatment improves cardiovascular clinical outcomes. However, results of several large randomized clinical trials have been conflicting (see discussion under "Fish Oils and Pure Eicosapentaenoic Acid").

PUFAs are metabolized by three pathway enzymes: cyclooxygenase (COX), lipoxygenase (LOX), and CypP450. n-3 FA include EPA (20:5, i.e., 20 carbons in length with 5 double bonds) and docosahexaenoic acid (DHA, 22:6). Alpha-linolenic acid (ALA) is metabolized into EPA, and EPA is modified into DHA. EPA and DHA are oxidized by COX and LOX enzymes to generate eicosanoid subfamilies including prostaglandins, prostacyclins, resolvins, and thromboxanes.[11] Certain n-3 derived eicosanoids have potent antiinflammatory and pro-resolving effects, independently, as well as by inhibiting proinflammatory n-6 PUFA-derived eicosanoids. EPA and DHA-derived eicosanoids compete for and inhibit arachidonic acid eicosanoid production and receptor stimulation (particularly in the COX pathway). EPA can also be metabolized into resolvin E1 which may be cardioprotective, or it can be elongated into the 22-carbon docosapentaenoic acid (DPA) which has resolvin-like antiinflammatory effects and can

shift arachidonic acid metabolism from COX to LOX pathway. DHA is thought to be cardioprotective after it is incorporated in cell membranes via mechanisms that improve receptor and ion channel function.[12] Genetic variants in fatty acid desaturases (*FADS*) – enzymes that modulate eicosanoid and other fatty acid levels – and in other genes encoding enzymes involved in eicosanoid metabolism (COX, LOX, and CypP450), also associate with CVD risk.[13] Deciphering the specific roles of n3-derived lipid metabolites in inflammatory and immune signaling would provide insight into their role as therapeutic and nutritional agents.

Lipoproteins, Apolipoproteins, Receptors, and Processing Enzymes

Lipoproteins are complex macromolecular structures coated by a water compatible envelope of phospholipids, free cholesterol, and apolipoproteins covering a hydrophobic core of cholesteryl esters and triglycerides (Fig. 27.2). Lipoproteins vary in size, density in the aqueous environment of plasma, and lipid and apolipoprotein content (see Table 27.1, Fig. 27.1B, *inset*). The classification of lipoproteins reflects their density in plasma (the density of plasma is 1.006 g/mL) as gauged by flotation in an ultracentrifuge. The TRLs, which consist of *chylomicrons*, *chylomicron remnants*, *very low-density lipoprotein* (VLDL) and *intermediate density lipoproteins* (IDL), have a density of less than 1.006 g/mL. The rest (bottom fraction) of the ultracentrifuged plasma consists of *LDL*, *HDL*, and *Lp(a)*.

Apolipoproteins have four major roles: (1) assembly and secretion of the lipoprotein (apoA-I, B100, and B48), (2) structural integrity of the lipoprotein (apo B, E, A-I, and A-II), (3) coactivators or inhibitors of enzymes (apoA-I, A-V, C-I, C-II, and C-III), and (4) binding or docking to

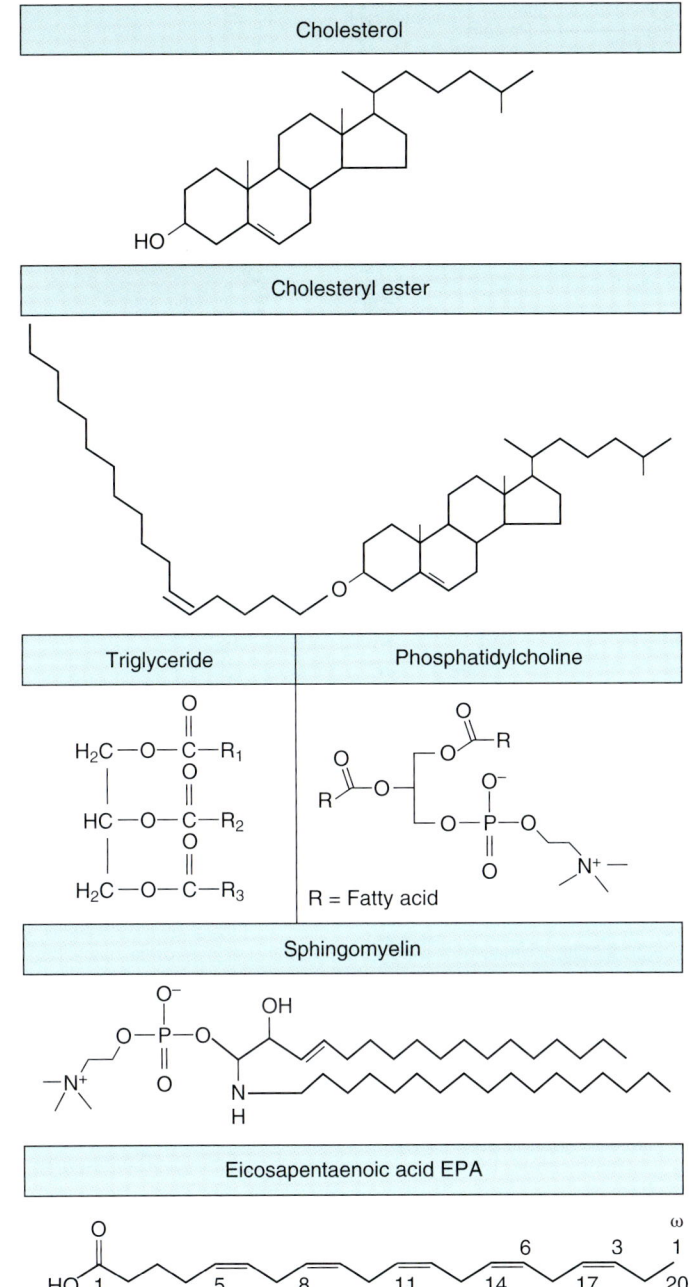

FIGURE 27.1 Biochemical structure of the major lipid molecules: cholesterol, cholesteryl esters, glycerolipids (triglycerides), and glycerophospholipids (e.g., phosphatidylcholine) and sphingomyelin. Eicosapentaenoic acid (EPA) is an essential polyunsaturated fatty acid. R indicates a fatty acyl chain.

uptake of chylomicron remnants and VLDL, preferentially recognizes apo E. LRP1 also interacts with hepatic lipase. The complex interaction between hepatocytes and the various lipoproteins containing apo E involves cell surface proteoglycans that provide scaffolding for lipolytic enzymes (lipoprotein lipase [LPL] and hepatic lipase) involved in recognition of remnant lipoproteins. Macrophages express receptors that bind modified (especially oxidized) lipoproteins. These scavenger lipoprotein receptors mediate the uptake of oxidatively modified LDL into macrophages. In contrast to the exquisitely regulated LDL-R, high cellular cholesterol content does not suppress scavenger receptors, thereby enabling intimal macrophages to accumulate abundant cholesterol, become foam cells, and form fatty streaks. Sterol accumulation in the endoplasmic reticulum may lead to cell apoptosis via the unfolded protein response. Endothelial cells can also take up modified lipoproteins through specific receptors such as the oxidized LDL-R, LOX-1.

At least three physiologically relevant receptors interact with HDL particles: the scavenger receptor class B (SR-B1) and the adenosine triphosphate (ATP)-binding cassette transporters A1 (ABCA1) and G1 (ABCG1). SR-B1 is a receptor for HDL (also for LDL and VLDL, but with less affinity). SR-B1 mediates the selective uptake of HDL cholesteryl esters in steroidogenic tissues, hepatocytes, and endothelium. ABCA1 mediates cellular phospholipid (and possibly cholesterol) efflux and HDL formation. The ABCG1 transporter transfers cellular cholesterol to already formed HDL particles.

Lipoprotein Metabolism and Transport

The lipoprotein transport system has two major roles: efficient transport of triglycerides from the intestine and liver to sites of utilization (fat tissue or muscle), and transport of cholesterol to peripheral tissues for membrane synthesis and steroid hormone production or to the liver for bile acid synthesis.

INTESTINAL PATHWAY (CHYLOMICRONS TO CHYLOMICRON REMNANTS)

Fat typically furnishes 20% to 40% of the daily calories. Triglycerides account for the major portion of ingested fats. For an individual consuming 2000 kcal/day, with 30% in the form of fat, this represents approximately 66 g of triglycerides and 250 mg (0.250 g) of cholesterol per day. The intestine has very efficient fat absorption mechanisms, probably evolved to maximize provision of the organism with nutrients under circumstances of limited or irregular availability of food.

On ingestion, lingual and pancreatic lipases hydrolyze triglycerides into FFAs and monoglycerides or diglycerides. Emulsification by bile salts leads to the formation of intestinal micelles. Micelles resemble lipoproteins insofar as they consist of phospholipids, free cholesterol, bile acids, diglycerides and monoglycerides, FFAs, and glycerol. The mechanism of micelle uptake by intestinal brush border cells still engenders debate. The Niemann-Pick C1-like 1 (NPC1L1) protein is part of an intestinal cholesterol transporter complex and the target for the selective cholesterol absorption inhibitor ezetimibe. After uptake into intestinal cells, fatty acids undergo re-esterification to form triglycerides and packaging into chylomicrons inside the intestinal cell and enter the portal circulation (Fig. 27.3, part 1). Chylomicrons contain apo B48, the amino-terminal component of apo B100. In the intestine, the apo B gene is modified during transcription into mRNA by substitution of a uracil for a cytosine via an apo B48–editing enzyme complex (ApoBec). This mechanism involves a cytosine deaminase and leads to a termination codon at residue 2153 and a truncated form of apo B. Only intestinal cells express ApoBec. Apo B48 does not bind to LDL-R. Intestinal cells absorb plant sterols (sitosterol, campesterol), sort these compounds into a separate cellular compartment, and re-secrete them into the intestinal lumen via the ABCG5/8 heterodimeric transporter. Mutations of the ABCG5/8 genes cause the rare disorder sitosterolemia.

Chylomicrons rapidly enter the plasma compartment after meals. In capillaries of adipose tissue or muscle cells in the peripheral circulation, chylomicrons encounter the enzyme LPL attached to heparan sulfate proteoglycans on the luminal surface of endothelial cells (see Fig. 27.3, part 2). Apo C-II and apo A-V activate, and apo C-III inhibits LPL activity. LPL has broad specificity for triglycerides; it cleaves all fatty acyl residues attached to glycerol and in the process generates three molecules of FFA for each molecule of glycerol. Muscle cells rapidly take up fatty acids.

specific receptors and proteins for cellular uptake of the entire particle or selective uptake of a lipid component (apoA-I, B100, and E) (see Table 27.2). The role of several apolipoproteins (A-IV, A-V, D, H, J, L, and M) remains incompletely understood.

Many proteins regulate the synthesis, secretion, and metabolic fate of lipoproteins; their characterization has provided insight into molecular cellular physiology and targets for drug development (see Table 27.3). Discovery of the LDL receptor (LDL-R) represented a landmark in understanding cholesterol metabolism and receptor-mediated endocytosis.[6] The LDL-R regulates the entry of cholesterol into cells, and tight control mechanisms alter its expression on the cell surface, depending on intracellular cholesterol. The LDL-R belongs to a superfamily of membrane receptors that include LDL-R, VLDL-R, LDL-R–mediated peptide type 1 (LRP1; apo E receptor), LRP1B, LRP4 (MGEF7), LRP5 and LRP6 (involved in the process of bone formation), LRP8 (apo E receptor-2), and LRP9. LRP1, which mediates the

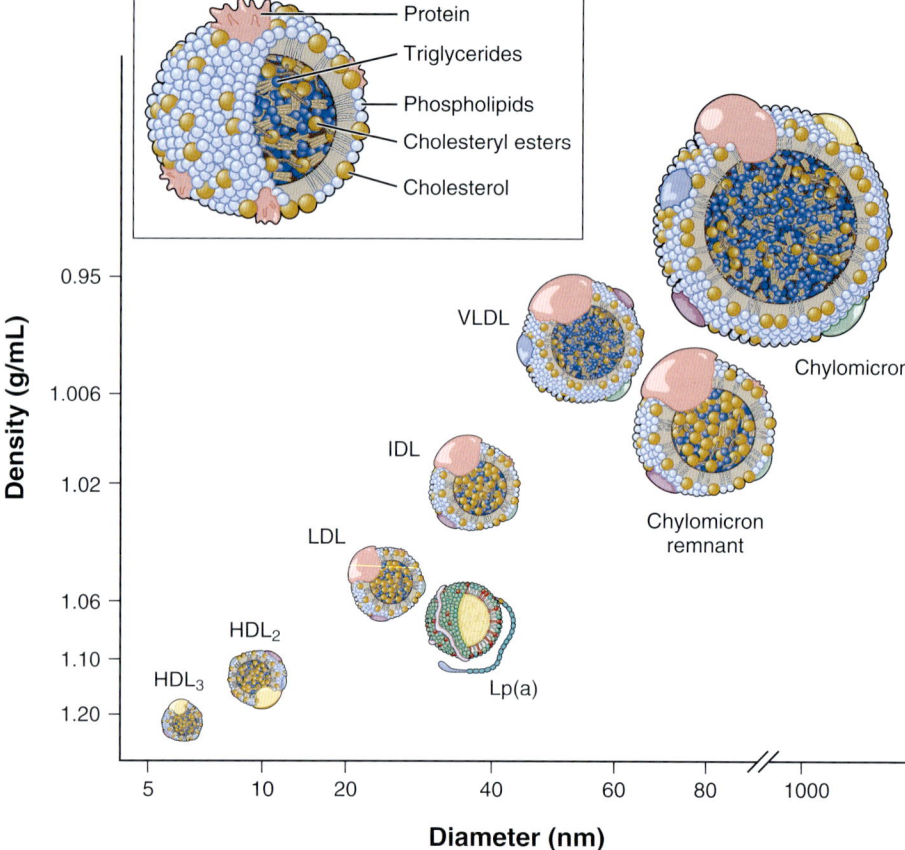

FIGURE 27.2 Relative size of plasma lipoproteins according to their hydrated density. The density of plasma is 1.006 g/mL. *Inset,* Structure of lipoproteins. Phospholipids are oriented with their polar group toward the aqueous environment of plasma. Free cholesterol is inserted within the phospholipid layer. The core of the lipoprotein is composed of cholesteryl esters and triglycerides. Apolipoproteins are involved in the secretion of lipoprotein, provide structural integrity, and act as cofactors for enzymes or as ligands for various receptors. *HDL,* High-density lipoprotein; *IDL,* intermediate-density lipoproteins; *LDL,* low-density lipoprotein; *Lp(a),* lipoprotein(a); *VLDL,* very-low-density lipoprotein.

Fatty acids provide the energy substrate for muscle contraction by the generation of ATP during beta-oxidation of fatty acyl residues in mitochondria. Adipose cells can store triglycerides made from fatty acids for energy utilization, a process that requires insulin. The triglyceride lipase hormone–sensitive lipase, that is activated by cyclic adenosine monophosphate (cAMP) in response to stress, releases stored fatty acids from adipose tissues. Fatty acids can also travel to the liver bound to fatty acid–binding proteins or albumin and undergo repackaging into VLDL. Peripheral resistance to insulin can thus increase the delivery of FFAs to the liver with a consequent increase in VLDL secretion and increased apo B particles in plasma, a characteristic of the "metabolic syndrome" and type 2 diabetes. The remnant particles, derived from chylomicrons following LPL action, contain apo E and enter the liver for degradation and reutilization of their core constituents (see Fig. 27.3, *part 3*).

HEPATIC PATHWAY (VERY LOW-DENSITY LIPOPROTEIN TO INTERMEDIATE-DENSITY LIPOPROTEIN)

Food is not always available, and dietary fat content varies. The body requires ready availability of triglyceride to meet energy demands. Hepatic secretion of VLDL particles serves this function (see Fig. 27.3, *part 4*). VLDLs are TRLs smaller than chylomicrons (see Table 27.1 and Fig. 27.2). They contain apo B100 as their main lipoprotein. As opposed to apo B48, apo B100 contains a domain recognized by LDL-R (the apo B/E receptor). VLDL particles follow the same catabolic pathway as chylomicrons through LPL (see Fig. 27.3, *part 2*).[14] During hydrolysis of TRLs by LPL, an exchange of proteins and lipids takes place: VLDL particles (and chylomicrons) acquire apo Cs and apo E, in part from HDL particles. VLDLs also exchange triglycerides for cholesteryl esters from HDL (mediated by cholesteryl ester transfer protein [CETP]) (see Fig. 27.3, *part 9*). Such bidirectional transfer of constituents between lipoproteins serves several purposes: acquisition of specific apolipoproteins by lipoproteins that will dictate their metabolic fate, transfer of phospholipids onto nascent HDL particles mediated by phospholipid transfer protein (PLTP) (during loss of the core triglycerides, the phospholipid envelope becomes redundant and sheds apoA-I to form new HDL particles), and transfer of cholesterol from HDL to VLDL remnants so that it can be metabolized in the liver. This exchange constitutes a major part of the "reverse cholesterol transport pathway."

Apo CIII, a small but important 79 amino acid peptide has a high affinity for TRLs and attenuates the activity of LPL and the clearance of TRLs, thus contributing to elevated triglycerides. Apo CIII also resides within HDL that seems to act as a "reservoir" for this apolipoprotein. Recent work identified an intracellular role for apo CIII for the assembly and secretion of VLDL.[15] Mendelian randomization experiments as well as epidemiologic studies have established that apo CIII can contribute causally to ASCVD.[16] This recognition has spurred therapeutic efforts to decrease apo CIII (see below).

After hydrolysis of triglycerides removes some triglycerides from VLDL, these particles have relatively more cholesterol, shed several apolipoproteins (especially the C apolipoproteins), and acquire apo E. The VLDL remnant lipoprotein, called intermediate-density lipoprotein (IDL), undergoes liver uptake via its apo E moiety (see Fig. 27.3, *part 3*) or further delipidation by hepatic lipase to form LDL particles (see Fig. 27.3, *part 6*). At least four receptors take up TRLs, TRL remnants, and apo B–containing lipoproteins: VLDL-R, the remnant receptor (apo ER2), LDL-R (also called the apo B/E receptor), and LRP1. Most hepatic receptors share the ability to recognize apo E, an engagement that mediates the uptake of several classes of lipoproteins, including VLDL and IDL. The complex interaction between apo E and its ligand involves the "docking" of TRLs on heparan sulfate proteoglycans to present the ligand to its receptor.

Low-Density Lipoproteins

LDL particles contain predominantly cholesteryl esters packaged with apo B100. Normally, triglycerides constitute only 4% to 8% of the LDL mass (see Table 27.1). In conditions with elevated plasma triglyceride concentrations, LDL particles can acquire triglycerides and deplete their core cholesteryl esters. Such changes in core constituents influence LDL particle size: an increase in triglycerides and a relative decrease in cholesteryl esters yields smaller, denser LDL particles.

Humans are unusual among mammals because they generate LDL as a cholesterol-rich lipoprotein. Nonhuman primates fed a cholesterol-enriched diet also carry cholesterol in LDL. In other mammals, such as rodents or rabbits, HDL particles transport most of the cholesterol. Cells can either make cholesterol from acyl CoA through enzymatic reactions

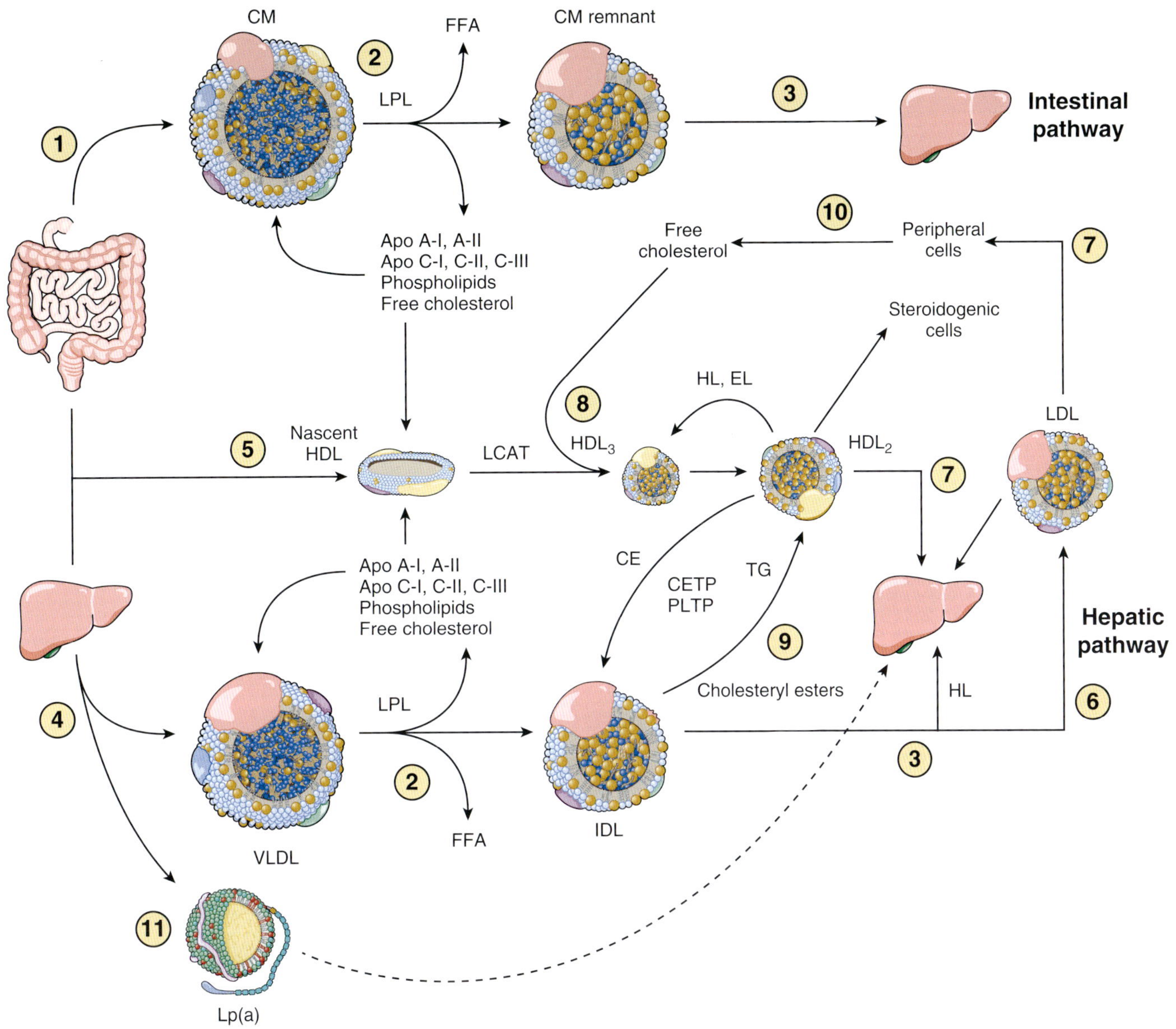

FIGURE 27.3 Schematic diagram of the lipid transport system. Numbers in circles refer to explanations in text. Refer to Tables 27.1–27.3 for abbreviations. *CM*, Chylomicron; *FFA*, free fatty acid.

requiring at least 33 enzymatic steps or obtain it as cholesteryl esters from HDL or LDL particles. Cells internalize LDL via LDL-R (Fig. 27.4).[6] LDL particles contain one molecule of apo B. Although several highly lipophilic domains of apo B associate with phospholipids, a region surrounding residue 3500 binds with high affinity to LDL-R. LDL-R localizes in a region of the plasma membrane rich in the protein clathrin (see Fig. 27.4; Fig. 27.3, *part 7*). Once bound to the receptor, clathrin polymerizes and forms an endosome that contains LDL bound to its receptor, a portion of the plasma membrane, and clathrin. This internalized particle then fuses with lysosomes whose hydrolytic enzymes (cholesteryl ester hydrolase, cathepsins) release free cholesterol and degrade apo B. LDL-R releases its ligand and can recycle to the plasma membrane. The chaperone proprotein convertase subtilisin/kexin type 9 (PCSK9), secreted by hepatocytes, undergoes auto-catalytic cleavage and binds to the LDL-R. Association with PCSK9 diverts the complex to the lysosomal degradative pathway, thus preventing the recycling of the LDL-R (Fig. 27.4). Gain-of-function mutations in the PCSK9 gene causes autosomal dominant hypercholesterolemia, whereas loss-of-function mutations increase LDL-R and lower LDL-C substantially.[17,18]

Cells regulate their cholesterol content tightly through highly conserved cellular pathways, including: (1) synthesis of cholesterol in the smooth endoplasmic reticulum (via the rate-limiting step hydroxymethylglutaryl-CoA [HMG-CoA] reductase), (2) receptor-mediated endocytosis of LDL (two mechanisms under the control of steroid-responsive element binding protein-2 [SREBP-2]), (3) efflux of cholesterol from the plasma membrane to cholesterol acceptor particles (predominantly apoA-I and HDL) via the ABCA1 and ABCG1 transporters, and (4) intracellular cholesterol esterification via the enzyme acetyl-CoA acetyltransferase (ACAT). SREBP-2 coordinately regulates the first two pathways at the level of gene transcription. Cellular cholesterol binds to SCAP (SREPB cholesterol-activated protein), which localizes on the endoplasmic reticulum. Cholesterol inhibits the interaction of SCAP with SREPB. In the absence of cholesterol, SCAP mediates the cleavage of SREBP at two sites by specific proteases with the release of an amino-terminal fragment of SREBP. This SREBP fragment migrates to the nucleus and increases the transcriptional activity of genes involved in cellular cholesterol and fatty acid homeostasis. The ACAT pathway regulates the cholesterol content in membranes. Humans express two separate forms of ACAT. ACAT1 and ACAT2 derive from different genes and mediate cholesterol esterification in cytoplasm and in the endoplasmic reticulum lumen for lipoprotein assembly and secretion.

FIGURE 27.4 Diagram of a hepatocyte expressing the low-density lipoprotein receptor (LDL-R). Top panel, In the absence (or mAb blockade) of PCSK9, the LDL-R recycles rapidly to the cell surface. LDL particles are cleared by LDL by receptor-mediated endocytosis, thereby lowering LDL-C concentration in the blood. Bottom panel, PCSK9 chaperones the internalized LDL-R/LDL particle complex to the endosome-lysosomal compartment, where it undergoes degradation. The consequent decrease in LDL-R impairs LDL clearance, yielding accumulation of cholesterol-rich LDL particles in the blood. *ER*, Endoplasmic reticulum; *TGN*, trans Golgi network.

High-Density Lipoprotein and Reverse Cholesterol Transport

Regulation of cholesterol efflux from cells depends in part on the ABCA1 pathway, controlled in turn by hydroxysterols (especially 24- and 27-OH cholesterol, which act as ligands for the liver-specific receptor [LXR] family of nuclear transcription factors). In conditions of cholesterol sufficiency, the cell can decrease cholesterol synthesis. The cell can also limit the amount of cholesterol that enters the cell via the LDL-R, thereby augmenting the amount stored as cholesteryl esters, and can promote cholesterol removal by increasing its movement to the plasma membrane for efflux.

Epidemiologic studies have consistently shown an inverse relationship between plasma levels of HDL-C and the presence of CAD[19]. HDL promotes reverse cholesterol transport and can prevent lipoprotein oxidation, and exert antiinflammatory actions in vitro, among many other seemingly salutary functions. Yet, Mendelian randomization analyses have cast doubt on the causal role of HDL as a protective cardiovascular risk factor.[20] Mutations of the genes for ABCA1 that cause lifelong HDL deficiency do not impart additional cardiovascular risk, and conversely, variants in genes that increase HDL-C do not associate with protection from cardiovascular events.

HDL has a complex and incompletely understood metabolism. The complexity arises because HDL particles acquire their components from several sources and these components undergo metabolism at different sites. In addition, steady-state levels of HDL in plasma may not reflect the dynamic nature of HDL-mediated cholesterol trafficking, in contrast to the situation with LDL. The intestine and liver synthesize apoA-I, the main protein of HDL. Approximately 80% of HDL originates from the liver and 20% from the intestine (see Fig. 27.3, *part 5*). Lipid-free apoA-I acquires phospholipids from cell membranes and from redundant phospholipids shed during the hydrolysis of TRLs. Lipid-free apoA-I binds to ABCA1 and promotes the transporter's phosphorylation via cAMP, which increases the net efflux of phospholipids and cholesterol onto apoA-I to form a nascent HDL particle (see Fig. 27.3, *part 10*). This particle contains apoA-I, phospholipids, and some free cholesterol. These nascent HDL particles will mediate further cellular efflux of cholesterol. Currently, standard laboratory tests do not measure these HDL precursors because they contain little or no cholesterol. On reaching a cell membrane, the nascent HDL particles capture membrane-associated cholesterol and promote the efflux of free cholesterol onto other HDL particles (see Fig. 27.3, *part 10*). Conceptually, the formation of HDL particles appears to involve two steps. The first step involves binding of HDL apoA-I to ABCA1 and generation of a specific membrane microdomain that allows the subsequent lipidation of apoA-I. Efflux of cellular cholesterol from peripheral cells, such as macrophages, does not contribute importantly to overall HDL-C mass but could export cholesterol from plaques. Macrophages can transfer cholesterol to apoA-I and apo E, to nascent discoid or ellipsoid HDL particles via the ABCA1 transporter. The ABCG1 transporter does not promote cellular cholesterol efflux to lipid-free or lipid-poor apoA-I but to mature HDL particles. In vitro assays can measure HDL-mediated cellular cholesterol efflux by plasma samples, a process that appears altered in many disease states, including diabetes and CAD. LCAT, an enzyme activated by apoA-I, then esterifies the free cholesterol (see Fig. 27.3, *part 8*). Such assays have proven useful in research but are not scalable or validated for clinical use. HDL also furnishes cholesterol to steroid hormone–producing tissues and the liver through *selective uptake of cholesterol* mediated by the scavenger receptor SR-B1.

Because of their hydrophobicity, cholesteryl esters move to the core of the lipoprotein, and the HDL particle now assumes a spherical configuration (a particle denoted HDL_3). With further cholesterol esterification, the HDL particle increases in size to become the more buoyant HDL_2. The cholesterol within HDL particles can transfer to TRLs via CETP, which mediates an equimolar exchange of cholesterol from HDL to TRL and movement of triglyceride from TRL onto HDL (see Fig. 27.3, *part 9*). Inhibition of CETP increases HDL-C in blood and has undergone exploration as a therapeutic target for prevention of ASCVD. However, in clinical trials, CETP inhibitors have failed to improve outcomes except for anacetrapib in the Randomized Evaluation of the Effects of Anacetrapib through Lipid Modification (REVEAL), an effect likely due to LDL-lowering properties of this drug rather than boosting HDL concentration.[21] Triglyceride-enriched HDLs are denoted HDL_{2b}. Hepatic lipase can hydrolyze triglycerides and endothelial lipase can hydrolyze phospholipids within these particles and thereby convert them back to HDL_3 particles.

Reverse cholesterol transport involves the uptake of cellular cholesterol from extrahepatic sources, such as lipid-laden macrophages, and its esterification by LCAT, transport by large HDL particles, and exchange for one triglyceride molecule by CETP. Hepatic receptors can now take up the cholesterol molecule originally on an HDL particle and residing in a TRL or LDL particle after this exchange. HDL particles therefore act as shuttles between tissue cholesterol, TRL, and the liver. Reverse cholesterol transport by HDL constitutes a small but potentially important portion of the plasma HDL mass. Indeed, selective inactivation of macrophage ABCA1 does not change HDL-C levels in mice but increases atherosclerosis. The protein component of HDL particles is exchangeable with lipoproteins of other classes. The kidneys appear to be a route of elimination of apoA-I and other HDL apolipoproteins.

LIPOPROTEIN DISORDERS

Definitions

Time and new knowledge have stimulated changes in the classification of lipoprotein disorders. The original classification of lipoprotein disorders by Fredrickson, Lees, and Levy (1967) which depended on analysis of lipoprotein patterns by ultracentrifugation or electrophoresis has fallen into disuse (see prior editions for details). Most clinicians now classify lipoprotein disorders by which specific lipoprotein lipid is elevated and, when sufficiently characterized, by the genetic defect, e.g., familial hypercholesterolemia (FH). For example, a young patient with eruptive xanthomas and a plasma triglyceride level of 22 mmol/L (2000 mg/dL) probably has familial hyperchylomicronemia as a result of LPL deficiency or other monogenic defects. A 38-year-old woman with a strong family history of ASCVD, tendinous xanthomas, and an untreated LDL-C of 240 mg/dL (6.4 mmol/L) likely has heterozygous familial hypercholesterolemia (HeFH). An obese, hypertensive middle-aged man with a cholesterol level of 6.4 mmol/L (245 mg/dL), a triglyceride level of 3.1 mmol/L (274 mg/dL), an HDL-C level of 0.8 mmol/L (31 mg/dL), and a calculated LDL-C level of 4.2 mmol/L (162 mg/dL) probably has metabolic syndrome, and this should trigger the clinician to seek other components of this cluster, including poor lifestyle, hypertension, and hyperglycemia. Conversely, an obese middle-aged man with a plasma triglyceride level of 7 mmol/L (620 mg/dL) probably has mutations in several genes associated with plasma triglyceride levels.

The clinical usefulness of apolipoprotein levels has stirred debate (see Chapter 25). Taken as a single measurement, the apo B level provides information on the number of potentially atherogenic particles and can be used as a goal of lipid-lowering therapy.[22] Similarly, LDL particle size correlates highly with plasma HDL-C and triglyceride levels, and most studies do not show it to be an independent cardiovascular risk factor in particular after adjusting for apo B or LDL particle concentration. Small, dense LDL particles tend to track with features of metabolic syndrome, which usually involves dyslipoproteinemia with elevated plasma triglyceride and reduced HDL-C levels. While there is some debate on the value of apo B or non-HDL-C as a better predictive biomarker of ASCVD, the Emerging Risk Factors Collaboration studies[19] and the UK Biobank (comprising 346,686 participants) have shown that measurement of non–HDL-C is equivalent to measurement of apo B in determination of cardiovascular risk.[22] The measurement of apoB remains a useful tool for cardiovascular risk prediction, especially in the primary prevention setting in the presence of features of the metabolic syndrome.[23] Similarly, HDL-C tracks as well with CVD risk as apoA-I does.[19]

Genetic Lipoprotein Disorders

Understanding of the genetics of lipoprotein metabolism has expanded rapidly (see Chapter 7). Classification of genetic lipoprotein disorders usually requires a biochemical phenotype in addition to a clinical phenotype. With the exception of FH, monogenic disorders tend to be very rare and constitute "orphan" diseases. Disorders considered heritable on careful family study may be difficult to characterize unambiguously because of age, sex, penetrance, and gene-gene and environmental

TABLE 27.4 Genetic Lipoprotein Disorders

DISORDER	GENE	FIGURE 27.3
LDL Particles		
• Autosomal dominant hypercholesterolemia (ADH)		
• Heterozygous Familial Hypercholesterolemia (HeFH)	LDLR	7
• Homozygous Familial Hypercholesterolemia (HoFH)	LDLR	7
• Familial defective apo B100	APOB	7
• Gain-of-function PCSK9 mutations	PCSK9	7
• Autosomal recessive hypercholesterolemia	LDLRAP1	7
• Abetalipoproteinemia	MTTP	
• Hypobetalipoproteinemia	APOB	
• Familial sitosterolemia	ABCG5/ABCG8	
• Familial Lp(a) hyperlipoproteinemia	APOA	11
Remnant Lipoproteins		
• Dysbetalipoproteinemia type III	APOE	3
Hepatic lipase deficiency	LIPC	6
Triglyceride-Rich Lipoproteins		
• Lipoprotein lipase deficiency (Familial Chylomicronemia Syndrome—FCS)	LPL	2
• Apo C-II deficiency	APOCII	2
• Apo A-V deficiency	APOAV	
• Familial hypertriglyceridemia	Polygenic	
• Familial combined hyperlipidemia	Polygenic	
High Density Lipoproteins		
• Apo A-I deficiency	APOAI	5
Tangier disease/familial HDL deficiency	ABCA1	10
Familial LCAT deficiency syndromes	LCAT	8
CETP deficiency	CETP	9
Niemann-Pick disease types A and B	SMPD1	
Niemann-Pick disease type C	NPC1	
Other		
• Cerebrotendinous xanthomatosis	CYP27A1	

CETP, Cholesteryl ester transfer protein; *LCAT*, lecithin-cholesterol acyltransferase.

interactions. Most common lipoprotein disorders encountered clinically result from the interaction of increasing age, lack of physical exercise, weight gain, and a suboptimal diet with individual genetic makeup. Genetic lipoprotein disorders can either raise or lower levels of LDL, Lp(a), remnant lipoproteins, TRLs (chylomicrons and VLDL), or HDL (Table 27.4).

Low-Density Lipoproteins
Familial Hypercholesterolemia

Elucidation of the pathway by which complex molecules enter the cell by receptor-mediated endocytosis and discovery of LDL-R represent landmarks in cell biology and clinical investigation.[6] Affected subjects have an elevated LDL-C level greater than the 95th percentile for age and sex, approximately 190 mg/dL (5.0 mmol/L) in adults. In adulthood, clinical manifestations include tendinous xanthomas over the extensor tendons (metacarpophalangeal joints, patellar, triceps, and Achilles tendons); corneal arcus and xanthelasma are less specific signs of FH. These clinical findings are increasingly rare, as biochemical testing enables earlier recognition and treatment. Transmission is autosomal codominant. The diagnosis of FH is usually made according to the Dutch Lipid Clinics Network or the Simon-Broome criteria. A new definition for FH relies on a simpler system combining LDL-C, family history of elevated cholesterol, or premature ASCVD.[24] These definitions are highly concordant and rely on the absolute levels of LDL-C, family history of premature ASCVD, family history of elevated LDL-C, cutaneous manifestations and, if available, DNA analysis. Heterozygous FH (HeFH) affects approximately 1 in 311,[25,26] with a higher prevalence in populations with a founder effect. Patients with FH have high risk for the development of CAD by the third to fourth decade in men and approximately 8 to 10 years later in women.[27] The presence of a mutation in a gene known to cause FH increases cardiovascular risk by greater than 10- to 20-fold.[28–30] Genetic testing for FH is now recommended to make a precise diagnosis and guide therapy, and to inform cascade testing of siblings and offspring.[31] Remarkably, prompt recognition in childhood or early adulthood and treatment (statins) can normalize life expectancy.[32]

LOW-DENSITY LIPOPROTEIN RECEPTOR GENE. Defects in the low-density lipoprotein receptor (*LDLR*) gene cause an accumulation of LDL particles in plasma and thus alter the function of the LDL-R protein and cause FH (see Fig. 27.3, *part 7*). Well in excess of 1700 mutations of the *LDLR* gene can cause FH.[27] For clinical purposes, *LDLR* gene mutations are characterized as defective (<20% to 30% residual activity) or null (0% activity). The severity of elevated LDL-C and age of onset of ASCVD correlates with the severity of the mutation.[33]

FAMILIAL DEFECTIVE APOLIPOPROTEIN B. Mutations within the apolipoprotein B *(APOB)* gene that lead to an abnormal ligand-receptor interaction can cause a form of autosomal dominant hypercholesterolemia clinically indistinguishable from FH. Several mutations at the postulated binding site to LDL-R cause familial defective apo B100 (see Fig. 27.3, *part 7*). The defective apo B has reduced affinity (20% to 30% of control) for LDL-R. LDL particles with defective apo B have a plasma half-life threefold to fourfold greater than the half-life of normal LDL. Because of their increased persistence, these LDL particles can more readily undergo oxidative modifications that can enhance their atherogenicity. Affected subjects usually have LDL-C levels elevated up to 400 mg/dL (10.4 mmol/L) but may also have normal levels. Familial defective apo B100 has a lower prevalence than *LDLR* mutations (approximately 1 in 500).

PROPROTEIN CONVERTASE SUBTILISIN/KEXIN TYPE 9. Gain-of-function mutations in the *PCSK9* gene decrease surface availability of the LDL-R protein and cause accumulation of LDL-C in plasma (see Fig. 27.4). A loss-of-function mutation in *PCSK9* confers lower LDL-C than in individuals without the mutation. Black Americans had a higher prevalence of this protective mutation than did whites in the ARIC (Atherosclerosis Risk in Communities) study, and subjects with life-long low LDL-C because of a mutation at the *PCSK9* gene locus had a marked reduction in coronary events,[18] thus confirming that genetically low LDL-C states lower cardiovascular risk.

Polygenic Hypercholesterolemia

In most cohorts of "definite" FH patients, as many as 20% do not have a mutation in the *LDLR*, *APOB* or *PCSK9* genes. While exome-wide sequencing has identified several other genes causing a phenocopy of FH, some patients have an accumulation of single nucleotide polymorphisms of genes known to elevate LDL-C in large-scale genome-wide association studies.[34]

AUTOSOMAL RECESSIVE HYPERCHOLESTEROLEMIA
An autosomal recessive form of FH identified in a kindred from Sardinia results from a mutation in the gene encoding the LDL-R adaptor protein (*LDL-RAP-1* gene), which encodes a protein involved in recycling of LDL-R. Other genes, including *APOE* del166LEU[35,36] and lysosomal acid lipase (LIPA) cause a phenocopy of FH. Other genes, such as STAP1 (Signal Transducing Adaptor Family Member 1) have been associated with FH, but careful studies performed on genetically modified animals dismissed this association, highlighting some of the limitations of exome-wide genetic association studies.[37]

HYPOBETALIPOPROTEINEMIA AND ABETALIPOPROTEINEMIA
Mutations within the *APOB* gene can lead to truncations of the mature apo B100 peptide. Many such mutations cause a syndrome characterized by reduced LDL-C and VLDL-C but few if any clinical manifestations and no known risk for ASCVD, a condition referred to as hypobetalipoproteinemia. Apo B truncated close to its amino terminus loses the ability to bind lipids, and produces a syndrome similar to abetalipoproteinemia, a rare recessive lipoprotein disorder of infancy that causes mental retardation and growth abnormalities. Abetalipoproteinemia results from a mutation in the gene coding for the microsomal triglyceride transfer protein (*MTTP*), which is required for assembly of apo B–containing lipoproteins in the liver and the intestine. The resulting lack of apo B–containing lipoproteins in plasma causes a lack of fat-soluble vitamins (A, D, E, and K) that circulate in lipoproteins. In turn, this deficiency result in mental and developmental retardation in affected children.

SITOSTEROLEMIA
A rare condition of increased intestinal absorption and decreased excretion of plant sterols (sitosterol and campesterol) can mimic severe FH with extensive xanthoma formation. Premature atherosclerosis, often apparent clinically well before adulthood, occurs in patients with sitosterolemia. Diagnosis requires specialized analysis of plasma sterols documenting an elevation in sitosterol, campesterol, cholestanol, sitostanol, and campestanol. Patients with sitosterolemia have normal or reduced plasma cholesterol levels, and normal triglyceride concentrations. Patients with sitosterolemia have rare homozygous (or compound heterozygous) mutations in the *ABCG5* and *ABCG8* genes. The gene products of ABCG5 and ABCG8 are half ABC transporters and form a heterodimer localized in the villous border of intestinal cells, that actively pumps plant sterols back into the intestinal lumen. A defect in either of the genes inactivates this transport mechanism, and net accumulation of plant sterols (because of impaired elimination) ensues.[38]

Lipoprotein(a) (Fig. 27.3)

Lp(a) (pronounced "lipoprotein little a") consists of an LDL particle linked covalently with one molecule of apo (a). The apo (a) moiety consists of a protein with a high degree of homology with plasminogen. The gene for apo (a) appears to have arisen from the plasminogen gene. The apo (a) gene has multiple repeats of one of the kringle motifs (kringle IV), which vary in number from 12 to more than 40 in each individual. Plasma Lp(a) levels depend almost entirely on genetics and correlate inversely with the number of kringle repeats and therefore with the molecular weight of apo (a). Human genetic data implicate Lp(a) as a causal cardiovascular risk factor.[39] Lp(a) concentrations follow a skewed distribution in the population, and African Americans tend to have higher Lp(a) levels than do other ethnic groups in the United States. Few environmental factors or medications modulate plasma Lp(a) levels. The pathogenesis of Lp(a) may result from an antifibrinolytic potential and/or ability to bind oxidized lipoproteins.[40] Statins do not decrease Lp(a) levels, in contrast to PCSK9 inhibitors which reduce Lp(a) levels modestly. A novel anti-sense RNA directed at the *LPA* gene mRNA has shown that long-term reduction of Lp(a) is feasible.[41] Ongoing phase 3 cardiovascular outcomes study will determine the usefulness of this approach. Genetic polymorphisms at the *LPA* gene have shown a strong association with aortic calcification and may have a causal role in aortic stenosis.[39,42]

Triglyceride-Rich Lipoproteins (see also Chapter 25)

TRLs are circulating apo B-carrying particles that carry predominantly hydrophobic triglycerides but also contain cholesterol ester, and include chylomicrons, VLDL, IDL, and remnant particles. In the fasting state, triglycerides are carried predominantly by VLDL particles and their remnants, while in the fed state triglycerides are additionally carried by chylomicrons and their remnants. Plasma triglycerides may arise from a higher TRL particle number (reflected by increased apo B, since each TRL carries one apoB moiety on it) and/or due to greater particle size.[43] Postprandial elevations in triglycerides and TRLs, often due to underlying abnormalities in TRL metabolism, may not be captured in the fasting state, hence guidelines have shifted to measuring nonfasting or fasting lipids for general risk screening or assessment.[44–46] Population studies have shown that nonfasting triglycerides are equally or even more strongly associated with cardiovascular endpoints than fasting levels.

Nonfasting triglycerides are higher than fasting levels (by approximately 0.3 mmol/L or 27 mg/dL), and guidelines consider nonfasting triglycerides ≥2 mmol/L (175 mg/dL) as abnormal, while for fasting triglycerides the corresponding level is ≥1.7 mmol/L (150 mg/dL). The 2018 American Heart Association/American College of Cardiology (AHA/ACC) cholesterol guideline and the 2019 AHA/ACC prevention guideline consider fasting or nonfasting triglycerides greater than 175 mg/dL as a risk enhancing factor that could prompt consideration for initiating or intensifying statin therapy.[46] There are some differences in the guideline cutpoints for severe hypertriglyceridemia, defined as fasting triglycerides greater than 10 mmol/L (885 mg/dL) in European guidelines[47] or ≥500 mg/dL (5.7 mmol/L) in US guidelines.[46] Because the triglyceride to cholesterol ratio in TRLs progressively increases as the hypertriglyceridemia becomes more severe, the Friedewald equation (which assumes a fixed triglyceride to cholesterol ratio of triglycerides/5 [mg/dL] or triglycerides/2.2 [mmol/L]) to calculate LDL-C is inaccurate when triglycerides are greater than 4.5 mmol/L (400 mg/dL), as it underestimates the true LDL-C at high triglyceride levels. Instead, it is preferable to use non-HDL-C or apo B instead of calculated LDL-C for LDL-related treatment decisions in patients with hypertriglyceridemia, as direct LDL-C assays may also be inaccurate.[23,45]

Hypertriglyceridemia correlates with risk of cardiovascular disease, and postprandial increase of TRL particles is an important factor in atherogenesis. However, it is less clear if triglycerides directly contribute to atherogenesis, or whether triglycerides are a marker of another atherogenic moiety of TRLs, such as the cholesterol (remnant/VLDL cholesterol) or apolipoproteins (e.g., apo B, apo CIII) that are also carried by these particles. Like LDL particles, all TRL particles carry one apo B per particle. While some studies found independent associations for triglycerides with cardiovascular disease risk, a meta-analysis of 68 prospective studies (>300,000 individuals) found that the association of triglycerides with cardiovascular risk was lost after adjusting for non-HDL-C or apo B.[19] Genetic studies suggest a causal association between plasma triglycerides and cardiovascular risk, but many genetic variants are pleiotropic and often also associate with differences in VLDL/remnant cholesterol, LDL-C, apo B, Lp(a), or HDL-C, making it challenging to identify the causal atherogenic moiety of TRLs. In a Mendelian randomization analysis of genetic scores composed of triglyceride-lowering variants in the LPL gene and LDL-C lowering variants in the LDLR gene, both sets of variants associated with similar risk of coronary disease per unit difference in apo B, suggesting that genetic variants that affect apoB are similarly atherogenic, regardless of differences in LDL-C or triglycerides.[42] In a meta-analysis of randomized trials (N = 374,358 from 25 statin trials and 24 nonstatin trials), triglyceride lowering associated with lower cardiovascular risk (approximately 15% lower risk per 1 mmol/L reduction in triglycerides), which was somewhat lower than for LDL-C (approximately 20% lower risk per 1 mmol/L reduction in LDL-C) and attenuated when the Reduction of Cardiovascular Events with Icosapent Ethyl-Intervention Trial (REDUCE-IT) was excluded.[48]

Clearance of TRL particles requires LPL, hepatic lipase, apoE and other catalytically active apolipoproteins, and functional LDL receptors and LRP1. Enzymatic hydrolysis of TRLs by LPL and acquisition of cholesteryl esters from HDL by CETP results in the formation of cholesterol-enriched remnant particles that are depleted of part of their triglyceride content (see Fig. 27.3, parts 2, 3, and 9). However, defective TRL clearance alone is often not sufficient (except in rare monogenic cases), and overproduction of TRL is usually necessary for hypertriglyceridemia.[43]

Severe hypertriglyceridemia can result from poorly controlled diabetes or from genetic disorders (polygenic or monogenic) of the processing enzymes or apolipoproteins, often in the context of secondary factors. Severe hypertriglyceridemia is often due to polygenic and nongenetic determinants, often exacerbated in the presence of secondary nongenetic factors, and less commonly due to monogenic conditions.[49,50] In patients with insulin resistance, metabolic syndrome, or diabetes, elevation of plasma triglyceride levels is usually mild to moderate and occurs most often in the presence of visceral (abdominal) obesity and a diet rich in calories, carbohydrates, and saturated fats. It is now recognized that the genetic basis for severe hypertriglyceridemia is multifactorial due to the combination of poor lifestyle on a background susceptibility of multiple genetic defects each of which raises triglycerides by only a fraction of a mmol/L, the cumulative sum of which produces a clinical phenotype (e.g., familial hypertriglyceridemia, familial combined hyperlipidemia, or type III dyslipidemia).[43] Thus, hypertriglyceridemia is best viewed as a complex disorder arising from the interaction of genetic and nongenetic factors. Primary causes of hypertriglyceridemia (Table 27.5) include the rare monogenic syndromes (homozygous or compound heterozygote mutations) in several canonical genes related to LPL, and the much more common polygenic or multifactorial cases, which could include contributions from rare heterozygote variants in these canonical genes and/or other common variants associated with elevated triglycerides.[50,51] Genetic screening of siblings of patients with monogenic disorders is suggested.[49]

Polygenic Hypertriglyceridemia (also Known as Familial Hypertriglyceridemia, Formerly Type IV Hyperlipoproteinemia)

Polygenic hypertriglyceridemia (formerly Type IV hyperlipidemia) results from both common and rare genetic variants that result in increased VLDL particles. This highly heterogeneous condition also has a strong environmental influence. The prevalence of polygenic hypertriglyceridemia ranges from 1 in 50 to 100. Hepatic overproduction of VLDL causes this condition (see Fig. 27.3, part 4); the catabolism (uptake) of VLDL particles can be normal or reduced. Lipolysis by LPL appears adequate under basal conditions, but not with excess

TABLE 27.5 Primary Causes of Hypertriglyceridemia

Mild-to-moderate HTG (TG 2.0–9.9 mmol/L)
Multifactorial or polygenic HTG (formerly HLP Type 4 or familial HTG)
Complex genetic susceptibility (see above)
Dysbetalipoproteinemia (formerly HLP Type 3 or dysbetalipoproteinemia)
Complex genetic susceptibility (see above), plus
APOE E2/E2 homozygosity or
APOE dominant rare variant heterozygosity
Combined hyperlipoproteinemia (formerly HLP Type 2B or familial combined hyperlipidemia)
Complex genetic susceptibility (see above), plus
Accumulation of common small effect LDL-C-raising polymorphisms
Severe HTG (TG >10 mmol/L)
Monogenic chylomicronemia (formerly HLP Type 1 or familial chylomicronemia syndrome)
Lipoprotein lipase deficiency (Bi-allelic LPL gene mutations)
Apo C-II deficiency (Bi-allelic APOC2 gene mutations)
Apo A-V deficiency (Bi-allelic APOA5 gene mutations)
Lipase maturation factor 1 deficiency (Bi-allelic LMF1 gene mutations)
GPIHBP1 deficiency (Bi-allelic GPIHBP1 gene mutations)
Multifactorial or polygenic chylomicronemia (formerly HLP Type 5 or mixed hyperlipidemia)
Complex genetic susceptibility, including
Heterozygous rare large-effect gene variants for monogenic chylomicronemia (see above); and/or
Accumulated common small-effect TG-raising polymorphisms (e.g., numerous GWAS loci including APOA1-C3-A4-A5; TRIB1, LPL, MLXIPL, GCKR, FADS1-2-3, NCAN, APOB, PLTP, ANGPTL3)
Other
Transient infantile HTG (glycerol-3-phosphate dehydrogenase 1 deficiency) from bi-allelic GPD1 gene mutations

Adapted from Laufs U, Parhofer KG, Ginsberg HN, Hegele RA. Clinical review on triglycerides. *Eur Heart J.* 2020;41(1):99–109.

triglyceride load, especially following fatty meals. Plasma triglycerides, VLDL-C, and VLDL triglycerides rise moderately to markedly; the LDL-C level is usually low, as is HDL-C. Total cholesterol is normal or elevated, depending on VLDL-C levels. Fasting plasma concentrations of triglycerides range between 2.3 to 5.7 mmol/L (200 to 500 mg/dL). After a meal, plasma triglycerides may exceed 11.3 mmol/L (1000 mg/dL). Polygenic hypertriglyceridemia does not associate with clinical signs such as corneal arcus, xanthoma, and xanthelasmas. This condition has a weaker relationship with CAD than combined hyperlipoproteinemia (familial combined hyperlipidemia), and not all studies support this association. The disorder clusters in first-degree relatives, but varies phenotypically depending on sex, age, hormone use (especially estrogens), and diet. Alcohol intake potently stimulates hypertriglyceridemia in these subjects, as does caloric or carbohydrate intake.

Human genetic studies have shown that many cases of severe hypertriglyceridemia result from mutations in one or more of the genes associated with triglyceride metabolism (see Table 27.4). Lifestyle modifications should be the first step in treatment, including weight reduction in overweight individuals, limiting alcohol intake, reducing caloric intake, increasing exercise and withdrawal of hormones (estrogens and progesterone or anabolic steroids).

An unrelated X-linked genetic disorder, familial glycerolemia, may mimic familial hypertriglyceridemia because most measurement techniques for triglycerides use the measurement of glycerol after enzymatic hydrolysis of triglycerides. Diagnosis of familial hyperglycerolemia requires ultracentrifugation of plasma and analysis of glycerol.

A less common subset of patients have more severe hypertriglyceridemia which is characterized by a more severe elevation in both VLDL and chylomicrons and are classified as having polygenic chylomicronemia (formerly Type V hyperlipidemia). The etiology is also multifactorial. Although they have the same genetic variants as patients with polygenic hypertriglyceridemia, they carry more of these variants and/or have stronger secondary or metabolic risk factors (e.g., fat-rich diet, obesity, or poorly controlled diabetes), which results in overproduction of both VLDL and chylomicrons and decreased catabolism of these particles.

Combined Hyperlipoproteinemia (also Known as Familial Combined Hyperlipidemia or Formerly Type 2B Hyperlipidemia)

Combined hyperlipoproteinemia (formerly familial combined hyperlipidemia) is common, with a prevalence of approximately 1 in 50 to 100, and accounts for 10% to 20% of patients with premature CAD, yet the diagnosis is often missed clinically because of overlap in the lipid profile with that of diabetes and metabolic syndrome.[52] Individuals with combined hyperlipoproteinemia have complex genetic susceptibility to elevated triglycerides, and in some patients also tendency to elevated LDL-C. Novel loci in the upstream transcription factor 1 (USF1) and stearoyl-CoA desaturase 1 genes are promising candidate genes. The description of loss of function in the angiopoietin-like protein-3 gene (ANGPTL3, a novel target for therapy) in a kindred with familial hypolipidemia renewed interest in the angiopoietin like proteins 3, 4 and 5 which modulate the activities of LPL and endothelial lipase (see Fig. 27.3, part 2). The phenotype is determined by interaction of multiple susceptibility genes and the environment. Modifying factors include gender, age at onset, and comorbid states such as obesity, lack of exercise, and diet.

Combined hyperlipoproteinemia is characterized by the presence of elevated total cholesterol and/or triglyceride levels based on arbitrary cut points in several members of the same family. Advances in analytic techniques have added measurement of LDL-C and apo B levels. Considerable overlap exists between combined hyperlipoproteinemia and other conditions (e.g., familial dyslipidemic hypertension, metabolic syndrome, and hyperapobetalipoproteinemia). The condition has few clinical signs; corneal arcus, xanthomas, and xanthelasmas occur infrequently. Biochemical abnormalities include elevation of plasma total cholesterol and LDL-C levels (>90th to 95th percentile) and/or elevation of plasma triglycerides (>90th to 95th percentile)—a type IIb lipoprotein phenotype, often associated with low HDL-C and elevated apo B levels; small, dense LDL particles occur frequently. The combination of apo B greater than 120 mg/dL and elevated triglycerides together with a family history of premature cardiovascular disease identifies patients who may have this condition. Underlying metabolic disorders include hepatic overproduction of apo B–containing lipoproteins, delayed postprandial clearance of TRLs, and increased flux of FFAs to the liver. Experimental data have shown that FFAs and cholesteryl esters drive hepatic apo B secretion. Increased delivery of FFAs to the liver, as occurs in states of insulin resistance and visceral obesity, leads to increased hepatic apo B secretion. In addition to lifestyle therapies, patients benefit from statins and other LDL-C lowering therapies.

Dysbetalipoproteinemia (Formerly Type III Hyperlipoproteinemia)

Dysbetalipoproteinemia is a rare genetic lipoprotein disorder that is characterized by accumulation of remnant lipoprotein particles in plasma and affects approximately 1 in 10,000. Similar to polygenic hypertriglyceridemia, it is now recognized that it also has a similar complex genetic predisposition but in addition these patients also carry the apo E2/2 genotype.[49] Apo E has three common alleles: E2, E3, and E4. The apo E2/2 genotype has a prevalence of approximately 0.7% to 1.0%, but dysbetalipoproteinemia only occurs in approximately 1% of subjects bearing the apo E2/2 genotype. Reasons for the relative rarity of dysbetalipoproteinemia are not fully understood. Other rare mutations of the gene for apo E or mutations in other genes associated with triglyceride metabolism contribute to the disease. The apo E2 allele has markedly decreased binding to the apo B/E receptor. The importance of the apo E gene and protein is underscored by the widespread use of the apo E–deficient mouse, which develops atherosclerosis. Diagnosis includes apo E genotyping or phenotyping, plasma ultracentrifugation for lipoprotein separation, or lipoprotein electrophoresis. Lipoprotein agarose gel electrophoresis shows a typical pattern of a broad band between the pre-beta (VLDL) and beta (LDL) lipoproteins, hence it was previously also referred to as "broad beta disease."

Clinical findings include pathognomonic tuberous xanthomas and palmar striated xanthomas. Patients with this disease have increased cardiovascular risk and are prone to premature coronary disease and peripheral arterial disease. The lipoprotein profile shows increased cholesterol and triglyceride levels and reduced HDL-C. Measuring apo B can differentiate it from mixed dyslipidemia. Remnant lipoproteins (partly catabolized chylomicrons and VLDL) accumulate in plasma and become enriched with cholesterol esters. The defect results from abnormal apo E, which does not bind to hepatic receptors that recognize apo E as a ligand (see Fig. 27.3, part 3). These patients have an elevated ratio of VLDL cholesterol to triglycerides, normally less than 0.7 (when measured in mmol/L; <0.30 in mg/dL), because of cholesteryl ester enrichment of remnant particles. Thus, calculation of LDL-C in such patients is unreliable. In general, patients respond well to dietary therapy, correction of other metabolic abnormalities (diabetes, obesity, hypothyroidism), and in cases requiring drug therapy, statins should be the drug of first choice.

Monogenic Chylomicronemia Syndrome (Formerly Familial Hyperchylomicronemia Syndrome or Type I Hyperlipidemia)

This rare (approximately 1 to 10 in a million) monogenic autosomal recessive disorder of severe hypertriglyceridemia elevates fasting plasma triglycerides (often to greater than 11.3 mmol/L, >1000 mg/dL) and VLDL cholesterol due to increased levels of chylomicrons, but usually with lower apo B concentrations (<75 mg/dL) than polygenic or multifactorial chylomicronemia.[52,53] Mutations of several genes involved in triglyceride metabolism elevate chylomicrons, and definitive diagnosis requires molecular detection of homozygous or compound heterozygous variants in 1 of 5 canonical genes that encode proteins needed for LPL-mediated lipolysis of chylomicrons: *LPL* (the most common of at least 100 mutations identified), *APOC2, APOA5, LMF1*, or *GPIHBP1*.[49] Populations with a founder effect can have a high prevalence of LPL mutations. The hypertriglyceridemia results from markedly reduced or absent LPL activity or, more rarely, absence of its activator apo C-II (see Fig. 27.3, part 2). These defects lead to impaired hydrolysis of chylomicrons and VLDL and their accumulation in plasma, especially after meals. Extreme elevations of plasma triglycerides (>113 mmol/L;>10,000 mg/dL) can result. Heterozygotes for the disorder tend to have an increase in fasting plasma triglycerides and smaller, denser LDL particles. Many patients with complete LPL deficiency exhibit failure to thrive in childhood and have recurrent bouts of pancreatitis. To underscore the importance of the role of LPL, *lpl* gene deficiency in the mouse leads to a perinatal lethal phenotype.

These patients have recurrent bouts of pancreatitis and eruptive xanthomas. Severe hypertriglyceridemia can also associate with lipemia retinalis, xerostomia, xerophthalmia, and behavioral abnormalities. Plasma from a patient with very high triglyceride levels is milky white, and a clear band of chylomicrons can be seen on top of the plasma after it stands overnight in a refrigerator. Treatment of acute pancreatitis includes intravenous hydration and avoidance of fat in the diet (including fat in parenteral nutrition), and only rarely requires plasma filtration. Chronic treatment includes avoidance of alcohol and dietary fat. Addition of short-chain fatty acids (which are not incorporated in chylomicrons) can increase palatability of the diet. Novel biologic agents are being evaluated and include therapies that target genes critical in the regulation of TRL, such as apo CIII, LPL, or intestinal diacylglycerol acyltransferase 1 (DGAT1) (see Novel Medications section).

High-Density Lipoproteins

Reduced plasma levels of HDL-C consistently correlate with the development or presence of ASCVD.[19] Most cases of reduced HDL-C accompany elevated plasma triglycerides and often keep company with other features of metabolic syndrome. Genetic disorders of HDL can result from decreased production or abnormal maturation and increased catabolism. Genetic lipoprotein disorders leading to moderate to severe elevations in plasma triglycerides cause a reduction in HDL-C levels. Monogenic hyperchylomicronemia, polygenic hypertriglyceridemia, and combined hyperlipoproteinemia all associate with reduced HDL-C levels. Plasma triglyceride and HDL-C levels vary inversely. Several mechanisms contribute to this association: (1) decreased lipolysis of TRLs decreases the availability of substrate (phospholipids) for HDL maturation, (2) HDL enriched with triglyceride has an increased catabolic rate and hence reduced plasma concentration, and (3) the augmented pool of TRLs saps cholesterol from the HDL compartment by CETP-mediated exchange.

Disorders of High-Density Lipoprotein Biogenesis
Apolipoprotein A-I Gene Defects
Primary defects affecting the production of HDL particles may be caused by mutations in the apo AI-CIII-AIV-AV gene complex. More than 50 mutations affect the structure of apoA-I and markedly reduce HDL-C levels. Not all these defects associate with premature CVD. Clinical findings can vary from extensive atypical xanthomatosis and corneal infiltration of lipids to no manifestations at all. Other mutations of apoA-I increased the catabolism of apoA-I and may not associate with CVD. One such mutation, apoA-I$_{Milano}$ (apoA-IArg173Cys), appears not to increase risk for CVD despite very low HDL levels.

Tangier Disease and Familial High-Density Lipoprotein Deficiency
A rare disorder of HDL deficiency, identified in a proband from Tangier Island in Virginia, Tangier disease and familial HDL deficiency result from mutations in the *ABCA1* gene, which encodes the ABCA1 transporter. More than 200 mutations in *ABCA1* can cause Tangier disease (homozygous or compound heterozygous mutations) or familial HDL deficiency (heterozygous mutations). Subjects with Tangier disease or familial HDL deficiency may have an increased risk for CAD, counterbalanced by their very low levels of LDL-C. Mendelian randomization analysis has not supported a causal relationship between mutations in the *ABCA1* gene and ASCVD.

Niemann-Pick type C disease is a disorder of lysosomal cholesterol transport. In patients with Niemann-Pick type C disease, mental retardation and neurologic manifestations occur frequently. The cellular phenotype involves markedly decreased cholesterol esterification and a defect in the cellular transport of cholesterol to the Golgi apparatus.

The gene for Niemann-Pick type C disease (*NPC1*) shuttles cholesterol between the late endosomal pathway and the plasma membrane. Niemann-Pick type C cells lack NPC1 protein; intracellular cholesterol sequestration suppresses ABCA1, impairing cellular cholesterol efflux and HDL assembly.

Disorders of High-Density Lipoprotein–Processing Enzymes
Lecithin-Cholesterol Acyltransferase Deficiency
Genetic defects in the HDL-processing enzymes give rise to interesting phenotypes. Deficiencies of LCAT, the enzyme that catalyzes the formation of cholesteryl esters in plasma, cause corneal infiltration of neutral lipids and hematologic abnormalities as a result of the abnormal constitution of red blood cell membranes. LCAT deficiency can lead to an entity called "fish eye disease" because of the characteristic pattern of corneal infiltration observed in affected individuals. Despite the profound HDL-C deficiency, LCAT deficiency does not appear to increase risk for CAD.

Cholesteryl Ester Transfer Protein Deficiency
Patients without CETP have very elevated levels of HDL-C, which is enriched in cholesteryl esters. Because CETP facilitates the transfer of HDL cholesteryl esters into TRLs, a deficiency of this enzyme causes accumulation of cholesteryl esters within HDL particles. CETP deficiency does not associate with premature CAD but may not afford protection against CAD.

Secondary Causes of Hyperlipidemia and Metabolic Syndrome (Table 27.6) (see also Chapter 25).
In clinical practice, many dyslipidemias, including the genetic forms, share important environmental factors. Lifestyle changes (diet, exercise, reduction of abdominal obesity) should form the foundation for the treatment. The effects of marked alterations in lifestyle, reduction in dietary fats, especially saturated fats, avoiding excessive carbohydrate and alcohol intake, and increasing physical activity improves lipids and other cardiovascular risk factors. Rigorous clinical data showing that these measures improve outcomes and implementing them in a sustained manner in practice, however, have proven more difficult. Laboratory screening for secondary causes includes evaluating for diabetes (fasting glucose, hemoglobin A1c), hypothyroidism (thyroid-stimulating hormone, TSH), liver disease (transaminases, bilirubin, alkaline phosphatase, gamma-glutamyl transferase), renal disease (creatinine, urinary albumin and albumin to creatinine ratio), and inflammatory or autoimmune diseases (C-reactive protein [CRP], serum rheumatoid factor, antinuclear antigen).[50]

Hormonal Causes
Hypothyroidism often elevates LDL-C, triglycerides, or both. An increased TSH provides the key to the diagnosis, and the lipoprotein abnormalities often revert to normal after correction of thyroid status. Rarely, hypothyroidism may uncover a genetic lipoprotein disorder. Estrogens can elevate plasma triglyceride and HDL-C levels, because of increases in both hepatic VLDL and apoA-I production. Oral contraceptives should be avoided in premenopausal women with hypercholesterolemia (LDL-C >4 mmol/L, 160 mg/dL), multiple risk factors, or at high thrombotic risk.[53] In postmenopausal women, estrogens may reduce LDL-C by up to 15%. Use of estrogens for the treatment of lipoprotein disorders is no longer recommended (see also Chapter 91).

Both cholesterol and triglycerides increase during pregnancy. Rarely, pregnancy (particularly in the third trimester) causes severe increases in triglycerides on a background of LPL deficiency or other genetic defects, even if such mutations do not result in dyslipidemia in the nonpregnant state. Such cases present a serious threat to mother and child and require referral to specialized centers. Male sex hormones and anabolic steroids can increase hepatic lipase activity and have been used for the treatment of hypertriglyceridemia in men; however, these agents can also contribute to an elevated triglyceride level, reduced HDL-C, increased blood pressure, and other features of metabolic syndrome. Growth hormone can reduce LDL-C and increase HDL-C but is not recommended for the treatment of lipoprotein disorders.

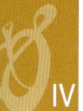

TABLE 27.6 Secondary Causes of Dyslipoproteinemias

CAUSE	DISORDER
Metabolic	Diabetes
	Lipodystrophy
	Glycogen storage disorders
Renal	Chronic renal failure
	Glomerulonephritis with nephritic syndrome
Hepatic	Cirrhosis
	Biliary obstruction
	Porphyria
	Primary biliary cirrhosis (with secondary lecithin-cholesterol acyltransferase [LCAT] deficiency)
Hormonal	Estrogens
	Progesterones
	Growth hormone
	Thyroid disorders (hypothyroidism)
	Corticosteroids
Lifestyle	Physical inactivity
	Obesity
	Diet rich in fats, saturated fats
	Alcohol intake
	Smoking
Medications	Retinoic acid derivatives
	Glucocorticoids
	Exogenous estrogens (including tamoxifen, raloxifene)
	Testosterone and other anabolizing steroids
	Thiazide diuretics
	Beta-adrenergic blockers (non-beta-1 selective)
	Bile acid sequestrants
	Immunosuppressive medications (cyclosporine, cyclophosphamide, interferon, tacrolimus, sirolimus)
	Antiviral medications (human immunodeficiency virus protease inhibitors)
	Antischizophrenic medications
	Rosiglitazone

Metabolic Causes

The most frequent secondary cause of dyslipoproteinemia is the constellation of metabolic abnormalities seen in patients with metabolic syndrome (see also Chapters 29 and 30). The finding of increased visceral fat (abdominal obesity), elevated blood pressure, and impaired glucose tolerance often clusters with increased plasma triglycerides and a reduced HDL-C level and represents the major components of metabolic syndrome. The main cause of dyslipoproteinemia in these patients is insulin resistance and associated increase in FFAs, the substrates for TRL synthesis. In addition, TRL and remnant clearance is impaired, in part because of the higher apo CIII concentrations.[52,53] Overt diabetes, especially type 2 diabetes, frequently elevates plasma triglycerides and reduces HDL-C. While LDL-C may be normal or nonelevated due to the excess of small dense LDL particles, increased concentrations of apo B or non-HDL-C are often present and result in a "discordant" lipid profile. These abnormalities have prognostic implications (see also Chapter 25). Poor control of diabetes, obesity, and moderate to severe hyperglycemia can yield severe hypertriglyceridemia with chylomicronemia and increased VLDL-C levels. Subjects with poorly controlled type 1 diabetes can also have severe hypertriglyceridemia. Familial lipodystrophy (complete or partial) may associate with increased VLDL secretion. Dunnigan lipodystrophy, a genetic disorder with features of metabolic syndrome, results from mutations within the lamin A/C gene and is associated with limb-girdle fat atrophy. Excess plasma triglycerides often accompany glycogen storage disorders.

Renal Disorders

In patients with glomerulonephritis and protein-losing nephropathies, a marked increase in secretion of hepatic lipoproteins can raise LDL-C, which may approach the levels seen in those with FH. By contrast, patients with chronic renal failure have a pattern of hypertriglyceridemia with reduced HDL-C and increased small dense LDL particles. Lp(a) may also be elevated. Patients with end-stage renal disease, including those undergoing hemodialysis or chronic ambulatory peritoneal dialysis, have a poor prognosis and accelerated atherosclerosis. In the Cholesterol Treatment Trialists meta-analysis of 28 trials of patients with varying degrees of renal impairment, statins reduced cardiovascular risk among patients with mild to moderate chronic kidney disease (estimated glomerular filtration rate ≥30 mL/min/1.73 m^2) with smaller benefit among patients with more advanced renal failure, and there was no benefit for patients with end-stage renal disease undergoing dialysis.[54] After organ transplantation, the immunosuppressive regimen (glucocorticoids and cyclosporine) typically elevates triglycerides and VLDL, reduces HDL-C, and increases small dense LDL particles. Because transplant recipients generally have an increase in cardiovascular risk, this secondary hyperlipidemia may warrant treatment. Patients receiving the combination of a statin plus cyclosporine merit careful dose titrations and monitoring for myopathy, since cyclosporine is metabolized through Cyp3A4. The Kidney Disease International Improving Outcomes (KDIGO) recommends statin or statin plus ezetimibe treatment for patients with chronic kidney disease but does not recommend lipid lowering treatment initiation in patients undergoing long-term dialysis.

Liver Disease

Obstructive liver disease, especially primary biliary cirrhosis, may lead to the formation of an abnormal lipoprotein termed *lipoprotein-x*. This type of lipoprotein, also associated with LCAT deficiency, consists of an LDL-like particle with a marked reduction in cholesteryl esters. Extensive xanthoma formation on the face and palmar areas can result from accumulation of lipoprotein-x.

Lifestyle (see also Chapters 25, 29 and 30)

Factors contributing to obesity, such as an imbalance between caloric intake and energy expenditure, lack of physical activity, and a diet rich in saturated fats and refined sugars, contribute in large part to the lipid and lipoprotein lipid levels within a population. Excessive alcohol intake stimulates chylomicron and VLDL secretion, VLDL overproduction, decreased LPL activity, and fatty acid oxidation. This results in TRL accumulation in the plasma and the liver, and increases hepatic fat accumulation and insulin resistance.

Alteration in Lipids by Medications

Several medications can alter lipoproteins (see Table 27.6). Thiazide diuretics can increase triglycerides. Beta-adrenergic blocking agents (beta blockers), especially non–beta1-selective agents, increase triglycerides and lower HDL-C. Retinoic acid and estrogens can increase triglyceride levels, sometimes dramatically. Corticosteroids and immunosuppressive agents can elevate triglycerides and lower HDL-C. Estrogens can increase plasma HDL-C and often raise triglycerides. Anabolic steroids, frequently used by endurance or body-building athletes, can cause hypertriglyceridemia and very low HDL-C. The exact composition, dosage, and frequency of use of anabolic steroids are often obscure. The use of atypical antipsychotic medications may lead to lipoprotein abnormalities, metabolic disorders, and weight gain. Highly active antiretroviral agents may cause severe lipoprotein disorders and an increase in CAD in patients with chronic human immunodeficiency virus infection (see also Chapter 85).

PHARMACOLOGIC MANAGEMENT OF LIPID RISK

Hydroxymethylglutaryl–Coenzyme A Reductase Inhibitors (Statins)

Mechanisms of Action

Statins inhibit cholesterol synthesis by inhibiting the enzyme HMG-CoA reductase and preventing the formation of mevalonate, the rate-limiting step of sterol synthesis. To maintain cellular cholesterol homeostasis, this reduction in intracellular cholesterol increases the expression of LDL-R on the surface of the hepatocyte and decreases hepatic production of VLDL and LDL. In addition to blocking the synthesis of cholesterol, statins also interfere with the synthesis of lipid intermediates with important biologic effects. Two of these intermediates, geranylgeranyl and farnesyl, participate in protein prenylation, the covalent attachment of a lipid moiety to a protein, thereby allowing anchoring into cell membranes and enhancing its biologic activity. Prenylated proteins important in cardiovascular signaling include the guanosine triphosphate–binding proteins Rho A, Rac, and Ras. Altered protein prenylation may also mediate some of the effects attributed to statins not related to LDL lowering. Atherosclerosis involves inflammation (see Chapter 24) and statins have anti-inflammatory effects. Statins decrease the inflammatory biomarker CRP independent of LDL-C lowering, augment the collagen content of atherosclerotic plaque, alter endothelial function, and decrease the inflammatory component of plaque.

Pharmacology and Lipid Effects (Table 27.7A and B)

Statins lower LDL-C in a dose-response manner which is nonlinear: for every doubling of the statin dose, LDL-C drops by about an additional 6%. Statin response should be monitored because there is wide variability in statin response for the same dose, which may relate partly to medication adherence, genetic variation (e.g., Asian individuals may have greater response), biologic variable and other factors including baseline LDL-C levels. Statins vary in intensity from high-intensity (atorvastatin 40 to 80 mg/day and rosuvastatin 20 to 40 mg/day; average lowering of LDL-C by ≥50%) to moderate-intensity (30% to 49%) and low-intensity (<30%). Statins reduce LDL-C and non-HDL-C more than reducing apo B (by 30%), triglycerides (by 10% to 20%, depending on baseline levels), and may increase HDL-C (by 1% to 10%). Statins do not reduce Lp(a).[55] Hence, patients who have elevated lipoprotein(a) (>50 mg/dL) may also have lower than expected LDL-C lowering with statins, and it has been recommended that Lp(a)-corrected LDL-C should be assessed at least once in patients with suspected or known high Lp(a), or if the patient shows a poor response to statin therapy.[23,45]

Statins differ in several aspects including their lipophilicity, plasma protein binding, and absorption, and many statins (except for pravastatin, rosuvastatin, and pitavastatin) undergo hepatic metabolism via cytochrome P450 isoenzymes. Concomitant drugs that interfere with the metabolism of statins by inhibiting the cytochrome P-450 3A4 (which metabolizes lovastatin, simvastatin, and atorvastatin) and 2C9 can increase plasma concentrations of statins. Common substances that may interact with statins include amiodarone, antibiotics (e.g., erythromycin, clarithromycin, rifampin), antifungal medications (e.g., azoles), certain antiviral drugs (e.g., lopinavir and ritonavir), grapefruit juice, calcium channel blockers, colchicine, cyclosporine, warfarin, and several others.

Safety, Tolerability, and Monitoring

Statins are generally well tolerated. The starting dose selected depends on the patient's cardiovascular risk, age, polypharmacy, and other clinical characteristics (renal function, liver function, hypothyroidism, prior history or family history of previous statin intolerance or muscle disorders, history of hemorrhagic stroke, Asian ancestry). Statin intolerance affects cardiovascular outcomes adversely. For patients who cannot tolerate daily statin, switching to an alternative appropriate statin with daily dosing (pravastatin, pitavastatin, and fluvastatin may have less muscle toxicity), or lowering the dose to a small dose of a

TABLE 27.7A Current Lipid-Lowering Medications

GENERIC NAME	TRADE NAME	RECOMMENDED DOSE RANGE
Statins		
Atorvastatin	Lipitor	10–80 mg
Fluvastatin	Lescol	20–80 mg
Lovastatin	Mevacor	20–80 mg
Pitavastatin	Livalo	2–4 mg
Pravastatin	Pravachol	10–40 mg
Rosuvastatin	Crestor	10–40 mg
Simvastatin	Zocor	10–80 mg
ATP-Citrate Lyase Inhibitor		
Bempedoic acid	Nexletol	180 mg
PCSK9 Inhibitors		
Evolocumab	Repatha	140 mg every 2 weeks or 420 mg once monthly
Alirocumab	Praluent	75 mg every 2 weeks or 300 mg once monthly
Inclisiran	Leqvio	300 mg twice yearly
Cholesterol Absorption Inhibitor		
Ezetimibe	Zetia (Ezetrol)	10 mg
Bile Acid Absorption Inhibitors		
Cholestyramine	Cholestyramine	Cholestyramine
Colestipol	Colestipol	Colestipol
Colesevelam	Colesevelam	Colesevelam
Fibrates		
Bezafibrate	Bezalip	400 mg
Fenofibrate	Tricor, Trilipix Lipidil (Micro, EZ)	40–200 mg
Gemfibrozil	Lopid	600–1200 mg
Niacin	**Niacin**	**1–3 g**
Nicotinic acid	Niaspan	1–2 g

high-intensity statin every other day or less frequently is usually tolerated and results in considerable LDL-C lowering although outcomes trials have not evaluated this alternate dosing approach.[56]

Before initiation of statin therapy, either a fasting or nonfasting lipid panel should be obtained along with baseline transaminase levels (alanine aminotransferase [ALT]) It is useful to also obtain a history of prior or current muscle symptoms and a baseline creatine kinase (CK) level for reference, especially among individuals at increased risk for adverse muscle events. The 2013 ACC/AHA cholesterol guidelines recommended against routine measurement of CK in all. After initiation of statin therapy, the response should be checked with a repeat lipid panel (fasting or nonfasting) within the first 1 to 3 months to determine the patient's adherence and response. Routine CK or transaminase measurements are not recommended in follow-up, unless the patient has muscle symptoms, fatigue, or symptoms of hepatotoxicity.[52,56] Mildly elevated ALT occurs in less than 2% of patients on statins and is not associated with hepatotoxicity. Clinically relevant ALT elevation is defined as greater than three times upper limit of normal on two consecutive occasions, and progression to liver failure is very rare. Percentage reduction in LDL-C is used in follow-up monitoring of patients to determine response. Follow-up visits, including by telemedicine, may encourage compliance and adherence to diet and lifestyle changes.

Statin side effects include adverse effects on muscle, glucose metabolism, and hemorrhagic stroke.[47,56] The unwanted effects of statins are muscle symptoms (statin-associated muscle symptoms [SAMS]) ranging from diffuse myalgias (normal CK without functional loss), seen in up to 10% to 15% of statin users, to myositis, defined as diffuse muscle pain with evidence of muscle inflammation and elevated CK levels, which necessitate discontinuation of use of these drugs in

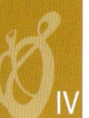

TABLE 27.7B Expected Decrease in Low-Density Lipoprotein Cholesterol in Response to Statins

DRUG	MEAN REDUCTION BY DOSE: % CHANGE FROM BASELINE				
	5 mg	10 mg	20 mg	40 mg	80 mg
Rosuvastatin	−40%	−46%	−52%	−55%	–
Atorvastatin	–	−37%	−43%	−48%	−51%
Simvastatin	−26%	−30%	−38%	−41%	−47%
Lovastatin	–	−21%	−27%	−31%	−40%
Pravastatin	–	−20%	−24%	−30%	−36%
Fluvastatin	–	–	−22%	−25%	−35%
Ezetimibe alone		−20%			
Bile acid sequestrants (Cholestyramine, Colestipol, Colesevelam): add a mean 15% decrease					

Adapted from Grundy SM, Stone NJ, Bailey AL, et al. 2018 AHA/ACC/AACVPR/AAPA/ABC/ACPM/ADA/AGS/APhA/ASPC/NLA/PCNA Guideline on the Management of Blood Cholesterol: A Report of the American College of Cardiology/American Heart Association Task Force on Clinical Practice Guidelines. *J Am Coll Cardiol.* 2019 Jun;73(24):e285–e350; and Mach F, Ray KK, Wiklund O, et al. Adverse effects of statin therapy: perception vs. the evidence—focus on glucose homeostasis, cognitive, renal and hepatic function, haemorrhagic stroke and cataract. *Eur Heart J.* 2018;39(27):2526–2539.

less than 1% of patients. A minority of statin users have increased CK levels, and a causal link with muscle symptoms requires rechallenge. In some cases of statin-associated myositis, a neuromuscular disease is identified (inclusion myositis and myopathies of genetic origin and spinal cord compression). Rarely, statin use associates with rhabdomyolysis. This life-threatening situation often associates with predisposing factors (advanced age, frailty, renal failure, shock, concomitant use of antifungal agents, antibiotics, the fibric acid derivative gemfibrozil, or hypothyroidism).

The use of statins is associated with a small but significant dose-dependent increase in new-onset diabetes of approximately 1 per thousand person-years. Genetic studies suggest that this effect is related to the mechanism of action of statins. Statins hasten the diagnosis almost exclusively in subjects with preexisting risk factors for the development of diabetes, such as baseline elevation of plasma glucose levels, metabolic syndrome/prediabetes, obesity, or family history of diabetes, and the risk is greater with high doses of potent statins. The overwhelming benefits of statins in subjects at high risk for or in the secondary prevention of ASCVD exceeds the small risk for development of diabetes. Nevertheless, statin therapy should accompany a diet and exercise program aimed at achieving a healthy diet and ideal body weight, and glucose should be monitored in statin-treated individuals with risk factors for diabetes.

Statins do not adversely affect cognitive function. Among patients with prior stroke, there has been a concern about a small increased risk of hemorrhagic stroke. However, the overall stroke benefit (from reduction of ischemic stroke) outweighs the small potential risk of hemorrhagic stroke. The Treating Stroke to Target trial was a parallel-group trial conducted among patients with recent ischemic stroke or transient ischemic attack (N = 2860) from France and South Korea assessing a target LDL-C of less than 70 mg/dL versus 90 to 110 mg/dL using statins and/or ezetimibe. The trial was stopped prematurely after 3.5 years due to lack of funding but showed a significant 22% risk reduction in cardiovascular events with the lower LDL-C target, with no increased risk of intracranial hemorrhage.[57]

The cumulative evidence from large-scale clinical outcomes trials supports the concept that reaching a low total cholesterol relates directly to lower cardiovascular risk. Some have expressed concern that low LDL-C could impair health. Several lines of evidence argue against this concern. (1) Most animals have little or no LDL-C and produce LDL particles only when dietary consumption of cholesterol and saturated fats increases. (2) Because of its importance in cellular functions, most (if not all) cell types have the cellular machinery to make cholesterol endogenously. (3) The HDL transport system, via the SR-B1 receptor, delivers cholesterol from hepatic sources to organs. (4) LDL deficiency states in humans, hypobetalipoproteinemia caused by mutations within the *APOB* gene, and loss-of-function mutations within the *PCSK9* gene, do not impair health but markedly reduce life-long cardiovascular events. The Cholesterol Treatment Trialists (CTT) meta-analysis of more than 170,000 patients treated with statins has shown long-term treatment with statins to be safe with low risk of clinically relevant adverse effects and no increase in cancer incidence or noncardiovascular mortality in patients treated to very low LDL-C with statins or nonstatins.[58,59]

Clinical Trials and Cardiovascular Outcomes (see also Chapter 25)

Clinical trials of LDL-lowering therapies across the spectrum of LDL-C have shown a significant relationship between on-treatment LDL-C levels and the reduction in risk of ASCVD events, supporting the principle that "lower is better."[46,59] On average, lowering of LDL-C by 1% corresponds to approximately 1% lower risk of cardiovascular events. Most of these trials have evaluated the effects of statin versus placebo or high- versus low-intensity statin on cardiovascular outcomes (reviewed in previous versions of this chapter and elsewhere). The Cholesterol Treatment Trialists meta-analysis included 27 randomized statin trials (N = 174,149 individuals, 27% women). It found for a 1 mmol/L (39 mg/dL) in LDL-C with statin versus placebo (22 trials), or more versus less intensive statin (5 trials), a 21% reduction in major vascular events over median follow-up of 4.9 years. There were significant risk reductions in all-cause mortality (10%) driven by reduction in vascular mortality (12%), major coronary events (23%), coronary revascularization (24%), and stroke (15%), with no effect on incident cancer or cancer mortality.[8] During the first year of statin treatment, the relative risk benefit was half as large as subsequent years. The relative risk reductions were similar for primary or secondary prevention populations, although individuals from primary prevention had lower absolute risks and hence lower absolute benefits. A Cochrane meta-analysis of 18 randomized trials of statin versus placebo on 56,934 individuals from primary prevention, yielded similar results, with 14% relative risk reduction in all-cause mortality and 25% reduction in vascular events.[60,61]

Use of Statins in Particular Populations

Adults with Diabetes (see also Chapter 31)

Cardiovascular disease is the leading cause of the increased morbidity and mortality in patients with diabetes, and statin therapy is first-line treatment for reducing cardiovascular risk. Data from the Cholesterol Treatment Trialists meta-analysis of statin trials in subjects with diabetes showed a 21% reduction in CVD events and a 9% all-cause mortality benefit in favor of statins. There was similar relative risk reduction among patients with or without diabetes, but since the absolute risk is higher for patients with diabetes, the absolute benefit is greater. The 2019 ACC/AHA guidelines recommend moderate-intensity statin for adults with diabetes age 40 to 75 years, and high intensity statin for adults with diabetes and multiple cardiovascular risk factors or with diabetes-specific risk enhancers (long diabetes duration, albuminuria, eGFR <60 mL/min/1.73 m^2, retinopathy, neuropathy, or ankle-brachial index <0.9).[62]

Older Adults
Elderly patients represent a special challenge; age accounts for most of the attributable cardiovascular risk in patients older than 75 or 80 years, and the predictive value of elevated cholesterol decreases with increasing age. In the Cholesterol Treatment Trialists meta-analysis of 186,854 individuals from 28 trials, a total of 14,483 individuals were older than 75 years at randomization. Over a median follow-up of 4.9 years, statin or more intensive statin reduced vascular events by 21% per 1 mmol/L reduction in LDL-C, with significant reductions in all age groups. Among individuals 70 to 75 years or older at baseline with no prior vascular disease, the relative risk reduction was smaller than those with manifest disease.[62] Starting statins in an otherwise healthy elderly subject requires clinical judgment and shared decision-making. Physicians must nevertheless exercise caution in implementing preventive strategies in older patients already taking multiple medications.

Women (see also Chapters 25 and 91)
Statins are contraindicated in pregnant or nursing women. In the Cholesterol Treatment Trialists meta-analysis of 27 randomized statin trials ($N = 174,149$ individuals, 27% women), statins had similar LDL-C lowering effects and similar relative risk reductions in cardiovascular events in women and men, including significant reduction in all-cause mortality (9% relative risk reduction in women and 10% in men) with no adverse effects on cancer or noncardiovascular mortality in women or men. Women had lower absolute risk for cardiovascular events compared with men, and hence a lower absolute benefit. But after adjusting for clinical differences, women and men with similar cardiovascular risk had similar benefit.[8]

Race and Ethnicity (see also Chapter 93)
Even though most studies under-represent nonwhite ethnic groups, current data provide no reason to think that lipid-lowering therapy will not reduce cardiovascular risk in various ethnic groups. The MEGA study included Japanese men and women. JUPITER included more than 4400 black or Hispanic individuals and showed no heterogeneity in response to statin therapy in comparison to white individuals. The Health Outcomes and Population Evaluation-3 (HOPE-3) study randomized 12,705 participants in 21 countries at intermediate risk of ASCVD to rosuvastatin 10 mg per day or placebo, resulting in 24% relative risk reductions in vascular events, with similar results by race and ethnicity.[63]

Advanced Heart Failure and Chronic Kidney Disease (see Chapter 101)
Statin therapy does not reduce cardiovascular morbidity or mortality in patients with advanced heart failure of ischemic or nonischemic cause. Among patients with chronic kidney disease, statin-related reductions in major vascular events became smaller with lower renal function. In the Cholesterol Treatment Trialists meta-analysis of 28 trials of patients with varying degrees of renal impairment, statins reduced cardiovascular risk among patients with mild to moderate chronic kidney disease (estimated glomerular filtration rate ≥30 mL/min per 1.73 m²), with smaller benefit among patients with more advanced renal failure, regardless of the level of cardiovascular risk. There was no benefit for patients with end-stage renal disease undergoing dialysis, despite these patients having very high risk for cardiovascular events and mortality.[54] Renal disease is a risk factor for statin-related myopathy, in particular with high statin doses, and clinical judgment must carefully weigh the benefits of such preventive measures in these patients.

Pro-Protein Convertase Subtilisin/Kexin Type 9 Inhibitors
Mechanisms of Action
In 2003, gain-of-function mutations in the PCSK9 gene were identified as causing autosomal dominant FH and early-onset coronary heart disease, present in approximately 1% of FH patients. PCSK9 is a protein that regulates the surface expression of the LDL-R on the hepatocyte (see Fig. 27.3). Elevated concentration or function of PCSK9 reduces LDL-R expression by binding to it and promoting lysosomal degradation of the LDL-R, resulting in higher circulating LDL. On the other hand, lower PCSK9 concentration or function increases the LDL-R expression and results in lower circulating LDL. PCSK9 also inhibits intracellular degradation of apo B, the main apolipoprotein on LDL and VLDL particles.

Inhibiting PCSK9 currently requires subcutaneous injection with either monoclonal antibodies (every two weeks or monthly) or with a small interfering RNA (every 3 to 6 months). Evolocumab and alirocumab are fully human monoclonal antibodies approved for clinical use based on clinical outcomes data. Alternatively, a liver-targeted small interfering (si) RNA (inclisiran) inhibits synthesis of PCSK9 by inhibiting the messenger RNA for PCSK9.[64] This RNA interference approach is appealing from a clinical standpoint as it requires infrequent dosing (twice a year), a strategy that is being evaluated in an outcomes trial (ORION-4) of 15,000 patients with known cardiovascular disease.

Effects on Lipids
The monoclonal antibodies (evolocumab [Repatha], and alirocumab [Praluent]) have demonstrated potent LDL-C-lowering capacity (50% to 60%), regardless of background therapy, in a wide variety of patients, including those on statins and statin-intolerant patients, as long as patients express LDL-R in the liver (including heterozygous FH), with less LDL-C lowering among homozygote FH with residual LDL-R expression.[52] They also moderately lower triglycerides (by approximately 25%) and may increase HDL-C. Unlike statins, they reduce Lp(a) levels by 25% to 30% through unclear mechanisms that may be contributing in part to their cardiovascular benefit. The siRNA inclisiran also lowered LDL-C and non-HDL-C in a dose-response manner by up to 50%, apo B (by 20% to 40%), with variable effects on lowering triglycerides and Lp(a).

Safety, Tolerability, and Monitoring
PCSK9 inhibition with the monoclonal antibodies (evolocumab or alirocumab) or RNA interference (inclisiran) is generally well-tolerated. Common side effects (approximately 5%) from the monoclonal antibodies include injection site reactions and flu-like symptoms; and injection site reactions are also seen with inclisiran. Autoantibodies have been rarely reported with the fully human monoclonal antibodies. In some earlier studies, there were reports of neurocognitive effects. Subsequently, the EBBINGHAUS trial examined the effect of evolocumab on cognitive function, tested formally in 1204 patients enrolled in FOURIER. After a mean follow-up of 20 months, there was no evidence of increased risk of cognitive events in patients treated with evolocumab, compared with placebo, including those who reached a very low LDL-C (<25 mg/dL, 0.7 mmol/L). Genetic studies suggested that PCSK9 inhibition, similar to statin therapy, may also result in increased risk for diabetes. Results so far from the randomized trials have shown no increased risk, at least during the duration of these trials. Loss-of-function mutations within the *PCSK9* gene associate with normal health and a marked reduction in life-long cardiovascular events. It is not clear yet if there are long-term safety concerns for blocking the intracellular PCSK9 pathway with the siRNA, and longer follow-up data is needed. For monitoring, lipids should be measured prior to initiation and 1 to 2 months after initiation of dose titration.

Clinical Outcomes Trials with Monoclonal Antibodies
Four outcome trials have evaluated safety and efficacy of monoclonal antibody inhibition in patients at high risk for cardiovascular disease. Two trials evaluating fully human antibodies (FOURIER: evolocumab, and ODYSSEY Outcomes: alirocumab) both showed similar 15% relative reductions in risk of cardiovascular events when added to statins ± ezetimibe, while the two other trials (SPIRE I and II, evaluating bococizumab, a monoclonal antibody that is not fully human) were stopped early due to development of high rates of antidrug neutralizing antibodies and attenuated LDL-C lowering. The FOURIER trial tested evolocumab (140 mg every 2 weeks or 420 mg monthly subcutaneously) versus placebo in 27,564 patients with cardiovascular disease plus additional risk factors on maximal statin ± ezetimibe

with starting LDL-C ≥70 mg/dL 1.8 mmol/L), or non-HDL-C ≥100 mg/dL (2.6 mmol/L).[65] The ODYSSEY Outcomes trial examined cardiovascular outcomes in 18,924 patients post–acute coronary syndrome treated with alirocumab versus placebo on top of baseline statin and LDL-C ≥70 mg/dL (1.8 mmol/L), non-HDL-C ≥100 mg/dL (2.6 mmol/L) or apoB ≥80 mg/dL. In an exploratory analysis, ODYSSEY Outcomes showed reduction in all-cause death (without reduction in cardiovascular death), while FOURIER did not find reduction in all-cause or cardiovascular death.[66]

In a meta-analysis of 66,478 patients from randomized trials (mean follow-up 2.3 years) evaluating alirocumab or evolocumab versus placebo or other lipid-lowering therapies, there was about 20% risk reduction in myocardial infarction and ischemic stroke with no significant reduction in all-cause or cardiovascular mortality and no significant increase in neurocognitive events, liver enzymes or new-onset diabetes.[67] In another meta-analysis of trials examining LDL-C lowering with statin or nonstatin therapies (including FOURIER with evolocumab, IMPROVE-IT with ezetimibe, and the REVEAL trial of the CETP inhibitor anacetrapib) of patients with starting LDL-C of 70 mg/dL (1.8 mmol/L), similar risk reductions (approximately 20% relative risk reduction per 1 mmol/L) in cardiovascular events were seen for statins or nonstatins, with similar results when ODYSSEY Outcomes was included.[67] There was no also increased risk of diabetes, myopathy, or cancer with nonstatin therapy versus control.[58]

Clinical Recommendations

Evolocumab and alirocumab have received approval for patients with established clinical ASCVD or FH and whose LDL-C remains above target despite maximally tolerated statin dosing ± ezetimibe. Approval is anticipated for inclisiran for LDL-C reduction before completion of the clinical outcomes ORION-4 trial based on its safety profile and efficacy in reducing LDL-C including among patients with heterozygous FH.

The 2018 ACC/AHA cholesterol guidelines state that it is reasonable to add PCSK9 inhibitors for patients on maximal statin and ezetimibe with elevated LDL-C (≥70 mg/dL, 1.8 mmol/L) or non-HDL-C (≥100 mg/dL, 2.6 mmol/L).[46,52] The 2019 European guidelines recommend combination therapy of statin with PCSK9 inhibitors for secondary prevention in patients at very high risk or for very–high-risk FH patients (with ASCVD or another major risk factor) not achieving their goals on maximum tolerated statin plus ezetimibe.[52] Nonetheless, costs have limited the access and widespread clinical use of PCSK9 inhibitors, even as prices have continued to decline. The use of PCSK9 inhibitors for secondary prevention of cardiovascular disease (in particular for nonfatal events) or for primary prevention among heterozygous FH patients on top of statin/ezetimibe requires a shared decision-making approach that takes into account the patient's absolute risk, the potential for improved clinical outcomes, and cost-effectiveness.

In statin-intolerant patients, evolocumab proved superior to ezetimibe in the carefully designed GAUSS-3 study. In GAUSS-3, only patients with statin intolerance who did not tolerate atorvastatin 20 mg, were randomized to ezetimibe or evolocumab. The mean percent LDL-C change on ezetimibe was −16.7% (95% CI, −20.5% to −12.9%), and −54.5% (95% CI, −57.2% to −51.8) on evolocumab ($P = 0.001$). Similar findings were reported in the ODYSSEY ALTERNATIVE randomized trial with alirocumab.

Ezetimibe

Ezetimibe inhibits cholesterol absorption via the Niemann-Pick C1-like protein 1 (NPC1L1). By reducing the amount of cholesterol that is delivered to the liver, the liver upregulates LDLR expression resulting in increased clearance of LDL from the circulation.[52] Ezetimibe monotherapy lowers LDL-C up to 20%, while ezetimibe added to statin reduces LDL-C by an additional 15% to 20%. Adding ezetimibe to statin did not result in increased elevations of CK levels or muscle adverse events compared with statin alone, and life-threatening liver failure is very rare. In the Improved Reduction of Outcomes: Vytorin Efficacy International Trial (IMPROVE-IT) of 18,144 patients after a recent acute coronary syndrome with baseline LDL-C levels of 50 to 125 mg/dL (1.3 to 3.2 mmol/L), adding ezetimibe 10 mg/day to statin therapy resulted in additional benefit of 6.4% relative risk reduction in ASCVD events (including coronary and stroke events) during a 7-year follow-up period. The median on-treatment LDL-C levels during the study was 54 mg/dL (1.4 mmol/L) in the combination group and 70 mg/dL (1.8 mmol/L) in the statin-only group.

Fibric Acid Derivatives (Fibrates)

Gemfibrozil (Lopid) lowers triglycerides but cannot be combined safely with statins due to a drug-drug interaction and has limited utility in current practice. Fenofibrate (TriCor, Trilipix, Lipidil Micro, Lipidil EZ) has a new formulation that is available to vary the dose from 40 mg (especially in patients with renal failure) to 267 mg/day. The US Food and Drug Administration (FDA) took the unusual step of withdrawing approval for fenofibric acid with statins to treat high cholesterol, citing a lack of cardiovascular benefit. Outside the United States, ciprofibrate (Lypanthyl, Lipanor), clofibrate (Atromid), and bezafibrate (Bezalip) are available.

Fibrates interact with the nuclear transcription factor PPAR-α, which regulates transcription of the LPL, apo C-III, and apoA-I genes. Side effects of fibrates include cutaneous manifestations, gastrointestinal effects (abdominal discomfort, increased bile lithogenicity), erectile dysfunction, elevated transaminase levels, interaction with oral anticoagulants, and elevated plasma homocysteine, especially with fenofibrate, and, to a lesser extent, with bezafibrate. Because fibrates increase LPL activity, LDL-C levels may rise in patients with hypertriglyceridemia treated with this class of medications. Fibrates, especially gemfibrozil, can inhibit the glucuronidation of statins and thus retard their elimination. Gemfibrozil combined with statins can increase the risk for myotoxicity, rendering this combination contraindicated. The clinical usefulness of fibrates is not well established, particularly in view of failure of the FIELD and ACCORD trials to achieve their primary endpoints. Subgroup analyses suggest a benefit of some fibrates in individuals with baseline high triglyceride levels, but no large endpoint study has tested this conjecture rigorously. Some advocate their use in very high-risk subjects such as diabetic patients with CVD and patients with renal failure.

Even though the overall effect of fibrates is neutral on cardiovascular mortality, subgroup analysis suggests that fibrates might be indicated in high-risk subjects with residual cardiovascular risk characterized by elevated triglyceride levels, reduced HDL-C, and elevated non–HDL-C who are receiving statin therapy. A clinical trial underway with a selective PPAR-α modulator (SPPARM-α), pemafibrate, targets residual cardiovascular risk remaining after treatment to reduce LDL-C in individuals with the type 2 diabetes mellitus and dyslipidemia.[68] The PROMINENT trial will randomize approximately 10,000 participants with type 2 diabetes, hypertriglyceridemia (TG: 200 to 499 mg/dL; 2.26 to 5.64 mmol/l) and low HDL-C (≤40 mg/dL; 1.03 mmol/L) to either pemafibrate (0.2 mg twice daily) or placebo. The average expected follow-up period will be 3.75 years. Participants must be receiving either moderate-to-high intensity statin therapy or meet specified LDL-C criteria. The study population is 1/3 primary and 2/3 secondary prevention (established ASCVD). The primary endpoint is a composite of nonfatal MI, nonfatal ischemic stroke, hospitalization for unstable angina requiring urgent coronary revascularization, and CV death.[69]

Another consideration with the use of fibrates is the theoretical prevention of pancreatitis in patients with severe hypertriglyceridemia (>11 mmol/L; 1000 mg/dL). Yet fibrates have little usefulness in LPL-deficient patients with hyperchylomicronemia. Lifestyle changes, including a marked reduction in fats, especially saturated fats, tight control of glycemia in diabetics, avoidance of alcohol, frequent small meals during the acute phase of a severe episode of hypertriglyceridemia, fish oil consumption, and avoidance of estrogens in women remain the fundamentals of prevention of pancreatitis in hypertriglyceridemic individuals.

Nicotinic Acid (Niacin)

Niacin increases HDL-C and lowers triglyceride levels but has more modest effects on LDL levels. Niacin requires doses in the range of 2000 to 3000 mg/day in three separate doses to maximize effects on lipid levels. An escalating dose schedule to reach the full dose in 2 to 3 weeks rather than starting with the full dose can help manage the adverse effects of this agent. Slow-release forms of niacin, including Niaspan (1 to 2 g/day), decrease the side effect profile of the drug. Daily aspirin intake can attenuate skin flushing, as does the prostaglandin D_2 receptor (DP1) antagonist laropiprant. Niacin decreases the hepatic secretion of VLDL and reduces FFA mobilization in the periphery. Side effects of niacin include flushing, hyperuricemia, hyperglycemia, hepatotoxicity, dysglycemia, bleeding, acanthosis nigricans, and gastritis. Recent clinical trials do not support the ability of niacin therapy to improve cardiovascular outcomes in patients receiving statins. As is the case for fibrates, the FDA withdrew approval for the combination of niacin with statins to treat high cholesterol, citing a lack of cardiovascular benefit.

Bile Acid–Binding Resins

Bile acid–binding resins interrupt the enterohepatic circulation of bile acids by inhibiting their reabsorption in the intestine (the site of reabsorption of more than 90% of bile acids). Currently, their main use is adjunctive therapy in patients with severe hypercholesterolemia secondary to increased LDL-C. Because bile acid–binding resins are not absorbed systemically (they remain in the intestine and are eliminated in stool), they are considered safe in children and in pregnant women. Cholestyramine (Questran) is used in 4-g unit doses as a powder, and colestipol (Colestid) is used in 5-g unit doses. Effective doses range from 2 to 6-unit doses/day, always taken with meals. The most important side effects are predominantly gastrointestinal: constipation, a sensation of fullness, and gastrointestinal discomfort. These drugs can cause hypertriglyceridemia. Decreased absorption of concomitantly administered drugs dictates careful scheduling of other medications 1 hour before or 4 hours after the patient takes bile acid–binding resins. Bile acid–binding resins can be used in combination with statins and/or cholesterol absorption inhibitors in cases of severe hypercholesterolemia.

Colesevelam is a bioengineered bile acid–binding resin that has roughly twice the capacity to bind cholesterol as cholestyramine does. In doses of 1.875 to 3.75 g/day, it can be a useful third-line therapy for patients not meeting their LDL-C targets or in whom the side effects of statins preclude their optimal use. Colesevelam can also decrease HbA1c, thus making this drug a potentially useful adjunct in the treatment of complicated diabetic patients. Even though relatively few drug-drug interactions have been reported with colesevelam, prudence still warrants a careful dosage schedule (4 hours), which makes the use of all bile acid–binding resins cumbersome in patients taking multiple medications.

Fish Oils and Pure Eicosapentaenoic Acid

Fish oils are rich in PUFAs and found in plants and marine oils. In the United States, there are currently several prescription n-3 treatments approved for treating hypertriglyceridemia, with various amounts, ratios, and bioavailability of EPA and DHA.[70] For over the counter fish oil supplements, the typical pill content is 180 mg for EPA and 120 mg for DHA, and the analytical content of EPA and DHA was found to be mostly consistent with the labeled amounts.[70] Absorption of n-3 fatty acids (in particular for ethyl esters) is improved by dietary fat. The dose-response curve for many favorable nonlipid n-3 fatty acid effects appears to plateau at n-3 doses of 0.5 to 1 g/day, including lowering heart rate, blood pressure, and arrhythmias, while other clinical effects such as triglyceride lowering or antithrombotic effects may require higher doses. The triglyceride-lowering response to fish oils depends on the dose, with up 10 g/day of EPA or DHA being required for maximal reduction of plasma triglycerides. Fish oils may raise LDL-C levels and have variable effects on HDL-C.

Multiple randomized trials have evaluated n-3 treatments in a variety of patient populations and found inconsistent results, which may be related to differences in cardiovascular risk (low vs. high), the specific formulation for the interventions, dose, presence or type of placebo, background diet, or clinical outcomes. With the exception of the VITamin D and OmegA-3 TriaL that was conducted in a generally older primary prevention US population at usual risk,[71] other trials were conducted in patients from secondary prevention or at high cardiovascular risk based on risk factors. Many of the trials conducted in secondary prevention or high cardiovascular risk populations did not find benefit for reducing risk of cardiovascular disease, but several of these trials found benefit.[70] Two early open-label trials found significant reductions in coronary events, specifically the Italian GISSI (Gruppo Italiano per lo Studio della Streptochinasi nell'Infarto) which tested 3.5 years of EPA+DHA (1 g/day) in 11,324 post recent myocardial infarction patients, and the Japanese JELIS (the Japan EPA Lipid Intervention Study), which tested 4.6 years of a purified EPA (1.8 g/day; containing 900 mg highly purified EPA ethyl ester) in 18,645 patients with hypercholesterolemia (approximately 20% secondary prevention) on top of statin treatment versus statin alone. Of the subsequent placebo-controlled secondary prevention trials, only two trials found significant cardiovascular benefit, namely the GISSI-Heart Failure of EPA+DHA (1 g/day) in chronic heart failure (NYHA II-IV, most with reduced ejection fraction), and REDUCE-IT (The Reduction of Cardiovascular Events with Icosapent Ethyl–Intervention Trial) trial which tested another highly purified EPA, icosapent ethyl (4 g/day) in 8,179 statin-treated patients with hypertriglyceridemia and either prior cardiovascular disease (approximately 70%) or diabetes plus other risk factors.[72] With the exception of REDUCE-IT which found benefit for both coronary and ischemic stroke events, none of the other trials found reduction in ischemic stroke, and benefit, if any, was mostly due to reductions in fatal coronary events.

Most meta-analyses conducted before 2019 that evaluated n-3 fatty acid supplementation found modest or no benefit for coronary death, and no benefit for stroke or major cardiovascular events. A 2018 meta-analysis from the Omega-3 Treatment Trialists' Collaboration from 10 n-3 fatty acid randomized trials (EPA dose ranged from 226 to 1800 mg/day; 9 trials tested combined EPA+DHA) conducted in high-risk populations (n = 77,917 individuals; 12,001 vascular events) and found no significant reduction in major cardiovascular or coronary events, with a trend toward 7% relative risk reduction in coronary deaths.[73]

In 2018, ASCEND (A Study of Cardiovascular Events in Diabetes) reported results of supplementation with 1 g/day fish oil capsule (840 mg EPA+DHA, same ratio and formulation as used in the VITAL trial) versus placebo in 15,480 UK patients with diabetes and no clinical evidence of cardiovascular disease.[74] There was no n-3 treatment-related reduction in the primary composite vascular endpoint over a 7.4-year follow-up period, although there was a significant reduction in vascular death (19%) driven by lower coronary death, with no reduction in stroke or stroke death. In a higher risk patient population than ASCEND, the REDUCE-IT trial examined a higher risk patient population of statin-treated patients (N = 8,179; 90% white), with elevated triglycerides (median baseline triglycerides 216 mg/dL [2.44 mmol/L], LDL cholesterol 75 mg/dL [1.94 mmol/L]) and known cardiovascular disease (70.7% of the study population) or high-risk patients diabetes plus one or more additional cardiovascular risk factors. The trial tested a high dose purified synthetic EPA (icosapent ethyl, [Vascepa] 4 g/day) versus placebo (paraffin, a mineral oil). Over a 5-year follow-up, there was a significant 26% reduction in major cardiovascular events, including significant reductions of 31%, 28%, and 20% in total MI, total stroke, and cardiovascular death, respectively, with significant benefit among patients treated with moderate or high dose statins. In the primary prevention diabetic cohort, there was 12% nonsignificant relative risk reduction in the primary endpoint (vs. 27% in the secondary prevention cohort), p for interaction 0.14. The n-3 intervention arm had more atrial fibrillation (5.3% vs. 3.9%) and a trend toward increased bleeding.

An updated meta-analysis of 30 trials of n-3 supplementation (N > 130,000) that included VITAL and ASCEND, but not REDUCE-IT, reported modest (7%) significant relative risk reductions for myocardial infarction and total coronary events with nonsignificant reduction in cardiovascular mortality and no reduction in stroke.[75] A subsequent meta-analysis of 13 marine n-3 trials (N = 127,477) included VITAL, ASCEND, and REDUCE-I.[76] Analyses that excluded REDUCE-IT found significant relative risk reductions (5% to 8%) in

MI, coronary heart disease, and coronary deaths, and significant reductions (3% to 5%) in total cardiovascular events and death from cardiovascular disease. After including REDUCE-IT the reduction in MI was greater (12% risk reduction), but with evidence of significant heterogeneity. Additional analyses suggested a linear dose-response association with cardiovascular events. Every 1 g/day of marine n-3 treatment corresponded to a 9% lower risk of myocardial infarction and 7% lower risk of total coronary events. There was no significant reduction in stroke risk.

STRENGTH (Statin Residual Risk Reduction With EpaNova in HiGh CV Risk PatienTs With Hypertriglyceridemia) tested a different high-dose purified formulation of n-3 carboxylic acids (Epanova 4 g/day, EPA+DHA, ratio 2.75:1) versus placebo (corn oil). The trial halted early in 2020 for futility in reducing major cardiovascular events in 13,086 patients with hypertriglyceridemia and low HDL cholesterol on maximally tolerated statins and with established atherosclerotic disease or at high cardiovascular risk. It is uncertain if the differences in outcome results for STRENGTH versus REDUCE-IT relate to differences in the n-3 formulations, placebo, the study populations, baseline diet, or other factors. With regards to other endpoints, trials of n-3 FAs have not found benefit for the prevention of recurrent atrial fibrillation or postoperative atrial fibrillation in cardiac surgery patients, nor for prevention of diabetes.[77] Finally, no study has yet compared EPA to DHA head-to-head.

In summary, for secondary prevention or high-risk primary prevention patients, high-dose EPA provides additional cardiovascular benefit among maximally statin-treated patients with high triglycerides and other risk factors. For usual risk primary prevention, it may be reasonable for adults with low fish consumption or among African Americans based on the VITAL trial results. Fish intake ≥2 servings/week should be encouraged for both primary and secondary prevention, in particular as part of an overall healthful diet such as the Mediterranean diet to replace less healthful foods (see also Chapters 25 and 29).

Phytosterols

Phytosterols are derivatives of cholesterol from plants and trees. They interfere with the formation of micelles in the intestine and prevent intestinal absorption of cholesterol. They are available as "nutraceuticals" and are incorporated in soft margarines. Sterols may prove useful for the adjunctive management of lipoprotein disorders. The safety of plant sterols has not been established.

Novel Medications[78]
Bempedoic Acid
A novel compound, bempedoic acid (Nexletol), inhibits ATP citrate lyase, which catalyzes a step in the biosynthesis of cholesterol upstream of HMG-CoA reductase, the target of statins. A randomized, double-blind, placebo-controlled clinical trial involving 779 patients with ASCVD, HeFH, or both and an LDL-C level greater than 70 mg/dL (1.8 mmol/L) despite maximally tolerated lipid-lowering therapy were randomized 2:1 to treatment with bempedoic acid (180 mg) ($n=522$) or placebo ($n=257$) once daily for 52 weeks. The primary end point was percent change from baseline in LDL-C level at week 12. Secondary measures included changes in levels of lipids, lipoproteins, and biomarkers. Bempedoic acid lowered LDL-C levels significantly more than placebo at week 12 (−15.1% vs. 2.4%, respectively; difference, −17.4% [95% CI, −21.0% to −13.9%]; $P < 0.001$). Side effects included a higher incidence of urinary tract infection (5.0% vs. 1.9%), and hyperuricemia (4.2% vs. 1.9%).[79] The CLEAR outcomes trial will determine if treatment with bempedoic acid decreases the risk of cardiovascular events in patients who are statin intolerant. The sample size is approximately 12,600 and study completion is expected in 2022.[80] In the United States, bempedoic acid is approved for the treatment of hypercholesterolemia in combination with diet and the highest tolerated statin therapy in adults with HeFH, or with established ASCVD, who need additional lowering of LDL-C. The EMA recommendation also includes the treatment of non-FH and mixed dyslipidemia, with or without statins or other lipid-lowering medications such as ezetimibe.

Rare diseases: Novel approaches for Homozygous Familial Hypercholesterolemia and Monogenic Chylomicronemia Syndrome

In homozygous FH, and in severe HeFH, several approaches have been approved to reduce LDL-C. Inhibition of MTTP with the small molecule lomitapide reduces LDL-C by approximately 30% to 50%.[81] Another approach is to inhibit apo B mRNA with phosphorothioate-linked antisense oligonucleotides. Mipomersen is the first such compound approved for limited use in patients with homozygous FH. Mipomersen reduces LDL-C by 20% to 30%. Although safety concerns were raised with these compounds, the severity of homozygous FH was deemed to warrant novel therapeutic avenues.[78,82] Inhibition of apo B synthesis and secretion is associated with accumulation of fat in the liver. Because of the small number of patients included in these trials, no outcome data are likely to become available. Nevertheless, the advent of lipoprotein apheresis and novel medication has dramatically increased survival in HoFH patients.[83]

Inhibition of APO CIII.

Apo CIII is an apolipoprotein that inhibits LPL activity, enhances the production and secretion of VLDL from the liver, and blocks the liver uptake of VLDL remnants, among other functions. It is found primarily on chylomicrons and VLDL but can be found on LDL and HDL particles. An anti-sense oligonucleotide (ASO) RNA inhibitor (volanesorsen, IONIS-APOCIIIRx) directed against apo CIII shows promise in the treatment of chylomicronemia syndromes or severe hypertriglyceridemia as it reduces triglycerides by 70% and apo C III by greater than 80%, with no change in LDL-C. Drug-induced thrombocytopenia is a common adverse event. Volanesorsen was conditionally approved in Europe in 2019 (but not in the United States) for monogenic hyperchylomicronemia syndrome as an adjunct to diet. Another ASO RNA inhibitor (AKCEA-APOCIII-LRx, Akcea/Novartis), which is a GalNAC-conjugated (liver targeted) ASO directed against apo CIII, showed 65% triglyceride lowering with no short-term safety signals.[78] Both agents require long-term safety assessment.

Inhibition of Angiopoietin-Like Protein 3 (ANGPTL3)

ANGPTL3 is a protein produced in the liver that regulates lipid metabolism by inhibiting LPL and endothelial lipase but also has LDL-C-lowering effects through possibly nonreceptor mechanisms.[84] An investigational fully human monoclonal anti-ANGPTL3 antibody (evinacumab, Regeneron) acts mainly in the circulation to bind ANGPTL3 and form immune complexes. Evinacumab reduces triglycerides by inhibiting ANGPTL3 which is critical for the clearance of TRLs.[49,85] This augments plasma lipase activity, reducing triglycerides (approximately 50% to 75%), LDL-C and non-HDL-C (approximately 50%), apo B (approximately 37%), and HDL-C, but not lipoprotein(a) or liver triglycerides.[84] ANGPTL3 can also be targeted in the liver with an ASO RNA inhibitor (vupanorsen or AKCEA-ANGPTL3-LRx) which is conjugated to GalNAC and inhibits hepatic production of ANGPTL3, thereby reducing triglycerides by 60% to 80%, and reducing liver triglycerides.[86] No short-term safety signals have been noted, but both agents require long-term safety and efficacy assessment. It is also unclear if both agents would have similar or different effects as the monoclonal antibody acts in the circulation while the conjugated ASO acts in the liver. Possible uses include chylomicronemia syndromes for lowering triglycerides, homozygous FH for lowering LDL-C, or treating hepatic steatosis (the latter only for the ASO).

Inhibition of Lp(a)

The use of a hepatic selective antisense oligonucleotide (AKCEA-APO[a]-L_{Rx}) was tested in patients ($n = 286$) with ASCVD and baseline Lp(a) levels of ≥60 mg% (150 nmol/L; mean baseline level >200 nmol/L) at doses of 20, 40, or 60 mg every 4 weeks; 20 mg every 2 weeks; or 20 mg every week. APO(a)-L_{Rx} resulted in dose-dependent decreases in Lp(a) levels, with mean % decreases of 35% at a dose of 20 mg every 4 weeks, 56% at 40 mg every 4 weeks, 58% at 20 mg every 2 weeks, 72% at 60 mg every 4 weeks, and 80% at 20 mg every week. There were no significant differences between any APO(a)-L_{Rx} dose and placebo with respect to platelet counts, liver and renal measures, or influenza-like symptoms. The most common adverse events were injection-site reactions. PCSK9 inhibitors result in modest reductions in Lp(a) which may contribute to the cardiovascular benefit related to PCSK9 inhibitors; it is not clear yet if there are safety concerns for blocking the intracellular PCSK9 pathway.[41,87] A phase 3 trial Lp(a)HORIZON is determining the effect of this agent on cardiovascular outcomes in over 7000 participants.

Gemcabene is a novel lipid-regulating drug that enhances the clearance of VLDL via the reduction of apoC-III mRNA. In the COBALT-1 study, 8 patients with HoFH were treated with gemcabene in an open-label study for 12 weeks. A decrease in LDL-C of 29% ($P = 0.001$) at the maximal dose of 900 mg per day was observed on top of conventional treatments.[88]

Gene therapy for HoFH was attempted in the 1990s with poor success. A new approach, using adeno-associated virus 8 (AAV8) is now being performed in phase 1 to 2 studies, and offers promise for long-term treatment.[89] However, increasing the expression of the membrane protein LDLR to a level sufficient to normalize LDL-C levels may be challenging given the number of hepatocytes required to be transduced via AAV gene therapy. It can be hypothesized that even a small increase in LDLR activity would lessen the severity of disease course in HoFH and potentially increase response to other therapies.[90] Gene editing technologies using CRISPR are under investigation as a method for targeting PCSK9.

CLINICAL APPROACH TO THE TREATMENT OF LIPOPROTEIN DISORDERS

Lifestyle Changes: Diet (see also Chapters 25, 29, and 30)

Diet was the leading risk factor for causes of death in the United States and has important impact on risk of coronary heart disease, stroke, neurocognitive health, hypertensive disorders, diabetes, lipids, obesity, and many cancers.[3] Many countries are in the midst of an obesity epidemic, and projected estimates are grim if current patterns continue. Diet accounted for more than half a million US deaths in 2016 alone, with the vast majority of these deaths due to cardiovascular disease. Only a few percent of US adults meet optimal dietary recommendations.[91] Modifying the diet to a healthier one, in a sustainable way, is a key component of improved long-term individual and population risk for cardiovascular and other chronic diseases.

While older guidelines had limits on dietary cholesterol (usually to <300 mg/day), recent guidelines do not recommend specific limits and avoid explicit guidance on dietary cholesterol, instead recommending one of a number of heart-healthy dietary patterns (Mediterranean-style pattern, DASH diet, or a healthy vegetarian diet).[46,52] These healthful dietary patterns emphasize fruits, vegetables, legumes, nuts, and whole grains, and are low in sodium, saturated fats, and refined carbohydrates. These diets typically contain less than 300 mg/day cholesterol, consistent with the typical US mean cholesterol daily intake. The Mediterranean diet is not a low-fat diet but has moderate intake of fat; however, the fats are mostly unsaturated (monounsaturated [extra virgin olive oil] or polyunsaturated).

Observational data does not show a strong or consistent association between dietary cholesterol and serum cholesterol, and the association often becomes null after adjusting for total caloric intake.[92] A meta-analysis of 40 studies found no significant association between dietary cholesterol and risk of coronary disease or stroke, although studies were heterogeneous.[93] In the 17 intervention trials included in the meta-analysis, there was a significant but modest positive association between dietary cholesterol and total cholesterol (+11 mg/dL), LDL-C (+7 mg/dL), and HDL-C (+3 mg/dL). Most foods contributing cholesterol to the diet also are high in or are consumed together with foods high in saturated fats, and replacing saturated fat with unsaturated fat may reduce LDL-C more than reducing dietary cholesterol alone. In an updated meta-regression analysis of controlled feeding intervention studies with similar ratio of polyunsaturated to saturated fats in the comparison diets, there remained a significant modest increase in total cholesterol with higher dietary cholesterol, but this effect was small.[92,94,95] Likewise, there is no consistent association for egg consumption with risk of coronary events or stroke. A recent meta-analysis of six US cohorts found positive association for both dietary cholesterol and egg consumption with cardiovascular disease risk. There was 17% higher risk for each 300 mg/day higher cholesterol intake, with 6% higher risk for each additional half-egg per day, but after adjustment for dietary cholesterol the association of egg intake with cardiovascular disease was no longer significant.[96] In another recent meta-analysis of greater than 400,000 European adults, a significant negative association (7% lower risk per 20 g/day) was noted for eggs with ischemic heart disease, which became nonsignificant after excluding the first 4 years of follow-up. However, there was a positive association for intake of red and processed meat with heart disease risk and with higher non-HDL-C and blood pressure.[94]

Individuals with dyslipoproteinemias, particularly those with diabetes or heart failure, should always adopt a healthful diet. For individuals with hypercholesterolemia, the National Lipid Association (NLA) recommends limiting dietary cholesterol intake to less than 200 mg/day to lower LDL-C and non-HDL-C, recognizing that there may be hypo- and hyper-responders. The 2013 AHA/ACC Lifestyle guidelines recommends that saturated fat intake should be less than 6% of energy intake. The 2019 AHA/ACC Prevention guideline recommends replacing dietary saturated fat with polyunsaturated or monounsaturated fat (but not with carbohydrates). High-risk subjects should have medications started concomitantly with a diet because in many cases, diet may not suffice to reach target levels. The diet should have three objectives. First, it should allow the patient to reach and maintain ideal body weight. Second, it should provide a well-balanced diet with fruits, vegetables, and whole grains, and third, it should be restricted in sodium, saturated fats, and refined carbohydrates. Dietary counseling should involve a professional dietitian. Frequently, the help of dietitians, weight loss programs, or diabetic outpatient centers can aid in achieving sustained weight loss.

Treatment of Combined Lipoprotein Disorders

Combined lipoprotein disorders, characterized by an increase in plasma total cholesterol and triglycerides, frequently occur in clinical practice and present difficult challenges. Patients with combined lipoprotein disorders have an increase in LDL-C and LDL particle number (as reflected by an increase in total or LDL apo B or non–HDL-C), small dense LDL particles, increased VLDL-C and VLDL triglycerides, and a reduced HDL-C level. The search for correctable causes (e.g., uncontrolled diabetes, obesity, hypothyroidism, and alcohol use) of combined dyslipoproteinemia and the benefit of lifestyle modifications require reemphasis (see Table 27.6). Patients with this pattern of combined dyslipoproteinemia often have obesity and metabolic syndrome. One in three US adults have metabolic syndrome, and the rates are increasing as the levels of overweight and obesity rise. Treatment should begin with lifestyle modification, which is the cornerstone of treatment, as it can improve about half of the deviation in lipid parameters. Lifestyle changes consist of dietary modification (in particular net caloric intake), reducing alcohol intake, smoking cessation, increasing habitual physical activity, and weight reduction.[51,53] Diet should be reduced in total calories and saturated fats, reduced dietary carbohydrates (particularly refined carbohydrates), replacing saturated fats with mono- or polyunsaturated fats, and increasing dietary fiber. Dietary fructose in particular increases triglycerides in a dose-dependent manner and should be avoided (e.g., sucrose). In individuals with hypertriglyceridemia, abstinence from alcohol could reduce triglycerides by up to 80%.[51] Weight loss reduces triglycerides by approximately 0.1 mmol/L (8 mg/dL) per kg of weight loss, while regular aerobic exercise and n-3 supplements reduce triglycerides by 10% to 20% (higher with higher doses of n-3).[51] Often, the help of dietitians, weight loss programs, or diabetic outpatient centers considerably aid management.

Drug treatment, when warranted, aims to correct the predominant lipoprotein abnormality. Statins, ezetimibe, and PCSK9 inhibitors have modest triglyceride-lowering effects (approximately 15% to 20%), with greater triglyceride lowering for fibrates and high-dose n-3 fatty acids

(at least 25% to 45%).[51] The 2018 AHA/ACC cholesterol guidelines and the 2019 AHA/ACC prevention guidelines consider metabolic syndrome as a risk enhancing factor for ASCVD that should prompt statin initiation or intensification. Statins can reduce plasma triglyceride levels, particularly in individuals with high baseline levels. The results of IMPROVE-IT support the combined use of a statin and ezetimibe. Fibrates can reduce triglycerides by up to 70% and may change the composition of LDL to larger and less dense particles. The combination of a statin with a fibrate, however, has proved effective in correcting the laboratory abnormalities that characterize the combined dyslipoproteinemias, but as noted earlier, currently available clinical trials have not established that this approach prevents cardiovascular events. In view of the effects of gemfibrozil on glucuronidation of statins, we advise against use of gemfibrozil in combination with statins. Patients taking a fibrate plus a statin merit close medical follow-up for evidence of hepatotoxicity or myositis within the first 6 weeks of therapy and every 6 months thereafter. The use of other combinations, including fibric acid derivatives with bile acid–binding resins or niacin lacks support from outcome trials, regulatory agencies, and requires care because of the risk of adverse effects such as hepatotoxicity and myositis. High-dose n-3 fatty acids (2 to 4 g/day), in particular with EPA (4 g/day of icosapent ethyl, Vascepa) as was evaluated in the REDUCE-IT trial, reduce triglycerides in a dose-dependent manner, although the cardiovascular benefit in REDUCE-IT appears unrelated to the triglyceride-lowering effects, since benefit was seen regardless of the baseline or on-treatment triglyceride levels. (See also section on Fish Oils and pure Eicosapentaenoic Acid.)

Residual Cardiovascular Risk (see also Chapter 25)

Patients with uncontrolled cardiometabolic risk factors or known ASCVD are at high risk of suffering from future cardiovascular events despite contemporary preventive therapies; this has been termed *residual risk*. Even with recent advances in cardiovascular interventions including statins, dual antiplatelet therapies, revascularization, and other therapies, cardiovascular event rates among patients with known cardiovascular disease remain high, ranging from 3% to 3.5% per year in recent clinical trials[97] and higher in real-world contemporary patient populations. There are also significant racial disparities, with African Americans having higher risk of recurrent events than whites.[91] Older patients with cardiovascular disease also have a high cumulative rate of readmissions and rehospitalizations for recurrent events, which is a substantial burden to patients and the health care system. Furthermore, patients with cardiovascular disease who experience recurrent events have lower quality of life, greater depression and psychosocial stress, and worse cognitive function than patients with first events. These factors impact compliance with medications, lifestyle changes, long-term prognosis, hospital readmissions, and health care costs.

Residual risk is multifactorial. Determinants of increased risk include traditional risk factors (older age, male gender, hypertension, diabetes, smoking, dyslipidemia, greater burden of clinical cardiovascular disease) and nontraditional cardiovascular risk factors (systemic inflammation, elevated Lp(a), remnant cholesterol, thrombosis).[98] Recognizing this, clinical guidelines have moved away from using LDL-C as the major criterion for identifying at-risk patients who would benefit from more intensive therapies, in particular since the benefits of statins and other therapies extend to patients across the spectrum of LDL-C. Instead, guidelines recommend tailoring the intensity of treatment to the patient's risk level, for both primary and secondary prevention. Until recently, secondary prevention strategies (e.g., statins, antiplatelets) were applied across the board to all patients with prior cardiovascular disease. However, with the recent development and approval or pending approval of novel therapeutics that confer benefit but at current high cost (e.g., PCSK9 inhibitors), it is important to estimate risk in patients with cardiovascular disease who would have the greatest absolute net benefit and value from the novel therapies. Hence, recent guidelines recommend risk stratification using a number of clinical risk factors to classify patients into average, high, and very high-risk categories.

Clinical Recommendations for Assessing Residual Risk

The 2018 AHA/ACC cholesterol guidelines recommend risk stratification of patients with cardiovascular disease using a number of clinical risk factors that clinicians could use to identify high and very high-risk patients.[46] (See the online chapter for tables with Guidelines summaries.) Very high-risk patients are those who have had multiple major ASCVD events or one major ASCVD event and multiple high-risk conditions. In 2019, an expert panel from the NLA conducted a systematic review and recommended further risk stratification of patients with ASCVD into extremely high, very high, and high-risk categories, including additional biomarkers and risk factors. For example, the NLA also included risk biomarkers such as CRP, Lp(a), and poorly controlled metabolic risk factors. Patients categorized into the average risk group are those who do not have these risk factors.

FUTURE PERSPECTIVES

The development of novel pharmaceutical agents for the treatment of lipoprotein disorders will probably continue because ASCVD secondary to atherosclerosis represents the largest burden of disease worldwide for the foreseeable future. Novel therapies, such as RNA therapeutics for PCSK9, apoCIII, Lp(a) and ANGPTL3, show promise for the long-term treatment of severe genetic lipoprotein disorders. These new agents will offer personalized medicine based on genotype and phenotype. Better targeting of high-risk individuals will allow optimization of expensive therapies.

Gene Therapy

Severe, homozygous, monogenic disorders may eventually be treated by gene therapy. The initial trials of gene therapy in patients with homozygous FH proved disappointing, Refinement in viral delivery vectors has rekindled interest in disease-specific gene therapy. Especially for HoFH, this approach could prove life-saving for a disease associated with considerable morbidity and premature mortality. Other diseases, such as abetalipoproteinemia, LPL deficiency, Niemann-Pick type C disease, sitosterolemia, and Tangier disease, may become targets for gene therapy. If the approach to correcting these disorders were successful, the more widespread application of gene-based therapies for the purpose of reducing potential cardiovascular risk will become a daunting medical, social, and ethical problem.

Gene editing techniques using the CRISPR/Cas9 system delivered the system by using AAV in a mouse model engineered to carry a human familial hypercholesterolemia null mutation (LdlrE208X). The mice that received the AAV-CRISPR-Cas9 system on a high-fat diet had significantly lower LDL-C levels and reduced aortic atherosclerosis compared to controls. Another potential approach is to correct the genetic defect in induced pluripotent stem cells (iPSCs), which are mature somatic cells that have been genetically reprogrammed into an embryonic-like state that can then differentiate into any other cell type. In a recent study, T cells isolated from a patient with HoFH were reprogrammed into iPSCs. After editing with CRISPR-Cas9, immunofluorescence staining found presence of the LDLR in the cell membrane, with improved LDL-C uptake. Such cells showed little immunogenicity and might be suitable for transplantation in the human host.[99]

Societal Changes

Drugs alone will not suffice to prevent and cure atherosclerosis. Societal changes aimed at encouraging healthful lifestyles and public health measures and infrastructure could provide overall, not just cardiovascular health benefits. Public health measures to reduce cigarette smoking have already reduced rates of myocardial infarction. As humanity continues to accommodate more than half the population in cities, organization of neighborhoods into local networks allowing less energy expenditure (rather than conservation via easy access to motorized transportation) will become necessary, especially in affluent countries. Personal changes with respect to food consumption and caloric intake will remain a major challenge. Indeed, the changes in diet and physical activity that have occurred in the past 50 years (now spreading globally) probably contributed to the epidemic of obesity and the increased prevalence of lipoprotein disorders, hypertension, and diabetes, with consequent ASCVD.

GUIDELINES

The Guidelines for Managing Dyslipidemias are presented in the online chapter.

REFERENCES

Lipids and Cardiovascular Risk

1. Collaborators GBDCD. Global, regional, and national age-sex-specific mortality for 282 causes of death in 195 countries and territories, 1980-2017: a systematic analysis for the Global Burden of Disease Study 2017. *Lancet*. 2018;392(10159):1736–1788.
2. GBD-NHLBI-JACC Global Burden of Cardiovascular Diseases Writing Group. Global burden of cardiovascular diseases and risk factors, 1990-2019: update from the GBD 2019 study. *J Am Coll Cardiol*. 2020;76(25):2982–3021.
3. Collaborators USBD, Mokdad AH, Ballestros K, et al. The state of US health, 1990-2016: burden of diseases, injuries, and risk factors among US states. *JAMA*. 2018;319(14):1444–1472.
4. Yusuf S, Joseph P, Rangarajan S, et al. Modifiable risk factors, cardiovascular disease, and mortality in 155 722 individuals from 21 high-income, middle-income, and low-income countries (PURE): a prospective cohort study. *Lancet*. 2020;395(10226):795–808.

Lipids and Lipoproteins

5. Burla B, Arita M, Arita M, et al. MS-based lipidomics of human blood plasma: a community-initiated position paper to develop accepted guidelines. *J Lipid Res*. 2018;59(10):2001–2017.
6. Goldstein JL, Brown MS. A century of cholesterol and coronaries: from plaques to genes to statins. *Cell*. 2015;161(1):161–172.
7. Ference BA, Ginsberg HN, Graham I, et al. Low-density lipoproteins cause atherosclerotic cardiovascular disease. 1. Evidence from genetic, epidemiologic, and clinical studies. A consensus statement from the European Atherosclerosis Society Consensus Panel. *Eur Heart J*. 2017;38(32):2459–2472.
8. Borén J, Chapman MJ, Krauss RM, et al. Low-density lipoproteins cause atherosclerotic cardiovascular disease: pathophysiological, genetic, and therapeutic insights: a consensus statement from the European Atherosclerosis Society Consensus Panel. Eur Heart J. 2020 41(24):2313-2330.
9. O'Donnell, VB Dennis EA, Wakelam MJO, Subramaniam S. Lipid maps: serving the next generation of lipid researchers with tools, resources, data, and training. *Sci Signal*. 2019;12(563).

Lipid Metabolism

10. Mason RP, Libby P, Bhatt DL. Emerging mechanisms of cardiovascular protection for the omega-3 fatty acid eicosapentaenoic acid. *Arterioscler Thromb Vasc Biol*. 2020;40(5):1135–1147.
11. Serhan CN, Levy BD. Resolvins in inflammation: emergence of the pro-resolving superfamily of mediators. *J Clin Invest*. 2018;128(7):2657–2669.
12. Dennis EA, Norris PC. Eicosanoid storm in infection and inflammation. *Nat Rev Immunol*. 2015;15(8):511–523.
13. Chilton FH, Dutta R, Reynolds LM, et al. Precision nutrition and omega-3 polyunsaturated fatty acids: a case for personalized supplementation approaches for the prevention and management of human diseases. *Nutrients*. 2017;9(11).
14. Basu D, Goldberg IJ. Regulation of lipoprotein lipase-mediated lipolysis of triglycerides. *Curr Opin Lipidol*. 2020;31(3):154–160.
15. Li D, Rodia CN, Johnson ZK, et al. Intestinal basolateral lipid substrate transport is linked to chylomicron secretion and is regulated by apoC-III. *J Lipid Res*. 2019;60(9):1503–1515.
16. Dron JS, Hegele RA. Genetics of triglycerides and the risk of atherosclerosis. *Curr Atheroscler Rep*. 2017;19(7):31.
17. Schulz R, Schlüter KD, Laufs U. Molecular and cellular function of the proprotein convertase subtilisin/kexin type 9 (PCSK9). *Basic Res Cardiol*. 2015 Mar;110(2):4.
18. Seidah NG, Abifadel M, Prost S, et al. The proprotein convertases in hypercholesterolemia and cardiovascular diseases: emphasis on proprotein convertase subtilisin/kexin 9. *Pharmacol Rev*. 2017;69(1):33–52.
19. Emerging Risk Factors Collaboration, Di Angelantonio E, Gao P, et al. Lipid-related markers and cardiovascular disease prediction. *JAMA*. 2012;307(23):2499–2506.
20. Rosenson RS, Brewer HB Jr, Barter PJ, et al. HDL and atherosclerotic cardiovascular disease: genetic insights into complex biology. *Nat Rev Cardiol*. 2018;15(1):9–19.
21. Tall AR, Rader DJ. Trials and tribulations of CETP inhibitors. *Circ Res*. 2018;122(1):106–112.
22. Welsh C, Celis-Morales CA, Brown R, et al. Comparison of conventional lipoprotein tests and apolipoproteins in the prediction of cardiovascular disease. *Circulation*. 2019;140(7):542–552.
23. Langlois MR, Chapman MJ, Cobbaert C, et al. European Atherosclerosis Society (EAS) and the European Federation of Clinical Chemistry and Laboratory Medicine (EFLM) joint consensus initiative. Quantifying atherogenic lipoproteins: current and future challenges in the era of personalized medicine and very low concentrations of LDL cholesterol. A consensus statement from EAS and EFLM. *Clin Chem*. 2018;64(7):1006–1103. 9;140(7):553-5.

Lipoprotein Disorders

24. Ruel I, Brisson D, Aljenedil S, et al. Simplified Canadian definition for familial hypercholesterolemia. *Can J Cardiol*. 2018;34(9):1210–1214.
25. Hu P, Dharmayat KI, Stevens CAT, et al. Prevalence of familial hypercholesterolemia among the general population and patients with atherosclerotic cardiovascular disease: a systematic review and meta-analysis. *Circulation*. 2020;141(22):1742–1759.
26. Beheshti SO, Madsen CM, Varbo A, Nordestgaard BG. Worldwide prevalence of familial hypercholesterolemia: meta-analyses of 11 million subjects. *J Am Coll Cardiol*. 2020;75(20):2553–2566.
27. Berberich AJ, Hegele RA. The complex molecular genetics of familial hypercholesterolaemia. *Nat Rev Cardiol*. 2019;16(1):9–20.
28. Khera AV, Won HH, Peloso GM, et al. Diagnostic yield and clinical utility of sequencing familial hypercholesterolemia genes in patients with severe hypercholesterolemia. *J Am Coll Cardiol*. 2016;67(22):2578–2589.
29. Abul-Husn NS, Manickam K, Jones LK, et al. Genetic identification of familial hypercholesterolemia within a single U.S. health care system. *Science*. 2016;354(6319).
30. Khera AV, Won H-H, Peloso GM, et al. Diagnostic yield of sequencing familial hypercholesterolemia genes in patients with severe hypercholesterolemia. *J Am Coll Cardiol*. 2016.
31. Sturm AC, Knowles JW, Gidding SS, et al. Clinical genetic testing for familial hypercholesterolemia: JACC scientific expert panel. *J Am Coll Cardiol*. 2018;72(6):662–680.
32. Nordestgaard BG, Chapman MJ, Humphries SE, et al. Familial hypercholesterolaemia is underdiagnosed and undertreated in the general population: guidance for clinicians to prevent coronary heart disease: consensus statement of the European Atherosclerosis Society. *Eur Heart J*. 2013;34(45):3478–3490a.
33. Lee S, Akioyamen LE, Aljenedil S, et al. Genetic testing for familial hypercholesterolemia: impact on diagnosis, treatment and cardiovascular risk. *Eur J Prev Cardiol*. 2019;26(12):1262–1270.
34. Trinder M, Francis GA, Brunham LR. Association of monogenic vs polygenic hypercholesterolemia with risk of atherosclerotic cardiovascular disease. *JAMA Cardiol*. 2020.
35. Marduel M, Ouguerram K, Serre V, et al. Description of a large family with autosomal dominant hypercholesterolemia associated with the APOE p.Leu167del mutation. *Hum Mutat*. 2013;34(1):83–87.
36. Awan Z, Choi HY, Stitziel N, et al. APOE p.Leu167del mutation in familial hypercholesterolemia. *Atherosclerosis*. 2013;231(2):218–222.
37. Loaiza N, Hartgers ML, Reeskamp LF, et al. Taking one step back in familial hypercholesterolemia: STAP1 does not alter plasma LDL (Low-Density Lipoprotein) cholesterol in mice and humans. *Arterioscler Thromb Vasc Biol*. 2020;40(4):973–985.
38. Mymin D, Salen G, Triggs-Raine B, et al. The natural history of phytosterolemia: observations on its homeostasis. *Atherosclerosis*. 2018;269:122–128.
39. Burgess S, Ference BA, Staley JR, et al. Association of LPA variants with risk of coronary disease and the implications for lipoprotein(a)-lowering therapies: a mendelian randomization analysis. *JAMA Cardiol*. 2018;3(7):619–627.
40. Nordestgaard BG, Chapman MJ, Ray K, et al. Lipoprotein(a) as a cardiovascular risk factor: current status. *Eur Heart J*. 2010;31(23):2844–2853.
41. Tsimikas S, Karwatowska-Prokopczuk E, Gouni-Berthold I, et al. Lipoprotein(a) reduction in persons with cardiovascular disease. *N Engl J Med*. 2020;382(3):244–255.
42. Ference BA, Bhatt DL, Catapano AL, et al. Association of genetic variants related to combined exposure to lower low-density lipoproteins and lower systolic blood pressure with lifetime risk of cardiovascular disease. *J Am Med Assoc*. 2019.
43. Lewis GF, Xiao C, Hegele RA. Hypertriglyceridemia in the genomic era: a new paradigm. *Endocr Rev*. 2015;36(1):131–147.
44. Nordestgaard BG, Langsted A, Mora S, et al. Fasting is not routinely required for determination of a lipid profile: clinical and laboratory implications including flagging at desirable concentration cut-points-a joint consensus statement from the European Atherosclerosis Society and European Federation of Clinical Chemistry and Laboratory Medicine. *Eur Heart J*. 2016;37(25):1944–1958.
45. Sniderman AD, Thanassoulis G, Glavinovic T, et al. Apolipoprotein B particles and cardiovascular disease: a narrative review. *JAMA Cardiol*. 2019 Dec 1;4(12):1287–1295.

Management of Lipid Risk

46. Grundy SM, Stone NJ, Bailey AL, et al. 2018 AHA/ACC/AACVPR/AAPA/ABC/ACPM/ADA/AGS/APhA/ASPC/NLA/PCNA guideline on the management of blood cholesterol: a report of the American College of Cardiology/American Heart Association task force on clinical practice guidelines. *Circulation*. 2019;139(25):e1082–e1143.
47. Mach F, Ray KK, Wiklund O, et al. Adverse effects of statin therapy: perception vs. the evidence - focus on glucose homeostasis, cognitive, renal and hepatic function, haemorrhagic stroke and cataract. *Eur Heart J*. 2018;39(27):2526–2539.
48. Marston NA, Giugliano RP, Im K, et al. Association between triglyceride lowering and reduction of cardiovascular risk across multiple lipid-lowering therapeutic classes: a systematic review and meta-regression analysis of randomized controlled trials. *Circulation*. 2019;140(16):1308–1317.
49. Hegele RA, Boren J, Ginsberg HN, et al. Rare dyslipidaemias, from phenotype to genotype to management: a European Atherosclerosis Society task force consensus statement. *Lancet Diabetes Endocrinol*. 2020;8(1):50–67.
50. Dron JS, Hegele RA. Genetics of hypertriglyceridemia. *Front Endocrinol*. 2020;24(11):455.
51. Laufs U, Parhofer KG, Ginsberg HN, Hegele RA. Clinical review on triglycerides. *Eur Heart J*. 2020;41(1):99–109c.
52. Mach F, Baigent C, Catapano AL, Koskinas KC, et al. 2019 ESC/EAS Guidelines for the management of dyslipidaemias: lipid modification to reduce cardiovascular risk. *Eur Heart J*. 2020;41(1):111–188.
53. Brown WV, Goldberg I, Duell B, Gaudet D. Roundtable discussion: familial chylomicronemia syndrome: diagnosis and management. *J Clin Lipidol*. 2018;12(2):254–263.
54. Herrington WG, Emberson J, Mihaylova B, et al. Are statins useful in patients with advanced chronic kidney disease? Authors' reply. *Lancet Diabetes Endocrinol*. 2016;4(12):971–972.
55. Willeit P, Ridker PM, Nestel PJ, et al. Baseline and on-statin treatment lipoprotein(a) levels for prediction of cardiovascular events: individual patient-data meta-analysis of statin outcome trials. *Lancet*. 2018;392(10155):1311–1320.
56. Mancini GB, Baker S, Bergeron J, et al. Diagnosis, prevention, and management of statin adverse effects and intolerance: Canadian consensus working group update (2016). *Can J Cardiol*. 2016;32(suppl 7):S35–S65.
57. Amarenco P, Kim JS, Labreuche J, et al. A comparison of two LDL cholesterol targets after ischemic stroke. *N Engl J Med*. 2020;382(1):9.
58. Sabatine MS, Wiviott SD, Im K, et al. Efficacy and safety of further lowering of low-density lipoprotein cholesterol in patients starting with very low levels: a meta-analysis. *JAMA Cardiol*. 2018;3(9):823–828.
59. Boekholdt SM, Hovingh GK, Mora S, et al. Very low levels of atherogenic lipoproteins and the risk for cardiovascular events: a meta-analysis of statin trials. *J Am Coll Cardiol*. 2014;64(5):485–494.
60. Byrne P, Cullinan J, Smith SM. Statins for primary prevention of cardiovascular disease. *BMJ*. 2019;367:l5674.
61. Arnett DK, Blumenthal RS, Albert MA, et al. 2019 ACC/AHA guideline on the primary prevention of cardiovascular disease: executive summary: a report of the American College of Cardiology/American Heart Association task force on clinical practice guidelines. *J Am Coll Cardiol*. 2019;74(10):1376–1414.
62. Cholesterol Treatment Trialists' Collaboration. Efficacy and safety of statin therapy in older people: a meta-analysis of individual participant data from 28 randomised controlled trials. *Lancet*. 2019;393(10170):407–415.
63. Yusuf S, Bosch J, Dagenais G, et al. Cholesterol lowering in intermediate-risk persons without cardiovascular disease. *N Engl J Med*. 2016;374(21):2021–2031.
64. Raal FJ, Kallend D, Ray KK, et al. Inclisiran for the treatment of heterozygous familial hypercholesterolemia. *N Engl J Med*. 2020;382(16):1520–1530.
65. Sabatine MS, Giugliano RP, Keech AC, et al. Evolocumab and clinical outcomes in patients with cardiovascular disease. *N Engl J Med*. 2017;376(18):1713–1722.
66. Schwartz GG, Steg PG, Szarek M, et al. Alirocumab and cardiovascular outcomes after acute coronary syndrome. *N Engl J Med*. 2018;379(22):2097–2107.
67. Guedeney P, Giustino G, Sorrentino S, et al. Efficacy and safety of alirocumab and evolocumab: a systematic review and meta-analysis of randomized controlled trials. *Eur Heart J*. 2019.
68. Araki E, Yamashita S, Arai H, et al. Effects of pemafibrate, a novel selective PPARalpha modulator, on lipid and glucose metabolism in patients with type 2 diabetes and hypertriglyceridemia: a randomized, double-blind, placebo-controlled, phase 3 trial. *Diabetes Care*. 2018;41(3):538–546.
69. Pradhan AD, Paynter NP, Everett BM, et al. Rationale and design of the pemafibrate to reduce cardiovascular outcomes by reducing triglycerides in patients with diabetes (PROMINENT) study. *Am Heart J*. 2018;206:80–93.
70. Siscovick DS, Barringer TA, Fretts AM, et al. Omega-3 polyunsaturated fatty acid (fish oil) supplementation and the prevention of clinical cardiovascular disease: a science advisory from the American Heart Association. *Circulation*. 2017;135(15):e867–e884.

71. Manson JE, Cook NR, Lee IM, et al. Marine n-3 fatty acids and prevention of cardiovascular disease and cancer. *N Engl J Med*. 2019;380(1):23–32.
72. Bhatt DL, Steg PG, Miller M. Cardiovascular risk reduction with icosapent ethyl. Reply. *N Engl J Med*. 2019;380(17):1678.
73. Aung T, Halsey J, Kromhout D, et al. Associations of omega-3 fatty acid supplement use with cardiovascular disease risks: meta-analysis of 10 trials involving 77917 individuals. *JAMA Cardiol*. 2018;3(3):225–234.
74. ASCEND Study Collaborative Group, Bowman L, Mafham M, et al. Effects of n-3 fatty acid supplements in diabetes mellitus. *N Engl J Med*. 2018;379(16):1540–1550.
75. Khan SU, Khan MU, Riaz H, et al. Effects of nutritional supplements and dietary interventions on cardiovascular outcomes: an umbrella review and evidence map. *Ann Intern Med*. 2019;171(3):190–198.
76. Hu Y, Hu FB, Manson JE. Marine omega-3 supplementation and cardiovascular disease: an updated meta-analysis of 13 randomized controlled trials involving 127 477 participants. *J Am Heart Assoc*. 2019;8(19):e013543.
77. Brown TJ, Brainard J, Song F, et al. Omega-3, omega-6, and total dietary polyunsaturated fat for prevention and treatment of type 2 diabetes mellitus: systematic review and meta-analysis of randomised controlled trials. *BMJ*. 2019;366:l4697.
78. Hegele RA, Tsimikas S. Lipid-lowering agents. *Circ Res*. 2019;124(3):386–404.
79. Niman S, Rana K, Reid J, et al. A review of the efficacy and tolerability of bempedoic acid in the treatment of hypercholesterolemia. *Am J Cardiovasc Drugs*. 2020.
80. Goldberg AC, Leiter LA, Stroes ESG, et al. Effect of bempedoic acid vs placebo added to maximally tolerated statins on low-density lipoprotein cholesterol in patients at high risk for cardiovascular disease: the CLEAR wisdom randomized clinical trial. *JAMA*. 2019;322(18):1780–1788.
81. Khoury E, Brisson D, Roy N, et al. Review of the long-term safety of lomitapide: a microsomal triglycerides transfer protein inhibitor for treating homozygous familial hypercholesterolemia. *Expert Opin Drug Saf*. 2019;18(5):403–414.
82. Blom DJ, Averna MR, Meagher EA, et al. Long-term efficacy and safety of the microsomal triglyceride transfer protein inhibitor lomitapide in patients with homozygous familial hypercholesterolemia. *Circulation*. 2017;136(3):332–335.
83. Belanger AM, Akioyamen L, Alothman L, Genest J. Evidence for improved survival with treatment of homozygous familial hypercholesterolemia. *Curr Opin Lipidol*. 2020.
84. Banerjee P, Chan KC, Tarabocchia M, et al. Functional analysis of LDLR (Low-Density Lipoprotein Receptor) variants in patient lymphocytes to assess the effect of evinacumab in homozygous familial hypercholesterolemia patients with a spectrum of LDLR activity. *Arterioscler Thromb Vasc Biol*. 2019;39(11):2248–2260.
85. Gaudet D, Gipe DA, Pordy R, et al. ANGPTL3 inhibition in homozygous familial hypercholesterolemia. *N Engl J Med*. 2017;377(3):296–297.
86. Gaudet D, Karwatowska-Prokopczuk E, Baum SJ, et al. Vupanorsen Study Investigators. Vupanorsen, an N-acetyl galactosamine-conjugated antisense drug to ANGPTL3 mRNA, lowers triglycerides and atherogenic lipoproteins in patients with diabetes, hepatic steatosis, and hypertriglyceridaemia. *Eur Heart J*. 2020;41(40):3936–3945.
87. Stiekema LCA, Prange KHM, Hoogeveen RM, et al. Potent lipoprotein(a) lowering following apolipoprotein(a) antisense treatment reduces the pro-inflammatory activation of circulating monocytes in patients with elevated lipoprotein(a). *Eur Heart J*. 2020;41(24):2262–2271.
88. Gaudet D, Durst R, Lepor N, et al. Usefulness of gemcabene in homozygous familial hypercholesterolemia (from COBALT-1). *Am J Cardiol*. 2019;124(12):1876–1880.

Future Perspectives

89. Rodriguez-Calvo R, Masana L. Review of the scientific evolution of gene therapy for the treatment of homozygous familial hypercholesterolaemia: past, present and future perspectives. *J Med Genet*. 2019;56(11):711.
90. Bajaj A, Cuchel M. Homozygous familial hypercholesterolemia: what treatments are on the horizon? *Curr Opin Lipidol*. 2020;31(3):119–124.
91. Virani SS, Alonso A, Benjamin EJ, et al. Heart disease and stroke statistics-2020 update: a report from the American Heart Association. *Circulation*. 2020;141(9):e139–e596.
92. Carson JAS, Lichtenstein AH, Anderson CAM, et al. Dietary cholesterol and cardiovascular risk: a science advisory from the American Heart Association. *Circulation*. 2020;141(3):e39–e53.
93. Berger S, Raman G, Vishwanathan R, et al. Dietary cholesterol and cardiovascular disease: a systematic review and meta-analysis. *Am J Clin Nutr*. 2015;102(2):276–294.
94. Key TJ, Appleby PN, Bradbury KE, et al. Consumption of meat, fish, dairy products, and eggs and risk of ischemic heart disease. *Circulation*. 2019;139(25):2835–2845.
95. Vincent MJ, Allen B, Palacios OM, et al. Meta-regression analysis of the effects of dietary cholesterol intake on LDL and HDL cholesterol. *Am J Clin Nutr*. 2019;109(1):7–16.
96. Zheng H, Yang R, Wang Z, et al. Characterization of pharmaceutic structured triacylglycerols by high-performance liquid chromatography/tandem high-resolution mass spectrometry and its application to structured fat emulsion injection. *Rapid Commun Mass Spectrom*. 2020;34(1):e8557.
97. Bonaca MP, Bhatt DL, Cohen M, et al. Long-term use of ticagrelor in patients with prior myocardial infarction. *N Engl J Med*. 2015;372(19):1791–1800.
98. Lawler PR, Bhatt DL, Godoy LC, et al. Targeting cardiovascular inflammation: next steps in clinical translation. *Eur Heart J*. 2020.
99. Okada H, Nakanishi C, Yoshida S, et al. Function and immunogenicity of gene-corrected iPSC-derived hepatocyte-like cells in restoring low density lipoprotein uptake in homozygous familial hypercholesterolemia. *Sci Rep*. 2019;9(1):4695.

28 Cardiovascular Disease Risk of Nicotine and Tobacco Products

ARUNI BHATNAGAR

HEALTH EFFECTS OF TOBACCO, 525
Cardiovascular Effects of Tobacco Products, 526

CLASSIC REFERENCES, 530

REFERENCES, 530

Wild plants belonging to the *Nicotiana* genus were first domesticated and cultivated in the Americas. They were used by Amer-Indians for many centuries in religious and healing practices. Early European settlers in the Americas learned to use tobacco from Amerindians and exported tobacco products to Europe in the 16th century, where their use spread quickly. By 1670, nearly half the adult male population of England was smoking tobacco daily, and by 1680, the Jamestown colony in America was producing over 25 million pounds of tobacco per year for sale in Europe.[1] In the 17th and the 18th century tobacco was widely chewed or smoked in pipes and cigars; however, paper cigarettes were introduced in the last decades of the 19th century. Because paper cigarettes are easier to manufacture, transport, carry, and use, they quickly became the most common form of tobacco use, and they remain so today. Nevertheless, tobacco continues to be used in many forms (hookah tobacco, chewing tobacco, cigars, pipes, bidis, and kreteks) and newer nicotine delivery devices (e-cigarettes, vape-pens, e-hookahs, and heated tobacco products [HTPs]) have been introduced in the market in the last decade.

EPIDEMIOLOGY OF TOBACCO PRODUCT USE

The use of tobacco in Europe and the United States continued to grow throughout the 18th and 19th century, and peaked after the World War II. However, even though the rates of smoking have declined since then, the absolute number of smokers across the globe has increased due to population growth. Currently, tobacco products are used by 1.3 billion people worldwide, and 6.5 trillion cigarettes are sold around the world each year. In the United States, 19.7% of the adults reported using tobacco products in 2018. Nearly 84% of current tobacco product users, use combustible products (Fig. 28.1), 3.9% report using cigars/cigarillos/filtered little cigars, and 3.2% report using e-cigarettes.[2] More men reported using tobacco products than women. Highest prevalence of tobacco product use is among those between 25 and 64 years of age (21% to 24%) than young adults of 18 to 24 years (17%), or older individuals who are more than 65 years old (12%). The prevalence of tobacco product use is similar between whites and Blacks, but lower among Asians and Hispanics (see Fig. 28.1). In the United States, the use of tobacco products also varies with region. In comparison with the Northeast and the West, tobacco product consumption is higher in the Midwestern and Southern states. The use of tobacco products is higher in those with a General Educational Diploma (GED; 41%) compared with those with no diploma (26%) or those with a high school or undergraduate degree (21% to 25%). It is much lower in those with a graduate degree (8.2%). Tobacco use also varies with income: 26% of those with income of less than $35,000 report using tobacco products, compared with only 14% of those making over $100,000 per year. Tobacco product use is much higher also in LGBTQ individuals (29.2%) than among those reporting a heterosexual orientation (19.5%). LGBTQ individuals are 1.5 times more likely to smoke cigarettes than those reporting a heterosexual orientation. Overall, there has been a substantial decrease in the use of tobacco products in the last decade. In 2005, nearly 21% adults reported using tobacco, which fell to 14% in 2018. Moreover, those who do report smoking report smoking fewer numbers of cigarettes than in the past. However, higher usage persists among individuals with low income or education, and among the LGBTQ community. This decrease, however, has been accompanied by a steep rise in the popularity electronic delivery devices, such as e-cigarettes, e-hookahs, or "vapes."

E-cigarettes were originally devised to aid smoking cessation and harm reduction in chronic smokers,[3] but they have become remarkably popular among youth and youth adults, and their use continues to grow. In 2016, the overall use of e-cigarettes in the United States was 4.5%, which remained stable in 2017, but increased to 5.4% in 2018. This translates to 11.2 million e-cigarette users in 2016, and 13.7 million in 2018.[4] The analysis of the National Youth Tobacco Survey shows that in 2019, 19.5% of high school students and 9.7% of middle school students reported ever using only e-cigarettes.[5] The escalating use of e-cigarettes among youth and young adults is a public health emergency because it threatens to erode gains in tobacco prevention over the last several decades, particularly because youth who use e-cigarettes are at a higher risk of transitioning to smoking combustible cigarettes.[6]

Like e-cigarettes, waterpipes/hookahs are also popular among youth and young adults. In a nationwide survey, 4.8% (95% confidence interval [CI] 4.1 to 5.7) of high school students in the United States reported smoking tobacco using a waterpipe in the prior 30 days, with similar rates among male and female students. Among adults, 7.5% (95% CI 6.8 to 8.2) report smoking waterpipe tobacco in the prior 30 days.[7] This rate was higher among those between 15 and 17 years of age, and among those who identify themselves as bisexual or gay/lesbian. Smoking tobacco using a hookah/waterpipe seems to be gaining popularity. In the United Kingdom, for example, waterpipe use among youth is twice as common as cigarette smoking.[7] However, most waterpipe/hookah use among youth is sporadic and in a social setting.

In addition to waterpipes and hookahs, cigars also remain popular tobacco products. Although their use seems to have declined in recent years, cigars, including little cigars and cigarillos, continue to remain in widespread use. In 2015, 12.5 million people in the United States aged 12 years or older were current cigar smokers. About 5.4% of adults reported ever use,[8] and 2.3% reported using cigars exclusively,[9] and 0.8% smoke cigars daily.[8] Most cigar users are male, and white, with at least some college education. In contrast, cigarette smoking is more concentrated among those with less than a college education.[8] Cigar smokers are also more likely to report nondaily use than cigarette users. In the United States, the prevalence of cigar smoking among adults is around 2.3%,[9] and it has remained essentially unchanged from 2000 to 2015, although there has been a slight increase among females and Blacks. This increase has coincided with changes in cigar flavor availability, pack sizes, and price. As with other tobacco products, the prevalence of cigar smoking also seems to be sensitive to changes in federal taxation.

HEALTH EFFECTS OF TOBACCO

Accumulating research over the last 8 decades has documented a wide array of adverse health effects associated with the use of tobacco products. For several decades, tobacco product use has remained the number one cause of preventable death worldwide. In 2019, tobacco product use was *the* leading risk factor for mortality in men, and the seventh leading risk factor for women. For both sexes combined, exposure to tobacco (smoking, secondhand smoke exposure, and chewing tobacco) accounted for 8.71 million deaths. Tobacco

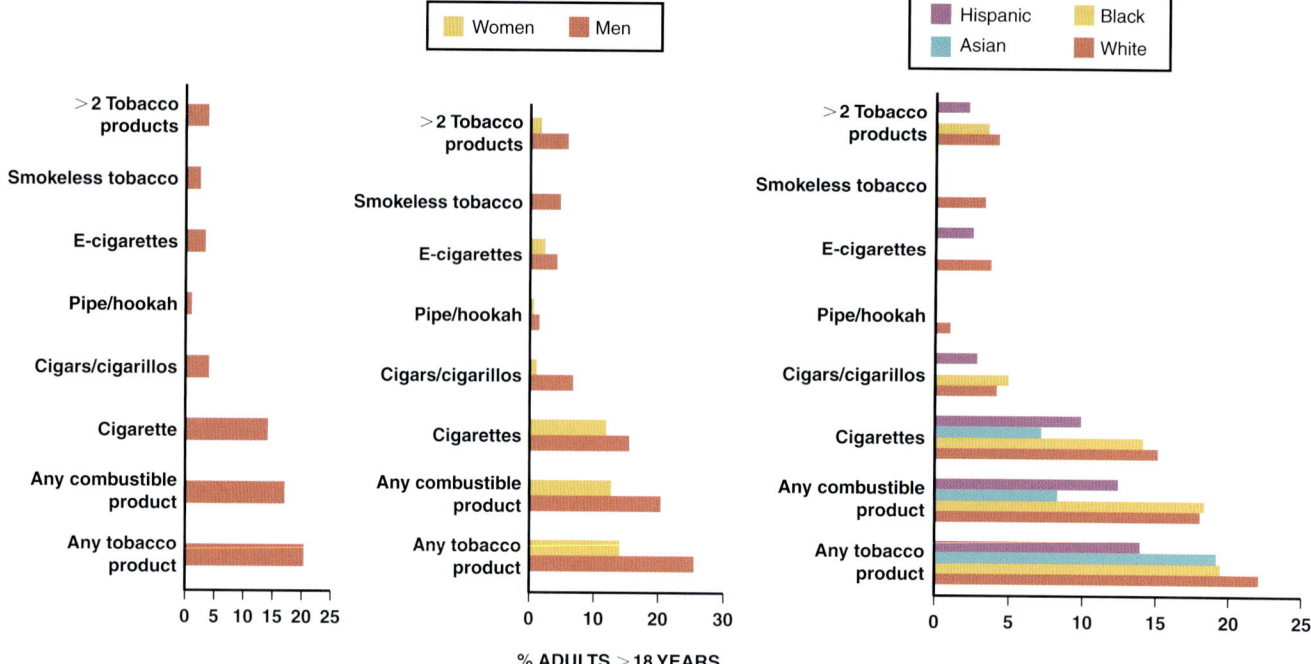

FIGURE 28.1 Tobacco product use among U.S. adults (2018). (From Creamer MR, et al. Tobacco product use and cessation indicators among adults—United States, 2018. MMWR Morb Mortal Wkly Rep 2019;68:1013-1019.)

accounted for 21.4% of all male deaths in the world that year. According to current estimates, the highest health burden imposed by tobacco use (estimated by disability adjusted life years [DALYs]) is in the Balkans, Poland, and Scotland, where the rates of smoking remain high. In these countries, nearly 20% of DALYs have been attributed to tobacco. In contrast, between 10% and 20% of DALYs in most other European countries could be attributed to tobacco. Canada, Russia, and many parts of Southeast Asia are also in the same category. For most of China, DALY estimates due to smoking are similar to that in Europe, except for a couple of provinces, where it exceeds 20%. In the United States, attributable burden is between 10% and 15% for most states, except for Kentucky and West Virginia, where DALY estimates vary between 17% and 20%.[10]

Tobacco use increases the risk of disease and disability. Smoking significantly and robustly increases the risk of premature mortality (hazard ratio [HR] = 1.98; 95% CI 1.93 to 2.02).[8] It harms nearly very organ system in the body; however, it does not affect all organs to the same extent. The lung and cardiovascular systems appear to be most vulnerable, and cardiovascular diseases (CVDs; including stroke) are the leading cause of death among smokers. These diseases kill more smokers over the age of 35 years (151,000) than lung cancer (127,700) or all respiratory diseases (chronic obstructive pulmonary disease [COPD], pneumonia, influenza, and tuberculosis, 113,100) combined. Despite reductions in the rate of smoking, tobacco use and secondhand smoke exposure remain major causes of cardiovascular mortality, contributing to approximately 17% of all cardiovascular deaths globally, about 3 million deaths per year.[11] In 2019, 35% to 36% mortality in both men and women tobacco users could be attributed to CVD, whereas neoplasms accounted for 32% of the mortality in male tobacco users and 16% in female tobacco users.[10]

Cardiovascular Effects of Tobacco Products
Cigarettes
Smoking cigarettes affects multiple forms of CVD. The risk of CVD due to smoking is in general lower than the risk of lung cancer. Individuals who smoke have a 9- to 10-fold higher risk of developing lung-cancer,[12] and a 4-fold higher risk of COPD.[13] In contrast, the relative CVD risk varies from 1.3 to 4. Nonetheless, smokers are at a particularly high risk of developing abdominal aortic aneurysm,[14] atrial fibrillation,[15] heart failure,[16] peripheral artery disease (see Classic References, Price et al.) and sudden cardiac death.[17] Patients with diabetes who smoke are also at greater risk as are individuals[18] who continue to smoke after a cardiovascular procedure such as percutaneous coronary intervention or coronary artery bypass surgery.[19] The relative risk (RR) for different cardiovascular conditions is shown in Table 28.1. In many cases, the effects of smoking appear to be dose-dependent; the relative risk (RR) of peripheral artery disease among heavy smokers is 3.94 in heavy smokers, but 1.87 to 1.70 in moderate smokers. Similarly, it has been reported that the risk of nonfatal acute myocardial infarction (MI) (odds ratio [OR] = 2.95) increases by 5.6% for every additional cigarette smoked.[20]

Although the adverse health effects of smoking are widely recognized, there is surprising lack of understanding of the mechanisms by which smoking impairs cardiovascular health and the specific harmful or potentially harmful substances (HPHCs) in tobacco smoke responsible for cardiovascular injury have not been clearly identified. Nonetheless, extensive evidence suggests that one of the key targets of smoking is the endothelium. In humans, smoking acutely causes endothelial cell damage (see Classic References, Blann et al.), diminishes endothelium-mediated relaxation, and long-term smoking is associated with impaired endothelium-dependent relaxation in conduit and coronary arteries (see Classic References, Barua et al. and Campisi et al.). These changes have been linked to a decrease in the bioavailability of nitric oxide in smokers.[21] Smoking-induced vascular dysfunction not only affects blood pressure regulation, but by altering the integrity of the vessel wall, it promotes the formation of atherosclerotic lesions as well. It has been found that cigarette smoking is an independent predictor of new coronary lesion formation and that smoking is associated with a consistent increase in intimal-medial thickness of the carotid artery.[21]

In addition to its hemodynamic and vascular effects, smoking could promote atherosclerosis also by affecting lipid metabolism. Many studies have shown that compared with nonsmokers, smokers have higher levels of serum cholesterol, triglycerides, and low-density lipoprotein (LDL)-cholesterol, but lower levels of high-density lipoprotein (HDL)-cholesterol (see Chapter 27).[21] But, because smoking is also associated with nutritional changes, it is unclear whether the changes in lipid profile are a direct effect of smoking or dietary differences between smokers and nonsmokers. The high-triglyceride/HDL ratio in smokers has

TABLE 28.1 Relative Risk of Cardiovascular Disease in Current and Former Smokers

CARDIOVASCULAR DISEASE	RELATIVE RISK OR ODDS RATIO	
	CURRENT SMOKER	FORMER SMOKER
Atrial fibrillation[a]	1.32 (1.12-1.56)	1.09 (1.0-1.18)
Abdominal aortic aneurysm[b]	4.87 (3.93-6.02)	2.10 (1.76-2.50)
Heart failure[c]	1.75 (1.54-1.99)	1.16 (1.01-1.96)
Sudden cardiac death[d]	3.06 (2.46-3.82)	1.38 (1.20-1.60)
Stroke[e]	1.92 (1.49-2.48)	1.30 (0.93-1.81)
Peripheral artery disease[f]	3.94 (2.04-7.62)*	
Nonfatal MI[g]	2.95 (2.77-3.14)	1.87 (1.55-2.24)
Ischemic heart disease mortality[h]	1.79 (1.59-2.02)	
Diabetes[i] all-cause mortality	1.48 (1.34-1.64)	
Cardiovascular mortality	1.36 (1.22-1.52)	
Coronary heart disease	1.54 (1.31-1.82)	
Stroke	1.52 (1.25-1.83)	
MI mortality after PCI/CABG[j]	1.15 (0.81-1.64)	1.19 (1.03-1.38)
Lung cancer[k]	8.93 (4.9-16.28)*	
COPD[l]	4.01 (3.18-5.05)	
Asthma[m]	1.61 (1.07-2.42)	

CABG, Coronary artery bypass grafting; COPD, chronic obstructive pulmonary disease; MI, myocardial infarction; PCI, percutaneous coronary intervention.
*For heavy smokers.
[a]Aune D, Schlesinger S, Norat T, Riboli E. Tobacco smoking and the risk of atrial fibrillation: A systematic review and meta-analysis of prospective studies. Eur J Prev Cardiol 2018;25:1437-1451.
[b]Aune D, Schlesinger S, Norat T, Riboli E. Tobacco smoking and the risk of abdominal aortic aneurysm: a systematic review and meta-analysis of prospective studies. Sci Rep 2018;8:14786.
[c]Aune D, Schlesinger S, Norat T, Riboli E. Tobacco smoking and the risk of heart failure: A systematic review and meta-analysis of prospective studies. Eur J Prev Cardiol 2019;26:279-288.
[d]Aune D, Schlesinger S, Norat T, Riboli E. Tobacco smoking and the risk of sudden cardiac death: A systematic review and meta-analysis of prospective studies. Eur J Epidemiol 2018;33:509-521.
[e]Pan B, Jin X, Jun L, Qiu S, et al. The relationship between smoking and stroke: A meta-analysis. Medicine (Baltimore) 2019;98:e14872.
[f]Price JF, Mowbray PI, Lee AJ, et al. Relationship between smoking and cardiovascular risk factors in the development of peripheral arterial disease and coronary artery disease: Edinburgh Artery Study. Eur Heart J 1999;20:344-353.
[g,h]Teo KK, Ounpuu, S, Hawken S, et al. Tobacco use and risk of myocardial infarction in 52 countries in the INTERHEART study: A case-control study. Lancet 2006;368:647-658.
[i]Qin R, Chen T, Lou Q, Yu D. Excess risk of mortality and cardiovascular events associated with smoking among patients with diabetes: Meta-analysis of observational prospective studies. Int J Cardiol 2013;167:342-350.
[j]Ma WQ, Wang Y, Sun XJ, et al. Impact of smoking on all-cause mortality and cardiovascular events in patients after coronary revascularization with a percutaneous coronary intervention or coronary artery bypass graft: A systematic review and meta-analysis. Coron Artery Dis 2019;30:367-376.
[k]O'Keeffe LM, Taylor G, Huxley RR, et al. Smoking as a risk factor for lung cancer in women and men: A systematic review and meta-analysis. BMJ Open 2018;8:e021611.
[l,m]Jayes L, Haslam PL, Gratziou CG, et al. SmokeHaz: Systematic reviews and meta-analyses of the effects of smoking on respiratory health. Chest 2016;150:164-179.

Despite extensive descriptions of the cardiovascular effects of smoking, the process that contributes to changes in vascular function, thrombosis, lipid metabolism, and atherogenesis in smokers remains unclear, and the specific constituents and chemicals that induce such injury have not been identified. Cigarette smoke, as well as smoke from combustible and HTPs, contains fine particulate matter (PM), which may be responsible for the cardiovascular risk of smoking. Indeed, a large body of work[24] has shown that exposure to ambient air PM leads to many of the cardiovascular changes seen with smoking, which suggests that adverse cardiovascular effects of smoking, at least in part, may be attributable to PM exposure. In addition to PM, both particulate and gaseous phases of tobacco smoke contain high levels of free radicals[21]; some of them are particularly long-lived and may be responsible for extensive tissue damage, oxidative stress, and inflammatory responses associated with smoking.

Cardiovascular injury caused by smoking may also be related to the gaseous phase of tobacco smoke. Tobacco smoke contains 3000 to 7000 different chemicals, many of which react avidly with a wide range of biomolecules. These chemicals include tobacco-specific nitrosamines, metals, gases such as carbon monoxide, and volatile organic compounds (VOCs) such as acrolein, formaldehyde, 1,3-butadiene, benzene, and acrylonitrile. The specific toxicologic profile of each of these chemicals remains uncertain and the contribution of each of these chemicals to the overall toxicity of cigarette smoke has not been well documented. Nevertheless, theoretical hazard estimates based on the toxicologic properties of individual constituents and their relative abundance in cigarette smoke suggest that a major portion of the toxicity of cigarettes could be attributed to VOCs such as acrolein.[25] This is significant because many of the newer tobacco products (e.g., e-cigarettes) do not generate high levels of tobacco-specific nitrosamines or carbon monoxide, but they do produce VOCs such as acrolein, which may be responsible for the residual toxicity associated with these products.

Even though combustion products, gases, and trace metals in tobacco smoke have received the most attention from toxicologists, the role of nicotine could not be entirely discounted. Because by itself nicotine is well tolerated and is often used for smoking cessation, it is widely believed that nicotine is relatively innocuous. This belief is fueled in part by the often-repeated phrase that "people smoke for nicotine, but they die from tar" (see Classic Reference, Russell). Nonetheless, nicotine is a potent sympathomimetic drug, which upon binding to very specific cholinergic receptors in nervous tissue elicits a wide range of metabolic and physiologic responses that could significantly affect vascular function, cardiac contractility, and lipid metabolism as shown in Fig. 28.2. These changes, brought about by acute nicotine delivery, could increase the risk of arrhythmias, plaque rupture, and sudden cardiac death.[26]

been suggested to be related to insulin resistance; however, the relationship between smoking and diabetes is complex,[22] and the effects of smoking on diabetes seem to vary with race and smoking intensity,[23] but mild-to-moderate insulin resistance may be a key link between cigarette smoking and CVD.[21]

Cigarette smoking can also increase the risk of CVD by affecting thrombosis and coagulation.[21] Smokers have higher circulating levels of fibrinogen, and platelets isolated from smokers show increased aggregation (see Chapter 95). Smoking also affects tissue factor (TF) and TF pathway inhibitor 1, and it increase blood viscosity, red blood cell counts, and hematocrit, thereby creating a prothrombotic state, which could increase the acute thrombotic responses upon plaque rupture.[21] In women, smoking has been associated with sudden cardiac death due to plaque erosion leading to the formation of a large occlusive thrombus (see Chapter 91).

Cigars/Cigarillos. The health effects associated with the use of cigars are similar to those observed with smoking. In contrast with never cigar smokers, former exclusive cigar users have higher risk of heart disease (adjusted disease prevalence ratios; aPR = 1.33, 95% CI 1.03 to 1.72) and stroke (aPR = 2.42, 95% CI 1.57 to 3.75) as well as all cancers (aPR = 1.44, 95% CI 1.09 to 1.88). It has been estimated that 65,000 heart conditions and 62,000 stroke cases among U.S. adults aged >35 years can be attributed to former or current exclusive cigar smoking.[9] Cigar smokers have a 20% higher all-cause mortality risk than never tobacco users.[8] Many cigar smokers use other tobacco products as well, so their disease risk may be additionally affected by the risk associated with these products. Because cigars, like cigarettes, generate complex aerosols consisting of PM, VOCs, and other HPHCs, the health effects of smoking cigars are likely to be similar to those observed with smoking. However, the relative health effects of the two nicotine delivery devices have not been directly compared.

Hookah/Waterpipe. Because both the side-stream and mainstream waterpipe tobaccos contain chemical and physical constituents similar to those generated by combustible cigarettes, the toxicity and the health effects of hookah are also similar to those seen with cigarette smoke. However, in a typical isolated session, hookah smokers inhale a systemic dose of nicotine equivalent to the smoking 2 to 3 cigarettes, but this results in 3 times higher levels of exposure to carbon monoxide, 27-fold higher levels of formaldehyde, 19-fold greater acrolein, and 20 to 50 times higher levels of polycyclic aromatic hydrocarbons.[7] As with

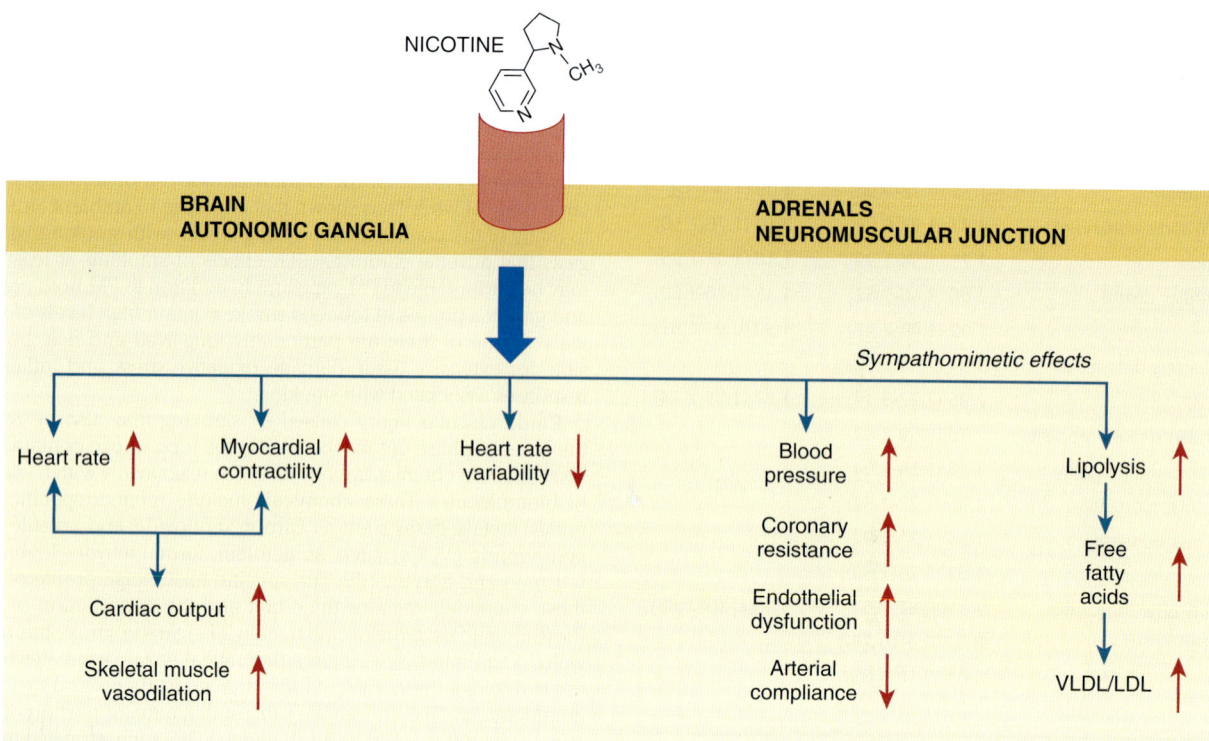

FIGURE 28.2 Physiologic effects of nicotine. By binding to the cholinergic receptor in several excitable tissues, nicotine triggers a series of physiologic responses that alter cardiovascular function and metabolism. In the long term, these physiologic changes could promote atherogenesis or contribute to arrhythmias, plaque rupture, and sudden death.

cigarette smoke, hookah smoking leads to transient increases in heart rate and blood pressure. Within 15 to 30 minutes of hookah smoking, the systolic blood pressure increases by 3 to 16 mm Hg and the diastolic blood pressure by 2 to 14 mm Hg. Heart rate increases by 6 to 13 beats/min. Hookah smoking increases myocardial oxygen demand and leads to a modest increase in coronary blood flow. It also leads to a significant increase in vascular resistance, and a decrease in forearm blood flow, venous outflow, and venous capacitance. Because hookah smoke contains a high level of carbon monoxide, many cases of acute carbon monoxide smoking have been reported among hookah smokers.[7]

The effects of hookah are related to decreased endothelial-dependent vasodilation and a hyperactive neurohormonal response. Long-term hookah use is associated with increased CVD risk, severity, and mortality. Chronic hookah use in several Asian countries is associated with hypertension, hyperlipidemia, and hyperglycemia. Long-term hookah use is associated with severe depression of vascular function, and lifetime exposure (exceeding 2 waterpipes per day for 20 years) is associated with a threefold increase in the odds of angiographically diagnosed coronary artery stenosis.[7] Coronary disease has been found to be much higher in waterpipe smokers than cigarette smokers or nonsmokers. Habitual waterpipe smokers who smoked hookah for most of their adult lives have a higher propensity for ST-segment elevation MI, poorer in-hospital outcomes with higher mortality, more frequent myocardial ischemia, and higher recurrent MI rates than cigarette smokers.[7]

Smokeless Tobacco. Smokeless tobacco was the most common form of tobacco use from the 17th to the 19th century. It was only displaced by paper cigarettes in the early 20th century. Nevertheless, even today smokeless tobacco continues to be used worldwide, particularly in Northern Europe and Southeast Asia. Both oral and nasal smokeless tobacco products are widely used and these include products like snus and snuff in Europe and the Americas, but also locally formulated chewing tobacco in Southeast Asian countries. Because of the wide variety of preparations, constituents, and use patterns, it is difficult to ascribe specific health effects to the use of individual products; nevertheless meta-analysis of several observational studies from Sweden and the United States show that the RR for fatal MI among smokeless tobacco product users is 1.13 (95% CI 1.06 to 1.21),[27] and it has been estimated that the 0.5% of MIs in the United States and 5.6% in Sweden could be attributed to the use of smokeless tobacco products.[27] Other global studies also indicate a similar level of risk of fatal coronary heart disease, with a RR of 1.10 (95% CI 1 to 1.2).[28] The risk persists, even after accounting for concurrent smoking.

Product-wise analysis shows that there is a positive association between fatal coronary heart disease and snus/snuff use (1.37; 95% CI 1.14 to 1.61).[28] That the use of snus/snuff is associated with risk for MI is consistent with previous work showing a reduction in post-MI mortality risk in snus quitters. Individuals who quit using snus after MI have been found to have half the mortality risk of post-MI that those who continue to use snus (HR = 0.51, 95% CI 0.29 to 0.91).[29] This level of risk reduction is similar to that estimated for people who quit smoking after MI.[29] In addition to MI, studies from both Sweden and the United States have reported that the use of smokeless tobacco is associated with an increase in the risk of fatal stroke (RR = 1.40, 95% CI 1.28 to 1.54),[27] and that the use of smokeless tobacco accounts for 1.7% and 5.4% of total stroke deaths.[27]

Although HPHCs in smokeless tobacco that contribute to CVD risk have not been identified, and likely to be highly variable, all preparations of smokeless tobacco contain nicotine, which has well-known effects on blood pressure and heart rate (see Fig. 28.2). Thus frequent intake of nicotine could create an adverse hemodynamic milieu, conducive to the development of atherosclerotic plaques or cardiocerebral events. Administration of smokeless tobacco products increases heart rate and blood pressure due to an increase in the levels of plasma epinephrine. Some studies show that smokeless tobacco users have higher systolic blood pressure than smokers, and that long-term use of smokeless tobacco products is associated with increased incidence of hypertension.[28] Data from animal models suggest that frequent exposure to smokeless tobacco decreases the levels of circulating angiogenic cells, and CD19+ B cells, CD4+ and CD8+ T cells, and CD11b+ monocytes, and it increases the levels of inflammatory cytokines such as tumor necrosis factor-alpha (TNF-α) in the plasma and liver.[30] These data suggest that the use of smokeless tobacco could establish a proinflammatory state that could exacerbate CVD.

Electronic Cigarettes

E-cigarettes are electronic nicotine delivery systems (ENDS) that aerosolize a solution of nicotine in propylene glycol and vegetable glycerin (PG:VG).[31] The basic design of an e-cigarette consists of a battery, a heating element, and a place to hold the liquid ("e-juice"). The first-generation e-cigarettes were designed to look like regular cigarettes ("cigalikes"), cigars, or pipes; however, newer devices resemble USB sticks and other everyday products like pens and watches. More than 400 different brands of e-cigarettes are currently on the market. These can be grouped into several basic types, such as cigalikes, eGos, mods, prefilled capsules, refillable tanks, rechargeable kits, and variable voltage e-cigarettes,[32] and they can be referred to as "e-cigs," "e-hookahs," "mods," "vape pens," "vapes," or "tank systems." Although most e-cigarettes contain nicotine, they can also be used to deliver marijuana and other drugs.

E-cigarettes were introduced in the market in 2007 as a safer alternative to smoking, ostensibly with the intent of reducing harm in long-term smokers.[31] However, because e-cigarettes do not generate foul-smelling combustion products, they were readily adopted by smokers to smoke in places where smoking was not permitted. Moreover, fueled in part by attractive designing, aggressive marketing, and enticing flavors, e-cigarettes found increasing acceptance among youth. In 2020, 4.4% of adults (11 million),[33] 19.6% of high school students (3.02 million) and 4.7% of middle school (550,000) students reported current use.[34] The rapid growth of e-cigarettes, especially among tobacco naive youth and young adults, has become a major public health concern.

By avoiding combustion, e-cigarettes generate lower levels of several toxic substances that are generated in combustible cigarettes. The major carcinogenic constituents of tar, benzopyrenes, and tobacco-specific nitrosamines are present only in trace quantities in e-cigarettes, and no carbon monoxide is produced.[31] Nonetheless, e-cigarette aerosols generate significant amounts of reactive volatile chemicals such as formaldehyde, acetaldehyde, and acrolein, which have been linked to cardiovascular injury,[35,36] and increased CVD risk.[37] In addition, e-cigarette aerosols produce aerosols that contain fine and ultrafine particles,[38] which can trigger cardiovascular events and promote the progression of pulmonary and cardiovascular disease.[39] Occasionally, e-cigarette aerosols also contain metals such as iron, nickel, copper, chromium, zinc, and lead, which are generated by the heating coil.[40] The presence of metals could further add to the toxicity of the aerosol.

Although the health effects due to long-term use of e-cigarettes have not been studied, acute use of e-cigarettes by smoking-naive healthy subjects has been shown to increase flow resistance, indicating obstruction of the conducting airways.[41] Those who use e-cigarettes regularly show inflammatory changes in their lungs, and their airways appear "friable and erythematous," indicating ongoing subclinical injury. Some studies have reported that daily use of e-cigarette decreases lung function (as measured by forced expiratory volume [FEV_1] and the ratio of FEV_1 and forced vital capacity). Whether e-cigarettes, like combustible cigarettes, increase the risk of lung cancer or COPD is not known, but in animal models, exposure to e-cigarette aerosol has been reported to lead to the development of lung adenocarcinomas and bladder urothelial hyperplasia,[42] and to the appearance of disorganization of alveolar and bronchial epithelium, suggesting incipient pulmonary injury.

In healthy adults, a single bout of e-cigarette use increases systolic and diastolic blood pressure as well as aortic stiffness.[41] The magnitude of these changes are similar to those observed with smoking a combustible cigarette. As in the case of cigarettes, these effects of e-cigarettes are accompanied by a marked shift in cardiac sympathovagal balance toward sympathetic predominance. Because such sympathomimetic effects are not seen in e-cigarettes without nicotine, it is likely that nicotine is the main constituent that elicits the hemodynamic changes seen after acute inhalation of e-cigarette aerosols. Habitual use of e-cigarettes has been found to be associated with a shift in cardiac autonomic balance toward sympathetic predominance, which can, over time, increase the risk of premature aging and CVD.

The use of e-cigarettes has also been shown to impair vascular function and to attenuate flow-mediated dilation, peak velocity, and the hyperemic index. It also leads to an increase in arterial stiffness, but a reduction in acetylcholine-mediated vasodilation.[41] The decrease in flow-mediated dilation observed in humans inhaling e-cigarette aerosol has been recapitulated in rats exposed to e-cigarette aerosols. Even though flow-mediated dilation changes in response to e-cigarettes are lower than those observed with combustible cigarettes, the observations that the use of e-cigarettes is associated with an increase in oxidative stress, decreased bioavailability of nitric oxide, and diminished rates of nitric oxide production from endothelial cells support the notion that e-cigarettes cause endothelial injury. Decreased nitric oxide production in endothelial cells has also been noted in endothelial cells exposed to flavoring agents used in e-cigarettes.[41]

A particularly striking example of the acute injury caused by e-cigarette use is provided by the cases of electronic cigarette or vaping-induced lung injury (EVALI) that were reported between 2019 and 2020, which led to more than 2000 cases of lung injury in the United States. A total of 2087 hospitalized cases or death have been reported by the Centers for Disease Control and Prevention.[41] Lung biopsies of EVALI patients showed signs of subacute lung injury, multifocal ground glass-opacity frequently with organizing consolidation, interlobular septal thickening, diffuse alveolar damage, and organizing pneumonia. These are all changes indicative of extensive lung damage, fluid accumulation, airway collapse, and fibrosis that often resulted in death. The specific constituents of e-cigarettes that led to the EVALI outbreak have not been identified, but because vitamin E acetate and tetrahydrocannabinol (THC) or its metabolites were identified in the bronchial lavage fluid from EVALI patients, it has been suggested that additives or cutting agents added to e-liquids may have been responsible for much of the observed lung injury. However, many EVALI patients reported using only nicotine-containing products,[43] so it is unclear whether the outbreak was related just to the toxicity of the additives in e-cigarette devices or the interaction of these chemicals with some preexisting conditions such as asthma, cardiac disease, or obesity that made some individuals more susceptible to pulmonary injury.

Heated Tobacco Products

Although HTPs were launched in the United States as early as 1988, they were removed from the market because they failed to gain a significant market share; however, after the success of e-cigarettes, HTPs were relaunched worldwide. An HTP device is a holder in which a heat stick is inserted and an electric heating element is activated by pressing a button for tobacco aerosolization without combustion, which is inhaled through a holder. Because there is no combustion in HTPs, the levels of HPHCs in HTP aerosols are 85% to 90% lower than those generated by a standard cigarette.[44] This reduction in exposure might be associated with lower health risks; however, the health effects of HTPs remain largely unknown. Despite reduction in the levels of several toxic substances, HTP emissions may have residual toxicity. These devices emit substantial levels of formaldehyde, acetaldehyde, and acrolein,[45] as well as reactive oxygen species[46] and tobacco-specific nitrosoamines,[47] albeit at levels much lower than those by combustible cigarettes. In animal models, exposure to HTPs has been shown to reduce flow-mediated dilation to an extent similar to that seen in combustible cigarettes, suggesting that the use of HTPs may not necessarily avoid the adverse cardiovascular effects of smoking combustible cigarettes.[48]

HARM REDUCTION AND CESSATION

A majority of the adverse cardiovascular effects of smoking have been attributed to HPHCs generated by combustion, therefore, noncombustible tobacco products that do not generate combustion products are considered by some to be safer than combustible cigarettes. Nonetheless, nicotine has a variety of strong cardiovascular effects (see Fig. 28.2), and, therefore, no tobacco product containing nicotine could be considered safe. Moreover, levels of other combustion and heating-related HPHCs vary from one product to another and with different use patterns. As a result, it remains unclear whether one product is less harmful than another. Importantly, a significant reduction in exposure does not necessary translate into proportional reduction in harm, because the dose-response relationship between smoking and CVD is nonlinear.[49] For example, smoking ≤3 cigarettes per day confers 80% of the risk of ischemic heart disease associated with smoking ≥20 cigarettes, suggesting that reducing exposure, e.g., by 80%, does not lead to an 80% reduction in harm. For the same reason, reducing cigarettes smoked per day has only a marginal effect on CVD risk, because even very light smoking is associated with significant excessive risk.[49] For instance, it has been reported that smoking even one cigarette per day has 46% of the excess RR of smoking 20 cigarettes. The corresponding estimate for 5 cigarettes per day is 57%.[50] Even those who smoke fewer than 1 or 1 to 10 cigarettes per day over their lifetime have higher all-cause mortality (RR = 1.87) relative to never smokers.[51] Moreover, even though CVD risk is diminished in those who transition from heavy to light smoking (RR = 0.78), it is unaffected in those who reduce smoking by 50% or switch from heavy to moderate smoking.[52] Therefore, it seems that full abstinence, rather than decreasing smoking intensity, is required to fully redeem the health benefits of withdrawing from tobacco use.

Many approaches have been used to promote tobacco cessation to varying degrees of success. Because tobacco is difficult to quit, unassisted cessation attempts fail often. Even with nicotine replacement therapy relapse rates remain high.[3] In contrast to nicotine replacement therapy alone, pharmacologic interventions have been found to be more effective; the 1-year abstinence rate with nicotine replacement therapy and bupropion is 20%, and the 24-week abstinence rate with varenicline has been reported to be 26%. In addition, e-cigarettes have been suggested to help adult smokers quit; however, it remains unclear whether their use facilitates smoking cessation.[3] In a randomized trial, the 1-year abstinence rate was double (18%) in those who used e-cigarettes than in those in the nicotine-replacement group (9%). However, 80% of those in the e-cigarette groups continued to use e-cigarettes compared with the 9% use of nicotine replacement patches in the nicotine replacement therapy group, suggesting that those using e-cigarettes find abstinence more difficult than those on nicotine patches. Moreover, the efficacy of e-cigarettes in promoting cessation was comparable or lower than that reported previously for other smoking cessation approaches, and because the success rate of nicotine replacement therapy was half that reported in other studies,[3] the difference between the e-cigarette and nicotine replacement groups may be higher in the trial than in the real world. In contrast, a meta-analysis of smoking cessation and e-cigarette use in the real world showed that as currently used, e-cigarettes are associated with significantly *less* quitting among smokers.[53] Nonetheless, in helping smokers quit, all avenues may need to be explored to develop a personalized cessation plan with the ultimate aim of complete withdrawal from any form of nicotine use. Cessation resources in the United States include the North American Quitline Consortium, National Cancer Institute; the World Health Organization also provides training and resources for cessation.

CLASSIC REFERENCES

Barua RS, Ambrose JA, Eales-Reynolds LJ, et al. Dysfunctional endothelial nitric oxide biosynthesis in healthy smokers with impaired endothelium-dependent vasodilatation. *Circulation*. 2001;104:1905–1910.

Blann AD, Kirkpatrick U, Devine C, et al. The influence of acute smoking on leucocytes, platelets and the endothelium. *Atherosclerosis*. 1998;141:133–1339.

Campisi R, Czernin J, Schoder H, et al. Effects of long-term smoking on myocardial blood flow, coronary vasomotion, and vasodilator capacity. *Circulation*. 1998;98:119–125.

Price JF, Mowbray PI, Lee AJ, et al. Relationship between smoking and cardiovascular risk factors in the development of peripheral arterial disease and coronary artery disease: Edinburgh Artery Study. *Eur Heart J*. 1999;20:344–353.

Russell MA. Low-tar medium-nicotine cigarettes: a new approach to safer smoking. *Br Med J*. 1976;1:1430–1433.

REFERENCES

Epidemiology of Tobacco Product Use

1. Brandt AM. *The Cigarette Century: The Rise, Fall, and Deadly Persistence of the Product that Defined America*. New York: Basic Books (AZ); 2007.
2. Creamer MR, Wang TW, Babb S, et al. Tobacco product use and cessation indicators among adults—United States, 2018. *MMWR Morb Mortal Wkly Rep*. 2019;68:1013–1019.
3. Bhatnagar A, Payne TJ, Robertson RM. Is there A role for electronic cigarettes in tobacco cessation? *J Am Heart Assoc*. 2019;8:e012742.
4. Obisesan OH, Osei AD, Uddin SI, et al. Trends in e-cigarette use in adults in the United States, 2016-2018. *JAMA Intern Med*. 2020;180:1394–1398.
5. Tam J. E-cigarette, combustible, and smokeless tobacco product use combinations among youth in the United States, 2014–2019. *Addict Behav*. 2020;112:106636.
6. Bhatnagar A, Whitsel LP, Blaha MJ, et al. New and emerging tobacco products and the nicotine endgame: the role of robust regulation and comprehensive tobacco control and prevention: a presidential advisory from the American Heart Association. *Circulation*. 2019;139:e937–e958.
7. Bhatnagar A, Maziak W, Eissenberg T, et al. Water pipe (hookah) smoking and cardiovascular disease risk: a scientific statement from the American Heart Association. *Circulation*. 2019;139:e917–e936.
8. Christensen CH, Rostron B, Cosgrove C, et al. Association of cigarette, cigar, and pipe use with mortality risk in the US population. *JAMA Intern Med*. 2018;178:469–476.
9. Rostron BL, Corey CG, Gindi RM. Cigar smoking prevalence and morbidity among US adults, 2000-2015. *Prev Med Rep*. 2019;14:100821.
10. GBP 2019 Risk Factors Collaborators. Global burden of 87 risk factors in 204 countries and territories, 1990-2019: a systematic analysis for the Global Burden of Disease. *Lancet*. 2020;396:1223–1249.
11. Institute for Health Metrics and Evaluation (IHME). GBD Compare Data Visualization. Seattle, WA: IHME, University of Washington, 2020. Available from: http://vizhub.healthdata.org/gbd-compare. (Accessed March 4, 2021)

Cigarettes

12. O'Keeffe LM, Taylor G, Huxley RR, et al. Smoking as a risk factor for lung cancer in women and men: a systematic review and meta-analysis. *BMJ Open*. 2018;8:e021611.
13. Jayes L, Haslam PL, Gratziou CG, et al. SmokeHaz: systematic reviews and meta-analyses of the effects of smoking on respiratory health. *Chest*. 2016;150:164–179.
14. Aune D, Schlesinger S, Norat T, Riboli E. Tobacco smoking and the risk of abdominal aortic aneurysm: a systematic review and meta-analysis of prospective studies. *Sci Rep*. 2018;8:14786.
15. Aune D, Schlesinger S, Norat T, Riboli E. Tobacco smoking and the risk of atrial fibrillation: a systematic review and meta-analysis of prospective studies. *Eur J Prev Cardiol*. 2018;25:1437–1451.
16. Aune D, Schlesinger S, Norat T, Riboli E. Tobacco smoking and the risk of heart failure: a systematic review and meta-analysis of prospective studies. *Eur J Prev Cardiol*. 2019;26:279–288.
17. Aune D, Schlesinger S, Norat T, Riboli E. Tobacco smoking and the risk of sudden cardiac death: a systematic review and meta-analysis of prospective studies. *Eur J Epidemiol*. 2018;33:509–521.
18. Qin R, Chen T, Lou Q, Yu D. Excess risk of mortality and cardiovascular events associated with smoking among patients with diabetes: meta-analysis of observational prospective studies. *Int J Cardiol*. 2013;167:342–350.
19. Ma WQ, Wang Y, Sun XJ, et al. Impact of smoking on all-cause mortality and cardiovascular events in patients after coronary revascularization with a percutaneous coronary intervention or coronary artery bypass graft: a systematic review and meta-analysis. *Coron Artery Dis*. 2019;30:367–376.
20. Teo KK, Ounpuu S, Hawken S, et al. Tobacco use and risk of myocardial infarction in 52 countries in the INTERHEART study: a case-control study. *Lancet*. 2006;368:647–658.
21. Ambrose JA, Barua RS. The pathophysiology of cigarette smoking and cardiovascular disease: an update. *J Am Coll Cardiol*. 2004;43:1731–1737.
22. Keith RJ, Al Rifai M, Carruba C, et al. Tobacco use, insulin resistance, and risk of type 2 diabetes: results from the multi-ethnic study of atherosclerosis. *PloS One*. 2016;11:e0157592.
23. White WB, Cain LR, Benjamin EJ, et al. High-intensity cigarette smoking is associated with incident diabetes mellitus in black adults: the Jackson Heart Study. *J Am Heart Assoc*. 2018;7:e007413.
24. Brook RD, Rajagopalan S, Pope CA, et al. Particulate matter air pollution and cardiovascular disease: an update to the scientific statement from the American Heart Association. *Circulation*. 2010;121:2331–2378.
25. Haussmann HJ. Use of hazard indices for a theoretical evaluation of cigarette smoke composition. *Chem Res Toxicol*. 2012;25:794–810.
26. Bhatnagar A. E-cigarettes and cardiovascular disease risk: evaluation of evidence, policy implications, and recommendations. *Curr Cardiovasc Risk Rep*. 2016;10:1–10.

Smokeless Tobacco

27. Boffetta P, Straif K. Use of smokeless tobacco and risk of myocardial infarction and stroke: systematic review with meta-analysis. *BMJ*. 2009;339:b3060.
28. Gupta R, Gupta S, Sharma S, et al. Risk of coronary heart disease among smokeless tobacco users: results of systematic review and meta-analysis of global data. *Nicotine Tob Res*. 2019;21:25–31.
29. Arefalk G, Hambraeus K, Lind L, et al. Discontinuation of smokeless tobacco and mortality risk after myocardial infarction. *Circulation*. 2014;130:325–332.
30. Malovichko MV, Zeller I, Krivokhizhina TV, et al. Systemic toxicity of smokeless tobacco products in mice. *Nicotine Tob Res*. 2019;21:101–110.

Electronic Cigarettes

31. Bhatnagar A, Whitsel LP, Ribisl KM, et al. Electronic cigarettes: a policy statement from the American Heart Association. *Circulation*. 2014;130:1418–1436.
32. Zhu SH, Sun JY, Bonnevie E, et al. Four hundred and sixty brands of e-cigarettes and counting: implications for product regulation. *Tob Control*. 2014;23. suppl 3:iii3-9.
33. National Center For Health Statistics. Selected Estimates Based on Data from the National Health Interview Survey. Available at: www.cdc.gov/nchs/nhis/erkeyindicators.htm.
34. Wang TW, Neff LJ, Park-Lee E, et al. E-cigarette use among middle and high school students - United States, 2020. *MMWR Morb Mortal Wkly Rep*. 2020;69:1310–1312.
35. Augenreich MA, Stickford JL, Stute N, et al. Vascular dysfunction and oxidative stress caused by acute formaldehyde exposure in female adults. *Am J Physiol Heart Circ Physiol*. 2020;319:H1369–H1379.
36. Srivastava S, Sithu SD, Vladykovskaya E, et al. Oral exposure to acrolein exacerbates atherosclerosis in apoE-null mice. *Atherosclerosis*. 2011;215:301–308.
37. DeJarnett N, Conklin DJ, Riggs DW, et al. Acrolein exposure is associated with increased cardiovascular disease risk. *J Am Heart Assoc*. 2014;3:e000934.
38. Schober W, Szendrei K, Matzen W, et al. Use of electronic cigarettes (e-cigarettes) impairs indoor air quality and increases FeNO levels of e-cigarette consumers. *Int J Hyg Environ Health*. 2014;217:628–637.
39. Kaufman JD, Elkind MSV, Bhatnagar A, et al. Guidance to reduce the cardiovascular burden of ambient air pollutants: a policy statement from the American Heart Association. *Circulation*. 2020;142:e432–437.
40. Olmedo P, Goessler W, Tanda S, et al. Metal concentrations in e-cigarette liquid and aerosol samples: the contribution of metallic coils. *Environ Health Perspect*. 2018;126:027010.
41. Keith R, Bhatnagar A. Cardiorespiratory and immunologic effects of electronic cigarettes. *Curr Addict Rep*. 2021;Mar 5:1–11.
42. Tang MS, Wu XR, Lee HW, et al. Electronic-cigarette smoke induces lung adenocarcinoma and bladder urothelial hyperplasia in mice. *Proc Natl Acad Sci USA*. 2019;116:21727–21731.

Heated Tobacco Products

43. Ghinai I, Navon L, Gunn JKL, et al. Characteristics of persons who report using only nicotine-containing products among interviewed patients with E-cigarette, or vaping, product use-associated lung injury - Illinois, August-December 2019. *MMWR Morb Mortal Wkly Rep*. 2020;69:84–89.
44. Zenzen V, Diekmann J, Gerstenberg B, et al. Reduced exposure evaluation of an electrically heated cigarette smoking system. Part 2: smoke chemistry and in vitro toxicological evaluation using smoking regimens reflecting human puffing behavior. *Regul Toxicol Pharmacol*. 2012;64:S11–S34.
45. Farsalinos KE, Yannovits N, Sarri T, et al. Carbonyl emissions from a novel heated tobacco product (IQOS): comparison with an e-cigarette and a tobacco cigarette. *Addiction*. 2018;113:2099–2106.
46. Salman R, Talih S, El-Hage R, et al. Free-base and total nicotine, reactive oxygen species, and carbonyl emissions from IQOS, a heated tobacco product. *Nicotine Tob Res*. 2019;21:1285–1288.
47. Leigh NJ, Palumbo MN, Marino AM, et al. Tobacco-Specific Nitrosamines (TSNA) in heated tobacco product IQOS. *Tob Control*. 2018;27:s37–s38.
48. Nabavizadeh P, Liu J, Havel CM, et al. Vascular endothelial function is impaired by aerosol from a single IQOS HeatStick to the same extent as by cigarette smoke. *Tob Control*. 2018;27:s13–s19.

Harm Reduction and Cessation

49. Pope 3rd CA, Burnett RT, Krewski D, et al. Cardiovascular mortality and exposure to airborne fine particulate matter and cigarette smoke: shape of the exposure-response relationship. *Circulation*. 2009;120:941–948.
50. Hackshaw A, Morris JK, Boniface S, et al. Low cigarette consumption and risk of coronary heart disease and stroke: meta-analysis of 141 cohort studies in 55 study reports. *BMJ*. 2018;360:j5855.
51. Inoue-Choi M, Liao LM, Reyes-Guzman C, et al. Association of long-term, low-intensity smoking with all-cause and cause-specific mortality in the National Institutes of Health-AARP Diet and Health Study. *JAMA Intern Med*. 2017;177:87–95.
52. Chang JT, Anic GM, Rostron BL, et al. Cigarette smoking reduction and health risks: a systematic review and meta-analysis. *Nicotine Tob Res*. 2021;23:635–642. https://doi.org/10.1093/ntr/ntaa156.
53. Kalkhoran S, Glantz SA. E-cigarettes and smoking cessation in real-world and clinical settings: a systematic review and meta-analysis. *Lancet Respir Med*. 2016;4:116–128.

29 Nutrition and Cardiovascular and Metabolic Diseases

DARIUSH MOZAFFARIAN

ENERGY BALANCE, 531

FOODS, 532
Fruits and Vegetables, 532
Nuts and Beans, 532
Whole Grains, Refined Grains, Starches, Sweets, 532
Fish, 534
Red Meats, 534
Poultry, Eggs, 535
Dairy, 535
Plant Oils, 535

BEVERAGES, 535
Sugar-Sweetened Beverages, 535
Milk, 535
Coffee, Tea, 535
Alcohol, 535

MACRONUTRIENTS, 535
Carbohydrates, 535
Fats, 536
Protein, 538

MICRONUTRIENTS, 539

Sodium, Potassium, 539

DIETARY PATTERNS, 539

EMERGING AREAS, 540
Food Processing, 540
Microbiome, 543
Personalized Nutrition, 543

CHANGING BEHAVIOR, 543

REFERENCES, 543

Together with physical activity, smoking cessation, sleep, and stress reduction, a healthy diet forms the foundation for prevention and treatment of cardiometabolic diseases, including coronary heart disease (CHD), stroke, type 2 diabetes mellitus (DM), obesity, and related conditions. Dietary factors represent 8 of the top 25 causes of global deaths, largely owing to effects on cardiometabolic diseases (see also Chapter 1). Insufficient intakes of healthy foods, such as fruits, nuts, whole grains, beans, vegetables, seafood, and yogurt, cause substantial burdens; as do excess intakes of salt, sugary beverages, and processed meats.[1] In the United States, suboptimal diet is the leading cause of poor health, estimated to cause approximately 1 in 4 overall deaths.[2]

Obesity, DM, and related conditions have increased in recent decades, owing to rapid social, cultural, and environmental transitions transmitted primarily through changes in diet and other lifestyle habits. Familiarity with the evidence for effects of different dietary factors, including controversies and uncertainties, is essential to prioritize interventions to improve eating habits and reduce diet-related diseases.

For much of the 20th century, research and policy focused on nutrient deficiency diseases (e.g., scurvy, pellagra) and increased agricultural production of inexpensive, shelf stable, starchy crops (e.g., rice, wheat, corn) to feed a rapidly growing world population.[3] These efforts were successful at achieving their goals, leading to a modern global food system that emphasizes commodity crops and shelf-stable, inexpensive packaged and processed foods rich in starch and sugar, preserved by salt, and fortified with vitamins. This legacy food system was built to address caloric hunger and vitamin deficiencies, not diet-related chronic diseases.

It was not until the 1980s that modern nutrition science turned to focus more on chronic conditions like cardiovascular disease (CVD), DM, and obesity. Over the last 40 years, the emerging science has rapidly advanced from less reliable ecologic (cross-national) comparisons, short-term experiments, and animal studies to more robust evidence from prospective cohort studies of disease endpoints, well-conducted metabolic trials of diverse risk markers and pathways, and randomized clinical trials of disease endpoints. Several new conclusions have emerged.[4] First, dietary habits influence not only blood cholesterol (a major focus of the 1980s) and obesity (a major current focus), but also multiple other established and emerging risk factors (Fig. 29.1). Consequently, health effects of any dietary factor cannot be inferred from effects on any single intermediate endpoint. Second, specific foods and overall dietary patterns, rather than isolated single nutrients, are most important for cardiometabolic health. Third, insufficient intakes of protective foods—e.g., minimally processed, phytonutrient-rich foods like fruits, seeds, nuts, beans, vegetables, and whole grains—produce similar or greater disease burdens than excess intakes of unhealthy factors.

This chapter reviews the evidence for effects of diet on cardiometabolic diseases, and highlights key knowledge gaps. Because translation of knowledge into action is essential, this chapter also briefly reviews effective behavior change strategies.

ENERGY BALANCE (SEE ALSO CHAPTER 30)

The global obesity epidemic is strikingly recent, commencing in the 1980s in the United States and many nations after decades of relative stability.[5] Abdominal adiposity, which produces largest metabolic harms, has also increased more than overall weight in many nations.[6] The breadth, depth, and pace of this epidemic, including in young children,[7] suggest strong environmental drivers, rather than purely behavioral or genetic explanations.

For years, the main scientific and policy responses to obesity have emphasized energy balance and calorie counting. Beyond the empiric failure of this approach to stem the obesity epidemic worldwide, new evidence indicates that the *quality* of food is the major driver of energy imbalance and weight gain.[8] Foods represent complex matrices of nutrients, ingredients, and processing characteristics, each with pleotropic effects on a range of pathways and tissues. More highly processed foods drive greater *ad libitum* energy intake (+508 kcal/day) and weight gain,[9] while carbohydrate quality and quantity also influence energy *expenditure*.[10] Diet quality is thus a major determinant of long-term energy imbalance, which can be considered a downstream mediator, not an upstream determinant, of the obesity epidemic. While nearly any popular diet can work for short-term weight loss, healthful food-based patterns appear most important for long-term weight maintenance.[11] Consequently, long-term obesogenic effects of foods should not be judged on the basis of calorie content alone, but also the molecular and physiologic effects that drive subsequent long-term energy intake and expenditure.

The evidence for effects of foods and diet patterns on obesity and weight control are described further in sections below. Mechanisms are being elucidated and involve, beyond conscious cues like hunger and satiety, unconscious drivers like brain craving and reward, glucose-insulin responses, hepatic fat synthesis, adipocyte function, visceral adiposity, metabolic expenditure, and the gut microbiome.[8,12,13]

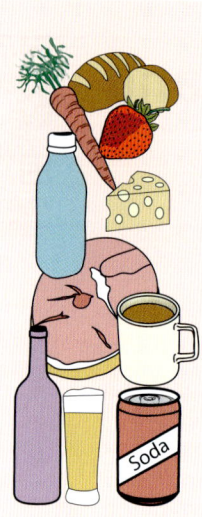

FIGURE 29.1 Diet and cardiovascular and metabolic risk—pathways and mechanisms. Most foods, nutrients, and other factors (e.g., additives, processing methods) have pleotropic effects on diverse pathways of risk. Thus, health effects can rarely be inferred from a single pathway (e.g., changes in blood cholesterol alone). Selected major effects are detailed in the text sections on each dietary factor. (From Mozaffarian D. Dietary and policy priorities for cardiovascular disease, diabetes, and obesity: a comprehensive review. *Circulation.* 2016;133:187–225.)

Other interacting factors include physical activity, industry marketing, TV watching, sleep duration, circadian alignment, and maternal-fetal (e.g., trans-generational) influences. For example, lower sleep duration and altered circadian rhythms alter hunger, food preferences toward "comfort foods" and leptin, ghrelin, insulin, and gut-peptide concentrations.[14] TV watching increases obesity and weight gain, but mediated by changes in diet (e.g., eating in front of the TV, less healthy choices due to TV marketing) rather than physical inactivity.[15–18] Liquid calories from sugary drinks and alcohol, larger portion sizes, and more meals away from home also associate with adiposity. Changes in social norms and networks, industry marketing, and local food availability also appear important.[19,20] Because habitual excess energy intakes as small as approximately 50 to 100 kcal/d may explain much of the obesity epidemic, subtle effects on these pathways are sufficient, when sustained, to account for population shifts in weight (see Fig. 25.4).

Notably, while global obesity has appropriately highlighted the central role of nutrition in health, a focus on obesity alone misses the many other health consequences of dietary habits (see Fig. 29.1). Changes in diet quality substantially improve cardiometabolic risk factors within 6 to 8 weeks, even without weight loss.[4] Thus, obesity should be considered only one mediating pathway for health effects of diet, and the main nutritional targets and metrics of success for individuals and populations should be for overall health, not weight.

FOODS

The successes of nutritional science and dietary guidelines in the 20th century to address vitamin deficiency diseases ensconced a reductionist approach to food that emphasized isolated single nutrients.[3] As chronic diseases emerged as a major public health problem in the 1980s, this scientific emphasis on single nutrients lingered. Thus, dietary fat was considered the major cause of obesity; and saturated fat and cholesterol, the major causes of heart disease. Advances in nutrition science demonstrate that, except for certain major additives like sodium, sugar, or trans fat, single nutrients in isolation are less relevant than food types and overall diet *patterns*—which comprise complex matrices of processing, carbohydrate types, fatty acids, proteins, micronutrients, and phytonutrients.[11,21]

Fruits and Vegetables

Higher fruit and vegetable intake associates with less long-term weight gain[22] and lower incidence of CHD and stroke (Fig. 29.2).[23,24] Total fruit or vegetable intake does not associate with DM, perhaps due to greater importance of certain subtypes.[25] 100% fruit juice similarly appears fairly neutral for glycemia and DM,[26,27] and associates with modestly lower risk of CVD.[28] In controlled trials lasting up to two years, diets including an emphasis on fruits and vegetables improve BP, lipid levels, insulin resistance, inflammation, adiposity, and endothelial function.[4] Such benefits likely derive from the combinations of micronutrients, phytonutrients, and fiber in fruits and vegetables, as well as their replacing less healthful foods. Together these studies provide consistent evidence that fruits and vegetables improve cardiometabolic health. Phytonutrient-rich fruits, such as berries, may have particular benefit.[22,29,30]

Nuts and Beans

Nuts are rich in unsaturated fats, vegetable protein, fiber, folate, minerals, tocopherols, and phenolic compounds. Consumption of nuts lowers total cholesterol, LDL-cholesterol, ApoB, triglycerides, and insulin resistance in trials;[31,32] associates with lower incidence of CHD in prospective studies (see Fig. 29.2);[25,33] and was a key component of a large Mediterranean diet trial that reduced abdominal obesity[34] and risk of hard CVD endpoints by 30%.[35] While their energy density has raised theoretical concerns for weight gain, nuts are rich in healthy fats, fiber, and phenolics, and both long-term observational studies and controlled trials demonstrate that nuts and seeds do not promote, and actually may reduce, weight gain and visceral adiposity.[15,36]

Cardiovascular effects of beans (used herein to include pulses [edible seeds] and legumes) are less well established. Like nuts, beans contain bioactive compounds including phenolics, minerals, and fiber; although also more starch, compared with unsaturated fat-rich nuts. In observational cohorts, bean intake inversely associates with total CVD, CHD, and incident hypertension, but not significantly with stroke or DM (see Fig. 29.2).[25,37] Meta-analyses of small trials of soy foods suggest modest improvements in blood cholesterol levels and arterial stiffness; and small to no effects on other risk factors such as glycemic control, blood pressure, inflammation, and body weight.[38–40] Based on available evidence, eating nuts is a priority for cardiometabolic health; legumes may also be beneficial.

Whole Grains, Refined Grains, Starches, Sweets

Carbohydrate-rich foods dominate most diets: bread, rice, white potatoes, breakfast cereals, crackers, pastas, chips and fries, salty snacks, muffins, sweet bakery products, sugar-sweetened beverages (SSBs),

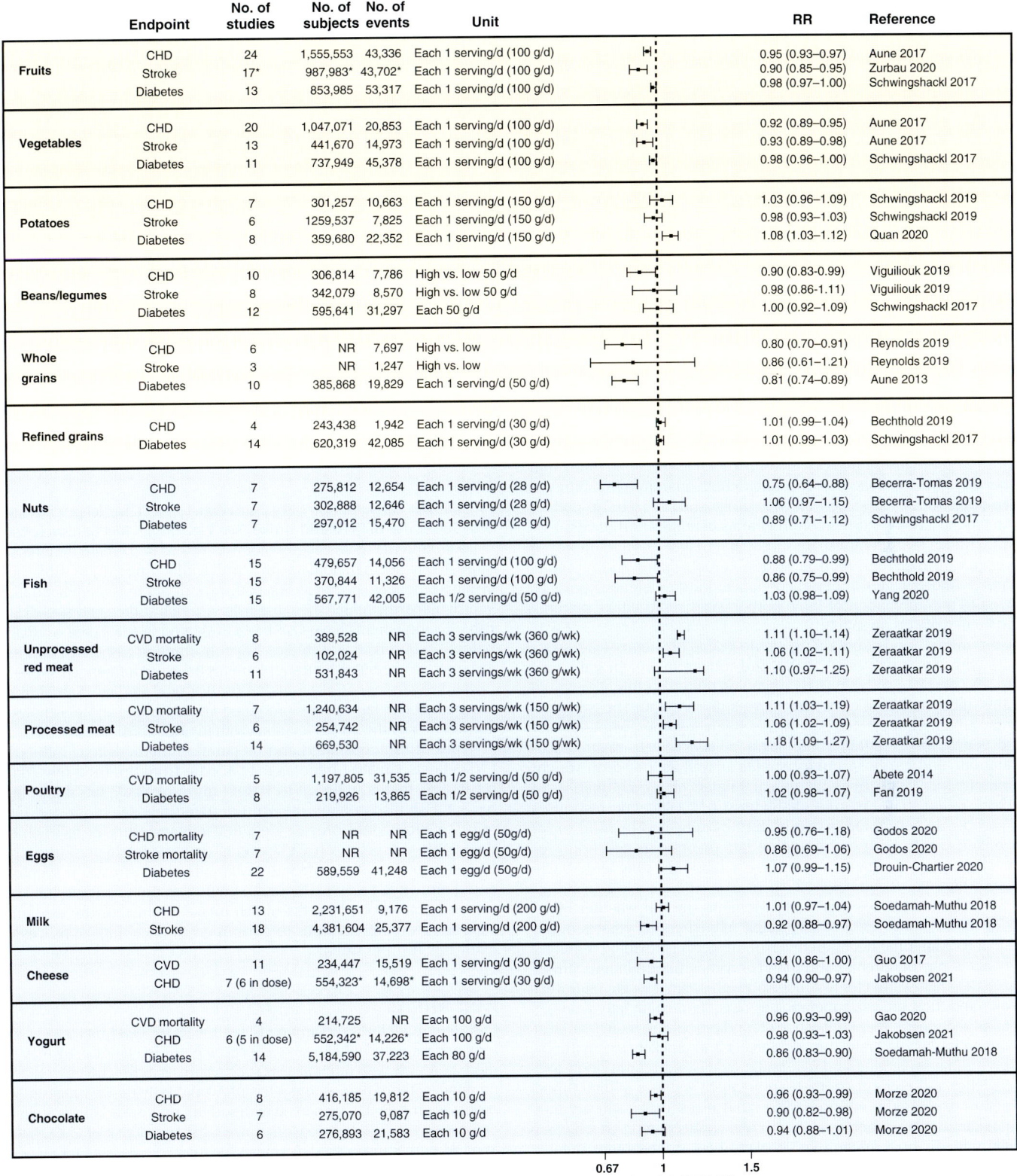

FIGURE 29.2 Meta-analyses of foods and associations with cardiometabolic outcomes. *CHD*, Coronary heart disease; *CVD*, cardiovascular disease; NR, not reported.

and candy. Health effects of such foods appear determined by several characteristics that only partly overlap: whole grain versus refined carbohydrate (starch+sugar) content, dietary fiber content, glycemic load, and food processing (Fig. 29.3).

A whole grain is a seed including its bran (exterior skin; providing fiber, B-vitamins, minerals, flavonoids, and tocopherols), endosperm (starchy interior; nearly all glucose), and germ (plant embryo; providing fatty acids, antioxidants, and phytonutrients). Refined carbohydrates include refined grains (e.g., white flour, white rice), stripped of their bran and germ to leave only starchy endosperm, and added sugars. All refined carbohydrates (sugars or starch) produce rapid, dose-dependent glycemic responses, with similar overall health harms.[4,15,41] Thus, refined carbohydrate (i.e., starch) in foods should be considered a "hidden sugar."

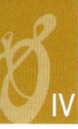

Endpoint		No. of studies	No. of subjects	No. of events	Unit	RR	Reference
100% fruit juice	CVD	2	65,018	4,087	2.3 servings/wk (18.7 oz/d) vs. none (non-linear)	0.90 (0.83–0.97)	D'Elia 2020
	Diabetes	11	407,288	34,549	Each 1 serving/d (8 oz/d)	1.06 (0.98–1.14)	Imamura 2015
SSB	CVD	10	198,388	16,999	Each 1 serving/day (8.5 oz/d)	1.08 (1.02–1.14)	Yin 2020
	Diabetes	7	464,937	38,253	Each 1 serving/day (8 oz/d)	1.27 (1.10–1.46)	Imamura 2015
Coffee	CVD mortality	29*	2,631,398 *	81,188 *	Each 1 cup/d	0.96 (0.95–0.97)	Kim 2019
	Diabetes	38	1,185,210	53,018	Each 1 cup/d	0.94 (0.93–0.95)	Carlstrom 2018
Tea	CHD	7	235,368	8,328	Each 1 cup/d	0.90 (0.81–0.996)	Zhang C 2015
	Stroke	13	407,068	NR	Each 1 cup/d	0.96 (0.93–0.99)	Chung 2020
	Diabetes	8	307,968	11,329	Each 1 cup/d	0.94 (0.90–0.97)	Zhang C 2015

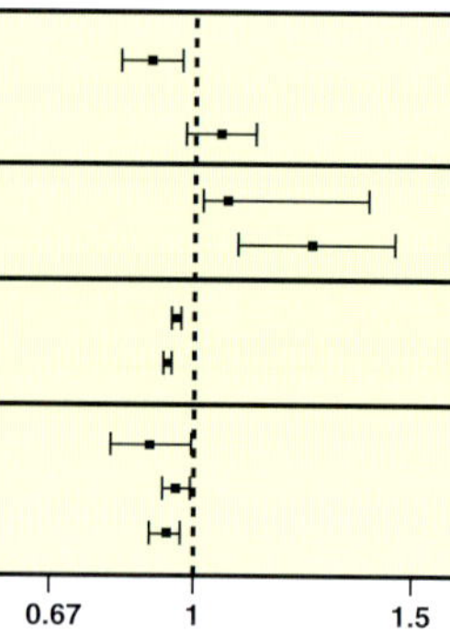

Relative risk (95% CI)

FIGURE 29.3 Meta-analyses of beverages and associations with cardiometabolic outcomes. *BMI*, Body mass index; *CHD*, coronary heart disease; *CVD*, cardiovascular disease; *NR*, not reported; *SSB*, sugar-sweetened beverage.

Foods rich in refined grains, starches, and added sugars associate with risk of long-term weight gain.[15] While the quantity of intake of refined grains does not significantly associate with CHD or DM (see Fig. 29.2), more discriminatory measures such as glycemic index and especially glycemic load, that account for both quantity and rapidity of digestion, strongly associate with CHD, stroke, and DM (see Fig. 29.3).[42–45] Metabolic feeding studies confirm harms of refined carbohydrates,[46] while clinical trials demonstrate substantial weight loss and improved glycemia on diets that reduce refined carbohydrates and glycemic load.[47–49] Added sugars in beverages appear most deleterious, perhaps owing to a combination of large portion sizes, rapid intake patterns, and limited effects on satiety.[4]

In contrast, foods containing whole grains or dietary fiber associate with lower risk of CVD, DM, and long-term weight gain (see Figs. 29.2 and 29.3).[8,50,51] In trials, replacing refined grains with whole grains improves blood cholesterol levels, glycemia, and possibly systemic inflammation.[52] Similarly, fruits, bean, legumes, whole grains, and yogurt also contain some sugar or starch, yet are linked to metabolic and cardiovascular benefits as well as long-term weight maintenance.[4] Such benefits appear related to a combination of factors, rather than any one characteristic.[4,53] Glycemic responses of carbohydrate-rich foods can be further mitigated by food order or mixed meals, such as by adding fats or proteins preceding or accompanying the meal, or even by a healthier long-term background diet.[54,55]

Several uncertainties exist. First, it remains unclear whether benefits of whole grains relate to displacing refined carbohydrates in the diet; or to additional health benefits of the germ (providing minerals, fatty acids, phytonutrients) and bran (providing fiber, minerals, phytonutrients). Dietary fiber, for instance, appears essential for gut microbial health and their bioactive metabolites (e.g., short-chain fatty acids).[56] Second, the independent relevance of food processing is unclear. Most commercial "whole grain" breads, cereals, and crackers are made by finely milling, separating, and reconstituting the endosperm, germ, and bran. Fiber and nutrient contents are retained, but loss of intact food structure exposes the endosperm to rapid digestion by salivary and pancreatic enzymes, increasing its glycemic index compared with less finely milled whole grains (e.g., steel-cut oats, stone-ground bread). Third, the best simple metric for selecting healthier grain products is uncertain (see Fig. 29.3). One pragmatic rule-of-thumb is to choose foods containing at least 1 g of fiber for every 10 g of carbohydrate per serving (carbohydrate:fiber ratio <10:1), which implicitly balances the relative proportions of starch, sugar, whole grain, bran, and added fiber.[57–60]

The relevance of personalization in carbohydrate responses is also of growing interest. Health effects of carbohydrate-rich foods can vary depending on insulin sensitivity, background diet, physical activity, or microbiome composition (see Microbiome and Personalization, below). Given the high rates of adiposity, prediabetes and DM, poor diet, and physical inactivity in most populations, reducing refined grains, starches, and added sugars should be a top priority for most individuals.

Fish

Regular fish consumption (1 to 2 servings/week) associates with modestly lower risk of CHD and stroke (see Fig. 29.2).[61] Mechanistic, observational, and trial data suggest that fish may have stronger benefits for fatal CHD rather than nonfatal myocardial infarction (MI) or stroke, suggesting potential specificity for pathways of acute ischemia-induced ventricular arrhythmia.[62] Because fish are a rich source of omega-3 fats, fish oil supplements have also been evaluated in trials (see n-3 PUFA, below). In observational studies, fish consumption associates with less ischemic stroke, but fish oil supplements have not influenced stroke in post-hoc analyses of CHD trials.[63] Observational studies of atrial fibrillation and heart failure have produced mixed findings.[64] Meta-analyses suggest no significant associations with incident DM.[65]

Types of fish consumed and preparation methods may influence CVD effects. Greatest benefits may accrue from nonfried oily (dark meat) fish, that contain up to 10-fold more omega-3 fats than other types.[64] Fish also contain other unsaturated fats, selenium, and vitamin D, which could provide benefit. Methylmercury in fish has no detectable influence on CVD events or incident hypertension.[66,67] Presence of persistent organic pollutants (e.g., dioxins, polychlorinated biphenyls) may partly reduce but does not appear to fully offset cardiometabolic benefits of fish intake.[68,69] In sum, the evidence supports recommendations to consume 1 to 2 servings of fish, especially oily fish, per week.

Red Meats

Prevalent guidelines recommend lean meats to lower dietary cholesterol and saturated fat. However, effects on cardiometabolic risk may be more complex, with other factors such as preservatives, heme iron, and cooking methods being more relevant. Available evidence suggests that processed meats (i.e., preserved with sodium or other additives, such as deli meats, sausage, hot dogs, bacon, etc.) increase risk of CVD, stroke, and DM; with unprocessed red meats having generally smaller associations, gram for gram, with these endpoints (see Fig. 29.2).[65,70,71] Because unprocessed versus processed meats contain similar average amounts of total fat, saturated fat, and cholesterol,[72] the stronger associations for processed meats suggest that sodium content—about 400% higher in processed meats—or other preservatives such as nitrites (hidden as "celery juice" in "nitrate-free" processed meats) may contribute.[73] Heme iron, a risk factor for DM in animal experiments, gestational DM, and inborn errors of iron metabolism such as hemochromatosis, may explain the higher risk of DM seen with both processed and unprocessed red meats.[74–76] Based on available evidence, processed meats should be avoided, and unprocessed meats eaten up to 1 to 2 servings/wk or less.

Poultry, Eggs

In prospective observational studies, poultry intake appears generally neutral for CVD and DM risk (see Fig. 29.2).[77,78] When combined with its relatively low content of bioactive nutrients, these findings suggest that poultry consumption has minimal cardiometabolic effects. Eggs appear similarly neutral for CVD risk in general populations (see Fig. 29.2).[79-81] Overall evidence suggests minimal cardiometabolic effects of poultry intake or occasional egg intake (e.g., up to 2 to 3 per week); consistent with recent similar conclusions on dietary cholesterol[11] (see Dietary Cholesterol, below).

Dairy

Cardiometabolic effects of dairy foods have generally been considered in relation to a limited set of nutrients: saturated fat, calcium, vitamin D. Yet, more diverse dairy nutrients and processing methods appear relevant. These include fermentation of yogurt and cheese (creating menaquinones), branch-chain, odd-chain, and medium-chain fatty acid contents, probiotics in yogurt, milk fat globule membrane content, and more.[82,83] In long-term cohorts, milk intake associates with lower risk of stroke, cheese with lower risk of CHD, and yogurt, cheese, and possibly butter with lower risk of DM (see Fig. 29.2).[84-86] In randomized trials, milk or total dairy consumption increases lean mass and reduces body fat and waist circumference.[87] In long-term observational studies, yogurt associates with relative weight loss,[15] potentially related to probiotic-microbiome interactions.[88-91]

In contrast, lower dairy fat content (reduced-fat or non-fat) does not consistently relate to lower cardiometabolic risk. Indeed, in a pooled analysis of 16 global cohorts, individuals with higher blood biomarkers of dairy fat consumption had significantly lower incidence of DM.[92] Recent experimental evidence suggests that odd-chain saturated fats such as 15:0, fairly unique to dairy fat, reduce inflammation and dyslipidemia by binding to key metabolic regulators and repairing mitochondrial function.[93] In sum, current evidence supports recommendations for modest dairy intake (2 to 3 servings/day), especially of yogurt and cheese, with more research needed to define the relevant active ingredients and health effects of dairy fat.

Plant Oils

While "industrial" or "refined" plant oils, especially those rich in n-6 PUFA, have been theorized to be harmful to health, little evidence supports this concern. The great majority of interventional and observational studies of total PUFA, n-6 PUFA, and MUFA have assessed industrialized plant oils like soybean, canola, and safflower oil. The cumulative evidence supports clear benefits of such plant oils (see Macronutrients, below). Whether virgin versions of these oils would have even greater benefits, for example due to greater concentrations of phenolics and phytosterols,[94,95] is possible and requires investigation. Few studies have evaluated tropical oils (e.g., palm, coconut), beyond their known effects on blood lipids (raising both LDL-cholesterol and HDL-cholesterol).[96-98]

BEVERAGES

Sugar-Sweetened Beverages

Ecologic data, prospective cohorts, and trials provide convincing evidence that SSB intake increases adiposity. In the United States, calories consumed from beverages rapidly increased after the 1960s, doubling to 21.0% of all calories consumed by 2002—an increase of 222 daily kcal per person.[99] This was largely due to increased SSBs (sodas, energy drinks, sweetened ice teas, fruit drinks), although that peak has been followed by gradual declines in SSB consumption thereafter.[100,101] Per serving, SSBs more strongly associate with long-term weight gain than nearly any other dietary factor.[15] Randomized trials confirm that reducing SSBs decreases weight gain and fat accumulation.[102,103] Calories in liquid form, compared with solid foods, appear to be less satiating and increase total calories consumed.[104] SSB intake also associates with significantly higher incidence of CVD and especially DM (see Fig. 29.3,[26,105] likely related to weight gain and other additional harms of the high sugar and glycemic load. Given clear evidence for harms, and multiple alternatives (e.g., water, seltzer, unsweetened tea, diet soda, milk), SSBs should be largely eliminated from the diet.

Alternative sweeteners can be artificial (e.g., saccharin, aspartame) or naturally low-calorie (e.g., stevia). Based on observational studies and clinical trials, alternative sweeteners are better for cardiometabolic health than added sugars.[15,106] Yet, alternative sweeteners may not be completely benign: animal experiments and limited human data suggest influences on brain reward, taste perception, oral-gastrointestinal taste receptors, glucose-insulin and energy homeostasis, metabolic hormones, and the gut microbiome.[107-111] For instance, if a child becomes accustomed to intense sweet tastes, will that reduce attractiveness of naturally sweet foods such as apples or carrots? In sum, alternative sweeteners can be a useful bridge to eliminate SSBs, but should not be considered innocuous; and subsequent shifts to non-sweetened drinks (e.g., seltzer, tea) should be encouraged.

Milk

See Dairy.

Coffee, Tea

While coffee and tea provide caffeine, these plant extracts—derived from beans and leaves—contain other bioactive compounds. Unrelated to caffeine content, frequent coffee intake (e.g., 3 to 4 cups/day) associates with less insulin resistance, DM, CVD, and in a few studies, heart failure (see Fig. 29.3).[112,113] Yet, clear physiologic benefits have not been established to support these observations. Acutely, caffeinated coffee worsens BP, insulin resistance, and glucose intolerance;[114,115] longer-term, habitual coffee intake does not affect BP, endothelial function, nor glucose metabolism, suggesting tachyphylaxis and/or other partly offsetting factors.[116,117] In mendelian randomization analyses, genetic variants linked to coffee intake do not associate with CHD, stroke, or DM.[118-120] Based on lack of physiologic benefits in trials or lower risk in mendelian randomization studies, the cardiometabolic benefits of coffee intake should still be considered questionable.

Like coffee, frequent tea drinking (e.g., 3+ cups/day) associates with lower CVD and DM, with borderline statistical significance (see Fig. 29.3).[121,122] In randomized trials, certain types of tea modestly lower BP (green, black, sour), LDL-cholesterol (green), and fasting glucose (green, sour).[116,123-126] In contrast to coffee, these physiologic effects support potential causal cardiometabolic benefits of tea, but larger and more rigorous studies are still needed.

Alcohol

See Chapter 84.

MACRONUTRIENTS

Carbohydrates

For decades, carbohydrates were recommended as the foundation of a healthful diet, e.g., grain products at the base of the 1992 Food Guide Pyramid. Current science makes clear that the quality and food source, rather than total amount, of carbohydrate is most relevant for cardiometabolic health (Fig. 29.4)[4] (also see Whole Grains, Refined Grains, Starches, Sweets). Because most carbohydrate in modern diets derives from refined starches and sugars, a "low-carb" diet will often produce metabolic benefit. Yet, healthful carbohydrate-containing foods like fruits, legumes, and minimally processed whole grains should not be avoided. For most patients with metabolic risk factors, a focus on reducing refined grains, starches, and added sugars should be a priority.[4,8,11]

While marketing claims are often made about different forms of sugars (disaccharides), major types (cane sugar, beet sugar, high-fructose corn syrup) are molecularly similar: about half glucose and half fructose. Thus, health differences between total free sugars, added sugars, or different subtypes of sugars have not been clearly demonstrated.[127-129]

Type	Processing and Structure	Examples
Intact whole grains	Whole grain with the bran, germ, and endosperm from the natural cereal intact	Barley, sorghum, millet, brown rice, bulgur wheat, amaranth, wheat berries
Minimally processed whole grains	Some processing is performed to improve palatability or digestibility, yet the bran and germ remain partially intact	Stone-ground whole wheat bread, cracked wheat, steel-cut oats
Milled whole grains	The whole grain, including bran, germ, and endosperm, is milled to fine flour	Most commercially available whole grain breads, whole grain breakfast cereals, whole grain pasta
Starchy vegetables*	Plants that have been bred or engineered to contain high levels of starch with relatively low dietary fiber and micronutrients	Potatoes, corn, green peas[†]
Refined grains*	The bran and germ are removed during processing, leaving the endosperm comprised largely of refined starch	White bread, white rice, most ready-to-eat breakfast cereals, instant oatmeal, regular pasta
Refined sugars*	Natural and industrially produced monosaccharides, disaccharides, and oligosaccharides, including sucrose, glucose, fructose, high-fructose corn syrup, maltose, dextrose, and maltodextrin	Candies, other sugars added to foods
Sweetened refined grains*	Refined grains with added refined sugars	Sweetened breakfast cereals, grain-based desserts (cakes, cookies, pies, doughnuts, sweet rolls, muffins)
Refined sugars in liquid form	Natural and industrially produced monosaccharides and disaccharides in liquid form	Sugar-sweetened beverages, including sodas, iced teas, sports drinks, and fruit drinks

FIGURE 29.4 A hierarchy of carbohydrate quality. Dietary fiber content, whole versus refined grain content, glycemic response to ingestion, and extent of processing of grains, cereals, and sugars can be separately altered, creating a complex hierarchy of effects from healthiest (*dark green*) to most harmful (*dark red*). *Simple and complex refined carbohydrates induce similarly high glycemic responses following ingestion and, in amounts typically consumed in Western diets, induce hepatic de novo lipogenesis, that is, synthesis of fat from carbohydrate. [†]Corn, peas, and certain potatoes provide reasonable fiber and modestly lower glycemic responses than white potatoes. Yams and sweet potatoes are not included here due to higher nutrient contents and lower glycemic responses.

The monosaccharides glucose and fructose—together forming sugar—have differing physiologic effects. When consumed at high, rapidly digested doses, both appear to cause metabolic harm. Glucose induces postprandial hyperglycemia, hyperinsulinemia, and related disturbances, as well as hepatic de novo lipogenesis at high levels; while fructose has little influence on blood glucose or insulin, but more directly stimulates hepatic de novo lipogenesis, hepatic and visceral adiposity, and uric acid production.[130,131] Such harms are avoided by modest, slowly digested doses of either glucose or fructose (e.g., as found in fruit or beans). Thus, the dose, rapidity of digestion, accompanying nutrients, and food structure (liquid, solid) may each modify health effects of sugars.

Resistant starches are of growing interest but understudied. Starches can be resistant to digestion due to physical inaccessibility (e.g., intact whole grains), crystalline form (e.g., raw potatoes, green bananas, high amylose maize), retrogradation (realignment of cooked, gelatinized starches during cooling, e.g. stale bread, cold rice), or chemical modification (e.g., many emulsifiers, stabilizers, thickening agents).[132] Like dietary fiber, resistant starches feed the microbiota in the large intestine, producing short-chain fatty acids and other microbial metabolites. Two recent meta-analyses identified only small, short-term trials of resistant starch, conducted in mixed patient populations.[133,134] Evaluating body weight, satiety, and glucose-insulin homeostasis, some benefits were identified, but these are of uncertain relevance given the small number of studies, heterogeneity, and uncertain risk of bias.

Fats
Total Fat
Whereas early ecologic (cross-national) studies suggested that fat intake increased cardiometabolic risk, prospective cohorts and randomized trials have established that the percent of total fat in foods or diets has negligible effects on CVD, DM (Fig. 29.5), or weight loss, weight gain, or overweight/obesity (*see* Energy Balance).[4,8,11,135,136] In contrast, different types of fats and fatty acids have important health effects. Conventionally, dietary fats are categorized based on chemistry—the number and position of double bonds—rather than physiologic effects. This classification obscures differences in dietary sources and biologic effects of individual fatty acids, which influence gene transcription, cell membrane fluidity, receptor function, and lipid metabolites and more importantly, their diverse food sources. This chapter follows the conventional categories but discusses effects of individual fatty acids where sufficient data exist.

Saturated Fats
Major sources include meats, dairy products, and tropical oils (e.g., palm, coconut). Based on ecologic comparisons, effects on LDL-cholesterol, and animal experiments, SFA intake would be expected to increase CHD risk. Yet, actual health effects are more complex. First, when replacing total carbohydrate, SFA increases LDL-cholesterol but at least partly due to increasing LDL-cholesterol particle size, rather than increasing ApoB; and SFA also reduces triglyceride-rich particles and lipoprotein(a) and raises HDL-cholesterol and Apo-A1.[137] In comparison to total carbohydrate, SFA has no significant effects on fasting glucose, HbA_{1c}, or insulin resistance.[135,138] These summed effects would predict relatively neutral effects of SFA on CVD events or DM, compared with carbohydrate or the average background diet. Prospective cohort studies confirm null associations with CHD and DM and possible inverse associations with stroke (see Fig. 29.5).[135,136,139] In a large randomized trial targeting total fat reduction, SFA intake was reduced by approximately 27%, largely replaced with carbohydrates, without effects on incident CHD (RR=0.98), stroke (RR=1.02), or DM

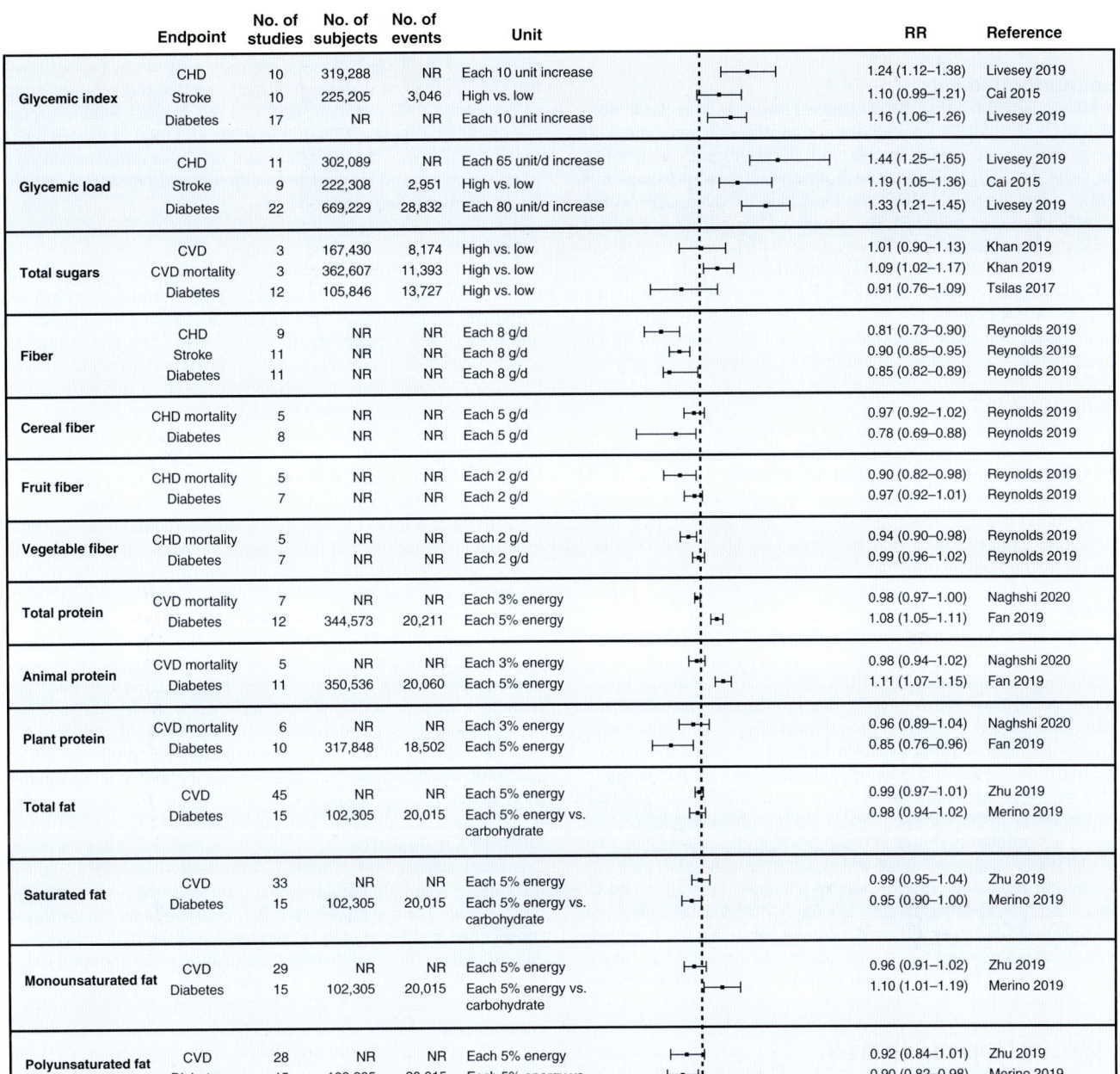

FIGURE 29.5 Meta-analyses of nutrients and associations with cardiometabolic outcomes. *CHD*, coronary heart disease; *CVD*, cardiovascular disease; *NR*, not reported.

(RR=0.96).[140,141] In the international PURE study,[142] very low SFA consumption was linked to higher risk of stroke, consistent with other reports.[139] Replacement of total SFA with polyunsaturated fats (PUFA) reduces CHD risk (see PUFA, below), but this appears largely attributable to benefits of PUFA, rather than harms of SFA.

Second, there are several different SFA: lauric (12:0), myristic (14:0), palmitic (16:0), and stearic (18:0) acid; odd-chain SFA in dairy (15:0, 17:0); and very long-chain SFA (20:0, 22:0, 24:0). Each of these has different effects on blood lipids; potential differing long-term health effects remain unclear.[137] Finally, health effects of SFA vary depending on the food source, with very different relationships for processed meats, unprocessed red meats, different types of dairy, plant oils, etc. (see Foods, above).

While major dietary guidelines continue to recommend a limit on SFA, guidance has shifted over time to specify replacement with PUFA, rather than carbohydrates or monounsaturated fats (MUFA).[11] Yet, the recommendation to limit total SFA is increasingly controversial, with many scientists stating that heterogeneity in health effects of different

SFA and their food sources indicates a need to move away from limits on total SFA and toward guidance on individual foods.[143,144]

Monounsaturated Fats

While MUFA favorably affect BP, cholesterol levels, and glycemic control in trials,[137,138,145] MUFA intake does not consistently associate with lower risk of CVD in cohort studies, and associates with higher risk of DM (see Fig. 29.5).[135,136] Because both animal fats and plant oils (e.g., olive, canola) provide MUFA, the food source may modify overall health effects, as seen with SFA. For instance, olive oil, but not mixed animal and plant sources of MUFA, associates with lower CHD;[146] while plant oil sources of MUFA reduce LDL proteoglycan binding, suggesting anti-atherogenic effects.[147] Thus, focusing on specific foods and oils, rather than MUFA content *per se*, may be most prudent. Extra-virgin olive oil, mixed nuts, avocados, and canola oil are sources of MUFA with reasonable evidence for cardiometabolic benefits.

Polyunsaturated Fats

PUFA are classified as n-6 or n-3, based on the carbon location of the first double bond. The predominant PUFA is n-6 linoleic acid (LA, 18:2n-6), derived principally from plant oils. Flaxseed, canola, walnuts, and soybeans provide alpha-linoleic acid (ALA, 18:3n-3); and seafood, eicosapentaenoic acid (EPA, 20:5n-3) and docosahexaenoic acid (DHA, 22:6n-3). Both LA and ALA are essential fatty acids—i.e., they cannot be synthesized by humans and must be derived from the diet.

n-6 PUFA

While harms of n-6 PUFA have been speculated upon, metabolic interventions, cohort studies, and clinical trials demonstrate health benefits. LA lowers LDL-cholesterol and triglyceride-rich lipoproteins, raises HDL-cholesterol, lowers HbA_{1c} and fasting insulin, and improves insulin secretion capacity.[137,138] While pro-inflammatory effects have been theorized, such effects are not seen in humans.[148,149] LA may actually reduce hepatic steatosis and systemic inflammation.[150,151] Arachidonic acid, the prototypical metabolite of LA, is commonly considered pro-inflammatory, but also gives rise to specialized proresolving mediators (SPMs) of inflammation,[152] and in prospective studies associates with lower CHD.[153] LA also associates with lower CHD and DM (see Fig. 29.5), whether replacing carbohydrate or saturated fat.[135,136,154] Objective blood biomarker levels of LA associate with lower incidence of CVD events and DM in pooled cohort studies, while AA levels do not associate with higher risk.[155,156] In meta-analysis of clinical trials, intake of n-6 rich plant oils like soybean oil, in place of animal fats, reduces CHD events.[157]

n-3 PUFA (see Chapters 25 and 27)

CVD effects of ALA, the plant-derived n-3 PUFA, remain inconclusive.[63,158,159] In a Dutch trial, an ALA-rich margarine did not significantly reduce total CVD events (RR=0.91; 95% CI: 0.78 to 1.05).[160] However, in a pooling project of 19 cohorts across 16 countries, blood biomarker levels of ALA associated with lower risk of fatal CHD, but not total CHD or nonfatal MI.[161] This is consistent with a reduction in cardiac arrhythmia in a meta-analysis of two trials of ALA supplementation.[63] More research is needed.

The long-chain n-3 PUFA EPA and DHA, derived from fish and shellfish, produce multiple physiologic benefits in human trials, improving heart rate, blood pressure, triglyceride-rich lipoproteins, endothelial function, adiponectin, cardiac function, and inflammatory responses.[64,162] In observational studies, dietary EPA+DHA most consistently associate with fatal CHD,[153,158,163] consistent with dog and primate experiments showing benefits for ischemia-induced ventricular fibrillation.[64] Similarly, in pooling projects of international cohorts, blood biomarker levels of long-chain n-3 PUFA associated with lower risk of fatal CHD, not total CHD or nonfatal MI; and lower risk of DM.[161,164]

Multiple clinical trials have evaluated CVD effects of n-3 PUFA supplements, most often in the form of fish oil.[63,64,165] Meta-analyses are most consistent with reduced risk of CHD mortality, similar to findings for dietary fish and EPA+DHA intake, but individual trial results have been conflicting.[63,165] In a recent trial of patients with elevated triglycerides, on statins, with either established CVD or diabetes plus other CVD risk factors (REDUCE-IT), supplementation with high-dose purified EPA (4 g/day) reduced combined CVD by 25% (HR 0.75; 95% CI 0.68 to 0.83).[166] A large primary prevention trial of low-dose fish oil (1 g/day) did not significantly reduce the primary endpoint of combined CVD (HR 0.92; 0.80 to 1.06), but did reduce secondary endpoints of total MI (HR 0.72; 0.59 to 0.90) and total CHD (HR 0.83; 0.71 to 0.97).[167] Reasons for the discrepant results of different fish oil trials remain unclear and may relate to differences in dose, population risk, background diet, and endpoints.

Trans Fats

Trans fats (TFA) are unsaturated fats with one or more double bonds in the *trans*, rather than *cis*, position. TFA cannot be synthesized by mammals. Natural sources include small amounts in ruminant meats and milk (formed by gut microorganisms in cows, sheep, and goats), which contribute minimally to diet (<0.5%E) and do not associate with CVD risk.[168] Indeed, higher blood levels of trans-16:1n-7, a natural TFA in dairy fat, associate with lower risk of DM.[92]

Much higher levels of industrial TFA, coming from partially hydrogenated vegetable oils, consistently associate with higher CVD (see Fig. 29.5).[136] Unique among dietary fats, TFA consumption raises LDL-cholesterol, ApoB, triglycerides, and lipoprotein(a), and lowers HDL-cholesterol and ApoA1.[169] TFA also exhibit non-lipid effects, promoting inflammation, endothelial dysfunction, insulin resistance, visceral adiposity, and arrhythmia, although strength of evidence for these non-lipid effects varies.[170] In sum, the implicated pathways suggest effects of TFA on adipocyte dysfunction and insulin resistance. Emerging evidence suggests that 18:2 TFA isomers may be most adverse, formed not only by partial hydrogenation but also other industrial processes such as oil deodorization and high-temperature cooking.[171,172] Because partially hydrogenated oils are food additives with clear adverse effects, their elimination is a public health priority. The Food and Drug Administration recently ruled that partially hydrogenated oils are no longer "generally regarded as safe," greatly reducing industrial TFA in the U.S. food supply.

Dietary Cholesterol

Dietary cholesterol raises both LDL-cholesterol and HDL-cholesterol, resulting in small net change in the total HDL-cholesterol ratio. In certain animals, dietary cholesterol is pro-atherogenic. Yet, in long-term prospective studies, dietary cholesterol and its major sources (e.g., eggs, shellfish) have inconsistent associations with incident CHD and stroke.[173-175] Among patients with prevalent DM, dietary cholesterol associates with higher CHD risk;[176] associations with incident DM appear mixed.[177,178] In sum, dietary cholesterol appears to have minor CVD effects in the general population, but may increase CVD among diabetic patients. Elucidation of reasons for this potential difference requires further investigation.

Protein

Increased dietary protein in combination with strength-training increases muscle mass more than strength-training alone in generally healthy middle-aged and older adults.[179,180] Given relevance of lean muscle mass for insulin sensitivity, this suggests protein consumption plus strength training could improve metabolic health. Yet, studies of dietary protein and satiety, weight control, or metabolic health show mixed findings. In meta-analysis of randomized trials, increased protein consumption had little effect on metabolic risk factors including adiposity, lipids, blood pressure, inflammation, or glucose.[181] In prospective cohorts, total protein intake has borderline associations with CVD and is associated with *higher* risk of diabetes (see Fig. 29.5).[78,182] When food sources were separately evaluated, animal protein sources were associated with higher DM risk; and plant protein sources, with lower risk. In interventional studies, high protein diets induce variable effects on the gut microbiome, again with differences for animal versus plant sources.[183] Given the broadly similar amino acid profiles of animal and plant proteins (indeed, the former are often more complete and bioavailable), these variable findings suggest that, like health effects of carbohydrates and fats, cardiometabolic effects of dietary protein depend on the food source and not the protein content per se.

MICRONUTRIENTS

Sodium, Potassium (see Chapter 26)

In Western countries, most sodium (approximately 75%) comes from packaged foods and restaurant meals (rather than home cooking or table salt); while in Asian countries, most comes from soy sauce or salt added during cooking or at the table.[184] Nearly every country in the world exceeds the recommended mean intake of 2000 mg/d.[185] Sodium raises BP in a dose-dependent fashion, with stronger effects among older individuals, hypertensives, and Blacks.[186] In meta-analyses, high sodium intakes associate most strongly with incident stroke (see Fig. 29.5).[187,188] Animal studies further suggest that habitually high dietary sodium induces long-term renal, myocardial, and vascular fibrosis.[189] While some observational studies suggest a potential J-shaped relation, with higher CVD risk at low intakes (e.g., <3000 g/day), specific biases related to sodium assessment in observational studies could produce a spurious J-shape.[190] The National Academies of Sciences, Engineering, and Medicine reviewed all the evidence and set the recommended intake at below 2300 mg/day.[191]

In trials, potassium lowers BP, with stronger effects among hypertensive individuals and when dietary sodium intake is high;[192] and potassium-rich diets associate with lower risk of stroke (see Fig. 29.5).[187,193,194] Potassium also attenuates, while insufficient dietary potassium exacerbates, the BP-raising effects of sodium. Overall, the evidence supports the importance of potassium-rich foods for reducing BP and CVD.

CALCIUM, MAGNESIUM

In short-term trials, calcium and magnesium supplements also modestly lower BP, although with substantial heterogeneity between studies. However, calcium supplements with or without vitamin D may increase risk of MI in controlled trials.[195] In observational analyses, dietary and blood Mg inversely associate with CVD and DM;[196,197] long-term trials have not been performed. Calcium and magnesium supplements cannot yet be recommended for general CVD prevention.

ANTIOXIDANT VITAMINS

Certain dietary vitamins and nutrients associate with lower CVD in observational studies, but fail to lower risk when given as supplements in trials, including folate, B-vitamins, beta-carotene, vitamin C, vitamin E, and selenium.[198] Most of these trials, for reasons of power, evaluated up to a few years of treatment in high-risk individuals or patients with established CVD. In contrast, most observational studies evaluated long-term or habitual intake among generally healthy people. Thus, discrepancies in findings could partly relate to different time periods of biologic sensitivity; for example, some vitamins and nutrients could be important only early in the disease course. Discrepancies may also relate to residual bias in observational studies from other behaviors (i.e., observed benefits are not due to diet) or due to other nutritional factors in vitamin-rich foods (i.e., observed benefits are due to diet but not to the specific isolated vitamin or mineral). Diets higher in antioxidant vitamins tend to be rich in fruits, vegetables, nuts, and whole grains, foods that contain multiple other beneficial factors including other vitamins, minerals, phytonutrients, and fiber, as well as replacing unhealthful foods. Thus, isolating limited nutrients in these foods as supplements may not produce similar effects as consuming the whole food.

VITAMIN D

Higher plasma vitamin D levels associate with lower CVD, but are largely driven by sun exposure, not diet. Meta-analysis of 21 large supplement trials shows no significant benefits,[199] nor do vitamin D supplements improve blood pressure or glycemic control.[200] Vitamin D supplementation is not indicated to improve cardiometabolic health.

POLYPHENOLS

Bioactive polyphenols include more than 5000 different flavanols (in onions, broccoli, tea, various fruits), flavones (parsley, celery, chamomile tea), flavanones (citrus fruits), flavanols (flavan-3-ols) such as catechins and procyanidins (cocoa, apples, grapes, red wine, tea), anthocyanidins (colored berries), and isoflavones (soy). In laboratory studies and randomized trials, flavonoid-rich cocoa or dark chocolate has small but measurable benefits on BP, endothelial function, insulin resistance, and blood lipids,[201,202] without increases in body weight or adiposity.[200] BP-lowering has been shown with as little as 6.3 g/day of dark chocolate and correlates with increased endothelial nitric oxide production.[203] Observational studies and trials of dietary flavan-3-ols also suggest cardiometabolic benefits.[204] In extra virgin olive oil, oleocanthal is an anti-inflammatory flavonoid that inhibits cyclooxygenase 1 and 2 isoenzymes and may partly explain health benefits.[205] Supplementation with flavonoids prevents diet-induced weight gain in several animal models, even on calorie-matched diets.[82] Some observational studies evaluating total or selected dietary flavonoids observe lower risk of cardiometabolic events;[82,204] one large clinical trial is ongoing. The heterogeneity of different flavonoids and their dietary sources limits inference for class effects, and clinical benefits and dose-responses remain unclear. Yet, many foods with evidence for cardiometabolic benefits—e.g., berries, nuts, extra-virgin olive oil—are rich in phenolics, and their physiologic and molecular effects are highly promising for further study.

DIETARY PATTERNS

Evidence-based healthful diet patterns, which represent overall combinations of foods consumed, share several key characteristics (Table 29.1): more minimally processed, bioactive-rich foods such as fruits, nuts or seeds, nonstarchy vegetables, beans, whole grains, seafood, yogurt, and plant oils; and fewer red meats, processed (sodium-preserved) meats, and processed and packaged foods rich in refined grains, starches, added sugars, salt, and trans fat. Two of the most studied, each with clear cardiometabolic benefits, are the traditional Mediterranean and DASH dietary patterns.[11]

Randomized trials in both primary and secondary prevention populations confirm significant cardiometabolic benefits of such healthful, food-based diet patterns.[35,206–208] This contrasts with small effects of nutrient-based approaches to dietary guidance, such as low-fat, low-saturated fat diets, in observational cohorts and randomized trials.[137,140,141,153] The main exceptions are additives, such as sodium, added sugar, and trans fats: because these can be added to or removed from otherwise similar foods and diet patterns, a specific nutrient focus on these additives is warranted. Focusing on overall diet patterns can lead to health benefits from modest changes across multiple foods, rather than large changes in a few factors, potentially increasing effectiveness and compliance. This flexibility can also facilitate behavioral counseling, permitting more room for more personalized focus (Table 29.2).[11]

People who follow vegetarian or vegan diets are often health-conscious and select healthier, minimally processed foods. Yet such diets can vary dramatically in their healthfulness, as much of what is harmful in modern foods—refined grains, starches, sugars, salt—is plant-based. A cardioprotective diet pattern is best characterized by being rich in specific healthful foods (see Table 29.1).

Newer popular dietary patterns include low-carbohydrate, ketogenic, and paleo diets. In a network meta-analysis of 56 randomized trials in patients with diabetes, Mediterranean, paleo, and vegetarian diets appeared most effective at reducing fasting glucose, while low-carb, Mediterranean, and paleo diets appeared most effective to reduce HbA_{1c}.[209] In exploratory subgroup analyses, low-carb diets appeared more effective in shorter-term studies, smaller studies, and older individuals (age 60+ years), while Mediterranean diets appeared more effective in longer-term studies, larger studies, and younger adults (age <60 years). For weight loss in diabetic patients, a meta-analysis of 20 randomized trials of various popular diets found significant weight loss only with a Mediterranean diet.[210] Nearly all of these trials did not exceed 1 year, raising questions about long-term effects.

Low-carbohydrate diets generally produce similar or greater weight loss than low-fat diets, with corresponding improvements in CVD risk factors,[47,211] and are superior to low-fat diets for glycemic control in diabetic patients.[49,212,213] A "low-carbohydrate" focus appears to be a simple rule to reduce selection of ultraprocessed foods rich in refined carbohydrates.[209] However, when minimally processed, phytonutrient-rich

TABLE 29.1 Food-Based Components of Dietary Patterns that Improve Cardiometabolic Health*

	GOAL[†]	SERVING SIZES
Consume More		
Fruits	3 servings per day	About 100 g, e.g., 1 medium-sized fruit; ½ cup of fresh, frozen, or canned fruit; ¼ cup of dried fruit; ½ cup of 100% juice. Goals should not be met with juice alone
Vegetables and beans	3–4 servings per day	About 100 g, e.g., 1 cup of raw leafy vegetable; ½ cup of cut-up raw vegetables, cooked vegetables, or 100% juice. Limit potatoes to ½ cup or less per day
Whole grains[‡]	3 servings per day, in place of refined grains	About 50 g, e.g., 1 slice of whole-grain bread; 1 cup of high-fiber whole-grain cereal; ½ cup cooked whole-grain rice, pasta, or cereal
Nuts	4–5 servings per week	About 28 g (1 oz)
Fish and shellfish	2+ servings per week, preferably oily	About 100 g (3.5 oz). Goals should not be met with commercially prepared deep-fried or breaded fish
Dairy products[§]	2–3 servings per day	1 cup of milk or yogurt; 1.5 oz of cheese
Plant oils	2–6 servings per day	About 1 teaspoon of oil, e.g., in cooking or salad dressing; or 1 tablespoon of vegetable spread
Consume Less		
Refined grains and starches	Minimize intake	1-oz equivalents, e.g., slice of bread, bowl of cereal
Processed meats (e.g., bacon, sausage, hot dogs, processed deli meats)	Avoid intake or at most modest intake, e.g., up to 1 serving per week	About 100 g (3.5 oz)
Foods containing partially hydrogenated plant oils (industrial trans fat)	Avoid intake	
Sugar-sweetened beverages, sweets, and bakery foods	Avoid intake or at most modest intake, e.g. up to 5 servings per week	8 oz of soda; 1 small cookie, doughnut, or muffin; 1 slice of cake or pie
Alcohol	Up to 2 daily drinks for men, 1 daily drink for women	5 oz wine; 12 oz beer; 1.5 oz spirits
Energy Balance	Eat healthy foods as above, reduce portion sizes of unhealthy foods, eat fewer fast-food and prepared meals, increase physical activity, limit TV watching, and ensure adequate (7–8 hr) sleep	

*Adapted from the evidence described in this chapter.
[†]Based on a 2000 kcal/day diet. Servings should be adjusted accordingly for higher or lower energy consumption.
[‡]A practical rule-of-thumb for selecting healthier grain or carbohydrate-rich products is to choose foods containing at least 1 g of dietary fiber for every 10 g of total carbohydrate per serving (a carb:fiber ratio<10:1), based on the Nutrition Facts Panel.
[§]Based on available evidence, the types of dairy (yogurt, cheese, milk, butter) appears more relevant than fat content (whole or reduced fat); yogurt and cheese seem most beneficial (see text for details).

foods are emphasized, low-carbohydrate and low-fat diets lead to similar weight loss, without caloric restriction.[9,214] Overall, a diet rich in minimally processed foods and healthy fats and low in ultraprocessed foods and refined grains, starches, and sugars appears optimal.

Extreme low-carbohydrate (i.e., ketogenic) diets can lead to meaningful weight loss and metabolic benefits.[215] However, such diets may be challenging to sustain and do not leverage health benefits of fruits, nonstarchy vegetables, beans/legumes, and minimally processed whole grains. Also, the biologic need for ketosis per se (vs. simply reducing refined starches and sugars) remains unclear. Extreme low-carb diets may be most useful for initial weight loss (e.g., over 6 to 12 months), followed by transitions toward slowly incorporating carbs from minimally processed, bioactive-rich foods as tolerated. Potential long-term health effects require further investigation.

Paleo diets aim to conform to foods consumed during human evolution over millennia. Benefits include avoidance of poor quality carbohydrates (refined starches, sugars) and other ultra-processed foods; and positive emphasis on nonstarchy vegetables, nuts, and fish; which together can produce weight loss and corresponding metabolic benefits.[216] Yet some interpretations of paleo diets include liberal intakes of red meats (including *non*-paleo processed meats), lard, and salt; plus avoidance of protective plant oils, legumes, and dairy; which may reduce net benefits.

EMERGING AREAS

Food Processing

Over the past 70 years, changes in plant and livestock breeding, agricultural practices, and food processing methods have transformed global food systems. The health implications of these changes are receiving increasing attention, with new food classification systems and even Brazil's national guidelines focusing on processing of foods.[8,9,217–220] Processing can increase palatability, nutrient bioavailability, shelf life, and convenience; and reduce food-borne pathogens. Processing can also reduce fiber, phenolics, minerals, fatty acids, vitamins, and other bioactives; increase the doses and flux of starch and sugar; and introduce compounds such as sodium, other preservatives and additives, trans fats, heterocyclic amines, and advanced glycation endproducts (AGEs). Food processing can also impact the microbiome (see below).

Processed meats and refined grains, starches, and added sugars are convincingly linked to cardiometabolic harms.[21] Yet, more "natural" foods such as eggs, butter, and unprocessed red meats do not improve metabolic health, while some processed products (e.g., yogurt, cheese, plant oils, margarines, canned fish, fruit- or nut-rich snacks) are beneficial. Because most foods must undergo some processing prior to consumption—for example, milling, refining, cooking, fermenting, etc.—more research is essential to understand which aspects of

TABLE 29.2 Effects of Food and Nutrients on Specific Cardiometabolic Risk Factors and Disease Endpoints

	STRENGTH OF EVIDENCE FOR BENEFITS*			INSUFFICIENT EVIDENCE FOR EFFECTS
	CONVINCING	**PROBABLE**	**POSSIBLE**	
Hypertension	Higher intakes of: Mediterranean- or DASH-type dietary pattern Dietary fiber Fruits and vegetables Fish or fish oil Cocoa or dark chocolate Potassium Lower intakes of: Sodium Alcohol	Higher intakes of: Tea Lower intakes of: Caffeine	Higher intakes of: Whole grains Magnesium Calcium Vitamin D Soy foods MUFA in place of SFA	Isoflavones Coffee or tea PUFA or carbohydrate in place of SFA
High LDL-cholesterol	Higher intakes of: MUFA or PUFA Dietary fiber Fruits and vegetables Green tea Soy protein Lower intakes of: Trans fat SFA (12:0–16:0) Dietary cholesterol	Higher intakes of: Butter Whole grains Soy foods Tea Lower intakes of: Unfiltered coffee	Higher intakes of: Cheese Yogurt Cream	
Atherogenic Dyslipidemia (low HDL-cholesterol, high triglycerides)	Higher intakes of: Mediterranean- or DASH-type dietary pattern MUFA or PUFA Fish or fish oil Lower intakes of: Simple or complex refined carbs (high GI or GL) Trans fat	Lower intakes of: Sugar-sweetened beverages	Higher intakes of: Fruits and vegetables Dairy	
Insulin Resistance, Type 2 Diabetes	Higher intakes of: Whole grains Dietary fiber PUFA or plant oils Lower intakes of: Processed meats Sugar-sweetened beverages Simple or complex refined carbs (high GL)	Higher intakes of: MUFA Yogurt Lower intakes of: Unprocessed meats	Higher intakes of: Fruits Beans Coffee Cheese Dairy fat Lower intake of: Eggs Dietary cholesterol Trans fat	Carbohydrate in place of SFA Vegetables Beans Poultry Fish or fish oil Milk Butter Tea
Obesity	Higher intakes of: Whole unprocessed foods (e.g., whole grains, nuts, fruits, vegetables, beans) Lower intakes of: Sugar-sweetened beverages Simple or complex refined carbs (high GL)	Higher intakes of: Dietary fiber Yogurt Lower intakes of: Ultra-processed foods Large portion sizes of unhealthy foods Red meats Processed meats Less television watching Greater sleep duration	Higher intakes of: Green tea Protein Lower intakes of: Deep-fried foods Meals from quick service restaurants Trans fat	Total fat (% E) SFA, MUFA, or PUFA

Continued

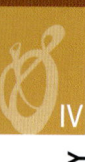

TABLE 29.2 Effects of Food and Nutrients on Specific Cardiometabolic Risk Factors and Disease Endpoints—cont'd

	STRENGTH OF EVIDENCE FOR BENEFITS*			
	CONVINCING	**PROBABLE**	**POSSIBLE**	**INSUFFICIENT EVIDENCE FOR EFFECTS**
Systemic Inflammation	Higher intakes of: Fruits and vegetables	Higher intakes of: Mediterranean- or DASH-type diet pattern Whole grains Fish oil (supplements). Lower intakes of: TFA	Higher intakes of: Fish, fish oil (diet), ALA PUFA Nuts Lower intakes of: Simple or complex refined carbs (high GI/GL)	SFA or MUFA
Coronary Heart Disease	Higher intakes of: Mediterranean- or DASH-type dietary pattern Fruits and vegetables Whole grains Nuts Dietary fiber PUFA in place of SFA Fish (CHD mortality) Lower intakes of: Trans fat Processed meats	Higher intakes of: Beans Lower intakes of: Simple or complex refined carbs (high GI or GL) Sodium Moderate alcohol use	Higher intakes of: Fish or fish oil (nonfatal CHD) Cheese ALA MUFA in place of SFA Vitamin D Lower intakes of: Unprocessed meats Dietary cholesterol in patients with DM	Total fat (% E) Carbohydrate in place of SFA Antioxidant or vitamin supplements Poultry Eggs Yogurt Milk Coffee or tea Dietary cholesterol in patients without DM
Ischemic Stroke	Higher intakes of: Mediterranean- or DASH-type dietary pattern Fruits Lower intakes of: Sodium		Higher intakes of: Whole grains Vegetables SFA Fish or fish oil Tea Cheese Lower intakes of: Processed meats Red meats	Poultry Eggs Milk ALA Antioxidant or vitamin supplements
Hemorrhagic Stroke		Higher intakes of: Whole grains Mediterranean- or DASH-type dietary pattern Lower intakes of: Sodium	Higher intakes of: Total fat SFA Animal protein Tea	Fish or fish oil
Heart Failure†	Lower intakes of: Heavy alcohol use		Higher intakes of: Mediterranean- or DASH-type dietary pattern Whole grains Fish Moderate alcohol use	
Atrial Fibrillation		Lower intakes of: Heavy alcohol use	Higher intakes of: Fish or fish oil	

*Strength of evidence based on Bradford-Hill and World Health Organization criteria. For most dietary factors, evidence is derived from controlled trials of risk factors plus long-term prospective cohorts of disease endpoints. For fish/EPA+DHA, n-6 PUFA, total fat, and Mediterranean-type dietary patterns, evidence is also derived from randomized clinical trials of clinical endpoints.
†Incidence. Limited data on dietary treatment for secondary prevention, except for one large, randomized trial of EPA+DHA supplementation that reduced total mortality, and clinical experience with sodium restriction to prevent fluid overload.

modern processing are detrimental and to define *optimal* processing of different foods for health.

Microbiome

Eating habits exert large, rapid effects on gut microbial composition and function, influencing host health.[221–224] Prebiotics like dietary fibers, fructans (e.g., inulin in chicory root), other oligosaccharides, resistant starch, and certain phenolics (e.g., cocoa-derived flavanols) feed the microbiome.[53,225,226] Probiotics—live bacteria or yeasts in fermented foods like yogurt, cheese, kefir, kimchi, kombucha, miso, natto, sauerkraut, and tempeh—can also alter gut microbial composition.[226] Trials of probiotic-containing foods and supplements demonstrate benefits on weight control, glycemia, and possibly nonalcoholic fatty liver disease.[88–91]

Food processing can adversely impact the microbiome.[8,219,227] Many processing methods (e.g., milling, refining) strip away key prebiotics. Even when reconstituted (e.g., added bran, fiber), loss of intact food structure (termed "acellular nutrition") may alter digestion and absorption in the proximal gut[219] and deprive the (dominant) distal gut microbiome of prebiotics.[227] In some animal models and limited human experiments, artificial sweeteners alter host microbial composition and adversely influence satiety, glucose-insulin homeostasis, caloric intake, and weight gain.[228,229] In some experiments, emulsifiers and thickeners influence the gut microbiome, gut mucosa, and related inflammatory pathways.[230,231] Further investigation of effects of different food processing applications on the microbiome is urgently needed.

Personalized Nutrition

While genetics as a predictor for personalized nutrition have shown disappointingly small effect sizes and reproducibility, sociodemographics, cultural factors, the microbiome, medical history, physiologic parameters, and epigenetics appear more promising.[12,13,232] Glycemic responses to carbohydrates and meats, for example, are influenced by both insulin resistance and the microbiome.[12,13,232–236] Patients with diabetes and atherogenic dyslipidemia may benefit most from reducing refined carbohydrates and increasing dietary fiber, proteins, and plant oils.[10,236–238] Personalized nutrition could theoretically inspire larger or more sustained behavioral changes than general recommendations.[12] This could include, for instance, assessing and incorporating a person's cognitive-behavioral stage and cultural and socioeconomic background[239]—although to date limited evidence supports this concept for nutrition behaviors.[240] Personalized interventions could also increase health disparities if they are costly or difficult to access due to required genomic, metabolomic, and other high-dimensional data.[232] Overall, personalized nutrition is a promising concept deserving of greater investigation.

CHANGING BEHAVIOR

Because changes in diet are low-risk, relatively low-cost, and broadly available, strategies for effective behavior change are essential. The massive, rapid global shifts in CVD, obesity, and diabetes across and within populations demonstrate the dominant influence of generalized environmental determinants. Population approaches to address these factors can have large impact as well as reduce health disparities.[19,241,242] For individual behavior change (e.g., in the clinic, with mobile apps), controlled trials have identified several effective and complementary strategies: set proximal targeted goals, self-monitor, provide regular feedback, use peer support, increase self-efficacy, and use motivational interviewing.[239,243] However, multi-faceted external influences on individual food preference, availability, access, and affordability are also powerful and must be addressed. Exciting strategies include "Food is Medicine" approaches to integrate food and nutrition into health care systems, such as producing Rx programs, medically tailored meals, and structured nutrition education for providers.[244] Effective policy and systems strategies have been identified to improve nutrition, such as within schools, worksites, federal feeding programs, the retail food environment, government structure and coordination, and business innovation and entrepreneurship.[245] Major scientific questions around food, nutrition, and health also remain uncertain and unanswered, requiring a new federal prioritization of coordination and investment in federal nutrition research.[246] For all of these strategies, a focus on foods, rather than single nutrients, facilitates dietary guidance and behavior change.

Such broader approaches are also essential to help reduce profound diet-related health disparities in the United States and globally. Ever-widening disparities in diet quality and diet-related chronic diseases are occurring by race/ethnicity, income, and education, further exacerbated by the COVID-19 pandemic.[246] Poor diets lead to a vicious cycle of lower academic achievement in school, lost productivity at work, increased chronic disease risk, increased out-of-pocket health costs, and poverty for the most vulnerable Americans.

The economic consequences of diet-related CVD, DM, obesity, and related conditions are a clarion call for action. Since 1970, US health care expenditures have risen from 6.9% to 17.9% of gross domestic product (GDP), largely owing to costs of chronic diseases. In constant 2017 dollars, health care spending per capita has skyrocketed from $1797 to $10,739 per year.[247] Much of this relates to management of diet-related chronic diseases,[248] with total economic costs of CVDs estimated at $316 billion/year; of diabetes, at $327 billion/year;[249] and of all obesity-related conditions, at $1.72 trillion/year.[250] These costs are straining budgets of governments, businesses, and families. The large impacts of the food and agricultural system on sustainability and climate change also have major implications for human health.[251,252] Given the core role of nutrition in cardiometabolic health, disparities, and health care costs, multi-sectoral approaches and policies for better nutrition should be a top priority for patients, clinicians, health systems, payers, businesses, and governments.

REFERENCES
Population Considerations

1. Lim SS, Vos T, Flaxman AD, et al. A comparative risk assessment of burden of disease and injury attributable to 67 risk factors and risk factor clusters in 21 regions, 1990-2010: a systematic analysis for the Global Burden of Disease Study 2010. *Lancet.* 2013;380:2224–2260.
2. US Burden of Disease Collaborators. The state of US health, 1990-2010: burden of diseases, injuries, and risk factors. *J Am Med Assoc.* 2013;310:591–608.
3. Mozaffarian D, Rosenberg I, Uauy R. History of modern nutrition science-implications for current research, dietary guidelines, and food policy. *BMJ.* 2018;361:k2392.
4. Mozaffarian D. Dietary and policy priorities for cardiovascular disease, diabetes, and obesity: a comprehensive review. *Circulation.* 2016;133:187–225.
5. NCD Risk Factor Collaboration (NCD-RisC). Rising rural body-mass index is the main driver of the global obesity epidemic in adults. *Nature.* 2019;569:260–264.
6. Albrecht SS, Gordon-Larsen P, Stern D, et al. Is waist circumference per body mass index rising differentially across the United States, England, China and Mexico? *Eur J Clin Nutr.* 2015.
7. Di Cesare M, Soric M, Bovet P, et al. The epidemiological burden of obesity in childhood: a worldwide epidemic requiring urgent action. *BMC Med.* 2019;17:212.
8. Mozaffarian D. Dietary and policy priorities to reduce the global crises of obesity and diabetes. *Nat Food.* 2020;1:38–50.

Foods

9. Hall KD, Ayuketah A, Brychta R, et al. Ultra-processed diets cause excess calorie intake and weight gain: an inpatient randomized controlled trial of ad libitum food intake. *Cell Metab.* 2019;30:226.
10. Ebbeling CB, Feldman HA, Klein GL, et al. Effects of a low carbohydrate diet on energy expenditure during weight loss maintenance: randomized trial. *BMJ.* 2018;363:k4583.
11. Dietary Guidelines Advisory Committee. *Scientific Report of the 2015 Dietary Guidelines Advisory Committee.* 2015; 2015.
12. de Toro-Martin J, Arsenault BJ, Despres JP, et al. Precision nutrition: a review of personalized nutritional approaches for the prevention and management of metabolic syndrome. *Nutrients.* 2017;9.
13. Christensen L, Roager HM, Astrup A, et al. Microbial enterotypes in personalized nutrition and obesity management. *Am J Clin Nutr.* 2018;108:645–651.
14. Gonnissen HK, Hulshof T, Westerterp-Plantenga MS. Chronobiology, endocrinology, and energy- and food-reward homeostasis. *Obes Rev.* 2013;14:405–416.
15. Mozaffarian D, Hao T, Rimm EB, et al. Changes in diet and lifestyle and long-term weight gain in women and men. *N Engl J Med.* 2011;364:2392–2404.
16. Haines J, McDonald J, O'Brien A, et al. Healthy habits, happy homes: randomized trial to improve household routines for obesity prevention among preschool-aged children. *JAMA Pediatr.* 2013;167:1072–1079.
17. Robinson TN. Reducing children's television viewing to prevent obesity: a randomized controlled trial. *J Am Med Assoc.* 1999;282:1561–1567.
18. Epstein LH, Roemmich JN, Robinson JL, et al. A randomized trial of the effects of reducing television viewing and computer use on body mass index in young children. *Arch Pediatr Adolesc Med.* 2008;162:239–245.
19. Mozaffarian D, Afshin A, Benowitz NL, et al. Population approaches to improve diet, physical activity, and smoking habits: a scientific statement from the American Heart Association. *Circulation.* 2012;126:1514–1563.
20. Christakis NA, Fowler JH. The spread of obesity in a large social network over 32 years. *N Engl J Med.* 2007;357:370–379.
21. Micha R, Shulkin ML, Penalvo JL, et al. Etiologic effects and optimal intakes of foods and nutrients for risk of cardiovascular diseases and diabetes: systematic reviews and meta-analyses from the Nutrition and Chronic Diseases Expert Group (NutriCoDE). *PloS One.* 2017;12:e0175149.

22. Bertoia ML, Mukamal KJ, Cahill LE, et al. Changes in intake of fruits and vegetables and weight change in United States men and women followed for up to 24 years: analysis from three prospective cohort studies. *PLoS Med*. 2015;12:e1001878.
23. Aune D, Giovannucci E, Boffetta P, et al. Fruit and vegetable intake and the risk of cardiovascular disease, total cancer and all-cause mortality-a systematic review and dose-response meta-analysis of prospective studies. *Int J Epidemiol*. 2017;46:1029–1056.
24. Zurbau A, Au-Yeung F, Blanco Mejia S, et al. Relation of different fruit and vegetable sources with incident cardiovascular outcomes: a systematic review and meta-analysis of prospective cohort studies. *J Am Heart Assoc*. 2020;9:e017728.
25. Schwingshackl L, Hoffmann G, Lampousi AM, et al. Food groups and risk of type 2 diabetes mellitus: a systematic review and meta-analysis of prospective studies. *Eur J Epidemiol*. 2017;32:363–375.
26. Imamura F, O'Connor L, Ye Z, et al. Consumption of sugar sweetened beverages, artificially sweetened beverages, and fruit juice and incidence of type 2 diabetes: systematic review, meta-analysis, and estimation of population attributable fraction. *BMJ*. 2015;351:h3576.
27. Murphy MM, Barrett EC, Bresnahan KA, et al. 100 % Fruit juice and measures of glucose control and insulin sensitivity: a systematic review and meta-analysis of randomised controlled trials. *J Nutr Sci*. 2017;6:e59.
28. D'Elia L, Dinu M, Sofi F, et al. 100% Fruit juice intake and cardiovascular risk: a systematic review and meta-analysis of prospective and randomised controlled studies. *Eur J Nutr*. 2020.
29. Guo X, Yang B, Tan J, et al. Associations of dietary intakes of anthocyanins and berry fruits with risk of type 2 diabetes mellitus: a systematic review and meta-analysis of prospective cohort studies. *Eur J Clin Nutr*. 2016.
30. Wang Y, Gallegos JL, Haskell-Ramsay C, et al. Effects of chronic consumption of specific fruit (berries, citrus and cherries) on CVD risk factors: a systematic review and meta-analysis of randomised controlled trials. *Eur J Nutr*. 2020.
31. Del Gobbo LC, Falk MC, Feldman R, et al. Effects of tree nuts on blood lipids, apolipoproteins, and blood pressure: systematic review, meta-analysis, and dose-response of 61 controlled intervention trials. *Am J Clin Nutr*. 2015;102:1347–1356.
32. Tindall AM, Johnston EA, Kris-Etherton PM, et al. The effect of nuts on markers of glycemic control: a systematic review and meta-analysis of randomized controlled trials. *Am J Clin Nutr*. 2019;109:297–314.
33. Becerra-Tomas N, Paz-Graniel I, Kendall CWC, et al. Nut consumption and incidence of cardiovascular diseases and cardiovascular disease mortality: a meta-analysis of prospective cohort studies. *Nutr Rev*. 2019;77:691–709.
34. Estruch R, Martinez-Gonzalez MA, Corella D, et al. Effect of a high-fat Mediterranean diet on bodyweight and waist circumference: a prespecified secondary outcomes analysis of the PREDIMED randomised controlled trial. *Lancet Diabetes Endocrinol*. 2016;4:666–676.
35. Estruch R, Ros E, Salas-Salvado J, et al. Primary prevention of cardiovascular disease with a Mediterranean diet. *N Engl J Med*. 2013.
36. Li H, Li X, Yuan S, et al. Nut consumption and risk of metabolic syndrome and overweight/obesity: a meta-analysis of prospective cohort studies and randomized trials. *Nutr Metab (Lond)*. 2018;15:46.
37. Viguiliouk E, Glenn AJ, Nishi SK, et al. Associations between dietary pulses alone or with other legumes and cardiometabolic disease outcomes: an umbrella review and updated systematic review and meta-analysis of prospective cohort studies. *Adv Nutr*. 2019;10:S308–S319.
38. Soltanipour S, Hasandokht T, Soleimani R, et al. Systematic review and meta-analysis of the effects of soy on glucose metabolism in patients with type 2 diabetes. *Rev Diabet Stud*. 2019;15:60–70.
39. Moradi M, Daneshzad E, Azadbakht L. The effects of isolated soy protein, isolated soy isoflavones and soy protein containing isoflavones on serum lipids in postmenopausal women: a systematic review and meta-analysis. *Crit Rev Food Sci Nutr*. 2019:1–15.
40. Man B, Cui C, Zhang X, et al. The effect of soy isoflavones on arterial stiffness: a systematic review and meta-analysis of randomized controlled trials. *Eur J Nutr*. 2020.
41. Vasilaras TH, Raben A, Astrup A. Twenty-four hour energy expenditure and substrate oxidation before and after 6 months' ad libitum intake of a diet rich in simple or complex carbohydrates or a habitual diet. *Int J Obes Relat Metab Disord*. 2001;25:954–965.
42. Cai X, Wang C, Wang S, et al. Carbohydrate intake, glycemic index, glycemic load, and stroke: a meta-analysis of prospective cohort studies. *Asia Pac J Public Health*. 2015;27:486–496.
43. Livesey G, Taylor R, Livesey HF, et al. Dietary glycemic index and load and the risk of type 2 diabetes: assessment of causal relations. *Nutrients*. 2019;11.
44. Livesey G, Taylor R, Livesey HF, et al. Dietary glycemic index and load and the risk of type 2 diabetes: a systematic review and updated meta-analyses of prospective cohort studies. *Nutrients*. 2019;11.
45. Livesey G, Livesey H. Coronary heart disease and dietary carbohydrate, glycemic index, and glycemic load: dose-response meta-analyses of prospective cohort studies. *Mayo Clin Proc Innov Qual Outcomes*. 2019;3:52–69.
46. Ludwig DS. *Always Hungry?* New York: Grand Central Life and Style; 2016.
47. Tobias DK, Chen M, Manson JE, et al. Effect of low-fat diet interventions versus other diet interventions on long-term weight change in adults: a systematic review and meta-analysis. *Lancet Diabetes Endocrinol*. 2015;3:968–979.
48. Viana LV, Gross JL, Azevedo MJ. Dietary intervention in patients with gestational diabetes mellitus: a systematic review and meta-analysis of randomized clinical trials on maternal and newborn outcomes. *Diabetes Care*. 2014;37:3345–3355.
49. Huntriss R, Campbell M, Bedwell C. The interpretation and effect of a low-carbohydrate diet in the management of type 2 diabetes: a systematic review and meta-analysis of randomised controlled trials. *Eur J Clin Nutr*. 2018;72:311–325.
50. Reynolds A, Mann J, Cummings J, et al. Carbohydrate quality and human health: a series of systematic reviews and meta-analyses. *Lancet*. 2019;393:434–445.
51. Aune D, Norat T, Romundstad P, et al. Whole grain and refined grain consumption and the risk of type 2 diabetes: a systematic review and dose-response meta-analysis of cohort studies. *Eur J Epidemiol*. 2013;28:845–858.
52. Marshall S, Petocz P, Duve E, et al. The effect of replacing refined grains with whole grains on cardiovascular risk factors: a systematic review and meta-analysis of randomized controlled trials with grade clinical recommendation. *J Acad Nutr Diet*. 2020;120:1859–1883.e31.
53. Weickert MO, Pfeiffer AFH. Impact of dietary fiber consumption on insulin resistance and the prevention of type 2 diabetes. *J Nutr*. 2018;148:7–12.
54. Shukla AP, Iliescu RG, Thomas CE, et al. Food order has a significant impact on postprandial glucose and insulin levels. *Diabetes Care*. 2015;38:e98–e99.
55. Kim Y, Keogh JB, Clifton PM. Differential effects of red meat/refined grain diet and dairy/chicken/nuts/whole grain diet on glucose, insulin and triglyceride in a randomized crossover study. *Nutrients*. 2016;8.
56. Kasubuchi M, Hasegawa S, Hiramatsu T, et al. Dietary gut microbial metabolites, short-chain fatty acids, and host metabolic regulation. *Nutrients*. 2015;7:2839–2849.
57. Mozaffarian RS, Lee RM, Kennedy MA, et al. Identifying whole grain foods: a comparison of different approaches for selecting more healthful whole grain products. *Public Health Nutr*. 2013;16:2255–2264.
58. Fontanelli MM, Micha R, Sales CH, et al. Application of the ≤ 10:1 carbohydrate to fiber ratio to identify healthy grain foods and its association with cardiometabolic risk factors. *Eur J Nutr*. 2019.
59. Ghodsian B, Madden AM. Evaluating the ≤ 10:1 wholegrain criterion in identifying nutrient quality and health implications of UK breads and breakfast cereals. *Public Health Nutr*. 2018;21:1186–1193.
60. Liu J, Rehm CD, Shi P, et al. A comparison of different practical indices for assessing carbohydrate quality among carbohydrate-rich processed products in the US. *PloS One*. 2020;15:e0231572.
61. Bechthold A, Boeing H, Schwedhelm C, et al. Food groups and risk of coronary heart disease, stroke and heart failure: a systematic review and dose-response meta-analysis of prospective studies. *Crit Rev Food Sci Nutr*. 2019;59:1071–1090.
62. Mozaffarian D. Fish, cardiovascular disease, and mortality-what is the global evidence? *JAMA Intern Med*. 2021.
63. Abdelhamid AS, Brown TJ, Brainard JS, et al. Omega-3 fatty acids for the primary and secondary prevention of cardiovascular disease. *Cochrane Database Syst Rev*. 2020;3:CD003177.
64. Mozaffarian D, Wu JH. Omega-3 fatty acids and cardiovascular disease: effects on risk factors, molecular pathways, and clinical events. *J Am Coll Cardiol*. 2011;58:2047–2067.
65. Yang X, Li Y, Wang C, et al. Meat and fish intake and type 2 diabetes: dose-response meta-analysis of prospective cohort studies. *Diabetes Metab*. 2020.
66. Mozaffarian D, Shi P, Morris JS, et al. Mercury exposure and risk of cardiovascular disease in two US cohorts. *N Engl J Med*. 2011;364:1116–1125.
67. Mozaffarian D, Shi P, Morris JS, et al. Mercury exposure and risk of hypertension in US men and women in two prospective cohorts. *Hypertension*. 2012;60:645–652.
68. Bergkvist C, Berglund M, Glynn A, et al. Dietary exposure to polychlorinated biphenyls and risk of myocardial infarction - a population-based prospective cohort study. *Int J Cardiol*. 2015;183:242–248.
69. Song Y, Chou EL, Baecker A, et al. Endocrine-disrupting chemicals, risk of type 2 diabetes, and diabetes-related metabolic traits: a systematic review and meta-analysis. *J Diabetes*. 2015.
70. Kim K, Hyeon J, Lee SA, et al. Role of total, red, processed, and white meat consumption in stroke incidence and mortality: a systematic review and meta-analysis of prospective cohort studies. *J Am Heart Assoc*. 2017;6.
71. Zeraatkar D, Han MA, Guyatt GH, et al. Red and processed meat consumption and risk for all-cause mortality and cardiometabolic outcomes: a systematic review and meta-analysis of cohort studies. *Ann Intern Med*. 2019;171:703–710.
72. Micha R, Wallace SK, Mozaffarian D. Red and processed meat consumption and risk of incident coronary heart disease, stroke, and diabetes mellitus: a systematic review and meta-analysis. *Circulation*. 2010;121:2271–2283.
73. Micha R, Michas G, Mozaffarian D. Unprocessed red and processed meats and risk of coronary artery disease and type 2 diabetes–an updated review of the evidence. *Curr Atheroscler Rep*. 2012;14:515–524.
74. Micha R, Michas G, Mozaffarian D. Unprocessed red and processed meats and risk of coronary artery disease and type 2 diabetes–an updated review of the evidence. *Curr Athero Rep*. 2012;14:515-524.
75. Fernandez-Real JM, McClain D, Manco M. Mechanisms linking glucose homeostasis and iron metabolism toward the onset and progression of type 2 diabetes. *Diabetes Care*. 2015;38:2169–2176.
76. Wang X, Fang X, Wang F. Pleiotropic actions of iron balance in diabetes mellitus. *Rev Endocr Metab Disord*. 2015;16:15–23.
77. Abete I, Romaguera D, Vieira AR, et al. Association between total, processed, red and white meat consumption and all-cause, CVD and IHD mortality: a meta-analysis of cohort studies. *Br J Nutr*. 2014;112:762–775.
78. Fan M, Li Y, Wang C, et al. Dietary protein consumption and the risk of type 2 diabetes: A dose-response meta-analysis of prospective studies. *Nutrients*. 2019;11.
79. Drouin-Chartier JP, Schwab AL, Chen S, et al. Egg consumption and risk of type 2 diabetes: findings from 3 large US cohort studies of men and women and a systematic review and meta-analysis of prospective cohort studies. *Am J Clin Nutr*. 2020.
80. Drouin-Chartier JP, Chen S, Li Y, et al. Egg consumption and risk of cardiovascular disease: three large prospective US cohort studies, systematic review, and updated meta-analysis. *BMJ*. 2020;368:m513.
81. Godos J, Micek A, Brzostek T, et al. Egg consumption and cardiovascular risk: a dose-response meta-analysis of prospective cohort studies. *Eur J Nutr*. 2020.
82. Mozaffarian D, Wu JHY. Flavonoids, dairy foods, and cardiovascular and metabolic health: a review of emerging biologic pathways. *Circ Res*. 2018;122:369–384.
83. Vors C, Joumard-Cubizolles L, Lecomte M, et al. Milk polar lipids reduce lipid cardiovascular risk factors in overweight postmenopausal women: towards a gut sphingomyelin-cholesterol interplay. *Gut*. 2020;69:487–501.
84. Pimpin L, Wu JH, Haskelberg H, et al. Is butter back? A systematic review and meta-analysis of butter consumption and risk of cardiovascular disease, diabetes, and total mortality. *PloS One*. 2016;11:e0158118.
85. Mishali M, Prizant-Passal S, Avrech T, et al. Association between dairy intake and the risk of contracting type 2 diabetes and cardiovascular diseases: a systematic review and meta-analysis with subgroup analysis of men versus women. *Nutr Rev*. 2019;77:417–429.
86. Sluijs I, Forouhi NG, Beulens JW, et al. The amount and type of dairy product intake and incident type 2 diabetes: results from the EPIC-InterAct Study. *Am J Clin Nutr*. 2012;96:382–390.
87. Geng T, Qi L, Huang T. Effects of dairy products consumption on body weight and body composition among adults: an updated meta-analysis of 37 randomized control trials. *Mol Nutr Food Res*. 2018;62.
88. Borgeraas H, Johnson LK, Skattebu J, et al. Effects of probiotics on body weight, body mass index, fat mass and fat percentage in subjects with overweight or obesity: a systematic review and meta-analysis of randomized controlled trials. *Obes Rev*. 2018;19:219–232.
89. Zhang Q, Wu Y, Fei X. Effect of probiotics on body weight and body-mass index: a systematic review and meta-analysis of randomized, controlled trials. *Int J Food Sci Nutr*. 2015;67:571–580.
90. Sun J, Buys NJ. Glucose- and glycaemic factor-lowering effects of probiotics on diabetes: a meta-analysis of randomised placebo-controlled trials. *Br J Nutr*. 2016;115:1167–1177.
91. Loman BR, Hernandez-Saavedra D, An R, et al. Prebiotic and probiotic treatment of nonalcoholic fatty liver disease: a systematic review and meta-analysis. *Nutr Rev*. 2018;76:822–839.
92. Imamura F, Fretts A, Marklund M, et al. Fatty acid biomarkers of dairy fat consumption and incidence of type 2 diabetes: a pooled analysis of prospective cohort studies. *PLoS Med*. 2018;15:e1002670.
93. Venn-Watson S, Lumpkin R, Dennis EA. Efficacy of dietary odd-chain saturated fatty acid pentadecanoic acid parallels broad associated health benefits in humans: could it be essential? *Sci Rep*. 2020;10:8161.
94. Kreps F, Vrbikova L, Schmidt S. Influence of industrial physical refining on tocopherol, chlorophyll and beta–carotene content in sunflower and rapeseed oil. *Eur J Lipid Sci Technol*. 2014;116:1572–1582.
95. Kraljic K, Skevin D, Barisic L, et al. Changes in 4-vinylsyringol and other phenolics during rapeseed oil refining. *Food Chem*. 2015;187:236–242.
96. Ismail SR, Maarof SK, Siedar AS, et al. Systematic review of palm oil consumption and the risk of cardiovascular disease. *PloS One*. 2018;13:e0193533.
97. Zulkiply SH, Balasubramaniam V, Abu Bakar NA, et al. Effects of palm oil consumption on biomarkers of glucose metabolism: a systematic review. *PloS One*. 2019;14:e0220877.

98. Neelakantan N, Seah JYH, van Dam RM. The effect of coconut oil consumption on cardiovascular risk factors: a systematic review and meta-analysis of clinical trials. *Circulation*. 2020;141:803–814.

Beverages

99. Duffey KJ, Popkin BM. Shifts in patterns and consumption of beverages between 1965 and 2002. *Obesity (Silver Spring, Md.)*. 2007;15:2739–2747.
100. Liu J, Rehm CD, Onopa J, et al. Trends in diet quality among youth in the United States, 1999-2016. *J Am Med Assoc*. 2020;323:1161–1174.
101. Rehm CD, Penalvo JL, Afshin A, et al. Dietary intake among US adults, 1999-2012. *J Am Med Assoc*. 2016;315:2542–2553.
102. Ebbeling CB, Feldman HA, Chomitz VR, et al. A randomized trial of sugar-sweetened beverages and adolescent body weight. *N Engl J Med*. 2012;367:1407–1416.
103. de Ruyter JC, Olthof MR, Seidell JC, et al. A trial of sugar-free or sugar-sweetened beverages and body weight in children. *N Engl J Med*. 2012;367:1397–1406.
104. Pan A, Hu FB. Effects of carbohydrates on satiety: differences between liquid and solid food. *Curr Opin Clin Nutr Metab Care*. 2011;14:385–390.
105. Yin J, Zhu Y, Malik V, et al. Intake of sugar-sweetened and low-calorie sweetened beverages and risk of cardiovascular disease: a meta-analysis and systematic review. *Adv Nutr*. 2021;12:89–101.
106. Laviada-Molina H, Molina-Segui F, Perez-Gaxiola G, et al. Effects of nonnutritive sweeteners on body weight and BMI in diverse clinical contexts: systematic review and meta-analysis. *Obes Rev*. 2020;21:e13020.
107. Johnson RK, Lichtenstein AH, Anderson CAM, et al. Low-calorie sweetened beverages and cardiometabolic health: a science advisory from the American Heart Association. *Circulation*. 2018;138:e126–e140.
108. Burke MV, Small DM. Physiological mechanisms by which non-nutritive sweeteners may impact body weight and metabolism. *Physiol Behav*. 2015.
109. Pepino MY. Metabolic effects of non-nutritive sweeteners. *Physiol Behav*. 2015;152:450–455.
110. Nichol AD, Holle MJ, An R. Glycemic impact of non-nutritive sweeteners: a systematic review and meta-analysis of randomized controlled trials. *Eur J Clin Nutr*. 2018;72:796–804.
111. Tey SL, Salleh NB, Henry J, et al. Effects of aspartame-, monk fruit-, stevia- and sucrose-sweetened beverages on postprandial glucose, insulin and energy intake. *Int J Obes*. 2017;41:450–457.
112. Carlstrom M, Larsson SC. Coffee consumption and reduced risk of developing type 2 diabetes: a systematic review with meta-analysis. *Nutr Rev*. 2018;76:395–417.
113. Kim Y, Je Y, Giovannucci E. Coffee consumption and all-cause and cause-specific mortality: a meta-analysis by potential modifiers. *Eur J Epidemiol*. 2019;34:731–752.
114. Moisey LL, Kacker S, Bickerton AC, et al. Caffeinated coffee consumption impairs blood glucose homeostasis in response to high and low glycemic index meals in healthy men. *Am J Clin Nutr*. 2008;87:1254–1261.
115. Beaudoin MS, Robinson LE, Graham TE. An oral lipid challenge and acute intake of caffeinated coffee additively decrease glucose tolerance in healthy men. *J Nutr*. 2011;141:574–581.
116. Kondo Y, Goto A, Noma H, et al. Effects of coffee and tea consumption on glucose metabolism: a systematic review and network meta-analysis. *Nutrients*. 2018;11.
117. Azad BJ, Heshmati J, Daneshzad E, et al. Effects of coffee consumption on arterial stiffness and endothelial function: a systematic review and meta-analysis of randomized clinical trials. *Crit Rev Food Sci Nutr*. 2020:1–14.
118. Nordestgaard AT, Thomsen M, Nordestgaard BG. Coffee intake and risk of obesity, metabolic syndrome and type 2 diabetes: a Mendelian randomization study. *Int J Epidemiol*. 2015;44:551–565.
119. Qian Y, Ye D, Huang H, et al. Coffee consumption and risk of stroke: a mendelian randomization study. *Ann Neurol*. 2020;87:525–532.
120. Said MA, van de Vegte YJ, Verweij N, et al. Associations of observational and genetically determined caffeine intake with coronary artery disease and diabetes mellitus. *J Am Heart Assoc*. 2020;9:e016808.
121. Yang WS, Wang WY, Fan WY, et al. Tea consumption and risk of type 2 diabetes: a dose-response meta-analysis of cohort studies. *Br J Nutr*. 2014;111:1329–1339.
122. Zhang C, Qin YY, Wei X, et al. Tea consumption and risk of cardiovascular outcomes and total mortality: a systematic review and meta-analysis of prospective observational studies. *Eur J Epidemiol*. 2015;30:103–113.
123. Araya-Quintanilla F, Gutierrez-Espinoza H, Moyano-Galvez V, et al. Effectiveness of black tea versus placebo in subjects with hypercholesterolemia: a PRISMA systematic review and meta-analysis. *Diabetes Metab Syndr*. 2019;13:2250–2258.
124. Xu R, Yang K, Ding J, et al. Effect of green tea supplementation on blood pressure: a systematic review and meta-analysis of randomized controlled trials. *Medicine*. 2020;99:e19047.
125. Najafpour Boushehri S, Karimbeiki R, Ghasempour S, et al. The efficacy of sour tea (Hibiscus sabdariffa L.) on selected cardiovascular disease risk factors: a systematic review and meta-analysis of randomized clinical trials. *Phytother Res*. 2020;34:329–339.
126. Mahdavi-Roshan M, Salari A, Ghorbani Z, et al. The effects of regular consumption of green or black tea beverage on blood pressure in those with elevated blood pressure or hypertension: a systematic review and meta-analysis. *Complement Ther Med*. 2020;51:102430.

Macronutrients

127. Choo VL, Viguiliouk E, Blanco Mejia S, et al. Food sources of fructose-containing sugars and glycaemic control: systematic review and meta-analysis of controlled intervention studies. *BMJ*. 2018;363:k4644.
128. Khan TA, Tayyiba M, Agarwal A, et al. Relation of total sugars, sucrose, fructose, and added sugars with the risk of cardiovascular disease: a systematic review and dose-response meta-analysis of prospective cohort studies. *Mayo Clin Proc*. 2019;94:2399–2414.
129. Tsilas CS, de Souza RJ, Mejia SB, et al. Relation of total sugars, fructose and sucrose with incident type 2 diabetes: a systematic review and meta-analysis of prospective cohort studies. *CMAJ*. 2017;189:E711–E720.
130. Evans RA, Frese M, Romero J, et al. Chronic fructose substitution for glucose or sucrose in food or beverages has little effect on fasting blood glucose, insulin, or triglycerides: a systematic review and meta-analysis. *Am J Clin Nutr*. 2017;106:519–529.
131. Evans RA, Frese M, Romero J, et al. Fructose replacement of glucose or sucrose in food or beverages lowers postprandial glucose and insulin without raising triglycerides: a systematic review and meta-analysis. *Am J Clin Nutr*. 2017;106:506–518.
132. Birt DF, Boylston T, Hendrich S, et al. Resistant starch: promise for improving human health. *Adv Nutr*. 2013;4:587–601.
133. Snelson M, Jong J, Manolas D, et al. Metabolic effects of resistant starch type 2: a systematic literature review and meta-analysis of randomized controlled trials. *Nutrients*. 2019;11.
134. Wang Y, Chen J, Song YH, et al. Effects of the resistant starch on glucose, insulin, insulin resistance, and lipid parameters in overweight or obese adults: a systematic review and meta-analysis. *Nutr Diabetes*. 2019;9:19.
135. Merino J, Guasch-Ferre M, Ellervik C, et al. Quality of dietary fat and genetic risk of type 2 diabetes: individual participant data meta-analysis. *BMJ*. 2019;366:l4292.
136. Zhu Y, Bo Y, Liu Y. Dietary total fat, fatty acids intake, and risk of cardiovascular disease: a dose-response meta-analysis of cohort studies. *Lipids Health Dis*. 2019;18:91.
137. Micha R, Mozaffarian D. Saturated fat and cardiometabolic risk factors, coronary heart disease, stroke, and diabetes: a fresh look at the evidence. *Lipids*. 2010;45:893–905.
138. Imamura F, Micha R, Wu JH, et al. Effects of saturated fat, polyunsaturated fat, monounsaturated fat, and carbohydrate on glucose-insulin homeostasis: a systematic review and meta-analysis of randomised controlled feeding trials. *PLoS Med*. 2016;13:e1002087.
139. Kang ZQ, Yang Y, Xiao B. Dietary saturated fat intake and risk of stroke: systematic review and dose-response meta-analysis of prospective cohort studies. *Nutr Metab Cardiovasc Dis*. 2020;30:179–189.
140. Howard BV, Van Horn L, Hsia J, et al. Low-fat dietary pattern and risk of cardiovascular disease: the women's health initiative randomized controlled dietary modification trial. *J Am Med Assoc*. 2006;295:655–666.
141. Tinker LF, Bonds DE, Margolis KL, et al. Low-fat dietary pattern and risk of treated diabetes mellitus in postmenopausal women: the Women's Health Initiative randomized controlled dietary modification trial. *Arch Intern Med*. 2008;168:1500–1511.
142. Dehghan M, Mente A, Zhang X, et al. Associations of fats and carbohydrate intake with cardiovascular disease and mortality in 18 countries from five continents (PURE): a prospective cohort study. *Lancet*. 2017;390:2050–2062.
143. Astrup A, Bertram HC, Bonjour JP, et al. WHO draft guidelines on dietary saturated and trans fatty acids: time for a new approach? *BMJ*. 2019;366:l4137.
144. Astrup A, Magkos F, Bier DM, et al. Saturated fats and health: a reassessment and proposal for food-based recommendations: JACC state-of-the-art review. *J Am Coll Cardiol*. 2020.
145. Schwingshackl L, Strasser B, Hoffmann G. Effects of monounsaturated fatty acids on cardiovascular risk factors: a systematic review and meta-analysis. *Ann Nutr Metabol*. 2011;59:176–186.
146. Schwingshackl L, Hoffmann G. Monounsaturated fatty acids, olive oil and health status: a systematic review and meta-analysis of cohort studies. *Lipids Health Dis*. 2014;13:154.
147. Jones PJ, MacKay DS, Senanayake VK, et al. High-oleic canola oil consumption enriches LDL particle cholesteryl oleate content and reduces LDL proteoglycan binding in humans. *Atherosclerosis*. 2015;238:231–238.
148. Su H, Liu R, Chang M, et al. Dietary linoleic acid intake and blood inflammatory markers: a systematic review and meta-analysis of randomized controlled trials. *Food Funct*. 2017;8:3091–3103.
149. Calder PC, Campoy C, Eilander A, et al. A systematic review of the effects of increasing arachidonic acid intake on PUFA status, metabolism and health-related outcomes in humans. *Br J Nutr*. 2019;121:1201–1214.
150. Bjermo H, Iggman D, Kullberg J, et al. Effects of n-6 PUFAs compared with SFAs on liver fat, lipoproteins, and inflammation in abdominal obesity: a randomized controlled trial. *Am J Clin Nutr*. 2012;95:1003–1012.
151. Rosqvist F, Iggman D, Kullberg J, et al. Overfeeding polyunsaturated and saturated fat causes distinct effects on liver and visceral fat accumulation in humans. *Diabetes*. 2014;63:2356–2368.
152. Spite M, Claria J, Serhan CN. Resolvins, specialized proresolving lipid mediators, and their potential roles in metabolic diseases. *Cell Metab*. 2014;19:21–36.
153. Chowdhury R, Warnakula S, Kunutsor S, et al. Association of dietary, circulating, and supplement fatty acids with coronary risk: a systematic review and meta-analysis. *Ann Intern Med*. 2014;160:398–406.
154. Farvid MS, Ding M, Pan A, et al. Dietary linoleic acid and risk of coronary heart disease: a systematic review and meta-analysis of prospective cohort studies. *Circulation*. 2014;130:1568–1578.
155. Marklund M, Wu JHY, Imamura F, et al. Biomarkers of dietary omega-6 fatty acids and incident cardiovascular disease and mortality: an individual-level pooled analysis of 30 cohort studies. *Circulation*. 2019.
156. Wu JHY, Marklund M, Imamura F, et al. Omega-6 fatty acid biomarkers and incident type 2 diabetes: pooled analysis of individual-level data for 39 740 adults from 20 prospective cohort studies. *Lancet Diabetes Endocrinol*. 2017;5:965–974.
157. Mozaffarian D, Micha R, Wallace S. Effects on coronary heart disease of increasing polyunsaturated fat in place of saturated fat: a systematic review and meta-analysis of randomized controlled trials. *PLoS Med*. 2010;7:e1000252.
158. Wu JH, Micha R, Imamura F, et al. Omega-3 fatty acids and incident type 2 diabetes: a systematic review and meta-analysis. *Br J Nutr*. 2012;107(suppl 2):S214–S227.
159. Jovanovski E, Li D, Thanh Ho HV, et al. The effect of alpha-linolenic acid on glycemic control in individuals with type 2 diabetes: a systematic review and meta-analysis of randomized controlled clinical trials. *Medicine*. 2017;96:e6531.
160. Kromhout D, Giltay EJ, Geleijnse JM, et al. n-3 fatty acids and cardiovascular events after myocardial infarction. *N Engl J Med*. 2010;363:2015–2026.
161. Del Gobbo LC, Imamura F, Aslibekyan S, et al. Omega-3 polyunsaturated fatty acid biomarkers and coronary heart disease: pooling project of 19 cohort studies. *JAMA Intern Med*. 2016;176:1155–1166.
162. Wu JH, Cahill LE, Mozaffarian D. Effect of fish oil on circulating adiponectin: a systematic review and meta-analysis of randomized controlled trials. *J Clin Endocrinol Metab*. 2013;98:2451–2459.
163. Larsson SC, Orsini N, Wolk A. Long-chain omega-3 polyunsaturated fatty acids and risk of stroke: a meta-analysis. *Eur J Epidemiol*. 2012;27:895–901.
164. Qian F, Ardisson Korat AV, Imamura F, et al. n-3 fatty acid biomarkers and incident type 2 diabetes: an individual participant-level pooling project of 20 prospective cohort studies. *Diabetes Care*. 2021.
165. Hu Y, Hu FB, Manson JE. Marine omega-3 supplementation and cardiovascular disease: an updated meta-analysis of 13 randomized controlled trials involving 127 477 participants. *J Am Heart Assoc*. 2019;8:e013543.
166. Bhatt DL, Steg PG, Miller M, et al. Cardiovascular risk reduction with icosapent ethyl for hypertriglyceridemia. *N Engl J Med*. 2019;380:11–22.
167. Manson JE, Cook NR, Lee IM, et al. Marine n-3 fatty acids and prevention of cardiovascular disease and cancer. *N Engl J Med*. 2019;380:23–32.
168. Mozaffarian D, Aro A, Willett WC. Health effects of trans-fatty acids: experimental and observational evidence. *Eur J Clin Nutr*. 2009;63(suppl 2):S5–S21.
169. Mozaffarian D, Clarke R. Quantitative effects on cardiovascular risk factors and coronary heart disease risk of replacing partially hydrogenated vegetable oils with other fats and oils. *Eur J Clin Nutr*. 2009;63(suppl 2):S22–S33.
170. Wallace SK, Mozaffarian D. Trans-fatty acids and nonlipid risk factors. *Curr Atheroscler Rep*. 2009;11:423–433.
171. Lambelet P, Grandgirard A, Gregoire S, et al. Formation of modified fatty acids and oxyphytosterols during refining of low erucic acid rapeseed oil. *J Agric Food Chem*. 2003;51:4284–4290.
172. Velasco J, Marmesat S, Bordeaux O, et al. Formation and evolution of monoepoxy fatty acids in thermoxidized olive and sunflower oils and quantitation in used frying oils from restaurants and fried-food outlets. *J Agric Food Chem*. 2004;52:4438–4443.
173. Berger S, Raman G, Vishwanathan R, et al. Dietary cholesterol and cardiovascular disease: a systematic review and meta-analysis. *Am J Clin Nutr*. 2015;102:276–294.
174. Cheng P, Pan J, Xia J, et al. Dietary cholesterol intake and stroke risk: a meta-analysis. *Oncotarget*. 2018;9:25698–25707.
175. Zhong VW, Van Horn L, Cornelis MC, et al. Associations of dietary cholesterol or egg consumption with incident cardiovascular disease and mortality. *J Am Med Assoc*. 2019;321:1081–1095.
176. Rong Y, Chen L, Zhu T, et al. Egg consumption and risk of coronary heart disease and stroke: dose-response meta-analysis of prospective cohort studies. *BMJ*. 2013;346:e8539.
177. Shin JY, Xun P, Nakamura Y, et al. Egg consumption in relation to risk of cardiovascular disease and diabetes: a systematic review and meta-analysis. *Am J Clin Nutr*. 2013;98:146–159.

178. Wallin A, Forouhi NG, Wolk A, et al. Egg consumption and risk of type 2 diabetes: a prospective study and dose-response meta-analysis. *Diabetologia*. 2016;59:1204–1213.
179. Morton RW, Murphy KT, McKellar SR, et al. A systematic review, meta-analysis and meta-regression of the effect of protein supplementation on resistance training-induced gains in muscle mass and strength in healthy adults. *Br J Sports Med*. 2018;52:376–384.
180. Liao CD, Tsauo JY, Wu YT, et al. Effects of protein supplementation combined with resistance exercise on body composition and physical function in older adults: a systematic review and meta-analysis. *Am J Clin Nutr*. 2017;106:1078–1091.
181. Schwingshackl L, Hoffmann G. Long-term effects of low-fat diets either low or high in protein on cardiovascular and metabolic risk factors: a systematic review and meta-analysis. *Nutr J*. 2013;12:48.
182. Naghshi S, Sadeghi O, Willett WC, et al. Dietary intake of total, animal, and plant proteins and risk of all cause, cardiovascular, and cancer mortality: systematic review and dose-response meta-analysis of prospective cohort studies. *BMJ*. 2020;370:m2412.
183. Blachier F, Beaumont M, Portune KJ, et al. High-protein diets for weight management: interactions with the intestinal microbiota and consequences for gut health. A position paper by the my new gut study group. *Clin Nutr*. 2019;38:1012–1022.

Micronutrients

184. Brown IJ, Tzoulaki I, Candeias V, et al. Salt intakes around the world: implications for public health. *Int J Epidemiol*. 2009;38:791–813.
185. Powles J, Fahimi S, Micha R, et al. Global, regional, and national sodium intakes in 1990 and 2010: a systematic analysis of 24 h urinary sodium excretion and dietary surveys worldwide. *BMJ Open*. 2013;3:e003733.
186. Mozaffarian D, Fahimi S, Singh GM, et al. Global sodium consumption and death from cardiovascular causes. *N Engl J Med*. 2014;371:624–634.
187. Jayedi A, Ghomashi F, Zargar MS, et al. Dietary sodium, sodium-to-potassium ratio, and risk of stroke: a systematic review and nonlinear dose-response meta-analysis. *Clin Nutr*. 2019;38:1092–1100.
188. Wang YJ, Yeh TL, Shih MC, et al. Dietary sodium intake and risk of cardiovascular disease: a systematic review and dose-response meta-analysis. *Nutrients*. 2020;12.
189. Susic D, Frohlich ED. Salt consumption and cardiovascular, renal, and hypertensive diseases: clinical and mechanistic aspects. *Curr Opin Lipidol*. 2012;23:11–16.
190. Cobb LK, Anderson CA, Elliott P, et al. Methodological issues in cohort studies that relate sodium intake to cardiovascular disease outcomes: a science advisory from the American Heart Association. *Circulation*. 2014;129:1173–1186.
191. National Academies of Sciences Engineering and Medicine. *Dietary Reference Intakes for Sodium and Potassium*; 2019.
192. Binia A, Jaeger J, Hu Y, et al. Daily potassium intake and sodium-to-potassium ratio in the reduction of blood pressure: a meta-analysis of randomized controlled trials. *J Hypertens*. 2015.
193. Vinceti M, Filippini T, Crippa A, et al. Meta-analysis of potassium intake and the risk of stroke. *J Am Heart Assoc*. 2016;5.
194. Adebamowo SN, Spiegelman D, Willett WC, et al. Association between intakes of magnesium, potassium, and calcium and risk of stroke: 2 cohorts of US women and updated meta-analyses. *Am J Clin Nutr*. 2015;101:1269–1277.
195. Yang C, Shi X, Xia H, et al. The evidence and controversy between dietary calcium intake and calcium supplementation and the risk of cardiovascular disease: a systematic review and meta-analysis of cohort studies and randomized controlled trials. *J Am Coll Nutr*. 2020;39:352–370.
196. Del Gobbo LC, Imamura F, Wu JH, et al. Circulating and dietary magnesium and risk of cardiovascular disease: a systematic review and meta-analysis of prospective studies. *Am J Clin Nutr*. 2013;98:160–173.
197. Zhao B, Zeng L, Zhao J, et al. Association of magnesium intake with type 2 diabetes and total stroke: an updated systematic review and meta-analysis. *BMJ Open*. 2020;10:e032240.
198. Ye Y, Li J, Yuan Z. Effect of antioxidant vitamin supplementation on cardiovascular outcomes: a meta-analysis of randomized controlled trials. *PloS One*. 2013;8:e56803.
199. Barbarawi M, Kheiri B, Zayed Y, et al. Vitamin D supplementation and cardiovascular disease risks in more than 83000 individuals in 21 randomized clinical trials: a meta-analysis. *JAMA Cardiol*. 2019;4:765–776.
200. Swart KM, Lips P, Brouwer IA, et al. Effects of vitamin D supplementation on markers for cardiovascular disease and type 2 diabetes: an individual participant data meta-analysis of randomized controlled trials. *Am J Clin Nutr*. 2018;107:1043–1053.
201. Hooper L, Kay C, Abdelhamid A, et al. Effects of chocolate, cocoa, and flavan-3-ols on cardiovascular health: a systematic review and meta-analysis of randomized trials. *Am J Clin Nutr*. 2012;95:740–751.
202. Lin X, Zhang I, Li A, et al. Cocoa flavanol intake and biomarkers for cardiometabolic health: a systematic review and meta-analysis of randomized controlled trials. *J Nutr*. 2016;146:2325–2333.
203. Taubert D, Roesen R, Lehmann C, et al. Effects of low habitual cocoa intake on blood pressure and bioactive nitric oxide: a randomized controlled trial. *J Am Med Assoc*. 2007;298:49–60.
204. Raman G, Avendano EE, Chen S, et al. Dietary intakes of flavan-3-ols and cardiometabolic health: systematic review and meta-analysis of randomized trials and prospective cohort studies. *Am J Clin Nutr*. 2019;110:1067–1078.
205. Scotece M, Conde J, Abella V, et al. New drugs from ancient natural foods. Oleocanthal, the natural occurring spicy compound of olive oil: a brief history. *Drug Discov Today*. 2015;20:406–410.
206. de Lorgeril M, Salen P, Martin JL, et al. Mediterranean diet, traditional risk factors, and the rate of cardiovascular complications after myocardial infarction: final report of the Lyon Diet Heart Study. *Circulation*. 1999;99:779–785.

Dietary Pattern

207. Estruch R, Martinez-Gonzalez MA, Corella D, et al. Effects of a Mediterranean-style diet on cardiovascular risk factors: a randomized trial. *Ann Intern Med*. 2006;145:1–11.
208. Salas-Salvado J, Bullo M, Estruch R, et al. Prevention of diabetes with Mediterranean diets: a subgroup analysis of a randomized trial. *Ann Intern Med*. 2014;160:1–10.
209. Schwingshackl L, Chaimani A, Hoffmann G, et al. A network meta-analysis on the comparative efficacy of different dietary approaches on glycaemic control in patients with type 2 diabetes mellitus. *Eur J Epidemiol*. 2018;33:157–170.
210. Ajala O, English P, Pinkney J. Systematic review and meta-analysis of different dietary approaches to the management of type 2 diabetes. *Am J Clin Nutr*. 2013;97:505–516.
211. Hu T, Mills KT, Yao L, et al. Effects of low-carbohydrate diets versus low-fat diets on metabolic risk factors: a meta-analysis of randomized controlled clinical trials. *Am J Epidemiol*. 2012;176(suppl 7):S44–S54.
212. Kodama S, Saito K, Tanaka S, et al. Influence of fat and carbohydrate proportions on the metabolic profile in patients with type 2 diabetes: a meta-analysis. *Diabetes Care*. 2009;32:959–965.
213. Schwingshackl L, Hoffmann G. Comparison of the long-term effects of high-fat v. low-fat diet consumption on cardiometabolic risk factors in subjects with abnormal glucose metabolism: a systematic review and meta-analysis. *Br J Nutr*. 2014;111:2047–2058.
214. Gardner CD, Trepanowski JF, Del Gobbo LC, et al. Effect of low-fat vs low-carbohydrate diet on 12-month weight loss in overweight adults and the association with genotype pattern or insulin secretion: the DIETFITS randomized clinical trial. *J Am Med Assoc*. 2018;319:667–679.
215. Hallberg SJ, McKenzie AL, Williams PT, et al. Effectiveness and safety of a novel care model for the management of type 2 diabetes at 1 year: an open-label, non-randomized, controlled study. *Diabetes Ther*. 2018.
216. Ghaedi E, Mohammadi M, Mohammadi H, et al. Effects of a paleolithic diet on cardiovascular disease risk factors: a systematic review and meta-analysis of randomized controlled trials. *Adv Nutr*. 2019;10:634–646.
217. Hoffman R, Gerber M. Food processing and the Mediterranean diet. *Nutrients*. 2015;7:7925–7964.
218. Dobarganes C, Marquez-Ruiz G. Possible adverse effects of frying with vegetable oils. *Br J Nutr*. 2015;113(suppl 2):S49–S57.

Emerging Area

219. Zinocker MK, Lindseth IA. The western diet-microbiome-host interaction and its role in metabolic disease. *Nutrients*. 2018;10.
220. Luevano-Contreras C, Gomez-Ojeda A, Macias-Cervantes MH, et al. Dietary advanced glycation end products and cardiometabolic risk. *Curr Diabetes Rep*. 2017;17:63.
221. Brunkwall L, Orho-Melander M. The gut microbiome as a target for prevention and treatment of hyperglycaemia in type 2 diabetes: from current human evidence to future possibilities. *Diabetologia*. 2017;60:943–951.
222. Rothschild D, Weissbrod O, Barkan E, et al. Environment dominates over host genetics in shaping human gut microbiota. *Nature*. 2018;555:210–215.
223. Canfora EE, Meex RCR, Venema K, et al. Gut microbial metabolites in obesity, NAFLD and T2DM. *Nat Rev Endocrinol*. 2019;15:261–273.
224. Valdes A, Walter J, Segal E, et al. Role of the gut microbiota in nutrition and health. *BMJ*. 2018;361:k2179.
225. Davani-Davari D, Negahdaripour M, Karimzadeh I, et al. Prebiotics: definition, types, sources, mechanisms, and clinical applications. *Foods*. 2019;8.
226. Yoo JY, Kim SS. Probiotics and prebiotics: present status and future perspectives on metabolic disorders. *Nutrients*. 2016;8:173.
227. Reese AT, Carmody RN. Thinking outside the cereal box: noncarbohydrate routes for dietary manipulation of the gut microbiota. *Appl Environ Microbiol*. 2019;85.
228. Suez J, Korem T, Zilberman-Schapira G, et al. Non-caloric artificial sweeteners and the microbiome: findings and challenges. *Gut Microbes*. 2015;6:149–155.
229. Pearlman M, Obert J, Casey L. The association between artificial sweeteners and obesity. *Curr Gastroenterol Rep*. 2017;19:64.
230. Chassaing B, Koren O, Goodrich JK, et al. Dietary emulsifiers impact the mouse gut microbiota promoting colitis and metabolic syndrome. *Nature*. 2015;519:92–96.
231. Halmos EP, Mack A, Gibson PR. Review article: emulsifiers in the food supply and implications for gastrointestinal disease. *Aliment Pharmacol Ther*. 2019;49:41–50.
232. Ordovas JM, Ferguson LR, Tai ES, et al. Personalised nutrition and health. *BMJ*. 2018;361: bmj.k2173.
233. Zeevi D, Korem T, Zmora N, et al. Personalized nutrition by prediction of glycemic responses. *Cell*. 2015;163:1079–1094.
234. Korem T, Zeevi D, Zmora N, et al. Bread affects clinical parameters and induces gut microbiome-associated personal glycemic responses. *Cell Metab*. 2017;25:1243–1253.e5.
235. Hjorth MF, Blaedel T, Bendtsen LQ, et al. Prevotella-to-Bacteroides ratio predicts body weight and fat loss success on 24-week diets varying in macronutrient composition and dietary fiber: results from a post-hoc analysis. *Int J Obes*. 2019;43:149–157.
236. Kabisch S, Meyer NMT, Honsek C, et al. Fasting glucose state determines metabolic response to supplementation with insoluble cereal fibre: a secondary analysis of the optimal fibre trial (OptiFiT). *Nutrients*. 2019;11.
237. Dong JY, Zhang ZL, Wang PY, et al. Effects of high-protein diets on body weight, glycaemic control, blood lipids and blood pressure in type 2 diabetes: meta-analysis of randomised controlled trials. *Br J Nutr*. 2013;110:781–789.
238. Hjorth MF, Bray GA, Zohar Y, et al. Pretreatment fasting glucose and insulin as determinants of weight loss on diets varying in macronutrients and dietary fibers-the POUNDS LOST study. *Nutrients*. 2019;11.
239. Artinian NT, Fletcher GF, Mozaffarian D, et al. Interventions to promote physical activity and dietary lifestyle changes for cardiovascular risk factor reduction in adults: a scientific statement from the American Heart Association. *Circulation*. 2010;122:406–441.
240. Celis-Morales C, Livingstone KM, Marsaux CF, et al. Effect of personalized nutrition on health-related behaviour change: evidence from the Food4Me European randomized controlled trial. *Int J Epidemiol*. 2017;46:578–588.
241. McGill R, Anwar E, Orton L, et al. Are interventions to promote healthy eating equally effective for all? Systematic review of socioeconomic inequalities in impact. *BMC Publ Health*. 2015;15:457.
242. Guzman-Castillo M, Ahmed R, Hawkins N, et al. The contribution of primary prevention medication and dietary change in coronary mortality reduction in England between 2000 and 2007: a modelling study. *BMJ Open*. 2015;5:e006070.
243. Afshin A, Babalola D, McLean M, et al. Information technology and lifestyle: a systematic evaluation of internet and mobile interventions for improving diet, physical activity, obesity, tobacco, and alcohol use. *J Am Heart Assoc*. 2016;5.
244. Downer S, Berkowitz SA, Harlan TS, et al. Food is medicine: actions to integrate food and nutrition into healthcare. *BMJ*. 2020;369:m2482.
245. Mande J, Willett W, Auerbach J, et al. *Report of the 50th Anniversary of the White House Conference on Food, Nutrition, and Health: Honoring the Past, Taking Actions for Our Future*; 2020.
246. Fleischhacker SE, et al. Strengthening national nutrition research: rationale and options for a new coordinated federal research effort and authority. *Am J Clin Nutr*. 2020 (in press).
247. Kamal R, Cox C. *How Has U.S. Spending on Healthcare Changed over Time?*; 2018.
248. Maresta A, Balduccelli M, Varani E, et al. Prevention of postcoronary angioplasty restenosis by omega-3 fatty acids: main results of the Esapent for Prevention of Restenosis Italian Study (ESPRIT). *Am Heart J*. 2002;143:E5.
249. American Diabetes Association. Economic costs of diabetes in the U.S. In 2017. *Diabetes Care*. 2018;41:917–928.
250. Waters H, Graf M. *America's Obesity Crisis: The Health and Economic Costs of Excess Weight*. Milken Institute; 2018.
251. Willett W, Rockstrom J, Loken B, et al. Food in the Anthropocene: the EAT-Lancet Commission on healthy diets from sustainable food systems. *Lancet*. 2019;393:447–492.
252. Haines A, Ebi K. The imperative for climate action to protect health. *N Eng J Med*. 2019;380:263–273.

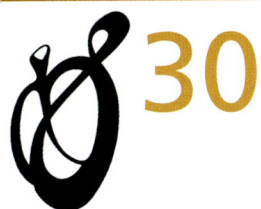

30 Obesity: Medical and Surgical Management

JEAN-PIERRE DESPRÉS, ERIC LAROSE, AND PAUL POIRIER

EPIDEMIOLOGY, 547
Traditional Definition of Obesity, 547
The Puzzling Relationship of Excess Body Weight and Fat with Cardiovascular Disease, 547
Risk Assessment in Overweight/Obese Patients: Waistline as a Vital Sign, 547
Evolving Focus from Adipose Tissue Mass to Quality and Functionality, 548

VISCERAL OBESITY, 549
Marker of Ectopic Fat Deposition, 549
Key Factors Associated with Visceral Obesity, 550
Clinical Tools to Identify Individuals at Cardiometabolic Risk, 551

CLINICAL MANAGEMENT OF CARDIOMETABOLIC RISK, 551
Key Nutritional Factors (Toward a Food-Based Approach, 551

Physical Activity and Exercise, 552
Sleep and Stress Management, 552
Pharmacotherapy, 552

SEVERE OBESITY: A RAPIDLY EXPANDING SUBGROUP OF OBESE PATIENTS, 552

SUMMARY AND PERSPECTIVES, 554

REFERENCES, 555

A medical perspective defines obesity as excess body fat associated with comorbid conditions and increasing mortality risk. This chapter discusses basic concepts on the cause of obesity as it relates to cardiovascular outcomes, including (1) fat accumulation in selective adipose depots and nonadipose tissues as related to various health outcomes, (2) the tools to assess the risk associated with the different forms of overweight and obesity, and (3) the options available in clinical practice to prevent or reduce the risk of cardiovascular disease (CVD) in overweight and obese patients.

EPIDEMIOLOGY

Traditional Definition of Obesity

Obesity increases risk of developing numerous health outcomes, including cardiovascular events[1] (Fig. 30.1). Clinical practice commonly uses body mass index (BMI, expressed in kg/m^2) to estimate adiposity.[1] Many population-based studies, including a recent international study pooling data of about 4 million individuals from 189 studies who were followed for an average of 13 years, have shown that a BMI value above approximately 25 kg/m^2 associates with a progressive increase in mortality rate and risk of chronic conditions.[2] A BMI of 25 kg/m^2 or higher defines *overweight*, BMI of 30 kg/m^2 or higher defines *obesity*, and BMI of 40 kg/m^2 or higher, or 35 kg/m^2 or higher with comorbidities, defines *severe obesity*.[1] The prevalence of obesity has increased worldwide, particularly since the early 1980s, with little evidence of plateauing.[3,4] The prevalence of severe obesity has reached epidemic proportions in the United States and elsewhere.[1,3,4]

The Puzzling Relationship of Excess Body Weight and Fat with Cardiovascular Disease

Although excess body weight or obesity associates with an increased risk of many health complications (see Fig. 30.1), equally overweight or obese patients display a remarkable heterogeneity in CVD risk (Fig. 30.2).[1,5,6] Thus, although an elevated BMI increases the risk of CVD or of other health complications, not every overweight/obese patient develops risk factors or health issues. Some investigators use the term "metabolically healthy" or "fit fat" obesity to refer to such individuals.[1,5,6] The existence of such metabolically healthy obese individuals has engendered debate. Indeed, there is no healthy pattern of increased weight.[1,7] Nevertheless, reasons for such major individual differences in the cardiometabolic risk profile of equally obese patients had remained unclear until imaging studies (computed tomography [CT] and then magnetic resonance imaging [MRI]) revealed marked individual differences in the way people store adipose tissue in the visceral depot.[1,5,6] For any given level of total body fat, individuals characterized by a low accumulation of abdominal visceral adipose tissue generally have a lower CVD risk profile than individuals closely matched for BMI or for total body fat but with high levels of visceral adipose tissue. Those with excessive visceral fat display a constellation of metabolic abnormalities, including insulin resistance, glucose intolerance leading to type 2 diabetes, atherogenic dyslipidemia (including increased triglyceride levels, increased concentrations of non-high-density lipoprotein [HDL] cholesterol and apolipoprotein B, low HDL cholesterol levels, small dense low-density lipoprotein [LDL] and HDL particles), elevated blood pressure (BP), subtle chronic inflammation, and a prothrombotic profile (see Fig. 30.2).[1,5-7] This risk cluster characterizes the so-called metabolic syndrome.[1,5-7]

In clinical practice, assessing CVD risk specifically related to obesity or excess adiposity has remained a challenge. After control for intermediate CVD risk factors (BP, lipids, diabetes), anthropometric adiposity indices such as BMI or waist circumference do not relate independently to CVD mortality.[1] However, very strong associations between adiposity indices and intermediate CVD risk factors are observed, suggesting that increased adiposity changes CVD risk.[1] Thus, the clinician must decide whether to reduce CVD risk by lowering BP, lipids (LDL cholesterol), and blood glucose with pharmacologic agents or to target weight loss. Whereas randomized trials have shown the clinical benefits of targeting BP, lipids, and glucose control (within certain limits), no weight loss drug specifically targeting obesity has proven unequivocally able to reduce cardiovascular events and mortality, with the exception of new diabetes drugs, which are not neutral in terms of body weight (see also Chapter 31).[8] A large well-conducted diet and weight loss trial in obese patients with type 2 diabetes (Look AHEAD) showed no reduction in CVD events as a result of an intensive lifestyle intervention that yielded weight loss, despite beneficial effects on some CVD risk factors and quality of life.[1] Various explanations may account for this result.[1]

Risk Assessment in Overweight/Obese Patients: Waistline as a Vital Sign

Because excess visceral adiposity exacerbates CVD risk in overweight and obese patients, a panel of international experts has recommended measurement of the patient's waist circumference in addition to BMI.[9] This variable should be assessed while the patient is standing, placing the tape just above the iliac crest. If a given patient has a large waistline for a given BMI, with altered risk factors, the CVD risk factor profile likely reflects excess abdominal visceral fat.[1,5,6,9,10] Simple clinical alterations (e.g., high-triglyceride low-HDL cholesterol dyslipidemia,

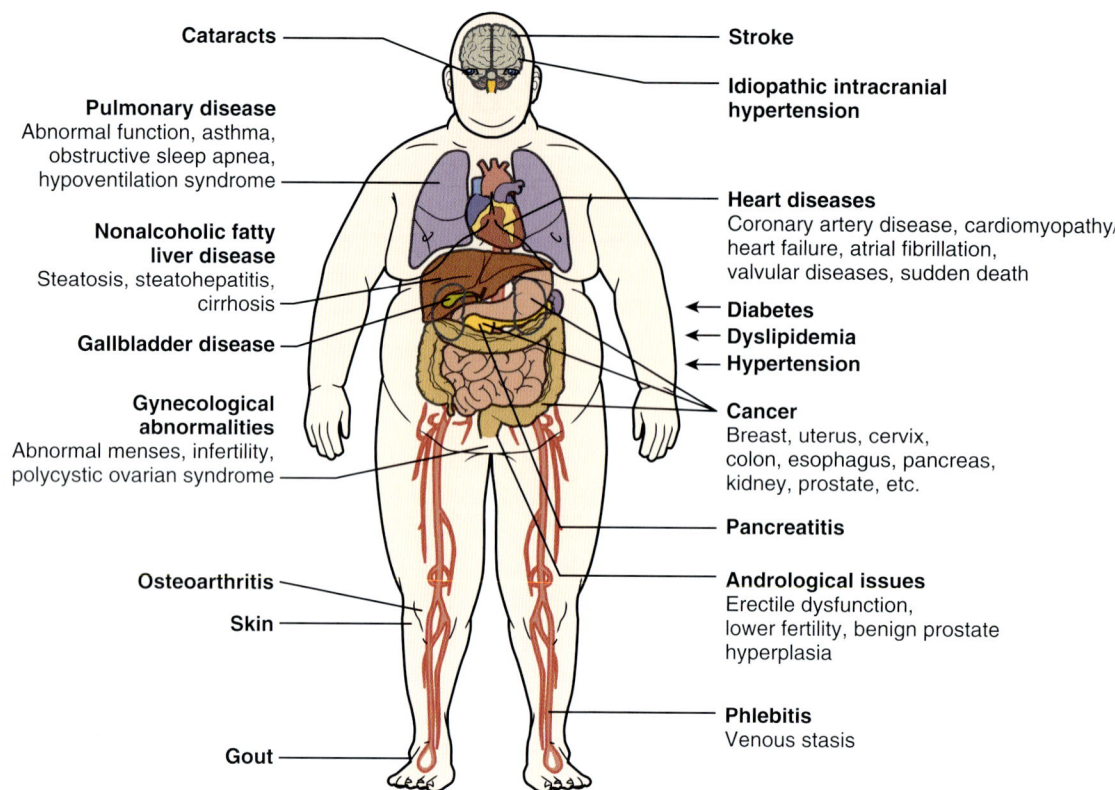

FIGURE 30.1 Some of the key medical complications associated with obesity.

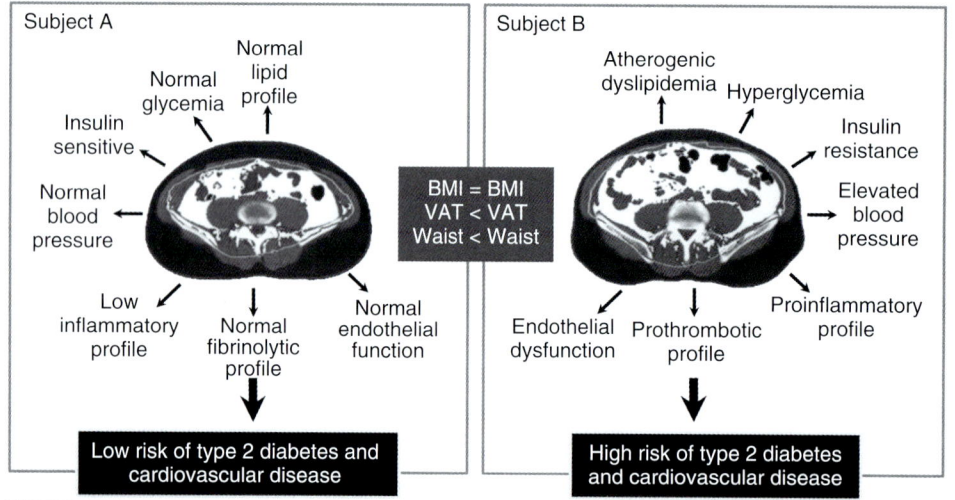

FIGURE 30.2 Marked differences in visceral adipose tissue (VAT) accumulation measured by computed tomography in two individuals having the same body mass index (BMI). However, subject B has a greater cross-sectional accumulation of VAT than subject A. This higher accumulation of VAT in subject B is associated with an altered cardiometabolic risk profile, increasing the risk of type 2 diabetes and cardiovascular disease compared to subject A.

elevated BP, increased fasting blood glucose levels) confirm a dysmetabolic state. Additional tests to confirm insulin resistance include fasting insulin, 2-hour glucose tolerance, hemoglobin (Hb) A_{1c} level, and high-sensitivity C-reactive protein (hsCRP) concentrations. In overweight or obese patients, the presence of these abnormalities along with an elevated waist circumference suggests an excess of abdominal visceral fat.[1,5,6,9,10]

Because the waistline and BMI correlate strongly, waist circumference alone largely reflects total adiposity. For any given BMI value, however, waist circumference can vary considerably and reflects CVD risk (Fig. 30.3).[9–11] Thus, although clinical guidelines have proposed waist cutoff values to define abdominal obesity, interpretation of these cutoffs requires caution. For example, a waist circumference of 105 cm reflects *abdominal* obesity in a man with a BMI of 26 kg/m². However, the same waistline value would simply reflect *overall* obesity in another individual with a BMI of 31 kg/m². Further work is required to refine clinically relevant BMI-specific waist cutoff values beyond those specified in current guidelines (Table 30.1).[1,9,12]

Evolving Focus from Adipose Tissue Mass to Quality and Functionality

As mentioned, the regional distribution of body fat is much more important than adipose tissue mass.[1,5,6,9,10] For example, excess accumulation of body fat in the lower part of the body (hips and thigh) does not associate with an increased risk of CVD or type 2 diabetes. Indeed, a large accumulation of lower body fat rather links with a reduced risk of developing these outcomes,[13] consistent with previous findings that hip and thigh fat are associated with a favorable CVD risk profile.[1,5] In contrast, excess abdominal fat, particularly *visceral adipose tissue*, confers heightened risk as previously detailed.[1,5,6] Imaging also showed substantial individual differences in the size of these inner fat depots, particularly the amount of fat in the abdominal cavity, which includes omental fat, mesenteric fat, and retroperitoneal adipose tissue.[1,5,6,10]

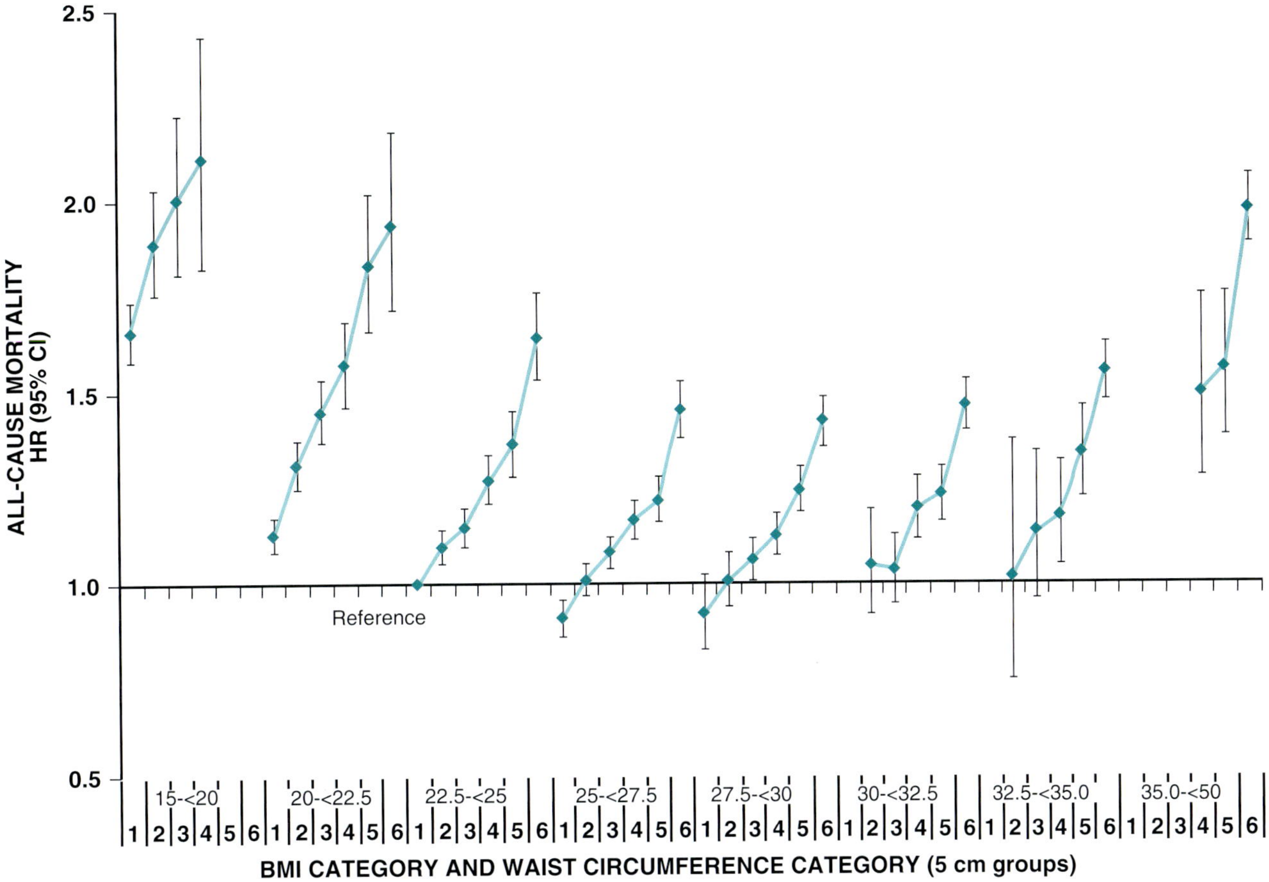

FIGURE 30.3 Hazard ratios (HR) and 95% confidence intervals (CI) for waist circumference in 5-cm increments* and all-cause mortality by body mass index (BMI) category (men and women combined), adjusted for education, marital status, smoking status, alcohol consumption, physical activity, and BMI. *Waist circumference cut points (cm) for men, less than 90.0, 90.0–94.9, 95.0–99.9, 100.0–104.9, 105.0–109.9, and 110.0+; and for women, less than 70.0, 70.0–74.9, 75.0–79.9, 80.0–84.9, 85.0–89.9, and 90.0+. (From Cerhan JR, Moore SC, Jacobs EJ, et al. A pooled analysis of waist circumference and mortality in 650,000 adults. *Mayo Clin Proc.* 2014;89:335–345.)

TABLE 30.1 Waist Circumference Thresholds

BMI CATEGORY (KG/M^2)	WAIST CIRCUMFERENCE (CM)*	
	WOMEN	MEN
Normal weight (18.5–24.9)	≥80	≥90
Overweight (25–29.9)	≥90	≥100
Obese I (30–34.9)	≥105	≥110
Obese II and III (≥35)	≥115	≥125

*Waist circumference threshold indicating increased health risk within each BMI category.
Table provides waist circumference thresholds stratified by body mass index (BMI) for white individuals; individuals with measurements higher than these values have a high risk of future coronary events (based on 10-year risk of coronary events or the presence of diabetes mellitus).
From Ross R, Neeland IJ, Yamashita S, et al. Waist circumference as a vital sign in clinical practice: a Consensus Statement from the IAS and ICCR Working Group on Visceral Obesity. *Nat Rev Endocrinol.* 2020;16:177–189. http://creativecommons.org/licenses/by/4.0/.

VISCERAL OBESITY

Marker of Ectopic Fat Deposition

The mechanisms underlying the independent association between excess visceral fat and cardiometabolic alterations remain unsettled. Three non–mutually exclusive scenarios may pertain: (1) the portal free fatty acid (FFA) hypothesis, (2) the endocrine functions of visceral adipose tissue, and (3) excess visceral adipose tissue as a marker of dysfunctional subcutaneous adipose tissue.[1,5,6]

Portal Free Fatty Acid Hypothesis

In vitro studies of the metabolic properties of visceral adipose tissue—mainly the omental fat depot drained by the portal vein—have shown that these omental adipocytes exhibit a hyperlipolytic state poorly inhibited by insulin compared to subcutaneous adipose tissue.[1,5,6] Therefore, the hypertrophied omental adipocytes in visceral adipose tissue deliver FFAs directly through the portal vein, leading to overproduction of triglyceride-rich lipoproteins, reduction of insulin extraction, and increased hepatic glucose production, hallmarks of obesity and type 2 diabetes. Despite its appeal, the finding that most circulatory FFAs originate from subcutaneous adipose tissue has challenged this hypothesis.

Visceral Adipose Tissue as an Endocrine Organ

The visceral adipose depot preferentially expands through adipose cell hypertrophy, generating very large fat cells that are prone to rupture and have a different FFA composition than subcutaneous adipose tissue.[1,5,6] Macrophages accumulate especially in visceral adipose tissue, contributing to local inflammation and an expanding list of "adipokines" that could exacerbate the metabolic risk profile of the patient with excess visceral adiposity.[1] Also, activation of the sympathetic nervous system may occur particularly in visceral adipose tissue.[1]

Visceral Adipose Tissue: Marker of Dysfunctional Subcutaneous Adipose Tissue?

Excess visceral adipose tissue may also accumulate when subcutaneous adipose tissue fails to expand in an energy surplus (Fig. 30.4).[1,5,6] Subcutaneous adipose tissue normally expands first by adipocyte hypertrophy, followed by proliferation of surrounding preadipocytes (hyperplasia).[1,5,6] If the hyperplastic response is adequate,

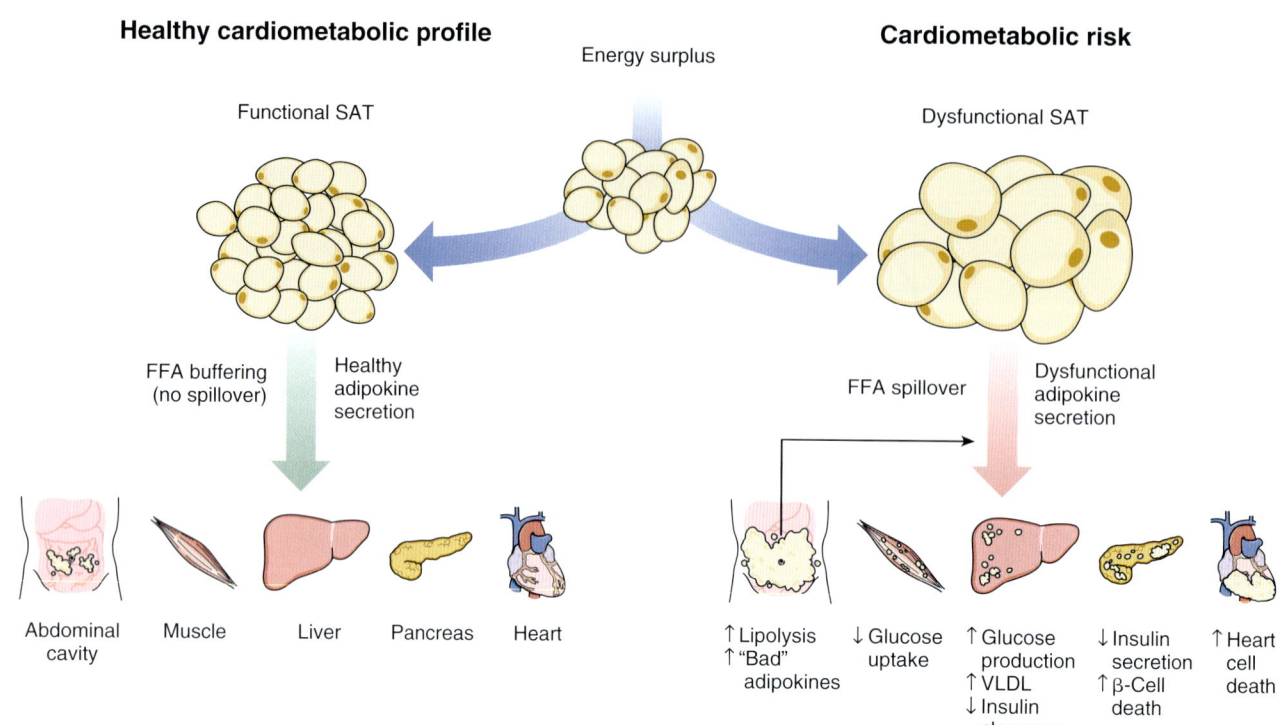

FIGURE 30.4 Overview of potential role of functional and dysfunctional adipose tissue contributing to increased cardiometabolic risk. As a consequence of the mobility of subcutaneous adipose tissue (SAT) to expand through generation of new fat cells, visceral adiposity and increased skeletal muscle, liver, pancreas, and epicardial, pericardial, and intra-myocardial fat generates a dysmetabolic profile increasing cardiovascular disease risk. *FFA*, Free fatty acid. (From Ross R, Neeland IJ, Yamashita S, et al. Waist circumference as a vital sign in clinical practice: a Consensus Statement from the IAS and ICCR Working Group on Visceral Obesity. *Nat Rev Endocrinol*. 2020;16:177–189. http://creativecommons.org/licenses/by/4.0/.)

subcutaneous adipose tissue will expand and act as a "sink" for excess calories[1,5,6] and will maintain autonomic balance.[14]

Genetic forms of lipodystrophy illustrate the importance of properly functioning and expanding (when required) adipose tissue.[1,5] Individuals lacking subcutaneous fat develop an excess of visceral adipose tissue as well as fat accumulation in normally lean tissues. Large cohort imaging studies have revealed that viscerally obese individuals have an increased accumulation of fat in lean tissues such as the liver, heart, skeletal muscle, and kidney, a phenomenon described as "ectopic fat deposition."[1,5,6,15] Thus, excess visceral adipose tissue may be a marker or consequence of the relative inability of subcutaneous adipose tissue to act as a protective "metabolic sink" and thus favor ectopic fat deposition (Fig. 30.5).

The extent to which each of these ectopic fat depots contributes to various cardiovascular outcomes is currently under investigation in several laboratories.[1,5,6,15] Considerable evidence suggest that excess liver fat is also a key abnormality responsible for the several cardiometabolic complications found in viscerally obese individuals.[15,16] Similar data also link excess epi/pericardial fat with various clinical outcomes.[17] On the other hand, the more favorable cardiometabolic risk profile and low levels of visceral/ectopic fat observed in premenopausal obese women with large hips and selective accumulation of lower body fat remain consistent with the protective role of lower body subcutaneous adipose tissue.[5]

Key Factors Associated with Visceral Obesity

The study of factors associated with the selective deposition of visceral/ectopic fat has generated considerable interest.[1,5,6,9]

Age and Sex

Age and sex show marked association with visceral adiposity. With age, visceral adipose tissue can accumulate and contribute to progressive cardiometabolic risk. Before menopause, women have on average 50% less visceral adipose tissue than men.[1,5] At menopause, the relative decline in some key sex steroids contributes to a progressive and selective deposition of visceral adipose tissue.[5] Such sex difference in visceral adipose tissue contributes to sex-dependent cardiometabolic risk. After menopause, because of the acceleration in visceral adipose tissue deposition, women progressively catch up to men (over 10 to 15 years), as can their cardiometabolic risk profile.

Sex Hormones

The major sex difference in visceral adiposity and cardiometabolic risk profile has stimulated exploration of the link between regional body fat distribution and sex hormones. The most informative intervention study supporting a major role of sex steroids involved transsexual patients. Male-to-female transsexuals receiving sex hormone therapy show substantial changes in regional body fat accumulation, with loss of visceral/ectopic fat and increase in the size of lower body fat.[5] Female-to-male transsexuals show the reverse pattern, with related deterioration in their cardiometabolic risk profile.[5]

Genetics

Genes can regulate susceptibility to visceral obesity.[5] Offspring of viscerally obese parents often develop the same pattern when they reach their 30s and 40s, a finding that may reflect both heritability and shared environmental factors. When exposed to the same standardized energy excess for 100 days, monozygotic twin pairs tend to show the same pattern of accumulation of visceral and subcutaneous adipose tissue. No major gene associated with this process has yet emerged despite intensive investigation.

Ethnicity

Ethnicity also associates with variations in visceral adiposity and ectopic fat.[1,5,6,18] Large imaging cardiometabolic studies have shown susceptibility to visceral adiposity/ectopic fat greatest in Asians, then Caucasians, and then African Americans.[1,5,6,18] Indeed, Asians develop diabetes because of excess visceral/ectopic fat at lower BMI values than whites or blacks.[1,5,6]

Hypothalamic-Pituitary-Adrenal Axis and Endocannabinoid System

The hypothalamic-pituitary-adrenal (HPA) axis and the endocannabinoid (EC) system can also modulate visceral adiposity/ectopic fat. Maladaptive responses to stress associate with chronic exposure of various tissues, including adipose tissue, to glucocorticoids, which can contribute to visceral and liver fat accumulation.[5] Adipose tissue contains EC receptors, and overactivation of the EC system may occur in visceral obesity, leading to altered metabolism of visceral adipocytes.[19] Lifestyle changes inducing weight loss can mitigate such overactivity of the EC system.[19] Drugs developed to reduce the activity of the EC system had shown promising results in inducing selective losses of visceral adipose tissue and liver fat, but their unwanted effects compromised their clinical use.[20]

Drugs

Clinicians should consider whether medications might contribute to a patient's excess weight and body fat.[21] Table 30.2 lists some key drugs that induce weight gain.[22]

Lifestyle: A Key Contributor to Visceral Obesity

Once identified, the overweight or obese patient with excess visceral/ectopic fat and increased CVD risk may benefit from pharmacotherapy, including antihypertensive and lipid-lowering agents, to improve risk factors, in accord with guidelines and the results of clinical trials.[23,24] Because excess body weight and obesity result largely from lifestyle, even for those with a genetic susceptibility, the clinician should also evaluate factors such as nutritional quality and level of physical activity.[1,7,9,21] Tools available for use in clinical practice have helped identify sedentary individuals and those with poor nutritional habits who could benefit substantially from improving lifestyle habits.[25,26] Lifestyle intervention studies have shown the value of targeting nutritional quality and sedentary behaviors to reduce waist circumference and improve cardiorespiratory fitness as well as CVD risk factors, irrespective of concomitant pharmacotherapy targeting intermediate CVD risk factors.[9] Patients in the waiting room may complete simple standardized questionnaires regarding diet and physical inactivity/activity. Food-based recommendations (less of some specific food categories and more of other, less-processed foods of high nutritional value and low energy density) combined with a written "lifestyle prescription" to reduce sedentary/sitting time and to introduce regular physical activity could contribute to substantially improving a patient's health profile.[25,26]

Clinical Tools to Identify Individuals at Cardiometabolic Risk

In clinical practice simple anthropometric tools can help to identify overweight and obese individuals with an excess of visceral adipose tissue/ectopic fat. As previously discussed, the simultaneous presence of an increased waistline for a given BMI and altered CVD risk factors should alert the clinician to the presence of excess visceral adiposity/ectopic fat.[9] However, a large waistline alone cannot distinguish excess subcutaneous from visceral adiposity. Another simple clinical marker, plasma triglyceride levels, suggests the presence of excess visceral adipose tissue, an association that we defined as "hypertriglyceridemic waist."[1,5,6] For example, the simultaneous presence of an increased waistline (≥90 cm in men, ≥85 cm in women) and high triglyceride levels (≥2.0 mmol/L in men, ≥1.5 mmol/L in women) predicted a 75% to 80% probability that a given individual had an excess of visceral adipose tissue and an altered cardiometabolic risk profile, a finding showing the importance of paying attention to these two markers.[1,6,27]

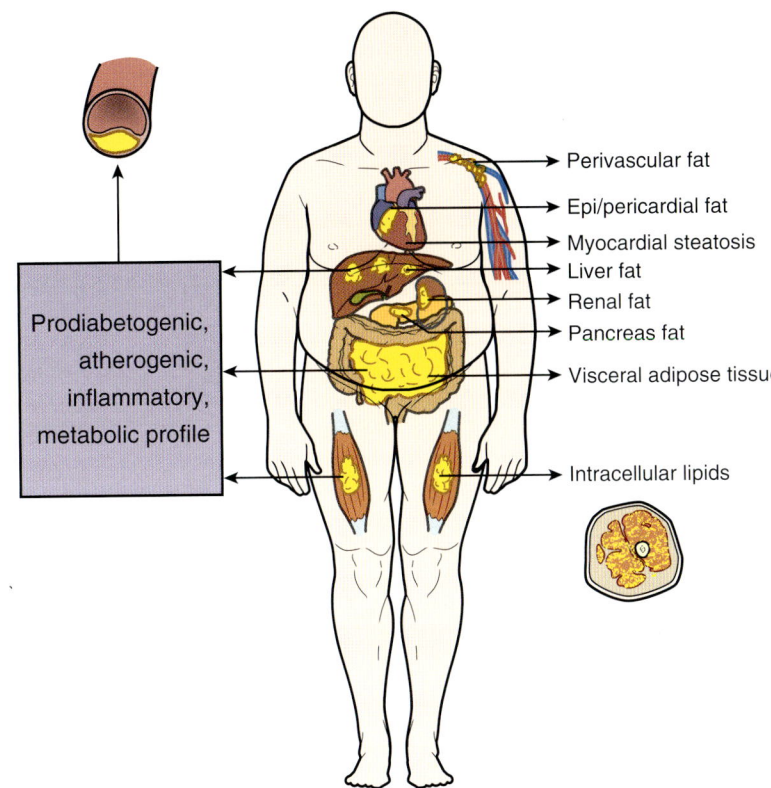

FIGURE 30.5 Working model for the classification of ectopic fat depots as a function of their putative systemic and local effects. (From Després JP. Body fat distribution and risk of cardiovascular disease: an update. *Circulation*. 2012;126:1301–1313.)

TABLE 30.2 Drugs That May Lead to Weight Gain

CATEGORY	DRUGS
Antidiabetics	Insulin, sulfonylureas (many), meglitinides (nateglinide, repaglinide), glitazones (pioglitazone, rosiglitazone)
Antidepressants or mood stabilizers	Monoamine oxidase inhibitors (many), tricyclics (some; e.g., doxepin), serotonin reuptake inhibitors (some; e.g., paroxetine), mirtazapine, lithium
Antipsychotics	Clozapine, risperidone, olanzapine, quetiapine, haloperidol, perphenazine
Anticonvulsants	Carbamazepine, gabapentin, valproate
Antihistamines	Cyproheptadine, diphenhydramine, doxepin
Adrenergic blockers	Propranolol, doxazosin
Adrenal steroids	Corticosteroids

From Bray GA, Frühbeck G, Ryan DH, Wilding JP. Management of obesity. *Lancet*. 2016;387:1947–1956.

CLINICAL MANAGEMENT OF CARDIOMETABOLIC RISK

Key Nutritional Factors (Toward a Food-Based Approach; see also Chapter 29)

Although excess visceral adiposity and ectopic fat has a genetic basis, diet clearly plays a pivotal role. A diet rich in added sugar, refined carbohydrates, and saturated fat may favor the selective accumulation

TABLE 30.3 International Chair on Cardiometabolic Risk "Eat Well, Drink Well, Move" Recommendations for Adults

Eat Well*

- Olive and vegetable oils, nuts, seeds, legumes, grains (mostly whole), fruits, vegetables
  Base every meal on these foods
- Eggs, poultry, cheese, yogurt, other dairy
  Daily to weekly
- Fish, seafood
  Often, at least two times per week
- Processed meat, red meat, sweets
  Less often

Drink Well†

- Water
  On several occasions daily
- Tea or coffee
  Daily
- Low-fat milk and soya-based beverages
  Daily to weekly
- Diet drinks and 100% fruit juices
  Occasionally
- Sugar-sweetened beverages
  Sparingly

Move

- Move as much as you can.
- Do at least 150 minutes of moderate-intensity aerobic physical activity weekly or 75 minutes of vigorous-intensity aerobic physical activity weekly or a mix of both.
- Do muscle-strengthening activities 2 or more days a week.
- Limit screen time and sitting time.

*Drink water to hydrate yourself. Drink wine in moderation. This healthy diet pattern is good for humans and for the planet.
†Sugar-sweetened beverages refer to any beverages with added sugar and include, but are not limited to, regular soda, sugar-sweetened fruit drinks such as fruit punch and lemonade, and sports or energy drinks. The 100% fruit juices contain natural fruit sugars. Tea and coffee should be consumed preferably unsweetened.

of visceral adipose tissue through as-yet poorly understood mechanisms.[28] Some simple precepts can guide clinician conversations with patients about dietary choices (Table 30.3). Recent guidelines and authoritative reviews have highlighted the potential of such an approach that is clearly more "user friendly" to patients than technical recommendations about diet macronutrient and fatty acid composition.[26,29] For example, the public health recommendation to decrease *saturated fat* in our diet, while still relevant, has unfortunately drifted to a reduction in *diet fat* content, which contributed to boost the intake of refined carbohydrates and of refined products with a considerable amount of added sugar. Thus the low dietary fat message likely contributed to the current epidemic of obesity and type 2 diabetes.[26,29] Accordingly, lifestyle intervention trials focused on reducing the fat content of the diet and on caloric restriction and weight loss have not improved cardiovascular outcomes.[26] On the other hand, a trial that used a simple approach in overweight and obese patients (50% with diabetes), giving participants olive oil and mixed nuts (PREDIMED), albeit revised, reported a significant reduction in cardiovascular outcomes, particularly the incidence of stroke.[30] The dietary intervention did not cause weight loss.[30] These results illustrate how improving overall nutritional quality can by itself reduce the risk of cardiovascular outcomes.

Physical Activity and Exercise

Physical inactivity and sedentary behaviors (for which sitting and screen time are good markers) predict increased risk of developing chronic diseases, including cardiovascular conditions.[31] This association does not depend solely on adiposity. Moderate- to vigorous-intensity physical activity or exercise increases cardiorespiratory fitness, one of the key predictors of the risk of developing CVD, independent of adiposity.[32] Therefore, practitioners should include assessment of physical inactivity/activity level in their patient evaluations. Advice regarding physical activity along with nutritional counseling can reduce visceral adiposity while improving all features of the cardiometabolic risk profile.[1,6,9,32] Furthermore, because physical activity and exercise can increase lean body mass, body weight may not always reflect beneficial changes in body composition, and thus an increase in lean body mass can balance the loss of harmful visceral/ectopic fat, an outcome particularly beneficial for the older frail patient. Weight loss should not be the sole target for CVD risk reduction in the management of overweight and obese patients.

Sleep and Stress Management (see also Chapters 89 and 99)

Sleep duration and quality can also influence energy balance and metabolism.[33] The most obvious group of patients with disturbed sleeping habits are those with *sleep apnea*, a condition frequently observed among sedentary overweight and obese patients, particularly those with an excess of visceral/ectopic fat.[33] The viscerally obese patient with sleep apnea or with episodes of apnea/hypopnea may enter a vicious cycle in which the fatigue associated with the poor quality of sleep may lead to additional inactivity, exacerbating their already disturbed cardiometabolic risk profile. Several mechanisms may link visceral adiposity/ectopic fat to sleep apnea, including physical obstruction of the upper airways by soft tissues infiltrated with fat.[34] Treatment of sleep apnea by positive-pressure devices may help progressively improve sleep quality of the viscerally obese patient and help break this cycle. Lifestyle intervention studies have also shown that weight loss in sleep apnea patients substantially improves their cardiometabolic risk profile.[33] In addition, because stress contributes to the selective accumulation of visceral/ectopic fat,[5] stress management strategies may constitute another measure to improve the lifestyle of these high-risk patients.

Pharmacotherapy

Pharmacologic tools to treat high-risk overweight and obese patients are limited by a lack of evidence for efficacy or long-term benefit.[21,22] Drugs currently specifically approved for the chronic management of obesity have not yet demonstrated improved cardiovascular outcomes or efficacy in reducing visceral adipose tissue or ectopic fat (Table 30.4).[22]

Contemporary trials of diabetes drugs with mechanisms that also impact energy balance and induce weight loss have shown, for the first time, a significant influence on reducing adverse cardiovascular outcomes.[8] Imaging studies could test to what extent the loss of visceral/ectopic fat that these drugs may cause could contribute to the observed reduction in CVD risk.

SEVERE OBESITY: A RAPIDLY EXPANDING SUBGROUP OF OBESE PATIENTS (SEE ALSO CHAPTERS 2 AND 25)

The terms overweight, obese, and severe obesity refer to a clinical continuum. Over the past four decades, the world has transitioned from an era when underweight prevalence was more than double that of obesity, to one in which more people are obese than underweight.[3] Numerous physiologic mechanisms regulate body weight and fat mass beyond voluntary food intake and physical exercise. A large body of clinical evidence has shown that voluntary attempts to eat less and exercise more render only modest effects on body weight in most individuals with severe obesity. Epidemiologic studies have shown substantial risks in people with severe obesity.[35]

TABLE 30.4 **Weight Loss Drugs Available in the United States* and European Union†**

DRUGS	MECHANISM OF ACTION
Phentermine* (15–30 mg orally)	Sympathomimetic
Orlistat*,† (120 mg orally three times a day before meals)	Pancreatic lipase inhibitor
Phentermine/Topiramate ER* (7.5 mg/46 mg or 15 mg/92 mg orally indicated as rescue; requires titration)	Sympathomimetic anticonvulsant (GABA receptor modulation, carbonic anhydrase inhibition, glutamate antagonism)
Naltrexone SR/bupropion SR*,† (32 mg/360 mg orally; requires titration)	Opioid receptor antagonist; dopamine and noradrenaline reuptake inhibitor
Liraglutide*,† (3.0 mg injection; requires titration)	GLP-1 receptor agonist

ER, Extended release; SR, sustained release; GLP, glucagon-likepeptide.
Adapted from Bray GA, Frühbeck G, Ryan DH, Wilding JP, et al. Management of obesity. *Lancet.* 2016;387:1947–1956. Please note that the Table was modified following the withdrawal of lorcaserin as recommended by the FDA.

Caucasian women 20 to 30 years old with BMI ≥ 45 kg/m² will lose 8 years of life and their male counterparts will lose 13 years.[36] The mean increases of BMI per decade (from 1975 to 2014) is equivalent to the world's population having gained on average more than 1.5 kg per decade. The global prevalence of severe obesity (BMI ≥ 40 kg/m²) was 0.64% in men and 1.6% in women in 2014; 58 million men and 126 million women were severely obese. High-income English-speaking countries contained an important share of the world's severely obese individuals (27.1%; 50 million), followed by 13.9% (26 million) in the Middle East and North Africa. More than one in four severely obese men and almost one in five severely obese women worldwide live in the United States.[3] If the current trends continue, severe obesity will surpass 9% in women and 6% in men.[3] Also, individuals with obesity who experience weight discrimination show higher levels of circulating CRP, cortisol, long-term cardiometabolic risk, and increased mortality compared with those who do not experience weight discrimination.[37]

There are often opposite views regarding the merits of prevention of obesity as a preferable alternative to treatments for established obesity, such as pharmacotherapy or bariatric surgery, which are more expensive. This is a misconception, framing prevention versus treatment as being mutually exclusive. These approaches generally target two distinct groups, with different but complementary needs. Available literature shows that in severe obesity, only bariatric surgery provides a significant substantial long-term weight loss and cures or durably improves comorbidities (Table 30.5). Currently, there are three principal treatments for severe obesity: (1) changes in lifestyle habits, (2) pharmacotherapy, and (3) bariatric surgery. Classically, bariatric surgery has been described as either restrictive or hybrid surgeries, which combines restriction and malabsorption (Fig. 30.6).[36] Several other procedures such as temporary intragastric balloons, gastric partitioning procedures and gastrointestinal liners, and embolization of the left gastric artery aim to mimic the effects of bariatric surgery. Bariatric surgery is often referred to as an easy way out, based on assumptions that these procedures mechanically restrict food intake compensating for the individuals who are not disciplined enough to accomplish it on their own. In contrast, evidence demonstrates that bariatric procedures modulate numerous metabolic effects opposite to the compensatory physiologic responses normally triggered by diet-induced weight reduction. Such mechanisms include a paradoxical decrease in appetite and increase in metabolic rate, contrary to changes in the opposite directions following most non-surgical weight loss.[1,37]

Although BMI has limitations as an index to assess the relationship between body weight and health of an individual due to its inability to assess body fat distribution, it is still considered the most useful screening tool at an individual level worldwide and is used as the cut-off for bariatric surgery eligibility. Almost 3 decades ago, the National Institutes of Health arbitrarily established that bariatric surgical therapy be proposed to those patients with a BMI greater than 40 or greater than 35 kg/m² with serious obesity-related comorbidities such as systemic hypertension, diabetes, or obstructive sleep apnea. Currently, several somewhat analogous guidelines furnish eligibility criteria for bariatric surgery. The American Diabetes Association[38] issued a consensus statement identifying bariatric surgery as the only proven effective option for sustainable weight loss and weight control inducing beneficial clinical outcomes in severe obesity. Bariatric surgery therapy should be proposed for adult patients with BMI ≥40 kg/m² or BMI ≥35 kg/m² with obesity-related comorbidities that are difficult to control with lifestyle and pharmacotherapy. Other guidelines discussed bariatric surgery for patients with class 1 obesity (see Table 30.1)[38,39] as well as for severely obese children and adolescents.[40] No guideline suggests a given procedure to be more appropriate than others for cardiac patients. Bariatric surgery is the most effective and cost-effective treatment, which not only leads to substantial weight loss but also results in higher remission rates of type 2 diabetes, hypertension, and hyperlipidemia. Data from a network of multiple randomized controlled trials showed no significant difference in weight loss (BMI reduction and percent of excess weight loss) between Roux-en-Y gastric bypass and sleeve gastrectomy, although they were both superior to laparoscopic adjustable gastric band.[41] Moreover, Roux-en-Y gastric bypass and sleeve gastrectomy resulted in a comparable rate of type 2 diabetes remission in studies with 2- to 5-year follow-up.[42] Weight regain unfortunately commonly occurs with all weight loss modalities. Its prevalence is estimated to range between 5% and 20%, whereas an amount of 5% to 10% of weight regain from the nadir is expected and considered normal after 18 to 24 months of bariatric surgery.[12] In the long term, patients who underwent bariatric surgery may experience weight regain resulting in frustration, depression, and return of obesity-related comorbidities. Overall, weight regain ranged from 23.7% to 38.3% in studies using higher weight regain cutoffs, in contrast with 39.3% to 59.6% in studies utilizing lower weight regain cutoffs.[43]

Retrospective and cohort studies have shown that bariatric surgery lowers the risk of all-cause mortality, myocardial infarction, stroke, and cancer in primary prevention. Other studies also revealed that bariatric surgery reduces the incidence of heart failure, angina, and new-onset atrial fibrillation, and significantly lowers emergency department visits and hospitalizations due to heart failure and coronary artery disease (CAD). These benefits all link to reduced subsequent health care costs.[44] In contrast with the clinical impacts of bariatric surgery in the setting of primary prevention, patients with severe obesity and CAD referred to bariatric surgery were at a higher risk of early and late (7.4 years) mortality (cardiac and noncardiac), myocardial infarction, stroke, and myocardial revascularization (MACCE) compared with non-CAD severely obese as reduced MACCE may be largely explained by lowering non-cardiac mortality with no significant effect on specific cardiovascular endpoints.[45] As is the case of new diabetes drugs that improve cardiovascular outcome, bariatric surgery is not readily accessible to most people in low-income and middle-income countries because of financial and health system barriers.[46] In addition, anatomical and physiologic alterations in the gastrointestinal tract following bariatric surgery modulate a wide variety of factors involved in oral drugs bioavailability. The majority of available data is based on Roux-en-Y gastric bypass and on the basis of current knowledge, predicting the pharmacokinetic change for a specific drug following bariatric surgery is challenging. Post-surgical monitoring is recommended in patients regarding clinical changes in response to medications.[47]

Surgical techniques differ in terms of morbidity and mortality rate, magnitude of weight loss, weight loss maintenance, and rate of resolution of comorbidities over time.[1,12,37] Early complications (<30 days) after bariatric surgery were reported to be under 10% and tend to be lower in restrictive surgeries compared to hybrid surgeries and 30-day operative mortality rates range from 0.1% to 1.2%.[37] Severe obesity disturbs the heart's structure and function as it associates with left

TABLE 30.5 Outcomes of Bariatric Surgery

	RESTRICTIVE PROCEDURES		HYBRID PROCEDURES	
	ADJUSTABLE GASTRIC BANDING	SLEEVE GASTRECTOMY	ROUX-EN-Y GASTRIC BYPASS	BILIOPANCREATIC DIVERSION WITH DUODENAL SWITCH
Mortality Rates				
<30-day	0%–0.10%	0.13%–0.50%	0.15%–1.15%	0.30%–1.20%
Complications	0.2%–20.0% (all procedures)			
Weight Loss				
1 year	14%–30%	20%–28%	23%–43%	38%–52%
2–5 years	17%–35%	21%	30%–42%	34%–53%
≥6 years	13%–14%	22%	25%–28%	36%–55%
Comorbidities Resolution				
Type 2 Diabetes				
1 year	23%–61%	37%–81%	17%–93%	59%–95%
2–5 years	20%–74%	14%–86%	50%–84%	90%–100%
Dyslipidemia				
1 year	17%	16%–83%	33%–47%	33%–65%
2–5 years	23%–61%	5%–48%	52%–97%	70%–100%
Hypertension				
1 year	19%–55%	15%–82%	20%–45%	24%–53%
2–5 years	17%–64%	25%–75%	29%–80%	57%–85%
Sleep Apnea				
1 year	78%	52%–100%	33%–100%	100%
2–5 years	33%–96%	39%–91%	67%–80%	74%–92%

From Piché ME, Auclair A, Harvey J, et al. How to choose and use bariatric surgery in 2015. *Can J Cardiol.* 2015;31:153–166.

ventricular (LV) remodeling and decreased LV systolic function, as well as LV diastolic dysfunction which may eventually lead to heart failure. Increased pulmonary vascular resistance and pulmonary artery pressure raising right ventricular (RV) afterload may also occur in severe obesity, leading to the development of RV dysfunction owing to RV hypertrophy and enlargement.[48] Data suggest that weight loss achieved by any means may improve cardiac structure and function (through reverse remodeling) and decreased cardiovascular risk but bariatric surgery also may reduce cardiac morbidity and mortality in patients with established cardiac disease. In addition, beneficial effects of bariatric surgery on cardiac imaging endpoints showed favorable improvements in cardiac geometry as well as diastolic and systolic functions.[48,49]

SUMMARY AND PERSPECTIVES

It is important to assess and manage high-risk overweight and obese patients in cardiovascular practice. Because of the increasing worldwide prevalence of overweight/obesity, cardiovascular specialists manage many overweight and obese patients, a number of whom also have excessive visceral adipose tissue/ectopic fat. Several simple metrics can alert practitioners to this metabolically dangerous condition, notably an elevated waistline (for a given BMI) and increased triglycerides. In addition, the clinician's evaluation should include simple lifestyle markers such as duration and quality of sleep, overall food-based nutritional quality, sedentary/sitting time, level of moderate/vigorous physical activity, and cardiorespiratory fitness, as well as identifying medications that promote weight gain.

Many current curricula provide only limited exposure of physicians and trainees to the importance of and tools for assessing and targeting lifestyle in overweight and obese patients. Physicians should never underestimate the potential impact they may exert on their patients' lifestyle as role models. A patient could be greatly influenced by a physician who would pay equal attention to his/her waistline, nutritional quality, physical activity level, and quality of sleep as to his/her cholesterol, BP, and blood glucose. Finally, we must recognize that the epidemic proportions reached by obesity and type 2 diabetes reflect societal conditions that extend beyond the traditional medical model. As key stakeholders, physicians can advocate for environments that promote human health rather than disease.

Restrictive Bariatric Surgeries

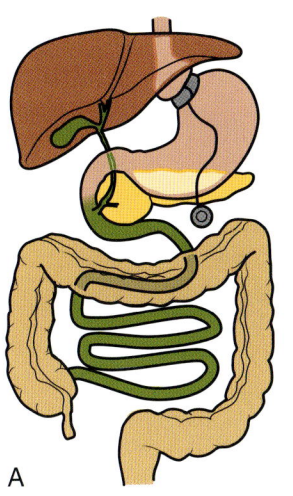
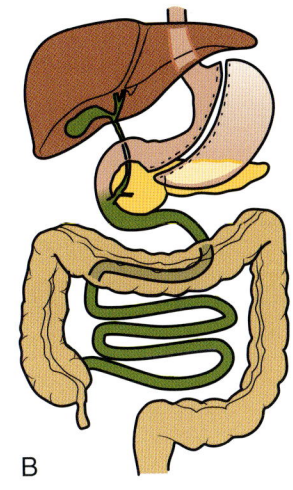

Hybrid Bariatric Surgeries

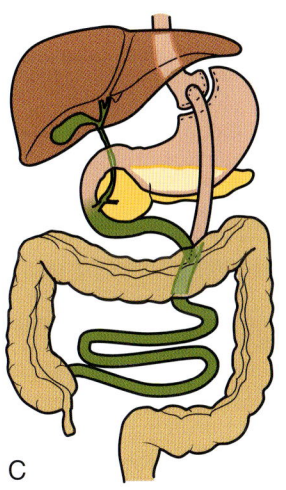
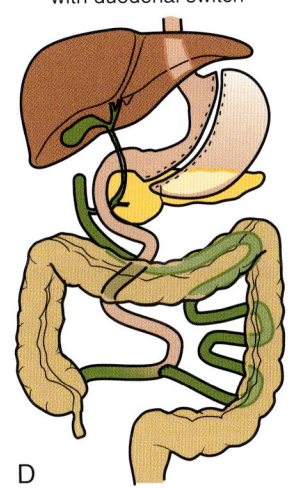

FIGURE 30.6 Restrictive (**A** and **B**) and hybrid (**C** and **D**) bariatric surgeries. *Dark pink,* Alimentary limb, food passage. *Light green,* Biliopancreatic limb, digestive juices from the stomach, bile, and pancreas. *Dark green,* Common limb, food mixed with digestive juices from the stomach, bile, and pancreas.

REFERENCES

Epidemiology

1. Piché ME, Tchernof A, Després JP. Obesity phenotypes, diabetes, and cardiovascular diseases. *Circ Res.* 2020;126:1477–1500.
2. Global BMI Mortality Collaboration, Di Angelantonio E, Bhupathiraju S, et al. Body-mass index and all-cause mortality: individual-participant-data meta-analysis of 239 prospective studies in four continents. *Lancet.* 2016;388:776–786.
3. NCD Risk Factor Collaboration. Trends in adult body-mass index in 200 countries from 1975 to 2014: a pooled analysis of 1698 population-based measurement studies with 19.2 million participants. *Lancet.* 2016;387:1377–1396.
4. Flegal KM, Kruszon-Moran D, Carroll MD, et al. Trends in obesity among adults in the United States, 2005 to 2014. *J Am Med Assoc.* 2016;315:2284–2291.

Relationship of Excess Body Weight and Fat with Cardiovascular Disease

5. Tchernof A, Després JP. Pathophysiology of human visceral obesity: an update. *Physiol Rev.* 2013;93:359–404.
6. Neeland IJ, Ross R, Després JP, et al. Visceral and ectopic fat, atherosclerosis, and cardiometabolic disease: a position statement. *Lancet Diabetes Endocrinol.* 2019;7:715–725.
7. Neeland IJ, Poirier P, Després JP. Cardiovascular and metabolic heterogeneity of obesity: clinical challenges and implications for management. *Circulation.* 2018;137:1391–1406.
8. Garg V, Verma S, Connelly K. Mechanistic insights regarding the role of SGLT2 inhibitors and GLP1 agonist drugs on cardiovascular disease in diabetes. *Prog Cardiovasc Dis.* 2019;62:349–357.

Visceral Obesity

9. Ross R, Neeland IJ, Yamashita S, et al. Waist circumference as a vital sign in clinical practice: a consensus statement from the IAS and ICCR working group on visceral obesity. *Nat Rev Endocrinol.* 2020;16:177–189.
10. Piché ME, Poirier P, Lemieux I, et al. Overview of epidemiology and contribution of obesity and body fat distribution to cardiovascular disease: an update. *Prog Cardiovasc Dis.* 2018;61:103–113.
11. Cerhan JR, Moore SC, Jacobs EJ, et al. A pooled analysis of waist circumference and mortality in 650,000 adults. *Mayo Clin Proc.* 2014;89:335–345.
12. Wharton S, Lau DCW, Vallis M, et al. Obesity in adults: a clinical practice guideline. *CMAJ.* 2020;192:E875–E891.
13. Neeland IJ, Turer AT, Ayers CR, et al. Body fat distribution and incident cardiovascular disease in obese adults. *J Am Coll Cardiol.* 2015;65:2150–2151.
14. Grenier A, Brassard P, Bertrand OF, et al. Rosiglitazone influences adipose tissue distribution without deleterious impact on heart rate variability in coronary heart disease patients with type 2 diabetes. *Clin Auton Res.* 2016;26:407–414.
15. Shulman GI. Ectopic fat in insulin resistance, dyslipidemia, and cardiometabolic disease. *N Engl J Med.* 2014;371:1131–1141.
16. Taskinen MR, Boren J. New insights into the pathophysiology of dyslipidemia in type 2 diabetes. *Atherosclerosis.* 2015;239:483–495.
17. Iacobellis G. Local and systemic effects of the multifaceted epicardial adipose tissue depot. *Nat Rev Endocrinol.* 2015;11:363–371.
18. Rao G, Powell-Wiley TM, Ancheta I, et al. Identification of obesity and cardiovascular risk in ethnically and racially diverse populations: a scientific statement from the American Heart Association. *Circulation.* 2015;132:457–472.
19. van Eenige R, van der Stelt M, Rensen PCN, et al. Regulation of adipose tissue metabolism by the endocannabinoid system. *Trends Endocrinol Metab.* 2018;29:326–337.

Clinical Management of Obesity

20. Cristino L, Becker T, Di Marzo V. Endocannabinoids and energy homeostasis: an update. *Biofactors.* 2014;40:389–397.
21. Heffron SP, Parham JS, Pendse J, et al. Treatment of obesity in mitigating metabolic risk. *Circ Res.* 2020;126:1646–1665.
22. Bray GA, Fruhbeck G, Ryan DH, et al. Management of obesity. *Lancet.* 2016;387:1947–1956.
23. Grundy SM, Stone NJ, Bailey AL, et al. 2018 AHA/ACC/AACVPR/AAPA/ABC/ACPM/ADA/AGS/APhA/ASPC/NLA/PCNA guideline on the management of blood cholesterol: a report of the American College of Cardiology/American Heart Association Task Force on Clinical Practice Guidelines. *Circulation.* 2019;139:e1082–e1143.
24. Whelton PK, Carey RM, Aronow WS, et al. 2017 ACC/AHA/AAPA/ABC/ACPM/AGS/APhA/ASH/ASPC/NMA/PCNA guideline for the prevention, detection, evaluation, and management of high blood pressure in adults: a report of the American College of Cardiology/American Heart Association Task Force on Clinical Practice Guidelines. *Hypertension.* 2018;71:e13–e115.
25. Ross R, Blair SN, Arena R, et al. Importance of assessing cardiorespiratory fitness in clinical practice: a case for fitness as a clinical vital sign: a scientific statement from the American Heart Association. *Circulation.* 2016;134:e653–e699.
26. Mozaffarian D. Dietary and policy priorities for cardiovascular disease, diabetes, and obesity: a comprehensive review. *Circulation.* 2016;133:187–225.
27. Ren Y, Luo X, Wang C, et al. Prevalence of hypertriglyceridemic waist and association with risk of type 2 diabetes mellitus: a meta-analysis. *Diabetes Metab Res Rev.* 2016;32:405–412.
28. Ma J, McKeown NM, Hwang SJ, et al. Sugar-sweetened beverage consumption is associated with change of visceral adipose tissue over 6 years of follow-up. *Circulation.* 2016;133:370–377.
29. Liu AG, Ford NA, Hu FB, et al. A healthy approach to dietary fats: understanding the science and taking action to reduce consumer confusion. *Nutr J.* 2017;16:53.
30. Estruch R, Ros E, Salas-Salvado J, et al. Primary prevention of cardiovascular disease with a Mediterranean diet supplemented with extra-virgin olive oil or nuts. *N Engl J Med.* 2018;378:e34.
31. Young DR, Hivert MF, et al. Sedentary behavior and cardiovascular morbidity and mortality: a science advisory from the American Heart Association. *Circulation.* 2016;134:e262–e279.
32. Lavie CJ, McAuley PA, Church TS, et al. Obesity and cardiovascular diseases: implications regarding fitness, fatness, and severity in the obesity paradox. *J Am Coll Cardiol.* 2014;63:1345–1354.
33. St-Onge MP, Grandner MA, Brown D, et al. Sleep duration and quality: impact on lifestyle behaviors and cardiometabolic health. A scientific statement from the American Heart Association. *Circulation.* 2016;134:e367–e386.
34. Kim AM, Keenan BT, Jackson N, et al. Tongue fat and its relationship to obstructive sleep apnea. *Sleep.* 2014;37:1639–1648.
35. Kitahara CM, Flint AJ, Berrington de Gonzalez A, et al. Association between class III obesity (BMI of 40-59 kg/m2) and mortality: a pooled analysis of 20 prospective studies. *PLoS Med.* 2014;11:e1001673.
36. Piché ME, Auclair A, Harvey J, et al. How to choose and use bariatric surgery in 2015. *Can J Cardiol.* 2015;31:153–166.
37. Rubino F, Puhl RM, Cummings DE, et al. Joint international consensus statement for ending stigma of obesity. *Nat Med.* 2020;26:485–497.
38. American Diabetes Association. 8. Obesity management for the treatment of type 2 diabetes: standards of medical care in diabetes-2020. *Diabetes Care.* 2020;43:S89–S97.
39. Aminian A, Chang J, Brethauer SA, et al. ASMBS updated position statement on bariatric surgery in class I obesity (BMI 30-35 kg/m(2)). *Surg Obes Relat Dis.* 2018;14:1071–1087.
40. Pratt JSA, Browne A, Browne NT, et al. ASMBS pediatric metabolic and bariatric surgery guidelines, 2018. *Surg Obes Relat Dis.* 2018;14:882–901.
41. Kang JH, Le QA. Effectiveness of bariatric surgical procedures: a systematic review and network meta-analysis of randomized controlled trials. *Medicine (Baltim).* 2017;96:e8632.
42. Borgeraas H, Hofso D, Hertel JK, et al. Comparison of the effect of Roux-en-Y gastric bypass and sleeve gastrectomy on remission of type 2 diabetes: a systematic review and meta-analysis of randomized controlled trials. *Obes Rev.* 2020;21:e13011.
43. Mauro MFFFP, Papelbaum M, Brasil MAA, et al. Is weight regain after bariatric surgery associated with psychiatric comorbidity? A systematic review and meta-analysis. *Obes Rev.* 2019;20:1413–1425.
44. Kuno T, Tanimoto E, Morita S, et al. Effects of bariatric surgery on cardiovascular disease: a concise update of recent advances. *Front Cardiovasc Med.* 2019;6:94.
45. Pirlet C, Biertho L, Poirier P, et al. Comparison of short and long term cardiovascular outcomes after bariatric surgery in patients with vs without coronary artery disease. *Am J Cardiol.* 2020;125:40–47.
46. Yusuf S, Joseph P, Rangarajan S, et al. Modifiable risk factors, cardiovascular disease, and mortality in 155 722 individuals from 21 high-income, middle-income, and low-income countries (PURE): a prospective cohort study. *Lancet.* 2020;395:795–808.
47. McLachlan LA, Chaar BB, Um IS. Pharmacokinetic changes post-bariatric surgery: a scoping review. *Obes Rev.* 2020;21:e12988.
48. Lascaris B, Pouwels S, Houthuizen P, et al. Cardiac structure and function before and after bariatric surgery: a clinical overview. *Clin Obes.* 2018;8:434–443.
49. Powell-Wiley TM, Poirier P, Burke L, et al. Obesity and cardiovascular disease: a scientific statement from the American Heart Association. *Circulation* 2021; 143. doi:10.1161/CIR.0000000000000973.

31 Diabetes and the Cardiovascular System

NIKOLAUS MARX, SILVIO E. INZUCCHI, AND DARREN K. MCGUIRE

SCOPE OF THE PROBLEM, 556
Diabetes Mellitus, 556
Atherosclerotic Vascular Disease, 556
Heart Failure, 556
Atrial Fibrillation, 556
Risk Stratification, 556

CORONARY HEART DISEASE IN THE PATIENT WITH DIABETES, 558
Mechanistic Considerations Linking Diabetes and Atherosclerosis, 558

Prevention and Treatment of Coronary Heart Disease and Its Complications in the Patient with Diabetes, 558
Acute Coronary Syndromes, 571
Coronary Revascularization Considerations, 573

HEART FAILURE IN THE PATIENT WITH DIABETES, 574
Scope of the Problem, 574
Mechanistic Considerations, 574

Prevention and Management of Heart Failure in Diabetes, 575
Atrial Fibrillation, 576

SUMMARY AND FUTURE PERSPECTIVES, 576

GUIDELINES, 577

REFERENCES, 577

SCOPE OF THE PROBLEM

Diabetes Mellitus

Diabetes mellitus (DM) involves insufficient production of insulin and/or failure to respond appropriately to insulin, resulting in hyperglycemia. Table 31.1 summarizes the current diagnostic criteria.[1] Type 2 DM is characterized by insulin resistance and relative insulin deficiency (>90% of all DM cases), whereas type 1 is defined by absolute insulin deficiency. This chapter focuses on type 2 DM, except when specifically indicated otherwise.

Diabetes, one of the most common chronic diseases in the world, affects an estimated 463 million adults in 2019 (Fig. 31.1).[2] The mounting incidence and prevalence of type 2 DM, driven by increasing population age, obesity, and physical inactivity, compound with its high global burden (see Chapters 2, 25, and 30), as does the increasing longevity of patients with the disease. DM will affect more than an estimated 700 million persons, 10.9% of the global adult population, by 2045.[2]

Cardiovascular disease (CVD) remains the principal comorbid condition and primary contributor to mortality in patients with DM, usually in the form of coronary heart disease (CHD), but also in the incremental risk associated with DM for cerebrovascular disease, peripheral vascular disease, heart failure (HF), and atrial fibrillation (AF). For these reasons, continuing effort toward mitigating the risk of CVD in DM remains a global public health imperative.

TABLE 31.1 American Diabetes Association Diagnostic Criteria for Diabetes Mellitus*

1. Fasting plasma glucose (FPG) ≥126 mg/dL (7.0 mmol/L). Fasting is defined as no caloric intake for at least 8 hr.
   Or
2. Two-hour plasma glucose ≥200 mg/dL (11.1 mmol/L) during an oral glucose tolerance test (OGTT). The test should be performed as described by the World Health Organization, using a glucose load containing the equivalent of 75 g anhydrous glucose dissolved in water.
   Or
3. Glycated hemoglobin (A_{1c}) ≥6.5% (48 mmol/mol). The test should be performed in a laboratory using a method that is National Glycohemoglobin Standardization Program (NGSP) certified and standardized to the Diabetes Control and Complications Trial (DCCT) assay.
   Or
4. In a patient with classic symptoms of hyperglycemia or hyperglycemic crisis, a random plasma glucose ≥200 mg/dL (11.1 mmol/L).

*Criteria 1 to 3 require confirmatory testing; criterion 4 does not.
Modified from American Diabetes Association. Classification and Diagnosis of Diabetes: Standards of Medical Care in Diabetes. *Diabetes Care*. 2020;43(suppl 1):S14–S31.

Atherosclerotic Vascular Disease

Patients with DM have a two- to fourfold increased risk for CHD, CV mortality, all-cause mortality, and CV hospitalization compared with those without DM (Fig. 31.2).[3,4] However, the CV risk and mortality in patients with DM remain substantially increased over those without DM, underscoring the unmet clinical need.[3,5]

Diabetes entails an increased risk for myocardial infarction (MI). Across the spectrum of acute coronary syndrome (ACS) events, in which DM may affect more than one in three patients, those with DM have worse CVD outcomes (see Chapters 36–39).[6] Despite overall improvements in outcomes during the past several decades for ACS patients with and without DM, the gradient of risk associated with DM persists (Fig. 31.3), although incremental in-hospital mortality risk associated with DM after ACS has declined (Fig. 31.4).[6] Furthermore, the graded association of increased risk in the setting of ACS extends to glucose values well below the DM threshold (Fig. 31.5).

In addition to CHD, DM increases the risks of stroke (twofold increase, see Chapter 45),[5] cerebrovascular disease, and peripheral arterial disease. Hyperglycemia affects approximately one in three patients with acute stroke and is associated to a two- to sixfold increased risk for adverse clinical outcomes.

Heart Failure

In the ambulatory setting, DM associates independently with a twofold to fivefold increased risk for HF over that in persons without DM, and patients with DM have worse outcomes once HF has developed.[7] HF in DM is a key driver of CV morbidity and mortality, leading to the inclusion of HF as a major endpoint in contemporary clinical trials.[7]

Atrial Fibrillation

It remains uncertain as to what degree DM independently augments AF risk, largely because of the difficulty in adjusting for risk factors common to both diseases. In patients with AF, DM increases stroke rate by 2% to 3.5% (see Chapter 66).[8] The CHA_2DS_2–VASc score includes DM and guidelines recommend anticoagulation for all DM patients who have AF.[8,9]

Risk Stratification

The high CV risk of patients with DM blurs the concept of primary versus secondary prevention. Recent guidelines classify patients with DM according to CV risk.[10] Very high risk patients are those with DM and established CVD, as well as those with target organ damage such as left ventricular hypertrophy or chronic kidney disease (CKD). Patients with

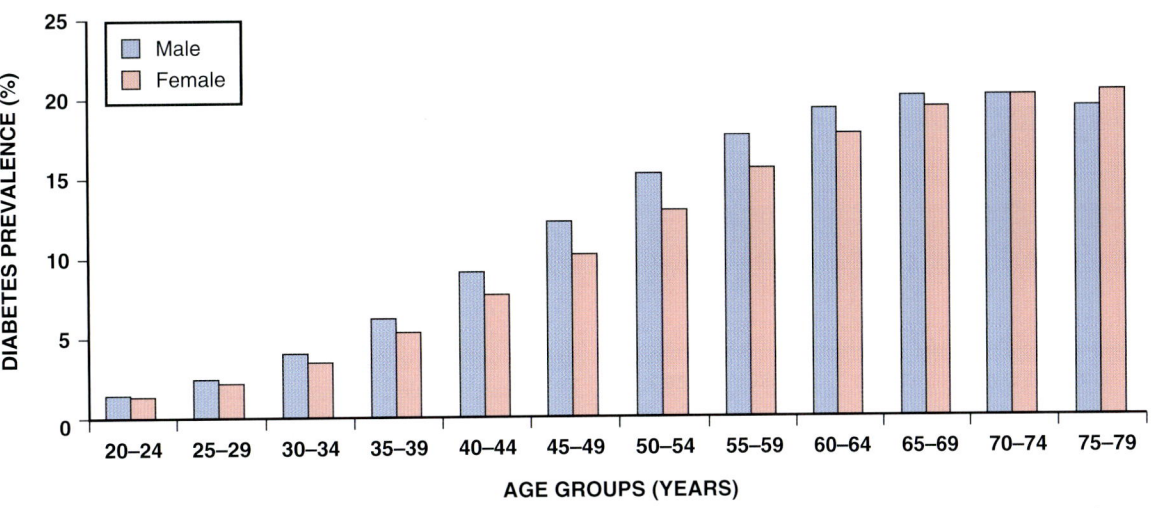

FIGURE 31.1 Diabetes mellitus prevalence by age and sex in 2019. (From Saeedi P, Petersohn I, Salpea P, et al. Global and regional DM prevalence estimates for 2019 and projections for 2030 and 2045: Results from the International DM Federation DM Atlas, 9th edition. *DM Res Clin Pract*. 2019;157:107843.)

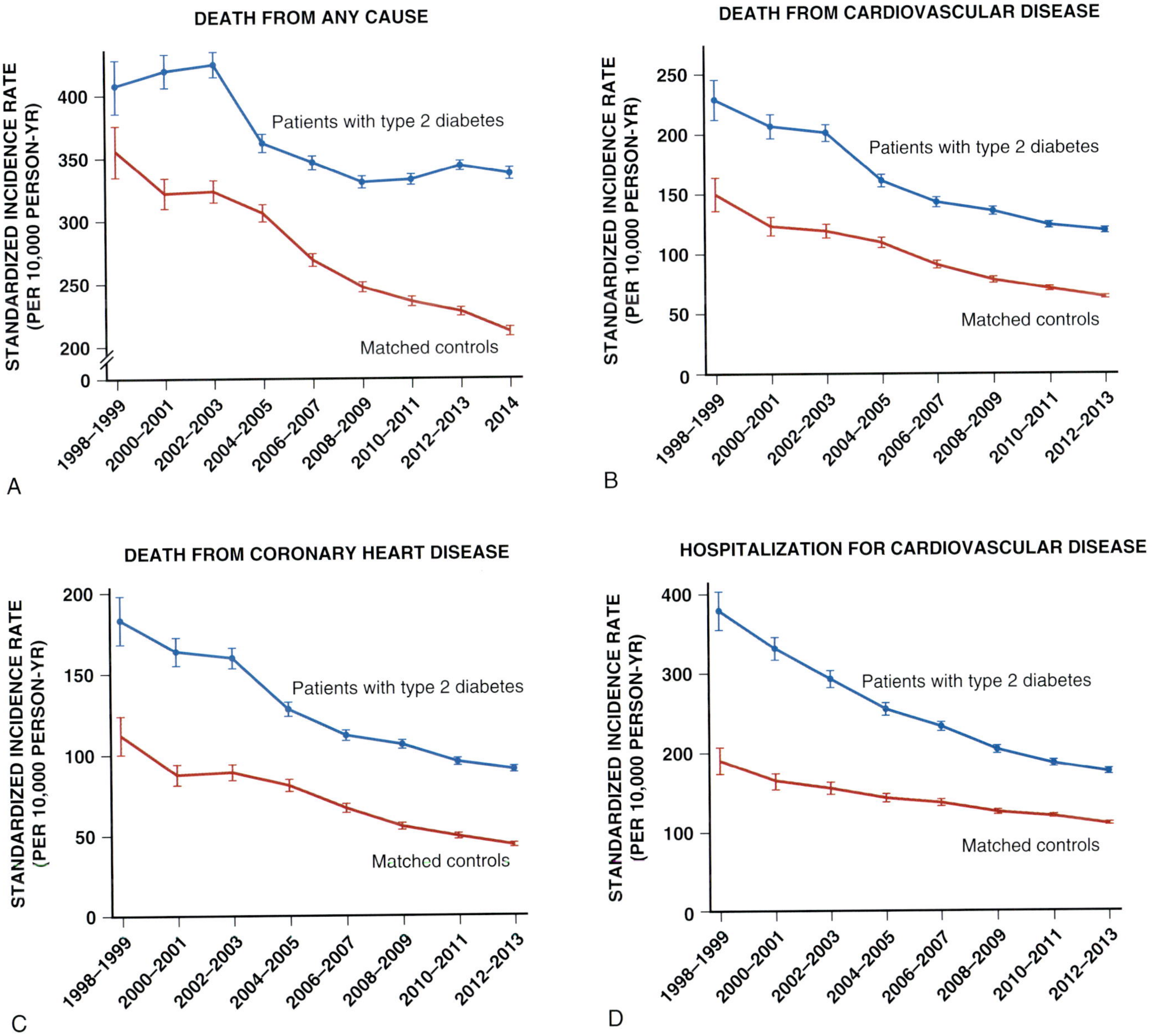

FIGURE 31.2 Major cardiovascular outcomes in patients with type 1 DM and matched controls. Controls were matched for age, sex, and country. I bars represent 95% confidence intervals. (From Rawshani A, Rawshani A, Franzen S, et al. Mortality and cardiovascular disease in type 1 and type 2 diabetes. *N Engl J Med*. 2017;376:1407–1418.)

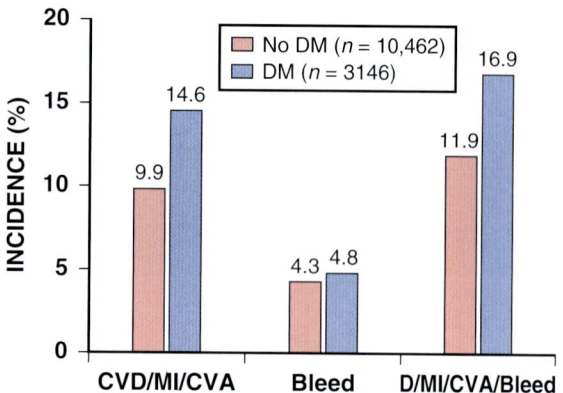

FIGURE 31.3 Adverse clinical outcomes after acute coronary syndromes during more than 1 year of follow-up, according to DM status, among patients participating in the TRITON–TIMI 38 randomized trial. *CVA*, Cerebrovascular accident; *CVD*, cardiovascular death; *D*, death; *DM*, diabetes mellitus; *MI*, myocardial infarction. (Modified from Wiviott SD, Braunwald E, McCabe CH, et al. Prasugrel versus clopidogrel in patients with acute coronary syndromes. *N Engl J Med.* 2007;357:2001–2015.)

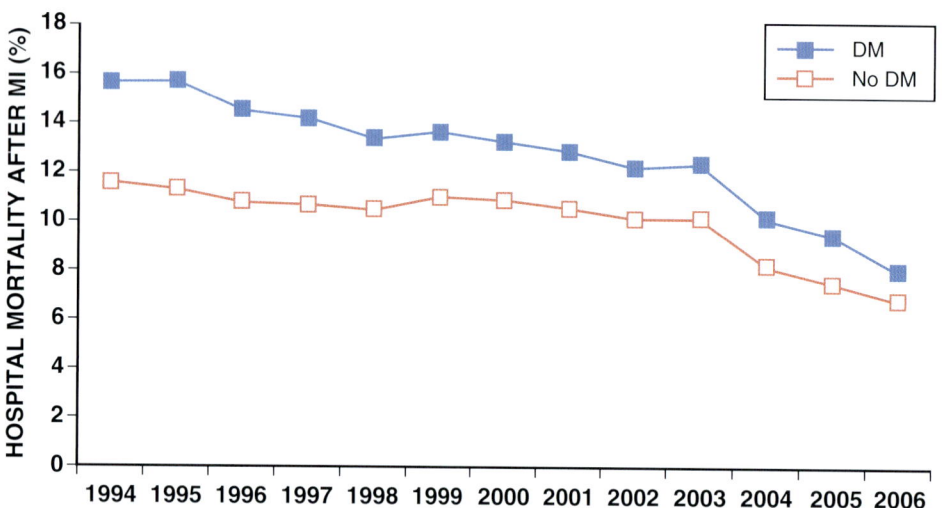

FIGURE 31.4 Unadjusted hospital mortality after myocardial infarction (MI) by year of study enrollment according to diabetes mellitus status (in-hospital deaths as percentage of total number of patients enrolled during each year of the study) among 1,734,431 patients with acute MI registered in the National Registry of Myocardial Infarction (NRMI) 1994 to 2006. (From Gore MO, Patel MJ, Kosiborod M, et al. Diabetes mellitus and trends in hospital survival after myocardial infarction, 1994 to 2006: data from the national registry of myocardial infarction. *Circulation Cardiovasc Qual Outcomes.* 2012;5:791–797.)

DM and three or more major risk factors are also considered to be at very high risk, as multiple risk factors in DM increase risk including CV death.[11] The high-risk category includes those with DM duration ≥10 years without target organ damage plus any other additional risk factors. Finally, younger patients (type 2 DM aged <50) with a DM duration less than 10 years and without other risk factors are considered at moderate risk.

CORONARY HEART DISEASE IN THE PATIENT WITH DIABETES

Mechanistic Considerations Linking Diabetes and Atherosclerosis

Traditional CHD risk factors such as hypertension, dyslipidemia, and adiposity cluster in patients with DM (see Chapters 25–30). However, this clustering does not completely account for the increased CHD risk observed among patients with DM (Table 31.2).[11]

The mechanisms of increased atherosclerotic risk remain poorly understood. The principal vascular perturbations linked to hyperglycemia include endothelial vasomotor dysfunction, vascular effects of advanced glycation end products (AGEs), adverse effects of circulating free fatty acids (FFAs), increased systemic inflammation, and a prothrombotic state. The myriad mechanisms contributing to endothelial dysfunction include abnormal nitric oxide biology, increased circulating endothelin and angiotensin II, and reduced prostacyclin (i.e., prostaglandin I_2) activity, all of which contribute to perturbations in the regulation of blood flow. Abnormalities in lipid metabolism also contribute to the increased atherosclerotic risk associated with DM (see Chapters 25 and 27). High triglyceride (TG) levels, low levels of high-density lipoprotein cholesterol (HDL-C), and increased small, dense low-density lipoprotein (LDL) particles characterize diabetic dyslipidemia, and contribute to aggravated atherosclerosis.

Perturbations in the coagulation and fibrinolytic pathways and in platelet biology add to the prothrombotic risk in DM.[8,12] These abnormalities include increased circulating tissue factor, factor VII, von Willebrand factor, and plasminogen activator inhibitor-1, and decreased levels of antithrombin III and protein C. Increased systemic inflammation accompanies DM and associates with increased oxidative stress and the accumulation of AGEs.[12]

Prevention and Treatment of Coronary Heart Disease and Its Complications in the Patient with Diabetes

Lifestyle interventions remain the pillar of prevention of the atherosclerotic complications in DM. As recommended by the American Diabetes Association (ADA), American Heart Association (AHA), European Society of Cardiology (ESC), and European Association for the Study of Diabetes (EASD), therapeutic lifestyle targets include smoking abstinence, 150 minutes or more of aerobic activity weekly, weight control, and healthy diet habits.[10,13,14] (See the Guidelines Tables 31G.1 through 31G.4 in the online chapter.)

Beyond lifestyle modifications, pharmacologic strategies effectively reduce CVD risk in DM.[10,13,14] Such interventions include assiduous blood pressure (BP) and LDL cholesterol (LDL-C) management for all patients, and for patients at highest risk and angiotensin-converting enzyme (ACE) inhibitors independent of BP. Daily aspirin therapy is no longer recommended for patients with DM without established atherosclerotic cardiovascular disease (ASCVD), except in those with a very high ASCVD risk.[10,13,14] The benefits of glucose control on macrovascular CVD risk mitigation remain far less robust.[13,15]

Lipid Management

Type 2 DM is associated with a characteristic pattern of dyslipidemia, reviewed in detail in Chapter 27. Each component of the diabetic dyslipidemia profile associates independently with CVD risk, including increased small, dense LDL particles, increased apolipoprotein B concentration, increased TG levels, and decreased HDL-C. Despite extensive research in modifying TG and HDL-C levels, the reduction of LDL-cholesterol remains the cornerstone of therapeutic lipid intervention in patients with DM.[10,13]

Statins

Contemporary guidelines for the management of diabetic dyslipidemia focus on the use of statins,[10,13,16,17] with estimates of numbers needed to treat (NNT) to prevent one major adverse CVD complication over 5 years in the setting of DM: 39 for patients without CVD and 19 among patients with prevalent CVD (see Chapters 25 and 27). These guidelines do not require an increased LDL-C to initiate statin therapy

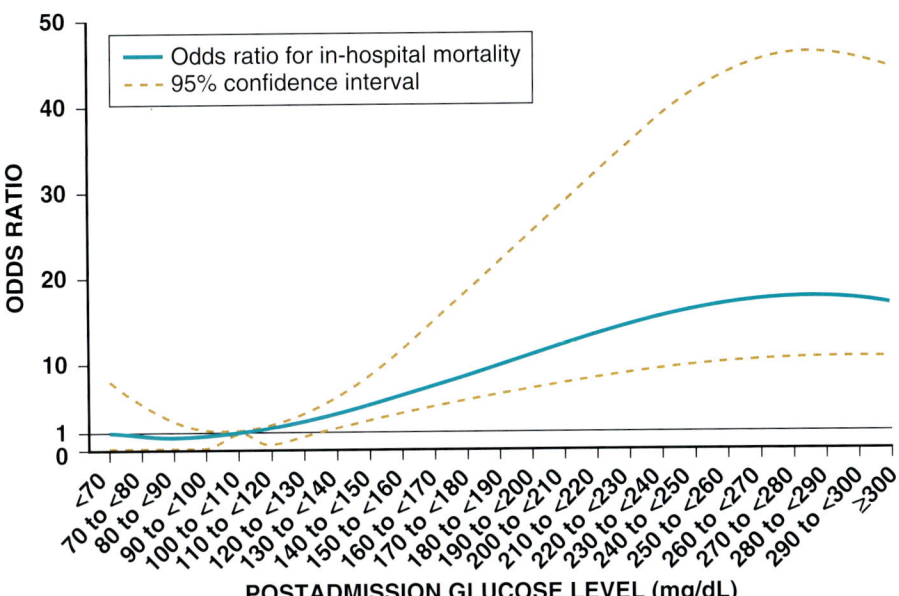

FIGURE 31.5 Postadmission glucose levels and mortality in a cohort of patients admitted for acute myocardial infarction (MI) with hyperglycemia on arrival, after multivariable adjustment (to convert glucose values to mmol/L multiply by 0.0555). (From Kosiborod M, McGuire DK. Glucose-lowering targets for patients with cardiovascular disease: focus on inpatient management of patients with acute coronary syndromes. *Circulation.* 2010;122:2736–2744.)

TABLE 31.2 Examples of Mechanisms Implicated in Diabetic Vascular Disease

Endothelium	↑ NF-κB activation
	↓ Nitric oxide production
	↓ Prostacyclin bioavailability
	↑ Endothelin 1 activity
	↑ Angiotensin II activity
	↑ Cyclooxygenase type 2 (COX-2) activity
	↑ Thromboxane A_2 activity
	↑ Reactive oxygen species
	↑ Lipid peroxidation products
	↓ Endothelium-dependent relaxation
	↑ RAGE expression
Vascular smooth muscle cells and vascular matrix	↑ Proliferation and migration into intima
	↑ Increased matrix degradation
	Altered matrix components
Inflammation	↑ IL-1β, IL-6, CD36, MCP-1
	↑ ICAMs, VCAMs, and selectins
	↑ Activity of protein kinase C
	↑ AGEs and AGE-RAGE interactions

AGEs, Advanced glycation end products; *ICAMs,* intracellular adhesion molecules; *IL,* interleukin; *MCP,* monocyte chemoattractant protein; *NF,* nuclear factor; *RAGE,* receptor for advanced glycation end products; *VCAMs,* vascular cell adhesion molecules.
Modified from Orasanu G, Plutzky J. The pathologic continuum of diabetic vascular disease. *J Am Coll Cardiol.* 2009;53:S35.

for patients with DM, and recommend treatment of all DM patients. The 2018 Guideline on the Management of Blood Cholesterol endorsed by multiple groups recommends moderate-intensity statin therapy in adults aged 40 to 75 years with DM regardless of estimated 10-year ASCVD risk. Adults with DM who have multiple ASCVD risk factors or prevalent ASCVD should receive a high-intensity statin with the aim to reduce LDL-C by 50%.

Statin therapy can hasten the onset of DM in patients at risk of developing DM.[18] Nevertheless, the benefits in terms of CV event reduction greatly exceed the risks of statin-induced DM. The ESC guidelines endorse a treat-to-target approach.[10] Diabetic patients with very high CVD risk should achieve an LDL-C target of less than 55 mg/dL or achieve a decrease in LDL-C of at least 50%. Most other patients with DM are categorized as "high risk," with an LDL-C target of at least less than 70 mg/dL.

EZETIMIBE. Ezetimibe inhibits the intestinal cholesterol transporter Niemann-Pick C1-like 1 (NPC1L1). The Improved Reduction of Outcomes: Vytorin Efficacy International Trial (IMPROVE-IT) assessed the effect of more intensive LDL-C targets with simvastatin/ezetimibe versus standard target control using simvastatin in 18,144 patients following ACS events.[19] After a mean follow-up of 5.7 years, ezetimibe/simvastatin yielded a significant 6.7% relative risk reduction (RRR) for the primary composite endpoint. In the subgroup of patients with DM, the beneficial effect on outcome was stronger than in patients without DM with a hazard ratio (HR) 0.85, 95% confidence interval (CI) 0.78 to 0.94.[20] The results in this subgroup were mainly due to a lower incidence of MI and ischemic stroke.

PCSK9 INHIBITORS. Inhibition of proprotein convertase subtilisin/kexin type 9 (PCSK9) with antibodies such as alirocumab or evolocumab reduce LDL-C by 40% to 60% over statins, with similar effects in patients with or without DM.[21,22] The FOURIER trial showed a significant 15% RRR for the primary composite endpoint of CV death, MI, stroke, hospitalization for unstable angina, or coronary revascularization with evolocumab versus placebo in 27,564 patients with clinically evident CVD.[23] At study baseline, 11,031 patients (40%) had DM. Evolocumab significantly and consistently reduced cardiovascular outcomes in patients with and without DM at baseline. Evolocumab did not increase the risk of new-onset DM in patients without DM at baseline (HR, 1.05, 0.94 to 1.17), including patients with prediabetes (HR, 1.00, 0.89 to 1.13).[23]

In the ODYSSEY OUTCOMES trial, alirocumab significantly reduced the risk of the primary composite endpoint (CV death, MI, stroke, or hospital admission for unstable angina) compared with placebo, with an HR of 0.85 (95% CI 0.78, 0.93).[24] In a subgroup analysis of patients with DM, alirocumab resulted in similar relative reductions in the incidence of the primary endpoint in each glycemic category, but a greater absolute risk reduction in the incidence of the primary outcome in patients with DM (2.3%, 95% CI 0.4 to 4.2) than in those with prediabetes (1.2%, 0.0 to 2.4) or normoglycemia (1.2%, −0.3 to 2.7; absolute risk reduction $p_{interaction}$=0.0019). Alirocumab did not increase the incidence of DM.[25]

FIBRIC ACID DERIVATIVES (FIBRATES). Fibrates are agonists of the nuclear transcriptional regulator peroxisome proliferator–activated receptor alpha (PPAR-α) that lower TGs and modestly increase HDL-C. Although fibrates favorably affect two of the fundamental abnormalities of diabetic dyslipidemia beyond LDL-C lowering by raising HDL-C and lowering TGs, the net CVD effects of this drug class remain uncertain, with no significant benefit observed in two CV outcomes trials of patients with type 2 DM, many of whom were treated with statins.[16] Sub-analyses of these trials suggest that the subset of patients with high baseline TGs concomitant with low HDL-C may derive incremental CVD risk reduction with fibrates added to background therapy—a hypothesis pending confirmation in a dedicated randomized trial.

OMEGA-3 FATTY ACIDS. Omega-3 fatty acids (fish oil) can reduce circulating TGs up to 40% (see Chapters 25, 27, and 29), and hold promise in the treatment of diabetic dyslipidemia. With no interactions with statins, prescription-grade n-3 fatty acids in high dose is attractive as an add-on therapy to statins for incremental TG reduction. The Outcome Reduction with an Initial Glargine Intervention (ORIGIN) trial randomized 12,536 patients with impaired fasting glucose, impaired glucose tolerance, or DM who randomly received either a 1-g capsule containing at least 900 mg (≥90%) of ethyl esters of n-3 fatty acids or a capsule containing 1 g of olive oil daily.[26] The primary outcome was CV mortality. Over a median follow-up of 6.2 years with 1155 CV deaths to analyze, there was no effect on the primary outcome with fish oil versus control (9.1% vs. 9.3%, respectively; $P = 0.72$). However, the REDUCE-IT trial examined a higher dose of highly purified eicosapentaenoic acid (icosapent ethyl, 2 g twice daily) in patients with established CVD or with DM and other risk factors, who had been receiving statin therapy and who had a fasting TG level of 135 to 499 mg/dL (1.52 to 5.63 mmol/L) and a LDL-C level of 41 to 100 mg/dL (1.06 to 2.59 mmol/L). Compared with placebo, icosapent ethyl significantly reduced the combined endpoint of CV death, non-fatal MI, or non-fatal stroke with a HR of 0.75; (95% CI, 0.68 to 0.83) in the overall population, with a similar benefit in the subgroup of patients with DM.[27]

INCLISIRAN. The subcutaneous injection of inclisiran, a small interfering RNA that targets PCSK9 mRNA offers a novel strategy to reduce LDL-C. In a phase 2, multicenter, double-blind, placebo-controlled, trial in patients at high risk for CVD,[28] inclisiran dose-dependently reduced PCSK9 and LDL-C levels. At day 180, the least-squares mean reductions in LDL-C levels were 27.9% to 41.9% after a single dose of inclisiran and 35.5% to 52.6% after two doses ($P < 0.001$ for all comparisons vs. placebo). In the ORION-1 trial inclisiran associated with marked declines in LDL-C in both patients without and with DM.[29]

Hypertension Management

Hypertension affects approximately 70% of patients with DM, with a steep-graded association between increasing BP and adverse CV outcomes (Fig. 31.6) (see Chapter 26).[30] Numerous classes of antihypertensive medications have reduced CVD risk in patients with DM.[30] BP targets for patients with DM have historically been more aggressive than for the overall population, with a goal of less than 130/80 mmHg in patients with DM, and a target of less than 140/80 mmHg in those not tolerating the lower goal.[10,13,30,31]

Renin-Angiotensin-Aldosterone System Antagonists

ACE inhibitors and angiotensin II receptor blockers (ARBs) are cornerstones of therapy for hypertension in DM because of their favorable effects on diabetic nephropathy and CVD outcomes.[13,14,30,31]

ANGIOTENSIN-CONVERTING ENZYME INHIBITORS. Data from randomized trials of patients with and without hypertension underpin the recommendation for ACE inhibitors as first-line agents for treatment of hypertension in the patient with DM. For example, the Heart Outcomes Prevention Evaluation (HOPE) trial compared ramipril (10 mg daily) with placebo in patients at increased risk for CVD and found that ramipril was superior to placebo in the DM subset of 3577 patients for the primary outcome of CV death, MI, and stroke (RRR, 25%; $P = 0.004$) and for overt nephropathy (RRR, 24%; $P = 0.027$).[30] The DM sub-analysis of the EUROPA (European Trial on Reduction of Cardiac Events with Perindopril in Stable Coronary Artery Disease) trial,[30] which tested perindopril versus placebo, showed an RRR of 19% among the 1502 participants with DM. These results and those from meta-analyses[30] support the consideration of ACE inhibitors for all patients with DM who have prevalent CVD, a clustering of CVD risk factors, or nephropathy with or without albuminuria.[10,13,31]

ANGIOTENSIN II RECEPTOR BLOCKERS. Data on CV outcomes with ARBs are much less robust than those on ACE inhibitors, particularly in patients with DM. The Telmisartan Randomized Assessment Study in ACE Intolerant Subjects with Cardiovascular Disease (TRANSCEND) trial enrolled 5926 patients with intolerance to ACE inhibitors, randomly assigned to receive telmisartan (80 mg daily) or placebo, 2118 of which had DM.[30] The overall trial failed to achieve statistical superiority for telmisartan versus placebo on the primary composite of CVD

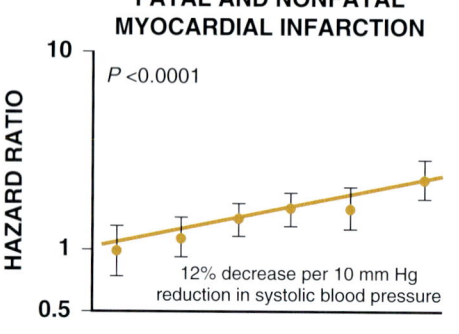
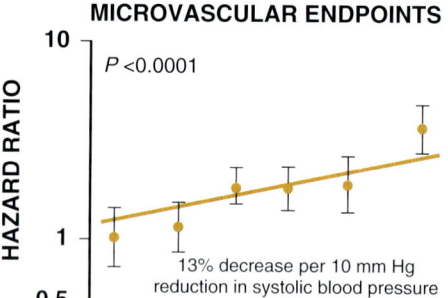
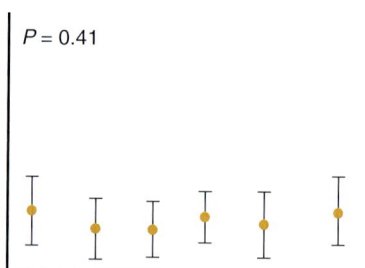
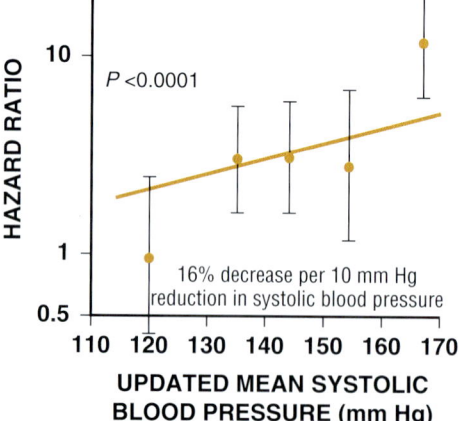
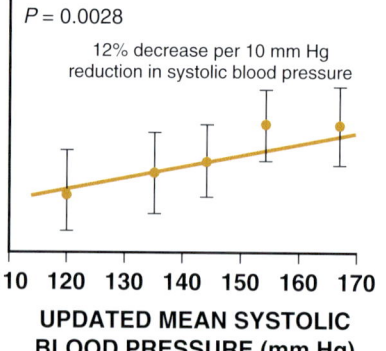

FIGURE 31.6 Hazard ratios (95% confidence intervals as floating absolute risks) as estimate of association between category of updated mean systolic blood pressure and myocardial infarction (MI), stroke, and heart failure (HF), with log linear scales. Reference category (hazard ratio of 1.0) is systolic pressure less than 120 mm Hg for MI and less than 130 mm Hg for stroke and HF; P values reflect contribution of systolic pressure to multivariable model. Data adjusted for age at diagnosis of diabetes mellitus (DM), ethnic group, smoking status, presence of albuminuria, hemoglobin A_{1c} (HbA_{1c}), high-density lipoprotein (HDL) and low-density lipoprotein (LDL) cholesterol, and triglyceride. (Modified from Adler AI, Stratton AM, Neil HA, et al. Association of systolic blood pressure with macrovascular and microvascular complications of type 2 diabetes (UKPDS 36): prospective observational study. BMJ. 2000;321:412.)

death, MI, stroke, and HF hospitalization (HR, 0.92; 95% CI 0.81 to 1.05), with a completely neutral point estimate in the subset with DM. Various guidelines have endorsed ARBs and ACE inhibitors in DM,[10,13,31] acknowledging the weaker evidence for ARBs. ACE inhibitors should remain first-line agents, with ARBs reserved for patients with intolerance to ACE inhibitors, and the two classes of medications should not be combined.[10,31]

Calcium Channel Blockers
Dihydropyridine calcium channel blockers (e.g., amlodipine, felodipine, nitrendipine, nisoldipine) are generally well tolerated and effectively lower BP. Analyses of data on DM subsets in randomized clinical trials suggest a magnitude of CVD clinical benefit similar to or greater than that observed in cohorts without DM.[30]

Thiazide Diuretics
Concern about the adverse glycemic and triglyceridemic effects of the thiazide diuretic types of medications, including hydrochlorothiazide, chlorthalidone, indapamide, and bendroflumethiazide, has led to some hesitancy regarding their use in patients with DM. However, randomized trials of chlorthalidone and indapamide that included substantial numbers of patients with DM have consistently demonstrated CVD benefits. In a sub-analysis of the Antihypertensive and Lipid-Lowering Treatment to Prevent Heart Attack Trial (ALLHAT), the CVD effects of chlorthalidone compared with both lisinopril and amlodipine were similar in patients with DM or impaired fasting glucose, despite modest but statistically significant increases in incident DM associated with chlorthalidone use.[32] Also, indapamide combined with perindopril in the Action in Diabetes and Vascular Disease: Preterax and Diamicron-MR Controlled Evaluation (ADVANCE) trial of 11,140 patients with DM showed superior CV outcomes.[33] A meta-analysis of randomized trials further supports the benefits of chlorthalidone and indapamide in the treatment of patients with DM.[30,32]

Beta Blockers
Beta blockers are rarely used as routine antihypertensive therapies in patients with DM.[10,31] Beta blockers offer no benefit over other evidence-based classes of medications, with some concern for increased risk for a composite of CV disease, stroke, and HF based on recent meta-analysis.[30] Therefore, use of beta blockers should be primarily limited to patients with HF with reduced ejection fraction (HFrEF) (carvedilol, metoprolol succinate, or bisoprolol) and after MI. Beta blockers have a place in therapy of angina and for rate control of AF.

Antihypertensive Therapy Summary
Four classes of antihypertensive medications reduce CVD risk in patients with DM: ACE inhibitors, ARBs, calcium channel blockers, and thiazide diuretics (specifically, chlorthalidone, indapamide). Other options in resistant hypertension, after eliminating secondary causes, include mineralocorticoid antagonists, alpha blockers, and centrally acting agents. Evidence supports a BP target of at least less than 140/80 mmHg for all patients with DM, with a more intensive systolic BP target of less than 130 mmHg for those patients who can achieve that target without excessive adverse effects.

Antiplatelet Therapy
Daily Aspirin
The ADA and AHA recommend daily aspirin (75 to 162 mg/day) for all patients with DM who have established ASCVD, with use for primary prevention no longer recommended, though it may be considered in those at very highest ASCVD risk.[10,13,34,35] Substantial evidence based on the setting of secondary ASCVD risk modification supports these recommendations, but a meta-analysis of primary prevention with aspirin in patients with DM failed to show significant benefit.[36] Two subsequent randomized clinical trials, ASCEND and ACCEPT-D underscore this finding. The ASCEND trial enrolled 15,480 patients with DM without established ASCVD, randomized to aspirin 100 mg daily versus placebo. There was a modest risk reduction for the primary composite of vascular death, MI, or stroke (RR 0.88; 95% CI, 0.79 to 0.97) in the context of increased risk for major bleeding (RR 1.29; 95% CI, 1.09 to 1.52), with bleeding hazard counterbalancing the benefits.[37]

P2Y$_{12}$ Receptor Antagonists
Though proven effective for patients following ACSs and coronary stenting, aspirin remains the preferred therapy over P2Y$_{12}$ receptor antagonists such as clopidogrel, prasugrel, or ticagrelor for chronic stable primary and secondary risk prevention. For patients with aspirin indication but with aspirin allergy or intolerance, a P2Y$_{12}$ receptor antagonist may be considered.[10] For patients with type 2 DM and prevalent coronary artery disease but without prior MI, results from the THEMIS randomized trial demonstrated the net clinical benefit of ticagrelor 60 mg twice daily added to low-dose aspirin versus low-dose aspirin alone in the large subset of patients with prior coronary stenting ($n = 11{,}154$), leading to the conclusion that ticagrelor should be considered as an add-on to aspirin in patients with DM and a history of percutaneous coronary intervention (PCI) who have tolerated antiplatelet therapy, have high ischemic risk, and low bleeding risk.[38] However, the reduction in the primary outcome was achieved at the expense of increased major bleeding, with a highly significant 2.3-fold increase in thrombolysis in myocardial infarction (TIMI) major bleeding, including intracranial bleeding.

Glucose Management
A total of 12 drug classes of glucose-lowering medications are presently available for type 2 DM (Table 31.3), with various mechanisms of action. Typically, two or three drugs simultaneously are used to reduce hyperglycemia.

Cardiovascular Effects of Selected Medications for Diabetes
Until 2008, the approval of drugs for DM depended almost exclusively on the demonstration of glucose lowering, without required proof of improved clinical outcomes. The regulatory landscape for DM drugs underwent major changes in 2008, such that all glucose-lowering agents for type 2 DM needed to demonstrate designated margins of CV safety to achieve and maintain regulatory approval.[39,40] This led to a rapid proliferation of CV outcome trials of glucose-lowering drugs which have provided rich datasets documenting either CV safety or actual efficacy in improving cardiac and/or renal outcomes (Table 31.4 and Fig. 31.7). Heretofore, the available data on the net CV impact of such medications had been quite limited, with older treatment guidelines essentially grounded on the proven microvascular disease benefits demonstrated through glucose control alone.[41,42] These new data spurred guidelines to endorse specific drug categories depending on patient characteristics, specifically the presence of CV or kidney disease. In 2020, the U.S. Food and Drug Administration (FDA) reversed course and will, going forward, no longer require extensive CV safety testing for new glucose-lowering medications in the absence of specific safety signals. Instead, when a new medication is proposed for glycemic control, its safety database from Phase 3 trials should include sufficient numbers of patients with established CVD, CKD, and age over 65 years, targeting at least 1200 patients with at least one of these conditions/states. Development program sponsors are also advised to use rigorous methods for the collection of adverse CV events and assess them by adjudication.

METFORMIN. Metformin, a biguanide, reduces blood glucose primarily by decreasing hepatic glucose output and perhaps by other mechanisms. Metformin, associated with modest initial weight reduction, has favorable effects on lipid levels, decrease in inflammatory markers, improvement in coagulation profiles, and low risk for hypoglycemia. In the United Kingdom Prospective Diabetes Study (UKPDS) of various glucose-lowering strategies in a population of patients with newly diagnosed type 2 DM, patients who were overweight at study entry were eligible for randomization to a policy of more intensive glucose control with metformin versus usual care. Those treated with metformin had statistically superior outcomes for all DM-related endpoints (RRR, 32%; 95% CI 13% to 47%), DM-related death (RRR, 42%; 95% CI 9% to 63%), and all-cause mortality (RRR, 36%; 95% CI 9% to 55%).[33] A second trial, the HOME study, randomized 390 patients with insulin-treated type 2 DM to metformin versus placebo.[33] The effect on the primary composite outcome, including micro- and macrovascular

TABLE 31.3 Characteristics of Glucose-Lowering Medications for Type 2 Diabetes Mellitus

CLASS	COMPOUND(S)	CELLULAR MECHANISM	MAIN PHYSIOLOGIC ACTION(S)	ADVANTAGES	DISADVANTAGES	COST
Biguanides	Metformin	Activates AMP-kinase ? Other	↓ Hepatic glucose production ? Other	Extensive experience No weight gain No hypoglycemia Likely ↓ CVD events (UKPDS)	GI side effects (diarrhea, abdominal cramping) Lactic acidosis risk (rare) Vitamin B$_{12}$ deficiency Multiple contraindications: advanced CKD, acidosis, hypoxia, dehydration, ethanol abuse, other	Low
Sulfonylureas	Second generation: Glyburide (glibenclamide) Glipizide Gliclazide*§ Glimepiride	Closes K$_{ATP}$ channels on beta cell plasma membranes	↑ Insulin secretion	Extensive experience ↓ Microvascular risk (UKPDS)	Hypoglycemia Weight gain ? Blunts myocardial ischemic preconditioning Low durability	Low
Meglitinides (glinides)	Repaglinide Nateglinide	Closes K$_{ATP}$ channels on beta cell plasma membranes	↑ Insulin secretion	↓ Postprandial glucose excursions Dosing flexibility	Hypoglycemia Weight gain ? Blunts myocardial ischemic preconditioning Frequent dosing schedule	High
Thiazolidinediones	Pioglitazone Rosiglitazone†	Activates the nuclear transcription factor PPAR-γ	↑ Insulin sensitivity	No hypoglycemia Durability ↑ HDL-C ↓ Triglycerides (pioglitazone) ↓ Albuminuria ? ↓ CVD events (pioglitazone)	Weight gain Edema/heart failure Bone fractures ↑ LDL-C (rosiglitazone) ? ↑ MI (meta-analyses, rosiglitazone)	Moderate
α-Glucosidase inhibitors‡	Acarbose Miglitol Voglibose*§	Inhibits intestinal α-Glucosidase	Slows intestinal carbohydrate digestion/absorption	No hypoglycemia ↓ Postprandial glucose excursions Nonsystemic	Generally modest HbA$_{1c}$ efficacy GI side effects (flatulence, diarrhea) Frequent dosing schedule	Moderate
DPP4 inhibitors	Vildagliptin* Sitagliptin Saxagliptin Alogliptin Linagliptin	Inhibits DPP4 activity, increasing postprandial active incretin (GLP-1, GIP) concentrations	↑ Insulin secretion (glucose dependent) ↓ Glucagon secretion (glucose-dependent)	No hypoglycemia Well tolerated	Generally modest HbA$_{1c}$ efficacy Urticaria/angioedema ? Pancreatitis Possible ↑ heart failure (saxagliptin; alogliptin)	High
Bile acid sequestrants‡	Colesevelam	Binds bile acids in intestinal tract, increasing hepatic bile acid production ? Activation of farnesoid receptor (FXR) in liver	Unknown ? ↓ Hepatic glucose production ? ↑ Incretin levels	No hypoglycemia ↓ LDL-C	Generally modest HbA$_{1c}$ efficacy Constipation ↑ Triglycerides May alter absorption of other medications	High
Dopamine-2 agonists‡	Bromocriptine (quick release)§	Activates dopaminergic receptors	Modulates hypothalamic regulation of metabolism ↑ Insulin sensitivity	No hypoglycemia ? ↓ CVD events (Cycloset Safety Trial)	Generally modest HbA$_{1c}$ efficacy Dizziness/syncope Nausea Fatigue Rhinitis	High

Continued

TABLE 31.3 Characteristics of Glucose-Lowering Medications for Type 2 Diabetes Mellitus—cont'd

CLASS	COMPOUND(S)	CELLULAR MECHANISM	MAIN PHYSIOLOGIC ACTION(S)	ADVANTAGES	DISADVANTAGES	COST
SGLT2 inhibitors	Dapagliflozin Canagliflozin Empagliflozin Ertugliflozin	Inhibits SGLT2 in the proximal renal tubule	Decreases glucose reabsorption, leading to glucosuria	Effective at all disease stages No hypoglycemia Weight loss ↓ Blood pressure r ↓ Albuminuria ↓ MACE (empa, cana) ↓ HF hospitalization (all) ↓ CV death (empa, cana) ↓ CKD progression (all but ertu)	Diabetic ketoacidosis Genitourinary infections Polyuria Volume depletion ↓ LDL-C Reversible ↓ eGFR ? Amputation risk (cana) ? Fracture risk (cana)	High
GLP-1 receptor agonists	Exenatide Exenatide (weekly) Liraglutide Albiglutide Dulaglutide Semaglutide Semaglutide (oral) Lixisenatide	Activates GLP-1 receptors	↑ Insulin secretion (glucose-dependent) ↓ Glucagon secretion (glucose-dependent) Slows gastric emptying ↑ Satiety	No hypoglycemia Weight reduction ↓ CV risk factors ↓ MACE (lira, sema, dula) ↓ CV death (lira) ↓ macroalbuminuria	GI side effects (nausea/vomiting) ↑ Pulse rate ↑ Gallbladder events ? Pancreatitis ? Mitogenicity/cancer risk Injectable Training requirements (injectables)	High
Amylin mimetics[=]	Pramlintide[§]	Activates amylin receptors	↓ Glucagon secretion Slows gastric emptying ↑ Satiety	↓ Postprandial glucose excursions Weight reduction	Generally modest HbA₁c efficacy GI side effects (nausea/vomiting) Hypoglycemia unless insulin dose is simultaneously reduced Injectable Training requirements Frequent dosing schedule	High
Insulins	Human NPH Human regular Lispro Aspart Glulisine Glargine Detemir Degludec Premixed (several types)	Activates insulin receptors	↑ Glucose disposal ↓ Hepatic glucose production	Universally effective Theoretically unlimited efficacy ↓ Microvascular risk (UKPDS)	Hypoglycemia Weight gain ? Mitogenicity/cancer risk Injectable Training requirements "Stigma" (for patients)	Variable[¶]

*Not licensed in the United States.
[†]Prescribing highly restricted in the United States; withdrawn in Europe.
[‡]Limited use in the United States/Europe.
[§]Not licensed in Europe.
[¶]Depends on type (analogues > human insulins) and dosage.

AMP, Adenosine monophosphate; *CKD*, chronic kidney disease; *CVD*, cardiovascular disease; *DPP4*, dipeptidyl peptidase 4; *eGFR*, estimated glomerular filtration rate; *GI*, gastrointestinal; *GIP*, glucose-dependent insulinotropic peptide; *GLP-1*, glucagon-like protein 1; *HDL-C*, high-density lipoprotein cholesterol; *LDL-C*, low-density lipoprotein cholesterol; *MACE*, major adverse cardiovascular event; *MI*, myocardial infarction; *SGLT2*, sodium-glucose cotransporter 2. *PROactive*, Prospective Pioglitazone Clinical Trial in Microvascular Events; *STOP-NIDDM*, Study to Prevent Non-Insulin-Dependent Diabetes Mellitus; *UKPDS*, United Kingdom Prospective Diabetes Study.

Modified and updated from Inzucchi SE, Bergenstal RM, Buse JB, et al. Management of hyperglycemia in type 2 diabetes, 2015: a patient-centered approach—update to a position statement of the American Diabetes Association and the European Association for the Study of Diabetes. *Diabetes Care.* 2015;38:141.

TABLE 31.4 Summary of Completed Cardiovascular Outcomes Trials of Medications for Type 2 Diabetes

TRIAL	DRUG*	PATIENTS (n)	STAGE	NCT
Completed Trials				
SAVOR-TIMI 53[60]	Saxagliptin	16,492	Completed	NCT01107886
EXAMINE[61]	Alogliptin	5,380	Completed	NCT00968708
TECOS[63]	Sitagliptin	14,671	Completed	NCT00790205
ELIXA[66]	Lixisenatide	6,068	Completed	NCT01147250
EMPA-REG-OUTCOME[75]	Empagliflozin	12,500	Completed	NCT01131676
LEADER[67]	Liraglutide	9,340	Completed	NCT01179048
SUSTAIN 6[70]	Semaglutide	3,299	Completed	NCT01720446
CANVAS[81]	Canagliflozin	4,330	Completed	NCT01032629
EXSCEL[68]	Exenatide LAR	14,752	Completed	NCT01144338
CV Outcomes-ITCA 650	Exenatide ITCA 650	4,156	Completed	NCT01455896
DEVOTE[59]	Insulin degludec	7,637	Completed	NCT01959529
CANVAS-R[81]	Canagliflozin	5,812	Completed	NCT01989754
CAROLINA[46]	Linagliptin versus glimepiride	6,000	Completed	NCT01243424
REWIND[72]	Dulaglutide	9,600	Completed	NCT01394952
VERTIS[85]	Ertugliflozin	8,246	Completed	NCT01986881
DECLARE-TIMI 58[82]	Dapagliflozin	17,160	Completed	NCT01730534
CARMELINA[47]	Linagliptin	6,980	Completed	NCT01897532
VERTIS CV[85]	Ertugliflozin	3,900	Completed	NCT01986881
CREDENCE[83]	Canagliflozin	3,627	Completed	NCT02065791
Ongoing Trials				
SOUL	Oral semaglutide	9,642	Started July, 2019	NCT03914326
SURPASS-CVOT	Tirzepatide vs. dulaglutide	12,500	Started May, 2020	NCT04255433

*All versus placebo except where noted.
NCT, National Clinical Trial [registration number].

complications, was neutral. However, the secondary outcome of major adverse CV events fell in the metformin group (RRR, 39%; 95% CI 6% to 60%), similar in magnitude to the macrovascular risk reductions seen in the UKPDS. Given the relatively small size and few CV events to analyze in both these trials, the CV efficacy of metformin remains uncertain, particularly in statin-treated patients.

Concerns about the potential of metformin to cause lactic acidosis delayed its regulatory approval in the United States and hindered its clinical uptake, stemming from earlier observations with another biguanide, phenformin, that clearly caused lactic acidemia and was removed from the market. In response to this concern, metformin was contraindicated for use in patients with impaired kidney function, for 48 to 72 hours after the administration of iodinated contrast, and in unstable HF. Despite widespread global use of metformin for more than five decades, however, and a substantial aggregated database of comparative clinical trials, no convincing signal for increased lactic acidemia with metformin treatment has emerged.[43,44]

Given this absence of data supporting the concern for lactic acidosis with metformin, in 2006 the FDA removed the product label warning for its use in patients with HF. More recently, the FDA also adjusted the prescribing guidelines for metformin products with regard to kidney contraindications.[45] Previously contraindicated with serum creatinine in men of 1.5 mg/dL or higher and in women of 1.4 mg/dL or higher, the updated recommendations allow for use in those with stable, mild-moderate CKD. The new cut points are based on the estimated glomerular filtration rate (eGFR) instead of serum creatinine. Metformin is now given to patients with an eGFR less than 60 mL/min/1.73 m^2, with safety reassessed for those taking metformin with an eGFR less than 45 mL/min/1.73 m^2, and with metformin contraindicated or to be stopped at an eGFR less than 30 mL/min/1.73 m^2. These changes should allow use of this effective, safe, and inexpensive medication to hundreds of thousands of patients in the United States alone. Regarding iodinated contrast administration, metformin need not be interrupted if the eGFR is greater than 60 mL/min/1.73 m^2, but should still be held in patients whose kidney function is below this level until no decrement in kidney function can be documented.

On the basis of safety, tolerability, low hypoglycemia risk, CV clinical outcomes data, and relatively low cost, metformin is widely considered the first-line drug for type 2 DM in the absence of contraindications or intolerance.[41,42] Metformin is the only oral antihyperglycemic medication routinely recommended to be continued in combination with insulin therapy.

SULFONYLUREAS. Sulfonylureas, in clinical use since the 1950s, are the oldest oral antihyperglycemic medications. They lower glucose by augmenting insulin release through inhibition of adenosine triphosphate (ATP)–dependent potassium (K_{ATP}) channels in pancreatic beta cells. Although sulfonylureas are well tolerated and are relatively potent, their use results in the highest rate of hypoglycemia of any available oral antihyperglycemic drug. They are also associated with weight gain. Although tolbutamide, a first-generation sulfonylurea, increased CV and all-cause mortality in an early randomized trial, no such adverse CV safety signals have emerged from subsequent randomized trials with assignment to second- and third-generation sulfonylureas.[33]

There had been concerns about the use of sulfonylureas in CVD cohorts, driven by their associated weight gain, increased risk for hypoglycemia and consequent stimulation of the adrenergic stress-response system with potential adverse CVD effects, and the potential of these drugs to inhibit so-called ischemic preconditioning through blockade of myocardial K_{ATP} channels. In experimental MI in animals, activation of myocardial K_{ATP} channels reduces infarct size, an effect termed ischemic preconditioning. The relevance of these observations in humans was always poorly understood, but this blocking effect is one potential explanation for the increased MI case-fatality rate observed in the more intensively treated patients in the ACCORD trial—a conjecture that remains unproved because of limited ability to analyze outcomes according to drug allocation in that trial.[33] Observations from the UKPDS trial counter the likelihood of such an effect, because an intensive glucose control policy with two different sulfonylureas, chlorpropamide and glibenclamide (glyburide in United States), yielded MI and CV death outcomes similar to those with insulin, metformin, and usual (diet) therapy.[33]

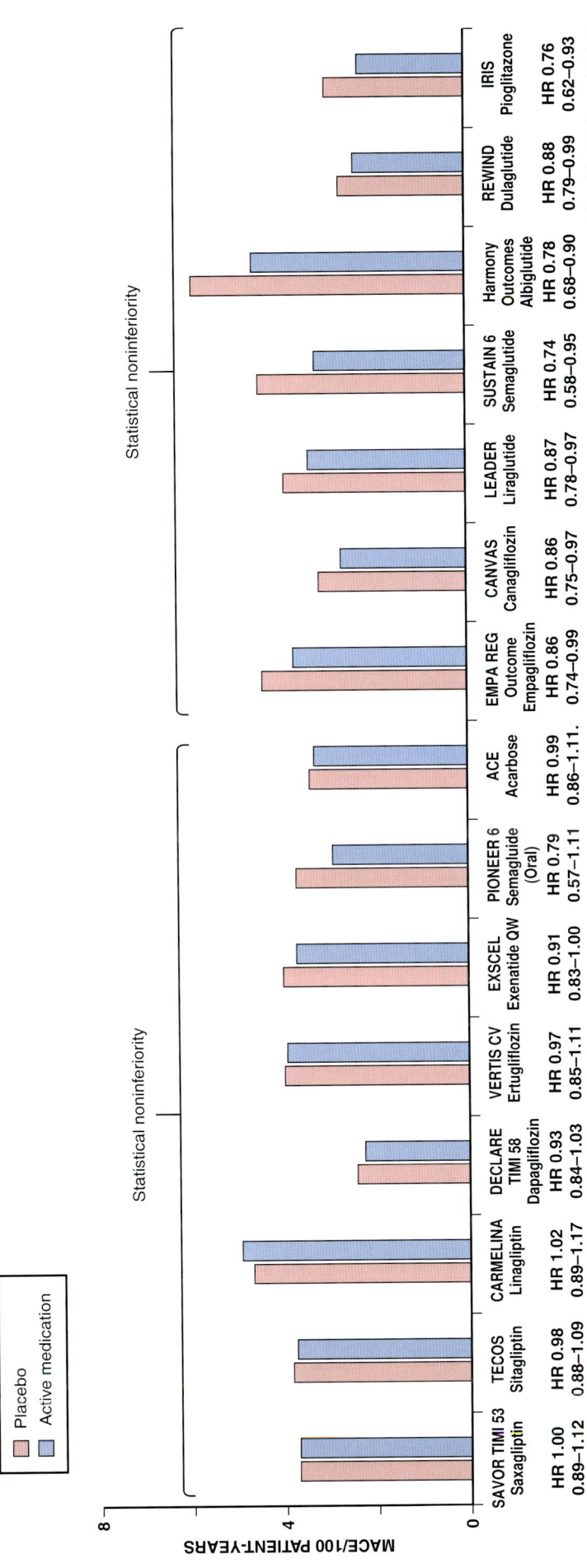

FIGURE 31.7 Summary results of the comparative incident rates (active medication vs. placebo) from large, randomized, placebo-controlled clinical trials of antihyperglycemic medications in patients with stable CV disease / CV risk factors using major adverse CV events (MACE) as primary outcomes. SAVOR TIMI 53 (Saxagliptin Assessment of Vascular Outcomes Recorded in Patients with Diabetes Mellitus–Thrombolysis in Myocardial Infarction); TECOS (Trial Evaluating Cardiovascular Outcomes With Sitagliptin); CARMELINA ((Cardiovascular and Renal Microvascular Outcome Study with Linagliptin in Patients with Type 2 Diabetes Mellitus); DECLARE TIMI 58 (Multicenter Trial to Evaluate the Effect of Dapagliflozin on the Incidence of Cardiovascular Events–Thrombolysis in Myocardial Infarction); VERTIS CV (Cardiovascular Outcomes Following Ertugliflozin Treatment in Type 2 Diabetes Mellitus Participants with Vascular Disease); EXSCEL (Exenatide Study of Cardiovascular Event Lowering Trial); PIONEER 6 (A Trial Investigating the Cardiovascular Safety of Oral Semaglutide in Subjects with Type 2 Diabetes); ACE (Acarbose Cardiovascular Evaluation Trial); EMPA REG Outcome (Empagliflozin Cardiovascular Outcome Event Trial in Type 2 Diabetes Mellitus Patients); CANVAS (Canagliflozin Cardiovascular Assessment Study); LEADER (Liraglutide Effect and Action in Diabetes: Evaluation of Cardiovascular Outcome Results); SUSTAIN 6 (Trial to Evaluate Cardiovascular and Other Long-term Outcomes with Semaglutide in Subjects with Type 2 Diabetes); Harmony Outcomes (Albiglutide and Cardiovascular Outcomes in Patients with Type 2 Diabetes and Cardiovascular Disease); REWIND (Researching Cardiovascular Events with a Weekly Incretin in Diabetes); IRIS (Insulin Resistance Intervention after Stroke). (Data from References 47, 52, 60, 63, 68, 70–73, 75, 81, 82, 85, 88.)

Due to these concerns, sulfonylureas that are relatively specific for pancreatic K_{ATP} channels were developed (e.g., glimepiride). In the CAROLINA trial,[46] while glimepiride was associated with significantly more hypoglycemia than the dipeptidyl peptidase 4 (DPP4) inhibitor (see below) linagliptin, major adverse CV events were equal between the two randomized groups. This finding is further evidence that glimepiride at least was safe for the heart, since as a group the DPP4 inhibitors are known to be safe themselves.[47] On the basis of the extensive clinical experience, the availability of low-cost generics, and the efficacy of glucose control demonstrated in several clinical trials, sulfonylureas constitute a category of second-line drugs (after metformin) for the treatment of type 2 DM, but certainly without the CV and/or renal advantages of some of the newer classes.[41]

Data from other observational studies have been inconsistent, however, with some[48-51] finding an association with adverse CV outcomes. This potential discrepancy between the apparent safety of sulfonylureas when studied in randomized trials versus their risk that emerges in observational studies has two explanations. First, the observational studies could be wrong, their findings influenced by confounders not assessable in the datasets, most importantly, indication. Second, under the careful observation of clinical trials the drugs could be safe, but their potential dangers may only emerge when used outside the research setting.

THIAZOLIDINEDIONES
Thiazolidinediones (e.g., rosiglitazone, pioglitazone) decrease glucose levels by increasing insulin sensitivity of target tissues and induce a wide variety of nonglycemic effects mediated through activation of the nuclear receptor PPAR-γ, including some favorable effects on intermediate markers of CVD and CVD risk. These findings engendered interest in their effects on CVD morbidity and mortality.[41] The Prospective Pioglitazone Clinical Trial in Macrovascular Events (the PROactive study) assessed the effect of a glucose-lowering medication on CV clinical outcomes. Treatment with pioglitazone yielded a significant 16% RRR for the prioritized secondary composite major adverse cardiovascular event (MACE) endpoint of all-cause mortality, nonfatal MI, and stroke compared with placebo in patients with type 2 DM and prevalent CVD at study entry, treated during a 34.5-month follow-up period, although the effect on the primary endpoint did not achieve statistical significance.[33] These data were considered hypothesis-generating because of failure to meet the primary outcome. More recently, in a 4.5-year study involving patients with insulin resistance but without DM who had a recent stroke or transient ischemic attack (TIA), pioglitazone versus placebo was associated with a 24% RRR in recurrent stroke or MI (HR, 0.76; 95% CI 0.62 to 0.93).[52] These data, admittedly in patients without DM, support the original PROactive MACE findings. In follow-up reports from IRIS, using updated international definitions, pioglitazone reduced ACS by 29%, type 1 MI by 38%,[53] and ischemic stroke alone by 28%.[54]

The TOSCA-IT study compared the CV effects of pioglitazone to several sulfonylureas in 3028 patients with type 2 DM not controlled on metformin monotherapy, most of whom did not have CVD.[55] The HR for the primary MACE outcome was 0.96 (95% CI 0.74 to 1.26), so no apparent benefit.

Rosiglitazone was at one point actually suspected of increasing MI risk.[41] These data from a controversial meta-analysis of phase 2 and 3 data initially led to severe product label restrictions for use in the United States and to withdrawal of rosiglitazone from the market elsewhere. However, a randomized open-label CV outcome trial, RECORD,[56] showed a neutral effect of rosiglitazone on CV outcomes in high-risk patients taking metformin or sulfonylureas. The rosiglitazone product label has since undergone updating to reflect this finding, but the drug remains infrequently used.

TZD increases the risk for peripheral edema, with a small but consistent increase in risk for new or worsening HF. The labels for these agents warn against their use in patients with HF, and are contraindicated in patients with New York Heart Association (NYHA) class III or IV HF and a caution against their use in any patient with HF. Although the mechanism of the observed increase in edema and HF remains unclear, it appears to result primarily from increased renal sodium reclamation and plasma volume expansion, with no evidence to date of pernicious cardiac effects of these drugs. Notably in insulin resistance intervention after stroke (IRIS), HF outcomes did not differ between the two randomized groups, likely a reflection of HF being an exclusion in the trial and on-trial protocols for study drug dose reduction if significant edema or excessive weight gain occurred.[57]

INSULIN. Early trials including those in both type 1 and type 2 DM suggest the CVD benefits with insulin but these studies all had limited statistical power to assess such effects. More recently the ORIGIN trial[58] randomly assigned 12,537 patients with CV risk factors plus impaired fasting glucose, impaired glucose tolerance, or prevalent type 2 DM to treatment with insulin glargine or standard care management. ORIGIN had dual primary trial outcomes of (1) nonfatal MI, nonfatal stroke, or death from CV causes, and (2) these events plus revascularization or hospitalization for HF. After a median follow-up of 6.2 years, insulin glargine and placebo groups showed no difference in first co-primary outcome (2.94 vs. 2.85 events per 100 patient-years; $P = 0.63$) or the second co-primary outcome (5.52 vs. 5.28 per 100 person-years; $P = 0.27$). Although ORIGIN did not demonstrate superiority of insulin glargine, the co-primary outcomes had point estimates of effect of 1.02 and 1.04, respectively, both with an upper confidence limit of 1.11—well within the current regulatory standard of upper confidence limit for CV effects of less than 1.3 to demonstrate CV safety of glucose-lowering drugs. As expected, insulin use is associated to more hypoglycemia and weight gain. Only one trial has assessed CV outcomes between two different types of basal insulins. DEVOTE randomized 7637 patients with T2DM to either insulin degludec or glargine or insulin.[59] The incidence of the primary MACE outcome proved similar at 8.5% versus 9.3% (HR, 0.91; 95%, CI 0.78 to 1.06). Fewer patients using degludec, however, experienced severe hypoglycemia (4.9% vs. 6.6%; rate ratio, 0.60; $P < 0.001$).

DIPEPTIDYL PEPTIDASE 4 INHIBITORS. The DPP4 inhibitors selectively inhibit the action of dipeptidyl peptidase 4, a circulating enzyme that degrades the endogenous incretin hormones glucagon-like protein (GLP)-1 and glucose-dependent insulinotropic polypeptide (GIP), which stimulate glucose-appropriate insulin secretion and/or inhibit glucagon release. Inhibiting DDP4 therefore potentiates GLP-1 and GIP action, reducing glucose levels. Four DPP inhibitors—saxagliptin, alogliptin, sitagliptin, and linagliptin—are available in the United States, with a fifth drug (vildagliptin) approved elsewhere. Each of these daily tablets have modest glucose-lowering potency and neutral effects on weight with low risk for hypoglycemia.

Randomized CV outcomes trials of four DPP4 inhibitors have been completed (see Table 31.4). In the Saxagliptin Assessment of Vascular Outcomes Recorded in Patients with Diabetes Mellitus (SAVOR)—TIMI 53 trial, 16,492 patients with type 2 DM or at increased risk for atherosclerotic CV disease randomly received blinded treatment with saxagliptin, 5 mg daily (or 2.5 mg daily in patients with eGFR ≤50 mL/min/1.73 m²) versus placebo.[60] Saxagliptin had no effect on the primary composite outcome of CV death, MI, and ischemic stroke , but unexpectedly increased hospitalization for HF (HR, 1.27; 95% CI 1.07 to 1.51), an observation that remains poorly understood and requires further exploration and assessment in the other outcomes trials evaluating the DPP4 inhibitors.

In the Examination of Cardiovascular Outcomes with Alogliptin versus Standard of Care (EXAMINE) trial, 5380 patients with type 2 DM and a recent ACS event randomly received alogliptin versus placebo.[61] Alogliptin had no effect on the primary composite outcome of CV death, MI, and stroke (HR, 0.96; upper 97.5% confidence limit = 1.16). In a subsequent report, HF hospitalization as the first event of an expanded MACE composite that included HF occurred similarly between patients assigned to alogliptin versus placebo (HR, 1.07; 95% CI 0.79 to 1.46), yet hospitalization for HF was statistically higher in alogliptin-treated patients without prevalent HF at trial entry (HR, 1.76; 95% CI 1.07 to 2.90).[62]

The Trial Examining Cardiovascular Outcomes with Sitagliptin (TECOS), assessed the CV effects of sitagliptin versus placebo in 14,671 patients with type 2 DM and prevalent ASCVD.[63] Sitagliptin had no effect on the primary composite outcome of CV death, MI, stroke, and hospitalization for unstable angina (HR, 0.98; 95% CI 0.88 to 1.09). In contrast to SAVOR and EXAMINE, the sitagliptin group did not experience increased HF hospitalization rates (HR, 1.0; 95% CI 83 to 1.20) in subgroups with or without HF at baseline.[64]

In the Cardiovascular and Renal Microvascular Outcome Study with Linagliptin (CARMELINA) trial,[47] involving 6979 patients and a median follow-up of 2.2 years, the primary MACE outcome occurred with equal frequency in the linagliptin and placebo groups (HR, 1.02; 95% CI, 0.89 to 1.17; $P < 0.001$ for noninferiority). Finally, the aforementioned Cardiovascular Outcome Study of Linagliptin Versus Glimepiride in Patients With Type 2 Diabetes (CAROLINA) was unique amongst recent type 2

DM CV outcomes trials using an active comparator, the sulfonylurea, glimepiride. With 6042 patients followed for a median of 6.3 years, the risk of developing the primary MACE outcome was equivalent between the treatment groups (HR, 0.98 [95.47% CI, 0.84 to 1.14]; $P < 0.001$ for noninferiority).

When data from the first 3 CV outcome trials were pooled, the HR for HF hospitalization with active therapy was 1.15 (0.98, 1.34), mainly driven by the outcomes in SAVOR-TIMI 53.[64] In a meta-analysis involving 84 DPP4 inhibition trials, the overall risk of HF hospitalization was greater in patients randomized to a DPP4 inhibitor compared with placebo or active comparator (odds ratio [OR], 1.19; 95% CI 1.03 to 1.37). In an observational study involving almost 60,000 patients with type 2 DM with average follow-up of 2.4 years, use of DPP4 inhibitors did not associate with increased HF ($OR_{adjusted}$, 0.88; 95% CI 0.63 to 1.22.).[65] Based on the randomized trial data, the FDA added an HF warning to the prescribing labels for both saxagliptin and alogliptin, but not sitagliptin nor linagliptin. Prescribers should consider stopping the medications if patients develop HF. In summary, the DDP4 inhibitors in relatively short-term clinical trials appear to have neutral effects on CV outcomes, with some concern about a modest increase in HF hospitalization rates with at least two DPP4 inhibitors, saxagliptin and alogliptin.

GLUCAGON LIKE PEPTIDE-1 RECEPTOR AGONISTS. The GLP-1 receptor agonists (RAs) are injectable agents that enhance the incretin system.[33] The incretin hormones GLP-1 and GIP are neuroendocrine hormones secreted by the intestine in response to meal ingestion. They stimulate glucose-dependent insulin secretion, suppress glucagon (also in a glucose-dependent fashion), slow gastric emptying, and enhance satiety. Therapeutic benefits with GLP-1 RAs in addition to glucose lowering include associated weight loss (typically 3 to 4 kg), and modest improvement in BP and lipid profiles. They do not increase the risk of hypoglycemia unless used with other drugs that themselves increase the risk (e.g., sulfonylureas, insulin).

The first GLP-1 RA CV outcomes trial, the Evaluation of Lixisenatide in Acute Coronary Syndrome (ELIXA), tested lixisenatide in 6068 patients with recent ACS and found no change in the primary composite MACE outcome (HR, 1.02; 95% CI 0.89 to 1.17).[66] However, in the second CV outcome trial of this class to report, Liraglutide Effect and Action in Diabetes: Evaluation of Cardiovascular Outcome Results (LEADER),[67] involving 9340 patients with a median follow-up of 3.8 years, liraglutide reduced the risk of MACE by 13% (HR, 0.87; 95% CI 0.78 to 0.97), with directionally concordant results for CV death (HR, 0.78; 95% CI 0.66 to 0.93), nonfatal MI (HR, 0.88; 95% CI 0.75 to 1.03), and stroke (HR, 0.89; 95% CI 0.72 to 1.11). In addition, the active therapy group had reduced all-cause mortality (HR, 0.85; 95% CI 0.74 to 0.97). HF hospitalization did not differ. Based on this trial, liraglutide was given a label indication for reducing MACE in type 2 DM patients with established CVD.

The results from other CV outcome trials involving this drug class have shown mixed but generally favorable results. In the Exenatide Study of Cardiovascular Event Lowering (EXSCEL) Trial ($N = 14,752$ over 3.2 years), exenatide once weekly proved neutral for MACE (HR, 0.91; 95% CI, 0.83 to 1.00; p = 0.061 for superiority), although adherence to the study drug was lower than in most trials and likely reduced the trial's power to detect a benefit.[68] All-cause mortality also reduced in the active therapy arm in this trial (HR, 0.86; CI, 0.77 to 0.91; $P = 0.016$). A post-hoc analysis of this study also suggested that drop-in sodium-glucose cotransporter (SGLT)2 inhibitor therapy (see below) may have attenuated the benefit of exenatide on MACE.[69] In the Trial to Evaluate Cardiovascular and Other Long-term Outcomes with Semaglutide in Subjects with Type 2 Diabetes (SUSTAIN-6),[70] 3297 patients were randomized to weekly semaglutide versus placebo and followed for a mean of 2.1 years. The risk of the primary MACE outcome fell by 26% in the active therapy group (HR, 0.74; 95% CI, 0.58 to 0.95; $P < 0.001$ for noninferiority), an effect driven predominately by a 26% RRR in MI and a 39% in stroke, but no apparent effect on CV death. In the Albiglutide and Cardiovascular Outcomes in Patients with Type 2 Diabetes and Cardiovascular Disease (Harmony Outcomes) trial ($N = 9463$ over 1.6 years), the RRR for MACE 22% lower in the albiglutide group (HR, 0.78, 95% CI, 0.68 to 0.90).[71] Albiglutide is no longer marketed, however.

In the Dulaglutide and Cardiovascular Outcomes in Type 2 Diabetes (REWIND) trial ($N = 9901$, 69% of whom had no established CVD at baseline, 5.4 years), dulaglutide showed a RRR of 12% (HR, 0.88, 95% CI 0.79 to 0.99) in MACE, with a 24% RRR in nonfatal stroke.[72] REWIND extended the benefits of GLP-1 RAs to primary prevention and garnered dulaglutide the first indication by the FDA of reducing CV events in patients with type 2 DM at high CV risk but not necessarily with overt CV disease.

Finally, in the first CV outcome trial involving an oral GLP-1 RA, PIONEER 6 (A Trial Investigating the Cardiovascular Safety of Oral Semaglutide in Subjects With Type 2 Diabetes) ($N = 3183$ over 16 months), there was a non-significant 21% RRR in MACE (HR, 0.79, 95% CI 0.57 to 1.11 $P < 0.001$ for noninferiority), with a large and significant reduction in CV death (HR, 0.49, 95% CI 0.27 to 0.92.).[73] The combined benefits from both injectable (SUSTAIN 6) and oral (PIONEER 6) earned the injectable formulation by the FDA a label indication to reduce MACE in type 2 DM patients with established CVD. The most comprehensive meta-analysis of GLP-1 RA CV outcome trials, found the category to have RRRs of 12% for MACE, 12% for CV death, 16% for stroke, and 9% for HF hospitalizations (Fig. 31.8).[74]

SODIUM-GLUCOSE COTRANSPORTER 2 INHIBITORS. Sodium-glucose cotransporter 2 (SGLT2) inhibitors, the newest class of antihyperglycemic drugs, block a SGLT in the proximal tubule of the kidney, increasing urinary excretion of glucose as well as sodium. This effect results not only in glucose lowering but also in modest reductions in body weight (approximately 2 kg) and BP (approximately 4/2 mmHg). The first completed CV outcome trial to assess the effect of an SGLT2 inhibitor, EMPA-REG OUTCOME, tested whether empagliflozin compared with placebo influences the incidence of CV events.[75] The study enrolled a high-risk population of patients with type 2 DM and prevalent ASCVD. It enrolled 7020 patients with longstanding DM (57% for >10 years) with mean follow-up of 3.1 years. The trial demonstrated a significant 14% RRR in the primary MACE (HR, 0.86; 95% CI 0.74 to 0.99). A 38% RRR in CV death (5.9% vs. 3.7%; HR, 0.62; 95% CI 0.49 to 0.77) drove this result. In addition, empagliflozin significantly reduced the risk of hospitalization for HF by 35% (HR, 0.65; 95% CI 0.50 to 0.85). The HF benefit applied to those without prior HF, suggesting that empagliflozin could prevent not only the clinical deterioration of HF but also its occurrence.[76] The event curves for both CV death and HF hospitalization outcomes diverged during the first few weeks of EMPA-REG OUTCOME, suggesting that the CV benefits likely did not arise due to an effect on atherosclerosis, but from other effects.[7,77,78] Empagliflozin also led to a 39% RRR in the progression of CKD (HR, 0.61, 95% CI 0.53 to 0.70), and post-hoc inquiries into the mediators of these effects have demonstrated that the benefits are largely independent of effects of the SGLT2 inhibitor on HbA_{1c}.[79,80]

The CANVAS program involved 10,142 patients with type 2 DM at high CV risk who were randomized to another SGLT2 inhibitor, canagliflozin, or placebo.[81] About two-thirds had established CVD while approximately one-third had risk factors only. The canagliflozin group experienced nearly identical risk reductions to those seen in EMPA-REG OUTCOME for MACE (HR, 0.86; 95% CI, 0.75 to 0.97), HF hospitalization (HR, 0.67; 95% CI, 0.52 to 0.87), and progression of CKD (HR, 0.60; 95% CI, 0.47 to 0.77). The estimate for CV mortality (HR, 0.87; 95% CI, 0.72 to 1.06) did not approach the major reduction observed in EMPA-REG OUTCOME. In addition, two adverse effects of canagliflozin were found in CANVAS: a doubling in the risk of lower limb amputations (HR, 1.97; 95% CI, 1.41 to 2.75) and a smaller increase in the risk of fracture (HR, 1.23; 95% CI, 1.04 to 1.52). The mechanisms behind these complications of therapy are unknown. Other SGLT2 inhibitors have not shown similar effects.

In the Multicenter Trial to Evaluate the Effect of Dapagliflozin on the Incidence of Cardiovascular Events (DECLARE-TIMI58),[82] 17,160 patients (59% of whom were without established CVD at baseline) received dapagliflozin or placebo. After a mean follow-up of 4.2 years, the MACE outcome proved equivalent between the two groups (HR, 0.93, 95% CI 0.84 to 1.03) but the other co-primary outcome of CV death and HF hospitalization fell significantly (RRR 17%; HR, 0.83, 95% CI 0.73 to 0.95), driven by a 27% reduction in the risk of HF hospitalization. CKD progression also occurred less often in the dapagliflozin group (HR = 0.76; 95% CI 0.67 to 0.87.)

	GLP–1 receptor agonist n/N (%)	Placebo n/N (%)	Hazard ratio (95% CI)	NNT (95% CI)	p value
Three-component MACE					
ELIXA	400/3034 (13%)	392/3034 (13%)	1.02 (0.89–1.17)		0.78
LEADER	608/4668 (13%)	694/4672 (15%)	0.87 (0.78–0.97)		0.015
SUSTAIN-6	108/1648 (7%)	146/1649 (9%)	0.74 (0.58–0.95)		0.016
EXSCEL	839/7356 (11%)	905/7396 (12%)	0.91 (0.83–1.00)		0.061
Harmony Outcomes	338/4731 (7%)	428/4732 (9%)	0.78 (0.68–0.90)		<0.001
REWIND	594/4949 (12%)	663/4952 (13%)	0.88 (0.79–0.99)		0.026
PIONEER 6	61/1591 (4%)	76/1592 (5%)	0.79 (0.57–1.11)		0.17
Overall (I^2=40.9%, p=0.118)	**2948/27977 (11%)**	**3304/28027 (12%)**	**0.88 (0.82–0.94)**	**75 (50–151)**	**<0.001**
Cardiovascular death					
ELIXA	156/3034 (5%)	158/3034 (5%)	0.98 (0.78–1.22)		0.85
LEADER	219/4668 (5%)	278/4672 (6%)	0.78 (0.66–0.93)		0.007
SUSTAIN-6	44/1648 (3%)	46/1649 (3%)	0.98 (0.65–1.48)		0.92
EXSCEL	340/7356 (5%)	383/7396 (5%)	0.88 (0.76–1.02)		0.096
Harmony Outcomes	122/4731 (3%)	130/4732 (3%)	0.93 (0.73–1.19)		0.58
REWIND	317/4949 (6%)	346/4952 (7%)	0.91 (0.78–1.06)		0.18
PIONEER 6	15/1591 (1%)	30/1592 (2%)	0.49 (0.27–0.92)		0.021
Overall (I^2=13.5%, p=0.327)	**1213/27977 (4%)**	**1371/28027 (5%)**	**0.88 (0.81–0.96)**	**175 (110–524)**	**0.003**
Fatal or non-fatal myocardial infarction					
ELIXA	270/3034 (9%)	261/3034 (9%)	1.03 (0.87–1.22)		0.71
LEADER	292/4668 (6%)	339/4672 (7%)	0.86 (0.73–1.00)		0.046
SUSTAIN-6	54/1648 (3%)	67/1649 (4%)	0.81 (0.57–1.16)		0.26
EXSCEL	483/7356 (7%)	493/7396 (7%)	0.97 (0.85–1.10)		0.62
Harmony Outcomes	181/4731 (4%)	240/4732 (5%)	0.75 (0.61–0.90)		0.003
REWIND	223/4949 (5%)	231/4952 (5%)	0.96 (0.79–1.15)		0·63
PIONEER 6	37/1591 (2%)	35/1592 (2%)	1.04 (0.66–1.66)		0·49
Overall (I^2=27.4%, p=0.219)	**1540/27977 (6%)**	**1666/28027 (6%)**	**0.91 (0.84–1.00)**	**193 (108–NA)**	**0·043**
Fatal or non-fatal stroke					
ELIXA	67/3034 (2%)	60/3034 (2%)	1.12 (0.79–1·58)		0.54
LEADER	173/4668 (4%)	199/4672 (4%)	0.86 (0.71–1·06)		0.16
SUSTAIN-6	30/1648 (2%)	46/1649 (3%)	0.65 (0.41–1.03)		0.066
EXSCEL	187/7356 (3%)	218/7396 (3%)	0.85 (0.70–1.03)		0.095
Harmony Outcomes	94/4731 (2%)	108/4732 (2%)	0.86 (0.66–1.14)		0.30
REWIND	158/4949 (3%)	205/4952 (4%)	0.76 (0.62–0.94)		0.01
PIONEER 6	13/1591 (1%)	17/1592 (1%)	0.76 (0.37–1.56)		0.43
Overall (I^2=0.0%, p=0.557)	**722/27977 (3%)**	**853/28027 (3%)**	**0.84 (0.76–0.93)**	**209 (139–477)**	**<0.001**

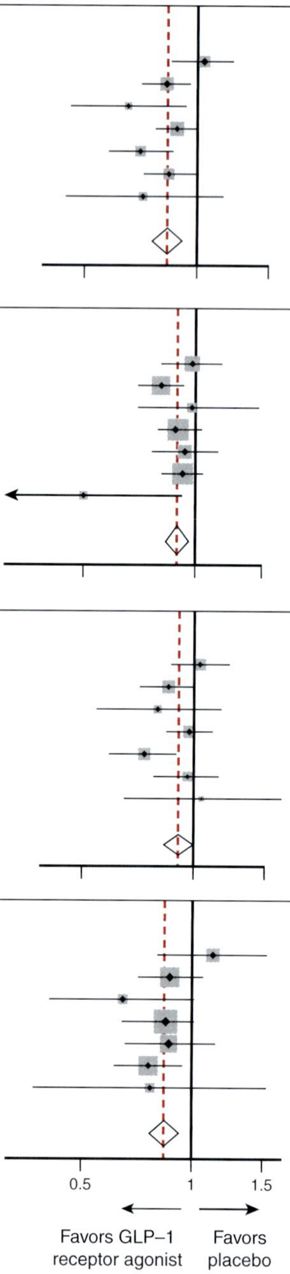

FIGURE 31.8 Meta-analysis of GLP-1 receptor agonist cardiovascular (CV) outcome trials (ELIXA, LEADER, SUSTAIN-6, ESXCEL, Harmony Outcomes, REWIND, PIONEER 6) with outcomes of 3-component major adverse CV events (MACE), CV death, fatal or non-fatal myocardial infarction, stroke, all-cause mortality, hospital admission for heart failure (HHF), composite kidney outcome (including macroalbuminuria), worsening of kidney function, and the composite for the progression of chronic kidney disease (CKD.) Hazard ratios (individual and overall) represent the comparison of the incidence rates in the active therapy versus the placebo groups. (From Kristensen SL, Rorth R, Jhund PS, et al. Cardiovascular, mortality, and kidney outcomes with GLP-1 receptor agonists in patients with type 2 diabetes: a systematic review and meta-analysis of cardiovascular outcome trials. *Lancet Diabetes Endocrinol.* 2019;7:776–785.)

The Evaluation of the Effects of Canagliflozin on Renal and Cardiovascular Outcomes in Participants With Diabetic Nephropathy (CREDENCE) trial primarily assessed the effect of canagliflozin on renal outcomes in 4401 type 2 DM patients with eGFR 30 to 90 mL/min/1.73 m^2 and prevalent macroalbuminuria.[83] The positive primary outcome in favor of canagliflozin, was a 30% RRR in CV death or end-stage kidney disease, a doubling of the creatinine level, or death from renal causes, with the risk of the renal-specific component of the broader composite reduced by 34%. The canagliflozin group also experienced a lower risk of MACE (HR, 0.80; 95% CI, 0.67 to 0.95.) and hospitalization for HF (HR, 0.61; 95% CI, 0.47 to 0.80.).

The Cardiovascular Outcomes Following Ertugliflozin Treatment in Type 2 Diabetes Mellitus Participants With Vascular Disease (VERTIS CV) trial,[84] compared ertugliflozin with placebo in 8238 patients with type 2 DM and established CVD. This was the only SLGT2i CV outcome trial to miss its primary superiority endpoint (MACE). HF hospitalizations occurred less frequently in the ertugliflozin group, however (HR, 0.70; 95% CI 0.54 to 0.090).[85]

The cardiovascular efficacy of the dual SGLT 1 and 2 inhibitor, sotagliflozin, has been studied in two large-scale randomized trials.[85a,85b] In SCORED, patients with type 2 diabetes and diabetic kidney disease were studied, and in SOLOIST patients with type 2 diabetes during or just after admission for decompensated heart failure were studied. Both trials demonstrated statistical superiority for sotagliflozin versus placebo on the primary composite outcome of CV death/hospitalization for heart failure/urgent heart failure visit, and in SCORED, sotagliflozin also significantly reduced the risk for the prioritized secondary outcome of MACE. Sotagliflozin has not been approved for clinical use

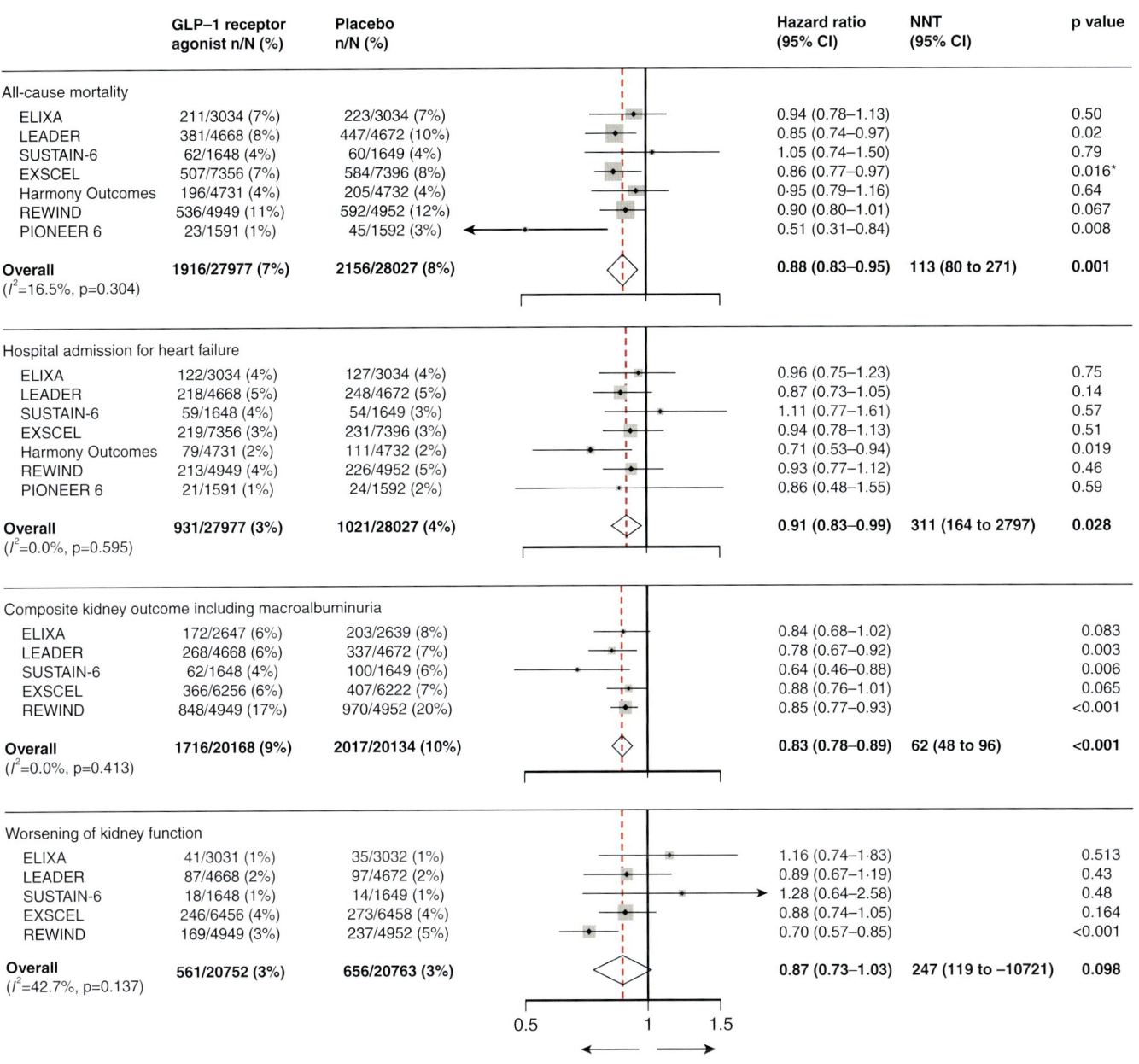

FIGURE 31.8 Continued

for patients with type 2 diabetes and has been approved but is not marketed in Europe for treatment of patients with type 1 diabetes.

In the most recent meta-analysis of SGLT2 inhibitor CV outcome trials,[86,87] RRRs for MACE, CV death, HF hospitalization, and CKD progression were estimated to be 10%, 15%, 32% and 38%, respectively (Fig. 31.9). The MACE benefit was significant only in those participants with established ASCVD. In contrast, for HF hospitalizations, patients both with and without ASCVD and with or without prior HF appeared to benefit. The greatest variability in the point estimates across trials was in CV death and the greatest consistency was in HF hospitalization. This class is now favored by treatment guidelines as preferred agents in patients with ASCVD, and especially in those with HF or mild-moderate CKD.

OTHER GLUCOSE-LOWERING MEDICATIONS (SEE TABLE 31.3). Data on CVD outcomes are generally limited for other less commonly used glucose-lowering medications.[33] These share the advantage of a very low risk for hypoglycemia, and almost are weight neutral. *Colesevelam*, a bile acid sequestrant initially approved for the treatment of hypercholesterolemia, is also approved for use as a glucose-lowering drug to treat type 2 DM, and *alpha-glucosidase inhibitors* impair intestinal carbohydrate absorption. The effects of these drugs on CV outcomes remain unknown, with the exception of a reduced incidence of MIs reported with *acarbose* in a DM prevention trial, STOP NIDDM.[33] However, in the larger ACE trial, involving 6522 Chinese patients with CHD and impaired glucose tolerance, acarbose had no effect to reduce a CV composite outcome.[88] Gastrointestinal intolerance has limited their clinical use.[41] The dopamine agonist, bromocriptine, activates hypothalamic control of insulin sensitivity, and has actually been demonstrated to be safe and potentially effective in an older CV outcome trial, but is rarely used.

Cardiovascular Effects of More Intensive Versus Less Intensive Glucose Control Strategies

The UKPDS trial randomly assigned 5102 patients with newly diagnosed type 2 DM to intensive glucose control with sulfonylurea or insulin or to management with diet alone; those overweight at study entry (n = 795) also could be randomized in the intensive arm to receive metformin.[33] In the insulin and sulfonylurea analyses, resulting

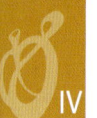

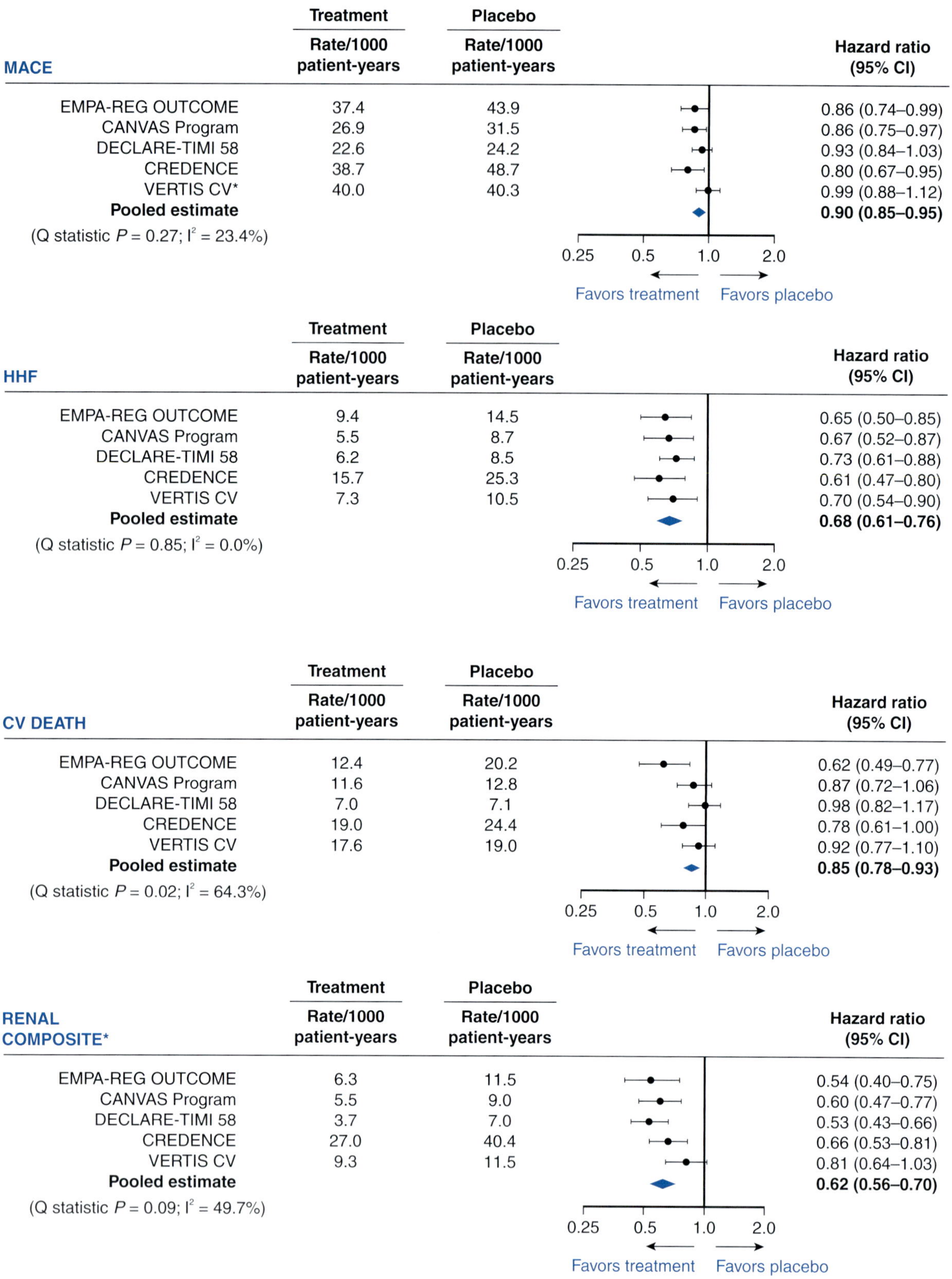

MACE	Treatment Rate/1000 patient-years	Placebo Rate/1000 patient-years		Hazard ratio (95% CI)
EMPA-REG OUTCOME	37.4	43.9		0.86 (0.74–0.99)
CANVAS Program	26.9	31.5		0.86 (0.75–0.97)
DECLARE-TIMI 58	22.6	24.2		0.93 (0.84–1.03)
CREDENCE	38.7	48.7		0.80 (0.67–0.95)
VERTIS CV*	40.0	40.3		0.99 (0.88–1.12)
Pooled estimate				**0.90 (0.85–0.95)**

(Q statistic $P = 0.27$; $I^2 = 23.4\%$)

HHF	Treatment Rate/1000 patient-years	Placebo Rate/1000 patient-years		Hazard ratio (95% CI)
EMPA-REG OUTCOME	9.4	14.5		0.65 (0.50–0.85)
CANVAS Program	5.5	8.7		0.67 (0.52–0.87)
DECLARE-TIMI 58	6.2	8.5		0.73 (0.61–0.88)
CREDENCE	15.7	25.3		0.61 (0.47–0.80)
VERTIS CV	7.3	10.5		0.70 (0.54–0.90)
Pooled estimate				**0.68 (0.61–0.76)**

(Q statistic $P = 0.85$; $I^2 = 0.0\%$)

CV DEATH	Treatment Rate/1000 patient-years	Placebo Rate/1000 patient-years		Hazard ratio (95% CI)
EMPA-REG OUTCOME	12.4	20.2		0.62 (0.49–0.77)
CANVAS Program	11.6	12.8		0.87 (0.72–1.06)
DECLARE-TIMI 58	7.0	7.1		0.98 (0.82–1.17)
CREDENCE	19.0	24.4		0.78 (0.61–1.00)
VERTIS CV	17.6	19.0		0.92 (0.77–1.10)
Pooled estimate				**0.85 (0.78–0.93)**

(Q statistic $P = 0.02$; $I^2 = 64.3\%$)

RENAL COMPOSITE*	Treatment Rate/1000 patient-years	Placebo Rate/1000 patient-years		Hazard ratio (95% CI)
EMPA-REG OUTCOME	6.3	11.5		0.54 (0.40–0.75)
CANVAS Program	5.5	9.0		0.60 (0.47–0.77)
DECLARE-TIMI 58	3.7	7.0		0.53 (0.43–0.66)
CREDENCE	27.0	40.4		0.66 (0.53–0.81)
VERTIS CV	9.3	11.5		0.81 (0.64–1.03)
Pooled estimate				**0.62 (0.56–0.70)**

(Q statistic $P = 0.09$; $I^2 = 49.7\%$)

FIGURE 31.9 Meta-analysis of SGLT2 inhibitor cardiovascular (CV) outcome trials (EMPA-REG OUTCOME, CANVAS, DECLARE, CREDENCE, and VERTIS CV) with outcomes of major adverse CV events (MACE), hospitalization for heart failure (HHF), CV death, and the composite for the progression of chronic kidney disease (CKD). Hazard ratios (individual and pooled) represent the comparisons of the incidence rates in the active therapy versus the placebo groups. (From McGuire DK. Metaanalysis Placeholder. 2020.)

in hemoglobin (Hb) A_{1c} levels of 7.0% versus 7.9%, respectively, during an average follow-up of 10 years, intensive control decreased risk for a composite endpoint of all DM-related complications (RRR, 12%; $P = 0.029$) and significantly improved microvascular disease risk (RRR, 25%; $P = 0.01$). Although intensive control showed a trend toward decreased risk of MI (14.8% vs. 16.8%; $P = 0.052$), the number of strokes was increased, although the difference did not achieve statistical significance (5.6% vs. 5.2%; $P = 0.52$). In overweight patients, metformin yielded better glucose control (HbA_{1c} 7.4% vs. 8.0%) and significantly decreased risk for MI (RRR, 39%; $P = 0.01$) and all-cause mortality (RRR, 36%; $P = 0.011$). The long-term follow-up of the UKPDS trial cohort has extended these observations to an average duration of 10 years,[33] during which glucose control converged rapidly after discontinuation of the study treatment. These analyses reveal a significantly reduced risk for MI in those originally randomly assigned to intensive control, both in the insulin and sulfonylurea group (RRR, 15%; $P = 0.01$) and in the metformin group (RRR, 33%; $P = 0.005$). The continued divergence of the CV event curves throughout the entire follow-up after randomized study treatment was discontinued, and despite rapid convergence of average glycemic control at study end, suggests a "legacy" of CV benefit of early assiduous glycemic control, a finding similarly observed in the long-term follow-up of the Diabetes Control and Complications Trial (DCCT) in patients with type 1 DM.[33] The biologic underpinnings of such an effect are not well understood.

Results from three trials assessed the CVD effects of more intensive versus standard glucose control among patients with type 2 DM at high CV risk.[33] Comprising more than 23,000 patients treated on study protocol from 3 to 5 years, this trio of trials showed no significant CVD benefit of intensified glucose control compared with contemporary glucose management.

The ACCORD trial compared intensive versus standard glucose control in 10,251 patients with type 2 DM who had high CVD risk, achieving a HbA_{1c} of 6.4% versus 7.5%.[33] This trial halted early due to an excess of all-cause mortality in the intensively treated group (257 vs. 203 events; $P = 0.04$), with no significant difference observed in the primary composite CVD endpoint of CV death, MI, and stroke (HR, 0.90; 95% CI 0.78 to 1.04). The initial trial observations persisted up to 17 months of follow-up in this cohort,[33] during which the primary composite outcome risks remained similar between groups. The risk of death from any cause was 19% higher in patients randomly assigned to the more intensive glucose control strategy in the trial ($P < 0.05$), and the HR for nonfatal MI was 0.83 ($P < 0.05$). The basis for the increased mortality remains unresolved; possible explanations include increased hypoglycemia precipitating CV death, pernicious effects of specific drugs or drug combinations, and a chance finding in the context of the other reported trials. The absence of randomization to specific therapies renders post-hoc analysis of cause especially difficult.

The ADVANCE trial enrolled 11,140 patients with type 2 DM who had CVD, microvascular disease, or another vascular risk factor at study entry.[33] Patients randomly received intensive glucose control with gliclazide plus other drugs in the intensive arm, compared with standard control with other drugs. Similar to the ACCORD trial, the ADVANCE trial did not show statistically significant improvement in the composite CVD outcome of CV death, MI, and stroke with intensive control (achieved HbA_{1c} of 6.4% vs. 7.0%), despite the ascertainment of 1147 events (RRR, 6%; 95% CI –6% to 16%). In contrast to the effects seen in UKPDS, 5-year follow-up data from ADVANCE did not show a reduction in macrovascular events in the group treated initially with intensive control.[89]

In the Veterans Affairs Diabetes Trial (VADT), 1791 U.S. veterans with type 2 DM and inadequate glucose control randomly received either intensive or standard glucose control.[33] Despite a wide separation in glucose control values (HbA_{1c} of 6.9% vs. 8.4%) and ascertainment of 499 primary MACEs, this trial also found no significant improvement in CV outcomes with intensive control (29.5% vs. 33.5%; $P = 0.14$). However, follow-up data obtained 3.3 years later in 78% of the initial study population suggest that intensive glucose control compared with standard therapy leads to a significant 17% reduction ($P = 0.04$) of the primary endpoint.[90]

From post-hoc analyses of data for each of these trials and supported by the long-term observations from UKPDS in patients with newly diagnosed DM at study entry, the concept has emerged that more intensive glycemic control may be safer and may have more favorable CV effects when used in patients earlier in the course of DM, particularly among those without prevalent CVD. The corollary to this strategy is that more liberal glycemic targets may be acceptable for selected patients at increased risk, such as very elderly patients and those with a high burden of underlying comorbidities, especially those with prevalent CVD. Although these hypotheses require confirmation in additional clinical trials, the most recent ADA/EASD guidelines for chronic glucose management for patients with type 2 DM endorse such a strategy of targeting intensity of glucose control in the context of global CVD risk, advocating HbA_{1c} target of 8% (or possibly higher) for selected patients, including those with moderate to severe CVD.[41,42] An overriding consideration of such an approach is the limited evidence of short-term benefits from any reduction in microvascular disease in those with limited life expectancy.

In summary, there is no clear incremental CV benefit with more intensive glucose control compared with contemporary targets, the analyses of the primary composite endpoints for each trial revealed point estimates of RRR ranging from 6% to 12%, each with upper 95% confidence limits of 1.04 to 1.06. Such results provide significant assurance of a margin of CV safety with more intensive glucose control, supported by recently published meta-analyses of the available data, demonstrating statistically significant reductions in MI (HR, 0.83; 95% CI 0.75 to 0.93), with no significant effects on stroke (HR, 0.93; 95% CI 0.81 to 1.06) or all-cause mortality (HR, 1.02; 95% CI 0.87 to 1.19). These observed upper confidence limits are well within the noninferiority margins recently adopted by US and European regulatory agencies for DM drug registration, to exclude the upper noninferiority 95% confidence limit of 1.3 (or 95% certainty of no greater than 30% worse than comparator) for CV safety.

Summary of Glucose Management and Treatment Guidelines

Intensive glucose control favorably affects microvascular disease risk, but its importance in CVD risk modification remains uncertain. Reflecting the accumulated data, the most recent guidelines from the ADA and EASD endorse a more individualized approach than previously recommended, with more liberal HbA_{1c} targets for patients with shorter expected life span and with significant comorbidity, including prevalent CVD (Fig. 31.10), suggesting a HbA_{1c} target of 8% (or higher).[41,42] Until recently, in the context of the paucity of clinical outcomes data for most antihyperglycemic therapies used for type 2 DM, the ordered addition of subsequent glucose-lowering medications after metformin was left to the discretion of the provider, taking individual patient and drug characteristics into such treatment determinations. The landmark findings from SGLT2 inhibitor and GLP-1 RA trials show that the method that lowers glucose levels matters, particularly those with established CVD. The benefits from SGLT2 inhibitors on HF hospitalization and CKD progression (but not MACE) appear to apply even in those without overt CVD. The MACE benefits of GLP-1 RAs also appear to apply in patients with multiple risk factors but no established CVD.

Current guidelines from professional organizations reflect these new findings.[10,13,15] The 2018 consensus report from the ADA and the EASD now advises the use of either a GLP-1 RA or an SGLT2 inhibitor after metformin monotherapy in those with established atherosclerotic CVD. For those in whom HF or CKD predominates the clinical picture, SGLT2 inhibitor would be favored. Importantly in the 2019 update to the consensus report, the addition of these medications is now advised irrespective of baseline HbA_{1c} or HbA_{1c} target.[15] This move away from the previous glucocentricity of these organizations is notable. From the cardiology community, both the American College of Cardiology and the ESC advise the use of one of these drug categories in those with type 2 DM and established CVD,[10,91] with the European group extending this to those at very high and high CV risk. In contrast to the ADA/EASD guidelines, the use of these medications should be considered as first line in those patients not taking metformin.[10]

Acute Coronary Syndromes

In view of the high risk associated with DM in the setting of ACS, much investigation has focused on this population. In general, as endorsed by the most recent ACS guidelines,[92,93] the treatment of patients with DM should mimic that of the overall population (see Chapters 37–39). Some specific therapies also are recommended for patients with DM.

Screening for Diabetes in Acute Coronary Syndrome Patients

One third of ACS patients have previously diagnosed DM.[6,94] Moreover, many patients present with an ACS event as the first complication of DM; previously undetected DM is also common, affecting up to an additional 20% to 25% of ACS patients.[94] Therefore, all patients with ACS events warrant screening for DM.[10,95,96] Given the stress hyperglycemia associated with ACS events that may confound blood glucose testing, screening should extend beyond assessment of fasting blood glucose and include HbA_{1C} testing and/or pre-discharge oral glucose tolerance

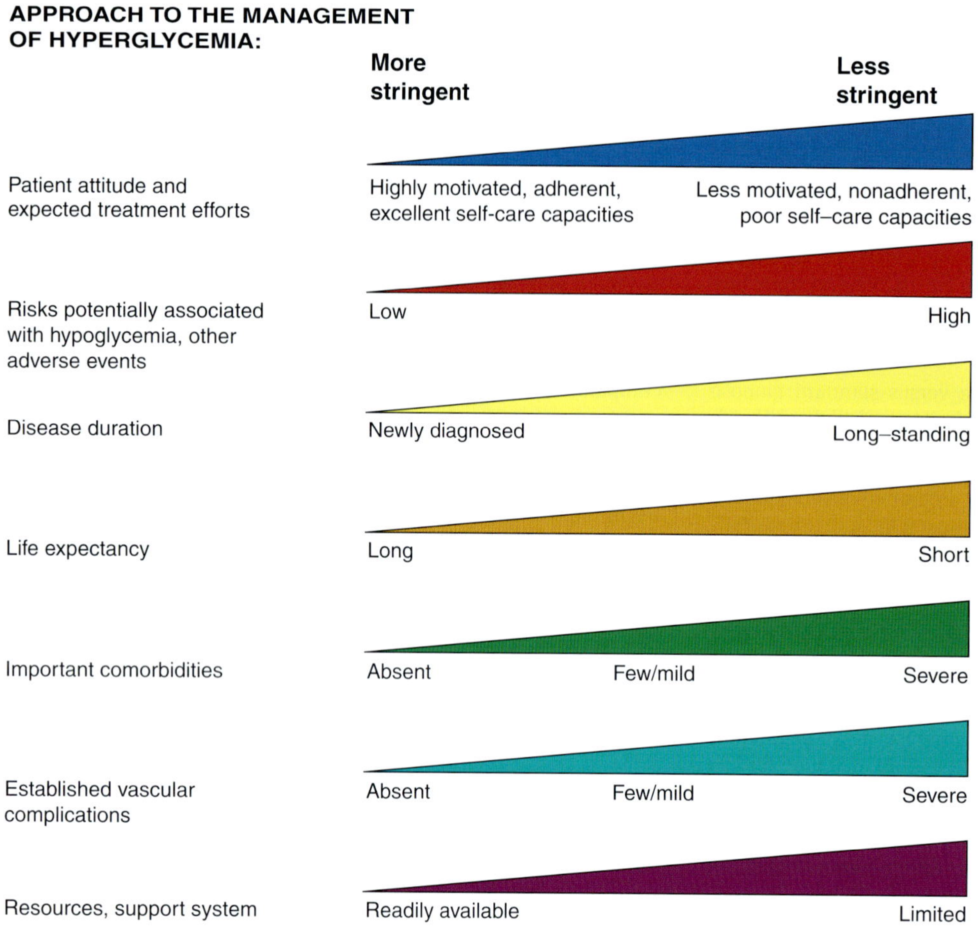

APPROACH TO THE MANAGEMENT OF HYPERGLYCEMIA:

	More stringent	Less stringent
Patient attitude and expected treatment efforts	Highly motivated, adherent, excellent self-care capacities	Less motivated, nonadherent, poor self-care capacities
Risks potentially associated with hypoglycemia, other adverse events	Low	High
Disease duration	Newly diagnosed	Long-standing
Life expectancy	Long	Short
Important comorbidities	Absent	Few/mild — Severe
Established vascular complications	Absent	Few/mild — Severe
Resources, support system	Readily available	Limited

FIGURE 31.10 Modulation of the intensiveness of glucose lowering in type 2 diabetes mellitus (DM). Depiction of patient and disease factors that may be used by the practitioner to determine optimal hemoglobin A_{1c} (HbA_{1c}) targets in patients with type 2 DM. Greater concerns regarding a particular domain are represented by increasing height of the corresponding ramp. Thus, characteristics/predicaments toward the left justify more stringent efforts to lower HbA_{1c}, whereas those toward the right suggest (indeed, sometimes mandate) less stringent efforts. Where possible, such decisions should be made with the patient, reflecting his or her preferences, needs, and values. This "scale" is not designed to be applied rigidly but to be used as a broad construct to guide clinical decision making. (From Inzucchi SE, Bergenstal RM, Buse JB, et al. Management of hyperglycemia in type 2 diabetes, 2015: a patient-centered approach: update to a position statement of the American Diabetes Association and the European Association for the Study of Diabetes. *Diabetes Care.* 2015;38:140–149.)

testing.[10,95] The diagnosis of DM early in the hospital course is important because it influences immediate and later therapeutic decisions.

Insulin Administration and Glucose Control

Research over decades has evaluated the role of myocardial metabolic modulation during ACS events, with insulin delivery as the primary focus of investigation. Almost all trials completed to date evaluating the role of intravenous (IV) insulin in ACS used very high insulin dosing supported by exogenous glucose administration to avoid hypoglycemia, with or without adjunctive delivery of potassium, so-called glucose-insulin-potassium (GIK) therapy. These protocols typically targeted permissive hyperglycemia of 126 to 200 mg/dL during the infusion. This strategy ultimately proved futile in contemporary ACS management in the CREATE ECLA GIK trial of 20,201 patients with ST-segment elevation MI (STEMI), randomized to GIK therapy versus usual care and accumulating 1980 mortality events—demonstrating no benefit of GIK therapy compared with usual care.[97] These results have led to the abandonment of GIK treatment for ACS patients.

No adequately powered clinical outcomes trial has been completed to date in the ACS setting evaluating targeted glucose control with IV insulin or any other therapy. The Diabetes Mellitus Insulin-Glucose Infusion in Acute Myocardial Infarction (DIGAMI) trial enrolled 620 patients with hyperglycemia at presentation with MI, randomly assigned to insulin infusion acutely, followed by multidose subcutaneous insulin injection or usual care, with significant mortality reduction demonstrated in the insulin-treated group during long-term follow-up.[97] DIGAMI used an acute infusion of high-dose insulin (5 units/hr), coupled with IV glucose administration with protocol-targeted permissive hyperglycemia of 126 to 198 mg/dL, an insulin-dosing protocol used in subsequent GIK trials, including the negative CREATE ECLA GIK trial previously summarized. Often misinterpreted as a trial of intensive glucose control, this study provided the basis of ACCF/AHA guideline recommendations for intensive glucose control in the management of ACS events since 2004. However, in the absence of evidence of beneficial effects of intensive glucose control in ACS populations, and a series of trials in other intensive care unit (ICU) settings demonstrating no significant benefit for the most part,[97] and increased mortality with intensive glucose control with IV insulin in the medical and surgical ICUs in the largest trial to date, guidelines for the management of hyperglycemia in the ACS setting have changed considerably.[97] More recently, both ACCF/AHA and ESC guidelines have omitted recommendations with regard to targeted glucose control during in the management of ACS events.[10,92,93] (See the Guidelines Tables 31G.1 through 31G.4 in the online chapter.)

Antiplatelet Medications

ACS patients with or without DM should receive aspirin. Various studies have tested the potential for more intensive antiplatelet therapies to provide particular benefit to ACS patients with DM.

$P2Y_{12}$ Receptor Antagonists

The incremental efficacy of adding thienopyridine and nonthienopyridine antagonists of the platelet receptor $P2Y_{12}$ (clopidogrel, prasugrel, and ticagrelor) to aspirin therapy in the treatment of ACS has been demonstrated in randomized clinical trials that included substantial numbers of patients with DM (see Chapters 38 and 39).[98-101] In the Clopidogrel in Unstable Angina to Prevent Recurrent Events (CURE) trial,[98] which included 2840 patients with DM, the estimate of treatment benefit of clopidogrel in this subpopulation of 15% RRR was numerically similar to the overall trial results (14.2% vs. 16.7%; $P > 0.05$). Prasugrel added to aspirin, compared with clopidogrel plus aspirin, significantly reduced the CVD risk in the DM subset of the Trial to Assess Improvement in Therapeutic Outcomes by Optimizing Platelet Inhibition with Prasugrel–Thrombolysis in Myocardial Infarction 38 (TRITON–TIMI 38) trial, including patients with ACS undergoing a primary invasive management strategy (12.2% vs. 17.0%; $P < 0.001$).[101,102] In the DM subset, prasugrel did not lead to a significant increase in major bleeding complications (2.6% vs. 2.5%). The Targeted Platelet Inhibition to Clarify the Optimal Strategy to Medically Manage Acute Coronary Syndromes (TRILOGY ACS) trial, however, which enrolled patients with MI treated medically without revascularization, randomly assigned to treatment with clopidogrel or prasugrel,[103] found no significant differences were between the groups in the primary composite outcome of CV death, MI, and stroke in the overall trial population, or in the DM subset, in which the interaction of treatment efficacy of prasugrel by DM status observed in the TRITON trial was not evident. In the Platelet Inhibition and Patient Outcomes (PLATO) trial, which enrolled 18,624 patients with an ACS, with or without ST-segment elevation, randomly assigned to receive ticagrelor or clopidogrel, ticagrelor (a nonthienopyridine

P2Y$_{12}$ antagonist) significantly reduced the primary composite outcome of death from vascular causes, MI, and stroke (9.8% vs. 11.7%; $P <$ 0.001).[101] Similar findings pertained to the subset of 4662 patients with DM at study entry.[99]

In aggregate, these observations support the incremental benefits of more potent antiplatelet treatment added to aspirin therapy in patients with DM with ACS events, with superiority of both prasugrel and ticagrelor over clopidogrel. The P2Y$_{12}$ receptor antagonists should be considered in the routine clinical management of patients with DM and ACS.

Renin-Angiotensin-Aldosterone System Antagonists
The ACE inhibitors have several favorable effects in ACS that may particularly benefit patients with DM. Observational data and sub-analyses of patients with DM in randomized trials, suggest greater beneficial effects on HF incidence and mortality in DM. Thus, the routine use of ACE inhibitors for patients with DM is a level I (A) recommendation in ACS.[10,92,93]

Although ARBs have similar effects on intermediate markers of myocardial structure and function to those of ACE inhibitors, the evidence base for their overall effects on clinical outcomes following an ACS event remains less robust, especially for the subset of patients with DM. For example, in the Optimal Trial in Myocardial Infarction with Angiotensin II Antagonist Losartan (OPTIMAAL), a randomized trial comprising patients with MI events complicated by HF, losartan versus captopril associated with a trend toward increased mortality (RR, 1.13; 95% CI 0.99 to 1.28), although the observed differences were not statistically significant.[30] In contrast, the Valsartan in Acute Myocardial Infarction Trial (VALIANT), which enrolled patients within 10 days of an acute MI complicated by HF, including 3400 patients with DM, showed no significant difference in mortality between patients randomly assigned to treatment with captopril and those treated with valsartan, and effects in the DM subset mirroring those observed in the overall study cohort.[30,104] Thus, ARBs should be considered an alternative only for patients intolerant of ACE inhibitors.

The Eplerenone Post–Acute Myocardial Infarction Heart Failure Efficacy and Survival Study (EPHESUS) compared the mineralocorticoid-selective aldosterone antagonist eplerenone to placebo, added to optimal therapy, in a population of 6632 patients with MI and decreased ejection fraction (EF) who had either clinical HF or, in the absence of manifest HF, DM.[105] In the overall study cohort, treatment with eplerenone compared with placebo reduced the risk of CV death by 17% (RR, 0.83; 95% CI 0.72 to 0.94), with numerically similar observations in the subset of 2232 patients with DM. On the basis of this trial, the use of an aldosterone antagonist for patients with DM and reduced EF (with or without clinical HF) after MI is recommended in ACS,[10,92,93] except in patients with impaired kidney function (creatinine >2.0 mg/dL) or hyperkalemia (potassium concentration [K$^+$] >5.0 mEq/L).

Beta-Adrenergic Blocking Agents
Despite evidence of their incremental effectiveness in the treatment of patients with DM after ACS events, beta blockers continue to be underprescribed in this group.[6,106] Biologic effects that support the incremental efficacy of beta blockers in the setting of DM include the restoration of the sympathovagal balance in patients with DM with autonomic neuropathy and decreasing fatty acid metabolism within the myocardium, reducing myocardial oxygen demand. Therefore, all patients with ACS should receive beta blockers, independent of their DM status, in the absence of contraindications.[10,92,93] The selection might consider the variable effects of available beta blockers on glycometabolic parameters, favorable for carvedilol and labetalol and unfavorable for others (e.g., metoprolol, atenolol), although these considerations have uncertain clinical relevance.[106]

Primary Invasive Strategy for Non–ST-Segment Elevation Acute Coronary Syndrome
In randomized trials comparing primary invasive versus noninvasive strategies for the treatment of ACS events, the subsets of patients with DM derived similar or greater benefits than those without DM associated with a primary invasive management strategy, although mortality and reinfarction rates were still higher in the groups with DM in both treatment arms (see Chapter 41).[96,107] Nonetheless, a primary invasive strategy for patients with DM continues to be underused in ACS patients with DM.[6]

Primary Reperfusion Therapy for ST-Segment Elevation Myocardial Infarction
Analyses from trials of primary PCI suggest greater benefit in patients with than in those without DM, with primary PCI proving superior to thrombolysis in these patients.[108] Similarly, in analyses of subsets with DM from randomized trials of thrombolytics, patients with DM derive greater absolute benefit from thrombolytic therapy than patients without DM.[93] Therefore, patients with DM and STEMI should undergo reperfusion therapy in the absence of contraindications, preferentially with a strategy of primary PCI when available (see Chapter 38).

Coronary Revascularization Considerations
In patients with DM, the anatomical pattern of CAD influences prognosis and the response to revascularization. Angiographic studies show that patients with DM are more likely to have left main and multivessel CAD, and diffuse and small vessel disease.[109] Current guidelines recommend medical treatment, including anti-ischemic drugs as first-line treatment for patients with DM and stable CAD. For patients requiring revascularization, the optimal strategy remains controversial.

Optimal Medical Therapy Versus Revascularization in Diabetes
Studies examining optimal medical therapy (OMT) versus a revascularization strategy in patients with DM with stable CAD are scarce. The largest such trial, the Bypass Angioplasty Revascularization Investigation 2 Diabetes (BARI-2D) trial, randomized 2368 patients with DM with obstructive CAD either to immediate revascularization (coronary artery bypass grafting [CABG] $n = 347$; PCI $n = 765$) in addition to OMT or OMT alone. After 5 years, no significant differences were noted in the combined endpoint of death, MI, or stroke between groups. However, the CABG stratum subgroup, despite having more advanced CAD, showed a significantly higher rate of freedom from major adverse cardiac and cerebrovascular events (MACCE) and death compared with OMT alone (77.5% vs. 69.6%; $P = 0.01$). In contrast, in the PCI stratum compared with OMT alone, there was no difference in freedom from MACCE (77% vs. 78.9%; $P = 0.15$).[108] Thus, BARI-2D demonstrated that OMT is a reasonable therapeutic option in patients with DM and less advanced CAD, independent of the presence of ischemia. Moreover, regarding the indirect comparison between CABG and PCI in this trial, overall mortality was significantly lower with CABG compared with PCI at 5-year follow-up (19.4% vs. 34.5%; $P = 0.003$).[108] Thus, in patients with more extensive CAD and proven ischemia, CABG may be preferred.

The ISCHEMIA trial assessed an initial invasive strategy (angiography and revascularization when feasible) and medical therapy or an initial conservative strategy of medical therapy alone and angiography if medical therapy failed in 5179 patients with CAD and moderate or severe ischemia including 2164 patients with DM.[110] The primary outcome was a composite of death from cardiovascular causes, MI, or hospitalization for unstable angina, HF, or resuscitated cardiac arrest. At 6 months, the cumulative event rate was 5.3% in the invasive-strategy group and 3.4% in the conservative-strategy group (difference, 1.9 percentage points; 95% CI, 0.8 to 3.0); at 5 years, the cumulative event rate was 16.4% and 18.2%, respectively (difference, −1.8 percentage points; 95% CI −4.7 to 1.0) suggesting that the initial invasive strategy did not reduce the risk of ischemic cardiovascular events or death from any cause. The results did not differ between patients with or without DM.

Percutaneous Coronary Intervention Versus Coronary Artery Bypass Grafting
Patients with DM have worse clinical outcomes after revascularization by either PCI or CABG than those without DM. Patients with DM have more recurrent CV events after PCI.[111] After CABG, patients with DM have elevated risk of wound infections, acute kidney injury, HF, and death.[108] The optimal strategy of coronary revascularization for patients with DM remains controversial.

Several large trials have compared PCI versus CABG,[112–115] but given technical advances in both interventional cardiology and coronary surgery over recent decades, the results of these trials may apply only partially today.[116] The Coronary Artery Revascularization in Diabetes

(CARDia) trial comparing PCI versus CABG in 510 patients with DM and multivessel CAD found no difference between groups for the primary composite endpoint of death or MI (PCI 13.0% versus CABG 10.5%; $P = 0.39$).[113] However, the addition of repeat revascularization to the composite outcome showed a benefit favoring CABG (11.3% vs. 19.3%; $P = 0.016$) at 1-year follow-up. Important limitations of the CARDia trial were the mixed use of bare-metal stents (BMS, 31%) and first-generation (sirolimus) drug-eluting stents (DES) in the PCI arm and the relatively small sample size.[113]

A subanalysis of the 452 patients with DM with left main or three-vessel CAD enrolled in the Synergy Between Percutaneous Coronary Intervention with Taxus and Cardiac Surgery (SYNTAX) trial of PCI versus CABG demonstrated higher rates of MACCE with PCI using paclitaxel-eluting stents (PES) compared with CABG at 1 year (26% vs. 14.2%; $P = 0.003$), and after 5 years of follow-up (46.5% vs. 29.6%; $P < 0.001$),[112] differences driven by more repeat revascularization in the PCI group at 1 year (PCI 20.3% vs. CABG 6.4%; $P < 0.001$) and at 5 years (PCI 35.3% vs. CABG 14.6%; $P < 0.001$). With respect to lesion complexity according to the SYNTAX score, only patients with DM with more complex disease (SYNTAX score ≥33) had a treatment benefit of CABG.[112]

In contrast to these studies, the Future Revascularization Evaluation in Patients with Diabetes Mellitus: Optimal Management of Multi-Vessel Disease (FREEDOM) trial studied a cohort of patients with type 2 DM and multivessel disease.[115] Among 1900 enrolled patients, the primary composite endpoint (death, MI, or stroke) was lower in patients treated with CABG versus PCI at 1 year (CABG 18.7% vs. PCI 26.6%; $P = 0.005$), and at 5 years of follow-up (CABG 11.8% vs. PCI 16.8%; $P = 0.004$).[115] Differences favoring CABG in death (CABG 10.9% vs. PCI 16.3%; $P = 0.049$) and MI (CABG 6.0% vs. PCI 13.9%; $P < 0.001$) at 5 years largely drove this result. Moreover, the incidence of repeat revascularization at 1 year after initial revascularization was significantly higher with PCI versus CABG (12.6% vs. 4.8%; $P < 0.01$). However, stroke risk was conversely higher in the CABG group (5.2% vs. 2.4%; $P = 0.03$), and CV mortality did not differ. Challenging contemporary generalizability, first-generation DES (sirolimus-eluting stent [SES] 51% and PES 43%) were used, and relatively low proportions of women (28.6%), patients with EF less than 40% (2.5%), and patients with less advanced CAD (SYNTAX score <22; 35.5%) were enrolled.[115] A collaborative, individual patient data pooled analysis of 11,518 patients with multivessel or LM CAD randomized to CABG or PCI with stents, demonstrated significantly lower all-cause death after CABG versus PCI,[117] a finding evident in patients with DM (10.7% vs. 15.7%, respectively; $P = 0.0001$) but not in patients without DM. Consequently, overall current evidence continues to favor CABG as the revascularization modality of choice for patients with DM and multivessel disease.

Based on these trials, the 2014 ACC/AHA guideline upgraded its previous recommendation in favor of CABG over PCI from class II (A) to class I (A) in patients with DM and stable CAD,[118] in particular if a left inferior mammary artery (LIMA) graft can be anastomosed to the left anterior ascending (LAD) artery, provided the patient is otherwise a good candidate for surgery. Similarly, the 2019 ESC Guidelines on Diabetes, prediabetes and CVD recommend CABG over PCI in patients with DM and triple-vessel disease. Both CABG and PCI receive a class I recommendation for patients with two-vessel disease with proximal LAD stenosis or left main stenosis with low complexity.[10]

HEART FAILURE IN THE PATIENT WITH DIABETES

Scope of the Problem

Diabetes independently predicts HF risk,[119] with an associated twofold to fivefold increased risk[7,120,121] (see Part VI, Heart Failure). Once HF is present, DM portends an especially adverse prognosis for subsequent morbidity and mortality.[7] In patients with DM and prevalent ASCVD observed in a registry over 4 years, HF at baseline independently associated with increased CV death (HR$_{adjusted}$ 2.5; 95% CI 2.2 to 2.8).[121] Even with state-of-the-art HF therapy like in the PARADIGM HF trial, 21% of all patients had died after median follow-up of 27 months, significantly more compared with patients without DM and a normal HbA$_{1c}$.[122]

Mechanistic Considerations

Patients with and without DM share common causes of HF, such as ischemic heart disease, hypertension, left ventricular hypertrophy, and AF. Yet, these common risk factors do not completely account for the incremental HF risk with DM,[119] suggesting increased myocardial vulnerability in the setting of DM and probable synergistic effects between such factors and DM that increase HF risk,[7] yielding the concept of "the ominous octet" of common conditions in DM that may underpin HF risk (Fig. 31.11).

Ischemic Heart Disease and Hypertension

Ischemic heart disease remains the principal risk factor for HF in DM patients. Contributors to this increased risk may include increased disease burden, prevalence of silent or atypical symptoms of ischemia delaying diagnosis and intervention, suboptimal use of therapeutic interventions, perturbed sympathovagal balance, a prothrombotic milieu, impaired coronary endothelial function, and abnormal myocardial metabolism.[64] Affecting both atherosclerosis and HF risk, hypertension prevalence exceeds 70% in populations with DM. Among patients with type 2 DM, risk of HF increases 12% to 14% for every increment of 10 mm Hg in systolic BP (see Fig. 31.6).[30]

MYOCARDIAL METABOLISM AND STRUCTURE

The direct effects of hyperglycemia and insulin resistance on myocardial cellular metabolism may contribute to cardiac dysfunction in DM,[7] with altered energy-substrate supply and impaired metabolic substrate switching under conditions of stress (see Chapters 46 and 47). The myocardium uses predominantly FFAs under aerobic conditions, but increasingly shifts to glycolysis and pyruvate oxidation during ischemia.[7,123] In T2DM, increased FFA levels activate PPAR-α, a nuclear receptor that controls transcripts of FFA metabolism, shifting energy metabolism towards anaerobic FFA utilization. Together with increasing insulin resistance, this phenomenon minimizes glucose utilization and makes the heart metabolically less flexible. The dominance of FFA utilization in diabetic hearts contributes to energetic inefficiency by augmenting oxygen demand for FFA oxidation compared to glucose oxidation and by mitochondrial uncoupling with associated deterioration of efficiency of ATP production.[123]

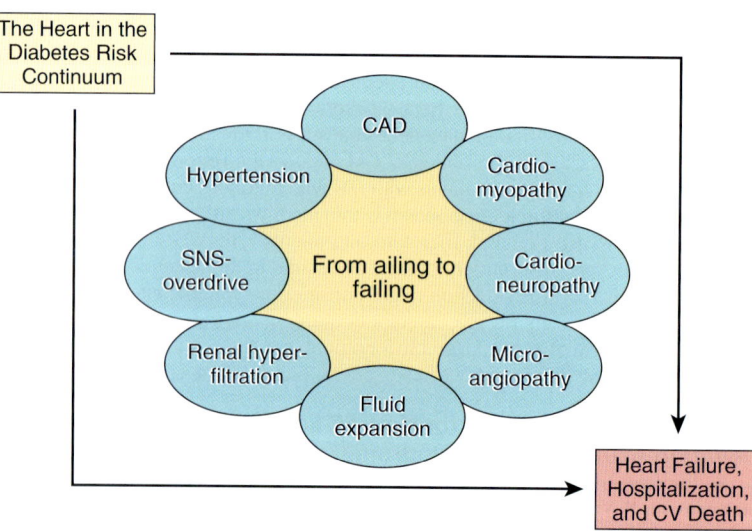

FIGURE 31.11 Heart failure in type 2 diabetes mellitus (DM): the ominous octet-multiple co-morbidities commonly associated with type 2 DM that individually and in aggregate contribute to the increased risk for heart failure in such patients. *CAD*, Coronary artery disease; *CV*, cardiovascular; *SNS*, sympathetic nervous system. (From Standl E, Schnell O, McGuire DK. Heart failure considerations of antihyperglycemic medications for type 2 diabetes. *Circ Res*. 2016;118:1830–1843.)

Diabetes causes a variety of morphologic changes in the myocardium, with abnormalities in myocytes, extracellular matrix (ECM), and microvasculature.[7] Whereas such abnormalities are usually present across causes of cardiomyopathy, they tend to be more common and severe in the setting of DM. In addition, more specific to DM, the myocardial accumulation of AGEs, including macromolecules nonenzymatically modified by glucose, the formation and accumulation of which depend on the severity of hyperglycemia, may contribute to HF risk. Deposition of AGEs within the myocardial ECM adversely affects both systolic and diastolic cardiac function, largely attributable to AGE cross-linking of matrix collagen.

Prevention and Management of Heart Failure in Diabetes

In general, drug therapies for HF generally have similar if not better efficacy in patients with compared with those without DM (see Part VI).

Therapy of Heart Failure with Preserved Ejection Fraction in Diabetes

There is currently no therapy proven to improve the prognosis of patients with HFpEF. The main goal of therapy is to preserve left ventricular function and treat comorbidities such as COPD, hypertension, obesity, AF, and risk for CKD, and consider treatment with RAAS blockers.

Therapy of Heart Failure with Reduced Ejection Fraction in Diabetes
Modulation of the Renin-Angiotensin-Aldosterone System
In patients with DM, meta-analysis of the effects of ACE inhibitors demonstrates a trend to reduce incident HF (RR, 0.87; 95% CI 0.72 to 1.06),[30] and in patients with moderate to severe systolic dysfunction, they significantly reduce mortality (RR, 0.84; 95% CI 0.7 to 1.0)[124,125]—numerically similar findings to patients without DM. Likewise, meta-analysis of placebo-controlled trials show reduced incident HF with ARBs (HR, 0.70; 95% CI 0.59 to 0.83).[30] Therefore, ACE inhibitors should be first-line agents for the prevention and treatment of HFrEF in patients with DM, with ARBs as alternatives for patients intolerant of ACE inhibitors.[124,125]

The effect of aldosterone antagonists (e.g., spironolactone, eplerenone) in patients with DM and HFrEF has not been extensively studied. EPHESUS (see above) showed efficacy of eplerenone in the DM subset of 2122 patients. Thus all patients with DM and acute MI with reduced EF should receive eplerenone, except in the presence of contraindications such as kidney dysfunction or hyperkalemia.[93,96,124]

Angiotensin Receptor-Neprilysin Inhibition (See Chapter 50)
PARADIGM HF compared sacubitril/valsartan to enalapril in patients with HFrEF.[126] The trial enrolled 8442 patients with class II to IV HF and with EF of 40%. Overall, sacubitril/valsartan significantly reduced the risk for composite outcome of HF hospitalization and CV death (HR, 0.80; 95% CI 0.73 to 0.87), death from any cause (HR, 0.84; 95% CI 0.76 to 0.93), and CV death (HR, 0.80; 95% CI 0.71 to 0.89). In the subset of 2907 patients with DM at baseline (39.4%), sacubitril/valsartan versus enalapril had comparable efficacy on the composite of HF hospitalization and CV death as observed in the overall trial, but there was heterogeneity of the effect on CV death. Morbidity seems to be improved by sacubitril/valsartan over enalapril in patients with or without DM, but there is no clear mortality benefit of sacubitril/valsartan over enalapril in patients with DM. Sacubitril/valsartan therapy led to a greater reduction in HbA_{1c} levels and a lower rate of insulin initiation over 3 years of follow-up compared with enalapril in patients with DM.[127]

Beta Blockers
Beta blockers and diuretic medications significantly reduce incident HF among patients with DM.[30] In addition, some beta blockers have demonstrated benefit independent of DM status in the setting of HFrEF (see Chapter 50).[10]

Heart Failure Considerations for Glucose Management Strategies and Antihyperglycemic Medications

Poor glycemic control is associated with risk of HF in patients with DM, with a stronger association in women than men. Whether dysglycemia is causal or simply an associated marker of underlying CVD risk remains uncertain. No trials to date have rigorously assessed the effect of targeting glucose control to any specific therapeutic levels, or the comparative effect of existing therapies alone or in combination with regard to their influence on major adverse HF events.[7] Meta-analyses of available data, however, demonstrate no significant effect of more versus less aggressive glucose control on the risk for HF. Therefore, the role of glucose control in the prevention and treatment of HF is unclear. It is therefore reasonable (as it is with other life-limiting comorbidities) to consider more liberal glycemic targets for patients with DM and advanced HF, such as HbA_{1c} target of less than 8% with the avoidance of hypoglycemia.[41]

Some specific considerations warrant attention with regard to drugs and strategies used to treat hyperglycemia in the setting of HF.[7] Avoidance of hypoglycemic episodes has particular importance in patients with DM and HFrEF, since the stress response to hypoglycemia stimulates the neurohormonal axis implicated in HF pathophysiology. Cautions regarding the use of metformin in the setting of HF were removed in 2006 on the basis of data showing no incremental risk for lactic acidemia,[43,44] and potential clinical benefit. The product label did retain a caution for use specifically in the setting of acute or decompensated HF. The best available evidence supports consideration of metformin in patients with stable and compensated HF, especially in the context of the available CVD outcomes data, low risk of hypoglycemia, low cost, and favorable tolerability profile. Limited data exist about the use of sulfonylureas in the setting of HF but so far, there are no data suggesting an increased risk of HF hospitalization in patients treated with sulfonylurea. The CAROLINA randomized trial showed similar HF hospitalization risk for glimepiride compared with linagliptin, the later having demonstrated neutrality for HF outcomes versus placebo in the CARMELINA trial.[46,128]

Thiazolidinedione medications have a propensity to increase plasma volume and to precipitate incident or worsening HF; their use requires caution in patients with any degree of HF, and they are contraindicated in patients with NYHA class III or IV HF.[129] Data from the aforementioned IRIS trial, however, suggest that with dose reduction/titration, pioglitazone may be used safely without increasing HF risk.[57]

Various cardiovascular outcome trials have assessed the effect of DPP4 inhibitors in patients with DM and high cardiovascular risk. As discussed above, SAVOR-TIMI 53 found that saxagliptin leads to an increased risk for HF hospitalization.[130] TECOS (sitagliptin) and CARMELINA (linagliptin) showed no such effect.[64,128] Alogliptin demonstrated a non-significant trend towards an increased HF hospitalization in the EXAMINE trial.[62] These data suggest that the increase in HF risk is not a class effect of the DPP4 inhibitors, but rather limited to saxagliptin.

As noted previously, SGLT2 inhibitors (empagliflozin, canagliflozin, dapagliflozin, and ertugliflozin) significantly reduced HF hospitalization in placebo-controlled CVOTs in patients with prevalent ASCVD or with risk factors. A meta-analysis of data from six trials of the four available SGLT2 inhibitors demonstrated a highly consistent significant reduction of risk for hospitalization for HF, irrespective of a history of HF at baseline and similar for those with established ASCVD or multiple risk factors (Fig. 31.12).[86] Data from the DAPA-HF and the EMPEROR-Reduced trials suggest that the beneficial effect of SGLT2 inhibitors in HFrEF extends to HF patients without DM.[120,131,132] The underlying mechanism of the beneficial effects of SGLT2 inhibitors on HF-related endpoints remain unclear, but may include plasma volume reduction without neurohumoral activation seen with traditional diuretics, effects on cardiac energetics through altered metabolic fuel supply, or direct effects on cardiac function through alterations in mitochondrial ion channels.[7,79,133,134] Insulin therapy remains an option in patients who fail to achieve benefit with conventional oral glucose-lowering therapies, although some concern persists based on the plausibility that insulin may exacerbate signs and symptoms of HF by increasing renal sodium reclamation, contributing to increased intravascular volume.[7] In the ORIGIN trial, patients randomly assigned to receive insulin glargine versus usual care tended to have fewer hospitalizations for HF, although this

	Treatment		Placebo			
	n/N	Rate/1000 patient-years	n/N	Rate/1000 patient-years	Weight (%)	Hazard ratio (95%CI)
Patients with history of heart failure						
EMPA-REG	75/462	63.6	49/244	85.5	13.27	0.72 (0.50, 1.04)
CANVAS Program	NA/803	35.4	NA/658	56.8	23.25	0.61 (0.46, 0.80)
DECLARE-TIMI 58	142/852	45.1	172/872	55.5	34.85	0.79 (0.63, 0.99)
VERTIS CV	164/1286	40.1	99/672	47.1	28.63	0.85 (0.66, 1.09)
Fixed effects model	(Q = 3.36, df = 3, p = 0.339; I^2 = 10.7%)					**0.75 (0.66, 0.86)**
Patients with no history of heart failure						
EMPA-REG	190/4225	15.5	149/2089	24.9	19.45	0.63 (0.51, 0.78)
CANVAS Program	NA/4992	13.6	NA/3689	15.2	23.48	0.87 (0.72, 1.06)
DECLARE-TIMI 58	275/7730	8.9	324/7706	10.5	34.63	0.84 (0.72, 0.99)
VERTIS CV	280/4213	18.8	151/2075	20.6	22.44	0.91 (0.75, 1.11)
Fixed effects model	(Q = 7.41, df = 3, p = 0.060; I^2 = 59.5%)					**0.82 (0.74, 0.90)**

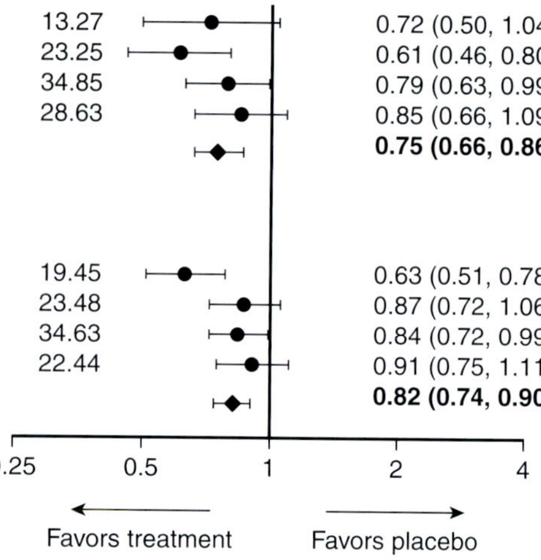

Favors treatment ← → Favors placebo

FIGURE 31.12 Meta-analysis of SGLT2 inhibitor cardiovascular (CV) outcome trials (EMPA-REG OUTCOME, CANVAS, DECLARE, and VERTIS CV) with outcome hospitalization for heart failure (HHF), stratified by the presence or absence of heart failure at baseline. Hazard ratios (individual and fixed effects model) represent the comparisons of the incidence rates in the active therapy versus the placebo groups. (From McGuire DK. Metaanalysis Placeholder. 2020.)

Drug	Effect on heart failure			
Thiazolidinediones/Glitazones	Unfavorable	🔴	⚪	⚪
DPP4 inhibitors	Saxagliptin: unfavorable	🔴	⚪	⚪
	Sitagliptin, Alogliptin, Linagliptin: neutral	⚪	🟡	⚪
GLP-1 receptor agonists	Lixisenatide, Liraglutide, Semaglutide, Exenatide: neutral	⚪	🟡	⚪
Insulin	Neutral	⚪	🟡	⚪
Sulfonylureas	Neutral	⚪	🟡	⚪
Alpha-Glucosidase inhibitors	Acarbose: neutral	⚪	🟡	⚪
Metformin	Neutral; potentially beneficial	⚪	⚪	🟢
SGLT2 inhibitors	Empagliflozin, Canagliflozin, Dapagliflozin, Ertugliflozin: beneficial	⚪	⚪	🟢

FIGURE 31.13 Effect of antidiabetic drugs on heart failure. (From Schütt K, Marx N. Heart failure and diabetes: management and open issues. *Herz.* 2019;44:203–209.)

difference was not statistically significant (4.9% vs. 5.5%; P = 0.16). Therefore, in patients with HF who fail to achieve acceptable HbA_{1c} targets with oral agents, insulin remains an acceptable option, if prescribed with caution to avoid hypoglycemia.[7] GLP-1 RAs lower blood glucose along and weight and BP as well.[74] The reduction of cardiovascular endpoints in the GLP-1 RA trials most likely resulted from reduced atherosclerosis-related events. GLP-1 RAs had neutral effects on HF hospitalization within each trial, but meta-analyses revealed a modest but significant 9% RRR. Two randomized trials of liraglutide versus placebo in patients with HFrEF, with or without DM, failed to demonstrate benefit and each had trends toward worse outcomes with liraglutide, so some caution is warranted with regard to GLP-1 RA use in moderate to severe HFrEF until further data are available.[135]

In summary, HF is common among patients with DM and associates with a worse prognosis; numerous abnormalities associated with DM may contribute to the increased HF risk.[7] HF therapy in patients with or without DM generally does not differ except with respect to the choice of antihyperglycemic agents. Thiazolidinediones and saxagliptin should be avoided, while HF patients should receive SGLT2 inhibitors preferentially. Other drugs, like metformin, SUs, insulin, and GLP-1 RA seem to be safe in most patients with DM and HF and can be used if intensification of glucose lowering is required (Fig. 31.13).[136]

Atrial Fibrillation

Type 2 DM associates independently with AF, and aggravates risk for stroke and systemic thromboembolism,[8,137] resulting in guideline recommendations for systemic anticoagulation for all patients with DM who have AF.[10] Although warfarin has historically been the mainstay of systemic anticoagulation for AF, the direct oral anticoagulants dabigatran, rivaroxaban, apixaban, and edoxaban now offer alternatives. For each therapy, the sub-analyses of efficacy and safety for patients with DM participating in the pivotal registration trials of these medications suggest similar or even favorably amplified benefit/risk balance.[8,10] In fact, with similar RRRs with the novel agents versus warfarin and the greater absolute risk for stroke observed in each trial, patients with versus without DM have more favorable NNT for benefit.

SUMMARY AND FUTURE PERSPECTIVES

Overall, DM increases risk for CVD events, notably ASCVD, HF, and AF. Virtually all the recent advances in the care of patients at risk for CVD complications apply to patients with DM, with similar or even greater benefit in this high-risk population. Nonetheless, the gradient of risk associated with DM persists. Further progress requires continued efforts in two areas: first, increased and optimal application of the existing evidence for CVD risk reduction has paramount importance, with studies consistently demonstrating a substantial gap between the accumulated evidence and its application in patients with DM. Second, continued investigation into specific therapies and strategies targeting the unique risks for CVD associated with DM remains a critical global public health imperative. In that light, largely driven by the regulatory evolution toward requiring CVD safety and efficacy evaluations for all antihyperglycemic medications developed for DM management, a proliferation of randomized CV clinical outcomes trials have recently provided us with substantial new information about reducing CV events in high-risk type 2 DM patients. Currently, members of two glucose-lowering medication classes, SGLT2 inhibitors and GLP-1 RA) have proven CV benefits.

GUIDELINES

See the Guidelines Tables 31G.1 through 31G.4 in the online chapter.

REFERENCES

Scope of the Problem

1. American Diabetes Association. 2. Classification and diagnosis of diabetes: standards of medical care in diabetes-2020. *Diabetes Care*. 2020;43:S14–S31.
2. Saeedi P, Petersohn I, Salpea P, et al. Global and regional diabetes prevalence estimates for 2019 and projections for 2030 and 2045: results from the International Diabetes Federation Diabetes Atlas, 9th edition. *Diabetes Res Clin Pract*. 2019;157:107843.
3. Rawshani A, Rawshani A, Franzen S, et al. Mortality and cardiovascular disease in type 1 and type 2 diabetes. *N Engl J Med*. 2017;376:1407–1418.
4. Gregg EW, Li Y, Wang J, et al. Changes in diabetes-related complications in the United States, 1990-2010. *N Engl J Med*. 2014;370:1514–1523.
5. Emerging Risk Factors C, Di Angelantonio E, Kaptoge S, et al. Association of cardiometabolic multimorbidity with mortality. *J Am Med Assoc*. 2015;314:52–60.

Coronary Heart Disease in the Patient with Diabetes

6. Gore MO, Patel MJ, Kosiborod M, et al. Diabetes mellitus and trends in hospital survival after myocardial infarction, 1994 to 2006: data from the national registry of myocardial infarction. *Circ Cardiovasc Qual Outcomes*. 2012;5:791–797.
7. Standl E, Schnell O, McGuire DK. Heart failure considerations of antihyperglycemic medications for type 2 diabetes. *Circ Res*. 2016;118:1830–1843.
8. Plitt A, McGuire DK, Giugliano RP. Atrial fibrillation, type 2 diabetes, and non-vitamin K antagonist oral anticoagulants: a review. *JAMA Cardiol*. 2017.
9. Ryden L, Grant PJ, Anker SD, et al. ESC Guidelines on diabetes, pre-diabetes, and cardiovascular diseases developed in collaboration with the EASD: the Task Force on diabetes, pre-diabetes, and cardiovascular diseases of the European Society of Cardiology (ESC) and developed in collaboration with the European Association for the Study of Diabetes (EASD). *Eur Heart J*. 2013;34:3035–3087.
10. Cosentino F, Grant PJ, Aboyans V, et al. 2019 ESC Guidelines on diabetes, pre-diabetes, and cardiovascular diseases developed in collaboration with the EASD. *Eur Heart J*. 2020;41:255–323.
11. Rawshani A, Rawshani A, Franzen S, et al. Risk factors, mortality, and cardiovascular outcomes in patients with type 2 diabetes. *N Engl J Med*. 2018;379:633–644.
12. Hess K, Grant PJ. Inflammation and thrombosis in diabetes. *Thromb Haemost*. 2011;105(suppl 1):S43–S54.
13. American Diabetes Association. Cardiovascular disease and risk management: standards of medical care in diabetes-2020. 10 *Diabetes Care*. 2020;43:S111–S134.
14. Fox CS, Golden SH, Anderson C, et al. Update on prevention of cardiovascular disease in adults with type 2 diabetes mellitus in light of recent evidence: a scientific statement from the American heart association and the American diabetes association. *Circulation*. 2015;132:691–718.
15. Buse JB, Wexler DJ, Tsapas A, et al. 2019 update to: management of hyperglycemia in type 2 diabetes, 2018. A consensus report by the American Diabetes Association (ADA) and the European Association for the Study of Diabetes (EASD). *Diabetes Care*. 2020;43:487–493.
16. Grundy SM, Stone NJ, Bailey AL, et al. 2018 AHA/ACC/AACVPR/AAPA/ABC/ACPM/ADA/AGS/APhA/ASPC/NLA/PCNA guideline on the management of blood cholesterol: a report of the American College of Cardiology/American Heart Association Task Force on clinical practice guidelines. *Circulation*. 2019;139:e1082–e1143.
17. Mach F, Baigent C, Catapano AL, et al. 2019 ESC/EAS Guidelines for the management of dyslipidaemias: lipid modification to reduce cardiovascular risk. *Eur Heart J*. 2020;41:111–188.
18. Crandall JP, Mather K, Rajpathak SN, et al. Statin use and risk of developing diabetes: results from the Diabetes Prevention Program. *BMJ Open Diabetes Res Care*. 2017;5:e000438.
19. Cannon CP, Blazing MA, Giugliano RP, et al. Ezetimibe added to statin therapy after acute coronary syndromes. *N Engl J Med*. 2015;372:2387–2397.
20. Giugliano RP, Cannon CP, Blazing MA, et al. Benefit of adding ezetimibe to statin therapy on cardiovascular outcomes and safety in patients with versus without diabetes mellitus: results from IMPROVE-IT (Improved Reduction of Outcomes: Vytorin Efficacy International Trial). *Circulation*. 2018;137:1571–1582.
21. Robinson JG, Farnier M, Krempf M, et al. Efficacy and safety of alirocumab in reducing lipids and cardiovascular events. *N Engl J Med*. 2015;372:1489–1499.
22. Sabatine MS, Giugliano RP, Wiviott SD, et al. Efficacy and safety of evolocumab in reducing lipids and cardiovascular events. *N Engl J Med*. 2015;372:1500–1509.
23. Sabatine MS, Giugliano RP, Keech AC, et al. Evolocumab and clinical outcomes in patients with cardiovascular disease. *N Engl J Med*. 2017;376:1713–1722.
24. Schwartz GG, Steg PG, Szarek M, et al. Alirocumab and cardiovascular outcomes after acute coronary syndrome. *N Engl J Med*. 2018;379:2097–2107.
25. Ray KK, Colhoun HM, Szarek M, et al. Effects of alirocumab on cardiovascular and metabolic outcomes after acute coronary syndrome in patients with or without diabetes: a prespecified analysis of the ODYSSEY OUTCOMES randomised controlled trial. *Lancet Diabetes Endocrinol*. 2019;7:618–628.
26. Origin Trial Investigators, Bosch J, Gerstein HC, et al. n-3 fatty acids and cardiovascular outcomes in patients with dysglycemia. *N Engl J Med*. 2012;367:309–318.
27. Bhatt DL, Steg PG, Miller M, et al. Cardiovascular risk reduction with icosapent ethyl for hypertriglyceridemia. *N Engl J Med*. 2019;380:11–22.
28. Ray KK, Landmesser U, Leiter LA, et al. Inclisiran in patients at high cardiovascular risk with elevated LDL cholesterol. *N Engl J Med*. 2017;376:1430–1440.
29. Leiter LA, Teoh H, Kallend D, et al. Inclisiran lowers LDL-C and PCSK9 irrespective of diabetes status: the ORION-1 randomized clinical trial. *Diabetes Care*. 2019;42:173–176.
30. Emdin CA, Rahimi K, Neal B, et al. Blood pressure lowering in type 2 diabetes: a systematic review and meta-analysis. *J Am Med Assoc*. 2015;313:603–615.
31. Whelton PK, Carey RM, Aronow WS, et al. 2017 ACC/AHA/AAPA/ABC/ACPM/AGS/APhA/ASH/ASPC/NMA/PCNA guideline for the prevention, detection, evaluation, and management of high blood pressure in adults: a report of the American College of Cardiology/American Heart Association Task Force on clinical practice guidelines. *Circulation*. 2018;138:e484–e594.
32. Krause T, Lovibond K, Caulfield M, et al. Management of hypertension: summary of NICE guidance. *BMJ*. 2011;343:d4891.

Cardiovascular Aspects of Therapy in Diabetic Patients

33. Lathief S, Inzucchi SE. Approach to diabetes management in patients with CVD. *Trends Cardiovasc Med*. 2016;26:165–179.
34. Arnett DK, Blumenthal RS, Albert MA, et al. 2019 ACC/AHA guideline on the primary prevention of cardiovascular disease: a report of the American College of Cardiology/American Heart Association Task Force on clinical practice guidelines. *Circulation*. 2019;140:e596–e646.
35. Marquis-Gravel G, Roe MT, et al. Revisiting the role of aspirin for the primary prevention of cardiovascular disease. *Circulation*. 2019;140:1115–1124.
36. Pignone M, Alberts MJ, Colwell JA, et al. Aspirin for primary prevention of cardiovascular events in people with diabetes: a position statement of the American Diabetes Association, a scientific statement of the American Heart Association, and an expert consensus document of the American College of Cardiology Foundation. *Circulation*. 2010;121:2694–2701.
37. Ascend Study Collaborative Group. Effects of aspirin for primary prevention in persons with diabetes mellitus. *N Engl J Med*. 2018;379:1529–1539.
38. Bhatt DL, Steg PG, Mehta SR, et al. Ticagrelor in patients with diabetes and stable coronary artery disease with a history of previous percutaneous coronary intervention (THEMIS-PCI): a phase 3, placebo-controlled, randomised trial. *Lancet*. 2019;394:1169–1180.
39. Gore MO, McGuire DK. Cardiovascular disease and type 2 diabetes mellitus: regulating glucose and regulating drugs. *Curr Cardiol Rep*. 2009;11:258–263.
40. McGuire DK, Marx N, Johansen OE, et al. FDA guidance on antihyperglycemic therapies for type 2 diabetes: one decade later. *Diabetes Obes Metab*. 2019;21:1073–1078.
41. Inzucchi SE, Bergenstal RM, Buse JB, et al. Management of hyperglycemia in type 2 diabetes, 2015: a patient-centered approach: update to a position statement of the American Diabetes Association and the European Association for the Study of Diabetes. *Diabetes Care*. 2015;38:140–149.
42. American Diabetes Association. Standards of medical care in diabetes –2015. *Diabetes Care*. 2015;38(Suppl):S1–S2.
43. Salpeter SR, Greyber E, Pasternak GA, et al. Risk of fatal and nonfatal lactic acidosis with metformin use in type 2 diabetes mellitus. *Cochrane Database of Syst Rev*. 2010:CD002967.
44. Inzucchi SE, Lipska KJ, Mayo H, et al. Metformin in patients with type 2 diabetes and kidney disease: a systematic review. *J Am Med Assoc*. 2014;312:2668–2675.
45. US Food and Drug Administration. *FDA Drug Safety Communication: FDA Revises Warnings Regarding Use of the Diabetes Medicine Metformin in Certain Patients with Reduced Kidney Function*; 2016. 2016.
46. Rosenstock J, Kahn SE, Johansen OE, et al. Effect of linagliptin vs glimepiride on major adverse cardiovascular outcomes in patients with type 2 diabetes: the CAROLINA randomized clinical trial. *J Am Med Assoc*. 2019.
47. Rosenstock J, Perkovic V, Johansen OE, et al. Effect of linagliptin vs placebo on major cardiovascular events in adults with type 2 diabetes and high cardiovascular and renal risk: the CARMELINA randomized clinical trial. *J Am Med Assoc*. 2019;321:69–79.
48. Schramm TK, Gislason GH, Vaag A, et al. Mortality and cardiovascular risk associated with different insulin secretagogues compared with metformin in type 2 diabetes, with or without a previous myocardial infarction: a nationwide study. *Eur Heart J*. 2011;32:1900–1908.
49. Monami M, Genovese S, Mannucci E. Cardiovascular safety of sulfonylureas: a meta-analysis of randomized clinical trials. *Diabetes Obes Metab*. 2013;15:938–953.
50. Varvaki Rados D, Catani Pinto L, Reck Remonti L, et al. The association between sulfonylurea use and all-cause and cardiovascular mortality: a meta-analysis with trial sequential analysis of randomized clinical trials. *PLoS Med*. 2016;13:e1001992.
51. Pladevall M, Riera-Guardia N, Margulis AV, et al. Cardiovascular risk associated with the use of glitazones, metformin and sulfonylureas: meta-analysis of published observational studies. *BMC Cardiovasc Disord*. 2016;16:14.
52. Kernan WN, Viscoli CM, Furie KL, et al. Pioglitazone after ischemic stroke or transient ischemic attack. *N Engl J Med*. 2016;374:1321–1331.
53. Young LH, Viscoli CM, Curtis JP, et al. Cardiac outcomes after ischemic stroke or transient ischemic attack: effects of pioglitazone in patients with insulin resistance without diabetes mellitus. *Circulation*. 2017;135:1882–1893.
54. Yaghi S, Furie KL, Viscoli CM, et al. Pioglitazone prevents stroke in patients with a recent transient ischemic attack or ischemic stroke: a planned secondary analysis of the IRIS trial (Insulin Resistance Intervention After Stroke). *Circulation*. 2018;137:455–463.
55. Vaccaro O, Masulli M, Nicolucci A, et al. Effects on the incidence of cardiovascular events of the addition of pioglitazone versus sulfonylureas in patients with type 2 diabetes inadequately controlled with metformin (TOSCA.IT): a randomised, multicentre trial. *Lancet Diabetes Endocrinol*. 2017;5:887–897.
56. Home PD, Pocock SJ, Beck-Nielsen H, et al. Rosiglitazone evaluated for cardiovascular outcomes in oral agent combination therapy for type 2 diabetes (RECORD): a multicentre, randomised, open-label trial. *Lancet*. 2009;373:2125–2135.
57. Young LH, Viscoli CM, Schwartz GG, et al. Heart failure after ischemic stroke or transient ischemic attack in insulin-resistant patients without diabetes mellitus treated with pioglitazone. *Circulation*. 2018;138:1210–1220.
58. Origin Trial Investigators, Gerstein HC, Bosch J, et al. Basal insulin and cardiovascular and other outcomes in dysglycemia. *N Engl J Med*. 2012;367:319–328.
59. Marso SP, McGuire DK, Zinman B, et al. Efficacy and safety of degludec versus glargine in type 2 diabetes. *N Engl J Med*. 2017;377:723–732.
60. Scirica BM, Bhatt DL, Braunwald E, et al. Saxagliptin and cardiovascular outcomes in patients with type 2 diabetes mellitus. *N Engl J Med*. 2013;369:1317–1326.
61. White WB, Cannon CP, Heller SR, et al. Alogliptin after acute coronary syndrome in patients with type 2 diabetes. *N Engl J Med*. 2013;369:1327–1335.
62. Zannad F, Cannon CP, Cushman WC, et al. Heart failure and mortality outcomes in patients with type 2 diabetes taking alogliptin versus placebo in EXAMINE: a multicentre, randomised, double-blind trial. *Lancet*. 2015;385:2067–2076.
63. Green JB, Bethel MA, Armstrong PW, et al. Effect of sitagliptin on cardiovascular outcomes in type 2 diabetes. *N Engl J Med*. 2015;373:232–242.
64. McGuire DK, Van de Werf F, Armstrong PW, et al. Association between sitagliptin use and heart failure hospitalization and related outcomes in type 2 diabetes mellitus: secondary analysis of a randomized clinical trial. *JAMA Cardiol*. 2016;1:126–135.
65. Yu OH, Filion KB, Azoulay L, et al. Incretin-based drugs and the risk of congestive heart failure. *Diabetes Care*. 2015;38:277–284.

66. Pfeffer MA, Claggett B, Diaz R, et al. Lixisenatide in patients with type 2 diabetes and acute coronary syndrome. *N Engl J Med*. 2015;373:2247–2257.
67. Marso SP, Daniels GH, Brown-Frandsen K, et al. Liraglutide and cardiovascular outcomes in type 2 diabetes. *N Engl J Med*. 2016;375:311–322.
68. Holman RR, Bethel MA, Mentz RJ, et al. Effects of once-weekly exenatide on cardiovascular outcomes in type 2 diabetes. *N Engl J Med*. 2017;377:1228–1239.
69. Clegg LE, Penland RC, Bachina S, et al. Effects of exenatide and open-label SGLT2 inhibitor treatment, given in parallel or sequentially, on mortality and cardiovascular and renal outcomes in type 2 diabetes: insights from the EXSCEL trial. *Cardiovasc Diabetol*. 2019;18:138.
70. Marso SP, Bain SC, Consoli A, et al. Semaglutide and cardiovascular outcomes in patients with type 2 diabetes. *N Engl J Med*. 2016;375:1834–1844.
71. Hernandez AF, Green JB, Janmohamed S, et al. Albiglutide and cardiovascular outcomes in patients with type 2 diabetes and cardiovascular disease (Harmony Outcomes): a double-blind, randomised placebo-controlled trial. *Lancet*. 2018;392:1519–1529.
72. Gerstein HC, Colhoun HM, Dagenais GR, et al. Dulaglutide and cardiovascular outcomes in type 2 diabetes (REWIND): a double-blind, randomised placebo-controlled trial. *Lancet*. 2019;394:121–130.
73. Husain M, Birkenfeld AL, Donsmark M, et al. Oral semaglutide and cardiovascular outcomes in patients with type 2 diabetes. *N Engl J Med*. 2019;381:841–851.
74. Kristensen SL, Rorth R, Jhund PS, et al. Cardiovascular, mortality, and kidney outcomes with GLP-1 receptor agonists in patients with type 2 diabetes: a systematic review and meta-analysis of cardiovascular outcome trials. *Lancet Diabetes Endocrinol*. 2019;7:776–785.
75. Zinman B, Wanner C, Lachin JM, et al. Empagliflozin, cardiovascular outcomes, and mortality in type 2 diabetes. *N Engl J Med*. 2015;373:2117–2128.
76. Fitchett D, Zinman B, Wanner C, et al. Heart failure outcomes with empagliflozin in patients with type 2 diabetes at high cardiovascular risk: results of the EMPA-REG OUTCOME(R) trial. *Eur Heart J*. 2016;37:1526–1534.
77. Heerspink HJ, Perkins BA, Fitchett DH, et al. Sodium glucose cotransporter 2 inhibitors in the treatment of diabetes mellitus: cardiovascular and kidney effects, potential mechanisms, and clinical applications. *Circulation*. 2016;134:752–772.
78. Marx N, McGuire DK. Sodium-glucose cotransporter-2 inhibition for the reduction of cardiovascular events in high-risk patients with diabetes mellitus. *Eur Heart J*. 2016;37:3192–3200.
79. Inzucchi SE, Zinman B, Fitchett D, et al. How does empagliflozin reduce cardiovascular mortality? Insights from a mediation analysis of the EMPA-REG OUTCOME trial. *Diabetes Care*. 2018;41:356–363.
80. Inzucchi SE, Kosiborod M, Fitchett D, et al. Improvement in cardiovascular outcomes with empagliflozin is independent of glycemic control. *Circulation*. 2018;138:1904–1907.
81. Neal B, Perkovic V, Mahaffey KW, et al. Canagliflozin and cardiovascular and renal events in type 2 diabetes. *N Engl J Med*. 2017;377:644–657.
82. Wiviott SD, Raz I, Bonaca MP, et al. Dapagliflozin and cardiovascular outcomes in type 2 diabetes. *N Engl J Med*. 2019;380:347–357.
83. Perkovic V, Jardine MJ, Neal B, et al. Canagliflozin and renal outcomes in type 2 diabetes and nephropathy. *N Engl J Med*. 2019;380:2295–2306.
84. Cannon CP, McGuire DK, Pratley R, et al. Design and baseline characteristics of the eValuation of ERTugliflozin efficacy and Safety CardioVascular outcomes trial (VERTIS-CV). *Am Heart J*. 2018;206:11–23.
85. Cannon CP, Pratley R, Dagogo-Jack S, et al. Cardiovascular outcomes with ertugliflozin in type 2 diabetes. *N Engl J Med*. 2020;383(15):1425–1435.
85a. Bhatt DL, Szarek M, Pitt B, et al. Sotagliflozin in patients with diabetes and chronic kidney disease. *N Engl J Med*. 2021;384(2):129–139.
85b. Bhatt DL, Szarek M, Steg PG, et al. Sotagliflozin in patients with diabetes and recent worsening heart failure. *N Engl J Med*. 2021;384(2):117–128.
86. McGuire DK, Shih WJ, Cosentino F, et al. Association of SGLT2 inhibitors with cardiovascular and kidney outcomes in patients with type 2 diabetes: a meta-analysis. *JAMA Cardiol*. 2021;6(2):148–158.
87. Arnott C, Li Q, Kang A, et al. Sodium-glucose cotransporter 2 inhibition for the prevention of cardiovascular events in patients with type 2 diabetes mellitus: a systematic review and meta-analysis. *J Am Heart Assoc*. 2020;9:e014908.
88. Holman RR, Coleman RL, Chan JCN, et al. Effects of acarbose on cardiovascular and diabetes outcomes in patients with coronary heart disease and impaired glucose tolerance (ACE): a randomised, double-blind, placebo-controlled trial. *Lancet Diabetes Endocrinol*. 2017;5:877–886.
89. Zoungas S, Chalmers J, Neal B, et al. Follow-up of blood-pressure lowering and glucose control in type 2 diabetes. *N Engl J Med*. 2014;371:1392–1406.
90. Hayward RA, Reaven PD, Wiitala WL, et al. Follow-up of glycemic control and cardiovascular outcomes in type 2 diabetes. *N Engl J Med*. 2015;372:2197–2206.
91. Das SR, Everett BM, Birtcher KK, et al. 2018 ACC expert consensus decision pathway on novel therapies for cardiovascular risk reduction in patients with type 2 diabetes and atherosclerotic cardiovascular disease: a report of the American College of Cardiology Task Force on expert consensus decision pathways. *J Am Coll Cardiol*. 2018;72:3200–3223.
92. Amsterdam EA, Wenger NK, Brindis RG, et al. 2014 AHA/ACC guideline for the management of patients with non-ST-elevation acute coronary syndromes: a report of the American College of Cardiology/American Heart Association Task Force on Practice Guidelines. *Circulation*. 2014;130:e344–e426.
93. O'Gara PT, Kushner FG, Ascheim DD, et al. 2013 ACCF/AHA guideline for the management of ST-elevation myocardial infarction: a report of the American College of Cardiology Foundation/American Heart Association Task Force on practice guidelines. *Circulation*. 2013;127:e362–e425.
94. Arnold SV, Lipska KJ, Li Y, et al. Prevalence of glucose abnormalities among patients presenting with an acute myocardial infarction. *Am Heart J*. 2014;168:466–470 e1.
95. Arnold SV, Lipska KJ, Inzucchi SE, et al. The reliability of in-hospital diagnoses of diabetes mellitus in the setting of an acute myocardial infarction. *BMJ Open Diabetes Res Care*. 2014;2:e000046.
96. Roffi M, Patrono C, Collet JP, et al. 2015 ESC guidelines for the management of acute coronary syndromes in patients presenting without persistent ST-segment elevation: Task Force for the management of acute coronary syndromes in patients presenting without persistent ST-segment elevation of the European Society of Cardiology (ESC). *Eur Heart J*. 2016;37:267–315.
97. Kosiborod M, McGuire DK. Glucose-lowering targets for patients with cardiovascular disease: focus on inpatient management of patients with acute coronary syndromes. *Circulation*. 2010;122:2736–2744.
98. Hall HM, Banerjee S, McGuire DK. Variability of clopidogrel response in patients with type 2 diabetes mellitus. *Diabetes Vasc Dis Res*. 2011;8:245–253.
99. James S, Angiolillo DJ, Cornel JH, et al. Ticagrelor vs. clopidogrel in patients with acute coronary syndromes and diabetes: a substudy from the PLATelet inhibition and patient Outcomes (PLATO) trial. *Eur Heart J*. 2010;31:3006–3016.
100. Wiviott SD, Braunwald E, McCabe CH, et al. Prasugrel versus clopidogrel in patients with acute coronary syndromes. *N Engl J Med*. 2007;357:2001–2015.
101. Kumbhani DJ, Marso SP, Alvarez CA, McGuire DK. State-of-the-Art: hypo-responsiveness to oral antiplatelet therapy in patients with type 2 diabetes mellitus. *Curr Cardiovasc Risk Rep*. 2015;9:4–22.
102. Wiviott SD, Braunwald E, Angiolillo DJ, et al. Greater clinical benefit of more intensive oral antiplatelet therapy with prasugrel in patients with diabetes mellitus in the trial to assess improvement in therapeutic outcomes by optimizing platelet inhibition with prasugrel-Thrombolysis in Myocardial Infarction 38. *Circulation*. 2008;118:1626–1636.
103. Roe MT, Armstrong PW, Fox KA, et al. Prasugrel versus clopidogrel for acute coronary syndromes without revascularization. *N Engl J Med*. 2012;367:1297–1309.
104. Bangalore S, Kumar S, Lobach I, Messerli FH. Blood pressure targets in subjects with type 2 diabetes mellitus/impaired fasting glucose: observations from traditional and bayesian random-effects meta-analyses of randomized trials. *Circulation*. 2011;123:2799–2810.
105. Yancy CW, Jessup M, Bozkurt B, et al. 2013 ACCF/AHA guideline for the management of heart failure: executive summary: a report of the American College of Cardiology Foundation/American Heart Association Task Force on practice guidelines. *Circulation*. 2013;128:1810–1852.
106. Arnold SV, Spertus JA, Lipska KJ, et al. Type of beta-blocker use among patients with versus without diabetes after myocardial infarction. *Am Heart J*. 2014;168:273–279 e1.
107. Jneid H, Anderson JL, Wright RS, et al. 2012 ACCF/AHA focused update of the guideline for the management of patients with unstable angina/Non-ST-elevation myocardial infarction (updating the 2007 guideline and replacing the 2011 focused update): a report of the American College of Cardiology Foundation/American Heart Association Task Force on practice guidelines. *Circulation*. 2012;126:875–910.
108. Levine GN, Bates ER, Blankenship JC, et al. 2011 ACCF/AHA/SCAI guideline for percutaneous coronary intervention: a report of the American College of Cardiology Foundation/American Heart Association Task Force on Practice Guidelines and the Society for Cardiovascular Angiography and Interventions. *Circulation*. 2011;124:e574–e651.
109. Piccolo R, Giustino G, Mehran R, Windecker S. Stable coronary artery disease: revascularisation and invasive strategies. *Lancet*. 2015;386:702–713.
110. Maron DJ, Hochman JS, Reynolds HR, et al. Initial invasive or conservative strategy for stable coronary disease. *N Engl J Med*. 2020;382:1395–1407.
111. Harskamp RE, Park DW. Percutaneous coronary intervention in diabetic patients: should choice of stents be influenced? *Expert Rev Cardiovasc Ther*. 2013;11:541–553.
112. Banning AP, Westaby S, Morice MC, et al. Diabetic and nondiabetic patients with left main and/or 3-vessel coronary artery disease: comparison of outcomes with cardiac surgery and paclitaxel-eluting stents. *J Am Coll Cardiol*. 2010;55:1067–1075.
113. Kapur A, Bartolini D, Finlay MC, et al. The Bypass Angioplasty Revascularization in Type 1 and Type 2 Diabetes Study: 5-year follow-up of revascularization with percutaneous coronary intervention versus coronary artery bypass grafting in diabetic patients with multivessel disease. *J Cardiovasc Med (Hagerstown)*. 2010;11:26–33.
114. Kamalesh M, Sharp TG, Tang XC, et al. Percutaneous coronary intervention versus coronary bypass surgery in United States veterans with diabetes. *J Am Coll Cardiol*. 2013;61:808–816.
115. Farkouh ME, Domanski M, Sleeper LA, et al. Strategies for multivessel revascularization in patients with diabetes. *N Engl J Med*. 2012;367:2375–2384.
116. Farkouh ME, Domanski M, Fuster V. Revascularization strategies in patients with diabetes. *N Engl J Med*. 2013;368:1455–1456.
117. Head SJ, Milojevic M, Daemen J, et al. Mortality after coronary artery bypass grafting versus percutaneous coronary intervention with stenting for coronary artery disease: a pooled analysis of individual patient data. *Lancet*. 2018;391:939–948.
118. Fihn SD, Blankenship JC, Alexander KP, et al. 2014 ACC/AHA/AATS/PCNA/SCAI/STS focused update of the guideline for the diagnosis and management of patients with stable ischemic heart disease: a report of the American College of Cardiology/American Heart Association Task Force on practice guidelines, and the American Association for Thoracic Surgery, Preventive Cardiovascular Nurses Association, Society for Cardiovascular Angiography and Interventions, and Society of Thoracic Surgeons. *Circulation*. 2014;130:1749–1767.
119. Rawshani A, Rawshani A, Sattar N, et al. Relative prognostic importance and optimal levels of risk factors for mortality and cardiovascular outcomes in type 1 diabetes mellitus. *Circulation*. 2019;139:1900–1912.

Heart Failure in the Patient with Diabetes

120. McMurray JJ, Gerstein HC, Holman RR, Pfeffer MA. Heart failure: a cardiovascular outcome in diabetes that can no longer be ignored. *Lancet Diabetes Endocrinol*. 2014;2:843–851.
121. Cavender MA, Steg PG, Smith Jr SC, et al. Impact of diabetes mellitus on hospitalization for heart failure, cardiovascular events, and death: outcomes at 4 Years from the Reduction of Atherothrombosis for Continued Health (REACH) registry. *Circulation*. 2015;132:923–931.
122. Kristensen SL, Preiss D, Jhund PS, et al. Risk related to pre-diabetes mellitus and diabetes mellitus in heart failure with reduced ejection fraction: insights from prospective comparison of ARNI with ACEI to determine impact on global mortality and morbidity in heart failure trial. *Circ Heart Fail*. 2016;9.
123. Maack C, Lehrke M, Backs J, et al. Heart failure and diabetes: metabolic alterations and therapeutic interventions: a state-of-the-art review from the translational research committee of the Heart Failure Association-European Society of Cardiology. *Eur Heart J*. 2018;39:4243–4254.
124. Ponikowski P, Voors AA, Anker SD, et al. 2016 ESC Guidelines for the diagnosis and treatment of acute and chronic heart failure: the Task Force for the diagnosis and treatment of acute and chronic heart failure of the European Society of Cardiology (ESC)Developed with the special contribution of the Heart Failure Association (HFA) of the ESC. *Eur Heart J*. 2016;37:2129–2200.
125. Yancy CW, Jessup M, Bozkurt B, et al. 2016 ACC/AHA/HFSA focused update on new pharmacological therapy for heart failure: an update of the 2013 ACCF/AHA guideline for the management of heart failure: a report of the American College of Cardiology/American Heart Association Task Force on Clinical Practice Guidelines and the Heart Failure Society of America. *Circulation*. 2016;134:e282–e293.
126. McMurray JJ, Packer M, Desai AS, et al. Angiotensin-neprilysin inhibition versus enalapril in heart failure. *N Engl J Med*. 2014;371:993–1004.
127. Seferovic JP, Claggett B, Seidelmann SB, et al. Effect of sacubitril/valsartan versus enalapril on glycaemic control in patients with heart failure and diabetes: a post-hoc analysis from the PARADIGM-HF trial. *Lancet Diabetes Endocrinol*. 2017;5:333–340.
128. McGuire DK, Alexander JH, Johansen OE, et al. Linagliptin effects on heart failure and related outcomes in individuals with type 2 diabetes mellitus at high cardiovascular and renal risk in CARMELINA. *Circulation*. 2019;139:351–361.
129. Monami M, Ahren B, Dicembrini I, Mannucci E. Dipeptidyl peptidase-4 inhibitors and cardiovascular risk: a meta-analysis of randomized clinical trials. *Diabetes Obes Metab*. 2013;15:112–120.
130. Scirica BM, Braunwald E, Raz I, et al. Heart failure, saxagliptin, and diabetes mellitus: observations from the SAVOR-TIMI 53 randomized trial. *Circulation*. 2014;130:1579–1588.
131. Packer M, Anker SD, Butler J, EMPEROR-Reduced Trial Investigators, et al. Cardiovascular and renal outcomes with empagliflozin in heart failure. *N Engl J Med*. 2020;383(15):1413–1424.
132. Anker SD, Butler J, Filippatos G, EMPEROR-Reduced Trial Investigators, et al. Effect of empagliflozin on cardiovascular and renal outcomes in patients with heart failure by baseline diabetes status: results from the EMPEROR-Reduced Trial. *Circulation*. 2021;143(4):337–349.
133. Griffin M, Rao VS, Ivey-Miranda J, et al. Empagliflozin in heart failure: diuretic and cardio-renal effects. *Circulation*. 2020.
134. Verma S, McMurray JJV. SGLT2 inhibitors and mechanisms of cardiovascular benefit: a state-of-the-art review. *Diabetologia*. 2018;61:2108–2117.
135. Khan MSFG, McGuire DK, Hernandez AF, et al. *GLP-1 MA Placeholder*; 2020.
136. Schütt K, Marx N. Heart failure and diabetes: management and open issues. *Herz*. 2019;44:203–209.
137. Seyed Ahmadi S, Svensson AM, Pivodic A, et al. Risk of atrial fibrillation in persons with type 2 diabetes and the excess risk in relation to glycaemic control and renal function: a Swedish cohort study. *Cardiovasc Diabetol*. 2020;19:9.

32 Exercise and Sports Cardiology

PAUL D. THOMPSON AND AARON L. BAGGISH

HISTORICAL PERSPECTIVE, 579

CARDIOVASCULAR RESPONSE TO EXERCISE AND EXERCISE TRAINING, 579

EFFECTS OF HABITUAL PHYSICAL ACTIVITY ON CARDIOVASCULAR RISK, 580

CARDIOVASCULAR RISKS OF EXERCISE, 581
The Pathology of Exercise-Related Cardiovascular Events, 581
The Relative and Absolute Risk of Exercise, 581

APPROACH TO COMMON CLINICAL PROBLEMS IN SPORTS CARDIOLOGY, 581
Decreased Exercise Capacity, 582
Abnormalities Found on Screening, 582
Cardiovascular Complaints in Athletes, 583

DETERMINING ATHLETIC ELIGIBILITY, 583
Advising Adult Athletes with Atherosclerotic Cardiovascular Disease, 583
Valve Disease, 584
Elevated "Cardiac Enzymes", 584

Atrial Fibrillation in Endurance Athletes, 584
Accelerated Atherosclerosis, 585
Myocardial Fibrosis, 585
Noncompaction Cardiomyopathy, 585
Exercise in Arrhythmogenic Right Ventricular Cardiomyopathy, 585

CONCLUSION, 586

REFERENCES, 586

This chapter presents basic exercise physiology, describes cardiovascular (CV) adaptations to exercise training, and addresses common clinical issues among physically active individuals. The goal is to help clinicians evaluate symptoms produced by exercise, manage questions and clinical problems in athletes and physically active people, and assess the risks and benefits of exercise for individual patients. The reader is referred to Chapter 15 for a discussion of Exercise Testing.

HISTORICAL PERSPECTIVE

Clinicians have long been interested in the CV risks and benefits of exercise. Herodicus (480 BC) was a Greek physician who advocated exercise in the practice of medicine, whereas F.C. Sky, a London surgeon, in 1867 equated the Oxford-Cambridge crew race to cruelty to animals and opined that such extreme exertion would cause heart disease. Concern about rowers', runners', and bicyclists' hearts emerged in the late 19th century, when these activities migrated from being occupational competitions among only the working classes to being sporting activities for the social elite. The normal CV adaptations to exercise training include resting bradycardia, global cardiac enlargement, and functional pulmonic and aortic valve flow murmurs. Evaluation of these normal adaptations by auscultation and cardiac percussion, the diagnostic tests of the day, led to their interpretation as signs of pathologic conduction disease, dilated cardiomyopathy, and valvular obstruction, respectively. Concerns about the risks associated with prolonged and vigorous exercise were commonplace in the 19th and early 20th centuries. Clarence DeMar, seven-time winner of the Boston Marathon, took a 5-year hiatus from competition during the peak of his competitive years, in part because, according to DeMar, "The frequent warnings of the doctors and fans of the danger to one's heart had left their impression."[1] Current concerns about the risks and benefits of exercise include the risk of exercise-related acute cardiac events, the effects of exercise training on cardiac structure, and whether or not long-term endurance exercise training has deleterious CV effects.[2]

CARDIOVASCULAR RESPONSE TO EXERCISE AND EXERCISE TRAINING

Physical activity acutely increases systemic oxygen (O_2) demand, which prompts the CV system to increase cardiac output (Q) and the arterial-venous (A-V) O_2 difference. The increase in Q is coupled to the energy required such that there is a 5- to 6-liter increase in Q for each 1-liter increase in oxygen consumption ($\dot{V}O_2$). Q is increased by augmentation of both the heart rate (HR) and stroke volume (SV). Several mechanisms increase the A-V O_2 difference, including shunting of blood from non-exercising tissue to working muscle, increased O_2 extraction by exercising muscle, and hemoconcentration. Myocardial oxygen (MO_2) demand depends in part on HR and systolic blood pressure (SBP) and therefore increases with exertion because both HR and SBP increase. This increase in MO_2 can produce ischemia in individuals with flow-limiting coronary artery lesions. In addition, the coronary arteries dilate in response to the myocardial metabolic demands of exertion, but inadequate vasodilation or frank vasoconstriction develops with exercise in some individuals with coronary atherosclerosis because of endothelial dysfunction.[3] Cardiac ischemia, induced by exercise, can contribute to cardiac events during exercise, as discussed later.

The CV response to exercise has both an external and internal work rate.[3] The *external work rate* is the $\dot{V}O_2$ required by the exercise task and, as mentioned, is a direct determinant of Q. $\dot{V}O_2$ can also be crudely estimated from treadmill speed and grade or from a stationary bicycle watt requirement. The *internal work rate* refers to the myocardial oxygen consumption (MO_2) required for the exercise task and relates directly to increases in HR. In contrast to Q, the HR response to exercise, and therefore MO_2, is not determined by the external work rate or $\dot{V}O_2$max but by the $\dot{V}O_2$ required relative to the individual's *maximal exercise capacity*, or $\dot{V}O_2$. Individuals with higher exercise capacity and a greater $\dot{V}O_2$max have a larger SV at any given external work rate, such that any exercise task, and $\dot{V}O_2$ demand, requires a slower HR to generate the same externally determined Q.

Repetitive aerobic exercise sessions and aerobic exercise training increase maximal exercise capacity, measured physiologically by an increase in $\dot{V}O_2$max. This increase in healthy individuals results from increases in both maximal Q and the maximal A-V O_2 difference.[3] Because maximal HR is largely immutable, determined by age, and minimally affected by exercise training, the increase in maximal Q results from an increase in maximal SV. The increase in SV means that performing the same exercise task or external work rate, which requires the same $\dot{V}O_2$max, can be performed at a slower HR and a lower MO_2 or internal work rate. The reduction in HR and thereby MO_2 contributes to the increase in exercise capacity in patients with angina pectoris after exercise training.[3] In addition to the increase in maximal exercise capacity, exercise training also increases *endurance capacity*, the ability to perform submaximal effort for a prolonged period. This effect contributes critically to the exercise training response because few work or recreational tasks require maximal CV effort.

Intense and prolonged aerobic exercise training produces an array of CV adaptations, commonly referred to as "athlete's heart" (Fig. 32.1).[3] Such changes include an increase in resting SV and a decrease in resting HR. The physiologic mediators of training-induced reductions

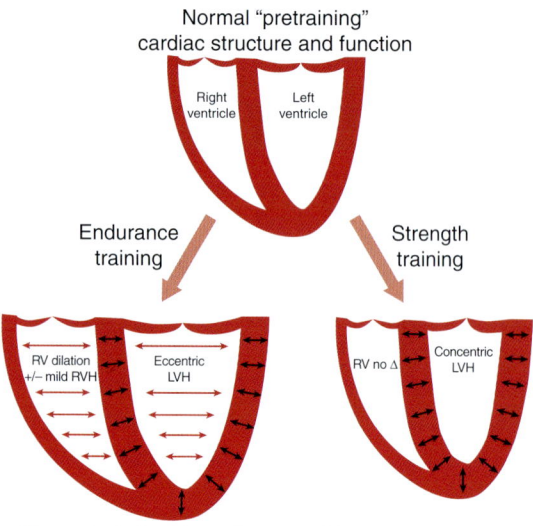

FIGURE 32.1 Summary of the ventricular remodeling that occurs with endurance and resistance exercise training. *LVEF*, Left ventricular ejection fraction; *LVH*, left ventricular hypertrophy; *RV no Δ*, no change in right ventricle; *RVH*, right ventricular hypertrophy. (From Weiner RB, Baggish AL. Exercise-induced cardiac remodeling. *Prog Cardiovasc Dis*. 2012;54:380.)

in resting HR are related in part to increased resting vagal tone and reduced resting sympathetic tone. However, the bradycardia persists in trained mice after autonomic blockade or sinus node denervation, suggesting that autonomic changes alone cannot explain the training effect on HR.[4] Indeed, trained mice show widespread remodeling of pacemaker ion channels, including downregulation of the I_f, or funny channel, mediated by microRNAs (miR-423-5p)[5] and blockade of I_f abolishing the reduced HR.[4] Highly trained endurance athletes often develop resting bradycardia, which may be associated with marked sinus arrhythmia, first-degree heart block, Mobitz I second-degree atrioventricular (AV) block, or even third-degree AV block during sleep. The reduced AV conduction velocity may make accessory conduction pathways, such as those of Wolff-Parkinson-White syndrome, more apparent. Athletes also have an increased prevalence of an early-repolarization ST-segment pattern and ST-T wave abnormalities, findings also historically attributed to increased vagal tone (Fig. 32.2).[6]

Four-chamber cardiac enlargement, often exceeding the standard upper limits of normal (ULN), develops in response to routine aerobic exercise training, whereas left ventricular (LV) wall thickness usually increases only mildly. Small increases in aortic root dimensions also occur, but increases in aortic size greater than expected for body size seldom occur in young athletes, even among those playing in the National Basketball Association.[7] The long-term effect of vigorous exercise on aortic dimensions is less clear. The aortic root diameter exceeded 40 mm in 41% of 152 asymptomatic, predominantly retired, Australian rugby players, and 58% had effacement of the sinotubular junction.[8] Similarly, among older runners and rowers (mean age ± SD of 61 ± 6 years) 31% of the men and 6% of the woman had an aortic diameter ≥40 mm.[9] Consequently, the possibility and significance of aortic enlargement in older, lifelong athletes requires additional study. In contrast to the extensive cardiac changes reported in endurance-trained athletes, strength exercise training produces modest increases in LV wall thickness with little change in chamber dimensions. Among 1300 elite Italian athletes, 45% exceeded the upper limit of normal (ULN) of 55 mm, with the most marked increases in LV size occurring

in the largest athletes and those with the slowest HR. In contrast, LV wall thickness rarely exceeds ULN among trained athletes. For example, among 947 national-caliber and international-caliber Italian athletes, only 16 had LV wall thickness greater than 12 mm.[3] Trained athletes usually have normal resting LV systolic function, most frequently measured as LV ejection fraction (LVEF), but may be near the lower limit of the normal range because large ventricles can meet resting metabolic demands with a lower LVEF.[10]

Cessation of exercise training, or "detraining," may help in clinically differentiating adaptations to exercise training from hypertrophic cardiomyopathy (HCM). Several studies have examined the effect of detraining in endurance athletes with eccentric LV hypertrophy (LVH), a geometric pattern characterized by concomitant LV wall thickening and chamber dilation. Regression of eccentric LVH can occur in highly trained athletes after 6 to 34 weeks (mean, 13 weeks) of abstinence from exercise. A detraining study of 40 Italian male athletes with eccentric LVH and peak fitness LV dimensions (mean ± SD) of 61.2 ± 2.9 mm and LV wall thickness of 12.0 ± 1.3 mm reported complete normalization of wall thickness and a significant but incomplete reduction in cavity dilation after 5.8 ± 3.6 years of detraining.[3] Because the LV wall thickening and concentric LVH common in strength-trained athletes can regress partially after 3 months and completely after 6 months of detraining, such diagnostic trials should last 6 months.[11]

EFFECTS OF HABITUAL PHYSICAL ACTIVITY ON CARDIOVASCULAR RISK

Multiple epidemiologic, cross-sectional studies examining the frequency of CV events in healthy individuals demonstrate that the more active participants have lower CV risk than their more sedentary counterparts. The reduction in risk in the most active versus the least active individuals is approximately 40%. Even small amounts of physical activity reduce CV risk. CV risk falls progressively with increasing physical activity until approximately 9.1 hours per week of moderate-intensity activity, such as brisk walking. After this level of exertion, there appears to be little additional benefit and, possibly diminution, of the beneficial effects.[12]

Cross-sectional studies, however, cannot prove that the reductions in CV risk result from physical activity alone. Individuals who engage in physical activity may inherit greater exercise capacity, thereby leading them to select active lifestyles and lower their CV risk. Physical activity contributes to the improvement in multiple CV risk factors including SBP, body weight (BW), blood glucose, and triglycerides. Nevertheless, there are no randomized clinical trials (RCTs) comparing the effects of physical activity or exercise training on CV outcomes in previously sedentary, healthy individuals, but there are multiple RCTs examining CV outcomes of exercise-based cardiac rehabilitation in patients with established disease. None of these studies was large enough to provide conclusive results alone, but a meta-analysis of 63 RCTs including 14,486 patients demonstrated a 26% decrease in CV mortality in the patients assigned to the exercise-based programs.[13] Such results, plus the plethora of epidemiologic and experimental evidence linking increased physical activity with lower CV risk have led to the acceptance of physical inactivity as a major modifiable CV risk factor. Epidemiologic data suggest that the largest reduction in CV risk with physical activity occurs at low levels of activity. Consequently, current American guidelines recommend 150 to 300 minutes weekly of moderate aerobic activity such as brisk walking or 75 to 100 minutes weekly of vigorous activity such as jogging, plus some resistance exercise twice weekly.[14]

Support for the possibility that habitual exercise and lower CV disease are genetically linked is provided by studies that have selected and bred rats over multiple generations for superior or reduced exercise performance. The animals that result from breeding for higher exercise capacity also developed lower CV "risk" profiles including less evidence of the metabolic syndrome, fewer CV complications, and greater longevity than rats bred for reduced exercise capacity even though CV risk factors were not considered in the breeding selection process.[3] Consequently, the same physiologic factors associated with increased exercise capacity may also be associated with reduced CV risk, and individuals choosing an active lifestyle may have lower CV risk independent of their exercise habits.

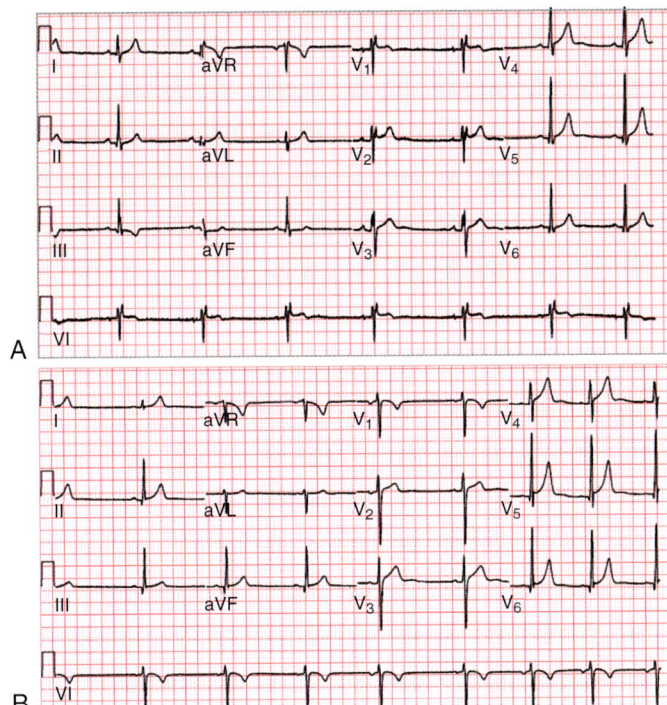

FIGURE 32.2 12-lead ECG tracings from asymptomatic athletes without structural or electrical diseases of the heart demonstrating common findings associated with exercise training. **A,** Sinus bradycardia and an incomplete right bundle branch block resulting from physiologic right ventricular dilation in a 23-year-old male professional hockey player. **B,** Sinus bradycardia with respirophasic sinus arrhythmia, precordial ST-segment elevation characteristic of benign normal early repolarization, and prominent precordial lead QRS voltage, often associated with underlying physiologic left ventricular hypertrophy, in a 19-year-old male distance runner.

CARDIOVASCULAR RISKS OF EXERCISE

The Pathology of Exercise-Related Cardiovascular Events

Despite the putative benefits of habitual physical activity, vigorous physical activity transiently increases the risk for sudden cardiac death (SCD) and acute myocardial infarction (AMI).[15] This conclusion is based on studies comparing the hourly cardiac event rate during vigorous exertion with rates during more sedentary activities. The pathologic substrate associated with these acute cardiac events varies by age, because the prevalence of cardiac conditions responsible for SCD also varies by age. Exercise-related SCD in young individuals, defined as age less than 30 or 40 years, has historically been attributed to inherited and congenital conditions, including HCM (see Chapters 54 and 70) and anomalous origin of the coronary arteries (AOCA), although acquired conditions such as myocarditis and cardiomyopathy can also cause exercise-related SCD in this group.[3]

Recent studies, however, have questioned the role of HCM as the leading cause of SCD in athletes. Autopsy data reveal no structural abnormality in up to 40% of SCDs in young athletes,[16] suggesting that many of these such deaths are due to the sudden arrhythmic death syndrome (SADS). Further, HCM and AOCA were found in only 6% and 5% of these cases respectively, thereby suggesting that other conditions, such as inherited channelopathies, may be more prevalent.[16] Each of these 357 cases was evaluated in a cardiac pathology referral center raising the possibility that definitively diagnosed cases of HCM and AOCA may have not been referred. Similar findings were generated by an analysis of SCD among National Collegiate Athletic Association (NCAA) athletes over a 10-year period in which HCM and AOCA were responsible for only 15% (79) of 514 deaths. There was no structural abnormality in 25% of the 64 autopsied cases, whereas only 5% and 11% were due to HCM and AOCA, respectively.[17] Similarly, a meta-analysis of 34 studies of SCD reported normal hearts in 23% of nonathletes and 18% of the athletes and HCM in 8% and 14% of the nonathletes and athletes, respectively.[18] These studies are difficult to compare because some included all SCDs in athletes, whereas others included only exercise-related SCDs. Consequently, it is not clear if this apparent shift in the causes of SCD during exertion is due to previous selected case ascertainment (because the earliest studies often originated from HCM centers), a true change in the causes of SCD because of more effective screening, diagnosis, and care of athletes with HCM, or to the inclusion of both exercise- and nonexercise-related SCDs in the analyses.

Atherosclerotic cardiovascular disease (ASCVD) causes most exercise-related AMI and SCD in adults,[15] although there are rare reports of spontaneous coronary artery dissection with vigorous exertion (more often in young, but occasionally in older individuals).[15] AMI in previously asymptomatic adults during exercise is usually associated with acute coronary arterial plaque disruption. However, malignant ventricular arrhythmias and SCD triggered by myocardial ischemia attributable to stable but obstructive coronary lesions also occur.[15] Several triggering mechanisms for plaque disruption may pertain, including increased flexing and bending of atherosclerotic coronary arteries.[3] Approximately 33% of SCDs in adults caused by ASCVD are associated with clinicopathologic findings of an acute coronary syndrome (ACS), whereas the remainder show evidence of nonacute ASCVD.[19]

The Relative and Absolute Risk of Exercise

Vigorous exercise increases the relative risk of cardiac events, but the absolute risk of exercise-related cardiac events is low, particularly among people who are habitually highly active.[15] Among young individuals, the increase in risk relative to SCD during exercise is greatest in the youngest age groups. Approximately 14% of SCD in individuals less than 35 years old in Portland, OR, were related to sport activity. In this cohort, SCDs occurred during sports in 39% of cases among individuals less than 18 years old, 13% of those aged 19 to 25, and 7% of those aged 25 to 34.[20]

This observed decline with increasing age is likely attributable to decreasing exercise intensity with increasing age, the rarity of non-exertion deaths in the youngest group, and the decrease in overall sport activity with increasing age. Importantly, the risk of exercise-related SCD appears higher in athletes than in nonathletes as evidenced by the fact that SCDs or cardiac arrests were ≈4.5-fold greater in French competitive athletes aged 10 to 35 than among recreational athletes of similar age.[3]

Estimates of the absolute risk of death among young competitive athletes are highly variable and depend on study design and the groups studied. The most consistent estimate for the absolute risk of sports-related SCD in the young is one death per year for every 200,000 athletes.[3] However, rates as high as one death per year for every 5100 Division 1 male NCAA basketball players[17] and every 14,704 male adolescent, elite soccer players (mean age ± SD; 16.4 ± 1.2 years) have been reported.[21] These rates are high compared to historical data, so additional studies are required to clarify this variability.

Between 4.4% and 13.6% of AMIs are associated with physical exertion[15] and approximately 5% of all SCDs are sports related.[19] Vigorous exertion increases the risk of SCD in adults between 3 and 17 times that of more sedentary activities.[15] Historical estimates of the absolute risk suggested that one exercise-related death occurred per year for every 15,000 to 18,000 previously healthy adult men,[3] but more recent estimates are markedly lower at between one death per year for every 50,000 to 300,000 individuals.[15] Most studies suggest that both young and older women have a much lower risk for exercise-related events

APPROACH TO COMMON CLINICAL PROBLEMS IN SPORTS CARDIOLOGY

Athletes and active individuals may seek CV evaluation for a multitude of reasons, but the following section discusses several common clinical complaints in athletic patients and the clinical approach to their management.

Decreased Exercise Capacity

Athletes with decreased exercise capacity are frequently referred to CV specialists for evaluation. SV contributes critically to Q and therefore to exercise capacity, but $\dot{V}o_2$max also requires maximal performance from its other CV components, HR and A-V O_2 difference, as well as from the central nervous system, lungs, and skeletal muscle. Decrements in any of these components can compromise exercise performance. An inappropriately fast HR at low levels of exertion as a result of hyperthyroidism or stimulant use can decrease exercise performance, as can exercise-induced asthma, diseases of skeletal muscle, and reduced O_2-carrying capacity from anemia (often resulting from iron deficiency in female endurance athletes who eat a vegetarian diet). Atrial fibrillation (AF) or frequent premature contractions during exercise can reduce exercise capacity. Recurrent pulmonary emboli are often not suspected in athletes because of their overall health and atypical presentation, but prolonged travel to competition, tissue trauma and immobility from injury, and factors such as genetic predisposition, birth control use, and dehydration can increase athletes' thrombotic risk.[25] Other conditions not directly related to the CV system, including viral illnesses (e.g., mononucleosis, hepatitis), hematologic malignancies, and autoimmune conditions, can initially be manifest in athletes as decreased exercise capacity or exercise intolerance.

These same issues can reduce exercise performance in older athletes but occult coronary disease with atypical symptoms always requires consideration first in older patients. Many adult athletes with reduced exercise capacity referred for expert evaluation have LV diastolic dysfunction because prior encounters have eliminated the more obvious diagnoses. This scenario often presents as a lifelong endurance athlete with "borderline hypertension" who avoided antihypertensive treatment. These patients frequently have mild-resting hypertension but exhibit an exaggerated blood pressure response to exercise.

Psychological factors and overtraining can cause decreased exercise capacity in athletes. Psychological issues generally occur in young athletes who have lost their desire to compete before their parents have lost interest in the child's sport. This diagnosis often becomes clear if parents or other key adults are included in the patient's assessment. Some athletes appear to find it easier to use a medical excuse for stopping sports participation rather than to admit that they have lost interest, want to pursue other interests, or "just aren't good enough" to continue.

Evaluation of athletes complaining of decreased exercise performance requires listening to the athlete's history carefully. Practitioners may dismiss many complaints in athletes because their exercise performance remains superior to that of nonathletes, but important cardiac conditions may present sooner in athletes because of the physical demands of their sport. Evaluating performance times, training diaries, and training/performance data captured by GPS-enabled wearable technology in endurance athletes often helps plot the time course of the complaint. The conditions mentioned earlier must be excluded, as must obvious cardiac disease. Exercise testing using protocols designed to mimic the athlete's sport frequently helps document the complaint and its cause. Exercise echocardiography and cardiopulmonary exercise testing with specific attention to the oxygen pulse curve are useful when the history suggests diastolic dysfunction. The oxygen pulse can be calculated by dividing $\dot{V}o_2$ by HR, and assuming no important change in the A-V O_2 difference, reflects SV. It can help determine when cardiac performance becomes a limiting factor during exercise. Long-term electrocardiographic monitoring, increasingly done using adhesive ambulatory monitoring patches and occasionally performed with implanted monitoring devices, can detect cardiac rhythm disorders in athletes with infrequent symptoms. Psychological and emotional issues should be diagnosed only after the exclusion of other medical conditions and require frank discussions with the athlete and family. Depression can frequently cause otherwise unexplained fatigue.

Overtraining is a complex interaction of psychological and physiologic fatigue in athletes that can occur after prolonged high-intensity training. The diagnosis of overtraining is made by careful history because there is no diagnostic test for this condition. Diminished exercise tolerance (sometimes with an elevated resting HR), the sensation of nocturnal fevers, and insomnia all characterize overtraining. The insomnia appears paradoxical because the athletes often experience extreme fatigue but find it difficult to sleep as a result of restlessness and sometimes involuntary muscle contractions. Overtraining should be diagnosed only when other conditions are excluded and frequently requires a therapeutic trial of markedly reduced training to see whether the symptoms resolve and performance improves. The optimal duration of prescribed detraining for overtrained athletes has yet to be defined but may be weeks to months depending on the duration and severity of the overtraining symptoms.

Abnormalities Found on Screening

Many athletes are referred to cardiologists because of CV abnormalities found on preparticipation screening. Both the American Heart Association (AHA) and the American College of Cardiology (ACC), as well as the European Society of Cardiology (ESC),[23] recommend preparticipation screening for athletes. The ESC recommends including a resting 12-lead electrocardiogram (ECG) as a mandatory and universal component of screening. In contrast, the most recent AHA/ACC recommendations endorse the use of ECG only in athlete cohorts surrounded by adequate expertise and resources to support this process. A scientific statement from the AHA argues strongly against mandatory and broad-based screening of young athletes (or nonathletes) using the ECG. However, these recommendations cautiously support the use of ECG screening in athlete cohorts under certain conditions and where there is adequate expertise and resources to support this process. The debates on CV screening in general, on screening athletes versus screening all children, and on the role of the ECG exceed the scope of this chapter.[24] A widely cited Italian study and recent evaluation of college athletes suggests that screening greatly reduces cardiac events in athletes, but other studies suggest that screening has no benefit.[24,25] A U.S. National Institutes of Health consensus conference concluded that the data were insufficient to recommend routine screening of the general population or athletes with an ECG.[26] Regardless of the scientific merit, many young athletes do undergo screening with an ECG, and abnormalities emerge.

Screening athletes with or without an ECG can detect a multitude of ECG variants that appear abnormal but are physiologic adaptations to exercise training. Well-trained endurance athletes have a slow HR and large SV, which can produce nonpathologic pulmonic flow murmurs in young athletes, especially if the athlete is examined in the supine position, which expands central blood volume. Pulmonic flow murmurs are soft systolic ejection murmurs heard best in the left second and third intercostal spaces in the supine position. Such murmurs typically diminish or disappear when the athlete assumes a sitting position. Older athletes with hemodynamically insignificant aortic sclerosis may have aortic flow murmurs. Athletes can also have ECG evidence of biatrial hypertrophy, LVH, incomplete or complete right bundle branch block, ST-T wave abnormalities, and conduction abnormalities. Most of these abnormalities occur in athletes undergoing intense endurance training. There are improved ECG criteria to separate the ECG patterns expected from exercise training from truly abnormal ECG tracings,[27] but even these "refined" criteria suggest a possible cardiac abnormality in 11% of black and 5% of white athletes.[27] Furthermore, ECGs are initially read by computer algorithms that are not yet sophisticated enough to identify these variants as normal, and clinicians often find it difficult to ignore the computer's interpretation. Similar ECG changes in endurance athletes with low training volumes or in strength-trained athletes should raise suspicion of a cardiac problem. A recent international conference proposed consensus criteria for interpretation of ECG in athletes.[28]

Most CV abnormalities found on screening are variants of normal, and most can be dismissed by a simple clinical examination and review of the ECG, with cardiac imaging procedures used to remove any residual doubt.[29] Some families and athletes have ongoing concern once a screening abnormality is identified, so having the athlete and family return in 3 to 6 months is sometimes useful, even when no abnormalities are found, to provide additional reassurance.

A common problem in athletes with a screening abnormality is what we have termed "diagnostic creep"—the finding of a minor abnormality on screening such as early ECG repolarization, which prompts a second diagnostic test such as echocardiography, which reveals another borderline finding such as mild LVH, which may prompt another diagnostic test such as cardiac magnetic resonance imaging (MRI). Sometimes, because of the CV adaptations that accompany exercise training, each diagnostic study reveals an additional borderline abnormality, thus making it difficult for a clinician to declare the athlete "normal." Screening abnormalities, especially if borderline abnormal, should be judged with less concern than definite abnormalities found in symptomatic athletes, because the screening abnormalities will most frequently represent normal variants.

Cardiovascular Complaints in Athletes

Athletes are sensitive to changes in their physical being and exercise performance and are more likely to note early CV abnormalities because of the CV demands of exercise training and competition. On the other hand, some athletes are excessively concerned about anything that may affect their performance and may seek evaluation for normal body sensations such as muscular aches produced by new training regimens. Nevertheless, possible CV complaints in athletes should cause greater concern than borderline abnormalities found on screening, and such complaints require careful evaluation with techniques appropriate for the differential diagnosis.

Chest pain is a common complaint in young and old athletes, possibly because the importance of chest pain in public perception, and because athletes have increasing concerns about the possible cardiac risks of exercise. Chest discomfort in athletes should never be dismissed summarily. Exertional chest pain may be the first sign of important cardiac diseases, including HCM, AOCA, or coronary artery atherosclerosis, but several issues pertain particularly to athletes. Chest pain that is reproducible with exercise and relieved by rest (i.e., typical angina), particularly when it occurs at a clear workload threshold that the athlete can identify, should be considered indicative of underlying cardiac pathology until proven otherwise. Determining the duration of chest pain is important because many athletes without underlying disease experience momentary chest pain. The sensation of momentary chest pain may accompany premature atrial or ventricular contractions, possibly because contraction against closed AV valves produces a momentary sensation of chest fullness. Fleeting chest pain with movement in athletes may also be related to muscle and joint issues. The relationship between chest pain and recent resistance exercise involving the chest muscles, such as push-ups and bench presses, is also important because such training is a frequent cause of chest discomfort in athletes. Some athletes who have died with AOCA had normal exercise stress test results,[3] indicating the importance of pursuing workups that include coronary imaging in athletes if the symptoms are worrisome, even when exercise testing yields normal results. Such an approach differs distinctly from what we advise in asymptomatic athletes with borderline test results.

Well-trained athletes often have *vasovagal syncope*, now formally referred to as "neurally mediated syncope," probably because of their resting bradycardia and large venous capacity, which permits sequestration of large amounts of blood when the athlete is upright and motionless.[30] Athletes also often have positive tilt-table tests as a result of the same physiologic changes thus limiting the diagnostic utility of this test in athletes. Neurally mediated syncope most often occurs in athletes immediately following exercise, particularly with abrupt termination of exercise. This common entity, "postexertional syncope," is benign and can frequently be managed by teaching the athlete avoidance techniques. The most important avoidance technique is for the athlete to keep moving after effort so that the muscle pump in the calf continues to return blood to the systemic circulation. Dietary sodium augmentation, aggressive pre-exercise hydration, and the use of commercially available compression socks may also prove useful. A key issue in evaluating syncope in athletes is to determine whether the syncope truly occurred during exertion. Syncope at rest or immediately after exercise under conditions consistent with vasovagal syncope or postural syncope is usually caused by these conditions. Neurally mediated syncope is also often followed by a period of confusion, whereas cardiac syncope generally has no cognitive sequelae.[31] Paradoxically, the athlete who feels fine after a syncopal episode and wants to return to the game immediately is the athlete most likely to have a cardiac condition. Consequently, syncope during exercise and syncope without post-syncope confusion should prompt a careful search for more serious problems, including inherited cardiomyopathies, aortic stenosis (AS), cardiac arrhythmia, or AOCA.[30]

DETERMINING ATHLETIC ELIGIBILITY

The AHA and ACC have developed eligibility and disqualification recommendations for cardiac conditions according to the advice of 15 task forces that created the guidelines based on literature review and expert opinion.[32] Guidelines are necessarily restrictive because they are used by a wide variety of clinicians, many of whom will have no special expertise in evaluating athletes. Guidelines often appear overly restrictive to clinicians with experience in evaluating athletes with minor variants of CV disease, but guidelines provide the best available consensus opinion on how to advise athletes regarding their risks during sports participation.

We use these guidelines as the basis for most of our recommendations but alter the final decision depending on multiple factors, including our perception of the athlete's risk given the severity of the lesion and symptoms, the importance of participation for the athlete's mental health, the danger to others, and the willingness of the athlete and family to share risk in making the decision. The diagnosis, its attendant risk, and the basis for any recommendations also require discussion (if the athlete agrees) with other key individuals, such as parents, school or team administrators, coaches, athletic trainers, and business agents. This process is best accomplished using a shared decision-making model and comprehensive recommendations pertaining to this approach have been previously published.[33] We use a similar decision-making approach with older athletes, although they usually have a greater ability to understand and assume personal risk.

Advising Adult Athletes with Atherosclerotic Cardiovascular Disease

Vigorous exercise increases the risk for SCD and AMI in adults with occult ASCVD, and individuals with diagnosed disease have greater increased risk with exercise. Many adults with ASCVD want to return to active athletic competition, often in demanding endurance events such as marathon running or long-distance cycling. Imaging techniques such as scanning for coronary artery calcification (CAC) have expanded the detection of asymptomatic and presymptomatic disease. All athletes with ASCVD require an explanation that vigorous exercise acutely increases their CV risk and that moderate amounts of exercise probably confer as much ASCVD reduction benefit as more intense activity.[12] Despite such discussion, many such athletes want to return to competition or intense exercise training. Plaque stability likely increases with decreasing lipid content of the plaque, and most plaque regression occurs within 2 years of aggressive lipid lowering (see Chapter 24). Consequently, in athletes strongly wanting to return to competition, we advise a minimum of 2 years of aggressive lipid treatment with the goal of achieving the greatest possible plaque regression before returning to competition. We also emphasize the importance of controlling other risk factors, as well as the need to report symptoms that may indicate progression of disease. Two years without competition is unacceptable to many middle-aged athletes so some negotiation of this time is often required. In these situations, many athletes find satisfaction in "participating" in competitive events like marathons or triathlons with prescribed intensity restrictions. This approach allows the athlete to maintain fitness and engagement in the social aspects of sport, retain hope for further unrestricted competition, and may motivate them to adhere to risk reduction strategies.

Adult athletes receiving lipid-lowering or antihypertensive treatment occasionally inquire whether their medications should be stopped before endurance athletic competition. We encourage athletes to continue aspirin and other antiplatelet medications under the assumption that they may help avoid an acute cardiac event if plaque disruption occurs. We continue therapy with a beta blocker to avoid the increase in adrenergic activity that occurs when use of these drugs is stopped abruptly. We generally discontinue other antihypertensive medications on the day of the athletic event or on days with unusually demanding training sessions depending on the severity of the athlete's hypertension, because exercise acutely reduces BP, and we want to avoid postexertional hypotension. We routinely discontinue statins for 5 to 7 days before endurance athletic competition because statins magnify the increase in creatine kinase (CK) that occurs with exercise,[34] and the combined effects of statins and exercise could lead to rhabdomyolysis.

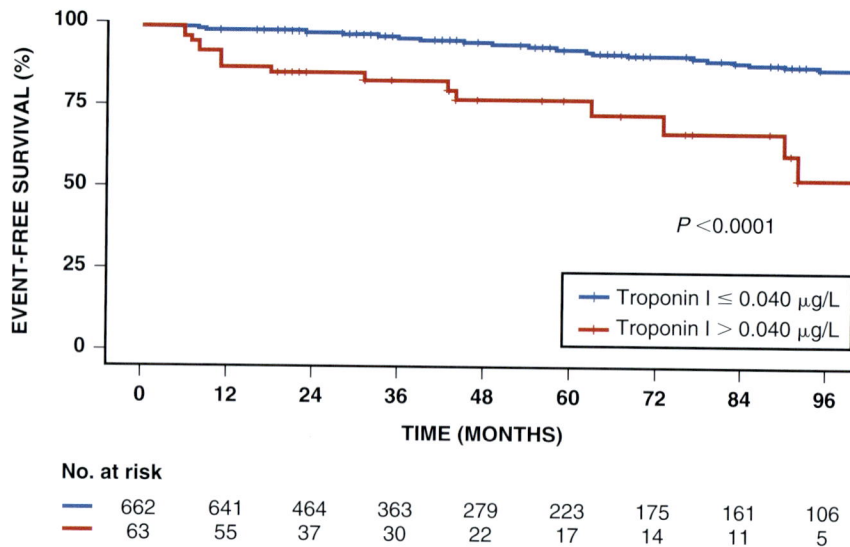

FIGURE 32.3 Kaplan-Meier unadjusted estimates for all-cause mortality and major adverse cardiovascular events in participants with or without troponin I concentrations greater than 0.04 μg/L after prolonged walking exercise. (From Aengevaeren VL, Hopman MTE, Thompson PD, et al. Exercise-induced cardiac troponin i increase and incident mortality and cardiovascular events. *Circulation.* 2019;140:804–814.)

Valve Disease

Valvular disease in athletes should be managed according to principles for the nonathletic population and AHA/ACC recommendations,[35] although several issues merit note. Athletes with echocardiographic evidence of critical AS should undergo careful evaluation for symptoms and maximal exercise stress testing that simulates as closely as possible the athlete's typical exercise training and competition. Many adult athletes with critical AS ignore important dyspnea at the start of exercise because it dissipates within 5 to 10 minutes, but this "warm-up dyspnea" frequently indicates clinically important AS. Among truly asymptomatic athletes being followed for severe AS, sudden reductions in exercise performance without alternative explanation often indicate that surgical intervention is warranted.

Athletes generally tolerate aortic regurgitation (AR) well, probably because the increased HR during exercise decreases diastole and regurgitant flow. Consequently, we rarely restrict athletic competition despite severe AR in the absence of evidence of ventricular deterioration, marked aneurysmal disease of the ascending aorta, or unexplained symptoms with exertion. We also rarely restrict resistance exercise in this group despite concern that this type of exercise increases AR, because we know of no data that indicate any benefit of such restriction.

Great concern exists regarding exercise and aortic dissection in athletes with a bicuspid aortic valve (BAV), and some clinicians have restricted participation in this group because of concern that athletics will contribute to aortic dilation (see Chapter 72).[3] Given the prevalence of BAV in approximately 1% of the population and the rarity of aortic dissection in young athletes, we do not restrict activity unless the aortic diameter exceeds 45 mm. The AHA/ACC Aortic Diseases Task Force recommends aortic root measurements biannually for individuals with aortic diameter greater than 40 mm in men and 36 mm in women.[36] Athletes found to have BAV should undergo imaging to determine proximal ascending aortic dimensions at diagnosis and then should be monitored by serial imaging during their years of competitive sport participation.

Elevated "Cardiac Enzymes"

Cardiac troponin (cTn) T and I are highly sensitive and specific biomarkers of myocardial necrosis. However, athletes can have increased cTn levels after prolonged exertion, such as a marathon run, or even after a brief intense treadmill run. Clinicians need to be aware that endurance athletes may have elevated cTn levels after exertion, and that the diagnosis of an acute cardiac event in an athlete requires confirmatory evidence of myocardial injury by either symptoms, ECG, or echocardiography. The increase in cTn after exercise resolves more rapidly than cTn increases attributable to pathologic acute myocardial injury. The cause of the cTn increase with exercise is not clear, but could represent mild myocardial injury or an increase in sarcolemmal permeability and release of free Tn not bound to tropomyosin.[37] Increased cTn levels after exertion are not necessarily benign. Men, aged 54 to 69 years, who walked 7.3 to 9.3 hours at 68% ± 10% of their predicted maximum HR (±SD) and who increased their cTnI levels greater than 99th percentile, experienced more subsequent CV events and deaths over a median of 43 months of follow-up compared to men with lower cTnI values.[38] Nevertheless, increased cTn levels after exercise are common[37] so that this observation of increased risk requires confirmation (Fig. 32.3).

Atrial Fibrillation in Endurance Athletes

The relationship between habitual exercise training and AF is complex and likely follows a U-shaped curve.[39] Low levels of physical activity and low exercise capacity are risk factors for AF. Few studies have examined how exercise training affects AF, but obese patients with AF participating in an exercise and weight loss intervention had the greatest reduction in AF if they lost ≥10% of their BW and increased their exercise capacity ≥7 mL O_2/kg/min.[40] Those who increased their exercise capacity, but did not lose greater than 10% BW also reduced recurrent AF more than those who neither lost greater than 10% BW nor increased their exercise capacity ≥7 mL O_2/kg/min. Such results suggest that exercise training alone can reduce AF.

In contrast, large amounts of exercise appear to increase the incidence of AF. A meta-analysis and review of studies of endurance athletes demonstrated an increase (up to fivefold) in AF.[41] Sweden's Vasaloppet Nordic ski race is an annual event with races from 30 to 90 km (18.6 to 55.8 miles) in distance and has provided some of the most provocative data on exercise and AF (Fig. 32.4).[42] A total of 208,654 participants in the 1989 to 2011 races were divided into performance groups based by finishing times. They were matched with 524,448 non-skiers, and their incidence of AF determined using Swedish national databases. Female skiers had less AF than non-skiers. AF was also not different in male skiers and non-skiers, but skiers were younger and had fewer AF risk factors. After adjusting for AF risk factors, male skiers had more AF, and those men who completed the most races and were the best performers had the highest rates of AF. Possible mechanisms include increased atrial size or changes in autonomic tone with training or acute increases in inflammation with exercise, and increased inflammation.[43]

Older athletes with AF should undergo the same evaluation as nonathletes to exclude cardiac disease, hyperthyroidism, alcohol excess, and sleep apnea. AF in young athletes is unusual and should prompt clinicians to question and confirm the diagnosis and to exclude issues like acute thyroiditis, use of performance-enhancing or other illicit substances, and structural cardiac abnormalities.

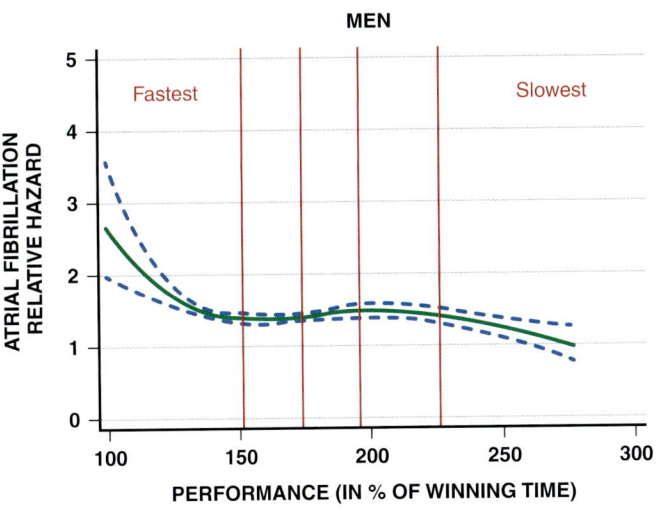
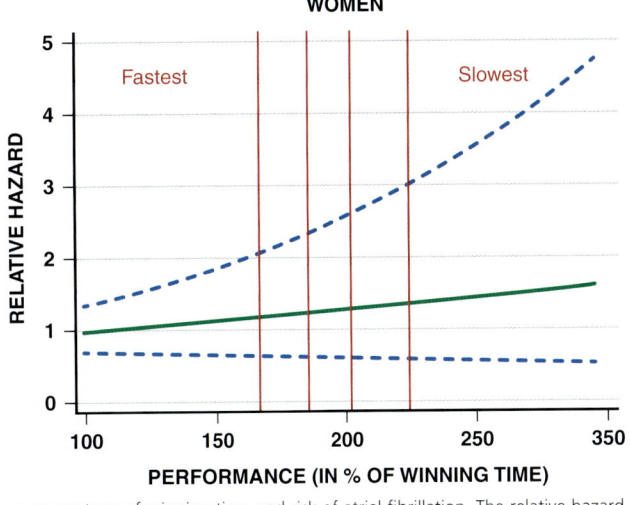

FIGURE 32.4 Relationship of performance in the Vasaloppet, a cross-country ski race, as a percentage of winning time and risk of atrial fibrillation. The relative hazard line of 1 represents the comparison group of non-skiers. Results are adjusted for age, income, education, time of inclusion, diabetes mellitus, hypertension, hyperthyroidism, and ischemic heart disease. Red lines indicate quintiles of performance. (From Niclas S, Sundström J, James S, et al. Long-term incidence of atrial fibrillation and stroke among cross-country skiers. *Circulation*. 2019;140:910–920.)

Accelerated Atherosclerosis

Several studies suggest that long-term endurance athletes have increased CAC scores compared to their sedentary counterparts (Fig. 32.5).[43] Coronary CT angiography (CCTA) demonstrates that the plaques in endurance athletes are primarily calcified and not the putatively more vulnerable mixed or non-calcified plaques.[43] This suggests that these plaques in athletes are less likely to rupture and to produce an acute cardiac event. On the other hand, four of eight participants in the Race Across America, a 140-day foot race, had coronary atherosclerosis at baseline determined by CCTA.[44] All four increased noncalcified plaque during the run. The observation of increased CAC scores in endurance athletes and the increase in atherosclerosis after prolonged exercise raises the possibility that vigorous exercise can increase atherosclerosis. This seems paradoxical because athletes typically have fewer cardiac events and enhanced longevity making the significance of high CAC scores in athletes unclear. Among athletes that come to us with elevated CAC scores, we evaluate for exercise-induced ischemia using maximal effort-limited exercise testing, treat ASCVD risk factors aggressively, especially with lipid-lowering agents, and provide reassurance that the significance of this finding is unknown and may be protective, rather than deleterious, because the plaque in athletes is predominantly calcified.

Myocardial Fibrosis

Myocardial fibrosis identified by late gadolinium enhancement (LGE) with cardiac MRI may result from a variety of insults, but myocardial fibrosis has also been found in healthy veteran endurance athletes.[45] Athletes with LGE had exercise-trained for much of their lives and had cardiac dimensions larger than comparison athletes. The LGE volume was small and often located where the right ventricle inserts into the interventricular septum, suggesting that it results from chronic right ventricular (RV) enlargement or RV dilatation during exercise.[45] The significance of this fibrosis is unclear, but clinicians should be aware of its presence in some athletes to avoid unnecessary, extensive evaluations. We do not routinely restrict athletes with incidentally detected myocardial fibrosis in the absence of concomitant structural heart disease or otherwise unexplained malignant arrhythmias.

Noncompaction Cardiomyopathy

The left ventricle is highly trabeculated during embryonic cardiac development to increase myocardial surface area and thus facilitate the delivery of oxygen and nutrients from intracavitary blood to the myocardium. These trabeculae regress and the myocardium becomes compacted during normal embryonic development. The degree of embryonic trabecular regression varies, and many healthy people have some trabecular tissue within the LV cavity. Noncompaction cardiomyopathy (NCCM) results from an arrest of this process characterized by a hypertrabeculated left ventricle with a thin, subepicardial, compacted layer. NCCM was first described in 1984 and named in 1990, so is a relatively new entity.[3] NCCM presenting in adults is inherited in an autosomal dominant pattern, but an X-linked pattern is seen in pediatric patients.[3] NCCM can produce myocardial dysfunction, systemic emboli from the deep ventricular pits, and SCD. There are various diagnostic criteria, but a ratio of noncompacted (NC) to compacted (C) myocardium greater than 2 is frequently used.[3] This cut point can be problematic for clinicians treating athletes, especially Black athletes, because 20% of 1146 athletes had increased trabeculations and 8% fulfilled criteria for NCCM,[3] and because Blacks have increased LV trabeculae even in the absence of exercise training. Referrals for possible NCCM in athletes have increased because of growing awareness of the condition, and because the expanded ECG screening of athletes has increased the number of athletes referred for echocardiography. Most of the individuals referred do not have NCCM but rather the benign, mildly trabeculated, normal LV variant previously described. We advise obtaining a careful family history and reviewing the myocardial images, with special attention to LV systolic function and thickness of the compacted layer. Patients with true NCCM that require sport restriction have decreased ventricular systolic function that is often most profound in the noncompacted wall segments and a thin, compacted layer of myocardium. The compacted layer is normal and can even be slightly thickened in athletes (see also Chapter 82.)

Exercise in Arrhythmogenic Right Ventricular Cardiomyopathy

Multiple studies since the 1990s have demonstrated that the right ventricle can dilate after prolonged endurance exercise, possibly because the relative increase in RV strain during exercise exceeds that of the left ventricle.[2] Physiologic RV dilation in the vast majority of athletes is benign. In contrast, genetically mediated arrhythmogenic RV cardiomyopathy/dysplasia results from defects in the genes that code for desmosomal proteins that facilitate connection of myocytes. Athletes with defects in desmosomal protein genes are more likely to satisfy the diagnostic criteria and to have a worse prognosis than similarly endowed nonathletes.[46] Individuals with confirmed genetic arrhythmogenic RV cardiomyopathy/dysplasia should be restricted from vigorous exercise training because it may increase the risk of incident arrhythmias and progression to heart failure (see Chapter 52).

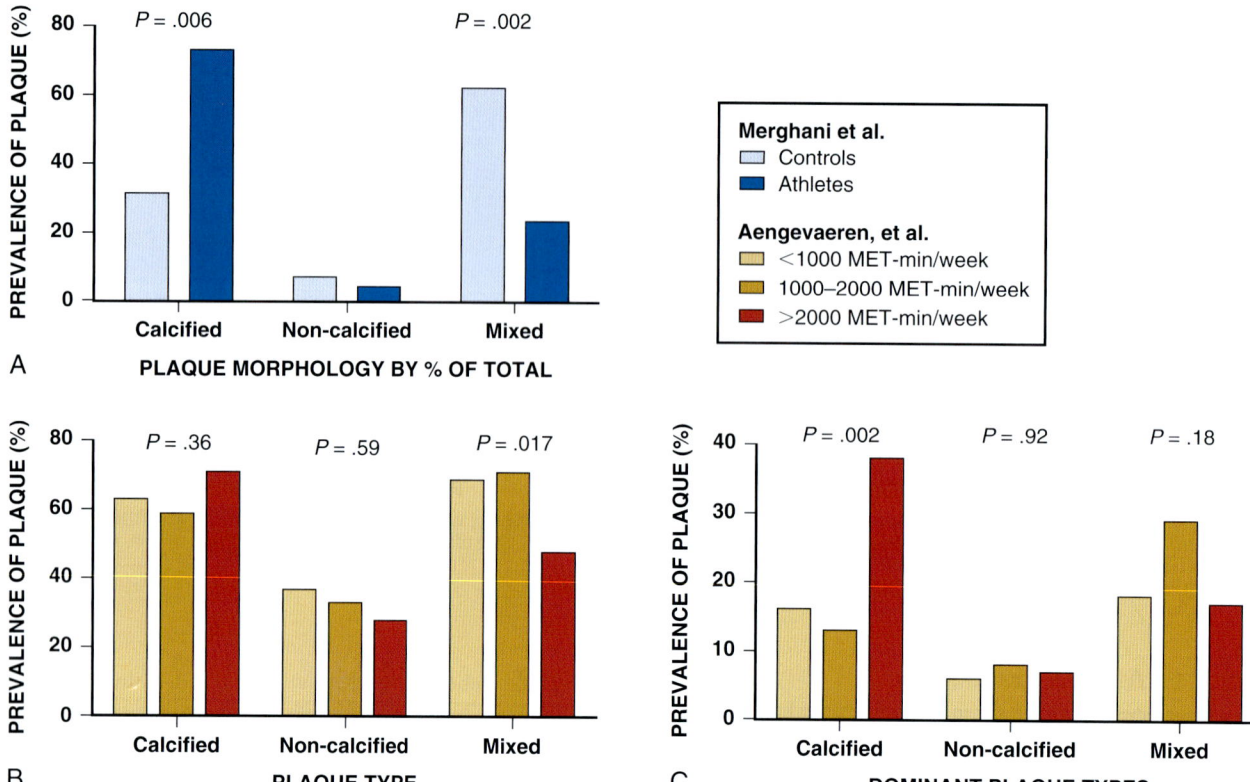

FIGURE 32.5 Coronary plaque characteristics in athletes. **A,** Plaque morphology of 99 plaques in athletes and 26 plaques in controls as reported by Merghani et al.[45] **B,** Percent of plaque morphology in athletes with plaque in each lifelong exercise group as reported by Aengevaeren et al.[48] **C,** Percent of athletes with only calcified, only non-calcified, and only mixed-type plaques. (From Aengevaeren VL, Mosterd A, Sharma S, et al. Exercise and coronary atherosclerosis: observations, explanations, relevance, and clinical management. Circulation. 2020;141:1338–1350.)

CONCLUSION

CV clinicians require a working knowledge of exercise physiology, the CV adaptations to exercise training, and the risks and benefits of exercise to advise and evaluate active patients appropriately. Clinicians should avoid overreacting to borderline findings detected on CV screening of asymptomatic athletes but should also avoid ignoring possible cardiac symptoms in active individuals. Sports cardiology has emerged as a subspecialty of cardiology, but general cardiologists can deal with many of the management issues and queries adequately if they understand the CV adaptations to exercise and the most common pathologic conditions that affect athletic patients.

REFERENCES

Historical Perspectives
1. Thompson PD. D Bruce Dill Historical lecture. Historical concepts of the athlete's heart. Med Sci Sports Exerc. 2004;36(3):363.
2. Eijsvogels TM, Fernandez AB, Thompson PD. Are there deleterious cardiac effects of acute and chronic endurance exercise? Physiol Rev. 2016;96(1):99–125.

Cardiovascular Response to Exercise and Effects of Habitual Exercise on CV Risk
3. Thompson PD, Baggish AL. Exercise and sports cardiology. In: Bonow RO, et al., ed. Braunwald's Heart Disease. 11th ed. Elsevier; 2016:1038–1045.
4. D'Souza A, Bucchi A, Anne BJ, et al. Exercise training reduces resting heart rate via downregulation of the funny channel HCN4. Nat Commun. 2014;5(1).
5. D'Souza A, Pearman CM, Wang Y, et al. Targeting miR-423-5p reverses exercise training-induced HCN4 channel remodeling and sinus bradycardia. Circ Res. 2017;121(9):1058–1068.
6. Noseworthy AP, Weiner JR, Kim JJ, et al. Early repolarization pattern in competitive athletes: clinical correlates and the effects of exercise training. Circ Arrhythm Electrophysiol. 2011;4(4):432–440.
7. Engel DJ, Schwartz A, Homma S. Athletic cardiac remodeling in US professional basketball players. JAMA Cardiol. 2016;1(1):80–87.
8. Kay S, Moore BM, Moore L, et al. Rugby player's aorta: Alarming prevalence of ascending aortic dilatation and effacement in elite rugby players. Heart Lung Circ. 2020;29(2):196–201.
9. Churchill TW, Groezinger E, Kim JH, et al. Association of ascending aortic dilatation and long-term endurance exercise among older masters-level athletes. JAMA Cardiol. 2020;5(5):522–531.
10. Churchill TW. Training-associated changes in ventricular volumes and function in elite female runners. Circ Cardiovasc Imaging. 2020;13(6):e010567.
11. Caruso MR, Garg L, Martinez MW. Cardiac imaging in the athlete: Shrinking the "gray zone". Curr Treat Options Cardiovasc Med. 2020;22(2):5.
12. Eijsvogels TM, Molossi S, Lee DC, et al. Exercise at the extremes: the amount of exercise to reduce cardiovascular events. J Am Coll Cardiol. 2016;67(3):316–329.
13. Anderson L, Oldridge N, Thompson DR, et al. Exercise-based cardiac rehabilitation for coronary heart disease: Cochrane systematic review and meta-analysis. J Am Coll Cardiol. 2016;67(1):1–12.
14. Piercy KL, Troiano RP, Ballard RM, et al. The physical activity guidelines for Americans. J Am Med Assoc. 2018;320(19):2020–2028.

Cardiovascular Risk of Exercise and Approach to Common Problems in Sports Cardiology
15. Franklin BA, Thompson PD, Al-Zaiti SS, et al. Exercise-related acute cardiovascular events and potential deleterious adaptations following long-term exercise training: Placing the risks into perspective-an update: a scientific statement from the American Heart Association. Circulation. 2020;141(13):e705–736.
16. Finocchiaro G, Papadakis M, Robertus JL, et al. Etiology of sudden death in sports: Insights from a United Kingdom regional registry. J Am Coll Cardiol. 2016;67(18):2108–2115.
17. Harmon KG, Asif IM, Maleszewski JJ, et al. Incidence, cause, and comparative frequency of sudden cardiac death in National Collegiate Athletic Association athletes: a decade in review. Circulation. 2015;132(1):10–19.
18. Ullal AJ, Abdelfattah RS, Ashley EA, Froelicher VF. Hypertrophic cardiomyopathy as a cause of sudden cardiac death in the young: a meta-analysis. Am J Med. 2016;129(5):486–496.e2.
19. Marijon E, Uy-Evanado A, Reinier K, et al. Sudden cardiac arrest during sports activity in middle age. Circulation. 2015;131(16):1384–1391.
20. Jayaraman R, Reinier K, Nair S, et al. Risk factors of sudden cardiac death in the young: Multiple-year community-wide assessment. Circulation. 2018;137(15):1561–1570.
21. Malhotra A, Dhutia H, Finocchiaro G, et al. Outcomes of cardiac screening in adolescent soccer players. N Engl J Med. 2018;379(6):524–534.
22. Taylor BA, Parducci PM, Zaleski AL, et al. Venous thromboemboli associated with acute aerobic exercise: a review of case report commonalities. Scand J Med Sci Sports. 2019;29(11):1749–1754.
23. Corrado D, Pelliccia A, Bjornstad HH, et al. Cardiovascular pre-participation screening of young competitive athletes for prevention of sudden death: Proposal for a common European protocol. Consensus statement of the study group of sport cardiology of the working group of cardiac rehabilitation and exercise physiology and the working group of myocardial and pericardial diseases of the European Society of Cardiology. Eur Heart J. 2005;26(5):516–524.
24. Thompson PD. The American approach to pre-participation screening. In: Thompson PD, Fernandez AB, eds. Exercise and Sports Cardiology—Volume 3: Exercise Risks, Cardiac Arrhythmia and Unusual Problems in Athletes. World Scientific Publishing Europe Ltd.; 2018:31–39.
25. Harmon KG, Suchsland MZ, Prutkin JM, et al. Comparison of cardiovascular screening in college athletes by history and physical Examination with and without an Electrocardiogram: Efficacy and Cost. Heart Rhythm. 2020;17(10):1649–1655.
26. Kaltman JR, Thompson PD, Lantos J, et al. Screening for sudden cardiac death in the young: report from a national heart, lung, and blood institute working group. Circulation. 2011;123(17):1911–1918.
27. Sheikh N, Papadakis M, Ghani S, et al. Comparison of electrocardiographic criteria for the detection of cardiac abnormalities in elite black and white athletes. Circulation. 2014;129(16):1637–1649.
28. Sharma S, Drezner JA, Baggish A, et al. International recommendations for electrocardiographic Interpretation in athletes. J Am Coll Cardiol. 2017;69:1057–1075.
29. Baggish AL, Battle RW, Beaver TA, et al. Recommendations on the use of multimodality cardiovascular imaging in young adult competitive athletes: a report from the American Society of Echocardiography in collaboration with the Society of Cardiovascular Computed Tomography and the Society for Cardiovascular Magnetic Resonance. J Am Soc Echocardiogr. 2020;33(5):523–549.
30. Mahowald MK, Fender EA, Prasad A, Nishimura RA. Exertional syncope in an athlete: the answer is in the history and exam. Circ Cardiovasc Imaging. 2020;13(4):e009992.

31. Christou GA, Christou KA, Kiortsis DN. Pathophysiology of noncardiac syncope in athletes. *Sports Med.* 2018;48(7):1561–1573.

Determining Athletic Eligibilty

32. Maron BJ, Udelson JE, Bonow RO, et al. Eligibility and disqualification recommendations for competitive athletes with cardiovascular abnormalities: Task force 3: Hypertrophic cardiomyopathy, arrhythmogenic right ventricular cardiomyopathy and other cardiomyopathies, and myocarditis: a scientific statement from the American Heart Association and American College of Cardiology. *Circulation.* 2015;132(22):e273–e280.
33. Baggish AL, Ackerman MJ, Putukian M, Lampert R. Shared decision making for athletes with cardiovascular disease: Practical considerations. *Curr Sports Med Rep.* 2019;18(3):76–81.
34. Noyes AM, Thompson PD. The effects of statins on exercise and physical activity. *J Clin Lipidol.* 2017;11(5):1134–1144.
35. Bonow RO, Nishimura RA, Thompson PD, Udelson JE. Eligibility and disqualification recommendations for competitive athletes with cardiovascular abnormalities: Task force 5: Valvular heart disease: a scientific statement from the American Heart Association and American College of Cardiology. *J Am Coll Cardiol.* 2015;66(21):2385–2392.
36. Braverman AC, Harris KM, Kovacs RJ, Maron BJ. Eligibility and disqualification recommendations for competitive athletes with cardiovascular abnormalities: Task force 7: aortic diseases, including Marfan syndrome: a scientific statement from the American Heart Association and American College of Cardiology. *J Am Coll Cardiol.* 2015;66(21):2398–2405.
37. Stavroulakis GA, George KP. Exercise-induced release of troponin. *Clin Cardiol.* 2020.
38. Aengevaeren VL, Hopman MTE, Thompson PD, et al. Exercise-induced cardiac troponin I increase and incident mortality and cardiovascular events. *Circulation.* 2019;140(10):804–814.
39. Thompson PD. Physical fitness, physical activity, exercise training, and atrial fibrillation: First the good news, then the bad. *J Am Coll Cardiol.* 2015;66(9):997–999.
40. Pathak RK, Elliott A, Middeldorp ME, et al. Impact of CARDIOrespiratory FITness on arrhythmia recurrence in obese individuals with atrial fibrillation: the CARDIO-FIT study. *J Am Coll Cardiol.* 2015;66(9):985–996.
41. Chung MK, et al. Lifestyle and risk factor modification for reduction of atrial fibrillation: a scientific statement from the American Heart Association. *Circulation.* 2020;141:e750–e772.
42. Svedberg N, Sundstrom J, James S, et al. Long-term incidence of atrial fibrillation and stroke among cross-country skiers. *Circulation.* 2019;140(11):910–920.
43. Aengevaeren VL, Mosterd A, Sharma S, et al. Exercise and coronary atherosclerosis: Observations, explanations, relevance, and clinical management. *Circulation.* 2020;141(16):1338–1350.
44. Lin J, DeLuca JR, Lu MT, et al. Extreme endurance exercise and progressive coronary artery disease. *J Am Coll Cardiol.* 2017;70(2):293–295.
45. Merghani A, Maestrini V, Rosmini S, et al. Prevalence of subclinical coronary artery disease in masters endurance athletes with a low atherosclerotic risk profile. *Circulation.* 2017;136(2):126–137.
46. van de Schoor FR, Aengevaeren VL, Hopman MT, et al. Myocardial fibrosis in athletes. *Mayo Clin Proc.* 2016;91(11):1617–1631.
47. James CA, Calkins H. Arrhythmogenic right ventricular cardiomyopathy: Progress toward personalized management. *Ann Rev Med.* 2020;70:1–18.
48. Aengevaeren VL, Mosterd A, Braber TL, et al. Relationship between lifelong exercise volume and coronary atherosclerosis in athletes. *Circulation.* 2017;136(2):138–148.

33 Comprehensive Cardiac Rehabilitation

RANDAL JAY THOMAS

EVOLUTION OF CARDIAC REHABILITATION, 588

ELEMENTS OF CARDIAC REHABILITATION PROGRAMS, 588
Structural Elements, 588

VALUE OF CARDIAC REHABILITATION, 589
Recovery from a Cardiovascular Disease Event, 589
Physiologic Improvements, 589

Cardiovascular Disease Risk Factor Control, 590
Cardiovascular Events, 590
Safety of Cardiac Rehabilitation, 590
Cost-Effectiveness of Cardiac Rehabilitation, 590

FUTURE DIRECTIONS FOR CARDIAC REHABILITATION, 591
Efforts to Reduce the Cardiac Rehabilitation Participation Gap, 591

Additional Patient Groups, 591
Improving the Cost-Effectiveness of Cardiac Rehabilitation, 591

SUMMARY, 591

CLASSIC REFERENCES, 591

REFERENCES, 591

For the past decades, a number of secondary preventive measures have been shown to help improve health and reduce recurrent cardiovascular events in individuals with known cardiovascular disease (CVD). Unfortunately, the delivery of these evidence-based therapies has been suboptimal in clinical practice. In a national study, only 50% of patients met goals for blood pressure control, 25% for physical activity, and 18% for lipid numbers.[1]

To help bridge gaps in the delivery of preventive therapies to patients with chronic health conditions like CVD, chronic care management principles have been developed, studied, and refined since the 1990s. This model seeks to coordinate health care and community resources to implement appropriate patient-centered, evidence-based treatment strategies, such as standardized protocols and case-management systems of care.[2]

A specific example of such an approach is cardiac rehabilitation (CR), a multidisciplinary, systematic approach to delivering evidence-based and personalized care management strategies to patients with known CVD. Despite its benefits, the scope of CR has been limited by a combination of patient, provider, health system, and societal barriers. Consequently, it can be reasonably argued that the gap in CR participation is one of the largest in the quality of care in cardiovascular medicine today. This chapter reviews the past and current context of CR, as well as explores future directions aimed at expanding its scope and impact.

EVOLUTION OF CARDIAC REHABILITATION

The roots of CR can be traced to the 1950s with the development of hospital-based regimens that were aimed at helping patients recover after a myocardial infarction (MI) event. At that time, prolonged bed rest was thought to help reduce stress and strain as the patient recovers. Eventually in-patient physical activity was found to be safe and helpful for patients recovering from the negative effects of MI as well as prolonged bed rest.

Additional studies in the outpatient CR setting involving patients recovering from a cardiac event showed the benefits of physical activity on functional capacity and quality of life. As more and more evidence was obtained in the 1980s and 1990s about the benefits of lifestyle and medication, CR began to evolve beyond exercise therapy alone as it involved effective lifestyle and medication. Today, CR programs are designed to be centers of secondary CVD prevention, applying evidence-based and guideline-directed medical therapies of known benefit with the help of a multidisciplinary team.

Early models of CR were offered only to patients recovering from MI, but as more evidence accumulated in other patient groups, the scope of the indications for CR expanded. The United States currently has seven patient groups for which CR is recommended in clinical practice guidelines and covered by the Centers for Medicare and Medicaid Services (CMS), as well as commercial insurance providers (Table 33.1). Those indications include: MI, percutaneous coronary intervention (PCI), coronary artery bypass graft surgery (CABG), stable angina, heart valve repair/replacement, heart transplantation, and heart failure with reduced ejection fraction (HFrEF). In addition, supervised exercise training is covered by CMS for patients with symptomatic peripheral arterial disease of the lower extremities (claudication).

ELEMENTS OF CARDIAC REHABILITATION PROGRAMS

Standards of practice for CR includes the following structural and procedural elements:

Structural Elements
Multidisciplinary Team
The CR care team is comprised of a multidisciplinary team of health care professionals including a physician medical director who oversees the safety and effectiveness of the CR program elements, and a team composed of nurses, exercise physiologists, physical therapists, dietitians, psychologists, social workers, and other professionals. The CR team members have appropriate training, skills, and certification to:
- Administer lifestyle therapies
- Assess and manage the underlying cardiovascular risk of a patient
- Coordinate the cardiovascular care for a patient's specific cardiovascular condition
- Identify and refer patients for appropriate care of their comorbid conditions
- Prevent and manage medical complications and emergencies that may occur during the course of a patient's CR program

Facilities, Equipment, and Technology Tools
Center-based CR programs utilize dedicated space, equipment, and technology tools that are appropriate for patient assessments, education and counseling, exercise training, and supervision. ECG telemetry can be used with higher-risk patients for dangerous arrhythmias

during CR. Clinical databases serve an important role in documenting patient care activities and outcomes, quality improvement, or research activities.

PROCESS ELEMENTS
Referral and Enrollment of Eligible Patients
Current insurance coverage policies for CR in the United States require that eligible patients be referred to a center-based CR program by a physician. A significant portion of patients are not referred to CR, and a significant number of those who are referred to CR do not enroll and participate in CR. These gaps occur for a variety of reasons (patient-, provider-, health-system- and community-based barriers). Systematic approaches to guide patient enrollment will overcome those barriers and promote greater participation of CR (Fig. 33.1).[3,4]

Patient Assessments
Patients undergo clinical assessments as they begin an outpatient CR program and at key checkpoints during the program. These assessments include a safety evaluation for high-risk cardiovascular conditions (e.g., unstable symptoms), a screening evaluation for comorbid conditions that may require additional evaluation and/or treatment (such as depression, diabetes), and an evaluation of clinical factors (such as functional capacity) that will be used by the CR staff and patients to formulate the individualized treatment plan (ITP), and to measure patient progress and outcomes.

Patient Care Activities. For center-based CR programs, patients ideally attend 36 in-person CR sessions over a period of 12 weeks or more, usually attending three sessions per week. With the help of the CR staff, the patient develops a patient-centered ITP that is followed in the CR center and also at home. The ITP includes patient actions that help the patient implement guideline-directed medical therapy and also appropriate lifestyle therapies, including physical activity and exercise training, nutritional therapy, smoking/tobacco cessation (if indicated), and psychological health management. The CR staff members review the ITP with patients regularly throughout their time in CR and reinforce the patient's goals with behavioral modification strategies and self-management skills.

Staff members educate patients about management of CVD and related symptoms. The CR staff members help coordinate a patient's CVD care with members of their health care team to assure that patients are receiving appropriate medications, that their CVD risk factors are under optimal control, and that any comorbid conditions are being addressed.

Quality Improvement Strategies. Quality improvement processes designed to assess adherence to appropriate clinical practice guidelines and performance measures, are an integral part of CR programs, to help meet standards for CR program certification by national organizations and to promote high-quality patient care and outcomes.

TABLE 33.1 Current Indications for Cardiac Rehabilitation in the United States

Indications
Myocardial infarction
Coronary artery bypass graft surgery
Percutaneous coronary intervention
Stable angina
Heart valve repair/replacement
Heart transplantation
Heart failure with reduced ejection fraction
*Peripheral artery disease with claudication

*Currently indicated for supervised exercise training.

VALUE OF CARDIAC REHABILITATION

An expanding body of evidence supports the value of CR, showing beneficial clinical, safety, and cost-benefit outcomes related to CR, including the following:

Recovery from a Cardiovascular Disease Event
Physical and psychological recovery after a CVD are enhanced for patients who participate in outpatient CR. Functional capacity improves 15% to 25% in CR participants compared to non-CR participants. Likewise, CR participation helps to significantly improve health-related quality of life and other measures of psychological health. Exercise training helps improve symptoms of depression, a common diagnosis in patients recovering from a CVD event.[5]

Physiologic Improvements (see Chapter 32)
Exercise training, nutritional therapy, weight loss, smoking cessation, stress management, CVD risk factor control, and improved adherence to preventive medications yield beneficial physiologic changes that reduce cardiovascular risk. Exercise training itself produces a number of beneficial physiologic adaptations including an increase in peak cardiopulmonary oxygen uptake and myocardial oxygen supply, a decrease in myocardial oxygen demand, and an improvement in endothelial function.[6]

Patients with HFrEF who undergo exercise training in CR also experience clinically meaningful improvements symptoms, functional capacity, hospital readmission rates, and health-related quality of life.[7] They experience improvements in cardiopulmonary efficiency and function, in skeletal muscle oxygen transport and utilization, and in various neurovascular mechanisms, such as an increase in heart rate variability, baroreceptor sensitivity, and a reduction neurohumoral factors.[8]

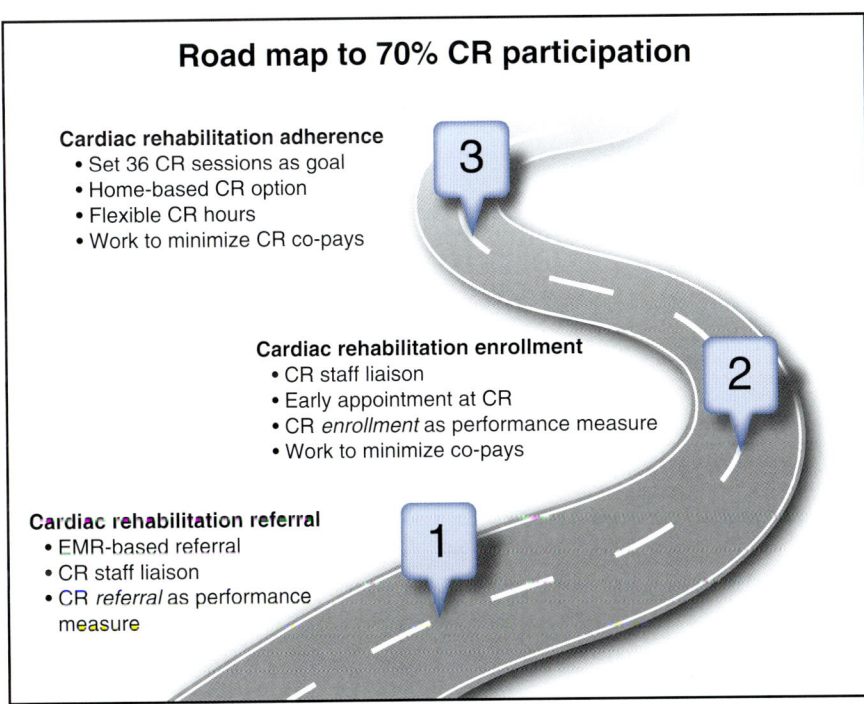

FIGURE 33.1 Evidence-based strategies to improve cardiac rehabilitation (CR) participation from current levels (20%) to more optimal levels (70%). (From Ades PA, Keteyian SJ, Wright JS, et al. Increasing cardiac rehabilitation participation from 20% to 70%: a road map from the Million Hearts Cardiac Rehabilitation Collaborative. Mayo Clin Proc. 2017;92:234–242.)

Cardiovascular Disease Risk Factor Control

Patients recovering from a CVD event who participate in CR are more likely to have their risk factors controlled than those who do not participate. This improved control is probably related to several factors related to CR participation, including the systematic use of protocols and other strategies to optimize the prescription of and adherence to guideline-directed lifestyle and medical therapies.

Cardiovascular Events

Hospital Readmission

Unplanned readmissions to the hospital several months following a CVD event are unwanted but common occurrences. While not all hospital readmissions are preventable, readmission rates are used as quality metrics for patient care. Participation in CR has been associated with 25% to 30% reduction in hospital readmission (both CVD and non-CVD readmissions) for patients recovering from a CVD event.[9]

Fatal and Non-Fatal Events

Longer-term randomized and observational studies have shown 20% to 45% reductions in all-cause and cardiovascular mortality in CR participants. One large study of Medicare patients found a dose-response effect between CR participation and mortality rates. A recent study of over 80,000 patients in the Netherlands found a 32% reduction in all-cause mortality in CR participants compared to non-CR participants (Fig. 33.2).[10] Most all-cause studies have been carried out in patients with coronary artery disease (i.e., MI, PCI, and/or coronary artery bypass surgery). However, in recent years studies have also reported a reduction in all-cause mortality associated with CR participation in patients recovering from heart valve repair/replacement[11] or heart transplantation.[12] Results of studies of the association between CR participation and subsequent MI or revascularization are unclear.

A few recent systematic reviews of randomized, controlled trials of CR have raised questions about the impact of CR on all-cause mortality, but these reviews are limited by their inclusion of several pivotal studies of shorter duration and that appear to have carried out ineffective CR intervention were not consistent with current CR standards of practice. Since the preponderance of evidence shows mortality benefit from CR participation, future randomized studies will need to compare outcomes of new models of CR to those of center-based cardiac rehabilitation (CBCR), the current standard of care (i.e., "usual care").

Safety of Cardiac Rehabilitation

Despite the inclusion of patients with relatively high CVD risk in CR programs and the use of exercise training as part of the program, the use of standardized safety protocols has helped CR programs maintain an excellent safety record, reporting very low rates of serious events (including in-center cardiac arrest, MI, or death). One study involving 65 CR centers reported one cardiac arrest, and no MI or deaths during 1.3 million patient-hours of CR.

Cost-Effectiveness of Cardiac Rehabilitation

The cost-benefit of CR has generally been reported to be favorable in the limited published studies on this topic. In a study from Canada, high levels of CR participation were associated with a significantly lower level of medical expenses per patient per year, with a yearly savings per patient of approximately $2920 (Canadian) or more in the CR participants compared to the non-CR participants (Fig. 33.3).[13] A systematic review involving 19 studies of the cost-benefits of CR showed that CR was cost-effective compared to non-CR with incremental cost-effectiveness ratios ranging from $1065 to $71,755 per quality-adjusted life-year.[14]

LIMITATIONS AND POTENTIAL SOLUTIONS TO CURRENT CARDIAC REHABILITATION MODELS

Key limitations to CR participation and their possible solutions include:

Low Patient Referral, Enrollment, and Participation Rates

Gaps in CR participation have been documented throughout the United States in all patient sub-groups, but the gap is even more notable in groups at highest risk for poor CVD outcomes (including in women, individuals older than 65 years of age, and individuals from racial/ethnic minority groups).[15]

Potential Solutions. A number of evidence-based solutions to barriers of CR participation are shown in Figure 33.1, and include such strategies as systematic CR referral and enrollment processes, and patient navigators to help patients enroll in CR even before leaving the hospital, to name a few. Centers that incorporate these solutions have reported significantly higher CR participation than the national average (60% to 70% versus 20% to 25%). The impact of implementing these strategies nationally and raising the CR participation rate to 70% would be to save an estimated 25,000 lives and to avoid 180,000 hospitalizations in the United States per year.[3] A study from Canada showed that the use of an automatic CR referral systematic combined with a patient navigator had significantly higher rates of CR referral (85% versus 32%, p < 0.05), and CR enrollment compared to usual care (78% vs. 29%, P < 0.05). Various types of incentives (monetary and nonmonetary) have been studied as possible ways to improve patient participation in CR, with initial results that are promising.

Lack of Sufficient Cardiac Rehabilitation Program Capacity

If all of the approximately 2500 CR programs in the United States were filled to maximum capacity, it is estimated that those programs would have the capacity to provide CR to less than half of the patients eligible for CR each year. This means that efforts to improve CR referral and enrollment alone would not be sufficient to achieve high rates of CR participation. Expansion of CR program capacity is therefore of great need.

Potential Solutions. To increase the capacity of CR services, it will be necessary to increase the capacity of existing CR centers, build new CR centers, and/or develop additional CR delivery models (community-based programs and home-based telehealth programs) that will effectively expand the scope and capacity of CR.

Longer-Term Maintenance of Cardiac Rehabilitation

While significant longer-term benefits accrue from the 12- to 18-week period of post-hospital CR, longer-term adherence to lifestyle and medical therapies after "graduation" from early outpatient CR is suboptimal for many patients.

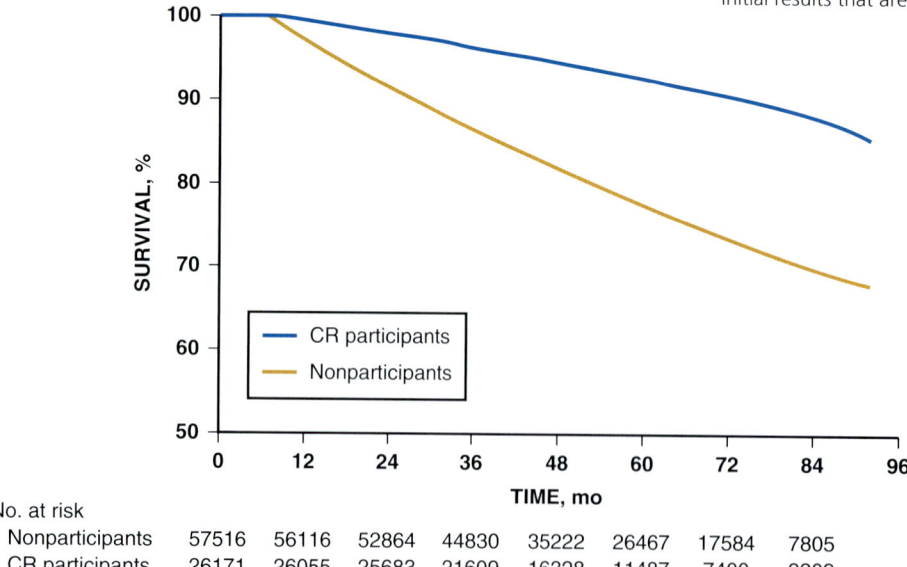

FIGURE 33.2 Event-free survival comparison for patients eligible for CR who did and who did not participate in CR (log-rank test comparing curves, P < 0.001 for overall survival). (From Eijsvogels TMH, Maessen MFH, Bakker EA, et al. Association of cardiac rehabilitation with all-cause mortality among patients with cardiovascular disease in the Netherlands. *JAMA Netw Open.* 2020;3:e2011686.)

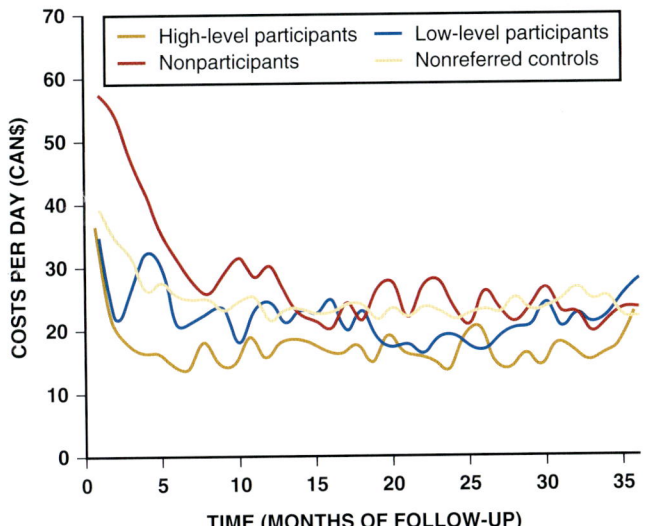

FIGURE 33.3 Health service utilization costs per patient per day in 36 months of follow-up, involving four groups of patients eligible for cardiac rehabilitation (CR): (1) patients not referred to CR, (2) patients referred to CR but who did not participate, (3) patients referred to CR and who participated in a low level of sessions, and (4) patients referred to CR and who participated in high level of sessions. (From Alter DA, Yu B, Bajaj RR, et al. Relationship between cardiac rehabilitation participation and health service expenditures within a universal health care system. *Mayo Clin Proc.* 2017;92:500–511.)

TABLE 33.2 Elements of Cardiac Rehabilitation

STRUCTURAL ELEMENTS	PROCESS ELEMENTS
Multidisciplinary team	Referral and enrollment of eligible patients
Facilities	Patient assessments
Equipment	Patient care activities
Technology tools	Quality of care strategies

Potential Solutions. There is a great need to identify more effective methods to optimize longer-term adherence to lifestyle and medical therapies than are currently utilized. Longer-term CR maintenance programs are offered in many settings and have been shown to help patients maintain their secondary CVD preventive therapies over time. In addition, social support groups, either in-person or virtual, and wearable devices with built-in-goal setting, feedback, and reminder options appear to be fruitful strategies to help improve longer-term maintenance of secondary CVD preventive efforts.

FUTURE DIRECTIONS FOR CARDIAC REHABILITATION

Since its inception over 60 years ago, CR has continually evolved to remain relevant and important in the spectrum of cardiovascular medicine. It will continue to remain relevant and important in the future as it focuses on the following directions:

Efforts to Reduce the Cardiac Rehabilitation Participation Gap

The need to reduce the gap in CR participation will continue into the future as a primary focus for clinical, research, and policy work. In addition, researchers will continue to explore new and better intervention strategies in CR to optimize patient receipt and adherence to guideline-directed lifestyle and medical therapies. Significant opportunities exist for new models of delivery to expand the capacity and reach of CR, especially into populations that are most underserved by current CR models, including women, individuals older than 65 years of age, and individuals from underserved racial and ethnic minority groups. Technologic developments (including wearable monitors, artificial intelligence-guided clinical tools, and improved patient-provider communication options) will enhance CR beyond the walls of CR centers.

Advances in options for home-based CR or non-center-based CR will likely play a prominent role in CR practice in the future. Many countries around the world currently utilize home-based CR, and its use gaining grounds in the United States. In home-based CR, staff members are linked to patients through virtual care and communication platforms, in real time (synchronous) or non-real-time (asynchronous) models. The same elements are utilized in home-based CR as in center-based CR (see Table 33.2). Short-term outcomes in low- to moderate-risk patients are similar in studies of home-based versus center-based CR, with some evidence of higher patient participation rates in home-based than in center-based CR. However, until additional longer-term research is available (showing similar or greater reductions in mortality and morbidity rates with home-based CR as with center-based CR), center-based programs will remain the first line of CR therapy, with home-based CR being used as an adjunct to center-based CR and/or as a secondary option for patients who are not able to participate in center-based CR.[16]

Additional Patient Groups

The future will also bring a continuing expansion of CR in the care of additional patient groups (patients with cardio-oncology disorders,[17] heart failure with preserved ejection fraction, atrial fibrillation,[18] or other chronic cardiovascular and noncardiovascular conditions) that could potentially benefit from system-based care management approaches such as CR.

Improving the Cost-Effectiveness of Cardiac Rehabilitation

Further research is needed to document the cost-effectiveness of CR (the cost-effectiveness of various CR models and elements). In addition, there is a need to provide affordable CR services worldwide, especially in areas with limited resources.[19] This will likely require a merging of simpler, lower-cost delivery models (home-based CR) with technology tools that can help improve efficiencies and effectiveness of CR (artificial intelligence assisted case management platforms).[20]

SUMMARY

CR is an evolving, evidence-based, valuable service for patients recovering from a CVD event. Participation in CR is cost-effective and is associated with a number of clinical benefits. The percentage of eligible patients who participate in CR is suboptimal, but strategies exist to improve that gap in participation. New directions, including an increased focus on home-based CR and the incorporation of new technology tools, will help expand the reach of CR and its beneficial impact on important patient outcomes.

CLASSIC REFERENCES

Grace SL, Russell KL, Reid RD, et al. Effect of cardiac rehabilitation referral strategies on utilization rates: a prospective, controlled study. *Arch Intern Med.* 2011;171:235–241.

Giannuzzi P, Temporelli PL, Marchioli R, et al. Global secondary prevention strategies to limit event recurrence after myocardial infarction: results of the GOSPEL study, a multicenter, randomized controlled trial from the Italian cardiac rehabilitation network. *Arch Intern Med.* 2008;168:2194–2204.

Hammill BG, Curtis LH, Schulman, Whellan DJ. Relationship between cardiac rehabilitation and long-term risks of death and myocardial infarction among elderly medicare beneficiaries. *Circulation.* 2010;121:63–70.

Pavy B, Iliou MC, Meurin P, et al. Safety of exercise training for cardiac patients: results of the French registry of complications during cardiac rehabilitation. *Arch Intern Med.* 2006;166:2329–2334.

Wagner EH, Austin BT, Von Korff M. Improving outcomes in chronic illness. *Manag Care Q.* 1996;4:12–25.

REFERENCES
Elements of Cardiac Rehabilitation

1. Brown TM, Voeks JH, Bittner V, et al. Achievement of optimal medical therapy goals for U.S. adults with coronary artery disease: results from the REGARDS Study (REasons for Geographic and Racial Differences in Stroke). *J Am Coll Cardiol.* 2014;63:1626–1633.

2. Schwal JD, McKee M, Huffman MD, Yusuf S. Resource effective strategies to prevent and treat cardiovascular disease. *Circulation*. 2016;133:742–755.
3. Ades PA, Keteyian SJ, Wright JS, et al. Increasing cardiac rehabilitation participation from 20% to 70%: a road map from the Million Hearts Cardiac Rehabilitation Collaborative. *Mayo Clin Proc*. 2017;92:234–242.
4. Candelaria D, Randall S, Ladek L, Gallagher R. Health-related quality of life and exercise-based cardiac rehabilitation in contemporary acute coronary syndrome patients: a systematic review and meta-analysis. *Qual Life Res*. 2020;29:579–592.

Value of Cardiac Rehabilitation

5. Belvederi Murri M, Ekkekakis P, Magagnoli M, et al. Physical exercise in major depression: reducing the mortality gap while improving clinical outcomes. *Front Psychiatry*. 2018;9:762.
6. Nystoriak MA, Bhatnagar A. Cardiovascular effects and benefits of exercise. *Front Cardiovasc Med*. 2018;5:135.
7. Taylor RS, Long L, Mordi IR, et al. Exercise-based rehabilitation for heart failure: cochrane systematic review, meta-analysis, and trial sequential analysis. *JACC Heart Fail*. 2019;7:691–705.
8. Fleg JL, Cooper LS, Borlaug BA, et al. Exercise training as therapy for heart failure: current status and future directions. *Circ Heart Fail*. 2015;8:209–220.
9. Dunlay SM, Pack QR, Thomas RJ, et al. Participation in cardiac rehabilitation, readmissions, and death after acute myocardial infarction. *Am J Med*. 2014;127:538–546.
10. Eijsvogels TMH, Maessen MFH, Bakker EA, et al. Association of cardiac rehabilitation with all-cause mortality among patients with cardiovascular disease in the Netherlands. *JAMA Netw Open*. 2020;3:e2011686.
11. Patel DK, Duncan MS, Shah AS, et al. Association of cardiac rehabilitation with decreased hospitalization and mortality risk after cardiac valve surgery. *JAMA Cardiol*. 2019;4:1250–1259.
12. Bachmann JM, Shah AS, Duncan MS, et al. Cardiac rehabilitation and readmissions after heart transplantation. *J Heart Lung Transplant*. 2018;37:467–476.
13. Alter DA, Yu B, Bajaj RR, Oh PI. Relationship between cardiac rehabilitation participation and health service expenditures within a universal health care system. *Mayo Clin Proc*. 2017;92:500–511.
14. Shields GE, Wells A, Doherty P, et al. Cost-effectiveness of cardiac rehabilitation: a systematic review. *Heart*. 2018;104:1403–1410.

Limitations, Potential Solutions and Future Directions

15. Li S, Fonarow GC, Mukamal K, et al. Sex and racial disparities in cardiac rehabilitation referral at hospital discharge and gaps in long-term mortality. *J Am Heart Assoc*. 2018;7.
16. Thomas RJ, Beatty AL, Beckie TM, et al. Home-based cardiac rehabilitation: a scientific statement from the American Association of Cardiovascular and Pulmonary Rehabilitation, the American Heart Association, and the American College of Cardiology. *Circulation*. 2019;140:e69–e89.
17. Gilchrist SC, Barac A, Ades PA, et al. Cardio-oncology rehabilitation to manage cardiovascular outcomes in cancer patients and survivors: a scientific statement from the American Heart Association. *Circulation*. 2019;139:e997–e1012.
18. Risom SS, Zwisler AD, Sibilitz KL, et al. Cardiac rehabilitation for patients treated for atrial fibrillation with ablation has long-term effects: 12-and 24-month follow-up results from the randomized CopenHeartRFA trial. *Arch Phys Med Rehabil*. 2020;101:1866–1877.
19. Grace SL, Turk-Adawi KI, Contractor A, et al. Cardiac rehabilitation delivery model for low-resource settings. *Heart*. 2016;102:1449–1455.
20. Gevaert AB, Adams V, Bahls M, et al. Towards a personalised approach in exercise-based cardiovascular rehabilitation: how can translational research help? A 'call to action' from the section on secondary prevention and cardiac rehabilitation of the European Association of Preventive Cardiology. *Eur J Prev Cardiol*. 2020;27:1369–1385.

34 Integrative Approaches to the Management of Patients with Heart Disease

STEPHEN DEVRIES

INTEGRATIVE CARDIOLOGY, 593
Utilization of Additional Therapies, 593
Why Is Integrative Cardiology Important?, 593
Need for Interprofessional Collaboration, 594

INTEGRATIVE STRATEGIES FOR SPECIFIC CARDIAC CONDITIONS, 594

Ischemic Heart Disease, 594
Hypertension, 595
Dyslipidemia, 595
Heart Failure, 596
Arrhythmias, 596

INTEGRATIVE SELF-CARE FOR THE CARDIOLOGIST, 597
CONCLUSION, 597
REFERENCES, 597

INTEGRATIVE CARDIOLOGY

Integrative cardiology is a philosophy of care rather than a description of a discrete set of practices, with a particular focus on prevention of disease and an emphasis on patient well-being and personal agency. Completely inclusive of guideline-based medical therapy, integrative cardiology seeks to empower patients to the greatest degree possible with the collaborative development of health goals and therapeutic plans (Fig. 34.1).

Utilization of Additional Therapies

In addition to a strong emphasis on nutrition and lifestyle-based interventions, integrative cardiology includes therapeutic modalities not typically used in conventional cardiac care. Examples include interventions focused on the connection between the mind and heart (i.e., breathing exercises, meditation, biofeedback, and guided imagery), acupuncture, and a select group of evidence-based over-the-counter products.

Cardiologists in particular need to be aware of these therapies frequently utilized by cardiac patients—often without disclosure of their use. Data from the 2017 National Health Interview Survey of over 26,000 adults documented that 31.8% of surveyed individuals with cardiovascular disease have used at least one form of "complementary" medicine within the previous 12 months.[1] The survey also found that patients who utilize complementary approaches do so as an adjunct rather than a replacement for conventional care—presumably to fill a gap perceived by the patient to be deficient or absent in usual care. Factors that predicted higher utilization of complementary therapies include female gender and higher levels of education, income, and health literacy.

Why Is Integrative Cardiology Important?

Integrative cardiology is important because it addresses unmet needs in conventional care.

A report from the Centers for Disease Control reveals that after years of consistent decline, the death rate from cardiovascular disease has begun to plateau.[2] This ebb in progress, despite advances in pharmacologic and procedural therapeutics, is largely attributed to unchecked increases in the prevalence of obesity and diabetes—diseases largely preventable through dietary intervention.

Paradoxically, despite the high burden of cardiovascular diseases rooted in diet and lifestyle, nutrition remains poorly emphasized in cardiology training and practice.[3] For example, in the current 56-page document from the Accreditation Council for Graduate Medical Education that contains very detailed procedural specifications for fellowship training in cardiovascular disease, there remains no requirement for nutrition education.[4] Accordingly, a recent survey found that 90% of cardiologists reported receiving minimal or no nutrition education in their training.[5] An integrative approach seeks to address this deficiency in both education and practice by highlighting nutrition and lifestyle as integral components of cardiac care.

One of the tenets of integrative cardiology is an emphasis on patient empowerment and shared decision making. Apart from the clear right of patients to determine their health priorities and goals, there is substantial evidence that patients who actively engage in decision making and self-care have greater insight into their condition and are more likely to adhere to a mutually agreed course of treatment. Recent Medicare policy has transformed shared decision making from a best practice to a payment necessity for select cardiac intervention, including implantation of cardioverter-defibrillators and left atrial appendage closure devices. Although likely fiscally driven initiatives, these policy changes are consistent with the patient-centered focus characteristic of integrative cardiology.

ASSOCIATED TREATMENT MODALITIES
Nutrition

Nutritional interventions are a foundation of integrative cardiac care for both the prevention and treatment of cardiovascular disease (see Chapter 29). Although current guidelines for cardiac care emphasize the primacy of diet and lifestyle interventions, the data show that dietary counseling currently plays a minimal role in cardiology practice.[5]

Mind/Body

In recognition of the strong influence of thoughts and emotional state on cardiovascular health, an integrative approach draws on this connection as a potential input for therapeutic intervention. In addition to the more traditional cognitive behavioral therapy and medication, modalities that might be recommended in an integrative model include meditation, breathing exercises, yoga, biofeedback, healing touch, and Reiki.

Acupuncture

Although acupuncture is most commonly used in the treatment of musculoskeletal pain, emerging data show promise for acupuncture to be used as adjunctive treatment for a range of cardiovascular conditions including hypertension.

Supplements/Botanicals

Integrative cardiology is open to the use of evidence-based supplements and botanicals, while rejecting those that have been disproven. Many physicians are understandably reluctant to consider the use of over-the-counter products, not only because of questions of efficacy, but also due to concerns regarding purity and safety. In recognition of

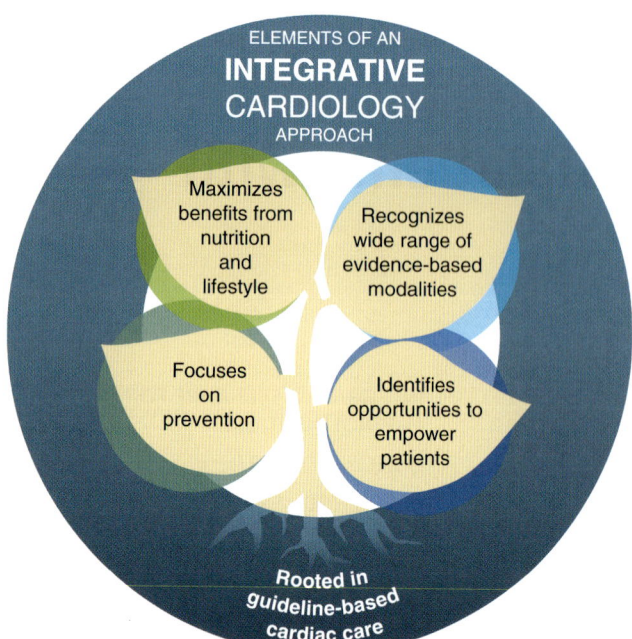

FIGURE 34.1 Key elements of an integrative cardiology approach.

TABLE 34.1 Resources for Evaluation of Supplements

- ConsumerLab.com
  http://www.ConsumerLab.com
- Natural Medicines Database
  http://www.naturaldatabase.com/
- National Institute of Health Office of Dietary Supplements
  http://ods.od.nih.gov
- U.S. National Library of Medicine MedlinePlus
  https://medlineplus.gov/druginfo/herb_All.html

these significant caveats, it is incumbent upon the cardiologist to be knowledgeable about the supplements most commonly used by cardiac patients and, most importantly, to be aware of trusted resources—as summarized in this chapter—that permit critical evaluation of the available science surrounding these compounds.

Although it is considered good medical practice to document all over-the-counter products taken by patients, this information has limited value if clinicians are unaware of the composition of these supplements and lack sufficient knowledge to credibly evaluate their potential benefits, risks, and interactions with medication.

Fortunately, several excellent resources are available to help clinicians learn about the science of supplements (Table 34.1), including the National Institutes of Health (NIH) Office of Dietary Supplements (http://ods.od.nih.gov), and a service of the U.S. National Library of Medicine, MedlinePlus (https://medlineplus.gov/druginfo/herb_All.html). The Natural Medicines Database (http://www.naturaldatabase.com/) is an independent group that provides an extensive fee-based literature review and assessment of the potential benefits and risks of a wide range of supplements. They also offer handouts to patients that summarize key facts in easy-to-understand language.

A valuable resource for clinicians to evaluate the chemical composition and purity of individual brands of supplements is ConsumerLab.com (http://www.ConsumerLab.com), a group that performs independent laboratory analyses on a wide range of commonly available products and offers detailed information on its web site for an annual fee. In addition, the scientific nonprofit US Pharmacopeial Convention has established quality standards recognized by a label that signifies compliance with these standards.

Need for Interprofessional Collaboration

Communication between cardiologists and allied health professionals, including those not typically associated with conventional medical care, has historically been challenging. Despite differences in language and perspectives, mutual respect and open communication between all health professionals, conventional and alternative, is essential for coordination of care and optimal outcomes.

INTEGRATIVE STRATEGIES FOR SPECIFIC CARDIAC CONDITIONS

The foundation of integrative cardiology is guideline-based therapy. In the following section, a select group of evidence-based approaches not often utilized in conventional management are described. These tools, added to guideline-based therapy, may extend its benefits, and provide additional opportunities to engage and empower patients.

Ischemic Heart Disease (See Chapter 40)
Nutrition
A recent analysis reveals that fully 45% of all cardiometabolic deaths are diet-related.[6] The foundational role of nutrition and lifestyle has been codified in the 2018 AHA/ACC Guideline on the Management of Blood Cholesterol, in which lifestyle interventions are positioned at the very apex of flowcharts for both primary and secondary prevention of atherosclerotic cardiovascular disease.[7]

Among the components of a cardioprotective diet, green leafy vegetables (including spinach and kale) appear to be especially beneficial. Combined data from the Nurses' Health Study and Health Professionals Follow-Up Study showed that each daily serving of green leafy vegetables significantly reduced the risk of coronary disease by 17% and ischemic stroke by 24%.[8]

Anthocyanins are dietary flavonoids that enhance endothelial function and have antioxidant and antihypertensive properties. Foods rich in anthocyanins, especially blueberries and strawberries, are strongly linked to cardiac health. During an 18-year follow-up of the Nurses' Health Study II that included 93,600 women, intake of four or more servings of blueberries and strawberries was associated with a 34% decreased risk of myocardial infarction.[9]

Nut consumption has consistently been found to reduce the risk of heart disease and improve longevity. The health-promoting properties of nuts are likely related to their rich content of magnesium, sterols, Vitamin E, fiber, and both polyunsaturated and monounsaturated fats. In addition to these cardioprotective nutrients, newer data suggest nuts have the added benefit of antiinflammatory properties and a beneficial impact on the gut microbiome.[10]

Mind/Heart Connection
There is no more vivid example of the connection between the mind and heart than Takotsubo syndrome, a condition of acute and severe left ventricular failure precipitated by psychological trauma (see Chapter 52). This syndrome is dramatic in its presentation and is one of the many manifestations of stress and emotional state on cardiac health. Not unexpectedly, the incidence of Takotsubo's cardiomyopathy significantly increased during the COVID-19 pandemic.[11]

Meditation
The link between mind and heart can be harnessed for prevention of ischemic heart disease. In a randomized, controlled study of meditation and conventional cardiac care in 201 individuals with coronary disease, the meditation group experienced a 48% (p= 0.025) reduced risk of a composite endpoint including all-cause mortality, myocardial infarction, and stroke.[12] The underlying mechanism of benefit is unclear but likely includes a favorable effect on blood pressure with possible additional salutary influences on endothelial function and inflammation. In acknowledgment of the data that support the value of meditation, the American Heart Association issued a scientific statement on meditation and cardiovascular risk reduction that included "…meditation may be considered as an adjunct to guideline-directed cardiovascular risk reduction by those interested in this lifestyle modification…".[12]

Tai Chi
Tai Chi is an ancient practice that consists of a sequence of smooth, slow-paced movements with coordinated breathing, often referred

to as a "meditation in motion." Because Tai Chi incorporates aspects of both physical activity and stress reduction, it has been studied for reduction of cardiovascular events.

Recognizing that over 60% of eligible patients do not participate in cardiac rehabilitation, an alternative program utilizing Tai Chi has been evaluated for patients with coronary disease. In a study of patients with coronary disease who refused traditional cardiac rehabilitation, those who participated in an extended program of Tai Chi (6 months compared to 3 months), experienced greater weight loss and improved quality of life.[13]

Supplements
Omega-3 (see also Chapters 25, 27, and 29)
A widely supported dietary recommendation is to consume at least two servings of omega-3 rich fish per week. Nevertheless, for those who cannot or choose not to eat fish, omega-3 supplements may be particularly beneficial. Several brands of prescription omega-3s are now available.

Over-the-counter fish oil supplements may also be prescribed, but dosing requires special attention. Many over-the-counter omega-3 supplements include a front-of-the-bottle label that describes total omega-3 content. The total omega-3 content can be misleading, as accurate dosing is dependent on docosahexaenoic acid (DHA) and eicosapentaenoic acid (EPA) content, which may be only a fraction of the total omega-3 amount listed on the front label. If, for example, 1000 mg of combined DHA and EPA are prescribed, patients should be advised to review the back label of an over-the-counter omega-3 product and take as many pills as needed to total 1000 mg of combined DHA and EPA. Despite a front label indicating 1000 mg of fish oil per pill, some omega-3 preparations require 2 or 3 pills daily to total 1000 mg of combined DHA and EPA. Current trial evidence primarily supports prescription eicosapentaenoic acid to reduce major adverse cardiovascular events.

Multivitamins
Approximately 30% of the United States population use multivitamins, often as a safeguard against dietary deficiencies, or with the goal of disease prevention. A review of 18 studies with mean follow-up of 11.6 years, showed no change in cardiovascular mortality with multivitamin use.[14] Baseline nutritional status, evaluated in a study with follow-up of 11.4 years, did not influence the effect of multivitamins on cardiovascular outcomes.[15]

A signal that the duration of multivitamin use might be important was noted in a study of over 18,000 men in Physicians' Health Study I cohort, which found a self-reported duration of multivitamin use of ≥20 years to be associated with reduced risk of a major cardiovascular event.[16]

Antioxidants
Although some early findings suggested benefit, a more comprehensive evaluation of antioxidant supplements, including vitamins A, C, E, beta-carotene, and selenium, has not shown benefit in reducing the occurrence of coronary heart disease or the development of cardiovascular events.[17] Although the results of antioxidants in supplement form have not been promising, the cardioprotective benefit of whole foods rich in antioxidants, especially vegetables and fruit, is well established.

Hypertension (see Chapter 26)
Nutrition
Dietary Approaches to Stop Hypertension (DASH): Diet, Potassium, and Sodium
Dietary approaches are extremely potent interventions in treating hypertension. The best-studied diet for blood pressure control is the DASH diet (Dietary Approaches to Stop Hypertension). The DASH diet, similar to a Mediterranean-style diet, includes 8 to 10 daily servings of combined vegetable and fruit in addition to low-fat dairy. An inverse relationship between potassium intake and blood pressure reduction is well established. The DASH diet was designed to boost potassium intake to approximately the 75th percentile of US consumption.

The sodium content of both the intervention and control arms of the original DASH diet were similar, approximately 3 g/day. In a follow-up study, DASH-Sodium, the blood pressure-lowering impact of the DASH diet and low sodium diets were studied separately and combined. Compared to the baseline diet, systolic blood pressure was reduced by 7.0 mm Hg with sodium restriction of 1150 mg/day, by 10.6 mm Hg by DASH diet, and 20.8 mm Hg with combined DASH diet and sodium restriction.[18]

Physical Activity
Aerobic exercise, involving high repetition movement of large muscle groups, is the form of physical activity best studied for blood pressure reduction. Less well appreciated is the potential for resistance exercise to aid in blood pressure reduction.

Isometric resistance, most commonly studied with handgrip exercises, has been documented in a meta-analysis to achieve a reduction in blood pressure of 7 mm Hg (systolic) and 3 mm Hg (diastolic).[19] Typical regimens consist of four repetitions of 2-minute periods of repetitive handgrips performed 3 times a week. The mechanism of blood pressure reduction with isometric resistance is likely related to stimulation of endothelial-dependent vasodilation.

Mind/Heart Connection
Breathing Exercises
Breathing exercises that include periods of slow, deep breaths help facilitate relaxation and are integral to meditation and yoga. More recently, device-guided slow-breathing protocols have also been shown to produce blood pressure-lowering effects. A meta-analysis of studies that evaluated the effect of slow-breathing exercises on blood pressure demonstrated a drop in both systolic and diastolic pressure of 6 mm Hg. Typical breathing exercises consisted of a total of 20 to 30 total minutes per day, divided into two daily sessions.[20] A wide range of instructions for self-directed breathing exercises are available on the web that are free of charge and accessible to all patients.

Meditation
Transcendental meditation has been studied for treatment of patients with established hypertension. A mindfulness-based program that included nine training sessions and 6-day-a-week practice of ≥45 minutes resulted in a reduction in systolic blood pressure at 1 year of 15 mm Hg for those with baseline hypertension.[21] The mechanism of benefit is not well defined, but likely involves a reduction in sympathetic nervous activation leading to lower heart rate and vascular tone. Individuals who are drawn to self-reflection may be especially interested in considering meditation as an adjunctive tool for blood pressure control.

Acupuncture
Acupuncture has been evaluated for treatment of hypertension. A recent meta-analysis found no change in blood pressure when acupuncture was used in isolation but showed significant incremental benefit for blood pressure reduction when acupuncture was added to pharmacologic therapy, with a further decline in blood pressure in the adjunctive acupuncture group of 7 mm Hg systolic and 4 mm Hg diastolic.[22]

Dyslipidemia (see Chapter 27)
Nutrition
As codified in the most recent Guideline on the Management of Blood Cholesterol, diet and lifestyle measures are foundational interventions for both primary and secondary prevention.[7] The 2019 ACC/AHA Guideline on the Primary Prevention of Cardiovascular Disease recommends a dietary pattern that emphasizes increased consumption of vegetables, fruit, nuts, whole grains, and fish, and minimizes intake of sugar-sweetened beverages, processed meat, and refined carbohydrates.[23]

A portfolio dietary pattern has been studied for treatment of dyslipidemia that combines four categories of foods with cholesterol-lowering properties. Foods in a typical portfolio plan based on a 2000 kcal/day diet include: (1) nuts (42 g); (2) plant protein from soy, beans, or lentils (50 g protein); (3) soluble fiber from oats, barley, psyllium, apples, oranges, or berries (20 g soluble fiber); and (4) plant sterols, often enriched in margarine (2 g plant sterols). A meta-analysis of seven trials of the portfolio diet showed a mean reduction in low-density lipoprotein cholesterol (LDL-C) of 17%.[24]

Physical Activity (see Chapter 32)
It has been estimated that nearly 20% of the reduction in cardiovascular disease from exercise is attributed to its beneficial effect on lipids. In adults, aerobic exercise has been shown to reduce LDL-C by 3 to 6 mg/dL. Resistance training is similarly effective, with an average reduction in LDL-C of 6 to 9 mg/dL when performed ≥3 days/week with three sets of nine exercises.[25]

STATIN INTOLERANCE
Many strategies exist to improve tolerance to statins in those with suspected adverse reactions, including a reduction in dose, an increase in dosing interval, and a change to a different statin formulation. Other options include switching to alternative lipid-lowering agents such as ezetimibe and PCSK9 inhibitors. However, for the patients in whom these strategies are not feasible, or for those who are philosophically opposed to taking prescription medication, over-the-counter supplements may be considered.

SUPPLEMENTS
Fiber
Fiber reduces cholesterol levels through inhibition of hepatic cholesterol synthesis and by induction of an increase in fecal excretion of cholesterol and bile acids. Studies of fiber supplementation show reductions in LDL-C by 5% to 15%.[26] Psyllium is the best-studied fiber supplement. In a meta-analysis of 28 trials, consumption of median dose of 10.2 g of psyllium (approximately 2 tsp/day, led to a reduction in LDL-C of 12.8 mg/dL, $P < 0.00001$.[27]

Stanols/Sterols
Stanols and sterols are compounds naturally present in many plant-sourced foods and are especially concentrated in seeds, nuts, and grain products. These compounds lower serum cholesterol by competing for intestinal absorption of cholesterol. The average daily intake from food is 200 to 400 mg/day. The most commonly studied dose for stanols and sterols in supplement form is approximately 2 g/day, effecting an LDL-C reduction in the 8% to 12% range.[26] Stanols and sterols can be used as monotherapy for treatment of hypercholesterolemia, or in combination with statins.

Red Yeast Rice
Red yeast rice is derived from the fermentation of rice with the yeast *Monascus purpureus*, yielding a series of cholesterol-lowering monacolins. The monacolin in highest concentration in red yeast rice is monacolin K, also known as lovastatin, the first FDA-approved HMG CoA reductase inhibitor. Typical dosages of red yeast rice (1200 to 2400 mg/day) result in an average reduction in LDL-C of 27%.[28] This degree of LDL-lowering is greater than expected based on the concentration of monacolin K alone, likely due to multiple cholesterol-lowering constituents contained in red yeast rice.

Red yeast rice has been studied as an alternative for patients intolerant of prescription statins. In a randomized study of 62 patients previously intolerant of prescription statins, red yeast rice (1800 mg twice daily) was well tolerated and resulted in a reduction of LDL-C of 21% compared to controls at 24 weeks.[26]

Outcomes data for red yeast rice are available from a study of 4870 patients with prior myocardial infarction. In this 5-year study, red yeast rice, compared to placebo, resulted in a 4.7% absolute and 45% relative risk reduction in the primary endpoint of nonfatal myocardial infarction and cardiac death, as well as a 33% decrease in total mortality.[26]

Brands of red yeast rice differ in both potency and purity. The concentration of total monacolins and monacolin K vary several-fold between manufacturers.[29] A few brands have been found to contain small amounts of citrinin, a nephrotoxin. Chemical analysis of various red yeast rice formulations, including analysis of monacolin and citrinin concentrations, is available through the independent group Consumer-Labs.com (http://www.Consumerlabs.com).

Because red yeast rice is a form of a statin, patients should be advised of precautions common to all statins and be monitored by a health care professional.

Coenzyme Q10
Coenzyme Q10 (CoQ10) is a fat-soluble coenzyme required for the production of cellular adenosine triphosphate (ATP). Statin therapy has been shown to reduce circulating levels of CoQ10, a finding that has been hypothesized as a possible etiology of statin-related adverse reactions, including myalgias.

Results of small studies that evaluated the efficacy of CoQ10 for improvement in statin-related myalgias have been inconsistent. However, a recent meta-analysis was performed of 12 randomized controlled studies with a total of 575 patients. Compared to placebo, CoQ10 was found to significantly reduce statin-associated muscle symptoms.[30] The benefit was independent of dose, which ranged between 100 and 600 mg/day, and duration of treatment, from 30 days to 3 months.

Heart Failure (See Chapters 50 and 51)
Nutrition and Lifestyle
Diet is integral to the development of congestive heart failure. A recent study evaluated the association between dietary patterns and incident congestive heart failure in a population without known coronary disease or prior heart failure.[31] The study examined over 16,000 participants with a median follow-up of 8.7 years. Individuals with the highest consumption of vegetables, fruit, beans, and fish, compared to the lowest quartile of intake, had a 41% lower risk of incident heart failure. Conversely, the group whose diet included the most organ meats, processed meats, eggs, added fat, and sugar-sweetened beverages, compared to those with the least consumption, experienced a 72% higher risk of incident heart failure.

The mechanism of benefit from the plant-sourced diet could not be determined but was postulated to include a rich supply of protective dietary phytochemicals with antiinflammatory and antioxidant properties.

Supplements
Coenzyme Q10
Myocardial levels of Coenzyme Q10, essential for mitochondrial ATP production, are depressed in patients with congestive heart failure in a graded manner that parallels both heart failure symptoms and the degree of systolic dysfunction. Accordingly, supplementation with CoQ10 has been studied as an adjunct to treatment of patients with systolic heart failure.

The efficacy of CoQ10 in patients with heart failure was evaluated in the Q-SYMBIO trial that included 420 patients with moderate to severe heart failure on conventional medical therapy randomized to CoQ10 300 mg/day or placebo.[32] No short-term benefits (16 weeks) were observed, but after 2 years, significant improvement was noted in the group receiving CoQ10. New York Heart Association (NYHA) function class increased by at least 1 grade in 58% receiving CoQ10, compared to 45% in the placebo group, p= 0.028. Cardiovascular mortality was also lower in those receiving CoQ10 compared to the placebo group (9% vs. 16%, p=0.039).

A subsequent meta-analysis of 14 randomized controlled trials with a total of 2149 patients with heart failure found that CoQ10 administration resulted in a 31% decrease in mortality, p=0.02, and a significant improvement in exercise capacity. No change in ejection fraction was identified.[33] Doses of CoQ10 studied were typically in the range of 100 to 300 mg/day.

Arrhythmias (See Chapter 61)
Comprehensive Lifestyle Approach
Following catheter ablation, a program of aggressive risk factor modifications program has been studied to reduce the recurrence of atrial fibrillation. A total of 281 consecutive patients treated with an ablation procedure for atrial fibrillation with a body mass index ≥ 27 kg/m² and at least one cardiac risk factor were entered into either a risk factor management group or a control group.[34] The risk factor management group received counseling regarding weight reduction and dietary salt restriction, began an exercise program, and were advised to take home blood pressure measurements.

At the 42-month follow-up, arrhythmia-free survival was 4.8 times as likely (p< 0.001) in the risk factor management group than in controls. This finding exemplifies the benefits of a truly integrative approach—the combination of low- and high-tech strategies to achieve optimal results.

Yoga

Yoga combines aspects of both physical activity and meditation, making it a promising candidate for reducing the burden of atrial fibrillation. A group of 52 patients with paroxysmal atrial fibrillation were enrolled in the Yoga My Heart Study. Participants were observed for 3 months, followed by 3 months of an intervention that consisted of twice-weekly yoga sessions. Following 3 months of yoga, symptomatic episodes of atrial fibrillation were reduced by 45% and asymptomatic episodes by 67%, p < 0.001 for both.[35]

INTEGRATIVE SELF-CARE FOR THE CARDIOLOGIST

The importance of an integrative approach in cardiology relates not only to patient care, but also extends to cardiologists' self-care. For example, a recent survey found that only 20% of cardiologists consume five or more servings of vegetables and fruit each day.[5] There is evidence linking dietary habits with physicians' sense of well-being,[36] a particularly relevant topic given recent data that reveal that more than one-quarter of cardiologists report feeling "burned out."[37]

At minimum, cardiologists may wish to consider as a personal goal the same dietary and physical activity recommendations described in the ACC/AHA Primary Prevention Guidelines that advise, at minimum, 150 minutes per week of moderate-intensity aerobic physical activity as well as diet that emphasizes intake of vegetables, fruits, legumes, nuts, whole grains, and fish.[23]

Greater attention to physician self-care also has implications for patient care, as data suggest that physicians who adopt healthier lifestyle practices are more likely to counsel their patients to do likewise.[38]

CONCLUSION

An integrative approach to heart health seeks to enlarge both the scope of available treatments and to enhance the level of patient engagement. As described in this chapter, an integrative approach opens the door to many low-risk, high-impact interventions that, when added to guideline-based therapy, can make a powerful difference to improve outcomes and satisfaction for both patients and physicians.

REFERENCES

Integrative Cardiology

1. Kohl WK, Dobos G, Cramer H. Conventional and complementary healthcare utilization among US adults with cardiovascular disease or cardiovascular risk factors: a nationally representative survey. *J Am Heart Assoc*. 2020;9:e014759.
2. Curtin SC. Trends in cancer and heart disease death rates among adults aged 45-64: United States, 1999-2017. *Nat Vital Stat Rep*. 2019;68:1–8.
3. Devries S, Willett W, Bonow RO. Nutrition education in medical school, residency training, and practice. *J Am Med Assoc*. 2019;321:1351–1352.
4. Accreditation Council for Graduate Medical Education. *ACGME Program Requirements for Graduate Medical Education in Cardiovascular Disease (Internal Medicine)*; 2020. https://www.acgme.org/Portals/0/PFAssets/ProgramRequirements/141_CardiovascularDisease_2020.pdf?ver=2020-02-14-154334-140. Published 2020. Accessed November 10, 2020.
5. Devries S, Agatston A, Aggarwal M, et al. A deficiency of nutrition education and practice in cardiology. *Am J Med*. 2017;130(11):1298–1305.

Ischemic Heart Disease

6. Micha R, Penalvo JL, Cudhea F, et al. Association between dietary factors and mortality from heart disease, stroke, and type 2 diabetes in the United States. *J Am Med Assoc*. 2017;317:912–924.

7. Grundy SM, Stone NJ, Bailey AL, et al. 2018 AHA/ACC/AACVPR/AAPA/ABC/ACPM/ADA/AGS/APhA/ASPC/NLA/PCNA guideline on the management of blood cholesterol: executive summary: a report of the American College of Cardiology/American Heart Association Task Force on Clinical Practice Guidelines. *Circulation*. 2019;139:e1046–e1081.
8. Blekkenhorst LC, Sim M, Bondonno CP, et al. Cardiovascular health benefits of specific vegetable types: a narrative review. *Nutrients*. 2018;10(5).
9. Kalt W, Cassidy A, Howard LR, et al. Recent research on the health benefits of blueberries and their anthocyanins. *Adv Nutr*. 2020;11:224–236.
10. Lamuel-Raventos RM, Onge MS. Prebiotic nut compounds and human microbiota. *Crit Rev Food Sci Nutr*. 2017;57:3154–3163.
11. Jabri A, Kalra A, Kumar A, et al. Incidence of stress cardiomyopathy during the Coronavirus Disease 2019 pandemic. *JAMA Netw Open*. 2020;3:e2014780.
12. Levine GN, Lange RA, Bairey-Merz CN, et al. Meditation and cardiovascular risk reduction: a scientific statement from the American Heart Association. *J Am Heart Assoc*. 2017;6. https://doi.org/10/1161/JAHA.117.002218.
13. Salmoirago-Blotcher E, Wayne PM, Dunsiger S, et al. Tai Chi is a promising exercise option for patients with coronary heart disease declining cardiac rehabilitation. *J Am Heart Assoc*. 2017;6. https://doi.org/10.1161/JAHA.117.006603.
14. Kim J, Choi J, Kwon SY, et al. Association of multivitamin and mineral supplementation and risk of cardiovascular disease: a systematic review and meta-analysis. *Circ Cardiovasc Qual Outcomes*. 2018;11:e004224.
15. Rautiainen S, Gaziano JM, Christen WG, et al. Effect of baseline nutritional status on long-term multivitamin use and cardiovascular disease risk: a secondary analysis of the Physicians' Health Study II randomized clinical trial. *JAMA Cardiol*. 2017;2:617–625.
16. Rautiainen S, Rist PM, Glynn RJ, et al. Multivitamin use and the risk of cardiovascular disease in men. *J Nutr*. 2016;146:1235–1240.
17. Jenkins DJA, Spence JD, Giovannucci EL, et al. Supplemental vitamins and minerals for CVD prevention and treatment. *J Am Coll Cardiol*. 2018;71:2570–2584.

Hypertension

18. Juraschek SP, Miller ER, Weaver CM, Appel LJ. Effects of sodium reduction and the DASH diet in relation to baseline blood pressure. *J Am Coll Cardiol*. 2017;70:2841–2848.
19. Smart NA, Way D, Carlson D, et al. Effects of isometric resistance training on resting blood pressure: individual participant data meta-analysis. *J Hypertens*. 2019;37:1927–1938.
20. Zou Y, Zhao X, Hou YY, et al. Meta-analysis of effects of voluntary slow breathing exercises for control of heart rate and blood pressure in patients with cardiovascular diseases. *Am J Cardiol*. 2017;120:148–153.
21. Loucks EB, Nardi WR, Gutman R, et al. Mindfulness-based blood pressure reduction (MB-BP): stage 1 single-arm clinical trial. *PloS One*. 2019;14(11):e0223095.
22. Zhao XF, Hu HT, Li JS, et al. Is acupuncture effective for hypertension? A systematic review and meta-analysis. *PloS One*. 2015;10(7):e0127019.

Dyslipidemia

23. Arnett DK, Blumenthal RS, Albert MA, et al. 2019 ACC/AHA guideline on the primary prevention of cardiovascular disease: a report of the American College of Cardiology/American Heart Association Task Force on Clinical Practice Guidelines. *Circulation*. 2019;140:e596–e646.
24. Chiavaroli L, Nishi SK, Khan TA, et al. Portfolio dietary pattern and cardiovascular disease: a systematic review and meta-analysis of controlled trials. *Prog Cardiovasc Dis*. 2018;61:43–53.
25. Eckel RH, Jakicic JM, Ard JD, et al. 2013 AHA/ACC guideline on lifestyle management to reduce cardiovascular risk: a report of the American College of Cardiology/American Heart Association Task Force on Practice Guidelines. *Circulation*. 2014;129(suppl 2):S76–S99.
26. Banach M, Patti AM, Giglio RV, et al. The role of nutraceuticals in statin intolerant patients. *J Am Coll Cardiol*. 2018;72:96–118.
27. Jovanovski E, Yashpal S, Komishon A, et al. Effect of psyllium (Plantago ovata) fiber on LDL cholesterol and alternative lipid targets, non-HDL cholesterol and apolipoprotein B: a systematic review and meta-analysis of randomized controlled trials. *Am J Clin Nutr*. 2018;108:922–932.
28. Moriarty PM, Roth EM, Karns A, et al. Effects of xuezhikang in patients with dyslipidemia: a multicenter, randomized, placebo-controlled study. *J Clin Lipidol*. 2014;8:568–575.
29. Cohen PA, Avula B, Khan IA. Variability in strength of red yeast rice supplements purchased from mainstream retailers. *Eur J Prev Cardiol*. 2017;24:1431–1434.
30. Qu H, Guo M, Chai H, et al. Effects of coenzyme Q10 on statin-induced myopathy: an updated meta-analysis of randomized controlled trials. *J Am Heart Assoc*. 2018;7(19):e009835.

Heart Failure and Arrhythmias

31. Lara KM, Levitan EB, Gutierrez OM, et al. Dietary patterns and incident heart failure in U.S. adults without known coronary disease. *J Am Coll Cardiol*. 2019;73:2036–2045.
32. Mortensen SA, Rosenfeldt F, Kumar A, et al. The effect of coenzyme Q10 on morbidity and mortality in chronic heart failure: results from Q-SYMBIO: a randomized double-blind trial. *JACC Heart Fail*. 2014;2:641–649.
33. Lei L, Liu Y. Efficacy of coenzyme Q10 in patients with cardiac failure: a meta-analysis of clinical trials. *BMC Cardiovasc Disord*. 2017;17:196.
34. Pathak RK, Middeldorp ME, Lau DH, et al. Aggressive risk factor reduction study for atrial fibrillation and implications for the outcome of ablation. *J Am Coll Cardiol*. 2014;64:2222–2231.
35. Akella K, Kanuri SH, Murtaza G, et al. Impact of yoga on cardiac autonomic function and arrhythmias. *J Atr Fibrillation*. 2020;13.2408.

Integrative Self-Care for the Cardiologist

36. Hamidi MS, Boggild MK, Cheung AM. Running on empty: a review of nutrition and physicians' well-being. *Postgrad Med J*. 2016;92:478–481.
37. Mehta LS, Lewis SJ, Duvernoy CS, et al. Burnout and career satisfaction among U.S. cardiologists. *J Am Coll Cardiol*. 2019;73:3345–3348.
38. Carlos S, Rico-Campa A, de la Fuente-Arrillaga C, et al. Do healthy doctors deliver better messages of health promotion to their patients?: data from the SUN cohort study. *Eur J Public Health*. 2020;30:466–472.

第五部分　动脉粥样硬化性心血管疾病

曹宇开　李悦　导读

动脉粥样硬化是冠心病（CAD）、缺血性脑卒中和周围动脉疾病（PAD）的主要原因。随着人口老龄化，动脉粥样硬化的危险因素随年龄逐渐增加，导致动脉粥样硬化性心血管疾病的发病率不断升高。

本部分将系统介绍动脉粥样硬化性心血管疾病，包括 CAD、主动脉疾病（第 42 章）、PAD（第 43、44 章）和缺血性脑卒中（第 45 章）等。其中以 CAD 为重点，从胸痛患者的处理（第 35 章）、冠状动脉血流与心肌缺血（第 36 章）、ST 段抬高型心肌梗死的病理生理学和临床进展（第 37 章）、ST 段抬高型心肌梗死的治疗（第 38 章）、非 ST 段抬高型急性冠脉综合征（第 39 章）、稳定型缺血性心脏病（SIHD，第 40 章）以及经皮冠状动脉介入治疗（PCI，第 41 章）等方面分别阐述。

冠状动脉粥样硬化所致急性冠脉综合征（ACS）可表现为急性胸痛，应根据胸痛特点、实验室及影像学检查结果与同样导致胸痛的其他疾病（如肺栓塞、主动脉夹层和张力性气胸等致命性胸痛及其他非致命性胸痛）进行鉴别诊断。ACS 包括 ST 段抬高型心肌梗死（STEMI）和非 ST 段抬高型急性冠脉综合征（NSTE-ACS），后者包括非 ST 段抬高型心肌梗死（NSTEMI）和不稳定型心绞痛（UA）。

在研究 CAD 的病理生理机制及对患者进行诊治之前，需要了解冠脉血流的调节、心肌耗氧量的决定因素以及缺血与收缩的相关性等知识。冠状动脉血流在心动周期的收缩期血流量达到最低点而舒张期血流增加。对于血流的变化，冠状动脉有自主调节能力，同时其舒缩有赖于功能正常的内皮，受到血管腔内物理作用力、神经-体液及代谢介质的调控。根据压力-血流关系，我们可以定量分析冠脉狭窄后的血流储备——绝对血流储备、相对血流储备和血流储备分数（FFR）。冠脉狭窄所致急性缺血可引起不可逆性心肌损伤，而可逆性反复缺血可引起慢性心肌顿抑、心肌冬眠等功能性结果。

应依据患者病史、临床症状及体征、心肌损伤标志物的变化、心电图及影像学检查结果做出 SIHD、NSTE-ACS 或 STEMI 诊断，指导后续治疗。明确 SIHD 病因及诊断后应治疗相关疾病、减少危险因素、启动药物防治，必要时进行血运重建。NSTE-ACS 治疗分为急性期治疗（重点关注临床症状和"罪犯"血管稳定性）及长期治疗（预防疾病进展和斑块破裂/侵蚀）。STEMI 治疗包括发病时治疗（院前护理、急诊室初始治疗和再灌注治疗）、住院治疗（药物治疗、并发症处理和出院准备）以及 STEMI 后早期二级预防。

随着诊疗流程的完善以及冠状动脉装置和手术技术的发展革新，PCI 在 CAD 中的应用越来越多。冠状动脉介入治疗器械包括球囊、支架以及为安全有效进行复杂冠状动脉血运重建所需的辅助装置。第 41 章详细介绍了 PCI 应用现状，以及冠状动脉介入治疗器械、血管入路及辅助抗栓治疗。

主动脉疾病包括主动脉瘤、急性主动脉综合征、主动脉炎综合征及原发性主动脉肿瘤等。第 42 章从发病机制、临床表现、辅助检查、诊断及治疗等方面详细介绍上述疾病。主动脉瘤是指病理性扩张的主动脉段，并且具有进一步扩张和破裂的倾向。急性主动脉综合征包括典型主动脉夹层、主动脉壁内血肿和穿透性粥样硬化性主动脉溃疡。而外伤、感染或者主动脉瘤、主动脉夹层或穿透性溃疡破裂可形成与主动脉腔相通的周围血肿，即假性动脉瘤。主动脉炎综合征即感染性主动脉瘤，病因包括邻近的胸部组织扩散、心内膜炎引起的脓毒症栓子及脓毒症或静脉注射药物滥用时细菌的血行播散。主动脉肿瘤多继发于邻近部位（尤其是肺和食管）肿瘤或转移瘤的直接侵袭，而原发性主动脉肉瘤非常罕见。

PAD通常指急性或慢性上肢或下肢动脉阻塞，严重者可造成肢体远端缺血及潜在的组织损伤；有时也包括颈动脉和肠系膜动脉等大、中动脉的疾病。第43章从流行病学、临床表现、辅助检查、治疗及预后等方面详细介绍PAD，并简要总结除动脉硬化性闭塞症之外其他类型PAD的发病机制、临床表现、诊断及治疗。第44章着重介绍了PAD及继发于慢性疾病的静脉疾病（下肢深静脉血栓及上腔静脉综合征）的经导管血管腔内治疗。

第45章聚焦于缺血性脑卒中及短暂性脑缺血发作（TIA）的病理生理机制、风险因素、预防及治疗措施。

PART V ATHEROSCLEROTIC CARDIOVASCULAR DISEASE

35 Approach to the Patient with Chest Pain

MARC P. BONACA AND MARC S. SABATINE

CAUSES OF ACUTE CHEST PAIN, 599
Myocardial Ischemia or Infarction, 599
Pericardial Disease, 600
Vascular Disease, 600
Pulmonary Conditions, 600
Gastrointestinal Conditions, 601

Musculoskeletal and Other Causes, 601
DIAGNOSTIC CONSIDERATIONS, 601
Clinical Evaluation, 601
Initial Assessment, 601
Decision Aids, 604

IMMEDIATE MANAGEMENT, 605
Chest Pain Protocols and Units, 605
Early Noninvasive Testing, 605
REFERENCES, 607

Acute chest pain remains one of the most common reasons for seeking care in the emergency department (ED), accounting for almost 10% of the approximately 100 million nontraumatic visits in the United States and representing the second most common complaint.[1] Such pain suggests acute coronary syndrome (ACS), but after diagnostic evaluation, only 10% to 15% of patients with acute chest pain actually have ACS.[2-5] It is difficult to differentiate patients with ACS or other life-threatening conditions from those with noncardiovascular, non-life-threatening chest pain. The diagnosis of ACS is missed in approximately 2% of patients, which can lead to substantial consequences—for example, the short-term mortality in patients with acute myocardial infarction (MI) who are mistakenly discharged from the ED is twofold higher than that expected for patients who are admitted to the hospital. However, for patients with a lower risk for complications, these concerns must be balanced against the cost and inconvenience of admission and against the risk for complications from tests and procedures with a low probability of improving patient outcomes.

There have been several advances in the accurate and efficient evaluation of patients with acute chest pain, including more specific blood markers for myocardial injury[6,7]; decision aids to stratify patients according to their risk of complications; early exercise testing[2,4,8]; radionuclide scanning for lower-risk patient subsets (see Chapter 18)[2,4,8]; multislice computed tomography for anatomic evaluation of coronary artery disease (CAD), pulmonary embolism (PE), and aortic dissection[9-11] (see Chapter 20); and the use of chest pain units[2,4,8,12,13] and critical pathways for efficient and rapid evaluation of lower-risk patients.[2,4,8,12,13]

CAUSES OF ACUTE CHEST PAIN

In a typical population of patients being evaluated for acute chest pain in EDs, about 10% to 15% have ACS.[1,14,15] A small percentage has other life-threatening problems, such as PE or acute aortic dissection, but most leave the ED without a diagnosis or with a diagnosis of a non–cardiac-related condition.[16] Such noncardiac conditions include musculoskeletal syndromes, disorders of the abdominal viscera (including gastroesophageal reflux disease), and psychological conditions (Table 35.1).

Myocardial Ischemia or Infarction

The most common serious cause of acute chest discomfort is myocardial ischemia or infarction (see Chapters 37–39), which occurs when the supply of myocardial oxygen is inadequate for the demand. MI usually occurs in the setting of coronary atherosclerosis, but it may also reflect dynamic components of coronary vascular resistance. Coronary spasm can occur in normal coronary arteries or, in patients with coronary disease surrounding atherosclerotic plaques, and in smaller coronary arteries (see Chapter 36). Other less common causes of impaired coronary blood flow include syndromes that compromise the orifices or lumina of the coronary arteries, such as coronary arteritis, proximal aortitis, spontaneous coronary dissection, proximal aortic dissection, coronary emboli from infectious or noninfectious endocarditis or thrombus in the left atrium or left ventricle, myocardial bridge, or a congenital abnormality of the coronary arteries (see Chapter 82).

The classic manifestation of ischemia is angina, which is usually described as a heavy chest pressure or squeezing, a burning feeling, or difficulty breathing. The discomfort often radiates to the left shoulder, neck, or arm. It typically builds in intensity over a period of a few minutes. The pain may begin with exercise or psychological stress, but ACS most commonly occurs without obvious precipitating factors.

Atypical descriptions of chest pain reduce the likelihood of myocardial ischemia or injury. The American College of Cardiology (ACC) and American Heart Association (AHA) guidelines list the following as pain descriptions uncharacteristic of myocardial ischemia[2]:

- Pleuritic pain (i.e., sharp or knifelike pain brought on by respiratory movements or coughing)
- Primary or sole location of the discomfort in the middle or lower abdominal region
- Pain that may be localized by the tip of one finger, particularly over the left ventricular apex
- Pain reproduced with movement or palpation of the chest wall or arms
- Constant pain that persists for many hours
- Very brief episodes of pain that last a few seconds or less
- Pain that radiates into the lower extremities

Nevertheless, data from large populations of patients with acute chest pain indicate that ACS occurs in those with atypical symptoms at sufficient frequency that no single factor suffices to exclude the diagnosis of acute ischemic heart disease. Clinicians should be mindful of "angina equivalents" such as jaw or shoulder pain in the absence of chest pain or dyspnea, nausea or vomiting, and diaphoresis. In particular, women, older persons, and individuals with diabetes may experience atypical symptoms of myocardial ischemia or infarction (see Chapter 91). Data from the National Registry of Myocardial Infarction demonstrate that among patients hospitalized with MI, women—particularly young women—less likely manifest chest pain than men.[17]

TABLE 35.1 Common Causes of Acute Chest Pain

SYSTEM	SYNDROME	CLINICAL DESCRIPTION	KEY DISTINGUISHING FEATURES
Cardiac	Angina	Retrosternal chest pressure, burning, or heaviness; radiating occasionally to the neck, jaw, epigastrium, shoulders, left arm	Precipitated by exercise, cold weather, or emotional stress; duration of 2–10 min
	Rest or unstable angina	Same as angina, but may be more severe	Typically <20 min; lower tolerance for exertion; crescendo pattern
	Acute myocardial infarction	Same as angina, but may be more severe	Sudden onset, usually lasting ≥30 min; often associated with shortness of breath, weakness, nausea, vomiting
	Pericarditis	Sharp, pleuritic pain aggravated by changes in position; highly variable duration	Pericardial friction rub
Vascular	Aortic dissection	Excruciating, ripping pain of sudden onset in the anterior aspect of the chest, often radiating to the back	Marked severity of unrelenting pain; usually occurs in the setting of hypertension or underlying connective tissue disorder such as Marfan syndrome
	Pulmonary embolism	Sudden onset of dyspnea and pain, usually pleuritic with pulmonary infarction	Dyspnea, tachypnea, tachycardia, signs of right-sided heart failure
	Pulmonary hypertension	Substernal chest pressure, exacerbated by exertion	Pain associated with dyspnea and signs of pulmonary hypertension
Pulmonary	Pleuritis and/or pneumonia	Pleuritic pain, usually brief, over the involved area	Pain pleuritic and lateral to the midline, associated with dyspnea
	Tracheobronchitis	Burning discomfort in the midline	Midline location, associated with coughing
	Spontaneous pneumothorax	Sudden onset of unilateral pleuritic pain, with dyspnea	Abrupt onset of dyspnea and pain
Gastrointestinal	Esophageal reflux	Burning substernal and epigastric discomfort, 10–60 min in duration	Aggravated by a large meal and postprandial recumbency; relieved by antacid
	Peptic ulcer	Prolonged epigastric or substernal burning	Relieved by antacid or food
	Gallbladder disease	Prolonged epigastric or right upper quadrant pain	Unprovoked or following a meal
	Pancreatitis	Prolonged, intense epigastric and substernal pain	Risk factors, including alcohol, hypertriglyceridemia, medications
Musculoskeletal	Costochondritis	Sudden onset of intense fleeting pain	May be reproduced by pressure over the affected joint; occasionally, swelling and inflammation over the costochondral joint
	Cervical disc disease	Sudden onset of fleeting pain	May be reproduced with movement of the neck
	Trauma or strain	Constant pain	Reproduced by palpation or movement of the chest wall or arms
Infectious	Herpes zoster	Prolonged burning pain in a dermatomal distribution	Vesicular rash, dermatomal distribution
Psychological	Panic disorder	Chest tightness or aching, often accompanied by dyspnea and lasting 30 min or more, unrelated to exertion or movement	Patient may have other evidence of an emotional disorder

Pericardial Disease

The visceral surface of the pericardium is insensitive to pain, as is most of the parietal surface. Therefore, noninfectious causes of pericarditis (e.g., uremia; see Chapter 86) usually cause little or no pain.[18] In contrast, infectious pericarditis almost always involves the surrounding pleura, so patients typically experience pleuritic pain with breathing, coughing, and changes in position.[19] Swallowing may induce the pain because of the proximity of the esophagus to the posterior portion of the heart. Because the central diaphragm receives its sensory supply from the phrenic nerve, which in turn arises from the third to fifth cervical segments of the spinal cord, pain from infectious pericarditis is frequently felt in the shoulders and neck. Involvement of the diaphragm more laterally can lead to symptoms in the upper part of the abdomen and back, and thus create confusion with pancreatitis or cholecystitis. Pericarditis occasionally causes a steady, crushing substernal pain resembling that of acute MI.[18]

Vascular Disease

Acute aortic dissection (see Chapter 42) usually causes a sudden onset of excruciating ripping pain, the location of which reflects the site and progression of the dissection.[20] Ascending aortic dissection manifests as pain in the midline of the anterior aspect of the chest, and posterior descending aortic dissection causes pain in the back of the chest. Aortic dissections are rare, with an estimated annual incidence of 3 per 100,000, and usually occur in the presence of risk factors, including Marfan and Ehlers-Danlos syndromes, bicuspid aortic valve, pregnancy (for proximal dissections), and hypertension (for distal dissections).[20]

Pulmonary emboli (see Chapter 87) often cause a sudden onset of dyspnea and pleuritic chest pain, although they may be asymptomatic.[21,22] Massive pulmonary emboli tend to cause severe and persistent substernal pain, likely due to distention of the pulmonary artery. Emboli that lead to pulmonary infarction can cause lateral pleuritic chest pain. Hemodynamically significant pulmonary emboli may cause hypotension, syncope, and signs of right-sided heart failure. Pulmonary hypertension (see Chapter 88) can result in chest pain similar to that of angina pectoris, presumably because of right-heart hypertrophy and ischemia.

Pulmonary Conditions

Pulmonary conditions that cause chest pain generally produce dyspnea and pleuritic symptoms, the location of which reflects the site of pulmonary disease. Tracheobronchitis tends to be associated with a burning midline pain, whereas pneumonia can cause pain over the involved lung. The pain in pneumothorax begins suddenly and is usually associated with dyspnea. Primary pneumothorax typically occurs in tall, thin young men; secondary pneumothorax occurs in the setting of pulmonary disease such as chronic obstructive pulmonary disease, asthma, or cystic fibrosis. Tension pneumothorax can be a life-threatening condition. Asthma exacerbations can be accompanied by chest discomfort, typically characterized as tightness.

Gastrointestinal Conditions

Irritation of the esophagus by acid reflux can produce a burning discomfort that may be exacerbated by intake of alcohol, aspirin, and some foods. Symptoms are often worsened by a recumbent position and are relieved by sitting upright and with acid-reducing therapies. Esophageal spasm can cause a squeezing chest discomfort similar to that of angina. Mallory-Weiss tears of the esophagus can occur in patients who have had prolonged vomiting episodes. Severe vomiting can also result in esophageal rupture (Boerhaave syndrome) with mediastinitis. Chest pain caused by peptic ulcer disease usually occurs 60 to 90 minutes after meals and typically responds rapidly to acid-reducing therapies. This pain is generally epigastric in location but can radiate to the chest and shoulders. Cholecystitis causes a wide range of pain syndromes and generally causes right upper quadrant abdominal pain, but chest and back pain is not unusual. The pain is frequently described as aching or colicky. Pancreatitis typically causes an intense, aching epigastric pain that may radiate to the back, with limited relief through acid-reducing therapies.

Musculoskeletal and Other Causes

Chest pain can arise from musculoskeletal disorders involving the chest wall (such as costochondritis), conditions affecting the nerves of the chest wall (such as cervical disc disease), by Herpes zoster, or following heavy exercise. Chest pain secondary to musculoskeletal causes is often elicited by direct pressure over the affected area or by movement of the patient's neck.[23] The pain itself can be fleeting, or it can be a dull ache that lasts for hours. Panic syndrome is a major cause of chest discomfort in ED patients. The symptoms typically include chest tightness, often accompanied by shortness of breath and a sense of anxiety, and generally last 30 minutes or longer.

DIAGNOSTIC CONSIDERATIONS

Clinical Evaluation

When evaluating patients with acute chest pain, clinicians must address a series of issues related to prognosis and immediate management.[2,24] Even before arriving at a definite diagnosis, high-priority questions include the following:
- *Clinical stability:* Does the patient need immediate treatment for actual or impending circulatory collapse or respiratory insufficiency?
- *Immediate prognosis:* If the patient is currently clinically stable, what is the risk that a life-threatening condition such as ACS, PE, or aortic dissection exists?
- *Safety of triage options:* If the risk for a life-threatening condition is low, is it safe to discharge the patient for outpatient management, or should further testing or observation to guide management be undertaken?

Initial Assessment

Evaluation of a patient with acute chest pain can begin before the physician sees the patient, and thus effectiveness may depend on the actions of the office staff and other nonphysician personnel. Guidelines from the ACC/AHA and European Society of Cardiology (ESC)[2,24] emphasize that patients with symptoms consistent with ACS should not be evaluated solely on the phone but should be referred to facilities to be evaluated by a physician and undergo a 12-lead electrocardiogram (ECG). These guidelines also recommend strong consideration of immediate referral to an ED or a specialized chest pain unit for patients with suspected ACS who experience chest discomfort at rest for longer than 20 minutes, hemodynamic instability, or recent syncope or near-syncope. Transport as a passenger in a private vehicle is considered an acceptable alternative to an emergency vehicle only if the wait would lead to a delay longer than 20 to 30 minutes.

Patients with the following chief complaints should undergo immediate assessment by triage nurses and be referred for further evaluation:
- Chest pain, pressure, tightness, or heaviness; pain that radiates to the neck, jaw, shoulders, back, or one or both arms
- Indigestion or heartburn; nausea and/or vomiting associated with chest discomfort
- Persistent shortness of breath
- Weakness, dizziness, lightheadedness, or loss of consciousness

For such patients, initial assessment involves taking a history, performing a physical examination, obtaining an ECG and chest radiograph, and measuring biomarkers of myocardial injury. Recent data suggest important sex-based disparities in the assessment and outcome of chest pain evaluations in emergency rooms.[25] In one analysis with over 54,000 patients, after adjusting for baseline differences, women were 18% less likely to be reviewed within 10 minutes and 16% less likely to be evaluated within an hour presentation.[25] Such observations underscore the need for more systematic and unbiased approaches to initially evaluate chest pain.

History

If the patient does not need immediate intervention because of impending or actual circulatory collapse or respiratory insufficiency, the physician's assessment should begin with a clinical history that captures the characteristics of the patient's pain, including its quality, location, and radiation; the time and tempo (abrupt or gradual) of onset; the duration of symptoms; provoking or palliating activities; and any associated symptoms, particularly those that are pulmonary or gastrointestinal.[2,14,24,26–28] ACS discomfort typically causes a diffuse substernal chest pressure that starts gradually, radiates to the jaw or arms, worsens with exertion, and is relieved by rest or nitroglycerin use. Because angina tends to be manifested in the same way in a given patient (at least if it is due to ischemia in the same territory), it is useful to compare the current episode with any previous documented episodes of angina. The response to nitroglycerin may not reliably discriminate cardiac chest pain from non–cardiac-related chest pain.[14] In contrast to the tempo of the chest pain in ACS, chest pain that is sudden and severe in onset characterizes PE, aortic dissection, and pneumothorax.[20,22,29] Moreover, pain that is pleuritic or positional in nature suggests PE, pericarditis, pneumonia, or a musculoskeletal condition. A review of the literature yielded eight factors from the chest pain history with a likelihood ratio for ACS significantly greater than 1 and six factors with a likelihood ratio significantly lower than 1 (Table 35.2).[2,14] Although chest pain severity should be elicited, it does not reliably predict myocardial ischemia.[30]

In addition to the characteristics of the acute episode, the presence of risk factors for atherosclerosis (e.g., advanced age, male sex, diabetes) increases the likelihood that the chest pain is resulting from myocardial ischemia. A history of MI communicates the presence of CAD and is associated with an increased risk for ACS and multivessel disease. Younger patients have a lower risk for ACS but should be screened with particular care for a history of recent cocaine use (see Chapter 84).[2,14,16,24] Although a thorough history is critical, clinician assessment alone does not suffice to rule in or rule out ACS. Combining the clinician assessment with physical exam and, more important, ECG and biomarkers greatly improves diagnostic assessment.[2,24,31,32]

Physical Examination (see Chapter 13)

The initial examination of patients with acute chest pain should aim at identifying potential precipitating causes of myocardial ischemia (e.g., uncontrolled hypertension), important comorbid conditions (e.g., chronic obstructive pulmonary disease), and evidence of hemodynamic complications (e.g., congestive heart failure, new mitral

TABLE 35.2 Value of Elements of the Chest Pain History for the Diagnosis of Acute Coronary Syndrome

PAIN DESCRIPTOR	POSITIVE LIKELIHOOD RATIO (95% CI)
Increased Likelihood of AMI	
Radiation to the right arm or shoulder	4.7 (1.9–12.0)
Radiation to both arms or shoulders	4.1 (2.5–6.5)
Associated with exertion	2.4 (1.5–3.8)
Radiation to the left arm	2.3 (1.7–3.1)
Associated with diaphoresis	2.0 (1.9–2.2)
Associated with nausea or vomiting	1.9 (1.7–2.3)
Worse than previous angina or similar to previous MI	1.8 (1.6–2.0)
Described as pressure	1.3 (1.2–1.5)
Decreased Likelihood of AMI	
Described as pleuritic	0.2 (0.1–0.3)
Described as positional	0.3 (0.2–0.5)
Described as sharp	0.3 (0.2–0.5)
Reproducible with palpation	0.3 (0.2–0.4)
Inframammary location	0.8 (0.7–0.9)
Not associated with exertion	0.8 (0.6–0.9)

AMI, Acute myocardial infarction; *CI*, confidence interval; *MI*, myocardial infarction.
Modified from Swap CJ, Nagurney JT. Value and limitations of chest pain history in the evaluation of patients with suspected acute coronary syndromes. *JAMA*. 2005;294:2623.

TABLE 35.3 Value of Electrocardiogram Findings for the Diagnosis of Acute Coronary Syndrome

ECG FINDING	POSITIVE LIKELIHOOD RATIO (95% CI WHERE AVAILABLE)
New ST-segment elevation ≥1 mm	5.7–53.9
New Q wave	5.3–24.8
Any ST-segment elevation	11.2 (7.1–17.8)
New conduction defect	6.3 (2.5–15.7)
New ST-segment depression	3.0–5.2
Any Q wave	3.9 (2.7–5.7)
Any ST-segment depression	3.2 (2.5–4.1)
T wave peaking and/or inversion ≥1 mm	3.1
New T wave inversion	2.4–2.8
Any conduction defect	2.7 (1.4–5.4)

CI, Confidence interval; *ECG*, electrocardiogram.
Modified from Panju AA, Hemmelgarn BR, Guyatt GH, Simel DL. The rational clinical examination. Is this patient having a myocardial infarction? *JAMA*. 1998;280:1256.

regurgitation, hypotension).[2,16,23,24,31,32] In addition to vital signs, examination of peripheral vessels should include assessing for the presence of bruits or absent pulses, which suggest extracardiac vascular disease (see Chapter 43).

For patients whose clinical findings do not suggest myocardial ischemia, the search for noncoronary causes of chest pain should focus first on potentially life-threatening issues (e.g., aortic dissection, PE) and then turn to the possibility of other cardiac diagnoses (e.g., pericarditis) and noncardiac diagnoses (e.g., esophageal discomfort).[14,31,32] Blood pressure or pulse disparities or a new murmur of aortic regurgitation accompanied by back or midline anterior chest pain suggests aortic dissection.[20] A friction rub may accompany pericarditis.[18] Differences in breath sounds in the presence of acute dyspnea and pleuritic chest pain raise the possibility of pneumothorax. Tachycardia, tachypnea, and an accentuated pulmonic component of the second heart sound (P_2) may be the major manifestations of PE on physical examination.[22]

Electrocardiography

For patients with ongoing chest discomfort, an ECG, which is a source of decisive data, should be obtained within 10 minutes after arrival, and as rapidly as possible for patients who have a history of chest discomfort consistent with ACS but whose discomfort has resolved by the time of evaluation so that patients who might benefit from immediate reperfusion therapy (mechanical or pharmacologic) can be identified (see Chapter 14).[2,24] To that end, obtaining a prehospital ECG decreases the door-to-diagnosis time and, for ST-segment elevation MI (STEMI), the door-to-balloon time. Importantly, these gains accrue without any prolongation of scene or transport times and, with a reduction in scene and transport times for patients with STEMI.[2,24] Wearables capable of recording and transmitting ECGs and other information may be useful in the triage of chest discomfort in the future (see Chapter 12).

The ECG aids in both diagnosis and prognosis. ST segment elevation ≥1 mm in ≥2 contiguous leads is required for the diagnosis of STEMI. ST segment depression as little as 0.5 mm is suggestive of ischemia. T wave inversions of at least 2 mm can also indicate ischemia but are less specific. The likelihood ratios for ACS with various findings on the ECG are shown in Table 35.3.[14] Completely normal findings on an ECG do not exclude the possibility of ACS; the risk for acute MI is approximately 4% in patients with a history of CAD and 2% in those with no such history. Patients with normal or nearly normal findings on an ECG, however, have a better prognosis than do those with clearly abnormal ECGs at initial evaluation. Moreover, a normal ECG has a negative predictive value of 80% to 90%, regardless of whether the patient was experiencing chest pain at the time that the ECG was obtained.[2,24] Diffuse ST-segment elevation and PR-segment depression suggest pericarditis. Right-axis deviation, right bundle branch block, T wave inversions in leads V_1 to V_4, and an S wave in lead I and Q wave and T wave inversions in lead III suggest PE.[22,29]

The availability of a previous ECG improves diagnostic accuracy and reduces the rate of admission for patients with abnormal baseline tracings. Serial electrocardiographic tracings improve the clinician's ability to diagnose acute MI, especially in the patient remains symptomatic and particularly if combined with serial measurement of cardiac biomarkers. Continuous electrocardiographic monitoring to detect ST-segment shifts is technically feasible but makes an uncertain contribution to patient management. Posterior leads can be useful for identifying ischemia in the territory supplied by the circumflex coronary artery, which is otherwise relatively silent on ECGs.

Chest Radiography (see also Chapter 17)

A chest radiograph is typically obtained for all patients with chest pain.[2,24] It is usually nondiagnostic in patients with ACS but can show pulmonary edema secondary to ischemia-induced diastolic or systolic dysfunction. It is more useful for diagnosing or suggesting other disorders; for example, it may show a widened mediastinum or aortic knob in patients with aortic dissection. The chest radiograph is generally normal in PE but can show atelectasis, an elevated hemidiaphragm, a pleural effusion, or more rarely, a Hampton hump or Westermark sign. The chest radiograph can reveal pneumonia or pneumothorax.

Biomarkers

Patients with chest discomfort possibly consistent with ACS should undergo measurement of biomarkers of myocardial injury. The preferred biomarker is cardiac troponin (cTn: T or I; cTnT or cTnI); creatine kinase MB isoenzyme (CK-MB) is less sensitive and is no longer recommended.[2,24] The advent of highly sensitive assays for cTn that enable earlier detection of MI have fundamentally changed the diagnostic approach to the patient with chest pain enabling early rule-out strategies and detection in a broader range of patients, including those with other causes of cTn elevation including structural heart disease.[2,6,24,33–38] In addition, there is an increased detection of MI (20% relative increase) with a reciprocal decrease in unstable angina (see also Chapters 37 to 39).[24]

Diagnostic Performance

Studies on the diagnostic performance of cTnI, cTnT, and CK-MB indicate that when any of these test findings are abnormal, the patient is likely to have ACS. It is inherently challenging to define the diagnostic performance of biomarkers for MI because part of the definition of MI includes the rise and fall of cardiac biomarkers of necrosis. In addition, the introduction of high-sensitivity cTn assays (hs-cTn) has enabled detection of a broader range of conditions and has redefined the epidemiology of MI.[24,38,39] Nevertheless, these assays are indispensable in the diagnosis of MI, and when the totality of clinical evidence is used as the reference standard for diagnosis, they have excellent sensitivity and specificity.

TROPONIN. Different genes encode troponins in cardiac muscle, slow skeletal muscle, and fast skeletal muscle; hence, assays for cardiac troponins are more specific for myocardial injury than assays for CK-MB, and cardiac troponin is the preferred diagnostic biomarker.[6,7,38] The high specificity of cardiac troponins for myocar-dium rarely gives false-positive increases (i.e., increase in the absence of myocardial injury). Rather, elevations in the absence of other clinical data consistent with ACS usually represent true myocardial damage from causes other than atherosclerotic plaque rupture. Type 2 MI occurs when there is clinical evidence of myocardial ischemia and an elevated biomarker of necrosis, but in the setting of stable cor-onary disease with either reduced myocardial oxygen supply (e.g., hypotension, vasospasm, severe anemia) or increased myocardial oxygen demand (e.g., hypertensive crisis, tachycardia, critical aortic stenosis, severe hypertrophic cardiomyopathy, extreme exercise).[38] Other patients may have an elevated troponin but without evidence of acute ischemia; this is termed "myocardial injury," and may be seen in direct myocyte injury, such as in myocarditis, myocardial contusion, or cardioversion or defibrillation.[17,38,40] Sepsis and acute viral infections including that due to SARS-CoV2 can precipitate type 2 MI. Myocardial injury can also occur in right ventricular strain as in PE, in other causes of acute pulmonary hypertension, or in cases of catechol excess such as in sepsis, stroke, or subarachnoid hemorrhage or other critical illness. Patients with renal disease can have stable but elevated levels of cardiac troponins.[6,7,40] The exact mechanism remains unclear, but in patients with a clinical history suggestive of ACS, an elevated cardiac troponin level conveys a similarly increased risk for ischemic complications across a broad range of renal function.[6,17,41] Sex may have a modest effect on hs-cTn concentrations (approximately 40%) although other factors such as age and renal dysfunction likely have greater impact (approximately 300% in healthy individuals).[24] Sex-specific cutpoints have been examined for troponin assays.[38] Studies evaluating sex-specific cutpoints including lower concentrations for women have found that such an approach may double the diagnosis of MI in women; however, the impact on outcomes of this approach is unclear.[42] Importantly, routine application of biomarkers to both men and women presenting with chest pain is also critical, with one study showing that women presenting with acute chest pain were 20% less likely than men to have a troponin test performed and were also less likely to be admitted to a specialized care unit and more likely to die.[25]

More recently, high-sensitivity assays have been developed with even lower limits of detection (e.g., <0.001 ng/mL or <1 pg/mL) and allow at least 50% (some ≥95%) of healthy individuals below the 99th percentile to have a measurable level of troponin. With the greater precision at the lower range, these assays allow one not only to determine if the level in the patient's blood is above the upper limit of normal, but also to detect reliably absolute changes in serial samples obtained at presentation and a few hours later.[6,34,43-47] By examining absolute levels and dynamic changes these assays can shorten the time interval to the next measurement to 1 to 2 hours and still achieve negative predictive values ≥ 99%.[6,34,43-47] Moreover, such assays may also permit the safe discharge of patients based on a single troponin value at presentation (see testing strategy below). Using a cutoff well below the 99th percentile and often the limit of detection, approximately 20% to 25% of patients will have such a low or undetectable level with a corresponding >99% negative predictive value.[6,34,43-47] The generalizability of these findings may also depend on the timing and nature of the presenting syndrome, with patients with a very short time from symptom onset to presentation needing serial sampling.[6,34,43-47]

CREATINE KINASE MB ISOENZYME. Until the advent of cardiac troponin assays, CK-MB was the biomarker of choice for the diagnosis of MI. Its major limitation is its relative lack of specificity because it can be found in the skeletal muscle, tongue, diaphragm, small intestine, uterus, and prostate.[2,24]

OTHER MARKERS

Several other biomarkers may be useful in the workup of a patient with chest pain including markers for noncoronary diagnoses. Myosin-binding protein C maybe useful in combination with hs-cTn but further studies are needed to establish its utility.[48] Copeptin is secreted from the pituitary gland early in the course of MI and is the C-terminal part of the vasopressin prohormone. It has shown substantial benefit as a stress marker in multiple medical conditions, including MI, when combined with prior generation cTn assays.[49] However, studies evaluating the incremental diagnostic contribution of copeptin added to high-sensitivity troponin showed no benefit in the negative predictive value for MI.[50-52]

Many patients with ACS, including those without evidence of myocyte necrosis, have elevated concentrations of inflammatory biomarkers such as C-reactive protein, serum amyloid A, myeloperoxidase, or interleukin-6. To date, no study has identified exact decision cutpoints or shown an incremental benefit with an admission or treatment strategy based on these new markers, thus limiting the clinical usefulness of these observations.[24]

D-dimer testing is useful for patients with chest pain to help rule out PE, because a negative enzyme-linked immunosorbent assay has a negative predictive value of greater than 99% in patients with a low clinical probability (patients with a higher clinical probability should undergo an imaging study).[53] Similarly, a negative D-dimer has a negative predictive value of 96% for aortic dissection.[54-56]

B-type natriuretic peptides (BNP and N-terminal pro-BNP) rise in the setting of increased ventricular wall stress. Natriuretic peptides commonly aid in the diagnosis of heart failure. BNP levels can rise in the setting of transient myocardial ischemia, and the magnitude of elevation in patients with ACS correlates with prognosis.[57] Although elevations are not specific for ACS, adding natriuretic peptide measurements to the diagnostic algorithm does improve discrimination and results in improved reclassification and is also associated with prognosis.[57]

Testing Strategy

Current practice guidelines recommend measuring biomarkers of cardiac injury in patients with symptoms that suggest ACS.[2,24] Patients with a very low probability of ACS should not undergo biomarker measurements because false-positive results could lead to unnecessary hospitalizations, tests, procedures, and complications.

The greater sensitivity of contemporary sensitive cardiac troponin assays has allowed the traditional serial biomarker sampling over 24 hours to be shortened considerably. European and U.S. guidelines are integrating the advantages of hs-cTn assays, with testing regimens that include measurements at presentation and 1 to 2 hours later, and examining both the absolute levels and change over time.[24,38] The specific cutpoints for initial concentration and change are specific to the assay, testing strategy, and duration of symptoms. However, the negative predictive value is approximately 99%. In some algorithms, a patient with a very low concentration (generally below the limit of detection) can be ruled out with a single hs-cTn measurement at least 3 hours after the onset of chest pain, whereas patients with a low concentration (assay-dependent but generally at or below the 99th percentile upper-reference limit) at baseline require a second sample but can be ruled out in the absence of changes meeting criteria for dynamic injury 1 or 2 hours later. Patients with elevated baseline levels or low or very low baseline levels with a subsequent increase exceeding the delta threshold are considered to have a high likelihood of non-ST elevation myocardial infarction (NSTEMI) and should continue with further workup and treatment. In centers where high-sensitivity assays are not available, serial testing at presentation, and 3 to 6 hours remains the standard of care.[2]

Decision Aids

An algorithm for the diagnostic evaluation of chest pain is presented in Figure 35.1. The history, physical examination, ECG, and biomarkers of myocardial injury can be integrated to allow the clinician to assess the likelihood of ACS and the risk for complications using contemporary risk scores (Tables 35.4 and 35.5). Furthermore, in terms of prognosis, multivariable algorithms have been developed and prospectively validated, with the goal of improving risk stratification in patients with acute chest pain. These algorithms can be used to estimate the probability of acute MI, unstable angina, or the risk for major cardiac complications in individual patients. They serve mainly to identify patients who are at low risk for complications and who therefore do not require admission to the hospital or coronary care unit. There exist decision aids for acute PE (see Chapter 87) and aortic dissection (see Chapter 42).

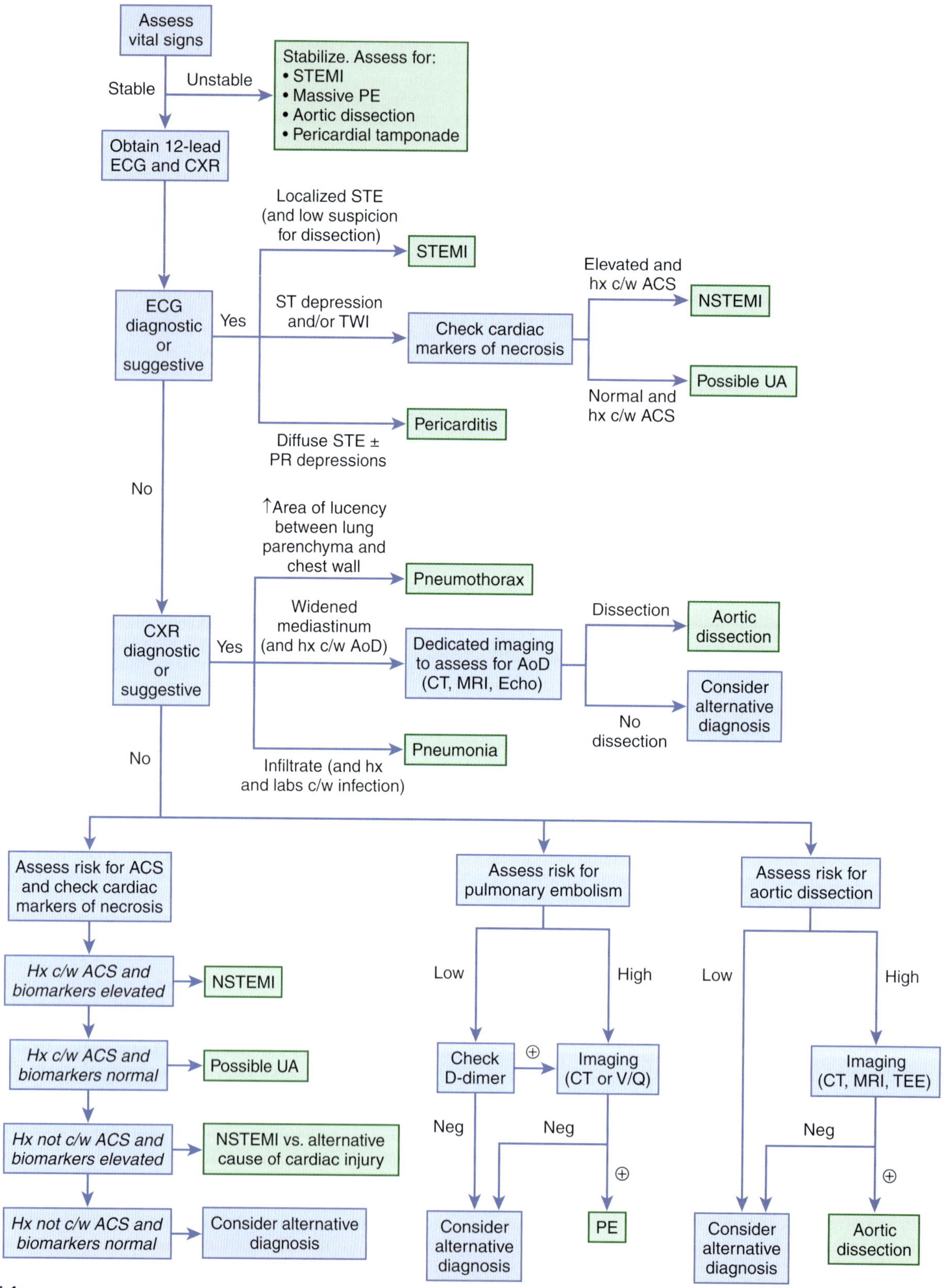

FIGURE 35.1 Algorithm for the initial diagnostic approach to a patient with chest pain. *AoD*, aortic dissection; *c/w*, consistent with; *CXR*, chest x-ray; *hx*, history; *STE*, ST elevation; *TEE*, transesophageal echocardiography; *UA*, unstable angina; *TWI*, T wave inversion; *V/A*, ventilation-perfusion scan.

The Thrombolysis in Myocardial Infarction (TIMI) Risk Score for unstable angina/NSTEMI has been derived and validated in patients enrolled in clinical trials with ACS (Table 35.4).[2] The HEART score uses similar components as the TIMI Risk score (Table 35.5). When combined with serial troponin measurements, it reduced the cardiac testing by 82%.[14] A subsequent evaluation of the HEART score and serial high-sensitivity troponin measurements at 0 and 3 hours in patients presenting with suspected ACS (HEART pathway) decreased testing at 30 days by 12.1%, decreased length of stay by 12 hours, and increased early discharges by 21%. At 30 days no patients identified for early discharge had cardiac events.[8]

IMMEDIATE MANAGEMENT

The ACC and AHA guidelines suggest an approach to the immediate management of patients with possible ACS that integrates information from the history, physical examination, 12-lead ECG, and initial cardiac marker tests to assign patients to four categories—noncardiac related diagnosis, chronic stable angina, possible ACS, and definite ACS (Fig. 35.2).[2] In this algorithm, patients with ST-segment elevations are triaged immediately for reperfusion therapy, in accordance with the ACC and AHA guidelines for STEMI. Patients with ACS who have ST wave or T wave changes, ongoing pain, positive cardiac markers, or hemodynamic abnormalities should be admitted to the hospital for the management of acute ischemia. For patients with possible or definite ACS who do not have diagnostic ECGs and whose initial serum cardiac markers are within normal limits, it is appropriate to observe them in a chest pain unit or other nonintensive care facility, with subsequent additional testing (see later). Similarly, the ESC guidelines suggest an approach based on clinical assessment, ECG, and biomarkers to enable triage for early discharge, observation, admission, or early intervention.[24]

Chest Pain Protocols and Units

According to the ACC/AHA and ESC recommendations, patients should have an assessment and patients with a low risk for ACS or associated complications can be observed while undergoing electrocardiographic monitoring and serial measurement of cardiac markers.[2,58] Patients in whom evidence of ischemia or other indicators of increased risk develop should be admitted to a cardiology service (step-down or coronary care unit) for further management. Patients in whom recurrent pain or other predictors of increased risk do not develop can either be discharged home if they are very low risk or be scheduled for early noninvasive testing (see later) before or after discharge. Specifically, as noted above, patients with normal troponin levels, no ECG abnormalities concerning for ischemia and a TIMI Risk Score of 0, or a History, Electrocardiogram, Age, Risk factors, and initial Troponin (HEART) score of ≤ 3 are at extremely low risk of adverse cardiovascular events and can be discharged. Noninvasive testing is reasonable in patients without biochemical or ECG evidence of ischemia but who are not at very low risk. Outpatient stress testing is a reasonable option if the patient is at low risk for ACS and if the testing can be accomplished within 72 hours; such a strategy has been shown to be safe. In such patients it is prudent to prescribe aspirin and possibly beta-adrenergic blocking agents (beta blockers) and to provide them with sublingual nitroglycerin.

To enhance the efficiency and reliability of implementation of such chest pain protocols, many hospitals send low-risk patients with chest pain to special chest pain units.[2,58] These units are often located adjacent to or within EDs. The rate of MI has been found to be approximately 1% to 2% in most such units, and they have proved to be safe and cost-saving sites of care for low-risk patients. Chest pain units are also sometimes used for intermediate-risk patients, such as those with a previous history of coronary disease but no other high-risk predictors. In one community-based randomized trial, patients with unstable angina and an overall intermediate risk for complications had similar outcomes and lower cost if they were triaged to a chest pain unit versus conventional hospital management.

Early Noninvasive Testing
Treadmill Electrocardiography
Treadmill exercise electrocardiography is inexpensive and available daily in many hospitals beyond traditional laboratory hours, and prospective data indicate that early exercise test results provide reliable prognostic information for low-risk patient populations.

TABLE 35.4 Thrombolysis in Myocardial Infarction Risk Score for Unstable Angina or Non-ST-Elevation Myocardial Infarction

FEATURE	ADD +1 FOR EACH COMPONENT
Age ≥65	Yes
Coronary risk factors (hypertension, hypercholesterolemia, diabetes, family history of coronary disease, current smoking)	≥3
Known coronary artery disease (stenosis ≥50%)	Yes
Aspirin use in the past 7 days	Yes
Severe angina (≥2 episodes in 24 hr)	Yes
ECG ST deviation ≥0.5 mm	Yes
Positive cardiac biomarker	Yes

Antman EM, Cohen M, Bernink PJ, et al: The TIMI risk score for unstable angina/non-ST elevation MI: A method for prognostication and therapeutic decision making. *JAMA* 2000;284(7):835-842.

TABLE 35.5 The HEART Score

FEATURE	ADD +2 FOR EACH COMPONENT	ADD +1 FOR EACH COMPONENT	ADD 0 FOR EACH COMPONENT
History	Highly suspicious	Moderately suspicious	Slightly suspicious
Electrocardiogram	Significant ST-segment deviation not due to left bundle branch block, left ventricular hypertrophy or digoxin	No ST-segment deviation but nonspecific repolarization disturbance	Normal
Age	>65	45–64	<45
Risk factors (hypertension, hypercholesterolemia, diabetes mellitus, body mass index >30 kg/m³, smoking, early family history, known atherosclerotic disease)	≥3	1–2	0
Initial troponin	>3× normal limit	1–3× normal limit	≤normal limit

Adapted from the HEART Score. Poldervaart JM, Reitsma JB, Six J, et al. Using the HEART score in patients with chest pain in the emergency department. *Ann Intern Med.* 2017;167(9):688; and Backus BE, Tolsma RT, Boogers MJ. The new era of chest pain evaluation in the Netherlands. *Eur J Emerg Med.* 2020;27(4):243–244.

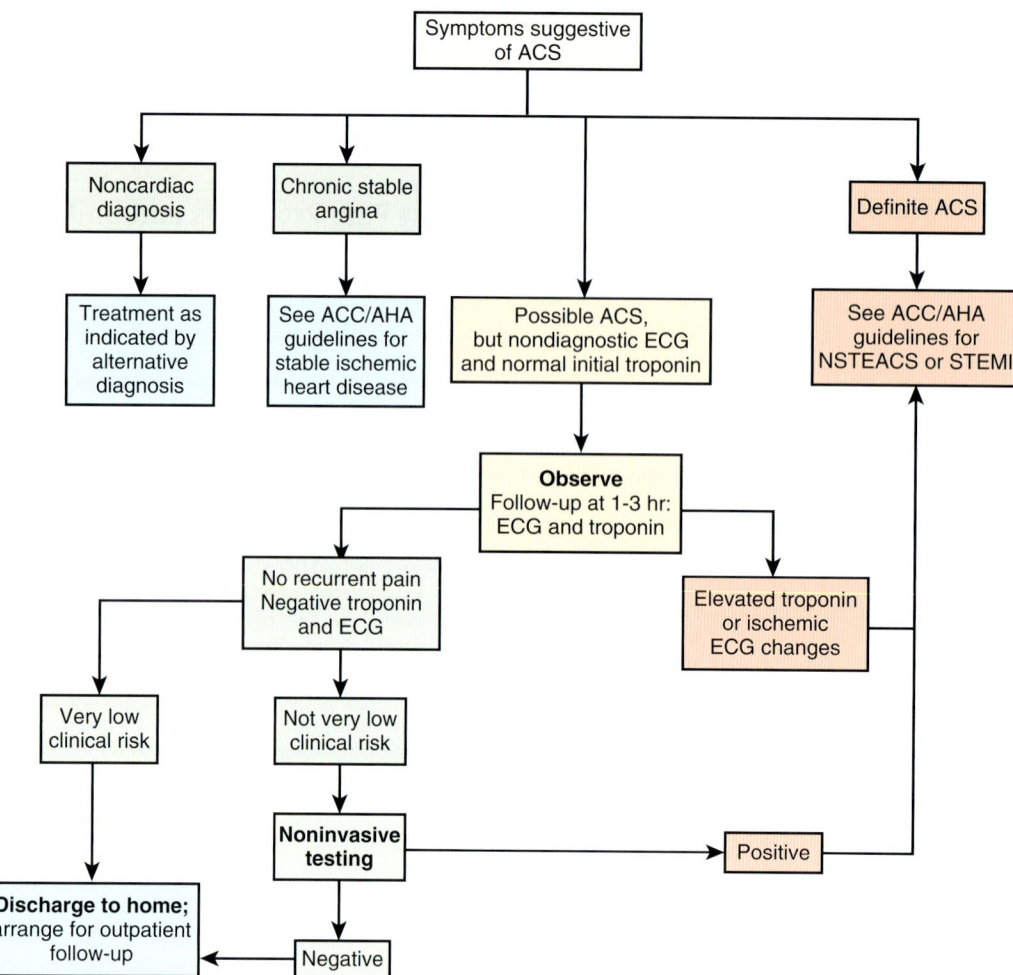

FIGURE 35.2 Algorithm for the evaluation and management of patients suspected of having ACS. (Adapted from Amsterdam EA, Wenger NK, Brindis RG, et al. 2014 AHA/ACC guideline for the management of patients with non-ST-elevation acute coronary syndromes: a report of the American College of Cardiology/American Heart Association Task Force on Practice Guidelines. *J Am Coll Cardiol.* 2014 Dec;64[24]:e139–e228.)

Most studies have used the Bruce or modified Bruce treadmill protocol. Multiple studies have demonstrated that in low-risk patients, exercise testing is safe and has a negative predictive value of typically greater than 99%, although the positive predictive value is frequently less than 50% (depending on the prevalence of ACS in the tested population).[2,24]

Patients with low clinical risk for complications can safely undergo exercise testing after their second negative troponin test (several hours later depending on testing strategy) and no other evidence of myocardial ischemia.[2,24] In general, protocols for early or immediate exercise testing exclude patients with electrocardiographic findings consistent with ischemia not recorded on previous tracings, ongoing chest pain, or evidence of congestive heart failure. The AHA/ACC guidelines note indications for and contraindications to exercise on electrocardiographic stress testing in the ED (Table 35.6).[2] For low-risk patients with no evidence of myocardial ischemia after serial ECGs and biomarkers, outpatient stress testing ideally within 24 hours, and no later than 72 hours, is safe.

Noninvasive Imaging Tests

Stress echocardiography or radionuclide scans are the preferred non-invasive functional testing modalities for patients who cannot undergo treadmill electrocardiographic testing because of physical disability or who have resting ECGs that confound interpretation. Imaging studies are less readily available and more expensive than exercise electrocardiography but are more sensitive in detecting coronary disease,

TABLE 35.6 Indications and Contraindications for Exercise Electrocardiographic Testing in the Emergency Department (ED)

Requirements before exercise electrocardiographic testing that should be considered in the ED setting:

- No evidence of myocardial injury by serial troponin (see section on biomarkers)
- ECG at the time of arrival and preexercise 12-lead ECG show no significant abnormality
- Absence of rest electrocardiographic abnormalities that would preclude accurate assessment of the exercise ECG
- From admission to the time that results are available from the second set of cardiac enzymes: patient asymptomatic, lessening chest pain symptoms, or persistent atypical symptoms
- Absence of ischemic chest pain at the time of exercise testing

Contraindications to exercise electrocardiographic testing in the ED setting:

- New or evolving electrocardiographic abnormalities on the rest tracing
- Abnormal cardiac enzyme levels
- Inability to perform exercise
- Worsening or persistent ischemic chest pain symptoms from admission to the time of exercise testing
- Clinical risk profiling indicating that imminent coronary angiography is likely

quantifying the extent of, and localizing the jeopardized myocardium. High-risk rest perfusion scans are associated with an increased risk for major cardiac complications, whereas patients with low-risk scans have low 30-day cardiac event rates (<2%).[10,59] The sensitivity of stress echocardiography appears to be comparable to that of myocardial perfusion imaging (85% to 90%), and its specificity is somewhat better (80% to 95% versus 75% to 90%).[10] As is the case for myocardial perfusion imaging, the results are less interpretable in patients with previous MI, in whom it is difficult to exclude whether the abnormalities are preexisting unless a prior study is available. Myocardial contrast-enhanced echocardiography using microbubble imaging agents offers reasonable (77%) concordance with radionuclide scanning, and the combination of regional wall motion abnormalities and reduced myocardial perfusion has a sensitivity of 80% to 90% and a specificity of 60% to 90% for ACS.[10]

In addition, echocardiography without stress in patients with active chest pain can be used to detect wall motion abnormalities consistent with myocardial ischemia or infarction. In addition, echocardiography in the acute setting may be helpful in identifying noncoronary etiologies of chest pain including right ventricular findings in PE, aortic dissection, pericardial effusion, and others. These findings are often not of adequate sensitivity or specificity on their own but will require subsequent testing to confirm those diagnoses (e.g., aortic CTA, PE CTA).[24] The presence of induced or baseline regional wall motion abnormalities correlates with a worse prognosis.

Likewise, in addition to stress imaging studies to detect provocable ischemia, rest radionuclide scans can also help determine whether a patient's symptoms is myocardial ischemia.[10,59] In a multicenter prospective randomized trial of 2475 adult ED patients with ongoing or recently resolved (<3 hours) chest pain or other symptoms suggestive of acute cardiac ischemia and with normal or nondiagnostic initial electrocardiographic results, patients were randomly assigned to receive the usual evaluation strategy or the usual strategy supplemented with results from acute resting myocardial perfusion imaging. The availability of scan results did not influence the management of patients with acute MI or unstable angina, but it reduced rates of hospitalization from 52% to 42% in patients without acute cardiac ischemia. Rest myocardial perfusion imaging is most sensitive if performed when a patient is experiencing ischemic symptoms, with its sensitivity progressively diminishing thereafter. Imaging should be performed within 2 hours of the resolution of symptoms, although data support its use for up to 4 hours.[53] It should be noted that perfusion defects seen at rest could represent either acute ischemia or previous infarction, which can be differentiated on subsequent pain-free rest imaging.

Cardiac magnetic resonance imaging (MRI) is also being explored for the assessment of patients with suspected ACS for anatomic (e.g., wall motion), perfusion, and angiography.[60-63] Similar to echocardiography, MRI can provide information on noncoronary etiologies of chest pain such as myocarditis. In a study that used cardiac MRI to quantify myocardial perfusion, ventricular function, and hyperenhancement in patients with chest pain, the sensitivity for ACS was 84% and the specificity was 85%. The addition of T2-weighted imaging, which can detect myocardial edema and thus help differentiate acute from chronic perfusion defects, improves the specificity to 96% without sacrificing sensitivity.[60] A randomized study of 1202 patients with suspected ACS found that cardiovascular MR resulted in a lower probability of unnecessary angiography within 12 months as compared to guideline-directed care with no difference in adverse cardiac outcomes.[64] Resource availability and time requirements may limit the common utilization of cardiac MRI in this setting.

Anatomic imaging with coronary computed tomographic angiography (CCTA) allows the visualization of the coronary arteries and other vascular territories (e.g., ascending aorta) and anatomic information on noncoronary structures such as the pericardium and lungs.[59] Using multidetector computed tomography, coronary CTA has a sensitivity of greater than 90% and a specificity of 65% to 90% for coronary stenosis greater than 50%.[24] Coronary CTA has been evaluated in patients presenting with suspected ACS. A meta-analysis of randomized trials testing coronary CTA versus usual care in chest pain patients judged to be at low-to-intermediate risk found that CTA use was associated with a reduction in ED costs and length of stay and no difference in death or rehospitalizations.[65] Most of these studies were performed using conventional (less sensitive) cTn assays and CTA and are associated with a greater use of invasive angiography.[24,65] A more recent study, however, in patients presenting with suspected MI found that upfront CCTA reduced the need for angiography.[63] An observational cohort study evaluated the combination of hs-cTn at presentation and CCTA looking at advanced features of CAD (≥50% stenosis, high-risk plaque features: positive remodeling, low <30-Hounsfield units plaque, napkin-ring sign, spotty calcium) relative to conventional troponin and CCTA looking at traditional features of CAD (no CAD, nonobstructive CAD, ≥50% stenosis) and found greater diagnostic accuracy for ACS using high-sensitivity troponin and advanced CTA assessment.[9] A subsequent study reported similar findings and reported a 90.9% negative predictive value for CCTA in patients with non-ST-elevation ACS.[66] In addition to diagnosis, CCTA can provide calcium scores providing prognostic information and potentially informing the need for additional cardiac testing.[67] The most recent ACC/AHA and ESC guidelines acknowledge CCTA as a reasonable alternative to stress testing in patients with low-to-intermediate clinical probability of CAD.[2,24]

Another advantage of CTA is that it is often the test of choice for PE and for aortic dissection (see Chapters 20, 42, and 87), and thus so-called triple-rule-out CTA can be performed to evaluate coronary disease, PE, and aortic dissection.[11,68] While this approach is accurate for detecting CAD, the low prevalence of PE and aortic dissection and the increased radiation and contrast exposure relative to traditional CCTA suggest it would be reasonable to restrict triple-rule-out scans to patients with a reasonable suspicion for PE or aortic dissection.[11,68,69] Another limitation is that the timing of contrast administration and imaging may not be optimized for all study components potentially limiting diagnostic accuracy. Ultimately, the traditional trifecta of a clinician's careful assessment of the prior probability of a cardiovascular origin for chest discomfort, the nature of the acute episode, and the physical examination should be coupled with even more precise objective data including serial ECGs, rapid biomarker testing, and tailored imaging to rapidly and optimally triage patients presenting with chest pain.

REFERENCES

Background

1. CDC. https://www.cdc.gov/nchs/fastats/emergency-department.htm. Web site. https://www.cdc.gov/nchs/fastats/emergency-department.htm. Accessed September 10, 2020.
2. Amsterdam EA, Wenger NK, Brindis RG, et al. AHA/ACC guideline for the management of patients with non-ST-elevation acute coronary syndromes: a report of the American College of Cardiology/American Heart Association Task Force on Practice Guidelines. *Circulation*. 2014;130(25):e344–e426.
3. Ko DT, Dattani ND, Austin PC, et al. Emergency department volume and outcomes for patients after chest pain assessment. *Circ Cardiovasc Qual Outcomes*. 2018;11(11):e004683.
4. Roffi M, Patrono C, Collet JP, et al. ESC guidelines for the management of acute coronary syndromes in patients presenting without persistent ST-segment elevation: Task Force for the management of acute coronary syndromes in patients presenting without persistent ST-segment elevation of the European Society of Cardiology (ESC). *Eur Heart J*. 2016;37(3):267–315. 2015.
5. Virani SS, Alonso A, Benjamin EJ, et al. Heart disease and stroke statistics-2020 update: a report from the American Heart Association. *Circulation*. 2020;141(9):e139–e596.
6. Morrow DA. Evidence-based algorithms using high-sensitivity cardiac troponin in the emergency department. *JAMA Cardiol*. 2016;1(4):379–381.
7. Morrow DA. Clinician's guide to early rule-out strategies with high-sensitivity cardiac troponin. *Circulation*. 2017;135(17):1612–1616.
8. Mahler SA, Riley RF, Hiestand BC, et al. The HEART Pathway randomized trial: identifying emergency department patients with acute chest pain for early discharge. *Circ Cardiovasc Qual Outcomes*. 2015;8(2):195–203.
9. Ferencik M, Liu T, Mayrhofer T, et al. Hs-troponin I followed by CT angiography improves acute coronary syndrome risk stratification accuracy and work-up in acute chest pain patients: results from ROMICAT II trial. *JACC Cardiovasc Imaging*. 2015;8(11):1272–1281.
10. Rybicki FJ, Udelson JE, Peacock WF, et al. ACR/ACC/AHA/AATS/ACEP/ASNC/NASCI/SAEM/SCCT/SCMR/SCPC/SNMMI/STR/STS appropriate utilization of cardiovascular imaging in emergency department patients with chest pain: a joint document of the American College of Radiology Appropriateness Criteria Committee and the American College of Cardiology Appropriate Use Criteria Task Force. *J Am Coll Cardiol*. 2016;67(7):853–879.
11. Whorowski AM, Halpern EJ. Diagnostic yield of triple-rule-out CT in an emergency setting. *AJR Am J Roentgenol*. 2016;207(2):295–301.
12. Poldervaart JM, Reitsma JB, Backus BE, et al. Effect of using the HEART score in patients with chest pain in the emergency department: a stepped-wedge, cluster randomized trial. *Ann Intern Med*. 2017;166(10):689–697.
13. Poldervaart JM, Reitsma JB, Six J, et al. Using the HEART score in patients with chest pain in the emergency department. *Ann Intern Med*. 2017;167(9):688.

Causes of Chest Pain

14. Bonaca MP, Sabatine MS. Approach to the patient with chest pain. In: Libby PL, ed. *Heart Disease*. Vol. 11. 2017:1059–1068.
15. Pickering JW, Greenslade JH, Cullen L, et al. Assessment of the European Society of Cardiology 0-hour/1-hour algorithm to rule-out and rule-in acute myocardial infarction. *Circulation*. 2016;134(20):1532–1541.

16. Fanaroff AC, Rymer JA, Goldstein SA, et al. Does this patient with chest pain have acute coronary syndrome?: the rational clinical examination systematic review. *J Am Med Assoc.* 2015;314(18):1955–1965.
17. Sandoval Y, Smith SW, Sexter A, et al. Clinical features and outcomes of emergency department patients with high-sensitivity cardiac troponin I concentrations within sex-specific reference intervals. *Circulation.* 2019;139(14):1753–1755.
18. McNamara N, Ibrahim A, Satti Z, et al. Acute pericarditis: a review of current diagnostic and management guidelines. *Future Cardiol.* 2019;15(2):119–126.
19. O'Connor MJ. Imaging the itis: endocarditis, myocarditis, and pericarditis. *Curr Opin Cardiol.* 2019;34(1):57–64.
20. Zhu Y, Lingala B, Baiocchi M, et al. Type A aortic dissection-experience over 5 decades: JACC historical breakthroughs in perspective. *J Am Coll Cardiol.* 2020;76(14):1703–1713.
21. Germini F, Zarabi S, Eventov M, et al. Pulmonary embolism prevalence among emergency department cohorts: a systematic review and meta-analysis by country of study. *J Thromb Haemost.* 2020.
22. Tomkiewicz EM, Kline JA. Concise review of the clinical approach to the exclusion and diagnosis of pulmonary embolism in 2020. *J Emerg Nurs.* 2020;46(4):527–538.
23. de Wolff JF, Fawcett KM. Non-cardiac chest pain. *Acute Med.* 2019;18(4):260.

Diagnostic Considerations and Testing Strategies

24. Collet JP, Thiele H, Barbato E, et al. ESC Guidelines for the management of acute coronary syndromes in patients presenting without persistent ST-segment elevation. *Eur Heart J.* 2020.
25. Mnatzaganian G, Hiller JE, Braitberg G, et al. Sex disparities in the assessment and outcomes of chest pain presentations in emergency departments. *Heart.* 2020;106(2):111–118.
26. Body R, Carley S, McDowell G, et al. The Manchester Acute Coronary Syndromes (MACS) decision rule for suspected cardiac chest pain: derivation and external validation. *Heart.* 2014;100(18):1462–1468.
27. Im DD, Jambaulikar GD, Kikut A, et al. Brief pain inventory-short form: a new method for assessing pain in the emergency department. *Pain Med.* 2020;21(12):3263–3269.
28. Kelly CR, Kirtane AJ, Stant J, et al. An updated protocol for evaluating chest pain and managing acute coronary syndromes. *Crit Pathw Cardiol.* 2017;16(1):7–14.
29. Stevenson A, Davis S, Murch N. Pulmonary embolism in acute medicine: a case-based review incorporating latest guidelines in the COVID-19 era. *Br J Hosp Med.* 2020;81(6):1–12.
30. Supinski D, Borg B, Schmitz K, et al. Chest pain severity rating is a poor predictive tool in the diagnosis of ST-segment elevation myocardial infarction. *Crit Pathw Cardiol.* 2020.
31. Barrabes JA, Bardaji A, Jimenez-Candil J, et al. Characteristics and outcomes of patients hospitalized with suspected acute coronary syndrome in whom the diagnosis is not confirmed. *Am J Cardiol.* 2018;122(10):1604–1609.
32. Body R, Cook G, Burrows G, et al. Can emergency physicians 'rule in' and 'rule out' acute myocardial infarction with clinical judgement? *Emerg Med J.* 2014;31(11):872–876.
33. Morrow A, Ahmad F, Steele C, et al. Treating the troponin: adverse consequences of over-treatment of elevated troponin in non-coronary presentations. *Scott Med J.* 2019;64(1):10–15.
34. Mueller C, Giannitsis E, Mockel M, et al. Rapid rule out of acute myocardial infarction: novel biomarker-based strategies. *Eur Heart J Acute Cardiovasc Care.* 2017;6(3):218–222.
35. Sandoval Y, Gunsolus IL, Smith SW, et al. Appropriateness of cardiac troponin testing: insights from the Use of TROPonin In Acute coronary syndromes (UTROPIA) study. *Am J Med.* 2019;132(7):869–874.
36. Sandoval Y, Smith SW, Shah AS, et al. Rapid rule-out of acute myocardial injury using a single high-sensitivity cardiac troponin I measurement. *Clin Chem.* 2017;63(1):369–376.
37. Shah ASV, Anand A, Strachan FE, et al. High-sensitivity troponin in the evaluation of patients with suspected acute coronary syndrome: a stepped-wedge, cluster-randomised controlled trial. *Lancet.* 2018;392(10151):919–928.
38. Thygesen K, Alpert JS, Jaffe AS, et al. Fourth universal definition of myocardial infarction (2018). *Circulation.* 2018;138(20):e618–e651.
39. Chapman AR, Lee KK, McAllister DA, et al. Association of high-sensitivity cardiac troponin I concentration with cardiac outcomes in patients with suspected acute coronary syndrome. *J Am Med Assoc.* 2017;318(19):1913–1924.
40. McCarthy CP, Raber I, Chapman AR, et al. Myocardial injury in the era of high-sensitivity cardiac troponin assays: a practical approach for clinicians. *JAMA Cardiol.* 2019;4(10):1034–1042.
41. Shah AS, Anand A, Sandoval Y, et al. High-sensitivity cardiac troponin I at presentation in patients with suspected acute coronary syndrome: a cohort study. *Lancet.* 2015;386(10012):2481–2488.
42. Shah AS, Griffiths M, Lee KK, et al. High sensitivity cardiac troponin and the under-diagnosis of myocardial infarction in women: prospective cohort study. *BMJ.* 2015;350:g7873.
43. Mueller C, Giannitsis E, Christ M, et al. Multicenter evaluation of a 0-hour/1-hour algorithm in the diagnosis of myocardial infarction using high-sensitivity cardiac troponin T. *Ann Emerg Med.* 2016;68(1):76–87.e74.
44. Peacock WF, Baumann BM, Bruton D, et al. Efficacy of high-sensitivity troponin T in identifying very-low-risk patients with possible acute coronary syndrome. *JAMA Cardiol.* 2018;3(2):104–111.
45. Pickering JW, Than MP, Cullen L, et al. Rapid rule-out of acute myocardial infarction with a single high-sensitivity cardiac troponin T measurement below the limit of detection: a collaborative meta-analysis. *Ann Intern Med.* 2017;166(10):715–724.
46. Reichlin T, Twerenbold R, Wildi K, et al. Prospective validation of a 1-hour algorithm to rule-out and rule-in acute myocardial infarction using a high-sensitivity cardiac troponin T assay. *CMAJ (Can Med Assoc J).* 2015;187(8):E243–E252.
47. Rottger E, de Vries-Spithoven S, Reitsma JB, et al. Safety of a 1-hour rule-out high-sensitive troponin T protocol in patients with chest pain at the emergency department. *Crit Pathw Cardiol.* 2017;16(4):129–134.
48. Kaier TE, Twerenbold R, Puelacher C, et al. Direct comparison of cardiac myosin-binding protein C with cardiac troponins for the early diagnosis of acute myocardial infarction. *Circulation.* 2017;136(16):1495–1508.
49. Mockel M, Searle J, Hamm C, et al. Early discharge using single cardiac troponin and copeptin testing in patients with suspected acute coronary syndrome (ACS): a randomized, controlled clinical process study. *Eur Heart J.* 2015;36(6):369–376.
50. Hillinger P, Twerenbold R, Jaeger C, et al. Optimizing early rule-out strategies for acute myocardial infarction: utility of 1-hour copeptin. *Clin Chem.* 2015;61(12):1466–1474.
51. Boeddinghaus J, Nestelberger T, Twerenbold R, et al. Direct comparison of 4 very early rule-out strategies for acute myocardial infarction using high-sensitivity cardiac troponin I. *Circulation.* 2017;135(17):1597–1611.
52. Mueller C, Mockel M, Giannitsis E, et al. Use of copeptin for rapid rule-out of acute myocardial infarction. *Eur Heart J Acute Cardiovasc Care.* 2018;7(6):570–576.
53. Crawford F, Andras A, Welch K, et al. D-dimer test for excluding the diagnosis of pulmonary embolism. *Cochrane Database Syst Rev.* 2016;8:CD010864.
54. Nazerian P, Mueller C, Soeiro AM, et al. Diagnostic accuracy of the aortic dissection detection risk score plus D-dimer for acute aortic syndromes: the ADvISED prospective multicenter study. *Circulation.* 2018;137(3):250–258.
55. Nitta K, Imamura H, Kashima Y, et al. Impact of a negative D-dimer result on the initial assessment of acute aortic dissection. *Int J Cardiol.* 2018;258:232–236.
56. Tsutsumi Y, Tsujimoto Y, Takahashi S, et al. Accuracy of aortic dissection detection risk score alone or with D-dimer: a systematic review and meta-analysis. *Eur Heart J Acute Cardiovasc Care.* 2020.2048872620901831.
57. Kavsak PA, Neumann JT, Cullen L, et al. Clinical chemistry score versus high-sensitivity cardiac troponin I and T tests alone to identify patients at low or high risk for myocardial infarction or death at presentation to the emergency department. *CMAJ (Can Med Assoc J).* 2018;190(33):E974–E984.

Chest Pain Protocols and Early Testing

58. Collet JP, Thiele H. The 'Ten Commandments' for the 2020 ESC Guidelines for the management of acute coronary syndromes in patients presenting without persistent ST-segment elevation. *Eur Heart J.* 2020;41(37):3495–3497.
59. Hoffmann U, Akers SR, Brown RK, et al. ACR appropriateness criteria acute nonspecific chest pain-low probability of coronary artery disease. *J Am Coll Radiol.* 2015;12(12 Pt A):1266–1271.
60. Bogaert J, Eitel I. Role of cardiovascular magnetic resonance in acute coronary syndrome. *Glob Cardiol Sci Pract.* 2015;2015(2):24.
61. De Filippo M, Capasso R. Coronary computed tomography angiography (CCTA) and cardiac magnetic resonance (CMR) imaging in the assessment of patients presenting with chest pain suspected for acute coronary syndrome. *Ann Transl Med.* 2016;4(13):255.
62. Garg P, Underwood SR, Senior R, et al. Noninvasive cardiac imaging in suspected acute coronary syndrome. *Nat Rev Cardiol.* 2016;13(5):266–275.
63. Smulders MW, Kietselaer B, Wildberger JE, et al. Initial imaging-guided strategy versus routine care in patients with non-ST-segment elevation myocardial infarction. *J Am Coll Cardiol.* 2019;74(20):2466–2477.
64. Greenwood JP, Ripley DP, Berry C, et al. Effect of care guided by cardiovascular magnetic resonance, myocardial perfusion scintigraphy, or NICE guidelines on subsequent unnecessary angiography rates: the CE-MARC 2 randomized clinical trial. *J Am Med Assoc.* 2016;316(10):1051–1060.
65. Siontis GC, Mavridis D, Greenwood JP, et al. Outcomes of non-invasive diagnostic modalities for the detection of coronary artery disease: network meta-analysis of diagnostic randomised controlled trials. *BMJ.* 2018;360:k504.
66. Linde JJ, Kelbaek H, Hansen TF, et al. Coronary CT angiography in patients with non-ST-segment elevation acute coronary syndrome. *J Am Coll Cardiol.* 2020;75(5):453–463.
67. Chaikriangkrai K, Shantha GPS, Jhun HY, et al. Prognostic value of coronary artery calcium score in acute chest pain patients without known coronary artery disease: systematic review and meta-analysis. *Ann Emerg Med.* 2016;68(6):659–670.
68. Hollander JE, Chang AM. Triple rule out CTA scans or the right test for the right patient. *JACC Cardiovasc Imaging.* 2015;8(7):826–827.
69. Burris 2nd AC, Boura JA, Raff GL, Chinnaiyan KM. Triple rule out versus coronary CT angiography in patients with acute chest pain: results from the ACIC consortium. *JACC Cardiovasc Imaging.* 2015;8(7):817–825.
70. Group TS. TIMI Risk Score Calculator for UA/NSTEMI. https://timi.org/calculators/timi-risk-score-calculator-for-ua-nstemi/.

36 Coronary Blood Flow and Myocardial Ischemia

DIRK J. DUNCKER AND JOHN M. CANTY JR.

CONTROL OF CORONARY BLOOD FLOW, 609
Determinants of Myocardial Oxygen Consumption, 609
Coronary Autoregulation, 609
Determinants of Coronary Vascular Resistance, 611
Endothelium-Dependent Modulation of Coronary Tone, 612
Paracrine Vasoactive Mediators and Coronary Vasospasm, 613
Structure and Function of the Coronary Microcirculation, 614

PHYSIOLOGIC ASSESSMENT OF CORONARY ARTERY STENOSES, 617
Stenosis Pressure-Flow Relation, 617
Interrelation Among Distal Coronary Pressure, Flow, and Stenosis Severity, 619
Flow- and Pressure-Derived Indices of Coronary Reserve, 619
Pathophysiologic States Affecting Microcirculatory Coronary Flow Reserve, 622

CORONARY COLLATERAL CIRCULATION, 627
Arteriogenesis and Angiogenesis, 628

Regulation of Collateral Resistance, 628

METABOLIC AND FUNCTIONAL CONSEQUENCES OF ISCHEMIA, 628
Irreversible Injury and Myocyte Death, 628
Reversible Ischemia and Perfusion-Contraction Matching, 629
Functional Consequences of Reversible Ischemia, 630

FUTURE PERSPECTIVES, 635

CLASSIC REFERENCES, 635

REFERENCES, 635

The coronary circulation is unique in that the heart is responsible for generating the arterial pressure that is required to perfuse the systemic circulation and yet, at the same time, has its own perfusion impeded during the systolic phase of the cardiac cycle. Because myocardial contraction is closely connected to coronary flow and oxygen delivery, the balance between oxygen supply and demand is a critical determinant of the normal beat-to-beat function of the heart (see Classic References, Feigl). When this relation is acutely disrupted by diseases affecting coronary blood flow, the resulting imbalance can immediately precipitate a vicious cycle whereby ischemia-induced contractile dysfunction precipitates hypotension and further myocardial ischemia. Thus, knowledge of the regulation of coronary blood flow, determinants of myocardial oxygen consumption, and the relation between ischemia and contraction is essential for understanding the pathophysiologic basis and management of many cardiovascular disorders (see Classic References, Hoffman and Spaan).

CONTROL OF CORONARY BLOOD FLOW

There are pronounced systolic and diastolic coronary flow variations throughout the cardiac cycle, with coronary arterial inflow out of phase with venous outflow (Fig. 36.1). Systolic contraction increases tissue pressure, redistributes perfusion from the subendocardial to the subepicardial layers of the heart, and impedes coronary arterial inflow, which reaches a nadir. At the same time, systolic compression reduces the diameter of intramyocardial microcirculatory vessels (arterioles, capillaries, and venules) and increases coronary venous outflow, which peaks during systole. During diastole, coronary arterial inflow increases with a transmural gradient that favors perfusion to the subendocardial vessels. At this time, coronary venous outflow falls.

Determinants of Myocardial Oxygen Consumption

In contrast to most other vascular beds, myocardial oxygen extraction is near-maximal at rest, averaging 70% to 80% of arterial oxygen content.[1,2] The ability to increase oxygen extraction as a means to increase oxygen delivery is limited to circumstances associated with sympathetic activation and acute subendocardial ischemia. Nevertheless, coronary venous oxygen tension (Pv_{O_2}) can only decrease from 25 mm Hg to approximately 15 mm Hg. Because of the high resting oxygen extraction, increases in myocardial oxygen consumption are primarily met by proportional increases in coronary flow and oxygen delivery[2]. In addition to coronary flow, oxygen delivery is directly determined by arterial oxygen content (Ca_{O_2}). This is equal to the product of hemoglobin concentration and arterial oxygen saturation plus a small amount of oxygen dissolved in plasma that is directly related to arterial oxygen tension (Pa_{O_2}). Thus, for any given flow level, anemia results in proportional reductions in oxygen delivery, whereas hypoxia, resulting from the nonlinear oxygen dissociation curve, results in relatively small reductions in oxygen content until Pa_{O_2} falls to the steep portion of the oxygen dissociation curve (below 50 mm Hg).

The major determinants of myocardial oxygen consumption are heart rate, systolic pressure (or myocardial wall stress), and left ventricular (LV) contractility (see Chapter 46). A twofold increase in any of these individual determinants of oxygen consumption requires an approximately 50% increase in coronary flow. Experimentally, the systolic pressure volume area is proportional to myocardial work and linearly related to myocardial oxygen consumption. The basal myocardial oxygen requirements needed to maintain critical membrane function are low (approximately 15% of resting oxygen consumption), and the cost of electrical activation is trivial when mechanical contraction ceases during diastolic arrest (as with cardioplegia) and diminishes during ischemia.

Coronary Autoregulation

Regional coronary blood flow remains constant as coronary artery pressure is reduced below aortic pressure over a wide range when the determinants of myocardial oxygen consumption are kept constant. This phenomenon is termed *autoregulation* (Fig. 36.2). When pressure falls to the lower limit of autoregulation, coronary resistance arteries are maximally vasodilated to intrinsic stimuli, and flow becomes pressure-dependent, resulting in the onset of subendocardial ischemia. Resting coronary blood flow under normal hemodynamic conditions averages 0.7 to 1.0 mL/min/g and can increase fourfold to fivefold during vasodilation. The ability to increase flow above resting values in response to pharmacologic vasodilation is termed *coronary flow reserve*. Flow in the maximally vasodilated heart is dependent on coronary arterial pressure. Maximum perfusion and coronary flow reserve are reduced when the diastolic time available for subendocardial perfusion is decreased (tachycardia) or the compressive determinants of diastolic perfusion (preload) are increased. Coronary reserve also is diminished by anything that increases resting flow, including increases in the hemodynamic determinants of oxygen consumption (systolic pressure, heart rate, and contractility) and reductions in arterial oxygen supply (anemia and hypoxia). Thus, circumstances can develop that precipitate subendocardial ischemia in the presence of normal coronary arteries (see Classic References, Hoffman and Spaan). Although initial studies suggested that the lower pressure limit of autoregulation is 70 mm Hg, it was later shown that coronary flow can be autoregulated to mean coronary pressures as low as 40 mm Hg (diastolic pressures of 30 mm Hg) in conscious dogs in the basal state (Fig. 36.3). These coronary pressure levels are similar to those recorded in humans without symptoms of ischemia, distal to chronic coronary occlusions, using pressure wire micromanometers. The lower autoregulatory pressure limit increases during tachycardia because of an increase in flow requirements, as well as a reduction in the time available for perfusion.

Figure 36.3 also illustrates important transmural variations in the lower autoregulatory pressure limit that result in increased vulnerability of the subendocardium to ischemia. Subendocardial flow occurs primarily in diastole and begins to decrease below a mean coronary pressure of 40 mm Hg. In contrast, subepicardial flow occurs throughout the cardiac cycle and is maintained until coronary pressure falls below 25 mm Hg. This difference arises from increased oxygen consumption in the subendocardium, requiring a higher resting flow level, as well as the more pronounced effects of systolic contraction on subendocardial vasodilator reserve. The transmural difference in the lower autoregulatory pressure limit results in vulnerability of the subendocardium to ischemia in the presence of a coronary stenosis. Although there is no pharmacologically recruitable flow reserve during ischemia

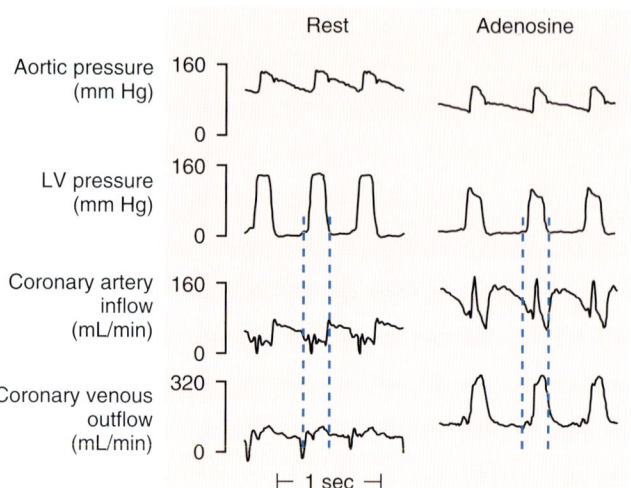

FIGURE 36.1 Phasic coronary arterial inflow and venous outflow at rest and during adenosine vasodilation. Arterial inflow primarily occurs during diastole. During systole (*dashed vertical lines*), arterial inflow declines as venous outflow peaks, reflecting the compression of microcirculatory vessels during systole. After adenosine administration, the phasic variations in venous outflow are more pronounced. *LV,* Left ventricular. (Modified from Canty JM Jr, Brooks A. Phasic volumetric coronary venous outflow patterns in conscious dogs. Am J Physiol 1990;258:H1457.)

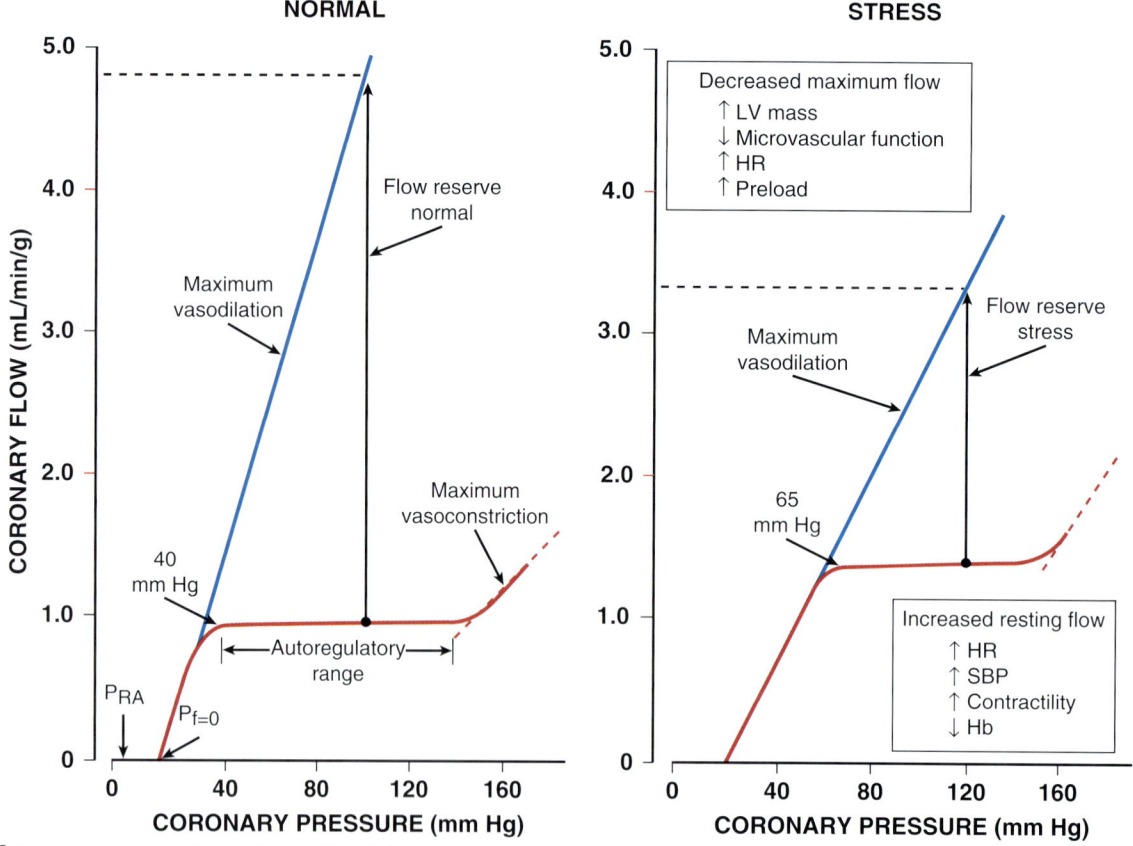

FIGURE 36.2 Autoregulatory relation under basal conditions and after metabolic stress (e.g., tachycardia). **Left,** The normal heart maintains coronary blood flow constant as regional coronary pressure is varied over a wide range when the global determinants of oxygen consumption are kept constant (*red lines*). Below the lower autoregulatory pressure limit (approximately 40 mm Hg), subendocardial vessels are maximally vasodilated and myocardial ischemia develops. During vasodilation (*blue lines*), flow increases four to five times above resting values at a normal arterial pressure. Coronary flow ceases at a pressure higher than right atrial pressure (P_{RA}), called *zero flow pressure* ($P_{f=0}$), which is the effective backpressure to flow in the absence of coronary collaterals. **Right,** During stress, tachycardia increases the compressive determinants of coronary resistance by decreasing the time available for diastolic perfusion and thus reduces maximum vasodilated flow. In addition, an increase in left ventricular (LV) preload, LV mass (i.e., LV hypertrophy) or a loss of microvascular function (e.g., in microvascular disease) all limit maximal blood flow per gram of myocardium. In addition, increases in myocardial oxygen demand or reductions in arterial oxygen content (e.g., from anemia or hypoxemia) increase resting flow. These changes reduce coronary flow reserve, the ratio between dilated and resting coronary flow, and cause ischemia to develop at higher coronary pressures. *Hb,* Hemoglobin; *HR,* heart rate; *SBP,* systolic blood pressure.

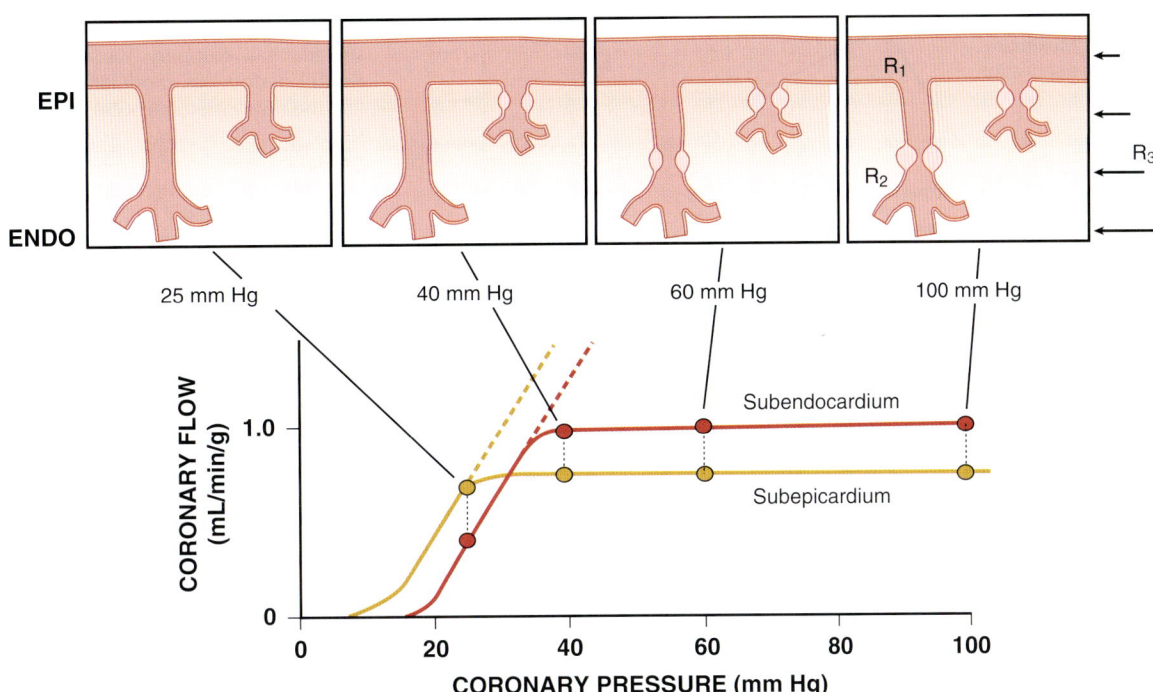

FIGURE 36.3 Transmural variations in coronary autoregulation and myocardial metabolism. Increased vulnerability of the subendocardium (ENDO, *red*) versus subepicardium (EPI, *gold*) to ischemia reflects the fact that autoregulation is exhausted at a higher coronary pressure (40 versus 25 mm Hg). This is the result of increased resting flow and oxygen consumption in the subendocardium and an increased sensitivity to systolic compressive effects, because subendocardial flow only occurs during diastole. Subendocardial vessels become maximally vasodilated before those in the subepicardium as coronary artery pressure is reduced. These transmural differences can be increased further during tachycardia or during conditions with elevated preload, which reduce maximum subendocardial perfusion. (Modified from Canty JM Jr. Coronary pressure-function and steady-state pressure-flow relations during autoregulation in the unanesthetized dog. Circ Res 1988;63:821-836.)

in the normal coronary circulation, reductions in coronary flow below the lower limit of autoregulation can occur in the presence of pharmacologically recruitable coronary flow reserve under certain circumstances, such as exercise (see Classic References, Duncker and Bache).

Determinants of Coronary Vascular Resistance

The resistance to coronary blood flow can be divided into three major components (see Figs. 36.3 and 36.4) (see Classic References, Klocke, 1976). Under normal circumstances, there is no measurable pressure drop in the epicardial arteries, indicating negligible conduit resistance (R_1). With the development of hemodynamically significant epicardial artery narrowing (>50% diameter reduction), the fixed conduit artery resistance begins to contribute an increasing component to total coronary resistance and, when severely narrowed (>90%), may reduce resting flow.

The second component of coronary resistance (R_2) is dynamic and arises primarily from microcirculatory resistance arteries and arterioles. This is distributed throughout the myocardium across a broad range of microcirculatory resistance vessel sizes (20 to 400 μm in diameter) and changes in response to physical forces (intraluminal pressure and shear stress), as well as the metabolic needs of the tissue. Normally, little resistance is contributed by coronary venules and capillaries, and their resistance remains fairly constant during changes in vasomotor tone. Even in the maximally vasodilated heart, capillary resistance accounts for no more than 20% of the microvascular resistance.[1] Thus a twofold increase in capillary density would increase maximal myocardial perfusion by only approximately 10%. Minimal coronary vascular resistance of the microcirculation is primarily determined by the size and density of arterial resistance vessels and results in substantial coronary flow reserve in the normal heart.

Extravascular Compressive Resistance. The third component, extravascular compressive resistance (R_3), varies with time throughout the cardiac cycle and is related to cardiac contraction and systolic pressure development within the left ventricle (see Fig. 36.4). In heart failure, compressive effects from elevated ventricular diastolic pressure also impede perfusion by passive compression of microcirculatory vessels from elevated extravascular tissue pressure during diastole. Increases in preload effectively raise the normal backpressure to coronary flow above coronary venous pressure levels. Compressive effects are most prominent in the subendocardium (see later).

During systole, cardiac contraction raises extravascular tissue pressure to values equal to LV pressure at the subendocardium. This declines to values near pleural pressure at the subepicardium. The increased effective backpressure during systole produces a time-varying reduction in the driving pressure for coronary flow that impedes perfusion to the subendocardium. Although this paradigm can explain variations in systolic coronary inflow, it is not able to account for the increase in coronary venous systolic outflow (see Fig. 36.1). To explain both impaired inflow and accelerated venous outflow, some investigators have proposed the concept of the intramyocardial pump (see Classic References, Hoffman and Spaan). In this model, microcirculatory vessels are compressed during systole and produce a capacitive discharge of blood that accelerates flow from the microcirculation to the coronary venous system (Fig. 36.5). At the same time, the upstream capacitive discharge impedes systolic coronary arterial inflow. Although this explains the phasic variations in coronary arterial inflow and venous outflow, as well as its transmural distribution in systole, vascular capacitance cannot explain compressive effects related to elevated tissue pressure during diastole. Thus, intramyocardial capacitance, compressive changes in effective coronary backpressure, increases in systolic coronary resistance, and a time-varying driving pressure all contribute to the compressive determinants of phasic systolic coronary blood flow.

Transmural Variations in Minimum Coronary Resistance (R_2) and Diastolic Driving Pressure. The subendocardial vulnerability to compressive determinants of vascular resistance is partially compensated by a reduced minimal resistance resulting from an increased arteriolar and capillary density. Because of this vascular gradient, subendocardial flow during maximal pharmacologic vasodilation of the nonbeating heart is greater than subepicardial perfusion. Coronary vascular resistance in the maximally vasodilated heart also is pressure dependent, reflecting passive distention of arterial resistance vessels. Thus, the instantaneous vasodilated value of coronary resistance obtained at a normal coronary distending pressure will be lower than that at a reduced pressure.

The precise determinants of the effective driving pressure for diastolic perfusion continue to be controversial. Most experimental studies demonstrate that the effective backpressure to flow in the heart is

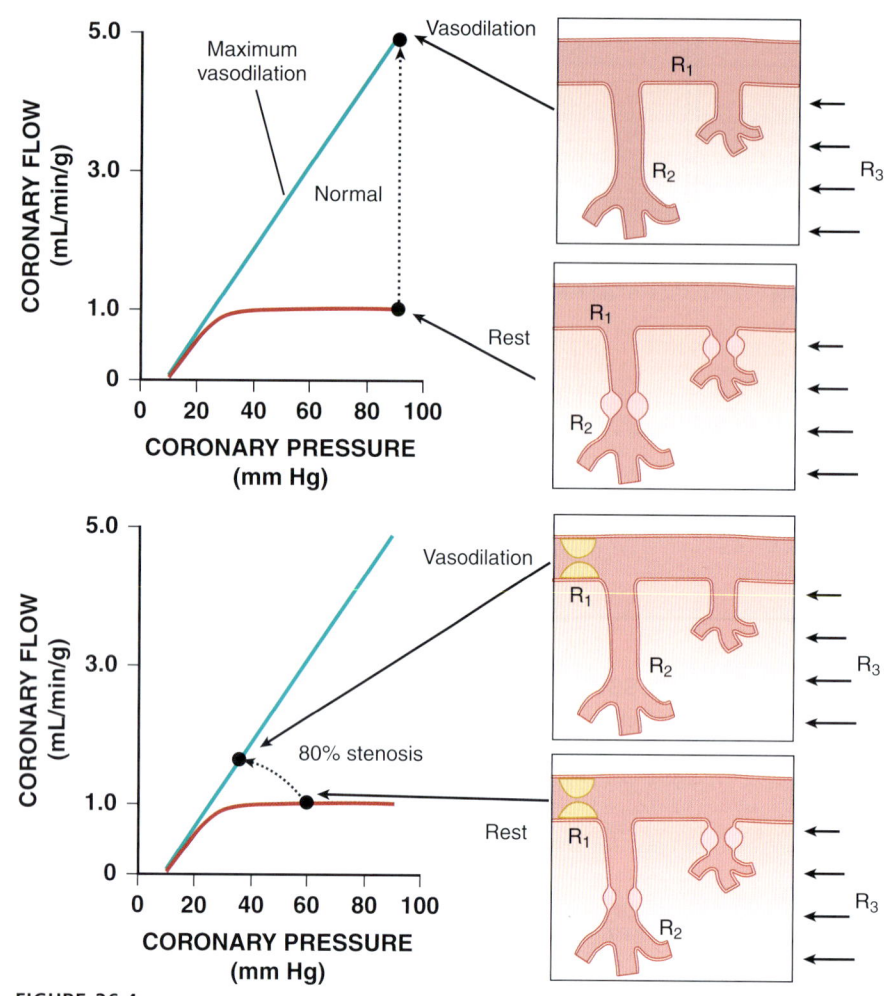

FIGURE 36.4 Schematic of components of coronary vascular resistance with and without a coronary stenosis. R_1 is epicardial conduit artery resistance, which normally is insignificant; R_2 is resistance secondary to metabolic and autoregulatory adjustments in flow and occurs in arterioles and small arteries; and R_3 is the time-varying compressive resistance that is higher in subendocardial than subepicardial layers. In the normal heart (upper panel), $R_2 > R_3 \gg R_1$. The development of a proximal stenosis or pharmacologic vasodilation reduces arteriolar resistance (R_2). In the presence of a severe epicardial stenosis (lower panel), $R_1 > R_3 > R_2$.

higher than right atrial pressure. This has been termed zero flow pressure ($P_{f=0}$) and its minimum value is approximately 10 mm Hg in the maximally vasodilated heart. This increases to values close to LV diastolic filling pressure when preload is elevated above 20 mm Hg. Elevated preload reduces coronary driving pressure and diminishes subendocardial perfusion. It is particularly important in determining flow when coronary pressure is reduced by a stenosis, as well as in the failing heart.

Endothelium-Dependent Modulation of Coronary Tone

Epicardial conduit arteries do not contribute significantly to coronary vascular resistance, yet arterial diameter is modulated by a wide variety of paracrine factors that can be released from platelets, as well as by circulating neurohormonal agonists, neural tone, and local control through vascular shear stress.[2] Figure 36.6 summarize the most common factors related to cardiovascular disease. The net effect of many of these agonists is critically dependent on whether a functional endothelium is present. Furchgott and Zawadzki (see Classic References) originally demonstrated that acetylcholine normally dilates arteries through an endothelium-dependent relaxing factor that was later identified to be nitric oxide (NO). This binds to guanylyl cyclase and increases cyclic guanosine monophosphate (cGMP), resulting in vascular smooth muscle relaxation. When the endothelium was removed, the dilation to acetylcholine was converted to vasoconstriction, reflecting the effect of muscarinic vascular smooth muscle

contraction. Subsequent studies have demonstrated that coronary resistance arteries also exhibit endothelial modulation of diameter, and that the response to physical forces such as shear stress, as well as paracrine mediators, vary with resistance vessel size.[1,3] The major endothelium-dependent biochemical pathways involved in regulating coronary epicardial and resistance artery diameter are discussed next.

Nitric Oxide (Endothelium-Derived Relaxing Factor)

Nitric oxide is produced in endothelial cells by the enzymatic conversion of L-arginine to citrulline via type III or endothelial nitric oxide synthase (eNOS). Endothelial NO diffuses abluminally into vascular smooth muscle, where it binds to guanylyl cyclase, increasing cGMP production and causing relaxation through a reduction in intracellular calcium. NO-mediated vasodilation is enhanced by cyclic or pulsatile changes in coronary shear stress. Chronic upregulation of eNOS occurs in response to episodic increases in coronary flow, such as during exercise training, which also potentiates the relaxation to various endothelium-dependent vasodilators. NO-mediated vasodilation is impaired in many disease states and in patients with one or more risk factors for coronary artery disease (CAD). This occurs via inactivation of NO by superoxide anion generated in response to oxidative stress. Such inactivation is the hallmark of impaired NO-mediated vasodilation in atherosclerosis, hypertension, and diabetes.

Endothelium-Dependent Hyperpolarizing Factor

Endothelium-dependent hyperpolarization is an additional endothelium-dependent mechanism for selected agonists (e.g., bradykinin), as well as shear stress–induced vasodilation, in the human coronary microcirculation. Endothelium-dependent hyperpolarizing factor (EDHF), produced by the endothelium, hyperpolarizes vascular smooth muscle and dilates arteries by opening calcium-activated potassium channels (K_{Ca}). The exact biochemical species of EDHF is still unclear, but prominent candidates are endothelium-derived hydrogen peroxide and epoxyeicosatrienoic acid, a metabolite of arachidonic acid metabolism produced by the cytochrome P-450 epoxygenase pathway.[4]

Prostacyclin

Metabolism of arachidonic acid via cyclooxygenase (COX) also can produce prostacyclin, which is a coronary vasodilator when administered exogenously. Although some evidence indicates that prostacyclin contributes to tonic coronary vasodilation, COX inhibitors fail to alter flow during ischemia distal to an acute stenosis or limit oxygen consumption in response to increases in metabolism. This suggests that it is overcome by other compensatory vasodilator pathways.[1,3] In contrast with the coronary resistance vasculature, vasodilator prostaglandins are very important determinants of coronary collateral vessel resistance, and inhibiting COX reduces collateral perfusion in dogs (see Classic References, Duncker and Bache).

Endothelin

The endothelins—ET-1, ET-2, and ET-3—are peptide endothelium-dependent constricting factors. ET-1 is a potent constrictor derived from the enzymatic cleavage of a larger precursor molecule (pre-pro–endothelin) via endothelin-converting enzyme. In contrast with the rapid vascular smooth muscle relaxation and recovery

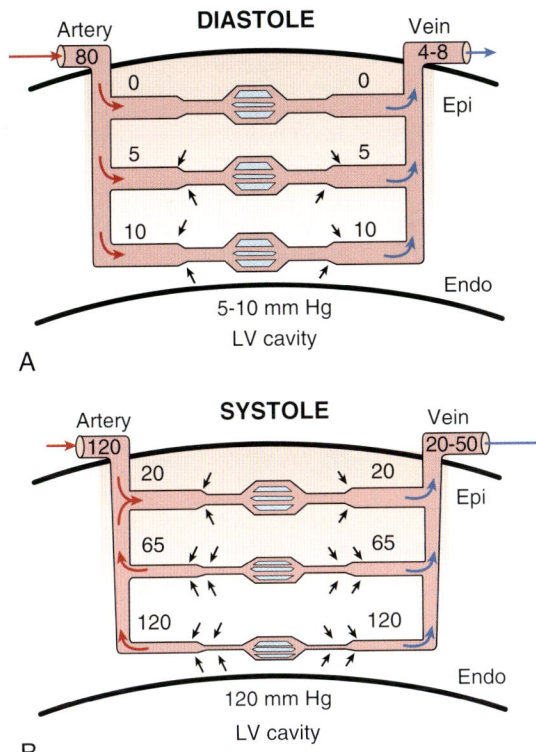

FIGURE 36.5 Effects of extravascular tissue pressure on transmural perfusion. **A,** Compressive effects during diastole are related to tissue pressures that decrease from the subendocardium (*Endo*) to subepicardium (*Epi*). At diastolic left ventricular (LV) pressures greater than 20 mm Hg, preload determines the effective backpressure to coronary diastolic perfusion. **B,** During systole, cardiac contraction increases intramyocardial tissue pressure surrounding compliant arterioles and venules. This produces a concealed arterial "backflow" that reduces systolic epicardial artery inflow, as depicted in Fig. 36.1. Compression of venules accelerates venous outflow. (Modified from Hoffman JI, Spaan JA. Pressure-flow relations in the coronary circulation. Physiol Rev 1990;70:331-390.)

characteristic of endothelium-derived vasodilators (NO, EDHF, and prostacyclin), the constriction to endothelin is prolonged. Changes in endothelin levels are largely mediated through transcriptional control and produce longer-term changes in coronary vasomotor tone. The effects of endothelin are mediated by binding to both ET_A and ET_B receptors. ET_A-mediated constriction is caused by the activation of protein kinase C in vascular smooth muscle. ET_B-mediated constriction is less pronounced and counterbalanced by ET_B-mediated endothelium-dependent NO production and vasodilation. Endothelin is only marginally involved in regulating coronary blood flow in the normal heart but can modulate vascular tone when interstitial and circulating concentrations increase in pathophysiologic states such as heart failure (HF).

Neurohumoral Control of Coronary Vascular Tone. Sympathetic and vagal nerves innervate coronary conduit arteries and segments of the resistance vasculature. Neural stimulation affects tone through mechanisms that alter vascular smooth muscle as well as by stimulating the release of NO from the endothelium. Diametrically opposite effects can occur in the presence of risk factors that impair endothelium-dependent vasodilation.

Cholinergic Innervation. Resistance arteries dilate to acetylcholine, resulting in increases in coronary flow. In conduit arteries, acetylcholine normally causes mild coronary vasodilation. This reflects the net action of a direct muscarinic constriction of vascular smooth muscle counterbalanced by an endothelium-dependent vasodilation caused by direct stimulation of eNOS and an increased flow-mediated dilation from concomitant resistance vessel vasodilation. The response in humans with atherosclerosis or risk factors for CAD is distinctly different. The resistance vessel dilation to acetylcholine is attenuated, and the reduction in flow-mediated NO production leads to net epicardial conduit artery vasoconstriction, which is particularly prominent in stenotic segments (Fig. 36.7A).

Sympathetic Innervation. Under basal conditions there is no resting sympathetic tone in the heart and thus no effect of denervation on resting perfusion. During sympathetic activation, coronary tone is modulated by norepinephrine released from myocardial sympathetic nerves, as well as by circulating norepinephrine and epinephrine.[1] In conduit arteries, sympathetic stimulation leads to alpha$_1$ constriction as well as beta-mediated vasodilation. The net effect is to dilate epicardial coronary arteries. This dilation is potentiated by concomitant flow-mediated vasodilation from metabolic vasodilation of coronary resistance vessels. When NO-mediated vasodilation is impaired, alpha$_1$ constriction predominates and can dynamically increase stenosis severity in asymmetric lesions where the stenosis is compliant. This is one of the mechanisms by which ischemia can be provoked during cold pressor testing (see Fig. 36.7B).

The effects of sympathetic activation on myocardial perfusion and coronary resistance vessel tone are complex and depend on the net actions of beta$_1$-mediated increases in myocardial oxygen consumption (resulting from increases in the determinants of myocardial oxygen consumption), direct beta$_2$-mediated coronary vasodilation, and alpha$_1$-mediated coronary constriction. Under normal conditions, exercise-induced beta$_2$-adrenergic "feed-forward" dilation predominates, resulting in a higher flow relative to the level of myocardial oxygen consumption.[1,2] This neural control mechanism produces transient vasodilation before the buildup of local metabolites during exercise and prevents the development of subendocardial ischemia during abrupt changes in demand. After nonselective beta blockade, sympathetic activation unmasks alpha$_1$-mediated coronary artery constriction. Although flow is mildly decreased, oxygen delivery is maintained by increased oxygen extraction and a reduction in coronary venous Po$_2$ at similar levels of cardiac workload. Intense alpha$_1$-adrenergic constriction can overcome intrinsic stimuli for metabolic vasodilation to result in ischemia in the presence of pharmacologic vasodilator reserve.[1,2] The role of presynaptic and postsynaptic alpha$_2$ responses is controversial. They appear to have a less significant role in controlling flow. This partly reflects the competing effects of presynaptic alpha$_2$ receptor stimulation, leading to reduced vasoconstriction by inhibiting norepinephrine release.

Paracrine Vasoactive Mediators and Coronary Vasospasm

Many paracrine factors can affect coronary tone in normal and pathophysiologic states that are unrelated to normal coronary circulatory control. The most important of these are summarized in Fig. 36.6. Paracrine factors are released from epicardial artery thrombi after activation of the thrombotic cascade initiated by plaque rupture. They can modulate epicardial tone in regions near eccentric ulcerated plaques still responsive to stimuli that alter smooth muscle relaxation and constriction, leading to dynamic changes in the physiologic significance of a stenosis. Paracrine mediators also can have differential effects on downstream vessel vasomotion that depend on vessel size (conduit arteries versus resistance arteries) as well as on the presence of a functionally normal endothelium, because many also stimulate the release of NO and EDHF.

Serotonin released from activated platelets causes vasoconstriction in normal and atherosclerotic conduit arteries and can increase the functional severity of a dynamic coronary stenosis through superimposed vasospasm. By contrast, it dilates coronary arterioles and increases coronary flow through the endothelium-dependent release of NO. In atherosclerosis or circumstances in which NO production is impaired, the direct effects on smooth muscle predominate, and the response of the microcirculation is converted to vasoconstriction. As a result, serotonin release generally exacerbates ischemia in CAD.

Thromboxane A$_2$ is a potent vasoconstrictor that is a product of endoperoxide metabolism and is released during platelet aggregation. It produces vasoconstriction of conduit arteries and isolated coronary resistance vessels and can accentuate acute myocardial ischemia.

Adenosine diphosphate (ADP) is another platelet-derived vasodilator that relaxes coronary microvessels and conduit arteries. It is mediated by NO and abolished by removing the endothelium.

Thrombin normally leads to vasodilation in vitro that is endothelium dependent and mediated by the release of prostacyclin and NO. In vivo,

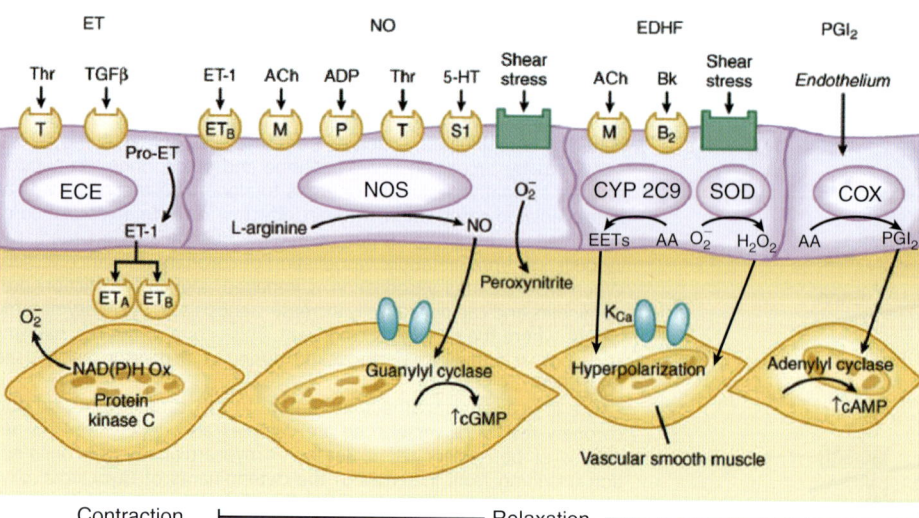

FIGURE 36.6 Endothelium-dependent control of vascular tone. In the normal coronary circulation, endothelium-dependent vasodilation occurs after increases in luminal flow or shear stress, as well as in response to agonists (e.g., released from platelets or cardiac nerves) that bind to receptors on the endothelial surface. These stimulate the production of nitric oxide (*NO*) and endothelium-dependent hyperpolarizing factor (*EDHF*), including epoxyeicosatrienoic acid products (*EETs*) and hydrogen peroxide (H_2O_2) released from mitochondria, which diffuse into vascular smooth muscle and cause relaxation. Prostacyclin, or prostaglandin I_2 (PGI_2), is produced in the coronary endothelium of collateral vessels and causes tonic vasodilation. The endothelium also produces endothelin (*ET*), which activates protein kinase C in vascular smooth muscle to produce coronary constriction and competes with endothelium-derived relaxing factors. Impaired endothelium-dependent vasodilation can result from the lack of production of relaxing factors (e.g., disrupted endothelium) or by inactivation of NO in disease states associated with oxidative stress and superoxide anion production (e.g., NO and O_2^- combining to produce peroxynitrite). In these circumstances, the effect of autacoids on vascular tone can be converted to vasoconstriction because of their direct effects on vascular smooth muscle (not shown). *AA*, Arachidonic acid; *Ach*, acetylcholine; *ADP*, adenosine diphosphate; *Bk*, bradykinin; *5-HT*, 5-hydroxytryptamine [serotonin]; K_{Ca}, calcium-activated potassium channel; *TGFβ*, transforming growth factor beta 1; *Thr*, thrombin. (Modified from Laughlin MH, et al. Peripheral circulation. Compr Physiol 2012;2:321-447.)

thrombin also releases thromboxane A_2, leading to vasoconstriction in epicardial stenoses in which endothelium-dependent vasodilation is impaired. In the coronary resistance vasculature, thrombin acts as an endothelium-dependent vasodilator and increases coronary flow.

Coronary Vasospasm

Coronary spasm results in transient functional occlusion of a coronary artery that is reversible with nitrate vasodilation. It most frequently occurs in the setting of a coronary stenosis, leading to dynamic stenosis behavior that can dissociate the effects on perfusion from anatomic stenosis severity (see Chapter 21). In CAD, endothelial disruption probably plays a role in focal vasospasm; the normal vasodilation from autacoids and sympathetic stimulation is converted into a vasoconstrictor response because of the lack of competing endothelium-dependent vasodilation. Nevertheless, although impaired endothelium-dependent vasodilation is a permissive factor for vasospasm, it is not causal, and a trigger is required (e.g., thrombus formation, sympathetic activation).

The mechanisms responsible for variant angina with normal coronary arteries, or Prinzmetal angina, are less clear. Data from animal models have pointed to sensitization of intrinsic vasoconstrictor mechanisms.[5] Coronary arteries demonstrate supersensitivity to vasoconstrictor agonists in vivo and in vitro, as well as reduced vasodilator responses. Some studies have demonstrated that Rho, a guanosine triphosphate (GTP)–binding protein, can sensitize vascular smooth muscle to calcium by inhibiting myosin phosphatase activity through the effector protein Rho kinase.

Pharmacologic Vasodilation. The effects of pharmacologic vasodilators on coronary flow reflect direct actions on vascular smooth muscle and secondary adjustments in resistance artery tone. Flow-mediated dilation can amplify the vasodilator response, whereas autoregulatory adjustments can overcome vasodilation in a segment of the microcirculation and restore flow to normal. The potent resistance vessel vasodilators are specifically used in assessing coronary stenosis severity.[6]

Nitroglycerin. Nitroglycerin dilates epicardial conduit arteries and small coronary resistance arteries but does not increase coronary blood flow in the normal heart (see Classic References, Duncker and Bache). The latter observation reflects the fact that transient arteriolar vasodilation is overcome by autoregulatory escape, which returns coronary resistance to control levels.[3] Although nitroglycerin does not increase coronary blood flow in the normal heart, it can produce vasodilation of larger coronary resistance arteries that improves the distribution of perfusion to the subendocardium when flow-mediated NO-dependent vasodilation is impaired. It also can improve subendocardial perfusion by reducing LV end-diastolic pressure through systemic venodilation in HF. Similarly, coronary collateral vessels dilate in response to nitroglycerin, and the reduction in collateral resistance can improve regional perfusion in some settings (see Classic References, Duncker and Bache).

Calcium Channel Blockers. All calcium channel blockers induce vascular smooth muscle relaxation and are, to various degrees, pharmacologic coronary vasodilators. In epicardial arteries the vasodilator response is similar to that of nitroglycerin and is effective in preventing coronary vasospasm superimposed on a coronary stenosis, as well as in normal arteries of patients with variant angina. Calcium channel blockers also submaximally vasodilate coronary resistance vessels. In this regard, dihydropyridine derivatives such as nifedipine are particularly potent and can sometimes precipitate subendocardial ischemia in the presence of a critical stenosis. This arises from a transmural redistribution of blood flow (coronary steal), as well as the tachycardia and hypotension that transiently occur with short half-life formulations of nifedipine.

Adenosine and A_2 Receptor Agonists. Adenosine dilates coronary arteries through activation of A_2 receptors on vascular smooth muscle and is independent of the endothelium in coronary arterioles isolated from humans with heart disease.[7] Experimentally, a differential sensitivity of the microcirculation to adenosine is observed, with the direct effects related to resistance vessel size and restricted primarily to vessels smaller than 100 μm. Larger upstream resistance arteries dilate through a NO-dependent mechanism from the increase in shear stress. Thus, in states in which endothelium-dependent vasodilation is impaired, maximal coronary flow responses to intravenous or intracoronary adenosine may be reduced in the absence of a stenosis (see Classic References, Duncker and Bache) and can be increased by interventions that improve NO-mediated vasodilation, such as lowering low-density lipoprotein (LDL) levels. Single-dose adenosine A_2 receptor agonists (e.g., regadenoson) are now more often employed in pharmacologic stress testing and are as effective as adenosine. These agents circumvent the need for continuous infusions during myocardial perfusion imaging[6] (see Chapter 18).

Dipyridamole. Dipyridamole produces vasodilation by inhibiting the myocyte reuptake of adenosine released from cardiac myocytes. It therefore has actions and mechanisms similar to those of adenosine, with the exception that the vasodilation is more prolonged. It can be reversed with the administration of the nonspecific adenosine receptor blocker aminophylline.

Papaverine. Papaverine is a short-acting coronary vasodilator that was the first agent used for intracoronary vasodilation. It causes vascular smooth muscle relaxation by inhibiting phosphodiesterase and increasing cyclic adenosine monophosphate (cAMP). After bolus injection, it has a rapid onset of action, but the vasodilation is somewhat more prolonged than after adenosine. Its actions are independent of the endothelium.

Structure and Function of the Coronary Microcirculation

The schematics in Figs. 36.3 and 36.4 suggest a fairly localized site for the control of coronary vascular resistance that is useful for conceptualizing

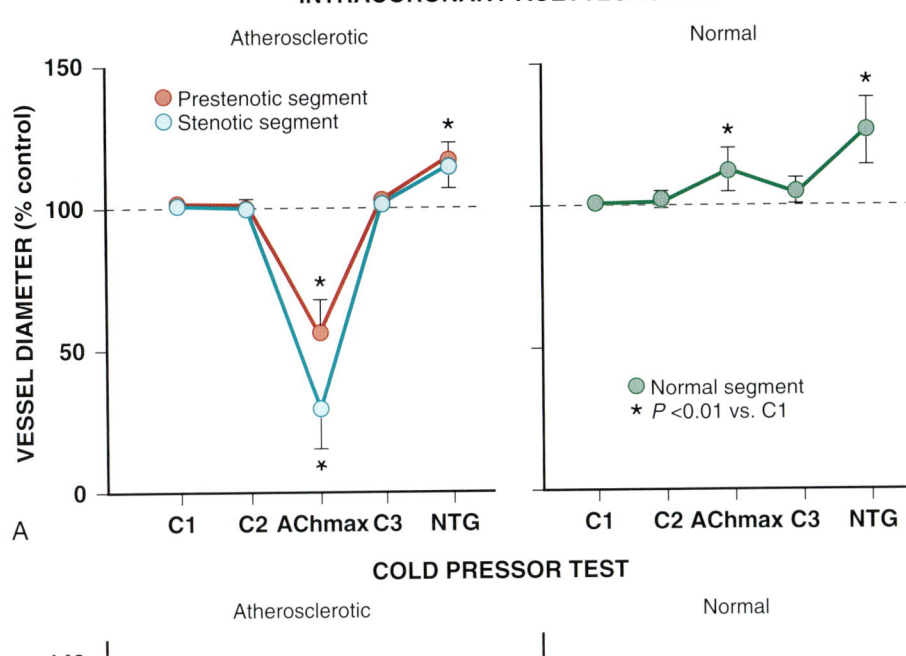
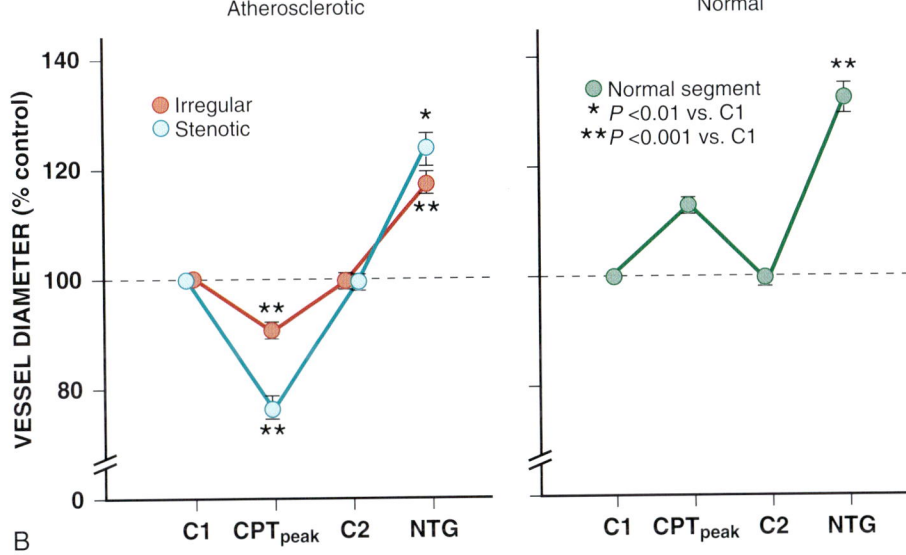

FIGURE 36.7 Differential conduit artery diameter responses in normal and atherosclerotic epicardial arteries. **A,** Acetylcholine. In normal arteries, acetylcholine elicits vasodilation, but there is vasoconstriction in the atherosclerotic artery, which is particularly pronounced in the stenosis. **B,** Cold pressor testing. Activation of sympathetic tone normally leads to net epicardial dilation, but vasoconstriction in irregular and stenotic coronary segments occurs in patients with atherosclerosis. *Ach,* Acetylcholine; *C,* control; *CPT,* cold pressor test (response); *NTG,* nitroglycerin. (**A** modified from Ludmer PL, et al. Paradoxical vasoconstriction induced by acetylcholine in atherosclerotic coronary arteries. N Engl J Med 1986;315:1046-1051; **B** modified from Nabel EG, et al. Dilation of normal and constriction of atherosclerotic coronary arteries caused by the cold pressor test. Circulation 1988;77:43-52.)

the major determinants of coronary vascular resistance. In fact, individual coronary resistance arteries are a longitudinally distributed network, and in vivo studies of the coronary microcirculation have demonstrated considerable spatial heterogeneity of specific resistance vessel control mechanisms[3,8] (Fig. 36.8). Each resistance vessel needs to dilate in an orchestrated fashion to meet the needs of the downstream vascular bed, which is frequently removed from the site of metabolic control of coronary resistance. This can be accomplished independently of metabolic signals by sensing physical forces such as intraluminal flow (shear stress–mediated control) or intraluminal pressure changes (myogenic control). Epicardial arteries (>400 μm in diameter) serve a conduit artery function, with diameter primarily regulated by shear stress, and contribute minimal pressure drop (<5%) over a wide range of coronary flow. Coronary arterial resistance vessels can be divided into small arteries (100 to 400 μm), which regulate their tone in response to local shear stress and luminal pressure changes (myogenic response), and arterioles (<100 μm), which are sensitive to changes in local tissue metabolism and directly control perfusion of the low-resistance coronary capillary bed[3] (see Fig. 36.8). Capillary density of the myocardium averages 3500/mm^2 (resulting in an average intercapillary distance of 17 μm), which is greater in the subendocardium than in the subepicardium.

Under resting conditions, most of the pressure drop in the microcirculation arises in resistance arteries between 50 and 200 μm, with minimal pressure drop occurring across capillaries and venules at normal flow levels. After pharmacologic vasodilation with dipyridamole, resistance artery vasodilation attenuates the precapillary pressure drop in arterial resistance vessels. At the same time, there is an increased pressure drop and redistribution of resistance to venular vessels, in which smooth muscle relaxation is limited and the already low resistance is fairly fixed.

Considerable heterogeneity in microcirculatory vasodilation is evident during physiologic adjustments in flow. For example, as pressure is reduced during autoregulation, dilation is accomplished primarily by arterioles smaller than 100 μm, whereas larger resistance arteries tend to constrict because of the reduction in perfusion pressure[3]. By contrast, metabolic vasodilation results from a more uniform vasodilation of resistance vessels of all sizes. Similar inhomogeneity in resistance vessel dilation occurs in response to endothelium-dependent agonists and pharmacologic vasodilators.

A unique component of subendocardial coronary resistance vessels is the transmural penetrating arteries that course from the epicardium to the subendocardial plexus.[3] These vessels not only are less sensitive to metabolic signals but also are removed from the metabolic stimuli that develop when ischemia is confined to the subendocardium. As a result, local control by altered shear stress and myogenic relaxation to local pressure become critical determinants of diameter in this "upstream" resistance segment. Even during maximal vasodilation, this segment creates an additional longitudinal component of coronary vascular resistance that must be traversed before the arteriolar microcirculation is reached. Because of this greater longitudinal pressure drop, the microcirculatory pressures in subendocardial coronary arterioles are lower than in the subepicardial arterioles.[3]

Intraluminal Physical Forces Regulating Coronary Resistance

Because much of the coronary resistance vasculature can be upstream from the effects of metabolic mediators of control, local vascular control mechanisms are critically important in orchestrating adequate regional tissue perfusion to the distal microcirculation. The differential expression of mechanisms is evident among different sizes and classes of coronary resistance vessels and coincides with their function.

Myogenic Regulation

The *myogenic response* refers to the ability of vascular smooth muscle to oppose changes in coronary arterial diameter.[1,3] Thus, vessels relax when distending pressure is decreased and constrict when distending pressure

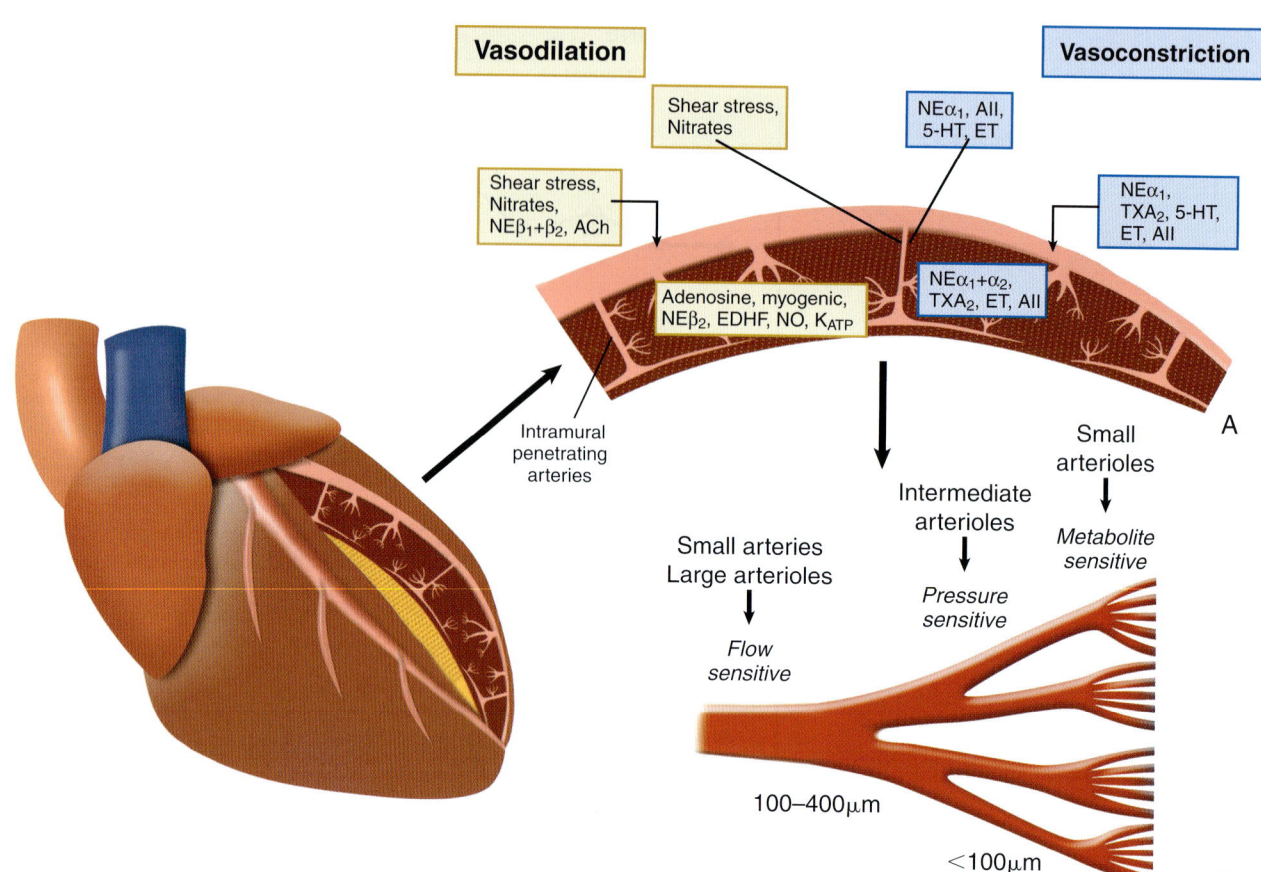

FIGURE 36.8 A, Transmural distribution of coronary resistance vessels—major vasodilator and vasoconstrictor mechanisms in epicardial conduit arteries and different sites of the microcirculation. The epicardial conduit arteries arborize into subepicardial and subendocardial resistance arteries. Intramural penetrating resistance arteries are unique in that they are removed from subendocardial metabolic stimuli and theoretically are more dependent on regulating their tone in response to shear stress and luminal pressure as mechanisms to produce dilation in response to changes in metabolism of the distal subendocardial arteriolar plexus. See text for further discussion. *AII,* Angiotensin II; *Ach,* acetylcholine; *EDHF,* endothelium-dependent hyperpolarizing factor; *ET,* endothelin; *5-HT,* 5-hydroxytryptamine (serotonin); K_{ATP}, ATP-dependent potassium channel; $NE\beta_1$, norepinephrine beta$_1$-adrenergic; $NE\alpha_1$, norepinephrine alpha$_1$-adrenergic; *NO,* nitric oxide; TXA_2, thromboxane A_2. **B,** Integrative regulation of coronary flow by ascending, metabolic, myogenic, and shear stress–induced mechanisms in response to metabolic activation. Small distal arterioles immediately before the capillaries are sensitive to tissue metabolites. Upstream intermediate arterioles are pressure sensitive, with myogenic mechanisms predominating. Small resistance arteries are removed from the metabolic milieu and primarily adjust local tone in response to shear stress and flow. Capillary and venular resistances are small and primarily considered to be fixed. (**A** modified from Duncker DJ, Bache RJ. Regulation of coronary vasomotor tone under normal conditions and during acute myocardial hypoperfusion. Pharmacol Ther 2000;86:87; **B** modified from Davis MJ, et al. Local regulation of microvascular perfusion. *In* Tuma RF et al., editors. Handbook of Physiology: Microcirculation. San Diego: Academic Press; 2008;161-284.)

is elevated (Fig. 36.9A). Myogenic tone is a property of vascular smooth muscle and occurs across a large size range of coronary resistance arteries in animals and in humans. Although the cellular mechanism is uncertain, it depends on vascular smooth muscle calcium entry, perhaps through stretch-activated L-type Ca^{2+} channels, eliciting cross-bridge activation. The resistance changes arising from the myogenic response tend to bring local coronary flow back to the original level. Myogenic regulation has been postulated as an important mechanism of the coronary autoregulatory response and in vivo appears to occur primarily in arterioles smaller than 100 μm.

Flow-Mediated Resistance Artery Control

Coronary small arteries and arterioles also regulate their diameter in response to changes in local shear stress (Fig. 36.9B). Flow-induced dilation in isolated coronary arterioles is endothelium dependent and mediated by NO, because it could be abolished with an L-arginine analog. By contrast, isolated atrial vessels from patients undergoing cardiac surgery exhibit flow-mediated vasodilation by EDHF.[7] The disparity with animal studies may reflect age or species variability in the relative importance of EDHF versus NO in the coronary circulation. The mechanisms also appear to vary as a function of vessel size, with studies in pigs demonstrating that hyperpolarization regulates epicardial conduit arteries, and NO predominates in the resistance vasculature.[3] In addition, EDHF may represent a compensatory pathway that normally is inhibited by NO and becomes upregulated in acquired disease states in which NO-mediated vasodilation is impaired.[7] More recent studies have demonstrated that this factor appears to be hydrogen peroxide.[9] Despite the variability in isolated vessels, blocking NOS with an L-arginine analog in the coronary circulation of humans reduces vasodilation to pharmacologic endothelium-dependent agonists and attenuates flow increases during metabolic vasodilation. This demonstrates that NO-mediated vasodilation plays a role in determining physiologic vascular tone in some segments of the coronary resistance vasculature.

Metabolic Mediators of Coronary Resistance Vessel Control. Although increasing knowledge has emerged regarding the distribution of coronary microvascular resistance, there is still no consensus regarding specific mediators of metabolic vasodilation.[10] Coronary resistance in any segment of the microcirculation represents the integration of local physical factors (e.g., pressure, flow), vasodilator metabolites (e.g., adenosine, P_{O_2}, pH), autacoids, and neural modulation. Each of these mechanisms contributes to net coronary vascular smooth muscle tone, which may ultimately be controlled by opening and closing vascular smooth muscle adenosine triphosphate (ATP)–sensitive K^+ (K_{ATP}) channels. There is considerable redundancy in the available local control mechanisms.[1,2] Because of this, blocking single mechanisms fails to alter coronary autoregulation or metabolic flow regulation at normal coronary pressures. This redundancy can, however, be unmasked by stressing the heart and evaluating flow regulation at reduced pressures distal to a coronary stenosis at rest or during exercise. Some of the candidates proposed and their role in metabolic resistance control and ischemia-induced vasodilation are summarized here (see Classic References, Duncker and Bache).

Adenosine. There has been a longstanding interest in the role of adenosine as a metabolic mediator of resistance artery control. It is released

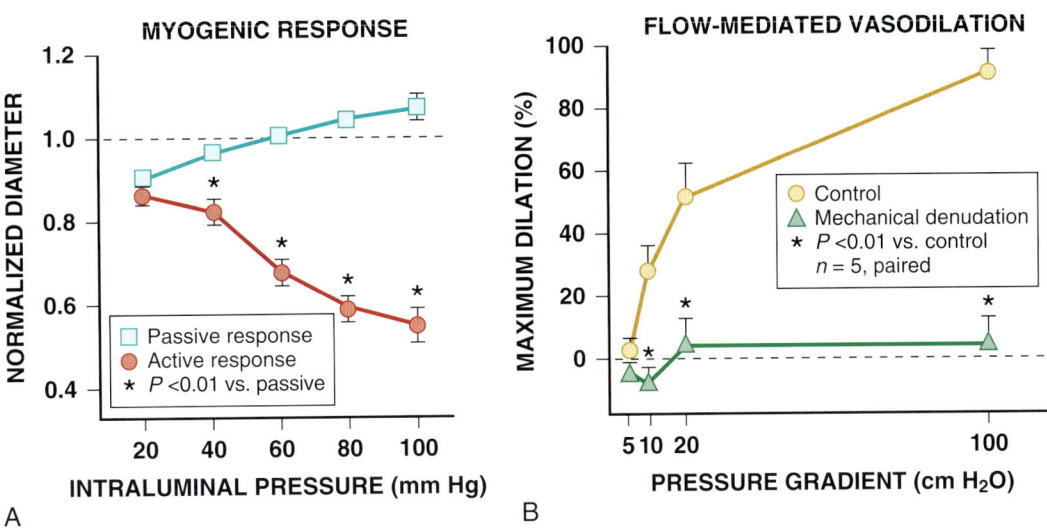

FIGURE 36.9 Effects of physical forces on coronary diameter in isolated human coronary resistance arteries (nominal diameter, 100 μm). **A,** As distending pressure is reduced from 100 mm Hg, progressive vasodilation occurs, consistent with myogenic regulation. Myogenic dilation reaches the maximum passive diameter of the vessel at 20 mm Hg. **B,** Flow-mediated vasodilation in cannulated human resistance arteries. As the pressure gradient across the isolated vessel is increased, intraluminal flow rises, causing progressive dilation that is abolished by removing the endothelium. Similar flow-mediated dilation occurs in most arterial vessels, including the coronary conduit arteries. (**A** modified from Miller FJ, et al. Myogenic constriction of human coronary arterioles. Am J Physiol 1997;273:H257-H264; **B** modified from Miura H, et al. Flow-induced dilation of human coronary arterioles: important role of Ca^{2+}-activated K^+ channels. Circulation 2001;103:1992-1998.)

from cardiac myocytes when the rate of ATP hydrolysis exceeds its synthesis during ischemia. Its production and release also increase with myocardial metabolism. Adenosine has an extremely short half-life (<10 seconds) as a result of its rapid inactivation by adenosine deaminase. It binds to A_2 receptors on vascular smooth muscle, increases cAMP, and opens K_{ATP} and intermediate calcium-activated potassium channels.[1,7] Adenosine has a differential effect on coronary resistance arteries, primarily dilating vessels smaller than 100 μm.[3] Although adenosine has no direct effect on larger resistance arteries and conduit arteries, these dilate through endothelium-dependent vasodilation from the concomitant increases in local shear stress as arteriolar resistance falls. Despite the attractiveness of adenosine as a local metabolic control mechanism, substantial in vivo experimental data have demonstrated convincingly that it is not required for adjusting coronary flow to increases in metabolism or autoregulation.[1,2] However, adenosine may contribute to vasodilation during hypoxia and during acute exercise-induced myocardial ischemia distal to a stenosis.[1]

ATP-Sensitive K^+ Channels. Coronary vascular smooth muscle K_{ATP} channels are tonically active, contributing to coronary vascular tone under resting conditions. Preventing K_{ATP} channel opening with glibenclamide causes constriction of arterioles smaller than 100 μm, reduces coronary flow, and accentuates myocardial ischemia distal to a coronary stenosis by overcoming intrinsic vasodilator mechanisms.[1] The K_{ATP} channels can modulate both coronary metabolic and autoregulatory responses. It is a potentially attractive mechanism, because many of the other candidates for metabolic flow regulation (e.g., adenosine, NO, beta$_2$-adrenoreceptors, prostacyclin) are ultimately affected by blocking this pathway. K_{ATP} channel opening is likely a common effector rather than sensor of metabolic activity or autoregulatory adjustments in flow. Also, reductions in coronary flow observed after blocking K_{ATP} channel vasodilation may be pharmacologic, caused by vasoconstriction of the microcirculation that overcomes intrinsic vasodilator stimuli, as seen when other potent vasoconstrictors (e.g., endothelin, vasopressin) are administered at pharmacologic doses.

Oxygen Sensing. Although Po_2 is a potent coronary vasodilator stimulus, its role in the regulation of arteriolar tone remains unresolved. Coronary flow increases in proportion to reductions in arterial oxygen content (reduced Po_2 or anemia), and there is a twofold increase in perfused capillary density in response to hypoxia. The underlying mechanism may involve the release of NO and ATP (which stimulates vascular endothelial P2 purinergic receptors to produce NO) from red blood cells, when intravascular Po_2 levels drop.[1] Studies demonstrating a direct effect of oxygen on metabolic or autoregulatory adjustments are lacking, however, and the vasodilator response to reduced arterial oxygen delivery may simply reflect the close relation between myocardial metabolism and flow.

Acidosis. Arterial hypercapnia and acidosis are potent stimuli shown to produce coronary vasodilation independent of hypoxia. Whereas their precise role in the local regulation of myocardial perfusion remains unclear,[1] it seems reasonable that some of the vasodilation occurring with increased myocardial metabolism could arise from increased myocardial carbon dioxide (CO_2) production and tissue acidosis in the setting of acute ischemia.

Right Coronary Artery Flow

Although the general concepts of coronary flow regulation developed for the left ventricle apply to the right ventricle, differences exist related to the extent of the right coronary artery (RCA) supply to the right ventricular (RV) free wall. This has been studied in dogs, in which the RCA is a nondominant vessel.[1] In terms of coronary flow reserve, arterial pressure supplying the RCA substantially exceeds RV pressure, minimizing the compressive determinants of coronary reserve. RV oxygen consumption is lower than LV consumption, and coronary venous oxygen saturations are higher than in the left coronary circulation. Because there is considerable oxygen extraction reserve, coronary flow decreases as pressure is reduced and oxygen delivery is maintained by increased extraction. These differences appear specific to the RV free wall. In humans, in whom the RCA is dominant and supplies much of the inferior left ventricle, factors affecting flow regulation to the LV myocardium are likely to predominate.

PHYSIOLOGIC ASSESSMENT OF CORONARY ARTERY STENOSES

The physiologic assessment of stenosis severity is a critical component of the management of patients with obstructive epicardial CAD[11] (see Chapter 21). Epicardial artery stenoses arising from atherosclerosis increase coronary resistance and reduce maximal myocardial perfusion. Abnormalities in coronary microcirculatory control also can contribute to causing myocardial ischemia in many patients. Separating the role of a stenosis from coronary resistance vessels can be accomplished by simultaneously assessing coronary flow and distal coronary pressure using intracoronary transducers currently available for clinical care[12] (see Chapters 21 and 41).

Stenosis Pressure-Flow Relation

The angiographically visible epicardial coronary arteries are normally able to accommodate large increases in coronary flow without producing any significant pressure drop and thus serve a conduit function to the coronary resistance vasculature. This changes dramatically in CAD, in which the epicardial artery resistance becomes dominant. This fixed component of resistance increases with stenosis severity and limits maximal myocardial perfusion.

As a starting point, it is helpful to consider the idealized relation among stenosis severity, pressure drop, and flow, as validated in animals and in humans studied under circumstances in which diffuse atherosclerosis and risk factors that can impair microcirculatory resistance vessel control are minimized. Fig. 36.10 summarizes the major determinants of stenosis energy losses. The relation between pressure drop across a stenosis and coronary flow for stenoses between 30% and 90% diameter reduction can be described using the Bernoulli principle. The total pressure drop across a stenosis is governed by three hydrodynamic factors—viscous losses, separation losses, and turbulence—although the last usually is a relatively minor component of pressure loss. The most important determinant of stenosis resistance for any given level of flow is the minimum lesional cross-sectional area within the stenosis (see Classic References, Klocke, 1983). Because resistance is inversely proportional to the square of the cross-sectional area, small dynamic changes in luminal area caused by thrombi or vasomotion in asymmetric lesions (in which vascular smooth muscle can relax or constrict in a portion of the stenosis) lead to major changes in the stenosis pressure-flow relation and reduce maximal perfusion during vasodilation. Separation losses determine the curvilinearity or "steepness" of the stenosis pressure-flow relation and become increasingly important as stenosis severity or flow rate increases. Stenosis length and changes in cross-sectional area distal to the stenosis are relatively minor determinants of resistance for most coronary lesions.

Diffuse abluminal outward remodeling with thickening of the arterial wall is common in coronary atherosclerosis but does not alter the pressure-flow characteristics of the stenosis for a given intraluminal geometry. By contrast, diffuse inward remodeling effectively reduces minimal lesion area along the length of the vessel and can lead to underestimation of stenosis severity using relative diameter or area measurements (see Chapter 21) and at the same time can contribute to a significant longitudinal pressure drop that also reduces maximum perfusion.[13]

Stenosis pressure drop and resistance increase exponentially as minimum lesional cross-sectional area decreases (Fig. 36.11). This reflects that the pressure drop becomes flow dependent and varies

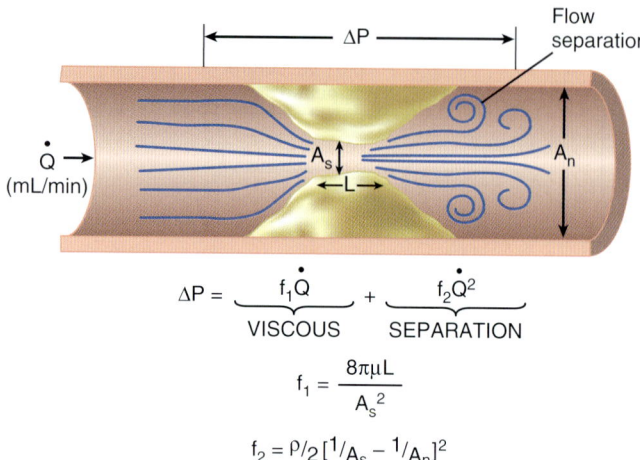

FIGURE 36.10 **Fluid mechanics of a stenosis.** The pressure drop across a stenosis can be predicted by the Bernoulli equation. It is inversely related to the minimum stenosis cross-sectional area and varies with the square of the flow rate as stenosis severity increases. A_n, Area of the normal segment; A_s, area of the stenosis; f_1, viscous coefficient; f_2, separation coefficient; L, stenosis length; μ, viscosity of blood; ρ, density of blood; ΔP, pressure drop; $\dot{Q}$, flow.

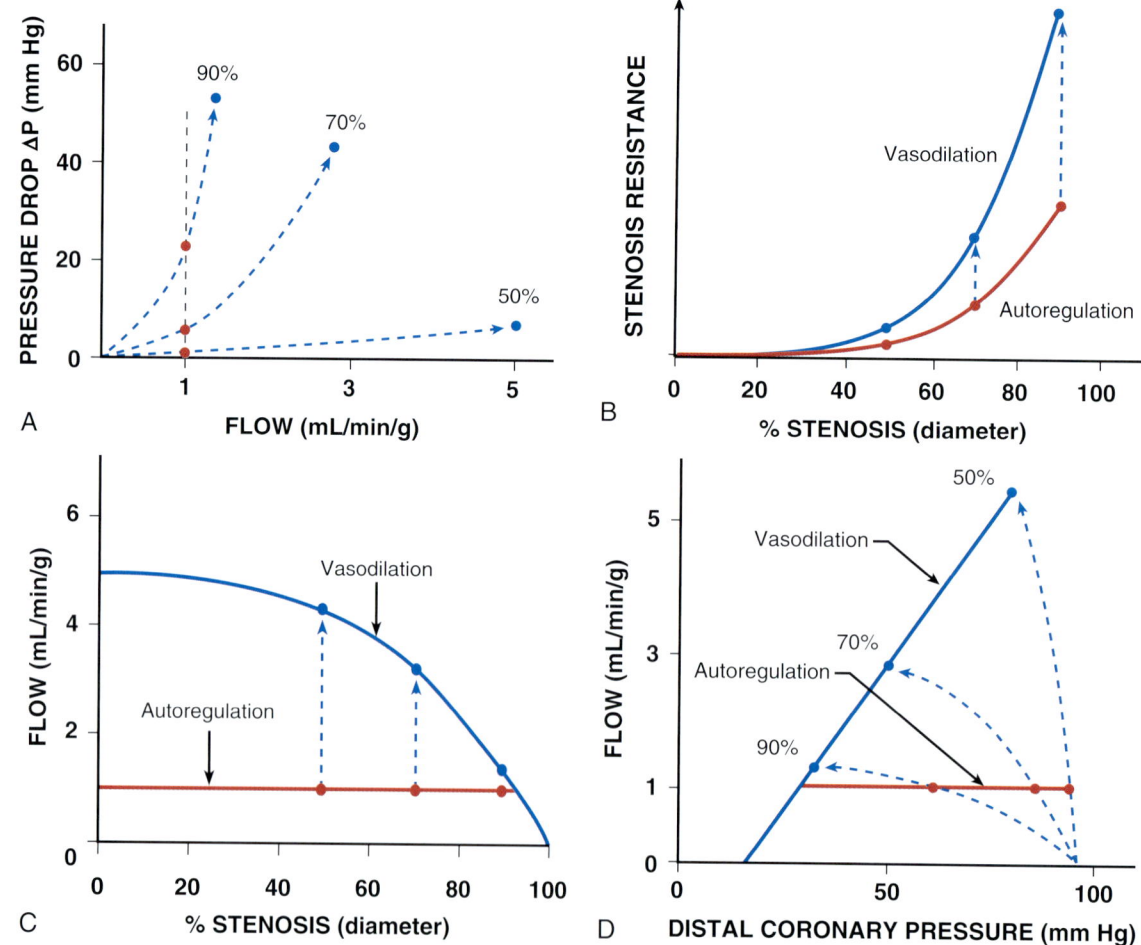

FIGURE 36.11 Interrelation of the epicardial artery stenosis pressure-flow relation **(A)**, stenosis resistance at the autoregulated resting and maximally vasodilated flow **(B)**, absolute coronary flow reserve **(C)**, and distal coronary pressure-flow relation **(D)**. *Red circles and lines* depict resting flow, and *blue circles and lines* show maximal vasodilation for stenoses of 50%, 70%, and 90% diameter reduction. As shown in **A**, the stenosis pressure-flow relation becomes extremely nonlinear as stenosis severity increases. **B**, Thus, the instantaneous resistance of the stenosis increases during vasodilation. As a result of the nonlinear stenosis pressure-flow behavior, very little pressure drop across a 50% stenosis is seen, and distal coronary pressure and vasodilated flow remain near normal. By contrast, a 90% stenosis critically impairs flow and, because of the steepness of the stenosis pressure-flow relation, causes a marked reduction in distal coronary pressure.

with the square of the flow or flow velocity. As a result, the instantaneous stenosis resistance progressively increases during vasodilation. This becomes particularly important in determining the stenosis pressure-flow behavior for severely narrowed arteries, leading to a situation in which small reductions in luminal area result in large reductions in poststenotic coronary pressure that limit maximum coronary perfusion of the distal microcirculation.

Interrelation Among Distal Coronary Pressure, Flow, and Stenosis Severity

Because maximum myocardial perfusion is ultimately determined by the coronary pressure distal to a stenosis, it is helpful to place the epicardial stenosis pressure-flow relation into the context of the coronary autoregulatory and vasodilated coronary pressure-flow relations. Similar relations have been validated in humans.[12,14] Figure 36.11 summarizes the effects of a stenosis on distal coronary pressure and flow at rest and after vasodilation for isolated lesions. Diffuse intraluminal narrowing is assumed to be absent, and minimal coronary microvascular resistance is normal. As illustrated in Fig. 36.11A, there is no significant pressure drop across a stenosis (ΔP) or stenosis-related alteration in maximal myocardial perfusion until stenosis severity exceeds a 50% diameter reduction (cross-sectional area reduction of 75%). As stenosis severity exceeds 50%, the pressure flow relation becomes curvilinear (Fig. 36.11B) and increases in stenosis resistance are accompanied by concomitant increases in ΔP across the stenosis that reduce distal coronary pressure. Because of coronary autoregulation, resting flow remains constant as stenosis severity increases (Fig. 36.11C and D). As a result, imaging resting perfusion cannot be used to identify hemodynamically significant stenoses (see Chapter 18). By contrast, the maximally vasodilated pressure-flow relation is much more sensitive to detect the effect of increases in stenosis severity on maximum myocardial perfusion. Normally, there is substantial coronary flow reserve, and flow can increase approximately five times the resting flow values in the absence of coronary microvascular dysfunction. A critical stenosis, one in which subendocardial flow reserve is completely exhausted at rest, usually develops when stenosis severity exceeds 90%. Under these circumstances, pharmacologic vasodilation of subepicardial resistance vessels results in a reduction in distal coronary pressure that actually redistributes flow away from the subendocardium, leading to a "transmural steal" phenomenon (see Classic References, Duncker and Bache).

Flow- and Pressure-Derived Indices of Coronary Reserve

Gould (see Classic References), originally proposed the concept of coronary flow reserve. It is possible to characterize this in humans using invasive catheter-based measurements of coronary flow (see Chapter 41), as well as with noninvasive imaging of myocardial perfusion with positron emission tomography (PET), single-photon emission computed tomography (SPECT), and, more recently, cardiac magnetic resonance (CMR) (see Chapters 18 and 19). The development of invasive approaches to assess distal coronary pressure and flow in humans using transducers placed on coronary guidewires have led to indices of coronary stenosis severity based on coronary flow reserve and resting and vasodilated distal coronary pressure. These have provided a more complete understanding of the role of epicardial coronary stenoses versus the coronary microcirculation in limiting myocardial perfusion[12] (Fig. 36.12). These have also demonstrated that abnormalities in coronary microcirculatory control contribute to the functional significance of isolated epicardial artery stenoses in many patients with CAD, as well as impairing coronary vasodilation in the presence of normal coronary arteries. Because of these complexities, multiple complementary approaches frequently are required to define limitations in myocardial perfusion that arise from stenosis severity versus

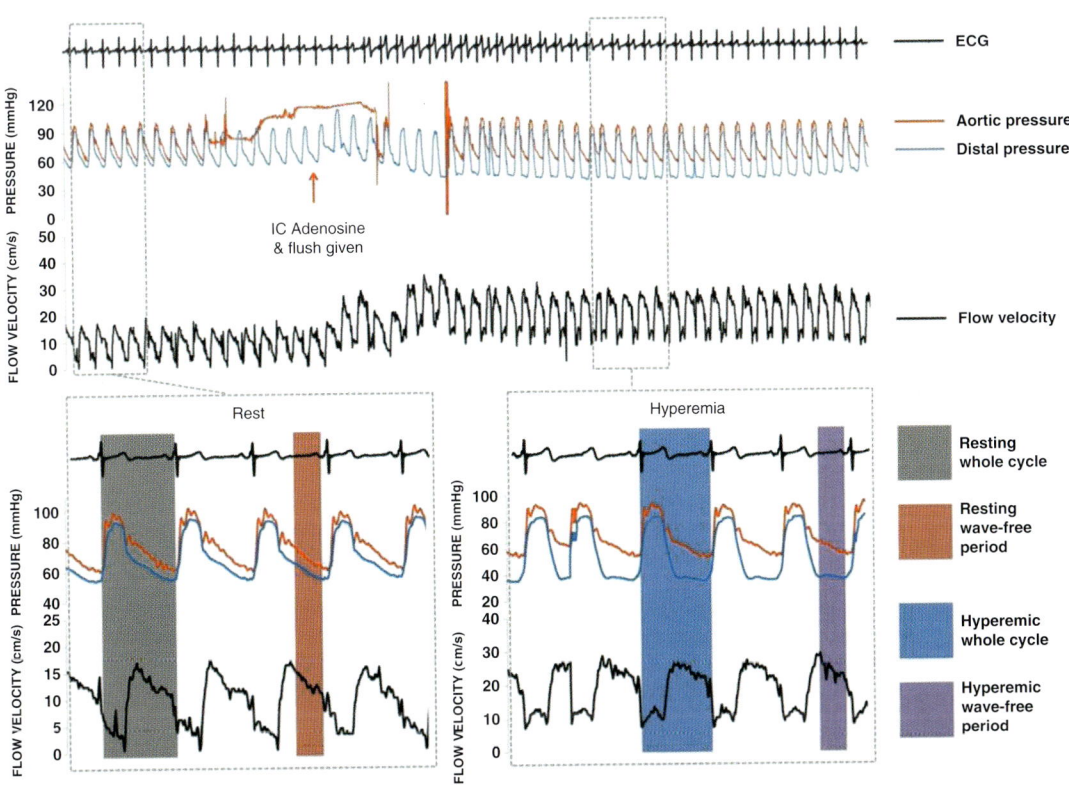

FIGURE 36.12 Coronary pressure and flow velocity tracings in a patient with a left anterior descending diameter stenosis of 69% by quantitative angiography with FFR of 0.79 are shown in the *upper panel*. The various phases of the cardiac cycle during which coronary flow velocities, mean distal coronary pressure (Pd) and aortic pressure (Pa) are measured in the resting and hyperemic state (intracoronary adenosine) are shown in the *lower panel*. Note the change in the flow velocity scale during hyperemia. After adenosine, there is an increase in pressure drop across the stenosis. This is particularly prominent during diastole when the effects of cardiac contraction are absent and phasic coronary flow is maximal (the "wave-free period"). As a result, distal coronary pressure during hyperemia is lower than that at rest. (Modified from Nijjer SS, et al. Coronary pressure and flow relationships in humans: phasic analysis of normal and pathological vessels and the implications for stenosis assessment: a report from the Iberian–Dutch–English (IDEAL) collaborators. Eur Heart J 2016;37:2069-2080.)

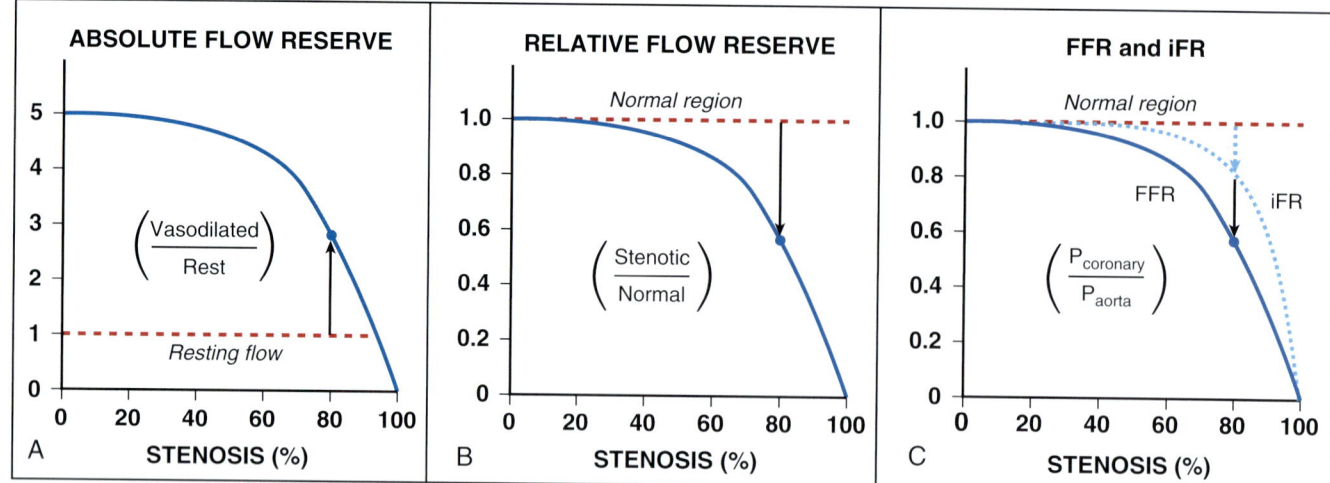

FIGURE 36.13 Interrelation of absolute flow reserve, relative flow reserve, fractional flow reserve (FFR), and instantaneous wave-free ratio (iFR). **A,** Absolute flow reserve is the ratio of coronary flow during vasodilation to the resting value. It can be obtained with invasive measurements of intracoronary flow velocity or quantitative kinetic perfusion measurements with positron emission tomography (PET). **B,** Relative flow reserve compares maximal vasodilated flow in a stenotic region with an assumed normal region in the same heart and is most commonly measured with perfusion imaging during stress. **C,** FFR (*dark blue solid line*) is conceptually similar to relative flow reserve and assesses maximal flow indirectly from coronary pressure measurements distal to a stenosis during vasodilation. *Panel C* also compares iFR, which is an index of the resting diastolic pressure gradient (*light blue dotted line*). For any given stenosis, reductions in iFR will be smaller than the vasodilated indices. Absolute flow reserve reflects the summed effects of a stenosis as well as abnormalities in the coronary microcirculation. By contrast, relative flow reserve and FFR (as well as iFR) identify the relative effects of a stenosis compared with a normal vessel. Unlike absolute flow reserve, none of the latter indices can identify the potential contribution of abnormalities in microcirculatory resistance control to the development of myocardial ischemia.

abnormalities of the coronary microcirculation. The three major indices currently used to quantify coronary flow reserve are absolute, relative, and fractional flow reserve (Fig. 36.13).

Perfusion-Based Indices of Stenosis Severity
Absolute Flow Reserve

Initial approaches to assess functional stenosis severity focused on assessing the relative increase in flow after ischemic vasodilation (reactive hyperemic response after transient occlusion of the coronary artery) or pharmacologic vasodilation of the microcirculation with intracoronary papaverine, adenosine, or intravenous dipyridamole. *Absolute flow reserve* can be quantified using intracoronary Doppler velocity or thermodilution flow measurements, as well as by quantitative approaches to image absolute tissue perfusion based on PET and magnetic resonance imaging (MRI). It is expressed as the ratio of maximally vasodilated flow to the corresponding resting flow value in a specific region of the heart and quantifies the ability of flow to increase above the resting value (see Fig. 36.13A). Clinically important reductions in maximum flow correlating with stress-induced ischemia on SPECT generally are associated with absolute flow reserve values below 2 (see Chapter 18). Absolute flow reserve is not only altered by factors that affect maximal coronary flow (e.g., stenosis severity, impaired microcirculatory control, arterial pressure, heart rate) but also by the corresponding resting flow value. As noted previously, resting flow can vary with hemoglobin content, baseline hemodynamics, and the resting oxygen extraction. Reductions in absolute flow reserve, therefore, can arise from inappropriate elevations in resting coronary flow as well as from reductions in maximal perfusion.

In the absence of diffuse atherosclerosis or LV hypertrophy, absolute flow reserve in conscious humans is similar to that measured in animals, with vasodilated flow reaching four to five times the value at rest. Thus, fairly good reduplication of the idealized relation between stenosis severity and absolute flow reserve occurs in patients with isolated one- or two-vessel CAD with intracoronary papaverine–induced vasodilation. By contrast, abnormalities in the coronary microcirculation as well as uncertainty in stenosis geometry or diffuse atherosclerosis leads to considerably more variability of the observed relation between stenosis severity and absolute flow reserve in patients with more extensive disease. Part of this reflects that patients with risk factors for CAD such as hypercholesterolemia and no significant coronary luminal narrowing have microcirculatory impairment in flow or attenuated vasodilator responsiveness, with absolute flow reserve using PET being lower than in normal individuals. Thus a significant limitation of absolute flow reserve measurements is that the importance of an epicardial stenosis cannot be dissociated from changes caused by functional abnormalities in the microcirculation that are common in patients with CAD (e.g., hypertrophy, impaired endothelium-dependent vasodilation). Likewise, primary coronary microvascular dysfunction is increasingly recognized as a cause of reduced coronary flow reserve (particularly in women) and can reflect structural and functional abnormalities of the microcirculation.[15]

Relative Flow Reserve

Relative coronary flow reserve measurements are the cornerstone of noninvasive identification of hemodynamically important coronary stenoses using nuclear perfusion imaging (see Chapter 18). In this approach, relative differences in regional perfusion (per gram of tissue) are assessed during maximal pharmacologic vasodilation or exercise stress and expressed as a fraction of flow to normal regions of the heart (see Fig. 36.13B). This approach compares relative perfusion states under the same hemodynamic conditions and is fairly insensitive to variations in mean arterial pressure, heart rate, and preload. An alternative approach uses invasive absolute flow reserve measurements and derives relative flow reserve by dividing absolute flow reserve in a stenotic vessel by absolute flow reserve in a remote normally perfused territory.[12]

Although widely used to identify hemodynamically significant stenoses, significant limitations arise in using imaging to quantify relative flow reserve. First, conventional SPECT imaging requires a normal reference segment within the left ventricle for comparison. Because of this, relative flow reserve measurements cannot accurately quantify stenosis severity when diffuse abnormalities in flow reserve related to either balanced multivessel CAD or impaired microcirculatory vasodilation are present. Moderately large differences in relative vasodilated flow are required to detect SPECT perfusion differences because nuclear tracers become diffusion limited and their myocardial uptake fails to increase proportionally with increases in vasodilated flow. As a result, differences in tracer deposition will variably underestimate the actual relative difference in perfusion. This problem can be overcome with use of PET tracers of perfusion and appropriate kinetic modeling to quantify flow. Finally, although prognostic data related to the perfusion deficit size are available, no imaging studies have been conducted to evaluate the quantitative severity of the stress or vasodilated flow reduction as a continuous outcome measure; conceptually, however, this should be similar to fractional flow reserve.

Indices of Stenosis Severity Based on Coronary Pressure
Vasodilated Pressure Measurements: Fractional Flow Reserve

Invasive point-of-care approaches use pressure measurements made distal to a coronary stenosis as an indirect index of stenosis severity[12] (see Fig. 36.12). This technique, pioneered by Pijls and Sels,[16] is based on the principle that the distal coronary pressure measured during vasodilation is directly proportional to maximum vasodilated perfusion (see Fig. 36.13C). *Fractional flow reserve* (FFR) is an indirect index determined by measuring the driving pressure for microcirculatory flow distal to the stenosis (distal coronary pressure minus coronary venous pressure) relative to the coronary driving pressure available in the absence of a stenosis (mean aortic pressure minus coronary venous pressure). The approach uses measurements of mean pressure averaged throughout the cardiac cycle. It assumes linearity of the vasodilated pressure-flow relation (which is known to be curvilinear at reduced coronary pressure[17]) and usually assumes that coronary venous pressure is zero. This results in the simplified clinical FFR index of mean distal coronary pressure/mean aortic pressure (P_d/P_{ao}). Although derived, the measurements are conceptually similar to those of relative coronary flow reserve because they only rely on minimum mean coronary pressure measurements during adenosine vasodilation (intracoronary or intravenous) and compare stenotic with normal regions under similar hemodynamic conditions. They are attractive for clinical use in that they can immediately assess the physiologic significance of an intermediate stenosis to help guide decisions regarding the need for percutaneous coronary intervention (PCI) and are unaffected by alterations in resting flow (see Chapter 41). Similarly, because they require only vasodilated coronary pressure determinations, FFR can be used to assess the functional effects of a residual lesion immediately after PCI.

A significant advantage of FFR is the availability of now-considerable prognostic information. The 15-year follow-up of a large prospective randomized study demonstrates that coronary lesions having FFR measurements greater than 0.75 are associated with excellent outcomes with deferred rather than prophylactic intervention in patients with stable ischemic heart disease.[18] Physiologically guided PCI using FFR versus angiographic criteria was safe and cost-effective and reduced the number of stents required to treat patients with multivessel CAD. Furthermore, a strategy based on assessing the physiologic severity of stenoses was accompanied by a significant reduction in major adverse cardiac events at 1 year (13.2% using FFR versus 18.3% in angiography-guided treatment).[17]

In subsequent trials, the same investigators showed that FFR-guided coronary intervention provided additional benefit over optimal medical therapy alone. Thus, patients with an FFR below 0.80 who underwent a coronary intervention in addition to optimal medical therapy displayed a reduction in major adverse cardiac events (Fig. 36.14) that was principally driven by a lesser need for urgent revascularization triggered by a myocardial infarction (MI) (or evidence of ischemia on an electrocardiogram (ECG).[19] A recent meta-analysis of three clinical trials further suggests a long-term impact on reducing the frequency of MI with this approach.[20] Collectively, these studies support the importance of functional stenosis severity in determining prognosis and the use of a physiologic-guided approach to determining the need for PCI in the patient with stable ischemic heart disease.

Unfortunately, FFR can assess only the functional significance of epicardial artery stenoses and cannot assess limitations in myocardial perfusion that arise from abnormalities in microcirculatory flow reserve in coronary resistance vessels. Although simple, FFR measurements are also critically dependent on achieving maximal pharmacologic vasodilation (underestimating stenosis severity if vasodilation is submaximal at the time of measurement). In addition, ignoring the backpressure to coronary flow by assuming that it is equal to zero and ignoring curvilinearity of the pressure-flow relation will cause the FFR to underestimate the physiologic significance of a stenosis.[17] This is

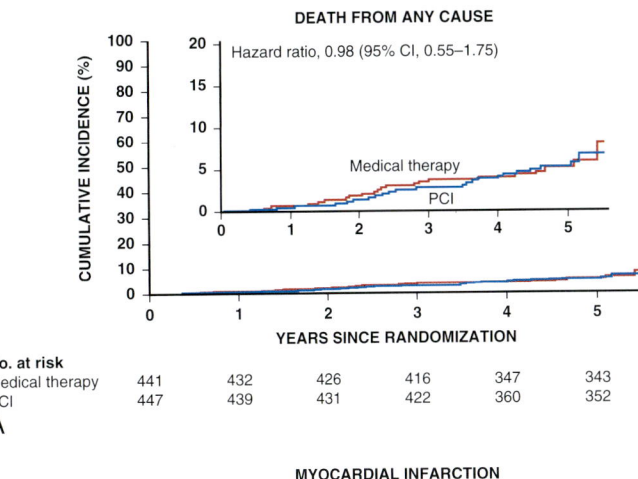

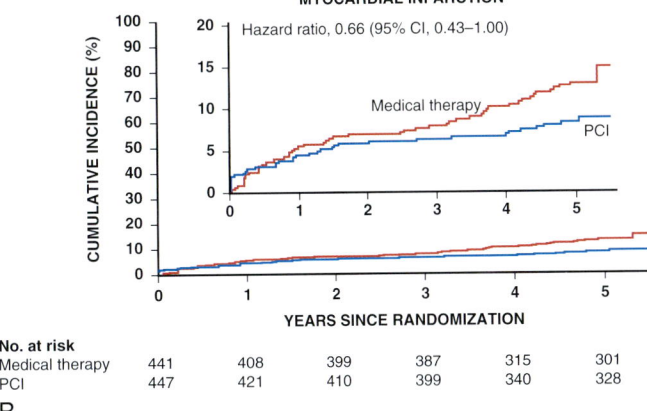

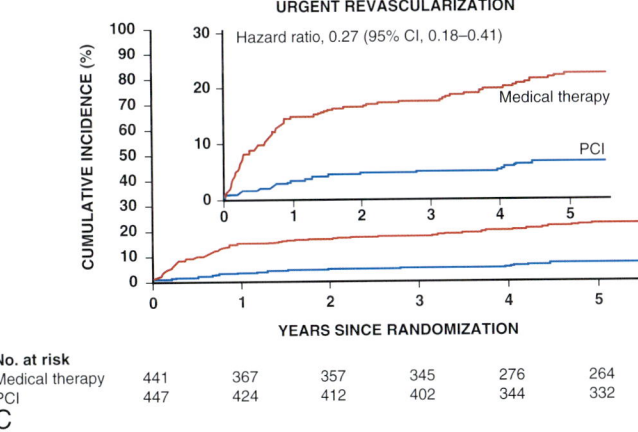

FIGURE 36.14 Patients with stable coronary artery disease with a fractional flow reserve (FFR) value of less than 0.80 randomized to percutaneous coronary intervention (PCI) plus optimal medical therapy versus optimal medical therapy alone have significantly lower rates of a composite end point of major adverse cardiovascular events. **A,** Although FFR-guided treatment did not affect survival, **(B)** there was a late effect on the incidence of myocardial infarction ($P = 0.05$), and **(C)** larger early effect on urgent revascularization ($P < 0.001$) compared to optimal medical therapy alone. Patients receiving FFR-guided PCI had an event rate similar to those in a registry who had no lesion with FFR less than 0.80 at enrollment. *CI,* Confidence interval. (From Xaplanteris P, et al. Five-year outcomes with PCI guided by fractional flow reserve. N Engl J Med 2018;379:250-259.)

particularly problematic at low coronary pressures and in assessing the functional significance of coronary collaterals, where venous pressure needs to be considered. Finally, inserting the pressure wire across a severe stenosis can lead to overestimation of stenosis severity in the presence of diffuse disease as well as small branch vessels. Despite these concerns and its invasive nature, determination of FFR can provide a rapid point-of-care assessment of the physiologic significance of individual coronary lesions.

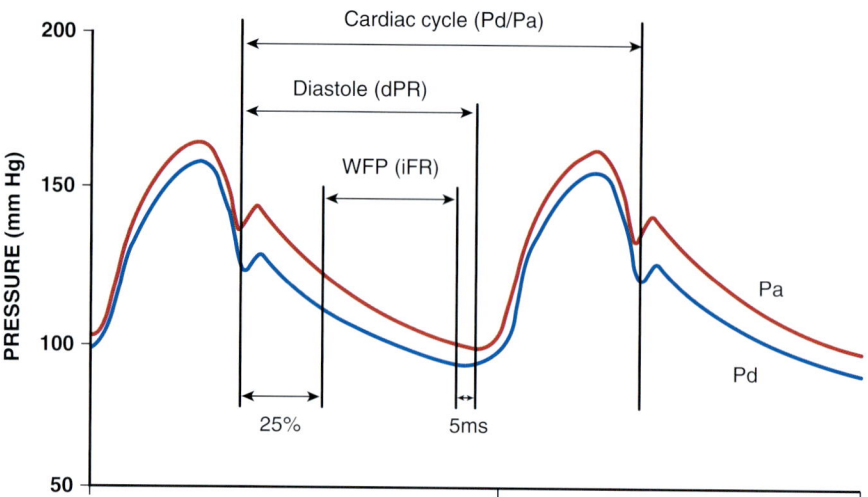

FIGURE 36.15 Pressure-derived indices to assess stenosis severity under basal resting conditions without pharmacologic vasodilation using the ratio of distal coronary pressure (Pd) to aortic pressure (Pa). Pd/Pa is defined as the ratio of mean distal coronary pressure (Pd) to mean aortic pressure (Pa) averaged over the full cardiac cycle; dPR is defined as the mean distal coronary pressure to mean aortic pressure ratio during the diastolic phase of the cardiac cycle; iFR (instantaneous wave-free ratio) is defined as the mean distal coronary pressure to mean aortic pressure ratio over the wave-free period (WFP). The WFP is defined as starting 25% into cardiac diastole and ending 5 ms before the end of diastole as illustrated. (Modified from van de Hoef TP, et al. Invasive coronary physiology: a Dutch tradition. Neth Heart J 2020;28:99-107.)

Resting Coronary Pressure Measurements: Instantaneous Wave-Free Ratio

Increased precision of pressure wire–based transducers has allowed resting distal coronary pressure to be used as an index of stenosis severity (see Fig 36.15). This is based on the finding that a resting pressure gradient does not develop until stenosis severity reaches a level that significantly affects maximal perfusion during vasodilation (see Fig. 36.11). A variety of indices have been studied with fairly similar results but the largest outcome data are based on the instantaneous wave-free ratio (iFR). This index reflects the ratio of distal coronary pressure to aortic pressure averaged throughout mid-diastole (i.e., the "wave-free period"). During mid-diastole, distal coronary resistance is free of the compressive effects of systole and phasic coronary flow and the stenosis diastolic pressure gradient are maximal (Fig. 36.15). Because the stenosis pressure gradient is smaller and distal coronary pressure higher at resting flow (see Fig. 36.11), the critical cutoff for iFR is a ratio of diastolic coronary to aortic pressure of 0.89 (versus 0.80 for FFR). Because iFR does not require pharmacologic vasodilation, it can be obtained rapidly and is not affected by abnormalities in the coronary microcirculation that can attenuate the vasodilator response to adenosine. On the other hand, iFR will overestimate the functional significance of a stenosis versus FFR in circumstances in which resting flow is abnormally elevated (e.g., anemia). Large clinical trials comparing both approaches have demonstrated that iFR is noninferior to FFR when employed to defer PCI of hemodynamically insignificant lesions[21,22] (Fig. 36.16). Nevertheless, a meta-analysis of these two trials suggests a borderline significant increase in the composite end point of death and MI using iFR versus FFR assessment.[23]

Noninvasive FFR_{CT} Using Computed Tomography and Computational Fluid Dynamics

Three-dimensional coronary imaging with coronary computed tomographic angiography (CTA) and modeling using computational fluid dynamics (CFD) allows coronary pressure gradients to be calculated throughout the entire coronary tree noninvasively[24] (see Chapter 20). These can be used to estimate FFR_{CT} throughout the entire heart. The major aspects of the procedure are illustrated in Fig 36.17; see also Fig. 20.12[25] The initial steps in the process create a patient-specific model of the coronary anatomy to provide luminal dimensions throughout the coronary tree. Next, total and vessel-specific absolute resting coronary flow are estimated using allometric scaling from measurements of LV mass to calculate microcirculatory resistance at rest. The effects of vasodilation are simulated by assuming a maximum reduction in the microcirculatory resistance index to 0.24 (i.e., approximately 4 times resting flow in nonstenotic arteries), which is typical of humans without coronary microvascular dysfunction. Using these data, three-dimensional CFD is used to estimate coronary pressure and calculate FFR_{CT} throughout the coronary tree during simulated pharmacologic vasodilation. Although this usually requires a separate analysis and considerable computational time and hardware, advances in computational techniques and machine learning are beginning to provide point-of-care analysis with desktop computing. Whether quantifying FFR_{CT} can provide prognostic information to defer coronary intervention such as invasive measurements has not yet been established. In addition, like other stenosis-based indices, FFR_{CT} cannot identify coronary microvascular dysfunction and in such circumstances, may overestimate the role of concomitant obstructive CAD in comparison to invasive measurements.

Advantages and Limitations of Coronary Flow Reserve Measurements. Assessing qualitative perfusion differences with noninvasive imaging is useful because relative perfusion deficit size is an important determinant of prognosis. Although the clinical role of invasive measurements available at the point of interventional care continue to evolve, FFR has been demonstrated to favorably affect postprocedural outcomes at reduced cost and safely defer interventions based solely on coronary anatomy. Incorporating these measurements into point of care decision making for PCI in patients with stable ischemic heart disease continues to increase.[12,26]

The major assumption common to all flow reserve measurements is that the administered pharmacologic vasodilator consistently achieves maximal vasodilation of the resistance vasculature in normal individuals and in patients with atherosclerotic disease and impaired endothelial function. The reductions in absolute flow reserve in humans with microvascular disease and angiographically insignificant stenoses, as well as variability in quantitative perfusion measurements with normal epicardial arteries and coronary risk factors, indicate that this may not always be the case.[15] The extent to which this variability is related to structural (e.g., caused by regional hypertrophy or vascular remodeling) versus functional (e.g., altered microcirculatory vasodilator response through impaired endothelium-dependent vasodilation) abnormalities in the microcirculation remains unclear (see later). A second limitation is that currently available approaches measure coronary flow reserve averaged across the entire wall of the heart. This is because they are based on epicardial coronary pressure distal to a stenosis (see Chapter 41) or, in the case of imaging (e.g., SPECT), have insufficient spatial resolution to assess transmural variations in flow (see Chapter 18). An imaging technique that could assess the physiologic significance of a stenosis in the subendocardial layers would be a major advance, because this region is most severely affected by an epicardial stenosis. This is now feasible with CMR but has yet to be incorporated broadly in clinical practice (see Chapter 19).

Pathophysiologic States Affecting Microcirculatory Coronary Flow Reserve

Various pathophysiologic states can accentuate the effects of a fixed-diameter coronary stenosis and may precipitate subendocardial ischemia during stress in the presence of normal coronary arteries.[15,27] Thus, it is important to consider measurements of stenosis severity in the context of coexisting abnormalities of coronary arterial resistance vessel control. In the former case, treatment will be directed at the epicardial stenosis, whereas in the latter, medical therapies designed to improve functional abnormalities in resistance vessel control will be required. The prognostic importance of abnormalities in coronary resistance vessel control is underscored by data in women evaluated for chest pain thought to be of ischemic origin.[27,28] Abnormalities in coronary flow reserve and endothelium-dependent vasodilation are common in women with insignificant epicardial coronary disease. They can variably produce metabolic evidence of myocardial ischemia as assessed by magnetic resonance spectroscopy (see Chapter 19) and negatively affect prognosis.[28,29] Common factors affecting microcirculatory resistance control independent of coronary stenosis severity in patients are LV hypertrophy, coronary microvascular disease, and impaired NO-mediated resistance vessel vasodilation, which is the result of many of the risk factors for CAD.[15,27,30]

Left Ventricular Hypertrophy. The effects of hypertrophy on coronary flow reserve are complex and must be seen in terms of the absolute flow level (e.g., measured with intracoronary Doppler probe) and the flow per gram of myocardial tissue[31] (Fig. 36.18). With acquired hypertrophy, resting flow per gram of myocardium remains constant, but the increase in LV mass necessitates an increase in the absolute level of resting flow (milliliters per minute) through the coronary artery (see Classic References, Bache). In terms of maximal perfusion, pathologic hypertrophy does not result in appreciable vascular proliferation (as opposed to physiologic hypertrophy produced by exercise training), and coronary resistance vessels remain essentially unchanged. Because maximum absolute flow (milliliters per minute) during vasodilation remains unchanged, the increase in LV mass in the absence of vascular proliferation reduces the maximum perfusion per gram of myocardium. The net effect of LV hypertrophy is that coronary flow reserve at any given coronary arterial pressure is reduced in a manner that is inversely related to the change in LV mass. For example, in the absence of a change in mean aortic pressure, a twofold increase in LV mass, as with severe LV hypertrophy, can reduce absolute coronary flow reserve in a nonstenotic artery from 4 to 2. This will increase the functional severity of any anatomic degree of coronary artery narrowing and can even precipitate subendocardial ischemia with normal coronary arteries.

Some degree of LV hypertrophy is common in patients with CAD, and it probably contributes to reductions in coronary flow reserve that are independent of coronary stenosis severity. The actual coronary flow reserve in hypertrophy will be critically dependent on the underlying cause of hypertrophy and its effects on coronary driving pressure.[30] A similar degree of hypertrophy caused by untreated systemic hypertension will be associated with a higher coronary flow reserve than in aortic stenosis, in which mean arterial pressure remains normal. Similarly, when hypertrophy results from systolic hypertension and increased pulse pressure is caused by reduced aortic compliance, the accompanying reduction in diastolic pressure can lower coronary reserve because myocardial perfusion occurs primarily in diastole.

Coronary Microvascular Disease and Dysfunction. The effects of primary coronary microvascular dysfunction (Fig. 36.19) on reducing coronary flow reserve are somewhat similar to those of LV hypertrophy but differ in terms of the effect on maximum coronary flow. As with hypertrophy, flow per gram of myocardium will be normal at rest and reduced during pharmacologic vasodilation. In contrast to hypertrophy, absolute flow remains normal at rest in microvascular disease, and the absolute vasodilated flow is reduced. Because absolute flow across the stenosis during vasodilation is the major determinant of the pressure drop and thus of distal coronary pressure, a similar stenosis will have a smaller pressure gradient and higher distal pressure in a patient with microvascular disease than in a patient with LV hypertrophy. Abnormalities in microvascular vasodilation may be functional rather than structural and, as discussed later, can arise from cumulative coronary risk factors that lead to endothelial dysfunction.

Measurements of coronary flow reserve in humans with risk factors for atherosclerosis (see Chapter 25) are systematically lower than in normal individuals without coronary risk factors, underscoring the importance of functional abnormalities in microvascular control in determining coronary flow reserve.[15,27] Perturbations in microvascular control may arise from abnormal local resistance vessel control through impaired endothelium-dependent vasodilation arising from NO inactivation associated with risk factors for CAD. Experimental hypercholesterolemia markedly attenuates the dilation of coronary arterioles in response to shear stress as well as pharmacologic agonists that stimulate NOS in the absence of epicardial stenoses (Fig. 36.20). This was reversed with L-arginine, suggesting that it reflects impaired NO synthesis or availability. CAD is associated with a shift from NO to the EDHF hydrogen peroxide (H_2O_2), which acts to compensate in part for the loss of NO.[9] This shift appears to be mediated by the sphingolipid ceramide (produced by neutral sphingomyelinase in patients with CAD), resulting in the endothelial production of reactive oxygen species, thereby reducing NO and increasing H_2O_2 levels.[7]

These in vitro abnormalities in NO-mediated vasodilation can be functionally significant and can impair the ability of the heart to autoregulate coronary blood flow. Fig. 36.21A shows the effects of inhibiting NO on the coronary autoregulatory relation in normal dogs. Although

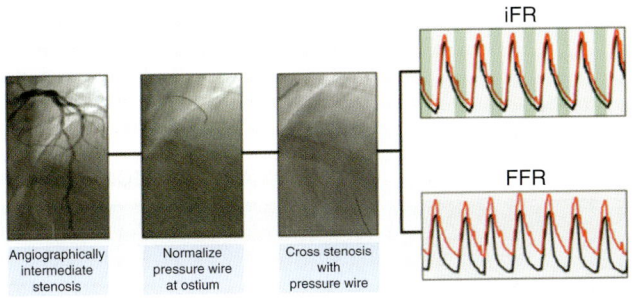

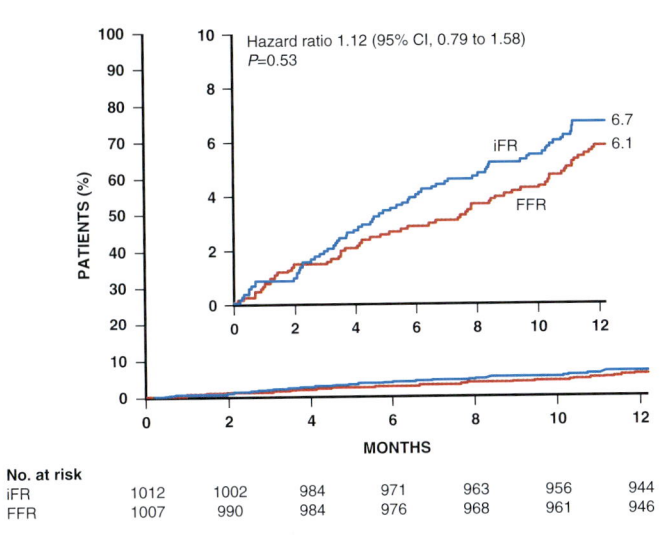

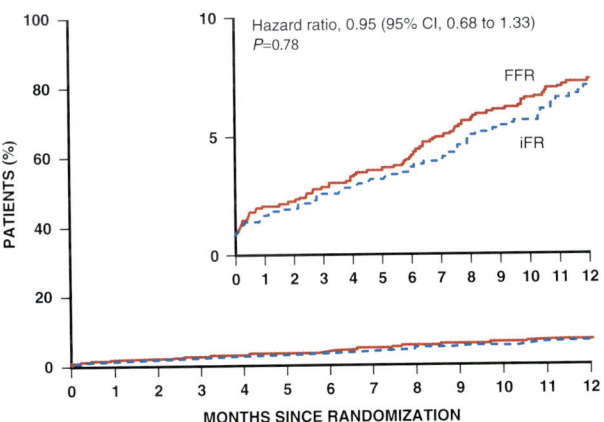

FIGURE 36.16 Functional outcome after percutaneous coronary intervention guided by instantaneous wave-free ratio (iFR) versus fractional flow reserve (FFR). **A,** Summary of the procedure. After inserting a pressure wire into the coronary artery (*left* angiogram) measurements from the pressure wire are normalized to aortic pressure (*middle* angiogram). The pressure wire is then advanced to measure pressure distal to the coronary stenosis (*right* angiogram). For iFR, measurements are taken at resting coronary flow and an algorithm automatically measures aortic and distal coronary pressure during diastole when the effects of systole on coronary flow are absent. This period is indicated by the vertical green bars (*top right panel*). For FFR, an intravenous infusion or intracoronary bolus of adenosine is used and FFR calculated as mean distal coronary pressure divided by mean aortic pressure in the guiding catheter. Whereas iFR is calculated based on measurements obtained during diastole, FFR is calculated based on measurements averaged over the entire cardiac cycle. **B, C,** Kaplan–Meier curves for the cumulative risk of the composite end point of death from any cause, nonfatal myocardial infarction, or unplanned revascularization at 1 year from two independent clinical trials. The *insets* show the same data on an enlarged y axis. There was no significant difference in outcomes with FFR versus iFR-guided revascularization in either study. (**A** and **B** from Götberg M, et al. Instantaneous wave-free ratio versus fractional flow reserve to guide PCI. N Engl J Med 2017;376:1813-1823; **C** from Davies JE, et al. Use of the instantaneous wave-free ratio or fractional flow reserve in PCI. N Engl J Med 2017;376:1824-1834.)

PATIENT-SPECIFIC ARTERIAL GEOMETRY BY CORONARY CTA

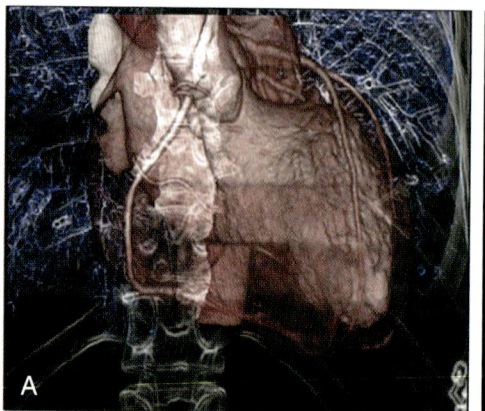

SUBVOXEL RESOLUTION EVALUATION

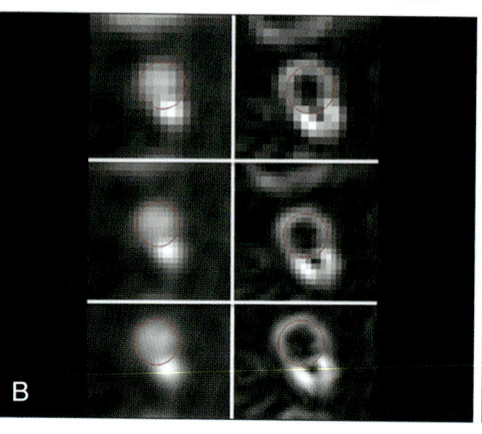

CORONARY ARTERY SEGMENTATION

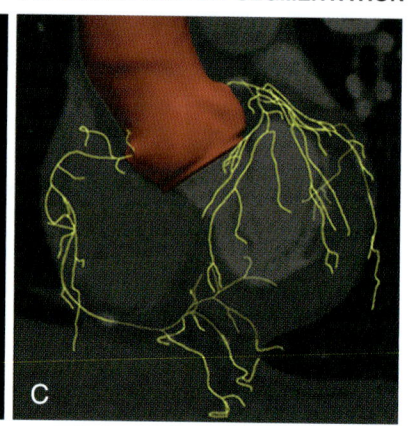

3D MESH GENERATION

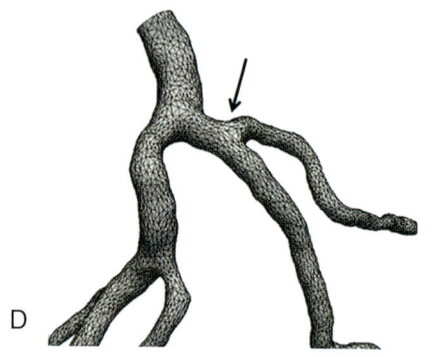

QUANTIFICATION OF REST CORONARY FLOW

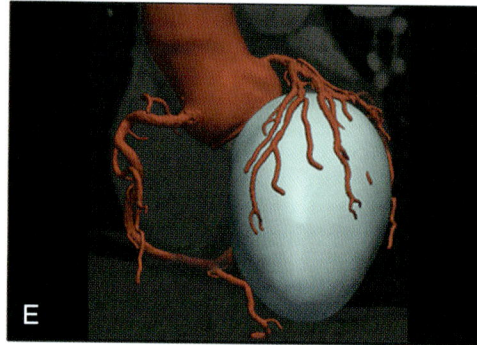

CALCULATION OF MICROVASCULAR RESISTANCE

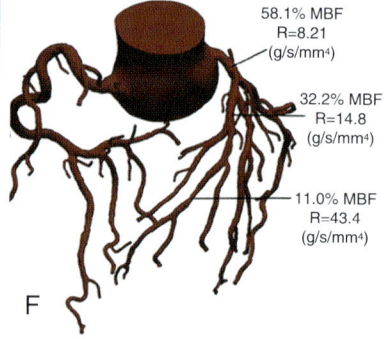

58.1% MBF
R=8.21
(g/s/mm⁴)

32.2% MBF
R=14.8
(g/s/mm⁴)

11.0% MBF
R=43.4
(g/s/mm⁴)

COMPUTATION OF HYPEREMIC CHANGES

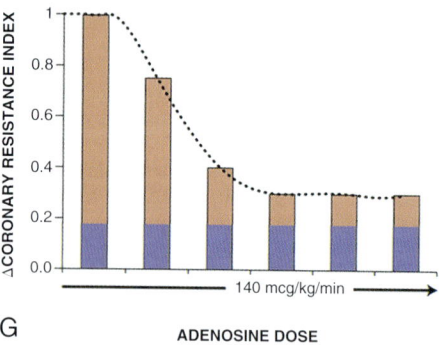

140 mcg/kg/min

ADENOSINE DOSE

COMPUTATIONAL FLUID DYNAMICS

Mass conservation (1 equation):

$$\frac{\partial v_x}{\partial x} + \frac{\partial v_y}{\partial y} + \frac{\partial v_z}{\partial z} = 0$$

Momentum balance (3 equations):

$$\rho \frac{\partial v_x}{\partial t} + \rho \left(v_x \frac{\partial v_x}{\partial x} + v_y \frac{\partial v_x}{\partial y} + v_z \frac{\partial v_x}{\partial z} \right) = -\frac{\partial p}{\partial x} + \mu \left(\frac{\partial^2 v_x}{\partial x^2} + \frac{\partial^2 v_x}{\partial y^2} + \frac{\partial^2 v_x}{\partial z^2} \right)$$

$$\rho \frac{\partial v_y}{\partial t} + \rho \left(v_x \frac{\partial v_y}{\partial x} + v_y \frac{\partial v_y}{\partial y} + v_z \frac{\partial v_y}{\partial z} \right) = -\frac{\partial p}{\partial y} + \mu \left(\frac{\partial^2 v_x}{\partial x^2} + \frac{\partial^2 v_y}{\partial y^2} + \frac{\partial^2 v_z}{\partial z^2} \right)$$

$$\rho \frac{\partial v_z}{\partial t} + \rho \left(v_x \frac{\partial v_z}{\partial x} + v_y \frac{\partial v_z}{\partial y} + v_z \frac{\partial v_z}{\partial z} \right) = -\frac{\partial p}{\partial z} + \mu \left(\frac{\partial^2 v_x}{\partial x^2} + \frac{\partial^2 v_y}{\partial y^2} + \frac{\partial^2 v_z}{\partial z^2} \right)$$

FFR$_{CT}$

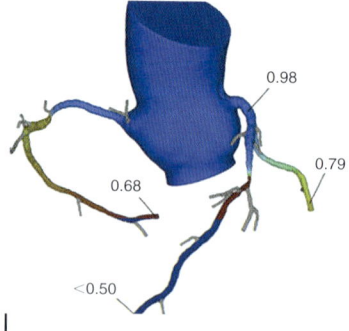

0.98
0.79
0.68
<0.50

FIGURE 36.17 Fractional flow reserve derived from multidetector CT (FFR$_{CT}$) involves the use of detailed three-dimensional anatomy and computational fluid dynamics to derive coronary pressure during vasodilation throughout the coronary tree. **A,** After the coronary computed tomography angiogram (CTA) is acquired, **(B)** it is subjected to subvoxel resolution techniques. Here, a typical cross-section of a coronary artery is shown, with image intensity data on the *left* and image-gradient data on the *right*. The coronary CTA is reconstructed with increasing image resolution *(middle and bottom images pairs)*. **C,** Next, coronary artery segmentation to second- and third-order vessels is performed. **D,** Discretization of mesh elements of the coronary vascular tree for subsequent computational fluid dynamics (CFD) at millions of points. **E,** The CT is used to characterize the relation between coronary artery size and the mass of myocardium subtended by each branch. **F,** These estimates are all combined to determine the relationship among coronary vessel caliber, flow, and resistance. **G,** The assumed relative reduction in coronary resistance index at an adenosine dose of 140 μg/kg/min. A major assumption is that the coronary microcirculation is normal with an approximately fourfold increase in coronary flow in the absence of a stenosis. **H,** Navier-Stokes equations that govern the fluid dynamics of blood (nonlinear partial differential equations related to mass conservation and momentum balance) are solved at multiple points in the reconstructed high-resolution three-dimensional coronary angiogram. **I,** Example of patient-specific FFR$_{CT}$ calculations. (From Min JK, et al. Noninvasive fractional flow reserve derived from coronary CT angiography clinical data and scientific principles. JACC Cardiovasc Imaging 2015;8:1209-1222.)

LEFT VENTRICULAR HYPERTROPHY

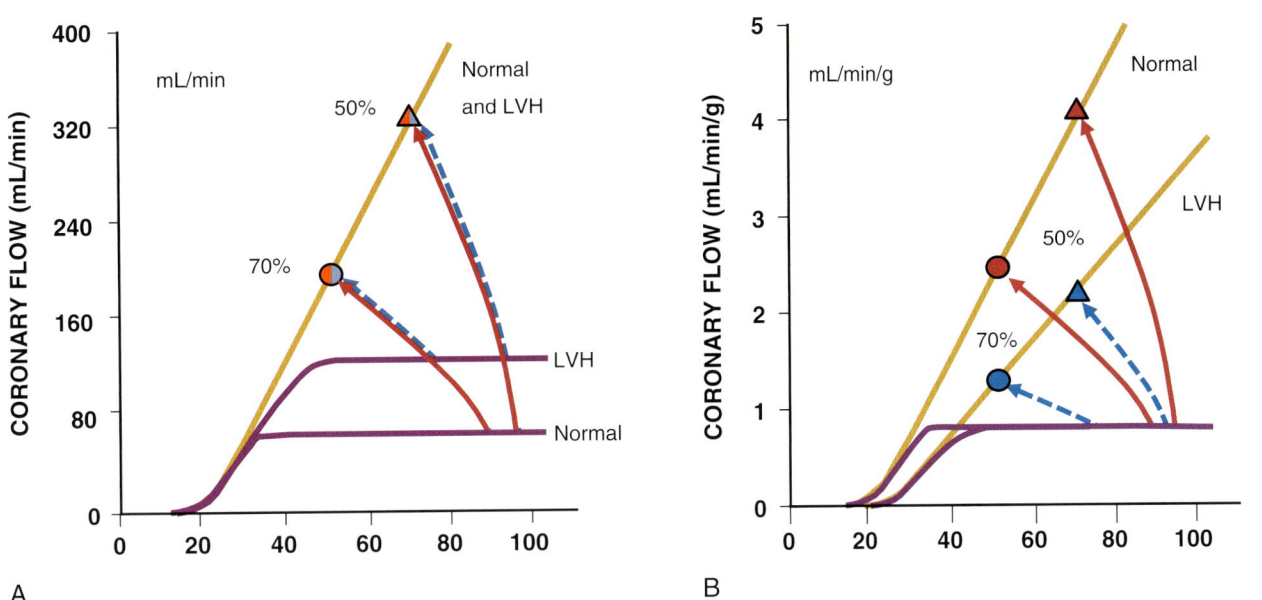

FIGURE 36.18 Effects of hypertrophy on absolute flow (mL/min) and flow per gram of tissue (mL/min/g). With acquired hypertrophy, myocardial mass increases without proliferation of the microcirculatory resistance arteries. **A**, The increase in left ventricular (LV) mass causes a proportional increase in absolute flow at rest (*purple lines*), while the maximum absolute flow per minute during vasodilation (*gold lines*) remains unchanged. **B**, When tissue perfusion is assessed using flow per gram of myocardium (e.g., as obtained using positron emission tomography [PET]), the maximum flow per gram of tissue (*gold lines*) falls inversely with the increase in LV mass. By contrast, the resting flow per gram of myocardium (*purple lines*) remains constant, because the increase in absolute resting flow is proportional to the increase in LV mass. Regardless of whether absolute flow or flow per gram is measured, the net effect of these opposing actions is to decrease coronary flow reserve at any coronary pressure in LV hypertrophy (LVH). As a result of the reduction in microcirculatory reserve in the absence of a coronary stenosis, the functional significance of a 50% stenosis (*triangles*) in the hypertrophied heart could approach a more severe stenosis (in the example, 70%, *circles*) in normal myocardium. This can even lead to ischemia with normal coronary arteries during stress.

CORONARY MICROVASCULAR DYSFUNCTION

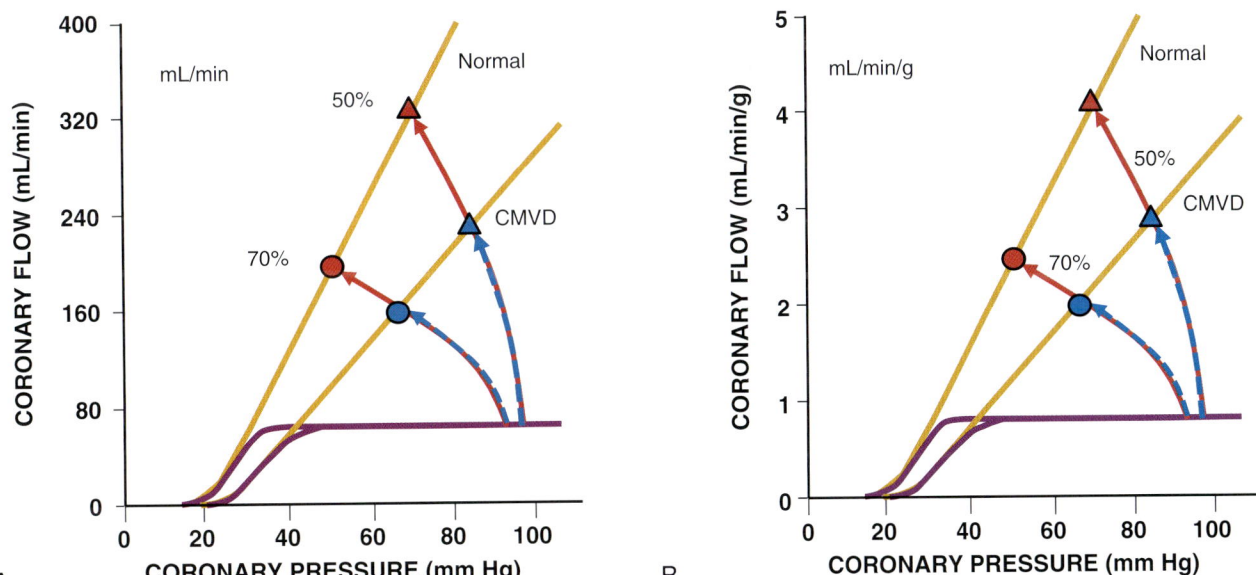

FIGURE 36.19 Effects of microvascular dysfunction on absolute flow (mL/min) and flow per gram of tissue (mL/min/g). In microvascular disease, resting flow and left ventricular mass remain normal. Thus, under resting conditions (*purple lines*), absolute flow and flow per gram of tissue are similar in patients with microvascular disease compared with normal subjects. By contrast, during maximum vasodilation (*gold lines*) **(A)** absolute flow and **(B)** flow per gram of tissue both are reduced in microvascular disease, reflecting a functional or structural abnormality of coronary resistance vessels. *CMVD*, Coronary microvascular dysfunction.

resting blood flow is not altered, there is a marked increase in the coronary pressure at which intrinsic autoregulatory adjustments become exhausted, with flow beginning to decrease at a distal coronary pressure of 60 versus 45 mm Hg, approximately similar to the shift occurring in response to a twofold increase in heart rate. In vivo microcirculatory studies have demonstrated that inhibiting NO production prevents resistance arteries from dilating maximally in response to shear stress.[3,7] This limiting effect probably reflects excess resistance in the transmural penetrating arteries, which are upstream of metabolic stimuli for vasodilation and extremely dependent on shear stress as a stimulus for local vasodilation. These functional abnormalities amplify the physiologic effects of a coronary stenosis, resulting in the development of subendocardial ischemia at a lower workload (Fig. 36.21B).

These observations in normal animals with impaired NO production appear to be relevant to pathophysiologic states associated with impaired endothelium-dependent vasodilation in humans. For example, coronary flow reserve is markedly reduced in the absence of a coronary stenosis in familial hypercholesterolemia, and improving endothelial

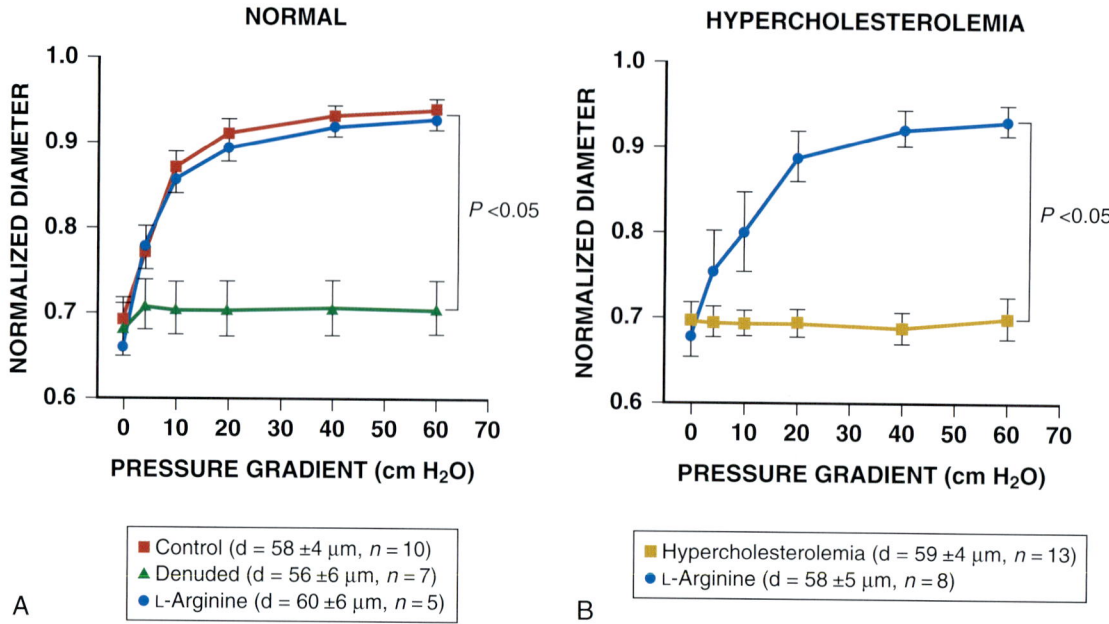

FIGURE 36.20 Flow-mediated vasodilation in coronary resistance arteries is abolished by dietary hypercholesterolemia in swine. **A,** In normal arterioles, increased flow (pressure gradient) elicits vasodilation that, similar to human vessels, is abolished by removing the endothelium (denuded). **B,** In animals with dietary hypercholesterolemia but no significant epicardial stenosis, flow-mediated vasodilation of arterioles is abolished. It was restored by administering L-arginine to increase NO production. Luminal diameters were normalized to the diameter at a luminal pressure of 60 cm H_2O in the presence of nitroprusside (10^{-4} M). Numbers of vessels (n) and average luminal diameter (d) with spontaneous tone in physiologic salt solution-albumin at 60 cm H_2O are shown. *Vertical bars* denote mean ± SEM. (Modified from Kuo L, et al. Pathophysiological consequences of atherosclerosis extend into the coronary microcirculation: restoration of endothelium-dependent responses by l-arginine. Circ Res 1992;70:465-476.)

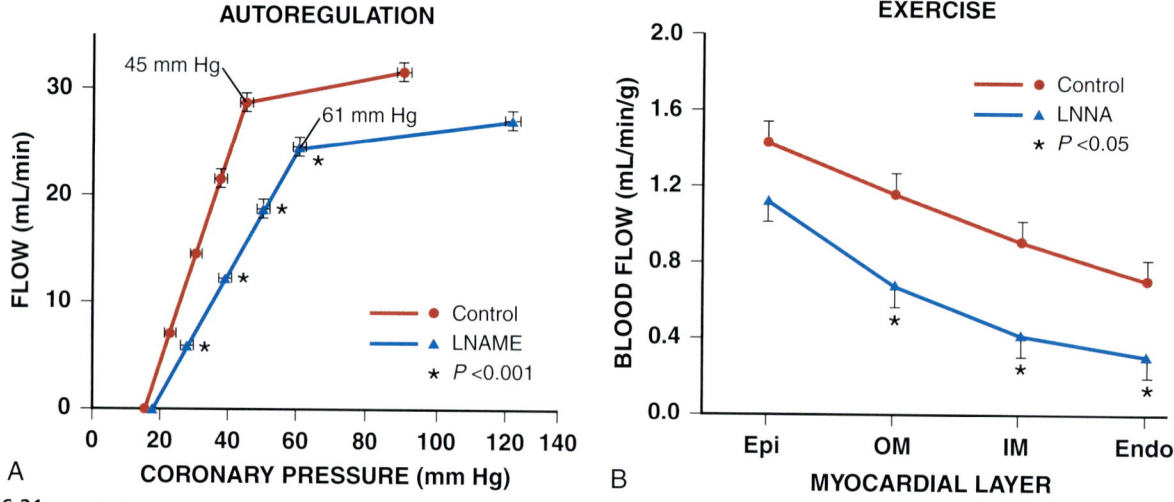

FIGURE 36.21 Impaired microcirculatory control with abnormal NO-mediated endothelium-dependent resistance artery dilation. **A,** Effects of blocking nitric oxide synthase (NOS) with the L-arginine analog LNAME in chronically instrumented dogs. There is an increase in the lower autoregulatory pressure limit, resulting in the onset of ischemia at a coronary pressure of 61 mm Hg versus 45 mm Hg under normal conditions that occurred without a change in heart rate. **B,** Transmural perfusion before and after blocking NO-mediated dilation with LNNA in exercising dogs subjected to a coronary stenosis. Although coronary pressure and hemodynamics were similar, blood flow was less in each layer of the heart after blocking NOS and was not overcome by metabolic dilator mechanisms during ischemia. Collectively, these experimental data support the notion that abnormalities in endothelium-dependent microvascular vasodilation can amplify the functional effects of a proximal coronary stenosis. *Endo,* Endocardium; *Epi,* epicardium; *IM,* inner mid; *OM,* outer mid; *LNAME,* Nω-nitro-L-arginine methyl ester; *LNNA,* Nω-nitro-L-arginine. (**A** modified from Smith TP Jr, Canty JM Jr. Modulation of coronary autoregulatory responses by nitric oxide: evidence for flow-dependent resistance adjustments in conscious dogs. Circ Res 1993;73:232; **B** modified from Duncker DJ, Bache RJ. Inhibition of nitric oxide production aggravates myocardial hypoperfusion during exercise in the presence of a coronary artery stenosis. Circ Res 1994;74:629-640.)

function by lowering elevated LDL levels with statins produces a delayed improvement in coronary flow reserve in normal and stenotic arteries and also ameliorates clinical signs of myocardial ischemia.[32] Impaired NO-mediated vasodilation probably affects the regulation of myocardial perfusion in other disease states in which endothelium-dependent vasodilation is impaired.

Impact of Microcirculatory Abnormalities on Physiologic Measures of Stenosis Severity.

If microcirculatory dysfunction is absent, quantitative measures of stenosis severity during vasodilation that are derived using absolute flow reserve, relative flow reserve, and FFR should all be closely related. Unfortunately, this is the exception rather than the rule, and microvascular dysfunction, variability in the microcirculatory response to pharmacologic vasodilation, and diffuse CAD dissociates the idealized relation between various indices of coronary flow reserve for a given stenosis severity. Fig. 36.22A shows the relation between paired invasive measurements of absolute flow reserve versus distal coronary pressure–derived FFR. Hemodynamically insignificant stenoses (FFR >0.8) can have an absolute flow reserve that varies from 1 to more than 5. Although this variability decreases when FFR is less than 0.8, it is still considerable until FFR falls below 0.5.

The variability in microvascular dysfunction and submaximal pharmacologic vasodilator responses can have a significant impact on assessing the physiologic significance of a coronary stenosis using FFR

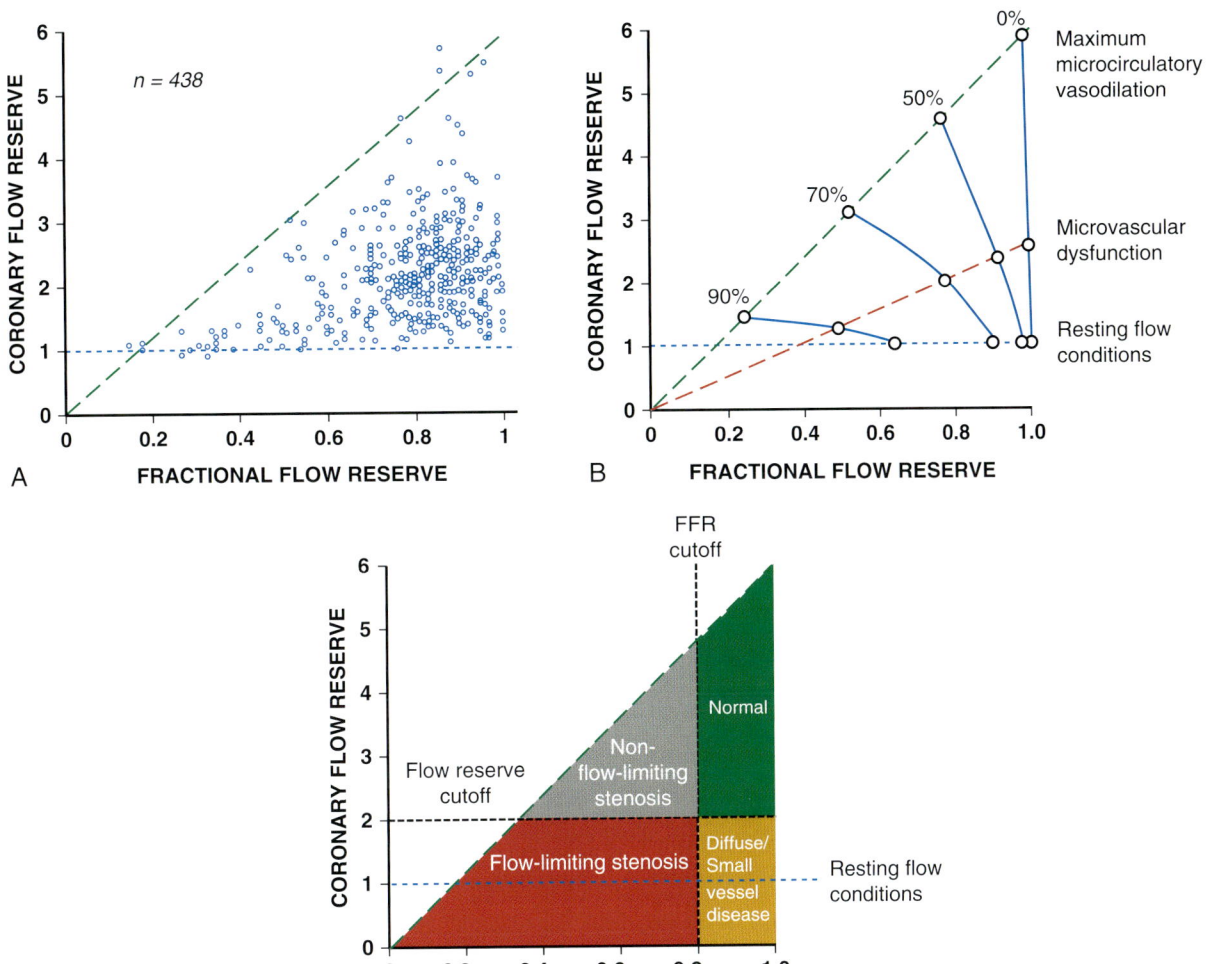

FIGURE 36.22 Wide variation in paired measurements of functional stenosis severity is observed with use of different indices of flow reserve in the same patient, suggesting the presence of coronary microvascular dysfunction. **A,** Simultaneous intracoronary catheter–based measurements of absolute coronary flow reserve (CFR) are compared with fractional flow reserve (FFR). This variability reflects differences in the contribution of the microcirculation and stenosis in individual patients. **B,** Effects of microvascular dysfunction on the stenosis pressure-flow relation and measurements of flow reserve. The *upper green dashed line* shows the idealized linear relation between CFR and FFR when the coronary microcirculation is normal and maximally vasodilated. The *lower red dashed line* indicates the relation between CFR and FFR, but there is microvascular dysfunction. Individual stenoses are illustrated by the *solid blue lines.* The *horizontal blue dashed line* indicates **(A)** a CFR of 1.0 or **(B)** the absolute resting flow conditions. The presence of microvascular dysfunction will limit vasodilation. Thus, absolute flow reserve will be reduced and will overestimate stenosis severity. By contrast, because distal coronary pressure is higher with submaximal vasodilation, FFR (and relative flow reserve) will underestimate stenosis severity. It is likely that these interactions contribute to the variability demonstrated in panel **A. C,** Four main quadrants can be identified by applying the clinically applied cutoff values for FFR and CFR, indicated by the *black dashed lines.* Patients in the *upper right green area* are characterized by concordantly normal FFR and CFR, and patients in the *lower left red area* are characterized by concordantly abnormal FFR and CFR. Patients in the *upper left gray area* and *lower right orange area* are characterized by discordant results between FFR and CFR. The combination of an abnormal FFR and a normal CFR indicates predominant focal epicardial, but non–flow-limiting, coronary artery disease. In contrast, the combination of a normal FFR and an abnormal CFR indicates coronary microvascular dysfunction or diffuse epicardial involvement in coronary artery disease. (**A** modified from Johnson NP, et al. Is discordance of coronary flow reserve and fractional flow reserve due to methodology or clinically relevant coronary pathophysiology? JACC Cardiovasc Imaging 2012;5:193-202; **B** modified from Duncker DJ, et al. Regulation of coronary blood flow in health and ischemic heart disease. Prog Cardiovasc Dis 2015;57:409-422; **C** modified from van de Hoef TP, et al. Invasive coronary physiology: a Dutch tradition. Neth Heart J 2020;28:99-107.)

(or relative perfusion with imaging). In Fig. 36.22B, the two dashed lines show idealized relations between absolute flow reserve and FFR (or relative flow reserve from perfusion imaging). Microvascular dysfunction in the presence of normal coronary arteries (0% stenosis) *attenuates* coronary flow reserve. Conversely, for any given stenosis, the FFR measured in the presence of microvascular disease will be *higher* than when vasodilator responses are normal. Thus, when maximum vasodilation is not achieved, FFR will underestimate the physiologic severity of the stenosis. This probably contributes to at least some of the discordance between FFR and absolute coronary flow reserve observed in clinical studies, underscoring the importance of combining both pressure- and flow-derived indices to assess vasodilator reserve of the total coronary vascular bed. Indeed, the availability of high-fidelity pressure and flow measurements on a single wire has now facilitated the development of approaches to assess the stenosis pressure-flow relation and abnormalities in microcirculatory reserve by determining FFR and absolute coronary flow reserve simultaneously. When assessed together, these measurements have the potential to identify circumstances in which mixed abnormalities from a stenosis and abnormal microcirculation contribute to the functional impact of a coronary stenosis[33] (Fig. 36.22C).

CORONARY COLLATERAL CIRCULATION

After a total coronary occlusion, residual perfusion to the myocardium persists through native coronary collateral channels that open with development of an intercoronary pressure gradient between the source and recipient vessel. In most animal species, the native collateral flow during occlusion is less than 10% of the resting flow levels and is insufficient to maintain tissue viability for longer than 20 minutes. Tremendous inter individual variability in the function of coronary collaterals is recognized among patients with chronic stenoses. In humans without coronary collaterals, coronary pressure during balloon angioplasty occlusion falls to approximately 10 mm Hg. In other patients, collaterals proliferate to the point at which they are sufficient not only to maintain resting perfusion at normal but also to prevent stress-induced ischemia at submaximal cardiac workloads. Ischemia does not develop during PCI balloon occlusion when FFR (based on coronary wedge pressure during occlusion minus venous pressure) is greater than 0.25.[34] A large observational cross-sectional study has demonstrated that patients with elevated distal coronary pressure arising from recruitable collaterals during transient total balloon occlusion (FFR >0.25) have a lower cardiovascular event rate and improved survival[34].

Arteriogenesis and Angiogenesis

Proliferation of coronary collaterals (see Chapters 21 and 24) occurs in response to repetitive stress-induced ischemia and the development of transient interarterial pressure gradients between the source and recipient vessel through a process termed *arteriogenesis* (see Classic References, Schaper). Resting distal coronary pressure consistently falls as stenosis severity exceeds 70% diameter reduction, and the resultant interarterial pressure gradient increases endothelial shear stress in preexisting collaterals smaller than 200 μm in diameter. This causes progressive enlargement of collaterals through a process dependent on physical forces and growth factors, particularly vascular endothelial growth factor (VEGF), that is mediated by NOS.[8] Thus, patients with impaired NO-mediated vasodilation caused by coronary risk factors may have a limited ability to develop coronary collaterals in response to a chronic coronary stenosis.

Most functional collateral flow arises from arteriogenesis in existing epicardial anastomoses that enlarge into mature vessels, which can reach 1 to 2 mm in diameter.[35] Collateral perfusion also can originate from de novo vessel growth, or *angiogenesis*, which refers to the sprouting of smaller, capillary-like structures from preexisting blood vessels. These vessels may provide nutritive collateral flow when they develop in the border between ischemic and nonischemic regions. Capillary angiogenesis may also occur within the ischemic region and can reduce the intercapillary distance for oxygen exchange. Nevertheless, because capillary resistance is already a small component of microcirculatory resistance, increases in capillary density in the absence of changes in arteriolar resistance will not significantly increase myocardial perfusion.

Great interest is currently directed toward experimental interventions to improve collateral flow (e.g., recombinant growth factors, in vivo gene transfer, adult progenitor cells). Although many interventions have been demonstrated to cause favorable angiogenesis of capillaries and improve myocardial function, few interventions have increased arteriogenesis in mature collaterals, and randomized human clinical trials have been disappointing.[35,36] Part of this limitation may arise from the fact that no intervention has resulted in measurable increases in maximum vasodilated myocardial perfusion or coronary flow reserve indices, the *sine qua non* of functional collateral formation. Improvements in myocardial function have been used as an end point, but such improvement may occur independently of increased perfusion and may arise from mechanisms that alter cardiac myocyte growth and repair rather than angiogenesis.[37]

Regulation of Collateral Resistance

The control of blood flow to collateral-dependent myocardium is governed by a series resistance arising from interarterial collateral anastomoses, largely epicardial, as well as the native downstream microcirculation. Collateral resistance is therefore the major determinant of perfusion, and coronary pressure distal to a chronic occlusion is already near the lower autoregulatory pressure limit. Consequently, subendocardial perfusion is critically dependent on mean aortic pressure and LV preload, with ischemia easily provoked by systemic hypotension, increases in LV end-diastolic pressure, and tachycardia. As with the distal resistance vessels, collaterals constrict when NO synthesis is blocked, which aggravates myocardial ischemia and can be overcome by nitroglycerin.[3] In contrast with the native coronary circulation, experimental studies have demonstrated that coronary collaterals are under tonic dilation from vasodilator prostaglandins, and blocking COX with aspirin exacerbates myocardial ischemia in dogs.[3] The role of prostanoids in human coronary collateral resistance regulation is unknown.

The distal microcirculatory resistance vasculature in collateral-dependent myocardium appears to be regulated by mechanisms similar to those present in the normal circulation, but it is characterized by impaired endothelium-dependent vasodilation compared with normal vessels.[3] Of interest, the remote normally perfused zone in collateralized hearts also shows alterations in coronary resistance vessel control, suggesting that abnormalities are not restricted to the collateral-dependent region. The extent to which these microcirculatory abnormalities alter the normal metabolic and coronary autoregulatory responses in collateral-dependent and remote myocardial regions is unknown.[3]

METABOLIC AND FUNCTIONAL CONSEQUENCES OF ISCHEMIA

Because oxygen delivery to the heart is closely related to coronary blood flow, a sudden cessation of regional perfusion after a thrombotic coronary occlusion quickly leads to the cessation of aerobic metabolism, depletion of creatine phosphate, and onset of anaerobic glycolysis. This is followed by the accumulation of tissue lactate, a progressive reduction in tissue ATP levels, and an accumulation of catabolites, including those of the adenine nucleotide pool. As ischemia continues, tissue acidosis develops and there is an efflux of potassium into the extracellular space. Subsequently, ATP levels fall below those required to maintain critical membrane function, resulting in the onset of myocyte death.

Irreversible Injury and Myocyte Death

The temporal evolution and extent of irreversible tissue injury after coronary occlusion are variable and depend on transmural location, residual coronary flow, and the hemodynamic determinants of oxygen consumption. Irreversible myocardial injury begins after 20 minutes of coronary occlusion in the absence of significant collaterals (Fig. 36.23). Irreversible injury starts in the subendocardium and progresses as a wavefront over time, from the subendocardial layers to the subepicardial layers. This reflects the higher oxygen consumption in the subendocardium and the redistribution of collateral flow to the outer layers of the heart by the compressive determinants of flow at reduced coronary pressure. In experimental infarction, the entire subendocardium is irreversibly injured within 1 hour of occlusion, and the transmural progression of infarction is largely completed within 4 to 6 hours after coronary occlusion. Factors that increase myocardial oxygen consumption (e.g., tachycardia) or reduce oxygen delivery (e.g., anemia, arterial hypotension) accelerate the progression of irreversible injury. By contrast, repetitive reversible ischemia or angina occurring before an occlusion can reduce irreversible injury through preconditioning.[38]

The magnitude of residual coronary flow through collaterals or through a subtotal coronary occlusion is the most important determinant of the actual time course of irreversible injury in patients with chronic CAD. The relation between infarct size and the area at risk of ischemia during a total occlusion is inversely related to collateral flow and likely explains the important role of collateral vessel function in determining prognosis.[34] When subendocardial collateral flow is more than approximately 30% of resting flow values, it prevents infarction after periods of ischemia lasting longer than 1 hour. More moderate subendocardial ischemia from a subtotal occlusion (e.g., flow reduced by no more than 50%) can persist for at least 5 hours without producing significant irreversible injury.[39] This explains why signs and symptoms of ischemia can be present for long periods without producing significant myocardial necrosis. It also explains the clinical observation that late coronary reperfusion with ongoing ischemia can salvage myocardium beyond the 6-hour time limit predicted from experimental models of MI.[38]

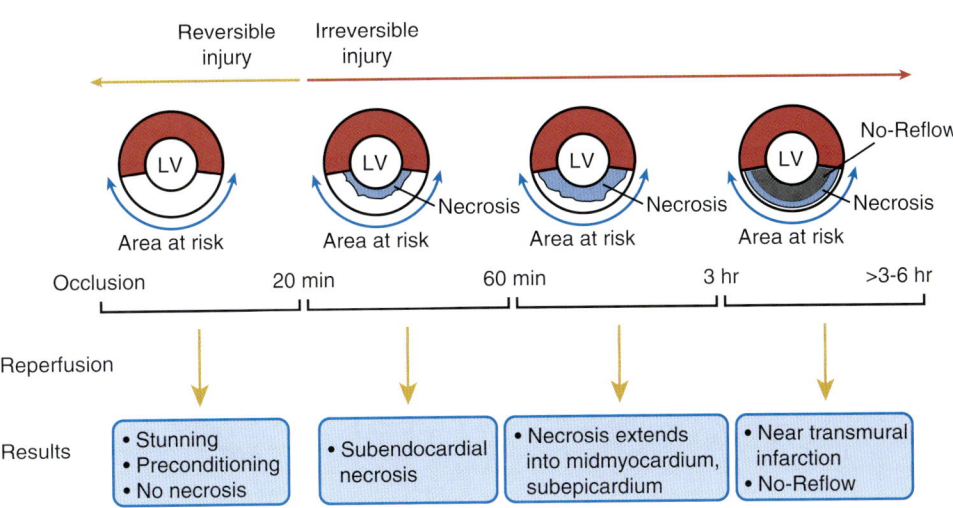

FIGURE 36.23 Wavefront of necrosis in infarction. Total coronary artery occlusions shorter than 20 minutes do not cause irreversible injury but can cause myocardial stunning and also precondition the heart and protect it against recurrent ischemic injury. Irreversible injury begins after 20 minutes and progresses as a wavefront from endocardium to epicardium. After 60 minutes, the inner third of the left ventricle (LV) wall is irreversibly injured. After 3 hours, only a subepicardial rim of tissue remains, with the transmural extent of infarction completed between 3 and 6 hours after occlusion. The most important factor delaying the progression of irreversible injury is the magnitude of collateral flow, which is directed primarily to the outer layers of the heart. Reperfusion after prolonged ischemia is accompanied by the development of no-reflow within the infarct area. (Modified from Kloner RA, Jennings RB. Consequences of brief ischemia: stunning, preconditioning, and their clinical implications: Part 1. Circulation 2001;104:2981-2989.)

Cell death arises from multiple mechanisms in MI[38] (see Chapter 37). Reperfusion immediately causes myocyte necrosis and sarcolemmal disruption, with the leakage of cell contents into the extracellular space. The injury may be further amplified by the reentry of leukocytes into the area of injury and by loss of coronary microvessel patency termed no-reflow. At later time points, myocytes initially salvaged can undergo programmed cell death or apoptosis, which can contribute to further delayed myocardial injury. *Apoptosis* is a coordinated involution of myocytes that circumvents the inflammation associated with necrotic cell death. Because apoptosis is an energy-dependent process, cells can be forced to switch to a necrotic pathway if energy levels are depleted below critical levels. In the setting of more chronic injury, autophagy can contribute to the mechanisms of myocyte death. Moreover, coronary no-reflow may impair wound healing and promote thinning and expansion of the infarct region, thus contributing to infarct adverse LV remodeling. Because of the temporal complexity of irreversible injury, the relative importance of each mechanism in MI continues to be controversial. Nevertheless, modulating mechanisms contributing to late cell death and coronary no-reflow could prevent deleterious LV remodeling.

Cardioprotection from Local and Remote Conditioning

Early reperfusion remains the best and only treatment that can clinically reduce myocardial infarct size. Although there are a wealth of studies supporting cardioprotective interventions in preclinical experimental studies, none have been translated to have an impact on outcomes in large randomized human clinical trials of MI.[38] Nevertheless, this continues to be an active area of investigation and the major aspects are reviewed in the following text.

Studies in the late 1980s serendipitously demonstrated that brief reversible ischemia preceding a prolonged coronary occlusion reduced infarct size, a phenomenon termed *acute preconditioning*[38] (Fig. 36.24). Because acute MI is frequently preceded by unstable angina, ischemic preconditioning is an endogenous mechanism that can delay the evolution of irreversible myocardial injury. It has been demonstrated in humans during angioplasty with reduced subjective and objective ischemia during successive coronary occlusions as an end point. Preconditioning also develops on a chronic basis (*delayed preconditioning*) and, once induced, persists for up to 4 days. It reduces MI size and also protects the heart from ischemia-induced stunning. *Myocardial postconditioning*[38] refers to the ability to engage cardiac protection by producing intermittent ischemia or administering pharmacologic agonists at reperfusion. It has the greatest clinical potential to affect irreversible injury because it can be induced after myocardial ischemia is established rather than requiring pretreatment (see Fig. 36.24). Finally, a number of experimental studies have demonstrated that ischemia in an extremity remote from the infarct can reduce infarct size. *Remote conditioning* is particularly attractive because it can be easily implemented using a blood pressure cuff and has been shown to experimentally reduce infarct size when administered before and after the onset of ischemia as well as at the time of reperfusion.[38]

There has been extensive investigation of the molecular mechanisms of protection arising from reversible ischemia and leading to a variety of pharmacologic agents that can reduce experimental infarct size.[38] Acute preconditioning can be induced using adenosine A_1 receptor agonists as well as agonists that stimulate protein kinase C or open mitochondrial K_{ATP} channels. The mechanisms of chronic preconditioning involve protein synthesis, with upregulation of the inducible form of NOS (iNOS), COX-2, and opening of the mitochondrial K_{ATP} channel. Protection from postconditioning occurs principally through activation of reperfusion injury salvage kinase pathways, thereby limiting opening of the mitochondrial permeability transition pore.[38] Remote ischemic preconditioning involves the systemic release of cardioprotective factors including nitric oxide and activation of the cardiosplenic axis via vagal efferents, suggesting a more complex integrative protective mechanism that may relate to inhibiting an inflammatory mechanism after myocardial reperfusion.[40]

Like preclinical studies of cardioprotection, many small clinical trials of ischemic and pharmacologic postconditioning and remote ischemic conditioning have shown promise.[41] Nevertheless, large randomized clinical trials of postconditioning and remote conditioning have failed to translate these into measurable impacts on clinical end points or infarct size. Thus, despite nearly 30 years of study since the original description, adjunctive cardioprotective strategies remain unproven.[41] Nevertheless, the study of combined remote and ischemic conditioning as well as newer approaches such as mechanical unloading before reperfusion with percutaneous LV assist devices are novel approaches under clinical investigation.[42]

Reversible Ischemia and Perfusion-Contraction Matching

Reversible ischemia is considerably more common than irreversible injury. *Supply-induced ischemia* can arise from transient coronary occlusion resulting from coronary vasospasm or transient thrombosis in a critically stenosed coronary artery, producing transmural ischemia similar to that present at the onset of MI. *Demand-induced ischemia* arises from an inability to increase flow in response to increases in myocardial oxygen consumption in which ischemia predominantly affects the subendocardium (see Chapter 40). These have fundamentally different effects on myocardial diastolic relaxation, with supply-induced ischemia increasing LV compliance and demand-induced ischemia reducing it. There is a fairly stereotypic sequence of physiologic changes that develop during an episode of spontaneous transmural ischemia. Coronary occlusion results in an immediate fall in coronary venous oxygen saturation, with a reduction in ATP production. This causes a decline in regional contraction within several beats, reaching dyskinesis within 1 minute. As regional contraction ceases, concomitant changes include a reduction in global LV contractility (dP/dt), a progressive rise in LV end-diastolic pressure, and a fall in systolic pressure. The magnitude of the systemic hemodynamic changes varies with the severity of ischemia and the amount of the left ventricle subjected to ischemia. Significant electrocardiographic ST-segment changes develop within 2 minutes as efflux of potassium into the extracellular space reaches a critical level. Symptoms of chest pain are variable and usually are the last event in the evolution of

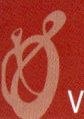

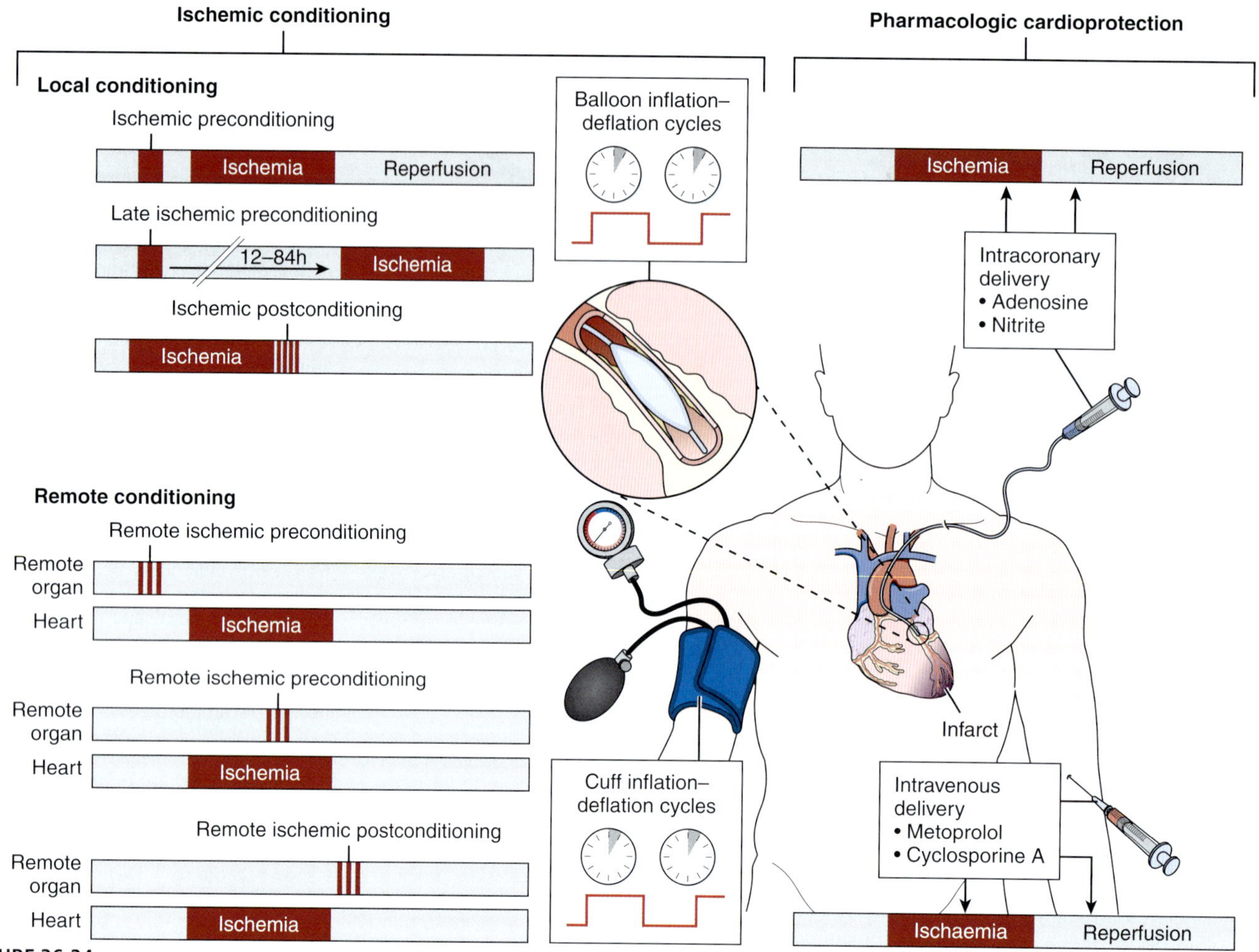

FIGURE 36.24 Experimental approaches for cardioprotective strategies for reperfused acute myocardial infarction. Strategies employing brief ischemia are summarized on the *left*. Brief episodes of reversible ischemia before infarction effectively reduce infarct size in preclinical studies and may afford some benefit to patients with infarction preceded by unstable angina. In contrast, ischemic postconditioning administers cycles of recurrent occlusion–reperfusion at the time of reperfusion. Unfortunately, recent large clinical trials investigating this have been negative. Another approach has been to employ remote ischemic conditioning by inflating and deflating a blood pressure cuff on a limb for example. This has been demonstrated to reduce experimental infarct size when initiated before as well as after the onset of ischemia. Clinical studies have yet to demonstrate an impact on outcomes. Pharmacological strategies are depicted on the *right*. Experimental studies have variably induced cardioprotection with intravenous drugs administered at the time of reperfusion (e.g., metoprolol and cyclosporine A) or intracoronary infusion (such as adenosine and nitrite) just before or at early reperfusion. Unfortunately, the results of intermediate-sized clinical trials have failed to demonstrate a clinical impact. This continues to be an area of active investigation. (Modified from Heusch G. Myocardial ischaemia–reperfusion injury and cardioprotection in perspective. Nat Rev Cardiol 2020;17:773-789.)

ischemia. On restoring perfusion, the sequence is reversed, with resolution of chest pain occurring before hemodynamic changes resolve, but regional contraction can remain depressed, reflecting the development of stunned myocardium. A similar temporal sequence of events occurs during exercise-induced ischemia, although the time frame of evolution can be more protracted because ischemia occurs primarily in the subendocardium. Because of the temporal delay in the development of angina and other factors, many episodes of ST-segment depression are symptomatically silent. It is also likely that very brief episodes of ischemia, as reflected by more sensitive indices, such as reduced regional contraction or elevations in end-diastolic pressure, can be electrocardiographically silent.

Acute Perfusion-Contraction Matching During Subendocardial Ischemia
When coronary pressure distal to a stenosis falls below the lower limit of autoregulation, flow reserve is exhausted, resulting in the onset of subendocardial ischemia. In this case, reductions in subendocardial flow are closely related to reductions in regional contractile function of the heart, as measured by sensitive approaches such as regional wall thickening.[39] An approximately linear relation has been shown between relative reductions in subendocardial blood flow and relative reductions in regional wall thickening at rest, during tachycardia, and during exercise-induced dysfunction distal to a critical stenosis[39] (Fig. 36.25). This forms the basis for using regional myocardial function as an index of the severity of subendocardial ischemia during stress imaging (see Chapters 15 and 16).

Short-Term Hibernation
In steady-state ischemia, the close matching between perfusion and contraction leads to a reduced regional oxygen consumption and energy utilization, a phenomenon termed *short-term hibernation*.[39,43] This reestablishes a balance between supply and demand, as reflected by regeneration of creatine phosphate and ATP with the resolution of lactate production, despite persistent hypoperfusion. Short-term hibernation is an extremely tenuous state, and small increases in the determinants of myocardial oxygen demand precipitate further ischemia and a rapid deterioration in function and metabolism.[43] Thus, the ability of short-term hibernation to prevent necrosis is limited by the severity and duration of ischemia, with irreversible injury developing frequently after periods longer than 12 to 24 hours.[44]

Functional Consequences of Reversible Ischemia
Various late consequences of ischemia have been documented after normal myocardial perfusion is reestablished. These reflect both acute and delayed effects of acute ischemia on regional function (Figs. 36.26 and 36.27) and in the most chronic state, they result in hibernating myocardium, characterized by chronic contractile dysfunction and regional cellular mechanisms that downregulate contractile and metabolic function of the heart so as to protect it from irreversible injury (Fig. 36.28). In clinical practice, it is difficult to separate all the various

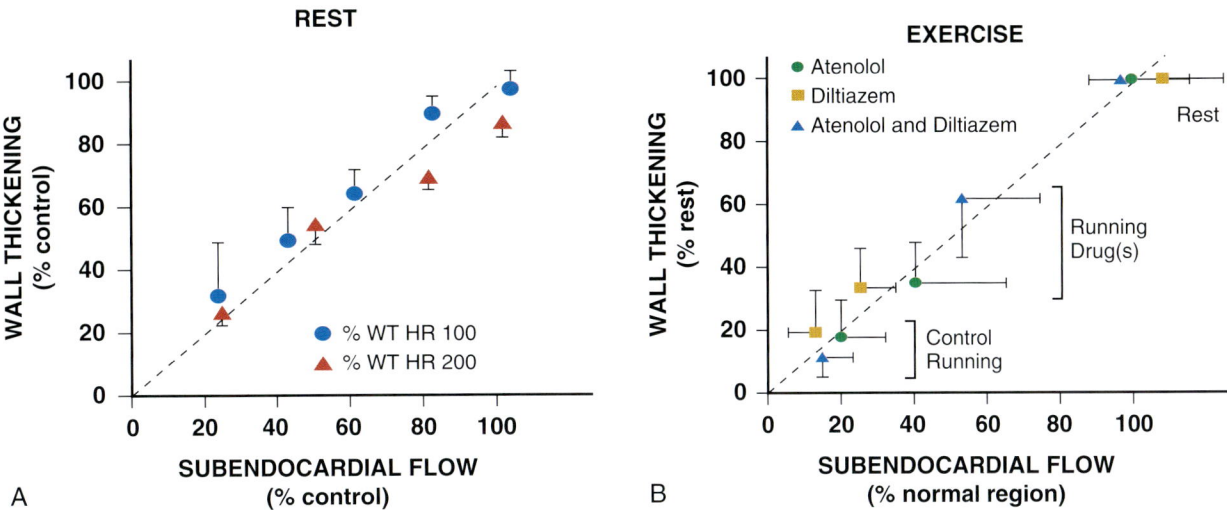

FIGURE 36.25 Perfusion-contraction matching during acute ischemia. Relative reductions in function (regional wall thickening) are proportional to the relative reduction in subendocardial flow measured with microspheres in conscious dogs. This relation is maintained **(A)** over a wide range of heart rates during autoregulation as well as **(B)** during exercise with a fixed coronary stenosis. In the latter case, medical interventions that ameliorate ischemia improve both subendocardial flow and wall thickening (WT) during exercise. *HR,* Heart rate. (**A** modified from Canty JM Jr. Coronary pressure-function and steady-state pressure-flow relations during autoregulation in the unanesthetized dog. Circ Res 1988;63:821-836; and Canty JM Jr, et al. Effect of tachycardia on regional function and transmural myocardial perfusion during graded coronary pressure reduction in conscious dogs. Circulation 1990;82:1815-1825; **B,** modified from Matsuzaki M, et al. Effect of the combination of diltiazem and atenolol on exercise-induced regional myocardial ischemia in conscious dogs. Circulation 1985;72:233-243.)

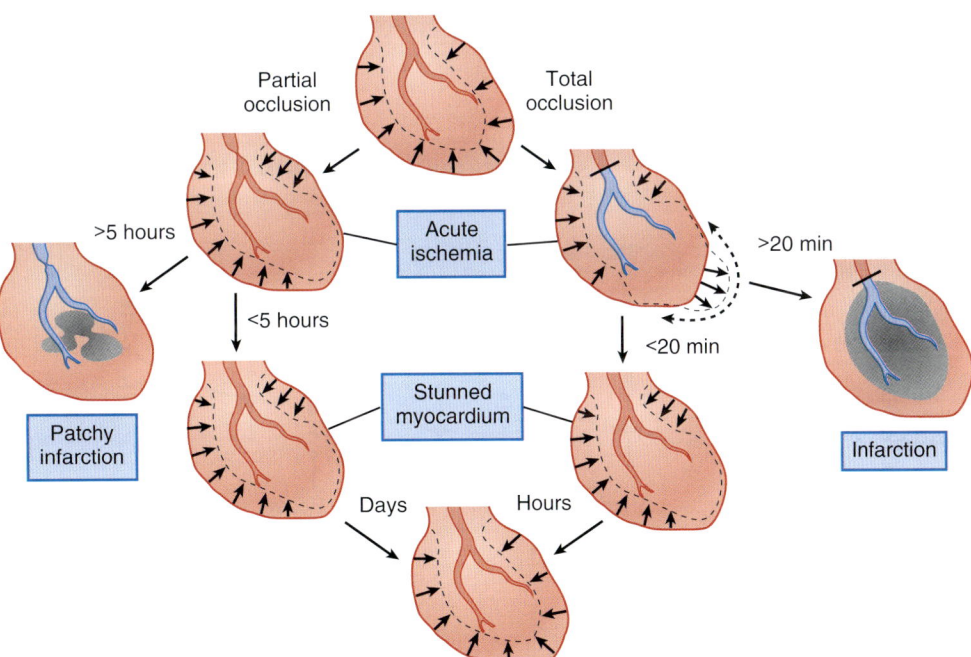

FIGURE 36.26 Consequences of acute ischemia on left ventricular function and irreversible injury. The ventriculograms illustrate contractile dysfunction (*dashed lines* and *arrows*). A brief total occlusion (*right*) or a prolonged partial occlusion (caused by an acute high-grade stenosis, *left*) leads to acute contractile dysfunction proportional to the reduction in blood flow. Irreversible injury begins after 20 minutes after a total occlusion but is delayed for up to 5 hours after a partial occlusion (or with significant collaterals) caused by short-term hibernation. When reperfusion is established before the onset of irreversible injury, stunned myocardium develops, and the time required for recovery of function is proportional to the duration and severity of ischemia. With prolonged ischemia, stunning in viable myocardium coexists with subendocardial infarction and accounts for a variable amount of irreversible dysfunction.

mechanisms involved in contributing to ischemia-induced viable dysfunctional myocardium, because they all may coexist to some extent in the same heart. They can be separated experimentally, however, and the important features and mechanisms from basic studies are summarized next.

Stunned Myocardium. Myocardial function normalizes rapidly after single episodes of ischemia lasting less than 2 minutes. As ischemia increases in duration and severity, a temporal delay in the recovery of function occurs despite that blood flow has been restored. Regional myocardial function remains depressed for up to 6 hours after resolution of ischemia following a 15-minute occlusion in the absence of tissue necrosis, a phenomenon called *myocardial stunning* (see Figs. 36.26 and 36.27). A defining feature of isolated myocardial stunning is that function remains depressed while resting myocardial perfusion is normal.[39,43] Thus, there is a dissociation of the usual close relation between subendocardial flow and function. Stunned myocardium also develops after demand-induced ischemia. For example, exercise-induced ischemia can result in depressed regional function distal to a coronary stenosis for hours after perfusion is restored, and repetitive ischemia can lead to cumulative stunning. Prolonged sublethal ischemia, as seen in short-term

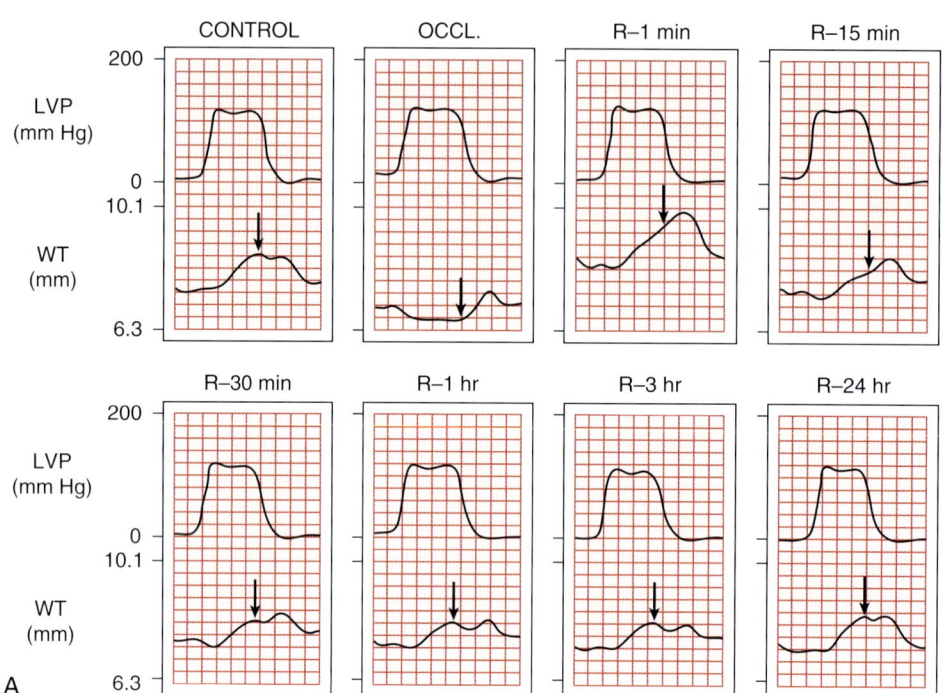
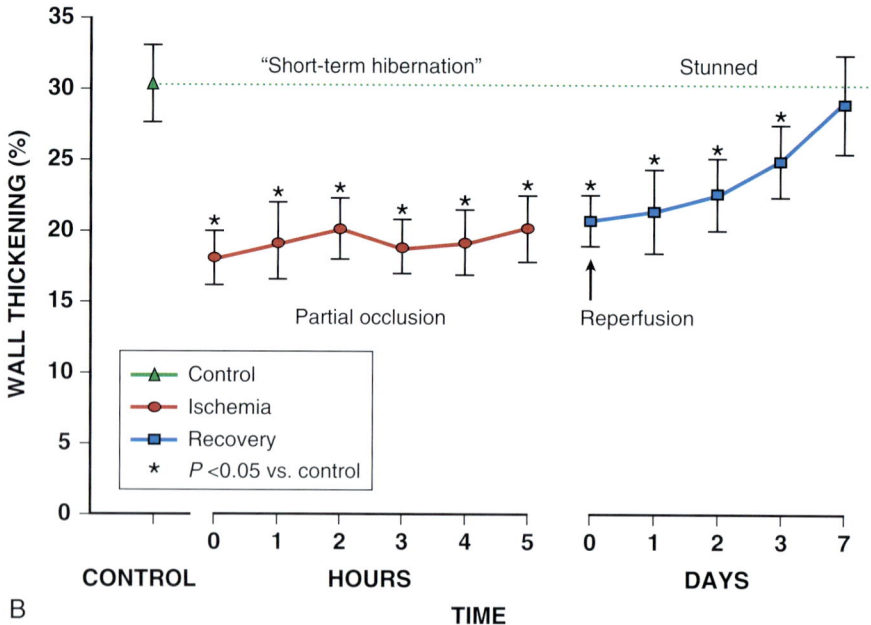

FIGURE 36.27 Stunned myocardium. A, Myocardial stunning after a brief total occlusion (OCCL.). Wall thickening (WT) measured by ultrasonic crystals is dyskinetic, with systolic thinning during occlusion. After reperfusion (R), function is completely normal after 24 hours. **B,** Myocardial stunning after a prolonged partial occlusion. During acute ischemia *(red circles),* there is short-term hibernation, reflecting an acute match between reduced flow, wall thickening, and metabolism. With reperfusion *(blue squares),* WT remains depressed and gradually returns to normal after 1 week. *LVP,* Left ventricular pressure. (**A** modified from Heyndrickx GR, et al. Depression of regional blood flow and wall thickening after brief coronary occlusions. Am J Physiol 1978;234:H653-H659; **B** modified from Matsuzaki M, et al. Sustained regional dysfunction produced by prolonged coronary stenosis: gradual recovery after reperfusion. Circulation 1983;68:170-182.)

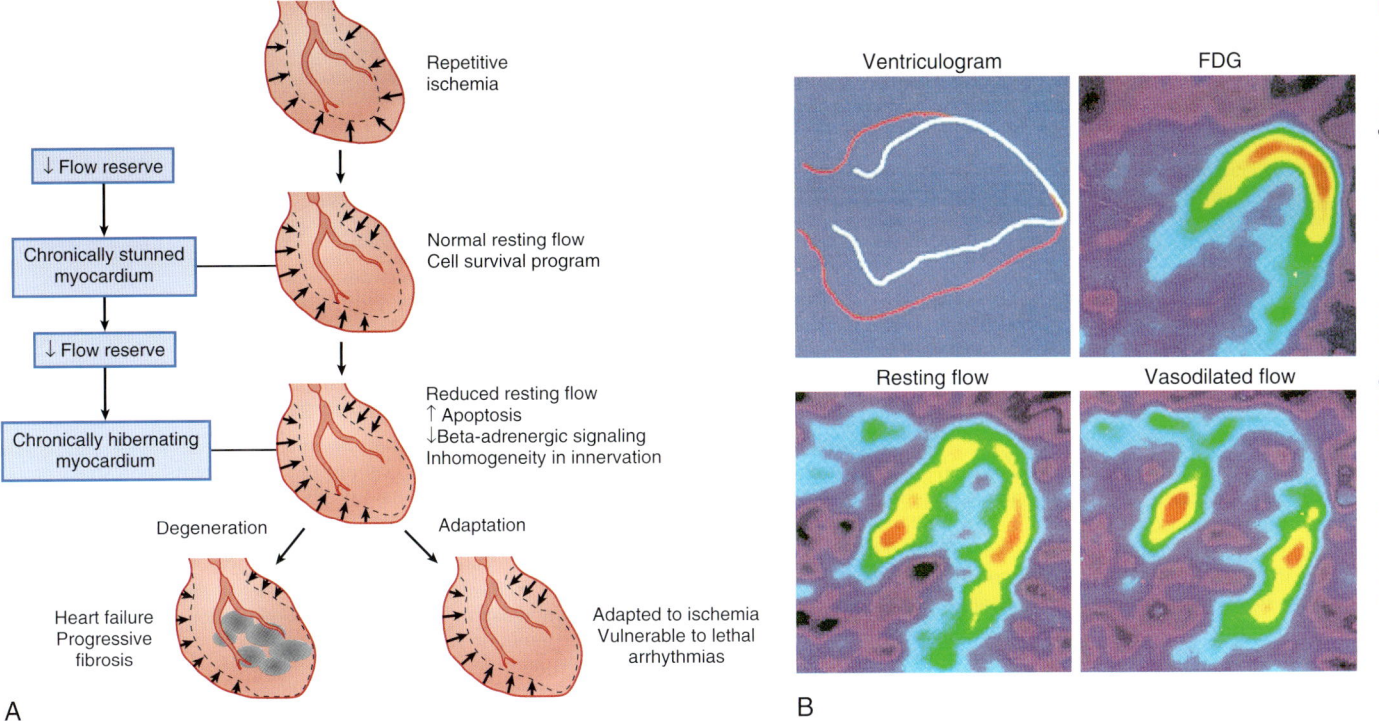

FIGURE 36.28 A, Consequences of chronic repetitive ischemia on function distal to a stenosis. As stenosis severity increases, coronary flow reserve decreases and the frequency of reversible ischemia increases. Reversible repetitive ischemia initially leads to chronic preconditioning against infarction and stunning (*not shown*). Subsequently, there is a gradual progression from contractile dysfunction with normal resting flow (chronically stunned myocardium) to contractile dysfunction with depressed resting flow (hibernating myocardium). This transition is related to the physiologic significance of a coronary stenosis and can occur in a time period as short as 1 week or develop chronically in the absence of severe angina. The cellular response during the progression to chronic hibernating myocardium is variable, with some patients exhibiting successful adaptation with little cell death and fibrosis and others developing degenerative changes difficult to distinguish from subendocardial infarction. **B,** Hibernating myocardium in humans with a chronic left anterior descending artery (LAD) occlusion and collateral-dependent myocardium. The right anterior oblique (RAO) tracing of the left ventriculogram shows anterior akinesis (*upper left*). Transaxial PET scans illustrate $^{13}NH_3$ flow measurements at rest (*lower left*) and after pharmacologic vasodilation with dipyridamole (*lower right*). Quantitative perfusion measurements showed LAD flow to be critically impaired. Viability (after an oral glucose load) is identified by increased ^{18}F-2-fluoro-2-deoxyglucose (FDG) uptake in the anterior wall (*upper right*). (**B** modified from Vanoverschelde JL, et al. Mechanisms of chronic regional postischemic dysfunction in humans: new insights from the study of noninfarcted collateral-dependent myocardium. Circulation 1993;87:1513-1523.)

hibernation, leads to stunning on restoration of perfusion that may take up to 1 week to resolve in the absence of necrosis (see Figs. 36.26 and 36.27). This may be an important cause of reversibly dysfunctional myocardium in the setting of an acute reduction in flow, as in an acute coronary syndrome. Stunned myocardium is also responsible for postoperative pump dysfunction after cardiopulmonary bypass. Further, areas of stunned myocardium can coexist with irreversibly injured myocardium, contributing to time-dependent improvements in function after MI.

Acutely stunned myocardium is clinically important to recognize because contractile function normalizes during stimulation with various inotropic agents, including beta-adrenergic agonists. In contrast with other dysfunctional states, function will spontaneously normalize within 1 week, provided that there is no recurrent ischemia. If repetitive episodes of reversible ischemia develop before function normalizes, they can cause a state of persistent dysfunction or chronic stunning. The cellular mechanism of stunning probably involves free radical–mediated myocardial injury and reduced myofilament calcium sensitivity.[43] In addition, although necrosis and pathologic evidence of infarction are absent in stunned myocardium, recent experimental studies have demonstrated that even brief ischemia leads to focal myocyte apoptosis and elevations in troponin I.[45]

Chronic Hibernating Myocardium

Viable dysfunctional myocardium is defined as any myocardial region in which contractile function improves after coronary revascularization (see Classic References, Rahimtoola). This broad definition of reversible dyssynergy includes three distinct categories with fairly diverse pathophysiologic mechanisms (Table 36.1). Complete normalization of function is the rule after acute ischemia but the exception in chronically dysfunctional myocardium. Brief occlusions or prolonged moderate ischemia (short-term hibernation) will result in postischemic stunning in the absence of infarction, with complete functional recovery occurring rapidly (within 1 week after reperfusion). The time course of improvement is somewhat dependent on the duration and severity of the ischemic episode. Reversible dyssynergy with delayed functional improvement can also arise from structural remodeling of the heart that is independent of ischemia or a coronary stenosis (e.g., remote myocardial remodeling in HF, reduced infarct volume over initial weeks after coronary reperfusion). The latter conditions can be readily identified when the clinical setting, coronary anatomy, and assessment of myocardial perfusion are taken into account. Many clinical studies have evaluated the presence of contractile reserve during dobutamine administration as a predictor of functional recovery. Although this identifies the likelihood of functional recovery (see Chapter 16), it cannot distinguish the diverse pathophysiologic states underlying reversible dyssynergy. Understanding the cause may be important to the extent that it affects the time course and magnitude of functional recovery after revascularization in patients undergoing revascularization to treat ischemic HF (see Classic References, Canty and Fallavollita).

Chronic segmental dysfunction arising from repetitive episodes of ischemia (frequently clinically silent) is common and present in at least one coronary distribution area in more than 60% of patients with ischemic cardiomyopathy (see Fig. 36.28). When resting flow relative to a remote region is normal in dysfunctional myocardium distal to a stenosis, the region is *chronically stunned*. In contrast, when relative resting flow is reduced in the absence of symptoms or signs of ischemia, *hibernating myocardium* is present. It is now clear that both entities can exist in patients and represent extremes in the spectrum of adaptive and maladaptive responses to chronic reversible ischemia. Viability studies are primarily required to distinguish infarction from hibernating myocardium because the myocardium is always viable when the resting flow is normal.[39,44]

TABLE 36.1 Viable Dysfunctional Myocardium: Patterns of Contractile Reserve, Resting Perfusion, and Temporal Recovery of Function after Revascularization

PARAMETER	CONTRACTILE RESERVE	RESTING FLOW	EXTENT OF FUNCTIONAL RECOVERY	TIME COURSE OF RECOVERY
Transient Reversible Ischemia				
Postischemic stunning	Present	Normal	Normalizes	<24 hr
Short-term hibernation	Present	Normal	Normalizes	<7 days
Chronic Repetitive Ischemia				
Chronic stunning	Present	Normal	Improves	Days to weeks
Chronic hibernating myocardium	Variable	Reduced	Improves	Up to 12 mo
Structural Remodeling				
Subendocardial infarction	Variable	Reduced	Variable	Weeks
Remodeled, tethered myocardium	Present	Normal	Improves	Months

It was originally thought that hibernating myocardium arose from a primary reduction in flow similar to experimental models of prolonged moderate ischemia and short-term hibernation. Whereas this is a plausible mechanism for the development of hibernating myocardium in association with an acute coronary syndrome, experimental studies have subsequently demonstrated that delayed subendocardial infarction is the rule rather than the exception when moderate flow reductions are maintained for more than 24 hours.[39] Many patients with hibernating myocardium present with LV dysfunction rather than symptomatic ischemia. Serial studies in animals (see Classic References, Canty and Fallavollita) have now demonstrated that the reductions in relative resting flow are a consequence rather than a cause of the contractile dysfunction.[39] This paradigm, relevant to chronic CAD, was proposed after experimental studies with a slowly progressive left anterior descending artery (LAD) stenosis demonstrated that dysfunction with normal resting flow, consistent with chronic stunning, precedes the development of hibernating myocardium after 3 months.[39,44] The progression from chronically stunned myocardium (with normal resting flow) to hibernating myocardium (with reduced resting flow) is related to the functional significance of the chronic stenosis supplying the LAD region and is probably a reflection of its propensity to produce repetitive supply- or demand-induced ischemia. This progression can be seen as soon as 1 week after placement of a critical stenosis that exhausts coronary flow reserve.[44] As regional dysfunction progresses from chronically stunned to hibernating myocardium, the myocyte takes on regional characteristics similar to those from an explanted heart with advanced failure. Normally perfused remote-zone cardiac myocytes can be normal or can take on structural alterations similar to the dysfunctional region. Some of the major cellular responses are summarized here.

Apoptosis, Myocyte Loss, and Myofibrillar Loss. The frequency of focal myocyte death from apoptosis varies during the development of viable dysfunctional myocardium and thus is probably responsible for the variability in the frequency of apoptosis when analyzing biopsies from patients.[44] Experimentally, apoptosis appears to arise from brief repetitive ischemia[45] and is particularly prominent during the transition from chronically stunned to hibernating myocardium resulting in a loss of approximately 30% of the regional myocytes. Pathologic findings in humans include small increases in interstitial connective tissue, myofibrillar loss (myolysis), increased glycogen deposition, and mini-mitochondria. Although experimental animal models of hibernating myocardium develop these structural changes, they also are present in remote, normally perfused regions of the heart.[39,44] Similar global cellular changes occur in the absence of coronary artery stenoses in humans suggesting that they may be the result of chronically elevated preload. This suggests that they are not causally related to the hibernating myocardium phenotype.[39,44]

Cell Survival and Antiapoptotic Program in Response to Repetitive Ischemia. Variability in the regulation of cell survival pathways in response to repetitive ischemia has been well documented. In experimental studies without HF, antiapoptotic and stress proteins such as heat shock protein (HSP)-70 have been found to be upregulated,[43] whereas increased proapoptotic proteins and a profile of progressive cell death and fibrosis have been reported in biopsies of patients with hibernating myocardium and HF.[44] This variability among reported studies probably reflects the frequency and severity of ischemia, modulation by neurohormonal activation in HF, and complexity of the temporal expression of adaptive and maladaptive responses in myocardium subjected to chronic repetitive ischemia. In this regard, the physiologic significance of a stenosis (i.e., coronary flow reserve) has been shown to be a major determinant of the intrinsic myocardial adaptations to ischemia.[46]

Metabolism and Energetics in Hibernating Myocardium. Once adapted, the metabolic and contractile response of hibernating myocardium appears to be dissociated from external determinants of workload. As a result, submaximal increases in oxygen consumption can occur without immediately leading to subendocardial ischemia.[44] Experimentally, the hibernating myocardial region appears to operate over a lower range of the normal myocardial supply-demand relation in a manner similar to that for the nonischemic failing heart. Although glycogen content is increased, maximum rates of glucose uptake during insulin stimulation are not altered. Studies of isolated mitochondria from swine with hibernating myocardium have demonstrated alterations in mitochondrial respiration, with downregulation of energy usage and oxygen consumption.[43] This slows ATP usage and presumably maintains cell viability during superimposed acute ischemia. Proteomic analysis has demonstrated a reduction in multiple proteins involved in oxidative metabolism and electron transport.[43] Some but not all of the molecular and cellular changes associated with hibernating reverse after revascularization, which can contribute to the failure of contractile function to normalize completely in the absence of MI.[47]

Inhomogeneity in Sympathetic Innervation, Beta-Adrenergic Responses, and Sudden Death. The contractile response of hibernating myocardium is blunted and partly related to a regional downregulation in beta-adrenergic adenylyl cyclase coupling, similar to that found globally in advanced HF. This effect may be related to local norepinephrine overflow and reduced presynaptic uptake of norepinephrine. The resultant inhomogeneity in myocardial sympathetic nerve function may be one of the reasons responsible for the vulnerability of experimental hibernating myocardium to develop lethal ventricular arrhythmias and ventricular fibrillation. Thus, reversing electrical instability and improving contractile dysfunction may account for the positive impact of coronary revascularization on survival.[44] Despite this effect, the extent of viable, denervated myocardium remains a strong predictor of arrhythmic death in patients with ischemic cardiomyopathy.[48]

Successful Adaptation Versus Degeneration in Hibernating Myocardium. There is considerable divergence among studies regarding the pathology of reversibly dyssynergic hibernating myocardium. At one extreme, some investigators think that the myocardium is destined to undergo irreversible myocyte death, which is supported by data showing large amounts of fibrosis (>30% of the tissue) and greatly abnormal high-energy phosphate metabolism, as well as by retrospective analysis suggesting that the degree of fibrosis is related to the duration of hibernating myocardium.[44] At the other extreme, in some circumstances, fibrosis is not a prominent feature with normal myocardial energetics at rest, suggesting that hibernating myocardium can be sustained for long periods without progressive degeneration (see Fig. 36.28). The factors that promote a path toward progressive degeneration versus adaptation are currently unknown but may be modulated by the superimposed neurohormonal activation and elevation in cytokine levels associated with advanced clinical HF, as well as intermittent irreversible injury that arises from intermittent reductions in coronary flow below the threshold required to maintain myocyte viability.

FUTURE PERSPECTIVES

The major factors determining myocardial perfusion and oxygen delivery that were established over the last 50 years have been incorporated into the current management of angina and have withstood the test of time. The basic understanding of the fluid mechanical behavior of coronary stenoses also has been translated to the cardiac catheterization laboratory, where measurements of coronary pressure distal to a stenosis and coronary flow are routinely obtained. These physiologic concepts now facilitate routine clinical decision making in a way that favorably affects outcomes.

Despite progress in advancing our mechanistic understanding of the coronary circulation and myocardial function in health and disease, important gaps remain in basic knowledge and in the translation of this knowledge to clinical care. For example, why some patients develop coronary collaterals or intrinsic adaptations to repetitive ischemia whereas others undergo progressive structural degeneration remains unclear. Basic research has identified the importance of physical factors such as shear stress and local coronary pressure in regulating isolated coronary resistance vessels, but how these interact in a complex vascular network to bring about the phenomenon of autoregulation and metabolic coronary vasodilation remains unanswered. Finally, although abnormalities in coronary microcirculatory control may be as important as stenosis severity in determining symptoms of myocardial ischemia and the risk for subsequent coronary events, our understanding of the physiologic and cellular mechanisms responsible for microvascular dysfunction is limited. Continued bench-to-bedside translational investigation in these and other areas is needed to advance our fundamental knowledge of coronary circulatory control and improve the care of patients with chronic ischemic heart disease.

CLASSIC REFERENCES

Bache RJ. Effects of hypertrophy on the coronary circulation. *Prog Cardiovasc Dis*. 1988;31:403–440.
Canty Jr JM, Fallavollita JA. Hibernating myocardium. *J Nucl Cardiol*. 2005;12:104–119.
Duncker DJ, Bache RJ. Regulation of coronary blood flow during exercise. *Physiol Rev*. 2008;88:1009–1086.
Feigl EO. Coronary physiology. *Physiol Rev*. 1983;63:1–205.
Furchgott RF, Zawadzki JV. The obligatory role of endothelial cells in the relaxation of arterial smooth muscle by acetylcholine. *Nature*. 1980;288:373–376.
Gould KL. Does coronary flow trump coronary anatomy? *JACC Cardiovasc Imaging*. 2009;2:1009–1023.
Hoffman JI, Spaan JA. Pressure-flow relations in coronary circulation. *Physiol Rev*. 1990;70:331–390.
Klocke FJ. Coronary blood flow in man. *Prog Cardiovasc Dis*. 1976;XIX:117–166.
Klocke FJ. Measurements of coronary blood flow and degree of stenosis: current clinical implications and continuing uncertainties. *J Am Coll Cardiol*. 1983;1:31–41.
Rahimtoola SH, Dilsizian V, Kramer CM, et al. Chronic ischemic left ventricular dysfunction: from pathophysiology to imaging and its integration into clinical practice. *JACC Cardiovasc Imaging*. 2008;1:536–555.
Schaper W. Collateral circulation: past and present. *Basic Res Cardiol*. 2009;104:5–21.

REFERENCES

Control of Coronary Blood Flow

1. Goodwill AG, Dick GM, Kiel AM, Tune JD. Regulation of coronary blood flow. *Compr Physiol*. 2017;7:321–382.
2. Duncker DJ, Bache RJ, Merkus D, Laughlin MH. Exercise and the coronary circulation. In: Zoladz JA, ed. *Muscle and Exercise Physiology*. London: Elsevier; 2019:467–503.
3. Duncker DJ, Koller A, Merkus D, Canty Jr JM. Regulation of coronary blood flow in health and ischemic heart disease. *Prog Cardiovasc Dis*. 2015;57:409–422.
4. Allaqaband H, Gutterman DD, Kadlec AO. Physiological consequences of coronary arteriolar dysfunction and its influence on cardiovascular disease. *Physiology*. 2018;33:338–347.
5. Lanza GA, Careri G, Crea F. Mechanisms of coronary artery spasm. *Circulation*. 2011;124:1774–1782.
6. Cademartiri F, Seitun S, Clemente A, et al. Myocardial blood flow quantification for evaluation of coronary artery disease by computed tomography. *Cardiovasc Diagn Ther*. 2017;7:129–150.
7. Gutterman DD, Chabowski DS, Kadlec AO, et al. The human microcirculation: regulation of flow and beyond. *Circ Res*. 2016;118:157–172.
8. Pries AR, Badimon L, Bugiardini R, et al. Coronary vascular regulation, remodelling, and collateralization: mechanisms and clinical implications on behalf of the working group on coronary pathophysiology and microcirculation. *Eur Heart J*. 2015;36:3134–3146.
9. Kadlec AO, Gutterman DD. Redox regulation of the microcirculation. *Compr Physiol*. 2019;10:229–259.
10. Tune JD, Goodwill AG, Kiel AM, et al. Disentangling the Gordian knot of local metabolic control of coronary blood flow. *Am J Physiol Heart Circ Physiol*. 2020;318:H11–H24.

Physiologic Assessment of Coronary Artery Stenosis

11. Johnson NP, Gould KL, Di Carli MF, Taqueti VR. Invasive FFR and noninvasive CFR in the evaluation of ischemia: what is the future? *J Am Coll Cardiol*. 2016;67:2772–2788.
12. Nijjer SS, de Waard GA, Sen S, et al. Coronary pressure and flow relationships in humans: phasic analysis of normal and pathological vessels and the implications for stenosis assessment: a report from the Iberian-Dutch-English (IDEAL) collaborators. *Eur Heart J*. 2016;37:2069–2080.
13. Johnson NP, Kirkeeide RL, Gould KL. Is discordance of coronary flow reserve and fractional flow reserve due to methodology or clinically relevant coronary pathophysiology? *JACC Cardiovasc Imaging*. 2012;5:193–202.
14. Lee JM, Hwang D, Park J, et al. Exploring coronary circulatory response to stenosis and its association with invasive physiologic indexes using absolute myocardial blood flow and coronary pressure. *Circulation*. 2017;136:1798–1808.
15. Padro T, Manfrini O, Bugiardini R, et al. ESC Working Group on Coronary Pathophysiology and Microcirculation position paper on 'coronary microvascular dysfunction in cardiovascular disease'. *Cardiovasc Res*. 2020;116:741–755.
16. Pijls NH, Sels JW. Functional measurement of coronary stenosis. *J Am Coll Cardiol*. 2012;59:1045–1057.
17. van de Hoef TP, Siebes M, Spaan JA, Piek JJ. Fundamentals in clinical coronary physiology: why coronary flow is more important than coronary pressure. *Eur Heart J*. 2015;36:3312–3319a.
18. Zimmermann FM, Ferrara A, Johnson NP, et al. Deferral vs. performance of percutaneous coronary intervention of functionally non-significant coronary stenosis: 15-year follow-up of the DEFER trial. *Eur Heart J*. 2015;36:3182–3188.
19. Xaplanteris P, Fournier S, Pijls NHJ, et al. Five-year outcomes with PCI guided by fractional flow reserve. *N Engl J Med*. 2018;379:250–259.
20. Zimmermann FM, Omerovic E, Fournier S, et al. Fractional flow reserve-guided percutaneous coronary intervention vs. medical therapy for patients with stable coronary lesions: meta-analysis of individual patient data. *Eur Heart J*. 2019;40:180–186.
21. Davies JE, Sen S, Dehbi HM, et al. Use of the instantaneous wave-free ratio or fractional flow reserve in PCI. *N Engl J Med*. 2017;376:1824–1834.
22. Götberg M, Cook CM, Sen S, et al. The evolving Future of instantaneous wave-free ratio and fractional flow reserve. *J Am Coll Cardiol*. 2017;70:1379–1402.
23. Berry C, Mcclure JD, Oldroyd KG. Meta-analysis of death and myocardial infarction in the DEFINE-FLAIR and iFR-SWEDEHEART trials. *Circulation*. 2017;136:2389–2391.
24. Taylor CA, Fonte TA, Min JK. Computational fluid dynamics applied to cardiac computed tomography for noninvasive quantification of fractional flow reserve: scientific basis. *J Am Coll Cardiol*. 2013;61:2233–2241.
25. Min JK, Taylor CA, Achenbach S, et al. Noninvasive fractional flow reserve derived from coronary CT angiography: clinical data and scientific principles. *JACC Cardiovasc Imaging*. 2015;8:1209–1222.
26. Kogame N, Ono M, Kawashima H, et al. The impact of coronary physiology on contemporary clinical decision making. *JACC Cardiovasc Interv*. 2020;13:1617–1638.
27. Kunadian V, Chieffo A, Camici PG, et al. An EAPCI Expert consensus document on ischaemia with non-obstructive coronary arteries in Collaboration with European Society of Cardiology working group on coronary pathophysiology & microcirculation endorsed by coronary vasomotor disorders International study group. *Eur Heart J*. 2020;41:3504–3520.
28. Pepine CJ, Ferdinand KC, Shaw LJ, et al. Emergence of nonobstructive coronary artery disease: a Woman's problem and need for change in definition on angiography. *J Am Coll Cardiol*. 2015;66:1918–1933.
29. Herscovici R, Sedlak T, Wei J, et al. Ischemia and No obstructive coronary artery disease (INOCA): what is the risk? *J Am Heart Assoc*. 2018;7:e008868.
30. Camici PG, Tschöpe C, Di Carli MF, et al. Coronary microvascular dysfunction in hypertrophy and heart failure. *Cardiovasc Res*. 2020;116:806–816.
31. Camici PG, d'Amati G, Rimoldi O. Coronary microvascular dysfunction: mechanisms and functional assessment. *Nat Rev Cardiol*. 2015;12:48–62.
32. Lardizabal JA, Deedwania PC. The anti-ischemic and anti-anginal properties of statins. *Curr Atheroscler Rep*. 2011;13:43–50.
33. van de Hoef TP, de Waard GA, Meuwissen M, et al. Invasive coronary physiology: a Dutch tradition. *Neth Heart J*. 2020;28:99–107.

Coronary Collateral Circulation

34. Seiler C, Meier P. Historical aspects and relevance of the human coronary collateral circulation. *Curr Cardiol Rev*. 2014;10:2–16.
35. Seiler C, Stoller M, Pitt B, Meier P. The human coronary collateral circulation: development and clinical importance. *Eur Heart J*. 2013;34:2674–2682.
36. Zimarino M, D'Andreamatteo M, Waksman R, et al. The dynamics of the coronary collateral circulation. *Nat Rev Cardiol*. 2014;11:191–197.
37. Weil BR, Suzuki G, Leiker MM, et al. Comparative Efficacy of intracoronary allogeneic mesenchymal stem cells and cardiosphere-derived cells in swine with hibernating myocardium. *Circ Res*. 2015;117:634–644.

Metabolic and Functional Consequences of Ischemia

38. Heusch G. Myocardial ischaemia-reperfusion injury and cardioprotection in perspective. *Nat Rev Cardiol*. 2020;17:773–789.
39. Canty Jr JM, Suzuki G. Myocardial perfusion and contraction in acute ischemia and chronic ischemic heart disease. *J Mol Cell Cardiol*. 2012;52:822–831.
40. Lieder HR, Kleinbongard P, Skyschally A, et al. Vago-splenic Axis in signal transduction of remote ischemic preconditioning in pigs and rats. *Circ Res*. 2018;123:1152–1163.
41. Heusch G, Gersh BJ. The pathophysiology of acute myocardial infarction and strategies of protection beyond reperfusion: a continual challenge. *Eur Heart J*. 2017;38:774–784.
42. Swain L, Reyelt L, Bhave S, et al. Transvalvular ventricular unloading before reperfusion in acute myocardial infarction. *J Am Coll Cardiol*. 2020;76:684–699.
43. Heusch G. Myocardial stunning and hibernation revisited. *Nat Rev Cardiol*. 2021;18:522–536.
44. Canty Jr JM, Fallavollita JA. Pathophysiologic basis of hibernating myocardium. In: Zaret BL, Beller GA, eds. *Clinical Nuclear Cardiology: State of the Art and Future Direction*. 4th ed. Philadelphia: Elsevier; 2010:577–593.
45. Weil BR, Young RF, Shen X, et al. Brief myocardial ischemia produces cardiac troponin I release and focal myocyte apoptosis in the absence of pathological infarction in swine. *JACC Basic Transl Sci*. 2017;2:105–114.
46. Page BJ, Young RF, Suzuki G, et al. The physiological significance of a coronary stenosis differentially affects contractility and mitochondrial function in viable chronically dysfunctional myocardium. *Basic Res Cardiol*. 2013;108:354.
47. Page BJ, Banas MD, Suzuki G, et al. Revascularization of chronic hibernating myocardium stimulates myocyte proliferation and partially reverses chronic adaptations to ischemia. *J Am Coll Cardiol*. 2015;65:684–697.
48. Fallavollita JA, Heavey BM, Luisi Jr AJ, et al. Regional myocardial sympathetic denervation predicts the risk of sudden cardiac arrest in ischemic cardiomyopathy. *J Am Coll Cardiol*. 2014;63:141–149.

37 ST-Elevation Myocardial Infarction: Pathophysiology and Clinical Evolution

BENJAMIN M. SCIRICA, PETER LIBBY, AND DAVID A. MORROW

CHANGING PATTERNS IN INCIDENCE AND CARE, 636

IMPROVEMENTS IN OUTCOME, 636
Limitations of Current Therapy, 636

PATHOLOGIC FINDINGS, 638
Plaque Formation and Disruption, 639
Heart Muscle, 639

PATHOPHYSIOLOGY, 649
Left Ventricular Function, 649
Ventricular Remodeling, 651
Pathophysiology of Other Organ Systems, 652

CLINICAL FEATURES, 653
Predisposing Factors, 653

History, 653
Physical Examination, 653
Laboratory Findings, 655

FUTURE PERSPECTIVES, 659

REFERENCES, 660

Myocardial infarction (MI) results from myocardial cell necrosis caused by an imbalance between oxygen supply and demand. Cardiac professional societies have jointly established criteria for the diagnosis of MI (Table 37.1). The universal definition of *myocardial infarction* classifies MI into five types, depending on the circumstances in which the MI occurs (Table 37.2).[1] Successive revisions to the definition of MI and a shift to more sensitive biomarkers of myocardial injury have had important implications for the clinical care of patients, epidemiologic monitoring, public policy, and clinical trials.[2]

Patients with unstable ischemic symptoms are considered to have an *acute coronary syndrome* (ACS), which encompasses unstable angina, non–ST-segment elevation MI (NSTEMI), and ST-segment elevation MI (STEMI) (Fig. 37.1). The 12-lead electrocardiogram (ECG) dichotomizes patients with suspected ACS into those with ST-segment elevation, the subject of this chapter and Chapter 38, and those without ST-segment elevation, the subject of Chapter 39.

CHANGING PATTERNS IN INCIDENCE AND CARE

Despite advances in the diagnosis and management, STEMI remains a major public health problem in the industrialized world and is on the rise in developing countries (see Chapter 2).[1] Each year in the United States alone, more than 1 million patients are hospitalized for an MI or coronary heart death.[3] The rate of MI rises sharply in both men and women with increasing age, and racial differences exist, with MI occurring more frequently in black men and women than white, regardless of age.[3] The proportion of patients with ACS events who have STEMI varies across observational studies but has declined over the past decade, in part due to the introduction of more sensitive assays of myocardial injury that increase the number of NSTEMI cases relative to STEMI; however, an overall reduction in the incidence of STEMI is noted across multiple registries in Europe and the United States.[3,4] This estimate does not include "silent" MI, which may not prompt hospitalization. Between 1999 and 2008, the proportion of patients with an ACS and STEMI declined by almost 50% (47.0% to 22.9%).[3,5] There is a shift towards patients presenting with more recurrent MI compared to incident, or first events, with fewer prehospital deaths.[6] Although hospitalizations for MI have declined for patients older than 55 years old, there has not been a similar decline in the rates for younger patients, in particular in women.[7-10] Of particular concern from a global perspective, the burden of coronary disease in low- and middle-income countries has reached the rate affecting more affluent countries.[11] The limited resources available to treat STEMI in low- and middle-income countries mandate major international efforts to strengthen primary prevention programs.[12]

IMPROVEMENTS IN OUTCOME

The overall number of deaths from STEMI has declined steadily over the past 30 years, but it has stabilized over the past decade. Both a decreased incidence of STEMI and a decline in the case-fatality rate after STEMI, which corresponds to greater implementation of guideline-directed care, contributes to this trend.[13] The short-term mortality rate of patients with STEMI ranges from 5% to 6% during the initial hospitalization and from 7% to 18% at 1 year.[4,14] In patients aged 65 years or older, the 30-day mortality declined from 20% to 12.4% and the 1-year recurrent MI decreased from 7.1% to 5.1%.[13] The highest risk of ischemic complications following MI occurs within 180 days, after which the risk becomes fairly linear. This pattern is most evident in patients older than 80 years (Fig. 37.2).[4,15] Mortality rates in clinical trial populations tend to be approximately half of those observed in registries of consecutive patients, most likely because of the exclusion of patients with more extensive comorbidities.

Improvements in the management of patients with STEMI have occurred in several phases. The "clinical observation phase" of coronary care consumed the first half of the 20th century and focused on detailed recording of physical and laboratory findings, with little active treatment of the infarction. The "coronary care unit phase" began in the mid-1960s and emphasized early detection and management of cardiac arrhythmias based on the development of monitoring and cardioversion/defibrillation capabilities. The "high-technology phase," heralded by the introduction of the pulmonary artery balloon flotation catheter, set the stage for bedside hemodynamic monitoring and directed hemodynamic management. The modern "reperfusion era" of STEMI care began with intracoronary and then intravenous (IV) fibrinolysis, increased use of aspirin (see Chapter 38), and subsequently the development and evolution of primary percutaneous coronary intervention (PCI) (Chapter 41).

Contemporary care of patients with STEMI has entered an "evidence-based coronary care phase," driven by professional society guidelines and performance measure benchmarks for clinical practice in conjunction with early reperfusion.[16,17] Implementation of guideline-directed medical treatment (GDMT) and regional quality initiatives has significantly decreased heterogeneity in care, increased compliance with evidence-based therapies, and improved outcomes.[4,18,19]

Limitations of Current Therapy

Rates of appropriate initiation of reperfusion therapy vary widely. Up to 30% of patients with STEMI who are eligible to receive reperfusion therapy do not benefit from this lifesaving treatment in some registries.[20] Care of another substantial proportion of patients does not meet the recommended door-to-reperfusion time.[21] This gap mandates

TABLE 37.1 Universal Definitions of Myocardial Injury and Myocardial Infarction: Summary

Criteria for myocardial injury

The term myocardial injury should be used when there is evidence of elevated cardiac troponin values (cTn) with at least one value above the 99th percentile upper reference limit (URL). The myocardial injury is considered acute if there is a rise and/or fall of cTn values.

Criteria for acute myocardial infarction (types 1, 2, and 3 MI)

The term acute myocardial infarction should be used when there is acute myocardial injury with clinical evidence of acute myocardial ischemia and with detection of a rise and/or fall of cTn values with at least one value above the 99th percentile URL and at least one of the following:
- Symptoms of myocardial ischemia
- New ischemic ECG changes
- Development of pathologic Q waves
- Imaging evidence of new loss of viable myocardium or new regional wall motion abnormality in a pattern consistent with an ischemic etiology
- Identification of a coronary thrombus by angiography or autopsy (not for type 2 or 3 MIs)

Postmortem demonstration of acute atherothrombosis in the artery supplying the infarcted myocardium meets criteria for *type 1 MI*.

Evidence of an imbalance between myocardial oxygen supply and demand unrelated to acute atherothrombosis meets criteria for *type 2 MI*.

Cardiac death in patients with symptoms suggestive of myocardial ischemia and presumed new ischemic ECG changes before cTn values become available or abnormal meets criteria for *type 3 MI*.

Criteria for coronary procedure-related myocardial infarction (types 4 and 5 MI)

Percutaneous coronary intervention (PCI)-related MI is termed *type 4a MI*.

Coronary artery bypass grafting (CABG) related MI is termed *type 5 MI*.

Coronary procedure–related MI ≤48 hr after the index procedure is arbitrarily defined by an elevation of cTn values >5 times for *type 4a MI* and >10 times for *type 5 MI* of the 99th percentile URL in patients with normal baseline values. Patients with elevated preprocedural cTn values, in whom the preprocedural cTn level is stable (≤20% variation) or falling, must meet the criteria for a >5- or >10-fold increase and manifest a change from the baseline value of >20%. In addition with at least one of the following:
- New ischemic ECG changes (this criterion is related to *type 4a MI* only)
- Development of new pathologic Q waves
- Imaging evidence of loss of viable myocardium that is presumed to be new and in a pattern consistent with an ischemic etiology
- Angiographic findings consistent with a procedural flow-limiting complication such as coronary dissection, occlusion of a major epicardial artery or graft, side-branch occlusion-thrombus, disruption of collateral flow, or distal embolization

Isolated development of new pathologic Q waves meets the *type 4a MI* or *type 5 MI* criteria with either revascularization procedure if cTn values are elevated and rising but less than the prespecified thresholds for PCI and CABG.

Other types of *type 4 MI* include *type 4b MI* stent thrombosis and *type 4c MI* restenosis that both meet *type 1 MI* criteria.

Postmortem demonstration of a procedure-related thrombus meets the *type 4a MI* criteria or *type 4b MI* criteria if associated with a stent.

Criteria for prior or silent/unrecognized myocardial infarction

Any one of the following criteria meets the diagnosis for prior or silent/unrecognized MI:
- Abnormal Q waves with or without symptoms in the absence of non-ischemic causes
- Imaging evidence of loss of viable myocardium in a pattern consistent with ischemic etiology
- Pathoanatomical findings of a prior MI.

CABG, Coronary artery bypass grafting; *cTn*, cardiac troponin; *ECG*, electrocardiogram; *MI*, myocardial infarction; *PCI*, percutaneous coronary intervention; *URL*, upper reference limit.
From Thygesen K, Alpert JS, Jaffe AS, et al. Fourth universal definition of myocardial infarction (2018). *J Am Coll Cardiol*. 2018;72:2231–2264.

TABLE 37.2 Causes of Myocardial Injury

Myocardial injury related to acute myocardial ischemia

Atherosclerotic plaque disruption with thrombosis

Myocardial injury related to acute myocardial ischemia because of oxygen supply/demand imbalance

Reduced myocardial perfusion
- Coronary artery spasm, microvascular dysfunction
- Coronary embolism
- Coronary artery dissection
- Sustained bradyarrhythmia
- Hypotension or shock
- Respiratory failure
- Severe anemia

Increased myocardial oxygen demand
- Sustained tachyarrhythmia
- Severe hypertension with or without left ventricular hypertrophy

Other causes of myocardial injury

Cardiac conditions
- Heart failure
- Myocarditis
- Cardiomyopathy (any type)
- Takotsubo syndrome
- Coronary revascularization procedure
- Cardiac procedure other than revascularization
- Catheter ablation
- Defibrillator shocks
- Cardiac contusion

Systemic conditions
- Sepsis, infectious disease
- Chronic kidney disease
- Stroke, subarachnoid hemorrhage
- Pulmonary embolism, pulmonary hypertension
- Infiltrative diseases, e.g., amyloidosis, sarcoidosis
- Chemotherapeutic agents
- Critically ill patients
- Strenuous exercise

From Thygesen K, Alpert JS, Jaffe AS, et al. Fourth universal definition of myocardial infarction (2018). *J Am Coll Cardiol*. 2018;72:2231–2264.

initiatives to increase timely administration of guideline-directed reperfusion therapy (see Chapter 38).[22]

Management and outcomes of patients with STEMI appear to vary substantially depending on the volume of such patients cared for within a hospital system.[23] Hospitals with a high clinical volume, a high rate of invasive procedures, and a top ranking in quality reports have lower STEMI mortality rates. Conversely, patients with STEMI not cared for by a cardiovascular specialist have higher mortality rates. Variation also occurs in the treatment patterns of certain population subgroups with STEMI, including elderly, women,[24,25] blacks,[10] and some high-risk patients (e.g., chronic kidney disease or presenting with cardiogenic shock).[26]

The advent of mandatory reporting for procedural complications and outcomes in STEMI has led to the establishment of benchmarks for procedural success and mortality rates and the ability to compare across different regions and hospitals.[18,19] However, public reporting of outcomes in STEMI may also have unintentionally led to lower rates of revascularization in the highest-risk patients, who would often benefit most from early revascularization (e.g., cardiogenic shock) because of the concern regarding higher case-fatality rates.[27,28]

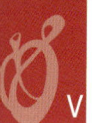

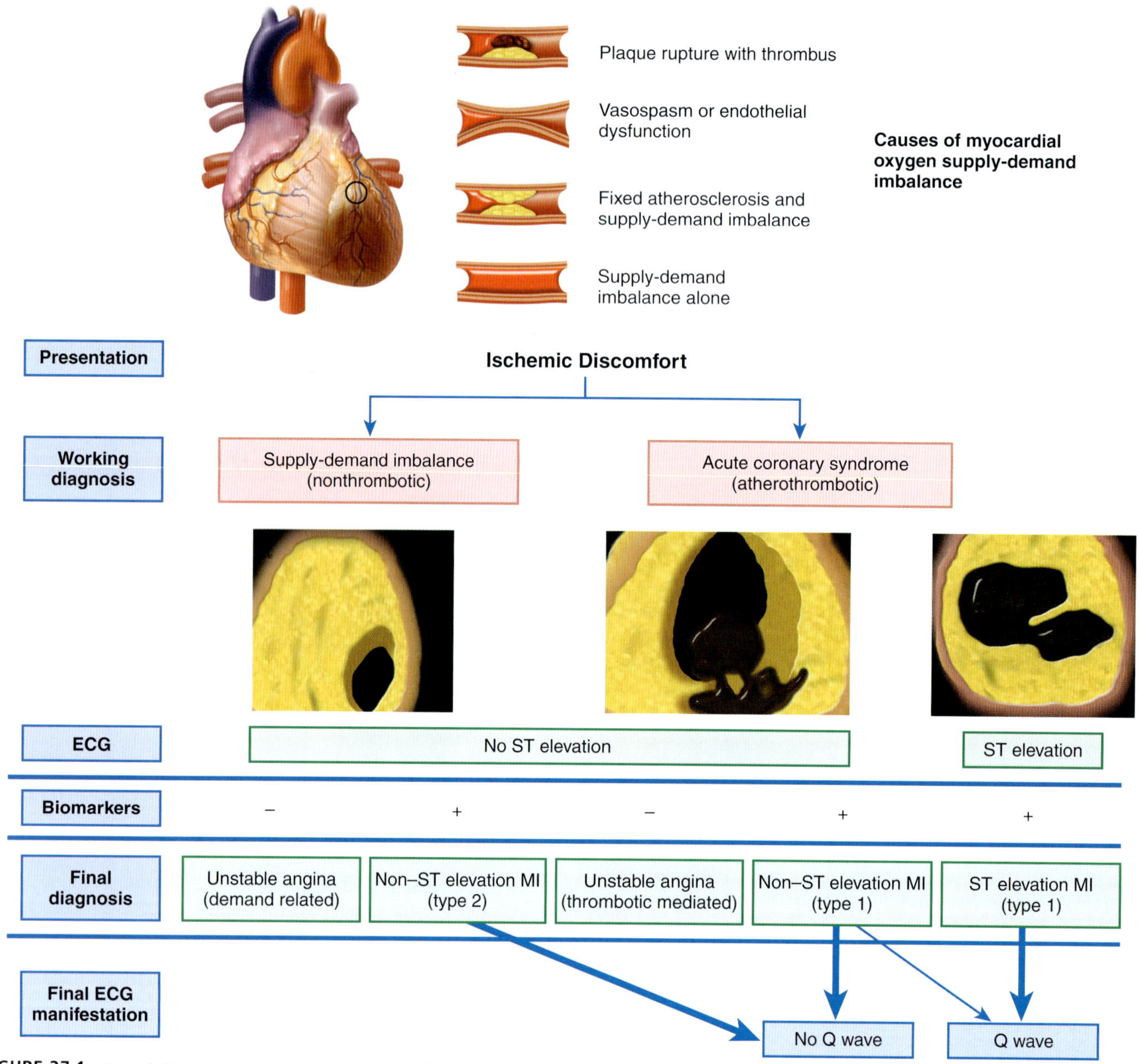

FIGURE 37.1 Myocardial ischemia and myocardial infarction (MI) can result from various coronary disease processes, including vasospasm, increased myocardial demand in the setting of a fixed coronary lesion, and erosion or rupture of vulnerable atherosclerotic plaque leading to acute thrombus formation and subsequent ischemia. All result in myocardial oxygen supply-demand mismatch and can precipitate ischemic symptoms, and all processes, when severe or prolonged, will lead to myocardial necrosis or infarction. Nonthrombotic-mediated events (*bottom half, left side*) typically occur without ST-segment elevation (STE) on the electrocardiogram (ECG) but can have elevated levels of cardiac biomarkers if the ischemia is severe and long enough, in which case they are classified as having type 2 MI. The atherothrombotic lesion is the hallmark pathobiologic event of an acute coronary syndrome (ACS). The reduction in flow may be caused by a completely occlusive thrombus (*bottom half, right side*) or by a subtotally occlusive thrombus (*bottom half, middle*). Ischemic discomfort may occur with or without STE on the ECG. Of patients with STE, Q wave MI ultimately develop in most, but not all patients, depending on the duration of ischemia and collateralization. Patients without STE have either unstable angina or non–ST-segment elevation MI (NSTEMI), a distinction that is ultimately made by the presence or absence of a serum or plasma cardiac marker (e.g., cardiac troponin) detected in blood. Non–Q wave MI ultimately develops in most patients with NSTEMI on the ECG; Q wave MI may develop in a few. MI that develops as the result of the atherothrombotic lesion of an ACS is classified as type 1 MI.

PATHOLOGIC FINDINGS

Most ACSs result from coronary atherosclerosis, generally with superimposed coronary thrombosis caused by rupture or erosion of an atherosclerotic lesion (see Chapter 24).[29] In the era of more widespread statin use, the proportion of ACS due to plaque erosions may be increasing.[30] Nonatherogenic forms of coronary artery disease (CAD) are discussed later in this chapter and causes of MI without coronary atherosclerosis are presented in Table 37.3.

When acute coronary atherothrombosis occurs, the resulting intracoronary thrombus may obstruct partially, which generally leads to myocardial ischemia in the absence of ST elevation, or occlude completely and cause more extensive myocardial ischemia and STEMI. Before the fibrinolytic era, clinicians typically divided patients with MI into Q wave versus non–Q wave MI based on evolution of the ECG pattern over several days. The term *Q wave infarction* was considered to be synonymous with "transmural infarction," whereas *non–Q wave infarctions* were often referred to as "subendocardial infarctions." Cardiac magnetic resonance imaging (CMR), though, indicates that the development of a Q wave depends more on the infarct size than on the depth of mural involvement. Thus, the use of *ACS* is the more appropriate, broad conceptual framework as it is anchored by the underlying unifying pathophysiology (see Fig. 37.1). Further classification of patients by the presence of ST-segment elevation (STEMI) or by its absence (non–ST-segment elevation ACS), rather than by the evolution of Q waves, permits immediate clinical triage decisions regarding the need for urgent revascularization (see Chapter 38).

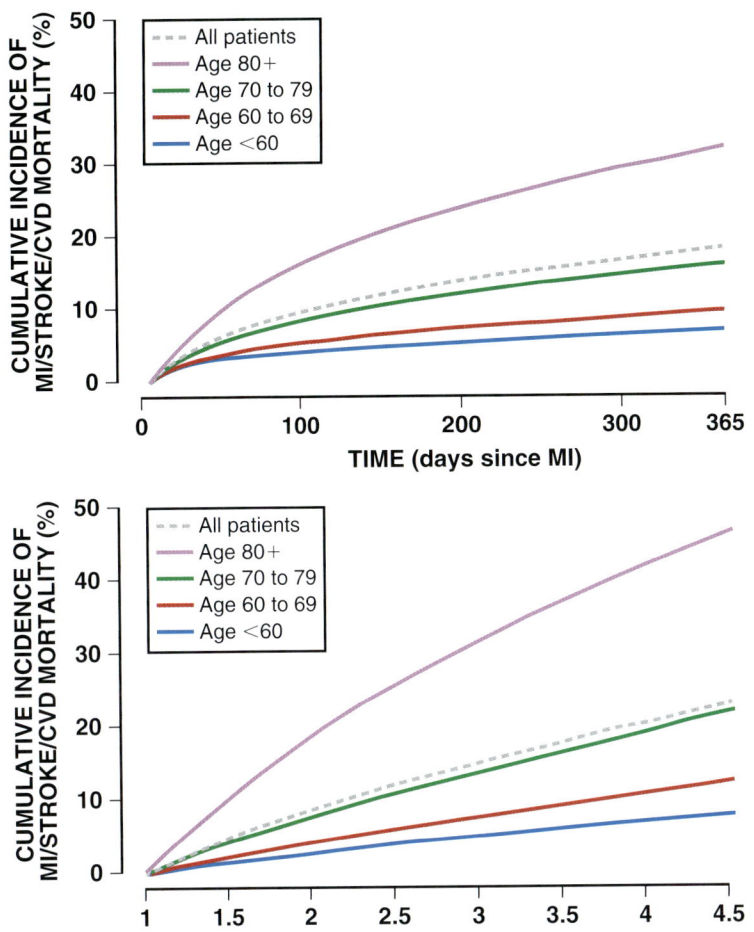

FIGURE 37.2 Cardiovascular risk after myocardial infarction (MI) by age. Kaplan-Meier estimate of the risk of the combined endpoint (MI, ischemic stroke, or cardiovascular disease mortality) during the first 365 days after the index MI *(top)* and after 1 year from the initial infarction *(bottom)*. (From Jernberg T, Hasvold P, Henriksson M, et al. Cardiovascular risk in post-myocardial infarction patients: nationwide real world data demonstrate the importance of a long-term perspective. *Eur Heart J.* 2015;36:1163–1170.)

completely occlusive thrombi lead to extensive injury to the ventricular wall in the myocardial bed subtended by the affected coronary artery (Fig. 37.4). Infarction alters the sequence of depolarization ultimately reflected as changes in the QRS-T complex. The most characteristic change in QRS that develops in most patients with STEMI is the evolution of Q waves in leads that interrogate the infarct zone. In a minority of patients with ST elevation, no Q waves develop but other abnormalities in the QRS complex occur frequently, such as diminution in R wave height and notching or splintering of the QRS (see Chapter 14). Patients who have ischemic symptoms without ST elevation are initially diagnosed as suffering either from unstable angina or, with evidence of myocardial necrosis, from NSTEMI.

Patients with persistent ST-segment elevation are candidates for reperfusion therapy (either catheter-based or if unavailable, pharmacologic) to restore flow in the occluded epicardial infarct-related artery.[16,17] Thus the 12-lead ECG remains at the center of the initial decision pathway for the management of patients with suspected ACS in order to distinguish between patients with ST elevation and those without it.

Heart Muscle
The cellular effects of ischemia commence within seconds of the onset of hypoxia with the loss of adenosine triphosphate (ATP) production and accumulation of toxic metabolites (e.g., lactic acid). Myocardial relaxation-contraction is compromised within a minute after the onset of severe ischemia with loss of systolic function, and irreversible cell injury begins within as early as 20 minutes. Irreversible cell death usually occurs in the ischemic region in 6 hours in the absence of reperfusion or sufficient collateral circulation (Fig. 37.5).

Gross Pathologic Findings
Gross alterations in the myocardium appear 6 to 12 hours after the onset of necrosis (Fig. 37.6), but a variety of histochemical stains can identify zones of necrosis after only 2 to 3 hours. Subsequently, the infarcted myocardium undergoes a sequence of gross pathologic changes (Fig. 37.7). Within hours of death from MI, the presence of an infarct can often be detected by immersing slices of myocardium in triphenyltetrazolium chloride (TTC), which turns noninfarcted myocardium a brick-red color due to preserved lactate dehydrogenase activity while the infarcted area remains unstained (Fig. 37.8). An MI can often be identified at 12 to 24 hours as a red-blue area of discoloration caused by edema and extravasated blood. By day 7, an infarct is rimmed by a zone of granulation tissue as it eventually evolves into a fibrous scar.

On gross inspection, MI falls into two major types: *transmural* infarcts, in which myocardial necrosis involves the full thickness (or almost full thickness) of the ventricular wall, and *subendocardial* (nontransmural) infarcts, in which the necrosis involves the subendocardium, the intramural myocardium, or both, without extending all the way through the ventricular wall to the epicardium (Fig. 37.9).

Occlusive coronary thrombosis appears to be much more common when the infarction is transmural and localized to the distribution of a single coronary artery (see Fig. 37.4). Nontransmural infarctions, however, frequently occur in the presence of severely narrowed but still patent coronary arteries, when the infarcted region has sufficient collateral circulation, or if the artery is only transiently occluded. Patchy nontransmural MI may arise secondary to fibrinolysis or PCI of an originally occlusive thrombus, with restoration of blood flow *before* the wavefront of necrosis has extended from the subendocardium across the full thickness of the ventricular wall.

Ultrastructural and Microscopic Findings of Ischemia
Ultrastructural changes appear within several minutes after the onset of ischemia. If reperfusion occurs, these early changes can

Plaque Formation and Disruption
Plaques that precipitate ACS usually provoke thrombi caused by fibrous cap rupture, superficial erosion, or occasionally vasospasm or disruption caused by a calcified nodule. Some cases of ACS lack an evident culprit thrombus (see Chapter 24). Current clinical data have challenged the more simplistic concept of the "vulnerable plaque." In a prospective study of 697 patients with ACS who underwent three-vessel coronary angiography and gray-scale radiofrequency intravascular ultrasonographic imaging after PCI found that less than 5% of plaques with ultrasound characteristics of a thin-capped fibroatheroma actually caused a clinical event during a 3.4-year follow-up (Fig. 37.3).[31] Thus, equating the lipid-rich, thin-capped plaque with "vulnerability" is a misnomer.[30] Other morphologic characteristics associated with rupture-prone plaque include expansive remodeling that minimizes luminal obstruction (mild stenosis by angiography), neovascularization (angiogenesis), plaque hemorrhage, adventitial inflammation, and a "spotty" pattern of calcification.[30,32]

Acute Coronary Syndromes
Plaque disruption or erosion exposes thrombogenic core and matrix material to the blood that then produce an extensive thrombus in the infarct-related artery (see Fig. 37.1). An adequate collateral network that prevents necrosis from occurring can result in clinically silent episodes of coronary occlusion; in addition, many plaque ruptures are asymptomatic if the thrombosis is not occlusive. Characteristically,

TABLE 37.3 Electrocardiographic Manifestations of Myocardial Infarction

Electrocardiographic Manifestations of Acute Myocardial Ischemia (in the Absence of Left Bundle Branch Block)

ST Elevation

New ST elevation at the J point in two contiguous leads with the following cut points:
- ≥0.1 mV in all leads (except V_2–V_3)
- In leads V_2–V_3 the following cut points apply:
  - ≥0.2 mV in men ≥40 years
  - ≥0.25 mV in men <40 years
  - ≥0.15 mV in women

ST Depression and T Wave Changes
- New horizontal or downsloping ST depression ≥0.05 mV in two contiguous leads
- T wave inversion ≥0.1 mV in two contiguous leads with a prominent R wave or R/S ratio >1

Electrocardiographic Manifestations of Ischemia in the Setting of Left Bundle Branch Block

Electrocardiographic Criterion	Points
ST-segment elevation ≥1 mm and concordant with the QRS complex	5
ST-segment depression ≥1 mm in lead V_1, V_2, or V_3	3
ST-segment elevation ≥5 mm and discordant with the QRS complex	2
A score of ≥3 had a specificity of 98% for acute MI	

Electrocardiographic Changes Associated With Previous Myocardial Infarction (in the Absence of Left Ventricular Hypertrophy and Left Bundle Block)

Any Q wave in leads V_2–V_3 ≥0.02 sec or a QS complex in leads V_2 and V_3

Q wave ≥0.03 sec and ≥0.1-mV deep or QS complex in leads I, II, aVL, aVF, or V_4–V_6 in any 2 leads of a contiguous lead grouping (I, aVL; V_1–V_6; II, III, aVF)

R wave ≥0.04 sec in V_1–V_2 and R/S ≥1 with a concordant positive T wave in absence of a conductions defect

Based on criteria from O'Gara PT, Kushner FG, Ascheim DD, et al. 2013 ACCF/AHA guideline for the management of ST-elevation myocardial infarction: a report of the American College of Cardiology Foundation/American Heart Association Task Force on Practice Guidelines. *J Am Coll Cardiol.* 2013;61:e78; and from Thygesen K, Alpert JS, Jaffe AS, et al. Fourth universal definition of myocardial infarction (2018). *J Am Coll Cardiol.* 2018;72:2231–2264.

reverse. Irreversible damage usually requires a reduction of flow to less than 10% of normal for 20 to 30 minutes. Disruption of the sarcolemma membrane is the earliest manifestation of myocyte necrosis, thus allowing the release of intracellular macromolecules (e.g., CKMB, troponin, myoglobin) into the microvasculature and lymphatics.

Histologic evaluation of MI reveals various stages of the acute injury and healing processes (see Figs. 37.6 and 37.7). In experimental infarction, the earliest ultrastructural changes in cardiac muscle after ligation of a coronary artery, noted within 20 minutes, is a reduction in the size and number of glycogen granules, myofibrillar relaxation, intracellular edema, and swelling and distortion of the transverse tubular system, sarcoplasmic reticulum, and mitochondria. Changes after 60 minutes of occlusion include myocyte swelling, swelling and internal disruption of mitochondria, development of amorphous (flocculent) aggregation and margination of nuclear chromatin, and relaxation of myofibrils. After 20 minutes to 2 hours of ischemia, the changes in some cells become irreversible.

Patterns of Myocardial Necrosis
Coagulation Necrosis

Coagulation necrosis results from severe, persistent ischemia and is usually present in the central region of infarcts. The tissue exhibits stretched myofibrils, many cells with pyknotic nuclei, congested microvessels, and phagocytosis of necrotic muscle cells (see Fig. 37.6). Mitochondrial damage occurs, but no calcification is evident.

Necrosis With Contraction Bands

This form of myocardial necrosis, also termed *contraction band necrosis* or *coagulative myocytolysis*, results primarily from severe ischemia followed by reflow. It is characterized by hypercontracted myofibrils with contraction bands and mitochondrial damage, frequently with calcification, marked vascular congestion, and healing by lysis of muscle cells. Necrosis with contraction bands results from increased influx of calcium ions (Ca^{2+}) into dying cells, which results in the arrest of cells in the contracted state in the periphery of large infarcts and, to a greater extent, in nontransmural than in transmural infarcts. The entire infarct may show this form of necrosis after reperfusion (see Figs. 37.6 and 37.7).

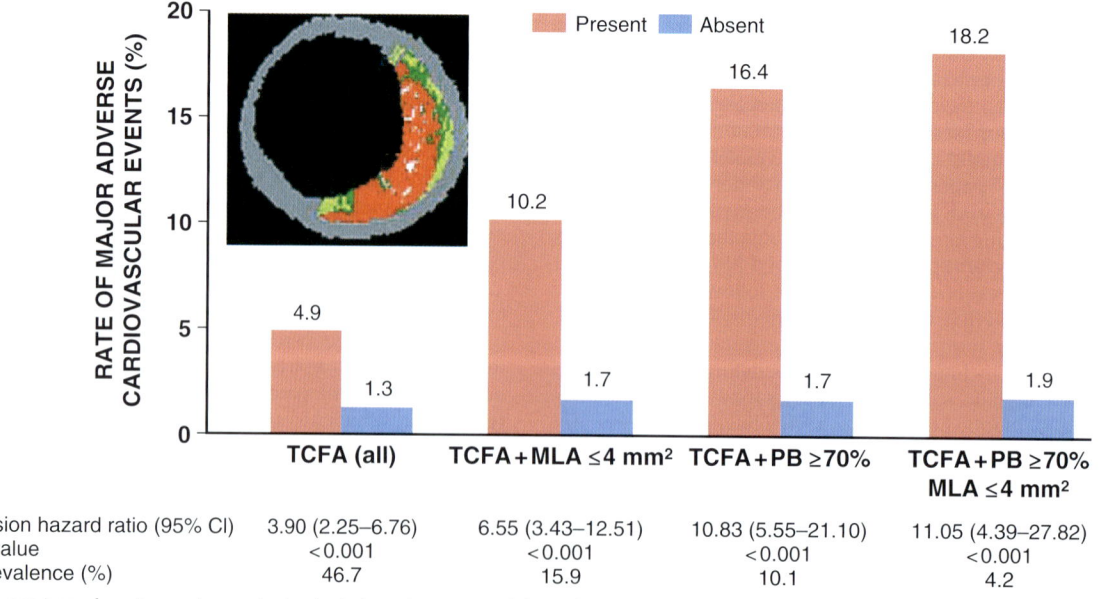

FIGURE 37.3 Comparison of cardiovascular event rates for lesions that were and those that were not thin-cap fibrothecomas (TCFAs). This figure shows the event rates associated with 595 non-culprit lesions that were characterized as TCFAs and 2114 that were not, by means of gray-scale radiofrequency intravascular ultrasonographic imaging according to minimal luminal area (MLA) and plaque burden (PB). Lesions that had a larger plaque burden, signifying greater atherosclerotic content, and smaller lumen were at greatest risk for subsequently triggering an acute coronary event. *Inset,* example of a TCFA imaged by radiofrequency ultrasonography. *Red* indicates necrotic core, *dark green* indicates fibrous tissue, *white* indicates confluent dense calcium, and *light green* indicates fibrofatty tissue. *CI,* Confidence interval. (From Stone GW, Maehara A, Lansky AJ, et al. A prospective natural-history study of coronary atherosclerosis. *N Engl J Med.* 2011;364:226.)

Myocytolysis

Ischemia without necrosis generally causes no acute changes visible on light microscopy, but severe prolonged ischemia can result in myocyte vacuolization, often termed *myocytolysis*. Prolonged severe ischemia, which is potentially reversible, causes cloudy swelling, as well as hydropic, vascular, and fatty degeneration.

Apoptosis

An additional pathway of myocyte death involves apoptosis, a form of programmed cell death. In contrast to coagulation necrosis, myocytes undergoing apoptosis exhibit shrinkage, and fragmentation of DNA without the usual cellular infiltrate indicative of inflammation. The role of apoptosis in the setting of MI is less well understood than

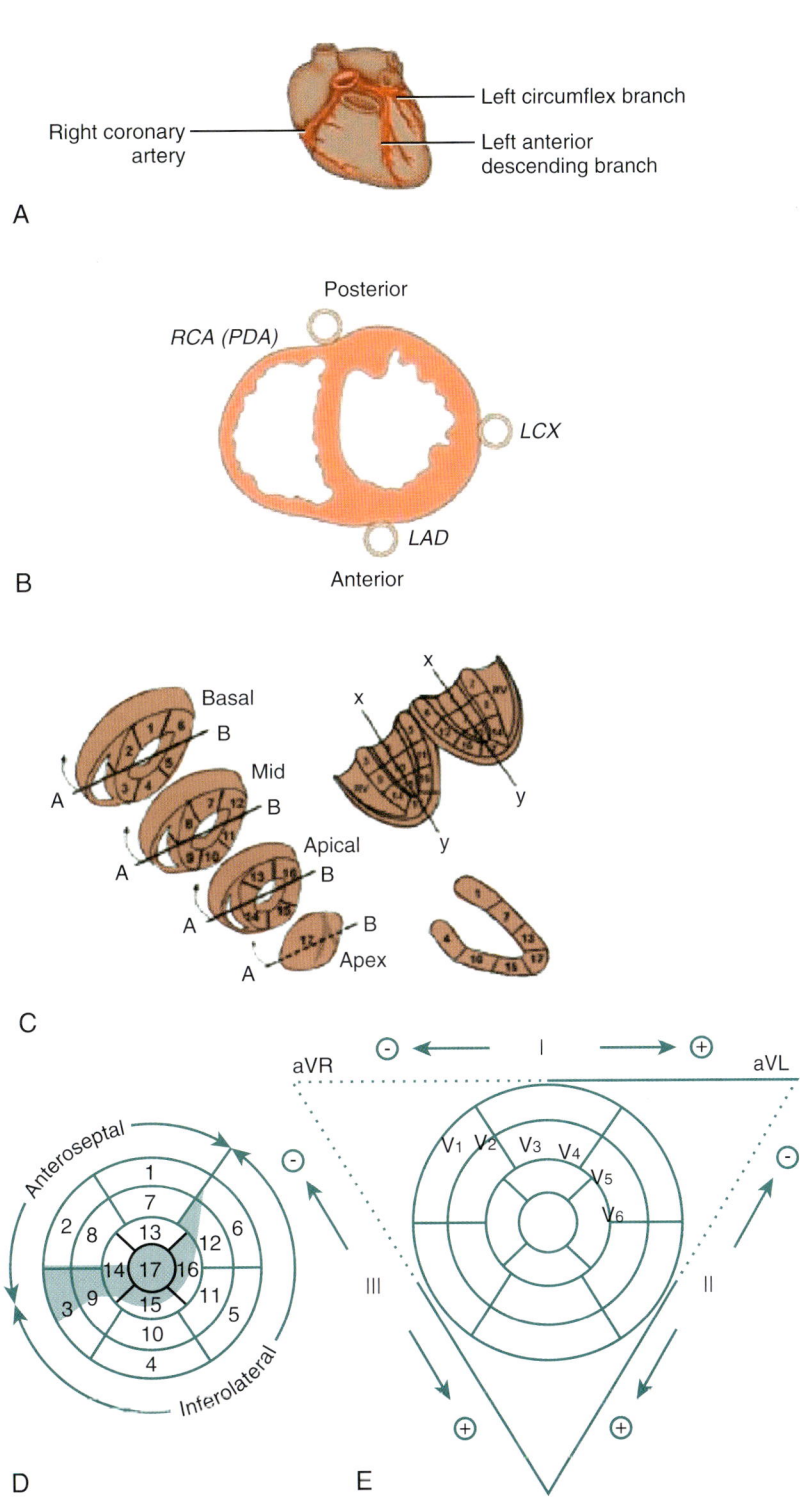

FIGURE 37.4 Correlation of sites of coronary occlusion, zones of necrosis, and abnormalities on the electrocardiogram (ECG). **A,** Schematic of the heart with location of major epicardial coronary arteries. **B,** Short-axis view of the left and right ventricles and approximate location of the left anterior descending (LAD), left circumflex (LCX), and right coronary (RCA) arteries; the RCA gives rise to the posterior descending artery (PDA) in most patients. **C,** The 17 myocardial segments in a polar map format. **D,** Position of the standard ECG leads relative to the polar map. **E,** Location of zones of necrosis after occlusion. The infarct artery can be deduced by identifying the leads that show ST elevation and referencing that polar map format (D).

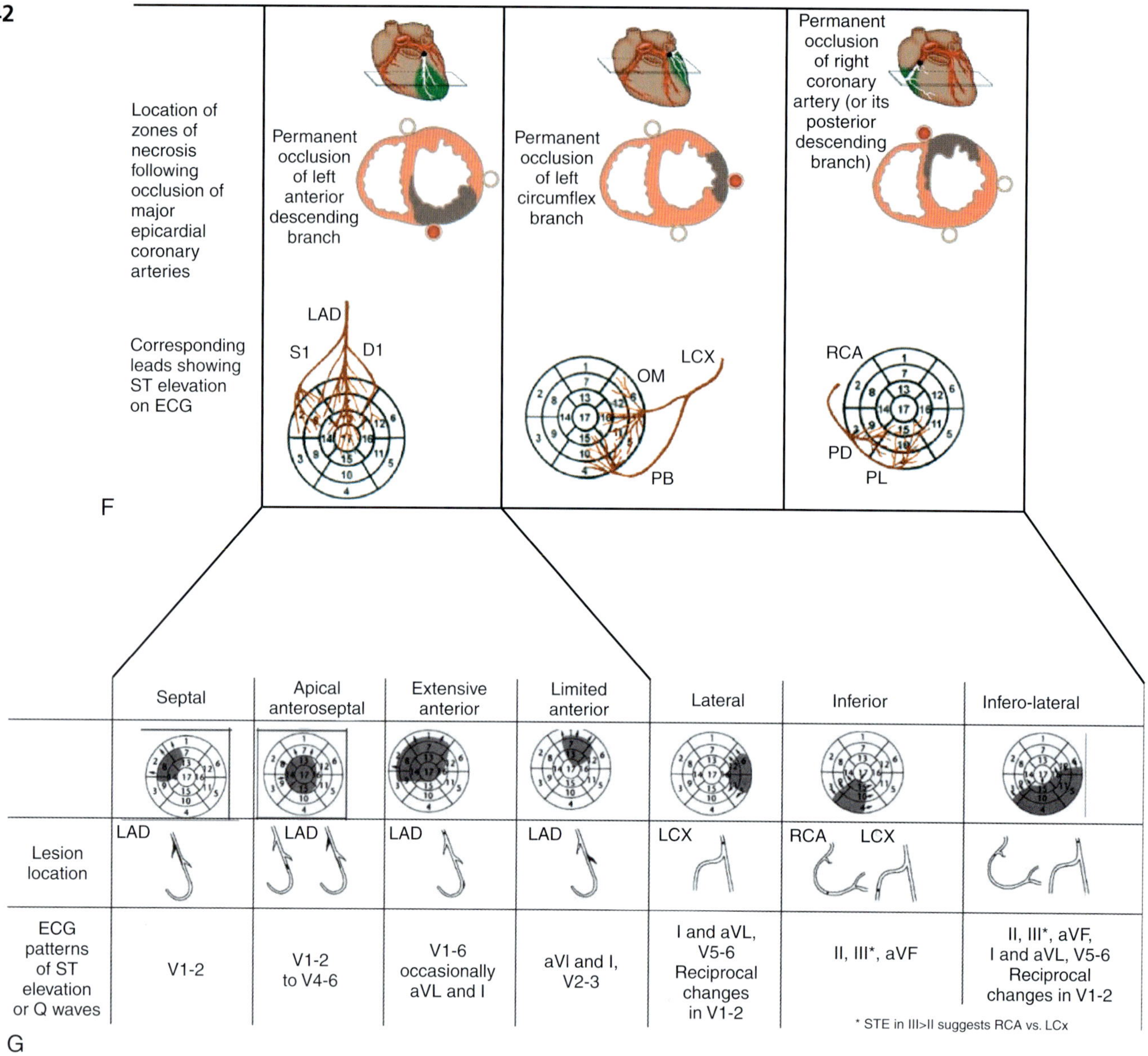

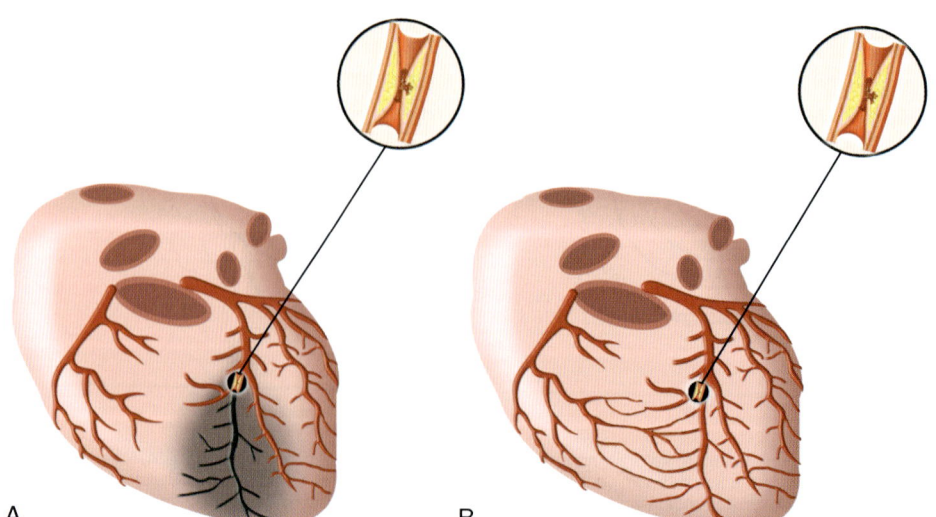

FIGURE 37.4 cont'd F, Identification of the infarct artery from the 12-lead ECG is shown for the arterial supply provided by the LAD, LCX, and RCA. For example, ST elevation seen most prominently in the leads overlying segments 1, 2, 7, 8, 13, 14, and 17 indicates that the LAD is the infarct artery. *D1*, First diagonal; *OM*, obtuse marginal; *PB*, posterobasal; *PD*, posterior descending; *PL*, posterolateral; *S1*, first septal. G, Further localization of culprit arteries via differential ECG patterns depends on the location of lesion (proximal versus distal) and branch artery inclusion. (Modified from Bayes-de-Luna A, Wagner G, Birnbaum Y, et al. A new terminology for the left ventricular walls and location of myocardial infarcts that present Q wave based on the standard of cardiac magnetic resonance imaging. *Circulation*. 2006;114:1755.)

FIGURE 37.5 Schematic drawing of the coronary artery circulation without (A) and with (B) interarterial anastomoses between the right coronary artery and the occluded left anterior descending artery (LAD) (occluded downstream of the third diagonal branch). A, Gray area indicates the ischemic area at risk for myocardial infarction (MI) (finally corresponding to infarct size) in the case of LAD occlusion and in the absence of collaterals. B, The area at risk for MI is equal to zero because of the extended collaterals. (From Traupe T, Gloekler S, de Marchi SF, et al. Assessment of the human coronary collateral circulation. *Circulation*. 2010;122:1210.)

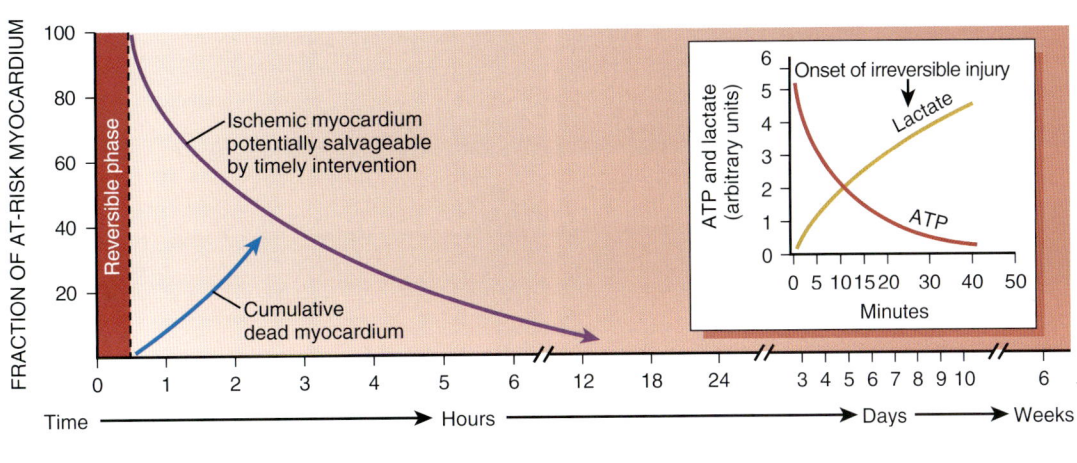
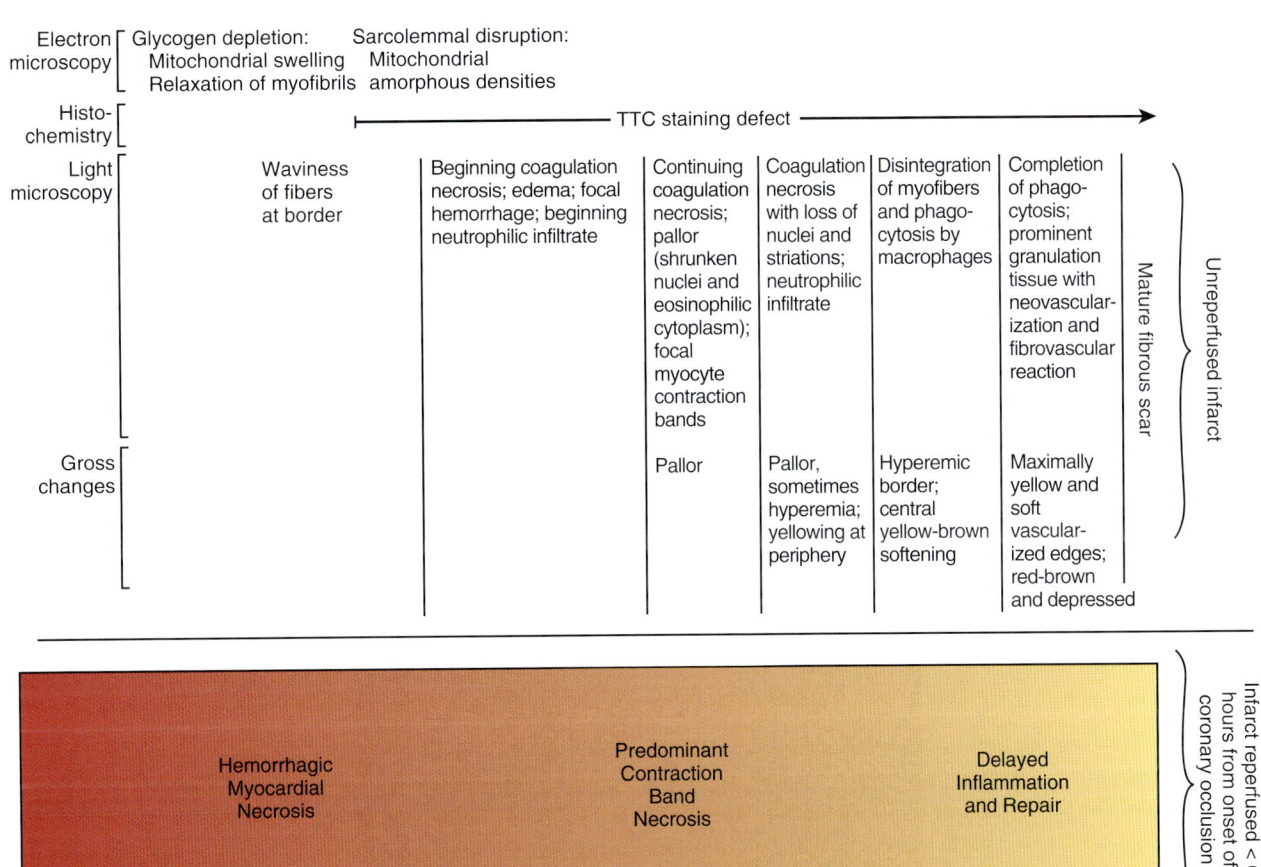

FIGURE 37.6 Temporal sequence of early biochemical, ultrastructural, histochemical, and histologic findings after the onset of myocardial infarction. Schematics of the time frames for early and late reperfusion of the myocardium supplied by an occluded coronary artery. For approximately 30 minutes after the onset of even the most severe ischemia, myocardial injury is potentially reversible; after this point, progressive loss of viability occurs and is complete by 6 to 12 hours. The benefits of reperfusion are greatest when it is achieved early, with progressively smaller benefits occurring as reperfusion is delayed. Note the alterations in the temporal sequence in the reperfused infarct. The pattern of pathologic findings following reperfusion varies depending on the timing of reperfusion, previous infarction, and collateral flow. *ATP*, Adenosine triphosphate; *TTC*, triphenyltetrazolium chloride. (From Schoen FJ. The heart. In Kumar V, et al., eds. *Robbins & Cotran Pathologic Basis of Disease*. 8th ed. Philadelphia: Saunders; 2009.)

that of classic coagulation necrosis. Apoptosis may occur shortly after the onset of myocardial ischemia, but its major impact appears to be on late myocyte loss and ventricular remodeling after MI.

Current Concepts of the Cellular Events During Myocardial Infarction and Healing

Classic studies defined the sequence of cellular events that occur during human MI by careful histologic studies.[33,34] Accumulation of granulocytes characterized the first days following MI, then mononuclear phagocytes accumulated in the infarct in tissue. Granulation tissue characterized by neovascularization and accumulation of extracellular matrix (fibrosis) followed. Experimental work in mice has delineated a sequence of accumulation of subpopulations of mononuclear phagocytes. The first wave, occurring during days 1 to 3 after coronary ligation, consists of a proinflammatory subset of monocytes characterized by high proteolytic and phagocytic capacity and

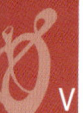

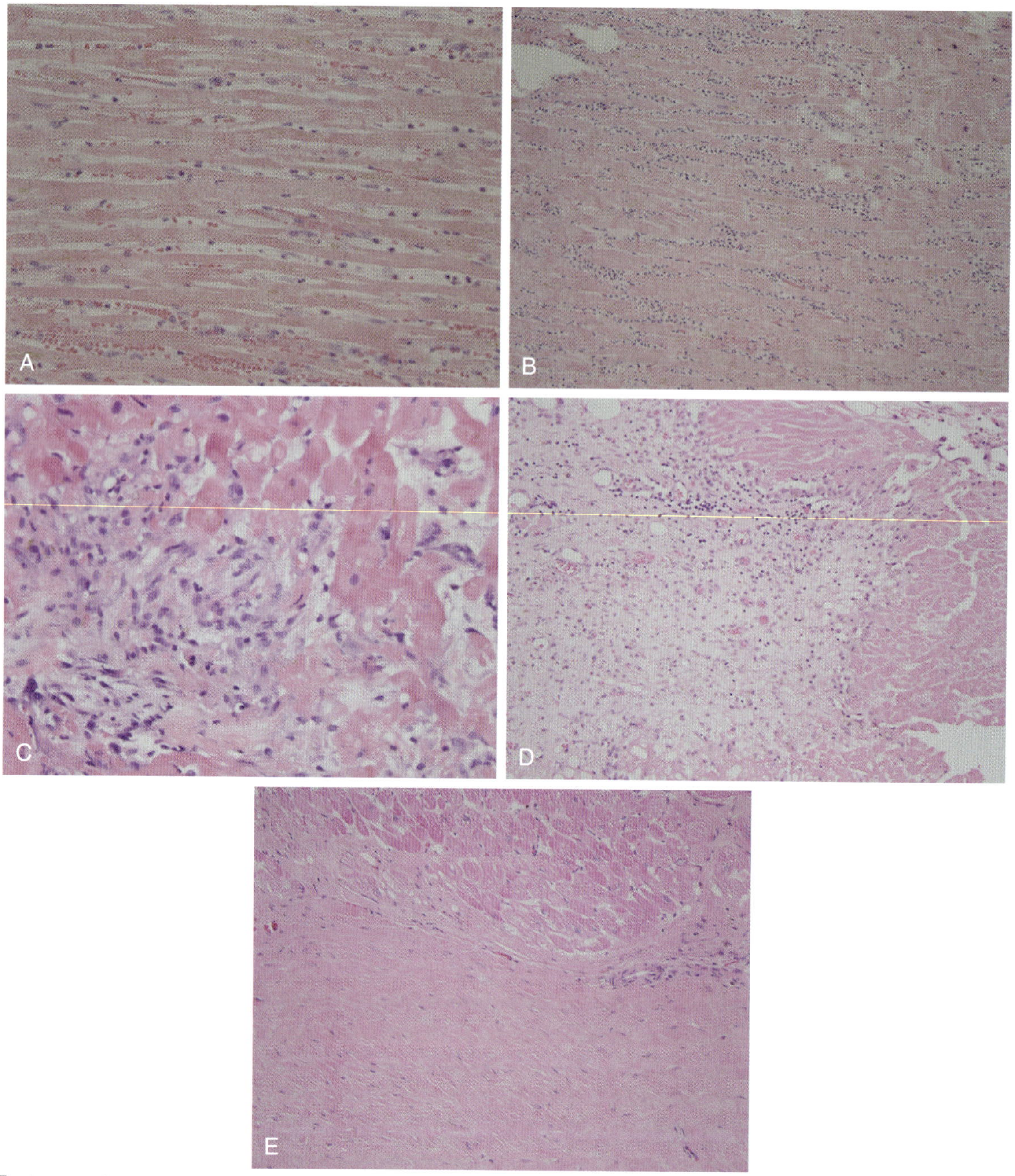

FIGURE 37.7 Microscopic features of myocardial infarction (MI). These histologic sections derived from the heart of a woman who suffered a stuttering reinfarction illustrate the histologic appearance of the injured myocardium and various phases of its healing. Times are estimated based on the clinical history and the typical pathologic findings of myocardial ischemic injury. **A,** At 8 hours post-MI, cross-striations are absent in some cardiac myocytes, and contraction bands are forming. There is myocardial interstitial edema, and leukocytes have begun to appear in the ischemically injured zone. **B,** At 36 hours post-MI, in the center of an ischemic area, most myocytes have lost cross-striations, contraction bands abound, and a predominantly polymorphonuclear leukocytic infiltrate has appeared. **C,** At 5 days post-MI, a few myocytes or fragments of myocytes persist with cross-striations. In the center of this micrograph, a predominantly monocytic leukocyte infiltrate surrounds the debris of dead myocytes. **D,** At 14 days following an acute ischemic insult, an island of granulation tissue has begun to form. There are numerous neovessels in areas of mononuclear cell accumulation. An organized extracellular matrix has begun to form. **E,** At 3 months following the acute ischemic event, an organized scar has formed in the matrix-rich and relatively hypocellular area on the bottom of this micrograph. Some surviving cardiac myocytes remain (*top* of micrograph). (Photomicrographs courtesy Dr. Robert F. Padera, Department of Pathology, Brigham and Women's Hospital, Boston.)

elaboration of proinflammatory cytokines. During a later phase (days 3 to 7), less inflammatory monocytes predominate and produce the angiogenic mediator vascular endothelial growth factor (VEGF) and the fibrogenic mediator transforming growth factor beta (TGF-β) (Fig. 37.10). This highly orchestrated sequential recruitment of subpopulations of monocytes probably plays an important role in myocardial healing. The granulocytes arriving on the scene of ischemic injury function as "first responders." They serve to initiate and amplify the acute local inflammatory response. The reactive oxygen species that they elaborate may contribute to endothelial damage, reperfusion injury, and the clinical phenomenon of "no-reflow." Experimental evidence in mice using single cell gene expression analysis discloses considerable functional diversity in the granulocyte populations that localize in acutely ischemic tissue.[35] The first wave of proinflammatory and phagocytically active mononuclear cells constitutes a "demolition crew" that can clear necrotic debris and pave the way for the second wave of less inflammatory monocytes, which contribute to healing by promoting the formation of granulation tissue (Fig. 37.11). These "repair" monocyte/macrophages elaborate a palette of mediators that stimulate angiogenesis and extracellular matrix production by surviving myocardial stromal cells. New microvessels and fibrosis are key constituents of granulation tissue, and these processes furnish the foundation for myocardial scar formation, ventricular remodeling, and infarct healing.

The elucidation of this tightly orchestrated response to myocardial ischemic injury provides new perspectives on the pathophysiology of infarction, suggesting novel therapeutic targets to "tune" this local inflammatory response in any way that can favor salutary myocardial healing and prevent the adverse remodeling of the infarcted left ventricle associated with ischemic cardiomyopathy and poor outcomes.[36] Experimental work has provided considerable new insight in this regard (Fig. 37.12). Sympathetic nervous activation caused by the pain and anxiety associated with the ACS can have far-reaching effects on the inflammatory response in addition to the well-recognized hemodynamic alterations produced by catecholamines. Beta-adrenergic stimulation can mobilize leukocyte progenitor cells from the bone marrow. Some of these cells can feed extramedullary hematopoiesis in the spleen. This "emergency hematopoiesis" can provide the leukocytes that participate in myocardial healing. In mice, mobilization of a preformed pool of proinflammatory monocytes from the spleen depends in part on the role of angiotensin in signaling. This experimental observation may provide a mechanistic understanding of the ability of angiotensin-converting enzyme (ACE) inhibitors to combat

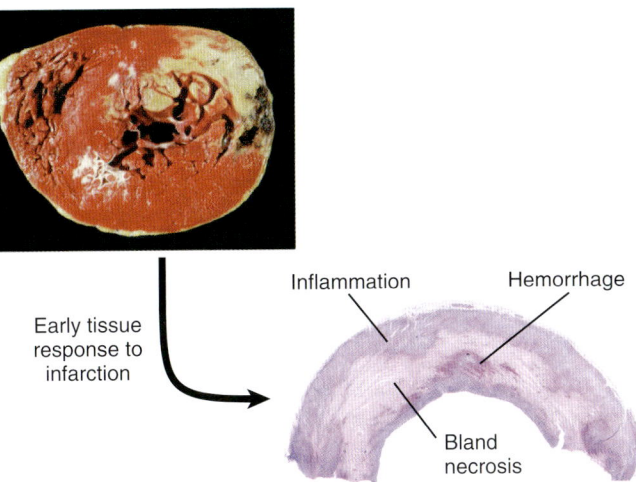

FIGURE 37.8 Top, Acute myocardial infarction, predominantly of the posterolateral left ventricle, demonstrated histochemically by lack of staining with triphenyltetrazolium chloride in areas of necrosis. The staining defect is caused by leakage of the enzyme following cell death. The myocardial hemorrhage at one edge of the infarct was associated with cardiac rupture, and the anterior scar *(lower left)* was indicative of an old infarct. The specimen was oriented with the posterior wall at the top. **Bottom,** The early tissue response to the infarction process involves a mixture of bland necrosis, inflammation, and hemorrhage. (From Schoen FJ. The heart. In Kumar V, et al., editors. *Robbins & Cotran Pathologic Basis of Disease.* 8th ed. Philadelphia: Saunders; 2009.)

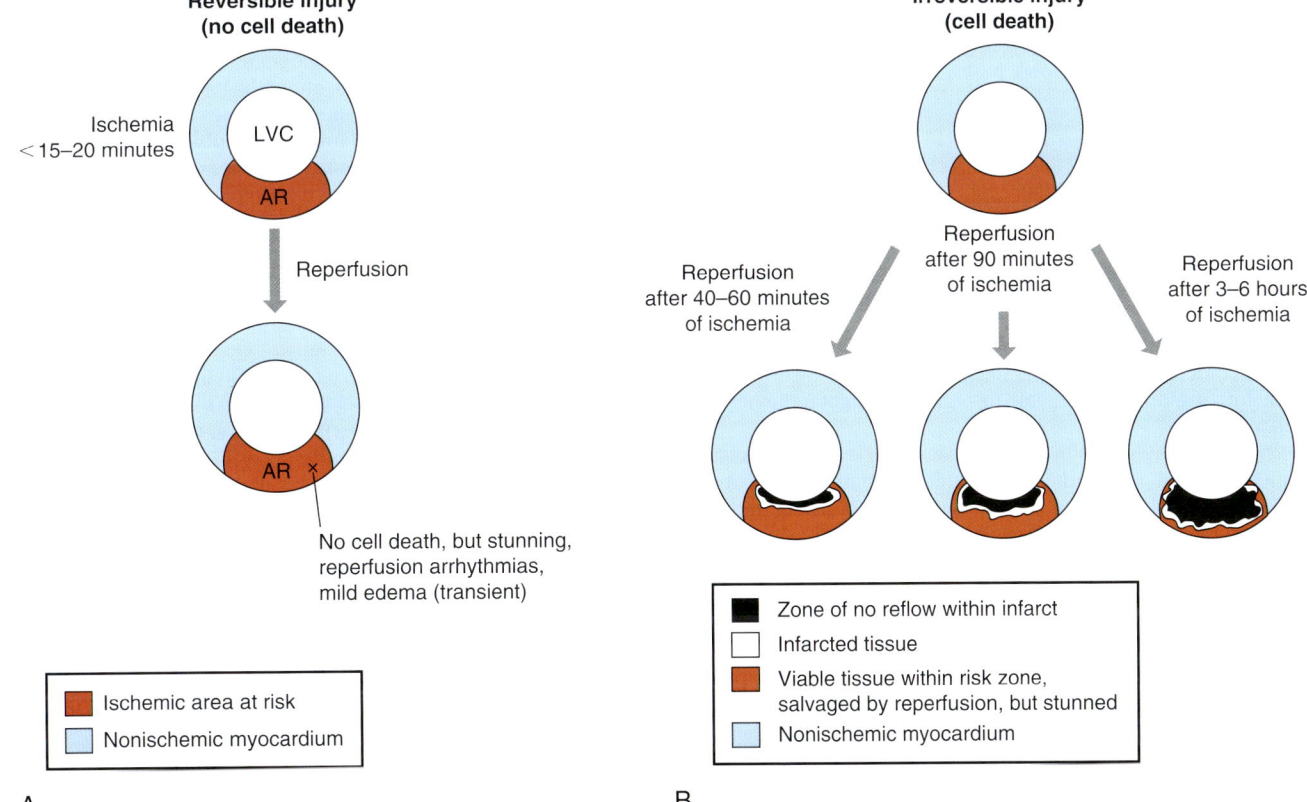

FIGURE 37.9 A, Schematic of a transmural section of the heart after a short period of ischemia (≤20 minutes). Cell death does not occur (reversible injury), but tissue is stunned and reperfusion arrhythmias might ensue. **B,** Schematic of a transmural section of the left ventricle derived from studies in the anesthetized canine model of proximal coronary occlusion and reperfusion. After 40 to 60 minutes of ischemia, irreversible cell damage is confined to the subendocardium. A smaller area of no-reflow is present within the necrotic region. If reperfusion is delayed to 90 minutes, the necrotic region expands from the subendocardium to the mid-myocardium within the ischemic risk zone, accompanied by an expansion of the no-reflow region. After 3 to 6 hours of ischemia, necrosis becomes nearly transmural, and the no-reflow region, although contained within the necrotic area, becomes larger. *AR,* Area at risk; *LVC,* left ventricular cavity. (From Kloner RA, Hale SL. Reperfusion injury. In Morrow, DA, ed. *Myocardial Infarction: A Companion to Braunwald's Heart Disease.* Philadelphia: Elsevier; 2017.)

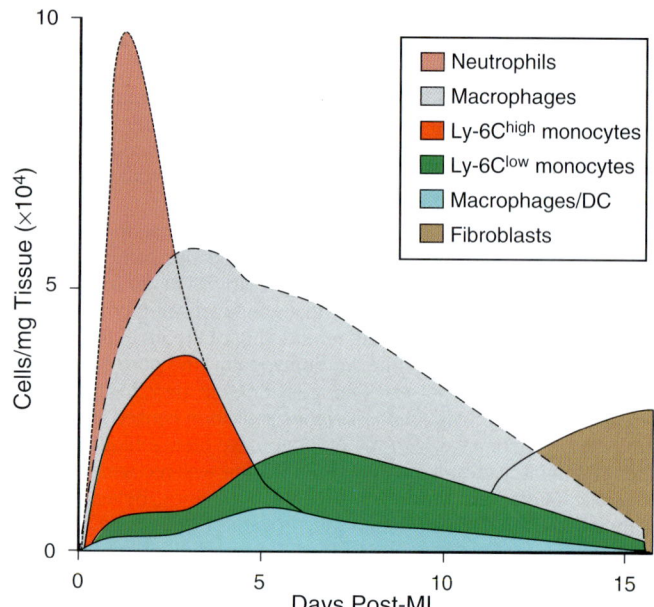

FIGURE 37.10 Sequencing waves of different cell types participate in myocardial infarction (MI) and healing. In the first hours to days following acute myocardial ischemia, neutrophils accumulate in the infarcting myocardium, as shown by the *salmon-colored* peak centered on days 1 and 2. Following this first wave of inflammatory cells, mononuclear phagocytes begin to accumulate in the ischemic tissue. Recent studies in mice have shown that in the early days of this monocytic infiltration, a particularly proinflammatory subset of mononuclear phagocytes characterized by high levels of the surface marker Ly-6C arrive first. In days 5 through 10, a reparative population of monocytes prevails *(green)*, marked by low surface expression of Ly-6C. As the accumulation of leukocytes in the injured myocardium wanes, fibroblasts and related mesenchymal cells synthesize extracellular matrix (ECM) macromolecules such as collagen. ECM production contributes to repair and scar formation during healing of the ischemically-injured heart tissue. *DC*, Dendritic cells. (From Nahrendorf M, et al. Mechanisms of myocardial ischemic injury, healing, and remodeling. In Morrow DA, ed. *Myocardial Infarction: A Companion to Braunwald's Heart Disease*. Philadelphia: Elsevier; 2017.)

adverse remodeling of the ischemic left ventricular (LV) myocardium. In addition to catecholamines, proinflammatory cytokines released during ACS can promote hematopoiesis and amplify the inflammatory response in the evolving infarct. In mice, interleukin (IL)-1β can mobilize precursors of leukocytes from the bone marrow. Inhibition of this proinflammatory cytokine does not change the size and experimental infarction but limits the decrement in contractile function in the infarcted ventricle.[37] This example illustrates how modulation of the inflammatory response in ischemic myocardium might influence the healing process.

Another insight bolstered by experimental work is the concept that inflammation in the myocardium can ignite inflammatory activity in remote atherosclerotic plaques, predisposing them to disrupt and provoke thrombosis. Such "echoes" of myocardial inflammation in plaques themselves may explain some of the early recurrent coronary events in patients with ACS. Moreover, this observation provides some mechanistic understanding of clinical observations that coronary atherosclerotic plaques remote from the culprit lesion exhibit inflammatory activation not only in the non–infarct-related artery, but also in other arterial beds, such as the carotid circulation. In mice, dampened leukocyte recruitment follows second infarction in a different territory. Thus, altered inflammatory responses, perhaps due to epigenetic changes, or "trained immunity" can also accompany a recurrent ACS.[38,39]

Although much of the information in Fig. 37.12 emerged from murine experiments, imaging observations in humans lend credence to their clinical applicability. Uptake of the glucose analogue ^{18}F-deoxyglucose (FDG) monitors metabolic activity. Patients with ACS show increased uptake of FDG in bone marrow and in the spleen compared to stable patients. These observations support the clinical translatability of the mouse experiments that revealed bone marrow activation following coronary artery ligation and boosted inflammatory processes in the spleen. Indeed, those with increased splenic FDG uptake appear to have a greater risk for recurrent events.[40] Thus a "cardiosplenic axis" of inflammatory signaling likely operates in humans and mice, furnishing new mechanistic insight into the pathogenesis of MI and uncovering novel therapeutic targets.

Modification of Pathologic Changes by Reperfusion

Early reperfusion of the myocardium evolving from ischemia to infarction (i.e., within 15 to 20 minutes) can prevent necrosis. Beyond this early stage, the number of salvaged myocytes—and therefore the amount of salvaged myocardial tissue (area of necrosis/area at risk)—relates directly to the duration of coronary artery occlusion, the level of myocardial oxygen consumption, and collateral blood flow (see Fig. 37.9). Reperfused infarcts typically show a mixture of necrosis, hemorrhage within zones of irreversibly injured myocytes, coagulative necrosis with contraction bands, and distorted architecture of cells in the reperfused zone. Reperfusion of infarcted myocardium accelerates the washout of leaked intracellular proteins, thereby producing an exaggerated and early peak value of substances such as cardiac-specific troponin T and I or the MB fraction of creatine kinase (CK-MB) (see later).[1]

While all patients who achieve reperfusion as soon as possible to preserve viable, but at risk, myocardium, the reperfusion of tissue perfusion can induce arrhythmias and potential for "reperfusion injury," which has been estimated to account for up to 50% of the ultimate infarct size. The physiology of reperfusion injury is likely multifactorial and includes release of cytotoxic mitochondrial content, myocyte hypercontractility due to Ca^{2+} excess, reactive oxygen species, leukocyte aggregation, and platelet and complement activation. Pathologic findings of reperfusion injury include widespread myocardial hemorrhage and contraction bands.

Coronary Anatomy and Location of Infarction

Approximately 90% of STEMI cases will have a total occlusion of the infarct-related vessel on initial angiogram. Spontaneous fibrinolysis of the thrombotic occlusion can occur in the period following the onset of MI and may account for some of the cases when no thrombosis is identified, but STEMI without any angiographically evident coronary disease is an increasingly recognized separate entity discussed below.

A STEMI with transmural necrosis typically occurs distal to an acutely totally occluded coronary artery with thrombus superimposed on an eroded or ruptured plaque (see Fig. 37.4). Yet, total occlusion of a coronary artery does not always cause MI. Collateral blood flow and other factors, such as the level of myocardial metabolism, presence and location of stenoses in other coronary arteries, rate of development of the obstruction, and quantity of myocardium supplied by the obstructed vessel, all influence the viability of myocardial cells distal to the occlusion.

Studies of patients in whom STEMI ultimately develops after having undergone coronary angiography at some time before its occurrence have helped clarify the extent of coronary disease before infarction. Although high-grade stenoses more frequently lead to STEMI than do less obstructive lesions, STEMI can result from sudden thrombotic occlusion at the site of disruption of previously noncritically stenosed plaque. When collateral vessels perfuse an area of the ventricle, an infarct may occur at a distance from a coronary occlusion. For example, following gradual obliteration of the lumen of the right coronary artery (RCA), collateral vessels arising from the left anterior descending coronary artery (LAD) can keep the inferior wall of the left ventricle viable. Later, an occlusion of LAD may cause infarction of the distal inferior wall.

Right Ventricular Infarction

Approximately 30% to 50% of patients with inferior infarction have some involvement of the right ventricle.[41] Right ventricular (RV) infarction almost invariably develops in association with a large infarction of the adjacent septum and inferior LV walls, but isolated infarction of the right ventricle is seen in just 3% to 5% of autopsy-proven cases of MI. RV infarction occurs less often than would be anticipated from the frequency of atherosclerotic lesions involving the RCA. The classic presentation of an RV infarct is hypotension, clear lung fields, and elevated

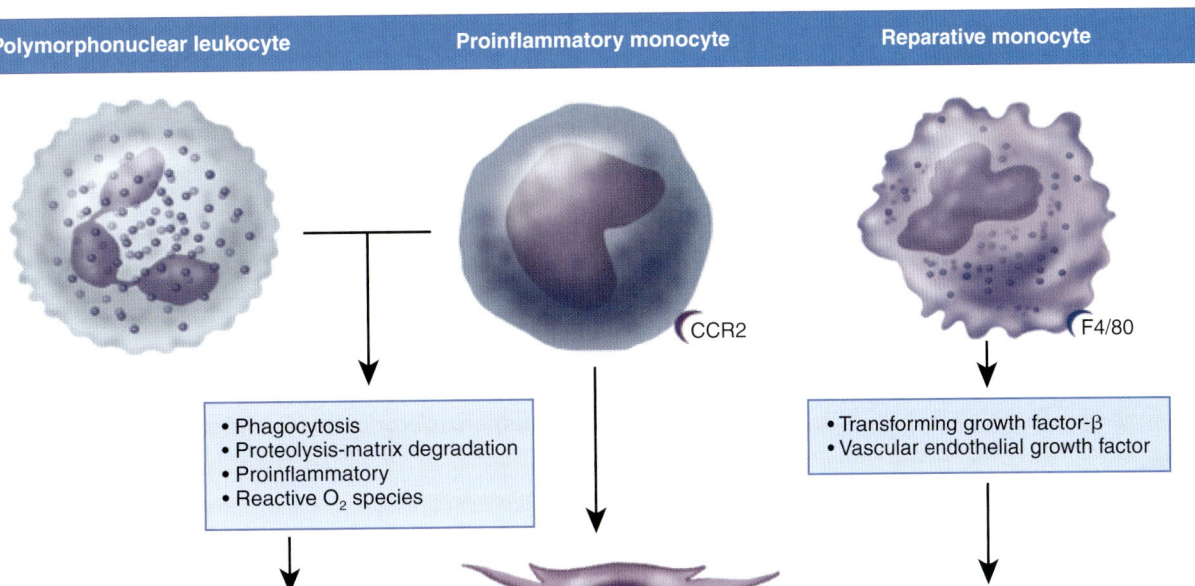

FIGURE 37.11 Regulation of the responses to myocardial ischemic injury. Immediate recruitment of polymorphonuclear leukocytes, the first responders, precede the accumulation of proinflammatory monocytes (typically bearing the chemokine receptor 2 [CCR2]). These phagocytic cells elaborate the mediators of the early phase of response to ischemic injury by clearing dead cells and debris and beckoning further inflammatory cells to enter the injured area. Reparative monocytes elaborate TGF-β that furnishes a strong stimulus to the production of extracellular matrix macromolecules that reinforce the cardiac skeleton during the healing phase. They also secrete VEGF, which stimulates microvessel formation characteristic of granulation tissue, the histologic hallmark of the reparative response in damaged tissues. The observation that monocytes can give rise to fibroblast-like cells capable of interstitial collagen synthesis adds a new dimension to understanding this healing response. By reinforcing repair of the myocardial skeleton, the extracellular matrix molecules manufactured by fibroblasts can forestall expansive remodeling of the infarct and myocardium, promoting a beneficial healing response associated with less risk for chronic heart failure. "Tuning" the balance between the damage clearance and the repair and healing functions provides an opportunity for therapeutic intervention to improve outcomes following acute coronary syndromes. *TGF,* Transforming growth factor; *VEGF,* vascular endothelial growth factor. (From Libby P, Swirski FK, Nahrendorf M, et al. The myocardium: more than myocytes. *J Am Coll Cardiol.* 2019 Dec 24;74[25]:3136–3138.)

jugular venous pressures. Acute management of RV infarction complicated by cardiogenic shock includes judicious volume replacement, early revascularization, maintenance of atrioventricular synchrony, and in refractory cases, mechanical circulatory support (see Chapter 59). In contrast to the left ventricle, the right ventricle can sustain long periods of ischemia but still demonstrate excellent recovery of contractile function after reperfusion.

Atrial Infarction
Infarction of the atria occurs in up to 10% of patients with STEMI if PR-segment displacement is used as the criterion.[42] Although less than 5% of patients with STEMI are felt to have isolated atrial infarction, it often occurs in conjunction with ventricular infarction, with an estimated incidence of approximately 15% all MI, and can rarely cause rupture of the atrial wall.[43] This type of infarction is more common on the right than the left side, occurs more frequently in the atrial appendages than in the lateral or posterior walls of the atrium, and can result in thrombus formation. Atrial arrhythmias frequently accompany atrial infarction. Reduced secretion of atrial natriuretic peptide may ensue and lead to a low–cardiac output syndrome when RV infarction coexists. Moreover, atrial infarction can lead to early atrial dilation, dysfunction, and fibrosis, and in the setting left atrial infarction, early occurrence of ischemic mitral regurgitation.[44]

Collateral Circulation in Acute Myocardial Infarction
Patients with occlusive CAD frequently have a particularly well-developed coronary collateral circulation, especially those with reduction of the luminal cross-sectional area by more than 75% in one or more major vessels; patients with chronic hypoxia, as occurs in severe anemia, chronic obstructive pulmonary disease (COPD), and cyanotic congenital heart disease; and those with LV hypertrophy (Fig. 37.5 and Chapter 36).

The magnitude of coronary collateral flow is a principal determinant of the infarct size. Indeed, patients with abundant collateral vessels may have totally occluded coronary arteries without evidence of infarction in the distribution of that artery; thus, survival of myocardium distal to such occlusions depends largely on collateral blood flow.[45,46] Even if the collateral perfusion existing at the time of coronary occlusion does not prevent infarction, it may still confer benefit by preventing the formation of LV aneurysms. The presence of a high-grade stenosis (90%), possibly with periods of intermittent total occlusion, probably permits the development of collateral vessels that remain only as potential conduits until a total occlusion occurs or recurs. Total occlusion then brings these channels into full operation. Patients with angiographic evidence of collateral formation have improved angiographic and clinical outcomes after MI.

Myocardial Infarction with Nonobstructive Coronary Arteries
Myocardial infarction with nonobstructive coronary arteries (MINOCA) is defined as the evidence of MI (positive cardiac biomarker and corroborative clinical evidence of infarction due to ischemia) with angiographically normal or near-normal coronary arteries (the absence of obstructive CAD on angiography [i.e., no coronary artery stenosis ≥50%] in any potential infarct-related artery), and no other explanation for the presentation.[47–49] It is estimated to be present

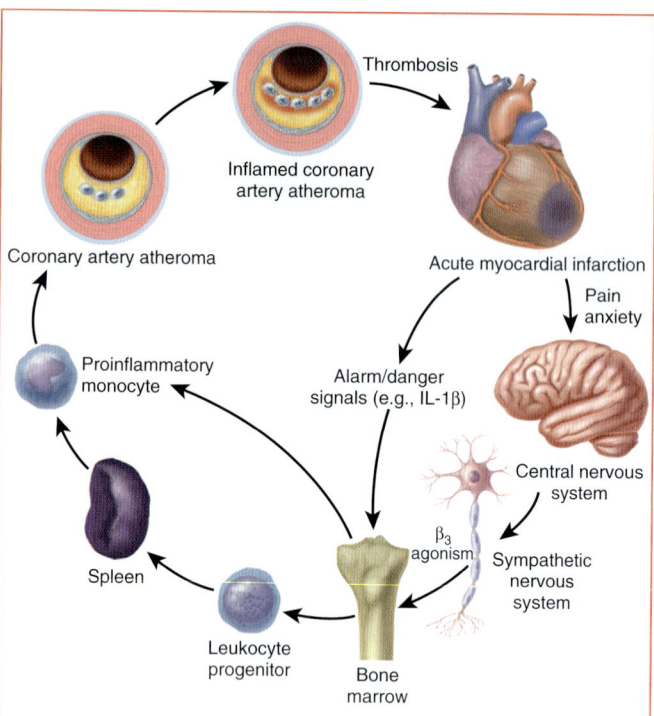

FIGURE 37.12 Leukocytes link local and systemic inflammation in ischemic cardiovascular disease. Myocardial infarction (MI) most often results from a disruption of a coronary artery atheroma that triggers thrombus formation. The sympathetic nervous system discharge in response to the pain and anxiety provoked by the acute MI evokes the mobilization of leukocyte progenitors from the bone marrow. Various humoral mediators, including the proinflammatory cytokine interleukin-1 beta (IL-1β) also help to recruit progenitor cells from the bone marrow. These progenitors can enter the bloodstream and make their way to the spleen, where they may engage in extramedullary leukopoiesis. The circulating proinflammatory monocytes can then home to atheromata that may localize remotely from the culprit lesion of the acute MI, setting the stage for a round of aggravated plaque evolution and recurrent events. This cyclic concept builds on the "cardiovascular continuum" concept promulgated by Dzau and Braunwald in 1991. (From Libby P, Nahrendorf M, Swirski FK. Leukocytes link local and systemic inflammation in ischemic cardiovascular disease: an expanded "cardiovascular continuum." *J Am Coll Cardiol*. 2016;67:1091–1103.)

in 5% to 10% of patients presenting with MI. The term MINOCA encompasses a variety of vascular and myocardial conditions that until recently, were poorly defined using standard electrocardiographic, angiographic, and imaging modalities. With greater sensitivity in techniques such as intravascular imaging (e.g., intravascular ultrasound [IVUS] and optical coherence tomography [OCT]) and magnetic resonance imaging (MRI), the underlying causes of MINOCA can be identified in a majority of patients. Coronary artery spasm, plaque erosion or rupture, and coronary dissection are common MINOCA etiologies affecting the epicardial arteries, as are plaque erosion and plaque rupture not discerned by standard angiography, whereas the two most common myocardial or microvascular mimickers of MI are acute myocarditis (see Chapter 55) and acute stress (takotsubo) cardiomyopathy. In one study of 301 women with MINOCA, an ischemic etiology was identified in 63.8% of women, a nonischemic etiology in 20.7%, and no mechanism in just 15.5%.[50] Based on these findings, MINOCA can include thrombotic-mediated ischemia and infarcts (Type 1 MI) or oxygen supply and demand mismatch infarcts (type 2 MI).

Compared to patients with atherosclerotic-mediated MI, patients with MINOCA tend to be younger, and more often female, black Maori or Pacific race, or Hispanic, with relatively few coronary risk factors except a history of cigarette smoking. One third of patients with MINOCA present with STEMI.[51] Usually, they have no history of angina pectoris before the infarction. These patients do not generally have a prodrome before infarction, but the clinical, laboratory, and electrocardiographic features of STEMI otherwise resemble those present in the overwhelming majority of patients with STEMI, who have classic obstructive atherosclerotic CAD. MINOCA should not be considered a final diagnosis per se, but rather a descriptive concept, or "working diagnosis" that should prompt more extensive evaluation to elucidate the underlying etiologies, which may then lead to distinct treatments such as antiplatelet therapy, statins, calcium channel blockers, or inhibitors of renin-angiotensin-aldosterone system (RAAS) based on the ultimate diagnosis (Fig. 37.13).

In general, patients who have survived STEMI without evidence of significant CAD have a smaller infarct sizes better long-term outlook than those with atherosclerotic-mediated STEMI; in-hospital mortality is approximately 60% lower, and 1-year mortality, 40% lower.[51] However, the subsequent risk for patients presenting with MINOCA is largely based on the underlying etiology and comorbidities and more recent observation.al data suggest the outcomes are similar to patients with atherosclerotic MI.[47,48,52]

Nonatherosclerotic Causes of Acute Myocardial Infarction

Numerous pathologic processes other than atherosclerosis can involve the coronary arteries and result in STEMI (see Table 37.3).[48]

Embolic/Thrombotic coronary arterial occlusions can result from embolization into a coronary artery. The causes of coronary embolism are numerous: infective endocarditis and nonbacterial thrombotic endocarditis (see Chapter 80), prolapsed mitral valve, or myxoma, mural thrombi, prosthetic valves, neoplasms, air introduced at cardiac surgery, and calcium deposits from manipulation of calcified valves at surgery. In situ thrombosis of coronary arteries can occur secondary to chest wall trauma or hypercoagulable states.

Spontaneous coronary artery dissection (SCAD), once thought to be a relatively rare event, is identified more frequently now with greater utilization of intracoronary imaging and may account for 25% to 33% of MIs in women younger than 50 years old.[53,54] The prevalence is much lower in men. The underlying cause is felt to be a medial dissection or rupture in the vasa vasorum, often in the setting of some physical or emotional stress in patients with some predisposition, that leads to intramural hemorrhage and subsequent coronary occlusion by the hematoma itself or a dissection flap. Initial triage and evaluation of patients with suspected SCAD should follow standard ACS algorithms. A clear dissection flap and thrombosis may be visible at angiography, but often there is only an intramural hematoma, which can be mistaken for vasospasm or an atherosclerotic plaque unless intracoronary imaging is used. SCAD is categorized angiographically into three or four types based on the lesion characteristics. Revascularization strategies for SCAD diverge from standard ACS recommendations. Conservative management with oral and IV antithrombotic therapy alone is recommended if coronary flow is preserved because of high rates of PCI-related complications. Revascularization with PCI or coronary artery bypass grafting (CABG) should be considered for occlusive lesions with ongoing ischemia, shock, or associated arrhythmias, recognizing a higher risk of complications.

Rarer causes include syphilitic aortitis, which can produce marked narrowing or occlusion of one or both coronary ostia, whereas Takayasu arteritis can result in obstruction of the coronary arteries. Necrotizing arteritis, polyarteritis nodosa, mucocutaneous lymph node syndrome (Kawasaki disease), systemic lupus erythematosus (see Chapter 97), and giant cell arteritis can cause coronary occlusion. Therapeutic levels of mediastinal radiation can result in coronary arteriosclerosis with subsequent infarction. MI can also result from coronary arterial involvement in patients with amyloidosis (see Chapter 53), Hurler syndrome, pseudoxanthoma elasticum, and homocystinuria. Cocaine can cause MI in patients with normal coronary arteries, preexisting MI, documented CAD, or coronary artery spasm (see Chapter 84).

Additional causes MI in the setting of normal-appearing coronary arteries include (1) CAD in vessels too small to be visualized on coronary arteriography or coronary arterial thrombosis with subsequent recanalization; (2) a hematologic disorder (e.g., polycythemia vera, cyanotic heart disease with polycythemia, sickle cell anemia, disseminated intravascular coagulation, thrombocytosis, thrombotic thrombocytopenic purpura) causing in situ thrombosis in the presence of normal coronary arteries; and (3) anatomic variations, such as anomalous origin of a coronary artery, coronary arteriovenous fistula, or a myocardial bridge.[55]

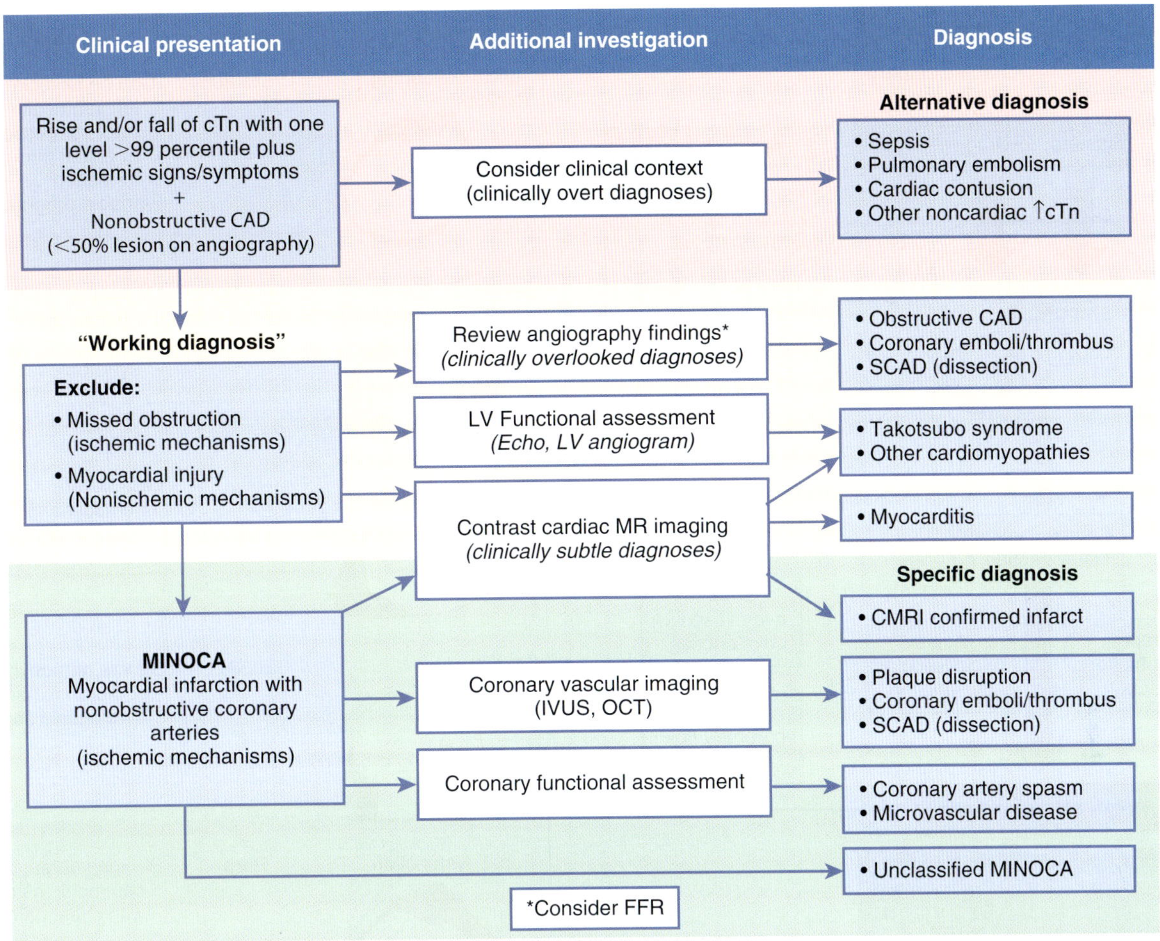

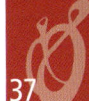

FIGURE 37.13 Clinical algorithm for the diagnosis of myocardial infarction in the absence of obstructive coronary artery disease (MINOCA). *CAD*, Coronary artery disease; *CMRI*, cardiac magnetic resonance imaging; *cTn*, cardiac troponin; *FFR*, fractional flow reserve; *IVUS*, intravascular ultrasound; *LV*, left ventricular; *MR*, magnetic resonance; *OCT*, optical coherence tomography; *SCAD*, spontaneous coronary artery dissection. *Consider FFR. (From Tamis-Holland JE, Jneid H, Reynolds HR, et al. Contemporary diagnosis and management of patients with myocardial infarction in the absence of obstructive coronary artery disease: a scientific statement from the American Heart Association. *Circulation.* 2019;139:e891–e908.)

Stress (Takotsubo) Cardiomyopathy

Acute stress cardiomyopathy, also termed *transient LV apical ballooning syndrome* or takotsubo cardiomyopathy, typically involves transient wall motion abnormalities involving the LV apex and midventricle (Fig. 37.14), although other patterns have been reported, including "reverse" takotsubo pattern.[56,57] This syndrome occurs in the absence of obstructive epicardial CAD and can mimic STEMI, but should not be considered a subtype of MINOCA as it has a specific pathophysiology that likely reflects neurocardiogenic myocardial stunning.[57] With greater recognition, its incidence is rising to 15 to 30 cases per 100,000 per year. Typically, an episode of physical or psychological stress precedes the development of takotsubo cardiomyopathy, although some cases lack an evident precipitant. More than half of patients presenting with takotsubo cardiomyopathy have an active or history of a neurologic or psychiatric disorder, potentially linking neurologic-mediated vasoconstriction. Initial ECGs demonstrate substantial and often diffuse ST-segment elevation, prompting, when coupled with the typical (frequently severe) chest discomfort, the appropriate immediate referral for coronary angiography.

The proposed diagnostic criteria typically include the presence of transient regional wall motion abnormalities, frequent (but not required) preceding stressful trigger, absence of culprit CAD lesion, abnormal electrocardiographic and biomarker findings, absence of myocarditis or pheochromocytoma, and recovery of ventricular function over subsequent weeks or months. One proposed ECG algorithm for differentiating stress cardiomyopathy from STEMI found that different patterns of ST elevations across the different coronary territories could distinguish stress cardiomyopathy from ACS with excellent specificity.[58] However, this observation requires validation and should not preclude urgent catheterization to exclude acute thrombotic lesions. A clinical score (InterTAK Diagnostic Score) assigns points for female sex, physical or emotional trigger, absence of ST-segment depression, known neurologic or psychiatric disorder, and QTc prolongation that can provide good specificity for stress myopathy or ACS in patients with high and low score, respectively.

The etiology of stress cardiomyopathy is not clear, but neurally activated or circulating catecholamine-mediated microvascular dysfunction, as well as myocardial stunning and injury, play important roles. Neuroimaging suggests increased blood flow in the hippocampus, brainstem, and basal ganglia in patients with stress cardiomyopathy. Central activation of these areas stimulates activation of brainstem noradrenergic neurons and other stimulatory neuropeptides, which with intense stress, may induce direct toxic effects on the epicardial and microvascular function. Elevated levels of circulating catecholamines (as opposed to neurally mediated stimulation) may lead to similar dysfunction. Most patients with stress cardiomyopathy will recover ventricular function rapidly, although more than 20% of patients do suffer inhospital complications, including heart failure (HF), arrhythmias, and death, at rates similar to patients with ACS.[55,56,59]

PATHOPHYSIOLOGY

Left Ventricular Function
Systolic Function
On interruption of antegrade flow in an epicardial coronary artery, the zone of myocardium supplied by that vessel immediately loses its ability to shorten and perform contractile work (Fig. 37.15). Four

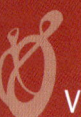

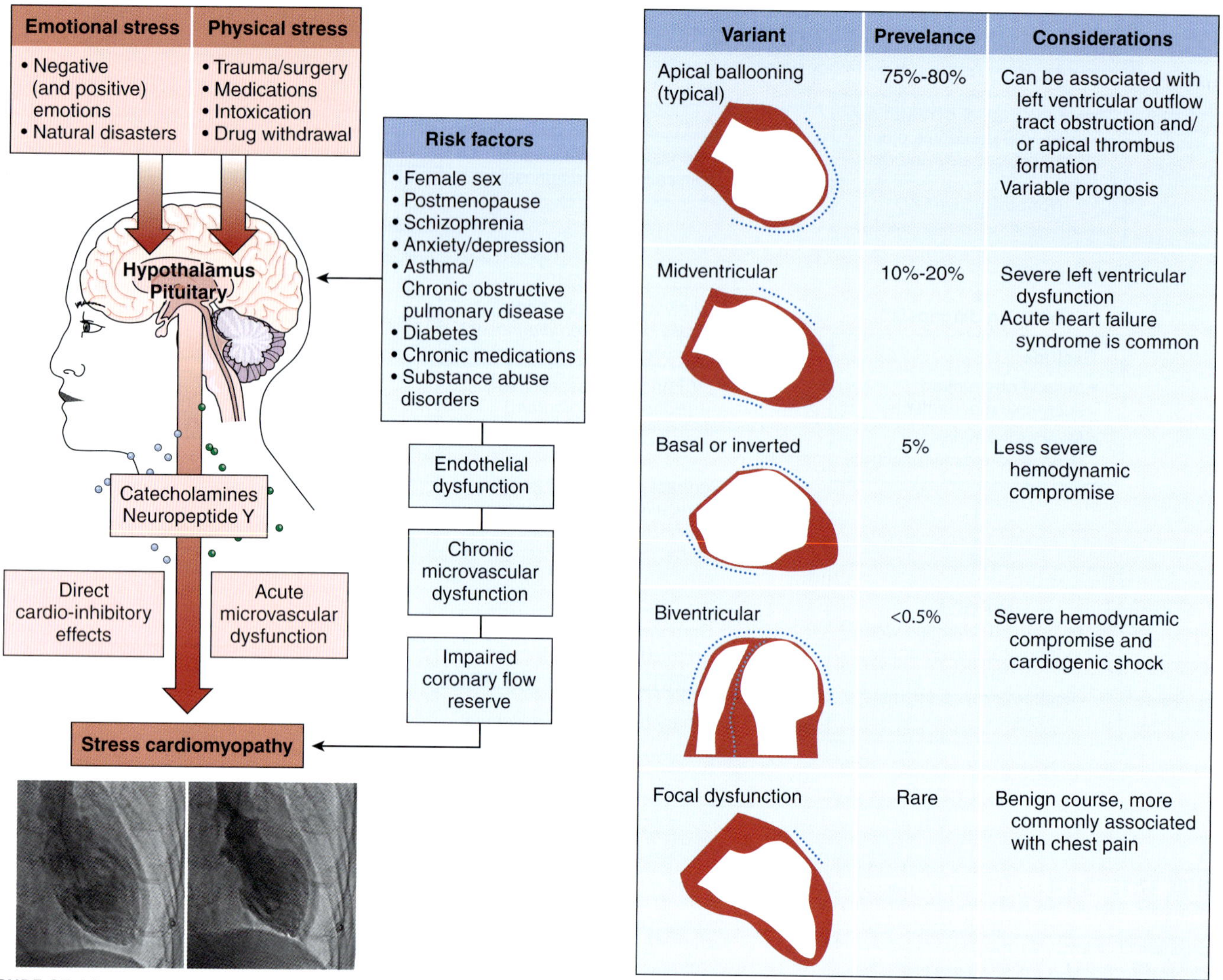

FIGURE 37.14 Left, Pathophysiology of stress cardiomyopathy. In a predisposed individual, who may have enrichment in neuropeptide Y/norepinephrine granules and risk factors for endothelial dysfunction, an intense stimulation for an adrenergic stimulation may be sufficient to trigger stress cardiomyopathy in response to emotional or physical stress. Stress-related neuropeptides stored in the presynaptic terminations of postganglionic neurons at level of the central autonomic nervous system may suddenly spill at myocardial level, and through a direct catecholamine toxicity and/or microvascular dysfunction, explain the prevailing theory of a neurogenic-mediated mechanism of myocardial stunning. **Right,** Anatomical variants of stress cardiomyopathy. (From Medina de Chazal H, Del Buono MG, Keyser-Marcus L, et al. Stress cardiomyopathy diagnosis and treatment: JACC state-of-the-art review. *J Am Coll Cardiol.* 2018;72[16]:1955–1971.)

abnormal contraction patterns develop in sequence: (1) *dyssynchrony,* or dissociation of the time course of contraction of adjacent segments, (2) *hypokinesis,* or a reduction in the extent of shortening, (3) *akinesis,* or cessation of shortening, and (4) *dyskinesis,* paradoxical expansion, and systolic bulging. Hyperkinesis of the remaining normal myocardium initially accompanies dysfunction of the infarct. The early hyperkinesis of the noninfarcted zones probably results from acute compensation, including increased activity of the sympathetic nervous system and the Frank-Starling mechanism. A portion of this compensatory hyperkinesis is ineffective work because contraction of the noninfarcted segments of myocardium causes dyskinesis of the infarct zone. The increased motion of the noninfarcted region subsides within 2 weeks of infarction, during which some degree of recovery often occurs in the infarct region as well, particularly if reperfusion of the infarcted area occurs and myocardial stunning diminishes.

Patients with STEMI may also have reduced myocardial contractile function in noninfarcted zones. This finding may result from previous obstruction of the coronary artery supplying the noninfarcted region of the ventricle and loss of collaterals from the freshly occluded infarct-related vessel, a condition termed *ischemia at a distance.* Conversely, the development of collaterals before STEMI occurs may allow greater preservation of regional systolic function in an area of distribution of the occluded artery and improvement in the LV ejection fraction (EF) early after infarction (see Fig. 37.5).[45,46]

If a sufficient quantity of myocardium undergoes ischemic injury (see Fig. 37.9), LV pump function becomes depressed; cardiac output, stroke volume, blood pressure (BP), and peak dP/dt decline; and end-systolic volume increases. The degree to which end-systolic volume increases is perhaps the most powerful hemodynamic predictor of mortality following STEMI. Paradoxical systolic expansion of an area of ventricular myocardium further decreases LV stroke volume.[60,61] As necrotic myocytes slip past each other, the infarct zone thins and elongates, especially in patients with large anterior infarcts, thereby leading to expansion of the infarct (see later). In some patients a vicious circle of dilation begetting further dilation ensues. Inhibitors of the RAAS can limit the degree of ventricular dilation, which depends closely on infarct size, patency of the infarct-related artery, and RAAS activation, even in the absence of symptomatic LV dysfunction.[62] With time, edema and ultimately fibrosis via mechanisms previously discussed (see Fig. 37.7) increase the stiffness of the infarcted myocardium back to and beyond preinfarct values. Increasing stiffness in the infarcted zone of myocardium improves LV function because it prevents paradoxical systolic wall motion (dyskinesia).

The likelihood of clinical symptoms developing correlates with specific parameters of LV function. The earliest abnormality is ventricular

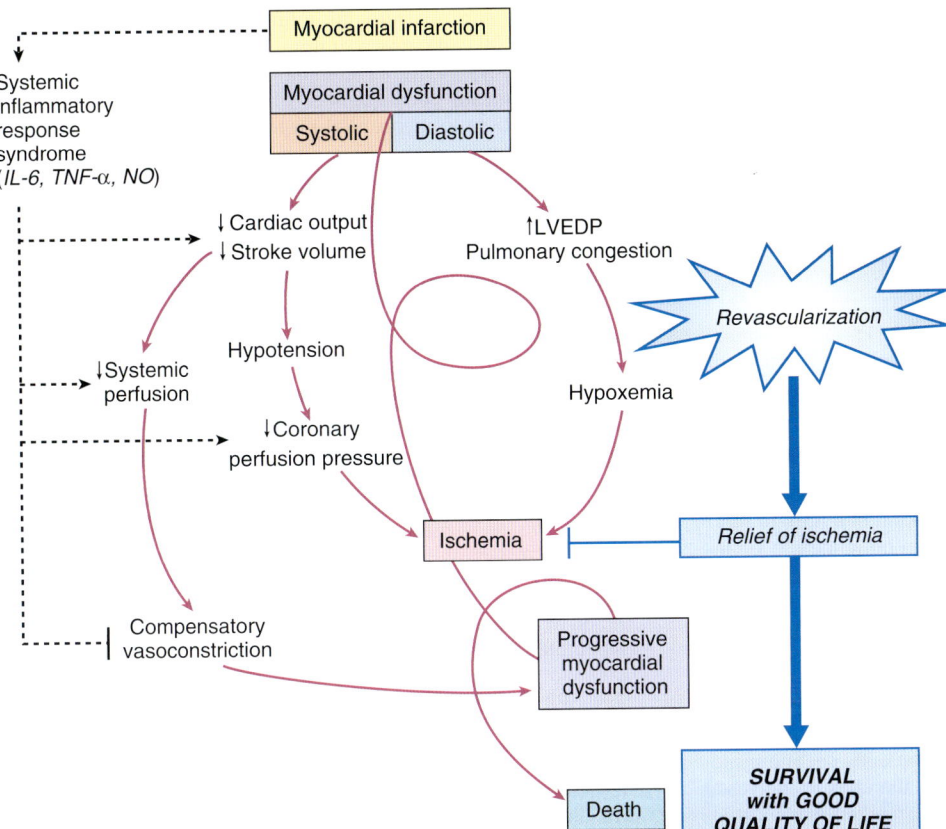

FIGURE 37.15 Pathophysiology of cardiogenic shock. Myocardial injury causes systolic and diastolic dysfunction. A decrease in cardiac output leads to a decrease in systemic and coronary perfusion. The decreased perfusion exacerbates ischemia and causes cell death in the infarct border zone and the remote zone of myocardium. Inadequate systemic perfusion triggers reflex vasoconstriction, which is usually insufficient. Systemic inflammation may play a role in limiting the peripheral vascular compensatory response and may contribute to the myocardial dysfunction. Whether inflammation plays a causal role or is only an epiphenomenon remains unclear. Revascularization leads to relief of ischemia. Demonstration of an increase in cardiac output or the left ventricular ejection fraction as the mechanism of benefit of revascularization has not been possible, but revascularization significantly increases the likelihood of survival with good quality of life. IL-6, Interleukin-6; LVEDP, left ventricular end-diastolic pressure; NO, nitric oxide; TNF, tumor necrosis factor. (From Reynolds HR, Hochman JS. Cardiogenic shock: current concepts and improving outcomes. Circulation. 2008;117:686.)

Circulatory Regulation

Patients with STEMI have an abnormality in circulatory regulation. The process begins with an anatomic or functional obstruction in the coronary vascular bed that results in regional myocardial ischemia and, if the ischemia persists, in MI. If the infarct is sufficiently large, it depresses overall LV function such that LV stroke volume declines and filling pressure increases. In the setting of acute MI, the relative reduction in stroke volume may be greater when compared to the reduction in EF because the ventricle has not dilated. A marked depression in LV stroke volume ultimately lowers aortic pressure and, together with increased LV end-diastolic pressure, further reducing coronary perfusion pressure. This condition may intensify myocardial ischemia and thereby initiate a vicious cycle (see Fig. 37.15), leading to cardiogenic shock, which occurs in 5% to 8% of patients with STEMI.[64,65]

Local myocardial injury leads to systemic inflammation due to the release of cytokines that contribute to the vasodilation and decreased systemic vascular resistance. The inability of the left ventricle to empty normally also increases left-sided preload; that is, it dilates the well-perfused, normally functioning portion of the left ventricle. This compensatory mechanism tends to restore stroke volume to normal levels, but at the expense of a reduced EF. Dilation of the left ventricle also elevates ventricular wall tension, because Laplace law dictates that at any given arterial pressure, the dilated ventricle must develop higher wall tension. This increased afterload not only depresses LV stroke volume but also elevates myocardial oxygen consumption, which in turn intensifies the myocardial ischemia. When regional myocardial dysfunction is limited and the function of the remainder of the left ventricle is normal, compensatory mechanisms—especially hyperkinesis of the nonaffected portion of the ventricle and an appropriate increase in heart rate—sustain overall LV function. Ventricular dilation also exacerbates functional mitral regurgitation due to tethered chordae and poor coaptation of the leaflets. If a large portion of the left ventricle ceases to function, pump failure ensues.

Ventricular Remodeling

As a consequence of STEMI, the changes in LV size, shape, and thickness involving both the infarcted and the noninfarcted segments of the ventricle described earlier occur and are collectively referred to as *ventricular remodeling*—which in turn can influence ventricular dimensions, function, and prognosis.[60,61,66] Changes in LV dilation combined with hypertrophy of residual noninfarcted myocardium cause remodeling. After infarct size, other important factors driving the process of LV dilation are ventricular volume, loading conditions, and infarct artery patency.[62] Elevated ventricular pressure contributes to increased wall stress and the risk for infarct expansion, but a patent infarct artery accelerates myocardial scar formation and increases tissue turgor in the infarct zone, thereby reducing the risk for infarct expansion and ventricular dilation. As discussed, inflammation is a key component in healing that may also govern the degree of adverse versus appropriate compensatory myocardial remodeling.[33] At immediate post-MI,

stiffness in diastole (see later), which occurs with infarcts involving only a small portion of the left ventricle. When the abnormally contracting segment exceeds 15% of the myocardium, the EF may decline, and LV end-diastolic pressure and volume may increase.[63] The risk for the development of physical signs and symptoms of LV failure also increases in proportion to increasing areas of abnormal LV wall motion. Clinical HF accompanies areas of abnormal contraction exceeding 25%, and loss of more than 40% of the LV myocardium usually leads to cardiogenic shock, often fatal.

Unless extension of the infarct occurs, some improvement in wall motion takes place during the healing phase, with recovery of function occurring in initially reversibly injured (stunned) myocardium (see Fig. 37.9). Regardless of the age of the infarct, patients who continue to demonstrate abnormal wall motion involving 20% to 25% of the left ventricle will probably manifest hemodynamic signs of LV failure, with its attendant poor prognosis for long-term survival.

Diastolic Function

The diastolic properties of the left ventricle change in ischemic and infarcted myocardium (see Chapters 46, 47, and 51). These alterations are associated with a decrease in the peak rate of decline in LV pressure (peak—dP/dt), an increase in the time constant of the fall in LV pressure, and an initial rise in LV end-diastolic pressure. Over several weeks, end-diastolic volume increases, and diastolic pressure begins to fall toward normal. As with impairment of systolic function, the magnitude of the diastolic abnormality appears to relate to the size of the infarct.

EF correlates only modestly with eventual LV volumes. Many large MIs do not lead to a poorly remodeled heart, while a subset of patients with relatively smaller infarcts progress to substantial adverse remodeling. Genetic or epigenetic differences in the regulation of the healing process resulting from a variable inflammatory response may explain in part the heterogeneous natural history of infarct healing.[66] Exaggerated ventricular dilation, for example, may result from an inflammatory process with excessive matrix degradation, whereas greater scar deposition and less dilation may follow an inflammatory process that preferentially stimulates a more profibrotic healing process.[67]

Infarct Expansion

An increase in the size of the infarcted segment, known as *infarct expansion*, is defined as "acute dilation and thinning of the area of infarction not explained by additional myocardial necrosis." Infarct expansion results from a combination of slippage between muscle bundles, which reduces the number of myocytes across the infarct wall, disruption of normal myocardial cells, and destruction of extracellular matrix within the necrotic zone. Infarct expansion involves thinning and dilation of the infarct zone before the formation of a firm, fibrotic scar. The degree of infarct expansion appears to be related to preinfarction wall thickness, with existing hypertrophy possibly protecting against infarct thinning.

On a cellular level, the degree of expansion and worsening remodeling depends on the intensity of the inflammatory response to the necrotic cells. Suppression of cytokine expression and stimulation may minimize the degree of inflammation and thus final infarct size.[33,37,66,67]

The apex, the thinnest region of the left ventricle, is particularly vulnerable to infarct expansion. Infarction of the apex secondary to LAD occlusion causes the radius of curvature at the apex to increase, thereby exposing this normally thin region to a marked elevation in wall stress.

Infarct expansion associates with both higher mortality and a higher incidence of nonfatal complications, such as HF and ventricular aneurysm. Infarct expansion is best recognized by elongation of the noncontractile region of the ventricle on echocardiography or CMR. When the expansion is severe enough to cause symptoms, the most characteristic clinical findings are deterioration of systolic function, new or worsening pulmonary congestion, and development of ventricular arrhythmias.

Ventricular Dilation

Although infarct expansion plays an important role in the ventricular remodeling that occurs early after MI, remodeling is also caused by dilation of the viable portion of the ventricle, which commences immediately after STEMI and progresses for months or years thereafter. A shift of the pressure-volume curve of the left ventricle to the right, which results in a larger LV volume at any given diastolic pressure and may accompany dilation. This dilation of the noninfarcted zone can be viewed as a compensatory mechanism that maintains stroke volume in the presence of a large infarction. This chronic dilation may also be a manifestation of a chronic inflammatory process affecting the myocardium that began at the time of the large infarct, but never fully resolved.[68] Large STEMIs place an extra load on the residual functioning myocardium, a burden that presumably causes the compensatory hypertrophy of the noninfarcted myocardium. This hypertrophy could help compensate for the functional impairment caused by the infarct and may be responsible for some of the hemodynamic improvement seen in some patients the months after infarction.

Effects of Treatment

Several factors can affect ventricular remodeling after STEMI, notably final infarct size (see Fig. 37.9).[69] Acute reperfusion and other measures to restrict the extent of myocardial necrosis limit the increase in ventricular volume after STEMI. Multiple pharmacologic agents that target reperfusion injury or regenerative therapies aimed at limiting infarct size have undergone evaluation in clinical trials, although few have produced significant results in adequately powered phase III investigations (see Chapter 38).[70] Appropriate and timely scar formation in the infarct also affects the degree of LV remodeling post-MI.

Glucocorticoids and nonsteroidal antiinflammatory drugs (NSAIDs) given early after MI can cause scar thinning and greater infarct expansion, whereas RAAS inhibitors attenuate the ventricular enlargement. Additional beneficial consequences of inhibition of angiotensin II that may contribute to myocardial protection include attenuation of endothelial dysfunction and direct antiatherogenic effects. Inhibition of aldosterone action may limit excessive fibrosis and decrease the development of ventricular arrhythmias. Whether other nonspecific or targeted anti-inflammatory agents can favorably modify remodeling and dilation still requires validation in larger clinical trials.[71]

Pathophysiology of Other Organ Systems

ENDOCRINE FUNCTION
Glucose Homeostasis (see Chapter 31)

Hyperglycemia is common in patients presenting with STEMI and associates with worse outcomes. Although patients with STEMI often have absolute concentrations of blood insulin in the normal range, these levels are usually inappropriately low for their blood sugar concentration, indicating insulin resistance.

Glucose permits the generation of ATP by anaerobic glycolysis, as opposed to free fatty acids (FFAs), which require aerobic conditions to furnish ATP. Because hypoxic heart muscle derives a considerable proportion of its energy from the metabolism of glucose (see Chapter 46), and because glucose uptake by the myocardium requires insulin, insulin deficiency can jeopardize the availability of energy. Despite these metabolic considerations, the most contemporary data indicate that maintaining glucose levels below 180 mg/dL, while avoiding hypoglycemia, is the safest post-MI glucose management strategy (see Chapter 38).

ACTIVATION OF THE RENIN-ANGIOTENSIN-ALDOSTERONE SYSTEM

Noninfarcted regions of the myocardium appear to exhibit activation of the tissue RAAS with increased production of angiotensin II. Both locally and systemically generated angiotensin II can stimulate the production of various growth factors, such as platelet-derived growth factor and TGF-β, that promote compensatory hypertrophy in the noninfarcted myocardium, as well as control the structure and tone of the infarct-related coronary and other myocardial vessels. Additional potential actions of angiotensin II that could aggravate infarction include the release of endothelin, plasminogen activator inhibitor (PAI)-1, and aldosterone, which may cause vasoconstriction, impair fibrinolysis, and increase sodium retention, respectively.[68]

THYROID GLAND

Although patients with STEMI are generally euthyroid clinically, serum triiodothyronine (T_3) levels can decrease transiently, a fall that is most marked on approximately the third day after the infarct. A rise in reverse T_3 usually accompanies this fall in T_3, with variable changes or no change in thyroxine (T_4) and thyroid-stimulating hormone levels.[68] The alteration in peripheral T_4 metabolism appears to correlate with infarct size and may result from the rise in endogenous levels of cortisol that accompanies STEMI.

HEMATOLOGIC ALTERATIONS
Platelets

STEMI generally occurs in the presence of extensive coronary and systemic atherosclerotic plaque, which may serve as the site for the formation of platelet aggregates—a sequence suggested as an early step in the process of coronary thrombosis, coronary occlusion, and subsequent MI. Platelets from patients with STEMI have an increased propensity for aggregation both systemically and locally in the area of disrupted plaque and release vasoactive substances. Thus, platelets are key therapeutic targets for the initial antithrombotic management in STEMI.

Hemostatic Markers

Elevated levels of serum fibrinogen degradation products, an end product of thrombosis, as well as release of distinctive proteins when platelets are activated (e.g., platelet factor 4, P-selectin), occur in some patients with STEMI. Fibrinopeptide A (FPA), a protein released from fibrin by thrombin, reflects ongoing thrombosis and increases during the early hours of STEMI. Marked elevation of hemostatic markers such as FPA, thrombin-antithrombin complex, and prothrombin fragment 1.2 associates with an increased risk for mortality in patients with STEMI.

CLINICAL FEATURES

Predisposing Factors
Up to one third of patients with STEMI have an identifiable precipitating trigger or prodromal symptoms. Unusually heavy exercise (particularly in fatigued or habitually inactive patients), emotional stress, and acute illness are the most frequent triggers.[72-74] Such infarctions could result from marked increases in myocardial oxygen consumption in the presence of severe coronary arterial narrowing (a type 2 MI), or the acute hemodynamic stress on a fragile plaque from a catecholamine or BP surge.

Accelerating angina and rest angina are two patterns of unstable angina that may culminate in STEMI (see Fig. 37.1). Noncardiac surgical procedures may also precede STEMI. Perioperative risk stratification and preventive measures may limit STEMI and cardiac-related mortality (see Chapter 23).[75] Reduced myocardial perfusion secondary to hypotension (e.g., hemorrhagic or septic shock) and the increased myocardial oxygen demands caused by aortic stenosis, fever, tachycardia, and agitation can also contribute to myocardial necrosis. Other factors reported to predispose to STEMI include respiratory infections, hypoxemia from any cause, pulmonary embolism, hypoglycemia, administration of ergot preparations, cocaine use, sympathomimetics, serum sickness, allergy, and rarely, wasp stings. In patients with Prinzmetal angina (see Chapter 40), STEMI may develop in the territory of the coronary artery that undergoes spasm.

Circadian Periodicity
The time of onset of STEMI has a pronounced circadian periodicity, with the peak incidence of events in the morning.[76] Circadian rhythms affect many physiologic and biochemical variables; plasma catecholamines and cortisol and platelet aggregability increase in the early morning hours. Patients receiving a beta-blocking agent or aspirin do not exhibit this characteristic circadian peak before the development of STEMI, consistent with precipitation by sympathetic stimuli or platelet activation. The concept of "triggering" a STEMI is complex and can involve the superimposition of multiple factors, such as the time of day, season, and the stress of natural disasters.

History
See also Chapters 13, 35, and 39.

Prodromal Symptoms
The patient's history remains crucial to diagnosing STEMI. Chest discomfort resembling classic angina pectoris usually characterizes the prodrome, but it occurs at rest or with less activity than usual. Yet the symptoms are often not disturbing enough to induce patients to seek immediate medical attention. A feeling of general malaise or frank exhaustion frequently accompanies other symptoms preceding STEMI.

Nature of the Pain
The symptoms associated with cardiac ischemia are reviewed in detail in Chapter 35. Pain in patients with STEMI varies in intensity; in most patients it is severe and in some instances is intolerable. The pain is prolonged—it generally lasts for more than 30 minutes and frequently for several hours if there is no reperfusion. In patients with preexisting angina pectoris, the pain of infarction generally resembles that of angina with respect to location, but it is normally much more severe, lasts longer, and is not relieved by rest or nitroglycerin.

STEMI pain may subside by the time that the physician first encounters the patient (or the patient reaches the hospital), or it may persist for many hours until adequate reperfusion (see Chapter 38). Both angina pectoris and STEMI pain likely arise from nerve endings in ischemic or injured, but not necrotic myocardium.

The pain often disappears suddenly and completely following restoration of blood flow to the infarct territory. Recurrent pain after initial reperfusion should prompt consideration of acute re-occlusion of the culprit lesion. Clinicians should *not* be complacent about ongoing plausibly ischemic pain. In some patients—particularly older adults, patients with diabetes, and heart transplant recipients—STEMI can manifest clinically not by chest discomfort but rather by symptoms of acute LV failure and chest tightness or by marked weakness or frank syncope.

Other Symptoms
Nausea and vomiting may occur, presumably because of activation of the vagal reflex or stimulation of LV receptors as part of the Bezold-Jarisch reflex. These symptoms occur more frequently in patients with inferior STEMI than with anterior STEMI. When the pain of STEMI is epigastric and associated with nausea and vomiting, the clinical picture can easily be confused with that of acute cholecystitis, gastritis, or peptic ulcer. Other symptoms include feelings of profound weakness, dizziness, palpitations, cold perspiration, and a sense of impending doom.

Differential Diagnosis
STEMI pain may overlap with that caused by acute pericarditis, acute aortic syndromes, pulmonary, and musculoskeletal discomfort, as discussed in detail in Chapter 35 (see Table 35.1).

"Silent" or Atypical Presentations of ST-Elevation Myocardial Infarction
STEMI can go unrecognized by the patient and may manifest only on subsequent routine electrocardiographic, imaging, or postmortem examination. Of these unrecognized infarctions, approximately half are truly silent, with patients unable to recall any symptoms. The other portion of patients with so-called silent infarction can recall an event characterized by symptoms compatible with acute MI in response to leading questions after finding ECG or imaging abnormalities. Unrecognized or silent infarction occurs more often in patients without antecedent angina pectoris and in patients with diabetes and hypertension and typically manifests as new wall motion abnormalities, fixed perfusion defects, or pathologic Q waves. Silent ischemia often follows silent STEMI (see Chapter 40). The prognosis of patients with silent and symptomatic manifestations of STEMI appears quite similar.[77,78]

Physical Examination (see also Chapters 13 and 38)

General Appearance
Patients suffering from STEMI often appear anxious and in considerable distress. An anguished facial expression is common, and—in contrast to patients with severe angina pectoris, who often lie, sit, or stand still because all forms of activity increase the discomfort—some patients suffering from STEMI may be restless and move about in an effort to find a comfortable position. They often massage or clutch their chests and frequently describe their pain with a clenched fist held against the sternum (Levine sign). In patients with LV failure and sympathetic stimulation, cold perspiration, and skin pallor may be evident; they typically sit or are propped up in bed and gasp for breath. Between breaths they may complain of chest discomfort or a feeling of suffocation. Cough producing frothy, pink, or blood-streaked sputum may occur if pulmonary edema is present. Patients in cardiogenic shock often lie listlessly and make few spontaneous movements. Their skin is cool and clammy, with a bluish or mottled color over the extremities, and there is marked facial pallor with severe cyanosis of the lips and nailbeds. Depending on the degree of cerebral perfusion, a patient in shock may converse normally or may be confused.

Heart Rate
The heart rate can vary from marked bradycardia to a rapid regular or irregular tachycardia, depending on the underlying rhythm and degree of LV failure. Typically, the pulse is rapid and regular initially (sinus tachycardia at 100 to 110 beats/min) and slows as the patient's pain and anxiety are relieved; premature ventricular contractions are common. Tachycardia at presentation associates with a higher risk for fatal complications of MI.

Blood Pressure

Most patients with uncomplicated STEMI are normotensive, although the reduced stroke volume accompanying the tachycardia can cause declines in systolic and pulse pressure and elevation of diastolic BP. In previously normotensive patients, a hypertensive response is occasionally seen during the first few hours, presumably because of adrenergic discharge due to pain, anxiety, and agitation. Previously hypertensive patients may become normotensive without treatment after STEMI, although many of them eventually regain their elevated BP levels, generally 3 to 6 months after infarction. In patients with massive infarction, the arterial pressure falls acutely because of LV dysfunction, and this drop may be exacerbated by morphine and/or nitrates, which cause venous pooling. During recovery, the arterial pressure tends to return to preinfarction levels.

Patients in cardiogenic shock by definition have systolic pressure below 90 mmHg and evidence of end-organ hypoperfusion.[65] Hypotension alone does not necessarily signify cardiogenic shock; some patients with inferior infarction and activation of the Bezold-Jarisch reflex may also transiently have a systolic BP below 90 mmHg. Their hypotension eventually resolves spontaneously, although IV atropine (0.5 to 1 mg) and adopting the Trendelenburg position can accelerate recovery. Other patients who are initially only slightly hypotensive may demonstrate gradually falling BP with a progressive reduction in cardiac output over several hours or days as cardiogenic shock develops because of ongoing ischemia or extension of infarction (see Fig. 37.15). Evidence of autonomic hyperactivity is common and varies with the type and location of the infarction. More than half of patients with inferior STEMI have evidence of excess parasympathetic stimulation, with hypotension, bradycardia, or both evident during initial evaluation, whereas approximately half of patients with anterior STEMI show signs of sympathetic excess and have hypertension, tachycardia, or both.

Temperature and Respiration

Fever, mediated by cytokine release from tissues undergoing necrosis, develops in most patients with extensive STEMI within 24 to 48 hours after the onset of infarction. Body temperature often begins to rise within 4 to 8 hours after onset of infarction, and rectal temperature may reach 38.3°C to 38.9°C (101°F to 102°F). The fever usually resolves by the fourth or fifth day after MI.

The respiratory rate may rise slightly after the development of STEMI; in patients without HF, it results from anxiety and pain and returns to normal after treating the physical and psychological discomfort. In patients with LV failure, the respiratory rate correlates with the severity of the failure; patients with significant pulmonary edema may have rates exceeding 40 breaths/min. However, the respiratory rate is not necessarily elevated in patients with cardiogenic shock. Cheyne-Stokes (periodic) respiration may occur in elderly individuals with cardiogenic shock or HF, particularly after opiate therapy or in the presence of cerebrovascular disease.

Jugular Venous Pulse

The jugular venous pulse is usually normal in STEMI involving the left ventricle. The *a*-wave may be prominent in patients with pulmonary hypertension secondary to LV failure or reduced compliance. In contrast, RV infarction (regardless of whether it accompanies LV infarction) often results in marked jugular venous distention and, if complicated by necrosis or ischemia of RV papillary muscles, in tall *c-v* waves of tricuspid regurgitation. Patients with STEMI and cardiogenic shock generally have elevated jugular venous pressure, although in the early phase, if RV function is relatively preserved, right-sided pressures may remain normal. In patients with STEMI, hypotension, and hypoperfusion (findings that may resemble those of patients with cardiogenic shock) without elevated jugular venous pressures, the depression in LV performance may be related to hypovolemia, at least in part. Assessing LV performance with echocardiography or by measuring LV filling pressure with a pulmonary artery catheter can help determine the cause of hypotension.

Carotid Pulse

Palpation of the carotid arterial pulse provides a clue to LV stroke volume: a small pulse suggests reduced stroke volume, whereas a sharp, brief upstroke often occurs in patients with mitral regurgitation or a ruptured ventricular septum with a left-to-right shunt. Pulsus alternans reflects severe LV dysfunction.

The Chest

Moist rales are audible in patients in whom LV failure or reduction in LV compliance leads to pulmonary edema. Diffuse wheezing can occur in patients with severe LV failure. Cough with hemoptysis, suggesting pulmonary embolism with infarction, can also occur. In 1967, Thomas Killip proposed a prognostic classification scheme on the basis of the presence and severity of rales in patients with STEMI. Class I patients have no rales and third heart sound (S_3). Class II patients have rales, but only to a mild to moderate degree (<50% of lung fields), and may or may not have an S_3. Class III patients have rales in more than half of each lung field and frequently have pulmonary edema. Class IV patients have cardiogenic shock. Despite the overall improvement in the mortality rate that applies to each category, the Killip classification still remains useful for prognostication.[65] Patients with RV infarct physiology or a ventricular septal defect can present with a relatively normal chest exam despite being in shock.

Cardiac Examination
Palpation

Palpation of the precordium may be normal, but in patients with transmural STEMI, it more often reveals a presystolic pulsation synchronous with an audible fourth heart sound (S_4), a finding reflecting vigorous left atrial contraction filling a ventricle with reduced compliance. Patients with LV systolic dysfunction may have a diffuse or dyskinetic LV impulse, or an outward movement of the left ventricle palpable in early diastole, coincident with an S_3.

Auscultation

HEART SOUNDS. The heart sounds, particularly the first sound, are frequently muffled and occasionally inaudible immediately after an infarct, and their intensity increases during convalescence. A soft first heart sound (S_1) may also reflect prolongation of the PR interval. Patients with marked ventricular dysfunction and/or left bundle branch block (LBBB) may have paradoxical splitting of the second heart sound (S_2). An S_4 is almost universally present in patients in sinus rhythm with STEMI, but it has limited diagnostic value because it is usually audible in most patients with chronic ischemic heart disease and is recordable, although not often audible, in many normal individuals older than 45. An S_3 in patients with STEMI reflect severe LV dysfunction with elevated ventricular filling pressure. It reflects rapid deceleration of transmitral blood flow during protodiastolic filling of the left ventricle and is typically heard in patients with large infarctions. S_3 is detected best at the apex with the patient in the left lateral recumbent position. An S_3 may result not only from LV failure but also from increased inflow into the left ventricle, as occurs when mitral regurgitation or a ventricular septal defect complicates STEMI. S_3 and S_4 emanating from the left ventricle are heard best at the apex, and in patients with RV infarcts, can be heard along the left sternal border and increase on inspiration.

MURMURS. Patients with STEMI typically have systolic murmurs, transient or persistent, that generally result from mitral regurgitation secondary to dysfunction of the mitral valve apparatus (papillary muscle dysfunction, or LV dilation). A new, prominent, apical holosystolic murmur accompanied by a thrill may represent rupture of a head of a papillary muscle. Rupture of the interventricular septum produces similar findings, although the murmur and thrill are usually most prominent along the left sternal border and may be audible at the right sternal border as well. The systolic murmur of tricuspid regurgitation (from RV failure caused by pulmonary hypertension or RV infarction, or from infarction of an RV papillary muscle) is also heard along the left sternal border. It is characteristically intensified by inspiration and is accompanied by a prominent *c-v* wave in the jugular venous pulse and an RV fourth sound.

FRICTION RUBS. Patients with STEMI may develop pericardial friction rubs. Rubs are notorious for their evanescence and thus are probably even more common than reported. Although friction rubs can be heard within 24 hours or as late as 2 weeks after onset of infarction, they occur most frequently on the second or third day. Occasionally, patients with extensive infarction can have a loud rub that lasts for many days. Patients with STEMI and a pericardial friction rub may have a pericardial effusion on echocardiographic study, but only rarely the classic ECG changes of pericarditis. Delayed onset of the rub and the associated discomfort of pericarditis (as late as 3 months after infarction) characterizes the now rare post-MI (Dressler) syndrome. Pericardial rubs are most readily audible along the left sternal border or just inside the apical impulse. Loud rubs may be audible over the entire precordium and even over the back. Occasionally, only the systolic portion of a rub is heard, which requires distinction from a systolic murmur, such as might result from rupture of the ventricular septum or mitral regurgitation.

Extremities

Coronary atherosclerosis is often associated with systemic atherosclerosis, and therefore patients with STEMI may have a history of intermittent claudication and may demonstrate the physical findings of peripheral vascular disease (see Chapter 43). Peripheral edema is a manifestation of RV failure and, as with congestive hepatomegaly, is unusual in patients with acute LV infarction. Cyanosis of the nailbeds is common in patients with severe LV failure and is particularly striking in patients with cardiogenic shock.

Neuropsychiatric Findings

Except for the altered mental status that occurs in patients with STEMI who have greatly reduced cardiac output and cerebral hypoperfusion, findings on neurologic examination are normal unless the patient has sustained a cerebral embolism secondary to mural thrombus. The association between these two conditions can be explained by systemic hypotension from STEMI precipitating a cerebral infarction, and vice versa, as well as by mural emboli from the left ventricle causing cerebral emboli. As discussed in Chapter 38, patients with STEMI frequently exhibit alterations in their emotional state, including intense anxiety, denial, and depression.

Laboratory Findings

Serum and Plasma Markers of Cardiac Damage

Proteins released into the blood from damaged myocardial cells can indicate myocardial injury. Ischemia leading to necrosis compromises the integrity of the sarcolemmal membrane. Intracellular macromolecules (serum and plasma cardiac markers) diffuse into the cardiac interstitium and ultimately into the microvasculature and lymphatics in the region of the infarct (Fig. 37.16; Table 37.3). The rate of appearance of these macromolecules in the peripheral circulation depends on several factors, including the degree of injury, the intracellular location, molecular weight, local blood and lymphatic flow, and the rate of elimination from blood.

Even though the availability of serum and plasma cardiac markers with greatly enhanced sensitivity for myocardial injury has enabled clinicians to identify much lower levels of injury, biochemical tests of myocardial injury provide no direct insight into the cause of the damage (Fig. 37.17).[1] Other nonischemic insults, such as myocarditis or direct myocardial toxins, may result in myocardial injury but should not be labeled MI. Moreover, the enhanced ability to detect myocardial damage has increased the number of cases of myocardial injury that result from non–plaque-related clinical events, thus necessitating the establishment of criteria for MI that place the injury in clinical context (see Tables 37.1 to 37.3).[1]

In patients with STEMI, clinicians should *not* wait for the results of biomarker assays to initiate treatment. Given the urgency for reperfusion in patients with STEMI, a rapid clinical assessment and the 12-lead ECG should serve to initiate such strategies. (A detailed review of markers of injury along with diagnostic decision making for patients with suspected ACS is presented in Chapter 35).

Recommendations for Measurement of Circulating Markers of Cardiac Injury in ST-Segment Elevation MI

All patients with suspected MI should undergo measurement of cardiac-specific troponin as soon as possible at the initial encounter (see Chapter 35). In patients with STEMI, the results of biomarker assessment should not delay interventions. From a cost-effectiveness perspective, measuring both a cardiac-specific troponin and CK-MB is unnecessary.[1]

Because of continuous release from a degenerating contractile apparatus in necrotic myocytes, elevations in cTnI may persist for 7 to 10 days after MI; elevations in cTnT may persist for up to 10 to 14 days (see Fig. 37.16). The prolonged time course of the elevation in cTnT and cTnI is advantageous for the late diagnosis of MI. Patients with STEMI who undergo successful recanalization of the infarct-related artery have a rapid release of cardiac troponins, which can indicate reperfusion (Fig. 37.18). It is not always necessary to repeatedly measure cTn levels after an MI until they reach their peak and decline. Due to the kinetics of cTn degradation, levels of cTn (and especially with high-sensitivity assays) may peak well after the infarct and remain elevated for days, in particular in large infarcts. Detecting reinfarctions should be based on the clinical scenario, ECG, and at least two serial tests. If the cTn concentrations are elevated but stable or declining at the time of the recurrent symptoms, then an elevation of greater than 20% indicates a reinfarction. If the initial concentration is normal, then the standard assay specific criteria and intervals for testing for MI should be used. Measuring concurrent CKMB may help identify early reinfarction because CKMB levels decline much faster than cTn.

Other Biomarkers (See Chapter 35)

Other biomarkers may be used noninvasively to assess the potential causes and identify patients at increased risk of complications of MI. Natriuretic peptides are released early after STEMI, with a peak at approximately 16 hours. The natriuretic peptides released from the left ventricle during STEMI originate both from the infarcted myocardium and from viable noninfarcted myocardium. The rise in B type natriuretic peptide (BNP) and N-terminal pro-B-type natriuretic peptide (NT-proBNP) after STEMI correlates with infarct size and regional wall motion abnormalities. Measurement of natriuretic peptides can provide useful information both early and late in the course of STEMI.[79,80] Although these additional biomarkers enhance risk assessment, no clear guidance is available on how to direct specific therapeutic maneuvers in the setting of STEMI based on these biomarkers. Future studies evaluating novel biomarkers should focus on unmet clinical scenarios such as earlier detection of MI, differentiation of type I from type 2 MI, distinguishing the mechanism of thrombosis (e.g., plaque rupture versus erosion), and improved risk stratification.

Other Laboratory Measurements

Serum Lipids

During the first 24 to 48 hours after admission, total cholesterol and high-density lipoprotein (HDL) cholesterol levels remain at or near baseline values, but they generally fall after that. The fall in HDL cholesterol after STEMI is greater than the fall in total cholesterol; thus, the ratio of total cholesterol to HDL cholesterol is no longer useful for risk assessment unless measured early after MI. All patients with STEMI admitted within 24 hours of symptom onset should have a lipid profile, although regardless of lipid levels and unless contraindicated, all patients with STEMI should receive high-intensity statin therapy. Lipid levels may still be clinically useful for patients admitted beyond 24 to 48 hours, but further measurements 4 to 8 weeks after MI provide more information on serum lipid concentrations. Increased triglycerides may offer additional risk stratification beyond LDL and HDL cholesterol levels (see Chapter 27).[81]

Hematologic Findings

Elevation of the white blood cell count usually develops within 2 hours after the onset of chest pain, reaches a peak 2 to 4 days after infarction, and returns to normal in 1 week; the peak leukocyte count generally ranges between 12 and 15 × 10³/mL but occasionally rises to as high as 20 × 10³/mL in patients with large STEMI. Frequently, there is an increase in the percentage of polymorphonuclear leukocytes and a left shift of the differential count. In epidemiologic studies, higher white blood cell

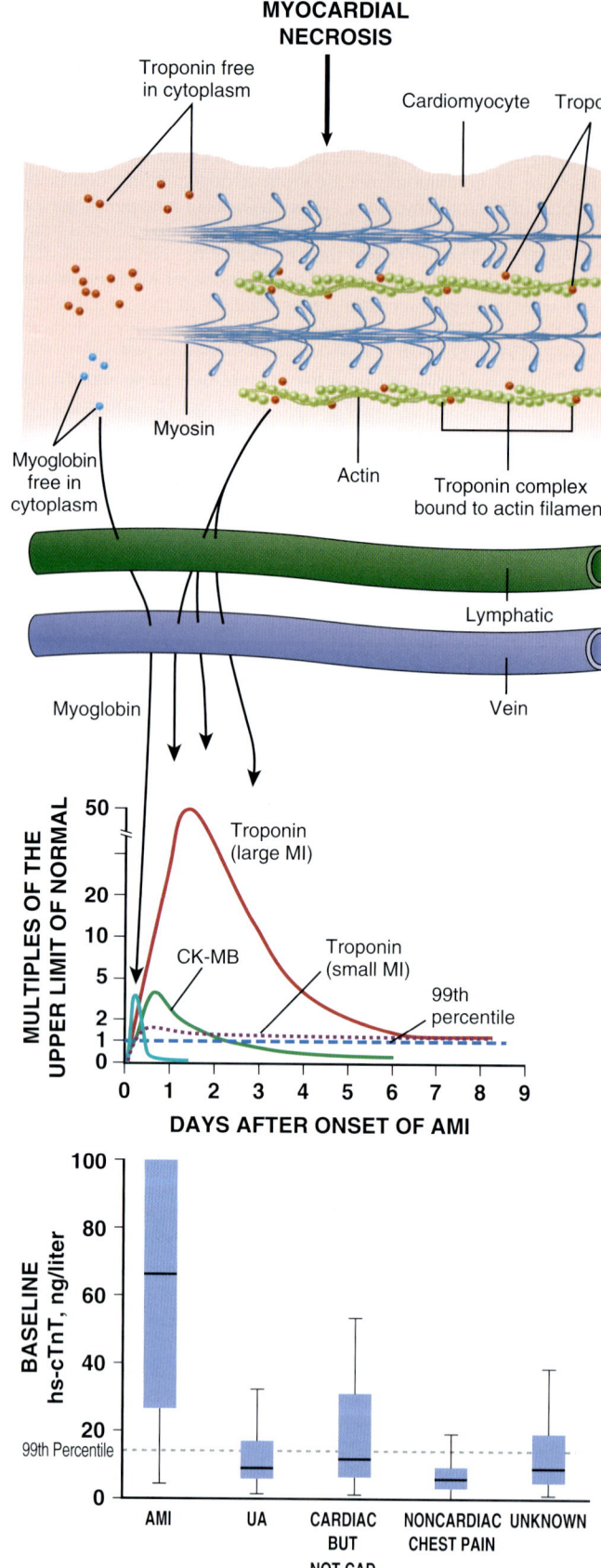

FIGURE 37.16 Release of biomarkers into the circulation begins with prolonged ischemia and subsequent necrosis that results in loss of integrity of the cellular membranes. After disruption of the sarcolemmal membrane of the cardiomyocyte, the cytoplasmic pool of biomarkers is released first (leftmost arrow in **bottom** portion of the **top panel**). Markers such as myoglobin are released rapidly, and blood levels rise quickly above the cutoff limit. More protracted release of biomarkers from the disintegrating myofilaments follows and may continue for several days (three-headed arrow). Cardiac troponin levels rise to substantially higher multiples of the upper reference limit (the 99th percentile of values in a reference control group) compared with CK-MB in patients with acute myocardial infarction (MI) and sustain sufficient myocardial necrosis that results in abnormally elevated levels of CK-MB. Clinicians can now diagnose MI by more sensitive assays that detect even small elevations in cardiac troponin above the upper reference limit, even though levels of CK-MB and troponin determined from older generations of assays may still be below the MI decision limit. Other causes of myocardial injury, such as renal failure or pulmonary embolism, can lead to detectable levels of cardiac troponin even without any coronary artery disease **(lower panel).** *AMI,* Acute myocardial infarction; *CAD,* coronary artery disease; *UA,* unstable angina. (Modified from Antman EM. Decision making with cardiac troponin tests. *N Engl J Med.* 2002;346:2079; Jaffe AS, Babuin L, Apple FS. Biomarkers in acute cardiac disease: the present and the future. *J Am Coll Cardiol.* 2006;48:1; and Reichlin T, Schindler C, Drexler B, et al. One-hour rule-out and rule-in of acute myocardial infarction using high-sensitivity cardiac troponin T. *Arch Intern Med.* 2012;172:1211.)

counts at initial evaluation in patients with an ACS associated with an increased risk for adverse clinical outcomes.[82] Experimental evidence suggests that the surge in catecholamines after coronary occlusion can mobilize leukocyte progenitors from bone marrow, thereby sustaining the inflammatory response following infarction.[33]

The hemoglobin value at initial evaluation of a patient with STEMI is strongly associated with the risk of recurrent major cardiovascular events following a J-shaped relationship. Cardiovascular mortality increases progressively as the initial hemoglobin value falls below 14 to 15 g/dL; conversely, it also rises as the hemoglobin level increases above 17 g/dL. The increased risk from anemia is probably related to diminished tissue delivery of oxygen, whereas the increased risk with polycythemia may be relates to an increase in blood viscosity.[83]

Electrocardiography

The ECG remains the most important diagnostic test in the evaluation of patients with suspected ischemic symptoms (see Chapter 14). Patients with chest pain and ECG changes consistent with or concerning for STEMI must be considered for immediate reperfusion. In addition to the typical ECG presentations of STEMI (see Table 37.3) there are atypical ECG presentations (Table 37.4). Because the right bundle is supplied by the septal perforators off the LAD, evidence of a new RBBB with a Q-wave in V1 in setting of STEMI is a specific but nonsensitive sign of an anteroseptal MI.[1,17]

Analysis of the constellation of ECG leads showing ST elevation may also be useful for identifying the site of occlusion in the infarct artery (see Fig. 37.4). The extent of ST deviation on the ECG, location of the infarction, and the QRS duration correlate with the risk for adverse outcomes. In addition to the diagnostic and prognostic information contained within the 12-lead ECG, the degree of ST-segment resolution provides valuable noninvasive information about the success of reperfusion for STEMI, regardless of whether it was achieved with fibrinolysis or primary coronary intervention (see Chapter 38).

Although general agreement exists on electrocardiographic and vectorcardiographic criteria for the recognition of infarction of the anterior and inferior myocardial walls, less agreement exists on criteria for lateral and posterior infarcts. Instead of "posterior," the descriptor "inferobasal" may be more appropriate given the segmental anatomy of the heart as it sits in the thorax and can often be identified with adding leads in the V_7 and V_8 position. Patients with an abnormal R wave in V_1 (0.04 second in duration and/or R/S ratio ≥1 in the absence of preexcitation or RV hypertrophy) and inferior or lateral Q waves have an increased incidence of isolated occlusion of a dominant left circumflex coronary artery without collateral circulation; such patients have a lower EF, increased end-systolic volume, and higher complication rate than do those with inferior infarction because of isolated occlusion of the RCA. ST-segment elevations in aVR, reflecting the basal intraventricular septum, can be observed in up to 30% of STEMIs and identifies patients with a higher likelihood of left main coronary artery or multivessel disease and worse outcomes.[84]

Serial changes on the ECG develop in most patients with STEMI, but many factors limit the usefulness of the ECG in diagnosing and localizing MI: the extent of myocardial injury, age of the infarct, its location,

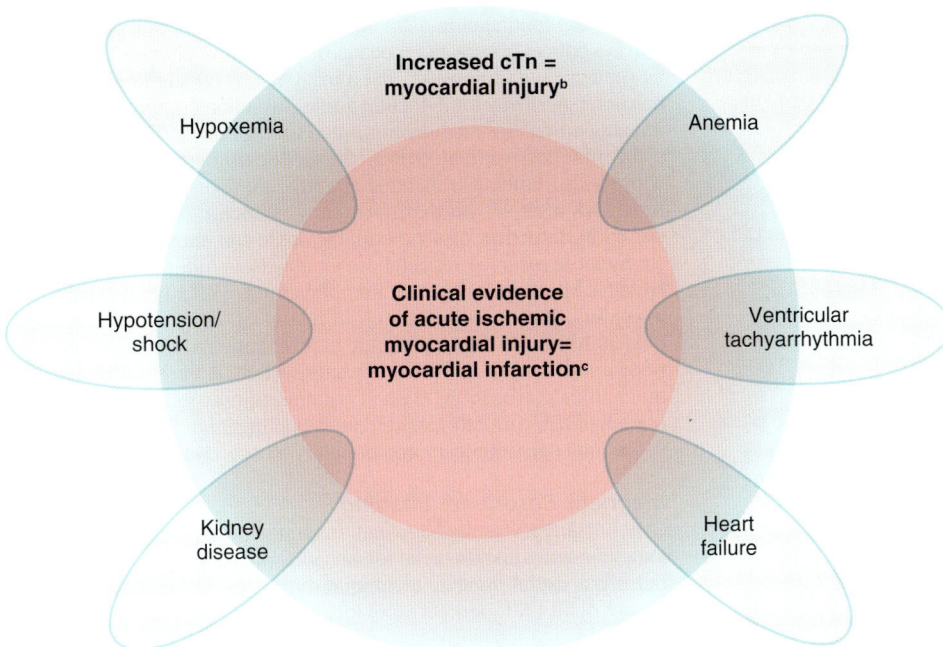

FIGURE 37.17 Spectrum of myocardial injury, ranging from no injury to myocardial infarction. Various clinical entities may involve these myocardial categories, for example, ventricular tachyarrhythmia, heart failure, kidney disease, hypotension/shock, hypoxemia, and anemia. cTn, cardiac troponin; URL, upper reference limit. [a]No myocardial injury = cTn values ≤99th percentile URL or not detectable. [b]Myocardial injury = cTn values >99th percentile URL. [c]Myocardial infarction = clinical evidence of myocardial ischemia and a rise and/or fall of cTn values >99th percentile URL. (From Thygesen K, Alpert JS, Jaffe AS, et al. Fourth universal definition of myocardial infarction (2018). *J Am Coll Cardiol.* 2018;72:2231–2264.)

presence of conduction defects, previous infarcts or acute pericarditis, and changes in electrolyte concentrations. Abnormalities in the ST segment and T wave can be quite nonspecific and may occur in a variety of conditions, including stable and unstable angina pectoris, ventricular hypertrophy, acute and chronic pericarditis, myocarditis, early repolarization, electrolyte imbalance, shock, and metabolic disorders, as well as after administration of digitalis. Serial ECGs help in differentiating these conditions from STEMI, although for early triage decisions, concurrent imaging may help distinguish potential STEMI from other etiologies. Many patients bear the stigmata of a STEMI on the ECG for the rest of their lives, particularly if Q waves evolve, but in a substantial minority the typical changes disappear, the Q waves regress, and findings on the ECG can even return to normal. Conditions that may mimic the electrocardiographic features of MI by producing a pattern of "pseudoinfarction" include ventricular hypertrophy, conduction disturbances, preexcitation, primary myocardial disease, pneumothorax, pulmonary embolism, amyloid heart disease, hypertrophic cardiomyopathy, primary and metastatic tumors of the heart, traumatic heart disease, intracranial hemorrhage, hyperkalemia, pericarditis, early repolarization, forms of muscular dystrophy, and cardiac sarcoidosis.

Q Wave and Non–Q Wave Infarction

The presence or absence of Q waves on the surface ECG does not reliably distinguish between transmural and nontransmural (subendocardial) MI. Q waves on the ECG signify abnormal electrical activity but do not imply irreversible myocardial damage, although Q waves associate with worse outcomes. Also, the absence of Q waves may simply reflect the insensitivity of the standard 12-lead ECG, especially in zones of the left ventricle supplied by the left circumflex artery (see Fig. 37.4).

Ischemia at a Distance

Patients with new Q waves and ST-segment elevation diagnostic of STEMI in one territory often have ST-segment depression in other territories. These additional ST-segment abnormalities, which imply a poor prognosis, result either from ischemia in a territory other than the area of infarction, termed *ischemia at a distance*, as noted above, or from reciprocal electrical phenomena. ST-segment depression in the anterior leads in the setting of acute inferior STEMI may be caused by concurrent anterior ischemia, inferolateral wall infarction, or true reciprocal changes. Although precordial ST-segment depression associates more often with extensive infarction of the lateral or inferior septal segments than with anterior wall subendocardial ischemia, echocardiography can evaluate the presence of an anterior wall motion abnormality.

Right Ventricular Infarction

ST-segment elevation in the right precordial leads (V_1, V_3R through V_6R) is a moderately sensitive and specific sign of RV infarction.[85] Occasionally, ST-segment elevation in V_2 and V_3 results from acute RV infarction; this appears to occur only when injury to the left inferior wall is minimal. Usually, the concurrent inferior wall injury suppresses this anterior ST-segment elevation resulting from RV injury. Similarly, RV infarction appears to reduce the anterior ST-segment depression often

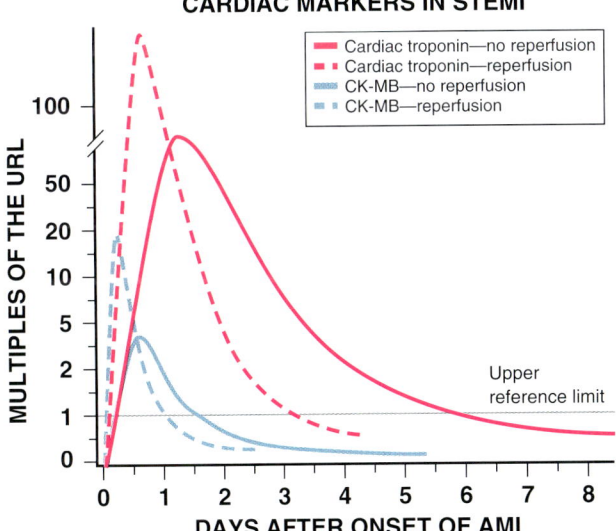

FIGURE 37.18 The kinetics of the release of CK-MB and cardiac troponin in patients who do not undergo reperfusion is shown in the *solid blue* and *red curves* as multiples of the upper reference limit (URL). When patients with ST-segment elevation myocardial infarction (STEMI) undergo reperfusion, as depicted in the *dashed blue* and *red curves,* the cardiac biomarkers are detected sooner and rise to a higher peak value but decline more rapidly, which results in a smaller area under the curve and limitation of infarct size. AMI, Acute myocardial infarction. (Modified from Antman EM, Anbe DT, Armstrong PW, et al. ACC/AHA guidelines for the management of patients with ST-elevation myocardial infarction: a report of the American College of Cardiology/American Heart Association Task Force on Practice Guidelines [Committee to Revise the 1999 Guidelines for the Management of Patients with Acute Myocardial Infarction]. *J Am Coll Cardiol* 2004;44:671–719.)

TABLE 37.4 Atypical Electrocardiographic Presentations That Should Prompt a Primary Percutaneous Coronary Intervention Strategy in Patients With Ongoing Symptoms Consistent With Myocardial Ischemia

Bundle Branch Block
Criteria that can be used to improve the diagnostic accuracy of STEMI in LBBB: • Concordant ST-segment elevation ≥1 mm in leads with a positive QRS complex   • Concordant ST-segment depression ≥1 mm in V_1–V_2 • Discordant ST-segment elevation ≥5 mm in leads with a negative QRS complex
The presence of RBBB may confound the diagnosis of STEMI
Ventricular Paced Rhythm
During RV pacing, the ECG also shows LBBB, and the above rules also apply for the diagnosis of myocardial infarction during pacing; however, they are less specific
Isolated Posterior Myocardial Infarction
Isolated ST depression ≥0.5 mm in leads V_1–V_2 and ST-segment elevation (≥0.5 mm) in posterior chest wall leads V_7–V_9
Ischemia Due to Left Main Coronary Artery Occlusion or Multivessel Disease
ST depression ≥1 mm in eight or more surface leads, coupled with ST-segment elevation in aVR and/or V_1, suggests left main-, or left main equivalent-coronary obstruction, or severe three vessel ischemia

ECG, Electrocardiogram; *LBBB*, left bundle branch block; *RBBB*, right bundle branch block; *RV*, right ventricular; *STEMI*, ST-segment deviation myocardial infarction.
From Thygesen K, Alpert JS, Jaffe AS, et al. Fourth universal definition of myocardial infarction (2018). *J Am Coll Cardiol.* 2018;72:2231–2264.

observed with inferior wall MI. A QS or QR pattern in V_3R and V_4R also suggests RV myocardial necrosis but has less predictive accuracy than ST-segment elevation in these leads.

Imaging

The value that noninvasive imaging provides in STEMI depends on the clinical timing and context. In most STEMI cases with a clear clinical history and unambiguous ECG, there is little role for noninvasive imaging as it only delays reperfusion. If the diagnosis of STEMI is not clear, then noninvasive imaging with echocardiography can provide useful diagnostic information to guide further evaluation or therapy. After the initial management of STEMI, imaging is key to determine the extent of the infarct, the presence of mechanical complications, and the overall function of the right and left ventricles.

Radiography

The initial chest radiograph in patients with STEMI is almost invariably a portable film obtained in the emergency department or cardiac intensive care unit (see Chapter 17). Chest imaging should not delay primary reperfusion strategies, unless there is a reason to evaluate a particular suspected pulmonary pathology. When present, prominent pulmonary vascular markings on the radiograph reflect elevated LV end-diastolic pressure, but significant temporal discrepancies can occur because of *diagnostic* and *post-therapeutic lags*. Up to 12 hours can elapse before pulmonary edema accumulates after ventricular filling pressure has increased. The post-therapeutic phase lag represents a longer interval; up to 2 days is required for pulmonary edema to resolve and the radiographic signs of pulmonary congestion to clear after ventricular filling pressure have returned toward normal. The degree of congestion and the size of the left side of the heart on the chest film are useful for defining groups of patients with STEMI who have an increased risk for fatal complications.

Echocardiography

The portability of echocardiographic equipment and point-of-care devices makes this technique ideal for the assessment of patients with suspected MI (see Chapter 16).[86] In patients with active chest pain compatible with ischemia but with a nondiagnostic ECG, the finding of a regional wall motion abnormality supports the diagnosis of myocardial ischemia. Echocardiography can also aid the evaluation of patients with chest pain and a nondiagnostic ECG who are suspected of having aortic dissection. Identification of an intimal flap consistent with aortic dissection is a critical observation because it would drive changes in therapeutic strategy (see Chapter 42), but transthoracic echocardiography (TTE) has poor sensitivity for detecting aortic dissection compared with other imaging modalities, such as computed tomography (CT) angiography.

LV function estimated from an echocardiogram correlates well with measurements from angiography and is useful in establishing prognosis after MI. Furthermore, early echocardiography can aid in the early detection of a potentially viable but stunned myocardium (contractile reserve), residual provocable ischemia, patients at risk for HF after MI, and mechanical complications of MI such as ventricular thrombus, acute mitral or tricuspid regurgitation, or ventricular septal defects. Although TTE is adequate in most patients, some patients have poor echocardiographic windows, especially if they are undergoing mechanical ventilation. In such patients, transesophageal echocardiography (TEE) or CMR can help in evaluating infarct size and location, ventricular septal defects, and papillary muscle dysfunction.

Magnetic Resonance Imaging

CMR imaging has limited application during the acute phase because of long scan-times and the need to transport patients with MI to the scanner, but it is a useful imaging technique during the subacute and chronic phases of MI. CMR permits exact localizing and sizing the area of infarction and a quantitative assessment of the severity of the ischemic insult (see Chapter 19). This modality is attractive because of its ability to assess perfusion of infarcted and noninfarcted tissue, as well as reperfused myocardium[87,88]; identify areas of jeopardized but not infarcted myocardium; identify myocardial edema, fibrosis, wall thinning, and hypertrophy; assess ventricular chamber size and segmental wall motion; and identify the temporal transition between ischemia and infarction (Fig. 37.19).[63,87,88] Because of these capabilities, CMR may be particularly useful in the diagnostic assessment of possible etiologies in MINOCA.[50]

Contrast-enhanced CMR with gadolinium can accurately define areas of myocardial necrosis. The transmural extent of late gadolinium enhancement (LGE) in regions of dysfunctional myocardium accurately predicts the likelihood of recovery of contractile function after successful restoration of coronary flow by mechanical revascularization.[89] Numerous clinical studies have also demonstrated the high sensitivity of LGE ("delayed hyperenhancement") in detecting small amounts of myonecrosis. LGE accurately identifies the infarct zone compared with histologic examination. The best predictor of return to normal ventricular wall thickening is less than 25% transmurality of LGE. LGE is also a sensitive technique for detecting RV infarcts.

In patients with a previous MI, estimation of the size of the peri-infarct zone by CMR with the delayed-enhancement technique provides incremental prognostic value beyond LV volume and EF. Besides detecting infarction, this imaging technique can characterize the presence and size of microvascular obstruction and intramyocardial hemorrhage as a result of infarction, which may be an even poorer prognostic finding than the extent of LGE.[88]

Nuclear Imaging

Radionuclide angiography, perfusion imaging, infarct-avid scintigraphy, and positron emission tomography (PET) can all evaluate patients with suspected ACS but have no role in the acute management of STEMI (see Chapter 18).[86] Nuclear cardiac imaging techniques can assess infarct size, collateral flow, and jeopardized myocardium ("myocardium at risk"); determine the effects of the infarct on ventricular function; and establish the prognosis of patients with STEMI.[90] However, echocardiography and CMR provide more relevant information regarding valvular and structural function than nuclear imaging.

Computed Tomography

CT can assess the cavity dimensions and wall thickness, can detect LV aneurysms, and—of particular importance in patients with STEMI—can identify intracardiac thrombi (see Chapter 20). Coronary CT angiography is sensitive in detecting coronary obstructions and may improve the diagnostic evaluation of patients with a low to intermediate probability of ACS, but it does not have a role in the management of suspected STEMI.[86]

Estimation of Infarct Size

Interest in limiting infarct size, largely because of the recognition that the quantity of infarcted myocardium has important prognostic implications, has focused attention on accurate determination of MI size. As reviewed earlier, the relationship between infarct size and subsequent changes in LV volumes and function is not directly linear. Other factors such as residual ischemia, inflammation, and therapy can affect eventual ventricular function and prognosis.[66] However, the degree of infarcted myocardium remains a strong predictor of subsequent outcomes.[69]

ELECTROCARDIOGRAPHY. The sum of ST-segment elevations measured from multiple precordial leads correlates with the extent of myocardial injury in patients with anterior MI. Moreover, a relationship exists between the number of ECG leads showing ST-segment elevation and the mortality rate: patients with 8 or 9 of 12 leads showing ST-segment elevation have three to four times the mortality of those with ST elevations in only 2 or 3.

CARDIAC MARKERS. Estimation of infarct size by analysis of serum or plasma cardiac markers of necrosis requires accounting for the quantity of the marker lost from the myocardium, its volume of distribution, and its release ratio. Serial measurements of proteins released by necrotic myocardium can help to determine MI size. Clinically, the peak troponin or CK-MB level provides an approximate estimate of infarct size.[91] Coronary artery reperfusion dramatically changes the washout kinetics of necrosis markers from myocardium, thereby resulting in early and exaggerated peak levels (see Fig. 37.18). Measuring cardiac-specific troponin level several days after STEMI, even in cases of successful reperfusion, may provide a reliable estimate of infarct size because such late troponin measurements reflect delayed release from the myofilament-bound pool in damaged myocytes.

NONINVASIVE IMAGING TECHNIQUES. The imaging modalities previously discussed can aid in experimental and clinical assessment of infarct size.[86] Echocardiography remains the most frequently used modality for assessing infarct size and LV function, although contrast-enhanced CMR can detect smaller degrees of ischemia and identify permanently damaged areas of the myocardium versus "stunned" regions, which may recover. Nuclear imaging and CMR can quantify the extent of infarct size more reliably than echocardiography. Even among patients undergoing primary PCI, the infarct size is associated strongly with worse outcomes, in particular during the first 6 months.[63,90] CMR can also discern the regional heterogeneity of infarction patterns in patients with persistently occluded infarct arteries or severe microvascular occlusion versus those with a successfully reperfused macrocirculation and microcirculation.

FUTURE PERSPECTIVES

The remarkable advances in understanding the cellular and molecular mechanisms of myocardial ischemic injury, coupled with recent insights into the mechanisms during repair and healing of the infarcted myocardium, have identified potential targets for "tuning" the healing response to optimize the repair process in ischemically injured myocardium and minimize adverse LV remodeling. We still triage patients who present with ACS on the basis of the ECG, but we should strive toward a more mechanistically based categorization of ACS that reflects the underlying biologic basis of the acute ischemic insult. To fill this gap, we need to seek, refine, and validate biomarkers of the different pathologic pathways that provoke acute myocardial ischemia and then apply at point of care, more mechanistically based therapies. Such biomarker-guided personalized therapy would thus achieve more precision in the care of ACS patients. For example, markers that distinguish fibrous cap rupture from superficial erosion as triggers to thrombus formation might inform different management strategies. This hypothesis would require rigorous validation but could lead to a more personalized management strategy.

We understand more clearly the different pathways in formation of coronary thrombi, but not all acute ischemic events result from clot formation. Past research centered on epicardial coronary artery spasm as a contributor to acute ischemic event, but we now recognize that dysfunction of smaller intramyocardial arteries may also provoke ischemia without necessarily causing evident thrombosis.[30] The spectrum of ischemic processes ranging from MINOCA and in the extreme stress (takotsubo) cardiomyopathy highlight the need for greater investigation into the microvasculature, to understand better the underlying mechanism of these diseases, and identify novel therapeutic strategies. Thus, although we have made considerable inroads in understanding and treating ACS in the last decades, the residual risk remains unacceptable. We must strive to expand our mechanistic understanding of the pathophysiology of ACS to address this residual burden and achieve the promise of precision medicine.

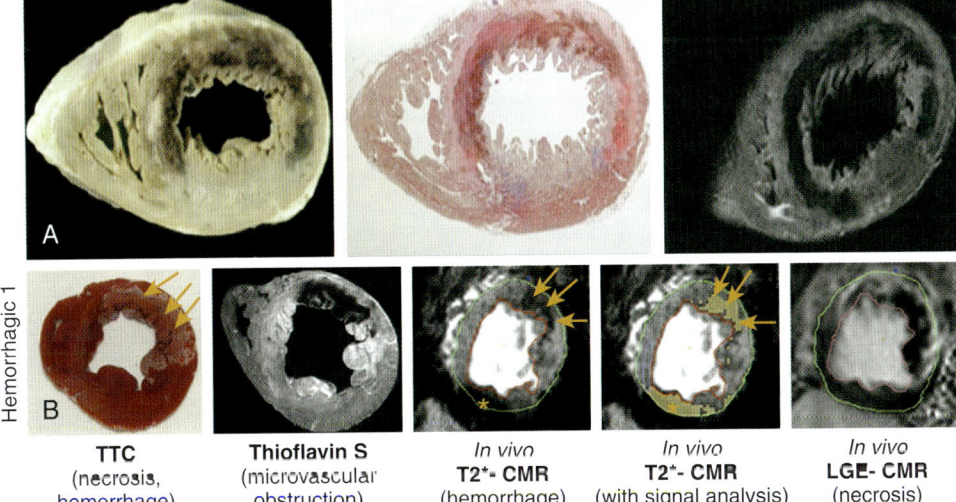

FIGURE 37.19 Cardiac magnetic resonance (CMR) images in myocardial infarction. **A,** *Left to right,* Gross anatomic image obtained at autopsy, histology image after staining with Heidenhain trichrome stain, and ex vivo T2-weighted CMR image from the short-axis slice. **B,** *Left to right,* Images from an experimentally induced MI in a dog. CMR was performed day 3 after reperfusion in which T2*-weighted gradient-echo imaging was performed. Ex vivo, thioflavin S imaging, and triphenyltetrazolium chloride (TTC) staining were performed to assess for microvascular obstruction (MVO), hemorrhage, and myocardial necrosis. *LGE,* Late gadolinium enhancement. (From Hamirani YS, Wong A, Kramer CM, et al. Effect of microvascular obstruction and intramyocardial hemorrhage by CMR on LV remodeling and outcomes after myocardial infarction: a systematic review and meta-analysis. *JACC Cardiovasc Imaging.* 2014;7:940–952.)

REFERENCES

Changing Patterns in Incidence and Care

1. Thygesen K, Alpert JS, Jaffe AS, et al. Fourth universal definition of myocardial infarction (2018). *J Am Coll Cardiol*. 2018;72(18):2231–2264.
2. Sandoval Y, Thygesen K, Jaffe AS. The universal definition of myocardial infarction: present and future. *Circulation*. 2020;141(18):1434–1436.
3. Virani SS, Alonso A, Benjamin EJ, et al. Heart disease and stroke statistics-2020 update: a report from the American Heart Association. *Circulation*. 2020;141(9):e139–e596.
4. Szummer K, Wallentin L, Lindhagen L, et al. Improved outcomes in patients with ST-elevation myocardial infarction during the last 20 years are related to implementation of evidence-based treatments: experiences from the SWEDEHEART registry 1995-2014. *Eur Heart J*. 2017;38(41):3056–3065.
5. Sacks NC, Ash AS, Ghosh K, et al. Trends in acute myocardial infarction hospitalizations: are we seeing the whole picture? *Am Heart J*. 2015;170(6):1211–1219.
6. Gerber Y, Weston SA, Jiang R, Roger VL. The changing epidemiology of myocardial infarction in Olmsted County, Minnesota, 1995-2012. *Am J Med*. 2015;128(2):144–151.
7. Wu WY, Berman AN, Biery DW, Blankstein R. Recent trends in acute myocardial infarction among the young. *Curr Opin Cardiol*. 2020;35(5):524–530.
8. DeFilippis EM, Collins BL, Singh A, et al. Women who experience a myocardial infarction at a young age have worse outcomes compared with men: the Mass General Brigham YOUNG-MI registry. *Eur Heart J*. 2020.
9. Arora S, Stouffer GA, Kucharska-Newton AM, et al. Twenty year trends and sex differences in young adults hospitalized with acute myocardial infarction. *Circulation*. 2019;139(8):1047–1056.
10. Sacks NC, Ash AS, Ghosh K, et al. Recent national trends in acute myocardial infarction hospitalizations in Medicare: shrinking declines and growing disparities. *Epidemiology*. 2015;26(4):e46–e47.
11. Roth GA, Huffman MD, Moran AE, et al. Global and regional patterns in cardiovascular mortality from 1990 to 2013. *Circulation*. 2015;132(17):1667–1678.
12. Kwan GF, Mayosi BM, Mocumbi AO, et al. Endemic cardiovascular diseases of the poorest billion. *Circulation*. 2016;133(24):2561–2575.
13. Krumholz HM, Normand ST, Wang Y. Twenty-year trends in outcomes for older adults with acute myocardial infarction in the United States. *JAMA Netw Open*. 2019;2(3):e191938.
14. Ford ES, Roger VL, Dunlay SM, et al. Challenges of ascertaining national trends in the incidence of coronary heart disease in the United States. *J Am Heart Assoc*. 2014;3(6):e001097.
15. Jernberg T, Hasvold P, Henriksson M, et al. Cardiovascular risk in post-myocardial infarction patients: nationwide real world data demonstrate the importance of a long-term perspective. *Eur Heart J*. 2015;36(19):1163–1170.
16. Levine GN, Bates ER, Blankenship JC, et al. 2015 ACC/AHA/SCAI focused update on primary percutaneous coronary intervention for patients with ST-elevation myocardial infarction: an update of the 2011 ACCF/AHA/SCAI guideline for percutaneous coronary intervention and the 2013 ACCF/AHA guideline for the management of ST-elevation myocardial infarction. *J Am Coll Cardiol*. 2016;67(10):1235–1250.
17. Ibanez B, James S, Agewall S, et al. 2017 ESC Guidelines for the management of acute myocardial infarction in patients presenting with ST-segment elevation: the Task Force for the Management of Acute Myocardial Infarction in Patients Presenting With ST-Segment Elevation of the European Society of Cardiology (ESC). *Eur Heart J*. 2018;39(2):119–177.
18. Wasfy JH, Borden WB, Secemsky EA, et al. Public reporting in cardiovascular medicine: accountability, unintended consequences, and promise for improvement. *Circulation*. 2015;131(17):1518–1527.
19. Granger CB, Bates ER, Jollis JG, et al. Improving care of STEMI in the United States 2008 to 2012. *J Am Heart Assoc*. 2019;8(1):e008096.
20. Chung SC, Gedeborg R, Nicholas O, et al. Acute myocardial infarction: a comparison of short-term survival in national outcome registries in Sweden and the UK. *Lancet*. 2014;383(9925):1305–1312.
21. Hira RS, Bhatt DL, Fonarow GC, et al. Temporal trends in care and outcomes of patients receiving fibrinolytic therapy compared to primary percutaneous coronary intervention: insights from the get with the Guidelines Coronary Artery Disease (GWTG-CAD) registry. *J Am Heart Assoc*. 2016;5(10).
22. Park J, Choi KH, Lee JM, et al. Prognostic implications of door-to-balloon time and onset-to-door time on mortality in patients with ST-segment-elevation myocardial infarction treated with primary percutaneous coronary intervention. *J Am Heart Assoc*. 2019;8(9):e012188.
23. Jolly SS, Cairns J, Yusuf S, et al. Procedural volume and outcomes with radial or femoral access for coronary angiography and intervention. *J Am Coll Cardiol*. 2014;63(10):954–963.
24. D'Onofrio G, Safdar B, Lichtman JH, et al. Sex differences in reperfusion in young patients with ST-segment-elevation myocardial infarction: results from the VIRGO study. *Circulation*. 2015;131(15):1324–1332.
25. Stehli J, Martin C, Brennan A, et al. Sex differences persist in time to presentation, revascularization, and mortality in myocardial infarction treated with percutaneous coronary intervention. *J Am Heart Assoc*. 2019;8(10):e012161.
26. Bagai A, Lu D, Lucas J, et al. Temporal trends in utilization of cardiac therapies and outcomes for myocardial infarction by degree of chronic kidney disease: a report from the NCDR chest pain-MI registry. *J Am Heart Assoc*. 2018;7(24):e010394.
27. McCabe JM, Waldo SW, Kennedy KF, Yeh RW. Treatment and outcomes of acute myocardial infarction complicated by shock after public reporting policy changes in New York. *JAMA Cardiol*. 2016.
28. Blumenthal DM, Valsdottir LR, Zhao Y, et al. A survey of interventional cardiologists' attitudes and beliefs about public reporting of percutaneous coronary intervention. *JAMA Cardiol*. 2018;3(7):629–634.

Pathophysiology

29. Tomaniak M, Katagiri Y, Modolo R, et al. Vulnerable plaques and patients: state-of-the-art. *Eur Heart J*. 2020;41(31):2997–3004.
30. Libby P, Pasterkamp G, Crea F, Jang IK. Reassessing the mechanisms of acute coronary syndromes. *Cir Res*. 2019;124(1):150–160.
31. Costopoulos C, Maehara A, Huang Y, et al. Heterogeneity of plaque structural stress is increased in plaques leading to MACE: insights from the PROSPECT study. *JACC Cardiovasc Imaging*. 2020;13(5):1206–1218.
32. Motoyama S, Ito H, Sarai M, et al. Plaque characterization by coronary computed tomography angiography and the likelihood of acute coronary events in mid-term follow-up. *J Am Coll Cardiol*. 2015;66(4):337–346.
33. Libby P, Nahrendorf M, Swirski FK. Leukocytes link local and systemic inflammation in ischemic cardiovascular disease: an expanded "cardiovascular continuum". *J Am Coll Cardiol*. 2016;67(9):1091–1103.
34. Libby P, Swirski FK, Nahrendorf M. The myocardium: more than myocytes. *J Am Coll Cardiol*. 2019;74(25):3136–3138.
35. Vafadarnejad E, Rizzo G, Krampert L, et al. Dynamics of cardiac neutrophil diversity in murine myocardial infarction. *Cir Res*. 2020;127(9):e232–e249.
36. Frangogiannis NG. Cardiac fibrosis. *Cardiovasc Res*. 2020; Nov2;cvaa324. https://doi.org/10.1093/cvr/cvaa324.
37. Sager HB, Heidt T, Hulsmans M, et al. Targeting interleukin-1beta reduces leukocyte production after acute myocardial infarction. *Circulation*. 2015;132(20):1880–1890.
38. Cremer S, Schloss MJ, Vinegoni C, et al. Diminished reactive hematopoiesis and cardiac inflammation in a mouse model of recurrent myocardial infarction. *J Am Coll Cardiol*. 2020;75(8):901–915.
39. Netea MG, Balkwill F, Chonchol M, et al. A guiding map for inflammation. *Nat Immunol*. 2017;18(8):826–831.
40. Emami H, Singh P, MacNabb M, et al. Splenic metabolic activity predicts risk of future cardiovascular events: demonstration of a cardiosplenic axis in humans. *JACC Cardiovasc Imaging*. 2015;8(2):121–130.
41. Namana V, Gupta SS, Abbasi AA, et al. Right ventricular infarction. *Cardiovasc Revasc Med*. 2018;19(1 Pt A):43–50.
42. Yildiz SS, Keskin K, Avsar M, et al. Electrocardiographic diagnosis of atrial infarction in patients with acute inferior ST-segment elevation myocardial infarction. *Clin Cardiol*. 2018;41(7):972–977.
43. Lu ML, De Venecia T, Patnaik S, Figueredo VM. Atrial myocardial infarction: a tale of the forgotten chamber. *Int J Cardiol*. 2016;202:904–909.
44. Aguero J, Galan-Arriola C, Fernandez-Jimenez R, et al. Atrial infarction and ischemic mitral regurgitation contribute to post-MI remodeling of the left atrium. *J Am Coll Cardiol*. 2017;70(23):2878–2889.
45. Elias J, Hoebers LPC, van Dongen IM, et al. Impact of collateral circulation on survival in ST-segment elevation myocardial infarction patients undergoing primary percutaneous coronary intervention with a concomitant chronic total occlusion. *JACC Cardiovasc Interv*. 2017;10(9):906–914.
46. van Dongen IM, Elias J, van Houwelingen KG, et al. Impact of collateralisation to a concomitant chronic total occlusion in patients with ST-elevation myocardial infarction: a subanalysis of the EXPLORE randomised controlled trial. *Open Heart*. 2018;5(2):e000810.
47. Tamis-Holland JE, Jneid H, Reynolds HR, et al. Contemporary diagnosis and management of patients with myocardial infarction in the absence of obstructive coronary artery disease: a scientific statement from the American Heart Association. *Circulation*. 2019;139(18):e891–e908.
48. Agewall S, Beltrame JF, Reynolds HR, et al. ESC working group position paper on myocardial infarction with non-obstructive coronary arteries. *Eur Heart J*. 2017;38(3):143–153.
49. Niccoli G, Scalone G, Crea F. Acute myocardial infarction with no obstructive coronary atherosclerosis: mechanisms and management. *Eur Heart J*. 2015;36(8):475–481.
50. Reynolds HR, Maehara A, Kwong RY, et al. Coronary optical coherence tomography and cardiac magnetic resonance imaging to determine underlying causes of myocardial infarction with non-obstructive coronary arteries in women. *Circulation*. 2021;16; 143(7):624–640.
51. Pasupathy S, Air T, Dreyer RP, et al. Systematic review of patients presenting with suspected myocardial infarction and nonobstructive coronary arteries. *Circulation*. 2015;131(10):861–870.
52. Grodzinsky A, Arnold SV, Gosch K, et al. Angina frequency after acute myocardial infarction in patients without obstructive coronary artery disease. *Eur Heart J Qual Care Clin Outcomes*. 2015;1(2):92–99.
53. Saw J, Humphries K, Aymong E, et al. Spontaneous coronary artery dissection: clinical outcomes and risk of recurrence. *J Am Coll Cardiol*. 2017;70(9):1148–1158.
54. Kim ESH. Spontaneous coronary-artery dissection. *N Eng J Med*. 2020;383(24):2358–2370.
55. Templin C, Ghadri JR, Diekmann J, et al. Clinical features and outcomes of takotsubo (stress) cardiomyopathy. *N Eng J Med*. 2015;373(10):929–938.
56. Lyon AR, Bossone E, Schneider B, et al. Current state of knowledge on takotsubo syndrome: a position statement from the Taskforce On Takotsubo Syndrome of the Heart Failure Association of the European Society of Cardiology. *Eur J Heart Fail*. 2016;18(1):8–27.
57. Medina de Chazal H, Del Buono MG, Keyser-Marcus L, et al. Stress cardiomyopathy diagnosis and treatment: JACC state-of-the-art review. *J Am Coll Cardiol*. 2018;72(16):1955–1971.
58. Frangieh AH, Obeid S, Ghadri JR, et al. ECG criteria to differentiate between takotsubo (stress) cardiomyopathy and myocardial infarction. *J Am Heart Assoc*. 2016;5(6).
59. Luscher TF, Templin C. Is takotsubo syndrome a microvascular acute coronary syndrome? Towards of a new definition. *Eur Heart J*. 2016.
60. Rodriguez-Palomares JF, Gavara J, Ferreira-Gonzalez I, et al. Prognostic value of initial left ventricular remodeling in patients with reperfused STEMI. *JACC Cardiovasc Imaging*. 2019;12(12):2445–2456.
61. Legallois D, Hodzic A, Alexandre J, et al. Definition of left ventricular remodelling following ST-elevation myocardial infarction: a systematic review of cardiac magnetic resonance studies in the past decade. *Heart Fail Rev*. 2020.
62. Garber L, McAndrew TC, Chung ES, et al. Predictors of left ventricular remodeling after myocardial infarction in patients with a patent infarct related coronary artery after percutaneous coronary intervention (from the Post-Myocardial Infarction Remodeling Prevention Therapy [PRomPT] trial). *Am J Cardiol*. 2018;121(11):1293–1298.
63. Stone GW, Selker HP, Thiele H, et al. Relationship between infarct size and outcomes following primary PCI: patient-level analysis from 10 randomized trials. *J Am Coll Cardiol*. 2016;67(14):1674–1683.
64. Shah RU, de Lemos JA, Wang TY, et al. Post-hospital outcomes of patients with acute myocardial infarction with cardiogenic shock: findings from the NCDR. *J Am Coll Cardiol*. 2016;67(7):739–747.
65. van Diepen S, Katz JN, Albert NM, et al. Contemporary management of cardiogenic shock: a scientific statement from the American Heart Association. *Circulation*. 2017;136(16):e232–e268.
66. Westman PC, Lipinski MJ, Luger D, et al. Inflammation as a driver of adverse left ventricular remodeling after acute myocardial infarction. *J Am Coll Cardiol*. 2016;67(17):2050–2060.
67. Frangogiannis NG. The inflammatory response in myocardial injury, repair, and remodelling. *Nat Rev Cardiol*. 2014;11(5):255–265.
68. Prabhu SD, Frangogiannis NG. The biological basis for cardiac repair after myocardial infarction: from inflammation to fibrosis. *Cir Res*. 2016;119(1):91–112.
69. Gibbons RJ, Araoz P. Does infarct size matter? *J Am Coll Cardiol*. 2016;67(14):1684–1686.
70. Hausenloy DJ, Botker HE, Engstrom T, et al. Targeting reperfusion injury in patients with ST-segment elevation myocardial infarction: trials and tribulations. *Eur Heart J*. 2016.
71. Libby P, Loscalzo J, Ridker PM, et al. Inflammation, immunity, and infection in atherothrombosis: JACC review topic of the week. *J Am Coll Cardiol*. 2018;72(17):2071–2081.
72. Smyth A, O'Donnell M, Lamelas P, et al. Physical activity and anger or emotional upset as triggers of acute myocardial infarction: the INTERHEART study. *Circulation*. 2016;134(15):1059–1067.
73. Mohammad MA, Karlsson S, Haddad J, et al. Christmas, national holidays, sport events, and time factors as triggers of acute myocardial infarction: SWEDEHEART observational study 1998-2013. *BMJ*. 2018;363:k4811.
74. Kwong JC, Schwartz KL, Campitelli MA, et al. Acute myocardial infarction after laboratory-confirmed influenza infection. *N Eng J Med*. 2018;378(4):345–353.
75. Fleisher LA, Fleischmann KE, Auerbach AD, et al. 2014 ACC/AHA guideline on perioperative cardiovascular evaluation and management of patients undergoing noncardiac surgery: a report of the American College of Cardiology/American Heart Association Task Force on Practice Guidelines. *J Am Coll Cardiol*. 2014;64(22):e77–e137.
76. Crnko S, Du Pre BC, Sluijter JPG, Van Laake LW. Circadian rhythms and the molecular clock in cardiovascular biology and disease. *Nat Rev Cardiol*. 2019;16(7):437–447.
77. Yang Y, Li W, Zhu H, et al. Prognosis of unrecognised myocardial infarction determined by electrocardiography or cardiac magnetic resonance imaging: systematic review and meta-analysis. *BMJ*. 2020;369:m1184.
78. Vahatalo JH, Huikuri HV, Holmstrom LTA, et al. Association of silent myocardial infarction and sudden cardiac death. *JAMA cardiol*. 2019;4(8):796–802.

Clinical Features

79. Kontos MC, Lanfear DE, Gosch K, et al. Prognostic value of serial N-terminal pro-brain natriuretic peptide testing in patients with acute myocardial infarction. *Am J Cardiol.* 2017;120(2):181–185.
80. Velders MA, Wallentin L, Becker RC, et al. Biomarkers for risk stratification of patients with ST-elevation myocardial infarction treated with primary percutaneous coronary intervention: insights from the Platelet Inhibition and Patient Outcomes trial. *Am Heart J.* 2015;169(6):879–889.e877.
81. Schwartz GG, Abt M, Bao W, et al. Fasting triglycerides predict recurrent ischemic events in patients with acute coronary syndrome treated with statins. *J Am Coll Cardiol.* 2015;65(21):2267–2275.
82. Ghaffari S, Nadiri M, Pourafkari L, et al. The predictive value of total neutrophil count and neutrophil/lymphocyte ratio in predicting in-hospital mortality and complications after STEMI. *J Cardiovasc Thor Res.* 2014;6(1):35–41.
83. Ketchum ES, Dickstein K, Kjekshus J, et al. The Seattle Post Myocardial Infarction Model (SPIM): prediction of mortality after acute myocardial infarction with left ventricular dysfunction. *Eur Heart J Acute Cardiovasc Care.* 2014;3(1):46–55.
84. Lee GK, Hsieh YP, Hsu SW, et al. Value of ST-segment change in lead aVR in diagnosing left main disease in Non-ST-elevation acute coronary syndrome-A meta-analysis. *Ann Noninvasive Electrocardiol.* 2019;24(6):e12692.
85. Albulushi A, Giannopoulos A, Kafkas N, et al. Acute right ventricular myocardial infarction. *Expert Rev Cardiovasc Ther.* 2018;16(7):455–464.
86. Rybicki FJ, Udelson JE, Peacock WF, et al. 2015 ACR/ACC/AHA/AATS/ACEP/ASNC/NASCI/SAEM/SCCT/SCMR/SCPC/SNMMI/STR/STS appropriate utilization of cardiovascular imaging in emergency department patients with chest pain: a joint document of the American College of Radiology Appropriateness Criteria Committee and the American College of Cardiology Appropriate Use Criteria Task Force. *J Am Coll Cardiol.* 2016;67(7):853–879.
87. Eitel I, de Waha S, Wohrle J, et al. Comprehensive prognosis assessment by CMR imaging after ST-segment elevation myocardial infarction. *J Am Coll Cardiol.* 2014;64(12):1217–1226.
88. Hamirani YS, Wong A, Kramer CM, Salerno M. Effect of microvascular obstruction and intramyocardial hemorrhage by CMR on LV remodeling and outcomes after myocardial infarction: a systematic review and meta-analysis. *JACC Cardiovasc Imaging.* 2014;7(9):940–952.
89. McAlindon E, Pufulete M, Lawton C, et al. Quantification of infarct size and myocardium at risk: evaluation of different techniques and its implications. *Eur Heart J Cardiovasc Imaging.* 2015;16(7):738–746.
90. Bulluck H, White SK, Frohlich GM, et al. Quantifying the area at risk in reperfused ST-segment-elevation myocardial infarction patients using hybrid cardiac positron emission tomography-magnetic resonance imaging. *Circ Cardiovasc Imaging.* 2016;9(3):e003900.
91. Mohammad MA, Koul S, Lønborg JT, et al. Usefulness of high sensitivity troponin T to predict long-term left ventricular dysfunction after ST-elevation myocardial infarction. *Am J Cardiol.* 2020;134:8–13.

38 ST-Elevation Myocardial Infarction: Management

ERIN A. BOHULA AND DAVID A. MORROW

PREHOSPITAL MANAGEMENT, 662
Prehospital Care, 662
Emergency Medical Service Systems, 663
Prehospital Fibrinolysis, 663

MANAGEMENT IN THE EMERGENCY DEPARTMENT, 664
General Treatment Measures, 665
Limitation of Infarct Size, 666

REPERFUSION THERAPY, 667
General Concepts, 667
Pathophysiology of Myocardial Reperfusion, 667
Fibrinolysis, 668
Effect of Fibrinolytic Therapy on Mortality, 669
Catheter-Based Reperfusion Strategies, 671
Selection of Reperfusion Strategy, 671
Anticoagulant and Antiplatelet Therapy, 675

HOSPITAL MANAGEMENT, 679
Coronary Care and Intermediate Care Units, 679
Pharmacologic Therapy, 680

HEMODYNAMIC DISTURBANCES, 684
Hemodynamic Assessment, 684
Left Ventricular Failure, 685
Cardiogenic Shock, 690
Right Ventricular Infarction, 694
Mechanical Causes of Heart Failure, 694

ARRHYTHMIAS, 699
Hemodynamic Consequences, 699
Ventricular Arrhythmias, 699
Bradyarrhythmias, 701
Supraventricular Tachyarrhythmias, 703

OTHER COMPLICATIONS, 703
Recurrent Chest Discomfort, 703

Pericardial Effusion and Pericarditis, 704
Venous Thrombosis and Pulmonary Embolism, 705
Left Ventricular Aneurysm, 705
Left Ventricular Thrombus and Arterial Embolism, 705

CONVALESCENCE, DISCHARGE, AND POST-MYOCARDIAL INFARCTION CARE, 705
Timing of Hospital Discharge, 705
Secondary Prevention After Acute Myocardial Infarction, 707

FUTURE PERSPECTIVES AND EMERGING THERAPIES, 710

REFERENCES, 710

The care of patients with ST-elevation myocardial infarction (STEMI) has transformed in conjunction with the shift in approach to reperfusion therapy from primarily pharmacologic to catheter-based strategies.[1-3] With simultaneous advances in medical therapy, the case-fatality rate for patients with STEMI has continued to decline (Fig. 38.1).[4,5] Nevertheless, optimal management of patients at high risk for or with established major complications of STEMI remains critical to the care of this condition. A discussion of the management of STEMI can follow the clinical course of the patient. Chapters 25 and 40 address primary and secondary prevention of coronary artery disease (CAD). Chapter 35 reviews the emergency evaluation of patients with chest pain. This chapter addresses treatment at the time of onset of STEMI (prehospital care, initial recognition and management in the emergency department (ED), and reperfusion), hospital management (medications, complications, and preparation for discharge), and early secondary prevention after STEMI. Chapter 41 discusses percutaneous coronary intervention (PCI) in patients with STEMI. Chapter 69 describes the use of implantable defibrillators for prevention of sudden cardiac death after myocardial infarction (MI). Chapter 40 discusses the long-term management of the patient with established stable ischemic heart disease, including patients with prior acute MI.

PREHOSPITAL MANAGEMENT

Given the progressive loss of functioning myocytes with persistent occlusion of the infarct-related artery in STEMI (see Chapter 37), initial management aims to restore blood flow to the infarct zone as rapidly as possible. Primary PCI is generally the preferred option, provided that an experienced operator and team can perform it in a timely fashion.[1-3,6] Missed opportunities for improvement in the care of STEMI include failure to deliver any form of reperfusion therapy in approximately 15% of patients and failure to minimize delays in reperfusion because of inefficient systems of care.[7,8] The "chain of survival" for STEMI involves a highly integrated strategy beginning with patient education about the symptoms of MI and early contact with the medical system, coordination of destination protocols in emergency medical service (EMS) systems, efficient practices in EDs to shorten door-to-reperfusion time, and expeditious implementation of the reperfusion strategy by a trained team.[8,9] The American Heart Association (AHA) has maintained a national initiative engineering improved health care delivery for STEMI, including implementation of systems that shorten total ischemic time while emphasizing overall quality of care for STEMI (Tables 38.1 and 38.2).[9]

Prehospital Care

The prehospital care of patients suspected of having STEMI bears directly on the likelihood of survival. Most deaths associated with STEMI occur within the first hour of its onset and usually result from ventricular fibrillation (VF) (see Chapter 70). Therefore, immediate implementation of resuscitative efforts and rapid transportation of the patient to a hospital have prime importance. Major components of the time from the onset of ischemic symptoms to reperfusion include (1) the time for the patient to recognize the problem and seek medical attention; (2) prehospital evaluation, treatment, and transportation; (3) the time for diagnostic measures and initiation of treatment in the hospital (e.g., "door-to-device" time for patients undergoing a catheter-based reperfusion strategy and "door-to-needle" time for patients receiving a fibrinolytic agent); and (4) the time from initiation of treatment to restoration of flow.

Patient-related factors that correlate with a longer delay until deciding to seek medical attention include older age; female sex; black race; low socioeconomic or uninsured status; history of angina, diabetes, or both; consulting a spouse or other relative; and consulting a physician.[1,8] Health care professionals should heighten the level of awareness of patients at risk for STEMI (e.g., those with hypertension, diabetes, history of angina pectoris). They should use elective patient encounters to review and reinforce with patients and their families the need to seek urgent medical attention for a pattern of symptoms that includes chest discomfort, or dyspnea. Patients should also be instructed in the proper use of sublingual nitroglycerin and to call emergency services if the ischemic-type discomfort persists for more than 5 minutes.[1]

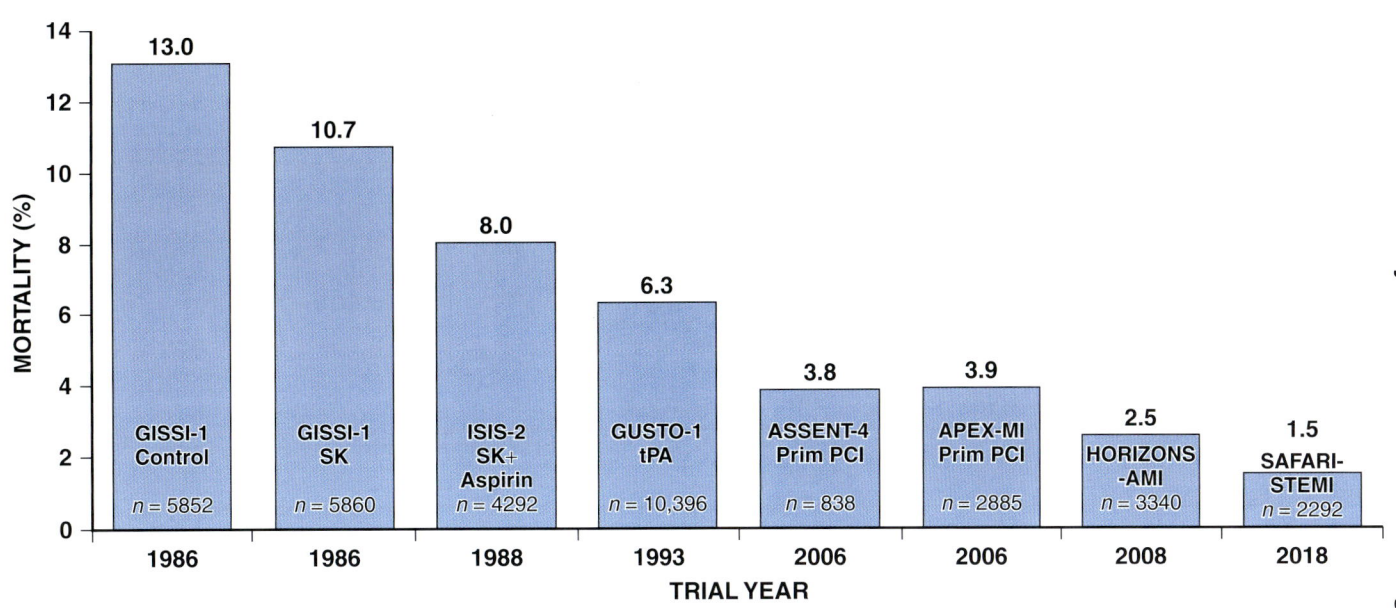

FIGURE 38.1 Early mortality rates have declined in major randomized trials of STEMI patients from 1986 to 2018 with the introduction and improvement in pharmacologic and/or mechanical reperfusion therapy. *Prim PCI*, Primary percutaneous coronary intervention; *SK*, streptokinase; *tPA*, tissue plasminogen activator. (From Van de Werf F. The history of coronary reperfusion. *Eur Heart J.* 2014;35;2510–2515; Le May et al. *JAMA Cardiol.* 2020;5:126–134.)

TABLE 38.1 Criteria for a System of Care for ST-Elevation Myocardial Infarction (STEMI)

1. The system should be registered with Mission: Lifeline.
2. Ongoing multidisciplinary team meetings should occur, including EMS, non-PCI hospitals/STEMI referral centers, and PCI hospitals/STEMI receiving centers, to evaluate outcomes and quality improvement data. Operational issues should be reviewed, problems identified, and solutions implemented.
3. Each STEMI system should include a process for prehospital identification and activation, destination protocols to STEMI receiving centers, and transfer for patients who arrive at STEMI referral centers and are primary PCI candidates, are ineligible for fibrinolytic therapy, and/or are in cardiogenic shock.
4. Each system should have a recognized system coordinator, physician champion, and EMS medical director.
5. Each system component (EMS, STEMI referral centers, and STEMI receiving centers) should meet the appropriate criteria.

EMS, Emergency medical services; *PCI*, percutaneous coronary intervention.

TABLE 38.2 Interventions to Improve Door-to-Device Times

1. A prehospital ECG for diagnosing STEMI is used to activate the PCI team while the patient is en route to the hospital.
2. Emergency physicians activate the PCI team.
3. A single call to a central page operator activates the PCI team.
4. A goal is set for the PCI team to arrive at the catheterization laboratory within 20 min after being paged.
5. Timely data feedback and analysis are provided to members of the STEMI care team.

ECG, Electrocardiogram; *PCI*, percutaneous coronary intervention; *STFMI*, ST-elevation myocardial infarction.
From O'Gara PT, Kushner FG, Ascheim DD, et al. 2013 ACCF/AHA guideline for the management of ST-elevation myocardial infarction: a report of the American College of Cardiology Foundation/American Heart Association Task Force on Practice Guidelines. *J Am Coll Cardiol.* 2013;61:e78.

Emergency Medical Service Systems

EMS systems have three major components: emergency medical dispatch, first response, and the EMS ambulance response (see Chapter 35). The expanded capability to record a prehospital 12-lead electrocardiogram (ECG) represents a major advance in EMS systems (see Table 38.2).[8,10,11] The ability to transmit such ECGs and to activate the STEMI care team before arrival at the hospital places EMS efforts at the center of the early response to STEMI.[8] Efforts to shorten the time until treatment of patients with STEMI include improvement in the medical dispatch component by expanding 911 coverage, providing automated external defibrillators to first responders, placing automated external defibrillators in critical public locations, and greater coordination of the EMS ambulance response. Well-equipped ambulances and helicopters staffed by personnel trained in the acute care of patients with STEMI allow definitive therapy to begin during transport to the hospital. Electronic transmission of the ECG to a medical control officer facilitates the triage of patients with STEMI (Fig. 38.2).

In addition to prompt defibrillation, the efficacy of prehospital care appears to depend on several factors, including early relief of pain with its deleterious physiologic sequelae, reduction of excessive activity of the autonomic nervous system, and treatment of arrhythmias such as ventricular tachycardia (VT)—but these efforts must not delay rapid transfer to the hospital (see Fig. 38.2).

Prehospital Fibrinolysis

Multiple observational studies and several randomized trials have evaluated the potential benefits of prehospital versus in-hospital fibrinolysis.[1,4] Although none of the individual trials showed a significant reduction in mortality with prehospital-initiated fibrinolytic therapy, earlier treatment generally provides greater benefit, and a meta-analysis of all the available trials demonstrated a 17% reduction in mortality.[1,2] In the STREAM (Strategic Reperfusion Early After Myocardial Infarction) trial, prehospital fibrinolysis offered similar efficacy to primary PCI in 1892 patients with STEMI who presented within 3 hours of symptom onset and who could not undergo primary PCI within 1 hour of first medical contact. The primary endpoint of death, shock, heart failure, or reinfarction at 30 days occurred in 12.4% of the fibrinolysis arm and 14.3% in the primary PCI arm (p = 0.21) (Fig. 38.3).[12] Rescue or urgent PCI was required in 36% of patients initially receiving fibrinolysis, with the remainder undergoing coronary angiography per protocol a median of 17 hours after randomization. The rate of intracranial hemorrhage was higher in the fibrinolysis group (1.0% versus 0.2%, p = 0.04), but non-intracranial bleeding rates were similar between the treatment groups. Prehospital fibrinolysis is reasonable in settings in which substantial time can be saved by prehospital treatment because of long transportation times (60 to 90 minutes or longer), and physicians are

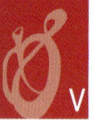

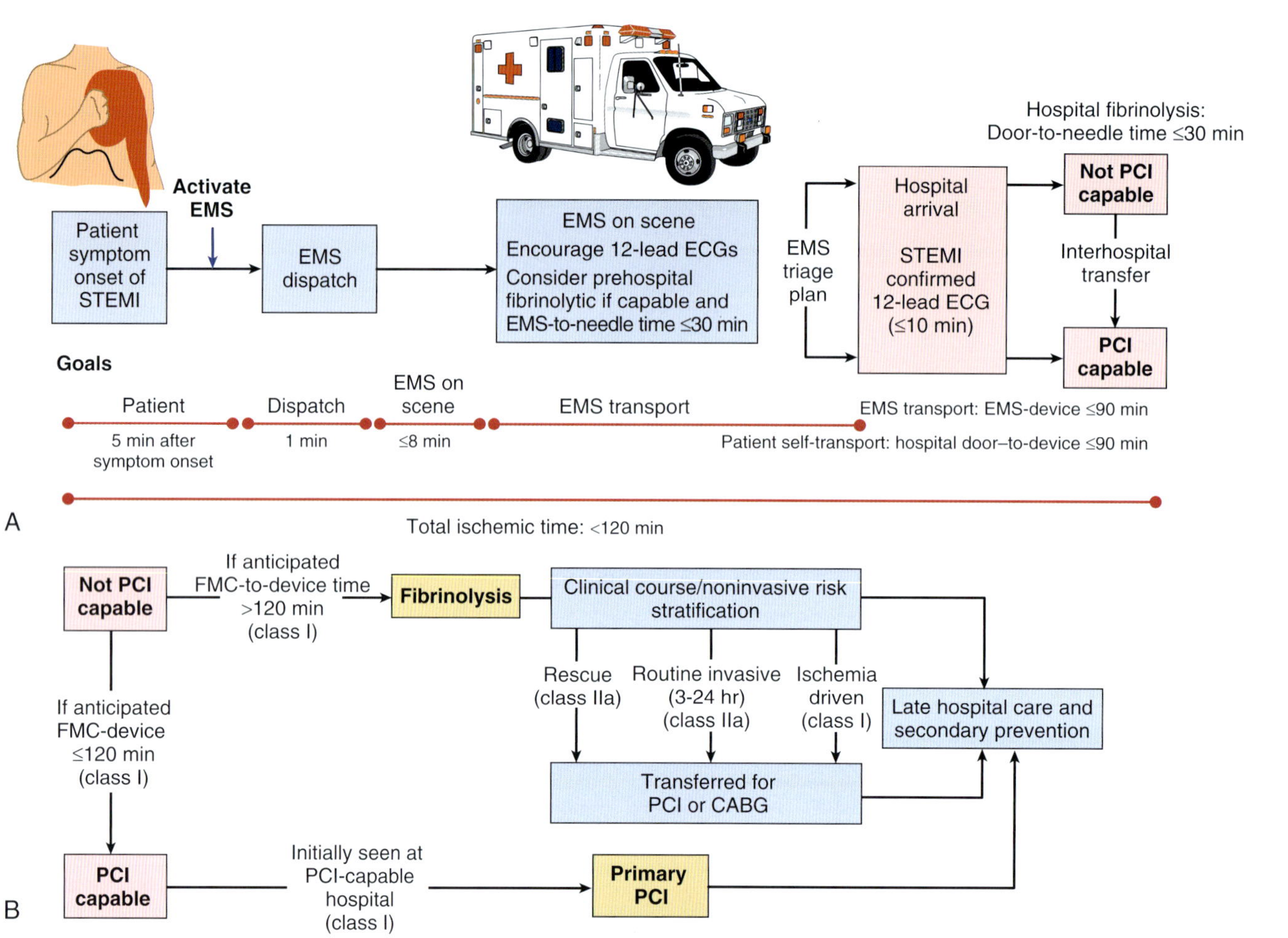

FIGURE 38.2 System goals and initial reperfusion treatment of patients with STEMI. Reperfusion in STEMI patients can be accomplished by pharmacologic (fibrinolysis) or catheter-based (primary PCI) approaches and may involve transfer from a non–PCI-capable to a primary PCI-capable center. **A,** Patient transported by the emergency medical services (EMS). The STEMI systems goal is to maintain a network of transportation and destination hospitals so that the total ischemic time is kept to less than 120 minutes. In addition to this overall goal, three additional time objectives exist. (1) If the EMS has fibrinolytic capability and the patient qualifies for therapy, prehospital fibrinolysis may be considered and, if used, should be started within 30 minutes of arrival of the EMS on scene. (2) For patients transported to a non–PCI-capable hospital where a fibrinolytic is to be administered, the hospital door-to-needle time should be 30 minutes or less. (3) If the patient is transported to a PCI-capable hospital, the time from first medical contact (FMC) to deployment of the first PCI device (FMC-to-device time) should be 90 minutes or less. Patient self-transportation is discouraged. If the patient arrives at a non–PCI-capable hospital and a fibrinolytic is to be administered, the door-to-needle time should be 30 minutes or less. If the patient arrives at a PCI-capable hospital, the door-to-balloon time should be 90 minutes or less. The treatment options and time recommendations after arrival at the hospital are the same. Consideration of emergency interhospital transfer of the patient to a PCI-capable hospital for mechanical revascularization is also appropriate if the use of a fibrinolytic is contraindicated or PCI can be initiated promptly (anticipated FMC-to-device time ≤120 minutes) or if fibrinolysis is unsuccessful (i.e., "rescue PCI"). Secondary nonemergency interhospital transfer can be considered for recurrent ischemia or routine invasive evaluation 3 to 24 hours after fibrinolysis. **B,** Reperfusion strategies for patients with STEMI, regardless of whether they go to a PCI-capable or to a non–PCI-capable hospital. The optimal strategy depends on the timing of the onset of symptoms, the patient's eligibility for fibrinolysis, and the options for timely transfer to a PCI-capable hospital. The denoted class I and class II recommendations are from the ACCF/AHA guidelines for the management of STEMI. For patients who receive fibrinolysis, noninvasive risk stratification is recommended to guide decisions regarding delayed coronary revascularization. *CABG,* Coronary artery bypass grafting. (Modified from Armstrong PW, Collen D, Antman E. Fibrinolysis for acute myocardial infarction: the future is here and now. *Circulation.* 2003;107:2533; and O'Gara PT, Kushner FG, Ascheim DD, et al. 2013 ACCF/AHA guideline for the management of ST-elevation myocardial infarction: a report of the American College of Cardiology Foundation/American Heart Association Task Force on Practice Guidelines. *J Am Coll Cardiol.* 2013;61:e78.)

present in the ambulance, or there is a well-organized EMS system with full-time paramedics who can obtain and transmit 12-lead ECG recordings from the field to an online medical command able to authorize prehospital fibrinolysis (see Fig. 38.2).[1-3]

MANAGEMENT IN THE EMERGENCY DEPARTMENT

When evaluating patients with chest pain in the ED, physicians must confront the difficult tasks of rapidly identifying patients who require urgent reperfusion therapy, triaging lower-risk patients to the appropriate setting within the hospital, and not discharging patients inappropriately while avoiding unnecessary admissions. A history of ischemic-type discomfort and the initial 12-lead ECG are the primary tools for screening patients with possible acute coronary syndrome (ACS) for STEMI (see Chapter 35). Because the 12-lead ECG is at the center of the decision pathway for initiation of reperfusion therapy, it should be obtained promptly (≤ 10 minutes after hospital arrival) in patients with suspected ischemic symptoms.[1] More extensive use of prehospital 12-lead ECGs has also facilitated early triage of patients with STEMI.[8,10,11] Because lethal arrhythmias can occur suddenly in patients with STEMI, all patients should have bedside monitoring of the ECG and intravenous (IV) access.

The presence of ST-segment elevation on the ECG in a patient with ischemic discomfort suggests thrombotic occlusion of an epicardial coronary artery and should trigger a well-rehearsed sequence of rapid assessment of the patient for initiation of a reperfusion strategy.[1] Critical factors that weigh into selection of a reperfusion strategy include the time elapsed since the onset of symptoms, the risk associated with STEMI, the time required to initiate an invasive strategy, and if that time is expected to be prolonged, the risk related to administering a fibrinolytic (see Fig. 38.2). In non–PCI-capable hospitals, the initial assessment should include evaluation of the contraindications to administration of a fibrinolytic (Table 38.3). Patients with an initial ECG that reveals ST-segment depression and/or T wave inversion

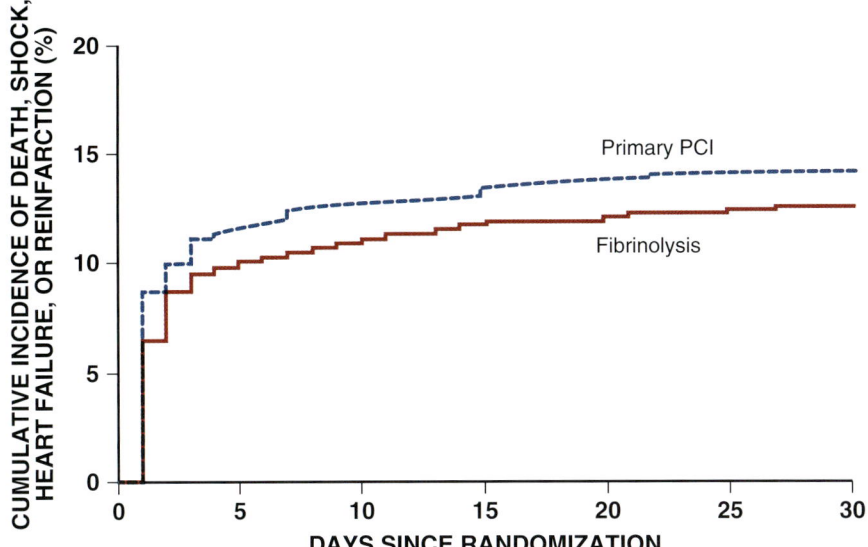

FIGURE 38.3 The STREAM (Strategic Reperfusion Early After Myocardial Infarction) study found that prehospital fibrinolysis offers similar efficacy to primary PCI in 1892 patients with STEMI who presented within 3 hours of symptom onset and who could not undergo primary PCI within 1 hour of FMC, where the primary endpoint of death, shock, heart failure, or reinfarction at 30 days occurred in 12.4% of the fibrinolysis arm and 14.3% in the primary PCI arm (hazard ratio, 0.86; confidence interval, 0.68 to 1.09; $P = 0.21$ by log-rank test). (Modified from Armstrong PW, Gershlick AH, Goldstein P, et al. Fibrinolysis or primary PCI in ST-segment elevation myocardial infarction. *N Engl J Med*. 2013;368(15):1379–1387.)

TABLE 38.3 Contraindications to and Cautions in the Use of Fibrinolytics for Treating ST-Elevation Myocardial Infarction*

Absolute Contraindications
Any previous intracranial hemorrhage
Known structural cerebral vascular lesion (e.g., arteriovenous malformation)
Known malignant intracranial neoplasm (primary or metastatic)
Ischemic stroke within 3 months *except* acute ischemic stroke within 4.5 hr
Suspected aortic dissection
Active bleeding or bleeding diathesis (excluding menses)
Significant closed-head or facial trauma within 3 months
Intracranial or intraspinal surgery within 2 months
Severe uncontrolled hypertension (unresponsive to emergency therapy)
For streptokinase, previous treatment within the previous 6 months
Relative Contraindications
History of chronic, severe, poorly controlled hypertension
Significant hypertension at initial evaluation (SBP >180 mm Hg or DBP >110 mm Hg)†
History of previous ischemic stroke >3 months
Dementia
Known intracranial pathology not covered in Absolute Contraindications
Traumatic or prolonged (>10 min) cardiopulmonary resuscitation
Major surgery (<3 weeks)
Recent (within 2 to 4 weeks) internal bleeding
Noncompressible vascular punctures
Pregnancy
Active peptic ulcer
Oral anticoagulant therapy

*Viewed as advisory for clinical decision making and may not be all-inclusive or definitive.
†Could be an absolute contraindication in low-risk patients with myocardial infarction.
DBP, Diastolic blood pressure; *SBP,* systolic blood pressure.
From O' Gara PT, Kushner FG, Ascheim DD, et al. 2013 ACCF/AHA guideline for the management of ST-elevation myocardial infarction: a report of the American College of Cardiology Foundation/American Heart Association Task Force on Practice Guidelines. *J Am Coll Cardiol*. 2013;61:e78.

without ST-segment elevation are not considered candidates for immediate reperfusion therapy unless a posterior (or inferobasal) injury current is suspected (see Chapter 14).

Given the importance of time to reperfusion,[4] emphasis has shifted to overall medical system goals, starting at the point of first medical contact with the patient.[1,2,9] Benchmarks for medical systems to use when assessing the quality of their performance are a door-to-needle time of 30 minutes or less for initiation of fibrinolytic therapy and a door-to-device time of 90 minutes or less for percutaneous coronary perfusion (see Fig. 38.2).[1,2] In patients with a clinical history suggestive of STEMI (see Chapter 35) and an initial nondiagnostic ECG (i.e., no ST-segment deviation or T wave inversion), serial tracings should be obtained during evaluation in the ED. ED staff can seek the sudden development of ST-segment elevation by periodic visual inspection of the bedside electrocardiographic monitor, by continuous ST-segment recording, or by auditory alarms when the ST-segment deviation exceeds programmed limits. Decision aids such as computer-based diagnostic algorithms, identification of high-risk clinical indicators, rapid determination of cardiac biomarkers, and echocardiographic evaluation for regional wall motion abnormalities have the greatest clinical usefulness when the findings on the ECG are not diagnostic.

General Treatment Measures

See also Chapter 39.

Aspirin

Aspirin is effective across the entire ACS spectrum and is part of the initial management strategy for patients with suspected STEMI. Because low doses take several days to achieve a full antiplatelet effect, 162 to 325 mg should be administered at the first opportunity after initial medical contact.[1] To achieve therapeutic blood levels rapidly, the patient should chew a non–enteric-coated tablet to promote buccal absorption bypassing the gastric mucosa.

Control of Cardiac Pain

Initial management of patients with STEMI should target relief of pain and its associated heightened sympathetic activity. Control of cardiac pain uses a combination of analgesics (e.g., morphine) and interventions to improve the balance of myocardial oxygen supply and demand, including oxygen (in the setting of hypoxia), nitrates, and in appropriately selected patients, beta-adrenergic receptor-blocking agents (beta blockers).[1]

Analgesics

Although a wide variety of analgesic agents, including meperidine, pentazocine, and morphine, can treat the pain associated with STEMI, morphine remains the drug of choice, except in patients with well-documented morphine hypersensitivity. An initial dose of 4 to 8 mg can be administered intravenously initially, followed by doses of 2 to 8 mg repeated at intervals of 5 to 15 minutes until the pain is relieved or side effects emerge—hypotension, depression of respiration, or vomiting.[1] Appropriate dosing of morphine sulfate will vary, however, depending on the patient's age, body size, blood pressure (BP), and heart rate (HR).

Reduction of anxiety with successful analgesia diminishes the patient's restlessness and the activity of the autonomic nervous system, with a consequent reduction in the heart's metabolic demands, and possible favorable effects on myocardial healing (see Chapter 37). Morphine has beneficial effects in patients with pulmonary edema as a result of peripheral arterial and venous dilation (particularly in those with excessive sympathoadrenal activity); it reduces the work of breathing and slows the HR secondary to combined withdrawal of sympathetic tone and augmentation of vagal tone. Counterbalancing these potential benefits, observational studies have suggested an association between the administration of morphine and adverse outcomes in patients with ACS, with the putative mechanism being a slowing of antiplatelet agent absorption.[13-15]

Maintaining the patient in a supine position and elevating the lower extremities if BP falls can minimize hypotension following the administration of nitroglycerin and morphine. Such positioning is undesirable in patients with pulmonary edema, but morphine rarely produces hypotension in these circumstances. IV administration of atropine may be helpful in treating excessive vagomimetic effects of morphine.

Nitrates

By virtue of their ability to enhance coronary blood flow by coronary vasodilation and to decrease ventricular preload by increasing venous capacitance, sublingual (SL) nitrates are indicated for most patients with an ACS. At present, the only groups of patients with STEMI in whom SL nitroglycerin should *not* be given are those with suspected right ventricular (RV) infarction or marked hypotension (e.g., systolic BP <90 mm Hg), especially if accompanied by bradycardia.

Once hypotension is excluded, an SL nitroglycerin tablet should be administered and the patient observed for improvement in symptoms or change in hemodynamics. If an initial dose is well tolerated and appears to be beneficial, further nitrates should be administered while monitoring vital signs. Even small doses can produce sudden hypotension and bradycardia, a reaction that can usually be reversed with IV atropine. Long-acting oral nitrate preparations should be avoided in the early course of STEMI because of the frequently changing hemodynamic status of the patient. In patients with a prolonged period of waxing and waning chest pain, continuous IV nitroglycerin infusion may help control the symptoms and lessen the ischemia, but this requires frequent BP monitoring. Initiation of a reperfusion strategy in patients with STEMI should not await assessing the patient's response to SL or IV nitrates.

Beta-Adrenergic Blocking Agents

Beta blockers aid in the relief of ischemic pain, reduce the need for analgesics in many patients, and reduce infarct size and life-threatening arrhythmias. Avoiding early IV beta blockers in patients with Killip class II or greater is important, however, because of the risk of precipitating cardiogenic shock.[1] Routine use of IV beta blockers is no longer recommended in patients with STEMI, but IV administration of a beta blocker at the initial evaluation of patients with STEMI who are hypertensive and have ongoing ischemia is reasonable.[1]

A practical protocol for use of a beta blocker is the following. First, exclude patients with heart failure (HF), hypotension (systolic BP <90 mm Hg), bradycardia (HR <60 beats/min), or significant atrioventricular (AV) block. Second, administer metoprolol in three 5-mg IV boluses. Third, observe the patient for 2 to 5 minutes after each bolus, and if HR falls below 60 beats/min or systolic BP falls below 100 mm Hg, do not administer any further drug. Fourth, if hemodynamic stability continues 15 minutes after the last IV dose, begin oral metoprolol tartrate, 25 to 50 mg every 6 hours for 2 to 3 days as tolerated and then switch to 100 mg twice daily.[1] Lower doses may be used in patients who have a partial decline in BP with the initial dosing or who appear to be at higher risk (e.g., larger infarction) for development of HF because of poor left ventricular (LV) performance. Infusion of an extremely short-acting beta blocker, such as esmolol, 50 to 250 μg/kg/min, may be useful in patients with relative contraindications to the administration of a beta blocker and in whom HR slowing is considered highly desirable.

Oxygen

Hypoxemia can occur in patients with STEMI and generally results from ventilation-perfusion abnormalities that are sequelae of LV failure; concomitant intrinsic pulmonary disease may also contribute to hypoxemia in some patients. Treating all patients hospitalized for STEMI with oxygen for at least 24 to 48 hours is an historical common practice based on the empiric assumption that increased oxygen in the inspired air may protect ischemic myocardium. However, augmentation of the fraction of oxygen in inspired air (FiO_2) does not elevate O_2 delivery significantly in patients who are not hypoxemic. Furthermore, it may increase systemic vascular resistance and arterial pressure, promote coronary vasoconstriction, and result in greater oxidative stress. Moreover, in a randomized trial comparing oxygen (8 L/min) with no supplemental oxygen in 441 patients with STEMI but without hypoxia, compared with the control therapy, supplemental O_2 therapy demonstrated a trend toward increased early myocardial injury measured with cardiac troponin.[16] In a secondary analysis, O_2 supplementation was associated with increased myocardial infarct size assessed by cardiac magnetic resonance imaging (CMR) at 6 months.

In view of these considerations, arterial oxygen saturation (SaO_2) can be estimated by pulse oximetry, and O_2 therapy can be omitted if the oximetric findings are normal. On the other hand, patients with STEMI and arterial hypoxemia (e.g., SaO_2 <90%) should receive oxygen.[1,2] In patients with severe pulmonary edema, endotracheal intubation and mechanical ventilation may be necessary to correct the hypoxemia and reduce the work of breathing.

Limitation of Infarct Size

Infarct size is an important determinant of prognosis in patients with STEMI.[17] Patients who succumb from cardiogenic shock generally exhibit either a single massive infarct or a moderate infarct superimposed on multiple previous infarctions. Survivors with large infarcts frequently exhibit late impairment of ventricular function, and their long-term mortality rate is higher than that of survivors with small infarcts.[17] In view of the prognostic importance of infarct size, the possibility of modifying infarct size has attracted much experimental and clinical attention (see Chapter 37).[4] Efforts to limit infarct size have used several different (sometimes overlapping) approaches: (1) early reperfusion, (2) reduction of myocardial energy demands, (3) manipulation of energy production sources in the myocardium, and (4) prevention of reperfusion injury.[18,19]

Dynamic Nature of Infarction

STEMI is a dynamic process that does not occur instantaneously but rather evolves over hours. The fate of jeopardized, ischemic tissue can be ameliorated by interventions that restore myocardial perfusion, reduce microvascular damage in the infarct zone, decrease myocardial oxygen requirements, inhibit accumulation or facilitate washout of noxious metabolites, augment the availability of substrate for anaerobic metabolism, or blunt the effects of mediators of injury that compromise the structure and function of intracellular organelles and constituents of cell membranes. Strong evidence in experimental animals and suggestive evidence in patients indicate that *ischemic preconditioning,* a form of endogenous protection against STEMI, before sustained coronary occlusion decreases infarct size and associates with a more favorable outcome, along with decreased risk for extension of infarction and recurrent ischemic events. Brief episodes of ischemia in one coronary vascular bed may precondition myocardium in a remote zone and thereby attenuate the size of infarction in the latter when sustained coronary occlusion occurs.[20]

Perfusion of myocardium in the infarct zone appears to fall maximally immediately following coronary occlusion. Spontaneous recanalization of an occluded infarct-related artery occurs in up to one-third of patients beginning at 12 to 24 hours. This delayed spontaneous reperfusion may enhance LV function because it improves healing of infarcted tissue, prevents ventricular remodeling, and reperfuses hibernating myocardium. Yet, strategies involving pharmacologically induced and catheter-based reperfusion of the infarct vessel can *maximize* the amount of salvaged myocardium by *accelerating* the process of reperfusion and also implementing it in patients who would otherwise have a persistently occluded infarct-related artery. An overarching concept that applies to all methods of reperfusion is the critical importance of time. The earlier the infarct artery is reperfused, the greater the reduction in mortality (Fig. 38.4).[1]

Additional factors that may limit infarct size during reperfusion include relief of coronary spasm, prevention of damage to the microvasculature, improved systemic hemodynamics (augmentation of coronary perfusion pressure and reduced LV end-diastolic pressure), and

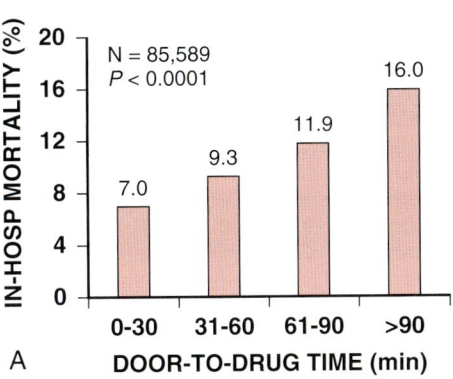
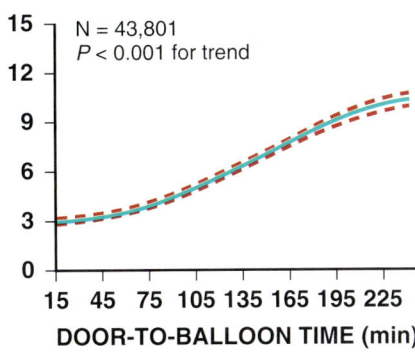

FIGURE 38.4 Importance of time to reperfusion in patients undergoing fibrinolysis (**A**) or primary PCI (**B**) for STEMI. **A,** Graph based on data from 85,589 patients treated with fibrinolysis. A progressive increase in the in-hospital mortality rate occurs for every 30-minute delay. **B,** Based on data from 43,801 patients, this graph depicts the adjusted in-hospital mortality rate as a function of door-to-balloon time. Estimated mortality ranged from 3% with a door-to-balloon time of 30 minutes to 10.3% in patients with a door-to-balloon time of 240 minutes. (Data from Cannon CP, Gibson CM, Lambrew CT, et al. Relationship of symptom-onset-to-balloon time and door-to-balloon time with mortality in patients undergoing angioplasty for acute myocardial infarction. JAMA. 2000;283:2941; and Rathore SS, Curtis JP, Chen J, et al. Association of door-to-balloon time and mortality in patients admitted to hospital with ST-elevation myocardial infarction: national cohort study. BMJ. 2009;338:b1807.)

Routine Measures for Limitation of Infarct Size

Although timely reperfusion of ischemic myocardium is the most important intervention to limit infarct size, several routine measures to accomplish this goal apply to all patients with STEMI, regardless of whether they receive reperfusion therapy.[1] The treatment strategies discussed in this section can be initiated at first medical contact and can be continued throughout the hospital phase of care.

Myocardial oxygen consumption should be minimized by maintaining the patient at rest both physically and emotionally and by using mild sedation and a quiet atmosphere—in addition to the interventions already discussed. Administration of adrenergic agonists should be avoided whenever possible. All forms of tachyarrhythmia require prompt treatment because they increase myocardial oxygen needs. HF should also be treated swiftly to minimize increases in adrenergic tone and hypoxemia (see later, Left Ventricular Failure). If ongoing ischemia occurs, severe anemia (hemoglobin <7 g/dL) can be corrected by the cautious administration of packed red blood cells, accompanied by a diuretic if there is any evidence of LV failure. Associated conditions, particularly infections and accompanying tachycardia, fever, and elevated myocardial oxygen needs, require management.

REPERFUSION THERAPY

General Concepts

Although late spontaneous reperfusion occurs in some patients, thrombotic occlusion persists in most patients with STEMI. Timely reperfusion of jeopardized myocardium is the most effective way of restoring the balance between myocardial oxygen supply and demand.[22] The dependence of myocardial salvage on the time elapsed until treatment pertains to patients treated with either fibrinolysis or PCI[1,23] (Fig. 38.5). The efficacy of fibrinolytic agents decreases as coronary thrombi mature over time.[1] Analyses have identified a linear relationship between delay to revascularization with PCI and mortality (see Fig. 38.4), with a greater increase in mortality for a given delay in patients presenting with out-of-hospital cardiac arrest or cardiogenic shock.[23]

In some patients, particularly those with cardiogenic shock, tissue damage occurs in a "stuttering" manner rather than abruptly. This scenario underscores the need for careful history taking to ascertain whether the patient appears to have had repetitive cycles of spontaneous reperfusion and reocclusion. Determining the precise time of onset of the infarction process in these patients, however, can be difficult and sometimes misleading. In such patients with waxing and waning ischemic discomfort, a rigid time interval from the first episode of pain should not be used when determining whether a patient is "outside the window" for benefit from acute reperfusion therapy.

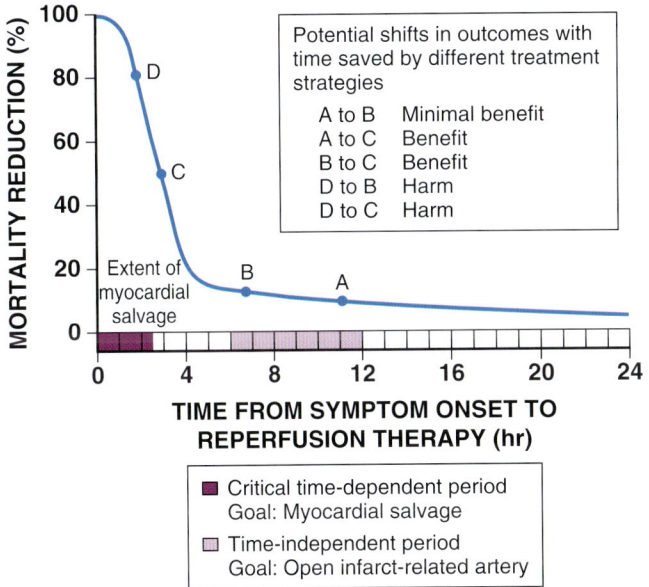

FIGURE 38.5 The reduction in mortality as a benefit of reperfusion therapy is greatest in the first 2 to 3 hours after the onset of symptoms of acute MI, most likely a consequence of myocardial salvage. The exact duration of this critical early period may be modified by several factors, including the presence of functioning collateral coronary arteries, ischemic preconditioning, myocardial oxygen demands, and the duration of sustained ischemia. After this early period, the magnitude of the mortality benefit is much reduced, and as the mortality reduction curve flattens, time to reperfusion therapy is less critical. The magnitude of the benefit depends on how far up the curve the patient can be shifted. The benefit of a shift from point A or B to point C would be substantial, but the benefit of a shift from point A to point B would be small. This schematic illustrates how a treatment strategy that delays therapy during the early critical period, such as transfer of a patient for PCI with a long transportation time, could be harmful (shift from point D to point C or point B). (Modified from Gersh BJ, Stone GW, White HD, Holmes DR Jr. Pharmacological facilitation of primary percutaneous coronary intervention for acute myocardial infarction: is the slope of the curve the shape of the future? JAMA. 2005;293:979.)

Pathophysiology of Myocardial Reperfusion

Prevention of cell death by restoration of blood flow depends on the severity and duration of the preexisting ischemia. Substantial experimental and clinical evidence indicates that the earlier blood flow is restored, the more favorable the recovery of LV systolic function, improvement in diastolic function, and reduction in overall mortality.[1] Collateral coronary vessels also appear to influence LV function after reperfusion.[24] They provide sufficient perfusion of myocardium to slow cell death and probably have greater importance in patients undergoing reperfusion later than 1 to 2 hours after coronary occlusion. Even after successful reperfusion and despite the absence of irreversible

collateral circulation. Prompt implementation of measures designed to protect ischemic myocardium and support myocardial perfusion may provide sufficient time for the development of compensatory mechanisms that limit the ultimate extent of infarction (see Chapter 37). Interventions designed to protect the ischemic myocardium during the initial event may also reduce the extension of infarction or early reinfarction. An area of active investigation includes LV unloading with a microaxial LV assist device prior to revascularization, attempting to reduce LV oxygen demands and therefore minimize ischemia and reperfusion injury.[21]

myocardial damage, a period of postischemic contractile dysfunction can occur—a phenomenon called *myocardial stunning*.[25]

Reperfusion Injury

Reperfusion, although beneficial in terms of myocardial salvage, may cause adverse sequelae described by the term *reperfusion injury* (see Chapter 37).[20,26] Several types of reperfusion injury occur in experimental animals: (1) *lethal* reperfusion injury, which refers to reperfusion-induced death of cells that were still viable at restoration of coronary blood flow; (2) *vascular* reperfusion injury, which is progressive damage to the microvasculature such that there is an expanding area of no-reflow and loss of coronary vasodilatory reserve; (3) *stunned myocardium*, in which salvaged myocytes display a prolonged period of contractile dysfunction after restoration of blood flow because of abnormalities in intracellular metabolism, leading to reduced energy production; and (4) *reperfusion arrhythmias*, which refer to bursts of VT (and occasionally VF) that occur within seconds of reperfusion.[8,20,26] Vascular reperfusion injury, stunning, and reperfusion arrhythmias can all occur in patients with STEMI. The concept of lethal reperfusion injury to potentially salvageable myocardium remains controversial, both in animals and in humans.[20,26]

> Microvasculature damage in the reperfused myocardium can lead to a hemorrhagic infarct (see Chapter 37). Fibrinolytic therapy appears more likely than catheter-based reperfusion to produce hemorrhagic infarction. Although there is a theoretical concern that this hemorrhage may lead to extension of the infarct, this does not appear to be the case. Histologic study of patients not surviving despite successful reperfusion has revealed hemorrhagic infarcts, but this hemorrhage does not usually extend beyond the area of necrosis.

PROTECTION AGAINST REPERFUSION INJURY
A variety of adjunctive therapies have been proposed to mitigate the injury that occurs after reperfusion, including modulators of nitric oxide (NO) and cyclic guanosine monophosphate (cGMP) signaling, such as atrial natriuretic peptide, exenatide, and NO, and inhibitors of mitochondrial permeability and dysfunction, such as cyclosporine A.[20,26] Also, using antiplatelet agents and antithrombins to minimize embolization of atheroembolic debris, and prevention of subsequent inflammatory damage may serve to maintain microvascular integrity. However, with the exception of antithrombotic therapy, at present, none of these interventions are recommended for clinical practice.

The effectiveness of interventions directed against reperfusion injury appears to decline rapidly the later that they are administered after reperfusion. In animals, no beneficial effect is detectable after 45 to 60 minutes of reperfusion has elapsed. Transient ischemia produced in other vascular beds may also reduce reperfusion injury, a concept called *remote ischemic conditioning* (RIC).[20,26] Application of this concept to patients undergoing coronary artery bypass grafting (CABG), using repeated cycles of prolonged BP cuff inflation on the upper extremity, reduced perioperative myocardial injury but did not improve clinical outcomes in two randomized trials.[26-28] Several studies have also identified a reduction in MI size in STEMI patients treated with RIC.[26] However, in a large study of 5401 STEMI patients undergoing primary PCI (CONDI2/ERIC-PPCI; Effect of Remote Ischaemic Conditioning on Clinical Outcomes in STEMI Patients Undergoing PPCI), remote ischemic preconditioning did not decrease the incidence of cardiovascular death or hospitalization for heart failure.[29,30]

An alternative experimental approach to protection against reperfusion injury is called *postconditioning*, which involves introducing brief, repetitive episodes of ischemia alternating with reperfusion.[20,26] This appears to activate the cellular protective mechanisms centering around pro-survival kinases.[26] Many of these protective kinases are also activated during ischemic preconditioning. Several clinical studies in patients with STEMI undergoing PCI have provided evidence that postconditioning associates with reduced infarct size and improvement in myocardial perfusion, but others have failed to show a benefit.[20,26] In a study of 1234 patients with STEMI and thrombolysis in MI (TIMI) flow grade 0 to 1, postconditioning failed to reduce the outcome of death or hospitalization for heart failure.[31] Despite the intense interest in pre- and postconditioning, the current clinical data do not support adoption in routine practice.

Reperfusion Arrhythmias
Transient sinus bradycardia occurs in many patients with inferior infarcts at the time of acute reperfusion, often accompanied by some degree of hypotension. This combination of hypotension and bradycardia with a sudden increase in coronary flow may involve activation of the Bezold-Jarisch reflex. Premature ventricular contractions (PVCs), accelerated idioventricular rhythm, and nonsustained VT also usually follow successful reperfusion. Although some investigators have postulated that early afterdepolarizations participate in the genesis of reperfusion-related ventricular arrhythmias, they are present during both ischemia and reperfusion and therefore not likely to be involved in the development of reperfusion-associated VT or VF.

When present, rhythm disturbances may actually indicate successful restoration of coronary flow, but their specificity for successful reperfusion is limited. In general, clinical features are inaccurate markers of reperfusion, with no single clinical finding or constellation of findings being reliably predictive of angiographically demonstrated coronary artery patency.[1] Although reperfusion arrhythmias may show a temporal clustering at restoration of coronary blood flow in patients after successful fibrinolysis, this brief "electrical storm" is generally innocuous and therefore does not warrant prophylactic antiarrhythmic therapy or specific treatment, except in rare cases of symptomatic or hemodynamically significant reperfusion arrhythmias.[1]

Late Establishment of Patency of the Infarct Vessel
The improved survival and ventricular function after successful reperfusion may not result entirely from limitation of infarct size. Poorly contracting or noncontracting myocardium in a zone that is supplied by a stenosed infarct-related artery with slow anterograde perfusion may still contain viable myocytes. PCI can augment flow in the infarct-related artery and thus improve the function of hibernating myocardium.[32]

Fibrinolysis
Although catheter-based reperfusion strategies for STEMI are preferable, when access is delayed or in practice environments where an invasive strategy is impractical, successful fibrinolysis can reduce infarct size and improves myocardial function and survival over both the short and the long term. Therefore, if the time from first medical contact to performing primary PCI is anticipated to exceed 120 minutes, administration of a fibrinolytic is indicated for the treatment of STEMI within 12 hours of onset in the absence of contraindications.[1] Patients treated within the first 1 to 2 hours after the onset of symptoms seem to have the greatest potential for long-term improvement in survival with fibrinolysis.[1]

ASSESSMENT OF REPERFUSION
Thrombolysis in Myocardial Infarction (TIMI) Flow Grade
To provide a level of standardization both for clinical communication and for studies comparing various reperfusion regimens, most clinicians and investigators describe the flow in the infarct vessel according to the TIMI trial grading system.[33] However, an angiographic snapshot in time does not reflect the fluctuating status of flow in the infarct vessel, which may undergo repeated cycles of patency and reocclusion before or during fibrinolysis. When assessed 60 to 90 minutes after the start of fibrinolytic therapy,[1] the finding of TIMI grade 3 flow is far superior to grade 2 in terms of the reduction of infarct size and both short-term and long-term mortality benefit. Therefore, TIMI grade 3 flow should be the goal for achieving reperfusion of the epicardial infarct artery.

Thrombolysis in Myocardial Infarction (TIMI) Frame Count
To provide a more quantitative statement of the briskness of coronary blood flow in the infarct artery and to account for differences in the size and length of vessels (e.g., left anterior descending versus right coronary artery) and interobserver variability, Gibson and coworkers developed the TIMI frame count—a simple count of the number of angiographic frames elapsed until the contrast material arrives in the distal bed of the vessel of interest.[34] This objective and quantitative index of coronary blood flow independently predicts in-hospital mortality from STEMI and also separates patients with TIMI grade 3 flow into low-risk and high-risk groups. The TIMI frame count can also be used to quantitate coronary blood flow (mL/sec), as calculated by:

$$21 \div (\text{Observed TIMI frame count}) \times 1.7$$

based on Doppler velocity wire data showing that normal flow equals 1.7 cm³/sec, which 21 frames encompass. The calculated coronary perfusion relates to mortality in patients treated with fibrinolytics or primary PCI and can be used to assess various modalities for reperfusion inpatientswithSTEMI.

Myocardial Perfusion
Even patients with TIMI grade 3 flow in the culprit artery may not always achieve adequate myocardial perfusion, especially if the delay between the onset of symptoms and restoration of epicardial flow is long.[34] The terms myocardial "no-reflow" and "coronary microvascular obstruction" describe a state of reduced myocardial perfusion after the opening of an epicardial infarct-related artery.[34] The four major impediments to normalization of myocardial perfusion are ischemia-related injury, reperfusion-related injury, distal embolization, and individual susceptibility of the microcirculation to injury (Fig. 38.6).[34] Obstruction of the distal microvasculature in the downstream bed of the infarct-related artery results from platelet or microparticle microemboli and thrombi. Fibrinolysis may exacerbate microembolization of platelet aggregates because of the exposure of clot-bound thrombin, an extremely potent platelet agonist. Spasm can also occur in the microvasculature as a result of the release of substances from activated platelets. Reperfusion injury results in endothelial cell edema, production of reactive oxygen species, and calcium overload. In addition, endothelial activation leads to the accumulation of neutrophils and inflammatory mediators that contribute to tissue injury.[34] Interstitial edema from ischemia and reperfusion injury can compress intramyocardial vessels, further compromising perfusion. Several techniques can evaluate the adequacy of myocardial perfusion.

Electrocardiography
Electrocardiographic ST-segment resolution, when present, has a high positive predictive value (PPV) of greater than 90% for infarct artery patency with, but persistent ST-segment elevation (i.e., lack of ST-segment resolution) is a poor predictor of infarct-related artery occlusion, with a negative predictive value (NPV) of approximately 50%. However, the persistence of ST-segment elevation after angiographically successful primary PCI identifies patients with a higher risk for LV dysfunction and mortality, presumably because of microvascular damage in the infarct zone.[35-37] Thus, the 12-lead ECG can reflect the biologic integrity of myocytes in the infarct zone and indicate inadequate myocardial perfusion even in the presence of TIMI grade 3 flow. The extent of ST-segment resolution provides powerful prognostic information early in the management of patients with STEMI.

Noninvasive Imaging
Defects in perfusion patterns seen with contrast-enhanced echocardiography correlate with regional wall motion abnormalities and lack of myocardial viability on dobutamine stress echocardiography (see Chapter 16).[38] Contrast-enhanced CMR can also identify regions of microvascular obstruction that associate with an adverse long-term prognosis (see Chapter19).[39]

Invasive Assessment
Doppler flow wire studies can also define abnormalities in myocardial perfusion. In addition, Gibson and colleagues developed an angiographic method for assessing myocardial perfusion: the TIMI myocardial perfusion (TMP) grade.[40] Abnormalities associated with increased myocardial perfusion, as assessed by the TMP grade, correlate with unfavorable ventricular remodeling and risk for mortality, even after adjusting for the presence of TIMI grade 3 flow or a normal TIMI frame count.[40]

Effect of Fibrinolytic Therapy on Mortality
Early IV fibrinolysis improves survival in patients with STEMI.[1] The Fibrinolytic Therapy Trialists' (FTT) Collaborative Group performed a comprehensive overview of nine trials of fibrinolytic therapy, and each of which enrolled more than 1000 patients. The overall results indicated an 18% reduction in short-term mortality, but as much as a 25% reduction in mortality in the subset of 45,000 patients with ST-segment elevation or bundle branch block. Two trials, LATE (Late Assessment of Thrombolytic Efficacy) and EMERAS (Estudio Multicéntrico Estreptoquinasa Repúblicas de América del Sur), when viewed together provide evidence that a reduction in mortality may still be observed in patients treated with thrombolytic agents between 6 and 12 hours after the onset of ischemic symptoms. These data form the basis for extending the window of treatment with fibrinolytics up to 12 hours after the onset of symptoms. Pooled analysis from more than 10 trials across six time categories from the onset of symptoms to randomization demonstrates a nonlinear relationship of treatment benefit to time, with the best outcome occurring in the first 1 to 2 hours after the onset of symptoms.[1]

The effect of fibrinolytic therapy on mortality in elderly patients has been controversial. Although patients older than 75 years were initially excluded from randomized trials of fibrinolytic therapy, they ultimately comprised approximately 15% of those studied in trials of fibrinolysis and 35% of those analyzed in registries of patients with STEMI.[1] Barriers to initiation of therapy in older patients with

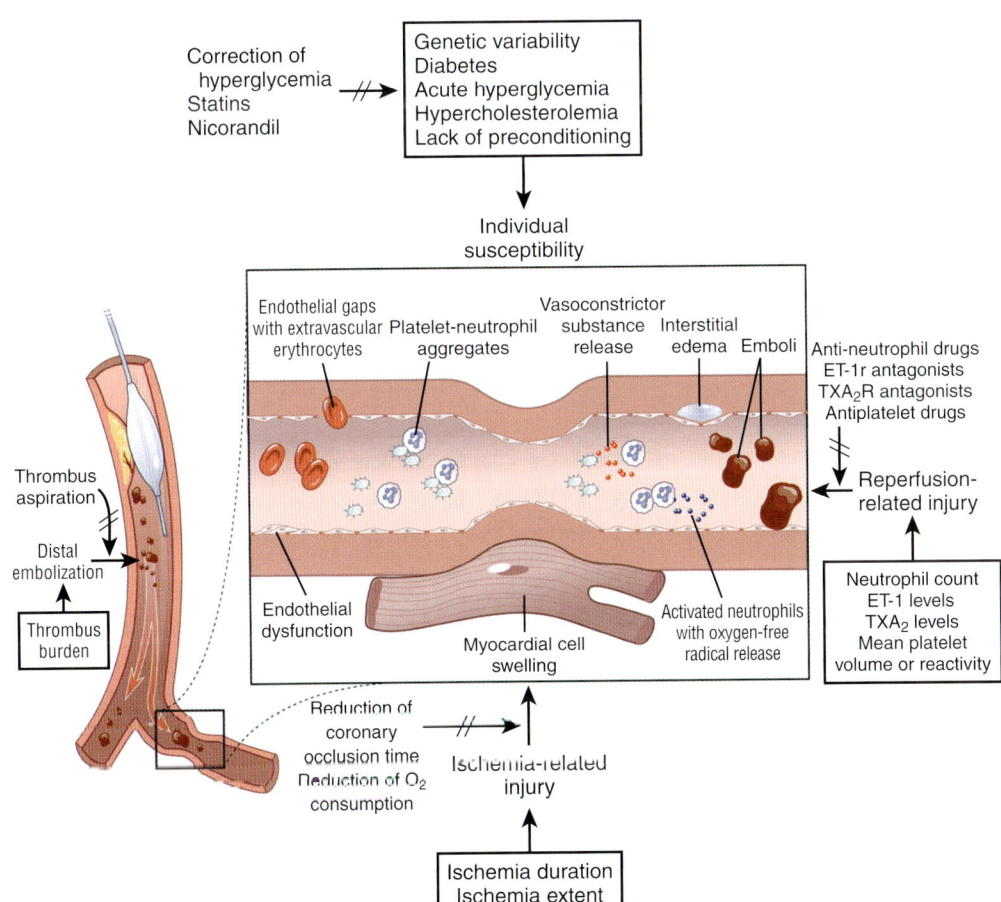

FIGURE 38.6 Multiple mechanisms involved in the pathogenesis of no-reflow that might be targeted by appropriate therapy. *ET*, Endothelin; *TXA₂*, thromboxane A₂. (Modified from Niccoli G, Burzotta F, Galiuto L, Crea F. Myocardial no-reflow in humans. *J Am Coll Cardiol.* 2009;54:281.)

STEMI include a protracted period of delay in seeking medical care, a lower incidence of ischemic discomfort and greater incidence of atypical symptoms and concomitant illnesses, and an increased incidence of nondiagnostic findings on the ECG.[1,31] Younger patients with STEMI achieved a slightly greater relative reduction in mortality than elderly patients, but the higher absolute mortality in elderly patients yielded similar absolute reductions in mortality. The STREAM (Strategic Reperfusion Early After Myocardial Infarction) study comparing an early pharmacoinvasive strategy to primary PCI found that a half-dose of tenecteplase had similar efficacy with lower rates of intracranial hemorrhage in patients 75 years or older.[12,41] This regimen, which has been incorporated into guidelines,[2] is being studied in an expanded population of patients 60 years or older in the STREAM-2 trial.[42]

Several models have integrated the many clinical variables available before the administration of fibrinolytic therapy that are associated with a patient's risk for death. A convenient, simple, bedside risk-scoring system predicts 30-day mortality at initial evaluation of fibrinolytic-eligible patients with STEMI.[1] Modeling of mortality risk cannot cover all clinical scenarios, however, and should only supplement clinical judgment in individual cases. For example, patients with inferior STEMI who might otherwise be considered to have a low risk for mortality, and for whom many physicians have questioned the benefits of fibrinolytic therapy, might be in a higher mortality risk subgroup if their inferior infarction is associated with RV infarction, precordial ST-segment depression, or ST-segment elevation in the lateral precordial leads. The short-term survival benefit enjoyed by patients who receive fibrinolytic therapy endures after 1 to 10 years. Advances in adjunctive antiplatelet and antithrombin therapies have led to reductions in the rate of reinfarction after fibrinolysis for STEMI.[4]

Comparison of Fibrinolytic Agents

Table 38.4 presents the comparative features of the approved fibrinolytic agents for IV therapy. All fibrinolytic agents exert their effect by converting the proenzyme plasminogen to the active enzyme plasmin. The so-called fibrin-specific fibrinolytics are those that are relatively inactive in the absence of fibrin but in its presence substantially increase their activity on plasminogen (see Chapter 95). The tissue plasminogen activator (t-PA) molecule contains five domains.[43] In the absence of fibrin, t-PA is a weak plasminogen activator; fibrin provides a scaffold on which t-PA and plasminogen are held in such a way that the catalytic efficiency of t-PA increases many-fold. A dose regimen of t-PA administered over a 90-minute period produces more rapid thrombolysis than a 3-hour fixed-rate infusion. Therefore, the recommended dosage for t-PA is the 90-minute "accelerated" regimen. Modifications in the native t-PA structure have yielded a group of fibrinolytic agents with prolonged clearance that allows them to be administered as a bolus (see Table 38.4).[43] Reteplase (double fixed-dose bolus) and tenecteplase (single weight-based bolus) confer mortality benefits similar to that achieved with accelerated t-PA, but with more convenient dosing. In one large trial, tenecteplase had a lower rate of major bleeding than accelerated t-PA or other regimens.[44] Streptokinase, a protein derived from streptococci, binds and activates human plasminogen and is an inexpensive and effective fibrinolytic agent that is still used in some regions of the world.

The choice of fibrinolytic in hospital systems is generally driven by the desire to establish consistent protocols within the health care system by weighing ease of dosing, cost, and other institutional preferences. In patients seen early with acceptable bleeding risk, a high-intensity fibrin-specific regimen, such as accelerated t-PA, reteplase, or tenecteplase, is usually preferable.[1] Bolus fibrinolytics have a lower chance of medication errors and are associated with less noncerebral bleeding—as well as offering the potential for prehospital treatment.[4,44]

Effect on Left Ventricular Function

As with survival, improvement in global LV function is related to the time of initiation of fibrinolytic treatment, with the greatest improvement occurring with the earliest therapy. Nevertheless, left ventricular ejection fraction (LVEF) is not adequate as a surrogate for infarct size because little difference is seen in EF between groups that show a significant difference in mortality. However, patients with smaller end-systolic volumes and better-preserved ventricular shape have better survival. The *myocardial salvage index* is defined as the difference between the initial perfusion defect (e.g., by CMR or sestamibi scintigraphy) and the final perfusion defect.[39,45] CMR can characterize LV volumes, the extent of the scar by gadolinium delayed hyperenhancement, and the presence of ischemia with stress perfusion imaging, providing significant incremental prognostic information over other clinical variables.[39,45]

Complications of Fibrinolytic Therapy

Bleeding complications are most common, and intracranial hemorrhage is the most serious complication of fibrinolytic therapy; its frequency is generally less than 1% but varies with the clinical characteristics of the patient and the fibrinolytic agent used (Fig. 38.7).[1] Intracranial bleeding in the setting of fibrinolysis for STEMI is associated with a high case-fatality rate. Nonintracranial bleeding can also increase morbidity, but whether it causes higher overall mortality after taking into account the higher-risk clinical characteristics that also predispose patients to bleeding during treatment of STEMI is uncertain.[1,2]

Reports have demonstrated an "early hazard" with fibrinolytic therapy—that is, an excess of deaths in the first 24 hours in fibrinolytic-treated patients compared with controls, especially in elderly patients treated more than 12 hours after symptom onset. However, this excess early mortality is more than offset by deaths prevented beyond the first day, with an average 18% (range, 13% to 23%) reduction in mortality by

TABLE 38.4 Comparison of Approved Fibrinolytic Agents

FIBRINOLYTIC AGENT	DOSE	FIBRIN SPECIFICITY *	FIBRINOGEN DEPLETION	ANTIGENIC	PATENCY RATE (90-MIN TIMI 2 OR 3 FLOW)
Fibrin Specific					
Tenecteplase (TNK)	Single IV weight-based bolus [†]	++++	Minimal	No	85%
Reteplase (r-PA)	10 units + 10-unit IV boluses given 30 min apart	++	Moderate	No	84%
Alteplase (t-PA)	90-min weight-based infusion [‡]	++	Mild	No	73–84%
Non-Fibrin Specific					
Streptokinase [§]	1.5 million units IV given over 30–60 min	No	Marked	Yes [¶]	60–68%

r-PA, Reteplase plasminogen activator; *t-PA*, tissue plasminogen activator.
*Strength of fibrin specificity: ++++ is stronger; ++ is less strong.
[†]Bolus of 30 mg for weight less than 60 kg, 35 mg for 60 to 69 kg, 40 mg for 70 to 79 kg, 45 mg for 80 to 89 kg, and 50 mg for 90 kg or greater.
[‡]Bolus of 15 mg, infusion of 0.75 mg/kg for 30 minutes (maximum, 50 mg), then 0.5 mg/kg (maximum, 35 mg) over the next 60 minutes; the total dose not to exceed 100 mg.
[§]Streptokinase is no longer marketed in the United States but is available in other countries.
[¶]Streptokinase is highly antigenic and absolutely contraindicated within 6 months of previous exposure because of the potential for serious allergic reaction.
From O'Gara PT, Kushner FG, Ascheim DD, et al. 2013 ACCF/AHA guideline for the management of ST-elevation myocardial infarction: a report of the American College of Cardiology Foundation/American Heart Association Task Force on Practice Guidelines. *J Am Coll Cardiol.* 2013;61:e78.

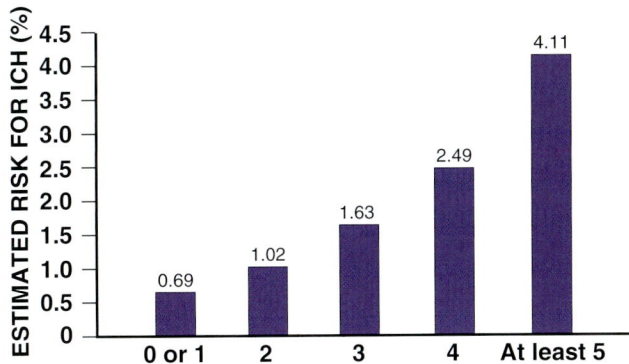

FIGURE 38.7 Estimation of risk for intracranial hemorrhage (ICH) with fibrinolysis. Common risk factors include increased age, low body weight, and hypertension on admission. See reference for further discussion. (Data from Brass LM, Lichtman JH, Wang Y, et al. Intracranial hemorrhage associated with thrombolytic therapy for elderly patients with acute myocardial infarction: results from the Cooperative Cardiovascular Project. *Stroke*. 2000;31:1802.)

35 days compared with offering no reperfusion therapy.[1] The mechanisms responsible for this early hazard are probably multiple, including an increased risk for myocardial rupture, fatal intracranial hemorrhage, and possibly myocardial reperfusion injury.

Recent exposure to streptococci or streptokinase produces some degree of antibody-mediated resistance to streptokinase (and anistreplase) in most patients. Although such resistance is only rarely of clinical consequence, patients should not receive streptokinase for STEMI if they have been treated with a streptokinase product within the past 6 months.

Late Therapy

No mortality benefit was demonstrated in the LATE and EMERAS trials when fibrinolytics were routinely administered to patients between 12 and 24 hours, although we believe that it is still reasonable to consider fibrinolytic therapy when PCI is not available for appropriately selected patients with clinical and electrocardiographic evidence of ongoing ischemia within 12 to 24 hours of symptom onset and a large area of myocardium at risk or hemodynamic instability. Because elderly patients treated with fibrinolytic agents more than 12 hours after the onset of symptoms have an increased risk for cardiac rupture, we believe that restricting late administration of a fibrinolytic to patients younger than 65 years with ongoing ischemia is preferable. An elderly patient with ongoing ischemic symptoms but initially seen late (>12 hours) is better managed with PCI than with fibrinolytic therapy.

Intracoronary Fibrinolysis

In contemporary practice, patients are more likely to be treated with PCI. This evolution has revived the concept of delivering fibrinolytic agents by the intracoronary route, but current efforts are largely restricted to adjunctive use during complicated PCI procedures.

Catheter-Based Reperfusion Strategies

Catheter-based strategies can also achieve reperfusion of the infarct artery. This approach has evolved from passage of a balloon catheter over a guidewire in the culprit vessel only to now include potent oral antiplatelet therapy, multiple options for anticoagulants, and coronary stents, with the possibility of multivessel revascularization.[1] PCI used as primary reperfusion therapy in patients with STEMI is referred to as direct or primary PCI (see Fig. 38.2). The approach to primary PCI, including device selection, the technical approach to percutaneous revascularization, and decision making regarding nonculprit vessel disease are discussed in more detail in Chapter 41. As an alternative to pharmacologic reperfusion therapy, primary PCI has evolved significantly. Several randomized trials have suggested use a strategy of multivessel PCI, either at the time of primary PCI or as a planned, staged procedure, may be safe and may improve outcomes in hemodynamically stable patients with STEMI (Fig. 38.8).[46-50] These findings have prompted a change in recommendation from class III to IIa[2] or IIb[6] for consideration of multivessel PCI in stable patients with STEMI. However, in patients with cardiogenic shock, immediate revascularization of only the infarct artery at the time of initial presentation is preferred based on improved outcomes for the composite of death or the need for renal replacement therapy in the CULPRIT-SHOCK study.[51] Aspiration thrombectomy at primary PCI has a class III recommendation based on trial data showing no improvement in cardiovascular (CV) outcomes and a possible increase in stroke risk.[2,6,52,53] Radial artery access is favored over femoral artery access in primary PCI based on the MATRIX (Minimizing Adverse Haemorrhagic Events by Transradial Access Site and Systemic Implementation of AngioX) trial, which demonstrated a reduction in bleeding and mortality (Fig. 38.9).[2,54] Finally, newer-generation drug-eluting stents (DESs) appear to result in lower rates of repeat revascularization with equivalent or lower rates of stent thrombosis compared to contemporary bare-metal stents (BMSs).[55-58]

Surgical Reperfusion

Providing surgical reperfusion in a timely fashion during STEMI is usually not logistically possible. Therefore, patients with STEMI who are candidates for reperfusion should undergo either immediate PCI or if not practical then fibrinolysis. However, patients with STEMI may be referred for CABG for persistent or recurrent ischemia after fibrinolysis or primary PCI with residual coronary disease not amenable to PCI, high-risk coronary anatomy (e.g., left main stenosis) discovered at initial catheterization or a complication of STEMI such as ventricular septal rupture or severe mitral regurgitation caused by papillary muscle dysfunction. STEMI patients with continued severe ischemic and hemodynamic instability will probably benefit from emergency revascularization.

Patients who successfully undergo fibrinolysis but have important residual stenoses and on anatomic grounds are more suitable for surgical revascularization than for PCI have undergone CABG with quite low rates of mortality (approximately 4%) and morbidity, provided that the procedure is carried out more than 24 hours after STEMI; patients requiring urgent or emergency CABG within 24 to 48 hours of STEMI have mortality rates between 12% and 15%.[1] Surgery performed under urgent conditions with active and ongoing ischemia or cardiogenic shock, are associated with higher operative mortality rates, in large part reflecting the patient's overall condition that necessitated emergency surgery.

Selection of Reperfusion Strategy

When performed rapidly after arrival at an experienced center, primary PCI is superior to pharmacologic reperfusion therapy.[1,4] However, registry and randomized data remind us that very early fibrinolysis may be at least as effective as primary PCI.[12,59] Improvements in catheterization laboratory facilities, new stents, evolution of adjunctive antithrombotic therapy, and development of collaborative systems for rapid transfer for invasive therapy have improved the efficacy and safety of primary PCI in patients with STEMI, including those being transferred for primary PCI (see Chapter 41).[8] Selection of the optimal form of reperfusion therapy therefore involves judgments regarding both system resources and individual patient characteristics.

For patients who arrive at an experienced primary PCI center, primary PCI should be performed in those with STEMI who present within 12 hours of symptom onset and those with later arrival who have ongoing ischemia, HF, or shock. In patients taken to centers that are not PCI capable, the primary consideration is the time required for transportation to a PCI-capable center. The greatest operational impediment to routine implementation of a PCI reperfusion strategy is the delay required for transportation to a skilled PCI center (see Fig. 38.2 and Table 38.1).[8] Trials conducted in health care systems with extremely short transportation and door-to-balloon times at PCI centers have demonstrated that referral to a PCI center can be superior to fibrinolysis administered at a local hospital.[8] If the delay to implementation of primary PCI is substantial, however, the mortality advantage over administration of a fibrin-specific agent is lost (Fig. 38.10). The best estimate of the time delay at which this advantage is lost is 1 to 2 hours, but it may vary depending on the timing of initial evaluation and the extent of myocardium at risk.[8]

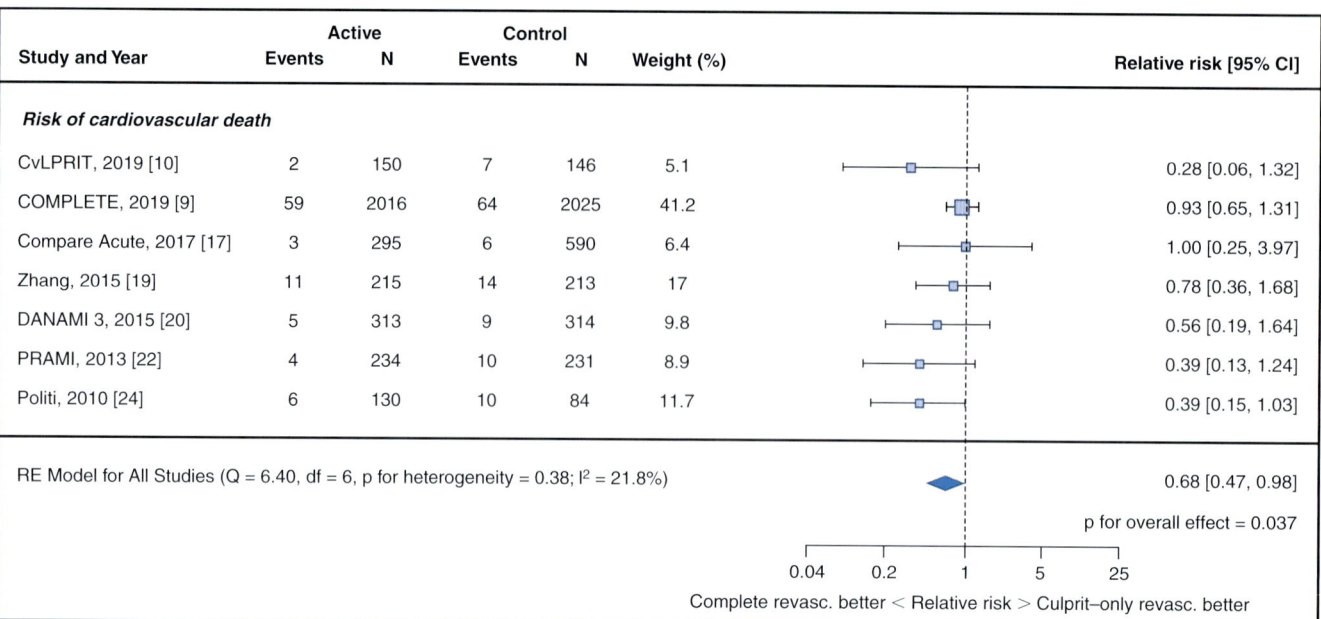

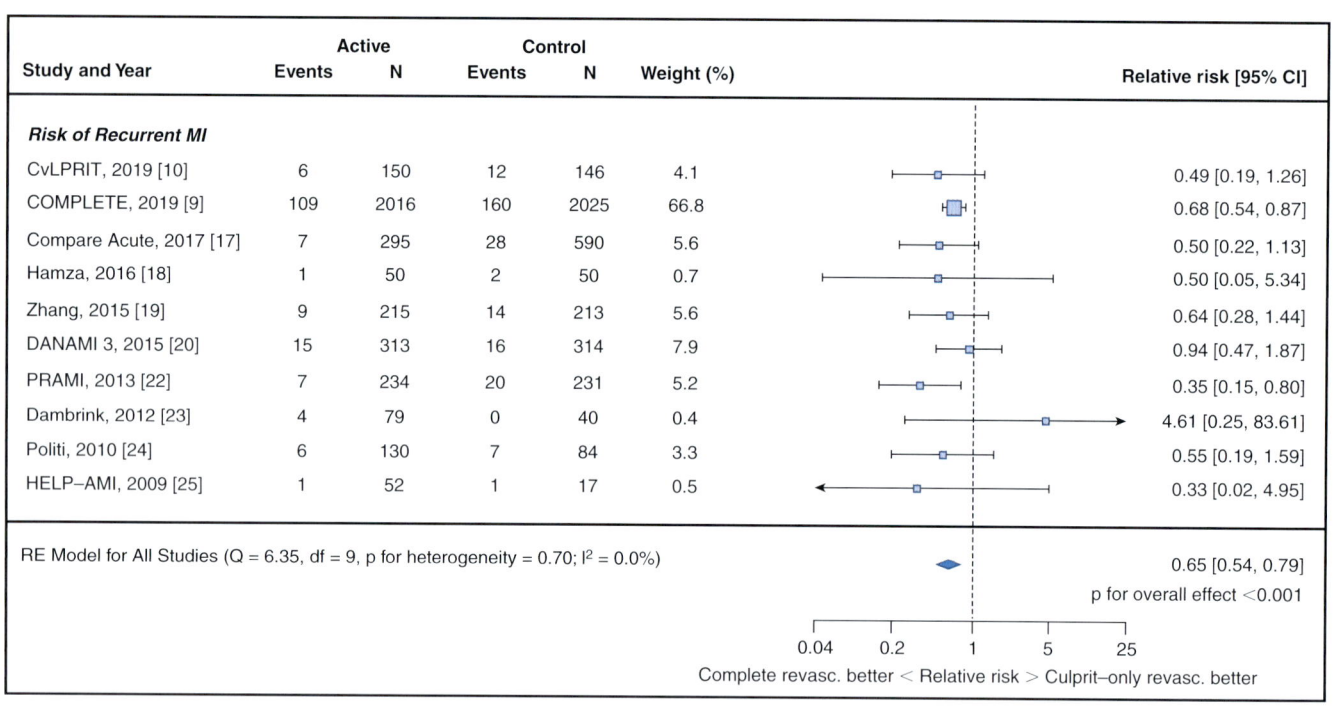

FIGURE 38.8 Meta-analysis of randomized controls trials comparing culprit-vessel only PCI and complete revascularization in patients with STEMI without shock for the endpoints of **(A)** cardiovascular death and **(B)** myocardial infarction. Compare Acute indicates Fractional Flow Reserve–Guided Multivessel Angioplasty in Myocardial Infarction; COMPLETE, Complete versus Culprit–Only Revascularization Strategies to Treat Multivessel Disease after Early PCI for STEMI; CvLPRIT, Complete Versus Lesion–Only Primary PCI trial; DANAMI 3 PRIMULTI, Complete revascularisation versus treatment of the culprit lesion only in patients with ST–segment–elevation myocardial infarction and multivessel disease; PRAMI, Preventive Angioplasty in Acute Myocardial Infarction. (From Ahmad Y, et al. *J Am Heart Assoc*. 2020;9[12]:e015263.)

If the time from first medical contact to PCI is expected to be more than 120 minutes, fibrinolysis is recommended in the absence of (1) significant contraindications to fibrinolysis, (2) shock or acute severe heart failure, or (3) late presentation. Otherwise, transfer for primary PCI is generally favored if any of these conditions are present, even if the delay to revascularization will be greater than 120 minutes (see Fig. 38.2 and Table 38.3):

1. *High risk for bleeding.* In patients with an increased risk for bleeding, particularly intracranial hemorrhage, therapeutic decision making strongly favors a PCI-based reperfusion strategy. If PCI is unavailable, the benefit of pharmacologic reperfusion should be balanced against the risk for bleeding. A decision analysis suggests that when PCI is not available, fibrinolytic therapy should still be favored over no reperfusion treatment until the risk for life-threatening bleeding exceeds 4%.
2. *Presence of shock or acute severe heart failure.* Patients in cardiogenic shock have improved survival if they are treated with an early revascularization strategy of PCI and/or CABG. Therefore, immediate transfer to a PCI-capable hospital is recommended in patients with shock or acute severe HF regardless of the time delay.[1,2,8]

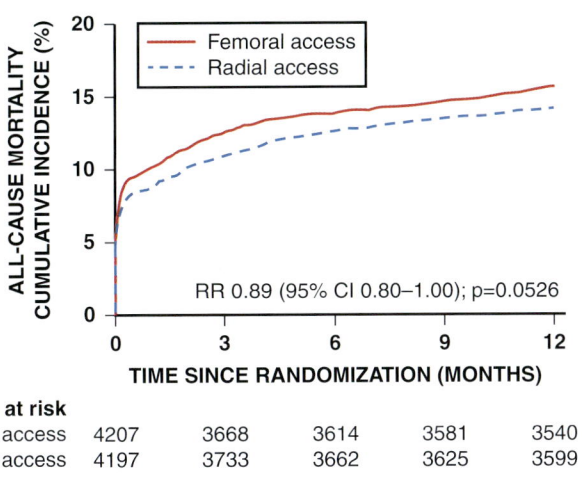

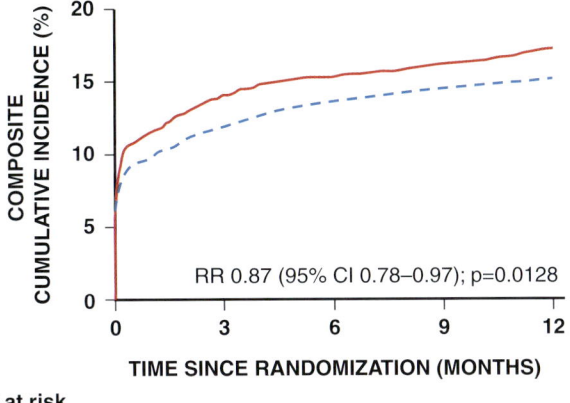

FIGURE 38.9 Comparison of radial versus femoral access for PCI in STEMI in the MATRIX study for the co-primary endpoints of **(A)** all-cause mortality, myocardial infarction or stroke and **(B)** all-cause mortality, myocardial infarction, stroke, or Bleeding Academic Research Consortium type 3 or 5 bleeding. (From Valgimigli et al. Lancet 2018;392:835–848.)

3. *Prolonged time from onset of symptoms to initiation of reperfusion therapy.* PCI is preferable in patients with late arrival, particularly those initially seen 12 to 24 hours after symptom onset. Fibrinolysis can be considered in the 12- to 24-hour window for patients with evidence of ongoing ischemia and where PCI is not available, although the benefit has not been established.[1]

When the diagnosis of STEMI is in doubt, an invasive strategy is clearly the preferred strategy because it not only provides key diagnostic information regarding the patient's symptoms but does so without the risk for intracranial hemorrhage associated with fibrinolysis.

Referral for Angiography with Intent of Revascularization after Initial Fibrinolysis

Patients with STEMI who are initially managed by fibrinolysis at a non–PCI-capable center should be transferred urgently to a PCI-capable center if the patient develops cardiogenic shock or severe HF or has failed reperfusion with a fibrinolytic. Transfer should also be considered (class IIa) as a part of a pharmacoinvasive strategy in stable patients with the intention of performing angiography, and PCI as necessary, 3 to 24 hours after fibrinolysis (Table 38.5; see Fig. 38.2).[1,2]

Patients undergoing angiography and PCI after the suspected failure of reperfusion with fibrinolysis tend to have a lower mortality rate and significantly lower rates of recurrent MI and HF compared with patients who continue medical therapy, including readministration of a fibrinolytic agent. In the REACT (Rapid Early Action for Coronary Treatment) study, patients with suspected failed reperfusion at 90 minutes by electrocardiographic criteria were randomly assigned to one of three treatment arms: rescue PCI, conservative care, or repeated fibrinolytic therapy. The composite of death, reinfarction, stroke, or severe HF at 6 months was significantly lower in patients randomly assigned to rescue PCI than in the two other treatment groups.[1] More minor bleeding, however, occurred in patients randomly assigned to rescue PCI. The option of administration of a fibrinolytic agent at non–PCI-capable hospitals, followed by routine transfer for angiography and PCI if indicated, has been advanced as an attractive strategy to offer timely reperfusion therapy and arrange a "nonemergency" transfer for subsequent procedures to reduce the risk for subsequent reinfarction. Retrospective analyses of trials of fibrinolytic therapy indirectly support this approach because they suggest a lower risk for recurrent MI and a lower 2-year mortality rate in patients who subsequently undergo early PCI. The limited randomized trials evaluating a strategy of routine catheterization after fibrinolysis have provided mixed results. Nevertheless, overall, these trials have suggested improvement in clinical outcomes in patients transferred for early catheterization, particularly those at higher risk for death and recurrent ischemia (Fig. 38.11).[1] In the largest of these studies, TRANSFER-AMI (Trial of Routine Angioplasty and Stenting after Fibrinolysis to Enhance Reperfusion in Acute Myocardial Infarction; $n = 1059$), immediate transfer for angiography versus conservative care reduced the composite endpoint of death, recurrent MI, recurrent ischemia, new or worsening HF, or shock at 30 days.[8] In a meta-analysis that included seven randomized trials of early transfer for catheterization, a strategy of routine early catheterization after fibrinolysis yielded a statistically significant 35% reduction in the incidence of death or MI at 30 days (odds ratio [OR], 0.65; 95% confidence interval [CI] 0.49 to 0.88) without an increase in the risk for major bleeding (see Fig. 38.11).[8,60]

Notably, the clinical trials that assessed routine invasive evaluation after initial fibrinolysis used a time window of 0 to 24 hours for the "early invasive" strategy, thus supporting earlier transfer after administration of fibrinolytic therapy, even for patients

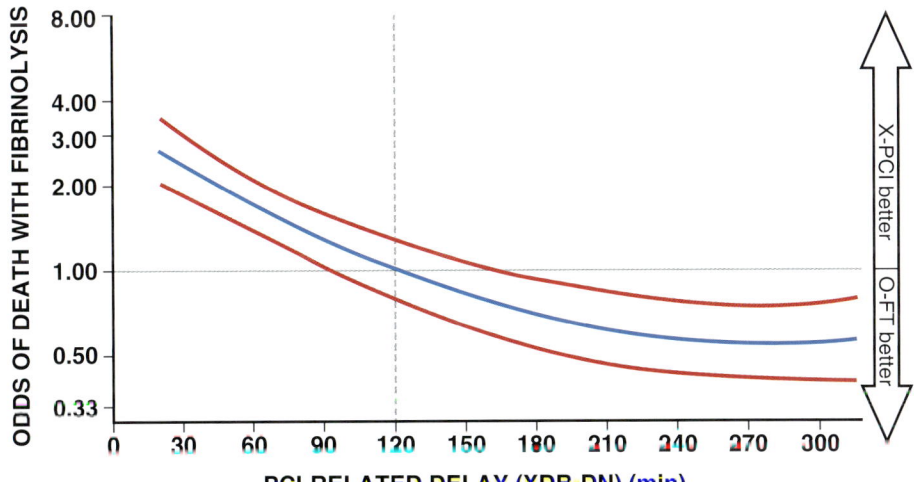

FIGURE 38.10 Relationship between PCI-related delay (minutes) during transfer from a non-PCI-capable hospital to a PCI-capable hospital and in-hospital mortality. The *red lines* represent 95% CIs. XDB-DN indicates transfer delay (transfer door-to-balloon minus door-to-needle time). With delays longer than 120 minutes between administration of a fibrinolytic on-site and balloon (or device) time at a receiving hospital, the on-site fibrinolytic strategy becomes preferable with respect to mortality risk when compared with transfer for PCI. *O-FT,* On-site fibrinolytic therapy; *X-PCI,* transfer PCI. (From Pinto DS, Frederick PD, Chakrabarti AK, et al. Benefit of transferring ST-segment-elevation myocardial infarction patients for percutaneous coronary intervention compared with administration of onsite fibrinolytic as delays increase. *Circulation.* 2011;124:2518.)

without high-risk features. Although we believe that there will probably be continued benefit even beyond 24 hours in patients with a patent but stenotic infarct artery after initial successful reperfusion, later time windows have not been directly examined. Because of the associated increased bleeding risk, very early (<2 to 3 hours) catheterization after the administration of fibrinolytic therapy with the intent to perform revascularization should be reserved for patients with evidence of failed fibrinolysis and significant myocardial jeopardy, for whom rescue PCI would be appropriate. In addition, when STEMI is suspected to have occurred by a mechanism other than thrombotic occlusion at the site of atherosclerotic plaque, coronary angiography may provide diagnostic information and direct specific therapy.

In summary, delayed coronary angiography with PCI of the infarct artery is indicated in patients initially treated with a noninvasive strategy (i.e., with fibrinolysis or without reperfusion therapy) who become unstable with cardiogenic shock, acute severe HF, or ongoing ischemia, provided that invasive management is not considered futile or inappropriate (see Table 38.5). Delayed PCI also appears to be reasonable in patients with failed fibrinolysis or reocclusion of the infarct artery or in those who demonstrate significant residual ischemia during hospitalization after initial noninvasive management. The benefits of routine (non-ischemia-driven) PCI on an angiographically significant stenosis in a patent infarct artery more than 24 hours after STEMI are less well established, and delayed PCI on a totally occluded infarct artery longer than 24 hours after STEMI should not be undertaken in clinically stable patients without evidence of severe ischemia.[1]

TABLE 38.5 Indications for Coronary Angiography in Patients Who Were Managed with Fibrinolytic Therapy or Who Did Not Receive Reperfusion Therapy

RECOMMENDATION	COR	LOE
Cardiogenic shock or acute severe heart failure that develops after initial evaluation	I	B
Intermediate- or high-risk findings on predischarge noninvasive ischemia testing	I	B
Spontaneous or easily provoked myocardial ischemia	I	C
Failed reperfusion or reocclusion after fibrinolytic therapy	IIa	B
Stable* patients after successful fibrinolysis—before discharge and ideally between 3 and 24 hours	IIa	B

COR, Class of recommendation; *LOE*, level of evidence.
*Although individual circumstances vary, *clinical stability* is defined as the absence of low output, hypotension, persistent tachycardia, apparent shock, high-grade ventricular or symptomatic supraventricular tachyarrhythmias, and spontaneous recurrent ischemia.
Modified from O'Gara PT, Kushner FG, Ascheim DD, et al. 2013 ACCF/AHA guideline for the management of ST-elevation myocardial infarction: a report of the American College of Cardiology Foundation/American Heart Association Task Force on Practice Guidelines. *J Am Coll Cardiol.* 2013;61:e78.

Patients Not Eligible for Reperfusion Therapy

Aspirin and antithrombin therapy can be prescribed for patients who are not candidates for acute reperfusion because of the lack of availability of PCI and contraindications to fibrinolysis. In the setting of absolute contraindications to fibrinolysis (see Table 38.3) and lack of access to PCI facilities, antithrombotic therapy should be initiated because of the slight chance (approximately 10%) of restoring TIMI

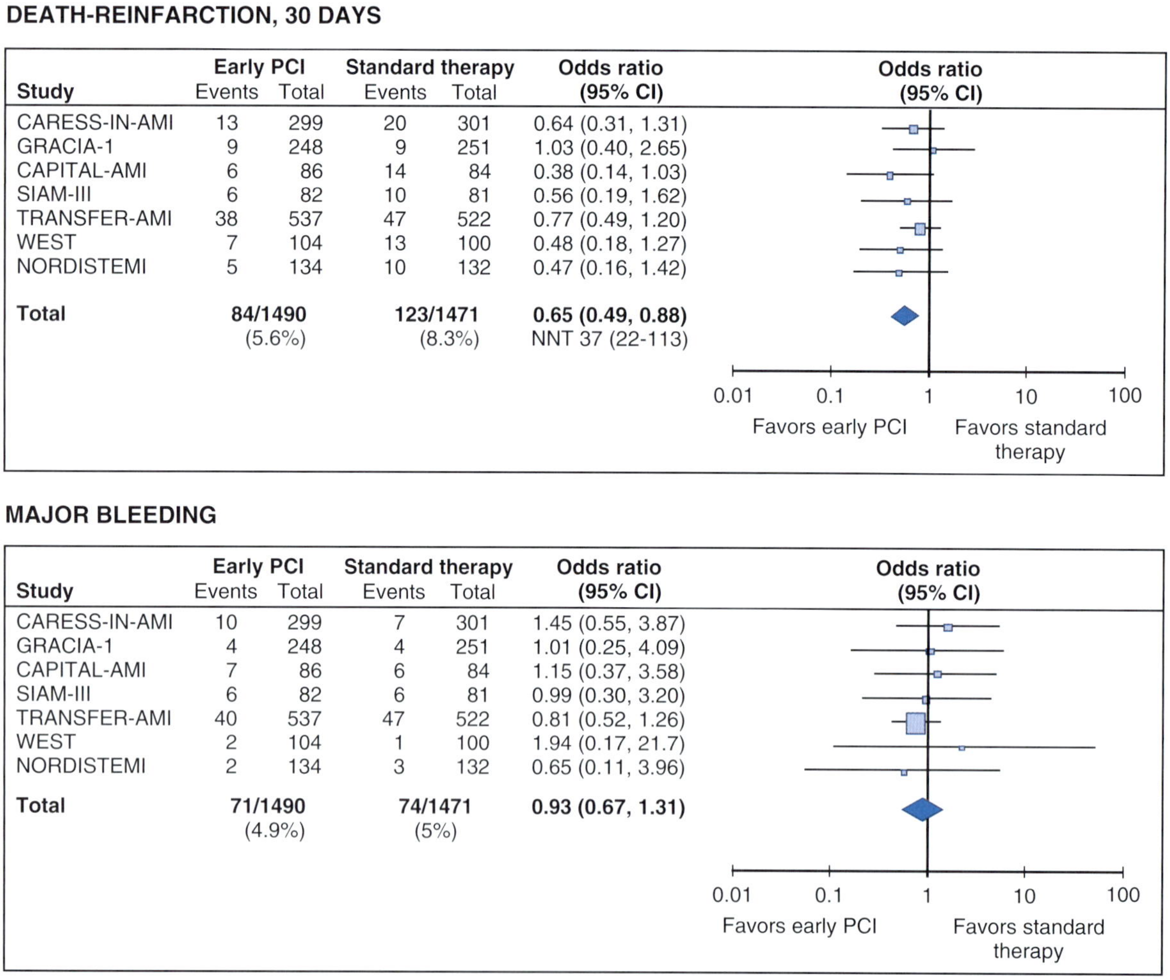

DEATH-REINFARCTION, 30 DAYS

Study	Early PCI Events	Total	Standard therapy Events	Total	Odds ratio (95% CI)
CARESS-IN-AMI	13	299	20	301	0.64 (0.31, 1.31)
GRACIA-1	9	248	9	251	1.03 (0.40, 2.65)
CAPITAL-AMI	6	86	14	84	0.38 (0.14, 1.03)
SIAM-III	6	82	10	81	0.56 (0.19, 1.62)
TRANSFER-AMI	38	537	47	522	0.77 (0.49, 1.20)
WEST	7	104	13	100	0.48 (0.18, 1.27)
NORDISTEMI	5	134	10	132	0.47 (0.16, 1.42)
Total	84/1490 (5.6%)		123/1471 (8.3%)		0.65 (0.49, 0.88) NNT 37 (22-113)

MAJOR BLEEDING

Study	Early PCI Events	Total	Standard therapy Events	Total	Odds ratio (95% CI)
CARESS-IN-AMI	10	299	7	301	1.45 (0.55, 3.87)
GRACIA-1	4	248	4	251	1.01 (0.25, 4.09)
CAPITAL-AMI	7	86	6	84	1.15 (0.37, 3.58)
SIAM-III	6	82	6	81	0.99 (0.30, 3.20)
TRANSFER-AMI	40	537	47	522	0.81 (0.52, 1.26)
WEST	2	104	1	100	1.94 (0.17, 21.7)
NORDISTEMI	2	134	3	132	0.65 (0.11, 3.96)
Total	71/1490 (4.9%)		74/1471 (5%)		0.93 (0.67, 1.31)

FIGURE 38.11 A meta-analysis of seven randomized trials of early transfer for catheterization, a strategy of routine early catheterization after fibrinolysis, was associated with a statistically significant 35% reduction in the incidence of death or MI at 30 days **(top)** with no increase in major bleeding **(bottom)**, for combined death-reinfarction and recurrent ischemia between early PCI and standard therapy. Size of data markers indicates the weight of each trial. (Modified from Borgia F, Goodman SG, Halvorsen S, et al. Early routine percutaneous coronary intervention after fibrinolysis versus standard therapy in ST-segment elevation myocardial infarction: a meta-analysis. *Eur Heart J.* 2010;31[17]:2156-69.)

grade 3 flow in the infarct vessel and decreasing the chance of complications of STEMI.

Anticoagulant and Antiplatelet Therapy
Anticoagulant Therapy
The rationale for administering anticoagulant therapy acutely to patients with STEMI includes establishing and maintaining patency of the infarct-related artery, regardless of whether a patient receives fibrinolytic therapy, and preventing deep venous thrombosis, pulmonary embolism, ventricular thrombus formation, and cerebral embolization.

Effect of Heparin on Mortality
Randomized trials of patients with STEMI conducted in the prefibrinolytic era showed a lower risk for reinfarction, pulmonary embolism, and stroke in those who received IV heparin, thus supporting the administration of heparin to STEMI patients not treated with fibrinolytic therapy. With the introduction of the fibrinolytic era and, importantly, after publication of the ISIS-2 (Second International Study of Infarct Survival) trial, the situation became more complicated because of strong evidence of a substantial reduction in mortality with aspirin alone and confusing and conflicting data regarding the risk/benefit ratio of heparin used as an adjunct to aspirin or in combination with aspirin and a fibrinolytic agent.[1] Nevertheless, a meta-analysis of trials in the fibrinolytic era suggested that for every 1000 patients treated with heparin versus aspirin alone, five fewer deaths ($P = 0.03$) and three fewer recurrent infarctions ($P = 0.04$) occur, but at the expense of three more major bleeding episodes ($P = 0.001$).[61]

OTHER EFFECTS OF HEPARIN. Several angiographic studies have examined the role of heparin therapy in establishing and maintaining patency of the infarct-related artery in patients with STEMI. Although evidence favoring the use of heparin in conjunction with a fibrin-specific fibrinolytic agent for enhancing patency of the infarct artery is not conclusive, the suggestion of a mortality benefit and amelioration of LV thrombi after STEMI supports the use of heparin for at least 48 hours after fibrinolysis.[1]

The most serious complication of anticoagulant therapy is bleeding (see Chapter 95), especially intracranial hemorrhage. Major hemorrhagic events occur more frequently in patients with low body weight, advanced age, female sex, marked prolongation of the activated partial thromboplastin time (APTT) (>90 to 100 seconds), and performance of invasive procedures.[62] Frequent monitoring of the APTT reduces the risk for major hemorrhagic complications in patients treated with heparin. During the first 12 hours after fibrinolytic therapy, however, the APTT may be elevated as a result of the fibrinolytic agent alone (particularly if streptokinase is administered), thus making it difficult to interpret accurately the effects of a heparin infusion on the patient's coagulation status.

DISADVANTAGES OF HEPARIN. Potential disadvantages of unfractionated heparin (UFH) include dependency on antithrombin III for inhibition of thrombin activity, sensitivity to platelet factor 4, inability to inhibit clot-bound thrombin, marked interpatient variability in therapeutic response, and the need for frequent monitoring of the APTT. Several alternative anticoagulants can circumvent these disadvantages of UFH.

Hirudin and Bivalirudin
In patients undergoing fibrinolysis, direct thrombin inhibitors such as hirudin or bivalirudin reduce the incidence of recurrent MI by 25% to 30% compared with heparin but have not reduced mortality. In addition, either hirudin or bivalirudin causes higher rates of major bleeding than heparin when used with fibrinolytic agents.[2] As direct thrombin inhibitors have not been studied with fibrin-specific agents, there is no evidence to guide recommendations on their use in fibrinolysis.[2]

In contrast, when administered for a short period as an adjunct to primary PCI in the HORIZONS-AMI (Harmonizing Outcomes with Revascularization and Stents in Acute Myocardial Infarction) trial, bivalirudin (open label), versus heparin plus glycoprotein (GP) IIb/IIIa inhibitors, reduced the 30-day rate of major bleeding or major adverse CV events, including death, reinfarction, target vessel revascularization for ischemia, and stroke (RR, 0.76; 95% CI 0.63 to 0.92; $P = 0.005$), driven by a significant 40% reduction in major bleeding. Treatment with bivalirudin significantly reduced mortality at 30 days and at 1 year but increased the early risk for stent thrombosis.[63] Similarly, in the EUROMAX (European Ambulance Acute Coronary Syndrome Angiography) trial, when started during transport for primary PCI in STEMI, bivalirudin reduced the primary outcome of death or major bleeding compared to heparin with optional GP IIb/IIIa, with a reduction in major bleeding but increase in stent thrombosis.[63] However, there was no significant difference in mortality. A meta-analysis of 16 randomized controlled trials (RCTs), including four with predominantly STEMI patients, reported an increased risk of major adverse cardiovascular events (MACE) (RR, 1.09; 95% CI 1.01 to 1.17; $P = 0.0204$) with bivalirudin, primarily from increases in MI, ischemia-driven revascularization, and acute stent thrombosis (Fig. 38.12).[64] There was no difference in mortality, and bleeding rates were generally lower with bivalirudin, with the magnitude of the reduction dependent on the rates of GP IIb/IIIa co-administration in the relevant trials.[64] The findings were consistent in the subset with STEMI.

Low-Molecular-Weight Heparins
Advantages of low-molecular-weight heparins (LMWHs) include a stable, reliable anticoagulant effect, high bioavailability permitting administration via the subcutaneous (SC) route, and a high anti-Xa/anti-IIa ratio producing blockade of the coagulation cascade in an upstream location and greatly reducing thrombin generation. The primary role of LMWH for the management of STEMI is as an adjunct to fibrinolytic therapy. Although LMWHs do not improve the rate of early (60 to 90 minutes) reperfusion of the infarct artery, LMWH reduces rates of reocclusion of the infarct artery, reinfarction, or recurrent ischemic events. This effect may underlie the significant reduction in recurrent MI with a strategy of extended anticoagulation with LMWHs, or a factor Xa antagonist versus standard therapy, in patients with STEMI undergoing fibrinolysis.

Moreover, in a placebo-controlled trial, an LMWH reduced the incidence of death, recurrent MI, or stroke at 30 days. This finding demonstrated not only that LMWHs are clinically effective in patients with STEMI, but also that anticoagulant therapy provides benefit as part of a fibrinolytic reperfusion strategy.

Several trials have compared an LMWH with UFH as part of a pharmacologic reperfusion strategy and demonstrated the LMWH to be superior.[65] In the ASSENT (Assessment of the Safety and Efficacy of a New Thrombolytic) 3 trial, enoxaparin (30-mg IV bolus, followed by SC injections of 1 mg/kg every 12 hours until discharge from the hospital)[65] reduced 30-day mortality, in-hospital reinfarction, or in-hospital refractory ischemia compared with UFH (RR, 0.74; 95% CI 0.63 to 0.87). The rate of intracranial hemorrhage was similar with UFH and enoxaparin (0.93% versus 0.88%; $P = 0.98$). In the ExTRACT-TIMI 25 (Enoxaparin and Thrombolysis Reperfusion for Acute Myocardial Infarction Treatment–Thrombolysis in Myocardial Infarction 25) trial, a strategy of enoxaparin administered for the duration of the index hospitalization was superior (Fig. 38.13A) to the conventional antithrombin strategy of UFH administration for 48 hours after fibrinolysis,[65] with a 33% reduction ($P = 0.001$) in reinfarction and a nonsignificant favorable trend on overall mortality ($P = 0.11$). This improvement in recurrent MI was balanced by an increase in the incidence of major bleeding (1.4% and 2.1%, $P = 0.001$). In a meta-analysis of trials of LMWH versus UFH, LMWH clearly reduced recurrent MI but with a pattern of increased bleeding (Fig. 38.13B).

Parenteral Factor Xa Antagonists
The OASIS-6 (Organization for the Assessment of Strategies for Ischemic Syndromes) trial evaluated the specific factor Xa antagonist fondaparinux (2.5 mg subcutaneously) in 12,092 patients with STEMI.[62] The trial design compared fondaparinux given for 8 days with placebo in patients when the treating physician thought that UFH was not indicated (stratum I) and with UFH for 48 hours when the treating physician thought that heparin was indicated (stratum II). Fondaparinux reduced the composite of death or reinfarction in stratum I (hazard

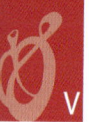

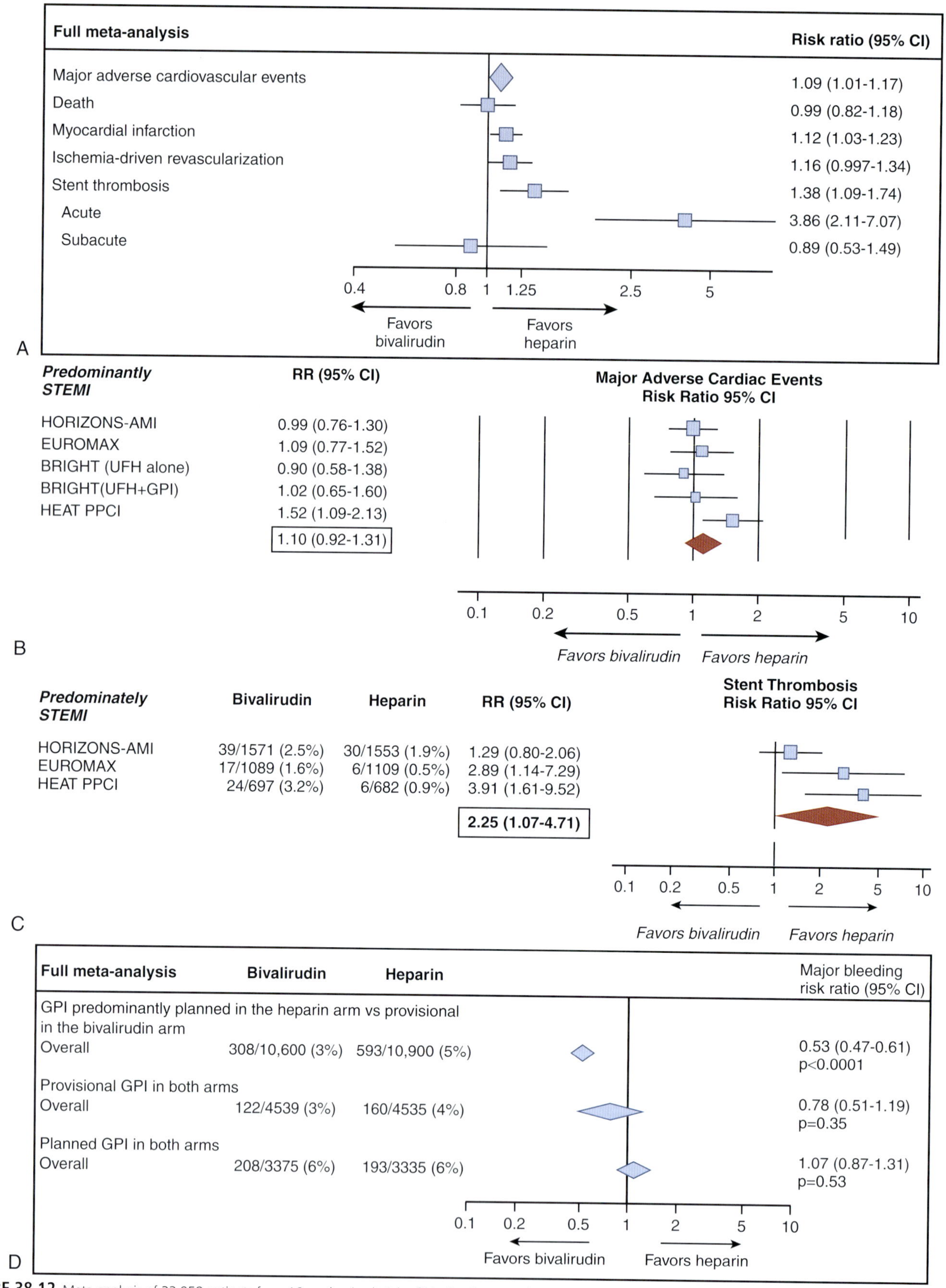

FIGURE 38.12 Meta-analysis of 33,958 patients from 16 randomized trials of bivalirudin versus heparin during PCI. There was an increase in the risk of major adverse cardiac events (MACE) at 30 days with bivalirudin-based regimens compared with heparin-based regimens (risk ratio, 1.09; 95% CI 1.01 to 1.17; $P = 0.0204$) in the overall study population **(A)**. While there was no difference in death or ischemia-driven revascularization, there was a significant increase in MI and acute stent thrombosis in the overall study population with bivalirudin-based regimens versus heparin-based regimens. There was a similar 10% increase in MACE **(B)** and numerically larger relative risk of stent thrombosis (risk ratio, 2.25; 95% CI 1.07 to 4.71) **(C)** in the four trials predominantly enrolling STEMI patients. Overall, bivalirudin-based regimens lowered the risk of major bleeding (risk ratio, 0.62; 95% CI 0.49 to 0.78; $P < 0.0001$), but the magnitude of this effect varied depending on whether glycoprotein IIb/IIIa inhibitors (GPI) were used predominantly in the heparin arm only, provisionally in both arms, or planned in both arms **(D)**. (Modified from Cavender M, Sabatine MS. Bivalirudin versus heparin in patients planned for percutaneous coronary intervention: a meta-analysis of randomised controlled trials. *Lancet.* 2014:384[9943]:599–606.)

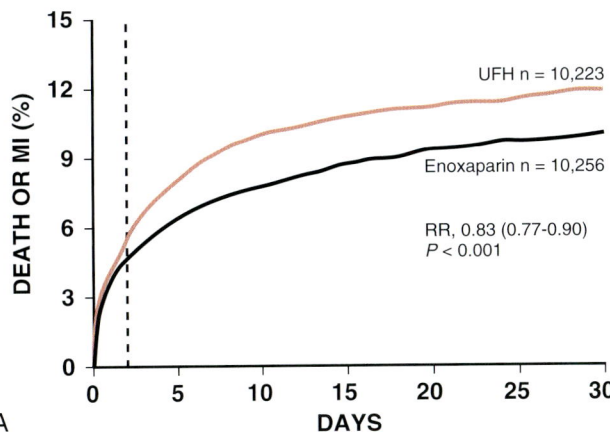

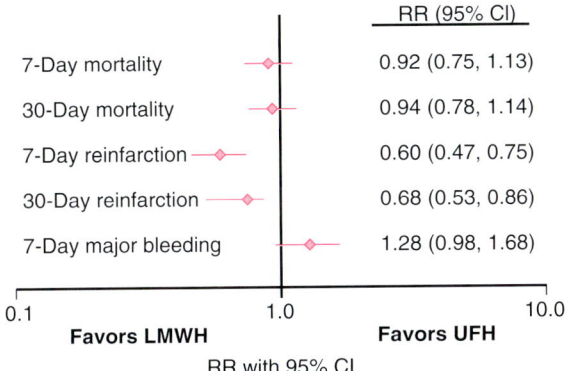

FIGURE 38.13 Comparison of enoxaparin with unfractionated heparin (UFH) as adjunctive therapy in patients with STEMI receiving fibrinolysis. **A,** Primary results from the ExTRACT-TIMI 25 trial showing that the rate of the primary endpoint (death or nonfatal MI) at 30 days was significantly lower in the enoxaparin group than in the UFH group (9.9% versus 12%, $P < 0.001$ by log-rank test). The *dashed vertical line* indicates the comparison at day 2 (direct pharmacologic comparison), at which time a trend in favor of enoxaparin was seen. **B,** Results of a meta-analysis of seven randomized controlled clinical trials of low-molecular-weight heparin (LMWH) versus UFH, including 27,577 patients with STEMI. Individual outcomes of all-cause death, reinfarction, and major bleeding are shown. (From Antman EM, Morrow DA, McCabe CH, et al. Enoxaparin versus unfractionated heparin with fibrinolysis for ST-elevation myocardial infarction. *N Engl J Med.* 2006;354:1477; and Singh S, Bahekar A, Molnar J, et al. Adjunctive low molecular weight heparin during fibrinolytic therapy in acute ST-elevation myocardial infarction: a meta-analysis of randomized control trials. *Clin Cardiol.* 2009;32:358.)

ratio [HR], 0.79; 95% CI, 0.68 to 0.92), but not in stratum II (HR, 0.96; 95% CI, 0.81 to 1.13). The outcome of patients in stratum II who underwent PCI tended to be worse with fondaparinux than with UFH probably because of an increased risk for catheter thrombosis.

Oral Factor IIa and Factor Xa Antagonists
See later section, Secondary Prevention of Acute Myocardial Infarction.

Recommendations for Anticoagulant Therapy
ADJUNCTIVE ANTICOAGULATION FOR PRIMARY PERCUTANEOUS CORONARY INTERVENTION (SEE CHAPTER 41). Either UFH or bivalirudin is recommended as an anticoagulant to support primary PCI, with a preference for bivalirudin or heparin without a concomitant GP IIb/IIIa inhibitor for patients at high risk for bleeding.[1,2,64] Fondaparinux is not recommended as the sole anticoagulant in this setting.[1] LMWH has not had sufficient evaluation in primary PCI to formulate recommendations for treatment. Some investigators who have used enoxaparin to support primary PCI for STEMI administer 0.5 mg/kg intravenously at the time of the procedure.

ANTICOAGULATION WITH FIBRINOLYSIS. Given the pivotal role of thrombin in the pathogenesis of STEMI, antithrombotic therapy remains an important intervention. A regimen of an IV UFH bolus of 60 units/kg to a maximum of 4000 units, followed by an initial infusion at 12 units/kg/hr to a maximum of 1000 units/hr for 48 hours, adjusted to maintain the APTT at 1.5 to 2 times control (approximately 50 to 70 seconds), is effective in patients receiving fibrinolytic therapy.[1]

Both the ExTRACT-TIMI 25 and the OASIS-6 trials indicated that prolonged administration of an anticoagulant for the duration of hospitalization is beneficial compared with the previous practice of administering UFH only for 48 hours unless clear-cut indications for discontinuing anticoagulation were present. Accordingly, patients managed with pharmacologic reperfusion therapy should receive anticoagulant therapy for a minimum of 48 hours and preferably for the duration of hospitalization after STEMI, up to 8 days. Enoxaparin or fondaparinux is preferred when the administration of an anticoagulant for longer than 48 hours is planned in patients with STEMI treated with a fibrinolytic.[1] Enoxaparin should be administered according to age, weight, and creatinine clearance and be given as an IV bolus, followed in 15 minutes by SC injection for the duration of the index hospitalization, up to 8 days or until revascularization. Fondaparinux should be administered as an initial IV dose, followed in 24 hours by daily SC injections if the estimated creatinine clearance is higher than 30 mL/min.[1,2] If PCI is performed in a patient treated with fondaparinux, co-administration of an additional antithrombin agent with anti-factor IIa activity is required to mitigate the risk of catheter-related thrombosis.

In patients with a known history of heparin-induced thrombocytopenia, bivalirudin in conjunction with streptokinase is a useful alternative to heparin.[1] For patients who are referred for CABG, UFH is the preferred antithrombin.

PATIENTS TREATED WITHOUT REPERFUSION THERAPY. Treatment with an anticoagulant is reasonable, and agents shown to be more effective than UFH in other groups with STEMI may be preferable. For example, in patients with STEMI not receiving reperfusion therapy, fondaparinux reduced the composite of death or recurrent MI without an increase in severe bleeding compared with placebo or UFH in the OASIS-6 trial.[62]

Antiplatelet Therapy
Platelets play a major role in the response to the disruption of coronary artery plaque, especially in the early phase of thrombus formation. Fibrinolysis can activate platelets, and platelet-rich thrombi resist fibrinolysis more than fibrin and erythrocyte-rich thrombi. Thus, a sound scientific basis exists for inhibiting platelet aggregation in *all* patients with STEMI, regardless of the reperfusion management strategy. The agent most extensively tested has been aspirin, and treatment with aspirin and a second antiplatelet agent, such as clopidogrel, prasugrel, ticagrelor, or cangrelor, has become the standard of care for patients with STEMI.

Antiplatelet Therapy for Percutaneous Coronary Intervention in ST-Elevation Myocardial Infarction
All patients with STEMI should receive aspirin as soon as possible after an initial encounter in the absence of contraindications. Adding the $P2Y_{12}$ inhibitor clopidogrel to aspirin appears to offer additional benefit in patients undergoing PCI after STEMI (Fig. 38.14). In patients undergoing either primary PCI or delayed PCI after initial therapy for STEMI, the more potent $P2Y_{12}$ inhibitor prasugrel was superior to clopidogrel in reducing the risk for CV death, MI, or stroke.[62] In the subgroup of patients with STEMI enrolled in TRITON-TIMI 38 (Trial to Assess Improvement in Therapeutic Outcomes by Optimizing Platelet Inhibition with Prasugrel–Thrombolysis in Myocardial Infarction; $n = 3534$), the primary endpoint was lowered by 32% at 30 days with prasugrel compared with aspirin (6.5% versus 9.5%, $P = 0.0017$) and by 21% at 15 months (10.0% versus 12.4%; $P = 0.022$) (Fig. 38.15).[62] Prasugrel reduced definite or probable stent thrombosis by 42% compared with clopidogrel. Analogously, in the PLATO (Platelet Inhibition and Patient Outcomes) trial, compared with clopidogrel, treatment with the reversible $P2Y_{12}$ inhibitor ticagrelor in patients with STEMI undergoing primary PCI ($n = 7544$) tended to reduce the primary endpoint of CV death, recurrent MI, or stroke by 13%, a magnitude similar to that for

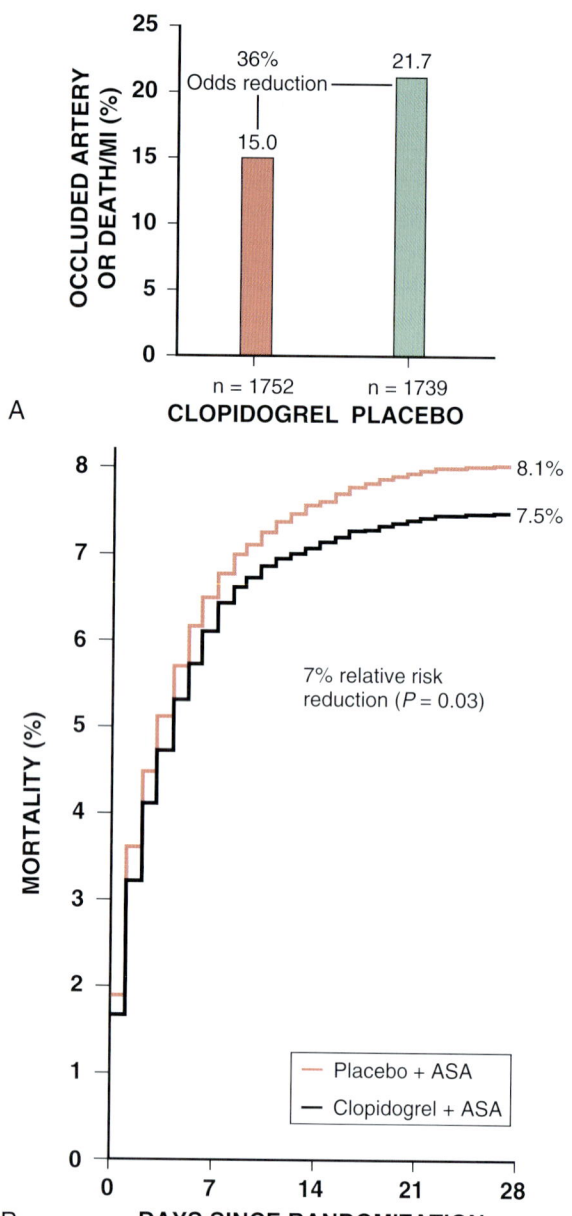

FIGURE 38.14 Impact of the addition of clopidogrel to aspirin (ASA) in patients with STEMI. **A,** Effects of the addition of clopidogrel in patients receiving fibrinolysis for STEMI. Patients in the clopidogrel group (n = 1752) had a 36% reduction in the odds of dying, sustaining a recurrent infarction, or having an occluded infarct artery compared with the placebo group (n = 1739) in the CLARITY-TIMI 28 trial. **B,** Effect of the addition of clopidogrel on in-hospital mortality after STEMI. These time-to-event curves show a 0.6% absolute reduction in mortality in the group receiving clopidogrel plus aspirin (n = 22,961) versus placebo plus aspirin (n = 22,891) in the COMMIT trial. (**A** modified from Sabatine MS, Cannon CP, Gibson CM, et al. Addition of clopidogrel to aspirin and fibrinolytic therapy for myocardial infarction with ST-segment elevation. *N Engl J Med.* 2005;352:1179; **B** modified from Chen ZM, Jiang LX, Chen, YP, et al. Addition of clopidogrel to aspirin in 45,852 patients with acute myocardial infarction: randomised placebo-controlled trial. *Lancet.* 2005;366:1607.)

elevation ACS.[1,62] In a subsequent meta-analysis that included data from randomized trials and registries, higher-risk STEMI patients had a lower risk for major coronary events with clopidogrel pretreatment, but not a reduction in mortality or an increase in bleeding.[67] Prehospital administration of ticagrelor did not improve the primary endpoint of coronary reperfusion but did reduce the secondary endpoint of stent thrombosis without any additional bleeding compared to in-hospital administration in patients with STEMI undergoing primary PCI in the ATLANTIC (Administration of Ticagrelor in the Cath Lab or in the Ambulance for New ST Elevation Myocardial Infarction to Open the Coronary Artery) trial.[68] Chapter 41 discusses the use of GP IIb/IIIa inhibitors as part of adjunctive therapy for patients with STEMI undergoing PCI.

Cangrelor, a potent, fast-acting reversible, IV P2Y12 inhibitor, can be used during PCI in patients who have not received a P2Y12 inhibitor before PCI based on CHAMPION-PHOENIX (A Clinical Trial Comparing Cangrelor to Clopidogrel Standard Therapy in Subjects Who Require Percutaneous Coronary Intervention) findings demonstrating a lower rate of death, MI, revascularization, or stent thrombosis, compared with clopidogrel in patients undergoing PCI, including primary PCI for STEMI.[69]

Antiplatelet Therapy with Fibrinolysis

The ISIS-2 study was the largest trial of aspirin in patients with STEMI; it provided the single strongest piece of evidence that aspirin reduces mortality in patients treated with or without fibrinolytic.[70] In contrast to the observations of a time-dependent mortality effect of fibrinolytic therapy, the reduction in mortality with aspirin was similar in patients treated within 4 hours (25% reduction in mortality), between 5 and 12 hours (21% reduction), and between 13 and 24 hours (21% reduction). An overall 23% reduction in mortality with aspirin occurred in ISIS-2 that was largely additive to the 25% reduction in mortality from streptokinase such that patients receiving both therapies experienced a 42% reduction in mortality. The reduction in mortality was as high as 53% in patients who received both aspirin and streptokinase within 6 hours of symptoms.

Obstructive platelet-rich arterial thrombi resist fibrinolysis and have an increased tendency for reocclusion after initial successful reperfusion in patients with STEMI. Despite inhibition of cyclooxygenase (COX) by aspirin, platelet activation leading to platelet aggregation and increased thrombin formation continues through thromboxane A_2–independent pathways. Adding other antiplatelet agents to aspirin has benefited patients with STEMI.[62] Inhibitors of the $P2Y_{12}$ adenosine diphosphate receptor help prevent the activation and aggregation of platelets. In the CLARITY-TIMI 28 trial, addition of the $P2Y_{12}$ inhibitor clopidogrel to background treatment with aspirin in patients with STEMI who were younger than 75 years and received fibrinolytic therapy reduced the risk for clinical events (death, reinfarction, stroke) and reocclusion of a successfully reperfused infarct artery (Fig. 38.14A).[62] An ST Resolution (STRes) electrocardiographic substudy from CLARITY-TIMI 28 provided insight into the mechanism of the benefit of clopidogrel in STEMI. No difference was seen in the rate of complete STRes between the clopidogrel and placebo groups at 90 minutes (38.4% versus 36.6%). When patients were stratified by STRes category, treatment with clopidogrel resulted in greater benefit in those with evidence of early STRes, with greater odds of having an open artery at late angiography in patients with partial or complete STRes, but no improvement in those with no STRes evident at 90 minutes. Thus, it appears that clopidogrel did not increase the rate of complete opening of occluded infarct arteries when fibrinolysis was administered but was effective in preventing reocclusion of an initially reperfused infarct artery.

In COMMIT (Clopidogrel and Metoprolol in Myocardial Infarction Trial), 45,852 patients with suspected MI were randomly assigned to clopidogrel, 75 mg/day (without a loading dose), or placebo in addition to aspirin, 162 mg/day (Fig. 38.14B).[62] Patients in the clopidogrel group had a lower rate of the composite endpoint of death, reinfarction, or stroke (9.2% versus 10.1%; $P = 0.002$). They also had a significantly lower rate of death (7.5% versus 8.1%; $P = 0.03$). No excessive bleeding with clopidogrel occurred in this trial.

the overall trial population (see Fig. 38.15); there was a 26% reduction in definite or probable stent thrombosis and an 18% reduction in all-cause mortality.[62]

Current evidence does not support initiation of $P2Y_{12}$ inhibitor therapy before PCI for STEMI unless the strategy is for delayed invasive evaluation. As part of the PCI-CLARITY (PCI-Clopidogrel as Adjunctive Reperfusion Therapy) study, the investigators performed a meta-analysis of PCI-CLARITY, PCI-CURE (PCI-Clopidogrel in Unstable angina to prevent Recurrent Events), and CREDO (Clopidogrel for the Reduction of Events During Observation) and found that pretreatment with clopidogrel significantly reduced the risk for 30-day CV death or MI in a population that included both patients with STEMI and non-ST

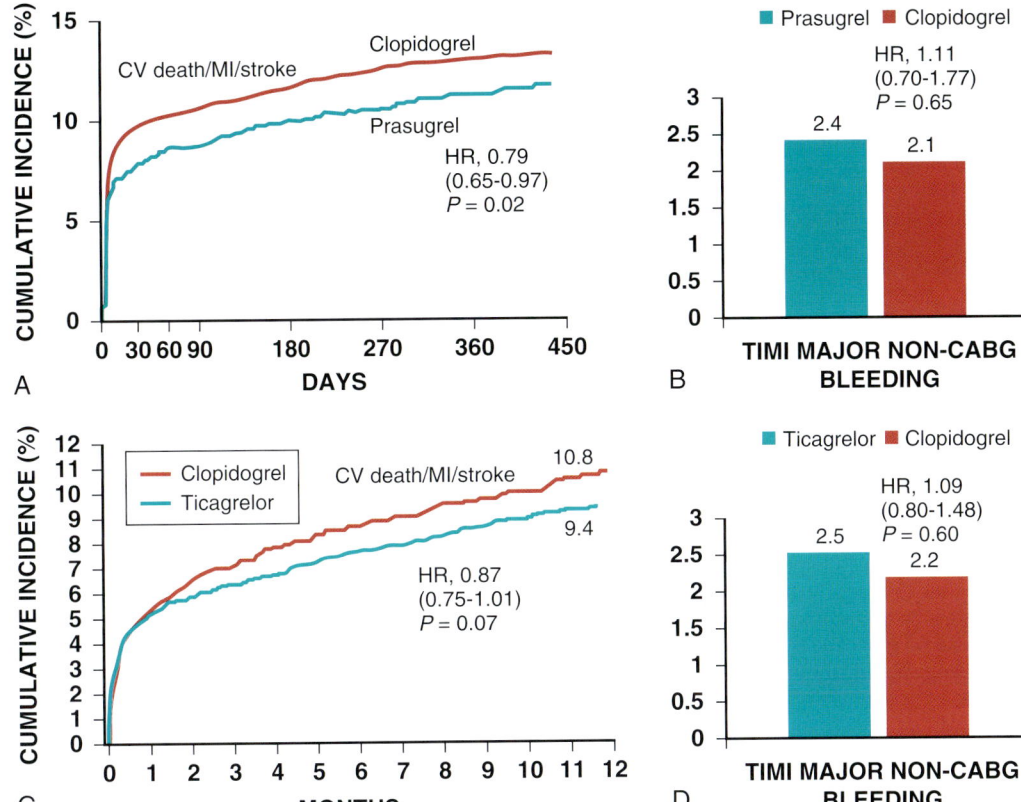

FIGURE 38.15 A, Efficacy of prasugrel in the subgroup of patients with STEMI enrolled in a randomized clinical trial of prasugrel versus clopidogrel in patients undergoing PCI after an ACS. Treatment with prasugrel associated with a 21% relative reduction in the risk for cardiovascular (CV) death, MI, or stroke during 15 months of follow-up. **B,** Major bleeding (TIMI non-CABG) increased with prasugrel in the trial overall but did not reach statistical significance in patients with STEMI. **C,** Efficacy results for ticagrelor (versus clopidogrel) in patients with STEMI enrolled in the PLATO trial. The effect of ticagrelor on the primary endpoint (incidence of MI, stroke, or CV death) was consistent with the superiority of ticagrelor versus clopidogrel in the overall trial. **D,** Rates of major bleeding (TIMI non-CABG) are shown. CABG, Coronary artery bypass grafting. (**A, B** from Montalescot G, Wiviott SD, Braunwald E, et al. Prasugrel compared with clopidogrel in patients undergoing percutaneous coronary intervention for ST-elevation myocardial infarction [TRITON-TIMI 38]: double-blind, randomised controlled trial. Lancet. 2009;373:723; **C, D** from Steg PG, James S, Harrington RA, et al. Ticagrelor versus clopidogrel in patients with ST-elevation acute coronary syndromes intended for reperfusion with primary percutaneous coronary intervention: a Platelet Inhibition and Patient Outcomes (PLATO) trial subgroup analysis. Circulation. 2010;122:2131.)

Combination Pharmacologic Reperfusion

Although trials of GP IIb/IIIa inhibitors combined with either full or reduced doses of fibrinolytics showed improvements in reperfusion, subsequent large outcomes trials revealed no significant effect on survival, and reductions in reinfarction were outweighed by the increases in bleeding.[2] Therefore, the combination of a GP IIb/IIIa inhibitor and a fibrinolytic as a pharmacologic reperfusion regimen is not recommended.[1]

Recommendations for Antiplatelet Therapy

Patients who have not taken aspirin before the development of STEMI should chew non-enteric-coated aspirin, and the dose should be 162 to 325 mg initially. During the maintenance phase of antiplatelet therapy following STEMI, the dose of aspirin should be reduced to 75 to 162 mg to minimize the risk of bleeding.[1] Lower doses are preferable because of the increased risk for bleeding with higher doses reported in several studies; the CURRENT-OASIS 7 trial did not find differences in terms of efficacy or safety in STEMI patients randomly assigned to 81 versus 325 mg of aspirin. If true aspirin allergy is present, other antiplatelet agents such as clopidogrel or ticlopidine can be substituted.

The addition of a $P2Y_{12}$ inhibitor to aspirin is warranted in most patients with STEMI.[1] Based on the results of the COMMIT and CLARITY-TIMI 28 trials, clopidogrel, 75 mg/day orally, is an option for all patients with STEMI regardless of whether they receive fibrinolytic therapy, undergo primary PCI, or do not receive reperfusion therapy. The data available suggest that a loading dose of 300 mg of clopidogrel should be given to patients younger than 75 years who receive fibrinolytic therapy. Data are insufficient in elderly patients to recommend a loading dose in those 75 years or older who receive a fibrinolytic; however, this is being addressed in an ongoing study of half-dose fibrinolytic in older patients.[42] When primary PCI is the mode of reperfusion therapy, an oral loading dose of 600 mg of clopidogrel before stent implantation is an established treatment, followed by 75 mg daily.[1,71] Interpatient variability in the response to clopidogrel can occur (see Chapters 9, 39, and 95), and individuals with lesser degrees of platelet inhibition have increased risk for death and ischemic complications.

Prasugrel and ticagrelor generally achieve greater degrees of platelet inhibition than clopidogrel and can be used to treat patients with STEMI. On the basis of the results of TRITON-TIMI 38, prasugrel administered as an oral loading dose of 60 and 10 mg daily thereafter demonstrated benefit in patients with STEMI but should not be used in patients with a history of cerebrovascular disease or who are at higher risk for life-threatening bleeding, including patients older than 75 years or those with low body weight.[1] Ticagrelor also reduced CV events compared with clopidogrel, and in PLATO, ticagrelor was administered as an oral loading dose of 180 mg and then 90 mg twice daily.[1,62] When using ticagrelor, the recommended maintenance dose of aspirin is 81 mg daily.[1] The duration of combined antiplatelet therapy for secondary prevention after STEMI is discussed in Chapter 41.

HOSPITAL MANAGEMENT

Coronary Care and Intermediate Care Units

Development of the coronary care unit (CCU) established the practice of continuously monitoring the cardiac rhythm by highly trained nurses with the skills and authority to initiate immediate treatment of arrhythmias in the absence of physicians and with the availability of specialized equipment (defibrillators, pacemakers).[72] The clustering of patients with STEMI in the CCU greatly enhanced efficient use of the trained personnel, facilities, and equipment to improve patient outcomes.[72] These benefits of geographic clustering with specialized nursing contribute to the optimal care of patients with STEMI, and in some hospitals, such care can be provided in "intermediate care" telemetry units with well-trained staff outside the CCU.[72] Such intermediate care units, when equipped with continuous electrocardiographic monitoring and resuscitation equipment, may be appropriate for initial admission of STEMI patients with a low risk for mortality and has become standard in many institutions for STEMI patients stable after primary PCI.[73] This strategy has proved cost-effective and may reduce CCU use by one-third, shorten hospital stays, and have no deleterious effect on patients' recovery.[1]

With increasing attention directed to limitations on resources and to the economic impact of intensive care, the proportion of appropriately selected patients with STEMI cared for in an intermediate care unit will likely increase. Nevertheless, a dedicated cardiac intensive care unit (CICU) plays a pivotal role in the management of patients with major complications of STEMI, which may require treatment of refractory arrhythmias, use of invasive hemodynamic monitoring, mechanical circulatory support, or with multiple organ failure.[72] In patients with STEMI managed in a CICU, those with an uncomplicated status, such as patients without HF, hypotension, heart block, hemodynamically compromising ventricular arrhythmias, or persistent ischemic-type discomfort, can be safely transferred out of the CICU within 24 to 36 hours. In patients with complicated STEMI, the duration of the CICU stay should be dictated by the need for "intensive" care—that is, hemodynamic monitoring, close nursing supervision, IV vasoactive drugs, and frequent changes in the medical regimen.

General Measures

The managing clinical staff should be sensitive to patient concerns about prognosis and future productivity. Beginning education on lifestyle changes, including dietary interventions, is an important component of an overall strategy for secondary prevention (see Chapter 40).

The results of laboratory tests should be scrutinized for any derangements potentially contributing to arrhythmias, such as disturbances in acid-base balance or electrolytes. Delirium can be provoked by medications frequently used in the hospital, including antiarrhythmic drugs, H_2 blockers, narcotics, and beta blockers. Use of potentially offending agents should be discontinued in patients with an abnormal mental status. Haloperidol, a butyrophenone, can be used safely in patients with STEMI.

Physical Activity

In the absence of complications, stabilized patients with STEMI need not be confined to bed for more than 12 hours, and unless they are hemodynamically compromised, they may use a bedside commode shortly after admission. Progression of activity should be individualized depending on the patient's clinical status, age, and physical capacity. In patients without hemodynamic compromise, early mobilization (e.g., sitting in a chair, standing, walking around the bed) does not usually cause important changes in HR, BP, or pulmonary wedge pressure. As long as BP and HR are monitored, early mobilization offers considerable psychological and physical benefit without any clear medical risk.

Pharmacologic Therapy

Beta Blockers

Use of beta blockers for the treatment of patients with STEMI can cause both immediate effects (when the drug is given early in the course of infarction) and long-term effects (secondary prevention), as discussed previously. Because beta-adrenergic blockade diminishes circulating levels of free fatty acids (FFAs) by antagonizing the lipolytic effects of catecholamines and because elevated FFA levels augment myocardial oxygen consumption and probably increase the incidence of arrhythmias, these metabolic actions of beta blockers may also benefit the ischemic heart. As noted earlier, because early administration of IV beta blockers can cause detrimental effects in some patients, the present guidelines omit this therapy for most patients.[1]

More than 52,000 patients have been randomly assigned to treatment in clinical trials studying beta-adrenergic blockade for acute MI.[1] These trials cover a range of beta blockers and timing of administration and were largely conducted in the era before reperfusion strategies were developed for STEMI. Data available in the pre-reperfusion era suggested favorable trends toward a reduction in mortality, reinfarction, and cardiac arrest. In the reperfusion era, adding an IV beta blocker to fibrinolytic therapy was not associated with a reduction in mortality but helped reduce the rate of recurrent ischemic events. Concern arose regarding the potential risk of provoking cardiogenic shock if early IV followed by oral beta-adrenergic blockade was routinely administered to all patients with STEMI. The largest trial of beta blockers in patients with acute MI was COMMIT, which randomly assigned 45,852 patients within 24 hours of MI to metoprolol given as sequential IV boluses of 5 mg up to 15 mg, followed by 200 mg/day orally, or to placebo.[1] The rate of the composite endpoint of death, reinfarction, or cardiac arrest in the metoprolol group (9.4%) did not differ from that in the placebo group (9.9%). Significant reductions occurred in reinfarction and episodes of VF in the metoprolol group, which translated into five fewer events for each of these endpoints per 1000 patients treated; yet, there were 11 more episodes of cardiogenic shock in the metoprolol group per 1000 patients treated. Risk for the development of cardiogenic shock (recorded as part of COMMIT protocol, in contrast to earlier studies) was greatest in patients with moderate to severe LV dysfunction (Killip class II or greater).

The combined results of the low-risk patients from COMMIT and data from earlier trials provide an overview of the effects of early IV therapy followed by oral therapy with beta blockers (Fig. 38.16). A 13% reduction occurred in all-cause mortality (7 lives saved per 1000 patients treated), along with a 22% reduction in reinfarction (5 fewer events per 1000 patients treated) and a 15% reduction in VF or cardiac arrest (5 fewer events per 1000 patients treated). To achieve these benefits safely, early administration of beta blockers to patients with relative contraindications should be avoided (Table 38.6).

Recommendations

Given the evidence of a benefit of early administration of beta blockers for STEMI, patients without a contraindication, regardless of the administration of concomitant fibrinolytic therapy or performance of primary PCI, should receive *oral* beta blockers within the first 24 hours (see Table 38.6). IV administration of beta-blocking therapy during this period is also reasonable if a tachyarrhythmia or hypertension is present, in the absence of signs of HF/low output, indicators of high risk for the development of shock, or other relative contraindications to beta blockers.[1]

Beta blockers are especially helpful in STEMI patients with significant residual unrevascularized CAD and evidence of recurrent ischemia or tachyarrhythmias early after the onset of infarction.[74] If adverse effects of beta blockers develop or if patients have complications of infarction that are contraindications to these agents, such as HF or heart block, beta blockers should be withheld. Unless there are contraindications (see Table 38.6), beta blockers probably should be continued in patients in whom STEMI develops. Moreover, patients who initially have contraindications to beta blockers, such as acute HF, should be reevaluated with respect to their candidacy for such therapy after 24 hours.[1]

Selection of Beta Blockers

Favorable effects have been reported with metoprolol, atenolol, carvedilol, timolol, and alprenolol; these benefits probably occur with propranolol and with esmolol, an ultrashort-acting agent, as well. In the absence of any favorable evidence supporting the benefit of agents with intrinsic sympathomimetic activity, such as pindolol and oxprenolol, and with some unfavorable evidence for these agents in secondary prevention, beta blockers with intrinsic sympathomimetic activity should probably not be chosen for the treatment of STEMI. The CAPRICORN (Carvedilol Post Infarction Survival Control in Left Ventricular Dysfunction) trial randomly assigned 1959 patients with MI and systolic dysfunction (EF <40%) to carvedilol or placebo in addition to contemporary pharmacotherapy, including angiotensin-converting enzyme (ACE) inhibitors in 98% of patients. All-cause mortality was reduced over a mean follow-up of 1.3 years by 23% with carvedilol compared to placebo ($P = 0.031$), with a similar pattern noted during the first 30 days.[75,76] Thus, CAPRICORN confirmed the benefit of administration of a beta blocker in addition to ACE inhibitor therapy in patients with transient or sustained LV dysfunction after MI.

Occasionally, clinicians may decide to proceed with therapy with a beta blocker even in patients with relative contraindications, such as a history of mild asthma, mild bradycardia, mild HF, or first-degree heart block. In this situation, a trial of esmolol may help determine whether the patient can tolerate beta-adrenergic blockade. Because the hemodynamic effects of this drug (half-life of 9 minutes) disappear in less

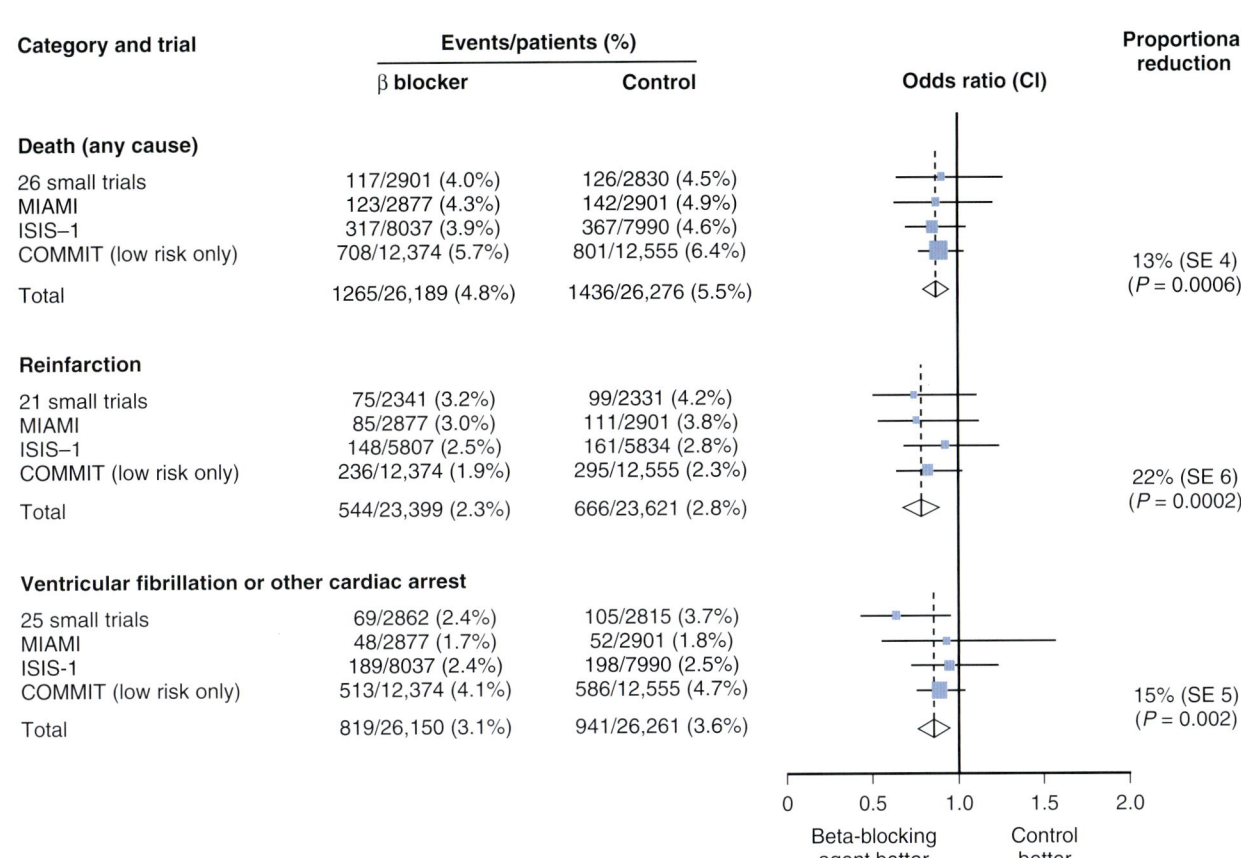

FIGURE 38.16 Meta-analysis of the effects of intravenous and then oral beta (β)-blocker therapy on death, reinfarction, and cardiac arrest during the scheduled treatment periods in 26 small randomized trials, MIAMI, ISIS-1, and the low-risk subset of COMMIT. For COMMIT, data are included only for patients with a systolic blood pressure higher than 105 mm Hg, a heart rate greater than 65 beats/min, and Killip class I (as in MIAMI). Five small trials included in the ISIS-1 report had no data on reinfarction. In the ISIS-1 trial, data on reinfarction in the hospital were available for the last three-quarters of the study and involved 11,641 patients. ORs (odd ratios) in each (*blue squares* with the area proportional to the number of events) were determined by comparing outcomes in patients allocated to β-blocker therapy with those in patients allocated to control, along with 99% CIs (confidence intervals) *(horizontal lines)*. Overall ORs and 95% CIs are plotted by the *diamonds,* with value and significance given alongside. (From Chen ZM, Pan HC, Chen YP, et al. Early intravenous then oral metoprolol in 45,852 patients with acute myocardial infarction: randomised placebo-controlled trial. *Lancet* .2005;366:1622.)

TABLE 38.6 Recommendations for Beta-Blocker Therapy for ST-Elevation Myocardial Infarction (STEMI)

RECOMMENDATION	COR	LOE
Oral beta blockers should be initiated in the first 24 hr in patients with STEMI who do not have any of the following: Signs of heart failure or evidence of a low-output state Increased risk for cardiogenic shock*: • Age >70 years • Systolic blood pressure <120 mm Hg • Sinus tachycardia >110 beats/min or heart rate <60 beats/min • Increased time since the onset of symptoms of STEMI Other relative contraindications to use of oral beta blockers: • PR interval longer than 0.24 second • Second- or third-degree heart block • Active asthma or reactive airways disease	I	B
Beta blockers should be continued during and after hospitalization for all patients with STEMI and no contraindications to their use.	I	B
Patients with initial contraindications to the use of beta blockers in the first 24 hours after STEMI should be reevaluated to determine their subsequent eligibility.	I	C
It is reasonable to administer IV beta blockers at initial encounter to patients with STEMI and no contraindications to their use who are hypertensive or have ongoing ischemia.	IIa	B

COR, Class of recommendation; *LOE,* level of evidence.
*The greater the number of risk factors present, the higher the risk for development of cardiogenic shock.
Modified from O'Gara PT, Kushner FG, Ascheim DD, et al. 2013 ACCF/AHA guideline for the management of ST-elevation myocardial infarction: a report of the American College of Cardiology Foundation/American Heart Association Task Force on Practice Guidelines. *J Am Coll Cardiol.* 2013;61:e78.

than 30 minutes, it offers an advantage over longer-acting agents when the risk for complications with a beta blocker is relatively high.

Inhibition of the Renin-Angiotensin-Aldosterone System

The rationale for inhibition of the renin-angiotensin-aldosterone system (RAAS) includes experimental and clinical evidence of a favorable impact on ventricular remodeling, improvement in hemodynamics, and a reduction in HF incidence. Unequivocal evidence from RCTs has shown that ACE inhibitors reduce mortality from STEMI.[1] These trials can be grouped into two categories. The first group *selected* MI patients for randomization on the basis of features indicative of increased mortality, such as LVEF lower than 40%, clinical signs and symptoms of HF, anterior location of infarction, and abnormal wall motion score index (Fig. 38.17). The second group consisted of *unselective* trials that

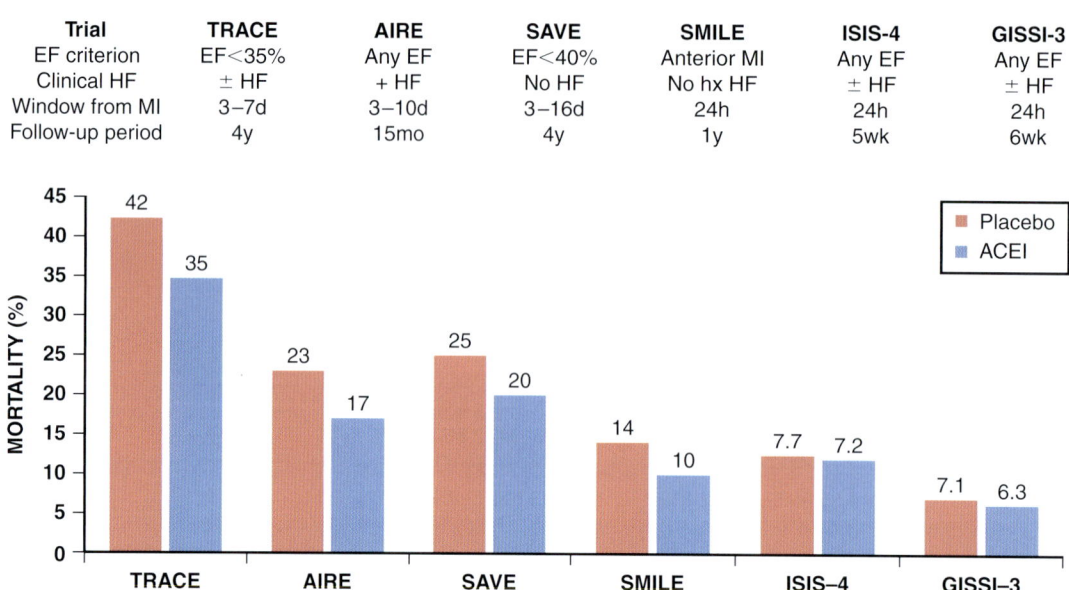

FIGURE 38.17 Effect of ACE inhibitors on mortality after MI. Data are from six randomized controlled trials of an ACE inhibitor versus placebo in patients with MI with varying criteria based on ejection fraction (EF), clinical history of heart failure (HF), and the timing of randomization after presentation with MI. Presented are the mortality rates for the specified follow-up interval and the absolute risk difference with ACE inhibitor therapy. *AIRE,* Acute Infarction Ramipril Efficacy; *d,* days; *GISSI,* Gruppo Italiano per lo Studio della Sopravvivenza nell'Infarto Miocardico; *h,* hours; *ISIS,* International Study of Infarct Survival; *SAVE,* Survival and Ventricular Enlargement; *SMILE,* Survival of Myocardial Infarction Long-term Evaluation; *TRACE,* Trandolapril Cardiac Evaluation; *wk,* weeks; *mo,* months; *y,* years.

Trial	Total No. in Study	OR	OR and 95% CI
CONSENSUS-II	6090	1.1	
GISSI-3	19,394	0.88	
SMILE	1556	0.67	
ISIS-4	58,050	0.94	
CCS-1	13,634	0.93	
All trials	98,724	0.93	

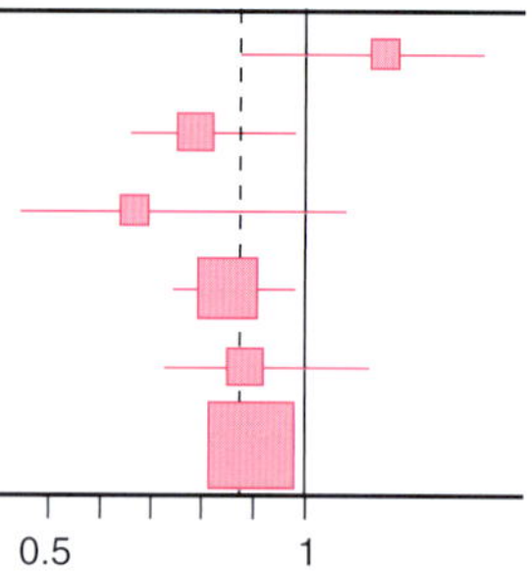

Risk reduction, 6.7%; *P* < 0.006
4.9 fewer deaths/1000 patients treated

FIGURE 38.18 Effects of ACE inhibitors on mortality after MI—results from short-term trials. (From Gornik H, O'Gara PT. Adjunctive medical therapy. In: Manson JE et al., eds. *Clinical Trials in Heart Disease: A Companion to Braunwald's Heart Disease.* Philadelphia: Saunders; 2004:114.)

randomized all patients with MI provided that they had a minimum systolic BP of approximately 100 mm Hg (ISIS-4, GISSI-3 [Gruppo Italiano per lo Studio della Sopravvivenza nell'infarto Miocardico], CONSENSUS II [Cooperative New Scandinavian Enalapril Survival Study II], and Chinese Captopril Study) (Fig. 38.18). All selective trials initiated ACE inhibitor therapy between 3 and 16 days (except for SMILE) and maintained it for 1 to 4 years, whereas the unselective trials all initiated treatment within the first 24 to 36 hours and maintained it for only 4 to 6 weeks.

A consistent survival benefit was observed in all the trials already noted, except for CONSENSUS II, the one study that used an IV preparation early in the course of MI. An estimate of the mortality benefit of ACE inhibitors in the unselective trials with a short duration of therapy was 5 lives saved per 1000 patients treated. Analysis of these unselective short-term trials indicates that approximately one-third of the lives saved occurred within the first 1 to 2 days. Certain subgroups, such as patients with anterior infarction, showed proportionately greater benefit with the early administration (11 lives saved per 1000) of ACE inhibitors. Not unexpectedly, greater survival benefits of 42 to 76 lives saved per 1000 patients treated were obtained in the selective trials with a long duration of therapy. Of note, a general 26% reduction in the risk for death attributable to ACE inhibitor treatment occurred in the selective trials. The reduction in mortality with ACE inhibitors was accompanied by significant reductions in the development of HF, thus supporting the underlying pathophysiologic rationale for administering this class of drugs to patients with STEMI.

The mortality benefits of ACE inhibitors add to those achieved with aspirin and beta blockers. The benefits of ACE inhibition appear to be a class effect because several agents reduce mortality and morbidity. To replicate these benefits in clinical practice, however, physicians should select a specific agent and prescribe the drug according to the protocols and dosages used in the clinical trials.[75] The major contraindications to ACE inhibitors in patients with STEMI include hypotension in the setting of adequate preload, known hypersensitivity, and pregnancy. Adverse reactions include hypotension, especially after the first dose, and intolerable cough; much less often, angioedema can occur.

An alternative method of pharmacologic inhibition of the RAAS is the administration of angiotensin II receptor-blocking agents (ARBs). The VALIANT (Valsartan in Acute Myocardial Infarction) trial compared the effects of the ARB valsartan, valsartan and captopril, and captopril alone on mortality in patients with acute MI complicated by LV systolic dysfunction and/or HF within 10 days of MI.[75,76] Mortality rates were similar in the three treatment groups: 19.9% with valsartan, 19.3% with valsartan plus captopril, and 19.5% with captopril alone. The combination of the ACE and the ARB caused more unwanted actions; thus, drugs from these classes should not be combined.

Aldosterone blockade is another pharmacologic strategy for inhibition of the RAAS. The EPHESUS (Eplerenone Post-AMI Heart Failure Efficacy and Survival) trial randomly assigned 6642 patients with acute MI *complicated by left ventricular dysfunction and heart failure* to the selective aldosterone-blocking agent eplerenone or placebo in conjunction with contemporary postinfarction pharmacotherapy.[76,77] During a mean follow-up of 16 months, a 15% reduction occurred in the RR for mortality in favor of eplerenone. Eplerenone also reduced CV mortality or hospitalization for CV events (Fig. 38.19). Serious hyperkalemia (serum potassium [K^+] concentration, 6 mmol/L) occurred in 5.5% of patients in the eplerenone group compared with 3.9% in the placebo group ($P = 0.002$). In contrast, in the ALBATROSS (Aldosterone Lethal Effects Blocked in Acute MI Treated with or without Reperfusion to Improve Outcome and Survival at Six Months Follow-up) trial, early mineralocorticoid antagonism versus placebo in an expanded population of patients with MI, *including both STEMI and non-ST*

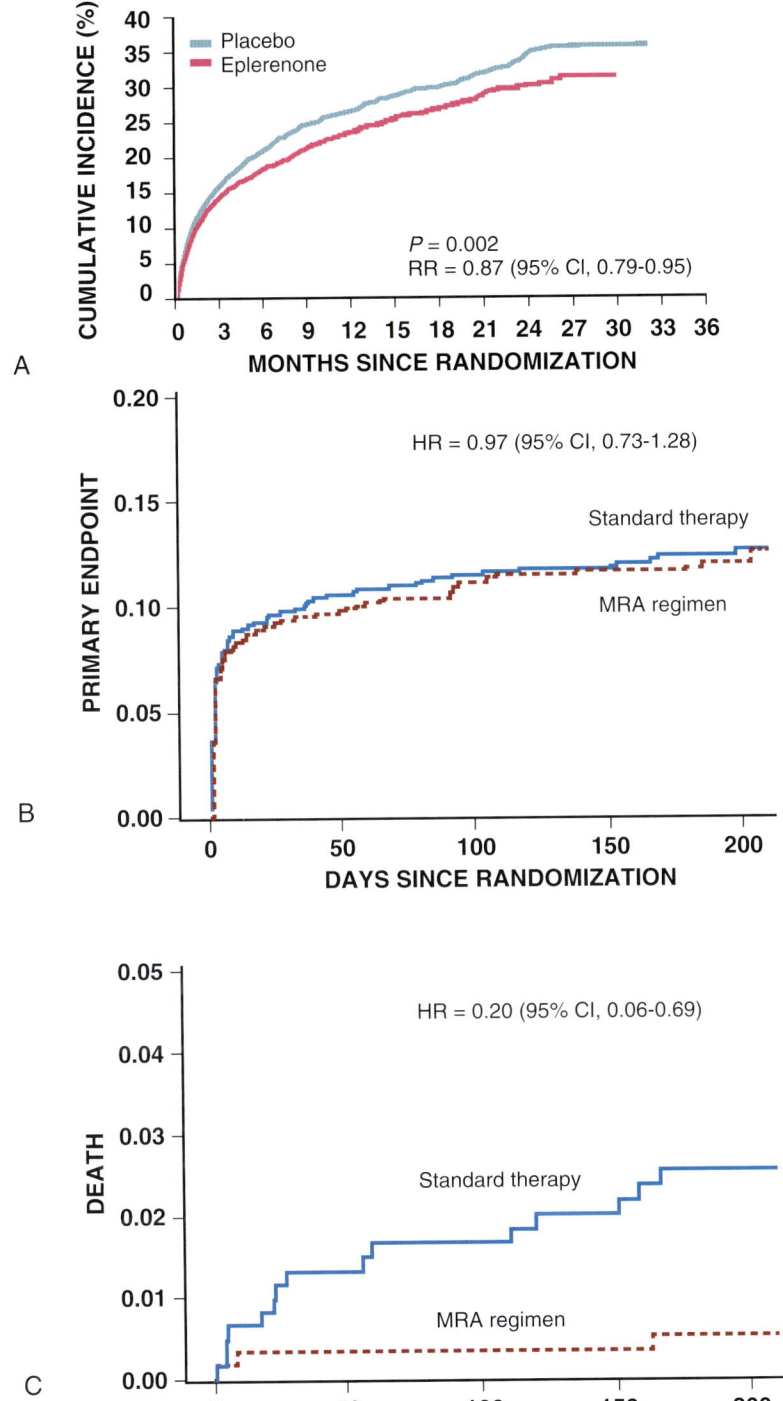

FIGURE 38.19 Mineralocorticoid receptor antagonism (MRA) following MI in patients with and without heart failure or left ventricular dysfunction. **A,** Eplerenone significantly reduced death from cardiovascular causes or hospitalization for cardiovascular events in the EPHESUS (Eplerenone Post-AMI Heart Failure Efficacy and Survival) trial in patients with acute MI *complicated by left ventricular dysfunction and heart failure*. **B,** The ALBATROSS (Aldosterone Lethal Effects Blocked in Acute MI Treated with or without Reperfusion to Improve Outcome and Survival at Six Months Follow-up) trial found no difference in the primary outcome of death, cardiac arrest, ventricular arrhythmia, ICD placement, or heart failure with early MRA versus placebo in acute MI *with or without left ventricular function or heart failure*. **C,** An exploratory subgroup analysis in patients with STEMI identified a reduction in all-cause death. (Modified from Pitt B, Remme W, Zannad F, et al. Eplerenone, a selective aldosterone blocker, in patients with left ventricular dysfunction after myocardial infarction. *N Engl J Med.* 2003;348:14, and Beygui F, Cayla G, Roule V, et al. Early aldosterone blockade in acute myocardial infarction: the ALBATROSS randomized clinical trial. *J Am Coll Cardiol.* 2016;67[16]:1917–1927.)

elevation MI, and patients without left ventricular function or heart failure, did not reduce the primary outcome of death, cardiac arrest, ventricular arrhythmia, implantable cardioverter-defibrillator (ICD) placement, or HF.[78] However, an exploratory analysis by MI type found a reduction in all-cause death (HR, 0.20; 95% CI 0.06 to 0.70) in the subgroup of patients with STEMI ($n = 1229$). Further studies are necessary to determine if a mineralocorticoid receptor antagonist (MRA) improves outcomes in all STEMI patients regardless of HF or LV dysfunction.[79]

Recommendations

After administration of aspirin and initiation of reperfusion strategies and, when appropriate, beta blockers, *all* patients with STEMI should be considered for inhibition of the RAAS. Although few disagree with the recommendation that high-risk STEMI patients (elderly, anterior infarction, previous infarction, Killip class II or greater, and asymptomatic patients with evidence of depressed global ventricular function on imaging) should receive lifelong treatment with ACE inhibitors, some have proposed short-term (4 to 6 weeks) therapy for a broader group of patients on the basis of the pooled results of the unselective mortality trials.[1]

Considering all the data available, we favor a strategy of an initial trial of oral ACE inhibitors in all patients with STEMI and HF, as well as in hemodynamically stable patients, commencing within the first 24 hours. ACE inhibition therapy should be continued indefinitely in patients with HF, evidence of a reduction in a global function, or a large regional wall motion abnormality. In patients without these findings, long-term treatment with ACE inhibitors is based on other considerations related to the potential benefits of secondary prevention. ARBs are a clinically effective alternative to ACE inhibitors. Although still being studied specifically among patients with acute MI,[80] an angiotensin receptor-neprilysin inhibitor (ARNI) can be considered over an ACE inhibitor or ARB for long-term management in patients with chronic symptomatic HF with reduced EF, including patients with ischemic cardiomyopathy from prior MI.[81] Finally, long-term aldosterone blockade should be instituted in high-risk patients following STEMI (EF <40%, clinical HF, diabetes mellitus) who are already receiving an ACE inhibitor and beta blocker and do not have contraindications. The small but definite increase in the risk for serious hyperkalemia when aldosterone blockade is prescribed, particularly when other measures for RAAS inhibition are used concurrently, warrants periodic monitoring of the serum K^+ level.

Nitrates

The potential for reductions in ventricular filling pressure, wall tension, and cardiac work, coupled with improvement in coronary blood flow, especially in ischemic zones, and antiplatelet effects, makes nitrates a logical and attractive pharmacologic intervention in patients with STEMI.[1] The administration of nitrates reduces pulmonary capillary wedge pressure (PCWP) and systemic arterial pressure, LV chamber volume, infarct size, and the incidence of mechanical complications. Nevertheless, routine administration of nitrates does not alter survival in patients with STEMI. Although a meta-analysis of 10 trials conducted in the prefibrinolytic era showed nitrate therapy to be associated with a reduction in mortality, two megatrials of nitrate therapy (GISSI-3 and ISIS-4) conducted in the reperfusion era demonstrated no benefit on major CV outcomes.[1]

With the aim of controlling hypertension or treating HF, IV nitroglycerin can be administered safely to patients with evolving STEMI as long as the dose is titrated to avoid induction of reflex tachycardia or systemic arterial hypotension.

Patients with inferior wall infarction may be sensitive to an excessive fall in preload, particularly with concurrent RV infarction.[1] In such cases, nitrate-induced venodilation could impair cardiac output and reduce coronary blood flow, thus worsening rather than improving myocardial oxygenation.

Clinically significant methemoglobinemia, although rare, can develop when unusually large doses of nitrates are administered. This problem is important not only for its potential to cause symptoms of lethargy and headache but also because elevated methemoglobin levels can impair the O_2-carrying capacity of blood and potentially exacerbate ischemia. Dilation of the pulmonary vasculature supplying poorly ventilated lung segments may produce a ventilation-perfusion mismatch. Tolerance to IV nitroglycerin (as manifested by increasing nitrate requirements) develops in many patients, often as soon as 12 hours after beginning the infusion.

Recommendations
Nitroglycerin is indicated for the relief of persistent pain and as a vasodilator in patients with infarction associated with LV failure or hypertension. In the absence of recurrent angina or HF, we do not routinely prescribe nitrates for patients with STEMI. Long-term nitrates have no clear benefit in asymptomatic patients, and we therefore do not prescribe them beyond the first 48 hours in patients without angina or LV failure.

Calcium Channel Antagonists
Despite sound experimental and clinical evidence of an anti-ischemic effect, calcium antagonists have not been helpful in the acute phase of STEMI, and several systematic overviews have raised concern about an increased risk for mortality when these agents, particularly short-acting dihydropyridines, are prescribed on a routine basis. Nondihydropyridine calcium channel-blocking agents (verapamil and diltiazem) can be given to slow a rapid ventricular response in atrial fibrillation in patients for whom beta blockers are ineffective. These agents should be avoided in patients with Killip class II or greater.

Other Therapies
Magnesium
A functional deficit in available magnesium may develop in patients with STEMI. Because of the risk for cardiac arrhythmias when electrolytes are deficient in the early phase of infarction, patients with STEMI should have their serum magnesium measured on admission. We advocate repleting magnesium deficits to maintain a serum magnesium level of 2 mEq/L or greater. In the presence of hypokalemia, the serum magnesium level should be rechecked and repleted if necessary because it is often difficult to correct a potassium deficit in the presence of a concurrent magnesium deficit. There is no indication for the routine IV administration of magnesium to patients with STEMI.

Glucose Control During ST-Elevation Myocardial Infarction
During the acute phase of STEMI, catecholamine levels increase in both the blood and ischemic myocardium. Insulin levels remain low, whereas cortisol, glucagon, and FFA levels increase. These factors may contribute to an elevation in the blood glucose level, which should be measured routinely on admission. Intensive insulin therapy to control blood glucose strictly is no longer recommended routinely for patients with MI. Blood glucose levels should be maintained below 180 mg/dL, if possible, while avoiding hypoglycemia[1] (see Chapter 31).

A series of small trials suggested that infusions of glucose-insulin-potassium (GIK) to patients with STEMI were beneficial, but the CREATE-ECLA (Clinical Trial of Metabolic Modulation in Acute Myocardial Infarction Treatment Evaluation–Estudios Cardiologicos Latinoamerica) investigators randomly assigned 20,201 patients with STEMI to GIK or placebo and found no impact on mortality.[82] In the contemporary era of management of STEMI treated with other effective therapies (reperfusion, antithrombotic therapy, ACE inhibitors), routine use of GIK infusions does not confer benefit.

Other Agents
Historically, adjunctive pharmacotherapies to prevent inflammatory damage in the infarct zone have been investigated but have not shown clinical benefit. For example, pexelizumab, a monoclonal antibody against the C5 component of complement, had no effect on infarct size in patients with STEMI treated with either fibrinolytics or PCI or on mortality in patients treated with primary PCI.[83] The anti-inflammatory agent losmapimod, a p38 mitogen-activated protein kinase (MAPK) inhibitor that reduces cytokine amplification in ACS, did not reduce the short-term risk of CV death, MI, or severe recurrent ischemia in 3503 patients with acute MI.[84] Similarly, darapladib, an oral, selective inhibitor of the lipoprotein-associated phospholipase A_2 enzyme, did not alter the composite of CV death, MI, or stroke in 13,026 patients with acute MI in the SOLID-TIMI 52 (Stabilization of Plaques Using Darapladib) trial.[85]

However, two anti-inflammatory agents have now shown benefit in patients with ischemic heart disease. Among 4745 patients within 30 days of an acute MI enrolled in COLCOT (Colchicine Cardiovascular Outcomes Trial), colchicine reduced the composite of CV death, resuscitated cardiac arrest, MI, stroke, or urgent coronary revascularization (HR 0.77; 0.61–0.96, p= 0.02) compared with placebo.[86] The primary endpoint of all-cause mortality, ACS, ischemia-driven urgent revascularization or ischemic stroke (6.1% vs 9.5%, p= 0.09) was not met in a smaller trial of colchicine in 795 patients with ACS.[87] These data are encouraging for the benefit of specific anti-inflammatory therapy in ACS and derive additional credence from studies of colchicine in stable ischemic heart disease (see Chapters 25 and 40) as well as of canakinumab, a monoclonal antibody targeting the inflammatory cytokine, interleukin-1β in the CANTOS (Canakinumab Antiinflammatory Thrombosis Outcome Study) trial, which identified a reduction in major adverse CV events in stable patients with atherosclerotic CV disease.[88]

HEMODYNAMIC DISTURBANCES

Hemodynamic Assessment
Patients with clinically uncomplicated STEMI do not require invasive hemodynamic monitoring because clinical evaluation can assess the status of the circulation. Routine assessments in patients with STEMI should include monitoring of the heart rate and rhythm, repeated measurement of systemic arterial pressure by the cuff, repeated auscultation of the lung fields for pulmonary congestion, measurement of urine output, examination of the skin for evidence of the adequacy of perfusion, and monitoring for hypoxemia.

In patients with STEMI who have clinical signs and symptoms of HF, assessment of the degree of hemodynamic compromise is important. Central venous pressure (CVP) reflects right rather than LV function. RV function—and therefore systemic venous pressure—may be normal or almost so in patients with substantial LV failure. Conversely, patients with RV failure caused by RV infarction may exhibit elevated right atrial (RA) pressure and CVP despite normal LV function. Low values for RA pressure and CVP imply hypovolemia, whereas elevated RA pressure usually results from RV failure secondary to LV failure, pulmonary hypertension, RV infarction, or less often, tricuspid regurgitation or pericardial tamponade.

In select patients with complicated STEMI, it may be useful to monitor invasively with an intra-arterial catheter and a pulmonary artery (PA) catheter for measurement of PA, PA occlusive, and RA pressures, as well as estimation of cardiac output. In patients with hypotension, a Foley catheter should be considered for continuous measurement of urine output.

Monitoring of Pulmonary Artery Pressure
Accurate determination of hemodynamics by clinical assessment can be difficult in critically ill patients. Use of a PA catheter thus often leads to important changes in therapy. Before inserting a PA catheter into a patient with STEMI, the physician must believe that the potential benefit of the information that can be obtained outweighs any potential risks. Major complications from PA catheters are uncommon, but severe problems can occur, including sepsis, pulmonary infarction, and PA rupture. Minimized duration of catheterization and strict adherence to aseptic techniques can diminish the risk. Using antiseptic-impregnated dressings can also reduce catheter-related bloodstream infections.

Evidence from settings other than STEMI suggests that routine invasive hemodynamic monitoring does not improve outcomes. The

TABLE 38.7 Indications for Hemodynamic Monitoring in Patients with ST-Elevation Myocardial Infarction

Management of complicated acute myocardial infarction
Shock with unclear clinical assessment of hemodynamics (e.g., filling pressures, vascular tone)
Ventricular septal rupture versus acute mitral regurgitation
Severe cardiogenic shock caused by right or left ventricular failure with a need for escalating vasopressor, inotropic, or mechanical circulatory support
Refractory ventricular tachycardia
Difficulty differentiating severe pulmonary disease from left ventricular failure with available noninvasive data
Assessment of cardiac tamponade

Data from Gore JM, Zwernet PL. Hemodynamic monitoring of acute myocardial infarction. In Francis GS, Alpert JS, eds. *Modern Coronary Care*. Boston: Little, Brown; 1990:138; and Yancy CW, Jessup M, Bozkurt B, et al. 2013 ACCF/AHA guideline for the management of heart failure: a report of the American College of Cardiology Foundation/American Heart Association Task Force on Practice Guidelines. *Circulation*. 2013;128(16):e240–327.

TABLE 38.8 Hemodynamic Classification of Patients with Acute Myocardial Infarction

A. BASED ON CLINICAL EXAMINATION		B. BASED ON INVASIVE MONITORING	
CLASS	DEFINITION	SUBSET	DEFINITION
I	Rales and S₃ absent	I	Normal hemodynamics PCWP <18, CI >2.2
II	Crackles, S₃ gallop, elevated jugular venous pressure	II	Pulmonary congestion PCWP >18, CI >2.2
III	Frank pulmonary edema	III	Peripheral hypoperfusion PCWP <18, CI <2.2
IV	Shock	IV	Pulmonary congestion and peripheral hypoperfusion PCWP >18, CI <2.2

CI, Cardiac index; *PCWP*, pulmonary capillary wedge pressure.
A modified from Killip T, Kimball J. Treatment of myocardial infarction in a coronary care unit: a two-year experience with 250 patients. *Am J Cardiol*. 1967;20:457; B from Forrester J, Diamond G, Chatterjee K, Swan HJ. Medical therapy of acute myocardial infarction by the application of hemodynamic subsets. *N Engl J Med*. 1976;295:1356.

Evaluation Study of Congestive Heart Failure and Pulmonary Artery Catheterization Effectiveness (ESCAPE) trial demonstrated no difference in death or hospitalization at 6 months, but increased rates of adverse events (21.9% versus 11.5%; $P = 0.04$) in 433 patients with HF not accompanied by shock randomly assigned to placement of a PA catheter or to noninvasive standard care.[76] A meta-analysis of data for 5051 patients from 13 RCTs of PA catheterization in patients undergoing surgery admitted to the ICU with advanced HF or diagnosed with acute respiratory distress syndrome (ARDS) and/or sepsis showed no difference in mortality.[76] In contrast, in a more recent multi-center, observational study identified an association between early PA catheter use and lower mortality in patients with cardiogenic shock, which many of whom presented with acute MI.[89]

Expert consensus recommends placement of a PA catheter in only a subset of patients, including those with presumed cardiogenic shock and need for escalating vasopressor therapy or mechanical circulatory support; those exhibiting clinical decompensation with equivocal findings on assessment of filling pressures, perfusion, and vascular tone (i.e., to assist with determination of shock type); and patients with ongoing significant symptoms or dependence on inotropes despite attempts at noninvasive optimization of recommended therapies (Table 38.7). In the setting of STEMI, PA catheterization is reasonable for diagnostic and management purposes in patients with mechanical lesions (or suspected lesions) such as severe mitral regurgitation, ruptured ventricular septum, or RV infarction.[76] Noninvasive methods of determination of cardiac output, such as pulse contour analysis and thoracic electrical bioimpedance, are also available.[90]

Hemodynamic Abnormalities

In 1976, Swan, Forrester, and associates measured cardiac output and wedge pressure simultaneously in a large series of patients with acute MI and identified four major hemodynamic subsets of patients (Table 38.8): (1) patients with normal systemic perfusion and without pulmonary congestion (normal cardiac output and normal wedge pressure), (2) patients with normal perfusion and pulmonary congestion (normal cardiac output and elevated wedge pressure), (3) patients with decreased perfusion but without pulmonary congestion (reduced cardiac output and normal wedge pressure), and (4) patients with decreased perfusion and pulmonary congestion (reduced cardiac output and elevated wedge pressure). This classification, which partly overlaps with a crude clinical classification proposed earlier by Killip and Kimball (see Table 38.8), has proved quite useful, but it should be noted that patients frequently pass from one category to another with therapy and sometimes apparently even spontaneously.

Hemodynamic Subsets

The hemodynamic groupings shown in Tables 38.8 and 38.9 allow rational approaches to therapy. The goals of hemodynamic therapy include maintenance of ventricular performance, BP support, and protection of jeopardized myocardium. Because these goals may occasionally be at cross-purposes, recognition of the hemodynamic profile, as assessed clinically or as available from hemodynamic monitoring, may be needed to design an optimal therapeutic management strategy.

Hypotension in the Prehospital Phase

Hypotension associated with bradycardia often reflects excessive vagotonia. Relative or absolute hypovolemia is often present when hypotension occurs with a normal or rapid HR. Marked diaphoresis, reduction of fluid intake, or vomiting during the period preceding and accompanying the onset of STEMI may contribute to the development of hypovolemia.

MANAGEMENT. In the absence of HF, when hypotension is suspected to result from excessive vagotonia, patients should be placed in the reverse Trendelenburg position. In patients with sinus bradycardia and hypotension, atropine should be administered (1 mg intravenously, repeated at 3- to 5-minute intervals, for a total dose of up to 3 mg). If these measures do not correct the hypotension, normal saline should be administered intravenously while monitoring for signs of HF. Because of the poor correlation between LV filling pressure and mean RA pressure, assessment of CVP can be of limited value as a guide to fluid therapy. Administration of positive inotropic or vasopressor agents is indicated during the prehospital phase if systemic hypotension persists despite correction of hypovolemia.

The Hyperdynamic State

When infarction is not complicated by hemodynamic impairment, no therapy other than general supportive measures and treatment of arrhythmias is necessary. However, if the hemodynamic profile involves a hyperdynamic state—that is, elevation of the sinus rate, arterial pressure, and CI, occurring singly or together in the presence of a normal or low LV filling pressure—treatment with beta blockers is indicated. Presumably, the increased HR and BP result from inappropriate activation of the sympathetic nervous system, possibly because of augmented release of catecholamines triggered by pain or anxiety.

Left Ventricular Failure

Left ventricular dysfunction is one of the most important predictors of mortality following STEMI[91] (Fig. 38.20). In patients with STEMI, either systolic dysfunction alone or both systolic and diastolic dysfunction

TABLE 38.9 Hemodynamic Patterns for Common Clinical Conditions

CARDIAC CONDITION	HEMODYNAMIC PARAMETER						
	RA	RV	PA	PAPI	PCW	CI	CPO
Normal	0–6	25/0–6	25/0–12	>1	6–12	≥2.5	>0.6
AMI without LVF	0–6	25/0–6	30/12–18	>1	≤18	≥2.5	>0.6
AMI with LVF	0–6	30–40/0–6	30–40/18–25	>1	>18	May be <2.0	<0.6
Biventricular failure	>6	50–60/>6	50–60/25	May be <1	18–25	May be <2.0	<0.6
RVMI	12–20	30/12–20	30/12	Often <1	≤12	May be <2.0	<0.6
Cardiac tamponade	12–16	25/12–16	25/12–16	Often <1	12–16	<2.0	<0.6
Acute Pulmonary embolism	12–20	30–50/12–20	30–50/12	Often <1	<12	<2.0	<0.6

AMI, Acute myocardial infarction; *CI*, cardiac index; *CPO*, cardiac power output (mean arterial pressure * cardiac output/451); *LVF*, left ventricular failure; *PA*, pulmonary artery; *PCW*, pulmonary capillary wedge; *RA*, right atrium; *RV*, right ventricle; *RVMI*, right ventricular myocardial infarction; *PAPI*, pulmonary artery pulsatility index ([PA systolic pressure minus pulmonary artery diastolic pressure]/RA);.
From Gore JM, Zwernet PL. Hemodynamic monitoring of acute myocardial infarction. In Francis GS, Alpert JS, eds. *Modern Coronary Care*. Boston: Little, Brown: 1990:139–64.

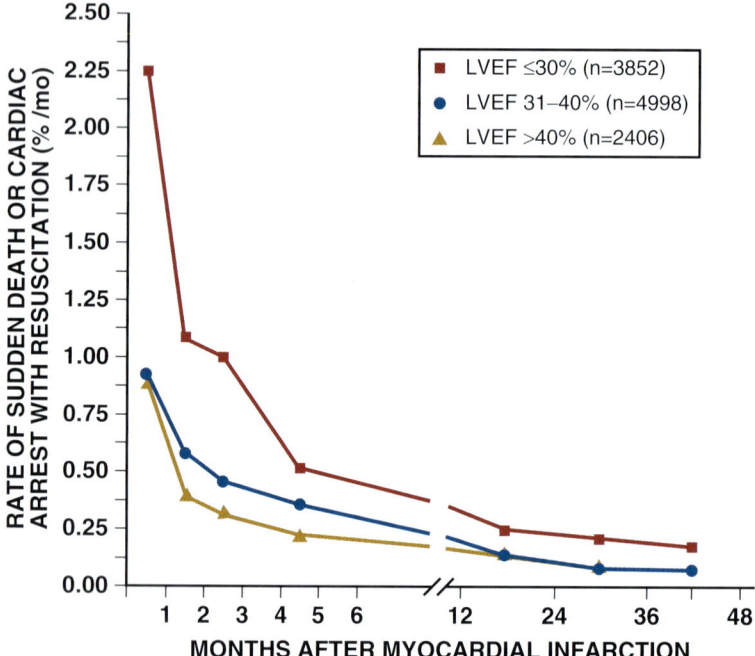

FIGURE 38.20 Rate of sudden death or cardiac arrest with resuscitation stratified by time from MI. The high rate of sudden death or cardiac arrest occurs within the first month after MI in all strata of left ventricular ejection fraction (LVEF) and declines exponentially to a plateau after 12 months. (From Zaman S, Kovoor P. Sudden cardiac death early after myocardial infarction: pathogenesis, risk stratification, and primary prevention. *Circulation*. 2014;129[23]:2426–2435.)

can occur. LV diastolic dysfunction leads to pulmonary venous hypertension and pulmonary congestion. Clinical manifestations of LV failure become more common as the extent of injury to the left ventricle increases. In addition to infarct size, other important predictors of the development of symptomatic LV dysfunction or cardiogenic shock include advanced age, dysglycemia, and delay to revascularization or unsuccessful revascularization.[92] Mortality increases in association with the severity of the hemodynamic deficit.[91]

Therapeutic Implications
Classification of patients with STEMI by hemodynamic subsets has therapeutic relevance. As already noted, patients with low to normal wedge pressure and hypoperfusion may benefit from an infusion of fluids because the peak stroke volume value is not usually attained until LV filling pressure reaches 18 to 24 mm Hg. However, a low level of LV filling pressure does not necessarily imply that the LV damage is slight. Such patients may be relatively hypovolemic or may have an RV infarct with or without severe LV damage.

Invasive hemodynamic monitoring can help guide therapy in patients with severe LV failure (PCWP >18 mm Hg and cardiac index <2.2 liters/min/m^2). Although positive inotropic agents can be useful, they do not represent the initial therapy of choice for patients with STEMI. Instead, HF, in the presence of elevated PCWP, is managed most effectively first by reducing ventricular preload and then, if possible, by lowering afterload. Arrhythmias can contribute to hemodynamic compromise and should be treated promptly in patients with LV failure.

Hypoxemia
In STEMI complicated by HF, a combination of pulmonary vascular engorgement (and in some cases, pulmonary interstitial edema), diminished vital capacity, and in some patients, contributory respiratory depression from narcotic analgesics may cause hypoxemia. Hypoxemia can impair the function of ischemic tissue at the margin of the infarct and thereby contribute to establishing or perpetuating the vicious cycle of ischemia. However, as noted, augmentation of F_{IO_2} in patients without hypoxemia may increase systemic vascular resistance (SVR) and arterial pressure, promote coronary vasoconstriction, and result in more oxidative stress and greater infarct size.[16] As a result, S_{aO_2} can be estimated by pulse oximetry, and O_2 therapy can be omitted if the oximetric findings are normal (see earlier, General Treatment Measures).[1] On the other hand, in patients with STEMI and arterial hypoxemia, increasing F_{IO_2} by facemask should be used initially, but if S_{aO_2} cannot be maintained above 85% to 90% with 100% F_{IO_2}, endotracheal intubation and positive-pressure ventilation should be considered. Positive end-expiratory pressure (PEEP) may diminish systemic venous return and reduce effective LV filling pressure. This effect may require reducing the PEEP amount, initiating normal saline infusions to maintain LV filling pressure, or adjusting the rate of infusion of vasodilators (e.g., nitroglycerin) in patients with relative hypovolemia. Because myocardial ischemia can occur during weaning of supported ventilation, the transition to unsupported spontaneous breathing should be accompanied by observation for signs of ischemia.

Diuretics
Mild HF in patients with STEMI frequently responds well to diuretics such as furosemide administered intravenously in doses of 10 to 40 mg, repeated at 3- to 4-hour intervals if necessary. The resultant lowering of LV wall tension that accompanies the reduction in LV diastolic volume diminishes myocardial oxygen requirements and may lead to improvement in contractility and augmentation of EF, stroke volume, and cardiac output. The reduction in LV filling pressure may also enhance myocardial oxygen delivery by diminishing the impedance to coronary perfusion attributable to the elevated ventricular wall tension.

It may also improve arterial oxygenation and dyspnea by reducing pulmonary vascular congestion.

IV furosemide reduces pulmonary vascular congestion and pulmonary venous pressure within 15 minutes, before renal excretion of sodium and water has occurred; presumably, this action results from a direct dilating effect of this drug on the systemic venous bed. LV filling pressure generally should not be reduced much below 18 mm Hg, the lower range being associated with optimal LV performance in patients with STEMI, because this may reduce cardiac output further and cause arterial hypotension. Excessive diuresis may also result in hypokalemia and magnesium loss.

Afterload Reduction

Myocardial oxygen requirements depend on LV wall stress, which in turn is proportional to the product of the peak developed LV pressure, volume, and wall thickness (Laplace's law). IV vasodilator therapy should be considered in patients with STEMI complicated by (1) HF unresponsive to treatment with diuretics, (2) hypertension, (3) mitral regurgitation (MR), or (4) ventricular septal defect (VSD). In these patients, treatment with vasodilator agents increases stroke volume and may reduce myocardial oxygen requirements and thereby lessen ischemia. Hemodynamic monitoring of systemic arterial pressure and in many cases PCWP and cardiac output in patients treated with these agents is generally indicated. Improvement in cardiac performance and energetics requires three simultaneous effects: (1) reduction of LV afterload, (2) avoidance of excessive systemic arterial hypotension to maintain effective coronary perfusion pressure, and (3) avoidance of excessive reduction of ventricular filling pressure with consequent diminution of cardiac output.

Vasodilator therapy is particularly useful when STEMI is complicated by MR or rupture of the ventricular septum. In such patients, vasodilators alone or in combination with intra-aortic balloon counterpulsation can sometimes provide sufficient hemodynamic stabilization to permit definitive studies, as well as to prepare the patient for early surgical or other intervention. Because of the precarious state of patients with complicated infarction and the need for meticulous adjustment of dosage, therapy is best initiated with agents that can be administered intravenously and have a short duration of action, such as nitroprusside or nitroglycerin.

Nitroglycerin

Animal experiments have shown this drug to be less likely than nitroprusside to produce "coronary steal" (i.e., diversion of blood flow from the ischemic to the nonischemic zone). Therefore, apart from consideration of its routine use in STEMI patients discussed earlier, it may be a particularly useful vasodilator in patients with STEMI complicated by LV failure. A dosage of 10 to 15 µg/min is infused, and the dose is increased by 10 µg/min every 5 minutes until the desired effect (improvement in hemodynamics or relief of ischemic chest pain) is achieved or a decline in systolic arterial pressure to 90 mm Hg or by more than 15 mm Hg has occurred. Although both nitroglycerin and nitroprusside lower systemic arterial pressure, SVR, and the heart rate–systolic blood pressure product, nitroglycerin produces a more prominent reduction in LV filling pressure because of its relatively greater effect than nitroprusside on venous capacitance vessels. Nevertheless, in patients with severe LV failure, cardiac output often increases despite the reduction in LV filling pressure produced by nitroglycerin.

Oral Vasodilators

The use of oral vasodilators for the treatment of chronic HF is discussed in Chapter 50. Patients with STEMI and persistent HF should receive long-term RAAS inhibition, including an ACE inhibitor or ARB, and an aldosterone antagonist.[1,76,81] Treatment with an ARNI may be indicated in patients with reduced EF who develop chronic HF after MI; however, patients with recent ACS were excluded from the pivotal trials of sacubitril/valsartan.[93,94] The reduced ventricular load achieved with RAAS inhibition decreases the left ventricle remodeling that typically occurs after STEMI and reduces the development of HF and risk for death.[76,81]

Glucose-Lowering Agents (see also Chapter 31)

Treatment with a sodium-glucose co-transporter-2 inhibitor (SGLT2i) may be indicated in patients with reduced EF who develop chronic HF after MI in those with and without diabetes to reduce the composite of hospitalization for heart failure or CV death as well as serious renal outcomes; however, patients with recent ACS were excluded from the trials of this class of agents.[95,96] Treatment with a glucagon-like peptide 1 receptor agonist (GLP1-RA) is indicated in patients with diabetes and stable, established ischemic heart disease or multiple CV risk factors for the prevention of MACE.[97,98] However, no benefit was observed in the ELIXA trial with the short-acting, exendin-4 based analog, lixisenatide, the only study conducted in patients shortly after an ACS.[99] As such, the benefit of both classes of agents is not proven in the acute setting after MI.

Digitalis (see Chapter 50)

Although digitalis increases the contractility and oxygen consumption of normal hearts, when HF is present, the diminution in heart size and wall tension frequently results in a net reduction of myocardial oxygen requirements. Although the issue is still controversial, digitalis glycosides may increase the incidence of arrhythmias when given to patients in the first few hours after the onset of STEMI, particularly in the presence of hypokalemia. Administration of digitalis to patients with STEMI in the hospital phase should generally be reserved for the management of supraventricular tachyarrhythmias, such as atrial flutter and fibrillation with rapid ventricular response despite standard therapies, in the setting of poor LV function and HF persisting despite treatment with diuretics or vasodilators.

Vasoactive Medications

In addition to early coronary reperfusion, preservation of cardiac output, BP, and end-organ perfusion is paramount in patients with acute MI complicated by cardiogenic shock. Inotropic agents and vasopressors may be administered with the goal of maintaining perfusion so as to preserve end-organ function. To achieve this goal, initial therapy should aim to support arterial pressure. Once BP is stabilized with resuscitation and vasopressor therapy, treatment can be tailored to address the underlying pathophysiology (e.g., addition of further inotropic support or vasodilator therapy). In general, the dose of vasopressor and inotropic therapy should be maintained at the minimal dose and duration of therapy necessary to achieve these aims because these agents can have adverse consequences (e.g., increased myocardial oxygen consumption, arrhythmias, or reduced organ perfusion).

Beta-Adrenergic Agonists

When LV failure is severe, as manifested by a marked reduction in the cardiac index (<2.2 liters/min/m^2), and PCWP is at optimal (18 to 24 mm Hg) or excessive (>24 mm Hg) levels despite therapy with diuretics, beta-adrenergic agonists are indicated.[100] Dopamine, norepinephrine, and epinephrine can be useful in hypotensive patients with STEMI and reduced cardiac output, increased LV filling pressure, and pulmonary vascular congestion.

Dopamine has dose-dependent stimulation of dopamine and beta$_1$ and alpha$_1$ receptors. At low doses, dopaminergic receptor stimulation predominates; at moderate doses, beta$_1$ activation results in augmentation of cardiac output and HR; at high doses, alpha$_1$ stimulation prevails, manifest as vasoconstriction (Table 38.10). Although "renal dosing" of dopamine was believed to improve urine output and renal protection in HF, this effect was not evident in an RCT of patients with acute HF and renal dysfunction in the overall population; however, a post-hoc analysis suggested potential benefit in the subgroup of patients with reduced EF.[101] Although dopamine is an important option as a vasopressor, particularly in patients with hypotension, it may cause tachycardia or tachyarrhythmias. Compared with norepinephrine, treatment with dopamine at doses up to 20 µg/kg/min was associated with a higher rate of tachyarrhythmias (24.1% versus 12.4%) among 1679 patients with shock in the SOAP (Sepsis Occurrence in Acutely Ill Patients) II trial.[100] In a subgroup analysis of patients with cardiogenic shock (280, 17% of total trial population), dopamine was not only associated with more arrhythmic events but also with increased mortality

TABLE 38.10 Inotropic and Vasopressor Agents: Indications, Dose Range, Receptor Binding, and Major Clinical Side Effects

DRUG	CLINICAL INDICATION	DOSE RANGE	RECEPTOR BINDING*				MAJOR SIDE EFFECTS
			A1	B1	B2	DA	
Catecholamines							
Dopamine	Shock (vasodilatory, cardiogenic) Symptomatic bradycardia unresponsive to atropine or pacing	2.0–20 (max 50) µg•kg⁻¹•min⁻¹	+++	++++	++	+++++	Severe hypertension (especially in patients taking nonselective beta blockers) Ventricular arrhythmias Cardiac ischemia Tissue ischemia, gangrene (high doses or caused by tissue extravasation)
Dobutamine	Low CO (decompensated HF, cardiogenic shock, sepsis-induced myocardial dysfunction) Symptomatic bradycardia unresponsive to atropine or pacing	2.0–20 (max 40) µg•kg⁻¹•min⁻¹	+	+++++	+++	N/A	Tachycardia Increased ventricular response rate in patients with atrial fibrillation Ventricular arrhythmias Cardiac ischemia Hypotension
Norepinephrine	Shock (vasodilatory, cardiogenic)	0.01–3 µg•kg⁻¹•min⁻¹	+++++	+++	++	N/A	Arrhythmias Bradycardia Peripheral (digital) ischemia Hypertension (especially nonselective beta-blocker patients)
Epinephrine	Cardiac arrest Anaphylaxis Shock (cardiogenic, vasodilatory)	Infusion: 0.01–0.10 µg•kg⁻¹•min⁻¹ Bolus: 1 mg IV every 3–5 min (max 0.2 mg/kg) IM: (1:1000):0.1–0.5 mg (max 1 mg)	+++++	++++	+++	N/A	Ventricular arrhythmias Severe hypertension Cardiac ischemia
Isoproterenol	Bradyarrhythmias (especially torsade des pointes) Brugada syndrome	2–10 µg/min	0	+++++	+++++	N/A	Ventricular arrhythmias Cardiac ischemia Hypertension
Phenylephrine	Hypotension (vagally mediated, medication induced) Increase MAP with aortic stenosis and hypotension Decrease left ventricular outflow tract gradient in HCM	Bolus: 0.1 to 0.5 mg IV every 10 to 15 min Infusion: 0.4 to 10 µg•kg⁻¹•min⁻¹	+++++	0	0	N/A	Reflex bradycardia Hypertension (especially with nonselective beta blockers) Severe peripheral and visceral vasoconstriction Tissue necrosis with extravasation

Continued

TABLE 38.10 Inotropic and Vasopressor Agents: Indications, Dose Range, Receptor Binding, and Major Clinical Side Effects—cont'd

DRUG	CLINICAL INDICATION	DOSE RANGE	RECEPTOR BINDING*				MAJOR SIDE EFFECTS
			A1	B1	B2	DA	
Phosphodiesterase Inhibitors (PDEIs)							
Milrinone	Low CO (decompensated HF, after cardiotomy)	Infusion: 0.375–0.75 µg•kg⁻¹•min⁻¹ (dose adjustment necessary for renal impairment)	N/A				Ventricular arrhythmias; Hypotension; Cardiac ischemia
Other Agents							
Vasopressin	Shock (vasodilatory, cardiogenic)	Infusion: 0.01–0.1 U/min (common fixed dose 0.04 U/min)	V1 receptors (vascular smooth muscle); V2 receptors (renal-collecting duct system)				Arrhythmias; Hypertension; Decreased CO (at doses >0.4 U/min); Cardiac ischemia; Severe peripheral vasoconstriction-causing ischemia (especially skin); Splanchnic vasoconstriction
	Cardiac arrest	Bolus: 40-U IV bolus					
Levosimendan	Decompensated HF	Loading dose: 12–24 µg/kg over 10 min; Infusion: 0.05–0.2 µg•kg⁻¹•min⁻¹	N/A				Tachycardia, enhanced AV conduction; Hypotension

A1, Alpha₁-adrenergic receptor; *AS*, aortic stenosis; *AV*, atrioventricular; *B1*, beta₁-adrenergic receptor; *B2*, beta₂-adrenergic receptor; *CO*, cardiac output; *DA*, dopamine receptors; *HCM*, hypertrophic cardiomyopathy; *HF*, heart failure; *IM*, intramuscular; *IV*, intravenous; *LVOT*, left ventricular outflow tract; *MAP*, mean arterial pressure; *max*, maximum.
*0, Zero significant receptor affinity; + to +++++, minimal to maximal relative receptor affinity; *N/A*, not applicable.
From Overgaard CB, Dzavik V. Inotropes and vasopressors: review of physiology and clinical use in cardiovascular disease. Circulation. 2008;118(10):1047–1056; and Van Diepen S, Katz JN, Albert NM, et al. Contemporary Management of Cardiogenic Shock: A Scientific Statement from the American Heart Association. Circulation. 2017;136:e232–3268.

(approximately 50% versus 40% at 28 days, log-rank P value = 0.03, P interaction by shock type = 0.87).[100]

Norepinephrine increases myocardial oxygen consumption because of its peripheral vasoconstrictor and positive inotropic actions and thus had previously been avoided in patients with MI and shock (see Table 38.10). However, based on the findings of SOAP-II, norepinephrine is generally recommended over dopamine, except in cases of relative bradycardia.[100]

Epinephrine is an activator of alpha- and beta-adrenergic receptors, resulting in increased HR, cardiac output, and vascular tone (see Table 38.10). It is generally reserved for refractory shock as a second- or third-line agent for cardiogenic shock or in the setting of anaphylaxis or during cardiac arrest. Although epinephrine is recommended during cardiac arrest according to the advanced CV life support algorithm, studies suggest that those who received epinephrine in the setting of out-of-hospital cardiac arrest had higher rates of return of spontaneous circulation, but equivalent or even worse survival and neurologic function.[102] A small randomized study of epinephrine versus norepinephrine in patients with cardiogenic shock after acute MI found no difference in hemodynamic effects but a higher rate of a post-hoc endpoint of refractory shock with epinephrine defined by sustained hypotension end-organ hypoperfusion or high-dose vasoactive agent requirements.[103] Well-powered studies are needed to determine the relative efficacy and safety of dopamine, norepinephrine, and epinephrine for the management of patients with cardiogenic shock and hypotension.

Other Positive Inotropic Agents

Dobutamine has a positive inotropic action comparable to that of dopamine, but a slightly less positive chronotropic effect, and vasodilatory rather than vasoconstrictor activity (see Table 38.10).[100] As a result, it is useful in select patients whose HF persists despite treatment with diuretics, who are not hypotensive, and who are likely to benefit from both an enhancement in contractility and afterload reduction. During the administration of dobutamine, heart rhythm and systemic arterial pressure should be continuously monitored. In patients with STEMI who develop cardiogenic shock warranting treatment with dobutamine, we also generally place a PA catheter for assessment of PCWP and for frequent estimation of cardiac output. The dose should be reduced if significant tachycardia develops, if supraventricular or ventricular tachyarrhythmias occur, or if ST-segment deviations increase.

Milrinone is a noncatecholamine, nonglycoside, phosphodiesterase inhibitor with inotropic and vasodilating actions (see Table 38.10).[100] Similar to dobutamine, it is useful in patients with cardiogenic shock without significant hypotension. Milrinone has a longer half-life than dobutamine (approximately 2.5 hours versus 2 minutes, with normal renal function) and also tends to correlate with greater pulmonary vasodilatation and fewer arrhythmic events. Calcium-sensitizing agents, such as levosimendan, may have some beneficial effects on CV outcomes, but these medications have shown little incremental value in randomized trials.[100]

Vasopressors

Vasopressor therapy may be required to stabilize BP in cardiogenic or mixed shock. *Vasopressin*, or antidiuretic hormone (ADH), results in arterial smooth muscle contraction through V1 receptor agonism on the systemic vasculature (see Table 38.10). Vasopressin is typically used for refractory vasodilatory shock, particularly septic shock. However, we also occasionally use vasopressin as a part of an "adrenergic-sparing" approach in patients with severe HF, particularly in the setting of mixed cardiogenic and vasodilatory shock, based on the hypothesis that endogenous vasopressin may be depleted over time in critically ill patients. Clinical trial data of outcomes are limited with vasopressin use in cardiogenic shock. *Phenylephrine*, a synthetic, selective alpha$_1$ agonist, is rarely used in cardiogenic shock because of potent vasoconstriction.

Cardiogenic Shock

Congestion and inadequate tissue or end-organ perfusion secondary to cardiac insufficiency characterize cardiogenic shock. This reduction in perfusion decreases O_2 and nutrient delivery to tissues, which if severe or protracted, can lead to multiorgan dysfunction and death. Cardiogenic shock complicating MI most often results from LV dysfunction (approximately 80%); the remainder have a mechanical defect (e.g., VSD, papillary muscle rupture) or predominant RV infarction (Fig. 38.21).[91] Patients with cardiogenic shock complicating STEMI

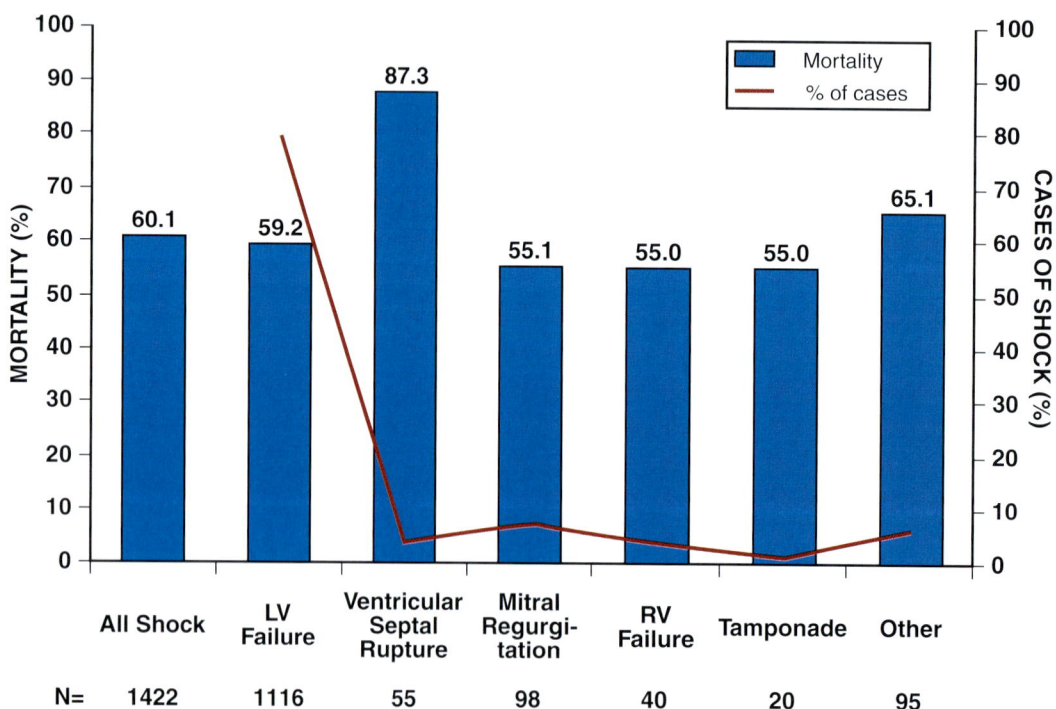

FIGURE 38.21 Mortality by etiology of cardiogenic shock following acute myocardial infarction (AMI). In-hospital mortality rates are shown for various primary etiologic conditions associated with death due to cardiogenic shock after AMI: left ventricular (LV) failure, ventricular septal rupture, acute severe mitral regurgitation, isolated right ventricular (RV) failure, cardiac tamponade/rupture (tamp), and "other" (includes previous severe valvular heart disease and excessive beta or calcium channel blockade). The proportion of patients in each category is shown *(red line).* (Modified from Hochman JS, Buller CE, Sleeper LA, et al. Cardiogenic shock complicating acute myocardial infarction—etiologies, management, and outcome: a report from the SHOCK Trial Registry. Should We Emergently Revascularize Occluded Coronaries for Cardiogenic Shock? *J Am Coll Cardiol.* 2000;36[3 Suppl A]:1063–1070.)

are more likely to be older; to have a history of diabetes mellitus, previous MI, or HF; and to have sustained an anterior infarction at the time of development of shock. In the past, cardiogenic shock occurred in up to 20% of patients with STEMI, but estimates from recent large trials and observational databases report an incidence rate of 5% to 10%.[100,104] When shock occurs, the prognosis remains poor, with in-hospital mortality rates of 30% to 50%, and few interventions, with the exception of prompt coronary revascularization of the infarct-related artery, conclusively provide benefit.[51,91,100]

Pathologic Findings
At autopsy, more than two-thirds of patients with cardiogenic shock demonstrate multivessel coronary disease, usually including the left anterior descending coronary artery (LAD). Almost all patients with cardiogenic shock exhibit thrombotic occlusion of the artery supplying the major region of recent infarction, with a loss of 40% or more of LV mass.[91] Patients who die of cardiogenic shock often have "piecemeal" necrosis, that is, progressive myocardial necrosis from marginal extension of the infarct into an ischemic zone bordering the infarction. Such extensions and focal lesions probably result in part from the shock state itself. The hydrodynamic force that develops during ventricular systole can disrupt necrotic myocardial muscle bundles, with resultant expansion and thinning of the akinetic zone of myocardium, which in turn contributes to deterioration of overall LV function.

Pathophysiology
The shock state in patients with STEMI appears to be the result of a vicious cycle, as demonstrated in Fig. 37.15.

Diagnosis
Generally accepted criteria for cardiogenic shock include (1) frank or relative hypotension, defined by a systolic BP below 80 or 90 mm Hg or a reduction in mean arterial pressure (MAP) of 30 mm Hg; (2) inadequate cardiac index, defined as less than 1.8 liters/min/m^2 without mechanical or pharmacologic support, or less than 2.2 liters/min/m^2 with support; (3) elevated end-diastolic pressures on the right (>10 to 15 mm Hg) and/or left (>18 mm Hg) side of the heart; and (4) evidence of end-organ hypoperfusion.[91,100] End-organ hypoperfusion may manifest as altered mental status, decreased urine output, acute kidney injury, cool or mottled extremities, acute liver injury, or lactic acidosis.

Spurious estimates of LV end-diastolic pressure based on measurements of PA wedge pressure can occur in patients with marked MR, in which the tall v wave in the left atrial (and PA wedge) pressure tracing elevates the mean atrial pressure above LV end-diastolic pressure. MR and other mechanical lesions (e.g., VSD, pseudoaneurysm) should be considered before making the diagnosis of cardiogenic shock caused by impairment of ventricular function. Mechanical complications should be suspected in any patient with STEMI in whom circulatory collapse occurs. Patients with cardiogenic shock merit immediate hemodynamic, angiographic, and echocardiographic evaluation. It is important to exclude mechanical complications because their treatment usually requires prompt invasive management with intervening mechanical support of the circulation.

Medical Management
In cardiogenic shock caused by impaired ventricular function, inotropic and vasopressor agents can provide pharmacologic support to maintain MAP and augment cardiac output; these agents should in principle be administered at the lowest possible doses. Although inotropic agents generally improve hemodynamics in these patients, they are not proven to improve hospital survival. Similarly, vasodilators may elevate cardiac output and reduce LV filling pressure, but lowering the already markedly reduced coronary perfusion pressure may further compromise myocardial perfusion and accelerate the vicious cycle illustrated in Fig. 37.15. Vasodilators may nonetheless be used in conjunction with mechanical circulatory support (see next section) and inotropic agents to increase cardiac output while sustaining or elevating coronary perfusion pressure.

Patients with cardiogenic shock usually have elevated SVR, although cardiogenic shock can be complicated by a systemic inflammatory response syndrome (SIRS) and a vasodilatory state, particularly with the shock of longer duration or more profound severity.[91,100,105] When SVR is lower than expected (e.g., <1200 dynes/sec/cm^5) in patients with cardiogenic shock, *inopressors*, or agents with inotropic and vasopressor properties (e.g. dopamine, norepinephrine, or epinephrine), can be useful to maintain perfusion through preservation of MAP and augmentation of cardiac output.

Mechanical Circulatory Support
The theoretical benefits of mechanical circulatory support (MCS) include the ability to (1) maintain end-organ perfusion and prevent progressive shock, (2) reduce intracardiac filling pressures and congestion, (3) reduce LV volumes, wall stress, and myocardial oxygen consumption, (4) augment coronary perfusion, (5) support the circulation during complex coronary interventions, (6) allow time for recovery of stunned or hibernating myocardium, and (7) limit infarct size (see Chapter 59).[106,107] No definitive evidence has yet established that MCS following MI improves outcomes, and data are lacking to define the optimal strategy for timing and choice of device.[106,107] Based primarily on expert consensus, early placement of MCS may be considered in those with cardiogenic shock who fail to stabilize quickly after initial interventions (e.g., reperfusion) and for those undergoing high-risk PCI (e.g., multivessel or unprotected left main) with severe HF or LV dysfunction (Fig. 38.22).[106]

Intra-Aortic Balloon Counterpulsation
In experimental animals, intra-aortic balloon (IAB) counterpulsation decreases preload, increases coronary blood flow, and improves cardiac performance. Unfortunately, the improvement is often only temporary in patients with cardiogenic shock. Although a response to IAB counterpulsation has correlated with better outcomes in observational studies and small randomized trials, in the largest and only adequately sized randomized trial conducted to date, IAB counterpulsation did not improve overall survival in patients with cardiogenic shock secondary to MI (Fig. 38.23).[108] Nor was benefit observed in any clinically relevant subgroup. Nevertheless, the 2013 ACCF/AHA Guideline for the Management of STEMI recommends that IAB counterpulsation can be useful (class IIa) in patients with cardiogenic shock whose condition does not stabilize with other interventions and as a bridge to recovery or more advanced therapies.[1] In contrast, the 2017 European Society of Cardiology (ESC) guideline for STEMI recommends that IAB counterpulsation be considered in patients with cardiogenic shock due to mechanical complications (class IIa) but not routinely for in patients with STEMI and shock (class III).[2]

Epidemiological studies demonstrate that IAB counterpulsation continues to be used for the treatment of STEMI in three groups of patients: (1) those with refractory ischemia that is not alleviated by other treatments, or who await definitive revascularization, (2) those with cardiogenic shock that does not respond to medical management, and occasionally (3) those with hemodynamic instability who require circulatory support for the performance of coronary angiography to assess lesions that are potentially correctable surgically or by PCI.[109–111a]

Percutaneous Left Ventricular Assist Devices
Several percutaneous temporary left ventricular assist devices (LVADs), often described as advanced temporary MCS to distinguish them from IAB counterpulsation, are available. However, none have rigorously demonstrated improved survival in patients with cardiogenic shock.

The most commonly used percutaneous advanced MCS is a microaxial pump that is placed across the aortic valve and delivers continuous non-pulsatile flow of blood (3 to 5 liters/min, depending on the system) from the left ventricle into the aorta, providing a larger increase in cardiac output and reduction in PCWP than IAB counterpulsation.[106,107] Extracorporeal membrane oxygenation (ECMO) is another percutaneous circulatory support option that provides biventricular support as well as oxygenation. Alternatively, a percutaneous LVAD using an external centrifugal pump may be placed by cannulation of the left femoral vein and advancement to the left atrium by transseptal puncture (see Fig. 38.22). Blood from the left atrium returns into

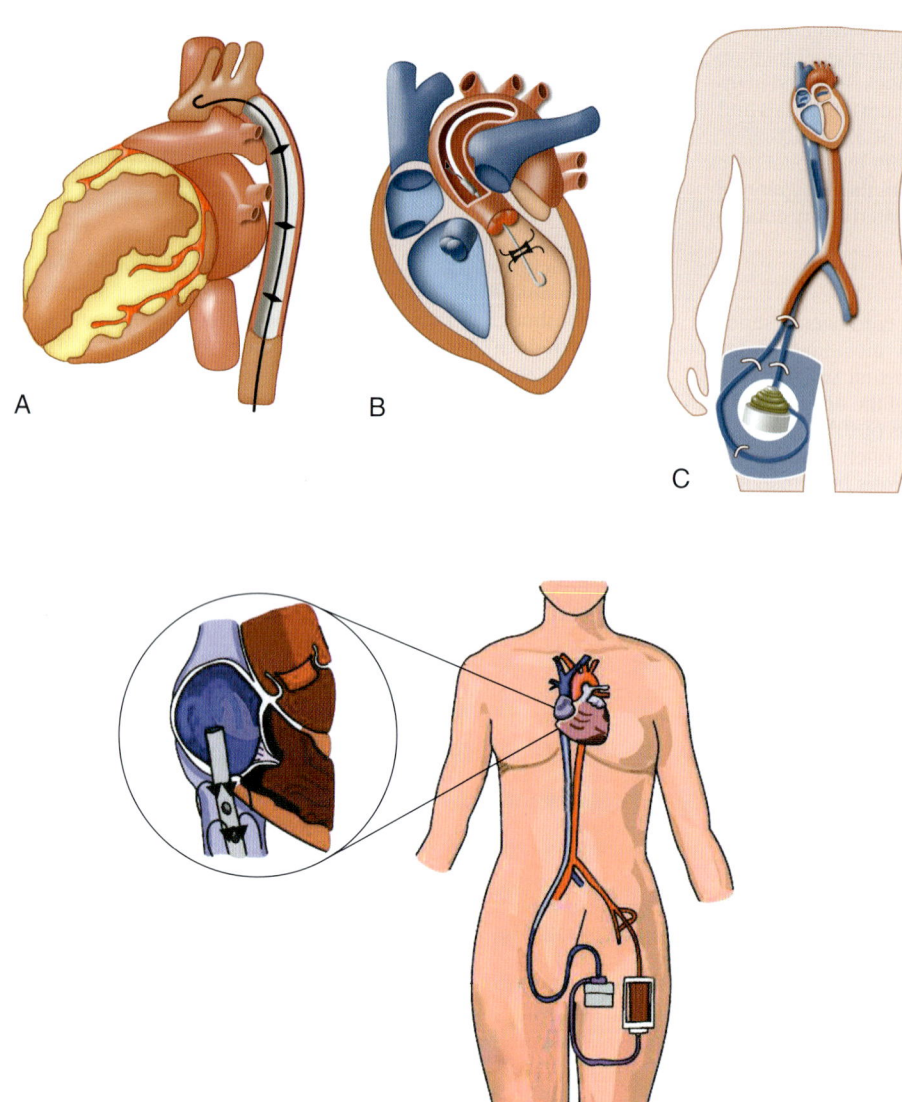

FIGURE 38.22 Schematic representation of examples of major categories of nonsurgical mechanical circulatory support. **A,** Intra-aortic balloon pump inserted into the descending aorta between the arch vessels and renal arteries. **B,** Impella Recover (Abiomed, Aachen, Germany). This rotational flow device is percutaneously inserted through the femoral artery and positioned across the aortic valve, with flow intake in the left ventricle and outflow in the aorta. **C,** TandemHeart (CardiacAssist, Pittsburgh). A cannula is inserted percutaneously through the right femoral vein and advanced toward the right atrium, where it is introduced into the left atrium by transatrial septal perforation, to establish inflow into an external rotational motor. A cannula in either femoral artery then provides the outflow. **D,** Extracorporeal membrane oxygenation (ECMO). A cannula is inserted percutaneously through the right internal jugular or either femoral vein and positioned near the right atrium. A cannula is placed in either femoral artery and then provides outflow after blood has passed through a nonpulsatile pump, and an oxygenation membrane. (Modified from Desai NR, Bhatt DL. Evaluating percutaneous support for cardiogenic shock: data shock and sticker shock. *Eur Heart J.* 2009;30:2073; and Combes A, et al. *Lancet.* 2020;396:199.)

the femoral artery via the nonpulsatile motor. This system may provide up to 5 liters/min of flow. Small randomized trials have not revealed any mortality advantage over IAB counterpulsation, but hemodynamic improvement is greater with this percutaneous LVAD.[106,107] Temporary advanced MCS aims to allow time for recovery of stunned or hibernating myocardium or for a bridge to more durable devices. Surgically placed LVADs as a bridge to transplantation or as a destination therapy are discussed in Chapter 59.

Complications
Complications of MCS include vascular damage, ischemia distal to the site of insertion for devices requiring femoral arterial cannulation, thrombocytopenia, hemolysis, athero- or thrombo-emboli, infection, mechanical failure, and bleeding in the setting of anticoagulation.

Revascularization
Of the five therapies frequently used to treat patients with cardiogenic shock—inotropes/vasopressors, MCS, fibrinolysis, PCI, and CABG—the first two are useful temporizing maneuvers. Revascularization, however, appears to improve survival.

The SHOCK (Should We Emergently Revascularize Occluded Coronaries for Cardiogenic Shock?) study evaluated early revascularization for the treatment of patients with MI complicated by cardiogenic shock.[91] Patients with shock caused by LV failure complicating STEMI were randomly assigned to emergency revascularization ($n = 152$), accomplished by either CABG or angioplasty, or to initial medical stabilization ($n = 150$). In 86% of patients in both groups, IAB counterpulsation was performed. The primary endpoint was all-cause mortality at 30 days; a secondary endpoint was mortality at 6 months. At 30 days, the overall mortality rate was 46.7% in the revascularization group, not significantly different from the 56% mortality observed in the medical therapy group ($P = 0.11$). Although the primary analysis was neutral, long-term survival improved significantly in patients with cardiogenic shock who underwent early revascularization (Fig. 38.24). Subgroups of patients in the SHOCK study who showed benefit from the early revascularization strategy (i.e., reduced 6-month mortality) were those younger than 75 years, those with a previous MI, and those randomly assigned less than 6 hours from the onset of infarction. A subsequent observational study of patients with MI complicated by shock indicated that well-selected elderly patients undergoing PCI had a 1-year survival similar to that in younger patients undergoing early revascularization.[112]

Multivessel disease affects 70% to 90% of patients with cardiogenic shock and acute MI, and the optimal extent of initial revascularization has undergone intense clinical investigation.[108] Multiple studies demonstrated robust reductions in recurrent CV events with multivessel or complete revascularization compared to infarct artery-only revascularization in patients with STEMI but without cardiogenic shock (see earlier, Catheter-Based Reperfusion Strategies).[46-50] However, in the pivotal randomized CULPRIT-SHOCK (Culprit Lesion Only PCI versus Multivessel PCI in Cardiogenic Shock) trial among 706 patients with cardiogenic shock onset within 12 hours in the setting of acute MI (ST- and non-ST-elevation MI), patients randomized to infarct artery-only compared with acute multivessel revascularization at index catheterization had a lower 30-day rate of death or severe renal failure leading to renal replacement therapy (RR 0.83; 95% CI 0.71 to 0.96; $P = 0.01$) (Fig. 38.25).[51] Moreover, the risk of death was lower in patients randomized to culprit-only PCI at the initial catheterization ($P = 0.03$).[51]

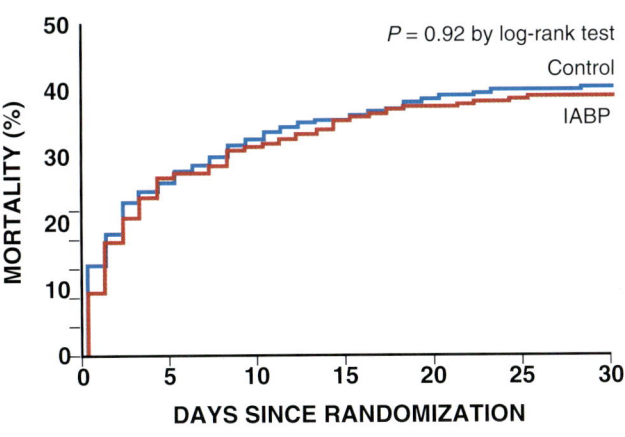

Baseline variable	No. of patients	IABP	Control	Relative risk (95% CI)	P value for interaction
		30-day mortality (%)			
Sex					0.61
Female	187	44.4	43.2	1.03 (0.74-1.43)	
Male	411	37.3	40.5	0.92 (0.72-1.18)	
Age					0.09
<50 yr	70	19.4	44.1	0.44 (0.21-0.95)	
50-75 yr	334	34.6	36.5	0.95 (0.71-1.27)	
>75 yr	194	53.7	50.0	1.07 (0.81-1.41)	
Diabetes					0.82
Yes	195	42.9	46.7	0.92 (0.67-1.26)	
No	399	37.2	38.9	0.96 (0.74-1.23)	
Hypertension					0.05
Yes	410	42.9	40.4	1.06 (0.84-1.34)	
No	183	28.9	43.0	0.67 (0.45-1.01)	
Type of MI					0.76
STEMI/LBBB	412	41.0	42.9	0.96 (0.77-1.21)	
Non-STEMI	177	37.5	38.3	0.98 (0.67-1.43)	
STEMI type					0.14
Anterior	216	35.4	43.7	0.81 (0.58-1.13)	
Nonanterior	196	48.3	42.2	1.16 (0.85-1.57)	
Previous infarction					0.04
Yes	131	47.9	33.3	1.44 (0.93-2.21)	
No	466	37.3	43.3	0.86 (0.39-1.07)	
Hypothermia					0.31
Yes	226	48.1	44.2	1.09 (0.82-1.44)	
No	372	35.1	39.3	0.89 (0.68-1.16)	
Blood pressure					0.76
<80 mm Hg	161	50.7	46.4	1.09 (0.79-1.50)	
≥80 mm Hg	432	35.9	39.2	0.92 (0.72-1.17)	

IABP better ← | → Control better

FIGURE 38.23 Primary result of a randomized trial of routine insertion of an intra-aortic balloon pump (IABP) versus standard care in patients with acute MI and cardiogenic shock. **A,** In this randomized trial of 600 patients, the primary endpoint of death from any cause did not differ between the randomized treatment groups. **B,** There was no convincing benefit of the routine use of IABP for shock in any of the major subgroups examined. LBBB, Left bundle branch block. (From Thiele H, et al. Intraaortic balloon support for myocardial infarction with cardiogenic shock. N Engl J Med. 2012;367:1287.)

Shock Teams

Many centers have created multidisciplinary shock teams to facilitate rapid assessment and optimal management of patients with cardiogenic shock.[100] These teams typically include representation from advanced heart failure, interventional cardiology, critical care cardiology, cardiac surgery, nursing, and other supportive services (e.g., social work and palliative care). Implementation of a multidisciplinary team-based, protocolized approach can improve outcomes.[113]

Recommendations

We recommend individualized assessment of patients to determine their desire for aggressive care and overall candidacy for further treatment (e.g., age, mental status, comorbid conditions). Suitable candidates should have revascularization of the culprit artery. Routine revascularization of nonculprit arteries in the same procedure as the primary PCI does not appear indicated and may worsen outcomes. In patients with STEMI and shock, in whom PCI or CABG is not suitable or accessible,

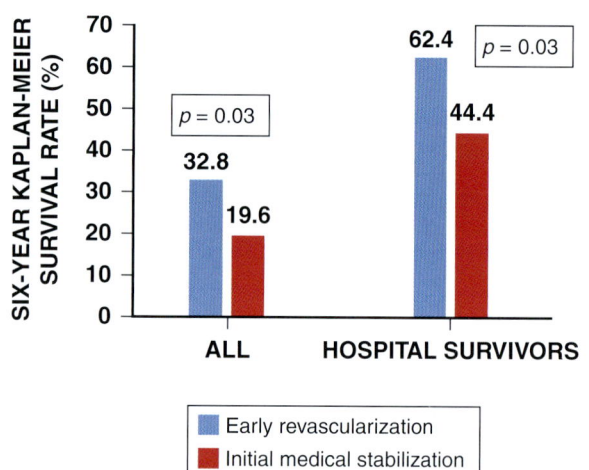

FIGURE 38.24 Impact of revascularization in patients in the SHOCK trial. Survival rates shown for all patients and among hospital survival in patients randomized to early revascularization and initial medical stabilization (IMS) groups at 6 years. (Data from Hochman JS, et al. JAMA 2006;295:2511.)

fibrinolytic agents can be given unless they have a contraindication.[1] Temporary LVADs may be used to bridge patients with refractory shock whose condition does not stabilize with other therapies to additional clinical decision making or advanced heart failure therapies.

Right Ventricular Infarction

The clinical features of RV infarction range from mild RV dysfunction to cardiogenic shock. Clinically significant RV infarction, which accompanies approximately one-third of inferior LV infarctions, produces characteristic electrocardiographic manifestations and hemodynamic patterns (Fig. 38.26). Right-sided heart filling pressures (CVP, RA, RV end-diastolic) are elevated, whereas LV filling pressure is normal or only slightly raised; RV systolic and pulse pressures are decreased, and cardiac output is often greatly depressed.

Diagnosis

Many patients with the combination of a normal LV filling pressure and depressed cardiac index have RV infarcts (with accompanying inferior LV infarcts). The hemodynamic picture may superficially resemble that seen in patients with pericardial disease (see Chapter 86) and includes elevated RV filling pressure; a steep, RA y descent; and an early diastolic drop and plateau (resembling the square root sign) in the RV pressure tracing. Moreover, patients with RV infarction may display the Kussmaul sign (increase in jugular venous pressure with inspiration) and pulsus paradoxus (decrease in systolic BP >10 mm Hg with inspiration) (Fig. 38.26C). In fact, the Kussmaul sign in the setting of inferior STEMI is highly predictive of RV involvement.

The ECG can provide the first clue to RV involvement in patients with inferior STEMI (Fig. 38.26B). Most patients with RV infarction have ST-segment elevation in lead V_4R (right precordial lead in the V_4 position).[1] Transient elevation of the ST segment in any of the right precordial leads can occur with RV MI, and the presence of ST-segment elevation of 0.1 mV or greater in any one or a combination of leads V_4R, V_5R, and V_6R in patients with the clinical picture of acute MI points to the diagnosis of RV MI. In addition to noting the presence or absence of convex upward ST elevation in V_4R, clinicians should determine whether the T wave is positive or negative; such distinctions help distinguish proximal versus distal occlusion of the right coronary artery versus occlusion of the left circumflex artery (Fig. 38.26B). Elevation of the ST segments in leads V_1 through V_4 caused by RV infarction can be confused with elevation caused by anteroseptal infarction. Although the elevated ST segments orient anteriorly in both cases, the frontal plane can provide important clues: the ST segments orient to the right with RV infarction (e.g., +120 degrees), whereas they orient to the left with anteroseptal infarction (e.g., −30 degrees).

Noninvasive Assessment

Echocardiography helps in the differential diagnosis because in patients with RV infarction, in contrast to pericardial tamponade, little or no pericardial fluid accumulates. The echocardiogram shows abnormal wall motion of the right ventricle, as well as RV dilation and depression of the RV wall motion.[114] MRI can also aid in recognition of RV infarction.[115] Impaired RV function delineated by either modality is associated with increased mortality after MI. Additionally, shock from isolated RV dysfunction carries almost as high a mortality risk as LV shock; serial studies have shown, however, some degree of ventricular recovery more frequently with RV infarction than with LV infarction.[115]

Treatment

Because of their ability to reduce preload, medications routinely prescribed for LV infarction may produce profound hypotension in patients with RV infarction. Specifically, nitrates, morphine, and diuretics should be avoided. In patients with hypotension caused by RV MI, hemodynamics can improve with a combination of expansion of plasma volume to augment RV preload and cardiac output and, when LV failure is present, arterial vasodilators.[1] If hypotension has not responded to brisk administration of 1 or more liters of fluid, however, consideration should be given to hemodynamic monitoring with a PA catheter because further volume infusion may be of little use and could produce pulmonary congestion. Arterial vasodilators reduce the impedance to LV outflow and, in turn, LV diastolic, left atrial, and pulmonary (arterial) pressure, thereby lowering impedance to RV outflow and enhancing RV output.

Right ventricular infarction is common in patients with inferior LV infarction. Therefore, otherwise unexplained systemic arterial hypotension with diminished cardiac output or marked hypotension in response to small doses of nitroglycerin in patients with inferior infarction should lead to prompt consideration of this diagnosis. In patients requiring pacing, ventricular pacing may fail to increase cardiac output, and AV sequential pacing may be needed. Successful reperfusion of the right coronary artery significantly improves RV mechanical function and lowers in-hospital mortality in patients with RV infarction.[115] Replacement of the tricuspid valve and repair of the valve with annuloplasty rings can treat severe tricuspid regurgitation caused by RV infarction.

Mechanical Causes of Heart Failure

The most dramatic complications of STEMI involve tearing or rupture of acutely infarcted tissue (Fig. 38.27). The clinical characteristics of these lesions vary considerably and depend on the site of rupture, which may involve the free wall of either ventricle, the interventricular septum, or the papillary muscles. The overall incidence of these complications, although difficult to assess because clinical and autopsy series differ considerably, appears to have decreased initially with the introduction of reperfusion therapy and subsequently decreased substantially with the widespread adoption of primary PCI.[116] Table 38.11 shows the comparative clinical profile of these complications, as gathered from different studies.

Free Wall Rupture

The clinical course of rupture varies from *catastrophic*, with an acute tear leading to tamponade and immediate death, to *subacute*, with nausea, hypotension, and pericardial discomfort the major clinical clues to its presence (see Fig. 38.27 and Table 38.11). The tear is usually preceded by a large infarct with subsequent expansion, sometimes with a dissecting hematoma, and occurs near the junction of the infarct and normal muscle. Rupture is more common in the left ventricle (specifically, the anterior or lateral wall) than in the right ventricle and seldom occurs in the atria. Other features associated with rupture include reperfusion with a fibrinolytic agent versus PCI, older age, female sex, hypertension, single-vessel disease without collateral circulation, and an anterior or first MI.[117] Mortality rates can be as high as 75% to 90% following free wall rupture. Survival depends on recognition of this complication, and most importantly, on prompt surgical repair.[1]

Pseudoaneurysm

Incomplete rupture of the heart may occur when organizing thrombus and hematoma, together with pericardium, seal a rupture of the left ventricle and thus prevent the development of hemopericardium. With time, this area of organized thrombus and pericardium can become a pseudoaneurysm (false aneurysm) that

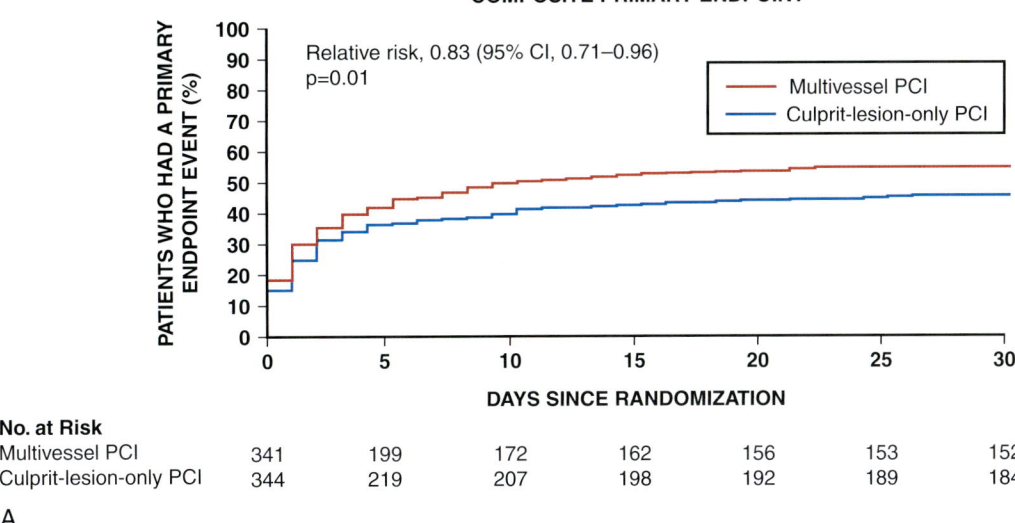

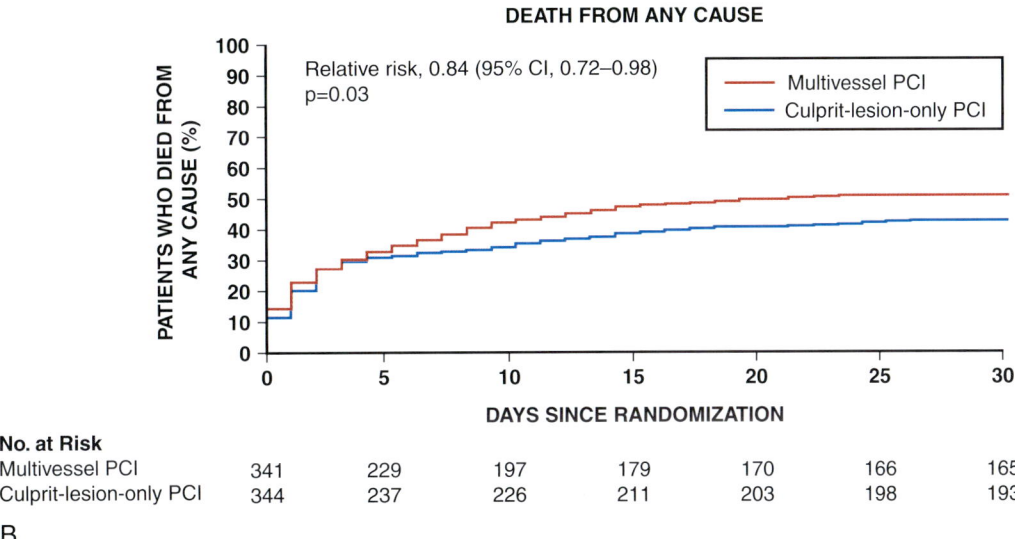

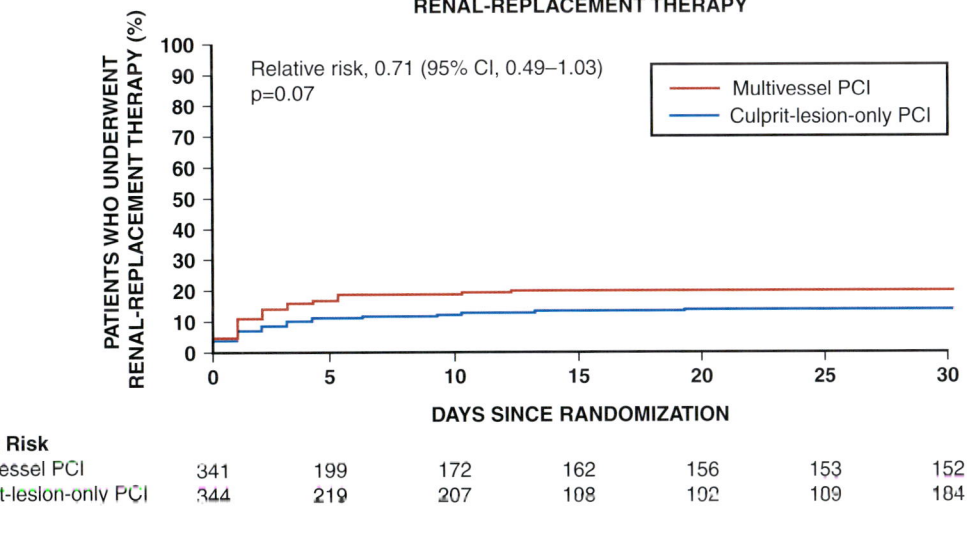

FIGURE 38.25 Randomized comparison of immediate multivessel versus culprit vessel-only PCI in patients with cardiogenic shock in the CULPRIT-Shock trial. **A,** Primary outcomes of all-cause death or severe renal failure leading to renal replacement therapy and individual components of **(B)** all-cause death and **(C)** renal replacement therapy at 30 days. (Data from Thiele H, et al. *N Engl J Med.* 2017;377:2419–2432.)

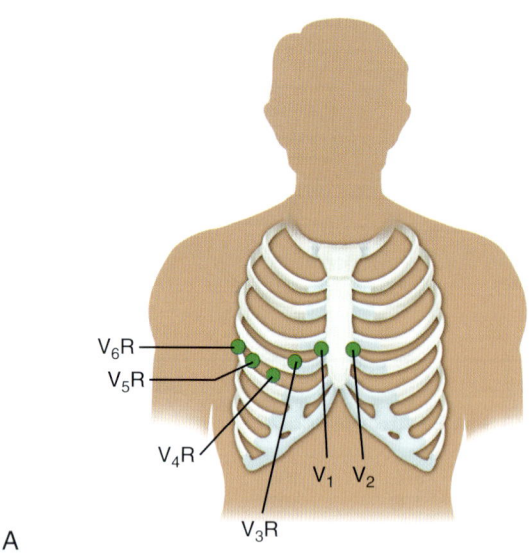
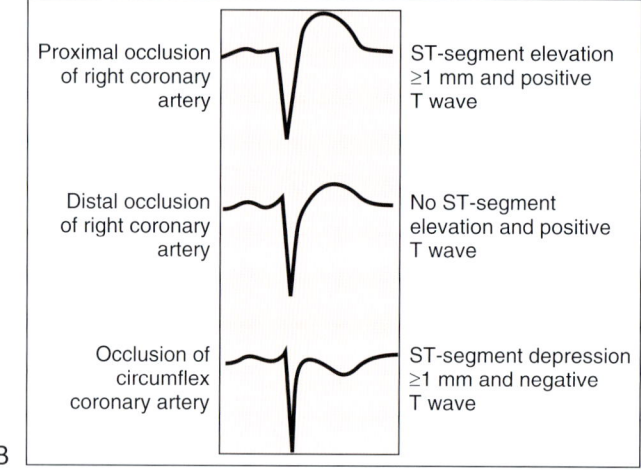

FIGURE 38.26 Right ventricular (RV) infarction: diagnosis, clinical features, and management. **A,** Placement of right-sided leads for electrocardiographic evaluation of RV infarction. **B,** ST elevation is seen in the right-sided ECG leads (e.g., V_4R), with variation in the repolarization pattern depending on the infarct artery and the location of the occlusion. **C,** Patients with hemodynamically significant RV infarction have shock but clear lungs and elevated jugular venous pressure (JVP). Management is directed at maintaining adequate RV preload and lowering pulmonary artery pressure to unload the right ventricle. Inotropic therapy may be necessary in some cases. *Echo,* Echocardiogram; *RA,* right atrial. (Modified from Wellens HJ. The value of the right precordial leads of the electrocardiogram. *N Engl J Med.* 1999;340:381; and Antman EM et al. ACC/AHA guidelines for the management of patients with ST-elevation myocardial infarction: a report of the American College of Cardiology/American Heart Association Task Force on Practice Guidelines [Committee to Revise the 1999 Guidelines for the Management of Patients with Acute Myocardial Infarction]. *J Am Coll Cardiol.* 2004;44(3):e1.)

maintains communication with the cavity of the left ventricle. In contrast to true aneurysms, which always contain some myocardial elements in their walls, the walls of pseudoaneurysms are composed of organized hematoma and pericardium and lack any elements of the original myocardial wall. Pseudoaneurysms can become quite large, even equaling the true ventricular cavity in size, and they communicate with the LV cavity through a narrow neck. Frequently, pseudoaneurysms contain old and recent thrombi, the superficial portions of which can cause arterial emboli. Pseudoaneurysms can drain off a portion of each ventricular stroke volume, exactly as do true aneurysms. The diagnosis of pseudoaneurysm can usually be made by echocardiography, contrast-enhanced angiography, CMR, or computed tomography (CT), although differentiation between a true aneurysm and a pseudoaneurysm can sometimes be difficult with any imaging technique.[118]

Diagnosis
Myocardial free wall rupture is usually accompanied by sudden profound shock, often rapidly leading to pulseless electrical activity caused by pericardial tamponade. Immediate pericardiocentesis can confirm the diagnosis. If the patient's condition is sufficiently stable, echocardiography can establish the diagnosis of tamponade.

Treatment
In patients with critically compromised hemodynamics, establishment of the diagnosis should be followed immediately by surgical resection of the necrotic and ruptured myocardium with primary reconstruction. When the rupture is subacute and a pseudoaneurysm is suspected or present, prompt elective surgery is indicated because the risk of rupture approaches 50% in untreated cases.[118]

Rupture of Interventricular Septum
As in rupture of the free wall of the ventricle, transmural infarction underlies rupture of the ventricular septum. The perforation can range in length from one to several centimeters (see Fig. 38.27). It can be a direct through-and-through opening or more irregular and serpiginous. Rupture of the septum with an anterior infarction tends to be apical in location, whereas inferior infarctions are associated with perforation of the basal septum and have a worse prognosis than those in an anterior location.

Clinical features associated with increased risk for rupture of the interventricular septum include lack of development of a collateral network, advanced age, female sex, and chronic kidney disease (see Table 38.11). A new, harsh, loud holosystolic murmur heard best at the lower left sternal border, usually accompanied by a thrill, characterizes a ruptured interventricular septum. Biventricular failure generally ensues within hours to days. The defect can also be recognized by echocardiography with color flow Doppler imaging (Fig. 38.28) or by insertion of a PA catheter to document the left-to-right shunt. Rupture of the interventricular septum after STEMI carries a poor prognosis, with mortality of 40% to 75%.[117] The likelihood of survival depends on the degree of impairment of ventricular function and the size of the defect, but because the rupture site can expand, prompt repair is necessary even in hemodynamically stable patients.[1] Septal rupture is most often repaired surgically, although transcatheter closure may be considered, particularly when the patient is deemed inoperable and the anatomy is amenable to the application of a closure device (Fig. 38.29).[119]

Rupture of a Papillary Muscle

Partial or total rupture of a papillary muscle is a rare but often fatal complication of transmural MI (see Fig. 38.21).[120] Complete transection of an LV papillary muscle is incompatible with life because the sudden massive MR that develops cannot be tolerated. Rupture of a portion of a papillary muscle, usually the tip or head of the muscle, that results in severe, although not necessarily overwhelming MR, is much more frequent and is not immediately fatal (Fig. 38.30). Inferior wall infarction can lead to rupture of the posteromedial papillary muscle, which because of its singular blood supply, occurs more frequently than rupture of the anterolateral muscle, a consequence of anterolateral MI. Unlike rupture of the ventricular septum, which occurs with large infarcts, papillary muscle rupture occurs with a relatively small infarction in approximately half of cases. These patients may have a modest extent of CAD as well. Rupture of an RV papillary muscle is unusual but can cause massive tricuspid regurgitation and RV failure. In a small number of patients, rupture of more than one cardiac structure is noted clinically or at postmortem examination; all possible combinations of rupture of the LV free wall, the interventricular septum, and the papillary muscles can occur.

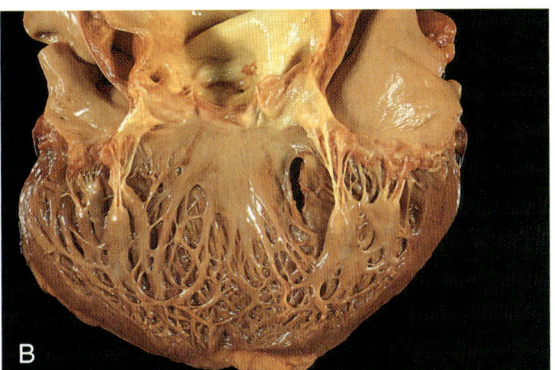
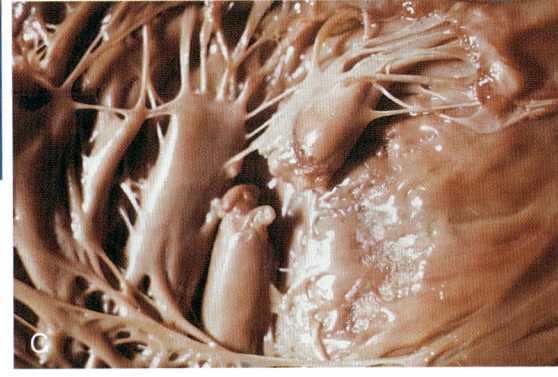

FIGURE 38.27 Cardiac rupture syndromes complicating STEMI. **A,** Anterior myocardial rupture in an acute infarct. **B,** Rupture of the ventricular septum. **C,** Complete rupture of a necrotic papillary muscle. (From Schoen FJ: The heart. In: Kumar V, et al, eds. *Robbins & Cotran Pathologic Basis of Disease*. 7th ed. Philadelphia: Saunders; 2005.)

TABLE 38.11 Characteristics of Ventricular Septal Rupture, Rupture of the Ventricular Free Wall, and Papillary Muscle Rupture

CHARACTERISTIC	VENTRICULAR SEPTAL RUPTURE	RUPTURE OF THE VENTRICULAR FREE WALL	PAPILLARY MUSCLE RUPTURE
Incidence	0.2–3% without reperfusion therapy, 0.2–0.3% with fibrinolytic therapy, 3.9% in patients with cardiogenic shock	Approximately 0.3–1%; fibrinolytic therapy does not reduce risk; primary PCI seems to reduce risk	Approximately 0.1–1% (posteromedial more frequent than anterolateral papillary muscle rupture)
Time course	Bimodal peak; within 24 hr and 3–5 days; range, 1–14 days	Bimodal peak; within 24 hr and 3–5 days; range, 1–14 days	Bimodal peak; within 24 hr and 3–5 days; range, 1–14 days
Clinical manifestations	Chest pain, shortness of breath, hypotension	Anginal, pleuritic, or pericardial chest pain; syncope; hypotension; restlessness; sudden death	Abrupt onset of shortness of breath and pulmonary edema; hypotension
Physical findings	Harsh holosystolic murmur, thrill, S_3, accentuated S_2, pulmonary edema, RV and LV failure, cardiogenic shock	Jugular venous distention (29% of patients), pulsus paradoxus (47%), electromechanical dissociation, cardiogenic shock	A soft murmur in some cases, no thrill, variable signs of RV overload, severe pulmonary edema, cardiogenic shock
Echocardiographic findings	Ventricular septal rupture, left-to-right shunt on color flow Doppler echocardiography through the ventricular septum, pattern of RV overload	>5 mm pericardial effusion not visualized in all cases; layered, high-acoustic echoes within the pericardium (blood clot); direct visualization of tear; signs of tamponade	Hypercontractile LV, torn papillary muscle or chordae tendineae, flail leaflet, severe mitral regurgitation on color flow Doppler echocardiography
Right-heart catheterization	Increase in oxygen saturation from the RA to RV, large v waves	Ventriculography insensitive, classic signs of tamponade not always present (equalization of diastolic pressures in the cardiac chambers)	No increase in oxygen saturation from the RA to RV, large v waves,* very high PCWP

LV, Left ventricle/left ventricular; *PCI*, percutaneous coronary intervention; *RA*, right atrium; *RV*, right ventricle/right ventricular.
*Large v waves are from the pulmonary capillary wedge pressure (PCWP).
Data from Antman EM, Anbe DT, Armstrong PW, et al. ACC/AHA guidelines for the management of patients with ST-elevation myocardial infarction: a report of the American College of Cardiology/American Heart Association Task Force on Practice Guidelines (Committee to Revise the 1999 Guidelines for the Management of Patients with Acute Myocardial Infarction). *Circulation*. 2004;110(9):e82; and Elbadawi A, Elgendy IY, Mahmoud K, et al. Temporal Trends and Outcomes of Mechanical Complications in Patients With Acute Myocardial Infarction. *JACC Cardiovasc Interv*. 2019;12:1825–1836.

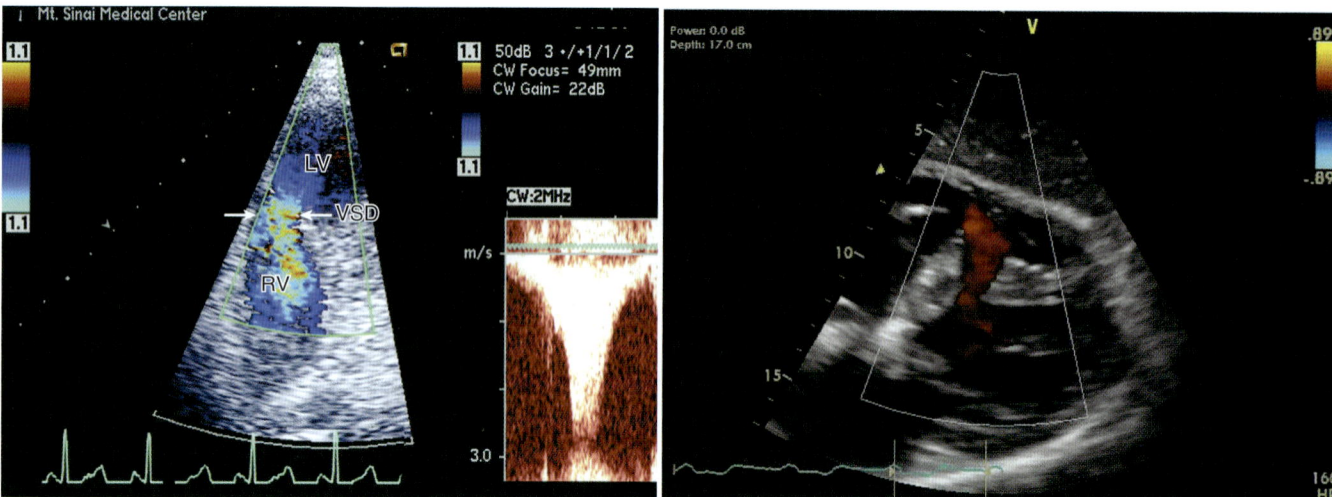

FIGURE 38.28 Echocardiography of two ventricular septal defects (VSDs) that developed after STEMI. A close-up of the ventricular septum demonstrates turbulent systolic color flow Doppler across a VSD (*white arrows*), and continuous-wave Doppler demonstrates systolic flow across a VSD **(left)**. A subcostal view demonstrates color flow Doppler across a VSD **(right)**. *LV,* Left ventricle; *RV,* right ventricle. (**Left** from Kamran M, Attari M, Webber G. Images in cardiovascular medicine. Ventricular septal defect complicating an acute myocardial infarction. *Circulation.* 2005;112:e337; **Right** from Brigham and Women's Hospital, 2013.)

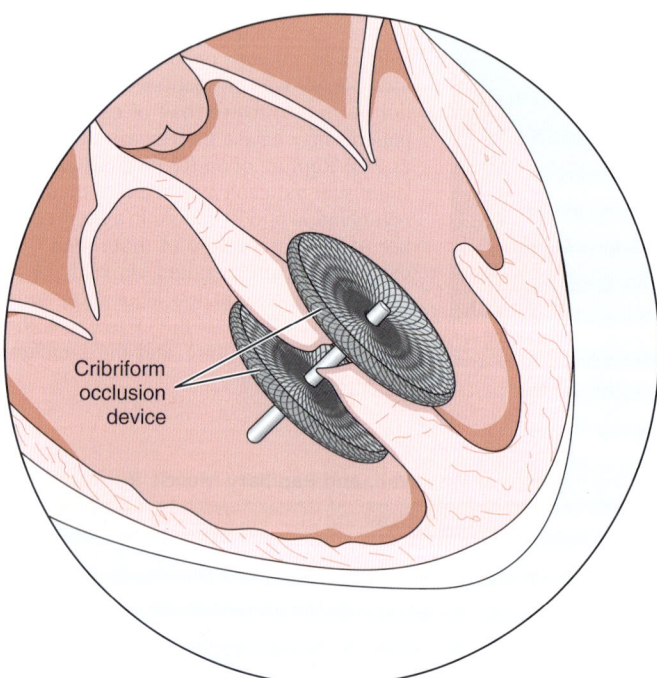

FIGURE 38.29 Schematic of a percutaneous, transcatheter closure of an ischemic ventricular septal defect using a cribriform occlusion device. (Redrawn from Kamioka N, et al. Circ Cardiovasc Interventions 2019;12[5]:e007788.)

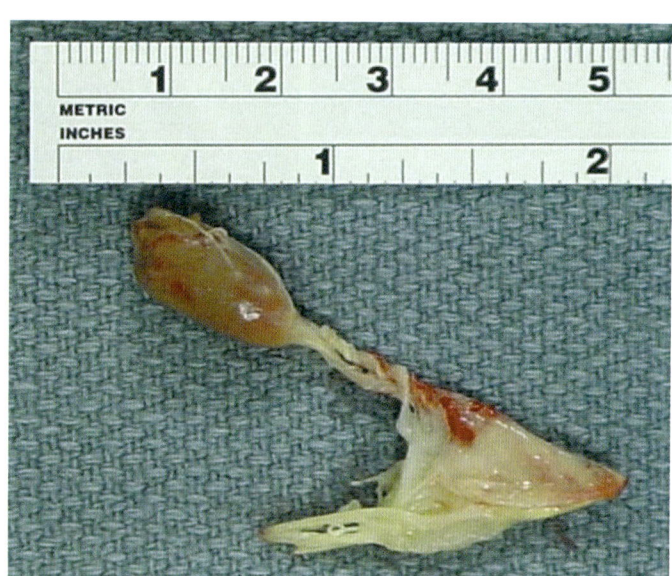

FIGURE 38.30 Surgical specimen showing a papillary muscle (*top left*), chordae, and anterior mitral leaflet (*bottom right*) from a patient who had a partial rupture of the papillary muscle and underwent mitral valve replacement for severe mitral regurgitation after STEMI. (Courtesy of Dr. Peter Libby, Brigham and Women's Hospital, Boston, MA.)

As with patients who have a ruptured VSD, those with papillary muscle rupture manifest with increasingly severe HF. These patients may also have a holosystolic murmur, but because of rapid equalization of pressures between the left atrium and ventricle, patients with torrential acute MR may have an unimpressive or absent murmur.[120] In either ventricular or papillary muscle rupture, the murmur may become softer or may disappear as arterial pressure falls. Echocardiography can promptly recognize MR secondary to partial or complete rupture of a papillary muscle and distinguish it from other, generally less severe forms of MR that occur with STEMI. Color flow Doppler imaging is particularly helpful in distinguishing acute MR from VSD in the setting of STEMI (see Table 38.11).[1] However, acute severe MR may be difficult to diagnose with transthoracic echocardiography (TTE) in cases with narrow eccentric jets with rapid equalization of pressures; therefore, transesophageal echocardiography (TEE) should be employed when suspicion is high because of its greater diagnostic accuracy.

Differentiation Between Ventricular Septal Rupture and Mitral Regurgitation

Distinguishing on clinical grounds between acute MR and rupture of the ventricular septum in patients with STEMI in whom a loud systolic murmur suddenly develops may be difficult. Such differentiation can be made most readily by color flow Doppler echocardiography. In addition, right-heart catheterization can readily distinguish between these two complications. Patients with ventricular septal rupture demonstrate a "step-up" in SaO in blood samples from the right ventricle and PA compared with those from the right atrium. Patients with acute MR lack this step-up; they may demonstrate tall *c-v* waves in both the pulmonary capillary and pulmonary arterial pressure tracings.

Management

We recommend the initiation of invasive monitoring in most cases once there is recognition of a major mechanical complication of STEMI. For acute MR and VSDs, unless systolic BP is below 90 mm Hg, vasodilator therapy, usually nitroglycerin or nitroprusside, should be instituted as soon as possible once hemodynamic monitoring is available. Inotropic agents may support adequate cardiac output. These interventions can prove critically important for stabilizing the patient's condition in preparation for further diagnostic studies and repair. If pharmacologic therapy is not tolerated or fails to achieve hemodynamic stability, MCS should be instituted rapidly as a bridge to definitive repair of the acute mechanical complication.

Operative intervention is most successful in patients with STEMI and circulatory collapse when a surgically correctable mechanical lesion (e.g., VSD, ruptured papillary muscle) can be identified and addressed (see Fig. 38.31). In most cases, surgery should not be delayed in patients with a correctable lesion who agree to an aggressive management strategy and require pharmacologic and mechanical support.[1] In such patients a serious complication frequently develops—infection, adult respiratory distress syndrome, extension of the infarct, or renal failure—if surgery is delayed. Early surgery, short duration of shock, and mild degrees of RV and LV impairment predict surgical survival.[1] In a subset of patients whose hemodynamic status remains stable, the operation may be postponed for 2 to 4 weeks to allow some healing of the infarct. Such complex decisions regarding the optimal timing of surgery require integration of multiple aspects of the clinical course and anatomy of the mechanical complication by a multidisciplinary "heart" team. These situations also require careful consideration of the goals of care with the patient or proxies to ensure respecting the patient's wishes and values, particularly in cases with a high degree of futility.

Catheter-based options for VSD repair may be appropriate in patients who are not candidates for early definitive surgical correction.[1,119] We sometimes undertake early catheter-based repair with the aim of temporizing the defect until a later definitive surgical repair when more infarct healing has occurred. However, because the initial closure of the defect is almost always incomplete, and the device requires time to thrombose and endothelialize, in most patients with hemodynamically significant mechanical complications, surgical management is the best option.[1,119]

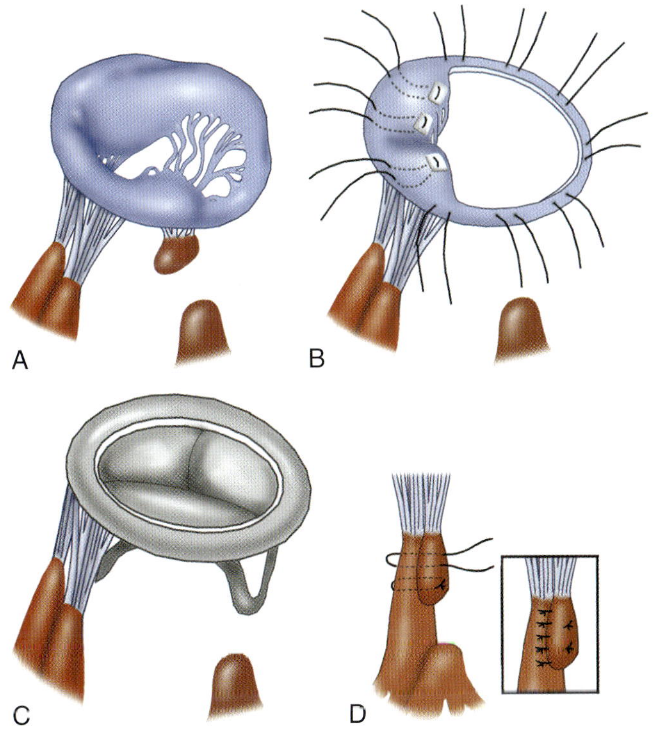

ARRHYTHMIAS

Arrhythmias can complicate the course of patients with STEMI (Table 38.12). Many serious arrhythmias develop before hospitalization. Some abnormality in cardiac rhythm also occurs in many patients with STEMI treated in the hospital. These arrhythmias can include both tachycardic and bradycardic episodes, either of which can provoke hemodynamic consequences (see also Part VII, Arrhythmias, Sudden Death, and Syncope).

Hemodynamic Consequences

Patients with LV dysfunction have a relatively fixed stroke volume and depend on changes in HR to alter cardiac output. However, the range of HR with maximal cardiac output is narrow: either faster or slower rates can cause reductions in output. Thus, all forms of tachycardia and bradycardia can depress cardiac output in patients with STEMI. Although optimal cardiac output may require a rate higher than 100 beats/min, because HR is one of the major determinants of myocardial oxygen consumption, more rapid HRs elevate myocardial energy needs to levels that can adversely affect ischemic myocardium. In patients with STEMI, therefore, the optimal rate is usually lower, in the range of 60 beats/min.

A second factor to consider in assessing the hemodynamic consequences of a particular arrhythmia is loss of the atrial contribution to ventricular preload. Studies of patients without STEMI have demonstrated that loss of atrial transport decreases LV output by 15% to 20%. In patients with reduced diastolic LV compliance of any cause (including STEMI), however, atrial systole is of greater importance for LV filling. In patients with STEMI, atrial systole boosts end-diastolic volume by approximately 15%, end-diastolic pressure by 30%, and stroke volume by 35%.

Ventricular Arrhythmias (see Chapter 67)
Ventricular Premature Depolarizations

Before the widespread use of reperfusion therapy, aspirin, and beta blockers for the management of STEMI, frequent ventricular premature complexes (VPCs) (>5/min), VPCs with a multiform configuration, early coupling ("R-on-T" phenomenon), and repetitive patterns in the form of couplets or salvoes were thought to presage VF. However, the number of patients who do not develop fibrillation who have such "warning arrhythmias" is similar to those who do. Primary VF (see later) can occur without antecedent warning arrhythmias and may even develop despite their suppression. Both primary VF and VPCs, especially R-on-T beats, occur during the early phase of STEMI, a period of considerable heterogeneity in electrical activity. Although R-on-T beats expose this heterogeneity and can precipitate VF in a small minority of patients, the ubiquitous nature of VPCs in patients with STEMI and the extremely infrequent nature of VF in the current era of STEMI management result in low sensitivity and specificity of the electrocardiographic patterns observed on monitoring systems for identifying patients at risk for VF.

Management
The incidence of VF in patients with STEMI seen in CICUs over the past three decades appears to have declined. The previous practice of prophylactic suppression of ventricular premature beats with antiarrhythmic drugs is not indicated and may actually increase the risk for fatal bradycardic and asystolic events.[1] Therefore, for patients with STEMI with VPCs, we do not routinely prescribe antiarrhythmic drugs, other than beta blockers, but instead correct any recurrent ischemia

FIGURE 38.31 Surgical management of mitral regurgitation (MR) caused by a ruptured papillary muscle. **A,** Acute papillary muscle rupture results in severe MR as a result of leaflet and commissural prolapse. Mitral valve replacement is usually necessary. **B,** Mitral débridement with retention of the unruptured commissural and leaflet segment is performed to preserve partial continuity of the annular papillary muscle. **C,** Mitral valve replacement is then performed. **D,** Occasionally, mitral valve repair can be performed by transfer of a papillary head to a non-ruptured segment. (Courtesy Dr. David Adams, Mt. Sinai Hospital, New York.)

TABLE 38.12 Cardiac Arrhythmias and Management During Acute Myocardial Infarction

CATEGORY	ARRHYTHMIA	OBJECTIVE OF TREATMENT	THERAPEUTIC OPTIONS
1. Electrical instability	Ventricular premature beats	Correction of electrolyte deficits and minimization of sympathetic tone	Potassium and magnesium solutions, beta blocker
	Ventricular tachycardia	Prophylaxis against ventricular fibrillation, restoration of hemodynamic stability	Antiarrhythmic agents, beta blocker; cardioversion/defibrillation; revascularization
	Ventricular fibrillation	Urgent reversion to sinus rhythm	Defibrillation; amiodarone, lidocaine; revascularization
	Accelerated idioventricular rhythm	Observation unless hemodynamic function is compromised	Increase sinus rate (atropine, atrial pacing); antiarrhythmic agents
	Nonparoxysmal atrioventricular junctional tachycardia	Search for precipitating cause (e.g., digitalis intoxication); suppress arrhythmia only if hemodynamic function is compromised	Atrial overdrive pacing; antiarrhythmic agents; cardioversion relatively contraindicated if digitalis intoxication present
2. Pump failure, excessive sympathetic stimulation	Sinus tachycardia	Reduce heart rate to diminish myocardial oxygen demands	Antipyretics; analgesics; consider beta blocker unless heart failure present
	Atrial fibrillation and/or atrial flutter	Reduce ventricular rate; restore sinus rhythm	Beta blocker unless heart failure present; Verapamil or diltiazem if LV systolic function preserved and no heart failure, digitalis glycosides; amiodarone; treat heart failure; cardioversion
	Paroxysmal supraventricular tachycardia	Reduce ventricular rate; restore sinus rhythm	Vagal maneuvers; beta blocker unless heart failure present; Verapamil or diltiazem if LV systolic function preserved and no heart failure, cardiac glycosides; cardioversion
3. Bradyarrhythmias, conduction disturbances	Sinus bradycardia	Acceleration of the heart rate only if hemodynamic function is compromised	Atropine; atrial pacing
	Junctional escape rhythm	Acceleration of the sinus rate only if loss of atrial "kick" causes hemodynamic compromise	Atropine; atrial pacing
	Atrioventricular block, intraventricular block		Insertion of a pacemaker

Modified from Antman EM, Rutherford JD, eds. *Coronary Care Medicine: A Practical Approach*. Boston: Martinus Nijhoff; 1986:78.

or electrolyte or metabolic disturbances.[1] When VPCs accompany sinus tachycardia at the inception of an infarction, augmented sympathoadrenal stimulation often contributes and can be treated by beta blockers. In fact, early administration of an IV beta blocker effectively reduces the incidence of VF in evolving MI.[121]

Accelerated Idioventricular Rhythm

An accelerated idioventricular rhythm typically occurs during the first 2 days with about equal frequency in anterior and inferior infarctions. Most episodes are brief. Accelerated idioventricular rhythm often follows successful reperfusion with fibrinolytic therapy. However, the frequent occurrence of this rhythm in patients without reperfusion limits its reliability as a marker of the restoration of patency of the infarct-related coronary artery and may have different implications following primary PCI.[122] In contrast to rapid VT, accelerated idioventricular rhythm is thought not to affect prognosis, and we do not routinely treat accelerated idioventricular rhythms.

Ventricular Tachycardia and Ventricular Fibrillation

A leading hypothesis for a major mechanism of ventricular arrhythmias in the acute phase of coronary occlusion is reentry caused by inhomogeneity of the electrical characteristics of ischemic myocardium (Fig. 38.32).[122] The cellular electrophysiologic mechanisms for reperfusion arrhythmias appear to include washout of various ions such as lactate and potassium and toxic substances that have accumulated in the ischemic zone. VT or VF occurring late in the course of STEMI is more common in patients with transmural infarction and LV dysfunction and associates more frequently with hemodynamic deterioration.

Prophylaxis

Because hypokalemia can increase the risk for development of VT, low serum potassium levels require prompt identification and treatment after admission for STEMI. Despite the lack of a consistent relationship between hypomagnesemia and ventricular arrhythmias, magnesium deficits may still link to risk because patients with STEMI have reduced intracellular magnesium levels not adequately reflected by serum measurements. As noted earlier, magnesium should be repleted to achieve a serum level of 2 mEq/L. Early beta-blocker use has reduced VF and can be instituted in patients who lack a contraindication.[1] Lidocaine prophylaxis to prevent primary VF is no longer advised.[1]

Management

Treatment of unstable VT or VF consists of electrical cardioversion implemented as rapidly as possible.[123] IV administration of amiodarone can also facilitate management of unstable ventricular arrhythmias or prevention of refractory recurrent episodes. After reversion to sinus rhythm, every effort should be made to correct any underlying abnormalities, such as hypoxia, hypotension, acid-base or electrolyte disturbances. Urgent revascularization is warranted if ventricular arrhythmias are ongoing and caused by ischemia. The use of extended antiarrhythmic therapy, such as amiodarone or lidocaine, is discussed in Chapter 67. In patients with sustained VT or VF at a time *after* successful reperfusion, we generally continue antiarrhythmic therapy, most often amiodarone, until a defibrillator is placed.

Prognosis

Among patients who underwent fibrinolytic therapy in the GUSTO-I (Global Utilization of Streptokinase and Tissue Plasminogen Activator for Occluded Coronary Arteries) study, approximately 10% experienced VT/VF. In the APEX-AMI (Assessment of Pexelizumab in Acute Myocardial Infarction) study, which included patients treated with primary PCI, sustained VT/VF developed in 5.7%. Patients with VT/VF had worse clinical outcomes than those without VT/VF. Additionally,

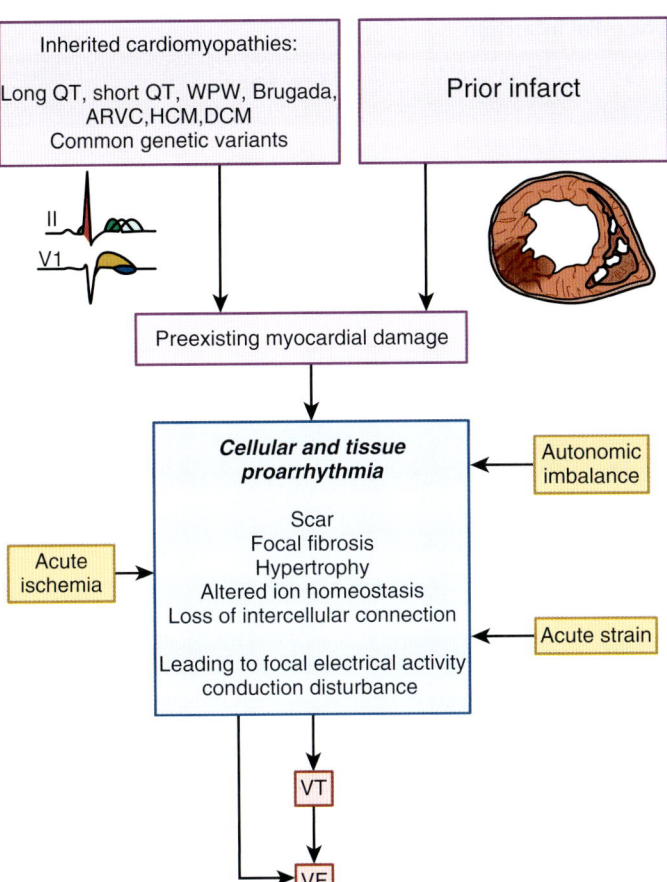

FIGURE 38.32 Drivers of arrhythmias in acute coronary syndromes. A preexisting substrate for ventricular arrhythmias, secondary to prior MI, cardiomyopathy, or a genetic predisposition, together with acute ischemia, autonomic tone, and acute ventricular strain, creates triggered activity and arrhythmias. ARVC, Arrhythmogenic right ventricular cardiomyopathy; DCM, dilated cardiomyopathy; HCM, hypertrophic cardiomyopathy; VF, ventricular fibrillation; VT, ventricular tachycardia; WPW, Wolf-Parkinson-White syndrome. (Adapted from Kirchhof P, et al. Primary prevention of sudden cardiac death. *Heart.* 2006;92:1873–8, Copyright BMJ Publishing Group Ltd; and from Basso C, Rizzo S, Thiene G. The metamorphosis of myocardial infarction following coronary recanalization. *Cardiovasc Pathol.* 2010;19:22–28.)

mortality rates were higher in those with late versus early VT/VF; specifically, when compared with patients without VT/VF, the adjusted risk of mortality at 90 days increased twofold or sixfold in patients with early or late VT/VF, respectively.[122] In patients in whom sustained VT/VF develops later in the course after STEMI (e.g., >48 hours) without evidence of a reversible cause, ICD therapy for secondary prevention should be considered before discharge.[1] This situation differs from that in patients with VT/VF *before* reperfusion therapy, in whom antiarrhythmic therapy other than a beta blocker is not indicated. Indications for insertion of an ICD for *primary* prevention in patients with a reduced LVEF after STEMI are discussed later.

Bradyarrhythmias (see Chapters 68 and 69)
Sinus Bradycardia
Sinus bradycardia frequently occurs during the early phases of STEMI, particularly in patients with inferior and posterior infarctions. On the basis of data from experimental infarction and some clinical observations, the increased vagal tone that produces sinus bradycardia during the early phase of STEMI may actually be beneficial, perhaps because it reduces myocardial oxygen demand. Thus, the acute mortality rate in patients with sinus bradycardia appears similar to that in those without this arrhythmia.[1]

Management
Isolated sinus bradycardia, unaccompanied by hypotension or ventricular ectopy, should be observed rather than treated. In the first 4 to 6 hours after infarction, if the sinus rate is extremely low (<40 to 50 beats/min) and associated with hypotension, IV atropine in doses of 1 mg every 3 to 5 minutes (maximum of 3 mg) can be administered to bring the heart rate up to approximately 60 beats/min.

Atrioventricular and Intraventricular Block
Ischemic injury can produce a conduction block at any level of the AV or intraventricular conduction system. Such blocks can occur in the AV node and the bundle of His and produce various grades of AV block in either the main bundle branch and produce a right or left bundle branch block and in the anterior and posterior divisions of the left bundle and produce left anterior or left posterior (fascicular) divisional blocks. Conduction disturbances can occur in various combinations. Table 38.13 summarizes the clinical features of proximal and distal AV conduction disturbances in patients with STEMI.

First-Degree Atrioventricular Block
A first-degree AV block does not generally require specific treatment. Beta blockers and calcium antagonists (other than dihydropyridines) prolong AV conduction and may be responsible for first-degree AV block as well, but discontinuation of the use of these drugs in the setting of STEMI could increase ischemia and ischemic injury. Therefore, we generally do not decrease the dosage of these drugs unless the PR interval is longer than 0.24 seconds. These agents should be stopped only if a higher-degree block or hemodynamic impairment occurs. If the block is a manifestation of excessive vagotonia and is associated with sinus bradycardia and hypotension, administration of atropine, as already outlined, may be helpful. Continued electrocardiographic monitoring is important in such patients in view of the possible progression to higher degrees of block.

Second-Degree Atrioventricular Block
First-degree and type I second-degree AV blocks do not appear to affect survival, are most often associated with occlusion of the right coronary artery and result from ischemia of the AV node (see Table 38.13). Specific therapy is not required in patients with type I second-degree AV block when the ventricular rate exceeds 50 beats/min and PVCs, HF, and bundle branch block are absent. If these complications develop, however, or if HR falls below approximately 50 beats/min and the patient is symptomatic, immediate treatment with atropine (1 mg) is indicated. Temporary pacing systems are almost never needed in the management of this arrhythmia.

Type II second-degree AV block in the setting of inferior or posterior STEMI is usually temporary and is manifested as a narrow-complex, junctional escape rhythm. These arrhythmias can typically be managed conservatively. With anterior or lateral STEMI, a type II second-degree AV block usually originates from a lesion in the conduction system below the bundle of His (see Table 38.13). Because of its potential for progression to complete heart block, patients with type II second-degree AV block in this setting should be treated with a temporary external or transvenous demand pacemaker.[1]

Complete (Third-Degree) Atrioventricular Block
Complete AV block can occur in patients with either inferior or anterior infarction, although it is more common in inferior than in anterior MI. Complete heart block in patients with inferior infarction usually develops gradually, often progressing from a first-degree or type I second-degree block.[122] The escape rhythm is typically stable without asystole and often junctional, with a rate exceeding 40 beats/min and a narrow QRS complex in 70% of cases and a slower rate and wide QRS complex in the others. This form of complete AV block is often transient, may respond to pharmacologic antagonism of adenosine with methylxanthines, and resolves in most patients within a few days (see Table 38.13).

Patients with inferior infarction often have concomitant ischemia or infarction of the AV node secondary to hypoperfusion of the AV node artery, but the His-Purkinje system usually escapes injury. Patients with inferior STEMI and AV block have larger infarcts and more depressed RV and LV function than patients with an inferior infarct and no AV

TABLE 38.13 Atrioventricular Conduction Disturbances in Acute Myocardial Infarction

	LOCATION OF ATRIOVENTRICULAR (AV) CONDUCTION DISTURBANCE	
	PROXIMAL	**DISTAL**
Site of block	Intranodal	Infranodal
Site of infarction	Inferoposterior	Anteroseptal
Compromised arterial supply	RCA (90%), LCX (10%)	Septal perforators of LAD
Pathogenesis	Ischemia, necrosis, hydropic cell swelling, excessive parasympathetic activity	Ischemia, necrosis, hydropic cell swelling
Predominant type of AV nodal block	First-degree (PR >200 msec)	Mobitz type II second-degree
	Mobitz type I second-degree	Third-degree
Common premonitory features of third-degree AV block	First- or second-degree AV block	Intraventricular conduction block
	Mobitz I pattern	Mobitz II pattern
Features of escape rhythm following third-degree block		
Location	Proximal conduction system (His bundle)	Distal conduction system (bundle branches)
QRS width	<0.12/sec*	>0.12/sec
Rate	45–60/min but may be as low as 30/min	Often <30/min
Stability of escape rhythm	Rate usually stable; asystole uncommon	Rate often unstable with moderate to high risk for ventricular asystole
Duration of high-grade AV block	Usually transient (2–3 days)	Usually transient but some form of AV conduction disturbance and/or intraventricular defect may persist
Associated mortality rate	Low unless associated with hypotension and/or with power failure or ventricular arrhythmias	High because of extensive infarction associated heart failure
Pacemaker therapy		
Temporary	Rarely required; may be considered for bradycardia associated with left ventricular power failure, syncope, or angina	Should be considered in patients with anteroseptal infarction and acute bifascicular block
Permanent	Almost never indicated because the conduction defect is usually transient	Indicated for patients with high-grade AV block and block in the His-Purkinje system and those with a transient advanced AV block and associated bundle branch block

LAD, Left anterior descending coronary artery; *LCX*, left circumflex coronary artery; *RCA*, right coronary artery.
*Some studies suggest that a wide QRS escape rhythm (>0.12 second) following high-grade AV block in inferior infarction is associated with a worse prognosis.
Modified from Antman EM, Rutherford JD, eds. *Coronary Care Medicine: A Practical Approach.* Boston: Martinus Nijhoff; 1986; and Dreifus LS, et al. Guidelines for implantation of cardiac pacemakers and antiarrhythmia devices. *J Am Coll Cardiol.* 1991;18:1.

block. As already noted, junctional escape rhythms with narrow QRS complexes occur frequently in this setting.

Pacing is not generally necessary in patients with inferior wall infarction and complete AV block because this is often transient in nature. Pacing is indicated, however, if symptoms related to a ventricular rate emerge, if ventricular arrhythmias or hypotension are present, or if pump failure develops. Atropine rarely proves adequate in these patients. Only when a complete heart block develops in less than 6 hours after the onset of symptoms is atropine likely to abolish the AV block or cause acceleration of the escape rhythm. In such cases, the AV block is more likely to be transient and related to increases in vagal tone, as opposed to the more persistent block seen later in the course of STEMI, which generally requires cardiac pacing.

In patients with anterior infarction, third-degree AV block can occur suddenly 12 to 24 hours after the onset of infarction, although it is usually preceded by intraventricular block and often a type II (not first-degree or type I) second-degree AV block. Such patients typically have unstable escape rhythms with wide QRS complexes and rates less than 40 beats/min, and ventricular asystole may occur quite suddenly. In patients with anterior infarction, AV block generally develops as a result of extensive septal necrosis involving the bundle branches. The high mortality rate in these patients with a slow idioventricular rhythm and wide QRS complex is caused by extensive myocardial necrosis resulting in severe LV failure and frequently shock (see Table 38.13).

Whether temporary transvenous pacing per se improves survival in patients with anterior STEMI remains controversial. Some physicians contend that ventricular pacing has limited efficacy when used to correct a complete AV block in patients with anterior infarction, in view of the poor prognosis in this group regardless of therapy. However, pacing protects against asystole and may protect against transient hypotension, with its attendant risks of extending the infarction and precipitating malignant ventricular tachyarrhythmias.

Intraventricular Block
The right bundle branch and the left posterior division have a dual blood supply from the left anterior descending and right coronary arteries, whereas the left anterior division is supplied by septal perforators originating from the LAD. Not all conduction blocks in patients with STEMI are complications of infarcts because almost half are already present at the first ECG recording and may represent antecedent conduction abnormalities. Compared with patients without conduction defects, those with STEMI and bundle branch blocks have higher peak biomarker levels, lower EF, and increased in-hospital and long-term mortality rates.[122,124,125] In the pre-fibrinolytic era, intraventricular conduction disturbances (i.e., block within one or more of the three subdivisions [fascicles] of the His-Purkinje system: anterior and posterior divisions of the left bundle and the right bundle) occurred in 5% to 10% of patients with STEMI. More recent series in the reperfusion era suggest that intraventricular blocks occur in approximately 2% to 5% of patients with MI.[1]

Isolated Fascicular Blocks
An isolated left anterior divisional block seldom progresses to complete AV block. Mortality is increased in these patients, although not as much as in those with other forms of conduction block. The posterior fascicle is larger than the anterior fascicle, and in general, a larger infarct is required to block it. As a consequence, mortality is markedly higher in patients who present with posterior fascicular block.

Complete AV block is an uncommon complication of either form of isolated divisional block.

Right Bundle Branch Block
Right bundle branch block (RBBB) alone can lead to AV block because it is often a new lesion associated with anteroseptal infarction. Isolated RBBB associates with increased mortality risk in patients with anterior STEMI, even if complete AV block does not occur, but this appears to be the case only if accompanied by HF.[124,125]

Bifascicular Block, Including Left Bundle Branch Block
The combination of RBBB with either left anterior or left posterior divisional block or the combination of left anterior and posterior divisional blocks (i.e., left bundle branch block [LBBB]) is known as *bidivisional* or *bifascicular block*. If a new block occurs in two of the three divisions of the conduction system, the risk for the development of a complete AV block is quite high. Mortality is also high because of the occurrence of severe pump failure secondary to the extensive myocardial necrosis required to produce such an extensive intraventricular block.[1]

Preexisting bundle branch block or divisional block is less often associated with the development of complete AV block in patients with STEMI than conduction defects acquired during the course of the infarct. Bidivisional block in the presence of prolongation of the PR interval (first-degree AV block) may indicate disease of the third subdivision rather than disease of the AV node and entails a greater risk for complete heart block than if first-degree AV block is absent.

Complete bundle branch block (either left or right), the combination of RBBB and left anterior divisional (fascicular) block, and any of the various forms of trifascicular block are all associated more often with anterior than with inferoposterior infarction. All these forms are more common with large infarcts and in older patients and have a higher incidence of other accompanying arrhythmias than seen in patients without bundle branch block.

Use of Pacemakers in Patients with Acute Myocardial Infarction (see Chapter 69)
Temporary Pacing
As with complete AV block, transvenous ventricular pacing has not resulted in a statistically demonstrable improvement in prognosis in STEMI patients who develop intraventricular conduction defects. Temporary pacing is advisable in some patients, however, because of the high risk for complete AV block. This category includes patients with new bilateral (bifascicular) bundle branch block (i.e., RBBB with left anterior or posterior divisional block and alternating right and left BBB); first-degree AV block adds to this risk. An isolated new block in only one of the three fascicles, even with PR prolongation and preexisting bifascicular block and a normal PR interval, poses somewhat less risk; these patients should be monitored closely, with insertion of a temporary pacemaker deferred unless a higher-degree AV block occurs.

Asystole
The presence of apparent ventricular asystole on monitor displays of continuously recorded ECGs may be misleading because the rhythm may actually be fine VF. The predominance of VF as the cause of cardiac arrest in this setting suggests electrical countershock as initial therapy, even if definitive electrocardiographic documentation of this arrhythmia is not available.

Permanent Pacing
The advisability of permanent pacemaker insertion is complicated because not all sudden deaths in patients with STEMI and conduction defects result from high-grade AV block. A high incidence of late VF occurs in survivors with anterior STEMI complicated by either RBBB or LBBB. Therefore, rather than asystole caused by failure of AV conduction and infranodal pacemakers, VF could be responsible for late sudden death.

Long-term pacing may be indicated when complete heart block persists throughout the hospital phase in a patient with STEMI, when sinus node function is greatly impaired, or when type II second-degree, high-grade atrioventricular block, alternating bundle branch block, or third-degree block persists or occurs intermittently after a waiting period.[126] Additional considerations that drive the decision to insert a permanent pacemaker include whether the patient is a candidate for an ICD or has severe HF that might be improved with biventricular pacing (see Chapters 50 and 69).

Supraventricular Tachyarrhythmias (see Chapters 65 and 66)
Sinus Tachycardia
Sinus tachycardia is typically associated with augmented sympathetic activity and may provoke transient hypertension or hypotension. Common causes are anxiety, persistent pain, LV failure, fever, pericarditis, hypovolemia, pulmonary embolism, and drugs (e.g., epinephrine, dopamine); rarely, it occurs in patients with atrial infarction. Sinus tachycardia is particularly common in patients with anterior infarction, especially in those with significant accompanying LV dysfunction. It is an undesirable rhythm in patients with STEMI because it augments myocardial oxygen consumption and reduces the time in diastole available for coronary perfusion, thereby intensifying the myocardial ischemia and external myocardial necrosis. Persistent sinus tachycardia can signify persistent HF and, in these circumstances, connotes a poor prognosis and excess mortality. An underlying cause should be sought and appropriate treatment instituted, such as analgesics for pain; diuretics for HF; oxygen, beta blockers, and nitroglycerin for ischemia; and aspirin for fever or pericarditis. Treating sinus tachycardia caused by pain, anxiety, or fever with beta blockers is reasonable, but these agents are contraindicated in patients who are tachycardic because of pump failure.

Atrial Flutter and Fibrillation
Atrial flutter and atrial fibrillation (AF) are usually transient in patients with STEMI; these arrhythmias typically result from augmented sympathetic stimulation of the atria and often occur in patients with LV failure, pulmonary emboli, or atrial infarction and aggravate the hemodynamic deterioration in these states (see Table 38.12). The increased ventricular rate and loss of the atrial contribution to LV filling can considerably reduce cardiac output. AF during STEMI is associated with increased mortality and stroke, particularly in patients with anterior infarction.[127,128] Because it is more common in patients with clinical and hemodynamic manifestations of extensive infarction, AF is probably a marker of a poor prognosis, and several studies have found at least a small, independent contribution to increased mortality.[127,128]

Management
Atrial flutter and AF in patients with STEMI are treated as in other settings (see Chapter 66). If the arrhythmia causes ongoing hypotension, ischemia, or HF, cardioversion should be considered. In stabilized patients and in the absence of contraindications, a beta blocker should be administered after STEMI; in addition to several other benefits, these agents help slow the ventricular rate should AF recur. Digitalis may also help slow the ventricular rate when AF develops after STEMI in the setting of ventricular dysfunction. In addition, amiodarone may aid management. Patients with recurrent episodes of AF should be treated with oral anticoagulants (to reduce the risk for stroke), even if sinus rhythm is present at hospital discharge.

OTHER COMPLICATIONS

Recurrent Chest Discomfort
Evaluation of postinfarction chest discomfort may be complicated by previous abnormalities on the ECG and the often vague nature of symptoms reported by patients in the early post-infarction and post-revascularization period. Clinicians face the critical task of distinguishing recurrent angina or infarction from nonischemic causes of discomfort that might result from infarct expansion, pericarditis, pulmonary

embolism, and non–cardiac-related conditions. Ischemic causes to consider include acute reocclusion of an initially recanalized or stented vessel, mechanical or thrombotic occlusion of a side branch or distal vessel during an initial PCI, new ischemia in a non-infarct-related coronary artery that was also stenosed but not occluded, and coronary spasm. Important diagnostic maneuvers include repeated physical examination, repeated ECG, and assessment of the response to SL nitroglycerin. (The use of noninvasive diagnostic evaluation for recurrent ischemia in patients whose symptoms appear only with moderate or higher levels of exertion is also discussed later in this chapter.)

Recurrent Ischemia and Reinfarction

Patients undergoing primary PCI for STEMI versus fibrinolysis have less postinfarction angina and reinfarction. Additionally, in high-risk patients with STEMI who were treated with fibrinolysis, transfer for PCI within 6 hours after fibrinolysis is also associated with significantly fewer ischemic complications than treatment with fibrinolysis alone.[8,60] Better stent design and interventional techniques as well as more effective antiplatelet and antithrombin therapies have also reduced the rate of recurrent ischemic events following STEMI.[1] Consequently, the incidence of early recurrent ischemic events in STEMI patients treated by immediate or delayed PCI now is less than 5%.[4]

Diagnosis

Extension of the original zone of necrosis or reinfarction into a separate myocardial zone can be a difficult diagnosis, especially within the first 24 hours after the index event. Diagnostic criteria have been established,[129] but discrimination of a new MI discrete from the initial STEMI is often challenging because cardiac markers may remain elevated as a result of the initial infarction, and distinguishing changes of the normal evolution after the index infarction from those caused by recurrent infarction may not be possible on the ECG. Recurrent infarction should be strongly considered, however, with dynamic recurrence of ST-segment elevation.

Pericarditis should also be considered in such patients. The presence of a rub and lack of responsiveness to nitroglycerin may be useful in distinguishing pericardial discomfort, but doing so on clinical grounds is frequently challenging, and diagnostic coronary angiography may be necessary to exclude acute native vessel or stent thrombosis. The predominant angiographic predictors of reinfarction in patients undergoing primary PCI include a final coronary stenosis greater than 30%, PCI-related coronary dissection or intracoronary thrombus, multivessel disease, and greater total stent length.[130]

Prognosis

Regardless of whether postinfarction angina is persistent or limited, its presence is important because of the associated higher short-term morbidity rate. Reinfarction links to higher rates of in-hospital complications (e.g., HF, AV block) and early and long-term mortality.[130]

Management

Patients with repeat ST-segment elevation and the appropriate clinical findings should undergo urgent catheterization and PCI unless pericarditis or other post-MI complications are the cause; repeated fibrinolysis can be considered if PCI is not available. In patients believed to have recurrent ischemia in the absence of ST elevation concerning for ongoing injury and who do not have evidence of hemodynamic compromise, an attempt should be made to control symptoms with SL or IV nitroglycerin and IV beta blocker to slow HR to 60 beats/min. Hypotension, HF, or ventricular arrhythmias developing during recurrent ischemia usually warrant urgent catheterization and revascularization.

High-risk patients with STEMI who undergo fibrinolysis may benefit from a strategy of routine referral for catheterization and revascularization (3 to 24 hours).[8,60] Clinicians should be alert to stent thrombosis as a cause of recurrent ischemia. Stent thrombosis can occur acutely (hours to days after stent deployment) or late (many months after stent deployment) (see Chapter 41).

Pericardial Effusion and Pericarditis (see Chapter 86)

Pericardial Effusion

Effusions are generally detected echocardiographically, and their incidence varies with imaging modality and technique, and criteria. Effusions are more common in patients with anterior or lateral STEMI, larger infarcts, more microvascular obstruction, greater LV dysfunction, no reperfusion, and higher rates of HF.[131-133] Most pericardial effusions after STEMI do not cause hemodynamic compromise. The reabsorption rate of a postinfarction pericardial effusion is slow, with resolution often taking several months. An effusion does not necessarily indicate pericarditis; although they may coexist, most effusions develop without other evidence of pericarditis. When tamponade does occur, it is usually caused by ventricular rupture or hemorrhagic pericarditis.[133]

Pericarditis

Although diminished in its incidence in the era of primary PCI, pericarditis can produce pain as early as the first day and as late as 8 weeks after STEMI. The pain of pericarditis may be confused with that resulting from postinfarction angina. An important distinguishing feature is radiation of the pain to either trapezius ridge, a finding that is almost pathognomonic of pericarditis and rarely seen with ischemic discomfort. Additionally, the discomfort of pericarditis usually worsens during a deep inspiration but can be relieved or diminished by sitting up and leaning forward.

Transmural MI, by definition, extends to the epicardial surface and can cause local pericardial inflammation. Acute fibrinous pericarditis, *pericarditis epistenocardica*, occurs frequently after transmural infarction, but most patients do not report any symptoms from this process. Although transient pericardial friction rubs are relatively common within the first 48 hours in patients with transmural infarction, pain or electrocardiographic changes occur much less often. The development of a pericardial rub, however, appears to correlate with a larger infarct and greater hemodynamic compromise.

Although anticoagulation clearly increases the risk for hemorrhagic pericarditis early after STEMI, this complication does not occur with sufficient frequency during heparinization or after fibrinolytic therapy to warrant absolute prohibition of such agents when a rub is present. Nevertheless, detection of a ≥1 cm on echocardiography or enlarging pericardial effusion usually should result in discontinuation of anticoagulation. Patients in whom continuation or initiation of anticoagulant therapy is strongly indicated should have heightened monitoring of clotting parameters and observation for clinical signs of possible tamponade. Late pericardial constriction caused by anticoagulant-induced hemopericardium can occur.

Traditional treatment of pericardial discomfort consists of aspirin, but usually in doses higher than prescribed routinely following infarction—doses of 650 mg orally as often as every 4 hours, together with a proton pump inhibitor.[1] However, practice is shifting to colchicine administration, particularly in light of the data supporting the protective effect for MACE following MI.[86] Nonsteroidal antiinflammatory drugs (NSAIDs) and steroids should be avoided because they may interfere with myocardial healing.[1,134]

Dressler Syndrome

Also known as *post-myocardial infarction syndrome*, Dressler syndrome usually occurs 1 to 8 weeks after infarction. Dressler cited an incidence of 3% to 4% of all patients with MI in 1957, but the incidence has decreased dramatically since that time. Clinically, patients with Dressler syndrome have malaise, fever, pericardial discomfort, leukocytosis, an elevated erythrocyte sedimentation rate (ESR), and a pericardial effusion. At autopsy, individuals with this syndrome usually demonstrate localized fibrinous pericarditis containing polymorphonuclear leukocytes (PMNs). The cause of post-MI syndrome is not clearly established, although detection of antibodies to cardiac tissue suggests an immunopathologic process. Treatment is with aspirin, 650 mg as often as every 4 hours, and colchicine may be effective.[1] Glucocorticosteroids and NSAIDs are best avoided in patients with Dressler syndrome within 4 weeks of STEMI because of their potential to impair infarct healing, cause ventricular rupture, and increase coronary vascular resistance.[1]

Venous Thrombosis and Pulmonary Embolism

Almost all peri-MI pulmonary emboli originate from thrombi in the veins of the lower extremities; much less frequently, they originate from mural thrombi overlying an area of RV infarction. Bed rest and HF predispose to venous thrombosis and subsequent pulmonary embolism (PE), circumstances that occur in patients with STEMI, particularly in those with large infarcts. At a time when patients with STEMI were routinely subjected to prolonged bed rest, more than 20% examined at autopsy had PE, and massive PE accounted for 10% of deaths from MI. In contemporary practice, with early mobilization and the widespread use of low-dose anticoagulant prophylaxis, PE has become an uncommon cause of death in patients with STEMI. When PE does occur in patients with STEMI, management is generally similar to that for patients without infarction (see Chapter 87).

Left Ventricular Aneurysm

The term *left ventricular aneurysm* (often called *true aneurysm*) is generally reserved for a discrete, dyskinetic area of the LV wall with a broad neck (to differentiate it from a pseudoaneurysm caused by a contained myocardial rupture). Dyskinetic or akinetic areas of the left ventricle are much more common than true aneurysms after STEMI. True LV aneurysms probably develop in less than 5% of all patients with STEMI.[1] The wall of a true aneurysm is thinner than that of the rest of the left ventricle, and it is usually composed of fibrous tissue, as well as necrotic muscle occasionally mixed with viable myocardium.

Pathogenesis

Total occlusion of a poorly collateralized LAD is associated with aneurysm formation after anterior STEMI. An aneurysm rarely occurs with multivessel disease with either extensive collaterals or a patent LAD. Aneurysms occur approximately four times more often at the apex and in the anterior wall than in the inferoposterior wall. The overlying pericardium generally adheres densely to the wall of the aneurysm, which may even become partially calcified after several years. True LV aneurysms (in contrast to pseudoaneurysms) rarely rupture.

Diagnosis

The presence of persistent ST-segment elevation in an electrocardiographic area of infarction, classically thought to suggest aneurysm formation, indicates a large infarct with a regional wall motion abnormality but does not necessarily imply an aneurysm. The diagnosis of aneurysm is best made by echocardiography, CMR, CT, or left ventriculography at cardiac catheterization.

Prognosis and Treatment

An LV aneurysm increases the risk for mortality, even compared with that in patients with a comparable LVEF. Death in these patients is frequently sudden and presumably related to the relatively high incidence of ventricular tachyarrhythmias that occur with aneurysms. With loss of shortening from the area of the aneurysm, the remainder of the ventricle may become hyperkinetic to compensate, but with relatively large aneurysms, complete compensation is impossible. Stroke volume falls, or if maintained, it is at the expense of an increase in end-diastolic volume, which in turn leads to increased wall tension and myocardial oxygen demand. Heart failure may ensue, and angina may appear or worsen.

Aggressive management of STEMI, including prompt reperfusion, may diminish the incidence of ventricular aneurysms. Surgical aneurysmectomy generally succeeds only if contractile performance in the nonaneurysmal portion of the left ventricle is relatively preserved. In such circumstances, when the operation is performed for worsening HF or angina, operative mortality is relatively low, and clinical improvement can be expected.[76] Compared with CABG alone, adding surgical ventricular reconstruction for patients with LVEF of 35% or less reduced LV volume but does not improve symptoms, exercise tolerance, or the endpoint of death or hospitalization for cardiac causes.[135] A transcatheter approach for aneurysm exclusion is currently under investigation; to date, device implantation has generally succeeded technically, but outcome data are limited.[136] Because of the risk for mural thrombosis and systemic embolization, patients with a residual LV aneurysm after STEMI may warrant long-term oral anticoagulation.[137]

Left Ventricular Thrombus and Arterial Embolism

Endocardial inflammation and the relative stasis of blood during the acute phase of infarction probably provide a thrombogenic surface for clots to form in the left ventricle. With extensive transmural infarction of the septum, however, mural thrombi may overlie infarcted myocardium in either ventricle. Using contemporary imaging modalities, including cardiac MRI, the incidence of LV thrombus formation after STEMI may be as much as 15% in patients with STEMI and 25% in patients with anterior MI.[137] Prospective studies have suggested that patients in whom a mural thrombus develops early (within 48 to 72 hours of infarction) have an extremely poor early prognosis, with a high rate of mortality from the complications of a large infarction (shock, reinfarction, rupture, and ventricular tachyarrhythmia), rather than emboli from the LV thrombus.

Even though a mural thrombus adheres to the endocardium overlying the infarcted myocardium, superficial portions can detach and embolize systemically. An observational study suggested that patients with an LV thrombus had a fourfold increased risk of embolic events, compared to matched controls without LV thrombus.[138] Echocardiographic risk factors for thrombus embolization include increased mobility and protrusion into the ventricular chamber, visualization on multiple views, and contiguous zones of akinesis and hyperkinesis. CMR can also characterize LV thrombi and assist in predicting the risk for embolism.

Management

A meta-analysis of multiple small studies suggested that anticoagulation reduces the development of LV thrombi by more than 50%. Fibrinolytic therapy also reduces the rate of thrombus formation. Few data from the era of dual-antiplatelet therapy after primary PCI are available to guide decisions. Recommendations for anticoagulation vary considerably; nevertheless, patients with STEMI and anterior apical akinesis or severe dyskinesis may merit a limited course of anticoagulant therapy to prevent LV thrombus formation.[1] Anticoagulation for 3 to 6 months is reasonable for many patients with demonstrable mural thrombi.

CONVALESCENCE, DISCHARGE, AND POST-MYOCARDIAL INFARCTION CARE

The transition to outpatient care after STEMI is a critical one. Posthospital systems of care designed to reduce hospital readmissions can facilitate coordinated, evidence-based outpatient care for all patients with STEMI (see also Chapter 33).[1]

Timing of Hospital Discharge

In practice, the timing of discharge from the hospital is variable. Patients with STEMI have risk for late in-hospital mortality from recurrent ischemia or infarction, hemodynamically significant ventricular arrhythmias, and severe HF. Risk indicators for mortality in the hospital include clinical HF, as evidenced by persistent sinus tachycardia and pulmonary congestion, recurrent VT and VF, new AF or atrial flutter, intraventricular conduction delays or heart block, anterior location of infarction, and recurrent episodes of angina with marked ST-segment abnormalities at low activity levels (see later, Risk Stratification after ST-Elevation Myocardial Infarction).

Aggressive reperfusion protocols with PCI or fibrinolytics can reduce the length of hospital stay without compromising survival after discharge. In patients with apparently successful reperfusion, absence of early sustained ventricular tachyarrhythmias, hypotension, or HF, coupled with a well-preserved LVEF, predicts a low risk for late complications in the hospital. Such patients appear to be suitable candidates for hospital discharge less than 5 days from the onset of symptoms; current practice in U.S. hospitals is discharge in 3 days or less for many STEMI patients who have undergone successful primary PCI.[139] Most complications that would preclude early discharge occur within the first 3 days of admission, permitting identification of patients suitable for expedited discharge early during the hospitalization. Several controlled trials and many uncontrolled trials of early discharge after STEMI have shown no increase in risk in patients appropriately selected for early discharge.[139]

Following STEMI, patients are often eager for information, anxious, in need of reassurance, confused by misinformation and previous impressions, and capable of counterproductive denial. The hospitalization after STEMI provides ample opportunities to begin the rehabilitation process. The decision regarding timing of discharge for patients with uncomplicated STEMI should consider the patient's psychological state after STEMI, the adequacy of dose titration for essential drugs such as beta blockers and RAAS inhibitors, and the availability and timing of follow-up with visiting nurses and the primary care physician. In patients who have experienced a complication, discharge is deferred until their condition has been stable for several days, and they clearly have responded appropriately to any interventions.

Counseling

Before discharge from the hospital, all patients should receive detailed instruction concerning physical activity. Initially, this should consist of walking at home but avoidance of isometric exercise such as lifting. The patient should be given fresh nitroglycerin tablets and instructed in their use (see Chapter 40). The patient should also be educated regarding all other medications prescribed. Graded resumption of activity should be encouraged, ideally as part of a monitored cardiac rehabilitation program (see Chapter 33). Many approaches have been used, ranging from formal rigid guidelines to general advice advocating moderation and avoidance of any activity that evokes symptoms. Sexual activity counseling, often overlooked during recovery from STEMI, should be included in the educational process.[140] In addition, physicians should explicitly discuss the risk associated with continued smoking and offer assistance in cessation, along with nicotine replacement therapy in appropriate patients.[1]

Some evidence indicates that behavioral alteration is possible after recovery from STEMI and may improve the prognosis. Patients with STEMI should be referred to a post-discharge cardiac rehabilitation program with supervised physical exercise and an educational component.[141] Given the relationship between depression and STEMI, psychosocial intervention programs can decrease symptoms of depression and are a useful adjunct to standard cardiac rehabilitation programs after STEMI[142] (see Chapters 33 and 99).

RISK STRATIFICATION AFTER ST-ELEVATION MYOCARDIAL INFARCTION

The process of risk stratification following STEMI occurs in several stages: initial findings, in-hospital course, and at hospital discharge. The tools used to form an integrated and dynamic assessment of the patient consist of baseline demographic information; serial ECGs and serum and plasma cardiac biomarker measurements; hemodynamic monitoring data; a variety of noninvasive tests; and if performed, the findings at cardiac catheterization. These findings, integrated with the occurrence of in-hospital complications, can provide information regarding survival.

Initial Findings

Certain demographic and historical factors portend a worse prognosis in patients with STEMI, including age older than 65, history of diabetes mellitus, previous angina pectoris, and previous MI. Diabetes mellitus, in particular, appears to confer a more than 40% increase in adjusted risk for death by 30 days (see Chapter 31). Surviving diabetic patients also experience a more complicated post-MI course, including a greater incidence of postinfarction angina, infarct extension, and HF. These higher rates of complications probably relate to the extensive accelerated atherosclerosis and higher risk for thrombosis and HF associated with diabetes mellitus.

In addition to playing a central role in the decision pathway for the management of patients with ACS based on the presence or absence of ST-segment elevation, the 12-lead ECG provides important prognostic information.[143] Mortality is greater in patients experiencing anterior wall STEMI than in those with inferior STEMI, even when corrected for infarct size. Patients with RV infarction complicating inferior infarction, as suggested by ST-segment elevation in V_4R, have higher mortality than patients sustaining an inferior infarction without RV involvement. Patients with multiple leads showing ST elevation and a high sum of ST-segment elevation have increased mortality, especially if their infarct is anterior. Patients whose ECGs demonstrate persistent advanced heart block (e.g., type II second-degree or third-degree AV block) or new intraventricular conduction abnormalities (bifascicular or trifascicular) in the course of STEMI have a worse prognosis than patients without these abnormalities (see earlier, Atrioventricular and Intraventricular Block). The influence of high degrees of heart block has particular importance in patients with RV infarction because such patients have greatly increased mortality risk.[143] Other electrocardiographic findings that augur poorly are persistent horizontal or downsloping ST-segment depression, Q waves in multiple leads, ST-segment depression in anterior leads in patients with inferior infarction, and atrial arrhythmias, especially AF.

Several validated clinical risk stratification tools may be used at initial evaluation to assess the short-term and long-term risk for death after MI.[143] In addition to the patient's age and historical factors such as diabetes and previous MI, clinical signs of HF, including tachycardia and hypotension, are common in many of these clinical risk assessment scores.

Hospital Course

Hospital mortality from STEMI depends directly on the severity of LV dysfunction. Risk stratification incorporating abnormalities of vital signs (e.g. HR, systolic BP); presence of HF, shock, or cardiac arrest; estimation of infarct size; and in appropriate patients, invasive hemodynamic monitoring provides an assessment of the likelihood of a complicated hospital course and may also identify important abnormalities, such as hemodynamically significant MR, that convey an adverse long-term prognosis (see Table 38.8).[144] In particular, the development of HF and LV dysfunction after MI entails a higher risk for sudden cardiac death.[145] Recurrent infarction and new stroke during hospitalization for STEMI also, not surprisingly, confer a higher risk for death.

Assessment at Hospital Discharge

Both short-term and long-term survival after STEMI depend on three major factors: resting LV function, residual potentially ischemic myocardium, and susceptibility to serious ventricular arrhythmias. The most important of these factors is the state of LV function (see Fig. 38.20).[143] The second most important factor is how the severity and extent of the obstructive lesions in the coronary vascular bed perfusing residual viable myocardium affect the risk for recurrent infarction and serious ventricular arrhythmias. Thus, survival is related to the quantity of myocardium that has become necrotic and the portion remaining in ischemic jeopardy. The third risk factor, susceptibility to serious arrhythmias, is reflected in ventricular ectopic activity and other indicators of electrical instability, such as reduced HR variability or baroreflex sensitivity and abnormal findings on a signal-averaged ECG.[143] All these factors identify patients at increased risk for death.

Assessment of Left Ventricular Function

The LVEF, a readily assessed measurement of LV function, is extremely useful for risk stratification. However, imaging of the left ventricle at rest may not adequately distinguish among infarcted, irreversibly damaged, and stunned or hibernating myocardium. To circumvent this difficulty, various techniques have been investigated to assess the extent of residual viable myocardium and degree of microvascular obstruction, including exercise and pharmacologic stress echocardiography, stress radionuclide perfusion imaging, positron emission tomography, and gadolinium-enhanced CMR.[2,146] Each of these techniques can be performed safely in postinfarction patients. Because no study has clearly shown one imaging modality to be superior to the others, clinicians should be guided in their selection of ventricular imaging technique by the availability and level of expertise with a given modality at their local institution.[2]

Assessment of Myocardial Ischemia

Because of the adverse consequences of recurrent MI after STEMI, assessing a patient's risk for future ischemia and infarction is important. Noninvasive testing for ischemia, usually before discharge, provides valuable information about the presence of residual ischemia in patients who might not have undergone coronary angiography during the initial management of STEMI. It may also be useful in assessing the functional significance of any coronary stenoses identified at angiography but not revascularized (see Table 38.5). In the latter case, stress imaging to localize ischemia may be useful.

EXERCISE TESTING. An exercise test also offers an opportunity to formulate a more precise exercise prescription and helps boost patients' confidence in their ability to conduct their daily activities after discharge. Patients who are incompletely revascularized and are unable to exercise can be evaluated by a pharmacologic stress protocol with echocardiography or perfusion imaging. Treadmill exercise testing after STEMI has traditionally used a submaximal protocol that requires the patient to exercise until symptoms of angina appear, electrocardiographic evidence of ischemia is seen, or a target workload (5 metabolic equivalents) has been reached, whichever comes first (see Chapters 15 and 33). Symptom-limited exercise tests can be performed safely before discharge in patients with an uncomplicated course after infarction. Variables derived from exercise tests after STEMI that have been evaluated for their ability to predict the occurrence of death or recurrent nonfatal infarction include the development and magnitude of ST-segment depression, the development of angina, exercise capacity, and the systolic BP response during exercise.[143]

Assessment for Electrical Instability

After STEMI, patients have the greatest risk for development of sudden cardiac death (SCD) from malignant ventricular arrhythmias in the first 1 to 2 years.[143] Multiple techniques may stratify patients into those who are at increased risk for SCD after STEMI. These include measurement of QT dispersion (variability in QT intervals between ECG leads), ambulatory ECGs for detection of ventricular arrhythmias (Holter monitoring), invasive electrophysiologic testing, recording of a signal-averaged ECG (a measure of delayed, fragmented conduction in the infarct zone), and measurement of HR variability (beat-to-beat variability in R-R intervals) or baroreflex sensitivity (slope of a line relating beat-to-beat change in the sinus rate in response to alteration of BP). However, none of these approaches has proved sufficiently useful for routine practice.[143]

Despite the increased risk for arrhythmic events following STEMI in patients who have abnormal results on one or more of the noninvasive tests described, several points merit emphasis. The low PPV (<30%) of the noninvasive screening tests limits their usefulness when viewed in isolation. Although the predictive value of screening tests can be improved by combining several tests, the therapeutic implications of an increased risk profile for arrhythmic events have not been established. The reductions in mortality achievable with the general use of beta blockers, ACE inhibitors, aspirin, and revascularization, when appropriate after infarction, coupled with concerns about the efficacy and safety of antiarrhythmic drugs and the cost of implanted defibrillators, leave considerable uncertainty about the therapeutic implications of an abnormal noninvasive test result for electrical instability in an asymptomatic patient. Action by clinicians on the results of an abnormal finding in asymptomatic patients should await additional data on patient outcomes. Management of patients with sustained, hemodynamically compromising arrhythmias is discussed in Part VII.

Prophylactic Antiarrhythmic Therapy

Although antiarrhythmic therapy can control atrial and ventricular arrhythmias effectively in many patients, routine use of prophylactic antiarrhythmic drug therapy, with the exception of beta blockers, does not improve outcome and with some agents increases the risk for death.[1] The most notable postinfarction trial in this area was CAST (Cardiac Arrhythmia Suppression Trial), which tested whether encainide, flecainide, or moricizine for suppression of ventricular arrhythmias detected on ambulatory electrocardiographic monitoring would reduce the risk for cardiac arrest and death; however, CAST was stopped prematurely because of increased mortality in the active treatment groups. The SWORD (Survival with Oral D-Sotalol) trial was similarly stopped prematurely because of increased mortality in the active treatment group. In contrast, CAMIAT (Canadian Amiodarone Myocardial Infarction Trial) showed that amiodarone reduces the frequency of ventricular premature depolarization in patients with recent MI and that this reduction correlated with lowering of arrhythmic death or resuscitation from VF. However, 42% of patients discontinued use of amiodarone during maintenance therapy in CAMIAT because of intolerable side effects. EMIAT (European Amiodarone Myocardial Infarction Trial) showed a reduction in arrhythmic death after MI in patients with depressed LV function, but total mortality and other CV-related mortality did not decrease.

The routine use of antiarrhythmic agents (including amiodarone) therefore cannot be recommended. Although trials that included post-STEMI patients in the study population have shown significant reductions in mortality in those randomly assigned to ICD implantation versus conventional medical therapy (see Chapter 69), early implantation of an ICD in the first few weeks after MI has not shown benefit.[147] Routine risk stratification to guide ICD placement early after STEMI is therefore not recommended; reassessment of LV function 40 days or longer after STEMI can guide consideration of an ICD for primary prevention of SCD[147] (Fig. 38.33). Wearable cardiac defibrillators can be considered in the immediate post-MI period (e.g., 40 days) in patients with LV dysfunction based on small studies demonstrating efficacy for detection and termination of VT/VF; however, the larger VEST (Vest Prevention of Early Sudden Death Trial) did not demonstrate a significant reduction in arrhythmic death[148] (Fig. 38.34).

Secondary Prevention After Acute Myocardial Infarction

Patients who survive the initial course of STEMI still have considerable risk for recurrent events, thus rendering preventive efforts imperative (see also Part IV, Preventive Cardiology).

Cardiac Rehabilitation (see Chapter 33)

Contemporary exercise-based cardiac rehabilitation after STEMI aims to increase functional capacity, reducing disability, improve quality of life, modify coronary risk factors, and limit morbidity and mortality.[141] The key components of cardiac rehabilitation include patient assessment; ongoing medical surveillance; nutritional counseling; management of hypertension, lipids, and diabetes mellitus; cessation of smoking; psychosocial counseling; physical activity counseling; exercise training; and pharmacologic treatment, as appropriate. When compared with usual care, cardiac rehabilitation is associated with lower total and cardiac mortality, but despite these outcomes, cardiac rehabilitation services remain vastly underused, particularly in women and minority populations.[149]

Lifestyle Modification (see also Part IV)

Efforts to improve survival and quality of life after MI are related to lifestyle modification of known risk factors. Of these, cessation of smoking and control of hypertension are probably the most important. Use of hospital-based smoking cessation programs and referral to cardiac rehabilitation programs have led to successful smoking cessation.[1]

Depression (see Chapter 99)

Physicians caring for patients following STEMI need to acknowledge the prevalence of major depression after infarction. This problem associates independently with higher mortality. In addition, lack of an emotionally supportive network in the patient's environment after discharge increases risk for recurrent cardiac events. The precise mechanisms relating depression and lack of social support to a worse prognosis after STEMI are not clear, but one possibility is lack of adherence to

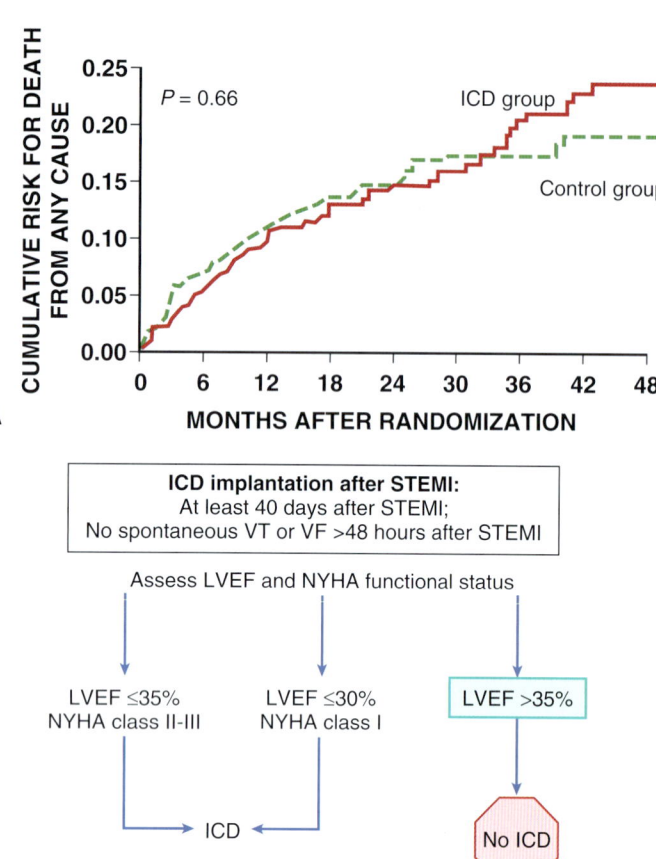

FIGURE 38.33 A, DINAMIT trial and algorithm for placement of an implantable cardioverter-defibrillator (ICD) in patients with STEMI but without ventricular fibrillation (VF) or sustained ventricular tachycardia (VT) more than 48 hours after STEMI. DINAMIT, a randomized, open-label study, compared ICD with no ICD therapy 6 to 40 days after an MI in 674 patients who also had a left ventricular ejection fraction (LVEF) of 35% or less and impaired cardiac autonomic function. The study concluded that ICD therapy reduced the rate of death from arrhythmias but that this advantage was offset by an increase in deaths from other causes. B, The appropriate management path is based on the measurement of LVEF; measurements obtained 3 days or less after STEMI should be repeated before proceeding with the algorithm. Patients with LVEF less than 35% at least 40 days after STEMI are referred for insertion of an ICD if they are in New York Heart Association (NYHA) Class II or III. Patients with a more depressed LVEF less than 30% are referred for ICD implantation even if they are NYHA Class I because of their increased risk for sudden cardiac death. Patients with LVEF less than 40% who have nonsustained VT and inducible VT on the electrophysiological study are discussed in Chapter 70. Patients with preserved left ventricular function (LVEF >40%) do not receive an ICD and are treated with medical therapy after STEMI. (A from Hohnloser SH, Kuck KH, Dorian P, et al. Prophylactic use of an implantable cardioverter-defibrillator after acute myocardial infarction. *N Engl J Med.* 2004;351:2481; B, modified from Al-Khatib SM, Stevenson WG, et al. 2017 AHA/ACC/HRS guideline for management of patients with ventricular arrhythmias and the prevention of sudden cardiac death: a report of the ACCF/AHA Task Force on Clinical Practice Guidelines and the Heart Rhythm Society. *J Am Coll Cardiol.* 2018;72:e91.)

prescribed treatments, a behavior associated with increased risk for post-MI mortality. Therefore, a comprehensive cardiac rehabilitation program that includes primary health care personnel who counsel patients and make home visits can reduce the rate of rehospitalization for recurrent ischemia and infarction.[149]

Modification of Lipid Profile (see Chapters 25 and 27)

Obtaining a lipid profile on admission is reasonable in all patients admitted with acute MI. Total cholesterol levels may fall 24 to 48 hours after infarction. We continue to ascribe to a long-term target low-density lipoprotein (LDL) cholesterol level ideally less than 55 mg/dL for patients who experience an ACS.[150,151] High-intensity statin therapy should be initiated or continued in all patients with STEMI and no contraindications to its use.[1] Ezetimibe, a nonstatin lipid-lowering agent, may be added during hospitalization for STEMI based on IMPROVE-IT (Improved Reduction of Outcome: Vytorin Efficacy International Trial), which demonstrated a reduction in recurrent CV events when added to statin therapy.[152–154] Bempedoic acid can lower LDL and avoid muscle complaints, but outcome data are not yet available (see Chapter 27). Proprotein convertase subtilisin/kexin type 9 (PCSK9) inhibitors result in decreased LDL receptor degradation and have demonstrated efficacy for CV event reduction in patients with a recent ACS or stable atherosclerotic CV disease.[155,156] Guidelines recommend addition of a PCSK9 inhibitor in high or very high risk individuals who have not met LDL cholesterol goals despite maximal possible dosing of other lipid-lowering therapies, such as a statin or ezetimibe.[150,151]

Another class of agents, omega-3 fatty acids that result in triglyceride lowering, have demonstrated mixed results in patients with hypertriglyceridemia. Two trials of purified, high dose eicosapentaenoic acid (EPA), a type of omega-3 fatty acid, reduced triglycerides and MACE in patients with elevated triglycerides and high CV risk.[157,158,160] Another large study of the combination of EPA and another omega-3 fatty acid, docosahexaenoic acid (DHA), did not alter the rate of MACE in a similar population.[159] The explanation for the differential findings remains unclear but may relate to the dosing and specific omega-3 fatty acid agent studied.[160]

Antiplatelet Agents (see Chapter 95)

On the basis of compelling data from the Antiplatelet Trialists' Collaboration of a 22% reduction in the risk for recurrent infarction, stroke, or vascular death in high-risk vascular patients receiving prolonged antiplatelet therapy, all patients with STEMI without contraindications should receive 75 to 325 mg of aspirin daily indefinitely, with 81 mg being the preferred maintenance dose.[1] Additional benefits of long-term aspirin therapy that can accrue in patients with STEMI include an increased likelihood of patency of the infarct artery and smaller infarcts if MI recurs. Patients with true aspirin allergy can receive clopidogrel (75 mg once daily). In the absence of contraindications, all patients after STEMI should receive a platelet inhibitor in addition to aspirin for 12 months according to one of the following regimens: clopidogrel (75 mg/day) in patients with STEMI treated with medical therapy alone, lytic therapy, or PCI; prasugrel (10 mg/day) in patients treated with PCI; or ticagrelor (90 mg twice daily) in patients treated with medical therapy alone or PCI.[1,71]

Aspirin therapy should be maintained indefinitely. In the absence of significant overt bleeding or risk factors for bleeding, it is reasonable to continue dual-antiplatelet therapy for more than 12 months based on the dual-antiplatelet therapy (DAPT) and PEGASUS-TIMI 54 (Prevention of Cardiovascular Events in Patients with Prior Heart Attack Using Ticagrelor Compared to Placebo on a Background of Aspirin) trials.[161,162] The PEGASUS-TIMI 54 study, which randomized 21,162 patients with MI in the preceding 1 to 3 years to ticagrelor versus placebo, demonstrated a reduction in the composite of CV death, MI, or stroke at the cost of increased bleeding.[162] The DAPT study demonstrated a reduction in death, MI, and stroke as well as stent thrombosis with continuation of a thienopyridine (clopidogrel or prasugrel) on background therapy with aspirin for 30 months versus 12 months in patients undergoing DES placement, including 1045 STEMI patients.[161] A large RCT of the thrombin receptor antagonist *vorapaxar* in stable patients with prior MI, ischemic stroke, or symptomatic peripheral artery disease provided additional evidence for a benefit of more potent oral antiplatelet therapy than aspirin alone for long-term secondary prevention.[163] A similar reduction in major atherothrombotic events with oral anticoagulants lends additional support to the concept of expanded antithrombotic therapy for long-term secondary prevention (see Anticoagulants). Risk stratification can aid in personalization of antiplatelet therapy in patients with stable ischemic heart disease based on balancing the risk of recurrent atherothrombotic events with the risk of bleeding.[164,165] In patients treated with PCI, prasugrel and ticagrelor have proved superior to clopidogrel and are recommended as preferred in some guidelines.[2,71]

Inhibition of the Renin-Angiotensin-Aldosterone System

To prevent late remodeling of the left ventricle and to decrease the likelihood of recurrent ischemic events, we advocate indefinite therapy with an ACE inhibitor in patients with HF, a moderate decrease in global EF, or a large regional wall motion abnormality, even in the

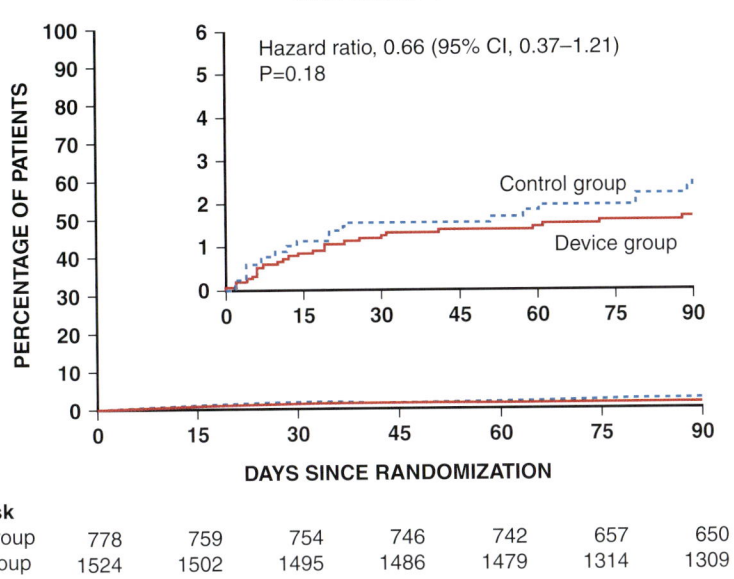

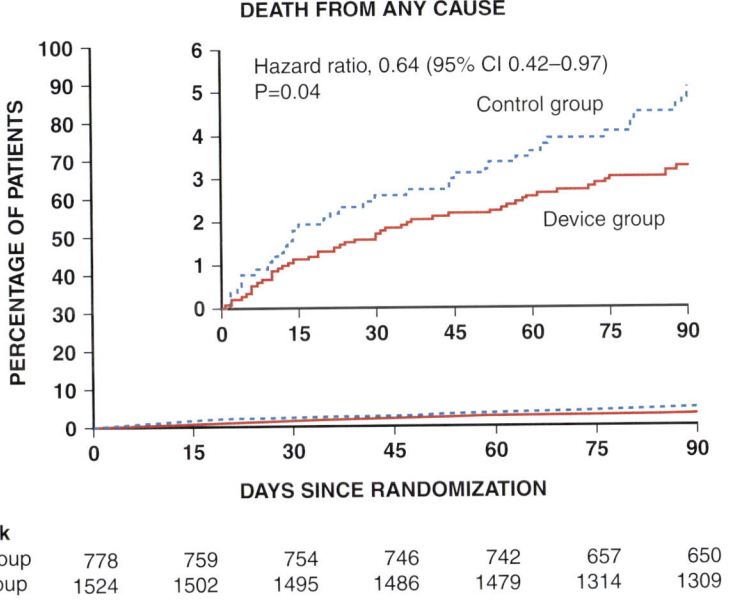

FIGURE 38.34 Comparison of wearable cardioverter-defibrillator versus guidelines-directed medical therapy only in patients with a recent acute coronary syndrome and left ventricular ejection fraction <35% in the VEST (Vest Prevention of Early Sudden Death Trial). **A,** Sudden death or death due to ventricular tachyarrhythmia and **(B)** all-cause death. (From Olgin JE, et al. *N Engl J Med*. 2018; 379:1205–1215.)

beta blockers (e.g., bradyarrhythmias) should undergo a monitored trial of therapy in the hospital. The dosage should be sufficient to blunt the HR response to stress or exercise. Much of the impact of beta blockers in preventing mortality occurs in the first weeks; consequently, treatment should commence as soon as possible. Programs that provide physician feedback to improve adherence to guidelines should be used.

Some controversy exists regarding how long patients should be treated. The collective data from five trials and a prospective observational registry on long-term follow-up of patients treated with beta blockers after infarction suggest that therapy should be continued for at least 2 to 3 years.[166] At that time, if the beta blocker is well tolerated and there is no reason to discontinue therapy, such therapy probably should be continued in most patients (see Chapter 40).

Nitrates
Although nitrates are suitable for the management of specific conditions after STEMI (e.g., recurrent angina) or as part of a treatment regimen for HF, little evidence indicates that nitrates reduce mortality over the long term when prescribed on a routine basis to all MI patients.

Anticoagulants (see Chapters 40 and 95)
After several decades of evaluation, the weight of evidence now suggests that anticoagulants have a favorable effect on late mortality, stroke, and reinfarction in patients hospitalized with STEMI. Nevertheless, given the multiple alternatives for antithrombotic therapy for long-term secondary prevention, clinicians must weigh the potential benefits of treatment with an OAC based on established indications for anticoagulation, the use of other antithrombotic therapies, including long-term DAPT, and the risk for bleeding.

At least three theoretical reasons exist for anticipating that anticoagulants might be beneficial in the long-term management of patients after STEMI. First, because the coronary occlusion responsible for STEMI is often caused by a thrombus, anticoagulants might be expected to halt progression, slow progression, or prevent the development of new thrombi elsewhere in the coronary arterial tree. Second, anticoagulants might be expected to diminish the formation of mural thrombi and resultant systemic embolization. Third, anticoagulants might reduce the incidence of venous thrombosis and pulmonary embolization.

Oral factor Xa inhibitors have undergone evaluation in patients with ACS, including STEMI. The ATLAS ACS 2-TIMI 51 (Anti-Xa Therapy to Lower Cardiovascular Events in Addition to Standard Therapy in Subjects with Acute Coronary Syndrome–Thrombolysis in Myocardial Infarction) trial tested two low doses of the oral factor Xa inhibitor rivaroxaban versus placebo. Rivaroxaban at doses of both 2.5 and 5 mg twice daily significantly reduced CV death, MI, or stroke compared to placebo (8.9% versus 10.7%; $P = 0.008$).[167] Both doses also reduced stent thrombosis. The group receiving the 2.5-mg dose demonstrated a significant reduction in CV mortality (2.7% versus 4.1%; $P = 0.002$) compared with placebo, which was not seen with 5 mg. Rivaroxaban resulted in an increase in major bleeding (2.1% versus 0.6%; $P < 0.001$) without a significant increase in fatal bleeding. In contrast with these findings, the APPRAISE-2 study, which tested apixaban versus placebo in patients following an ACS, was terminated early because of an increase in major bleeding without a significant improvement in efficacy.[62,167] The divergent results of the ATLAS ACS 2-TIMI 51 and APPRAISE-2 studies may relate to a higher baseline risk of the patients and concordant

presence of a normal global EF. (See earlier, Pharmacologic Therapy, Inhibition of the Renin-Angiotensin-Aldosterone System.)

Beta-Adrenergic Blocking Agents
Meta-analyses of trials from the pre-thrombolytic era involving more than 24,000 patients who received beta blockers in the convalescent phase of STEMI have shown a 23% reduction in long-term mortality. In most patients who have beta blocker administration initiated during the convalescent phase of STEMI, the reduction in long-term mortality probably results from the combination of an antiarrhythmic effect (prevention of SCD) and prevention of reinfarction.

Despite the well-documented benefits of therapy with a beta blocker, this treatment continues to be underused, especially in high-risk groups such as older adults. Patients with a relative contraindication to competing risks, the inclusion of patients with previous stroke or transient ischemic attack, and higher degrees of anticoagulation in APPRAISE-2.

The risk-benefit profile of low-dose oral anticoagulant therapy for secondary prevention after STEMI has been supplemented by the results of a large trial of secondary prevention in patients with stable atherosclerosis, including prior MI. In the COMPASS (Cardiovascular OutcoMes for People Using Anticoagulation StrategieS) trial, 27,395 patients with established stable CAD or peripheral artery disease were randomized to treatment with rivaroxaban (2.5 mg twice daily) plus aspirin (100 mg once daily), rivaroxaban (5 mg twice daily), or aspirin (100 mg once daily).[168] Patients with CAD qualified for participation with either a history of MI in the past 20 years or multivessel CAD. Compared with aspirin alone, rivaroxaban 2.5 mg twice daily plus aspirin reduced the risk of CV death, MI, or stroke by 24% (HR 0.76; 95% CI, 0.66 to 0.86; P < 0.001). Major bleeding was increased by the addition of rivaroxaban from 1.9% to 3.1% (HR 1.70; 95% CI, 1.40 to 2.05; P < 0.001). However, there were fewer deaths overall in the rivaroxaban 2.5 mg twice daily plus aspirin group compared with aspirin alone (HR 0.82; 95% CI, 0.71 to 0.96; nominal P = 0.01). Rivaroxaban 5 mg twice daily without aspirin did not significantly reduce the primary endpoint compared with aspirin alone. COMPASS did not study patients receiving an ADP antagonist in any treatment arm. The role of the available options for long-term antithrombotic therapy in addition to aspirin (e.g., ticagrelor, or rivaroxaban) is likely to be refined with clinical experience, additional research, and review by professional society guidelines committees.[169]

Calcium Channel Antagonists

We do *not* recommend the routine use of calcium antagonists for the secondary prevention of MI. A possible exception is a patient who cannot tolerate a beta blocker because of adverse effects on bronchospastic lung disease but who has well-preserved LV function. Such patients may be candidates for a rate-slowing calcium antagonist such as diltiazem or verapamil.

Hormone Therapy (see Chapters 25 and 91)

The decision to prescribe hormone therapy is often complex and involves the desire to suppress postmenopausal symptoms versus the risk for breast and endometrial cancer and vascular events. At present, we recommend that hormone therapy with estrogen plus progestin should *not* be started after STEMI and should be discontinued in postmenopausal women after STEMI.

Nonsteroidal Antiinflammatory Drugs

COX-2–selective drugs and NSAIDs with varying COX-1/COX-2 inhibitory ratios appear to promote a prothrombotic state, and their use is associated with an increased risk for atherothrombotic events.[1] Given the desire not to interfere with the beneficial pharmacologic actions of low-dose aspirin after STEMI, and reports of increased mortality and reinfarction when NSAIDs are used after MI, clinicians should avoid prescribing NSAIDs to patients recovering from STEMI.[1] If NSAIDs must be prescribed for relief of pain, the lowest dose required to control symptoms should be administered for the shortest time required.

FUTURE PERSPECTIVES AND EMERGING THERAPIES

Although the case-fatality rate of patients with STEMI has declined substantially, considerable opportunities for improvement remain. Of these, we emphasize three major directions: (1) mitigation of reperfusion injury and impaired myocardial tissue perfusion, (2) management of cardiogenic shock after STEMI, and (3) amelioration of the adverse remodeling.

Although PCI usually restores flow through epicardial arteries, many patients do not achieve adequate nutrient flow at the myocardial level in the infarct zone because of impaired microvascular flow (see Fig. 38.6). Despite effective restoration of flow in the culprit epicardial artery, patients with impaired microvascular reperfusion have reduced survival.[34] Identification of therapies that reliably improve microvascular perfusion in the setting of primary PCI and pharmacologic reperfusion has proved challenging. For example, although thrombus aspiration was hypothesized to improve outcomes through a reduction in microvascular obstruction due to distal embolization, improvements in ST-segment resolution did not translate to a reduction in recurrent CV events.[52,53,170]

Reperfusion injury to the microvasculature can also extend myocardial injury beyond the initial ischemic zone. To date, multiple candidate interventions to reduce reperfusion injury that appeared promising in initial studies have failed in definitive randomized trials. Amelioration of the reperfusion injury that contributes to long-term myocardial dysfunction remains an unmet clinical need. Therefore, therapies that target microvascular obstruction and reperfusion injury merit ongoing investigation.[20,34]

Even if reperfusion were achieved in a timely fashion and microvascular obstruction was minimized, patients with STEMI inevitably lose some myocytes. When ventricular failure or severe mechanical disruption results, cardiogenic shock may ensue. Mortality from cardiogenic shock remains in excess of 30%. Improvement in the outcomes of patients in whom shock develops after STEMI remains a vexing clinical challenge.[91] The disappointing results of trials of percutaneous mechanical support have challenged common clinical assumptions.[106] Novel therapies and strategies for the management of shock are an area of unmet clinical need.

In addition to the early risk for ventricular failure because of acute myocardial injury, secondary damage to the left ventricle can also occur in the long term as a result of ventricular remodeling after STEMI. Treatments to minimize ventricular remodeling include the standard approaches to disruption of the RAAS, reducing the amount of central nervous system generation of aldosterone, enhancing the synthesis of endothelial nitric oxide synthase, modulating beta-adrenergic signaling, and minimizing the processes that lead to cardiac apoptosis. Novel approaches using biological and mechanical interventions to improve ventricular structure are under investigation.[171] Moreover, myocytes may be capable of entering the cell cycle and dividing.[172,173] Cardiac regenerative measures merit rigorous evaluation regarding efficacy in ameliorating the adverse ventricular remodeling or myocardial repair by use of either endogenous or exogenous sources of cells that give rise to myocytes have not yet proven clinically effective.[173]

REFERENCES

Guidelines and Temporal Trends

1. O'Gara PT, Kushner FG, Ascheim DD, et al. 2013 ACCF/AHA guideline for the management of ST-elevation myocardial infarction: a report of the American College of Cardiology Foundation/American Heart Association task force on practice guidelines. *J Am Coll Cardiol.* 2013;61:e78–e140.
2. Ibanez B, James S, Agewall S, et al. 2017 ESC guidelines for the management of acute myocardial infarction in patients presenting with ST-segment elevation: the Task Force for the management of acute myocardial infarction in patients presenting with ST-segment elevation of the European Society of Cardiology (ESC). *Eur Heart J.* 2018;39:119–177.
3. Anderson JL, Morrow DA. Acute myocardial infarction. *N Engl J Med.* 2017;376:2053–2064.
4. Van de Werf F. The history of coronary reperfusion. *Eur Heart J.* 2014;35:2510–2515.
5. Le May M, Wells G, So D, et al. Safety and efficacy of femoral access vs radial access in ST-segment elevation myocardial infarction: the SAFARI-STEMI randomized clinical trial. *JAMA Cardiol.* 2020;5:126–134.
6. Levine GN, Bates ER, Blankenship JC, et al. 2015 ACC/AHA/SCAI focused update on primary percutaneous coronary intervention for patients with ST-elevation myocardial infarction: an update of the 2011 ACCF/AHA/SCAI guideline for percutaneous coronary intervention and the 2013 ACCF/AHA guideline for the management of ST-elevation myocardial infarction. *J Am Coll Cardiol.* 2016;67:1235–1250.

Prehospital Management and Emergency Care

7. Dasari TW, Hamilton S, Chen AY, et al. Non-eligibility for reperfusion therapy in patients presenting with ST-segment elevation myocardial infarction: contemporary insights from the National Cardiovascular Data Registry (NCDR). *Am Heart J.* 2016;172:1–8.
8. Bagai A, Dangas GD, Stone GW, Granger CB. Reperfusion strategies in acute coronary syndromes. *Circ Res.* 2014;114:1918–1928.
9. American Heart Association Mission Lifeline.
10. Squire BT, Tamayo-Sarver JH, Rashi P, et al. Effect of prehospital cardiac catheterization lab activation on door-to-balloon time, mortality, and false-positive activation. *Prehosp Emerg Care.* 2014;18:1–8.
11. Langabeer 2nd JR, Dellifraine J, Fowler R, et al. Emergency medical services as a strategy for improving ST-elevation myocardial infarction system treatment times. *J Emerg Med.* 2014;46:355–362.
12. Sinnaeve PR, Armstrong PW, Gershlick AH, et al. ST-segment-elevation myocardial infarction patients randomized to a pharmaco-invasive strategy or primary percutaneous coronary intervention: strategic reperfusion early after myocardial infarction (STREAM) 1-year mortality follow-up. *Circulation.* 2014;130:1139–1145.
13. Hobl EL, Stimpfl T, Ebner J, et al. Morphine decreases clopidogrel concentrations and effects: a randomized, double-blind, placebo-controlled trial. *J Am Coll Cardiol.* 2014;63:630–635.

14. Kubica J, Adamski P, Ostrowska M, et al. Morphine delays and attenuates ticagrelor exposure and action in patients with myocardial infarction: the randomized, double-blind, placebo-controlled IMPRESSION trial. *Eur Heart J.* 2016;37:245–252.
15. Furtado RHM, Nicolau JC, Guo J, et al. Morphine and cardiovascular outcomes among patients with non-ST-segment elevation acute coronary syndromes undergoing coronary angiography. *J Am Coll Cardiol.* 2020;75:289–300.
16. Stub D, Smith K, Bernard S, et al. Air versus oxygen in ST-segment-elevation myocardial infarction. *Circulation.* 2015;131:2143–2150.

Limitation of Infarct Size

17. Stone GW, Selker HP, Thiele H, et al. Relationship between infarct size and outcomes following primary PCI: patient-level analysis from 10 randomized trials. *J Am Coll Cardiol.* 2016;67:1674–1683.
18. Ibanez B, Heusch G, Ovize M, et al. Evolving therapies for myocardial ischemia/reperfusion injury. *J Am Coll Cardiol.* 2015;65:1454–1471.
19. Heusch G. Myocardial ischaemia-reperfusion injury and cardioprotection in perspective. *Nat Rev Cardiol.* 2020;17:773–789.
20. Hausenloy DJ, Yellon DM. Ischaemic conditioning and reperfusion injury. *Nat Rev Cardiol.* 2016;13:193–209.
21. Kapur NK, Alkhouli MA, DeMartini TJ, et al. Unloading the left ventricle before reperfusion in patients with anterior ST-segment-elevation myocardial infarction. *Circulation.* 2019;139:337–346.

Reperfusion Therapy

22. Frampton J, Devries JT, Welch TD, Gersh BJ. Modern management of ST-segment elevation myocardial infarction. *Curr Prob Cardiol.* 2020;45:100393.
23. Scholz KH, Maier SKG, Maier LS, et al. Impact of treatment delay on mortality in ST-segment elevation myocardial infarction (STEMI) patients presenting with and without haemodynamic instability: results from the German prospective, multicentre FITT-STEMI trial. *Eur Heart J.* 2018;39:1065–1074.
24. Kim EK, Choi JH, Song YB, et al. A protective role of early collateral blood flow in patients with ST-segment elevation myocardial infarction. *Am Heart J.* 2016;171:56–63.
25. Kloner RA, Hale HL. Reperfusion injury: prevention and management. In: Morrow D, ed. *Myocardial Infarction: A Companion to Braunwald's Heart Disease.* St. Louis: Elsevier; 2016:286–294.
26. Hausenloy DJ, Botker HE, Engstrom T, et al. Targeting reperfusion injury in patients with ST-segment elevation myocardial infarction: trials and tribulations. *Eur Heart J.* 2017;38:935–941.
27. Meybohm P, Bein B, Brosteanu O, et al. A multicenter trial of remote ischemic preconditioning for heart surgery. *N Engl J Med.* 2015;373:1397–1407.
28. Hausenloy DJ, Candilio L, Evans R, et al. Remote ischemic preconditioning and outcomes of cardiac surgery. *N Engl J Med.* 2015;373:1408–1417.
29. Hausenloy DJ, Kharbanda RK, Moller UK, et al. Effect of remote ischaemic conditioning on clinical outcomes in patients with acute myocardial infarction (CONDI-2/ERIC-PPCI): a single-blind randomised controlled trial. *Lancet.* 2019;394:1415–1424.
30. Hausenloy DJ, Ntsekhe M, Yellon DM. A future for remote ischaemic conditioning in high-risk patients. *Basic Res Cardiol.* 2020;115:35.
31. Engstrom T, Kelbaek H, Helqvist S, et al. Effect of ischemic postconditioning during primary percutaneous coronary intervention for patients with ST-segment elevation myocardial infarction: a randomized clinical trial. *JAMA Cardiol.* 2017;2:490–497.
32. Kloner RA. Stunned and hibernating myocardium: where are we nearly 4 decades later? *J Am Heart Assoc.* 2020;9:e015502.
33. Group TS. The Thrombolysis In Myocardial Infarction (TIMI) trial. Phase I findings. *N Engl J Med.* 1985;312:932–936.
34. Niccoli G, Scalone G, Lerman A, Crea F. Coronary microvascular obstruction in acute myocardial infarction. *Eur Heart J.* 2016;37:1024–1033.
35. Lonborg J, Kelbaek H, Holmvang L, et al. Comparison of outcome of patients with ST-segment elevation myocardial infarction and complete versus incomplete ST-resolution before primary percutaneous coronary intervention. *Am J Cardiol.* 2016;117:1735–1740.
36. Spitaleri G, Brugaletta S, Scalone G, et al. Role of ST-segment resolution in patients with ST-segment elevation myocardial infarction treated with primary percutaneous coronary intervention (from the 5-year outcomes of the EXAMINATION [Evaluation of the Xience-V Stent in Acute Myocardial Infarction] trial). *Am J Cardiol.* 2018;121:1039–1045.
37. Dizon JM, Brener SJ, Maehara A, et al. Relationship between ST-segment resolution and anterior infarct size after primary percutaneous coronary intervention: analysis from the INFUSE-AMI trial. *Eur Heart J Acute Cardiovasc Care.* 2014;3:78–83.
38. Pradhan J, Senior R. Assessment of myocardial viability by myocardial contrast echocardiography: current perspectives. *Curr Opin Cardiol.* 2019;34:495–501.
39. Reinstadler SJ, Thiele H, Eitel I. Risk stratification by cardiac magnetic resonance imaging after ST-elevation myocardial infarction. *Curr Opin Cardiol.* 2015;30:681–689.
40. Allencherril J, Jneid H, Atar D, et al. Pathophysiology, diagnosis, and management of the No-reflow phenomenon. *Cardiovasc Drugs Ther.* 2019;33:589–597.
41. Armstrong PW, Zheng Y, Westerhout CM, et al. Reduced dose tenecteplase and outcomes in elderly ST-segment elevation myocardial infarction patients: insights from the Strategic Reperfusion Early After Myocardial Infarction trial. *Am Heart J.* 2015;169:890–898.e1.
42. Armstrong PW, Bogaerts K, Welsh R, et al. The Second Strategic Reperfusion Early after Myocardial Infarction (STREAM-2) study optimizing pharmacoinvasive reperfusion strategy in older ST-elevation myocardial infarction patients. *Am Heart J.* 2020;226:140–146.
43. Lin H, Xu L, Yu S, et al. Therapeutics targeting the fibrinolytic system. *Exp Mol Med.* 2020;52:367–379.
44. Jinatongthai P, Kongwatcharapong J, Foo CY, et al. Comparative efficacy and safety of reperfusion therapy with fibrinolytic agents in patients with ST-segment elevation myocardial infarction: a systematic review and network meta-analysis. *Lancet.* 2017;390:747–759.
45. Arcari LB-DC, Francone M, Agati L. Myocardial salvage imaging: where are we and where are we heading? A cardiac magnetic resonance perspective. *Curr Cardiovasc Imaging Rep.* 2018;11.
46. Engstrom T, Kelbaek H, Helqvist S, et al. Complete revascularisation versus treatment of the culprit lesion only in patients with ST-segment elevation myocardial infarction and multivessel disease (DANAMI-3-PRIMULTI): an open-label, randomised controlled trial. *Lancet.* 2015;386:665–671.
47. Wald DS, Morris JK, Wald NJ, Investigators P. Preventive angioplasty in myocardial infarction. *N Engl J Med.* 2014;370:283.
48. Gershlick AH, Khan JN, Kelly DJ, et al. Randomized trial of complete versus lesion-only revascularization in patients undergoing primary percutaneous coronary intervention for STEMI and multivessel disease: the CvLPRIT trial. *J Am Coll Cardiol.* 2015;65:963–972.
49. Mehta SR, Wood DA, Storey RF, et al. Complete revascularization with multivessel PCI for myocardial infarction. *N Engl J Med.* 2019;381:1411–1421.
50. Smits PC, Abdel-Wahab M, Neumann FJ, et al. Fractional flow reserve-guided multivessel angioplasty in myocardial infarction. *N Engl J Med.* 2017;376:1234–1244.
51. Thiele H, Akin I, Sandri M, et al. PCI strategies in patients with acute myocardial infarction and cardiogenic shock. *N Engl J Med.* 2017;377:2419–2432.
52. Jolly SS, Cairns JA, Yusuf S, et al. Stroke in the TOTAL trial: a randomized trial of routine thrombectomy vs. percutaneous coronary intervention alone in ST elevation myocardial infarction. *Eur Heart J.* 2015;36:2364–2372.
53. Lagerqvist B, Frobert O, Olivecrona GK, et al. Outcomes 1 year after thrombus aspiration for myocardial infarction. *N Engl J Med.* 2014;371:1111–1120.
54. Valgimigli M, Gagnor A, Calabro P, et al. Radial versus femoral access in patients with acute coronary syndromes undergoing invasive management: a randomised multicentre trial. *Lancet.* 2015;385:2465–2476.
55. Bonaa KH, Mannsverk J, Wiseth R, et al. Drug-eluting or bare-metal stents for coronary artery disease. *N Engl J Med.* 2016;375:1242–1252.
56. Raber L, Yamaji K, Kelbaek H, et al. Five-year clinical outcomes and intracoronary imaging findings of the COMFORTABLE AMI trial: randomized comparison of biodegradable polymer-based biolimus-eluting stents with bare-metal stents in patients with acute ST-segment elevation myocardial infarction. *Eur Heart J.* 2019;40:1909–1919.
57. Sabate M, Brugaletta S, Cequier A, et al. The EXAMINATION trial (Everolimus-Eluting stents versus bare-metal stents in ST-segment elevation myocardial infarction): 2-year results from a multicenter randomized controlled trial. *JACC Cardiovasc Interv.* 2014;7:64–71.
58. Sabate M, Brugaletta S, Cequier A, et al. Clinical outcomes in patients with ST-segment elevation myocardial infarction treated with everolimus-eluting stents versus bare-metal stents (EXAMINATION): 5-year results of a randomised trial. *Lancet.* 2016;387:357–366.
59. Danchin N, Puymirat E, Steg PG, et al. Five-year survival in patients with ST-segment-elevation myocardial infarction according to modalities of reperfusion therapy: the French Registry on Acute ST-Elevation and Non-ST-Elevation Myocardial Infarction (FAST-MI) 2005 Cohort. *Circulation.* 2014;129:1629–1636.
60. Siddiqi TJ, Usman MS, Khan MS, et al. Meta-analysis comparing primary percutaneous coronary intervention versus pharmacoinvasive therapy in transfer patients with ST-elevation myocardial infarction. *Am J Cardiol.* 2018;122:542–547.

Anticoagulant and Antiplatelet Therapy

61. Kushner FG, Bates ER. ST-segment elevation myocardial infarction. In: Antman EM, Sabatine MS, eds. *Cardiovascular Therapeutics.* 4th ed. Philadelphia, PA: Elsevier; 2013:178–213.
62. Bhatt DL, Hulot JS, Moliterno DJ, Harrington RA. Antiplatelet and anticoagulation therapy for acute coronary syndromes. *Circ Res.* 2014;114:1929–1943.
63. Stone GW, Mehran R, Goldstein P, et al. Bivalirudin versus heparin with or without glycoprotein IIb/IIIa inhibitors in patients with STEMI undergoing primary percutaneous coronary intervention: pooled patient-level analysis from the HORIZONS-AMI and EUROMAX trials. *J Am Coll Cardiol.* 2015;65:27–38.
64. Cavender MA, Sabatine MS. Bivalirudin versus heparin in patients planned for percutaneous coronary intervention: a meta-analysis of randomised controlled trials. *Lancet.* 2014;384:599–606.
65. Onwordi EN, Gamal A, Zaman A. Anticoagulant therapy for acute coronary syndromes. *Interv Cardiol.* 2018;13:87–92.
66. Montecucco F, Carbone F, Schindler TH. Pathophysiology of ST-segment elevation myocardial infarction: novel mechanisms and treatments. *Eur Heart J.* 2016;37:1268–1283.
67. Bellemain-Appaix A, O'Connor SA, Silvain J, et al. Association of clopidogrel pretreatment with mortality, cardiovascular events, and major bleeding among patients undergoing percutaneous coronary intervention: a systematic review and meta-analysis. *J Am Med Assoc.* 2012;308:2507–2516.
68. Montalescot G, van 't Hof AW. Prehospital ticagrelor in ST-segment elevation myocardial infarction. *N Engl J Med.* 2014;371:2339.
69. Bhatt DL, Stone GW, Mahaffey KW, et al. Effect of platelet inhibition with cangrelor during PCI on ischemic events. *N Engl J Med.* 2013;368:1303–1313.
70. Kandan SR, Johnson TW. Contemporary antiplatelet strategies in the treatment of STEMI using primary percutaneous coronary intervention. *Interv Cardiol.* 2015;10:26–31.
71. Levine GN, Bates ER, Bittl JA, et al. 2016 ACC/AHA guideline focused update on duration of dual antiplatelet therapy in patients with coronary artery disease: a report of the American College of Cardiology/American Heart Association task force on clinical practice guidelines: an update of the 2011 ACCF/AHA/SCAI guideline for percutaneous coronary intervention, 2011 ACCF/AHA guideline for coronary artery bypass graft surgery, 2012 ACC/AHA/ACP/AATS/PCNA/SCAI/STS guideline for the diagnosis and management of patients with stable ischemic heart disease, 2013 ACCF/AHA guideline for the management of ST-elevation myocardial infarction, 2014 AHA/ACC guideline for the management of patients with non-ST-elevation acute coronary syndromes, and 2014 ACC/AHA guideline on perioperative cardiovascular evaluation and management of patients undergoing noncardiac surgery. *Circulation.* 2016;134:e123–e155.

Hospital Management and Other Pharmacotherapy

72. Silverman MG, Morrow DA. Hospital triage of acute myocardial infarction: is admission to the coronary care unit still necessary? *Am Heart J.* 2016;175:172–174.
73. Shavadia JS, Chen AY, Fanaroff AC, et al. Intensive care utilization in stable patients with ST-segment elevation myocardial infarction treated with rapid reperfusion. *JACC Cardiovasc Interv.* 2019;12:709–717.
74. Priori SG, Blomstrom-Lundqvist C, Mazzanti A, et al. 2015 ESC guidelines for the management of patients with ventricular arrhythmias and the prevention of sudden cardiac death: the task force for the management of patients with ventricular arrhythmias and the prevention of sudden cardiac death of the European Society of Cardiology (ESC). Endorsed By: Association for European Paediatric and Congenital Cardiology (AEPC). *Eur Heart J.* 2015;36:2793–2867.
75. Yancy CW, Jessup M, Bozkurt B, et al. 2017 ACC/AHA/HFSA focused update of the 2013 ACCF/AHA guideline for the management of heart failure: a report of the American College of Cardiology/American Heart Association task force on clinical practice guidelines and the heart failure society of America. *Circulation.* 2017;136:e137–e161.
76. Yancy CW, Jessup M, Bozkurt B, et al. 2013 ACCF/AHA guideline for the management of heart failure: executive summary: a report of the American College of Cardiology Foundation/American Heart Association Task Force on practice guidelines. *Circulation.* 2013;128:1810–1852.
77. Parviz Y, Iqbal J, Pitt B, et al. Emerging cardiovascular indications of mineralocorticoid receptor antagonists. *Trends Endocrinol Metab.* 2015;26:201–211.
78. Beygui F, Cayla G, Roule V, et al. Early aldosterone blockade in acute myocardial infarction: the ALBATROSS randomized clinical trial. *J Am Coll Cardiol.* 2016;67:1917–1927.
79. Dahal K, Hendrani A, Sharma SP, et al. Aldosterone antagonist therapy and mortality in patients with ST-segment elevation myocardial infarction without heart failure: a systematic review and meta-analysis. *JAMA Intern Med.* 2018;178:913–920.
80. Prospective ARNI vs ACE Inhibitor Trial to Determine Superiority in Reducing Heart Failure Events after MI (PARADISE-MI).
81. Writing Committee M, Yancy CW, Jessup M, et al. 2016 ACC/AHA/HFSA focused update on new pharmacological therapy for heart failure: an update of the 2013 ACCF/AHA guideline for the management of heart failure: a report of the American College of Cardiology/American Heart Association task force on clinical practice guidelines and the Heart Failure Society of America. *Circulation.* 2016;134:e282–e293.
82. Jin PY, Zhang HS, Guo XY, et al. Glucose-insulin-potassium therapy in patients with acute coronary syndrome: a meta-analysis of randomized controlled trials. *BMC Cardiovasc Disord.* 2014;14:169.
83. Seropian IM, Toldo S, Van Tassell BW, Abbate A. Anti-inflammatory strategies for ventricular remodeling following ST-segment elevation acute myocardial infarction. *J Am Coll Cardiol.* 2014;63:1593–1603.

84. O'Donoghue ML, Glaser R, Cavender MA, et al. Effect of losmapimod on cardiovascular outcomes in patients hospitalized with acute myocardial infarction: a randomized clinical trial. *J Am Med Assoc*. 2016;315:1591–1599.
85. O'Donoghue ML, Braunwald E, White HD, et al. Effect of darapladib on major coronary events after an acute coronary syndrome: the SOLID-TIMI 52 randomized clinical trial. *J Am Med Assoc*. 2014;312:1006–1015.
86. Tardif JC, Kouz S, Waters DD, et al. Efficacy and safety of low-dose colchicine after myocardial infarction. *N Engl J Med*. 2019;381:2497–2505.
87. Tong DC, Quinn S, Nasis A, et al. Colchicine in patients with acute coronary syndrome: the Australian COPS randomized clinical trial. *Circulation*. 2020;142:1890–1900.
88. Ridker PM, Everett BM, Thuren T, et al. Antiinflammatory therapy with canakinumab for atherosclerotic disease. *N Engl J Med*. 2017;377:1119–1131.

Hemodynamic Monitoring and Structural Complications

89. Garan AR, Kanwar M, Thayer KL, et al. Complete hemodynamic profiling with pulmonary artery catheters in cardiogenic shock is associated with lower in-hospital mortality. *JACC Heart Fail*. 2020;8:903–913.
90. Nguyen LS, Squara P. Non-invasive monitoring of cardiac output in critical care medicine. *Front Med*. 2017;4:200.
91. Thiele H, Ohman EM, Desch S, et al. Management of cardiogenic shock. *Eur Heart J*. 2015;36:1223–1230.
92. Auffret V, Cottin Y, Leurent G, et al. Predicting the development of in-hospital cardiogenic shock in patients with ST-segment elevation myocardial infarction treated by primary percutaneous coronary intervention: the ORBI risk score. *Eur Heart J*. 2018;39:2090–2102.
93. McMurray JJ, Packer M, Desai AS, et al. Angiotensin-neprilysin inhibition versus enalapril in heart failure. *N Engl J Med*. 2014;371:993–1004.
94. Velazquez EJ, Morrow DA, DeVore AD, et al. Angiotensin-neprilysin inhibition in acute decompensated heart failure. *N Engl J Med*. 2019;380:539–548.
95. McMurray JJV, Solomon SD, Inzucchi SE, et al. Dapagliflozin in patients with heart failure and reduced ejection fraction. *N Engl J Med*. 2019;381:1995–2008.
96. Packer M, Anker SD, Butler J, et al. Cardiovascular and renal outcomes with empagliflozin in heart failure. *N Engl J Med*. 2020;383:1413–1424.
97. Kristensen SL, Rorth R, Jhund PS, et al. Cardiovascular, mortality, and kidney outcomes with GLP-1 receptor agonists in patients with type 2 diabetes: a systematic review and meta-analysis of cardiovascular outcome trials. *Lancet Diabetes Endocrinol*. 2019;7:776–785.
98. Cosentino F, Grant PJ, Aboyans V, et al. 2019 ESC guidelines on diabetes, pre-diabetes, and cardiovascular diseases developed in collaboration with the EASD. *Eur Heart J*. 2020;41:255–323.
99. Pfeffer MA, Claggett B, Diaz R, et al. Lixisenatide in patients with type 2 diabetes and acute coronary syndrome. *N Engl J Med*. 2015;373:2247–2257.
100. van Diepen S, Katz JN, Albert NM, et al. Contemporary management of cardiogenic shock: a scientific statement from the American Heart Association. *Circulation*. 2017;136:e232–e268.
101. Wan SH, Stevens SR, Borlaug BA, et al. Differential response to low-dose dopamine or low-dose nesiritide in acute heart failure with reduced or preserved ejection fraction: results from the ROSE AHF trial (renal optimization strategies evaluation in acute heart failure). *Circ Heart Fail*. 2016;9.
102. Dumas F, Bougouin W, Geri G, et al. Is epinephrine during cardiac arrest associated with worse outcomes in resuscitated patients? *J Am Coll Cardiol*. 2014;64:2360–2367.
103. Levy B, Clere-Jehl R, Legras A, et al. Epinephrine versus norepinephrine for cardiogenic shock after acute myocardial infarction. *J Am Coll Cardiol*. 2018;72:173–182.
104. Kolte D, Khera S, Aronow WS, et al. Trends in incidence, management, and outcomes of cardiogenic shock complicating ST-elevation myocardial infarction in the United States. *J Am Heart Assoc*. 2014;3:e000590.
105. Berg DD, Bohula EA, van Diepen S, et al. Epidemiology of shock in contemporary cardiac intensive care units. *Cir Cardiovasc Qual Outcomes*. 2019;12:e005618.
106. Rihal CS, Naidu SS, Givertz MM, et al. 2015 SCAI/ACC/HFSA/STS clinical expert consensus statement on the use of percutaneous mechanical circulatory support devices in cardiovascular care: endorsed by the American Heart Association, The Cardiological Society of India, and Sociedad Latino Americana De Cardiologia Intervencionista; Affirmation of Value by the Canadian Association of Interventional Cardiology-Association Canadienne De Cardiologie D'intervention. *J Am Coll Cardiol*. 2015;65:2140–2141.
107. Combes A, Price S, Slutsky AS, Brodie D. Temporary circulatory support for cardiogenic shock. *Lancet*. 2020;396:199–212.
108. Thiele H, Zeymer U, Thelemann N, et al. Intraaortic balloon pump in cardiogenic shock complicating acute myocardial infarction: long-term 6-year outcome of the randomized IABP-SHOCK II trial. *Circulation*. 2018.
109. Berg DD, Barnett CF, Kenigsberg BB, et al. Clinical practice patterns in temporary mechanical circulatory support for shock in the Critical Care Cardiology Trials Network (CCCTN) registry. *Cir Heart Fail*. 2019;12:e006635.
110. Sandhu A, McCoy LA, Negi SI, et al. Use of mechanical circulatory support in patients undergoing percutaneous coronary intervention: insights from the National Cardiovascular Data Registry. *Circulation*. 2015;132:1243–1251.
111. Amin AP, Spertus JA, Curtis JP, et al. The evolving landscape of impella use in the United States among patients undergoing percutaneous coronary intervention with mechanical circulatory support. *Circulation*. 2020;141:273–284.
111a. Henry TD, Tomey MI, Tamis-Holland JE, et al. American Heart Association Interventional Cardiovascular Care Committee of the Council on Clinical Cardiology; Council on Arteriosclerosis, Thrombosis and Vascular Biology; and Council on Cardiovascular and Stroke Nursing. Invasive Management of Acute Myocardial Infarction Complicated by Cardiogenic Shock: A Scientific Statement From the American Heart Association. *Circulation*. 2021;143(15):e815–e829.
112. Kumar S, McDaniel M, Samady H, Forouzandeh F. Contemporary revascularization dilemmas in older adults. *J Am Heart Assoc*. 2020;9:e014477.
113. Tehrani BN, Truesdell AG, Sherwood MW, et al. Standardized team-based care for cardiogenic shock. *J Am Coll Cardiol*. 2019;73:1659–1669.
114. Rallidis LS, Makavos G, Nihoyannopoulos P. Right ventricular involvement in coronary artery disease: role of echocardiography for diagnosis and prognosis. *J Am Soc Echocardiogr*. 2014;27:223–229.
115. Albulushi A, Giannopoulos A, Kafkas N, et al. Acute right ventricular myocardial infarction. *Expert Rev Cardiovasc Ther*. 2018;16:455–464.
116. Elbadawi A, Elgendy IY, Mahmoud K, et al. Temporal trends and outcomes of mechanical complications in patients with acute myocardial infarction. *JACC Cardiovasc Interv*. 2019;12:1825–1836.
117. Bates ER. Reperfusion therapy reduces the risk of myocardial rupture complicating ST-elevation myocardial infarction. *J Am Heart Assoc*. 2014;3:e001368.
118. Arsanjani R, Lohrmann G, Allen S, et al. A multi-modality approach to left ventricular aneurysms: true vs false. *Am J Med*. 2016;129:e113–e116.
119. Schlotter F, de Waha S, Eitel I, et al. Interventional post-myocardial infarction ventricular septal defect closure: a systematic review of current evidence. *EuroIntervention*. 2016;12:94–102.
120. Nishimura RA, Otto CM, Bonow RO, et al. 2014 AHA/ACC guideline for the management of patients with valvular heart disease: executive summary: a report of the American College of Cardiology/American Heart Association task force on practice guidelines. *Circulation*. 2014;129:2440–2492.

Arrhythmias

121. Roolvink V, Ibanez B, Ottervanger JP, et al. Early intravenous beta-blockers in patients with ST-segment elevation myocardial infarction before primary percutaneous coronary intervention. *J Am Coll Cardiol*. 2016;67:2705–2715.
122. Gorenek B, Lundqvist CB, Terradellas JB, et al. Cardiac arrhythmias in acute coronary syndromes: position paper from the joint EHRA, ACCA, and EAPCI task force. *Eur Heart J Acute Cardiovasc Care*. 2015;4:386.
123. Link MS, Berkow LC, Kudenchuk PJ, et al. Part 7: adult advanced cardiovascular life support: 2015 American Heart Association guidelines update for cardiopulmonary resuscitation and emergency cardiovascular care. *Circulation*. 2015;132:S444–S464.
124. Chan WK, Goodman SG, Brieger D, et al. Clinical characteristics, management, and outcomes of acute coronary syndrome in patients with right bundle branch block on presentation. *Am J Cardiol*. 2016;117:754–759.
125. Xiong Y, Wang L, Liu W, et al. The prognostic significance of right bundle branch block: a meta-analysis of prospective cohort studies. *Clin Cardiol*. 2015;38:604–613.
126. Kusumoto FM, Schoenfeld MH, Barrett C, et al. 2018 ACC/AHA/HRS guideline on the evaluation and management of patients with bradycardia and cardiac conduction delay: executive summary: a report of the American College of Cardiology/American Heart Association task force on clinical practice guidelines, and the heart rhythm society. *J Am Coll Cardiol*. 2019;74:932–987.
127. Kundu A, O'Day K, Shaikh AY, et al. Relation of atrial fibrillation in acute myocardial infarction to in-hospital complications and early hospital readmission. *Am J Cardiol*. 2016;117:1213–1218.
128. Rene AG, Genereux P, Ezekowitz M, et al. Impact of atrial fibrillation in patients with ST-elevation myocardial infarction treated with percutaneous coronary intervention (from the HORIZONS-AMI [Harmonizing Outcomes with Revascularization and Stents in Acute Myocardial Infarction] trial). *Am J Cardiol*. 2014;113:236–242.

Other Complications

129. Thygesen K, Alpert JS, Jaffe AS, et al. Fourth universal definition of myocardial infarction (2018). *J Am Coll Cardiol*. 2018;72:2231–2264.
130. Stone SG, Serrao GW, Mehran R, et al. Incidence, predictors, and implications of reinfarction after primary percutaneous coronary intervention in ST-segment-elevation myocardial infarction: the Harmonizing Outcomes with Revascularization and Stents in Acute Myocardial Infarction Trial. *Circ Cardiovasc Interv*. 2014;7:543–551.
131. Biere L, Mateus V, Clerfond G, et al. Predictive factors of pericardial effusion after a first acute myocardial infarction and successful reperfusion. *Am J Cardiol*. 2015;116:497–503.
132. Jobs A, Eitel C, Poss J, et al. Effect of pericardial effusion complicating ST-elevation myocardial infarction as predictor of extensive myocardial damage and prognosis. *Am J Cardiol*. 2015;116:1010–1016.
133. Figueras J, Barrabes JA, Lidon RM, et al. Predictors of moderate-to-severe pericardial effusion, cardiac tamponade, and electromechanical dissociation in patients with ST-elevation myocardial infarction. *Am J Cardiol*. 2014;113:1291–1296.
134. Adler Y, Charron P, Imazio M, et al. 2015 ESC guidelines for the diagnosis and management of pericardial diseases: the task force for the diagnosis and management of pericardial diseases of the European Society of Cardiology (ESC) endorsed by: the European Association for Cardio-Thoracic Surgery (EACTS). *Eur Heart J*. 2015;36:2921–2964.
135. Jones RH, Velazquez EJ, Michler RE, et al. Coronary bypass surgery with or without surgical ventricular reconstruction. *N Engl J Med*. 2009;360:1705–1717.
136. Costa MA, Mazzaferri Jr EL, Sievert H, Abraham WT. Percutaneous ventricular restoration using the parachute device in patients with ischemic heart failure: three-year outcomes of the PARACHUTE first-in-human study. *Circ Heart Fail*. 2014;7:752–758.
137. McCarthy CP, Vaduganathan M, McCarthy KJ, et al. Left ventricular thrombus after acute myocardial infarction: screening, prevention, and treatment. *JAMA Cardiol*. 2018;3:642–649.
138. Velangi PS, Choo C, Chen KA, et al. Long-term embolic outcomes after detection of left ventricular thrombus by late gadolinium enhancement cardiovascular magnetic resonance imaging: a matched cohort study. *Circ Cardiovasc Imaging*. 2019;12:e009723.

Secondary Prevention

139. Jang SJ, Yeo I, Feldman DN, et al. Associations between hospital length of stay, 30-day readmission, and costs in ST-segment-elevation myocardial infarction after primary percutaneous coronary intervention: a nationwide readmissions database analysis. *J Am Heart Assoc*. 2020;9:e015503.
140. Rothenbacher D, Dallmeier D, Mons U, et al. Sexual activity patterns before myocardial infarction and risk of subsequent cardiovascular adverse events. *J Am Coll Cardiol*. 2015;66:1516–1517.
141. Anderson L, Oldridge N, Thompson DR, et al. Exercise-based cardiac rehabilitation for coronary heart disease: cochrane systematic review and meta-analysis. *J Am Coll Cardiol*. 2016;67:1–12.
142. Smolderen KG, Buchanan DM, Gosch K, et al. Depression treatment and 1-year mortality after acute myocardial infarction: insights from the TRIUMPH registry (translational research investigating underlying disparities in acute myocardial infarction patients' health status). *Circulation*. 2017;135:1681–1689.
143. Morrow DA. Cardiovascular risk prediction in patients with stable and unstable coronary heart disease. *Circulation*. 2010;121:2681–2691.
144. McNamara RL, Kennedy KF, Cohen DJ, et al. Predicting in-hospital mortality in patients with acute myocardial infarction. *J Am Coll Cardiol*. 2016;68:626–635.
145. Zaman S, Kovoor P. Sudden cardiac death early after myocardial infarction: pathogenesis, risk stratification, and primary prevention. *Circulation*. 2014;129:2426–2435.
146. van Kranenburg M, Magro M, Thiele H, et al. Prognostic value of microvascular obstruction and infarct size, as measured by CMR in STEMI patients. *JACC Cardiovasc Imaging*. 2014;7:930–939.
147. Kusumoto FM, Calkins H, Boehmer J, et al. HRS/ACC/AHA expert consensus statement on the use of implantable cardioverter-defibrillator therapy in patients who are not included or not well represented in clinical trials. *Circulation*. 2014;130:94–125.
148. Olgin JE, Pletcher MJ, Vittinghoff E, et al. Wearable cardioverter-defibrillator after myocardial infarction. *N Engl J Med*. 2018;379:1205–1215.
149. Sandesara PB, Lambert CT, Gordon NF, et al. Cardiac rehabilitation and risk reduction: time to "rebrand and reinvigorate. *J Am Coll Cardiol*. 2015;65:389–395.
150. Grundy SM, Stone NJ, Bailey AL, et al. 2018 AHA/ACC/AACVPR/AAPA/ABC/ACPM/ADA/AGS/APhA/ASPC/NLA/PCNA guideline on the management of blood cholesterol: executive summary: a report of the American College of Cardiology/American Heart Association task force on clinical practice guidelines. *Circulation*. 2019;139:e1046–e1081.
151. Mach F, Baigent C, Catapano AL, et al. 2019 ESC/EAS Guidelines for the management of dyslipidaemias: lipid modification to reduce cardiovascular risk. *Eur Heart J*. 2020;41:111–188.
152. Cannon CP, Blazing MA, Giugliano RP, et al. Ezetimibe added to statin therapy after acute coronary syndromes. *N Engl J Med*. 2015;372:2387–2397.
153. Giugliano RP, Wiviott SD, Blazing MA, et al. Long-term safety and efficacy of achieving very low levels of low-density lipoprotein cholesterol: a prespecified analysis of the IMPROVE-IT trial. *JAMA Cardiol*. 2017;2:547–555.
154. Murphy SA, Cannon CP, Blazing MA, et al. Reduction in total cardiovascular events with ezetimibe/simvastatin post-acute coronary syndrome: the IMPROVE-IT trial. *J Am Coll Cardiol*. 2016;67:353–361.
155. Sabatine MS, Giugliano RP, Keech AC, et al. Evolocumab and clinical outcomes in patients with cardiovascular disease. *N Engl J Med*. 2017;376:1713–1722.

156. Schwartz GG, Steg PG, Szarek M, et al. Alirocumab and cardiovascular outcomes after acute coronary syndrome. *N Engl J Med.* 2018;379:2097–2107.
157. Bhatt DL, Steg PG, Miller M, et al. Cardiovascular risk reduction with icosapent ethyl for hypertriglyceridemia. *N Engl J Med.* 2019;380:11–22.
158. Boden WE, Bhatt DL, Toth PP, et al. Profound reductions in first and total cardiovascular events with icosapent ethyl in the REDUCE-IT trial: why these results usher in a new era in dyslipidaemia therapeutics. *Eur Heart J.* 2020;41:2304–2312.
159. Nicholls SJ, Lincoff AM, Garcia M, et al. Effect of high-dose omega-3 fatty acids vs corn oil on major adverse cardiovascular events in patients at high cardiovascular risk: the STRENGTH randomized clinical trial. *J Am Med Assoc.* 2020;324:2268–2280.
160. Sharma G, Martin SS, Blumenthal RS. Effects of omega-3 fatty acids on major adverse cardiovascular events: what matters most: the drug, the dose, or the placebo? *J Am Med Assoc.* 2020;324:2262–2264.
161. Mauri L, Kereiakes DJ, Yeh RW, et al. Twelve or 30 months of dual antiplatelet therapy after drug-eluting stents. *N Engl J Med.* 2014;371:2155–2166.
162. Bonaca MP, Bhatt DL, Cohen M, et al. Long-term use of ticagrelor in patients with prior myocardial infarction. *N Engl J Med.* 2015;372:1791–1800.
163. Frampton JE. Vorapaxar: a review of its use in the long-term secondary prevention of atherothrombotic events. *Drugs.* 2015;75:797–808.
164. Bohula EA, Bonaca MP, Braunwald E, et al. Atherothrombotic risk stratification and the efficacy and safety of vorapaxar in patients with stable ischemic heart disease and previous myocardial infarction. *Circulation.* 2016;134:304–313.
165. Yeh RW, Secemsky EA, Kereiakes DJ, et al. Development and validation of a prediction rule for benefit and harm of dual antiplatelet therapy beyond 1 year after percutaneous coronary intervention. *J Am Med Assoc.* 2016;315:1735–1749.
166. Sorbets E, Steg PG, Young R, et al. beta-blockers, calcium antagonists, and mortality in stable coronary artery disease: an international cohort study. *Eur Heart J.* 2019;40:1399–1407.
167. Harrison RW, Newby LK. Rivaroxaban in acute coronary syndromes: we have a compass and an atlas, but where are we headed? *J Am Heart Assoc.* 2019;8:e012014.
168. Eikelboom JW, Connolly SJ, Bosch J, et al. Rivaroxaban with or without aspirin in stable cardiovascular disease. *N Engl J Med.* 2017;377:1319–1330.
169. Knuuti J, Wijns W, Saraste A, et al. 2019 ESC Guidelines for the diagnosis and management of chronic coronary syndromes. *Eur Heart J.* 2020;41:407–477.
170. Jolly SS, Cairns JA, Yusuf S, et al. Outcomes after thrombus aspiration for ST elevation myocardial infarction: 1-year follow-up of the prospective randomised TOTAL trial. *Lancet.* 2016;387:127–135.
171. Bhatt AS, Ambrosy AP, Velazquez EJ. Adverse remodeling and reverse remodeling after myocardial infarction. *Curr Cardiol Rep.* 2017;19:71.
172. Bergmann O, Jovinge S. Cardiac regeneration in vivo: mending the heart from within? *Stem Cell Res.* 2014;13:523–531.
173. Lee RT, Walsh K. The future of cardiovascular regenerative medicine. *Circulation.* 2016;133:2618–2625.

39 Non–ST Elevation Acute Coronary Syndromes

ROBERT P. GIUGLIANO AND EUGENE BRAUNWALD

EPIDEMIOLOGY, 714
PATHOPHYSIOLOGY, 714
CLINICAL ASSESSMENT, 715
History, 715
Physical Examination, 716
Electrocardiography, 716
Laboratory Testing: Biomarkers, 717
IMAGING, 718
Noninvasive Testing, 718
Invasive Imaging, 719
RISK ASSESSMENT, 720
Residual Risk, 720
Natural History, 720
Risk Assessment Scores, 720

MANAGEMENT, 721
General Measures, 721
Anti-Ischemic Therapy, 721
Antiplatelet Therapy, 723
Anticoagulant Therapy, 726
Patients with Indications for Both Oral Anticoagulant and Antiplatelet Therapy, 727
Bleeding: Risk Assessment, Prevention, and Treatment, 728
Anti-Inflammatory Therapies, 728
Invasive Versus Conservative Management, 728
Lipid-Lowering Therapy, 731
Discharge and Posthospital Care, 732

GROUPS OF SPECIAL INTEREST, 732
Older Adults, 732
Women, 733
Diabetes Mellitus and Glucose Intolerance, 733
Heart Failure, 734
Vasospastic Angina, 734
Cardiac Syndrome X, 735
Cocaine, Amphetamines, and Psychoactive Substances, 735
FUTURE PERSPECTIVES, 735
REFERENCES, 736

Ischemic heart disease may manifest clinically as either chronic stable angina (see Chapter 40) or an acute coronary syndrome (ACS).[1] The spectrum of ACS includes ST-segment elevation myocardial infarction (STEMI) (see Chapters 37 and 38) and the non–ST elevation acute coronary syndromes (NSTE-ACS). The latter consist of non–ST elevation myocardial infarction (NSTEMI) and unstable angina (UA) (Fig. 39.1), which have indistinguishable clinical presentations at the initial evaluation.

Several features help to differentiate ACS from chronic stable angina, including (1) sudden onset of symptoms at rest (or with minimal exertion) that last at least 10 minutes unless treated promptly; (2) severe pain, pressure, or discomfort in the chest; and (3) an accelerating pattern of angina that develops more frequently, with greater severity, or that awakens the patient from sleep. The 12-lead electrocardiogram (ECG) and markers of myocardial necrosis are essential tools in distinguishing between the three types of ACS mentioned previously. Patients with typical symptoms *without* persistent (>20 minutes) ST-segment elevation in at least two contiguous electrocardiographic leads, but with elevation of myocardial biomarkers (>99% of the normal range), are classified as having NSTEMI. Patients with typical symptoms and serial negative markers of myocardial necrosis are classified as having UA, a diagnosis that carries a better prognosis.

EPIDEMIOLOGY

Despite the decline in age-adjusted cardiovascular disease (CVD) mortality over the past three decades, ischemic heart disease remains the leading cause of death worldwide, affecting 197 million individuals and is responsible for 9.14 million deaths annually with more disability life-years lost (182 million) than any other cause worldwide in 2019.[1] In the United States in 2020, it is estimated that more than 1 million patients will experience a coronary heart disease event, of whom 76% will have an MI.[2] The fraction of ACS attributed to NSTEMI continues to increase, while that for STEMI is declining, for several reasons: (1) wider use of preventive measures such as aspirin, statins, and smoking cessation; (2) aging of the population, with greater prevalence of diabetes and chronic kidney disease (CKD); (3) wider use of cardiac troponin (cTn) (see later) assays with higher sensitivity for myocardial necrosis, which shifts the diagnosis from UA to NSTEMI; and (4) wider implementation of the universal definition of MI.[3]

PATHOPHYSIOLOGY

The pathogenesis of NSTE-ACS involves five processes operating singly or in various combinations: (1) disruption of an unstable atheromatous plaque, (2) erosion of an atheromatous plaque (Fig. 39.2; Table 39.1), (3) coronary arterial vasoconstriction, (4) gradual intraluminal narrowing of an epicardial coronary artery caused by progressive atherosclerosis or restenosis after percutaneous coronary intervention (PCI), and (5) oxygen supply-demand mismatch (see Chapter 36). Our understanding of the complex interactions between these pathways continues to evolve. For example, studies have implicated a role for matrix metalloproteinase-9 (MMP-9) in T-cell hyperactivity and dysregulation during the acute phase of ACS by its cleavage of the transmembrane glycoprotein adhesion molecule CD31 leading to lymphocyte activation.[4] In addition to serving as useful biomarkers in ACS, better understanding of the pathophysiology of ACS could identify molecular targets for anti-inflammatory therapies in patients with this condition.

Three mechanisms may lead to plaque disruption: plaque fissure with inflammation, plaque fissure without inflammation, or plaque erosion. Although plaque rupture remains the most common mechanism of ACS, plaque erosion is increasing in frequency and is present in up to 40% of ACS cases[5] (Fig. 39.3). Plaques that rupture characteristically have large lipid pools with foam cells and a thin fibrous cap. Increasing use of high-intensity lipid-lowering therapies that can deplete intimal lipid collections can halt progression or even cause regression of plaques.[6] Plaques that are lipid poor with few macrophages but rich

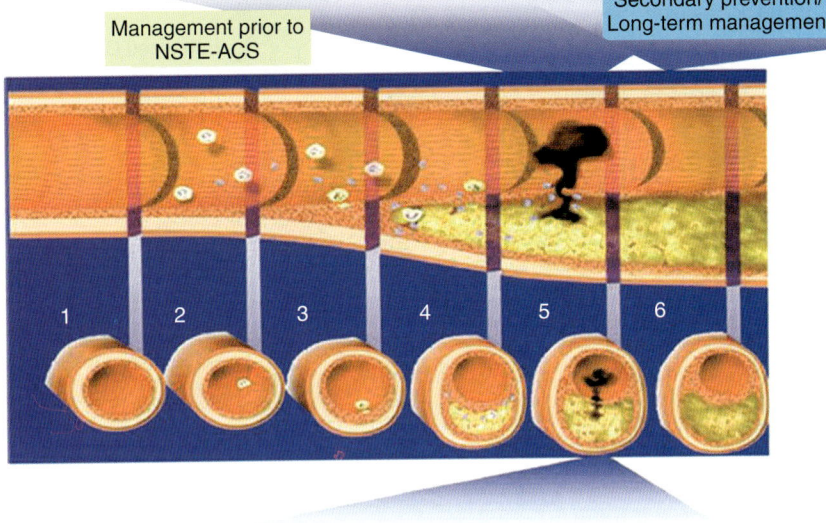

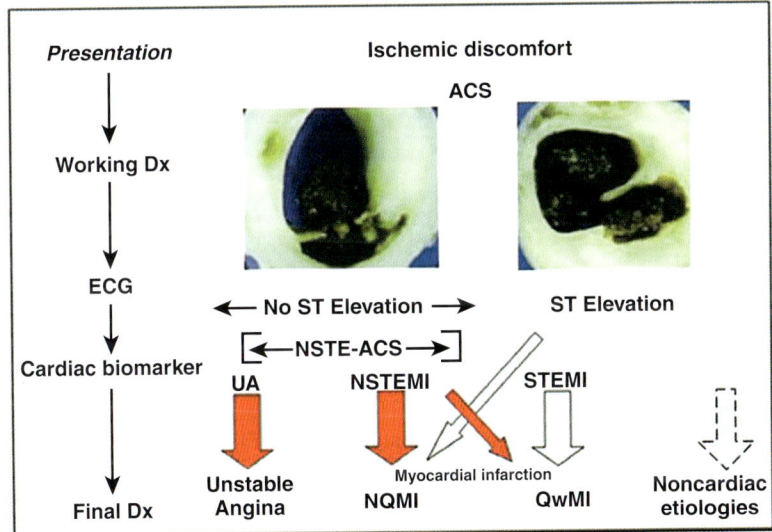

FIGURE 39.1 Acute coronary syndrome. *Top:* Progression of plaque formation and onset and complications of NSTE-ACS. The numbered section of an artery depicts atherogenesis from (1) normal artery to (2) extracellular lipid to (3) fibrofatty stage to (4) procoagulant expression and weakening of the fibrous cap. ACS develops with (5) disruption of the fibrous cap, which is the stimulus for thrombogenesis. (6) Thrombus resorption may be followed by collagen accumulation and smooth muscle cell growth. Thrombus formation reduces blood flow in the affected coronary artery and causes ischemic chest pain. *Bottom:* The clinical, pathologic, electrocardiographic, and biomarker correlates in ACS and approach to management. Flow reduction may be related to a completely occlusive thrombus or subtotally occlusive thrombus. Most patients with ST elevation *(thick white arrow in bottom panel)* develop Q wave myocardial infarction (QwMI), and a few *(thin white arrow)* develop non–Q wave myocardial infarction (NQMI). Those without ST elevation have either UA or NSTEMI *(thick red arrows)*, a distinction based on cardiac biomarkers. Most patients presenting with NSTEMI develop NQMI; a few may develop QwMI. CPG, Clinical practice guideline; *Dx*, diagnosis. (From Amsterdam E, et al. 2014 ACC/AHA Non-ST-Segment Elevation ACS Guideline. J Am Coll Cardiol. 2014;64(24):e139–e228, and Libby P. Current concepts of the pathogenesis of the acute coronary syndromes. Circulation 2001;104:365–372.)

in matrix are more prone to erosion[7] and are increasingly common. In addition, plaque rupture leads to fibrin-rich red thrombi; plaque erosion is associated with white platelet-rich thrombi. Whether this distinction has therapeutic implications is an area of ongoing investigation. Vasoconstriction causing dynamic obstruction of coronary arterial flow may result from spasm of epicardial coronary arteries (Prinzmetal's vasospastic angina [see later]) or from constriction of small, intramural muscular coronary arteries. The latter may result from vasoconstrictors released by platelets, from endothelial dysfunction, adrenergic stimuli, cold temperature, cocaine, or amphetamines (see later). More than one of these mechanisms may operate simultaneously.

Activation of the coagulation cascade and of platelets play central roles in the formation of thrombus following plaque disruption or erosion (see Chapter 95). The key steps in thrombus formation include (1) *adhesion* of platelets to the arterial wall, (2) platelet *activation*, (3) platelet degranulation and *further activation*, and (4) parallel expression of tissue factor with *activation of the coagulation cascade*.

Four observations support the central role of coronary artery thrombosis in the pathogenesis of NSTE-ACS: (1) autopsy findings of thrombi in the coronary arteries typically localized to a ruptured or eroded atherosclerotic plaque; (2) visualization by optical coherence tomography (OCT), invasive coronary arteriography, or coronary computed tomographic angiography (CCTA) of plaque ulceration and/or irregularities in the fibrous cap of atherosclerotic plaque, consistent with plaque rupture and thrombus formation; (3) elevation of serum markers of platelet activity, thrombin generation, and fibrin formation; and (4) improvement in clinical outcome with antiplatelet and anticoagulant therapies.

CLINICAL ASSESSMENT

History

NSTE-ACS resulting from atherosclerosis is relatively uncommon in men <40 years and women <50 in the absence of genetic disorders such as familial hypercholesterolemia, but the incidence rises steadily thereafter. Patients with ACS frequently have traditional risk factors for coronary artery disease (CAD) (see Chapters 25 and 27). However, while coronary risk factors reliably assess risk in populations, they are less helpful in the assessment of individual patients.

The initial symptom of NSTE-ACS is typically described as retrosternal pressure, heaviness, or frank pain, and although it resembles stable exertional angina, it is usually more intense and lasts longer (>10 minutes). Radiation to the ulnar aspect of the upper left arm, either shoulder, the neck, or the jaw is common, but symptoms may localize anywhere between the ear and epigastrium.[8] Diaphoresis, nausea, abdominal pain, dyspnea, and syncope may accompany the discomfort. Features that support the diagnosis include exacerbation of symptoms by physical exertion and precipitation by severe anemia, infection, inflammation, fever, or metabolic or endocrinologic (e.g., thyroid) disorders. Atypical manifestations, such as dyspnea without chest discomfort and pain limited to the epigastrium or indigestion, represent "anginal equivalents." These atypical findings are more prevalent in women, older adults, and patients with diabetes mellitus (DM), CKD, or dementia and can lead to under recognition, undertreatment, and worse outcomes ("chest pain that is pleuritic, positional, or described as "stabbing" is generally not caused by myocardial ischemia. The clinical manifestations may appear suddenly, with severe, new-onset symptoms occurring during minimal exertion (Canadian Cardiovascular Society Class [CCSC] III) or at rest (CCSC IV), an accelerating pattern of angina (more frequent, more intense, longer lasting), or angina occurring shortly after a completed MI.[9]

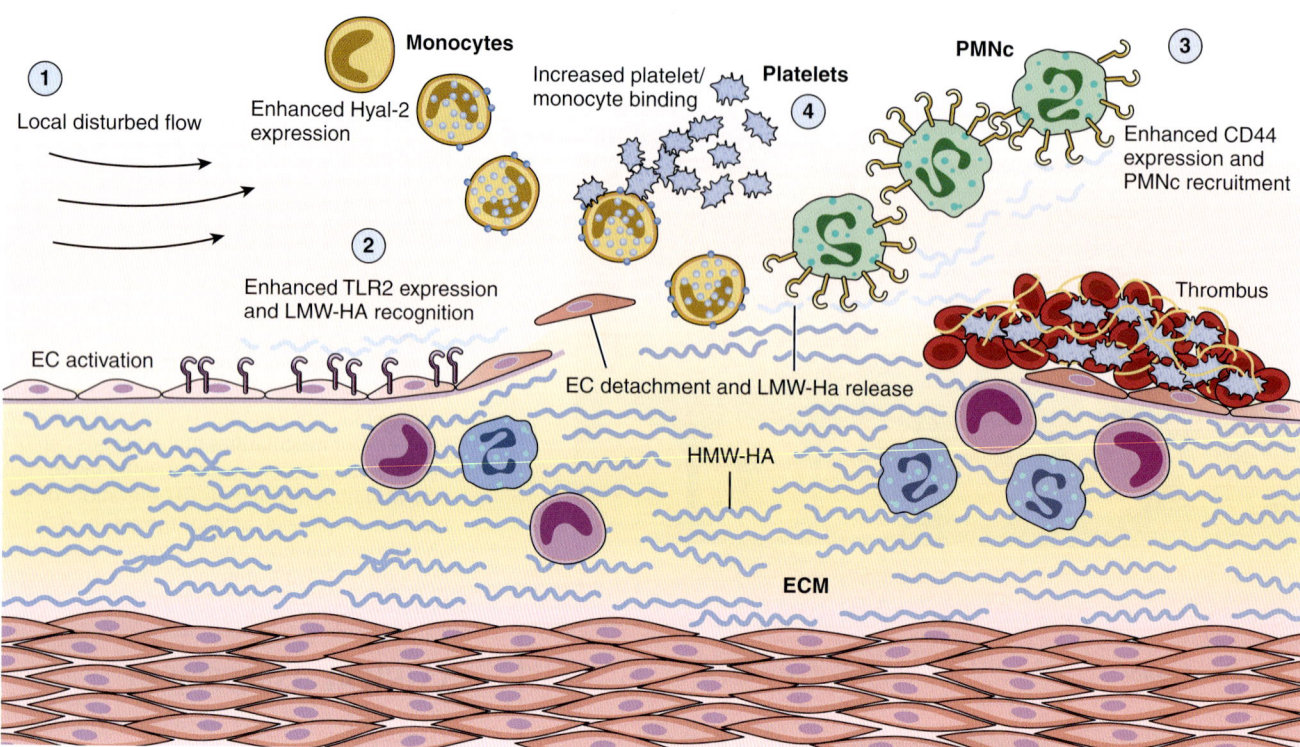

FIGURE 39.2 **Model of plaque erosion.** The driving hypothesis that derives from postmortem studies on plaque erosion. Overexpression of hyaluronidase 2 (Hyal-2) in peripheral blood mononuclear cells (membrane, cytoplasm, and nuclei) under conditions of increased shear stress (1) leads to degradation of high-molecular-weight hyaluronan to proinflammatory low-molecular-weight hyaluronan, which, in turn, promotes endothelial activation and detachment via TLR3 stimulation (2), as well as neutrophil recruitment (3), the latter amplified by overexpression of CD44, which is necessary for adhesion of neutrophils to low-molecular-weight hyaluronan. Finally, low-molecular-weight hyaluronan induces increased platelet-monocyte binding, thus promoting thrombus formation (4). Inflammatory cells are found in the intima, close to the site of erosion (T cells in green and foam cells). *EC*, Endothelial cell; *ECM*, extracellular matrix; *HA*, hyaluronan; *HMW-HA*, high-molecular-weight hyaluronan; *LMW-HA*, low-molecular-weight hyaluronan; *PBMC*, peripheral blood mononuclear cell; *PMNc*, polymorphonuclear cell. (From Pedicino D, et al. Alterations of hyaluronan metabolism in acute coronary syndrome: implications for plaque erosion. J Am Coll Cardiol 2018;72:1490–1503.)

TABLE 39.1 **Main Characteristics of Plaque Rupture and Superficial Erosion**

PLAQUE RUPTURE	PLAQUE EROSION
Lipid rich	Lipid poor
Collagen poor, thin fibrous cap	Proteoglycan and glycosaminoglycan rich
Interstitial collagen breakdown	Nonfibrillar collagen breakdown
Abundant inflammation	Few inflammatory cells
Smooth muscle cell apoptosis	Endothelial cell apoptosis
Macrophage predominance	Secondary neutrophil involvement
Less expression of hyaluronidase-2 and of the hyaluronan-receptor CD44	Profound alteration of hyaluronan metabolism resulting in hyaluronan accumulation
Larger number of nonculprit plaques and greater panvascular instability	Smaller number of nonculprit plaques and less panvascular instability
Male predominance	Female predominance
High level of low-density lipoprotein cholesterol	High level of triglycerides

Modified from Libby P, Pasterkamp G. Requiem for the "vulnerable plaque." Eur Heart J 2015;36:2984–2987.

Physical Examination

The physical examination may be normal, although patients with large territories of myocardial ischemia may have audible third and/or fourth heart sounds or pulmonary rales. Rarely, hypotension, pale cool skin, sinus tachycardia, or frank cardiogenic shock can occur; these findings are much more common with STEMI than with NSTE-ACS. Potential precipitating causes of ACS, such as fever, resistant or inadequately treated hypertension, tachycardia, profound bradycardia, thyroid disease, and gastrointestinal (GI) bleeding, can sometimes be identified. Pulse deficits, tachypnea, and tachycardia in the presence of clear lung fields and pulsus paradoxus with jugular venous distention may lead to alternative life-threatening diagnoses, such as aortic dissection, pulmonary embolism, or cardiac tamponade.

Electrocardiography

The most common abnormalities on the 12-lead ECG are ST-segment depression and T wave inversion, which are more likely to be present while the patient is symptomatic. If possible, comparison with a recent ECG is important because dynamic ST-segment depression as little as 0.05 mV is a sensitive (but not specific) marker for NSTE-ACS. Deep (>0.2 mV) T wave inversions are compatible with, but not necessarily diagnostic of, NSTE-ACS, whereas isolated T wave inversions of lesser magnitude are not particularly helpful given their low specificity. When present in patients with established NSTE-ACS, new T wave abnormalities are strongly associated with myocardial edema on T2-weighted images on MRI.[10] Dynamic ST and T wave changes that are associated with clinical symptoms in patients with an elevated cTn may be helpful in identifying acute MI, although myocardial injury due to myocarditis or Takotsubo cardiomyopathy may mimic these changes[3] (see later). Greater degrees of ST-segment depression predict poorer outcomes. Transient ST-segment elevation lasting less than 20 minutes occurs in up to 10% of patients and suggests either UA or coronary vasospasm.

More than half of patients with NSTE-ACS may have normal or nondiagnostic ECGs. Because ischemia may occur in a territory that is not

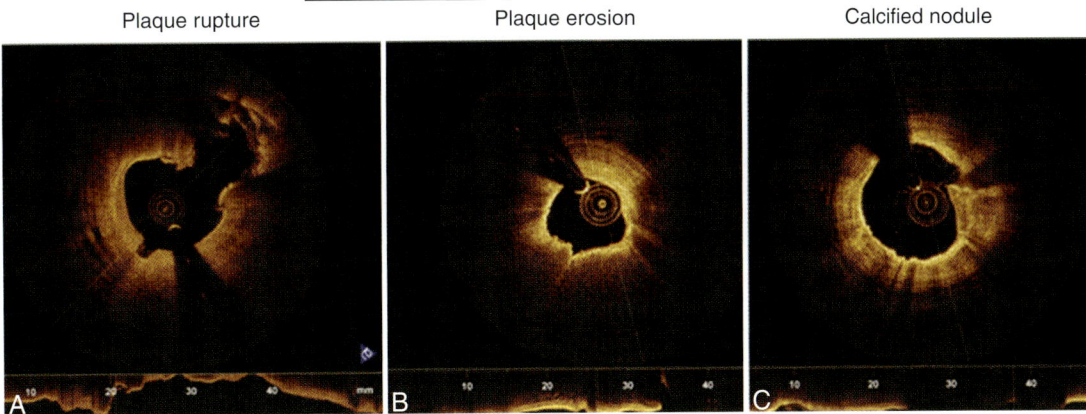

FIGURE 39.3 Representative optical coherence tomography images of underlying plaque. **A,** Plaque rupture. **B,** Plaque erosion. **C,** Calcified nodule. **A,** Plaque rupture of a necrotic core with an overlying thin-ruptured cap represents the most frequent pathophysiologic process leading to an acute coronary syndrome. **B,** Plaque erosion with a thrombus in direct contact with an intimal plaque that is rich in smooth muscle cells and proteoglycan matrix is shown. **C,** The least common plaque morphology is the calcified nodule, which is a heavily calcified plaque with a surrounding area of fibrosis. There are breaks in the calcified plate of the plaque with bone formation and interspersed fibrin, with a disrupted fibrous cap and overlying thrombus. A calcified nodule as the basis of an acute coronary syndrome is more common in older men than in women or younger patients. *mm,* millimeters; *sec,* seconds. (From Eisen A, et al. Updates on acute coronary syndrome: a review. JAMA Cardiol 2016;1:718–730; images provided by Ik-Kyung Jang, MD, PhD, Massachusetts General Hospital, Boston.)

well represented on the standard 12-lead ECG (see later), or because the patient may have episodic ischemia that is missed on the initial ECG, tracings should be repeated every 20 to 30 minutes until the symptoms resolve, or the diagnosis of MI is established or excluded.

Patients with baseline conduction disturbances and paced rhythms represent particular challenges for diagnosing myocardial ischemia by ECG. Comparison with a prior tracing when the patient was asymptomatic and recording an ECG with the pacing function temporarily switched off (in patients who are not pacemaker dependent) may be helpful.

Coronary angiography identifies a culprit lesion in the circumflex coronary artery in one-third of patients with high-risk NSTE-ACS. Because the standard 12-lead ECG does not represent the territory supplied by the circumflex coronary artery well, assessment of posterior leads V_7 through V_9 (with the gain increased to 20 mm/mV) should be considered in patients with a history suggestive of ACS and a nondiagnostic initial ECG. Similarly, ACS caused by isolated involvement of an acute marginal branch of the right coronary artery is often not apparent on the standard 12-lead ECG but may be suspected from leads V_3R and V_4R. Therefore, it is useful to obtain these extra leads in patients suspected of having ACS but with normal findings on a 12-lead ECG. Continuous monitoring of the ECG in the days following NSTE-ACS can identify patients at higher risk for recurrent events. ST-segment depressions noted on such monitoring within the first week after NSTE-ACS are associated with an increased risk for reinfarction and death.

Laboratory Testing: Biomarkers

A number of biomarkers reflecting the diverse causes of NSTE-ACS are useful for prognostication. These include markers of myocyte necrosis, hemodynamic stress, vascular damage (particularly renovascular), acceleration of atherosclerosis, and inflammation (Fig. 39.4). Cardiac-specific troponins I (cTnI) and T (cTnT) are the biomarkers of choice to identify myocardial injury, thus distinguishing between NSTE-ACS and UA. Because the sensitivities of different Tn assays in clinical practice vary, the consensus recommendation is to define injury by an elevation in cTnI or cTnT >99th percentile of the normal range of the specific assay used,[3,11] with a typical temporal rise and fall indicating acute injury (Fig. 39.5). The diagnosis of acute MI is appropriate in patients with acute MI and a clinical presentation and/or ECG findings consistent with ACS. However, a number of other cardiac and systemic causes may lead to myocardial injury (Table 39.2); these can be distinguished from acute MI depending on the clinical context and information from imaging studies.

As high-sensitivity troponin (hsTn) assays[11] that can detect ultralow concentrations of troponin in approximately >90% of healthy individuals become increasingly available, consideration of the clinical context of a troponin elevation will become even more important in avoiding misdiagnosis and improper triage in patient management. Noncardiac factors such as anemia, hypoxemia, kidney disease, shock, and CV conditions (e.g., heart failure [HF], tachyarrhythmia) may lead to myocardial injury in the absence of acute MI (see Chapter 36).

The assessment of patients with suspected ACS begins with integration of the cTn results at presentation with the clinical assessment and ECG findings. New hsTn assays can permit exclusion of acute MI with

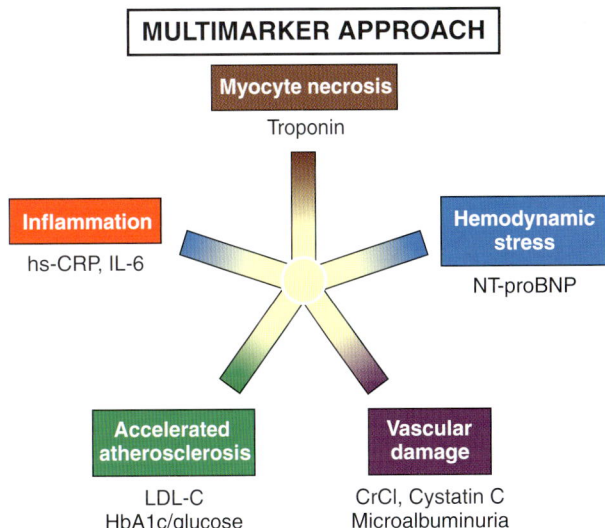

Biomarker	Independent predictor of risk	Useful as a component in a multimarker strategy	Therapeutic implication
Troponin	+++	++	+++
NT-proBNP	+++	++	+
LDL-C	+++	+++	+++
Renal dysfunction	++	+	+
HgbA1c/glucose	+	0	+
hs-CRP	++	++	++

FIGURE 39.4 Multimarker approach for risk stratification in ACSs. Glucose metabolism: hyperglycemia or elevated glycated hemoglobin (HbA$_{1c}$). *CrCl,* creatinine clearance; *GDF15,* Growth differentiation factor 15; *hs-CRP,* high-sensitivity C-reactive protein; *IL-6,* interleukin-6; *LDL-C,* low density lipoprotein cholesterol *NT-proBNP,* N-terminal brain natriuretic peptide. (Modified from Morrow DA, Braunwald E. Future of biomarkers in acute coronary syndromes. Circulation 2003;108:250.)

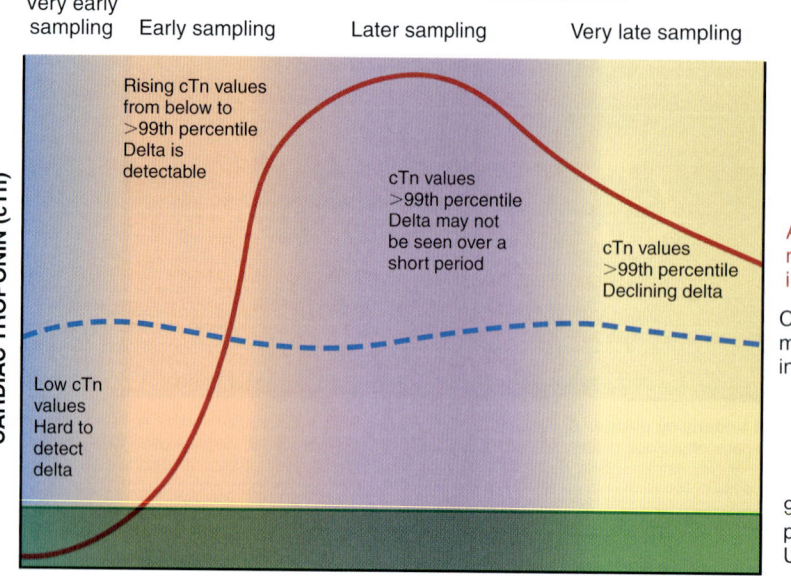

FIGURE 39.5 The timing of biomarker release into the circulation is dependent on blood flow and how soon after the onset of symptoms samples are obtained. Thus the ability to consider small changes as diagnostic can be problematic. Many comorbidities increase cTn values and, in particular, high-sensitivity cardiac troponin (hs-cTn) values, so that elevations can be present at baseline even in those with MI who present early after symptom onset. Changes in cTn values or deltas can be used to define acute compared with chronic events, and the ability to detect these is indicated in the figure. Increased cTn values can often be detected for days after an acute event. *URL*, Upper reference limit. (From Thygesen K, et al. Fourth universal definition of myocardial infarction. J Am Coll Cardiol 2018;72:2231–2249.)

a single measurement in patients with symptom onset >3 hours before presentation or with two measurements performed at presentation and 1 hour later (the so-called "0/1" approach) in patients who present within 3 hours of symptom onset. In such patients both the absolute and the change in hsTn concentration from hour 0 to hour 1 should be considered. In both scenarios, the cut points for absolute and change in cTn used are assay specific.

With serial measurements of hsTn at 0/1 hours, 60% of patients presenting to the emergency department (ED) with acute chest pain were ruled out MI with 100% sensitivity and negative predictive value (NPV).[12] This allows for more rapid discharge from the ED and high specificity and positive predictive value for MI (97% and 84%, respectively). Large independent validation studies in patients presenting to the ED demonstrated NPVs of 99.1% to 100%[13] with a 0/1 hour approach using hsTn. Some patients with intermediate absolute and/or change in hsTn at 1 hour may require an additional hsTn at 3 hours. A comparison of accelerated diagnostic protocols to rule-in or rule-out MI are shown in Table 39.3.[14]

Studies comparing a 0/1 with 0/3 hour algorithms concluded that the 0/1 hour was preferable as it provided a more favorable combination of safety (NPV) with diagnostic accuracy.[15,16] In some high-risk subgroups (e.g., elderly, CKD) the specificity of hsTn is substantially lower, and thus slightly higher cutoff concentrations may be needed.[15,16] The HEART (*H*istory, *E*CG, *A*ge, *R*isk factors, and *T*roponin) pathway is an algorithm that combines a clinical score with a serial troponin and identified 31% of patients as low risk with an NPV of 99.6% for 30-day death or MI.[17] Prognostication can be improved by use of a multimarker approach or coronary imaging with CCTA for patients at low-intermediate likelihood, or by invasive coronary angiography in patients with high clinical suspicion for MI. It is not recommended to measure additional biomarkers of necrosis (creatine kinase, creatine kinase myocardial band, fatty acid binding protein, or copeptin) in addition to hsTn.[18]

Several other biomarkers may be useful in estimating prognosis and helping to guide care. Of these, the natriuretic peptides (NPs; i.e., brain natriuretic peptide [BNP] and N-terminal pro-BNP) have been most widely used and endorsed by guidelines.[18] NPs rise in proportion to the degree of ventricular distention (strain) and correlate with the risk of adverse events, including death, HF, and MI, in a graded fashion. More importantly, elevation of a baseline NP identifies patients who are more likely to benefit from more intensive anti-ischemic and lipid-lowering regimens as well as early coronary revascularization.

Similarly, high-sensitivity C-reactive protein (hs-CRP), a marker of inflammation, is elevated following NSTE-ACS, and the degree of elevation correlates with long-term CV outcomes.[19] In addition, serials increases in hs-CRP may identify patients with NSTE-ACS who require more intensive management of risk factors (e.g., lipids, glucose, blood pressure (BP), and weight) and/or targeted anti-inflammatory therapy.[20] Growth differentiation factor (GDF)-15 independently predicted death and CV events when added to a model that included clinical risk factors and left ventricular ejection fraction (EF), both early and late (5 years median follow-up) after ACS.[21]

Multimarker approaches (e.g., simultaneous assessment of hsTn, hs-CRP, BNP, GDF-15, and cystatin-C) as well as serial assessments of hsTn and hs-CRP[18] can improve risk stratification of patients with NSTE-ACS.[22] While lipid measurements are less helpful for individual prognostication, assessment of the low-density lipoprotein cholesterol (LDL-C) and triglycerides, along with glucose or hemoglobin (Hb) A_{1c}, can identify uncontrolled risk factors that, with proper management, could reduce the risk of future CV events. Assessments of arterial oxygenation, hematocrit, and thyroid function may identify treatable conditions that can cause secondary ACS.

IMAGING

Noninvasive Testing

Noninvasive testing in patients with established or suspected NSTE-ACS has been shown to play several important roles: (1) establishing the presence (or absence) of significant CAD, (2) diagnosing CAD as the cause of cTn elevation in patients who may have other explanations (see previous section), (3) evaluating the extent of residual ischemia after initiation of medical therapy to guide management, (4) localizing the territory of ischemia before revascularization in patients with multivessel disease, and (5) assessing left ventricular (LV) function.

The safety of early stress testing in patients with NSTE-ACS has been debated, but symptom-limited or pharmacologic stress testing appears to be safe after at least 24 hours of stabilization without symptoms of active ischemia or other signs of hemodynamic or electrical instability. For most patients, electrocardiographic exercise stress testing is recommended if the ECG at rest lacks significant baseline abnormalities (e.g., ST depressions, bundle-branch block, electronic pacing) (see Chapter 69). If significant baseline ECG abnormalities are present, stress perfusion or echocardiographic imaging should be performed before and immediately after exercise. In patients who cannot achieve a significant workload during exercise, pharmacologic stress testing with imaging is recommended. Exercise stress myocardial perfusion imaging with nuclear isotopes and stress echocardiography with dobutamine have greater sensitivity than electrocardiographic exercise stress testing without imaging (see Chapters 14, 16 and 18). High-risk findings on the stress test (e.g., severe ischemia as reflected by ST-segment depression ≥0.2 mV before stage 3, hypotension with exercise, ventricular tachyarrhythmia, new or worsening LV dysfunction) are indications to proceed rapidly with coronary angiography with the intent to perform coronary revascularization, if possible.

TABLE 39.2 Reasons for the Elevation of Cardiac Troponin Values Because of Myocardial Injury

Myocardial Injury Related to Acute Myocardial Ischemia

Atherosclerotic plaque disruption with thrombosis

Myocardial Injury Related to Acute Myocardial Ischemia Because of Oxygen Supply/Demand Imbalance

Reduced myocardial perfusion:
- Coronary artery spasm, microvascular dysfunction
- Coronary embolism
- Coronary artery dissection
- Hypotension or shock
- Respiratory failure
- Severe anemia
- Sustained bradyarrhythmia

Increased myocardial oxygen demand:
- Severe hypertension with or without left ventricular hypertrophy
- Sustained tachyarrhythmia

Other Causes of Myocardial Injury
- Cardiac contusion
- Cardiac procedure other than revascularization (e.g., ablation, pacing, cardioversion, or endomyocardial biopsy)
- Cardiomyopathy (any type)
- Catheter ablation
- Coronary revascularization procedure
- Defibrillator shocks
- Heart failure
- Myocarditis
- Takotsubo syndrome
- Valvular heart disease (e.g., aortic stenosis)

Systemic conditions:
- Aortic dissection
- Chemotherapeutic agents (e.g., doxorubicin, %-fluorouracil, Herceptin)
- Chronic kidney disease
- Critically ill patients
- Hypo- and hyperthyroidism
- Infiltrative diseases (e.g., amyloidosis, hemochromatosis, sarcoidosis, scleroderma)
- Poisons or toxins (e.g., snake venom)
- Pulmonary embolism, pulmonary hypertension
- Renal dysfunction
- Rhabdomyolysis (e.g., with extreme endurance efforts)
- Sepsis
- Strenuous exercise
- Stroke, subarachnoid hemorrhage

From Thygesen K, et al. Fourth universal definition of myocardial infarction. J Am Coll Cardiol 2018;72:2231–2264; and Collet J-P, et al. 2020 ESC Guideline for the management of acute coronary syndromes in patients presenting without persistent ST-segment elevation. Eur Heart J 2020;42(14):1289–1367.

---

which vessel(s) have obstruction, and (3) assist in risk stratification and prognosis (see Chapter 20). Three large randomized trials have shown that CCTA compared with standard evaluation (which could include functional and imaging studies other than CCTA) expedites the triage of patients presenting with chest discomfort in the ED, thereby shortening length of stay.[23] Additional benefits include reductions in costs and of return visits to the ED. A randomized trial comparing standard of care with or without CCTA in patients with suspected angina demonstrated that CCTA better clarified the diagnosis of angina due to CAD, reduced the need for stress testing, but increased the use of coronary angiography.[24] These studies and others led to Class 1 recommendations to use of CCTA in the ED in patients with chest discomfort and suspected ACS who are at low risk at presentation[18,25] (Table 39.4). Some studies have suggested that CCTA may improve risk stratification in patients in whom hsTn levels do not conclusively rule MI in or out.[25]

The benefits of CCTA may extend beyond the ED, permitting more rapid and accurate identification of high-risk patients who may benefit from early, intensive therapies, including invasive coronary angiography and revascularization.[24]

Cardiac magnetic resonance (CMR) imaging using a rapid-scan protocol can provide precise measurements of ventricular volumes and function, detect and assess ventricular wall edema, identify areas of infarcted versus viable hibernating myocardium, establish the presence of myocardial perfusion, quantify wall motion, and identify myocardium at risk in patients with NSTE-ACS (see Chapter 19). Addition of high-resolution late gadolinium enhanced imaging can help provide this information when CMR alone is inconclusive. Detailed assessments by noninvasive cardiac imaging can help guide coronary revascularization in several common clinical scenarios, such as when the stenosis is of borderline significance, the culprit lesion is uncertain because of multivessel disease, or when myocardial viability in a territory at risk requires clarification.

Invasive Imaging

Invasive coronary angiography has been the standard technique for imaging the coronary arterial tree for nearly six decades. The culprit lesion in NSTE-ACS typically exhibits an eccentric stenosis with scalloped or overhanging edges and a narrow neck (see Chapter 21). These angiographic findings may represent disrupted atherosclerotic plaque or thrombus. Features suggesting thrombus include globular intraluminal masses with a rounded or polypoid shape; "haziness" of a lesion suggests the presence of thrombus, but this finding is not specific.

Approximately 90% of patients with a clinical diagnosis of NSTE-ACS have significant coronary obstruction, i.e., >50% stenosis of luminal diameter in at least one major coronary artery.[26] Most have obstructive disease in multiple epicardial arteries (approximately 10% have left main [LM] CAD) often accompanied by multivessel CAD. Among patients without LM disease, about 35% have three-vessel disease, and 25% two-vessel disease, whereas only approximately 20% have single-vessel disease. The remaining 10% have no significant coronary obstruction, a finding that is more common in women and minorities than in white men.[26] In such patients, NSTE-ACS may be related to microvascular coronary obstruction, endothelial dysfunction, or coronary artery spasm and may have a more favorable prognosis. In 37,101 patients enrolled in eight clinical trials of NSTE-ACS, the 30-day rate of death or MI was 2.2% in those with no obstructive CAD compared with 13.3% in patients with obstructive disease.[26]

Intravascular ultrasound (IVUS) and OCT are two invasive cross-sectional imaging techniques that can provide details regarding plaque morphology (see Fig. 39.3). In the clinical setting, IVUS or OCT are used most commonly to guide coronary stent placement (see Chapter 41). These techniques and others (e.g., near-infrared spectroscopy, intravascular CMR, angioscopy) can provide detailed plaque morphology and establish the pathophysiologic etiology of ACS, although the clinical utility of such additional information is uncertain.

Echocardiography (see Chapters 14 and 16) is useful in the assessment of LV systolic and diastolic function and can also identify left atrial dilation, functional mitral regurgitation, tricuspid annular plane systolic excursion, diastolic dysfunction, ventricular mechanical dyssynchrony, and ultrasound "lung comets" (extravascular lung fluid observed on thoracic ultrasound scanning). Each of these is associated with an adverse prognosis in patients with NSTE-ACS.

CCTA in patients with or suspected of having NSTE-ACS can help to (1) recognize or exclude the presence of epicardial CAD, (2) identify

TABLE 39.3 Summary of hsTn Rapid Rule-Out and Rule-In Accelerated Diagnostic Panels

	0/3 h	HIGH STEACS	0/2 h	0/1 h
Rule-Out Criteria				
hs-cTnT	<14 ng/L at 0 and 3 h* and GRACE score <140	NA	<14 ng/L at 0 and 2 h and Δ <4 ng/L	<12 ng/L at 0 and 1 h Δ <3 ng/L
hs-cTnI†	<26 ng/L at 0 and 3 h* and GRACE score <140	<5 ng/L at 0 h or a 3-h value: <16 ng/L in women <34 ng/L in men and Δ <3 ng/L	<6 ng/L at 0 and 2 h and Δ <2 ng/L	<5 ng/L at 0 and 1 h Δ <2 ng/L
NPV for MI	98.3%–100%	99.5%	99.4%–99.9%	98.9%–100%
Sensitivity for MI	98.9%–100%	97.7%	96.0%–99.6%	96.7%–100%
Proportion ruled out	39.8%–49.1%	74.2%	56.0%–77.8%	47.9%–64.2%
Rule-In Criteria				
hs-cTnT	>14 ng/L at 0 or 3 h	NA	≥53 ng/L at 0 h or ≥10 ng/L Δ at 2 h	≥52 ng/L at 0 h or 1 h Δ ≥ 5 ng/L
hs-cTnI	>26 ng/L at 0 or 3 h	>16 ng/L in women >34 ng/L in men at 0 or 3 h	≥64 ng/L at 0 h or ≥15 ng/L Δ at 2 h	≥52 ng/L at 0 h or 1 h Δ ≥ 6 ng/L
PPV for MI	72.0%–83.5%	59.5%	75.8%–85.0%	63.4%–84.0%
Specificity for MI	96.7%–98.2%	87.6%	95.2%–99.0%	93.8%–97%
Proportion ruled-in	9.7%–38.2%	22.0%	7.7%–16.7%	13.1%–23.0%

0/1h, accelerated diagnostic protocol to rule out MI in patients presenting >3 h from symptoms using a single hs-cTn measurement at presentation, whereas for other patients, an absolute hs-cTn at presentation and 1-h Δ are used to rule out or rule in MI or to place patients in an observational zone; *0/2h*, accelerated diagnostic protocol that uses maximal levels and absolute Δ hs-cTnI or T concentrations at 0 and 2 h to rule out or rule in MI or place patients in an observational zone; *0/3h*, accelerated diagnostic protocol that incorporates hs-cTn at 0 and 3 h, hs-cTn change, and time since pain onset to determine which patients are appropriate for discharge or stress testing versus invasive management; *GRACE*, Global Registry of Acute Coronary Events; *High STEACS*, High-Sensitivity Troponin in the Evaluation of Patients with Acute Coronary Syndrome; *hs-cTnI*, high-sensitivity cardiac troponin I; *hs-cTnT*, high-sensitivity cardiac troponin T; *NA*, not applicable; *NPV*, negative predictive value; *PPV*, positive predictive value.
*In patients with ≥6 h of pain, only a single value below this threshold is required.
†Abbott ARCHITECT hs-cTnI.
From Januzzi JL Jr, et al. Recommendations for Institutions Transitioning to High-Sensitivity Troponin Testing: JACC Scientific Expert Panel. J Am Coll Cardiol 2019;73:1059–1077.

RISK ASSESSMENT

Residual Risk

The risk for recurrent ischemic events following an episode of ACS depends as much on the presence and stability of multifocal lesions as on the culprit lesion responsible for the initial event. A new broad conceptual framework to address residual risk from atherosclerotic disease has been proposed that includes five domains: lipoproteins, inflammation, obesity and glucose metabolism, platelets, and coagulation.[27] Aggressive medical management targeting the domains that have not been optimized is required to treat the remaining plaques and prevent new ones, thus reducing the risk of recurrent events.

Natural History

Patients with UA have lower short-term mortality (<2.0% at 30 days) than do those with NSTEMI or STEMI. However, with the increasing use of hsTn, the fraction of patients with NSTE-ACS diagnosed with UA is declining.[3,28] The early mortality risk with NSTEMI is related to the extent of myocardial damage and resulting hemodynamic compromise and is lower than in patients with STEMI, who usually have larger infarcts. In an analysis of 66,252 patients with NSTEMI enrolled in 14 Thrombolysis in Myocardial Ischemia (TIMI) trials, 85% of the deaths in the first 30 days were CV, of which recurrent MI and HF were the most common causes.[29] After 30 days, sudden cardiac death (SCD) was the most common mode of CV death.

In contrast, patients with STEMI have higher rates of early mortality, while long-term outcomes with respect to both mortality and nonfatal events are worse in patients with NSTE-ACS. This finding probably results from the greater age, extent of CAD, history of a previous MI, comorbid condition (e.g., diabetes, impaired renal function), and likelihood of recurrence of ACS in patients with NSTE-ACS than in those with STEMI. In the aforementioned analysis of the TIMI trials, an analysis of causes of death after 30 days showed that CV deaths represented 70% of the total; sudden death (46%) was more than twice as common as any other CV cause.[29]

Risk Assessment Scores

Several risk scores that integrate clinical variables and findings on the ECG and from serum biomarkers have been developed for patients with NSTE-ACS.[30-32] The TIMI risk score for UA/NSTEMI identifies seven independent risk factors; their sum correlates directly with death or recurrent ischemic events[30] (Fig. 39.6A). This simple, rapid assessment at the initial evaluation identifies high-risk patients who can derive benefit from an early invasive strategy and more intensive antithrombotic therapy. The Global Registry of Acute Coronary Events (GRACE) risk score[32] uses a larger number of weighted risk factors to predict mortality after NSTE-ACS; however, it is more complex than the TIMI risk score and is not easily calculated by hand. For longer-term prognostication in patients following ACS, a risk score based on nine independent clinical predictors identifies a gradient of risk for recurrent atherothrombotic events called the TIMI stable ischemic CAD risk score[33] (see Fig. 39.6B). It distinguishes patients with greater absolute benefit with more intensive antithrombotic[33] and lipid-lowering therapies.[34] A risk score evaluated in 23,489 patients who survived hospitalization for ACS had excellent discrimination (c-statistic 0.80) to predict 2-year mortality using 17 variables, including quality-of-life, educational level, and geographic region in addition to typical CV risk factors. This score may be helpful for the identification of patients at higher risk and tailor secondary prevention measures.[35]

TABLE 39.4 Appropriateness of Coronary Computed Tomographic Angiography in Patients with Acute Chest Pain Syndromes

Appropriate Indications
- Electrocardiogram negative or indeterminate for myocardial ischemia
- Low-intermediate pretest likelihood by risk stratification tools
- TIMI risk score of 0-2 (low risk) ideal or TIMI score of 3-4 (intermediate) in some cases
- HEART score <3
- ≥1 negative troponin value, including point-of-care assays
- Equivocal or inadequate previous functional testing during index ED or within previous 6 months

Equivocal Indications
- High clinical likelihood of ACS by clinical assessment and standard risk criteria (e.g., TIMI score >4)
- Previously known coronary artery disease
- Known calcium score ≥400

Relative Contraindications
- History of allergic reaction to iodinated contrast
- eGFR 30 to <60 mL/min/1.73 m²
- Factors likely to lead to nondiagnostic scans; specific will vary with scanner technology and site capabilities
- Heart rate greater than site maximum for reliably diagnostic scans after beta blockers (usually 70-80 beats/min)
- Contraindications to beta blockers and heart rate not controlled
- Atrial fibrillation or other markedly irregular rhythm
- Body mass index >39 kg/m²

Absolute Contraindications
- Known acute coronary syndromes
- eGFR <30 unless on long-term dialysis
- Previous anaphylaxis after iodinated contrast administration
- Previous episode of contrast allergy after adequate steroid/antihistamine preparation
- Pregnancy or uncertain pregnancy status in premenopausal women

TIMI, Thrombolysis in myocardial infarction.
Modified from Hollander JE, et al. State-of-the-art evaluation of emergency department patients presenting with potential acute coronary syndromes. Circulation 2016;134:547–564.

MANAGEMENT

Management of patients with NSTE-ACS consists of an acute phase focused on relief of the clinical symptoms and stabilization of the culprit lesion(s) and a long-term phase that involves therapies directed at the prevention of disease progression and future plaque rupture/erosion. Retrospective angiographic studies and a prospective natural history study of patients with NSTE-ACS managed with PCI have shown that plaques that cause more severe stenosis have a higher risk of rupture leading to an ACS event. However, since plaques with less severe stenosis are more prevalent, these less obstructive lesions are responsible for about half of the future ACS events.

General Measures

Patients with new or worsening chest discomfort or an anginal equivalent symptom suggestive of ACS should be transported rapidly to the ED by ambulance, if possible, and evaluated immediately. The initial evaluation should include a directed history and physical examination and ECG performed within 10 minutes of arrival.[18] If possible, the ECG should be recorded in the ambulance. Blood specimens for cTn or, if possible, hsTn assay should be obtained immediately with expedited assessment through either a point-of-care device or laboratory measurement that can provide results within 60 minutes. Additional laboratory studies, such as a complete blood count, serum electrolytes, creatinine, and glucose, can help guide early management treatments and strategy.

Patients with elevated cTn or new ST-segment abnormalities or are deemed to be at moderate or high risk based on a validated risk score (e.g., TIMI, GRACE, see earlier) should be admitted to a specialized cardiovascular care unit. Patients with UA but without elevated cTn and ischemic electrocardiographic changes should be admitted to a monitored bed, preferably in a CV step-down unit.[8] In these settings, continuous ECG monitoring with telemetry is recommended for 24 hours or until revascularization[18] to detect tachyarrhythmias, alterations in atrioventricular (AV) and intraventricular conduction, and changes in ST-segment deviation. Patients should be placed on bed rest and inhaled oxygen in those patients with arterial oxygen saturation (SaO_2) less than 90% and/or those with HF and pulmonary rales. Routine oxygen in patients with suspected ACS without hypoxemia or HF is of unclear benefit.[36] Ambulation, as tolerated, is permitted if the patient has been stable without recurrent chest discomfort or ECG changes for at least 12 to 24 hours.

Anti-Ischemic Therapy

Guidelines emphasize the early use of anti-ischemic therapies to improve the balance between oxygen supply and demand.[8,18] The goals of anti-ischemic therapy include relief of symptoms and prevention of early sequelae of ACS, including recurrent MI, HF, arrhythmias, and death. Table 39.5 summarizes traditional and newer/experimental pharmacologic anti-ischemic therapies.

Nitrates

Nitrates are vasodilators that increase myocardial blood flow and reduce myocardial oxygen requirements by lowering cardiac preload (systemic venodilation) and afterload (systemic arterial dilation), thereby diminishing ventricular wall stress, and they may have a mild antiplatelet effect. Reflex increases in heart rate and myocardial contractility by nitrates that increase myocardial O_2 demand can be mitigated by concomitant use of a beta blocker. Well-controlled clinical trials have not shown a reduction in cardiac events with nitrates; however, the rationale for nitrate use in NSTE-ACS is extrapolated from pathophysiologic principles and extensive clinical observations demonstrating their clinical effectiveness in relief of pain or other discomfort caused by myocardial ischemia.

In symptomatic patients without hypotension, the initial administration of rapidly acting nitroglycerin (sublingual [SL] or buccal, 0.3 to 0.6 mg at 5-minute intervals), beginning before hospital arrival whenever possible, is recommended. Intravenous (IV) nitroglycerin (5 to 10 μg/min, titrated to a maximum of 200 μg/min as needed) should be initiated in patients with hypertension and in patients with persistent or recurrent ischemic symptoms or HF, provided that the systolic blood pressure (SBP) is at least 90 to 100 mm Hg. Tolerance to nitrates may develop within 12 to 24 hours and can be mitigated by nitrate-free intervals or increasing the dose if symptoms persist. Abrupt discontinuation of high doses of IV nitrates is not advised because it may precipitate recurrent ischemia and/or rebound hypertension; instead, IV nitrates should be weaned over several hours.

Important contraindications to nitrates include hypotension and use within 24 hours of a phosphodiesterase type 5 (PDE-5) inhibitor, sildenafil or vardenafil, or tadalafil within 48 hours. Since the catalytic site of PDE-5 normally degrades cyclic guanosine monophosphate, inhibitors of PDE-5 potentiate the endogenous levels of cyclic guanosine monophosphate, possibly resulting in exaggerated, prolonged, and dangerous vasodilatory effects of nitrates. Relative contraindications to nitrates include hypotension (SBP <90 mm Hg), severe obstruction to LV outflow, large right ventricular infarction, or hemodynamically significant pulmonary embolism. In such patients, nitrates should be used with caution, if at all.

Beta-Adrenergic Receptor–Blocking Agents

Beta blockers inhibit the O_2 oxygen consumption by lowering heart rate, BP, and myocardial contractility (see Chapters 38 and 40). They may be initiated intravenously for rapid onset, followed by long-term oral use. The evidence supporting beta blockers derives largely from older studies of patients with acute MI (generally STEMI) or new left bundle branch block, before the current era of reperfusion therapy. In

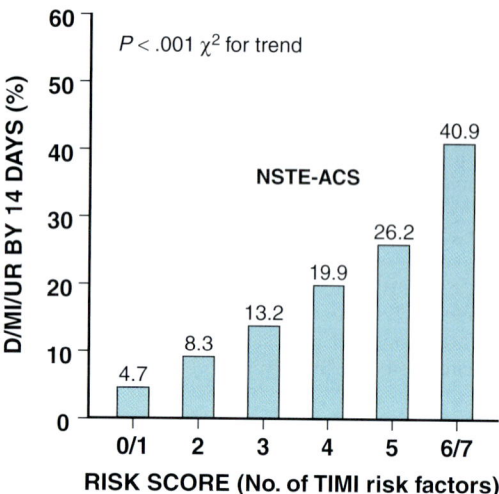
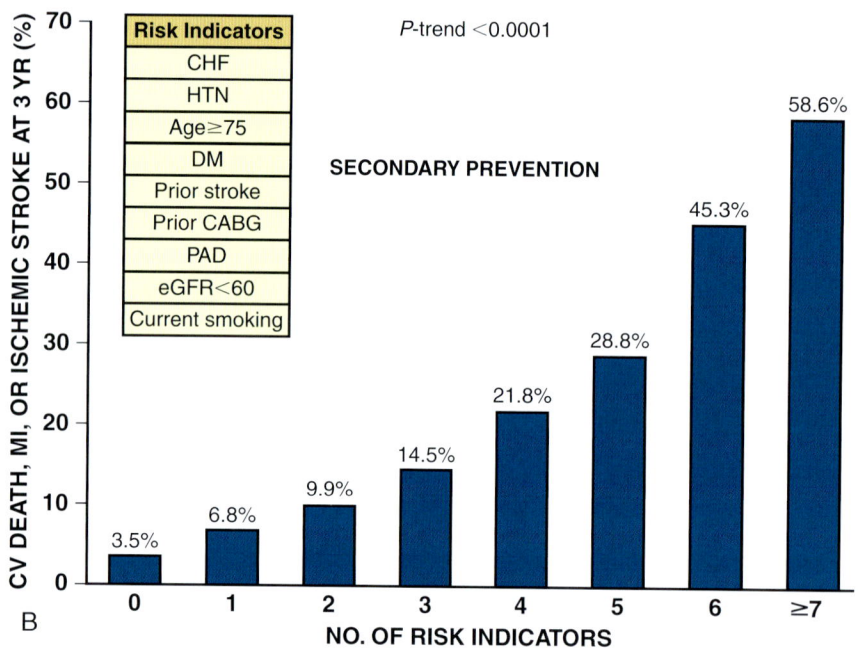

FIGURE 39.6 A, TIMI risk score for NSTE-ACS. The number of risk factors present is counted. **B,** TIMI risk score for secondary prevention Long-term risk stratification after MI. Nine independent factors when combined in a simple long-term risk score can identify a broad range of future risk of the composite of cardiovascular death, MI, or ischemic stroke. (**A** adapted from Antman EM, et al. The TIMI risk score for unstable angina/non-ST elevation MI: a method for prognostication and therapeutic decision making. JAMA 2000;284:835; **B** from Bohula EA, et al. Atherothrombotic risk stratification and the efficacy and safety of vorapaxar in patients with stable ischemic heart disease and prior myocardial infarction. Circulation 2016;134:304–313.)

clinical trials of patients with acute MI, both early IV administration and long-term oral beta blockers have been shown to reduce reinfarction, ventricular arrhythmias, and death.[37] The findings from these trials, most on patients with STEMI (see Chapter 38), have been extrapolated to patients with UA and NSTEMI.

A systematic review that pooled data on approximately 4700 patients with UA from five trials performed before 1986 showed that beta blockers reduced the risk for progression to MI.[38] Whether beta blockers would have similar efficacy in the modern era of intensive pharmacologic management with an early invasive strategy is unclear.

Intravenous Beta Blockers
If ischemia persists despite IV nitrate therapy, IV beta blockers (e.g., metoprolol 5 mg over 1 to 2 min, repeated every 5 min for a total initial dose of 15 mg) may be used cautiously, and generally followed by initiation of oral administration. Beta blockers should be avoided in patients with (1) acute or severe HF, (2) low cardiac output, (3) hypotension, (4) contraindications to beta blocker therapy (e.g., high-degree AV block, active bronchospasm), and (5) coronary vasospasm or acute intoxication with cocaine or methamphetamine because unopposed alpha-mediated coronary vasoconstriction may occur, worsening coronary spasm. IV beta blockers have been shown to increase mortality in patients with or at high risk for developing cardiogenic shock.[39]

Oral Beta Blockers
Oral beta blockers in doses used for chronic stable angina (e.g., metoprolol tartrate 25 mg every 6 hours; see Chapter 40) should be initiated within the first 24 hours in the absence of the previously mentioned scenarios.[8,18] Patients with initial contraindications to beta blockers should be reevaluated to determine subsequent eligibility to receive one of these agents. Beta blockers with intrinsic sympathomimetic activity (e.g., acebutolol, pindolol) should be avoided because they may increase the risk of ventricular tachycardia and fibrillation.

Morphine. If there is ongoing ischemic discomfort or pain despite treatment with maximally tolerated anti-ischemic medications (nitrates, beta blockers), in the absence of contraindications (e.g., hypotension, allergy, history of opiate addiction), it is reasonable to administer IV morphine (1 to 5 mg), with the caveat that morphine may slow intestinal absorption of oral platelet inhibitors. Data suggest that coadministration of morphine and clopidogrel may blunt the antiplatelet effect of clopidogrel and is associated with an increase short-term risk of ischemic events.[40] The morphine dose may be repeated every 5 to 30 minutes to relieve symptoms and maintain the patient's comfort. Morphine may act as both an analgesic and an anxiolytic; its venodilator effects may be beneficial by reducing preload (particularly in patients who have experienced acute pulmonary edema), and mildly reduces heart rate and BP by increasing vagal tone. Morphine may cause hypotension; supine positioning and IV saline may be used to restore BP. Naloxone (0.4 to 2.0 mg IV) may be administered for morphine overdose with respiratory or circulatory depression. In patients with morphine allergy, meperidine can be substituted.

Calcium Channel Blockers
Calcium channel blockers (CCBs) have vasodilatory effects and reduce arterial pressure. Some CCBs, such as verapamil and diltiazem, also slow heart rate, reduce myocardial contractility, thereby reducing myocardial oxygen requirements. CCBs have been effective in reducing ischemia in patients with NSTE-ACS and persistent ischemia despite treatment with full-dose nitrates and beta blockers, as well as in patients with contraindications to beta blockers and in patients with hypertension.[8,18] Such patients should receive nondihydropyridine CCBs that lower heart rate. The short-acting formulation of the dihydropyridine nifedipine, which

TABLE 39.5 Pharmacologic Anti-Ischemic Therapies in Non–ST Elevation Acute Coronary Syndromes

CLASS OF MEDICATION	MECHANISM OF ACTION	CLINICAL EFFECTS IN NSTE-ACS
Traditional Therapies		
Beta blockers	Decrease heart rate, blood pressure, and contractility through antagonism of beta$_1$ receptors	Decrease mortality[51]
Nitrates	Decrease preload through venodilation; vasodilate coronary arteries	No benefit on mortality
Calcium channel blockers	May vasodilate, reduce heart rate, or decrease contractility depending on specific drug	No clear benefit on mortality or reinfarction. Increased reinfarction rate when short-acting nifedipine is used alone
Newer and Experimental Therapies		
Ranolazine	Inhibits late inward sodium current	Decreases recurrent ischemia and arrhythmias
Trimetazidine	Shifts myocardial metabolism from fatty acid to glucose use	Decreases short-term mortality
Nicorandil	Activates ATP-sensitive K$^+$ channels and dilates arterioles; may have ischemic precondition-like effect	Decreases arrhythmias and transient ischemia

From Soukoulis V, et al. Nonantithrombotic medical options in acute coronary syndromes: old agents and new lines on the horizon. Circ Res 2014;114:1944–1958.

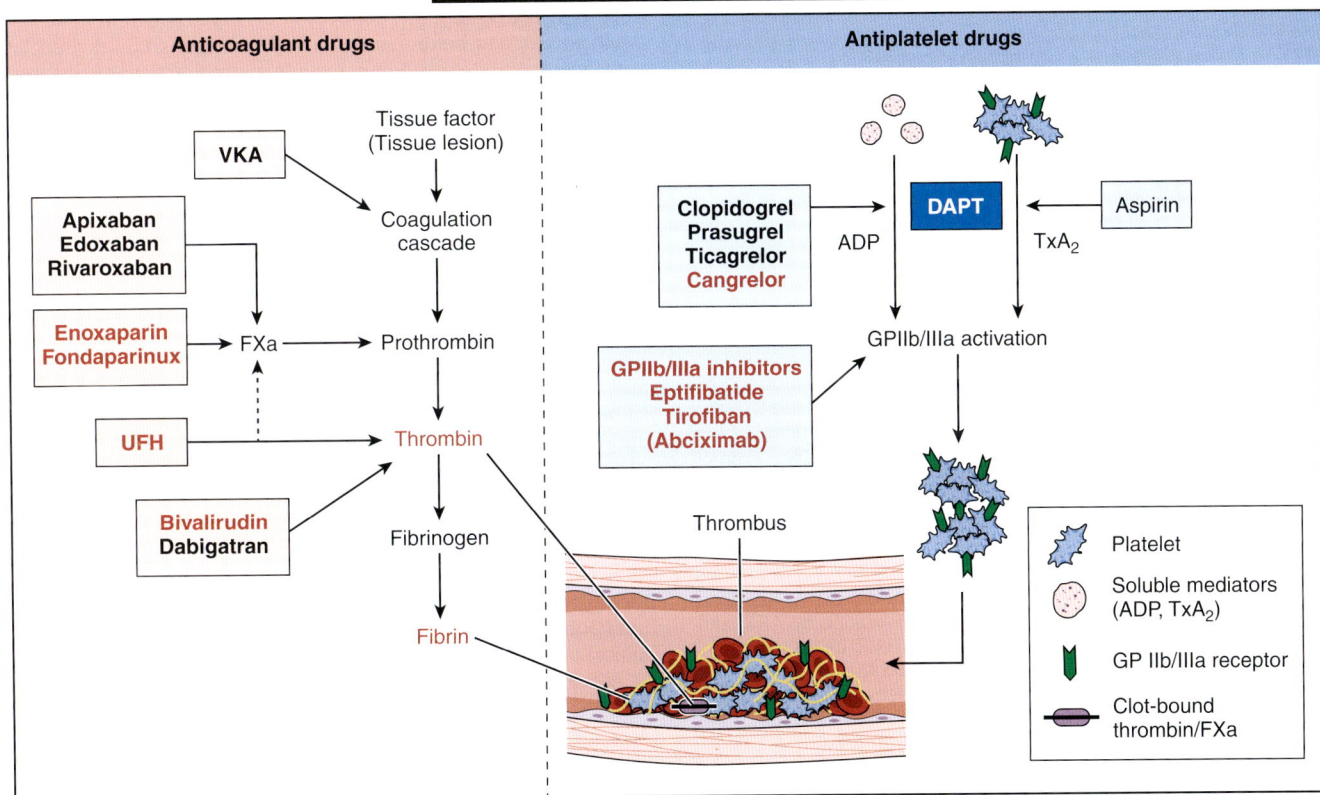

FIGURE 39.7 Antithrombotic treatments in non–ST-segment elevation acute coronary syndrome patients: pharmacologic targets. Drugs with oral administration are shown in black type and drugs with parenteral administration are in red. *FXA,* Factor Xa; *Tx,* thromboxane. (From Collet J-P, et al. 2020 ESC guidelines for the management of acute coronary syndromes in patients presenting without persistent ST-segment elevation. Eur Heart J 2020;42(14):1289–1367.)

accelerates heart rate, can cause harm in patients with ACS when not co-administered with a beta blocker and should be avoided. No harm has been observed with long-term treatment with the long-acting dihydropyridines, amlodipine and felodipine, in patients with documented LV dysfunction and CAD, suggesting that these agents may be safe in patients with NSTE ACS and LV dysfunction. However, use of dihydropyridines in the absence of beta blocker remains controversial in ACS.[41] Contraindications to nondihydropyridine CCBs include significant LV dysfunction, increased risk of cardiogenic shock, PR interval longer than 0.24 second, and high-degree AV block.

Antiplatelet Therapy (see Chapter 95)

See Fig. 39.7, Table 39.6.

Oral Antiplatelet Drugs

Aspirin (acetylsalicylic acid [ASA]) acetylates platelet cyclooxygenase 1 (COX-1), thereby blocking the synthesis and release of thromboxane A$_2$ (TxA$_2$), a platelet activator, and reducing platelet aggregation and arterial thrombus formation. Because the inhibition of COX-1 by ASA is irreversible, the antiplatelet effects last for the lifetime of the platelets, approximately 7 to 10 days. Several placebo-controlled trials have demonstrated the benefit of ASA in patients with NSTE-ACS.[42] In addition to reducing adverse clinical events in the first months of treatment, ASA also reduces the frequency of ischemic events in secondary prevention. It is a cornerstone of antiplatelet therapy in patients with all forms of ACS, as well as those with chronic CAD.

TABLE 39.6 Antithrombotic Therapy in Patients on Chronic Oral Anticoagulation Who Present with an NSTE-ACS

1. Aspirin: All patients should immediately receive aspirin (150 to 300 mg) oral loading dose (or 75 to 150 mg intravenously).
2. Parenteral anticoagulation before PCI:
   - UFH or enoxaparin preferred. Bivalirudin may be considered. Avoid fondaparinux.
   - Patients on VKA: Uninterrupted anticoagulation with VKA therapy is preferred, as interruption of VKA with use of bridging parenteral anticoagulation is associated with increased bleeding.
   - Patients on NOAC: Stop NOAC and start parenteral anticoagulation with UFH or LMWH, regardless of the timing of the last NOAC dose.
3. Anticoagulation during PCI:
   - If immediate PCI (<2 h from symptom onset), use low-dose intravenous anticoagulation, regardless of the last dose of oral anticoagulant. Options include UFH 60 IU/kg or enoxaparin 0.5 mg/kg intravenously.
   - For PCI >2 h from symptom onset:
     - Patients on VKA: Perform PCI without interruption of VKA if the INR is >2.5 without additional parenteral anticoagulation. Low-dose (if INR 2.0-2.5) or standard dose UFH or enoxaparin (if INR <2.0) may be used otherwise.
     - Patients on NOAC: Use additional intraprocedural low-dose parenteral anticoagulation, irrespective of timing of last dose of NOAC.
4. $P2Y_{12}$ inhibitors: To reduce the risk of bleeding, consider:
   - Postpone administration of $P2Y_{12}$ inhibitors until the coronary anatomy is known, and PCI is planned.
   - Use clopidogrel instead of ticagrelor or prasugrel.
5. GP IIb/IIIa inhibitors: avoid use unless for bail-out.
6. Stent selection: Do not use bioabsorbable vascular scaffolds due to a higher thrombotic risk and need for longer DAPT duration.

Even though doses of ASA have ranged from 50 to 1300 mg/day in randomized trials, there does not appear to be a dose-response effect on efficacy, but GI bleeding is increased at higher doses.[42] The CURRENT OASIS-7 trial[43] randomized patients with ACS to high-dose (300 to 325 mg/day) or low-dose (75 to 100 mg/day) ASA for 30 days (and to high-dose versus regular-dose clopidogrel; see later). No difference in the risk for CV death, MI, or stroke was observed between the two doses of ASA, but GI bleeding increased with the higher dose. Guidelines recommend that in patients with NSTE-ACS who have not been taking ASA, the initial loading dose should be 162 to 325 mg of non–enteric-coated ASA, followed by a maintenance dose of 75 to 100 mg daily.[44] Enteric-coated ASA should be avoided initially because it delays and reduces absorption. Most nonsteroidal anti-inflammatory drugs (NSAIDs) bind reversibly to COX-1, preventing this enzyme's inhibition by ASA, and may cause prothrombotic effects; thus NSAIDs should be avoided.

So-called ASA resistance may occur during chronic therapy, with 2% to 8% of patients exhibiting a limited antiplatelet effect resulting in a greater risk of recurrent cardiac events. Causes of ASA resistance are varied and include poor compliance (pseudoresistance), use of enteric-coated forms, reduced absorption, interaction with ibuprofen or other NSAIDs, and overexpression of COX-2 mRNA.

Contraindications to ASA include documented allergy (e.g., ASA-induced asthma), nasal polyps, active bleeding, or a known platelet disorder. Dyspepsia or other GI symptoms with long-term ASA therapy (i.e., ASA intolerance) do not usually preclude therapy in the short term. In patients who have an allergy to ASA, desensitization or substituting clopidogrel, prasugrel, or ticagrelor is recommended.[8] Clopidogrel may be substituted in place of ASA in patients who cannot tolerate ASA because of GI bleeding.

$P2Y_{12}$ Inhibitors

Management of ACS now routinely includes dual-antiplatelet therapy (DAPT) consisting of both ASA and a $P2Y_{12}$ inhibitor, which blocks the $P2Y_{12}$ receptor and blocks adenosine diphosphate (ADP) binding to the surface of the platelets (see Table 39.6). The latter includes the oral thienopyridines (clopidogrel, prasugrel), which are irreversible blockers, as well as a cyclopentyltriazolopyrimidine (ticagrelor), which is a reversible $P2Y_{12}$ inhibitor. Thienopyridines are prodrugs that require oxidation by the hepatic cytochrome P-450 (CYP) system to form the active metabolites. Thus drugs that inhibit the CYP system reduce the formation of the active form of thienopyridines, unlike ticagrelor, which does not depend on the CYP system. In addition to inhibition of platelet activation and aggregation, thienopyridines also reduce fibrinogen, blood viscosity, and erythrocyte deformability and aggregability through mechanisms that appear to be independent of ADP.

Clopidogrel

Clopidogrel was the first thienopyridine to be widely studied in patients with CAD, NSTE-ACS, and patients undergoing PCI. For over a decade, clopidogrel, used in combination with ASA, was the preferred oral antiplatelet drug combination in multiple guidelines. With the development of more potent antiplatelet drugs (prasugrel, ticagrelor), clopidogrel has been in part supplanted, although it is still frequently used in patients who are at very high risk of bleeding and in patients with contraindications or difficulty accessing the newer agents.

In the CURE trial, patients with NSTE-ACS who were treated with ASA, were randomized to either clopidogrel or placebo.[45] The addition of clopidogrel to ASA reduced CV death, MI, or stroke by 20% in both low- and high-risk patients, regardless of whether they were managed with medical therapy, PCI, or coronary artery bypass grafting (CABG). Benefit was seen as early as 24 hours, with Kaplan-Meier curves beginning to diverge after just 2 hours. Moreover, the reduction in MI or CV death was similar before and after PCI.[46] Clopidogrel was associated with an increase in bleeding, including nonsignificant increases in both life-threatening and fatal bleeding.[45]

Current guidelines recommend clopidogrel (600 mg loading dose, 75 mg daily maintenance dose) in addition to aspirin in patients with NSTE-ACS who cannot receive ticagrelor or prasugrel (e.g., due to intolerance or very high risk of bleeding due to a prior intracranial hemorrhage or indication for full-dose oral anticoagulation or cost).[44] Use of a 600-mg loading dose achieves a steady-state level of platelet inhibition after 2 hours, more rapidly than the 300-mg dose. Two strategies for initiating clopidogrel therapy in patients with NSTE-ACS have evolved: (1) starting clopidogrel at arrival or hospital admission or (2) delaying treatment with clopidogrel until after coronary angiography and then administering the drug on the catheterization table if PCI is to be performed. The early treatment strategy is preferred because it affords the benefits of reducing early ischemic events, but at the cost of an increase in bleeding in the minority of patients who undergo CABG instead of PCI, and thus is no longer recommended in patients in whom the coronary anatomy is not known and an early invasive approach is planned.[18] In patients undergoing CABG, those who had received clopidogrel within 5 days of surgery had an increased risk for major bleeding and the need for reoperation, which led to the recommendation that clopidogrel be discontinued at least 5 days before major surgery, if possible.[47]

Although DAPT reduces recurrent ischemic events in patients with NSTE-ACS compared with ASA alone, up to 10% of patients treated with ASA and clopidogrel have events within the first year of ACS, including stent thrombosis in up to 2% of patients at 1 year.[48]

As with ASA, hyporesponders to clopidogrel have been identified and are at higher risk for recurrent cardiac events, including stent thrombosis, MI, and death. The incidence of patients not achieving the expected pharmacologic response to clopidogrel ranges from 5% to 30%, depending on the population and the definition used to assess response. Hyporesponsiveness to clopidogrel is more common in patients with DM, obesity, advanced age, and certain genetic polymorphisms of the CYP system. Patients with a minimal antiplatelet response to clopidogrel have lower concentrations of the active metabolite, thus indicating failure of necessary conversion of the prodrug to the active drug.

Several polymorphisms of the gene encoding for the CYP2C19 enzyme have been associated with reduced production of the active metabolite of clopidogrel (see Chapter 9). These polymorphisms (especially the reduced-function *C2 allele) occur in approximately one-third of white individuals and up to half of Asians and have been associated with increased adverse clinical outcomes in patients treated with clopidogrel.[49] In other studies, reduced-function alleles are associated with increased stent thrombosis. Testing for these polymorphisms in patients who are candidates for thienopyridine treatment can identify those who are likely to be unresponsive or hyporesponsive to the standard dose of clopidogrel and are candidates for alternative antiplatelet regimens.

Proton pump inhibitors (PPIs) modestly reduce the antiplatelet effect of clopidogrel because of competition for metabolism by the CYP3A4 enzyme. The clinical significance of this interaction remains uncertain as the addition of omeprazole to clopidogrel did not increase CV events compared with placebo plus clopidogrel, but omeprazole did decrease adverse GI outcomes in a randomized, double-blind trial.[50]

Prasugrel

Like clopidogrel, prasugrel is a prodrug requiring hepatic oxidation to form an active metabolite that irreversibly inhibits the platelet $P2Y_{12}$ receptor. However, unlike clopidogrel, formation of the active metabolite of prasugrel requires only one step and is generated within 30 minutes of ingestion. While the active metabolites of clopidogrel and prasugrel exert equal antiplatelet effects in vitro, the generation of the prasugrel metabolite is approximately 10 times as great as the clopidogrel metabolite.

Prasugrel (60-mg loading dose, 10-mg daily maintenance dose) was compared with clopidogrel in patients with NSTE-ACS with known coronary anatomy in the TRITON-TIMI 38 trial.[51] The primary composite of CV death, MI, or stroke was reduced significantly by 19% in the patients randomized to prasugrel through 15 months of follow-up (Fig. 39.8). This benefit was driven by a significant 24% reduction in MI and was particularly striking in patients with diabetes (30% reduction).[52] In addition, prasugrel markedly reduced the rate of definite or probable stent thrombosis (by 52%), particularly in patients with drug-eluting stents (DESs) (64%)[53]; thus prasugrel should be considered in patients who present with stent thrombosis despite compliance with clopidogrel therapy.[18]

Severe bleeding complications were more common with prasugrel than clopidogrel, including non-CABG major (see Fig. 39.8), spontaneous, and fatal bleeding. Prasugrel is contraindicated in patients with prior stroke or transient ischemic attack due to evidence of net harm in this group in TRITON-TIMI 38. Bleeding rates were especially high in elderly patients (≥75 years) and those with reduced body weight (<60 kg [132 lb]). Thus prasugrel should be avoided in such patients unless they are at high risk for thrombosis, in which case a 5-mg maintenance dose is preferred. In patients younger than 75 years who weighed at least 60 kg and had no prior stroke or transient ischemic attack, the "core" group of patients for whom the U.S. Food and Drug Administration (FDA) approved its use, prasugrel was associated with a 26% reduction in the primary end point.[54] Prasugrel should be discontinued at least 7 days before cardiac surgery whenever possible.[47]

Prasugrel (10-mg daily) was compared with clopidogrel (75 mg daily) on a background of ASA and other standard therapies in patients with NSTE-ACS managed with an ischemia-guided strategy in the TRILOGY ACS randomized trial.[55] There was no benefit of treatment with prasugrel over clopidogrel, and bleeding rates were similar. The ACCOAST trial of high-risk patients with NSTE-ACS managed with an early invasive strategy was randomized to prasugrel or clopidogrel prior to angiography.[56] There was no significant difference in the composite primary efficacy endpoint, but prasugrel did increase bleeding compared with clopidogrel. Given the totality of the evidence from these three randomized trials, prasugrel (60-mg loading dose, 10-mg daily maintenance) in addition to ASA is most suitable in patients with NSTE-ACS <75 years without a prior stroke or transient ischemic attack who have had coronary angiography and in whom PCI is planned. Prasugrel is not recommended for use in patients with NSTE-ACS before the coronary anatomy is known.[44]

Ticagrelor

Ticagrelor is the first nonthienopyridine ADP blocker approved for use. It is a reversible inhibitor (half-life approximately 12 hours) of the $P2Y_{12}$ platelet receptor, in contrast to the thienopyridines, which are irreversible inhibitors. Both the parent drug and its metabolite are active and have similar potency; thus similar to prasugrel, inhibition of $P2Y_{12}$-mediated platelet aggregation is nearly complete and more rapid than with clopidogrel. Because ticagrelor does not require metabolism via the CYP2C19 pathway to generate an active metabolite, the variability of antiplatelet activity described with clopidogrel does not apply to ticagrelor.

The phase 3 PLATO trial compared ticagrelor (180-mg loading dose, 90-mg twice-daily maintenance dose) with clopidogrel (300- or 600-mg loading dose, 75-mg daily maintenance dose) on a background of ASA. In PLATO, 11,067 (59%) of the 18,624 patients had NSTE-ACS.[57] Ticagrelor significantly reduced the primary endpoint (CV death, MI, or stroke) by 16% (see Fig. 39.8) and also reduced stent thrombosis by 33%, CV death by 21%, and total mortality by 22%. A broad array of subgroups demonstrated consistent benefit with ticagrelor over clopidogrel, including patients age ≥75 years, weight <60 kg, with a prior history of stroke or transient ischemic attack, and those managed with a noninvasive strategy. However, there was no benefit of ticagrelor in patients enrolled in the United States, in whom the dose of ASA was higher on average than in other countries.[58] Whether this finding is related to chance, to more frequent use of higher-dose ASA (e.g., 325 mg daily), or some other aspect of care that

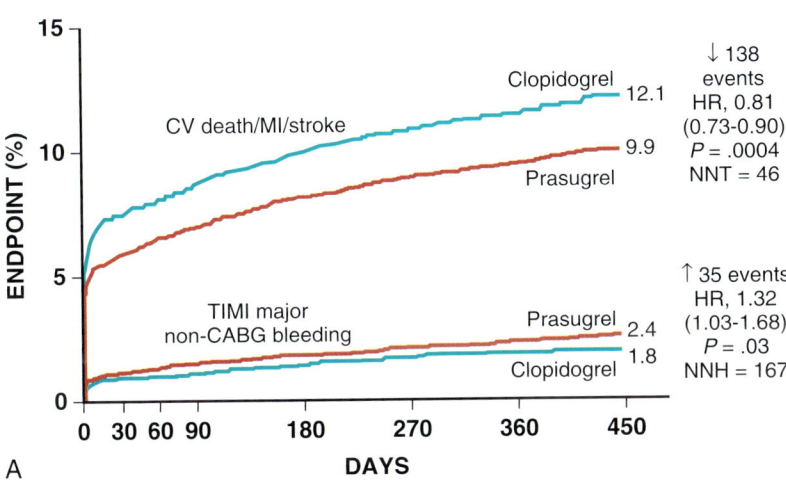

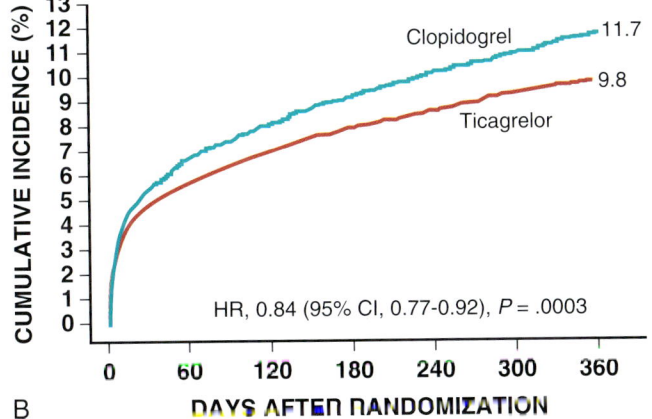

FIGURE 39.8 Comparison of newer ADP inhibitors with clopidogrel. **A,** Comparison of the efficacy and safety of prasugrel versus clopidogrel in the TRITON-TIMI 38 trial in patients with ACS undergoing PCI. **B,** The primary endpoint of the PLATO trial, a composite of death from vascular causes, MI, or stroke, occurred significantly less often in the ticagrelor group than in the clopidogrel group. *CV,* Cardiovascular; *HR,* hazard ratio; *KM,* Kaplan-Meier; *NNT,* number of patients needed to prevent one primary endpoint event; *NNH,* number of patients needed to be treated to cause harm (TIMI major bleeding). (**A** from Wiviott SD, et al. Prasugrel versus clopidogrel in patients with acute coronary syndromes. N Engl J Med. 2007;347:2001-2015; **B** from Wallentin L, et al. Ticagrelor versus clopidogrel in patients with acute coronary syndromes. N Engl J Med 2009;361:1045-1057.)

differed in the United States remains uncertain. Nevertheless, the FDA has recommended that low-dose ASA (75 to 100 mg daily) be used in combination with ticagrelor.

Safety events were similar between ticagrelor and clopidogrel, with three important differences that were significantly more common with ticagrelor: non–CABG-related major bleeding (4.5% vs. 3.8%), dyspnea (13.8% vs. 7.8%), and pauses in sinus rates in the first week lasting longer than 3 seconds (5.8% vs. 3.6%).[57] Although a reversible P2Y[12] inhibitor with a shorter effective half-life than clopidogrel, ticagrelor achieves a higher level of platelet inhibition and thus should be discontinued at least 5 days before major surgery.[47]

Long-term use of ticagrelor with ASA in patients who had experienced MI 1 to 3 years earlier was evaluated in the PEGASUS-TIMI 54 trial.[59] Compared with placebo, both the standard maintenance dose of ticagrelor (90 mg twice daily) and a lower dose (60 mg twice daily) reduced the rate of the primary composite endpoint (CV death, MI, or stroke) by 15% and 16%, respectively. Although the rates of TIMI major bleeding were higher with ticagrelor, rates of intracranial and fatal bleeding were not increased. Major bleeding rates were lower and tolerability better with the 60-mg twice-daily dose,[60] which was FDA approved for the prevention of CV death, MI, and stroke in stable patients with a history of MI.

TICAGRELOR VS. PRASUGREL

The ISAR-REACT 5 trial[61] was an open-label, multicenter, randomized trial that compared a ticagrelor-based strategy with a prasugrel-based strategy in patients who presented with ACS (59% had NSTE-ACS) in whom an invasive evaluation was planned. The trial demonstrated a ~40% relative reduction in patients with NSTE-ACS randomized to prasugrel versus ticagrelor in the primary composite endpoint of death, MI, or stroke at 1 year. Bleeding rates were similar between the treatment arms. Despite limitations in the study design and conduct, including the lack of a double-dummy design, and the high rate of early drug discontinuation, some have advocated for the preferential selection of prasugrel over ticagrelor in patients who are eligible for both.[62]

SELECTION AND DURATION OF DAPT REGIMEN AND NSTE-ACS TREATMENT STRATEGY. Patients with NSTE-ACS are most commonly managed with PCI (50% to 70%) (see later) or medical therapy without revascularization (30% to 50%), with a declining use of CABG during the index admission (5% to 15%), and with wide variation between hospitals and countries.[63] The selection of the DAPT regimen and its duration post-ACS are complex decisions that include factors such as the relative risks of bleeding and ischemia, decision to revascularize, type of revascularization (CABG vs. PCI, type of stent), and use of oral anticoagulation (see later).

In most patients with NSTE-ACS a duration of 6 to 12 months of DAPT is appropriate. Patients at low risk of ischemic complications who are either at high risk of bleeding or also receiving concomitant oral anticoagulation should receive shorter duration DAPT (1 to 3 months). The TWILIGHT trial[64] randomized high-risk patients with NSTE-ACS who had received 3 months of ASA + ticagrelor post-PCI to either continued DAPT versus ticagrelor alone in a double-blinded study. The primary bleeding endpoint at 1 year was reduced from 7.6% to 3.6% with ticagrelor monotherapy, while there was no significant difference in the efficacy composite (4.3% vs. 4.4%). These contemporary results provide additional support to shortening DAPT to 3 months in stable patients after NSTE-ACS treated with PCI to reduce the risk of bleeding.

On the other hand, for patients who have tolerated DAPT without a bleeding complication, continuation of DAPT for longer than 12 months may be considered[18,59,65] in patients with high ischemic risk (e.g., ≥65 years, diabetes, >1 prior spontaneous MIs, multivessel CAD, CKD). In such patients, ticagrelor 60 mg twice daily with aspirin for longer than 12 months may be preferred over clopidogrel or prasugrel.[44]

SWITCHING BETWEEN ORAL P2Y[12] INHIBITORS. Three common clinical scenarios in which switching between oral P2Y[12] inhibitors may arise include (1) patients who have recurrent ACS despite DAPT with chronic clopidogrel and ASA, (2) patients who experience intolerance or side effects, or (3) excessive cost. Because of differences in binding sites, speed of onset/offset, and half-life, switching between agents should be made with care. In patients on ASA and clopidogrel who experience ACS, switching from clopidogrel to ticagrelor at a loading dose of 180 mg followed by 90 mg twice daily early after hospital admission, is a Class I recommendation[44] based on an analysis from the PLATO trial.[48] An international expert consensus document provided details on how to safely switch between P2Y[12] inhibitors.[66]

Intravenous Antiplatelet Agents

Cangrelor is an IV direct-acting P2Y[12] inhibitor that blocks ADP-induced platelet activation and aggregation with an almost immediate onset of action and short half-life of 3 to 6 minutes. Three large outcome trials have evaluated cangrelor in more than 25,000 patients undergoing PCI across a broad spectrum of clinical presentations (stable angina, UA, NSTEMI, STEMI). In a patient-level meta-analysis, cangrelor reduced the risk of the primary composite outcome of death, MI, ischemia-driven revascularization, and stent thrombosis at 48 hours by 18% ($P = 0.04$) relative to the control arms among the patients who underwent PCI after NSTE-ACS.[67] There was an excess of 3 per 1000 non-CABG bleeds with cangrelor.

Because cangrelor is administered intravenously and has a rapid onset and offset of action, it has the potential to overcome several practical limitations of oral P2Y[12] inhibitors in patients with NSTE-ACS undergoing PCI. These limitations include (1) a slower onset action with oral delivery, (2) delayed absorption of oral agents in patients who have decreased GI perfusion, nausea, or receive opiates, and (3) the need to postpone CABG for 5 to 7 days after an oral P2Y[12] inhibitor to reduce the risk of bleeding.

GLYCOPROTEIN IIB/IIIA INHIBITORS

The glycoprotein (GP) IIb/IIIa inhibitors block the final common pathway of platelet aggregation, fibrinogen-mediated cross-linkage of platelets, caused by a variety of stimuli (e.g., thrombin, ADP, collagen, serotonin) (see Fig. 39.7) and were more frequently used in the era before the introduction of potent oral and IV P2Y[12] inhibitors. Three agents in this class are available: abciximab, a monoclonal antibody approved in patients undergoing PCI, and eptifibatide and tirofiban, both of which are reversible small-molecule inhibitors approved for use in patients with ACS and in those undergoing PCI.

Several trials, mostly on a background of ASA without P2Y[12] inhibitor, have shown benefit of GP IIb/IIIa inhibition in the management of patients with NSTE-ACS, with an overall small (9%) but statistically significant relative reduction in death or MI at 30 days in a large meta-analysis, with greater benefit in high-risk patients with ST-segment changes and/or elevated troponin concentration or diabetes.[68] However, the rates of major hemorrhage were significantly higher in patients treated with GP IIb/IIIa inhibitors, occurring in 2.4% compared with 1.4% of those given placebo, and severe thrombocytopenia was also increased.[69]

Two large trials have examined routine early administration at initial evaluation versus delayed provisional use of GP IIb/IIIa inhibitors just before PCI in patients who also received a P2Y[12] inhibitor (most commonly pre-PCI); the GP IIb/IIIa showed no significant benefit with an increased risk of bleeding.[70,71] Based on the totality of the evidence, the routine administration of GP IIb/IIIa inhibitors to patients with NSTE-ACS who receive DAPT with ASA and a P2Y[12] inhibitor (i.e., triple-antiplatelet therapy) is *not* recommended. However, in patients with or at high risk for thrombotic complications during PCI, such as those with diabetes or angiographic evidence of thrombus, and who are at low risk for bleeding, selective use of GP IIb/IIIa inhibitors remains a reasonable option.

Anticoagulant Therapy (see Chapter 95)

Once the diagnosis of NSTE-ACS has been established, a parenteral anticoagulant should be initiated in addition to DAPT, unless the patient has an absolute contraindication (e.g., uncontrolled bleeding)[8,18] (see Fig. 39.7).

Heparin

Unfractionated heparin (UFH) is a mixture of polysaccharide chains of different lengths that prevent coagulation by blocking thrombin (factor IIa) and factor Xa. UFH also binds to circulating plasma proteins, acute-phase reactants, and endothelial cells and thus has an unpredictable anticoagulant effect. Because of its short half-life, UFH must be administered as an IV infusion to ensure a stable level of anticoagulation.

A meta-analysis of 1353 patients in six trials showed a 33% reduction in death or MI with UFH plus ASA versus ASA alone.[72] A weight-adjusted dose of UFH (60-unit/kg bolus and 12-unit/kg/hr infusion), with monitoring of the anticoagulant response via the activated partial thromboplastin time (APTT) and titrations of the infusion rate according to a standardized nomogram to achieve an APTT of 50 to 70 seconds or 1.5 to 2.5 times control.[8,18] Prolonged infusions of UFH increase the risk of an immunogenic heparin-induced thrombocytopenia (HIT), which is an infrequent but serious complication that can cause thrombosis and bleeding and may even be fatal. In patients with HIT, a direct thrombin inhibitor (e.g., bivalirudin [see later] to achieve APTT 1.5 to 2.5 times control) or fondaparinux (see later) should be substituted.[18]

Low-Molecular-Weight Heparin

The low-molecular-weight forms of heparin (LMWH) are enriched with shorter polysaccharide chains, which results in a more predictable anticoagulant effect than does UFH. LMWH has several potential advantages over UFH: (1) its greater anti–FXa activity (relative to factor IIa) inhibits thrombin generation more effectively; (2) it induces greater release of tissue factor pathway inhibitor than UFH, and it is not neutralized by platelet factor 4; (3) it causes HIT less frequently than UFH; (4) the high and consistent bioavailability of LMWH allows subcutaneous (SC) administration; (5) monitoring of the anticoagulation level is not necessary; and (6) LMWH binds less avidly to plasma proteins than UFH and therefore has a more consistent anticoagulant effect.

Although several LMWHs have been approved, the weight of evidence supports the choice of *enoxaparin* in patients with ACS.[8,18] The standard dose is 1 mg/kg subcutaneously every 12 hours, with dosing only once daily for patients with a creatinine clearance (CrCl) <30 mL/min. Administration of enoxaparin for up to 8 days (or until hospital discharge) was found to be effective in patients with ACS, whereas extending therapy to 6 weeks did not reduce ischemic events further.[73] In a meta-analysis of 21,945 patients from six trials of patients with NSTE-ACS in which enoxaparin was compared with UFH, new or recurrent MI occurred significantly less frequently with enoxaparin, whereas the rate of major bleeding was similar between these agents.[74] LMWH should not be used in patients with a history of HIT.

Heparin Reversal

Protamine sulfate binds heparin to form a stable salt, thus quickly reversing the anticoagulant effect of UFH. Because the half-life of UFH is approximately 1 to 1.5 hours, the dose of protamine necessary to reverse an infusion of UFH should be based on the total UFH dose administered in the preceding 2 to 3 hours. Approximately 1 mg neutralizes 100 units of UFH. A slow IV infusion is recommended to avoid hypotension or bradycardia. Protamine reverses approximately 60% of the anticoagulant effect of LMWH but does not completely neutralize its anti-Xa activity, and it is not effective to reverse pure factor Xa (FXa) inhibitors such as fondaparinux and the oral FXa inhibitors.

Direct Thrombin Inhibitors

The direct thrombin inhibitors have a potential advantage over indirect thrombin inhibitors such as UFH or LMWH in that they do not require antithrombin and can inhibit clot-bound thrombin. Direct thrombin inhibitors do not interact with plasma proteins, provide a very stable level of anticoagulation, and do not cause thrombocytopenia, thus making them an excellent choice for anticoagulation in patients with a history of HIT.

Bivalirudin, the drug in this class most widely used in patients with ACS or undergoing PCI, binds reversibly to thrombin and has a half-life of approximately 25 minutes. In earlier trials of patients with ACS undergoing PCI, patients randomized to bivalirudin without a GP IIb/IIIa inhibitor experienced less bleeding compared with the combination of a GP IIb/IIIa inhibitor with either UFH or enoxaparin. However, there were no differences in major bleeding between anticoagulants (UFH or enoxaparin vs. bivalirudin) in patients taking a GP IIb/IIIa inhibitor, and there were no differences in ischemic events between the three treatment arms.[75] A meta-analysis of four trials enrolling predominantly patients with NSTE-ACS showed that heparin-based regimens reduced major adverse cardiovascular events (MACEs) slightly compared with bivalirudin-based regimens.[76]

Subsequent trials[77] comparing bivalirudin with UFH in a contemporary setting of radial arterial access and limited use of GP IIb/IIIa inhibitors (both of which reduce bleeding), demonstrated a similar risk for both ischemia and bleeding between these two anticoagulants. Current European guidelines consider the use of bivalirudin (with ASA and a $P2Y_{12}$ inhibitor) an acceptable second-line alternative to heparin-based regimens in patients with NSTE-ACS managed with an early invasive strategy.[47] In patients with NSTE-ACS before angiography, the recommended dose of bivalirudin is a 0.10-mg/kg IV bolus followed by an infusion of 0.25 mg/kg/hr. If started during the procedure, a 0.75-mg/kg bolus dose of bivalirudin should be administered, followed by an infusion at 1.75 mg/kg/hr during PCI.[8] It may be discontinued shortly after PCI to permit removal of arterial access sheaths.

FACTOR XA INHIBITORS

Both parenteral and oral FXa inhibitors have been studied in patients with NSTE-ACS.

Fondaparinux

This synthetic pentasaccharide indirectly inhibits factor Xa and requires the presence of antithrombin for its action. The OASIS-5 trial compared daily SC fondaparinux (2.5 mg) with standard-dose enoxaparin in patients with high-risk NSTE-ACS.[78] No difference was found in the primary ischemic composite through 9 days, although fondaparinux did reduce major bleeding by nearly one half, and mortality at 30 days tended to be lower with fondaparinux. In patients undergoing PCI, however, fondaparinux was associated with a greater than threefold increased risk for catheter-related thrombi. Supplemental UFH at catheterization (85 units/kg if no GP IIb/IIIa inhibitor is used; 60 units/kg with concomitant GP IIb/IIIa inhibitor) appeared to minimize the risk of this problem with fondaparinux.[79] Thus, fondaparinux is an alternative for patients with NSTE-ACS managed noninvasively, particularly in patients at high risk for bleeding.[8,18]

Oral Factor Xa Inhibitors

Two oral direct factor Xa inhibitors, rivaroxaban and apixaban, have been studied in phase 3 trials of patients with ACS who do not have another indication for full-dose oral anticoagulation (e.g., AF, recent venothromboembolism). In the ATLAS ACS 2-TIMI 51 trial, low-dose rivaroxaban (5 mg twice daily) and very-low-dose rivaroxaban (2.5 mg twice daily) reduced the primary composite (death, MI, or stroke) significantly by 16% compared with placebo on a background of DAPT.[80] Bleeding, including intracranial hemorrhage, was significantly increased with the addition of rivaroxaban to DAPT. Because the 2.5-mg twice-daily dose had a more favorable safety profile and also significantly reduced death, it was approved by the European Medicines Agency for the prevention of atherothrombotic events in post–acute MI patients. However, rivaroxaban has not been approved for use after ACS by the FDA.

Patients with Indications for Both Oral Anticoagulant and Antiplatelet Therapy

Combination of Chronic Oral Anticoagulant and Antiplatelet Therapy Post NSTE-ACS

Approximately 10% of patients presenting with NSTE-ACS have an indication for ongoing oral anticoagulation, such as AF, mechanical heart valve, or recent venous thromboembolism. In a nationwide cohort from Denmark of 272,315 patients with atrial fibrillation, the combination of oral anticoagulation with DAPT is associated with an incidence of major bleeding of 10% per year, with patients ≥90 years of age, prior major bleeding, or CHADS-VASc 6 or higher experiencing annualized rates of 17% to 23%.[81] Each of the four newer oral anticoagulants (NOACs) approved for prevention of stroke and systemic embolism in patients with AF has been compared with vitamin K agonist (VKA) (most commonly warfarin) in moderate-sized trials of patients with AF undergoing PCI, the majority of whom had ACS. These trials were designed and powered to compare NOAC-based antithrombotic regimens with VKA + DAPT.[82] A meta-analysis of 7890 patients included in the arms comparing NOAC + $P2Y_{12}$ inhibitor with VKA + DAPT from the aforementioned 4 trials demonstrated a 38% reduction in major or clinically relevant non-major bleeding favoring NOAC + $P2Y_{12}$ inhibitor.[82]

However, there were unfavorable trends toward increased risk of stent thrombosis (hazard ratio [HR] 1.55, 95% confidence interval [CI] 0.99-2.41) and MI (HR 1.18, 95% CI 0.93 to 1.52) with NOAC + $P2Y_{12}$ inhibitor that may have been related to the early events in the absence of aspirin post randomization. No differences were observed between the NOAC- and VKA-based strategies for all-cause mortality, stroke, or MACEs.

Current consensus statements[83,84] in patients with AF and ACS who undergo PCI provide variable recommendations, generally ranging from 1 to 12 months for and the combination of antiplatelet and anticoagulation therapy, depending on the bleeding and thromboembolic risk and type of coronary stent. Given the data from large randomized trials of patients with AF and venous thromboembolism, as well as the studies of patients with AF who experience NSTE-ACS or undergo PCI cited earlier,[82] NOACs are now preferred over VKA due to the lower risk of bleeding (especially intracranial) and ease of use.

Guidance for managing antithrombotic therapy in patients with AF, ACS, and PCI that allows for tailored approaches depending on the balance between bleeding and ischemic risks have been provided.[18,84] The major concepts include (1) a short initial course of triple therapy with NOAC + $P2Y_{12}$ inhibitor + aspirin 75 to 100 mg (up to 1 week,[18] after which aspirin is discontinued); (2) dual therapy with a NOAC + $P2Y_{12}$ inhibitor until 1 year; (3) NOAC monotherapy after the first year; (4) options to shorten the duration and intensity (e.g., use of clopidogrel instead of more potent $P2Y_{12}$ inhibitors, continuing aspirin in favor of a $P2Y_{12}$ inhibitor) combination therapy in patients with uncorrectable bleeding risk factors who are at low atherothrombotic risk; and (5) options to increase the duration of intensity combination therapy in patients at high atherothrombotic risk (e.g., due to anatomic complexity of coronary stenting, prior stent thrombosis, multiple recurrent MIs) and low bleeding risk[85] (Fig. 39.9).

Acute Antithrombotic Therapy for NSTE-ACS in Patients on a Chronic Oral Anticoagulant

There are limited data, and no large randomized trials available to guide the selection of anticoagulant and antiplatelet therapy in patients on chronic oral anticoagulation who develop NSTE-ACS.

Recent NSTE-ACS With an Indication for Oral Anticoagulation

Some patients with a recent (<6 to 12 months) NSTE-ACS receiving DAPT may develop AF or acute venous thromboembolism requiring full-dose anticoagulation. In them, the risk of bleeding with the addition of an oral anticoagulant needs to be carefully balanced with the risk of stent thrombosis and recurrent MI.[83] A NOAC (rather than VKA) should be started in such patients with one or more risk factors for stroke (other than the known vascular disease) or who develop an acute venous thromboembolism. Algorithms have been published to help guide decisions regarding the timing of cessation of concomitant antiplatelet therapies.[84] In some patients whose only stroke risk factor is vascular disease, it may be possible to omit full-dose anticoagulation; however, given the safety profile of NOACs, risk-benefit balance tends to favor NOAC in most patients.[85]

Bleeding: Risk Assessment, Prevention, and Treatment

Severe bleeding is the most common complication of antithrombotic therapy. Efforts to minimize the risk of bleeding include (1) assessment of bleeding (and ischemic) risk using established risk scores[18,30-32] to identify and manage modifiable risk factors and to select the most appropriate antithrombotic treatment regimen and duration; (2) selection of the anticoagulant and antiplatelet(s) therapies with a lower risk of bleeding; (3) appropriate dose adjustment of antithrombotic drugs according to age, body weight, renal function, and use of concomitant medications that increase drug exposure (e.g., verapamil, dronedarone), especially in women and older patients; (4) avoidance of other therapies that increase the risk for bleeding (e.g., NSAIDs); and (5) radial arterial approach as default vascular access, smaller sheath sizes, timely removal of arterial sheaths, and femoral closure devices.[86]

Other steps that should be considered to reduce the risk of bleeding include use of bare-metal stents (BMSs) to permit a shorter duration (1 month) of DAPT and prophylactic administration of gastroprotective agents such as PPIs[44] (particularly in patients at increased risk of upper GI bleeding such as the elderly or with dyspepsia, gastroesophageal reflux disease, *Helicobacter pylori* infection, or chronic alcohol use). New recommendations from the 2020 European Guidelines[18] include performing PCI without interruption of preadmission oral anticoagulant; not administering UFH in patients on VKAs with an international normalized ratio (INR) >2.5, and in patients on NOACs; adding low-dose parenteral anticoagulation (e.g., enoxaparin 0.5 mg/kg intravenously or UFH 60 IU/kg) regardless of the timing of the last administration of the last NOAC dose; avoiding routine pretreatment with P2Y12 inhibitors; and restricting use of GP IIb/IIIa inhibitors for bailout or periprocedural complications only. Routine platelet function testing to adjust antiplatelet therapy before or after stenting is not recommended, as it has not been demonstrated to reduce the risk of bleeding.[44]

In case of major bleeding, the European Society of Cardiology (ESC) provides the following recommendations[18]: (1) interrupt both anticoagulant and antiplatelet therapies, unless bleeding can be adequately controlled by specific hemostatic measures; (2) neutralize anticoagulant therapy; (3) consider platelet transfusion to neutralize antiplatelet agents; (4) because blood transfusions may have deleterious effects on outcome, transfusions should usually be withheld in hemodynamically stable patients with Hb above 7 g/dL; (5) erythropoietin is not indicated as a treatment for acute anemia or blood loss, because it may increase the risk of arterial or venous thromboembolism; and (6) minor bleeding should be managed if possible without interruption of antithrombotic therapies.

Anti-Inflammatory Therapies

Given the important role that inflammation plays in the development of ACS, therapies targeting inflammation have been highly sought after. In addition to standard therapies such as ASA and statins that have anti-inflammatory effects and proven benefit to reduce CV events post NSTE-ACS, two novel approaches deserve mention. Oral colchicine was studied in the double-blind COLCOT trial[87] involving 4745 patients randomized within 30 days of MI to either low-dose colchicine (0.5 mg daily) or placebo. After a median of 23 months, colchicine significantly reduced a broad CV composite compared with placebo (HR 0.77). Pneumonia occurred more frequently with colchicine (0.9% vs. 0.4%).

The CANTOS trial[88] of a monoclonal antibody targeting interleukin-1β (canakinumab) versus placebo in 10,061 patients with prior MI demonstrated significant reduction in recurrent CV events. Fatal infections were increased slightly with canakinumab and further development of this drug for an indication in patients with CAD was paused. Although patients with ACS <30 days were not eligible for the CANTOS trial, this trial suggests that future therapies that target inflammation/immune pathways, such as interleukin-1β, maybeeffective.

Invasive Versus Conservative Management

Three general approaches to cardiac catheterization and revascularization can be used to manage patients with NSTE-ACS: (1) an early invasive strategy involving routine early (within 48 hours of initial evaluation) cardiac catheterization, followed by PCI, CABG, or continuing medical therapy, depending on the coronary anatomy; (2) a delayed invasive approach (coronary angiography >48 hours after presentation); and (3) an ischemia-guided (or selective invasive) approach, with initial medical management and catheterization reserved for patients with hemodynamic instability or recurrent ischemia, either at rest or on a noninvasive stress test, followed by revascularization if the anatomy is suitable. An early invasive strategy is *not* recommended in patients with extensive comorbidities in whom the risks of revascularization outweigh the potential benefits, or in patients with acute chest pain with low clinical likelihood of ACS and a negative troponin assay[8] (Fig. 39.10).

A meta-analysis of seven trials confirmed an overall significant 25% reduction in mortality and a 17% reduction in nonfatal MI after 2 years of follow-up in patients managed with an early invasive strategy

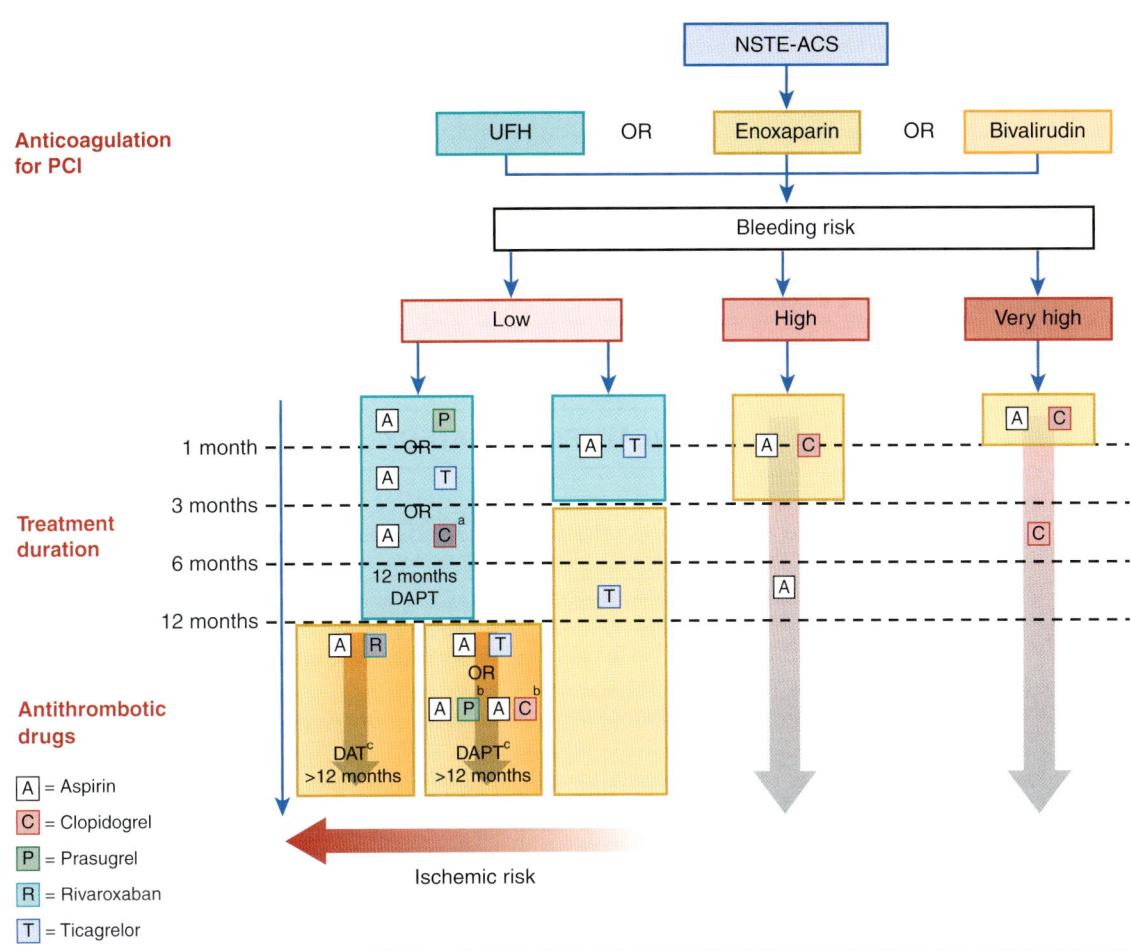
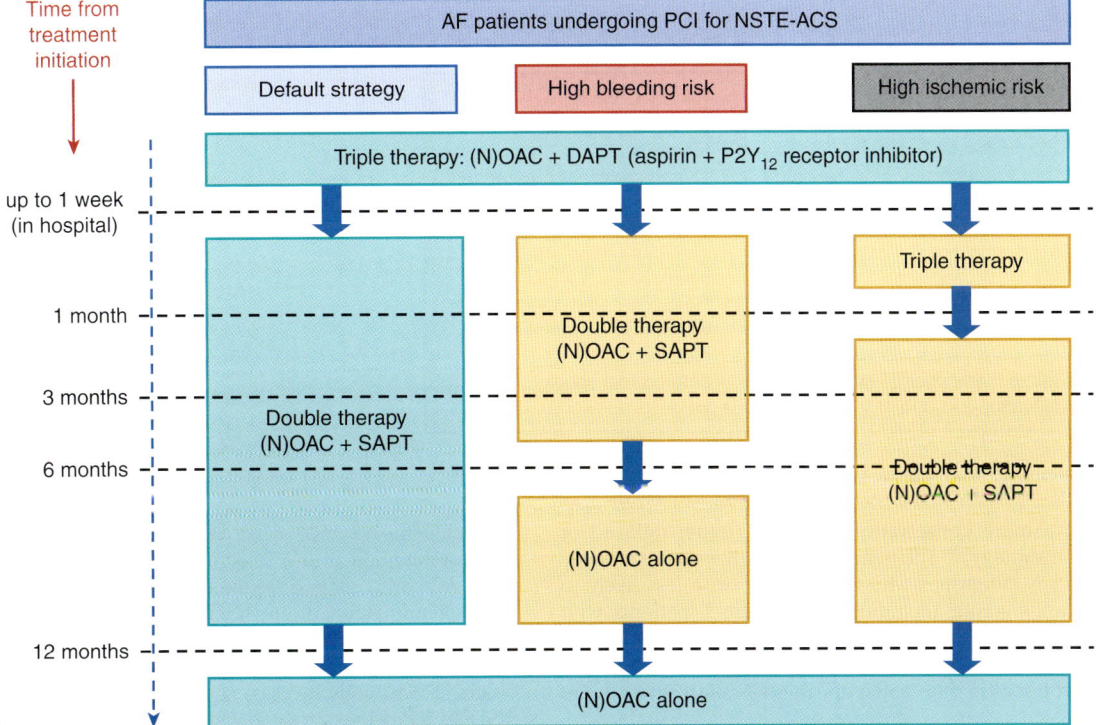

FIGURE 39.9 For legend see top of next page

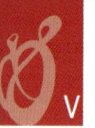

FIGURE 39.9 A, Algorithm for antithrombotic therapy in non–ST-segment elevation acute coronary syndrome patients without atrial fibrillation undergoing percutaneous coronary intervention. High bleeding risk (HBR) is considered as an increased risk of spontaneous bleeding during DAPT. Color-coding refers to the ESC classes of recommendations (*green, class I; yellow, class IIa; orange, class IIb*). Very HBR is defined as recent bleeding in the past month and/or not deferrable planned surgery. *DAT,* Dual antithrombotic therapy (here: aspirin + rivaroxaban). [a]Clopidogrel during 12 months of DAPT if patient is not eligible for treatment with prasugrel or ticagrelor or in a setting of DAPT de-escalation with a switch to clopidogrel (class IIb). [b]Clopidogrel or prasugrel if patient is not eligible for treatment with ticagrelor. Class IIa indication for DAT or DAPT >12 months in patients at high risk for ischemic events and without increased risk of major bleeding (= prior history of intracranial hemorrhage or ischemic stroke, history of other intracranial pathology, recent gastrointestinal bleeding, or anemia caused by possible gastrointestinal blood loss, other gastrointestinal pathology associated with increased bleeding risk, liver failure, bleeding diathesis or coagulopathy, extreme old age or frailty, renal failure requiring dialysis, or with eGFR <15 mL/min/1.73 m^2); Class IIb indication for DAT or DAPT >12 months in patients with moderately increased risk of ischemic events and without increased risk of major bleeding. **B,** Algorithm for antithrombotic therapy in non–ST-segment elevation acute coronary syndrome patients with atrial fibrillation undergoing percutaneous coronary intervention or medical management. *Green* (class I) and *yellow* (class IIa) colors denote the classes of recommendation. OAC: preference for a NOAC over VKA for the default strategy and in all other scenarios if no contraindications. For both TAT and DAT regimens, the recommended doses for the NOACs are as follows: (1) apixaban 5 mg b.i.d., (2) dabigatran 110 mg or 150 mg b.i.d., (3) edoxaban 60 mg/day, (4) rivaroxaban 15 mg or 20 mg/day. NOAC dose reductions are recommended in patients with renal failure and may be considered in patients with ARC-HBR1. SAPT: preference for a P2Y$_{12}$ receptor inhibitor over aspirin. Ticagrelor may be considered in patients with high ischemic risk and low bleeding risk. Treatment >1 month: OAC + DAPT (TAT) may be considered for up to 6 months in selected patients with high ischemic risk (IIa C). Treatment >12 months: OAC + SAPT may be considered in selected patients with high ischemic risk: ARC-HBR and in addition with a PRECISE-DAPT score of > 25. *A,* Aspirin; *AF,* atrial fibrillation; *ARC-HBR,* Academic Research Consortium High Bleeding Risk; *b.i.d.,* twice a day; *C,* clopidogrel; *DAT,* dual antithrombotic therapy; *NOAC,* non-vitamin K antagonist oral anticoagulant; *OAC,* oral anticoagulation/anticoagulant; *P,* prasugrel; *PRECISE-DAPT,* PREdicting bleeding Complications In patients undergoing Stent implantation and subsEquent Dual Anti Platelet Therapy; *R,* rivaroxaban; *SAPT,* single antiplatelet therapy; *T,* ticagrelor; *TAT,* triple antithrombotic therapy; (**A, B** adapted from Collet J-P, et al. 2020 ESC Guideline for the management of acute coronary syndromes in patients presenting without persistent ST-segment elevation. Eur Heart J 2020;42(14):1289–1367.)

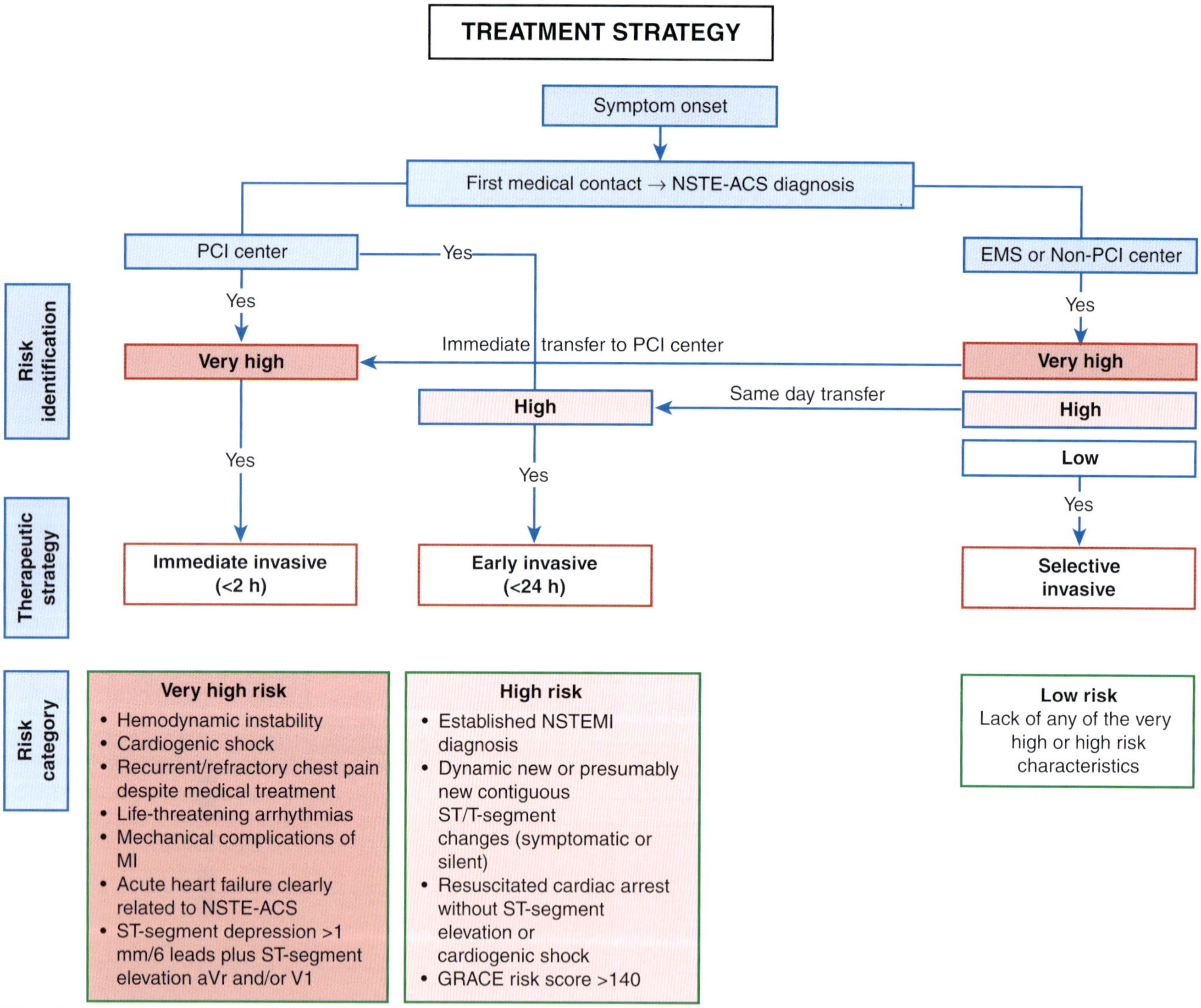

FIGURE 39.10 Selection of non–ST-segment elevation acute coronary syndrome treatment strategy and timing according to initial risk stratification. (Adapted from Collet J-P, et al. 2020 ESC Guideline for the management of acute coronary syndromes in patients presenting without persistent ST-segment elevation. Eur Heart J 2020; 42(14):1289–1367.)

compared with a more conservative approach (either delayed or selective invasive strategy).[89] The benefit of an early invasive strategy also applied to key subgroups who traditionally were less likely to undergo early angiography, including older adults,[90] patients with CKD, and women (except those at low risk).[91] At 10 years, the benefits between an early invasive versus selective strategy were no longer apparent, in part because of a "catch-up" in revascularization in the latter group.[92]

Thus, in the absence of a contraindication, an early invasive strategy is recommended over a selective invasive approach in patients with NSTE-ACS who have ST-segment changes and/or positive troponin assay on admission, or in whom these high-risk features develop over the subsequent 24 hours. Other high-risk indicators, such as recurrent ischemia or evidence of congestive HF, also favor an early invasive strategy.[8,18] An early invasive strategy is also advised in patients with NSTE-ACS previously treated with CABG[8] and in patients who have had

NSTE-ACS within 6 months of a previous PCI and in whom restenosis may be responsible.[18] Indications for an initial conservative strategy include patients with life-threatening comorbid conditions or in low-risk patients without recurrent symptoms and in whom the risks outweigh the potential benefits.[8,18]

Timing of an Invasive Approach

The timing of an invasive approach may be divided into three groups: (1) immediate invasive (<2 hours of hospital presentation) in patients at very high risk, (2) early invasive (<24 hours) in patients at high risk, and (3) delayed invasive approach (>48 hours) in patients at intermediate risk. Fig. 39.10 summarizes the guideline recommendations[47] regarding timing of an invasive approach.

A meta-analysis of 13 randomized controlled trials in 11,972 patients comparing outcomes in patients with early versus delayed angiography demonstrated a significant 15% reduction in MI in long-term follow-up after an early invasive approach.[91] No difference in mortality was observed. In a prespecified subgroup analysis of 6 trials with available GRACE risk scores, patients with a score >140 who underwent an early invasive approach had a significant 12% reduction in major adverse cardiac events, whereas those with a low GRACE score showed no clear benefit.

Although relatively uncommon (<3% incidence), patients with NSTEMI who develop cardiogenic shock represent a particularly high-risk subgroup, with an in-hospital mortality of 35% in a U.S. national database of over 2.2 million patients with NSTEMI.[93] The risk-adjusted mortality was reduced by more than 50% with an invasive strategy in these patients. However, a delayed, as opposed to an immediate, invasive approach should be considered in patients who are hemodynamically stable without ST-segment elevation successfully resuscitated after an out-of-hospital cardiac arrest.[18]

Predischarge Risk Stratification in Patients Managed with an Ischemia-Guided Strategy

In stable patients managed with an ischemia-guided strategy, non-invasive stress testing is recommended after at least 12 to 24 hours following the most recent symptoms.[8] Options include exercise testing (in patients without resting ST-segment abnormalities), exercise testing with imaging modalities in patients with ST-segment changes, or pharmacologic stress testing in patients unable to exercise. An additional benefit of imaging studies is the assessment of LV function, which should be ascertained in patients with definite ACS.[8]

Percutaneous Coronary Intervention (see Chapter 41)

Angiographic success (TIMI epicardial grade 2 or 3 flow) can be achieved in a large majority (95%) of patients with NSTE-ACS who undergo PCI, even in those considered to be at high risk.[94] However, the development of intraprocedural complications, such as transient or sustained loss of a side branch, abrupt closure, distal embolization, or development of the no-reflow phenomenon, may substantially increase risk of death or MI over the next 30 days.[94] Although use of DESs has reduced the risk for restenosis, there is a risk for late stent thrombosis following DES implantation, especially when DAPT (i.e., ASA and a $P2Y_{12}$ inhibitor) is discontinued early. This serious complication can be reduced in patients with DESs, by continuing DAPT beyond 12 months after stenting.[59,65]

The newer-generation DES have demonstrated consistent benefits compared with earlier-generation stents coated with sirolimus or paclitaxel and to BMSs).[95] Given reductions in stent thrombosis, restenosis, and other ischemic events following placement of a new-generation DES, the need for prolonged (≥12 months) DAPT is less clear, and shorter durations of DAPT may be possible. Ongoing innovation in stent technology,[96] including DES with thinner struts, new scaffold designs to improve the delivery of polymer, polymers with varying durability or that can degrade, and the introduction of new antiproliferative coatings have led to >30 available types of DES. Data from large-scale randomized trials comparing different DES in patients with NSTE-ACS are needed to guide stent selection.

With continued improvements in coronary interventions, the question of whether complete or culprit-only lesion intervention should be performed in patients with ACS has arisen. Data from an observational cohort study of 21,857 patients with NSTEMI and multivessel disease treated at 8 London cardiac centers demonstrated a 10% reduction in mortality favoring complete revascularization.[97] Contemporary randomized trials in patients with NSTE-ACS, as have been performed in STEMI, are needed. Current guidelines state that complete revascularization should be considered in patients without cardiogenic shock and with multivessel disease.[18]

Percutaneous Coronary Intervention Versus Coronary Artery Bypass Grafting

Several trials have compared PCI and CABG in patients with stable CAD, but no large studies have randomized patients with NSTE-ACS to different modes of revascularization. Based on the results from patients with stable CAD, CABG has been the recommended method of revascularization in patients with disease of the left main coronary artery (LMA), as well as for those with multivessel disease (involving all three major epicardial vessels or the proximal left anterior descending artery plus a second artery) and a left ventricular ejection fraction (LVEF) less than 40% and/or DM. However, data from the EXCEL trial comparing CABG with DES in patients with LMA stenosis with low or intermediate anatomical complexity suggest that PCI may be a viable option.[98]

For patients with less severe CAD, and with suitable coronary anatomy, although PCI is associated with slightly lower initial morbidity and mortality and lower rates of stroke than CABG, it is associated with a higher need for repeat PCI, less complete revascularization, and somewhat less relief of angina.[99] However, it is associated with a much more rapid recovery than CABG.

Both North American[8] and European[47] guidelines recommend using a "heart team" approach to guide decisions regarding revascularization, which includes input from interventional cardiologists and cardiothoracic surgeon in patients with CAD including LMA. Factors that favor CABG include (1) clinical factors such as DM, LVEF <35%, and contraindication to DAPT, (2) anatomic features, such as diffuse in-stent restenosis, severe coronary calcification, and inability to achieve complete revascularization with PCI; and (3) other surgical indications, such as need for valve or aortic surgery.[47]

Lipid-Lowering Therapy (see Chapters 27 and 40)

A prespecified subgroup of 3260 patients with UA in the LIPID trial experienced a 26% reduction in total mortality with pravastatin compared with placebo.[100] However, intensive statin (atorvastatin, 80 mg) was even more effective than pravastatin (40 mg) in the 2724 patients post–NSTE-ACS enrolled in the PROVE IT-TIMI 22 trial,[101] reducing the composite of CV death, MACE, or stroke by 20% relative (5% absolute reduction) over an average of 2 years of follow-up. Atorvastatin (80 mg) not only achieved a lower on-treatment LDL than pravastatin (40 mg), but was also more effective in reducing hs-CRP, which may have contributed to the early divergence of the event curves beginning 2 weeks after randomization.[102] In a meta-analysis of 13 randomized controlled trials involving 17,963 patients with ACS (a mixture of STEMI and NSTE-ACS), early (on average 4 days after admission), intensive statin therapy compared with control, usually placebo, decreased the rate of death and CV events over 2 years of follow-up significantly by 19%.[103]

The U.S. Multisociety Cholesterol[104] and European Dyslipidemia[105] Guidelines both support use of a maximally tolerated statin able to achieve >50% reduction in LDL-C in patients with NSTE-ACS. The U.S. Guidelines recommend a target of <70 mg/dL,[101] whereas the European guidelines recommend a goal LDL-C <55 mg/dL.[105] In patients with recurrent atherosclerotic CV events within 2 years, the European guidelines recommend that an even lower goal of <40 mg/dL may be considered.[105]

The IMPROVE-IT trial demonstrated the added clinical benefit of adding a nonstatin therapy (*ezetimibe*, a cholesterol absorption inhibitor) to background statin therapy. In 18,144 patients following

ACS (71% of whom had NSTE-ACS), ezetimibe significantly reduced the risk of CV death, MACE, or stroke by 6.4%) at 7 years.[106] MI and stroke fell significantly by 13% and 21%, respectively. In the 12,941 patients with NSTE-ACS at presentation, ezetimibe was well tolerated with no increase in serious side effects, even among patients achieving an LDL-C <30 mg/dL who were followed for an average of 6 years.[107] The benefits of ezetimibe were most prominent in post-ACS patients at high risk of MACE, including patients older than 75 years,[108] those with DM,[109] prior CABG,[110] or an elevated risk score.[33] On the basis of the IMPROVE-IT results, both U.S.[104] and European[105] guidelines recommended ezetimibe in patients with NSTE-ACS who are at very high risk and in whom LDL-C remains elevated (≥70 mg U.S. guideline, ≥55 mg/dL European guideline) despite maximally tolerated statin.

Subsequently, drugs targeting the proprotein convertase subtilisin kexin type-9 (PCSK9) protein were developed and have been shown to reduce LDL-C by 40% to 60% regardless of background lipid therapy in a variety of populations with hyperlipidemia.[111] Two monoclonal antibodies to PCSK9 (evolocumab, alirocumab) have been approved for reducing LDL-C and prevent CV events, while a small interfering (si) RNA (inclisiran) is undergoing regulatory review in the United States and Europe[112] (Fig. 39.11). In 5711 patients with a recent (<12 months) MI enrolled in the FOURIER trial, evolocumab significantly reduced the risk of adverse CV events by 19% and the key secondary endpoint of CV death, MI, or stroke by 25% compared with placebo after follow-up of 2.2 years[113] (see Fig. 39.11). The largest experience with PCSK9 inhibition in patients with recent ACS in the ODYSSEY OUTCOMES[114] trial that randomized 18,924 with ACS (65% with NSTE-ACS) 1 to 12 months before enrollment to either alirocumab or placebo every 2 weeks added to a high-intensity statin. After a median of 2.8 years the primary endpoint was reduced significantly by 15% with alirocumab (see Fig. 39.11). The reductions in CV events were consistent across the spectrum of ACS, including the 9175 patients with NSTEMI and the 3182 patients with UA. With both evolocumab and alirocumab, the only adverse event that occurred significantly more frequently with the PCSK9 inhibitor was local injection site reactions, most of which were minor and did not lead to drug discontinuation.

PCSK9 inhibitors are recommended in patients with NSTE-ACS at very high risk in whom the LDL-C remains elevated (see earlier) despite maximal tolerated statin and ezetimibe. Because of their higher cost compared with statins and ezetimibe (which are now available as generic preparations), the National Lipid Association recommends targeting the use of PCSK9 inhibitors to the highest risk patients for whom reasonable cost-effectiveness might be expected,[115] including patients with a recent NSTE-ACS with LDL-C ≥70 mg/dL with extensive burden of or active atherosclerotic CV disease or those with poorly controlled cardiometabolic risk factors.

The previously mentioned findings underscore the importance of initiating intensive lipid-lowering therapy as soon as possible after hospital admission in patients with NSTE-ACS to achieve a ≥50% reduction in LDL-C. Given the ongoing benefit seen during follow-up in the ACS trials, lipid-lowering therapy should be continued indefinitely, without dose reduction in patients who are tolerating the therapy regardless of the LDL-C decline, given the lack of adverse effects even among patients achieving an LDL-C <20 mg/dL.[116]

Discharge and Posthospital Care

The period just before hospital discharge following ACS is a potential "teachable moment" for the patient, in which the physician and staff can review and optimize the medical regimen for long-term secondary prevention (see Chapters 27 and 40).

GROUPS OF SPECIAL INTEREST

Older Adults (see Chapter 90)

Patients age ≥75 have a higher incidence and prevalence of adverse outcomes when experiencing NSTE-ACS. Advanced age is accompanied by a greater degree of comorbidity; age- and disease-related changes in physiology can affect pharmacokinetics/dynamics, volume of distribution, drug sensitivity, and polypharmacy (increasing the risk of drug-drug interactions), each of which poses additional challenges in the management of NSTE-ACS. Elderly patients are more likely to present with atypical symptoms (e.g., dyspnea rather than chest pain or discomfort), and with ECG abnormalities that are less diagnostic than those seen in younger patients.[8,18] Nevertheless, elderly patients with NSTE-ACS derive similar or even greater absolute benefits from guideline-directed therapies including DAPT,[117] an earlier invasive approach,[118] DES instead of BMS,[119] and intensive lipid lowering,[111,120] than younger patients, yet, paradoxically, they are less likely to receive such proven therapies.[121] Several suggestions can reduce the risk of bleeding, which is more common in the elderly: (1) exclusive use of low-dose maintenance ASA, 75 to

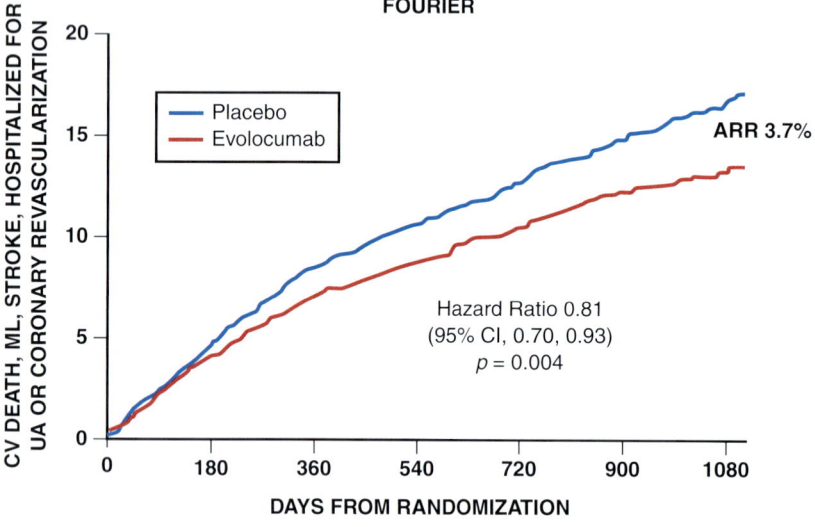

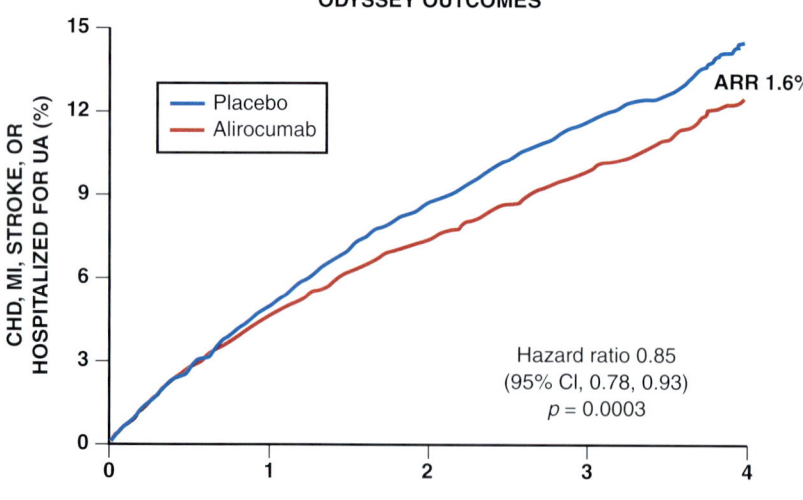

FIGURE 39.11 PCSK9 inhibitors in patients with recent MI (<12 months). **A,** FOURIER. **B,** ODYSSEY OUTCOMES. (**A** from Gencer B, et al. Efficacy of evolocumab on cardiovascular outcomes in patients with recent myocardial infarction a prespecified secondary analysis from the FOURIER Trial. JAMA Cardiol. 2020; e200882; and **B,** from Schwartz GG, et al. Alirocumab and cardiovascular outcomes after acute coronary syndrome. N Engl J Med 2018;379:2097–2107.)

100 mg; (2) use of clopidogrel as the P2Y$_{12}$ inhibitor; (3) avoidance of concomitant medications that increase the risk of bleeding or dose reduction of more potent agents; and (4) avoidance of abciximab (see earlier) if a GP IIb/IIIa inhibitor is needed to manage a peri-PCI thrombotic complication.

In addition, it is critically important to dose-adjust therapies according to body weight and renal function to avoid excess dosing of antithrombotics in older patients, which can lead to excess bleeding.[18] Reliance on the serum creatinine alone may underestimate the true extent of renal dysfunction, because age contributes importantly to determining CrCl. Guidelines recommend assessment of renal function in all patients at the time of ACS and during long-term follow-up at an interval in months equal to the CrCl (in mL/min) divided by 10 (e.g., for a CrCl of 30 mg/dL, reassess renal function in 30/10 = 3 months).[84]

Because older patients are more likely to have more severe and extensive CAD, they are more likely to have coronary anatomy amenable to revascularization than younger patients with NSTE-ACS. However, because elderly patients are at higher risk for procedural complications and bleeding, patients and physicians often exercise more caution, resulting in lower rates of revascularization. A collaborative meta-analysis[118] including 1282 (24%) patients age ≥75 from 8 trials suggested that in the elderly early intervention was associated with a significant reduction in mortality compared with a delayed invasive approach. Barring comorbidities that prove to be contraindications, advanced age should not deter otherwise indicated comprehensive treatment of NSTE-ACS, including the use of an early invasive strategy and revascularization.[8]

Women (see Chapter 91)

Heart disease is the leading cause of death in women worldwide including the United States,[122] yet women continue to be understudied, underdiagnosed, and undertreated. In an analysis of 68,730 patients with NSTE-ACS enrolled in 10 TIMI trials, the 19,827 (29%) women were on average older and more frequently had hypertension, diabetes, prior HF, and renal impairment than did the men.[123]

However, women are more likely to have atypical symptoms and nonatherosclerotic causes of angina, such as microvascular dysfunction and abnormal vascular reactivity.[8] Women have a different proteomic profile (higher concentrations of adipokines, inflammatory markers, and BNP, but lower concentrations of markers of fibrosis, platelet reactivity, and myocardial necrosis).[124] Nevertheless, women with NSTE-ACS should receive the same pharmacologic therapy as men in both the acute care and the secondary prevention phases, and women with NSTE-ACS with high-risk features should undergo an early invasive strategy.[8] In a pooled analysis of 3550 patients with NSTE-ACS from 8 trials, women were found to be more likely than men to have nonobstructive CAD on coronary angiography.[25] Although rates of MACE are lower in patients with nonobstructive disease compared with those with obstructive CAD, they are not negligible, and are similar in women and men.[125] Therefore secondary preventive measures (see later) should not be withheld either in women or men with nonobstructive CAD.

Because women on average have lower body weight and are older than men with NSTE-ACS, they are more likely to have impaired renal function and are at greater risk for excess dosing of antithrombotic therapies that require renal dose adjustment. Data from the Minimizing Adverse Haemorrhagic Events by Transradial Access Site and Systemic Implementation of Angiox trial[126] demonstrated a similar advantage of radial over femoral arterial access in women as in men. Furthermore, analyses from ACS registries suggest that the poorer outcomes in women were associated with lower rates of evidence-based care than men[127]; however, the gap appears to be narrowing over time.[128] A sex-specific meta-analysis of 7 randomized trials in 87,840 patients (28% women) demonstrated comparable relative efficacy and safety outcomes with potent P2Y$_{12}$ inhibitors (prasugrel, ticagrelor, and cangrelor) in women as in men.[129] Thus strategies to promote guideline adherence and greater awareness of the similar CV risk in patients with NSTE-ACS, regardless of sex, are needed.[130]

Diabetes Mellitus and Glucose Intolerance (see Chapter 31)

More than 34 million Americans (13% of all adults) have DM, and approximately 30% of U.S. adults have prediabetes.[131] CAD is responsible for 75% of deaths in patients with DM. Since more than 30% of patients with NSTE-ACS in the United States have DM[132] and such patients have higher rates of adverse CV outcomes, all patients presenting with NSTE-ACS should be screened for DM during hospitalization. Patients with known DM or glucose intolerance should receive the medical therapies established in those with normal glucose metabolism, but in addition, should have frequent glucose monitoring through discharge. Patients with persistent glucose levels >180 mg/dL should be considered for insulin therapy to achieve a target range of 140 to 180 mg/dL during hospitalization.[133] Because of the U-shaped relationship between glucose levels and outcomes in patients with DM and ACS, hypoglycemia (<90 mg/dL) should be avoided.[8] Patients with DM have a blunted response to standard antiplatelet regimens, including clopidogrel and ASA.[134] Subgroup analyses comparing outcomes in patients with and without DM have suggested incrementally greater benefit of some more potent antiplatelet agents, including prasugrel[52] and GP IIb/IIIa inhibitors,[68] in patients with DM.

With regard to revascularization, the ESC NSTE-ACS guidelines[18] recommend an early invasive strategy and a preference for CABG over PCI in patients with DM and complex (e.g., multivessel or LMA) CAD.[135] When PCI is selected, a newer-generation DES should be employed. Renal function should be closely monitored for 2 to 3 days after coronary angiography or PCI in patients with renal dysfunction or who are treated with metformin. If renal function deteriorates, metformin should be held for at least 48 hours until renal function improves.

A pooled analysis of 15,459 patients with NSTE-ACS enrolled in 11 TIMI trials demonstrated that DM is associated independently with a significantly higher risk of mortality at 30 days and at 1 year.[136] This increased risk also extended to patients with previously undiagnosed DM and those with pre-diabetes.[137]

Chronic Kidney Disease (see Chapter 101)

According to current estimates, 15% of U.S. adults (37 million) have CKD.[138] Patients with impaired renal function and NSTE-ACS are older on average and more likely to have additional comorbid conditions, including DM, peripheral arterial disease (PAD), and HF. Thus they have increased risk for recurrent ischemic events, including stent thrombosis, post-PCI ischemic events, and treatment complications.[139] They are underrepresented in clinical trials and are often undertreated in clinical practice. All patients admitted with NSTE-ACS should have a glomerular filtration rate (GFR) estimated at presentation to permit informed decisions regarding management and proper dosing of antithrombotic agents.

In an observational study of nearly 4.5 million patients admitted to hospital with NSTEMI in the United States from 2004 to 2014, the use of PCI, as renal function worsened, decreased from 32% (no CKD) to 14% to 22% (CKD grades 3 to 5), while adjusted rates of in-hospital mortality and bleeding were greater in patients with more severe CKD regardless of treatment strategy.[140] Randomized data on patients with advanced CKD (stages 4 or 5) and ACS are limited as most trials excluded patients with estimated glomerular filtration rate (eGFR) <30 mL/min/1.73 m^2. A meta-analysis of five trials of 1453 patients with NSTE-ACS and CKD with eGFR <60 mL/min/1.73 m^2 demonstrated favorable trends in all-cause mortality, the composite of death or nonfatal MI, and rehospitalization with an early invasive strategy compared with conservative management.[141] Thus coronary angiography should be considered in patients with NSTE-ACS and CKD, and the benefits of prompt revascularization should be weighed against the risks of bleeding and contrast induced nephropathy. In patients with CKD undergoing PCI, newer-generation DESs are preferred over BMSs. In patients with multivessel CAD, acceptable surgical risk, and life expectancy exceeding 1 year, CABG is preferred over PCI, whereas in patients with high surgical risk or shorter life expectancy, PCI is recommended.[18]

Patients with CKD have a greater risk of bleeding because of impaired platelet function. In patients with CKD, the dosage of

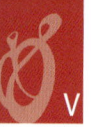

renally cleared medications requires adjustment; such medications include enoxaparin, bivalirudin, eptifibatide, and tirofiban. In addition, patients with CKD have increased risk for contrast-induced nephropathy following angiography and revascularization. Current guidelines recommend that the risk for contrast-induced nephropathy be assessed by measurement of the ratio of contrast volume to eGFR and that this ratio not exceed 3.7.[47] Adequate hydration with isotonic saline from 12 hours before to 24 hours after dye exposure is essential.

Heart Failure (see Chapters 49 to 51)

An estimated 6.2 million adult Americans have HF, with projections showing that the prevalence will increase by 46% over the next decade.[2] Both the American Heart Association (AHA)/American College of Cardiology (ACC)[8] and ESC[18] guidelines provide specific new recommendations regarding patients with NSTE-ACS complicated by HF. An early invasive approach is recommended because these patients are at increased risk of major morbidity and death; revascularization, particularly CABG, improves outcomes.[47] The revascularization strategy should be determined by coronary anatomy and degree of LV and valvular dysfunction as assessed by imaging studies. If there is a large territory of myocardial ischemia and severe LV systolic dysfunction, LV support (e.g., percutaneous ventricular assist devices) may be necessary for hemodynamic support peri-PCI.

Although cardiogenic shock is less common in patients with NSTEMI-ACS than in patients with STEMI, in NSTEMI, the shock tends to occur later in the hospitalization and in patients with more comorbidities, common extensive CAD, and recurrent ischemia/infarction. When possible, immediate revascularization with PCI is recommended; emergency CABG is recommended if the coronary anatomy is not suitable for PCI. Short-term use of mechanical circulatory support should be considered in patients with hemodynamic instability caused by mechanical complications. However, routine use of intra-aortic balloon counterpulsation in patients without mechanical complications is not recommended,[47] given the lack of proven benefit.[142] A percutaneous LV assist device (LVAD) may be considered in selected patients as a bridge to cardiac transplantation or to an implanted LVAD. Patients who emerge from the acute episode stable, but with persistent LV systolic dysfunction, should receive management as outlined in Chapter 50.

Vasospastic Angina

In 1959, Prinzmetal and colleagues described a syndrome of ischemic pain that occurred at rest, accompanied by ST-segment elevation.[143] The syndrome was named Prinzmetal's variant angina but it is now known as vasospastic angina (VA). Spasm of one or more proximal coronary arteries with resultant transmural ischemia and abnormalities in LV function are the diagnostic hallmarks of VA, which may be associated with acute MI, ventricular tachycardia, ventricular fibrillation, and SCD.[144] Patients with VA tend to be younger than those with NSTE-ACS attributable to coronary atherosclerosis, and many do not exhibit the classic coronary risk factors, except they are frequently heavy cigarette smokers. Angina at rest is often extremely severe, tends to cluster between midnight and 8 AM, and may be accompanied by syncope related to AV block, asystole, or ventricular tachyarrhythmia.[144] Increased QT dispersion appears to be a risk marker for SCD in these patients.

Approximately one-third of patients with VA also exhibit severe fixed coronary obstruction and may have a combination of exertion-induced angina with ST-segment depression and episodes of angina at rest with ST-segment elevation. Rarely, VA appears to be a manifestation of a generalized vasospastic disorder associated with migraine and/or Raynaud phenomenon. VA can also develop in association with aspirin-induced asthma and administration of 5-fluorouracil and cyclophosphamide. The ergot derivatives used to treat migraine headache and serotonin antagonists used to treat depression can precipitate episodes of VA. The incidence of VA has always been greater in Japan and South Korea than in Western countries, but across the world, the incidence appears to have fallen markedly over the past 3 decades, possibly related in part to the widespread use of calcium antagonists and nitrates.

The key to diagnosis of VA lies in the detection of episodic ST-segment elevation, often accompanied by severe chest pain, usually occurring at rest. Multiple asymptomatic episodes of (silent) ST-segment elevation occur in many patients. ST-segment deviations may be present in any leads, depending on the artery involved. Patients with no or mild fixed coronary obstruction tend to experience a more benign course than do patients with VA and associated severe obstructive lesions.[144] Coronary Vasomotion Disorders International Study Group (COVADIS) developed international diagnostic standards for VA.[145] These standards consisted of (1) nitrate-responsive angina during spontaneous episodes, (2) transient ischemic ECG changes (ST-segment elevation or depression ≥0.1 mV, and (3) coronary artery spasm, defined as transient coronary artery occlusion "with angina and ECG changes either spontaneously or in response to a provocative stimulus."

Three provocative tests for coronary spasm can be performed at coronary angiography, hyperventilation, intracoronary acetylcholine, and intracoronary ergonovine, although the latter test is no longer available in the United States. These provocative maneuvers should be used only in patients without obstructive CAD and in whom VA is suspected, but not yet confirmed. In patients with MI with nonobstructive CAD who are suspected to have coronary vasomotor abnormalities, guidelines endorse the use of provocative testing for spasm to identify a high-risk subgroup of patients, establish its cause, and permit appropriate treatment.[146,147]

Coronary microvascular obstruction has been reported to accompany VA.[148] It can be detected by CMR imaging or positron emission tomography.[149]

Management

Patients with VA should be urged strongly to discontinue smoking. The mainstay of therapy is a calcium antagonist, alone or preferably in combination with a long-acting nitrate. SL or IV nitroglycerin often abolishes attacks of VA promptly, while the long-acting nitrates are useful in preventing attacks. The response to beta blockade in patients with VA is variable. Some patients, particularly those with associated fixed obstructions, show a reduction in the frequency of exertion-induced angina caused primarily by augmentation of myocardial oxygen requirements. In others, however, nonselective beta-blocking agents may actually be detrimental because blockade of beta$_2$ receptors, which mediate coronary dilation, may allow unopposed alpha receptor–mediated coronary vasoconstriction. In a study of 640 Japanese patients with VA confirmed by acetylcholine provocation testing and no significant coronary stenosis, statin therapy significantly reduced the risk of MACE.[150] Prevention of plaque formation or progression may explain part of the benefit of statins, but the pleiotropic effects of statins, such as the amelioration of endothelial dysfunction, suppression of inflammation, and inhibition of the Rho A/Rho-kinase pathway, may also pertain.

PCI and occasionally CABG may be indicated in patients with VA associated with discrete, proximal, fixed obstructive lesions, but revascularization is contraindicated in patients with isolated coronary artery spasm without accompanying fixed obstructive disease. Patients who have experienced ischemia-associated ventricular fibrillation and continue to manifest ischemic episodes despite maximal medical treatment should receive an implantable cardioverter-defibrillator (ICD).

Many patients with VA pass through an acute, active phase, with frequent episodes of angina and cardiac events occurring during the first 6 months after diagnosis. The extent and severity of the underlying CAD and the tempo of the syndrome have a major effect on the incidence of late mortality and MI. Remission occurs more frequently in patients without significant fixed coronary artery stenoses and in those who have discontinued smoking. For unclear reasons, some patients, after a relatively quiescent period of months or even years, experience a recrudescence of vasospastic activity with frequent and severe episodes of ischemia. Fortunately, these patients generally respond to retreatment with calcium antagonists and nitrates. Clinical outcomes are excellent in patients with isolated coronary spasm and no underlying CAD, with no cardiac death occurring in 76 patients monitored for 3 years in the CAS-PAR study, although about half these patients experienced angina frequently.[145,151]

Cardiac Syndrome X

Approximately 10% to 25% of patients with UA and 6% to 10% of patients with acute MI may present with nonobstructive (<50% stenosis) epicardial coronary disease,[152] although they may have evidence of myocardial ischemia by electrocardiography or myocardial perfusion imaging. This condition is sometimes still referred to as "cardiac syndrome X or MINOCA (Myocardial Infarction with Nonobstructive Coronary Arteries)." It must be distinguished from metabolic syndrome (Chapter 31).

Cocaine, Amphetamines, and Psychoactive Substances (see Chapter 84)

Cocaine use causes a marked increase in sympathetic tone by blocking the reuptake of norepinephrine from synapses by preganglionic neurons, thereby resulting in increased myocardial oxygen demand and decreased supply. This may cause acute myocardial ischemia and may manifest as ACS. This condition, which has similar findings as amphetamine abuse, occurs more frequently in younger persons and should be especially considered in males younger than 30 years. Among 2097 patients age ≤50 years with first MI (47% with NSTEMI), cocaine and/or marijuana use was present in 10% and was associated with worse all-cause and CV mortality.[153]

The use of novel psychoactive "street" drugs, including "bath salts" that contain synthetic cathinones and synthetic cannabinoids (known as "K2" in the United States and "spice" in Europe) have cocaine-like actions. They may also cause CV complications, including ischemic stroke and ACS.[154]

Patients with NSTE-ACS and a recent history of cocaine, methamphetamine, or novel psychoactive substance use should be treated similar to those without recent stimulant use, except that patients with signs of acute intoxication (e.g., euphoria, tachycardia, hypertension) should not receive beta blockers because of the risk of coronary spasm.[8] Vasodilators and CCBs are preferred agents, and benzodiazepines alone or in combination with nitroglycerin may also be used to manage hypertension.

FUTURE PERSPECTIVES

NSTE-ACS is a heterogeneous syndrome, not a specific disease. Subgroups of patients who respond to specific therapies should be identified. Specifically, there is considerable variation in the responses to antiplatelet agents and anticoagulants, in terms of both efficacy and safety, and the optimal duration and intensity of treatment. Predictors of responses to these agents and their risks deserve further study. In addition to phenotypic subgroups of patients with NSTE-ACS, the "omics" technologies, especially genomics, proteomics, and metabolomics, will play critically important roles in this effort. For example, the inflammatory biomarker hs-CRP is used to identify patients with NSTE-ACS with active or persistent inflammation. These patients are at substantially higher risk of recurrent ACS and should receive intensive secondary prevention. Because inflammation appears to play a key role in the development of unstable atherosclerotic plaques and studies with some anti-inflammatory drugs (colchicine, canakinumab) have shown promise in patients with prior MI or stable CAD while others have not (e.g., methotrexate), further studies in patients with NSTE-ACS are needed.

TABLE 39.7 Key Unanswered Questions in Non–ST Elevation Acute Coronary Syndromes

Pathophysiology
- Will superficial plaque erosion continue to rise to become the dominant pathophysiology?
- Should patients be treated differently based on their underlying pathophysiology?
- What are the critical determinants that cause one vulnerable plaque to cause a clinical event but another vulnerable plaque to be silent and heal?

Diagnosis
- What will be the role of concomitant use of coronary computed tomographic angiography and high-sensitivity troponin (hsTn) assays in evaluating patients with suspected ACS?
- Will shorter rule-out algorithms with hsTn assays improve patient outcomes?
- What will be the role of genetic testing to individualize treatment and improve patient outcomes?

Acute Treatment
- What is the preferred antithrombotic regimen peri- and post-PCI?
- What is the optimal combination of and timing for administering high-potency lipid-lowering therapies?
- What is the optimal timing and dosing for administering beta blockers?
- What is the optimal timing of oral antiplatelet administration in patients undergoing an early invasive strategy?
- What are the indications for and timing of revascularization of obstructed nonculprit lesions?
- What is the role of fractional flow reserve–guided PCI?
- What are the contemporary benefits of CABG versus PCI in patients with multivessel disease?
- Will novel pharmacologic and mechanical circulatory support strategies improve survival in patients with cardiogenic shock?
- What is the desired hemoglobin level, and what is the optimal timing for blood transfusion?

Chronic Treatment
- What is the optimal duration and regimen of antiplatelet therapy, and how does this differ if an oral anticoagulant is needed?
- Will newer-generation stents allow shortening of the duration of antiplatelet therapy?
- Can dual-antiplatelet therapy be replaced by a single potent $P2Y_{12}$ inhibitor?
- What is the role of PCSK9 inhibitors in patients admitted with ACS?

Prognosis and Secondary Prevention
- Can we improve prediction of the risk of sudden cardiac death and identify who might benefit more from prevention strategies?
- How can the rate of recurrent ischemic cardiovascular events be further reduced?
- What is the role of cardiac regenerative medicine in patients with left ventricular dysfunction after MI?

Modified from Eisen A, et al. Updates on acute coronary syndrome: A review. JAMA Cardiol 2016;1(6):718–730.

As the number of proven therapies continues to grow resulting in increasingly complex clinical guidelines, continued research exploring how to best leverage electronic medical records and "smart" technology to guide clinical decision making and medical education is a high priority. Table 39.7 summarizes important additional unanswered questions regarding NSTE-ACS.

The guidelines for non–ST elevation acute coronary syndromes are presented in the online chapter.

REFERENCES

Epidemiology

1. Roth GA, Mensah GA, Johnson CO, et al. Global burden of cardiovascular diseases and risk factors, 1990-2019. *J Am Coll Cardiol*. 2020;76:2982–3021.
2. Virani SS, Alonso A, Aparicio HJ, et al. Heart disease and stroke statistics-2021 update: a report from the American Heart Association. *Circulation*. 2021;143:e254–e743.
3. Chapman AR, Adamson PD, Shah ASV, et al. High-sensitivity cardiac troponin and the universal definition of myocardial infarction. *Circulation*. 2020;141:161–171.
4. Angelini G, Flego D, Vinci R, et al. Matrix metalloproteinase-9 might affect adaptive immunity in non-ST segment elevation acute coronary syndromes by increasing CD31 cleavage on CD4+ T-cells. *Eur Heart J*. 2018;39:1089–1097.
5. Sugiyama T, Yamamoto E, Fracassi F, et al. Calcified plaques in patients with acute coronary syndromes. *JACC Cardiovasc Interv*. 2019;12:531–540.
6. Ahmadi A, Argulian E, Leipsic J, et al. From subclinical atherosclerosis to plaque progression and acute coronary events: JACC state-of-the-art review. *J Am Coll Cardiol*. 2019;74:1608–1617.
7. Libby P, Pasterkamp G, Crea F, et al. Reassessing the mechanisms of acute coronary syndromes. *Circ Res*. 2019;124:150–160.
8. Amsterdam EA, Wenger NK, Brindis RG, et al. 2014 AHA/ACC guideline for the management of patients with non-ST-elevation acute coronary syndromes: a report of the American College of Cardiology/American Heart Association task force on practice guidelines. *J Am Coll Cardiol*. 2014;64:e139–e228.
9. Braunwald E. Unstable angina and non-ST elevation myocardial infarction. *Am J Respir Crit Care Med*. 2012;185:924–932.
10. Cardona A, Zareba KM, Nagaraja HN, et al. T-wave abnormality as electrocardiographic signature of myocardial edema in non-ST-elevation acute coronary syndromes. *J Am Heart Assoc*. 2018;7.
11. Thygesen K, Alpert JS, Jaffe AS, et al. Fourth universal definition of myocardial infarction (2018). *J Am Coll Cardiol*. 2018;72:2231–2264.
12. Reichlin T, Schindler C, Drexler B, et al. One-hour rule-out and rule-in of acute myocardial infarction using high-sensitivity cardiac troponin T. *Arch Intern Med*. 2012;172:1211–1218.
13. Chew DP, Lambrakis K, Blyth A, et al. A randomized trial of a 1-hour troponin T protocol in suspected acute coronary syndromes: the rapid assessment of possible acute coronary syndrome in the emergency department with high-sensitivity troponin T study (RAPID-TnT). *Circulation*. 2019;140:1543–1556.
14. Januzzi Jr JL, Mahler SA, Christenson RH, et al. Recommendations for Institutions transitioning to high-sensitivity troponin testing: JACC scientific expert panel. *J Am Coll Cardiol*. 2019;73:1059–1077.
15. Badertscher P, Boeddinghaus J, Twerenbold R, et al. Direct comparison of the 0/1h and 0/3h algorithms for early rule-out of acute myocardial infarction. *Circulation*. 2018;137:2536–2538.
16. Twerenbold R, Costabel JP, Nestelberger T, et al. Outcome of applying the ESC 0/1-hour algorithm in patients with suspected myocardial infarction. *J Am Coll Cardiol*. 2019;74:483–494.
17. Mahler SA, Lenoir KM, Wells BJ, et al. Safely identifying emergency department patients with acute chest pain for early discharge. *Circulation*. 2018;138:2456–2468.
18. Collet J-P, Thiele H, Barbato E, et al. 2020 ESC Guideline for the management of acute coronary syndromes in patients presenting without persistent ST-segment elevation. *Eur Heart J*. 2020;00,1–79. https://doi.org/10.1093/eurheartj/ehaa575.
19. Qamar A, Giugliano RP, Bohula EA, et al. Biomarkers and clinical cardiovascular outcomes with ezetimibe in the IMPROVE-IT trial. *J Am Coll Cardiol*. 2019;74:1057–1068.
20. Mani P, Puri R, Schwartz GG, et al. Association of initial and serial C-reactive protein levels with adverse cardiovascular events and death after acute coronary syndrome: a secondary analysis of the VISTA-16 trial. *JAMA Cardiol*. 2019;4:314–320.
21. Peiro OM, Garcia-Osuna A, Ordonez-Llanos J, et al. Long-term prognostic value of growth differentiation factor-15 in acute coronary syndromes. *Clin Biochem*. 2019;73:62–69.
22. Lindholm D, James SK, Gabrysch K, et al. Association of multiple biomarkers with risk of all-cause and cause-specific mortality after acute coronary syndromes: a secondary analysis of the PLATO biomarker study. *JAMA Cardiol*. 2018;3:1160–1166.

Imaging

23. Garg P, Underwood SR, Senior R, et al. Noninvasive cardiac imaging in suspected acute coronary syndrome. *Nat Rev Cardiol*. 2016;13:266–275.
24. SCOT-HEART investigators. CT coronary angiography in patients with suspected angina due to coronary heart disease (SCOT-HEART): an open-label, parallel-group, multicentre trial. *Lancet*. 2015;385:2383–2391.
25. Ferencik M, Hoffmann U, Bamberg F, et al. Highly sensitive troponin and coronary computed tomography angiography in the evaluation of suspected acute coronary syndrome in the emergency department. *Eur Heart J*. 2016;37:2397–2405.

Risk Assessment

26. De Ferrari GM, Fox KA, White JA, et al. Outcomes among non-ST-segment elevation acute coronary syndromes patients with no angiographically obstructive coronary artery disease: observations from 37,101 patients. *Eur Heart J Acute Cardiovasc Care*. 2014;3:37–45.
27. Patel KV, Pandey A, de Lemos JA. Conceptual framework for addressing residual atherosclerotic cardiovascular disease risk in the era of precision medicine. *Circulation*. 2018;137:2551–2553.
28. Braunwald E, Morrow DA. Unstable angina: is it time for a requiem? *Circulation*. 2013;127:2452–2457.
29. Berg DD, Wiviott SD, Braunwald E, et al. Modes and timing of death in 66 252 patients with non-ST-segment elevation acute coronary syndromes enrolled in 14 TIMI trials. *Eur Heart J*. 2018;39:3810–3820.
30. Antman EM, Cohen M, Bernink PJ, et al. The TIMI risk score for unstable angina/non-ST elevation MI: a method for prognostication and therapeutic decision making. *J Am Med Assoc*. 2000;284:835–842.
31. Boersma E, Pieper KS, Steyerberg EW, et al. Predictors of outcome in patients with acute coronary syndromes without persistent ST-segment elevation. Results from an international trial of 9461 patients. The PURSUIT Investigators. *Circulation*. 2000;101:2557–2567.
32. Fox KA, Dabbous OH, Goldberg RJ, et al. Prediction of risk of death and myocardial infarction in the six months after presentation with acute coronary syndrome: prospective multinational observational study (GRACE). *BMJ*. 2006;333:1091.
33. Bohula EA, Bonaca MP, Braunwald E, et al. Atherothrombotic risk stratification and the efficacy and safety of vorapaxar in patients with stable ischemic heart disease and previous myocardial infarction. *Circulation*. 2016;134:304–313.
34. Bohula EA, Morrow DA, Giugliano RP, et al. Atherothrombotic risk stratification and ezetimibe for secondary prevention. *J Am Coll Cardiol*. 2017;69:911–921.
35. Pocock SJ, Huo Y, Van de Werf F, et al. Predicting two-year mortality from discharge after acute coronary syndrome: an internationally-based risk score. *Eur Heart J Acute Cardiovasc Care*. 2019;8:727–737.

Management

36. Hofmann R, James SK, Jernberg T, et al. Oxygen therapy in suspected acute myocardial infarction. *N Engl J Med*. 2017;377:1240–1249
37. Chatterjee S, Chaudhuri D, Vedanthan R, et al. Early intravenous beta-blockers in patients with acute coronary syndrome–a meta-analysis of randomized trials. *Int J Cardiol*. 2013;168:915–921.
38. Yusuf S, Wittes J, Friedman L. Overview of results of randomized clinical trials in heart disease. I. Treatments following myocardial infarction. *J Am Med Assoc*. 1988;260:2088–2093.
39. Kontos MC, Diercks DB, Ho PM, et al. Treatment and outcomes in patients with myocardial infarction treated with acute beta-blocker therapy: results from the American College of Cardiology's NCDR((R)). *Am Heart J*. 2011;161:864–870.
40. Furtado RHM, Nicolau JC, Guo J, et al. Morphine and cardiovascular outcomes among patients with non-ST-segment elevation acute coronary syndromes undergoing coronary angiography. *J Am Coll Cardiol*. 2020;75:289–300.
41. Rodriguez F, Mahaffey KW. Management of patients with NSTE-ACS: a comparison of the recent AHA/ACC and ESC guidelines. *J Am Coll Cardiol*. 2016;68:313–321.
42. Antithrombotic Trialists' Collaboration. Collaborative meta-analysis of randomised trials of antiplatelet therapy for prevention of death, myocardial infarction, and stroke in high risk patients. *BMJ*. 2002;324:71–86.
43. Mehta SR, Bassand JP, Chrolavicius S, et al. Dose comparisons of clopidogrel and aspirin in acute coronary syndromes. *N Engl J Med*. 2010;363:930–942.
44. Valgimigli M, Bueno H, Byrne RA, et al. 2017 ESC focused update on dual antiplatelet therapy in coronary artery disease developed in collaboration with EACTS: the Task Force for dual antiplatelet therapy in coronary artery disease of the European Society of Cardiology (ESC) and of the European Association for Cardio-Thoracic Surgery (EACTS). *Eur Heart J*. 2018;39:213–260.
45. Yusuf S, Zhao F, Mehta SR, et al. Effects of clopidogrel in addition to aspirin in patients with acute coronary syndromes without ST-segment elevation. *N Engl J Med*. 2001;345:494–502.
46. Mehta SR, Yusuf S, Peters RJ, et al. Effects of pretreatment with clopidogrel and aspirin followed by long-term therapy in patients undergoing percutaneous coronary intervention: the PCI-CURE study. *Lancet*. 2001;358:527–533.
47. Neumann FJ, Sousa-Uva M, Ahlsson A, et al. 2018 ESC/EACTS Guidelines on myocardial revascularization. *Eur Heart J*. 2019;40:87–165.
48. Cannon CP, Harrington RA, James S, et al. Comparison of ticagrelor with clopidogrel in patients with a planned invasive strategy for acute coronary syndromes (PLATO): a randomised double-blind study. *Lancet*. 2010;375:283–293.
49. Jeong YH, Tantry US, Kim IS, et al. Effect of CYP2C19*2 and *3 loss-of-function alleles on platelet reactivity and adverse clinical events in East Asian acute myocardial infarction survivors treated with clopidogrel and aspirin. *Circ Cardiovasc Interv*. 2011.
50. Bhatt DL, Cryer BL, Contant CF, et al. Clopidogrel with or without omeprazole in coronary artery disease. *N Engl J Med*. 2010;363:1909–1917.
51. Wiviott SD, Braunwald E, McCabe CH, et al. Prasugrel versus clopidogrel in patients with acute coronary syndromes. *N Engl J Med*. 2007;357:2001–2015.
52. Wiviott SD, Braunwald E, Angiolillo DJ, et al. Greater clinical benefit of more intensive oral antiplatelet therapy with prasugrel in patients with diabetes mellitus in the trial to assess improvement in therapeutic outcomes by optimizing platelet inhibition with prasugrel-Thrombolysis in Myocardial Infarction 38. *Circulation*. 2008;118:1626–1636.
53. Wiviott SD, Braunwald E, McCabe CH, et al. Intensive oral antiplatelet therapy for reduction of ischaemic events including stent thrombosis in patients with acute coronary syndromes treated with percutaneous coronary intervention and stenting in the TRITON-TIMI 38 trial: a subanalysis of a randomised trial. *Lancet*. 2008;371:1353–1363.
54. Wiviott SD, Desai N, Murphy SA, et al. Efficacy and safety of intensive antiplatelet therapy with prasugrel from TRITON-TIMI 38 in a core clinical cohort defined by worldwide regulatory agencies. *Am J Cardiol*. 2011;108:905–911.
55. Roe MT, Armstrong PW, Fox KA, et al. Prasugrel versus clopidogrel for acute coronary syndromes without revascularization. *N Engl J Med*. 2012;367:1297–1309.
56. Montalescot G, Bolognese L, Dudek D, et al. Pretreatment with prasugrel in non-ST-segment elevation acute coronary syndromes. *N Engl J Med*. 2013;369:999–1010.
57. Wallentin L, Becker RC, Budaj A, et al. Ticagrelor versus clopidogrel in patients with acute coronary syndromes. *N Engl J Med*. 2009;361:1045–1057.
58. Mahaffey KW, Wojdyla DM, Carroll K, et al. Ticagrelor compared with clopidogrel by geographic region in the Platelet Inhibition and Patient Outcomes (PLATO) trial. *Circulation*. 2011;124:544–554.
59. Bonaca MP, Bhatt DL, Cohen M, et al. Long-term use of ticagrelor in patients with prior myocardial infarction. *N Engl J Med*. 2015;372:1791–1800.
60. Storey RF, Angiolillo DJ, Bonaca MP, et al. Platelet inhibition with ticagrelor 60 mg versus 90 mg twice daily in the PEGASUS-TIMI 54 trial. *J Am Coll Cardiol*. 2016;67:1145–1154.
61. Schupke S, Neumann FJ, Menichelli M, et al. Ticagrelor or prasugrel in patients with acute coronary syndromes. *N Engl J Med*. 2019;381:1524–1534.
62. Jneid H. Ticagrelor or prasugrel in acute coronary syndromes - the Winner Takes it all? *N Engl J Med*. 2019;381:1582–1585.
63. Bueno H, Rossello X, Pocock SJ, et al. In-hospital coronary revascularization rates and post-discharge mortality risk in non-ST-segment elevation acute coronary syndrome. *J Am Coll Cardiol*. 2019;74:1454–1461.
64. Mehran R, Baber U, Sharma SK, et al. Ticagrelor with or without aspirin in high-risk patients after PCI. *N Engl J Med*. 2019;381:2032–2042.
65. Mauri L, Kereiakes DJ, Yeh RW, et al. Twelve or 30 months of dual antiplatelet therapy after drug-eluting stents. *N Engl J Med*. 2014;371:2155–2166.
66. Angiolillo DJ, Rollini F, Storey RF, et al. International expert consensus on switching platelet P2Y12 receptor-Inhibiting therapies. *Circulation*. 2017;136:1955–1975.
67. Steg PG, Bhatt DL, Hamm CW, et al. Effect of cangrelor on periprocedural outcomes in percutaneous coronary interventions: a pooled analysis of patient-level data. *Lancet*. 2013;382:1981–1992.
68. Boersma E, Harrington RA, Moliterno DJ, et al. Platelet glycoprotein IIb/IIIa inhibitors in acute coronary syndromes: a meta-analysis of all major randomised clinical trials. *Lancet*. 2002;359:189–198.
69. Wessler JD, Giugliano RP. Risk of thrombocytopenia with glycoprotein IIb/IIIa inhibitors across drugs and patient populations: a meta-analysis of 29 large placebo-controlled randomized trials. *Eur Heart J Cardiovasc Pharmacother*. 2015;1:97–106.
70. Giugliano RP, White JA, Bode C, et al. Early versus delayed, provisional eptifibatide in acute coronary syndromes. *N Engl J Med*. 2009;360:2176–2190.
71. Stone GW, Bertrand ME, Moses JW, et al. Routine upstream initiation vs deferred selective use of glycoprotein IIb/IIIa inhibitors in acute coronary syndromes: the ACUITY Timing trial. *J Am Med Assoc*. 2007;297:591–602.
72. Eikelboom JW, Anand SS, Malmberg K, et al. Unfractionated heparin and low-molecular-weight heparin in acute coronary syndrome without ST elevation: a meta-analysis [see comments]. *Lancet*. 2000;355:1936–1942.
73. Antman EM, McCabe CH, Gurfinkel EP, et al. Enoxaparin prevents death and cardiac ischemic events in unstable angina/non-Q-wave myocardial infarction. Results of the thrombolysis in myocardial infarction (TIMI) 11B trial [see comments]. *Circulation*. 1999;100:1593–1601.
74. Murphy SA, Gibson CM, Morrow DA, et al. Efficacy and safety of the low-molecular weight heparin enoxaparin compared with unfractionated heparin across the acute coronary syndrome spectrum: a meta-analysis. *Eur Heart J*. 2007;28:2077–2086.
75. Stone GW, McLaurin BT, Cox DA, et al. Bivalirudin for patients with acute coronary syndromes. *N Engl J Med*. 2006;355:2203–2216.
76. Cavender MA, Sabatine MS. Bivalirudin versus heparin in patients planned for percutaneous coronary intervention: a meta-analysis of randomised controlled trials. *Lancet*. 2014;384:599–606.

77. Erlinge D, Omerovic E, Frobert O, et al. Bivalirudin versus heparin monotherapy in myocardial infarction. *N Engl J Med.* 2017;377:1132–1142.
78. Yusuf S, Mehta SR, Chrolavicius S, et al. Effects of fondaparinux on mortality and reinfarction in patients with acute ST-segment elevation myocardial infarction: the OASIS-6 randomized trial. *J Am Med Assoc.* 2006;295:1519–1530.
79. Steg PG, Jolly SS, Mehta SR, et al. Low-dose vs standard-dose unfractionated heparin for percutaneous coronary intervention in acute coronary syndromes treated with fondaparinux: the FUTURA/OASIS-8 randomized trial. *J Am Med Assoc.* 2010;304:1339–1349.
80. Mega JL, Braunwald E, Wiviott SD, et al. Rivaroxaban in patients with a recent acute coronary syndrome. *N Engl J Med.* 2012;366:9–19.
81. van Rein N, Heide-Jorgensen U, Lijfering WM, et al. Major bleeding rates in atrial fibrillation patients on single, dual, or triple antithrombotic therapy. *Circulation.* 2019;139:775–786.
82. Vranckx P, Valgimigli M, Eckardt L, et al. Edoxaban-based versus vitamin K antagonist-based antithrombotic regimen after successful coronary stenting in patients with atrial fibrillation (ENTRUST-AF PCI): a randomised, open-label, phase 3b trial. *Lancet.* 2019;394:1335–1343.
83. Lip GYH, Collet JP, Haude M, et al. 2018 Joint European consensus document on the management of antithrombotic therapy in atrial fibrillation patients presenting with acute coronary syndrome and/or undergoing percutaneous cardiovascular interventions: a joint consensus document of the European Heart Rhythm Association (EHRA), European Society of Cardiology working group on thrombosis, European Association of Percutaneous Cardiovascular Interventions (EAPCI), and European Association of Acute Cardiac Care (ACCA) endorsed by the Heart Rhythm Society (HRS), Asia-Pacific Heart Rhythm Society (APHRS), Latin America Heart Rhythm Society (LAHRS), and Cardiac Arrhythmia Society of Southern Africa (CASSA). *Europace.* 2019;21:192–193.
84. Steffel J, Collins R, Antz M, et al. 2021 European Heart Rhythm Association Practical Guide on the Use of Non-Vitamin K Antagonist Oral Anticoagulants in Patients with Atrial Fibrillation. *Europace.* 2021;00:1–65. doi:10.1093/europace/euab065.
85. Sulzgruber P, Wassmann S, Semb AG, et al. Oral anticoagulation in patients with non-valvular atrial fibrillation and a CHA2DS2-VASc score of 1: a current opinion of the European Society of Cardiology working group on cardiovascular Pharmacotherapy and European Society of Cardiology Council on stroke. *Eur Heart J Cardiovasc Pharmacother.* 2019;5:171–180.
86. Mason PJ, Shah B, Tamis-Holland JE, et al. An update on radial artery access and best practices for transradial coronary angiography and intervention in acute coronary syndrome: a Scientific statement from the American Heart Association. *Circ Cardiovasc Interv.* 2018;11:e000035.
87. Tardif JC, Kouz S, Waters DD, et al. Efficacy and safety of low-dose colchicine after myocardial infarction. *N Engl J Med.* 2019;381:2497–2505.
88. Ridker PM, Everett BM, Thuren T, et al. Antiinflammatory therapy with canakinumab for atherosclerotic disease. *N Engl J Med.* 2017;377:1119–1131.
89. Bavry AA, Kumbhani DJ, Rassi AN, et al. Benefit of early invasive therapy in acute coronary syndromes: a meta-analysis of contemporary randomized clinical trials. *J Am Coll Cardiol.* 2006;48:1319–1325.
90. Savonitto S, Cavallini C, Petronio AS, et al. Early aggressive versus initially conservative treatment in elderly patients with non-ST-segment elevation acute coronary syndrome: a randomized controlled trial. *JACC Cardiovasc Interv.* 2012;5:906–916.
91. O'Donoghue M, Boden WE, Braunwald E, et al. Early invasive vs conservative treatment strategies in women and men with unstable angina and non-ST-segment elevation myocardial infarction: a meta-analysis. *J Am Med Assoc.* 2008;300:71–80.
92. Hoedemaker NPG, Damman P, Woudstra P, et al. Early invasive versus selective strategy for non-ST-segment elevation acute coronary syndrome: the ICTUS trial. *J Am Coll Cardiol.* 2017;69:1883–1893.
93. Kolte D, Khera S, Dabhadkar KC, et al. Trends in coronary angiography, revascularization, and outcomes of cardiogenic shock complicating non-ST-elevation myocardial infarction. *Am J Cardiol.* 2016;117:1–9.
94. Pride YB, Mohanavelu S, Zorkun C, et al. Association between angiographic complications and clinical outcomes among patients with acute coronary syndrome undergoing percutaneous coronary intervention: an EARLY ACS (Early Glycoprotein IIb/IIIa Inhibition in Non-ST-Segment Elevation Acute Coronary Syndrome) angiographic substudy. *JACC Cardiovasc Interv.* 2012;5:927–935.
95. Piccolo R, Bonaa KH, Efthimiou O, et al. Drug-eluting or bare-metal stents for percutaneous coronary intervention: a systematic review and individual patient data meta-analysis of randomised clinical trials. *Lancet.* 2019;393:2503–2510.
96. Torii S, Jinnouchi H, Sakamoto A, et al. Drug-eluting coronary stents: insights from preclinical and pathology studies. *Nat Rev Cardiol.* 2020;17:37–51.
97. Rathod KS, Beirne AM, Bogle R, et al. Prior coronary artery bypass graft surgery and outcome after percutaneous coronary intervention: an observational study from the Pan-London percutaneous coronary intervention Registry. *J Am Heart Assoc.* 2020;9:e014409.
98. Stone GW, Kappetein AP, Sabik JF, et al. Five-year outcomes after PCI or CABG for left main coronary disease. *N Engl J Med.* 2019;381:1820–1830.
99. Spadaccio C, Benedetto U. Coronary artery bypass grafting (CABG) vs. percutaneous coronary intervention (PCI) in the treatment of multivessel coronary disease: quo vadis? -a review of the evidences on coronary artery disease. *Ann Cardiothorac Surg.* 2018;7:506–515.
100. Tonkin AM, Colquhoun D, Emberson J, et al. Effects of pravastatin in 3260 patients with unstable angina: results from the LIPID study. *Lancet.* 2000;356:1871–1875.
101. Cannon CP, Braunwald E, McCabe CH, et al. Intensive versus moderate lipid lowering with statins after acute coronary syndromes. *N Engl J Med.* 2004;350:1495–1504.
102. Ray KK, Cannon CP, McCabe CH, et al. Early and late benefits of high-dose atorvastatin in patients with acute coronary syndromes: results from the PROVE IT-TIMI 22 trial. *J Am Coll Cardiol.* 2005;46:1405–1410.
103. Hulten E, Jackson JL, Douglas K, et al. The effect of early, intensive statin therapy on acute coronary syndrome: a meta-analysis of randomized controlled trials. *Arch Intern Med.* 2006;166:1814–1821.
104. Grundy SM, Stone NJ, Bailey AL, et al. 2018 AHA/ACC/AACVPR/AAPA/ABC/ACPM/ADA/AGS/APhA/ASPC/NLA/PCNA guideline on the management of blood cholesterol: Executive summary: a report of the American College of Cardiology/American heart association task force on clinical practice guidelines. *Circulation.* 2019;139:e1046–e1081.
105. Mach F, Baigent C, Catapano AL, et al. 2019 ESC/EAS Guidelines for the management of dyslipidaemias: lipid modification to reduce cardiovascular risk. *Eur Heart J.* 2020;41:111–188.
106. Cannon CP, Blazing MA, Giugliano RP, et al. Ezetimibe added to statin therapy after acute coronary syndromes. *N Engl J Med.* 2015;372:2387–2397.
107. Giugliano RP, Wiviott SD, Blazing MA, et al. Long-term safety and efficacy of achieving very low levels of low-density lipoprotein cholesterol: a prespecified analysis of the IMPROVE-IT trial. *JAMA Cardiol.* 2017;2:547–555.
108. Bach RG, Cannon CP, Giugliano RP, et al. Effect of Simvastatin-ezetimibe compared with Simvastatin monotherapy after acute coronary syndrome among patients 75 Years or older: a secondary analysis of a randomized clinical trial. *JAMA Cardiol.* 2019;4:846–854.
109. Giugliano RP, Cannon CP, Blazing MA, et al. Benefit of adding ezetimibe to statin therapy on cardiovascular outcomes and safety in patients with versus without diabetes mellitus: results from IMPROVE-IT (Improved Reduction of Outcomes: Vytorin Efficacy International Trial). *Circulation.* 2018;137:1571–1582.
110. Eisen A, Cannon CP, Blazing MA, et al. The benefit of adding ezetimibe to statin therapy in patients with prior coronary artery bypass graft surgery and acute coronary syndrome in the IMPROVE-IT trial. *Eur Heart J.* 2016;37:3576–3584.
111. Giugliano RP, Sabatine MS. Are PCSK9 inhibitors the next breakthrough in the cardiovascular field? *J Am Coll Cardiol.* 2015;65:2638–2651.
112. Dyrbus K, Gasior M, Penson P, et al. Inclisiran-New hope in the management of lipid disorders? *J Clin Lipidol.* 2020;14:16–27.
113. Gencer B, Mach F, Murphy SA, et al. Efficacy of evolocumab on cardiovascular outcomes in patients with recent myocardial infarction: a prespecified secondary analysis from the FOURIER trial. *JAMA Cardiol.* 2020.
114. Schwartz GG, Steg PG, Szarek M, et al. Alirocumab and cardiovascular outcomes after acute coronary syndrome. *N Engl J Med.* 2018;379:2097–2107.
115. Robinson JG, Jayanna MB, Brown AS, et al. Enhancing the value of PCSK9 monoclonal antibodies by identifying patients most likely to benefit. A consensus statement from the National Lipid Association. *J Clin Lipidol.* 2019;13:525–537.
116. Giugliano RP, Pedersen TR, Park JG, et al. Clinical efficacy and safety of achieving very low LDL-cholesterol concentrations with the PCSK9 inhibitor evolocumab: a prespecified secondary analysis of the FOURIER trial. *Lancet.* 2017;390:1962–1971.
117. Tarantini G, Ueshima D, D'Amico G, et al. Efficacy and safety of potent platelet P2Y12 receptor inhibitors in elderly versus nonelderly patients with acute coronary syndrome: a systematic review and meta-analysis. *Am Heart J.* 2018;195:78–85.
118. Jobs A, Mehta SR, Montalescot G, et al. Optimal timing of an invasive strategy in patients with non-ST-elevation acute coronary syndrome: a meta-analysis of randomised trials. *Lancet.* 2017;390:737–746.

Special Groups

119. Varenne O, Cook S, Sideris G, et al. Drug-eluting stents in elderly patients with coronary artery disease (SENIOR): a randomised single-blind trial. *Lancet.* 2018;391:41–50.
120. Cholesterol Treatment Trialists C. Efficacy and safety of statin therapy in older people: a meta-analysis of individual participant data from 28 randomised controlled trials. *Lancet.* 2019;393:407–415.
121. Engberding N, Wenger NK. Acute coronary syndromes in the elderly. *F1000Res.* 2017;6:1791.
122. Heron M. Deaths: leading causes for 2017. *Natl Vital Stat Rep.* 2019;68:1–77.
123. Sarma AA, Braunwald E, Cannon CP, et al. Outcomes of women compared with men after non-ST-segment elevation acute coronary syndromes. *J Am Coll Cardiol.* 2019;74:3013–3022.
124. Lau ES, Paniagua SM, Guseh JS, et al. Sex differences in circulating biomarkers of cardiovascular disease. *J Am Coll Cardiol.* 2019;74:1543–1553.
125. Ouellette ML, Loffler AI, Beller GA, et al. Clinical Characteristics, sex differences, and outcomes in patients with normal or near-normal coronary arteries, non-obstructive or obstructive coronary artery disease. *J Am Heart Assoc.* 2018;7.
126. Gargiulo G, Ariotti S, Vranckx P, et al. Impact of sex on Comparative outcomes of radial versus femoral access in patients with acute coronary syndromes undergoing invasive management: data from the randomized MATRIX-access trial. *JACC Cardiovasc Interv.* 2018;11:36–50.
127. Izadnegahdar M, Mackay M, Lee MK, et al. Sex and Ethnic differences in outcomes of acute coronary syndrome and stable Angina patients with obstructive coronary artery disease. *Circ Cardiovasc Qual Outcomes.* 2016;9:S26–S35.
128. Porter A, Paradkar A, Goldenberg I, et al. Temporal trends analysis of the Characteristics, management, and outcomes of women with Acute Coronary Syndrome (ACS): ACS Israeli Survey Registry 2000-2016. *J Am Heart Assoc.* 2020;9:e014721.
129. Lau ES, Braunwald E, Murphy SA, et al. Potent P2Y12 inhibitors in men versus women: a collaborative meta-analysis of randomized trials. *J Am Coll Cardiol.* 2017;69:1549–1559.
130. Mehta LS, Beckie TM, DeVon HA, et al. Acute myocardial infarction in women: a Scientific statement from the American Heart Association. *Circulation.* 2016;133:916–947.
131. Centers for Disease Control and Prevention. *National Diabetes Statistics Report;* 2020.
132. Malta Hansen C, Wang TY, Chen AY, et al. Contemporary patterns of early coronary angiography use in patients with non-ST-segment elevation myocardial infarction in the United States: insights from the national cardiovascular data Registry acute coronary treatment and intervention outcomes Network Registry. *JACC Cardiovasc Interv.* 2018;11:369–380.
133. American Diabetes Association. Diabetes care in the hospital: standards of medical care in diabetes-2020. *Diabetes Care.* 2020;43:S193–S202.
134. Locane S, Pucite E, Miglane E, et al. Antiplatelet resistance in patients with atherosclerosis. *Proc Latv Acad Sci.* 2019;73:373–378.
135. Farkouh ME, Domanski M, Sleeper LA, et al. Strategies for multivessel revascularization in patients with diabetes. *N Engl J Med.* 2012;367(25):2375–2384.
136. Donahoe SM, Stewart GC, McCabe CH, et al. Diabetes and mortality following acute coronary syndromes. *J Am Med Assoc.* 2007;298:765–775.
137. Giraldez RR, Clare RM, Lopes RD, et al. Prevalence and clinical outcomes of undiagnosed diabetes mellitus and prediabetes among patients with high-risk non-ST-segment elevation acute coronary syndrome. *Am Heart J.* 2013;165:918–925.e912.
138. Centers for Disease Control and Prevention. *Chronic Kidney Disease in the United States, 2019.* Atlanta, GA: US Department of Health and Human Services, Centers for Disease Control and Prevention; 2019.
139. Navarro MA, Gosch KL, Spertus JA, et al. Chronic kidney disease and Health Status outcomes following acute myocardial infarction. *J Am Heart Assoc.* 2016;23(5):e002772.
140. Bhatia S, Arora S, Bhatia SM, et al. Non-ST-segment-elevation myocardial infarction among patients with chronic kidney disease: a Propensity score-Matched comparison of percutaneous coronary intervention versus conservative management. *J Am Heart Assoc.* 2018;7:e007920.
141. Charytan DM, Wallentin L, Lagerqvist B, et al. Early angiography in patients with chronic kidney disease: a collaborative systematic review. *Clin J Am Soc Nephrol.* 2009;4:1032–1043.
142. Thiele H, Desch S, Piek JJ, et al. Multivessel versus culprit lesion only percutaneous revascularization plus potential staged revascularization in patients with acute myocardial infarction complicated by cardiogenic shock: design and rationale of CULPRIT-SHOCK trial. *Am Heart J.* 2016;172:160–169.
143. Prinzmetal M, Kennamer R, Merliss R, et al. Angina pectoris. I. A variant form of angina pectoris; preliminary report. *Am J Med.* 1959;27:375–388.
144. de Luna AB, Cygankiewicz I, Baranchuk A, et al. Prinzmetal angina: ECG changes and clinical considerations: a consensus paper. *Ann Noninvasive Electrocardiol.* 2014;19:442–453.
145. Beltrame JF, Crea F, Kaski JC, et al. International standardization of diagnostic criteria for vasospastic angina. *Eur Heart J.* 2017;38:2565–2568.
146. Ibanez B, James S, Agewall S, et al. 2017 ESC Guidelines for the management of acute myocardial infarction in patients presenting with ST-segment elevation: the Task Force for the management of acute myocardial infarction in patients presenting with ST-segment elevation of the European Society of Cardiology (ESC). *Eur Heart J.* 2018;39:119–177.
147. Montone RA, Niccoli G, Fracassi F, et al. Patients with acute myocardial infarction and non-obstructive coronary arteries: safety and prognostic relevance of invasive coronary provocative tests. *Eur Heart J.* 2018;39:91–98.
148. Suda A, Takahashi J, Hao K, et al. Coronary functional abnormalities in patients with angina and nonobstructive coronary artery disease. *J Am Coll Cardiol.* 2019;74:2350–2360.

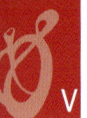

149. Taqueti VR. Coronary microvascular dysfunction in vasospastic angina: provocative role for the Microcirculation in Macrovessel disease prognosis. *J Am Coll Cardiol.* 2019;74:2361–2364.
150. Ishii M, Kaikita K, Sato K, et al. Impact of statin therapy on clinical outcome in patients with coronary spasm. *J Am Heart Assoc.* 2016;5:e003426.
151. Ong P, Athanasiadis A, Borgulya G, et al. 3-year follow-up of patients with coronary artery spasm as cause of acute coronary syndrome: the CASPAR (coronary artery spasm in patients with acute coronary syndrome) study follow-up. *J Am Coll Cardiol.* 2011;57:147–152.
152. Manolis AS, Manolis AA, Manolis TA, et al. Acute coronary syndromes in patients with angiographically normal or near normal (non-obstructive) coronary arteries. *Trends Cardiovasc Med.* 2018;28:541–551.
153. DeFilippis EM, Singh A, Divakaran S, et al. Cocaine and marijuana Use among Young adults with myocardial infarction. *J Am Coll Cardiol.* 2018;71:2540–2551.
154. Lisowska A, Makarewicz-Wujec M, Kozlowska-Wojciechowska M. Can "Legal highs" Trigger myocardial infarction? Patients' Characteristics based on published cases. *Subst Use Misuse.* 2017;52:1712–1720.

Future Perspectives

155. Collet J-P, Thiele H. The 'Ten Commandments' for the 2020 ESC Guidelines for the management of acute coronary syndromes in patients presenting without persistent ST-segment elevation. *Eur Heart J.* 2020;41:3495–3497.
156. Eckel RH, Jakicic JM, Ard JD, et al. 2013 AHA/ACC guideline on lifestyle management to reduce cardiovascular risk: a report of the American College of Cardiology/American Heart Association task force on practice guidelines. *Circulation.* 2014;129:S76–S99.
157. Matanock A, Lee G, Gierke R, et al. Use of 13-Valent pneumococcal Conjugate vaccine and 23-Valent pneumococcal polysaccharide vaccine among adults aged ≥65 Years: updated recommendations of the advisory Committee on Immunization practices. *MMWR Morb Mortal Wkly Rep.* 2019;68:1069–1075.
158. Kaier TE, Twerenbold R, Puelacher C, et al. Direct comparison of cardiac Myosin-binding protein C with cardiac troponins for the early diagnosis of acute myocardial infarction. *Circulation.* 2017;136:1495–1508.
159. Kraaijeveld AO, de Jager SC, de Jager WJ, et al. CC chemokine ligand-5 (CCL5/RANTES) and CC chemokine ligand-18 (CCL18/PARC) are specific markers of refractory unstable angina pectoris and are transiently raised during severe ischemic symptoms. *Circulation.* 2007;116:1931–1941.
160. Klingenberg R, Aghlmandi S, Liebetrau C, et al. Cysteine-rich angiogenic inducer 61 (Cyr61): a novel soluble biomarker of acute myocardial injury improves risk stratification after acute coronary syndromes. *Eur Heart J.* 2017;38:3493–3502.
161. Sumaya W, Wallentin L, James SK, et al. Fibrin clot properties independently predict adverse clinical outcome following acute coronary syndrome: a PLATO substudy. *Eur Heart J.* 2018;39:1078–1085.
162. Kato ET, Morrow DA, Cannon CP, et al. Growth Differentiation Factor-15 (GDF-15) for risk stratification in patients after an acute coronary syndrome: insights from the SOLID-TIMI 52 trial. *Circulation.* 2015;132:A14844.
163. Viswanathan K, Kilcullen N, Morrell C, et al. Heart-type fatty acid-binding protein predicts long-term mortality and re-infarction in consecutive patients with suspected acute coronary syndrome who are troponin-negative. *J Am Coll Cardiol.* 2010;55:2590–2598.
164. Beygui F, Silvain J, Pena A, et al. Usefulness of biomarker strategy to improve GRACE score's prediction performance in patients with non-ST-segment elevation acute coronary syndrome and low event rates. *Am J Cardiol.* 2010;106:650–658.
165. Simon T, Taleb S, Danchin N, et al. Circulating levels of interleukin-17 and cardiovascular outcomes in patients with acute myocardial infarction. *Eur Heart J.* 2013;34:570–577.
166. Lindberg S, Pedersen SH, Mogelvang R, et al. Soluble form of membrane attack complex independently predicts mortality and cardiovascular events in patients with ST-elevation myocardial infarction treated with primary percutaneous coronary intervention. *Am Heart J.* 2012;164:786–792.
167. Morrow DA, Sabatine MS, Brennan ML, et al. Concurrent evaluation of novel cardiac biomarkers in acute coronary syndrome: myeloperoxidase and soluble CD40 ligand and the risk of recurrent ischaemic events in TACTICS-TIMI 18. *Eur Heart J.* 2008;29:1096–1102.
168. Koga S, Ikeda S, Yoshida T, et al. Elevated levels of systemic pentraxin 3 are associated with thin-cap fibroatheroma in coronary culprit lesions: assessment by optical coherence tomography and intravascular ultrasound. *JACC Cardiovasc Interv.* 2013;6:945–954.
169. Lenderink T, Heeschen C, Fichtlscherer S, et al. Elevated placental growth factor levels are associated with adverse outcomes at four-year follow-up in patients with acute coronary syndromes. *J Am Coll Cardiol.* 2006;47:307–311.
170. Bonaca MP, Scirica BM, Sabatine MS, et al. Prospective evaluation of pregnancy-associated plasma protein-a and outcomes in patients with acute coronary syndromes. *J Am Coll Cardiol.* 2012;60:332–338.
171. Samman Tahhan A, Hammadah M, Raad M, et al. Progenitor cells and clinical outcomes in patients with acute coronary syndromes. *Circ Res.* 2018;122:1565–1575.
172. Mallat Z, Steg PG, Benessiano J, et al. Circulating secretory phospholipase A2 activity predicts recurrent events in patients with severe acute coronary syndromes. *J Am Coll Cardiol.* 2005;46:1249–1257.
173. Gerber Y, Weston SA, Enriquez-Sarano M, et al. Contemporary risk stratification after myocardial infarction in the Community: performance of scores and incremental value of soluble suppression of Tumorigenicity-2. *J Am Heart Assoc.* 2017;6:e005958.
174. Wang YK, Tang JN, Shen YL, et al. Prognostic utility of soluble TREM-1 in predicting mortality and cardiovascular events in patients with acute myocardial infarction. *J Am Heart Assoc.* 2018;7:e008985.
175. Li XS, Obeid S, Wang Z, et al. Trimethyllysine, a trimethylamine N-oxide precursor, provides near- and long-term prognostic value in patients presenting with acute coronary syndromes. *Eur Heart J.* 2019;40:2700–2709.
176. O'Malley RG, Bonaca MP, Scirica BM, et al. Prognostic performance of multiple biomarkers in patients with non-ST-segment elevation acute coronary syndrome: analysis from the MERLIN-TIMI 36 trial (metabolic Efficiency with Ranolazine for less ischemia in non-ST-elevation acute coronary syndromes-thrombolysis in myocardial infarction 36). *J Am Coll Cardiol.* 2014;63:1644–1653.
177. Asleh R, Enriquez-Sarano M, Jaffe AS, et al. Galectin-3 levels and outcomes after myocardial infarction: a population-based study. *J Am Coll Cardiol.* 2019;73:2286–2295.
178. Nazer B, Ray KK, Sloan S, et al. Prognostic utility of neopterin and risk of heart failure hospitalization after an acute coronary syndrome. *Eur Heart J.* 2011;32:1390–1397.
179. Omland T, Ueland T, Jansson AM, et al. Circulating osteoprotegerin levels and long-term prognosis in patients with acute coronary syndromes. *J Am Coll Cardiol.* 2008;51:627–633.
180. Ueland T, Akerblom A, Ghukasyan T, et al. Osteoprotegerin is associated with major bleeding but not with cardiovascular outcomes in patients with acute coronary syndromes: insights from the PLATO (Platelet Inhibition and Patient Outcomes) trial. *J Am Heart Assoc.* 2018;7:e007009.

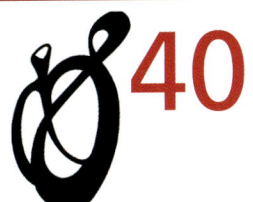

40 Stable Ischemic Heart Disease

DAVID A. MORROW AND JAMES DE LEMOS

扫描二维码阅读
第40章中文导读

MAGNITUDE OF THE PROBLEM, 739

STABLE ANGINA PECTORIS, 739
Clinical Manifestations, 739
Differential Diagnosis of Chest Pain, 740
Pathophysiology, 741

EVALUATION AND MANAGEMENT, 742
Biochemical Tests, 742
Noninvasive Testing, 744
Invasive Assessment, 748
Natural History and Risk Stratification, 749

Medical Management, 749
Pharmacologic Management of Angina, 757
Revascularization Approaches in Stable Ischemic Heart Disease, 764
Percutaneous Coronary Intervention, 766
Restenosis and Late Stent Thrombosis, 766
Coronary Artery Bypass Grafting, 770

OTHER MANIFESTATIONS OF CORONARY ARTERY DISEASE, 777
Prinzmetal (Variant) Angina, 777

Angina and Ischemia Without Obstructive Epicardial CAD, 777
Silent Myocardial Ischemia, 779
Heart Failure in Ischemic Heart Disease, 779

FUTURE PERSPECTIVES, 781

REFERENCES, 781

The spectrum of stable ischemic heart disease (SIHD) is broad and includes individuals with chronic stable angina, asymptomatic ischemia, prior myocardial infarction, and prior coronary revascularization, as well as individuals with nonobstructive coronary atherosclerosis, including microvascular disease. Because this spectrum of ischemic heart disease may unpredictably become unstable, some experts prefer the term chronic coronary syndrome.[1] While underscoring the concept that patients with SIHD are always at some degree of risk for acute periods of instability and therefore warrant preventive management discussed in this chapter, we will continue to use the term SIHD to discriminate this population of individuals from those presenting with acutely unstable ischemic heart disease (IHD), including unstable angina and acute myocardial infarction (see Chapters 37 to 39).

SIHD is most commonly caused by atheromatous plaque that obstructs or gradually narrows the epicardial coronary arteries. The pathogenesis of atherosclerosis is described in Chapter 24. However, other contributors, such as endothelial dysfunction, microvascular disease, and vasospasm, may also exist alone or in combination with coronary atherosclerosis and may be the dominant cause of myocardial ischemia in some patients (Fig. 40.1). Thus, the concept that IHD is synonymous with obstructive coronary atherosclerosis is an overly simplified view.[2,3]

Factors that predispose to coronary atherosclerosis are discussed in Chapters 25 and 27, control of coronary blood flow in Chapter 36, percutaneous coronary revascularization in Chapter 41, ST-segment elevation myocardial infarction (MI) in Chapters 37 and 38, non–ST-segment elevation acute coronary syndromes (ACSs) in Chapter 39, and sudden cardiac death, another significant consequence of IHD, in Chapter 70.

The presenting symptoms in patients with IHD are highly variable. Chest discomfort is usually the predominant symptom in chronic (stable) angina, unstable angina, Prinzmetal (variant) angina, microvascular angina, and acute MI. However, manifestations of IHD also occur in which chest discomfort is absent or not prominent, such as heart failure, asymptomatic (silent) myocardial ischemia, cardiac arrhythmias, and sudden death. Notably, IHD may also present with anginal equivalents such as midepigastric discomfort, dyspnea, effort intolerance, and excessive fatigue, which are observed more frequently in women, older adults, and individuals with diabetes.

Coronary arteries may also become obstructed by nonatherosclerotic mechanisms, including extrinsic compression, myocardial bridging, embolism, coronary arteritis in association with systemic vasculitis, and radiation-induced coronary artery disease (CAD). Myocardial ischemia and angina pectoris may also occur in the setting of extreme myocardial O_2 demand with or without underlying obstructive CAD, as in the case of aortic valve disease (see Chapter 72), hypertrophic cardiomyopathy (see Chapter 54), dilated nonischemic cardiomyopathies (see Chapter 52), or pulmonary hypertension (see Chapter 88).

MAGNITUDE OF THE PROBLEM

The importance of IHD in contemporary society is attested to by the large number of persons afflicted (see Chapter 2). It is estimated that 18,200,000 Americans have IHD, of whom 9,400,000 have angina pectoris and 8,400,000 have had MI.[4] Based on data from the Framingham Heart Study, the lifetime risk for IHD among individuals with an optimal risk factor profile has been estimated as 3.6% for men and <1% for women; whereas among individuals with two or more major risk factors, the lifetime risk is 37.5% for men and 18.3% for women. In 2017, CAD accounted for 43% of all deaths caused by cardiovascular disease and was the single most frequent cause of death in American men and women, resulting in more than one in seven deaths in the United States. The economic cost of IHD is formidable, and in the United States in 2014 to 2015 it was estimated to be $218.7 billion per year. Despite a steady decline in age-specific mortality from CAD over the past several decades, IHD is the leading cause of death worldwide, and it is expected that the worldwide prevalence of CAD will increase in the coming decades. Moreover, with a decline in case-fatality of MI, the prevalence of survivors with SIHD has increased despite a relatively stable rate of incident MI. At the same time, the burden of IHD is shifting progressively to lower socioeconomic groups with contributory factors that include aging of the population, increases in prevalent obesity and type 2 diabetes, and a rise in cardiovascular risk factors in younger generations. The World Health Organization has estimated that by 2030, the global number of deaths from IHD will have risen from 7.4 million in 2012 to 9.2 million (see Chapter 2).

STABLE ANGINA PECTORIS

Clinical Manifestations

Characteristics of Angina (see Chapter 35)

Angina pectoris is a discomfort in the chest or adjacent areas caused by myocardial ischemia. It is usually precipitated by exertion but may also be initiated by other stressors that increase myocardial O_2 demand, including emotional distress. Angina that is prolonged, occurs at rest or occurs in an accelerating pattern of increasing frequency and tempo is indicative of unstable angina or acute MI. Heberden's initial description of angina as conveying a sense of "strangling and anxiety" is still remarkably pertinent. Other adjectives frequently used to describe this distress include constricting, suffocating, crushing, heavy,

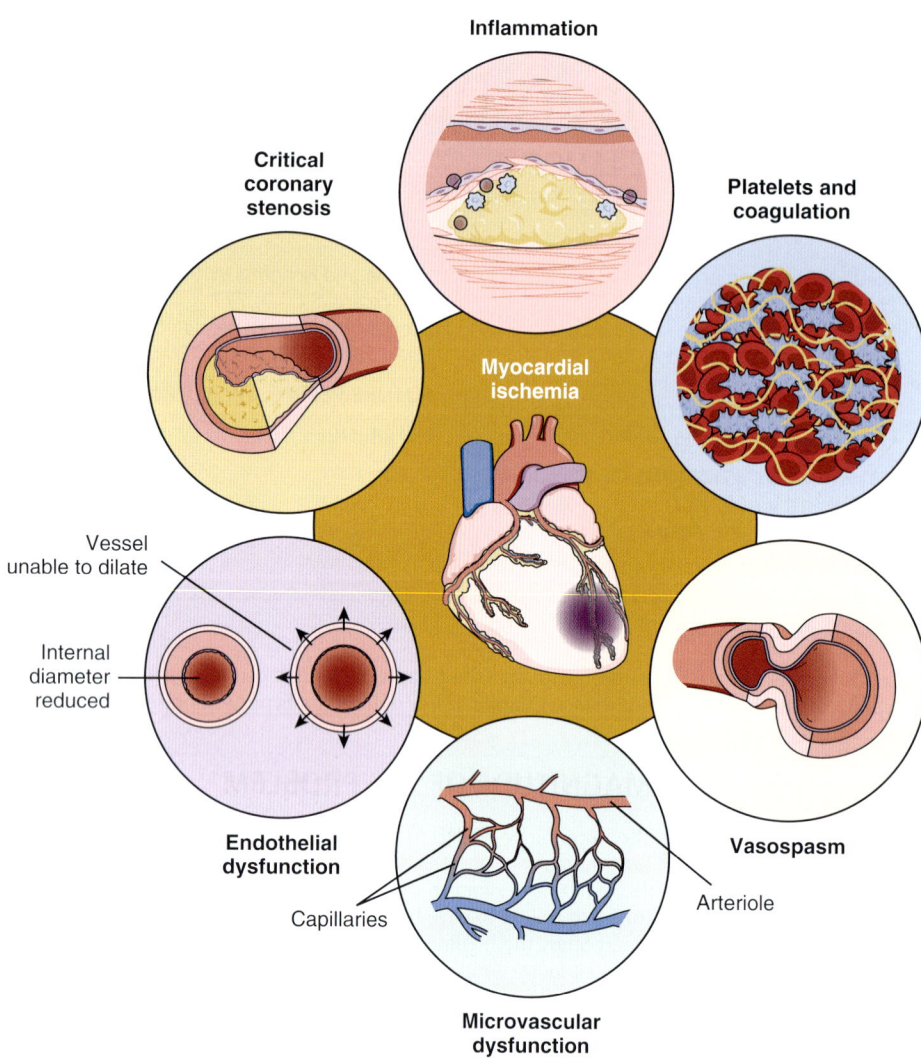

FIGURE 40.1 Pathophysiology of ischemic heart disease. The notion that ischemic heart disease is synonymous with critical stenoses of epicardial coronary arteries is overly simplified. The potential contributors to ischemic heart disease are multiple.

and squeezing. In other patients, the quality of the sensation can be vague and described as a mild pressure-like discomfort, tightness, an uncomfortable numbness, or a burning sensation. The site of the discomfort is usually retrosternal, but radiation is common and generally occurs down the ulnar surface of the left arm; the right arm and the outer surfaces of both arms may also be involved, as can the neck, back, or jaw. Epigastric discomfort alone or in association with chest pressure may occur and can masquerade as indigestion. Anginal discomfort above the mandible or below the epigastrium is rare. Anginal equivalents (i.e., symptoms of myocardial ischemia other than angina), such as dyspnea, faintness, fatigue, and frequent belching, are more commonly seen in women and older adults. A history of abnormal exertional dyspnea may be an indicator of IHD even when angina is absent. Nocturnal angina may be a manifestation of unstable angina but should also raise suspicion of sleep apnea (see Chapter 89). Postprandial angina, presumably caused by redistribution of coronary blood flow to the splanchnic circulation, may be a marker of severe IHD.

The typical episode of angina pectoris usually begins gradually and reaches its maximum intensity over a period of minutes before dissipating. It is unusual for angina pectoris to reach its maximum severity within seconds, and it is characteristic that patients with angina generally prefer to rest, sit, or stop walking during episodes. Chest discomfort while walking in the cold or uphill is suggestive of angina. Features inconsistent with angina pectoris include pain that is pleuritic, sharp, or stabbing in quality or reproduced by movement or palpation of the chest wall or arms. Constant pain lasting many hours or, alternatively, very brief episodes of pain lasting seconds are also unlikely to be due to angina. Typical angina pectoris is relieved within minutes by rest or the use of shortacting nitroglycerin. Response to the latter is often a useful diagnostic tool, although it should be remembered that esophageal pain may also respond to nitroglycerin. A delay of more than 5 to 10 minutes before relief is obtained with rest and nitroglycerin suggests that the symptoms are either not caused by ischemia or are caused by severe ischemia, as with acute MI or unstable angina. The phenomenon of warm-up angina is used to describe the ability of some patients to be able to exercise at higher intensity without angina after an intervening period of rest. This attenuation of myocardial ischemia observed with repeated exertion has been postulated to be caused by ischemic preconditioning (see Chapter 36).

Assessment and Classification of Angina Pectoris

A system of grading the severity of angina pectoris proposed by the Canadian Cardiovascular Society (CCS) is widely used (see Table 11.1). The system is a modification of the New York Heart Association (NYHA) functional classification and allows patients to be categorized in more specific terms. Functional estimates based on the CCS criteria have shown a reproducibility that is only moderate and do not correlate well with objective measures of exercise performance.

More objective measures of the impact of angina on quality of life are available, using either general instruments such as the Medical Outcomes Study 36-Item Short Form Health Survey (SF-36) or the disease-specific Seattle Angina Questionnaire (SAQ). The SAQ is a validated 19 item self-administered questionnaire that assesses domains of anginal frequency and stability, physical limitation, treatment satisfaction, and disease perception.[5] It can be measured serially to assess the impact of medical therapies and revascularization on angina-related quality of life and has emerged as the preferred instrument for assessment of quality of life in clinical trials.[6]

Although these objective measurements have typically been applied in the research setting, a short seven-question version of the SAQ may be practical for the clinical setting. In the future, embedding simple, objective, patient-centered disease measurements into the clinical encounter is likely to become increasingly important for chronic diseases like SIHD. Understanding the impact of angina on quality of life is a necessary prerequisite for shared decision making, which plays a larger role in SIHD than in many other cardiovascular diseases.

Differential Diagnosis of Chest Pain
Esophageal Disorders

Common disorders that may simulate or coexist with angina pectoris are gastroesophageal reflux and disorders of esophageal motility, including diffuse spasm. To compound the difficulty in distinguishing between angina and esophageal pain, both may be relieved by nitroglycerin. However, esophageal pain is often relieved by milk, antacids, foods, or occasionally warm liquids.

Biliary Colic
Although visceral symptoms are commonly associated with myocardial ischemia (particularly acute inferior MI; see Chapters 37 and 38), biliary colic and related hepatobiliary disorders may also mimic ischemia. Biliary pain is steady, usually lasts 2 to 4 hours, and subsides spontaneously, without any symptoms between attacks. It is generally most intense in the right upper abdominal area but may also be felt in the epigastrium or precordium. This discomfort is often referred to the scapula and may radiate around the costal margin to the back.

Costochondritis
In 1921 Tietze first described a syndrome of local pain and tenderness, generally limited to the anterior chest wall and associated with swelling of costal cartilage. The full-blown Tietze syndrome (i.e., pain associated with tender swelling of the costochondral junctions) is uncommon, whereas costochondritis causing tenderness of the costochondral junctions (without swelling) is relatively common. Pain on palpation of these joints is usually well localized and is a useful clinical sign, although deep palpation may elicit pain in the absence of costochondritis. Although palpation of the chest wall often reproduces pain in patients with various musculoskeletal conditions, it should be appreciated that chest wall tenderness does not exclude symptomatic CAD.

Other Neurologic and Musculoskeletal Disorders
Cervical radiculopathy may be confused with angina. This condition may occur as a constant ache, worsened with neck movement, and sometimes results in a sensory deficit. Occasionally, pain mimicking angina can be caused by compression of the brachial plexus by the cervical ribs, and tendinitis or bursitis involving the left shoulder may also cause angina-like pain. Physical examination may also detect pain brought about by movement of an arthritic shoulder or a calcified shoulder tendon. Herpes zoster, caused by recrudescence of the varicella-zoster virus, can manifest by pain across the chest and should be recognized by its dermatomal distribution and associated blistering or crusting rash. Postherpetic neuralgia may persist in the absence of a rash.

Other Causes of Angina-Like Pain
Severe pulmonary hypertension may be associated with exertional chest pain with the characteristics of angina pectoris, and indeed, this pain is thought to be caused by right ventricular ischemia that develops during exertion (see Chapter 88). Other associated symptoms include exertional dyspnea, dizziness, and syncope. Related findings are commonly seen on physical examination, such as a parasternal lift, a palpable and loud pulmonary component of the second heart sound, and right ventricular hypertrophy on the ECG.

Pulmonary embolism is initially characterized by dyspnea as the cardinal symptom, but chest pain may also be present (see Chapter 87). Pleuritic pain suggests pulmonary infarction, and a history of exacerbation of the pain with inspiration, along with a pleural friction rub, if present, helps distinguish it from angina pectoris.

The pain of acute pericarditis (see Chapter 86) may at times be difficult to distinguish from angina pectoris. Recognition of pericarditis may be facilitated by the combination of chest pain not relieved by rest or nitroglycerin and exacerbated by movement, deep inspiration, and lying flat; a pericardial friction rub, which may be evanescent; and changes on the ECG (notably PR-segment depression or diffuse ST elevation).

The classic symptom of aortic dissection is a severe, often sharp pain that radiates to the back (see Chapter 42).

Physical Examination
Most patients with SIHD have normal findings on cardiac examination, and thus the single best clue to the diagnosis of angina is the clinical history. Nonetheless, careful examination can exclude other conditions that mimic angina and may reveal atherosclerosis in noncoronary vascular territories, evidence of risk factors for coronary atherosclerosis (i.e., acanthosis nigricans or tendon xanthomas) or the consequences of myocardial ischemia (see Chapter 13).

Pathophysiology
Angina pectoris results from myocardial ischemia, which is caused by an imbalance between myocardial O_2 requirements and myocardial O_2 supply. The former may be elevated by increases in heart rate, left ventricular (LV) wall stress, and contractility (see Chapter 36); the latter is determined by coronary blood flow and coronary arterial O_2 content (Fig. 40.2). The clinical precipitants and manifestations of supply-demand imbalance are discussed in this section. The pathobiology of atherosclerosis is discussed in Chapter 24. see Angina and Ischemia Without Obstructive Epicardial CAD in this chapter and Chapter 36 for discussion of other abnormalities in coronary function and contributors to myocardial ischemia in the absence of critical coronary obstruction.

Angina Caused by Increased Myocardial O_2 Requirements
In this condition, sometimes termed *demand angina*, the myocardial O_2 requirement increases in the presence of a constant and usually restricted O_2 supply. The increased O_2 requirement commonly stems from a physiologic response to exertion, emotional duress, or mental stress. Of great importance to the myocardial O_2 requirement is the rate and intensity at which any physical task is carried out. Mental and emotional stress may also precipitate angina, presumably by increased hemodynamic and catecholamine responses to stress, increased adrenergic tone, and reduced vagal activity. The combination of physical exertion and emotion in association with sexual activity may precipitate angina. Other precipitants of angina include physical exertion after a heavy meal and the excessive metabolic demands imposed by

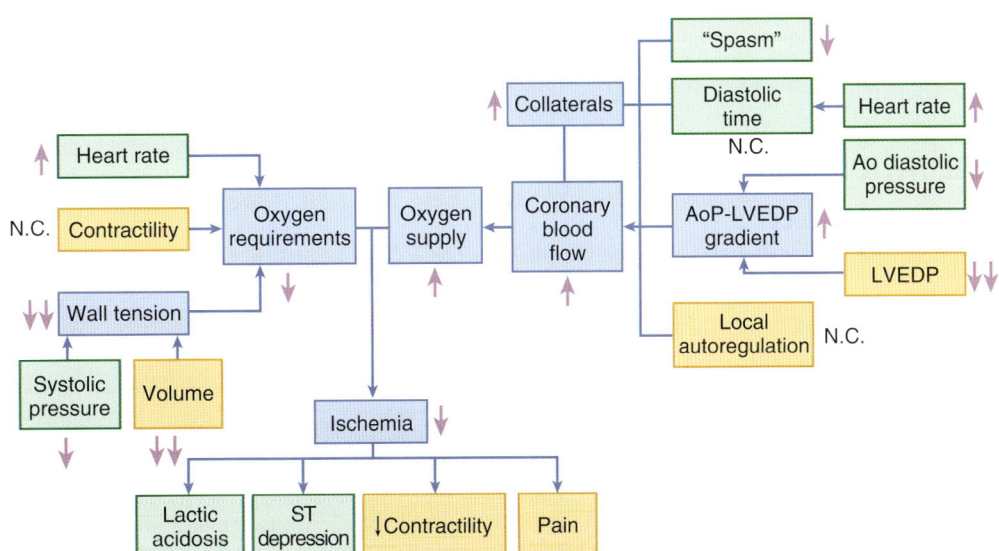

FIGURE 40.2 Factors influencing the balance between myocardial O_2 demand (*left side*) and supply (*right side*). Arrows indicate effects of nitrates. In relieving angina pectoris, nitrates exert favorable effects by reducing O_2 requirements and increasing supply. Although a reflex increase in heart rate would tend to reduce the time for coronary flow, dilation of collaterals and enhancement of the pressure gradient for flow to occur as left ventricular end-diastolic pressure (LVEDP) falls tend to increase coronary flow. Ao, aortic; LVEDP, left ventricular end diastolic pressure; *AoP-LVEDP*, aortic pressure minus LVEDP; *N.C.*, no change. (From Frishman WH. Pharmacology of the nitrates in angina pectoris. Am J Cardiol 1985;56:8I.)

fever, thyrotoxicosis, tachycardia from any cause, uncontrolled hypertension, and exposure to the cold.

Angina Caused by Transiently Decreased O_2 Supply

Like unstable angina, stable angina may be caused by transient reductions in O_2 supply, a condition sometimes termed *supply angina*, as a consequence of coronary vasoconstriction that results in dynamic stenosis. In the presence of atherosclerotic stenoses, platelet thrombi and leukocytes may elaborate vasoconstrictor substances such as serotonin and thromboxane A_2. In addition, endothelial damage in atherosclerotic coronary arteries decreases production of vasodilator substances such as nitric oxide, resulting in an abnormal vasoconstrictor response to exercise and other stimuli. A variable threshold of myocardial ischemia in patients with chronic stable angina may be caused by dynamic changes in smooth muscle tone and also by constriction of arteries distal to the stenosis. Patients with resulting "variable-threshold angina" may have good days, when they are capable of substantial physical activity, as well as bad days, when even minimal activity can cause clinical and/or electrocardiographic evidence of myocardial ischemia or angina at rest. They often complain of a circadian variation in angina that is more common in the morning. Angina on exertion and sometimes even at rest may be precipitated by cold temperature, emotion, and mental stress. Other factors that reduce myocardial oxygen delivery, such as hypoxemia and anemia, may precipitate angina or lower the anginal threshold.

In rare instances, severe dynamic obstruction may develop in patients without organic obstructing lesions and can cause myocardial ischemia and angina at rest (see Chapters 36 and 37). On the other hand, in patients with severe fixed obstruction in one or more epicardial coronary arteries, only a minor increase in dynamic obstruction is necessary for coronary blood flow to fall below a critical level and cause myocardial ischemia.

Importance of Pathophysiologic Considerations in Configuring Therapy

The pathophysiologic and clinical contributions to ischemia in patients with SIHD may have important implications for the selection of anti-ischemic agents, as well as for their timing. The greater the contribution from increased myocardial O_2 demand associated with tachycardia or increased contractility, the greater the likelihood that beta-blocking agents will be effective; nitrates and calcium channel–blocking agents, at least hypothetically, are more likely to be effective in episodes caused primarily by coronary vasoconstriction. The finding that an increase in myocardial O_2 requirement precedes episodes of ischemia in most patients with stable angina—that is, that they have demand angina—argues in favor of controlling the heart rate and blood pressure as a primary therapeutic approach.

EVALUATION AND MANAGEMENT

Biochemical Tests

In patients with SIHD, metabolic abnormalities that are risk factors for the development of CAD are frequently detected. Such abnormalities include dyslipidemia (see Chapter 27) and insulin resistance. Moreover, chronic kidney disease is strongly associated with risk for atherosclerotic vascular disease (see Chapter 101). All patients with established or suspected CAD warrant evaluation of total cholesterol, low-density lipoprotein (LDL) cholesterol, high-density lipoprotein (HDL) cholesterol, triglyceride, serum creatinine or cystatin-C (for estimating glomerular filtration rate [eGFR]), fasting blood glucose levels, and hemoglobin A1c.

Measurement of other lipid elements that are particularly atherogenic, such as apolipoprotein B and small dense LDL, appears to add prognostic information to the measurement of total cholesterol and LDL and may be considered a secondary target for therapy in patients who have achieved therapeutic targets for LDL.[7,8] However, no consensus has been reached regarding routine measurement, and a simple approach based on calculation of non-HDL cholesterol (particularly in patients with triglyceride levels >200 mg/dL) may capture most of the important information related to other atherogenic lipid particles.

Lipoprotein(a) (Lp[a]) is a highly heritable lipid-related risk factor that should be considered for measurement in selected individuals with premature CAD, or a strong family history of CAD, and may be reasonable to measure at least once among any individual with CAD.[8,9] After decades of study, large genetic studies have now clearly established Lp(a) as a causal risk factor for CAD.[10] Although niacin can lower Lp(a), it should not be used for this purpose given the absence of benefit from niacin in randomized trials. Proprotein convertase subtilisin–kexin type 9 (PCSK9) inhibitors also lower Lp(a), possibly contributing to the therapeutic benefit of this class of agents.[11,12] More recently, antisense oligonucleotide and small interfering RNA (siRNA) compounds directly targeting Lp(a) synthesis have been developed, which lower Lp(a) by more than 50%.[13] These are now entering phase 3 clinical trials for patients with IHD.

Although homocysteine has also been linked to atherogenesis, prospective studies suggest, at most, a modest increase in risk associated with elevated homocysteine levels and have not consistently demonstrated a relationship independent of traditional risk factors. Moreover, placebo-controlled trials have failed to demonstrate clinical benefit associated with interventions to mitigate the adverse effects of homocysteine.[14] Therefore general screening for elevated homocysteine levels is not recommended.

Biomarkers of Myocyte Injury, Ischemia, and Hemodynamic Stress

Multiple circulating biomarkers reflecting myocardial injury, inflammation, fibrosis, and wall stress demonstrate associations with the risk of major cardiovascular events in patients with SIHD (Fig. 40.3). Blood levels of cardiac troponins T and I are typically used to differentiate patients with acute MI from those with SIHD. However, with the development of high-sensitivity assays, low levels of circulating troponins are now detectable in most patients with SIHD, consistent with chronic myocardial injury, and higher concentrations demonstrate a graded relationship with the subsequent risk for cardiovascular mortality and heart failure.[15-17] Moreover, patients with SIHD who have increases in high sensitivity troponin levels over time are at increased risk for adverse outcomes, even in the absence of an evident change in clinical status. Although the prognostic importance of chronic myocardial injury is now clear, the therapeutic implications remain an important area for study. Emerging data suggest that more intensive lifestyle and preventive therapies, including higher levels of physical activity and fitness, tighter blood pressure control, and possibly use of sodium-glucose cotransporter 2 (SGLT2) inhibitors among patients with type 2 diabetes mellitus, may attenuate either chronic injury or the risk for adverse events associated with elevated troponin levels.[18] In addition, measuring cardiac troponin may be useful for identifying patients with sufficiently high risk to fall into a population recommended to receive the most intense lipid lowering strategies or patients who don't meet clinical criteria for blood pressure lowering agents but are sufficiently high risk to warrant antihypertensive therapy.[19,20,20a] Moreover, high-intensity statin and intensive blood pressure lowering regimens reduce risk in those with elevated troponin, with absolute risk reductions that are heightened given the high risk status of these patients.[15,19,21]

Biomarkers of neurohormonal activation have also been extensively studied in patients with SIHD. For example, the plasma concentration of brain natriuretic peptide (BNP) increases in response to spontaneous or provoked ischemia. Although BNP and N-terminal pro-BNP (NT-proBNP) do not have sufficient specificity to aid in the diagnosis of SIHD, higher concentrations of these peptides are strongly associated with risk for cardiovascular events in those at risk for and with established CAD. As has been shown with high sensitivity troponin, serial measurements of natriuretic peptides also provide incremental prognostic information in patients with SIHD, suggesting a potential role of outpatient monitoring with these tests.[22] Similar to cardiac troponins, higher levels of NT-proBNP identifies patients with hypertension with greater absolute risk reduction for death and heart failure with more intensive blood pressure lowering, with greatest risk reduction among patients with elevation in both biomarkers.[21] Given the strong

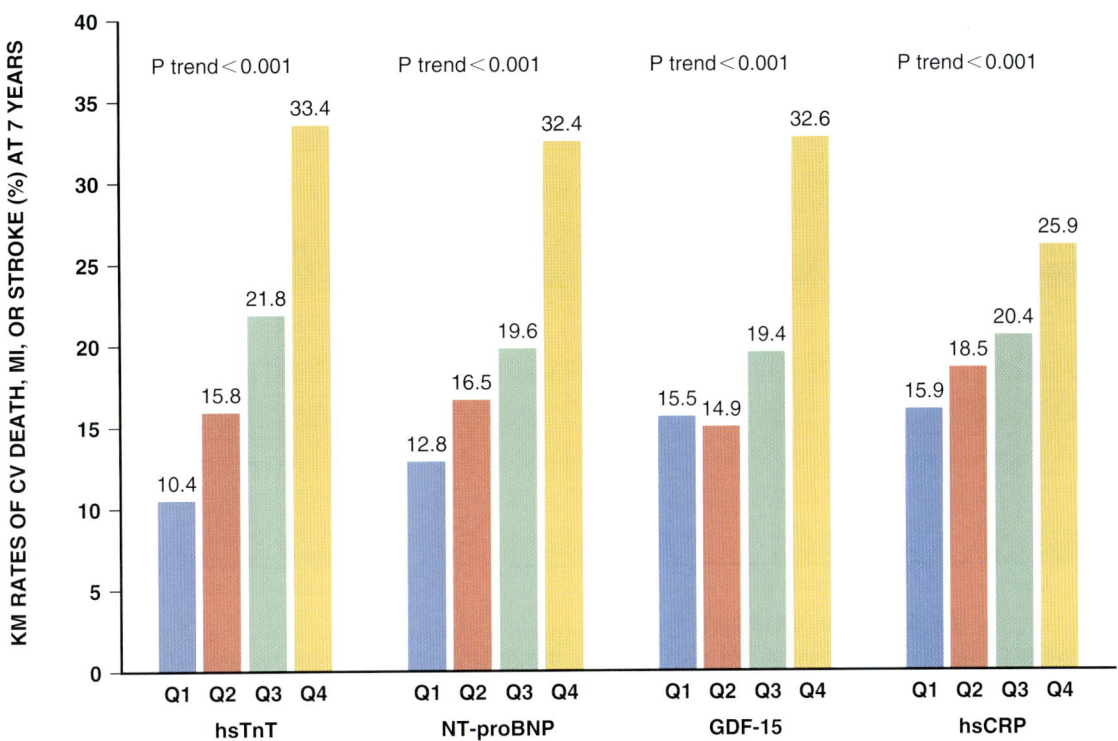

FIGURE 40.3 Incidence of cardiovascular death, myocardial infarction, or stroke according to the concentration of high-sensitivity troponin T (hsTnT), N-terminal pro–B–type natriuretic peptide (NT-proBNP), growth differentiation factor (GDF)-15, and high-sensitivity C-reactive protein (hsCRP) in 7195 patients with established ischemic heart disease subgrouped by quartiles of biomarker concentration. Each biomarker showed a significant graded association with major cardiovascular events. (From Qamar A, et al. Biomarkers and clinical cardiovascular outcomes with ezetimibe in the IMPROVE-IT Trial. J Am Coll Cardiol 2019;74:1061.)

association of natriuretic peptides and high-sensitivity troponins with pathologic cardiac remodeling, consideration of echocardiography is reasonable for patients with abnormal levels of these biomarkers, particularly when increasing over time. However, evaluation for ischemia is generally not indicated as these biomarkers are more strongly associated with structural cardiac abnormalities than ischemia. Given the promising results of studies to date, selective measurement of cardiac troponin and natriuretic peptides is emerging as a consideration to guide the intensity of preventive therapies. However, routine measurement of these biomarkers is not yet warranted in patients with SIHD.

Growth differentiation factor-15, ST2, fibroblast growth factor-23, and galectin-3 are also biomarkers that may putatively reflect myocardial ischemia or its consequences and have been associated with cardiovascular outcomes in clinical studies of patients with SIHD.[22] However, insufficient information is available to demonstrate that these measurements provide robust incremental information beyond natriuretic peptide and high-sensitivity troponin measurements, which have emerged as the strongest candidate biomarkers for disease surveillance in patients with SIHD.

Inflammatory Biomarkers

Understanding of the inflammatory contributions to the pathobiology of atherothrombosis (see Chapter 24) established interest in inflammatory biomarkers as noninvasive indicators of underlying atherosclerosis and cardiovascular risk. Moreover, demonstration of improved clinical outcomes for patients with SIHD treated with the anti-inflammatory therapies canakinumab and colchicine have provided additional evidence for the importance of chronic inflammation and its potential modification.[23,24]

The blood concentration of the acute-phase protein high-sensitivity C-reactive protein (hsCRP) correlates with the risk for incident cardiovascular events in patients with SIHD or at risk for its development (see Chapter 25). The prognostic value of hsCRP is additive to traditional risk factors, including lipids; however, its incremental clinical value for screening among individuals without known vascular disease continues to be debated. Multiple studies also confirm independent associations of hsCRP with adverse cardiac events among individuals with established SIHD.[25] In addition, hsCRP may be an important biomarker reflecting residual risk among patients following ACS or with established SIHD who are treated to low LDL goals with lipid-lowering therapy.[25,26] Patients who achieve low LDL cholesterol levels (<70 mg/dL) but with hsCRP levels above 2 mg/L are at higher risk for subsequent ischemic events than patients with low levels of both LDL and hsCRP. Interleukin (IL)-1β, a cytokine that is activated by the Nod-like receptor (NLR)P3 inflammasome, and IL-6, which stimulates hepatic production of CRP, are also both associated with first and recurrent atherothrombotic events.[27] Measurement of their downstream signal manifest by CRP is more practical as CRP is easier to measure and levels are more stable over time; however, with the emerging potential of therapies directed at the IL-1β pathway and other components of NLRP3-inflammasone activation,[23] a rationale for direct measurement of these cytokines may also arise.[28,29]

Although other biomarkers of inflammation, such as trimethylamine N-oxide,[30] growth factors, cytokines, and metalloproteinases, remain under study as potential biomarkers reflecting inflammatory pathways contributing to atherosclerosis, given their lack of cardiac specificity, they appear unlikely to emerge as clinically useful biomarkers.

Genetic and Transcriptomic Biomarkers

Large-scale genetic mapping programs, utilizing genome-wide association studies (GWAS) and more recently next-generation genome sequencing have identified >50 unique genetic variants contributing to IHD (see Chapter 7). These studies have contributed to the identification of many new potential pathogenic targets and have made feasible testing for large numbers of genetic variations simultaneously at relatively low cost. Because the genes contributing to IHD individually explain only a small amount of the variation in disease, combining multiple variants in genetic risk scores is presently thought to be the only viable strategy by which genetic risk prediction could enter clinical practice. Polygenic risk scores can help predict the risk of major adverse cardiovascular event (MACE) in both primary and secondary prevention populations. However, in individuals without known IHD, when compared with conventional predictors, polygenic risk scores appear to only modestly improve discrimination and risk

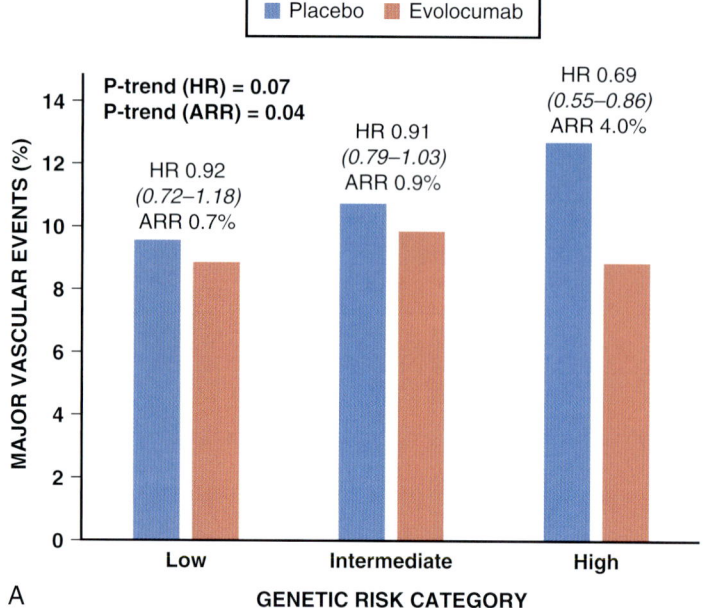
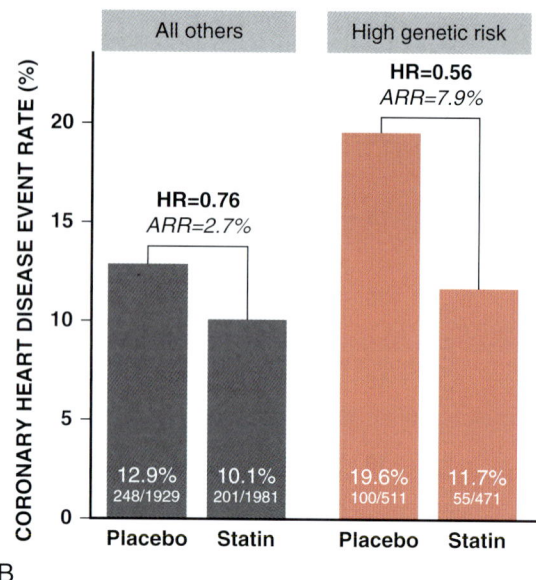

FIGURE 40.4 Relative and absolute risk reductions of lipid lowering agents stratified by genetic risk scores for atherosclerotic vascular events. **A**, Among 14,298 patients with atherosclerotic cardiovascular disease in the FOURIER trial (Further Cardiovascular Outcomes Research With PCSK9 Inhibition in Subjects With Elevated Risk), a 27–single-nucleotide polymorphism genetic risk score was used to defined low (quintile 1), intermediate (quintiles 2 to 4), and high (quintile 5) genetic risk. Higher genetic risk identified patients more likely to benefit from the PCSK9 inhibitor, evolocumab, compared with placebo. **B**, In a randomized controlled trial of primary prevention with statin therapy in 4910 participants in the West of Scotland Coronary Prevention Study (WOSCOPS), researchers studied a polygenic risk score derived from up to 57 common DNA sequence variants previously associated with coronary heart disease. Among patients at high genetic risk, pravastatin was associated with a relative risk reduction of 44% (95% CI, 22 to 60; $P < 0.001$), whereas in all others, the relative risk reduction was 24% (95% CI, 8 to 37; $P = 0.004$). (**A** from Marson NA, et al. Predicting benefit from evolocumab therapy in patients with atherosclerotic disease using a genetic risk score. Circulation 2020;141:620.) (**B** from Natarajan P, et al. Polygenic risk score identifies subgroup with higher burden of atherosclerosis and greater relative benefit from statin therapy in the primary prevention setting. Circulation 2017;135:2093.)

reclassification, if at all.[31] The findings have been similar in patients with previous CAD. As an example, in a study of a genome-wide polygenic risk score for CAD in ~47,000 individuals, while the top 20% of estimated polygenic risk had a 1.9-fold higher odds of developing CAD, only an additional 4.1% of primary prevention candidates might have qualified for statin therapy if a high risk score were considered to be a risk-enhancing factor.[32] It is possible that continued evolution of larger genetic risk scores, incorporating additional variants identified with finer gene mapping strategies, may improve their performance.[33] It is more likely that genetic testing will enter routine practice as a tool to guide therapeutic drug selection (see Chapter 9). Several studies have demonstrated that individuals with high genetic risk scores identifying a genetic predisposition to IHD derive greater reduction in risk with intensive lipid-lowering therapy than do individuals with low genetic risk scores (Fig. 40.4).[34,35]

Noninvasive Testing
Resting Electrocardiogram

Findings on the resting electrocardiogram (ECG) (see Chapter 14) are normal in approximately half of patients with SIHD, and even patients with severe CAD may have a normal tracing at rest. A normal resting ECG suggests the presence of normal resting LV function and is an unusual finding in a patient with an extensive previous MI. The most common abnormalities on the ECG in patients with SIHD are nonspecific ST-T wave abnormalities with or without abnormal Q waves. In patients with known CAD, however, the occurrence of ST-T wave abnormalities on the resting ECG (particularly if obtained during an episode of angina) correlate with the severity of the underlying heart disease and are associated with prognosis. In contrast, a normal resting ECG is a more favorable long-term prognostic sign in patients with suspected or definite CAD.

Interval ECGs may reveal the development of Q wave MIs that have gone unrecognized clinically. Various conduction disturbances, most frequently left bundle branch block and left anterior fascicular block, may occur in patients with SIHD. They are often associated with impairment of LV function, reflect multivessel CAD, and are an indicator of a relatively poor prognosis. Various arrhythmias, especially ventricular premature beats, may be present on the ECG, but they too have low sensitivity and specificity for accurately detecting CAD. LV hypertrophy on the ECG is associated with a worse prognosis in patients with chronic stable angina. This finding implies the presence of underlying hypertension, aortic stenosis, hypertrophic cardiomyopathy, or previous MI with remodeling and warrants further evaluation, such as echocardiography to assess LV size, wall thickness, and function.

During an episode of angina pectoris, findings on the ECG become abnormal in 50% or more of patients with normal resting ECGs. The most common finding is ST-segment depression, although ST-segment elevation and normalization of previous resting ST-T wave depression or inversion (pseudonormalization) may develop.

Resting Echocardiography (see Chapter 16)

Assessment of global LV function is one of the most valuable aspects of echocardiography. Identification of regional wall motion abnormalities may be suggestive of CAD, whereas other findings such as valvular stenosis or pulmonary hypertension may suggest alternative diagnoses. U.S. and European guidelines differ notably regarding recommendations for routine echocardiography in patients with SIHD. European Society of Cardiology (ESC) guidelines recommend routine echocardiography (class I, LOE B) for patients with SIHD[1] whereas U.S. guidelines do not recommend routine echocardiography for all patients with angina pectoris (class III, LOE C); rather echocardiography is recommended for patients with a history of MI, ST-T wave changes, or conduction defects or Q waves on the ECG (class I, LOE B).[36] We also believe echocardiography is appropriate for patients with persistent elevation in cardiac biomarkers such as BNP (or NT-proBNP) or cardiac troponin.

Chest Roentgenography (see Chapter 17)

The chest roentgenogram is generally within normal limits in patients with SIHD, particularly if they have normal findings on the resting ECG and have not experienced MI. If cardiomegaly is present, it is indicative of severe CAD with previous MI, preexisting hypertension, or an associated nonischemic condition such as concomitant valvular heart disease or cardiomyopathy.

TABLE 40.1 Pretest Likelihood of Coronary Artery Disease in Symptomatic Patients According to Age, Sex, and Symptom Quality

AGE	PROBABILITY OF CAD BY AGE, GENDER, AND SYMPTOMS					
	NONANGINAL PAIN		ATYPICAL ANGINA		TYPICAL ANGINA	
	WOMEN	MEN	WOMEN	MEN	WOMEN	MEN
30-39	5%	18%	10%	29%	28%	59%
40-49	8%	25%	14%	38%	37%	69%
50-59	12%	34%	20%	49%	47%	77%
60-69	17%	44%	28%	59%	58%	84%
70-79	24%	54%	37%	69%	68%	89%
>80	32%	65%	47%	78%	76%	93%

(Adapted from Genders TS, et al. A clinical prediction rule for the diagnosis of coronary artery disease: validation, updating, and extension. *Eur Heart J* 2011 Jun;32:1316-1330.)

Stress Testing (see Chapters 15 and 18)

Noninvasive stress testing can provide useful information to establish the diagnosis and estimate the prognosis in patients with suspected stable angina. However, appropriate application of any noninvasive testing for SIHD requires consideration of Bayesian principles, which state that the negative and positive predictive values of any test are defined not only by its sensitivity and specificity but also by the prevalence of disease (or pretest probability) in the population under study. The value of noninvasive stress testing is greatest when the pretest likelihood is intermediate because the test result is likely to have the greatest effect on the post-test probability of CAD. Moreover, noninvasive testing should be performed only if the incremental information provided by a test is likely to alter the planned management strategy.

A classification scheme developed by Diamond and Forrester over 40 years ago that incorporates age, sex, and whether symptoms are typical, atypical, or nonanginal to estimate the pretest probability of CAD has been replaced by newer algorithms.[37] These newer algorithms for predicting CAD have been developed and calibrated in more modern cohorts. The two CAD Consortium scores, a basic score (Table 40.1) and a more detailed clinical score, are now recommended in the ESC Guidelines on the management of chronic coronary syndromes.[1] A head-to-head comparison of the Diamond-Forrester and CAD Consortium scores demonstrated substantial improvement in the prediction of obstructive CAD with the two newer scores, suggesting that use of these scores could reduce unnecessary referrals for diagnostic testing.[38]

Exercise Electrocardiography (see also Chapter 15)

Diagnosis of Coronary Artery Disease. The exercise ECG is particularly helpful in patients with chest pain syndromes who are considered to have a moderate probability of CAD and in whom the resting ECG is normal, provided that they are capable of achieving an adequate workload.[39] Although the incremental diagnostic value of exercise testing is limited in patients in whom the estimated prevalence of CAD is high or low, the test provides useful additional information about the degree of functional limitation in both groups of patients and about the severity of ischemia and prognosis in patients with a high pretest probability of CAD. Interpretation of the exercise test should include consideration of the patient's exercise capacity (duration and metabolic equivalents) and clinical, hemodynamic, and electrocardiographic responses.

Asymptomatic Persons. Exercise testing in asymptomatic individuals without known CAD is not recommended, with the possible exception of asymptomatic individuals at high cardiac risk who plan to begin vigorous exercise. Exercise testing is not required before initiating moderate exercise, even for high-risk individuals.

Risk Stratification. One of the most important and consistent prognostic markers is maximal exercise capacity, regardless of whether it is measured by exercise duration or by workload achieved or whether the test was terminated because of dyspnea, fatigue, or angina. After adjustment for age, the peak exercise capacity measured in metabolic equivalents is among the strongest predictors of mortality in patients with cardiovascular disease. Other factors identified with exercise treadmill testing associated with a poor prognosis in patients with SIHD include the presence and magnitude of ST depression and abnormal heart rate and blood pressure response.

Regardless of the severity of symptoms, patients with high-risk stress test results should undergo either a coronary computed tomography angiography (CTA) or invasive angiogram. Such patients, even if asymptomatic, are at risk for left main or triple-vessel CAD, and many have impaired LV function. By contrast, patients with clearly negative exercise test results, regardless of symptoms, have an excellent prognosis that cannot usually be improved by revascularization. If they do not have other high-risk features or refractory symptoms, additional testing is not generally indicated. Similarly, patients in whom objective evidence of mild ischemia (e.g., 1-mm ST-segment depression) develops at a high workload (e.g., >9 to 10 minutes on a Bruce protocol) do not require coronary arteriography before an adequate trial of medical therapy is first administered.

Influence of Antianginal Therapy. Antianginal therapy may reduce the sensitivity of exercise testing as a screening tool. If the purpose of the exercise test is to *diagnose* ischemia, it should be performed, if possible, in the absence of antianginal medications, particularly long-acting beta-blocking agents, which should be omitted for 2 to 3 days before testing. For long-acting nitrates, calcium antagonists, and short-acting beta blockers, discontinuing use of the medications the day before testing usually suffices. If the test is being performed for *risk stratification* in a patient with known CAD, discontinuation of medications is not necessary.

Sex Differences in Exercise Testing for the Diagnosis of Coronary Artery Disease (see Chapter 91). On the basis of earlier studies that indicated a much higher frequency of false-positive stress test results in women than in men, it is generally accepted that electrocardiographic stress testing is not as reliable in women.[39,40] However, the prevalence of CAD in women in the patient populations under study was low, and the lower positive predictive value of an exercise ECG in women can be accounted for, in large part, on the basis of Bayesian principles (see Table 40.1). Once men and women are stratified appropriately according to the pretest prevalence of disease, the results of stress testing are similar, although the specificity is probably slightly less in women. Exercise imaging modalities have greater diagnostic accuracy than does exercise electrocardiography in men and women.[41,42]

Nuclear Cardiology Techniques (see Chapter 18)

Stress Myocardial Perfusion Imaging. Exercise myocardial perfusion imaging (MPI) with simultaneous ECG recording is generally considered to be superior to an exercise ECG alone in detecting CAD, in identifying multivessel CAD, in localizing diseased vessels, and in determining the magnitude of ischemic and infarcted myocardium. Exercise single-photon emission computed tomography (SPECT) yields higher sensitivity and specificity than exercise electrocardiography alone (Table 40.2).

Stress MPI is particularly helpful in the diagnosis of CAD in patients with abnormal resting ECGs and in those in whom ST-segment responses cannot be interpreted accurately, such as patients with repolarization abnormalities caused by LV hypertrophy and those receiving digitalis. Because stress MPI is a relatively expensive test (three to four times the cost of an exercise ECG) and is associated with radiation exposure, stress MPI should *not* be used as a screening test in patients in whom the prevalence of CAD is low.[43]

Myocardial Perfusion Imaging with Pharmacologic Vasodilator Stress

For patients unable to exercise adequately, pharmacologic vasodilator stress with adenosine derivatives (and rarely dipyridamole) may be used. As a general rule, a patient should be able to walk up two flights of stairs without stopping to complete a standard exercise stress test. The need for pharmacologic stress should be considered among patients who are

TABLE 40.2 Selected Sensitivities and Specificities of Noninvasive Tests for the Detection of Coronary Artery Disease

	SENSITIVITY (95% CI)	SPECIFICITY (95% CI)
Exercise ECG	0.58 (0.45-0.69)	0.62 (0.54-0.69)
Stress Echo	0.85 (0.80-0.89)	0.82 (0.72-0.89)
Stress MPI	0.87 (0.83-0.90)	0.70 (0.53-0.76)
PET	0.83 (0.70-0.93)	0.89 (0.86-0.91)
CMRI	0.88 (0.80-0.93)	0.89 (0.85-0.93)
CCTA	0.97 (0.93-0.99)	0.78 (0.67-0.86)

CCTA, Coronary computed tomography angiography; *CMRI*, cardiac magnetic resonance imaging; *ECG*, electrocardiogram; *MPI*, myocardial perfusion imaging; *PET*, positron emission tomography.
Data from meta-analyses of studies using outcome of anatomically significant CAD by coronary angiography.

TABLE 40.3 Risk Stratification Based on Noninvasive Testing

High Risk (>3% Annual Risk For Death or Myocardial Infarction)

1. Severe resting left ventricular dysfunction (LVEF <35%) not readily explained by noncoronary causes
2. Resting perfusion abnormalities involving ≥10% of the myocardium without previous known MI
3. High-risk stress findings on the ECG, including
   - ≥2-mm ST-segment depression at low workload or persisting into recovery
   - Exercise-induced ST-segment elevation
   - Exercise-induced VT/VF
4. Severe stress-induced LV dysfunction (peak exercise LVEF <45% or drop in LVEF with stress ≥10%)
5. Stress-induced perfusion abnormalities involving ≥10% of the myocardium or stress segmental scores indicating multiple vascular territories with abnormalities
6. Stress-induced LV dilation
7. Inducible wall motion abnormality (involving >2 segments or 2 coronary beds)
8. Wall motion abnormality developing at a low dose of dobutamine (≤10 mg/kg/min) or at a low heart rate (<120 beats/min)
9. Multivessel obstructive CAD (≥70% stenosis) or left main stenosis (≥50% stenosis) on CCTA

Intermediate Risk (1%-3% Annual Risk For Death or Myocardial Infarction)

1. Mild to moderate resting LV dysfunction (LVEF of 35%-49%) not readily explained by noncoronary causes
2. Resting perfusion abnormalities involving 5%-9.9% of the myocardium in patients without a history or previous evidence of MI
3. ≥1-mm ST-segment depression occurring with exertional symptoms
4. Stress-induced perfusion abnormalities encumbering 5%-9.9% of the myocardium or stress segmental scores (in multiple segments) indicating one vascular territory with abnormalities but without LV dilation
5. Small wall motion abnormality involving one to two segments and only one coronary bed
6. One-vessel CAD with ≥70% stenosis or moderate CAD stenosis (50%-69% stenosis) in ≥2 arteries on CCTA

Low Risk (<1% Annual Risk For Death or Myocardial Infarction)

1. Low-risk treadmill score (score ≥5) or no new ST-segment changes or exercise-induced chest pain symptoms when achieving maximal levels of exercise
2. Normal or small myocardial perfusion defect at rest or with stress encumbering ≥5% of the myocardium*
3. Normal stress or no change in limited resting wall motion abnormalities during stress
4. No coronary stenosis >50% on CCTA

*Although the published data are limited, patients with these findings will probably not be at low risk in the presence of either a high-risk treadmill score or severe resting LV dysfunction (LVEF <35%).
Assessment of coronary artery calcium can also be used to contribute to risk assessment.
CCTA, Cardiac computed tomography angiography; *LVEF*, left ventricular ejection fraction; *VF*, ventricular fibrillation; *VT*, ventricular tachycardia.
(Modified from Fihn SD, et al. 2012 ACCF/AHA/ACP/AATS/PCNA/SCAI/STS guideline for the diagnosis and management of patients with stable ischemic heart disease: A report of the American College of Cardiology Foundation/American Heart Association Task Force on Practice Guidelines, and the American College of Physicians, American Association for Thoracic Surgery, Preventive Cardiovascular Nurses Association, Society for Cardiovascular Angiography and Interventions, and Society of Thoracic Surgeons. Circulation 2012;126:e354.)

older or have claudication, pulmonary disease, orthopedic problems, or severe obesity. In most nuclear cardiology laboratories, vasodilator studies account for approximately 40% to 50% of those referred for perfusion imaging. Although the diagnostic accuracy of pharmacologic vasodilator stress perfusion imaging is comparable to that achieved with exercise perfusion imaging (see Table 40.2), treadmill testing is preferred for patients who are capable of exercising because the exercise component of the test provides additional diagnostic and prognostic information, including ST-segment changes, effort tolerance, symptomatic response, and heart rate and blood pressure response (Table 40.3). For patients unable to tolerate adenosine or regadenoson, dobutamine MPI can be performed.

Vasodilator stress agents are also used with PET to diagnose CAD and determine its severity. PET is associated with improved diagnostic accuracy compared with SPECT (see Table 40.2), as well as lower radiation dose, due to the shorter half-life of the radiotracers commonly used.[43] However, PET is less widely available. Both SPECT and PET are valuable for assessing myocardial viability in patients with regional or global LV dysfunction and as such may be useful to help identify candidates with ischemic cardiomyopathy who will most benefit from revascularization (see section Myocardial Hibernation).[44]

High-Risk Findings on Myocardial Perfusion Imaging. The prognostic value of stress MPI is well established. MPI can stratify patients into low (<1% risk for future cardiovascular events with a normal MPI study), intermediate (1% to 5%), or high (>5%) risk categories (see Table 40.3). The prognostic data obtained from MPI, which include left ventricular ejection fraction (LVEF) as well as the size and distribution of perfusion abnormalities, are incremental to clinical and treadmill exercise data in predicting future cardiac events.[45]

Stress Echocardiography (See Chapter 16)

Two-dimensional echocardiography is useful for the evaluation of patients with chronic CAD because it can be used to assess global and regional LV function under basal conditions and during ischemia, as well as to detect LV hypertrophy and associated valve disease. Stress echocardiography may be performed with exercise or pharmacologic stress with dobutamine and allows detection of regional ischemia by identifying wall motion abnormalities induced by ischemia. Adequate images can be obtained in more than 85% of patients, and the test is highly reproducible in expert centers. Numerous studies have shown that exercise echocardiography can detect the presence of CAD with an accuracy similar to that of stress MPI and is superior to exercise electrocardiography alone (see Table 40.2).[46] Stress echocardiography is also valuable in localizing and quantifying ischemic myocardium. Limitations imposed by poor visualization of endocardial borders in a sizable subset of patients have been reduced by use of myocardial contrast agents, three-dimensional imaging, and strain-rate echocardiography. Although less expensive than nuclear perfusion imaging, stress echocardiography is more expensive than and not as widely available as exercise electrocardiography.

As with perfusion imaging, stress echocardiography also provides important prognostic information about patients with known or suspected CAD. The presence or absence of inducible regional wall motion abnormalities and the response of the ejection fraction to exercise or pharmacologic stress provide incremental prognostic information to that provided by the resting echo. Moreover, a negative stress echocardiographic result portends a low risk for future events (<1% per person-year; see Table 40.3).

Computed Tomography (see Chapter 20)

Coronary artery calcification (CAC) can be detected with a rapid noncontrast CT that utilizes only low doses of ionizing radiation. CAC screening does not have a role in the diagnosis of obstructive CAD among symptomatic patients. However, screening of *asymptomatic* individuals at intermediate risk for CAD can be useful to guide decisions about initiation and titration of preventive therapies such as statins and aspirin (see Chapter 20).[7,47]

Coronary CTA is a noninvasive method for angiography of the coronary arterial tree and quantification of ventricular function. CT technology has progressed such that high-quality images of the coronary arteries can be obtained in most patients at relatively low overall radiation exposure. Coronary CTA has become a first-line test for evaluation of symptomatic patients with indications for diagnostic testing who do not have known CAD.[48] Sensitivity and specificity of coronary CTA compare favorably to other noninvasive techniques (see Table 40.2). Compared with nuclear MPI, a comprehensive anatomic evaluation with coronary CTA offers superior accuracy for the prediction of an abnormal invasive fractional flow reserve (FFR).[49]

The accuracy of coronary CTA for estimating the severity of luminal stenosis is limited in patients with tachycardia unable to be controlled adequately with beta blockers, heavy coronary calcification, or in the region of previously placed coronary stents. For these reasons, stress testing with adjunctive imaging is preferred over CTA for patients with known CAD. In the randomized PROMISE (Prospective Multicenter Imaging Study for Evaluation of Chest Pain) trial among 10,003 symptomatic patients without known CAD, coronary CTA was compared with functional testing as an initial evaluation strategy. Clinical outcomes and costs were similar in the CTA and functional testing arms over a median follow-up of 2 years (Fig. 40.5). Patients randomized to coronary CTA underwent more cardiac catheterizations but were less likely to be found to have no obstructive disease on invasive angiography.[50] An important finding from this study was the low rate of cardiovascular events in both treatment arms, highlighting the possibility that deferral of all testing may be reasonable for many lower-risk individuals.

An important advantage of CTA over stress testing is the ability to detect nonobstructive plaque. This capacity has important prognostic and therapeutic implications. In the PROMISE trial, for example, more than half of the coronary events occurred among individuals with <70% stenosis by CTA, many of whom would not be detected with nuclear perfusion imaging. In the SCOT HEART (Scottish Computed Tomography of the Heart) trial, the detection of nonobstructive CAD led to increased administration of preventive therapies in patients undergoing CTA vs patients in the standard of care stress testing arm.[51,52] It is possible that augmented secondary prevention therapies contributed to the apparent long-term benefit favoring CTA over usual care in SCOT HEART.

Stress myocardial CT perfusion imaging is an emerging technique that provides both anatomic and physiologic information that can be combined with CT angiography in a single protocol with a radiation dose similar to that of nuclear perfusion imaging.[53] In a study of 381 patients across 16 centers, CT perfusion imaging sensitivity and specificity for the diagnosis of CAD (>50% stenosis) were 88% and 55%, respectively, compared with 62% and 67% for SPECT with overall superior accuracy for CT (0.74 versus 0.64, p= 0.001).[53]

In experienced centers with advanced technology, CT has also been used to characterize plaque composition and, when paired with PET in a hybrid PET/CT scanner, can offer an assessment of coronary anatomy concurrent with information regarding myocardial blood flow and metabolism.[54] Nevertheless, the capacity of CT for determination of plaque composition is currently not sufficient for routine application.[55] Fractional flow reserve can also now be estimated from CT angiogram images using complex computational algorithms (CTA-FFR), but these currently require off-line processing using proprietary software.[56] The

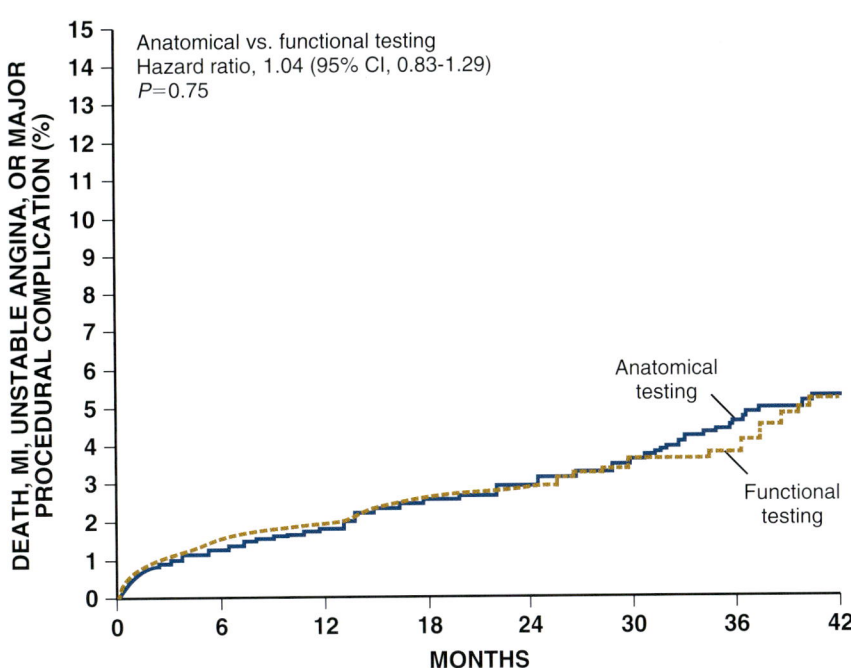

FIGURE 40.5 Among 10,003 patients with symptoms suggestive of coronary artery disease randomized to a strategy of initial anatomical testing (coronary computed tomographic angiography) or to functional testing (exercise electrocardiography, nuclear stress testing, or stress echocardiography), the composite primary end point of death, myocardial infarction, hospitalization for unstable angina, or major procedural complication did not differ between the two diagnostic strategies. (Adapted from Douglas PS, et al. Outcomes of anatomical versus functional testing for coronary artery disease. N Engl J Med 2015;372:1298.)

PLATFORM study compared patient care guided by CTA + CTA-FFR versus usual care and reported a reduction in the probability of finding no obstructive CAD in the group that underwent CTA-FFR before angiography.[57]

Currently, the clinical strength of CT angiography remains its ability to exclude significant CAD with a high negative predictive value and identify low-risk patients with no stenosis and no plaque. In the ISCHEMIA trial, all patients without contraindications underwent a blinded screening CTA before enrollment to ensure significant CAD was present and exclude patients with significant left main CAD. The study, which compared coronary revascularization with initial medical therapy for patients with SIHD and noninvasive evidence of ischemia, did not demonstrate benefit of revascularization despite evidence of substantial ischemia in the study population (see Comparisons between Percutaneous Coronary Intervention and Medical Therapy).[58] Among the many important implications of the ISCHEMIA trial, one is that a strategy using coronary CTA as the initial diagnostic test for patients with angina to exclude severe left main disease before initiating medical therapy for angina can support good outcomes without a need for invasive management.[59] An important corollary is that use of noninvasive stress testing, with or without imaging, is likely to decrease. Since revascularization does not appear to improve outcomes in patients with stable CAD and severe ischemia, the rationale for assessing ischemia before initiating medical therapy for established CAD is questionable.

Cardiac Magnetic Resonance Imaging (see Chapter 19)

Cardiac magnetic resonance imaging (CMRI) is established as a valuable clinical tool for imaging the aorta and cerebral and peripheral arterial vasculature. It is also a versatile noninvasive cardiac imaging modality that has multiple potential applications in patients with SIHD.[60] CMRI has emerged as highly useful for assessment of myocardial viability because of evidence demonstrating its ability to predict functional recovery after percutaneous or surgical revascularization and good correlation with PET. Pharmacologic stress perfusion imaging with CMRI compares favorably with SPECT (see Table 40.2) and also offers accurate characterization of LV function, as well as delineation of patterns of myocardial disease that are often useful in discriminating ischemic from nonischemic myocardial dysfunction.[61,62] In an unblinded, randomized, clinical-effectiveness trial of CMRI MPI versus invasive FFR among 918 patients with suspected CAD, patients allocated to CMRI were less likely to undergo coronary revascularization (35.7% versus 45.0%; $P = 0.005$) and CMRI was noninferior compared with invasive FFR for MACE (3.6% versus 3.7%).[63] However, from a viewpoint of practical implementation, availability is limited compared with most other stress imaging modalities.

CMRI coronary angiography in humans has not demonstrated sufficient accuracy to support clinical application.[64] However, it is established as a modality to characterize congenital coronary anomalies (see Chapters 19 and 82).

Invasive Assessment
Catheterization and Coronary Angiography
The clinical examination and noninvasive techniques described earlier are extremely valuable in establishing the diagnosis of CAD and are indispensable to the overall assessment of patients with this condition. Currently, however, precise assessment of the anatomic severity of CAD still requires invasive coronary angiography (see Chapters 19 and 82). Nevertheless, it should be remembered that myocardial ischemia may occur in the absence of epicardial CAD (see Angina and Ischemia Without Obstructive Epicardial CAD).[3,65] In a report from the National Cardiovascular Data Registry (NCDR) that included almost 400,000 patients without known CAD, the proportion of individuals who reported angina but had no obstructive disease on coronary angiography approached 50%.[3] In contrast, in a large clinical trial population enrolled on the basis of moderate to severe ischemia on functional testing with or without imaging, after exclusion of patients with left main CAD by coronary CT (1%), 6.4% had no coronary stenoses >50%, 22.3% had single-vessel disease, 31.7% had two-vessel disease, and 39.6% had three-vessel disease.[58]

LV function can be assessed by contrast ventriculography (see Chapter 21). Global abnormalities in LV systolic function are reflected by elevations in LV end-diastolic and end-systolic volume and depression of the ejection fraction. Abnormalities in regional wall motion (e.g., hypokinesis, akinesis, dyskinesis) may reflect the consequences of CAD.

Limitations of Angiography
Coronary angiography provides information principally about the degree of luminal stenosis of the coronary arteries. However, coronary angiography is not a reliable indicator of the functional significance of stenosis. Furthermore, coronary angiographic determinants of the severity of stenosis are based on a decrease in the caliber of the lumen at the site of the lesion relative to adjacent reference segments, which are considered, often erroneously, to be relatively free of disease. This approach may lead to significant underestimation of the severity and extent of atherosclerosis. The recent evolution in invasive diagnostics that frequently includes measurement of FFR and instantaneous wavefree ratio (iFR) to assess the functional severity of lesions, and to guide revascularization, is an important step addressing this limitation of coronary angiography.

The most serious limitation to the routine use of coronary angiography for prognosis in patients with SIHD is its inability to identify which coronary lesions can be considered to be at high risk for future events, such as MI or sudden death. Lesions causing mild obstruction can rupture, thrombose, and occlude, thereby leading to MI and sudden death. In fact, most acute MIs emanate from antecedent coronary stenoses that obstruct less than 50% of the luminal diameter. Approaches to quantifying the extent of CAD, inclusive of nonobstructive lesions, appear to offer additional prognostic information.

Advanced Structural Coronary Imaging
Advanced invasive imaging techniques such as intravascular ultrasound (IVUS) provide a more comprehensive evaluation of the coronary wall and have substantially enhanced the detection and quantification of coronary atherosclerosis, as well helping to characterize the vulnerability of coronary atheroma to rupture (see Chapter 21). Studies incorporating both coronary angiography and IVUS have demonstrated that IVUS detects the presence of atherosclerosis missed by angiography alone. Although clinical use of IVUS for assessment of borderline stenoses has been largely supplanted by FFR measurement, IVUS continues to have a role in assessing left main coronary stenoses, and bifurcation lesions, and in optimizing stent deployment.[66] Virtual-histology intravascular ultrasound (VH-IVUS) uses IVUS backscatter data to identify plaque components, including calcification, fibrous, and fibrofatty tissue. In several studies, VH-IVUS–defined thin-capped fibroatheroma (VH-TCFA) was associated with future MACE.[67,68]

Intravascular optical coherence tomography (OCT) is a light-based technology that provides much higher resolution images of the coronary atheroma (10 to 15 microns, versus 100 to 150 microns with IVUS) but penetration is limited to 1 to 3 mm in depth. OCT is particularly useful for measuring fibrous cap thickness and endothelial coverage of stent struts.[69] The major current clinical role for OCT is evaluating patients with acute MI and no evidence of coronary obstruction by angiography, where OCT may detect occult plaque rupture and spontaneous coronary dissection unrecognized on the coronary angiogram.[70]

Functional Assessment
FFR has emerged as the most important invasive tool to complement coronary angiography, providing a functional assessment of the hemodynamic impact of a coronary stenosis.[71] The measurement is simple to perform and highly reproducible. The primary role of FFR is in guiding decisions regarding percutaneous coronary intervention (PCI) for stenoses that appear intermediate in severity by angiography. FFR is determined as the ratio of pressure distal to a stenosis/pressure before the stenosis under conditions of maximal hyperemia, which is usually achieved with adenosine. For practical purposes the proximal pressure measurement is performed in the aorta using the guiding catheter. A stenosis with an FFR value <0.75 is highly likely to be associated with ischemia on nuclear perfusion imaging, whereas stenoses with FFR >0.8 are rarely associated with ischemia; 0.75 to 0.8 represents a "grey zone."

The iFR has been developed as an alternative to FFR that does not require administration of a vasodilator and thus avoids adverse effects from adenosine and is simpler to perform in the catheterization laboratory.[72] An iFR of >0.89 is commonly used as an analogous threshold to FFR >0.8 as a threshold above which PCI can be deferred. Two large randomized controlled trials comparing PCI guided by iFR versus by FFR show similar outcomes but fewer adverse symptoms and shorter procedural times with iFR (see Fractional Flow Reserve and Chapter 41).[73,74]

Additional options for functional assessment include measurement of coronary flow reserve (maximum hyperemic coronary flow divided by resting flow) and endothelial function; these measurements frequently produce abnormal results in patients with CAD and play an important role in detecting microvascular dysfunction, particularly in those without obstructive epicardial disease.[72,75] The index of microcirculatory resistance (IMR) is a newer tool to interrogate the coronary microcirculation. These techniques are discussed in Chapters 18 and 20 (see also Patient Selection for Revascularization).

Integrated Invasive Assessment in Patients Without Obstructive CAD
For patients with angina and evidence of ischemia on noninvasive testing, and no obvious epicardial obstructive CAD, symptom burden may be substantial (see Angina and Ischemia Without Obstructive Epicardial CAD). In such patients an integrated functional assessment is possible to identify potential causal pathophysiology.[3] For example, FFR or iFR can be performed to exclude hemodynamically significant diffuse CAD that is underappreciated by angiography. Next, CFR or IMR can be used to interrogate the coronary microcirculation. Finally, acetylcholine can be given at low doses to assess coronary endothelial function and at higher dosages to evaluate for coronary spasm. While such a comprehensive evaluation is currently limited to specialized

centers, in a pilot study the CorMicA investigators studied 151 patients with angina and no obstructive CAD with an integrated functional assessment and then randomized them to providing the information to the clinician or blinding the information. The results of the functional assessment were used to stratify patients into endotypes (microvascular angina, coronary spasm, both, or noncardiac pain) with treatment in the randomized group based on the underlying pathophysiology. At 6 months and 1 year, the intervention group had significantly improved SAQ and other health status scores.[76] Additional studies are needed to demonstrate the feasibility of this approach in a broader group of catheterization laboratory practices.

Other Angiographic Findings
Coronary artery ectasia, coronary artery aneurysms, coronary collaterals, and myocardial bridging.

Natural History and Risk Stratification
Up to 30% of patients with a history of stable angina experience angina one or more times per week. Stable angina is associated with physical limitation and worse quality of life. The frequency of reported angina varies substantially between providers, suggesting significant heterogeneity in identifying, characterizing, and managing angina.[79] Women have a similar incidence of stable angina as men, and angina in both sexes is associated with higher risk for mortality than in the general population. Data from the Framingham Study, obtained before the widespread use of aspirin, beta-blocking agents, and aggressive modification of risk factors, revealed an average annual mortality rate of 4% in patients with SIHD. The combination of these treatments has improved the prognosis, with a current annual mortality rate of 1% to 3% and an annual rate of major ischemic events of 1% to 2%. For example, among 38,602 outpatients with SIHD enrolled in the REACH Registry, the 1-year rate of cardiovascular death was 1.9% (95% confidence interval [CI], 1.7% to 2.1%), that of all-cause mortality was 2.9% (95% CI, 2.6% to 3.2%), and that of cardiovascular death, MI, or stroke was 4.5% (95% CI, 4.2% to 4.8%). Clinical, noninvasive, and invasive tools are useful for refining the estimated risk in individual patients with SIHD. Moreover, noninvasively acquired information is valuable in identifying patients who are candidates for invasive evaluation with cardiac catheterization.

Risk Stratification and Risk Models
Risk stratification is an integral component of the assessment and management of patients with SIHD. Risk assessment should be considered an iterative process, by which the estimation of risk is continually updated as new clinical or test information becomes available or symptoms change. Clinical characteristics, including older age, male sex, diabetes mellitus, previous MI, and the presence of symptoms typical of angina, are predictive of the presence of CAD and associated with a higher risk of major cardiovascular events in patients with SIHD. Left ventricular dysfunction and clinical heart failure are important adverse prognostic indicators in patients with SIHD. The severity of angina, especially the tempo of intensification, and the presence of dyspnea are also important predictors of outcome. Each of the noninvasive and invasive tests that assess the extent of CAD, burden of ischemia, and LV function, also provide powerful prognostic information (see Noninvasive Testing and Invasive Assessment).

Several risk scores that integrate widely available clinical risk indicators have been developed to aid in prognostication with the aim of directing follow-up and therapeutic decision making. Patients with SIHD and prior MI vary in their risk for recurrent cardiovascular (CV) events. The TIMI Risk Score for Secondary Prevention (TRS 2°P) is a pragmatic integer score based on nine routinely assessed clinical characteristics (age, diabetes, hypertension, smoking, peripheral arterial disease, prior stroke, prior coronary artery bypass grafting (CABG), history of heart failure, and renal dysfunction) that demonstrated a graded relationship with the risk for cardiovascular death, MI, or ischemic stroke in a population of 8598 patients with established coronary or peripheral atherosclerosis (Fig. 40.6A).[80] As well, this risk score distinguished a pattern of increasing absolute benefit from treatment with the novel platelet inhibitor vorapaxar. In a second validation cohort in the IMPROVE IT trial of ezetimibe, the TRS 2°P performed similarly for risk stratification and also identified patients with a significantly greater absolute and relative risk reduction with the addition of ezetimibe to simvastatin (Fig. 40.6B).[81] Although the discriminatory capacity of the TRS 2°P was only moderate (c-statistic 0.68) in both datasets, the demonstrated role for estimating benefit from more than one specific therapy lends clinical relevance.

In addition, at least three risk scores have been developed for patients who have undergone PCI to aid in decision making regarding the duration of dual antiplatelet therapy.[82] The DAPT risk score estimates net clinical outcome (balancing reductions in ischemia with increases in bleeding) with extending the duration of dual antiplatelet therapy from 12 to 30 months after stenting. The PARIS risk score was developed as a weighted integer score to predict new coronary thrombotic events (MI or stent thrombosis) in patients who had undergone PCI. The PARIS risk variables are similar to those in the TRS 2°P, including PCI for acute coronary syndrome, revascularization before the qualifying PCI, diabetes mellitus, renal dysfunction, and current smoking. Patients are stratified into three bins of coronary thrombotic risk ranging from 1.8% to 10% at 2 years. The PRECISE-DAPT scores a simple five-item risk score, using age, creatinine clearance, hemoglobin, white blood cell count, and previous spontaneous bleeding, that predicts out-of-hospital bleeding during DAPT.

Medical Management
Comprehensive management of SIHD has five aspects: (1) identification and treatment of associated diseases that can precipitate or worsen angina and ischemia, (2) improvement of coronary risk factors, (3) application of pharmacologic and nonpharmacologic interventions for secondary prevention, (4) pharmacologic management of angina, and (5) revascularization by catheter-based PCI or by CABG, when indicated. Although discussed individually in this chapter, all five of these approaches must be considered, often simultaneously, in each patient. Of the medical therapies, aspirin, statins, and angiotensin-converting enzyme (ACE) inhibitors— and in selected patients $P2Y_{12}$ inhibitors, ezetimibe, PCSK9 inhibitors, and high-dose eicosapentaenoic acid (EPA)—have been shown to reduce mortality or morbidity in patients with SIHD. Colchicine has also been shown to reduce major cardiovascular events in patients with SIHD but does not appear to lower all-cause mortality.[24] Other therapies such as nitrates, beta blockers, calcium antagonists, and ranolazine have been shown to improve symptoms and exercise performance, but their effect, if any, on survival in patients with SIHD has not been demonstrated.[83,84]

In stable patients with LV dysfunction following MI, ACE inhibitors and beta-blocking agents reduce both mortality and the risk for repeat MI, and these agents are recommended in all such patients, with or without chronic angina, along with aspirin, statins, and in selected individuals aldosterone antagonists.

Treatment of Associated Diseases
Several common medical conditions that can increase myocardial O_2 demand or reduce O_2 delivery may contribute to the onset of new angina pectoris or exacerbation of previously stable angina. Such conditions include anemia, occult thyrotoxicosis, fever, infections, and tachycardia. Cocaine, which can cause acute coronary spasm and MI, is discussed in Chapter 84. Heart failure, by causing cardiac dilation, increases in filling pressures or tachyarrhythmias (including sinus tachycardia), can increase myocardial O_2 need, and increase the frequency and severity of angina in patients with CAD. Identification and treatment of these conditions are critical to the management of SIHD.

Reduction of Coronary Risk Factors
Hypertension (see Chapter 26)
Epidemiologic links between increased blood pressure and CAD severity and mortality are well established. For individuals 40 to 70 years

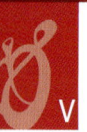

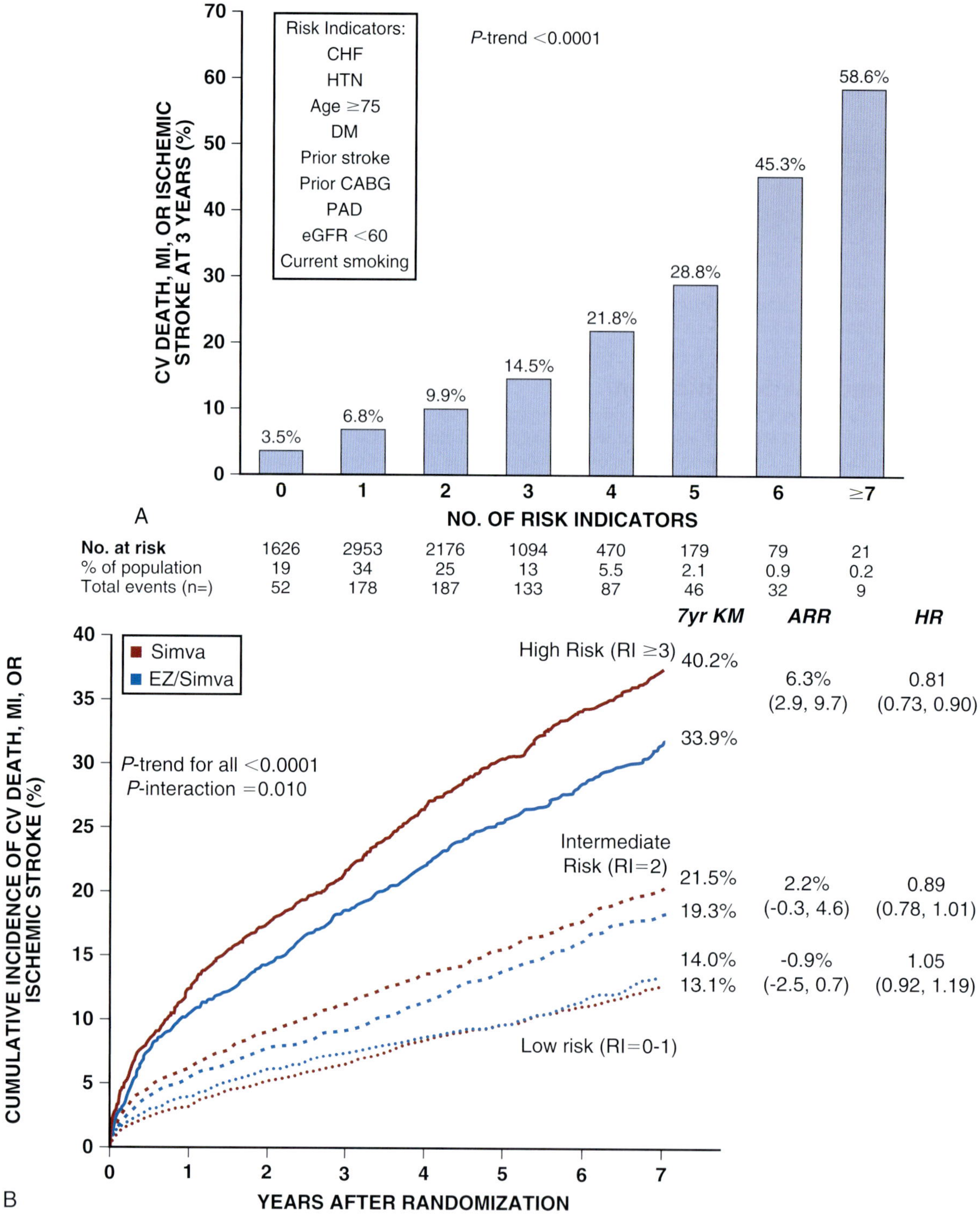

FIGURE 40.6 The TIMI Risk Score for Secondary Prevention (https://timi.org/timi-risk-score-for-2p/) was developed as a pragmatic nine-variable risk stratification tool among 8589 stable patients with a history of prior MI, prior stroke, or symptomatic peripheral artery disease. **A,** The 3-year risk of cardiovascular death, MI, or ischemic stroke is shown by risk score group along with the proportion of the development population that fell within each group. **B,** The risk score was applied prospectively to 17,717 patients stabilized after an acute coronary syndrome and randomized to ezetimibe/simvastatin (EZ/simva) or simvastatin (Simva) alone. The cumulative incidence of cardiovascular death, MI, or ischemic stroke is shown by risk category and treatment group, demonstrating a pattern of increasing benefit with higher risk categories defined by the score. ARR, absolute risk reduction; HR, hazard ratio. (**A** from Bohula EA, et al. Atherothrombotic Risk Stratification and the Efficacy and Safety of Vorapaxar in Patients With Stable Ischemic Heart Disease and Previous Myocardial Infarction. Circulation 2016;134:304-313; **B** from Bohula EA, et al. Atherothrombotic risk stratification and ezetimibe use in IMPROVE-IT. J Am Coll Cardiol 2016;67:2129.)

of age, risk for IHD doubles for each 20–mm Hg increment in systolic blood pressure across the entire range of 115 to 185 mm Hg.[7,85] Hypertension predisposes to vascular injury, accelerates the development of atherosclerosis, increases myocardial O_2 demand, and intensifies ischemia in patients with preexisting obstructive CAD. A meta-analysis of clinical trials of treatment of mild to moderate hypertension has shown a statistically significant 16% reduction in CAD events and mortality in patients receiving antihypertensive therapy. This treatment effect is almost twice as great in older as in younger persons. It is logical to extend these observations about the benefits of antihypertensive therapy to patients with established CAD. Moreover, the number of individuals treated to avoid one death is lower in patients with established cardiovascular disease. Therefore, blood pressure control is an essential component of the management of patients with SIHD, with a goal of less than 130/80 mm Hg.[7,85,86] However, there is also evidence for a "J"-shaped risk relationship for diastolic blood pressure, reflecting adverse outcomes in patients with a very low diastolic blood pressure on therapy.[87] Therefore, in patients who have CAD with evidence of myocardial ischemia, the BP should be lowered slowly and, given concern of an increase risk at low ranges of diastolic BP, it is recommended to avoid diastolic BP <60 mm Hg in the elderly. Newer and emerging options for the treatment of hypertension are discussed in Chapter 26.

Although there has been an assumed incremental risk for increased cardiovascular events in hypertensive patients with SIHD and a belief that more intensive blood pressure lowering would reduce clinical events, the data from randomized trials that have examined systolic blood pressure targets <140 mm Hg have had mixed results. Among patients with SIHD and diabetes mellitus, the ACCORD-BP study did not reveal an additional benefit of lowering systolic blood pressure below 120 mm Hg in persons with type 2 diabetes mellitus as compared with lowering blood pressure to less than 140 mm Hg. However, in the Systolic Blood Pressure Intervention Trial (SPRINT), among 9361 patients with hypertension and a high risk indicator other than diabetes, patients randomized to a systolic blood pressure target <120 mm Hg compared with <140 mm Hg had a significantly reduced rate of the primary endpoint of acute coronary syndrome, stroke, heart failure, or death (1.65%/year versus 2.19%/year, HR 0.75; 95% CI, 0.64 to 0.89) as well as all-cause mortality (hazard ratio [HR] 0.73; 95% CI 0.60 to 0.90).[88] In the U.S. 2017 Guideline for the Prevention, Detection, Evaluation, and Management of High Blood Pressure in Adults, pharmacologic therapy to lower blood pressure is recommended in addition to lifestyle modification for patients with atherosclerotic vascular disease and a BP >130/80 mm Hg, with a BP goal of <130/80 mm Hg.[86]

Cigarette Smoking

Smoking remains one of the most powerful risk factors for the development of CAD in all age groups (see Chapter 28). In patients with CAD, cigarette smokers have a higher 5-year risk for sudden death, MI, and all-cause mortality than do those who have stopped smoking. Cigarette smoking may also acutely aggravate angina by increasing myocardial O_2 demand and reducing coronary blood flow by means of an alpha-adrenergically–mediated increase in coronary artery tone. Moreover, passive exposure to cigarette smoke has adverse cardiovascular effects that are almost as large as those of active smoking. Smoking cessation lessens the risk for adverse coronary events in patients with established CAD and is one of the most effective and cost-saving approaches to prevention of disease progression.[7] Strategies for smoking cessation are discussed in Chapter 25. Studies of nicotine medications and smokeless tobacco suggest that the risks of nicotine without tobacco combustion products are lower compared with cigarette smoking but are still of concern in people with cardiovascular disease.[7] The health implications of electronic cigarette use and vaping are discussed in Chapter 28.[89-91] While the long-term direct cardiovascular effects of e-cigarettes remain uncertain, the available evidence suggests that while e-cigarettes may be modestly safer than smoked tobacco, they should not be regarded as safe from a cardiovascular perspective.[89,91,92]

Management of Dyslipidemia (see Chapter 27)

Results from secondary prevention trials of patients with a history of SIHD, unstable angina, or previous MI have provided convincing evidence that effective lipid-lowering therapy significantly improves overall survival and reduces cardiovascular mortality in patients with CAD, regardless of baseline cholesterol levels.[8,9] Moreover, results from trials of intensive-versus moderate-dose statin therapy in patients with established IHD have provided evidence of greater reduction in major cardiovascular events with intensive compared with moderate-dose statin therapy. In the aggregate, angiographic and IVUS trials of intensive cholesterol lowering in patients with chronic CAD have shown that effects on coronary obstruction are achievable but modest compared with the substantive reduction in cardiovascular events, thus demonstrating that regression of atherosclerosis is not the primary mechanism of benefit. Furthermore, lipid-lowering with statins significantly improves endothelium-mediated responses in the coronary and systemic arteries of patients with hypercholesterolemia or known atherosclerosis, reduces circulating levels of hsCRP, decreases thrombogenicity, and favorably alters the collagen and inflammatory components of arterial atheroma.

Multiple studies of LDL-lowering agents other than statins have established their efficacy for secondary prevention of major atherosclerotic vascular events. In the IMPROVE-IT trial, 18,144 patients stabilized after an ACS with a baseline LDL-C level between 50 and 100 mg/dL were randomized to simvastatin (40 mg) plus ezetimibe or simvastatin (40 mg) alone. The addition of ezetimibe lowered the composite of cardiovascular death, MI, unstable angina requiring hospitalization, or coronary revascularization by a relative 6.4% (2% absolute difference at 7 years; p= 0.016).[93] In addition, two large clinical outcome trials of PCSK9 inhibitors in patients post-ACS or with chronic CAD have demonstrated that these agents improve cardiovascular outcomes when added to guideline based statin therapy.[94,95] In the FOURIER trial that included 27,564 patients with SIHD treated with maximally tolerated statin, compared with placebo, evolocumab reduced the primary outcome of MACE at 48 weeks from 11.3% to 9.8% (HR 0.85; 95% CI, 0.79 to 0.92), with no significant difference in all-cause mortality.[94] In the ODYSSEY OUTCOMES trial of 18,924 patients with ACS in the prior 1 to 12 months, addition of alirocumab to statin therapy resulted in a significant 15% relative reduction in the composite MACE outcome and a similar 15% relative reduction in all-cause mortality (3.5% versus 4.1%; HR 0.85; 95% CI, 0.73 to 0.98).[95] Both trials demonstrated favorable safety and side effect profiles, and a long-term neurocognitive follow-up study demonstrated no effects of PCSK9 inhibition on cognitive function.[96]

After moving away from LDL-C treatment goals with the 2013 ACC/AHA Cholesterol Guidelines, the 2018 ACC/AHA Cholesterol Guidelines pivoted back to an LDL-C goal-based approach for patients with established CAD.[8] This step was necessary to guide appropriate use of ezetimibe and PCSK9 inhibitors on top of high-intensity statin therapy. If LDL-C is ≥70 mg/dL (1.8 mmol/L) on maximally tolerated therapy, the guideline recommends addition of ezetimibe. If the patient is falls into a very high-risk category and LDL-C remains ≥70 mg/dL (1.8 mmol/L) on statin + ezetimibe (or the patient is intolerant to one or both of these therapies), a PCSK9 inhibitor is recommended. Very high risk of atherothrombotic events is defined by multiple prior atherosclerotic vascular events, or one prior event with multiple high-risk conditions such as ≥65 years, family history of premature CAD, prior CABG/PCI, diabetes mellitus, hypertension, chronic kidney disease, current smoking, LDL ≥100 mg/dL, or HF. Elevated Lp(a) may also be an important factor to guide selected use of PCSK9 inhibitors in patients on maximally tolerated statins. PCSK9 inhibitors lower Lp(a) and subgroup analyses from the large PCSK9 inhibitor outcomes trials demonstrated greater reduction in coronary, peripheral arterial, and venous thromboembolic events with PCSK9 inhibitors among patients with high compared with normal Lp(a).[11,97]

The ESC takes an even more aggressive position on adding additional agents to statins, recommending ezetimibe and/or PCSK9 for high-risk individuals with LDL-C ≥55 mg/dL (1.4 mmol/L).[9]

LOW HIGH-DENSITY LIPOPROTEIN CHOLESTEROL. Patients with established CAD and low levels of HDL cholesterol represent a subgroup at considerable risk for future coronary events, even when LDL cholesterol is low.[7,8] Low HDL levels are often associated with obesity, hypertriglyceridemia, insulin resistance, and hypertension. The constellation of these findings—often referred to as metabolic syndrome—typically signifies the presence of small lipoprotein remnants and small, dense, LDL particles, which are thought to be particularly atherogenic (see Chapter 27). Therapies to raise HDL have focused on diet and exercise, as well as smoking cessation. Whether HDL itself should be a target for pharmacologic therapies remains a controversial question.[98] Data on fibric acid derivatives, which lower triglycerides and raise HDL, have provided conflicting results, and no benefit was seen in the most contemporary trial that combined fenofibrate with statin therapy.[99,100] Moreover, two randomized trials of extended-release niacin failed to show benefit when this agent was added to contemporary therapy, despite marked increases in HDL-C among niacin-treated patients.[99,100] Inhibitors of cholesterol ester transport protein (CETP) have also been disappointing despite large increases in HDL-C with these agents. Four large randomized trials testing torcetrapib, dalcetrapib, evacetrapib, and anacetrapib have provided somewhat conflicting but ultimately disappointing results,[99-102] Although additional study of HDL mimetics is ongoing, the multitude of negative studies with HDL-C raising compounds challenges HDL cholesterol as a target for secondary prevention.

HIGH TRIGLYCERIDES. Hypertriglyceridemia (TG >150 mg/dL [1.7 mmol/L]) is commonly associated with obesity, physical inactivity insulin resistance, hypothyroidism, and type 2 diabetes, particularly when diabetes is poorly controlled. Although some of the vascular risk associated with high triglycerides (TG) is mediated by these factors, mendelian randomization studies implicating apo C-III and ANGPTL3 in vascular risk provide support for a direct causal role of TG-rich lipoproteins in atherosclerotic vascular disease. Severe hypertriglyceridemia (TG >500 mg/dL) merits treatment to prevent pancreatitis, whereas treatment of moderate TG elevation (150 to 500 mg/dL) can be considered to lower atherosclerotic vascular disease risk.

First-line treatments for high TGs include lifestyle interventions such as weight loss, aerobic exercise, carbohydrate restriction, and limitation of alcohol intake. Statins, which have modest TG-lowering properties, are first-line pharmacologic agents. Although fibrates lower TGs and may be useful for patients with very high levels to prevent pancreatitis, when administered in combination with statins, fibrates have not been shown to improve cardiovascular outcomes. Omega-3 polyunsaturated fatty acids (PUFAs), which are commonly present in fish oil preparations, increase clearance and reduce synthesis of TG-rich lipoproteins, and high-dose preparations are well tolerated TG-lowering agents.[103] However, clinical outcome studies evaluating PUFA show varied results. Multiple randomized trials of balanced fish oil preparations that contain both EPA and docosahexaenoic acid (DHA) have reported no benefit from these agents on cardiac events.[104-106] In contrast, in the JELIS trial, a purified EPA compound (1.8 g/day) reduced MACE events when added to statin monotherapy. Subsequently, in the much larger Reduction of Cardiovascular Events with Icosapent Ethyl–Intervention Trial (REDUCE-IT), high-dose purified EPA (4 g/day) was compared with placebo in 8179 patients at high risk or with established CAD on statin therapy, with controlled LDL-C and TG >150 mg/dL.[107] In this trial, EPA lowered TG by 45% and reduced MACE (17.2% versus 22.0%; HR 0.75; 95% CI, 0.68 to 0.83) and CV mortality (4.3% versus 5.2%; HR 0.80; 95% CI, 0.66 to 0.98) when compared with mineral oil placebo. Subsequent analyses also demonstrated robust reductions in coronary revascularization events (HR 0.64; 95% CI, 0.56 to 0.74).[108] It is not clear to what extent the benefit of high-dose purified EPA observed in REDUCE-IT was due to TG lowering versus other, pleiotropic effects of the drug. Although these data from randomized trials are mixed and have contributed to some uncertainty regarding the possible mechanisms, high-dose EPA is a new and important secondary prevention agent for patients with SIHD and moderate TG elevation after statin initiation and titration.

MANAGEMENT OF DIABETES MELLITUS (SEE CHAPTER 31). Patients with diabetes mellitus are at significantly higher risk for atherosclerotic vascular disease. Weight management, physical activity, blood pressure control, and lipid management are recommended for all patients with SIHD and diabetes mellitus.[36] Additional considerations related to managing diabetes mellitus in patients with SIHD include both managing hyperglycemia as a potential therapeutic target and the efficacy and safety of specific classes of oral hypoglycemic agents with respect to cardiovascular outcomes in patients with diabetes mellitus and established atherosclerotic vascular disease.[109,110]

Although a favorable impact of control of glycemia as a therapeutic target on microvascular complications of diabetes has been established, the effect on macrovascular complications (including CAD) is unclear. During a mean follow-up of 17 years in participants in the Diabetes Control and Complications Trial, patients with type 1 diabetes assigned to intensive glycemic therapy were at lower risk for cardiovascular complications. However, the results of studies of glycemic therapy with a shorter duration of follow-up, principally in subjects with type 2 diabetes, are mixed. Moreover, three large randomized trials comparing tight versus standard glucose control strategies failed to demonstrate benefit of more aggressive treatment, including one trial stopped prematurely due to excess mortality in the group randomized to tight glucose control. Thus, although a near normal HbA$_{1C}$ level (i.e., below 6.5% [53 mmol/L]) is optimal to minimize microvascular complications, for older patients and those with preexisting CV disease a less stringent HbA$_{1C}$ target of ≤8% is recommended.[111]

A series of randomized trials have firmly established the efficacy and safety of several newer classes of oral hypoglycemic agents for secondary prevention of atherosclerotic vascular events and heart failure in patients with diabetes mellitus.[109,110,112,113] Given the lack of cardiovascular benefit and reported CV risks of some prior generations of oral hypoglycemic agents, U.S. and European regulatory authorities have required that large outcomes trials be performed to establish the CV safety of new agents. Thus, a wealth of new data has become available on the CV effects of these drugs, several of which have shown improvements in CV outcomes. The SGLT2 inhibitors lower blood glucose by promoting glucosuria with concurrent diuretic and natriuretic effects.[114] The EMPA-REG Outcomes trial compared two doses of empagliflozin versus placebo in 7020 patients with type 2 diabetes mellitus and established CV disease and was the first large outcomes trial to demonstrate a CV benefit of the class of SGLT2 inhibitors.[115] The primary endpoint of CV death, MI, and stroke was reduced by 14% in the combined empagliflozin groups, a finding driven by a 38% reduction in CV death (HR 0.62; 95% CI, 0.49 to 0.78, p< 0.001). Significant reductions were also seen in all-cause mortality (5.7% versus 8.3%; HR 0.68; 95% CI, 0.57 to 0.82) and heart failure hospitalization (HR 0.65; 95% CI, 0.50 to 0.85, p< 0.001). Subsequent trials with dapagliflozin and canagliflozin have shown similar cardiovascular benefits with these agents.[116-118] A meta-analysis of these trials supports the conclusion that SGLT2 inhibitors have moderate benefits on atherosclerotic events that seem confined to patients with established atherosclerotic cardiovascular disease rather than patients with diabetes and CV risk factors alone. However, the SGLT2 inhibitors have robust benefits on reducing hospitalization for heart failure and progression of renal disease regardless of existing atherosclerotic cardiovascular disease.[118]

Cardiovascular benefits have also emerged with the glucagon-like peptide (GLP-1) receptor agonists liraglutide and semaglutide. In the Liraglutide Effect and Action in Diabetes: Evaluation of Cardiovascular Outcome Results—A Long Term Evaluation (LEADER) trial, subcutaneous liraglutide reduced MACE by a relative 13% (HR 0.87; 95% CI, 0.78 to 0.97; $P < 0.001$) and cardiovascular death by 22% (HR 0.78; 95% CI, 0.66 to 0.93; $P = 0.007$) among 9340 patients with type 2 diabetes and elevated cardiovascular risk.[119] Weekly subcutaneous administration of semaglutide also demonstrated CVD benefit in a modest-sized randomized trial,[120] and definitive outcomes trials are underway with this agent, including a large CV outcomes trial of an oral formulation (ClinicalTrials.gov Identifier: NCT03914326). The GLP-1 agonists are associated with more gastrointestinal (GI) side effects than the SGLT2 inhibitors and have not been demonstrated to lower heart failure risk.

The American Diabetes Association Standards of Medical Care in Diabetes 2020 recommend metformin as the first-line therapy for all patients with type 2 diabetes mellitus. Thereafter, among patients with established atherosclerotic cardiovascular disease, a SGLT2 inhibitor or GLP-1 receptor agonist with demonstrated cardiovascular disease benefit is recommended as part of the patient's glucose-lowering regimen independent of the A$_{1C}$ concentration.[112] In contrast, the European Society of Cardiology guidelines recommend either a SGLT2 inhibitor or GLP-1 receptor agonist as first-line monotherapy for patients with atherosclerotic vascular disease or at high CV risk.[110]

ESTROGEN THERAPY. In view of the collective data from randomized clinical trials, it is *not* advised that hormone replacement therapy be initiated or continued for secondary cardiovascular prevention in women with CAD (see Chapter 91).[36]

Exercise (see Chapters 25, 32, and 33)

The conditioning effect of exercise on skeletal muscles allows a greater workload at any level of total-body O$_2$ consumption. By decreasing the heart rate at any level of exertion, higher cardiac output can be achieved at any level of myocardial O$_2$ consumption. The combination of these two effects of exercise conditioning permits patients with stable angina to increase physical performance substantially following institution of a continuing exercise program.

Most of the information about the physiologic effects of exercise and their effect on prognosis in patients with IHD has come from studies on patients entered into cardiac rehabilitation programs, many of whom previously sustained an MI.[121] Less information is available on the benefits of exercise in patients with SIHD without a previous MI. Collectively, small randomized trials evaluating exercise training in patients with SIHD indicate improved effort tolerance, O_2 consumption, and quality of life and reduced evidence of ischemia on MPI. In addition, exercise training reduces hospitalizations and revascularization procedures and is associated with favorable changes in inflammatory and hemostatic mediators of cardiovascular risk in proportion to the intensity of exercise. Whether exercise accelerates the development of collateral vessels in patients with chronic CAD is unclear.

Exercise is safe if increased gradually, and if survivors of MI can be used as a yardstick, it is probably cost-effective.[122] Exercise may improve well-being scores and positive affect scores. In addition, patients who are involved in exercise programs are also more likely to be health conscious, to pay attention to diet and weight, and to discontinue cigarette smoking.[123] Overall physical activity is associated with better survival in individuals with and without CV disease.[124] For all these reasons, patients should be urged to participate in regular exercise programs, usually walking, in conjunction with their drug therapy.[122] Moreover, the Centers for Medicare and Medicaid Services (CMS) has determined that cardiac rehabilitation is reasonable and necessary in patients with stable angina, including in the absence of prior MI, CABG, or PCI. Home-based cardiac rehabilitation may enhance adherence compared with center-based programs.[121,125]

Obesity (see Chapters 29 and 30)

Obesity is both an independent contributor to the risk for IHD and associated with a constellation of other risk factors, including hypertension, dyslipidemia, and abnormal glucose metabolism.[126] Weight loss can improve or prevent many of the metabolic consequences of obesity.[127,128] However, the association of obesity with outcomes among patients with established SIHD is complex, with the most favorable outcomes consistently seen among individuals with overweight or mild-moderate obesity, and worse outcomes among normal weight individuals and those with extreme obesity (BMI ≥40 kg/m²). The explanation for the "obesity paradox" by which mild-moderate obesity appears protective in observational studies has not been fully elucidated.

Safety concerns with pharmacologic agents used to facilitate weight loss, such as phentermine, had previously limited the role of weight loss pharmacotherapy in patients with SIDH. However, several pharmacologic agents recently have demonstrated both efficacy for weight loss, as well as cardiovascular safety, including lorcaserin, liraglutide, and semaglutide.[129,130] These and other agents in development may play a larger role in the future with regard to obesity management in patients with SIHD. Bariatric surgery is substantially more effective than weight loss drugs and has been demonstrated to prevent incident CVD events, but data are limited in patients with established IHD. A recent large observational study performed within the SWEEDHEART Registry compared outcomes between 509 patients with prior MI undergoing bariatric surgery (mostly Roux-en Y gastric bypass) versus 509 matched controls with prior MI not undergoing metabolic surgery. Postoperative complications occurred in 8.4% of patients, with 3.8% judged serious. Over 8 years of follow-up, cardiac event rates were significantly lower among individuals undergoing bariatric surgery than in controls (18.7% versus 36.2%; adjusted HR 0.44; 95% CI, 0.32 to 0.61), as was all-cause mortality (adjusted HR 0.45; 95% CI, 0.29 to 0.70).[131] These data suggest a potentially favorable risk/benefit profile for bariatric surgery in severely obese patients with IHD, but randomized controlled trials are needed to adequately evaluate safety and efficacy.

Inflammation (see Chapters 24 and 25)

Atherothrombosis has long been thought to be an inflammatory disease.[132,133] However, only in the past few years have trials of therapeutic interventions established inflammation as a modifiable contributor. Three important trials of pharmacotherapies targeting inflammation alone—without also targeting lipids—have demonstrated clinical benefit in patients with IHD. In Canakinumab Antiinflammatory Thrombosis Outcome Study (CANTOS), three different doses of canakinumab, a monoclonal antibody targeting IL-1β, were tested versus placebo in 10,061 patients with prior MI and hsCRP >2 mg/L.[23] The drug lowered hsCRP and IL-6, but did not affect lipids and significantly reduced rates of the composite outcome of CV death, MI, and stroke. The drug did not lower all-cause mortality and caused a significant excess of fatal infections, highlighting clinical challenges with potent anti-inflammatory agents. Canakinumab will not move forward for clinical development for a cardiovascular indication. A second trial testing low-dose methotrexate did not demonstrate cardiovascular benefit, but conclusions are limited as no effect of the drug at this dose was seen on inflammatory biomarkers.[134]

The most promising agent for current clinical application is low-dose colchicine. After favorable preliminary studies, two large outcome trials have demonstrated clinical benefit of this agent among patients with IHD. The Colchicine Cardiovascular Outcomes Trial (COLCOT) randomized 4745 patients within 30 days of MI to colchicine at a dose of 0.5 mg/day or placebo.[135] The primary ischemic endpoint occurred at approximately 2 years in 7.1% of placebo-treated patients and 5.5% of colchicine-treated patients (HR 0.77; 95% CI, 0.61 to 0.96). The drug was well tolerated but the risk of pneumonia was higher with colchicine and no benefit was seen in all-cause mortality. The Low Dose Colchicine for Secondary Prevention of Cardiovascular Disease (LoDoCo)-2 trial enrolled 5522 patients with SIHD, randomizing them to 0.5 mg of colchicine orally once daily versus placebo and treating for an average of approximately 3 years.[24] The primary composite endpoint was significantly reduced in the colchicine arm (HR 0.69; 95% CI, 0.57 to 0.83; $P < 0.001$; Fig. 40.7). Although the drug was well tolerated, an excess in non-CVD deaths was observed (0.7 versus 0.5 events/100

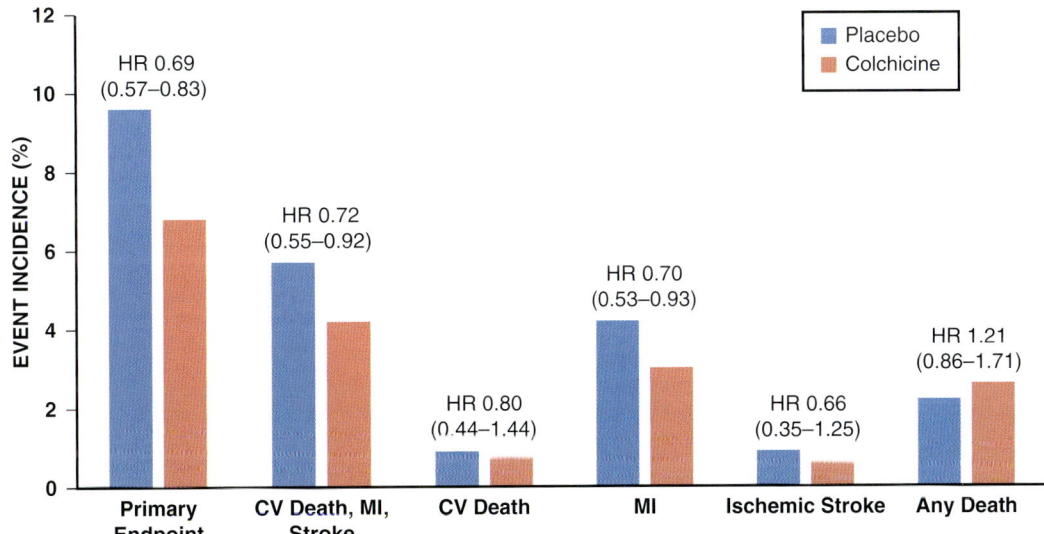

FIGURE 40.7 Event rates after a median duration of 28.6 months of follow-up among 5522 patients with chronic coronary artery disease randomized to colchicine 0.5 mg orally once daily versus matched placebo. Colchicine significantly reduced the primary endpoint of cardiovascular death, spontaneous myocardial infarction, ischemic stroke, or ischemia-driven coronary revascularization, as well as a composite of cardiovascular death, spontaneous myocardial infarction, or ischemic stroke, with a consistent pattern for each element of this composite. However, deaths from any cause trended in the opposite direction with a nonsignificant excess with colchicine. (Data from Nidorf SM, et al. Colchicine in patients with chronic coronary disease. N Engl J Med 2020;383:1838-1847.)

person-years; HR 1.51; 95% CI, 0.99 to 2.31), neutralizing the benefit seen for CVD mortality.[24]

Together, these studies provide compelling evidence that targeting inflammation is a viable strategy for reducing CVD risk. However, to date, none of these anti-inflammatory agents have demonstrated reduction in all-cause mortality and all have reported signals of adverse effects on non-CVD outcomes that may mitigate benefit to some extent. Although colchicine is the most promising agent for current clinical use, additional study is needed to identify patients more likely to suffer infectious or other noncardiac adverse effects from this agent. This area has re-emerged as a priority area for therapeutic development, and additional agents targeting specific inflammatory pathways are being developed and tested.

PHARMACOTHERAPY FOR SECONDARY PREVENTION
Aspirin (see Chapters 24, 40, and 41)

Aspirin reduces the incidence of major cardiovascular events in men and women with previous MI or stroke and after CABG. Moreover, small studies have supported the benefit of aspirin in patients with chronic stable angina but without a history of MI.[36] Therefore administration of aspirin daily is advisable in patients with SIHD and no contraindications to this drug. Dosing at 75 to 162 mg daily appears to have comparable effects on secondary prevention as dosing at 160 to 325 mg daily and is associated with lower bleeding risk. Even among patients with intracoronary stenting, low-dose aspirin has been showed to be preferable to higher-dose aspirin. Thus aspirin, 75 to 162 mg daily, is preferred for secondary prevention.[36]

$P2Y_{12}$ Inhibitors

Other orally acting antiplatelet agents have been studied in patients with SIHD, including patients with or without a prior MI and patients managed with or without prior coronary stenting. Clopidogrel, a thienopyridine derivative, may be substituted for aspirin in patients with aspirin hypersensitivity or in those who cannot tolerate aspirin (see Chapter 41).[36] In a randomized comparison between clopidogrel and aspirin in patients with established atherosclerotic vascular disease (the Clopidogrel versus Aspirin in Patients at Risk of Ischemic Events [CAPRIE] trial), treatment with clopidogrel resulted in a modest 8.7% relative reduction in the risk for vascular death, ischemic stroke, or MI ($P = 0.043$) over a period of 2 years. A meta-analysis of nine randomized trials of aspirin or $P2Y_{12}$ inhibitor therapy as monotherapy in patients with atherosclerotic vascular disease was consistent with the results of CAPRIE, demonstrating a relative 19% lower odds of MI.[136]

Studies evaluating the addition of adenosine diphosphate receptor antagonists such as clopidogrel, prasugrel, and ticagrelor, to aspirin in patients with ACS or after PCI have demonstrated important risk reductions. Therefore, dual-antiplatelet therapy (DAPT) combining aspirin with one of these agents is routine in patients with ACS (see Chapters 38 and 39). In contrast, the treatment of patients with SIHD with DAPT should be more individualized, as the clinical data suggest important risk/benefit tradeoffs.[137] The selection and duration of antiplatelet therapy after PCI is discussed in Chapter 41.

When studied in a population that included patients with clinically evident cardiovascular disease ($n = 12,153$) or asymptomatic subjects with multiple risk factors ($n = 3284$) enrolled in the CHARISMA (Clopidogrel for High Atherothrombotic Risk and Ischemic Stabilization Management and Avoidance) trial, the addition of clopidogrel to aspirin showed no significant benefit with respect to the primary endpoint of cardiovascular death, MI, or stroke over a median of 28 months. However, in the large subgroup of those with established vascular disease, the addition of clopidogrel was associated with a 1% absolute reduction in these events (6.9% versus 7.9%; $P = 0.046$), thus supporting the hypothesis of a potential benefit from clopidogrel in patients with SIHD taking aspirin.[138] In a subsequent study, patients who had received a coronary stent were randomized to discontinuation of thienopyridine therapy at 12 months or continuation of DAPT through 30 months. Continuation of long-term DAPT reduced the risk of death, MI, or stroke by 13% (absolute difference 1.6%) and stent thrombosis by 72% (absolute 1%) at the cost of a significant increase in bleeding (0.9%). The balance of ischemia reduction and bleeding was more favorable among individuals in this trial who underwent PCI for ACS event than those who underwent elective PCI for SIHD.[139]

Two trials of ticagrelor have demonstrated a reduction of ischemic vascular events in patients with SIHD, but at a cost of increased bleeding. In a randomized placebo-controlled trial of ticagrelor in patients who were 1 to 3 years after a prior MI, whether managed medically or with revascularization, the addition of ticagrelor to aspirin reduced the rate of cardiovascular death, MI, or stroke, balanced against an increased rate of bleeding.[140] Ticagrelor 60 mg twice daily offered similar efficacy with less bleeding than 90 mg twice daily, the dose used in the first year after ACS. A combined analysis of these and other trials of long-term DAPT, predominantly in patients with prior ACS, revealed a significant reduction in cardiovascular mortality.[141] In a subsequent trial among ~19,000 patients with diabetes mellitus and established SIHD without a prior known MI, ticagrelor added to aspirin reduced the incidence of cardiovascular death, MI, or stroke by a relative 10% (7.7% versus 8.5%; HR 0.90; 95% CI, 0.81 to 0.99). However, major bleeding was increased by more than twofold (2.2% versus 1.0%; HR 2.32; 95% CI, 1.81 to 2.94).[142] As such, treatment with long-term DAPT may be reasonable for selected SIHD patients at high risk of recurrent thrombosis, particularly those with a prior ACS event, provided they have an acceptable risk of bleeding.[137]

Importantly, patients at lower risk for ischemic events, including most patients undergoing PCI for SIHD symptoms who have not had a prior ACS, may not have a favorable balance of risk/benefit with extending the duration of DAPT. Indeed, studies evaluating optimal DAPT duration for elective stenting for SIHD have suggested that *shorter* durations than 1 year are associated with expectedly lower rates of bleeding than longer durations of treatment.[143] Several studies have examined the discontinuation of aspirin rather than a $P2Y_{12}$ inhibitor for longer-term antiplatelet monotherapy.[144] A network meta-analysis of 79,000 patients from 24 trials with different durations of DAPT after PCI with drug eluting stents supports the conclusion that compared with 12-months of DAPT, short-term DAPT followed by $P2Y_{12}$ inhibitor monotherapy reduces major bleeding after PCI with drug eluting stents, while extended-term DAPT reduces MI at the cost of more bleeding.[145] As such, the 2016 DAPT guideline from the ACC/AHA recommended that the standard duration of DAPT be at least 6 months for most patients receiving stents for SIHD.[137] Since then, some experts have advocated for even shorter durations of DAPT in some patients post-PCI.[146] Risk scores aimed at weighing these competing risks for ischemic events and bleeding may be useful in decision making (see Risk Stratification and Risk Models).[80,147,148] Patients who are at higher risk of atherothrombotic events with acceptable bleeding risk may be considered for durations of DAPT longer than 6 to 12 months.[80,147,148]

Vorapaxar, an antagonist of the platelet-activating action of thrombin, reduces the risk for recurrent atherothrombosis in patients with SIHD with a prior MI. However, because of a significant increase in the risk for bleeding with vorapaxar, clinical use has been limited and mostly among patients with concomitant peripheral artery disease.

Oral Anticoagulation

Oral anticoagulants (OAC) may be used in patients with SIHD either for secondary prevention of atherothrombosis or because of other indications for chronic anticoagulation, including atrial fibrillation, venous thromboembolic disease, or mechanical heart valves (see also Chapter 95). Decisions regarding combined antiplatelet and anticoagulant therapy necessarily take into account the risk of bleeding versus potential antithrombotic benefit. The addition of a single antiplatelet agent to an OAC increases major bleeding rates by >50%, whereas bleeding is more than doubled among those requiring "triple therapy" with OAC, aspirin, and clopidogrel.[149]

Among patients without an indication for OAC for another indication, the addition of a low-dose of the direct OAC rivaroxaban to low-dose aspirin significantly reduced the risk of major cardiovascular events. In the Cardiovascular Outcomes for People Using Anticoagulation Strategies (COMPASS) trial, 27395 patients with stable atherosclerotic vascular disease of whom 24824 patients had stable CAD were randomized to receive rivaroxaban 2.5 mg twice daily by mouth plus aspirin or rivaroxaban 5 mg twice daily, or aspirin alone.[150] Patients who qualified for the trial because of CAD who were younger than 65 years of age were also required to have atherosclerosis involving at least two vascular beds or to have at least two additional risk factors for vascular events (current smoking, diabetes mellitus, an eGFR <60 mL per minute, heart failure, or nonlacunar ischemic stroke ≥1 month earlier). Patients receiving a $P2Y_{12}$ inhibitor were excluded from participation. In the cohort with SIHD, compared with the aspirin-only group, those allocated to rivaroxaban plus aspirin experienced a 26% relative reduction in the risk of cardiovascular death, MI, or stroke ($P < 0.001$). Major bleeding was increased with rivaroxaban-plus-aspirin (3% versus 2%, $P < 0.001$). In contrast, rivaroxaban 5 mg twice daily without aspirin did not significantly reduce the rate of major cardiovascular events but did increase the risk of bleeding.[150] Rivaroxaban plus aspirin also reduced mortality when compared with aspirin alone (3% versus 4%; HR 0.77; 95% CI, 0.65 to 0.90, $p= 0.0012$). Based on these results, the ESC guidelines for the management of chronic coronary syndromes (class IIa) recommend considering the addition of a second antithrombotic drug to aspirin for long-term secondary prevention in patients with a high risk of ischemic events and without high bleeding risk. The second antithrombotic drug may be either a P2Y$_{12}$ inhibitor or rivaroxaban 2.5 mg twice daily.[1]

For SIHD patients with indications for *full*-dose OAC who are at relatively low ischemic risk (i.e., no recent MI or stent), it appears reasonable to omit antiplatelet therapy altogether, particularly if bleeding risk is increased. The AFIRE trial randomized patients with atrial fibrillation and stable CAD coronary revascularization >1 year previously) to rivaroxaban monotherapy or rivaroxaban in combination with a single antiplatelet agent. The combination therapy group had higher rates of bleeding, ischemic events, and mortality than the rivaroxaban monotherapy group.[151]

For patients with atrial fibrillation who have indications for DAPT due to recent ACS or coronary stenting, reassessment of the risks and benefits of OAC should be performed after considering the increased bleeding risk associated with combination therapy. For example, among patients at lower stroke risk it may be preferable to defer OAC after MI and/or stenting, and re-initiate OAC once the patient can safely be withdrawn from DAPT. When triple therapy is necessary, recommendations include (1) limiting exposure to triple therapy to the shortest possible duration, (2) targeting the lower range of international normalized ratio (INR) for warfarin, (3) avoiding the more potent P2Y$_{12}$ antagonist of prasugrel and ticagrelor (i.e., clopidogrel is preferred in combination with OAC), and (4) routinely administering proton pump inhibitors to prevent GI bleeding. Multiple studies have assessed withdrawal of aspirin from triple therapy and demonstrated a favorable effect on the incidence of bleeding without significant loss of efficacy on stroke and systemic embolism and stent thrombosis/MI compared with triple therapy.[152] However, it should be acknowledged that none of the key trials were adequately powered to detect small to moderate increases in ischemic events. The possible regimens and timing of withdrawal of aspirin after PCI in patients with CAD and atrial fibrillation are discussed in Chapter 41.[153] In general, for patients with atrial fibrillation and indications for DAPT, current evidence supports shortening the course of aspirin, continuing clopidogrel and using a DOAC instead of warfarin.

Beta-Blocking Agents

Beta adrenoceptor–blocking drugs (beta-blocking agents) reduce death and recurrent MI in patients who have experienced MI (see Chapters 38 and 39) and are useful for managing angina.[83] However, the optimal duration of treatment after MI is not clear, particularly for patients without LV dysfunction. Moreover, whether these drugs are also of value in preventing MI and sudden death in patients with SIHD without previous MI is less certain, and there have been no prospective controlled trials involving placebo.[84] Findings from observational studies are mixed, with one of the largest studies reporting no reduction in mortality in patients with SIHD receiving beta-blocking agents (Fig. 40.8).[154] However, such observational studies are limited by the high potential for uncontrolled confounding. Moreover, it is plausible that the favorable effects of beta blockers on ischemia and arrhythmias evident in randomized trials among patients with prior MI or reduced LVEF may extend to other patients with SIHD. Therefore, although the use of beta blockers as first-line therapy for uncomplicated hypertension has been questioned, it is sensible to use these drugs when angina, hypertension, or both are present in patients with SIHD and when these drugs are well tolerated.[1,36,84]

Angiotensin-Converting Enzyme Inhibitors and Angiotensin Receptor Blockers

Although inhibitors of the renin-angiotensin-aldosterone system are not indicated for the treatment of angina, these drugs appear to have important benefits in reducing the risk for future ischemic events in some patients with cardiovascular disease.[1,36,155] Potentially beneficial effects of ACE inhibitors include reductions in LV hypertrophy, progression of atherosclerosis, plaque rupture, and thrombosis, in addition to a potentially favorable influence on myocardial O$_2$ supply-and-demand relationships, cardiac hemodynamics, sympathetic activity, and coronary endothelial function.

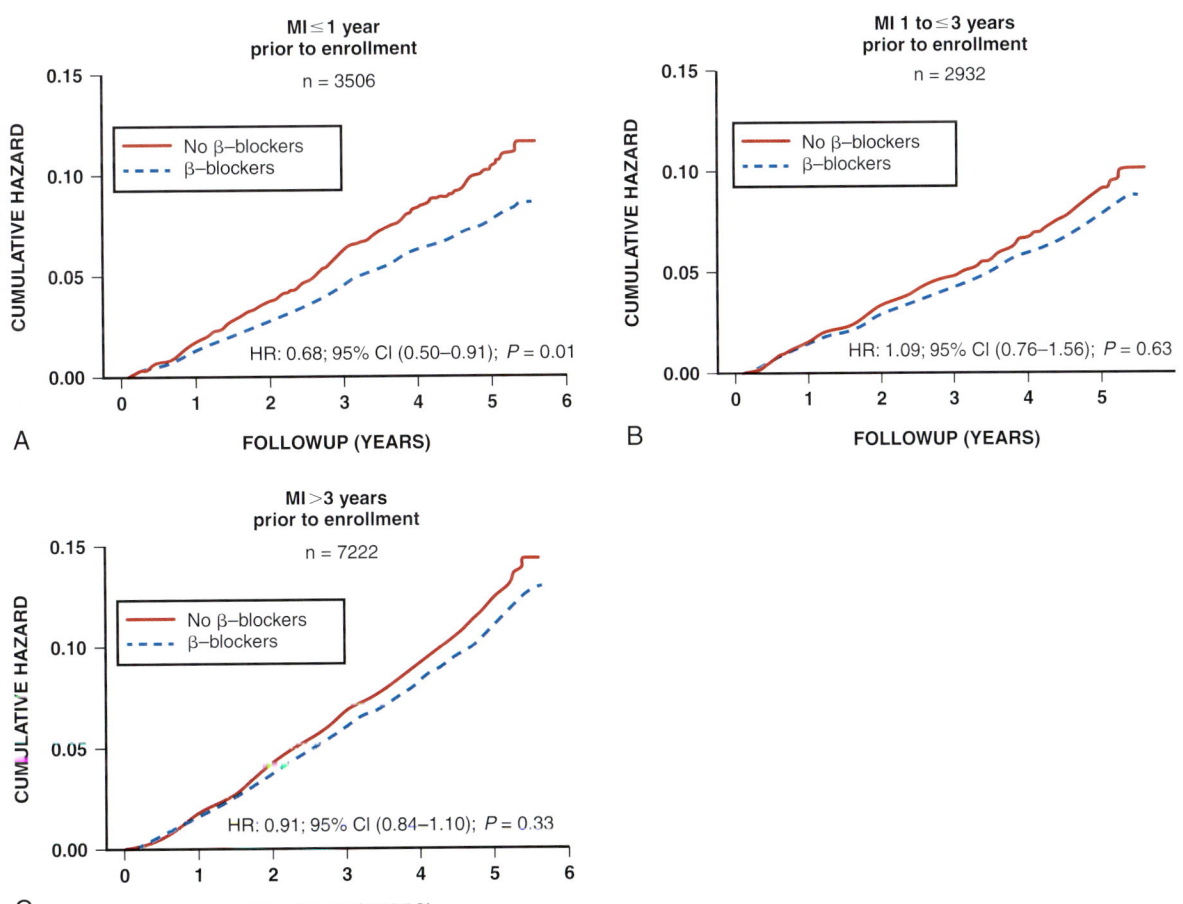

FIGURE 40.8 Cumulative incidence of death in patients with stable ischemic heart disease (SIHD) treated with a beta blocker versus patients treated without a beta blocker categorized by the time since a prior myocardial infarction (MI). This nonrandomized observational analysis was performed among the subgroup of patients with a prior myocardial infarction followed annually to 5 years in the CLARIFY registry. The hazard ratios are adjusted for the REACH risk score, systolic blood pressure, left ventricular ejection fraction, history of coronary revascularization, peripheral artery disease, and asthma or obstructive pulmonary disease. (From Sorbets E, et al. Eur Heart J 2019;40:1399-1402.)

Two trials provided strong evidence supporting the therapeutic benefit of ACE inhibitors in patients with normal LV function and absence of heart failure. In the HOPE (Heart Outcomes Prevention Evaluation) study, ramipril significantly decreased the risk for major vascular events by a relative 22% in 9297 patients with atherosclerotic vascular disease or diabetes mellitus. EUROPA (European Trial on Reduction of Cardiac Events with Perindopril in Stable CAD) similarly showed a 20% relative reduction in the risk for cardiovascular death, MI, or cardiac arrest in 13,655 patients with stable CAD in the absence of heart failure. In contrast, in the PEACE (Prevention of Events with Angiotensin Converting Enzyme Inhibition) trial, trandolapril showed no effect on the risk for cardiovascular death, MI, or coronary revascularization or all-cause mortality alone in 8290 patients with stable CAD and preserved LV function receiving intensive preventive therapy (see Fig. 40.9).[1,36,155] ACE inhibitors are recommended for all patients with CAD and LV dysfunction and for those with hypertension, diabetes, or chronic kidney disease. ACE inhibitors may be considered for optional use in all other patients with SIHD, including those with a normal LV ejection fraction and well-controlled cardiovascular risk factors.[1,36] In patients with established vascular disease or high-risk diabetes, angiotensin receptor blockers (ARBs) appear to provide similar secondary prevention benefits as ACE inhibitors, and thus are suitable alternatives for patients intolerant to ACE inhibitors. However, they should generally not be used in combination with ACE inhibitors as the combination provides no additional benefit over the individual agents and results in an increased rate of complications.[156]

Antioxidants and Vitamins (see Chapter 25)

Oxidized LDL particles are strongly linked to the pathophysiology of atherogenesis, and observational studies have suggested that high dietary intake of antioxidant vitamins (A, C, and beta-carotene) and flavonoids (polyphenolic antioxidants), naturally present in vegetables, fruits, tea, and wine, is associated with a decrease in CAD events. However, in multiple large randomized trials of antioxidant supplements, including vitamin E, vitamin C, beta-carotene, folic acid, and vitamins B_6 and B_{12}, the risk for major cardiovascular events was not reduced. Similarly, despite multiple observational studies suggesting that low levels of vitamin D are associated with increased CV risk, randomized trials have failed to show reduction in cardiovascular disease with vitamin D supplementation.[157,158] Thus, there is no basis for recommending that individuals with IHD take supplemental folate, vitamins C, D, or E, or beta-carotene for the purpose of improving cardiovascular outcomes.[36]

Counseling and Changes in Lifestyle (see Chapter 25)

The psychosocial issues faced by patients with angina are similar to, although usually less intense than, those experienced by patients with acute MI. Depressive symptoms are strongly associated with health status as reported by the patient, including the burden of symptoms and overall quality of life, independent of LV function, and the presence of ischemia.[159] In addition, the association between depressive symptoms and IHD may reflect a causal relationship between the former and atherothrombosis inasmuch as depressive symptoms are associated with higher levels of circulating biomarkers of inflammation. Moreover, a genetic predisposition to depression has been associated with risk for CAD.[160] In conjunction with counseling, treatment with a selective serotonin reuptake inhibitor appears to be safe and effective in managing depression in patients with IHD.[159] Thus, effort to evaluate and treat depression in patients with SIHD is an important element of the overall management of such patients. Moreover, psychosocial stress at work, home, or both is associated with an increased risk for MI and may be a target for preventive interventions. Physical exercise may complement antidepressant pharmacotherapy in reducing depressive symptoms.

An important aspect of the physician's role is to counsel patients with respect to dietary habits, goals for physical activity, the types of work that they can do, and their leisure activities.[161,162] Certain changes in lifestyle may be helpful, such as modifying strenuous activities if they produce angina. A history of stable angina should not preclude physical exertion, either for recreational activities and lifestyle or when physical exertion is required in employment. However, isometric activities such as weightlifting and other activities such as snow shoveling, which involves an energy expenditure of between 60% and 65% of peak O_2 consumption, and cross-country skiing may be undesirable. In addition, these latter activities expose the individual to the detrimental effects of cold on the O_2 supply-and-demand relationship.

Eliminating or reducing the factors that precipitate anginal episodes is of obvious importance. Patients learn their usual threshold by trial and error. Patients should avoid sudden bursts of activity, particularly after long periods of rest or inactivity, after meals, and in cold weather. Both chronic angina and unstable angina exhibit a circadian rhythm characterized by a peak shortly after arising. The stress of sexual intercourse is approximately equal to that of climbing one flight of stairs at a normal pace or any activity that induces a heart rate of approximately 120 beats/min. Most patients with stable angina are able to continue satisfactory sexual activity. Patients with SIHD may use sildenafil and other phosphodiesterase inhibitors to treat organic impotence, but these agents cannot be used in conjunction with nitrates as this combination may promote life-threatening hypotension.

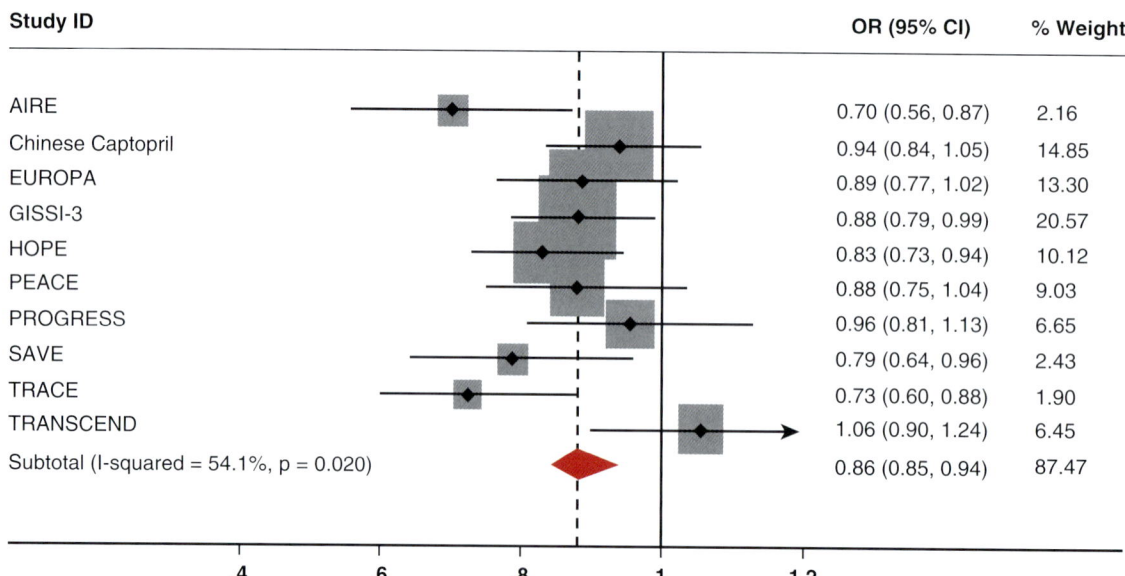

FIGURE 40.9 Meta-analysis of the results for the endpoint of all-cause death from randomized trials of angiotensin-converting enzyme inhibitors in patients with atherosclerotic vascular disease. In randomized trials, angiotensin-converting enzyme inhibitors/angiotensin receptor blockers reduced mortality in individuals with atherosclerotic vascular disease by 11%. *AIRE,* Acute Infarction Ramipril Efficacy; *CI,* confidence interval; *EUROPA,* EURopean trial On reduction of cardiac events with Perindopril in stable coronary Artery disease; *HOPE,* Heart Outcomes Prevention Evaluation; *OR,* odds ratio; *PEACE,* Prevention of Events with Angiotensin Converting Enzyme Inhibition; *PROGRESS,* Perindopril protection against recurrent stroke study; SAVE, Survival and Ventricular Enlargement; *TRANSCEND,* Telmisartan Randomised Assessment Study in ACE-I Intolerant Subjects with Cardiovascular Disease. (Modified from Leong DP, et al. From ACE Inhibitors/ARBs to ARNIs in coronary artery disease and heart failure (Part 2/5). J Am Coll Cardiol 2019;74:693.)

Although from a perspective of both quality of life and avoiding prolonged ischemia, it is desirable to minimize the number of bouts of angina, occasional angina is not to be feared. If there is a clear pattern of effort angina, prophylactic use of short-acting nitrates several minutes before engaging in the offending activity may provide sufficient vasodilation to prevent an anginal episode.

Pharmacologic Management of Angina
Beta Adrenoceptor–Blocking Agents

Beta-blocking agents remain a cornerstone of therapy for angina.[163] In addition to their anti-ischemic properties, beta-blocking agents are modestly effective antihypertensives (see Chapter 26) and antiarrhythmics (see Chapter 64). They have also been shown to reduce mortality and reinfarction in patients after MI and to reduce mortality in patients with heart failure with reduced ejection fraction (see Chapter 50).

Beta blockers reduce the frequency of anginal episodes and raise the anginal threshold, both when given alone and when added to other antianginal agents. This combination of actions makes them extremely useful in the management of SIHD.

The beneficial actions of these drugs depend on their ability to competitively inhibit the effects of neuronally released and circulating catecholamines on beta adrenoceptors (Tables 40.4 and 40.5). Beta blockade reduces myocardial O_2 requirements, primarily by slowing the heart rate; the slower heart rate in turn increases the duration of diastole, with a corresponding increase in the time available for coronary perfusion (Fig. 40.10; see also Table 40.4). In addition, these drugs reduce exercise-induced increases in blood pressure and contractility. Thus beta-blocking agents reduce myocardial O_2 demand primarily during activity or excitement, when surges of increased sympathetic activity occur. These effects of beta blockers on myocardial O_2 demand may favorably alter the

TABLE 40.4 Effects of Antianginal Agents on Indices of Myocardial Oxygen Supply and Demand

INDEX	NITRATES	BETA ADRENOCEPTOR–BLOCKING AGENTS				CALCIUM ANTAGONISTS		
		ISA		CARDIOSELECTIVE		NIFEDIPINE	VERAPAMIL	DILTIAZEM
		NO	YES	NO	YES			
Supply								
Coronary Resistance								
Vascular tone	↓↓	↑	0	↑	0↑	↓↓↓	↓↓↓	↓↓↓
Intramyocardial diastolic tension	↓↓↓	↑	0	↑	↑	↓↓	0↑	0
Coronary collateral blood flow	↑	0	0	0	0	↑	0	↑
Duration of diastole	0 (↓)	↑↑↑	0↓	↑↑↑	↑↑↑	0↑ (↓↓)	↑↑↑ (↓)	↑↑ (↓)
Demand								
Intramyocardial Systolic Tension								
Preload	↓↓↓	↑	0	↑	↑	↓0	↑0↓	0↓
Afterload (peripheral vascular resistance)	↓	↑	↑	↑↑	↑	↓↓	↓	↓
Contractility	0 (↑)	↓↓↓	↓	↓↓↓	↓↓↓	↓ (↑↑)*	↓↓ (↑)*	↓ (↑)*
Heart rate	0 (↑)	↓↓↓	0↓	↓↓↓	↓↓↓	0 (↑↑)	↓↓ (↑)	↓↓ (↑)

↑ = increase; ↓ = decrease; 0 = little or no definite effect. The number of arrows represents the relative intensity of effect. Symbols in parentheses indicate reflex-mediated effects.
ISA, Intrinsic sympathomimetic activity.
*Effect of calcium entry on LV contractility, as assessed in the intact animal model. The net effect on LV performance is variable because it is influenced by alterations in afterload, reflex cardiac stimulation, and the underlying state of the myocardium.
From Shub C, et al. Selection of optimal drug therapy for the patient with angina pectoris. Mayo Clin Proc 1985;60:539.

TABLE 40.5 Physiologic Actions of Beta-Adrenergic Receptors

ORGAN	RECEPTOR TYPE	RESPONSE TO STIMULUS
Heart		
Sinoatrial node	Beta$_1$	Increased heart rate
Atria	Beta$_1$	Increased contractility and conduction velocity
AV node	Beta$_1$	Increased automaticity and conduction velocity
His-Purkinje system	Beta$_1$	Increased automaticity and system conduction velocity
Ventricles	Beta$_1$	Increased automaticity, contractility, and conduction velocity
Arteries		
Peripheral	Beta$_2$	Dilation
Coronary	Beta$_2$	Dilation
Carotid	Beta$_2$	Dilation
Other	Beta$_2$	Increased insulin release
		Increased liver and muscle glycogenolysis
Lungs	Beta$_2$	Dilation of bronchi
Uterus	Beta$_2$	Smooth muscle relaxation

From Abrams J. Medical therapy of stable angina pectoris. In Beller G, Braunwald E, editors. Chronic Ischemic Heart Disease. Atlas of Heart Disease. Vol 5. Philadelphia: WB Saunders; 1995, p 7.19.

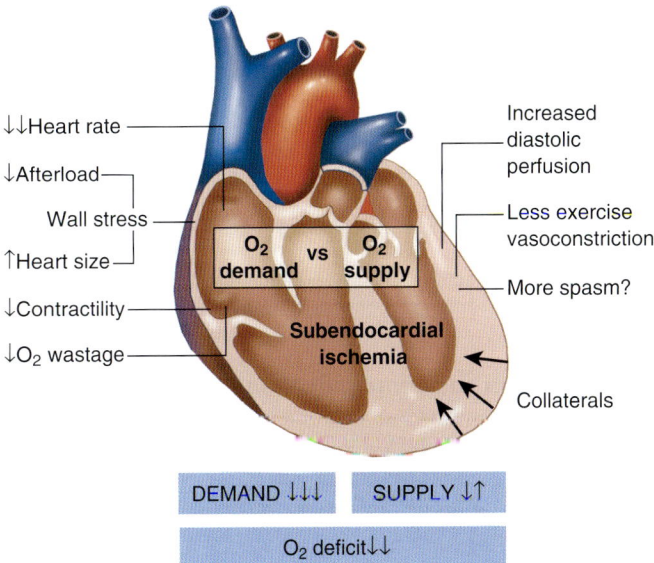

FIGURE 40.10 Effects of beta blockade on an ischemic heart. Beta blockade has a beneficial effect on ischemic myocardium unless (1) the preload rises substantially, as in left-sided heart failure or (2) vasospastic angina is present, in which case spasm may be promoted in some patients. Note the suggestion that beta blockade may diminish exercise-induced vasoconstriction. (Modified from Opie LH: Drugs for the Heart. 4th ed. Philadelphia: WB Saunders; 1995, p 6.)

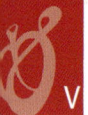

TABLE 40.6 Pharmacokinetics and Pharmacology of Some Beta Adrenoceptor–Blocking Agents

CHARACTERISTIC	ATENOLOL	METOPROLOL/XL	NADOLOL	PINDOLOL	PROPRANOLOL/LA	TIMOLOL	ACEBUTOLOL	LABETALOL
Extent of absorption (%)	≈50	>95	≈30	>90	>90	>90	≈70	>90
Extent of bioavailability (% of dose)	≈40	≈50/77	≈30	≈90	≈30/20	75	≈50	≈25
Beta-blocking plasma concentration	0.2-0.5 μg/mL	50-100 ng/mL	50-100 ng/mL	50-100 ng/mL	50-100 ng/mL	50-100 ng/mL	0.2-2.0 μg/mL	0.7-3.0 μg/mL
Protein binding (%)	<5	12	≈30	57	93	≈10	30-40	≈50
Lipophilicity*	Low	Moderate	Low	Moderate	High	Low	Low	Low
Elimination half-life (hour)	6-9	3-7	14-25	3-4	3.5-6/8-11	3-4	3-4†	≈6
Drug accumulation in renal disease	Yes	No	Yes	No	No	No	Yes‡	No
Route of elimination	RE (mostly unchanged)	HM	RE	RE (40% unchanged and HM)	HM	RE (20% unchanged and HM)	HM‡	HM
Beta-blockade potency ratio (propranolol = 1)	1.0	1	1.0	6.0	1	6.0	0.3	0.3
Adrenergic receptor–blocking activity	β_1‖	β_1‖	β_1/β_2	β_1/β_2	β_1/β_2	β_1/β_2	β_1‖	$\beta_1/\beta_2/\alpha_1$
Intrinsic sympathetic activity	0	0	0	+	0	0	+	0
Membrane-stabilizing activity	0	0	0	+	++	0	+	0
Usual maintenance dose	50-100 mg/day	50-100 mg bid-qid/50-400 mg/day	40-80 mg/day	10-40 mg/day (bid-tid)	80-320 mg/day (bid-tid)/80-160 mg/day	10-30 mg bid	200-600 mg bid	100-400 mg bid
FDA-Approved Indications								
Hypertension	Yes	Yes/Yes	Yes	Yes	Yes/Yes	Yes	Yes	Yes
Angina	Yes	Yes/Yes	Yes	No	Yes/Yes	No	No	No
After MI	Yes	Yes/No	No	No	Yes/No	Yes	No	No
Heart failure	No	Yes/Yes	No	No	No/No	No	No	No

*Determined by the distribution ratio between octanol and water.
†The half-life of the active metabolite diacetolol is 12 to 15 hours.
‡Acebutolol is eliminated mainly by the liver, but its major metabolite diacetolol is excreted by the kidney.
§Rapid metabolism by esterases in the cytosol of red blood cells.
‖Beta$_1$ selectivity is maintained at lower doses, but beta$_2$ receptors are inhibited at higher doses.
FDA, U.S. Food and Drug Administration; HM, hepatic metabolism; ND, no data; RE, renal excretion.

imbalance between supply and demand and thereby mitigate ischemia.

Beta-blocking agents may reduce blood flow to most organs by means of the combination of unopposed alpha-adrenergic vasoconstriction and beta$_2$ receptor blockade (see Table 40.5). Complications are relatively minor, but in patients with peripheral vascular disease, the reduction in blood flow to skeletal muscles with the use of nonselective beta-blocking agents may decrease maximal exercise capacity.

The receptor selectivity, relative potency, lipid solubility, and other characteristics of different beta-blocking agents are summarized in Table 40.6.

Adverse Effects and Contraindications

Most of the adverse effects of beta-blocking agents occur as a consequence of the known properties of these drugs and include cardiac effects (e.g., severe sinus bradycardia, sinus arrest, AV block, reduced LV contractility), bronchoconstriction, fatigue, mental depression, nightmares, sexual dysfunction, and intensification of insulin-induced hypoglycemia (Table 40.7; see also Table 40.5). Lethargy, weakness, and fatigue may be caused by reduced cardiac output or may arise from a direct effect on the central nervous system. In patients who already have impaired LV function, heart failure may be exacerbated. Pindolol, because of its ISA activity, may be preferable in patients with sinus node dysfunction. Carvedilol has been shown to exhibit modest insulin-sensitizing properties and can relieve some manifestations of metabolic syndrome. Blockade of beta$_2$ receptors also inhibits the vasodilating effects of catecholamines in peripheral blood vessels and leaves the constrictor (alpha-adrenergic) receptors unopposed, thereby enhancing vasoconstriction. Noncardioselective beta blockers may precipitate episodes of Raynaud phenomenon in patients with this condition. Reduced flow to the limbs may also occur in patients with peripheral vascular disease.

Abrupt withdrawal of beta blockers after prolonged administration can result in increased total ischemic activity in patients with chronic stable angina. Chronic beta blocker therapy can be safely discontinued by slowly withdrawing the drug in a stepwise manner over the course of 2 to 3 weeks. If abrupt withdrawal of beta blockers is required, patients should be instructed to reduce exertion and manage angina episodes with sublingual nitroglycerin and/or substitute a calcium antagonist.

Calcium Antagonists

The critical role of calcium ions in the normal contraction of cardiac and vascular smooth muscle is discussed in Chapters 36 and 47. The calcium antagonists are a heterogeneous group of compounds that inhibit movement of calcium ions through slow channels in cardiac and smooth muscle membranes by noncompetitive blockade of voltage-sensitive L-type calcium channels. The three major classes of calcium antagonists are the dihydropyridines (nifedipine is the prototype), the phenylalkylamines (verapamil is the prototype), and the modified benzothiazepines (diltiazem is the prototype). Amlodipine and felodipine are additional dihydropyridines that are among the

CHARACTERISTIC	BISOPROLOL	BETAXOLOL	CARTEOLOL	PENBUTOLOL	CARVEDILOL/ CARVEDILOL CR	ESMOLOL (IV)	SOTALOL
Extent of absorption (%)	>90	>90	>90	100	ND	ND	ND
Extent of bioavailability (% of dose)	80	90	85	100	≈30/~25	100	>90
Beta-blocking plasma concentration	0.01-0.1 µg/mL	20-50 ng/mL	40-160 ng/mL	ND	ND	0.15-2.0 µg/mL	ND
Protein binding (%)	30	50-60	23-30	80-98	95-98	55	0
Lipophilicity*	Moderate	Moderate	Low	High	High	Low	Low
Elimination half-life (hour)	7-15	12-22	5-7	17-26	6-10/11	4.5 min	12
Drug accumulation in renal disease	Yes	Yes	Yes	Yes	No	No	Yes
Route of elimination	HM 50%; RE 50%	HM	RE	HM	HM	§	RE
Beta-blockade potency ratio (propranolol = 1)	10	4	10	1	10	0.02	0.3
Adrenergic receptor–blocking activity	β_1'	β_1'	β_1/β_2	β_1/β_2	$\beta_1/\beta_2/\alpha_1$	β_1'	β_1/β_2
Intrinsic sympathetic activity	0	0	+	+	0	0	0
Membrane-stabilizing activity	0	0	0	0	+	0	0
Usual maintenance dose	5-20 mg/day	5-20 mg/day	2.5-10 mg/day	10-40 mg/day	3.125-50 mg bid/10-18 mg/day	Bolus of 500 µg/kg; infusion at 50-200 µg/kg/min	80-160 mg bid
FDA-Approved Indications							
Hypertension	Yes	Yes	Yes	Yes	Yes/Yes	Yes	No
Angina	No	No	No	No	No/No	No	No
After MI	No	No	No	No	No/No	Yes	No
Heart failure	No	No	No	No	Yes/Yes	No	No

most commonly used calcium antagonists in the United States. The two predominant effects of calcium antagonists result from blocking the entry of calcium ions and slowing recovery of the channel. Phenylalkylamines have a marked effect on recovery of the channel and thereby exert depressant effects on cardiac pacemakers and conduction, whereas dihydropyridines, which do not impair channel recovery, have little effect on the conduction system.

Mechanism of Action

The efficacy of calcium antagonists in patients with angina pectoris is related to the reduction in myocardial O_2 demand and the increase in O_2 supply that they induce (see Table 40.4). The latter effect is particularly important in patients with conditions in which a prominent vasospastic or vasoconstrictor component may be present, such as Prinzmetal (variant) angina. Calcium antagonists may be effective on their own or in combination with beta-blocking agents and nitrates in patients with stable angina. Several calcium antagonists are effective for the treatment of angina pectoris (Table 40.8). Each relaxes vascular smooth muscle in the systemic arterial and coronary arterial beds. In addition, blockade of the entry of calcium into myocytes results in a negative inotropic effect, which is counteracted to some extent by peripheral vascular dilation and by activation of the sympathetic nervous system in response to drug-induced hypotension. However, the negative inotropic effect must be taken into consideration in patients with significant LV dysfunction.

First-Generation Calcium Antagonists

NIFEDIPINE. Nifedipine, a dihydropyridine, is a particularly effective dilator of vascular smooth muscle and is a more potent vasodilator than diltiazem or verapamil. The beneficial effects of nifedipine in the treatment of angina result from its capacity to reduce myocardial O_2 requirements because of its afterload-reducing effect and to increase myocardial O_2 delivery as a result of its dilating action on the coronary vascular bed (see Table 40.4). Because immediate-release formulations can precipitate hypotension and adverse events, an extended-release formulation should be used when nifedipine is administered. A meta-analysis of 15 studies of long-acting calcium channel antagonists, including nifedipine, in patients with CAD demonstrated significant reductions in angina, stroke, and heart failure, with no improvement in other cardiovascular outcomes. Long-acting nifedipine should be considered an effective and safe antianginal drug for the treatment of symptomatic patients with angina who are already receiving beta-blocking agents, with or without nitrates.

ADVERSE EFFECTS. These occur in 15% to 20% of patients and require discontinuation of medication in approximately 5%. Most adverse effects are related to systemic vasodilation and include headache, dizziness, palpitations, flushing, hypotension, and leg edema (unrelated to heart failure). In rare cases in patients with extremely severe fixed coronary obstructions, nifedipine aggravates angina, presumably by lowering arterial pressure excessively with subsequent reflex tachycardia. For this reason, combined treatment of angina with nifedipine

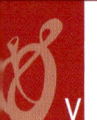

TABLE 40.7 Candidates for Use of Beta-Blocking Agents for Angina

Ideal Candidates
Prominent relationship of physical activity to attacks of angina
Coexistent hypertension
History of supraventricular or ventricular arrhythmias
Previous MI
LV systolic dysfunction
Mild to moderate heart failure symptoms (NYHA functional classes II, III)
Prominent anxiety state

Poor Candidates
Asthma or reversible airway component in patients with chronic lung disease
Severe LV dysfunction with severe heart failure symptoms (NYHA functional class IV)
History of severe depression
Raynaud phenomenon
Symptomatic peripheral vascular disease
Severe bradycardia or heart block
Diabetes with frequent hypoglycemic episodes

and a beta-blocking agent is particularly effective and superior to nifedipine alone. Nifedipine has been reported to worsen heart failure in patients with preexisting chronic heart failure and is contraindicated in patients who are hypotensive or have severe aortic valve stenosis.

VERAPAMIL. Verapamil dilates systemic and coronary resistance vessels and large coronary conductance vessels. It slows the heart rate and reduces myocardial contractility. This combination of actions results in a reduction in the myocardial O_2 requirement, which is the basis for the drug's efficacy in the management of chronic stable angina (see Table 40.8). A strategy combining sustained-release verapamil and trandolapril versus atenolol and a diuretic for the treatment of patients with hypertension and CAD, including those with previous MI, showed equivalent outcomes with respect to death, MI, or stroke.

In patients with cardiac dysfunction, verapamil may reduce cardiac output, increase LV filling pressure, and cause clinical heart failure. Verapamil slows the heart rate and AV conduction. Therefore, it is contraindicated in patients with preexisting AV nodal disease, sick sinus syndrome, or systolic heart failure. Verapamil should generally not be used together with a beta-blocking agent due to the risk for bradycardia or heart block. It is contraindicated in patients with suspected digitalis toxicity. The bioavailability of verapamil is increased by cimetidine and carbamazepine, whereas verapamil may increase plasma levels of cyclosporine and digoxin.

Adverse effects of verapamil are noted in approximately 10% of patients and are related to systemic vasodilation (hypotension and facial flushing), GI symptoms (constipation and nausea), and central nervous system reactions such as headache and dizziness. A rare side effect is gingival hyperplasia, which appears after 1 to 9 months of therapy.

DILTIAZEM. Diltiazem's actions are intermediate between those of nifedipine and verapamil. In clinically useful doses its vasodilator effects are less profound than those of nifedipine, and its cardiac depressant action on the sinoatrial and AV nodes and myocardium is less than that of verapamil. This profile may explain the low incidence of adverse effects of diltiazem. Diltiazem is a systemic vasodilator that lowers arterial pressure at rest and during exertion and increases the workload required to produce myocardial ischemia, but it may also increase myocardial O_2 delivery. Although this drug causes little vasodilation of epicardial coronary arteries under basal conditions, it may enhance perfusion of the subendocardium distal to a flow-limiting coronary stenosis; it also blocks exercise-induced coronary vasoconstriction.

Major side effects are similar to those of the other calcium channel–blocking agents and are related to vasodilation, but they are relatively infrequent, particularly if the dosage does not exceed 240 mg daily. As is the case with verapamil, diltiazem should be prescribed with caution for patients with sick sinus syndrome or AV block. In patients with preexisting LV dysfunction, diltiazem may exacerbate or precipitate heart failure.

Diltiazem interacts with other drugs, including beta-blocking agents (causing enhanced negative inotropic, chronotropic, and dromotropic effects), flecainide, and cimetidine (which increases the bioavailability of diltiazem). Diltiazem has been associated with increased plasma levels of substrates of cytochrome P-450 (CYP3A4), including apixaban, atorvastatin, simvastatin, cilostazol, dofetilide, ivabradine, and ranolazine, as well as non-CYP3A4 substrates including carbamazepine and cyclosporin. Diltiazem may reduce digoxin clearance, especially in patients with renal failure (see Chapter 9).

Second-Generation Calcium Antagonists

The second-generation calcium antagonists (e.g., nicardipine, amlodipine, felodipine) are mainly dihydropyridine derivatives, with nifedipine being the prototypic agent. The second-generation calcium antagonists differ in potency, tissue specificity, and pharmacokinetics and, in general, are potent vasodilators because of the greater vascular selectivity than seen with the first-generation antagonists (e.g., verapamil, nifedipine, diltiazem).

AMLODIPINE. This agent, which is less lipid soluble than nifedipine, has a slow, smooth onset and ultralong duration of action (plasma half-life of 36 hours). It causes marked coronary and peripheral dilation and is useful in the treatment of patients with angina accompanied by hypertension. It may be used as a once-daily antihypertensive or antianginal agent. In a series of randomized placebo-controlled studies in patients with exercise-induced angina pectoris, amlodipine was effective and well tolerated. In two trials involving patients with established CAD, amlodipine reduced the risk for major cardiovascular events. Amlodipine has little, if any negative inotropic action and may be useful in patients with stable angina and LV dysfunction.

The usual dosage of amlodipine is 5 to 10 mg once daily. Downward adjustment of the starting dose is appropriate for patients with liver disease and the elderly. Significant changes in blood pressure are typically not evident until 24 to 48 hours after initiation. Steady-state serum levels are achieved at 7 to 8 days. Amlodipine should not be co-administered with simvastatin as it increases drug levels of this statin and may increase risk for myopathy.

NICARDIPINE. This drug has a half-life similar to that of nifedipine (2 to 4 hours) but appears to have greater vascular selectivity. Nicardipine may be used as an antianginal and antihypertensive agent and requires administration three times daily, although a sustained-release formulation is available for twice-daily dosing in patients with hypertension. For stable angina pectoris, it appears to be as effective as verapamil or diltiazem, and its efficacy is enhanced when combined with a beta-blocking agent.

FELODIPINE AND ISRADIPINE. In the United States, both of these drugs are approved by the U.S. Food and Drug Administration for the treatment of hypertension but not for angina pectoris. Felodipine has similar efficacy to nifedipine in patients with stable angina. Felodipine has also been reported to be more vascular selective than nifedipine and to have a mild positive inotropic effect as a result of calcium channel agonist properties. Isradipine has a longer half-life than nifedipine and demonstrates greater vascular sensitivity.

Nitrates
Mechanism of Action

The action of nitrates is to relax vascular smooth muscle. The vasodilator effects of nitrates are evident in systemic (including coronary) arteries and veins, but they appear to be predominant in the venous circulation. The venodilator effect reduces ventricular preload, which in turn reduces myocardial wall tension and O_2 requirements. The action of nitrates in reducing preload and afterload makes them useful in the treatment of heart failure (see Fig. 40.2), as well as angina. By reducing the heart's mechanical activity, volume, and O_2 consumption, nitrates increase exercise capacity in patients with IHD, thereby allowing greater total-body workload to be achieved before the angina threshold is reached. Thus, in patients with stable angina, nitrates improve exercise tolerance and time to ST-segment depression during treadmill exercise tests. When used in combination with calcium channel–blocking agents and/or betablocking agents, the antianginal effects appear to be greater.[36]

TABLE 40.8 Pharmacokinetics of Some Calcium Antagonists Used for Angina Pectoris

CHARACTERISTIC	DILTIAZEM/SR	NICARDIPINE	NIFEDIPINE/SR	VERAPAMIL/SR	AMLODIPINE	FELODIPINE	ISRADIPINE	NISOLDIPINE
Usual adult dose	30-90 mg tid-qid SR: 60-180 mg bid CD: 120-480 mg/day	20-40 mg tid SR: 30-60 mg bid	IR: 10-30 mg tid SR: 90 mg/day	80-120 mg tid-qid SR: 180-480 mg/day	2.5-10 mg/day	SR: 2.5-10 mg/day	CR: 2.5-10 mg bid	SR: 10-40 mg/day
Extent of absorption (%)	80-90	100	90	90	>90	>90	>90	ND
Extent of bioavailability (%)	40-70	30	65-75/86	20-35	60-90	20	25	5
Onset of action	30-60 min	20 min	20 min	30 min	30-60 min	2 hr	20 min	1-3 hr
Time to peak serum concentration (hr)	2-3/6-11	0.5-2.0	0.5/6	IV: 3-5 min Oral: 1-2 SR: 7-9	6-12	2-5	1.5	6-12
Therapeutic serum levels (ng/mL)	50-200	30-50	25-100	80-300	5-20	1-5	2-10	ND
Elimination half-life (hr)	3.5/5-7	2.0-4.0	2.0-5.0	3.0-7.0*	30-50	11-16	8	7-12
Elimination pass, hepatic	60% metabolized by the liver; remainder excreted by the kidneys	High first-pass hepatic metabolism	High first-pass hepatic metabolism	85% eliminated by first-pass hepatic metabolism	Hepatic	High first-pass hepatic metabolism	High first-pass hepatic metabolism	Hepatic
Heart rate	↓	↑	↑↑	↓	0	↑	0	0
Peripheral vascular resistance	↓	↓↓↓	↓↓↓	↓↓	↓↓↓	↓↓↓	↓↓↓	↓↓↓
FDA-approved indications	IR, SR		IR, SR	IR, SR				
Hypertension	No	Yes†	Yes	Yes	Yes	Yes	Yes	Yes
Angina	Yes	Yes	Yes	Yes	Yes	No	No	Yes
Coronary spasm	Yes	No	Yes	No	Yes	No	No	No

*Half-life of 4.5 to 12 hours with multiple dosing; may be prolonged in older adults.
†The sustained-release formulation may be preferred for hypertension.
CD, Combination drug; CR, controlled release; FDA, U.S. Food and Drug Administration; IR, immediate release; ND, no data; SR, sustained release.

TABLE 40.9 Recommended Dosing Regimens for Long-Term Nitrate Therapy

PREPARATION OF AGENT	DOSE	SCHEDULE
Nitroglycerin*		
Ointment	0.5-2 inches	2-3 times daily
Transdermal patch	0.2-0.8 mg/hr	q24 hr; remove at bedtime for 12-14 hr
Sublingual tablet	0.3-0.6 mg	As needed, up to 3 doses 5 min apart
Spray	1 or 2 sprays	As needed, up to 3 doses 5 min apart
Isosorbide Dinitrate*		
Oral	10-40 mg	2 or 3 times daily
Oral sustained release	80-120 mg	Once or twice daily (eccentric schedule)
Isosorbide 5-Mononitrate		
Oral	20 mg	Twice daily (given 7-8 hr apart)
Oral sustained release	30-240 mg	Once daily

*A 10- to 12-hour nitrate-free interval is recommended.

Types of Preparations and Routes of Administration

Short-acting nitroglycerin administered sublingually (either by tablet or spray) remains the drug of choice for the treatment of acute angina episodes (Table 40.9). Because sublingual administration avoids first-pass hepatic metabolism, a transient but effective concentration of the drug rapidly appears in the circulation. Within 30 to 60 minutes, hepatic breakdown has abolished the hemodynamic and clinical effects. Sublingual nitroglycerin is also useful when taken prophylactically shortly before undertaking physical activities that are likely to cause angina. When used for this purpose, it may prevent angina for up to 40 minutes.

ADVERSE REACTIONS. Adverse reactions are common and include headache, flushing, and hypotension. The last is rarely severe, but in some patients with volume depletion and in an upright posture, nitrate-induced hypotension is accompanied by a paradoxical bradycardia, consistent with a vasovagal or vasodepressor response. This reaction is more common in older adults, who are less able to tolerate hypovolemia, and may be magnified in hot weather.

PREPARATIONS

SHORT-ACTING NITROGLYCERIN (NITROGLYCERIN TABLETS AND ORAL SPRAY). Nitrate preparations are available in sublingual, buccal, oral, spray, and ointment forms (see Table 40.9). A nitroglycerin spray that dispenses metered, aerosolized doses of 0.4 mg may be better absorbed than the sublingual tablet in patients with dry mucosal membranes. For prophylaxis the spray should be used 5 to 10 minutes before angina-provoking activities. An additional advantage of the pump spray preparation is a longer shelf-life (up to 2 years) than that of sublingual nitroglycerin (which is approximately 6 months).

ISOSORBIDE DINITRATE. This drug is available in tablets for sublingual use, in chewable form, in tablets for oral use, and in sustained-release capsules. Partial or complete nitrate tolerance (see later) develops with regimens of isosorbide dinitrate administered as 30 mg three or four times daily. A dosage schedule should be adopted that allows a ≥12-hour nitrate-free interval. If the drug is administered on a three-times-daily schedule (e.g., at 8 AM, 1 PM, and 6 PM), the antianginal benefit lasts for approximately 6 hours, and the magnitude of the antianginal benefit decreases with each successive dose.

ISOSORBIDE 5-MONONITRATE. Plasma levels of isosorbide 5-mononitrate reach their peak between 30 minutes and 2 hours after ingestion, and the drug has a plasma half-life of 4 to 6 hours. Tolerance has not been demonstrated with once-daily or eccentric dosing intervals but does occur with a twice-daily dosing regimen at 12-hour intervals. The only sustained-release preparation of isosorbide 5-mononitrate is Imdur, which is given once daily at a dosage of 30 to 240 mg. Presumably, this preparation avoids tolerance by providing a sufficiently low nitrate level or a duration of action of 12 hours or less.

Once-daily dosing of oral nitrates improves compliance and may offer better efficacy in reducing angina.

TOPICAL NITROGLYCERIN. Nitroglycerin may be applied as a transdermal patch. Application of a silicone gel or polymer matrix impregnated with nitroglycerin results in absorption for 24 to 48 hours at a rate determined by various methods of preparation of the patch. Transdermal nitroglycerin therapy has been shown to increase exercise duration and maintain its anti-ischemic effects for 12 hours after patch application throughout 30 days of therapy, without significant evidence of nitrate tolerance or rebound phenomena, provided that the patch is not applied for more than 12 of 24 hours.

Other Issues Related to Oral Nitrates

INTERACTION WITH CYCLIC GUANOSINE MONOPHOSPHATE–SPECIFIC PHOSPHODIESTERASE TYPE 5 INHIBITORS. The combination of nitrates and phosphodiesterase type 5 (PDE5) inhibitors (sildenafil, tadalafil, and vardenafil) may cause serious, prolonged, and potentially life-threatening hypotension. Nitrate therapy is an absolute contraindication to the use of these agents, and vice versa. Patients who wish to take a PDE5 inhibitor should be aware of the serious nature of this adverse drug interaction and be warned about taking any of these agents within 24 hours of any nitrate preparation, including short-acting sublingual nitroglycerin tablets.

Other Pharmacologic Agents
Ranolazine

Ranolazine is a piperazine derivative that is available in the United States for use in patients with stable angina.[163] Ranolazine is distinct among available antianginals in that its anti-ischemic effects are achieved without a clinically meaningful change in heart rate or blood pressure. When studied at high concentrations in in vitro experiments, ranolazine was shown to shift myocardial substrate uptake from fatty acid to glucose and thus was considered to be a potential myocardial metabolic modulator. However, subsequent studies at concentrations of ranolazine consistent with doses tested in clinical trials indicate that ranolazine exerts favorable effects on ischemia through a reduction in calcium overload in ischemic myocytes via inhibition of the late inward sodium current (I_{Na}). In animal models of ischemia and reperfusion, ranolazine preserves tissue levels of adenosine triphosphate (ATP) and improves myocardial contractile function.

A sustained-release formulation of ranolazine has been studied in four randomized placebo-controlled clinical trials and improved exercise performance and increased the time to ischemia during exercise treadmill testing when used as monotherapy or in combination with the most frequently used doses of atenolol, amlodipine, or diltiazem. Ranolazine also decreases angina frequency and nitroglycerin use when used in conjunction with a beta-blocking agent or calcium channel–blocking agent and in patients with diabetes mellitus.[164]

Despite the favorable effect of ranolazine on ischemic symptoms, in two multinational, randomized, placebo-controlled outcomes trials, ranolazine has not reduced major cardiovascular events. When studied in 6560 patients with non-ST-segment elevation ACS, ranolazine, administered for an average of approximately 1 year, reduced the incidence of recurrent ischemia but did not prevent major cardiovascular events. Consistent with previous studies, the reduction in angina and improvement in exercise performance were evident only in patients with a history of chronic angina. When studied in 2651 patients with incomplete revascularization after PCI, ranolazine had no demonstrable effect on ischemia-driven revascularization or hospitalization (HR 0.95; 95% CI, 0.82 to 1.10; p= 0.48)[165] or on quality of life.[166]

Because of its proposed mechanism of action on cardiac myocytes rather than modulation of the heart rate or blood pressure, ranolazine has been studied in patients with angina and ischemia without obstructive epicardial CAD. In a pilot study of 20 women with angina and no obstructive CAD but with impaired coronary flow reserve on CMRI, ranolazine reduced symptoms with evidence of an improved myocardial perfusion reserve index. However, a subsequent study in 128 women with evidence of microvascular dysfunction in the absence of obstructive CAD showed no benefit of ranolazine with respect to symptoms or myocardial perfusion abnormalities.[167,168]

The half-life of the sustained-release formulation of ranolazine is approximately 7 hours. A steady state is generally achieved within 3 days of twice-daily dosing. Ranolazine is metabolized primarily through the CYP3A4 pathway, and thus the plasma concentration is increased if administered in combination with moderate (e.g., diltiazem) or strong (e.g., ketoconazole and macrolide antibiotic) inhibitors of this system. Verapamil increases the absorption of ranolazine by inhibition of P-glycoprotein. Plasma concentrations of simvastatin are increased approximately twofold after the administration of ranolazine, and it should not be co-administered with ranolazine in doses greater than 20 mg daily.

Ranolazine should be started at 500 mg twice daily and may be increased to a maximum of 1000 mg twice daily in patients with persistent angina. The most commonly reported adverse effects in clinical studies are nausea, generalized weakness, and constipation. Dizziness has also been reported, as has a small dose-related increase in the corrected QT (QTc) interval, an average of 2 to 5 milliseconds in the dosage range of 500 to 1000 mg twice daily. In contrast to beta blockers and calcium antagonists, ranolazine does not have adverse effects on LV contractility.

The electrophysiologic effects of ranolazine include inhibition of the delayed rectifier current and inhibition of I_{Na}; the net effect is to shorten the action potential duration and suppress early after depolarizations.[169,170] Thus ranolazine does not have the electrophysiologic profile that has been observed with QT-prolonging drugs associated with torsade de pointes. Rather, ranolazine appears to have favorable electrophysiologic effects on ventricular and atrial arrhythmias. For example, in patients with recent ACS, ranolazine reduced the incidence of arrhythmias detected on ambulatory electrocardiographic monitoring when compared with placebo. Subsequent experimental and small human studies have revealed possible favorable effects on atrial fibrillation, suppression of torsade de pointes, and recurrence of internal defibrillator discharges. Ranolazine has been investigated for its potential clinical antiarrhythmic effects alone and in combination with other agents.[171,172] Nevertheless, because of its effect on the QT interval, ranolazine is contraindicated in patients with preexisting QT prolongation, in patients receiving other QT-prolonging medications, or in those with hepatic impairment, which has been associated with a steeper relationship between ranolazine and the QTc.

In addition to these electrophysiologic effects, ranolazine also appears to have favorable glycometabolic effects, including a modest reduction in hemoglobin A1c. Moreover, there is preliminary suggestion that the clinical antianginal effects of ranolazine may be modestly greater among individuals with higher hemoglobin A1c.[173]

Other Antianginal Therapies
Ivabradine, nicorandil, and trimetazidine are discussed in the online version of this chapter.

Other Considerations of Medical Management of Angina Pectoris
Choice of Initial Therapy
Selection of initial therapy for angina pectoris should be based on an individualized approach that considers other cardiovascular conditions such as hypertension, tachyarrhythmias, conduction system disease, peripheral artery disease, and LV dysfunction, as well as other non–cardiac-related medical conditions such as severe reactive airways disease, diabetes, or depression. Comparative studies of antianginal agents have not shown any meaningful difference in efficacy to differentiate one specific class of agents from another for patients with SIHD and no previous MI. Rather, selection of the optimal agent is usually based on overall consideration of the management of coexisting conditions, tolerability, and cost. For most patients, beta-blocking agents or calcium channel antagonists, which are effective and low cost, remain the first line of therapy.

Relative Advantages of Beta-Blocking Agents and Calcium Antagonists (Table 40.10)
The choice between a beta-blocking agent and a calcium channel antagonist as initial therapy in patients with chronic stable angina is controversial because both classes of agents are effective in relieving symptoms and reducing ischemia.[1,36,79] Trials comparing beta blockers and calcium antagonists have not shown any difference in the rate

TABLE 40.10 Recommended Use of Beta-Blocking Agents or Calcium Antagonists in Patients Who Have Angina in Conjunction with Other Medical Conditions

CLINICAL CONDITION	RECOMMENDED DRUG*
Cardiac Arrhythmia or Conduction Disturbance	
Sinus bradycardia	Nifedipine, amlodipine
Sinus tachycardia (not caused by cardiac failure)	Beta-blocking agent
Supraventricular tachycardia	Beta-blocking agent, verapamil, or diltiazem
AV block	Nifedipine or amlodipine
Rapid atrial fibrillation	Beta-blocking agent, verapamil, or diltiazem
Ventricular arrhythmia	Beta-blocking agent
Left Ventricular Dysfunction	
Heart failure	Beta-blocking agent
Miscellaneous Medical Conditions	
Systemic hypertension	Beta-blocking agent or calcium antagonist
Severe preexisting migraine headaches	Beta-blocking agent, verapamil, or diltiazem
COPD with bronchospasm or asthma	Nifedipine, amlodipine, verapamil, or diltiazem
Hyperthyroidism	Beta-blocking agent
Raynaud syndrome	Nifedipine or amlodipine
Claudication	Calcium antagonist
Severe depression	Calcium antagonist

COPD, Chronic obstructive pulmonary disease.

of death or MI, although in some studies beta blockers appeared to have greater antianginal efficacy. Because long-term administration of beta blockers has been demonstrated to prolong life in patients after acute MI, whereas calcium blockers have not, U.S. guidelines recommend beta blockers over calcium antagonists as the agents of choice in treating patients with SIHD.[36] Nevertheless, as highlighted by a large observational study, evidence to support a preference for beta blockers in SIHD without recent MI or LV dysfunction is weak.[83,154]

Selection of Therapy
The choice of initial drug therapy for management of angina is influenced by a number of clinical factors (see Table 40.10).[1,36]

1. In patients with a history of asthma or chronic obstructive lung disease with wheezing on clinical examination, in whom beta-blocking agents, even relatively selective agents, may not be tolerated, calcium antagonists or nitrates are preferred and ranolazine is an option. A trial of a beta blocker should be considered if the patient has a history of previous MI or LV dysfunction.
2. Amlodipine, nifedipine (long acting) and nicardipine are the calcium antagonists of choice in patients with chronic stable angina and sick sinus syndrome, sinus bradycardia, or significant AV conduction disturbances, whereas beta blockers and verapamil should be used only with caution in such patients. In patients with symptomatic conduction disease, neither a beta blocker nor a heart rate–lowering calcium antagonist should be used unless a pacemaker is in place. If a beta blocker is required in patients with asymptomatic evidence of conduction disease, pindolol, which has the greatest ISA, is useful. In the case of calcium channel–blocking agents in patients with conduction system disease, amlodipine, nifedipine, or nicardipine are preferable to verapamil and diltiazem. Nitrates and ranolazine are alternatives.
3. Calcium antagonists or long-acting nitrates are preferred for patients with suspected Prinzmetal (variant) angina; beta blockers may even aggravate angina under these circumstances.
4. Calcium antagonists may be preferred over beta blockers in patients with symptomatic peripheral arterial disease because the latter may cause peripheral vasoconstriction.
5. Beta-blocking agents should usually be avoided in patients with a history of significant depressive illness and should be avoided or monitored for exacerbation of symptoms in patients with sexual dysfunction, sleep disturbance, nightmares, fatigue, or lethargy.

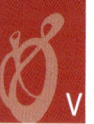

6. The beneficial effects of beta blockers on survival in patients with LV dysfunction after MI, coupled with their beneficial effects on survival and LV performance in patients with heart failure, have established beta-blocking agents as the drug class of choice for the treatment of angina in patients with LV dysfunction, with or without symptoms of heart failure, together with ACE inhibitors or ARBs. If a beta blocker is not tolerated or angina persists despite beta blockade and nitrates, amlodipine can be administered. Ranolazine is also an option for such patients. In countries where it is available, ivabradine may be considered in patients with angina in conjunction with LV dysfunction and an HR >70 beats/min on beta blocker therapy. Verapamil, nifedipine, and diltiazem should be avoided.
7. Hypertensive patients with angina pectoris can be treated with either beta blockers or calcium antagonists because both have antihypertensive effects, and an ACE inhibitor should strongly be considered for all patients with CAD and hypertension. Although less effective as antihypertensive agents, present professional society guidelines favor use of beta blockers in patients with angina and hypertension, with nondihydropyridine calcium channel blockers as an alternative if symptom relief or control of hypertension is inadequate with the beta blocker. Carvedilol has a more robust effect than metoprolol on blood pressure and is better tolerated than labetalol, and thus may be the preferred beta blocker for patients with angina and hypertension.

Combination Therapy

A combination of multiple agents is widely used for the management of stable angina, with options that include a beta blocker, calcium antagonist, long-acting nitrate, or ranolazine. Ranolazine may be particularly useful when heart rate, blood pressure, or LV dysfunction limit escalation of other therapy. In patients with severe hypertension and angina, the combination of amlodipine and carvedilol may be particularly effective to achieve both angina relief and potent BP reduction. In patients with moderate or severe LV dysfunction, sinus bradycardia, or AV conduction disturbances, combination therapy with nondihydropyridine calcium antagonists and beta blockers should be avoided or should be initiated with caution. The negative inotropic effects of calcium antagonists are not usually a problem in combined therapy with low doses of beta blockers but can become significant with higher doses. With such doses, amlodipine is the calcium antagonist of choice, but it should be used cautiously. Ranolazine may be useful in such patients who do not tolerate other agents.

Synthesis of an Integrated Approach to Management of Patients with Stable Angina

This approach is as follows:
1. Identify and treat precipitating factors, such as anemia, uncontrolled hypertension, thyrotoxicosis, tachyarrhythmias, uncontrolled heart failure, and concomitant valvular heart disease.
2. Initiate risk factor modification, physical exercise, diet, and lifestyle counseling. Commence therapy with a high-intensity statin regimen and low dose aspirin (or clopidogrel).
3. Initiate a shared decision-making discussion with the patient to determine the frequency and duration of angina and the impact on the patient's quality of life. Explain the complementary role of antianginal medical therapy and revascularization for angina relief, making sure the patient is fully aware of the limited role of revascularization for improvement of hard clinical outcomes. For patients with high anginal burden, particularly at low workload, and those who prefer not to take additional antianginal medications, it is not unreasonable to offer revascularization as first-line therapy for symptom relief, provided the patient understands the risks of the procedure and that the benefits would only be expected on quality of life and not death or MI outcomes.
4. For most patients, begin pharmacotherapy with a beta blocker or calcium antagonist. Initiate an ACE inhibitor or ARB in all patients with an LV ejection fraction of 0.40 or lower and in those with hypertension, diabetes, or chronic kidney disease. In addition, an ACE inhibitor may be considered for all other patients.
5. Use sublingual nitroglycerin for alleviation of anginal symptoms and for prophylaxis, if needed.
6. If angina persists, the next step is usually the addition of a second agent: a calcium antagonist or beta blocker, or long-acting nitrate via dosing schedules that prevent nitrate tolerance. The need to treat concomitant hypertension or the presence of LV dysfunction and symptoms of heart failure may be an indication for the use of one of these agents, even in patients in whom episodes of symptomatic angina are infrequent. Ranolazine is an alternative for some patients, particularly those in whom initiation or titration of other agents is limited by low heart rate or blood pressure.
7. If angina persists despite two antianginal agents (usually a beta blocker with a long-acting nitrate preparation or a calcium antagonist), add a third antianginal agent. Selection of the agent will be guided by potential side effects and the presence or absence of concomitant hypertension, relative hypotension, conduction system disease, tachyarrhythmias, or LV dysfunction. As well, shared decision making with the patient ought to guide consideration of escalation of multidrug antianginal therapy versus coronary revascularization.
8. Coronary angiography, with a view to considering coronary revascularization, is indicated in patients with refractory symptoms after titration of medical antianginal therapy. As noted above, referral to coronary angiography in patients without refractory symptoms is reasonable as part of shared decision making.

NONPHARMACOLOGIC TREATMENT APPROACHES. These therapies are generally considered only for patients who have refractory ischemic symptoms after failing medical therapy with multiple agents and coronary revascularization. These methods, which include enhanced external counterpulsation and spinal cord stimulation, are discussed in the online version of this chapter. See also Revascularization Approaches in Stable Ischemic Heart Disease.

Revascularization Approaches in Stable Ischemic Heart Disease (see Chapter 41)

Approach to Decision Making Regarding Revascularization

IHD represents as a dynamic continuum of disease with a variable natural history that may, over decades, encompass many phases of clinical expression ranging from asymptomatic periods, development of chronic exertional angina, subsequent quiescent periods, progression to accelerating angina, and culmination in unstable angina, acute MI, heart failure, or sudden cardiac death. Therefore, the approach to treatment should be tailored to the individual patient's clinical status and symptom burden. Atherosclerosis is typically a diffuse or multifocal process that requires a comprehensive systemic approach to management. Moreover, myocardial ischemia may also occur in the absence of obstructive CAD. In general, the principles guiding patient management are predicated on addressing two simultaneous goals, if possible: (1) use of disease-modifying therapies or approaches to prolong life and reduce major cardiovascular events such as acute MI, hospitalization for ACS, or heart failure and (2) optimization of the patient's health status, quality of life, and functional capacity such that angina or ischemia do not have an adverse impact on activities of daily living.[36]

Revascularization should be considered an important component of an overall management strategy that includes guideline-directed medical therapy (GDMT) and lifestyle management. While lifestyle modification and GDMT should be initiated in all patients with SIHD, revascularization is indicated for the subsets of patients with either particular high-risk features (typically extensive CAD, particularly with LV dysfunction), or limiting angina after optimizing antianginal therapy. Decisions regarding the best mode of revascularization (catheter-based or surgical) should follow a thoughtful assessment of whether and when revascularization is necessary to achieve these goals of therapy. When coronary anatomy is complex or when comorbidity burden is high, decisions should be informed by a multidisciplinary heart team that includes a noninterventional cardiologist, an interventional cardiologist, and a cardiac surgeon.[181] Since most revascularization procedures in SIHD are done to relieve angina and improve quality of life, patients are essential participants in decision making, and shared decision making is critical to ensure optimal use of revascularization in SIHD.[182,183]

Patient Selection for Revascularization
Each of the following considerations may be used to guide decisions regarding the indications for (as well as the approach to) revascularization: (1) the presence and severity of symptoms, (2) physiologic significance of the coronary lesions and other anatomic considerations, (3) results of functional testing, (4) the presence of LV dysfunction, and (5) other medical conditions that influence the risks associated with percutaneous or surgical revascularization and longevity after revascularization.

Presence and Severity of Symptoms
Coronary revascularization (catheter-based or surgical) should be considered if ischemic symptoms persist after intensification of medical therapy and impair functional status or quality of life, or if unacceptable side effects or the patient's therapeutic preferences limit antianginal therapy (see Assessment and Classification of Angina). The impact of angina on quality of life varies substantially between patients based on activity level, pain threshold and other comorbidities that also may impair functional status and quality of life. For example, patients who are physically limited due to lung disease, arthritis, or peripheral artery disease may not achieve improvement in overall functional status with successful revascularization due to other competing comorbidities.

Significance of Coronary Lesions (and Other Anatomic Considerations)
Seventy percent or greater stenosis of an epicardial coronary artery is considered to be anatomically significant (≥50% for left main coronary stenosis). Thus, the professional guidelines that have influenced clinical practice regarding revascularization have historically been framed principally around these anatomic criteria (number of diseased vessels and severity of anatomic disease), together with functional considerations (magnitude and distribution of ischemia and the amount of threatened myocardium).[36] However, data from the large, prospective COURAGE randomized trial of PCI versus medical therapy in patients without left main CAD or LV dysfunction revealed that, contrary to conventional wisdom, no anatomic subset of CAD stenosis severity (including patients with 70% to 90% narrowing and >90% narrowing of the LAD coronary artery) benefitted from PCI versus medical therapy with respect to long-term clinical events.[36] Similar findings have been reported in the ISCHEMIA trial, in which severe ischemia, more extensive CAD, and proximal LAD stenosis did not identify patients with clinical benefit from revascularization.[58,184]

Clinicians also fairly commonly face uncertainty regarding the potential clinical significance of "borderline" visual coronary stenoses, nominally defined as lesions in the 50% to 70% range. It is widely acknowledged that angiographically determined stenosis severity expressed as the percentage of luminal narrowing is often an inaccurate measure of a lesion's functional significance.[65,185] Even though cardiac surgeons have considered 50% or greater stenosis as the criterion for "significant," many factors other than visual stenosis severity (e.g., lesion eccentricity, tortuosity, presence of plaque rupture or asymmetric luminal filling defects, presence of additional serial lesions) can potentially render a 50% to 70% stenosis "functionally or hemodynamically significant." Additional techniques, such as IVUS, OCT, and coronary pressure and flow measurements (see Invasive Assessment and see Chapters 20, 21, and 41), provide enhanced assessment of the anatomic and functional significance of specific coronary lesions.

Other anatomic features, in addition to lesion severity, also influence the likelihood of success and the approach to revascularization for a given patient. Such features include vessel size, extent of calcification, tortuosity, and relationships to side branches. Patients with diffuse severe disease of the distal coronary arteries may be poor candidates for any revascularization procedure.

Fractional Flow Reserve (see Invasive Assessment; see Chapters 20 and 41)
Measurement of FFR is extremely useful for guiding appropriate decisions regarding revascularization of intermediate stenoses.[186,187] In a study of 325 patients with an intermediate stenosis scheduled for PCI, patients with an FFR higher than 0.75 (56%) were randomly assigned to PCI or medical therapy. Patients managed medically had a risk for cardiac death or MI that was less than 1% per year over the first 5 years and was not increased relative to the group that underwent stenting through 15 years of follow-up.[188,189] Subsequently, FFR was evaluated in the FAME (Fractional Flow Reserve versus Angiography for Multivessel Evaluation) trial, in which patients were randomly assigned to conventional PCI guided by visual assessment of the angiogram, or FFR-guided PCI (with PCI performed only in lesions in which the FFR was 0.8 or less). The results showed a lower 2-year rate of death or MI with the FFR-guided strategy. From 2 years to 5 years, the risks with the two strategies were similar. Therefore, at 5 years, outcomes in the two treatment groups were also similar; however, the FFR-guided group had a lower number of stented arteries and less resource use.[190] Nonetheless, the FAME trial did not include a comparison group that received GDMT without revascularization. The FAME 2 trial, which did include a comparison group receiving GDMT without revascularization,[191] is discussed in the section Comparisons between Percutaneous Coronary Intervention and Medical Therapy. The FAME 3 trial is testing use of FFR to guide multivessel PCI and is comparing FFR-guided PCI with contemporary drug-eluting stents to CABG in patients with three-vessel disease.[192]

Presence of Left Ventricular Dysfunction and Extent of Ischemia
The three major determinants of risk in patients with CAD are LV function, the burden of ischemia, and extent of coronary disease. The magnitude of the benefit with revascularization versus medical therapy is enhanced in the setting of LV dysfunction. Moreover, the greatest survival benefits of CABG, as well as symptomatic and functional improvements, are evident in patients with impaired LV function (generally defined as an ejection fraction <0.40). In contrast, while the extent of ischemia on noninvasive testing is associated with risk for subsequent adverse outcomes, randomized trials have not shown that revascularization provides clinical benefit over that of medical therapy beyond the relief of symptoms in those with moderate ischemia.[58]

Risks Associated with the Procedure
Patients with SIHD commonly have other medical conditions, such as renal dysfunction, peripheral atherosclerosis, or pulmonary disease, that may influence the patient's suitability for surgical or percutaneous revascularization. For example, a patient with three-vessel CAD and impaired LV function who might derive a more durable survival benefit from CABG may be too high risk clinically to undergo surgery and might be a better candidate for multivessel PCI.

In addition, some general principles regarding the choice of treatment in patients with SIHD should be considered:

1. For most patients with stable angina, revascularization should not constitute the initial management strategy before evidence-based medical therapy (pharmacologic antianginal therapy, disease-modifying treatments, and therapeutic lifestyle intervention) is initiated and optimized.[36]
2. When improvement in survival is not a relevant consideration, the severity of angina or impairment in health status should guide shared decision making to determine whether revascularization is appropriate to enhance quality of life.
3. In some patients it may be difficult to reliably ascertain whether symptoms such as exertional dyspnea or fatigue are a direct manifestation of underlying IHD, especially in patients with significant obesity, those who are sedentary, or those who may have coexisting chronic obstructive pulmonary disease. In such settings, symptoms that are atypical for obstructive CAD may not necessarily improve with revascularization, even when they coexist with physiologically significant CAD.
4. The decision to proceed with revascularization in a patient with SIHD should entail a thoughtful, transparent discussion of all potential treatment options, with full disclosure of the anticipated benefits and potential risks associated with PCI or CABG relative to GDMT. Since the short-term risks in SIHD are generally low, these discussions can occur over several office visits to allow patients and families time to weigh options and also to facilitate a more complete assessment of symptom burden and response to therapy. Use of a "heart team" is prudent and clinically appropriate in complex patients. Although it is common to undertake ad hoc PCI once the

patient's coronary anatomy is defined in the catheterization laboratory, it is frequently difficult to have the type of discussion that would involve a complete review of the potential risks and benefits of all treatment options by the heart team in this setting.

5. In summary, treatment decisions must be individualized according to the specific clinical features and personal preferences of a given patient (often in collaboration with family members and the patient's referring physician), along with informed discussion about the potential risks and benefits of all three therapeutic options.

Percutaneous Coronary Intervention (see Chapter 41)

PCI, which includes percutaneous transluminal coronary angioplasty (PTCA), intracoronary stenting, and related techniques, continues to evolve. PTCA was almost completely supplanted by bare metal stents (BMSs) in the mid-1990s, followed by the introduction of drug-eluting stents (DESs) in 2003 with subsequent evolutions in stent design to include thinner struts and improved drug-eluting platforms and delivery systems to minimize both restenosis and stent thrombosis. Additional technical and procedural advances allow PCI to be performed successfully by experienced operators in highly complex lesions, including chronic total occlusions (CTO). Moreover, adjunctive pharmacotherapy continues to evolve as stents have become safer and less thrombogenic. Use of radial vascular access allows PCI to be performed with lower risk of vascular complications and bleeding, greater patient comfort, and shortened length of stay, including same day discharge for some low-risk patients. PCI is an important treatment modality in patients with SIHD, particularly in those with chronic angina who remain symptomatic despite optimal GDMT. The technical aspects, early outcomes, and long-term outcomes of PCI are discussed in Chapter 41. This section focuses on comparisons of PCI with medical therapy and when to select PCI as part of a therapeutic strategy.

> Among the desirable features of PCI is the fact that it can be performed during the same clinical encounter as diagnostic angiography. Stable patients can often be discharged on the same or next day. In many instances, relief of symptoms may be immediate and dramatic.
> **Early Outcome.** Continued improvement in the technical aspects of PCI has had a favorable impact on the rate of primary success and the rate of reductions in complications. The ACC National Cardiovascular Data Registry (ACC-NCDR) has reported an angiographic success rate of 96% and a procedural success rate (angiographic success without death, MI, or emergency revascularization) of 93% in patients undergoing PCI. The incidence of death before hospital discharge is less than 1%, and emergency CABG is required in 0.3% of cases. The ACC-NCDR has also reported a periprocedural MI rate of 1%. Finally, with modern generation DES, the rate of restenosis is now <10%. Outcomes in specific challenging subgroups of patients, such as those with CTO, are discussed in Chapter 41. Advances in technology have improved success rates to >80% for PCI of CTO, supporting this approach as a reasonable alternative (class IIa) in patients with appropriate clinical indications and suitable anatomy when performed by experienced operators.[193]
> **Long-Term Outcome**
> *Stenting versus Angioplasty.* Compared with balloon angioplasty, coronary stenting reduces major adverse cardiac events by approximately 40% as a result of reduced repeat revascularization without a detectable decrease in mortality or the rate of MI.

Restenosis and Late Stent Thrombosis (see Chapter 41)

Comparisons between Percutaneous Coronary Intervention and Medical Therapy

Studies comparing balloon angioplasty with medical therapy are of limited clinical relevance in the contemporary era. Randomized trials and meta-analysis comparing PCI versus medical therapy for patients with SIHD provide more relevant data to guide current clinical practice (Fig. 40.11).

Between 1999 and 2004, 2287 patients with objective evidence of ischemia and proximal angiographic CAD (≥70% visual stenosis) were randomized to optimal medical therapy (OMT) with or without PCI in the COURAGE (Clinical Outcomes Utilization Revascularization and Aggressive DruG Evaluation) trial.[1,36] During a median follow-up of 4.6 years, death or MI occurred with similar frequency in both arms (HR for PCI + OMT versus OMT, 1.05; 95% CI, 0.87 to 1.27; $P = 0.62$). Thus, the main study findings indicated that as an initial management strategy in patients with SIHD, PCI did not reduce death, MI, or other major cardiovascular events when added to OMT. Patients initially treated with PCI had less angina at 1 and 3 years, but not at 5 years, than did patients initially treated without initial PCI. As expected, in patients who received OMT without initial PCI, subsequent PCI was performed more frequently than in those initially treated with PCI, although only 16.5% of OMT patients required revascularization during the first year of follow-up whereas the remaining 16.1% of patients crossed over to revascularization between years 1 and 7. Subgroup analyses revealed consistency among clinically relevant special populations: no difference between PCI plus OMT versus OMT in patients with multivessel CAD, low LV ejection fraction, CCS class II or III angina, or diabetes. The primary endpoint (death or MI) was similar in the two treatment groups for the subsets with either no to mild ischemia (18% and 19%, respectively, $P = 0.92$) or moderate to severe ischemia (19% and 22%, respectively, $P = 0.53$, interaction P value = 0.65). Moreover, there was no gradient increase in events for the overall cohort based on the extent of ischemia.

The subsequent ISCHEMIA (International Study of Comparative Health Effectiveness with Medical and Invasive Approaches) trial compared initial invasive with conservative management among 5179 patients with stable CAD and at least moderate ischemia on stress testing with imaging (or severe ischemia on stress testing without imaging).[58] Patients were enrolled before coronary angiography, a feature that enhances generalizability compared with studies like COURAGE. Before randomization, patients without contraindications underwent blinded CCTA to exclude patients with >50% left main stenosis and those without obstructive CAD. An important strength of the trial was close protocol adherence and a relatively low rate of crossover between arms: In the invasive arm, coronary angiography was performed in 96% and revascularization in 79% versus only 26% undergoing angiography and 21% revascularization during follow-up in the conservative arm. Of the revascularizations performed, approximately 25% were CABG and 75% PCI.

The primary composite outcome of CV death, MI, resuscitated cardiac arrest, hospitalization for unstable angina or heart failure at 5 years was not significantly different between the invasive (16.4%) and conservative (18.2%) arms (absolute difference −1.8%; 95% CI, −4.7% to 1.0%). There was also no difference in the key secondary outcome of CV death or nonfatal MI (14.2% versus 16.5%; absolute difference, −2.3%; 95% CI, −5.0% to 0.4%). All-cause mortality was similar between groups (HR, 1.05; 95% CI, 0.83 to 1.32), but the interpretation of MI was more complex. Higher rates of procedural MI were seen early in the invasive arm. In contrast lower rates of spontaneous MI emerged over time in the invasive arm, with the balance leading to no significant difference total MI at 5 years (10.3% versus 11.9%; absolute difference −1.6; 95% CI, −3.9% to 0.7%).

The effect on anginal symptoms was assessed using the SAQ. SAQ summary scores were modestly improved in the invasive arm relative to the conservative arm, with greater benefit on angina-related quality of life among those with worse angina at baseline.[6]

A recent meta-analysis comparing routine revascularization with medical therapy in SIHD, combined 14 RCTs (including ISCHEMIA and ISCHEMIA CKD) with 14,877 patients and a weighted mean of 4.5 years of follow-up (see Fig. 40.11). Compared with medical therapy, revascularization was associated with similar rates of death (RR = 0.99, 95% CI, 0.90 to 1.09), lower nonprocedural MI (RR = 0.76; 95% CI, 0.67 to 0.85) but higher procedural MI (RR = 2.48; 95% CI, 1.86 to 3.31) resulting in no difference in overall MI (RR = 0.93; 95% CI, 0.83 to 1.03). Unstable angina was reduced (RR = 0.64; 95% CI, 0.45 to 0.92); freedom from angina increased (RR = 1.10; 95% CI, 1.05 to 1.15) with revascularization.[184]

An important issue with the interpretation of improved angina from these RCTs is that the PCI was not blinded.[194] The ORBITA trial was a small, short-term, randomized, blinded and sham placebo-controlled

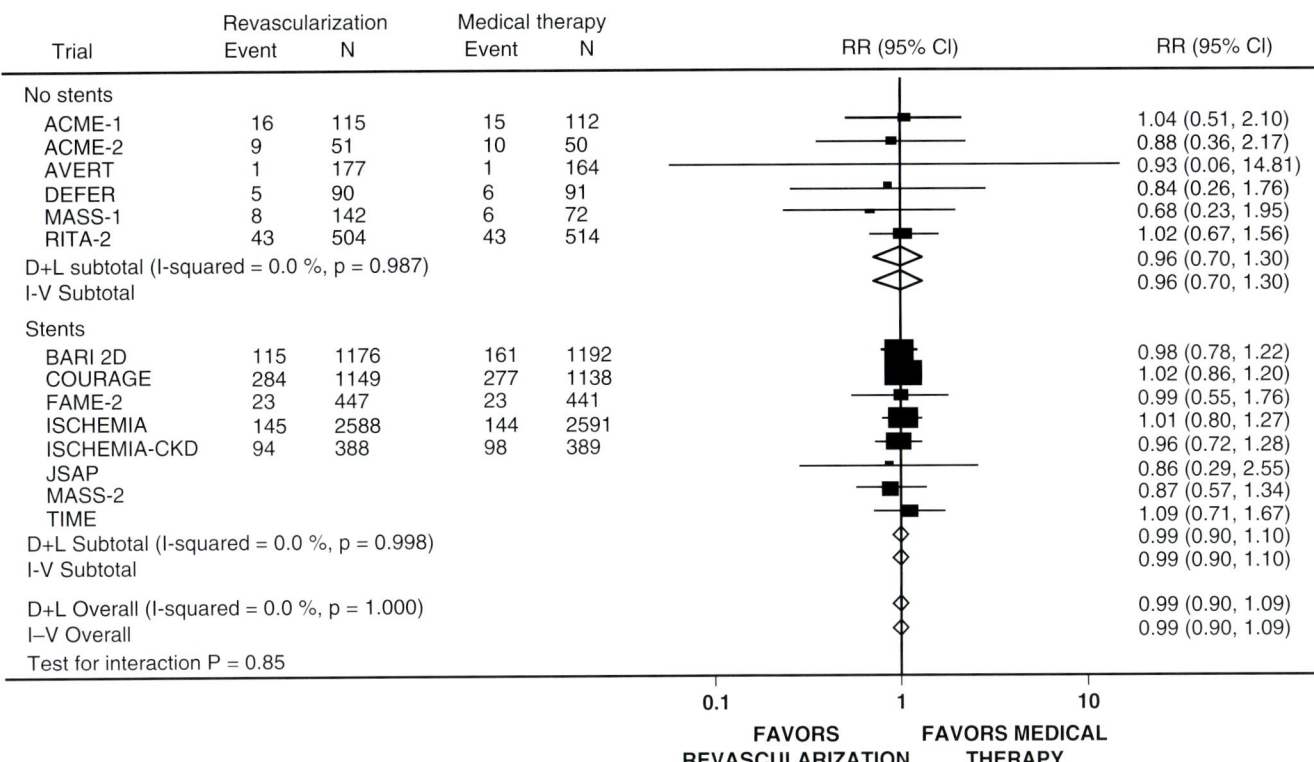

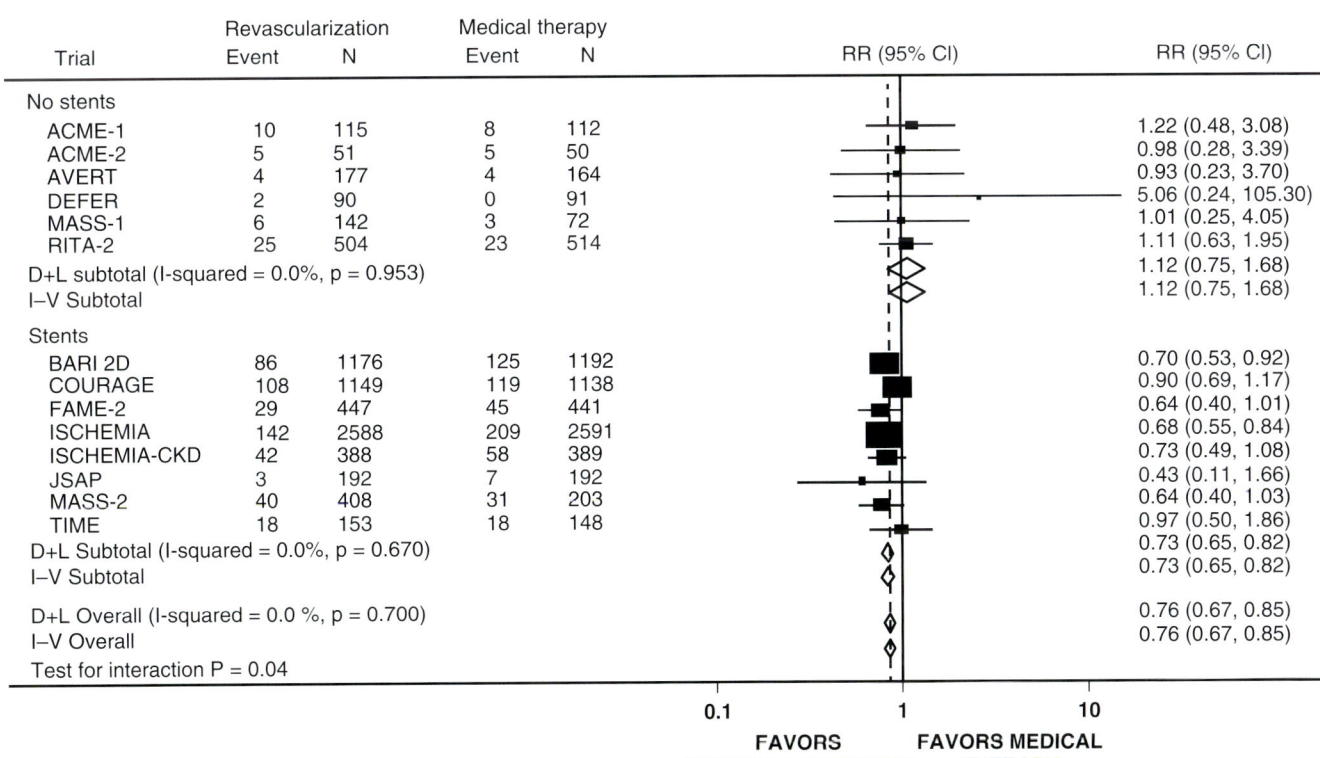

FIGURE 40.11 Meta-analysis of routine revascularization versus an initial conservative strategy within 14 trials that enrolled 14,877 patients followed for a weighted mean of 4.5 years. There was no evidence of benefit of routine revascularization compared with an initial conservative strategy for prevention of death. A favorable effect of revascularization on nonprocedural myocardial infarction was counterbalanced by an increase in procedural myocardial infarction. Routine revascularization resulted in an increase in freedom from angina. *D+L*, DerSimonian and Laird methodology; *I-V*, inverse-variance. (Adapted from Bangalore S, et al. Routine revascularization versus initial medical therapy for stable ischemic heart disease. Circulation 2020;142:850-851.)

Procedural MI

Trial	Revascularization Event	N	Medical therapy Event	N	RR (95% CI)
No stents					
ACME-1	4	115	0	112	8.77 (0.47, 162.80)
ACME-2	1	51	1	50	0.98 (0.06, 15.67)
AVERT	1	177	0	164	2.78 (0.11, 68.23)
DEFER	3	90	0	91	7.08 (0.37, 137.02)
MASS-1	2	142	0	72	2.54 (0.12, 52.81)
RITA-2	7	504	0	514	15.30 (0.87, 267.84)
D+L subtotal (I-squared = 0.0%, p = 0.796)					4.32 (1.29, 14.40)
I–V Subtotal					4.32 (1.29, 14.40)
Stents					
BARI 2D	32	1176	13	1192	2.50 (1.31, 4.75)
COURAGE	35	1149	9	1138	3.85 (1.85, 8.01)
FAME-2	7	447	9	441	0.77 (0.29, 2.06)
ISCHEMIA	70	2588	25	2591	2.80 (1.78, 4.43)
ISCHEMIA-CKD	7	388	4	389	1.75 (0.51, 5.99)
JSAP	0	192	0	192	1.00 (0.02, 50.40)
MASS-2	4	408	0	203	4.48 (0.24, 83.17)
TIME	3	153	3	148	0.97 (0.20, 4.79)
D+L Subtotal (I-squared = 22.5%, p = 0.250)					2.26 (1.55, 3.31)
I–V Subtotal					2.40 (1.78, 3.23)
D+L Overall (I-squared = 0.0%, p = 0.506)					2.48 (1.86, 3.31)
I–V Overall					2.48 (1.86, 3.31)
Test for interaction P = 0.35					

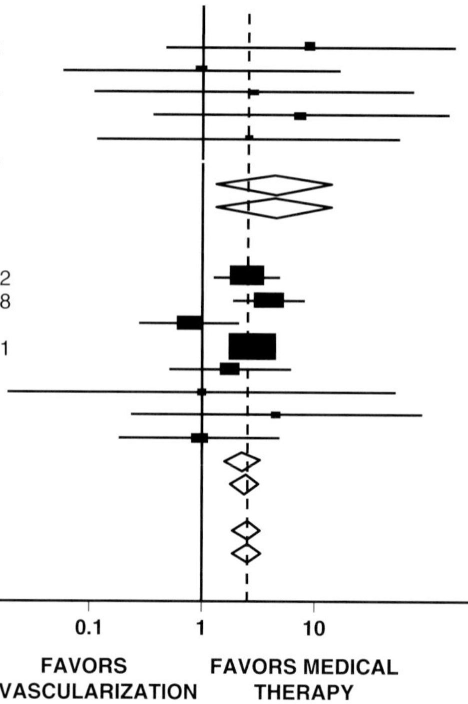

0.1 — 1 — 10
FAVORS REVASCULARIZATION | FAVORS MEDICAL THERAPY

Freedom from angina

Trial	Revascularization Event	N	Medical therapy Event	N	RR (95% CI)
No stents					
ACME-1	53	115	42	112	1.23 (0.82, 1.84)
ACME-2	27	51	18	50	1.47 (0.81, 2.67)
AVERT	95	177	67	164	1.31 (0.96, 1.80)
DEFER	51	90	61	91	0.85 (0.58, 1.23)
MASS-1	92	142	17	72	2.74 (1.64, 4.60)
RITA-2	252	504	231	514	1.11 (0.93, 1.33)
D+L subtotal (I-squared = 66.0%, p = 0.012)					1.29 (1.00, 1.66)
I–V Subtotal					1.20 (1.05, 1.36)
Stents					
BARI 2D	800	1176	715	1192	1.13 (1.03, 1.25)
COURAGE	316	1149	296	1138	1.06 (0.90, 1.24)
FAME-2	326	447	308	441	1.04 (0.89, 1.22)
ISCHEMIA	1707	2588	1588	2591	1.08 (1.01, 1.15)
ISCHEMIA-CKD	249	388	254	389	0.98 (0.83, 1.17)
MASS-2	245	408	92	203	1.32 (1.04, 1.68)
D+L Subtotal (I-squared = 0.6%, p = 0.412)					1.09 (1.03, 1.14)
I–V Subtotal					1.09 (1.04, 1.14)
D+L Overall (I-squared = 49.3%, p = 0.027)					1.12 (1.04, 1.21)
I–V Overall					1.10 (1.05, 1.15)
Test for interaction P = 0.20					

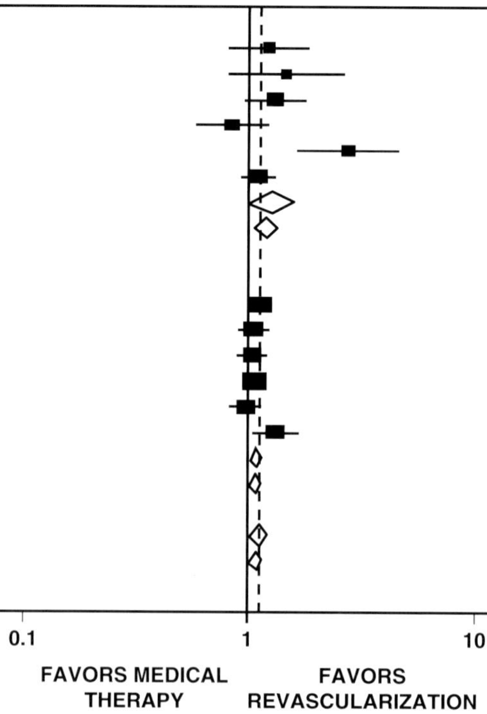

0.1 — 1 — 10
FAVORS MEDICAL THERAPY | FAVORS REVASCULARIZATION

FIGURE 40.11—cont'd

trial of PCI for stable angina.[195] No difference was seen in ORBITA with PCI versus sham placebo on change in exercise time (the primary endpoint), or SAQ and CCS angina scales (secondary endpoints). In contrast, secondary analyses showed PCI led to greater freedom from angina and lower angina frequency among patients with greater baseline ischemia.[196] ORBITA should remind clinicians about an important placebo effect from PCI in some patients, but still supports benefits of PCI on angina relief among individuals with high burden of symptoms or ischemia.

PCI Guided by Coronary Artery Hemodynamic Data
An FFR-guided PCI strategy plus medical therapy was compared with medical therapy alone in the FAME 2 trial.[191] In this trial, patients with an FFR of 0.8 or less in one or more visually stenotic coronary arteries (≥50% stenosis) were randomly assigned to medical therapy alone or PCI plus medical therapy. The trial was terminated prematurely after enrollment of 888 patients (about half of the planned enrollment) because of a highly significant reduction in the composite primary endpoint of death, MI, or urgent revascularization (HR, 0.32; 95% CI, 0.19 to 0.53; $P < 0.001$). Notably, the difference in this open label trial was driven solely by a lower rate of urgent revascularization in the PCI group than in the medical therapy group (1.6% versus 11.1%; HR, 0.13; 95% CI, 0.06 to 0.30; $P < 0.001$), with no significant difference in death or MI (Fig. 40.12).[189] These findings are broadly consistent the larger and longer-duration COURAGE and ISCHEMIA studies showing that in patients with SIHD, PCI reduces ischemic symptoms and the need for future revascularization, but not death or MI. Although FAME 2 did not test use of FFR versus no FFR, the findings lend indirect support to current guidelines for the selective use of FFR to guide PCI decision making for borderline visual lesions (≈50% to 70% stenosis).

Several subsequent trials compared PCI guided by iFR, an alternative measure for hemodynamic assessment of coronary lesions that does not require vasodilator administration, with PCI guided by FFR. In the DEFINE-FLAIR (n = 2492) and iFR-SWEDEHEART (n = 2037) trials, rates of MACE were noninferior (and similar) with the iFR-guided approach (iFR ≤0.89), and side effects were lower with iFR, given the absence of adenosine.[73,74] In both trials, fewer lesions were deemed significant with iFR than FFR, leading to fewer PCIs performed. Procedure time was also shorter with iFR.

Selection of Percutaneous Coronary Intervention for Revascularization
At present, based on the best available data from randomized trials, it appears reasonable to pursue a strategy of initial medical therapy for most patients with SIHD and to reserve revascularization for those with persistent lifestyle limiting symptoms despite OMT and those with LV dysfunction. Whether to refer patients with very high-risk criteria on noninvasive testing, such as inducible ischemia involving a large territory of myocardium[36] or severe ischemia at low workload, is controversial in light of null findings described above from the COURAGE and ISCHEMIA trials. However, observational studies have consistently identified such individuals at high risk when treated without revascularization, and the proportions of these very high-risk patients enrolled in the revascularization trials is small. Patients with significant left main CAD have also been excluded from the relevant contemporary randomized trials of revascularization plus medical therapy versus medical therapy alone and should be referred for coronary revascularization.

In addition to general considerations regarding the indications and approach to revascularization (see Approach to Decision Making Regarding Revascularization), additional factors that need to be weighed in selecting PCI as an option for therapy include the following:
1. The likelihood of successful catheter-based revascularization based on the angiographic characteristics of the lesion
2. The ability to achieve complete revascularization based on the extent of CAD and the volume of myocardium and the severity of ischemia in the distribution of the artery or arteries amenable to PCI
3. Although advances in technology have significantly reduced the rates of both acute failure of PCI and target lesion restenosis, consideration of these risks and their potential consequences remain relevant to decision making regarding PCI. The diffuseness and anatomic complexity of CAD, including specific angiographic factors such as small vessel diameter, long lesion length, total occlusion, and saphenous vein graft disease, may be relevant to the potential risks and benefit of PCI (see Chapter 41).

PERCUTANEOUS CORONARY INTERVENTION IN SPECIFIC SUBGROUPS OF PATIENTS WITH STABLE ISCHEMIC HEART DISEASE

Diabetes Mellitus
Patients with diabetes are at substantially higher risk for complications after PCI (see Chapter 31). Possible explanations for the higher rate of adverse outcomes include a greater burden of coronary atherosclerosis, an altered vascular biologic response to balloon and/or stent injury, rapid progression of disease in nonrevascularized segments, and higher platelet reactivity. The diabetic atherosclerotic milieu is characterized by a procoagulant state, decreased fibrinolytic activity, increased proliferation, and inflammation. Restenosis is more frequent in patients with diabetes, as is disease progression. For this reason, CABG, which bypasses most of the vessel instead of a specific lesion, may offer a better intermediate- to long-term outcome. The optimal strategy for revascularization in patients with diabetes is discussed later in this chapter. A strategy of initial OMT appears to be reasonable for most patients with diabetes and SIHD.[109]

Left Ventricular Dysfunction
Despite advances in interventional cardiology, LV dysfunction remains independently associated with higher in-hospital and long-term mortality after PCI. Specifically, in patients with stable CAD and estimated ejection fractions of 40% or less, 41% to 49%, and 50% or higher in the NHLBI Dynamic Registry, mortality at 1 year after PCI was 11.0%, 4.5%, and 1.9%, respectively. Contemporary trials of PCI versus medical therapy have included too few patients with impaired LV function to guide therapeutic decision making in this important subset of patients. Observational studies have not revealed any benefit of PCI in addition to medical therapy.[197]

Women and Older Patients
Specific issues related to PCI in women and older adults are discussed in Chapters 90 and 91. Observational studies have shown higher rates of complications, particularly bleeding, among women compared with men undergoing invasive management. A post hoc study from the COURAGE trial showed that the 40% of the patients who were 65 years or older had a twofold higher rate of death or MI than did younger patients, although no age-related differences in clinical outcomes were noted in patients randomly assigned to PCI or GDMT. Of note, despite the potential increased risk for complications in older patients undergoing PCI, no such increased rate of comorbid conditions (e.g., local vascular complications, worsening renal function, bleeding) was noted.[198]

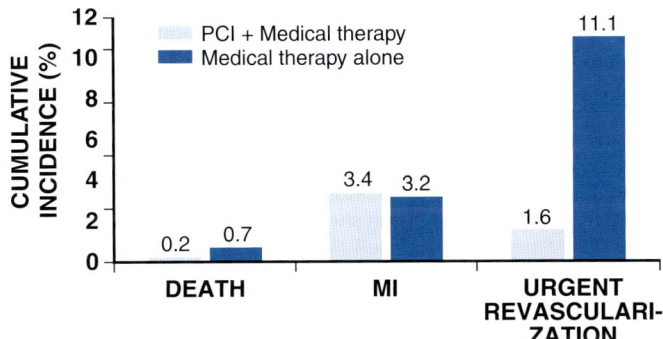

FIGURE 40.12 Outcome of death, MI, or urgent revascularization in 888 patients with stable CAD for whom PCI was being considered. The patients underwent assessment of all stenoses by fractional flow reserve (FFR) and were randomly assigned to FFR-guided PCI plus best available medical therapy or the best available medical therapy alone. Enrollment was halted prematurely because of a significant reduction in the primary endpoint in patients treated with an FFR-guided revascularization strategy: 4.3% in the PCI group and 12.7% in the medical therapy group (HR with PCI, 0.32; 95% CI, 0.19 to 0.53; $P < 0.001$). However, this effect on the primary endpoint was driven entirely by a reduction in unplanned revascularization rather than by death or MI. (Modified from De Bruyne B, et al. Fractional flow reserve–guided PCI versus medical therapy in stable coronary disease. N Engl J Med 2012;367:998.)

Renal Dysfunction

Patients with impaired renal function (generally those with an eGFR <60 mL/min), particularly those with diabetes, are at increased risk for worsening azotemia, and this is often an important consideration in the physician's decision of whether to proceed with coronary angiography and PCI in such patients.

The ISCHEMIA-CKD trial is the largest trial of coronary revascularization performed in patients with CKD.[199] This trial, performed concurrently with the ISCHEMIA trial, randomized 777 patients with advanced CKD (eGFR < 30 mL/min/1.73 m²) and moderate to severe ischemia on stress testing to initial revascularization or initial medical therapy. The design was similar to ISCHEMIA except screening CTA was not performed routinely due to the risks of contrast nephropathy. Catheterization and revascularization were performed in 85% and 50% of patients in the invasive therapy group versus 32% and 20% in the conservative arm. Multivessel CAD was present in 51% and nonobstructive CAD in 26% in the invasive arm. Among those undergoing revascularization, PCI was performed in 85% and CABG in 15%. The primary outcome of death or MI at 3 years did not differ between the treatment arms (36.4% versus 36.7%; adjusted HR, 1.01; 95% CI, 0.79 to 1.29). However, the stroke rate was higher (HR 3.76; 95% CI, 1.52 to 9.32) as was the composite of death or new dialysis initiation (HR 1.48; 95% CI, 1.04 to 2.11) with invasive therapy. Additionally, unlike the ISCHEMIA trial, improvement in SAQ and other quality of life metrics was not seen with invasive therapy in ISCHEMIA-CKD.[200] These data highlight continued poor contemporary outcomes for patients with SIHD and advanced CKD and support a limited role of coronary revascularization in this population. In patients with severe CKD, coronary revascularization may be best reserved for patients with ACS or refractory symptoms and perhaps in those with LV dysfunction.

Coronary Artery Bypass Grafting

In 1964, Garrett, Dennis, and DeBakey first used CABG as a "bailout" procedure. Use of an internal mammary artery (IMA) graft was pioneered by Kolessov in 1967 and by Green and colleagues in 1970. CABG has evolved progressively since then and today remains an important treatment modality for many patients with SIHD. Most bypass operations continue to be performed through a median sternotomy with the use of cardiopulmonary bypass (CPB) and cardioplegic cardiac arrest, with a smaller number performed without bypass on a beating heart. Less invasive approaches have been developed for selected patients who may be appropriate candidates for more limited coronary revascularization, including anterior and lateral thoracotomies, partial sternotomies, and epigastric incisions.[201] The technical goal of bypass surgery is to achieve, whenever possible, complete revascularization by grafting all coronary arteries of sufficient caliber that have physiologically significant proximal stenoses. CABG has been documented to prolong survival, relieve angina, and improve quality of life in specific subgroups of patients with CAD.[202]

The annual number of CABG operations in the United States rose steadily over the first three decades, with a peak in the late 1990s. Since then, rates of CABG have steadily declined, related to growth of the use of PCI, particularly in patients with multivessel CAD.[203] CABG provides excellent short- and intermediate-term results in the management of SIHD; its long-term results are affected by failure of venous grafts. Long-term data with totally arterial surgical revascularization (i.e., using bilateral IMA grafts) are few.[204]

Minimally Invasive Coronary Artery Bypass Surgery

Less invasive or minimally invasive approaches may be divided into four major categories based on the approach and use of CPB.[201,202] Port-access CABG is performed through limited incisions with femoral-femoral CPB and cardioplegic arrest. Port-access technology has also now enabled totally endoscopic robotically assisted CABG (TECAB) surgery performed on the arrested heart. Off-pump CABG (OPCAB) is performed by using a standard median sternotomy, with generally small skin incisions, and stabilization devices to reduce motion of the target vessels while anastomoses are performed without CPB.[205-207] Finally, minimally invasive direct coronary artery bypass (MIDCAB) is performed through a left anterior thoracotomy without CPB. Thus off-pump approaches to CABG include both OPCAB and MIDCAB techniques.

Potential advantages of the minimally invasive approaches include reduced postoperative patient discomfort, minimized risk for wound infection, and shorter recovery times. However, the findings from three major trials of off-pump versus on-pump CABG have produced similar findings with more incomplete revascularization and a higher need for repeat revascularization with the off-pump technique.[206] In the ROOBY (Randomized On/Off Bypass) trial of OPCAB versus CABG in 2203 patients, in particular, there was also worse graft patency, and a higher incidence of death, MI, or repeat revascularization at 1 year among patients who underwent off-pump CABG (9.9% versus 7.4%, respectively, $P = 0.04$). Five-year results of two of these trials are now available with discordant results. In the ROOBY follow-up study, the 5-year rate of death was higher in the OPCAB versus CABG group (15.2% versus 11.9%; $P = 0.02$).[207] In contrast, in 5-year results from the CORONARY (CABG Off or On Pump Revascularization Study) trial in 4752 patients randomly assigned to OPCAB versus traditional CABG, there was no significant difference in the rates of death, stroke, MI, renal failure, or repeat revascularization.[208] It is possible that the experience of the surgeons played a role in the discrepant results of these trials.[209] Nevertheless, a concern remains that poorer graft patency and incomplete revascularization may contribute to a hazard associated with OPCAB.[210,211] However, with appropriate patient selection, OPCAB continues to play a role in some centers.[206,212]

Novel approaches to coronary revascularization combine a minimally invasive surgical CABG procedure on the LAD coronary artery (i.e., a left IMA implant to the proximal LAD coronary artery using OPCAB) with PCI on the remaining vessels. Additional experience with these so-called hybrid revascularization procedures is needed to further clarify appropriate selection criteria and to determine whether this strategy offers important advantages over multivessel CABG alone. Despite initial enthusiasm for TECAB, robotic-assisted CABG remains less than 1% of total CABG volume.[213]

Arterial and Venous Conduits

The current standard for bypass grafting advocates routine use of an IMA for grafting the LAD coronary artery and supplemental saphenous vein grafts to other vessels.[214,215] Although the benefits of a single IMA graft over a saphenous vein graft alone are not in dispute, the superiority of bilateral IMA grafts over a single IMA graft is less well accepted.[215] Initial enthusiasm for the use of bilateral IMA grafts was tempered by a higher rate of postoperative complications, including bleeding, wound infection, and prolonged ventilatory support. Wound infection, most notably deep sternal wound infection, has been of particular concern but remains modest in frequency (<3%), except in patients who are obese or have diabetes or those who require prolonged ventilatory support. In a randomized trial of 3102 patients undergoing CABG, the use of bilateral IMA grafts conferred similar cardiovascular outcomes at 30 days, 1 year, 5 years, and 10 years as the use of a single IMA graft, but higher rates of sternal complications.[216] The interpretation of the ARTS trial is limited by several features of the trial, including greater use of radial conduits in the single IMA group and high rates of crossover from bilateral IMA to LIMA only.[215] In an as-treated analysis that assigned ARTS patients based on which grafts they actually received, the composite of death, MI, and stroke (adjusted HR 0.80; 95% CI, 0.69 to 0.93) and mortality (adjusted HR 0.81; 95% CI, 0.68 to 0.95) were lower among those who received multiple vs a single arterial graft.[216] These results are supported by a large propensity matched analysis from >50,000 patients undergoing CABG in Canada with ≥8 years of follow-up demonstrated an association of multi-arterial grafting (either bilateral IMA or LIMA + radial) with lower MACE (adjusted HR 0.82; 95% CI, 0.77 to 0.88) and mortality (adjusted HR 0.80; 95% CI, 0.73 to 0.88). No difference was seen between those receiving three versus two arterial grafts.[217] Current professional society guidelines recommend use of bilateral IMA grafts as reasonable (class IIa) in younger patients in the absence of excessive risk of sternal complications.[182,214] Nevertheless, given the increased technical demands and longer operative times of bilateral IMA grafting, it has not been adopted widely.

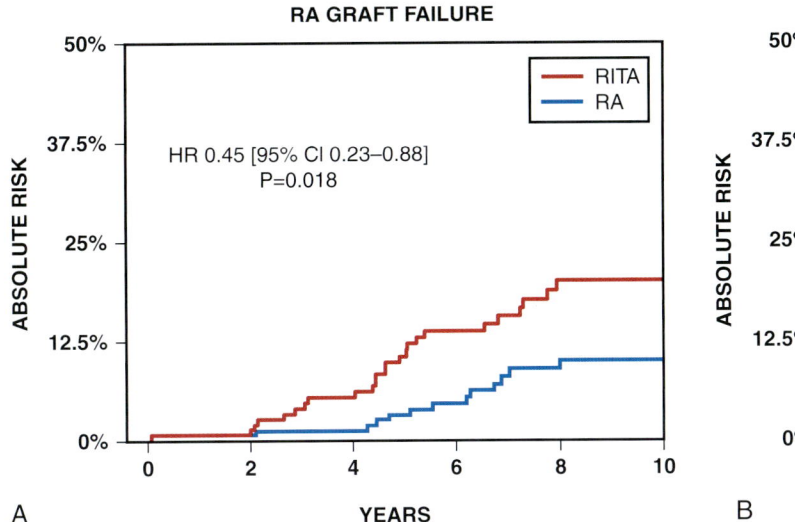
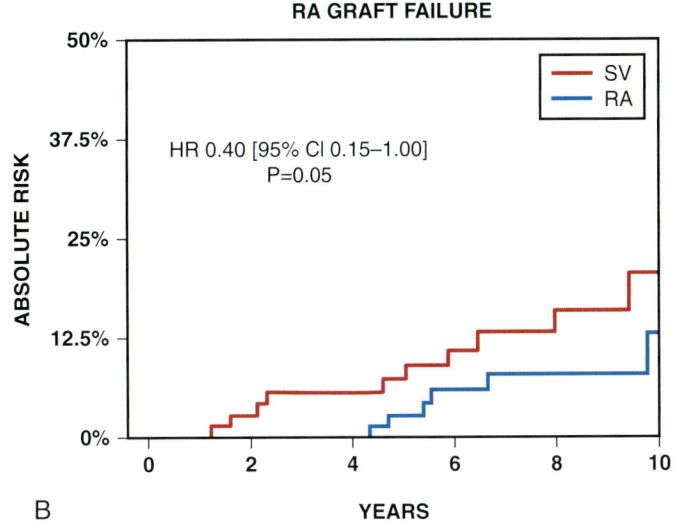

FIGURE 40.13 Rates of graft failure at 10 years in the Radial Artery Patency and Clinical Outcomes-Right Internal Thoracic Artery (RAPCO-RITA) and RAPCO-Saphenous Vein (RAPCO-SV) trials. In both trials, patients undergoing coronary artery bypass graft (CABG) surgery received a left internal thoracic artery graft and were randomized to a second graft. **A,** RAPCO-RITA randomized 394 patients to either a RITA or radial artery (RA) conduit. **B,** RAPCO-SVG randomized 225 patients to either RA or SV conduits. Ten-year graft failure was significantly lower for the radial artery conduit in both trials. (Adapted from Buxton BF, et al. Long-term results of the RAPCO trials. Circulation 2020;142:1330-1338.)

The radial artery conduit may be emerging as the preferred second arterial conduit after the IMA. In a patient-level analysis of six randomized trials, patients treated with radial-artery grafts compared with saphenous vein grafts had a significantly lower rate of the composite of death, MI, or repeat revascularization at five years (HR 0.67; 95% CI, 0.49 to 0.90), as well as a higher rate of great patency.[218] At 10 years' follow-up in the Radial Artery Patency and Clinical Outcomes -Right Internal Thoracic Artery (RAPCO-RITA) trial ($n = 394$) patency was higher with the radial artery than the right internal thoracic artery (89% versus 80%; HR for graft failure 0.45; 95% CI, 0.23 to 0.88; $n = 394$), as was survival (91% versus 84%; HR 0.53; 95% CI, 0.30 to 0.95) (Fig. 40.13). A potential limitation of this trial was the use of a free rather than in situ RITA graft. However, prior studies have showed that patency of free RITA is similar to in situ RITA. In the parallel RAPCO-Saphenous Vein Graft (SVG) trial ($n = 225$), 10-year patency was 85% for the radial artery versus 71% for the SV (HR for graft failure 0.40; 95% CI, 0.15 to 1.00) and survival was 73% for the radial artery versus 65% for the SV (HR 0.76; 95% CI, 0.47 to 1.22) (see Fig. 40.13). The lower patency and survival in RAPCO-SVG versus RAPCO-RITA reflects different entry criteria: RAPCO-RITA was restricted to patients <70 (<60 if diabetic).[204] However, uncertainty in the selection of optimal arterial conduits is reflected in the variability in the strength of existing recommendation from professional societies ranging from class IIb to class I,[182] with a class IIa recommendation in the 2015 guidelines from the Society of Thoracic Surgeons that does not yet reflect consideration of more recent trials.[214]

PATENCY OF VENOUS AND ARTERIAL GRAFTS. Early occlusion (before hospital discharge) occurs in 8% to 12% of venous grafts, and by 1 year, 15% to 30% of vein grafts have become occluded. After the first year the annual occlusion rate is 2% and rises to approximately 4% annually between years 6 and 10. Patency rates with arterial grafts are vastly superior.[219] The individual patient meta-analysis described above reported clear advantages of the radial artery over saphenous vein conduit for patency at 5 years. (HR for graft failure 0.67; 95% CI, 0.49 to 0.90).[218] Arterial grafts are more susceptible to failure due to competitive flow from native blood vessels than SVGs; thus, arterial grafts should not be used to revascularize borderline stenoses without clear evidence of flow limitation.

DISTAL VASCULATURE. The state of the distal coronary vasculature is important for the fate of bypass grafts. Late patency of grafts is related to coronary arterial runoff as determined by the diameter of the coronary artery into which the graft is inserted, the size of the distal vascular bed, and the severity of coronary atherosclerosis distal to the site of insertion of the graft. The highest graft patency rates are found when the lumina of vessels distal to the graft insertion are larger than 1.5 mm in diameter, perfuse a large vascular bed, and are free of atheroma obstructing more than 25% of the vessel lumen. For saphenous veins, optimal patency rates are achieved with a lumen of 2.0 mm or larger.

Progression of Disease in Native Arteries

The rate of disease progression appears to be highest in arterial segments already showing evidence of disease, and it is between three and six times higher in grafted native coronary arteries than in nongrafted native vessels. These data have suggested that bypassing an artery with minimal disease, even if initially successful, may ultimately be harmful to patients, who incur both a risk for graft closure and an increased risk for accelerated obstruction of native vessels. Lesions in the native vessel that are long (>10 mm) and greater than 70% in diameter are at increased risk for progressing to total occlusion.

EFFECTS OF THERAPY ON VEIN GRAFT OCCLUSION AND NATIVE VESSEL PROGRESSION. Measures aimed at enhancing long-term patency are generally directed at delaying the overall process of atherosclerosis, and thus they may have several additional benefits. Secondary preventive therapy, in particular aspirin and lipid-lowering treatment, is important in reducing the risk for failure of venous grafts. Chronic anticoagulant therapy has not been convincingly shown to alter outcomes.

Antiplatelet Therapy

Several trials have demonstrated the efficacy of aspirin therapy for maintaining early graft patency when started within 24 hours preoperatively, but the benefit is lost when aspirin is started more than 48 hours postoperatively. Aspirin, 75 to 325 mg daily, should be continued indefinitely for long-term secondary prevention. Although the addition of clopidogrel to aspirin is indicated after CABG for patients with ACS, results for P2Y12 inhibitors after CABG in SIHD are mixed. In a trial of 500 patients undergoing elective CABG in China and randomized 1:1:1 to ticagrelor plus aspirin, ticagrelor alone, and aspirin alone, 1-year patency rates (by CTA or coronary angiography) were 88.7%, 82.8%, and 76.5%, respectively, with differences between ticagrelor + aspirin versus aspirin alone statistically significant (absolute difference 12.2%; $p < 0.001$).[220] In contrast, in a placebo-controlled trial of 499 patients undergoing CABG, randomization to ticagrelor + aspirin versus aspirin alone found no benefit of ticagrelor on graft patency at 1 year, with 10.5% of grafts occluded in the ticagrelor arm and 9.1% in the placebo arm (odds ratio [OR] 1.29; 95% CI, 0.73 to 2.30).[221] In aggregate, these data do not provide compelling support for routine use of dual antiplatelet therapy after CABG in patients with SIHD (without ACS). Clopidogrel monotherapy should be used for patients who have an allergy or are intolerant to aspirin.

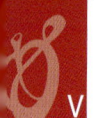

Lipid-Lowering Therapy

Three randomized trials of lipid-lowering therapy have shown a favorable impact on the development of graft disease. High-intensity statin therapy is indicated for post-CABG patients, as clinical trials comparing intensive with moderate statin doses confirm similar relative benefit in subgroups with prior CABG.

Patient Selection

Indications for CABG are centered on evidence demonstrating improvement in the quality and/or duration of life.[182,222] The decision to perform revascularization with PCI or CABG is determined largely from the coronary anatomy, LV function, other medical comorbid conditions that may affect the patient's risk associated with either revascularization procedure and patient preference (see Approach to Decision Making Regarding Revascularization and Choosing between Percutaneous Coronary Intervention, Coronary Artery Bypass Surgery, and Medical Therapy). CABG is indicated, regardless of symptoms, for patients with CAD in whom survival is likely to be prolonged. Patients with more extensive and severe CAD have an increasing magnitude of benefit from CABG over medical therapy. Patients with left main and/or three-vessel CAD and, in particular those with multivessel CAD and LV systolic dysfunction, should be considered candidates for CABG to prolong life, whereas similar data support the benefits of CABG in diabetic patients with multivessel CAD if revascularization is needed. Other factors that must always be considered in the decision are general health and noncoronary-related comorbid conditions that influence both the risks associated with surgery and the likelihood of durable functional benefit.

Surgical Outcomes and Long-Term Results

The patient population undergoing CABG has been changing over time, particularly with the wider use of PCI. When compared with the 1970s, patients undergoing CABG today are older, include a higher percentage of women, and are sicker in that a greater proportion have unstable angina, three-vessel CAD, previous coronary revascularization with either CABG or PCI, LV dysfunction, and comorbid conditions, including hypertension, diabetes, and peripheral vascular disease. Despite the increasing risk profile of this population, outcomes with CABG have generally remained stable or have improved.

Operative Mortality

Robust multivariable models have been developed and refined with the objective of predicting perioperative mortality. In particular, the Society of Thoracic Surgeons (STS) risk estimator (riskcalc.sts.org) and the European System for Cardiac Operative Risk Evaluation (EuroSCORE, www.euroscore.org) are well validated risk estimation tools that are available with convenient online calculators. Risk indicators for death following CABG that are shared across the available risk tools include (1) preoperative cardiovascular factors including the number of coronary vessels diseases, the presence of left main CAD, recent acute MI or ACS event, prior CABG, hemodynamic instability, LV dysfunction, concomitant valvular heart disease, pulmonary hypertension with or without right heart failure, and associated carotid or peripheral vascular disease; (2) preoperative noncardiac comorbid conditions and demographic factors such as older age at surgery, female sex, diabetes mellitus, and pulmonary and renal disease as well as overall frailty; (3) intraoperative factors such as intraoperative ischemic damage and failure to use IMA grafts.

The cumulative mortality in approximately 1.5 million isolated CABG operations recorded in the STS database declined from 3.05% between 1997 and 1999 to approximately 2% in 2008 and has remained at approximately that rate through 2017, with an upward trend from 2015 to 2017.[223] Moreover, CABG-related mortality has declined substantially over the past two decades when adjusted for changes in clinical risk profile.

Perioperative Complications

The perioperative complications of CABG that include but are not limited to MI, stroke, atrial fibrillation, and renal failure.

Relief of Angina

All the major randomized trials have demonstrated greater relief of angina, better exercise performance, and a lower requirement for antianginal medications at 5 years in surgically treated than in medically treated patients. Independent predictors of recurrence of angina include female sex, obesity, and lack of use of the IMA as a conduit. In patients with three-vessel CAD undergoing CABG, the completeness of revascularization is a significant determinant of the relief of symptoms at 1 year and over a 5-year period. After 5 years, approximately 75% of surgically treated patients can be predicted to be free of an ischemic event, sudden death, occurrence of MI, or recurrence of angina; approximately 50% remain free for approximately 10 years and around 15% for 15 or more years.

Effects on Survival

Clinical practice has been shaped by three major randomized trials of CABG versus medical therapy in which patients were enrolled between 1972 and 1984: the Veterans Affairs (VA) trial, the European Cardiac Society Study (ECSS), and the National Heart, Lung, and Blood Institute (NHLBI)-supported CASS (see eFig. 40.6).[182,202,222] The evidence base consists of data from 2649 patients participating in these and several smaller trials and has important limitations with respect to application to current practice because the risk profile of patients referred for surgery, as well as the available surgical and medical interventions, have evolved substantially since these trials were conducted. In particular, these trials antedated the widespread use of IMAs and the disease-modifying therapies that currently comprise GDMT.

Nevertheless, major points guiding clinical practice have been drawn from a meta-analysis of these trials. In each of the trials, a survival benefit of CABG emerged during midterm follow-up (2 to 6 years), an advantage that eroded during long-term follow-up. Considered together, the results of these trials supported a reduction in long-term mortality (10 years), an absolute 4.1% lowering of mortality rates with CABG compared secondary preventive medical therapy at the time. Subgroup analyses revealed several high-risk criteria that identify patients who are likely to sustain a more substantial survival benefit: (1) left main CAD; (2) single- or double-vessel CAD with proximal LAD disease; (3) LV systolic dysfunction; and (4) a composite evaluation that indicates high risk, including severity of symptoms, high-risk exercise tolerance test, history of previous MI, and the presence of ST depression on the resting ECG.

Taken together, the results of all the trials and registries indicate that the higher the risk of the patient—based on the presence of diabetes mellitus, the number of vessels diseased, and the presence of LV dysfunction—the greater the benefit of surgical over medical therapy on survival. In these practice-guiding trials, CABG prolonged survival compared with medical therapy alone in patients with significant left main CAD irrespective of symptoms. Subsequent trials of medical therapy versus revascularization have excluded patients with critical left main CAD. The preponderance of evidence indicates that surgical therapy prolongs life in patients with impaired LV function with three-vessel and two-vessel CAD, particularly with proximal narrowing of one or more coronary arteries and severe angina.

PATIENTS WITH DEPRESSED LEFT VENTRICULAR FUNCTION (SEE CHAPTER 50)

Depressed LV function is one of the most powerful predictors of perioperative and late mortality.[234-236] For example, in the New York State CABG registry, an ejection fraction of 25% or less was associated with 6.5% in-hospital mortality compared with 1.4% in those with an ejection fraction greater than 40%. In the CABG Patch trial confined to patients with an ejection fraction of 35% or less, perioperative mortality was 3.5% for patients without clinical signs of heart failure versus 7.7% for those with heart failure. Although the effect of a reduced ejection fraction on operative mortality cannot be eliminated, careful attention to intraoperative metabolic, inotropic, and mechanical support may decrease perioperative mortality relative to the mortality rates expected from prediction models. Thus, in experienced centers, in-hospital mortality for patients with severe LV dysfunction is less than 4% to 5%.

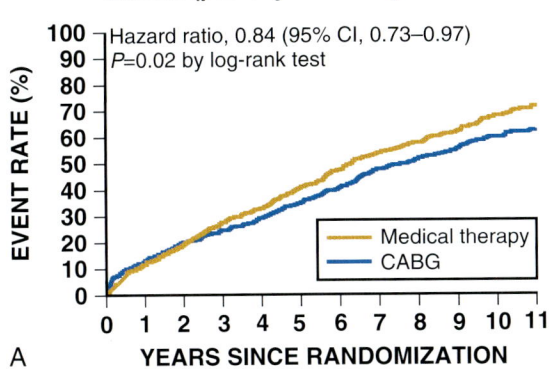
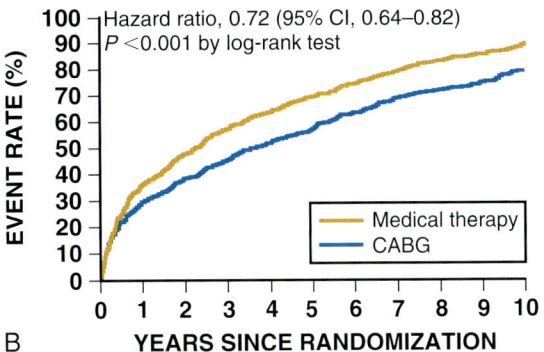

FIGURE 40.14 The Surgical Treatment for Ischemic Heart Failure (STICH) trial included 1212 patients with an ejection fraction of 35% or less and coronary artery disease amenable to CABG who were randomly assigned to undergo CABG plus medical therapy or medical therapy alone. In the STITCH extension study (STITCHES), patients were followed for 10 years. **A,** Death from any cause occurred in 58.9% of the CABG group and 66.1% in the medical-therapy group (HR 0.84; 95% CI, 0.73 to 0.97; P = 0.02 by log-rank test). **B,** Death from any cause or cardiovascular hospitalization was similarly reduced by CABG compared with medical therapy alone. (Adapted from Velazquez EJ, et al. Coronary-artery bypass surgery in patients with ischemic cardiomyopathy. N Engl J Med 2016;374:1511-1520.)

Although preoperative LV dysfunction is associated with higher perioperative risk, ischemic LV dysfunction is also a potential indication for CABG.[222,237] This approach is supported by large contemporary registries with long-term follow-up of patients with LV dysfunction as well as randomized trials of CABG plus medical therapy versus medical therapy alone. In a propensity-adjusted observational analysis comparing 10-year survival with CABG versus medical therapy in patients with an LV ejection fraction less than 35% and no left main stenosis greater than 50%, CABG was associated with a survival advantage. Moreover, in a large meta-analysis of randomized trials of CABG versus medical therapy, the most striking survival benefits of CABG, as well as symptomatic and functional improvements, were shown by patients with impaired LV function, in whom the prognosis with medical therapy is poor.[236]

In the randomized STICH (Surgical Treatment for Ischemic Heart Failure) trial of predominantly on-pump CABG versus medical therapy in 1212 patients with CAD amenable to revascularization and an ejection fraction of 35% or less in the absence of left main CAD or severe (class III) angina, the rate of death from any cause at an average of 56 months after randomization was 36% in patients assigned to CABG and 41% in those assigned to medical therapy (HR, 0.86; 95% CI, 0.72 to 1.04; P = 0.12). However, the combined endpoint of death or hospitalization for cardiovascular causes was significantly lower (58%) in the CABG group than in the medical therapy group (68%; HR, 0.74; 95% CI, 0.64 to 0.85; P < 0.001). Moreover, in the STITCH Extension Study (STICHES), in which follow-up was extended to 10 years, a significant benefit with respect to mortality emerged favoring the CABG arm (58.9% versus 66.1%; HR 0.84; 95% CI, 0.73 to 0.97; P = 0.02) (Fig. 40.14).[238,239]

Although preoperative LV dysfunction creates the potential for significant benefit, the perioperative risk must be considered and weighed in shared decision making with the patient.[237] Despite the absence of a clear impact of myocardial viability on outcomes with CABG in the STICH trial,[240] selective evaluation of patients for viable myocardium may be a reasonable strategy when considering CABG for high-risk patients with severe LV dysfunction.[44,241]

Myocardial Hibernation (See Chapter 36)

Successful reperfusion of viable but noncontractile or poorly contracting myocardium is a goal of coronary revascularization in patients with LV dysfunction. Two related pathophysiologic conditions have been described to explain reversible ischemic contractile dysfunction: (1) myocardial stunning, which describes prolonged but temporary post-ischemic LV dysfunction without myocardial necrosis and (2) myocardial hibernation, or persistent LV dysfunction due either to chronically reduced myocardial perfusion or to repetitive stunning.[242] The reduction in myocardial contractility in hibernating myocardium conserves metabolic demands and may be protective, but more prolonged and severe hibernation may lead to severe ultrastructural abnormalities, irreversible loss of contractile units, and apoptosis.

Hibernating myocardium can cause abnormal systolic or diastolic LV function, or both. Several clinical and imaging markers may be used to determine the likelihood that a dysfunctional myocardial segment is viable or nonviable (Table 40.11).[242] Whereas a severe reduction in the diastolic wall thickness of dysfunctional LV segments is indicative of scarring, akinetic or dyskinetic segments with preserved diastolic wall thickness may represent a mixture of scarred and viable myocardium. Imaging tools that may be used for assessment of myocardial hibernation and viability (dobutamine echocardiography, PET, contrast-enhanced CMRI, CT, and thallium rest-redistribution imaging) are discussed in Chapters 18 to 20. Studies involving PET, thallium-201, and dobutamine echocardiography have demonstrated that patients with LV dysfunction and evidence of hibernating myocardium have a high mortality rate when treated with medical therapy alone.

TABLE 40.11 Markers of Viable Myocardium

CLINICAL INDICATOR	FEATURE SUGGESTING VIABILITY/NON-VIABILITY	DIAGNOSTIC TEST	ALTERNATIVE TEST
Diastolic wall thickness	Wall thickness <6 mm highly suggestive of nonviable scar	Standard echo	CT, CMRI
Regional wall motion	Improved wall motion after stimulation with low-dose dobutamine (i.e., contractile reserve) suggests viability	Low-dose dobutamine echo	CT, CMRI, gated SPECT
Regional blood flow	Late redistribution or redistribution with second tracer injection suggest viability	SPECT	PET, CMRI
Myocardial metabolism	Mismatch between flow (low) and metabolism (active) suggests viability	PET	SPECT
Myocardial fibrosis	Scar limited to subendocardium suggests viability while transmural or near-transmural scar indicates non-viability	CMRI	CT

CT, computed tomography; CMRI, cardiac magnetic resonance imaging; echo, echocardiography; SPECT, single photon emission computed tomography; PET, positron emission tomography.

Surgical Treatment in Special Groups
Women (see Chapter 91)

Women are less likely than men to be referred for coronary angiography and subsequent revascularization. In some studies, sex-based differences in referral for revascularization are explained fully by clinical factors. Moreover, it has not been established whether sex-based differences represent underuse of CABG in women, overuse in men, or both. When compared with men, women who undergo CABG are sicker, as defined by age, comorbid conditions, severity of angina, and history of heart failure. In-hospital mortality and perioperative morbidity after CABG have remained, on average, 1.5 to 2 times higher in women than in men. However, when adjusted for the greater risk profile of women referred for CABG, short-term mortality rates and long-term outcomes are similar to those for men in most but not all studies, with similar advantages of CABG over multivessel PCI.[243] With generally similar long-term outcomes after surgical revascularization after risk-adjustment, female sex should not be a significant factor in decisions regarding whether to offer CABG.

Older Patients (See Chapter 90)
The aging of the population, in combination with marked improvement in perioperative care and in the outcomes of CABG has resulted in a burgeoning population of older patients with extensive CAD undergoing such surgery.[244] The number of individuals older than 75 years in the United States is expected to quadruple in the next 50 years, with cardiovascular disease being the leading cause of morbidity and mortality in this population. Many such individuals are likely to become candidates for CABG.

Older patients are sicker than their younger counterparts in that they have a greater frequency of comorbid conditions, including peripheral vascular and cerebrovascular disease, more extensive triple-vessel and left main CAD, and a higher frequency of LV dysfunction and history of heart failure. Not unexpectedly, these differences translate into higher perioperative mortality and complication rates, with a sharp increase in the slope of the curve relating mortality to age in patients older than 70 years. Despite these differences, in-hospital mortality for older adults has declined over time and has been reported to be as low as 3% to 4% in the subgroup of octogenarians without significant medical comorbid conditions. However, elderly patients with high indices of frailty and disability are at significantly higher risk for major morbidity and mortality during CABG. Given the marked variation in outcomes in older patients undergoing revascularization, decisions should be based on individual risk and needs assessment.

Renal Disease
Cardiovascular disease is the major cause of mortality in patients with end-stage renal disease (ESRD) and accounts for >50% of deaths. Patients with ESRD, as well as those with less severe renal insufficiency, have numerous risk factors that not only accelerate the development of CAD but also complicate its medical management.[199] These risk factors include diabetes, hypertension with LV hypertrophy, systolic and diastolic dysfunction, abnormal lipid metabolism, anemia, and increased homocysteine levels. Therefore, mild or more severe renal dysfunction is prevalent in as many as 50% of patients undergoing CABG. Coronary revascularization with PCI or CABG is commonly performed in patients with ESRD, but mortality and complication rates are increased. Patients with milder degrees of renal insufficiency who are not dependent on dialysis are also at higher risk for major perioperative complications, longer recovery times, and lower rates of short-term and midterm survival. Observational data have suggested that in patients undergoing chronic dialysis, CABG may be the preferred strategy for revascularization over PCI for patients with multivessel CAD.[245] However, randomized data are few, and 30-day mortality in patients with ESRD undergoing CABG ranges from 9% to as high as 20%.

Patients with Diabetes (See Chapter 31)
Diabetes is an important independent predictor of mortality in patients undergoing surgical revascularization. Patients with diabetes have smaller distal vessels, which are deemed to be poorer targets for bypass grafting. Nevertheless, the patency of arterial and venous grafts appears to be similar in diabetic and nondiabetic patients. Despite these higher risks with operative intervention, because of the potential long-term benefits of CABG in patients with diabetes and severe CAD, such patients should be considered candidates for CABG (see Comparisons between Percutaneous Coronary Intervention and Coronary Artery Bypass Surgery and Choosing between Percutaneous Coronary Intervention, Coronary Artery Bypass Surgery, and Medical Therapy).

PATIENTS WITH ASSOCIATED OTHER VASCULAR DISEASE. The management of patients with peripheral artery disease and cerebrovascular disease are discussed in the online version of this chapter.

Patients Requiring Reoperation
An estimated 5% to 10% of isolated CABG surgeries are cardiac reoperations, with the major indication for reoperation being late disease of saphenous vein grafts.[247] An added factor underlying recurrent symptoms is progression of disease in native vessels between the first and second operations. Several series have emphasized the sicker preoperative status of patients undergoing reoperation, including older age, more serious comorbid conditions, associated valvular heart disease, and a greater prevalence of LV dysfunction and greater extent of ischemic jeopardized myocardium.

Not unexpectedly, the mortality associated with reoperation is significantly higher than that of initial CABG procedures. At a time when mortality in STS was 2.6% for urgent and 6% for emergency first CABG operations, the corresponding rates were 7.4% and 13.5% in patients undergoing repeated CABG. As a result of the higher risk and operative complexity of redo CABG, PCI is increasingly being considered as the first-line option in patients with SVG failure.[248] In such cases, PCI of the native coronary vessels is preferred to SVG PCI due to lower complication rates and better long-term patency. When the native coronary artery has a CTO, revascularization decisions can be challenging. Many CTOs, which previously required redo CABG, can now be successfully revascularized by expert PCI operators in specialized referral centers. However, it has not been demonstrated that CTO PCI improves clinical outcomes.

Comparisons between Percutaneous Coronary Intervention and Coronary Artery Bypass Surgery
Observational Studies
Observational studies comparing CABG with coronary stenting have had mixed results. For example, in an analysis of approximately 600,000 patients with multivessel CAD enrolled in the ACC-NCDR and STS databases, the observed 1-year mortality rates were similar between patients who underwent CABG and those who underwent PCI. However, 4-year mortality was significantly lower in the CABG group in multiple sensitivity analyses aimed at addressing potential confounders.[249] In contrast, a propensity-matched analysis of approximately 18,000 patients with multivessel CAD who underwent PCI with second-generation DES (everolimus) or CABG showed similar risk of death in the two groups but a higher risk of MI and need for repeat revascularization among patients treated with PCI.[250] In a similar propensity-matched analysis comparing PCI with second- and third-generation stents with CABG for multivessel disease in the United Kingdom ($n = 6383$), PCI was associated with higher 5-year mortality rate (adjusted HR for PCI versus CABG 1.74; 95% CI, 1.41 to 2.16; $P < 0.001$).[251] However, the potential for residual confounding in observational studies has underscored the importance of randomized trials.

Randomized Trials
Overall, the findings from randomized trials indicate that in selected patients with multivessel or left main CAD and preserved ejection fraction, when compared with multivessel PCI, CABG results in fewer repeat revascularizations and fewer symptoms with a heterogenous effect on survival depending on the extent and complexity of underlying CAD, the presence of diabetes, and the duration of follow-up.[252-255] In patients with greater complexity of coronary atherosclerosis followed over 5 to 10 years, CABG has had a more favorable survival than multivessel PCI.[256-258]

PERCUTANEOUS CORONARY INTERVENTION VERSUS CORONARY ARTERY BYPASS SURGERY IN PATIENTS WITH MULTIVESSEL DISEASE
At least 10 published randomized studies have compared PCI with CABG in patients with multivessel CAD. Despite the heterogeneity of the trials in regard to design, methods, and the patient

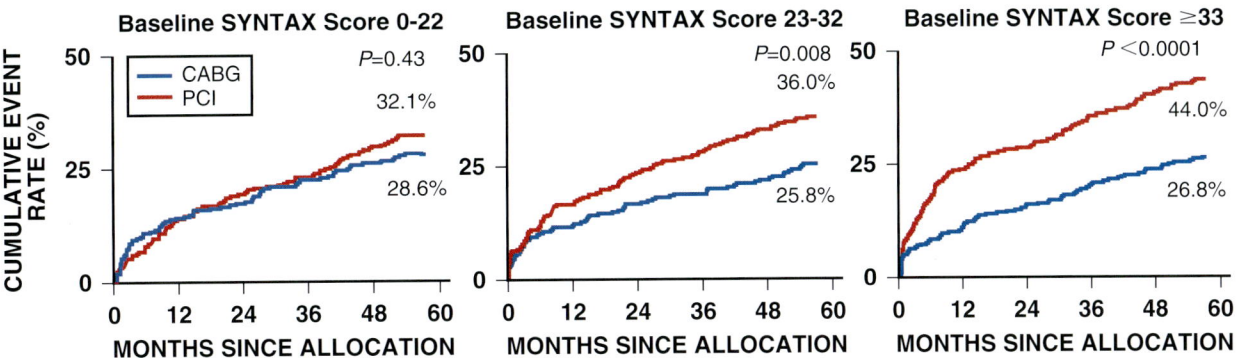

FIGURE 40.15 Major adverse cardiac and cerebral events at 5 years' follow-up in the SYNergy between percutaneous coronary intervention with TAXus and cardiac surgery (SYNTAX) trial, stratified by baseline SYNTAX score tertiles. The SYNTAX trial compared coronary artery bypass graft (CABG) surgery with percutaneous coronary intervention (PCI) in patient with left main or three-vessel coronary artery disease (CAD). The SYNTAX score describes the location, extent, and complexity of angiographic CAD, with low scores reflecting less complex disease and high scores more complex disease. CABG and PCI yielded similar outcomes among individuals in the lowest SYNTAX score tertile, but CABG was superior among individuals in the upper two tertiles, with the largest difference favoring CABG seen among patients with the most complex disease. (Adapted from Mohr FW, et al. Coronary artery bypass graft surgery versus percutaneous coronary intervention in patients with three-vessel disease and left main coronary disease: 5-year follow-up of the randomised, clinical SYNTAX trial. Lancet 2013;381:629-38.)

population enrolled, the results are generally comparable and provide a consistent perspective of CABG and PCI in selected patients with multivessel CAD. Nevertheless, there are limitations that should be recognized. Conducted over several decades, the trials evolved substantially with respect to the technology used for both procedures and disease-modifying preventive therapy. Moreover, most patients entered into the trials had preserved LV function.[36]

With progressive improvements in stent technology, patients with higher-risk coronary anatomy have been enrolled in trials. In the SYNTAX trial conducted between 2005 and 2007, 1800 patients with three-vessel or left main CAD were randomly assigned to undergo CABG or PCI after a "multidisciplinary team" consisting of a local cardiac surgeon and interventional cardiologist determined that equivalent anatomic revascularization could be achieved with either treatment.[253] The primary outcome measure was a noninferiority comparison of the two groups for major adverse cardiac or cerebrovascular events (i.e., death from any cause, stroke, MI, or repeat revascularization) during the 12-month period after randomization. Long-term follow-up of this trial has revealed important new information over time. At 12 months, the rate of the primary outcome was significantly higher in the PCI group (17.8% versus 12.4% for CABG; $P = 0.002$), in large part because of an increased rate of repeat revascularization (13.5% versus 5.9%; $P < 0.001$) with a similar rate of death and MI between the two groups. However, stroke was significantly more likely to occur with CABG (2.2% versus 0.6% with PCI; $P = 0.003$). At 5 years, rates of MI (3.8% with CABG versus 9.7% with PCI; $P < 0.0001$) and repeat revascularization (13.7% with CABG versus 25.9% with PCI; $P < 0.0001$) were significantly lower in the CABG group, whereas all-cause mortality (11.4% with CABG versus 13.9% with PCI; $P = 0.10$) did not differ significantly between groups. However, by 10 years of follow-up, significant heterogeneity was apparent between patients with underlying left main CAD versus multivessel disease. While 10-year mortality did not differ between PCI and CABG for patients with left main CAD, a survival advantage was suggested with CABG for patients with multivessel CAD (21% with CABG versus 28% with PCI; adjusted HR for PCI versus CABG 1.42; 95% CI, 1.11 to 1.81).[253]

The comparative effectiveness of CABG versus PCI differs based on the anatomic complexity and severity of the CAD, as determined by the SYNTAX score.[252] This score considers the number, location, and complexity of the coronary stenoses. Among patients with intermediate or high SYNTAX scores, CABG was clearly superior to PCI for major cardiovascular events, but among those with low scores, outcomes were similar (Fig. 40.15). Therefore, CABG should remain the standard of care for patients with complex coronary lesions (high or intermediate SYNTAX scores), whereas for patients with less complex CAD (low SYNTAX scores) or left main CAD (with low or intermediate SYNTAX scores), PCI remains an acceptable alternative.[255] In a meta-analysis of 11 randomized trials, long-term mortality was more favorable with CABG versus PCI in most subgroups with multivessel CAD; particularly in patients with diabetes or more complex disease.[252] Moreover, patients with diabetes with multivessel disease and low surgical risk may be appropriate candidates for CABG with increasing benefit with longer follow-up time. Inhospital costs are lower for patients undergoing PCI, but the need for recurrent hospitalization and repeat revascularization procedures over the long term contributes to an increase in postdischarge cost in patients treated with PCI, which resulted in similar overall cost over a 3- to 5-year period.

Patients with Diabetes (See Chapter 31)

An initially unexpected finding in the BARI (Bypass Angioplasty Revascularization Investigation) trial was that patients with previously treated diabetes who underwent PTCA had a 5-year mortality of 34.5% versus 19.4% for those who underwent CABG ($P = 0.003$). In a collaborative meta-analysis of individual patient data from 7812 patients in 10 trials of PCI versus CABG, total mortality was significantly reduced by 30% with CABG in the subset of 1233 diabetic patients—findings that persisted even after exclusion of the BARI trial.[259] The FREEDOM (Future REvascularization Evaluation in patients with Diabetes mellitus: Optimal management of Multivessel disease) trial of 1900 patients with diabetes and multivessel CAD who were randomly assigned to either DES treatment or CABG showed a convincing clinical benefit from CABG versus PCI. In particular, the trial findings showed significant reductions in all-cause mortality and the composite of death or MI in CABG-treated diabetic patients.[260,261] The results of the FREEDOM trial contributed substantially to the accumulated evidence that patients with SIHD and diabetes, especially those with three-vessel CAD, have better long-term clinical outcomes with CABG than with PCI, even when using DES.[252,256] A potential advantage of CABG over PCI is that bypass grafts to the mid-coronary vessel both treat the culprit lesion (regardless of anatomic complexity) and may afford prophylaxis against new proximal disease progression, whereas stents treat only localized stenotic segments with no benefit against the development of new disease. Based on the findings of BARI-2D, FREEDOM, and meta-analyses, CABG is regarded as the preferred revascularization approach in patients with multivessel CAD and diabetes when reduction of clinical events is the principal goal of treatment (Fig. 40.16).

Choosing between Percutaneous Coronary Intervention, Coronary Artery Bypass Surgery, and Medical Therapy

Optimal medical therapy for SIHD involves a reduction in reversible risk factors, counseling in lifestyle alteration, treatment of conditions that intensify angina, and pharmacologic management of ischemia. Unlike the situation in ACS patients, revascularization has not been shown to reduce the rate of death or MI when used in patients with SIHD (with the exception of CABG in patients meeting specific anatomic criteria). Moreover, patients with LV dysfunction have been excluded from randomized trials of PCI versus CABG.[262]

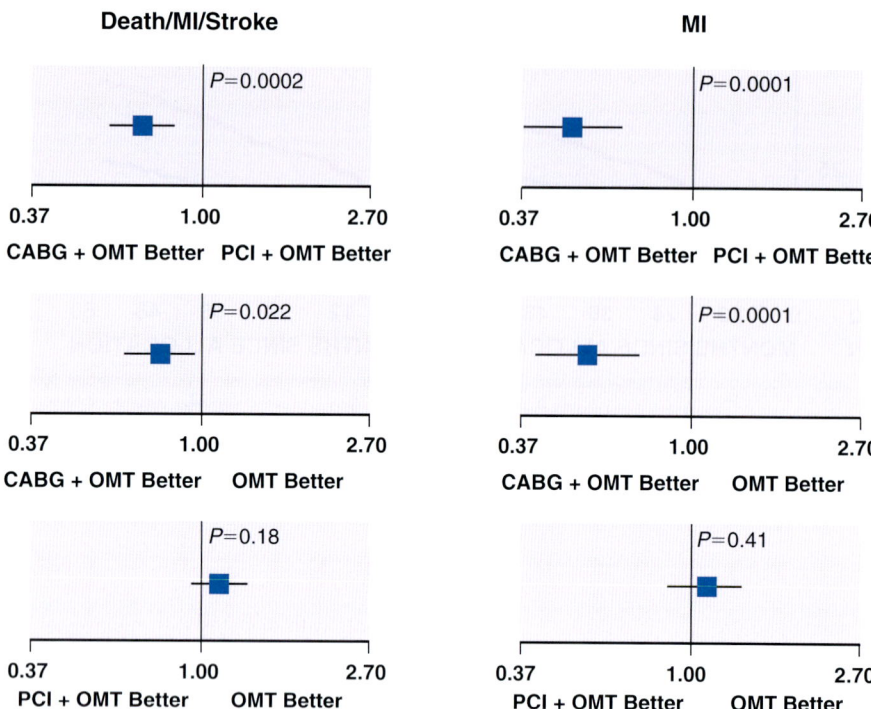

FIGURE 40.16 Meta-analysis of randomized trials comparing different revascularization strategies for patients with coronary artery disease and type 2 diabetes mellitus. Trial-adjusted hazard ratios are reported for comparisons of coronary artery bypass graft (CABG) surgery versus percutaneous coronary intervention (PCI), CABG versus optimal medical therapy (OMT), and PCI versus OMT. CABG was superior to PCI and to OMT for both the composite outcome as well as the individual MI endpoint. In contrast, PCI was not superior to OMT for either outcome. (From Mancini GB, et al. Medical treatment and revascularization options in patients with type 2 diabetes and coronary disease. J Am Coll Cardiol 2016;68:985-995.)

with PCI or CABG. Additional anatomic factors, such as the presence of severe proximal LAD disease, should also be considered and weigh in favor of surgery. For patients with severe three-vessel CAD and LV dysfunction,[252,263] CABG is generally the best approach and is recommended (class I) in professional society guidelines.[36,182]

The approach to left main CAD in patients with preserved LV function is evolving.[264] In selected patients with left main CAD, randomized trial have shown that excellent technical and clinical results can be obtained with PCI, but with a greater need for repeated revascularization procedures than with CABG.[265,266] With newer generation DES, outcomes for left main PCI have improved, and PCI represents a suitable alternative to CABG if anatomic features are favorable (i.e., diffuse CAD is not present). PCI for unprotected left main disease is an alternative to CABG (class I) in patients for whom the coronary anatomy is consistent with a low risk of PCI procedural complications and a high likelihood of good long-term outcome (e.g., a low SYNTAX score of ≤ 22, ostial or trunk left main CAD), particularly if the risk of adverse surgical outcomes is high (e.g., STS-predicted risk of operative mortality ≥ 5%).[264,267-269] In patients, with moderate disease complexity (e.g. SYNTAX 23-32), PCI is a reasonable alternative to CABG; however, PCI is not recommended in patients with more complex CAD.[182] In general, for all patients with complex multivessel CAD for whom revascularization is being contemplated, there should be a thorough review and discussion of treatment options with the patient by a team that includes a cardiac surgeon and interventional cardiologist to reach a consensus on which approach is best suited for a particular patient.[181]

Recommendations for either PCI or CABG should be based on the severity of anginal symptoms or functional impairment, with consideration of the extent and severity of ischemia (by noninvasive stress testing or by invasive assessment of the hemodynamic significance of anatomic stenosis). When an unacceptable level of angina persists despite medical management, the patient has troubling side effects from the anti-ischemic drugs, the coronary anatomy should be defined to allow selection of the appropriate technique for revascularization. Shared decision making with the patient is essential. After elucidation of the coronary anatomy, selection of the technique of revascularization should be made as follows.[182,222]

Single-Vessel Disease
In patients with single-vessel disease in whom revascularization is deemed necessary and the lesion is anatomically suitable, PCI is almost always preferred over CABG.

Multivessel Disease
The first step is to assess the extent of CAD and its complexity while considering whether the patient falls into a subset of patients for whom surgical revascularization may confer a survival benefit. Over a 5-year horizon in patients with preserved LV function, PCI and CABG offer similar survival in patients without highly complex CAD (e.g., patients with SYNTAX score <22); however, rates of MI and repeat revascularization are higher in patients treated with PCI as is long-term mortality in patients with highly complex CAD.

For patients who either refuse surgery or are not deemed suitable candidates for CABG, PCI remains a reasonable treatment option versus medical therapy, provided that the patient accepts the possibility of symptom recurrence and the need for repeat revascularization. Patients with focal stenoses in each affected vessel (i.e., low SYNTAX score) and preserved LV function generally have similar outcomes

Need for Complete Revascularization
Complete revascularization is an important goal in patients with LV dysfunction and/or multivessel CAD. The major advantage of CABG over PCI is its greater ability to achieve complete revascularization, particularly in patients with triple-vessel CAD, in addition to providing a conduit to the distal native vessel downstream of future de novo coronary stenoses.[254] In a pooled patient-level analysis across three randomized trials of CABG versus PCI for patients with multivessel CAD, five-year survival was similar in patients with complete revascularization (achieved in 67% of patients treated with CABG and 57% of patients treated with PCI). However, CABG was superior if revascularization was incomplete.[270] In patients with borderline LV function (ejection fraction between 0.40 and 0.50) and milder degrees of ischemia, PCI may provide adequate revascularization, even if it is not complete anatomically.

In many patients, either method of revascularization is suitable. Other factors to be considered include the following:
1. Access to a high-quality team and operator (surgeon or interventional cardiologist).
2. Patient preference—some patients are reluctant to remain at risk for recurrence of symptoms and reintervention; such patients are better candidates for surgical treatment. Other patients are attracted by the less invasive nature and more rapid recovery from PCI; these patients prefer to have PCI as their initial revascularization with the idea of undergoing CABG if the symptoms persist and/or excellent revascularization has not been achieved.
3. Advanced patient age and comorbidity—frail, very elderly patients and those with comorbid conditions are often better candidates for PCI.

OTHER MANIFESTATIONS OF CORONARY ARTERY DISEASE

Prinzmetal (Variant) Angina
See Chapter 36.

Angina and Ischemia Without Obstructive Epicardial CAD

The syndrome of angina or angina-like chest discomfort with no obstructive coronary disease, previously termed *syndrome X* (to be differentiated from "metabolic syndrome X"), is an important clinical entity that is often associated with clinical and electrocardiographic evidence of myocardial ischemia and has previously been underrecognized. This syndrome, sometimes referred to as INOCA (**I**schemia with **N**o **O**bstructive **C**oronary **A**rtery Disease) was generally regarded as having a benign long-term prognosis but is now recognized to be associated with an increased risk for adverse outcomes in certain subsets of patients.[3,65,271,272] Potential explanations for angina in the absence of flow-limiting CAD that have historically been offered include misinterpretation of the coronary angiogram, potential misdiagnosis of flush (or stump) coronary occlusions at sites of major arterial bifurcations, coronary vasospasm, increased subendocardial pressure leading to coronary artery compression, or hyperdynamic ventricular contraction with an elevated ejection fraction resulting in a supply-demand imbalance. In some patients, particularly premenopausal women, when exercise-induced ST-segment depression during treadmill exercise triggered referral for diagnostic coronary angiography that resulted in normal angiographic findings, these abnormal noninvasive test results were dismissed as being "false-positives." However, steady accumulation of experimental and clinical data has provided a sound scientific basis for recognizing that myocardial ischemia may occur without critical coronary stenosis and may be explained by overlapping effects of concealed diffuse coronary atherosclerosis revealed by FFR, iFR or IVUS, endothelial dysfunction, microvascular dysfunction, coronary spasm, and, in some cases, myocardial bridging (Fig. 40.17).[72,273,274]

Patients with chest pain and normal findings on coronary arteriography may represent as many as 10% to 30% of those undergoing coronary arteriography because of clinical suspicion of angina. This proportion may be substantially higher in women. For example, in the initial WISE (Women's Ischemic Syndrome Evaluation) study, approximately two-thirds of women with chest pain and other findings suggestive of SIHD had no critical coronary stenoses detected with angiography.[275] Data from 388 U.S. hospitals participating in the ACC-NCDR revealed that at least 50% of women and 30% of men referred for coronary angiography had no obstructive CAD. True myocardial ischemia, as reflected by the production of lactate by the myocardium during exercise or pacing, is present in some of these patients. In addition, coronary artery reactivity testing demonstrates evidence of endothelial and microvascular dysfunction in a substantial proportion of such individuals.[274] The incidence of coronary calcification on CT is significantly higher than that in normal controls (53% versus 20%) but lower than that in patients with angina secondary to obstructive CAD (96%). Moreover, observational data have established that their outcome is not as uniformly excellent as suggested by early cohort studies.[65] In addition, abnormal measures of endothelial and microvascular function in these patients are associated with a higher risk for death, MI, or hospitalization for heart failure.

The causes of the syndrome are heterogeneous across individuals.[2,72,76,273,274] Vascular (endothelial and microvascular) dysfunction, coronary vasospasm, and myocardial metabolic abnormalities, as noted above, have each been implicated. Included in this syndrome are patients in whom angina may be the direct consequence of subendocardial ischemia as a result of abnormalities in the coronary microvasculature (or arteriolar resistance vessels), the small caliber of which would be beyond the resolution of coronary angiography. Alternatively, in some individuals, chest discomfort without ischemia may be caused by abnormal pain perception or sensitivity. Furthermore, IVUS studies have demonstrated anatomic and physiologic heterogeneity in patients with INOCA with a spectrum ranging from completely normal epicardial coronary arteries to vessels with intimal thickening and atheromatous plaque and non–flow-limiting obstructions (10% to 30% diameter reductions) that are insufficient to cause angina on the basis of coronary luminal narrowing alone, but which may result in ischemia in the setting of superimposed dynamic coronary vasomotor tone. Finally, it may be difficult to distinguish patients with angina and normal findings on coronary arteriography in whom chest pain is caused by ischemia from patients with noncardiac pain. However, an approach of assuming a favorable prognosis and dismissing symptoms in all such patients is clearly not justified by the evidence.[272]

Microvascular Dysfunction

The Coronary Vasomotion Disorders International Study Group definition of microvascular angina includes (1) symptoms suggestive of myocardial ischemia, (2) objective evidence of myocardial ischemia, (3) absence of obstructive CAD (no stenosis with >50% diameter reduction and/or FFR >0.80), and (4) documentation of reduced CFR and/or inducible microvascular spasm.[276] In the CorMicA trial, microvascular dysfunction was the most common abnormality detected when integrated invasive functional assessments were performed among patients with INOCA.[76,277] Two endotypes of coronary microvascular dysfunction have recently been described on the basis of detailed exercise hemodynamic studies incorporating intracoronary Doppler and perfusion MRI. Structural microvascular dysfunction (MVD) was characterized by high vascular tone at rest, potentially due to capillary rarefaction, fibrosis, and LV hypertrophy, whereas functional MVD, the more common endotype, was characterized by normal vascular tone at rest. Patients with structural MVD were more likely to have hypertension, diabetes, and elevated NT-proBNP than those with functional MVD.[278]

Abnormal endothelium-dependent vasoreactivity has been associated with regional myocardial perfusion defects on SPECT, PET, and CMRI. Patients with angina and angiographically normal coronary anatomy may also have impaired vasodilator reserve in forearm vessels and airway hyperresponsiveness, suggesting that the smooth muscle of systemic arteries and other organs may be affected in addition to that of the coronary circulation.

Endothelial dysfunction and endothelial cell activation, reported in patients with microvascular angina, may participate in the release of cellular adhesion molecules, proinflammatory cytokines, and constricting mediators that induce changes in the arterial wall and result in microvascular coronary dysfunction and higher risk for the future development of obstructive CAD.

Evidence of Ischemia

Despite the general acceptance that microvascular and/or endothelial dysfunction is present in many patients with angina and normal findings on coronary arteriography, whether ischemia is in fact the putative cause of the symptoms in all patients is not clear. Studies of transmyocardial production of lactate have generated mixed results. In contrast, the development of LV dysfunction and electrocardiographic or scintigraphic abnormalities during exercise in some of these patients supports an ischemic cause. Moreover, stress echocardiography with dobutamine detects regional contraction abnormalities consistent with ischemia in a subset of patients. More sensitive techniques, such as perfusion analysis with CMRI, have demonstrated that subendocardial perfusion abnormalities in particular may be associated with angina with normal angiographic findings.

Abnormal Pain Perception

The lack of definitive evidence of ischemia in many patients with angina and normal coronary angiographic findings has focused attention on alternative nonischemic causes of cardiac-related pain, including a decreased threshold for visceral pain perception. This hypersensitivity may result in an awareness of chest pain in response to stimuli such as arterial

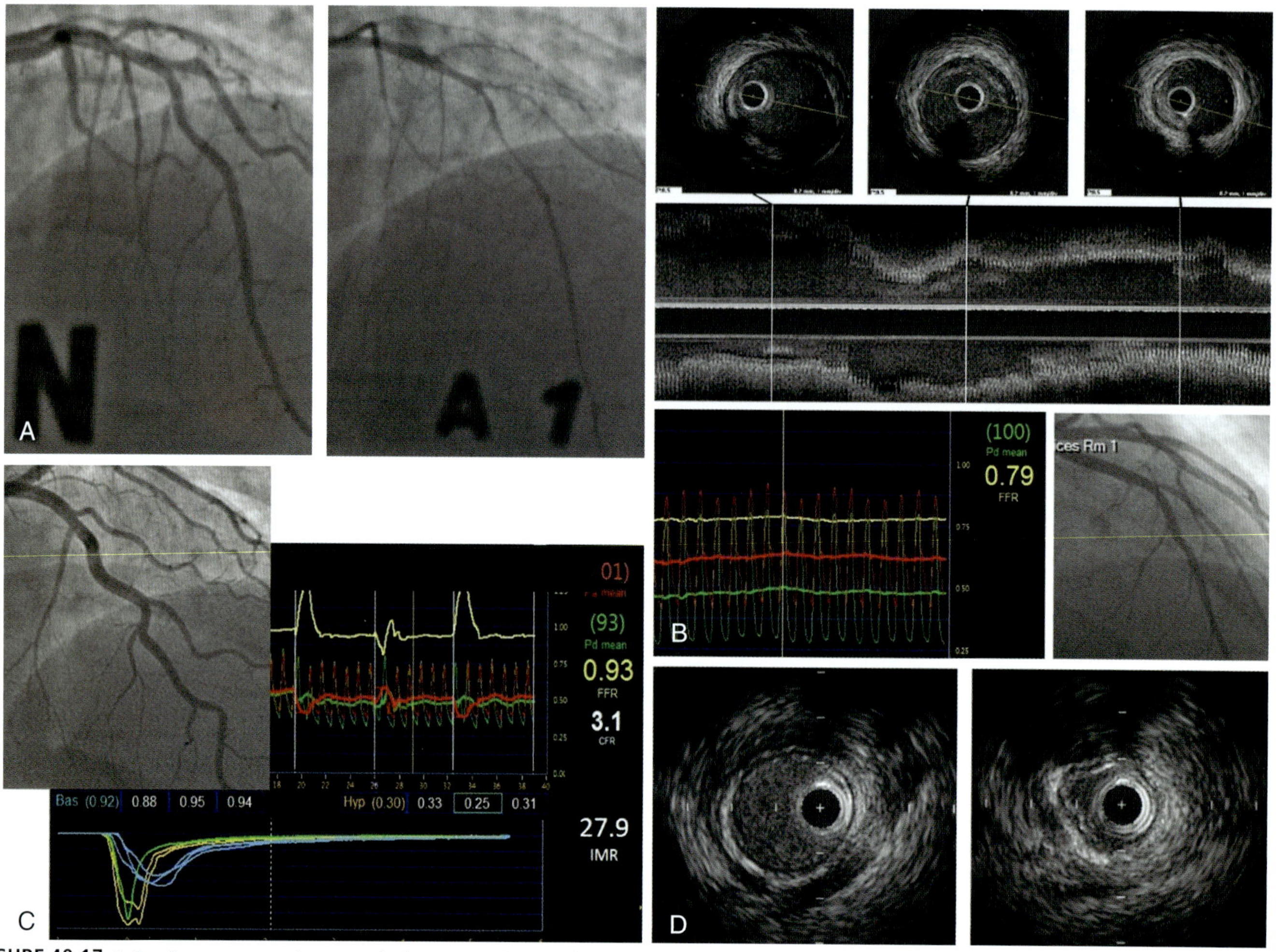

FIGURE 40.17 A, Baseline coronary angiogram and subsequent angiogram after intracoronary acetylcholine demonstrating diffuse endothelial dysfunction with vasoconstriction. **B,** Cross-sectional and longitudinal intravascular ultrasound images demonstrating diffuse atherosclerosis and coronary pressure tracing revealing an abnormal fractional flow reserve in a normal appearing left anterior descending coronary artery on angiography. **C,** Coronary angiogram revealing a normal left anterior descending coronary artery with a pressure tracing showing an abnormal index of microcirculatory resistance. **D,** Cross-sectional intravascular ultrasound images of a myocardial bridge segment. (From Lee BK, et al. Invasive evaluation of patients with angina in the absence of obstructive coronary artery disease. Circulation 2015;131:1054-060.)

stretch or changes in heart rate, rhythm, or contractility. A sympathovagal imbalance with sympathetic predominance in some of these patients has also been postulated. At the time of cardiac catheterization, some patients with angina are unusually sensitive to intracardiac instrumentation, with the typical chest pain being consistently produced by direct right atrial stimulation and saline infusion. Measurements of regional cerebral blood flow at rest and during chest pain have suggested differential handling of afferent stimuli between such patients and those with obstructive CAD.

Clinical Features

The syndrome of angina or angina-like chest pain with no obstructive disease of the epicardial arteries occurs more frequently in women, many of whom are premenopausal, whereas obstructive CAD is found more commonly in men and postmenopausal women.[271] Similarly to women with critical epicardial CAD, many women with microvascular angina may experience dyspnea or fatigue or may have a preponderance of symptoms such as nausea and midepigastric pain. Although the features are frequently atypical of myocardial ischemia, the chest pain may nonetheless be severe and disabling. Angina in the absence of obstructive CAD may have markedly adverse effects on quality of life, employment, and use of health care resources.

Clinical and Diagnostic Assessment

Abnormal physical findings reflecting ischemia are uncommon in these patients. The resting ECG may be normal, but nonspecific ST-T wave abnormalities are often observed, sometimes occurring in association with the chest pain. Approximately 20% to 30% of patients with chest pain and normal coronary angiographic findings have positive exercise test results. However, many patients with this syndrome do not complete the exercise test because of fatigue or mild chest discomfort. LV function is usually normal at rest and during stress, unlike the situation in obstructive CAD, in which function often becomes impaired during stress.

Comprehensive invasive assessment of patients with evidence for myocardial ischemia on noninvasive testing can provide diagnostic information in more than 75% of patients without obstructive CAD (see also Microvascular Dysfunction and Evidence of Ischemia in this section).[65] Such a comprehensive invasive assessment may include FFR or IFR to evaluate diffuse epicardial obstructive disease that was not apparent from the angiogram, endothelial function, and spasm testing with acetylcholine; CFR and/or IMR testing with adenosine; and IVUS to assess for diffuse structural abnormalities and myocardial bridging (Table 40.12). Such findings may be useful to guide management (see also Integrated Invasive Assessment in Patients Without Obstructive CAD).

Prognosis

Accumulating data suggest that the prognosis in patients with chest pain without obstructive CAD is more heterogeneous than once thought. In patients with an ejection fraction of 50% or greater in the CASS registry, the 7-year survival rate was 96% for patients with normal arteriographic findings and 92% for those whose arteriographic study revealed mild CAD (50% luminal stenosis). However, subsequent studies have shown that the prognosis is not as favorable in some groups of patients. For example, an ischemic response to exercise is associated with increased mortality. Moreover, in

TABLE 40.12 Techniques for Functional Assessment of Coronary Vascular Function in Patients without Obstructive Coronary Artery Disease

FUNCTIONAL ASSESSMENT	TECHNIQUE USED	CLINICAL USE IN INOCA
Fractional flow reserve (FFR)	Intracoronary pressure wire with (FFR) or without (iFR) administration adenosine or other vasodilator	Identify hemodynamic impact of diffuse coronary stenoses
Instantaneous wave-free ratio (iFR)		
Coronary flow reserve (CFR)	Intracoronary Doppler wire; MRI; PET; administration of adenosine or other vasodilator	Diagnose coronary microvascular dysfunction in the absence of epicardial CAD
Index of microvascular resistance (IMR)	Intracoronary pressure wire and temperature sensor	Diagnose coronary microvascular dysfunction in the presence of epicardial CAD
Endothelial function testing	Quantitative coronary angiography after administration of low-dose acetylcholine	Diagnose endothelial dysfunction
Provocative testing for coronary spasm	Quantitative coronary angiography after administration of high-dose acetylcholine or ergonovine; 12-lead ECG	Diagnose coronary vasospasm

women with angina and no obstructive CAD enrolled in the WISE investigations, persistence of symptoms was associated with more than a twofold higher risk for cardiovascular events. Such patients may be appropriate candidates for formal studies of vascular function and aggressive risk factor modification.

Management

No specific guideline-recommended therapy is available for patients with signs and symptoms of IHD who do not have obstructive CAD.[272] Risk factors for atherosclerotic vascular disease should be managed and for those with established atherosclerosis, even if nonobstructive, GDMT should be instituted. For those with ischemic symptoms, a trial of anti-ischemic therapy with nitrates, calcium antagonists, and beta-blocking agents is logical, but the response to this therapy is variable. Perhaps because of the heterogeneity of this population, studies testing these antianginal therapies have produced conflicting results. For example, beta blockers may be most effective in such patients who also have evidence of a hyperadrenergic state characterized by increased sympathetic nervous system activity (e.g., hypertension, tachycardia, and reduced heart rate variability). Sublingual nitroglycerin has shown paradoxical (negative) effects on blood flow and exercise tolerance in some studies and beneficial effects in others. Observational studies of calcium antagonists have in general resulted in disappointing outcomes with respect to amelioration of symptoms. Although a small pilot study of women with well-documented microvascular angina and myocardial ischemia treated with ranolazine showed an improvement in functional status and quality of life, no benefit from ranolazine was seen in a subsequent placebo-controlled trial performed in patients with angina and MRI evidence of impaired coronary flow reserve.[167,168]

ACE inhibitors have favorable effects on endothelial function, vascular remodeling, and sympathetic tone that may be relevant to the pathophysiology of the underlying myocardial ischemia in some of these patients. Preliminary data on ACE inhibitors in this population are promising. Similarly, estrogen has been shown to attenuate vasoconstrictor responses to acetylcholine, increase coronary blood flow, and potentiate endothelium-dependent vasodilation in postmenopausal women. Studies of estrogen replacement in postmenopausal women with angina but without critical epicardial CAD have demonstrated improvement in symptoms and/or exercise performance; however, the role of exogenous estrogen in treatment of this group remains in question. Finally, treatment with imipramine (50 mg daily) and structured psychological intervention targeted to the altered somatic and visceral pain perception experienced by certain patients have been reported to be helpful in some.

Silent Myocardial Ischemia

Epidemiologic studies of sudden death (see Chapter 70), as well as clinical and postmortem studies of patients with silent MI, have suggested that many patients with severe IHD never experience angina pectoris. These patients may be considered to have a defective anginal warning system in that they may not be subjectively aware of myocardial ischemia when it is present. In addition, up to a third of patients with chronic stable angina also exhibit episodes of silent (asymptomatic) ischemia. Analysis of ambulatory electrocardiographic recordings in patients with CAD who had both symptomatic and silent myocardial ischemia has shown that 85% of ambulant ischemic episodes occur without chest pain and 66% of angina reports were unaccompanied by ST-segment depression. The total ischemic burden in these patients refers to the total period of ischemia, both symptomatic and asymptomatic. In the context of the results of the ISCHEMIA trial, the value of seeking to quantify asymptomatic ischemia has come into question.

Heart Failure in Ischemic Heart Disease (See Chapter 50)

Currently, the leading cause of heart failure in developed countries is CAD. In the United States, CAD and its complications account for two-thirds to three-fourths of all cases of heart failure. In many patients the progressive nature of heart failure reflects the advancing nature of the underlying CAD. The term *ischemic cardiomyopathy* is used for the clinical syndrome in which one or more of the pathophysiologic features just discussed result in LV dysfunction and heart failure symptoms. This condition is the predominant form of heart failure related to CAD.[280] Additional complications of CAD that may become superimposed on ischemic cardiomyopathy and precipitate heart failure are the development of an LV aneurysm and mitral regurgitation caused by papillary muscle dysfunction.

Ischemic Cardiomyopathy

Symptoms of heart failure caused by ischemic myocardial dysfunction and hibernation, diffuse fibrosis, or multiple MIs, alone or in combination, may dominate the clinical picture of CAD, with symptoms indistinguishable from those of dilated cardiomyopathy. In some patients with chronic CAD, angina may be the principal clinical manifestation at one time, but later this symptom diminishes or even disappears as heart failure becomes more prominent. Other patients with ischemic cardiomyopathy have no history of angina or MI, and it is in this subgroup that ischemic cardiomyopathy is most often confused with dilated cardiomyopathy. When angina coexists with ischemic cardiomyopathy, outcomes appear particularly poor. In patients with ischemic cardiomyopathy, symptoms resulting from chronic LV dysfunction may result from necrotic and scarred myocardium or from a reversible ischemic process (see Myocardial Hibernation).[242]

The outlook for patients with ischemic cardiomyopathy treated medically is poor, and revascularization or cardiac transplantation may be considered.[280] The prognosis is particularly poor for patients in whom ischemic cardiomyopathy is caused by recurrent MIs, in those with associated ventricular arrhythmias, and in those with an extensive amount of hibernating myocardium. The key to management of patients with ischemic cardiomyopathy, in addition to providing evidence-based medical therapy for heart failure, is to carefully select patients who may be appropriate candidates for revascularization (see Coronary Artery Bypass Grafting: Patients with Depressed Left Ventricular Function).

Although seemingly of intuitive value, the role of viability testing to guide revascularization decisions in patients with ischemic cardiomyopathy is not clear.[44,240,281] Observational studies had suggested that patients with ischemic cardiomyopathy who have extensive multivessel CAD and viable myocardium may derive a survival advantage with CABG. Nonetheless, in the randomized STICH trial (see Coronary Artery Bypass Grafting: Patients with Depressed Left Ventricular Function), viability testing did not appear to identify patients in whom CABG provided incremental survival benefit.[240] Similarly, the small PET and Recovery Following Revascularization-2 (PARR-2) study of 430 patients randomly assigned to PET-guided management versus standard care did not demonstrate an advantage of revascularization when viability testing was used as a guide.[241] Additional, rigorous, adequately sized observational studies and randomized controlled trials are needed to define the role of viability testing.

Mitral Regurgitation Secondary to Coronary Artery Disease

Mitral regurgitation is an important cause of heart failure in some patients with CAD. Rupture of a papillary muscle or the head of a papillary muscle usually causes severe acute mitral regurgitation in the course of acute MI. The cause of chronic mitral regurgitation in patients with CAD is multifactorial, and the geometric determinants are complex; these include papillary muscle dysfunction from ischemia and fibrosis in conjunction with a wall motion abnormality and changes in LV shape in the region of the papillary muscle and/or dilation of the mitral annulus. Enlargement of the mitral annulus at end-systole is asymmetric, with lengthening primarily involving the posterior annular segments and leading to prolapse of leaflet tissue tethered by the posterior papillary muscle and restriction of leaflet tissue attached to the anterior leaflet. Most patients with SIHD and mitral regurgitation have previously suffered an MI. Clinical features that help identify mitral regurgitation secondary to papillary muscle dysfunction as the cause of acute pulmonary edema or of milder symptoms of left-sided heart failure include a loud systolic murmur and demonstration of a flail mitral valve leaflet on echocardiography. In some patients with severe mitral regurgitation into a small, noncompliant left atrium, the murmur may be unimpressive or inaudible. Doppler echocardiography is helpful in assessing the severity of the regurgitation. As in mitral regurgitation of other causes, the left atrium is not usually greatly enlarged unless mitral regurgitation has been present for more than 6 months. The ECG is nonspecific, and most patients have angiographic evidence of multivessel CAD.

Management

In patients with severe mitral regurgitation, the indications for surgical correction, usually in association with CABG, are fairly clear-cut. Because of progression of underlying LV dysfunction and resultant structural abnormalities, mitral valve repair is not always durable.[285] In a randomized trial from the NHLBI Cardiothoracic Surgery Network (CTSN), mitral replacement was equivalent to repair in producing reverse LV remodeling and resulted in more durable correction.[286] The decision for mitral valve surgery is based on the anatomic characteristics of the structures forming the mitral valve apparatus, the urgency of the need for surgery, and the severity of LV dysfunction.

A more complex and frequently encountered problem has involved the indications for mitral valve surgery in patients undergoing a CABG procedure in whom the severity of mitral regurgitation is moderate. In a trial comparing CABG alone with CABG plus mitral-valve repair in 301 patients with moderate ischemic mitral regurgitation, mitral valve repair reduced the 2-year rate of moderate or severe residual mitral regurgitation (11.2% versus 32.3%, $P < 0.001$) but did not result in a significant difference in the LV end-systolic volume index (LVESVI) or survival at 1 year or 2 years of follow-up (HR 0.90; 95% CI, 0.45 to 1.83; $P = 0.78$).[286] Individual treatment decisions require balancing the risks of an increased rate of adverse perioperative events with combined surgery against uncertain benefits of a lower incidence of postoperative moderate or severe mitral regurgitation.

The average mortality associated with combined CABG and mitral valve repair is less than 6%.[223] Predictors of early mortality include the need for replacement versus repair (in some but not all series) but, in addition, may include other variables such as age, comorbid conditions, the urgency of surgery, and LV function. Late results are strongly influenced by the pathophysiologic mechanisms underlying mitral regurgitation and are poorer in patients with regurgitation resulting from annular dilation or restrictive leaflet motion than in patients with chordal or papillary muscle rupture. It is encouraging that despite the relatively high operative mortality, long-term outcomes of hospital survivors are excellent. In patients with very poor LV function and dilation of the mitral annulus, mitral regurgitation can intensify the severity of LV failure. In such patients the risk associated with surgery is high and the long-term benefit is not established, and a trial of intensive medical therapy, including afterload reduction and beta blockade, and biventricular pacing in patients with prolonged QRS duration on the 12-lead ECG may be worthwhile because favorable remodeling may reduce the severity of mitral regurgitation without the need for surgery.[285,287] For patients undergoing CABG, the procedural risks associated with combined CABG and mitral valve repair may outweigh the benefit of reduced mitral regurgitation in those at highest perioperative risk.

Among patients with ischemic mitral regurgitation at high risk for surgery, transcatheter mitral valve repair may be a consideration. The role of transcatheter-based procedures for mitral valve disease is rapidly evolving. The most commonly performed percutaneous mitral procedure is the edge-to-edge repair with the MitraClip. This procedure provides an alternative to surgical mitral repair when surgical risk is prohibitive, but it is associated with less complete and less durable results than surgical.

CARDIAC ARRHYTHMIAS

In some patients with CAD, cardiac arrhythmias are the dominant clinical manifestation of the disease. Various degrees and forms of ventricular ectopic activity are the most common arrhythmias in patients with CAD, but serious ventricular arrhythmias may be a major component of the clinical findings in other subgroups. The clinical features of arrhythmias and their management in patients with CAD are discussed in Part VII.

NONATHEROMATOUS CORONARY ARTERY DISEASE

Although atherosclerosis is by far the most common cause of CAD, other conditions may also be responsible. These include congenital abnormalities in the origin or distribution of the coronary arteries (see Chapters 20, 21, and 82), the most important of which are anomalous origin of a coronary artery (usually the left) from the pulmonary artery, origin of both coronary arteries from either the right or the left sinus of Valsalva, and coronary arteriovenous fistula. An anomalous origin of the left main coronary artery or right coronary artery from the aorta, with subsequent coursing between the aorta and pulmonary trunk, is a rare and sometimes fatal coronary arterial anomaly. Coronary anomalies are reported to cause between 12% and 19% of sports-related deaths in U.S. high school and college athletes and account for a third of cardiac anomalies in military recruits with non-traumatic sudden death.

MYOCARDIAL BRIDGING

This cause of systolic compression of the LAD coronary artery is a well-recognized angiographic phenomenon of questionable clinical significance.[78]

CONNECTIVE TISSUE DISORDERS
Several inherited connective tissue disorders are associated with myocardial ischemia, including Marfan syndrome (causing aortic and coronary artery dissection), Hurler syndrome (causing coronary obstruction), Ehlers-Danlos syndrome (causing coronary artery dissection), and pseudoxanthoma elasticum (causing accelerated CAD).

SPONTANEOUS CORONARY DISSECTION
This is a rare cause of MI and sudden cardiac death that is much more common in women than men and is often unrecognized or misdiagnosed.[288,289] Chronic dissection manifesting as heart failure has been described. Some cases are associated with atherosclerosis. Emerging data suggests that fibromuscular dysplasia may be an important cause of this syndrome and screening of the renal arteries with angiography or CTA is recommended. Other contributing factors include estrogen use and hypertension. In the acute phase, a conservative strategy is recommended as PCI failure rates are high, iatrogenic dissection is common, and complete healing may lead to a favorable outcome without intervention.[288,289] In one study, angiographic healing was apparent in 95% of patients undergoing repeat angiography more than 30 days post-spontaneous dissection.[290] In survivors of spontaneous coronary artery dissection, the subsequent 3-year mortality is about 20%, and 10% to 15% of patients suffer a recurrent dissection.

CORONARY VASCULITIS AND VASCULOPATHY
Connective tissue diseases or autoimmune forms of vasculitis, including polyarteritis nodosa, giant cell (temporal) arteritis, or vasculopathy, such as scleroderma, can involve the coronary arteries (see Chapter 97). Kawasaki disease, a mucocutaneous lymph node syndrome, may cause coronary artery aneurysms and IHD in children. Coronary arteritis is seen at autopsy in approximately 20% of patients with rheumatoid arthritis but is rarely associated with clinical manifestations. The incidence of CAD is increased in women with systemic lupus erythematosus (SLE). In patients with SLE, CAD has been attributed to vasculitis, immune complex–mediated endothelial damage, and coronary thrombosis from antiphospholipid antibodies, as well as accelerated atherosclerosis. Antiphospholipid syndrome, characterized by arterial and venous thrombosis and the presence of antiphospholipid antibodies, may be associated with MI, angina, and diffuse LV dysfunction. Luetic aortitis may also produce myocardial ischemia by causing coronary ostial obstruction.

TAKAYASU ARTERITIS
In rare cases (see Chapter 97), this condition is associated with angina, MI, and cardiac failure in patients younger than 40 years. Coronary blood flow may be decreased by involvement of the ostia or proximal segments of the coronary arteries, but disease in distal coronary segments is rare. The average age at the onset of symptoms is 24 years, and the event-free survival rate 10 years after diagnosis is approximately 60%. CT angiography has been shown to be useful in detecting involvement of the coronary arteries in Takayasu arteritis.

POSTMEDIASTINAL IRRADIATION
The occurrence of CAD and morbid cardiac events in young individuals after mediastinal irradiation is highly suggestive of a cause-and-effect relationship. Pathologic changes include adventitial scarring and medial hypertrophy with severe intimal atherosclerotic disease. Radiation injury may be latent and may not be manifested clinically for many years after therapy. Contributory factors include higher doses than those currently administered and the presence of cardiac risk factors. In patients without risk factors who receive an intermediate total dose of 30 to 40 Gy, the risk for cardiac death and MI is low.

Cardiac Transplantation–Associated Coronary Arteriopathy
See Chapters 24 and 60.

FUTURE PERSPECTIVES
Despite the fact that Heberden aptly described angina almost two and a half centuries ago, our understanding of the syndrome, its causes, and optimal management continue to evolve. We wish to highlight three major areas in need of continued investigation. First, given evolving insight into the heterogenous causes of myocardial ischemia in the absence of obstructive epicardial coronary disease, research should move forward to elucidate therapies that are more clearly effective for this set of conditions. Preclinical, translational, and clinical epidemiologic data have all demonstrated abnormalities in coronary artery function that may result in myocardial ischemia in the absence of atherosclerotic obstruction. However, as yet, therapies proposed to address this important syndrome appear to be insufficient. Second, although it is now clear that a strategy of routine revascularization does not improve intermediate-term survival compared with OMT alone in most patients with SIHD, including patients with moderate or severe ischemia on noninvasive testing, the emergence of a possible late reduction in nonprocedural MI in the ISCHEMIA trial has raised the possibility that a survival benefit may emerge with longer-term follow-up. Moreover, the results of the ISCHEMIA trial, in which even severe ischemia did not identify patients who benefited from initial revascularization, prompts a reappraisal of the role of functional testing for risk stratification and clinical decision making in patients with suspected CAD. Third, recent positive clinical trials of anti-inflammatory therapies that do not modify lipids, such as canakinumab and colchicine, have provided much needed proof to support the inflammatory hypothesis of atherosclerosis. However, the benefits of these therapies may be partially countered by increased risk for infection and other complications. Thus, additional investigation of these and other anti-inflammatory therapies in needed to more fully characterize their risk-benefit profile and to establish their role in patients with SIHD.

REFERENCES
Guideline Overview
1. Knuuti J, Wijns W, Saraste A, et al. 2019 ESC Guidelines for the diagnosis and management of chronic coronary syndromes. *Eur Heart J.* 2020;41:407–477.
2. Pepine CJ. Multiple causes for ischemia without obstructive coronary artery disease: not a short list. *Circulation.* 2015;131:1044–1046.
3. Marzilli M, Crea F, Morrone D, et al. Myocardial ischemia: from disease to syndrome. *Int J Cardiol.* 2020;314:32–35.
4. Virani SS, Alonso A, Aparicio HJ, et al. Heart Disease and Stroke Statistics-2021 update: a report from the American Heart Association. *Circulation.* 2021;143:s254–e743.
5. Spertus JA, Arnold SV. The evolution of patient-reported outcomes in clinical trials and management of patients with coronary artery disease: 20 Years with the Seattle angina questionnaire. *JAMA Cardiol.* 2018;3:1035–1036.
6. Spertus JA, Jones PG, Maron DJ, et al. Health-status outcomes with invasive or conservative care in coronary disease. *N Engl J Med.* 2020;382:1408–1419.
7. Arnett DK, Blumenthal RS, Albert MA, et al. 2019 ACC/AHA guideline on the primary prevention of cardiovascular disease: a report of the American College of Cardiology/American Heart Association task force on clinical practice guidelines. *J Am Coll Cardiol.* 2019;74:e177–e232.
8. Grundy SM, Stone NJ, Bailey AL, et al. 2018 AHA/ACC/AACVPR/AAPA/ABC/ACPM/ADA/AGS/APhA/ASPC/NLA/PCNA guideline on the management of blood cholesterol: a report of the American College of Cardiology/American Heart Association task force on clinical practice guidelines. *Circulation.* 2019;139:e1082–e1143.
9. Mach F, Baigent C, Catapano AL, et al. 2019 ESC/EAS Guidelines for the management of dyslipidaemias: lipid modification to reduce cardiovascular risk. *Eur Heart J.* 2020;41:111–188.

Evaluation and Medical Management
10. Burgess S, Ference BA, Staley JR, et al. Association of LPA variants with risk of coronary disease and the implications for lipoprotein(a)-lowering therapies: a mendelian randomization analysis. *JAMA Cardiol.* 2018;3:619–627.
11. O'Donoghue ML, Fazio S, Giugliano RP, et al. Lipoprotein(a), PCSK9 inhibition, and cardiovascular risk. *Circulation.* 2019;139:1483–1492.
12. Bittner VA, Szarek M, Aylward PE, et al. Effect of alirocumab on lipoprotein(a) and cardiovascular risk after acute coronary syndrome. *J Am Coll Cardiol.* 2020;75:133–144.
13. Tsimikas S, Karwatowska-Prokopczuk E, Gouni-Berthold I, et al. Lipoprotein(a) reduction in persons with cardiovascular disease. *N Engl J Med.* 2020;382:244–255.
14. Chrysant SG, Chrysant GS. The current status of homocysteine as a risk factor for cardiovascular disease: a mini review. *Expert Rev Cardiovasc Ther.* 2018;16:559–565.
15. Bonaca MP, O'Malley RG, Jarolim P, et al. Serial cardiac troponin measured using a high-sensitivity assay in stable patients with ischemic heart disease. *J Am Coll Cardiol.* 2016;68:322–323.
16. Cavender MA, White WB, Jarolim P, et al. Serial measurement of high-sensitivity troponin I and cardiovascular outcomes in patients with type 2 diabetes mellitus in the EXAMINE trial (examination of cardiovascular outcomes with alogliptin versus standard of care). *Circulation.* 2017;135:1911–1921.
17. Eisen A, Bonaca MP, Jarolim P, et al. High-sensitivity troponin I in stable patients with atherosclerotic disease in the TRA 2 degrees P - TIMI 50 trial. *Clin Chem.* 2017;63:307–315.
18. Januzzi Jr JL, Butler J, Jarolim P, et al. Effects of canagliflozin on cardiovascular biomarkers in older adults with type 2 diabetes. *J Am Coll Cardiol.* 2017;70:704–712.
19. Marston NA, Bonaca MP, Jarolim P, et al. Clinical application of high-sensitivity troponin testing in the atherosclerotic cardiovascular disease framework of the current cholesterol guidelines. *JAMA Cardiol.* 2020;5:1255–1262.
20. Pandey A, Patel KV, Vongpatanasin W, et al. Incorporation of biomarkers into risk assessment for allocation of antihypertensive medication according to the 2017 ACC/AHA high blood pressure guideline: a pooled cohort analysis. *Circulation.* 2019;140:2076–2088.
20a. Marston NA, Oyama K, Jarolim p, et al. Combining high-sensitivity troponin with the AHA/ACC cholesterol guidelines to guide evolocumab therapy. *Circulation.* 2021;144(3):249–251.
21. Berry JD, Nambi V, Ambrosius W, et al. Associations of high sensitivity troponin and natriuretic peptide levels with outcomes after intensive blood pressure lowering: findings from SPRINT. *JAMA Cardioln.* 2021 (in press).

22. Omland T, White HD. State of the art: blood biomarkers for risk stratification in patients with stable ischemic heart disease. Clin Chem. 2017;63:165–176.
23. Ridker PM, Everett BM, Thuren T, et al. Antiinflammatory therapy with canakinumab for atherosclerotic disease. N Engl J Med. 2017;377:1119–1131.
24. Nidorf SM, Fiolet ATL, Mosterd A, et al. Colchicine in patients with chronic coronary disease. N Engl J Med. 2020;383:1838–1847.
25. Bohula EA, Giugliano RP, Leiter LA, et al. Inflammatory and cholesterol risk in the FOURIER trial. Circulation. 2018;138:131–140.
26. Ridker PM, MacFadyen JG, Everett BM, et al. Relationship of C-reactive protein reduction to cardiovascular event reduction following treatment with canakinumab: a secondary analysis from the CANTOS randomised controlled trial. Lancet. 2018;391:319–328.
27. Fanola CL, Morrow DA, Cannon CP, et al. Interleukin-6 and the risk of adverse outcomes in patients after an acute coronary syndrome: observations from the SOLID-TIMI 52 (Stabilization of Plaque using Darapladib-Thrombolysis in Myocardial Infarction 52) trial. J Am Heart Assoc. 2017;6:e005637.
28. Ridker PM, MacFadyen JG, Glynn RJ, et al. Comparison of interleukin-6, C-reactive protein, and low-density lipoprotein cholesterol as biomarkers of residual risk in contemporary practice: secondary analyses from the Cardiovascular Inflammation Reduction Trial. Eur Heart J. 2020;41:2952–2961.
29. Ridker PM, MacFadyen JG, Thuren T, et al. Residual inflammatory risk associated with interleukin-18 and interleukin-6 after successful interleukin-1beta inhibition with canakinumab: further rationale for the development of targeted anti-cytokine therapies for the treatment of atherothrombosis. Eur Heart J. 2020;41:2153–2163.
30. Tang WHW, Backhed F, Landmesser U, et al. Intestinal microbiota in cardiovascular health and disease: JACC state-of-the-art review. J Am Coll Cardiol. 2019;73:2089–2105.
31. Khan SS, Cooper R, Greenland P. Do polygenic risk scores improve patient selection for prevention of coronary artery disease? J Am Med Assoc. 2020;323:614–615.
32. Aragam KG, Dobbyn A, Judy R, et al. Limitations of contemporary guidelines for managing patients at high genetic risk of coronary artery disease. J Am Coll Cardiol. 2020;75:2769–2780.
33. Labos C, Thanassoulis G. Genetic risk prediction for primary and secondary prevention of atherosclerotic cardiovascular disease: an update. Curr Cardiol Rep. 2018;20:36.
34. Mega JL, Stitziel NO, Smith JG, et al. Genetic risk, coronary heart disease events, and the clinical benefit of statin therapy: an analysis of primary and secondary prevention trials. Lancet. 2015;385:2264–2271.
35. Marston NA, Kamanu FK, Nordio F, et al. Predicting benefit from evolocumab therapy in patients with atherosclerotic disease using a genetic risk score: results from the FOURIER trial. Circulation. 2020;141:616–623.
36. Fihn SD, Blankenship JC, Alexander KP, et al. 2014 ACC/AHA/AATS/PCNA/SCAI/STS focused update of the guideline for the diagnosis and management of patients with stable ischemic heart disease: a report of the American College of Cardiology/American Heart Association task force on practice guidelines, and the American Association for Thoracic Surgery, Preventive Cardiovascular Nurses Association, Society for Cardiovascular Angiography and Interventions, and Society of Thoracic Surgeons. J Am Coll Cardiol. 2014;64:1929–1949.
37. Gulati M, Levy PD, Mukherjee D, et al. AHA/ACC/ASE/CHEST/SAEM/SCCT/SCMR guideline for the evaluation and diagnosis of chest pain: a report of the American College of Cardiology/American Heart Association Joint Committee on Clinical Practice Guidelines. J Am Coll Cardiol. 2021.
38. Bittencourt MS, Hulten E, Polonsky TS, et al. European Society of Cardiology-recommended coronary artery disease consortium pretest probability scores more accurately predict obstructive coronary disease and cardiovascular events than the Diamond and Forrester score: the partners registry. Circulation. 2016;134:201–211.
39. Polonsky TS, Blankstein R. Exercise treadmill testing. J Am Med Assoc. 2015;314:1968–1969.
40. Mieres JH, Bonow RO. Ischemic heart disease in women: a need for sex-specific diagnostic algorithms. JACC Cardiovasc Imaging. 2016;9:347–349.
41. Baldassarre LA, Raman SV, Min JK, et al. Noninvasive imaging to evaluate women with stable ischemic heart disease. JACC Cardiovasc Imaging. 2016;9:421–435.
42. Aggarwal NR, Bond RM, Mieres JH. The role of imaging in women with ischemic heart disease. Clin Cardiol. 2018;41:194–202.
43. Schindler TH, Bateman TM, Berman DS, et al. Appropriate use criteria for PET myocardial perfusion imaging. J Nucl Med. 2020;61:1221–1265.
44. Garcia MJ, Kwong RY, Scherrer-Crosbie M, et al. State of the art: imaging for myocardial viability: a scientific statement from the American Heart Association. Circ Cardiovasc Imaging. 2020;13:e000053.
45. Di Carli MF. Challenges and opportunities for nuclear cardiology. J Nucl Cardiol. 2019;26:1043–1046.
46. Pellikka PA, Arruda-Olson A, Chaudhry FA, et al. Guidelines for performance, interpretation, and application of stress echocardiography in ischemic heart disease: from the American Society of Echocardiography. J Am Soc Echocardiogr. 2020;33:1–41.e48.
47. Blankstein R, Shaw LJ, Nasir K. The not so secret power of cardiac CT: prevention and value. J Cardiovasc Comput Tomogr. 2020;14:289–290.
48. Shaw L, Kwong RY, Nagel E, et al. Cardiac imaging in the post-ISCHEMIA trial era: a multisociety viewpoint. JACC Cardiovasc Imaging. 2020;13:1815–1833.
49. Stuijfzand WJ, van Rosendael AR, Lin FY, et al. Stress myocardial perfusion imaging vs coronary computed tomographic angiography for diagnosis of invasive vessel-specific coronary physiology: predictive modeling results from the Computed Tomographic Evaluation of Atherosclerotic Determinants of Myocardial Ischemia (CREDENCE) trial. JAMA Cardiol. 2020;5:1338–1348.
50. Douglas PS, Hoffmann U, Patel MR, et al. Outcomes of anatomical versus functional testing for coronary artery disease. N Engl J Med. 2015;372:1291–1300.
51. Scot-Heart Investigators, Newby DE, Adamson PD, et al. Coronary CT angiography and 5-year risk of myocardial infarction. N Engl J Med. 2018;379:924–933.
52. Adamson PD, Williams MC, Dweck MR, et al. Guiding therapy by coronary CT angiography improves outcomes in patients with stable chest pain. J Am Coll Cardiol. 2019;74:2058–2070.
53. Patel AR, Bamberg F, Branch K, et al. Society of cardiovascular computed tomography expert consensus document on myocardial computed tomography perfusion imaging. J Cardiovasc Comput Tomogr. 2020;14:87–100.
54. Di Carli MF, Geva T, Davidoff R. The future of cardiovascular imaging. Circulation. 2016;133:2640–2661.
55. Daghem M, Bing R, Fayad ZA, et al. Noninvasive imaging to assess atherosclerotic plaque composition and disease activity: coronary and carotid applications. JACC Cardiovasc Imaging. 2020;13:1055–1068.
56. van den Hoogen IJ, van Rosendael AR, Lin FY, et al. Coronary computed tomography angiography as a gatekeeper to coronary revascularization: emphasizing atherosclerosis findings beyond stenosis. Curr Cardiovasc Imaging Rep. 2019;12:24.
57. Zhuang B, Wang S, Zhao S, et al. Computed Tomography Angiography-Derived Fractional Flow Reserve (CT-FFR) for the detection of myocardial ischemia with invasive fractional flow reserve as reference: systematic review and meta-analysis. Eur Radiol. 2020;30:712–725.
58. Maron DJ, Hochman JS, Reynolds HR, et al. Initial invasive or conservative strategy for stable coronary disease. N Engl J Med. 2020;382:1395–1407.
59. Blankstein R, Shaw LJ. Ischemia trial: implications for coronary CT angiography. J Cardiovasc Comput Tomogr. 2020;14:1–2.

60. Greenwood JP, Walker S. Stress CMR imaging for stable chest pain syndromes: underused and undervalued? JACC Cardiovasc Imaging. 2020;13:1518–1520.
61. Kwong RY, Ge Y, Steel K, et al. Cardiac magnetic resonance stress perfusion imaging for evaluation of patients with chest pain. J Am Coll Cardiol. 2019;74:1741–1755.
62. Antiochos P, Ge Y, Steel K, et al. Evaluation of stress cardiac magnetic resonance imaging in risk reclassification of patients with suspected coronary artery disease. JAMA Cardiol. 2020.
63. Nagel E, Greenwood JP, McCann GP, et al. Magnetic resonance perfusion or fractional flow reserve in coronary disease. N Engl J Med. 2019;380:2418–2428.
64. Hajhosseiny R, Bustin A, Munoz C, et al. Coronary magnetic resonance angiography: technical innovations leading us to the promised land? JACC Cardiovasc Imaging. 2020;13:2653–2672.
65. Bairey Merz CN, Pepine CJ, Walsh MN, et al. Ischemia and No Obstructive Coronary Artery Disease (INOCA): developing evidence-based therapies and research agenda for the next decade. Circulation. 2017;135:1075–1092.
66. Malik AH, Yandrapalli S, Aronow WS, et al. Intravascular ultrasound-guided stent implantation reduces cardiovascular mortality - updated meta-analysis of randomized controlled trials. Int J Cardiol. 2020;299:100–105.
67. Hirai T, Chen Z, Zhang L, et al. Evaluation of variable thin-cap fibroatheroma definitions and association of virtual histology-intravascular ultrasound findings with cavity rupture size. Am J Cardiol. 2016;118:162–169.
68. Waksman R, Di Mario C, Torguson R, et al. Identification of patients and plaques vulnerable to future coronary events with near-infrared spectroscopy intravascular ultrasound imaging: a prospective, cohort study. Lancet. 2019;394:1629–1637.
69. Ramasamy A, Chen Y, Zanchin T, et al. Optical coherence tomography enables more accurate detection of functionally significant intermediate non-left main coronary artery stenoses than intravascular ultrasound: a meta-analysis of 6919 patients and 7537 lesions. Int J Cardiol. 2020;301:226–234.
70. Reynolds HR. Coronary optical coherence tomography and cardiac magnetic resonance imaging to determine underlying causes of myocardial infarction with nonobstructive coronary arteries in women. Circulation. 2021;143:624–640.
71. Kogame N, Ono M, Kawashima H, et al. The impact of coronary physiology on contemporary clinical decision making. JACC Cardiovasc Interv. 2020;13:1617–1638.
72. De Maria GL, Garcia-Garcia HM, Scarsini R, et al. Novel indices of coronary physiology: do we need alternatives to fractional flow reserve? Circ Cardiovasc Interv. 2020;13:e008487.
73. Davies JE, Sen S, Dehbi HM, et al. Use of the instantaneous wave-free ratio or fractional flow reserve in PCI. N Engl J Med. 2017;376:1824–1834.
74. Gotberg M, Christiansen EH, Gudmundsdottir IJ, et al. Instantaneous wave-free ratio versus fractional flow reserve to guide PCI. N Engl J Med. 2017;376:1813–1823.
75. De Bruyne B, Oldroyd KG, Pijls NH. Microvascular (Dys)Function and clinical outcome in stable coronary disease. J Am Coll Cardiol. 2016;67:1170–1172.
76. Ford TJ, Stanley B, Sidik N, et al. 1-Year outcomes of angina management guided by invasive coronary function testing (CorMicA). JACC Cardiovasc Interv. 2020;13:33–45.
77. Kawsara A, Nunez Gil IJ, Alqahtani F, et al. Management of coronary artery aneurysms. JACC Cardiovasc Interv. 2018;11:1211–1223.
78. Murtaza G, Mukherjee D, Gharacholou SM, et al. An updated review on myocardial bridging. Cardiovasc Revasc Med. 2020;21:1169–1179.
79. Ohman EM. Chronic stable angina. N Engl J Med. 2016;374:1167–1176.
80. Bohula EA, Bonaca MP, Braunwald E, et al. Atherothrombotic risk stratification and the efficacy and safety of vorapaxar in patients with stable ischemic heart disease and previous myocardial infarction. Circulation. 2016;134:304–313.
81. Bohula EA, Morrow DA, Cannon CP, et al. Atherothrombotic risk stratification and ezetimibe use in improve-it. J Am Coll Cardiol. 2016;67:2129.
82. Urban P, Mehran R, Colleran R, et al. Defining high bleeding risk in patients undergoing percutaneous coronary intervention. Circulation. 2019;140:240–261.
83. Sorbets E, Steg PG, Young R, et al. Beta-blockers, calcium antagonists, and mortality in stable coronary artery disease: an international cohort study. Eur Heart J. 2019;40:1399–1407.
84. Joseph P, Swedberg K, Leong DP, et al. The evolution of beta-blockers in coronary artery disease and heart failure (Part 1/5). J Am Coll Cardiol. 2019;74:672–682.
85. Rosendorff C, Lackland DT, Allison M, et al. Treatment of hypertension in patients with coronary artery disease: a scientific statement from the American Heart Association, American College of Cardiology, and American Society of Hypertension. Circulation. 2015;131:e435–e470.
86. Whelton PK, Carey RM, Aronow WS, et al. 2017 ACC/AHA/AAPA/ABC/ACPM/AGS/APhA/ASH/ASPC/NMA/PCNA guideline for the prevention, detection, evaluation, and management of high blood pressure in adults: a report of the American College of Cardiology/American Heart Association task force on clinical practice guidelines. Hypertension. 2018;71:e13–e115.
87. Bohm M, Schumacher H, Teo KK, et al. Achieved diastolic blood pressure and pulse pressure at target systolic blood pressure (120-140 mmHg) and cardiovascular outcomes in high-risk patients: results from ONTARGET and TRANSCEND trials. Eur Heart J. 2018;39:3105–3114.
88. The SPRINT Research Group. A randomized trial of intensive versus standard blood-pressure control. N Engl J Med. 2015;373:2103–2116.
89. Dinakar C, O'Connor GT. The health effects of electronic cigarettes. N Engl J Med. 2016;375:1372–1381.
90. King BA, Jones CM, Baldwin GT, et al. The EVALI and youth vaping epidemics - implications for public health. N Engl J Med. 2020;382:689–691.
91. Buchanan ND, Grimmer JA, Tanwar V, et al. Cardiovascular risk of electronic cigarettes: a review of preclinical and clinical studies. Cardiovasc Res. 2020;116:40–50.
92. Kavousi M, Pisinger C, Barthelemy JC, et al. Electronic cigarettes and health with special focus on cardiovascular effects: position paper of the European Association of Preventive Cardiology (EAPC). Eur J Prev Cardiol. 2020. 2047487320941993.
93. Cannon CP, Blazing MA, Giugliano RP, et al. Ezetimibe added to statin therapy after acute coronary syndromes. N Engl J Med. 2015;372:2387–2397.
94. Sabatine MS, Giugliano RP, Keech AC, et al. Evolocumab and clinical outcomes in patients with cardiovascular disease. N Engl J Med. 2017;376:1713–1722.
95. Schwartz GG, Steg PG, Szarek M, et al. Alirocumab and cardiovascular outcomes after acute coronary syndrome. N Engl J Med. 2018;379:2097–2107.
96. Giugliano RP, Mach F, Zavitz K, et al. Cognitive function in a randomized trial of evolocumab. N Engl J Med. 2017;377:633–643.
97. Schwartz GG, Steg PG, Szarek M, et al. Peripheral artery disease and venous thromboembolic events after acute coronary syndrome: role of lipoprotein(a) and modification by alirocumab: prespecified analysis of the ODYSSEY OUTCOMES randomized clinical trial. Circulation. 2020;141:1608–1617.
98. Allard-Ratick MP, Kindya BR, Khambhati J, et al. HDL: fact, fiction, or function? HDL cholesterol and cardiovascular risk. Eur J Prev Cardiol. 2019. 2047487319848214.
99. Wilson PWF, Polonsky TS, Miedema MD, et al. Systematic review for the 2018 AHA/ACC/AACVPR/AAPA/ABC/ACPM/ADA/AGS/APhA/ASPC/NLA/PCNA guideline on the management of blood cholesterol: a report of the American College of Cardiology/American Heart Association task force on clinical practice guidelines. J Am Coll Cardiol. 2019;73:3210–3227.
100. Riaz H, Khan SU, Rahman H, et al. Effects of high-density lipoprotein targeting treatments on cardiovascular outcomes: a systematic review and meta-analysis. Eur J Prev Cardiol. 2019;26:533–543.

101. Lincoff AM, Nicholls SJ, Riesmeyer JS, et al. Evacetrapib and cardiovascular outcomes in high-risk vascular disease. *N Engl J Med*. 2017;376:1933–1942.
102. HPS3/TIMI55-REVEAL Collaborative Group, Bowman L, Hopewell JC, et al. Effects of anacetrapib in patients with atherosclerotic vascular disease. *N Engl J Med*. 2017;377:1217–1227.
103. Mason RP, Libby P, Bhatt DL. Emerging mechanisms of cardiovascular protection for the omega-3 fatty acid eicosapentaenoic acid. *Arterioscler Thromb Vasc Biol*. 2020;40:1135–1147.
104. Ascend Study Collaborative Group, Bowman L, Mafham M, et al. Effects of n-3 fatty acid supplements in diabetes mellitus. *N Engl J Med*. 2018;379:1540–1550.
105. Manson JE, Cook NR, Lee IM, et al. Marine n-3 fatty acids and prevention of cardiovascular disease and cancer. *N Engl J Med*. 2019;380:23–32.
106. Nicholls SJ. Effect of high-dose omega-3 fatty acids vs corn oil on major adverse cardiovascular events in patients at high cardiovascular risk: the STRENGTH randomized clinical trial. *J Am Med Assoc*. 2020;324:2268–2280.
107. Bhatt DL, Steg PG, Miller M, et al. Cardiovascular risk reduction with icosapent ethyl for hypertriglyceridemia. *N Engl J Med*. 2019;380:11–22.
108. Peterson BE, Bhatt DL, Steg PG, et al. Reduction in revascularization with icosapent ethyl: insights from REDUCE-IT REVASC. *Circulation*. 2020;143:33–44.
109. Arnold SV, Bhatt DL, Barsness GW, et al. Clinical management of stable coronary artery disease in patients with type 2 diabetes mellitus: a scientific statement from the American Heart Association. *Circulation*. 2020;141:e779–e806.
110. Cosentino F, Grant PJ, Aboyans V, et al. 2019 ESC Guidelines on diabetes, pre-diabetes, and cardiovascular diseases developed in collaboration with the EASD. *Eur Heart J*. 2020;41:255–323.
111. American Diabetes Association 6. Glycemic targets: standards of medical care in diabetes-2020. *Diabetes Care*. 2020;43:S66–S76.
112. American Diabetes Association. 9. Pharmacologic approaches to glycemic treatment: standards of medical care in diabetes-2020. *Diabetes Care*. 2020;43:S98–S110.
113. Das SR, Everett BM, Birtcher KK, et al. 2020 expert consensus decision pathway on novel therapies for cardiovascular risk reduction in patients with type 2 diabetes: a report of the American College of Cardiology Solution Set Oversight Committee. *J Am Coll Cardiol*. 2020;76:1117–1145.
114. Zelniker TA, Braunwald E. Cardiac and renal effects of sodium-glucose Co-transporter 2 inhibitors in diabetes: JACC state-of-the-art review. *J Am Coll Cardiol*. 2018;72:1845–1855.
115. Zinman B, Wanner C, Lachin JM, et al. Empagliflozin, cardiovascular outcomes, and mortality in type 2 diabetes. *N Engl J Med*. 2015;373:2117–2128.
116. Neal B, Perkovic V, Matthews DR. Canagliflozin and cardiovascular and renal events in type 2 diabetes. *N Engl J Med*. 2017;377:2099.
117. Wiviott SD, Raz I, Bonaca MP, et al. Dapagliflozin and cardiovascular outcomes in type 2 diabetes. *N Engl J Med*. 2019;380:347–357.
118. Zelniker TA, Wiviott SD, Raz I, et al. SGLT2 inhibitors for primary and secondary prevention of cardiovascular and renal outcomes in type 2 diabetes: a systematic review and meta-analysis of cardiovascular outcome trials. *Lancet*. 2019;393:31–39.
119. Marso SP, Daniels GH, Brown-Frandsen K, et al. Liraglutide and cardiovascular outcomes in type 2 diabetes. *N Engl J Med*. 2016;375:311–322.
120. Marso SP, Bain SC, Consoli A, et al. Semaglutide and cardiovascular outcomes in patients with type 2 diabetes. *N Engl J Med*. 2016;375:1834–1844.
121. Lavie CJ, Pack QR, Levine GN. Expanding traditional cardiac rehabilitation in the 21st century. *J Am Coll Cardiol*. 2020;75:1562–1564.
122. Anderson L, Oldridge N, Thompson DR, et al. Exercise-based cardiac rehabilitation for coronary heart disease: Cochrane systematic review and meta-analysis. *J Am Coll Cardiol*. 2016;67:1–12.
123. Lavie CJ, Ozemek C, Kachur S. Promoting physical activity in primary and secondary prevention. *Eur Heart J*. 2019;40:3556–3558.
124. Jeong SW, Kim SH, Kang SH, et al. Mortality reduction with physical activity in patients with and without cardiovascular disease. *Eur Heart J*. 2019;40:3547–3555.
125. Thomas RJ, Beatty AL, Beckie TM, et al. Home-based cardiac rehabilitation: a scientific statement from the American Association of Cardiovascular and Pulmonary Rehabilitation, the American Heart Association, and the American College of Cardiology. *Circulation*. 2019;140:e69–e89.
126. Jaacks LM, Vandevijvere S, Pan A, et al. The obesity transition: stages of the global epidemic. *Lancet Diabetes Endocrinol*. 2019;7:231–240.
127. Mozaffarian D. Dietary and policy priorities for cardiovascular disease, diabetes, and obesity: a comprehensive review. *Circulation*. 2016;133:187–225.
128. Angell SY, McConnell MV, Anderson CAM, et al. The American Heart Association 2030 impact goal: a presidential advisory from the American Heart Association. *Circulation*. 2020;141:e120–e138.
129. Bohula EA, Wiviott SD, McGuire DK, et al. Cardiovascular safety of lorcaserin in overweight or obese patients. *N Engl J Med*. 2018;379:1107–1117.
130. Singh AK, Singh R. Pharmacotherapy in obesity: a systematic review and meta-analysis of randomized controlled trials of anti-obesity drugs. *Expert Rev Clin Pharmacol*. 2020;13:53–64.
131. Naslund E, Stenberg E, Hofmann R, et al. Association of metabolic surgery with major adverse cardiovascular outcomes in patients with previous myocardial infarction and severe obesity: a nationwide cohort study. *Circulation*. 2021;143:1458–1467.
132. Libby P, Hansson GK. Inflammation and immunity in diseases of the arterial tree: players and layers. *Circ Res*. 2015;116:307–311.
133. Libby P, Nahrendorf M, Swirski FK. Leukocytes link local and systemic inflammation in ischemic cardiovascular disease: an expanded "cardiovascular continuum". *J Am Coll Cardiol*. 2016;67:1091–1103.
134. Ridker PM, Everett BM, Pradhan A, et al. Low-dose methotrexate for the prevention of atherosclerotic events. *N Engl J Med*. 2019;380:752–762.
135. Tardif JC, Kouz S, Waters DD, et al. Efficacy and safety of low-dose colchicine after myocardial infarction. *N Engl J Med*. 2019;381:2497–2505.
136. Chiarito M, Sanz-Sanchez J, Cannata F, et al. Monotherapy with a P2Y12 inhibitor or aspirin for secondary prevention in patients with established atherosclerosis: a systematic review and meta-analysis. *Lancet*. 2020;395:1487–1495.
137. Levine GN, Bates ER, Bittl JA, et al. 2016 ACC/AHA guideline focused update on duration of dual antiplatelet therapy in patients with coronary artery disease: a report of the American College of Cardiology/American Heart Association task force on clinical practice guidelines. *Circulation*. 2016;134:e123–55.
138. Donadini MP, Bellesini M, Squizzato A. Aspirin plus clopidogrel vs aspirin alone for preventing cardiovascular events among patients at high risk for cardiovascular events. *J Am Med Assoc*. 2018;320:593–594.
139. Yeh RW, Kereiakes DJ, Steg PG, et al. Benefits and risks of extended duration dual antiplatelet therapy after PCI in patients with and without acute myocardial infarction. *J Am Coll Cardiol*. 2015;65:2211–2221.
140. Bonaca MP, Bhatt DL, Cohen M, et al. Long-term use of ticagrelor in patients with prior myocardial infarction. *N Engl J Med*. 2015;372:1791–1800.
141. Udell JA, Bonaca MP, Collet JP, et al. Long-term dual antiplatelet therapy for secondary prevention of cardiovascular events in the subgroup of patients with previous myocardial infarction: a collaborative meta-analysis of randomized trials. *Eur Heart J*. 2016;37:390–399.
142. Steg PG, Bhatt DL, Simon T, et al. Ticagrelor in patients with stable coronary disease and diabetes. *N Engl J Med*. 2019;381:1309–1320.
143. Bittl JA, Baber U, Bradley SM, et al. Duration of dual antiplatelet therapy: a systematic review for the 2016 ACC/AHA guideline focused update on duration of dual antiplatelet therapy in patients with coronary artery disease: a report of the American College of Cardiology/American Heart Association task force on clinical practice guidelines. *Circulation*. 2016;134:e156–e178.
144. Ziada KM, Moliterno DJ. Dual antiplatelet therapy: is it time to cut the cord with aspirin? *J Am Med Assoc*. 2019;321:2409–2411.
145. Khan SU, Singh M, Valavoor S, et al. Dual antiplatelet therapy after percutaneous coronary intervention and drug-eluting stents: a systematic review and network meta-analysis. *Circulation*. 2020;142:1425–1436.
146. Valgimigli M, Bueno H, Byrne RA, et al. 2017 ESC focused update on dual antiplatelet therapy in coronary artery disease developed in collaboration with EACTS: the task force for dual antiplatelet therapy in coronary artery disease of the European Society of Cardiology (ESC) and of the European Association for Cardio-Thoracic Surgery (EACTS). *Eur Heart J*. 2018;39:213–260.
147. Yeh RW, Secemsky EA, Kereiakes DJ, et al. Development and validation of a prediction rule for benefit and harm of dual antiplatelet therapy beyond 1 Year after percutaneous coronary intervention. *J Am Med Assoc*. 2016;315:1735–1749.
148. Baber U, Mehran R, Giustino G, et al. Coronary thrombosis and major bleeding after PCI with drug-eluting stents: risk scores from PARIS. *J Am Coll Cardiol*. 2016;67:2224–2234.
149. Fox KAA, Velentgas P, Camm AJ, et al. Outcomes associated with oral anticoagulants plus antiplatelets in patients with newly diagnosed atrial fibrillation. *JAMA Netw Open*. 2020;3:e200107.
150. Connolly SJ, Eikelboom JW, Bosch J, et al. Rivaroxaban with or without aspirin in patients with stable coronary artery disease: an international, randomised, double-blind, placebo-controlled trial. *Lancet*. 2018;391:205–218.
151. Yasuda S, Kaikita K, Akao M, et al. Antithrombotic therapy for atrial fibrillation with stable coronary disease. *N Engl J Med*. 2019;381:1103–1113.
152. Lopes RD, Hong H, Harskamp RE, et al. Optimal antithrombotic regimens for patients with atrial fibrillation undergoing percutaneous coronary intervention: an updated network meta-analysis. *JAMA Cardiol*. 2020;5:582–589.
153. Verheugt FWA, Ten Berg JM, Storey RF, et al. Antithrombotics: from aspirin to DOACs in coronary artery disease and atrial fibrillation (Part 3/5). *J Am Coll Cardiol*. 2019;74:699–711.
154. Dahl Aarvik M, Sandven I, Dondo TB, et al. Effect of oral beta-blocker treatment on mortality in contemporary post-myocardial infarction patients: a systematic review and meta-analysis. *Eur Heart J Cardiovasc Pharmacother*. 2019;5:12–20.
155. Leong DP, McMurray JJV, Joseph PG, et al. From ACE Inhibitors/ARBs to ARNIs in coronary artery disease and heart failure (Part 2/5). *J Am Coll Cardiol*. 2019;74:683–698.
156. Mann JF, Bohm M. Dual renin-angiotensin system blockade and outcome benefits in hypertension: a narrative review. *Curr Opin Cardiol*. 2015;30:373–377.
157. Manson JE, Cook NR, Lee IM, et al. Vitamin D supplements and prevention of cancer and cardiovascular disease. *N Engl J Med*. 2019;380:33–44.
158. Barbarawi M, Kheiri B, Zayed Y, et al. Vitamin D supplementation and cardiovascular disease risks in more than 83000 individuals in 21 randomized clinical trials: a meta-analysis. *JAMA Cardiol*. 2019;4:765–776.
159. Jha MK, Qamar A, Vaduganathan M, et al. Screening and management of depression in patients with cardiovascular disease: JACC state-of-the-art review. *J Am Coll Cardiol*. 2019;73:1827–1845.
160. Tang B, Yuan S, Xiong Y, et al. Major depressive disorder and cardiometabolic diseases: a bidirectional Mendelian randomisation study. *Diabetologia*. 2020;63:1305–1311.
161. Aspry KE, Van Horn L, Carson JAS, et al. Medical nutrition education, training, and competencies to advance guideline-based diet counseling by physicians: a science advisory from the American Heart Association. *Circulation*. 2018;137:e821–e841.
162. Lobelo F, Rohm Young D, Sallis R, et al. Routine assessment and promotion of physical activity in healthcare settings: a scientific statement from the American Heart Association. *Circulation*. 2018;137:e495–e522.
163. Ferrari R, Pavasini R, Camici PG, et al. Anti-anginal drugs-beliefs and evidence: systematic review covering 50 years of medical treatment. *Eur Heart J*. 2019;40:190–194.
164. Rosano GM, Vitale C, Volterrani M. Pharmacological management of chronic stable angina: focus on ranolazine. *Cardiovasc Drugs Ther*. 2016;30:393–398.
165. Weisz G, Genereux P, Iniguez A, et al. Ranolazine in patients with incomplete revascularisation after percutaneous coronary intervention (RIVER-PCI): a multicentre, randomised, double-blind, placebo-controlled trial. *Lancet*. 2016;387:136–145.
166. Alexander KP, Weisz G, Prather K, et al. Effects of ranolazine on angina and quality of life after percutaneous coronary intervention with incomplete revascularization: results from the ranolazine for incomplete vessel revascularization (RIVER-PCI) trial. *Circulation*. 2016;133:39–47.
167. Bairey Merz CN, Handberg EM, Shufelt CL, et al. A randomized, placebo-controlled trial of late Na current inhibition (ranolazine) in Coronary Microvascular Dysfunction (CMD): impact on angina and myocardial perfusion reserve. *Eur Heart J*. 2016;37:1504–1513.
168. Rambarat CA, Elgendy IY, Handberg EM, et al. Late sodium channel blockade improves angina and myocardial perfusion in patients with severe coronary microvascular dysfunction: women's ischemia syndrome evaluation-coronary vascular dysfunction ancillary study. *Int J Cardiol*. 2019;276:8–13.
169. Scirica BM, Belardinelli L, Chaitman BR, et al. Effect of ranolazine on atrial fibrillation in patients with non-ST elevation acute coronary syndromes: observations from the MERLIN-TIMI 36 trial. *Europace*. 2015;17:32–37.
170. Hartmann N, Mason FE, Braun I, et al. The combined effects of ranolazine and dronedarone on human atrial and ventricular electrophysiology. *J Mol Cell Cardiol*. 2016;94:95–106.
171. De Ferrari GM, Maier LS, Mont L, et al. Ranolazine in the treatment of atrial fibrillation: results of the dose-ranging RAFFAELLO (Ranolazine in Atrial Fibrillation Following An ELectricaL CardiOversion) study. *Heart Rhythm*. 2015;12:872–878.
172. Reiffel JA, Camm AJ, Belardinelli L, et al. The HARMONY trial: combined ranolazine and dronedarone in the management of paroxysmal atrial fibrillation: mechanistic and therapeutic synergism. *Circ Arrhythm Electrophysiol*. 2015;8:1048–1056.
173. Fanaroff AC, James SK, Weisz G, et al. Ranolazine after incomplete percutaneous coronary revascularization in patients with versus without diabetes mellitus: RIVER-PCI trial. *J Am Coll Cardiol*. 2017;69:2304–2313.
174. Santucci A, Riccini C, Cavallini C. Treatment of stable ischaemic heart disease: the old and the new. *Eur Heart J Suppl*. 2020;22:E54–E59.
175. Tarkin JM, Kaski JC. Vasodilator therapy: nitrates and nicorandil. *Cardiovasc Drugs Ther*. 2016;30:367–378.
176. Pisano U, Deosaran J, Leslie SJ, et al. Nicorandil, gastrointestinal adverse drug reactions and ulcerations: a systematic review. *Adv Ther*. 2016;33:320–344.
177. Marzilli M, Vinereanu D, Lopaschuk G, et al. Trimetazidine in cardiovascular medicine. *Int J Cardiol*. 2019;293:39–44.
178. Ferrari R, Ford I, Fox K, et al. A randomized, double-blind, placebo-controlled trial to assess the efficAcy and safety of Trimetazidine in patients with angina pectoris having been treated by percutaneous coronary intervention (ATPCI study): rationale, design, and baseline characteristics. *Am Heart J*. 2019;210:98–107.
179. Ferrari R, Ford I, Fox K, et al. Efficacy and safety of trimetazidine after percutaneous coronary intervention (ATPCI): a randomised, double-blind, placebo-controlled trial. *Lancet*. 2020;396:830–838.
180. Qin X, Deng Y, Wu D, et al. Does Enhanced External Counterpulsation (EECP) significantly affect myocardial perfusion?: a systematic review & meta-analysis. *PloS One*. 2016;11:e0151822.

181. Riley RF, Henry TD, Mahmud E, et al. SCAI position statement on optimal percutaneous coronary interventional therapy for complex coronary artery disease. *Catheter Cardiovasc Interv*. 2020;96:346–362.

Invasive Management

182. Neumann FJ, Sousa-Uva M, Ahlsson A, et al. 2018 ESC/EACTS Guidelines on myocardial revascularization. *Eur Heart J*. 2019;40:87–165.
183. Reardon MJ, Leon MB, Popma JJ, et al. Heart team 2.0. *EuroIntervention*. 2019;15:825–827.
184. Bangalore S, Maron DJ, Stone GW, et al. Routine revascularization versus initial medical therapy for stable ischemic heart disease: a systematic review and meta-analysis of randomized trials. *Circulation*. 2020;142:841–857.
185. Kaski JC, Crea F, Gersh BJ, et al. Reappraisal of ischemic heart disease. *Circulation*. 2018;138:1463–1480.
186. Fearon WF, De Bruyne B. The shifting sands of coronary microvascular dysfunction. *Circulation*. 2019;140:1817–1819.
187. Parikh RV, Liu G, Plomondon ME, et al. Utilization and outcomes of measuring fractional flow reserve in patients with stable ischemic heart disease. *J Am Coll Cardiol*. 2020;75:409–419.
188. Zimmermann FM, Ferrara A, Johnson NP, et al. Deferral vs. performance of percutaneous coronary intervention of functionally non-significant coronary stenosis: 15-year follow-up of the DEFER trial. *Eur Heart J*. 2015;36:3182–3188.
189. Zimmermann FM, Omerovic E, Fournier S, et al. Fractional flow reserve-guided percutaneous coronary intervention vs. medical therapy for patients with stable coronary lesions: meta-analysis of individual patient data. *Eur Heart J*. 2019;40:180–186.
190. van Nunen LX, Zimmermann FM, Tonino PA, et al. Fractional flow reserve versus angiography for guidance of PCI in patients with multivessel coronary artery disease (FAME): 5-year follow-up of a randomised controlled trial. *Lancet*. 2015;386:1853–1860.
191. Xaplanteris P, Fournier S, Pijls NHJ, et al. Five-year outcomes with PCI guided by fractional flow reserve. *N Engl J Med*. 2018;379:250–259.
192. Zimmermann FM, De Bruyne B, Pijls NH, et al. Rationale and design of the Fractional Flow Reserve versus Angiography for Multivessel Evaluation (FAME) 3 Trial: a comparison of fractional flow reserve-guided percutaneous coronary intervention and coronary artery bypass graft surgery in patients with multivessel coronary artery disease. *Am Heart J*. 2015;170:619–626 e612.
193. Brilakis ES, Mashayekhi K, Tsuchikane E, et al. Guiding principles for chronic total occlusion percutaneous coronary intervention. *Circulation*. 2019;140:420–433.
194. Joshi PH, de Lemos JA. Diagnosis and management of stable angina: a review. *JAMA*. 2021;325:1765–1778.
195. Al-Lamee R, Thompson D, Dehbi HM, et al. Percutaneous coronary intervention in stable angina (ORBITA): a double-blind, randomised controlled trial. *Lancet*. 2018;391:31–40.
196. Al-Lamee RK, Shun-Shin MJ, Howard JP, et al. Dobutamine stress echocardiography ischemia as a predictor of the placebo-controlled efficacy of percutaneous coronary intervention in stable coronary artery disease: the stress echocardiography-stratified analysis of ORBITA. *Circulation*. 2019;140:1971–1980.
197. DeVore AD, Yow E, Krucoff MW, et al. Percutaneous coronary intervention outcomes in patients with stable coronary disease and left ventricular systolic dysfunction. *ESC Heart Fail*. 2019;6:1233–1242.
198. Madhavan MV, Gersh BJ, Alexander KP, et al. Coronary artery disease in patients >/=80 Years of age. *J Am Coll Cardiol*. 2018;71:2015–2040.
199. Bangalore S, Maron DJ, O'Brien SM, et al. Management of coronary disease in patients with advanced kidney disease. *N Engl J Med*. 2020;382:1608–1618.
200. Spertus JA, Jones PG, Maron DJ, et al. Health status after invasive or conservative care in coronary and advanced kidney disease. *N Engl J Med*. 2020;382:1619–1628.
201. Gaudino MFL, Spadaccio C, Taggart DP. State-of-the-Art coronary artery bypass grafting: patient selection, graft selection, and optimizing outcomes. *Interv Cardiol Clin*. 2019;8:173–198.
202. Alexander JH, Smith PK. Coronary-artery bypass grafting. *N Engl J Med*. 2016;374:1954–1964.
203. Mozaffarian D, Benjamin EJ, Go AS, et al. Heart disease and stroke statistics-2016 update: a report from the American Heart Association. *Circulation*. 2016;133:e38–e60.
204. Buxton BF, Hayward PA, Raman J, et al. Long-term results of the RAPCO trials. *Circulation*. 2020;142:1330–1338.
205. Kowalewski M, Pawliszak W, Malvindi PG, et al. Off-pump coronary artery bypass grafting improves short-term outcomes in high-risk patients compared with on-pump coronary artery bypass grafting: meta-analysis. *J Thorac Cardiovasc Surg*. 2016;151:60–77. e61–e58.
206. Blackstone EH, Sabik 3rd JF 3rd. Changing the discussion about on-pump versus off-pump CABG. *N Engl J Med*. 2017;377:692–693.
207. Shroyer AL, Hattler B, Wagner TH, et al. Five-year outcomes after on-pump and off-pump coronary-artery bypass. *N Engl J Med*. 2017;377:623–632.
208. Lamy A, Devereaux PJ, Prabhakaran D, et al. Five-year outcomes after off-pump or on-pump coronary-artery bypass grafting. *N Engl J Med*. 2016;375:2359–2368.
209. Puskas JD, Gaudino M, Taggart DP. Experience is crucial in off-pump coronary artery bypass grafting. *Circulation*. 2019;139:1872–1875.
210. Benedetto U, Puskas J, Kappetein AP, et al. Off-pump versus on-pump bypass surgery for left main coronary artery disease. *J Am Coll Cardiol*. 2019;74:729–740.
211. Thakur U, Nerlekar N, Muthalaly RG, et al. Off- vs. On-pump coronary artery bypass grafting long-term survival is driven by incompleteness of revascularisation. *Heart Lung Circ*. 2020;29:149–155.
212. Wahba A, Milojevic M, Boer C, et al. 2019 EACTS/EACTA/EBCP guidelines on cardiopulmonary bypass in adult cardiac surgery. *Eur J Cardio Thorac Surg*. 2020;57:210–251.
213. Whellan DJ, McCarey MM, Taylor BS, et al. Trends in robotic-assisted coronary artery bypass grafts: a study of the society of thoracic surgeons adult cardiac surgery database, 2006 to 2012. *Ann Thorac Surg*. 2016;102:140–146.
214. Aldea GS, Bakaeen FG, Pal J, et al. The society of thoracic surgeons clinical practice guidelines on arterial conduits for coronary artery bypass grafting. *Ann Thorac Surg*. 2016;101:801–809.
215. Gaudino M, Bakaeen FG, Benedetto U, et al. Arterial grafts for coronary bypass: a critical review after the publication of ART and RADIAL. *Circulation*. 2019;140:1273–1284.
216. Taggart DP, Benedetto U, Gerry S, et al. Bilateral versus single internal-thoracic-artery grafts at 10 years. *N Engl J Med*. 2019;380:437–446.
217. Rocha RV, Tam DY, Karkhanis R, et al. Multiple arterial grafting is associated with better outcomes for coronary artery bypass grafting patients. *Circulation*. 2018;138:2081–2090.
218. Gaudino M, Benedetto U, Fremes S, et al. Radial-artery or saphenous-vein grafts in coronary-artery bypass surgery. *N Engl J Med*. 2018;378:2069–2077.
219. Gaudino M, Benedetto U, Fremes SE, et al. Angiographic outcome of coronary artery bypass grafts: the radial artery database International Alliance. *Ann Thorac Surg*. 2020;109:688–694.
220. Zhao Q, Zhu Y, Xu Z, et al. Effect of ticagrelor plus aspirin, ticagrelor alone, or aspirin alone on saphenous vein graft patency 1 Year after coronary artery bypass grafting: a randomized clinical trial. *J Am Med Assoc*. 2018;319:1677–1686.
221. Willemsen LM, Janssen PWA, Peper J, et al. The effect of adding ticagrelor to standard aspirin on saphenous vein graft patency in patients undergoing Coronary Artery Bypass Grafting (POPular CABG): a randomized, double-blind, placebo-controlled trial. *Circulation*. 2020;142:1799–1807.
222. Hillis LD, Smith PK, Anderson JL, et al. 2011 ACCF/AHA guideline for coronary artery bypass graft surgery: a report of the American College of Cardiology Foundation/American Heart Association task force on practice guidelines. *Circulation*. 2011;124:e652–e735.
223. Society of thoracic surgeons database. Available at: www.sts.org. Accessed September ,2020.
224. Fernandez FG, Shahian DM, Kormos R, et al. The society of thoracic surgeons National Database 2019 Annual Report. *Ann Thorac Surg*. 2019;108:1625–1632.
225. Ben-Yehuda O, Chen S, Redfors B, et al. Impact of large periprocedural myocardial infarction on mortality after percutaneous coronary intervention and coronary artery bypass grafting for left main disease: an analysis from the EXCEL trial. *Eur Heart J*. 2019;40:1930–1941.
226. Thygesen K, Alpert JS, Jaffe AS, et al. Fourth universal definition of myocardial infarction (2018). *J Am Coll Cardiol*. 2018;72:2231–2264.
227. Gaudino M, Angiolillo DJ, Di Franco A, et al. Stroke after coronary artery bypass grafting and percutaneous coronary intervention: incidence, pathogenesis, and outcomes. *J Am Heart Assoc*. 2019;8:e013032.
228. Lorusso R, Moscarelli M, Di Franco A, et al. Association between coronary artery bypass surgical techniques and postoperative stroke. *J Am Heart Assoc*. 2019;8:e013650.
229. Kerwin M, Saado J, Pan J, et al. New-onset atrial fibrillation and outcomes following isolated coronary artery bypass surgery: a systematic review and meta-analysis. *Clin Cardiol*. 2020;43:928–934.
230. Gillinov AM, Bagiella E, Moskowitz AJ, et al. Rate control versus rhythm control for atrial fibrillation after cardiac surgery. *N Engl J Med*. 2016;374:1911–1921.
231. Benedetto U, Gaudino MF, Dimagli A, et al. Postoperative atrial fibrillation and long-term risk of stroke after isolated coronary artery bypass graft surgery. *Circulation*. 2020;142:1320–1329.
232. Butt JH, Xian Y, Peterson ED, et al. Long-term thromboembolic risk in patients with postoperative atrial fibrillation after coronary artery bypass graft surgery and patients with nonvalvular atrial fibrillation. *JAMA Cardiol*. 2018;3:417–424.
233. Nadim MK, Forni LG, Bihorac A, et al. Cardiac and vascular surgery-associated acute kidney injury: the 20th international consensus conference of the ADQI (Acute Disease Quality Initiative) group. *J Am Heart Assoc*. 2018;7.
234. Thuijs D, Milojevic M, Stone GW, et al. Impact of left ventricular ejection fraction on clinical outcomes after left main coronary artery revascularization: results from the randomized EXCEL trial. *Eur J Heart Fail*. 2020;22:871–879.
235. Omer S, Adeseye A, Jimenez E, et al. Low left ventricular ejection fraction, complication rescue, and long-term survival after coronary artery bypass grafting. *J Thorac Cardiovasc Surg*. 2020.
236. Yanagawa B, Lee J, Puskas JD, et al. Revascularization in left ventricular dysfunction: an update. *Curr Opin Cardiol*. 2019;34:536–542.
237. Guyton RA, Smith AL. Coronary bypass-survival benefit in heart failure. *N Engl J Med*. 2016;374:1576–1577.
238. Velazquez EJ, Lee KL, Jones RH, et al. Coronary-artery bypass surgery in patients with ischemic cardiomyopathy. *N Engl J Med*. 2016;374:1511–1520.
239. Howlett JG, Stebbins A, Petrie MC, et al. CABG improves outcomes in patients with ischemic cardiomyopathy: 10-year follow-up of the STICH trial. *JACC Heart Fail*. 2019;7:878–887.
240. Panza JA, Ellis AM, Al-Khalidi HR, et al. Myocardial viability and long-term outcomes in ischemic cardiomyopathy. *N Engl J Med*. 2019;381:739–748.
241. Anavekar NS, Chareonthaitawee P, Narula J, et al. Revascularization in patients with severe left ventricular dysfunction: is the assessment of viability still viable? *J Am Coll Cardiol*. 2016;67:2874–2887.
242. Kloner RA. Stunned and hibernating myocardium: where are we nearly 4 decades later? *J Am Heart Assoc*. 2020;9:e015502.
243. Huckaby LV, Seese LM, Sultan I, et al. The impact of sex on outcomes after revascularization for multivessel coronary disease. *Ann Thorac Surg*. 2020.
244. Lemaire A, Soto C, Salgueiro L, et al. The impact of age on outcomes of coronary artery bypass grafting. *J Cardiothorac Surg*. 2020;15:158.
245. Bangalore S, Guo Y, Samadashvili Z, et al. Revascularization in patients with multivessel coronary artery disease and chronic kidney disease: everolimus-eluting stents versus coronary artery bypass graft surgery. *J Am Coll Cardiol*. 2015;66:1209–1220.
246. Tzoumas A, Giannopoulos S, Texakalidis P, et al. Synchronous versus staged carotid endarterectomy and coronary artery bypass graft for patients with concomitant severe coronary and carotid artery stenosis: a systematic review and meta-analysis. *Ann Vasc Surg*. 2020;63:427–438. e421.
247. Mohamed MO, Shoaib A, Gogas B, et al. Trends of repeat revascularization choice in patients with prior coronary artery bypass surgery. *Catheter Cardiovasc Interv*. 2020.
248. Maltais S, Widmer RJ, Bell MR, et al. Reoperation for coronary artery bypass grafting surgery: outcomes and considerations for expanding interventional procedures. *Ann Thorac Surg*. 2017;103:1886–1892.
249. Weintraub WS. Role of big data in cardiovascular research. *J Am Heart Assoc*. 2019;8:e012791.
250. Bangalore S, Guo Y, Samadashvili Z, et al. Everolimus-eluting stents or bypass surgery for multivessel coronary disease. *N Engl J Med*. 2015;372:1213–1222.
251. Panoulas VF, Ilsley CJ, Kalogeras K, et al. Coronary artery bypass confers intermediate-term survival benefit over percutaneous coronary intervention with new-generation stents in real-world patients with multivessel coronary artery disease, including left main disease: a retrospective analysis of 6383 patients. *Eur J Cardio Thorac Surg*. 2019;56:911–918.
252. Head SJ, Milojevic M, Daemen J, et al. Mortality after coronary artery bypass grafting versus percutaneous coronary intervention with stenting for coronary artery disease: a pooled analysis of individual patient data. *Lancet*. 2018;391:939–948.
253. Thuijs D, Kappetein AP, Serruys PW, et al. Percutaneous coronary intervention versus coronary artery bypass grafting in patients with three-vessel or left main coronary artery disease: 10-year follow-up of the multicentre randomised controlled SYNTAX trial. *Lancet*. 2019;394:1325–1334.
254. Doenst T, Haverich A, Serruys P, et al. PCI and CABG for treating stable coronary artery disease: JACC review topic of the week. *J Am Coll Cardiol*. 2019;73:964–976.
255. Windecker S, Neumann FJ, Juni P, et al. Considerations for the choice between coronary artery bypass grafting and percutaneous coronary intervention as revascularization strategies in major categories of patients with stable multivessel coronary artery disease: an accompanying article of the task force of the 2018 ESC/EACTS guidelines on myocardial revascularization. *Eur Heart J*. 2019;40:204–212.
256. Farkouh ME, Domanski M, Dangas GD, et al. Long-term survival following multivessel revascularization in patients with diabetes: the FREEDOM follow-on study. *J Am Coll Cardiol*. 2019;73:629–638.
257. Park DW, Ahn JM, Yun SC, et al. 10-Year outcomes of stents versus coronary artery bypass grafting for left main coronary artery disease. *J Am Coll Cardiol*. 2018;72:2813–2822.
258. Gaudino M, Taggart DP. Percutaneous coronary intervention vs coronary artery bypass grafting: a surgical perspective. *JAMA Cardiol*. 2019;4:505–506.
259. Tu B, Rich B, Labos C, et al. Coronary revascularization in diabetic patients: a systematic review and Bayesian network meta-analysis. *Ann Intern Med*. 2014;161:724–732.
260. Tam DY, Dharma C, Rocha R, et al. Long-term survival after surgical or percutaneous revascularization in patients with diabetes and multivessel coronary disease. *J Am Coll Cardiol*. 2020;76:1153–1164.
261. Puri R, Brophy JM, Mack MJ. Revascularizing diabetic multivessel coronary artery disease in the 2020s: forever surgically sweet? *J Am Coll Cardiol*. 2020;76:1165–1167.
262. Velazquez EJ. Percutaneous coronary intervention or coronary artery bypass grafting to treat ischemic cardiomyopathy? *JAMA Cardiol*. 2020;5:641–642.
263. Sun LY, Gaudino M, Chen RJ, et al. Long-term outcomes in patients with severely reduced left ventricular ejection fraction undergoing percutaneous coronary intervention vs coronary artery bypass grafting. *JAMA Cardiol*. 2020;5:631–641.
264. Ullah W, Sattar Y, Ullah I, et al. Percutaneous intervention or bypass graft for left main coronary artery disease? A systematic review and meta-analysis. *J Interv Cardiol*. 2020. 4081642.

265. Gershlick AH, Kandzari DE, Banning A, et al. Outcomes after left main percutaneous coronary intervention versus coronary artery bypass grafting according to lesion site: results from the EXCEL trial. *JACC Cardiovasc Interv*. 2018;11:1224–1233.
266. Stone GW, Kappetein AP, Sabik JF, et al. Five-year outcomes after PCI or CABG for left main coronary disease. *N Engl J Med*. 2019;381:1820–1830.
267. Milojevic M, Serruys PW, Sabik 3rd JF, et al. Bypass surgery or stenting for left main coronary artery disease in patients with diabetes. *J Am Coll Cardiol*. 2019;73:1616–1628.
268. Modolo R, Chichareon P, Kogame N, et al. Contemporary outcomes following coronary artery bypass graft surgery for left main disease. *J Am Coll Cardiol*. 2019;73:1877–1886.
269. Shlofmitz E, Genereux P, Chen S, et al. Left main coronary artery disease revascularization according to the SYNTAX score. *Circ Cardiovasc Interv*. 2019;12:e008007.
270. Ahn JM, Park DW, Lee CW, et al. Comparison of stenting versus bypass surgery according to the completeness of revascularization in severe coronary artery disease: patient-level pooled analysis of the SYNTAX, PRECOMBAT, and BEST trials. *JACC Cardiovasc Interv*. 2017;10:1415–1424.

Microvascular Angina and Other Considerations

271. Waheed N, Elias-Smale S, Malas W, et al. Sex differences in non-obstructive coronary artery disease. *Cardiovasc Res*. 2020;116:829–840.
272. Bairey Merz CN, Pepine CJ, Shimokawa H, et al. Treatment of coronary microvascular dysfunction. *Cardiovasc Res*. 2020;116:856–870.
273. Anderson RD, Petersen JW, Mehta PK, et al. Prevalence of coronary endothelial and microvascular dysfunction in women with symptoms of ischemia and No obstructive coronary artery disease is confirmed by a new cohort: the NHLBI-Sponsored Women's Ischemia Syndrome Evaluation-Coronary Vascular Dysfunction (WISE-CVD). *J Interv Cardiol*. 2019:7169275.
274. Pepine CJ, Elgendy IY. Invasive functional assessment in patients with angina and coronary microvascular dysfunction: a plea for more. *J Am Coll Cardiol*. 2020;75:2550–2552.
275. Barsky L, Merz CNB, Wei J, et al. Even "WISE-R?"-an update on the NHLBI-Sponsored Women's ischemia syndrome evaluation. *Curr Atheroscler Rep*. 2020;22:35.
276. Ong P, Camici PG, Beltrame JF, et al. International standardization of diagnostic criteria for microvascular angina. *Int J Cardiol*. 2018;250:16–20.
277. Ford TJ, Stanley B, Good R, et al. Stratified medical therapy using invasive coronary function testing in angina: the CorMicA trial. *J Am Coll Cardiol*. 2018;72:2841–2855.
278. Rahman H, Ryan M, Lumley M, et al. Coronary microvascular dysfunction is associated with myocardial ischemia and abnormal coronary perfusion during exercise. *Circulation*. 2019;140:1805–1816.
279. Fearon WF. The prognostic importance of silent ischemia. *Int J Cardiol*. 2019;291:27–28.
280. Yancy CW, Jessup M, Bozkurt B, et al. 2017 ACC/AHA/HFSA focused update of the 2013 ACCF/AHA guideline for the management of heart failure: a report of the American College of Cardiology/American Heart Association task force on clinical practice guidelines and the Heart Failure Society of America. *J Am Coll Cardiol*. 2017;70:776–803.
281. Redfors B, Stone GW. Myocardial viability and CABG surgery: a Bayesian appraisal of STICH. *Nat Rev Cardiol*. 2019;16:702–703.
282. Castelvecchio S, Garatti A, Gagliardotto PV, et al. Surgical ventricular reconstruction for ischaemic heart failure: state of the art. *Eur Heart J Suppl*. 2016;18:E8–E14.
283. Hui DS, Restrepo CS, Calhoon JH. How to do it: surgical decision-making for left ventricular aneurysmectomy. *Ann Thorac Surg*. 2020.
284. Doulamis IP, Perrea DN, Chloroyiannis IA. Left ventricular reconstruction surgery in ischemic heart disease: a systematic review of the past two decades. *J Cardiovasc Surg*. 2019;60:422–430.
285. Nappi F, Avtaar Singh SS, Padala M, et al. The choice of treatment in ischemic mitral regurgitation with reduced left ventricular function. *Ann Thorac Surg*. 2019;108:1901–1912.
286. O'Gara PT, Mack MJ. Secondary mitral regurgitation. *N Engl J Med*. 2020;383:1458–1467.
287. Nappi F, Antoniou GA, Nenna A, et al. Treatment options for ischemic mitral regurgitation: a meta-analysis. *J Thorac Cardiovasc Surg*. 2020.
288. Hayes SN, Kim ESH, Saw J, et al. Spontaneous coronary artery dissection: current state of the science: a scientific statement from the American Heart Association. *Circulation*. 2018;137:e523–e557.
289. Krittanawong C, Saw J, Olin JW. Updates in spontaneous coronary artery dissection. *Curr Cardiol Rep*. 2020;22:123.
290. Hassan S, Prakash R, Starovoytov A, et al. Natural history of spontaneous coronary artery dissection with spontaneous angiographic healing. *JACC Cardiovasc Interv*. 2019;12:518–527.

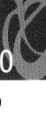

41 Percutaneous Coronary Intervention

DHARAM J. KUMBHANI AND DEEPAK L. BHATT

BACKGROUND, 786

INDICATIONS, 786
Clinical Presentations, 786
Patient-Specific Considerations, 787

CORONARY DEVICES, 793
Balloon Angioplasty, 793
Coronary Stents, 793
Coronary Atherectomy, 794
Thrombectomy and Aspiration Devices, 795
Embolic Protection Devices, 795
Drug-Coated Balloons, 795
Coronary Physiology, 795
Intravascular Imaging, 796

MECHANICAL CIRCULATORY SUPPORT, 796

VASCULAR ACCESS, 798
Complications, 799
Vascular Closure Devices, 799

ANTIPLATELET AGENTS, 799
Aspirin, 799
Adenosine Diphosphate (ADP) Receptor Antagonists, 799
Glycoprotein IIb/IIIa Inhibitors, 800

ANTITHROMBIN AGENTS, 801
Unfractionated Heparin, 801
Low-Molecular-Weight Heparin, 801

Bivalirudin, 801
Factor Xa Inhibitors, 801

OUTCOMES AFTER PERCUTANEOUS CORONARY INTERVENTION, 801
Early Clinical Outcomes, 801
Late Clinical Outcomes, 802
Outcomes Benchmarking and Procedural Volumes, 803

FUTURE PERSPECTIVES, 803

ACKNOWLEDGMENTS, 803

REFERENCES, 803

BACKGROUND

The first balloon angioplasty in humans was performed by Dr. Andreas Gruentzig in 1977 in Zurich, Switzerland, when he passed a prototype, fixed-wire balloon catheter across a severe lesion in the left anterior descending artery (LAD).[1] Much has changed since then. This is driven by relentless innovation and robust data from randomized controlled trials. Coronary stents, introduced in the 1990s, dramatically improved upon angioplasty's efficacy and reduced periprocedural complications. Bare-metal stents gave way to drug-eluting stents that addressed the problem of in-stent restenosis, and the diversity of lesions treatable with percutaneous coronary intervention (PCI) has increased exponentially over the past two to three decades. In addition, to these and other technical innovations on the procedural side, there have also been significant improvements in peri- and post-procedural medications, widespread availability of mechanical circulatory devices for very high-risk patients, as well as systematic adoption of care-delivery pathways. All of these have led to improvements in outcomes post-PCI in a synergistic fashion and enabled operators to tackle even the most complex and high-risk patients and lesions successfully. Currently, the number of PCI procedures done for revascularization far exceeds the number of coronary artery bypass graft surgeries (CABG) done for the same indication worldwide. In fact, cardiac surgeons and interventional cardiologists have come a full circle—many PCIs in the contemporary era are now performed on surgical turndowns. Interestingly, widespread use of effective risk factor modification strategies, prevention of restenosis with drug-eluting stents, and a better understanding of the patients who will benefit from revascularization have resulted in a slowing in PCI volume growth, and an increase in PCI complexity.[2,3] The number of PCIs is expected to grow modestly (1% to 5%) over the next decade as a result of the aging U.S. population and an increased frequency of risk factors including obesity and diabetes.

INDICATIONS

Clinical Presentations

The major value of percutaneous or surgical coronary revascularization is relief of the symptoms and signs of ischemic CAD. PCI reduces the risk for mortality and subsequent myocardial infarction (MI) compared with medical therapy in patients with acute coronary syndromes (ACS). On the other hand, optimal medical therapy (OMT) appears to be as effective as PCI in reducing death and MI in patients with stable angina, although relief of symptoms and improvement of ischemia are better with PCI. Greater than 5% improvement in the ischemic burden is achieved more often with PCI, and the magnitude of the residual ischemia correlates with less frequent death and MI.

Stable Ischemic Heart Disease and Stable Angina

ACME (Angioplasty Compared to Medicine) was the first randomized study comparing PTCA with conventional medical therapy to be published, where PTCA resulted in an improvement in exercise duration and freedom from angina. Since then, both angioplasty and medical management have come a long way. More recently, studies such as COURAGE, FAME-2, ORBITA and ISCHEMIA have added significantly to our understanding of stable ischemic heart disease (SIHD) and stable angina management (see Chapter 40).[3-6]

A meta-analysis of all major SIHD trials (14 RCTs, 14,877 patients, weighted mean duration of follow-up: 4.5 years) suggested that, compared with medical therapy alone, revascularization alone was not associated with a reduced risk of death (relative risk [RR], 0.99 [95% CI, 0.90 to 1.09]). Revascularization was associated with a reduced nonprocedural MI (RR, 0.76 [95% CI, 0.67 to 0.85]) but also with increased procedural MI (RR, 2.48 [95% CI, 1.86 to 3.31]) with no difference in overall MI (RR, 0.93 [95% CI, 0.83 to 1.03]). A significant reduction in unstable angina (UA; RR, 0.64 [95% CI, 0.45 to 0.92]) and increase in freedom from angina (RR, 1.10 [95% CI, 1.05 to 1.15]) was also observed with revascularization.[7] This seems to be a reasonable summary of the available evidence for revascularization for SIHD/stable angina. In addition, among patients with either heart failure (HF) or left ventricular (LV) dysfunction (EF 35% to 45%) at baseline in ISCHEMIA (7.7% of total cohort), a salutary effect of early revascularization was noted for the primary endpoint at 4 years (p for interaction = 0.055), as well for CV death or MI.[6] Irrespective of the indication for revascularization, PCI should be coupled with OMT after the procedure, such as control of hypertension and diabetes, exercise, and smoking cessation. Lipid management, particularly statin use, is also an important component of OMT.

Compared with PCI alone, CABG is associated with a late mortality benefit in certain high-risk medical and anatomic subsets, such as patients with left main disease, three-vessel CAD, and extensive markers of higher anatomic risk for PCI, such as determined by a SYNTAX (Synergy Between PCI with TAXUS and Cardiac Surgery) score,[8] or patients with diabetes and significant multivessel disease.[9,10] These benefits are manifested beyond 1 year after treatment and for up to 5 years of follow-up, but the early periprocedural risks, particularly for stroke, are higher with CABG, and patients have a longer in-hospital recovery period. The risks and benefits associated with coronary revascularization therefore need careful review with the patient and family, and the relative options of PCI, CABG, or OMT should be discussed before performing these procedures. Patients with left main or multivessel disease benefit from joint consultation with a cardiac surgeon, an interventional cardiologist, and the referring cardiologist, and consideration of patient preferences in weighing diverse factors is valuable. A task force of the American College of Cardiology (ACC) and American Heart Association (AHA) has published guidelines for the performance of PCI and CABG procedures,[11] and a multispecialty writing committee has developed appropriate use criteria for revascularization in several clinical and lesion-specific subsets.[12,13]

Acute Coronary Syndromes

Early cardiac catheterization and coronary revascularization in moderate- to high-risk patients with UA or non–ST-segment elevation MI (NSTEMI) may improve mortality and reduce the rate of reinfarction.[14] In a meta-analysis of seven trials with 8375 patients monitored for up to 2 years, the all-cause mortality rate was 4.9% in the early invasive group versus 6.5% in the conservative group (risk ratio [RR], 0.75; $P = 0.001$). The 2-year incidence of nonfatal MI was 7.6% in the invasive group and 9.1% in the conservative group (RR, 0.83; $P = 0.012$). At a mean of 13 months of follow-up, rehospitalization for UA was reduced as well (RR, 0.69; $P < 0.0001$).[15] Current guidelines suggest that an early invasive strategy (typically within 48-72 hours) should be pursued in patients with recurrent ischemia despite therapy, elevated troponin levels, new ST-segment depression, new or worsening symptoms of HF, depressed LV function, hemodynamic instability, sustained ventricular tachycardia (VT), or a recent PCI or CABG procedure.[14] For patients at very high risk for adverse cardiovascular events (for example, a GRACE risk score >140, age ≥ 75 years), a very early invasive approach (within 12 hours) can be considered. The predominant benefit appears to be a reduction in refractory ischemia, but a mortality signal may exist for high-risk subgroups.[16-18]

Specific clinical recommendations pertain to patients with STEMI, including primary PCI, rescue PCI, facilitated PCI, and PCI following successful thrombolysis are listed in Chapters 37 and 38 (also see the online chapter).[19,20] Timely PCI in patients with STEMI improves survival over that achieved with medical therapy, provided that it is performed by a physician who routinely performs PCI, and that the hospital has sufficient PCI volume to support its proficiency. Patients with cardiogenic shock or severe HF also benefit from primary PCI, regardless of their age at initial evaluation (see "Preoperative Considerations").

Asymptomatic or Minimally Symptomatic Patients

Asymptomatic patients or those who have only mild symptoms are generally best treated with medical therapy unless one or more high-grade lesions subtend a moderate to large area of viable myocardium, the patient prefers to maintain a very active lifestyle or has a high-risk occupation, and the procedure can be performed with a high chance of success and low likelihood of complications. Patients who are minimally symptomatic or asymptomatic should not undergo coronary revascularization if only a small area of myocardium is at risk, if no objective evidence of ischemia can be detected, or if the likelihood of success is low or the chance of complications is high.[12,13]

Preoperative Considerations (see Chapter 23)

Patients scheduled to undergo noncardiac surgery should have an assessment of the risk of a cardiovascular perioperative cardiac event. In general, revascularization should be considered for similar clinical indications as discussed above (i.e., even if they were not undergoing surgery). The 2014 ACC/AHA guidelines suggest an important role for the patient's functional capacity to help with decision making. For higher risk patients (mortality >1%) with poor or unclear exercise tolerance (<4 METs), pharmacological stress testing is indicated. If positive, coronary angiography and revascularization where appropriate may be indicated.[21]

Patient-Specific Considerations

Assessment of the potential risks and benefits of PCI must address five fundamental patient-specific risk factors: extent of jeopardized myocardium, baseline lesion morphology, underlying cardiac function (e.g., LV function, rhythm stability, coexisting valvular heart disease), presence of renal dysfunction, and preexisting medical comorbid conditions that may place the patient at higher risk for PCI. Each of these factors contributes independently to the risks and benefits attributable to PCI. Proper planning for a PCI procedure requires careful attention to each of these factors.

Extent of Jeopardized Myocardium

The proportion of viable myocardium subtended by the treated coronary artery is the principal consideration in assessing the acute risk associated with the PCI procedure. PCI interrupts coronary blood flow for a period of seconds to minutes, and the ability of patients to hemodynamically tolerate a sustained coronary occlusion depends on both the extent of "downstream" viable myocardium and the presence and grade of collaterals to the ischemic region. Although the risk for abrupt closure has been reduced substantially with the availability of coronary stents, when other procedural complications develop—such as a large side branch occlusion, distal embolization, perforation, or no-reflow—rapid clinical deterioration may occur that is proportionate to the extent of jeopardized myocardium. In the unlikely event that out-of-hospital stent thrombosis develops, the clinical sequelae of the episode are related to the extent of myocardium subtended by the occluded stent. Predictors of cardiovascular collapse with a failed PCI include the magnitude of myocardium at risk, the severity of the baseline stenosis, multivessel CAD, and the presence of diffuse disease.

Specific Lesion Subsets

Several angiographic findings increase the technical complexity of PCI and elevate the risk for acute and long-term complications. The SYNTAX angiographic scoring system, when combined with clinical factors, has become a method of deciding between complex PCI and CABG. An online calculator is available (www.syntaxscore.com).

Left Main Disease

Left main coronary artery disease may be present in approximately 6% of patients who undergo coronary angiography overall, and in 12% of subjects presenting with ACS. It is further associated with multivessel disease in a large proportion. LM disease is associated with a poor prognosis with medical therapy, given the large myocardial territory at risk (ranging from 75% to 100% of the myocardium depending on the coronary dominance). Revascularization is recommended by current guidelines for patients with an LM stenosis greater than or equal to 50%, regardless of symptomatic status or associated ischemic burden.[11] Traditionally, CABG has represented the gold standard for LM revascularization.

The major trials are listed in Table 41.1. In the prespecified and stratified LM subgroup of the SYNTAX trial, MACCE rates at 5 years were 36.9% versus 31.0% in PCI versus CABG patients ($P = 0.12$). Mortality rates were 12.8% versus 14.6% (HR 0.88; 95% CI, 0.58 to 1.32; $P = 0.53$), while repeat revascularization was greater in the PCI arm (26.7% vs. 15.5%, respectively; HR 1.82; 95% CI, 1.28 to 2.57; $P < 0.01$).[22,23] Results with PCI were slightly better for left main only or left main + one-vessel disease, compared with left main + two or three-vessel disease. A recently published extended follow-up report (SYNTAX—Extended Survival) showed no differences in the primary endpoint of 10-year

TABLE 41.1 Important Randomized Controlled Trials in Specific Populations

STUDY OR AUTHOR	COMPARATORS	STUDY POPULATION	OUTCOMES OF INTEREST	RESULTS
Left Main PCI				
SYNTAX (n =1800)[8,22-24]	1st generation (paclitaxel-eluting) stent vs. CABG	Left main (n = 705) or multivessel disease (n = 1709)	MACCE (all-cause death, stroke, myocardial infarction, or repeat revascularization)	Rates higher with PCI vs. CABG at 12 months (17.8% vs. 12.4%; p = 0.002) driven by repeat revascularization (13.5% vs. 5.9%, respectively; $P < 0.001$). PCI did not meet criteria for noninferiority. Death and MI similar, stroke rate higher with CABG. Among patients with low scores (≤22), there was no significant difference in the primary outcome between PCI and CABG patients, but with intermediate or with high scores (>33), MACCE rates were lower with CABG.
				LM subset: MACCE at 5 years: 36.9% vs. 31.0%; p = 0.12; mortality (12.8% vs. 14.6%, p = 0.53); repeat revascularization higher in PCI arm (26.7% vs. 15.5%; HR 1.82; 95% CI, 1.28–2.57; I < 0.01).
				Results with PCI were slightly better for left main only or left main + one-vessel disease, compared with left main + two or three-vessel disease.
				Five-year outcomes similar.
PRECOMBAT (n = 600)[26,27]	1st generation (sirolimus-eluting) stent vs. CABG	Unprotected left main	MACCE (all-cause death, stroke, MI, or ischemia-driven target-vessel revascularization)	MACCE at 5 years for PCI vs. CABG: 17.5% vs. 14.3%; $P = 0.26$ with higher ID-TLR rates with PCI than with CABG (11.4% vs. 5.5%; $P = 0.012$).
				Similar results reported at 10-year follow-up.
NOBLE (n = 1201)[28,29]	2nd generation DES vs. CABG. DES were primarily biolimus-eluting stents; approximately 10% received first-generation DES	Unprotected left main. Median SYNTAX score 22.5; 52% had low SYNTAX scores	MACCE (all-cause death, stroke, MI, or ischemia-driven target-vessel revascularization)	MACCE at 5 years for PCI vs. CABG: 28% vs. 19%, $p_{superiority} = 0.002$. Mortality rates were similar (9% vs. 9%, $p = 0.68$), while non-procedural MI and any revascularization were all higher with PCI.
EXCEL (n = 1905)[25]	2nd-generation DES (everolimus-eluting) vs. CABG.	Unprotected left main. Low SYNTAX score in 60.5%, intermediate in rest. Distal LM: 80.5%, multivessel CAD: 51%	Death, MI, or stroke	At 3-year follow-up, death, MI, or stroke occurred with similar frequency in the PCI and CABG groups (15.4% vs. 14.7%, $P = 0.98$), meeting the noninferiority assumption for PCI compared with CABG. Mortality at 3 years similar (8.2% vs. 5.9%, p= 0.11), while ischemia-driven revascularization was higher with PCI (12.6% vs. 7.5%, p < 0.0001). On the other hand, stent thrombosis or graft occlusion were lower with PCI (0.7% vs. 5.4%, p< 0.001).[30]
				At 5 years, no differences were noted for PCI vs. CABG for the primary endpoint (22.0% vs. 19.2%, $P = 0.13$) However, all-cause mortality (13% vs. 9.9%), non-procedural MI (6.8% vs. 3.5%) and ID-TLR rates (16.9% vs. 10%) were higher with PCI compared with CABG.
PCI of Chronic Total Occlusions				
EXPLORE (n = 304)[37]	CTO PCI vs. no CTO PCI	Post-PCI STEMI patients with concurrent CTO	LVEF and LVEDV assessed on cMRI at 4 months	No difference between groups (44.1 ± 12.2% vs. 44.8 ± 11.9%; p = 0.60)
DECISION-CTO (n = 834)[38]	CTO PCI + OMT vs. OMT alone	Stable angina, non-symptomatic ischemia, or ACS with CTO	Death, MI, stroke, or repeat revascularization at 3 years	No difference between groups for primary endpoint (22.3% vs. 22.4%, p = 0.86)
				SAQ-angina similar
EURO-CTO (n = 396)[39]	CTO PCI + OMT vs. OMT alone	Stable angina or equivalent with CTO in viable territory	QOL by SAQ score (primary)	Improved QOL in CTO PCI arm (primary)
			1 year death or non-fatal MI (secondary)	No difference between groups in death or MI

Continued

TABLE 41.1 Important Randomized Controlled Trials in Specific Populations—cont'd

STUDY OR AUTHOR	COMPARATORS	STUDY POPULATION	OUTCOMES OF INTEREST	RESULTS
PCI of Saphenous Vein Grafts				
ISAR-CABG (n = 610)[45]	1st generation DES vs. BMS	Stable angina (61%), acute MI (15%)	MACE (death, MI, TLR, stent thrombosis)	MACE at 1 year lower with DES (15.4% vs. 22.1%, $p = 0.03$), primarily due to reduction in TLR.
				MACE at 5 years similar for DES vs. BMS, with higher TLR in DES arm beyond 1 year
DIVA (n = 597)[46]	2nd generation DES vs. BMS (9% received 1st generation DES)	Stable angina or ACS (no STEMIs)	Target vessel failure	No difference between groups at 12 months for primary endpoint (17% vs. 19%, $p = 0.7$). No difference over median 2.7 years follow-up (37% vs. 34%, $p = 0.44$)
FFR-guided PCI of Non-Culprit Vessels in STEMI				
DANAMI-3-PRIMULTI (n = 627)[97]	Immediate non-culprit vessel PCI vs. FFR-guided staged complete revascularization of non-culprit vessels	STEMI	Mortality, MI, ID-TLR of non-infarct vessel	Primary endpoint lower at median of 27 months with FFR guided PCI vs. immediate PCI (13% vs. 22%, $p = 0.004$)
COMPARE-ACUTE (n = 885)[98]	Complete FFR-guided revascularization of non-infarct vessel vs. no intervention with blinded FFR assessment	STEMI	Death from any cause, nonfatal myocardial infarction, revascularization, and cerebrovascular events	Primary endpoint lower in FFR-guided PCI arm, mostly driven by reduction in need for repeat revascularization

ACS, Acute coronary syndrome; *BMS*, bare-metal stent; *CABG*, coronary artery bypass graft; *cMRI*, cardiac magnetic resonance imaging; *CTO*, chronic total occlusion; *DES*, drug-eluting stent; *FFR*, fractional flow reserve; *ID-TLR*, ischemia-driven target lesion revascularization; *LVEDV*, left ventricular end-diastolic volume; *LVEF*, left ventricular ejection fraction; *MACCE*, major adverse cardiac or cerebrovascular events; *MACE*, major adverse cardiovascular event; *MI*, myocardial infarction; *OMT*, optimal medical therapy; *PCI*, percutaneous coronary intervention; *QOL*, quality of life; *SAQ*, Seattle angina questionnaire; *STEMI*, ST elevation myocardial infarction; *TLR*, target lesion revascularization.

all-cause death between PCI and CABG in patients with LM disease (26% vs. 28%, respectively; HR 0.90; 95% CI, 0.68 to 1.20).[24]

The EXCEL trial randomized 1905 patients with significant LM disease and a SYNTAX score of less than 32 to CABG or PCI with a second-generation DES (Xience, Abbott Vascular, Santa Clara, CA). At 5 years, no differences were noted for PCI versus CABG for the primary endpoint (22.0% vs. 19.2%, P = 0.13). However, all-cause mortality (13.0% vs. 9.9%), non-procedural MI (6.8% vs. 3.5%) and ID-TLR rates (16.9% vs. 10%) were higher with PCI compared with CABG.[25] Due to violation of proportional hazards, a piecemeal hazard model analysis was used. During the first 30 days after revascularization, PCI was associated with a lower risk of the primary endpoint (HR 0.61; 95% CI, 0.42 to 0.88), which was driven by a lower incidence of (procedural) MI (HR 0.63; 95% CI, 0.42 to 0.94). Between 30 days and 1 year, the primary endpoint rates between PCI and CABG were similar (HR 1.07; 95% CI, 0.68 to 1.70), as were each of its individual components. Between 1 year and 5 years, the risk for the primary endpoint was higher in the PCI arm (HR 1.61; 95% CI, 1.23 to 2.12) (Fig. 41.1).

Taken together,[26–29] these results suggest that CABG may still be superior to PCI for patients with LM disease. Patients with ostial or isolated shaft lesions and low SYNTAX score may do well with PCI. The EXCEL trial also suggests a role for shared decision making among patients with LM disease. From a PCI standpoint, intravascular imaging using intravascular ultrasound (IVUS) or optical coherence tomography (OCT) should be considered as standard of care for LM PCI optimization. In addition, for distal LM lesions, a double kiss (DK) crush 2-stent strategy is superior to provisional stenting or Culotte stenting, with significant reductions in MACE, repeat revascularization and stent thrombosis.[30,31]

Multivessel Disease

Although there is a fair amount of overlap with patients who have diabetes mellitus (DM; see below), the summary of data seems to indicate that CABG is superior to PCI for patients with multivessel disease (i.e., two or three-vessel disease), particularly in the setting of higher SYNTAX scores.[32] For instance, in the SYNTAX trial, among patients with triple vessel disease, MACCE rates at 5 years were higher in the PCI arm compared with CABG (37.5% vs. 24.2%, p< 0.001), including a higher risk of all-cause mortality (14.6% vs. 9.2%, p = 0.006), MI (9.2% vs. 4.0%, p = 0.001), and repeat revascularization (25.4% vs. 12.6%, p< 0.001), with a similar risk of stroke (3.0% vs. 3.5%). When stratified by SYNTAX score, patients with low (0 to 22) SYNTAX scores had comparable MACCE rates with PCI or CABG (33.3% vs. 26.8%, p = 0.21), with a higher rate of repeat revascularization (25.4% vs. 12.6%, p = 0.038) with PCI.[33-34]

For multivessel PCI in STEMI, see Chapter 38, and for cardiogenic shock, see "Cardiomyopathy/Left Ventricular Dysfunction".

Chronic Total Occlusions

Chronic coronary occlusions occur in many patients with severe (>70% stenosis) CAD and are the most important factor leading to referral for CABG procedures rather than PCI. The four main aspects of CTO anatomy that are important are (1) proximal cap morphology; (2) occlusion length, course, and composition (e.g., calcium); (3) quality of the distal vessel; and (4) characteristics of the collateral circulation.[35] In addition, tools such as the J-CTO score (Multicenter CTO Registry of Japan) have been developed to estimate the likelihood of successful antegrade guidewire crossing.[36] Once the chronic total occlusion (CTO) has been crossed, DESs may be used to reduce late clinical recurrence, with liberal use of intravascular imaging to optimize stent deployment.

Few clinical trials have compared CTO PCI to medical management head-to-head (see Table 41.1).[37–39] Over an intermediate duration of follow-up, CTO PCI does not improve hard outcomes, but may provide reductions in angina frequency. Other trials, including a sham-controlled trial are ongoing, and will further inform this field in the future.[35]

Saphenous Vein Grafts (Fig.41.2)

SVGs are unique in that three distinct pathophysiologic processes lead to SVG failure: thrombosis and technical failure is the predominant mechanism within the first week and during the first month after CABG, followed by intimal hyperplasia (due to "arterialization" of the venous conduit) from 1 month to 1 year, and atherosclerosis beyond 1 year.[40] There are two major considerations: (1) distal embolization and no-reflow in the acute phase and (2) high rates of restenosis during follow-up.

SVG-PCI can be challenging because they typically have extensive plaque burden predisposing to distal embolism of friable atheromatous material during PCI; slow and no-reflow rates can be as high as 15% to 20%, and are substantially higher than native coronary artery

PCI.[41] Strategies to minimize slow/no-reflow include direct stenting rather than predilation, appropriate stent sizing (minimizing oversizing) and the use of embolic protection devices (EPDs) when feasible.[42] The 2011 ACC/AHA PCI guidelines recommend EPDs for SVG-PCI as a class I recommendation, while the 2018 ESC/EACTS guidelines recommend them as a class IIa recommendation.[11,43] When no-reflow occurs, administration of arterial vasodilators (e.g., nitroprusside, verapamil, adenosine) into the SVG may improve flow into the distal native circulation, but the risk for death or MI is still substantially increased.

As far as choice of revascularization strategy, lower rates of restenosis in SVG lesions occur after coronary stent placement than after balloon angioplasty. In contrast to coronary PCI, trials comparing BMS and DES for SVG PCI are less clear in terms of DES superiority, although DES may have lower restenosis rates, mostly in the short to intermediate term (see Table 41.1).[44-46]

Bifurcation Lesions

Bifurcation lesions comprise 15% to 18% of all lesions treated with PCI. They can be technically quite challenging, and restenosis and TLR rates are higher than for non-bifurcation PCI. The goals in approaching bifurcation lesions are to (1) Maximize flow in both the parent vessel while maintaining flow in the side branch; (2) prevent side branch occlusion or compromise; (3) maximize long-term patency of both parent vessel and side branch; and (4) minimize procedure time and radiation.

Robust data from clinical trials suggest that a "provisional approach"—stenting of the main vessel with optional side branch treatment—remains the best option for most bifurcation lesions.[47,48] This is also endorsed as a class I recommendation in the 2018 ESC/EACTS myocardial revascularization guidelines.[43] A variety of two-stent techniques may be helpful when needed, including T, T with small protrusion (TAP), mini-Crush and Culotte. It is important to note that side-branch "pinching" after main vessel stenting occurs not just due to "snowplowing" of plaque, but also due to a change in geometry of the bifurcation itself. Accordingly, FFR assessment of an angiographically narrowed side branch can be useful in guiding decision-making regarding the need for another stent in the side branch.[49] When a two-stent strategy is felt to be necessary upfront, the double-kissing crush technique appears to have the best angiographic and clinical

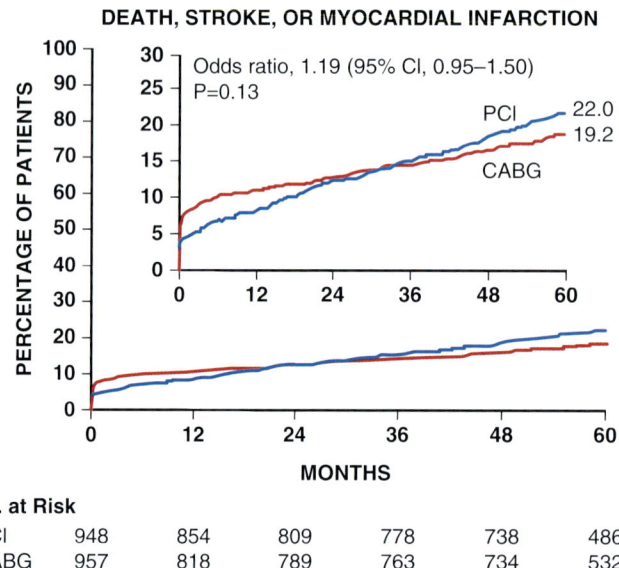

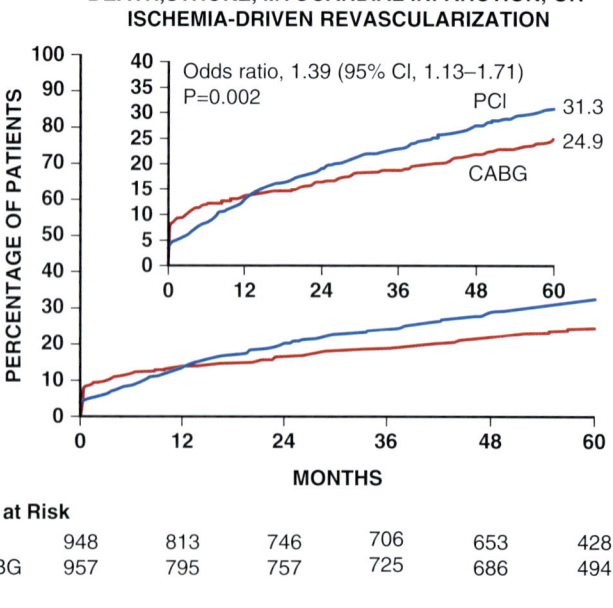

A

FIGURE 41.1 Time-to-first-event curves for the primary and secondary composite outcomes (**A**) and for components of the primary and secondary composite outcomes (**B**) through 5-year follow-up in EXCEL. (From Stone GW, Kappetein AP, Sabik JF, et al. Five-Year Outcomes after PCI or CABG for Left Main Coronary Disease. *N Engl J Med.* 2019;381:1820–1830.)

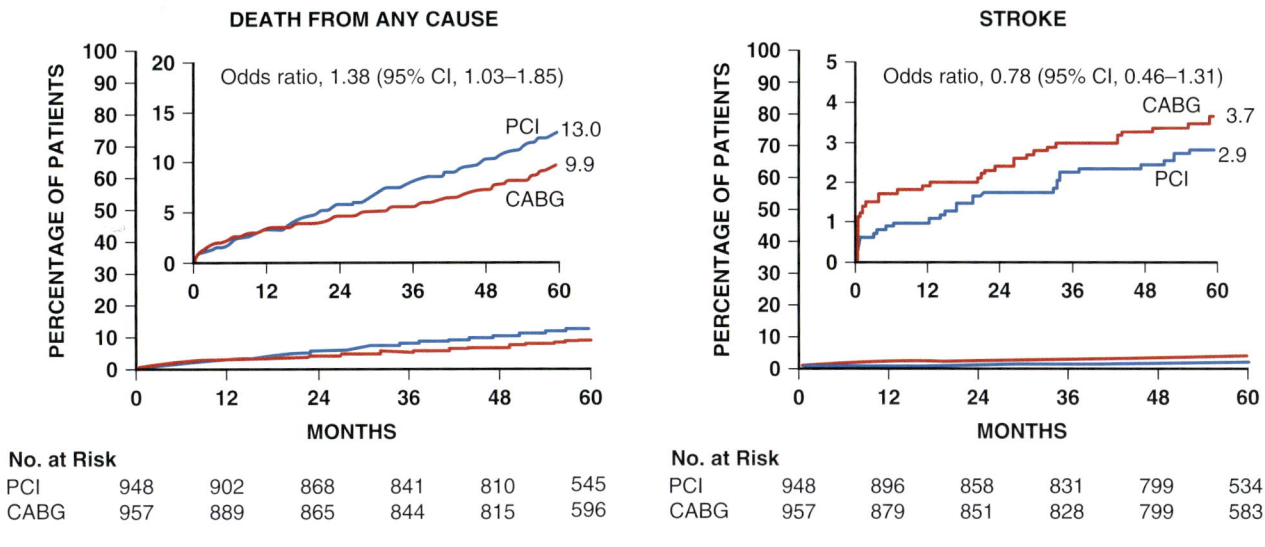
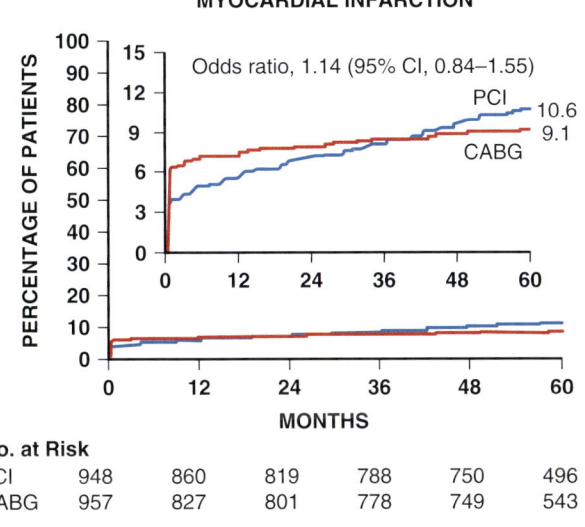
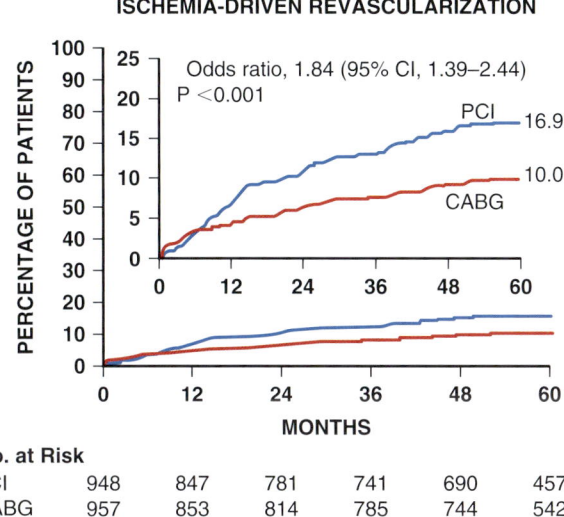

FIGURE 41.1 cont'd

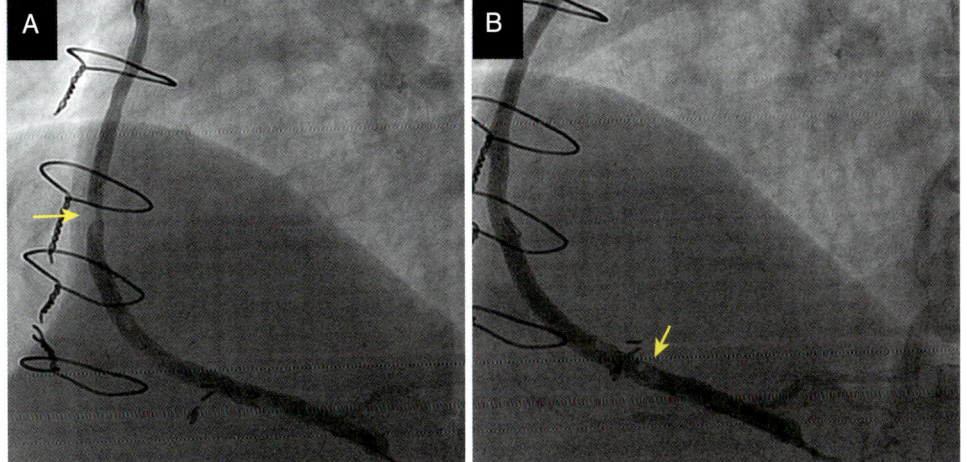

FIGURE 41.2 Examples of debris capture by a filter. **A,** FilterWire placed distally to eccentric saphenous vein graft body lesion. **B,** During PCI, debris embolized distally and was captured within the filter. (From Brilakis ES, Banerjee S. Bypass graft interventions. In: Bhatt DL, ed. *Cardiovascular Intervention: A Companion to Braunwald's Heart Disease*. Philadelphia: Elsevier; 2016.)

outcomes, but requires a higher level of skill and expertise.[30] This is particularly important for bifurcation PCI subtending large areas of myocardium such as the distal left main.

Lesion Calcification

The presence of extensive coronary calcification poses unique challenges for PCI because calcium in the vessel wall leads to irregular and inflexible lumens, thus making delivery of guidewires, balloons, and stents much more challenging. Extensive coronary calcification also renders the vessel wall rigid, which necessitates higher balloon inflation pressure to achieve complete stent expansion and, on occasion, leads to "undilatable" lesions that resist any balloon expansion pressure that can be achieved. In this setting, atherectomy can address vessel wall calcification and facilitate stent delivery and complete stent expansion (see "Coronary Atherectomy").

Thrombotic Lesions

Conventional angiography has poor sensitivity for the detection of coronary thrombus, but the presence of a large, angiographically apparent coronary thrombus heightens the risk for procedural complications. Large coronary thrombi may fragment and embolize during PCI or may extrude through gaps between stent struts placed in the vessel, thereby risking lumen compromise or thrombus propagation and acute thrombosis of the treated vessel. In addition, large coronary thrombi can embolize to other coronary branches or vessels or dislodge and compromise the cerebral or other vascular beds. In the setting of contemporary primary PCI for STEMI, routine manual catheter aspiration of thrombus appears to have no significant effect on mortality and may increase the risk of stroke,[50] but it may be helpful in select patients.[51,52] (see "Thrombectomy and Aspiration Devices").

Diabetes Mellitus (see Chapter 31)

Diabetes is one of the most common comorbidities among patients with CAD; ischemic heart disease remains the biggest cause of mortality and morbidity in this patient population. The largest trial to date devoted to studying outcomes after revascularization in patients with DM and multivessel disease is FREEDOM (Future Revascularization Evaluation in Patients with Diabetes Mellitus: Optimal Management of Multivessel Disease) that compared the outcomes of PCI and CABG in patients with DM and multivessel disease. The primary outcome (all-cause mortality, nonfatal MI, or nonfatal stroke) at 5 years was worse in patients treated with PCI than in those who underwent CABG (26.6% vs. 18.7%; $P = 0.005$). There was a significantly increased long-term risk for all-cause mortality and nonfatal MI with PCI as opposed to CABG. CABG, however, was associated with an increased risk for nonfatal stroke, and the severity of strokes in the CABG group was twice as likely to disable a patient severely as were strokes occurring in the PCI group.[53] On subgroup analysis, the incidence of the primary endpoint was higher among PCI patients irrespective of SYNTAX score.[54]

The results of the FREEDOM trial have largely validated smaller studies, subgroup analyses, and meta-analyses attempting to compare methods of revascularization in diabetic patients with multivessel disease. The recommendations from contemporary guidelines favor CABG over PCI as the optimal revascularization strategy in patients with DM and multivessel disease. Despite this, a significant proportion of patients with diabetes and multivessel disease in the United States continue to undergo PCI rather than CABG.[10]

Cardiomyopathy/Left Ventricular Dysfunction
Ischemic Cardiomyopathy

Like DM, there is an overlap between patients with multivessel disease and ischemic cardiomyopathy/LV systolic dysfunction. Ischemic cardiomyopathy remains the main cause of congestive HF in the developed world (see Chapters 47 and 50). According to the 2018 ESC/EACTS guidelines, coronary revascularization has a class I recommendation for patients with impaired LV function (LVEF ≤35%) and significant two or three–vessel disease to improve prognosis.[43] There are no good randomized controlled data on the utility of PCI for chronic LV dysfunction. The STICH (Surgical Treatment for Ischemic Heart Failure) trial compared surgical revascularization with medical therapy in 1212 patients with LVEF ≤35%. Over 6 years of follow-up, the primary outcome of all-cause mortality was similar between the CABG + medical therapy versus medical therapy arms (36% vs. 41%, p = 0.12). However, CV mortality was lower in the CABG + medical therapy arm (28% vs. 33%, HR = 0.81, 95% CI 0.66 to 1.00, p = 0.05), as was all-cause mortality or CV hospitalization (58% vs. 68%, HR = 0.74, 95% CI 0.64 to 0.85, p < 0.001).[55] At 10 years, a mortality benefit was noted for CABG + medical therapy (58.9% vs. 66.1%, HR = 0.84, 95% CI 0.73 to 0.97, p = 0.02).[56] Although commonly utilized, the value of viability testing for prognostic improvement in patients with LV dysfunction is unclear.[57] In several situations with excessive surgical morbidity (frailty, chronic kidney dysfunction, severe respiratory disorders), where the surgical outcomes might be less optimal, a more precise evaluation of non–viable myocardium might be helpful. Under these circumstances, viability studies can help to determine the potential risks and benefits of revascularization and guide the decision-making process.

Role of Left Ventricular Dysfunction in PCI

LV function is an important predictor of outcome during PCI. For each 10% decrement in resting LV ejection fraction (EF), the risk for in-hospital mortality following PCI increases approximately two-fold. Associated valvular disease or ventricular arrhythmia further increases the risk associated with PCI in the setting of LV dysfunction. A more extreme scenario is cardiogenic shock, which is defined as a state in which ineffective cardiac output caused by a primary cardiac disorder results in both clinical and biochemical manifestations of inadequate tissue perfusion, most commonly caused by acute MI resulting in acute LV dysfunction. Objectively, this has been defined as a pulmonary capillary wedge pressure (PCWP) higher than 18 mm Hg and a cardiac index (CI) lower than 2.2 L/min/m^2, typically with a systolic blood pressure ≤ 90 mm Hg.[58,59] Patients with cardiogenic shock have very high mortality; post-MI cardiogenic shock has a prevalence of 3% to 13%, and is associated with 30-day mortality rates from 30% to 50%.[59,60] An important consideration is that cardiogenic shock is a heterogeneous entity, and patients with cardiac arrest have the worst outcomes. More recently, classifications such as the Society for Cardiovascular Angiography and Interventions (SCAI) shock system have been proposed for better risk stratification.[61] Treatment efforts to reduce mortality have focused on improvement of hemodynamic parameters by mechanical circulatory support (MCS) devices (also see "Mechanical Circulatory Support").[62]

Role of PCI in Cardiogenic Shock

Approximately 70% to 80% of patients with cardiogenic shock present with multivessel disease defined as additional stenoses/occlusions in addition to the infarct related artery.[62] The landmark SHOCK trial showed that early revascularization (87% overall, including angioplasty in 54.5% [bare-metal stent use 35.7% overall], CABG in 37.5%) resulted in a mortality benefit at 6 months in patients presenting with post-MI shock (although this was not noted at 30 days).[63] This benefit was sustained out to 6 years of follow-up. Several registries have confirmed the significant decrease in mortality with early revascularization, from about 70% to 80% in earlier years to about 40% to 50% in the current era.[64] Both, US and European guidelines recommend emergent angiography as a class I recommendation for patients with MI-shock.[19,43,65] Further, till recently, guidelines encouraged operators to perform multivessel PCI of all critical stenosis, in addition to the culprit lesion for patients with MI-shock (class IIa recommendation).[19,65]

CULPRIT-SHOCK (Culprit Lesion Only PCI versus Multivessel PCI in Cardiogenic Shock) trial showed a significant clinical benefit of a culprit-lesion-only strategy compared with immediate multi-vessel PCI, with a reduction in the primary endpoint of 30-day mortality or renal replacement therapy (45.9% vs. 55.4%; RR 0.83; 95% CI 0.71 to 0.96; p = 0.01). 30-day mortality was also reduced with culprit-vessel only PCI (43.3% vs. 51.5%; p= 0.03).[66] At 1 year, the difference in all-cause mortality between the two strategies was nominally significant (50.0% vs. 56.9%, RR 0.88, 95% CI 0.76 to 1.01), while rates of recurrent infarction were similar (1.7% vs. 2.1%). Repeat revascularization was performed at a greater than three-fold higher rate in the culprit-only arm (32.3% vs. 9.4%, RR 3.44, 95% CI 2.39 to 4.95). Based on this trial, the ESC 2018 revascularization guidelines now advise against routine immediate multivessel PCI (Class IIIB recommendation); no updates to the US guidelines have been issued yet.[43] CABG is rarely performed in cardiogenic shock with rates less than 5% in registries and randomized trials.[62,64,67]

Renal Dysfunction and Other Comorbidities

The morbidity and mortality associated with PCI are directly related to the extent of baseline renal disease (see also Chapter 101). Patients with evidence of mild renal dysfunction have a 20% higher risk for death at 1 year following PCI than do those with preserved renal function. Renal dysfunction following PCI may be related to hemodynamic instability, contrast-induced nephropathy, cholesterol embolization syndrome, or a combination of these. The risk for nephropathy is dependent on the dose of the contrast agents used, hydration status at the time of the procedure, preexisting renal function of the patient, age, hemodynamic stability, anemia, and diabetes. The risk for cholesterol embolization syndrome is related to manipulation of the catheter in an ascending or descending atherosclerotic aorta from which cholesterol crystals are released. Although the risk associated with hemodialysis is less than 3% in cases of uncomplicated contrast-induced nephropathy, in-hospital mortality in the setting of hemodialysis exceeds 30%. Mild renal dysfunction is associated with an up to fourfold increased risk for death at 1 year after PCI compared with patients with preserved renal function, although this association is probably not causal.[68]

Other important comorbidities that can affect post-PCI outcomes include concomitant liver disease, bleeding diatheses, and peripheral vascular disease, to name a few. A special higher-risk subset is patients needing concomitant oral anticoagulation for atrial fibrillation, venous thromboembolic disease, etc (see "Antithrombin Agents").[69]

A recent development in the interventional field is specialization in so-called "CHIP" (Complex High Risk and Indicated Procedures) interventions.[70] These patients typically have multiple comorbidities, poor ventricular function, or grossly deranged hemodynamics, in addition to anatomically complex, atypical, or high-risk coronary disease (i.e., CTOs, single remaining coronary vessel, severe calcification, multivessel disease and proximal bifurcations). Operators are skilled in performing complex PCI typically with utilization of MCS devices in various clinical settings. Dedicated training programs have been created, although the overall acceptance of this concept is low as its utility outside of large academic centers remains unclear.

CORONARY DEVICES

Over the past few decades, steady improvements in the equipment used for coronary revascularization (e.g., reductions in device profile and improvements in catheter flexibility) have been supplemented by the introduction of periodic "transformational technology," such as drug-eluting stents, which have dramatically extended the scope and breadth of clinical practice.

Balloon Angioplasty

Balloon angioplasty expands the coronary lumen by stretching and tearing the atherosclerotic plaque and vessel wall and, to a lesser extent, by redistributing atherosclerotic plaque along its longitudinal axis. This results in a localized dissection of the intima, and sometimes the media. The dissection is covered by platelet-rich thrombus and later by new intimal layers. Elastic recoil of the stretched vessel wall generally leaves a 30% to 35% residual diameter stenosis, and the vessel expansion can result in propagation of coronary dissections and lead to abrupt vessel closure in 5% to 8% of patients. Restenosis rates at 6 months are as high as 30% to 49%.[71] Current indications for stand-alone balloon angioplasty are rare.

Coronary Stents

Coronary stents have emerged as the predominant form of PCI and are currently used in more than 90% of PCI procedures worldwide. They act as scaffolds for arterial dissection flaps, thereby lowering the incidence of vessel closure and need for emergency CABG; they also lessen the frequency of restenosis because of their effect in preventing arterial recoil, which is the primary mechanism of restenosis with balloon angioplasty. To overcome restenosis due to intimal hyperplasia in metal-only stents, they are coated with a pharmacologic agent on their abluminal surface (so-called, "drug-coated" or "drug-eluting" stents [DES]; see below); accordingly, the earlier stents are now referred to as "bare-metal" stents (BMS).

Drug-Eluting Stents
The three components of a conventional DES (also called durable polymer [DP]-DES) are a balloon-expandable metallic stent, a durable or resorbable polymer coating that provides sustained drug delivery, and the pharmacologic agent used to limit intimal hyperplasia. DP-DES have proven efficacy in patients with virtually every lesion type. First-generation DES (sirolimus- and paclitaxel-eluting stents) were associated with a significantly elevated risk of late and very late stent thrombosis, compared with BMS, with a median thrombosis time that was 1 to 14 months longer than late BMS thrombosis.[72] Both of these stents are not clinically available in the United States. Current DP-DES show lower risk of stent thrombosis than the first DES and consistent prevention of restenosis compared with BMS, as well as improved deliverability because of lower-profile materials.[73] Stent thrombosis is now rare compared with risk of MI unrelated to prior stents. Stent thrombosis rates with contemporary DP-DES are as low as 0.4% to 0.5% at 1 year, and less than 1% at 5 years.

With current DES, contemporary guidelines recommend 6 months or longer of dual-antiplatelet therapy (DAPT) in patients without ACS who are not at high risk of bleeding and who tolerated DAPT without a bleeding complication. Guidelines have also been updated regarding longer-duration DAPT based on recently published trials and indicate that 12 months or longer may be reasonable for patients who do not have a high risk of bleeding and who have tolerated DAPT without a bleeding complication.[74,75] Although low stent thrombosis risks with DES are further reduced with extended therapy, the recommendations are largely based on reduction in the risk of late MI unrelated to the stent, rather than stent thrombosis.[75]

Zotarolimus-Eluting Stents
Zotarolimus (also known as ABT-578) is a rapamycin analogue released from a phosphorylcholine-coated stent that was initially evaluated in the Endeavor stent (Medtronic Vascular, Santa Rosa, California).[76] Late lumen loss was higher with the Endeavor stent compared with both first-generation DES.[77] This was felt to be a stent design issue rather than a drug-failure issue as zotarolimus was eluted within a few weeks from the polymer, with 95% of the drug released within about two weeks. Accordingly, Endeavor-ZES was redesigned as Resolute-ZES with an alternative polymer that extended the delivery of zotarolimus (85% within 60 days and the remainder by 180 days). In the RESOLUTE All Comers Trial of 2292 patients, the Resolute zotarolimus-eluting stent was found to be noninferior to everolimus-eluting stents for the primary endpoint of target-lesion failure (8.2% vs. 8.3%, respectively; p < 0.001 for noninferiority).[78] At 5 years of follow-up, there were no significant differences between the two second-generation DP-DES in target-lesion failure, its components, or stent thrombosis.

Resolute-ZES has since been replaced by Resolute Onyx. The biggest difference is thinner struts in Resolute Onyx (81 [for stents ≤4.0 mm] vs. 91 μm) and improved radiographic visibility. Resolute Onyx DES has US FDA approval for a new 1-month DAPT labeling among patients at high bleeding risk. Resolute Onyx is also the only DES that is available for PCI in very small (2.0 mm) or very large (5.0 mm) vessels.

Everolimus-Eluting Stents
Everolimus is a semisynthetic analogue of sirolimus (rapamycin), with both immunosuppressive and antiproliferative effects. Two versions of everolimus-eluting stents with a DP are available: one with cobalt chromium (Xience, Abbott Vascular, Chicago, Illinois) and one with platinum chromium (Promus, Boston Scientific, Marlborough, Massachusetts). The polymer is the same in both stents (PBMA/PVDF-HFP). These fluoropolymers are more biocompatible, with reduced vascular injury and inflammation, faster endothelialization, reduced neointimal proliferation and lower thrombogenicity.[79] Strut thickness for both stents is 81 μm; thinner struts afford greater flexibility and deliverability, and also reduce stent-induced arterial injury and inflammation and facilitate faster endothelialization.[79]

In a 2012 network meta-analysis from 76 randomized controlled trials with 117,762 patient-years of follow-up, short-term (up to 1 year) target vessel revascularization (TVR) rates were lowest for sirolimus (4.1%), everolimus (4.4%) and Resolute-ZES (4.9%), with higher rates for Endeavor-ZES (7.6%), paclitaxel (7.4%) and bare-metal stents (15.8%). Definite/probable stent thrombosis rates were lowest for everolimus (0.04%; 86.3% likelihood of having lowest stent thrombosis rates), followed by Resolute-ZES (0.07%) and sirolimus (0.08%); rates for paclitaxel (0.17%) bare-metal (0.18%) and Endeavor-ZES (0.19%) were higher. Longer-term stent thrombosis rates also seemed to be best for everolimus-eluting stents.[73] Five-year event rates for repeat revascularization and stent thrombosis appear to be comparable for the Xience and Promus stent platforms.

Bioabsorbable Polymer Drug-ElutingStents

Bioabsorbable polymers have the potential benefit of no polymer remaining after the period required for drug suppression of neointimal hyperplasia, therefore limiting possible vascular reaction and toxicity. There are two stent designs that incorporate bioabsorbable polymers: (i) bioabsorbable polymer drug-eluting stents (BP-DES), where the drug and polymer are both eluted/degraded over a period of time, leaving behind a BMS in the vessel, and (ii) bioresorbable vascular scaffold (BVS), where the polymer and stent scaffold are both resorbed once the drug has been eluted, thus leaving nothing behind in the vessel. A third design is polymer-free stents, where the drug is coated directly onto the stent frame, and elutes over a month or so, leaving behind a BMS after that. These stents are also called drug-coated stent.

Currently, the two most widely used BP-DES in the United States are Synergy BP-DES (Boston Scientific) or Orsiro (Biotronik, Bülach, Switzerland). In both stents, the drug elutes over 3 to 4 months, and the polymer over 4 (Synergy) to 24 (Orsiro) months. Other BP-DES such as the biolimus-eluting Nobori stent, and sirolimus-eluting MiStent, have also shown no difference in 12-month TLR and stent thrombosis when compared to current-generation DP-DES. An important distinguishing factor appears to be strut thickness—the ultra-thin strut BP-DES (strut thickness less than 70 μm; for example, Orsiro) have lower rates of target lesion failure and MI compared with thicker-strut BP-DES or DP-DES.[80] The BioFreedom stent (Biosensors Europe, Morges, Switzerland) is a polymer-free DCS that transfers umirolimus (biolimus A9) into the vessel wall over 1 month (approximately 90% within 48 hours). Its efficacy is felt to be intermediate between BMS and contemporary DES.[81,82]

Bioresorbable Vascular Scaffolds

It was felt that a BVS stent would address the following issues with non-absorbable scaffolding: very-late stent thrombosis thought to be due to uncovered stent struts; impaired coronary vasomotion due to retention of obstructive scaffolding; decreased luminal size due to retained scaffolding, and chronic inflammation due to retained foreign-body metal. Abbott (Santa Clara, California) was one of the first to enter this realm, with the creation of its ABSORB BVS. The stent scaffolding is made of poly-L-lactide (PLLA), which also degrades to lactic acid and carbon dioxide over time. IVUS examinations of PLLA scaffolds have shown complete resorption by three years in most patients. When compared with cobalt-chromium and stainless-steel scaffolding, however, PLAA has less radial strength, necessitating much thicker stent struts in order to match the strength of current-generation DES; the first-generation ABSORB BVS has a strut thickness of 156 μm.[83]

In the ABSORB III trial, the primary endpoint of target-lesion failure at 1 year occurred in 7.8% of patients treated with an everolimus-eluting bioabsorbable scaffold (ABSORB) and in 6.1% of patients treated with a DP everolimus-eluting stent (Xience) (noninferiority P = 0.007; difference P = 0.16).[84] The stent was approved for clinical use by the US FDA in 2015. The findings were not maintained over time, however, as further studies showed inferior performance of the ABSORB stent when compared to Cobalt-Chromium EES, with a particularly concerning signal for scaffold thrombosis. Given the safety concerns of the ABSORB BVS, in addition to the cost-limiting market penetration, Abbott pulled the product from European and North American markets in 2017. Although no BVS are currently available in the United States, the development of future-generation BVS continues; efforts have focused on reductions of strut size to decrease thrombogenicity, polymers other than PLLA and other anti-restenotic drugs.[85]

Coronary Atherectomy

Atherectomy refers to removal (rather than simple displacement) of the obstructing atherosclerotic plaque. By removing plaque or improving lesion wall compliance in severely calcified or fibrotic lesions, atherectomy can provide a larger final minimal lumen diameter than can be achieved by balloon angioplasty alone. Fewer than 5% of current PCI procedures involve the use of atherectomy. There are two main forms of atherectomy: rotational and orbital. Excimer laser angioplasty involves utilizing predominantly the photoacoustic effects of laser energy to cause tissue absorption, and thereby plaque ablation (Fig. 41.3).

In recent years, the lithotripsy concept (ultrasonic waves to treat renal calculi) has been adopted for treating calcified coronary lesions. The Intravascular Lithotripsy (IVL) System (Shockwave Medical Inc, Santa Clara, California) has multiple lithotripsy emitters that are mounted on a traditional catheter platform and transforms electrical energy into mechanical energy during low-pressure balloon inflation. In contrast to debulking and atherectomy techniques, the calcium fragments resulting from the IVL therapy remain *in situ*, thus reducing the likelihood of distal embolization.

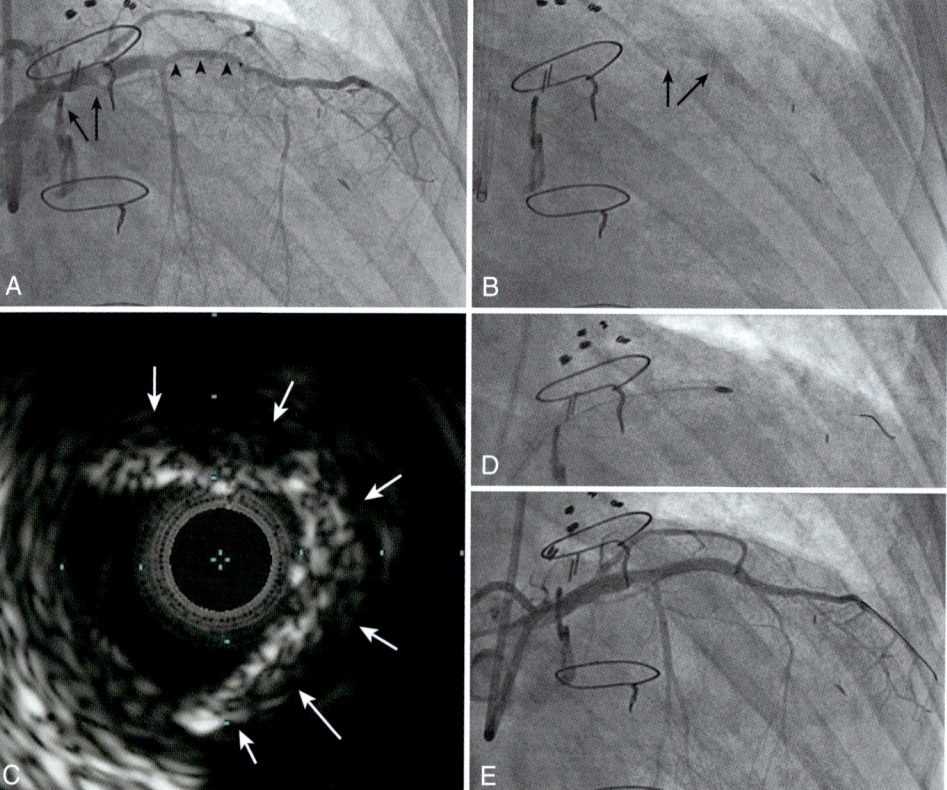

FIGURE 41.3 Rotational atherectomy of the left anterior descending coronary artery (LAD)/diagonal. **A,** Initial angiogram demonstrates severe calcified stenosis in the proximal (*arrows*) and mid-LAD (*arrowheads*) extending to the diagonal. **B,** Fluoroscopy alone shows the severe calcification (*arrows*). **C,** Intravascular ultrasound demonstrates 270-degree calcification (*arrows*) with echo dropout behind the calcium. **D,** Rotaburr in the mid-LAD. **E,** Final angiogram after stent placement. (From Krishnaswamy A, Whitlow PL. Calcified lesions. In: Bhatt DL, ed. *Cardiovascular Intervention: A Companion to Braunwald's Heart Disease*. Philadelphia: Elsevier; 2016.)

DISRUPT CAD (Disrupt Coronary Artery Disease)—II was a single-arm study in 120 patients with severe calcified de novo coronary lesions. Clinical success was high, and residual stenosis was 32% immediately after IVL and 7.8% after further DES implantation. 30-day MACE rate was 7.6%, driven mostly by peri-procedural MIs.[86] These results were confirmed in the recently presented larger DISRUPT III trial, which enrolled 431 patients with severely calcified *de novo* coronary artery lesions ≤40 mm in length, and noted similar safety and efficacy.

Thrombectomy and Aspiration Devices

There are two main types of thrombectomy/aspiration devices for coronary lesions, mainly for primary PCI during STEMI: simple catheter aspiration (such as Export and Pronto catheters), and mechanical aspiration (such as AngioJet and X-Sizer). In the TAPAS (Thrombus Aspiration during Percutaneous Coronary Intervention in Acute Myocardial Infarction Study) trial, there were significant reductions in all-cause (4.7% vs. 7.6%, p= 0.04) and cardiovascular (3.6% vs. 6.7%, p = 0.02) mortality at 1 year, with a trend towards reduction in subacute and late stent thrombosis with adjunctive aspiration thrombectomy compared with conventional PCI alone.[87] This led to a class IIa recommendation for use in the 2009 and 2013 ACC/AHA STEMI guidelines.[19,88] However, subsequent trials did not show a benefit with aspiration thrombectomy during primary PCI. TOTAL was the largest of these (n = 10,732). No differences in clinical outcomes were observed at 6 months in favor of aspiration thrombectomy compared with conventional primary PCI, including in the primary MACE outcome (6.9% vs. 7.0%, p = 0.86), cardiovascular death (3.1% vs. 3.5%, p = 0.34) or stent thrombosis (1.5% vs. 1.7%, p = 0.42); stroke rates were higher with aspiration thrombectomy (0.7% vs. 0.3%, p= 0.02).[50] Based on this evidence, routine aspiration thrombectomy was downgraded to a class III recommendation in the 2015 ACC/AHA STEMI guidelines.[20]

Embolic Protection Devices (also see section on Specific Lesion Subsets on Saphenous Vein Grafts PCI)

The advent of embolic protection systems has reduced the risk for postprocedural adverse events following SVG PCI. In particular, distal embolization causes postprocedural elevation of cardiac enzymes in almost 20% of patients after SVG PCI, and this enzyme elevation can be associated with substantial morbidity and mortality. Currently only two distal embolic protection devices are available in the United States—the FilterWireEZ (Boston Scientific, Natick, Massachusetts) and the SpiderFx (Medtronic).

These filters are advanced across the target lesion in their smaller collapsed state, and withdrawal of the retaining sheath allows the filters to open and expand against the vessel wall. The filters then remain in place to catch any liberated embolic material larger than the pore size (usually 120 to 150 μm) of the filter during intervention. At the end of the intervention the filters are collapsed by using a sheath, and the captured embolic material is removed from the body. This type of device has the advantage of maintaining anterograde flow during the procedure and allowing intermittent injection of contrast material to visualize the underlying anatomy, but it has the potential disadvantage of allowing debris with a diameter smaller than the pore size of the filter to pass.

Drug-Coated Balloons

Although DES significantly reduced the incidence of ISR as compared with BMS, the treatment of ISR is challenging. The treatment of in-stent restenosis with a DES has also raised concerns about an increased risk of stent thrombosis given the presence of two or more layers of metal in a native coronary artery. A few trials have sought to study the efficacy of drug-coated angioplasty balloons (DCBs), primarily paclitaxel-coated balloons, for the treatment of in-stent restenosis. The comparison groups in these trials have been balloon angioplasty repeat stenting with BMS or paclitaxel-eluting stents, but not contemporary DES.[89,90] These balloons are not currently commercially available for coronary use in the United States.

Coronary Physiology (see Chapter 36)

Coronary angiography provides limited information regarding the functional significance of a given coronary stenosis. In addition, relying on diagnostic angiography alone to decide functional severity and need for guide revascularization (typical angiographic threshold ≥70% stenosis) can be unreliable with significant inter-observer variability.[91]

Fractional flow reserve (FFR) is an accurate and lesion-specific physiologic test that provides a functional assessment of the presence of a reduction in flow, and correlates well with ischemia as detected by nuclear scintigraphy. The FFR technique involves placement of a pressure wire across a potentially significant lesion, and maximal vasodilation/hyperemia is achieved with either intravenous or intracoronary administration of vasodilators such as adenosine. It is defined as the ratio of coronary pressure distal to a coronary artery stenosis (P_d) and aortic pressure (P_a) under conditions of maximal hyperemia (range 0 to 1, normal value 0.94 to 1).[92] An FFR value less than 0.75 is considered flow-limiting and typically associated with ischemia, and therefore appropriate for revascularization (sensitivity 88%, specificity 100%). In contrast, an FFR value greater than 0.8 excludes ischemia in greater than 90% of patients, with a low cardiac event rate (<1%/year) with medical therapy alone. Although an FFR value between 0.75 and 0.8 is sometimes considered a gray zone, more recent outcomes trials have utilized 0.8 as the ischemic threshold for revascularization and is the routinely used cutoff value in clinical practice as well.[93,94] FFR is helpful in several lesion types, including intermediate, serial, diffuse and long, side branch, and multivessel disease.[95,96] In addition, post-PCI FFR may have prognostic value as well. The use of FFR is endorsed as a class IIa recommendation for patients with SIHD and intermediate lesions in the 2011 ACC/AHA/SCAI PCI guidelines (Fig. 41.4).[11]

The FAME (Fractional Flow Reserve versus Angiography for Multivessel Evaluation) trial compared angiography with FFR guidance for selection of lesions in 1005 patients with multivessel disease (1/3 with UA, the rest with SIHD), with PCI reserved for a lesion in the FFR arm if ≤0.8. FFR guidance resulted in fewer overall stented lesions. MACE at 1 year, a composite of death, MI, repeat revascularization, was significantly lower in the FFR group (13.2% vs. 18.3%, p= 0.02), with a reduction in death and MI at 1 year as well (7.3% vs. 11.1%, p = 0.04).[93] These results were sustained out to 5 years of follow-up (see "Stable Ischemic Heart Disease and Stable Angina" and "FAME-2 and SIHD" in the online chapter).

Although the use of FFR is most established among patients presenting with stable angina/SIHD, revascularization of non-infarct-related coronary arteries at the time of an acute myocardial infarction (AMI) remains a hotly debated topic. Two recent randomized trials add to the growing body of evidence supporting FFR-guided revascularization of the non-infarct-related artery in this patient population (see Table 41.1).[97,98]

Despite its strengths for lesion assessment over angiography alone, the interventional community was slow to adopt FFR for reasons that included additional time, cost, loss of procedural reimbursement, and use of adenosine. A new concept, the instantaneous wave-free ratio (iFR) was introduced in 2012, which uses wave intensity analysis. This is a resting translesional pressure ratio taken during a specific diastolic interval in which the natural microvascular resistance is constant and low, and therefore meets the criteria of FFR without inducing hyperemia (i.e., without the need for adenosine). FFR and iFR appear to have good correlation (0.8).[99] The exact cutoffs for iFR and the optimal way to use iFR are controversial, but iFR less than 0.86 is judged positive and iFR greater than 0.94 as negative, and standard FFR can be measured to classify stenoses with iFR falling between 0.86 and 0.94.[99] In practice, an iFR ≤0.89 is frequently considered as positive, and greater than 0.89 as negative, to minimize the need for adenosine/FFR.

DEFINE-FLAIR (Functional Lesion Assessment of Intermediate Stenosis to Guide Revascularisation) (n = 2492) and iFR-SWEDEHEART

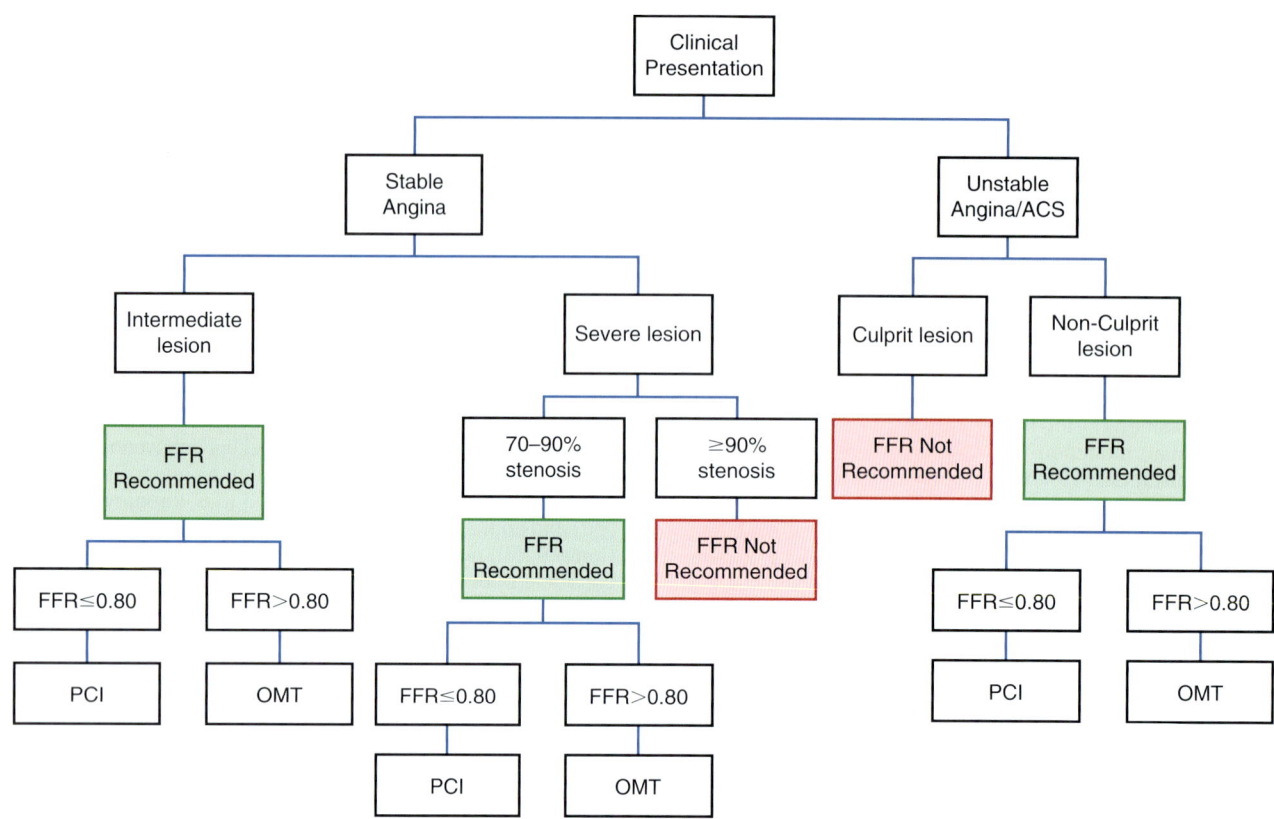

FIGURE 41.4 Algorithm for physiologic lesion assessment. (From Jeremias A, Kirtane AJ, Stone GW. A Test in Context: Fractional Flow Reserve: Accuracy, Prognostic Implications, and Limitations. *J Am Coll Cardiol*. 2017;69:2748–2758.)

(Evaluation of iFR vs FFR in Stable Angina or Acute Coronary Syndrome) (n = 2109) tested whether iFR-guided coronary revascularization strategy was noninferior to an FFR-guided strategy. The two trials had nearly identical trial designs (including iFR threshold of 0.89) and used the same primary composite end point of all-cause mortality, nonfatal MI, and unplanned revascularization. At 12 months, both studies demonstrated noninferiority to FFR (DEFINE-FLAIR 6.8% versus 7.0% for iFR versus FFR, noninferiority $P < 0.001$; iFR SWEDEHEART 6.7% versus 6.1%, noninferiority P= 0.007).[100,101]

Over the past few years, a variety of different physiologic indices, both invasive and noninvasive, have been proposed. The invasive indices use a pressure wire and are non-hyperemic, but they differ regarding the phase of the cardiac cycle in which the measurement takes place. These include phase-specific indices such as DFR (diastolic hyperemia-free ratio), DPR (diastolic pressure ratio), and whole cardiac-cycle indices such as resting Pd/Pa, contrast FFR, and RFR (resting full-cycle ratio). There are also angiography-based FFR simulations, such as QFR (quantitative flow ratio), vFFR (vessel FFR) and FFR_{angio}.[102]

Intravascular Imaging (see Chapter 21)

There are two main methods of intravascular imaging: IVUS and OCT. The advantage of both these techniques is that they are able to directly image the vessel and vessel wall in 3D, compared with the 2D nature of coronary angiography (Fig 41.5). These imaging modalities help interventionalists optimize stent implantation in multiple ways, including need for lesion preparation, stent sizing, and identifying acute complications.[103] Both modalities may also help with identification of flowlimiting stenoses. For instance, a minimum luminal area (MLA) of less than 6 mm² in the left main on IVUS correlates with an FFR value of less than 0.75 to 0.8 (Table 41.2).[104]

The IVUS catheter uses ultrasound (approximately 40 mm wavelength at 40 MHz), either by means of a mechanical transducer system (single piezoelectric crystal) or a multielement electronic array system (solid-state system, 64 piezoelectric crystals). Currently available IVUS systems (20 to 45 Hz) have an axial resolution of 100 μm and lateral resolution of 250 μm. OCT, on the other hand, uses infrared light (1.3-mm wavelength), which confers significantly greater resolution but at a cost of lower tissue penetration. Because the wavelength of OCT is shorter than the 8-mm diameter of a red blood cell, backscattering from blood occurs with OCT such that the vessel wall cannot be seen without blood clearance (typically, with simultaneous contrast injection). The combination of better resolution and clearance of blood during OCT imaging provides a much clearer interface between lumen and plaque surface, enabling accurate automatic lumen measurements[103] Fig. 41.6 illustrate some of the important differences between IVUS and OCT.

IVUS and OCT-guided stent optimization has been shown to improve PCI outcomes compared with angiography alone.[105–107] This is particularly helpful for complex lesions, including PCI of left main, long, and heavily calcified lesions. Intravascular imaging is felt to be *sine qua non* for BVS optimization.

MECHANICAL CIRCULATORY SUPPORT (ALSO SEE FIG. 41.7 AND "ROLE OF LEFT VENTRICULAR DYSFUNCTION IN PCI"; SEE CHAPTER 59)

Although used extensively for patients in cardiogenic shock, inotropes and vasopressors have several limitations, such as worsening ischemia, arrhythmogenic potential, vasoconstriction resulting in increased afterload.[108] In addition, they are frequently unable to consistently maintain adequate perfusion pressures, and prevent or reverse multisystem failure. Accordingly, a number of MCS are currently available for clinical use, primarily for temporary support. However, despite an increasing number of different percutaneous MCS devices for either LV or RV support, data derived from randomized clinical trials on the effectiveness, safety, differential indications for different devices, and optimal timing are still limited. The use in CS remains high, particularly for AMI-CS (approximately 25% to 50%). MCS selection should be based

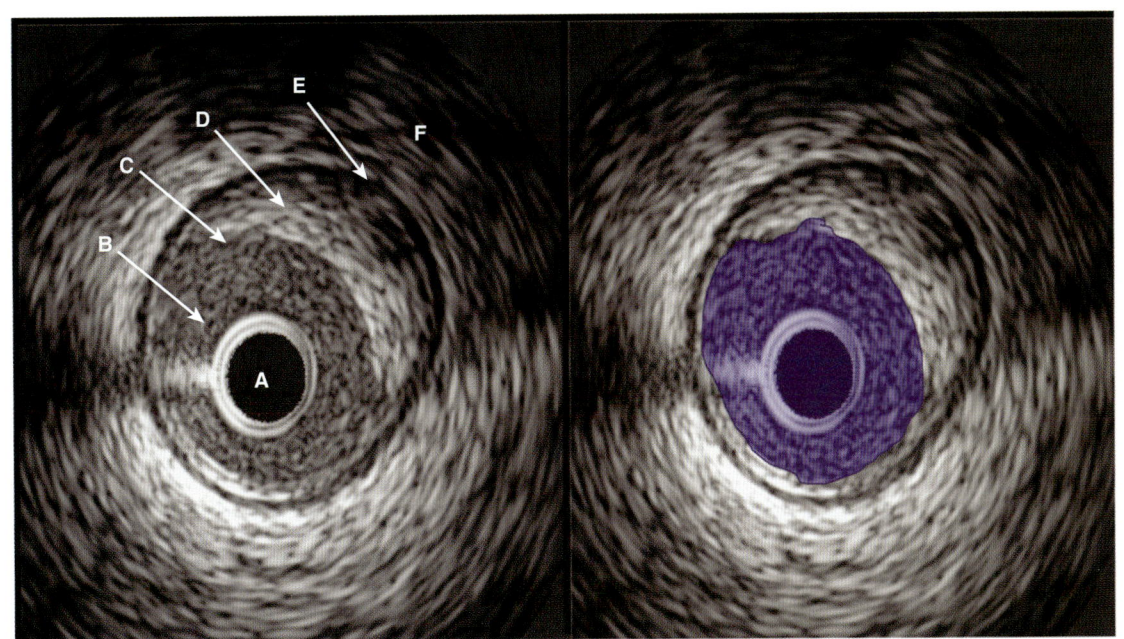

FIGURE 41.5 Basic IVUS measurements: IVUS catheter (*A*), arterial lumen (*B*), interface between intima and media (*C*). Note, the intima is only one cell layer thick (i.e., the endothelium). *D*, Atheromatous plaque within the media. *E*, External elastic membrane, which is the interface between the media and adventitia. *F*, Adventitia. The right panel highlights the minimal luminal area (MLA). (From Bavry AA, Kumbhani DJ. Indications and Techniques of Percutaneous Procedures. Springer 2012.)

TABLE 41.2 Intravascular Ultrasound Criteria for Functionally Significant Stenosis

	IVUS MLD, mm	IVUS MLA, mm²	CFR	FFR
Ischemia detection (native CAD other than LM)	≤1.8	<2.7–4.0	<2.0	<0.75–0.80
Ischemia detection (LM)	<2.8	<6.0	<2.0	<0.75–0.80
Adequacy of stenting	...	>9.0 (>80% reference area)	...	≥0.90

CAD, Coronary artery disease; *CFR*, coronary flow reserve; *FFR*, fractional flow reserve; *IVUS*, intravascular ultrasound; *LM*, left main; *MLA*, minimal lumen cross-sectional area; *MLD*, minimal lumen diameter.
Bangalore S, Bhatt DL. Coronary intravascular ultrasound. *Circulation*. 2013;127:e868–e874.

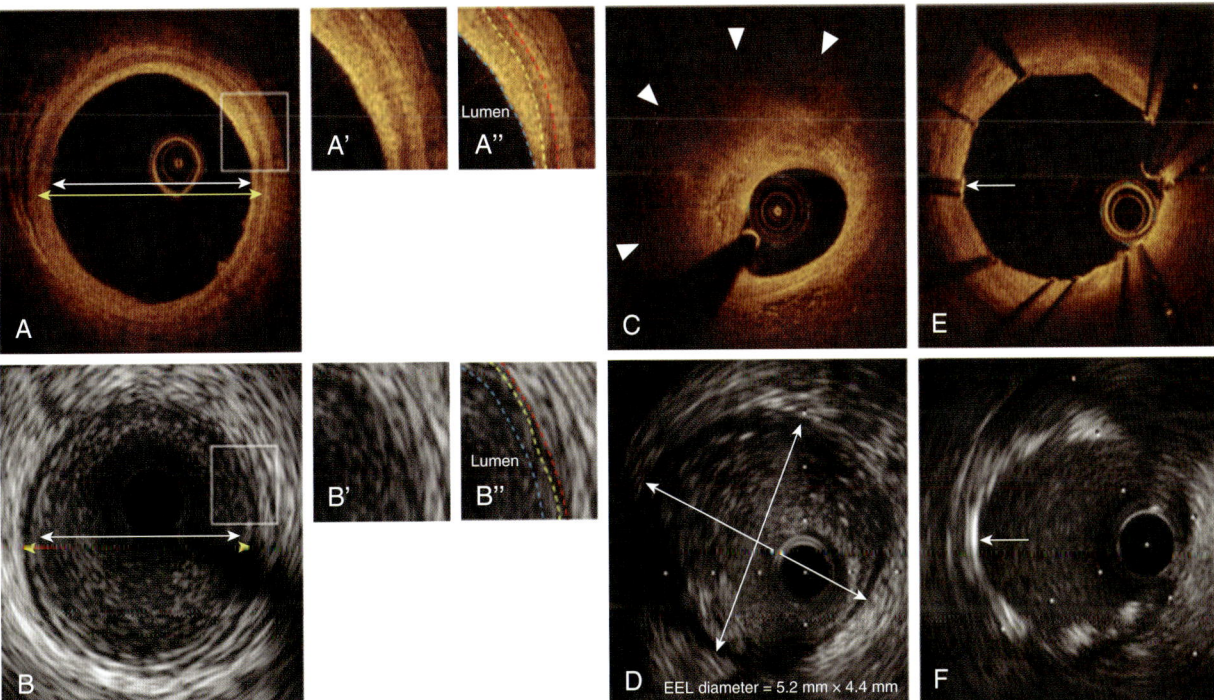

FIGURE 41.6 Differences in lumen and stent measurements between OCT and IVUS. Matched OCT and IVUS images from the same lesions are shown. Lumen area measured 8.40 mm² by OCT (**A**) and 8.83 mm² by IVUS (**B**). Magnification of selected squares in **A** and **B** are shown in (**A′**) and (**A″**) (OCT) and in (**B′**) and (**B″**) (IVUS), and include the EEL (*red dotted line*), internal elastic lamina (*yellow dotted line*), and lumen surface (*blue dotted line*). EEL diameter (*yellow arrow*) measured 3.86 mm by OCT and 4.09 mm by IVUS. Lumen diameter (*white arrow*) measured 3.28 mm by OCT and 3.54 mm by IVUS. At the lesion, although EEL diameter by IVUS (**D**) was visible (*arrows*, 5.2 × 4.4 mm), OCT (**C**) failed to show the EEL border (*arrowheads*) due to attenuation of plaque and limited penetration depth. Stent area measured 8.10 mm² by OCT (**E**) and 8.24 mm² by IVUS (**F**). Arrow indicates stent strut. The difference of area measurement between OCT and IVUS was less in stented segments than in nonstented segments. EEL, external elastic lamina. (From Maehara A, Matsumura M, Ali ZA, et al. IVUS-Guided Versus OCT-Guided Coronary Stent Implantation: A Critical Appraisal. *JACC Cardiovasc Imaging*. 2017;10:1487–1150.)

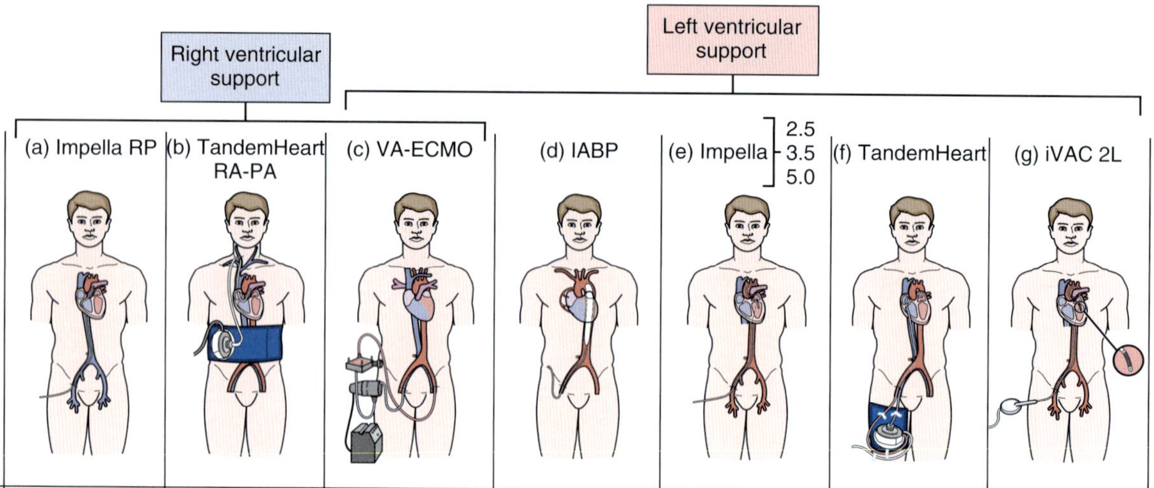

	(a) Impella RP	(b) TandemHeart RA-PA	(c) VA-ECMO	(d) IABP	(e) Impella 2.5 / 3.5 / 5.0	(f) TandemHeart	(g) iVAC 2L
Flow:	max. 4.0 L	max. 4.0 L	max. 7.0 L		2.5-5.0 L	max. 4.0 L	max. 2.8 L
Pump speed:	33.000 rpm	max. 7.500 rpm	max. 5000 rpm		max. 51.000 rpm	max. 7.500 rpm	40 ml/beat
Cannula size:	22 F	29 F	14-19 F arterial 17-21 F venous	7-8 F	12-14 F	14-19 F arterial 21 F venous	17 F
Insertion/Placement	Femoral vein	Internal jugular vein	Femoral artery Femoral vein	Femoral artery	Femoral artery	Femoral vein for LA access	Femoral artery
LV Unloading	−	−	−	(+)	+ − ++	++	+
RV Unloading	+	+	++	−	−	−	−

FIGURE 41.7 Current percutaneous mechanical support devices for cardiogenic shock with technical features. On the left are devices for right ventricular support and on the right are those for left ventricular support. (a) Impella RP, (b) TandemHeart RA-PA (right atrium–pulmonary artery), (c) VA extracorporeal membrane oxygenation (ECMO), (d) Intra-aortic balloon pump, (e) Impella, (f) TandemHeart, and (g) iVAC 2L. (From Thiele H, Ohman EM, de Waha-Thiele S, et al. Management of cardiogenic shock complicating myocardial infarction: an update 2019. *Eur Heart J*. 2019;40:2671–2683.)

on device availability, multidisciplinary team familiarity, and patient-specific needs.[58]

The IABP is still the most widely used MCS device in CS, primarily due to ease of use and widespread availability. It is a 7 to 8 Fr device that is positioned in the descending thoracic aorta just distal to the left subclavian artery and timed to inflate and deflate in concert with the cardiac cycle, thereby increasing the diastolic blood pressure and reducing the SBP. IABP support may be useful when LV function is severely compromised or when the PCI target lesion supplies a substantial portion of viable myocardium. Routine use of IABPs appears to have no benefit in patients with STEMI and cardiogenic shock, although they are still routinely used for patients with cardiogenic shock.[58,67] European guidelines have downgraded IABP use for cardiogenic shock from a previous class I to a class III recommendation.[43,65] In the US guidelines, IABP use has been downgraded to a class IIb recommendation.[19] A variety of more potent percutaneous cardiopulmonary support devices are also available and widely used, but with limited data from clinical trials (Fig. 41.7). Impella is a micro-axial flow device, and an impeller pump is located towards the distal end of the catheter. The inflow is placed retrogradely across the aortic valve into the left ventricle. A pump revolving at high speeds draws blood out of the left ventricle and ejects it proximally into the ascending aorta. Currently, the Impella system is available in three sizes—2.5, CP and 5.0; the latter has to be placed surgically via the subclavian cutdown. Sheath sizes required for these devices are large; for instance, 13 and 14 Fr for Impella 2.5 and CP, respectively. TandemHeart is a left atrium-to-aorta assist device with a centrifugal pump. Placement of this device requires the operator to be facile with trans-septal access, in addition to large bore peripheral access (15 to 19 Fr arterial access, 21 Fr venous access). There has also been a rapid uptake in the use of extracorporeal life support systems (for instance, venoarterial extracorporeal membrane oxygenation [VA-ECMO]) for this indication in recent years. An ECMO device provides biventricular support along with oxygenation capability, thus providing the ability to bypass the lungs as well, when used in a standard VA format. A common issue related to peripheral insertion is the resulting increase in LV afterload, which may lead to inadequate unloading of the LV. In these cases, combining VA-ECMO with IABP, Impella support (so called "ECPELLA"), atrial septostomy, or other venting maneuvers may help to achieve more complete LV unloading.[109] All of these devices may permit very-high-risk PCI with less chance of hemodynamic collapse during the procedure, although current data do not show them to be superior to IABPs. In addition, their use may be associated with a higher risk of complications including stroke and vascular injury.

MCS options for the temporary management of RV failure (including RV infarction) are currently also available but need more clinical data regarding utility. The Impella RP (Abiomed) is inserted percutaneously though the femoral vein. When properly positioned, this catheter can deliver blood from the inlet area (in the inferior vena cava), through the cannula, and into the pulmonary artery with an intent to reduce RV workload, and to allow cardiac recovery. Similarly, Protek Duo is a dual lumen cannula designed for RV support that is used in conjunction with the TandemHeart pump.

VASCULAR ACCESS

The most frequently used vascular access sites for PCI include the common femoral or radial arteries, and infrequently the brachial or ulnar arteries (see Chapter 21). The femoral approach (either right or left sided) is the most commonly used vascular access site in the United States and provides the advantages of large vessel size (typical common femoral artery diameter is 6 to 8 mm) and the ability to accommodate larger (>6 Fr) sheath sizes, including MCS. In addition, because of the typically straight path from the femoral artery to the ascending aorta, the femoral approach provides excellent guide catheter support and manipulability and access to the venous system through the adjacent femoral vein. The presence of severe peripheral arterial disease or peripheral vascular bypass grafts and the requirement for immobilization after the procedure limit use of the femoral approach in some patients. Using ultrasound guidance for femoral access may help reduce vascular complications, time to access and venipuncture sticks.[110]

The radial approach has gained in popularity and is increasingly becoming the *de facto* site of access for many catheterization laboratories across the world. It is also an attractive option as an alternative to femoral access in patients with significant peripheral vascular disease, particularly in obese patients. The radial approach provides direct access to the ascending aorta and has the unique advantage of allowing immediate mobilization following PCI. Although the modified Allen's and/or Barbeau's tests were routinely used to test for ulnopalmar patency prior to radial access at one time, this practice remains contentious, and has mostly fallen out of favor with most operators in the current era.[110] Tortuosity of the brachiocephalic trunk may limit use of the radial approach in 2% to 3% of patients; crossover rates to femoral access are around 5%. The small size of the radial artery limits the size of guiding catheters that can be used during PCI (typically 5 or 6 Fr for women and 7 Fr for men, although larger, sheathless guides are now available). Transradial access is associated with a generally lower rate (2%) of vascular complications. In the RIVAL (Radial vs Femoral Access for Coronary Intervention) trial, 7021 patients with ACS undergoing PCI were randomly assigned to either femoral or radial access. Although the overall trial was negative for a benefit of radial over femoral access for the primary endpoint at 30 days, there was a significant reduction among STEMI patients (n = 1958; 30-day death, MI, stroke for radial vs. femoral: 3.1% vs. 5.2%, p = 0.026; p for interaction = 0.025), and in the highest volume radial centers. Major vascular complications and ACUITY major bleeding were lower in the radial arm, but the prespecified safety endpoint of non-CABG-related TIMI major bleeding was similar.[111] A meta-analysis suggested that radial access reduced major adverse events, including potentially mortality, in comparison to femoral access.[112]

The brachial approach was historically used as the principal alternative to femoral access, but because the brachial artery provides the only circulation to the forearm and hand (i.e., it is a functional endartery), any compromise to it can lead to severe ischemic complications in the hand. Other approaches such as distal radial (puncture site immediately above the scaphoid or trapezium bones in the hand, typically in the "anatomical snuffbox") or ulnar access have been considered recently for arterial access as well.

Vascular Closure Devices

Vascular access closure devices were introduced in the mid-1990s as a way of managing access sites following femoral access procedures. Vascular closure devices reduce the time to ambulation, increase patient comfort after PCI, and facilitate efficient case flow in the catheterization laboratory. Currently approved vascular closure devices fall into three categories: (1) sealant devices, including collagen-based and thrombin-based systems, which leave no mechanical anchor inside or outside the vessel; (2) mechanical closure devices, including suture-mediated and nitinol clip–based systems, which provide immediate secure closure to the vessel; and (3) hybrid closure devices, such as the dissolvable AngioSeal device (St. Jude Medical, Minneapolis, Minnesota), which use a combination of collagen sealant and internal mechanical closure to induce rapid hemostasis. Although each device has proved to be relatively safe and effective, a lack of comparative data prohibits evaluation of the RRs and benefits associated with each device. Meta-analyses have concluded that vascular closure devices do not lower the risk of vascular complications compared with manual hemostasis, but infections may occur more often with suture-based closure devices, and occlusions are found more often with hybrid devices.[113] Previous reports reveal that closure devices reduce bleeding complications in selected patients, but randomized clinical trials are necessary to validate this finding.[114,115] For large-bore access, such as for TAVR, specialized closure devices have been developed, but suture-based devices (ProGlide, Abbott Vascular, Abbott Park, Illinois) remain the primary mode of closure.

ANTIPLATELET AGENTS (SEE ALSO CHAPTERS 9, 38, 39, 40)

Currently available antiplatelet agents include aspirin, thienopyridines, GP IIb/IIIa inhibitors, and others such as cilostazol and dipyridamole. While a number of oral GP IIb/IIIa inhibitors have been investigated in ACS, only intravenous preparations are approved for use in the United States as of today, owing to a lack of demonstrable efficacy and a higher risk of bleeding with oral agents.

Aspirin

Aspirin, or acetyl salicylic acid (ASA), is the most widely used and costeffective drug in the prevention of platelet aggregation. Aspirin irreversibly inhibits cyclooxygenase (COX) and thus blocks the synthesis of thromboxane A2 (TxA2), a vasoconstriction agent that promotes platelet aggregation.[116] Since it inhibits only one pathway by which platelet activation and aggregation occur (other agonists can directly stimulate the glycoprotein IIb/IIIa receptor, for example, thereby bypassing the arachidonic acid–thromboxane pathway), it is a relatively weak antiplatelet agent. Studies indicate that aspirin substantially reduces periprocedural MI caused by thrombotic occlusions compared with placebo and is standard for all patients undergoing PCI. The inhibitory effect of aspirin occurs within 30 to 60 minutes, and its effect on platelets lasts for up to 7 days after discontinuation. Although the minimum effective aspirin dosage in the setting of PCI remains uncertain, patients maintained on a regimen of daily chronic aspirin therapy should receive 81 to 325 mg of aspirin before PCI. Patients not already taking daily long-term aspirin therapy should be given 325 mg of aspirin at least 2 hours and preferably 24 hours before PCI is performed. After PCI, aspirin should be continued indefinitely in patients without allergy, and a lower dose (e.g., 81 mg) may be preferable to decrease the risk for gastrointestinal bleeding risk. Recent trials such as TWILIGHT suggest that stopping aspirin after a short duration of dual antiplatelet therapy (for instance, 3 months in TWILIGHT) may be feasible post-PCI.[117]

Adenosine Diphosphate (ADP) Receptor Antagonists

Adenosine diphosphate (ADP) receptor antagonists are broadly classified as thienopyridines (ticlopidine, clopidogrel, prasugrel) and non-thienopyridines (ticagrelor, cangrelor). Because aspirin and the ADP receptor antagonists have distinct mechanisms of action, their combination inhibits platelet aggregation to a greater extent than either agent alone.

The thienopyridines cause irreversible platelet inhibition through their effects on the P2Y12 ADP receptor, which can activate the glycoprotein IIb/IIIa complex.[118,119] Both clopidogrel and prasugrel are pro-drugs that require metabolic conversion to their active metabolites in the liver.[120] Prasugrel demonstrates less variability than clopidogrel in antiplatelet efficacy, presumptively due to more predictable conversion of pro-drug to active metabolite of prasugrel requiring a single cytochrome p450 metabolic step contrasted with clopidogrel requiring two sequential steps. Use of the combination of aspirin and clopidogrel (or in older studies, ticlopidine) for 14 to 28 days was essential to prevent stent thrombosis after BMS placement. The combination of aspirin and clopidogrel was also found to reduce death, MI, and urgent revascularization within 12 months in patients undergoing PCI in the setting of NSTEMI and UA and in those undergoing elective PCI. In the case of clopidogrel, maximal inhibition of ADP-induced platelet aggregation occurs three to five days after the initiation of a standard dose (75 mg daily). A loading dose of 600 mg of clopidogrel rather than 300 mg results in more rapid (<2 hours) platelet inhibition and improved clinical outcomes, including lower rates of stent thrombosis.[119] Additional clopidogrel loading with 300 or 600 mg may also be used in patients being treated with chronic maintenance clopidogrel therapy, although whether this actually improves clinical outcomes is unclear. The need for pretreatment with clopidogrel among ACS patients is more controversial in that the improved clinical outcomes need to be balanced against the potential risk for bleeding should CABG be necessary. For patients receiving clopidogrel, current guidelines recommend that a 600-mg loading dose of clopidogrel be administered before or during PCI. For SIHD patients undergoing DES PCI, clopidogrel remains the preferred P2Y12 inhibitor, and dual antiplatelet therapy (with low-dose aspirin) should be continued for at least 6 months if they do not have a high risk for bleeding. For post-PCI patients receiving a BMS, current guidelines recommend clopidogrel for a minimum of 1 month and ideally up to 12 months (unless the patient has an increased risk for bleeding, in whom it should be given for a minimum of 2 weeks).[74] However, recent studies comparing BMS with current DES do not indicate greater safety with BMS, with similar or higher risks of stent thrombosis and higher risks of repeat revascularization within 12 months.

Prasugrel, a thienopyridine, is a more potent P2Y12 ADP receptor inhibitor with a more rapid onset of action and higher levels of platelet inhibition than higher-dose clopidogrel.[121] In the TRITON-TIMI 38 trial, 13,608 patients with moderate- to high-risk ACS undergoing scheduled PCI were randomly assigned to receive prasugrel (60-mg loading dose and 10-mg daily maintenance dose) or clopidogrel (300-mg loading dose and 75-mg daily maintenance dose) for 6 to 15 months. The primary efficacy endpoint—a composite of death from cardiovascular causes, nonfatal MI, or nonfatal stroke—occurred in 12.1% of patients receiving clopidogrel and in 9.9% of those receiving prasugrel ($P < 0.001$). Prasugrel was also associated with significant reductions in rates of MI (9.7% for clopidogrel versus 7.4% for prasugrel; $P < 0.001$), urgent target-vessel revascularization (3.7% versus 2.5%; $P < 0.001$), and stent thrombosis (2.4% vs. 1.1%; $P < 0.001$). On the other hand, major bleeding was observed in 2.4% of patients receiving prasugrel and in 1.8% of patients receiving clopidogrel ($P = 0.03$), with more frequent rates of life-threatening bleeding occurring in the prasugrel group (1.4% vs. 0.9% with clopidogrel; $P = 0.01$), including fatal bleeding (0.4% vs. 0.1%, respectively; $P = 0.002$).[122,123] Prasugrel does not however appear to have a role in the treatment of medically managed patients with ACS, and may increase bleeding risk without an ischemic benefit.[124] Among patients treated with clopidogrel, carriers of reduced-function CYP2C19 alleles had high rates of "non-responsiveness", with significantly lower levels of active metabolite, diminished platelet inhibition, and higher rates of adverse cardiovascular events.[125] Such a relationship was not found in patients treated with prasugrel. Further research will be necessary to determine whether point-of-care platelet assays or determination of genetic polymorphisms can help in allocating therapy, although to date this type of testing does not appear to be clinically useful.

Ticagrelor is an orally active non-thienopyridine that belongs to the cyclopentyltriazolopyrimidine class. It is a reversible P2Y12 receptor antagonist, and provides faster, greater, and more consistent ADP receptor inhibition than clopidogrel. In PLATO, 18,624 patients with ACS, with or without ST-segment elevation, were randomly assigned to treatment with ticagrelor (180-mg loading dose, then 90 mg twice daily) or clopidogrel (300- to 600-mg loading dose, then 75 mg daily) for 12 months. The primary endpoint—a composite of death from vascular causes, MI, or stroke at 12 months—occurred in 9.8% of patients receiving ticagrelor and in 11.7% of those receiving clopidogrel (hazard ratio, 0.84; $P < 0.001$). Ticagrelor was also associated with significant reductions in MI alone (5.8% vs. 6.9% in clopidogrel group; $P = 0.005$) and in death from vascular causes (4.0% vs. 5.1%, respectively; $P = 0.001$). No significant difference in overall rates of major bleeding was observed between the ticagrelor and clopidogrel groups (11.6% and 11.2%, respectively; $P = 0.43$), but ticagrelor was associated with a higher rate of major bleeding not related to CABG (4.5% vs. 3.8%; $P = 0.03$).[126]

Current US guidelines recommend DAPT for at least 12 months after DES PCI for an ACS indication. Either clopidogrel or ticagrelor are recommended for all patients with NSTE-ACS without contraindications who are treated with either an early invasive or ischemia-guided strategy (ticagrelor preferred over clopidogrel as a class IIa recommendation); prasugrel is only indicated for ACS patients undergoing PCI. The PRECISE-DAPT score was developed to help further refine individualized treatment by determining which patients are most likely to benefit from or be harmed by continuation of DAPT beyond 12 months.[127,128]

Prolonged ADP receptor antagonist therapy not only reduces late stent thrombosis but also prevents MI remote from the initial intervention.[129] Nonetheless, in patients with elevated bleeding risk, it may be reasonable to consider shorter durations of therapy (6 months) with current DES. Indefinite aspirin and clopidogrel therapy is recommended in patients undergoing brachytherapy, and long-term higher doses (150 mg daily) of clopidogrel, or alternatively, prasugrel or ticagrelor, may be considered in patients in whom stent thrombosis may be catastrophic, such as those with unprotected left main coronary artery stenting or with stenting of the last remaining vessel. A complex subgroup is patients with PCI also needing anticoagulation for AF or VTE. These patients were historically treated with an AC and dual antiplatelet therapy—so called "triple therapy." This however significantly increases the risk of bleeding. Recent data from randomized controlled trials suggests that for patients requiring both an AC and APT, the default strategy after recent PCI should be dual antithrombotic therapy consisting of an AC and a P2Y12i.[60] If the patient is perceived to be at particularly high risk for coronary thrombosis and bleeding risk is judged to be low, aspirin may be added to a P2Y12i and an AC for up to 30 days following PCI.[130] In such scenarios, clopidogrel is the preferred P2Y12i of choice, and a DOAC is the preferred AC of choice.

Cangrelor is an intravenous adenosine triphosphate (ATP) analogue that binds reversibly and with high affinity to the platelet P2Y12 recep-tor and has a short plasma half-life (<10 minutes).[131] It produces a highly effective inhibition of ADP-induced platelet aggregation immediately after bolus administration and allows for restoration of platelet function within 1 to 2 hours of infusion discontinuation in NSTE-ACS patients. A pooled analysis of the CHAMPION studies (69% of patients with PCI for ACS) noted a 19% relative risk reduction (RRR) in periprocedural death, MI, ischemia-driven revascularization, and stent thrombosis with a 39% RRR in stent thrombosis alone (cangrelor vs. clopidogrel 0.5% vs. 0.8%; p = 0.008). The combination of TIMI major and minor bleeds was increased but there was no increase in the rate of transfusions.[132–135]

Glycoprotein IIb/IIIa Inhibitors

Thrombin and collagen are potent platelet agonists that can cause release of ADP and serotonin and activate GP IIb/IIIa receptors on the platelet surface. Functionally active GP IIb/IIIa has a role in the "final common pathway" of platelet aggregation by binding fibrinogen and other adhesive proteins that bridge adjacent platelets. Three intravenous GP IIb/IIIa inhibitors are approved for clinical use. Studies supporting the use of these agents during PCI were performed before the widespread use of DAPT, however, and use of these agents has been reevaluated in this context. Overall, the GP IIb/IIIa inhibitors have demonstrated improvement in clinical outcomes within the first 30 days after PCI, primarily by reducing ischemic complications, including periprocedural MI and recurrent ischemia. They are particularly useful in patients with troponin-positive ACS but have no consistent effect in reducing late restenosis. Although GP IIb/IIIa inhibitors differ in their structure, reversibility, and duration, two meta-analyses found no difference between their clinical effects in patients undergoing primary PCI.[136,137] Bleeding is the major risk associated with GP IIb/IIIa inhibitors, and therefore downward adjustment of the unfractionated heparin (UFH) dose has been recommended. GP IIb/IIIa inhibitors are recommended in patients with NSTEMI and UA who are not pretreated with clopidogrel, and it is reasonable to administer them to patients with troponin-positive ACS who have also been pretreated with clopidogrel.[138,139]

ANTITHROMBIN AGENTS (SEE CHAPTERS 9, 38, AND 39)

Unfractionated Heparin

UFH is the most commonly used thrombin inhibitor during PCI. UFH consists of a mixture of polysaccharide chains that exert an anticoagulant effect by facilitating activation of antithrombin III, which in turn inactivates factors IIa (thrombin), IXa, and Xa. Point-of-care activated clotting time (ACT) monitoring has facilitated heparin dose titration during PCI, and retrospective studies on balloon angioplasty have related the ACT value to clinical outcome after PCI. An ACT in the range of 350-375 seconds provided the lowest composite ischemic event rate, although any level of ACT longer than 250 seconds was not associated with any further reductions in ischemic complications with the concomitant use of GP IIb/IIIa inhibitors. More recent studies in the thienopyridine era have failed to correlate ischemic outcomes with the level of anticoagulation achieved with UFH during coronary stent placement. Weight-adjusted heparin dosing regimens of 50 to 70 IU/kg help avoid "overshooting" the ACT. Sufficient UFH should be administered during PCI to achieve an ACT longer than 250 to 300 seconds if no GP IIb/IIIa inhibitor is given, and longer than 200 to 250 seconds if a GP IIb/IIIa inhibitor is given. Routine use of IV heparin after PCI is no longer indicated. If no closure device has been used, early sheath removal is encouraged when the ACT falls to less than 150 to 180 seconds.

Low-Molecular-Weight Heparin

Enoxaparin is considered a reasonable alternative to UFH in patients with non–ST-segment elevation ACS undergoing PCI, but difficulty monitoring the levels of anticoagulation in the event that PCI is performed has limited its clinical use at many centers.[140] When enoxaparin is given before PCI, empiric dose algorithms have been designed to guide additional anticoagulation therapy during PCI. If the last dose of enoxaparin was administered less than 8 hours before PCI, no additional antithrombin is needed. If the last dose of enoxaparin was given between 8 and 12 hours, a 0.3 mg/kg bolus of IV enoxaparin should be administered. If the dose was administrated more than 12 hours before PCI, conventional anticoagulation therapy is indicated.[14] If enoxaparin is used as primary anticoagulant, it should be given as a 0.5 to 0.75 mg/kg IV bolus. This will typically result in a peak anti-Xa level of >0.5 IU/mL.

Bivalirudin

Bivalirudin is a direct thrombin inhibitor that has been used as an alternative to UFH in patients undergoing PCI. Bivalirudin generally causes fewer bleeding complications than UFH because of its shorter half-life (25 minutes) and more predictable bioavailability. Bivalirudin is also accessible to clot-bound thrombin, because its anticoagulant effect does not depend on binding with antithrombin. Bivalirudin was not inferior to the combination of UFH and GP IIb/IIIa inhibitor in 6010 "low-risk" patients undergoing urgent or elective PCI in the REPLACE-2 (Second Randomized Evaluation in PCI Linking Angiomax to Reduced Clinical Events) trial.[141] In ACUITY, 13,819 patients with UA and NSTEMI were randomized to bivalirudin monotherapy, bivalirudin plus a GP IIb/IIIa inhibitor, or heparin plus a GP IIb/IIIa inhibitor. Using a composite ischemia endpoint of death, MI, or unplanned revascularization for ischemia and major bleeding to determine the net clinical benefit, bivalirudin monotherapy versus heparin plus a GP IIb/IIIa inhibitor showed non-inferiority in the composite ischemia endpoint (7.8% and 7.3%, respectively) and significantly reduced rates of major bleeding (3.0% vs. 5.7%; $P < 0.001$), which resulted in a better net clinical outcome (10.1% vs. 11.7%; $P = 0.02$).[142] More recent trials have sought to compare bivalirudin to UFH in a more head-to-head fashion (GP inhibitor reserved for "bailout" only), although mostly in a primary PCI population.

A recent meta-analysis included 16 trials with 33,958 patients randomized to bivalirudin-based or heparin-based regimens. The former was associated with a significant increase in the risk of major adverse cardiac events (risk ratio 1.09, p = 0.02), mainly due to an increase in MI, particularly due to acute stent thrombosis in patients undergoing primary PCI for STEMI (risk ratio 1.38, p = 0.0074). Bivalirudin seemed to reduce the risk of bleeding compared with heparin-based regimens, mostly in the setting of concomitant GP inhibitor use.[143]

Factor Xa Inhibitors

Fondaparinux is a pentasaccharide that has anti–factor Xa activity without effects on factor IIa and may cause less bleeding when used to treat patients with ACS. Potential limitations include the relatively long half-life of fondaparinux and the need for adjunctive anticoagulation with heparin during PCI to avoid the development of catheter thrombi. Fondaparinux is not effective in reducing ischemic events in patients undergoing primary PCI for STEMI.

OUTCOMES AFTER PERCUTANEOUS CORONARY INTERVENTION

Early Clinical Outcomes

Anatomic (or angiographic) success after PCI is defined as attainment of a residual diameter stenosis of less than 50%, which is generally associated with at least a 20% improvement in diameter stenosis and relief of ischemia. With the widespread use of coronary stents, the angiographic criterion for success is ≤20% stenosis when stents are used. Procedural success is defined as angiographic success without the occurrence of major complications (death, MI, or CABG) within 30 days of the procedure. Clinical success is defined as procedural success without the need for urgent repeated PCI or surgical revascularization within the first 30 days of the procedure. Several clinical, angiographic, and technical variables can be used to predict the risk for procedural failure in patients undergoing PCI. Major complications include death, MI, or stroke, and minor complications include transient ischemic attacks, vascular complications, contrast-induced nephropathy, and angiographic complications.

Mortality

Although mortality after PCI is rare (approximately 1%), it is higher in the setting of STEMI, in cardiogenic shock, and in patients with previously poor LV function in whom an occlusion develops. Several risk factors for early mortality after PCI have been identified.[144]

Myocardial Infarction

Periprocedural MI is one of the most common complications of PCI. The 2018 Fourth Universal Definition of Myocardial Infarction defines a periprocedural MI as an elevation of cTn values more than five times the 99th percentile upper reference limit (URL) in patients with normal baseline values. In patients with elevated pre-procedure cTn, in whom the cTn levels are stable (≤20% variation) or falling, the postprocedure cTn must rise by greater than 20%. However, the absolute postprocedural value must still be at least five times the 99th percentile URL.[145] In addition, one of the following is required:

- New ischemic ECG changes.
- Development of new pathologic Q waves
- Imaging evidence of new loss of viable myocardium or new regional wall motion abnormality in a pattern consistent with an ischemic etiology.
- Angiographic findings consistent with a procedural flow-limiting complication such as coronary dissection, occlusion of a major epicardial artery or a side branch occlusion/thrombus, disruption of collateral flow, or distal embolization.

The SCAI definition is more stringent, and defines a clinically relevant MI post – PCI as elevation in CK – MB to ≥ 10 × ULN or cTn (I or T) to ≥ 70 × ULN (or by CK – MB to ≥ 5 × ULN or cTn to ≥ 35 × ULN plus the development of new pathologic Q-waves in ≥ 2 contiguous leads or LBBB).[146] A systematic consensus definition for standardizing reporting from clinical trials was recently proposed by the Academic Research Consortium (ARC).[147]

In clinical practice, asymptomatic CK-MB elevation (less than five times the upper limit of normal) occurs after 3% to 11% of technically successful PCIs and has little apparent clinical consequence. Troponin T and I elevations occur more often than CK-MB elevations, but their prognostic significance over that of CK-MB elevation is not as well established. Larger degrees of myonecrosis are associated with higher 1-year mortality rates and should be considered a periprocedural MI.[148] Many of these clinically silent infarcts may reflect a higher atherosclerotic burden in patients with such events and may not be truly causal. Spontaneous MI after PCI has much more prognostic importance than periprocedural enzyme elevation.[149]

Urgent Revascularization

Emergency or urgent CABG following PCI is now uncommon and, in the era of coronary stents, results from catastrophic complications during PCI, such as coronary perforation or severe dissection and abrupt closure. Chest pain after PCI is relatively common, and evaluation requires an immediate 12-lead ECG. Recurrent ischemia after PCI, as manifested by chest pain, ECG abnormalities, and elevated levels of cardiac biomarkers, may result from acute or subacute stent thrombosis, residual dissections, plaque prolapse, side branch occlusion, or thrombus at the treatment site or may be related to residual disease not treated during the initial procedure. In the presence of suspected recurrent ischemia, coronary angiography is the most expeditious way to identify the cause of the residual ischemia.

Angiographic Complications

Complications that occur during PCI, depending on their severity and duration, may result in periprocedural MI. If coronary dissections that extend deeper into the media or adventitia begin to compromise the true lumen of the vessel, clinical ischemia may develop. Even though most intraprocedural dissections can be treated promptly by stenting, significant residual dissections of the treated artery occur in 1.7% of patients. These residual dissections increase the risk for postprocedural MI, need for emergency CABG, and the incidence of stent thrombosis and increase mortality three-fold. In addition to barotrauma-induced dissections, dissections attributable to the guiding catheter represent another mechanism for disrupting the coronary vessel and compromising distal flow.

Coronary perforation develops in 0.2% to 0.5% of patients undergoing PCI and is more common with atheroablative devices and hydrophilic wires than with balloon angioplasty or conventional guidewires. Depending on the rate of flow through the vessel perforation, cardiac tamponade and hemodynamic collapse can occur within minutes, thus requiring immediate recognition and treatment of the perforation.

No-reflow is defined as reduced anterograde perfusion in the absence of a flow-limiting stenosis and occurs in up to 2% to 3% of PCI procedures, typically during interventions on degenerated SVGs, during rotational atherectomy, and during acute MI interventions. No-reflow is probably caused by distal embolization of atheromatous and thrombotic debris dislodged by balloon inflation, atherectomy, or stent implantation. Once it occurs, no-reflow can cause severe short- and long-term consequences, including a fivefold increased risk for periprocedural MI and a threefold increased risk for death. Although numerous pharmacologic strategies (e.g., intracoronary sodium nitroprusside) have been used to treat no-reflow, their efficacy in reducing the frequency of subsequent adverse events is still debated.

Stent Thrombosis

With the routine use of a high-pressure stent post- dilation and DAPT after stent implantation, the rate of stent thrombosis has declined to approximately 1% within the first year after stenting, although it can be higher in patients with STEMI or after complex PCI. Certain clinical, angiographic, and procedural factors predispose to its development. Lesion-specific factors that increase the likelihood of stent thrombosis include a residual dissection at the margin of the stent, impaired flow into or out of the stent, small stent diameter (<3 mm), long stent length, and treatment of acute MI. Patient noncompliance with DAPT, resistance to the antiplatelet effects of aspirin and clopidogrel, and hypercoagulability may also play important roles in the development of stent thrombosis.

The timing of stent thrombosis is defined as *acute* (<24 hours), *subacute* (24 hours to 30 days), *late* (30 days to 1 year), and *very late* (>1 year). Traditional definitions of stent thrombosis have included only episodes associated with an ACS and angiographic or pathologic demonstration of thrombosis within the stent or its margins. The ARC group has proposed criteria for documentation of all possible stent thrombosis in clinical studies, including the categories of definite, probable, and possible.

Early reports suggested a low rate of very late stent thrombosis (0.2% to 0.5% per year) occurring 1 year or longer after contemporary DES implantation.[72,73,80] Inhibition of endothelialization caused by the potent antiproliferative effect of the drugs delivered by DES may significantly prolong the period of risk for the development of stent thrombosis. Although concerning, these events have not yet been shown to cause a significant increase in late morbidity or mortality, probably because of the benefits of DES in reducing the need for repeated revascularization procedures and avoidance of the complications associated with the development of in-stent restenosis. Ongoing evaluation of the long-term safety of DES has engendered intense investigation, with efforts focused on determining whether patient- and lesion-specific risk factors, such as insensitivity to aspirin or clopidogrel, may contribute; whether these risks are device-specific or drug-specific phenomena; and whether prolonged DAPT may ameliorate these risks.

The not-infrequent scenario of a patient requiring noncardiac surgery in the weeks following PCI can markedly increase the risk for stent thrombosis. Studies of outcomes in patients undergoing noncardiac surgery soon after BMS PCI have documented high stent thrombosis occurring in the first 2 weeks after PCI, with risks declining to baseline rates by 8 weeks. This increased risk probably results from the frequent cessation of ADP receptor antagonist treatment before surgery, as well as the hypercoagulable state in the perioperative period. The PARIS reg-istry noted a trend towards higher MACE and stent thrombosis rates after DAPT interruption (as for urgent noncardiac surgery) compared with DAPT continuation. In this registry, patients who stopped DAPT due to noncompliance or bleeding ("disruption") had the highest MACE and stent thrombosis rates, particularly within the first 7 days.[150]

Late Clinical Outcomes

Ischemic events within the first year after PCI result from one of three processes. Lumen renarrowing requiring repeated target-lesion revascularization occurs in 20% to 30% of patients undergoing balloon angioplasty because of reparative arterial constriction, also known as "negative remodeling." Clinical restenosis after stent implantation is less common (10% to 20%) and attributable to intimal hyperplasia within the stent. Clinical recurrence caused by restenosis is least common (3% to 5%) after DES placement because of focal tissue growth within the stent or at its margins.[151,152] Yet another cause of clinical events after PCI is progression of coronary atherosclerosis at a site remote from that treated earlier by PCI.[153] Death and MI can also result from sudden rupture of a plaque that is remote from the site of the initial intervention.

These processes can be partially distinguished by the timing of their occurrence. Clinical restenosis resulting from lumen renarrowing at the site of PCI generally develops within the first 6 to 9 months after PCI, whereas death and MI because of plaque instability may occur at any point after PCI at a low but constant rate (1% to 2% risk per year, but higher for ACS vs. SIHD PCI). Predictors of higher risk for all-cause late mortality include advanced age, reduced LV function, congestive HF, DM, a higher number of diseased vessels, inoperable disease, or severe comorbid conditions. A 95% 10-year survival rate can be expected in patients with single-vessel CAD, and an 80% survival rate after PCI can be achieved in those with multivessel CAD.

A somewhat recent discovery is the phenomenon of neoatherosclerosis following stent implantation. This refers to accumulation of lipid-laden foamy macrophages within the neointima after stent implantation, with or without necrotic core formation and/or calcification.[154] OCT is currently the best imaging modality to detect neoatherosclerosis, but the resolution is not high enough to detect foamy macrophages consistently. It appears to have a role in both stent restenosis and thrombosis.[155]

Outcomes Benchmarking and Procedural Volumes

Along with CABG, PCI ranks among the most studied of all procedures in the United States. National structured outcomes registries, such as the National Heart, Lung and Blood Institute (NHLBI) Dynamic Registry and the ACC National Cardiovascular Data Repository (NCDR), have been examined. The NCDR CathPCI registry also provides contemporary risk-adjusted outcomes benchmarked to hundreds of participating institutions. Participants in such national, regional, or statewide outcomes-reporting initiatives can compare their risk-adjusted clinical outcomes with those at institutions with similar patient mix and size. The detailed nature of these datasets, in which the data collected span the range of patient clinical characteristics, lesion descriptors, and device-level information, provides centers with a comprehensive comparison of their practice patterns and outcomes with those at peer institutions. More than 50% of U.S. hospitals participate in the NCDR CathPCI registry. Participation in a prospective quality assessment and outcomes registry is recommended for centers performing PCI.

In the United States, the COCATS Task Force of the ACC recommends that physicians undergo a 3-year comprehensive cardiac training program with at least 6 months of training in diagnostic catheterization, during which the trainee performs 300 diagnostic catheterizations.[156] Interventional training requires a fourth year of training, including more than 250 interventional coronary procedures, a level that is also required for physicians to be eligible for the American Board of Internal Medicine certifying examination in interventional cardiology.[157]

There are also specific volume requirements, although these have been the topic of much debate.[60,158-160] Considerations include annual operator volume, annual hospital volumes and lifetime operator volumes (experience).[158] Current US guidelines recommend that operators perform at least 50 PCIs/year.[11,157]

Although PCI has traditionally been performed at centers that offer on-site surgical backup, more recent analyses have shown that PCI for STEMI and elective PCI can be performed safely, provided that PCI is performed by high-volume operators with minimal institutional volume requirements.[161,162] Off-site PCI is best suited for underserved areas that are geographically far removed from major centers.

Institutions must have a system for quality measurement and improvement that includes valid peer review. The guidelines recommend that quality assessment reviews take into consideration risk adjustment, statistical power, and national benchmark statistics. They should also include tabulation of adverse event rates for comparison with benchmark values, as well as case review of complicated procedures and some uncomplicated procedures.

FUTURE PERSPECTIVES

After four decades of rapid growth and dissemination of coronary interventional techniques and the associated dramatic refinement in the devices used for revascularization, many challenges still remain for the percutaneous treatment of CAD. For instance, further investigation into the optimal management and methodology for treating complex lesions such as unprotected left main, complex bifurcation lesion and CTOs must continue. Determination of the optimal duration of antiplatelet therapy following DES deployment requires ongoing study.

DES design is continually evolving in an attempt to optimize effective early endothelialization of the stented segment without sacrificing the long-term benefits of DES in reducing target-lesion revascularization. Theoretically, advances in stent, polymer, and drug design could lead to improvements in restenosis and thrombosis rates, which in turn may reduce rates of MI and even death. Of course, this concept would need to be tested prospectively in adequately powered trials of sufficient duration, but it could lead to reexamination of the relative merits of PCI versus medical therapy or CABG in a variety of settings.

Early investigations of myocardial regeneration following acute MI by percutaneous delivery of autologous stem cell or progenitor cell lines have generated great interest in the potential of such therapies to improve myocardial recovery, but more clinical data are needed.

Continued refinement of ventricular support devices offers hope for myocardial recovery in the patient with severe myocardial dysfunction.

ACKNOWLEDGMENTS

The authors acknowledge the late Donald Baim, MD, Fred Resnic, MD, Jeff Popma, MD, and Laura Mauri, MD, for their previous contributions to this chapter, and Thomas Lee, MD, for his previous contribution to the Guidelines section.

REFERENCES

Background and Indication

1. Gruntzig A. Transluminal dilatation of coronary-artery stenosis. *Lancet*. 1978;1:263.
2. Hochman JS, Rutherford JD. Clinical studies in myocardial revascularization. *Circulation*. 2019;139:1007–1011.
3. Maron DJ, Hochman JS, Reynolds HR, et al. Initial invasive or conservative strategy for stable coronary disease. *N Engl J Med*. 2020;382:1395–1407.
4. De Bruyne B, Pijls NH, Kalesan B, et al. Fractional flow reserve-guided PCI versus medical therapy in stable coronary disease. *N Engl J Med*. 2012;367:991–1001.
5. Al-Lamee R, Thompson D, Dehbi HM, et al. Percutaneous coronary intervention in stable angina (ORBITA): a double-blind, randomised controlled trial. *Lancet*. 2018;391:31–40.
6. Lopes RD, Alexander KP, Stevens SR, et al. Initial invasive versus conservative management of stable ischemic heart disease patients with a history of heart failure or left ventricular dysfunction: insights from the ISCHEMIA trial. *Circulation*. 2020.
7. Bangalore S, Maron DJ, Stone GW, Hochman JS. Routine revascularization versus initial medical therapy for stable ischemic heart disease: a systematic review and meta-analysis of randomized trials. *Circulation*. 2020;142:841–857.
8. Serruys PW, Morice MC, Kappetein AP, et al. Percutaneous coronary intervention versus coronary-artery bypass grafting for severe coronary artery disease. *N Engl J Med*. 2009;360:961–972.
9. BARI 2D Study Group, Frye RL, August P, et al. A randomized trial of therapies for type 2 diabetes and coronary artery disease. *N Engl J Med*. 2009;360:2503–2515.
10. Pandey A, McGuire DK, de Lemos JA, et al. Revascularization trends in patients with diabetes mellitus and multivessel coronary artery disease presenting with non-ST elevation myocardial infarction: insights from the National Cardiovascular Data Registry Acute Coronary Treatment and Intervention Outcomes Network Registry-Get With the Guidelines (NCDR ACTION registry-GWTG). *Circ Cardiovasc Qual Outcomes*. 2016;9:197–205.
11. Levine GN, Bates ER, Blankenship JC, et al. 2011 ACCF/AHA/SCAI guideline for percutaneous coronary intervention: a report of the American College of Cardiology Foundation/American Heart Association task force on practice guidelines and the Society for Cardiovascular Angiography and Interventions. *Circulation*. 2011;124:e574–e651.
12. Patel MR, Dehmer GJ, Hirshfeld JW, et al. ACCF/SCAI/STS/AATS/AHA/ASNC 2009 appropriateness criteria for coronary revascularization: a report by the American College of Cardiology Foundation appropriateness criteria task force, Society for Cardiovascular Angiography and Interventions, Society of Thoracic Surgeons, American Association for Thoracic Surgery, American Heart Association, and the American Society of Nuclear Cardiology endorsed by the American Society of Echocardiography, the Heart Failure Society of America, and the Society of Cardiovascular Computed Tomography. *J Am Coll Cardiol*. 2009;53:530–553.
13. Patel MR, Dehmer GJ, Hirshfeld JW, Smith PK, Spertus JA. ACCF/SCAI/STS/AATS/AHA/ASNC/HFSA/SCCT 2012 appropriate use criteria for coronary revascularization focused update: a report of the American College of Cardiology Foundation appropriate use criteria task force, Society for Cardiovascular Angiography and Interventions, Society of Thoracic Surgeons, American Association for Thoracic Surgery, American Heart Association, American Society of Nuclear Cardiology, and the Society of Cardiovascular Computed Tomography. *J Am Coll Cardiol*. 2012;59:857–881.
14. Amsterdam EA, Wenger NK, Brindis RG, et al. 2014 AHA/ACC guideline for the management of patients with non-ST-elevation acute coronary syndromes: a report of the American College of Cardiology/American Heart Association task force on practice guidelines. *J Am Coll Cardiol*. 2014;64:e139–e228.
15. Bavry AA, Kumbhani DJ, Rassi AN, et al. Benefit of early invasive therapy in acute coronary syndromes: a meta-analysis of contemporary randomized clinical trials. *J Am Coll Cardiol*. 2006;48:1319–1325.
16. Jobs A, Mehta SR, Montalescot G, et al. Optimal timing of an invasive strategy in patients with non-ST-elevation acute coronary syndrome: a meta-analysis of randomised trials. *Lancet*. 2017;390:737–746.
17. Mehta SR, Granger CB, Boden WE, et al. Early versus delayed invasive intervention in acute coronary syndromes. *N Engl J Med*. 2009;360:2165–2175.
18. Kofoed KF, Kelbaek H, Hansen PR, et al. Early versus standard care invasive examination and treatment of patients with non-ST-segment elevation acute coronary syndrome. *Circulation*. 2018;138:2741–2750.
19. O'Gara PT, Kushner FG, Ascheim DD, et al. 2013 ACCF/AHA guideline for the management of ST-elevation myocardial infarction: a report of the American College of Cardiology Foundation/American Heart Association task force on practice guidelines. *Circulation*. 2013;127:e362–425.
20. Levine GN, Bates ER, Blankenship JC, et al. 2015 ACC/AHA/SCAI focused update on primary percutaneous coronary intervention for patients with ST-elevation myocardial infarction: an update of the 2011 ACCF/AHA/SCAI guideline for percutaneous coronary intervention and the 2013 ACCF/AHA guideline for the management of ST-elevation myocardial infarction. *J Am Coll Cardiol*. 2016;67:1235–1250.
21. Fleisher LA, Fleischmann KE, Auerbach AD, et al. 2014 ACC/AHA guideline on perioperative cardiovascular evaluation and management of patients undergoing noncardiac surgery: a report of the American College of Cardiology/American Heart Association Task Force on practice guidelines. *J Am Coll Cardiol*. 2014;64:e77–137.

Outcomes

22. Morice MC, Serruys PW, Kappetein AP, et al. Five-year outcomes in patients with left main disease treated with either percutaneous coronary intervention or coronary artery bypass grafting in the synergy between percutaneous coronary intervention with taxus and cardiac surgery trial. *Circulation*. 2014;129:2388–2394.
23. Mohr FW, Morice MC, Kappetein AP, et al. Coronary artery bypass graft surgery versus percutaneous coronary intervention in patients with three-vessel disease and left main coronary disease: 5-year follow-up of the randomised, clinical SYNTAX trial. *Lancet*. 2013;381:629–638.
24. Thuijs D, Kappetein AP, Serruys PW, et al. Percutaneous coronary intervention versus coronary artery bypass grafting in patients with three-vessel or left main coronary artery disease: 10-year follow-up of the multicentre randomised controlled SYNTAX trial. *Lancet*. 2019;394:1325–1334.

25. Stone GW, Kappetein AP, Sabik JF, et al. Five-year outcomes after PCI or CABG for left main coronary disease. *N Engl J Med*. 2019;381:1820–1830.
26. Ahn JM, Roh JH, Kim YH, et al. Randomized trial of stents versus bypass surgery for left main coronary artery disease: 5-year outcomes of the PRECOMBAT study. *J Am Coll Cardiol*. 2015;65:2198–2206.
27. Park DW, Ahn JM, Park H, et al. Ten-year outcomes after drug-eluting stents versus coronary artery bypass grafting for left main coronary disease: extended follow-up of the PRECOMBAT trial. *Circulation*. 2020;141:1437–1446.
28. Makikallio T, Holm NR, Lindsay M, et al. Percutaneous coronary angioplasty versus coronary artery bypass grafting in treatment of unprotected left main stenosis (NOBLE): a prospective, randomised, open-label, non-inferiority trial. *Lancet*. 2016;388:2743–2752.
29. Holm NR, Makikallio T, Lindsay MM, et al. Percutaneous coronary angioplasty versus coronary artery bypass grafting in the treatment of unprotected left main stenosis: updated 5-year outcomes from the randomised, non-inferiority NOBLE trial. *Lancet*. 2020;395:191–199.
30. Chen SL, Zhang JJ, Han Y, et al. Double kissing crush versus provisional stenting for left main distal bifurcation lesions: DKCRUSH-V randomized trial. *J Am Coll Cardiol*. 2017;70:2605–2617.
31. Chen SL, Xu B, Han YL, et al. Comparison of double kissing crush versus Culotte stenting for unprotected distal left main bifurcation lesions: results from a multicenter, randomized, prospective DKCRUSH-III study. *J Am Coll Cardiol*. 2013;61:1482–1488.
32. Bhatt DL. CABG the clear choice for patients with diabetes and multivessel disease. *Lancet*. 2018;391:913–914.
33. Head SJ, Davierwala PM, Serruys PW, et al. Coronary artery bypass grafting vs. percutaneous coronary intervention for patients with three-vessel disease: final five-year follow-up of the SYNTAX trial. *Eur Heart J*. 2014;35:2821–2830.
34. Park SJ, Ahn JM, Kim YH, et al. Trial of everolimus-eluting stents or bypass surgery for coronary disease. *N Engl J Med*. 2015;372:1204–1212.
35. Brilakis ES, Mashayekhi K, Tsuchikane E, et al. Guiding principles for chronic total occlusion percutaneous coronary intervention. *Circulation*. 2019;140:420–433.
36. Morino Y, Abe M, Morimoto T, et al. Predicting successful guidewire crossing through chronic total occlusion of native coronary lesions within 30 minutes: the J-CTO (Multicenter CTO Registry in Japan) score as a difficulty grading and time assessment tool. *JACC Cardiovasc Interv*. 2011;4:213–221.
37. Henriques JP, Hoebers LP, Ramunddal T, et al. Percutaneous intervention for concurrent chronic total occlusions in patients with STEMI: the EXPLORE trial. *J Am Coll Cardiol*. 2016;68:1622–1632.
38. Lee SW, Lee PH, Ahn JM, et al. Randomized trial evaluating percutaneous coronary intervention for the treatment of chronic total occlusion. *Circulation*. 2019;139:1674–1683.
39. Werner GS, Martin-Yuste V, Hildick-Smith D, et al. A randomized multicentre trial to compare revascularization with optimal medical therapy for the treatment of chronic total coronary occlusions. *Eur Heart J*. 2018;39:2484–2493.
40. Caliskan E, de Souza DR, Boning A, et al. Saphenous vein grafts in contemporary coronary artery bypass graft surgery. *Nat Rev Cardiol*. 2020;17:155–169.
41. Brilakis ES, Rao SV, Banerjee S, et al. Percutaneous coronary intervention in native arteries versus bypass grafts in prior coronary artery bypass grafting patients: a report from the National Cardiovascular Data Registry. *JACC Cardiovasc Interv*. 2011;4:844–850.
42. Stone GW, Rogers C, Hermiller J, et al. Randomized comparison of distal protection with a filter-based catheter and a balloon occlusion and aspiration system during percutaneous intervention of diseased saphenous vein aorto-coronary bypass grafts. *Circulation*. 2003;108:548–553.
43. Neumann FJ, Sousa-Uva M, Ahlsson A, et al. 2018 ESC/EACTS guidelines on myocardial revascularization. *Eur Heart J*. 2019;40:87–165.

Coronary Devices

44. Colleran R, Kufner S, Mehilli J, et al. Efficacy over time with drug-eluting stents in saphenous vein graft lesions. *J Am Coll Cardiol*. 2018;71:1973–1982.
45. Mehilli J, Pache J, Abdel-Wahab M, et al. Drug-eluting versus bare-metal stents in saphenous vein graft lesions (ISAR-CABG): a randomised controlled superiority trial. *Lancet*. 2011;378:1071–1078.
46. Brilakis ES, Edson R, Bhatt DL, et al. Drug-eluting stents versus bare-metal stents in saphenous vein grafts: a double-blind, randomised trial. *Lancet*. 2018;391:1997–2007.
47. Steigen TK, Maeng M, Wiseth R, et al. Randomized study on simple versus complex stenting of coronary artery bifurcation lesions: the Nordic bifurcation study. *Circulation*. 2006;114:1955–1961.
48. Colombo A, Bramucci E, Sacca S, et al. Randomized study of the crush technique versus provisional side-branch stenting in true coronary bifurcations: the CACTUS (coronary bifurcations: application of the crushing technique using sirolimus-eluting stents) study. *Circulation*. 2009;119:71–78.
49. Koo BK, Waseda K, Kang HJ, et al. Anatomic and functional evaluation of bifurcation lesions undergoing percutaneous coronary intervention. *Circ Cardiovasc Interv*. 2010;3:113–119.
50. Jolly SS, Cairns JA, Yusuf S, et al. Randomized trial of primary PCI with or without routine manual thrombectomy. *N Engl J Med*. 2015;372:1389–1398.
51. Kumbhani DJ, Bavry AA, Desai MY, Bangalore S, Bhatt DL. Role of aspiration and mechanical thrombectomy in patients with acute myocardial infarction undergoing primary angioplasty: an updated meta-analysis of randomized trials. *J Am Coll Cardiol*. 2013;62:1409–1418.
52. Kumbhani DJ, Bavry AA. The rise and fall of aspiration thrombectomy. *JACC Cardiovasc Interv*. 2016;9:135–137.
53. Farkouh ME, Domanski M, Sleeper LA, et al. Strategies for multivessel revascularization in patients with diabetes. *N Engl J Med*. 2012;367:2375–2384.
54. Esper RB, Farkouh ME, Ribeiro EE, et al. SYNTAX score in patients with diabetes undergoing coronary revascularization in the FREEDOM trial. *J Am Coll Cardiol*. 2018;72:2826–2837.
55. Velazquez EJ, Lee KL, Deja MA, et al. Coronary-artery bypass surgery in patients with left ventricular dysfunction. *N Engl J Med*. 2011;364:1607–1616.
56. Velazquez EJ, Lee KL, Jones RH, et al. Coronary-artery bypass surgery in patients with ischemic cardiomyopathy. *N Engl J Med*. 2016;374:1511–1520.
57. Bonow RO, Maurer G, Lee KL, et al. Myocardial viability and survival in ischemic left ventricular dysfunction. *N Engl J Med*. 2011;364:1617–1625.
58. van Diepen S, Katz JN, Albert NM, et al. Contemporary management of cardiogenic shock: a scientific statement from the American Heart Association. *Circulation*. 2017;136:e232–e268.
59. Wayangankar SA, Bangalore S, McCoy LA, et al. Temporal trends and outcomes of patients undergoing percutaneous coronary interventions for cardiogenic shock in the setting of acute myocardial infarction: a report from the CathPCI registry. *JACC Cardiovasc Interv*. 2016;9:341–351.
60. Kumbhani DJ, Cannon CP, Fonarow GC, et al. Association of hospital primary angioplasty volume in ST-segment elevation myocardial infarction with quality and outcomes. *J Am Med Assoc*. 2009;302:2207–2213.
61. Baran DA, Grines CL, Bailey S, et al. SCAI clinical expert consensus statement on the classification of cardiogenic shock: this document was endorsed by the American College of Cardiology (ACC), the American Heart Association (AHA), the Society of Critical Care Medicine (SCCM), and the Society of Thoracic Surgeons (STS) in April 2019. *Catheter Cardiovasc Interv*. 2019;94:29–37.
62. Thiele H, Ohman EM, de Waha-Thiele S, et al. Management of cardiogenic shock complicating myocardial infarction: an update 2019. *Eur Heart J*. 2019;40:2671–2683.
63. Hochman JS, Sleeper LA, Webb JG, et al. Early revascularization in acute myocardial infarction complicated by cardiogenic shock. SHOCK investigators. should we emergently revascularize occluded coronaries for cardiogenic shock. *N Engl J Med*. 1999;341:625–634.
64. Jeger RV, Radovanovic D, Hunziker PR, et al. Ten-year trends in the incidence and treatment of cardiogenic shock. *Ann Intern Med*. 2008;149:618–626.
65. Ibanez B, James S, Agewall S, et al. 2017 ESC guidelines for the management of acute myocardial infarction in patients presenting with ST-segment elevation: the Task Force for the management of acute myocardial infarction in patients presenting with ST-segment elevation of the European Society of Cardiology (ESC). *Eur Heart J*. 2018;39:119–177.
66. Thiele H, Akin I, Sandri M, et al. PCI strategies in patients with acute myocardial infarction and cardiogenic shock. *N Engl J Med*. 2017;377:2419–2432.
67. Thiele H, Zeymer U, Neumann FJ, et al. Intraaortic balloon support for myocardial infarction with cardiogenic shock. *N Engl J Med*. 2012;367:1287–1296.
68. Giacoppo D, Madhavan MV, Baber U, et al. Impact of contrast-induced acute kidney injury after percutaneous coronary intervention on short- and long-term outcomes: pooled analysis from the HORIZONS-AMI and ACUITY trials. *Circ Cardiovasc Interv*. 2015;8:e002475.
69. Kumbhani DJ, Cannon CP, Beavers C, et al. 2020 ACC expert consensus decision pathway for anticoagulant and antiplatelet therapy in patients with atrial fibrillation or venous thromboembolism undergoing percutaneous coronary intervention or with atherosclerotic cardiovascular disease: a report of the American College of Cardiology Solution Set Oversight Committee. *J Am Coll Cardiol*. 2020.
70. Kirtane AJ, Doshi D, Leon MB, et al. Treatment of higher-risk patients with an indication for revascularization: evolution within the field of contemporary percutaneous coronary intervention. *Circulation*. 2016;134:422–431.
71. Ellis SG, Cowley MJ, Whitlow PL, et al. Prospective case-control comparison of percutaneous transluminal coronary revascularization in patients with multivessel disease treated in 1986-1987 versus 1991: improved in-hospital and 12-month results. Multivessel Angioplasty Prognosis Study (MAPS) Group. *J Am Coll Cardiol*. 1995;25:1137–1142.
72. Bavry AA, Kumbhani DJ, Helton TJ, et al. Late thrombosis of drug-eluting stents: a meta-analysis of randomized clinical trials. *Am J Med*. 2006;119:1056–1061.
73. Bangalore S, Kumar S, Fusaro M, et al. Short- and long-term outcomes with drug-eluting and bare-metal coronary stents: a mixed-treatment comparison analysis of 117 762 patient-years of follow-up from randomized trials. *Circulation*. 2012;125:2873–2891.

Antiplatelet Agents

74. Levine GN, Bates ER, Bittl JA, et al. 2016 ACC/AHA guideline focused update on duration of dual antiplatelet therapy in patients with coronary artery disease: a report of the American College of Cardiology/American Heart Association task force on clinical practice guidelines: an update of the 2011 ACCF/AHA/SCAI guideline for percutaneous coronary intervention, 2011 ACCF/AHA guideline for coronary artery bypass graft surgery, 2012 ACC/AHA/ACP/AATS/PCNA/SCAI/STS guideline for the diagnosis and management of patients with stable ischemic heart disease, 2013 ACCF/AHA guideline for the management of ST-elevation myocardial infarction, 2014 AHA/ACC guideline for the management of patients with non-ST-elevation acute coronary syndromes, and 2014 ACC/AHA guideline on perioperative cardiovascular evaluation and management of patients undergoing noncardiac surgery. *Circulation*. 2016;134:e123–e155.
75. Mauri L, Yeh RW, Kereiakes DJ. Duration of dual antiplatelet therapy after drug-eluting stents. *N Engl J Med*. 2015;372:1373–1374.
76. Fajadet J, Wijns W, Laarman GJ, et al. Randomized, double-blind, multicenter study of the Endeavor zotarolimus-eluting phosphorylcholine-encapsulated stent for treatment of native coronary artery lesions: clinical and angiographic results of the ENDEAVOR II trial. *Circulation*. 2006;114:798–806.
77. Kandzari DE, Leon MB, Popma JJ, et al. Comparison of zotarolimus-eluting and sirolimus-eluting stents in patients with native coronary artery disease: a randomized controlled trial. *J Am Coll Cardiol*. 2006;48:2440–2447.
78. Serruys PW, Silber S, Garg S, et al. Comparison of zotarolimus-eluting and everolimus-eluting coronary stents. *N Engl J Med*. 2010.
79. Kolandaivelu K, Swaminathan R, Gibson WJ, et al. Stent thrombogenicity early in high-risk interventional settings is driven by stent design and deployment and protected by polymer-drug coatings. *Circulation*. 2011;123:1400–1409.
80. Bangalore S, Toklu B, Patel N, et al. Newer-generation ultrathin strut drug-eluting stents versus older second-generation thicker strut drug-eluting stents for coronary artery disease. *Circulation*. 2018;138:2216–2226.
81. Urban P, Meredith IT, Abizaid A, et al. Polymer-free drug-coated coronary stents in patients at high bleeding risk. *N Engl J Med*. 2015;373:2038–2047.
82. Jensen LO, Maeng M, Raungaard B, et al. Randomized comparison of the polymer-free biolimus-coated BioFreedom stent with the ultrathin strut biodegradable polymer sirolimus-eluting Orsiro stent in an all-comers population treated with percutaneous coronary intervention: the SORT OUT IX trial. *Circulation*. 2020;141:2052–2063.
83. Kereiakes DJ, Onuma Y, Serruys PW, Stone GW. Bioresorbable vascular scaffolds for coronary revascularization. *Circulation*. 2016;134:168–182.
84. Ellis SG, Kereiakes DJ, Metzger DC, et al. Everolimus-eluting bioresorbable scaffolds for coronary artery disease. *N Engl J Med*. 2015;373:1905–1915.
85. Omar WA, Kumbhani DJ. The current literature on bioabsorbable stents: a review. *Curr Atheroscler Rep*. 2019;21:54.
86. Ali ZA, Nef H, Escaned J, et al. Safety and effectiveness of coronary intravascular lithotripsy for treatment of severely calcified coronary stenoses: the disrupt CAD II study. *Circ Cardiovasc Interv*. 2019;12:e008434.
87. Vlaar PJ, Svilaas T, van der Horst IC, et al. Cardiac death and reinfarction after 1 year in the Thrombus Aspiration during Percutaneous coronary intervention in Acute myocardial infarction Study (TAPAS): a 1-year follow-up study. *Lancet*. 2008;371:1915–1920.
88. Kushner FG, Hand M, Smith Jr SC, et al. 2009 focused updates: ACC/AHA guidelines for the management of patients with ST-elevation myocardial infarction (updating the 2004 guideline and 2007 focused update) and ACC/AHA/SCAI guidelines on percutaneous coronary intervention (updating the 2005 guideline and 2007 focused update): a report of the American College of Cardiology Foundation/American Heart Association task force on practice guidelines. *Circulation*. 2009;120:2271–2306.
89. Scheller B, Hehrlein C, Bocksch W, et al. Treatment of coronary in-stent restenosis with a paclitaxel-coated balloon catheter. *N Engl J Med*. 2006;355:2113–2124.
90. Jeger RV, Farah A, Ohlow MA, et al. Drug-coated balloons for small coronary artery disease (BASKET-SMALL 2): an open-label randomised non-inferiority trial. *Lancet*. 2018;392:849–856.

Functional Assessment

91. Nallamothu BK, Spertus JA, Lansky AJ, et al. Comparison of clinical interpretation with visual assessment and quantitative coronary angiography in patients undergoing percutaneous coronary intervention in contemporary practice: the Assessing Angiography (A2) project. *Circulation*. 2013;127:1793–1800.
92. Pijls NH, De Bruyne B, Peels K, et al. Measurement of fractional flow reserve to assess the functional severity of coronary-artery stenoses. *N Engl J Med*. 1996;334:1703–1708.
93. Tonino PA, De Bruyne B, Pijls NH, et al. Fractional flow reserve versus angiography for guiding percutaneous coronary intervention. *N Engl J Med*. 2009;360:213–224.
94. De Bruyne B, Fearon WF, Pijls NH, et al. Fractional flow reserve-guided PCI for stable coronary artery disease. *N Engl J Med*. 2014;371:1208–1217.
95. Kumbhani DJ, Bhatt DL. Fractional flow reserve in serial coronary artery stenoses. *JAMA Cardiol*. 2016;1:359–360.

96. Jeremias A, Kirtane AJ, Stone GW. A test in context: fractional flow reserve: accuracy, prognostic implications, and limitations. *J Am Coll Cardiol.* 2017;69:2748–2758.
97. Engstrom T, Kelbaek H, Helqvist S, et al. Complete revascularisation versus treatment of the culprit lesion only in patients with ST-segment elevation myocardial infarction and multivessel disease (DANAMI-3-PRIMULTI): an open-label, randomised controlled trial. *Lancet.* 2015;386:665–671.
98. Smits PC, Abdel-Wahab M, Neumann FJ, et al. Fractional flow reserve-guided multivessel angioplasty in myocardial infarction. *N Engl J Med.* 2017;376:1234–1244.
99. De Rosa S, Polimeni A, Petraco R, et al. Diagnostic performance of the instantaneous wave-free ratio: comparison with fractional flow reserve. *Circ Cardiovasc Interv.* 2018;11:e004613.
100. Davies JE, Sen S, Dehbi HM, et al. Use of the instantaneous wave-free ratio or fractional flow reserve in PCI. *N Engl J Med.* 2017;376:1824–1834.
101. Gotberg M, Christiansen EH, Gudmundsdottir IJ, et al. Instantaneous wave-free ratio versus fractional flow reserve to guide PCI. *N Engl J Med.* 2017;376:1813–1823.
102. De Maria GL, Garcia-Garcia HM, Scarsini R, et al. Novel indices of coronary physiology: do we need alternatives to fractional flow reserve? *Circ Cardiovasc Interv.* 2020;13:e008487.
103. Maehara A, Matsumura M, Ali ZA, et al. IVUS-guided versus OCT-guided coronary stent implantation: a critical appraisal. *JACC Cardiovasc Imaging.* 2017;10:1487–1503.

Management Concerns

104. Bangalore S, Bhatt DL. Coronary intravascular ultrasound. *Circulation.* 2013;127:e868–e874.
105. Zhang J, Gao X, Kan J, et al. Intravascular ultrasound versus angiography-guided drug-eluting stent implantation: the ULTIMATE trial. *J Am Coll Cardiol.* 2018;72:3126–3137.
106. Elgendy IY, Mahmoud AN, Elgendy AY, Bavry AA. Outcomes with intravascular ultrasound-guided stent implantation: a meta-analysis of randomized trials in the era of drug-eluting stents. *Circ Cardiovasc Interv.* 2016;9:e003700.
107. Ali ZA, Maehara A, Genereux P, et al. Optical coherence tomography compared with intravascular ultrasound and with angiography to guide coronary stent implantation (ILUMIEN III: optimize PCI): a randomised controlled trial. *Lancet.* 2016;388:2618–2628.
108. De Backer D, Biston P, Devriendt J, et al. Comparison of dopamine and norepinephrine in the treatment of shock. *N Engl J Med.* 2010;362:779–789.
109. van Diepen S. Routine unloading in patients treated with extracorporeal membrane oxygenation for cardiogenic shock: mixed outcomes set the stage for future trials. *Circulation.* 2020;142:2107–2109.
110. Sandoval Y, Burke MN, Lobo AS, et al. Contemporary arterial access in the cardiac catheterization laboratory. *JACC Cardiovasc Interv.* 2017;10:2233–2241.
111. Jolly SS, Yusuf S, Cairns J, et al. Radial versus femoral access for coronary angiography and intervention in patients with acute coronary syndromes (RIVAL): a randomised, parallel group, multicentre trial. *Lancet.* 2011;377:1409–1420.
112. Ferrante G, Rao SV, Juni P, et al. Radial versus femoral access for coronary interventions across the entire spectrum of patients with coronary artery disease: a meta-analysis of randomized trials. *JACC Cardiovasc Interv.* 2016;9:1419–1434.
113. Bangalore S, Bhatt DL. Femoral arterial access and closure. *Circulation.* 2011;124:e147–e156.
114. Chhatriwalla AK, Amin AP, Kennedy KF, et al. Association between bleeding events and in-hospital mortality after percutaneous coronary intervention. *J Am Med Assoc.* 2013;309:1022–1029.
115. Bhatt DL. Advancing the care of cardiac patients using registry data: going where randomized clinical trials dare not. *J Am Med Assoc.* 2010;303:2188–2189.
116. Roth GJ, Stanford N, Majerus PW. Acetylation of prostaglandin synthase by aspirin. *Proc Natl Acad Sci U S A.* 1975;72:3073–3076.
117. Mehran R, Baber U, Sharma SK, et al. Ticagrelor with or without aspirin in high-risk patients after PCI. *N Engl J Med.* 2019;381:2032–2042.
118. Hollopeter G, Jantzen HM, Vincent D, et al. Identification of the platelet ADP receptor targeted by antithrombotic drugs. *Nature.* 2001;409:202–207.
119. Desai NR, Bhatt DL. The state of periprocedural antiplatelet therapy after recent trials. *JACC Cardiovasc Interv.* 2010;3:571–583.
120. Schomig A. Ticagrelor–is there need for a new player in the antiplatelet-therapy field? *N Engl J Med.* 2009;361:1108–1111.
121. Wiviott SD, Trenk D, Frelinger AL, et al. Prasugrel compared with high loading- and maintenance-dose clopidogrel in patients with planned percutaneous coronary intervention: the prasugrel in comparison to clopidogrel for inhibition of platelet activation and aggregation-thrombolysis in myocardial infarction 44 trial. *Circulation.* 2007;116:2923–2932.
122. Wiviott SD, Braunwald E, McCabe CH, et al. Prasugrel versus clopidogrel in patients with acute coronary syndromes. *N Engl J Med.* 2007;357:2001–2015.
123. Bhatt DL. Intensifying platelet inhibition–navigating between Scylla and Charybdis. *N Engl J Med.* 2007;357:2078–2081.
124. Roe MT, Ohman EM, TRILOGY ACS Investigators. Prasugrel versus clopidogrel for acute coronary syndromes. *N Engl J Med.* 2013;368:188–189.
125. Bhatt DL. Tailoring antiplatelet therapy based on pharmacogenomics: how well do the data fit? *J Am Med Assoc.* 2009;302:896–897.
126. Wallentin L, Becker RC, Budaj A, et al. Ticagrelor versus clopidogrel in patients with acute coronary syndromes. *N Engl J Med.* 2009;361:1045–1057.
127. Costa F, van Klaveren D, James S, et al. Derivation and validation of the predicting bleeding complications in patients undergoing stent implantation and subsequent dual antiplatelet therapy (PRECISE-DAPT) score: a pooled analysis of individual-patient datasets from clinical trials. *Lancet.* 2017;389:1025–1034.
128. Khan SU, Singh M, Valavoor S, et al. Dual antiplatelet therapy after percutaneous coronary intervention and drug-eluting stents: a systematic review and network meta-analysis. *Circulation.* 2020;142:1425–1436.
129. Bonaca MP, Bhatt DL, Cohen M, et al. Long-term use of ticagrelor in patients with prior myocardial infarction. *N Engl J Med.* 2015;372:1791–1800.
130. Lopes RD, Leonardi S, Wojdyla DM, et al. Stent thrombosis in patients with atrial fibrillation undergoing coronary stenting in the AUGUSTUS trial. *Circulation.* 2020;141:781–783.
131. Roffi M, Patrono C, Collet JP, et al. 2015 ESC guidelines for the management of acute coronary syndromes in patients presenting without persistent ST-segment elevation: task force for the management of acute coronary syndromes in patients presenting without persistent ST-segment elevation of the European Society of Cardiology (ESC). *Eur Heart J.* 2016;37:267–315.
132. Harrington RA, Stone GW, McNulty S, et al. Platelet inhibition with cangrelor in patients undergoing PCI. *N Engl J Med.* 2009;361:2318–2329.
133. Bhatt DL, Lincoff AM, Gibson CM, et al. Intravenous platelet blockade with cangrelor during PCI. *N Engl J Med.* 2009;361:2330–2341.
134. Bhatt DL, Stone GW, Mahaffey KW, et al. Effect of platelet inhibition with cangrelor during PCI on ischemic events. *N Engl J Med.* 2013;368:1303–1313.
135. Steg PG, Bhatt DL, Hamm CW, et al. Effect of cangrelor on periprocedural outcomes in percutaneous coronary interventions: a pooled analysis of patient-level data. *Lancet.* 2013;382:1981–1992.
136. Gurm HS, Tamhane U, Meier P, et al. A comparison of abciximab and small-molecule glycoprotein IIb/IIIa inhibitors in patients undergoing primary percutaneous coronary intervention: a meta-analysis of contemporary randomized controlled trials. *Circ Cardiovasc Interv.* 2009;2:230–236.
137. De Luca G, Ucci G, Cassetti E, Marino P. Benefits from small molecule administration as compared with abciximab among patients with ST-segment elevation myocardial infarction treated with primary angioplasty: a meta-analysis. *J Am Coll Cardiol.* 2009;53:1668–1673.
138. Mehilli J, Kastrati A, Schulz S, et al. Abciximab in patients with acute ST-segment-elevation myocardial infarction undergoing primary percutaneous coronary intervention after clopidogrel loading: a randomized double-blind trial. *Circulation.* 2009;119:1933–1940.
139. Gutierrez A, Bhatt DL. Balancing the risks of stent thrombosis and major bleeding during primary percutaneous coronary intervention. *Eur Heart J.* 2014;35:2448–2451.
140. Bhatt DL, Hulot JS, Moliterno DJ, Harrington RA. Antiplatelet and anticoagulation therapy for acute coronary syndromes. *Circ Res.* 2014;114:1929–1943.
141. Lincoff AM, Bittl JA, Harrington RA, et al. Bivalirudin and provisional glycoprotein IIb/IIIa blockade compared with heparin and planned glycoprotein IIb/IIIa blockade during percutaneous coronary intervention: REPLACE-2 randomized trial. *J Am Med Assoc.* 2003;289:853–863.
142. Stone GW, McLaurin BT, Cox DA, et al. Bivalirudin for patients with acute coronary syndromes. *N Engl J Med.* 2006;355:2203–2216.
143. Cavender MA, Sabatine MS. Bivalirudin versus heparin in patients planned for percutaneous coronary intervention: a meta-analysis of randomised controlled trials. *Lancet.* 2014;384:599–606.
144. Brennan JM, Curtis JP, Dai D, et al. Enhanced mortality risk prediction with a focus on high-risk percutaneous coronary intervention: results from 1,208,137 procedures in the NCDR (National Cardiovascular Data Registry). *JACC Cardiovasc Interv.* 2013;6:790–799.
145. Thygesen K, Alpert JS, Jaffe AS, et al. Fourth universal definition of myocardial infarction (2018). *J Am Coll Cardiol.* 2018;72:2231–2264.
146. Moussa ID, Klein LW, Shah B, et al. Consideration of a new definition of clinically relevant myocardial infarction after coronary revascularization: an expert consensus document from the Society for Cardiovascular Angiography and Interventions (SCAI). *Catheter Cardiovasc Interv.* 2014;83:27–36.
147. Garcia-Garcia HM, McFadden EP, Farb A, et al. Standardized end point definitions for coronary intervention trials: the academic research consortium-2 consensus document. *Circulation.* 2018;137:2635–2650.
148. Olivier CB, Sundaram V, Bhatt DL, et al. Definitions of peri-procedural myocardial infarction and the association with one-year mortality: Insights from CHAMPION trials. *Int J Cardiol.* 2018;270:96–101.
149. Prasad A, Gersh BJ, Bertrand ME, et al. Prognostic significance of periprocedural versus spontaneously occurring myocardial infarction after percutaneous coronary intervention in patients with acute coronary syndromes: an analysis from the ACUITY (Acute Catheterization and Urgent Intervention Triage Strategy) trial. *J Am Coll Cardiol.* 2009;54:477–486.
150. Mehran R, Baber U, Steg PG, et al. Cessation of dual antiplatelet treatment and cardiac events after percutaneous coronary intervention (PARIS): 2 year results from a prospective observational study. *Lancet.* 2013;382:1714–1722.
151. Mehran R, Dangas G, Abizaid AS, et al. Angiographic patterns of in-stent restenosis: classification and implications for long-term outcome. *Circulation.* 1999;100:1872–1878.
152. Dangas GD, Claessen BE, Caixeta A, et al. In-stent restenosis in the drug-eluting stent era. *J Am Coll Cardiol.* 2010;56:1897–1907.
153. Stone GW, Maehara A, Lansky AJ, et al. A prospective natural-history study of coronary atherosclerosis. *N Engl J Med.* 2011;364:226–235.
154. Nakazawa G, Otsuka F, Nakano M, et al. The pathology of neoatherosclerosis in human coronary implants bare-metal and drug-eluting stents. *J Am Coll Cardiol.* 2011;57:1314–1322.
155. Otsuka F, Vorpahl M, Nakano M, et al. Pathology of second-generation everolimus-eluting stents versus first-generation sirolimus- and paclitaxel-eluting stents in humans. *Circulation.* 2014;129:211–223.
156. King SB, Babb JD, Bates ER, et al. COCATS 4 task force 10: training in cardiac catheterization. *J Am Coll Cardiol.* 2015;65:1844–1853.
157. Harold JG, Bass TA, Bashore TM, et al. ACCF/AHA/SCAI 2013 update of the clinical competence statement on coronary artery interventional procedures: a report of the American College of Cardiology Foundation/American Heart Association/American College of physicians task force on clinical competence and training (writing committee to revise the 2007 clinical competence statement on cardiac interventional procedures). *J Am Coll Cardiol.* 2013;62:357–396.
158. Kumbhani DJ, Bhatt DL. A new dimension in the relationship between procedural volumes and quality. *Circulation.* 2019;139:473–476.
159. Kumbhani DJ, Nallamothu BK. PCI volume benchmarks: still adequate for quality assessment in 2017? *J Am Coll Cardiol.* 2017;69:2925–2928.
160. Kumbhani DJ. *Training Program Guidelines, Case Numbers, and Recertification.* CathSAP; 2019.
161. Aversano T, Lemmon CC, Liu L, Atlantic CPORT Investigators. Outcomes of PCI at hospitals with or without on-site cardiac surgery. *N Engl J Med.* 2012;366:1792–1802.
162. Jacobs AK, Normand SL, Massaro JM, et al. Nonemergency PCI at hospitals with or without on-site cardiac surgery. *N Engl J Med.* 2013;368:1498–1508.

42 Diseases of the Aorta

ALAN C. BRAVERMAN AND MARC SCHERMERHORN

THE NORMAL AORTA, 806
Anatomy and Physiology, 806
Evaluation of the Aorta, 806

AORTIC ANEURYSMS, 806
Abdominal Aortic Aneurysms, 807
Thoracic Aortic Aneurysms, 810

AORTIC DISSECTION, 818
Classification, 819
Cause and Pathogenesis, 819

Clinical Manifestations, 821
Diagnostic Techniques, 823
Integrated Diagnostic Evaluation and Management Algorithms, 824
Long-Term Therapy and Follow-Up, 830

AORTIC DISSECTION VARIANTS, 831
Aortic Intramural Hematoma, 831
Penetrating Atherosclerotic Aortic Ulcer, 831

AORTOARTERITIS SYNDROMES, 832
Bacterial Infections of the Aorta, 832

PRIMARY TUMORS OF THE AORTA, 834

FUTURE PERSPECTIVES, 834

REFERENCES, 835

THE NORMAL AORTA

Anatomy and Physiology

The aorta, the largest artery in the body, has thoracic and abdominal components (Fig. 42.1). The thoracic aorta is divided into the ascending, arch, and descending segments, and the abdominal aorta into the suprarenal and infrarenal segments. The ascending aorta has two distinct portions. The *aortic root* begins at the aortic valve and extends to the sinotubular junction. The aortic root supports the bases of the aortic valve leaflets. The right and left coronary arteries arise from the sinuses of Valsalva. The upper portion of the ascending aorta begins at the sinotubular junction and rises to join the aortic arch. The proximal portion of the ascending aorta lies within the pericardial cavity, anterior to the pulmonary artery bifurcation. The aortic arch gives rise to the innominate artery, the left common carotid artery, and the left subclavian artery. The descending thoracic aorta begins distal to the left subclavian artery. The ligamentum arteriosum marks the point at which the aortic arch joins the descending aorta, denoted the *aortic isthmus*. The aortic isthmus marks the site of transition between the relatively mobile ascending aorta and the fixed descending aorta making it vulnerable to deceleration trauma. The descending aorta gives rise to posterior paired intercostal arteries at multiple levels of the spine. Distally, the thoracic aorta passes through the diaphragm becoming the abdominal aorta. The abdominal aorta gives rise to the celiac artery and the superior mesenteric artery anteriorly, followed by the posterolateral origins of the left and anterolateral right renal arteries. This segment of the aorta is called the suprarenal or visceral segment. The infrarenal aorta lies anterior to the lumbar spine, where paired lumbar artery branches arise posteriorly. The aorta ends by bifurcation into common iliac arteries.

MICROSCOPIC STRUCTURE

The aortic wall includes three layers: the *intima*, the *tunica media*, and the *tunica adventitia* (Fig. 42.2) (see also Chapter 24). The internal elastic lamina demarcates the intima, lined by endothelial cells, from the media. The media has concentric layers of elastic fibers alternating with vascular smooth muscle cells (SMCs). Each layer of elastin and SMCs constitutes a "lamellar unit." The media gives the aorta its circumferential resilience (elasticity), which resists hemodynamic stress. The external elastic lamina delineates the abluminal portion of the media from the adventitia. The adventitia contains collagen fibers, fibroblasts, nerves, and vasa vasorum. The adventitial collagen fibers govern the tensile strength of the aortic wall.

The ascending aorta normally contains about 55 to 60 elastic lamellae, with a gradual decrease in the number of elastic lamellae down the length of the aorta to roughly 26 at the aortic bifurcation. Oxygen and nutrients reach the aortic wall by simple diffusion from the lumen, at least in segments of the aorta that contain up to approximately 29 elastic lamellae. In the proximal aortic segments, the *vasa vasorum* supply additional nutrients to the outer third of the thoracic aortic media. The infrarenal aorta normally lacks an independent microvascular supply.

The compliance of the aortic wall under normal conditions results from reversible extension of the elastic lamellar units in the media. At mechanical strain levels that exceed the extensile capacity of the medial elastic fibers, aortic tensile strength becomes dependent on the collagen fiber meshwork of the media and adventitia. Although not functionally significant under normal circumstances or in systemic hypertension, the dependence on adventitial collagen in accommodating greater hemodynamic stress can contribute to abdominal aortic aneurysms (AAAs), in which the wall tension within the dilated segment may exceed by orders of magnitude higher than in a normal aorta. In AAAs, collagen fibers reorganize to accommodate higher degrees of tensile stress.

Physiology

The aorta as an elastic conduit transmits pulsatile arterial blood pressure to all points in the arterial tree. The biomechanical properties of the aorta, including resilience to cyclical deformation, derive from the elastin and collagen in the media and adventitia. The aortic wall pressure-diameter relationship is nonlinear; a more distensible component is demonstrated at lower pressures and a stiffer component at higher pressures, with the transition from distensible to stiff behavior occurring at pressures higher than 80 mm Hg.

The pressure-diameter curve of the aorta becomes less steep with increasing age (i.e., the aorta stiffens and aortic diameter increases). The aortic diameter is generally less than 40 mm at the root and becomes smaller distally. Aortic diameters depend upon age, sex, body size, and blood pressure and increase in size by about 1 mm per decade.[1]

Evaluation of the Aorta

In some individuals, the aorta can be palpated in the midabdominal region. The bifurcation typically occurs at the level of the umbilicus and the L4 vertebral body. Plain radiography is insensitive in evaluating the thoracic and abdominal aorta, but diagnostic detail can be obtained with ultrasound (including echocardiography), computed tomography (CT), magnetic resonance imaging (MRI), and less frequently, aortography.

AORTIC ANEURYSMS

The term *aortic aneurysm* refers to a pathologic segment of aortic dilatation that expands and can eventually rupture or dissect. One criterion for abnormal aortic dilatation is a diameter of at least 50% greater than

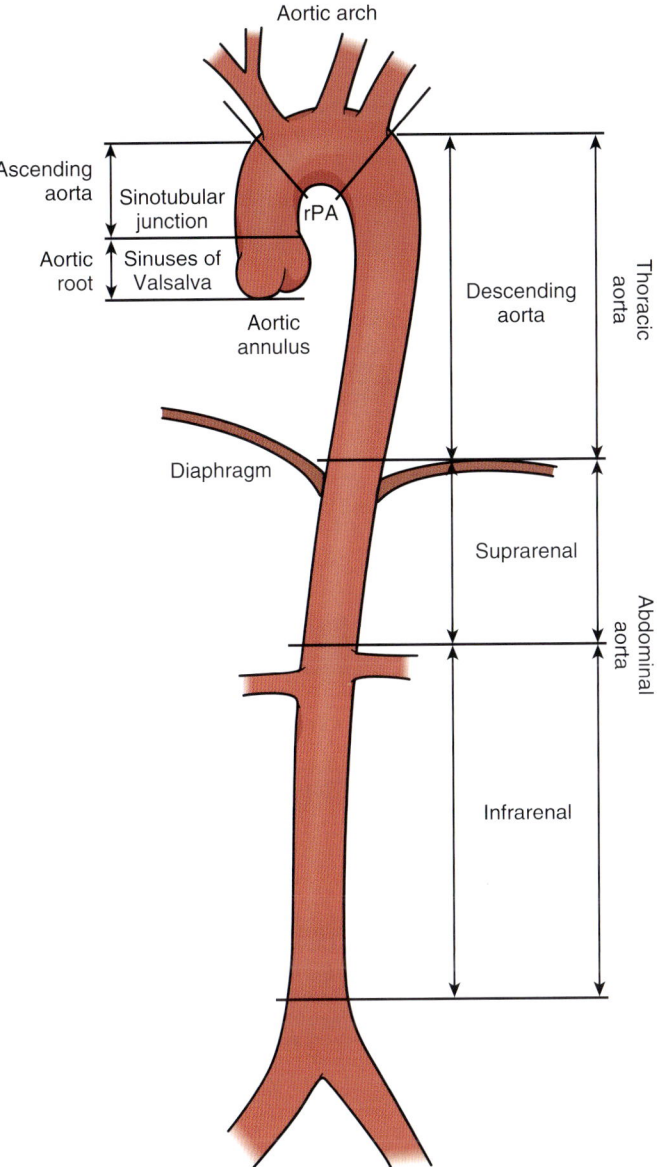

FIGURE 42.1 Anatomical segments of the aorta. *rPA*, Right pulmonary artery. (From Erbel R, Aboyans V, Boileau C, et al. 2014 ESC Guidelines on the diagnosis and treatment of aortic diseases: document covering acute and chronic aortic diseases of the thoracic and abdominal aorta of the adult. The Task Force for the Diagnosis and Treatment of Aortic Diseases of the European Society of Cardiology (ESC). *Eur Heart J.* 2014;35:2873–2926.)

expected for the same aortic segment in unaffected individuals of the same age and sex, or for a focal dilation 50% greater than the adjacent normal aorta. Aortic aneurysms are described by their size, location, morphology, and cause. Aortic aneurysms can be either *fusiform* or *saccular*. Fusiform aneurysms, the more common type, are symmetrically dilated with involvement of the entire aortic circumference. Saccular aneurysms exhibit a focal outpouching. These both are "true" aneurysms with an intact aortic wall involving all layers. In contrast, in pseudoaneurysms (false aneurysms) bleeding has occurred through the aortic wall resulting in a contained periaortic hematoma in continuity with the aortic lumen. Pseudoaneurysms may result from trauma, infection or contained rupture of an aortic aneurysm, dissection, or penetrating ulcer.

Abdominal Aortic Aneurysms

AAAs are defined by an abdominal aorta greater than 3.0 cm in diameter, with lower thresholds possibly appropriate for women and some Asian populations.[2] AAAs are the most common form of aortic aneurysms, being present in 2.3% of those 75 to 79 years old.[2] Most AAAs (>80%) arise in the infrarenal aorta, but up to 10% may involve the pararenal or visceral aorta and may extend into the thoracoabdominal segment. AAAs are approximately five times more prevalent in men than in women, and are associated strongly with age, with most occurring in those older than 60 years and even higher risk in those older than 75 years.[3] AAAs strongly are associated with cigarette smoking and current smokers are seven times more likely to have an AAA than nonsmokers, with duration and quantity of smoking increasing risk.[3] Smoking also increases AAA growth rate.[3] Other risk factors include emphysema, hypertension, and hyperlipidemia. A family history is a potent risk factor for AAA being present in about 20% of patients, denoting an important heritable component. The major complication of AAA is acute rupture, estimated to cause 150,000 to 200,000 deaths each year worldwide.[4]

Pathogenesis

AAA formation associates with chronic aortic wall inflammation, increased local expression of proteinases, and degradation of structural connective tissue proteins.[4] Aneurysmal dilation and rupture result from mechanical failure of medial elastin and adventitial collagen. Inflammatory cells commonly infiltrate the aortic wall and "inflammatory AAAs" may exhibit extension of this process to the periaortic retroperitoneal tissues. Matrix-degrading enzymes released by inflammatory cells lead to medial degeneration and play a role in dilation and rupture. Inflammatory cells may enter the media in response to signals resulting from hemodynamic stress, ischemia, autoimmune processes, or extension of intimal atherosclerosis. A combination of environmental and genetic factors stimulating an immune response in the aorta may underlie AAA.[4] Destruction of and reduced concentration of medial elastin characterize AAAs. The aortic wall tensile strength results principally from interstitial collagen and AAAs are associated with increased collagen content. Enzymes including matrix metalloproteinases (MMPs) and elastolytic cathepsins degrade arterial matrix constituents contributing to aneurysm expansion and rupture.[5] Tetracyclines and other MMP inhibitors can suppress experimental aneurysm formation in animal models, but do not reduce AAA growth in humans.[5,6]

The natural history of AAAs involves a balance between degradative and reparative processes. Medial SMC loss characterizes AAAs with mechanisms including apoptosis, which may be initiated by medial ischemia, signaling molecules, or cellular immune responses. In the absence of vasa vasorum, the nutrient supply to the media of the distal aorta depends on diffusion from the lumen, which may be jeopardized by intimal thickening and atherosclerotic plaque.

Clinical Features

AAAs develop insidiously over a period of several years and rarely cause symptoms in the absence of distal thromboembolism, rapid expansion, or rupture. Although large AAAs are at substantial risk of rupturing, the vast majority of AAAs are small. Most AAAs are detected by screening studies or as an incidental finding on imaging studies performed for another purpose.

Physical examination is insensitive in detecting AAAs, but abdominal palpation may reveal a pulsatile epigastric or periumbilical mass. Only 30% to 40% of AAAs are noted on physical examination, although aneurysms larger than 5 cm can be detected in approximately 75% of patients, depending on body habitus.[3] Symptoms may occur due to impending rupture or expansion and include pain radiating to the back or genitals or distal embolization from mural thrombus. Because AAA is present in up to 85% of patients with a femoral artery aneurysm and 60% of patients with a popliteal artery aneurysm, screening for AAA in these patients is indicated.[3] Patients with AAA may have coexisting TAA disease (25%) and have an increased prevalence of iliac and popliteal aneurysms.[1,3]

Diagnostic Imaging

Ultrasound/Computed Tomography/Magnetic Resonance Imaging/Aortography

Abdominal ultrasound can detect AAAs with high accuracy and is preferred over CT in screening for AAAs because it is inexpensive,

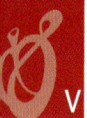

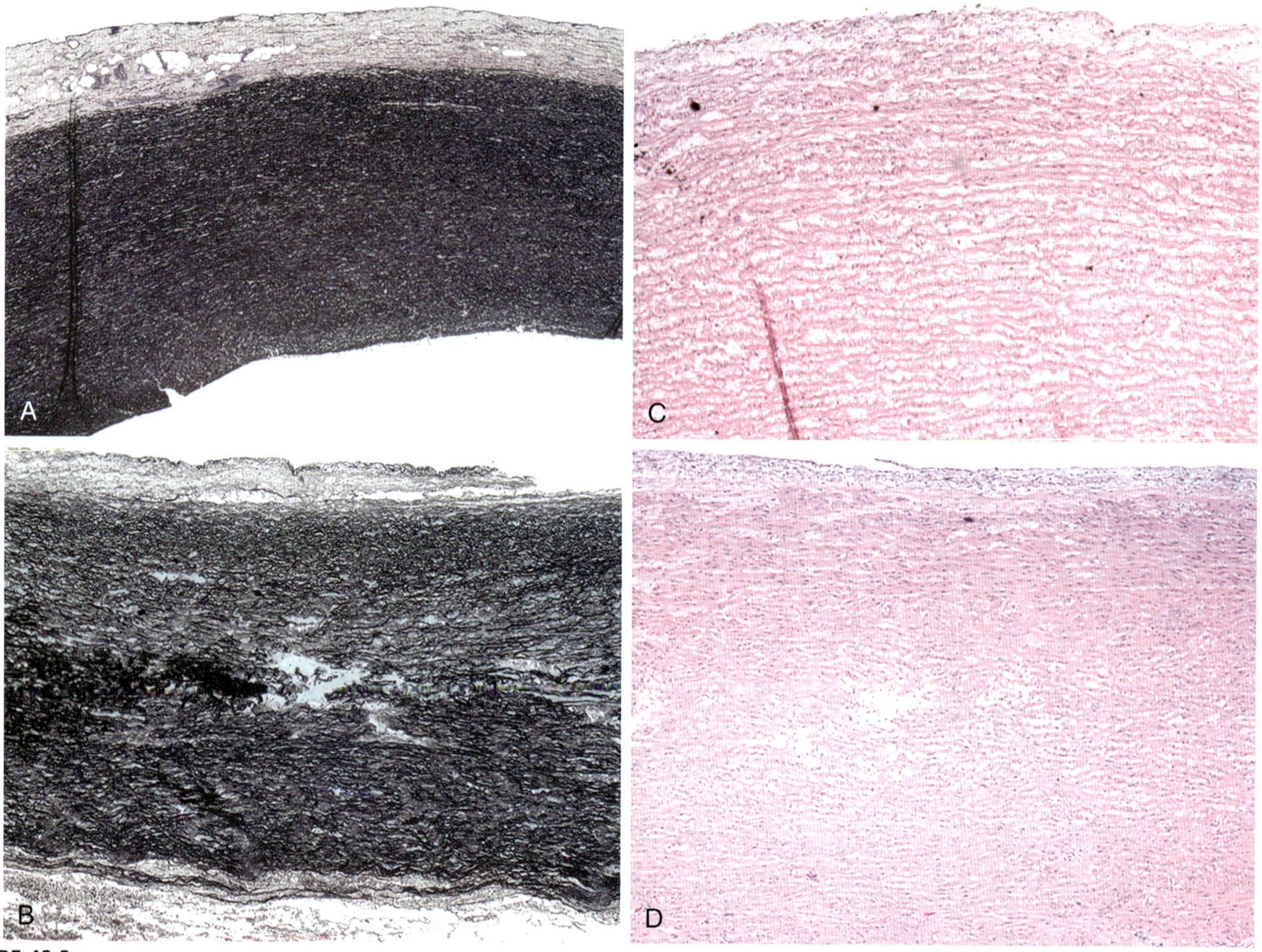

FIGURE 42.2 Histology of ascending aortas. **A,** Normal ascending aorta showing dense elastic fibers in a young adult (Movat pentachrome, original magnification, ×10). **B,** Ascending aorta with cystic medial degeneration (CMD) and elastic fiber loss, characteristic of many genetic forms of aortic disease (Movat pentachrome, original magnification, ×10). **C,** Ascending aorta from a subject with Loeys-Dietz syndrome with generalized widening of intralamellar spaces, typical of diffuse medial degeneration (DMD) (hematoxylin–eosin, original magnification, ×15). **D,** Ascending aorta with CMD secondary to focal interlamellar degeneration (hematoxylin–eosin, original magnification, ×10). (From Jain D, Dietz HC, Oswald GL, et al. Causes and histopathology of ascending aortic disease in children and young adults. *Cardiovasc Path*. 2011;20:15–25.)

noninvasive, and avoids radiation and contrast agents.[2,3] Because ultrasound-derived measurements of AAA diameter are less accurate than by CT or MRI, many use ultrasound for follow-up of small AAAs and CT or MRI for larger AAAs. When combined with radiographic contrast enhancement, with outer wall-to-outer wall measurements perpendicular to the centerline of the aorta, CT angiography (CTA) is more accurate than ultrasound. CTA is especially useful in demonstrating the relationship of the AAA to the renal, visceral, and iliac arteries and patterns of mural thrombus, calcification, or coexisting occlusive atherosclerosis, which might influence AAA repair. Three-dimensional reconstructions enhance visualization of the AAA before endovascular aneurysm repair (EVAR). CT can also assess AAA variants, such as inflammatory AAAs and mycotic aneurysms. Magnetic resonance angiography (MRA) has high accuracy in detecting AAAs, measuring aneurysm diameter, and planning treatment. MRA avoids exposure to radiation and iodine-based contrast material. CTA has superseded aortography in the evaluation and management of AAAs. Aortography is an initial step in EVAR and in subsequent interventions following EVAR, such as embolization of the lumbar or iliac artery branches.

Screening

While AAA probability is low in the general population, it is significantly higher when risk factors are present. Screening for AAAs with ultrasound, coupled with repair of AAAs above a size threshold, has reduced risk of AAA rupture and AAA-related deaths.[2,3] The incidence of screening-detected AAAs ranges from 1 per 1000 in adults younger than 60 years but it may be as high as 10% in those with risk factors such as older age, male sex, smoking, family history, history of other aneurysms, hypertension, and atherosclerosis. Despite the cost-effectiveness of AAA screening in men 65 to 74 years of age, routine screening for AAAs in women remains controversial, and has not demonstrated a survival benefit, although the single study that included women was likely underpowered to detect a difference in that subgroup and took place before the advent of endovascular AAA repair.[3] AAAs occur about 10 years later in women than men, and rates of rupture and mortality from rupture are both higher in women. The U.S. Preventive Services Task Force recommends a one-time ultrasound screening for AAAs in men 65 to 75 years of age with a history of smoking and selective screening for those who never smoked.[3] The Society for Vascular Surgery (SVS) recommends a one-time screening for AAAs in all men ≥65 years and for women ≥65 years with a history of tobacco use or a family history of AAAs.[3] The Centers for Medicare and Medicaid Services will currently reimburse screening for men 65 to 75 who ever smoked and men and women 65 to 75 with a family history of AAA.

Genetics/Molecular Genetics

Several genetic disorders are associated with thoracic aortic aneurysms (TAAs), including Marfan syndrome (MFS), Loeys-Dietz syndrome (LDS), and vascular Ehlers-Danlos syndrome (vEDS), but less commonly with aneurysms of the abdominal aorta. Up to 20% of patients with an infrarenal AAA have a family history of AAAs, suggesting an inherited component. Genetic variants, SNP loci, and epigenetic differences may underlie additional individual predilection for AAA.[4,7]

Natural History

AAAs expand gradually and variably with an average growth rate of 2.2 mm (range 1 to 5 mm) per year and larger aortas grow more rapidly.[3] While AAA diameter is most important in predicting rupture, size alone may not predict risk for rupture.[3] Factors associated with risk of AAA rupture include current smoking, female gender, emphysema, HTN, and immunotherapy after organ transplantation.[3] The aortic size indexed to body size may predict risk better in women. The risk of rupture is 5.3% per year for AAAs between 5.5 and 7.0 cm. In a study of those unfit for repair, the risk of rupture was 9% per year for AAA between 5.5 and 5.9 cm, 10% for those 5.0 to 6.9 cm, and 33% for those 7.0 cm or greater, but recent reports suggest a lower risk of rupture.[3] The rate of growth, wall stiffness, and wall tension may be more sensitive measures of rupture risk.[3]

Ruptured Abdominal Aortic Aneurysm

Symptoms from AAAs usually relate to rupture of the aneurysm or rapid expansion and impending rupture. Rupture of AAAs into the peritoneal cavity results in acute hemorrhage, severe abdominal pain, and hypotension due to exsanguination (Fig. 42.3). Rupture into the retroperitoneum may result in a temporarily contained periaortic hematoma, with severe abdominal or back pain that may radiate to the flank or groin. A tender pulsatile abdominal or flank mass may be present, along with hypotension and/or syncope. Approximately 30% to 50% of patients with ruptured AAAs die before hospitalization, and an additional 30% to 40% die after reaching a hospital but before treatment.[3] Stable patients with symptomatic but apparently unruptured AAAs should undergo CT to determine whether rupture has occurred. Because emergency repair entails a much higher mortality rate, in the absence of rupture, it may be prudent in certain cases to delay surgical repair for 4 to 24 hours to optimize conditions under close monitoring.[3]

Management

Surveillance/Medical Therapy

Patients with small AAAs can be observed safely with imaging surveillance. In a study of men 65 years and older, 14% of aortas initially measuring 2.6 to 2.9 cm exceeded 5.5 cm at 10-year follow-up.[3] In general, repair should be considered for asymptomatic aneurysms greater than 5.0 to 5.5 cm in diameter.[2,3] Symptomatic aneurysms and those with rapid growth (>1 cm/year) require more urgent consideration. AAA repair at smaller size (closer to 5 cm) should be considered for women due to increased risk of rupture.[2] In patients with AAAs larger than 4.5 cm, CT is preferred over ultrasound for more accurate measurement. The following surveillance imaging strategy for AAAs of various sizes has been proposed: 2.5 to 2.9 cm, every 7 years; 3.0 to 3.9 cm, every 3 years; 4.0 to 4.9 cm, every 12 months; and 5.0 to 5.4 cm, every 3 to 6 months.[2,3] Current smokers and women may require more frequent imaging. Young, healthy patients—especially women—with AAAs between 5 and 5.4 cm may benefit from early repair.[2,3]

Several steps are recommended to help minimize the risk for aneurysm expansion. Smoking cessation is critical as ongoing tobacco use links with increased AAA expansion and rupture risk. Patients with AAAs and coexisting atherosclerotic disease benefit from statin therapy,[3] and statin therapy after AAA repair associates with improved long-term survival.[8] Patients with small AAAs should exercise regularly because moderate physical activity does not adversely influence the risk for rupture and may limit AAA growth.[2,3]

Surgery

The decision to undergo elective repair of an asymptomatic AAA depends on life expectancy and the estimated risk for rupture, balanced against the estimated risks associated with AAA repair. In general, repair of AAA is recommended when the diameter exceeds 5.4 cm with earlier repair considered for those with rapid expansion, young age, and in women.[3] The 5-year survival after successful AAA repair is below 70% with cardiovascular and pulmonary diseases the leading causes of death.[3] In the absence of recent symptoms or an acute cardiac condition, further noninvasive testing is indicated only if it will change management.[2,3] Some patients benefit from preoperative evaluation for coronary ischemia and treatment (see also Chapter 23). Perioperative medical management to reduce cardiac risk may include continuation of beta blockers, statins, and/or aspirin. AAA is treated surgically by either open surgical repair (OSR) or EVAR, with EVAR associated with a threefold less perioperative mortality (1.5% with EVAR vs. 4.2% to 5.2% for OSR).[3] Selection of the approach depends on the AAA anatomy, age, and risks associated with anesthesia and surgery, with most patients currently undergoing EVAR.[2,3] Better outcomes are reported in high-volume centers for both OSR and EVAR and in ruptured AAA.[2]

TECHNIQUES AND OUTCOMES. For OSR of infrarenal AAAs, the abdominal aorta is approached through either a transperitoneal or a left retroperitoneal exposure using a tube or bifurcated prosthetic graft. The operative mortality rate for OSR ranges from 1% to 4% in reports from single-institution centers of excellence, and mortality rates in large databases range from 4% to 8%.[3] Operative complication rates range from 10% to 30%, with morbidity being related to cardiac, pulmonary, and renal complications and colonic ischemia. Because outcomes with OSR relate to hospital and surgeon volumes, OSR for AAAs should optimally be performed at centers with demonstrable operative mortality rates lower than 5%. Late complications develop in as many as 15% to 30% of patients after OSR for AAAs, including hernia and bowel obstruction, perianastomotic aneurysms (including pseudoaneurysms at suture lines and true aneurysms proximally), graft infection, graft-enteric fistula, and graft limb occlusions with lower extremity ischemia. Late aneurysm formation at anastomotic sites after OSR is uncommon and affects 1%, 5%, and 20% of patients, respectively, at 5, 10, and 20 years postoperatively and is more common with a distal anastomosis to the femoral artery as opposed to the aorta or iliac.[3] After OSR patients should generally have annual clinical follow-up with CT at 5-year intervals, or more frequently if there are small aneurysms in adjacent vessels such as the iliacs or suprarenal aorta that were not repaired.

ENDOVASCULAR ABDOMINAL AORTIC ANEURYSM REPAIR. In patients with suitable anatomy, EVAR offers a less invasive alternative to OSR. EVAR requires adequate nonaneurysmal proximal and distal attachment sites. Randomized controlled trials (RCTs) comparing EVAR with OSR for asymptomatic infrarenal AAAs have demonstrated

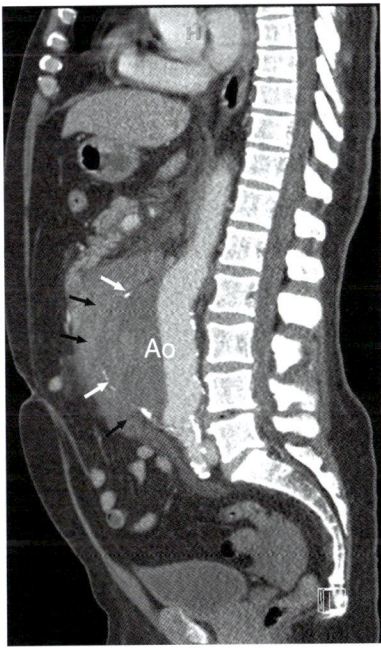

FIGURE 42.3 Contrast CT scan demonstrated ruptured infrarenal abdominal aortic aneurysm. The *white arrows* denote intimal calcification in the outer wall of aneurysm with a large amount of mural thrombus; *black arrows* denote rupture of the aneurysm with hemoperitoneum. *Ao,* Aorta.

a lower 30-day mortality rate with EVAR than with OSR (Table 42.1).[2,3,9] A significantly higher number of aneurysm ruptures and repeated interventions occur in the EVAR group.[2,3] In a large Medicare sample, EVAR had a similar early benefit in perioperative mortality (1.6% vs. 5.2%) and complications.[9] At long-term (≈8-year) follow-up, AAA-related or all-cause mortality did not differ significantly between EVAR and OSR.[2,3,9]

Observational studies report a mortality benefit of EVAR over OSR in ruptured AAA.[2,3] Although RCTs have yet to demonstrate a survival benefit of EVAR for ruptured AAA, guidelines recommend treatment of ruptured AAA in centers with a protocol for rapid evaluation and management preferentially with EVAR for suitable patients.[3]

Appropriate patient selection permits low perioperative mortality (1% to 2%) and complication (10% to 15%) rates with EVAR for elective AAA repair.[3] Currently, the options of EVAR and OSR are considered in "medically fit" patients with suitable anatomy. At follow-up after 6 and 8 years in the DREAM and EVAR-1 studies, EVAR had more late complications and secondary reinterventions, and the initial reduction in mortality with EVAR did not persist after a few years.[3] It is reasonable to consider an OSR first strategy for younger, low-risk patients with long life expectancy.[2]

"Endoleaks" (persistent blood flow in the aneurysm sac outside the endograft) develop in almost 25% of patients at follow-up with many requiring subsequent therapy; they can also cause aortic rupture after EVAR.[3] Type I endoleaks, which result from loss of complete sealing at the proximal (type IA) or distal (type IB) end of the stent graft, lead to increased pressure in the aneurysm sac and are associated with increased risk for rupture and therefore warrant repair.[10] Type II endoleaks, the most common, result from retrograde filling of the aneurysm sac by aortic branch vessels, usually by the lumbar or inferior mesenteric arteries. Type III endoleaks are caused by separation of components or disruption of the endograft fabric and require treatment, usually by re-lining with a stent graft. Type IV endoleaks are related to blood seeping through porous graft material and are self-limited. Endotension, an enlarging AAA after EVAR without a demonstrated endoleak and with a diameter increased to greater than 10 mm, usually requires repair. Late complications of EVAR (endograft migration, limb thrombosis), implant-related complications, and graft infection can occur. Monitoring the repair requires long-term radiographic surveillance. Imaging with contrast-enhanced CTA is typically performed at one month and annually after implantation of the device.[3] The presence of endoleak may mandate more frequent surveillance. Color duplex ultrasonography to detect endoleaks and AAA enlargement may be used in those with stable imaging findings after one year. When IV contrast is contraindicated, duplex ultrasound may be combined with noncontrast CT.

Widespread use of EVAR has demonstrated a reduction in early morbidity and mortality in patients with AAAs, especially in older adults. This advantage does not persist in long-term follow-up, however. EVAR should be performed at centers with very low in-hospital mortality and a low conversion rate to OSR for elective repair.[3] The development of fenestrated and branched endografts is extending EVAR to increasingly challenging aneurysms that extend more proximally to involve the renal and mesenteric vessels. However, long-term data are needed to support the widespread use of these technologies.

Thoracic Aortic Aneurysms

The expected size of the thoracic aorta depends upon one's age, sex, body size, and height with nomograms to index aortic size to populations and aortic diameters greater than 40 mm in adults generally considered to be enlarged.[1] Prolonged endurance exercise is associated with an increased prevalence of ascending aortic dilatation.[11] TAAs have an estimated incidence of at least 5 to 10 per 100,000 person-years.[12] The cause, natural history, and treatment vary depending on the location of the TAA. Aortic root or ascending aortic aneurysms are most common (approximately 60%), followed by aneurysms of the descending aorta (approximately 35%) and aortic arch (<10%).[12] *Thoracoabdominal aortic aneurysm* (approximately 10%) refers to descending thoracic aneurysms that extend distally to involve the abdominal aorta.

Cause and Pathogenesis

Causes of TAAs include heritable disorders, congenital disorders, degenerative (atherosclerotic), mechanical, inflammatory, and infectious diseases. Many of the heritable disorders preferentially involve the aortic root and ascending aorta, but some may involve the arch and descending aorta. Risk factors for TAAs include smoking, hypertension, age, chronic obstructive pulmonary disease (COPD), coronary disease, and family history. Up to 25% of patients with AAA have either synchronous or metachronous TAA.[1] Cystic medial degeneration (CMD) describes degeneration and fragmentation of elastic fibers, loss of SMCs, increase in deposition of collagen, and interstitial "cysts" of mucoid-appearing basophilic-staining extracellular matrix (see Fig. 42.2). Patients with MFS and many other heritable TAA diseases have aortic CMD. Aging associates with some degree of CMD, a process that may be accelerated by hypertension. These changes lead to progressive weakening of the aortic wall and may result in dilation and aneurysm formation.

Genetically Triggered Thoracic Aortic Aneurysm Diseases

Many disorders of the thoracic aorta are related to a genetic or heritable condition (also called heritable TAA [HTAD]), some of which are associated with multisystem features (*syndromic*) and others with thoracic aortic disease and branch vessel disease alone (*nonsyndromic*) (Table 42.2).[7] Syndromic HTADs include MFS, LDS, and vEDS. Nonsyndromic HTADs (also called familial TAA disorders) are due to mutations in multiple genes.[7] Up to 20% of individuals with a TAA will have a family history of TAA or will have an affected first-degree relative. These disorders are associated with abnormalities in the aortic media, extracellular matrix proteins, vascular SMCs, or contractile proteins (Fig. 42.4).[7] Clinical features may increase the likelihood of a genetic predisposition to TAA disease (Table 42.3).[13] Turner syndrome (TS), due to a defect in the X chromosome, associates with TAA.[14] Bicuspid aortic valve (BAV), which may be familial, frequently leads to TAA.[15] The timing of prophylactic surgery for aneurysm disease depends on

TABLE 42.1 Randomized Controlled Trials of Endovascular Repair and Open Surgical Repair for Abdominal Aortic Aneurysms

STUDY	RECRUITMENT DATES	PATIENTS (N)	OUTCOMES
EVAR1	1999–2003	1082	Perioperative mortality lower with EVAR (1.7% vs. 4.7%); similar survival after 2 years with higher AAA-related mortality after 8 years in EVAR group
DREAM	2000–2003	351	Perioperative mortality lower with EVAR (1.2% vs. 4.6%); similar long-term survival after 1 year with higher repeat interventions in EVAR group
OVER	2002–2008	881	Perioperative mortality lower with EVAR (0.5% vs. 3%); after 3 years, early survival benefit lost in EVAR group
ACE	2003–2008	316	Perioperative mortality similar (EVAR 1.3%, OSR 0.6%); no difference in 3-year survival

AAAs, Abdominal aortic aneurysms; *EVAR*, endovascular aneurysm repair; *OSR*, open surgical repair.
Modified from Wanhainen A, Verzini F, Van Herzeele I, et al. Editor's Choice—European Society for Vascular Surgery (ESVS) 2019 Clinical Practice Guidelines on the Management of Abdominal Aorto-iliac Artery Aneurysms. *Eur J Vasc Endovasc Surg.* 2019;57(1):8–93.

TABLE 42.2 Thoracic Aortic Aneurysm Syndromes and Conditions Due to a Heritable or Genetic Cause

CONDITION	GENE	CLINICAL FEATURES
Syndromic HTAD*		
Marfan syndrome	FBN1	Aortic root aneurysm, AD, TAA, MVP, long bone overgrowth, scoliosis, pectus deformities, ectopia lentis, myopia, tall stature, PTX, dural ectasia
Loeys-Dietz syndrome	TGFBR1, TGFBR2, *SMAD3, TGFB2, TGFB3, SMAD2	TAA, branch vessel aneurysms, AD, arterial tortuosity, MVP, craniosynostosis, hypertelorism, bluish sclera, bifid/broad uvula, translucent skin, visible veins, club feet, dural ectasia, *premature osteoarthritis
Vascular Ehlers-Danlos syndrome	COL3A1	TAA, AAA, arterial rupture, AD, MVP, bowel and uterine rupture, PTX, translucent skin, atrophic scars, small joint hypermobility, easy bruising, carotid-cavernous fistula
Arterial tortuosity syndrome	SLC2A10	Tortuous large-and medium-sized arteries, aortic dilatation, craniofacial, skin and skeletal features
Shprintzen-Goldberg syndrome	SKI	Craniosynostosis, skeletal features, aortic dilatation
Congenital contractural arachnodactyly (Beals syndrome)	FBN2	MVP, arachnodactyly, Marfanoid habitus, digital contractures, mild aortic dilatation
Cutis laxa	EFEMP2 (Fibulin-4)	TAA, arterial tortuosity, arterial stenosis, hypertelorism, arachnodactyly
EDS with periventricular nodular heterotopia (PVNH)	FLNA (filamin A)	X-linked, PVNH, TAA, BAV, MV disease, PDA, VSD, seizures, joint hypermobility
Meester-Loeys syndrome	BGN	X-linked, TAA, AD, skeletal abnormalities
LOX-related TAA	LOX (lysyl oxidase)	TAA, BAV, AD, Marfanoid habitus in some
Nonsyndromic HTAD (Familial TAA)		
FTAA	ACTA2 (α-smooth muscle actin)	TAA, AD, BAV, Moya-Moya, premature CAD and CVD, livedo reticularis, iris flocculi
FTAA	MYH11 (Myosin heavy chain-11)	TAA, AD, PDA
FTAA	MYLK (Myosin light chain kinase)	AD at relatively small aortic size
FTAA	PRKG1 (Protein kinase cGMP-dependent)	Aortic root aneurysm and AD
FTAA	MAT2A (MAT IIα)	TAA, AD, BAV
FTAA	MFAP5 (microfibrillar-associated protein 5)	TAA, AD, skeletal features may be present
FTAA	FOXE3 (forkhead transcription factor)	TAA, AD
Bicuspid Aortic Valve/Associated Ascending Aortic Aneurysm		
Familial BAV/AS and TAA	NOTCH1 (NOTCH1)	Aortic stenosis, TAA
TGFBR1, TGFBR2, TGFB2, TGFB3, ACTA2, MAT2A, GATA5, SMAD6, LOX, ROBO4, TBX20	BAV with TAA	Syndromic and nonsyndromic FTAA with an increased frequency of BAV
Turner syndrome	XO, Xp	BAV, COA, TAA, AD, short stature, lymphedema, webbed neck, premature ovarian failure, affects 1 in 2500 live-born girls

*Some individuals with pathogenic variants in a gene which can lead to syndromic HTAD have very few or no syndromic features and variants in some genes causing syndromic HTAD may also lead to nonsyndromic HTAD.

AAA, Abdominal aortic aneurysm; *AAT*, aortic aneurysm syndrome; *AD*, aortic dissection; *BAV*, bicuspid aortic valve; *CAD*, coronary artery disease; *COA*, coarctation of the aorta; *CVD*, cerebrovascular disease; *EDS*, Ehlers-Danlos syndrome; *FTAA*, familial thoracic aortic aneurysm (and dissection) syndrome; *HTAD*, heritable TAA; *LDS*, Loeys-Dietz syndrome; *MFS*, Marfan syndrome; *MV*, mitral valve; *MVP*, mitral valve prolapse; *PDA*, patent ductus arteriosus; *PTX*, pneumothorax; *TAA*, thoracic aortic aneurysm; *TGF*, transforming growth factor; *VSD*, ventricular septal defect.

the specific condition and other factors including genetic mutation, aortic diameter, rate of aortic growth, family history, age, sex, and patient and physician preferences (Table 42.4).

MFS, an autosomal dominant disorder of connective tissue, results from abnormal fibrillin-1 due to mutations in the *FBN1* gene.[7] Aortic dilation in MFS affects most prominently the sinuses of Valsalva (Fig. 42.5), but distal aortic aneurysms and dissections may occur. Fibrillin-1 is the major component of the microfibril, a primary component of the extracellular matrix, and by interaction with lysyl oxidase (encoded by *LOX*), promotes vascular SMC adhesion and elastin support.[7] Abnormal fibrillin-1 in MFS leads to structural deterioration and abnormalities in TGF-β signaling, which contributes to the pathogenesis of MFS and related aortopathies (see Fig. 42.4).[16,17] Angiotensin interrelates with TGF-β signaling, and blocking TGF-β by the angiotensin receptor blocker (ARB) losartan attenuates or prevents aortic aneurysm formation in MFS mice.[16] However, in randomized trials, there was no significant difference in the rate of aortic dilatation in Marfan patients treated with either atenolol or losartan.[17] At present, the maximal dose of beta blocker and/or ARB treatment in MFS is recommended to lessen aortic growth rate. A combination of beta blocker and ARB (in the AIMS study) may be beneficial.[17]

LDS, due to mutations in multiple genes in the TGF-β signaling pathway (see Table 42.2), leads to craniofacial abnormalities (hypertelorism, bifid/broad uvula [Fig. 42.6], cleft palate, craniosynostosis), arterial tortuosity, and aneurysms and dissections of the aorta and branch vessels.[1,7,12,18] Cutaneous features include easy bruisability, visible veins, widened scars, and facial milia. LDS has a more aggressive vascular phenotype than MFS, with dissections occurring at smaller sizes and younger ages. *TGFBR2* mutations may have a more aggressive phenotype than *TGFBR1* mutations and aortic surgery is recommended at aortic root dimensions of 4 to 4.5 cm.[18] Severe craniofacial features and arterial tortuosity may inform vascular risk.[1,12,18] Aneurysms-osteoarthritis syndrome (AOS or LDS3), due to *SMAD3* mutations, involves severe osteoarthritis and osteochondritis dissecans, in addition to the vascular, skeletal, and cutaneous features of LDS and may merit aortic surgery at relatively small aortic root diameters and mutations in *TGFB2* share features of MFS and LDS.[1,7] In the absence of outcomes data, many experts recommend treatment of LDS with beta blockers and ARBs.

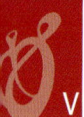

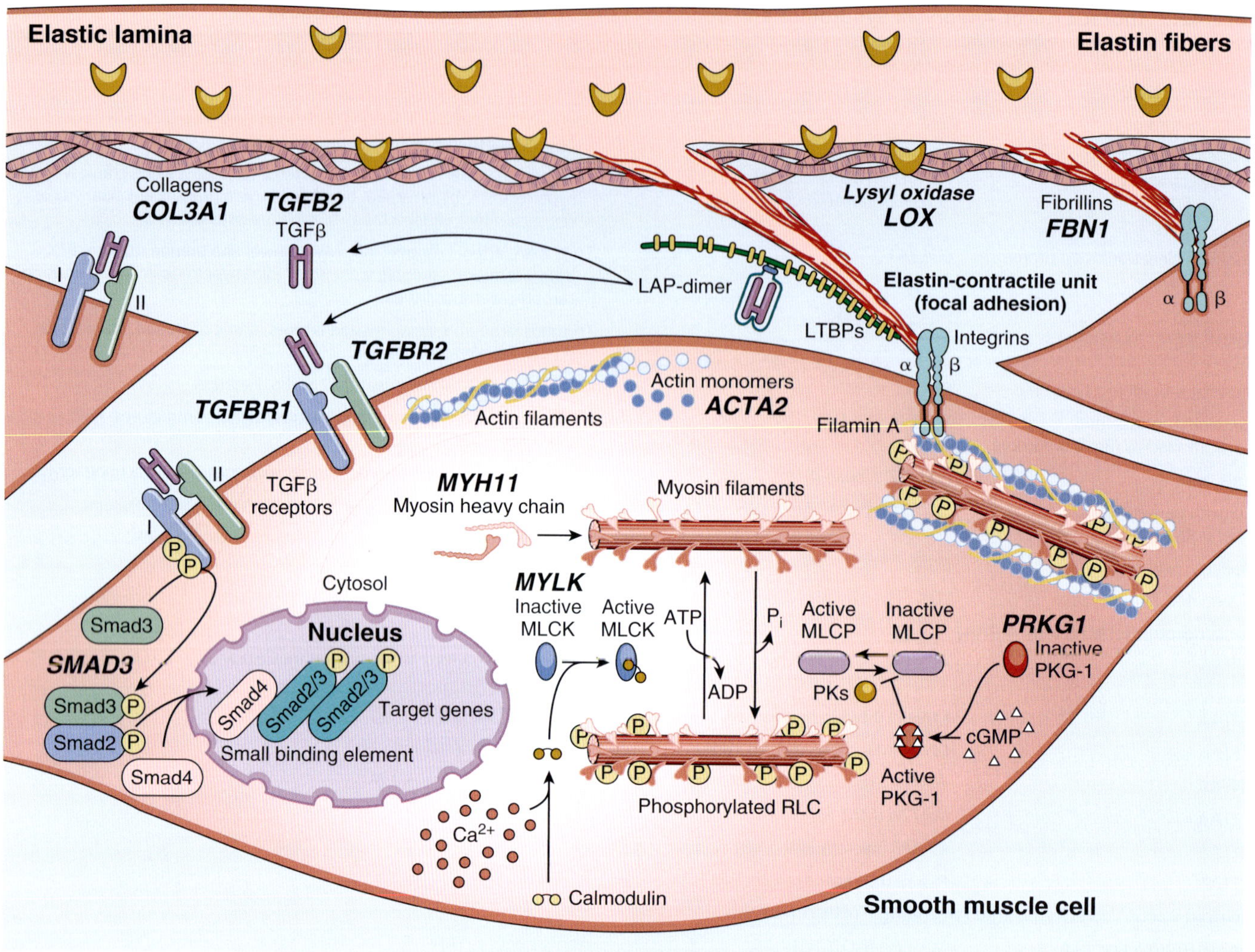

FIGURE 42.4 Schematic representation of elastin lamellae and smooth muscle cells (SMCs) highlighting the proteins that are disrupted by mutations in genes, leading to heritable thoracic aortic disease. Extensions from the elastin lamellae with fibrillin-1–containing microfibrils at the end link to integrin receptors on the cell surface of SMCs. The integrin receptors then link to the contractile filaments inside the cells, thus forming the elastin-contractile unit. Also illustrated are the proteins involved in canonical TGF (transforming growth factor)-β signaling that are disrupted by mutations in the corresponding genes to also lead to heritable thoracic aortic disease. The validated genes predisposing to thoracic aortic disease are shown in red and are adjacent to their corresponding protein. *LAP,* Latency-associated peptide; *LTBP,* latent TGF-β binding protein; *MLCK,* myosin light chain kinase; *MLCP,* myosin light chain phosphatase; *PK,* protein kinase; *PKG-1,* type I cGMP-dependent protein kinase; *RLC,* regulatory light chains; *Smad,* mothers against decapentaplegic drosophila homolog. (Illustration Credit: Ben Smith. From Pinard A, Jones GT, Milewicz DM. Genetics of thoracic and abdominal aortic diseases. *Circ Res.* 2019;124:588–606.)

vEDS, due to mutations in *COL3A1* causing abnormal type III procollagen synthesis, associates with aortic and branch vessel aneurysm, rupture, and/or dissection and rupture of visceral organs at a young age leading to reduced lifespan.[19] Individuals with vEDS have risk for spontaneous arterial dissection and rupture, often involving medium-sized arteries that did not exhibit significant dilation. Aortic root disease is less common, with more frequent involvement of the descending and abdominal aorta and branch vessels. Unlike MFS and LDS, the abnormal arteries in patients with vEDS are friable, thus making surgical repair difficult, but with improving outcomes recently.[19]

Nonsyndromic HTADs (familial TAA) are inherited as an autosomal dominant trait with decreased penetrance and variable expression (especially in women) and are more common than syndromic aortopathies. Pathogenic variants in multiple genes cause familial TAA, some of which also are associated with cerebral aneurysm (see Table 42.2).[7] Genetic testing identifies mutations in only 20% to 25% of nonsyndromic HTAD and a negative test does not exclude a genetic predisposition.[7,13] Mutations in genes coding for proteins affecting SMC contractile function and kinases (*ACTA2, MYH11, MYLK,* and *PRKG1*) lead to aortic aneurysm and dissection (see Fig. 42.4).[7] Fibrillin-1 microfibrils contribute to mechanotransduction in vascular SMCs, linking matrix protein fibrillin-1 to intracellular actin filaments (see Fig. 42.4).[7] Mutations in *ACTA2* are associated with livedo reticularis, iris flocculi, and premature coronary and cerebrovascular disease.[7] Aortic dissection at diameters less than 5 cm are described and approximately 50% of *ACTA2* patients had aortic events with a cumulative risk estimated at 76% by age 85 years.[7,12] First-degree relatives of individuals with unexplained TAA or dissection should undergo aortic imaging or genetic testing when a mutation is present in the family.[13]

BAV, affecting 1% of the population, associates with ascending aortic aneurysm, coarctation of the aorta, and aortic dissection.[15] The BAV exhibits abnormal leaflet folding, wrinkling, and increased leaflet doming, which can result in turbulence even in the absence of a stenotic or regurgitant lesion. Abnormal aortic wall shear stress due to helical flow patterns in the setting of BAVs may underlie the aortopathy of BAV disease (Fig. 42.7).[15] Ascending TAAs associated with BAVs may develop independent of valve function and may develop late after aortic valve replacement (AVR). There are multiple aortic phenotypes in BAV aortopathy and the root phenotype (present in 10%) may have a higher aortic risk.[15] The aortic dilatation in BAV disease occurs most often in the proximal to mid-ascending aorta, making imaging of the entire ascending aorta important in patients with BAVs.[12] CMD underlies the aortic aneurysm and risk for dissection associated with BAVs.[15] When BAV and TAA coexist, CMD is more pronounced in regurgitant than stenotic BAV.[15] The lifetime risk of aortic dissection for the BAV patient is 4 to 8 times higher than the risk in the general population, but the absolute risk is very low unless aortic aneurysm is present.[15] BAVs and ascending aortic aneurysm may be familial, inherited as an autosomal dominant

TABLE 42.3 Clinical Features Increasing the Likelihood of a Genetic Predisposition for Thoracic Aortic Aneurysm Disease

1. Aortic dilatation (especially >45 mm)
   a. Consideration for 40–45 mm (or z-score >3), especially when dilated sinuses of Valsalva, or in the young (<50 years old), or when associated with a +FH
2. Positive family history of TAA (and/or cerebral aneurysm disease)
   a. First-degree and/or second-degree relative with:
      i. TAA or aortic dissection
      ii. Aneurysm or dissection in the arterial tree, diagnosed below 60 years old*
      iii. Bicuspid aortic valve
      iv. Patent ductus arteriosus
      v. Sudden (unexplained) death below 50 years old
3. Syndromic features
   a. Craniofacial features (craniosynostosis, hypertelorism, cleft palate, bifid uvula)
   b. Ocular features (lens dislocation, retinal detachment, high myopia [-6 diopters or higher], iris flocculi
   c. Cardiovascular features (MVP, arterial tortuosity, multiple aneurysms/dissections, BAV, PDA)
4. Musculoskeletal features
   a. Pectus deformities
   b. Disproportionately elongated fingers, toes, arms, legs
   c. Joint dislocations, hypermobility, or contractures
   d. Severe, early-onset osteoarthritis
   e. Severe scoliosis or kyphosis
   f. Lumbosacral dural ectasia
5. Cutaneous features
   a. Translucent skin with visible veins
   b. Livedo reticularis
   c. Abnormal striae not related to weight gain
   d. Widened scars
   e. Facial milia
6. Other features
   a. Spontaneous pneumothorax
   b. Recurrent hernias
   c. Spontaneous rupture of internal organs

*There may be a wide variability in the age of onset or recognition of aneurysm disease in heritable thoracic aortic disease.
BAV, Bicuspid aortic valve; *FH*, family history; *MVP*, mitral valve prolapse; *PDA*, patent ductus arteriosus; *TAA*, thoracic aortic aneurysm.
Adapted from Verhagen JMA, Kempers M, Cozijnsen L, et al. Expert consensus recommendations on the cardiogenetic care for patients with thoracic aortic disease and their first-degree relatives. Int J Cardiol. 2018;258:243–248.

TABLE 42.4 Size Threshold for Prophylactic Aortic Root or Ascending Aortic Aneurysm Resection for Various Conditions

CONDITION	SIZE THRESHOLD FOR PROPHYLACTIC AORTIC ROOT OR ASCENDING ANEURYSM RESECTION*
Degenerative aneurysm	≥5.5 cm
Bicuspid aortic valve	≥5.5 cm
Bicuspid aortic valve with risk factors or low surgical risk[†]	≥5.0 cm
Bicuspid aortic valve requiring aortic valve replacement	≥4.5 cm
Marfan syndrome	≥5.0 cm
Marfan syndrome with risk factors[‡]	≥4.5 cm
Loeys-Dietz syndrome[§]	4.0–4.5 cm
Familial thoracic aortic aneurysm syndromes[¶]	4.5–5.0 cm
Turner syndrome**	>2.5 cm/m^2

*Lower thresholds for intervention may be considered according to body surface area in patients of small stature or in the case of rapid growth of the aorta. Age, body size, rapid growth, family history, risk of surgery, and patient and physician preferences may influence aortic size threshold.
[†]Family history of aortic dissection or aortic growth rate ≥0.5 cm per year or if the patient is at low surgical risk (<4%) and the surgery is performed by an experienced aortic surgical team in a center with established expertise in these procedures. Other risk factors for aortic dissection include coarctation of the aorta, hypertension, and the root phenotype of BAV.
[‡]Family history of aortic dissection or rapid aortic growth (>3 mm per year), severe aortic or mitral regurgitation. If pregnancy desired, consider prophylactic aortic surgery for aortic diameter of ≥4.0 to 4.5 cm.
[§]It is reasonable to consider surgical repair of the aorta in adults with Loeys-Dietz syndrome (LDS) or a confirmed *TGFBR1* or *TGFBR2* mutation with aortic diameter of ≥4.2 cm by transesophageal echocardiogram or ≥4.4 to 4.6 cm by CT or MRI. Aortic surgery at smaller diameters (>4 cm) may be recommended when there are severe craniofacial features, marked arterial tortuosity, rapid growth or a family history of aortic dissection. LDS due to *SMAD3* mutations may be treated similarly and less information is available for LDS related to *TGFB2* and *TGFB3* mutations.
[¶]Surgical thresholds vary depending upon the specific gene mutation involved. TAA due to *ACTA2*, *SMAD3*, and *MYLK* may lead to aortic dissection at relatively small aortic diameters and smaller size thresholds may be indicated.
**AHA Scientific Statement (Silberbach M, et al., 2018) recommends prophylactic surgery at ASI greater than 2.5 cm/m^2, whereas ESC 2014 Guidelines (Erbel R, et al., 2014) recommend prophylactic surgery at ASI ≥2.75 cm/m^2.
Adapted from Erbel R, Aboyans V, Boileau C, et al. 2014 ESC Guidelines on the diagnosis and treatment of aortic diseases: document covering acute and chronic aortic diseases of the thoracic and abdominal aorta of the adult. The Task Force for the Diagnosis and Treatment of Aortic Diseases of the European Society of Cardiology (ESC). Eur Heart J. 2014;35:2873–2926; Hiratzka LF, Bakris GL, Beckman JA, et al. 2010 ACCF/AHA/AATS/ACR/ASA/SCA/SCAI/SIR/STS/SVM guidelines for the diagnosis and management of patients with Thoracic Aortic Disease. Circulation. 2010;121:e266–e369; Hiratzka LF, Creager MA, Isselbacher EM, et al. Surgery for aortic dilatation in patients with bicuspid aortic valves: a statement of clarification from the American College of Cardiology/American Heart Association Task Force on Clinical Practice Guidelines. J Am Coll Cardiol. 2016;67:724–731. Silberbach M, Roos-Hesselink JW, Andersen NH, et al. Cardiovascular Health in Turner Syndrome: A Scientific statement from the American Heart Association. Circ Genom Precis Med. 2018 Oct;11(10):e000048.

disorder with variable expressivity and incomplete penetrance. While certain HTAD have a higher prevalence of BAV (especially with root phenotype), the vast majority of individuals with BAV do not have a recognized genetic mutation.[15] Gene mutations associated with BAV and TAA are listed in Table 42.2. First-degree relatives of a patient with BAV, especially with aortopathy, should undergo evaluation for BAVs and ascending TAA.[12]

TS, which affects 1 in 2500 live-born girls, results from complete or partial loss of a second sex chromosome (XO, Xp). Approximately 50% of patients with TS have cardiovascular defects, including BAVs in 15% to 30%, coarctation of the aorta in 7% to 18%, elongation of the transverse arch in 30%, and ascending aortic dilatation 33%.[14] Patients with TS have an estimated 100-fold greater risk for aortic dissection than do age-matched controls.[14] Most women with TS who suffer aortic dissection have risk factors, including aortic dilatation, BAV, coarctation of the aorta, or hypertension. Women with TS but without risk factors for aortic dissection should undergo reevaluation of the aorta every 5 to 10 years or when clinically indicated (such as when contemplating pregnancy).[14] Women with risk factors or known cardiovascular defects require more frequent imaging. Because patients with TS have short stature, ascending aortic dimensions should be evaluated in relation to body surface area. TS patients have increased aortic diameter relative to body surface area and a higher risk for dissection at smaller absolute aortic diameters.[14]

Aortic enlargement and CMD are associated with other congenital heart diseases, including coarctation of the aorta, tetralogy of Fallot,

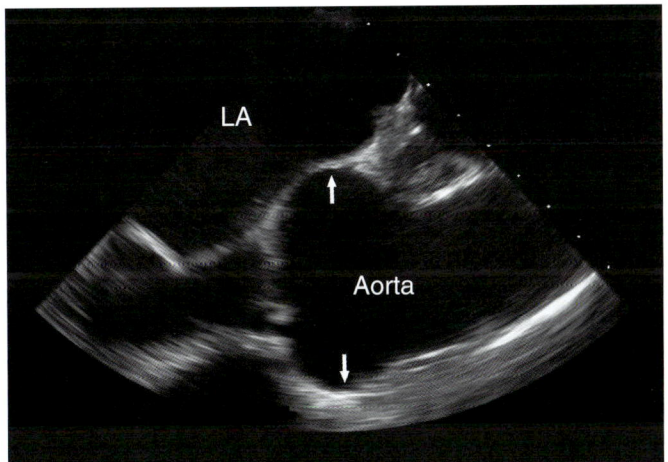

FIGURE 42.5 Transesophageal echocardiogram demonstrating an aortic root aneurysm of 53 mm (arrows) in an individual with Marfan syndrome. LA, Left atrium.

transposition of the great vessels, truncus arteriosus, ventricular septal defect, and tetralogy of Fallot.

Degenerative Aneurysms

Degenerative TAAs occur most commonly in the descending aorta, have a male predominance (1.7 to 1), present at an average age of 65 years, and are associated with aortic atherosclerosis.[20] Descending TAA and thoracoabdominal aortic aneurysms have an incidence of 6 to 10 cases per 100,000 person-years.[20] Isolated arch aneurysms may be degenerative or related to penetrating aortic ulcers, CMD, and rarely, syphilis or other infections. Most descending TAAs are degenerative but may also result from genetic disorders. These aneurysms tend to originate just distal to the origin of the left subclavian artery, may be either fusiform or saccular, and may extend into the abdominal aorta or coexist with AAAs.

Aortic Dissection

Dissection is a common cause of aneurysm of the descending thoracic aorta and the arch. Frequently, aneurysm formation develops during the chronic stage of dissection, being most common in the proximal descending aorta (see below).

Kommerell Diverticulum

Kommerell diverticulum is the embryologic remnant located at the origin of an aberrant subclavian artery that may lead to aneurysmal dilatation, rupture, or aortic dissection. Surgical intervention is considered when the diverticulum diameter exceeds 30 mm and/or the diameter of the descending aorta adjacent to the diverticulum exceeds 50 to 55 mm.[20,21]

Syphilis and Aortitis

Cardiovascular syphilis occurs in the tertiary stage and typically involves the ascending aorta and arch. Aortitis rarely occurs today because of antibiotic treatment of syphilis early in its course. Cardiovascular syphilis becomes evident after a latent period of at least 10 to 25 years. Pathologic features include lymphocytic and plasma cell inflammation in the adventitia, with the classic appearance of a "tree bark" or wrinkled appearance of the aortic intima. Ascending aortic aneurysm formation occurs in 40% of cases. Tertiary syphilis may cause aortic valvulitis, aortic regurgitation (AR), and coronary ostial stenosis.

Infectious aortitis (typically bacterial, less commonly fungal) is discussed later in this chapter (see also Chapter 80). Other causes of TAAs include noninfectious aortitis such as giant cell arteritis, other vasculitides, and idiopathic aortitis and IgG4 disease. Noninfectious aortitis may underlie aortic aneurysms in 2% to 8% of TAAs and is discussed in other chapters.

Clinical Manifestations

Most TAA are asymptomatic and are discovered incidentally. Physical findings such as AR may suggest TAA. Symptoms of TAAs usually relate to a local mass effect, progressive AR, systemic embolization due to mural thrombus or atheroembolism, or related to acute dissection or rupture. Obstruction of the superior vena cava or innominate vein may result from ascending aorta or arch aneurysms. TAAs may compress the trachea, bronchus, or esophagus or lead to hoarseness from laryngeal nerve compression. Persistent chest or back pain may occur because of a direct mass effect from the TAA, with compression of intrathoracic structures or erosion into bones. The most serious complications of TAAs are rupture and dissection (Fig. 42.8). Aortic rupture leads to sudden severe chest or back pain. Rupture into the pleural cavity (usually left) or into the mediastinum is associated with hypotension, rupture into the esophagus leads to hematemesis, and rupture into the bronchus or trachea leads to hemoptysis. Infected TAAs are associated with pain, fever, and fistulas. Acute aortic expansion, contained rupture, and pseudoaneurysm can cause chest or back pain. Thoracic aortic dissection (discussed later) is more common than rupture.

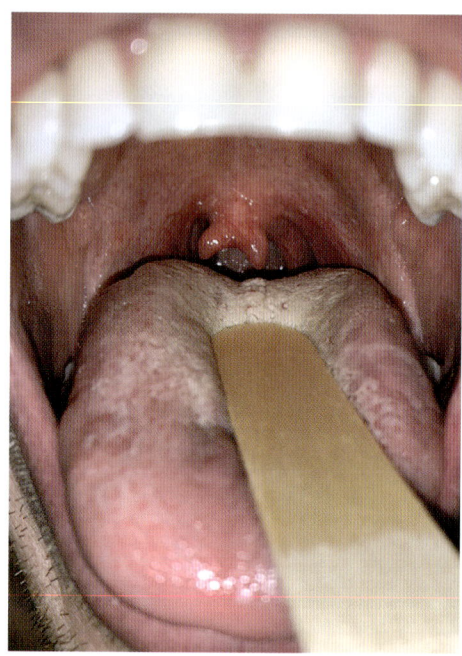

FIGURE 42.6 Bifid uvula in Loeys-Dietz syndrome in an individual with familial aortopathy and a *TGFBR2* pathogenic variant.

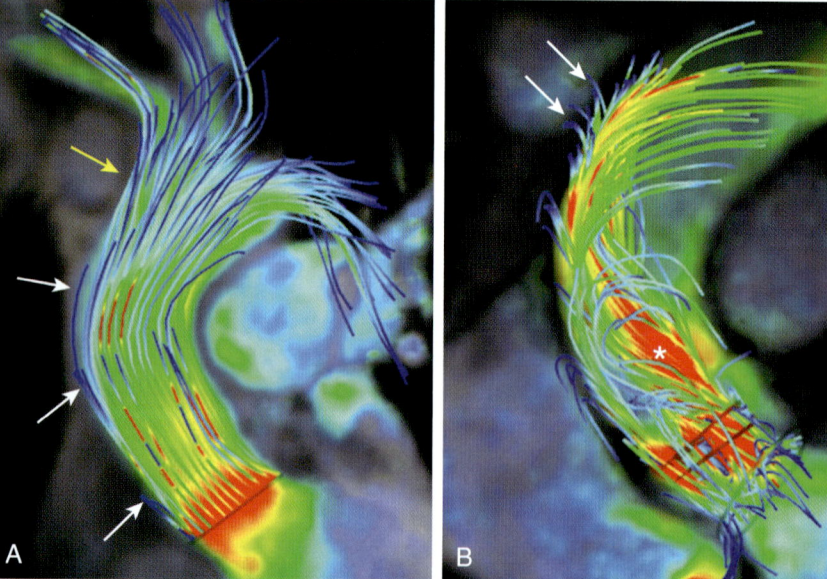

FIGURE 42.7 Abnormal ascending aortic flow patterns related to bicuspid aortic valve (BAV). **A,** Healthy subject with normal 3-cusp aortic valve. Streamline visualization demonstrates normal laminar flow in the ascending aorta (*white arrows*) and proximal arch (*yellow arrow*), with color scale representing flow velocity (blue indicates low velocity, red indicates high velocity). **B,** Subject with BAV without stenosis or regurgitation or ascending aortic dilation. Streamlines illustrate eccentric, helical flow in the ascending aorta with high-velocity systolic flow jet (*asterisk*) impacting the aortic wall in the region of the greater curvature (*white arrows*). (Courtesy Dr. Nicholas Burris. From Bhave NM, Nienaber CA, Clough RE, Eagle KA. Multimodality imaging of thoracic aortic diseases in adults. *JACC Cardiovasc Imaging*. 2018;11:902–919.)

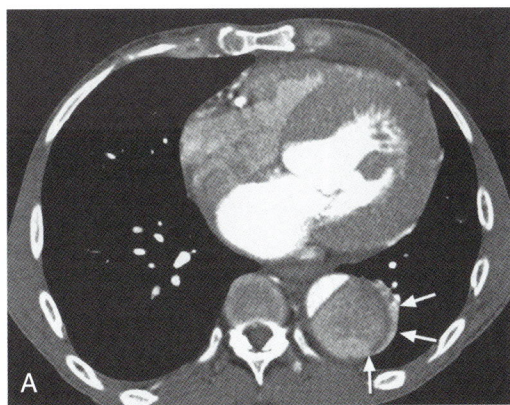
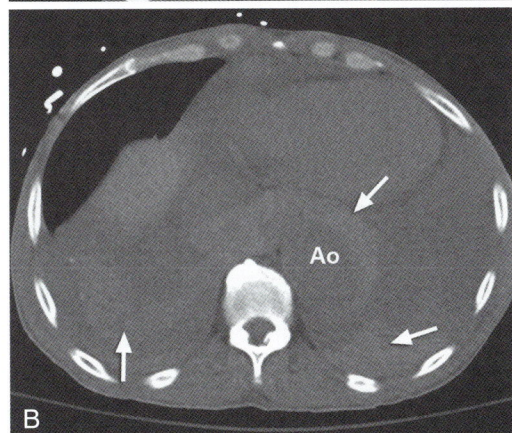
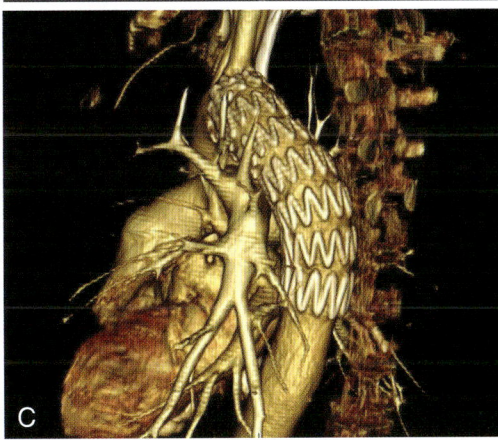

FIGURE 42.8 Rupture of type B aortic dissection. **A,** Contrast-enhanced CT demonstrating early leakage of blood from the dilated false lumen *(arrows)*. The small true lumen is densely opacified with contrast material. **B,** Non-contrast-enhanced CT demonstrating acute hemorrhage from the ruptured type B dissection *(arrows)*. *Ao,* Aorta **C,** Three-dimensional reconstruction of the descending thoracic aorta after emergency endovascular repair of the ruptured aortic dissection.

Diagnosis

Some TAAs are evident on chest x-rays, with features including a widened mediastinum, prominent aortic knob, or displaced trachea, but smaller TAAs may not be visible. Aneurysms involving the sinuses of Valsalva, being "hidden" behind the sternum, mediastinal structures, and vertebrae, may not be seen on chest x-ray. Aortic tortuosity and unfolding in older adults may also mimic or mask TAAs. Thus, chest x-rays cannot exclude TAA.

Transthoracic echocardiography (TTE) can visualize TAAs involving the sinuses of Valsalva and often the proximal ascending aorta, aortic arch, and proximal descending aorta. Aortic root size varies with age, height or body surface area, and sex, and nomograms provide normal ranges.[12] Although TTE does not thoroughly characterize the aortic arch and descending TAAs, transesophageal echocardiography (TEE) can image most of the thoracic aorta.

Contrast-enhanced CT and MRA provide outstanding detail of aortic and branch vessel anatomy in TAA disease.[22,23] In the setting of a tortuous aorta, axial images alone can be misleading and may "overstate" the true dimension of the aorta. When the axial images cut through the descending aorta at a plane that is off axis, it results in a falsely large aortic diameter. Multidetector CTA and MRA allow reconstruction of the axial data into three-dimensional images, permitting aortic measurement in a double oblique technique to obtain an accurate diameter (Fig. 42.9). One must specify location of measurements, as sinus-to-sinus are about 2 mm larger than commissure-to-cusp measurements.[22] The echocardiogram measures the internal diameter, whereas CT and/or MR measure the external diameter of the aorta, which is expected to be 0.2 to 0.4 cm larger than the internal diameter.[12] Interobserver variability in aortic measurements of up to 2 mm may occur, emphasizing the importance of careful image acquisition, measuring, and reporting.

Natural History

Many factors influence the natural history of TAAs. Individuals with genetic aortopathies have a more rapid aneurysm growth rate than do those with degenerative aneurysms.[24] The location and size of the TAA also affect its rate of growth and likelihood of rupture or dissection. TAAs are relatively indolent, with a growth rate of approximately 1 to 2 mm/year and marked individual variability.[1,24–26] Larger aneurysms grow faster than smaller ones.[25] Dissected TAAs grow more rapidly than those without dissection.[24]

Rupture and acute dissection are the major complications of TAAs (see Fig. 42.8). Less than half of patients with rupture arrive at the hospital alive; mortality at 24 hours reaches 75%. The risk of aortic dissection, rupture, and death increases with enlarging aortic diameters with "hinge points" at aortic diameters greater than 5.25 to 5.75 cm for ascending aortic aneurysms[26] (Fig. 42.10) and above 6.0 cm for descending aortic aneurysms (Fig. 42.11).[25] A low risk of acute type A dissection is reported among people with MFS and aortic root diameters less than 4.5 to 5 cm undergoing imaging, taking beta blockers (or ARB), and avoiding strenuous exercise.[27,28] For LDS, familial TAA syndromes, and vascular EDS, the aortic diameter is less predictive and dissection may occur at smaller aortic sizes.[1,7,12,18,19] In patients with degenerative descending TAA or TAAAs, the estimated risks of aortic dissection, rupture, and death increase when the aorta diameter exceeds 6 cm.[25] Untreated 6 cm descending TAA are reported as having a 3.7% per year risk for rupture.[20] Saccular aneurysms may carry higher risk.[20]

Risk factors for increased growth and rupture of TAAs include older age, hypertension, cigarette smoking, COPD, rapid aneurysm growth, aortic dissection, and a positive family history.[12,20] Aortic diameter is the most important risk factor for aneurysm complications, but other factors influence this risk including sex, body surface area and height, and indexing of aortic size in certain populations may inform risk.[12,25,26] Ascending aortic elongation may also be predictive.[29]

Surgical thresholds for TAA repair depend upon the disease present and patient-specific factors (see Table 42.4).[1,12,18,30,31] For degenerative aneurysms, surgical replacement of the aorta is recommended when the aortic root or ascending aortic diameter reaches 5.5 cm; the arch greater than 5.5 to 6 cm; and the descending or thoracoabdominal aorta reaches greater than 5.5 to 6 cm.[1,12] Surgery is recommended in MFS when the aortic root diameter is ≥50 mm, with a lower threshold for those with rapid aortic growth or a family history of aortic dissection[1,12,27,28]; in familial TAA syndromes at 4.5 to 5 cm[1,12]; in BAV aneurysm at ≥5.5 cm; and at ≥5.0 cm if there are risk factors for aortic dissection (family history of dissection, rapid aortic growth (>3 to 5 mm/year), coarctation of the aorta, or hypertension) or if the patient is at low surgical risk.[15,30,31] If surgery is being performed on the BAV, aortic aneurysm surgery may be performed in acceptable candidates at aortic diameters greater than 4.5 cm.[31] Adults with LDS should have surgery when the aortic root measures 4.0 to 4.5 cm, although some recommend surgery in patients with LDS once the aortic root is greater than 4 cm, especially when accompanied by a high craniofacial index.[12,18]

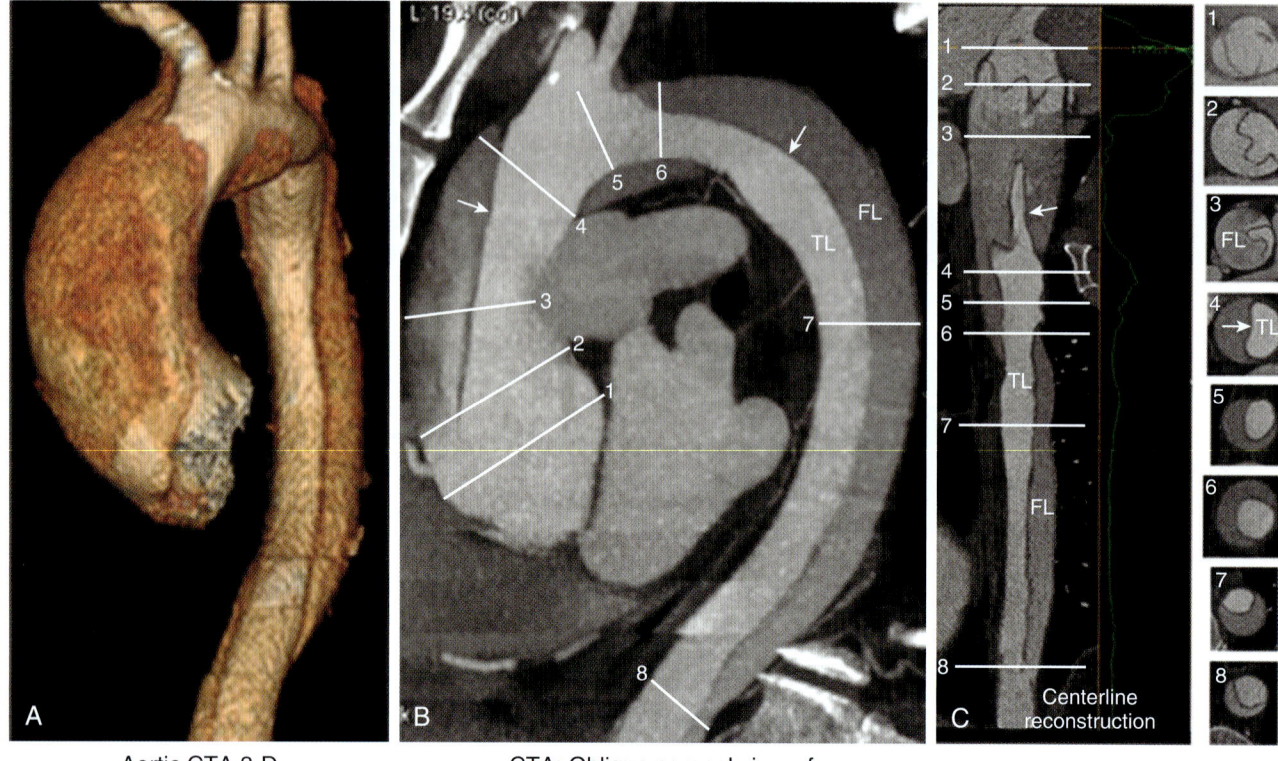

FIGURE 42.9 Computed tomographic angiography (CTA) of the thoracic aorta. **A,** Three-dimensional volume rendering. **B,** Oblique coronal view of the aorta. Note linear gating artifacts. **C,** Centerline reconstruction of the aorta as a straight vessel, eliminating tortuosity and allowing for measurement in true short axis (*right panel*). Corresponding levels of measurements are shown on **B** and **C**: *1,* Sinuses of Valsalva; *2,* sinotubular junction; *3,* proximal ascending aorta; *4,* distal ascending aorta; *5,* aortic arch; *6,* aortic isthmus; *7,* mid–descending aorta; *8,* distal descending aorta at diaphragm. Type A aortic dissection flap *(arrows),* true lumen *(TL),* and false lumen *(FL)* are shown in **B** and **C**. (From Mongeon FP, Marcotte F, Terrone DG. Multimodality noninvasive imaging of thoracic aortic aneurysms: time to standardize? *Can J Cardiol.* 2016;32:48–59.)

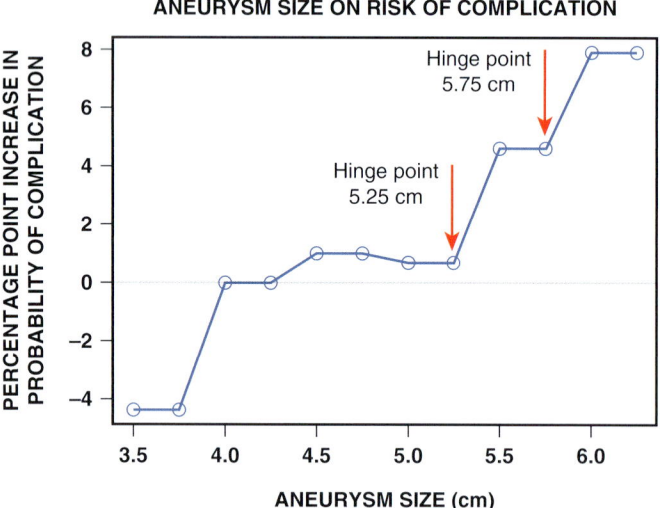

FIGURE 42.10 Estimated probability of rupture or dissection of the ascending aorta by aneurysm size. (From Zafar MA, Li Y, Rizzo JA, et al. Height alone, rather than body surface area, suffices for risk estimation in ascending aortic aneurysm. *J Thorac Cardiovasc Surg.* 2018;155[5]:1938–1950.)

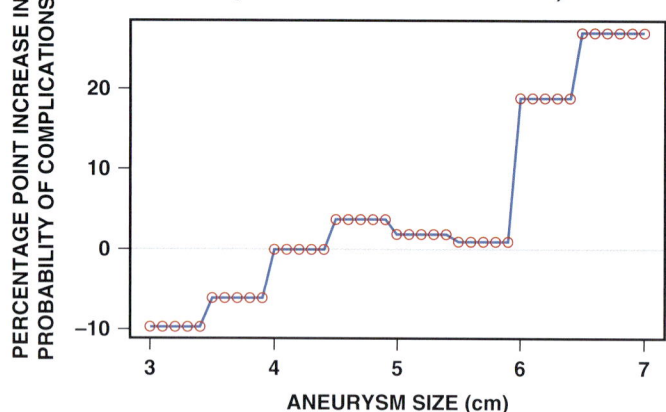

FIGURE 42.11 Probability of rupture or aortic death of the descending thoracic/thoracoabdominal aorta by aneurysm size. Analysis of the predicted probability of fatal complications (i.e., rupture or aortic death) revealed that the risk increased sharply at 2 hinge points: 6.0 cm and 6.50 cm. (From Zafar MA, Chen JF, Wu J, et al. Natural history of descending thoracic and thoracoabdominal aortic aneurysms. *J Thorac Cardiovasc Surg.* 2019;161[2]:498–511.e1.)

In TS, prophylactic surgery should be considered when the ascending aortic size index is ≥2.5 cm/m^2.[14] The indication for surgery on an isolated arch aneurysm depends upon the underlying condition and state of the adjacent aortic segments and is considered at a diameter of 55 mm.[12,32] For descending TAA, repair (typically thoracic endovascular aortic repair [TEVAR]) is recommended at 60 mm and may be considered in appropriate candidates when greater than 55 mm (and may be considered in those with heritable diseases [with OSR] at 50 to 55 mm).[23] Surgical timing also depends on the family history, sex, rate of aneurysm growth, body size, coexisting aortic valve disease, need for other heart surgery, comorbid conditions, and patient and physician preference. Because aortic complications occur at diameters lower than surgical thresholds, one must individualize management based on surgical risk and other factors. Endovascular approaches may lead to earlier therapy for appropriate candidates.

Management

Surgical Treatment

ASCENDING THORACIC AORTIC ANEURYSMS. Treatment of ascending TAAs involves opening the ascending aorta and placement of a prosthetic graft with or without concomitant AVR. A composite graft consisting of a Dacron tube with a prosthetic aortic valve sewn into one end (the modified Bentall procedure) is generally the method of choice in treating ascending TAAs involving the root and associated with significant aortic valve disease. The valve and graft are sewn directly into the aortic annulus, and the coronary arteries are reimplanted into the Dacron graft. For elective aneurysm repair, the risk for death or stroke ranges from 1% to 5% depending on the disease, patient population, and surgical experience.[1,12] The risk for morbidity and mortality increases with the need for arch replacement. Emergency operations on the proximal aorta carry much higher risk. Patients with structurally normal aortic valve leaflets and those whose AR is secondary to dilation of the sinotubular junction or aortic annulus may be able to undergo a valve-sparing root replacement—reimplanting the native valve within a Dacron graft (David procedure) or by remodeling the aortic root (Yacoub procedure).[33] The reimplantation technique is preferable to the remodeling technique (especially in genetic aortopathy) because it stabilizes the annulus and limits aortic dilation and late AR.[33] Personalized external aortic root support (PEARS), involving surgical implantation of an individualized mesh support around the aortic root and ascending aorta, has been developed in Europe to treat aortic root aneurysm in selected cases of MFS and related conditions.[34]

A pulmonary autograft (the Ross procedure) is an alternative to a composite aortic graft in appropriate candidates. This procedure involves replacing the native aortic valve and root with the patient's own pulmonary root, inserted into the aortic position.[35] The pulmonary root is replaced with a cryopreserved homograft root. The Ross procedure carries risks of late autograft aneurysm formation and should not be used in patients with genetically triggered aortic root diseases. Methods to support or replace the aorta lessen late aneurysm formation.[35] Another alternative is the use of cryopreserved aortic allografts (cadaveric aortic root and proximal ascending aorta), but durability issues and late aortic calcification limit this choice. Estimates of risk for mortality for thoracic aortic elective repair are composite valve graft, 1% to 5%; separate AVR and ascending aortic repair, 1% to 5%; valve-sparing root replacement, less than 1% to 1.5%; and BAV and ascending aortic repair, 1.5%.[12]

AORTIC ARCH ANEURYSMS. Aortic arch aneurysms are more difficult to treat surgically because reconstruction of the aortic arch vessels requires interruption of blood flow to these vessels.[1,12,21] One approach uses a hemiarch resection—the arch vessels remain intact, with the upper aortic arch as a roof, and the remaining arch is replaced. Extended arch resection requires either removing the entire arch and using branched grafts to replace the arch and great vessels, by using bypasses constructed to each great vessel, or less often reimplanting an island of arch tissue that includes the origins of the great vessels.[21] Cerebral protection during arch surgery can use several methods, now shifting to moderate hypothermic circulatory arrest.[21] Because the aortic disease often extends distally, the polyester graft can be extended as an elephant trunk into the descending aorta, and necessitates a second procedure to complete the repair. In this procedure, the distal anastomosis is created to the midportion of a graft and the distal graft is within the lumen of the aorta and thus can be retrieved without manipulation of the arch. A modification of this procedure uses a covered endovascular stent graft attached to a vascular graft to allow fixation of the stent graft within the descending aorta and vascular graft reconstruction of the aortic arch.[12,21] This "frozen elephant trunk" procedure allows total replacement of the arch and descending aorta in a single stage for complex aneurysms and also the treatment of acute type A dissection.[1,12,21] Spinal cord injury occurs in 5% to 9% of frozen elephant trunk procedures.[1,12,21] Arch aneurysm surgery has a morbidity and mortality rate of 2% to 7% risk for both death and stroke.[1,12,21] Surgery for arch aneurysms is considered when aneurysm diameter is greater than 55 mm.[21] Increased operative risk merits consideration of endovascular techniques using debranching procedures and extra-anatomic reconstructions to treat complex aortic arch aneurysms and complete elephant trunk procedures.[21] Commercially made branched endografts to replace the aortic arch are currently under investigation in the United States.

DESCENDING THORACIC ANEURYSMS. Treatment paradigms for descending TAAs have changed due to the rapid development of TEVAR with endovascular repair recommended when feasible and appropriate.[1,23] The mortality rate for descending TAA repair is lower early after TEVAR compared to OSR, whereas mid-term survival rates are similar for either technique.[1] The European Society for Vascular Surgery Guidelines recommend that repair should be considered when descending TAA reaches 60 mm and may be considered for aneurysms of 56 to 59 mm, with lower thresholds to be considered in women and in those with heritable aortic disease.[23] The Society for Vascular Surgery Guidelines recommend TEVAR for low-risk individuals with descending TAA diameter greater than 55 mm.[20] TEVAR has a higher risk of complications in MFS and heritable aortopathies, and is typically reserved for urgent complications, high-risk patients, or when there are proximal and distal hand-sutured grafts in which to "land" the endograft.[1,36] OSR of descending TAAs involves replacement of the aneurysmal segment with a polyester graft. The procedures are performed with partial femorofemoral bypass or atriofemoral bypass to maintain retrograde perfusion to critical arterial branches; they are associated with a perioperative mortality of 10% (5% to 22%) and a paraplegia rate of approximately 2% to 6%, depending on the extent of repair and the expertise of the center.[20,23] Five-year survival rates after descending TAA resection approach 70%. TEVAR is discussed later. Ruptured descending TAA is often fatal before hospital arrival and has a mortality rate of 33% in those who undergo OSR and 19% in those undergoing TEVAR.[23]

THORACOABDOMINAL ANEURYSMS. Thoracoabdominal aneurysms (TAAAs) can extend from the subclavian artery to the iliac vessels. The Crawford classification (modified by Safi) describes the extent of the aneurysm, and this predicts morbidity, mortality, and risk for paralysis with repair.[23] Because of the risk of the procedure, in general, surgical repair is considered for low- to moderate-risk patients with TAAA greater than 60 mm (less for those with heritable aortic disease, rapid growth [>10 mm/year], or with symptoms).[23]

> Crawford type I involves the entire thoracic aorta and the upper abdominal aorta extending from the proximal descending aorta above the T6 vertebra to the level of the renal arteries (approximately 25 of TAAAs); type II is the highest-risk group, with the aneurysm involving the entire thoracic and most or all of the abdominal aorta extending from the proximal descending aorta above T6 to below the renal arteries, often to the iliac bifurcation (30% of TAAAs); type III aneurysms involve the distal half of the descending thoracic aorta below T6 and extend into the abdominal aorta (<25% of TAAAs); and type IV extends from the diaphragm and involves most of the abdominal aorta to the aortic bifurcation (<25% of TAAAs). Crawford type V aneurysms arise in the distal half of the descending aorta (below T6) and extend into the abdominal aorta, but are limited to the visceral segment.[12] Repair of Crawford types I to III aneurysms is complex and usually performed through an extensive thoracoabdominal incision. The procedure requires bypass to maintain perfusion of the lower extremities and the mesenteric vessels. Spinal fluid drainage and other techniques, as for thoracic aneurysms, may diminish the risk for paraplegia and paraparesis.[12,23] The mortality rate in low-risk patients is 3% to 10% (with lower rates in high-volume centers), with a paraplegia rate of 3% to 10%, depending on the extent of the repair.[12,23] Morbidity and mortality with repair of Crawford type IV aneurysms is intermediate between AAA and type I to III TAAA. Hybrid repairs and branched endografts may allow less extensive operations.[23]

ENDOVASCULAR REPAIR OF THORACIC ANEURYSMS. TEVAR, a far less invasive alternative to OSR of descending TAAs, has lower morbidity and mortality rates than OSR and is preferable when feasible.[20] For TEVAR, the aorta must have adequate proximal and distal landing zones of at least 20 to 25 mm in length and diameters that accommodate the endograft and adequate vascular access.[23] TEVAR for descending TAA has a lower 30-day mortality rate than OSR (5.6% vs. 17%) and a lower risk of stroke and paraplegia. Stroke risk in TEVAR for TAA disease is 3% to 6%.[20] The anatomic configuration of the ascending aorta and transverse arch makes applying these techniques and devices challenging in these proximal segments. Hybrid techniques using extra-anatomic bypass procedures can create an appropriate proximal landing zone for the endovascular graft without the need for major open surgery.[21] Branched and fenestrated arch endografts allow endovascular repair in appropriate patients.[21] In 10% to 50% of TEVAR procedures, the stent graft intentionally covers the left subclavian artery, but this associates with an increased risk of stroke, spinal cord ischemia, and upper extremity ischemia.[23] Transposition of the left subclavian artery or a left carotid-to-subclavian bypass is recommended before TEVAR when covering the left subclavian is required to lessen ischemic risk.[12,23] If all the branches of the aortic arch need to be excluded for appropriate endovascular repair of an arch aneurysm, other options are available. Complete extra-anatomic aortic arch debranching can be performed, with reconstruction of the arch branches and subsequent carotid and subclavian bypasses as necessary. Another option is to perform an elephant trunk procedure under cardiopulmonary arrest; a prosthetic graft is sutured to the healthy portion of the ascending aorta and aortic arch, and branches of the aortic arch are left intact. This approach creates a proximal attachment zone that can be extended distally with an endovascular graft to complete the aneurysm repair. Bypasses to all the aortic arch branches can also be performed from the proximal ascending aortic arch in selected patients, with a healthy portion left in the ascending aorta for attachment and seal of an endovascular graft. Branched devices developed to manage patients with complex thoracic and TAAAs are undergoing early evaluation. Debranching procedures involving visceral vessels may be performed before proceeding with endograft implantation although the morbidity and mortality of this hybrid approach has not been found to be lower than standard OSR for the visceral aorta.[12,23] Open and endovascular repair of TAAs is associated with a variety of significant risks, including cardiac, pulmonary, renal, and cerebrovascular complications.[23] Spinal cord dysfunction with the development of paraparesis or paraplegia is a major source of morbidity. Drainage of cerebrospinal fluid has been used in combination with a mean arterial pressure of at least 70 mm Hg (>90 mm Hg in those at high risk) to lessen spinal cord complications.[12,20] Rescue protocols typically use these measures combined with supplemental oxygen, flat positioning in bed, and blood transfusion to hemoglobin greater than 10 mg/dL to improve oxygen delivery to the spinal cord. However, placement of a spinal drain is also associated with complications and routine use is typically not recommended unless there are risk factors such as coverage greater than 15 cm of descending thoracic aorta, or loss of the left subclavian, hypogastric, or lumbar arteries from prior or concomitant aortic surgery or occlusive disease.[20,23]

Serial imaging surveillance is required after TEVAR to evaluate for complications (endoleak, migration, collapse) and to assess aneurysm dimensions with imaging at 1 and 12 months, and then yearly, with more frequent imaging if abnormalities detected.[20,23] Up to 10% of device-related complications take place in the first 30 days after TEVAR.[12] Endoleaks are the most common complication of endovascular repairs and occur in 10% to 20% of patients.[12,20]

Medical Management
Treating hypertension and smoking cessation are important because they are risk factors for TAA development, expansion, and rupture.[1,12] Patients with degenerative TAAs should receive cholesterol-lowering therapy. Beta blockers or ARBs are recommended for patients with MFS.[1,12] Many use beta blockers and/or ARBs in other genetic aortopathies based upon animal models, altered TGF-β signaling, and limited clinical information.

Long-term imaging surveillance of the aorta is imperative. After discovery of an aneurysm, patients should be reevaluated in 6 months to assess the aneurysm status. In general, for degenerative TAAs, annual imaging is recommended when the aorta is between 4.0 and 4.5 cm, and imaging at 6- to 12-month intervals for aneurysms of 4.5 to 5.4 cm, depending upon size and growth rate. For relatively small aneurysms that are stable from year to year, imaging may be performed every 2 to 3 years.[12] In patients with MFS and familial TAAD, annual imaging is recommended for aortic sizes of 3.5 to 4.4 cm and annual or biannual imaging for aortic sizes of 4.5 to 5 cm. For BAV with aortic

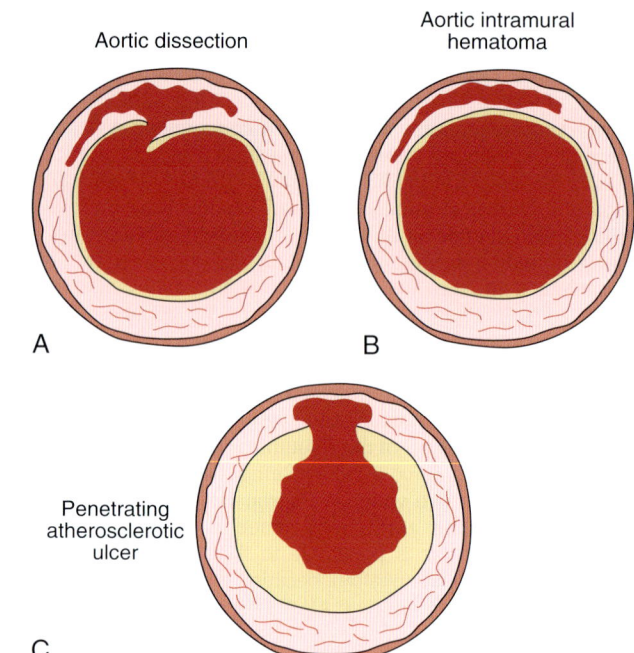

FIGURE 42.12 Acute aortic syndromes. **A,** Classic aortic dissection. There is a tear in the intima with blood entering the media and a dissecting cleavage plane propagating for variable distances anterograde (and occasionally retrograde) throughout the aortic wall. **B,** Aortic intramural hematoma. Acute hemorrhage occurs in the aortic media in the absence of a visible intimal tear or intimal flap. **C,** Penetrating atherosclerotic aortic ulcer. An ulcerated aortic plaque ruptures into the media leading to an outpouching or ulceration in the aortic wall. This may be associated with intramural hematoma formation, pseudoaneurysm, or a focal, thick-walled aortic dissection.

dilatation annual imaging is recommended, depending upon size. In LDS and in some familial TAA diseases, imaging from the head to the pelvis is recommended because of the potential for widespread aneurysms.[1,7,12,18]

Lifestyle modification is important for living with TAAs, including awareness of the condition and the risk for aortic dissection and rupture. Aortic events have been associated with fluoroquinolone use and avoidance of this antibiotic class is recommended for those with or at risk for aneurysm disease.[37] Avoidance of strenuous physical activity, especially isometric exercise and weightlifting, is important and this restriction may impact work-related recommendations.[38,39] Pregnancy associates with an increased risk for aortic dissection in those with aortopathy conditions and management strategies must encompass this risk.[40] When a known genetic mutation underlies TAA disease (see Table 42.2), first-degree relatives should undergo counseling and genetic testing.[12,13] Then only relatives with the genetic mutation should undergo aortic imaging. In the absence of an identified mutation, first-degree relatives should have evaluation and aortic imaging (see Table 42.3). If a first-degree relative has aneurysm disease, second-degree relatives should also be screened.[12,13]

AORTIC DISSECTION

Acute aortic syndromes include aortic dissection, aortic intramural hematoma (IMH), and penetrating atherosclerotic aortic ulcer (PAU) (Fig. 42.12).[1,12,23,41–43] In 80% to 90% of acute aortic syndromes, aortic dissection is present, with intimal disruption leading to a dissection plane in the media that may propagate anterograde (or less often, retrograde) throughout the length of the aorta (Figs. 42.8 and 42.9). Adventitial disruption may occur leading to rupture, or more commonly, distal tear(s) results in blood reentering the aortic lumen. In aortic dissection, an intimal flap exists between the two lumens (true and false lumens). Ten to 20% of acute aortic syndromes result from IMH, where bleeding in the aortic wall occurs without imaging evidence of an intimal tear or dissection flap.[41,42] PAUs also lead to acute aortic syndromes in approximately 5% of cases.

TABLE 42.5 Classification Schemes of Acute Aortic Dissection

DeBakey Classification

Type I dissection originates in the ascending aorta and extends at least to the aortic arch and typically to the descending aorta (and beyond)

Type II dissection only in the ascending aorta

Type III dissection originates in the descending aorta, usually just distal to the left subclavian artery, and extends distally

Type IIIa dissection tear limited to the descending aorta

Type IIIb dissection tear extends below the diaphragm

Stanford Classification

Type A dissection involves the ascending aorta (with or without extension into the descending aorta)

Type B dissection does not involve the ascending aorta (includes arch dissection)

Society for Vascular Surgery/Society of Thoracic Surgeons (SVS/STS) Aortic Dissection Classification System

Type A Entry tear originates only in the ascending aorta (zone 0)

Type B Entry tear originates distal to the ascending aorta (zone 1 or beyond). The distal extent of a type A dissection is further characterized by zone. The distal extent of a type B dissection is further characterized by two subscripts (the proximal zone of involved aorta and the distal zone of involved aorta).

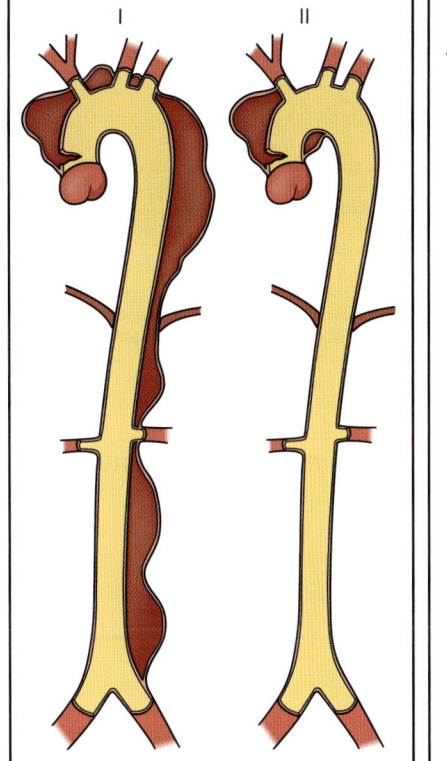

FIGURE 42.13 Classification schemes of acute aortic dissection. **DeBakey Classification:** Type I dissection originates in the ascending aorta and extends at least to the aortic arch and typically to the descending aorta (and beyond). Type II dissection only in the ascending aorta. Type III dissection originates in the descending aorta, usually just distal to the left subclavian artery, and extends distally. Type IIIa dissection tear limited to the descending aorta. Type IIIb dissection tear extends below the diaphragm. **Stanford Classification:** Type A dissection involves the ascending aorta (with or without extension into the descending aorta). Type B dissection does not involve the ascending aorta (includes arch dissection). (From Braverman AC. Aortic dissection: prompt diagnosis and emergency treatment are critical. *Cleve Clin J Med.* 2011;78:1695–1704.)

Establishing the incidence of aortic dissection is difficult as many patients (18% to 49%) die before the condition is recognized.[44] Population studies estimate the incidence of acute aortic syndrome to range from 2.6 to 7.7 cases per 100,000 person-years,[1,42,45] with 15 cases per 100,000 in the middle-aged.[43] In autopsy series, the prevalence of aortic dissection ranges from 0.2% to 0.8%.[1,12] Two thirds of aortic dissections occur in men.[41] Acute aortic dissection has a very high early mortality, with up to a 1% per hour death rate in the first hours after acute type A dissection.[12,46] Type A aortic dissection (see later) occurs most commonly in individuals between 50 and 60 years of age, and type B (see later) dissection at a peak of 60 to 70 years of age. Women present at older ages than men.[41]

The main hypothesis for acute aortic dissection is a primary entry tear in the aortic intima with blood penetrating into the diseased media and leading to propagation of the dissection and creation of the true and false lumens. Primary rupture of the vasa vasorum with resultant intimal disruption is a second hypothesis. Distention of the false lumen with blood causes the intimal flap to compress the true lumen and narrow its caliber and may lead to malperfusion syndromes.

Classification

There are two major classification schemes for aortic dissection—the DeBakey classification and the Stanford classification. The DeBakey classification divides dissections into types I, II, and III based upon the origin and extent of the dissection and the Stanford classification is based upon whether or not the ascending aorta is involved in the dissection (Table 42.5, Fig. 42.13). Dissections involving the aortic arch but not the ascending aorta are categorized as type B in the Stanford classification, whereas others classify this type as "non-A, non-B."[47] The new Society for Vascular Surgery/Society for Thoracic Surgery Aortic Classification System characterize dissections based upon the location of the primary entry tear and extent of the dissection.[48]

Most type A dissections begin within a few centimeters of the aortic valve, and most type B dissections begin just distal to the left subclavian artery. Approximately 65% of intimal tears occur in the ascending aorta, 30% in the descending aorta, less than 10% in the aortic arch, and approximately 1% in the abdominal aorta. Aortic dissection is classified according to its duration with recent classifications highlighting hyperacute, acute, subacute, and chronic (Table 42.6),[1,12,46,48] emphasizing variable risk periods (Fig. 42.14). Classification including type of dissection, location of the entry tear, and malperfusion may aid in decision making and predict outcomes.[47]

Cause and Pathogenesis

Several conditions predispose the aorta to dissection (Table 42.7), most due to disruption of the integrity of the aortic wall or marked increases in aortic wall circumferential stress (see earlier discussion in the section on TAAs). Some 75% of all patients with aortic dissection have hypertension.[41] Hypertension may affect arterial elastic properties and increase stiffness predisposing to aneurysm or dissection. However, hypertension alone is not usually associated with significant aortic dilation, and only a small minority of hypertensive patients suffer aortic dissection. In the IRAD, conditions associated with dissection included: hypertension (77%), atherosclerosis (27%), previous cardiac surgery (16%), known aortic aneurysm (16%), MFS (5%), iatrogenic (3%), and cocaine use (1.8%).[41]

Heritable thoracic aortic aneurysm disease (HTAD) (both syndromic and nonsyndromic), certain congenital heart diseases, inflammatory and infectious aortitis, and cocaine and methamphetamine use are all risk factors for aortic dissection. CMD is often present in aortic dissection but does not elucidate the cause (see Fig. 42.2). Perturbations in cellular signaling pathways and alterations in SMC contractile elements and their environment due to genetic mutations underlie many HTAD at risk for aortic dissection (see Table 42.2 and Fig. 42.4).[7] Patients with MFS and other HTAD have a high risk for aortic root and ascending aortic aneurysm and especially for type A aortic dissection. While only present in 1 in 5000 individuals, MFS accounts for approximately 5% of all aortic dissections and a large proportion of aortic dissection in young patients.[12,41] Type B dissection may also complicate HTAD, may be the first presentation of the disease, and is more common after prior root replacement.[23,49,50]

TABLE 42.6 Aortic Dissection Classification Based Upon Duration from Symptom Onset

CLASSICAL DEFINITION	TAD GUIDELINES*	IRAD CLASSIFICATION†	ESC GUIDELINES‡	SVS/STS REPORT§
Acute: <14 days	Acute: <14 days	Hyperacute: <24 hr	Acute: <14 days	Hyperacute: <24 hr
Chronic: >14 days	Subacute: <2–6 weeks	Acute: 2–7 days	Subacute: 14–90 days	Acute: 1–14 days
	Chronic: >6 weeks	Subacute: 8–30 days	Chronic: >90 days	Subacute: 15–90 days
		Chronic: >30 days		Chronic: >90 days

*Hiratzka LF, Bakris GL, Beckman JA, et al. Guidelines for the diagnosis and management of patients with thoracic aortic disease: a report of the American College of Cardiology Foundation/American Heart Association Task Force on Practice Guidelines, American Association for Thoracic Surgery, American College of Radiology, American Stroke Association, Society of Cardiovascular Anesthesiologists, Society for Cardiovascular Angiography and Interventions, Society of Interventional Radiology, Society of Thoracic Surgeons, and Society for Vascular Medicine. *Circulation*. 2010;121:e266–e369.
†Booher AM, Isselbacher EM, Nienaber CA, et al. The IRAD classification system for characterizing survival after aortic dissection. *Am J Med*. 2013;126:730 e19–e24.
‡Erbel R, Aboyans V, Boileau C, et al. 2014 ESC Guidelines on the diagnosis and treatment of aortic diseases: document covering acute and chronic aortic diseases of the thoracic and abdominal aorta of the adult. The Task Force for the Diagnosis and Treatment of Aortic Diseases of the European Society of Cardiology (ESC). *Eur Heart J*. 2014;35:2873–2926.
§Lombardi JV, Hughes GC, Appoo JJ, et al. Society for Vascular Surgery (SVS) and Society of Thoracic Surgeons (STS) reporting standards for Type B aortic dissections. *Ann Thorac Surg*. 2020;109:959–981.
ESC, European Society of Cardiology; *IRAD*, International Registry of Acute Aortic Dissection; *TAD*, thoracic aortic diseases.

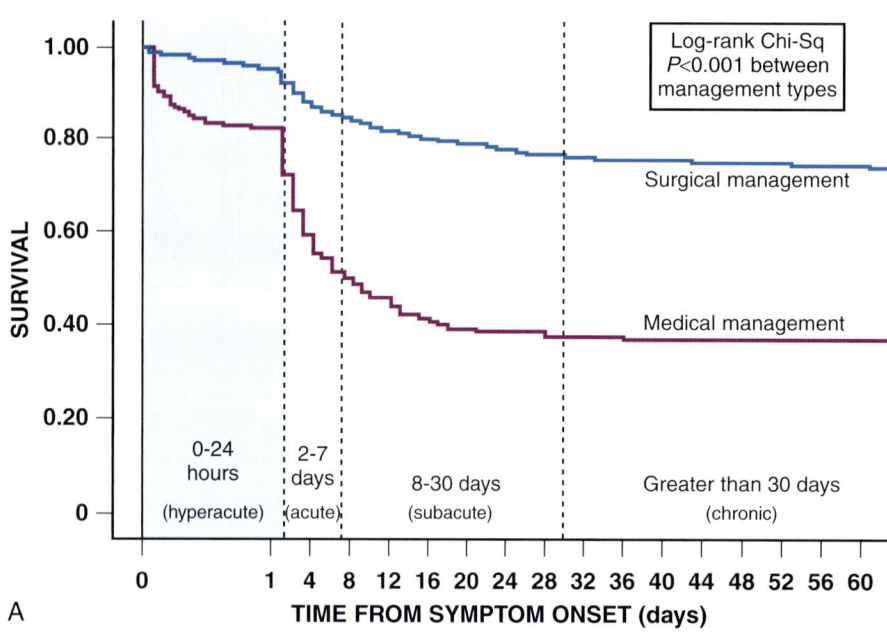

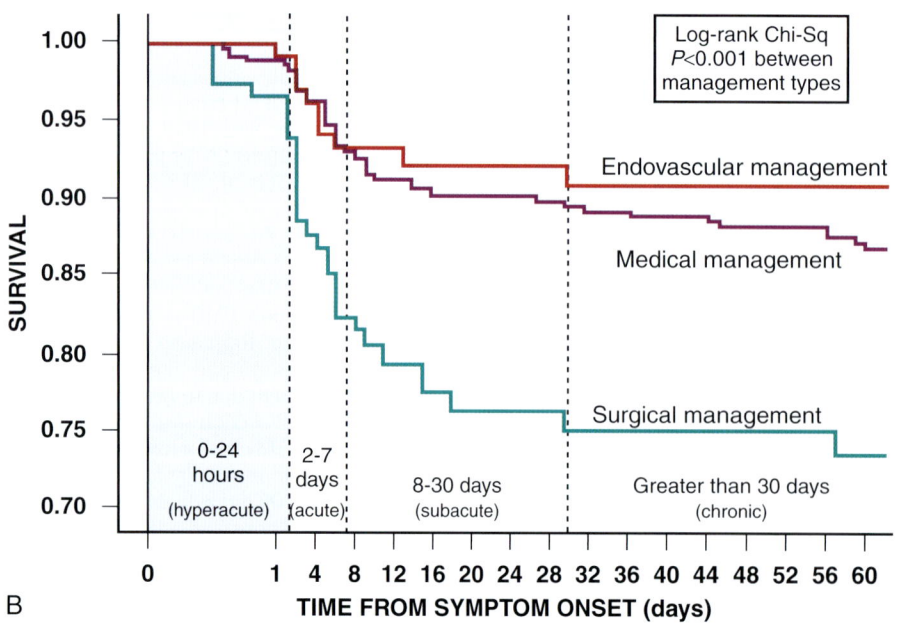

FIGURE 42.14 International Registry of Acute Aortic Dissection (IRAD) classification system of survival after aortic dissection. **A**, Kaplan-Meier survival curve for type A dissection stratified by treatment type. **B**, Kaplan-Meier survival curve for type B dissection stratified by treatment type. (From Booher AM, Isselbacher EM, Nienaber CA, et al. The IRAD classification system for characterizing survival after aortic dissection. *Am J Med*. 2013;126:730 e719–724.)

TABLE 42.7 Risk Factors for Aortic Dissection

Hypertension
Heritable thoracic aortic conditions and syndromes (see Table 47.2)
Marfan syndrome
Loeys-Dietz syndrome
Vascular Ehlers-Danlos syndrome
Nonsyndromic heritable thoracic aortic disease
Congenital conditions
Bicuspid aortic valve
Coarctation of the aorta
Turner syndrome
Tetralogy of Fallot
Atherosclerosis
Penetrating atherosclerotic ulcer
Trauma, blunt or iatrogenic
Coronary artery bypass grafting/aortic valve replacement/TAVR
Endovascular aneurysm repair (EVAR, TEVAR)
Catheter/guidewire/intra-aortic balloon pump
Aortic/vascular surgery
Motor vehicle accident
Cocaine/methamphetamine use
Inflammatory/infectious diseases
Giant cell arteritis
Takayasu's arteritis
Behçet disease
Aortitis/IgG4-related disease
Syphilis
Pregnancy (with underlying aortopathy)
Weightlifting (with underlying aortopathy)

EVAR, Endovascular aneurysm repair; *TAVR*, transcatheter aortic valve replacement; *TEVAR*, thoracic endovascular aneurysm repair.

BAV is an important risk factor for ascending aortic aneurysm and dissection (see Fig. 42.7).[15,51] Aortic dissection also associates with unicuspid aortic valve, supravalvular aortic stenosis, aberrant right subclavian artery, Kommerell diverticulum, right-sided aortic arch, polycystic kidney disease, and Alport syndrome (in men).[1,12]

Aortic dissection may complicate aortitis, particularly giant cell arteritis. Nonspecific aortitis, Takayasu arteritis, IgG4-related aortitis, and Behçet disease all are associated with aortic dissection. Syphilitic aortitis is a rare cause of dissection. Cocaine-related aortic dissection is more commonly type B, often presenting with hypertension and small aortic diameters.[41] Aortic dissection may occur with intense weightlifting, but generally in the setting of an underlying aortopathy or aneurysm.

Aortic dissection can occur during pregnancy or postpartum and relates to hemodynamic factors and hormonal changes in women with aortopathy.[40] Although most pregnancy-related aortic dissections are due to underlying aortopathy, the condition is often not diagnosed until after dissection.[40] Women with MFS, LDS, nonsyndromic HTAD, vEDS, TS, and BAV with aneurysm have increased risk for acute aortic dissection related to pregnancy.[12,14,40] In MFS, the risk for type A dissection increases related to aortic size and is estimated at 1% when the aortic diameter is less than 40 mm and higher in patients with larger aortic sizes, rapid dilation, or previous aortic dissection.[40] After aortic root replacement, pregnancy in aortopathy conditions still carries a risk of distal dissection.[40]

Blunt aortic trauma may cause localized tears or periaortic or frank aortic transection, but rarely causes aortic dissection. Iatrogenic causes account for 3% of aortic dissections.[41] Arterial catheterization and interventions may induce aortic dissection by intimal disruption. Iatrogenic type A dissection related to coronary artery interventions are rare and when limited and stable by imaging, may often be treated conservatively.[42] Cardiac surgery entails a very small risk for acute aortic dissection related to aortic cannulation, crossclamps, aortic anastomosis, and retrograde dissection after femoral cannulation. Aortic dissection may occur late (months to years) after cardiac surgery, with those undergoing AVR or with a previous aneurysm or dissection having higher risk. Aortic injuries may follow TEVAR including stent graft-induced new entry (SINE) proximally leading to retrograde type A dissection (associating with high mortality) and distally (which may lead to antegrade false lumen reperfusion).[52]

Individuals with TAA have risk for aortic dissection, with higher risk for dissection and rupture as aortic size increases. However, many aortic dissections occur in patients with aortic dimensions that are not markedly dilated and are below thresholds for prophylactic aortic repair.[25,26,41] Of type A aortic dissections in the IRAD, aortic diameter averaged 5.3 cm, with 60% having aortic diameters less than 5.5 cm and 40% having aortic diameters less than 5.0 cm.[41] In addition to aortic diameter, age, sex, body size, genetics, rate of aortic growth, and mechanical and hemodynamic factors also play a role. The mechanisms responsible for individual susceptibility to aortic dissection at a specific aortic diameter are not well understood.

Clinical Manifestations
Symptoms
The symptoms of aortic dissection are variable and may mimic those of more common conditions, thus highlighting the importance of a high index of suspicion. Abrupt onset of severe chest or back pain is the most classic feature.[1,41] Distinct from the discomfort of coronary ischemia, the pain is described as severe in approximately 90% of patients and usually of sudden onset, with maximum intensity occurring at its inception. Some patients describe a "sense of doom." The pain quality is most often described as "sharp," "severe," or "stabbing," and descriptors such as "tearing" or "ripping" are less common.[1,12,41,42] Symptoms highly suggestive of aortic dissection, such as a feeling of being "stabbed in the chest with a knife" or "hit in the back with a baseball bat," may be reported, but some describe less severe chest burning, pressure, or pleuritic pain. The symptoms may relate to a complication (such as syncope, heart failure, or stroke) dominating the presentation or the pain may not be mentioned or is downplayed. The pain may lessen or resolve, making diagnosis even more challenging. Factors associated with delay in diagnosis include predominant abdominal pain, female sex, heart failure presentation, transfer from another hospital, fever, and normal blood pressure.[41,43]

The pain of aortic dissection may radiate from the chest to the back or vice versa and is migratory in approximately 17% of cases, following the path of the dissection through the aorta.[1,41,42] Pain in the neck, throat, jaw, or head predicts involvement of the ascending aorta (and often the great vessels),[53] whereas pain in the back, abdomen, or lower extremities usually indicates descending aortic involvement.

Other clinical features at presentation include congestive heart failure (CHF) (<10%), syncope (9%), acute stroke (6%), acute MI, paraplegia, and cardiac arrest or sudden death.[1,42,43] Acute CHF related to type A dissection may result from acute severe AR.[41] Syncope in patients with type A dissection usually associates with hemopericardium, rupture, arch vessel involvement, or stroke.[41] Patients with aortic dissection may have predominantly abdominal pain, which may lead to delays in diagnosis.[41] "Painless" aortic dissection occurs in 6% of patients and associates with syncope, stroke, previous aortic aneurysm, and prior cardiac surgery.[41]

Physical Findings
Findings on physical examination and organ system complications in patients with acute aortic dissection are highly variable ranging from unremarkable to cardiac arrest due to hemopericardium or rupture. The findings may demonstrate complications related to the dissection, such as AR, abnormal peripheral pulses, stroke, or CHF (Table 42.8). The presence of these findings must heighten clinical suspicion for aortic dissection, but their absence does not exclude dissection and should not dissuade pursuit of the diagnosis when suspected. While greater than 70% of individuals with aortic dissection have a history of hypertension, elevated BP on presentation is present in 80% of type B dissections and 36% of type A dissections, with most with type A presenting normotensive or hypotensive.[1,12,41,48] Hypotension complicating acute dissection may result from cardiac tamponade, acute aortic rupture, or CHF related to acute severe AR.

TABLE 42.8 Organ System Complications of Acute Aortic Dissection

Cardiovascular	Aortic regurgitation
	Congestive heart failure
	Syncope
	Coronary ischemia or acute myocardial infarction
	Hemopericardium or cardiac tamponade
	Pericarditis
	Cardiac arrest
Pulmonary	Pleural effusion
	Hemothorax
	Hemoptysis (from an aortotracheal or bronchial fistula)
Renal	Renal ischemia or infarction
	Acute renal failure
	Renovascular hypertension
Neurologic	Stroke
	Transient ischemic attack
	Paraparesis or paraplegia
	Encephalopathy
	Coma
	Ischemic neuropathy
Gastrointestinal	Mesenteric ischemia or infarction
	Ileus/abdominal pain
	Pancreatitis
	Hemorrhage (from mucosal ischemia or an aortoenteric fistula)
Peripheral vascular	Upper-or lower-extremity ischemia
Systemic	Fever

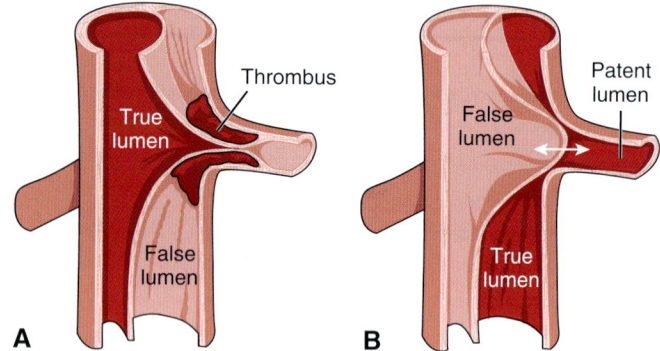

FIGURE 42.15 Static and dynamic obstruction in malperfusion syndrome complicating acute aortic dissection. This figure depicts two causes of malperfusion syndrome: (A) static and (B) dynamic obstruction. Static obstruction is the result of any fixed obstruction, and the most common cause, dissection of the branch vessel and thrombosis of the false lumen, is shown here. Dynamic obstruction is the more common cause of malperfusion syndrome and occurs when the branch vessel ostium is intermittently blocked by the dissection flap. (From Tadros RO, Tang GHL, Barnes HJ, et al. Optimal treatment of uncomplicated Type B aortic dissection: JACC review topic of the week. *J Am Coll Cardiol.* 2019;74[11]:1494–1504.)

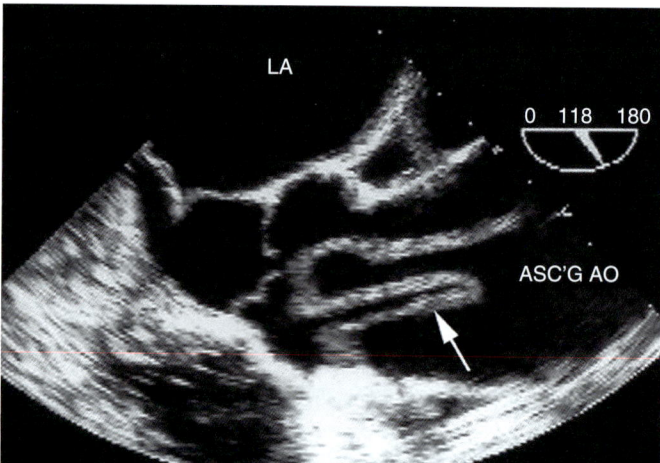

FIGURE 42.16 Stanford type-A aortic dissection. During aortic assessment with transesophageal echocardiography, there is an intimal flap *(arrow)*, consistent with type- A dissection. ASC'G AO, Ascending aorta; LA, left atrium. (From Patel PA, Bavaria JE, Ghadimi K, et al. Aortic regurgitation in acute Type-A aortic dissection: a clinical classification for the perioperative echocardiographer in the era of the functional aortic annulus. *J Cardiothorac Vasc Anesth.* 2018;32[1]:586–597.)

A pulse deficit is reported in 30% of type A dissections and 20% of type B dissections with frank limb ischemia less common.[1,12,41] Malperfusion, occurring in up to 30%, is the most common dynamic, but may be static or mixed.[54] Dynamic malperfusion results from the pressurized false lumen pushing the septum toward the true lumen leading to collapse of the true lumen, obstructing branch vessels. Static malperfusion results from stenosis or occlusion of a branch artery due to the dissection flap, hematoma, embolism, or thrombosis (Fig.42.15).[12,54]

AR occurs in 41% to 76% of patients with type A dissection, with a diastolic murmur audible in 40%.[12,41] The murmur of AR varies in intensity, depending on blood pressure and the degree of heart failure, and may be inaudible. Mechanisms of AR relate to the functional aortic annulus and aortic valve and may be due to acute dilation of the aortic sinuses and/or sinotubular junction, commissural disruption, restrictive cusp mobility, aortic leaflet prolapse, circumferential dehiscing intimal flap prolapsing into the left ventricular outflow tract during diastole interfering with valve coaptation (Fig. 42.16), or preexisting AR due to a preexisting aortic root aneurysm or BAV.[55,56]

Neurologic manifestations occur in 15% to 40% of patients with aortic dissection and are more common with type A dissections.[57,58] Neurologic syndromes include persistent or transient ischemic stroke, spinal cord ischemia, ischemic neuropathy, and hypoxic encephalopathy and are related to malperfusion of one or more branches supplying the brain, spinal cord, or peripheral nerves. Ischemic stroke occurs in approximately 6% of patients with type A dissection.[12] Less common neurologic features include seizures, ischemic neuropathy, disturbances in consciousness and coma, and paraparesis or paraplegia related to spinal cord ischemia. Coma and cerebral malperfusion are associated with worse outcomes,[58] but some studies have failed to identify brain malperfusion as an independent risk factor for an adverse outcome after surgical repair.[12,41]

Coronary ischemia is present in 5% to 10% of patients with type A dissection and ST-segment elevation myocardial infarction (STEMI) occurs in approximately 2% (most commonly affecting the right cor-onary artery).[1,56,59] Type A aortic dissection was the cause in 0.5% of STEMI cases in one center.[59] Coronary malperfusion may be due to the false lumen involving the coronary ostium, dissection flap extending into the coronary, or avulsion of the coronary artery. Troponin elevations and nonspecific ST-T changes in acute dissection may also be due to demand ischemia and lack of suspicion of dissection may lead to inappropriate therapy and delay in diagnosis and treatment of dissection.[1,12,59] One should consider aortic dissection in the differential diagnosis of patients with acute coronary ischemia or infarction, especially when their risk factors, symptoms, or findings on examination (or echocardiogram) are compatible with this diagnosis. When coronary angiography in a patient with ST-segment elevation MI shows no culprit lesion, aortic dissection should be excluded.[12]

Aortic dissection may extend into the abdominal aorta and result in vascular complications and malperfusion. Renal artery involvement occurs in at least 5% to 10% of patients and may lead to renal ischemia, infarction, or renal insufficiency or refractory hypertension. Mesenteric ischemia occurs in less than 5% of dissection and associates with a marked increase in mortality. The symptoms may be insidious, associated with nonspecific abdominal complaints, and a

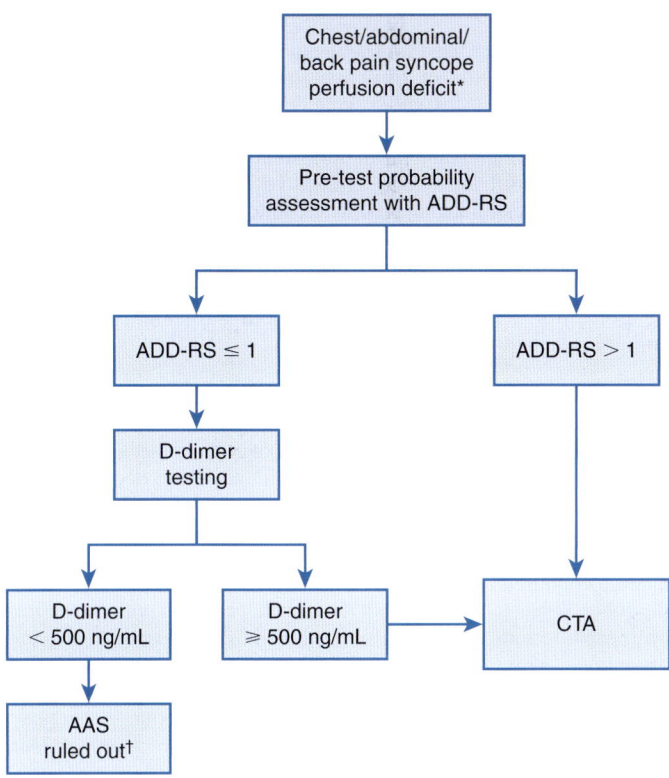

FIGURE 42.17 Proposed diagnostic algorithm for acute aortic dissection based on pretest probability assessment and D-dimer. *AAS*, Acute aortic syndrome; *ADD-RS*, aortic dissection detection risk score (see discussion under "Integrated Diagnostic Evaluation and Management Algorithms" in text); *CTA*, computed tomography angiography. *AAS in differential diagnosis. †Caution in patients with early presentation (≤ 2 hours) or long-lasting symptoms (≥ 1 week).

elastin fragments), MMPs, sST2, TGF-β, and fibrin degradation products occurs after aortic dissection.[60] These markers have limited usefulness because of sensitivity, specificity, or time delay and are not currently appropriate for clinical use. Patients with acute aortic dissection have elevated D-dimer levels making this a very useful biomarker for classic acute dissection.[1,41] In patients seen within the first 24 hours of onset, a D-dimer level lower than 500 ng/mL had a negative likelihood ratio of 0.07 and a negative predictive value of 95%. D-dimer is reported as having a sensitivity of 97% and a specificity of 47%.[1,41] Notably, normal D-dimer levels can occur with aortic dissection and a thrombosed false lumen, as well as with aortic IMH and PAU.[12] Additionally, patients may initially be seen longer than 24 hours after symptom onset, which affects D-dimer levels. Among very low-suspicion patients (aortic dissection score of ≤1), a negative D-dimer has a very low failure rate of detection (0.3%), missing 1 in 300 cases of acute aortic syndrome (Fig. 42.17). (See section below: Integrated Diagnostic Evaluation and Management Algorithms.)[60] However, among those with higher risk of dissection (i.e., aortic dissection risk score [see below] of >1), a normal D-dimer has a higher failure rate (4%) and cannot be used to "rule out" acute aortic syndrome in these patients.[12,60]

Diagnostic Techniques

When aortic dissection is suspected, expedient and accurate confirmation of the diagnosis is important. Diagnostic methods available to diagnose aortic dissection include contrast-enhanced CT, MRI, TEE, and TTE. TEE, helical CT, and MRI have very high diagnostic accuracy for suspected aortic dissection.[1,12] Each modality has advantages and disadvantages with respect to diagnostic ability, speed, convenience, and risk.[22,42,43] The choice of imaging study depends on the availability and expertise in the individual institution. If the probability of dissection is high and initial testing is negative or nondiagnostic, a second diagnostic test should be performed. Besides diagnosing the type and location of dissection, additional useful information includes anatomic features and complications related to the dissection, including its extent, entry sites, and reentry sites; patency of the false lumen; involvement of branch vessels; severity of AR; hemopericardium; coronary artery involvement; malperfusion; and rupture.

Computed Tomography

Contrast-enhanced CTA is the modality most commonly used for evaluating aortic dissection and is best performed with an ECG-gated, multidetector scanner, which may eliminate aortic pulsation motion artifacts (see also Chapter 20).[22] On CTA, aortic dissection is diagnosed by the presence of two distinct lumens with a visible intimal flap or by detection of two lumens by their differing rates of opacification with contrast material (Fig. 42.18). If the false lumen is completely thrombosed, it demonstrates low attenuation. The false lumen usually has slower flow and a larger diameter than the true lumen.[1,22] Contrast-enhanced CT has a sensitivity and specificity of 98% to 100% in diagnosing aortic dissection, but false-negative results may occur with inadequate contrast bolus.[12,22] CTA allows three-dimensional reconstruction for evaluation of the dissection and branch vessels and is critical for endovascular repair. CTA requires intravenous (IV) contrast, and without contrast enhancement, aortic dissection may go undetected. CT can identify the presence of thrombus in the false lumen and detect hemopericardium, aortic rupture, branch vessel involvement, and blood supply from the true and false lumens. Findings including aortic aneurysm, hemopericardium, hemomediastinum, high-attenuation aortic wall thickening (indicating IMH), and internal displacement of intimal calcification greatly increase the likelihood of acute aortic syndrome.[22] Major limitations of CT include complications associated with the use of contrast agents, especially nephropathy (see Chapter 101).

Magnetic Resonance Imaging

MRI is less often used for initial evaluation of acute aortic syndromes due to longer scanning times, contraindications with metallic implants, and less overall availability (see Chapter 19). MRI is highly accurate in diagnosing acute dissection with a sensitivity and specificity of 98% and does not require IV iodinated contrast material or ionizing

high index of suspicion must be maintained for this complication.[12] Aortic dissection may lead to a left-sided bland or inflammatory pleural effusion, but hemothorax may occur from aortic rupture. Type A aortic dissection may lead to acute pericarditis, but more commonly a bland pericardial effusion. Hemopericardium with acute cardiac tamponade from rupture complicates 9% of type A dissections and is related to worse outcomes.[12] Isolated abdominal aortic dissection is rare and associates with an existing AAA or an iatrogenic cause.

Laboratory Findings

The chest x-ray may increase suspicion of aortic dissection, but the findings are nonspecific and, in many cases, completely normal. The dissected aorta may not be dilated and its image may not be displaced or widened on x-ray. The most common abnormalities are abnormal aortic contour or widening of the aortic silhouette, appearing in approximately 70% to 80% of cases (83% of type A; 72% of type B).[41] Pleural effusions occur in approximately 20% of dissections. Notably, normal chest x-ray findings were reported in 29% of type A and 36% of type B dissections.[41] Therefore, a normal chest x-ray cannot exclude an aortic dissection. Laboratory tests important to evaluate for complications of aortic dissection include complete blood count, comprehensive metabolic profile, lactic acid, troponin, lactate dehydrogenase, and creatine kinase levels.

The electrocardiographic findings with aortic dissection are nonspecific but may indicate acute complications such as myocardial ischemia or infarction related to coronary artery involvement or low-voltage QRS complexes related to hemopericardium. Electrocardiogram (ECG) changes of ischemia may be present in type A or type B dissection and acute STEMI complicates approximately 2% of type A dissection.[1,41,42,59]

BIOMARKERS
Reliable biomarkers for the diagnosis or exclusion of acute aortic dissection have provoked great interest. Due to the dissection process, release of smooth muscle and interstitial proteins (myosin heavy chain, calponin,

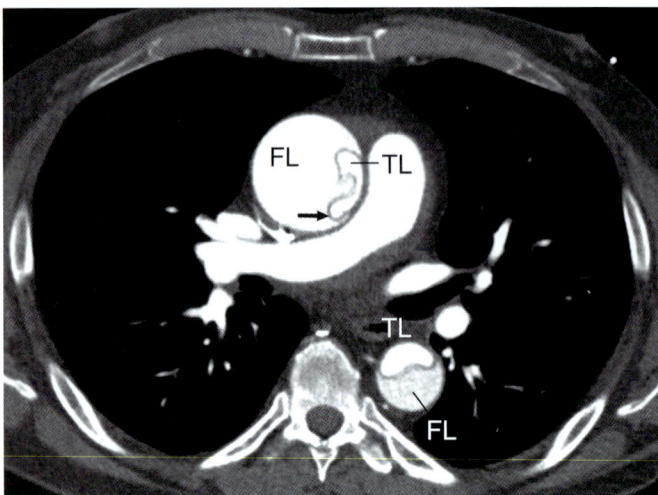

FIGURE 42.18 Contrast CT scan of an acute type A aortic dissection. The ascending aorta is dilated and a dissection flap *(arrow)* and the compressed and smaller true lumen *(TL)* and the expanded false lumen *(FL)* are visualized in the ascending aorta. In the descending aorta, the smaller true lumen demonstrates increased contrast enhancement as compared to the false lumen.

radiation.[22] MRI permits multiplanar imaging with threedimensional reconstruction and cine-MRI for visualization of blood flow, differentiation of slow flow and clot, evaluation of intimal flap mobility, and detection and quantification of AR. MRI can assess branch vessel morphology when combined with contrast-enhanced MRA. Characteristic features of the aortic wall on MRI sequences can differentiate IMH from mural thrombus.[22] MRI is highly accurate to detect pericardial effusion, aortic rupture, and entry and exit points. Gadolinium contrast must be used with caution in those with reduced kidney function due to risk of nephrogenic systemic fibrosis.

Echocardiogram (see also Chapter 16)
The echocardiogram (and ultrasound) diagnosis of aortic dissection is based on the presence of an undulating intimal flap with independent motion within the aortic lumen that separates the true and false lumens.[1,22] Color-flow Doppler demonstrates differential flow in the two lumens and can detect intimal tears. When the false lumen is thrombosed, displacement of intimal calcification or thickening of the aortic wall suggests aortic dissection.

Transthoracic Echocardiography
TTE can be performed quickly at the bedside and in the ER, and in the setting of an acute type A aortic dissection may have a sensitivity to detect type A dissection as high as approximately 85% to 90%,[22] but is much less sensitive than other modalities for the diagnosis of type B aortic dissection ([TBAD]).[12] Because TTE has a reduced sensitivity for detection, negative findings do not exclude acute aortic dissection, but certain clues, including a dilated aorta, AR, or hemopericardium, may heighten diagnostic suspicion.

Transesophageal Echocardiography
TEE, being operator dependent, is highly accurate in the evaluation and diagnosis of acute aortic dissection (sensitivity, ≈98%; specificity, ≈95%) (see Fig. 42.16).[1,12,22] TEE may not adequately visualize the distal ascending aorta and proximal aortic arch, but it interrogates the remaining thoracic aortic segments well. TEE may visualize the intimal tear, differentiate the true and false lumens, and identify fenestrations in the intimal flap. Features of the true lumen on TEE include a smaller lumen, systolic expansion, systolic anterograde flow, communication from the true to the false lumen in systole, and early and fast contrast-enhanced echocardiographic flow. TEE evaluates the mechanism and severity of AR (see Videos 42.8–42.12, and 42.16) and provides information about left ventricular function, the proximal coronary arteries, and hemopericardium.

Aortography
Aortography is rarely used for the diagnosis of suspected acute aortic dissection but may detect dissection after coronary angiography was performed in patients for whom acute coronary syndrome was initially (incorrectly) suspected. Findings of dissection on aortography include two lumens or an intimal flap, an undulating deformation of the aortic lumen, aortic wall thickening, branch vessel involvement, and AR. Compared to other imaging modalities, aortography is less accurate in diagnosing aortic dissection. A falsenegative aortogram may result from thrombosis of the false lumen, from equal opacification of both the true and false lumens, and from IMH. Intravascular ultrasound may be useful in selected cases for diagnosis and is routinely used during endovascular treatment of aortic dissection.

Selecting an Imaging Modality
Because of its availability on an emergency basis, contrast-enhanced CT is usually the first choice for the diagnosis of aortic dissection. The risk for contrast-induced nephropathy may complicate the decision about which test to perform when TEE or MRI is unavailable. Importantly, a non–contrast-enhanced CT might fail to diagnose aortic dissection. Non–contrast-enhanced MRA may diagnose aortic dissection when gadolinium contrast is contraindicated. TTE may be able to diagnose aortic dissection (especially type A) but does not have a high enough sensitivity to exclude aortic dissection. When there is a high suspicion of acute dissection, if TEE or MRI is not available on an urgent basis, one must accept the risks associated with IV contrast material given the potential fatal consequences of failing to diagnose aortic dissection.

The Role of Coronary Angiography
Routine coronary angiography is not recommended before surgery for acute type A aortic dissection because of concern about delay in emergency surgery.[12] In addition to the time delay incurred, coronary angiography may be technically difficult in the setting of dissection. Arterial access may fail to gain entry into the true lumen, and injury to the aorta from the catheter or guidewire may cause extension of the dissection or perforation of the aorta. In patients undergoing surgery for acute type A dissection, coronary artery involvement by the dissection can most often be corrected intraoperatively,[61] and angiography is not required.

Integrated Diagnostic Evaluation and Management Algorithms
Acute aortic syndromes lead to a small fraction of acute chest pain syndromes, but have a high mortality rate, especially when undiagnosed. The Thoracic Aortic Disease guidelines provide an algorithm for the management of patients with presentations compatible with acute aortic dissection (Fig.42.19).[12,62] A bedside risk assessment (Aortic Dissection Detection [ADD] Risk Score) stratifies patients into low (score 0), intermediate (score 1), and high (score 2 to 3) risk groups depending upon predisposing conditions, pain characteristics, and clinical features and considers: (1) *high-risk condition* (MFS or related disorder, family history of aortic disease, known aortic valve disease [such as BAV], recent aortic manipulation, or known TAA); (2) *high-risk pain features*, including chest, back, or abdominal pain described as abrupt in onset, severe in intensity, and of ripping/tearing/sharp or stabbing quality; and (3) *high-risk examination features*, including perfusion deficit (pulse deficit, blood pressure differential, focal neurologic deficit), murmur of AR, or hypotension/shock. The presence of two or more ADD strongly suggests aortic dissection. Patients considered highly likely to have acute aortic dissection undergo emergency surgical consultation and expedited imaging. Patients with presentations suggesting aortic dissection and who do not have an alternative diagnosis require expedited imaging. Those with lower-risk profiles are evaluated for alternative diagnoses, but when none are considered likely or are confirmed, aortic imaging is recommended. Integrating D-dimer testing (see earlier) may assist with excluding dissection in very low-suspicion patients (ADD score ≤ 1) but cannot exclude dissection among those with higher pretest probability.[60] Prospective evaluation of the ADD score is necessary for applicability to emergency departments and other sites.

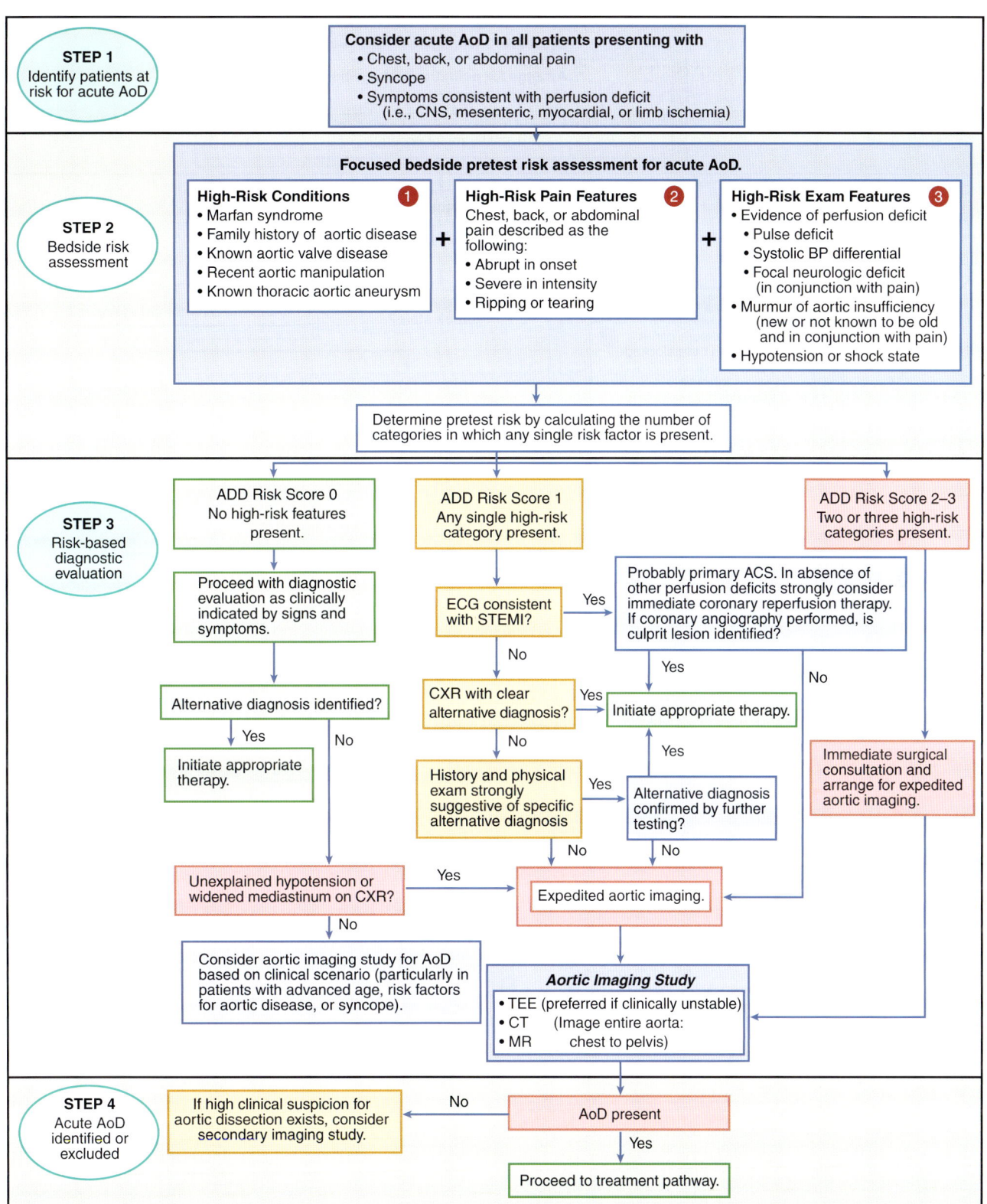

FIGURE 42.19 Evaluation pathway for aortic dissection (AoD). *ACS,* Acute coronary syndrome; *ADD,* aortic dissection detection; *BP,* blood pressure; *CNS,* central nervous system; *CXR,* chest x-ray; *STEMI,* ST-segment elevation myocardial infarction. (Modified from 2010 American College of Cardiology/American Heart Association Thoracic Aortic disease guidelines. From Rogers AM, Hermann LK, Booher AM, et al. Sensitivity of the aortic dissection detection risk score, a novel guideline-based tool for identification of acute aortic dissection at initial presentation: results from the international registry of acute aortic dissection. *Circulation.* 2011;123:2213.)

Management

The Thoracic Aortic Disease guidelines suggest a management pathway for patients with acute aortic dissection (Fig. 42.20).[12] Initial medical management includes stabilizing the patient, controlling pain, and lowering blood pressure with beta blockers to reduce the rate of rise in the force (dP/dt) of left ventricular contraction. These measures should commence immediately while the patient is undergoing diagnostic evaluation. Lowering blood pressure may help prevent further propagation of the dissection and lessen the risk for aortic rupture. Aortic dissection has a high mortality rate. Historically, medical management of acute type A dissection had a mortality of 20% at 24 hours and 30% by 48 hours.[41] Recently, the IRAD reported

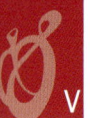

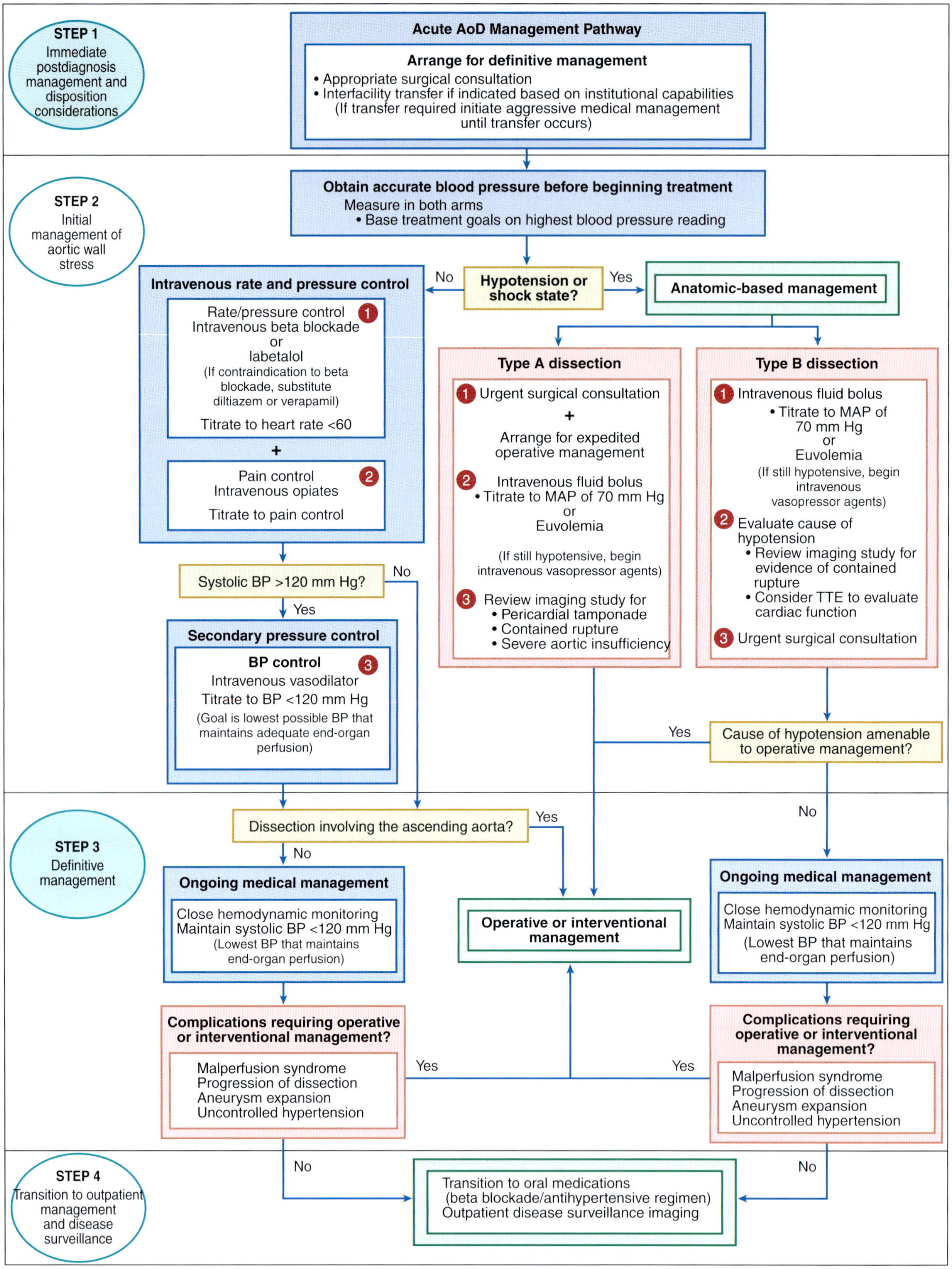

FIGURE 42.20 Management pathway for acute aortic dissection. *AoD*, Aortic dissection; *BP*, blood pressure; *MAP*, mean arterial pressure. (From Hiratzka LF, Bakris GL, Beckman JA, et al. 2010 ACCF/AHA/AATS/ACR/ASA/SCA/SCAI/SIR/STS/SVM guidelines for the diagnosis and management of patients with thoracic aortic disease: Executive summary. A report of the American College of Cardiology Foundation/American Heart Association Task Force on Practice Guidelines, American Association for Thoracic Surgery, American College of Radiology, American Stroke Association, Society of Cardiovascular Anesthesiologists, Society for Cardiovascular Angiography and Interventions, Society of Interventional Radiology, Society of Thoracic Surgeons, and Society for Vascular Medicine. *J Am Coll Cardiol*. 2010;55:e27–e129.)

survival for medically managed type A dissections to be 82% at 24 hours; 51% at 7 days; 40% at 30 days; and 38% at 60 days.[46] Emergency surgery improves survival for acute type A dissections with an 18% in-hospital mortality for surgically treated and 56% mortality for medically treated patients (see Fig. 42.14).[41] Even among the much older adults, surgical management associates with lower mortality and age alone is not an exclusion for surgery[12,41] Emergency transfer to a tertiary medical center with access to cardiovascular surgery, vascular surgery, interventional radiology, and cardiology is recommended for patients with acute dissection.[1,12] Hospitals and surgeons with higher procedural volumes for patients with acute type A dissections may have lower mortality rates.[1,63]

Blood Pressure Reduction
Reduction of systolic blood pressure to 100 to 120 mm Hg or the lowest level necessary for adequate perfusion and a heart rate of 60 to 80 beats/min is recommended.[1] Beta blockers should be administered even if the patient does not have hypertension. For rapid administration of agents to reduce the rate of rise in ventricular force (dP/dt) and stress on the aorta, IV beta blockers may be given. Selected IV pharmacotherapy in acute dissection is listed in Table 42.9. When encountering refractory hypertension in acute dissection one must consider renal artery malperfusion (especially with signs of renal ischemia). The need for multiple antihypertensive agents to control blood pressure acutely may wane after the first several days.

Management of Cardiac Tamponade
Cardiac tamponade, which occurs in 8% to 31% of acute type A dissections, is one of the most common mechanisms of death in patients with dissection.[1,12,41] Patients with tamponade may present with hypotension, syncope, or altered mental status and have twice as high an in-hospital mortality rate as do those without tamponade (54% vs. 25%).[64] Pericardiocentesis for acute hemopericardium in patients with dissection can result in recurrent bleeding and acute hemodynamic collapse, especially if a larger volume of fluid is removed and increased blood pressure causes further brisk bleeding into the pericardial space. In a relatively stable patient with acute type A dissection and cardiac tamponade, the risks associated with pericardiocentesis probably outweigh its benefits. Hypotension or shock from hemopericardium secondary to ascending dissection requires emergency aortic surgery. In patients with persistent hypotension or shock from hemopericardium due to type A dissection who will not survive open surgery, careful aspiration of small volumes of pericardial fluid associates with improved blood pressure and may be lifesaving and should be considered in this setting.[12,65]

Definitive Therapy
Definitive therapy for acute aortic dissection includes emergency surgery for type A dissection in patients considered surgical candidates (Fig. 42.21). Patients with acute type A aortic dissection are at risk for aortic rupture, AR with heart failure, stroke, cardiac tamponade, and visceral ischemia. Compared to medical therapy, immediate surgical treatment improves survival in patients with acute type A aortic dissection.[1,12,41,46] In large registries, the mortality rate of patients with type A aortic dissection undergoing surgery was 18%, as opposed to 56% in those treated medically (typically because of advanced age and comorbid conditions) (see Fig. 24.14).[41,46] In experienced centers, 30-day surgical mortality for acute type A dissection is between 10% and 25%.[57] Factors associated with mortality include shock, heart failure, cardiac tamponade, MI, renal failure, age, extent of dissection, and malperfusion.[12,41,57,66] Age alone should not deter operative therapy and type A aortic dissection surgery had a mortality rate of 16% in septuagenarians and 35% in octogenarians.[57] While shock in type A dissection associates with a high mortality rate, survivors demonstrate favorable outcomes.[67] Major brain injury complicates approximately 10% of type A dissection,[41] cerebral malperfusion and neurologic deficits occur in 15%,[58] and arch vessel involvement and stroke or coma are associated with much higher mortality, whereas medical therapy alone with these complications have poor outcomes.[41] Brain function may recover after surgery and preoperative brain injury should not preclude surgery.[41,58] Risk prediction tools from IRAD and other large registries permit estimation of the mortality rate associated with surgery for acute type A aortic dissection.[41,47,66]

TABLE 42.9 Selected Pharmacologic Therapy for Acute Aortic Dissection*

Intravenous Beta-Blocker (Preferred Negative Inotrope)
• **Esmolol**: Bolus 250–500 μg/kg IV, then continuous IV infusion at 50–100 μg/kg/min, titrated to effect with maximum dose of 200 μg/kg/min
• **Labetalol**: Bolus 20 mg IV over 2 min, then 20–80 mg IV every 10 min until adequate response (maximum 300 mg), then continuous IV infusion at 0.5–2 mg/min IV, titrated to effect
• **Metoprolol**: Give 2.5–15 mg IV followed by 2.5–15 mg IV every 3–6 hr
Intravenous Calcium Channel Blocker (Secondary Negative Inotrope)
• **Diltiazem**: Initial bolus of 0.25–0.35 mg/kg IV, then continuous IV infusion of 5–20 mg/hr
• **Verapamil**: 5–10 mg IV and may repeat after 5–10 min
Intravenous Vasodilator (*After* Initiation of Negative Inotrope)
• **Clevidipine**: Give 1–2 mg/hr; can double dose up to maximum dose of 16–32 mg/hr
• **Sodium nitroprusside**: Start continuous infusion at 0.25–0.5 μg/kg/min, titrated to a maximum of 8–10 μg/min. Use only in presence of beta blockers 　• *Caution*: Thiocyanate toxicity may occur in patients with renal impairment or prolonged infusions
• **Nicardipine**: Give 2.5–5 mg/hr and titrate up to a maximum of 15 mg/hr
• **Nitroglycerin**: Initial 5 μg/min, up to 200 μg/min as an IV infusion
• **Enalaprilat**: Give 1.25 mg, then 1.25–5 mg IV every 6 hr, titrated to effect
• **Fenoldopam**: Give 0.1 μg/kg/min and titrate up to a maximum of 1.6 μg/kg/min

*Goal of therapy is heart rate less than 70 beats/min and blood pressure 100–120 mm Hg or as low as possible without compromising organ perfusion.

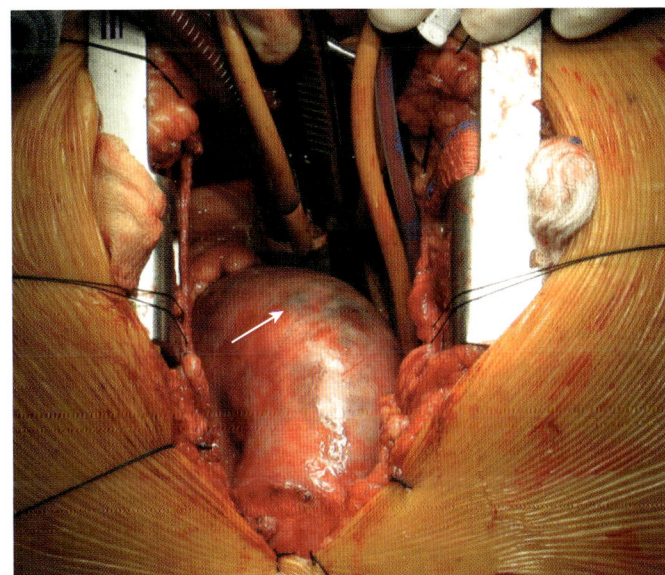

FIGURE 42.21 Intraoperative photograph of acute ascending aortic dissection demonstrating a dilated aortic root and ascending aorta. The aorta has a bluish discoloration *(arrow)* typical of underlying aortic dissection. (Photograph courtesy Dr. Nicholas Kouchoukos.)

Selected patients with type A dissection considered high risk for OSR have undergone TEVAR and hybrid treatment, but more data are required in this area due to technical and anatomical restrictions.[68] Acute retrograde type A dissection with a primary intimal tear in the descending aorta is usually treated surgically. A favorable outcome is reported for carefully selected patients treated with initial medical therapy and timely interventions when the ascending aortic extension is thrombosed and not aneurysmal and with TEVAR to cover entry distal tears with retrograde type A IMH with type B dissection.[69]

Patients with acute TBAD have a lower acute mortality rate than do those with acute type A dissection, with overall in-hospital mortality rates of approximately 10% (see Fig. 42.14).[41,46,48,70] The in-hospital mortality rate is lower for uncomplicated type B dissection, reported as 1% to 6% in those requiring only medical therapy[71,72]—but is much higher for complicated type B dissection, especially when accompanied by shock or malperfusion.[41–43,54,70] Increasing age, female gender, periaortic hematoma, aortic diameter greater than 5.5 cm, and malperfusion are associated with increased mortality rates.[70] In a recent IRAD series, 57% of patients with acute type B dissection were treated medically, 32% endovascular, and 7% with open surgery, with in-hospital mortality rates of 10%, 14%, and 21% in each group, respectively (see Fig. 42.14).[41] Indications for TEVAR (or less commonly OSR when TEVAR is not feasible) in complicated TBAD include visceral or limb ischemia, rupture or impending rupture, rapid aortic expansion, uncontrollable pain, or retrograde extension of the dissection into the ascending aorta (Figs. 42.22 and 42.23, Table 42.10).[1] However, extra-anatomic bypass may be used to restore flow to an ischemic limb (femorofemoral bypass), or renal or mesenteric vessel, typically with a take-off from an uninvolved artery (most commonly iliac). Alternatively, endovascular fenestration of the dissection membrane will usually improve flow to vessels that are compromised and is more commonly used at centers with experience with these techniques. This is an important technique to consider when type B dissection is complicated by spinal ischemia as TEVAR may worsen this both by covering intercostals and diverting flow away from the false lumen which commonly supplies the intercostals.

Acute aortic dissection with entry tears in the arch (also called "non-A, non-B" dissections) represent 4% to 10% of dissections and their management must be individualized.[32,73] When the dissection extends retrograde to involve the ascending aorta, surgical intervention (often with arch replacement) is recommended, whereas when uncomplicated and the ascending aorta is spared, the majority are treated medically (or with TEVAR, as indicated).[32] Surgical repair of acute arch dissection has a mortality rate between 15% and 29%.[32] Type B dissections that extend retrograde into the arch occur in 16% and are managed variably, including medical therapy (53%), endovascular (33%), or OSR (12%), depending upon complications.[32] Isolated abdominal aortic dissections are rare, and are associated with hypertension, penetrating aortic ulcers, preexisting aneurysm disease, or genetic conditions. Most are spontaneous, but some relate to trauma or iatrogenic causes.

SURGICAL MANAGEMENT
Operative therapy for acute aortic dissection is technically very demanding (see Fig. 42.21). The aortic wall is thin and friable, and Teflon felt and sutures with pledgets are used to buttress the wall and prevent the sutures from tearing the fragile aortic wall.

TYPE A AORTIC DISSECTION
Open surgery, performed as expediently as possible, is the treatment of choice for acute type A aortic dissection to prevent life-threatening complications.[1,12] There is an inverse relationship between hospital/surgeon volume and operative mortality for patients with acute type A dissection.[1,63] Expedient transfer to a center of excellence is often required. Surgical therapy aims to treat or prevent complications of dissection, including cardiac tamponade, AR, aortic rupture, stroke, and visceral ischemia. Surgical goals are to excise the intimal tear; to restore flow in the true lumen and obliterate the false channel by oversewing the edges of the aorta; and to reconstitute the aorta with placement of an interposition graft. In type A dissection, AR is treated by resuspension of the aortic valve leaflets or by prosthetic AVR. Although some controversy exists regarding the timing of directly treating malperfusion, the general consensus when this complication accompanies acute type A dissection is to repair the proximal aorta first because this will correct the malperfusion in most patients.[1,12,44] An individualized approach is necessary in critically ill patients when patient-specific therapeutic decisions must be made depending upon the mechanism of malperfusion.[74] When severe malperfusion syndrome due to mesenteric ischemia or descending aortic pseudocoarctation is present and there are no acute proximal aortic complications, initial endovascular therapy to the descending aorta may be performed with delayed proximal surgery, recognizing the risk of interim rupture.[74]

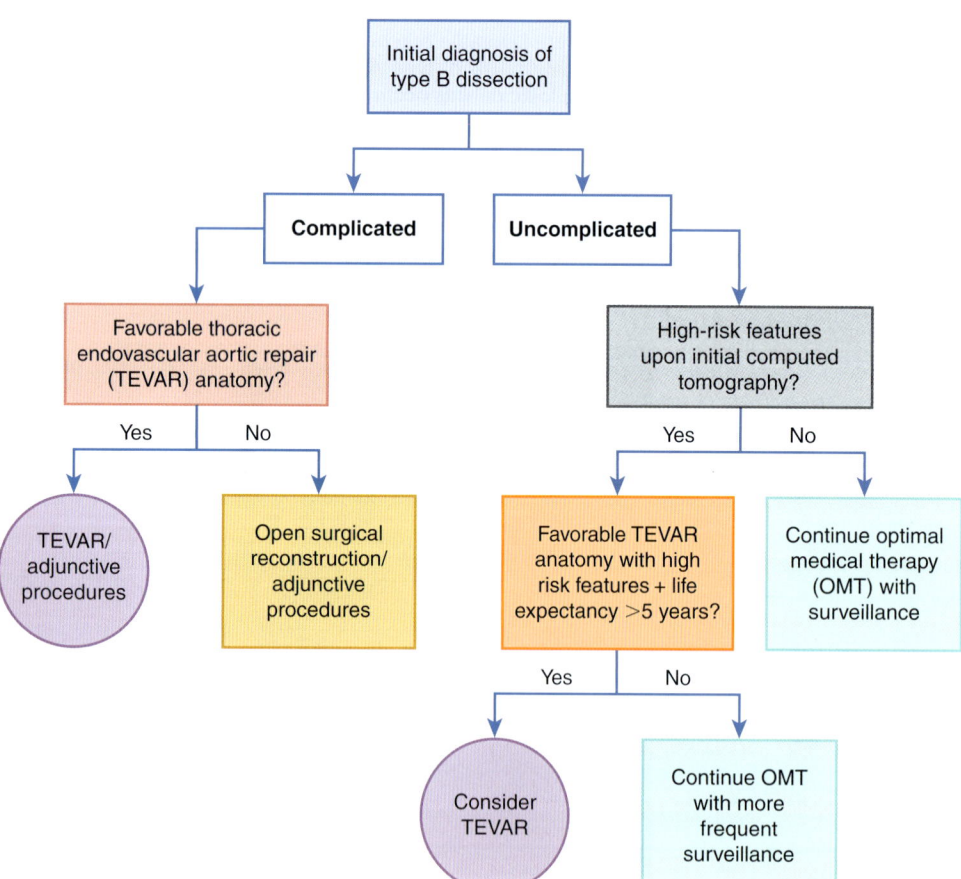

FIGURE 42.22 Management algorithm for acute type B aortic dissection. Adjunctive procedures are, for example, endovascular fenestration, surgical revascularization, coil embolization, and selective branch vessel stenting. High-risk features include primary entry tear diameter greater than 10 mm, initial aortic diameter greater than 40 mm, false lumen diameter greater than 22 mm, partially thrombosed false lumen, and saccular false lumen formation. *OMT*, Optimal medical therapy; *TEVAR*, thoracic endovascular aortic repair. (From Tadros RO, Tang GHL, Barnes HJ, et al. Optimal treatment of uncomplicated Type B aortic dissection: JACC review topic of the week. *J Am Coll Cardiol.* 2019;74:1494–1504.)

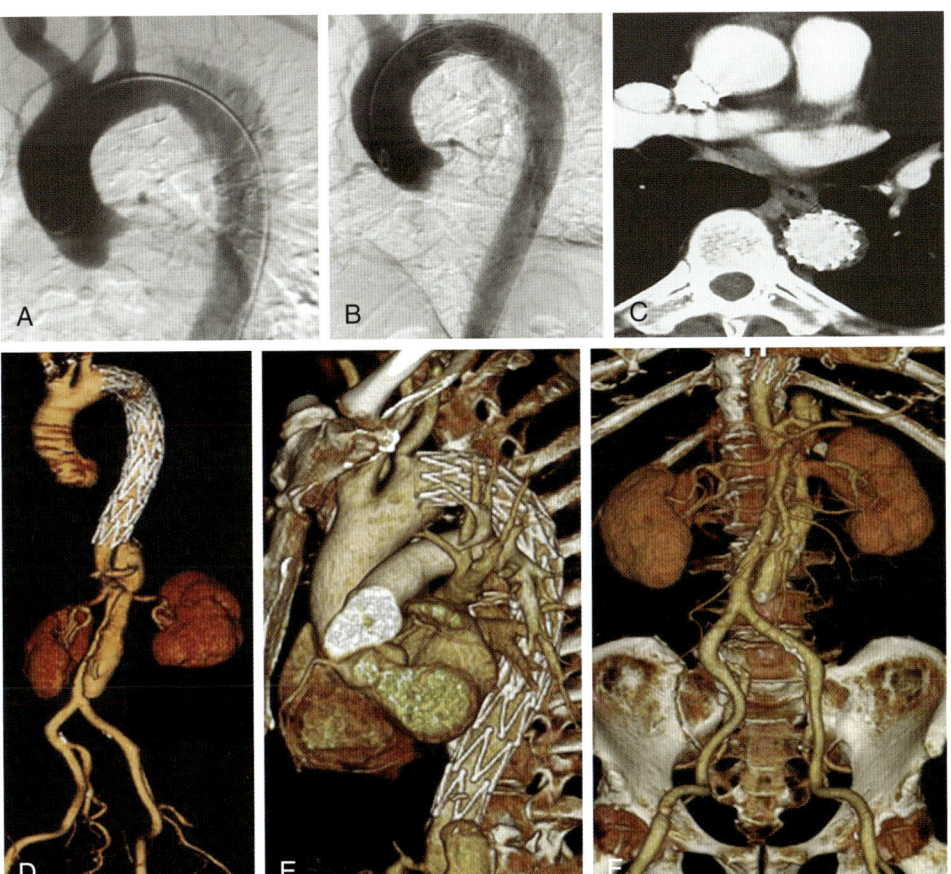

FIGURE 42.23 Long-term follow-up of thoracic endovascular aortic repair (TEVAR) for management of type B aortic dissection. **A,** Left anterior oblique projection from thoracic aortogram documents type B aortic dissection in 49-year-old man with acute abdominal and back pain. **B,** Repeat aortogram post stent-graft placement without antegrade opacification of the false lumen. **C,** Axial CT image at mid-thoracic level 20 months post-TEVAR shows stent-graft within true lumen and complete thrombosis of the false lumen which appears now as only a crescentic remnant along the posterolateral aortic border. **D,** Three-dimensional reconstruction CT data set obtained 8 years after TEVAR details stable appearance to thoracic aorta and residual patency of the abdominal false lumen without interval enlargement. **E** and **F,** Rendering of thoracic and abdominal CT scan performed 22 years after original TEVAR depicts stable appearance without interval disease progression. (From Thakkar D, Dake MD. Management of type B aortic dissections: treatment of acute dissections and acute complications from chronic dissections. *Tech Vasc Interventional Rad.* 2018;21:124–130.)

TABLE 42.10 Indications for Thoracic Endovascular Aortic Repair for Complicated Type B Aortic Dissection (or Open Surgical Repair if Anatomy Is Unsuitable for Thoracic Endovascular Aortic Repair)

Rupture/Impending rupture
Malperfusion
Hemothorax
Refractory pain
Refractory hypertension
Aneurysmal dilatation (>55 mm)
Rapid increase in aortic diameter
Recurrent symptoms

A median sternotomy is performed, and cannulation for cardiopulmonary bypass generally involves the right axillary/subclavian artery or less commonly, the femoral approach, to avoid trauma to the weakened aortic wall and risk of malperfusion through the dissected aorta.[1,12,75] Methods for cerebral and organ protection include cerebral perfusion techniques and variable hypothermia protocols. A vascular graft replaces the ascending aorta, and surgeon-specific methods to support the anastomosis are used (see Fig. 42.19).[75]

Most patients are treated by obliteration of the false lumen by placement of (supported by Teflon felt and BioGlue) supracoronary interposition grafting and resuspension of the native aortic valve. Intraoperative aortic valve inspection and TEE guidance assist in managing the aortic valve in patients with proximal aortic dissection.[55] When AR complicates dissection, repair of the aortic wall, decompression of the false lumen, and resuspension of the commissures to the aortic wall usually restores valve competence. However, root dilation or progressive AR may develop late and require AVR or root replacement. When aortic leaflet disease precludes repair, AVR plus associated ascending aortic replacement is indicated. When the sinuses are dilated, composite valve and root replacement is often performed via the modified Bentall procedure. If the sinus of Valsalva is involved by dissection, it is preferable to replace the aortic root to prevent late AR.[1] When the aortic root is dilated but the aortic leaflets are normal, many have achieved success by performing a reimplantation valve-sparing root replacement.[12] This is a longer procedure requiring surgical expertise, and for many, composite valve and root replacement is more appropriate. For dissections with a tear localized to the ascending aorta with a normal size arch without distal malperfusion, surgical repair involves a hemiarch replacement with an open distal anastomosis under circulatory arrest.[75]

The aortic arch is dissected in more than 70% of type A dissections, and arch vessel involvement in the dissection process is reported in 28% to 73%.[1,12,75] Arch replacement, under hypothermic circulatory arrest, is also performed when there is extensive intimal tear throughout the arch and arch vessels that is not amenable to primary resection, if the aortic arch is aneurysmal or ruptured, if a primary arch tear is identified at the time of surgery, and in some with heritable aneurysm disease. Prolonged circulatory arrest times increase morbidity and mortality. Branched graft techniques are preferred in managing arch vessels involved.[75] More extensive open and hybrid arch and distal aortic repairs lessen risk of future interventions,[21] but these more complex and higher-risk procedures are typically performed in dedicated aortic centers by experienced surgeons. Extended distal repair using a frozen elephant trunk may be performed to seal tears extending to the descending aorta (or with retrograde type A dissections) and to improve malperfusion distally and are being used more extensively in dedicated aortic centers.[44] Complications of surgery for type A dissection include coagulopathy/bleeding, neurologic injury, and complications (cardiac, visceral, renal) from malperfusion.[44]

TYPE B AORTIC DISSECTION

Uncomplicated TBAD is treated medically with anti-impulse blood pressure control, but approximately 25% to 30% present with complications, including malperfusion syndromes, associating with high morbidity and mortality (see Fig. 42.22).[23,41,54] TEVAR is recommended for TBAD complicated by malperfusion, aortic rupture, intractable pain, or rapid aortic enlargement having much lower morbidity and mortality than OSR (Fig. 42.23).[1,41,54] In patients with type B dissection in IRAD, 63% were treated medically with a mortality rate of 8.7%; 23% received endovascular repair with a mortality rate of 12%; and 13% underwent OSR with a mortality rate of 17%.[41,42] In other studies, OSR for complicated TBAD has a mortality rate of approximately 30%.[23] In acute complicated TBAD, TEVAR associates with 30-day mortality rates of 5% to 10%, stroke rates of 7% to 9%, and paraplegia/paraparesis rates of 6% to 9%, demonstrating favorable late aortic remodeling and 5-year survival.[23,48]

TEVAR covers the area of the primary intimal tear and redirects flow to the true lumen promoting thrombosis of the false lumen and allowing aortic remodeling. This treatment often corrects malperfusion syndromes and branch vessel ischemia and is useful in the treatment of enlarging symptomatic dissections and ruptured aortas. At present, endovascular devices are approved for the treatment of type B dissections (acute, chronic, complicated, or uncomplicated). Up to two-thirds of patients so treated have persistence of a perfused false lumen, which can require reintervention and surgical conversion. If malperfusion of a branch vessel persists, branch vessel stenting or the technique of provisional extension to induce complete attachment (PETTICOAT)—in which the entry point is sealed with an endograft and a bare stents are implanted distally—may correct the problem.[23] Fenestration of the dissection membrane may be useful when TEVAR is not feasible or in addition to TEVAR if the distal bare stents are not available. Hybrid approaches (TEVAR and OSR) to dissections involving the arch and descending aorta have lower risk than open surgery. Retrograde ascending dissection is a potentially lethal complication that may occur during TEVAR for TBAD, emphasizing the requirement for an open repair team at institutions performing TEVAR for aortic dissection.[12]

Patients with uncomplicated TBAD are at risk for long-term complications, including aneurysmal dilation (in 30% to 40%) and late rupture.[54] Whether early TEVAR of subacute/chronic stable TBAD alters its natural history is being studied. The ADSORB trial compared TEVAR with medical therapy in uncomplicated TBAD and found TEVAR to improve aortic remodeling, but no difference in overall mortality after 1 year.[23,48,54] The INSTEAD trial reported no difference in 2-year mortality between patients with uncomplicated subacute/chronic TBAD treated with TEVAR versus medical therapy.[54] Those receiving TEVAR had more favorable aortic remodeling, including false lumen thrombosis and true lumen expansion (91% vs. 19% for TEVAR vs. medical therapy), and at 5 years had improved aortic outcomes.[54] Reimaging 14 to 30 days after TBAD may detect features indicating high risk to allow selective TEVAR while aortic plasticity is optimal. Imaging characteristics predict late aortic complications in initially uncomplicated TBAD, being related to pressurizing the false lumen, whereas a thrombosed false lumen, multiple entry tears, and outer curvature false lumen are associated with less aortic growth.[54] TheIRAD reported improved outcomes in nonrandomized patients with TBAD treated with TEVAR compared to medical therapy.[41] TEVARin initially uncomplicated TBAD does carry risks including retrograde dissection, stroke, spinal cord ischemia, post-implantation syndrome, and continued perigraft flow. Because endografts reside within the true lumen and typically do not oppose to the outer aortic wall distally, perigraft flow is described differently than for endoleaks after aneurysm repair.[48]

Typical indications for TEVAR (or OSR) in chronic type B AD include progressive aortic enlargement (>5 to 10 mm/year), aneurysmal enlargement (>55 to 60 mm), malperfusion syndromes, or recurrent pain.[1,23,48] Extensive aneurysms lead to less favorable endovascular therapy and may require open and hybrid procedures and re-interventions. Stent-graft new entry (SINE), a new tear caused by the TEVAR, can occur early or late, is most common distally, and is related to oversizing of the distal stent compared to the true lumen diameter.[48] Repair of chronic type B AD demonstrates high rates of operative mortality (OSR 6% to 20%, TEVAR <5%, 0% to 14%), complications (stroke OSR 0% to 13%, TEVAR approximately 1% [0% to 10%], and spinal cord ischemia OSR 3% to 12%, TEVAR approximately 1% [0% to 10%]).[23,76] Reintervention rates were also high (OSR 6% to 29%, TEVAR 4% to 47%).[76] Currently, OSR is reserved for patients with aortic diameters greater than 55 to 60 mm who are good surgical candidates, including those with heritable/genetic aortic conditions, and at greater than 60 mm for reasonable candidates, whereas those at high surgical risk should be considered for TEVAR at dedicated centers.[23]

Long-Term Therapy and Follow-Up

Short- and long-term survival rates for type A aortic dissection for those discharged from hospital historically have ranged between 52% and 94% at 1 year and between 45% and 88% at 5 years.[12] Recently, IRAD reported survival after discharge to be 96% and 90% at 1 and 3 years, respectively.[41] Others report that patients with type A dissection who survive surgery have survival rates of 85% at 5 years, 65% at 10 years, and up to 38% at 30 years.[44]

Medically treated patients with type A aortic dissection have a very high mortality rate, with death rates in excess of 20% by 24 hours and 50% in the first week early after diagnosis.[41,46] Nonoperative therapy is chosen in approximately 10% of type A dissection due to advanced age, comorbidities, and complications upon presentation. The IRAD reported a 38% survival rate at 60 days for medically managed type A aortic dissections.[46] A few patients are initially seen when in the subacute stage, and they should undergo surgery. On occasion, patients are incidentally discovered to have a chronic type A dissection during evaluation for AR or a dilated ascending aorta. Surgical treatment is recommended for appropriate candidates with chronic type A dissection, especially younger patients and those with an ascending aortic aneurysm greater than 5 to 5.5 cm, AR, or symptoms.[77]

Outcomes after TBAD depend upon preexisting comorbidities and presenting complications and in IRAD, 75% to 80% of discharged patients survive 3 years.[41] Findings at long-term follow-up after TBAD are worse than after type A dissection. Previous studies have demonstrated that many deaths in follow-up are related to subsequent aortic complications such as rupture, extension of the dissection, and the risks associated with subsequent aortic and vascular surgery. In a nonrandomized study, patients with TBAD receiving endovascular repair (typically for complications) had a lower 5-year death rate (16% vs. 29%) than those treated medically.[41]

Long-term management after aortic dissection includes blood pressure control, screening the patient and first-degree relatives for heritable disorders associated with aortic dissection (see Tables 42.2 and 42.3), serial imaging of the aorta, lifestyle modifications, education, and psychosocial support.[13,38]

Treating hypertension, with a blood pressure goal of lower than 120/80 mm Hg, often requires multiple medications, making compliance difficult. Poorly controlled hypertension associates with an increase in late morbidity and mortality.[12,48] Randomized trials comparing medications in aortic dissection are lacking. Beta blockers, the most commonly used drugs after dissection, are the drugs of first choice because of their effect on aortic stress and dP/dt and are recommended even without hypertension as they are associated with improved survival (specifically with type A dissection) and may lessen the requirement for late surgery.[1,12,41] Calcium channel blockers may improve survival after type B dissection and ACE inhibitors are associated with lower late aortic events.[41] Smoking cessation and risk factor modification for atherosclerotic disease are emphasized.[12]

Many patients with dissection will eventually be found to have an underlying genetic predisposition or have a family history of aortic disease. Some have syndromic features recognized as MFS or LDS (see Fig. 42.6); features of these disorders should be sought on examination (see TAA section and Tables 42.2 and 42.3).[13] Recognition of dural ectasia—widening or enlargement of the dural canal, usually in the lumbosacral spine on CT or MRI—may indicate an underlying heritable aortic condition (such as MFS or LDS). Some patients will have an underlying BAV, a familial condition in 9% of cases,[15] whereas other patients will have nonsyndromic heritable thoracic aortic disease.[7] It is recognized that 20% of individuals with a TAA or dissection will have a first-degree relative with thoracic aortic disease, hence the importance of screening all first-degree relatives for aortic disease.[13]

Long-term management after dissection requires serial imaging of the aorta and its branches for complications, especially aneurysmal enlargement. The distal arch and the proximal descending aorta are the areas at highest risk for aneurysm formation after aortic dissection. Between 5% and 18% of patients require reoperation within 5 years (with much higher risk among those with genetic aortopathy).[44] Typical imaging after acute dissection includes CT or MRA at 1 to 3, 6, and 12 months and annually thereafter, with intervals depending on aortic size and rate of change over time.[1,12,44] MRA should be considered for long-term follow-up to avoid repeated radiation exposure, whereas some favor CTA.[48]

Risk factors for late aneurysm formation and poorer outcomes include aortic dilation, hypertension, larger false lumen diameter (>22 mm), entry tear diameter greater than 10 mm, and partial false lumen thrombosis.[23,41,48] Many late deaths following surgery for aortic dissection result from rupture of the aorta at the site of previous dissection or from rupture of another aneurysm at a remote site.[23] Aneurysms related to expansion of the false lumen have relatively thin walls and are at higher risk for rupture than degenerative aneurysms are. Rapid aortic growth (>5 mm/year) or aortic diameter greater than 60 mm are risk factors for rupture. The timing of repair for aneurysmal involvement of the residual aorta depends on several factors, including the patient's age and general medical condition, comorbid conditions, underlying disease process, rate of aneurysmal enlargement, and absolute size of the aorta. In general, patients with descending aorta diameter after dissection that exceeds 5.5 to 6 cm or if the rate of aortic expansion exceeds 1 cm/year should have evaluation for repair.[1,12] For patients at relatively lower risk and in those with heritable thoracic aortic disease, OSR at a smaller aortic diameter is appropriate.

Lifestyle modifications are necessary after aortic dissection. Isometric activities, including weightlifting, lead to increased blood pressure and aortic wall stress.[38] Many have to modify work or physical activities and for some, permanent disability is required due to the aortic dissection or aortopathy. Quality of life after aortic dissection is reported as lower than the general population with depression, anxiety, and post-traumatic stress reported in many.[41,44] Low to moderate levels of many types of physical activity, including sexual relations, are considered low-risk and participation in exercise may lessen depression and lower blood pressure.[38,41] Participation in modified cardiac rehabilitation programs and involvement in support groups may improve exercise tolerance and quality of life.

AORTIC DISSECTION VARIANTS

In addition to acute aortic dissection, aortic IMH and PAU are included in the acute aortic syndromes (see Fig. 42.12). These disorders may be identical to classic aortic dissection in their manifestations and cause acute chest or back pain, but they have important differences in their imaging and management. IMH is associated with many of the same risk factors as classic aortic dissection, whereas PAU is more common in the descending aorta and is associated with heavy calcification and atherosclerosis.

Aortic Intramural Hematoma

Aortic IMH, representing 10% to 20% of acute aortic syndromes (and higher incidence [30%] in Asia), is defined as a hematoma in the medial layer of the aortic wall without identifiable communication between the lumen and hematoma and no evidence of an intimal flap or false lumen.[1,12,23,41,48,78] IMH involves the ascending aorta in 30%, the arch in 10%, and the descending aorta in 60% to 70%. IMH may result from rupture of the vasa vasorum and subsequent mural hemorrhage. Supporting this theory is the location of IMH in the outer aortic media in distinction to the inner medial location of a classic dissection. However, improved imaging technology can identify micro-intimal tears or focal intimal disruptions in 20% to 60% of cases of IMH that may initiate or complicate the process.[78–80]

IMH is classified as type A or type B as for classic aortic dissection. Symptoms and risk factors of IMH resemble those of aortic dissection, with acute chest and/or back pain predominating. Ascending IMH may lead to AR, hemopericardium, or rupture, but malperfusion is less common. The proximity of the IMH to the adventitia may explain the frequent coexistence of pleural effusion, pericardial effusion, and periaortic hematoma and underlies the higher risk for aortic rupture.[1,12,42,78,80]

Imaging studies useful for the diagnosis of IMH include TEE, CT, and MRI.[22,56,78] TTE has a very low sensitivity. Crescentic or circumferential wall thickening without a visible intimal flap is the hallmark. On non–contrast-enhanced CT, IMH appears as an area of high attenuation (due to bleeding) in the aortic wall, whereas on contrast-enhanced CT, the aortic wall demonstrates low attenuation (because no contrast material enters the wall) (Fig. 42.24). TEE features of IMH include focal crescentic or circumferential aortic wall thickening ≥ 5 mm (Fig. 42.25), an eccentric aortic lumen, displaced intimal calcification, and areas of echolucency within the aortic wall and no intimal flap or flow in the aortic wall.[56,78] MRI demonstrates focal thickening and absence of blood flow with pulse sequences allowing definition of blood within the aortic wall. Tiny intimal disruptions frequently occur and may resolve.[78] Focal intimal disruptions and ulcer-like projections (ULP) (a localized blood-filled pouch protruding into the hematoma in the aortic wall which may be due to micro-intimal defects), focal contrast enhancement (intramural blood pools) within the hematoma, thick hematoma, and a large aortic diameter are associated with higher complication risk.[78–80]

Distinct from an aneurysm with mural thrombus, IMH has a smooth lumen and curvilinear wall (see Figs. 42.23 and 42.25). In certain cases, differentiating IMH from aortic dissection with thrombosis of the false lumen, mural thrombus within an aortic aneurysm, or aortic atherosclerosis may be difficult. On TEE, identifying the intima—often calcified and echodense—helps in making this distinction. Thickening beneath the intima suggests IMH, whereas thickening above the intima (on the luminal side) occurs with mural thrombus. In contrast to aortic atherosclerosis, IMH is not typically associated with diffuse intimal irregularities unless related to a penetrating ulcer.

Current guidelines recommend surgery for type A IMH, especially in the setting of hemodynamic instability, hemopericardium, rupture, or proximal aortic complications, and medical therapy for type B IMH.[1,12,41] In North America and Europe, open surgery is performed in greater than 80% of type A IMH and compared to medical therapy, and associates with improved survival (24% vs. 40%).[41–43] In Asia (South Korea/Japan), stable patients with type A IMH are often managed medically with close observation and frequent imaging, with resolution of the IMH in 40% and low mortality (10%).[80] However, serious complications may occur within the first days to weeks after onset, including aortic dissection (25% to 50%), hemopericardium, and rupture, and surgical therapy is required in 30-50% of patients receiving initial medical therapy.[80] Given the potential for unpredictable and catastrophic complications, surgical therapy is recommended for most type A IMH and medical management for patients with type B IMH.[1,12,41,78,80]

Type B IMH is treated medically in the vast majority with endovascular procedures performed for complications (Fig. 42.26).[23,48,78] Management of localized arch IMH must be individualized, with initial medical therapy often used for this group. Complete resolution of type B IMH occurs in greater than 50%, whereas some progress to frank dissection (5%), localized dissection or ULP (25%), rupture (4%), or late aneurysm formation (27%).[1,78,80] Frequent imaging follow-up is recommended, especially when ULP is visualized. Predictors of resolution of type B IMH have included younger age, smaller aortic diameter (<4 to 4.5 cm), hematoma thickness less than 1 cm, and use of beta blockers.[1,81,82] Aortic diameter greater than 45 mm is a poor prognostic feature.[78] TEVAR (or less often, OSR) in type B IMH is reserved for complications such as persistent pain, aortic aneurysm, progression, impending rupture, or rupture.[1,48,78,80] The average 30-day mortality rate in type B IMH is 4% in medically treated patients, 2% to 6% with TEVAR, and 16% in those requiring surgery.[80] Mortality at 3 years was 14% in medically treated patients and 23% for surgically treated patients.[1]

Penetrating Atherosclerotic Aortic Ulcer

PAU, representing approximately 5% of acute aortic syndromes, is an atherosclerotic plaque that penetrates through the internal elastic lamina into the media and often associates with a variable degree of IMH.[1,78,83] PAUs may lead to pseudoaneurysm, aortic rupture, or late aneurysm. Aortic ulcers may be single or multiple and range from 5 to

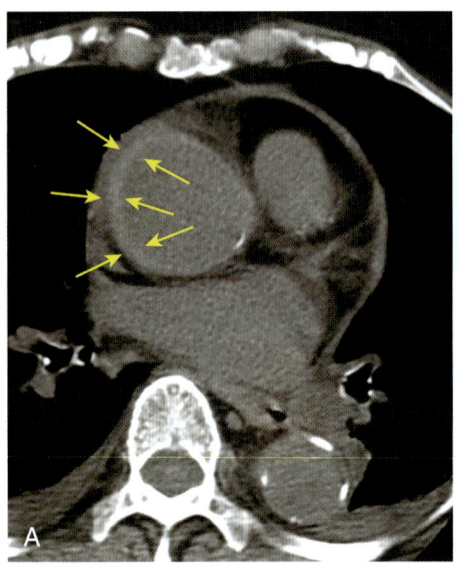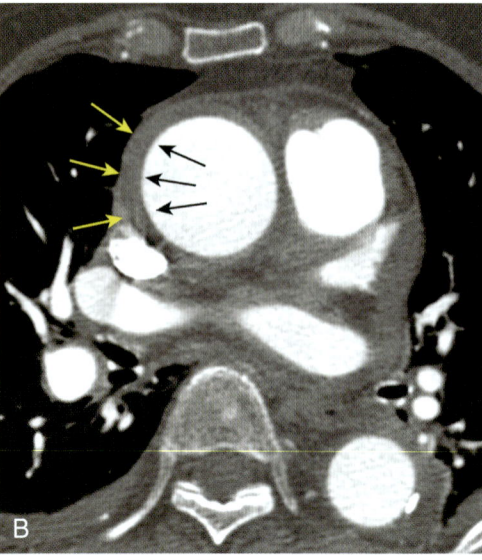

FIGURE 42.24 Crescentic ascending aortic intramural hematoma, indicated with arrows, on precontrast **(A)** and postcontrast **(B)** computed tomographic angiography. On precontrast images, high-attenuation blood products are discernible within the arterial media. If postcontrast imaging alone were performed, these might be mistaken for non-calcified atherosclerotic plaque or intraluminal thrombus. (Images courtesy Dr. Smita Patel. From Bhave NM, Nienaber CA, Clough RE, Eagle KA, et al. Multimodality imaging of thoracic aortic diseases in adults. *JACC Cardiovasc Imaging.* 2018;11[6]:902–919.)

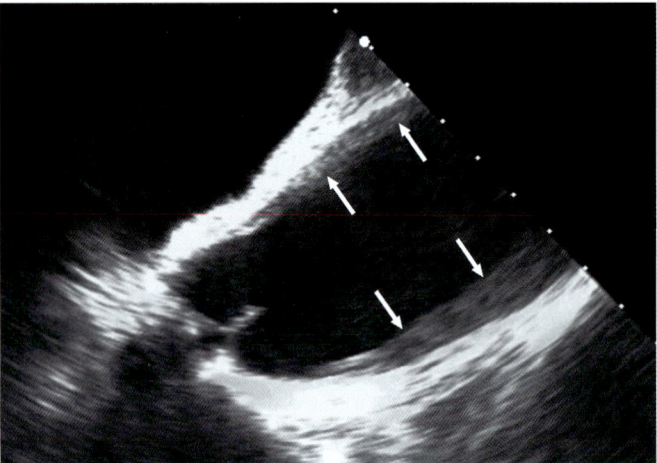

FIGURE 42.25 Acute type A intramural hematoma of the aorta. Transesophageal echocardiogram shows thickening of the ascending aorta due to intramural hemorrhage *(arrows).*

25 mm in diameter and 4 to 30 mm in depth. PAUs are more common in the mid-to distal descending aorta than in the arch or ascending or abdominal aorta.[1,78,83] Patients with PAUs are typically older adults with coexisting vascular disease and many have concomitant aneurysmal dilation of the aorta elsewhere, especially in the abdominal aorta. While 25% of PAUs are found incidentally on imaging studies, typical symptoms of PAUs include acute chest or back pain, similar in description to that of classic aortic dissection. Although PAUs may lead to aortic dissection, most patients do not have AR, pulse deficits, or visceral ischemia.

Imaging techniques for PAUs include CT, MRI, TEE, and aortography. Findings on CT include focal aortic ulceration, associated IMH, and a calcified, displaced intima (Fig. 42.27).[56,78,83,84] Typically, a crater-like outpouching with irregular edges occurs in the setting of heavy atherosclerosis. In some cases, it may be difficult to differentiate PAU with an IMH from an IMH with ULP. CT may also demonstrate pleural effusions, mediastinal hemorrhage, coexisting aneurysms, contained rupture, pseudoaneurysm, and frank rupture. Most patients have some degree of IMH formation. When a PAU is associated with aortic dissection, the dissection often involves a short segment of aorta and has a thick intimal flap. MRI findings in patients with PAUs include localized areas of high signal intensity in the aorta wall consistent with IMH, focal intimal thickening, and ULP.[78] TEE demonstrates aortic atherosclerosis with focal ulceration of the intima, often with hematoma (see Fig. 42.27).[78,84]

PAUs have an uncertain natural history, with variability in the literature depending on patient selection. A PAU may "stabilize" or lead to complications, including IMH, distal embolization, aortic rupture, pseudoaneurysm (contained rupture), aortic dissection, or development of a saccular or fusiform aneurysm.[1] Larger and deeper ulcers and those with saccular aneurysms are often progressive and associated IMH carries a worse prognosis.[83] Some studies report gradual aortic enlargement and a low incidence of life-threatening complications, whereas others report a high incidence of acute complications.[1,78,83] In general, patients with ascending PAUs undergo surgical resection. Stable patients with type B PAUs may be managed medically, with close follow-up and serial imaging. When an asymptomatic PAU is discovered, serial imaging studies are required to document stability.[1,83] Patients with refractory or recurrent pain, overlying IMH or periaortic hemorrhage, or rapid increase in size are at increased risk of rupture and should undergo TEVAR, if feasible.[1,23,48,83] Indications for TEVAR (or less often, surgery) may include hemorrhage, periaortic hematoma, expanding pseudoaneurysm, saccular aneurysm formation, continued pain, or rupture. Predictors of disease progression include increasing aortic wall thickness, ulcer craters greater than 15 to 20 mm in diameter or greater than 10 mm in depth, increasing aortic hematoma, and increasing pleural effusion.[23,78,83] The short segment involved and the high-risk patient population make TEVAR preferred over OSR.[23,83] In-hospital mortality in TEVAR-treated descending aortic PAU is 4% to 11%.[85] Endoleak risk may be mitigated using endovascular techniques.[85]

AORTOARTERITIS SYNDROMES

Bacterial Infections of the Aorta (see Chapter 80)

Infected aortic aneurysms (*mycotic aneurysms*) are a rare but lethal condition and account for 0.6% to 2% of all aortic aneurysms.[86] Infection may result from contiguous spread from adjacent tissues, such as mediastinitis, abscess, infected lymph nodes, empyema, or paravertebral abscess. Other causes include septic emboli from endocarditis and hematogenous dissemination of bacteria in the setting of sepsis or IV drug abuse. Infection most often arises in a diseased aorta, whether aneurysmal, atherosclerotic, or traumatized from previous aortic cannulation or suturing. Although the disease may be insidious in onset, it may also be fulminant with frequent aneurysm rupture (44%) and a high mortality rate (>25% to 50%).[86]

The classic triad of an infected aortic aneurysm includes fever (67%); pain (77%) in the abdomen, back, or chest; and a pulsatile tender mass, but only a minority present with this triad.[87] Patients have elevated markers of inflammation. Bacteremia is common (present in 50% to 75%), but blood cultures may be negative, especially after antibiotics, and in some the organism is established only during surgery by culture and Gram stain of the aortic wall.[86,88] Patients often have comorbid conditions, including diabetes, immunocompromised states (41%), or chronic steroid therapy. Many have recently undergone gastrointestinal operations or invasive procedures. Infected aneurysms most commonly involve the infrarenal aorta (60%) and the descending aorta.[86,88] Infected TAAs are less common, most commonly affect

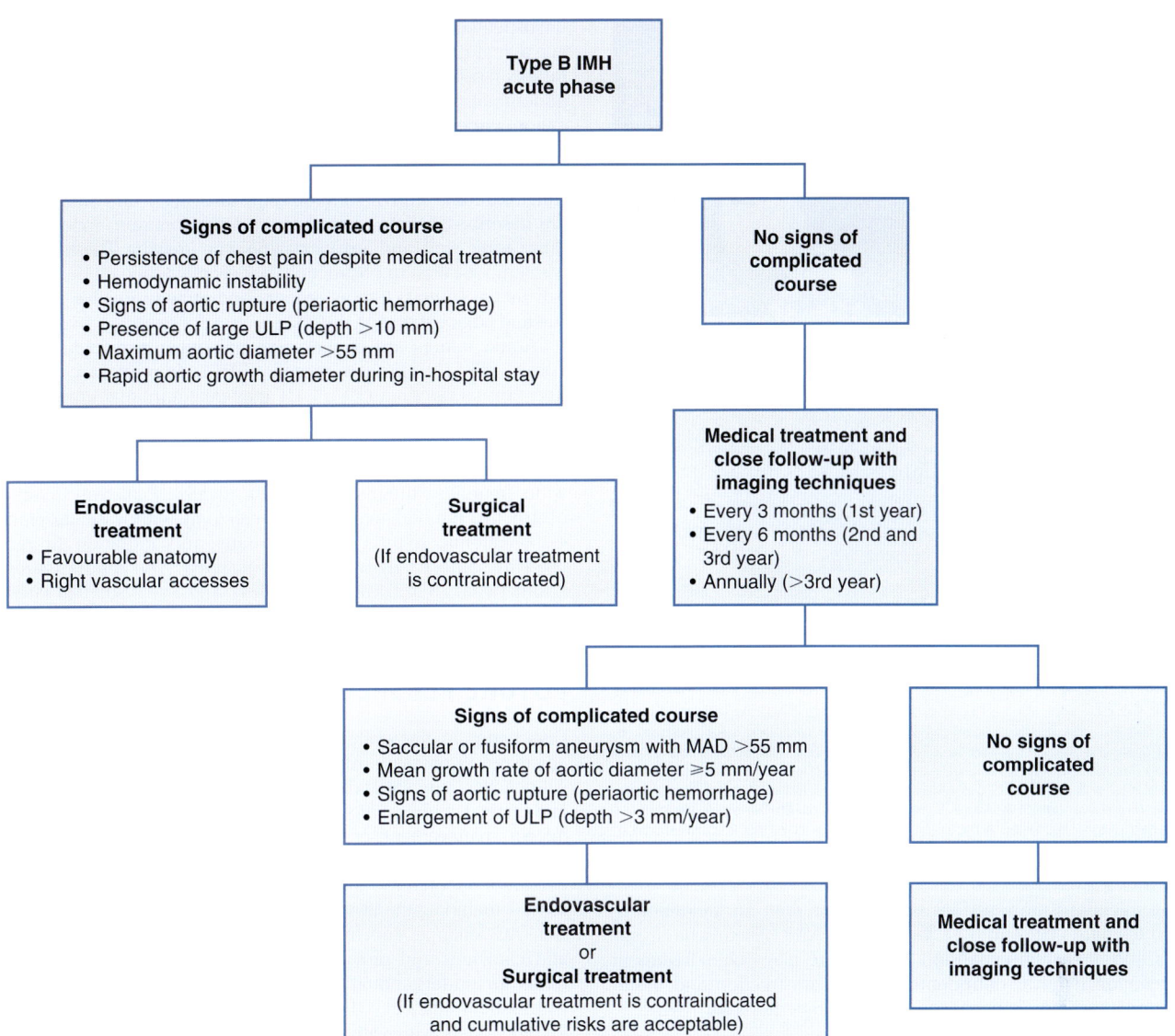

FIGURE 42.26 Acute and chronic management pathway for type B intramural hematoma (IMH). *MAD,* Maximum aortic diameter; *ULP,* ulcer-like projection. (From Evangelista A, Czerny M, Nienaber C, et al. Interdisciplinary expert consensus on management of type B intramural haematoma and penetrating aortic ulcer. *Eur J Cardiothorac Surg.* 2015;47[2]:209–217.)

the descending aorta, and are often accompanied by rupture (in 44%) or pseudoaneurysm.[86]

The most common microorganisms associated with infected aortic aneurysms include *Staphylococcus aureus,* streptococcal, and *Salmonella* species, but infections with gram-negative bacilli and fungi can occur.[86,87] *Salmonella* may directly penetrate an intact intima of a normal aortic wall and lead to arteritis and aneurysm formation. Thus, suspicion for aortic seeding is prudent when *Salmonella* bacteremia occurs.

CT, MRI, and aortography may be diagnostic in patients with infected aortic aneurysms (Fig. 42.28).[2,86] Saccular aneurysms due to rapid focal arterial wall degeneration are present in greater than 90%.[70,86] Features on CT include disruption of calcification, irregular wall thickening, periaortic mass, rim enhancement, and periaortic stranding. The presence of gas and vertebral body erosion is highly suggestive of infection. MRI features of infected aneurysms include a soft tissue mass, stranding, and rim enhancement. Radiotraced WBC scans may be suggestive of infection. Fluorodeoxyglucose positron emission tomography (FDG-PET) may assist in diagnosing mycotic aneurysms and graft infections by detecting hypermetabolic activity and can monitor response to antibiotic therapy.[86]

Untreated infected aortic aneurysms generally expand and eventually rupture, often with rapid progression. *Salmonella* and other gram-negative infections have a greater tendency for early rupture and death. Overall mortality from infected aortic aneurysms ranges from 50% to 100% with medical therapy alone.[86] OSR of infected AAAs involves excision and debridement or exclusion of the infected aortic tissue, revascularization (in situ or extra-anatomic bypass), and prolonged antibiotic therapy. (T)EVAR for mycotic aneurysms has been considered a temporizing measure.[20] Recently, about 60% infected aneurysms (and an even higher percentage of descending mycotic TAAs) have been treated by endovascular techniques.[86,88] Mortality rates depend upon the aortic segment infected and the surgical approach.[86,88] The 30- to 90-day mortality rates for mycotic aneurysms of the infrarenal aorta and iliac arteries was 3% to 9% for EVAR and 5% to 23% for OSR and for thoracic aortic mycotic aneurysms was 15% for TEVAR and 7% to 20% for OSR.[86,88] Subsequent graft infections complicate approximately 20% of cases with extra-anatomic bypass having worse outcomes compared to in situ repair.[86,88] While EVAR may not include debridement, EVAR was not associated with a higher rate of infections or reoperations when compared to OSR.[86,88] TEVAR for mycotic descending TAA has favorable short- and long-term survival compared to OSR cohorts (see Fig. 42.28).[88] Mycotic aneurysm associated with a 19% death rate at 6 months in one series,[87] whereas in a Swedish study, survival was 92% at 30 days, 78% at one year, and 71% at 5 years.[88] Development of microbe-resistant and antibiotic-bonded stent grafts may improve outcomes.[86]

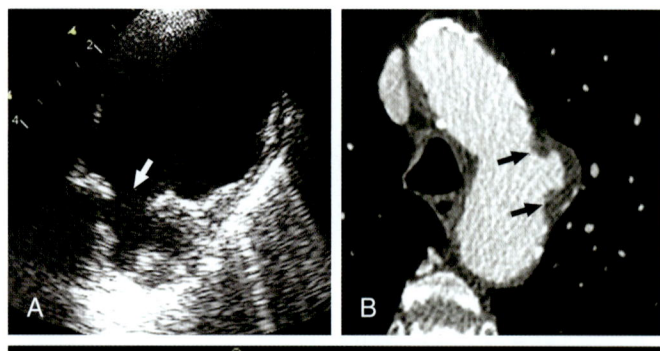
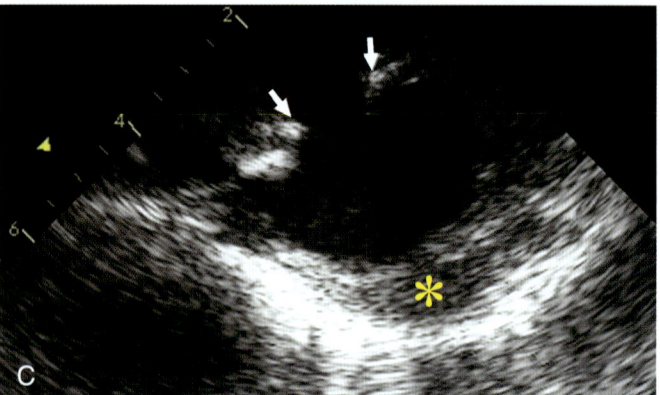

FIGURE 42.27 Penetrating atherosclerotic aortic ulcers (PAU). **A,** Transesophageal echocardiogram view in the descending thoracic aorta depicting a PAU *(arrow)*. **B,** Axial CT scan in aortic arch showing a PAU with significant atherosclerosis around the lesion *(arrows)*. **C,** Transesophageal echocardiogram view in aortic arch demonstrating a PAU with calcified edges *(arrows)* and associated intramural hemorrhage *(asterisk)*. (From Evangelista A, Moral S, Ballesteros E, Castillo-Gandía A. Beyond the term penetrating aortic ulcer: a morphologic descriptor covering a constellation of entities with different prognoses. *Prog Cardiovasc Dis.* 2020;63:488–495.)

Graft infections are a serious complication with an incidence of 0.3% to 6% after OSR and 0.2% to 1% after EVAR.[2] Pseudoaneurysm, fistulas, and aneurysm expansion and rupture may occur. Treatment includes graft removal, debridement and reconstruction and in-situ repair, or extra-anatomic bypass and possible omentoplasty.[2]

PRIMARY TUMORS OF THE AORTA

Tumors affecting the aorta most commonly arise secondarily from direct invasion by adjacent cancer or metastases, especially from the lung and esophagus. Primary aortic sarcomas are very rare, typically unsuspected until histopathology reveals malignancy.[23,89] The average age at diagnosis is 60 years, with a male preponderance.[89] These tumors most commonly localize in the descending thoracic (38%) and abdominal (43%) aorta.[89] Symptoms include pain, embolism, claudication, visceral ischemia, or constitutional symptoms. Less commonly, these tumors may cause hemorrhage or invade adjacent structures. Metastatic disease at diagnosis (56%) is common.[89] Intimal tumors (angiosarcoma and myofibroblastic sarcomas) and mural sarcomas are described. Intimal sarcomas are most common, spread along the inner aortic wall, and appear polypoid on imaging. These may present with embolization or obstruction. Widely metastatic emboli may occur. Adventitial (mural) tumors are rare and grow to involve periaortic tissue and adjacent organs.

Aortic tumors are of mesenchymal origin and include angiosarcoma (37%), intima sarcoma (31%), leiomyosarcoma (11%), and fibrous sarcoma (7%).[89] CT may detect intimal tumors, but MRI may better differentiate between tumor and atheromatous material. If no metastases are present, resection with prosthetic graft replacement is recommended. Because of difficulty in achieving wide margins, tumors may recur locally. Palliative treatment of obstructive tumors includes endarterectomy, endovascular grafts, and extra-anatomic bypass. Chemotherapy and radiation therapy are used in some cases with limited success. The median survival is about 1 year (3 to 24 months) with 1- and 3-year survival rates being 26% and 8% respectively.[89]

FUTURE PERSPECTIVES

Discoveries in the evaluation and treatment of aortic disease have advanced through innovations in basic science, molecular and clinical genetics, surgical and endovascular therapy, translational research, and clinical studies. Targeted therapy based upon animal models may inform management of genetic aortopathies. Recent management guidelines for abdominal and thoracic aortic disease provide up-to-date information for evaluation and treatment. Large registries and consortia—including the IRAD, GERAADA, Montalcino Aortic Consortium, GenTAC Alliance, and others—bring together stakeholders, scientists, and clinicians and provide important clinical and translational platforms for understanding of aortic disease. International partnerships with patient advocacy organizations improve awareness and support for individuals living with aortic disease.

Advanced imaging platforms to understand the biology and biomechanics of the aortic wall, improvements in endovascular techniques to allow treatment of complex conditions, and enhanced awareness of the important genetic component of aortic aneurysm (and dissection) disease will lead to further increases in the quality of life and lifespan for individuals and families with aortic disease.

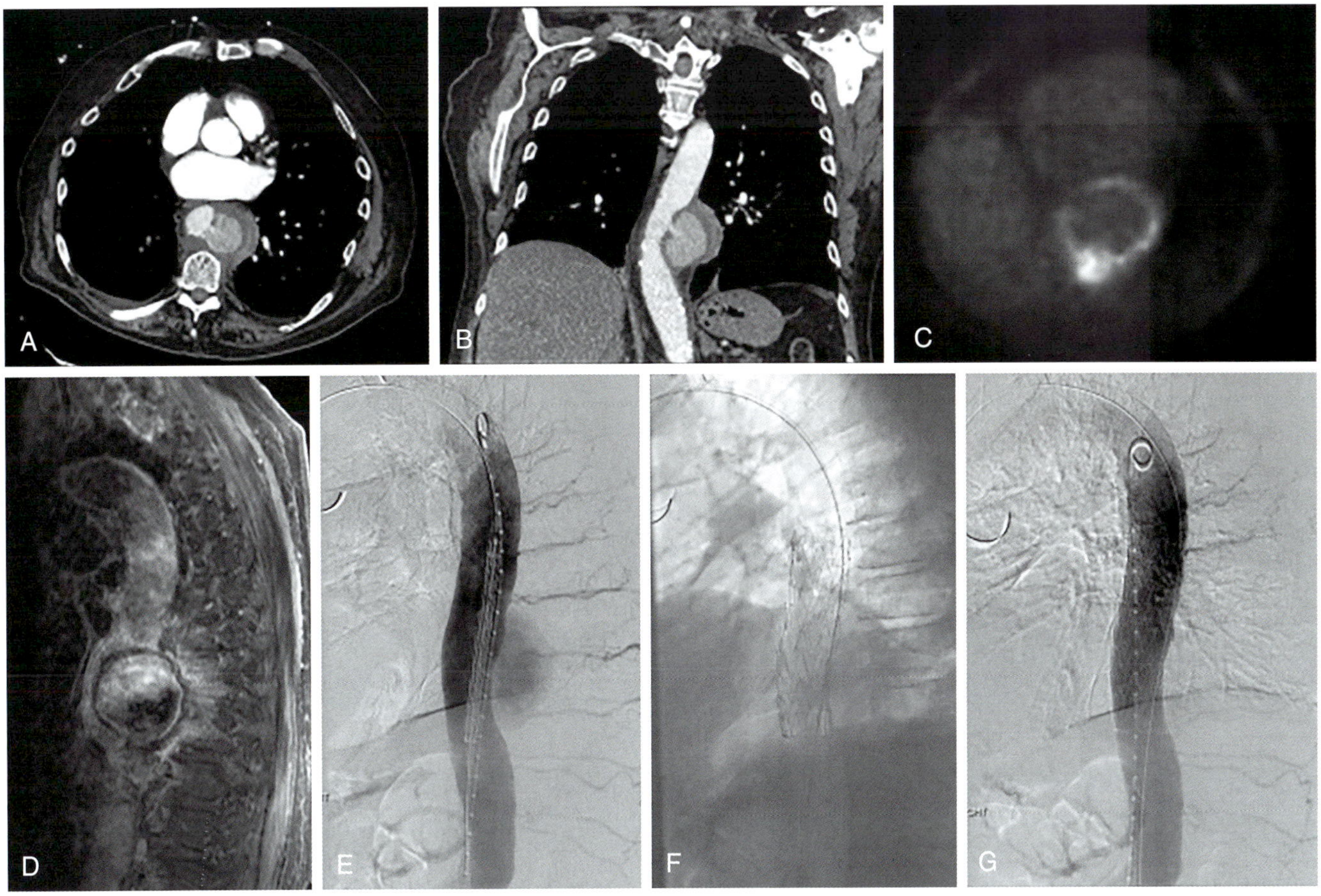

FIGURE 42.28 Example of mycotic aortic aneurysm treated with endovascular repair. Axial **(A)** and coronal **(B)** contrast-enhanced CT images demonstrate a focal saccular outpouching, with surrounding inflammatory changes and rupture. **C,** Positron emission tomography CT demonstrates uptake in the aortic wall and in an adjacent vertebral body concerning for extension of infection. **D,** Sagittal T2-weighted MRI shows high signal in the adjacent vertebrae and discs, consistent with associated discitis-osteomyelitis. Again, MA is shown as a focal saccular outpouching with inflammatory changes. **E,** Aortogram demonstrates filling of the focal outpouching in the distal thoracic aorta. A stent graft is in position, just prior to being deployed. **F,** The covered stent has been deployed and postdilated. **G,** Completion aortogram demonstrates exclusion of the aneurysm by the stent. (From Deipolyi AR, Bailin A, Khademhosseini A, Oklu R. Imaging findings, diagnosis, and clinical outcomes in patients with mycotic aneurysms: single center experience. *Clin Imaging.* 2016;40:512–516.)

REFERENCES

The Normal Aorta
1. Erbel R, Aboyans V, Boileau C, et al. 2014 ESC Guidelines on the diagnosis and treatment of aortic diseases: document covering acute and chronic aortic diseases of the thoracic and abdominal aorta of the adult. The Task Force for the Diagnosis and Treatment of Aortic Diseases of the European Society of Cardiology (ESC). *Eur Heart J.* 2014;35(41):2873–2926.

Aortic Aneurysms
2. Wanhainen A, Verzini F, Van Herzeele I, et al. Editor's choice—European Society for Vascular Surgery (ESVS) 2019 clinical practice guidelines on the management of abdominal aorto-iliac artery aneurysms. *Eur J Vasc Endovasc Surg.* 2019;57(1):8–93.
3. Chaikof EL, Dalman RL, Eskandari MK, et al. The Society for Vascular Surgery practice guidelines on the care of patients with an abdominal aortic aneurysm. *J Vasc Surg.* 2018;67(1):2–77.e72.
4. Golledge J. Abdominal aortic aneurysm: update on pathogenesis and medical treatments. *Nat Rev Cardiol.* 2019;16(4):225–242.
5. Davis FM, Rateri DL, Daugherty A. Mechanisms of aortic aneurysm formation: translating preclinical studies into clinical therapies. *Heart.* 2014;100(19):1498–1505.
6. Baxter BT, Matsumura J, Curci JA, et al. Effect of doxycycline on aneurysm growth among patients with small infrarenal abdominal aortic aneurysms: a randomized clinical trial. *J Am Med Assoc.* 2020;323(20):2029–2038.
7. Pinard A, Jones GT, Milewicz DM. Genetics of thoracic and abdominal aortic diseases. *Circ Res.* 2019;124(4):588–606.
8. O'Donnell TFX, Deery SE, Shean KE, et al. Statin therapy is associated with higher long-term but not perioperative survival after abdominal aortic aneurysm repair. *J Vasc Surg.* 2018;68(2):392–399.
9. Schermerhorn ML, Buck DB, O'Malley AJ, et al. Long-term outcomes of abdominal aortic aneurysm in the Medicare population. *N Engl J Med.* 2015;373(4):328–338.
10. Moll FL, Powell JT, Fraedrich G, et al. Management of abdominal aortic aneurysms clinical practice guidelines of the European society for Vascular Surgery. *Eur J Vasc Endovasc Surg.* 2011;41(suppl 1):S1–S58.
11. Churchill TW, Groezinger E, Kim JH, et al. Association of ascending aortic dilatation and long-term endurance exercise among older masters-level athletes. *JAMA Cardiol.* 2020.
12. Hiratzka LF, Bakris GL, Beckman JA, et al. 2010 ACCF/AHA/AATS/ACR/ASA/SCA/SCAI/SIR/STS/SVM guidelines for the diagnosis and management of patients with thoracic aortic disease. A report of the American College of Cardiology Foundation/American Heart Association Task Force on Practice Guidelines, American Association for Thoracic Surgery, American College of Radiology, American Stroke Association, Society of Cardiovascular Anesthesiologists, Society for Cardiovascular Angiography and Interventions, Society of Interventional Radiology, Society of Thoracic Surgeons, and Society for Vascular Medicine. *J Am Coll Cardiol.* 2010;55(14):e27–e129.
13. Verhagen JMA, Kempers M, Cozijnsen L, et al. Expert consensus recommendations on the cardiogenetic care for patients with thoracic aortic disease and their first-degree relatives. *Int J Cardiol.* 2018;258:243–248.
14. Silberbach M, Roos-Hesselink JW, Andersen NH, et al. Cardiovascular health in Turner syndrome: a scientific statement from the American Heart Association. *Circ Genom Precis Med.* 2018;11(10):e000048.
15. Braverman AC. Aortic replacement for bicuspid aortic valve aortopathy: when and why? *J Thorac Cardiovasc Surg.* 2019;157(2):520–525.
16. Milewicz DM, Ramirez F. Therapies for thoracic aortic aneurysms and acute aortic dissections. *Arterioscler Thromb Vasc Biol.* 2019;39(2):126–136.
17. Hofmann Bowman MA, Eagle KA, Milewicz DM. Update on clinical trials of losartan with and without beta-blockers to block aneurysm growth in patients with Marfan syndrome: a review. *JAMA Cardiol.* 2019;4(7):702–707.
18. Jondeau G, Ropers J, Regalado E, et al. International registry of patients carrying TGFBR1 or TGFBR2 mutations: results of the MAC (Montalcino Aortic Consortium). *Circ Cardiovasc Genet.* 2016;9(6):548–558.
19. Shalhub S, Byers PH, Hicks KL, et al. A multi-institutional experience in the aortic and arterial pathology in individuals with genetically confirmed vascular Ehlers-Danlos syndrome. *J Vasc Surg.* 2019;70(5):1543–1554.
20. Upchurch Jr GR, Escobar GC, Azizzdeh A, et al. Society for vascular surgery clinical practice guidelines for thoracic endovascular aneurysm repair (TEVAR). *J Vasc Surg.* 2020.
21. Czerny M, Schmidli J, Adler S, et al. Current options and recommendations for the treatment of thoracic aortic pathologies involving the aortic arch: an expert consensus document of the European Association for Cardio-Thoracic surgery (EACTS) and the European Society for Vascular Surgery (ESVS). *Eur J Cardio Thorac Surg.* 2019;55(1):133–162.
22. Bhave NM, Nienaber CA, Clough RE, Eagle KA. Multimodality imaging of thoracic aortic diseases in adults. *JACC Cardiovasc Imaging.* 2018;11(6):902–919.
23. Riambau V, Bockler D, Brunkwall J, et al. Editor's choice—management of descending thoracic aorta diseases: clinical practice guidelines of the European Society for Vascular Surgery (ESVS). *Eur J Vasc Endovasc Surg.* 2017;53(1):4–52.
24. Oladokun D, Patterson BO, Sobocinski J, et al. Systematic review of the growth rates and influencing factors in thoracic aortic aneurysms. *Eur J Vasc Endovasc Surg.* 2016;51(5):674–681.
25. Zafar MA, Chen JF, Wu J, et al. Natural history of descending thoracic and thoracoabdominal aortic aneurysms. *J Thorac Cardiovasc Surg.* 2019.
26. Zafar MA, Li Y, Rizzo, et al. Height alone, rather than body surface area, suffices for risk estimation in ascending aortic aneurysm. *J Thorac Cardiovasc Surg.* 2018;155(5):1938–1950.
27. Milleron O, Arnoult F, Delorme G, et al. Pathogenic FBN1 genetic variation and aortic dissection in patients with marfan syndrome. *J Am Coll Cardiol.* 2020;75(8):843–853.
28. Martin C, Evangelista A, Serrano-Fiz S, et al. Aortic complications in Marfan syndrome: should we anticipate preventive aortic root surgery? *Ann Thorac Surg.* 2020;109(6):1850–1857.
29. Wu J, Zafar MA, Li Y, et al. Ascending aortic length and risk of aortic adverse events: the neglected dimension. *J Am Coll Cardiol.* 2019;74(15):1883–1894.
30. Borger MA, Fedak PWM, Stephens EH, et al. The American Association for Thoracic Surgery consensus guidelines on bicuspid aortic valve-related aortopathy: full online-only version. *J Thorac Cardiovasc Surg.* 2018;156(2):e41–e74.

31. Hiratzka LF, Creager MA, Isselbacher EM, et al. Surgery for aortic dilatation in patients with bicuspid aortic valves: a statement of clarification from the American College of Cardiology/American Heart Association Task Force on Clinical Practice Guidelines. *J Am Coll Cardiol.* 2016;67(6):724–731.
32. Trimarchi S, de Beaufort HWL, Tolenaar JL, et al. Acute aortic dissections with entry tear in the arch: a report from the International Registry of Acute Aortic Dissection. *J Thorac Cardiovasc Surg.* 2019;157(1):66–73.
33. David TE. Aortic valve sparing in different aortic valve and aortic root conditions. *J Am Coll Cardiol.* 2016;68(6):654–664.
34. Izgi C, Newsome S, Alpendurada F, et al. External aortic root support to prevent aortic dilatation in patients with marfan syndrome. *J Am Coll Cardiol.* 2018;72(10):1095–1105.
35. Mazine A, El-Hamamsy I, Verma S, et al. Ross procedure in adults for cardiologists and cardiac surgeons: JACC state-of-the-art review. *J Am Coll Cardiol.* 2018;72(22):2761–2777.
36. Pellenc Q, Girault A, Roussel A, et al. Optimising aortic endovascular repair in patients with marfan syndrome. *Eur J Vasc Endovasc Surg.* 2020;59(4):577–585.
37. Lee CC, Lee MG, Hsieh R, et al. Oral fluoroquinolone and the risk of aortic dissection. *J Am Coll Cardiol.* 2018;72(12):1369–1378.
38. Chaddha A, Eagle KA, Braverman AC, et al. Exercise and physical activity for the post-aortic dissection patient: the clinician's conundrum. *Clin Cardiol.* 2015;38(11):647–651.
39. Braverman AC, Harris KM, Kovacs RJ, et al. Eligibility and disqualification recommendations for competitive athletes with cardiovascular abnormalities: Task force 7: aortic diseases, including marfan syndrome: a scientific statement from the American Heart Association and American College of Cardiology. *Circulation.* 2015;132(22):e303–e309.
40. Braverman AC, Mittauer E, Harris KM, et al. Aortic dissection related to pregnancy: results from the International Registry of Acute Aortic Dissection (IRAD). *JAMA Cardiol.* 2020 (in press).

Aortic Dissection

41. Evangelista A, Isselbacher EM, Bossone E, et al. Insights from the international registry of acute aortic dissection: a 20-year experience of collaborative clinical research. *Circulation.* 2018;137(17):1846–1860.
42. Bossone E, LaBounty TM, Eagle KA. Acute aortic syndromes: diagnosis and management, an update. *Eur Heart J.* 2018;39(9):739d–749d.
43. Mussa FF, Horton JD, Moridzadeh R, et al. Acute aortic dissection and intramural hematoma: a systematic review. *J Am Med Assoc.* 2016;316(7):754–763.
44. Gudbjartsson T, Ahlsson A, Geirsson A, et al. Acute type A aortic dissection—a review. *Scand Cardiovasc J.* 2020;54(1):1–13.
45. DeMartino RR, Sen I, Huang Y, et al. Population-based assessment of the incidence of aortic dissection, intramural hematoma, and penetrating ulcer, and its associated mortality from 1995 to 2015. *Circ Cardiovasc Qual Outcomes.* 2018;11(8):e004689.
46. Booher AM, Isselbacher EM, Nienaber CA, et al. The IRAD classification system for characterizing survival after aortic dissection. *Am J Med.* 2013;126(8):730.e719-e724.
47. Sievers HH, Rylski B, Czerny M, et al. Aortic dissection reconsidered: type, entry site, malperfusion classification adding clarity and enabling outcome prediction. *Interact Cardiovasc Thorac Surg.* 2020;30(3):451–457.
48. Lombardi JV, Hughes GC, Appoo JJ, et al. Society for Vascular Surgery (SVS) and Society of Thoracic Surgeons (STS) reporting standards for type B aortic dissections. *Ann Thorac Surg.* 2020;109(3):959–981.
49. den Hartog AW, Franken R, Zwinderman AH, et al. The risk for type B aortic dissection in Marfan syndrome. *J Am Coll Cardiol.* 2015;65(3):246–254.
50. de Beaufort HWL, Trimarchi S, Korach A, et al. Aortic dissection in patients with Marfan syndrome based on the IRAD data. *Ann Cardiothorac Surg.* 2017;6(6):633–641.
51. Kreibich M, Rylski B, Czerny M, et al. Type A aortic dissection in patients with bicuspid aortic valve aortopathy. *Ann Thorac Surg.* 2020;109(1):94–100.
52. Czerny M, Eggebrecht H, Rousseau H, et al. Distal stent-graft induced new entry after TEVAR or FET—insights into a new disease from EuREC. *Ann Thorac Surg.* 2020.
53. Philip S, Missov E, Gilon D, et al. Head and neck pain in patients presenting with acute aortic dissection. *Aorta (Stamford).* 2018;6(6):130–138.
54. Tadros RO, Tang GHL, Barnes HJ, et al. Optimal treatment of uncomplicated type B aortic dissection: JACC review topic of the week. *J Am Coll Cardiol.* 2019;74(11):1494–1504.
55. Patel PA, Bavaria JE, Ghadimi K, et al. Aortic regurgitation in acute type-A aortic dissection: a clinical classification for the perioperative echocardiographer in the era of the functional aortic annulus. *J Cardiothorac Vasc Anesth.* 2018;32(1):586–597.
56. Carroll BJ, Schermerhorn ML, Manning WJ. Imaging for acute aortic syndromes. *Heart.* 2020;106(3):182–189.
57. Conzelmann LO, Weigang E, Mehlhorn U, et al. Mortality in patients with acute aortic dissection type A: analysis of pre- and intraoperative risk factors from the German Registry for Acute Aortic Dissection Type A (GERAADA). *Eur J Cardio Thorac Surg.* 2016;49(2):e44–e52.
58. Sultan I, Bianco V, Patel HJ, et al. Surgery for type A aortic dissection in patients with cerebral malperfusion: results from the international registry of acute aortic dissection. *J Thorac Cardiovasc Surg.* 2019.
59. Zhu QY, Tai S, Tang L, et al. STEMI could be the primary presentation of acute aortic dissection. *Am J Emerg Med.* 2017;35(11):1713–1717.
60. Nazerian P, Mueller C, Soeiro AM, et al. Diagnostic accuracy of the aortic dissection detection risk score plus D-dimer for acute aortic syndromes: the ADvISED prospective multicenter study. *Circulation.* 2018;137(3):250–258.
61. Kreibich M, Bavaria JE, Branchetti E, et al. Management of patients with coronary artery malperfusion secondary to type A aortic dissection. *Ann Thorac Surg.* 2019;107(4):1174–1180.
62. Rogers AM, Hermann LK, Booher AM, et al. Sensitivity of the aortic dissection detection risk score, a novel guideline-based tool for identification of acute aortic dissection at initial presentation: results from the international registry of acute aortic dissection. *Circulation.* 2011;123(20):2213–2218.
63. Umana-Pizano JB, Nissen AP, Sandhu HK, et al. Acute type A dissection repair by high-volume vs low-volume surgeons at a high-volume Aortic center. *Ann Thorac Surg.* 2019;108(5):1330–1336.
64. Cruz I, Stuart B, Caldeira D, et al. Controlled pericardiocentesis in patients with cardiac tamponade complicating aortic dissection: experience of a centre without cardiothoracic surgery. *Eur Heart J Acute Cardiovasc Care.* 2015;4(2):124–128.
65. Nakai C, Izumi S, Haraguchi T, et al. Long-term outcomes after controlled pericardial drainage for acute type A aortic dissection. *Ann Thorac Surg.* 2020.
66. Czerny M, Siepe M, Beyersdorf F, et al. Prediction of mortality rate in acute type A dissecti case ID: 00562704 and 00571627on: the German Registry for Acute Type A aortic dissection score. *Eur J Cardio Thorac Surg.* 2020.
67. Bossone E, Pyeritz RE, Braverman AC, et al. Shock complicating type A acute aortic dissection: clinical correlates, management, and outcomes. *Am Heart J.* 2016;176:93–99.
68. Roselli EE, Idrees JJ, Johnston DR, et al. Zone zero thoracic endovascular aortic repair: a proposed modification to the classification of landing zones. *J Thorac Cardiovasc Surg.* 2018;155(4):1381–1389.
69. Nauta F, de Beaufort H, Mussa FF, et al. Management of retrograde type A IMH with acute arch tear/type B dissection. *Ann Cardiothorac Surg.* 2019;8(5):531–539.
70. Tolenaar JL, Froehlich W, Jonker FH, et al. Predicting in-hospital mortality in acute type B aortic dissection: evidence from International Registry of Acute Aortic Dissection. *Circulation.* 2014;130(11 suppl 1):S45–S50.
71. Pape LA, Awais M, Woznicki EM, et al. Presentation, diagnosis, and outcomes of acute aortic dissection: 17-year trends from the International Registry of Acute Aortic Dissection. *J Am Coll Cardiol.* 2015;66(4):350–358.
72. Nienaber CA, Clough RE. Management of acute aortic dissection. *Lancet.* 2015;385(9970):800–811.
73. Rylski B, Perez M, Beyersdorf F, et al. Acute non-A non-B aortic dissection: incidence, treatment and outcome. *Eur J Cardio Thorac Surg.* 2017;52(6):1111–1117.
74. Yang B, Rosati CM, Norton EL, et al. Endovascular fenestration/stenting first followed by delayed open aortic repair for acute type A aortic dissection with malperfusion syndrome. *Circulation.* 2018;138(19):2091–2103.
75. El-Hamamsy I, Ouzounian M, Demers P, et al. State-of-the-art surgical management of acute type A aortic dissection. *Can J Cardiol.* 2016;32(1):100–109.
76. Kamman AV, de Beaufort HW, van Bogerijen GH, et al. Contemporary management strategies for chronic type B aortic dissections: a systematic review. *PLoS One.* 2016;11(5):e0154930.
77. Kim WK, Park SJ, Kim HJ, et al. The fate of unrepaired chronic type A aortic dissection. *J Thorac Cardiovasc Surg.* 2019;158(4):996–1004 e1003.

Aortic Dissection Variants

78. Evangelista A, Maldonado G, Moral S, et al. Intramural hematoma and penetrating ulcer in the descending aorta: differences and similarities. *Ann Cardiothorac Surg.* 2019;8(4):456–470.
79. Moral S, Cuellar H, Avegliano G, et al. Clinical implications of focal intimal disruption in patients with type B intramural hematoma. *J Am Coll Cardiol.* 2017;69(1):28–39.
80. Maslow A, Atalay MK, Sodha N. Intramural hematoma. *J Cardiothorac Vasc Anesth.* 2018;32(3):1341–1362.
81. Evangelista A, Czerny M, Nienaber C, et al. Interdisciplinary expert consensus on management of type B intramural haematoma and penetrating aortic ulcer. *Eur J Cardio Thorac Surg.* 2015;47(2):209–217.
82. Harris KM, Braverman AC, Eagle KA, et al. Acute aortic intramural hematoma: an analysis from the International Registry of Acute Aortic Dissection. *Circulation.* 2012;126(11 suppl 1):S91–S96.
83. Oderich GS, Karkkainen JM, Reed NR, et al. Penetrating aortic ulcer and intramural hematoma. *Cardiovasc Intervent Radiol.* 2019;42(3):321–334.
84. Evangelista A, Moral S, Ballesteros E, Castillo-Gandia A. Beyond the term penetrating aortic ulcer: a morphologic descriptor covering a constellation of entities with different prognoses. *Prog Cardiovasc Dis.* 2020.
85. Janosi RA, Gorla R, Tsagakis K, et al. Thoracic endovascular repair of complicated penetrating aortic ulcer: an 11-year single-center experience. *J Endovasc Ther.* 2016;23(1):150–159.

Aortoarteritis Syndromes and Primary Tumors of the Aorta

86. Sorelius K, Budtz-Lilly J, Mani K, Wanhainen A. Systematic review of the management of mycotic aortic aneurysms. *Eur J Vasc Endovasc Surg.* 2019;58(3):426–435.
87. Deipolyi AR, Bailin A, Khademhosseini A, Oklu R. Imaging findings, diagnosis, and clinical outcomes in patients with mycotic aneurysms: single center experience. *Clin Imaging.* 2016;40(3):512–516.
88. Sorelius K, Wanhainen A, Wahlgren CM, et al. Nationwide study on treatment of mycotic thoracic aortic aneurysms. *Eur J Vasc Endovasc Surg.* 2019;57(2):239–246.
89. Vacirca A, Faggioli G, Pini R, et al. Predictors of survival in malignant aortic tumors. *J Vasc Surg.* 2020;71(5):1771–1780.

43 Peripheral Artery Diseases

MARC P. BONACA AND MARK A. CREAGER

EPIDEMIOLOGY, 837
Risk Factors for Peripheral Artery Disease, 838
Pathophysiology of Peripheral Artery Disease, 838
Skeletal Muscle Structure and Metabolic Function, 839

CLINICAL FEATURES, 840
Symptoms, 840
Physical Findings, 841
Categorization, 841

TESTING FOR PERIPHERAL ARTERY DISEASE, 842
Segmental Pressure Measurement, 842
Ankle-Brachial Index, 843
Treadmill Exercise Testing, 843
Pulse Volume Recording, 843
Doppler Ultrasonography, 844
Duplex Ultrasound Imaging, 844
Magnetic Resonance Angiography, 844
Computed Tomographic Angiography, 845
Contrast-Enhanced Angiography, 845

OTHER MEASUREMENT TOOLS, 845

PROGNOSIS, 845

TREATMENT, 847
Risk Factor Modification, 847
Diet, 847
Smoking Cessation, 847
Treatment of Diabetes, 847
Lipid-Lowering Therapy, 848
Antithrombotic Therapy for Reduction of Major Adverse Cardiovascular and Limb Events, 848

TREATMENT OF SYMPTOMS AND PREVENTION OF LIMB VASCULAR EVENTS, 849
Smoking Cessation, 849
Supervised and Home-Based Exercise Training, 850
Pharmacotherapy to Improve Claudication, 850
Percutaneous Transluminal Angioplasty and Stents, 851

Peripheral Artery Surgery, 851

VASCULITIS, 851
Thromboangiitis Obliterans, 851

TAKAYASU ARTERITIS AND GIANT CELL ARTERITIS, 853
Fibromuscular Dysplasia, 853

POPLITEAL ARTERY ENTRAPMENT SYNDROME, 853

ACUTE LIMB ISCHEMIA, 854
Prognosis, 854
Pathogenesis, 854
Diagnostic Tests, 854
Treatment, 854

ATHEROEMBOLISM, 855
Pathogenesis, 855
Clinical Features, 856

ACKNOWLEDGEMENT, 856

REFERENCES, 856

Peripheral artery disease (PAD) generally refers to acute or chronic obstruction of the arteries supplying the lower or upper extremities that, when severe, results in downstream ischemia and potentially tissue loss.[1,2] Most often caused by atherosclerosis, PAD may also result from thrombosis, embolism, vasculitis, fibromuscular dysplasia (FMD), or entrapment. The term *peripheral vascular disease* is less specific because it encompasses a group of diseases affecting blood vessels that include other atherosclerotic conditions, such as renal artery disease and carotid artery disease, as well as vasculitides, vasospasm, venous thrombosis, venous insufficiency, and lymphatic disorders.

The primary morbidity in patients with PAD relates to limb symptoms and ischemic limb complications including intermittent claudication, chronic critical limb ischemia (CLI), acute limb ischemia (ALI), and tissue loss.[3–5] The majority of patients with PAD suffer from functional limitation even though a minority report typical claudication.[2] This limb morbidity impacts quality of life and independence and, in its severe forms, associates with increased mortality.[6,7] In addition to limb morbidity, patients with atherosclerotic PAD have a heightened risk of major adverse cardiovascular events (MACEs) similar to patients with prior myocardial infarction or stroke, and this risk is increased in patients with symptomatic disease in multiple territories, called polyvascular disease.[8–10]

Due to lower rates of public recognition relative to coronary artery disease (CAD) and stroke as well as underrecognition of atypical claudication symptoms, PAD is underdiagnosed. A telephone survey of more than 2500 people found that only 26% knew about PAD relative to more than 65% who were familiar with coronary heart disease, stroke, and heart failure and only 14% recognized that PAD could lead to amputation.[2] Even in patients with a diagnosis of PAD, preventive therapies are underused overall and relative to patients with CAD.[11] These observations may explain in part why rates of CLI and related hospitalizations are stable or increasing.[12] Clinicians treating patients with PAD not only must be skilled in application of strategies to reduce systemic ischemic risk but also must know how to characterize the severity of limb disease and use therapies to optimize function and reduce the risk of tissue loss. This chapter provides a framework for the diagnosis and management of patients with PAD.

EPIDEMIOLOGY

The prevalence of PAD varies according to the population studied, the diagnostic method used, and whether symptoms are included to derive estimates. Most epidemiologic studies have used a noninvasive measurement, the *ankle-brachial index* (ABI), to diagnose PAD. The ABI is the ratio of ankle to brachial systolic blood pressure (SBP) (see later). The prevalence of PAD based on abnormal ABI values ranges from approximately 6% in persons 40 years and older to 15% to 20% in those 65 years and older.[7,13] Claims data suggest that the annual incidence and prevalence of PAD are 2.69% and 12.02%, respectively.[14] PAD affects some 8 to 10 million individuals in the United States and more than 200 million people worldwide.[6] The prevalence of PAD is greater in men than in women in most studies. Taking into consideration the total number of women and men in the U.S. population, however, there are more women than men with PAD.[6,7] Blacks have a higher prevalence of PAD than non-Hispanic whites, as well as higher rates of amputation.[6]

Questionnaires specifically designed to elicit symptoms of intermittent claudication can serve to assess the prevalence of symptomatic disease in these populations. Overall, the estimated prevalence of claudication ranges from 1.0% to 4.5% in a population older than 40 years.[1,2,7] The prevalence and incidence of claudication increase with age and are greater in men than in women in most studies.[15] Estimates vary by age and sex but generally indicate that 10% to 30% of patients with PAD have claudication. The incidence of CLI is approximately 0.35%, and the prevalence is 1.33% in an insured population, with an annualized incidence of CLI in patients with known PAD of 11.08%.[6,12,14,16] The incidence of ALI in patients with PAD is estimated to be approximately 1% to 2% per year, with higher rates in patients with a history of lower extremity

Risk Factors for Peripheral Artery Disease

The well-known modifiable risk factors associated with coronary atherosclerosis also contribute to atherosclerosis of the peripheral arteries; however, the impact of risk predictors is not identical (see Chapter 25).[6] Risk factors are listed in Table 43.1. For example, cigarette smoking has an age- and sex-adjusted odds ratio (OR) of 3.94 for PAD and 1.66 for coronary heart disease. Smoking, type 2 diabetes mellitus (DM), hypertension, and hypercholesterolemia account for about 75% of the risk of developing PAD. Other risk factors include inflammation as measured by C-reactive protein (CRP), chronic kidney disease (CKD), diet, and sedentary lifestyle. Data from several observational studies indicate a twofold to fourfold increase in the prevalence of PAD in current smokers in comparison to never smokers, with smoking cessation associated with better outcomes. In the Women's Health Study, the hazard ratio for incident symptomatic PAD in smokers of more than 15 cigarettes per day was 17 (95% confidence interval [CI] 11 to 27); the risk decreased following smoking cessation.

Diabetes and metabolic syndrome similarly associate strongly with incident PAD.[6,20] Diet also associates with incident PAD.[21] Patients with DM often have extensive and severe PAD and a greater propensity for distal disease and arterial calcification. Involvement of the femoral and popliteal arteries resembles that in nondiabetic persons, but distal disease affecting the tibial and peroneal arteries occurs more frequently. Among patients with PAD, diabetic patients are more likely than nondiabetic patients to have CLI or to undergo an amputation, and microvascular disease may be a compounding problem to conduit artery disease in this population.[22,23] In addition, concomitant DM independently associates with increased MACE risk in patients with PAD even after adjusting for other risk factors.[24]

Abnormalities in lipid metabolism associate with PAD. Elevations in total or low-density lipoprotein (LDL) cholesterol increase the risk for PAD and claudication in most studies.[1,2,25] Hypertriglyceridemia predicts risk for PAD when considered as an independent variable, but its effect diminishes when adjusted for other lipid fractions.[7,16] In addition, lipoprotein(a) associates with both incident PAD as well as higher risk of adverse limb outcomes and amputation in patients with PAD.[26-28]

The pathobiology of PAD involves inflammation, as does atherosclerosis in other tissue beds; however, inflammation may be increased in PAD patients beyond that observed in stable CAD.[29,30] High concentrations of fibrinogen associate with an increased risk of developing PAD, most likely a reflection of increased inflammation rather than a procoagulant effect. Levels of leukocyte adhesion molecules and characteristics of leukocyte-platelet aggregates correlate with the development and extent of PAD.[31-34] Levels of CRP, monocytes, and lipoprotein-associated phospholipase A_2 in peripheral blood are independently associated with PAD, consistent with a role of innate immunity and chronic inflammation in its pathogenesis.[31,33–35] Inflammation provides the mechanistic link between many of the common risk factors for atherosclerosis and the pathophysiologic processes in the arterial wall that lead to PAD (see also Chapter 24).

Genetic factors affect both incident PAD and adverse outcomes in PAD. Monogenic diseases relating to lipid metabolism and homocysteine associate with PAD. In addition, genome-wide association studies (GWASs) have identified several loci associated with PAD including 9p21 and DAB2 interaction protein (DAB21P).[36] A large study involving the Million Veteran Program and replicated in the UK biobank identified 19 autosomal dominant loci including four variants that appeared specific for PAD (relative to coronary or cerebrovascular disease) including F5 p.R506Q, known to be associated with thrombosis risk.[37]

Pathophysiology of Peripheral Artery Disease

Intermittent claudication results from an oxygen (O_2) supply-demand mismatch analogous to angina in patients with stable angina. Impairment in O_2 delivery capacity coupled with dysfunction in O_2 extraction and utilization at the muscular level result in ischemic pain through activation of local sensory receptors by accumulation of lactate or other metabolites (Fig. 43.1). Patients with intermittent claudication may have single or multiple occlusive lesions in the arteries supplying the limb. Blood flow and leg O_2 consumption are normal at rest, but the obstructive lesions limit blood flow and O_2 delivery during exercise such that the metabolic needs of the exercising muscle outstrip the available supply of O_2 and nutrients. Patients with CLI typically have multiple occlusive lesions such that even the resting blood supply cannot meet the nutritional needs of the limb, leading to rest pain and tissue loss. In addition, there is considerable heterogeneity in patterns of occlusive disease including medial artery calcification and a predominance of below knee disease particularly in patients with diabetes and/or CKD.[38] In addition, there is increasing evidence that thrombosis plays a key role not only in the pathophysiology of ALI but also in the development of chronic CLI, suggesting a complex interplay between progressive atherosclerosis and subacute thrombosis leading to worsening ischemia.[39,40]

Factors Regulating Blood Supply

Flow through an artery is directly related to perfusion pressure and inversely related to vascular resistance. Stenoses reduce flow through the artery (Fig. 43.2), as described in the Poiseuille equation:

$$Q = \frac{\Delta P \pi r^4}{8 \eta l}$$

TABLE 43.1 Odds Ratio of Peripheral Artery Disease in Persons With Risk Factors

RISK FACTOR	ODDS RATIO (95% CI)
Cigarette smoking	4.46 (2.25–8.84)
Diabetes mellitus	2.71 (1.03–7.12)
Hypertension	1.75 (0.97–3.13)
Hypercholesterolemia	1.68 (1.09–2.57)
Hyperhomocysteinemia	1.92 (0.95–3.88)
Chronic kidney disease	2.00 (1.08–3.70)
Insulin resistance	2.06 (1.10–4.00)
C-reactive protein	2.20 (1.30–3.60)

Data derived from reports of the National Health and Nutrition Examination Survey (NHANES): Selvin E, Erlinger TP. Prevalence of and risk factors for peripheral arterial disease in the United States: results from NHANES, 1999–2000. *Circulation.* 2004;110:738; Pande RL, Perlstein TS, Beckman JA, Creager MA. Association of insulin resistance and inflammation with peripheral arterial disease: the National Health and Nutrition Examination Survey, 1999 to 2004. *Circulation.* 2008;118:33; O'Hare AM, Glidden DV, Fox CS, Hsu CY. High prevalence of peripheral arterial disease in persons with renal insufficiency: results from NHANES, 1999–2000. *Circulation.* 2004;109:320; and Guallar E, Silbergeld EK, Navas-Acien A, et al. Confounding of the relation between homocysteine and peripheral arterial disease by lead, cadmium, and renal function. *Am J Epidemiol.* 2006;163:700.

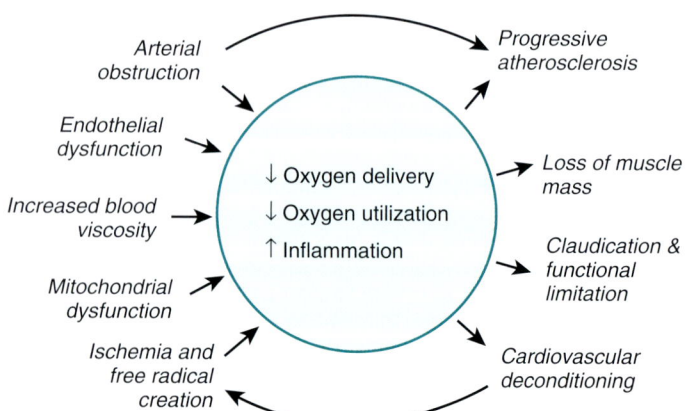

FIGURE 43.1 Mechanisms for functional limitations in PAD. (Adapted from Bonaca MP, Creager MA. Pharmacological treatment and current management of peripheral artery disease. *Circ Res.* 2015;116:1579–1598.)

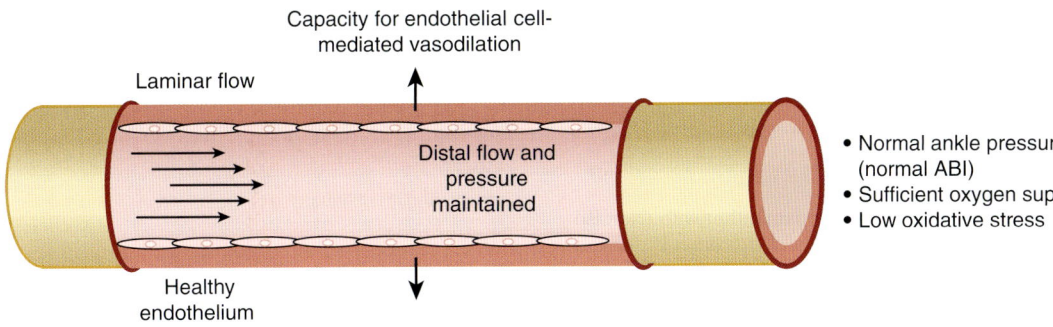

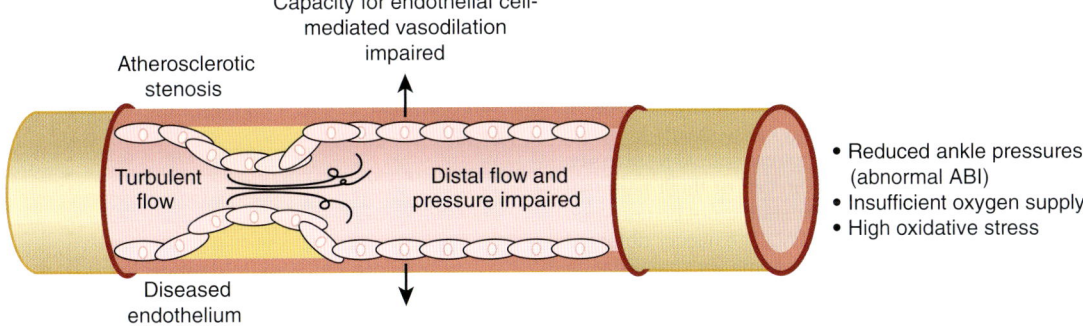

FIGURE 43.2 Effects of atherosclerotic obstruction on flow and downstream hemodynamics, oxygen supply, and oxidative stress. (Adapted from Hiatt WR, Brass EP. Pathophysiology of intermittent claudication. In: Creager MA, Beckman J, Loscalzo J, eds. *Vascular Medicine. A Companion to Braunwald's Heart Disease*. 2nd ed. Philadelphia: Elsevier; 2013.)

where ΔP is the pressure gradient across the stenosis, r is the radius of the residual lumen, η is blood viscosity, and l is the length of the vessel affected by the stenosis. As the severity of a stenotic lesion increases, flow falls progressively. The pressure gradient across the stenosis increases in a nonlinear manner, thus emphasizing the importance of a stenosis at high blood flow rates. Usually, a blood pressure (BP) gradient exists at rest if the stenosis reduces the diameter of the lumen by more than 50% because as distorted flow develops, kinetic energy is lost. A stenosis that does not cause a pressure gradient at rest may cause one during exercise when blood flow increases because of the higher cardiac output and decreased vascular resistance. Consequently, as flow through a stenosis increases, distal perfusion pressure drops. As the metabolic demand of exercising muscle outstrips its blood supply, local metabolites (including adenosine, nitric oxide [NO], potassium [K^+], and hydrogen ion [H^+]) accumulate, and peripheral resistance vessels dilate. Perfusion pressure then drops further because the stenosis limits flow. In addition, intramuscular pressure rises during exercise and may exceed the arterial pressure distal to an occlusion and halt blood flow. Flow through collateral blood vessels can usually meet the resting metabolic needs of skeletal muscle tissue at rest but does not suffice during exercise.

Functional abnormalities in vasomotor reactivity may also interfere with blood flow. Patients with peripheral atherosclerosis have reduced vasodilator capability of both conduit and resistance vessels. Normally, arteries dilate in response to pharmacologic and biochemical stimuli, such as acetylcholine, serotonin, thrombin, and bradykinin, as well as in response to shear stress induced by increases in blood flow. This vasodilator response results from the release of biologically active substances from the endothelium, particularly NO. The relaxation of a conduit vessel that occurs after a flow stimulus, such as that induced by exercise, may facilitate the delivery of blood to exercising muscles in healthy persons. The atherosclerotic femoral arteries and calf resistance vessels of patients with PAD have impaired endothelium-dependent vasodilation in response to flow or pharmacologic stimuli. This failure of vasodilation might prevent an increase in blood supply to exercising muscle because endothelium-derived NO can contribute to hyperemic blood flow after an ischemic stimulus.

Abnormalities in the microcirculation also contribute to the pathophysiology of CLI. Patients with severe limb ischemia have a reduced number of perfused skin capillaries. Observational studies have observed that microvascular disease associates with amputation independently of conduit artery disease or concomitant diabetes.[22] Other potential causes of decreased capillary perfusion in CLI include reduced red blood cell deformability, increased leukocyte adhesiveness, platelet aggregates, fibrinogen, microvascular thrombosis, excessive vasoconstriction, and interstitial edema. Intravascular pressure may also decrease because of precapillary arteriolar dilation secondary to locally released vasoactive metabolites.[41]

Skeletal Muscle Structure and Metabolic Function

Electrophysiologic and histopathologic examination has found evidence of partial axonal denervation of skeletal muscle in legs affected by PAD. Type I, oxidative slow-twitch fibers are preserved, but type II, glycolytic fast-twitch fibers are lost in the skeletal muscle of patients with PAD. The loss of type II fibers correlates with decreased muscle strength and reduced exercise capacity. In skeletal muscle distal to PAD, the shift to anaerobic metabolism occurs earlier during exercise and persists longer after exercise. Patients with claudication have increased lactate release and accumulation of acylcarnitines during exercise and slowed O_2 desaturation kinetics, indicative of ineffective oxidative metabolism. Moreover, mitochondrial respiratory activity and phosphocreatine and adenosine triphosphate (ATP) recovery time are delayed in the calf muscles of PAD patients, as assessed after submaximal exercise by ^{31}P magnetic resonance spectroscopy.[41,42]

CLINICAL FEATURES

The American College of Cardiology/American Heart Association (ACC/AHA) Guideline recommendations for clinical assessment and testing are outlined online in Tables 43G.1 to Table 43G.3 and Table 43G.6.

Symptoms

The cardinal symptoms of PAD include limb pain either with exercise (intermittent claudication) or at rest. The term *claudication* is derived from the Latin *claudicare*, "to limp." Intermittent claudication refers to a pain, ache, sense of fatigue, or other discomfort that occurs in the affected muscle group with exercise, particularly walking, and resolves with rest. The location of the symptom is often related to the site of the most proximal stenosis. Buttock, hip, or thigh claudication typically occurs in patients with obstruction of the aorta and iliac arteries. Calf claudication is caused by femoral or popliteal artery stenoses. The gastrocnemius muscle consumes more oxygen during walking than other muscle groups in the leg do and thus causes the most frequent symptoms reported by patients. Ankle or foot claudication occurs in patients with tibial and peroneal artery disease. Similarly, stenoses of the subclavian, axillary, or brachial arteries may cause shoulder, biceps, or forearm claudication, respectively. The symptoms should resolve several minutes after cessation of effort. Episodic calf or thigh pain that occurs during rest, such as nocturnal cramps, should not be confused with claudication and are not symptoms of PAD. The history obtained from persons reporting claudication should note the walking distance, speed, and incline that precipitate claudication. Such baseline assessment serves to evaluate disability and provides an initial qualitative measure with which to determine stability, improvement, or deterioration during subsequent encounters with the patient. PAD may result in functional limitations beyond those caused by pain. Patients with PAD walk more slowly and have less walking endurance than do patients without PAD.[43]

Several questionnaires serve to assess the presence and severity of claudication. The Rose Questionnaire was developed initially to diagnose both angina and intermittent claudication in epidemiologic surveys. It queries whether pain develops in either calf with walking and whether the pain occurs at rest, while walking at an ordinary or hurried pace, or on walking uphill. Several modifications of this questionnaire have been developed, including the Edinburgh Claudication Questionnaire and the San Diego Claudication Questionnaire,[43] both of which are more sensitive and specific than a physician's diagnosis of intermittent claudication based on walking distance, walking speed, and nature of the symptoms. Another validated instrument, the Walking Impairment Questionnaire, asks a series of questions and derives a point score based on walking distance, walking speed, and nature of the symptoms.[41,43,44]

Symptoms resembling limb claudication occasionally result from nonatherosclerotic causes of artery obstruction (Table 43.2), including arterial embolism; vasculitides such as thromboangiitis obliterans (TAO), Takayasu arteritis, and giant cell arteritis; aortic coarctation; FMD; irradiation; endofibrosis of the external iliac artery; and extravascular compression as a result of arterial entrapment or an adventitial cyst (see Chapter 97). Several nonvascular causes of exertional leg pain should be considered in the differential diagnosis of intermittent claudication. Lumbosacral radiculopathy resulting from degenerative joint disease, spinal stenosis, and herniated discs can cause pain in the buttock, hip, thigh, calf, or foot with walking, often after very short distances or even with standing. This symptom has been called *neurogenic pseudoclaudication*. Lumbosacral spine disease and PAD both preferentially affect the elderly population and thus may coexist in the same individual. Positional changes in symptoms or attenuation of pain while walking stooped forward, such as with a shopping cart, are suggestive of a neurogenic rather than a vascular cause of symptoms. Arthritis of the hips and knees also provokes leg pain with walking. Typically, the pain is localized to the affected joint and can be elicited on physical examination by palpation and range-of-motion maneuvers. *Exertional compartment syndrome* most often occurs in athletes with large calf muscles; increased tissue pressure during exercise limits microvascular flow and results in calf pain or tightness. Symptoms improve after cessation of exercise. Rarely, skeletal muscle disorders such as myositis can cause exertional leg pain. *Glycogen storage disease type V*, also known as McArdle syndrome, in which skeletal muscle phosphorylase is deficient, can cause symptoms mimicking the claudication of PAD. Patients with chronic venous insufficiency sometimes report leg discomfort with exertion, a condition designated *venous claudication*. Venous hypertension during exercise increases arterial resistance in the affected limb and limits blood flow. In the case of venous insufficiency, elevated extravascular pressure caused by interstitial edema further diminishes capillary perfusion. Peripheral edema, venous stasis pigmentation, and occasionally venous varicosities demonstrated on physical examination may provide clues for this unusual cause of exertional leg pain.

Symptoms or tissue loss occur at rest in patients with CLI. Typically, patients complain of pain or paresthesias in the foot or toes of the affected extremity. This discomfort worsens with leg elevation and improves with leg dependency, as might be anticipated by the effect of gravity on perfusion pressure. The pain can be particularly severe at sites of skin fissuring, ulceration, or necrosis. Frequently, the skin is very sensitive, and even the weight of bedclothes or sheets elicits pain. Patients may sit on the edge of the bed and dangle their legs to alleviate the discomfort. Patients with neuropathy, however, can experience little or no pain despite the presence of severe ischemia.

CLI and digital ischemia can result from arterial occlusions from a variety of etiologies in addition to atherosclerosis, including conditions such as TAO, vasculitides such as systemic lupus erythematosus (SLE) or scleroderma, vasospasm, atheromatous embolism, and acute arterial occlusion secondary to thrombosis or embolism (see later). Acute gouty arthritis, trauma, and sensory neuropathy such as that caused by DM, lumbosacral radiculopathies, and complex regional pain syndrome (previously known as "reflex sympathetic dystrophy") can

TABLE 43.2 Differential Diagnosis of Exertional Leg Pain

Vascular Causes
Atherosclerosis
Thrombosis
Embolism
Vasculitis
Thromboangiitis obliterans
Takayasu arteritis
Giant cell arteritis
Aortic coarctation
Fibromuscular dysplasia
Irradiation
Endofibrosis of the external iliac artery
Extravascular compression
Arterial entrapment (e.g., popliteal artery entrapment, thoracic outlet syndrome)
Adventitial cysts
Nonvascular Causes
Lumbosacral radiculopathy
Degenerative arthritis
Spinal stenosis
Herniated disc
Arthritis
Hips, knees
Venous insufficiency
Myositis
Glycogen storage disease type V (McArdle syndrome)

cause foot pain. Leg ulcers also occur in patients with venous insufficiency or sensory neuropathy, particularly that related to diabetes. These ulcers appear to be distinct from those caused by PAD. The ulcer of venous insufficiency usually localizes near the medial malleolus and has an irregular border and a pink base with granulation tissue. In general, they produce milder pain than those caused by PAD. *Neurotrophic ulcers* occur at sites of pressure or trauma, usually on the sole of the foot. These ulcers are deep, frequently infected, and not generally painful because of the loss of sensation. In patients with PAD, concomitant diabetes associates with increased risk of ulcer and tissue loss, and the etiology is multifactorial including chronic ischemia and infection in the setting of impaired perfusion, microcirculatory disease, and increased susceptibility to infection.[45]

Physical Findings

A complete CV examination includes palpation of the peripheral pulses, inspection of the extremities, including the feet, and auscultation of accessible arteries for bruits. Pulse abnormalities and bruits increase the likelihood of PAD.[1,2,43] Readily palpable pulses in healthy individuals include the brachial, radial, and ulnar arteries in the upper extremities and the femoral, popliteal, dorsalis pedis, and posterior tibial arteries in the lower extremities. The aorta can also be palpated in thin people. A decreased or absent pulse indicates diminished pressure from a more proximal stenosis. For example, a normal right femoral pulse but absent left femoral pulse suggests the presence of left iliofemoral arterial stenosis. A normal femoral artery pulse but absent popliteal artery pulse would indicate a stenosis in the superficial femoral artery or proximal popliteal artery. A palpable popliteal artery pulse with absent dorsalis pedis or posterior tibial artery pulses indicates disease of the anterior and posterior tibial arteries, respectively.

Bruits are often a sign of accelerated blood flow velocity and flow disturbance at sites of stenosis. A stethoscope should be used to auscultate the supraclavicular and infraclavicular fossae for evidence of subclavian artery stenosis; the abdomen, flank, and pelvis for evidence of stenoses in the aorta and its branch vessels; and the inguinal region for evidence of femoral artery stenoses. Pallor can be elicited on the soles of the feet of some patients with PAD by performing a maneuver in which the feet are elevated above the level of the heart and the calf muscles are exercised by repeated dorsiflexion and plantar flexion of the ankle. The legs are then placed in the dependent position, and the time until the onset of hyperemia by evident rubor and venous distention is measured. Each of these variables depends on the rate of blood flow, which in turn reflects the severity of stenosis and adequacy of collateral vessels.

The legs of patients with chronic aortoiliac disease may show muscle atrophy. Additional signs of chronic low-grade ischemia include hair loss, dystrophic, thickened and brittle toenails, smooth and shiny skin, and atrophy of the subcutaneous fat of the digital pads. Patients with severe limb ischemia have cool skin and may also have petechiae, persistent cyanosis or pallor, dependent rubor, pedal edema resulting from prolonged dependency, skin fissures, ulceration, or gangrene. The ulcers caused by PAD typically have a pale base with irregular borders and usually involve the tips of the toes or the heel of the foot or develop at sites of pressure (Fig. 43.3). These ulcers vary in size and may be as small as 3 to 5 mm.

Categorization

Classification of patients with PAD depends on the severity of the symptoms and abnormalities detected on physical examination. Categorization of the clinical manifestations of PAD helps to characterize risk and provides a basis for the types and intensity of therapeutic intervention. Fontaine described one widely used scheme that classifies patients into one of four stages, progressing from asymptomatic to CLI (Table 43.3), a term first used in 1982. Several professional vascular societies have adopted the Rutherford scale, a contemporary, more descriptive classification that includes asymptomatic patients, three grades of claudication, and three grades of CLI ranging from rest pain alone to minor and major tissue loss (Table 43.4).[1,2,43]

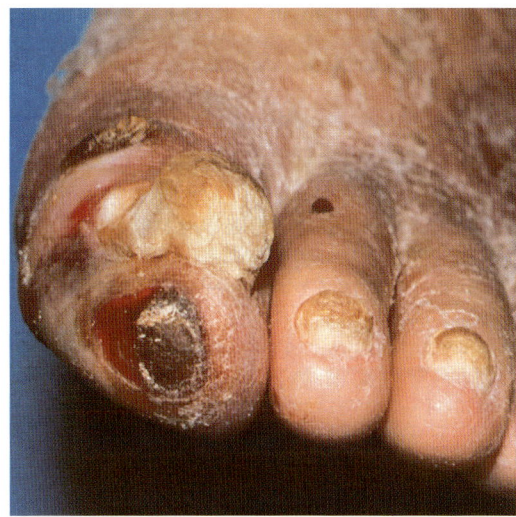

FIGURE 43.3 Typical arterial ulcer. Discrete, circumscribed, necrotic ulcer located on the great toe.

TABLE 43.3 Fontaine Classification of Peripheral Artery Disease

STAGE		SYMPTOMS
I		Asymptomatic
II		Intermittent claudication
	IIa	Pain free, claudication walking >200 m
	IIb	Pain free, claudication walking <200 m
III		Rest and nocturnal pain
IV		Necrosis, gangrene

TABLE 43.4 Rutherford Categories of Chronic Limb Ischemia

GRADE	CATEGORY	CLINICAL DESCRIPTION
	0	Asymptomatic
I	1	Mild claudication
	2	Moderate claudication
	3	Severe claudication
II	4	Ischemic rest pain
	5	Minor tissue loss: nonhealing ulcer, focal gangrene with diffuse pedal ulcer
III	6	Major tissue loss extending above the transmetatarsal level, functional foot no longer salvageable

Modified from Rutherford RB, Baker JD, Ernst C, et al. Recommended standards for reports dealing with lower extremity ischemia: revised version. *J Vasc Surg.* 1997;26:517.

The term CLI is also in evolution and it has been modified by the Global Vascular Guidelines writing group to "chronic limb-threatening ischemia" or CLTI. The definition of CLTI is "advanced PAD with rest pain, gangrene, or ulceration of greater than 2 weeks."[46] These guidelines also endorse the WIFI (Wound, Ischemia, and Foot Infection) classification, which acknowledges and evaluates the multifactorial nature of wounds in patients with PAD including wound characteristics, infection, and ischemia (Table 43.5–43.7).[47] The WIFI classification is associated with outcomes and has been validated in observational cohorts.[48] The pathobiologic complexity implicit in the definition of CLTI and the WIFI classification reflects that tissue loss in PAD is often not driven by acute ischemia but rather the complex interplay between chronic ischemia and infection, particularly in patients with diabetes.

TABLE 43.5 Wound Grading in Wound, Ischemia, and Foot Infection (WIFI) Classification

GRADE	ULCER	GANGRENE
0	No ulcer	No gangrene
	Clinical description: ischemic rest pain (requires typical symptoms + ischemia grade 3); no wound	
1	Small, shallow ulcer on distal leg or foot; no exposed bone, unless limited to distal phalanx	No gangrene
	Clinical description: minor tissue loss. Salvageable with simple digital amputation (1 or 2 digits) or skin coverage	
2	Deeper ulcer with exposed bone, joint, or tendon; generally not involving the heel; shallow heel ulcer, without calcaneal involvement	Gangrenous changes limited to digits
	Clinical description: major tissue loss salvageable with multiple (3 or more) digital amputations or standard transmetatarsal amputation with or without skin coverage	
3	Extensive, deep ulcer involving forefoot and/or midfoot; deep, full-thickness heel ulcer ± calcaneal involvement	Extensive gangrene involving forefoot and/or midfoot; full-thickness heel necrosis ± calcaneal involvement
	Clinical description: extensive tissue loss salvageable only with a complex foot reconstruction (nontraditional transmetatarsal, Chopart, or Lisfranc amputation); flap coverage or complex wound management needed for large soft tissue defect.	

Modified from Conte MS, Bradbury AW, Kolh P, et al. Global vascular guidelines on the management of chronic limb-threatening ischemia. *J Vasc Surg.* 2019;69:3S–125S.e40.

TABLE 43.6 Ischemia Grading in Wound, Ischemia, and Foot Infection (WIFI) Classification

GRADE	ANKLE BRACHIAL INDEX	ANKLE SYSTOLIC PRESSURE	TOE PRESSURE, TcPO$_2$
0	≥ 0.80	>100 mm Hg	≥ 60 mm Hg
1	0.60–0.79	70–100 mm Hg	40–59 mm Hg
2	0.40–0.59	50–70 mm Hg	30–39 mm Hg
3	≤ 0.39	<50 mm Hg	<30 mm Hg

Modified from Conte S, Bradbury AW, Kolh P, et al. Global vascular guidelines on the management of chronic limb-threatening ischemia. *J Vasc Surg.* 2019;69:3S–125S.e40.

TABLE 43.7 Infection Grading in Wound, Ischemia, and Foot Infection (WIFI) Classification

CLINICAL MANIFESTATION OF INFECTION	SVS GRADE	INFECTION SEVERITY
No symptoms or signs of infection	0	Uninfected
Infection present but involving the skin and subcutaneous tissue only	1	Mild
Local infection involving structures deeper than skin and subcutaneous tissues	2	Moderate
Local infection with signs of systemic inflammatory response syndrome	3	Severe

SVS, Society for Vascular Surgery. Modified from Conte S, Bradbury AW, Kolh P, et al. Global vascular guidelines on the management of chronic limb-threatening ischemia. *J Vasc Surg.* 2019;69:3S–125S.e40.

TESTING FOR PERIPHERAL ARTERY DISEASE

Patients with signs or symptoms suggestive of PAD should have testing to confirm the diagnosis and to characterize the distribution and severity of disease. In patients with risk factors, clinicians should be aware of atypical symptoms, perform a vascular physical examination, and perform diagnostic testing in those with a history or examination suggestive of PAD. Many patients with PAD are asymptomatic or have unrecognized symptoms, and appropriate testing should be considered in high-risk individuals after careful history taking.[1,2,49] One randomized trial of men aged 65 to 74 years found that screening for PAD, as well as hypertension and abdominal aortic aneurysm, had a mortality benefit.[50]

Segmental Pressure Measurement

Measurement of SBP along sequential segments of each extremity is one of the simplest noninvasive measures for ascertaining the presence and severity of stenoses in the peripheral arteries. In the lower extremities, pneumatic cuffs are placed on the upper and lower portions of the thigh, on the calf, above the ankle, and often over the metatarsal area of the foot. Similarly, for the upper extremities, pneumatic cuffs are placed on the upper part of the arm over the biceps, on the forearm below the elbow, and at the wrist. SBP at each respective limb segment is measured by first inflating the pneumatic cuff to suprasystolic pressure and then determining the pressure at which blood flow occurs during deflation of the cuff. The onset of flow is assessed by placing a Doppler ultrasound flow probe over an artery distal to the cuff. In the lower extremities, it is most convenient to place the Doppler probe on the foot over the posterior tibial artery, because it courses inferior and posterior to the medial malleolus, or over the dorsalis pedis artery on the dorsum of the metatarsal arch. In the upper extremities the Doppler probe can be placed over the brachial artery in the antecubital fossa or over the radial and ulnar arteries at the wrist.

Left ventricular contraction imparts kinetic energy to blood, which is maintained throughout the large- and medium-sized vessels. SBP may be higher in the more distal vessels than in the aorta and proximal vessels because of amplification and reflection of BP waves. A stenosis can cause loss of pressure energy because of increased frictional forces and disturbance of flow at the site of the stenosis. Approximately 90% of the cross-sectional area of the aorta must be narrowed before a pressure gradient develops. In smaller vessels, such as the iliac and femoral arteries, a 70% to 90% decrease in cross-sectional area will cause a resting pressure gradient sufficient to decrease SBP distal to the stenosis. Taking into consideration the precision of this noninvasive method and the variability in BP during even short periods, a BP gradient in excess of 20 mm Hg between successive cuffs is generally used as evidence of arterial stenosis in the lower extremity, whereas a gradient of 10 mm Hg indicates a stenosis between sequential cuffs in the upper extremity. SBP in the toes and fingers is approximately 60% of SBP at the ankle and wrist, respectively, because pressure diminishes further in the smaller distal vessels. Fig. 43.4 provides examples of leg segmental BP measurements in a patient with left calf claudication. In the right leg, there are no pressure gradients between the upper and lower parts of the thigh or between the calf and ankle. In the left leg, pressure gradients between the upper and lower parts of the thigh, between the lower part of the thigh and calf, and between the calf and ankle indicate an ankle SBP less than 55 mm Hg predicts poor ulcer healing. Leg BP recordings are not reliable in patients with calcified vessels, as might occur in those with DM or renal insufficiency. Inflation of the pneumatic cuff cannot compress the calcified vessel; the Doppler probe consequently indicates continuous blood flow, even when the cuff pressure exceeds 250 mm Hg. An ABI higher than 1.40 indicates a noncompressible artery, and the test is not informative for either confirming or excluding PAD. In this case, a *toe-brachial index* (TBI) may be informative, with a ratio of 0.70 or higher reflecting normal perfusion pressure.[1,2]

Treadmill Exercise Testing (see Chapter 15)

Treadmill exercise testing can be used to evaluate the clinical significance of peripheral artery stenoses and provide objective evidence of the patient's walking capacity. The claudication onset time is when symptoms of claudication first develop, and the peak walking time occurs when the patient can no longer continue walking because of severe leg discomfort. This standardized and more objective measure of walking capacity supplements the patient's history and provides a quantitative assessment of the patient's disability, as well as a metric for monitoring therapeutic interventions. Treadmill exercise protocols use a motorized treadmill that incorporates fixed or progressive speeds and angles of incline. A fixed workload test usually maintains a constant grade of 12% and a speed of 1.5 to 2.0 mph. A progressive, or graded, treadmill protocol typically maintains a constant speed of 2 mph while the grade gradually increases by 2% every 2 to 3 minutes. Repeated treadmill test results have better reproducibility with progressive than with constant-grade protocols.

Treadmill testing can determine whether arterial stenoses contribute to the patient's symptoms of exertional leg pain. During exercise, blood flow through a stenosis increases as vascular resistance falls in the exercising muscle. According to the Poiseuille equation, described previously, the pressure gradient across the stenosis increases in direct proportion to flow. Thus, ankle and brachial SBP is measured during resting conditions before treadmill exercise, within 1 minute after exercise, and repeatedly until baseline values are reestablished. Normally, the BP increase that occurs during exercise should be the same in both the upper and the lower extremities, with a constant ABI of 1.0 or greater being maintained. In the presence of peripheral artery stenoses, however, the ABI decreases because the BP increase observed in the arm is not matched by a comparable increase in ankle BP. A 25% or greater decrease in the ABI after exercise in a patient whose walking capacity is limited by claudication is considered diagnostic and implicates PAD as a cause of the patient's symptoms. This provocative test should be considered in patients with risk factors and symptoms suggestive of vascular claudication but with normal resting ABI, as may occur in those with proximal disease.[52,53]

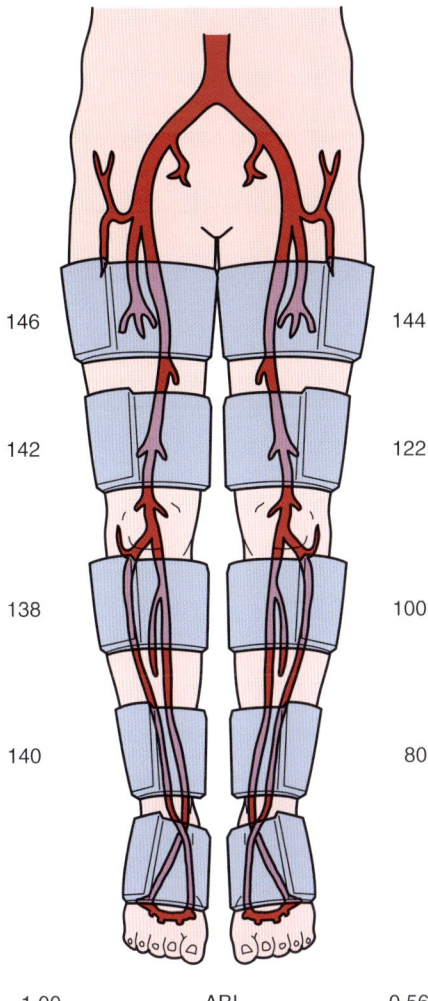

FIGURE 43.4 Segmental pressure measurements in a patient with intermittent claudication of the left calf. A pressure gradient is present between the left upper and lower thigh cuffs, lower thigh and calf cuffs, and calf and ankle cuffs, consistent with multisegmental disease affecting the femoral-popliteal and tibial arteries. The left ABI is 0.56, which is abnormal. Segmental pressure measurements and the ABI in the right leg are normal.

stenoses in the superficial femoral and popliteal arteries and in the tibioperoneal arteries.

Ankle-Brachial Index

Determination of the ABI is a simplified application of leg segmental BP measurements that can readily be used at the bedside. This index is the ratio of SBP measured at the ankle to SBP measured at the brachial artery.[1,2] A pneumatic cuff placed around the ankle is inflated to suprasystolic pressure and subsequently deflated while the onset of flow is detected with a Doppler ultrasound probe placed over the dorsalis pedis and posterior tibial arteries, thus denoting ankle SBP. Brachial artery SBP can be assessed in a routine manner with either a stethoscope to listen for the first Korotkoff sound or a Doppler probe to listen for the onset of flow during cuff deflation. The *normal* ABI range is 1.00 to 1.40. An ABI value of 0.91 to 0.99 is *borderline*, and an ABI of 0.90 or less is *abnormal*.[1,2] An ABI of 0.90 or lower has a specificity of 83% to 99% and a sensitivity of 69% to 73% in detecting stenoses greater than 50%.[1,2] The sensitivity of an ABI less than 1.0 approaches 100%. The ABI is often used to gauge the severity of PAD. Patients with symptoms of leg claudication often have an ABI ranging from 0.5 to 0.8, and patients with CLI usually have an ABI lower than 0.5. A low ABI is associated with shorter walking distance and lower speed. Less than 40% of patients whose ABI is lower than 0.40 can complete a 6-minute walk.[41,43,51] In patients with skin ulcerations,

Pulse Volume Recording

The pulse volume recording graphically illustrates the volumetric change in a segment of the limb that occurs with each pulse. Plethysmographic instruments, typically using strain gauges or pneumatic cuffs, can transduce volumetric changes in the limb, which can be displayed on a graphic recorder. These transducers, placed strategically along the limb, record the pulse volume in its different segments, such as the thigh, calf, ankle, metatarsal region, and toes, or the upper part of the arm, forearm, and fingers. The normal pulse volume contour depends on both local arterial pressure and vascular wall distensibility and resembles a BP waveform. It consists of a sharp systolic upstroke rising rapidly to a peak, a dicrotic notch, and a concave downslope that drops off gradually toward the baseline. The contour of the pulse wave changes distal to a stenosis, with loss of the dicrotic notch, a slower rate of rise, a more rounded peak, and a slower descent. The amplitude becomes lower with increasing severity of disease, and the pulse wave may not be recordable at all in a critically ischemic limb. Segmental analysis of the pulse wave may indicate the location of an arterial stenosis, which probably resides in the artery between a normal and an abnormal pulse volume recording. The pulse volume wave also provides information about the integrity of blood flow when BP measurements cannot be obtained accurately because of noncompressible vessels.

Doppler Ultrasonography

Continuous-wave and pulsed-wave Doppler systems transmit and receive high-frequency ultrasound signals. The Doppler frequency shift caused by moving red blood cells varies directly with the velocity of blood flow. Typically, the perceived frequency shift is between 1 and 20 kHz and is within the audible range of the human ear. Therefore, placement of a Doppler probe along an artery enables the examiner to hear whether blood flow is present and the vessel is patent. Processing and graphic recording of the Doppler signal permit a more detailed analysis of the frequency components.

Doppler instruments can be used without or with gray-scale imaging to evaluate an artery for the presence of stenoses. The Doppler probe is positioned at approximately a 60-degree angle over the common femoral, superficial femoral, popliteal, dorsalis pedis, and posterior tibial arteries. The normal Doppler waveform has three components: a rapid forward-flow component during systole, a transient flow reversal during early diastole, and a slow anterograde component during late diastole. The Doppler waveform becomes altered if the probe is placed distal to an arterial stenosis and is characterized by deceleration of systolic flow, loss of the early diastolic reversal, and diminished peak frequencies. Arteries in a limb with critical ischemia may not show any Doppler frequency shift. As with pulse volume recordings, change from a normal to an abnormal Doppler waveform as the artery is interrogated more distally suggests the location of a stenosis.

Duplex Ultrasound Imaging

Duplex ultrasound imaging provides a direct, noninvasive means of assessing both the anatomic characteristics of peripheral arteries and the functional significance of arterial stenoses. The methodology incorporates gray-scale B-mode ultrasound imaging, pulsed Doppler velocity measurements, and color coding of the Doppler shift information (Fig. 43.5). Real-time ultrasonographic scanners emit and receive high-frequency sound waves, typically ranging from 2 to 10 MHz, to construct an image. The acoustic properties of the vascular wall differ from those of the surrounding tissue, thus enabling them to easily be imaged. Atherosclerotic plaque may be present and visible on gray-scale images. Pulsed-wave Doppler systems emit ultrasound beams at precise times and can therefore sample the reflected ultrasound waves at specific depths to enable the examiner to determine blood cell velocity within the lumen of the artery. By positioning the pulsed Doppler beam at a known angle, the examiner can calculate blood flow velocity according to the following equation:

$$Df = 2VF \cos \theta / C$$

where Df is the frequency shift, V is the velocity, F is the frequency of the transmitted sound, θ is the angle between the transmitted sound and the velocity vector, and C is the velocity of sound and tissue. For optimal measurements, the angle of the pulsed Doppler beam should be less than 60 degrees. With color Doppler, the frequency shift information within the entire field sampled by the ultrasound beam can be superimposed on the gray-scale image. This approach provides a composite real-time display of flow velocity within the vessel.

Color-assisted duplex ultrasound imaging is an effective means of localizing peripheral arterial stenoses (Fig. 43.6). Normal arteries have laminar flow, with the highest velocity occurring at the center of the artery. The corresponding color image is usually homogeneous with relatively constant hue and intensity. In the presence of an arterial stenosis, blood flow velocity increases through the narrowed lumen. As the velocity increases, there is progressive desaturation of the color display, and flow disturbance distal to the stenosis causes changes in hue and color. Pulsed Doppler velocity measurements can be made along the length of the artery and particularly at areas of flow abnormalities

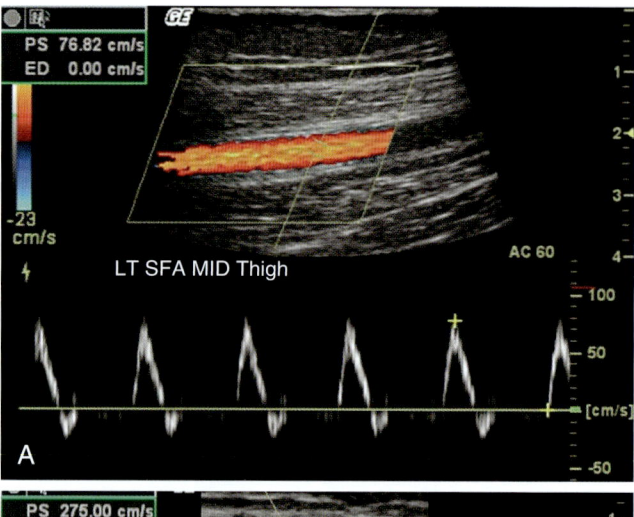

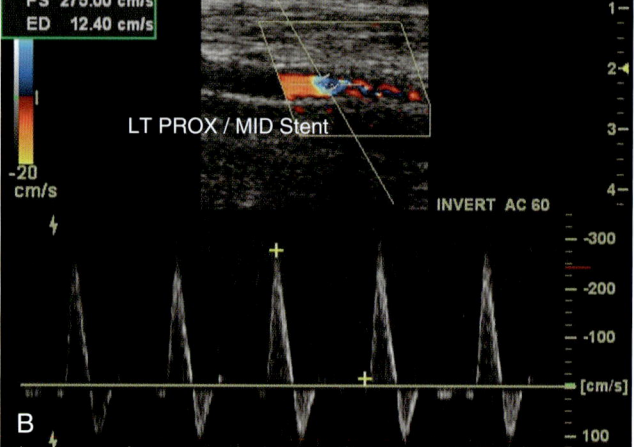

FIGURE 43.5 Duplex ultrasonogram of the common femoral artery (CFA) bifurcation into the superficial femoral artery (SFA) and deep femoral artery. **A,** Normal gray-scale image of the artery in which the intima is not thickened and the lumen is widely patent. **B,** Recording of the pulse Doppler velocity sampled from the superficial femoral artery. The triphasic profile is apparent, the envelope is thin, and peak systolic velocity is within normal limits.

suggested by the color images. A twofold or greater increase in peak systolic velocity at the site of an atherosclerotic plaque indicates a 50% or greater stenosis (see Fig. 43.6). A threefold increase in velocity suggests a 75% or greater stenosis. An occluded artery generates no Doppler signal. Duplex ultrasound imaging for identification of sites of arterial stenosis has approximately 89% to 99% specificity and 80% to 98% sensitivity.[1,2] Measurement of sequential peak systolic velocities enables evaluation of restenosis of peripheral stents or bypass grafts and to determine the need to consider reintervention to preserve vessel patency.[54] Assessment of peak systolic velocities postendovascular intervention also may be used to determine hemodynamic improvement.[55]

Magnetic Resonance Angiography (see Chapter 19)

Magnetic resonance angiography (MRA) can visualize the aorta and peripheral arteries noninvasively. Resolution of the vascular anatomy with gadolinium-enhanced MRA approaches that of conventional contrast-enhanced digital subtraction angiography (DSA). Comparison of MRA with intra-arterial DSA found a sensitivity of 95% and a specificity of 96% for detecting segmental stenotic and occlusive lesions.[1,2] MRA currently has its greatest usefulness in the evaluation of symptomatic patients to assist in decision making before endovascular and surgical intervention or in patients at risk for renal, allergic, or other complications during conventional angiography.

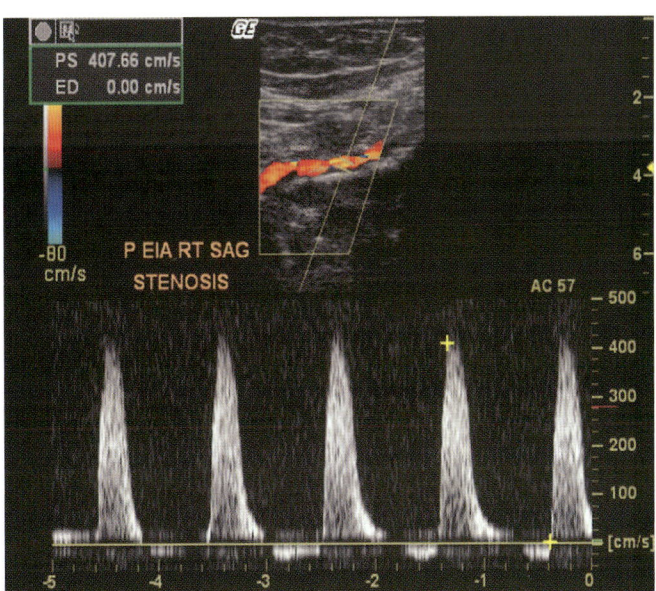

FIGURE 43.6 Duplex ultrasonogram of the external iliac artery. **Top,** Color image of the artery in which there is heterogeneity and desaturation of color, indicative of high-velocity flow through a stenosis. **Bottom,** Recording of the pulse Doppler velocity sampled from the right external iliac artery. The peak velocity of 350 cm/sec is elevated. These features are consistent with a significant stenosis.

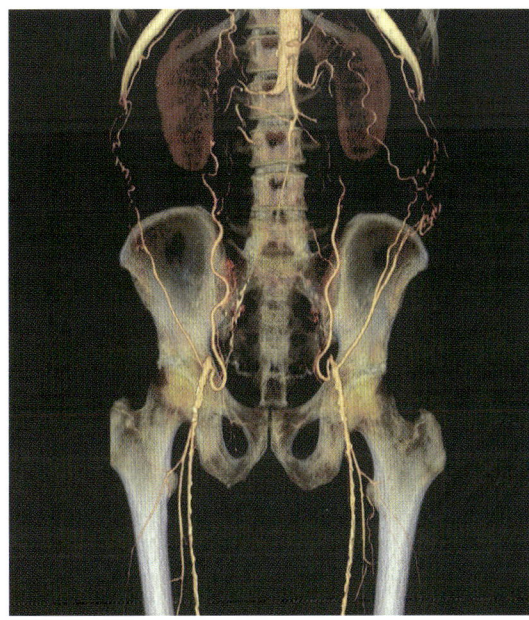

FIGURE 43.7 CTA in a patient with complete occlusion of the aorta and both iliac arteries. The common femoral arteries have been reconstituted. (Courtesy of the 3D and Image Processing Center of Brigham and Women's Hospital, Boston, MA.)

Computed Tomographic Angiography (see Chapter 20)

Computed tomography (CT) permits imaging of peripheral arteries with excellent spatial resolution during a relatively short time and with limited amounts of radiocontrast material (Fig. 43.7). Image reconstructions in three dimensions permit rotation to optimize visualization of arterial stenoses. Compared with conventional contrast-enhanced angiography, the sensitivity and specificity for stenoses greater than 50% or occlusion reported for computed tomographic angiography (CTA) using multidetector technology are 95% and 96%, respectively.[1,2] CTA offers advantages over MRA because it can be used in patients with stents, metal clips, and pacemakers, although it has the disadvantage of requiring radiocontrast material and ionizing radiation.

Contrast-Enhanced Angiography

Conventional angiography can aid in evaluation of the arterial anatomy before a revascularization procedure. It still has occasional usefulness when the diagnosis is in doubt. Most contemporary angiography laboratories use digital subtraction techniques after intra-arterial administration of contrast material to enhance resolution. Injection of the contrast material into the aorta permits visualization of the aorta and iliac arteries, and injection of contrast material into the iliofemoral segment of the involved leg permits optimal visualization of the femoral, popliteal, tibial, and peroneal arteries (Fig. 43.8).

OTHER MEASUREMENT TOOLS

Other measures of flow and perfusion are available to assess flow and perfusion in PAD.[56] One such technology is near-infrared fluorescence imaging (NIR), used also for imaging retinal vessels, which uses near-infrared laser light to produce fluorescence of an intravenously injected dye. Detection and measurement of this fluorescence evaluates perfusion. Meta-analyses report a sensitivity of 67% to 100% and specificity of 72% to 100% for diagnosing PAD.[57] Indications for using NIR include diagnosis, monitoring in revascularization, assessment for potential amputation, and visualization of perfusion. NIR may be helpful in selected circumstances and is technique used in research. Transcutaneous oxygen pressure measurement ($TcpO_2$), contrast-enhanced ultrasound (CEUS), and scintigraphy has utility primarily in research, particularly in patients with PAD and diabetes.[58] The use of $TcpO_2$ has been adopted particularly in patients with CLI to assess the likelihood of healing after amputation, particularly where toe wounds or forefoot amputation may prohibit toe pressure measurement.[56] A normal $TcPO_2$ is above 55 mm Hg with levels below 30 mm Hg associated with low probability of wound healing. Studies have reported a sensitivity of 98% and a specificity of 44% for predicting resolution of limb salvage problems.[56] Venous occlusion plethysmography (VOP) has been around for more than 100 years and can quantify limb blood flow and hemodynamic compromise in PAD.[59] In addition, data are emerging supporting positron emission tomography (PET) both to understand plaque characteristics as well as perfusion and muscle function.[60]

PROGNOSIS

Patients with PAD have, by definition, a heightened risk of severe ischemic limb complications as well as loss of function. In addition, by nature of their underlying atherosclerotic disease, which frequently affects multiple territories (called polyvascular disease), they have risk for adverse CV events with rates as high or higher than patients with CAD and no PAD (Fig. 43.9).[10] Overall, PAD associates with high rates of CV complications and mortality, with a strong inverse relationship between ABI (excluding noncompressibility) and mortality for both men and women. The specificity of an abnormal ABI in predicting future CV events is approximately 90%.[1]

Worsening symptoms develop in approximately 25% of patients with claudication, and over 3 years, approximately 20% will require an intervention to improve lower extremity perfusion (see Fig. 43.9). Moreover, loss of mobility occurs more often in patients with PAD than in those without PAD, even in patients without classic symptoms of claudication.[43] Both smoking and DM independently predict progression of disease.[1,24] Those with DM have at least a 12-fold higher likelihood of amputation than nondiabetic persons.[13] The risk for limb loss is higher in PAD patients with CLI in whom revascularization fails or is not feasible and approximates 40% by 6 months.[16]

Due to complex comorbidities and advanced age of many patients with PAD, causes of death are as likely to be non-CV as they are CV.[61] Patients with PAD have heterogeneous risk profiles. Those patients

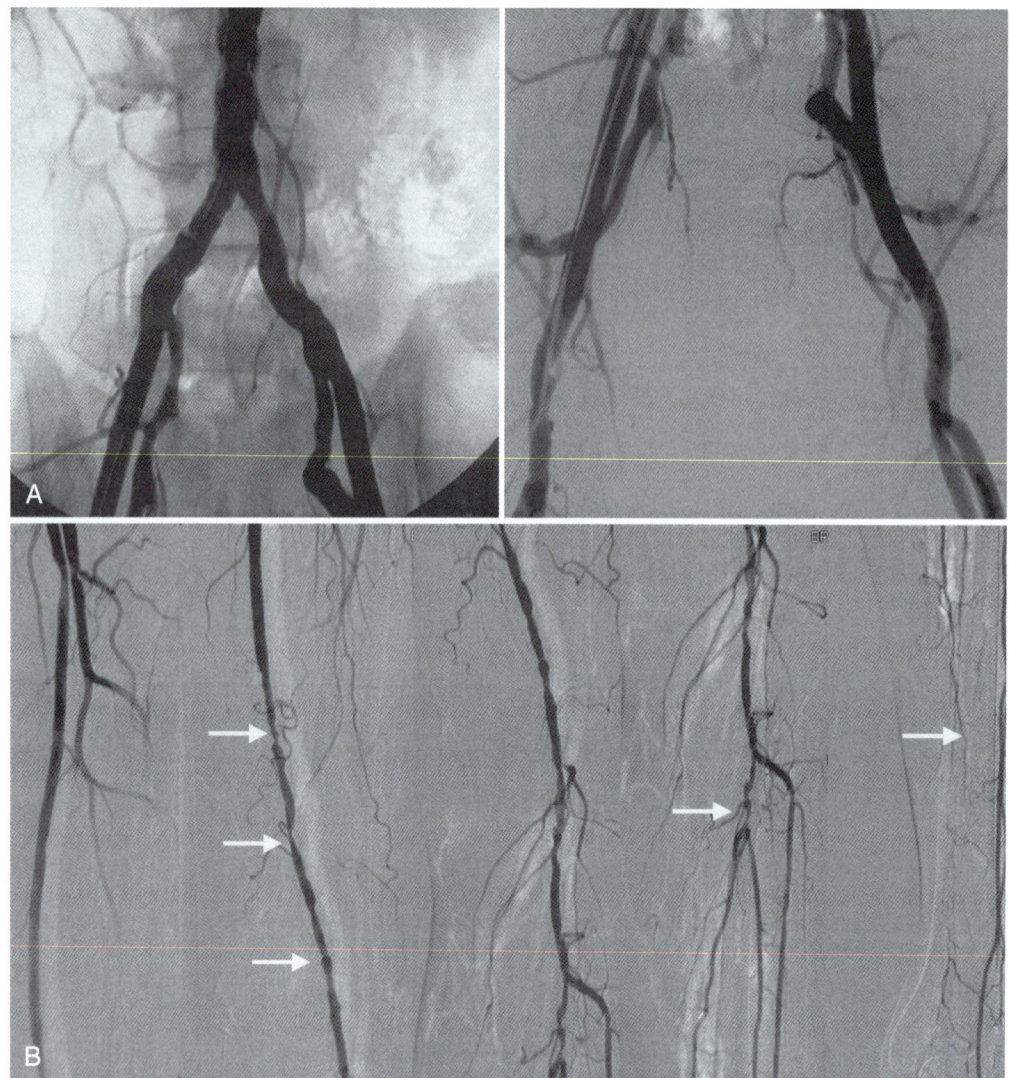

FIGURE 43.8 Angiogram of a patient with disabling left calf claudication. **A,** The aorta and bilateral common iliac arteries are patent. **B,** The left superficial femoral artery has multiple stenotic lesions (*left arrows*). Significant stenosis of the left tibioperoneal trunk and left posterior tibial artery (*right arrows*) is present.

with multiple symptomatic territories, or polyvascular disease, particularly involving the coronary bed have a very high risk of MACEs even beyond those with CAD alone.[4,9,28] Patients with PAD and prior myocardial infarction have a particularly poor CV prognosis, with a 3-year risk of CV death, myocardial infarction, or stroke approaching 20%, reflecting a 60% increase in risk relative to those with prior myocardial infarction but no PAD.[17,62] Given the systemic manifestations of atherosclerosis, many patients with PAD have coronary atherosclerosis; however, in recent clinical trials of patients with PAD only a third have symptomatic CAD.[61,63]

Patients with PAD who have had severe enough symptoms to necessitate revascularization appear to be at particularly high risk of future limb complications such as ALI, even long-term after intervention.[3,4,19,63] Those with the most severe symptoms of PAD, notably those with CLI, have the worst prognosis with high rates of amputation and mortality. Patients with PAD and concomitant DM have increasing rates of amputation in spite of lower rates of myocardial infarction and stroke over the same period.[24,64,65] It is also increasingly recognized that the etiologies of amputation in those with PAD and DM are often multifactorial, including infection and ischemia.[45]

Prognosis in PAD is heterogenous based on geography, socioeconomic factors and race. Black patients with PAD face higher amputation rates.[66] In addition, PAD incidence and hospitalizations are associated with socioeconomic status.[67] Disparities in

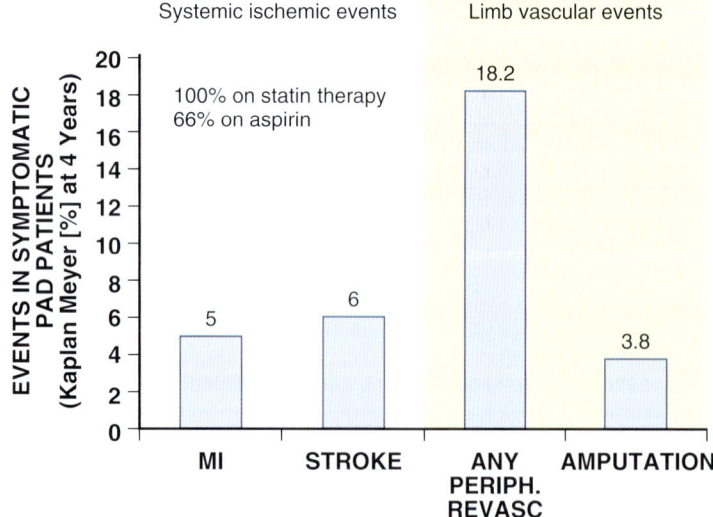

FIGURE 43.9 Event rates in patients with PAD at 4 years in the REACH registry. (Adapted from Kumbhani DJ, Steg PG, Cannon CP, et al. Statin therapy and long-term adverse limb outcomes in patients with peripheral artery disease: insights from the REACH registry. *Eur Heart J.* 2014;35:2864–2872.)

socioeconomic factors and health care delivery are important factors in the prognosis of patients with PAD.

TREATMENT

The ACC/AHA Guidelines for Medical Management of PAD are summarized in online Table 43G.1 to Table 43G.8. The goals of treatment in PAD are to improve quality of life and function as well as to reduce the risk of ischemic limb and CV complications. Therapeutic considerations therefore include modification of risk factors by alterations in lifestyle and use of pharmacologic therapy to reduce the risk for adverse limb outcomes as well as CV events, such as myocardial infarction, stroke, and death, There has been increasing appreciation of the frequency and morbidity of major adverse limb outcomes (MALEs) including ALI and major amputation, as well as the role of medical therapies in reducing these risks.[68] Increasing data suggest heterogeneity in the risk of MALEs in patients with PAD with the greatest risk in those with prior LER or amputation.[3,18,19,69,70] This risk appears particularly high in the acute postrevascularization setting.[3,63] Unfortunately, secondary prevention in PAD is underused, particularly when compared with other manifestations of atherosclerosis such as CAD.[11] Screening programs demonstrating improved outcomes may in part result in greater use of preventive strategies through increased diagnosis, education, and awareness.[50]

Symptoms of claudication improve with exercise and selected pharmacotherapies. Optimal management of CLI often includes endovascular interventions or surgical reconstruction to improve blood supply and maintain limb viability. Revascularization can aid some patients with disabling symptoms of claudication that persist despite exercise therapy and pharmacotherapy.[1,2]

Risk Factor Modification (see also Chapter 25)

Strategies for risk factor modification are consistent with those generally used for patients with atherosclerosis, including diet modification and weight optimization, exercise, smoking cessation, and optimization of risk factors such as hypertension and dyslipidemia. Intensive management of risk factors is critical in patients with PAD to reduce CV risks with glucose management critical for the prevention of microvascular complications, including neuropathy and amputation.

Diet

A secondary analysis of a randomized trial evaluating the efficacy of the Mediterranean diet demonstrated a lower risk of incident PAD in those on the diet versus control.[21] Dietary interventions that help optimize body weight and reduce sodium associate with improvements in metabolic parameters and BP.[1,2]

Smoking Cessation

Prospective trials examining the benefits of smoking cessation are lacking, but observational evidence unequivocally shows that cigarette smoking increases the risk for atherosclerosis and its clinical sequelae including PAD.[71] Nonsmokers with PAD have lower rates of myocardial infarction and mortality than those who have smoked or continue to smoke, and PAD patients who discontinue smoking have approximately twice the 5-year survival rate of those who continue to smoke. In addition to frequent physician advice, pharmacologic interventions that effectively promote smoking cessation include nicotine replacement therapy, bupropion, and varenicline.[1,2]

Treatment of Diabetes (see also Chapter 31)

Aggressive treatment of diabetes decreases the risk for microangiopathic events such as nephropathy and retinopathy, but until recently, most classes of glucose-lowering drugs have not shown a reduction of macrovascular events.[72] In several trials, intensive glucose control versus standard therapy has not reduced ischemic risk associated with increased mortality.[73] Target-specific therapies, however, have shown important CV benefits for MACE and heart failure in patients with atherosclerosis including PAD. In the EMPA-REG trial, the sodium glucose transporter 2 (SGLT2) inhibitor *empagliflozin* reduced all-cause mortality by 32% in patients with type 2 DM at increased risk of CV events, including more than 600 patients with PAD.[74,75] The observations of increased rates of leg and foot amputation in ongoing studies with a related agent, however, raised concerns for safety PAD with subsequent observations regarding BP and limb outcomes suggesting a potential mechanism.[76,77] Subsequent studies, however, have not confirmed this risk and have shown consistent and robust benefits of SGLT2 inhibitors, particularly for heart failure and renal outcomes in patients with diabetes and PAD.[45,78,79] The glucagon-like protein (GLP)-1 agonists liraglutide and semaglutide improved macrovascular outcomes in patients with type 2 DM and either established CV disease or at heightened CV risk.[80,81] Current guidelines recognize the importance of these agents in patients with vascular disease, including atherosclerotic vascular disease (ASCVD), beyond glucose lowering alone.[73]

Because of multiple drivers of amputation in patients with PAD and diabetes and the important role of wounds and infection, reducing the risk of adverse limb outcomes requires a multifactorial approach.[22,45,65] Although long-term glucose reduction reduces microvascular disease and associated complications including amputation, novel antidiabetic agents may reduce amputation through similar antiischemic mechanisms underlying their benefits for preventing myocardial infarction and stroke. A subanalysis of the LEADER trial observed a reduction in amputations with liraglutide in patients with diabetes and vascular disease.[82] This observation renders GLP-1 agonists particularly attractive in patients with diabetes and concomitant PAD. Dedicated trials of these agents in patients selected on the basis of PAD are ongoing and will further elucidate limb-specific benefits.

Blood Pressure Control

Antihypertensive therapy reduces the risk for stroke, CAD, and vascular death (see Chapter 26). In patients with PAD, the intensity of antihypertensive treatment must take into consideration benefits of reduced risk of CV events and the potential to exacerbate limb symptoms. Although several studies have suggested that intensive BP control (versus moderate BP control) reduces CV events in diabetic patients with PAD, data with regard to specific targets are mixed.[1,2] A post-hoc analysis of the International Verapamil-SR/Trandolapril study found that PAD was associated with higher ischemic risk, but there appeared to be a J-shaped relationship between SBP and outcome, suggesting that patients with PAD might require specific BP targets. In the SPRINT trial, a target SBP of 120 mm Hg or less resulted in a significant reduction in CV events, but few patients with PAD were included.[83] More recently an analysis from the ALLHAT trial including 33,357 patients followed for a median of 4.3 years observed, SBP less than 120 mm Hg was associated with a 26% higher hazard of PAD events with a similar observation for SBP ≥ 160 mm Hg relative to those with an SBP of 120 to 129.[77] The authors also observed a relationship between diastolic blood pressure (DBP) and PAD events with a 72% increased hazard in those with a DBP less than 60 mm Hg versus ≥ 60 mm Hg. A U-shaped relationship was observed between pulse pressure and PAD events.[77] These data raise the question of whether more specific BP targets in patients with PAD are needed. There are no comparative studies of specific antihypertensive agents in patients with PAD, but findings from several clinical trials support the use of angiotensin-converting enzyme (ACE) inhibitors and angiotensin receptor blockers (ARBs) in patients with atherosclerosis, including those with PAD. In the HOPE (Heart Outcomes Prevention Evaluation) study, the ACE inhibitor ramipril decreased the risk for vascular death, myocardial infarction, or stroke by 22%, with 44% having PAD.[84] Other ACE inhibitors as well as ARBs have shown similar benefits.[84] Although in theory, beta blockers could worsen lower extremity symptoms in PAD, a systematic review that included six studies of beta blocker therapy found no significant impairment of walking capacity.[84] Recent registry analyses have not observed increased risk of CV events or amputation with beta blockers after hospitalization.[85] Thus, if clinically indicated for other conditions, these drugs should not be withheld in patients with PAD.

Lipid-Lowering Therapy (see also Chapter 27)

Genetic studies support the role of lipids in the pathogenesis of PAD and PAD outcomes.[37] Therapies to lower LDL cholesterol reduce the risk of CV events.[86] Clinical trials supporting the importance of achieving very low levels of LDL cholesterol in patients with PAD have included statins, ezetimibe, and proprotein convertase subtilisin/kexin type 9 (PCSK9) inhibitors.[9,10,28,84] LDL-lowering agents improve PAD outcomes even in patients with no known coronary or cerebrovascular disease.[10] Therefore, management of dyslipidemia, particularly lowering of LDL cholesterol, is of key importance in patients with PAD, with recent guidelines recommending achievement of very low LDL targets using combination therapies when necessary.[86]

A growing body of evidence supports the role of lipid-lowering agents in modifying limb outcomes in PAD. The Heart Protection Study, a randomized trial of simvastatin versus placebo in patients with atherosclerotic vascular disease including PAD, reported that simvastatin reduced the risk of a first acute peripheral vascular event, defined retrospectively as the first occurrence of a noncoronary revascularization, aneurysm repair, major amputation, or death from PAD.[84] In the TREADMILL (Treatment of Peripheral Atherosclerotic Disease with Moderate or Intensive Lipid Lowering) trial, atorvastatin (80 mg) increased pain-free walking distance by more than 60% versus a 38% increase with placebo.[84] A propensity-adjusted analysis in an observational dataset described a reduction in amputations with statin use in patients with PAD.[87] Limb outcomes have been described in subanalyses of two randomized trials of PCSK9 inhibitors in populations with atherosclerosis. The FOURIER trial observed an approximately 50% reduction MALE with evolocumab overall with consistent effects in patients with PAD but no coronary disease or stroke.[10] There was a consistent benefit for MALE reduction with lower achieved LDL cholesterol extending to levels less than 10 mg/dL. Similarly, in the ODYSSEY trial, which randomized patients to alirocumab or placebo after acute coronary syndrome, showed a consistent reduction in MALE.[28,88] Both trials observed a magnitude of benefit per mmol/L reduction in LDL cholesterol greater than that observed for MACE and greater than those observed for statins. Although this observation should be interpreted with caution due to low numbers, it does raise the hypothesis of pleiotropic effects. Specifically, lipoprotein(a) associates with PAD risk and adverse outcomes and is lowered by PCSK9 inhibition. In fact, the limb benefits in ODYSSEY appeared driven primarily by Lp(a) reduction rather than LDL reduction.[28] Novel agents targeting Lp(a) are currently under investigation and will clarify the role of inhibition of Lp(a) and limb outcomes in PAD.

Antithrombotic Therapy for Reduction of Major Adverse Cardiovascular and Limb Events

Substantial evidence supports the use of antithrombotic agents to reduce atherothrombotic MACE in patients with atherosclerosis, particularly those with CAD (see Chapter 25). The benefits of antithrombotic therapy for MACE reduction and, particularly, more intensive strategies may be greatest in those with PAD and concomitant symptomatic CAD versus PAD without symptomatic CAD. A growing body of evidence, however, now supports the importance of more potent antithrombic strategies in reducing MALE, particularly in patients with prior lower-extremity intervention.

Antiplatelet Monotherapy

The Antithrombotic Trialists' (ATT) Collaboration Meta-analysis of more than 9000 patients with symptomatic PAD showed a 23% reduction in vascular death, myocardial infarction, or stroke with antiplatelet monotherapy.[1,2] There were no reported benefits for MALE. Although the findings are often taken as evidence supporting the use of aspirin, the trials included several classes of antiplatelet agents (e.g., aspirin, thienopyridines, dipyridamole, picotamide). The benefits were counterbalanced by a 60% increase in major extracranial bleeding. Moreover, any conclusions regarding aspirin therapy from this analysis cannot be extrapolated to patients who have asymptomatic PAD. Both the POPADAD (Prevention of Progression of Arterial Disease And Diabetes) and AAA (Aspirin for Asymptomatic Atherosclerosis) trials found no difference in CV outcomes with long-term aspirin in patients with an abnormal ABI but no symptoms other symptoms of atherosclerosis.[84]

The CAPRIE (Clopidogrel versus Aspirin in Patients at Risk of Ischemic Events) trial compared clopidogrel with aspirin in reducing ischemic events in patients with recent myocardial infarction, recent ischemic stroke, or PAD. Overall, clopidogrel reduced vascular death, myocardial infarction, or stroke by 8.7% versus aspirin.[84] Notably, among the 6452 patients in the PAD subgroup, clopidogrel treatment appeared to be associated with a greater 23.8% relative risk reduction. The EUCLID (Examining Use of Ticagrelor in PAD) trial evaluated ticagrelor, a novel potent $P2Y_{12}$ inhibitor, relative to clopidogrel in patients selected on the basis of PAD, with approximately one third having concomitant established CAD. In contrast to findings in the Study of Platelet Inhibition and Patient Outcomes (PLATO) trial, which showed superiority for ticagrelor versus clopidogrel for MACE in patients with acute coronary syndrome including those with PAD, EUCLID was neutral overall, showing no difference in outcome between ticagrelor and clopidogrel.[61,89,90] Although unexpected, there was statistical heterogeneity with apparent benefit of ticagrelor in some patients with PAD and CAD, including those with prior PCI or CABG.[61] Taken together, these data demonstrate that antiplatelet monotherapy reduces CV risk in patients with symptomatic PAD, but it is of uncertain benefit in those with a marginally low ABI and no symptoms.

Although CAPRIE supports the use of clopidogrel monotherapy for MACE reduction, the effects of $P2Y_{12}$ monotherapy for MALE reduction have been mixed. In a small trial of ticlopidine, a first-generation $P2Y_{12}$ inhibitor, versus placebo in patients with PAD showed that it reduced limb events and mortality.[84] In CAPRIE, however, there were numerically more amputations with clopidogrel (52 versus 47) than aspirin.[84] EUCLID showed no reduction in ALI or limb events with ticagrelor versus clopidogrel in patients without prior revascularization.[19,61] It therefore has not been shown that $P2Y_{12}$ inhibitor monotherapy or aspirin reduces MALE.

Dual Antiplatelet Therapy with Aspirin and $P2Y_{12}$ Inhibition

The benefits and risks of dual antiplatelet therapy (DAPT) have been investigated in several trials. The CHARISMA (Clopidogrel for High Atherothrombotic Risk and Ischemic Stabilization, Management, and Avoidance) trial evaluated the addition of clopidogrel to aspirin versus aspirin alone in patients with established CAD, cerebrovascular disease, or PAD, as well as in patients with multiple risk factors. Although neutral overall, a post-hoc analysis suggested benefit in those with established CV disease, particularly prior myocardial infarction.[1,2] Although there was no reported benefit for MALEs, there was a reduction in hospitalizations that may have been attributed to limb ischemic events.

The suggested benefits of DAPT as well as the heterogeneity of response in patients with PAD were further clarified in trials of patients with coronary disease examining subgroups with concomitant PAD (polyvascular disease). The PEGASUS-TIMI 54 trial (Prevention of Cardiovascular Events in Patients with Prior Heart Attack Using Ticagrelor Compared to Placebo on a Background of Aspirin) tested addition of ticagrelor, 60 mg twice daily, to aspirin versus aspirin alone in patients with prior myocardial infarction. In the subgroup with concomitant PAD, ticagrelor resulted in a 5.2% absolute risk reduction in CV death, myocardial infarction, or stroke, with significant reductions in both CV and all-cause mortality in patients with PAD and prior myocardial infarction.[17] In addition to these benefits for MACE, there was a significant reduction in adjudicated MALE including a reduction in ALI by 35%.[17] The Effect of Ticagrelor on Health Outcomes in Diabetes Mellitus Patients Intervention Study (THEMIS) studied the same regimen in patients with DM and stable coronary disease but no history of myocardial infarction and found ticagrelor superior to placebo for MACE reduction. THEMIS confirmed the benefits of the combination of aspirin and ticagrelor for reducing MALEs captured through prospectively adjudication. There was a statistically significant, approximately 50% reduction in the composite of ALI or major amputation of a vascular etiology; however, event rates were low as a minority of patients had PAD.[91] A third trial of DAPT in patients with CAD with a PAD subgroup was the PRODIGY trial, which investigated prolonged DAPT after coronary stenting, showed benefit including lower mortality with extended $P2Y_{12}$ inhibition in those with PAD and CAD.[62] Limb outcomes were not reported.

The most common application of DAPT in patients with PAD is in the postintervention setting where benefits after endovascular intervention have been largely extrapolated from the coronary setting. In fact, the only randomized trial of DAPT after revascularization was the CASPAR (Clopidogrel and Acetylsalicylic Acid in Bypass Surgery for Peripheral Artery Disease) trial. In CASPAR, DAPT versus aspirin did not reduce the primary composite endpoint of graft occlusion, revascularization, amputation, or death in patients undergoing below-knee bypass surgery for PAD and moderate or severe bleeding was increased.[1,2] An analogous trial after endovascular intervention called CAMPER never completed.[1,2]

Overall, there are data to support antiplatelet monotherapy for MACE reduction in PAD, but data for MALE benefit are mixed. The efficacy of DAPT is supported for the reduction of MACEs and MALEs in patients with both PAD and CAD (polyvascular disease), although there is increased bleeding risk.[92] Although DAPT is commonly used, there are a paucity of randomized data to support DAPT use for the reduction of MALEs after intervention.

Combination Antiplatelet and Anticoagulant Therapy
The WAVE (Warfarin Antiplatelet Vascular Evaluation) trial compared combination antiplatelet and therapeutic vitamin K antagonist (VKA) therapy with antiplatelet therapy alone in patients with PAD.[1,2] Anticoagulation with warfarin did not reduce the primary composite endpoint of myocardial infarction, stroke, or CV death, but there was a greater than threefold increase in life-threatening bleeding resulting in a recommendation against use of this strategy for MACE reduction in patients with PAD in current guidelines.[1,2] There was no benefit for MALE with warfarin in WAVE. Therapeutic warfarin has been used after bypass surgery to reduce the risk of graft thrombosis. The Dutch Bypass Oral Anticoagulants or Aspirin Study examined this question in patients after bypass surgery but found no benefit in limb outcomes with warfarin after infrainguinal bypass surgery but a significant increase in hemorrhagic stroke.[1,2] Although used in selected patients felt to be at high risk of graft thrombosis, the routine use of therapeutic VKA therapy with antiplatelet therapy in PAD has not been shown to be efficacious and increases bleeding.

Factor Xa inhibition with very low doses of rivaroxaban has been evaluated in the Cardiovascular Outcomes for People Using Anticoagulation Strategies (COMPASS) and the Vascular Outcomes Study of ASA Along with Rivaroxaban in Endovascular or Surgical Limb Revascularizations for Peripheral Artery Disease (VOYAGER PAD) trials.[63,93,94] The COMPASS trial randomized 27,359 patients with stable atherosclerotic vascular disease, including lower extremity PAD to rivaroxaban 2.5 twice daily with aspirin, rivaroxaban 2.5 mg twice daily, or aspirin monotherapy. The majority of patients with PAD had concomitant CAD (polyvascular disease). The trial was ended early for overwhelming benefit and demonstrated a 24% reduction in MACEs for the rivaroxaban plus aspirin arm versus aspirin alone, while the rivaroxaban only arm did not show superiority. The benefits extended to reductions in CV death and all-cause mortality. The benefit was accompanied by a 70% increase in major bleeding but no statistically significant increase in intracranial hemorrhage or fatal bleeding. A subgroup analysis of 7470 patients with noncoronary vascular disease, including a subgroup with lower extremity PAD, demonstrated consistent efficacy and safety with the overall trial.[93] The majority of patients (>90%) in COMPASS had concomitant coronary disease, therefore demonstrating the clearest benefit for patients with both symptomatic CAD and PAD. In addition to benefits for MACEs, rivaroxaban significantly reduced the secondary endpoint of MALEs by approximately 45% with consistent effects for ALI and major vascular amputation. The greatest absolute benefits for reducing MALEs in COMPASS were observed in patients with symptomatic PAD with a history of prior revascularization relative to those with no history of revascularization, with little absolute benefit in those with asymptomatic PAD detected by a low ABI.[69,95]

The VOYAGER PAD trial tested the same strategy of aspirin and rivaroxaban 2.5 mg twice daily versus aspirin alone in a broader PAD population selected only on the basis of symptomatic lower extremity PAD requiring intervention.[63] In contrast to COMPASS, only approximately one third had coronary disease and approximately 10% had a prior myocardial infarction. The endpoint also differed and was a 5-point composite including ALI, major amputation of a vascular etiology, myocardial infarction, ischemic stroke, or CV death. Consistent with the COMPASS results, the combination of aspirin and rivaroxaban 2.5 twice daily was superior to aspirin alone, with a 15% relative risk reduction and 2.6% absolute risk reduction at 3 years. There was a 43% relative increase and 0.78% absolute increase in major bleeding at 3 years but no increase in intracranial hemorrhage or fatal bleeding. The benefits of rivaroxaban in VOYAGER PAD appeared greatest for limb outcomes, although there was consistency among the components with the exception of CV death where there was no apparent benefit. Together, COMPASS and VOYAGER PAD explored the efficacy and safety of rivaroxaban 2.5 mg twice daily plus aspirin versus aspirin alone across the spectrum of PAD. The MACE benefits were greatest in the COMPASS population and the subgroup of VOYAGER PAD patients with concomitant CAD (polyvascular disease) while the limb benefits were greatest in VOYAGER PAD and the subset of COMPASS with prior LER. Although rivaroxaban increased bleeding, there was a net benefit in both studies with a 6:1 benefit-risk ratio in VOYAGER PAD.

Other Combination Therapies
The TRA2°P-TIMI 50 trial studied vorapaxar, an antagonist of protease-activated receptor 1 (PAR-1), which is the platelet receptor for thrombin, in addition to aspirin and/or clopidogrel, in stable patients with established atherosclerosis. Overall, vorapaxar reduced the risk of myocardial infarction, stroke, and CV death but was associated with an increase in moderate or severe bleeding.[96] Benefit was greatest in patients with myocardial infarction or PAD, whereas there was overall harm in patients with prior stroke. Subsequent analyses have shown that in patients with PAD, the benefit of vorapaxar for MACEs was isolated to those with concomitant CAD rather than PAD without CAD.[4] In TRA2°P-TIMI 50, vorapaxar, added to aspirin, clopidogrel, or DAPT, decreased ALI by 42%, with associated reductions in risk of graft thrombosis, stent thrombosis, and de novo thrombosis and the greatest benefit in patients with prior revascularization.[4,18]

TREATMENT OF SYMPTOMS AND PREVENTION OF LIMB VASCULAR EVENTS

The morbidity in patients with symptomatic PAD includes progressive decline in functional status as well as limb-threatening events such as ALI and CLI, both of which frequently result in amputation. Therefore, a primary focus in the care of patients with PAD should be measures that improve functional capacity, alleviate symptoms, preserve limb viability, and reduce the risk of limb loss.

Smoking Cessation
Smoking cessation reduces the risk for developing symptomatic PAD and lessens the risk of progression to CLI and amputation in those with PAD.[12] In addition, smoking intensity is associated with outcomes after revascularization. An observational study of 693 PAD patients after surgical revascularization observed a 48% increase in the risk of amputation and death after surgery in those that smoked more than 1 pack per day even after adjustment for baseline differences.[97]

Supervised and Home-Based Exercise Training

Exercise training is the most effective noninvasive intervention for improving limb-related symptoms. The evidence supporting exercise therapy in PAD was first demonstrated for peak walking time in 1966.[98] Postulated mechanisms of benefit include the formation of collateral vessels and improvement in endothelium-dependent vasodilation, hemorheology, muscle structure and metabolism, and walking efficiency (Fig. 43.10).[43,98,99] Exercise increases the expression of angiogenic factors, particularly in hypoxic tissue. Improvement in calf blood flow has not been demonstrated consistently in patients with claudication; however, some studies have found that exercise training increased capillary density in calf muscle and that this change preceded the improvement in maximal O_2 consumption.

Much of the benefit of exercise training likely results from changes in skeletal muscle structure or function, such as increased muscle mitochondrial enzyme activity, oxidative metabolism, and ATP production rate (see Fig. 43.10). Improvement in exercise performance is associated with a decrease in plasma and skeletal muscle short-chain acylcarnitine concentrations, which indicates improvement in oxidative metabolism and increased peak O_2 consumption. Higher physical activity levels are associated with greater calf muscle area and density.[41,43] Training may also enhance biomechanical performance and enable patients to walk more efficiently with less energy expenditure. Supervised exercise training increases maximal walking time by 50% to 200%.[43,98] Exercise therapy is effective and durable, with the best results achieved with supervised exercise followed by home-based programs (Fig. 43.11). The greatest benefit occurs when sessions are at least 30 minutes in duration, when sessions take place at least three times per week for 6 months, and when walking is the mode of exercise. Home-based exercise training, when governed with a step-activated monitor, also improves walking time in patients with claudication (see Fig. 43.11).[41,43] Leg strength training improves walking time, although not as much as does treadmill exercise training. Arm ergometry also improves walking performance.[41,43] In the CLEVER (Claudication Exercise versus Endoluminal Revascularization) trial of patients with iliac artery stenosis, supervised exercise training improved mean walking time more than endovascular intervention, and both were more effective than optimal medical therapy; however, quality-of-life measures improved more in the endovascular intervention group.[1,2] In the ERASE (Endovascular Revascularization and Supervised Exercise) trial, the combination of endovascular revascularization and exercise in patients with femoropopliteal disease was superior to exercise alone.[1,2] Current guidelines recommend that patients with intermittent claudication undergo supervised exercise rehabilitation as initial therapy.[1,2,98] Translation of these recommendations is anticipated to increase in the United States with recent determinations with regard to reimbursement.[100]

Pharmacotherapy to Improve Claudication

Both pentoxifylline and cilostazol are available for the treatment of claudication in patients with PAD. *Pentoxifylline* is a xanthine derivative with benefits thought to be mediated through its hemorheologic properties, including

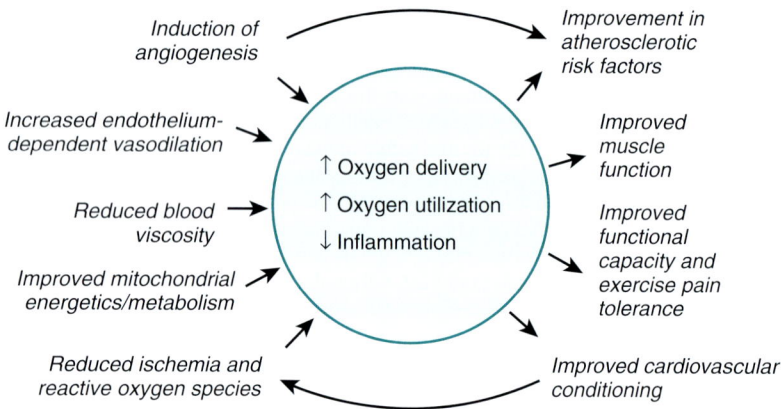

FIGURE 43.10 Mechanisms underlying the benefit of exercise in PAD. (Adapted from Bonaca MP, Creager MA. Pharmacological treatment and current management of peripheral artery disease. *Circ Res.* 2015;116:1579–1598.)

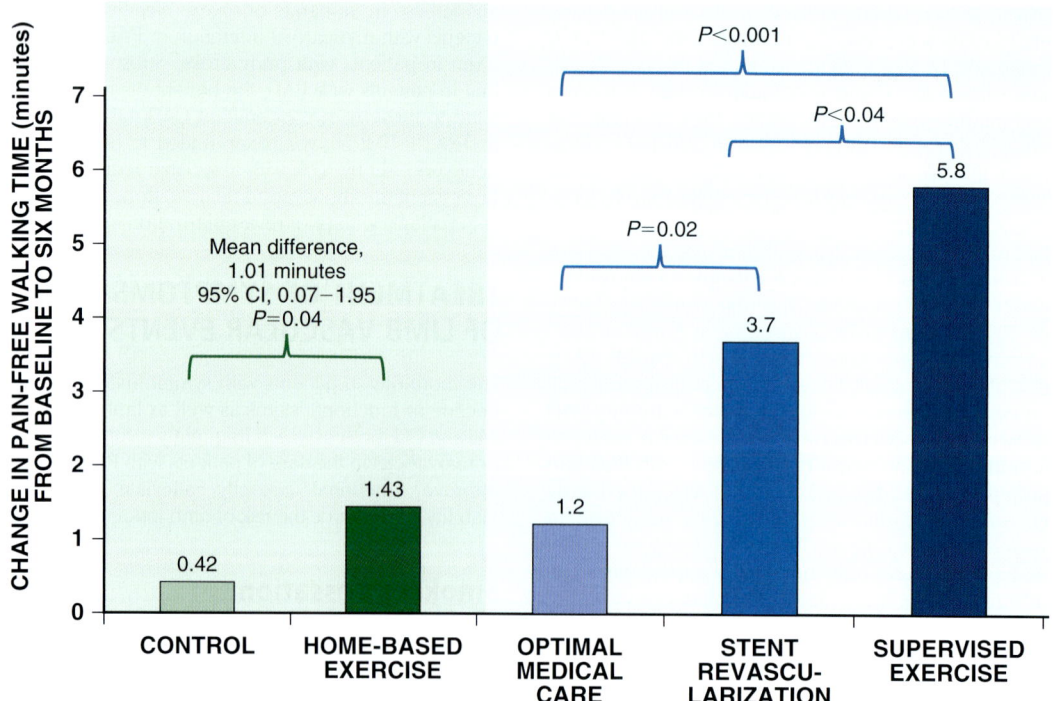

FIGURE 43.11 The relative efficacy of medical care alone, home-based exercise, supervised exercise, and stent revascularization in patients with PAD. (Adapted from McDermott MM, Liu K, Guralnik JM, et al. Home-based walking exercise intervention in peripheral artery disease: a randomized clinical trial. *JAMA.* 2013;310:57–65; and Murphy TP, Cutlip DE, Regensteiner JG, et al. Supervised exercise versus primary stenting for claudication resulting from aortoiliac peripheral artery disease: six-month outcomes from the claudication: exercise versus endoluminal revascularization (CLEVER) study. *Circulation.* 2012;125:130–139.)

its ability to decrease blood viscosity and to improve erythrocyte flexibility, although it likely has marginal efficacy.[1,2,84] *Cilostazol* is a quinolinone derivative that inhibits phosphodiesterase 3 (PDE3), thereby decreasing degradation of cyclic adenosine monophosphate and increasing its concentration in platelets and blood vessels. Although cilostazol inhibits platelet aggregation and causes vasodilation in experimental animals, its mechanism of action in patients with PAD is not known. Meta-analyses have found that cilostazol improves absolute claudication distance by 40% to 50% in comparison to placebo.[1,2,84] Quality-of-life measures, as assessed by the 36-Item Short-Form Medical Outcomes Scale (SF-36) and Walking Impairment Questionnaire, also demonstrate improvement. A U.S. Food and Drug Administration (FDA) advisory states that cilostazol should not be used in patients with congestive heart failure because other PDE3 inhibitors decrease survival in these patients. A long-term safety trial found that cilostazol (versus placebo) did not increase the risk for total or CV mortality, but the study was limited because more than 60% of the patients discontinued treatment before completion of the study.[1,2,84]

Vasodilators
Most studies of vasodilators have failed to demonstrate any efficacy in patients with intermittent claudication. Several pathophysiologic explanations may account for the failure of vasodilator therapy in patients with PAD. During exercise, resistance vessels distal to a stenosis dilate in response to ischemia. Vasodilators would have minimal if any effect on these endogenously dilated vessels but would decrease resistance in other vessels and create a relative steal phenomenon, thereby reducing blood flow and perfusion pressure to the affected leg. Moreover, in contrast to their effects on myocardial O_2 consumption in patients with CAD (because of afterload reduction), vasodilators do not reduce skeletal muscle O_2 demand.

Other Medical Therapies
Other classes of drugs, including serotonin (5-HT_2) antagonists, alpha-adrenergic antagonists, L-arginine, carnitine derivatives, vasodilator prostaglandins, antibiotics, and angiogenic growth factors, have been studied for the treatment of either claudication or CLI.[84] Overall, these therapies have not proved useful in improving PAD symptoms.[1,2] Angiogenic growth factors yielded encouraging preliminary findings in patients with CLI. However, large phase 3 clinical trials did not demonstrate improvement in the rate of amputation-free survival in patients with CLI or improvement in walking time in patients with intermittent claudication. In initial reports, stem cell–based therapies for PAD improved ABI, rest pain, and pain-free walking time and prevented amputation in some patients with chronic limb ischemia.[101] The response to cell therapy, however, may depend on patient selection, with some suggestion that patients with advanced CLI are poor candidates.[102] The findings from these preliminary trials require confirmation with additional clinical trials.

Percutaneous Transluminal Angioplasty and Stents (see Chapter 44)
Peripheral catheter–based interventions are indicated for selected patients with lifestyle-limiting claudication despite a trial of exercise rehabilitation or pharmacotherapy.[1,2] Drug-coated products increase long-term patency and reduce the need for recurrent revascularizations.[103,104] Recently, there has been concern raised regarding the safety of these products; however, there has been ongoing debate. Patients with CLI with anatomy amenable to catheter-based therapy may also be candidates for endovascular intervention. A large clinical trial is comparing the efficacy of endovascular intervention with surgical revascularization on limb outcomes in patients with CLI.[105]

Peripheral Artery Surgery
The ACC/AHA management of intervention is summarized in Table 43G.7. Surgical revascularization improves symptoms in patients with disabling claudication and is indicated to relieve rest pain and preserve limb viability in patients with CLI that is not amenable to percutaneous interventions. The specific operation must take into account the anatomic location of the arterial lesions and the presence of comorbid conditions. Planning for surgical procedures requires identification of the arterial obstruction by imaging to ensure sufficient arterial inflow to and outflow from the graft to maintain patency. Surgical approaches include endarterectomy, bypass, and hybrid approaches (endovascular and surgical).[106] *Aortobifemoral bypass* is the most frequent open surgical operation performed in patients with aortoiliac disease. Typically, a knitted or woven prosthesis made of Dacron or polytetrafluoroethylene (PTFE) is anastomosed proximally to the aorta and distally to each common femoral artery.[106] On occasion the iliac artery is used for the distal anastomosis to maintain anterograde flow into at least one hypogastric artery. A systematic review of 29 studies from 1970 to 2007 that compared 5738 patients who underwent aortobifemoral bypass surgery found an operative mortality rate of 4%, although high-volume centers in the United States report lower mortality rates. Five-year patency rates for aortobifemoral bypass grafts exceed 80%.

Extra-anatomic surgical reconstructive procedures for aortoiliac disease include axillobifemoral bypass, iliobifemoral bypass, and femoral-femoral bypass. These bypass grafts circumvent the aorta and iliac arteries and are generally used in high-risk patients with CLI. Five-year patency rates range from 50% to 70% for axillobifemoral bypass operations and from 70% to 80% for femoral-femoral bypass grafts.[106] The operative mortality rate for extra-anatomic bypass procedures is 3% to 5% and reflects, in part, the serious comorbid conditions and advanced atherosclerosis in many of the patients who undergo these procedures.

Reconstructive surgery for infrainguinal arterial disease includes femoral-popliteal and femoral-tibial or femoral-peroneal artery bypass. Infrainguinal bypass uses in situ or reversed autologous saphenous veins or synthetic grafts made of PTFE as conduits. Patency rates for autologous saphenous vein bypass grafts exceed those with PTFE grafts.[106] Grafts with the distal anastomosis placed in the popliteal artery above the knee have better patency rates than those placed below the knee. Five-year primary patency rates for femoral-popliteal reconstruction in patients with claudication are approximately 80% and 75% for autogenous vein grafts and PTFE grafts, respectively, and approximately 65% and 45%, respectively, in patients with CLI. For femoral below-knee bypass, including tibioperoneal artery reconstruction, the 5-year patency rates for saphenous vein grafts in patients with claudication or CLI are similar to those for femoral-popliteal above-knee grafts (60% to 80%). The 5-year patency rate for PTFE grafts in the infrapopliteal position is considerably lower, approximately 65% in patients with claudication and 33% in patients with CLI. The operative mortality rate for infrainguinal bypass operations is 2% to 3%.

Graft stenoses can result from technical errors at surgery, such as retained valve cuffs or intimal flap or valvotome injury; from fibrous intimal hyperplasia, usually within 6 months of surgery; or from atherosclerosis, which usually occurs within the vein graft at least 1 to 2 years after surgery. Institution of graft surveillance protocols with the use of color-assisted duplex ultrasonography has enabled the identification of graft stenoses, thereby prompting graft revision and avoiding complete graft failure. Routine ultrasonographic surveillance improves graft outcome.[106] Ongoing challenges include control of neointimal hyperplasia and lack of adequate autogenous conduit requiring use of prosthetics and associated suboptimal outcomes.[106]

Figure 43.12 provides an overview of medical therapy for patients with PAD.

VASCULITIS (SEE ALSO CHAPTER 97)

Thromboangiitis Obliterans
TAO, a segmental vasculitis that involves the distal arteries, veins, and nerves of the upper and lower extremities, typically affects younger persons who smoke.[107]

Pathology and Pathogenesis
TAO primarily affects the medium and small vessels of the arms, including the radial, ulnar, palmar, and digital arteries, and their counterparts in the legs, including the tibial, peroneal, plantar, and digital arteries. Involvement can extend to the cerebral, coronary, renal, mesenteric, aortoiliac,

Axis of therapy	Symptomatic PAD No prior revascularization No CAD No CVD	Symptomatic PAD Prior revascularization Or Polyvascular disease
Lifestyle	Smoking cessation, diet, exercise	Smoking cessation, diet, exercise
Antithrombotic	Antiplatelet monotherapy	Antiplatelet monotherapy if at high bleeding risk If at low bleeding risk then add rivaroxaban to aspirin. Vorapaxar can be added to aspirin as an alternative. DAPT with a P2Y12 can be used if CAD/prior MI.
Lipid modifying	High-intensity statin + eze and/or PCSK9i (target LDL-C goal) in selected patients	High-intensity Statin + eze and/or PCSK9i (target LDL-C goal) in selected patients
Angiotensin inhibition	If HTN then ACEi preferred	If HTN then ACEi preferred
Glucose lowering	If T2DM then GLP1 agonist and/or SGLT2i depending on patient risk profile	If T2DM then GLP1 agonist and/or SGLT2i depending on patient risk profile
For symptoms	Exercise, cilostazol	Exercise, cilostazol

FIGURE 43.12 A summary of medical management of patients with PAD. EZE, ezetimibe; PCSK9, proprotein convertase subtilisin/kexin type 9; T2DM, type 2 diabetes mellitus; GLP-1, glucagon-like peptide 1; HTN, hypertension; ACE1, angiotensin-converting enzyme 1; DAPT, dual antiplatelet therapy; Vora, vorapaxar (Adapted from Bonaca MP, Creager MA. Pharmacological treatment and current management of peripheral artery disease. Circ Res. 2015;116:1579–1598.)

and pulmonary arteries.[107] Pathologic findings include an occlusive, highly cellular thrombus that incorporates polymorphonuclear leukocytes, microabscesses, and occasionally multinucleated giant cells. The inflammatory infiltrate can also affect the vascular wall, but the internal elastic membrane remains intact. In the chronic phase of the disease, the thrombus becomes organized and the vascular wall becomes fibrotic.

The precise cause of TAO is not known. Tobacco use or exposure is present in virtually every patient. Hypercoagulability, immunologic mechanisms, and endothelial dysfunction may contribute to the pathogenesis of TAO. Potential immunologic mechanisms include increased cellular sensitivity to types I and III collagen and the presence of antiendothelial cell antibodies. CD4+ T cells have been identified in the cellular infiltrates of vessels of patients with TAO.[107] Decreased endothelium-dependent vasodilation can occur in both the affected and the unaffected limbs of patients with TAO. Some reports have found increased frequency of a prothrombin gene mutation, elevated plasma homocysteine concentration, or increased levels of anticardiolipin antibodies in patients with TAO.

Clinical Features

The prevalence of TAO is greater in Asia than in North America or Western Europe. In the United States, TAO occurs in approximately 13 per 100,000 persons. Symptoms develop in most before 45 years of age, and 75% to 90% are men. Patients can have claudication of the hands, forearms, feet, or calves. Most patients with TAO have pain at rest and digital ulcerations; frequently, more than one extremity is affected. Raynaud phenomenon occurs in approximately 45% of patients, and superficial thrombophlebitis, which may be migratory, develops in approximately 40%. The risk for amputation within 5 years is approximately 25%.[107] The radial, ulnar, dorsalis pedis, and posterior tibial pulses may be absent. Two thirds of patients have abnormal Allen test results. The distal aspects of the extremities may have discrete, tender, erythematous subcutaneous cords, indicative of superficial thrombophlebitis.

Diagnosis

No specific laboratory tests, other than biopsy, can diagnose TAO. Most tests therefore aim to exclude other diseases that might have similar clinical features, including autoimmune diseases such as scleroderma or SLE, hypercoagulable states, DM, and acute arterial occlusion secondary to embolism. Acute-phase indicators, such as the erythrocyte sedimentation rate (ESR) or CRP, are usually normal. Serum immunologic markers, including antinuclear antibodies and rheumatoid factor, should not be present, and serum complement levels should be normal. If clinically indicated, a proximal source of embolism should be excluded by imaging. Arteriography of an affected limb supports the diagnosis of TAO if there is segmental occlusion of small and medium arteries, absence of atherosclerosis, and corkscrew collateral vessels circumventing the occlusion (Fig. 43.13). These same findings, however, can occur in patients with scleroderma, SLE, mixed connective tissue disease, and antiphospholipid antibody syndrome. The conclusive test is a biopsy specimen showing the classic pathologic findings. However, this procedure is rarely indicated, and biopsy sites may fail to heal because of severe ischemia. The diagnosis therefore usually depends on an age at onset of younger than 45 years, a history of tobacco use, physical examination demonstrating distal limb ischemia, exclusion of other diseases, and, if necessary, angiographic demonstration of typical lesions.

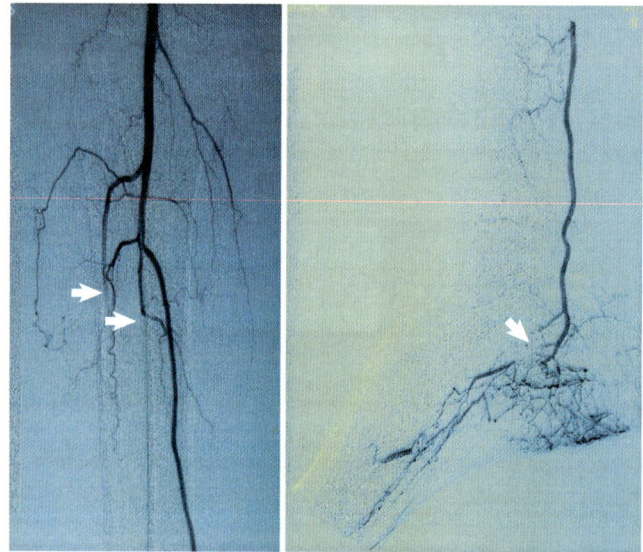

FIGURE 43.13 Angiogram of a young woman with thromboangiitis obliterans. **Left,** Occlusion of the anterior tibial and peroneal arteries (*arrows*). **Right,** Occlusion of the distal portion of the posterior tibial artery (*arrow*) with bridging collateral vessels.

Treatment

The cornerstone of TAO treatment is cessation of tobacco use. Patients without gangrene who stop smoking rarely require amputation.[107] In contrast, one or more amputations may ultimately be required in 40% to 45% of those who continue to smoke. Trigger avoidance beyond smoking cessation is recommended including avoidance of cold exposures as well as other chemical or mechanical sources of injury. Proper skin hygiene and daily foot checks are recommended. No definitive drug therapy is available for TAO. Intravenous iloprost, a prostacyclin analogue, may be more effective than aspirin for rest pain and ischemic ulcers, but oral iloprost is not effective.[108] There is insufficient evidence to support the use of other vasodilator prostaglandin analogues in this setting.[108] Vascular reconstructive surgery is not usually a viable option because of the segmental nature of this disease and the involvement of distal vessels. An autogenous saphenous vein bypass graft can be considered if a target vessel for the distal anastomosis is available. Sympathectomy may improve some symptoms of TAO. Hyperbaric oxygen therapy may improve healing and reduce amputations although reports are limited to small patient numbers.[109] In severe refractory cases, bosentan can be considered based on observed healing in a case series.[110]

TAKAYASU ARTERITIS AND GIANT CELL ARTERITIS (SEE CHAPTER 97)

Fibromuscular Dysplasia

FMD is a noninflammatory disorder that affects medium and large arteries, typically the renal, carotid, and vertebral arteries. It also may involve the arteries supplying the leg, particularly the iliac arteries and less often the femoral, popliteal, tibial, and peroneal arteries.[111,112] FMD rarely causes intermittent claudication or CLI. It most often affects women but can occur at any age in both sexes. Although traditionally thought to occur in young women, recent registries have described occurrence primarily in middle-aged women.[111,112] In addition, while historically described as affecting the renal arteries with the highest frequency, registries describe similar involvement of the carotid, vertebral, and renal arteries, with approximately 65% of patients having multivessel involvement. Aneurysm or dissection is present in more than 40% of patients at diagnosis.[113] Spontaneous coronary artery dissection (SCAD) is an uncommon presentation of FMD. The most frequent presenting signs and symptoms are hypertension, headache, pulsatile tinnitus, and dizziness illustrating clinical scenarios that should prompt consideration of FMD (Table 43.8).[114]

In patients with suspected FMD, the diagnosis is confirmed by imaging including CT, magnetic resonance imaging (MRI), and duplex ultrasound. DSA is generally reserved for patients with a high clinical suspicion and nondiagnostic noninvasive imaging. FMD can be distinguished from atherosclerosis by imaging and patient characteristics (younger, lack of atherosclerosis risk factors) and from vasculitis by the absence of clinical signs, symptoms, or testing suggesting inflammation (e.g., elevated ESR or CRP).

Histopathologic examination shows fibroplasia most often affecting the media, but it can involve the intima or adventitia. The histologic classification of FMD includes the medial subtypes (medial fibroplasia, perimedial fibroplasia, and medial hyperplasia), as well as intimal fibroplasia and adventitial hyperplasia.[111] Depending on the histopathologic type, stenosis results from hyperplasia of the fibrous or muscular components of the vessel wall. Angiographic findings can be classified into two subtypes. The first, *multifocal* FMD, is more common and presents with the classic "string of beads" and has been pathologically associated with intimal fibroplasia, medial hyperplasia, and to perimedial fibroplasia. The second, *focal* FMD, appears as a tubular stenosis, is less common, and is pathologically associated with medial hyperplasia and periarterial hyperplasia (Fig. 43.14). As many as one third of cases cannot be classified using angiographic criteria, and the pathologic subtypes overlap considerably. The lack of routine histopathology in the clinical setting and limitations of angiographic criteria have prompted consideration of alternative classification systems.[111]

Symptomatic FMD patients can undergo angioplasty. All patients should receive medical therapy to treat any conventional risk factors (e.g., antihypertensive medications) and should have serial clinical evaluations with laboratory testing and/or imaging when indicated, based on clinical assessment. Smoking is associated with worse outcomes, underscoring the importance of cessation.[115]

TABLE 43.8 Clinical Circumstances Prompting Consideration of Fibromuscular Dysplasia

Hypertension <35 years old or resistant hypertension at any age
Epigastric bruit and hypertension
Transient ischemic attack, stroke, or cervical bruit in a patient <60 years old
Symptomatic PAD in a woman <60 years old without atherosclerotic risk factors
Subarachnoid hemorrhage
Pulsatile tinnitus
Severe and recurrent headaches
Peripheral artery dissection or spontaneous coronary artery dissection
Visceral or intracranial aneurysm
Aortic aneurysm in a patient <60 years old
Renal infarction

Modified from Olin JW, Froehlich J, Gu X, et al. The United States Registry for Fibromuscular Dysplasia: results in the first 447 patients. *Circulation.* 2012;125:3182–3190.

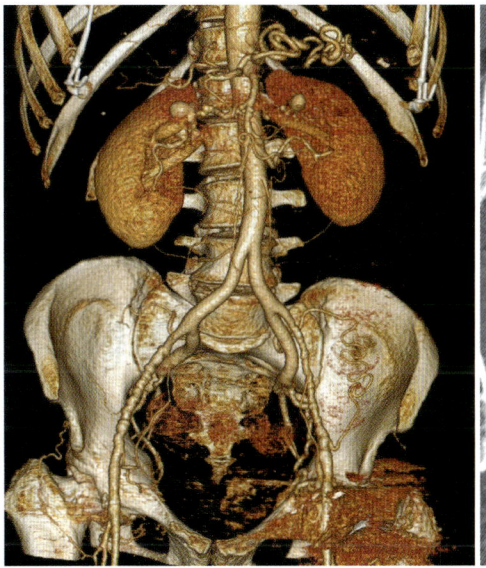 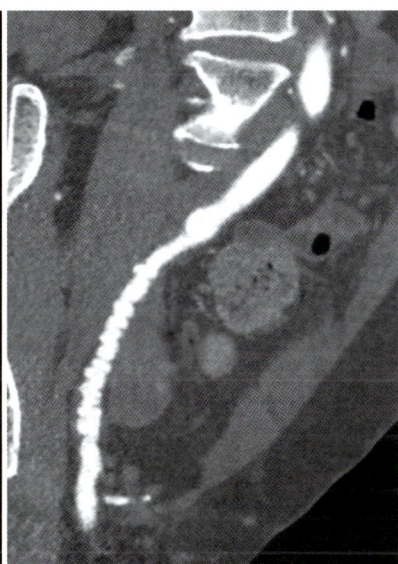

FIGURE 43.14 Angiogram of a patient with FMD. **Left,** 3D volume rendered demonstrating bilateral external iliac FMD. **Right,** Maximum intensity projection of the external iliac. (Images courtesy of Jeffrey Olin, MD.)

POPLITEAL ARTERY ENTRAPMENT SYNDROME

Popliteal artery entrapment syndrome is an uncommon cause of intermittent claudication. It occurs when an anatomic variation in the configuration or insertion of the medial head of the gastrocnemius muscle compresses the popliteal artery.[116,117] The popliteus muscle also can compress the popliteal artery and cause this syndrome. Popliteal artery entrapment is bilateral in approximately one third of affected patients. It should be suspected when a young, typically athletic, usually male person is evaluated for claudication. Potential consequences include popliteal artery thrombosis, embolism, and aneurysm formation.

Findings on peripheral pulse examination may be normal unless provocative maneuvers are performed. Walking or repeated ankle dorsiflexion and plantar flexion maneuvers may cause attenuation or disappearance of the pedal pulses and a decrease in the ABI in patients with popliteal artery entrapment. Imaging studies such as duplex ultrasonography, CTA, MRA, or conventional angiography, performed at rest and during ankle flexion maneuvers, can confirm the diagnosis. Treatment of popliteal artery entrapment syndrome involves release of the popliteal artery, which may require division and reattachment of the medial head of the gastrocnemius muscle. On occasion, occlusion of the popliteal artery requires surgical bypass. Five-year patency rates for surgical treatment exceed 80%.[118]

ACUTE LIMB ISCHEMIA

ALI occurs when an arterial occlusion suddenly reduces blood flow to the arm or leg.[119] The metabolic needs of the tissue outstrip perfusion, thereby jeopardizing limb viability. Pain may develop quickly and affect the part of the extremity distal to the site of obstruction. It is not necessarily confined to the foot or toes or the hand or fingers, as is usually the case with chronic critical limb ischemia (CLI). Concurrent ischemia of peripheral nerves causes sensory loss and motor dysfunction. Findings on physical examination can include absence of pulses distal to the occlusion, cool skin, pallor, delayed capillary return and venous filling, diminished or absent sensory perception, and muscle weakness or paralysis. This constellation of symptoms and signs is often recalled as the "six Ps": pain, paresthesias, pallor, pulselessness, poikilothermia, and paralysis.

Prognosis

Patients with ALI usually have comorbid CV disorders, which may even be responsible for the ischemia. The risk for limb loss depends on the severity of the ischemia and the time elapsed before revascularization. Among patients with atherosclerosis presenting with ALI in recent studies, approximately 18% required amputation, and 15% either died or were unable to return home after hospitalization.[18,95] The Society for Vascular Surgery and the International Society for Cardiovascular Surgery developed a classification that takes into consideration the severity of ischemia and the viability of the limb, along with related neurologic findings and Doppler signals.[2]

Pathogenesis

Causes of ALI include embolism, thrombosis in situ, dissection, and trauma. A large proportion are embolic (Fig. 43.15).[120] Most arterial emboli arise from thrombotic sources in the heart, as occurs in atrial fibrillation, or other sources such as prosthetic cardiac valves, paradoxical embolism, and cardiac tumors such as left atrial myxomas. Aneurysms of the aorta or peripheral arteries may lead to embolization of thrombus to more distal arterial sites and usually lodge at branch points where the artery decreases in size. In patients with established PAD, causes of ALI include in situ atherothrombosis, graft thrombosis, or stent thrombosis[18,95] (see Fig. 43.15). Thrombosis in situ occurs in atherosclerotic peripheral arteries, infrainguinal bypass grafts, peripheral artery aneurysms, and normal arteries of patients with hypercoagulable states. In patients with PAD, thrombosis in situ may complicate plaque rupture and cause acute arterial occlusion and limb ischemia, as occurs in the coronary arteries of patients with acute MI. One of the most common causes of ALI in patients with PAD is thrombotic occlusion of an infrainguinal bypass graft. Acute thrombotic occlusion of a normal artery is unusual but may occur in patients with acquired thrombophilic disorders such as antiphospholipid antibody syndrome, heparin-induced thrombocytopenia, disseminated intravascular coagulation, and myeloproliferative diseases. There is limited evidence that inherited thrombophilic disorders such as activated protein C resistance (factor V Leiden), prothrombin *G20210* gene mutation, or deficiencies of antithrombin III and protein C and S increase the risk for acute peripheral arterial thrombosis.

Diagnostic Tests

The history and physical examination usually establish the diagnosis of ALI. Tests should not delay urgent revascularization procedures to rescue a limb with threatened viability. Pressure in the affected limb and corresponding ABI can be measured if flow is detectable by Doppler ultrasonography. A Doppler probe can assess the presence of blood flow in peripheral arteries, even when pulses are not palpable. Color-assisted duplex ultrasonography can determine the site of occlusion, particularly to evaluate the patency of infrainguinal bypass grafts. MRA, CTA, and conventional arteriography can demonstrate the site of occlusion and provide an anatomic guide for revascularization. Assessment of limb status according to the ACC/AHA guidelines as summarized in Table 43G.9.

Treatment

For patients with acute leg ischemia, the bed should be positioned such that the feet are lower than chest level, thereby increasing limb perfusion pressure by hydrostatic effects. Effort should be made to reduce pressure on the heels, on bone prominences, and between the toes by appropriate placement of soft material on the bed (e.g., sheepskin) and between the toes (e.g., lambswool). Heparin should be administered intravenously immediately.[1,2] The dose should maintain the partial thromboplastin time at 2.0 to 2.5 times control values or titrated to factor Xa levels depending on local practice and with a goal to prevent propagation of thrombi or recurrent embolism.

Revascularization is indicated when the viability of the limb is threatened or when symptoms of ischemia persist (Fig. 43.16). Options

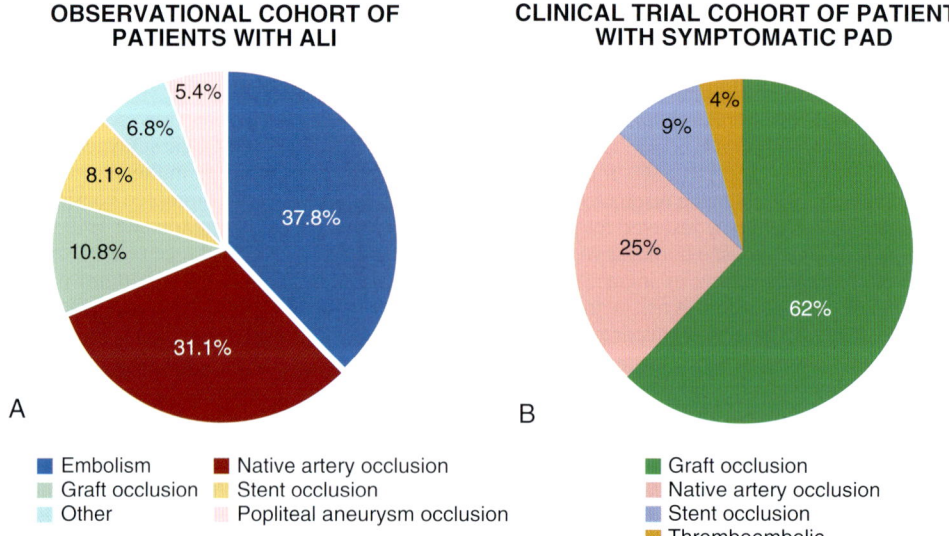

FIGURE 43.15 Etiologies of acute limb ischemia (ALI) in an all-comers registry (**A**) and in patients with symptomatic PAD not requiring anticoagulation (**B**). (**A** adapted from Duval S, Keo HH, Oldenburg NC, et al. The impact of prolonged lower limb ischemia on amputation, mortality, and functional status: the FRIENDS registry. *Am Heart J*. 2014;168:577–587; **B** adapted from Bonaca MP, Gutierrez JA, Creager MA, et al. Acute Limb Ischemia and Outcomes With Vorapaxar in Patients With Peripheral Artery Disease: Results From the Trial to Assess the Effects of Vorapaxar in Preventing Heart Attack and Stroke in Patients With Atherosclerosis-Thrombolysis in Myocardial Infarction 50 (TRA2°P-TIMI 50). *Circulation*. 2016;133:997–1005.)

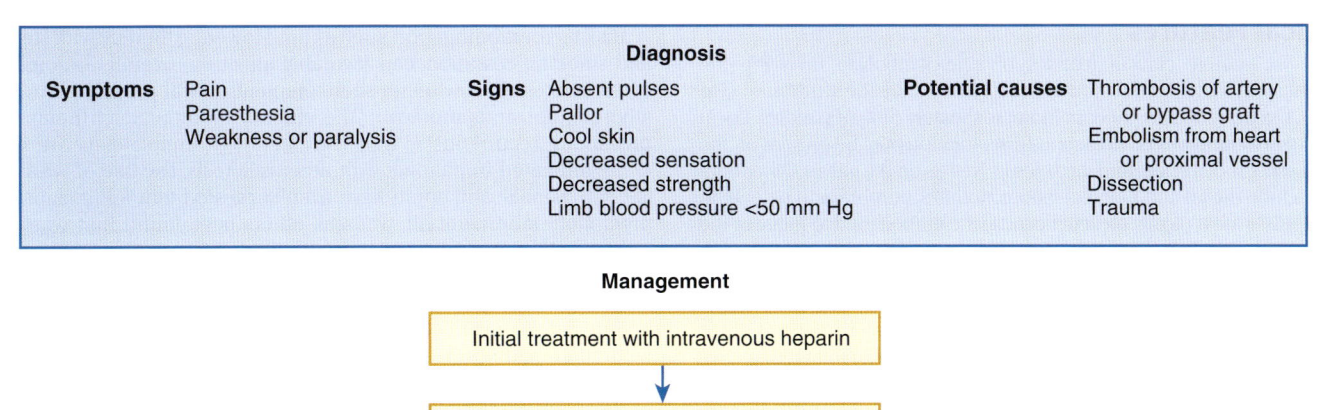
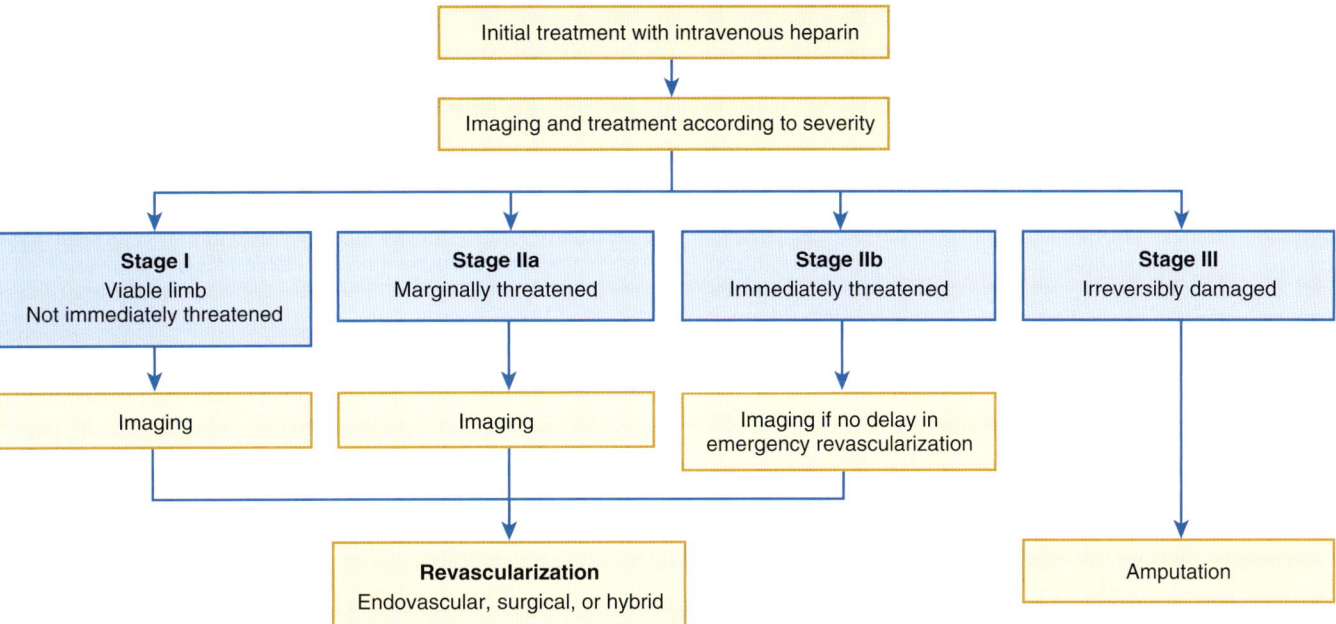

FIGURE 43.16 Diagnostic and treatment approach for patients presenting with acute limb ischemia.

for restoration of blood flow include endovascular revascularization, intra-arterial thrombolytic therapy, and surgical revascularization. Catheter-directed intra-arterial thrombolysis plus thrombectomy is an initial treatment option for patients with either category I or II ALI if they have no contraindication to thrombolysis.[1,2] Identification and repair of a graft stenosis after successful thrombolysis improve long-term graft patency. The thrombolytic regimens currently used include the recombinant tissue plasminogen activators alteplase, reteplase, and tenecteplase. Catheter-based thrombolytic therapy should generally be continued for 24 to 48 hours to achieve optimal benefit and to limit the risk for bleeding. Adjuvant use of platelet glycoprotein IIb/IIIa inhibitors shortens thrombolysis time but does not improve outcome. Percutaneous, catheter-based mechanical thrombectomy, with devices that remove thrombus via aspiration, fragmentation, or high-energy ultrasound, can be used alone or in addition to pharmacologic thrombolysis to treat patients with ALI. Surgical revascularization, including thromboembolectomy and bypass of the occluded area, is an option for restoration of blood flow to an ischemic limb. Five prospective randomized trials have compared the benefits and risks of thrombolysis and surgical reconstruction in ALI patients. Overall, the two interventions did not differ in the rate of death or amputation during the 1 year between, although patients undergoing thrombolysis had a greater risk for major bleeding. Findings from the individual trials suggest that catheter-based thrombolysis is an appropriate initial option in patients with viable or marginally threatened limbs and when the ischemia is of less than 14 days' duration, whereas surgical revascularization is more appropriate in those with immediately threatened limbs and in those whose symptoms have lasted for more than 14 days. Patients with irreversible injury require amputation (see Fig. 43.16).

The optimal long-term antithrombotic strategy in patients with ALI remains uncertain. Long-term anticoagulant therapy is usually indicated for patients with an embolic source, such as atrial fibrillation.

For patients with symptomatic PAD who develop ALI from thrombotic complications in the limbs (e.g., graft occlusion, stent thrombosis, in situ thrombosis), intensive antithrombotic therapy may be more effective than aspirin alone in reducing recurrent events particularly if treated with revascularization.[1,2,63] Warfarin has not proven beneficial in secondary prevention of nonembolic ALI and is generally only indicated based on the underlying etiology (e.g., atrial fibrillation).

ATHEROEMBOLISM

Atheroembolism refers to occlusion of arteries resulting from detachment and embolization of atheromatous debris, including fibrin, platelets, cholesterol crystals, and calcium fragments. Other terms include *atherogenic embolism* and *cholesterol embolism*. Atheroemboli originate most frequently from "shaggy," protruding atheroma of the aorta and less frequently from atherosclerotic branch arteries. The atheroemboli typically occlude small downstream arteries and arterioles of the skin, extremities, brain, eyes, kidneys, or mesentery. Most affected individuals are men older than 60 years with clinical evidence of atherosclerosis.

Pathogenesis

Patients with aortic atherosclerosis characterized by large complex atheromas have the greatest risk for atheroembolism. Identification of large, protruding atheromas by transesophageal ultrasound predicts future embolic events. Catheter manipulation may also cause atheroemboli in approximately 1% to 2% of patients undergoing endovascular procedures. Similarly, surgical manipulation of the aorta during cardiac or vascular operations may precipitate atheroembolism. Controversy remains whether anticoagulants or thrombolytic drugs contribute to atheroembolism.

Clinical Features

The most notable clinical features of atheroembolism involving the extremities include painful cyanotic toes, called "blue toe syndrome" (Fig. 43.17). Livedo reticularis occurs in approximately 50% of patients. Local areas of erythematous or violaceous discoloration may be present on the lateral aspects of the feet and the soles, as well as on the calves. Other findings include digital and foot ulcerations, nodules, purpura, and petechiae. Pedal pulses are typically present because the emboli tend to lodge in the more distal digital arteries and arterioles. Symptoms and signs indicating additional organ involvement with atheroemboli should be sought. Renal involvement, manifested by increased BP and azotemia, typically occurs in patients with peripheral atheroemboli. Patients also sometimes show evidence of mesenteric or bladder ischemia and splenic infarction.

The clinical setting and findings usually suffice for the diagnosis of atheroembolism, but other diseases may have some of the manifestations of atheroemboli. Hypersensitivity vasculitides secondary to connective tissue diseases, infections, drugs, polyarteritis nodosa, or cryoglobulinemia generally involve multiple organ systems and cause cutaneous findings of purpura, ulcers, and digital ischemia, similar to those resulting from atheroemboli (see Chapter 97). Procoagulant disorders such as antiphospholipid antibody syndrome, heparin-induced thrombocytopenia, and myeloproliferative disorders such as essential thrombocythemia can cause digital artery thrombosis with resultant digital ischemia, cyanosis, and ulceration.

Diagnostic Tests

Laboratory findings consistent with atheroembolism include an elevated ESR, eosinophilia, and eosinophiluria. Other findings may include anemia, thrombocytopenia, hypocomplementemia, and azotemia. Imaging of the aorta with transesophageal echocardiography (TEE), MRA, or CTA may identify sites of severe atherosclerosis indicating a source of the atheroemboli. The only definitive test for atheroembolism is pathologic confirmation on skin or muscle biopsy specimens. Pathognomonic findings include elongated needle-shaped clefts in small arteries caused by cholesterol crystals and often accompanied by inflammatory infiltrates composed of lymphocytes and possibly giant cells and eosinophils, intimal thickening, and perivascular fibrosis.

Treatment

No definitive treatment has been established for atheroembolism. Local foot care should be provided as with ALI. It may be necessary to excise or amputate necrotic areas.

Risk factor modification, such as lipid-lowering therapy with statins and smoking cessation, can favorably affect the overall outcome of atherosclerosis, but whether such intervention will prevent recurrent atheroembolism is unknown. The efficacy of antiplatelet therapy in preventing recurrence is unknown, although antiplatelets are generally indicated in patients with atherosclerosis. The use of warfarin is controversial, and some have even suggested that anticoagulants precipitate atheroemboli, whereas others have found that warfarin reduces atheroembolic events, particularly in patients with mobile aortic atheroma. The use of corticosteroids to treat atheroembolism is also controversial.

Surgical removal of the source should be considered in patients with atheroembolism, particularly in those with recurrence. Surgical procedures include excision and replacement of affected portions of the aorta, endarterectomy, and bypass operations. Operative intervention targets the site of the aorta and iliac or femoral arteries with aneurysm formation or evidence for mobile atherosclerotic plaque. Frequently, diffuse aortic disease makes it difficult to identify the precise segment responsible for the atheroembolism. Several small case series have reported endovascular placement of stents and stent grafts to prevent recurrent atheroembolism (Table 43G.7).

ACKNOWLEDGMENT

The authors thank Dr. Peter Libby, co-author of this chapter in editions 6 to 10, for his contributions and mentorship.

REFERENCES

Background and Epidemiology

1. Aboyans V, Ricco JB, Bartelink MEL, et al. 2017 ESC guidelines on the diagnosis and treatment of peripheral arterial diseases, in collaboration with the European Society for Vascular Surgery (ESVS): document covering atherosclerotic disease of extracranial carotid and vertebral, mesenteric, renal, upper and lower extremity arteries. Endorsed by: the European Stroke Organization (ESO) the task force for the diagnosis and treatment of peripheral arterial diseases of the European Society of Cardiology (ESC) and of the European Society for Vascular Surgery (ESVS). Eur Heart J. 2018;39:763–816.
2. Gerhard-Herman MD, Gornik HL, Barrett C, et al. 2016 AHA/ACC guideline on the management of patients with lower extremity peripheral artery disease: a report of the American College of Cardiology/American Heart Association task force on clinical practice guidelines. Circulation. 2017;135:e726–e779.
3. Hess CN, Rogers RK, Wang TY, et al. Major adverse limb events and 1-year outcomes after peripheral artery revascularization. J Am Coll Cardiol. 2018;72:999–1011.
4. Qamar A, Morrow DA, Creager MA, et al. Effect of vorapaxar on cardiovascular and limb outcomes in patients with peripheral artery disease with and without coronary artery disease: analysis from the TRA2°P-TIMI 50 trial. Vasc Med. 2020;25:124–132.
5. Kumbhani DJ, Steg PG, Cannon CP, et al. Statin therapy and long-term adverse limb outcomes in patients with peripheral artery disease: insights from the REACH registry. Eur Heart J. 2014;35:2864–2872.
6. Virani SS, Alonso A, Benjamin EJ, et al. Heart disease and stroke statistics-2020 update: a report from the American Heart Association. Circulation. 2020;141:e139–e596.
7. Fowkes FG, Aboyans V, Fowkes FJ, et al. Peripheral artery disease: epidemiology and global perspectives. Nat Rev Cardiol. 2017;14:156–170.
8. Berger JS, Abramson BL, Lopes RD, et al. Ticagrelor versus clopidogrel in patients with symptomatic peripheral artery disease and prior coronary artery disease: insights from the EUCLID trial. Vasc Med. 2018;23:523–530.
9. Bonaca MP, Gutierrez JA, Cannon C, et al. Polyvascular disease, type 2 diabetes, and long-term vascular risk: a secondary analysis of the IMPROVE-IT trial. Lancet Diabetes Endocrinol. 2018;6:934–943.
10. Bonaca MP, Nault P, Giugliano RP, et al. Low-density lipoprotein cholesterol lowering with evolocumab and outcomes in patients with peripheral artery disease: insights from the FOURIER trial (further cardiovascular outcomes research with PCSK9 inhibition in subjects with elevated risk). Circulation. 2018;137:338–350.
11. Colantonio LD, Hubbard D, Monda KL, et al. Atherosclerotic risk and statin use among patients with peripheral artery disease. J Am Coll Cardiol. 2020;76:251–264.
12. Agarwal S, Sud K, Shishehbor MH. Nationwide trends of hospital admission and outcomes among critical limb ischemia patients: from 2003-2011. J Am Coll Cardiol. 2016;67:1901–1913.
13. Criqui MH, Aboyans V. Epidemiology of peripheral artery disease. Circ Res. 2015;116:1509–1526.
14. Nehler MR, Duval S, Diao L, et al. Epidemiology of peripheral arterial disease and critical limb ischemia in an insured national population. J Vasc Surg. 2014;60:686–695.e2.
15. Forbang NI, Criqui MH, Allison MA, et al. Sex and ethnic differences in the associations between lipoprotein(a) and peripheral arterial disease in the Multi-Ethnic Study of Atherosclerosis. J Vasc Surg. 2016;63:453–458.
16. Howard DP, Banerjee A, Fairhead JF, et al. Population-based study of incidence, risk factors, outcome, and prognosis of ischemic peripheral arterial events: implications for prevention. Circulation. 2015;132:1805–1815.
17. Bonaca MP, Bhatt DL, Storey RF, et al. Ticagrelor for prevention of ischemic events after myocardial infarction in patients with peripheral artery disease. J Am Coll Cardiol. 2016;67:2719–2728.
18. Bonaca MP, Gutierrez JA, Creager MA, et al. Acute limb ischemia and outcomes with vorapaxar in patients with peripheral artery disease: results from the trial to assess the effects of vorapaxar in preventing heart attack and stroke in patients with atherosclerosis-thrombolysis in myocardial infarction 50 (TRA2°P-TIMI 50). Circulation. 2016;133:997–1005.
19. Jones WS, Baumgartner I, Hiatt WR, et al. Ticagrelor compared with clopidogrel in patients with prior lower extremity revascularization for peripheral artery disease. Circulation. 2017;135:241–250.

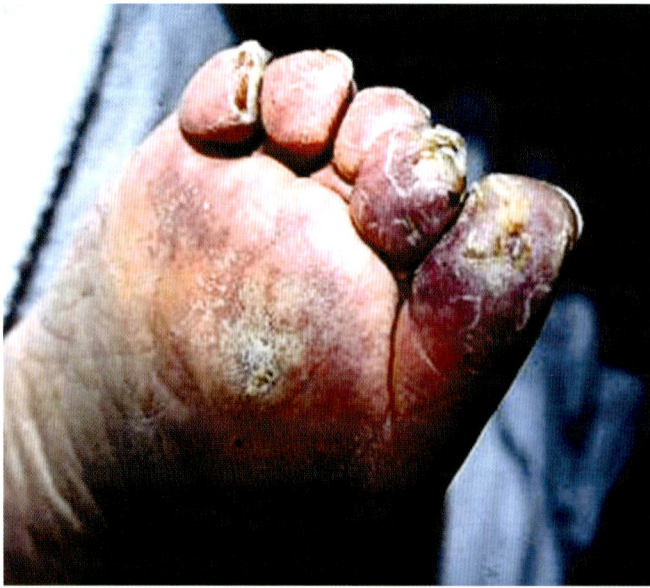

FIGURE 43.17 Atheroemboli involving the foot, or "blue toe syndrome." There is cyanotic discoloration of the toes along with localized areas of violaceous discoloration. (Modified from Beckman JA, Creager MA. Peripheral artery disease: clinical evaluation. In: Creager MA, Beckman JA, Loscalzo J, eds. *Vascular Medicine: A Companion to Braunwald's Heart Disease.* 2nd ed. Philadelphia: Elsevier; 2013:231.)

Risk Factors

20. Garg PK, Biggs ML, Carnethon M, et al. Metabolic syndrome and risk of incident peripheral artery disease: the cardiovascular health study. *Hypertension*. 2014;63:413–419.
21. Ruiz-Canela M, Estruch R, Corella D, et al. Association of Mediterranean diet with peripheral artery disease: the PREDIMED randomized trial. *J Am Med Assoc*. 2014;311:415–417.
22. Beckman JA, Duncan MS, Damrauer SM, et al. Microvascular disease, peripheral artery disease, and amputation. *Circulation*. 2019;140:449–458.
23. Vidula H, Liu K, Criqui MH, et al. Metabolic syndrome and incident peripheral artery disease - the Multi-Ethnic Study of Atherosclerosis. *Atherosclerosis*. 2015;243:198–203.
24. Low Wang CC, Blomster JI, Heizer G, et al. Cardiovascular and limb outcomes in patients with diabetes and peripheral artery disease: the EUCLID trial. *J Am Coll Cardiol*. 2018;72:3274–3284.
25. Benjamin EJ, Muntner P, Alonso A, et al. Heart disease and stroke statistics-2019 update: a report from the American Heart Association. *Circulation*. 2019;139:e56–e528.
26. Gurdasani D, Sjouke B, Tsimikas S, et al. Lipoprotein(a) and risk of coronary, cerebrovascular, and peripheral artery disease: the EPIC-Norfolk prospective population study. *Arterioscler Thromb Vasc Biol*. 2012;32:3058–3065.
27. Laschkolnig A, Kollerits B, Lamina C, et al. Lipoprotein (a) concentrations, apolipoprotein (a) phenotypes, and peripheral arterial disease in three independent cohorts. *Cardiovasc Res*. 2014;103:28–36.
28. Schwartz GG, Steg PG, Szarek M, et al. Peripheral artery disease and venous thromboembolic events after acute coronary syndrome: role of lipoprotein(a) and modification by alirocumab: prespecified analysis of the ODYSSEY OUTCOMES randomized clinical trial. *Circulation*. 2020;141:1608–1617.
29. Ding N, Yang C, Ballew SH, et al. Fibrosis and inflammatory markers and long-term risk of peripheral artery disease: the ARIC study. *Arterioscler Thromb Vasc Biol*. 2020:ATVBAHA120314824.
30. Rein P, Saely CH, Silbernagel G, et al. Systemic inflammation is higher in peripheral artery disease than in stable coronary artery disease. *Atherosclerosis*. 2015;239:299–303.
31. Berardi C, Wassel CL, Decker PA, et al. Elevated levels of adhesion proteins are associated with low ankle-brachial index. *Angiology*. 2017;68:322–329.
32. Brevetti G, Giugliano G, Brevetti L, Hiatt WR. Inflammation in peripheral artery disease. *Circulation*. 2010;122:1862–1875.
33. Dopheide JF, Rubrech J, Trumpp A, et al. Leukocyte-platelet aggregates-a phenotypic characterization of different stages of peripheral arterial disease. *Platelets*. 2016;27:658–667.
34. Gardner AW, Montgomery PS, Wang M, et al. Vascular inflammation, calf muscle oxygen saturation, and blood glucose are associated with exercise pressor response in symptomatic peripheral artery disease. *Angiology*. 2019;70:747–755.
35. McDermott MM, Liu K, Green D, et al. Changes in D-dimer and inflammatory biomarkers before ischemic events in patients with peripheral artery disease: the BRAVO Study. *Vasc Med*. 2016;21:12–20.
36. Kullo IJ, Leeper NJ. The genetic basis of peripheral arterial disease: current knowledge, challenges, and future directions. *Circ Res*. 2015;116:1551–1560.
37. Klarin D, Lynch J, Aragam K, et al. Genome-wide association study of peripheral artery disease in the Million Veteran Program. *Nat Med*. 2019;25:1274–1279.

Pathophysiology

38. Ho CY, Shanahan CM. Medial arterial calcification: an overlooked player in peripheral arterial disease. *Arterioscler Thromb Vasc Biol*. 2016;36:1475–1482.
39. Narula N, Dannenberg AJ, Olin JW, et al. Pathology of peripheral artery disease in patients with critical limb ischemia. *J Am Coll Cardiol*. 2018;72:2152–2163.
40. Narula N, Olin JW, Narula N. Pathologic Disparities between peripheral artery disease and coronary artery disease. *Arterioscler Thromb Vasc Biol*. 2020:ATVBAHA119312864.
41. Hiatt WR, Armstrong EJ, Larson CJ, Brass EP. Pathogenesis of the limb manifestations and exercise limitations in peripheral artery disease. *Circ Res*. 2015;116:1527–1539.
42. Hart CR, Layec G, Trinity JD, et al. Increased skeletal muscle mitochondrial free radical production in peripheral arterial disease despite preserved mitochondrial respiratory capacity. *Exp Physiol*. 2018;103:838–850.
43. McDermott MM. Lower extremity manifestations of peripheral artery disease: the pathophysiologic and functional implications of leg ischemia. *Circ Res*. 2015;116:1540–1550.
44. Henni S, Ammi M, Sempore Y, et al. Treadmill measured vs. Questionnaire estimated changes in walking ability in patients with peripheral artery disease. *Eur J Vasc Endovasc Surg*. 2019;57:676–684.
45. Bonaca MP, Wiviott SD, Zelniker TA, et al. Dapagliflozin and cardiac, kidney, and limb outcomes in patients with and without peripheral artery disease in DECLARE-TIMI 58. *Circulation*. 2020;142:734–747.

Physical Findings, Categorization, and Testing

46. Conte MS, Bradbury AW, Kolh P, et al. Global vascular guidelines on the management of chronic limb-threatening ischemia. *J Vasc Surg*. 2019;69:3S–125S.e40.
47. Mills JL, Sr, Conte MS, Armstrong DG, et al. The society for vascular surgery lower extremity threatened limb classification system: risk stratification based on wound, ischemia, and foot infection (WIfI). *J Vasc Surg*. 2014;59:220–234.e1-2.
48. Mills JL, Sr. Update and validation of the Society for Vascular Surgery wound, ischemia, and foot infection threatened limb classification system. *Semin Vasc Surg*. 2014;27:16–22.
49. Beckman JA. ABI: the goal line is in sight. *Vasc Med*. 2018;23:107–108.
50. Lindholt JS, Sogaard R. Population screening and intervention for vascular disease in Danish men (VIVA): a randomised controlled trial. *Lancet*. 2017;390:2256–2265.
51. McDermott MM, Guralnik JM, Criqui MH, et al. Six-minute walk is a better outcome measure than treadmill walking tests in therapeutic trials of patients with peripheral artery disease. *Circulation*. 2014;130:61–68.
52. Aday AW, Kinlay S, Gerhard-Herman MD. Comparison of different exercise ankle pressure indices in the diagnosis of peripheral artery disease. *Vasc Med*. 2018;23:541–548.
53. Hammad TA, Strefling JA, Zellers PR, et al. The effect of post-exercise ankle-brachial index on lower extremity revascularization. *JACC Cardiovasc Interv*. 2015;8:1238–1244.
54. Zierler RE, Jordan WD, Lal BK, et al. The Society for Vascular Surgery practice guidelines on follow-up after vascular surgery arterial procedures. *J Vasc Surg*. 2018;68:256–284.
55. Wilson DG, Harris SK, Barton C, et al. Tibial artery duplex ultrasound-derived peak systolic velocities may be an objective performance measure after above-knee endovascular therapy for arterial stenosis. *J Vasc Surg*. 2018;68:481–486.
56. Misra S, Shishehbor MH, Takahashi EA, et al. Perfusion assessment in critical limb ischemia: principles for understanding and the development of evidence and evaluation of devices: a Scientific Statement from the American Heart Association. *Circulation*. 2019;140:e657–e672.
57. van den Hoven P, Ooms S, van Manen L, et al. A systematic review of the use of near-infrared fluorescence imaging in patients with peripheral artery disease. *J Vasc Surg*. 2019;70:286–297.e1.
58. Eiken FL, Pedersen BL, Baekgaard N, Eiberg JP. Diagnostic methods for measurement of peripheral blood flow during exercise in patients with type 2 diabetes and peripheral artery disease: a systematic review. *Int Angiol*. 2019;38:62–69.
59. Salisbury DL, Brown RJ, Bronas UG, et al. Measurement of peripheral blood flow in patients with peripheral artery disease: methods and considerations. *Vasc Med*. 2018;23:163–171.
60. Dregely I, Koppara T, Nekolla SG, et al. Observations with simultaneous 18F-FDG PET and MR imaging in peripheral artery disease. *JACC Cardiovasc Imaging*. 2017;10:709–711.

Prognosis

61. Hiatt WR, Fowkes FG, Heizer G, et al. Ticagrelor versus clopidogrel in symptomatic peripheral artery disease. *N Engl J Med*. 2017;376:32–40.
62. Franzone A, Piccolo R, Gargiulo G, et al. Prolonged vs short duration of dual antiplatelet therapy after percutaneous coronary intervention in patients with or without peripheral arterial disease: a subgroup analysis of the PRODIGY randomized clinical trial. *JAMA Cardiol*. 2016;1:795–803.
63. Bonaca MP, Bauersachs RM, Anand SS, et al. Rivaroxaban in peripheral artery disease after revascularization. *N Engl J Med*. 2020;382:1994–2004.
64. Geiss LS, Li Y, Hora I, Albright A, et al. Resurgence of diabetes-related nontraumatic lower-extremity amputation in the young and middle-aged adult U.S. population. *Diabetes Care*. 2019;42:50–54.
65. Barnes JA, Eid MA, Creager MA, Goodney PP. Epidemiology and risk of amputation in patients with diabetes mellitus and peripheral artery disease. *Arterioscler Thromb Vasc Biol*. 2020;40:1808–1817.
66. Arya S, Binney Z, Khakharia A, et al. Race and socioeconomic status independently affect risk of major amputation in peripheral artery disease. *J Am Heart Assoc*. 2018;7.
67. Vart P, Coresh J, Kwak L, et al. Socioeconomic status and incidence of hospitalization with lower-extremity peripheral artery disease: atherosclerosis risk in communities study. *J Am Heart Assoc*. 2017;6.

Treatment

68. Creager MA. A bon VOYAGER for peripheral artery disease. *N Engl J Med*. 2020;382:2047–2048.
69. Bonaca MP, Creager MA. Antithrombotic therapy and major adverse limb events in peripheral artery disease: a step forward. *J Am Coll Cardiol*. 2018;71:2316–2318.
70. Bonaca MP, Creager MA, Olin J, et al. Peripheral revascularization in patients with peripheral artery disease with vorapaxar: insights from the TRA2°P-TIMI 50 trial. *JACC Cardiovasc Interv*. 2016;9:2157–2164.
71. Clark 3rd D, Cain LR, Blaha MJ, et al. Cigarette smoking and subclinical peripheral arterial disease in Blacks of the Jackson heart study. *J Am Heart Assoc*. 2019;8:e010674.
72. Ghosh-Swaby OR, Goodman SG, Leiter LA, et al. Glucose-lowering drugs or strategies, atherosclerotic cardiovascular events, and heart failure in people with or at risk of type 2 diabetes: an updated systematic review and meta-analysis of randomised cardiovascular outcome trials. *Lancet Diabetes Endocrinol*. 2020;8:418–435.
73. Grant PJ, Cosentino F. The 2019 ESC guidelines on diabetes, pre-diabetes, and cardiovascular diseases developed in collaboration with the EASD: new features and the 'ten commandments' of the 2019 guidelines are discussed by professor Peter J. Grant and Professor Francesco Cosentino, the task force chairmen. *Eur Heart J*. 2019;40:3215–3217.
74. Zinman B, Wanner C, Lachin JM, et al. Empagliflozin, cardiovascular outcomes, and mortality in type 2 diabetes. *N Engl J Med*. 2015;373:2117–2128.
75. Verma S, Mazer CD, Al-Omran M, et al. Cardiovascular outcomes and safety of empagliflozin in patients with type 2 diabetes mellitus and peripheral artery disease: a subanalysis of EMPA-REG outcome. *Circulation*. 2018;137:405–407.
76. Matthews DR, Li Q, Perkovic V, et al. Effects of canagliflozin on amputation risk in type 2 diabetes: the CANVAS Program. *Diabetologia*. 2019;62:926–938.
77. Itoga NK, Tawfik DS, Lee CK, et al. Association of blood pressure measurements with peripheral artery disease events. *Circulation*. 2018;138:1805–1814.
78. Perkovic V, Jardine MJ, Neal B, et al. Canagliflozin and renal outcomes in type 2 diabetes and nephropathy. *N Engl J Med*. 2019;380:2295–2306.
79. Zelniker TA, Wiviott SD, Raz I, et al. SGLT2 inhibitors for primary and secondary prevention of cardiovascular and renal outcomes in type 2 diabetes: a systematic review and meta-analysis of cardiovascular outcome trials. *Lancet*. 2019;393:31–39.
80. Verma S, Bhatt DL, Bain SC, et al. Effect of liraglutide on cardiovascular events in patients with type 2 diabetes mellitus and polyvascular disease: results of the LEADER trial. *Circulation*. 2018;137:2179–2183.
81. Zelniker TA, Wiviott SD, Raz I, et al. Comparison of the effects of glucagon-like peptide receptor agonists and sodium-glucose cotransporter 2 inhibitors for prevention of major adverse cardiovascular and renal outcomes in type 2 diabetes mellitus. *Circulation*. 2019;139:2022–2031.
82. Dhatariya K, Bain SC, Buse JB, et al. The impact of liraglutide on diabetes-related foot ulceration and associated complications in patients with type 2 diabetes at high risk for cardiovascular events: results from the LEADER trial. *Diabetes Care*. 2018;41:2229–2235.
83. Group SR, Wright Jr JT, Williamson JD, et al. A randomized trial of intensive versus standard blood-pressure control. *N Engl J Med*. 2015;373:2103–2116.
84. Bonaca MP, Creager MA. Pharmacological treatment and current management of peripheral artery disease. *Circ Res*. 2015;116:1579–1598.
85. Mirault T, Galloula A, Cambou JP, et al. Impact of betablockers on general and local outcome in patients hospitalized for lower extremity peripheral artery disease: the COPART Registry. *Medicine (Baltim)*. 2017;96:e5916.
86. Mach F, Baigent C, Catapano AL, et al. 2019 ESC/EAS Guidelines for the management of dyslipidaemias: lipid modification to reduce cardiovascular risk. *Eur Heart J*. 2020;41:111–188.
87. Arya S, Khakharia A, Binney ZO, et al. Association of statin dose with amputation and survival in patients with peripheral artery disease. *Circulation*. 2018;137:1435–1446.
88. Schwartz GG, Steg PG, Szarek M, et al. Alirocumab and cardiovascular outcomes after acute coronary syndrome. *N Engl J Med*. 2018;379:2097–2107.
89. Patel MR, Becker RC, Wojdyla DM, et al. Cardiovascular events in acute coronary syndrome patients with peripheral arterial disease treated with ticagrelor compared with clopidogrel: data from the PLATO Trial. *Eur J Prev Cardiol*. 2015;22:734–742.
90. Wallentin L, Becker RC, Budaj A, et al. Ticagrelor versus clopidogrel in patients with acute coronary syndromes. *N Engl J Med*. 2009;361:1045–1057.
91. Steg PG, Bhatt DL, Simon T, et al. Ticagrelor in patients with stable coronary disease and diabetes. *N Engl J Med*. 2019;381:1309–1320.
92. Knuuti J, Wijns W, Saraste A, et al. 2019 ESC Guidelines for the diagnosis and management of chronic coronary syndromes. *Eur Heart J*. 2020;41:407–477.
93. Anand SS, Bosch J, Eikelboom JW, et al. Rivaroxaban with or without aspirin in patients with stable peripheral or carotid artery disease: an international, randomised, double-blind, placebo-controlled trial. *Lancet*. 2018;391:219–229.
94. Eikelboom JW, Connolly SJ, Yusuf S. Rivaroxaban in stable cardiovascular disease. *N Engl J Med*. 2018;378:397–398.
95. Anand SS, Caron F, Eikelboom JW, et al. Major adverse limb events and mortality in patients with peripheral artery disease: the COMPASS trial. *J Am Coll Cardiol*. 2018;71:2306–2315.
96. Morrow DA, Braunwald E, Bonaca MP, et al. Vorapaxar in the secondary prevention of atherothrombotic events. *N Engl J Med*. 2012;366:1404–1413.
97. Young JC, Paul NJ, Karatas TB, et al. Cigarette smoking intensity informs outcomes after open revascularization for peripheral artery disease. *J Vasc Surg*. 2019;70:1973–1983.e5.
98. Treat-Jacobson D, McDermott MM, Bronas UG, et al. Optimal exercise programs for patients with peripheral artery disease: a scientific statement from the American Heart Association. *Circulation*. 2019;139:e10–e33.
99. Olin JW, White CJ, Armstrong EJ, et al. Peripheral artery disease: evolving role of exercise, medical therapy, and endovascular options. *J Am Coll Cardiol*. 2016;67:1338–1357.

100. Network ML. *Supervised Exercise Therapy (SET) for Symptomatic Peripheral Artery Disease (PAD)*; 2017.
101. Iyer SR, Annex BH. Therapeutic angiogenesis for peripheral artery disease: lessons learned in translational science. *JACC Basic Transl Sci*. 2017;2:503–512.
102. Madaric J, Klepanec A, Valachovicova M, et al. Characteristics of responders to autologous bone marrow cell therapy for no-option critical limb ischemia. *Stem Cell Res Ther*. 2016;7:116.
103. Rosenfield K, Jaff MR, White CJ, et al. Trial of a paclitaxel-coated balloon for femoropopliteal artery disease. *N Engl J Med*. 2015;373:145–153.
104. Rosenfield K, Metzger DC, Scheinert D. A paclitaxel-coated balloon for femoropopliteal artery disease. *N Engl J Med*. 2015;373:1785–1786.
105. Menard MT, Farber A, Assmann SF, et al. Design and rationale of the Best Endovascular Versus Best Surgical Therapy for Patients with Critical Limb Ischemia (BEST-CLI) trial. *J Am Heart Assoc*. 2016;5.
106. Vartanian SM, Conte MS. Surgical intervention for peripheral arterial disease. *Circ Res*. 2015;116:1614–1628.

Thromboangiitis Obliterans

107. Rivera-Chavarria IJ, Brenes-Gutierrez JD. Thromboangiitis obliterans (Buerger's disease). *Ann Med Surg (Lond)*. 2016;7:79–82.
108. Cacione DG, Macedo CR, Baptista-Silva JC. Pharmacological treatment for Buerger's disease. *Cochrane Database Syst Rev*. 2016;3:CD011033.
109. Hemsinli D, Altun G, Kaplan ST, et al. Hyperbaric oxygen treatment in thromboangiitis obliterans: a retrospective clinical audit. *Diving Hyperb Med*. 2018;48:31–35.
110. Narvaez J, Garcia-Gomez C, Alvarez L, et al. Efficacy of bosentan in patients with refractory thromboangiitis obliterans (Buerger disease): a case series and review of the literature. *Medicine (Baltim)*. 2016;95:e5511.

Fibromuscular Dysplasia

111. Gornik HL, Persu A, Adlam D, et al. First international consensus on the diagnosis and management of fibromuscular dysplasia. *J Hypertens*. 2019;37:229–252.
112. Narula N, Kadian-Dodov D, Olin JW. Fibromuscular dysplasia: contemporary concepts and future directions. *Prog Cardiovasc Dis*. 2018;60:580–585.
113. Kadian-Dodov D, Gornik HL, Gu X, et al. Dissection and aneurysm in patients with fibromuscular dysplasia: findings from the U.S. Registry for FMD. *J Am Coll Cardiol*. 2016;68:176–185.
114. Wells BJ, Modi RD, Gu X, et al. Clinical associations of headaches among patients with fibromuscular dysplasia: a report from the US Registry for Fibromuscular Dysplasia. *Vasc Med*. 2020;25:348–350.
115. O'Connor S, Gornik HL, Froehlich JB, et al. Smoking and adverse outcomes in fibromuscular dysplasia: U.S. Registry report. *J Am Coll Cardiol*. 2016;67:1750–1751.

Popliteal Entrapment Syndrome

116. Shahi N, Arosemena M, Kwon J, et al. Functional popliteal artery entrapment syndrome: a review of diagnosis and management. *Ann Vasc Surg*. 2019;59:259–267.
117. Hicks CW, Black 3rd JH, Ratchford EV. Popliteal artery entrapment syndrome. *Vasc Med*. 2019;24:190–194.
118. Lavingia KS, Dua A, Rothenberg KA, et al. Surgical management of functional popliteal entrapment syndrome in athletes. *J Vasc Surg*. 2019;70:1555–1562.

Acute Limb Ischemia

119. Creager MA, Kaufman JA, Conte MS. Clinical practice. Acute limb ischemia. *N Engl J Med*. 2012;366:2198–2206.
120. Duval S, Keo HH, Oldenburg NC, et al. The impact of prolonged lower limb ischemia on amputation, mortality, and functional status: the FRIENDS registry. *Am Heart J*. 2014;168:577–587.

44 Treatment of Noncoronary Obstructive Vascular Disease

SCOTT KINLAY AND DEEPAK L. BHATT

APPROACH TO THE PATIENT WITH PERIPHERAL ARTERY DISEASE, 859
Quality of Evidence Evaluating Endovascular Treatments, 860

ENDOVASCULAR TECHNOLOGIES, 860
Balloon Angioplasty, 860
Bare-Metal Stents, 860
Drug-Eluting Peripheral Stents, 860
Drug-Coated Balloons, 861

Covered Stents, 862
Thrombolysis, 862

PLANNING AN INTERVENTION, 863
Vascular Imaging, 863
Vascular Access, 864

ENDOVASCULAR TREATMENT OF ARTERIAL DISEASE, 864
Peripheral Artery Disease of the Lower Extremities, 864

Cervical Artery Disease, 865
Mesenteric and Renal Artery Disease, 867

ENDOVASCULAR TREATMENT OF VENOUS DISEASE, 867
Extremity Deep Venous Thrombosis, 867
Superior Vena Cava Syndrome, 868

FUTURE PERSPECTIVES, 868

REFERENCES, 868

Peripheral vascular disease is a general term that includes pathologic processes affecting arteries, veins, and lymphatics (see Chapter 43). This chapter focuses on catheter-based endovascular treatment of large- and medium-sized arteries predominantly affected by atherosclerosis, as well as large-vein obstruction secondary to chronic disease. Although *peripheral artery disease* (PAD) refers to lower limb arterial disease, sometimes the term is used to describe disease in the large and medium arteries of the upper limbs, neck, and aortomesenteric arteries. The incidence and prevalence of PAD increase with age and with other risk factors for atherosclerosis. Thus, these two demographic forces will likely lead to a global increase in PAD (see Chapter 2).

Increasing awareness of PAD, the impact that PAD has on cardiovascular (CV) risk and quality of life, and the rapid development of percutaneous techniques for revascularization continue to accelerate the number of endovascular procedures for PAD. Appropriate use of this expensive technology requires a clear understanding of the goals of medical and revascularization therapies.

APPROACH TO THE PATIENT WITH PERIPHERAL ARTERY DISEASE

Chronic PAD may be asymptomatic or may manifest as claudication, critical limb ischemia (CLI), or embolic infarction of a distal organ (e.g., stroke). Asymptomatic disease is common. In the lower extremities, asymptomatic disease occurs in at least half and in as many as 80% of patients with abnormal functional test results indicative of obstructive arterial disease (e.g., abnormal ankle-brachial index [ABI]). Even asymptomatic disease indicates elevated CV risk.[1-4] These considerations warrant intensive modification of atherosclerosis risk factors as a prime goal of therapy to reduce the risk for myocardial infarction (MI) and stroke, the most common causes of death in patients with PAD.[1,3,5,6]

Claudication classically refers to leg discomfort, weakness, or pain related to exercise and relieved by rest, but it also describes discomfort in the upper limbs caused by effort-related ischemia. Claudication affects function (the ability to walk or use a limb) and quality of life. Therefore, treatment of claudication aims to improve function and reduce discomfort at the maximum level of activity desired by a patient. Stopping cigarette smoking and starting a regular walking regimen are the two most important lifestyle interventions for claudication. Supervised exercise training consisting of 1-hour sessions two to three times a week for 12 weeks is particularly useful at improving walking, with or without endovascular intervention (see Chapter 43).[1,3,7,8] Together, these interventions reduce the mechanisms responsible for the progression of disease and favorably change arterial biologic state, including vasodilator function, muscle metabolism, and angiogenesis.[1,3,5,6,9] It is important to tell patients that the pain or discomfort associated with claudication is not harmful, and that once this discomfort abates with rest, they should continue to push their activity again to improve endurance. Revascularization strategies aim to improve arterial blood flow in obstructed large- and medium-sized arteries when noninvasive therapies fail. Catheter-based interventions, when indicated, should be deployed together with lifestyle and medical treatment.[1,3,10]

Critical limb ischemia, also referred to as critical limb-threatening ischemia, refers to PAD with ischemic pain at rest or tissue loss (e.g., ulcer or gangrene).[1,3,11] This scenario has clinical urgency because of near-term risk for limb jeopardy requiring major amputation. *Major* amputation in the lower limbs refers to amputation at or above the level of the ankle and requires a prosthesis for the patient to walk.[11] Amputation is disfiguring and at higher levels (above versus below knee amputation) has greater impact on functional independence of the patient. In contrast, *minor* amputations (e.g., toe or transmetatarsal) usually have little impact on the patient's ability to walk. Catheter-based therapies for CLI are used to improve blood flow and heal ischemic tissue, to salvage the limb (prevent major amputation), or to enable a lower level of amputation that might have less impact on the patient's ability to walk.

Acute limb ischemia (ALI) is a sudden loss of limb perfusion (defined as within 14 days) typically caused by embolus or in situ thrombus. Thrombolysis may be indicated for acute thrombosis with a threatened but viable extremity, but an immediately threatened limb (e.g., with sensory or early motor deficits) is more often treated by surgical revascularization,[1,3,12] which offers more rapid reperfusion, the ability to débride devitalized tissue, and the opportunity to relieve compartment syndromes (see Chapter 43).

Cervical carotid, vertebral, and subclavian disease, although often asymptomatic, can lead to artery-to-artery embolism with transient ischemic attack (TIA) and stroke. The risk for major stroke is high shortly after a symptomatic event but declines to the level of asymptomatic disease after approximately 3 months.[1] Mesenteric and renal artery disease affects organ function. Chronic ischemia of the gut causes postprandial abdominal discomfort and food avoidance leading to weight loss, but it may progress to frank mesenteric infarction with a high mortality rate.[13] Renal artery stenosis can precipitate hypertensive crises associated with pulmonary edema, hypertension resistant to treatment, and rapidly worsening renal dysfunction.[14]

Symptomatic disease that threatens a distal organ (e.g., CLI, TIA, mesenteric angina) justifies a more aggressive approach because these manifestations entail the highest risk for functional loss and death without treatment. PAD associated with less-threatening clinical scenarios (e.g.,

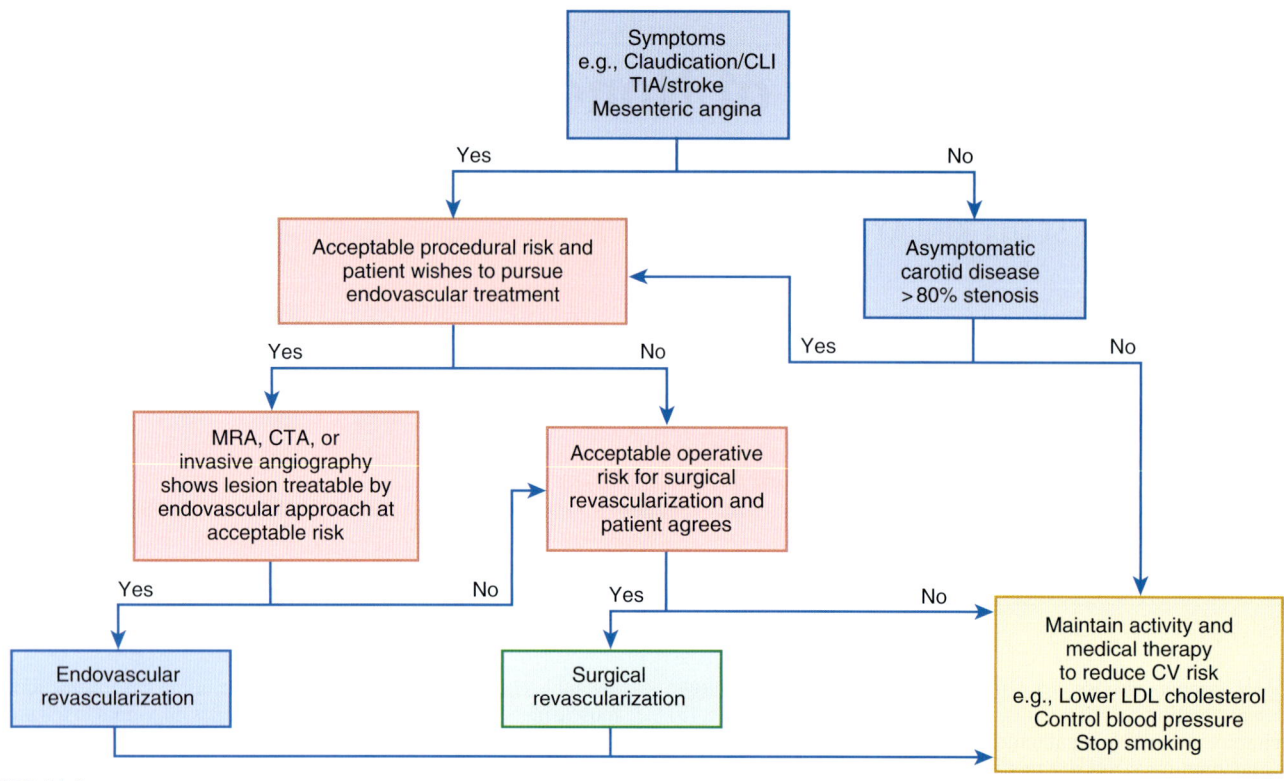

FIGURE 44.1 Approach to a patient with peripheral artery disease. This strategy is based on assessment of the risk for adverse events with and without treatment by taking into consideration procedural or operative risks and the patient's informed decision to proceed with revascularization. *CLI,* Critical limb ischemia; *CTA,* computed tomographic angiography; *CV,* cardiovascular; *LDL,* low-density lipoprotein; *MRA,* magnetic resonance angiography; *TIA,* transient ischemic attack.

claudication) may allow a less aggressive approach, with more time to assess the response to lifestyle and medical therapies (Fig. 44.1). There is rarely justification for catheter-based or surgical revascularization of asymptomatic lower or upper limb PAD, mesenteric disease, or subclavian or vertebral artery disease. Revascularizing asymptomatic extracranial carotid disease beyond medical therapy has uncertain value, although guidelines support such interventions for patients at higher risk for stroke and low risk for periprocedural adverse events.[1,15]

Quality of Evidence Evaluating Endovascular Treatments

Increasingly, well-controlled randomized-controlled studies are used to evaluate endovascular treatment of PAD and venous disease. However, many studies are single arm, and most focus on patency (lack of restenosis) and repeated revascularization over a relatively short period. Although these endpoints provide information on the mechanisms likely to lead to improved control of symptoms, function, quality of life, and tissue preservation, they do not provide direct guidance on symptoms and function in patients with claudication or CLI. Interventionalists should recognize the limitations in many studies and encourage future studies to address patient-oriented endpoints and adjudicated CV outcomes.[16]

ENDOVASCULAR TECHNOLOGIES

Balloon Angioplasty

Balloon angioplasty remains the mainstay of endovascular intervention for PAD and venous disease[12] (Fig. 44.2). Angioplasty remodels the artery by expansion and accommodates the atherosclerotic plaque to expand the vessel lumen. This procedure usually causes dissection of the plaque that may or may not impair blood flow. Angioplasty is limited in the short term by acute recoil of the artery and flow-limiting dissections, which may cause abrupt closure of the artery. In the intermediate time frame, overexuberant neointimal hyperplasia and negative remodeling of the artery may lead to symptomatic restenosis. Despite these limitations, balloon angioplasty can achieve durable results, particularly with shorter lesions, and is less likely than stenting to obstruct side branches associated with the lesion. Most operators use prolonged inflations (at least 1 minute or more). Both rapid-exchange and over-the-wire platforms are available, as well as short and long shaft lengths for lesions close to or farther from the access site.

Bare-Metal Stents

Bare-metal stents (BMSs) come in two types: balloon-expandable stents (Fig. 44.3) and self-expanding stents[12]. Stent implantation requires aspirin therapy and an adenosine receptor antagonist (i.e., clopidogrel), although the evidence for dual-antiplatelet therapy (DAPT) is largely derived by extrapolation from the coronary stent literature.

Balloon-expandable stents have greater radial strength and are less likely to move on deployment, which is important for ostial placement. Such stents can be crushed by external compression and are therefore avoided outside the torso. They are sometimes used to treat tibial disease, but only for CLI, for which long-term patency may be less of an issue once tissue healing has occurred.

Self-expanding stents were originally made of stainless steel but are now usually made of nitinol. Nitinol stents reexpand on compression and are therefore used outside the torso, where external compression is more likely to occur. They may also be used in tortuous arteries, where they probably conform better than balloon-expandable stents. Their lower radial strength, however, increases the risk for recoil. Contemporary self-expanding stent designs are more durable and less likely to fracture than older designs.[12] Nitinol stents cannot be overdilated if the stent is undersized for the artery, which may lead to stent malapposition or even embolization.

Drug-Eluting Peripheral Stents

Drug coated self-expanding stents using a polymer[17] or polymer-free coating[18] of paclitaxel offer lower rates of restenosis than bare-metal self-expanding stents. The 5-year follow-up of the Zilver PTX study

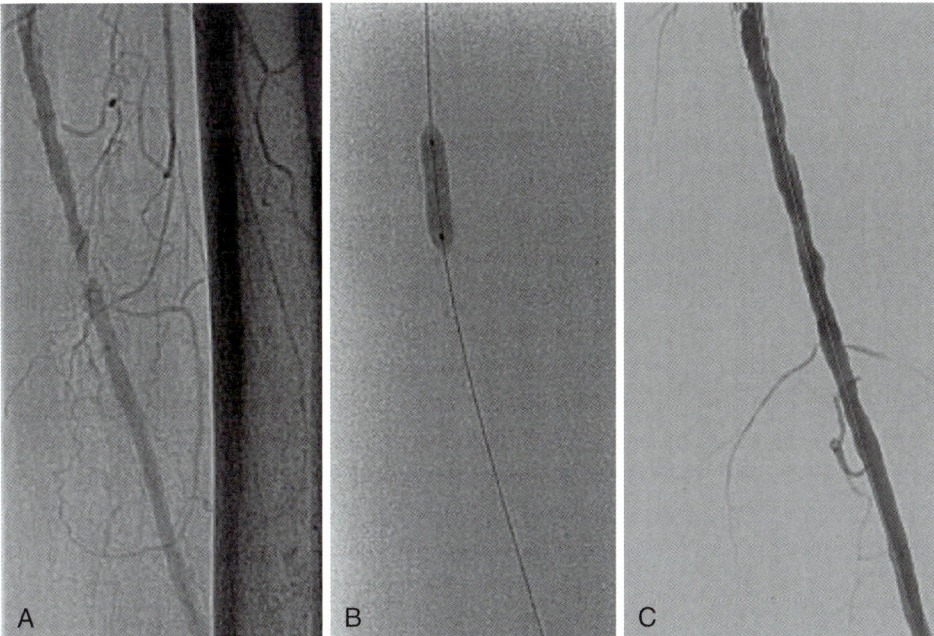

FIGURE 44.2 Treatment of a mid–superficial femoral artery stenosis **(A),** with balloon angioplasty alone **(B),** with an excellent final result **(C).**

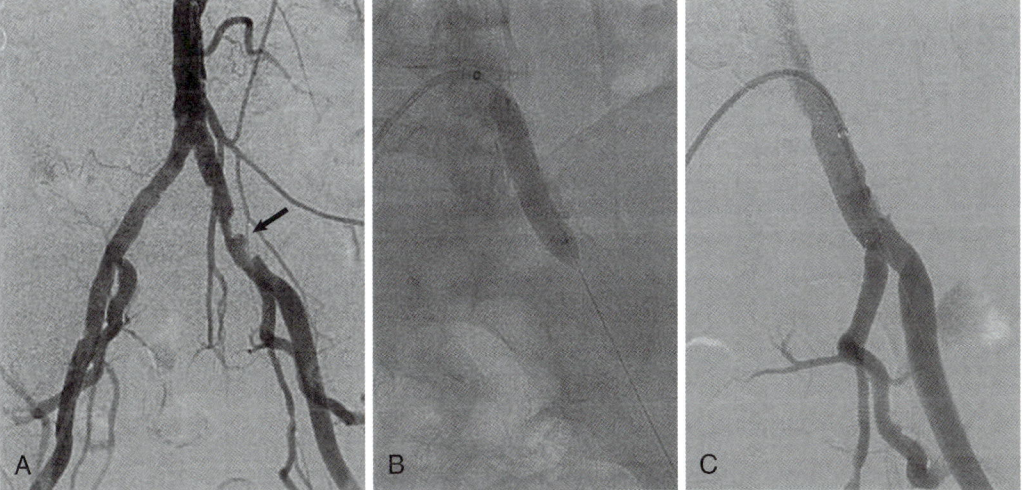

FIGURE 44.3 Treatment of left common iliac stenosis with a balloon-expandable stent from the contralateral right femoral artery. **A,** Serial stenoses in the left common iliac artery *(arrow).* **B,** Balloon-expandable stent deployment. **C,** Final angiogram.

demonstrated a sustained benefit from self-expanding drug-eluting stents (DESs) over balloon angioplasty and BMSs on freedom from clinical symptoms of ischemia (80% versus 59%) and repeat revascularization (66% versus 43%) in femoral-popliteal arteries.[17] In the IMPERIAL study, a polymer-coated paclitaxel stent had similar 12 months of efficacy and safety outcomes to a polymer-free paclitaxel stent,[18] and a single-arm cohort study suggested no "catch-up" target vessel revascularization over 3 years with this device.[19] In one trial, drug-coated self-expanding stents had similar patency and target lesion revascularization at 12 months with lower complication rates and shorter lengths of hospital stay than surgical bypass with prosthetic graft.[20] The duration of DAPT required for these stents is uncertain, but recent randomized trials have generally used 2 to 6 months of treatment with an adenosine receptor antagonist.[17,18]

Drug-Coated Balloons

Balloons coated with antirestenosis agents (drug-eluting balloons) are designed to decrease restenosis without the use of stents. This technology uses a non–stent-related method to deliver drugs such as paclitaxel into the arterial wall after angioplasty or atherectomy. Compared with plain balloon angioplasty, drug-coated balloons have less restenosis and repeat revascularization in the femoral-popliteal arteries,[21-25] and similar patency to drug-coated self-expanding stents.[26,27] Drug-coated balloons also offer a lower risk of restenosis at 1 year compared with plain balloon angioplasty for treating in-stent restenosis lesions.[27-30] Late follow-up of two randomized trials at 2 and 5 years shows a sustained benefit on patency and repeat revascularization with drug-coated versus plain balloon angioplasty in femoral-popliteal arteries, without concerns of aneurysm or late stenoses.[23,31] The duration of DAPT with drug-coated balloons in the femoral-popliteal arteries is uncertain but varies between 1 and 6 months in most randomized trials.

The effect of drug-coated balloons in below-knee angioplasty, primarily for CLI, is less certain. A meta-analysis of eight randomized controlled trials (RCTs) compared drug-coated balloon angioplasty to plain balloon angioplasty in tibial arteries.[32] Overall, there was a significant decrease in target vessel repeat revascularization with drug-coated balloons, but an increased risk of death or amputation, although with significant heterogeneity in some of the outcomes in this meta-analysis. Currently the paclitaxel drug-coated technologies are under increased scrutiny due to some meta-analyses suggesting higher rates of all-cause mortality 3 to 5 years after treatment (see later).

Controversy About Paclitaxel-Coated Balloons and Stents

Lesion length is a key determinant of restenosis,[12,33] and a meta-analysis suggests that long lesions have less restenosis and need for target revascularization with paclitaxel drug-coated balloons and stents.[34] However, in 2018 a group-level meta-analysis of randomized trials suggested that patients treated with paclitaxel drug-coated balloons or stents for femoral-popliteal disease had higher rates of mortality 2 to 5 years after their procedure compared with non-paclitaxel balloons and stents.[35] In a subsequent meta-analysis, drug-coated balloons for infrapopliteal disease[32] were associated with increased all-cause mortality two or more years after treatment. Meta-regression analyses in both studies suggested greater risks from devices with higher doses of paclitaxel coating. In response to these reports, investigators of the clinical trials reported patient-level long-term outcomes data and meta-analyses refuting the higher late mortality risk 3 to 5 years after treatment with DESs or balloons in the femoral-popliteal artery.[36-39] Analyses of large administrative databases from Medicare/Medicaid in the United States[40] and Germany[41] suggested lower mortality and amputation at 5 years after drug-coated balloons or stents for CLI or intermittent claudication. Furthermore, late mortality risks were not observed with drug-coated balloons used to treat coronary artery disease.[42]

The group-level meta-analyses were limited by the relatively small number of deaths in studies that were not powered to assess mortality, and the lack of trials with long follow-up beyond 1 to 2 years. Until more data are available, the Federal Drug Agency recommends discussing the potential long-term risks with patients, using alternative technologies if possible, and reserving paclitaxel technologies for patients at very high risk of restenosis. Currently, drug-coated devices that deliver the limus class of drugs are under investigation and may replace paclitaxel devices if they have improved efficacy and safety.

Covered Stents

Stents covered with or sandwiching a polymer such as polytetrafluoroethylene (PTFE) are very useful for treating perforations related to endovascular treatment or excluding aneurysms. Results from randomized trials and meta-analyses of covered stents compared with BMSs are inconsistent for the out-come of restenosis at 1 year and found no difference in limb salvage or survival.[34,43,44] In one series, covered stents that cross the knee joint were associated with higher rates of occlusion and major amputation than those deployed above the knee (34% versus 10%).[45] Potential disadvantages of covered stents include unintentional occlusion of important branch vessels, concerns about the risk for late stent thrombosis, and whether restenosis was merely delayed rather than prevented.

Thrombolysis

Catheter-directed thrombolysis is an important adjunctive therapy for arterial thrombosis, stent thrombosis, and occlusive thrombotic venous disease. Thrombolysis may be indicated for acute thrombosis with a threatened but viable extremity, but an immediately threatened limb (e.g., with sensory or early motor deficits) is more often treated by surgical revascularization.[1,3,12] Much of the experience with catheter-based thrombolysis comes from its use for ALI, venous thrombosis, or pulmonary embolism. It serves as an adjunctive treatment of semiacute manifestations such as peripheral stent thrombosis. Long-term results tend to be better when thrombolysis reveals an anatomic stenosis that probably precipitated the thrombosis and is treatable, for example, by repeated angioplasty.

Catheter-directed thrombolysis is more effective than intravenous thrombolysis only if an infusion catheter (with multiple infusion holes) is inserted into the thrombosed vessel (Fig. 44.4). It is also less effective if given more than 14 days after thrombosis.[1,3,12] Typi-cally, the infusion continues for 12 to 24 hours, because treatment over 48 hours is associated with depletion of circulating fibrinogen and a higher risk for major bleeding. A meta-analysis comparing catheter and mechanically assisted thrombolysis versus surgical thrombectomy showed no difference in limb salvage but higher bleeding rates with thrombolysis.[46] Lower dose thrombolysis regimens may offer a lower risk of bleeding complications, but may require a longer treatment duration.[47] Catheter-based thrombolysis with or without angioplasty or stenting also reduces the incidence of post-thrombotic syndrome in patients with proximal (iliac) deep venous thrombosis (DVT),[48] and it is used as adjunctive therapy for massive pulmonary emboli (see Chapter 87).

Any thrombolysis regimen increases risk for fatal or major bleeding. Absolute contraindications to thrombolysis include (1) a cerebrovascular event less than 2 months previously, (2) active bleeding, (3) gastrointestinal bleeding less than 10 days previously, and (4) neurosurgery (intracranial or spinal surgery) or trauma less than 3 months previously. Relative contraindications include (1) cardiopulmonary resuscitation less than 10 days previously, (2) nonvascular surgery or trauma less than 10 days previously, (3) uncontrolled hypertension (sustained systolic blood pressure [BP] >180 mm Hg or diastolic BP >110 mm Hg), (4) puncture of a noncompressible vessel, (5) intracranial tumor, and (6) recent eye surgery.

Mechanical and Aspiration Thrombectomy

Mechanical and aspiration thrombectomy are used with and without thrombolytic agents. At this stage, the quality of studies comparing these methods to catheter-based thrombolytic infusion does not allow any firm conclusions to assess their incremental benefit.[46,49] Catheter aspiration thrombectomy designed initially for aspirating thrombi in coronary arteries uses 5 to 7 French (F) catheters with a rapid-exchange port to direct the catheter to the thrombus and an aspiration port to aspirate the catheter with a large syringe (e.g., Export Advance catheter, Medtronic, Minneapolis; Pronto catheter, Vascular Solutions, Minneapolis). These catheters can aspirate smaller thrombi but are generally inadequate for a large burden of thrombus (e.g., long femoral stent thrombosis). The Inari flow retriever system (Inari Medical, Irvine, CA) uses a much larger catheter (up to 24F) and is designed mainly for venous thromboembolism, but case reports show large thrombi extracted with this system.

The Penumbra Indigo (Penumbra, Almeda, CA) aspiration system uses a mechanical aspirator and a range of 3 to 8F catheters to generate a greater suction than manual aspiration catheters. This was initially developed for aspirating intracranial arterial emboli, but has peripheral vascular catheters designed to aspirate peripheral arterial and venous thrombi.

Other mechanical thrombectomy devices break up a clot before aspiration and may use adjunctive locally delivered thrombolytic

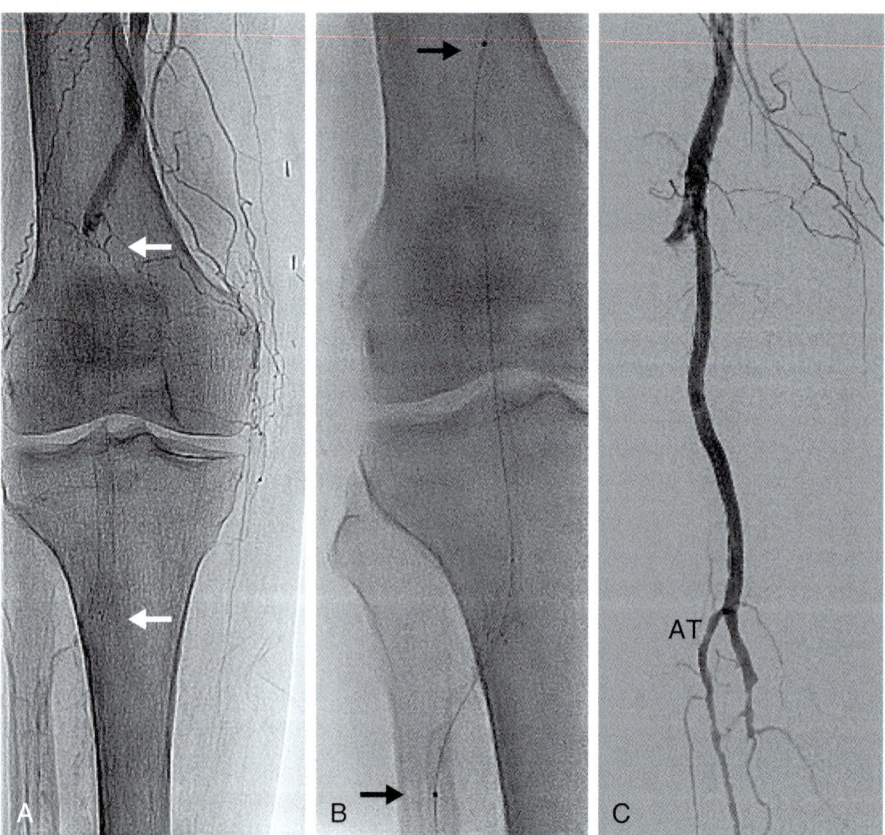

FIGURE 44.4 Catheter-based thrombolysis of a thrombosed and occluded right popliteal artery stent. **A,** Thrombosed right popliteal artery stent with *white arrows* indicating the proximal and distal edges of the stent. **B,** Multiholed infusion catheter placed with proximal and distal markers of the infusion segment indicated with *arrows*. **C,** Angiogram 24 hours later showing a patent popliteal stent and outflow into the anterior tibial artery (AT).

agents before extraction. These include the AngioJet device (Boston Scientific, Marlborough, MA), which uses a Venturi effect to break up and aspirate a thrombus. The Jetstream (Boston Scientific, Marlborough, MA) is primarily a rotational atherectomy device but also aspirates debris and is used for atherectomy and aspiration of a thrombus. Mechanical thrombectomy is a more rapid treatment than catheter-directed thrombolysis; embolization can occlude the distal arterial bed and lead to infarction and tissue loss, although combination with an embolic protection device might theoretically reduce this risk.

Rotational, Orbital, and Directional Atherectomy

Atherectomy devices, although conceptually attractive, have not proved better than angioplasty in direct comparisons in most arterial beds.[4,12] A Cochrane review of four trials comparing atherectomy to established treatments for PAD found no evidence to support atherectomy as an alternative to balloon angioplasty.[50] Atherectomy is one of several niche tools and serves best in heavily calcified arteries to improve balloon and stent expansion or in regions where vessels encounter repetitive flexion or torsion, such as over joints, and where stents are avoided (because of kinking and increased fracture). In these settings, atherectomy may improve the distensibility of an artery to permit adequate expansion by balloon angioplasty without flow-limiting dissection. There is renewed interest in drug-eluting balloons for this technology because they may reduce the contribution of excessive intimal hyperplasia to restenosis.

Rotational atherectomy devices include the Rotablator and the Jetstream devices. The Rotablator (Boston Scientific, Marlborough, MA) is generally too small for the larger peripheral arteries, and it is uncertain how a large amount of plaque ablated from a long peripheral lesion would affect the downstream microcirculation. However, for the smaller popliteal artery rotational atherectomy may allow balloon dilation without stenting. The Jetstream has a cutting head and blades mounted just behind the head that are folded down on initial passes, but it can stand up when rotated in the opposite direction to increase the cutting diameter from 2.0 mm to 3.1 and 3.5 mm, depending on the catheter.

The Diamondback360 (Cardiovascular Systems, Inc., St. Paul, MN) is an *orbital* atherectomy device. This has an eccentrically mounted cutting crown on the drive cable that encourages an orbital path around the wire to increase the diameter of the cutting arc.

Directional atherectomy devices include the SilverHawk device. All the peripheral devices have a tendency to embolize plaque into microvessels. Distal embolic protection devices may reduce this complication.

Laser Atherectomy

Excimer *laser atherectomy* uses high-energy monochromatic ultraviolet light to vaporize tissue in contact with the catheter tip and debulk de novo and restenotic lesions in peripheral arteries.[51] Laser ablates tissue by breaking down mechanical carbon-carbon bonds in tissue (photoablation), thermal energy effects (photothermal), and generation of a vapor bubble that produces kinetic energy to disrupt tissue (photomechanical). Laser catheters are advanced over a 0.014-inch guidewire. As blood absorbs some of the laser energy, laser runs are accompanied with a slow saline flush. The saline flushes constrain the size of the vapor bubble to avoid excessive mechanical injury to the artery. The repetition rate of pulses and the energy delivered per pulse (fluence) are adjusted to increase the ablation. Some operators will use a short puff of dilute contrast with laser runs to increase the size of the vapor bubble. This can increase mechanical forces on the artery to aid subsequent balloon expansion but can lead to artery injury or slow flow in the artery.

Cryoplasty and Intravascular Lithotripsy

Cryoplasty involves the use of proprietary balloon and inflation technology to inflate the balloon with nitrous oxide, which chills on expansion to −10°C. Network meta-analyses comparing multiple different therapies suggest cryoplasty is inferior to other technologies with a higher rate of restenosis.[34,43]

Intravascular lithotripsy (Shockwave Medical, Santa Clara, CA) uses a balloon with up to five pressure-emitting nodes along the balloon shaft to generate waves of pressure into the artery wall during a low-pressure balloon inflation. The pressure waves create microfractures in intravascular calcium deposits to permit arterial dilation at pressures lower than without lithotripsy. There are no randomized trials assessing this technology, but a meta-analysis of cohort studies of calcified lesions in the leg arteries indicates acute improvements in stenosis severity with acute adverse events of dissection, perforation, no reflow, or embolization of about 1% to 2% of cases.[52] This technology may be an adjunctive treatment for large calcified arteries resistant to balloon dilation.

Medical Therapy to Improve Endovascular Durability

Supervised exercise training is a proven treatment for walking function in patients with claudication. Supervised exercise training after endovascular interventions may also improve maximum walking distance over endovascular interventions alone and should be considered as an adjunctive therapy.[1,3,7,8] *Cilostazol* is a phosphodiesterase inhibitor that improves walking function in some patients with intermittent claudication. Small meta-analyses suggest cilostazol used after endovascular therapy may improve walking function[7] and decrease the risk for restenosis, repeat revascularization, and major amputation.[53] In the VOYAGER trial, antithrombotic therapy with low-dose rivaroxaban 2.5 mg twice a day with aspirin decreased the risk of a combined endpoint of vascular, cardiac, and cerebrovascular ischemic events with an increase in major bleeding.[54] This regimen may be considered in patients with a favorable balance of bleeding and ischemic risk (see Chapter 43).

PLANNING AN INTERVENTION

Vascular Imaging

Vascular imaging is the first stage of planning an endovascular intervention[1,3,11,12]. Traditionally, invasive angiography served to determine the extent and severity of obstructive disease. Conventional angiography can use lower frame rates than needed for coronary angiography because most peripheral arteries are relatively static. *Digital subtraction angiography* images remove bone and soft tissue from the image while leaving the contrast-enhanced image of the artery for more clarity, provided that the limb remains still during acquisition. *Carbon dioxide* can be used as a substitute for iodinated contrast with digital subtraction angiography in patients with chronic kidney disease to avoid contrast nephropathy. Vapor lock in the aorta due to delayed elimination in a tortuous aorta or contamination of carbon dioxide with air are thought responsible for more serious complications including mesenteric infarction and death.[55] *Noninvasive imaging* is often used to plan the vascular access and the tools required for the procedure.[11,12] Magnetic resonance imaging (MRI) uses gadolinium or other contrast agents or time-of-flight techniques. Time of flight relies on laminar blood flow to image arteries and has the advantage of not requiring contrast material, which can rarely cause serious adverse effects in patients with renal insufficiency (e.g., nephrogenic sclerosing fibrosis). However, time-of-flight techniques may overestimate the severity of disease in regions of disturbed flow near obstructive or nonobstructive plaque. Computed tomographic angiography (CTA) using iodinated contrast material provides more rapid imaging, but heavy calcification can mask stenoses and make interpretation of lesion severity more difficult. Iodinated contrast agents can cause adverse reactions or impair renal function.

MRI cannot be used in patients who have retained ferric metals (e.g., some pacemakers, shrapnel). Most contemporary stents are compatible with MRI but leave a flow void that does not allow interpretation of obstructive disease. High-resolution contrast-enhanced CT scans offers advantages for assessing stent patency.

Duplex ultrasound is very useful for imaging arteries in the limbs and the cervical arteries and veins. This modality does require considerable time to map out large arterial systems, however, explaining the

Vascular Access

Vascular access can use either antegrade or retrograde approaches. The contralateral common femoral artery (CFA) is the most common vascular access for the lower limb. A catheter enters the access side over the bifurcation of the aorta and into the target iliac arteries through a support wire. A sheath is directed up and over the aortic bifurcation and pointed into the target iliac artery. This approach accesses the CFA at its most superficial location and allows compression of the artery against the femoral head to aid in manual hemostasis after removal of the sheath.

The anterograde femoral approach involves skin access several cen-timeters cranial to the CFA and angles toward the femoral head. This approach offers greater pushability for total occlusions and is closer to distal tibial lesions, but it is difficult in overweight patients, in whom the access needle must traverse a large depot of subcutaneous fat.

Retrograde access from the popliteal artery, superficial femoral artery (SFA), or from a tibial artery can assist in crossing a total occlusion that cannot be crossed from an anterograde approach[11,12]. Retrograde access has the disadvantages of the potential to cause injury to the distal access site because of the smaller artery size (tibial arteries) or more difficult hemostasis from a deeper location (popliteal). Techniques that combine retrograde and anterograde approaches can assist in crossing difficult total occlusions. An unsuccessful procedure from a retrograde access site, however, could lead to a nonhealing ulcer.

Most balloons and devices are based on shaft lengths of 130 to 150 cm and offer limited utility for leg interventions from the brachial or radial access sites, and usually are not able to treat lesions distal to the common femoral arteries. The brachial artery requires a longer compression time after removal of the sheath and has higher rates of vascular complications compared with the radial artery. The rapid adoption of the radial approach for coronary angiography has stimulated the development of long sheaths, and balloons and stents on longer shafts (up to 200 cm) permitting treatment of the SFA from the radial artery. Drug-coated technologies and other adjunctive devices are likely to be designed for the radial approach in the future. Long sheaths or guides used from the radial and brachial approaches often provide better support for interventions in the mesenteric arteries, as these arteries typically have a caudal angulation and can assist or be primary access sites for arm interventions.

ENDOVASCULAR TREATMENT OF ARTERIAL DISEASE

Peripheral Artery Disease of the Lower Extremities

The clinical history and physical examination can generally differentiate PAD from other causes of leg discomfort. Physiologic tests such as the ABI are quick and easy to perform, but segmental leg pressures can indicate the level of obstructive disease (see Chapter 43). Infrainguinal disease usually diminishes distal pulses and impairs the resting ABI. Typical symptoms of PAD with a normal resting ABI should raise suspicion for iliac or aortic disease, in which case an exercise ABI is generally abnormal (see Chapter 43).[56] More advanced imaging such as MRA, CTA, or invasive angiography is generally indicated only if revascularization is considered. MRI or CT can help identify the level, extent, and severity of PAD and help indicate the likelihood of endovascular success versus surgical treatment, as well as access site and adjunctive endovascular technologies. In general, treatment of proximal disease offers higher long-term durability than does treatment of distal disease.

Aortoiliac Disease

Aortoiliac disease is approached from the ipsilateral femoral artery, contralateral femoral artery, the radial artery, or brachial artery. An ipsilateral femoral approach is more direct and associated with greater wire pushability through an occlusion. Many operators will often use a second arterial access (e.g., contralateral femoral) to provide quick access to the aorta or proximal iliac artery for temporary balloon occlusion in the event of perforation and rapid hemorrhage. Although plain balloon angioplasty produces a very durable result, balloon-expandable stents are now pre-ferred for their better long-term durability, particularly with long lesions.[1,3,4] "Kissing stents" are a well-described option for disease involving the distal aorta, but in many cases of iliac disease, landing stents at the ostium of the iliac artery yields a good response and preserves contralateral access if arterial interventions are required for a leg in the future. Balloon-expandable stents are usually preferable for most lesions involving ostia because of their greater radial strength and precision of placement, but self-expanding stents may be better in more tortuous lesions. Although covered stents prevent plaque prolapse, they have uncertain added value and the potential disadvantage of occluding the opposite iliac artery if deployed too high or occluding the ipsilateral internal iliac artery if deployed too low. They also appear to have a higher risk of thrombosis. Covered stents are useful for treating aneurysms and potentially lifesaving for treating vessel rupture or perforation.[12] Occlusions involving the distal aorta often undergo surgical treatment, although percutaneous transluminal angioplasty and stenting offer an option to patients with prohibitive surgical risk.

The external iliac artery rises out of the pelvis and joins the CFA just above the femoral head. This ascent out of the pelvis is deceptive on angiography, which may be related to the higher risk for perforation or dissection with endovascular treatment. Once the artery leaves the pelvis, it can undergo external compression, prompting consideration of self-expanding stents. Endovascular angioplasty and stenting, particularly for shorter and common iliac lesions, has very good technical success with excellent durability (>80% patency) over a 5-year period, similar to results with surgical revascularization.[1,3,4]

Femoral-Popliteal Artery Disease

Obstructive atherosclerosis is more common in the SFA than the popliteal artery or the CFA. Usually, the profunda femoris serves as an important source of collateral blood flow to the leg in patients with obstructive SFA disease. The CFA is more difficult to treat because it is subject to greater flexion and extension with movement of the hip, and complications that occlude the CFA are likely to lead to an acutely threatened limb as a result of obstruction of the profunda and SFAs. Even though balloon angioplasty can successfully treat obstructive CFA disease secondary to atherosclerosis or complications of CFA access for other procedures, surgical repair with patch angioplasty is the standard of care for most patients with acceptable surgical risk. Balloon-expandable stents should not be used in this location because of repetitive compression during movement of the hip. In patients with a prohibitive surgical risk, balloon angioplasty with or without atherectomy is used for CFA lesions, along with bail-out self-expanding stents for flow-limiting dissections.[57] The profunda femoris is a smaller artery with a thinner wall than the SFA, and the risk for complications and evidence of long-term success with catheter-based intervention are uncertain.

Most percutaneous femoral interventions involve the SFA and popliteal artery, and interventional techniques are similar with both arteries. The distal SFA and particularly the popliteal artery are subject to torsion, stretch, and kinking with movement of the leg. For this reason, stents are generally avoided below the level of the top of the patella and above the tibial metaphyseal plate when viewed with the leg straight. Stenting between this region subjects stents to extreme flexion, compression, and torsion and is associated with stent fracture, restenosis, and poor long-term durability, although specific helical mesh stents may be more durable than other self-expanding stents in this location. Most operators only consider stenting the popliteal artery across the knee in patients with CLI and a poor angioplasty result and in those with prohibitive surgical risk.

Acute procedural success rates with catheter-based interventions now approach 90%, in part because of a wide variety of wires, crossing catheters, reentry catheters, and combined antegrade and retrograde approaches for difficult total occlusions.

Restenosis rates are higher than in the iliac artery and may require repeated interventions. Catheter-based therapies should be considered part of a long-term strategy of surveillance for recurrent and new disease and repeated interventions when needed.[12] Balloon angioplasty alone has durability similar to that of primary stenting for short lesions (<50 to 100 mm in length),[12] and in this setting, provisional stenting for abrupt closure, flow-limiting dissection, or poor expansion (residual stenosis >50%) is an acceptable strategy. For longer lesions (>100 mm), primary stenting with self-expanding nitinol stents offer better durability and walking function than balloon angioplasty with provisional stenting[12] (Fig. 44.4). Drug-eluting nitinol self-expanding stents offer less restenosis than does balloon angioplasty with and without provisional stenting with nitinol BMSs.[17,18] In one study, the benefits of drug-eluting self-expanding stents were maintained over 5 years after the index procedure.[17]

Interventionalists need to establish systems to monitor patients for recurrent or new disease and treat atherosclerosis risk factors intensively. Collaboration with surgical colleagues and vascular medicine specialists should improve outcomes.

Tibial Disease
The popliteal artery divides into three tibial arteries: the anterior tibial, which becomes the dorsalis pedis in the foot; the posterior tibial, which forms the pedal arcade with the anterior tibial artery; and the peroneal artery, which usually ends just above the ankle but can be an important collateral to the foot. In general, claudication is rare with loss of even two of the three tibial arteries. Catheter-based interventions have high rates of restenosis, in part because of the small diameter and long lesion length, and they are rarely justified in patients with claudication. Frequently, correction of obstructive proximal disease will often resolve the claudication even with extensive residual tibial disease.

In contrast, treating severe tibial disease in patients with CLI can promote wound healing, resolve pain at rest, and prevent major amputation. Vascular access is more limited for distal tibial disease, because a contralateral femoral approach or an arm approach is often too distant for the shaft length of most devices. Antegrade CFA access can allow equipment to reach the foot if needed and often gives greater pushability to drive through long occlusions. The retrograde pedal approach uses noninvasive ultrasound and a micropuncture needle to access one of the tibial arteries at the foot or ankle. Access from above (e.g., antegrade CFA) allows a retrograde wire from the foot to be snared and exteriorized and provides a rigid rail for angioplasty balloons. A pedal access site may become a nonhealing ulcer if the intervention is unsuccessful.

Angiosome-directed revascularization refers to revascularization of a tibial artery that supplies the area of a nonhealing ulcer or gangrene.[11] The value of angiosome-directed revascularization versus restoring any straight flow to the foot is debated. In observational studies, wound healing was better and amputation lower with angiosome-directed rather than indirect (nonangiosome) tibial revascularization.[58] These observations may be confounded, however, because indirect revascularization may be a marker for more complex tibial disease and poorer limb outcomes.[11] In one study, changes in foot microcirculation assessed by skin perfusion pressures improved to a similar degree in angiosome and nonangiosome tibial revascularization.[59]

Tibial disease is most often treated by prolonged balloon inflation, but stents are used as bail-out treatment of flow-limiting dissection. Although balloon-expandable coronary stents are used, they are prone to external compression. Randomized trials of coronary DESs offer greater patency and less reintervention for restenosis than BMSs, plain balloon angioplasty, or drug-coated balloon angioplasty.[4,60] Most of these studies are underpowered to show an effect on major amputation or survival.

Multiple catheter-based interventions over several months may be required to heal an ulcer because restenosis slows healing. Once healed, however, restenosis may be less of an issue, given the use of adequate foot care and protection to prevent skin breakdown. Managing CLI with ulceration or gangrene requires close follow-up to débride dead tissue in ulcerated areas and aid healing. Gangrenous toes can be left dry until they mummify and autoamputate or can be surgically amputated once viable and devitalized tissue are clearly demarcated. Infected gangrene does require surgical amputation to avoid osteomyelitis. These complexities mandate a team approach to care that includes wound specialists, podiatrists, surgeons, and prosthesis specialists for optimum management.

Cervical Artery Disease
Extracranial Carotid Disease
Extracranial disease of the internal and common carotid artery is a potential source of artery-to-artery embolism, one of the causes of ischemic stroke (see Chapter 45). Over the last two decades, improvements in catheter-based techniques have enabled patients at increased risk for stroke from this cause to be treated with outcomes similar to those of traditional carotid endarterectomy, particularly in patients younger than 70 years of age.[15,61]

Symptoms are the most important factor related to the risk for disabling stroke and the indication for revascularization. "Symptomatic disease" refers to patients with a minor stroke or TIA. In the carotid circulation, symptoms are typically dysphasia, contralateral hemiparesis or hemiparesthesia, or ipsilateral transient monocular blindness (amaurosis fugax). Symptoms lasting less than 24 hours and without infarction noted on imaging are classified as TIAs. Minor strokes are classified as "mild clinical deficits" or "no clinical residual deficits" with evidence of infarction on imaging. The higher sensitivity of newer imaging techniques (e.g., diffusion-weighted MRI) compared with older technologies may have increased the likelihood of finding small infarcts with no residual clinical deficits.[1,15]

In older trials of endarterectomy versus medical therapy, patients with recent symptoms and a stenosis of 50% to 99% had higher risk of stroke and a greater benefit from endarterectomy within the first week after symptoms. The risk of stroke declines rapidly after this time, with a smaller net benefit from revascularization especially more than 3 months after symptoms.[1] Compared with carotid endarterectomy, carotid stenting in symptomatic patients is associated with a higher risk of death or stroke over the following 30 days in patients over 70 years of age, but patients younger than 70 years of age had similar outcomes, and the risk of MI and cranial nerve injury was lower with stenting in all age groups.[61] Outcomes over the longer time frame up to 3 years are similar between both techniques.[61] Carotid stenting for patients with a 50% to 99% stenosis and recent TIA or minor stroke symptoms may be considered in patients with good anatomy for stenting and with high risk of MI or poor surgical outcomes with endarterectomy (Tables 44.1 and 44.2).[15,61]

In *asymptomatic* patients, the *severity of stenosis* determines risk, with stenoses greater than 80% increasing the risk of stroke. The reduction in risk with revascularization accrues slowly over the long term and needs to offset the small but important periprocedural/operative risk. This benefit usually takes several years to accrue, and asymptomatic patients need to have reasonable 5-year survival for a realistic chance of achieving a net benefit from revascularization. Improved medical therapy with intensive lipid-lowering and antiplatelet agents has likely decreased the benefit-to-risk ratio. These therapies were increasingly used in the medical-treated arms of the carotid endarterectomy trials,

TABLE 44.1 Factors Associated with Increased Risk for Complications with Carotid Artery Stent Placement

Tortuous aortic arch
Platelet or clotting disorder
Difficult vascular access
Lesion or heavy vessel calcification
Visible thrombus
Advanced age (>75-80 years)*

*The risk for a cerebrovascular accident (stroke) with carotid artery stent placement is increased, and the risk for myocardial infarction with carotid endarterectomy is increased.

and coincided with a decline in the annual stroke risk of 60% to 70% over the years from 1995 to 2010 to approximately 1% per year.[1] As a result, the net benefit of carotid surgery or stenting is maximized by identifying patients at low procedural risk and higher risk of stroke (for example, rapidly increasing stenosis severity over time may indicate a higher risk of stroke) (see Tables 44.1 and 44.2). Patients older than 80 years have a higher risk for perioperative adverse events with stenting or surgery. The primary outcome of the CREST study of patients at average surgical risk suggested no difference in outcomes at 10 years with stenting versus surgery.[62] The 2020 Cochrane Review also suggested no significant differences in long-term outcomes between carotid stenting and surgery for asymptomatic patients.[61] For asymptomatic patients, indications for carotid stenting include 80% to 99% stenosis in those with a periprocedural risk for stroke or death of less than 3%.[1]

Carotid stenting starts with access to the common carotid artery with a diagnostic catheter and then a delivery sheath. Embolic protection consists of distal protection using filters or obstructive balloons deployed distal to the carotid stenosis or proximal occlusion devices deployed proximal to the stenosis. Filters allow blood flow to the brain to continue and theoretically lead to less brain ischemia if the circle of Willis is incomplete. Self-expanding stents using delivery systems on a 0.014-inch platform resist external compression (Fig. 44.5).

Vertebral and Subclavian Artery Disease

The left and right vertebral arteries usually arise from the left and right subclavian arteries, course through the upper vertebrae into the posterior of the skull, and join together as the basilar artery. One vertebral artery is often larger (dominant) than the other, and loss of one such artery is usually well tolerated. Diagnosis of vertebrobasilar insufficiency is clinical with symptoms affecting the brainstem and cerebellum, including dizziness, ataxia, diplopia, and syncope. Atherosclerosis usually affects the proximal vertebral arteries, but more extensive proximal disease in the subclavian or brachiocephalic arteries can cause vertebrobasilar insufficiency. Patients with vertebrobasilar insufficiency have a 5-year risk for stroke of approximately 30% without any treatment.[1,15]

Medical treatment of vertebral artery disease includes antiplatelet agents and statins. BP control to reduce ischemic stroke requires careful titration to avoid hypotension and hypoperfusion, which can precipitate symptoms. Surgical therapy consisting of transection and reimplantation into an adjacent subclavian artery entails considerable morbidity, including Horner syndrome, lymphocele, and thrombosis. Extracranial percutaneous treatment, particularly with stenting, has much lower morbidity and short-term mortality. Two randomized trials of intracranial or extracranial vertebral artery stenting for symptomatic vertebral artery disease showed no significant reduction in stroke compared with medical therapy; however, both trials were stopped early.[63,64] Subgroup analyses showed a much higher periprocedural stroke rate with intracranial vertebral stenting (20%) versus extracranial vertebral stenting (1% to 2%). There was a trend to lower stroke rates over 3.5 years with stenting extracranial vertebral disease in one trial,[64] but larger trials are needed to assess the value of this therapy for stroke prevention. Observational studies of extracranial vertebral stenting for symptomatic vertebral stenoses report lower subsequent stroke rates (2% at 1 year) than historical studies (approximately 6% per year); however, the improved medical therapy may account for some of this difference.[15]

Subclavian stenosis more often affects the left subclavian origin than the brachiocephalic or right subclavian arteries. This predilection may result from more disturbed blood flow at the origin of the left subclavian artery. Subclavian stenosis usually causes a 15 mm Hg or greater difference in noninvasive brachial BP between the two arms,[1] in the absence of significant bilateral disease. Most subclavian stenosis, however, is asymptomatic and does not need investigation or revascularization. Symptoms from subclavian stenosis include arm claudication with activity, angina in patients with a left internal mammary/thoracic artery graft from previous coronary artery bypass surgery, vertebrobasilar insufficiency with arm activity because of vertebral steal, or ischemic (hand) steal syndrome in patients with a dialysis fistula. Although noninvasive imaging can identify reverse flow in the vertebral artery distal to a subclavian stenosis, this physiologic abnormality does not always lead to symptoms, particularly if it involves a nondominant vertebral artery or blood flow in the contralateral vertebral artery is not impeded. Thus, physiologic reversal

TABLE 44.2 Factors Associated with Increased Risk from Carotid Artery Surgery

Anatomic Criteria
High cervical or intrathoracic lesion
Previous neck surgery or radiation therapy
Contralateral carotid artery occlusion
Previous ipsilateral carotid endarterectomy
Contralateral laryngeal nerve palsy
Tracheostomy
Medical Comorbidities
Age >80 years*
Class III or IV congestive heart failure
Class III or IV angina pectoris
Left main coronary disease
Two- or three-vessel coronary artery disease
Need for open heart surgery
Ejection fraction ≤30%
Recent myocardial infarction
Severe chronic obstructive lung disease

*The risk for a cerebrovascular accident (stroke) with carotid artery stent placement is increased, and the risk for myocardial infarction with carotid endarterectomy is increased.

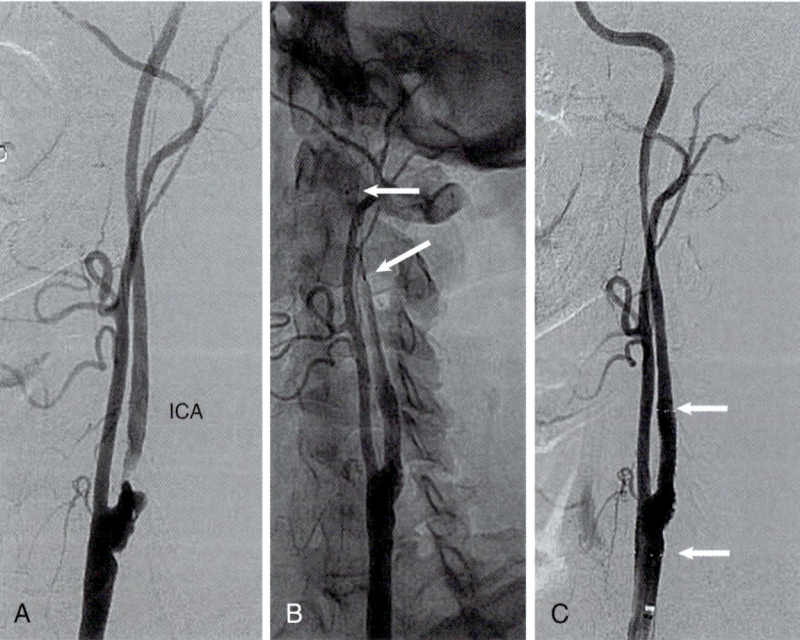

FIGURE 44.5 Carotid stenting for symptomatic carotid stenosis. **A,** Stenosis at origin of left internal carotid artery. **B,** Stent deployed. *Arrows* indicate markers of embolic protection filter. **C,** Final angiogram with *arrows* indicating the margins of the stent.

of flow in the vertebral artery without symptoms is not an indication for revascularization.

Medical therapy targets the progression of atherosclerosis (e.g., antiplatelet agents, statins, BP control). Because most subclavian disease is proximal or ostial, surgical revascularization usually involves subclavian-to-common carotid bypass. More commonly, symptomatic subclavian artery disease is treated with the less morbid procedure of subclavian artery stenting. Both treatments have low periprocedural risks of stroke (1% to 2%).[1] Balloon-expandable stents are generally used because they allow more precise placement to cover the ostium of the artery and avoid the vertebral and left internal mammary artery origins. Embolic stroke is rare, possibly because of reverse flow down the vertebral artery during balloon dilation and stenting. Thus, embolic protection is infrequently used for vertebral and subclavian artery stenting. The long-term results of stenting subclavian and brachiocephalic disease are excellent (>80% overall patency).[1]

Mesenteric and Renal Artery Disease

Mesenteric Artery

Three arteries supply the mesenteric viscera: celiac, superior mesenteric, and inferior mesenteric. Although advanced atherosclerosis of the aorta is common, mesenteric angina or infarction is very uncommon, probably because of the multiple collateral networks in the mesentery. Acute mesenteric ischemia with infarction is a surgical emergency because it is usually associated with infarction of the small or large intestine.[13] An embolus (e.g., from thrombus in the heart associated with atrial fibrillation) is a common cause and typically lodges in the proximal mesenteric artery (usually the superior mesenteric artery). Although some cases can be treated by endovascular techniques, clinical signs of peritonitis or CT findings of pneumatosis, free intra-abdominal air, or portal venous gas indicate bowel necrosis and need for open surgery. In this situation, urgent surgery within 24 hours is required to resect dead bowel and revascularize ischemic bowel, with death in virtually all cases treated beyond this time.

Chronic mesenteric ischemia is a more insidious syndrome that causes abdominal discomfort or pain 30 to 60 minutes after eating, early satiety, and substantial weight loss because of food fear or avoidance.[13] Classically, more than two mesenteric arteries are stenosed or occluded. The disease is usually adjacent and involves advanced atherosclerosis of the aorta and origins of the mesenteric arteries. Asymptomatic disease of the mesenteric arteries does not require revascularization.

Bowel endoscopy can detect changes associated with chronic ischemia, but noninvasive arterial imaging with duplex ultrasound or MRA or CTA generally identifies the extent of disease. Invasive angiography usually requires a lateral aortogram to identify clearly the origins of the mesenteric arteries. Surgical revascularization with reimplantation of the arteries has high mortality and morbidity (10% to 15%) because of the advanced age and other vascular comorbid conditions. Percutaneous angioplasty with stenting has lower mortality (<5%) and morbidity and achieves good resolution of symptoms in about 70% to 80% of patients over several years[13]. Restenosis may require further intervention and can be identified by duplex ultrasound and CTA.

Renal Artery

Renal artery stenosis can cause secondary hypertension or rapidly deteriorating renal function. Clinical clues to the diagnosis of renal artery stenosis include onset of hypertension before 55 years of age, resistant or malignant hypertension (particularly in a previously well-controlled patient), rapidly increasing creatinine level over a several-month period or earlier, and sudden pulmonary edema without a clear cardiac cause (e.g., because of sudden hypertension with or without acute mitral regurgitation). Imaging with duplex ultrasound or with MRA, CTA, or invasive angiography can identify renal artery stenosis.

Although renal artery stenosis is relatively common, determining whether it is a reversible cause of hypertension or declining renal function is difficult. Screening outside the aforementioned clinical scenarios probably offers low yield and justification because treatment does not usually impact BP control or renal function.[65,66] Even though many operators use embolic protection devices during renal stenting, these devices have unknown value in preventing atheroemboli or worsening renal function.

Three randomized trials of stenting renal arteries with greater than 40% to 60% stenosis by angiography to control resistant hypertension or preserve renal function showed no effect on BP control, preservation of renal function, or CV events.[66,67] In the CORAL study, even the subgroup of participants with a renal artery stenosis of at least 80% did not benefit from renal artery stenting.[67] As a result, the enthusiasm for renal artery stenting has waned considerably, although there is still some support for stenting renal artery stenosis in the presence of "flash" pulmonary edema without cardiac causes, rapidly decreasing renal function, and some cases of accelerating or resistant hypertension, based mainly on case reports and case series.[68]

Fibromuscular dysplasia (FMD) is a rarer cause of renal artery stenosis and hypertension more often seen in younger patients, with a higher prevalence in women.[69] Although defined histologically in the past, this is now superseded by a classification based on imaging (multifocal "beading" versus focal disease). FMD typically involves the middle or distal renal artery, whereas atherosclerosis usually involves the ostium or proximal renal artery. FMD often accompanies similar disease in other arterial beds (e.g., carotid arteries).[69] This diagnosis has particular importance in that balloon angioplasty without stenting often very effectively controls BP with a durable response.

Resistant hypertension despite multiple antihypertensive agents is a marker of elevated CV risk.[70] Recognition that the rich plexus of sympathetic nerves in the adventitia of renal arteries may contribute to resistant hypertension led to a number of catheter-based technologies to ablate the sympathetic nerves to lower BP and CV risk (see Chapter 26). Several randomized sham-controlled trials show on average a modest effect on systolic BP after catheter-based renal sympathetic denervation. In early studies, this procedure decreased systolic BP by an average 2 mm Hg, with second-generation devices lowering systolic BP by an average of 6 mm Hg.[71] However, the later studies did not require treatment-resistant hypertension and there is wide variability in the BP response. Future studies will need to determine the factors that predict a greater effect.

ENDOVASCULAR TREATMENT OF VENOUS DISEASE

Extremity Deep Venous Thrombosis

Upper and lower extremity DVT results from multiple factors often encompassed in the Virchow triad: abnormalities in coagulation, hemodynamic flow, and endothelial injury (see Chapter 87). Such factors include hypercoagulable states, venous stasis, external obstruction, scarring or congenital abnormalities of veins, or injury to veins.

Lower extremity DVT is treated primarily medically with anticoagulation,[72] but endovascular treatment is an option for patients with proximal venous thrombosis defined as being at the level of the common femoral vein or higher. Thrombosis at this site occurs in about one third of all cases of lower extremity DVT and obstructs venous return from the lower limb. Proximal DVT occurs more frequently in the left leg as a result of compression of the left iliac vein by the overlying right iliac artery (May-Thurner syndrome). Acute severe proximal deep venous occlusion, characterized by a blue limb, pain, and limb ischemia (phlegmasia cerulea dolens) is often associated with malignancy. Chronic post-thrombotic syndrome occurs over several years in about half the patients with iliofemoral DVT[48] and involves limb swelling, heaviness, and pain. Medical treatment includes compression stockings and anticoagulation. Endovascular treatment of proximal DVT by catheter-directed thrombolysis with or without balloon angioplasty and self-expanding stents reduces the incidence of post-thrombotic syndrome by about 30%.[48]

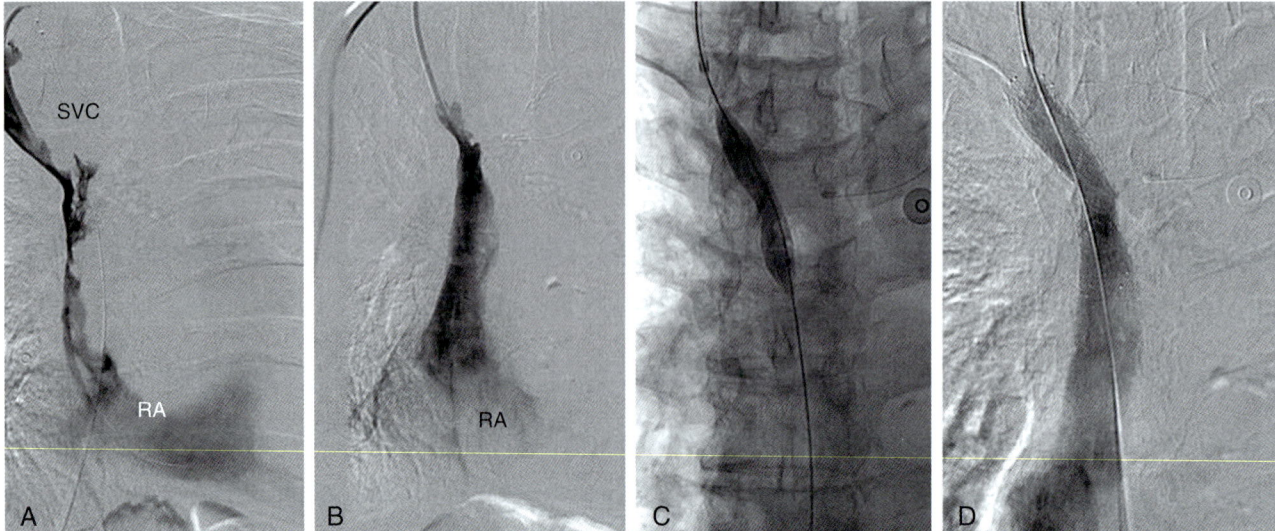

FIGURE 44.6 Superior vena cava (SVC) syndrome secondary to external compression of the SVC by a lung tumor and thrombosis of the SVC. **A,** Initial venogram showing compression of the SVC and filling defects because of thrombus; *RA,* right atrium. **B,** Venogram after 24 hours of catheter-directed thrombolysis with resolution of the thrombus but residual stenosis. **C,** Balloon venoplasty. **D,** Final angiogram after deployment of a self-expanding stent.

Upper extremity DVT is related to effort-related proximal vein thrombosis in athletes (Paget-Schroetter syndrome), venous thoracic outlet syndrome, catheter-related thrombosis, or malignancy.[73] Effort-related thrombosis is usually associated with vigorous arm exercise (e.g., weightlifting). *Venous thoracic outlet syndrome* is related to compression of the subclavian vein as it exits the thoracic cage between the clavicle, first rib, costoclavicular ligament, and subclavian and anterior scalene muscles. Catheter-related thrombosis is associated with indwelling catheters, ports, and pacemaker or defibrillator leads. Malignancy with external obstruction is more frequently associated with superior vena cava syndrome (see next). Anticoagulation is the most common treatment of upper extremity DVT, but endovascular therapy can provide relief from post-thrombotic syndrome. Endovascular therapy includes catheter-directed thrombolysis and treatment of any precipitating cause. For example, thoracic outlet syndrome generally requires surgical decompression (resection of the first rib or other structures) and venoplasty soon after thrombolysis because stents usually crush or fracture in this location.[73] Central venous catheters should be removed if they are no longer required, or the patient should be maintained on a long-term anticoagulation regimen.

Superior Vena Cava Syndrome

Superior vena cava syndrome results from obstruction of the superior vena cava with impairment of venous return from the head and upper limbs (see Chapters 95 and 98). Typical causes include external compression, invasion from a tumor, or thrombosis related to an indwelling central catheter (e.g., for chemotherapy) or leads from pacemakers or defibrillators. Symptoms include swelling and fullness in the head, headache, dyspnea, and a sense of choking. Angioplasty alone rarely relieves this condition successfully because of vessel recoil, but stenting very effectively reduces symptoms. Thrombosis often accompanies stenosis and requires catheter-directed thrombolytic therapy before balloon and stent therapy (Fig. 44.6). The stent should be oversized and extended well above and partly below the lesion so that it has an hourglass shape to help keep it anchored and less likely to embolize. Anticoagulation is generally prescribed, often indefinitely for superior vena cava obstruction or thrombosis associated with malignancy. Symptoms usually respond rapidly within 24 hours. Indwelling catheters and pacemaker leads should be removed before stenting and reimplanted afterward if required. Long-term outcomes depend more on the cause of the superior vena cava obstruction, but in nonmalignant cases, resolution of symptoms occurs in more than 70% of cases.[74]

FUTURE PERSPECTIVES

New technologies have advanced endovascular treatment of noncoronary vascular disease into the mainstream. In many cases, adapting techniques from interventional cardiology has revolutionized the ability to treat patients with complex peripheral vascular disease through minimally invasive endovascular means. In coming years, an even greater proportion of peripheral vascular disease may be treated in the angiography suite instead of in the operating room.

REFERENCES

1. Aboyans V, Ricco JB, Bartelink MEL, et al. ESC guidelines on the diagnosis and treatment of peripheral arterial diseases, in collaboration with the European Society for Vascular Surgery (ESVS): document covering atherosclerotic disease of extracranial carotid and vertebral, mesenteric, renal, upper and lower extremity arteries. Endorsed by: the European Stroke Organization (ESO)the Task force for the diagnosis and treatment of peripheral arterial diseases of the European Society of Cardiology (ESC) and of the European Society for Vascular Surgery (ESVS). *Eur Heart J.* 2017;39:763–816. 2018.
2. Gerhard-Herman MD, Gornik HL, Barrett C, et al. 2016 AHA/ACC guideline on the management of patients with lower extremity peripheral artery disease: a report of the American College of Cardiology/American Heart Association task force on clinical practice guidelines. *Circulation.* 2017;135:e726–e779.
3. Gerhard-Herman MD, Gornik HL, Barrett C, et al. 2016 AHA/ACC guideline on the management of patients with lower extremity peripheral artery disease: Executive summary: a report of the American College of Cardiology/American Heart Association task force on clinical practice guidelines. *Circulation.* 2017;135:e686–e725.
4. Jaff MR, White CJ, Hiatt WR, et al. An update on methods for revascularization and expansion of the TASC lesion classification to include below-the-knee arteries: a supplement to the intersociety consensus for the management of peripheral arterial disease (TASC II): the TASC steering committee. *Catheter Cardiovasc Interv.* 2015;86:611–625.
5. Kullo IJ, Rooke TW. CLINICAL PRACTICE. Peripheral artery disease. *N Engl J Med.* 2016;374:861–871.
6. Olin JW, White CJ, Armstrong EJ, et al. Peripheral artery disease: evolving role of exercise, medical therapy, and endovascular options. *J Am Coll Cardiol.* 2016;67:1338–1357.
7. Fakhry F, Fokkenrood HJ, Spronk S, et al. Endovascular revascularisation versus conservative management for intermittent claudication. *Cochrane Database Syst Rev.* 2018;3:CD010512.
8. Saratzis A, Paraskevopoulos I, Patel S, et al. Supervised exercise therapy and revascularization for intermittent claudication: network meta-analysis of randomized controlled trials. *JACC Cardiovasc Interv.* 2019;12:1125–1136.
9. Golledge J, Singh TP, Alahakoon C, et al. Meta-analysis of clinical trials examining the benefit of structured home exercise in patients with peripheral artery disease. *Br J Surg.* 2019;106:319–331.
10. Fakhry F, Spronk S, van der Laan L, et al. Endovascular revascularization and supervised exercise for peripheral artery disease and intermittent claudication: a randomized clinical trial. *J Am Med Assoc.* 2015;314:1936–1944.
11. Kinlay S. Management of critical limb ischemia. *Circ Cardiovasc Interv.* 2016;9:e001946.
12. Thukkani AK, Kinlay S. Endovascular intervention for peripheral artery disease. *Circ Res.* 2015;116:1599–1613.
13. Clair DG, Beach JM. Mesenteric ischemia. *N Engl J Med.* 2016;374:959–968.
14. Jennings CG, Houston JG, Severn A, et al. Renal artery stenosis-when to screen, what to stent? *Curr Atheroscler Rep.* 2014;16:416.
15. Powers WJ, Rabinstein AA, Ackerson T, et al. 2018 Guidelines for the early management of patients with acute ischemic stroke: a guideline for healthcare professionals from the American Heart Association/American Stroke Association. *Stroke.* 2018;49:e46–e110.
16. Calvert M, Kyte D, Mercieca-Bebber R, et al. Guidelines for inclusion of patient-reported outcomes in clinical trial protocols: the SPIRIT-PRO extension. *J Am Med Assoc.* 2018;319:483–494.
17. Dake MD, Ansel GM, Jaff MR, et al. Durable clinical effectiveness with paclitaxel-eluting stents in the femoropopliteal artery: 5-year results of the Zilver PTX randomized trial. *Circulation.* 2016;133:1472–1483; discussion 1483.

18. Gray WA, Keirse K, Soga Y, et al. A polymer-coated, paclitaxel-eluting stent (Eluvia) versus a polymer-free, paclitaxel-coated stent (Zilver PTX) for endovascular femoropopliteal intervention (IMPERIAL): a randomised, non-inferiority trial. *Lancet*. 2018;392:1541–1551.
19. Muller-Hulsbeck S, Keirse K, Zeller T, et al. Long-term results from the MAJESTIC trial of the eluvia paclitaxel-eluting stent for femoropopliteal treatment: 3-year follow-up. *Cardiovasc Intervent Radiol*. 2017;40:1832–1838.
20. Bosiers M, Setacci C, De Donato G, et al. ZILVERPASS study: ZILVER PTX stent vs bypass surgery in femoropopliteal lesions. *J Endovasc Ther*. 2020;27:287–295.
21. Rosenfield K, Jaff MR, White CJ, et al. Trial of a paclitaxel-coated balloon for femoropopliteal artery disease. *N Engl J Med*. 2015;373:145–153.
22. Scheinert D, Duda S, Zeller T, et al. The LEVANT I (Lutonix paclitaxel-coated balloon for the prevention of femoropopliteal restenosis) trial for femoropopliteal revascularization: first-in-human randomized trial of low-dose drug-coated balloon versus uncoated balloon angioplasty. *JACC Cardiovasc Interv*. 2014;7:10–19.
23. Schneider PA, Laird JR, Tepe G, et al. Treatment effect of drug-coated balloons is durable to 3 years in the femoropopliteal arteries: long-term results of the IN.PACT SFA randomized trial. *Circ Cardiovasc Interv*. 2018;11:e005891.
24. Tepe G, Laird J, Schneider P, et al. Drug-coated balloon versus standard percutaneous transluminal angioplasty for the treatment of superficial femoral and popliteal peripheral artery disease: 12-month results from the IN.PACT SFA randomized trial. *Circulation*. 2015;131:495–502.
25. Zeller T, Rastan A, Macharzina R, et al. Drug-coated balloons vs. drug-eluting stents for treatment of long femoropopliteal lesions. *J Endovasc Ther*. 2014;21:359–368.
26. Bausback Y, Wittig T, Schmidt A, et al. Drug-eluting stent versus drug-coated balloon revascularization in patients with femoropopliteal arterial disease. *J Am Coll Cardiol*. 2019;73:667–679.
27. Liistro F, Angioli P, Porto I, et al. Drug-eluting balloon versus drug-eluting stent for complex femoropopliteal arterial lesions: the DRASTICO study. *J Am Coll Cardiol*. 2019;74:205–215.
28. Cassese S, Wolf F, Ingwersen M, et al. Drug-coated balloon angioplasty for femoropopliteal in-stent restenosis. *Circ Cardiovasc Interv*. 2018;11:e007055.
29. Krankenberg H, Tubler T, Ingwersen M, et al. Drug-coated balloon versus standard balloon for superficial femoral artery in-stent restenosis: the randomized Femoral Artery In-Stent Restenosis (FAIR) trial. *Circulation*. 2015;132:2230–2236.
30. Ott I, Cassese S, Groha P, et al. ISAR-PEBIS (Paclitaxel-Eluting balloon versus conventional balloon angioplasty for in-stent restenosis of superficial femoral artery): a randomized trial. *J Am Heart Assoc*. 2017;6:e006321.
31. Tepe G, Schnorr B, Albrecht T, et al. Angioplasty of femoral-popliteal arteries with drug-coated balloons: 5-year follow-up of the THUNDER trial. *JACC Cardiovasc Interv*. 2015;8:102–108.
32. Katsanos K, Spiliopoulos S, Kitrou P, et al. Risk of death and amputation with use of paclitaxel-coated balloons in the infrapopliteal arteries for treatment of critical limb ischemia: a systematic review and meta-analysis of randomized controlled trials. *J Vasc Interv Radiol*. 2020;31:202–212.
33. Rocha-Singh KJ, Beckman JA, Ansel G, et al. Patient-level meta-analysis of 999 claudicants undergoing primary femoropopliteal nitinol stent implantation. *Catheter Cardiovasc Interv*. 2017;89:1250–1256.
34. Koifman E, Lipinski MJ, Buchanan K, et al. Comparison of treatment strategies for femoropopliteal disease: a network meta-analysis. *Catheter Cardiovasc Interv*. 2018;91:1320–1328.
35. Katsanos K, Spiliopoulos S, Kitrou P, et al. Risk of death following application of paclitaxel-coated balloons and stents in the femoropopliteal artery of the leg: a systematic review and meta-analysis of randomized controlled trials. *J Am Heart Assoc*. 2018;7:e011245.
36. Bittl JA, He Y, Baber U, et al. Bayes factor meta-analysis of the mortality claim for peripheral paclitaxel-eluting devices. *JACC Cardiovasc Interv*. 2019;12:2528–2537.
37. Gray WA, Jaff MR, Parikh SA, et al. Mortality assessment of paclitaxel-coated balloons: patient-level meta-analysis of the ILLUMENATE clinical program at 3 years. *Circulation*. 2019;140:1145–1155.
38. Ouriel K, Adelman MA, Rosenfield K, et al. Safety of paclitaxel-coated balloon angioplasty for femoropopliteal peripheral artery disease. *JACC Cardiovasc Interv*. 2019;12:2515–2524.
39. Schneider PA, Laird JR, Doros G, et al. Mortality not correlated with paclitaxel exposure: an independent patient-level meta-analysis of a drug-coated balloon. *J Am Coll Cardiol*. 2019;73:2550–2563.
40. Secemsky EA, Kundi H, Weinberg I, et al. Association of survival with femoropopliteal artery revascularization with drug-coated devices. *JAMA Cardiol*. 2019;4:332–340.
41. Behrendt CA, Sedrakyan A, Peters F, et al. Editor's choice - long term survival after femoropopliteal artery revascularisation with paclitaxel coated devices: a propensity score matched cohort analysis. *Eur J Vasc Endovasc Surg*. 2020;59:587–596.
42. Scheller B, Vukadinovic D, Jeger R, et al. Survival after coronary revascularization with paclitaxel-coated balloons. *J Am Coll Cardiol*. 2020;75:1017–1028.
43. Antonopoulos CN, Mylonas SN, Moulakakis KG, et al. A network meta-analysis of randomized controlled trials comparing treatment modalities for de novo superficial femoral artery occlusive lesions. *J Vasc Surg*. 2017;65:234–245.e11.
44. Hajibandeh S, Hajibandeh S, Antoniou SA, et al. Covered vs uncovered stents for aortoiliac and femoropopliteal arterial disease: a systematic review and meta-analysis. *J Endovasc Ther*. 2016;23:442–452.
45. Shackles C, Rundback JH, Herman K, et al. Above and below knee femoropopliteal VIABAHN(R). *Catheter Cardiovasc Interv*. 2015;85:859–867.
46. Veenstra EB, van der Laan MJ, Zeebregts CJ, et al. A systematic review and meta-analysis of endovascular and surgical revascularization techniques in acute limb ischemia. *J Vasc Surg*. 2020;71:654–668.e3.
47. Ebben HP, Jongkind V, Wisselink W, et al. Catheter directed thrombolysis protocols for peripheral arterial occlusions: a systematic review. *Eur J Vasc Endovasc Surg*. 2019;57:667–675.
48. Watson L, Broderick C, Armon MP. Thrombolysis for acute deep vein thrombosis. *Cochrane Database Syst Rev*. 2016;11:CD002783.
49. Robertson L, McBride O, Burdess A. Pharmacomechanical thrombectomy for iliofemoral deep vein thrombosis. *Cochrane Database Syst Rev*. 2016;11:CD011536.
50. Ambler GK, Radwan R, Hayes PD, et al. Atherectomy for peripheral arterial disease. *Cochrane Database Syst Rev*. 2014:CD006680.
51. Dippel EJ, Makam P, Kovach R, et al. Randomized controlled study of excimer laser atherectomy for treatment of femoropopliteal in-stent restenosis: initial results from the EXCITE ISR trial (EXCImer Laser Randomized Controlled Study for Treatment of FemoropopliTEal In-Stent Restenosis). *JACC Cardiovasc Interv*. 2015;8:92–101.
52. Madhavan MV, Shahim B, Mena-Hurtado C, et al. Efficacy and safety of intravascular lithotripsy for the treatment of peripheral arterial disease: an individual patient-level pooled data analysis. *Catheter Cardiovasc Interv*. 2020;5:959–968.
53. Megaly M, Abraham B, Saad M, et al. Outcomes with cilostazol after endovascular therapy of peripheral artery disease. *Vasc Med*. 2019;24:313–323.
54. Bonaca MP, Bauersachs RM, Anand SS, et al. Rivaroxaban in peripheral artery disease after revascularization. *N Engl J Med*. 2020;382:1994–2004.
55. Sharafuddin MJ, Marjan AE. Current status of carbon dioxide angiography. *J Vasc Surg*. 2017;66:618–637.
56. Aday AW, Kinlay S, Gerhard-Herman MD. Comparison of different exercise ankle pressure indices in the diagnosis of peripheral artery disease. *Vasc Med*. 2018;23:541–548.
57. Goueffic Y, Della Schiava N, Thaveau F, et al. Stenting or surgery for de novo common femoral artery stenosis. *JACC Cardiovasc Interv*. 2017;10:1344–1354.
58. Biancari F, Juvonen T. Angiosome-targeted lower limb revascularization for ischemic foot wounds: systematic review and meta-analysis. *Eur J Vasc Endovasc Surg*. 2014;47:517–522.
59. Kawarada O, Yasuda S, Nishimura K, et al. Effect of single tibial artery revascularization on microcirculation in the setting of critical limb ischemia. *Circ Cardiovasc Interv*. 2014;7:684–691.
60. Spreen MI, Martens JM, Knippenberg B, et al. Long-term follow-up of the PADI trial: Percutaneous transluminal angioplasty versus drug-eluting stents for infrapopliteal lesions in critical limb ischemia. *J Am Heart Assoc*. 2017;6:e004877.
61. Muller MD, Lyrer P, Brown MM, et al. Carotid artery stenting versus endarterectomy for treatment of carotid artery stenosis. *Cochrane Database Syst Rev*. 2020;2:CD000515.
62. Brott TG, Howard G, Roubin GS, et al. Long-term results of stenting versus endarterectomy for carotid-artery stenosis. *N Engl J Med*. 2016;374:1021–1031.
63. Compter A, van der Worp HB, Schonewille WJ, et al. Stenting versus medical treatment in patients with symptomatic vertebral artery stenosis: a randomised open-label phase 2 trial. *Lancet Neurol*. 2015;14:606–614.
64. Markus HS, Larsson SC, Kuker W, et al. Stenting for symptomatic vertebral artery stenosis: The vertebral artery ischaemia stenting trial. *Neurology*. 2017;89:1229–1236.
65. Bohlke M, Barcellos FC. From the 1990s to CORAL (Cardiovascular Outcomes in Renal Atherosclerotic Lesions) trial results and beyond: does stenting have a role in ischemic nephropathy? *Am J Kidney Dis*. 2015;65:611–622.
66. Jenks S, Yeoh SE, Conway BR. Balloon angioplasty, with and without stenting, versus medical therapy for hypertensive patients with renal artery stenosis. *Cochrane Database Syst Rev*. 2014:CD002944.
67. Cooper CJ, Murphy TP, Cutlip DE, et al. Stenting and medical therapy for atherosclerotic renal-artery stenosis. *N Engl J Med*. 2014;370:13–22.
68. Parikh SA, Shishehbor MH, Gray BH, et al. SCAI expert consensus statement for renal artery stenting appropriate use. *Catheter Cardiovasc Interv*. 2014;84:1163–1171.
69. Gornik HL, Persu A, Adlam D, et al. First International Consensus on the diagnosis and management of fibromuscular dysplasia. *Vasc Med*. 2019;24:164–189.
70. Whelton PK, Carey RM, Aronow WS, et al. 2017 ACC/AHA/AAPA/ABC/ACPM/AGS/APhA/ASH/ASPC/NMA/PCNA guideline for the prevention, detection, evaluation, and management of high blood pressure in adults: executive summary: a report of the American College of Cardiology/American Heart Association task force on clinical practice guidelines. *Circulation*. 2018;138:e426–e483.
71. Sardar P, Bhatt DL, Kirtane AJ, et al. Sham-controlled randomized trials of catheter-based renal denervation in patients with hypertension. *J Am Coll Cardiol*. 2019;73:1633–1642.
72. Serhal M, Barnes GD. Venous thromboembolism: a clinician update. *Vasc Med*. 2019;24:122–131.
73. Cai TY, Rajendran S, Saha P, et al. Paget-Schroetter syndrome: a contemporary review of the controversies in management. *Phlebology*. 2020:268355519898920.
74. Sfyroeras GS, Antonopoulos CN, Mantas G, et al. A review of open and endovascular treatment of superior vena cava syndrome of benign aetiology. *Eur J Vasc Endovasc Surg*. 2017;53:238–254.

45 Prevention and Management of Ischemic Stroke

MARK J. ALBERTS

CLASSIFICATION OF ISCHEMIC STROKE, 870
STROKE RISK FACTORS AND PREVENTION, 873
Hypertension, 874
Hyperlipidemia, 875
Diabetes, 876
Smoking, 876
Nutrition, 876
Obesity, 876
Exercise, 876
Sleep Apnea, 876
Other Risk Factors, 876

ANTITHROMBOTIC AGENTS FOR STROKE PREVENTION, 877
Antiplatelet Therapy for Primary Prevention, 877
Stroke Prevention in Atrial Fibrillation, 877
Secondary Prevention of Ischemic Stroke, 878
MANAGEMENT OF ACUTE ISCHEMIC STROKE, 879
Intravenous Recombinant Tissue Plasminogen Activator, 880
Endovascular Therapy, 881
Anticoagulation Therapy for Acute Ischemic Stroke, 883

Other Modalities for Treatment of Acute Ischemic Stroke, 885
Management of Specific Causes of Stroke, 885
DIAGNOSIS AND TREATMENT OF PATIENTS WITH A TRANSIENT ISCHEMIC ATTACK, 886
FUTURE DIRECTIONS, 886
CONCLUSIONS, 887
CLASSIC REFERENCES, 887
REFERENCES, 887

Each year, almost 800,000 Americans have a stroke, and between 200,000 and 500,000 have a transient ischemic attack (TIA). Data from 2020 show that about 610,000 of these strokes are new and 185,000 are recurrent.[1] Overall the incidence of stroke has declined in adults from the 1980s to 2010, although this was somewhat uneven in various patient subgroups.[1] Approximately 146,000 people in the United States die of a stroke each year, making stroke the fifth leading cause of death. (Globally, stroke is the second leading cause of death.) Stroke kills more women than men, mainly because there are more elderly women than men in the United States. About 1 out of every 19 deaths in the United States is due to a stroke, of which the majority (63%) occur outside of an acute care hospital.[1] Although ischemic strokes are most common, the mortality associated with an acute ischemic stroke is much lower (about 15%) than with a hemorrhagic stroke (mortality of 40% to 45%). The overall number of deaths from stroke has declined 30-40% from the 1980s to 2010. This likely reflects improved stroke prevention as well as improvements in acute care. The decline is similar in men and women but is more pronounced in an older population (65 and above) compared with younger groups.[2]

Overall, the incidence of stroke is lower in women than in men in most age groups. However, the impact of cardiovascular disease (CVD) risk factors (high blood pressure [BP], diabetes, heart disease) on stroke risk is higher in women than in men in most age groups.[2] Although stroke incidence may be declining in some groups, aging of the population combined with more CVD risk factors may be contributing to an increased lifetime risk of having a stroke. Approximately 6.8 million Americans age 20 years or older have had a stroke, which is a leading cause of severe, long-term disability. Stroke disproportionately affects some minority populations (see Chapter 93). Black and Hispanic populations (compared with whites) have a higher incidence and mortality from stroke.[3] This disparity likely results in part from more stroke risk factors, more severe risk factors, and undertreatment of these risk factors in certain groups and populations. Environmental factors as well as socioeconomic disparities also play a role in the differential impact of some risk factors on various populations, leading to higher mortality.

Strokes are generally classified as ischemic or hemorrhagic (Fig. 45.1). This chapter will focus primarily on ischemic stroke and TIAs and will begin by discussing the various types of ischemic strokes and TIAs and the pathophysiology leading to a stroke (Table 45.1). The next section will review approaches for primary and secondary stroke prevention. The third section will focus on acute therapy for patients with ischemic stroke and TIA. The important topic of rehabilitation will not be discussed in this chapter because of space limitations but is discussed in Chapter 33.

CLASSIFICATION OF ISCHEMIC STROKE

Ischemic stroke is a heterogeneous condition with a common pathway of injury, namely reduced or obstructed arterial blood flow to one or more parts of the brain (which includes the retina and spinal cord). Even among ischemic strokes, there are a variety of underlying mechanisms that can lead to reduced blood flow (see Table 45.1). (There are a few rare processes that do not follow this common pathway, e.g., mitochondrial encephalomyopathy, lactic acidosis, and stroke-like episodes [MELAS] and cerebral autosomal dominant arteriopathy with subcortical infarcts and leukoencephalopathy [CADASIL][4].)

Atherothrombosis is the most common underlying mechanism for an ischemic stroke. It can affect large vessels (aorta, carotid artery, vertebral and basilar arteries), medium-sized vessels (middle, anterior, posterior cerebral arteries), and small vessels deep in the brain (and the retina). It is important to understand that atherothrombosis is a systemic disorder affecting blood vessels in many different locations throughout the body (heart, kidneys, major vessels such as the aorta and femoral artery, etc.) (see Chapter 24).[5,6] It is typically mediated by a host of cardiovascular disease risk factors, as discussed later. Therefore, the prevention and treatment of atherothrombosis should be viewed from a systemic perspective.

Atherothrombosis of the carotid artery can cause a hemispheric stroke as well as areas of watershed ischemia involving parts of the hemisphere. If the process involves the basilar artery, it can produce a devastating brainstem stroke. Atherothrombotic lesions can also act as a source of artery-to-artery emboli whereby parts of a proximal lesion embolize downstream to produce a smaller stroke (see Chapter 25).

Embolization from a central source such as the heart (or aorta) is another very common stroke mechanism. Cardiac emboli can affect almost any part of the body, although the brain is the most sensitive to this type of insult. Such emboli typically lodge in medium to small-sized vessels. Common underlying etiologies include atrial fibrillation (AF), valvular disease, recent myocardial infarction (MI), mural thrombus, infective endocarditis, paradoxical emboli, and others (see Chapters 37, 41, 66, 74, 75, and 79).

Lacunar strokes account for about 20% to 24% of all ischemic strokes. They involve a tiny artery (200 μm) deep in the brain and produce one of five common lacunar stroke syndrome (Table 45.2). The underlying pathology is either a hypertrophic proliferation of the vessel wall (lipohyalinosis) or microatheroma in the penetrating vessels.[5] It is noteworthy that rupture of the same vessels in the same location can also produce a hypertensive cerebral hemorrhage.

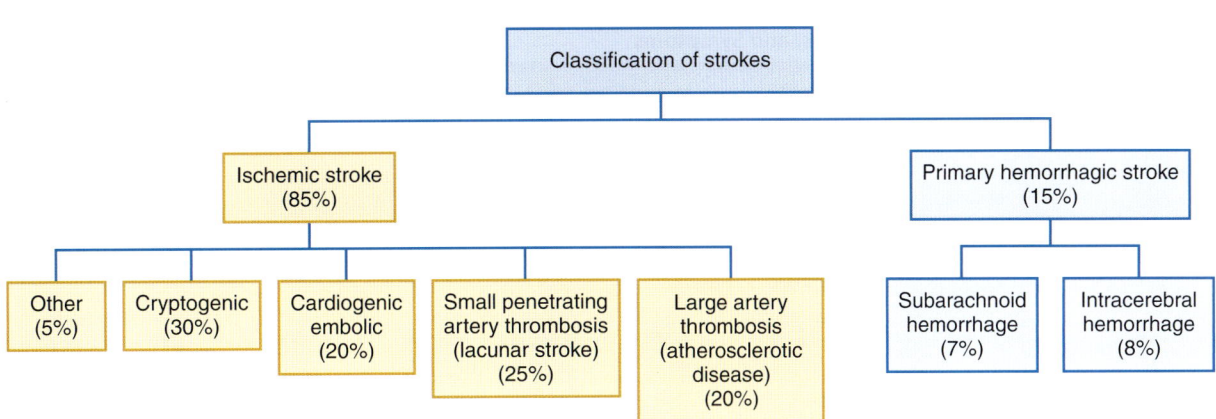

FIGURE 45.1 Broad classification of different types of stroke.

TABLE 45.1 Overview of Ischemic Stroke Etiologies, Mechanisms, and Treatments

STROKE MECHANISM	VESSEL TYPE	STROKE TYPE/SYNDROME	ACUTE THERAPY	SECONDARY PREVENTION	COMMENT
Atherothrombotic	Variable small, medium, large	Highly variable; large hemispheric to tiny lacunar; brainstem also	IV lytics, EVT if large/medium vessel	CVD risk factors control; antiplatelet agents consider surgery or stent	Most common etiology; highly variable presentation
Cardioembolic	Variable; MCA or MCA branch is typical	Cortical or hemispheric syndrome	IV lytics, could be EVT if large/medium vessel	Consider anticoagulation if AF	Other etiologies besides AF; endocarditis, valve disease, PFO
Artery-to-artery embolization	Typically small or medium vessel	Cortical branch syndrome	IV lytics	Medical therapy; consider CEA or stent	Identify proximal atherostenotic lesion
Hypercoagulable state	Typically small or medium vessel	Cortical branch syndrome	IV alteplase	Anticoagulation	Rule out underlying cancer
Inflammatory vasculopathy	Small or medium vessel	Any vessel; could impact retina, spinal cord	Consider steroids	Immunosuppressive therapy	May be due to systemic autoimmune disease or isolate to CNS
Structural vasculopathy/dissection	Vertebral or internal carotid artery	Vessel occlusion or artery-to-artery emboli	Anticoagulation, stent, antiplatelets		
Venous thrombosis	Sagittal or transverse sinus, jugular vein; not in a typical arterial territory	Hemorrhagic infarction; increased intracranial pressure	Anticoagulation	Address underlying process	Typically due to underlying hypercoagulable state; common in pregnancy

AF, Atrial fibrillation; *CEA,* carotid endarterectomy; *CNS,* central nervous system; *CVD,* cardiovascular disease; *EVT,* endovascular therapy; *IV,* intravenous; *MCA,* middle cerebral artery; *PFO,* patent foramen ovale.

TABLE 45.2 Types of Lacunar Strokes

LACUNAR SYNDROME	ANATOMY	TYPICAL SYMPTOMS
Pure motor hemiparesis	Internal capsule	Hemiparesis affecting face/arm/leg about equally
Hemisensory loss	Thalamus	Loss of sensation affecting face, arm, trunk, and leg
Ataxic-hemiparesis	Basis pontis or posterior limp of internal capsule	Ataxia > weakness involving leg > arm; no dysarthria
Mixed motor-sensory syndrome	Internal capsule or centrum semiovale	Mixed motor and sensory symptoms
Dysarthria-clumsy hand	Internal capsule, basis-pontis	Dysarthria, ataxia/dysdiadochokinesia

In the hyperacute setting it may not be possible to precisely determine the underlying etiology of a stroke or TIA because of time constraints. However, for effective secondary prevention, understanding the underlying mechanism and etiology is often very important.

In any type of stroke, the symptoms will be dependent on the vessel involved and the territory of infarcted tissue (Table 45.3). The rapidity of onset may also be a clue to the stroke mechanism. Atherothrombotic and lacunar strokes typically display a gradual or stepwise onset of symptoms, with evolution spanning minutes to an hour or more. An embolic mechanism typically will have maximum symptoms at once, which may lessen a bit over ensuing minutes to hours in some cases.

Cryptogenic strokes account for 15% to 20% of all ischemic strokes (Table 45.4). Recent studies of these patients have identified some common mechanisms that may help to better define the underlying etiology in some of these patients (see Tables 45.3 and 45.4). Paroxysmal AF has been identified in at least 12% of such patients after 1 year of cardiac monitoring (see Chapter 66). A patent foramen ovale (PFO) is also found in 5% to 10% of such patients, particularly those <50 years of age (see Chapter 82). Less common mechanisms for ischemic stroke include vasculopathies (inflammatory, structural) and a hypercoagulable state. Atherosclerotic plaques without a high-grade stenosis may be an underappreciated etiology for cryptogenic strokes. Patients may have entities such as antiphospholipid antibodies/anticardiolipin antibodies or a lupus anticoagulant (see Chapter 95). Some patients may have a hypercoagulable state due to an underlying malignancy, which is often occult. Rare genetic disorders (e.g., CADASIL, cerebral autosomal recessive arteriopathy with subcortical infarcts and leukoencephalopathy [CARASIL] CARASIL[4]) are other uncommon etiologies. The diagnosis and treatment of such patients may be problematic.[4,7,8]

There is another uncommon stroke type or mechanism, a cerebral venous/sinus thrombosis (CVST).[8a] The sinus does not refer to nasal structures; rather the term "sinus" refers to large venous pathways typically at the base or surface of the brain. When one of the veins (i.e., superior sagittal sinus, transverse sinus, internal jugular vein) becomes occluded, it often leads to obstruction of venous outflow (Fig. 45.2A). Arterial inflow will then back up, leading to congestion of cerebral arteries and veins, increased intracranial pressure, headaches, and venous infarction. Such infarcts typically display substantial edema and mass effects and often undergo hemorrhagic transformation

TABLE 45.3 Vascular Anatomy, Stroke Patterns, and Symptoms

INVOLVED VESSEL	BRAIN REGION	COMMON MECHANISM	TYPICAL SYMPTOMS	COMMENT
Carotid artery	Hemisphere	Atherothrombotic or dissection	Complete hemiplegia + aphasia or neglect syndrome	May develop ipsilateral Horner syndrome
Middle cerebral artery	Portions of hemisphere	Embolic	Partial hemiparesis (face, arm > leg); aphasia if dominant hemisphere; neglect syndrome and apraxia if nondominant	Symptoms dependent on artery involved
Anterior cerebral artery	Frontal lobe	Atherothrombotic or embolic	Weakness leg > arm > face; apraxia	May display abulic behavior
Basilar artery	Brainstem	Atherothrombotic	Possible loss of consciousness, bilateral weakness; abnormal ocular movements; ataxia	May develop crossed sensory deficits, Horner syndrome
Posterior cerebral artery	Occipital lobe	Embolic	Visual field cut; unable to read	May develop visual neglect if tracts involved; unable to read
Lacunar syndrome	Deep in hemisphere or brainstem	Lipohyalinosis or small vessel atheroma	• Pure motor hemiparesis • Hemisensory loss • Mixed motor/sensory lesion • Dysarthria clumsy hand • Ataxia hemiparesis	• Internal capsule • Thalamus • Deep white matter/internal capsule • Basis pontis

TABLE 45.4 Rare and Cryptogenic Stroke Etiologies

PRESUMED ETIOLOGY/ MECHANISM	DIAGNOSTIC TEST	COMMENT
Inflammatory vasculitis	Cerebral angiogram	May not be associated with a systemic inflammatory condition; often associated with prominent or new headaches
New or occult hypercoagulable condition	Full coagulation panel + genetic tests	Look for systemic clotting features (deep vein thrombosis, pulmonary embolism); may be seen with an occult malignancy
Cardioembolic	Implantable cardiac monitor to evaluate for paroxysmal atrial fibrillation; consider cardiac CT or MRI	Consider blood cultures to rule out endocarditis; cardiac imaging rule out fibroelastoma
Pulmonary arteriovenous malformation	Chest CT scan	May be associated with hereditary hemorrhagic telangiectasia
Genetic disorder	Family history; specific gene testing	Gene testing is commercially available; look for systemic signs of disease
Occult drug abuse	Complete toxicology screen	Patients often not forthcoming about drug abuse

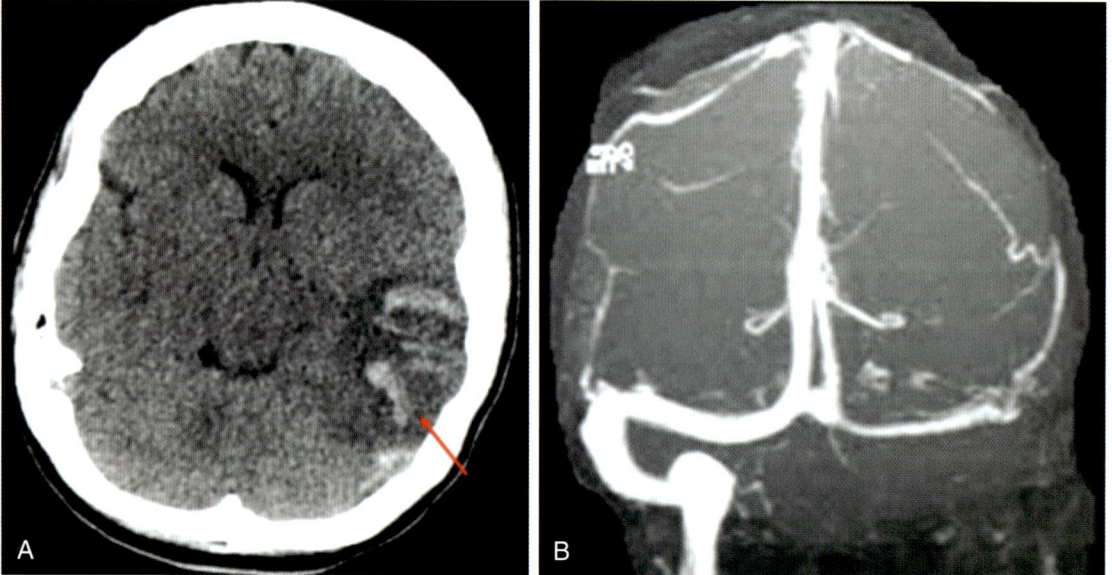

FIGURE 45.2 Cerebral venous thrombosis. **A,** Typical hemorrhagic infarction (involving the left temporal-parietal region) due to cerebral venous sinus thrombosis. **B,** Magnetic resonance venogram showing attenuation of the left transverse sinus and occlusion of the left sigmoid and jugular veins.

(Fig. 45.2B). They often do not follow usual arterial territories. Risk factors include pregnancy or postpartum state, sickle cell disease, dehydration, cancer, and hypercoagulable states. CVST has also been associated on rare occasions with adenovirus vector COVID-19 vaccines (see Chapter 94). CVST can be difficult to diagnose and visualize, especially if it involves the deep venous system. Magnetic resonance imaging (MRI) and magnetic resonance venography are key for making the diagnosis. Systemic anticoagulation is the initial treatment of choice.[9,10]

This chapter will next focus on the risk factors and prevention strategies for ischemic stroke and TIA, followed by the acute care of these patients. Readers are directed to American Heart Association guidelines reviewing the use of carotid endarterectomy and angioplasty/stenting for primary and secondary prevention of stroke[11-13] and for the chapters noted earlier for the treatment of common cardiac diseases such as AF, acute MI, and related conditions that can cause a stroke.

STROKE RISK FACTORS AND PREVENTION

This section will begin by focusing on identifying stroke risk factors, assessing their impact, and reviewing treatment options. Chapters 25, 26, 27, and 31 also address common CVD risk factors and their treatment.

Approximately 78% of strokes are first events, which makes primary prevention of paramount importance.[1] Approximately 18% of survivors will have a second stroke within 4 years. Various studies have suggested that up to 80% to 90% of all strokes could theoretically be prevented with proper identification and optimal use of medications and behavior modification. Of course, identification of risk factors in asymptomatic patients represents a significant challenge in part because of a lack of access to healthcare, screenings for risk factors, the need for high levels of compliance, and the resources for adequate long-term treatment. This strategy also implies treatment of many asymptomatic patients for years to accrue the benefit of stroke prevention. Such an approach is challenging because of the long-term commitment needed, the high expense, and the lack of an immediate benefit.

Some common and clinically important risk factors are listed in Table 45.5. These mirror some risk factors for CVD and coronary artery disease (CAD). These risk factors can be divided into modifiable (i.e., hypertension, diabetes, smoking, diet) and nonmodifiable (i.e., age, race, inherited/genetic conditions and traits (Table 45.6). Other environmental risk factors (secondhand smoke, place of residence [such as the Stroke Belt]) are also modifiable, but not in the traditional way via medications or daily behaviors. In the past few years, additional and novel risk factors for stroke have been identified (see Table 45.5); these include sleep apnea, acute COVID-19 infection, and acquired hypercoagulable states. (see Chapters 89, 94, and 95).

Overall, the modifiable risk factors for stroke largely mirror those for CAD and peripheral artery disease (PAD), although the impacts of these risk factors are not always equivalent. The American Heart Association/American Stroke Association (AHA/ASA) and other groups provide detailed, current evidence-based guidelines for prevention of a first stroke.[14,15]

In general, the identification and treatment of these risk factors do not differ very much from a primary versus secondary prevention perspective. Although some studies have failed to show convincing evidence that treating certain risk factors impacts the primary prevention of stroke, there is considerable cross-risk among stroke, CAD, and PAD. Therefore, treating the systemic risk factors almost always has a positive impact on disease prevention. Hence, primary and secondary prevention will be discussed together.

Modifiable risk factors are a focus for primary and secondary stroke prevention. High-priority areas include improving physical activity, treatment of dyslipidemia with statins and other agents (as well as diet), diet and nutrition, glycemic control, hypertension, treatment for obesity, and smoking cessation. The international INTERSTROKE study is an important resource to understand risk factors for all types of stroke.[16] More than 13,000 patients with an acute stroke and 13,000

TABLE 45.5 Common Risk Factors for Cerebrovascular Disease and Stroke

RISK FACTOR	STROKE TYPE/VESSEL	TREATMENT OPTIONS	COMMENT
Elevated blood pressure	All types and vessels	Antihypertensive medications; diet, weight loss	Most modifiable risk factor
Diabetes	Small vessel > large vessel	Blood glucose control with medications; weight loss; diet; exercise	Requires long-term treatment; unclear benefits for primary prevention
Atrial fibrillation	Cardioembolic; medium and small vessels	Anticoagulation	Often asymptomatic
Hyperlipidemia	Large > small vessels	Diet, statins	Impacts large vessel strokes
Smoking/tobacco use	All types and vessels	Behavioral modification; medications	Applies to any use of tobacco; especially powerful for subarachnoid hemorrhage
Physical inactivity	All types and vessels	Behavior modification	Very common
Nutrition	All types and vessels	Change diet	Mediterranean diet helpful
Kidney disease	Small/medium > large vessel	Treat CVD risk factors	Related to glomerular filtration rate
Pregnancy	Medium/small vessel; venous infarction	Treat elevated blood pressure; possible coagulation disorder	Highest risk in third trimester and postpartum
Hormone therapy/OCPs	Small and medium vessels; venous thrombosis	Avoid if possible	Risk of ischemic stroke and venous thrombosis
Migraine headaches	Small and medium vessels	Avoid hormone therapy, smoking, vasoconstrictive agents	Highest risk if >30, complicated migraine, hormone replacement therapy use
Obstructive sleep apnea	All types	Sleep posture control, weight loss, CPAP	Underrecognized and undertreated
Psychosocial issues	All types	Treat underlying depression, stress	Address environmental factors
Inherited disorders	Variable	Variable	See Tables 45.6 and 45.10
COVID-19 infection	All types and venous infarction	Possible anticoagulants	Evolving science
Geographic factors (Stroke Belt)	Small and medium vessel	Address CVD risk factors; consider moving	Complex environmental interactions
Air pollution	All types	Filters	Complex public health issue
Drug abuse	Large/medium vessels	Cessation of drug abuse	Cocaine can cause vasospasm and a vasculitis

CPAP, Continuous positive airway pressure; *CVD*, cardiovascular disease; *HRT*, hormone replacement therapy; *OCPs*, oral contraceptive pills.

controls were used to identify major risk factors for stroke. Ten risk factors were estimated to account for about 90% of the modifiable risks for stroke (Table 45.7). Because of how INTERSTROKE was designed, these 10 risk factors differ from other common risk factors; however, both are relevant in certain clinical circumstances (i.e., pregnancy, migraine headaches). Although these risk factors varied by region, they do provide a reasonable starting point to identify opportunities and targets for treatment.

When discussing the various risk factors, we must be aware that the risk factors are not just present or absent, as the severity and duration of the exposure have a significant impact. One approach to optimize primary (as well as secondary) prevention is to use the population attributable risk (PAR) to identify which risk factors will result in the largest number of prevented strokes.

As shown in Table 45.7, the most prominent modifiable stroke risk factor with the highest PAR (48) is hypertension.[17] This is consistent with many other epidemiologic studies of stroke. Other factors with high PARs include lack of physical activity (PAR 35.8), apolipoprotein ratios (26.8), diet (23.2), psychosocial factors (17.4), and smoking (12.4). Other well-recognized risk factors seem to have a lower impact on PAR; these include cardiac etiologies (PAR 9.1), heavy alcohol use (5.8), and diabetes (3.9). Fortunately, many of these factors can be modified with proper medical interventions such as the use of antihypertensives, weight loss, and exercise. Reducing BP has more of an impact in hemorrhagic stroke than ischemic stroke, but it clearly reduces the risks of all types of stroke.

Hypertension

Because hypertension is such a pervasive and important risk factor for all types of stroke, this chapter will provide additional details about its diagnosis and treatment (see Chapters 2 and 26). Overall, the prevalence of hypertension is 45.7 among non-Hispanic whites, 59.0 among non-Hispanic Blacks, 46.1 for Mexican Americans, and 45.2 for people of other races and ethnicities in the United States (see Chapter 93).[1] This somewhat mirrors the stroke risk for different populations. In NHANES, the overall study population had BPs of 122.4/70.7 mm Hg. Among the patients with hypertension, the average BPs were 133.0/74.4 mm Hg for non-Hispanic whites, 136.8/76.1 mm Hg for non-Hispanic Blacks, and 134.8/76.1 mm Hg for Mexican Americans.[18] This overall pattern closely matches the risks of stroke among the various groups. The risk of all CV events is further increased by the presence of additional CVD risk factors. The INTERSTROKE study found that untreated hypertension was associated with a higher risk of ischemic stroke (odds ratio [OR] 4.76, confidence interval [CI] 3.99 to 5.68), and a younger age at onset for all strokes (61.4 versus 65.4 years).

The 2020 International Society of Hypertension (ISH) guidelines recommend that for BPs in the <130/85 mm Hg range, monitoring every 3 years is reasonable.[19] For patients with BPs in the 135/85 to 150/99 mm Hg range, confirmation with repeated measurements is recommended. If the BP is >160/100 mm Hg, confirmation within a few days is now recommended. Because >50% of patients with hypertension have other CVD risk factors, an assessment for these other factors (diabetes, hyperlipidemia, etc.) is recommended.[19]

The ISH guidelines are somewhat different from the 2017 AHA/ACC hypertension guidelines. The 2017 guidelines, based largely on the results of the SPRINT (Systolic Blood Pressure Intervention Trial) study, redefined a normal BP as less than 120/80 mm Hg.[20,21] A BP of 120 to 129 mm Hg systolic and diastolic >80 mm Hg is now defined as "elevated BP." Stage 1 hypertension is now defined as a systolic BP of 130 to 139 mm Hg or diastolic BP of 80 to 89 mm Hg (Table 45.8). This has implications for hypertension awareness, treatment, and potential risk reduction in large populations.

Although a specific antihypertensive regimen must be individualized, the actual reduction in BP is generally more important than the specific agent or agents used. SPRINT compared the benefit of treatment of systolic BP to a target of lower than 120 mm Hg with treatment to a target of lower than 140 mm Hg in patients at increased risk of CVD events who had systolic BP of 130 to 180 mm Hg. Stroke occurrence fell from 1.5% to 1.3% annually, but the difference was not significant (HR, 0.89; 95% CI 0.63 to 1.25; $P = 0.50$).[21]

Although the landmark SPRINT trial did show the benefits of aggressive BP reduction to <120/80 mm Hg in patients at high risk for CVD events, there did not appear to be an overt benefit in terms of stroke reduction. This may have been due in part to the exclusion of patients with a prior stroke from the SPRINT trial.[21] Other factors might have

TABLE 45.6 General Categories and Types of Risk Factors for Ischemic Stroke and TIA

ACQUIRED DISEASES (MODIFIABLE)	NON-MODIFIABLE	INHERITED DISORDERS	OTHER
Hypertension	Age	Vasculopathy	Place of residence
Diabetes	Gender	Fabry's disease	Medications (ethical and drug abuse)
Hyperlipidemia	Race	Hematologic	COVID-19 infection
Cardiac disease	Ethnicity	Clotting disorders	Sleep apnea
Smoking/secondhand smoke	Genetic	Cardiac disorders	
Obesity/lack of exercise		Many acquired disorders may often have a genetic component (i.e., some forms of hypertension, diabetes, lipid disorders)	

TABLE 45.7 Stroke Risk Factors from the INTERSTROKE Global Study

RISK FACTOR	ODDS RATIO	PAR (99% CI)	COMMENT
Hypertension	2.64	48 (45-51)	Most important treatable risk factor
Current smoking	2.09	12 (10-15)	
Waist to hip ratio	1.65	19 (13-25)	Obesity is a growing concern
Diet risk score	1.35	23 (18-29)	Underappreciated
Physical activity	0.65	36 (28-45)	Underappreciated
Diabetes mellitus	1.36	4 (2-8)	Less impact on stroke
Alcohol intake	1.51	6 (3-10)	More important in men than women
Psychosocial stress/depression	1.30-1.35	17 (13-23)	Various definitions
Cardiac disease	2.38	9 (8-10)	
Ratio of apolipoprotein B to A1	1.89	27 (22-42)	May be a biomarker of obesity

PAR, Population attributable risk.
From O'Donnell MJ, et al. Risk factors for ischaemic and intracerebral haemorrhagic stroke in 22 countries (the INTERSTROKE study): a case-control study. Lancet. 2010;376:112-123; PAR data from Hankey GJ. Population impact of potentially modifiable risk factors for stroke. Stroke. 2020;51:719-728.

TABLE 45.8 Updated Definitions of Blood Pressure Levels

BLOOD PRESSURE READING (MM HG)	CLASSIFICATION
<130 SBP and <85 DPB	Normal BP
130-139 SBP and/or 85-89 DBP	High-normal BP
140-159 SBP and/or 90-99	Grade 1 hypertension
≥160 SBP and/or >100 DBP	Grade 2 hypertension

DBP, Diastolic blood pressure; *SBP*, systolic blood pressure.
Modified from Linger T, et al. 2020 International Society of Hypertension global hypertension practice guidelines. Hypertension. 2020;75:1334-1357.

been the relatively small number of stroke events in the study, choice of medications, and duration of follow-up. Otherwise, CVD death, overall mortality, and heart failure were all significantly reduced with BP reductions.[22]

The HOPE-3 trial also evaluated an antihypertensive in people at intermediate risk but without CVD; no overall benefit for stroke reduction was found.[23] Explanations for this neutral result might include the choice of antihypertensives (candesartan and hydrochlorothiazide) and the small reduction in BP with treatment (mean, 6/3 mm Hg).

A large meta-analysis (>300,000 patients) of BP reduction for the primary prevention of stroke and other major CVD outcomes, along with other large analyses, did show a benefit for stroke prevention. There was a clear association between the magnitude of the benefit and the baseline BP.[24] Patients with the highest BP (defined as >160 mm Hg systolic) showed the most significant benefit of BP reduction on primary stroke prevention. People with lower baseline BPs showed only marginal benefits for stroke prevention. However, benefit was found for the prevention of other CVD events. Nonetheless, because stroke patients have a high risk of other CVD events and related outcomes, treatment of hypertension is supported by neurologists (and especially vascular neurologists).

Treatment of patients with hypertension to prevent CVD and strokes is centered on lifestyle modification (Table 45.9), avoidance of drugs that might exacerbate high BP (some nonsteroidal anti-inflammatory drugs, oral contraceptives, etc.) and specific pharmacologic interventions. Several classes of antihypertensive medications have shown efficacy for stroke prevention; these include thiazide type diuretics, angiotensin converting enzyme (ACE) inhibitors, angiotensin receptor blockers, and calcium channel blockers.

A systematic review of seven studies and eight control groups using a variety of BP reduction agents found overall a 23% to 25% reduction in recurrent stroke, fatal stroke, and MI, but no reduction in vascular or all-cause mortality (see Rashid, Classic References). The overall sample size was 15,527 patients.

Whether ACE inhibitors have a specific benefit in reducing recurrent stroke risk also remains uncertain. The HOPE study compared the effects of an ACE inhibitor and placebo in high-risk persons and reported a 24% reduction in the risk for stroke, MI, or vascular death in 1013 patients with a history of stroke or TIA (see Yusuf, Classic References). The PROGRESS (Perindopril Protection Against Recurrent Stroke Study) study tested the effects of a BP-lowering regimen, including an ACE inhibitor, in 6105 patients with stroke or TIA within the previous 5 years (see PROGRESS, Classic References). Randomization was stratified by intention to use single (ACE inhibitor) or combination therapy (ACE inhibitor plus the diuretic indapamide) in hypertensive (>160 mm Hg systolic or >90 mm Hg diastolic) and in normotensive patients. The combination, which reduced BP by an average of 12/5 mm Hg, led to a 43% reduction in recurrent stroke and a 40% reduction in major CVD events. This effect was present in both hypertensive and normotensive groups. Monotherapy with either agent showed no significant benefit. Specific patient characteristics and comorbid conditions should guide the choice of a specific antihypertensive regimen.

A more recent analysis of 93 trials examined BP reduction with various agents. The combined studies had >504,000 enrolled subjects who were followed for an average of 3.3 years. Using pairwise comparisons, relative benefits were seen for calcium channel blockers over ACE inhibitor, and combination therapy, particularly ACE inhibitor plus a calcium channel blocker, showed significant efficacy.[25]

TABLE 45.9 Lifestyle Modifications to Address Hypertension and Reduce Stroke

RISK REDUCTION STRATEGY	COMMENT
Reduce salt intake	Modify diet, additives
Eat healthy diet	High in grains, fruits, vegetables
Healthy drinks	Moderate use of coffee and tea; beet juice, cocoa OK
Moderate alcohol consumption	2 drinks per day for men; 1 drink per day for women
Weight reduction	Ethnic specific guidance
Smoking cessation	Specific programs, medications
Reduce stress	Meditation daily if possible
Reduce exposure to air pollution	Air filters, rural environment

In clinical practice we often encounter patients with resistant hypertension despite treatment with three or more medications. In addition to optimizing adherence to current medications and maximizing lifestyle changes, such patients may warrant additional medical interventions. These might include adding medications such as a mineralocorticoid receptor antagonist, a beta- or alpha-adrenergic receptor antagonist, and minoxidil. Consultation with a hypertension specialist is warranted if multiple medications are needed for BP control (see Chapter 26).

Hyperlipidemia

Elevated low-density lipoprotein (LDL) cholesterol is an important risk factor for ischemic stroke in a primary or secondary prevention setting. This is especially true in patients with diabetes and other CVD risk factors. Lifestyle modification is a key component to reduce the risk of strokes. The use of statin agents has the potential to significantly reduce stroke risk in a primary-prevention population (see Chapter 27). Treatment of patients with coronary heart disease (CHD) or those at elevated risk for CHD with hydroxymethylglutaryl–coenzyme A reductase inhibitors (statins) reduces not only cardiac events but also the risk for a first stroke. A meta-analysis of statin therapy has shown that for each 39 mg/dL decrease in LDL cholesterol there is a 21% decline in the relative risk of a first ischemic stroke.[26,27] Statin therapy did not appear to be associated with a significant increase in the occurrence of intracerebral hemorrhage (ICH).

JUPITER (Justification for the Use of Statin in Prevention: An Intervention Trial Evaluating Rosuvastatin) evaluated the effect of a statin in persons with higher than median (>2 mg/dL) level of high-sensitivity C-reactive protein who were not otherwise candidates for statin treatment. In this group, treatment with rosuvastatin 20 mg daily reduced stroke by approximately 50%.[28] The benefit of stroke reduction with statin therapy may extend to those at lower (5% to 10% 5-year) risk for vascular events. The HOPE-3 trial assessed the effect of rosuvastatin (10 mg daily) in CVD-free patients at intermediate risk (approximately 1% per year). Over 5.6 years, randomization to treatment led to a reduction in death from CVD causes, nonfatal MI, or nonfatal stroke from 4.8% to 3.7% (HR, 0.76; 95% CI 0.64 to 0.9; $P = 0.002$).[26]

The HPS (Heart Protection Study) included 3280 patients with a history of stroke (including 1820 with stroke and no history of CHD) who were treated with either a statin or placebo (see Collins, Classic References). In those with a previous history of stroke, statin treatment reduced the frequency of major vascular events (MI, stroke, revascularization procedure, or vascular death) by 20%, but did not lower the risk for recurrent stroke (occurring in 10.5% of placebo versus 10.4% of statin group). The most reasonable explanation might be that patients were randomized an average of approximately 4 years after the index event. Most recurrent strokes occur soon (within the first few years), so those randomized in the HPS had a relatively low risk for recurrent stroke. More recent studies have shown clear benefits for stroke reduction (see later).

The SPARCL (Stroke Prevention with Aggressive Reduction in Cholesterol Levels) trial randomly assigned more than 4700 patients within 6 months of a noncardioembolic stroke or TIA and no known CHD to high-dose statin (atorvastatin 80 mg daily) or placebo for a primary endpoint of the first occurrence of a nonfatal or fatal stroke (see Amarenco, Classic References). Those randomized to high-dose statin treatment had a 16% relative reduction in nonfatal or fatal stroke as well as a 35% relative reduction in major coronary events. Added to the previous data on prevention of a first stroke, SPARCL showed that treatment with a high-dose statin can reduce the risk for recurrent stroke after stroke or TIA. On the basis of this trial, patients with atherosclerotic ischemic stroke or TIA and without known CHD should receive high-intensity statin therapy to reduce the risk for stroke and other CV events.[29]

In the FOURIER (Further Cardiovascular Outcomes Research with PCSK9 Inhibition in Subjects with Elevated Risk) trial, adding the PCSK9 inhibitor evolocumab to standard therapy in patients with evidence of atherosclerotic disease significantly reduced the risk of a first or recurrent ischemic stroke (but there was no effect on hemorrhagic stroke).[30] The risk of ischemic stroke was reduced by 25%, and the risk of stroke or TIA was reduced by 23%. Interestingly, the use of other lipid-lowering agents such as fibrates, niacin, and ezetimibe, as well as dietary modifications, did not impact stroke rates (although such interventions did reduce rates of other CV events in some populations).[30]

The mechanism(s) by which statin therapy might reduce stroke rates include reducing intima-media thickness growth, slowing plaque progression, and reducing arterial inflammation. Despite some concerns about myalgias and the rare occurrence of significant myopathy, overall statin therapy is well tolerated and widely accepted as a mainstay of primary and secondary stroke prevention.

Diabetes

Diabetes is a common and major risk factor for all types of cardiovascular disease, including stroke (see Chapter 31). Currently >30 million adults in the United States have diabetes, and more than 84 million have prediabetes, which is a major precursor to diabetes. It is associated with a 2 to 6 times increased risk of stroke compared with nondiabetic patients. A recent meta-analysis of more than 100 studies of diabetes has shown that diabetic patients have a 2.3 times increased risk of ischemic stroke and 1.6 times increased risk of hemorrhagic stroke.[31] Almost a quarter (24%) of people with diabetes are unaware they even have the disease.

Aggressive medical therapies as well as lifestyle changes are recommended to mitigate elevated blood glucose, prevent diabetic complications, and reduce the risk of cardiovascular events including death and stroke. However, numerous studies of patients with diabetes for the primary prevention of strokes have not shown an overwhelming positive effect. For example, the Euro Heart Survey on Diabetes and the Heart, the UK Prospective Diabetes Study, the ACCORD Study, the Veterans Affairs Diabetes Study, and the DCCT/EDIC study, among others, did not show evidence of a reduction in stroke as an isolated endpoint (although other CVD endpoints were reduced). An analysis of 9 large studies with more than 59,000 patients treated with intensive glycemic control did not find evidence for a reduction in stroke. Based on these data, aggressive treatment of diabetes and/or intensive glycemic control does not appear to have a significant impact on stroke reduction—although it is beneficial for the reduction of other CV events.[32]

There is evidence that tight control of diabetes decreases stroke risk in a secondary prevention setting. As previously reviewed, management of BP and use of statins reduce stroke risk in patients with diabetes. The Insulin Resistance Intervention after Stroke (IRIS) trial tested the hypothesis that pioglitazone reduces the rates of stroke and MI after ischemic stroke or TIA in patients without diabetes who have insulin resistance. Over 4.8 years, stroke or MI occurred in 9.0% of the pioglitazone group and 11.8% of the placebo group (RR of 24%).[33] The primary complications of treatment were a greater frequency of more than 4.5 kg weight gain, peripheral edema (35.6% versus 24.9%), and bone fracture requiring surgery or hospitalization (5.1% versus 3.2%).

What might explain this dichotomy between an effect on many CVD events and outcomes, but not stroke, for primary prevention? One factor may be the heterogeneity of stroke etiologies. Ischemic strokes can be due to atherothrombosis of small and large cerebral and cervical arteries, emboli from a cardiac source or the aorta, carotid dissection, hypercoagulable states, etc. Perhaps only some of these processes are directly related to diabetes and respond to glycemic control. See Chapter 31 for a discussion of newer diabetic medications that can reduce cardiovascular events and may do so by mechanisms that do not depend on glucose-lowering per se.

Smoking

Cigarette smoking appears to increase the risk of stroke in a dose-dependent manner based on the number of pack-years of exposure (see Chapter 28). It is now well established that smoking cigarettes increases the risk of subarachnoid hemorrhage and possibly ICH although the data are somewhat conflicting. Secondhand smoke is a recently identified risk factor for stroke also. The good news is that within 2 to 4 years of smoking cessation, the risk of stroke related to smoking appears to return to a baseline level.[34] Smoking cessation can be achieved via various behavioral modification programs and counseling, with or without specific pharmacologic interventions. Specific medications that are effective for smoking cessation include nicotine replacement therapies, bupropion, and varenicline. Furthermore, community and state restrictions on smoking appear to reduce smoking rates and related complications.

Nutrition

Diet and nutrition play an important role in stroke risk (see Chapters 29 and 34). This may be mediated in part via impacts of diet on important stroke risk factors such as hypertension, lipid levels, and diabetes. Although data proving specific cause and effect relationships directly between diet and stroke may be lacking, there are some general recommendations that appear reasonable to address this important lifestyle modification (see Table 45.9). Some recommendations such as reducing sodium intake, increasing potassium intake, and using a DASH diet may improve outcomes in some high-risk populations such as Blacks and people with hypertension.[35,36]

Obesity

Being overweight (BMI 25 to 29) or obese (BMI >30) are both associated with an increased risk of stroke, particularly ischemic stroke. This is being seen with increased frequency in young adults, where obesity and CVD risk factors are increasing (see Chapter 30). A reduction in BMI and weight has been associated with a reduction in BP and in some cases a reduced risk of stroke. It is difficult to separate the effects of weight loss on various stroke risk factors such as BP, lipid status, exercise, etc. But overall aggressive weight loss combined with a healthy diet and exercise may mitigate some of the stroke risk in a general population.[37]

Exercise

Lack of physical activity and a sedentary lifestyle have been associated with an increased risk of stroke (see Chapter 32). Although rigorous randomized studies have not proven that exercise reduces the incidence of a primary stroke, current AHA/ASA recommendations support vigorous exercise 3 to 4 days/week for at least 40 minutes to combat the negative effects of physical inactivity.[38] To the extent that lack of exercise leads to weight gain, obesity, diabetes, and other detrimental cardiovascular outcomes, the AHA recommendations are quite reasonable. A summary of lifestyle interventions to reduce stroke are shown in Table 45.9.

Sleep Apnea

Obstructive sleep apnea (OSA) is emerging as a common risk factor for stroke as well as for ischemic heart disease and all-cause mortality (see Chapter 89). However, it is often not recognized, not diagnosed, or not properly treated. OSA is related to obesity as well as CVD and related conditions such as diabetes. Furthermore, there appears to be a dose-effect relationship, with more severe OSA being associated with high rates of stroke, CVD events, and death.[39] Patients with severe sleep apnea appear to have worse outcomes after a stroke.[40] OSA can be treated using weight loss, continuous positive airway pressure, and other devices and approaches. Research is underway to determine how treatment of OSA may affect primary and secondary stroke prevention.

Other Risk Factors

Stroke incidence and mortality are elevated on the Stroke Belt region of the United States, which generally encompasses the southeast region from Washington, DC to Florida and west to Texas. Within the Stroke Belt, there is a "belt buckle" that is generally defined as eastern regions of North Carolina, South Carolina, and Georgia. Studies have determined that demographic imbalances, an excess of CVD risk factors, and socioeconomic factors largely explain the excess stroke risk in the Stroke Belt.[41]

Elevated homocysteine is associated with an increased risk of cardiovascular ischemic events, including ischemic stroke. Mutations in the *MTHFR* gene can lead to elevated homocysteine levels that are associated with an increased risk of ischemic vascular events such as stroke and MI.[42] Elevated homocysteine can occur without an underlying gene mutation. Detailed analysis of this association after controlling for confounding factors has shown that it is most pronounced in younger patients with hypertension. Although treatment with multivitamins such as B_6, B_{12}, and folate is successful in reducing homocysteine levels, it is unclear if this leads to a reduction in ischemic vascular events. The recent Chinese Stroke Primary Prevention Trial did show some benefits of folate or B_{12} supplements in some groups who had not received folate or B_{12} supplements in the past.[43]

There are a number of generally nonmodifiable risk factors for stroke (see Table 45.6). They include age, low birth weight, race/ethnicity, and a host of genetic factors (Table 45.10).[4] Age is the most important nonmodifiable stroke risk factor. Studies have shown that in general the risk of stroke doubles every 10 years above the age of 55 in men and women. However, there are also trends toward more strokes occurring at somewhat younger ages. This may reflect earlier onset of stroke risk factors as well as environmental influences. Approximately 10% of strokes occur in persons 18 to 50 years of age.[1]

There are some genetic factors and diseases that increase stroke risk and may be amenable to therapy. These are listed in Table 45.10. Genetic factors also play a variable role in some traditional risk factors such as hypertension, diabetes, and hyperlipidemia, among others. Specific mutations may lead to the premature development of a risk factor, or a severe form of the phenotype. In other cases, a gene mutation leads to a specific disease that directly causes a stroke. Examples include CADASIL, Fabry disease, and sickle cell disease. Other disorders such as hypercoagulable conditions may be inherited or sporadic. Sickle cell disease is common in Black patients and carries an increased risk of ischemic and hemorrhagic stroke. The judicious use of regular blood transfusions may reduce the risk of strokes. Gene therapy is also being explored for the long-term treatment of patients with sickle cell disease.

An acute or recent infection with COVID-19 appears to be a newly appreciated stroke risk factor (see Chapter 94). Stroke (mostly ischemic) can be seen in up to 1% of patients with an acute COVID-19 infection. Overall, about 75% of the strokes are ischemic, 21% hemorrhagic, and 4% CVST. The ischemic strokes tend to be large vessel, but all sizes are possible. Most of the strokes occur while the patient is hospitalized for severe COVID disease.[44] The mechanism in some cases is thought to be increased coagulability and/or inflammation. The use of some COVID-19 vaccines (those with an adenovirus vector) is associated with rare cases of CVST and thrombocytopenia, perhaps mediated by antibodies to platelet factor 4.[45]

ANTITHROMBOTIC AGENTS FOR STROKE PREVENTION

Antithrombotic agents (antiplatelet therapy and anticoagulation) are key for the acute therapy, primary prevention, and secondary prevention of ischemic stroke. This section will address these various scenarios.

Antiplatelet Therapy for Primary Prevention

The use of antiplatelet agents for preventing a first stroke has generated renewed controversy and uncertainty. There have been several individual studies as well as meta-analyses of studies that have closely examined the benefits and risks of low-dose aspirin for primary stroke prevention in a variety of populations (Table 45.11). The ARRIVE study[46] examined the efficacy and safety of aspirin in people of moderate or high risk of CVD events. The ASPREE study[47] enrolled patients who were older (i.e., >70 years), and the ASCEND study[48] enrolled patients at high risk due to diabetes. Although specific enrollment criterion varied somewhat, the summary of these various studies was quite consistent. Overall, aspirin was successful in preventing ischemic CVD events, including ischemic stroke. But this benefit was counterbalanced by an increase in hemorrhagic events, including hemorrhagic stroke. Overall, there was no net benefit in all-cause mortality for the aspirin-treated patients compared with controls.

The Women's Health Study randomized healthy women to 100 mg every other day of ASA versus placebo for 10 years of treatment (see Ridker, Classic References). Although there was no significant effect on the combined endpoint of MI, CVD death, and stroke, there was a significant 24% reduction in ischemic stroke (and a nonsignificant increase in cerebral hemorrhage). Serious gastrointestinal (GI) bleeding was increased significantly in the ASA-treated patients. This benefit for stroke occurred primarily in women who had stroke risk factors (e.g., hypertension, diabetes). Thus, aspirin may be considered for primary stroke prevention in women whose risk for stroke outweighs its associated bleeding risk.[14]

Based on these new studies and meta-analyses, aspirin is no longer recommended for the primary prevention of ischemic stroke in people at low or medium risk for CVD. This is reflected in guidelines, which have been changed to reflect these new data about aspirin. The benefit of aspirin for primary CVD prophylaxis outweighs its associated risk for bleeding complications in persons with a 10-year risk of CVD greater than 10%. There is no evidence that antiplatelet therapy reduces the risk for stroke in persons at low risk, or in those with diabetes in the absence of other major risk factors, and aspirin is not recommended for these purposes (see Chapter 95).

Stroke Prevention in Atrial Fibrillation

Patients with atrial fibrillation (AF) should generally receive anticoagulation for primary prevention of stroke (see Chapters 66 and 95). The CHADS-VASC score may be used to stratify high-risk patients.[49] In general, treatment with a direct oral anticoagulant (DOAC) agent is preferred over warfarin for primary prevention (this is addressed in recent guidelines).[50] Aspirin or the combination of aspirin and clopidogrel is inferior to warfarin or DOACs for stroke prevention in patients with AF and should be considered only in people who cannot take anticoagulants.[51]

TABLE 45.10 Genetic Disorders Associated with Ischemic Stroke and TIA*

VASCULOPATHIES	CLOTTING	BLOOD DISEASES	METABOLIC	OTHER
CADASIL	Prothrombin gene mutation	Sickle cell disease	Hyperhomocysteinemia	Fabry disease
CARASIL	Factor V mutation	Hemoglobinopathies (thalassemia)	Diabetes	MELAS
RVCL	Antiphospholipid antibodies and lupus anticoagulants**		Hyperlipidemia	Marfan syndrome
Moya-moya disease	Protein C and S deficiency			Renal artery stenosis
	Antithrombin III deficiency			

*Only the most common genetic disorders are listed. Clotting disorders are typically more common with venous (not arterial) mechanisms.
**Usually sporadic but may be inherited.
CADASIL, cerebral autosomal dominant arteriopathy with subcortical infarcts and leukoencephalopathy; CARASIL, cerebral autosomal recessive arteriopathy with subcortical infarcts and leukoencephalopathy; RVCL, retinal vasculopathy with cerebral leukoencephalopathy.

TABLE 45.11 New and Updated Randomized Trials of Aspirin for Primary Prevention of Stroke

STUDY	PATIENTS (NO.)	POPULATION TYPE	ASPIRIN DOSE	MEAN FOLLOW-UP (YEARS)	STROKE OUTCOMES (RELATIVE RISK ASPIRIN VS CONTROL)	ALL CAUSE DEATH (RELATIVE RISK ASPIRIN VS CONTROL)	MAJOR BLEEDING (RELATIVE RISK ASPIRIN VS CONTROL)	COMMENT
ASPREE	9525/9589	Age 70+ or 65+ in Blacks+Hispanics	100 mg/day	4.7	0.97	1.14	1.37	Increase in ICH
ARRIVE	6270/6276	Age 55+ (M) or 65+ (F) AND 2+ risk factors	100 mg/day	5	1.12	0.99	2.72	No change in ICH
ASCEND	7740/7740	Age 40+ and diabetes	100 mg/day	7.4	0.91	0.94	1.28	Increase in ICH

ICH, intracerebral hemorrhage.
From Gaziano JM, et al. Use of aspirin to reduce risk of initial vascular events in patients at moderate risk of cardiovascular disease (ARRIVE): a randomised, double-blind, placebo-controlled trial. Lancet. 2018;392:1036-1046; McNeil JJ, et al. Effect of aspirin on cardiovascular events and bleeding in the healthy elderly. N Engl J Med. 2018;379:1509-1518; The ASCEND Study Collaborative Group. Effects of aspirin for primary prevention in persons with diabetes mellitus. N Engl J Med. 2018;379:1529-1539.

Secondary Prevention of Ischemic Stroke

Antiplatelet Therapy

A recurrent stroke, or a stroke after a TIA, is a common and serious event. The risk of a recurrent stroke is typically in the range of 5% to 7% after 1 year and 16% after 5 years. Mortality after a recurrent stroke is quite high, ranging from 16% in whites and 21% in Blacks.[52,53] The risk of a stroke after a TIA is typically in the range of 3% to 5% after 2 days and up to 5% to 7% after 90 days. Most importantly, a TIA or stroke is a signal of underling cerebrovascular and cardiovascular disease, and puts the patient at a higher risk of other CVD events (MI, vascular death, etc.).[54,55]

As noted earlier, antiplatelet agents reduce the risk for recurrent stroke in patients with a history of ischemic stroke or TIA. *Aspirin* reduces the risk of recurrent stroke after a stroke or TIA by approximately 12% to 17%, and reduced death and disability by about 5%. The risk reduction is more pronounced in the first few days and week after the initial event.[56,57]

Clopidogrel monotherapy given to patients with a history of MI, stroke, or symptomatic PAD reduces the combined risk of MI, stroke, or vascular death by 8.7% (95% CI 0.3% to 16.5%; $P = 0.043$) compared with aspirin. The combination of clopidogrel and aspirin does reduce the rate of MI, stroke, or cardiovascular death more than aspirin alone in patients with CVD (including stroke) or multiple risk factors. When tested specifically in patients with a history of stroke, the combination of clopidogrel and aspirin was associated with an increase in bleeding complications without a reduction in ischemic stroke. SPS3 (Stroke Prevention Study 3) similarly found a higher risk for hemorrhage with no reduction in ischemic events after lacunar stroke in those treated with the combination versus aspirin alone.[56]

A direct comparison study (ProFESS) found that aspirin plus dipyridamole was comparable to clopidogrel monotherapy for secondary stroke prevention in patients with noncardioembolic stroke.[58] However, aspirin plus dipyridamole was associated with increased GI side effects as well as bleeding; thus this combination is rarely used in the United States for secondary stroke prevention.

The Clopidogrel in High-Risk Patients with Acute Nondisabling Cerebrovascular Events (CHANCE) trial, conducted in China, compared clopidogrel plus aspirin versus aspirin alone starting within 24 hours of minor ischemic stroke or high-risk TIA, with the combination continued for 21 days. The combination reduced the risk of stroke (8.2% versus 11.7%; hazard ratio [HR], 0.68; 95% CI 0.57 to 0.81; $P < 0.001$) with no difference in hemorrhage.[59] Whether these results extend to other populations is uncertain. A secondary analysis of data from CHANCE found that the benefit of clopidogrel (a prodrug) was limited to those who were not carriers of the *CYP2C19* loss-of-function allele (i.e., those who could activate clopidogrel).[60] Population-based differences in allele frequency could lead to different trial results in different regions. Genetic testing for these alleles is not generally recommended.

The POINT study focused on patients with an acute mild ischemic stroke or TIA. Patients were randomized to aspirin alone versus aspirin combined with clopidogrel (after a loading dose) for 90 days of therapy.[61] The primary endpoint was ischemic stroke, MI, or vascular death. The event rates were 5% with combination therapy versus 6.5% for aspirin alone (Fig. 45.3). Rates of major hemorrhages were higher with combination therapy (0.9%) versus monotherapy (0.4%). Most of the benefits were seen in the first few weeks of therapy.[61] Overall there was a clear net benefit with combination therapy. Based on these results a short course of clopidogrel and aspirin started within 24 hours after a TIA or minor noncardioembolic stroke is recommended in most guidelines. Long-term clopidogrel plus aspirin therapy should not be used routinely for stroke prevention in patients with a recent stroke due to an elevated long-term risk of bleeding.

The THALES study examined acute combination antiplatelet therapy in patients with a minor stroke or TIA, comparing aspirin plus ticagrelor (90 mg twice daily) versus aspirin alone for 30 days of therapy.[62] The rate of stroke and death (the primary endpoint) was 5.5% with combination therapy versus 6.6% with aspirin alone (Fig. 45.4). The rate of major bleeding was 0.5% with combination therapy versus 0.1% for aspirin alone, and the occurrence of disability was equal in both groups.[62] Ticagrelor has a more consistent antiplatelet response compared with clopidogrel, which is a prodrug and must be metabolized into its active form.

The results of these more recent studies continue a common theme for the use of combination antiplatelet therapy in the setting of acute ischemic cerebral events, namely shorter durations of therapy provide protection for ischemic events, but with a slight increase in hemorrhagic complications.

No prospective randomized trials have assessed different antithrombotic regimens in patients who have a recurrent event while receiving an antiplatelet drug. In routine clinical practice it is common to add a second antiplatelet agent for a few (1 to 3) months in patients who fail monotherapy. The supposition is that an inflamed plaque will heal in a few months, form a new fibrous cap, and be less likely to stimulate platelet aggregation.

Anticoagulant Therapy

Evidence supporting the use of anticoagulation for prevention of recurrent stroke in patients without AF or other high-risk cardiogenic

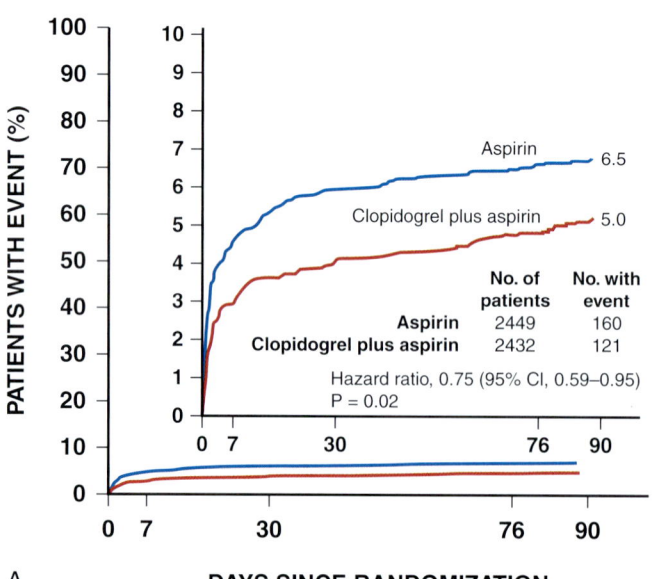
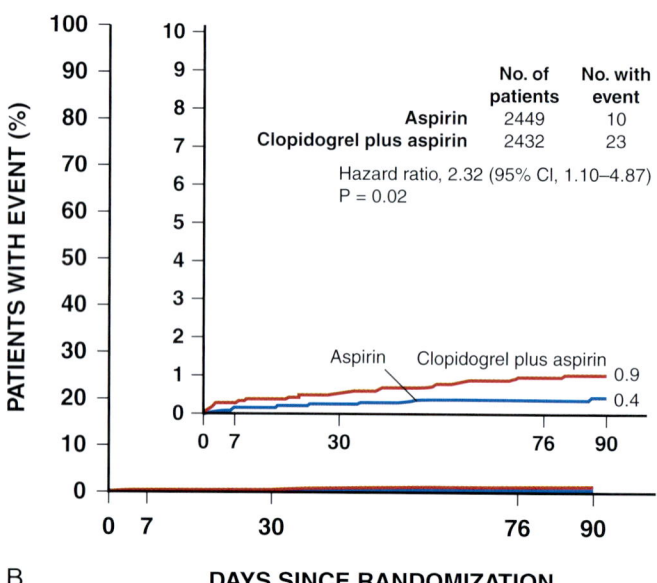

FIGURE 45.3 Overall results of the POINT trial of acute dual antiplatelet agents (aspirin plus clopidogrel) versus aspirin alone in patients with a TIA or minor stroke. **A,** Efficacy results. **B,** Safety results. (From Johnston SC, et al. Clopidogrel and aspirin in acute ischemic stroke and high-risk TIA. N Engl J Med. 2018;379:215-225.)

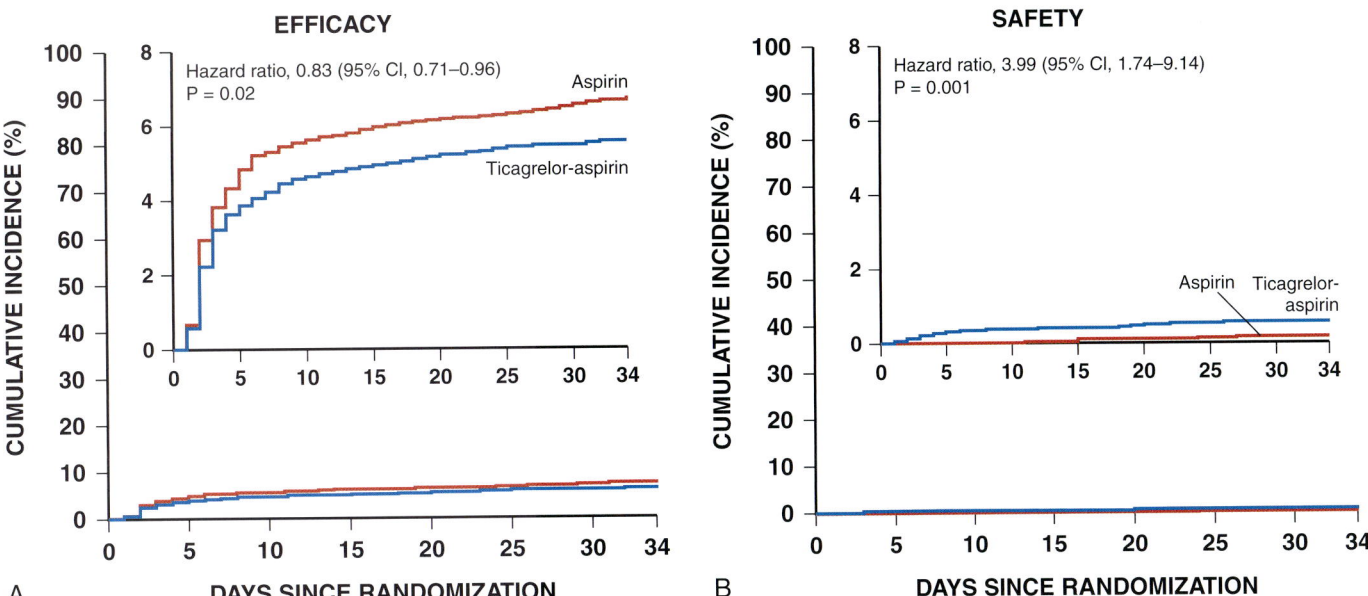

FIGURE 45.4 Overall results of the THALES trial of acute dual antiplatelet therapy (aspirin plus ticagrelor) versus aspirin alone in patients with a TIA or minor stroke. **A,** Efficacy results. **B,** Safety results. (From Johnston SC, et al. Ticagrelor and aspirin or aspirin alone in acute ischemic stroke or TIA. N Engl J Med. 2020;383:207-217.)

sources is uncertain, or the evidence suggests that the benefit does not outweigh the risk for warfarin-associated bleeding complications. Thus, patients who have had a noncardioembolic ischemic stroke or TIA should receive antiplatelet agents rather than oral anticoagulation to reduce the risk for recurrent stroke and other CV events.[63]

The WASID (Warfarin-Aspirin Symptomatic Intracranial Disease) trial compared warfarin (international normalized ratio [INR] of 2 to 3) with aspirin (1300 mg/day) in patients with >50% symptomatic intracranial stenosis (see Chimowitz, Classic References). The rate of recurrent ischemic stroke, ICH or non–stroke-related vascular death did not differ between the two treatment regimens (22% with warfarin versus 21% with aspirin; P = 0.83), but the rate of major hemorrhage was higher with warfarin (8.3% versus 3.2%; P = 0.01). Because of a lack of efficacy and a higher rate of bleeding complications, warfarin should not generally be used for patients with symptomatic large-vessel intracranial stenoocclusive disease.

The SAMMPRIS (Stenting and Aggressive Medical Management for Preventing Recurrent Stroke in Intracranial Stenosis) trial enrolled patients with high-grade symptomatic intracranial stenosis. Most patients had 70% to 99% stenosis of the internal carotid or middle cerebral artery (MCA). The results showed that aggressive medical management was superior to angioplasty/stenting for the endpoint of stroke or death.[64] There was an elevated risk of early stroke with endovascular treatment. Further work shows that intracranial atherosclerotic stenosis can regress with modern medical therapy.

Congestive heart failure (CHF) is associated with an increased risk of stroke, although the exact mechanism of stroke is unclear (due to the presence of AF and other CVD risk factors in many of these patients). Data from several large prospective randomized trials have not identified the optimal antithrombotic therapy for these patients.

The WATCH (Warfarin and Antiplatelet Therapy in Chronic Heart Failure) trial compared open-label warfarin (target INR of 2.5 to 3.0) and double-blind treatment with either clopidogrel or aspirin in patients with chronic CHF (ejection fraction [EF] <35%).[65] No differences were found between warfarin and aspirin (HR, 0.98; 95% CI 0.86 to 1.12; P = 0.77), between warfarin and clopidogrel (HR, 0.89; 95% CI 0.68 to 1.16; P = 0.39), or between clopidogrel and aspirin (HR, 1.08; 95% CI 0.83 to 1.40; P = 0.57) for the primary outcome (time until nonfatal stroke, nonfatal MI, or death).

The WARCEF trial compared warfarin (target INR of 2.0 to 3.5) with aspirin (325 mg/day) in patients in normal sinus rhythm who had a reduced left ventricular ejection fraction. Ischemic stroke, ICH or death from any cause (primary outcome) occurred at a rate of 7.47 events per 100 patient-years with warfarin versus 7.93 with aspirin. A reduction in ischemic stroke with warfarin was balanced by an increase in intracranial hemorrhage.[66] The recent COMMANDER HR study using low-dose rivaroxaban twice a day versus antiplatelet therapy did not show an overall benefit for the composite endpoint of stroke, MI, and all-cause mortality.[67] There did appear to be a significant reduction in stroke rates, including disabling stroke.

The various inherited coagulopathies (e.g., protein C, protein S, or antithrombin III deficiency; factor V Leiden; prothrombin G20210A mutation) and acquired conditions (e.g., lupus anticoagulant, anticardiolipin or antiphospholipid antibodies) are more often associated with venous than arterial thrombosis (see Chapter 95). Despite clear instances in which these types of disorders associate with ischemic stroke, particularly in children or young adults, causal relationships remain controversial. For example, in APASS (Antiphospholipid Antibody Stroke Study), a substudy of WARSS, 41% of 1770 participants were positive for one or more antiphospholipid antibody (see Levine, Classic References). Rates of recurrent thromboembolic events were somewhat higher in persons positive for antiphospholipid antibody, but outcomes did not differ between antibody-positive patients treated with warfarin or with aspirin. Nonetheless, in some patients with cryptogenic strokes, one of these disorders may be found after an extensive workup and no viable alternative explanation. In such a setting, some clinicians may use a short course (3 to 6 months) of anticoagulation.

MANAGEMENT OF ACUTE ISCHEMIC STROKE

Approaches to manage a patient with a stroke begin with recognition that a stroke is occurring. Studies by large emergency medical systems (EMS) have shown in up to 38% of cases the stroke was not recognized by the EMS personnel, and approximately 30% of patients diagnosed acutely with a stroke did not actually have a stroke after a full evaluation.[68] Failure to rapidly recognize, diagnose, and treat such patients will lead to worse outcomes. There are several processes and diseases that are well recognized as "stroke mimics" (Table 45.12). This is an important issue, as treating patients with a complicated migraine or another stroke mimic with IV alteplase is unlikely to be beneficial and may lead to serious complications.

In the setting of an acute ischemic stroke, almost 2,000,000 neurons die each minute of the event. Hence, time is of the essence when implementing acute therapy. The rapid recognition and field triage of a patient with a potential stroke is a key step in the care paradigm. EMS should call the destination emergency department once they are en route in an effort to reduce any delays in acute therapy. Such "prenotification" can improve treatment times and increase the use of IV alteplase in eligible patients. Various prehospital assessment scales are being used by EMS to screen patients in the field for a stroke. These scales include CPSS, LAPSS, and RACE.

In the United States there are networks of hospitals (stroke centers) with various designations (Table 45.13) that form the foundation for

TABLE 45.12 Common and Important Stroke Mimics

STROKE MIMIC	COMMENT
Focal seizure/postictal state	Check for prior seizure history
Metabolic disturbance	Test for hypoglycemia, hyperglycemia, others
Complicated migraine	History of migraine, precipitating factors
Brain tumor, other mass lesion	Gradual symptom onset
Drug abuse	Check toxicology screen
Cervical spine process	No symptoms above the neck
Hysteria/functional process	History of prior psychological disease; increase in stress factors

TABLE 45.13 Types, Characteristics, and Capabilities of Various Levels of Stroke Centers

TYPE OF STROKE CENTER	TYPICAL LOCATION	CAPABILITIES	COMMENT
Acute stroke ready	Rural, small urban	Initial diagnosis, stabilization; able to use IV alteplase	Typically will not admit most patients; likely to transfer patient to a PSC
Primary stroke center	Wide variety	Diagnose and treat most patients with uncomplicated strokes	Stroke unit required; most common type of stroke center; >1500 in the United States
Thrombectomy capable stroke center	Urban and metropolitan	24/7 capability for EVT for LVO strokes and some ICHs	Growing use based on emergence of EVT and physicians trained in INR
Comprehensive stroke center	Large urban and metropolitan	Able to treat all types of patients with all types of stroke and CVD	About 200-250 in the United States; stringent certification criterion

Estimated total number of stroke centers as of 2020: acute stroke ready 200-300; primary stroke center (PSC) >1500; thrombectomy capable stroke center 200-300; comprehensive stroke center 200-250. *CVD*, cardiovascular disease; *EVT*, Endovascular therapy; *ICH*, intracerebral hemorrhage; *LVO*, large vessel occlusion.

TABLE 45.14 Key Elements of a Primary Stroke Center

ELEMENT	COMMENT
Continuum of care	EMS, ED, stroke unit, stroke ward, rehabilitation
Stroke unit	Varies by hospital size; typical range is three to 12 beds
Dedicated professional staff for leadership	Neurologists, neurosurgeons, radiology/neuroradiology, emergency medicine, nursing, therapy
Detailed treatment protocols	Avoid aspiration, deep vein thrombosis, etc.
Quality improvement programs	Should include acute care, ward services, continuum of care
Close monitoring of vital signs and neurologic status	Frequent nursing assessments, NIHSS, automated telemetry
Multidisciplinary care teams	MDs/advanced practice providers/nursing, physical therapy/occupational therapy/speech/social worker/discharge planner
Medical education requirements	Continuing medical education hours/year

NIHSS, National Institutes of Health Stroke Scale.

acute stroke care[69,70] (see also Alberts, Classic References). This hospital infrastructure, when combined with EMS for initial prehospital care and recognition, and rehabilitation for postacute care, are part of what is often called a Stroke System of Care (SSOC).[71] Depending on the type of stroke and its severity, as well as the location of other hospitals, patients may be transported to the nearest facility initially, or they might bypass the nearest hospital to go to a facility better equipped to provide acute stroke care. Several cities and large metropolitan areas are using mobile stroke units (MSUs) to more efficiently triage these patients and begin some care (i.e., IV alteplase) in the field. Emerging data has shown that the MSU does reduce door to needle times for IV alteplase.[72] The operational features of a SSOC are complex and will vary depending on population density, travel times, hospital capabilities and capacities, and coverage paradigms. The AHA and others have published some broad concepts for developing a SSOC.[71]

Several key elements of a primary stroke center (PSC) have particular impact in terms of ensuring rapid acute care, accurate diagnosis, reduction of complications, and prevention of another stroke (Table 45.14). This is also true for a comprehensive stroke center (CSC), which cares for the most complex patients, including those with ischemic and hemorrhagic stroke.

There is a formal and rigorous process to certify a hospital as a PSC (as well as an acute stroke ready hospital, thrombectomy capable stroke center [TSC], and CSC). This involves the training and expertise of the staff, ongoing education via a continuing medical education process, availability of appropriate personnel and infrastructure, tracking complications and patient outcomes, a site visit, and a review of patient records. Several national organizations such as the Joint Commission and the AHA are leading these certification programs. To date there are approximately 1500 certified PSCs in the United States and 200 to 250 CSCs. Many PSC and CSCss use the Get-With-the-Guidelines-Stroke (GWTG) database to track and report processes of care and patient outcomes.[73]

In the hyperacute setting, because the time to reperfusion is a key determinant of functional outcomes, a complete workup is not feasible. Basic steps such as stabilization of vital signs, checking blood glucose, and a head computed tomography (CT) scan are needed to establish a presumed diagnosis of stroke. Vascular imaging, especially computed tomographic angiography (CTA), is useful for determining if a large vessel occlusion (LVO) exists (because such patients may require transfer to a TSC or CSC for thrombectomy). A CTA is also helpful if there are concerns about a high-grade carotid lesion, aneurysm, vasculitis, or questions about collateral flow patterns. (MRI and magnetic resonance angiography [MRA] may be done instead of CT and CTA.) Obtaining a summary of past major medical problems, the time the patient was last known to be well (last known well), current medications, major and recent bleeding or surgical events, and a baseline NIH Stroke Score are the key elements that are needed to begin therapy.

Immediately following the brief assessment outlined earlier, and assuming a tentative diagnosis of an acute ischemic stroke, the patient should be considered for reperfusion therapy using IV alteplase or another lytic agent, mechanical thrombectomy, or a combination of these two therapies.

Intravenous Recombinant Tissue Plasminogen Activator

The FDA approval of IV alteplase in 1996 ushered in an era of acute stroke therapy rather than just diagnosis. As a lytic agent, alteplase is presumed to work by lysing a clot that is occluding or limiting blood flow to a brain region. By restoring flow, it is hoped that ischemic brain can be salvaged (partially or completely) and prevent cerebral infarction. IV alteplase is FDA approved for use within 3 hours of stroke onset or time last known well. Current guidelines have

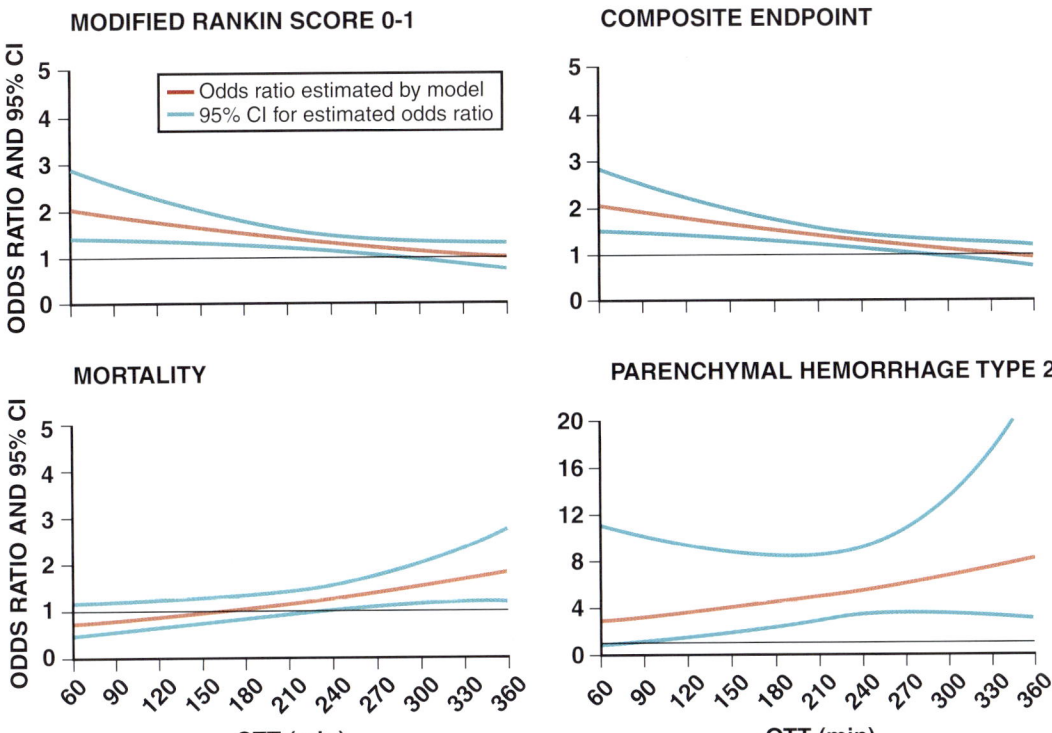

FIGURE 45.5 Benefits of IV alteplase versus time for various neurologic outcomes (comparison is standard medical therapy). *OTT*, Onset to start of treatment. (From Lees KR, et al. Time to treatment with intravenous alteplase and outcome in stroke: an updated pooled analysis of ECASS, ATLANTIS, NINDS, and EPITHET trials. Lancet. 2010;375:1695-1703.)

expanded the treatment time window to 4.5 hours.[63] Compared with placebo, alteplase results in a 12% to 13% absolute increase (and 32% relative increase) in the number of patients who are neurologically normal (defined as a modified Rankin score [mRS] of 0 to 1) at 90 days. Included in this outcome are the 6% of patients who have a symptomatic ICH. This benefit was present in essentially all types of ischemic stroke mechanisms, although those with small vessel occlusion may have a better outcome. In addition to cerebral hemorrhage, the major or common side effects of alteplase are systemic hemorrhagic and rare cases of angioedema. The clinical benefits of IV alteplase are more pronounced the sooner it is administered after stroke onset (Fig. 45.5).[74] National guidelines seek to have a "door to needle" time for IV alteplase of 60 minutes or less. Recent quality improvement efforts seek to reduce this time to 30 to 45 minutes in at least 50% of patients.

Clinical guidelines for treatment with IV tissue plasminogen activator (t-PA) initially reflected a strict protocol that closely followed those used in the clinical trials on which the use of alteplase was based. These guidelines have been revised based on subsequent data and clinical experience.[63] Furthermore, guideline-based recommendations do not align completely with the FDA product labeling. Various conditions that were initially contraindications for IV alteplase have been modified so that they are now only warnings or cautions.[63]

There are a number of recent developments related to the use of IV lytics for acute ischemic stroke. Tenecteplase (TNK) has been studied as an alternative to alteplase. Tenecteplase is more fibrin specific than alteplase, has a faster onset of action, and can be administered as a brief bolus; thus it is easier to use than IV alteplase, which requires a 60-minute infusion. The safety and efficacy of TNK appear similar to those of IV alteplase.[75] The dose of TNK that appears optimal in terms of safety and efficacy is 0.25 mg/kg with a maximum dose of 25 mg.[63,76] To date the use of IV tenecteplase as a replacement for IV alteplase has been limited. Meta-analyses have not shown superiority of TNK over alteplase. Although TNK is recommended in AHA/ASA guidelines, it is not FDA approved for this indication. In addition, the cost of TNK versus alteplase is about $3000 less per dose.

Using TNK (versus alteplase) as bridging therapy for endovascular therapy (EVT) is another area of active investigation. Compared with alteplase, TNK may achieve a higher rate of recanalization and reperfusion.[77] It remains unclear if this translates into improved 3-month clinical outcomes. The use of TNK is not associated with an increase in ICH compared with alteplase. Bridging therapy is discussed later in more detail.

Other recent developments are attempts to extend the time window for IV alteplase using imaging-based criteria, including MRI diffusion/fluid-attenuated inversion recovery (FLAIR) imaging to identify ischemic lesions on diffusion-weighted imaging (DWI) with no hyperintensity on FLAIR, indicating that the stroke occurred within approximately 4.5 hours (Fig. 45.6). Two trials, WAKE UP and EXTEND, and a meta-analysis have used advanced imaging techniques to select patients for IV alteplase treatment up to 9 hours after presumed stroke onset (Table 45.15).[78,79] The WAKE UP trial selected 503 patients with MRI diffusion/FLAIR mismatch indicating stroke onset within the past 4.5 hours but unknown precise time of onset.[78] There was an absolute benefit in efficacy, defined as an mRS of 0 to 1, of >11% for alteplase versus placebo. Treated patients were more likely to have a variety of cerebral hemorrhages (2% versus 0.4%); but these are included in the primary outcome.

The second trial, EXTEND, used imaging paradigms very similar to the DEFUSE3 and DAWN studies for patient selection (see Endovascular Therapy for details). Patients were enrolled 4.5 to 9 hours after symptom onset or time last known well. There was a 6% absolute increase in efficacy (defined as mRS 0 to 1 at 90 days) compared with placebo, and a 5% increase in symptomatic ICH (see Table 45.15).[79] This was a small study with only 225 randomized patients; the study was stopped early based on the results of the WAKE UP trial. WAKE UP was also followed by two other small alteplase trials, THAWS[80] and ECASS-4[81], with 131 and 119 patients, respectively, both using MRI for selection of patients with strokes >4.5 hours after symptom onset. These latter two trials failed to show treatment benefit, but a meta-analysis of all four trials concluded that IV alteplase resulted in better functional outcome at 90 days than placebo or standard care, with net benefit for all functional outcomes despite an increased risk hemorrhage.[82]

Based on the mixed results of these four small trials, currently there has not been wide adoption of expanding the IV alteplase time window to 6 or 9 hours. Although using imaging and tissue-based selection processes make biologic sense, the currently existing narrow treatment time window (4.5 hours) is well established in emergency departments and hospital protocols. It might require more than a few small studies to affect a major change in current treatment paradigms. Furthermore, the sophisticated imaging required may not be widely available at many PSCs and other hospitals on a 24/7 basis. Despite these concerns, recent AHA and European Stroke Organization (ESO) guidelines (Fig. 45.7) do support the use of alteplase beyond the 4.5-hour time window.[63,83]

Endovascular Therapy

Catheter-based endovascular approaches (i.e., thrombectomy, EVT) for acute reperfusion of patients with LVO has shown significant efficacy and a very positive safety profile. The use of newer catheter systems with a smaller profile and the ability to either stent an intracranial vessel or retrieve a clot (i.e., stent retriever or aspiration catheter) have proven very successful. The target lesions are typically clots in the

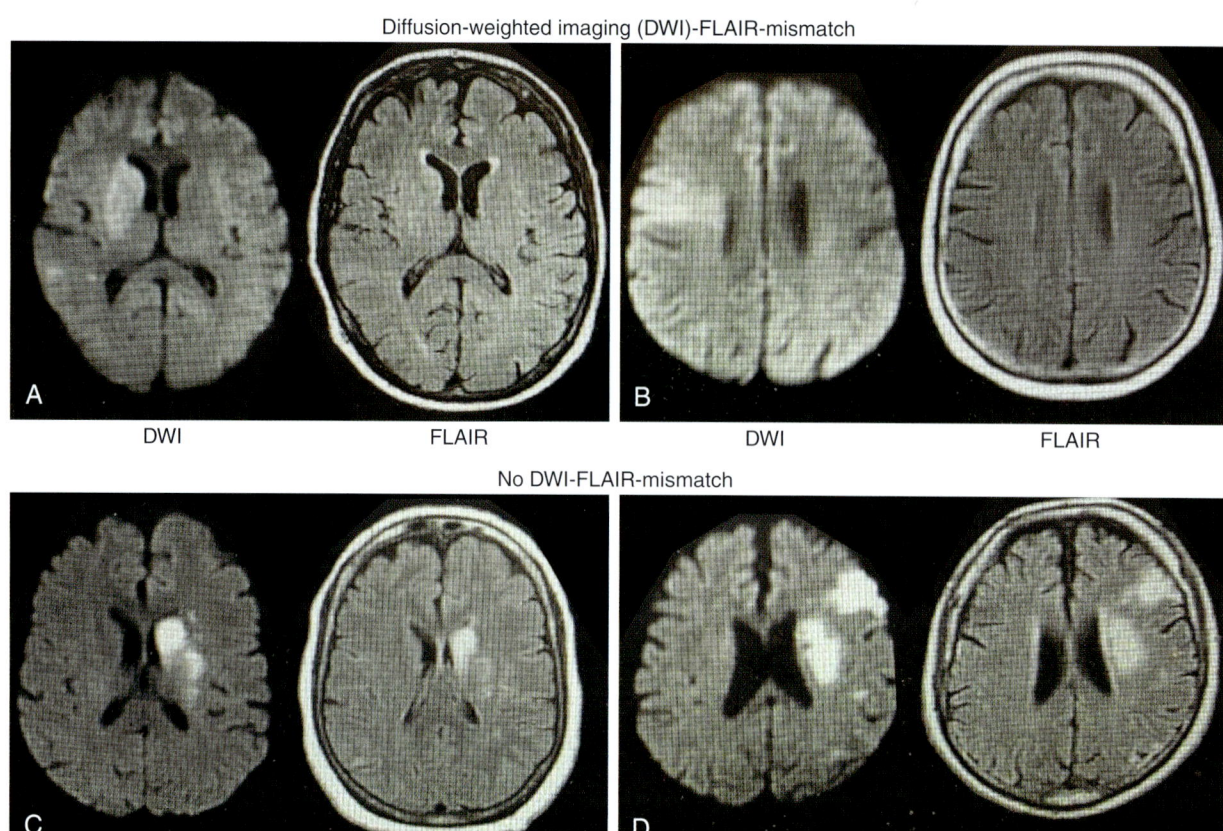

FIGURE 45.6 MRI examples of diffusion-FLAIR mismatch **(A, B)** in patients with clinical evidence of a possible ischemic stroke, compared with patients with diffusion-FLAIR match **(C, D)**. *FLAIR*, fluid attenuated inversion recovery.

TABLE 45.15 Comparison of EXTEND and WAKE-UP Trials

	EXTEND	WAKE-UP
Time window	4.5-9.0 hours	>4.5 hours
Number enrolled (Rx versus placebo)	113 vs 112	254 vs 249
Imaging	CTP or MRP penumbra	FLAIR/DWI mismatch
Positive clinical outcome*	35.4% vs 29.5%	53.3% vs 41.8%
Symptomatic ICH (alteplase versus placebo)**	6.2% vs 0.9%	4% vs 0.4%

Numbers represent treatment versus placebo/standard therapy groups.
CTP, Computed tomographic perfusion; *DWI*, diffusion weighted MRI; *FLAIR*, fluid-attenuated inversion recovery; *ICH*, intracerebral hemorrhage; *MRP*, magnetic resonance perfusion.
*Positive clinical outcome defined as a modified Rankin score of 0 to 1 at 90 days in both studies.
**Symptomatic ICH was defined as a parenchymal hemorrhage 2 (PH2) in both studies.
From Thomalla G, et al. MRI-guided thrombolysis for stroke with unknown time of onset. N Engl J Med. 2018;379:611-622; Ma H, et al. Thrombolysis guided by perfusion imaging up to 9 hours after onset of stroke. N Engl J Med. 2019;380:1795-1803.

intracranial internal carotid artery or proximal MCA, basilar artery, or tandem lesions (cervical carotid artery plus an intracranial lesion). Clots in small arteries (i.e., anterior cerebral, posterior cerebral) are sometimes treated based on the clinical deficit and technical feasibility.

Initial studies treated patients within 6 to 12 hours of stroke onset and demonstrated modest efficacy and reasonable safety.[84-88] The landscape for acute EVT changed dramatically with the publication of the landmark DAWN and DEFUSE3 trials.[89,90] Both used advanced imaging, mainly MR diffusion/perfusion mismatch or CT-based perfusion data, to identify patients without large cores of infarcted tissue but with an ischemic penumbra who might benefit from acute thrombectomy (Fig. 45.8). Patients were enrolled up to 24 hours after symptom onset or time last known well in DAWN and 16 hours in DEFUSE3 (Table 45.16).

Both DAWN and DEFUSE 3 enrolled patients with relatively small infarct cores (7 to 9 mL median volumes), although the ischemic penumbra was often larger. The use of IV alteplase was <10% in both studies (due in large part to the later time window of enrollment). Both studies showed very impressive efficacy as determined by an mRS of 0 to 2, which is defined as functionally independent. The absolute benefit for functional independence at 90 days (compared with standard medical therapy) was 28% in DEFUSE 3 and 36% in DAWN. Each study showed that EVT was surprisingly safe up to 24 hours after stroke onset, with low rates of symptomatic ICH (6% versus 3% in DAWN, and 7% versus 4% in DEFUSE 3) and no significant cerebral edema.[89,90]

Since the publication of DAWN and DEFUSE, numerous follow-up studies, case series, and registries have replicated these impressive results in the United States and globally.[91,92] The issue of pretreatment with IV alteplase before EVT remains unsettled, with some studies showing benefits, while others have not reported a significant impact. A recent meta-analysis of 35 studies suggests that initial treatment with IV alteplase is associated with some benefits, but the results were not definitive.[93] A major complicating factor is the earlier treatment times for patients who receive IV alteplase compared with EVT alone. In up to 20% of potential EVT patients, the occlusion resolves after IV alteplase therapy.

The EVT treatment paradigm has now evolved and is focused on improved identification of patients in the field (by EMS) so that patients who might benefit from EVT can be rapidly identified and transferred to stroke centers capable of performing EVT.[94] Several recent studies have investigated different triage paradigms to determine if patients with an LVO should be taken first to a PSC to receive IV alteplase, or if they should be transported directly to a center capable of performing EVT.[95] This is a complex treatment algorithm that is impacted by distances, hospital capabilities and expertise, and patient characteristics (Fig. 45.9). It has also led to more hospitals developing the capability to perform EVT. There does not appear to be a "one size fits all" answer that would apply to all cities and regions. The Joint Commission has

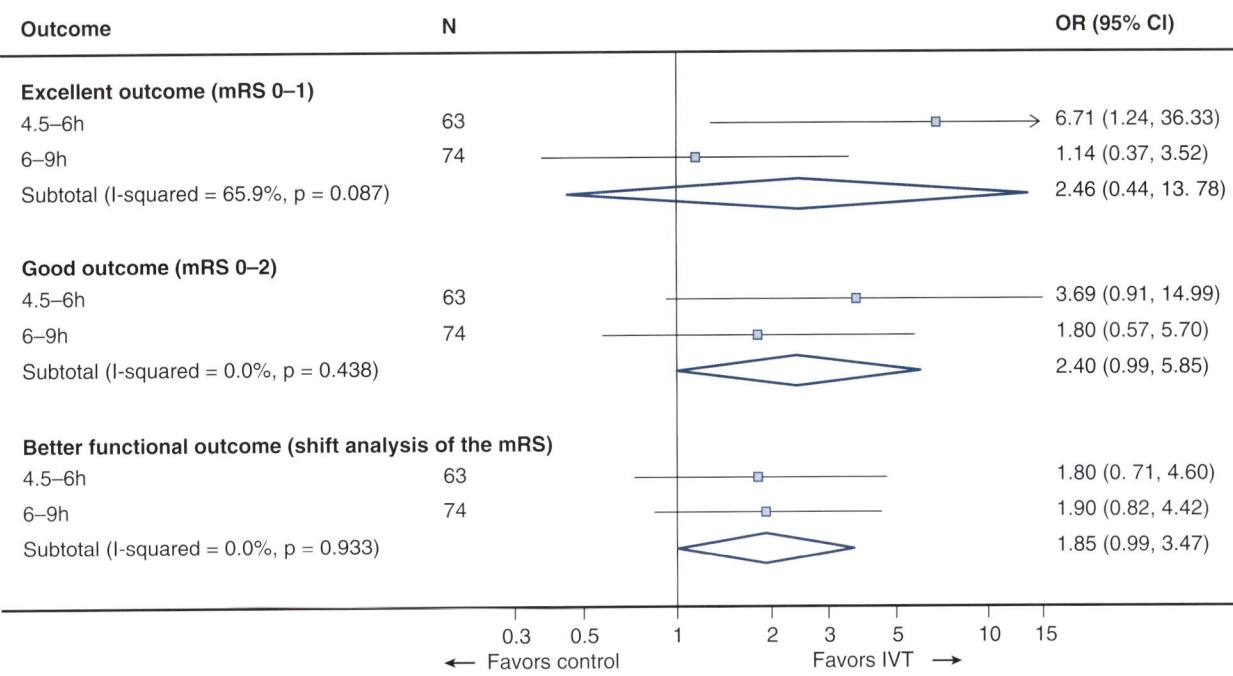

FIGURE 45.7 **Benefits of IV alteplase administered >4.5 hours after stroke onset as reported in the 2021 European Stroke Association guidelines.** Outcomes are based on modified Rankin score (mRS). Pooled odds ratio for excellent outcome (mRS 0 to 1), good outcome (mRS 0 to 2) and better functional outcome (common OR across the whole range of the mRS) in patients with ischemic stroke of 4.5 to 9 hours duration (known onset time) treated with IV thrombolysis versus control. The numbers and the ORs for the 4.5- to 6-hour and 6- to 9-hour time windows (adjusted on age and baseline NIH Stroke Score) are taken from the individual patient data meta-analysis by Campbell BCV, Ma H, Ringleb PA, et al. Extending thrombolysis to 4.5 to 9 hours and wake-up stroke using perfusion imaging: a systematic review and meta-analysis of individual patient data from Berge E, et al. European Stroke Organisation (ESO) guidelines on intravenous thrombolysis for acute ischaemic stroke. Eur Stroke J. 2021;6:I-LXII.

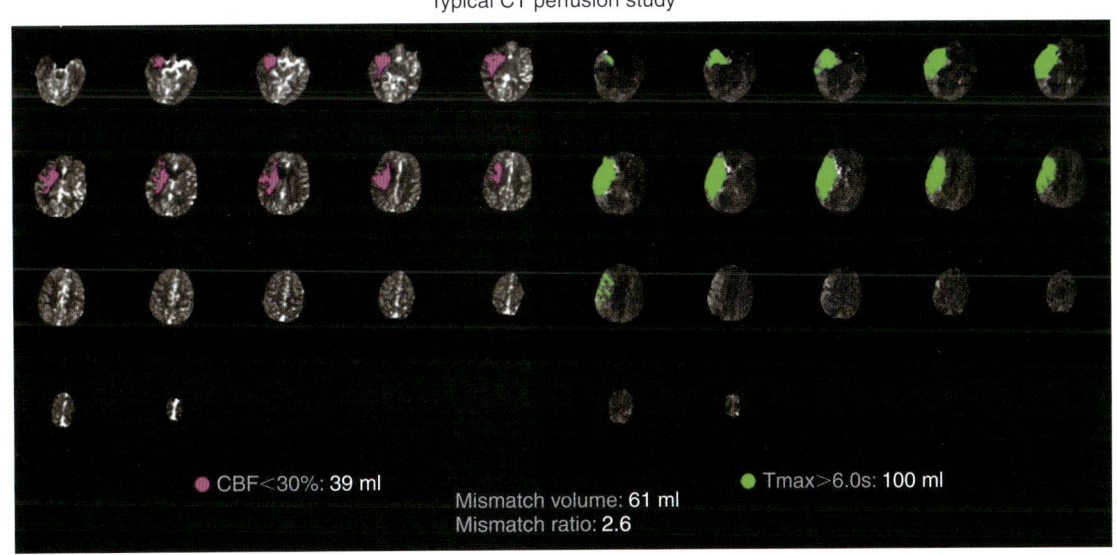

FIGURE 45.8 **CT perfusion images of a patient with an acute deficit consistent with a middle cerebral artery ischemic stroke.** Purple areas (*left*) depict a region of likely infarcted brain; green areas (*right*) are presumed ischemic penumbra that might be salvaged with reperfusion therapy (typically a thrombectomy).

defined a new level of stroke center, a TSC, that has these capabilities (see Table 45.13).

Anticoagulation Therapy for Acute Ischemic Stroke

The indications for acute anticoagulation of patients with ischemic stroke are extremely limited. The most recent AHA guidelines reflect this view and specifically advise against acute anticoagulation for improving neurologic outcomes or preventing early recurrent stroke in patients with acute ischemic stroke.[63] This caution is based on the risk of causing hemorrhagic transformation of an acute ischemic stroke. Such transformation may be minor and microscopic or could be major and produce significant neurologic worsening. Furthermore, systemic anticoagulation is essentially prohibited within 24 hours of treatment with IV alteplase.

When to begin anticoagulation after an acute ischemic stroke in the setting of nonvalvular AF is a common question and clinical conundrum. One has to balance the benefit of early initiation of anticoagulation for stroke prevention against increased central nervous system (CNS) bleeding risks, versus waiting for days or weeks and incurring the risk an early recurrent ischemic stroke. This is a complex clinical decision-making process. One approach, which I generally use and support, adds additional imaging and clinical data to the decision-making equation (Fig. 45.10). The risk for early recurrence in patients with stroke related to AF is generally low (0.3% to 0.5%/day for first

TABLE 45.16 Comparison of DAWN and DEFUSE 3 Studies

STUDY	DAWN	DEFUSE3	COMMENT
Enrollment (total)	206	182	Enrollment in DEFUSE 3 stopped early based on data analysis
Selection criteria	Mismatch between infarct volume and clinical deficit based on DWI or CT perfusion scans	Mismatch on MR DWI and perfusion scans or CT perfusion scans	Enrollment was based on patient age and size of infarct and penumbra; varied by study
Time window	6-24 hours	6-16 hours	
Infarct size	Variable based on age, NIHSS score	<70 cc	Median infarct volume was 7.6 cc in DAWN; 9.4 cc in DEFUSE3
mRS 0-2 (thrombectomy versus medical therapy)	49% vs 13%	45% vs 17%	
Symptomatic intracerebral hemorrhage	6% vs 3%	7% vs 4%	5% treated with alteplase in DAWN; 11% in DEFUSE3
Mortality	19% vs 18%	14% vs 26%	

CT, Computed tomography; *DWI*, diffusion weighted imaging; *MR*, magnetic resonance; *mRS*, modified Rankin Score
Numbers represent EVT versus standard medical care groups.

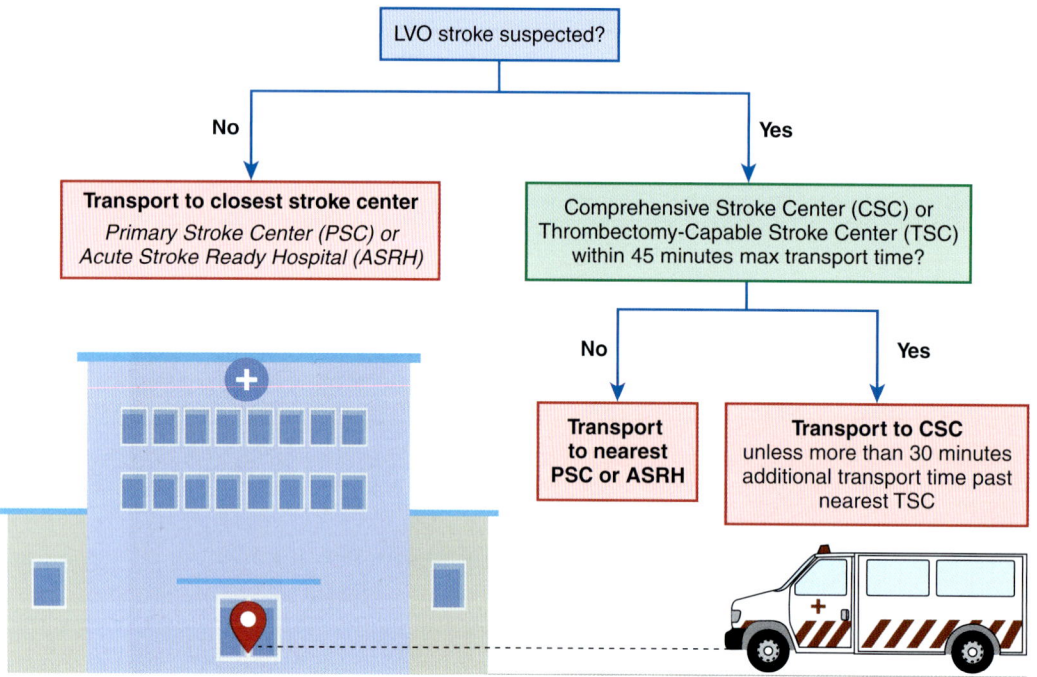

FIGURE 45.9 A typical triage algorithm that might be applicable in a suburban setting for patients with large vessel occlusion (LVO) stroke. (Based on recommendations by Adeoye O, et al. Recommendations for the establishment of stroke systems of care: a 2019 update. Stroke. 2019;50:e187-e210.)

2 weeks), so the timing of initiation of anticoagulation needs to be balanced against the risk for bleeding.[96] Information about stroke size and bleeding as well as brain and cardiac imaging is helpful to determine the timing of acute anticoagulation. BP levels and control are also important considerations.

In patients with a large stroke, especially those with MRI evidence of some hemorrhagic transformation and no evidence of a thrombus in the cardiac chambers, there is likely no need for early anticoagulation because the risk of bleeding is relatively high and the risk of an early recurrent stroke is low. Conversely, patients with a small stroke (and no hemorrhagic transformation on MRI) but who might have evidence of a left atrial thrombus may benefit from early anticoagulation since the bleeding risk is low, but the risk of a recurrent stroke is elevated.

There are a few other scenarios where acute anticoagulation might be considered. Although not supported by rigorous clinical studies, many clinicians might consider acute anticoagulation in the following circumstances: (1) strokes due to an intraluminal clot (typically in a major vessel; carotid, basilar artery), (2) acute dissection of a major cerebral vessel (often with a superimposed thrombus), (3) CVST, and (4) an intracardiac thrombus.[63] Recurrent strokes of unclear etiology despite aggressive antiplatelet therapy is another scenario that may warrant the use of acute systemic anticoagulation.

Those with large strokes (especially due to a cardioembolic event or infection) and those with uncontrolled hypertension generally have the highest risk for spontaneous hemorrhagic transformation of an ischemic stroke and are not typically treated with systemic anticoagulation in the acute (first 5 to 7 days) setting.

Infective Endocarditis

Infective endocarditis is associated with numerous neurologic complications including meningitis, encephalitis, ischemic and hemorrhagic strokes, abscesses, venous thrombosis, and seizures.[97] The use of anticoagulants in patients with stroke related to infective endocarditis is problematic (see Chapter 80). Systemic embolization occurs in 22% to 50% of patients with infective endocarditis, with up to 65% of emboli affecting the CNS, most of which (90%) involve the MCA.[97] Anticoagulation has shown no benefit in patients with native valve endocarditis, and it is not generally recommended for at least the first 2 weeks of antibiotic therapy in patients with stroke related to *Staphylococcus aureus* prosthetic valve endocarditis. These patients are at high risk of hemorrhagic transformation if systemic anticoagulation is used.

In patients with infective endocarditis and an acute ischemic stroke, the use of systemic thrombolytic therapy is associated with an increased risk of cerebral hemorrhage.[98] Mechanical thrombectomy, if there is a large vessel occlusion, may be a safer option and also offer good efficacy.[99]

Of particular concern is the possible development of mycotic intracranial aneurysms in the setting of infective endocarditis. These aneurysms are often multiple and can be either asymptomatic, associated with focal neurologic signs or, because they most commonly affect distal branches of the MCA, associated with signs and symptoms of subarachnoid hemorrhage or a sterile meningitis.[100] Although CTA or MRA can screen patients with symptoms suggesting the presence of a mycotic

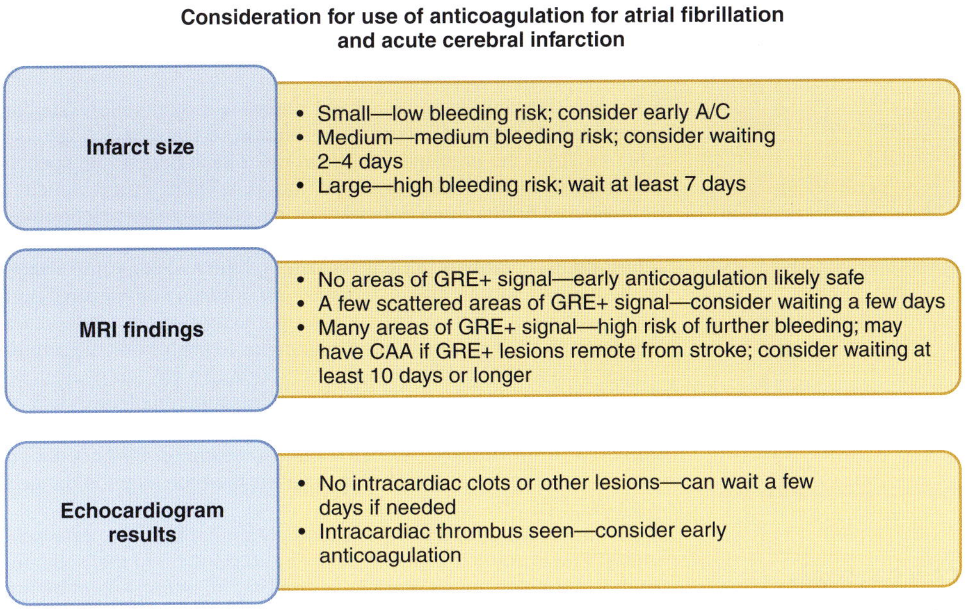

Consideration for use of anticoagulation for atrial fibrillation and acute cerebral infarction

Infarct size
- Small—low bleeding risk; consider early A/C
- Medium—medium bleeding risk; consider waiting 2–4 days
- Large—high bleeding risk; wait at least 7 days

MRI findings
- No areas of GRE+ signal—early anticoagulation likely safe
- A few scattered areas of GRE+ signal—consider waiting a few days
- Many areas of GRE+ signal—high risk of further bleeding; may have CAA if GRE+ lesions remote from stroke; consider waiting at least 10 days or longer

Echocardiogram results
- No intracardiac clots or other lesions—can wait a few days if needed
- Intracardiac thrombus seen—consider early anticoagulation

FIGURE 45.10 Treatment algorithm for determining the use and timing of anticoagulation (A/C) in the setting of an acute ischemic stroke and atrial fibrillation. GRE, gradient echo; CAA, cerebral amyloid angiopathy.

aneurysm, because distal portions of the artery are most commonly affected, catheter-based angiography remains the definitive modality for detection of these lesions (distal portions of MCA can be difficult to visualize with CTA or MRA). Many intracranial mycotic aneurysms regress with antibiotic treatment. Surgical clipping or endovascular obliteration may also be considered. Anticoagulation should be avoided in these patients, as mycotic aneurysms have a propensity to rupture.[97]

Other Modalities for Treatment of Acute Ischemic Stroke

There are other elements of acute stroke care. Most patients should adhere to bed rest for the initial 24 hours after hospital admission. A small but definite group of patients (i.e., those with large artery occlusions or high-grade stenosis or labile BP) may experience worsening of their stroke symptoms if mobilized too early. Gradual mobilization after that time appears to be safe for most patients. Precautions should be taken to avoid dysphagia-related aspiration pneumonia, deep venous thrombosis due to prolonged bed rest, pulmonary embolism, and concomitant cardiac ischemia (which can complicate 2% to 5% of acute strokes).[63]

It is common for BP to be markedly elevated in the hyperacute setting of an ischemic stroke. It typically falls spontaneously to its baseline level within the initial 48 hours, though that is often still elevated. Unless the patient has been treated with IV alteplase or tenecteplase, in most cases the BP should not be aggressively treated in the acute setting. The China Antihypertensive Trial in Acute Ischemic Stroke (CATIS) randomly assigned more than 4000 patients to receive antihypertensive treatment (target reduction of 10% to 25% within the first 24 hours) or to discontinue all antihypertensive medications during hospitalization. BP reduction did not reduce death or major disability at 14 days or hospital discharge.[101] Exceptions include BP that is either very elevated (>220 mm Hg diastolic) or very low (<110 mm Hg systolic).[63] Long-term BP control is a key factor to reduce the risk of a recurrent stroke.

Two of the most common and feared complications of acute ischemic stroke are CNS hemorrhage and cerebral edema with potential for herniation. Hemorrhagic transformation of an ischemic stroke can be mild or even microscopic, moderate, or severe. Underlying factors such as stroke size, underlying etiology (cardioembolic), use of anticoagulation or lytics, and CVD risk factors (especially hypertension and diabetes) play important roles in determining bleeding risk.[102]

Cerebral edema after an acute ischemic stroke can be very difficult to prevent and treat. Unlike the vasogenic edema seen around a brain tumor or cerebral abscess, the cytotoxic edema caused by an ischemic stroke does not respond to steroids and is somewhat resistance to osmotic therapy such as hypertonic saline and mannitol. Drainage of cerebrospinal fluid may be needed, along with a craniotomy to directly relieve increased pressure within the cranial vault. The actual removal of infarcted brain tissue may also be needed if the aforementioned medical measures are ineffective.[103]

Several other important questions often arise in the management of patients with acute ischemic stroke, as well as regarding the use of other interventions that lack definitive supporting data. A key issue is determining the underlying mechanism of the stroke (see Table 45.1). Although identifying and treating common CVD risk factors (hypertension, diabetes, smoking, hyperlipidemia, lack of exercise) is recommended in essentially all of the guidelines, there is still a need to understand the underling stroke mechanism, as this may determine the optimal approaches for secondary prevention. There may be unusual etiologies that mandate atypical therapies as highlighted in Table 45.4. Examples include steroids for a CNS vasculitis, anticoagulation for an inherited coagulopathy, stenting for a carotid dissection, and so forth.

Because thrombophilias (especially the genetic forms previously listed) are more frequently associated with venous thrombosis, cryptogenic stroke in this setting should prompt an evaluation for potential sources of paradoxical embolism. The yield of MRI of the pelvis and lower extremities is higher than that of Doppler ultrasound, and MRI or magnetic resonance venography (MRV) should be considered in patients with a presumed paradoxical embolus (and a PFO). However, the vast majority of such studies fail to identify a venous source of clots.

MANAGEMENT OF SPECIFIC CAUSES OF STROKE
Patent Foramen Ovale

A PFO is found in about 20% to 25% of people in the general population. It is seen more commonly in patients with a cryptogenic stroke and in those younger than 60 years. The presumed mechanism is via a paradoxical embolism migrating from the legs or a pelvic vein to a cerebral artery via the PFO. Other sources include clots in the right atrium or other "right-sided" sources (vena cava, liver, etc.). In rare cases a clot might form in or near the actual PFO or a septal aneurysm between the atria. However, it is often the case that a PFO is found without clear evidence of a right-sided venous clot or probable source.

PFOs can be detected by a transthoracic echocardiography (see Chapter 16), which should be part of the workup for most patients with a new stroke. Sometimes a transesophageal echocardiogram can provide additional information about the PFO morphology, presence of an atrial septal aneurysm, aortic arch plaque, and other intracardiac lesions. The injection of IV contrast can be used to improve the detection of a right-to-left intracardiac shunt. A transcranial Doppler study can be used to detect signals of an embolic event in the brain.

A complete workup for other stroke etiologies is part of this assessment. The RoPE score (Table 45.17) is one tool to define patients with PFOs that may benefit from treatment. It can be used to stratify those patients with a PFO in whom the PFO may play a causative role in a stroke or TIA, thus justifying consideration of PFO closure. It is recommended that a multidisciplinary team including neurologists and cardiologists evaluate patients before PFO closure to ensure proper patient selection. With these caveats, recent guidelines are recommending PFO closure in carefully selected patients with a stroke.

There are a variety of PFO closure devices that can be inserted percutaneously (see Chapter 82). Initial studies showed fewer recurrent strokes after device insertion, but the benefits were not statistically significant. More recent studies (RESPECT, REDUCE, CLOSE, DEFENSE PRO) have shown benefits of PFO closure in carefully selected patients with cryptogenic strokes, with stroke relative risk reductions in the 50% to 75% range (compared with aspirin therapy).[104]

These studies had longer follow-up periods and more enrolled patients than initial studies. They also enrolled high-risk patients, defined as those with larger PFOs and with atrial septal aneurysms.

The major complication of PFO closure via insertion of a percutaneous device is the occurrence of AF, which can be seen in 1% to 6% of patients.[104] Although it is typically transient, a small group of patients will develop chronic AF that may require cardioversion or chronic anticoagulation. This raises the interesting question of whether these patients actually had paroxysmal AF as the cause of the initial or recurrent stroke, which might have been unmasked by the PFO closure

TABLE 45.17 Risk of Paradoxical Embolism (RoPE) Score

CLINICAL CHARACTERISTIC	POINTS
No history of hypertension	+1
No history of diabetes	+1
No history of stroke or TIA	+1
Nonsmoker	+1
Cortical infarct on imaging	+1
Age	
18-29	+5
30-39	+4
40-49	+3
50-59	+2
60-69	+1
>70	+0

TABLE 45.18 Comparison of ABCD2 and ABCD3-I Scores

CLINICAL DATA	ABCD2	ABCD3-I
Age >60 = 1 point	X	X
Blood pressure >140/90 mm Hg = 1 point	X	X
Clinical features Unilateral weakness = 2 points Speech change = 1 point	X	X
Duration of TIA >60 minutes = 2 points 10-59 minutes = 1 point	X	X
History of diabetes = 1 point	X	X
Dual TIAs within 7 days = 2 points		X
Imaging >50% ipsilateral ICA stenosis = 2 points Acute DWI lesion = 2 points		X

DWI, diffusion weighted imaging; *ICA*, internal carotid artery.

procedure. Overall, in these randomized studies there was no significant impact of PFO closure on major bleeding and death.

Stroke After Percutaneous Coronary Interventions and Thrombolytic Treatment of Myocardial Infarction

Although infrequent, stroke can complicate percutaneous coronary interventions (PCIs) (see Chapter 41). The most common mechanism is embolic, with the clot embolism originating from an aortic plaque or catheter tip. The same principles outlined for the management of acute ischemic stroke in other settings apply. The patient could receive IV alteplase and could be evaluated for endovascular therapy, provided that all the other inclusion criteria are met and the patient has no other contraindications to the therapy. It is important to establish systems to ensure the rapid evaluation and treatment of patients with stroke after PCI.

Intracerebral or subarachnoid hemorrhage following administration of a thrombolytic agent for acute MI or pulmonary embolism is a serious and potentially fatal complication. The lytic (or heparin) infusion should be discontinued immediately in any patient in whom acute neurologic symptoms develop. Because these symptoms might result from either hemorrhage or ischemia, a brain imaging study is mandatory before proceeding with further treatment.

Treatments to reduce the amount of thrombolytic-associated intracerebral hemorrhage once it has occurred are not well established. Options include the rapid administration of cryoprecipitate, aminocaproic acid, prothrombin complex concentrate, platelets, and recombinant factor VII[105] and/or fresh-frozen plasma has been advocated. Heparin can be reversed by protamine injection. Those with brainstem compression related to cerebellar hemorrhage may benefit from surgical evacuation of the hematoma. Such patients require prompt transfer to a setting with expertise in neurologic intensive care.

DIAGNOSIS AND TREATMENT OF PATIENTS WITH A TRANSIENT ISCHEMIC ATTACK

A TIA is a transient event with focal neurologic dysfunction (similar to a stroke), but with spontaneous resolution of symptoms. A key feature of a TIA is the presence of a focal neurologic deficit (i.e., speech disturbance, focal weakness, facial droop, specific visual deficits). Defining and finding such deficits can be a challenge for practitioners not trained in the neurosciences. Patients with vague symptoms (headaches, diffuse numbers, global weakness, blurry vision) are always challenging. Metabolic derangements, drug intoxication, seizures, and migraine headaches may produce similar symptoms in some cases (see Table 45.12). This can be very challenging in the hyperacute setting.

Based on a 2009 publication, the definition of a TIA has evolved so that it is now based on imaging results, not the duration of the deficit or the presence of specific symptoms.[106] Therefore a TIA-like event is now defined as a stroke if the MRI shows a new lesion on DWI consistent with an acute stroke. If the DWI is negative, then the event is defined as a TIA.

The mechanisms of a TIA are essentially similar to those of an ischemic stroke. In some patients the extent and duration of the ischemic insult is not sufficient to produce a cerebral infarction—thereby the DWI is negative and it is a TIA. If the patient cannot get an MRI (due to a pacemaker, severe claustrophobia, etc.), then a repeat head CT in 48 hours is reasonable to detect new areas of infarction.

The risk of a stroke or other vascular event (MI, vascular death) after a TIA has evolved over time based the study population and treatment approaches, with more recent studies showing lower event rates. Earlier studies reported an 11% risk of stroke at 90 days, with about half of strokes occurring within 2 days.[1] A larger study of 3847 patients found a 5-year risk of stroke and other vascular events of 13%, of which half occurred in the first year, and the remainder in years 2 to 5.[107] Risk factors for a subsequent event included ipsilateral carotid atherosclerosis, cardioembolic event, and an elevated ABCD2 score. The ABCD2 score was developed to help assess the short-term risk for stroke in patients with TIA (Table 45.18).[108] The risk for stroke within 2 days is low (1%) in those with a score of 0 to 3, moderate (4%) in those with a score of 4 to 5, and high (8%) in those with a score of 6 to 7.

Adding the results of emergent brain imaging studies can be used to better predict short-term stroke risk. The ABCD3-I score uses both a time- and tissue-based definition of TIA to predict early and late stroke occurrence.[109] Specific components of ABCD3-I are shown in Table 45.17. Tissue-based imaging with ABCD3-I enhances risk stratification of short-term stroke risk (Fig. 45.11).

The treatment of patients with a TIA is medically similar to that for an ischemic stroke in terms of risk factor control and antiplatelet therapy. Short-term treatment with dual antiplatelet therapy, as supported by the POINT and THALES studies (see Antiplatelet Therapy and Figs. 45.4 and 45.5), is now the standard of care. Such patients should be evaluated for the presence of CAD, as this is a common cause of death long term.

FUTURE DIRECTIONS

The best way to treat a stroke is to prevent the stroke. Using megadata approaches has the potential to help develop tools that can more accurately predict which patients are at high versus low risk of an event. Using individual patient data from large databases improves predictive stroke models from about 60% up to 80%. Such improvements will better help practitioners target patients and resources to achieve optimal prevention interventions.

The trend for acute therapy is expanding treatment time windows by using enhanced imaging tools and techniques. Using mobile stroke units to triage patients in the field is one approach to reduce treatment times and improve outcomes. Expanding stroke centers to more hospitals will provide optimal care to larger segments of the population, including underserved communities and disadvantaged individuals. More sensitive brain imaging to better differentiate ischemic from infarcted tissue may increase the benefits of reperfusion therapies while reducing their risk. Research continues into the identification of neuroprotective agents (beyond hypothermia) that can reduce cell death in the setting of acute ischemia.

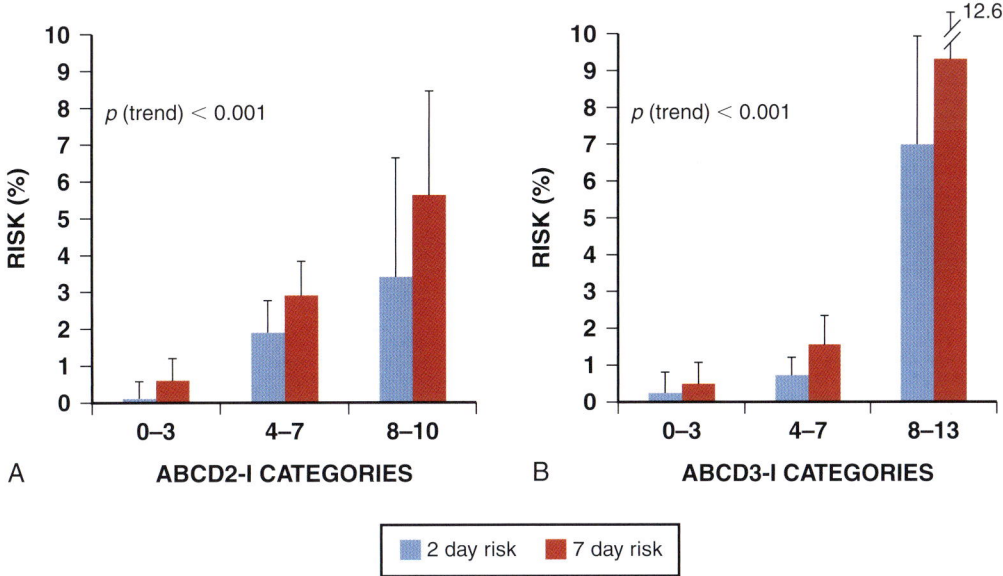

FIGURE 45.11 Stroke risk after TIA stratified by ABCD2-I and ABCD3-I categories. **A,** Stroke risk stratified by ABCD2-I categories at 2 days and 7 days. **B,** Stroke risk stratified by ABCD3-I categories. Error bars indicate 95% CIs. (From Kelly PJ, et al. Validation and comparison of imaging-based scores for prediction of early stroke risk after transient ischaemic attack: a pooled analysis of individual-patient data from cohort studies. Lancet Neurol. 2016;15:1238-1247.)

CONCLUSIONS

Significant progress has been made since 1996 on preventing strokes and improving acute treatments, all with the goal of reducing death and disability related to stroke and cerebrovascular disease. A multidisciplinary approach is needed to maximize both primary and secondary prevention, and the use of reperfusion strategies within a stroke system of care has the potential to improve outcomes if prevention fails. However, as the population ages there will likely be more patients with stroke in the upcoming decades. This will necessitate more effective strategies for both prevention and acute care.

CLASSIC REFERENCES

Alberts MJ, Latchaw RE, Selman WR, et al. Recommendations for comprehensive stroke centers: a consensus statement from the Brain Attack Coalition. *Stroke*. 2005;36:1597–1616.
Amarenco P, Bogousslavsky J, Callahan 3rd A, et al. High-dose atorvastatin after stroke or transient ischemic attack. *N Engl J Med*. 2006;355:549–559.
Chimowitz MI, Lynn MJ, Howlett-Smith H, et al. Comparison of warfarin and aspirin for symptomatic intracranial arterial stenosis. *N Engl J Med*. 2005;352:1305–1316.
Collins R, Armitage J, Parish S, et al. Effects of cholesterol-lowering with simvastatin on stroke and other major vascular events in 20536 people with cerebrovascular disease or other high-risk conditions. *Lancet*. 2004;363:757–767.
Levine SR, Brey RL, Tilley BC, et al. Antiphospholipid antibodies and subsequent thrombo-occlusive events in patients with ischemic stroke. *JAMA*. 2004;291:576–584.
PROGRESS Collaborative Group. Randomised trial of a perindopril-based blood-pressure-lowering regimen among 6,105 individuals with previous stroke or transient ischaemic attack. *Lancet*. 2001;358:1033–1041.
Rashid P, Leonardi-Bee J, Bath P. Blood pressure reduction and secondary prevention of stroke and other vascular events: a systematic review. *Stroke*. 2003;34:2741–2748.
Ridker PM, Cook NR, Lee IM, et al. A randomized trial of low-dose aspirin in the primary prevention of cardiovascular disease in women. *N Engl J Med*. 2005;352:1293–1304.
Yusuf S, Sleight P, Pogue J, Bosch J, Davies R, et al. Effects of an angiotensin-converting-enzyme inhibitor, ramipril, on cardiovascular events in high-risk patients. *N Engl J Med*. 2000;342:145–153.

REFERENCES

1. Virani SS, Alonso A, Benjamin EJ, et al. Heart disease and stroke statistics-2020 update: a report from the American Heart Association. *Circulation*. 2020;141:e139–e596.
2. Howard VJ, Madsen TE, Kleindorfer DO, et al. Sex and race differences in the association of incident ischemic stroke with risk factors. *JAMA Neurol*. 2019;76:179–186.
3. Gardener H, Sacco RL, Rundek T, et al. Race and ethnic disparities in stroke incidence in the Northern Manhattan Study. *Stroke*. 2020;51:1064–1069.
4. Bersano A, Kraemer M, Burlina A, et al. Heritable and non-heritable uncommon causes of stroke. *J Neurol*. 2021;268:2780–2807.

Classification of Ischemic Stroke

5. Regenhardt RW, Das AS, Lo EH, Caplan LR. Advances in understanding the pathophysiology of lacunar stroke: a review. *JAMA Neurol*. 2018;75:1273–1281.
6. Rennert RC, Wali AR, Steinberg JA, et al. Epidemiology, natural history, and clinical presentation of large vessel ischemic stroke. *Neurosurgery*. 2019;85:S4–S8.
7. Kamel H, Navi BB, Merkler AE, et al. Reclassification of ischemic stroke etiological subtypes on the basis of high-risk nonstenosing carotid plaque. *Stroke*. 2020;51:504–510.
8. Navi BB, Mathias R, Sherman CP, et al. Cancer-related ischemic stroke has a distinct blood mRNA expression profile. *Stroke*. 2019;50:3259–3264.
8a. Ropper AH, Klein JP. Central venous thrombosis. *N Engl J Med*. 2021;385:59–64.
9. Capecchi M, Abbattista M, Martinelli I. Cerebral venous sinus thrombosis. *J Thromb Haemost*. 2018;16:1918–1931.
10. Sader N, de Lotbiniere-Bassett M, Tso MK, Hamilton M. Management of venous sinus thrombosis. *Neurosurg Clin N Am*. 2018;29:585–594.
11. Paraskevas KI, Veith FJ, AbuRahma AF, et al. A comparison of the society for vascular surgery and the European Society for Vascular Surgery guidelines to identify which asymptomatic carotid patients should be offered a carotid endarterectomy. *J Vasc Surg*. 2020;72:2149–2152.
12. Neequaye SK, Halliday AW. Carotid artery stenting: the 2011 NICE guidelines. *Heart*. 2012;98:274–275.
13. Bladin C, Chambers B, New G, et al. Guidelines for patient selection and performance of carotid artery stenting. *ANZ J Surg*. 2010;80:398–405.

Stroke Risk Factors and Prevention

14. Meschia JF, Bushnell C, Boden-Albala B, et al. Guidelines for the primary prevention of stroke: a statement for healthcare professionals from the American Heart Association/American Stroke Association. *Stroke*. 2014;45:3754–3832.
15. Tsivgoulis G, Safouris A, Kim DE, Alexandrov AV. Recent advances in primary and secondary prevention of atherosclerotic stroke. *J Stroke*. 2018;20:145–166.
16. O'Donnell MJ, Xavier D, Liu L, et al. Risk factors for ischaemic and intracerebral haemorrhagic stroke in 22 countries (the INTERSTROKE study): a case-control study. *Lancet*. 2010;376:112–123.
17. Hankey GJ. Population impact of potentially modifiable risk factors for stroke. *Stroke*. 2020;51:719–728.
18. Al Kibria GM. Racial/ethnic disparities in prevalence, treatment, and control of hypertension among us adults following application of the 2017 American College of Cardiology/American Heart Association guideline. *Prev Med Rep*. 2019;14:100850.
19. Unger T, Borghi C, Charchar F, et al. 2020 International Society of Hypertension global hypertension practice guidelines. *Hypertension*. 2020;75:1334–1357.
20. Whelton PK, Carey RM, Aronow WS, et al. 2017 ACC/AHA/AAPA/ABC/ACPM/AGS/APhA/ASH/ASPC/NMA/PCNA guideline for the prevention, detection, evaluation, and management of high blood pressure in adults: executive summary: a report of the American College of Cardiology/American Heart Association task force on clinical practice guidelines. *Circulation*. 2018;138:e426–e483.
21. Group SR, Wright Jr JT, Williamson JD, et al. A randomized trial of intensive versus standard blood-pressure control. *N Engl J Med*. 2015;373:2103–2116.
22. The Sprint Research Group. Final report of a trial of intensive versus standard blood-pressure control. *N Engl J Med*. 2021;384:1921–1930.
23. Lonn EM, Jung H, Yusuf S. Blood-pressure and cholesterol lowering in the hope-3 trial. *N Engl J Med*. 2016;375:1193–1194.
24. Katsanos AH, Filippatou A, Manios E, et al. Blood pressure reduction and secondary stroke prevention: a systematic review and metaregression analysis of randomized clinical trials. *Hypertension*. 2017;69:171–179.
25. Zhong XL, Dong Y, Xu W, et al. Role of blood pressure management in stroke prevention: a systematic review and network meta-analysis of 93 randomized controlled trials. *J Stroke*. 2021;23:1–11.
26. Yusuf S, Bosch J, Dagenais G, et al. Cholesterol lowering in intermediate-risk persons without cardiovascular disease. *N Engl J Med*. 2016;374:2021–2031.
27. Amarenco P, Labreuche J. Lipid management in the prevention of stroke: review and updated meta-analysis of statins for stroke prevention. *Lancet Neurol*. 2009;8:453–463.
28. Ridker PM, Danielson E, Fonseca FA, et al. Rosuvastatin to prevent vascular events in men and women with elevated c-reactive protein. *N Engl J Med*. 2008;359:2195–2207.
29. Kleindorfer DO, Towfighi A, Chaturvedi S, et al. 2021 Guideline for the prevention of stroke in patients with stroke and transient ischemic attack: a guideline from the American Heart Association/American Stroke Association. *Stroke*. 2021;52:e364–e467.
30. Giugliano RP, Pedersen TR, Saver JL, et al. Stroke prevention with the PCSK9 (proprotein convertase subtilisin-kexin type 9) inhibitor evolocumab added to statin in high-risk patients with stable atherosclerosis. *Stroke*. 2020;51:1546–1554.
31. Tun NN, Arunagirinathan G, Munshi SK, Pappachan JM. Diabetes mellitus and stroke: a clinical update. *World J Diabetes*. 2017;8:235–248.
32. Skyler JS, Bergenstal R, Bonow RO, et al. Intensive glycemic control and the prevention of cardiovascular events: implications of the ACCORD, ADVANCE, and VA Diabetes trials: a position statement of the American Diabetes Association and a scientific statement of the American College of Cardiology Foundation and the American Heart Association. *J Am Coll Cardiol*. 2009;53:298–304.

33. Kernan WN, Viscoli CM, Furie KL, et al. Pioglitazone after ischemic stroke or transient ischemic attack. *N Engl J Med*. 2016;374:1321–1331.
34. Epstein KA, Viscoli CM, Spence JD, et al. Smoking cessation and outcome after ischemic stroke or tia. *Neurology*. 2017;89:1723–1729.
35. Larsson SC, Wallin A, Wolk A. Dietary approaches to stop hypertension diet and incidence of stroke: results from 2 prospective cohorts. *Stroke*. 2016;47:986–990.
36. Pandian JD, Gall SL, Kate MP, et al. Prevention of stroke: a global perspective. *Lancet*. 2018;392:1269–1278.
37. Mitchell AB, Cole JW, McArdle PF, et al. Obesity increases risk of ischemic stroke in young adults. *Stroke*. 2015;46:1690–1692.
38. Lobelo F, Rohm Young D, et al. Routine assessment and promotion of physical activity in healthcare settings: a scientific statement from the American Heart Association. *Circulation*. 2018;137:e495–e522.
39. McDermott M, Brown DL. Sleep apnea and stroke. *Curr Opin Neurol*. 2020;33:4–9.
40. Lisabeth LD, Sanchez BN, Lim D, et al. Sleep-disordered breathing and poststroke outcomes. *Ann Neurol*. 2019;86:241–250.
41. Howard G, Howard VJ. Twenty years of progress toward understanding the stroke belt. *Stroke*. 2020;51:742–750.
42. Feng Y, Kang K, Xue Q, et al. Value of plasma homocysteine to predict stroke, cardiovascular diseases, and new-onset hypertension: a retrospective cohort study. *Medicine (Baltim)*. 2020;99:e21541.
43. Spence JD. Homocysteine lowering for stroke prevention: unravelling the complexity of the evidence. *Int J Stroke*. 2016;11:744–747.
44. Shahjouei S, Tsivgoulis G, Farahmand G, et al. SARS-COV-2 and stroke characteristics: a report from the multinational COVID-19 Stroke Study Group. *Stroke*. 2021;52:e117–e130.
45. Schultz NH, Sorvoll IH, Michelsen AE, et al. Thrombosis and thrombocytopenia after ChAdOx1 nCoV-19 vaccination. *N Engl J Med*. 2021.

Antithrombotic Agents For Stroke Prevention

46. Gaziano JM, Brotons C, Coppolecchia R, et al. Use of aspirin to reduce risk of initial vascular events in patients at moderate risk of cardiovascular disease (ARRIVE): a randomised, double-blind, placebo-controlled trial. *Lancet*. 2018;392:1036–1046.
47. McNeil JJ, Wolfe R, Woods RL, et al. Effect of aspirin on cardiovascular events and bleeding in the healthy elderly. *N Engl J Med*. 2018;379:1509–1518.
48. The ASCEND Study Collaborative Group. Effects of aspirin for primary prevention in persons with diabetes mellitus. *N Engl J Med*. 2018;379:1529–1539.
49. January CT, Wann LS, Calkins H, et al. 2019 AHA/ACC/HTS focused update of the 2014 AHA/ACC/HRS guideline for the management of patients with atrial fibrillation: a report of the American College of Cardiology/American Heart Association task force on clinical practice guidelines and the Heart Rhythm Society. *J Am Coll Cardiol*. 2019;74:104–132.
50. January CT, Wann LS, Calkins H, et al. 2019 AHA/ACC/HRS focused update of the 2014 AHA/ACC/HRS guideline for the management of patients with atrial fibrillation: a report of the American College of Cardiology/American Heart Association task force on clinical practice guidelines and the heart rhythm society. *Heart Rhythm*. 2019;16:e66–e93.
51. Chao TF, Nedeljkovic MA, Lip GYH, Potpara TS. Stroke prevention in atrial fibrillation: comparison of recent international guidelines. *Eur Heart J Suppl*. 2020;22:O53–O60.
52. Chandratheva A, Mehta Z, Geraghty OC, et al. Population-based study of risk and predictors of stroke in the first few hours after a TIA. *Neurology*. 2009;72:1941–1947.
53. Pendlebury ST, Rothwell PM. Risk of recurrent stroke, other vascular events and dementia after transient ischaemic attack and stroke. *Cerebrovasc Dis*. 2009;27(suppl 3):1–11.
54. Alberts MJ, Bhatt DL, Mas JL, et al. Three-year follow-up and event rates in the international reduction of atherothrombosis for continued Health registry. *Eur Heart J*. 2009;30:2318–2326.
55. Rother J, Alberts MJ, Touze E, et al. Risk factor profile and management of cerebrovascular patients in the reach registry. *Cerebrovasc Dis*. 2008;25:366–374.
56. Sandercock PA, Counsell C, Tseng MC, Cecconi E. Oral antiplatelet therapy for acute ischaemic stroke. *Cochrane Database Syst Rev*. 2014:CD000029.
57. Rothwell PM, Algra A, Chen Z, et al. Effects of aspirin on risk and severity of early recurrent stroke after transient ischaemic attack and ischaemic stroke: time-course analysis of randomised trials. *Lancet*. 2016;388:365–375.
58. Sacco RL, Diener HC, Yusuf S, et al. Aspirin and extended-release dipyridamole versus clopidogrel for recurrent stroke. *N Engl J Med*. 2008;359:1238–1251.
59. Wang Y, Johnston SC, Wang Y. Clopidogrel with aspirin in minor stroke or transient ischemic attack. *N Engl J Med*. 2013;369:1376–1377.
60. Wang Y, Zhao X, Lin j, et al. Association between CYP2C19 loss-of-function allele stutus and efficacy of clopidogrel for risk reduction among patients with minor stroke or transient ischemic attack. *J Am Med Assoc*. 2016;316:70–78.
61. Johnston SC, Easton JD, Farrant M, et al. Clopidogrel and aspirin in acute ischemic stroke and high-risk TIA. *N Engl J Med*. 2018;379:215–225.
62. Johnston SC, Amarenco P, Dennision H, et al. Ticagrelor and aspirin or aspirin alone in acute ischemic stroke or TIA. *N Engl J Med*. 2020;383:207–217.
63. Powers WJ, Rabinstein AA, Ackerson T, et al. Guidelines for the early management of patients with acute ischemic stroke: 2019 update to the 2018 guidelines for the early management of acute ischemic stroke: a guideline for healthcare professionals from the American Heart Association/American Stroke Association. *Stroke*. 2019;50:e344–e418.
64. Chimowitz MI, Lynn MJ, Derdeyn CP, et al. Stenting versus aggressive medical therapy for intracranial arterial stenosis. *N Engl J Med*. 2011;365:993–1003.
65. Massie BM, Collins JF, Ammon SE, et al. Randomized trial of warfarin, aspirin, and clopidogrel in patients with chronic heart failure: the Warfarin and Antiplatelet Therapy in Chronic Heart Failure (WATCH) trial. *Circulation*. 2009;119:1616–1624.
66. Homma S, Thompson JL, Pullicino PM, et al. Warfarin and aspirin in patients with heart failure and sinus rhythm. *N Engl J Med*. 2012;366:1859–1869.
67. Zannad F, Anker SD, Byra WM, et al. Rivaroxaban in patients with heart failure, sinus rhythm, and coronary disease. *N Engl J Med*. 2018;379:1332–1342.

Management of Acute Ischemic Stroke

68. Brandler ES, Sharma M, McCullough F, et al. Prehospital stroke identification: factors associated with diagnostic accuracy. *J Stroke Cerebrovasc Dis*. 2015;24:2161–2166.
69. Alberts MJ, Latchaw RE, Jagoda A, et al. Revised and updated recommendations for the establishment of primary stroke centers: a summary statement from the Brain Attack Coalition. *Stroke*. 2011;42:2651–2665.
70. Alberts MJ, Wechsler LR, Jensen ME, et al. Formation and function of acute stroke-ready hospitals within a stroke system of care recommendations from the Brain Attack Coalition. *Stroke*. 2013;44:3382–3393.
71. Adeoye O, Nystrom KV, Yavagal DR, et al. Recommendations for the establishment of stroke systems of care: a 2019 update. *Stroke*. 2019;50:e187–e210.
72. Freitag E, Kaffes M, Weber JE, Audebert HJ. How to set up a successfully running mobile stroke unit program. *Stroke*. 2021;52:e107–e110.
73. Man S, Zhao X, Uchino K, et al. Comparison of acute ischemic stroke care and outcomes between comprehensive stroke centers and primary stroke centers in the United States. *Circ Cardiovasc Qual Outcomes*. 2018;11:e004512.

Management of Acute Ischemic Stroke: Thrombolytic Therapy

74. Lees KR, Bluhmki E, von Kummer R, et al. Time to treatment with intravenous alteplase and outcome in stroke: an updated pooled analysis of ECASS, ATLANTIS, NINDS, and EPITHET trials. *Lancet*. 2010;375:1695–1703.
75. Parsons M, Spratt N, Bivard A, et al. A randomized trial of tenecteplase versus alteplase for acute ischemic stroke. *N Engl J Med*. 2012;366:1099–1107.
76. Coutts SB, Berge E, Campbell BC, et al. Tenecteplase for the treatment of acute ischemic stroke: a review of completed and ongoing randomized controlled trials. *Int J Stroke*. 2018;13:885–892.
77. Campbell BCV, Mitchell PJ, Churilov L, et al. Tenecteplase versus alteplase before thrombectomy for ischemic stroke. *N Engl J Med*. 2018;378:1573–1582.
78. Thomalla G, Simonsen CZ, Boutitie F, et al. MRI-guided thrombolysis for stroke with unknown time of onset. *N Engl J Med*. 2018;379:611–622.
79. Ma H, Campbell BCV, Parsons MW, et al. Thrombolysis guided by perfusion imaging up to 9 hours after onset of stroke. *N Engl J Med*. 2019;380:1795–1803.
80. Koga M, Yamamoto H, Inoue M, et al. Thrombolysis with alteplase at 0.6 mg/kg for stroke with unknown time of onset: a randomized controlled trial. *Stroke*. 2020;51:1530–1538.
81. Ringleb P, Bendszus M, Bluhmki E, et al. Extending the time window for intravenous thrombolysis in acute ischemic stroke using magnetic resonance imaging-based patient selection. *Int J Stroke*. 2019;14:483–490.
82. Thomalla G, Boutitie F, Ma H, et al. Intravenous alteplase for stroke with unknown time of onset guided by advanced imaging: systematic review and meta-analysis of individual patient data. *Lancet*. 2020;396:1574–1584.
83. Berge E, Whiteley W, Audebert H, et al. European Stroke Organisation (ESO) guidelines on intravenous thrombolysis for acute ischaemic stroke. *Eur Stroke J*. 2021;6:I–LXII.

Management of Acute Ischemic Stroke: Endovascular Therapy

84. Campbell BC, Mitchell PJ, Kleinig TJ, et al. Endovascular therapy for ischemic stroke with perfusion-imaging selection. *N Engl J Med*. 2015;372:1009–1018.
85. Furlan AJ. Endovascular therapy for stroke: it's about time. *N Engl J Med*. 2015;372:2347–2349.
86. Goyal M, Demchuk AM, Menon BK, et al. Randomized assessment of rapid endovascular treatment of ischemic stroke. *N Engl J Med*. 2015;372:1019–1030.
87. Jovin TG, Chamorro A, Cobo E, et al. Thrombectomy within 8 hours after symptom onset in ischemic stroke. *N Engl J Med*. 2015;372:2296–2306.
88. Saver JL, Goyal M, Bonafe A, et al. Stent-retriever thrombectomy after intravenous t-PA vs. t-PA alone in stroke. *N Engl J Med*. 2015;372:2285–2295.
89. Nogueira RG, Jadhav AP, Haussen DC, et al. Thrombectomy 6 to 24 hours after stroke with a mismatch between deficit and infarct. *N Engl J Med*. 2018;378:11–21.
90. Albers GW, Marks MP, Kemp S, et al. Thrombectomy for stroke at 6 to 16 hours with selection by perfusion imaging. *N Engl J Med*. 2018;378:708–718.
91. Bosson N, Gausche-Hill M, Saver JL, et al. Increased access to and use of endovascular therapy following implementation of a 2-tiered regional stroke system. *Stroke*. 2020;51:908–913.
92. Casetta I, Fainardi E, Saia V, et al. Endovascular thrombectomy for acute ischemic stroke beyond 6 hours from onset: a real-world experience. *Stroke*. 2020;51:2051–2057.
93. Vidale S, Romoli M, Consoli D, Agostoni EC. Bridging versus direct mechanical thrombectomy in acute ischemic stroke: a subgroup pooled meta-analysis for time of intervention, eligibility, and study design. *Cerebrovasc Dis*. 2020;49:223–232.
94. McTaggart RA, Holodinsky JK, Ospel JM, et al. Leaving no large vessel occlusion stroke behind: reorganizing stroke systems of care to improve timely access to endovascular therapy. *Stroke*. 2020;51:1951–1960.
95. Sarraj A, Savitz S, Pujara D, et al. Endovascular thrombectomy for acute ischemic strokes: current US access paradigms and optimization methodology. *Stroke*. 2020;51:1207–1217.

Management of Acute Ischemic Stroke: Anticoagulation and Other Treatments

96. Paciaroni M, Agnelli G, Falocci N, et al. Early recurrence and cerebral bleeding in patients with acute ischemic stroke and atrial fibrillation: effect of anticoagulation and its timing: the RAF study. *Stroke*. 2015;46:2175–2182.
97. Sotero FD, Rosario M, Fonseca AC, Ferro JM. Neurological complications of infective endocarditis. *Curr Neurol Neurosci Rep*. 2019;19:23.
98. Marquardt RJ, Cho SM, Thatikunta P, et al. Acute ischemic stroke therapy in infective endocarditis: case series and systematic review. *J Stroke Cerebrovasc Dis*. 2019;28:2207–2212.
99. Bettencourt S, Ferro JM. Acute ischemic stroke treatment in infective endocarditis: systematic review. *J Stroke Cerebrovasc Dis*. 2020;29:104598.
100. Salaun E, Touil A, Hubert S, et al. Intracranial haemorrhage in infective endocarditis. *Arch Cardiovasc Dis*. 2018;111:712–721.
101. He J, Zhang Y, Xu T, et al. Effects of immediate blood pressure reduction on death and major disability in patients with acute ischemic stroke: the CATIS randomized clinical trial. *J Am Med Assoc*. 2014;311:479–489.
102. Paciaroni M, Agnelli G, Corea F, et al. Early hemorrhagic transformation of brain infarction: rate, predictive factors, and influence on clinical outcome: results of a prospective multicenter study. *Stroke*. 2008;39:2249–2256.
103. Cook AM, Morgan Jones G, Hawryluk GWJ, et al. Guidelines for the acute treatment of cerebral edema in neurocritical care patients. *Neurocrit Care*. 2020;32:647–666.
104. Alkhouli M, Sievert H, Holmes DR. Patent foramen ovale closure for secondary stroke prevention. *Eur Heart J*. 2019;40:2339–2350.
105. Yaghi S, Eisenberger A, Willey JZ. Symptomatic intracerebral hemorrhage in acute ischemic stroke after thrombolysis with intravenous recombinant tissue plasminogen activator: a review of natural history and treatment. *JAMA Neurol*. 2014;71:1181–1185.

Diagnosis and Management of TIA

106. Easton JD, Saver JL, Albers GW, et al. Definition and evaluation of transient ischemic attack: a scientific statement for healthcare professionals from the American Heart Association/American Stroke Association Stroke council; council on cardiovascular surgery and anesthesia; council on cardiovascular radiology and intervention; council on cardiovascular nursing; and the interdisciplinary council on peripheral vascular disease. The American Academy of Neurology affirms the value of this statement as an educational tool for neurologists. *Stroke*. 2009;40:2276–2293.
107. Amarenco P, Lavallee PC, Monteiro Tavares L, et al. Five-year risk of stroke after TIA or minor ischemic stroke. *N Engl J Med*. 2018;378:2182–2190.
108. Johnston SC, Rothwell PM, Nguyen-Huynh MN, et al. Validation and refinement of scores to predict very early stroke risk after transient ischaemic attack. *Lancet*. 2007;369:283–292.
109. Kelly PJ, Albers GW, Chatzikonstantinou A, et al. Validation and comparison of imaging-based scores for prediction of early stroke risk after transient ischaemic attack: a pooled analysis of individual-patient data from cohort studies. *Lancet Neurol*. 2016;15:1238–1247.

第12版

下册

BRAUNWALD'S
HEART DISEASE
A TEXTBOOK OF CARDIOVASCULAR MEDICINE

BRAUNWALD
心脏病学
（影印中文导读版）

第12版

下册

BRAUNWALD'S
HEART DISEASE
A TEXTBOOK OF CARDIOVASCULAR MEDICINE

BRAUNWALD

心脏病学

(影印中文导读版)

编审委员会顾问专家　高润霖
编审委员会主任委员　吴永健　张　健　姚　焰

Edited by

PETER LIBBY, MD
Mallinckrodt Professor of Medicine
Harvard Medical School
Brigham and Women's Hospital
Boston, Massachusetts

ROBERT O. BONOW, MD
Max and Lilly Goldberg Distinguished Professor of Cardiology
Department of Medicine
Northwestern University Feinberg School of Medicine
Chicago, Illinois

DOUGLAS L. MANN, MD
Lewin Distinguished Professor of Cardiovascular Disease
Washington University School of Medicine in St. Louis
Saint Louis, Missouri

GORDON F. TOMASELLI, MD
Professor of Medicine (Cardiology)
The Marilyn and Stanley M. Katz Dean
Albert Einstein College of Medicine
Executive Vice President and Chief Academic Officer
Montefiore Medicine
Bronx, New York

DEEPAK L. BHATT, MD, MPH
Executive Director of Interventional Cardiovascular Programs
Brigham and Women's Hospital
Senior Physician
Brigham and Women's Hospital
Professor of Medicine
Harvard Medical School
Boston, Massachusetts

SCOTT D. SOLOMON, MD
The Edward D. Frohlich Distinguished Chair
Professor of Medicine
Harvard Medical School
Senior Physician
Brigham and Women's Hospital
Boston, Massachusetts

Founding Editor and Online Editor

**EUGENE BRAUNWALD, MD,
MD(Hon), ScD(Hon), FRCP**
Distinguished Hersey Professor of Medicine
Harvard Medical School
Founding Chairman, TIMI Study Group
Brigham and Women's Hospital
Boston, Massachusetts

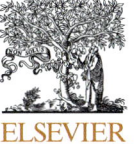

ELSEVIER

Braunwald XINZANGBINGXUE（DI 12 BAN）（YINGYIN ZHONGWEN DAODUBAN）（XIACE）

图书在版编目（CIP）数据

Braunwald 心脏病学：第 12 版：影印中文导读版：上下册＝ Braunwald's Heart Disease：A Textbook of Cardiovascular Medicine，12th edition：英文 /（美）彼得·利贝（Peter Libby）等原著 . —北京：北京大学医学出版社，2023.3
ISBN 978-7-5659-2805-5

Ⅰ. ① B… Ⅱ. ①彼… Ⅲ. ①心脏病学－英文 Ⅳ. ① R541

中国国家版本馆 CIP 数据核字（2023）第 019315 号

北京市版权局著作权合同登记号：图字：01-2022-6707

Elsevier (Singapore) Pte Ltd.
3 Killiney Road, #08-01 Winsland House I, Singapore 239519
Tel: (65) 6349-0200; Fax: (65) 6733-1817

Braunwald's Heart Disease: A Textbook of Cardiovascular Medicine, 12th edition
Copyright © 2022 by Elsevier Inc. All rights reserved.
Previous editions copyrighted 2019, 2015, 2012, 2008, 2005, 2001, 1997, 1992, 1988, 1984, 1980 by Elsevier Inc.
ISBN-13: 9780323824682

This English Adaptation of Braunwald's Heart Disease: A Textbook of Cardiovascular Medicine, 12th edition by Peter Libby, Robert O. Bonow, Douglas L. Mann, Gordon F. Tomaselli, Deepak L. Bhatt, Scott D. Solomon was undertaken by Peking University Medical Press and is published by arrangement with Elsevier (Singapore) Pte Ltd.
Braunwald's Heart Disease: A Textbook of Cardiovascular Medicine, 12th edition by Peter Libby, Robert O. Bonow, Douglas L. Mann, Gordon F. Tomaselli, Deepak L. Bhatt, Scott D. Solomon 由北京大学医学出版社进行改编影印，并根据北京大学医学出版社与爱思唯尔（新加坡）私人有限公司的协议约定出版。

ISBN: 978-7-5659-2805-5
Copyright © 2023 by Elsevier (Singapore) Pte Ltd. and Peking University Medical Press.
All rights reserved. No part of this publication may be reproduced or transmitted in any form or by any means, electronic or mechanical, including photocopying, recording, or any information storage and retrieval system, without permission in writing from Elsevier (Singapore) Pte Ltd. and Peking University Medical Press.
Online resources are not available with this adaptation. 本书不包含英文原版配套电子资源。

Notice
The adaptation has been undertaken by Peking University Medical Press at its sole responsibility. Practitioners and researchers must always rely on their own experience and knowledge in evaluating and using any information, methods, compounds or experiments described herein. Because of rapid advances in the medical sciences, in particular, independent verification of diagnoses and drug dosages should be made. To the fullest extent of the law, no responsibility is assumed by Elsevier, authors, editors or contributors in relation to the adaptation or for any injury and/or damage to persons or property as a matter of products liability, negligence or otherwise, or from any use or operation of any methods, products, instructions, or ideas contained in the material herein.

Published in China by Peking University Medical Press under special arrangement with Elsevier (Singapore) Pte Ltd. This edition is authorized for sale in the People's Republic of China only, excluding Hong Kong SAR, Macau SAR and Taiwan. Unauthorized export of this edition is a violation of the contract.

Braunwald 心脏病学（第 12 版）（影印中文导读版）（下册）

原　　著：Peter Libby　Robert O. Bonow　Douglas L. Mann　Gordon F. Tomaselli　Deepak L. Bhatt　Scott D. Solomon
出版发行：北京大学医学出版社
地　　址：（100191）北京市海淀区学院路 38 号　北京大学医学部院内
电　　话：发行部 010-82802230；图书邮购 010-82802495
网　　址：http://www.pumpress.com.cn
E - m a i l：booksale@bjmu.edu.cn
印　　刷：北京信彩瑞禾印刷厂
经　　销：新华书店
责任编辑：高　瑾　　责任校对：靳新强　　责任印制：李　啸
开　　本：889 mm×1194 mm　1/16　印张：127.75　字数：4100 千字
版　　次：2023 年 3 月第 1 版　2023 年 3 月第 1 次印刷
书　　号：ISBN 978-7-5659-2805-5
定　　价：980.00 元（上下册）
版权所有，违者必究
（凡属质量问题请与本社发行部联系退换）

BRAUNWALD 心脏病学
第 12 版（影印中文导读版）
编审委员会

编审委员会顾问专家

高润霖　　中国医学科学院阜外医院

编审委员会主任委员

吴永健　　中国医学科学院阜外医院
张　健　　中国医学科学院阜外医院
姚　焰　　中国医学科学院阜外医院

编审委员会副主任委员

蒋雄京　　中国医学科学院阜外医院
柳志红　　中国医学科学院阜外医院
唐熠达　　北京大学第三医院
杨　清　　天津医科大学总医院
程　翔　　华中科技大学同济医学院附属协和医院
陶　凌　　空军军医大学西京医院
李　悦　　哈尔滨医科大学附属第一医院
张　力　　上海交通大学医学院附属新华医院

编审委员会委员

吴永健　　中国医学科学院阜外医院
王　媛　　首都医科大学附属北京友谊医院
武德崴　　首都医科大学宣武医院
张丽华　　中国医学科学院阜外医院
王宇彬　　首都医科大学宣武医院
王彬成　　中国医学科学院阜外医院
王墨扬　　中国医学科学院阜外医院
牛冠男　　中国医学科学院阜外医院

周　政　　中国医学科学院阜外医院
陈　阳　　中国医学科学院阜外医院
丰德京　　中国医学科学院阜外医院
张宇轩　　中国医学科学院阜外医院
张　健　　**中国医学科学院阜外医院**
贺春晖　　中国医学科学院阜外医院
冉　君　　中国医学科学院阜外医院
靳晓萌　　中国医学科学院阜外医院
李心晴　　中国医学科学院阜外医院
齐　晨　　中国医学科学院阜外医院
辛桉燃　　中国医学科学院阜外医院
陈安天　　中国医学科学院阜外医院
姚　焰　　**中国医学科学院阜外医院**
吴灵敏　　中国医学科学院阜外医院
张筑欣　　中国医学科学院阜外医院
范思洋　　首都医科大学附属北京朝阳医院
李　乐　　中国医学科学院阜外医院
杜忠鹏　　中国医学科学院阜外医院深圳医院
李晓飞　　中国医学科学院阜外医院
蒋雄京　　**中国医学科学院阜外医院**
董　徽　　中国医学科学院阜外医院
李弘武　　中国医学科学院阜外医院
柳志红　　**中国医学科学院阜外医院**
赵　青　　中国医学科学院阜外医院
胡美曦　　中国医学科学院阜外医院
罗　勤　　中国医学科学院阜外医院
高璐阳　　中国医学科学院阜外医院
张　毅　　中国医学科学院阜外医院
章思铖　　中国医学科学院阜外医院
赵智慧　　中国医学科学院阜外医院
李　欣　　中国医学科学院阜外医院
段安琪　　中国医学科学院阜外医院
黄志华　　中国医学科学院阜外医院
唐熠达　　**北京大学第三医院**
汪京嘉　　北京大学第三医院

温　军　　　北京大学第三医院
张　阔　　　北京大学第三医院
王远耕硕　　北京大学第三医院
王旭梁　　　北京大学第三医院
孟祥彬　　　北京大学第三医院
王文尧　　　北京大学第三医院
李　晨　　　北京大学第三医院
郑一天　　　北京大学第三医院
杨　杰　　　北京大学第三医院
祁　雨　　　北京大学第三医院
郑济林　　　北京大学第三医院
曹宝山　　　北京大学第三医院
高　峻　　　北京大学第三医院
宋璟景　　　北京大学第三医院
任佳梦　　　北京大学第三医院

杨　清　　　天津医科大学总医院
周　欣　　　天津医科大学总医院
孙蓬飞　　　天津医科大学总医院
韩　旭　　　天津医科大学总医院
陶西西　　　天津医科大学总医院
孙浩楠　　　天津医科大学总医院
吴肇贵　　　天津医科大学总医院
李　晟　　　天津医科大学总医院
陈晓智　　　天津医科大学总医院
刘文楠　　　天津医科大学总医院
李　治　　　天津医科大学总医院
王卓群　　　天津医科大学总医院
宋习文　　　天津医科大学总医院
裴崇哲　　　天津医科大学总医院

程　翔　　　华中科技大学同济医学院附属协和医院
卢玉枝　　　华中科技大学同济医学院附属协和医院
苏冠华　　　华中科技大学同济医学院附属协和医院
王　亚　　　华中科技大学同济医学院附属协和医院
江　颖　　　华中科技大学同济医学院附属协和医院
张凌雪　　　华中科技大学同济医学院附属协和医院

陈　儒　　华中科技大学同济医学院附属协和医院
余刘玉　　华中科技大学同济医学院附属协和医院
杨　芬　　华中科技大学同济医学院附属协和医院
毛小香　　华中科技大学同济医学院附属协和医院
潘雅杰　　华中科技大学同济医学院附属协和医院
黄丹丹　　华中科技大学同济医学院附属协和医院

陶　凌　　空军军医大学西京医院
王汝涛　　空军军医大学西京医院

李　悦　　哈尔滨医科大学附属第一医院
曹宇开　　哈尔滨医科大学附属第一医院
洪　勇　　哈尔滨医科大学附属第一医院
高　强　　哈尔滨医科大学附属第一医院
虞　辉　　哈尔滨医科大学附属第一医院

张　力　　上海交通大学医学院附属新华医院
徐肖磊　　上海交通大学医学院附属新华医院

原著者名单

Keith D. Aaronson, MD, MS
Bertram Pitt MD Collegiate Professor of Cardiovascular Medicine
Professor of Internal Medicine
Division of Cardiovascular Medicine
University of Michigan
Ann Arbor, Michigan
Chapter 59. Mechanical Circulatory Support

Michael J. Ackerman, MD, PhD
Windland Smith Rice Cardiovascular Genomics Research Professor
Professor of Medicine, Pediatrics, and Pharmacology
Mayo Clinic College of Medicine and Science
Department of Cardiovascular Medicine (Division of Heart Rhythm Services and the Windland Smith Rice Genetic Heart Rhythm Clinic)
Department of Molecular Pharmacology & Experimental Therapeutics (Windland Smith Rice Sudden Death Genomics Laboratory)
Department of Pediatric and Adolescent Medicine (Division of Pediatric Cardiology)
Mayo Clinic
Rochester, Minnesota
Chapter 63. Genetics of Cardiac Arrhythmias

Philip A. Ades, MD
Endowed Professor of Medicine
Division of Cardiology
University of Vermont College of Medicine
Director, Cardiac Rehabilitation and Prevention
University of Vermont Medical Center
Burlington, Vermont
Chapter 15. Exercise Physiology and Exercise Electrocardiographic Testing

Christine M. Albert, MD
Chair and Professor of Cardiology
Smidt Heart Institute, Cedars-Sinai Medical Center
Los Angeles, California
Chapter 70. Cardiac Arrest and Sudden Cardiac Death

Michelle A. Albert, MD, MPH
Professor of Medicine
Director, Center for the Study of Adversity and Cardiovascular Disease (NURTURE Center)
University of California at San Francisco
San Francisco, California
Chapter 93. Heart Disease in Racially and Ethnically Diverse Populations

Mark J. Alberts, MD
Chief of Neurology
Hartford Hospital
Hartford, Connecticut;
Co-Physician-in-Chief
Ayer Neuroscience Institute
Hartford HealthCare
Professor of Neurology
University of Connecticut
Storrs, Connecticut
Chapter 45. Prevention and Management of Ischemic Stroke

Sadeer Al-Kindi, MD
Assistant Professor of Medicine
Case Western Reserve University
Harrington Heart and Vascular Institute
University Hospitals Cleveland Medical Center
Cleveland, Ohio
Chapter 3. Impact of the Environment on Cardiovascular Health

Nandan S. Anavekar, MBBCh
Professor of Medicine
Department of Cardiovascular Diseases
Department of Radiology
Mayo Clinic College of Medicine and Science
Rochester, Minnesota
Chapter 80. Infectious Endocarditis and Infections of Indwelling Devices

Zachi Attia, PhD
Department of Cardiovascular Medicine
Mayo Clinic College of Medicine and Science
Rochester, Minnesota
Chapter 11. Artificial Intelligence in Cardiovascular Medicine

Sonya V. Babu-Narayan, MBBS, BSc, PhD, FRCP
Adult Congenital Heart Disease
Royal Brompton Hospital
Reader, National Heart and Lung Institute
Imperial College London
London, United Kingdom
Chapter 82. Congenital Heart Disease in the Adolescent and Adult

Larry M. Baddour, MD
Professor of Medicine
Mayo Clinic College of Medicine and Science
Rochester, Minnesota
Chapter 80. Infectious Endocarditis and Infections of Indwelling Devices

Aaron L. Baggish, MD
Associate Professor of Medicine
Harvard Medical School
Director, Cardiovascular Performance Program
Massachusetts General Hospital
Boston, Massachusetts
Chapter 32. Exercise and Sports Cardiology

C. Noel Bairey Merz, MD
Women's Guild Endowed Chair in Women's Health
Director, Barbra Streisand Women's Heart Center
Erika J. Glazer Women's Heart Research Initiative Director
Director, Linda Joy Pollin Women's Heart Health Program
Barbra Streisand Women's Heart Center
Cedars-Sinai Heart Institute
Los Angeles, California
Chapter 91. Cardiovascular Disease in Women

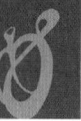

George L. Bakris, MD, MA
Professor of Medicine
Section of Endocrinology, Diabetes and Metabolism
Director, American Heart Association Comprehensive Hypertension Center
UChicago Medicine
Chicago, Illinois
Chapter 26. Systemic Hypertension: Mechanisms, Diagnosis, and Treatment

Gary J. Balady, MD
Professor of Medicine
Boston University School of Medicine
Director, Non-Invasive Cardiovascular Laboratories
Boston Medical Center
Boston, Massachusetts
Chapter 15. Exercise Physiology and Exercise Electrocardiographic Testing

David T. Balzer, MD
Professor of Pediatrics
Division of Pediatric Cardiology
Washington University School of Medicine in St. Louis
Saint Louis, Missouri
Chapter 83. Catheter-Based Treatment of Congenital Heart Disease in Adults

Joshua A. Beckman, MD
Professor of Medicine
Division of Cardiovascular Medicine
Vanderbilt University College of Medicine
Director, Section of Vascular Medicine
Vanderbilt University Medical Center
Nashville, Tennessee
Chapter 23. Anesthesia and Noncardiac Surgery in Patients with Heart Disease

Donald M. Bers, PhD
Distinguished Professor and Chair
Department of Pharmacology
University of California, Davis
Davis, California
Chapter 46. Mechanisms of Cardiac Contraction and Relaxation

Aruni Bhatnagar, PhD
Professor of Medicine
University of Louisville
Louisville, Kentucky
Chapter 28. Cardiovascular Disease Risk of Nicotine and Tobacco Products

Deepak L. Bhatt, MD, MPH
Executive Director of Interventional Cardiovascular Programs
Brigham and Women's Hospital
Senior Physician
Brigham and Women's Hospital
Professor of Medicine
Harvard Medical School
Boston, Massachusetts
Chapter 41. Percutaneous Coronary Intervention
Chapter 44. Treatment of Noncoronary Obstructive Vascular Disease

Bernadette Biondi, MD
Professor of Internal Medicine
Department of Clinical Medicine and Surgery
Federico II University
Naples, Italy
Chapter 96. Endocrine Disorders and Cardiovascular Disease

Ron Blankstein, MD
Associate Director, Cardiovascular Imaging Program
Director, Cardiac Computed Tomography
Co-Director, Cardiovascular Imaging Training Program
Brigham and Women's Hospital
Professor of Medicine and Radiology
Harvard Medical School
Boston, Massachusetts
Chapter 20. Cardiac Computed Tomography

Erin A. Bohula, MD, DPhil
TIMI Study Group and Division of Cardiology
Brigham and Women's Hospital
Harvard Medical School
Boston, Massachusetts
Chapter 38. ST-Elevation Myocardial Infarction: Management

Marc P. Bonaca, MD, MPH
Executive Director
CPC Clinical Research
Professor of Medicine
Cardiology and Vascular Medicine
University of Colorado
Aurora, Colorado
Chapter 35. Approach to the Patient with Chest Pain
Chapter 43. Peripheral Artery Diseases

Robert O. Bonow, MD
Max and Lilly Goldberg Distinguished Professor of Cardiology
Department of Medicine
Northwestern University Feinberg School of Medicine
Chicago, Illinois
Chapter 72. Aortic Valve Stenosis
Chapter 73. Aortic Regurgitation
Chapter 76. Mitral Regurgitation

Barry A. Borlaug, MD
Professor of Medicine
Mayo Medical School
Director, Circulatory Failure Research
Consultant, Cardiovascular Diseases
Mayo Clinic College of Medicine and Science
Rochester, Minnesota
Chapter 46. Mechanisms of Cardiac Contraction and Relaxation

Jason S. Bradfield, MD
Associate Professor of Medicine
Director, Specialized Program for Ventricular Tachycardia
UCLA Cardiac Arrhythmia Center
Ronald Reagan UCLA Medical Center
Los Angeles, California
Chapter 102. Cardiovascular Manifestations of Autonomic Disorders

Eugene Braunwald, MD, MD(Hon), ScD(Hon), FRCP
Distinguished Hersey Professor of Medicine
Harvard Medical School
Founding Chairman, TIMI Study Group
Brigham and Women's Hospital
Boston, Massachusetts
Chapter 1. Cardiovascular Disease: Past, Present, and Future
Chapter 39. Non-ST Elevation Acute Coronary Syndromes

Alan C. Braverman, MD
Alumni Endowed Professor in Cardiovascular Diseases
Director, Marfan Syndrome and Aortopathy Clinic
Washington University School of Medicine in St. Louis
Director, Inpatient Cardiology Firm
Barnes-Jewish Hospital
Saint Louis, Missouri
Chapter 42. Diseases of the Aorta

John E. Brush Jr., MD
Senior Medical Director
Sentara Health Research Center
Sentara Healthcare
Professor of Medicine
Department of Internal Medicine
Eastern Virginia Medical School
Norfolk, Virginia
Chapter 5. Clinical Decision-Making in Cardiology

Hugh Calkins, MD
Catherine Ellen Poindexter Professor of Cardiology
Professor of Medicine
Director, Cardiac Arrhythmia Service
The Johns Hopkins Medical Institutions
Baltimore, Maryland
Chapter 66. Atrial Fibrillation: Clinical Features, Mechanisms, and Management
Chapter 71. Hypotension and Syncope

John M. Canty Jr., MD
SUNY Distinguished and Albert and Elizabeth Rekate Professor of Medicine
Division of Cardiovascular Medicine
Jacobs School of Medicine and Biomedical Sciences
University at Buffalo
Buffalo, New York
Chapter 36. Coronary Blood Flow and Myocardial Ischemia

Robert M. Carney, PhD
Professor of Psychiatry
Washington University School of Medicine in St. Louis
Saint Louis, Missouri
Chapter 99. Psychiatric and Psychosocial Aspects of Cardiovascular Disease

Y.S. Chandrashekhar, MD
Professor of Medicine
Division of Cardiology
University of Minnesota
Chief of Cardiology
VA Medical Center
Minneapolis, Minnesota
Chapter 75. Mitral Stenosis

Peng-Shen Chen, MD
Cedars-Sinai Medical Center
Los Angeles, California
Chapter 71. Hypotension and Syncope

Mina K. Chung, MD
Professor of Medicine
Cardiovascular and Metabolic Sciences
Lerner Research Institute
Cleveland Clinic Lerner College of Medicine of Case Western Reserve University
Staff, Cardiovascular Medicine
Cleveland Clinic
Cleveland, Ohio
Chapter 69. Pacemakers and Implantable Cardioverter-Defibrillators

Leslie T. Cooper Jr., MD
Professor of Medicine
Chair, Department of Vascular Medicine
Mayo Clinic
Jacksonville, Florida
Chapter 55. Myocarditis

Mark A. Creager, MD
Professor of Medicine and Surgery
Geisel School of Medicine at Dartmouth
Hanover, New Hampshire;
Director, Heart and Vascular Center
Heart and Vascular Center
Dartmouth-Hitchcock Medical Center
Lebanon, New Hampshire
Chapter 43. Peripheral Artery Diseases

Paul C. Cremer, MD
Assistant Professor of Medicine
Cleveland Clinic Lerner College of Medicine of Case Western Reserve University
Associate Director of Cardiovascular Training Program
Cleveland Clinic Foundation
Cleveland Clinic
Cleveland, Ohio
Chapter 86. Pericardial Diseases

Juan A. Crestanello, MD
Professor of Surgery
Mayo Clinic College of Medicine and Science
Rochester, Minnesota
Chapter 80. Infectious Endocarditis and Infections of Indwelling Devices

Anne B. Curtis, MD
Charles and Mary Bauer Professor and Chair
SUNY Distinguished Professor
Department of Medicine
Jacobs School of Medicine and Biomedical Sciences
University at Buffalo
Buffalo, New York
Chapter 61. Approach to the Patient with Cardiac Arrhythmias

George D. Dangas, MD, PhD
Professor of Medicine (Cardiology)
Zena and Michael A Wiener Cardiovascular Institute
Icahn School of Medicine at Mount Sinai
New York, New York
Chapter 21. Coronary Angiography and Intravascular Imaging

James P. Daubert, MD
Professor of Medicine
Cardiology (Electrophysiology)
Duke University Medical Center
Durham, North Carolina
Chapter 69. Pacemakers and Implantable Cardioverter-Defibrillators

James A. de Lemos, MD
Professor of Medicine
Sweetheart Ball-Kern Wildenthal MD PhD Distinguished Chair in Cardiology
UT Southwestern Medical Center
Dallas, Texas
Chapter 40. Stable Ischemic Heart Disease

Jean-Pierre Després, PhD
Professor
Kinesiology Department
Université Laval
Scientific Director
VITAM – Centre de recherche en santé durable
Centre intégré universitaire de santé et de services sociaux de la Capitale-Nationale
Québec City, Québec, Canada
Chapter 30. Obesity: Medical and Surgical Management

Stephen Devries, MD
Executive Director
Gaples Institute for Integrative Cardiology
Deerfield, Illinois;
Division of Cardiology
Northwestern University Feinberg School of Medicine
Chicago, Illinois
Chapter 34. Integrative Approaches to the Management of Patients with Heart Disease

Marcelo F. Di Carli, MD
Seltzer Family Professor of Radiology and Medicine
Harvard Medical School
Executive Director, Cardiovascular Imaging Program
Chief, Division of Nuclear Medicine and Molecular Imaging
Brigham and Women's Hospital
Boston, Massachusetts
Chapter 18. Nuclear Cardiology

Sharmila Dorbala, MD, MPH
Professor of Radiology
Harvard Medical School
Director, Nuclear Cardiology
Division of Nuclear Medicine and Molecular Imaging
Brigham and Women's Hospital
Boston, Massachusetts
Chapter 18. Nuclear Cardiology

Adam L. Dorfman, MD
Professor
Departments of Pediatrics and Radiology
Director, Non-Invasive Imaging, Division of Pediatric Cardiology
University of Michigan Medical School
C.S. Mott Children's Hospital
Ann Arbor, Michigan
Chapter 82. Congenital Heart Disease in the Adolescent and Adult

Dirk J. Duncker, MD, PhD
Professor of Experimental Cardiology
Department of Cardiology
Erasmus MC, University Medical Center Rotterdam
Rotterdam, The Netherlands
Chapter 36. Coronary Blood Flow and Myocardial Ischemia

Kenneth A. Ellenbogen, MD
Martha M. and Harold W. Kimmerling Professor of Cardiology
Director, Electrophysiology and Pacing
Virginia Commonwealth University School of Medicine
Richmond, Virginia
Chapter 64. Therapy for Cardiac Arrhythmias

Thomas H. Everett IV, PhD
Associate Professor of Medicine
The Krannert Institute of Cardiology and Division of Cardiology
Indiana University School of Medicine
Indianapolis, Indiana
Chapter 71. Hypotension and Syncope

James C. Fang, MD
Professor of Medicine
Division of Cardiovascular Medicine
University of Utah
Executive Director, Cardiovascular Service Line
University of Utah Health Sciences
Salt Lake City, Utah
Chapter 13. History and Physical Examination: An Evidence-Based Approach

G. Michael Felker, MD, MHS
Professor of Medicine
Vice Chief for Clinical Research
Division of Cardiology
Duke University School of Medicine
Director, Cardiovascular Research
Duke Clinical Research Institute
Durham, North Carolina
Chapter 49. Diagnosis and Management of Acute Heart Failure

Jerome L. Fleg, MD
Medical Officer
Division of Cardiovascular Sciences
National Heart, Lung, and Blood Institute
Bethesda, Maryland
Chapter 90. Cardiovascular Disease in Older Adults

Lee A. Fleisher, MD
Professor
Anesthesiology and Critical Care
Professor of Medicine
University of Pennsylvania Perelman School of Medicine
Philadelphia, Pennsylvania
Chapter 23. Anesthesia and Noncardiac Surgery in Patients with Heart Disease

Daniel E. Forman, MD
Professor of Medicine
University of Pittsburgh
Chair, Section of Geriatric Cardiology
Divisions of Geriatrics and Cardiology
University of Pittsburgh Medical Center
Director, Cardiac Rehabilitation
VA Pittsburgh Healthcare System
Pittsburgh, Pennsylvania
Chapter 90. Cardiovascular Disease in Older Adults

Kenneth E. Freedland, PhD
Professor of Psychiatry
Washington University School of Medicine in St. Louis
Saint Louis, Missouri
Chapter 99. Psychiatric and Psychosocial Aspects of Cardiovascular Disease

Paul Friedman, MD
Norman Blane & Billie Jean Harty Chair
Mayo Clinic Department of Cardiovascular Medicine Honoring Robert L. Frye, MD
Professor of Medicine
Mayo Clinic College of Medicine and Science
Rochester, Minnesota
Chapter 11. Artificial Intelligence in Cardiovascular Medicine

J. Michael Gaziano, MD, MPH
Professor of Medicine
Harvard Medical School
Chief, Division of Aging
Brigham and Women's Hospital
Director, Preventive Cardiology
VA Boston Healthcare System
Boston, Massachusetts
Chapter 2. Global Burden of Cardiovascular Disease

Thomas A. Gaziano, MD, MSc
Associate Professor
Harvard Medical School
Physician
Cardiovascular Medicine Division
Brigham & Women's Hospital
Boston, Massachusetts
Chapter 2. Global Burden of Cardiovascular Disease

Jacques Genest, MD
Professor of Medicine
Faculty of Medicine
McGill University
Research Institute of the McGill University Health Centre
Montreal, Quebec, Canada
Chapter 27. Lipoprotein Disorders and Cardiovascular Disease

Robert Gerszten, MD
Herman Dana Professor of Medicine
Harvard Medical School
Chief, Division of Cardiovascular Medicine
Beth Israel Deaconess Medical Center
Boston, Massachusetts
Chapter 8. Proteomics and Metabolomics in Cardiovascular Medicine

Linda D. Gillam, MD, MPH
Dorothy and Lloyd Huck Chair
Department of Cardiovascular Medicine
Morristown Medical Center
Morristown, New Jersey;
Professor of Medicine
Thomas Jefferson University
Philadelphia, Pennsylvania
Chapter 16. Echocardiography

John R. Giudicessi, MD, PhD
Assistant Professor of Medicine
Department of Cardiovascular Medicine (Division of Heart Rhythm Services and the Windland Smith Rice Genetic Heart Rhythm Clinic)
Mayo Clinic College of Medicine and Science
Rochester, Minnesota
Chapter 63. Genetics of Cardiac Arrhythmias

Robert P. Giugliano, MD, SM
Staff Physician
Cardiovascular Medicine
Brigham and Women's Hospital
Professor of Medicine
Harvard Medical School
Boston, Massachusetts
Chapter 39. Non-ST Elevation Acute Coronary Syndromes

Ary L. Goldberger, MD
Professor of Medicine
Harvard Medical School
Department of Medicine
Beth Israel Deaconess Medical Center
Boston, Massachusetts
Chapter 14. Electrocardiography

Jeffrey J. Goldberger, MD, MBA
Professor of Medicine
Chief, Cardiovascular Division
University of Miami Miller School of Medicine
Miami, Florida
Chapter 70. Cardiac Arrest and Sudden Cardiac Death

Samuel Z. Goldhaber, MD
Professor of Medicine
Harvard Medical School
Director, Thrombosis Research Group
Associate Chief and Clinical Director
Division of Cardiovascular Medicine
Brigham and Women's Hospital
Boston, Massachusetts
Chapter 87. Pulmonary Embolism and Deep Vein Thrombosis

William J. Groh, MD, MPH
Clinical Professor of Medicine
Medical University of South Carolina
Chief of Medicine
Ralph H. Johnson VAMC
Charleston, South Carolina
Chapter 100. Neuromuscular Disorders and Cardiovascular Disease

Martha Gulati, MD, MS
Chief of Cardiology
Professor of Medicine
University of Arizona–Phoenix
Phoenix, Arizona
Chapter 91. Cardiovascular Disease in Women

Rebecca Tung Hahn, MD
Director of Interventional Echocardiography
Center for Interventional and Vascular Therapy
Columbia University Medical Center
New York, New York
Chapter 76. Mitral Regurgitation

Gerd Hasenfuss, MD
Professor of Medicine
Chair, Department of Cardiology and Pneumology
University of Göttingen Medical Center
Göttingen, Germany
Chapter 47. Pathophysiology of Heart Failure

Howard C. Herrmann, MD
John W. Bryfogle Jr. Professor of Cardiovascular Medicine
Division of Cardiovascular Medicine
University of Pennsylvania Perelman School of Medicine
Health System Director for Interventional Cardiology
Hospital of the University of Pennsylvania
Philadelphia, Pennsylvania
Chapter 78. Transcatheter Therapies for Mitral and Tricuspid Valvular Heart Disease

Joerg Herrmann, MD
Professor of Medicine
Department of Cardiovascular Medicine
Mayo Clinic
Rochester, Minnesota
Chapter 22. Invasive Hemodynamic Diagnosis of Cardiac Disease
Chapter 57. Cardio-Oncology: Approach to the Patient

Ray E. Hershberger, MD
Professor of Internal Medicine
Director, Division of Human Genetics
Division of Cardiovascular Medicine
Section of Heart Failure and Cardiac Transplantation
Dorothy M. Davis Heart and Lung Research Institute
Wexner Medical Center at the Ohio State University
Columbus, Ohio
Chapter 52. The Dilated, Restrictive, and Infiltrative Cardiomyopathies

Carolyn Y. Ho, MD
Associate Professor of Medicine
Cardiovascular Division
Brigham and Women's Hospital
Boston, Massachusetts
Chapter 54. Hypertrophic Cardiomyopathy

Priscilla Y. Hsue, MD
Professor
Department of Medicine
University of California, San Francisco
San Francisco, California
Chapter 85. Cardiovascular Abnormalities in HIV-Infected Individuals

W. Gregory Hundley, MD
Professor of Medicine
Chairman, Cardiology Division
VCU School of Medicine
Director, Pauley Heart Center
Virginia Commonwealth University Health
Richmond, Virginia
Chapter 98. Tumors Affecting the Cardiovascular System

Silvio E. Inzucchi, MD
Professor, Internal Medicine (Endocrinology)
Yale University School of Medicine
Clinical Chief, Endocrinology
Director, Yale Diabetes Center
Yale-New Haven Hospital
New Haven, Connecticut
Chapter 31. Diabetes and the Cardiovascular System

Francine L. Jacobson, MD, MPH
Thoracic Radiologist
Brigham and Women's Hospital
Harvard Medical School
Boston, Massachusetts
Chapter 17. Chest Radiography in Cardiovascular Disease

James L. Januzzi Jr., MD
Physician
Cardiology Division
Massachusetts General Hospital
Hutter Family Professor of Medicine
Harvard Medical School
Boston, Massachusetts
Chapter 48. Approach to the Patient with Heart Failure

Karen E. Joynt Maddox, MD, MPH
Associate Professor of Medicine
Cardiovascular Division
Washington University School of Medicine in St. Louis
Co-Director, Center for Health Economics and Policy
Institute for Public Health at Washington University
Saint Louis, Missouri
Chapter 6. Impact of Health Care Policy on Quality, Outcomes, and Equity in Cardiovascular Disease

Jonathan M. Kalman, MBBS, PhD
Director of Cardiac Electrophysiology
Department of Cardiology
Royal Melbourne Hospital, Melbourne
Professor of Medicine
University of Melbourne
Melbourne, Victoria, Australia
Chapter 65. Supraventricular Tachycardias

Suraj Kapa, MD
Assistant Professor of Medicine
Cardiovascular Diseases
Mayo Clinic College of Medicine and Science
Rochester, Minnesota
Chapter 11. Artificial Intelligence in Cardiovascular Medicine

Morton J. Kern, MD
Professor of Medicine
University California, Irvine
Orange, California;
Chief of Medicine and Cardiology
Veterans Administration Long Beach Healthcare System
Long Beach, California
Chapter 22. Invasive Hemodynamic Diagnosis of Cardiac Disease

Scott Kinlay, MBBS, PhD
Chief, Cardiology (acting)
Director Cardiac Catheterization Laboratory and Vascular Medicine
VA Boston Healthcare System
West Roxbury, Massachusetts
Physician, Cardiovascular Division
Brigham and Women's Hospital
Associate Professor in Medicine
Harvard Medical School
Adjunct Associate Professor in Medicine
Boston University Medical School
Boston, Massachusetts
Chapter 44. Treatment of Noncoronary Obstructive Vascular Disease

Allan L. Klein, MD, FRCP(C)
Professor of Medicine
Cleveland Clinic Lerner College of Medicine of Case Western Reserve University
Director, Center for the Diagnosis and Treatment of Pericardial Diseases
Department of Cardiovascular Medicine
Heart, Vascular and Thoracic Institute
Cleveland Clinic
Cleveland, Ohio
Chapter 86. Pericardial Diseases

Robert A. Kloner, MD, PhD
Professor of Medicine (Clinical Scholar)
Cardiovascular Division
Keck School of Medicine of University of Southern California
Los Angeles, California;
Chief Science Officer
Scientific Director of Cardiovascular Research Institute
Huntington Medical Research Institutes
Pasadena, California
Chapter 84. Cardiomyopathies Induced by Drugs or Toxins

Kirk U. Knowlton, MD
Director of Cardiovascular Research
Intermountain Healthcare Heart Institute
Adjunct Professor
Department of Medicine
University of Utah
Salt Lake City, Utah;
Professor Emeritus of Medicine
University of California, San Diego
La Jolla, California
Chapter 55. Myocarditis

Eric V. Krieger, MD
Professor of Medicine
Division of Cardiology
University of Washington School of Medicine
Director, Adult Congenital Heart Service
University of Washington Medical Center
Seattle Children's Hospital
Seattle, Washington
Chapter 82. Congenital Heart Disease in the Adolescent and Adult

Harlan M. Krumholz, MD, SM
Harold H. Hines, Jr. Professor of Medicine
Section of Cardiovascular Medicine
Department of Medicine
Department of Health Policy and Management
School of Public Health
Yale School of Medicine
Center for Outcomes Research and Evaluation
Yale New Haven Hospital
New Haven, Connecticut
Chapter 5. Clinical Decision-Making in Cardiology

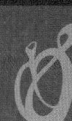

Dharam J. Kumbhani, MD, SM
Associate Professor of Medicine
Section Chief, Interventional Cardiology
Department of Internal Medicine
University of Texas Southwestern Medical Center
Dallas, Texas
Chapter 41. Percutaneous Coronary Intervention

Raymond Y. Kwong, MD, MPH
Professor of Medicine
Harvard Medical School
Director of Cardiac Magnetic Resonance Imaging
Cardiovascular Division
Brigham and Women's Hospital
Boston, Massachusetts
Chapter 19. Cardiovascular Magnetic Resonance Imaging

Bonnie Ky, MD, MSCE
Associate Professor of Medicine and Epidemiology
Division of Cardiovascular Medicine
Senior Scholar
Department of Biostatistics, Epidemiology and Informatics
University of Pennsylvania School of Medicine
Philadelphia, Pennsylvania
Chapter 56. Cardio-Oncology: Managing Cardiotoxic Effects of Cancer Therapies

Carolyn S.P. Lam, MBBS, PhD, MRCP, MS
Professor
Cardiovascular Academic Clinical Program
Duke–National University of Singapore
Senior Consultant Cardiologist
National Heart Centre Singapore
Singapore
Chapter 51. Heart Failure with Preserved and Mildly Reduced Ejection Fraction

Eric Larose, DVM, MD, FRCPC
Professor and Head of Cardiology Division
Department of Medicine
Chair of Research & Innovation in Cardiovascular Imaging
Université Laval
Cardiologist, Institut universitaire de cardiologie et de pneumologie de Québec – Université Laval
Quebec City, Quebec, Canada
Chapter 30. Obesity: Medical and Surgical Management

John M. Lasala, MD, PhD
Professor of Medicine
Director, Structural Heart Disease Program
Cardiology Division
Washington University School of Medicine in St. Louis
Saint Louis, Missouri
Chapter 83. Catheter-Based Treatment of Congenital Heart Disease in Adults

Daniel J. Lenihan, MD
President, International Cardio-Oncology Society
Professor of Medicine
Director, Cardio-Oncology Center of Excellence
Cardiovascular Division
Washington University School of Medicine in St. Louis
Saint Louis, Missouri
Chapter 98. Tumors Affecting the Cardiovascular System

Eric J. Lenze, MD
Professor of Psychiatry
Washington University School of Medicine in St. Louis
Saint Louis, Missouri
Chapter 99. Psychiatric and Psychosocial Aspects of Cardiovascular Disease

Martin B. Leon, MD
The Mallah Family Professor of Cardiology
Director, Center for Interventional Vascular Therapy
Columbia University Irving Medical Center
NY Presbyterian Hospital
Founder and Chairman Emeritus
Cardiovascular Research Foundation
New York, New York
Chapter 74. Transcatheter Aortic Valve Replacement

Martin M. LeWinter, MD
Professor Emeritus of Medicine and Molecular Physiology and Biophysics
Larner College of Medicine at the University of Vermont
Attending Cardiologist
University of Vermont Medical Center
Burlington, Vermont
Chapter 86. Pericardial Diseases

Peter Libby, MD
Mallinckrodt Professor of Medicine
Harvard Medical School
Brigham and Women's Hospital
Boston, Massachusetts
Chapter 10. Biomarkers and Use in Precision Medicine
Chapter 24. The Vascular Biology of Atherosclerosis
Chapter 25. Primary Prevention of Cardiovascular Disease
Chapter 27. Lipoprotein Disorders and Cardiovascular Disease
Chapter 37. ST-Elevation Myocardial Infarction: Pathophysiology and Clinical Evolution

JoAnn Lindenfeld, MD
Professor of Medicine
Samuel S Riven MD Directorship in Cardiology
Vanderbilt University Medical Center
Nashville, Tennessee
Chapter 58. Devices for Monitoring and Managing Heart Failure

Brian R. Lindman, MD, MSc
Associate Professor of Medicine
Medical Director, Structural Heart and Valve Center
Cardiovascular Division
Vanderbilt University Medical Center
Nashville, Tennessee
Chapter 72. Aortic Valve Stenosis

Michael J. Mack, MD
Chair, Cardiovascular Service Line
Baylor Scott & White Health
President, Baylor Scott & White Research Institute
Dallas, Texas
Chapter 74. Transcatheter Aortic Valve Replacement

Mohammad Madjid, MD, MS
Associate Professor of Medicine
McGovern Medical School
University of Texas Health Science Center at Houston
Interventional Cardiologist
Heart and Vascular Institute
Memorial Hermann Hospital
Houston, Texas
Chapter 94. Endemic and Pandemic Viral Illnesses and Cardiovascular Disease: Influenza and COVID-19

Douglas L. Mann, MD
Lewin Distinguished Professor of Cardiovascular Disease
Washington University School of Medicine
Saint Louis, Missouri
Chapter 47. Pathophysiology of Heart Failure
Chapter 48. Approach to the Patient With Heart Failure
Chapter 50. Management of Heart Failure Patients with Reduced Ejection Fraction

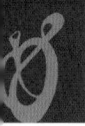

Bradley A. Maron, MD
Associate Professor of Medicine
Division of Cardiovascular Medicine
Brigham and Women's Hospital
Harvard Medical School
Department of Cardiology
Boston VA Healthcare System
Boston, Massachusetts
Chapter 88. Pulmonary Hypertension

Nikolaus Marx, MD
Professor of Medicine / Cardiology
Head of the Department of Internal Medicine I
University Hospital Aachen
Aachen, Germany
Chapter 31. Diabetes and the Cardiovascular System

Justin C. Mason, PhD, FRCP
Professor of Vascular Rheumatology
Vascular Sciences and Rheumatology
Imperial College London
London, United Kingdom
Chapter 97. Rheumatic Diseases and the Cardiovascular System

Mathew S. Maurer, MD
Arnold and Arlene Goldstein Professor of Cardiology
Professor of Medicine
Columbia University College of Physicians and Surgeons
Center for Advanced Cardiac Care
Columbia University Medical Center
Director, Clinical Cardiovascular Research Laboratory for the Elderly
New York, New York
Chapter 53. Cardiac Amyloidosis

Peter A. McCullough, MD, MPH
Consultant Cardiologist
Clinical Professor of Medicine
Department of Internal Medicine
Texas A&M College of Medicine
Dallas, Texas
Chapter 101. Interface Between Renal Disease and Cardiovascular Illness

Darren K. McGuire, MD, MHSc
Professor, Internal Medicine
Division of Cardiology
University of Texas Southwestern Medical Center
Dallas, Texas
Chapter 31. Diabetes and the Cardiovascular System

John McMurray, OBE BSc (Hons), MB ChB (Hons), MD, FRCP
Professor of Medical Cardiology
Deputy-Director (Clinical), Institute of Cardiovascular and Medical Sciences
BHF Cardiovascular Research Centre
University of Glasgow
Honorary Consultant Cardiologist
Queen Elizabeth University Hospital
Glasgow, Scotland, United Kingdom
Chapter 4. Clinical Trials in Cardiovascular Medicine

Elizabeth M. McNally, MD, PhD
Director, Center for Genetic Medicine
Northwestern University Feinberg School of Medicine
Chicago, Illinois
Chapter 100. Neuromuscular Disorders and Cardiovascular Disease

Roxana Mehran, MD
Professor of Medicine (Cardiology)
Director of Interventional Cardiovascular Research and Clinical Trials
Zena and Michael A. Wiener Cardiovascular Institute
Icahn School of Medicine at Mount Sinai
New York, New York
Chapter 21. Coronary Angiography and Intravascular Imaging

John M. Miller, MD
Professor of Medicine
Indiana University School of Medicine
Director, Cardiac Electrophysiology Services
Indiana University Health
Indianapolis, Indiana
Chapter 64. Therapy for Cardiac Arrhythmias

David M. Mirvis, MD
Professor Emeritus
Preventive Medicine
University of Tennessee College of Medicine
Memphis, Tennessee
Chapter 14. Electrocardiography

Ana Olga Mocumbi, MD, PhD
Associate Professor
Internal Medicine
Universidade Eduardo Mondlane
Head of Division
Non Communicable Diseases
Instituto Nacional de Saúde
Maputo, Mozambique
Chapter 81. Rheumatic Fever

Samia Mora, MD
Associate Professor of Medicine
Harvard Medical School
Associate Physician
Brigham and Women's Hospital
Boston, Massachusetts
Chapter 25. Primary Prevention of Cardiovascular Disease
Chapter 27. Lipoprotein Disorders and Cardiovascular Disease

Fred Morady, MD
McKay Professor of Cardiovascular Disease
Department of Medicine
University of Michigan
Ann Arbor, Michigan
Chapter 66. Atrial Fibrillation: Clinical Features, Mechanisms, and Management

Alanna A. Morris, MD, MSc
Associate Professor of Medicine
Director, Heart Failure Research
Emory University School of Medicine
Atlanta, Georgia
Chapter 93. Heart Disease in Racially and Ethnically Diverse Populations

David A. Morrow, MD, MPH
Professor of Medicine
Harvard Medical School
Boston, Massachusetts
Chapter 37. ST-Elevation Myocardial Infarction: Pathophysiology and Clinical Evolution
Chapter 38. ST-Elevation Myocardial Infarction: Management
Chapter 40. Stable Ischemic Heart Disease

Dariush Mozaffarian, MD, DrPH
Dean, Friedman School of Nutrition Science & Policy
Jean Mayer Professor of Nutrition
Tufts University School of Medicine
Boston, Massachusetts
Chapter 29. Nutrition and Cardiovascular and Metabolic Diseases

Kiran Musunuru, MD, PhD, MPH, ML
Professor of Cardiovascular Medicine and Genetics
Cardiovascular Institute
University of Pennsylvania Perelman School of Medicine
Philadelphia, Pennsylvania
Chapter 7. Applications of Genetics to Cardiovascular Medicine

Robert J. Myerburg, MD
Professor of Medicine and Physiology
Department of Medicine
University of Miami Miller School of Medicine
Miami, Florida
Chapter 70. Cardiac Arrest and Sudden Cardiac Death

Pradeep Natarajan, MD, MMSc
Director of Preventive Cardiology
Massachusetts General Hospital
Assistant Professor of Medicine
Harvard Medical School
Boston, Massachusetts;
Associate Member
Program in Medical and Population Genetics
Broad Institute of Harvard and MIT
Cambridge, Massachusetts
Chapter 7. Applications of Genetics to Cardiovascular Medicine

Stanley Nattel, MDCM
Professor
Department of Medicine
Paul-David Chair in Cardiovascular Electrophysiology
Montreal Heart Institute
University of Montreal
Montreal, Quebec, Canada
Chapter 62. Mechanisms of Cardiac Arrhythmias

Rick A. Nishimura, MD
Judd and Mary Morris Leighton Professor of Cardiovascular Diseases
Department of Cardiovascular Medicine
Mayo Clinic College of Medicine and Science
Rochester, Minnesota
Chapter 73. Aortic Regurgitation

Vuyisile T. Nkomo, MD, MPH
Cardiologist
Professor of Medicine
Department of Cardiovascular Medicine
Mayo Clinic College of Medicine and Science
Rochester, Minnesota
Chapter 77. Tricuspid, Pulmonic, and Multivalvular Disease

Peter Noseworthy, MD
Consultant
Cardiovascular Diseases
Mayo Clinic College of Medicine and Science
Rochester, Minnesota
Chapter 11. Artificial Intelligence in Cardiovascular Medicine

Patrick T. O'Gara, MD
Professor of Medicine
Harvard Medical School
Senior Physician
Cardiovascular Division
Brigham and Women's Hospital
Boston, Massachusetts
Chapter 13. History and Physical Examination: An Evidence-Based Approach
Chapter 79. Prosthetic Heart Valves

Jeffrey E. Olgin, MD
Gallo-Chatterjee Distinguished Professor
Chief, Division of Cardiology
University of California, San Francisco
San Francisco, California
Chapter 68. Bradyarrhythmias and Atrioventricular Block

Steve R. Ommen, MD
Division of Cardiovascular Diseases
Mayo Clinic College of Medicine and Science
Rochester, Minnesota
Chapter 54. Hypertrophic Cardiomyopathy

Catherine M. Otto, MD
Professor of Medicine
J. Ward Kennedy-Hamilton Endowed Chair in Cardiology
Division of Cardiology
University of Washington School of Medicine
Director, Heart Valve Clinic
Associate Director, Echocardiography
University of Washington Medical Center
Seattle, Washington
Chapter 72. Aortic Valve Stenosis

Francis D. Pagani, MD, PhD
Otto Gago MD Endowed Professor of Cardiac Surgery
Department of Cardiac Surgery
University of Michigan
Ann Arbor, Michigan
Chapter 59. Mechanical Circulatory Support

Kristen K. Patton, MD
Professor of Medicine
Division of Cardiology
University of Washington
Seattle, Washington
Chapter 68. Bradyarrhythmias and Atrioventricular Block

Patricia A. Pellikka, MD
The Betty Knight Scripps Professor of Medicine
Mayo Clinic College of Medicine and Science
Vice Chair, Academic Affairs and Faculty Development
Consultant, Department of Cardiovascular Medicine
Director, Ultrasound Research Center
Mayo Clinic
Rochester, Minnesota
Chapter 77. Tricuspid, Pulmonic, and Multivalvular Disease

Gregory Piazza, MD, MS
Staff Physician
Cardiovascular Division
Department of Medicine
Section Head, Vascular Medicine
Brigham and Women's Hospital
Boston, Massachusetts
Chapter 87. Pulmonary Embolism and Deep Vein Thrombosis

Philippe Pibarot, DVM, PhD
Professor
Department of Medicine
Québec Heart & Lung Institute
Université Laval
Québec City, Quebec, Canada
Chapter 79. Prosthetic Heart Valves

Paul Poirier, MD, PhD, FRCPC
Chief, Cardiac Prevention/Rehabilitation
Institut universitaire de cardiologie et de pneumologie de Québec – Université Laval
Professor
Faculty of Pharmacy
Université Laval
Quebec City, Quebec, Canada
Chapter 30. Obesity: Medical and Surgical Management

Dorairaj Prabhakaran, MD, DM (Cardiology), MSc, FRCP
Vice President, Research and Policy
Public Health Foundation of India
Executive Director, Centre for Chronic Disease Control
Gurgaon, Haryana, India;
Professor
Department of Epidemiology
London School of Hygiene and Tropical Medicine
London, United Kingdom
Chapter 2. Global Burden of Cardiovascular Disease

Sanjay Rajagopalan, MD
Professor of Medicine
Director, Case Cardiovascular Research Institute
Case Western Reserve University
Chief, Division of Cardiovascular Medicine
Harrington Heart and Vascular Institute
University Hospitals Cleveland Medical Center
Cleveland, Ohio
Chapter 3. Impact of the Environment on Cardiovascular Health

Michael J. Reardon, MD
Professor of Cardiothoracic Surgery
Department of Cardiovascular Surgery
Houston Methodist Hospital
Houston, Texas
Chapter 78. Transcatheter Therapies for Mitral and Tricuspid Valvular Heart Disease
Chapter 98. Tumors Affecting the Cardiovascular System

Susan Redline, MD, MPH
Peter C. Farrell Professor of Sleep Medicine
Harvard Medical School
Senior Physician
Division of Sleep and Circadian Disorders
Departments of Medicine and Neurology
Brigham and Women's Hospital
Boston, Massachusetts
Chapter 89. Sleep-Disordered Breathing and Cardiac Disease

Shereif Rezkalla, MD
Adjunct Professor of Medicine
University of Wisconsin
Madison, Wisconsin;
Department of Cardiology and Cardiovascular Research
Marshfield Clinic Health System
Marshfield, Wisconsin
Chapter 84. Cardiomyopathies Induced by Drugs or Toxins

Michael W. Rich, MD
Professor of Medicine
Division of Cardiology
Washington University School of Medicine in St. Louis
Saint Louis, Missouri
Chapter 90. Cardiovascular Disease in Older Adults
Chapter 99. Psychiatric and Psychosocial Aspects of Cardiovascular Disease

Paul M Ridker, MD, MPH
Eugene Braunwald Professor of Medicine
Harvard Medical School
Director, Center for Cardiovascular Disease Prevention
Brigham and Women's Hospital
Boston, Massachusetts
Chapter 10. Biomarkers and Use in Precision Medicine
Chapter 25. Primary Prevention of Cardiovascular Disease

Dan M. Roden, MD
Professor of Medicine, Pharmacology, and Biomedical Informatics
Senior Vice President for Personalized Medicine
Vanderbilt University School of Medicine
Nashville, Tennessee
Chapter 9. Principles of Drug Therapeutics, Pharmacogenomics, and Biologics

Frederick L. Ruberg, MD
Associate Professor of Medicine
Section of Cardiovascular Medicine
Department of Medicine and Amyloidosis Center
Boston Medical Center
Boston University School of Medicine
Boston, Massachusetts
Chapter 53. Cardiac Amyloidosis

Marc S. Sabatine, MD, MPH
Chair, TIMI Study Group
Lewis Dexter MD Distinguished Chair in Cardiovascular Medicine
Brigham and Women's Hospital
Professor of Medicine
Harvard Medical School
Boston, Massachusetts
Chapter 35. Approach to the Patient with Chest Pain

Prashanthan Sanders, MBBS, PhD
Director, Centre for Heart Rhythm Disorders
School of Medicine
University of Adelaide
Director, Cardiac Electrophysiology and Pacing
Department of Cardiology
Royal Adelaide Hospital
Director, Heart Rhythm Group
Heart Health
South Australian Health and Medical Research Institute
Adelaide, Australia
Chapter 65. Supraventricular Tachycardias

Marc Schermerhorn, MD
George H. A. Clowes Jr. Professor of Surgery
Harvard Medical School
Chief, Division of Vascular and Endovascular Surgery
Beth Israel Deaconess Medical Center
Boston, Massachusetts
Chapter 42. Diseases of the Aorta

Benjamin M. Scirica, MD, MPH
Associate Professor of Medicine
Harvard Medical School
Senior Investigator, TIMI Study Group
Associate Physician, Cardiovascular Division
Brigham and Women's Hospital
Boston, Massachusetts
Chapter 37. ST-Elevation Myocardial Infarction: Pathophysiology and Clinical Evolution

Arnold H. Seto, MD, MPA
Associate Clinical Professor
University of California, Irvine
Cardiologist
Veterans Administration Long Beach Healthcare System
Long Beach, California
Chapter 22. Invasive Hemodynamic Diagnosis of Cardiac Disease

Sanjiv J. Shah, MD
Neil Stone MD Professor of Medicine
Division of Cardiology
Northwestern University Feinberg School of Medicine
Chicago, Illinois
Chapter 51. Heart Failure with Preserved and Mildly Reduced Ejection Fraction

Shabana Shahanavaz, MBBS
Associate Professor of Pediatrics
Director, Cardiac Catheterization Laboratory
The Heart Institute
Cincinnati Children's Hospital
Cincinnati, Ohio
Chapter 83. Catheter-Based Treatment of Congenital Heart Disease in Adults

Kalyanam Shivkumar, MD, PhD
Professor of Medicine (Cardiology), Radiology, and Bioengineering
Director, UCLA Cardiac Arrhythmia Center and Electrophysiology Programs
Director, Adult Cardiac Catheterization Laboratories
Ronald Reagan UCLA Medical Center
Los Angeles, California
Chapter 102. Cardiovascular Manifestations of Autonomic Disorders

Candice K. Silversides, SM, MD
Professor of Medicine
University of Toronto Pregnancy and Heart Disease Program
Toronto, Ontario, Canada
Chapter 92. Pregnancy and Heart Disease

Samuel C. Siu, MD, SM, MBA
Professor of Medicine
Division of Cardiology
Schulich School of Medicine and Dentistry
Western University
London, Ontario, Canada
Chapter 92. Pregnancy and Heart Disease

Scott D. Solomon, MD
The Edward D. Frohlich Distinguished Chair
Professor of Medicine
Harvard Medical School
Senior Physician
Brigham and Women's Hospital
Boston, Massachusetts
Chapter 4. Clinical Trials in Cardiovascular Medicine
Chapter 16. Echocardiography
Chapter 51. Heart Failure with Preserved and Mildly Reduced Ejection Fraction
Chapter 94. Endemic and Pandemic Viral Illnesses and Cardiovascular Disease: Influenza and COVID-19

Matthew J. Sorrentino, MD
Professor of Medicine
Section of Cardiology
UChicago Medicine
Chicago, Illinois
Chapter 26. Systemic Hypertension: Mechanisms, Diagnosis, and Treatment

Randall C. Starling, MD, MPH
Professor of Medicine
Kaufman Center for Heart Failure
Heart, Thoracic and Vascular Institute
Cleveland Clinic
Cleveland, Ohio
Chapter 60. Cardiac Transplantation

William G. Stevenson, MD
Professor of Medicine
Division of Cardiology
Vanderbilt University Medical Center
Nashville, Tennessee
Chapter 67. Ventricular Arrhythmias

John R. Teerlink, MD, FRCP(UK)
Professor of Medicine
University of California School of Medicine, San Francisco, Director, Heart Failure
Director, Echocardiography
Section of Cardiology
San Francisco Veteran Affairs Medical Center
San Francisco, California
Chapter 49. Diagnosis and Management of Acute Heart Failure

David J. Tester, BS
Associate Professor of Medicine
Mayo Clinic College of Medicine and Science
Department of Molecular Pharmacology & Experimental Therapeutics (Windland Smith Rice Sudden Death Genomics Laboratory)
Mayo Clinic
Rochester, Minnesota
Chapter 63. Genetics of Cardiac Arrhythmias

Randal Jay Thomas, MD, MS
Professor of Medicine
Mayo Clinic Alix School of Medicine
Medical Director, Cardiac Rehabilitation Program
Division of Preventive Cardiology
Department of Cardiovascular Medicine
Mayo Clinic
Rochester, Minnesota
Chapter 33. Comprehensive Cardiac Rehabilitation

Paul D. Thompson, MD
Chief of Cardiology, Emeritus
Hartford Hospital
Hartford, Connecticut
Chapter 32. Exercise and Sports Cardiology

Gordon F. Tomaselli, MD
Professor of Medicine (Cardiology)
The Marilyn and Stanley M. Katz Dean
Albert Einstein College of Medicine
Executive Vice President and Chief Academic Officer
Montefiore Medicine
Bronx, New York
Chapter 61. Approach to the Patient with Cardiac Arrhythmias
Chapter 62. Mechanisms of Cardiac Arrhythmias
Chapter 66. Atrial Fibrillation: Clinical Features, Mechanisms, and Management
Chapter 100. Neuromuscular Disorders and Cardiovascular Disease

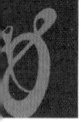

Mintu P. Turakhia, MD, MAS
Associate Professor of Medicine (Cardiovascular Medicine)
Executive Director, Center for Digital Health
Stanford University
Stanford, California;
Chief, Cardiac Electrophysiology
VA Palo Alto Health Care System
Palo Alto, California
Chapter 12. Wearable Devices in Cardiovascular Medicine

Anne Marie Valente, MD
Associate Professor
Pediatrics and Internal Medicine
Harvard Medical School
Director, Boston Adult Congenital Heart Program
Children's Hospital Boston
Brigham and Women's Hospital
Boston, Massachusetts
Chapter 82. Congenital Heart Disease in the Adolescent and Adult

Orly Vardeny, PharmD, MS
Associate Professor of Medicine
Center for Care Delivery and Outcomes Research
Minneapolis VA Health Care System and University of Minnesota
Minneapolis, Minnesota
Chapter 94. Endemic and Pandemic Viral Illnesses and Cardiovascular Disease: Influenza and COVID-19

David D. Waters, MD
Professor Emeritus
Department of Medicine
University of California, San Francisco
San Francisco, California
Chapter 85. Cardiovascular Abnormalities in HIV-Infected Individuals

Jeffrey I. Weitz, MD, FRCP(C)
Professor of Medicine and Biochemistry
McMaster University
Executive Director
Thrombosis and Atherosclerosis Research Institute
Hamilton, Ontario, Canada
Chapter 95. Hemostasis, Thrombosis, Fibrinolysis, and Cardiovascular Disease

Nanette Kass Wenger, MD
Professor of Medicine (Cardiology) Emeritus
Emory University School of Medicine
Consultant, Emory Heart and Vascular Center
Atlanta, Georgia
Chapter 90. Cardiovascular Disease in Older Adults

Walter R. Wilson, MD
Professor of Medicine
Mayo Clinic College of Medicine and Science
Rochester, Minnesota
Chapter 80. Infectious Endocarditis and Infections of Indwelling Devices

Justina C. Wu, MD, PhD
Assistant Professor of Medicine
Harvard Medical School
Director of Echocardiography
Brigham and Women's Hospital
Boston, Massachusetts
Chapter 16. Echocardiography

Katja Zeppenfeld, MD, PhD
Professor of Cardiology
Leiden University Medical Centre
Leiden, The Netherlands
Chapter 67. Ventricular Arrhythmias

Michael R. Zile, MD
Charles Ezra Daniels Professor of Medicine
Division of Cardiology
Medical University of South Carolina
Charleston, South Carolina
Chapter 58. Devices for Monitoring and Managing Heart Failure

To
Beryl, Oliver, and Brigitte
Pat, Rob, Sam, Laura, and Yoko
Benjamin Tan
Charlene, Sarah, Emily, and Matthew
Shanthala, Vinayak, Arjun, Ram, and Raj
Caren, Will and Lyz, Katie and Zach, and Dan

《Braunwald 心脏病学》中文导读版序言

《Braunwald 心脏病学》是培育全球心血管病医师的经典教科书，是心血管病医师的权威参考书。其内容完整、详实，既有丰富的历史沿革，又有不断更新的当代进展。从心血管病的基础研究到临床实践，用简洁明了的语言，客观生动的表述，清晰明了的图表，丰富全面的引文，充分展现了现代心血管病学的全貌。全书的每一个章节都由该领域全球最优秀的专家撰写，自出版以来，已经成为心血管病专业最具影响力和代表性的教科书和参考书，也是中国心血管病医生的必读书目。

我有幸通过参加 Braunwald 教授主持的 TIMI 全球研究等工作，直接深刻地感受到他高尚的人格和严谨的学风，科学的态度和孜孜不倦的精神。他于办公室赠送予我第 8 版《Braunwald 心脏病学》的照片作为珍贵纪念一直摆放在我的案头。陈灏珠院士曾经主持翻译了这部巨著的第 5 版，对推动我国心血管内科医师的专业教育起到了重要作用。今天非常高兴地看到由吴永健、张健、姚焰教授组织全国百位专家共同导读的《Braunwald 心脏病学》第 12 版（影印中文导读版）付梓出版，这是一种很好的、崭新的尝试。一方面凝练的导读介绍，会给读者一个相关内容的核心理念；另一方面完整保留了原文，让读者能够细致学习、品味原著的精髓；其三，之后还将根据学术进展更新电子资源中的导读内容或配上对应的中文视频讲解。多种形式、深入浅出地阐述核心内容将带给大家耳目一新的感受，有效地提高学习积极性和效果。

当代心血管病学的基础和临床研究日新月异，飞速进步。流行病学、遗传学、各种组学、影像学和生物标志物等方面的研究不断揭示和夯实了心血管病的发病机制，完善了评价体系；新药研究、新器械开发、生物工程学应用等方面的不断进展，进一步提升了心血管病治疗学的水平和能力。的确，这是一个知识爆炸的时代，也是一个充满挑战和希望的时代。我国中青年一代心血管病研究和临床工作者既要满怀热情和理想，又要踏踏实实地潜心读书，从事科学研究和临床实践。《Braunwald 心脏病学》无疑将成为我们学习心血管病学的基石，成为我们从事心血管病专业的最重要的教科书和参考书。希望此"中文导读版"对读者更好地理解原著有所裨益。

于中国医学科学院　北京协和医学院　阜外医院
国家心血管病中心
2023 年 2 月

《Braunwald 心脏病学》中文导读版前言

心血管病学是过去数十年间发展最快的学科之一，新理念、新知识、新技术层出不穷，令人目不暇接，稍有懈怠就跟不上学科发展。在浩如烟海的各种教科书和学术刊物中，《Braunwald 心脏病学》一直是经典巨著，它教育了一代又一代心血管病医生。Braunwald 本人是当代心脏病学之父。年近九旬的他依然活跃在世界心脏病领域。他主导的 TIMI 系列研究几乎代表了现代心脏病学的发展。如今在西方国家，《Braunwald 心脏病学》是心脏科医生成长的必读之书。其内容涵盖了心血管疾病的方方面面。所有参与编写的作者都是在其编写的章节领域的全世界最权威专家。该书另外一个最大的特点就是帮助年轻医生建立心脏病学的整体理念。如它会帮助您了解心脏病学发展的历史、全球心脏病的状况、环境因素和生活方式对心血管疾病的影响、心血管疾病基础和临床研究的方法和模式、医疗卫生政策与人群心血管疾病以及教您学会心血管疾病的诊治理念。

《Braunwald 心脏病学》对于中国医生同样是最好的教科书。陈灏珠教授曾经组织中国的专家将《Braunwald's HEART DISEASE》第 7 版全书翻译成中文，形成中文版的《Braunwald 心脏病学》，对于很多中国医生的成长发挥了重要的作用。随着心脏病学在各个方面的快速发展，该书反复再版，如今已是第十二版，体现了目前心脏病领域的最新进展。众多中国心脏科医生都渴望能获得此书，以作为工作中的指导和陪伴。有鉴于此，北京大学医学出版社引进出版了中文导读影印版的《Braunwald 心脏病学》，并联合玲珑医学共同组织中国的专家对每一章节进行中文导读，这样可以让阅读者快速了解该章节的大致内容，如果读者对其中的内容感兴趣，可以继续阅读原文。很多重要章节的后面配有编译者制作的中文幻灯和编译者的影像版讲解，由此提供更多、更灵活的学习形式。

受玲珑医学的委托，遵循北京大学出版社的要求，本次参与《Braunwald 心脏病学》编译的专家主要来自中国医学科学院阜外医院，同时邀请了部分兄弟医院的专家。由于这是初次尝试一种全新的编译方式，缺乏经验和参考，问题和不足在所难免，还望广大读者朋友提出批评和建议。但编译委员会相信，我国心脏科医生的英文阅读能力均有了大幅度提高，采取编译的方式也许对于我国读者来说是一种更好的尝试。我们衷心地期待这种形式能够帮助中国医生的成长，同时也希望它成为心脏科医生的好帮手。

吴永健　张健　姚焰
2023 年 1 月

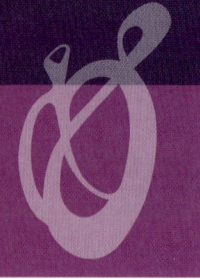

Preface

The knowledge relevant to the practice of cardiology continues to grow by leaps and bounds. Scientific and clinical advances have occurred at such a rapid pace that clinicians often suffer information overload. Communications about advances in cardiovascular medicine inundate practitioners on a seemingly minute-to-minute basis through journals, mailings, text messages, newsletters, social media, webinars, advertisements, and other electronic and print media. How can a practitioner or trainee sift through this cacophony to discern reliable, durable, and important information critical for practice?

This textbook of cardiovascular medicine offers a solution to this quandary. The 12th edition of *Braunwald's Heart Disease* provides a comprehensive, carefully curated, balanced, and unbiased distillation not only of the tried and true, but especially the latest advances in our field. This volume should serve the novice and experienced practitioner alike. Trainees and those preparing for certification or recertification examinations can use this text for an overall review of contemporary cardiovascular medicine. Practitioners confronting a particular clinical problem can consult the appropriate section of the book on an as-needed basis to answer the clinical question at hand to aid on-the-spot clinical decision making. While not a basic science textbook, this volume builds on Dr. Braunwald's founding vision and reviews fundamental pathophysiologic mechanisms to furnish a foundation for informed practice where appropriate.

Cardiovascular medicine has expanded so enormously that few if any individuals can maintain mastery of the entire scope of practice. Sub-specialization and even sub-sub-specialization have increased. Yet, each of us encounters issues within these super-specialized areas when we care for and counsel our own patients. The palette of patients' problems often overlaps the fine divisions our specialty has developed. This book aims to provide a ready reference so that we can update our knowledge with recent and authoritative information in areas of cardiovascular medicine afield from our own primary areas of expertise. Indeed, with the addition of companion volumes, the *Heart Disease* family has become a living learning system and comprehensive reference.

As necessitated by evolution and progress in cardiovascular medicine, in planning this 12th edition the editors have carefully reviewed the content to reflect current knowledge. This edition has 14 totally new chapters. For example, we have added chapters on artificial intelligence in cardiology and on the use of wearables in cardiovascular medicine. These two topics will doubtless change our practices profoundly. We expect that future editions will continue to build on these and other novel areas that will provide us with innovative tools to confront our patients' problems.

We have added a new chapter, "Impact of the Environment on Cardiovascular Health," as we recognize increasingly the clinical importance of this critical interface. Another new chapter, "Cardiovascular Disease Risk of Nicotine and Tobacco Products," highlights the concerning increase in smokeless tobacco use among youth. The burgeoning field of cardio-oncology has expanded coverage in the 12th edition, with two chapters devoted to different aspects of this topic. Expanded coverage of valvular heart disease includes a new chapter on interventions for mitral and tricuspid valvulopathies, which complements an updated chapter on percutaneous interventions for the aortic valve. These additions acknowledge the growing role of structural heart disease interventions in tackling these conditions.

The period of planning and preparation of this 12th edition coincided with the pandemic caused by SARS-CoV-2. We would be remiss not to include an expanded discussion of viral heart diseases in a new chapter, as our specialty needs to prepare for likely future viral pandemics, as well as deal with the potentially long-term cardiovascular consequences of COVID-19. Of course, each and every chapter in the book has undergone extensive updating and revision to reflect advances since the last edition. To this end, a number of chapters are completely written de novo by new authors. Indeed, the 12th edition boasts almost 80 new authors, reflecting our commitment to continuous refreshment and review of the content.

Our field can take considerable pride in the rapid advances in both basic and clinical investigation that this book highlights. Yet, we face a disconnect between these advances and their application to practice. To this end we include a new chapter, "Impact of Health Care Policy on Quality and Outcomes of Cardiovascular Disease," that focuses on practical societal approaches to ensure that our patients can benefit from the clinical and basic scientific advances in our field. Moreover, closing gaps in offering progress in cardiovascular medicine to racially, ethnically, geographically diverse, or underserved populations presents a global challenge. We focus on cardiovascular conditions in particular segments of the population—women, people with diabetes, and those with HIV/AIDS—that may require specialized approaches; each of these and others have been accorded a separate chapter. The global pandemic has placed disparities and inequities in health care in stark relief, locally and globally. To address this problem, a new chapter, "Heart Disease in Racially and Ethnically Diverse Populations," deals with cardiovascular conditions that confront disadvantaged segments of our population.

Finally, the Editors were fortunate to enlist Professor Eugene Braunwald, the founder of this textbook, to contribute an opening chapter, "Cardiovascular Disease: Past, Present, and Future," which shares his vision from his uniquely broad perspective. We have striven to uphold the standards that he set for this textbook from the first five editions that he edited solo. We have aimed to emulate his editorial prowess and example of refreshing every page of this textbook in each edition to maximize its utility for all who care for patients with or at risk of developing cardiovascular disease.

Peter Libby
Robert O. Bonow
Douglas L. Mann
Gordon F. Tomaselli
Deepak L. Bhatt
Scott D. Solomon

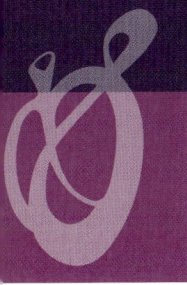

Preface to the First Edition

Cardiovascular disease is the greatest scourge affecting the industrialized nations. As with previous scourges — bubonic plague, yellow fever, and small pox — cardiovascular disease not only strikes down a significant fraction of the population without warning but also causes prolonged suffering and disability in an even larger number. In the United States alone, despite recent encouraging declines, cardiovascular disease is still responsible for almost 1 million fatalities each year and more than half of all deaths; almost 5 million persons afflicted with cardiovascular disease are hospitalized each year. The cost of these diseases in terms of human suffering and material resources is almost incalculable.

Fortunately, research focusing on the prevention, causes, diagnosis, and treatment of heart disease is moving ahead rapidly. Since the early part of the twentieth century, clinical cardiology has had a particularly strong foundation in the basic sciences of physiology and pharmacology. More recently, the disciplines of molecular biology, genetics, developmental biology, biophysics, biochemistry, experimental pathology and bioengineering have also begun to provide critically important information about cardiac function and malfunction.

In the past 25 years, in particular, we have witnessed an explosive expansion of our understanding of the structure and function of the cardiovascular system—both normal and abnormal—and of our ability to evaluate these parameters in the living patient, sometimes by means of techniques that require penetration of the skin but also with increasing accuracy, by noninvasive methods. Simultaneously, remarkable progress has been made in preventing and treating cardiovascular disease by medical and surgical means. Indeed, in the United States, a steady reduction in mortality from cardiovascular disease during the past decade suggests that the effective application of this increased knowledge is beginning to prolong human life span, the most valued resource on earth.

To provide a comprehensive, authoritative text in a field that has become as broad and deep as cardiovascular medicine, I enlisted the aid of a number of able colleagues. However, I hoped that my personal involvement in the writing of about half of the book would make it possible to minimize the fragmentation, gaps, inconsistencies, organizational difficulties, and impersonal tone that sometimes plague multiauthored texts. Although *Heart Disease: A Textbook of Cardiovascular Medicine* is primarily a clinical treatise and not a textbook of fundamental cardiovascular science, an effort has been made to explain, in some detail, the scientific bases of cardiovascular diseases.

To the extent that this book proves useful to those who wish to broaden their knowledge of cardiovascular medicine and thereby aids in the care of patients afflicted with heart disease, credit must be given to the many talented and dedicated persons involved in its preparation. I offer my deepest appreciation to my fellow contributors for their professional expertise, knowledge, and devoted scholarship, which has so enriched this book. I am deeply indebted to them for their cooperation and willingness to deal with a demanding editor.

Eugene Braunwald
1980

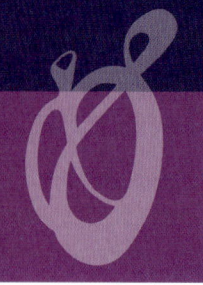

Acknowledgments

The conception and creation of this textbook of over 100 chapters and almost 2000 pages required the expertise, assistance, and skills of many dedicated individuals. We thank the contributors who have authored the chapters that comprise this textbook. We recognize the leadership of Ms. Dolores Meloni, executive content strategist at Elsevier, for her guidance and assistance at all stages of the planning and preparation of this volume. Ms. Anne Snyder, senior content development specialist, provided invaluable and detailed assistance on a daily basis. The editors owe her a great debt of gratitude. Mr. John Casey, senior project manager, cheerfully worked with the authors and the editors in executing the composition and proofing of this tome and accommodating last-minute additions and alterations to make the print edition as accurate and up to date as possible. The editors would not have been able to produce this book and ensure its quality without all of these contributions.

We also thank colleagues the world over who provided suggestions on how to improve *Braunwald's Heart Disease* and identified points that could use clarification. We welcome such input that will enable us to improve this edition in subsequent printings and plan future editions to meet our readers' needs even better.

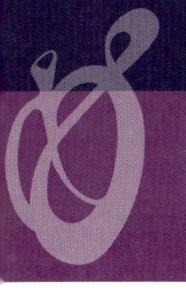

目录

第一部分　心血管医学基础
（吴永健　导读）

PART I　FOUNDATIONS OF CARDIOVASCULAR MEDICINE

1. Cardiovascular Disease: Past, Present, and Future, 1
   EUGENE BRAUNWALD

2. Global Burden of Cardiovascular Disease, 14
   THOMAS A. GAZIANO, DORAIRAJ PRABHAKARAN, AND J. MICHAEL GAZIANO

3. Impact of the Environment on Cardiovascular Health, 31
   SADEER AL-KINDI AND SANJAY RAJAGOPALAN

4. Clinical Trials in Cardiovascular Medicine, 42
   SCOTT D. SOLOMON AND JOHN MCMURRAY

5. Clinical Decision-Making in Cardiology, 53
   JOHN E. BRUSH JR. AND HARLAN M. KRUMHOLZ

6. Impact of Health Care Policy on Quality, Outcomes, and Equity in Cardiovascular Disease, 62
   KAREN E. JOYNT MADDOX

第二部分　心血管疾病的个体化诊疗
（周欣　杨清　导读）

PART II　INDIVIDUALIZING APPROACHES TO CARDIOVASCULAR DISEASE

7. Applications of Genetics to Cardiovascular Medicine, 71
   PRADEEP NATARAJAN AND KIRAN MUSUNURU

8. Proteomics and Metabolomics in Cardiovascular Medicine, 87
   ROBERT GERSZTEN

9. Principles of Drug Therapeutics, Pharmacogenomics, and Biologics, 92
   DAN M. RODEN

10. Biomarkers and Use in Precision Medicine, 102
    PETER LIBBY AND PAUL M RIDKER

11. Artificial Intelligence in Cardiovascular Medicine, 109
    ZACHI ATTIA, SURAJ KAPA, PETER NOSEWORTHY, AND PAUL FRIEDMAN

12. Wearable Devices in Cardiovascular Medicine, 117
    MINTU P. TURAKHIA

第三部分　患者的评估
（张力　导读）

PART III　EVALUATION OF THE PATIENT

13. History and Physical Examination: An Evidence-Based Approach, 123
    JAMES C. FANG AND PATRICK T. O'GARA

14. Electrocardiography, 141
    DAVID M. MIRVIS AND ARY L. GOLDBERGER

15. Exercise Physiology and Exercise Electrocardiographic Testing, 175
    GARY J. BALADY AND PHILIP A. ADES

16. Echocardiography, 196
    JUSTINA C. WU, LINDA D. GILLAM, AND SCOTT D. SOLOMON
    ILLUSTRATED BY BERNARD BULWER

17. Chest Radiography in Cardiovascular Disease, 268
    FRANCINE L. JACOBSON

18. Nuclear Cardiology, 277
    SHARMILA DORBALA AND MARCELO F. DI CARLI

19. Cardiovascular Magnetic Resonance Imaging, 314
    RAYMOND Y. KWONG

20. Cardiac Computed Tomography, 335
    RON BLANKSTEIN

21. Coronary Angiography and Intravascular Imaging, 363
    GEORGE D. DANGAS AND ROXANA MEHRAN

22. Invasive Hemodynamic Diagnosis of Cardiac Disease, 385
    MORTON J. KERN, ARNOLD H. SETO, AND JOERG HERRMANN

23 **Anesthesia and Noncardiac Surgery in Patients with Heart Disease, 410**
LEE A. FLEISHER AND JOSHUA A. BECKMAN

第四部分　预防心脏病学
（卢玉枝　苏冠华　程翔　导读）

PART IV　PREVENTIVE CARDIOLOGY

24 **The Vascular Biology of Atherosclerosis, 425**
PETER LIBBY

25 **Primary Prevention of Cardiovascular Disease, 442**
SAMIA MORA, PETER LIBBY, AND PAUL M RIDKER

26 **Systemic Hypertension: Mechanisms, Diagnosis, and Treatment, 471**
GEORGE L. BAKRIS AND MATTHEW J. SORRENTINO

27 **Lipoprotein Disorders and Cardiovascular Disease, 502**
JACQUES GENEST, SAMIA MORA, AND PETER LIBBY

28 **Cardiovascular Disease Risk of Nicotine and Tobacco Products, 525**
ARUNI BHATNAGAR

29 **Nutrition and Cardiovascular and Metabolic Diseases, 531**
DARIUSH MOZAFFARIAN

30 **Obesity: Medical and Surgical Management, 547**
JEAN-PIERRE DESPRÉS, ERIC LAROSE, AND PAUL POIRIER

31 **Diabetes and the Cardiovascular System, 556**
NIKOLAUS MARX, SILVIO E. INZUCCHI, AND DARREN K. MCGUIRE

32 **Exercise and Sports Cardiology, 579**
PAUL D. THOMPSON AND AARON L. BAGGISH

33 **Comprehensive Cardiac Rehabilitation, 588**
RANDAL JAY THOMAS

34 **Integrative Approaches to the Management of Patients with Heart Disease, 593**
STEPHEN DEVRIES

第五部分　动脉粥样硬化性心血管疾病
（曹宇开　李悦　导读）

PART V　ATHEROSCLEROTIC CARDIOVASCULAR DISEASE

35 **Approach to the Patient with Chest Pain, 599**
MARC P. BONACA AND MARC S. SABATINE

36 **Coronary Blood Flow and Myocardial Ischemia, 609**
DIRK J. DUNCKER AND JOHN M. CANTY JR.

37 **ST-Elevation Myocardial Infarction: Pathophysiology and Clinical Evolution, 636**
BENJAMIN M. SCIRICA, PETER LIBBY, AND DAVID A. MORROW

38 **ST-Elevation Myocardial Infarction: Management, 662**
ERIN A. BOHULA AND DAVID A. MORROW

39 **Non–ST Elevation Acute Coronary Syndromes, 714**
ROBERT P. GIUGLIANO AND EUGENE BRAUNWALD

40 **Stable Ischemic Heart Disease, 739**
DAVID A. MORROW AND JAMES DE LEMOS

41 **Percutaneous Coronary Intervention, 786**
DHARAM J. KUMBHANI AND DEEPAK L. BHATT

42 **Diseases of the Aorta, 806**
ALAN C. BRAVERMAN AND MARC SCHERMERHORN

43 **Peripheral Artery Diseases, 837**
MARC P. BONACA AND MARK A. CREAGER

44 **Treatment of Noncoronary Obstructive Vascular Disease, 859**
SCOTT KINLAY AND DEEPAK L. BHATT

45 **Prevention and Management of Ischemic Stroke, 870**
MARK J. ALBERTS

第六部分　心力衰竭
（贺春晖　张健　导读）

PART VI　HEART FAILURE

46 **Mechanisms of Cardiac Contraction and Relaxation, 889**
DONALD M. BERS AND BARRY A. BORLAUG

47 **Pathophysiology of Heart Failure, 913**
GERD HASENFUSS AND DOUGLAS L. MANN

48 **Approach to the Patient with Heart Failure, 933**
JAMES L. JANUZZI JR. AND DOUGLAS L. MANN

49 **Diagnosis and Management of Acute Heart Failure, 946**
G. MICHAEL FELKER AND JOHN R. TEERLINK

50	**Management of Heart Failure Patients with Reduced Ejection Fraction, 975** DOUGLAS L. MANN
51	**Heart Failure with Preserved and Mildly Reduced Ejection Fraction, 1007** CAROLYN S.P. LAM, SANJIV J. SHAH, AND SCOTT D. SOLOMON
52	**The Dilated, Restrictive, and Infiltrative Cardiomyopathies, 1031** RAY E. HERSHBERGER
53	**Cardiac Amyloidosis, 1052** FREDERICK L. RUBERG AND MATHEW S. MAURER
54	**Hypertrophic Cardiomyopathy, 1062** CAROLYN Y. HO AND STEVE R. OMMEN
55	**Myocarditis, 1077** LESLIE T. COOPER JR. AND KIRK U. KNOWLTON
56	**Cardio-Oncology: Managing Cardiotoxic Effects of Cancer Therapies, 1091** BONNIE KY
57	**Cardio-Oncology: Approach to the Patient, 1099** JOERG HERRMANN
58	**Devices for Monitoring and Managing Heart Failure, 1107** JOANN LINDENFELD AND MICHAEL R. ZILE
59	**Mechanical Circulatory Support, 1119** KEITH D. AARONSON AND FRANCIS D. PAGANI
60	**Cardiac Transplantation, 1132** RANDALL C. STARLING

第七部分　心律失常
（吴灵敏　姚焰　导读）

PART VII　ARRHYTHMIAS, SUDDEN DEATH, AND SYNCOPE

61	**Approach to the Patient with Cardiac Arrhythmias, 1145** ANNE B. CURTIS AND GORDON F. TOMASELLI
62	**Mechanisms of Cardiac Arrhythmias, 1163** STANLEY NATTEL AND GORDON F. TOMASELLI
63	**Genetics of Cardiac Arrhythmias, 1191** JOHN R. GIUDICESSI, DAVID J. TESTER, AND MICHAEL J. ACKERMAN
64	**Therapy for Cardiac Arrhythmias, 1208** JOHN M. MILLER AND KENNETH A. ELLENBOGEN
65	**Supraventricular Tachycardias, 1245** JONATHAN M. KALMAN AND PRASHANTHAN SANDERS
66	**Atrial Fibrillation: Clinical Features, Mechanisms, and Management, 1272** HUGH CALKINS, GORDON F. TOMASELLI, AND FRED MORADY
67	**Ventricular Arrhythmias, 1288** WILLIAM G. STEVENSON AND KATJA ZEPPENFELD
68	**Bradyarrhythmias and Atrioventricular Block, 1312** KRISTEN K. PATTON AND JEFFREY E. OLGIN
69	**Pacemakers and Implantable Cardioverter-Defibrillators, 1321** MINA K. CHUNG AND JAMES P. DAUBERT
70	**Cardiac Arrest and Sudden Cardiac Death, 1349** JEFFREY J. GOLDBERGER, CHRISTINE M. ALBERT, AND ROBERT J. MYERBURG
71	**Hypotension and Syncope, 1387** HUGH CALKINS, THOMAS H. EVERETT IV, AND PENG-SHENG CHEN

第八部分　心脏瓣膜疾病
（王墨扬　吴永健　导读）

PART VIII　DISEASES OF THE HEART VALVES

72	**Aortic Valve Stenosis, 1399** BRIAN R. LINDMAN, ROBERT O. BONOW, AND CATHERINE M. OTTO
73	**Aortic Regurgitation, 1419** ROBERT O. BONOW AND RICK A. NISHIMURA
74	**Transcatheter Aortic Valve Replacement, 1430** MARTIN B. LEON AND MICHAEL J. MACK
75	**Mitral Stenosis, 1441** Y. S. CHANDRASHEKHAR
76	**Mitral Regurgitation, 1455** REBECCA TUNG HAHN AND ROBERT O. BONOW
77	**Tricuspid, Pulmonic, and Multivalvular Disease, 1473** PATRICIA A. PELLIKKA AND VUYISILE T. NKOMO
78	**Transcatheter Therapies for Mitral and Tricuspid Valvular Heart Disease, 1484** HOWARD C. HERRMANN AND MICHAEL J. REARDON
79	**Prosthetic Heart Valves, 1495** PHILIPPE PIBAROT AND PATRICK T. O'GARA

- 80 **Infectious Endocarditis and Infections of Indwelling Devices, 1505**
  LARRY M. BADDOUR, NANDAN S. ANAVEKAR, JUAN A. CRESTANELLO, AND WALTER R. WILSON

- 81 **Rheumatic Fever, 1531**
  ANA OLGA MOCUMBI

第九部分　心肌、心包和肺血管系统疾病
（赵青　柳志红　导读）

PART IX　DISEASES OF THE MYOCARDIUM, PERICARDIUM, AND PULMONARY VASCULATURE BED

- 82 **Congenital Heart Disease in the Adolescent and Adult, 1541**
  ANNE MARIE VALENTE, ADAM L. DORFMAN, SONYA V. BABU-NARAYAN, AND ERIC V. KRIEGER

- 83 **Catheter-Based Treatment of Congenital Heart Disease in Adults, 1587**
  SHABANA SHAHANAVAZ, JOHN M. LASALA, AND DAVID T. BALZER

- 84 **Cardiomyopathies Induced by Drugs or Toxins, 1593**
  ROBERT A. KLONER AND SHEREIF REZKALLA

- 85 **Cardiovascular Abnormalities in HIV-Infected Individuals, 1603**
  PRISCILLA Y. HSUE AND DAVID D. WATERS

- 86 **Pericardial Diseases, 1615**
  MARTIN M. LEWINTER, PAUL C. CREMER, AND ALLAN L. KLEIN

- 87 **Pulmonary Embolism and Deep Vein Thrombosis, 1635**
  SAMUEL Z. GOLDHABER AND GREGORY PIAZZA

- 88 **Pulmonary Hypertension, 1656**
  BRADLEY A. MARON

- 89 **Sleep-Disordered Breathing and Cardiac Disease, 1678**
  SUSAN REDLINE

第十部分　特定人群的心血管疾病
（王汝涛　陶凌　导读）

PART X　CARDIOVASCULAR DISEASE IN SELECT POPULATIONS

- 90 **Cardiovascular Disease in Older Adults, 1687**
  DANIEL E. FORMAN, JEROME L. FLEG, NANETTE KASS WENGER, AND MICHAEL W. RICH

- 91 **Cardiovascular Disease in Women, 1710**
  MARTHA GULATI AND C. NOEL BAIREY MERZ

- 92 **Pregnancy and Heart Disease, 1723**
  SAMUEL C. SIU AND CANDICE K. SILVERSIDES

- 93 **Heart Disease in Racially and Ethnically Diverse Populations, 1743**
  ALANNA A. MORRIS AND MICHELLE A. ALBERT

第十一部分　心血管疾病和其他器官疾病
（王文尧　唐熠达　导读）

PART XI　CARDIOVASCULAR DISEASE AND DISORDERS OF OTHER ORGANS

- 94 **Endemic and Pandemic Viral Illnesses and Cardiovascular Disease: Influenza and COVID-19, 1751**
  ORLY VARDENY, MOHAMMAD MADJID, AND SCOTT D. SOLOMON

- 95 **Hemostasis, Thrombosis, Fibrinolysis, and Cardiovascular Disease, 1766**
  JEFFREY I. WEITZ

- 96 **Endocrine Disorders and Cardiovascular Disease, 1791**
  BERNADETTE BIONDI

- 97 **Rheumatic Diseases and the Cardiovascular System, 1809**
  JUSTIN C. MASON

- 98 **Tumors Affecting the Cardiovascular System, 1829**
  DANIEL J. LENIHAN, MICHAEL J. REARDON, AND W. GREGORY HUNDLEY

- 99 **Psychiatric and Psychosocial Aspects of Cardiovascular Disease, 1841**
  KENNETH E. FREEDLAND, ROBERT M. CARNEY, ERIC J. LENZE, AND MICHAEL W. RICH

- 100 **Neuromuscular Disorders and Cardiovascular Disease, 1853**
  WILLIAM J. GROH, ELIZABETH M. MCNALLY, AND GORDON F. TOMASELLI

- 101 **Interface Between Renal Disease and Cardiovascular Illness, 1873**
  PETER A. MCCULLOUGH

- 102 **Cardiovascular Manifestations of Autonomic Disorders, 1893**
  JASON S. BRADFIELD AND KALYANAM SHIVKUMAR

第六部分　心力衰竭

贺春晖　张健　导读

心力衰竭（心衰）是由心室结构和功能障碍导致心室充盈或射血异常，从而引起的一种复杂临床综合征。心衰的临床综合征可能是因心脏结构和功能的各个方面异常或紊乱所导致，但大多数患者的心肌功能都出现损害——从正常的心室大小及功能到明显的扩张和功能减弱。心衰的症状通常取决于左心或右心充盈压力的升高，但"充血性"心衰一词不再被推崇——评估的许多患者并无明显充血，但其症状可能因心排血量减少所致。

在全球范围内，心衰影响近2300万人。美国最新流行病学数据表明，620万美国成年人患有心衰，到2030年患病率将增加46%。北美和欧洲40岁以上人群患心衰的风险约为1/5，危险因素包括缺血性心脏病、心肌梗死、心肌炎、心脏瓣膜疾病、心动过速、糖尿病、与先天性心脏病相关的结构性心脏病、睡眠呼吸暂停、药物过量或酗酒及肥胖。约30%～40%的非缺血性心衰被认为与遗传相关。随着全球人口老龄化趋势加速，高血压和冠心病治疗水平显著提高，人群预期寿命延长，这些因素决定了心衰必然会成为本世纪全球心血管疾病领域的突出问题。

随着心衰病理生理机制研究的不断深入，其成果逐渐转化并应用到临床，心衰的治疗方法也取得长足进展。目前，治疗方面的突出进展是调节神经内分泌系统药物的应用，主要是血管紧张素转化酶抑制剂（ACEI）、血管紧张素Ⅱ受体抑制剂（ARB）、醛固酮受体拮抗剂、β受体阻滞剂和钠-葡萄糖协同转运蛋白2（SGLT2）抑制剂等。一些新的心衰监测和辅助器械的研发也已经显示出器械治疗在心衰发生发展中的潜在作用，这让我们看到了发展治疗心衰新器械和新方法的希望。

《Braunwald心脏病学》中的第46～60章为心衰部分。力图较全面反映心衰的发病机制、基础知识和临床诊治等方面内容以及近年来的进展。在机制方面，第46章主要从心脏的收缩和舒张生理机制出发，从收缩细胞和蛋白质的显微解剖学、心脏收缩-舒张周期中的钙离子流、肌纤维膜对Ca^{2+}和Na^+的控制、肾上腺素能信号系统、胆碱能和一氧化氮信号、心脏的收缩性能及展望未来等方面详细阐述。第47章主要介绍了心衰的病理生理学，从心衰的发病机制和左室重构可逆性与左室功能恢复两方面进行详述。第48章开始从临床角度出发，对心衰患者的处理方法深入讲解，包括心衰的定义和流行病学、病史和体格检查、常规实验室评估、预后风险评分、右心导管检查、心内膜心肌活检、合并症情况、生活质量评估、心肺运动试验、在心衰患者诊断和管理中的影像学方法的使用、晚期心衰转诊时间等。第49章围绕急性心衰的诊断和处理，从流行病学、病理生理学、急性心衰患者的评价、急性心衰患者的管理及未来展望方面进行论述。第50和51章根据射血分数将心衰分为射血分数降低的心衰（HFrEF）、射血分数保留的心衰（HFpEF）和射血分数轻度降低的心衰（HFmrEF），根据目前的研究结果针对各自疾病的特点，有针对性地进行了详细阐述。如针对HFrEF从病因、预后、处理方法、液体潴留治疗、预防疾病进展、对有症状患者的管理、药物基因组学/个性化医学、动脉粥样硬化疾病的管理、瓣膜疾病的管理、特殊人群的管理、抗凝和抗血小板治疗、心律失常的处理、器械治疗、睡眠呼吸障碍、疾病综合管理、难治性终末期心衰患者（D期）的管理、将姑息治疗融入心衰护理等方面详述。针对HFpEF和HFmrEF从流行病学、诊断、病理生理学和治疗方面做了相应阐述。第52章对扩张型、限制型和浸润型心肌病从各自的临床特点分别做了详述。第53章针对心脏淀粉样变的流行病学、病理生理学、临床特征和预后、诊断、临床管理进行详述。第54章针对肥厚型心肌病，从肥厚型心肌病的诊断、形态学和病因学，病理生理学，自然病程，基因检测和家庭管理，临床管理，是否存在梗阻，及临床试验和新兴疗法等角度进行了探讨。第55章针对心肌炎，从概述和定义、流行病学、特异性病原体、病毒性心肌炎的发病机制、临床综合征、诊断方法、预后和治疗等方面详述。第56和57章针对心脏肿瘤学，分别从管理癌症治疗的心脏毒性效应和处理患者的方法两方面进行了深入探讨。第58章针对近年来蓬勃发展的监测和管理心衰的器械进行了介绍，包括心室不同步情况下心脏再同步化治疗的靶点，慢性心衰患者的心脏性猝死，HFrEF患者心脏再同步化和植入式心脏复律除颤器应用指南，新型植入式心衰治疗器械，监测心衰的植入式器械，以及药物和器械之间的相互作用。第59章针对心衰患者机械循环支持进行详细介绍，包括适应证、策略和器械选择，心室辅助装置设计，患者选择、共病和干预时机，患者结局及机械辅助循环支持跨机构登记研究等。第60章针对心脏移植，从其历史沿革、流行病学、潜在受者评估、捐献者分配制度、心脏捐献者、手术注意事项、免疫抑制和排斥、心脏移植后结局、感染、医疗并发症和共存疾病等方面做了深入分析。

近年来医学科学飞速发展，在心衰的基础和临床研究的各个领域都取得了丰硕成果。我们亟需将心衰的最新知识和研究成果尽快转化到临床应用与教学，为我国心衰的研究和临床实践提供一份精神食粮。希望这本书能够成为临床医生、科研人员的好助手。

PART VI HEART FAILURE

46 Mechanisms of Cardiac Contraction and Relaxation

DONALD M. BERS AND BARRY A. BORLAUG

MICROANATOMY OF CONTRACTILE CELLS AND PROTEINS, 889
Ultrastructure of Contractile Cells, 889
Mitochondrial Morphology and Function, 891
Contractile Proteins, 892
Graded Effects of $[Ca^{2+}]_i$ on Cross-Bridge Cycle, 894

CALCIUM ION FLUXES IN CARDIAC CONTRACTION-RELAXATION CYCLE, 895
Calcium Movements and Excitation-Contraction Coupling, 895
Calcium Release and Uptake by Sarcoplasmic Reticulum, 896
Calcium Uptake into Sarcoplasmic Reticulum by Sarcoendoplasmic Reticulum Ca^{2+}–Adenosine Triphosphatase, 897

SARCOLEMMAL CONTROL OF Ca^{2+} AND Na^+, 898
Calcium and Sodium Channels, 898
Ion Exchangers and Pumps, 899

ADRENERGIC SIGNALING SYSTEMS, 899
Physiologic Fight-or-Flight Response, 899
Beta-Adrenergic Receptor Subtypes, 900
Alpha-Adrenergic Receptor Subtypes, 901
G Proteins, 901
Cyclic Adenosine Monophosphate and Protein Kinase A, 901
Ca^{2+}/Calmodulin-Dependent Protein Kinase II, 903

CHOLINERGIC AND NITRIC OXIDE SIGNALING, 903
Cholinergic Signaling, 903
Nitric Oxide, 904

CONTRACTILE PERFORMANCE OF THE HEART, 904
The Cardiac Cycle, 904
Contractility Versus Loading Conditions, 906
Starling's Law of the Heart, 906
Wall Stress, 907
Heart Rate and Force-Frequency Relationship, 908
Myocardial Oxygen Uptake, 909
Measurements of Contractile Function, 910
Left Ventricular Relaxation and Diastolic Dysfunction, 910
Right Ventricular Function, 911
Atrial Function, 911

FUTURE PERSPECTIVES, 911

ACKNOWLEDGMENT, 911

REFERENCES, 911

MICROANATOMY OF CONTRACTILE CELLS AND PROTEINS

Ultrastructure of Contractile Cells

The major function of cardiac muscle cells (*cardiomyocytes* or *myocytes*) is to execute cardiac excitation-contraction-relaxation that depends on the electrical calcium ion (Ca^{2+}) transport and contractile properties.[1,2] Cardiomyocytes constitute approximately 75% of total ventricular volume and weight, but only one third of the total number of cells there.[1-4] Approximately half of each ventricular myocyte is occupied by myofibrils of the myofibers and 30% by mitochondria (Fig. 46.1 and Table 46.1). A *myofiber* is a group of cardiomyocytes held together by surrounding collagen connective tissue, the latter being a major component of the extracellular matrix. Further strands of collagen connect myofibers to each other.

Ventricular myocytes are roughly brick shaped, typically 150 × 20 × 12 μm (see Table 46.1), and are connected at the long ends by specialized junctions that mechanically and electrically couple the myocytes with each other. Atrial myocytes are smaller and more spindle shaped (<10 μm in diameter and <100 μm in length). When examined under a light microscope, atrial and ventricular myocytes have cross striations and are often branched. Each myocyte is bounded by a complex cell membrane, the *sarcolemma* (muscle plasma membrane), and is filled with rodlike bundles of *myofibrils* containing the contractile elements. The sarcolemma invaginates to form an extensive transverse tubular network (*transverse tubules* [T tubules]) that extends the extracellular space into the interior of the cell (see Figs. 46.1 and 46.2). Ventricular myocytes are typically binucleate, and these nuclei contain most of the cell's genetic information. Some smaller or more juvenile myocytes have one nucleus and some up to three to four nuclei. Rows of mitochondria are located between the myofibrils and also immediately beneath the sarcolemma. Mitochondria function mainly to generate the energy, in the form of adenosine triphosphate (ATP), that is needed to maintain cardiac contractile function and the associated ion gradients. The *sarcoplasmic reticulum* (SR) is a specialized form of endoplasmic reticulum that is critical for calcium (Ca^{2+}) cycling, which is the on-off switch for contraction. When the wave of electrical excitation reaches the T tubules, voltage-gated Ca^{2+} channels open to provide relatively small entry of Ca^{2+}, which triggers additional release of Ca^{2+} from the SR via closely apposed Ca^{2+} release channels. This is the Ca^{2+} that initiates myocardial contraction. Ca^{2+} sequestration by the SR and extrusion from the myocyte causes relaxation (diastole).

Anatomically, the SR is a lipid membrane–bounded, fine interconnected network spreading throughout the myocytes. The Ca^{2+} release channels (or ryanodine receptors [RyRs]) are concentrated at the part of the SR that is in very close apposition to the T tubular Ca^{2+} channel. These are called terminal cisternae or the junctional sarcoplasmic reticulum (jSR). The second part of the SR, the longitudinal, free, or network SR, consists of ramifying tubules that surround the myofilaments (see Fig. 46.1) that take Ca^{2+} back up into the SR and thus drive relaxation. Such Ca^{2+} uptake is achieved by the ATP-consuming Ca^{2+} pump known as SERCA (sarcoendoplasmic reticulum Ca^{2+}–adenosine triphosphatase, or SR Ca-ATPase). The Ca^{2+} taken up into the SR is then stored at high concentration, in part bound to Ca^{2+}-buffering proteins, including calsequestrin, before being released again in response to the next wave of depolarization. Cytoplasm or sarcoplasm refers to the intracellular fluid and proteins therein, but excludes the contents of organelles such as the mitochondria, nucleus, and SR. The cytoplasm is crowded with myofilaments, but this is the fluid within which the concentration of Ca^{2+} rises and falls to cause cardiac contraction and relaxation.

Subcellular Microarchitecture

There are many microdomains and even nanometer-scale nanodomains involved in molecular signaling that convey messages within

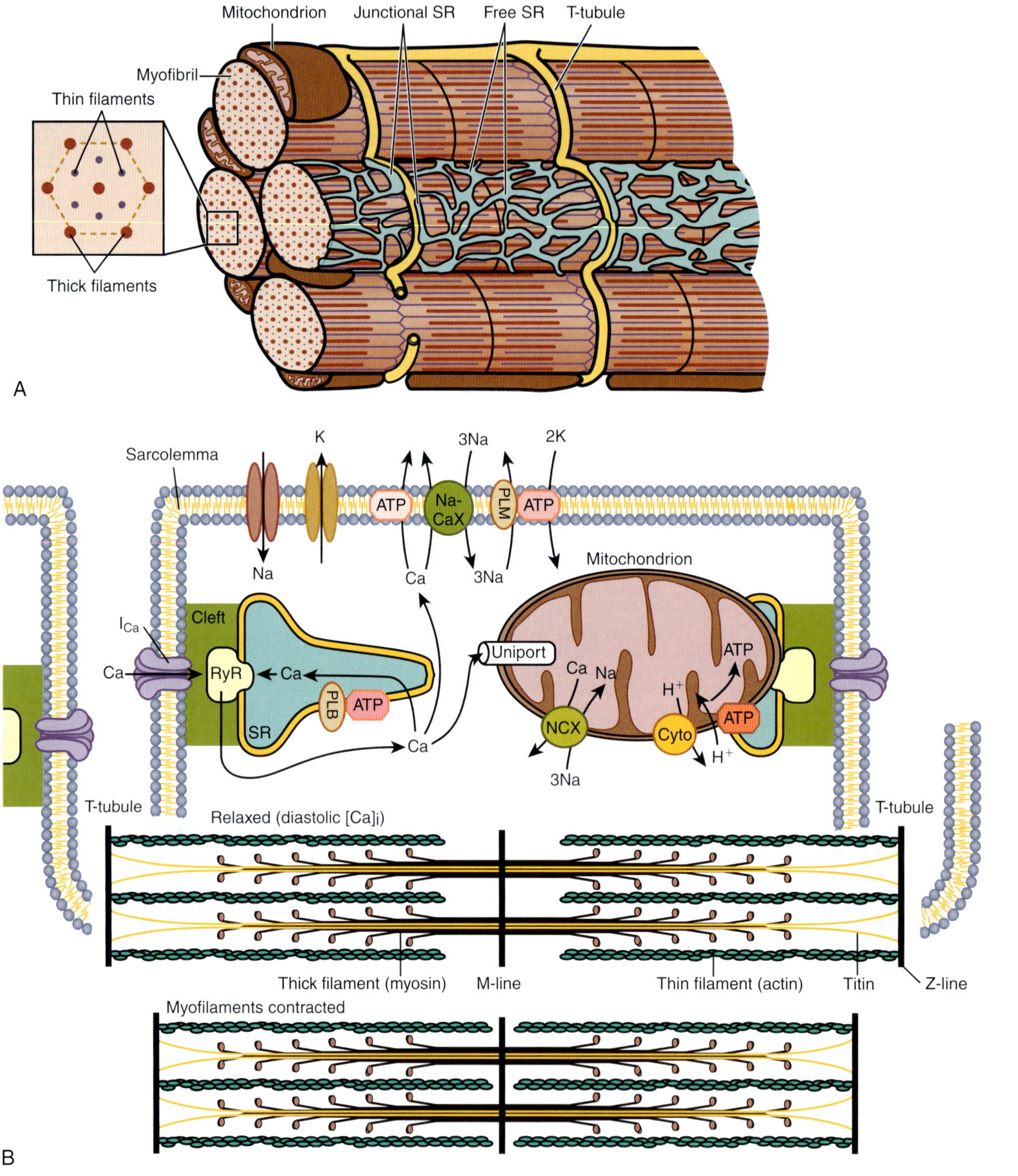

FIGURE 46.1 Ultrastructural components of excitation-contraction coupling in ventricular myocytes, viewed anatomically (**A,** with *inset* showing an end-on view of thick and thin filament organization) and schematically (**B**). The action potential is conducted along the surface sarcolemma and sarcolemma that extends into the T tubules. Ca^{2+} current (I_{Ca}) at sites of junctional SR clefts trigger local Ca^{2+} release, and the Ca^{2+} diffuses throughout the cytosol to activate myofilament contraction. The $[Ca^{2+}]_i$ quickly declines at each beat because of Ca^{2+} uptake via the SR Ca^{2+}-ATPase (ATP/PLB), extrusion via sarcolemmal Na^+/Ca^{2+} exchange (NCX) and Ca^{2+}-ATPase (and mitochondrial Ca^{2+} uniport), allowing relaxation (diastole) to proceed. The myofibrils are bundles of contractile proteins that are organized into a regular sarcomeric array, bounded longitudinally by Z-lines that are immediately adjacent to T tubules that run in parallel. In diastole (*bottom*) the thin filaments (containing mainly actin) create a cage around the thick filaments (containing mainly myosin) that have cross-bridges (myosin heads) that extend toward the thin filament. Myosin molecule tails all face the center of the sarcomere, creating a zone around the M-line devoid of myosin heads. During systole, the myosin cross-bridges pull the thin filament "cage" toward the M-line, thus shortening the sarcomere length (additional details are in subsequent figures). *ATP,* Adenosine triphosphate; *PLB,* phospholamban; *SR,* sarcoplasmic reticulum; *T tubules,* transverse tubules. (**A** Redrawn, based on a classic sketch by Fawcett DW, McNutt NS: The ultrastructure of the cat myocardium: I. Ventricular papillary muscle [*J Cell Biol*. 1969;42:1–45].)

TABLE 46.1 Characteristics of Cardiac Cells, Organelles, and Contractile Proteins

MICROANATOMY OF HEART CELLS			
	VENTRICULAR MYOCYTE	ATRIAL MYOCYTE	PURKINJE CELLS
Shape	Long and narrow	Elliptical	Long and broad
Length (μm)	75–170	20–100	150–200
Diameter (μm)	15–30	5–6	35–40
Volume (μm³)	15,000–100,000	400–1500	135,000–250,000
T tubules	Plentiful	Rare or none	Absent
Intercalated disc	Prominent end-to-end transmission	Side-to-side as well as end-to-end transmission	Very prominent abundant gap junctions Fast; end-to-end transmission
General appearance	Mitochondria and sarcomeres very abundant Rectangular branching bundles with little interstitial collagen	Bundles of atrial tissue separated by wide areas of collagen	Fewer sarcomeres, paler

COMPOSITION AND FUNCTION OF VENTRICULAR CELL		
ORGANELLE	PERCENTAGE OF CELL VOLUME	FUNCTION
Myofibril	≈50–60	Interaction of thick and thin filaments during contraction cycle
Mitochondria	16 in neonate 33 in adult rat 23 in adult man	Provide ATP chiefly for contraction
T-system	≈1	Transmission of electrical signal from sarcolemma to cell interior
SR	10 in neonate 2–3 in adult	Takes up and releases Ca^{2+} during contraction cycle
SR terminal cisternae	0.33 in adult	Site of calcium storage and release
Rest of network of SR	Rest of volume	Site of calcium uptake en route to cisternae
Sarcolemma	Very low	Control of ionic gradients, channels for ions (action potential), maintenance of cell integrity, receptors for drugs and hormones
Nucleus	≈3	Transcription
Lysosomes	Very low	Intracellular digestion and proteolysis
Sarcoplasm (= cytoplasm) (includes myofibril but not mitochondria or SR)	~60	Cytosolic volume within which $[Ca^{2+}]_i$ rises and falls

ATP, Adenosine triphosphate; *SR*, sarcoplasmic reticulum.

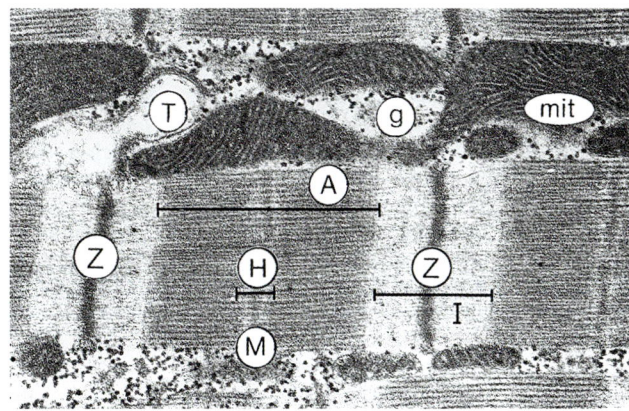

FIGURE 46.2 The sarcomere is the distance between the two Z-lines. Note the presence of numerous mitochondria (*mit*) sandwiched between the myofibrils and the presence of T tubules (*T*), which penetrate into the muscle at the level of the Z-lines. This two-dimensional picture should not disguise the fact that the Z-line is really a "Z-disc," as is the M-line (*M*), also shown in Figure 46.1. *A*, Band of actin-myosin overlap; *g*, glycogen granules; *H*, central clear zone containing only myosin filament bodies and the M-line; *I*, band of actin filaments, titin, and Z-line (rat papillary muscle, 32,000×). (Courtesy Dr. J. Moravec, Dijon, France.)

Mitochondrial Ca and Na Transport: Connection to Metabolism

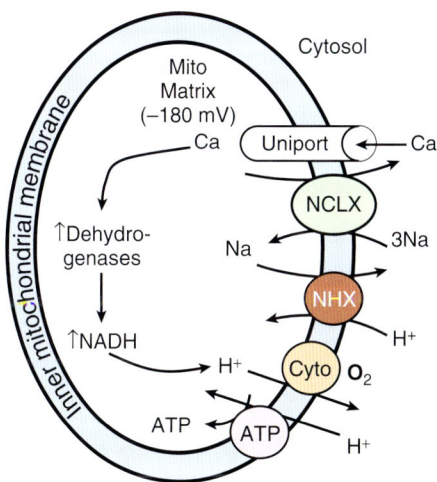

FIGURE 46.3 Mitochondrial Ca^{2+} regulation. The intramitochondrial matrix is very negative with respect to the cytosol (−180 mV). Ca^{2+} enters mitochondria via the Ca^{2+} uniporter in the inner mitochondrial membrane and is extruded by Na^+/Ca^{2+} exchange (*NCLX*). Na^+ is extruded via Na^+/H^+ exchange (NHX). Protons (H^+) are pumped out of mitochondria by the cytochrome (*Cyto*) systems, thereby allowing H^+ to enter via F_0F_1 ATP synthase (*ATP*). When mitochondrial [Ca] is increased, it activates mitochondrial dehydrogenases, which increase NADH levels and provide additional reducing equivalent protons to the electron transport chain. (Modified from Bers DM. *Excitation-Contraction Coupling and Cardiac Contractile Force*. Dordrecht, Netherlands: Kluwer Academic; 2001.)

myocytes. These include the jSR-T-tubule junctions where T-tubular Ca^{2+} channels are within 10 nm of a cluster of RyR channels in the jSR membrane to produce the synchronous Ca^{2+} transients that control contraction. There are also sarcolemmal receptor complexes, such as beta-adrenergic receptors that have specific molecular partners (more below) that produce second messengers (cyclic nucleotides) that can diffuse to other functional targets in the myocyte. *Caveolae* (small, flask-shaped sarcolemmal invaginations) are also microdomains with key localized signaling cascades. *Scaffolding proteins* such as caveolin, A-kinase anchoring proteins (AKAPs), and the RyR itself bring interacting molecules closely together at these locations. These complexes can also release components that translocate and signal elsewhere in the cell, such as the nucleus, where they can signal for myocyte growth. Another type of subcellular shuttling is involved in transporting the ATP produced in mitochondria to sites where it is used (e.g., myofilaments), which is facilitated by the location of creatine kinase, an enzyme that converts creatine phosphate to ATP.

Mitochondrial Morphology and Function

The typical ventricular myocyte has approximately 8000 mitochondria, each of which is ovate with a long axis measuring 1 to 2 μm and short axis of 300 to 500 nm. Mitochondria have two membranes: outer and inner mitochondrial membranes (OMM and IMM; Figs. 46.1 and 46.3).

The IMM is "crumpled" into folds called cristae, which provide a large surface area within a small volume. The IMM also contains the cytochrome complexes that make up the respiratory chain, including F_0-F_1 ATP synthase. The space within the IMM, the mitochondrial matrix, contains enzymes of the tricarboxylic acid (TCA) cycle and other key metabolic components. These components provide reducing equivalent protons that are pumped out of the matrix by the cytochromes, and it is this proton pumping that creates the very negative voltage with respect to cytosol ($\psi_m = -180$ mV). The proton pumping out of the matrix also creates a trans-IMM [H$^+$] gradient, which together with the very negative ψ_m creates a strong electrochemical gradient for protons to enter the matrix. The energy from this "downhill" proton flux is used by the F_0 F_1 ATP synthase to make ATP. However, in the absence of the normal proton and ψ_m, this elegant F_0-F_1 ATP synthase runs backward, consuming ATP. The ATP produced in the matrix is transported across the IMM by an adenine nucleotide transporter that exchanges mitochondrial ATP for cytosolic adenosine diphosphate (ADP). This system is exquisitely regulated to maintain cytosolic [ATP] and [ADP] constant during dramatic changes in cardiac workload.[5] The multiple control mechanisms involved in this process are not fully understood, but one is relevant to excitation-contraction coupling. Increased cardiac work in a physiologic setting is usually driven by higher-amplitude and/or more frequent Ca^{2+} transients. This elevation in average intracellular [Ca^{2+}] ([Ca^{2+}]$_i$) also increases mitochondrial matrix [Ca^{2+}] ([Ca^{2+}]$_m$), which activates key dehydrogenases in the TCA cycle and also pyruvate dehydrogenase to restore levels of reduced nicotinamide adenine dinucleotide (NADH), which drives cytochrome activity and helps restore (ATP) toward normal.

This raises the issue of how mitochondria regulate [Ca^{2+}]$_m$, because there is also a huge electrochemical gradient favoring entry of Ca^{2+} into mitochondria.[2] Indeed, [Ca^{2+}]$_m$ is typically similar to [Ca^{2+}]$_i$ and is kept at that level by a mitochondrial Na/Ca exchanger (NCLX), which uses the also steep Na$^+$ electrochemical gradient to pump Ca^{2+} out of the mitochondria.[2] However, this would load the mitochondria with Na$^+$, so Na$^+$ must also be extruded from the mitochondria. This is accomplished by the mitochondrial Na/H exchanger in the IMM, but a consequence is that this influx of H$^+$ costs energy. That is, these protons could have entered the mitochondria via the F_0-F_1 ATP synthase making ATP, but instead they were used to extrude Na$^+$ and Ca^{2+}. Thus in a sense the mitochondrion can make ATP or extrude Ca^{2+}. This becomes important when myocytes (or other cells) experience Ca^{2+} overload. In the short term, mitochondria can take up large amounts of Ca^{2+} to protect the cell from short-term Ca^{2+} overload, but chronic high [Ca^{2+}]$_i$ has dire consequences. First, this Ca^{2+} uptake can diminish ψ_m and occurs at the expense of ATP production (as noted), thus hampering energetic recovery from such stress. Second, elevated [Ca^{2+}]$_i$ and [Ca^{2+}]$_m$ can facilitate opening of the mitochondrial permeability transition pore, which immediately dissipates ψ_m, results in the F_0 F_1 ATP synthase consuming rather than making ATP, and allows the matrix contents to be released to the cytosol. This is usually the death knell for individual mitochondria, as well as the cells that rely on their robust function.

Thus, mitochondria can rapidly become agents of cell death as just described, as well as by producing excessive reactive oxygen species (ROS), which can promote necrotic cell death through the mitochondrial permeability transition pore and release of proapoptotic proteins (see Chapter 47).[6] Mitochondria can also induce mitochondrial autophagy, or *mitophagy*, which selectively and adaptively clears damaged mitochondria. Increased oxidative stress and apoptotic proteases can inactivate mitophagy and thereby cause cell death.[7] Mitochondria can also undergo fission, sometimes with one daughter mitochondrion being less healthy and targeted for mitophagy. They can also undergo fusion, to merge smaller ones into a larger mitochondrion. Fission, fusion and mitophagy are normal and healthy parts of mitochondrial life, and dysfunction of any of these can have pathologic consequences.

Contractile Proteins

The two chief contractile proteins are the motor protein *myosin* on the thick filament and *actin* on the thin filament (see Figs. 46.1B and 46.2). Ca^{2+} initiates the contraction cycle by binding to the thin filament regulatory protein *troponin C* to relieve the inhibition otherwise exerted by this troponin complex (Fig. 46.4). The thin actin filaments are connected to the *Z-lines* at either end of the *sarcomere*, which is the functional contractile unit that is repeated through the filaments. The sarcomere is limited on either side by a Z-line, which with the thin filaments creates a "cage" around the thick myosin filament that extends from the center of the sarcomere outward toward the Z-line. During contraction, the myosin heads grab onto actin and pull the

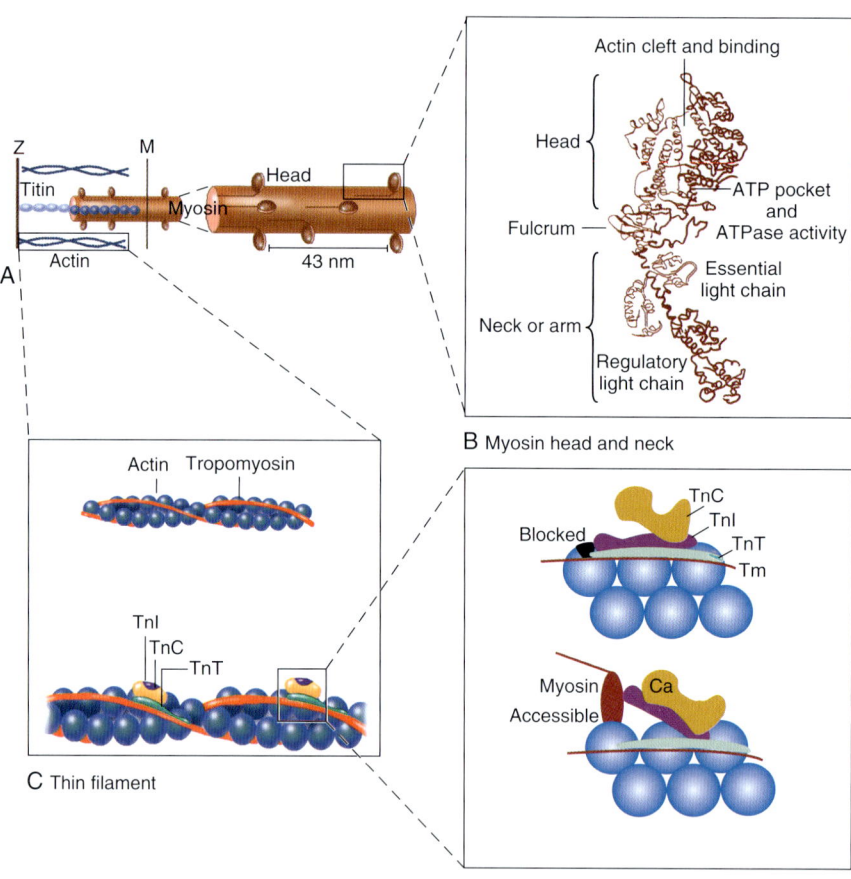

FIGURE 46.4 Key contractile protein interactions. The thin actin filament **(A)** interacts with the myosin head **(B)** when Ca^{2+} ions arrive at troponin C (*TnC*) **(C)**. This causes troponin-tropomyosin shifts to expose the actin site to which a myosin head can attach. **A**, The thin actin filament contains TnC and its Ca^{2+} binding sites. When TnC is not activated by Ca^{2+}, troponin I (*TnI*) stabilizes troponin T (*TnT*) and tropomyosin (*Tm*) along the actin filament to block myosin cross-bridge binding **(D)**. **B**, The molecular structure of the myosin head, based on Rayment and colleagues,[8] is composed of heavy and light chains. The heavy head chain in turn has two major domains: one of 70 kDa (i.e., 70,000 molecular weight) that interacts with actin at the actin cleft and has an ATP binding pocket. The "neck" domain of 20 kDa, also called the "lever," is an elongated alpha helix that extends and bends and has two light chains surrounding it as a collar. The essential light chain is part of the structure. The other regulatory light chain may respond to phosphorylation to influence the extent of the actin-myosin interaction. **C**, TnC with sites in the regulatory domain for activation by calcium and for interaction with TnI. **D**, Binding of calcium to TnC causes TnI to shift binding from TnT to TnC, allowing the TnT-Tm complex to shift deeper into the actin groove and expose the myosin binding domain on actin. (Modified from Opie LH. *Heart Physiology, from Cell to Circulation*. Philadelphia: Lippincott Williams & Wilkins; 2004. Figure copyright L. H. Opie, 2004. **D**, Modified from Solaro RJ, Van Eyk J. Altered interactions among thin filament proteins modulate cardiac function. *J Mol Cell Cardiol*. 1999;28:217.)

actin filaments toward the center of the sarcomere. The thin and thick filaments can thus slide over each other to shorten the sarcomere and cell length, without the individual actin or myosin molecules actually changing length (see Fig. 46.1B). The interaction of the myosin heads with actin filaments that is switched on when Ca^{2+} arrives is called cross-bridge cycling. As the actin filaments move inward toward the center of the sarcomere, they draw the Z-lines closer together so that the sarcomere length shortens. The energy for contraction is provided by breakdown of ATP (myosin is an ATPase).

Titin and Length Sensing

Titin is a giant molecule, the largest protein yet described. It is extraordinarily long, elastic, and slender (Fig. 46.5). Titin extends from the Z-line into the thick filament, approaching the M-line, and connects the thick filament to the Z-line (see Fig. 46.1). Titin has two distinct segments: an inextensible anchoring segment and an extensible elastic segment that stretches as sarcomere length increases. Thus the titin molecule can stretch between 0.6 and 1.2 μm in length and has multiple functions. First, it tethers myosin and thick filaments to the Z-line, thereby stabilizing sarcomeric structure. Second, as it stretches and relaxes, its elasticity contributes to the stress-strain relationship of cardiac and skeletal muscle. At short sarcomere lengths, the elastic domain is coiled up on itself to generate restoring force (see Fig. 46.5), similar to a spring, helping to relengthen the sarcomere and aid early diastolic filling. These changes in titin help explain the *series elastic element* that was inferred from mechanics studies as elasticity in series with the myosin filaments. Third, the increased diastolic stretch of titin as the length of the sarcomere in cardiac muscle is increased causes the enfolded part of the titin molecule to straighten. This stretched molecular spring then limits overstretching of sarcomeres and end-diastolic volume (EDV) and returns some potential energy during systole as the sarcomeres shorten during cardiac ejection.[4] Fourth, titin may transduce mechanical stretch into growth signals. Sustained diastolic stretch, as in volume overload, can cause titin-dependent signaling to muscle LIM protein (MLP) attached to the Z-line end of titin.[8] MLP is proposed to be a stretch sensor that transmits the signals that result in the myocyte growth pattern characteristic of volume overload, and it may be defective in a subset of human dilated cardiomyopathy.[9]

Molecular Basis of Muscular Contraction

Although the molecular level details underlying the cross-bridge cycle are complex, cross bridges appear to exist in either a strong or a weak binding state (but a super-relaxed state also exists).[10] During diastole, myosin heads normally have ATP bound (Fig. 46.6B) and hydrolyzed to ADP plus inorganic phosphate (Pi), although ADP-Pi is not yet released and the energy of ATP is not yet fully consumed (Fig. 46.6C). Thus the cross bridges are poised and ready to bind to actin. This interaction is permitted when Ca^{2+} arrives and binds to troponin C, shifting the position of the troponin-tropomyosin complex on the actin filament (see Fig. 46.4C, D). This enables the poised myosin heads to form strong binding cross bridges with actin molecules (Fig. 46.6D) and use the energy stored in myosin-ADP-P$_i$ to rotate the myosin head while bound to actin in the *power stroke* (and release P$_i$) while still in the strong binding state (Fig. 46.6D and E). Once a particular cross bridge proceeds through the power stroke (using the energy previously stored in the ATP molecule), it will remain in the strong binding or *rigor* state (Fig. 46.6A) until ATP binds again to myosin, causing a shift back to the weak binding state and allowing cross-bridge detachment and ATP hydrolysis (Fig. 46.6C). As long as $[Ca^{2+}]_i$ and [ATP] remain high, the cycle can continue with myosin-ADP-Pi binding to a new actin molecule. The weak binding state predominates when $[Ca^{2+}]_i$ falls and Ca^{2+} dissociates from troponin C, allowing relaxation during diastole. If intracellular [ATP] declines too far (e.g., during ischemia), ATP cannot bind and disrupt the rigor linkage, leaving cross bridges locked in the strong binding state (as in rigor mortis).

Actin and Troponin Complex

The Ca^{2+} on-switch of cross-bridge cycling is mediated by a series of interactions within the troponin, tropomyosin, and actin complex (see Fig. 46.4C, D). Thin filaments are composed of two helical intertwining actin filaments, with a long tropomyosin molecule that spans seven actin monomers located in the groove between the two actin filaments. Also, at every seventh actin molecule (38.5 nm along this structure) there is a three-protein regulatory *troponin complex:* troponin C (Ca^{2+} binding), I (inhibitory), and T (tropomyosin binding).

When $[Ca^{2+}]_i$ is low, the position of tropomyosin blocks the myosin heads from interacting effectively with actin. As a result, most cross bridges are in the "blocked position," with a few visiting the weak binding state. Ca^{2+} binding with troponin C causes troponin C to bind more tightly to troponin I (see Fig. 46.4D), which allows tropomyosin to roll deeper into the thin filament groove,[1] thereby opening access to allow myosin binding to actin. This allows the cross-bridge cycle to proceed (see Fig. 46.6). As they form, strong cross bridges can nudge tropomyosin deeper into the actin groove, allowing cross-bridge attachment at one site to enhance actin-myosin at its "nearest-neighbor" sites. This cooperatively spreads activation farther along the myofilaments.[1,4]

Myosin Structure and Function

Each myosin head is the terminal part of the myosin heavy chain molecule. The other ends of two myosin molecules (tails) intertwine as a coil that forms the bulk of the thick filament. Also, a short "neck" leads to the myosin head that protrudes out from the filament (see Fig. 46.4). According to the Rayment model, the base of the head and/or neck region changes configuration during the power stroke previously described.[8] Each head has an *ATP-binding pocket* and a narrow cleft that extends from the base of this pocket to the actin-binding face (see Fig. 46.6).[11]

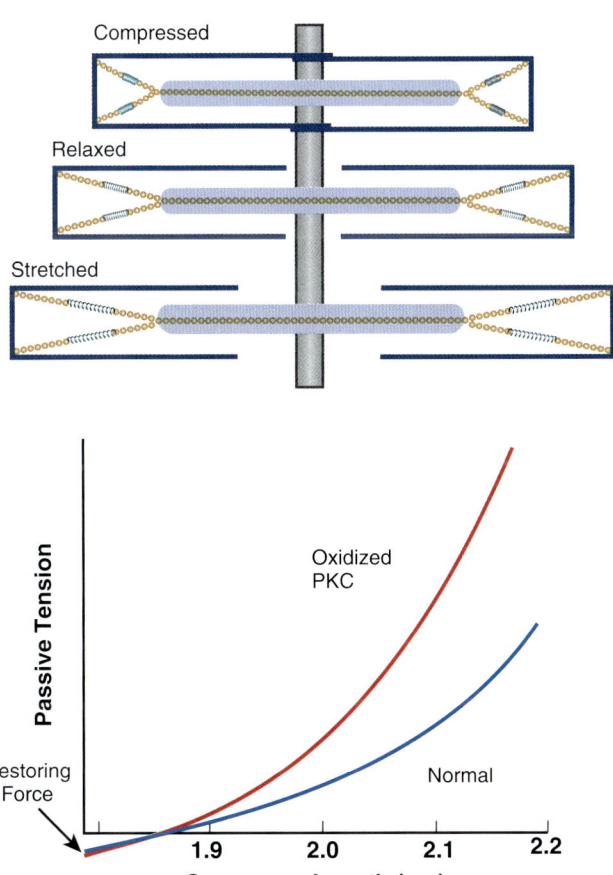

FIGURE 46.5 Titin is a huge elastic elongated protein that connects myosin and the M-line to the Z-line. It is a bidirectional spring that develops passive force in stretched sarcomeres and resting force in shortened sarcomeres. **Upper panel,** As the sarcomere is stretched to its maximum physiologic diastolic length of 2.2 μm, titin stretches and increases passive force generated (contributing to end-diastolic pressure). At short lengths (*top*), which may reflect end-systole, substantial restoring force is generated, shown as negative tension **(lower panel).** Note that oxidation and PKC-dependent phosphorylation increase titin stiffness. (Modified with permission of the American Heart Association, from Lewinter MM, Granzier HL. Titin is a major human disease gene. *Circulation.* 2013;127:938–944.)

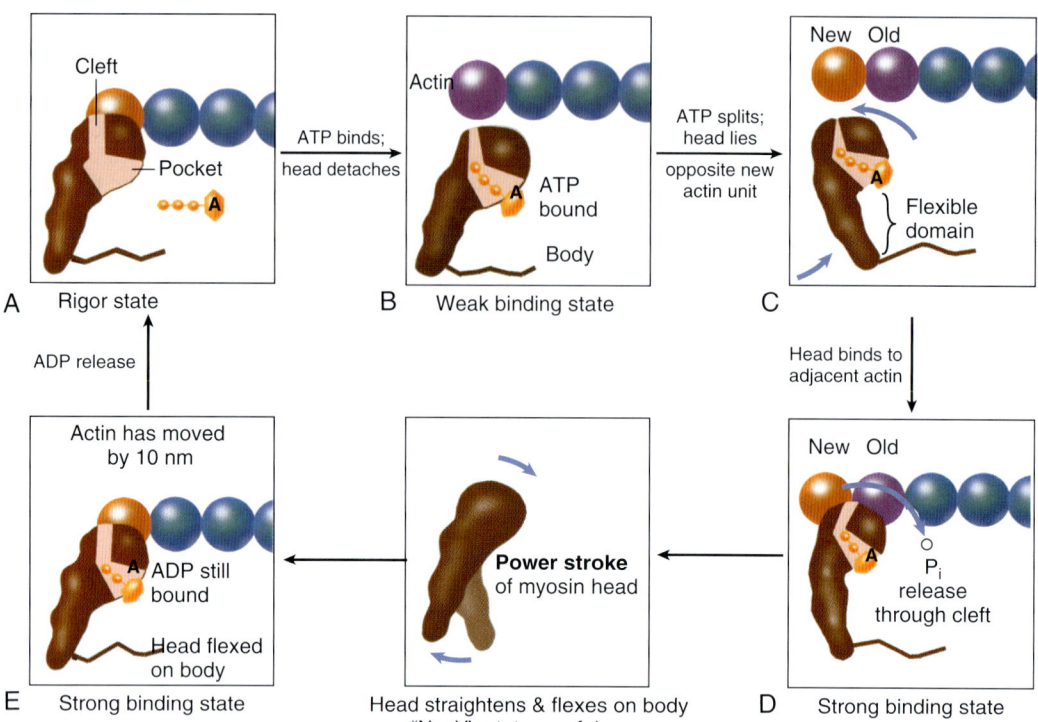

FIGURE 46.6 Cross-bridge cycling molecular model. The cross-bridge (only one myosin head depicted) is pear shaped, and the catalytic motor domain interacts with the actin molecule and is attached to an extended alpha helical "neck region," which acts as a lever arm. The nucleotide pocket that binds adenosine triphosphate (ATP) is in the catalytic domain. The actin binding cleft bisects the catalytic motor domain. Starting with the rigor state **(A)**, binding of ATP to the pocket **(B)** is followed by ATP hydrolysis **(C)**, which alters the actin binding domain, favoring release from actin. The binding to actin is enhanced when phosphate is released, and the myosin head strongly attaches to actin to induce the power stroke **(D** and **E)**. During the power stroke the head rotates around the head-neck fulcrum. As the head flexes, the actin filament can be displaced by approximately 10 nm **(E)**, causing shortening (although during isometric contraction the neck region stretches and bears force). In this process, ADP is also released, so the binding pocket becomes vacant, resulting in the rigor state again **(A)** until ATP binds to release the cross bridge.

During the power stroke when there is no mechanical load on the muscle, the myosin head flexes and can move the actin filament by approximately 10 nm.[1] When the pocket releases ADP and binds ATP, the cross bridge releases back to an orientation more perpendicular to the direction of the thin and thick filaments. During isometric (or isovolumic) contraction, the cross bridges rotate but cannot fully move the actin filament, and the stretched strong binding cross bridges bear force. During shortening (ejection), the actin filament moves during the power stroke, accompanied by decreases in sarcomere length and ventricular volume.

Note that myosin heads stick out from the thick filament in six directions in an organized array to allow interactions with each of six actin filaments that surround each thick filament (see Fig. 46.1A). The myosin molecules are also oriented in reversed longitudinal directions on either side of the M-line (which itself contains only myosin tails), such that each side is trying to pull the Z-lines toward the center. That is, when cross bridges are in the strong binding or rigor linkages, they form "chevrons" (or *arrows*) pointing toward the Z-line on that side of the M-line.

Each cycle of the cross bridge consumes one molecule of ATP, and this *myosin ATPase activity* is the major site of ATP consumption in the beating heart. Thus, when the heart is more strongly activated, the level of ATP consumption is similarly increased. The two myosin heads that stick out from an intertwined pair of myosin molecules seem to work through a hand-over-hand action such that the myosin dimer never fully releases the thin filament during the activation period.[12] There are also two main myosin isoforms in cardiac myocytes, alpha and beta, which have similar molecular weight but exhibit substantially different cross-bridge cycle and ATPase rates. The beta-myosin heavy chain (β-MHC) isoform exhibits a slower ATPase rate and is the predominant form in adult humans. In small mammals (rats and mice), the faster α-MHC form normally predominates but shifts to the β-MHC pattern during chronic stress and heart failure.[4] β-MHC has been targeted therapeutically using both gain and loss of function approaches. Mavacamten is a novel therapeutic myosin inhibitor that targets the excessive contractility and impaired relaxation, myocardial energetics and compliance in patients with obstructive hypertrophic cardiomyopathy (oHCM). In the PIONEER clinical trial (NCT03470545), mavacamten improved exercise capacity, left ventricular (LV) outflow tract obstruction, New York Heart Association (NYHA) functional class, and health status in patients with oHCM (see also Chapter 54). Omecamtiv mecarbil is a novel therapeutic that activates myosin ATPase and enhances myosin cross-bridge formation and duration, thereby prolonging myocardial contraction. The GALACTIC-HF trial demonstrated that treatment with the selective cardiac myosin activator omecamtiv mecarbil reduced the incidence of a composite of a heart-failure event or death from cardiovascular causes in patients with heart failure and reduced EF[12a] (see also Chapter 49).

Each myosin molecule neck also has two light chains (see Fig. 46.4A). The *essential myosin light chain* (MLC-1) is more proximal to the myosin head and may limit the contractile process by interaction with actin. The *regulatory myosin light chain* (MLC-2) is a potential site for phosphorylation (e.g., in response to beta-adrenergic stimulation) and may promote cross-bridge cycling.[13] In vascular smooth muscle, which lacks the troponin-tropomyosin complex, contraction is activated by the Ca^{2+}-dependent myosin light chain kinase (MLCK) rather than by Ca^{2+} binding to troponin C (as in striated muscle). Myosin-binding protein C appears to traverse the myosin molecules in the A-band, thereby potentially tethering the myosin molecules and stabilizing the myosin head with respect to the thick and thin filaments. Defects in myosin, myosin-binding protein C, and several other myofilament proteins are genetically linked to familial hypertrophic cardiomyopathy.[14]

Graded Effects of $[Ca^{2+}]_i$ on Cross-Bridge Cycle

The myofilaments are activated in a graded rather than all-or-none manner as a function of $[Ca^{2+}]_i$ (Fig. 46.7), such that as $[Ca^{2+}]_i$ rises force of contraction increases going up the curve. Then as $[Ca^{2+}]_i$ declines relaxation proceeds (back to the diastolic point). The dynamics and regulation of Ca^{2+} transients in cardiac myocytes are discussed in the following section, but a major physiologic mechanism for regulating cardiac contractility (e.g., during sympathetic activity) is to increase peak $[Ca^{2+}]_i$ and more fully activate the myofilaments. The higher the

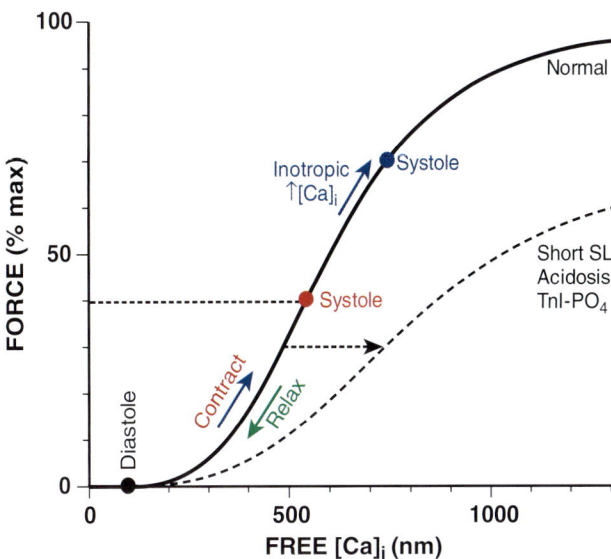

FIGURE 46.7 Myofilament Ca^{2+} sensitivity. Active force development in cardiac muscle depends on the cytosolic free $[Ca]_i$. As $[Ca]_i$ rises during systole, force develops as dictated by the sigmoidal myofilament Ca^{2+} sensitivity curve (*solid curve*; Force = $100/(1+[600\ nm]/[Ca]_i)^4$). As $[Ca]_i$ declines relaxation ensues and force declines. If peak $[Ca]_i$ increases (as in inotropy) the peak force can reach a higher value. At shorter sarcomere length (SL), acidosis, and troponin I (TnI) phosphorylation, the myofilament Ca^{2+} sensitivity is reduced, and the former two also decrease maximal force (*dashed curve*).

$[Ca^{2+}]_i$, the more fully saturated are the Ca^{2+} binding sites on troponin C, and consequently, more sites are available for cross bridges to form. When more cross bridges are working in parallel, the myocyte (and heart) can develop greater force (or ventricular pressure). There is high cooperativity in this process, in large part because of the "nearest-neighbor" effect mentioned earlier. That is, Ca^{2+} bound to a single troponin C molecule encourages local cross-bridge formation, and both Ca^{2+} binding and cross-bridge formation directly enhance the likelihood of cross-bridge formation in the seven actin molecules controlled by one tropomyosin molecule. Furthermore, the openness of that domain directly enhances that of the neighboring domain with respect to both Ca^{2+} binding and cross-bridge formation. This cooperativity means that a small change in $[Ca^{2+}]_i$ can have a great effect on the strength of contraction.

Length-Dependent Activation and the Frank-Starling Effect

Besides $[Ca^{2+}]_i$, the other major factor influencing the strength of contraction is sarcomere length at the end of diastole (preload), just before the onset of systole. Both Otto Frank and Ernest Starling observed that the more the diastolic filling of the heart, the greater the strength of the heartbeat. The increased heart volume translates into increased sarcomere length, which acts by a length-sensing mechanism. A part of this Frank-Starling effect has historically been ascribed to increasingly optimal overlap between the actin and myosin filaments. Clearly, however, there is also a substantial increase in myofilament Ca^{2+} sensitivity with an increase in sarcomere length (see Fig. 46.7).[1] A plausible mechanism for this regulatory change may reside in the decreasing interfilament spacing as heart muscle is stretched. That is, the myocyte is at constant volume (over the cardiac cycle), so as the cell shortens, it must thicken, and conversely, when it is stretched, the cell becomes thinner and filament spacing becomes narrower. This attractive lattice-dependent explanation for the Frank-Starling relationship has been challenged by careful x-ray diffraction studies,[4] which found that reducing sarcomere lattice spacing by osmotic compression failed to influence myofilament Ca^{2+} sensitivity. Although several mechanisms could contribute to myofilament Ca^{2+} sensitization at longer sarcomere length, the issue is unresolved.

When changes in diastolic length (or preload) are the cause of altered contractile strength, it is said to be a Frank-Starling (or Starling) effect. Conditions in which contraction is strengthened independent of sarcomere length (e.g., typically by increased Ca^{2+} transient amplitude) are referred to as positive *inotropic states* or enhanced *contractility*. The distinction between these heterometric (Starling) and homeometric (inotropic) mechanisms of altered cardiac strength is functionally and therapeutically important.

Cross-Bridge Cycling Differs from Cardiac Contraction-Relaxation Cycle

The cardiac cycle of Wiggers (see Fig. 46.16) must be distinguished from the cross-bridge cycle. The cardiac cycle reflects the overall changes in pressure in the left ventricle, whereas the cross-bridge cycle is the repetitive interaction between myosin heads and actin. During isovolumic contraction (before aortic valve opening), the sarcomeres do not shorten appreciably, but cross bridges are developing force, although not all simultaneously. That is, at any given moment, some myosin heads will be flexing or flexed (resulting in force generation), some will be extending or extended, and some will be attached weakly to actin and some detached from actin. Numerous such cross-bridge cycles, each lasting microseconds, are integrated to produce the resulting force (and pressure). When ventricular pressure (sum of cross-bridge forces) reaches aortic pressure (afterload), ejection begins and is associated with the cross bridges actively moving the thin actin filaments toward the center of the sarcomere (M-line), thereby shortening the sarcomere. Note that as ejection proceeds (and sarcomeres shorten), myofilament Ca^{2+} sensitivity declines (see Fig. 46.7). Thus, both $[Ca^{2+}]_i$ decline and shortening cause a progressive decline in the contractile state as systole gives way to diastole. Both the Ca^{2+} transient properties and the myofilament Ca^{2+} sensitivity and cross-bridge cycling rate are altered under physiologic conditions, such as sympathetic stimulation and local acidosis or ischemia, as discussed later.

Force Transmission

Volume and pressure overload may have different effects on myocardial growth because of different patterns of force transmission.[4] Whereas increased diastolic force is transmitted longitudinally by titin to reach MLP, the postulated sensor (see earlier), increased systolic force may be transmitted laterally (i.e., at right angles) by the Z-disc and cytoplasmic actin to reach the cytoskeletal proteins and cell-to-matrix junctions, such as the focal adhesion complex. This mechanical force is translated into signals by the dystrophin and integrin protein complexes that mediate force transmission between the intracellular cytoskeleton, the extracellular matrix, and neighboring cells. These can activate intrinsic short-term adaptive such as the Anrep effect, as well as signaling to the nucleus to activate the growth pathways via altered gene regulation, as addressed in other chapters.

> **CONTRACTILE PROTEIN DEFECTS AND CARDIOMYOPATHY**
>
> Genetic-based hypertrophic and dilated cardiomyopathies not only produce hearts that look and behave very differently but also have diverse molecular causes. These cardiomyopathies in general are linked to mutant genes that cause abnormalities in the force-generating system, such as β-MHC, MLCs, myosin-binding protein C, troponin subunits, and tropomyosin (see Chapter 52). One hypothesis is that mutations that increase myofilament calcium sensitivity, contractility, and energy demand result in concentric hypertrophy,[15] whereas mutations that reduce myofilament calcium sensitivity or force generation or that result in non–force-generating cytoskeletal proteins (e.g., dystrophin, nuclear lamin, cytoplasmic actin, titin) lead to a dilated cardiomyopathy. Although useful, such broad distinction between the two types of cardiomyopathy is oversimplified, with several examples of overlapping mechanisms.

CALCIUM ION FLUXES IN CARDIAC CONTRACTION-RELAXATION CYCLE

Calcium Movements and Excitation-Contraction Coupling

Ca^{2+} is central to cardiac contraction and relaxation, and the associated Ca^{2+} fluxes that link contraction to the wave of excitation (excitation-contraction coupling) are now well understood and accepted.[1,2] Each QRS complex in the electrocardiogram (ECG) represents the synchronization of ventricular myocyte action potentials (APs) that trigger Ca^{2+} transients and consequent contraction-relaxation in each myocyte (Fig. 46.8A). Relatively small amounts of Ca^{2+} (trigger Ca^{2+}) enter and leave the cardiomyocyte during each cardiac cycle, with larger amounts being released and taken back up by the SR (see Fig. 46.8B). Each AP depolarization opens voltage-gated L-type Ca^{2+} channels in the T tubules that are physically near the junctional SR, and that local Ca^{2+} influx activates SR Ca^{2+} release channels (RyRs) to release additional Ca^{2+} which can diffuse to cause a whole-cell Ca^{2+} transient that activates contraction. In this Ca^{2+}-induced Ca^{2+} release mechanism, a smaller amount of Ca^{2+} entering via the calcium current (I_{Ca}) triggers the release of a larger amount of Ca^{2+} into the cytosol.[1,4] In the human ventricle and large mammals, SR Ca^{2+} release is three to four times larger than Ca^{2+} influx by I_{Ca}. In rat and mouse myocytes, however, SR Ca^{2+} cycling is more than 10 times greater than sarcolemmal Ca^{2+} flux.[1] The combined Ca^{2+} release and influx elevates $[Ca^{2+}]_i$ and promotes binding of Ca^{2+} to troponin C and thus contractile activation. Contraction is terminated mainly by Ca^{2+} reuptake into the SR by SERCA and extrusion from the myocyte by Na^+/Ca^{2+} exchange (NCX) which return $[Ca^{2+}]_i$ to the diastolic level.

Calcium Release and Uptake by Sarcoplasmic Reticulum

Sarcoplasmic Reticulum Network and Ca^{2+} Movements

Electron and fluorescence microscopy studies show that the SR is a continuous network surrounding the myofilaments with connections across Z-lines and transversely between myofibrils. Moreover, the lumens of the entire SR network and nuclear envelope are connected in adult cardiac myocytes. This allows relatively rapid diffusion of Ca^{2+} within the SR to balance free $[Ca^{2+}]$ within the SR ($[Ca^{2+}]_{SR}$).[16,17] The total SR Ca^{2+} content is the sum of $[Ca^{2+}]_{SR}$ plus Ca^{2+} bound to intra-SR Ca^{2+} buffers (especially calsequestrin). SR Ca^{2+} content is critical to normal cardiac function and electrophysiology, and its abnormalities contribute to systolic and diastolic dysfunction and arrhythmias. $[Ca^{2+}]_{SR}$ dictates the SR Ca^{2+} content and driving force for Ca^{2+} release and also regulates RyR release channel gating.[17]

Junctional Sarcoplasmic Reticulum and Ryanodine Receptor

The RyR channels that mediate SR Ca^{2+} release are mainly located in the jSR membrane at the junctions with the T tubule.[1] Each junction has 50 to 250 RyR channels on the jSR that are directly under and nearly touching a cluster of 20 to 40 sarcolemmal L-type Ca^{2+} channels across a 15-nm junctional gap (that is crowded with protein). RyR2 (the cardiac isoform) functions both as a Ca^{2+} channel and as a scaffolding protein that localizes numerous key regulatory proteins to the jSR.[1,4] On the large cytosolic side, these include proteins that can stabilize RyR gating (e.g., calmodulin [CaM], FK-506 binding protein [FKBP-12.6]); kinases that can regulate RyR gating by phosphorylation (e.g., protein kinase A [PKA], Ca^{2+}/CaM-dependent protein kinase II [CaMKII]); and the protein phosphatases PP1 and PP2A, which dephosphorylate the RyR. Inside the SR, the RyR also couples to several proteins (e.g., junctin, triadin, and via these, calsequestrin) that similarly regulate RyR gating and, in the case of calsequestrin, provides a local reservoir of buffered Ca^{2+} close to the release channel. The actual RyR channel is made up of a symmetric tetramer of RyR molecules, each of which may have the aforementioned regulatory proteins associated with it. Thus the RyR receptor complex is very large (>7000 kDa; Fig. 46.8).[18] When the T tubule is depolarized, one or more L-type Ca^{2+} channels open, and local cleft $[Ca^{2+}]$ increases sufficiently to activate at least one local jSR RyR (multiple channels here ensure high-fidelity signaling). The Ca^{2+} released from these first openings recruit additional RyRs in the junction through Ca^{2+}-induced Ca^{2+} release to amplify release of Ca^{2+} into the junctional space. The Ca^{2+} diffuses out of this space throughout the sarcomere to activate contraction. Each of the approximately 20,000 jSR regions in the typical ventricular myocyte seems to function independently in response to local activation by I_{Ca}. Thus the global Ca^{2+} transient in the myocyte at each beat is the spatiotemporal summation of SR Ca^{2+} release events from thousands of jSR regions, synchronized by the upstroke of the AP and activation of I_{Ca} at each junction.

Turning Off Ca^{2+} Release: Breaking Positive Feedback

Ca^{2+}-induced Ca^{2+} release is a positive feedback process, but it is now known that SR Ca^{2+} release turns off when $[Ca]_{SR}$ drops by approximately 50% (i.e., from a diastolic value of 1 mM to a nadir of 400 μM).[13] Elegant studies have documented how I_{Ca} is inactivated by high local $[Ca^{2+}]$, and

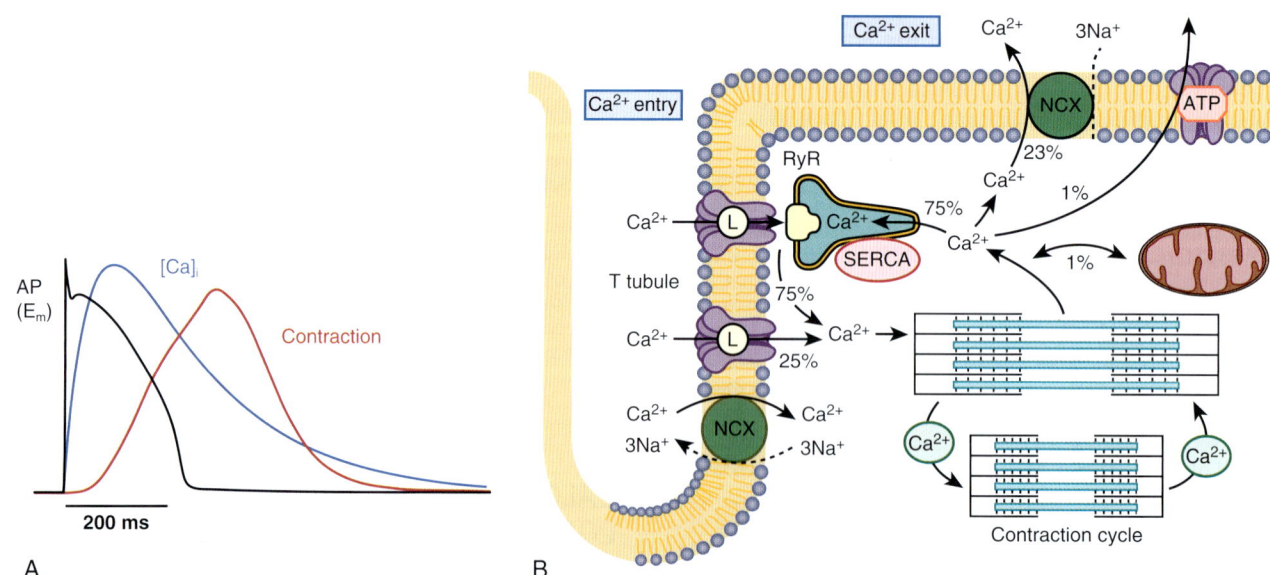

FIGURE 46.8 Myocyte Ca^{2+} fluxes during excitation-contraction (E–C) coupling. Rapid depolarization during the action potential (AP) triggers the Ca^{2+} transient that activates contraction **(A)**. **B,** Crucial features are (1) Ca^{2+} entry via the voltage-activated L-type Ca^{2+} channels, which triggers release of more Ca^{2+} from the SR; (2) a tiny amount of Ca^{2+} may enter via Na^+/Ca^{2+} exchange early in the action potential; and (3) removal of Ca^{2+} ions from the cytosol is mainly via the SR Ca-ATPase (SERCA; 75%) and Na^+/Ca^{2+} exchange (24%), with tiny amounts transported by mitochondrial Ca^{2+} uniport and the sarcolemmal Ca-ATPase (1%). The sodium pump (Na^+/K^+-ATPase) extrudes the Na^+ ions that entered during Na^+ current and Na^+/Ca^{2+} exchange action. Note that extracellular and intra-SR $[Ca^{2+}]$ (1 to 2 mM) is much higher than diastolic $[Ca^{2+}]_i$ (0.10 μM). Mitochondria can act as a buffer against excessive changes in cytosolic Ca^{2+}. (**B** modified from diagram by Bers DM. Cardiac excitation-contraction coupling. *Nature.* 2002;415:198.)

this robust calcium-dependent inactivation is mediated by binding of Ca^{2+} to the CaM that is already associated with that channel. When Ca^{2+} binds to CaM, it alters channel conformation such that I_{Ca} inactivation is favored. I_{Ca} is also subject to voltage-dependent inactivation during the AP plateau, and thus inactivation limits further entry of Ca^{2+} into the cell.

As for Ca^{2+}-dependent RyR activation, several mechanisms may contribute to breaking its inherent positive feedback. Although not necessarily most compelling, one mechanism is analogous to Ca^{2+}/CaM-dependent inactivation of I_{Ca}. That is, binding of Ca^{2+} to CaM that is prebound to RyR2 favors closure of RyR channels and inhibits reopening (Fig. 46.9).[19] A second mechanism, undoubtedly important, is that RyR2 gating is also sensitive to luminal $[Ca^{2+}]_{SR}$ such that high $[Ca^{2+}]_{SR}$ favors opening and low $[Ca^{2+}]_{SR}$ favors closure.[20] Indeed, release of Ca^{2+} from the SR during normal Ca^{2+} transients is robustly turned off when $[Ca^{2+}]_{SR}$ falls to approximately half its normal value (400 µM, which is still 500 times higher than bulk $[Ca^{2+}]_i$), almost regardless of the rate of SR Ca^{2+} release.[15,16] A third and related mechanism is that as Ca^{2+} release proceeds and $[Ca^{2+}]_{SR}$ declines, Ca^{2+} flux through the RyR falls and junctional $[Ca^{2+}]$ also falls, all of which tend to disrupt the positive feedback. That is, the RyR is less sensitive to activating Ca^{2+} (because $[Ca^{2+}]_{SR}$ is low) and lower $[Ca^{2+}]$ on the cytosolic side also activates more weakly.[21]

CALMODULIN: VERSATILE MEDIATOR OF Ca^{2+} SIGNALING

CaM has four Ca^{2+}-binding sites, resembles troponin C, and participates in many different cellular pathways, from ion channels to transcriptional regulation.[19] In many cases (e.g., L-type Ca^{2+}, Na^+, and some K^+ channels; RyR and inositol 1,4,5-triphosphate receptors), CaM is already prebound or "dedicated" such that elevation of local $[Ca^{2+}]_i$ can rapidly induce Ca^{2+}-CaM effects on their gating (see Fig. 46.9).[22,23] Indeed, more than 90% of the CaM in myocytes is already bound to cellular targets before Ca^{2+} binds to and activates it. Nevertheless, many myocyte CaM targets (e.g., CaMKII, calcineurin, nitric oxide synthase [NOS]) compete for this limited pool of "promiscuous" CaM. Thus, CaM signaling in myocytes is complex and is further complicated by the effects of CaMKII, which influences some of the same targets and processes as CaM itself does.[19,23]

CALCIUM SPARKS AND WAVES

In addition to SR Ca^{2+} release triggered by I_{Ca} during normal excitation-contraction coupling, there is a finite probability that a given RyR will open stochastically. Because of local Ca^{2+}-induced Ca^{2+} release in the junctional cleft, this can lead to spontaneous local SR Ca^{2+} release events known as Ca^{2+} sparks.[21,24] Under normal resting conditions, these Ca^{2+} sparks have a low probability (approximately 10^{-4}), which means that at any moment there might be one or two Ca^{2+} sparks per myocyte. Because local $[Ca^{2+}]_i$ declines rapidly as Ca^{2+} diffuses away from the initiating cleft, the resulting local $[Ca^{2+}]_i$ at the next cleft (1 to 2 µm away) is normally too low to trigger that neighboring site. Thus, Ca^{2+} sparks are very local events (within 2 µm in the cell). However, the probability of Ca^{2+} sparks is greatly enhanced when $[Ca^{2+}]_i$ or $[Ca^{2+}]_{SR}$ is elevated or under conditions in which the RyR is otherwise sensitized (e.g., by oxidation or CaMKII). These conditions can greatly enhance the likelihood that SR Ca^{2+} release from one junction will be sufficient to trigger neighboring junctions 1 to 2 µm away and result in propagating Ca^{2+} waves throughout the whole myocyte. These Ca^{2+} waves can be arrhythmogenic. The Ca^{2+} wave can activate substantial inward current through NCX (see later), which can depolarize the membrane potential and contribute to both early and delayed afterdepolarizations (EADs and DADs) during the AP plateau or during diastole, respectively. EADs result in prolongation of the AP duration, and DADs can initiate premature ventricular complexes (PVCs).

Calcium Uptake into Sarcoplasmic Reticulum by Sarcoendoplasmic Reticulum Ca^{2+}–Adenosine Triphosphatase

Ca^{2+} is transported into the SR by SERCA, which constitutes nearly 90% of the SR protein. Its molecular weight is 115 kDa, with 10 transmembrane domains and large cytosolic and small SR-luminal domains. Three isoforms exist, but in cardiac myocytes the dominant form is SERCA2a. For each molecule of ATP hydrolyzed by this enzyme, two calcium ions are taken up into the SR (Fig. 46.10; see also Fig. 46.9). SR Ca^{2+} uptake is the primary driver of cardiac myocyte relaxation, and reuptake starts as soon as $[Ca^{2+}]_i$ begins to rise. Because Ca^{2+} removal is slower than Ca^{2+} influx and release, a characteristic rise and fall in $[Ca^{2+}]_i$ called the Ca^{2+} transient takes place. As $[Ca^{2+}]_i$ falls, Ca^{2+} dissociates from troponin C, which progressively switches off the myofilaments. A reduction in SERCA expression or function (as seen in heart failure or energetic limitations) can thus directly result in slower rates of cardiac relaxation. In addition, the strength of SR Ca^{2+} uptake directly influences the diastolic SR Ca^{2+} content and $[Ca^{2+}]_{SR}$, which dictates both the sensitivity of the RyR and the flux rate of SR Ca^{2+} release. Thus, SR Ca^{2+} uptake and release are an integrated system.

Phospholamban (PLB) was so named by its discoverers Tada and Katz[25] to mean "phosphate receiver." PLB is a single-transmembrane pass protein that binds directly to SERCA2a. Under basal conditions, this reduces the affinity of SERCA for cytosolic Ca^{2+}, which results in slower SR Ca^{2+} uptake at any given $[Ca^{2+}]_i$. However, when PLB is phosphorylated by either PKA or CaMKII (at Ser16 or Thr17, respectively), the inhibitory effect is relieved, thereby resulting in increased rates of SR Ca^{2+} uptake, cardiac relaxation (lusitropic effect), and increased SR Ca^{2+} content, which drives stronger contraction (inotropic effect; see Fig. 46.10).

The Ca^{2+} taken up into the SR is stored within the SR before the next release. Calsequestrin is a highly charged, low-affinity Ca^{2+} buffer (K_d = 600 µM) found primarily inside the jSR, where it enhances the local availability of Ca^{2+} for release through the nearby RyR. Calreticulin is another Ca^{2+}-storing protein that is similar to calsequestrin in structure and function. There is also evidence that calsequestrin and two other proteins located in the SR membrane (junctin and triadin) may regulate the properties of the RyR and be part of the mechanism by which higher $[Ca]_{SR}$ enhances RyR opening.[20] Reuptake by SERCA occurs everywhere

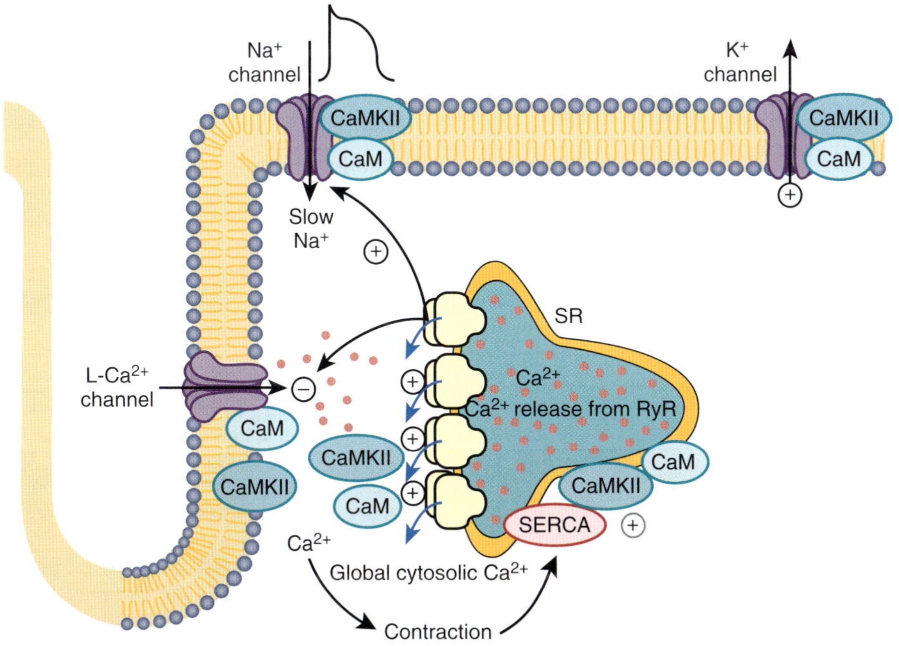

FIGURE 46.9 Role of CaM and CaMKII in regulating intracellular $[Ca^{2+}]$. The rising cytosolic Ca^{2+} concentration in systole activates the Ca^{2+} regulatory system whereby Ca^{2+}-CaM causes inactivation of L-type Ca^{2+} current and RyR release. This negative feedback system limits cellular Ca^{2+} gain. The effects of CaMKII can also modulate these systems.[22] For example, (1) CaMKII limits the extent of Ca^{2+}-dependent inactivation and enhances Ca^{2+} current amplitude, (2) it increases the fraction of SR Ca^{2+} released from the RyR in response to the Ca^{2+} current trigger (which can be arrhythmogenic), (3) it phosphorylates PLB to enhance SR Ca^{2+} uptake by SERCA, and (4) it can modulate Na^+ and K^+ channel gating in ways that are also proarrhythmic.[22,23]

in the SR membrane, including the network SR that surrounds the myofilaments. Diffusion of Ca^{2+} within the SR is relatively fast, which allows restoration of [Ca^{2+}]$_{SR}$ at the jSR to occur quickly after Ca^{2+} is taken back up everywhere.[26] Indeed, during normal Ca^{2+} release, intra-SR Ca^{2+} diffusion is rapid enough to limit Ca^{2+} gradients between SR release sites in the jSR and the Ca^{2+} uptake sites. This diffusion also ensures that [Ca^{2+}]$_{SR}$ is relatively uniform throughout the myocyte, which facilitates the uniformity of SR Ca^{2+} release and myofilament activation throughout the cell.

SARCOLEMMAL CONTROL OF Ca^{2+} AND Na$^+$

Calcium and Sodium Channels

Excitation-contraction coupling is initiated by voltage-induced opening of the sarcolemmal L-type Ca^{2+} channels. The channels are pore-forming macromolecular proteins that span the sarcolemmal lipid bilayer to allow a highly selective pathway for transfer of ions into the heart cell when the channel changes from a closed to an open state. Ion channels have two major properties: gating and permeation. Ca^{2+} and Na$^+$ channels have two functional "gates," activation and inactivation. At the normal resting membrane potential, the activation gates are closed and the inactivation gate is open, so the channels are available to open on depolarization in their characteristic voltage-gated manner. On activation, the inactivation gate starts to close, and the kinetics of inactivation depends on voltage, time, and local [Ca^{2+}]$_i$. Recovery from inactivation (which makes the channels available for activation again) is also time, voltage, and Ca^{2+} dependent. Thus, after the AP ends, time is required for the Ca^{2+} and Na$^+$ channels to recover from inactivation.

Permeation (or conductance) refers to the actual flow of ions or current through the open channel. Ca^{2+} and Na$^+$ channels are highly selective for Ca^{2+} and Na$^+$, respectively, relative to other physiologic ions. However, nonphysiologic ions can also permeate; barium (Ba^{2+}) and strontium (Sr^{2+}) readily permeate Ca^{2+} channels, and lithium (Li$^+$) permeates Na$^+$ channels, and these ions are sometimes used experimentally to study I_{Ca} and I_{Na}. The concentration of the permeant ion influences the conductance, and in simple Ohm's law terms ($I_{Ca} = g_{Ca}[E_m - E_{Ca}]$), current is the product of conductance (g_{Ca}; which depends on gating and permeation) times the electrochemical driving force ($E_m - E_{Ca}$), which is the difference between the membrane potential (E_m) and the potential that exactly counterbalances the transmembrane [Ca^{2+}] gradient (E_{Ca}, typically +120 mV but changes as [Ca]$_i$ changes). Thus, depolarization activates both Ca^{2+} and Na$^+$ channels but also decreases the driving force for the currents.

Molecular Structure of Ca^{2+} and Na$^+$ Channels

Both Ca^{2+} and Na$^+$ channels contain a major alpha subunit with four transmembrane domains (I to IV), each of which has six transmembrane helices (S1 to S6) and a pore loop between S5 and S6. Each channel also has associated auxiliary subunits ($\alpha 2\delta$, β, and γ for Ca^{2+} channels) that may influence trafficking and gating.[1] Activation is now understood in molecular terms as outward movement of the charged S4 transmembrane segment (called the *voltage sensor*) in each of the four domains of Na$^+$ and Ca^{2+} channels. This S4 voltage dependence differs among channels, and Na$^+$ channels are activated at more negative E_m than are Ca^{2+} channels. *Inactivation* is more complex and involves multiple channel domains, and channels accumulate in this state during prolonged depolarization. The open state is typically the last of a sequence of multiple molecular closed conformations. However, there is typically a binary switch between closed and open such that the single-channel conductance is either near zero or at a constant open conductance. This stochastic nature means that it is often better to speak of the *probability of channel opening* for a single channel, while the whole-cell current integrates flux through all the stochastic channels.

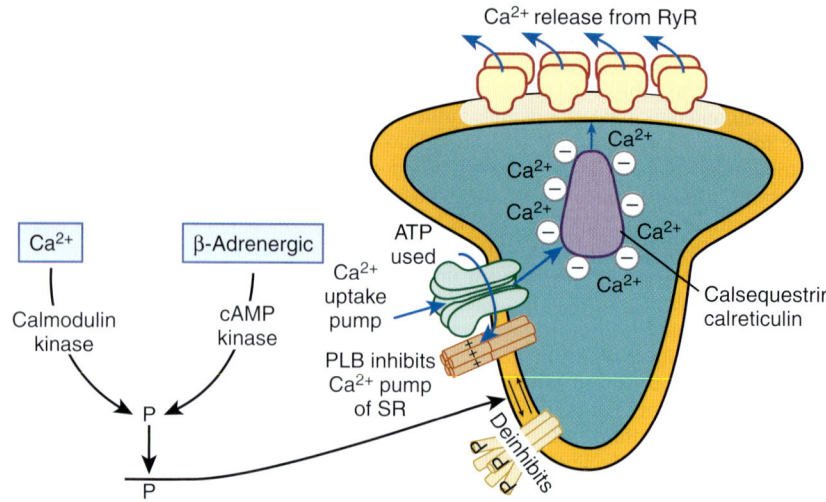

FIGURE 46.10 Ca^{2+} uptake into the SR by SERCA2a. An increased rate of uptake of Ca^{2+} into the SR enhances the rate of relaxation (*lusitropic effect*). PLB, when phosphorylated (*P*), removes the inhibition exerted on the Ca^{2+} pump by its dephosphorylated form. Thereby, Ca^{2+} uptake is increased either in response to enhanced cytosolic [Ca^{2+}] or in response to beta-adrenergic agonists or CaMKII activation (which can be secondary to the beta-adrenergic system).[1,23,32]

T-Versus L-Type Ca^{2+} Channels

The cardiovascular system has two major types of sarcolemmal Ca^{2+} channels, T-type and L-type channels. T (transient)–type channels open at a more negative voltage, have short bursts of opening, and do not interact with conventional Ca^{2+} antagonist drugs.[1] In adult ventricular myocytes, there is normally little T-type I_{Ca} (except under pathophysiologic conditions). Even when expressed in ventricular myocytes, T-type channels do not seem to target the regions where RyRs are, and consequently do not participate in excitation-contraction coupling per se. However, measurable T-type I_{Ca} is present in neonatal ventricular myocytes, Purkinje fibers, and some atrial cells (especially pacemaker cells). In these locations the negative activation voltages may allow T-type I_{Ca} to contribute to pacemaker function. Thus, in ventricular myocytes, L-type currents predominate.

L-Type Ca^{2+} Channel Localization and Regulation

L (long-lasting)–type Ca^{2+} channels are concentrated in the T tubules at jSR sites, where they are positioned for Ca^{2+}-induced Ca^{2+} release from the RyR. A fraction of L-type Ca^{2+} channels are also localized in caveolae, where they may participate in local Ca^{2+} signaling, which is distinct from triggering of SR Ca^{2+} release. L-type Ca^{2+} channels are inhibited by Ca^{2+} channel blockers such as verapamil, diltiazem, and the dihydropyridines. I_{Ca} is rapidly activated during the rising phase of the AP, but the combination of Ca^{2+} influx via I_{Ca} itself and local SR Ca^{2+} release causes rapid Ca^{2+}-dependent inactivation of I_{Ca}. Voltage-dependent inactivation also contributes to I_{Ca} decline during the AP, but I_{Ca} continues at low levels throughout the AP.[27] Inward I_{Ca} is an important contributor to the plateau phase of the cardiac AP, and excess I_{Ca} or failure of inactivation can prolong the duration of the AP and participate in EADs.

During beta-adrenergic stimulation, cyclic adenosine monophosphate (cAMP) and PKA activity increases and results in phosphorylation of the Ca^{2+} channel and alteration of its gating properties. Notably, most of the molecular components of this beta-adrenergic receptor–cAMP-PKA and phosphatase pathway are localized directly at the L-type Ca^{2+} channel, which facilitates rapid sympathetic activation of I_{Ca}. PKA-dependent phosphorylation of the channel shifts activation (and inactivation) to more negative voltages and increases the open time of the channel. This combination can greatly increase I_{Ca}, which increases both the fraction of SR Ca^{2+} release and the Ca^{2+} load of the cell and SR (to enhance further the Ca^{2+} transient amplitude and inotropic state).

Sodium Channels

Voltage-gated cardiac Na$^+$ current is carried mainly by the Nav1.5 *cardiac* isoform, but a minor component is attributed to several other, *neuronal* isoforms. The Nav1.5 channels are especially concentrated at the ends of the myocyte near intercalated discs, but the overall density of I_{Na} is relatively uniform between the T tubule and surface membrane.[28] Depolarization activates I_{Na}, and peak I_{Na} is very large and drives the upstroke of the cardiac AP. Voltage-dependent inactivation of I_{Na} is very rapid, and under normal conditions, Na+ channels inactivate within 4 milliseconds of depolarization. However, a tiny fraction of Na+ channels remain open (or reopen), thereby creating a small but persistent influx of Na+ throughout the plateau of the AP. This so-called late sodium current (I_{NaL}) is characterized by ultraslow, voltage-independent inactivation and reactivation.[29] Although the amplitude of I_{NaL} is small (<1% of peak I_{Na}), because peak I_{Na} is so large, this I_{NaL} still constitutes a significant inward current during the plateau phase of the AP. Under pathophysiologic conditions, the amount of I_{NaL} can increase significantly, which can result in acquired long-QT (LQT) syndrome and also cause Na+ and Ca2+ loading of myocytes, which carries additional arrhythmogenic potential. Thus, I_{NaL} has emerged as a potentially important therapeutic target.[22,30]

Ca2+/CALMODULIN-DEPENDENT PROTEIN KINASE II ALTERS GATING OF I_{Na}, I_{Ca}, AND OTHER CHANNELS

CaMKII is known to be upregulated and chronically activated in numerous pathophysiologic conditions (e.g., ischemia-reperfusion, heart failure, ROS). Also, CaMKII-dependent Na+ channel phosphorylation causes increased I_{NaL}, which may produce an acquired form of LQT3 syndrome in patients with genetically normal Na+ channels (see Fig. 46.9).[22,30] At the same time, CaMKII also shifts Na+ channel availability to more negative voltages, enhances intermediate inactivation, and slows recovery from inactivation, all loss-of-function effects that could cause an acquired Brugada syndrome–like condition. Indeed, this can foster both phenotypes, depending on the heart rate (HR): LQT syndrome at a lower HR and Brugada syndrome at a higher HR.[22] CaMKII also modulates Ca2+ and potassium (K+) channel currents, which can further promote arrhythmogenesis through EADs and enhanced transmural dispersion of repolarization.[22]

Ion Exchangers and Pumps

To maintain steady-state Ca2+ and Na+ balance, the amount of Ca2+ and Na+ entering during each AP must be exactly balanced by efflux before the next beat. This is the definition of steady state. For Ca2+, Na+/Ca2+ exchange (NCX) is responsible for extruding most of the Ca2+ that entered by I_{Ca} and NCX, whereas a very small fraction is extruded by the plasma membrane Ca2+-ATPase (PMCA). NCX uses the inward [Na+] electrochemical gradient from 3 Na+ ions to pump each Ca2+ ion into the extracellular space against a large electrochemical gradient (and PMCA uses 1 ATP to pump each Ca2+ ion). The main mechanism for extruding Na+ from the cell is Na+,K+-ATPase, which pumps 3 Na+ ions out for each ATP consumed. Note that NCX also indirectly uses the energy from Na+,K+-ATPase to perform its function.

Sodium-Calcium Exchanger

During relaxation, SR Ca2+-ATPase and NCX compete for the removal of cytosolic Ca2+, with the SR pump normally being dominant.[1,4] NCX is reversible, so the direction of Ca2+ flux depends on the membrane potential and [Na+] and [Ca2+] on both sides of the sarcolemma. The E_m at which the inward electrochemical potential is the same for 3 Na+ ions as for 1 Ca2+ ion to enter is the reversal or equilibrium potential (E_{NCX}, similar to that for ion channels). When E_m is higher than this voltage, entry of Ca2+ is favored, whereas for E_m below E_{NCX}, the Ca2+ efflux mode is thermodynamically favored. During diastole (E_m = −80 mV), NCX normally extrudes Ca2+, but because [Ca2+]$_i$ is low during diastole, the Ca2+ flux rate is low (low substrate concentration). As the AP rises to a peak, E_m normally exceeds E_{NCX} and Ca2+ influx is favored, but this occurs only briefly because the high local [Ca2+]$_i$ near the membrane drives NCX back into the Ca2+ extrusion mode. When the AP repolarizes, the negative E_m further enhances the Ca2+ extrusion flux, and at this time, [Ca2+]$_i$ is above the diastolic level, so NCX can transport Ca2+ effectively. Note that if SR Ca2+ release is small and/or I_{Ca} is small or [Na+]$_i$ is abnormally high (as occurs in heart failure), NCX can continue to bring Ca2+ into the cell during much of the AP duration and in that sense can partially compensate for the lack of I_{Ca} or SR Ca2+ release.[1] NCX is also allosterically activated by increasing [Ca2+]$_i$.[31] Although such regulation is time dependent, it may provide a mechanism to enhance the cell's ability to extrude Ca2+ when [Ca2+]$_i$ is chronically high, as well as to keep NCX from driving [Ca2+]$_i$ and indirectly [Ca2+]$_{SR}$ to inappropriately low levels when cytosolic Ca2+ is in short supply.

Under normal conditions in human or rabbit ventricular myocytes, the steady-state condition occurs when the relative Ca2+ removal from the cytosol by SERCA and NCX is 70% to 75% and 20% to 25%, respectively, with PMCA contributing 1% or less (see Fig. 46.8). In heart failure, in which SERCA is downregulated and NCX may be upregulated, the SERCA and NCX contributions are closer to the same. In the mouse and rat ventricle, the difference is larger (92% SERCA, 7% NCX). This steady state involves all the various Ca2+ transport systems dynamically, but the relative rates of Ca2+ flux by SERCA and NCX at physiologic [Ca2+]$_i$ are useful. These removal fluxes must also pertain to the integrated Ca2+ fluxes into the cytosol. That is, the combination of Ca2+ entry by I_{Ca} and NCX in human and mouse ventricle would be 25% and 8%, respectively. In other words, amplification of the Ca2+ transient by SR Ca2+ release is only approximately fourfold for human or rabbit ventricle (and less in heart failure) but approximately 12-fold for mouse or rat ventricle.

HEART RATE AND Na+/Ca2+ EXCHANGE

NCX participates in the force-frequency relationship (treppe or Bowditch phenomenon).[1] An increasing HR (independent of sympathetic activation) increases the amount of Na+ and Ca2+ entry per unit time and also diminishes the time available for extrusion of Na+ and Ca2+. This will tend to increase the amount of Ca2+ in the SR simply because of more frequent I_{Ca} pulses and less time for removal of Ca2+ from the cell. However, the same happens for Na+, and the elevation in [Na+]$_i$ also limits the ability of NCX to extrude Ca2+, which further increases the amount of Ca2+ in the myocyte and SR when the cell achieves a new steady state. This NCX effect (once referred to as the "sodium pump lag" hypothesis) thus amplifies the intrinsic inotropic effect of an increase in HR.

Sodium Pump (Na+,K+–Adenosine Triphosphatase)

During the normal heartbeat, Na+ enters the myocyte mainly by Na+ channels and NCX, with NCX being quantitatively most important.[32] Na+/H+ exchange also mediates significant Na+ influx, particularly when cells are acidotic. In the steady state, this Na+ influx is matched by an equal Na+ efflux, mediated mainly by sarcolemmal Na+,K+-ATPase (the Na+ pump). The Na+ pump is activated by internal Na+ or external K+ and transports 3 Na+ ions out and 2 K+ ions in per ATP molecule used. During this process, one positive charge leaves the cell, and thus Na+,K+-ATPase is electrogenic and carries an outward current.[32] Na+,K+-ATPase in the heart is modulated by the endogenous accessory protein *phospholemman* (PLM), which works in a manner analogous to the PLB-SERCA2a mechanism. That is, at baseline, PLM reduces the intracellular Na+ affinity of Na+,K+-ATPase, but when it is phosphorylated (by either PKA or protein kinase C [PKC]), that inhibitory effect is relieved.[32] Thus, during sympathetic activation, Na+,K+-ATPase activity is increased at any given [Na+]$_i$ to keep up better with the higher rates of Na+ influx that occur under this condition.

Digitalis glycosides inhibit Na+,K+-ATPase and have been used for more than 200 years as a cardiac inotropic drug for the treatment of heart failure, although their use has diminished in recent years (see also Chapter 50). Partial inhibition of Na+,K+-ATPase causes an increase in [Na+]$_i$ in myocytes, which limits the ability of NCX to extrude Ca2+, resulting in enhanced myocyte and SR Ca2+ loading and release. A limitation with this approach is the narrow therapeutic range, and too much inhibition can lead to myocyte Ca2+ overload and trigger arrhythmias. However, this emphasizes the close interrelationship between Na+ and Ca2+ regulation mediated by the powerful NCX present in cardiac myocytes.

ADRENERGIC SIGNALING SYSTEMS

Physiologic Fight-or-Flight Response

During the classic adrenergic fight-or-flight response, cardiac myocyte beta-adrenergic receptors are activated, which leads to increased cAMP production and PKA activation and consequent phosphorylation and altered function of numerous myocyte targets. This results in an increased HR (*positive chronotropy*), increased contractility (*positive inotropy*), faster cardiac relaxation (*positive lusitropy*), and enhanced conduction velocity through the conduction system (*positive dromotropy*). These events enhance cardiac output by enhancing the HR, stroke volume, and diastolic filling. Thus, the adrenergic response is a key physiologic mechanism for increasing cardiac output in response to increased metabolic and hemodynamic demands.

During the adrenergic response, norepinephrine is released by sympathetic neurons at small swellings on small end-branches, or *varicosities*, into the local myocyte environment (Fig. 46.11), analogous to synaptic transmission. Norepinephrine is synthesized in the varicosities from dopa and dopamine and the amino acid tyrosine and stored within the terminals in *storage granules* (or *vesicles*) for release upon adrenergic nervous impulse. Thus, when central stimulation increases during excitement or exercise, an increased number of sympathetic nerve impulses liberate an increased amount of norepinephrine from the terminals into the close vicinity of myocyte surface (akin to neuronal synaptic clefts). Most of the released norepinephrine is taken back up by the nerve terminal varicosities to reenter the storage vesicles or to be metabolized. The released norepinephrine at these *synaptic clefts* interacts with both alpha- and beta-adrenergic receptors on myocytes and also alpha-adrenergic receptors in arterioles (Table 46.2). The beta-adrenergic effects on the sinoatrial (SA) node and conduction system contribute to the chronotropic and dromotropic effects mentioned earlier, whereas those on myocytes are responsible mainly for the inotropic and lusitropic effects. These effects can also be modulated by coactivation of myocyte alpha-adrenergic receptors. Increased alpha-adrenergic activity causes arteriolar constriction and increased vascular impedance, although local metabolic control of arteriolar resistance is strong in the heart and dominates in controlling coronary resistance in arterioles. Parasympathetic (vagal) innervation is strongest in the conduction system, where local release of acetylcholine (ACh) activates muscarinic receptors and tends to slow the HR and conduction velocity (see Fig. 46.11). In these conditions the HR and blood pressure fall. The influence of these main effector pathways is also modulated by numerous other signaling factors, such as local adenosine and nitric oxide (NO) and the powerful neuromodulator angiotensin II, which can also potentiate release of norepinephrine and vasoconstriction. Both alpha- and beta-adrenergic receptors are part of the family of seven–transmembrane domain G protein–coupled receptors (GPCRs).

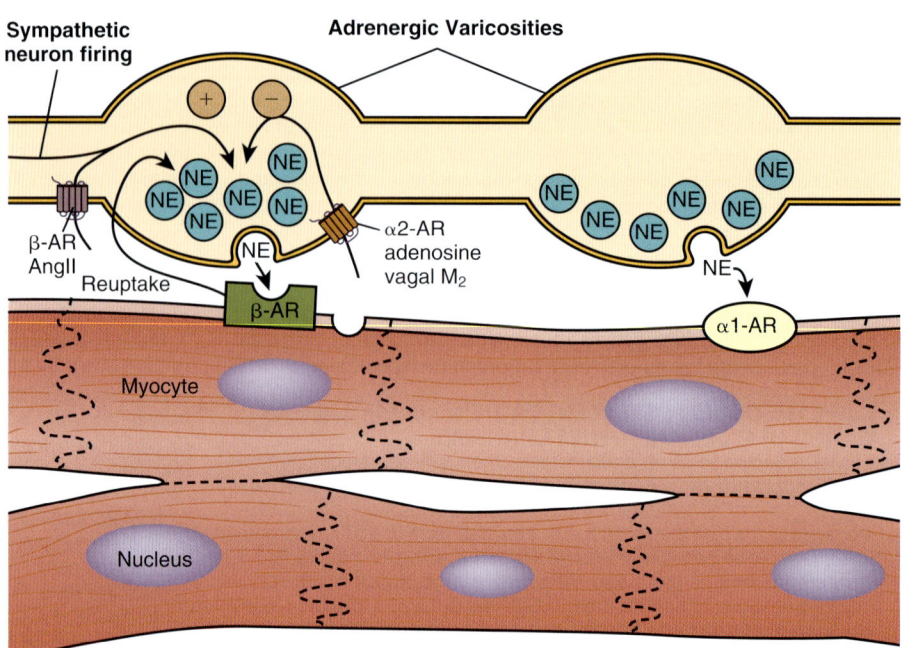

FIGURE 46.11 Norepinephrine (NE) release from sympathetic neurons. NE is released from storage granules in adrenergic varicosities into narrow, synapse-like spaces near its receptors in the sarcolemma of the cardiac and smooth muscle myocytes of the heart and arterial walls. In cardiomyocytes, beta-adrenergic receptor (βAR) activation increases heart rate (chronotropy), contractile force (inotropy) and relaxation (lusitropy), and conduction (dromotropy). However, NE also activates cardiac myocyte alpha$_1$-adrenergic receptors, which can further modulate contractility and myocyte signaling cascades. In arterioles, NE predominantly causes vasoconstriction via postsynaptic alpha$_1$ receptors. NE also stimulates presynaptic alpha$_2$ receptors to invoke feedback inhibition that can limit its own release. Circulating epinephrine stimulates vascular vasodilatory beta$_2$ receptors but also presynaptic receptors on the nerve terminal, which promotes NE release. Angiotensin II (AngII) is also powerfully vasoconstrictive and acts both by stimulation of NE release (presynaptic receptors, as indicated schematically) and directly on arteriolar AngII receptors. M$_2$ is muscarinic receptor, subtype two.

Beta-Adrenergic Receptor Subtypes

Cardiac beta-adrenergic receptors are chiefly (80%) the beta$_1$ subtype, with 20% being beta$_2$ in the left ventricle. Most noncardiac receptors are beta$_2$. Whereas beta$_1$ receptors are linked to the stimulatory G protein G$_s$, a component of the G protein–adenylyl cyclase system, beta$_2$ receptors are linked to both G$_s$ and the inhibitory protein G$_i$ (Fig. 46.12), so their signaling pathway bifurcates at the first postreceptor step.[4] In humans the main positive inotropic response to adrenergic activation is mediated via beta$_1$ adrenergic receptors. Some beta$_2$ stimulation by salbutamol (albuterol) can appear to be inotropic but may at least in part be through beta$_2$ receptors on the terminal neurons of cardiac sympathetic nerves, thereby causing norepinephrine release which in turn exerts dominant beta$_1$ effects.[4] Indirect evidence suggests that the G$_i$ pathway is relatively augmented in heart failure, whereas the strength of the G$_s$ path is lessened because of uncoupling of G$_s$ from the beta receptor (see Chapter 47). There also appears to be a small

TABLE 46.2 Comparative Cardiovascular Effects of Alpha- and Beta-Adrenergic Receptor Stimulation

	ALPHA1 MEDIATED	BETA MEDIATED
Electrophysiologic effects	±	++
		Conduction
		Pacemaker
		Heart rate
		– AP duration
Myocardial mechanics	±	++
		Contractility, lusitropy
		Stroke volume
		Cardiac output
Myocardial metabolism	±	++
	Glycolysis	O$_2$ uptake ↑
		ATP consumption
Signal systems	GPCR, can activate PKC and MAPK	GPCR, activates cAMP and PKA
Coronary arterioles	++	+ Direct dilation
	Constriction	+++ Indirect dilation (metabolic)
Peripheral arterioles	+++	+
	Constriction	Dilation
	SVR ↑	SVR ↓
	SBP ↑	SBP ↓

AP, Action potential; *cAMP*, cyclic adenosine monophosphate; *GPCR*, G protein–coupled receptor; *MAPK*, mitogen-activated protein kinase; *PK*, protein kinase; *PKC*, protein kinase C; *SBP*, systolic blood pressure; *SVR*, systemic vascular resistance.
Modified from Opie LH. *Heart Physiology, from Cell to Circulation*. 4th ed. Philadelphia: Lippincott, Williams & Wilkins; 2004.

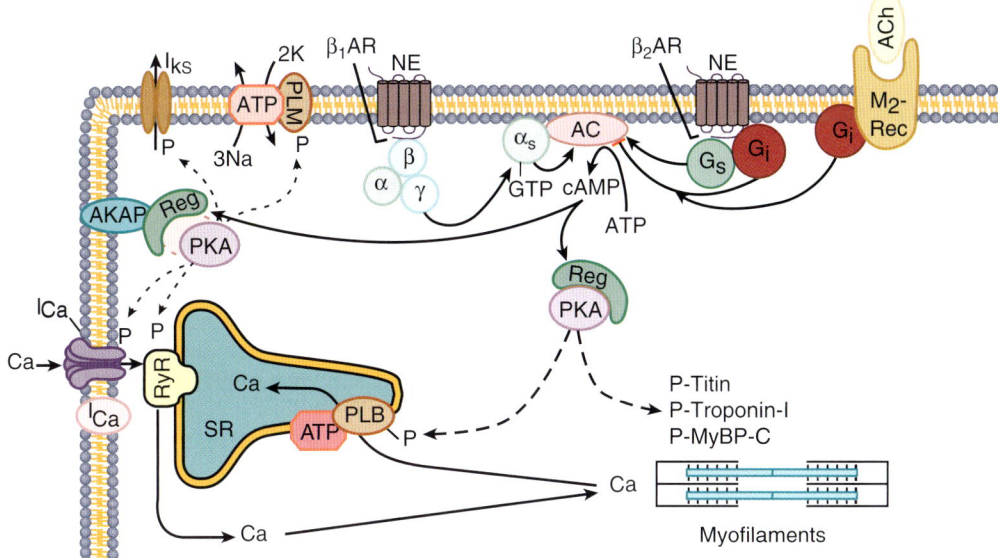

FIGURE 46.12 Beta-adrenergic and muscarinic activation in cardiac myocytes interact. Activation of beta$_1$-adrenergic receptors (β_1AR) activate adenylyl cyclase (*AC*) via G$_s$ (via the activated alpha subunit (α_s) dissociation from the beta and gamma subunits (β and γ). AC produces cAMP, which activates protein kinase A (*PKA*), which phosphorylates (*P*) several key functional targets (*broken arrows*). β_2-AR activate both G$_s$ and G$_i$, which activate or inhibit AC, respectively. Activation of muscarinic M$_2$ receptors (M_2-Rec) by acetylcholine (*ACh*) from parasympathetic neurons inhibits AC via G$_i$. *PLB*, Phospholamban; *PLM*, phospholemman; *Reg*, regulatory subunit of PKA. (Modified from Bers DM. *Excitation-Contraction Coupling and Cardiac Contractile Force*. Dordrecht, Netherlands: Kluwer Academic; 2001.)

THE STIMULATORY G PROTEIN G$_s$

The G protein itself is a heterotrimer composed of G$_\alpha$, G$_\beta$, and G$_\gamma$, which on receptor stimulation splits into the alpha subunit that is bound to GTP and the beta-gamma subunit. Either of these subunits may regulate different effectors such as adenylyl cyclase, phospholipase C, and ion channels. The activity of adenylyl cyclase is controlled by two different G protein complexes, namely, G$_s$, which stimulates, and G$_i$, which inhibits. The alpha subunit of G$_s$ (α_s) combines with GTP and then separates from the other two subunits to enhance the activity of adenylyl cyclase. The beta and gamma subunits (beta-gamma) appear to be linked structurally and functionally.

THE INHIBITORY G PROTEIN G$_i$

In contrast, a second trimeric GTP-binding protein, G$_i$, is responsible for inhibition of adenylyl cyclase.[4] During stimulation of muscarinic and some beta$_2$-adrenergic receptors, GTP binds to the inhibitory alpha subunit α_i. The latter then dissociates from the beta-gamma subunits. The beta-gamma subunits act as follows. By stimulating the enzyme guanosine triphosphatase (GTPase), they break down the active α_s subunit (α_s-GTP) to limit activation of adenylyl cyclase which occurs in response to G$_s$ stimulation. Furthermore, the beta-gamma subunit activates the K$_{ACh}$ channel, which can slow SA node firing and thereby contribute to the bradycardic effect of cholinergic stimulation. The α_i subunit may also activate another potassium channel (K$_{ATP}$) that stabilizes the diastolic membrane potential. The major physiologic stimulus for G$_i$ is thought to be vagal muscarinic receptor stimulation (although beta$_2$-adrenergic receptors may contribute as well). In addition, adenosine, by interaction with A$_1$ receptors, couples to G$_i$ to inhibit contraction and HR. The adenosine A$_2$ receptor paradoxically increases cAMP. The latter effect, only of ancillary significance in the myocardium, is of major importance in vascular smooth muscle, where it induces vasorelaxation. Pathologically, G$_i$ is increased in experimental postinfarct heart failure[4] and in donor hearts before cardiac transplantation.[4]

A THIRD G PROTEIN, G$_q$

This protein links a group of GPCRs, including the alpha-adrenergic receptor and those for angiotensin II and endothelin-1, to another membrane-associated enzyme, phospholipase C, and then to PKC and PKD (and IP$_3$-induced Ca^{2+} mobilization). G$_q$ has at least four isoforms, two of which have been found in the heart. This G protein, unlike G$_i$, is not susceptible to inhibition by pertussis toxin. Overexpression of G$_q$ in mice induces a dilated cardiomyopathy,[4] which is of interest because angiotensin II and endothelin, which act through G$_q$, are overactive in human heart failure. Conversely, when the activity of G$_q$ is genetically inhibited, the hypertrophic response to pressure overload is attenuated, wall stress increases, but cardiac function is relatively well maintained.

number of beta$_3$-adrenergic receptors in cardiac myocytes that seem to produce more G$_i$-mediated negative inotropic signaling, mediated in part by NO, but this pathway is not as well understood. The beta-adrenergic receptor site is highly stereospecific, the best fit among catecholamines being achieved with the synthetic agent isoproterenol rather than with the naturally occurring catecholamines norepinephrine and epinephrine. In the case of beta$_1$ receptors, the order of agonist activity is isoproterenol > epinephrine = norepinephrine, whereas in the case of beta$_2$ receptors, the order is isoproterenol > epinephrine > norepinephrine. Human beta$_1$ and beta$_2$ receptors have been cloned and studied extensively.[4] The transmembrane domains are the site of agonist and antagonist binding, whereas the cytoplasmic domains interact with G proteins.

Alpha-Adrenergic Receptor Subtypes

The two alpha-adrenergic receptor isoforms are alpha$_1$ and alpha$_2$. Those on the sarcolemma of vascular smooth muscle are vasoconstrictor alpha$_1$ receptors, whereas those situated on the terminal varicosities are alpha$_2$-adrenergic receptors that feed back (see Fig. 46.11) to inhibit release of norepinephrine. Pharmacologically, an alpha$_2$-adrenergic receptor mediates a response in which the effects resemble those of the pharmacologic agent phenylephrine. Among catecholamines, the relative potencies of alpha$_1$-agonists are norepinephrine > epinephrine > isoproterenol. Physiologically, norepinephrine liberated from nerve terminals is the chief stimulus to vascular alpha$_1$-adrenergic activity. Both alpha$_1$ and alpha$_2$ receptors are also found in cardiac myocytes, where their activation can fine-tune Ca^{2+} transients, ionic currents, and myofilament properties acutely, but they are also known to be important modulators of cardiac remodeling (in both adaptive and maladaptive contexts).[33]

G Proteins

G proteins are a superfamily of proteins that bind guanine triphosphate (GTP) and other guanine nucleotides. G proteins are crucial in carrying the signal onward from the agonist and its receptor to the activity of the membrane-bound enzyme system that produces the second messenger cAMP (Fig. 46.13; see also Fig. 46.12).[4] Thus the combination of the beta receptor, G protein complex, and adenylyl cyclase is the crux of beta-adrenergic signaling.

Cyclic Adenosine Monophosphate and Protein Kinase A

Adenylyl Cyclase

Adenylyl cyclase (also called adenylate or adenyl cyclase) catalyzes formation of the second messenger cAMP. Several isoforms exist, but AC5 and AC6 are most prominent in cardiac myocytes, and these isoforms are partially inhibited by high [Ca^{2+}]$_i$. Adenylyl cyclase, when stimulated by G$_s$, produces cAMP, which acts through multiple intracellular signals (including importantly PKA) to mediate the chronotropic, inotropic, lusitropic, and dromotropic effects of cardiac beta-adrenergic agonists. In contrast, cholinergic (and vagal) stimulation can inhibit adenylyl cyclase through G$_i$, to slow HR, but also limit cAMP formation downstream of G$_s$ activation.

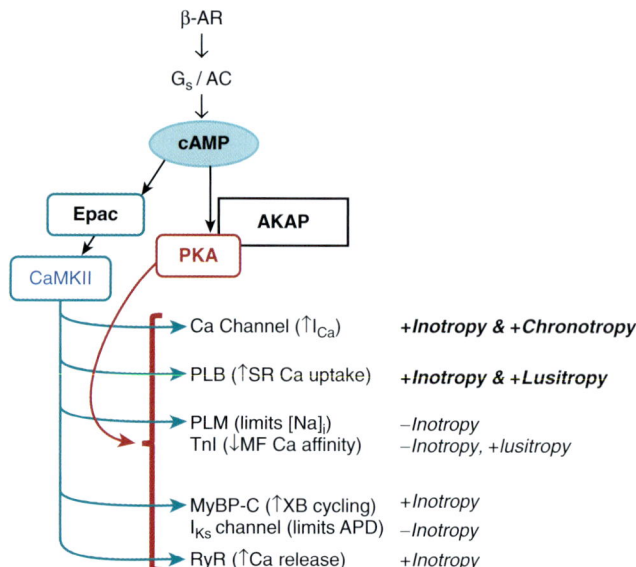

FIGURE 46.13 Key roles of PKA (and CaMKII) in beta-adrenergic responses. Major intracellular effects of beta-agonist catecholamines are via the formation of cyclic adenosine monophosphate (cAMP), which increases the activity of PKA and also Epac (exchange protein activated by cAMP). PKA is localized by A-kinase anchoring proteins (AKAPs) that target PKA function to local nanodomains. Epac also activates CaMKII which can phosphorylate and modulate function of some of the same targets as PKA (often by phosphorylation at different amino acids).

Adenylyl cyclase is the only enzyme that produces cAMP, using low concentrations of Mg^{2+}-ATP as substrate. It is a transmembrane enzyme, with most mass on the cytoplasmic side where G proteins interact. Cyclic guanosine monophosphate (cGMP) is a related second messenger that often antagonizes cAMP effects. cAMP has very rapid turnover as a result of a constant dynamic balance between its formation by adenylyl cyclase and conversion to AMP by phosphodiesterases (PDEs). Several major PDE isoforms have different substrate specificity (cAMP versus cGMP) and are differentially regulated by cyclic nucleotides and Ca^{2+}/calmodulin.[34] In general, directional changes in the tissue content of cAMP can be related to directional changes in cardiac contractile activity, but local subcellular domains may have differential cAMP and PKA regulation that depends in part on PDE isoform localization. For example, while beta-adrenergic stimulation increases both cAMP and PKA target phosphorylation, differences may occur at ion channel and myofilament target sites.[35] *Forskolin* is a potent direct adenylyl cyclase activator, and isobutyl methylxanthine (*IBMX*) is a PDE inhibitor that inhibits all PDE isoforms. These are widely used agents experimentally, but isoform-specific PDE inhibitors are being explored as more targeted therapeutic strategies. A number of hormones or peptides can couple to myocardial adenylyl cyclase independent of the beta-adrenergic receptor. These include glucagon, thyroid hormone, prostacyclin, and calcitonin gene–related peptide.

There is also a GTP *e*xchange *p*rotein directly *a*ctivated by *c*AMP (*Epac*) that is activated in parallel to cAMP-dependent PKA activation. This allows additional parallel signaling downstream of beta-adrenergic activation. For example, beta-adrenergic activation of SR Ca^{2+} release is mediated by cAMP-Epac–dependent signaling to CaMKII and consequent RyR2 phosphorylation,[36] and not by PKA activation.

Protein Kinase A

PKA occurs in two isoforms, but PKA-II predominates in cardiac cells. It is now clear that many key cAMP effects are mediated by activation of PKA and phosphorylation of key proteins.[37] Each PKA complex is composed of two regulatory (R) and two catalytic (C) subunits, the latter of which transfers the terminal phosphate of ATP to serine and threonine residues of the protein substrates. When cAMP interacts with the inactive protein kinase, it binds to the R subunits, causing partial release and activation of the C subunits. A former dogma was that the C subunits were completely released from the R subunits, but more recent evidence suggests that a loose tethering likely remains when PKA is active. The R subunits are bound to specific AKAPs that target PKA-dependent phosphorylation at specific subcellular targets.[38] This helps to explain the local compartmentalization of cAMP and PKA signaling. Indeed, there is good evidence that beta-adrenergic receptors, G proteins, adenylyl cyclase, PKA, AKAP, PDE, and phosphatases can all complex at targets such as the L-type Ca^{2+} channel and RyR2 to facilitate local PKA-dependent signaling (see Fig. 46.13).[16,39,40]

Beta$_1$-Adrenergic and Protein Kinase A Signaling in Ventricular Myocytes

The sequence of events for PKA activation is as follows (see Fig. 46.12): catecholamine stimulation → beta receptor → molecular changes → binding of GTP to the α_s subunit of G protein → GTP-α_s subunit stimulating adenylyl cyclase → formation of cAMP from ATP → activation of cAMP-dependent PKA, locally bound by an AKAP → phosphorylation of the target proteins. The L-type Ca^{2+} channel is rapidly phosphorylated by this cascade, which results in both a large increase in the amount of peak I_{Ca} and a shift in the activation voltage to more negative potentials. This increases the amount of Ca^{2+} that enters the cell at each beat and also enhances excitability (including in pacemaker cells). In addition, the higher I_{Ca} triggers more SR Ca^{2+} release, but the higher peak I_{Ca} and SR Ca^{2+} release also enhance Ca-dependent inactivation of I_{Ca}, which limits the total amount of Ca^{2+} entry during the AP. This contributes to an increased Ca^{2+} transient amplitude, the inotropic effect, and also the chronotropic and dromotropic effects of PKA in heart (Figs. 46.12–46.14).

Another major contributor to the inotropic effect of PKA in the heart is phosphorylation of PLB. PLB is associated with SERCA2 and at baseline inhibits the Ca^{2+} pump by reducing its affinity for Ca^{2+}. On phosphorylation of PLB by PKA (or CaMKII), the inhibitory effect is relieved and the Ca^{2+} pumping function greatly enhanced. This allows more Ca^{2+} to accumulate inside the SR during the cardiac cycle, which enhances the amount that can then be released (thereby contributing to inotropy). The faster rate of SR Ca^{2+} uptake is also the major factor in accelerating relaxation, the lusitropic effect of PKA. This occurs because twitch $[Ca^{2+}]_i$ decline is faster, which allows faster Ca^{2+} dissociation from the myofilaments.

Phosphorylation of troponin I by PKA also contributes to the enhanced lusitropic effect of beta-adrenergic agonists (see Fig. 46.13). PKA-dependent troponin I phosphorylation reduces myofilament sensitivity for calcium, which is intrinsically negatively inotropic, but has the benefit of faster dissociation of Ca^{2+} from myofilaments, which hastens relaxation and diastolic filling. In addition, myosin-binding protein C is also a target for PKA, and its phosphorylation appears to be responsible for accelerating the cross-bridge turnover rate. This effect also serves largely to offset the negative inotropic effect of troponin I phosphorylation and also may hasten the rate of sarcomere shortening at a given $[Ca^{2+}]$ and mechanical load, which could enhance stroke volume.[41]

PKA also phosphorylates the RyR, although the impact of this effect is controversial.[42] One group has suggested that this displaces the immunophilin FKBP-12.6 from its binding to RyR2, thereby activating RyR openings, and that this is an important part of the beta-adrenergic inotropy and cardiac dysfunction in heart failure.[43] However, this idea has been strongly challenged by extensive mechanistic experimental data and theoretical arguments from numerous groups worldwide.[42] Although the effects of PKA on the cardiac RyR may enhance the rate of RyR activation during excitation-contraction coupling, it does not seem to increase the amount released (for a given I_{Ca} trigger and SR Ca^{2+} load),[44] nor does it directly enhance the likelihood of spontaneous SR Ca^{2+} release events.[45] Moreover, even when the RyR is sensitized, it causes enhanced SR Ca^{2+} release only for several beats, which then drives greater efflux of Ca^{2+} from the cell (by NCX) and reduces the SR Ca^{2+} content such that it cannot explain the enhanced Ca^{2+} transients during beta-adrenergic activation.[46]

PKA also phosphorylates PLM, a small PLB-like protein that regulates Na^+,K^+-ATPase (see earlier).[32] This is actually a sensible integral part of the fight-or-flight response because the increase in HR incurs more frequent I_{Na} pulses and Ca^{2+} influx (by I_{Ca}) that causes more Na^+ influx by NCX, resulting in a major increase in $[Na^+]_i$. This Na^+,K^+-ATPase activation limits the rise in $[Na^+]_i$ during sympathetic activation and thus allows NCX to remain functional in removing Ca^{2+} from the myocyte.

The increase in Na$^+$,K$^+$-ATPase function thus is somewhat negatively inotropic (by limiting [Na$^+$]$_i$). This is opposite the effect mediated by inhibition of Na$^+$,K$^+$-ATPase by digitalis cardiac glycosides. Notably, digitalis toxicity is associated with cellular Ca^{2+} overload and arrhythmogenesis. Consequently, Na$^+$,K$^+$-ATPase stimulation may limit these arrhythmogenic consequences associated with higher Ca^{2+} loading.

BETA-ADRENERGIC RECEPTOR DESENSITIZATION

There is a potent and rapid feedback mechanism whereby beta-adrenergic receptor stimulation can be muted so that the signal can be turned off (see Fig. 46.14). Physiologically, this mechanism of beta-adrenergic receptor desensitization occurs within minutes. Sustained beta-agonist stimulation recruits a G protein–coupled receptor kinase (GRK2; also called beta-adrenergic receptor kinase 1 [βARK1]). GRK2 phosphorylates a site on the carboxyl-terminal of the beta-adrenergic receptor, which by itself does not switch off signaling. However, GRK2 activity increases beta receptor affinity for arrestins, which uncouple receptor signaling. Beta-arrestin is a scaffolding and signaling protein that links to one of the cytoplasmic loops of the beta-adrenergic receptor and lessens activation of adenylyl cyclase, thereby inhibiting receptor function. Furthermore, beta-arrestin can switch agonist coupling from G$_s$ to G$_i$ and also lead to internalization of the beta-adrenergic receptor.[4] Resensitization of the receptor occurs if the phosphate groups are removed by a phosphatase, and the receptor then more readily linked to G$_s$ (or by recycling the internalized receptor to the surface). Beta-arrestin signaling can also evoke an alternative protective path by activating the epidermal growth factor receptor (EGFR), which leads to the protective extracellular signal–related kinase (ERK)/MAPK pathway (see Fig. 46.14).[47] Although the GRK2-arrestin effects are best described for the beta$_2$ receptor, they also occur with the beta$_1$ receptor. Prolonged beta receptor stimulation, as in hyperadrenergic conditions, is linked to adverse end results in that it both impairs contractile function and enhances adverse signaling. As discussed in Chapter 47, this mechanism also plays a role in long-term desensitization of the beta-adrenergic receptor as in heart failure, and transgenic mice overexpressing GRK2 are protected from heart failure.[48]

Ca^{2+}/Calmodulin-Dependent Protein Kinase II

CaMKII is a serine/threonine-specific protein kinase that is regulated by the Ca^{2+}/CaM complex. CaMKII is involved in many signaling cascades in the heart, and several of the key proteins that are phosphorylated by PKA are also phosphorylated by CaMKII (see Fig. 46.13), typically at different amino acids. Moreover, there is good evidence that CaMKII is activated during beta-adrenergic stimulation.[23] Thus, CaMKII signaling is often coactivated with PKA and can synergize at downstream targets.[23,49] CaMKII activates L-type Ca^{2+} channels (I$_{Ca}$ facilitation), which results in increased peak I$_{Ca}$ and also slows down inactivation, thereby boosting total Ca^{2+} influx by I$_{Ca}$. CaMKII also phosphorylates PLB at Thr17 (vs. at Ser16 by PKA) and, by the same mechanism as for PKA, can enhance SR Ca^{2+} uptake. However, the CaMKII effects on I$_{Ca}$ and SERCA/PLB are typically smaller in magnitude than the effects of PKA activation, so PKA is probably dominant physiologically at these targets. CaMKII can also phosphorylate RyR2 at Ser2814, close to a recognized PKA target site (2808). In contrast to PKA, it is more universally agreed that CaMKII strongly activates the RyR and that this effect may be important in causing a diastolic SR Ca^{2+} leak, which can both reduce the SR Ca^{2+} content (contributing to both systolic and diastolic dysfunction) and contribute to triggered arrhythmias.[22,23,42] CaMKII can also phosphorylate cardiac Na$^+$ and K$^+$ channels and lead to arrhythmogenic consequences.[22,23] CaMKII-dependent activation of the late Na$^+$ current may also lead to elevated intracellular [Na$^+$] and [Ca^{2+}], which can create Ca^{2+} overload and trigger arrhythmias. Myofilament proteins are also targets for CaMKII (e.g., myosin-binding protein C and titin),[50] but the relative functional importance of this effect is not yet fully resolved. The chronic activation of CaMKII in pathologic states such as heart failure makes these pathways important to keep in mind.

CHOLINERGIC AND NITRIC OXIDE SIGNALING

Cholinergic Signaling

Parasympathetic stimulation reduces the HR and is negatively inotropic. As in adrenergic signaling, there is an extracellular messenger (ACh), a GPCR (the *cholinergic* muscarinic receptor in heart; M$_2$), and a sarcolemmal signaling system (G protein system, specifically G$_i$; see Fig. 46.12). Receptor stimulation produces a negative chronotropic response that is inhibited by atropine. NO, also formed by beta$_3$-adrenergic signaling,[51] facilitates cholinergic signaling at two levels, the nerve terminal and myocyte enzyme system that produces the second messenger cGMP. *Neuregulins* are growth factors that maintain the activity of the muscarinic receptor, thereby indirectly helping to balance the normal parasympathetic modulation of excess beta-adrenergic stimulation.[52,53]

Muscarinic G$_i$ activation also inhibits adenylyl cyclase, which functionally integrates the input from activating G$_s$ (e.g., from beta$_1$-adrenergic and other receptors) and the inhibitory effects of G$_i$ (from M$_2$ muscarinic and other receptors; Fig. 46.12). As a result, vagal stimulation also limits [cAMP] resulting from ambient sympathetic tone. The net effect is slowing of the HR. This is partly because cardiac vagal innervation is highest in the SA and atrioventricular (AV) nodes, with lower density in atrial myocardium and the lowest density in ventricular myocardium. Consequently, vagal activity has less strong effects on atrial or ventricular myocyte electrophysiology, Ca^{2+} transients, or contractility than on conduction system cells, but that is also because these cells lack major pacemaker function and have higher inward rectifier I$_{K1}$ channels that already stabilize diastolic membrane potential at more negative values. Nevertheless, vagal activation can shorten the AP duration in the atria and, to a lesser degree, in the ventricles (primarily by I$_{K(ACh)}$ activation).

CYCLIC GUANOSINE MONOPHOSPHATE SIGNALING IN THE HEART

The second messenger cGMP typically has negative inotropic effects in the heart, in contrast to its cyclic nucleotide cousin cAMP. Cyclic GMP is produced from GTP in cardiac myocytes mainly by soluble and particulate guanylyl cyclases, which are activated downstream of NO and natriuretic peptide receptor activation, respectively (Fig. 46.15), and possibly by cholinergic effects. Local subcellular microdomains in which NO and cGMP signaling take place are also likely to exist.[39] When local [cGMP]

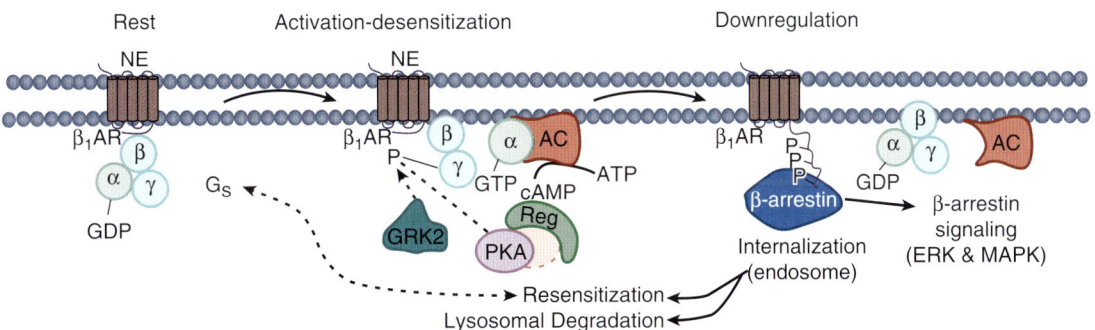

FIGURE 46.14 Beta$_1$-adrenergic receptor (β$_1$AR) activation, desensitization, downregulation, and recycling. Prolonged β$_1$AR activation causes recruitment of a G-protein receptor kinase (GRK2) that phosphorylates the receptor and favors recruitment of beta-arrestin (β-arrestin). β-arrestin promotes its own signaling cascades (e.g. via extracellular receptor and MAP kinase (ERK and MAPK) as well as internalization of the β$_1$AR into endosomes. From there β$_1$AR can either be degraded or recycled to the cell surface. (Modified from Bers DM. *Excitation-Contraction Coupling and Cardiac Contractile Force*. Dordrecht, Netherlands: Kluwer Academic; 2001.)

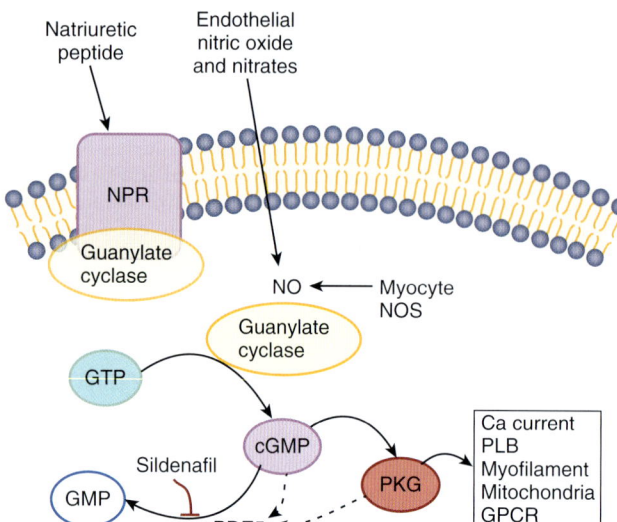

FIGURE 46.15 Nitric oxide (NO) and the natriuretic peptide receptor (NPR) activate guanylate cyclase (via particulate and soluble cyclases, respectively), resulting in production of cyclic guanosine monophosphate (cGMP) and activation of protein kinase G (PKG). PKG can phosphorylate numerous myocyte targets that tend to counteract cyclic adenosine monophosphate (cAMP) and PKA effects at some targets (with some exceptions). Phosphodiesterase 5 (PDE5) breaks down cGMP, and PDE5 inhibitors (e.g., sildenafil) can thus increase cGMP levels. Notably, high cGMP and PKG levels promote vasodilation and negative inotropic effects, and antianginal nitrates promote vasodilation by this mechanism.

is elevated, it can stimulate protein kinase G (PKG), which results in inhibitory cardiac effects such as a decreased HR and negative inotropic response. These effects are largely achieved by modulation of Ca^{2+} entry through L-type Ca^{2+} channels and through alteration of internal Ca^{2+} cycling.[53,54] PKG has also been suggested to be a critical suppressor of pathophysiologic hypertrophy.[55]

cGMP is broken down by PDE, and seven PDE isoforms are expressed in the heart, some of which break down both cAMP and cGMP (PDE1 to PDE3), whereas PDE4 is cAMP specific and PDE5 is cGMP specific.[54] Cell-permeable analogues of cGMP have antiadrenergic effects, potentially by activating PDE2 that also breaks down cAMP. PDE5 has achieved prominence as a result of its inhibition by sildenafil and related compounds that all enhance penile vasodilation. Emerging data show wider therapeutic potential. Thus sildenafil, by accumulation of cGMP, combats the harmful excessive adrenergic stimulation of contractile function. Furthermore, through cGMP, sildenafil can inhibit excess LV growth in response to aortic constriction.[56] Conversely, in human cardiac hypertrophy and heart failure, PDE5 is more highly expressed, which may exacerbate adverse remodeling. The key target of cGMP, PKG, as with its counterpart PKA, colocalizes with its targets to control substrate phosphorylation.[57] The anchoring protein for PKG may be the same AKAP as for PKA, thus allowing tight subcellular colocalization and regulation of the counterpoised activities of cAMP and cGMP and of their respective upstream signaling cascades.[54]

Nitric Oxide

The focus of the Nobel Prize Award for 1998, NO is a unique messenger in that it is formed in so many tissues, is a gas, and is a physiologic free radical. NO is generated in the heart by one of three isoenzymes.[53] All three isoforms are present in the heart. NOS1 (nNOS, or neuronal NOS) and NOS3 (eNOS, or endothelial NOS) are always present, whereas NOS2 (iNOS, or inducible NOS) expression is induced in pathological conditions.[58,59] Both NOS1 and NOS3 are activated by local Ca^{2+}-CaM, where relatively low concentrations of Ca^{2+}-CaM suffice to activate NOS activation. In contrast, NOS2 constitutively produces NO, independent of Ca^{2+}-CaM activation. NO can directly activate soluble guanylate cyclase (see Fig. 46.15), feeding into the cGMP signaling system, but many other myocyte proteins are S-nitrosylated by NO which can modulate their function, including CaMKII.[59,60]

CONTRACTILE PERFORMANCE OF THE HEART

There are five main determinants of ventricular mechanical performance: preload (or Frank-Starling mechanism), afterload, contractility, lusitropy (diastolic function), and HR. This section describes the cardiac cycle and then the determinants of LV function.

The Cardiac Cycle

The cardiac cycle, fully assembled by Lewis[61] but first conceived by Wiggers,[62] yields important information on the temporal sequence of events (Fig. 46.16). The three basic events with respect to the left ventricle are LV contraction, LV relaxation, and LV filling (Table 46.3). Similar mechanical events occur in the right ventricle.

Left Ventricular Contraction

LV pressure increases as Ca^{2+} arrives at the contractile proteins after cellular depolarization, triggering actin-myosin interaction.[4] This occurs shortly after the upstroke of the ventricular AP, indicated by the QRS complex of the ECG (Fig. 46.16). When LV pressure exceeds pressure in the left atrium (normally 8 to 15 mm Hg), the mitral valve closes, causing the mitral component of the first sound, M_1. Right ventricular (RV) pressure changes are usually slightly delayed because of electrical conduction, such that tricuspid valve closure (T_1) follows M_1. The phase of LV contraction after mitral closure and before aortic opening when the LV volume is fixed is referred to as *isovolumic contraction*. As more myofibers become activated, LV pressure proceeds to increase until it exceeds aortic pressure, causing the aortic valve to open (usually a clinically silent event). Opening of the aortic valve is followed by the phase of *rapid ejection*. The rate of ejection is determined by the pressure gradient across the aortic valve, as well as the elastic properties of the aorta and the arterial tree, which undergo systolic expansion. LV pressure rises to a peak and then starts to fall.

Left Ventricular Relaxation

As myocyte $[Ca^{2+}]_i$ starts to decline because of SR Ca^{2+} uptake, Ca^{2+} dissociates from troponin C, thereby preventing further cross-bridge formation.[4] As this state of relaxation progresses, the rate of LV ejection of blood into the aorta falls (*phase of reduced ejection*). During this phase, blood flow from the left ventricle to the aorta rapidly diminishes but is maintained by aortic recoil—the Windkessel effect.[4] When the pressure in the aorta significantly exceeds the falling LV pressure, the aortic valve closes, which creates the first component of the second sound, A_2 (the second component, P_2, results from closure of the pulmonic valve as pulmonary artery pressure exceeds RV pressure). Thereafter, the ventricle continues to relax. Because the mitral valve is still closed during this phase after aortic closure, LV volume does not change (*isovolumic relaxation*). The rate of pressure decay during isovolumic relaxation is related to the magnitude of systolic shortening in the preceding contraction, similar to a spring compressed below its unstressed slack length.[63] When LV pressure falls to below that in the left atrium, the mitral valve opens (normally silent), and the filling phase of the cardiac cycle restarts (see Fig. 46.16).

Left Ventricular Filling Phases

Following mitral valve opening, the phase of rapid or early filling occurs and accounts for most of the increase in LV volume during diastole.[4] Under normal circumstances, this is caused by a negative pressure gradient from atrium to the LV apex, creating a suction effect, especially during exercise, when LV filling rates must be augmented to increase cardiac output.[63] Such rapid filling may cause the physiologic third heart sound (S_3), when there is a hyperkinetic circulation, or a pathologic S_3 when left atrial (LA) and LV diastolic pressures are elevated in congestive heart failure.[4] As pressures in the atrium and ventricle equalize, LV filling virtually stops (diastasis, separation). Renewed filling requires that atrial pressure exceed LV pressure. This is achieved by atrial systole (or the "LA kick"), which is especially important at a high

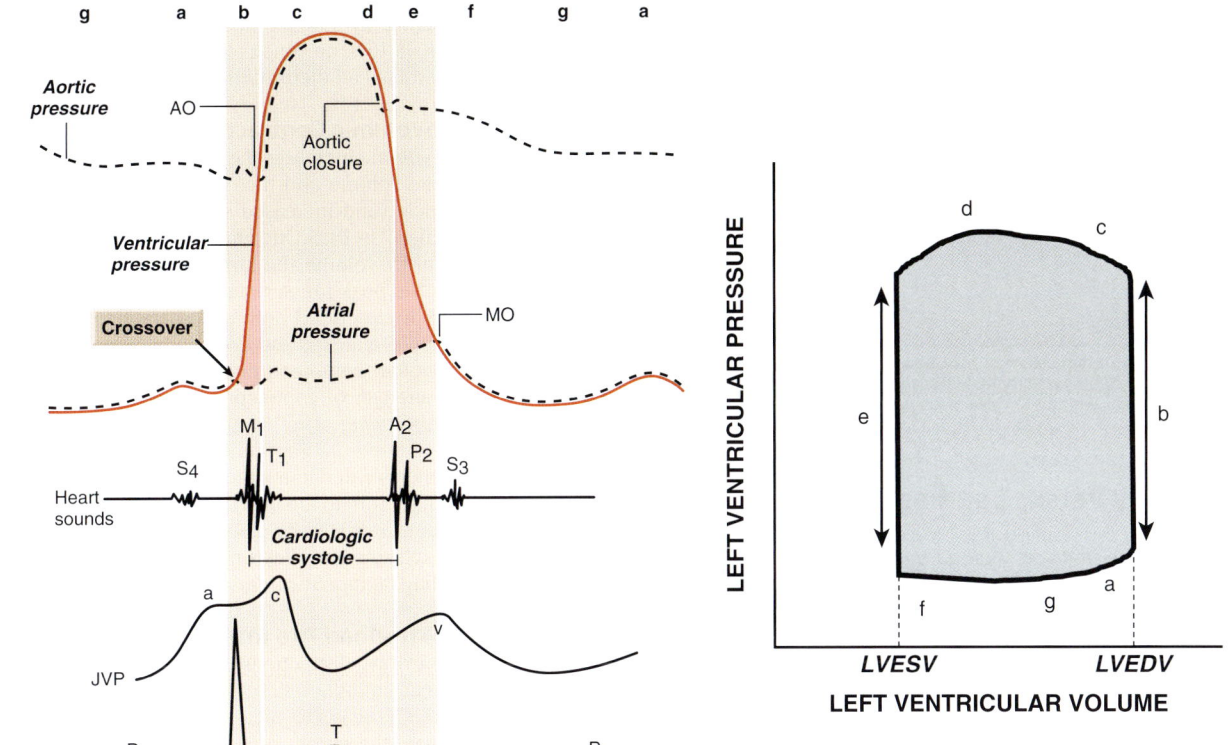

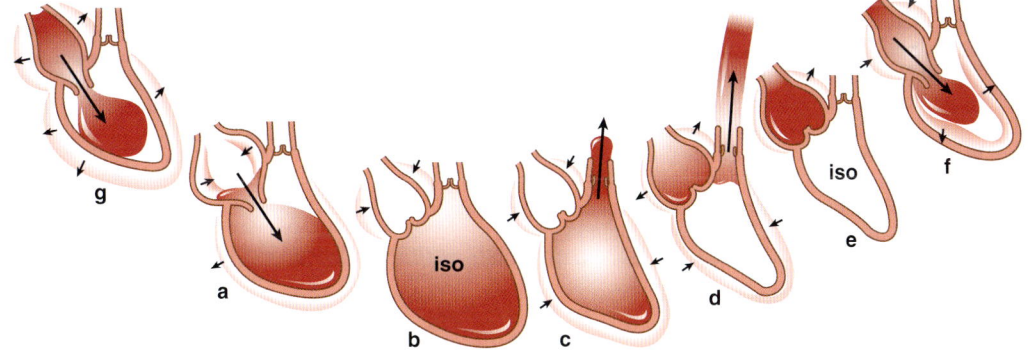

FIGURE 46.16 Mechanical events in the cardiac cycle depicted as pressure versus time (**upper left**) and left ventricular pressure versus volume (**upper right**). The visual phases of the ventricular cycle are shown in the **bottom panel**. For an explanation of phases a to g in upper right and bottom panels, see Table 46.3. *a*, Wave produced by right atrial contraction; A_2, aortic valve closure, aortic component of the second sound; *AO*, aortic valve opening, normally inaudible; *c*, carotid wave artifact during the rapid LV ejection phase; *ECG*, electrocardiogram; *JVP*, jugular venous pressure; *LVEDV*, left ventricular end-diastolic volume; *LVESV*, left ventricular end-systolic volume; M_1, mitral component of the first sound at the time of mitral valve closure; *MO*, mitral valve opening, may be audible in mitral stenosis as the opening snap; P_2, pulmonary component of the second sound, pulmonary valve closure; S_3, third heart sound; S_4, fourth heart sound; T_1, tricuspid valve closure, second component of the first heart sound; *v*, venous return wave, which causes pressure to rise with the tricuspid valve closed. (Modified from Opie LH. *Heart Physiology, from Cell to Circulation*. Philadelphia: Lippincott, Williams & Wilkins; 2004. Figure copyright L.H. Opie, 2004. **Bottom panel** modified from Shepherd JT, Vanhoutte PM. *The Human Cardiovascular System*. New York: Raven Press; 1979:68.)

HR, as during exercise, or when the left ventricle fails to relax normally, as in patients with LV hypertrophy or increased chamber stiffness.[4]

DEFINITIONS OF SYSTOLE AND DIASTOLE

In Greek, systole means "contraction" and diastole means "to send apart." The start of systole can be regarded as the beginning of isovolumic contraction, when LV pressure exceeds the atrial pressure, or as mitral valve closure (M_1). Physiologic systole lasts from the start of isovolumic contraction to the peak of the ejection phase (see Fig. 46.16 and Table 46.3). Physiologic diastole commences as Ca^{2+} is taken back into the SR, so that myocyte relaxation dominates over contraction, and as the LV pressure starts to fall, as shown on the pressure-volume curve. In contrast, cardiologic systole is longer than physiologic systole and is demarcated by the interval between the first heart sound (M_1) to the closure of the aortic valve (A_2). The remainder of the cardiac cycle automatically becomes cardiologic diastole. For the cardiologist, protodiastole is the early phase of rapid filling, the time when S_3 can be heard (also referred to as a protodiastolic gallop). This sound probably reflects ventricular wall vibrations during rapid filling and becomes audible with an increase in LV diastolic pressure, wall stiffness, or rate of filling.

TABLE 46.3 The Cardiac Cycle

Left Ventricular Contraction
Isovolumic contraction (b)
Maximal ejection (c)
Left Ventricular Relaxation
Start of relaxation and reduced ejection (d)
Isovolumic relaxation (e)
LV filling: rapid phase (f)
Slow LV filling (diastasis) (g)
Atrial systole or kick (a)

The letters a to g refer to the phases of the cardiac cycle shown in Wiggers' diagram (see Fig. 46.16). These letters are arbitrarily allocated so that atrial systole (a) coincides with the A wave and (c) with the C wave of jugular venous pressure.

Contractility Versus Loading Conditions
Contractility
Contractility, or the *inotropic state of the heart*, reflects the inherent capacity of the myocardium to contract independently of changes in preload or afterload.[63] These are key terms in the language of cardiology. At the molecular level, an increased inotropic state is usually explained by either enhanced Ca^{2+} transients or enhanced myofilament Ca^{2+} sensitivity and typically results in a greater rate of contraction to reach a greater peak force. Frequently, increased contractile function is associated with enhanced rates of relaxation, or a lusitropic effect (e.g., as during beta-adrenergic activation). Contractile function is an important regulator of myocardial oxygen (O_2) uptake. Factors that increase contractility include exercise, adrenergic stimulation, digitalis, and other inotropic agents.

Preload
It is important to stress that any change in the contractility should be independent of the loading conditions. An increase in stroke volume that is caused by an increase in preload alone may not reflect an increase in contractility per se. Ventricular preload describes the degree of myocardial stretch or distention before contraction has started and is best represented at the chamber level by the LV EDV. Because volume is difficult to measure accurately and precisely in practice, preload is often estimated by LV end-diastolic pressure (EDP), but it is important to remember that the relationship between EDP and EDV varies between patients, especially when diastolic dysfunction or ventricular interdependence are present. In such patients, a higher EDP is required to achieve a given EDV, meaning that preload may be normal or even low despite elevated intracardiac filling pressures.

Afterload
Afterload refers in a broad sense to the forces opposing LV ejection.[4,63] Afterload is often oversimplified as being equal to aortic blood pressure but is more accurately described as aortic *impedance* or *elastance*, which incorporates steady and oscillatory components of cardiac load. LV afterload can also be expressed by the wall stress that exists during systole. When preload increases, the stroke volume rises according to Starling's law if all other factors are held constant. Conversely, when afterload increases, stroke volume drops.

Starling's Law of the Heart
Venous Filling Pressure and Heart Volume
In 1918, Starling related the venous pressure in the right atrium to the heart volume in a dog heart-lung preparation.[4] He proposed that, within physiologic limits, the larger the volume of the heart, the greater the energy of its contraction and the amount of chemical change at each contraction. Starling did not, however, measure sarcomere length. He could only relate *LV volume* to cardiac output. In practice the LV volume is not often measured, rather making use of a variety of surrogate measures, such as LVEDP or the pulmonary capillary wedge pressure (PCWP). The relation between LVEDV and LVEDP is curvilinear, with the slope reflecting LV compliance (bottom portion of pressure-volume loop, Fig. 46.16). The venous filling pressure can be measured in humans by cardiac catheterization, as can the stroke volume.

Frank and Isovolumic Contraction
If a larger heart volume increases the initial length of the muscle fiber, to increase stroke volume and thus cardiac output, diastolic stretch of the left ventricle (and increased sarcomere length) increases the force of contraction.[4] In 1895, Otto Frank had already reported that the greater the initial LV volume, the more rapid the rate of rise in pressure, the greater the peak pressure reached, and the faster the rate of relaxation. Thus, he described both a positive *inotropic effect* and an increased lusitropic effect. These complementary findings of Frank and Starling are often combined into the *Frank-Starling law*. Thus an increase in the strength of contraction can generally be categorized as either a *Frank-Starling effect* (increased sarcomere length) or an inotropic effect (altered Ca^{2+} transient or myofilament Ca^{2+} sensitivity), although both effects can occur simultaneously, as with physical exercise, where venous return to the heart is increased while β-1 adrenergic receptors are being activated by catecholamines to augment the Ca^{2+} transient. Being able to parse effects mechanistically in this way can be helpful in selecting therapeutic interventions.

Preload and Afterload Are Interlinked
Although the previous distinctions between preload and afterload are useful, one can influence the other. By the Frank-Starling law, an increased LV volume leads to increased contractile function, which in turn will increase the systolic aortic pressure and thus the afterload in the subsequent contraction cycle. During LV ejection, sarcomere length progressively declines, decreasing both myofilament Ca^{2+} sensitivity and maximal force, which along with progressive $[Ca^{2+}]_i$ decline, reduces contractile force. Afterload also dynamically changes during ejection and declines as ejection wanes.

PRELOAD AND DIASTOLIC PRESSURES MAY BECOME UNCOUPLED IN DISEASED HEARTS
LV pressure and volume are nonlinearly related because of myocardial compliance variations. In patients with reduced diastolic LV compliance, a higher EDP is required to achieve a similar EDV (preload). While the left and right ventricles influence each another in series (right ventricle pumps blood to left ventricle), factors in the right heart and pericardium also may influence LV pressure when there is enhanced ventricular interdependence, for example, with RV dilation from acute infarction or pulmonary embolism, or pericardial restraint caused by fibrotic constrictive pericarditis.[64] In these situations, EDP may be high even when EDV is normal or low, because the right heart and pericardium are applying "external pressure" that uncouples pressure from preload volume.

The true "distending" pressure that determines LV preload volume is referred to as the LV transmural pressure and can be calculated by EDP minus the external pericardial pressure. Pericardial pressure is approximated by right atrial pressure; thus transmural pressure can be estimated by the difference between EDP (or PCWP) and right atrial pressure.[64]

Force-Length Relationships and Ca^{2+} Transients
Acute changes in sarcomere length do not alter the Ca^{2+} transient appreciably. Thus the favored explanation for the steep length-tension relationship of cardiac muscles is enhanced myofilament Ca^{2+} sensitivity as the initial sarcomere length increases (via the Frank-Starling effect) (Fig. 46.17).

Anrep Effect: Abrupt Increase in Afterload
When the aortic pressure is elevated abruptly, ejection is limiting, tending to increase EDV, which acutely increases force and pressure at the next beat by the Frank-Starling effect. However, in a slower adaptation that takes seconds to minutes, the inotropic state of the heart increases (and Ca^{2+} transients are larger). Both phases of this can be readily recapitulated in isolated muscle strips from the heart. This slow force response or adaptation is referred to as the *Anrep effect*. Extensive study has implicated stretch-induced activation of several important

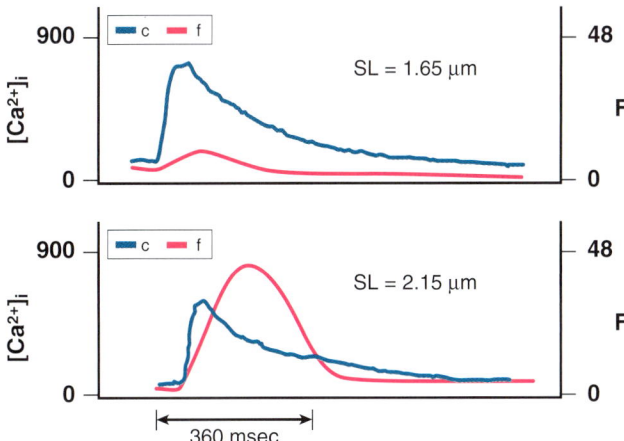

FIGURE 46.17 Length-dependent enhancement of myofilament Ca sensitivity. In the **top panel,** sarcomere length (SL) is 1.65 μm, which produces modest developed force (f). In the **bottom panel,** at near-maximal sarcomere length (2.15 μm), the Ca^{2+} transient (c) is almost unchanged, but causes much greater force development. (Modified from Backx PH, ter Keurs HEDJ. Fluorescent properties of rat cardiac trabeculae microinjected with fura-2 salt. *Am J Physiol.* 1993;264:H1098.)

autocrine/paracrine myocyte signaling pathways in this slowly developing inotropic effect. Recent work suggests that increased afterload causes a NOS1- and CaMKII-dependent increase in Ca^{2+} transients to cause this myocyte-intrinsic gradual inotropic effect.[65,66]

Wall Stress

Wall stress develops when tension is applied to a cross-sectional area, and the units are force per unit area (Fig. 46.18). According to Laplace's law, wall stress = (pressure × radius)/(2 × wall thickness). This equation, although an oversimplification, emphasizes two points. First, the larger the LV size and radius, the higher is the wall stress.[4] Second, at any given radius (LV size), the greater the pressure developed by the left ventricle, the greater is the wall stress. An increase in wall stress achieved by either of these two mechanisms (LV size or intraventricular pressure) will increase myocardial O$_2$ uptake, because a greater rate of ATP use is required for the myofibrils to develop more tension.

In cardiac hypertrophy, Laplace's law explains the effects of changes in wall thickness on wall stress (see Fig. 46.18). The increased wall thickness from hypertrophy balances the increased pressure, and wall stress remains unchanged during the phase of compensatory hypertrophy.[4] The concept that this change is compensatory and beneficial has been challenged by a mouse model in which the process of hypertrophy was genetically inhibited so that wall stress increased in response to a pressure load, yet these mice had better cardiac mechanical function than did the wild-type mice in which compensatory hypertrophy developed.[4] Another clinically useful concept is that in congestive heart failure, the heart dilates so that the increased radius elevates wall stress. Furthermore, because ejection of blood is inadequate, the radius stays too large throughout the contractile cycle, and both end-diastolic and end-systolic wall stress is higher. This decreases LV efficiency, increases myocardial O$_2$ demand, and augments release of natriuretic peptide levels. The overall reduction in heart size decreases wall stress and improves LV function.[4]

WALL STRESS, PRELOAD, AND AFTERLOAD

This definition brings in both the volume and the fiber length that define the radius.[4] Preload can be defined as the wall stretch at the end of diastole, and therefore at the maximal resting length of the sarcomere (see Fig. 46.18). Measurement of wall stress in vivo is difficult because use of the radius of the left ventricle (see the preceding sections) neglects the confounding influence of the complex LV anatomy. Surrogate preload indices include LVEDP or dimensions (the latter being the major and minor axes of the heart in a two-dimensional echocardiographic view). Afterload, being the load on the contracting myocardium, is also the wall stress during LV ejection. Increased afterload means that increased intraventricular pressure has to be generated first to open the aortic

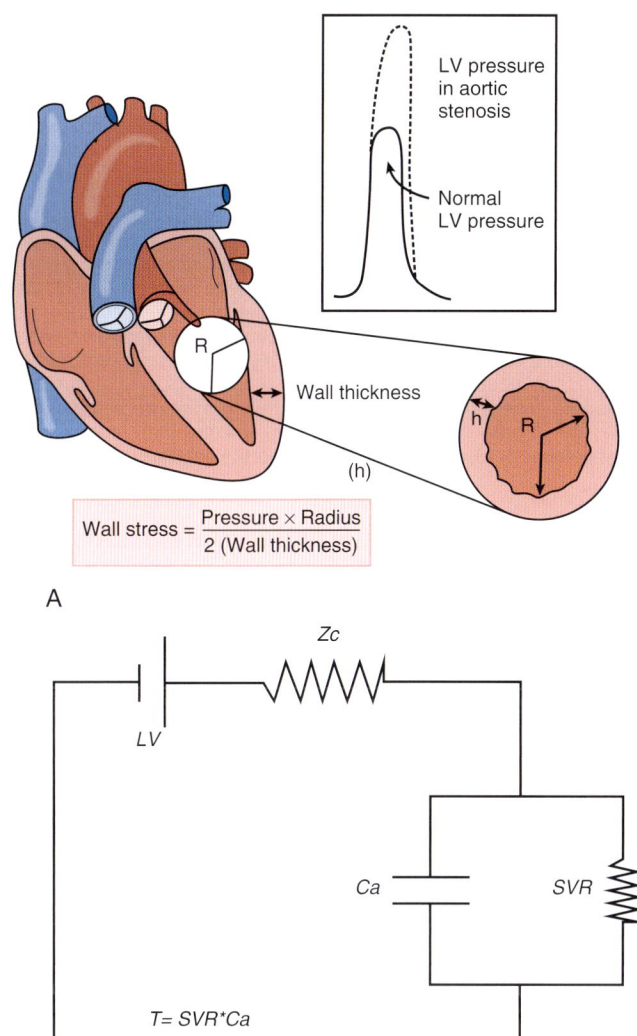

FIGURE 46.18 A, Wall stress increases as afterload increases. The formula shown is derived from Laplace's law. The increased left ventricular (LV) pressure in aortic stenosis is compensated for by LV wall hypertrophy, which decreases the denominator on the right side of the equation. **B,** Electrical circuit analog of the arterial system as it relates to LV afterload, based on the three-element Windkessel model. The LV generates current (flow, cardiac output) that is ejected through an upstream impedance in the proximal aorta (characteristic impedance, Zc) upstream of total arterial compliance (Ca) and systemic vascular resistance (SVR) that arranged in parallel. Effective arterial elastance (Ea) is a lumped measure of net arterial "stiffness" that is related to each of these components and can be estimated by the ratio of end-systolic LV pressure (ESP) to stroke volume (SV). Ea (and thus arterial afterload) increases as Zc or SVR increases or as Ca decreases. R, Radius. (**A** from Opie LH. *Heart Physiology, from Cell to Circulation.* Philadelphia: Lippincott Williams & Wilkins; 2004. Figure copyright L.H. Opie, 2004; **B** from Borlaug BA, Kass DA. Ventricular-vascular interaction in heart failure. *Heart Fail Clin* 2008; 4:23-36.)

valve and then during the ejection phase. These increases will translate into increased myocardial wall stress, which can be measured either as an average value or at end-systole.

Peak systolic wall stress reflects the three major components of afterload: peripheral resistance, arterial compliance, and peak intraventricular pressure.[4] Decreased arterial compliance and increased afterload can be anticipated with aortic remodeling and dilation, as in severe systemic hypertension or in older adult patients. The systolic timing of the afterload can also influence LV relaxation. In experimental and human studies, a late systolic load, as when the aorta has stiffened, is associated with impaired LV systolic shortening and diastolic relaxation.[67,68] This is why it is crucial to consider both afterload and preload when evaluating indices of LV function based on the velocity or extent of tissue motion using echocardiography.[68]

Aortic impedance or elastance gives another accurate measure of LV afterload (see Fig. 46.18). The advantage of impedance/elastance compared to wall stress is that this measure is totally independent of heart size or wall thickness. The aortic impedance reflects the ratio of aortic pressure to flow across different frequency harmonics. During systole, when the aortic valve is open, an increased afterload will communicate itself to the ventricles by increasing wall stress. In LV failure, aortic impedance is augmented not only by peripheral vasoconstriction (high systemic vascular resistance), but also by decreases in aortic compliance (ability of aorta to "yield" during systole), especially with aging. The problem with the clinical measurement of aortic impedance is that it is expressed in the frequency domain, which is cumbersome to relate to time-domain measures of LV function. An alternative index of LV afterload is the *arterial elastance* (Ea), estimated by the relationship between end-systolic LV pressure and stroke volume (see Fig. 46.18). Ea is derived from the Windkessel model of the arterial system, which includes upstream characteristic impedance (Zc) and a downstream resistance and capacitor that are situated in parallel. Thus, Ea incorporates both mean resistive components of load along with HR and aortic compliance.

Heart Rate and Force-Frequency Relationship
Treppe or Bowditch Effect
An increased HR progressively enhances the force of ventricular muscle contraction, even in isolated papillary muscle preparations and isolated myocytes, the *Bowditch staircase phenomenon*.[4] Alternative names are the *treppe* (German, "steps") phenomenon, positive inotropic effect of activation, or force-frequency relationship (Fig. 46.19A). Conversely, a decreased HR has a negative staircase effect. However, at a very high HR, force progressively decreases. These effects at the myocyte level

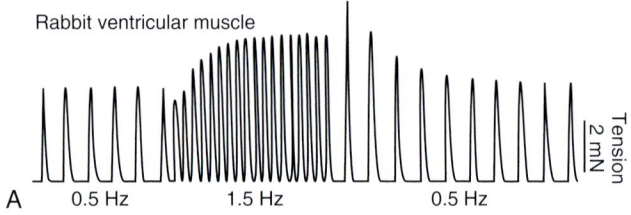

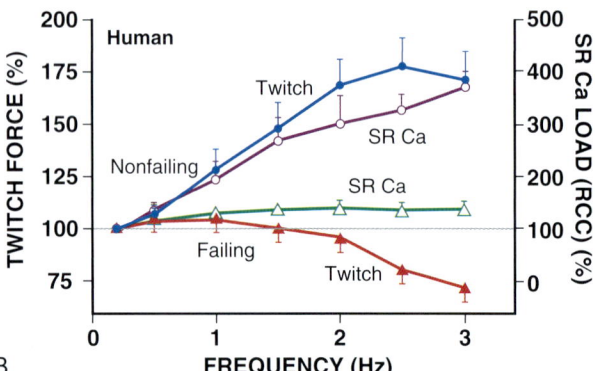

FIGURE 46.19 Heart rate dependence on contraction: Bowditch staircase or *treppe* phenomenon. **A,** An increased stimulation rate increases the force of contraction. The tension developed by rabbit ventricular muscle is shown in mN. During the first shortened diastolic interval the first beat is smaller, an effect caused mainly by refractoriness of the SR Ca^{2+} release channel. As the 1.5-Hz stimulation approaches a steady state, the contraction is progressively increased, an effect attributable to the gain in myocyte Na^+ and Ca^{2+} and enhanced SR Ca^{2+} content. When the diastolic interval is prolonged (first beat at 0.5 Hz), the first beat is especially large because the SR Ca^{2+} load is still elevated and there is more time for the RyR to recover from refractoriness. The larger Ca^{2+} transient then drives higher extrusion of Ca^{2+} from the cell as the initial 0.5-Hz steady state is eventually achieved. **B,** With an increasing heart rate, normal nonfailing ventricular muscle exhibits a progressive increase in SR Ca^{2+} content (*SR Ca*) and a positive force-frequency relationship that peaks at approximately 2.5 Hz. The decline at 3 Hz is caused by reduced fractional SR Ca^{2+} release. In failing human ventricular muscle, the SR fails to increase its Ca^{2+} content appreciably at higher heart rates; this results in a negative force-frequency relationship (which is dominated by the refractoriness, but here is not compensated by increased SR Ca^{2+}). SR Ca^{2+} in these experiments was assessed by rapid-cooling contractures (*RCC*). (From Bers DM. *Excitation-Contraction Coupling and Cardiac Contractile Force*. Dordrecht, Netherlands: Kluwer Academic; 2001.)

are largely attributable to changes in Na^+ and Ca^{2+} in the myocyte. At a higher HR, there is more Na^+ and Ca^{2+} entry per unit time and less time for the cell to extrude these ions, which results in higher $[Na^+]_i$ and cellular and SR Ca^{2+} content.[1] The increase in SR Ca^{2+} content increases the amount of Ca^{2+} released during the AP, the primary cause of the increase in contractility at higher HRs. The elevation in $[Na^+]_i$ also further reduces the efficacy of NCX in extruding Ca^{2+} during the cardiac cycle, thereby leading to further gains in cellular (and SR) Ca^{2+}. A new steady-state Ca^{2+} load will be achieved when the increased Ca^{2+} transients cause Ca^{2+} extrusion by NCX to match the amount of Ca^{2+} influx at each beat (and similarly when Na^+,K^+-ATPase extrudes the amount of Na^+ that enters per beat). This is the definition of steady state, with no net gain or loss of cellular Ca^{2+} (or Na^+) from beat to beat.

To the extent that the SR can take up this extra Ca^{2+} load at a higher HR, diastolic $[Ca^{2+}]_i$ and stiffness remain low. This is helped by an increase in the rate of SR Ca^{2+} uptake at a higher HR (known as "frequency-dependent acceleration of relaxation") mediated by faster SR Ca^{2+} uptake function (although the mechanism is not fully resolved).[1] However, if SR Ca^{2+}-ATPase and NCX are unable to remove Ca^{2+} sufficiently from the cytoplasm during the time between beats, an increase in diastolic $[Ca^{2+}]_i$ and force/stiffness will occur. This is an important contributor to prolongation of relaxation and elevation in cardiac filling pressures as occurs in patients with ventricular hypertrophy or heart failure.[69]

Systolic function is also limited at increasing HRs. The primary reason for this at physiologic HRs is that the SR Ca^{2+} release process has refractoriness that is reminiscent of that seen with voltage-gated Na^+ and Ca^{2+} channels. Thus, at higher HRs, even when a normal AP and Ca^{2+} current signal occurs, the fraction of SR Ca^{2+} released can be reduced (see Fig. 46.19B).[1] In a sense, the resulting Ca^{2+} transient and contraction at increasing HRs can be seen as the product of the increasing SR Ca^{2+} content times the declining fractional SR Ca^{2+} release, with the former factor being dominant (especially at more moderate HR) but the latter being progressively limiting.

In the intact heart this scenario is complicated by alterations in filling time and consequent changes in preload. That is, at higher HRs there will also be a reduced filling time that will limit preload (EDV), and thus a negative Frank-Starling effect will modulate the positive and negative inotropic effects to limit the overall strength of LV contraction. In addition, higher aortic elastance (Ea) at increased HRs will also increase cardiac afterload and limit the ability of the left ventricle to eject blood. Thus, both fundamental myocyte and hemodynamic properties combine to influence net cardiac function at increased HRs.

Premature ventricular complexes (PVCs) or *extrasystoles* can also modulate contraction in understandable ways. When a PVC occurs during the time when SR Ca^{2+} release is partially refractory and the left ventricle has not been refilled, the strength of that PVC will be very weak and may even fail to open the aortic valve. However, because the PVC had low SR Ca^{2+} release, less Ca^{2+} current inactivation and less Ca^{2+} extrusion from the cell occur and result in much higher SR Ca^{2+} release at the next (postextrasystolic) beat following the usual compensatory pause (because of AV node refractoriness during the next sinus node beat). Similarly, by the time the postextrasystolic beat occurs, the much smaller LV ejection and continued LV filling result in greater preload, reduced afterload, and a larger Ca^{2+} transient. These cellular and hemodynamic effects combine to cause an extremely strong, postextrasystolic potentiation beat that a person can often sense as the heart "skipping a beat." Patients with greater postextrasystolic potentiation have increased risk for adverse outcomes, probably because the greater potentiation reflects more severe abnormalities in Ca^{2+} handling within cardiac myocytes in the diseased heart.[70]

Physiologic Force-Frequency Relationship and Optimal Heart Rate
When the HR increases under physiologic conditions, it is usually accompanied and partially mediated by sympathetic beta-adrenergic activation at myocytes throughout the heart. As discussed earlier, this will increase Ca^{2+} current influx, the rate of SR Ca^{2+} uptake, and the amount of SR Ca^{2+} released during the beat, which greatly amplifies the inotropic and lusitropic effects associated with alteration of the HR without sympathetic

activation. However, the beta-adrenergic system also enhances Na$^+$,K$^+$-ATPase activity to limit the rise in [Na$^+$]$_i$ that occurs at the higher HR, and this would temper the overall inotropic effect. Normally, peak contractile force at a fixed muscle length (isometric contraction) increases, and a peak is reached at about 150 to 180 beats/min (see Fig. 46.19B).[1,4] In situ, the optimal HR is also dependent on the previous hemodynamic factors and a functioning sympathetic system, so the exact value of the HR when cardiac output starts to decrease rather than increase is more difficult to specify and likely varies among people. Pacing rates of up to 150 beats/min can be tolerated, whereas higher rates cannot because of the development of AV block. In contrast, during exercise, indices of LV function still increase up to a maximum HR of about 170 beats/min, presumably because of enhanced contractile function and peripheral vasodilation.[4] The critical HR associated with a fall-off in LV function likely occurs at lower values in diseased hearts, but this is not well understood and likely varies between patients.

Myocardial Oxygen Uptake

Myocardial O$_2$ demand can be increased by elevations in HR, preload, or afterload (Fig. 46.20), factors that can all precipitate myocardial ischemia in those with coronary artery disease (CAD). Because myocardial O$_2$ uptake ultimately reflects the rate of mitochondrial metabolism and thus ATP production, any increase in ATP requirement will be reflected in increased O$_2$ uptake. In general, factors increasing wall stress will increase O$_2$ uptake. Increased afterload causes increased systolic wall stress, which requires greater O$_2$ uptake. Increased diastolic wall stress, resulting from increased preload (EDV), will also require more oxygen because the greater stroke volume must be ejected against the afterload. In states of enhanced contractile function, the rate of change in wall stress is increased. Because systolic blood pressure (SBP) is an important correlate of afterload, a practical index of O$_2$ uptake is SBP × HR, the *double product*. The concept of wall stress in relation to O$_2$ uptake also explains why heart size is such an important determinant of myocardial O$_2$ uptake (because a larger radius increases wall stress). In patients with heart failure, the increase in myocardial O$_2$ demand during exercise outstrips the ability to augment myocardial O$_2$ supply, contributing to ischemia which is associated with an increase in myocyte injury.[71]

Work of the Heart

External work (pressure × volume) is done by the heart, with stroke volume (or cardiac output) being the volume moved against arterial blood pressure. *Volume work* (associated with increased stroke volume) requires less oxygen than *pressure work* does (increased pressure or HR), and one might suppose that external work is not an important determinant of myocardial O$_2$ uptake. However, three determinants of myocardial O$_2$ uptake are involved: preload (because this helps determine stroke volume), afterload (in part determined by blood pressure), and HR. *Minute work* can be defined as the product of SBP, stroke volume, and HR (SBP × SV × HR). Not surprisingly, heart work is related to O$_2$ uptake. This *pressure-work index* takes into account both the double product (SBP × HR) and HR × SV (i.e., cardiac output). The *pressure-volume area* is another index of cardiac work or O$_2$ uptake but requires invasive monitoring for accurate measurements (see Fig. 46.18). External cardiac work can account for up to 40% of the total myocardial O$_2$ uptake.

INTERNAL WORK (POTENTIAL ENERGY)

Total O$_2$ consumption is related to the total work of the heart (area *abcd* in Fig. 46.21), which means that both external work (area *abce*) and the volume-pressure triangle joining the end-systolic volume-pressure point

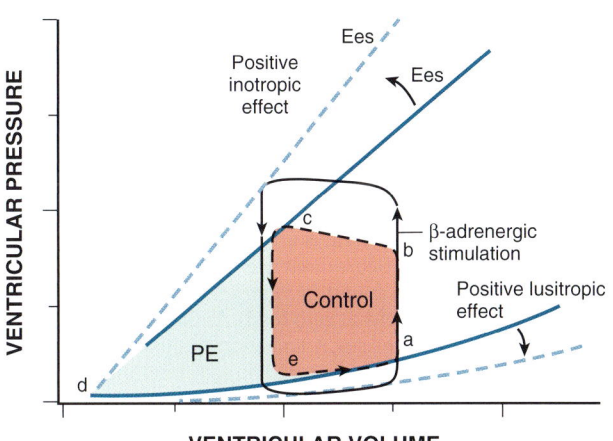

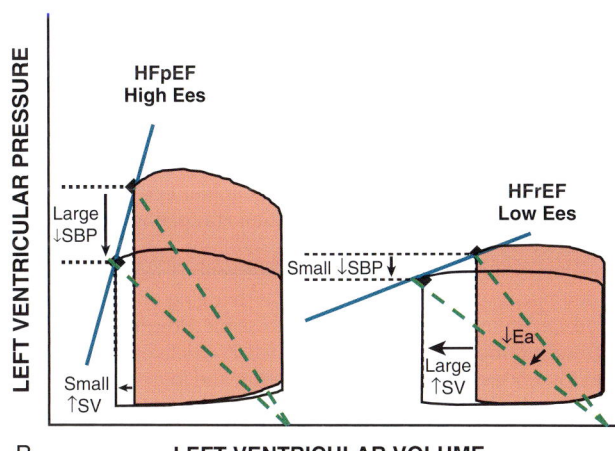

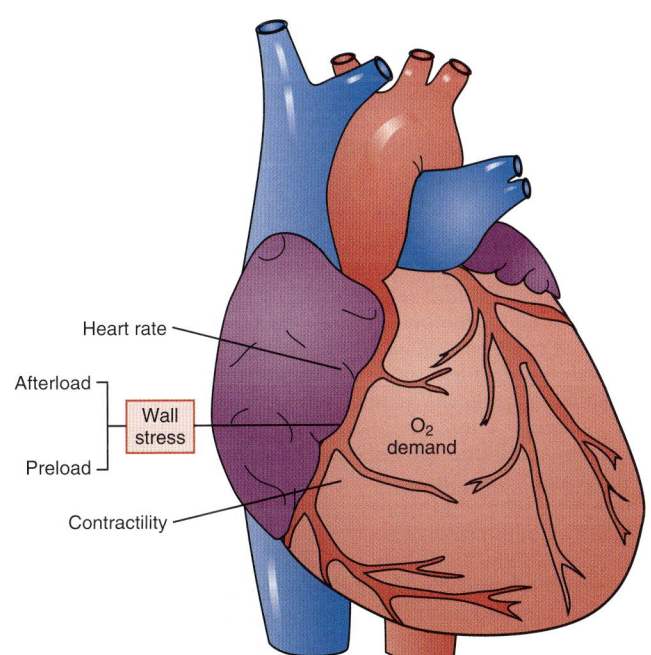

FIGURE 46.20 Major determinants of the O$_2$ demand of the normal heart: heart rate, wall stress, and contractile function. (Modified with permission from Opie LH. *Heart Physiology, from Cell to Circulation*. Philadelphia: Lippincott Williams & Wilkins; 2004. Figure copyright L.H. Opie, 2004.)

FIGURE 46.21 Pressure-volume loop of the left ventricle. **A,** Note the effects of beta-adrenergic catecholamines with both positive inotropic (increased slope of line *Ees*) and increased lusitropic (relaxant) effects. *Ees* is slope of the pressure-volume relationship. The total pressure-volume area (for the control area, see *abcd*) is closely related to myocardial O$_2$ uptake. The area *cde* is the component of work spent in generating potential energy (*PE*). **B,** Representative left ventricular (LV) pressure-volume loops in a patient with heart failure and preserved ejection fraction (HFpEF, *left*) and heart failure with reduced ejection fraction (HFrEF, *right*) demonstrating the differential effects of vasodilator therapy. In HFpEF, the end-systolic pressure volume relationship is steep, Ees is high, and reductions in arterial afterload or elastance (*Ea*) from acute vasodilator therapy (in this case, nitroprusside infusion) lead to dramatic reductions in systolic blood pressure (*SBP*) and modest increases in stroke volume (*SV*, defined by the width of the pressure-volume loop). In the patient with HFrEF, contractility is depressed, Ees is low, and the end-systolic pressure volume relationship is accordingly shallow. Thus the same degree of vasodilation (reduction in Ea) causes much less reduction in SBP and much more increase in forward SV. (**A** modified from Opie LH. *Heart Physiology, from Cell to Circulation*. Philadelphia: Lippincott, Williams & Wilkins; 2004. Figure copyright L.H. Opie, 2004; **B** modified from Schwartzenberg S, Redfield MM, From AM, Sorajja P, Nishimura RA, Borlaug BA. Effects of vasodilation in heart failure with preserved or reduced ejection fraction implications of distinct pathophysiologies on response to therapy. J Am Coll Cardiol 2012; 59:442-51.)

to the origin (area *cde*; marked PE).[72] Although this area has been called internal work, more strictly it should be called the "potential energy" that is generated within each contraction cycle but not converted to external work. Such potential energy at the end of systole (point c) may be likened to the potential energy of a compressed spring.

Efficiency of work is the relationship between the work performed and myocardial O_2 uptake.[4] Metabolically, efficiency is increased by promotion of glucose rather than fatty acids as the major myocardial fuel, as oxidation of glucose produces more ATP relative to O_2 consumed (higher P/O ratio). Conversely, heart failure decreases the efficiency of work, although the basis is not fully understood. Because as little as 12% to 14% of O_2 uptake may be converted to external work,[4] it is probably the "internal work" that becomes less demanding. Ion fluxes ($Na^+/K^+/Ca^{2+}$) account for approximately 20% to 30% of the ATP requirement of the heart, so most ATP is spent on actin-myosin interaction and much of that on the generation of heat rather than on external work. An increased initial muscle length sensitizes the contractile apparatus to Ca^{2+}, thereby theoretically increasing the efficiency of contraction by diminishing the amount of Ca^{2+} flux required.

Measurements of Contractile Function
Force-Velocity Relationship and Maximum Contractile Function in Muscle Models

If contractility is truly independent of load and the HR, unloaded heart muscle stimulated at a fixed rate should have a maximum value of contractile function for any given magnitude of the cytosolic Ca^{2+} transient. This value, the V_{max} of muscle contraction, is defined as the *maximal velocity of contraction* when there is no afterload to prevent maximal rates of cardiac ejection.[4] Beta-adrenergic stimulation increases V_{max}, and converse changes are found in failing myocardium. V_{max} is also termed V_0 (maximum velocity at zero load). As the load increases, the velocity of shortening decreases. A limitation of this relatively simple concept is that V_{max} cannot be measured directly but must be extrapolated from the *force-velocity relationship* to the velocity axis intercept. The other extreme condition is zero muscle shortening, with all the energy going into the development of pressure (P_0) or force (F_0). This situation is an example of *isometric contraction* (with internal cross-bridge stretching).

Isometric Versus Isotonic Contraction

Data for P_0 are obtained under isometric conditions (length unchanged). When muscle is allowed to shorten against a steady load, the conditions are *isotonic* (*tonic*, "contractile force").[4] Thus the force-velocity curve may be a combination of initial isometric conditions followed by isotonic contraction and then abrupt and total unloading to measure V_{max}. Although isometric conditions can be found in the whole heart (e.g., during isovolumic contraction), isotonic conditions are rare because afterload is constantly changing during the ejection period, and complete unloading is impossible. However, as shortening progresses during ejection, the maximal P_0 declines and velocity is lower for any given nonzero load. Therefore the force-velocity relationship is heuristically useful, but measurements in vivo are limited.

Pressure-Volume Loops

Accordingly, measurements of pressure-volume loops are among the best of the current approaches for assessment of the contractile behavior of the intact heart (see Figs. 46.18 and 46.21). A crucial measurement is the *end-systolic elastance* (Ees) from the pressure-volume relationship.[4] When the loading conditions are changed, alterations in the slope of this line joining the different E_s points (the end-systolic pressure-volume relationship [ESPVR]) are generally a good load-independent index of the contractile performance of the heart. In clinical practice, the need to change the loading conditions and the requirement for invasive monitoring for the full pressure-volume loop lessen the usefulness of this index. Measurement of LV volume adequately and continuously throughout the cardiac cycle is not easy. During a positive inotropic intervention, the pressure-volume loop changes in characteristic ways, resulting in a smaller end-systolic volume and a higher end-systolic pressure, so the slope of the pressure-volume relationship (E_s) has moved upward and to the left (see Fig. 46.21A). When the positive inotropic intervention consists of beta-adrenergic stimulation, the enhanced relaxation (lusitropic effect) may result in a lower pressure-volume curve during ventricular filling.

VENTRICULAR FUNCTION IN HEART FAILURE (SEE ALSO CHAPTER 47)

In patients with heart failure and reduced ejection fraction (HFrEF), the ventricle is dilated, EF is low, and contractility is severely depressed.[73] As such, the pressure-volume loop is shifted to the far right on the volume axis, and the (ESPVR, contractility) is very shallow (see Fig. 46.21B). In this setting, a reduction in arterial afterload (Ea) produces modest reductions in blood pressure despite often dramatic increases in stroke volume. This heightened "afterload dependence" of the LV in HFrEF serves as the hemodynamic basis for aggressive use of vasodilators in this disease. In contrast, patients with heart failure and preserved ejection fraction (HFpEF) display an increased Ees (steep ESPVR). In this patient, the same degree of afterload reduction (decrease in Ea) using a vasodilator causes a much more dramatic drop in blood pressure, with little improvement in forward stroke volume.

Limitations of the Concept of Contractility

Despite all the previous procedures that can be adopted in an attempt to measure true contractility (or the inotropic state), the concept has at least two serious defects: (1) the absence of any noninvasive index that can be measured unequivocally and (2) the impossibility of separating the cellular and chamber-level mechanisms of changes in contractile function from those of load or the HR. Thus an increased HR, by the changes in Na^+ and Ca^{2+} handling noted earlier, gives rise to increased cytosolic Ca^{2+} transients and contraction, which is clearly an inotropic effect. However, the simultaneous changes in preload and afterload also involve Frank-Starling effects, which complicates this picture in the clinical setting. Similarly, increased preload involves increased fiber stretch, which in turn causes enhanced myofilament Ca^{2+} sensitivity, a factor that in a sense is built into the Frank-Starling effect. However, additional changes in myofilament Ca^{2+} sensitivity (e.g., during acidosis or alpha-adrenergic activation) would be attributed to inotropic changes. *So there is a clear overlap between contractility, which should be independent of load or HR, and the effects of load and HR on the cellular mechanisms.*[3,4] Even though this does not undermine the importance of the intrinsic mechanistic distinctions between contractility/inotropy and Frank-Starling mechanisms, the distinction can be blurred by the clinical context and available measurements. For example, in humans with atrial fibrillation and constantly varying ventricular frequency, contractility inferred from pressure-volume loops constantly changes from beat to beat. It is then more difficult to infer a "true" change in LV contractility versus operation of the Frank-Starling mechanism because of varying diastolic filling times.[4]

Left Ventricular Relaxation and Diastolic Dysfunction

Normal diastolic function allows the ventricle to fill adequately during rest and exercise, without an abnormal increase in LA pressure.[63] The phases of diastole are isovolumic pressure decline and filling. The filling phase is divided into early rapid filling, diastasis, and atrial systole. Early rapid filling contributes 70% to 80% of LV filling in normal individuals. Early diastolic filling is driven by the LA-to-LV pressure gradient, which is dependent on a complex interplay of factors, including myocardial relaxation, LV elastic recoil, LV diastolic stiffness, LA pressure, ventricular interaction, pericardial constraint, pulmonary vein properties, and mitral orifice area. Diastasis occurs in mid-diastole when LA and LV pressures equalize and transmitral flow becomes nil. In normal persons, atrial systole contributes 15% to 25% of LV diastolic filling. This contribution depends on the PR interval, atrial inotropic state, atrial preload, atrial afterload, autonomic tone, and HR. In patients with atrial fibrillation this component is lost. Chapter 51 further details the basic mechanisms of LV relaxation, as well as measurements of LV relaxation. In addition to being important in heart failure, abnormalities in diastolic relaxation and stiffness develop as part of normal aging, and this cardiac aging process seems to be accelerated in the presence of obesity.[74]

Right Ventricular Function

Most of the foregoing principles and discussions also apply to the right ventricle, and the differences are not discussed in any detail here. RV myocytes are fundamentally the same as those in the left ventricle, with some minor, mainly quantitative differences in their ion channel, electrophysiology, Ca^{2+} handling, and myofilament properties. The most important functional differences are in the chamber geometry related to Laplace's law and the normal levels of pressure developed (lower pressure in the right ventricle and pulmonary circulation).[75] The right ventricle has a larger radius of curvature, which would tend to increase wall tension, but it normally develops much lower pressure, which greatly reduces wall tension (wall tension = [radius × pressure]/[2 × thickness]). RV wall thickness is also lower such that the normal characteristics of RV shape and size are functionally matched to the different prevailing conditions on the right ventricle. The right ventricle is poorly suited to eject against high pressures, as in pulmonary hypertension, and this heightened afterload-dependence is further accentuated in patients with heart failure.[76]

Atrial Function

The left atrium has five main functions.[4,77] First and best known, the left atrium functions as a blood-receiving reservoir chamber. Second, it also is a contractile chamber that by presystolic contraction helps complete LV filling with an atrial kick. Third, the left atrium functions as a conduit that empties its contents into the left ventricle down a pressure gradient after the mitral valve opens. Fourth, it is a *blood volume sensor* in the heart and releases atrial natriuretic peptide (ANP) in response to stretch so that ANP-induced diuresis can help restore blood volume to normal. Notably, in congestive heart failure, when the renin-angiotensin system causes fluid retention and exacerbates the elevation in LA pressure and volume, ANP secretion is elevated. Fifth, the left atrium contains receptors for the afferent arms of various reflexes, including mechanoreceptors that increase the sinus discharge rate, thereby contributing to the tachycardia of exercise as venous return increases (Bainbridge reflex).[3,4]

The atrial pressure-volume loop is very different in shape from that of the ventricles in that it resembles a figure 8. The atria have a number of differences in structure and function from the ventricles, including smaller myocytes with fewer T tubules, a shorter AP duration, and more fetal myosin isoforms (both heavy and light chains).[78] The more rapid atrial repolarization is caused by increased outward potassium currents, such as I_{to}, and also has faster Ca^{2+} transient kinetics. In general, these histologic and physiologic changes might be related to the decreased need for the atria to generate high intrachamber pressures, rather than being sensitive to changes in volume while retaining enough contractile action to help with LV filling and to respond to inotropic stimuli. *Atrial remodeling* refers to a variety of ionic, structural, contractile, and metabolic changes that are induced by insults such as chronic atrial tachyarrhythmias, including atrial fibrillation,[78] or by LA stretch and enlargement. Cellular mechanisms include decreased L-type Ca^{2+} channel activity,[78] increased abnormal collagen,[79] and probably adverse stretch-induced signaling. The results include poor contractile performance and increased initiation and perpetuation of atrial fibrillation. Atrial remodeling and deterioration in LA function lead to worsening pulmonary hypertension and secondary RV dysfunction in patients with heart failure.[77,80]

FUTURE PERSPECTIVES

During the last 20 years we have gained tremendous molecular and cellular insight into a much richer, quantitatively detailed understanding of the individual steps in the overall excitation-contraction-relaxation process. In addition, there is a greatly enhanced understanding about how all these processes interact at the cellular and tissue level, how they are regulated by numerous interacting signaling pathways, and what goes wrong during certain cardiac pathologies. This is a very complex system, and diseases such as heart failure are also extremely complex. In the coming 5 years we can expect further clarification of all these systems, likely with a better understanding of signaling in local microdomains and protein complexes. At present, however, we must use this rich mechanistic knowledge to test novel therapeutic strategies for heart failure (e.g., SERCA2 overexpression, RyR inhibitors, GRK2 inhibitors, myofilament enhancers). This work may provide novel effective therapies but will also help us better understand how the fundamental systems impacted by these approaches integrate into the behavior of the whole system. This emphasizes how critical it is to integrate our knowledge of these many systems that dynamically regulate contraction and relaxation over multiple physical scales (molecules to cell to heart to animal) and time scales (milliseconds to seconds, minutes, hours, days, and years), as well as in multiple disciplinary and methodologic perspectives, to help bring the entire system to a higher level of understanding. In this way the therapeutic strategies that we must also continue to test are likely to improve.

ACKNOWLEDGMENT

We honor the memory of Dr. Lionel H. Opie who contributed to previous versions of this chapter over the years.

REFERENCES

Microanatomy of Contractile Cells and Proteins

1. Bers DM. *Excitation-Contraction Coupling and Cardiac Contractile Force*. Dordrecht, Netherlands: Kluwer Academic Press; 2001.
2. Bers DM. Calcium cycling and signaling in cardiac myocytes. *Annu Rev Physiol*. 2008;70:23–49.
3. Opie LH. *Heart Physiology, from Cell to Circulation*. 4th ed. Philadelphia: Lippincott Williams & Wilkins; 2004.
4. Opie LH, Bers DM. Mechanisms of cardiac contraction and relaxation. In: Mann DL, Zipes DP, Libby P, Bonow RO, eds. *Braunwald's Heart Disease: a Textbook of Cardiovascular Medicine*. 10th ed. Philadelphia: Elsevier Saunders; 2015:429–453.
5. Covian R, Balaban RS. Cardiac mitochondrial matrix and respiratory complex protein phosphorylation. *Am J Physiol Heart Circ Physiol*. 2012;303:H940–H966.
6. Dorn GW Jr, Kitsis RN. The mitochondrial dynamism-mitophagy-cell death interactome: multiple roles performed by members of a mitochondrial molecular ensemble. *Circ Res*. 2015;116:167–182.
7. Kubli DA, Gustafsson AB. Mitochondria and mitophagy: the yin and yang of cell death control. *Circ Res*. 2012;111:1208–1221.
8. Rayment I, Holden HM, Whittaker M. Structure of the actin-myosin complex and its implications for muscle contraction. *Science*. 1993;261:58–65.
9. Gigli M, Begay RL, Morea G, et al. A review of the giant protein titin in clinical molecular diagnostics of cardiomyopathies. *Front Cardiovasc Med*. 2016;3:21.
10. Hooijman P, Stewart MA, Cooke R. A new state of cardiac myosin with very slow ATP turnover: a potential cardioprotective mechanism in the heart. *Biophys J*. 2011;100:1969–1976.
11. Knoll R, Hoshijima M, Hoffman HM, et al. The cardiac mechanical stretch sensor machinery involves a Z disc complex that is defective in a subset of human dilated cardiomyopathy. *Cell*. 2002;111:943–955.
12. Beausang JF, Shroder DY, Nelson PC, Goldman YE. Tilting and wobble of myosin V by high-speed single-molecule polarized fluorescence microscopy. *Biophys J*. 2013;104:1263–1273.
12a. Teerlink JR, Diaz R, Felker GM, et al; GALACTIC-HF Investigators. Cardiac myosin activation with omecamtiv mecarbil in systolic heart failure. *N Engl J Med*. 2021;384(2):105–116.
13. Warren SA, Briggs LE, Zeng H, et al. Myosin light chain phosphorylation is critical for adaptation to cardiac stress. *Circulation*. 2012;126:2575–2588.
14. McNally EM, Golbus JR, Puckelwartz MJ. Genetic mutations and mechanisms in dilated cardiomyopathy. *J Clin Invest*. 2013;123:19–26.
15. Bers DM, Shannon TR. Calcium movements inside the sarcoplasmic reticulum of cardiac myocytes. *J Mol Cell Cardiol*. 2013;58:59–66.

Calcium Fluxes in Cardiac Contraction-Relaxation Cycle

16. Zima AV, Picht E, Bers DM, Blatter LA. Termination of cardiac Ca^{2+} sparks: role of intra-SR $[Ca^{2+}]$, release flux, and intra-SR Ca^{2+} diffusion. *Circ Res*. 2008;103:e105–e115.
17. Bers DM. Cardiac sarcoplasmic reticulum calcium leak: basis and roles in cardiac dysfunction. *Annu Rev Physiol*. 2014;76:107–127.
18. Bers DM. Macromolecular complexes regulating cardiac ryanodine receptor function. *J Mol Cell Cardiol*. 2004;37:417–429.
19. Saucerman JJ, Bers DM. Calmodulin binding proteins provide domains of local Ca^{2+} signaling in cardiac myocytes. *J Mol Cell Cardiol*. 2012;52:312–316.
20. Radwanski PB, Belevych AE, Brunello L, et al. Store-dependent deactivation: cooling the chain-reaction of myocardial calcium signaling. *J Mol Cell Cardiol*. 2013;58:77–83.
21. Sato D, Bers DM. How does stochastic ryanodine receptor-mediated Ca leak fail to initiate a Ca spark? *Biophys J*. 2011;101:2370–2379.
22. Bers DM, Grandi E. Calcium/calmodulin-dependent kinase II regulation of cardiac ion channels. *J Cardiovasc Pharmacol*. 2009;54:180–187.
23. Anderson ME, Brown JH, Bers DM. Camkii in myocardial hypertrophy and heart failure. *J Mol Cell Cardiol*. 2011;51:468–473.
24. Cheng H, Lederer WJ. Calcium sparks. *Physiol Rev*. 2008;88:1491–1545.
25. Tada M, Katz AM. Phosphorylation of the sarcoplasmic reticulum and sarcolemma. *Annu Rev Physiol*. 1982;44:401–423.
26. Picht E, Zima AV, Shannon TR, et al. Dynamic calcium movement inside cardiac sarcoplasmic reticulum during release. *Circ Res*. 2011;108:847–856.

Sarcolemmal Control of Ca^{2+} and Na^+

27. Morotti S, Grandi E, Summa A, et al. Theoretical study of L-type Ca^{2+} current inactivation kinetics during action potential repolarization and early afterdepolarizations. *J Physiol*. 2012;590:4465–4481.
28. Orchard C, Brette F. T-tubules and sarcoplasmic reticulum function in cardiac ventricular myocytes. *Cardiovasc Res*. 2008;77:237–244.
29. Maltsev VA, Reznikov V, Undrovinas NA, et al. Modulation of late sodium current by Ca^{2+}, calmodulin, and CaMKII in normal and failing dog cardiomyocytes: similarities and differences. *Am J Physiol Heart Circ Physiol*. 2008;294:H1597–H1608.
30. Wimmer NJ, Stone PH. Anti-anginal and anti-ischemic effects of late sodium current inhibition. *Cardiovasc Drugs Ther*. 2013;27:69–77.

31. Ginsburg KS, Weber CR, Bers DM. Cardiac Na$^+$-Ca^{2+} exchanger: dynamics of Ca^{2+}-dependent activation and deactivation in intact myocytes. *J Physiol*. 2013;591:2067–2086.
32. Despa S, Bers DM. Na$^+$ transport in the normal and failing heart—remember the balance. *J Mol Cell Cardiol*. 2013;61:2–10.

Adrenergic Signaling Systems

33. Woodcock EA, Du XJ, Reichelt ME, Graham RM. Cardiac alpha 1-adrenergic drive in pathological remodelling. *Cardiovasc Res*. 2008;77:452–462.
34. Mika D, Leroy J, Fischmeister R, Vandecasteele G. Role of cyclic nucleotide phosphodiesterases type 3 and 4 in cardiac excitation-contraction coupling and arrhythmias. *Med Sci (Paris)*. 2013;29:617–622.
35. Barbagallo F, Xu B, Reddy GR, et al. Genetically encoded biosensors reveal PKA hyperphosphorylation on the myofilaments in rabbit heart failure. *Circ Res*. 2016;119:931–943.
36. Pereira L, Cheng H, Lao DH, et al. Epac2 mediates cardiac beta1-adrenergic-dependent sarcoplasmic reticulum Ca^{2+} leak and arrhythmia. *Circulation*. 2013;127:913–922.
37. Bers DM. Cardiac excitation-contraction coupling. *Nature*. 2002;415:198–205.
38. Kritzer MD, Li J, Dodge-Kafka K, Kapiloff MS. AKAPs: the architectural underpinnings of local cAMP signaling. *J Mol Cell Cardiol*. 2012;52:351–358.
39. Castro LR, Verde I, Cooper DM, Fischmeister R. Cyclic guanosine monophosphate compartmentation in rat cardiac myocytes. *Circulation*. 2006;113:2221–2228.
40. Harvey RD, Hell JW. Cav1.2 signaling complexes in the heart. *J Mol Cell Cardiol*. 2013;58:143–152.
41. Negroni JA, Morotti S, Lascano EC, et al. Beta-adrenergic effects on cardiac myofilaments and contraction in an integrated rabbit ventricular myocyte model. *J Mol Cell Cardiol*. 2015;81:162–175.
42. Bers DM. Ryanodine receptor S2808 phosphorylation in heart failure: smoking gun or red herring? *Circ Res*. 2012;110:796–799.
43. Marks AR. Calcium cycling proteins and heart failure: mechanisms and therapeutics. *J Clin Invest*. 2013;123:46–52.
44. Ginsburg KS, Bers DM. Modulation of excitation-contraction coupling by isoproterenol in cardiomyocytes with controlled SR Ca^{2+} load and Ca^{2+} current trigger. *J Physiol*. 2004;556:463–480.
45. Valdivia HH, Kaplan JH, Ellis-Davies GC, Lederer WJ. Rapid adaptation of cardiac ryanodine receptors: modulation by Mg^{2+} and phosphorylation. *Science*. 1995;267:1997–2000.
46. Eisner DA, Kashimura T, O'Neill SC, et al. What role does modulation of the ryanodine receptor play in cardiac inotropy and arrhythmogenesis? *J Mol Cell Cardiol*. 2009;46:474–481.
47. Engelhardt S. Alternative signaling: cardiomyocyte beta1-adrenergic receptors signal through EGFRs. *J Clin Invest*. 2007;117:2396–2398.
48. Sato PY, Chuprun JK, Schwartz M, Koch WJ. The evolving impact of G protein-coupled receptor kinases in cardiac health and disease. *Physiol Rev*. 2015;95:377–404.
49. Hegyi B, Bers DM, Bossuyt J. CaMKII signaling in heart diseases: emerging role in diabetic cardiomyopathy. *J Mol Cell Cardiol*. 2019;127:246–259.
50. Bardswell SC, Cuello F, Kentish JC, Avkiran M. CMYBP-C as a promiscuous substrate: phosphorylation by non-PKA kinases and its potential significance. *J Muscle Res Cell Motil*. 2012;33:53–60.

Cholinergic and Nitric Oxide Signaling

51. Niu X, Watts VL, Cingolani OH, et al. Cardioprotective effect of beta-3 adrenergic receptor agonism: role of neuronal nitric oxide synthase. *J Am Coll Cardiol*. 2012;59:1979–1987.
52. Okoshi K, Nakayama M, Yan X, et al. Neuregulins regulate cardiac parasympathetic activity: muscarinic modulation of beta-adrenergic activity in myocytes from mice with neuregulin-1 gene deletion. *Circulation*. 2004;110:713–717.
53. Ziolo MT, Bers DM. The real estate of NOS signaling: location, location, location. *Circ Res*. 2003;92:1279–1281.
54. Takimoto E. Cyclic GMP-dependent signaling in cardiac myocytes. *Circ J*. 2012;76:1819–1825.
55. Zhang M, Takimoto E, Lee DI, et al. Pathological cardiac hypertrophy alters intracellular targeting of phosphodiesterase type 5 from nitric oxide synthase-3 to natriuretic peptide signaling. *Circulation*. 2012;126:942–951.
56. Takimoto E, Champion HC, Li M, et al. Chronic inhibition of cyclic GMP phosphodiesterase 5a prevents and reverses cardiac hypertrophy. *Nat Med*. 2005;11:214–222.
57. Dodge-Kafka KL, Langeberg L, Scott JD. Compartmentation of cyclic nucleotide signaling in the heart: the role of A-kinase anchoring proteins. *Circ Res*. 2006;98:993–1001.
58. Zhang YH, Casadei B. Sub-cellular targeting of constitutive NOS in health and disease. *J Mol Cell Cardiol*. 2012;52:341–350.
59. Murphy E, Kohr M, Menazza S, et al. Signaling by S-nitrosylation in the heart. *J Mol Cell Cardiol*. 2014;73:18–25.
60. Erickson JR, Nichols CB, Uchinoumi H, et al. S-nitrosylation induces both autonomous activation and inhibition of calcium/calmodulin-dependent protein kinase II. *J Biol Chem*. 2015;290:25646–25656.

Contractile Performance of Intact Hearts

61. Lewis T. *The Mechanism and Graphic Registration of the Heart Beat*. London: Shaw & Sons; 1920.
62. Wiggers CJ. *Modern Aspects of Circulation in Health and Disease*. Philadelphia: Lea & Febiger; 1915.
63. Borlaug BA. The pathophysiology of heart failure with preserved ejection fraction. *Nat Rev Cardiol*. 2014;11:507–515.
64. Borlaug BA, Reddy YNV. The role of the pericardium in heart failure: implications for pathophysiology and treatment. *JACC Heart Fail*. 2019;574–585.
65. Konstam MA, Kiernan MS, Bernstein D, et al. Evaluation and management of right-sided heart failure: a scientific statement from the American Heart Association. *Circulation*. 2018;137:e578–e622.
66. Jian Z, Han H, Zhang T, et al. Mechanochemotransduction during cardiomyocyte contraction is mediated by localized nitric oxide signaling. *Sci Signal*. 2014;7:ra27.
67. Chirinos JA, Segers P, Rietzschel ER, et al. Early and late systolic wall stress differentially relate to myocardial contraction and relaxation in middle-aged adults: the ASKLEPIOS study. *Hypertension*. 2013;61:296–303.
68. Borlaug BA, Melenovsky V, Redfield MM, et al. Impact of arterial load and loading sequence on left ventricular tissue velocities in humans. *J Am Coll Cardiol*. 2007;50:1570–1577.
69. Runte KE, Bell SP, Selby DE, et al. Relaxation and the role of calcium in isolated contracting myocardium from patients with hypertensive heart disease and heart failure with preserved ejection fraction. *Circ Heart Fail*. 2017;8:e004311.
70. Sinnecker D, Dirschinger RJ, Barthel P, et al. Postextrasystolic blood pressure potentiation predicts poor outcome of cardiac patients. *J Am Heart Assoc*. 2014;3:e000857.
71. Obokata M, Reddy YNV, Melenovsky V, et al. Myocardial injury and cardiac reserve in patients with heart failure and preserved ejection fraction. *J Am Coll Cardiol*. 2018;72:29–40.
72. Suga H, Hisano R, Hirata S, et al. Mechanism of higher oxygen consumption rate: pressure-loaded vs volume-loaded heart. *Am J Physiol*. 1982;242:H942–H948.
73. Schwartzenberg S, Redfield MM, From AM, et al. Effects of vasodilation in heart failure with preserved or reduced ejection fraction implications of distinct pathophysiologies on response to therapy. *J Am Coll Cardiol*. 2012;59:442–451.
74. Wohlfahrt P, Redfield MM, Lopez-Jimenez F, et al. Impact of general and central adiposity on ventricular-arterial aging in women and men. *JACC Heart Fail*. 2014;2:489–499.
75. Konstam MA, Kiernan MS, Bernstein D, et al. Evaluation and management of right-sided heart failure: a scientific statement from the American Heart Association. *Circulation*. 2018;137:e578–e622.
76. Melenovsky V, Hwang SJ, Lin G, et al. Right heart dysfunction in heart failure with preserved ejection fraction. *Eur Heart J*. 2014;35:3452–3462.
77. Reddy YNV, Obokata M, Verbrugge FH, et al. Atrial dysfunction in patients with heart failure with preserved ejection fraction and atrial fibrillation. *J Am Coll Cardiol*. 2020;76(9):1051–1064.
78. Grandi E, Pandit SV, Voigt N, et al. Human atrial action potential and Ca^{2+} model: sinus rhythm and chronic atrial fibrillation. *Circ Res*. 2011;109:1055–1066.
79. Maillet M, van Berlo JH, Molkentin JD. Molecular basis of physiological heart growth: fundamental concepts and new players. *Nat Rev Mol Cell Biol*. 2013;14:38–48.
80. Melenovsky V, Hwang SJ, Redfield MM, et al. Left atrial remodeling and function in advanced heart failure with preserved or reduced ejection fraction. *Circ Heart Fail*. 2015;8:295–303.

47 Pathophysiology of Heart Failure

GERD HASENFUSS AND DOUGLAS L. MANN

PATHOGENESIS, 913
Neurohormonal Mechanisms, 913
Left Ventricular Remodeling, 921

REVERSIBILITY OF LEFT VENTRICULAR REMODELING AND RECOVERY OF LEFT VENTRICULAR FUNCTION, 930

FUTURE PERSPECTIVES, 931
REFERENCES, 931

This chapter focuses on the molecular and cellular changes that underlie heart failure with a reduced ejection fraction (HFrEF), with an emphasis on the role of neurohormonal activation and left ventricular (LV) remodeling as the primary determinants for disease progression in HF. The hemodynamic, contractile, and wall motion disorders in HF are discussed in the chapters on cardiac contraction and relaxation (Chapter 46), echocardiography (Chapter 16), cardiac catheterization (Chapter 22), and radionuclide imaging (Chapter 18). The clinical assessment of patients with HF is discussed in Chapter 48, and Chapter 51 discusses the pathogenesis of HF with preserved ejection fraction.

PATHOGENESIS

As shown in Figure 47.1A, HFrEF is initiated after an index event either damages the heart muscle, with a resultant loss of functioning cardiac myocytes or, alternatively, disrupts the ability of the myocardium to generate force, thereby preventing the heart from contracting normally. This index event may have an abrupt onset, as in the case of a myocardial infarction (MI); it may have a gradual or insidious onset, as in the case of hemodynamic pressure or volume overloading; or it may be hereditary, as in the case of many of the genetic cardiomyopathies. Regardless of the nature of the inciting event, the feature that is common to each of these index events is that they all, in some manner, produce a decline in pumping capacity of the heart. The circulatory changes that arise from impaired myocardial pump function are sensed by peripheral arterial baroreceptors as "underfilling" of the circulation. These sensory and other peripheral receptors (e.g., metaboreceptors and ergoreceptors) activate a series of compensatory mechanisms discussed below that lead to changes in heart rate and cardiac contractility, salt and water retention, and constriction of the peripheral blood vessels.[1]

In some patients LV function will recover spontaneously after resolution or removal of the inciting stress that compromised myocardial function; however, in a significant proportion of patients LV function will remain depressed. Some patients with LV dysfunction will remain asymptomatic or minimally symptomatic after the initial decline in pumping capacity of the heart, or symptoms develop only after the dysfunction has been present for some time. The precise reasons why patients with LV dysfunction remain asymptomatic are not known. One potential explanation is that a number of compensatory mechanisms that become activated in the setting of cardiac injury or depressed cardiac output are sufficient to modulate LV function within a physiologic/homeostatic range, such that the patient's functional capacity is preserved or is depressed only minimally. However, sustained activation of neurohormonal systems leads to peripheral vasoconstriction, salt and water retention by the kidney, as well as a series of end-organ changes within the myocardium that contribute to worsening LV dilation (referred to as LV remodeling) and LV dysfunction (Fig. 47.1B). As HF progresses patients undergo the transition from asymptomatic to symptomatic HF.

Neurohormonal Mechanisms

A growing body of experimental and clinical evidence suggests that HF progresses as a result of the overexpression of biologically active molecules that are capable of exerting deleterious effects on the heart and circulation (see Fig. 47.1B).[1] The portfolio of compensatory mechanisms that have been described thus far includes activation of the sympathetic nervous system (SNS) and the renin-angiotensin aldosterone system (RAAS), which are responsible for maintaining cardiac output through increased retention of salt and water; peripheral arterial vasoconstriction and increased contractility; and inflammatory mediators that are responsible for mediating cardiac repair and remodeling. It bears emphasis that *neurohormone* is largely a historical term, reflecting the original observation that many of the molecules that were elaborated in HF were produced by the neuroendocrine system and thus acted on the heart in an endocrine manner. It has since become apparent, however, that a great many of the so-called classic neurohormones such as norepinephrine (NE) and angiotensin II are synthesized directly within the myocardium by myocytes and thus act in an autocrine and paracrine manner. Nonetheless, the important unifying concept that arises from the neurohormonal model is that the overexpression of portfolios of biologically active molecules contributes to disease progression by virtue of the deleterious effects these molecules exert on the heart and circulation.

Activation of Sympathetic Nervous System

The decrease in cardiac output in HF activates a series of compensatory adaptations that are intended to maintain cardiovascular homeostasis. One of the most important adaptations is activation of the sympathetic (adrenergic) nervous system, which occurs early in the course of HF. Activation of the SNS in HF is accompanied by a concomitant withdrawal of parasympathetic tone. Although these disturbances in autonomic control initially were attributed to loss of the inhibitory input from arterial or cardiopulmonary baroreceptor reflexes, increasing evidence indicates that excitatory reflexes also may participate in the autonomic imbalance that occurs in HF.[2] In healthy persons, "high-pressure" carotid sinus and aortic arch baroreceptors and "low-pressure" cardiopulmonary mechanoreceptors provide inhibitory signals to the central nervous system (CNS) that repress the sympathetic outflow to the heart and peripheral circulation. Under normal conditions, inhibitory inputs from high-pressure carotid sinus and aortic arch baroreceptors and the low-pressure cardiopulmonary mechanoreceptors are the principal inhibitors of sympathetic outflow, whereas discharge from the nonbaroreflex peripheral chemoreceptors and from muscle *metaboreceptors* are the major excitatory inputs to sympathetic outflow. The vagal limb of the baroreceptor heart rate reflex also is responsive to arterial baroreceptor afferent inhibitory input. Healthy persons display low sympathetic discharge at rest and have a high heart rate variability. In patients with HF, however, inhibitory input from baroreceptors and mechanoreceptors decreases and excitatory input increases, with the net result that there is a generalized increase in sympathetic nerve traffic and blunted parasympathetic nerve traffic, leading to loss of heart rate variability and increased peripheral vascular resistance.[3]

As a result of the increase in sympathetic tone, there is an increase in circulating levels of NE, a potent adrenergic neurotransmitter. The elevated levels of circulating NE result from a combination of increased release of NE from adrenergic nerve endings and its

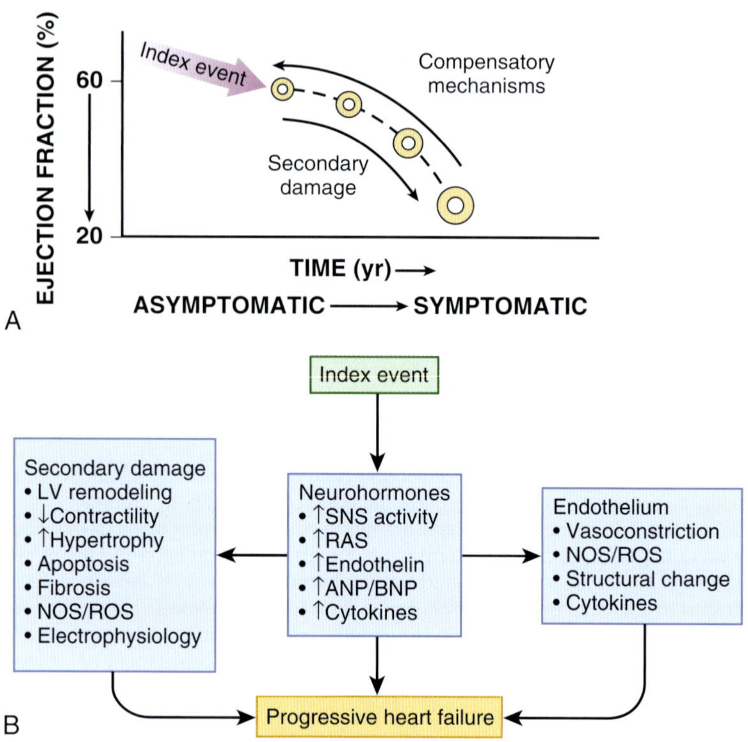

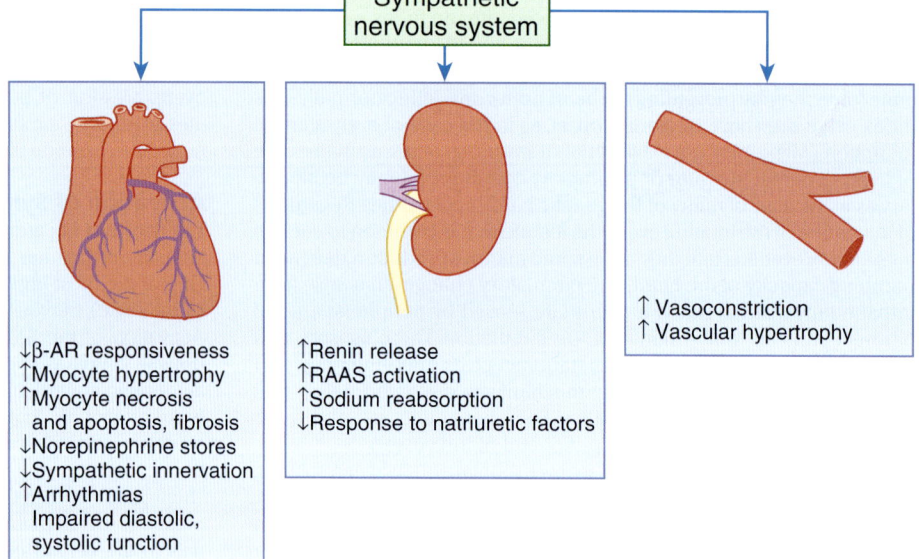

FIGURE 47.1 Pathogenesis of heart failure (HF). **A,** HF begins after a so-called index event produces an initial decline in pumping capacity of the heart. **B,** After this initial decline in pumping capacity, a variety of compensatory mechanisms are activated, including the adrenergic nervous system, the renin-angiotensin system (RAS), and the cytokine systems. In the short term, these systems are able to restore cardiovascular function to a normal homeostatic range, with the result that the patient remains asymptomatic. With time, however, the sustained activation of these systems can lead to secondary end-organ damage within the ventricle, with worsening LV remodeling and subsequent cardiac decompensation. As a result of these changes, patients undergo the transition from asymptomatic to symptomatic HF. *ANP/BNP*, Atrial/brain-type natriuretic peptide; *NOS*, nitric oxide synthase; *ROS*, reactive oxygen species; *SNS*, sympathetic nervous system. (From Mann DL. Mechanisms and models in HF: a combinatorial approach. *Circulation*. 199;100:99; and Kaye DM, Krum H. Drug discovery for heart failure: a new era or the end of the pipeline? *Nat Rev Drug Discov*. 2007;6:127.)

FIGURE 47.2 Activation of the sympathetic nervous system. Increased sympathetic nervous system (SNS) activity may contribute to the pathophysiology of congestive heart failure (HF) by multiple mechanisms involving cardiac, renal, and vascular function. In the heart, increased SNS outflow may lead to desensitization of beta-adrenergic receptors (β-ARs), myocyte hypertrophy, necrosis, apoptosis, and fibrosis. In the kidneys, increased SNS activation induces arterial and venous vasoconstriction, activation of the renin-angiotensin-aldosterone system (RAAS), increase in salt and water retention, and an attenuated response to natriuretic factors. In the peripheral vessels, neurogenic vasoconstriction and vascular hypertrophy are induced by increased SNS activity. (From Nohria A, et al. Neurohormonal, renal and vascular adjustments in heart failure. In Colucci WS, editor. *Atlas of Heart Failure*. 4th ed. Philadelphia: Current Medicine; 2008:106.)

consequent "spillover" into the plasma, as well as reduced uptake of NE by adrenergic nerve endings. In patients with advanced HF, the circulating levels of NE in resting patients are two to three times those found in normal persons. Indeed, plasma levels of NE predict mortality in patients with HF. Whereas the normal heart usually extracts NE from the arterial blood, in patients with moderate HF the coronary sinus NE concentration exceeds the arterial concentration, indicating increased adrenergic stimulation of the heart. However, as HF progresses there is a significant decrease in the myocardial concentration of NE. The mechanism responsible for cardiac NE depletion in severe HF is not clear and may relate to an "exhaustion" phenomenon resulting from the prolonged adrenergic activation of the cardiac adrenergic nerves in HF. In addition, there is decreased activity of myocardial tyrosine hydroxylase, which is the rate-limiting enzyme in the synthesis of NE. In patients with cardiomyopathy, iodine 131 (^{131}I)–labeled metaiodobenzylguanidine (MIBG), a radiopharmaceutical that is taken up by adrenergic nerve endings, is not taken up normally, suggesting that NE reuptake is also depressed.

Increased sympathetic activation of the beta$_1$-adrenergic receptor results in increased heart rate and force of myocardial contraction, with a resultant increase in cardiac output (see Chapter 46). In addition, the heightened activity of the adrenergic nervous system leads to stimulation of myocardial alpha$_1$-adrenergic receptors, which elicits a modest positive inotropic effect, as well as peripheral arterial vasoconstriction (Fig. 47.2). Although NE enhances both contraction and relaxation and maintains blood pressure, myocardial energy requirements are augmented, which can intensify ischemia when myocardial oxygen (O_2) delivery is restricted. The augmented adrenergic outflow from the CNS also may trigger ventricular tachycardia or even sudden cardiac death, particularly in the presence of myocardial ischemia. Thus, activation of the SNS provides short-term support that has the potential to become maladaptive over the long term. Moreover, increasing evidence suggests

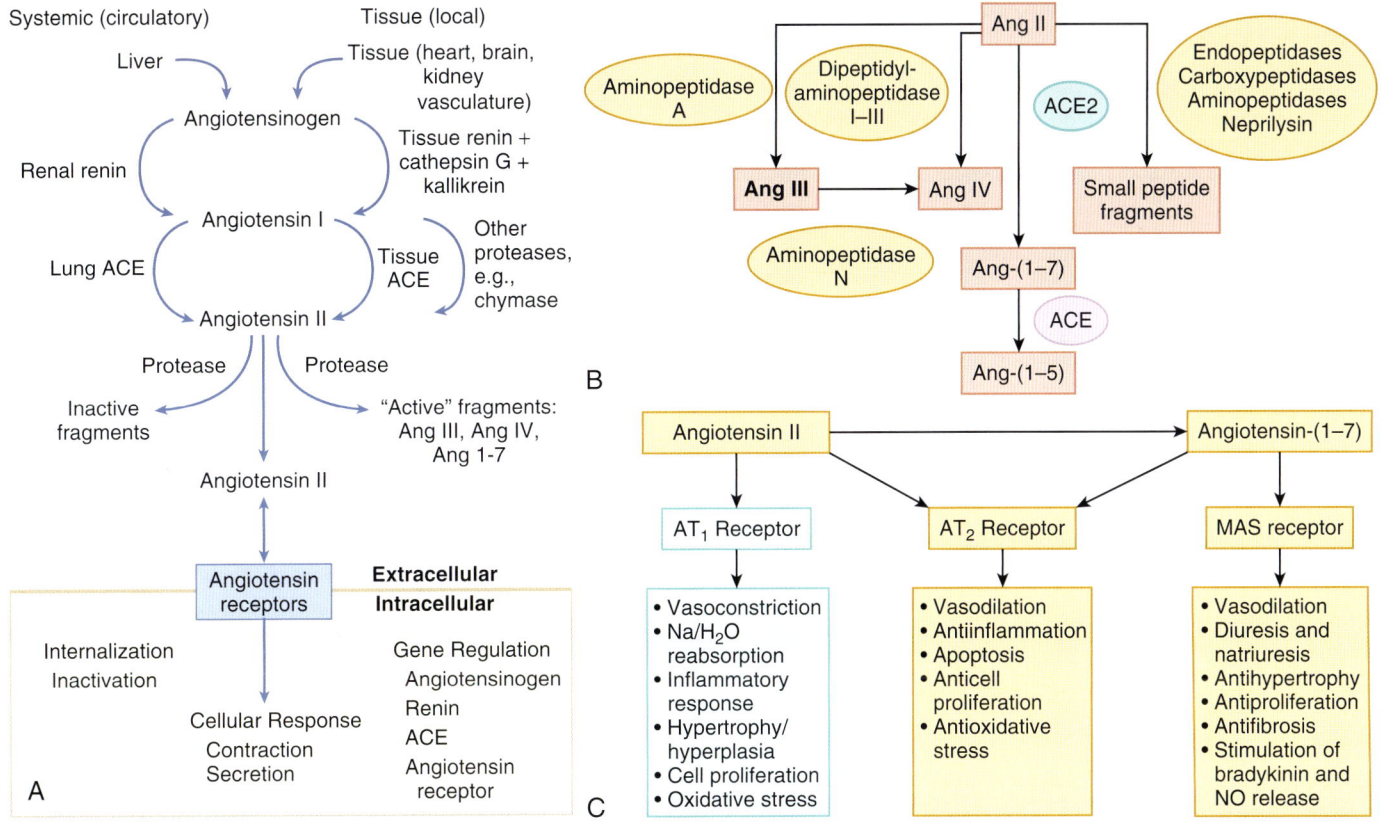

FIGURE 47.3 A, The systemic and tissue components of the renin-angiotensin system (RAS). Several tissues, including myocardium, vasculature, kidney, and brain, have the capacity to generate angiotensin II independent of the circulating RAS. Angiotensin II produced at the tissue level may play an important role in the pathophysiology of heart failure (HF). *ACE,* Angiotensin-converting enzyme; *Ang,* angiotensin. **B,** Angiotensin II degradation pathways. Angiotensin II is degraded by angiotensin-converting enzyme 2 (ACE2) to form Ang-(1–7), which subsequently can be degraded by ACE to form Ang-(1–5). Other pathways of angiotensin II degradation include aminopeptidase A to Ang-(2–8), dipeptidyl-aminopeptidase I–III to Ang IV, and neprilysin and various peptidases to other small peptide products. Ang-(2–8) and Ang IV may also be reversibly interchanged via aminopeptidase N. **C,** Action of angiotensin II type 1 (AT_1) and type 2 (AT_2) receptors and MAS-mediated signaling. *NO,* Nitric oxide. (**A,** Modified from Timmermans PB, Wong PC, Chiu AT, et al. Angiotensin II receptors and angiotensin II receptor antagonists. *Pharmacol Rev.* 1993;45:205; **B,** Modified from Batlle D, Wysocki J, Soler MJ, Ranganath K, et al. Angiotensin-converting enzyme 2: enhancing the degradation of angiotensin II as a potential therapy for diabetic nephropathy. *Kidney Int.* 2012;81:520–528; and **C,** Modified from Iwai M, Horiuchi M. Devil and angel in the renin-angiotensin system. *Hypertens Res.* 2009;32:533–536.)

that apart from the deleterious effects of sympathetic activation, parasympathetic withdrawal also may contribute to the pathogenesis of HF. Withdrawal of parasympathetic nerve stimulation has been associated with decreased nitric oxide (NO) levels, increased inflammation, increased sympathetic activity, and worsening LV remodeling. Several clinical trials with direct vagal nerve stimulation did not meet their primary endpoint but additional studies are ongoing.[4]

Activation of the Renin-Angiotensin System

In contrast with the SNS, the components of the renin-angiotensin system (RAS) are activated comparatively later in HF. The presumptive mechanisms for RAS activation in HF include renal hypoperfusion, decreased filtered sodium reaching the macula densa in the distal tubule, and increased sympathetic stimulation of the kidney, leading to increased renin release from juxtaglomerular apparatus. As shown in Figure 47.3, renin cleaves four amino acids from circulating angiotensinogen, which is synthesized in the liver, to form the biologically inactive decapeptide angiotensin I. Angiotensin-converting enzyme (ACE) cleaves two amino acids from angiotensin I to form the biologically active octapeptide (1 to 8) angiotensin II. Most ACE activity (approaching 90%) in the body is found in tissues; the remaining 10% is found in a soluble (non–membrane-bound) form in the interstitium of the heart and vessel wall. The importance of tissue ACE activity in HF is suggested by the observation that ACE messenger RNA (mRNA) and ACE-binding sites and ACE activity are increased in explanted human hearts.[5] Angiotensin II also can be synthesized using renin-independent pathways through the enzymatic conversion of angiotensinogen to angiotensin I by kallikrein and cathepsin G (Fig. 47.3A). The tissue production of angiotensin II also may occur along ACE-independent pathways, through the activation of chymase. This latter pathway may be of major importance in the myocardium, particularly when the levels of renin and angiotensin I are increased by the use of ACE inhibitors. Angiotensin II itself can undergo further proteolysis to generate three biologically active fragments: angiotensin III (2 to 8), angiotensin IV (3 to 8), and angiotensin 1 to 7 (Fig. 47.3B). The latter results mainly from angiotensin II cleavage by angiotensin converting enzyme 2 (ACE2), which is a type I transmembrane carboxypeptidase with 40% homology to ACE. ACE2 has also been identified as the cellular receptor of SARS-CoV-2 (see also Chapter 94).[5]

Angiotensin II exerts its effects by binding to two G protein–coupled receptors (GPCRs), the angiotensin type 1 (AT_1) and angiotensin type 2 (AT_2) receptors. The predominant angiotensin receptor in the vasculature is the AT_1 receptor. Although both AT_1 and AT_2 receptor subtypes are present in human myocardium, the AT_2 receptor predominates in a 2:1 molar ratio. Cellular localization of the AT_1 receptor in the heart is most abundant in nerves distributed in the myocardium, whereas the AT_2 receptor is localized more specifically in fibroblasts and the interstitium. Activation of the AT_1 receptor leads to vasoconstriction, cell growth, aldosterone secretion, and catecholamine release, whereas activation of the AT_2 receptor leads to vasodilation, inhibition of cell growth, natriuresis, and bradykinin release (Fig. 47.3C). Studies have shown that the AT_1 receptor and mRNA levels are downregulated in failing human hearts, whereas AT_2 receptor density is increased or unchanged, so that the ratio of AT_1 to AT_2 receptors decreases. The MAS receptor is a GPCR that is expressed primarily in the brain and testes but also in the heart (see Fig. 47.3C).

Angiotensin II has several important actions that are critical to maintaining short-term circulatory homeostasis. The sustained expression of angiotensin II is maladaptive, however, leading to fibrosis of the heart, kidneys, and other organs. Angiotensin II can also lead to worsening neurohormonal activation by enhancing the release of NE from sympathetic nerve endings, as well as stimulating the zona glomerulosa of the adrenal cortex to produce aldosterone. Analogous to angiotensin II, aldosterone provides short-term support to the circulation by promoting the reabsorption of sodium in exchange for potassium in the distal segments of the nephron. However, the sustained expression of aldosterone may exert harmful effects by provoking hypertrophy and fibrosis within the vasculature and the myocardium, contributing to reduced vascular compliance and increased ventricular stiffness. In addition, aldosterone provokes endothelial cell dysfunction, baroreceptor dysfunction, and inhibition of NE uptake, any of which may lead to worsening HF. The mechanism of action of aldosterone in the cardiovascular system appears to involve oxidative stress, with resultant inflammation in target tissue. Although the exact role of angiotensin III (2 to 8), angiotensin IV (3 to 8), and angiotensin 1 to 7 in HF are not known, experimental studies suggest that angiotensin 1 to 7 counteracts the effects of angiotensin II, and attenuates LV remodeling.[1] In contrast, angiotensin III directly stimulates the zona glomerulosa of the adrenal glands to produce aldosterone,[6] which promotes sodium resorption in the distal collecting duct of the kidney. Angiotensin III also has an important role in vasopressin release in the brain, which controls water retention in the distal collecting duct of the kidney. Angiotensin III in the brain can also modulate cardiac nervous sympathetic hyperactivity, as well as LV remodeling after MI.[1]

OXIDATIVE STRESS

Reactive oxygen species (ROS) are a normal byproduct of aerobic metabolism. In the heart, the potential sources for ROS include the mitochondria, xanthine oxidase, and nicotinamide-adenine dinucleotide phosphate (NADPH) oxidase (Fig. 47.4). ROS can modulate the activity of a variety of intracellular proteins and signaling pathways, including essential proteins involved in myocardial excitation-contraction coupling, such as ion channels, sarcoplasmic reticulum (SR) calcium release channels, and myofilament proteins, as well as signaling pathways that are coupled to myocyte growth.[7] "Oxidative stress" occurs when the production of ROS exceeds the buffering capacity of antioxidant defense systems, leading to an excess of ROS within the cell. Substantial evidence indicates that the level of oxidative stress is increased both systemically and in the myocardium of patients with HF. Oxidative stress in the heart may be caused by reduced antioxidant capacity and increased production of ROS, which may arise secondary to mechanical strain of the myocardium, neurohormonal stimulation (angiotensin II, alpha-adrenergic agonists, endothelin-1 [ET-1]), or inflammatory cytokines (tumor necrosis factor [TNF], interleukin [IL]-1). Excessive mitochondria-derived ROS in cardiac myocytes have been demonstrated in experimental models of HF and may contribute to contractile dysfunction in advanced HF. Increased xanthine oxidase expression and activity have been reported in canine rapid pacing–induced HF and patients with end-stage HF. Moreover, increased expression and activity of myocardial NADPH oxidases have been demonstrated in both experimental and human HF in cultured cardiac myocytes,[7] ROS stimulate myocyte hypertrophy, reexpression of fetal gene programs, and apoptosis. ROS also can modulate fibroblast proliferation and collagen synthesis and trigger increased matrix metalloproteinase (MMP) abundance and activation. ROS also can affect the peripheral vasculature in HF by decreasing the bioavailability of NO. These and other observations have led to the suggestion that strategies to reduce ROS may be of therapeutic value in patients with HF. However, xanthine oxidase inhibition with allopurinol to reduce oxidative stress in hyperuremic patients with HF did not improve clinical status or cardiac function in a clinical trial.[8]

The importance of aldosterone, independent of angiotensin II, has been demonstrated by clinical trials (see Chapter 50) showing that low-dose spironolactone increased the survival of patients with New York Heart Association (NYHA) class II to IV systolic HF, as well as improved survival after MI, independent of changes in volume or electrolyte status.[9]

Neurohormonal Alterations of Renal Function

One of the signatures of advancing HF is increased salt and water retention by the kidneys. Traditional theories have ascribed this increase to either "forward" failure, which attributes sodium retention to inadequate renal perfusion as a consequence of impaired cardiac output, or "backward" failure, which emphasizes the importance of increased venous pressure in favoring transudation of salt and water from the intravascular to the extracellular compartment. These mechanisms have largely been supplanted by the concept of decreased *effective arterial blood volume*, which postulates that despite blood volume expansion in HF, inadequate cardiac output sensed by baroreceptors in the vascular tree leads to a series of compensatory neurohormonal adaptations that resemble the homeostatic response to acute blood loss.[6] As illustrated in Figure 47.5, a falling cardiac output or redistribution of the circulating blood volume is sensed by baroreceptors in the left ventricle, aortic arch, carotid sinus, and renal afferent arterioles. The loss of inhibitory input from arterial or cardiopulmonary baroreceptor reflexes leads to sustained activation of the SNS and the RAS. An implantable barostimulation device that activates the carotid

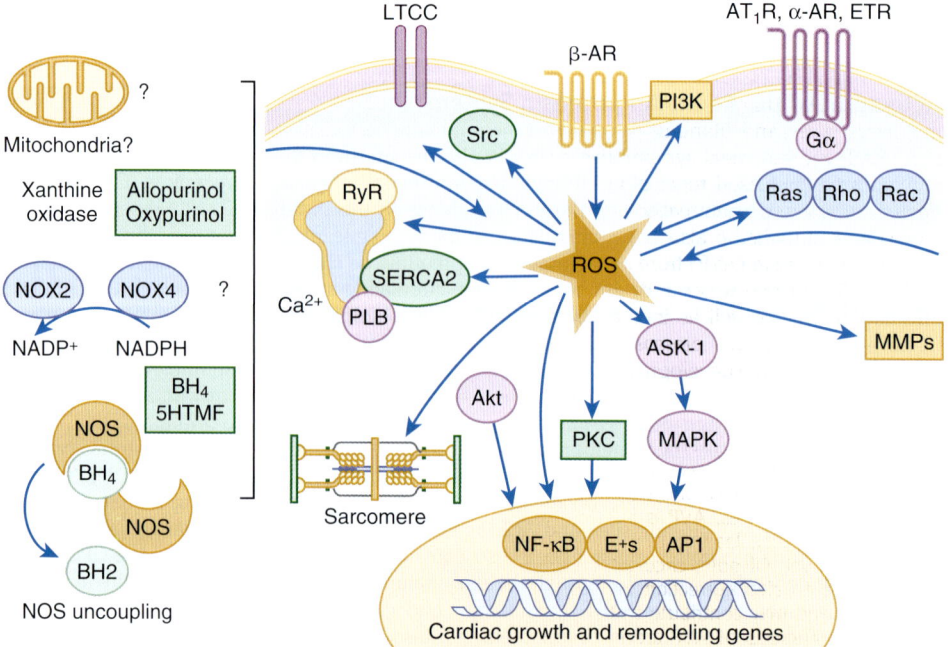

FIGURE 47.4 Cellular sources of reactive oxygen species (ROS) and ROS signaling in cardiac hypertrophy. ROS-generating systems are shown on the *left* and include xanthine oxidase, nicotinamide-adenine dinucleotide phosphate (NADPH) oxidases (NOX2, NOX4), nitric oxide synthase (NOS), and mitochondrial complexes. ROS activation has protean effects on calcium handling, myofilament function, matrix activation, kinase and phosphatase stimulation, and transcriptional regulation of matrix metalloproteinases (MMPs). *Akt*, Protein kinase B; *ASK-1*, apoptosis signal-regulating kinase 1; *ETR*, endothelin receptor; *5HTMF*, 5-hydrotetramethylpholate; *LTCC*, L-type calcium channel; *MAPK*, mitogen-activated protein kinase; *NF-κB*, nuclear factor-kappaB; *PKC*, protein kinase C; *PI3K*, phosphatidylinositol 3-kinase; *PLB*, phospholamban; *RyR*, ryanodine receptor; *SERCA2*, sarcoendoplasmic reticulum Ca^{2+}-ATPase. (Modified from McKinsey TA, Kass DA. Small-molecule therapies for cardiac hypertrophy: moving beneath the cell surface. *Nat Rev Drug Discov*. 2007;6:617.)

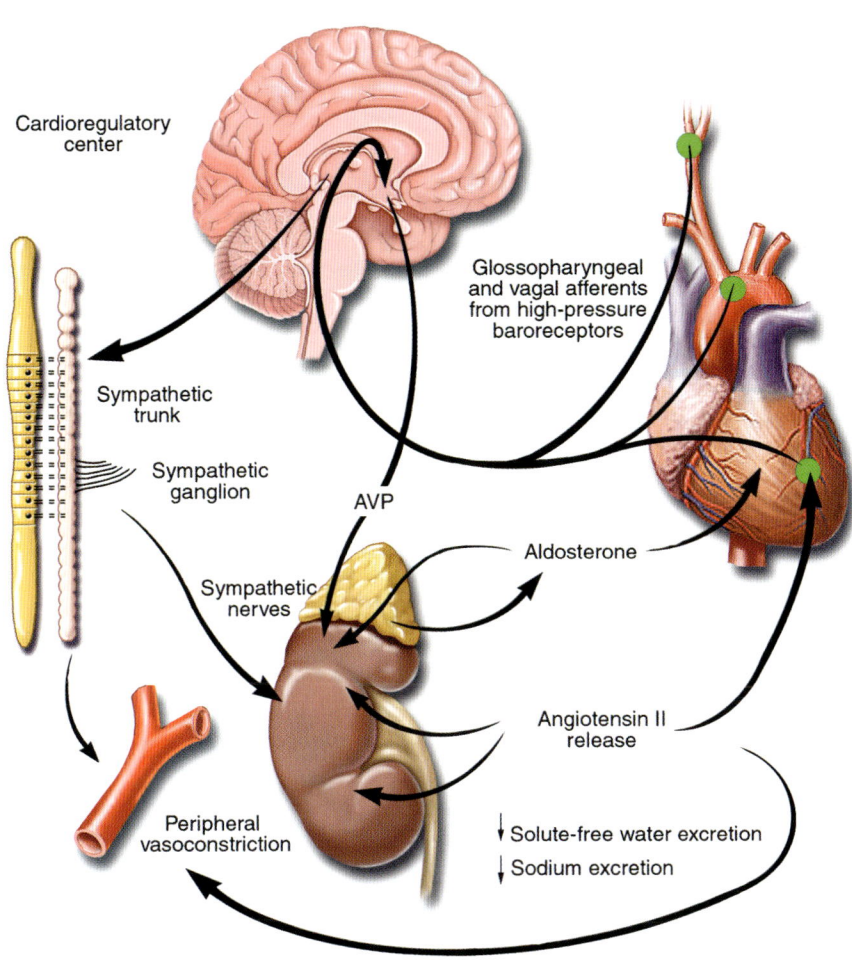

FIGURE 47.5 Unloading of high-pressure baroceptors (*green circles*) in the left ventricle, carotid sinus, and aortic arch generates afferent signals that stimulate cardioregulatory centers in the brain, resulting in the activation of efferent pathways in the sympathetic nervous system. The sympathetic nervous system (SNS) appears to be the primary integrator of the neurohumoral vasoconstrictor response to arterial underfilling. Activation of renal sympathetic nerves stimulates the release of arginine vasopressin (AVP). Sympathetic activation also causes peripheral and renal vasoconstriction, as does angiotensin II. Angiotensin II constricts blood vessels and stimulates the release of aldosterone from the adrenal gland, and it also increases tubular sodium reabsorption and causes remodeling of cardiac myocytes. Aldosterone also may have direct cardiac effects, in addition to increasing the reabsorption of sodium and the secretion of potassium (K+) and hydrogen (H+) ions in the collecting duct. The *black arrows* designate circulating hormones. (Modified from Schrier RW, Abraham WT. Hormones and hemodynamics in heart failure. *N Engl J Med*. 1999;341:577.)

baroreceptors to decrease sympathetic activation and increase vagal tone improved quality of life, exercise capacity, and NT-proBNP in patients with symptomatic HF in the BeAT-HF (Barostimulation for Heart Failure).[10]

There is little evidence to suggest that a primary renal abnormality is responsible for the initial sodium retention in the heart; however, there is mounting evidence that secondary changes in the kidney contribute importantly to volume overload as HF progresses. Volume overload in HF is multifactorial and is secondary, at least in part, to several factors that have the potential to cause increased sodium reabsorption, including activation of the SNS, activation of RAS, reduced renal perfusion pressures, and blunting of renal responsiveness to natriuretic peptides. Increased renal sympathetic nerve–mediated vasoconstriction leads to decreased renal blood flow, as well as increased renal tubular sodium and water reabsorption throughout the nephron. Renal sympathetic stimulation also can lead to the nonosmotic release of arginine vasopressin (AVP) from the posterior pituitary, which reduces the excretion of free water and contributes to worsening peripheral vasoconstriction, as well as increased endothelin (ET) production.[1] Increased renal venous pressure can also lead to renal interstitial hypertension, with the development of tubular injury and renal fibrosis.

ARGININE VASOPRESSIN

AVP is a pituitary hormone that plays a central role in the regulation of free water clearance and plasma osmolality (see Fig. 47.5). Under normal circumstances, AVP is released in response to an increase in plasma osmolality, leading to increased retention of water from the collecting duct. Of note, circulating AVP is elevated in many patients with HF, even after correction for plasma osmolality (i.e., nonosmotic release),[1] and may contribute to the hyponatremia that occurs in HF. The cellular effects of AVP are mediated mainly by interactions with three types of receptors, termed V_1, V_2, and V_3 (previously V_{1b}). The V_1 receptor, the most widespread subtype, is found primarily in vascular smooth muscle cells. The V_3 receptor has a more limited distribution and is located mainly in the CNS. The V_2 receptors are found primarily in the epithelial cells in the renal collecting duct and the thick ascending limb. AVP receptors are members of the GPCRs. The V_1 receptors mediate vasoconstriction, platelet aggregation, and stimulation of myocardial growth factors, whereas V_3 modulates adrenocorticotropic hormone (ACTH) secretion from the anterior pituitary. The V_2 receptor mediates antidiuretic effects by stimulating adenyl cyclase to increase the rate of insertion of water channel–containing vesicles into the apical membrane. Because the vesicles contain preformed functional water channels, termed *aquaporins*, their localization in the apical membranes in response to V_2 stimulation increases the water permeability of the apical membrane, leading to water retention. The "vaptans," vasopressin receptor antagonists with V_1 (relcovaptan) or V_2 (tolvaptan, lixivaptan) selectivity or nonselective V_1/V_2 activity (conivaptan), have been shown to reduce body weight and reduce hyponatremia in clinical trials (see Chapters 49 and 50).

Increased renal sympathetic activity leads to increased renin production by the kidneys, with a resultant sustained activation of RAAS, despite an expanded extracellular volume. Angiotensin II facilitates retention of sodium and water by multiple renal mechanisms, including a direct proximal tubular effect, as well as through activation of aldosterone, which leads to increased sodium resorption in the distal tubule. Angiotensin II also stimulates the thirst center of the brain and provokes the release of AVP and aldosterone, both of which can lead to further dysregulation of salt and water homeostasis.

A number of counterregulatory neurohormonal systems become activated in HF to offset the deleterious effects of the vasoconstricting neurohormones. Metabolites of vasodilatory prostaglandins, including prostaglandin E_2 (PGE_2) and prostacyclin

(PGI$_2$), are elevated in patients with HF. In addition to being a vasodilator, PGE$_2$ enhances renal sodium excretion and modulates the antidiuretic action of AVP. One class of the most important counterregulatory neurohormonal systems that become activated in HF are the natriuretic peptides, including ANP and brain (B-type) natriuretic peptide (BNP). Under physiologic conditions, ANP and BNP function as natriuretic hormones that are released in response to increases in atrial and myocardial stretch, often secondary to excessive sodium intake. Once released, these cardiac peptides act on the kidney and peripheral circulation to unload the heart, through increased excretion of sodium and water, while inhibiting the release of renin and aldosterone (Fig. 47.6). In the setting of RAAS activation, the release of ANP and BNP may serve as an important counterregulatory mechanism that maintains sodium and water homeostasis. However, for reasons that are not entirely clear, the renal effects of the natriuretic peptides appear to become blunted with advancing HF, leaving the effects of RAAS unopposed.[11] Potential reasons for this blunting include low renal perfusion pressure, relative deficiency or altered molecular forms of the natriuretic peptides, and decreased levels of natriuretic peptide receptors.

NATRIURETIC PEPTIDES

The natriuretic peptide system consists of five structurally similar peptides: ANP, urodilatin (an isoform of ANP), BNP, C-type natriuretic peptide (CNP), and dendroaspis natriuretic peptide (DNP) (Fig. 47.6A).[12] ANP, a 28–amino acid peptide hormone, is produced principally in the cardiac atria, whereas BNP, a 32–amino acid peptide originally isolated from porcine brain, was later identified as a hormone that was primarily produced in the cardiac ventricles. Both ANP and BNP are secreted in response to increasing cardiac wall tension; however, other factors such as neurohormones (e.g., angiotensin II, ET-1, catecholamines) or physiologic factors (e.g., age, gender, renal function) may also play a role in their regulation. The biosynthesis, secretion, and clearance of BNP differs from ANP, suggesting that these two natriuretic peptides have discrete physiologic and pathophysiologic roles. Whereas ANP is secreted in short bursts in response to acute changes in atrial pressure, the activation of BNP is regulated transcriptionally in response to chronic

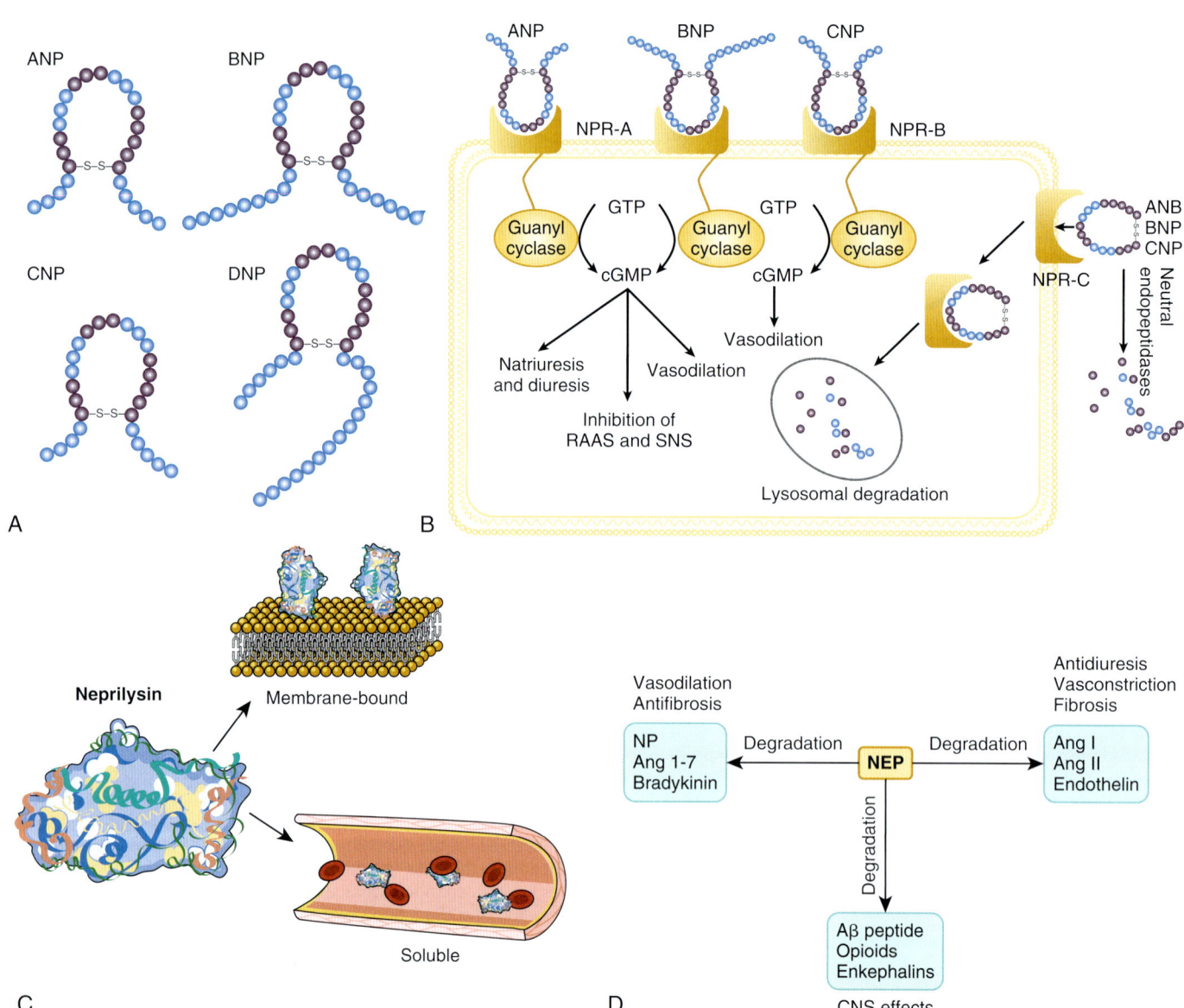

FIGURE 47.6 Natriuretic peptides. **A,** The similar 17–amino acid disulfide ring in natriuretic peptides A, B, C, and D. Identical amino acid sequences are marked in *purple*. **B,** Action and clearance of the natriuretic peptides. **C,** Neprilysin is a membrane-bound enzyme that can be released from the cell surface, producing a soluble form that can be detected in the blood. **D,** Neutral endopeptidases (*NEP*) degrade a variety of different peptides. *NP,* natriuretic peptide. (**B** modified from Gardner RS, Chong KS, McDonagh TA, et al. B-type natriuretic peptides in heart failure. *Biomark Med.* 2007;1:243; **C** modified from Bayes-Genis A, Barallat J, Galán A, et al. Soluble neprilysin is predictive of cardiovascular death and heart failure hospitalizations in heart failure patients. *J Am Coll Cardiol.* 2015;65:657–665; **D** modified from Volpe M, Carnovali M, Mastromarino V. The natriuretic peptides system in the pathophysiology of heart failure: from molecular basis to treatment. *Clin Sci (Lond)* 2016;130:57.)

increases in atrial/ventricular pressure. ANP and BNP initially are synthesized as prohormones that are subsequently proteolytically cleaved, respectively, by corin and furin, to yield large, biologically inactive N-terminal fragments (NT-ANP and NT-BNP) and smaller, biologically active peptides (i.e., ANP and BNP). ANP has a relatively short half-life of approximately 3 minutes, whereas BNP has a plasma half-life of approximately 20 minutes. CNP, which is located primarily in the vasculature, also is released as a prohormone that is cleaved into biologically inactive form (NT-CNP) and a 22–amino acid, biologically active form (i.e., CNP).

Figure 47.6B illustrates the signaling pathway of the natriuretic peptide system. The natriuretic peptides stimulate the production of the intracellular second-messenger cyclic guanosine monophosphate (cGMP), via binding to the natriuretic peptide A receptor (NPR-A), which preferentially binds ANP and BNP, and the natriuretic peptide B receptor (NPR-B), which preferentially binds CNP. Both NPR-A and NPR-B are coupled to particulate guanylate cyclase. Activation of NPR-A and NPR-B results in natriuresis, vasorelaxation, inhibition of renin and aldosterone, inhibition of fibrosis, and increased lusitropy. The natriuretic peptide C receptor (NPR-C) is not linked to cGMP and serves as a clearance receptor for the natriuretic peptides.

All three natriuretic peptides are degraded by two major mechanisms: NPR-C–mediated internalization, followed by lysosomal degradation and enzymatic degradation by neutral endopeptidase (NEP) 24.11 (neprilysin), which is widely expressed in multiple tissues, where it often is colocalized with ACE. Both ACE and NEP are membrane-bound zinc-containing metallopeptidases involved in the metabolism of a variety of biologic peptides.[13]

Neprilysin, like many other membrane-bound metalloproteases, can be released from the cell surface, producing a non–membrane-associated soluble form that retains catalytic activity. NEP preferentially cleaves small peptides on the N-terminal side of hydrophobic residues (Fig. 47.6C). NEP has a wide range of tissue distribution, including vascular endothelium, smooth muscle cells, myocytes, fibroblasts, kidney tubule cells, and nerve cells. NEP degrades multiple peptides, including natriuretic peptides (Fig. 47.6D), angiotensin I, angiotensin II, ET-I, adrenomedullin, opioids, bradykinin, chemotactic peptides, enkephalins, and a ^{14}myoid-β peptide (Aβ). NEP inhibition of degradation of natriuretic peptides results in vasorelaxation, natriuresis, inhibition of hypertrophy, and fibrosis. On the other hand, inhibition of degradation of other vasoactive peptides, such as angiotensin II, angiotensin 1 to 7, and ET, opposes the vasodilatory effects of natriuretic peptides. Accordingly, NEP inhibition has variable effects on blood pressure. NEP inhibition increases urinary kinin levels, which may contribute to its natriuretic effects. NEP plays an important role in clearance of amyloid peptides in the brain. In particular, NEP is of major relevance for degrading the amyloid-beta peptides (Aβ), which play a significant role in neurotoxicity, and formation of amyloid plaques from Aβ aggregates in complex with other proteins is a hallmark of Alzheimer disease. Overexpression of neprilysin ameliorated the development of Alzheimer disease, and disruption of the neprilysin gene induces cognitive dysfunction in a mouse model of Alzheimer disease. Because of the potentially beneficial effects of natriuretic peptides in HF, NEP inhibition was pursued as a rational approach for HF therapy. The early use of omapatrilat, a dual vasopeptidase inhibitor that inhibits both ACE and NEP, was not shown to be more effective than ACE inhibition alone in HF patients.[14] However, the use of a combined AT$_1$ receptor antagonist and a neprilysin inhibitor (valsartan/sacubitril, LCZ696) was shown to have a favorable impact on HF outcome, including quality of life, exercise capacity, and more importantly, HF hospitalization and total mortality, in the PARADIGM-HF trial (see Chapter 50).

The biologic importance of the natriuretic peptides in renal sodium handling has been demonstrated in multiple studies using NPR antagonists, as well as overexpression of ANP or BNP. In experimental HF models, either acute blockade of NPR-A and NPR-B or chronic genetic disruption of NPR-A blunts the renal natriuretic response to acute volume expansion, demonstrating the renal protective action of natriuretic peptide activation. The infusion of a recombinant human ANP and BNP exerts beneficial hemodynamic effects, characterized by decreases in arterial and venous pressures, increase in cardiac output, and suppression of neurohormonal activation in humans, resulting in their clinical development as therapeutic agents for human HF (see Chapter 49). In addition to their important biologic role, the natriuretic peptides have provided important diagnostic and prognostic information in HF (see Chapter 48).

Neurohormonal Alterations in the Peripheral Vasculature

In patients with HF, the complex interactions between the autonomic nervous system and local autoregulatory mechanisms tend to preserve circulation to the brain and heart while decreasing blood flow to the skin, skeletal muscles, splanchnic organs, and kidneys. This intense visceral vasoconstriction during exercise helps to divert the limited cardiac output to exercising muscle but contributes to hypoperfusion of the gut and kidneys. The most powerful stimulus for peripheral vasoconstriction is sympathetic activation, which releases the potent vasoconstrictor NE. Other vasoconstrictors that contribute to maintaining circulatory homeostasis include angiotensin II, ET, neuropeptide Y, urotensin II, thromboxane A$_2$, and AVP. The increased sympathetic adrenergic stimulation of the peripheral arteries and the increased concentrations of circulating vasoconstrictors contribute to the arteriolar vasoconstriction and to the maintenance of arterial pressure. The sympathetic stimulation of the veins contributes to an increase in venous tone, which helps to maintain venous return and ventricular filling and to support cardiac performance by Starling's law of the heart (see Chapter 46).

As noted, the vasoconstricting neurohormones activate counterregulatory vasodilator responses, including release of natriuretic peptides, NO, bradykinin, adrenomedullin, apelin, and vasodilating PGI$_2$ and PGE$_2$. Under normal circumstances, the continuous release of NO (endothelium-derived relaxing factor) from the endothelium counteracts these vasoconstricting factors and allows for appropriate vasodilatory responses during exercise. As HF advances, however, the endothelial cell–mediated vasodilatory responsiveness is lost, which contributes to the excessive peripheral arterial vasoconstriction that is emblematic of advanced HF. Of interest, the vasodilator response can be restored by the administration of L-arginine, a precursor of endothelium-derived NO.

Nitric Oxide

The free radical gas NO is produced by three isoforms of NO synthase (NOS). All three isoforms are present in the heart, including NOS1 (neuronal NOS [nNOS]), NOS2 (inducible NOS [iNOS]) and NOS3 (so-called endothelial-constitutive NOS [eNOS]). NOS1 has been detected in cardiac conduction tissue, in intracardiac neurons, and in the SR of cardiac myocytes. NOS2 is an inducible isoform that is not normally expressed in the myocardium but is synthesized de novo in virtually all cells in the heart in response to inflammatory cytokines. NOS3 is expressed in coronary endothelium and endocardium and in the sarcolemma and transverse (T)-tubule membranes of cardiac myocytes. NOS1 and NOS3 can be activated by calcium or calmodulin, whereas the induction of NOS2 is calcium independent. NO activates soluble guanylate cyclase. Vericiguat, an oral soluble guanylate cyclase stimulator, reduced the composite of death from cardiovascular causes and first HF hospitalization in the VICTORIA (Vericiguat Global Study in Subjects with Heart Failure with Reduced Ejection Fraction) trial (see Chapter 50).[15]

Under normal circumstances, the continuous release of NO (endothelium-derived relaxing factor) from the endothelium counteracts the vasoconstricting factors and allows for appropriate vasodilatory responses during exercise. This activation leads to the production of cGMP, which in turn activates protein kinase G (PKG) and cascade of different signaling events. In normal persons, NO released by endothelial cells mediates vasodilation in the peripheral vasculature through cGMP-mediated relaxation of vascular smooth muscle. In patients with HF, endothelium-dependent NO-mediated dilation of the peripheral vasculature is blunted, which has been attributed to decreased NOS3 expression and activity.

The actions of NO on the myocardium are complex and include both short-term alterations in function and energetics and longer-term effects on structure. NO modulates the activity of several key calcium channels involved in excitation-contraction coupling as well as mitochondrial respiratory complexes. This type of regulation is accomplished by spatial localization of different NOS isoforms in distinct cellular microdomains involved in excitation-contraction coupling. Specifically, NOS1 localizes to the SR in proximity to the ryanodine receptor (RyR) and sarcoendoplasmic reticulum calcium–adenosine triphosphatase (SR Ca^{2+}-ATPase, SERCA2a), and NOS3 is found in sarcolemmal caveolae compartmentalized with cell surface receptors and the L-type Ca^{2+} channel. NO also participates in mitochondrial respiration, the process that fuels excitation-contraction coupling. The different NOS isoforms also may participate in the process of cardiac remodeling. LV remodeling was ameliorated and survival improved after MI in transgenic mice deficient in NOS2. By contrast, overexpression of NOS3 resulted in improved remodeling after MI. These contrasting effects of NOS2 and NOS3 may reflect the differences in amount of NO produced, which is much higher with NOS2. Emerging evidence indicates an imbalance between increasing free radical production and decreased NO generation in HF, which has been termed the "nitroso-redox imbalance." NOS uncoupling secondary to a deficiency of tetrahydrobiopterin may further contribute to the nitroso-redox imbalance.[16] The nitroso-redox imbalance probably contributes to disease progression in HF secondary to increased oxidative stress, as well as loss of the peripheral vasodilatory effects of NO.

BRADYKININ

Kinins are vasodilators that are released from inactive protein precursors (kininogens) through the action of proteolytic enzymes termed *kallikreins*. The biologic actions of the kinins are mediated by binding to B_1 and B_2 receptors. Most cardiovascular actions are initiated by the B_2 receptor, which is distributed widely in tissues, where it binds bradykinin and kallidin. The B_1 receptor binds the metabolites of bradykinin and kallidin. Stimulation of the B_2 receptor leads to vasodilation, which is mediated by the activation of NOS3, phospholipase A_2, and adenylyl cyclase. Studies suggest that bradykinin plays an important role in the regulation of vascular tone in HF.[17] The breakdown of bradykinin is catalyzed by ACE and neprilysin, so these enzymes not only lead to the formation of a potent vasoconstrictor (angiotensin II) but also mediate the breakdown of a vasodilator (bradykinin). The augmentation of bradykinin levels likely contributes to the beneficial actions of ACE inhibitors and NEP inhibitors (see Chapter 50).

ADRENOMEDULLIN

Adrenomedullin is a 52-amino acid vasodilatory peptide that originally was discovered in human pheochromocytoma tissue. Subsequently, high levels of adrenomedullin immunoreactivity were detected in cardiac atrium and adrenal and pituitary glands, with lower levels detected in the ventricle, kidney, and vasculature.[18] Adrenomedullin binds to a number of G-protein coupled receptors (GPRCs) that are present in multiple cell types, including on endothelial and vascular smooth muscle cells. Circulating concentrations of adrenomedullin are elevated in cardiovascular disease and HF in proportion to the severity of cardiac and hemodynamic impairment. Increasing evidence suggests that adrenomedullin may play a compensatory role in HF by offsetting the deleterious effects of excessive peripheral vasoconstriction. For example, the excretion of adrenomedullin that is stimulated by volume overload is thought to be protective by preserving endothelial barrier function. Moreover, adrenomedullin inhibits the renin-angiotensin-aldosterone system. Recently, a new immunoassay that specifically measures the biologically active form of adrenomedullin has been developed and may become a biomarker for tissue congestion.[19]

APELIN

Apelin is a vasoactive peptide that is an endogenous ligand for the GPCR APJ. The *APJ* gene encodes a receptor that most closely resembles the angiotensin receptor AT_1. However, the APJ receptor does not bind angiotensin II. In the cardiovascular system, apelin elicits endothelium-dependent, NO-mediated vasorelaxation and reduces arterial blood pressure. In addition, apelin demonstrates potent inotropic activity without stimulating concomitant cardiac myocyte hypertrophy. Apelin also produces diuresis by inhibition of AVP activity. In experimental animals, apelin concentrations are significantly lower in failing hearts and are increased after treatment with an angiotensin receptor blocking agent. Furthermore, apelin levels are significantly reduced in patients with HF compared with controls and are significantly increased after cardiac resynchronization. The APJ receptor is a bifunctional GPCR that conveys cytoprotective signals after endogenous ligand stimulation and also acts as a mechanosensor to decrease cardiac hypertrophy after hemodynamic pressure overload.[20] Recently, the apelin receptor has been shown to be activated by a novel endogenous peptide ligand referred to as Apela/Elabela/Toddler (ELA).[21] In contrast to apelin, the expression of ELA is mainly enriched in stem cells, the kidney, prostate, and vascular endothelium. ELA exerts similar cardiovascular effects as apelin and may be more potent than apelin. ELA is also downregulated in experimental models and humans with HF. The ELP-AJP axis is currently being evaluated as a therapeutic target in patients with chronic HF.[21]

ADIPOKINES

Although adipose tissue was once considered a simple storage depot for fat, it is now known to synthesize and secrete a family of proteins collectively referred to as adipokines. Adipokines include adiponectin, TNF, plasminogen activator inhibitor type 1 (PAI-1), transforming growth factor-β, and resistin. Leptin is a 16-kDa protein hormone that plays a key role in regulating energy intake and energy expenditure. The product of the ob gene, leptin is predominantly synthesized and secreted by adipocytes, although the heart is also a site of leptin synthesis. The initial role of leptin was thought to decrease appetite through hypothalamic stimulation and thus regulation of food intake. However, elevated circulating levels of leptin and soluble leptin receptor, which act via activating a family of receptor (ob.R) isoforms, are markedly elevated in patients with HF.[22] Leptin may affect myocardial function by promoting activation of both the SNS and the RAS. Moreover, leptin can stimulate the secretion of aldosterone.[22] Several studies suggest that leptin directly induces hypertrophy in both human and rodent cardiac myocytes.[23] Leptin resistance may lead to an accumulation of lipids in non-adipose peripheral tissues, resulting in a variety of "lipotoxic" effects, including cardiac myocyte apoptosis.

Adiponectin is a 224–amino acid polypeptide that modulates a number of metabolic processes, including glucose regulation and fatty acid oxidation. Although adiponectin initially was thought to be exclusively produced by adipose tissue, recent studies have demonstrated adiponectin expression in the heart. Studies in adiponectin-deficient mice demonstrated progressive cardiac remodeling after hemodynamic pressure overloading, whereas administration of adiponectin diminished infarct size, apoptosis, and TNF production after myocardial ischemia-reperfusion in both wild-type and adiponectin-deficient mice. Adiponectin inhibits cardiac hypertrophy, inflammation, and fibrosis. Moreover, adiponectin suppresses aldosterone secretion. Thus, adiponectin has been proposed as a potential biomarker of HF, as well as a potential therapeutic target for the treatment of HF.[23]

INFLAMMATORY MEDIATORS

As shown in Figure 47.7 myocardial injury leads to the activation of the innate and adaptive immune systems in the heart. Whereas the innate immune system provides a global, nonspecific defense against tissue injury, the adaptive immune system provides a highly specific response mediated by B cells and T cells.[24] The innate immune system is activated by transmembrane and cytosolic receptors that recognize molecular motifs from endogenous material released by dying or stressed cells (damage-associated molecular patterns [DAMPs]). These receptors, referred to as pattern recognition receptors (PRRs), are expressed by cells residing in the heart, including cardiac myocytes, endothelial cells, and tissue-resident immune cells. PRRs in the heart include Toll-like receptors (TLRs), RIG-I-like receptors (retinoic acid-inducible), NOD-like receptors (NLRs), the NLRP3 inflammasome, pentraxins, and C-type lectin receptors. Transcriptional profiling of human heart samples showed that failing and non-failing hearts have distinct expression profiles of genes related to innate immune responses, and the expression profiles of these genes were different in samples from patients with ischemic and non-ischemic HF.[24] Activation of PRRs by DAMPs initiates downstream signaling cascades that regulate the expression of ensembles of genes encoding pro-inflammatory cytokines, including TNF, IL-1β, and IL-6, as well as chemokines, both of which serve as downstream "effectors" of the innate immune system. Activation of the innate immune system can lead subsequently to the activation of humoral immunity, through recruitment and stimulation of B cells and T cells. Activation of innate and adaptive immune responses provides the heart with a short-term adaptation to increased stress (physiologic inflammation). However, this inflammatory response can become dysregulated and result in chronic inflammation that leads to LV dysfunction and LV remodeling. Circulating levels of proinflammatory cytokines (e.g., CRP, TNF, IL-1β, IL-6) are increased in patients with HF and correlate with adverse patient outcomes.[25] As shown in Table 47.1, the sustained expression of inflammatory mediators is sufficient to recapitulate virtually all aspects of the HF phenotype, by provoking deleterious changes in cardiac myocytes and nonmyocytes, as well as changes in the myocardial extracellular matrix (ECM). The clinical relevance of these findings is suggested by a prespecified analysis of the CANTOS (Cardiovascular Risk Reduction Study) trial, which showed that targeted anti-cytokine therapy with canakinumab (a monoclonal antibody against IL-1β) reduced HF-related hospitalizations and mortality in patients with previous MI. Importantly, canakinumab-treated patients who achieved on-treatment hsCRP

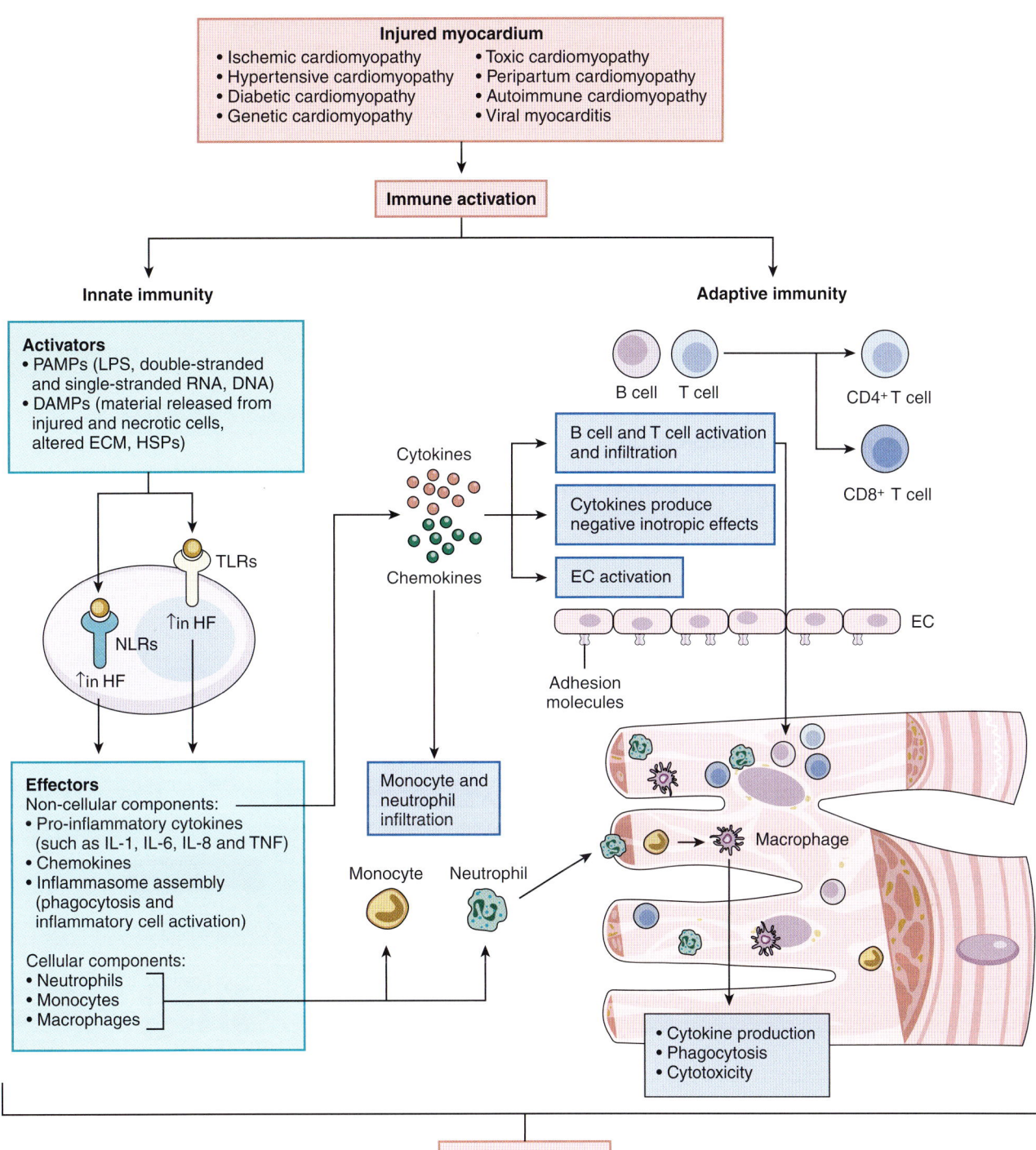

FIGURE 47.7 The innate and adaptive immune systems in heart failure. A variety of cardiac disease states that lead to cardiac injury can activate the innate immune response in the heart through binding of pathogen-associated molecular patterns (PAMPs) or damage-associated molecular patterns (DAMPs) to pattern-recognition receptors (PRRs), such as Toll-like receptors (TLRs) and NOD-like receptors (NLRs), present on cardiomyocytes and tissue-resident immune cells. Activation of PRRs induces a variety of non-cellular effectors in the heart, including pro-inflammatory cytokines and chemokines and activation of the complement system, which lead to endothelial cell (EC) activation and recruitment of monocytes and neutrophils. Activation of the innate immune system triggers the activation of the adaptive immune response through the recruitment of B cells and T cells to the injured myocardium. *ECM*, Extracellular matrix; *HF*, heart failure; *HSP*, heat shock protein; *LPS*, lipopolysaccharide; *TNF*, tumor necrosis factor. (From Adamo L, Rocha-Resende C, Prabhu SD, Mann DL. Reappraising the role of inflammation in heart failure. *Nat Rev Cardiol*. 220;5:269–285.)

concentrations of less than 2 mg/L had significant reductions in the risk of HF related outcomes, including all-cause death when compared with patients receiving placebo, suggesting that inflammation contributes to the progression of HF.[26]

Left Ventricular Remodeling

Although the neurohormonal concept explains many aspects of disease progression in the failing heart, increasing clinical evidence suggests that current neurohormonal models fail to completely explain the basis for this progression. That is, although neurohormonal antagonists stabilize and in some cases reverse certain aspects of the disease process in HF, in the overwhelming majority of patients, it will progress, albeit more slowly. It has been suggested that LV remodeling is directly related to future deterioration in LV performance and a less favorable clinical course in HFrEF patients. LV remodeling is influenced by hemodynamic, neurohormonal, epigenetic, and genetic factors,[27] as well as by comorbid conditions. Although the complex changes that occur in the heart during LV remodeling have traditionally been described in anatomic terms, the process of LV remodeling also has an important impact on the biology of the cardiac myocyte, on changes in the volume of myocyte and nonmyocyte components of the myocardium, and on the geometry and architecture of the LV chamber (Table 47.2).

Alterations in Biology of Cardiac Myocyte

Numerous studies have suggested that failing human cardiac myocytes undergo a number of important changes that might be expected to lead to a progressive loss of contractile function. These include decreased alpha-myosin heavy chain gene expression with a concomitant increase in beta-myosin heavy chain expression, progressive loss of myofilaments in cardiac myocytes, alterations in cytoskeletal proteins, and alterations in excitation-contraction coupling and in energy metabolism, as well as desensitization of beta-adrenergic signaling (see Table 47.2).

TABLE 47.1 Effects of Inflammatory Mediators on Left Ventricular Remodeling

Alterations in the Biology of the Myocyte
Myocyte hypertrophy
Fetal gene expression
Negative inotropic effects
Increased oxidative stress
Alterations in the Biology of Nonmyocytes
Conversion of fibroblasts to myofibroblasts
Upregulation of AT_1 receptors on fibroblasts
Increased matrix metalloproteinase secretion by fibroblasts
Alterations in the Extracellular Matrix
Degradation of the matrix
Myocardial fibrosis
Progressive Myocyte Loss
Necrosis
Apoptosis

TABLE 47.2 Overview of Left Ventricular Remodeling

Alterations in Myocyte Biology
Excitation-contraction coupling
Myosin heavy chain (fetal) gene expression
Beta-adrenergic desensitization
Hypertrophy
Myocytolysis
Cytoskeletal proteins
Myocardial Changes
Myocyte loss
Necrosis
Apoptosis
Autosis
Alterations in extracellular matrix
Matrix degradation
Myocardial fibrosis
Alterations in Left Ventricular Chamber Geometry
Left ventricular (LV) dilation
Increased LV sphericity
LV wall thinning
Mitral valve incompetence

Cardiac Myocyte Hypertrophy

Two basic patterns of cardiac hypertrophy occur in response to hemodynamic overload (Fig. 47.8). In pressure overload hypertrophy (e.g., with aortic stenosis or hypertension), increased systolic wall stress leads to the addition of sarcomeres in parallel, an increase in myocyte cross-sectional area, and increased LV wall thickening. This pattern of remodeling has been referred to as "concentric" hypertrophy (Fig. 47.8A) and has been linked with alterations in Ca^{2+}/calmodulin-dependent protein

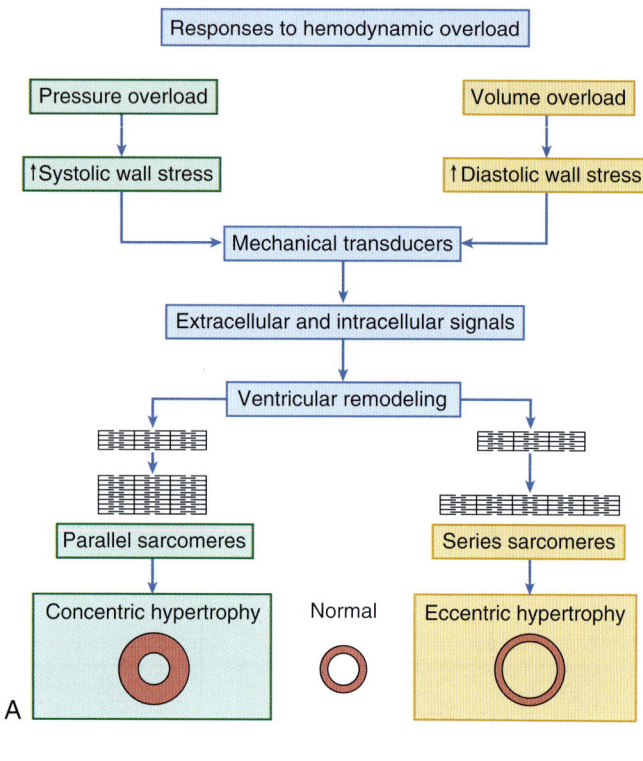

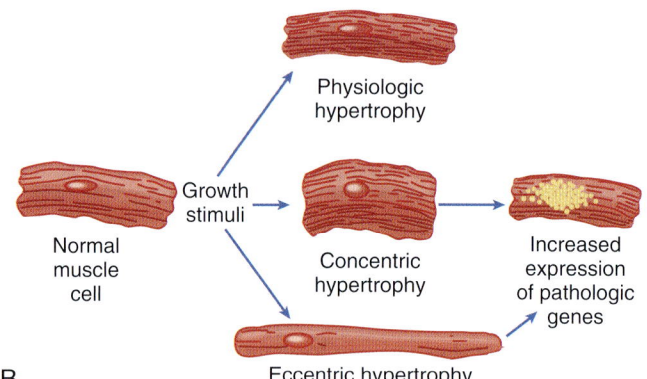

FIGURE 47.8 The pattern of cardiac and cellular remodeling that occurs in response to hemodynamic overloading depends on the nature of the inciting stimulus. **A,** When the overload is predominantly due to an increase in pressure (e.g., with systemic hypertension or aortic stenosis), the increase in systolic wall stress leads to the parallel addition of sarcomeres and widening of the cardiac myocytes, resulting in "concentric" cardiac hypertrophy. When the overload is predominantly due to an increase in ventricular volume, the increase in diastolic wall stress leads to the series addition of sarcomeres, lengthening of cardiac myocytes, and left ventricular (LV) dilation, which is referred to as "eccentric" chamber hypertrophy. **B,** Phenotypically distinct changes occur in the morphology of myocytes in response to the type of hemodynamic overload that is superimposed. When the overload is predominantly due to an increase in pressure, the increase in systolic wall stress leads to the parallel addition of sarcomeres and widening of the cardiac myocytes. When the hemodynamic overload is predominantly due to an increase in ventricular volume, the increase in diastolic wall stress leads to the series addition of sarcomeres with consequent lengthening of cardiac myocytes. The expression of maladaptive genes is increased in both eccentric and concentric hypertrophy, but not in physiologic myocyte hypertrophy as occurs with exercise (see Table 47.2). (**A** from Colucci WS, ed. *Heart Failure: Cardiac Function and Dysfunction*. 2nd ed. Philadelphia: Current Medicine; 1999:4.2. **B** modified from Hunter JJ, Chien KR. Signaling pathways for cardiac hypertrophy and failure. *N Engl J Med*. 1999;341:1276.)

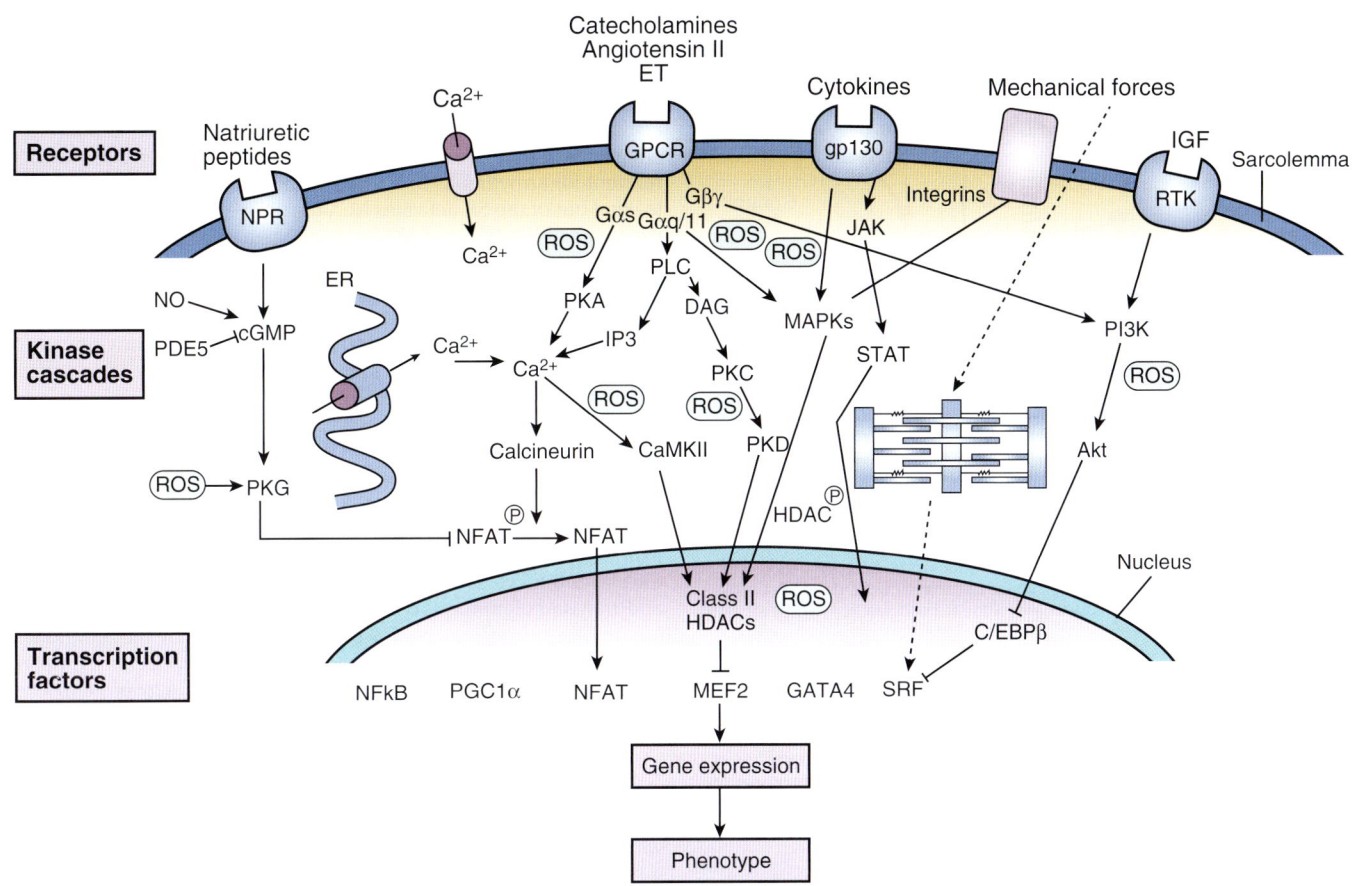

FIGURE 47.9 Cellular signaling pathways in cardiac myocyte hypertrophy. Many signaling pathways have the potential to regulate the growth of cardiac cells acting through an increasingly complex network of intracellular signaling cascades. Agonists for α-adrenergic, angiotensin, and endothelin (*ET*) receptors couple to phospholipase C (*PLC*) and calcium influx channels by way of G proteins. Activation of PLC results in the generation of two second messengers, inositol triphosphate (*IP3*) and diacylglycerol (*DAG*). IP3 causes the release of calcium from intracellular stores, and DAG activates protein kinase C (*PKC*). Changes in intracellular calcium stores can activate Ca^{2+}/calmodulin-dependent kinases (*CaMKII*), as well as calcineurin, which can affect gene expression in multiple ways. PKC and G proteins can affect gene expression by activating mitogen-activated protein kinase (*MAPK*) cascades. Histone deacetylase complexes (*HDACs*) are emerging as important negative regulators of genes involved in cardiac hypertrophy. Cytokines and peptide growth factors, such as insulin-like growth factor (*IGF*), can be elaborated by various cells within the heart and may act in an autocrine or paracrine manner. These growth factors activate cellular receptors that usually possess receptor tyrosine kinase (*RTK*) activity and are coupled to a cascade of protein kinase. Mechanical deformation of cardiac myocytes through matrix-integrin interactions can lead to activation or modulation of several signaling pathways, at least in part through autocrine action of released agonists such as angiotensin. Both nitric oxide (NO) and oxidative stress may be induced after stimulation of signaling pathways and modulate the activity of kinase cascades and transcription factors leading to alterations in contractile phenotype, growth, and death in myocytes. *Akt*, Protein kinase B; *C/EBPβ*, CCAAT/enhancer binding protein-β; *ER*, endoplasmic reticulum; *GATA4*, GATA-binding protein; *gp130*, glycoprotein 130; *GPCR*, G protein–coupled receptor; *JAK*, Janus kinase; *MEF2*, myocyte enhancer factor; *NFAT*, nuclear factor of activated T cells; *NFκB*, nuclear factor-kappaB cells; *NPR*, natriuretic peptide receptor; *P*, phosphorylation; *PDE5*, phosphodiesterase type 5; *PGC1α*, peroxisome proliferator–activated receptor gamma, coactivator 1 alpha; *PKA, PKD, PKG*, protein kinases A, D, G; *STAT*, signal transducer and activator of transcription; *SRF*, serum response factor. (From Shah AM, Mann DL. In search of new therapeutic targets and strategies for heart failure: recent advances in basic science. *Lancet.* 2011;378:704.)

kinase II–dependent signaling (Fig. 47.9).[28] By contrast, in volume overload hypertrophy (e.g., with aortic and mitral regurgitation), increased diastolic wall stress leads to an increase in myocyte length with the addition of sarcomeres in series, thereby engendering increased LV ventricular dilation. This pattern of remodeling has been referred to as "eccentric" hypertrophy (because of the position of the heart in the chest), or a "dilated" phenotype (see Fig. 47.7A), and has been linked with protein kinase B (Akt) activation (see Fig. 47.8).[28] Patients with HF classically present with a dilated left ventricle with or without LV wall thinning. The myocytes from these failing ventricles have an elongated appearance that is characteristic of myocytes obtained from hearts subjected to chronic volume overload.

Cardiac myocyte hypertrophy also leads to changes in the biologic phenotype of the myocyte that are secondary to reactivation of portfolios of genes normally not expressed postnatally. The reactivation of these fetal genes, the so-called fetal gene program, also is accompanied by decreased expression of a number of genes that are normally expressed in the adult heart. As discussed later, activation of the fetal gene program may contribute to the contractile dysfunction that develops in the failing myocyte. As shown in Figure 47.9, the stimuli for the genetic reprogramming of the myocyte include mechanical stretch/strain of the myocyte, neurohormones (e.g., NE, angiotensin II), inflammatory cytokines (e.g., TNF, IL-1β, IL-6), other peptides and growth factors (e.g., ET), and ROS (e.g., superoxide, NO). These stimuli occur both locally within the myocardium, where they exert autocrine/paracrine effects, and systemically, where they exert endocrine effects.

The early stage of cardiac myocyte hypertrophy is characterized morphologically by increases in the number of myofibrils and mitochondria, as well as enlargement of mitochondria and nuclei. At this stage, the cardiac myocytes are larger than normal, but with preservation of cellular organization. As hypertrophy continues, there is an increase in the number of mitochondria, as well as the addition of new contractile elements in localized areas of the cell. Cells subjected to longstanding hypertrophy show more obvious disruptions in cellular organization, such as extremely enlarged nuclei with highly lobulated membranes, accompanied by the displacement of adjacent myofibrils with loss of the normal registration of the Z-bands. The late stage of hypertrophy is characterized by loss of contractile elements (myocytolysis) with marked disruption of Z-bands and severe disruption of the normal parallel arrangement of the sarcomeres, accompanied by dilation and increased tortuosity of T tubules.

Alterations in Excitation-Contraction Coupling

As discussed in Chapter 46, excitation-contraction coupling refers to the cascade of biologic events that begins with the cardiac action potential and ends with myocyte contraction and relaxation. Impaired

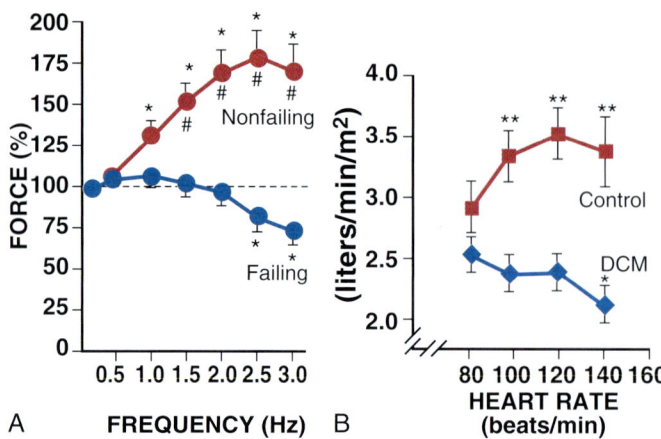

FIGURE 47.10 Relationship between contraction frequency and cardiac performance (force-frequency relation) in heart failure. **A**, Relationship between stimulation frequency and force generation of isolated muscle strip preparations from nonfailing and failing human hearts. In nonfailing myocardium, contractile force increases up to a stimulation rate of approximately 2.5 Hz (150 beats/min), whereas contractile force does not significantly increase in failing myocardium. (*indicates $P < 0.05$ versus 0.25 Hz; # indicates $P < 0.05$ between failing and nonfailing myocardium.) **B**, Cardiac index versus heart rate in patients with and without heart failure (HF). Heart rate was changed by temporary pacing during cardiac catheterization, and cardiac output was measured by thermodilution. In patients without HF, cardiac index increases with higher heart rates up to 120 beats/min, but it declines continuously in patients with HF. (*indicates $P < 0.05$ and **$P < 0.01$ versus lowest pacing rate.) DCM, Dilated cardiomyopathy. (**A**, Modified from Pieske B, Maier LS, Bers DM, Hasenfuss G. Ca2+ handling and sarcoplasmic reticulum Ca2+ content in isolated failing and nonfailing human myocardium. Circ Res. 1999;85:38; and **B**, modified from Hasenfuss G, Holubarsch C, Hermann HP, et al. Influence of the force-frequency relationship on haemodynamics and left ventricular function in patients with non-failing hearts and in patients with dilated cardiomyopathy. Eur Heart J. 1994;15:164.)

contraction and relaxation of the failing heart is most prominent at high heart rates, which results in a depressed force-frequency relationship. This has been demonstrated both in isolated strips of human myocardium and in clinical observations of patients (Fig. 47.10). Normally, higher contraction frequency increases cardiac performance because of a frequency-dependent augmentation of intracellular Ca^{2+} transients. By contrast, in the failing myocardium, a decline in force generation is seen with higher heart rates that is secondary to a decrease in amplitude of intracellular Ca^{2+}, a prolonged decline of the Ca^{2+} transient, and increased levels of diastolic calcium. The reduced intracellular Ca^{2+} transient is secondary to depletion of Ca^{2+} from the SR, the result of three major defects in calcium cycling that occur in the failing heart: (1) increased Ca^{2+} leak through RyRs, (2) impaired SR Ca^{2+} uptake from reduced SERCA2a (SR calcium pump) protein levels and function, and (3) increased expression and function of the sarcolemmal Na^+/Ca^{2+} exchanger (NCX).

Increased Ca^{2+} Leak

Ca^{2+} enters the cell during the action potential through L-type calcium channels and triggers a release of a much larger amount of calcium from the SR through RyRs. Although controversy surrounds the expression levels of RyRs in HF, as well as the coupling of RyRs to L-type Ca^{2+} channels, there is general agreement that the diastolic Ca^{2+} leak in HF is the result of RyR opening during diastole.[29] The resultant release of calcium from the SR event is referred to as a "Ca^{2+}-spark." The pathophysiologic mechanism underlying the diastolic Ca^{2+} leak in HF has been attributed to increased phosphorylation of the RyR by protein kinase A (PKA), Ca^{2+}/calmodulin-dependent protein kinase II (CaMKII), and decreased binding of the RyR stabilizing protein calstabin (FKBP12.6). Experimental studies suggest that PKA-dependent phosphorylation of the RyR may provoke Ca^{2+} leak by destabilizing the association between calstabin and FKB (see Chapter 46). Interestingly, in dogs, beta-adrenergic blockers prevent the development of Ca^{2+} leak by restoring RyR stabilization by FKBP12.6.[29] This observation has led to the suggestion that the increase in contractile function following treatment with beta blockers is secondary to RyR stabilization. The role of excess PKA-dependent RyR phosphorylation in the cause of HF appears somewhat paradoxical, in that the β-receptor is downregulated in HF. One current proposal is that there are microdomains in close proximity to the RyR where there is increased PKA phosphorylation and more cyclic adenosine monophosphate (cAMP) and decreased activity of the type 4 phosphodiesterase (PDE4D3).[30] In addition to its contribution to reduced SR Ca^{2+} content, increased leak seems to be relevant for arrhythmias in HF. This results from activation of NCX: Ca^{2+} leaking out of the SR activates NCX to remove Ca^{2+} from the cytosol in exchange of Na^+. Because NCX is electrogenic (3 Na^+ versus 1 Ca^{2+}), the increased influx of Na^+ results in a net inward current generating the so-called delayed afterdepolarizations (DADs), which serve as a trigger of arrhythmias. A recent study suggests that the increased leak may have a dominant role for the induction of ventricular arrhythmias and sudden cardiac death rather than for the development of contractile failure.[31]

Sarcoplasmic Reticulum Ca^{2+} Reuptake and Sarcolemmal Ca^{2+} Elimination

Relaxation of the contractile proteins occurs after dissociation of Ca^{2+} from troponin C and Ca^{2+} elimination from the cytosol. In the human heart, there are two main mechanisms responsible for elimination of Ca^{2+} from the cytosol: SR uptake of Ca^{2+} by the SERCA2a Ca^{2+} pump and transsarcolemmal Ca^{2+} elimination through NCX. Under normal conditions, approximately 75% of Ca^{2+} is taken up by the SR and 25% extruded from the cell through NCX. In HF there is decreased uptake of Ca^{2+} by the SR secondary to decreased SERCA2a protein levels and SERCA2a function. In addition, phosphorylation of phospholamban (PLB) is reduced in the failing heart, resulting in increased PLB-dependent inhibition of the SR Ca^{2+} pump.[32] In addition to PLB, the activity of SERCA is inhibited by the binding of small transmembrane micropeptides, myoregulin and dwarf open reading frame (DWORF), which lower the affinity of SERCA for Ca^{2+} and decrease the rate of Ca^{2+} reuptake into the SR.[33] The decrease of SR Ca^{2+} uptake in the failing heart results in a relative increase of transsarcolemmal Ca^{2+} elimination by the NCX, which is most likely secondary to increased expression of NCX protein. Restoring deficient SERCA2a by gene transfer has been shown to improve contractile function and restore electrical stability experimentally. However, the CUPID trial failed to show clinical benefit of SERCA2a gene transfer in patients with HF.[34] Although the increase in NCX activity may result in increased Ca^{2+} elimination from the myocyte, thereby preserving diastolic calcium levels and preventing diastolic dysfunction when SR calcium uptake is reduced, increased NCX activity may further reduce SR Ca^{2+} accumulation/content and may therefore reduce Ca^{2+} activation of contractile proteins. As noted, electrogenic NCX activity induces DADs and arrhythmias.

ALTERATIONS IN T-TUBULES

Cardiac excitation–contraction coupling occurs primarily at the sites of T-tubule/SR junctions (see Chapter 46). Organization of the T-tubule network is essential for coordinated excitation and synchronous activation of Ca^{2+} release from the SR. The L-type Ca^{2+} channels are located mainly on the T-tubule membrane in close proximity to RyRs on the SR. Studies have shown that there is extensive remodeling of the T-tubule system in experimental models of HF, as well as myocardial samples from failing human hearts.[35] T-tubule remodeling within cardiac myocytes leads to loss of coordinated Ca^{2+} release and contraction of ventricular cardiac myocytes, which could contribute to worsening LV dysfunction in HF. Junctophilin-2 (JP2) has been identified as an important protein that serves to bridge the physical gap between T-tubules and the SR, and thus is essential for maintaining EC coupling. Loss of JP2 expression has been demonstrated in failing human hearts and several HF models.[35]

Action Potential Duration and Sodium Handling

Several factors contribute to the prolongation of the action potential duration, which is a ubiquitous finding in failing hearts.[36] The transient outward potassium current (Ito) and the inward rectifier potassium current (Ik1) both are reduced in HF. In addition, the increased inward Na^+ current through the NCX and persistent activity of the sodium channel also may contribute to prolongation of the action potential.

The latter mechanism, also termed the "late sodium current," may be important in the pathogenesis of cardiac arrhythmias in HF. As discussed in Chapter 46, the voltage-gated Na⁺ channels are activated on depolarization of the cell membrane, leading to rapid influx of Na⁺ that is responsible for the fast upstroke of the action potential. Under normal conditions, Na⁺ channels inactivate a few milliseconds after depolarization. However, it is now recognized that some Na⁺ channels remain open (or reopen), leading to a small but persistent influx of Na⁺ throughout the plateau of the action potential, which generates a "late" sodium current (INa).[37] Late INa is sufficient to lead to a substantial influx of Na⁺ into the cell in HF, with consequent prolongation of the action potential and early afterdepolarizations (EADs), which may be a significant source of increased arrhythmias in HF. High levels of intracellular Na⁺ also may lead to cellular acidosis secondary to increased sodium-proton exchange activity. Increased intracellular Na⁺ also influences the electrogenic driving forces for the NCX, thereby reducing Ca²⁺ extrusion through the forward mode of the NCX, which when combined with reduced activity of the SERCA2a pump, may be a cause of the elevated diastolic cytosolic calcium levels and disturbed diastolic function in HF. Inhibition of the late Na⁺ current with the inhibitor ranolazine can improve disturbed diastolic function in isolated myocardium from failing human hearts and also may exhibit antiarrhythmic properties.[38] Of note, the different contributions to altered Ca²⁺ handling may vary significantly from patient to patient, which may explain some of the heterogeneity among different HF phenotypes. If SERCA2a expression is decreased and intracellular sodium is high, both systolic and diastolic function will be impaired. By contrast, higher NCX expression with moderately elevated intracellular Na⁺ will result in excess transsarcolemmal calcium elimination, and diastolic function will be preserved. However, this may be associated with increased arrhythmias secondary to increased NCX activity.

Abnormalities in Contractile and Regulatory Proteins

Early studies showed that the activity of myofibrillar ATPase was reduced in the hearts of patients who died of HF. Furthermore, reductions in the activity of myofibrillar ATPase, actomyosin ATPase, or myosin ATPase have been demonstrated in several animal models of HF. Subsequent studies showed that these abnormalities in ATPase activity could be explained by a shift to the fetal isoform of myosin heavy chain (MHC) in cardiac hypertrophy and failure. In rodents the predominant MHC is the "fast" V1 isoform (alpha-MHC [MYHC6]), which has high ATPase activity. With pressure-induced hypertrophy or after MI in rodents, re-expression of the "slow" V3 fetal isoform of MHC that has low ATPase activity (beta-MHC [MYHC7]) and decreased expression of the V1 isoform have been observed. Although translating this information to human HF proved to be more challenging, because the predominant MHC isoform in humans is the slower V3 isoform (MYHC7), polymerase chain reaction (PCR) techniques have shown that MYHC6 accounts for approximately 33% of MHC mRNA in normal human myocardium, whereas MYHC6 mRNA abundance decreases to approximately 2% in failing hearts. Furthermore, when myocardial biopsy was performed in patients receiving beta blockers, reciprocal changes were observed in the levels of MYHC6 (increase) and MYHC7 (decrease) mRNA, and an increase in the MYHC6/MYHC7 ratio was noted in those who demonstrated an improvement in LV function. However, these changes in myosin isoform shifts did not occur in HF patients who showed no improvement in LV function with beta blockers. Thus the decreased expression of MYHC6 may play a significant role in the pathophysiology of dilated cardiomyopathy (DCM).

Another important modification of contractile proteins that contributes to contractile dysfunction is proteolysis of the myofilaments themselves (myocytolysis). Myocardial biopsy samples from patients with advanced LV dysfunction show a significant reduction in the volume of myofibrils per cell, which may contribute to the development of cardiac decompensation.

Alterations in the expression and/or activity of myofilament regulatory proteins also have been proposed as a potential mechanism for the decrease in cardiac contractile function in HF (Table 47.3), including the myosin light chains, the troponin-tropomyosin complex, and titin. Changes in myosin light chain isoforms have been observed in the

TABLE 47.3 Changes in the Biology of the Failing Myocyte

PROTEIN	CHANGE IN HUMAN HEART FAILURE
Plasma Membrane	
L-type calcium channels	Decreased*,†
Sodium/calcium exchanger	Increased*,†
Sodium pump	Reexpression of fetal isoforms
Beta₁-adrenergic receptor	Decreased*,†
Beta₂-adrenergic receptor	Increased*
Alpha₁-adrenergic receptor	Increased*
Contractile Proteins	
Myosin heavy chain (MHC)	Reversion to fetal isoform (↓MYHC6/MYHC7)
Myosin light chain (MLC)	Reversion to fetal isoform
Actin	Normal*
Titin	Isoform switch (↑N2BA/N2B), hypophosphorylated
Troponin I	Normal*, hypo- and hyperphosphorylated‡
Troponin T	Isoform switch, hyperphosphorylated‡
Troponin C	Normal*
Tropomyosin	Normal*
Sarcoplasmic Reticulum	
SERCA2a	Decreased*,†
Phospholamban	Hypophosphorylated
Ryanodine receptor	Hyperphosphorylated†
Calsequestrin	Normal*
Calreticulin	Normal*

*Refers to protein level.
†Refers to functional activity.
‡Hyperphosphorylation results in decreased Ca²⁺ sensitivity.
Modified from Katz AM. *Physiology of the Heart*. Philadelphia: Lippincott Williams & Wilkins; 2001.

atria and ventricles of patients whose hearts have been subjected to mechanical overload. Although changes in the abundance and/or isoforms of troponins TnI and TnC have not been reported in HF, isoform shifts have been reported in TnT (see Chapter 46). In normal adult myocardium, TnT is expressed as a single isoform (cTnT3). In myocardium samples from patients with end-stage HF, however, both the fetal cTnT1 and the cTnT4 isoforms are expressed at increased levels, which might be expected to lead to a decrease in maximal active tension. Changes in the titin (*TTN*) isoform from N2B, which is expressed postnatally and is stiffer, to N2BA, the more distensible fetal isoform, have been associated with increased compliance in hearts from patients with HF. As discussed in Chapter 52, truncating variants in *TTN* are common, and are associated with 10% to 20% of cases of DCM depending upon cohort studied (Fig. 52.4).

Abnormalities in Cytoskeletal Proteins

The cytoskeleton of cardiac myocytes consists of actin, the intermediate filament desmin, the sarcomeric protein titin (see Chapter 46), and alpha- and beta-tubulin, which form the microtubules by polymerization. Vinculin, talin, dystrophin, and spectrin constitute a separate group of membrane-associated proteins. In numerous experimental studies, a role for cytoskeletal and membrane-associated proteins has been implicated in the pathogenesis of HF. In patients with DCM, titin is downregulated, and the cytoskeletal proteins desmin and membrane-associated proteins such as vinculin and dystrophin are upregulated. Proteolytic digestion of the dystrophin molecule has been identified as a possible reversible cause of HF. Loss of integrity of the cytoskeleton and its linkage of the sarcomere to the sarcolemma and ECM would be expected to lead to contractile dysfunction at the myocyte level, as well as at the myocardial level.

Beta-Adrenergic Desensitization

Ventricles obtained from HF patients demonstrate a marked reduction in beta-adrenergic receptor density, isoproterenol-mediated adenyl cyclase stimulation, and the contractile response to beta-adrenergic agonists.[39] The downregulation of beta-adrenergic receptors is likely mediated by increased levels of NE in the vicinity of the receptor. In patients with DCM, this reduction in receptor density involves primarily the beta1-receptor protein and mRNA and is proportional to the severity of HF. In contrast, the level of beta2-adrenergic receptor protein and mRNA are unchanged or increased. In addition, there are increases in the expression of beta-adrenergic receptor kinase 1 (βARK1, also called G protein–coupled receptor kinase 2 [GRK2]), a member of the family of GPCR kinases, in failing human hearts. As noted in Chapter 46, βARK phosphorylates the cytoplasmic loops of both beta1- and beta2-adrenergic receptors and increases the affinity of these receptors for a scaffolding protein termed beta-arrestin (see Fig. 46.14). The binding of beta-arrestins to the cytoplasmic tail of the beta receptor not only uncouples the receptor from heterotrimeric G proteins, but also targets the receptor for internalization in clathrin-coated vesicles. Although this internalization fosters receptor dephosphorylation and serves as a prelude to recycling the beta receptor to the surface for reactivation, at some point receptor entry via endocytosis is not followed by recycling, but rather leads to receptor trafficking to lysosomes and receptor degradation. Increased βARK (GRK2) activity may therefore contribute to the desensitization of both beta1 and beta2 receptors in patients with HF. Desensitization of the beta receptors can be both beneficial and deleterious in HF; by reducing LV contractility, desensitization may be deleterious. However, by reducing energy expenditure of the energy-starved myocardium and protecting the myocyte from the deleterious effects of sustained adrenergic stimulation, this adaptive response is beneficial. Interestingly, lymphocyte GRK2 protein levels were shown to be independent predictors of cardiovascular mortality in patients with HF and added prognostic and clinical value over demographic and clinical variables.[40]

Alterations in the Myocardium

The changes that occur in failing myocardium may be categorized broadly into those that occur in the volume of cardiac myocytes and those that occur in the volume and composition of the ECM. For changes in the myocyte component of the myocardium, increasing evidence suggests that progressive myocyte loss, through necrotic, apoptotic, or cell death pathways linked to autophagy, may contribute to progressive cardiac dysfunction and LV remodeling.

NECROSIS

Although necrosis initially was thought to be a "passive" form of cell death, emerging evidence indicates that necrotic cell death also is "regulated."[41] The relative proportion of unregulated versus regulated necrotic death in the heart is not currently known; however, regulated necrosis is an important component of MI, HF, and cerebrovascular accident (stroke). The hallmark features of necrosis are loss of plasma membrane integrity and depletion of cellular adenosine triphosphate (ATP). Dysfunction of the plasma membrane in necrotic cells leads to cell swelling and rupture. There is also swelling of organelles such as the mitochondria. In the heart, increased plasma membrane permeability allows Ca^{2+} to leak into the cell, exposing the contractile proteins to very high concentrations of this activator, which in turn initiates extreme interactions between the myofilaments (contraction bands), further contributing to disruption of the cellular membrane. Necrotic myocyte death occurs in ischemic heart disease, myocardial injury, toxin exposure (e.g., daunorubicin; see Chapter 56), infection, and inflammation. Neurohormonal activation also can lead to necrotic cell death. For example, concentrations of NE available within myocardial tissue, as well as circulating levels in patients with advanced HF, are sufficient to provoke myocyte necrosis in experimental model systems. Moreover, excessive stimulation with angiotensin II, ET, or TNF has been shown to provoke myocyte necrosis in experimental models.

In contrast with apoptosis, the rupture of cell membranes with cell necrosis releases intracellular contents, which include the release of so-called danger-associated molecular patterns (DAMPs) that are sufficient to evoke an intense inflammatory reaction, leading to the influx of granulocytes, macrophages, and collagen-secreting fibroblasts into the area of injury. The final result is a fibrotic scar, which may alter the structural and functional properties of the myocardium.[42] The regulated cell death pathways that have been studied thus far include TNF signaling through the type 1 TNF receptor (TNFR1) and opening of the mitochondrial permeability transition pore (MPTP) in the inner mitochondrial membrane, resulting in loss of the electrical potential difference ($\Delta\Psi m$) across the inner mitochondrial membrane, leading to ATP depletion.

APOPTOSIS

Apoptosis, or programmed cell death, is an evolutionarily conserved process that allows multicellular organisms to selectively remove cells through a highly regulated program of cell suicide. Apoptosis is mediated by two pathways. The extrinsic pathway uses cell surface receptors, whereas the intrinsic pathway involves the mitochondria and endoplasmic reticulum (ER), and each of these pathways leads to caspase activation. In addition, connections between the pathways amplify signals, increasing the efficiency of killing. The intrinsic pathway is responsible for transducing most apoptotic stimuli, including those caused by inadequate nutrients or survival factors, hypoxia, oxidative stress, nutrient stress, proteotoxic stress, DNA damage, and chemical and physical toxins. These stimuli ultimately converge at the mitochondria to trigger the release of apoptogenic proteins, such as cytochrome c, and at the ER to stimulate the release of luminal Ca^{2+}.[43] Apoptosis plays important roles in development and in postnatal life, when it is critical for tissue homeostasis and surveillance for damaged or transformed cells. However, under pathologic circumstances, such as acute ischemia and in DCM, the apoptotic program can be triggered inappropriately, resulting in inadvertent cell death that can lead to organ failure. In contrast with the cell swelling that characterizes necrosis, during apoptosis the cell shrinks and eventually breaks up into small, membrane-surrounded fragments. The latter often contain bits of condensed chromatin referred to as *apoptotic bodies*. Maintenance of plasma membrane integrity until late in the apoptotic process allows the dying cell to be engulfed by macrophages, which prevents the release of the reactive intracellular contents, thereby preventing an inflammatory reaction.

Cardiac myocyte apoptosis has been shown to occur in failing human hearts.[44] Indeed, many of the factors implicated in the pathogenesis of HF, including catecholamines acting through beta$_1$-adrenergic receptor, angiotensin II, ROS including NO, inflammatory cytokines (e.g., TNF), and mechanical strain, have been shown to trigger apoptosis in vitro. Moreover, activation of either the extrinsic or the intrinsic cell death pathway provokes progressive LV dilation and decompensation in transgenic mice.[45] Nonetheless, the exact physiologic significance and consequence(s) of apoptosis in human HF have been difficult to determine because of the uncertainty about the actual rate of cardiac myocyte apoptosis in the failing human heart.[44] The aggregate clinical and experimental data, however, suggest that apoptosis is likely to play an important role in HF.

AUTOPHAGY

Autophagy refers to the homeostatic cellular process of sequestering organelles, proteins, and lipids in a double-membrane vesicle inside the cell (autophagosome), where the contents are subsequently delivered to the lysosome for degradation. Unlike necrosis and apoptosis, autophagy is primarily a survival mechanism that regulates the quality and abundance of intracellular proteins and organelles. In mammalian cells, autophagy serves two physiologic purposes: one is to continuously degrade intracellular proteins at low levels, referred to as "basal or constitutive autophagy," which is responsible for clearance of excess or damaged organelles thereby maintaining the quality of essential intracellular components. The second purpose is to supply amino acids that are requisite for cell survival during conditions of environmental stress (e.g., nutrient deprivation), referred to as "adaptive autophagy." Prior studies have established a critical role for basal autophagy in the heart.[46] Accumulation of autophagosomes and autophagic substrates are increased in human HF.[47] Insufficient autophagy in the heart can lead to shortage of properly functioning intracellular organelles; moreover, accumulation of damaged mitochondria and damaged proteins can lead, respectively, to increased oxidative stress and increased ER stress. Autophagy can also induce cell death with distinctive morphologic characteristics and mechanisms of regulation, referred to as autosis.[48] Autosis has several unique morphologic features that differentiate it from necrosis and apoptosis, including increased autophagosomes/autolysosomes, as well as focal swelling of the perinuclear space at late stages. Experimental studies have shown that autosis contributes to cardiac myocyte cell death and increased myocardial injury following ischemia reperfusion injury in the heart.[48] Of note autosis is inhibited by in vitro and in vivo by Na+,K+-ATPase antagonists, such as cardiac glycosides. The role of autosis in the pathogenesis of HF remains to be determined.

Although the distinction between necrosis and apoptosis is apparent in certain circumstances, it often is less clear in the failing heart. Indeed, similar mechanisms can operate in both types of cell death. Thus, instead of the existence of distinct types of cell death in HF, a more likely scenario is a continuum of cell death responses that contribute to progressive myocyte loss and disease progression.

Alterations in the ECM constitute the second important myocardial adaptation that occurs during cardiac remodeling. The myocardial ECM consists of a basement membrane, a fibrillar collagen network that surrounds the myocytes, proteoglycans and glycosaminoglycans, and specialized proteins such as matricellular proteins. The major fibrillar collagens in the heart are types I and III, with a type I/III ratio of approximately 1.3:1 to 1.9:1. The organization of myocardial fibrillar type I and type III collagen ensures the structural integrity of adjoining myocytes and is essential for maintaining alignment of myofibrils within the myocyte through the interaction of collagen and integrins and the cytoskeletal proteins (Fig. 47.11A). *Matricellular proteins* are a class of nonstructural ECM proteins exerting regulatory functions, most likely through their interactions with cell surface receptors, the structural proteins, and soluble extracellular factors such as growth factors and cytokines. *Osteopontin* (OPN [Eta-1]) is a matricellular protein that is expressed in various cell types, including cardiac myocytes and fibroblasts and myofibroblasts (Fig. 47.11B). Because of its localization and molecular properties, OPN is likely to be involved in the communication between the ECM and cardiac myocytes, which implies a role in cardiac remodeling after hemodynamic overloading. OPN is markedly upregulated in animal models of cardiac hypertrophy and failure and myocardial ischemia and in the hearts of patients with DCM. OPN is elevated in the peripheral circulation of patients in direct relation to HF disease severity.[49]

During cardiac remodeling, important alterations in the ECM include changes in fibrillar collagen synthesis and degradation (Fig. 47.12) and in the degree of collagen cross-linking, as well as loss of collagen struts that connect the individual cardiac myocytes. Markers of collagen turnover have been shown to be increased in patients with DCM compared with age-matched controls.[50] In patients with idiopathic or ischemic DCM, serum N-terminal peptide type III collagen propeptide (PIIINP) levels have been shown to be independent predictors of mortality.[51] In the RALES trial (see Chapter 50), serum C-terminal peptide type I collagen propeptide (PIP) and PIIINP were decreased in the spironolactone-treated patients but not in the placebo group, suggesting that aldosterone may play an important role in ECM synthesis. Moreover, it is becoming increasingly apparent that the three-dimensional organization of the ECM plays an important role in regulating cardiac structure and function in HF.

CARDIAC FIBROBLASTS AND MAST CELLS

The cardiac fibroblast, which accounts for almost 90% of nonmyocyte cells in the heart, is the primary cell type that is responsible for the secretion of a majority of ECM components in the heart, such as collagens I, III, and IV and laminin and fibronectin. In response to mechanical stress and neurohormonal activation and inflammation, a subset of fibroblasts undergoes phenotypic conversion to myofibroblasts that are characterized by increased expression of α-smooth muscle actin and enhanced secretory activity. Recent studies have shown that myofibroblasts, which are responsible for the collagen secretion and contraction/realignment of the nascent collagen fibers, arise from tissue-resident fibroblasts that become activated after tissue injury.[52] Myofibroblasts migrate into the area surrounding tissue and play an important role in the final scar formation. Cardiac myofibroblasts also may regulate the phenotype of cardiac myocytes through multiple paracrine signaling pathways (Fig. 47.11B). Several lines of evidence suggest that cardiac fibroblasts and myocytes release proteins that regulate neighboring cells.[53] The proteins that have been implicated thus far include transforming growth factor-β1 (TGF-β1), fibroblast growth factor-2 (FGF2), members of the IL-6 family, and the recently discovered cytokine IL-33. Increasing evidence also suggests that mast cells, which are bone marrow–derived cells that "home" to and reside in the myocardium, also play an important role in remodeling of the

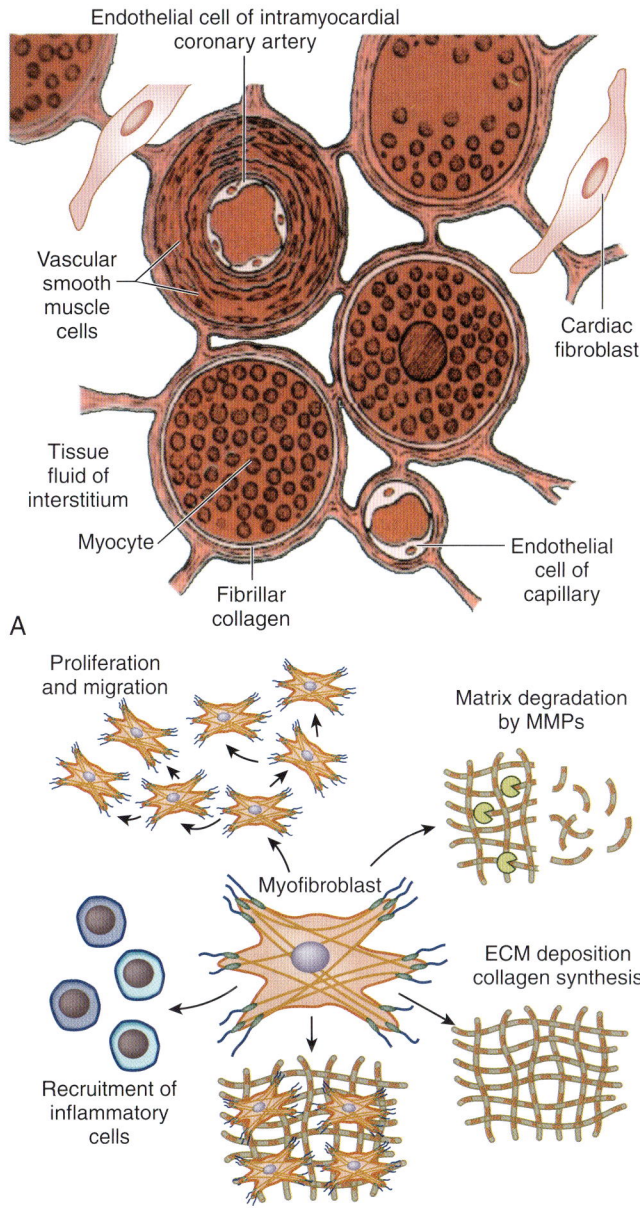

FIGURE 47.11 Extracellular matrix in heart failure. **A,** Although myocytes are the major components of heart on the basis of mass, they represent only a minority on the basis of number. Nonmyocyte cellular constituents of the myocardium include fibroblasts, smooth muscle cells, and endothelial cells. Myocytes and nonmyocytes are interconnected by a complex of connective tissue and extracellular matrix (ECM). Components of ECM include collagens, proteoglycans, glycoproteins (e.g., fibronectin), several peptide growth factors, and proteases (e.g., plasminogen activators) and collagenases (e.g., matrix metalloproteinases [MMPs]). **B,** Interactions among cardiac fibroblasts, myocytes, and ECM. In response to biomechanical stress, peptide growth factors in ECM and adjacent cardiac fibroblasts release an ensemble of peptide growth factors that activate hypertrophic signaling pathways in cardiac myocytes. Activated cardiac myofibroblasts express elevated levels of various proinflammatory and profibrotic factors that directly contribute to inflammatory cell infiltration and fibroblast proliferation, secrete high levels of MMPs and other ECM-degrading enzymes that facilitate fibroblast migration, and contribute to the deposition of collagen and other ECM proteins, leading to scar formation. (**A** modified from Weber KT, Brilla CG. Pathological hypertrophy and cardiac interstitium. *Circulation.* 1991;83:1849; **B** from Travers JG, Kamal FA, Robbins J, et al. Cardiac fibrosis: the fibroblast awakens. *Circ Res.* 2016;118:1021–1240. Copyright 2016 American Heart Association.)

ECM. Myocardial mast cells are located mainly around blood vessels and between myocytes, where they are capable of releasing profibrotic cytokines and growth factors that influence ECM remodeling. In experimental studies, mast cells that are recruited to the heart during inflammation were responsible for TGF-β1–mediated fibroblast activation, myocardial fibrosis, and LV diastolic dysfunction.[54]

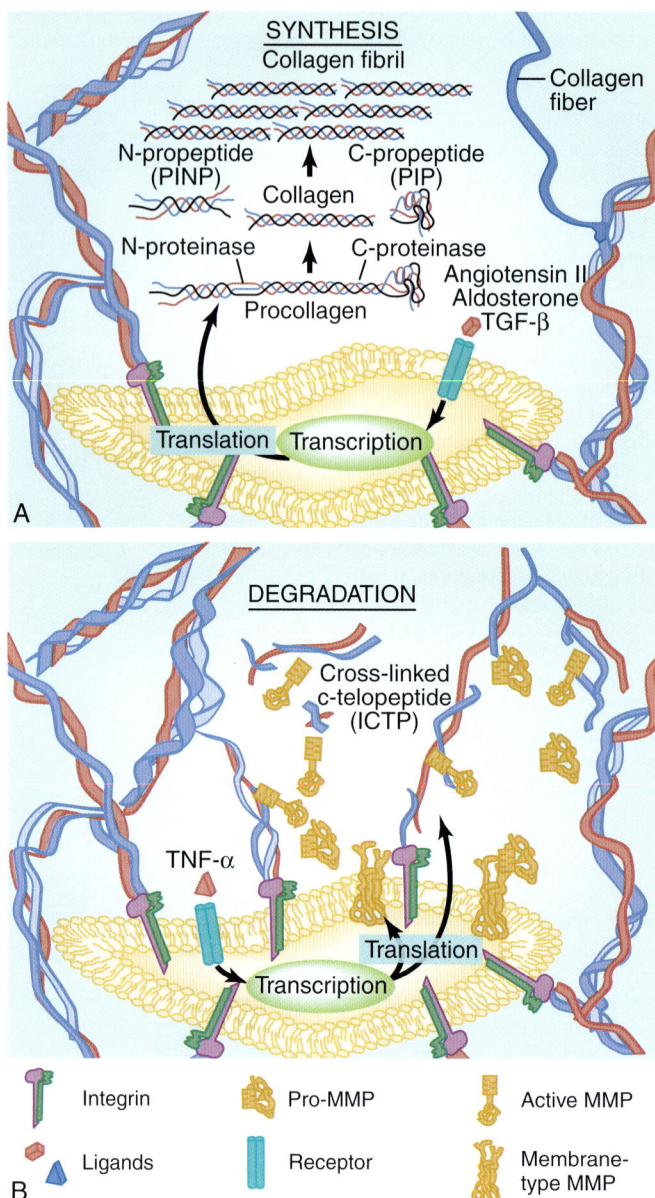

FIGURE 47.12 Collagen synthesis and degradation. **A,** Intracellular signals generated by neurohormonal and/or mechanical stimulation of cardiac fibroblasts results in transcription and translation of nascent collagen proteins containing amino terminal (N-terminal) and carboxyl terminal (C-terminal) propeptides that prevent collagen from assembling into mature fibrils. Once secreted into the interstitium, these propeptides are cleaved by N- and C-proteinases, yielding two procollagen fragments and a mature triple-stranded collagen molecule. In the case of collagen type I, these propeptides are referred to as N-terminal peptide type I collagen propeptide (PINP) and C-terminal peptide type I collagen propeptide (PIP). Removal of the propeptide sequences allows the secreted collagen molecule to integrate into growing collagen fibrils, which can then further assemble into collagen fibers. After the collagen fibrils form in the extracellular space, their tensile strength is greatly strengthened by the formation of covalent cross-links between the lysine residues on the collagen molecules. **B,** The degradation of the collagen matrix within the myocardium entails a number of biochemical events involving several protease systems. Degradation of collagen fibrils occurs through catalytic cleavage of the three collagen alpha chains at a single locus by interstitial collagenase, yielding 36-kDa and 12-kDa collagen telopeptides that maintain their helical structure and thus are resistant to further proteolytic degradation. The large 36-kDa telopeptide spontaneously denatures into nonhelical gelatin derivatives, which in turn are completely degraded by interstitial gelatinases. The small 12-kDa pyridinoline cross-linked C-terminal telopeptide resulting from the cleavage of collagen type I (ICTP) is found intact in blood, where it appears to be derived from tissues, with a stoichiometric ratio of 1:1 between the number of collagen type I molecules degraded and that of ICTP released. (From Deschamps AM, Spinale FG. Extracellular matrix. In: Walsh RA, ed. *Molecular Mechanisms of Cardiac Hypertrophy and Failure.* Boca Raton, FL: Taylor & Francis; 2005:101–116.)

As noted earlier, one of the histologic signatures of advancing HF is the progressive increase in collagen content of the heart (myocardial fibrosis). Studies in failing human myocardium have shown a quantitative increase in collagen types I, III, VI, and IV, along with fibronectin, laminin, and vimentin, and a decrease in the type I/III collagen ratio in patients with ischemic cardiomyopathy. Moreover, clinical studies show a progressive loss of cross-linking of collagen in the failing heart, as well as loss of connectivity of the collagen network with individual myocytes, which would be expected to result in profound alterations in LV structure and function. Furthermore, loss of cross-linking of the fibrillar collagen has been associated with progressive LV dilation after myocardial injury. The accumulation of collagen can occur on a "reactive" basis around intramural coronary arteries and arterioles (perivascular fibrosis) or in the interstitial space (interstitial fibrosis) and does not require myocyte cell death. Alternatively, collagen accumulation can occur as a result of microscopic scarring, which develops in response to cardiac myocyte cell death. This scarring or "replacement fibrosis" is an adaptation to the loss of parenchyma and is therefore critical to preserve the structural integrity of the heart. The increased fibrous tissue would be expected to lead to increased myocardial stiffness, which presumably would result in decreased myocardial shortening for a given degree of afterload. In addition, myocardial fibrosis may provide the structural substrate for atrial and ventricular arrhythmias, thus potentially contributing to inhomogeneous activation, bundle branch block, and dyssynchrony, as well as sudden death (see Chapter 70). Although the full complement of molecules responsible for fibroblast activation is not known, many of the classic neurohormones (e.g., angiotensin II, aldosterone) and cytokines (ET, TGF-β, cardiotrophin-1) that are expressed in HF are sufficient to provoke fibroblast activation. Studies in patients with aortic valve replacement for aortic stenosis have shown that the baseline burden of myocardial fibrosis was associated with worse LV function, a greater degree of pathologic LV remodeling, and more pronounced HF symptoms. Moreover, burden of myocardial fibrosis was an independent predictor of all-cause and cardiovascular mortality after transcatheter aortic valve implantation.[55] Indeed, the use of ACE inhibitors, beta blockers, and aldosterone receptor antagonists has been associated with a decrease in myocardial fibrosis in experimental HF models and in human HF.[56]

Although the fibrillar collagen matrix initially was thought to form a relatively static complex, it is now recognized that these structural proteins can undergo rapid turnover. A major development in understanding the pathogenesis of cardiac remodeling was the discovery that a family of collagenolytic enzymes, the *matrix metalloproteinases*, is activated within the failing myocardium. Conceptually, ECM disruption would be expected to lead to LV dilation and wall thinning as a result of mural realignment of myocyte bundles and within the LV wall, as well as LV dysfunction as a result of dyssynchronous contraction of the left ventricle. Although the precise biochemical triggers responsible for activation of MMPs are not known, TNF and other cytokines and peptide growth factors expressed within the failing myocardium are capable of activating MMPs.

However, the biology of matrix remodeling in HF is likely to be much more complex than the simple presence or absence of MMP activation because degradation of the matrix also is controlled by glycoproteins termed *tissue inhibitors of matrix metalloproteinases (TIMPs)*. TIMPs are capable of regulating the activation of MMPs by binding to and preventing these enzymes from degrading the collagen matrix of the heart. The TIMP family at present consists of four distinct members, TIMP-1, -2, -3, and -4, each of which is constitutively expressed in the heart by fibroblasts as well as myocytes. TIMPs are secreted proteins that act as the natural inhibitors of active forms of all MMPs, although the efficiency of MMP inhibition varies among the different members. The extant literature suggests that MMP activation can lead to progressive LV dilation, whereas TIMP expression favors progressive myocardial fibrosis.

NONCODING RNAS

Once considered "transcriptional noise," noncoding RNAs have emerged as potential biomarkers as well as therapeutic targets in HF. The noncoding portion of the genome is actively transcribed, generating thousands of regulatory short and long noncoding RNAs that are capable of regulating gene networks. Noncoding RNAs are classified based on their length. Small noncoding RNAs are less than 200 nucleotides in size and include both small interfering RNAs (siRNAs) and microRNAs (miRNAs). Transcripts larger than 200 nucleotides are called long noncoding RNAs (lncRNAs). MicroRNAs are involved in virtually all cellular processes. The lncRNAs also regulate gene and protein levels but through more complicated and diverse mechanisms.

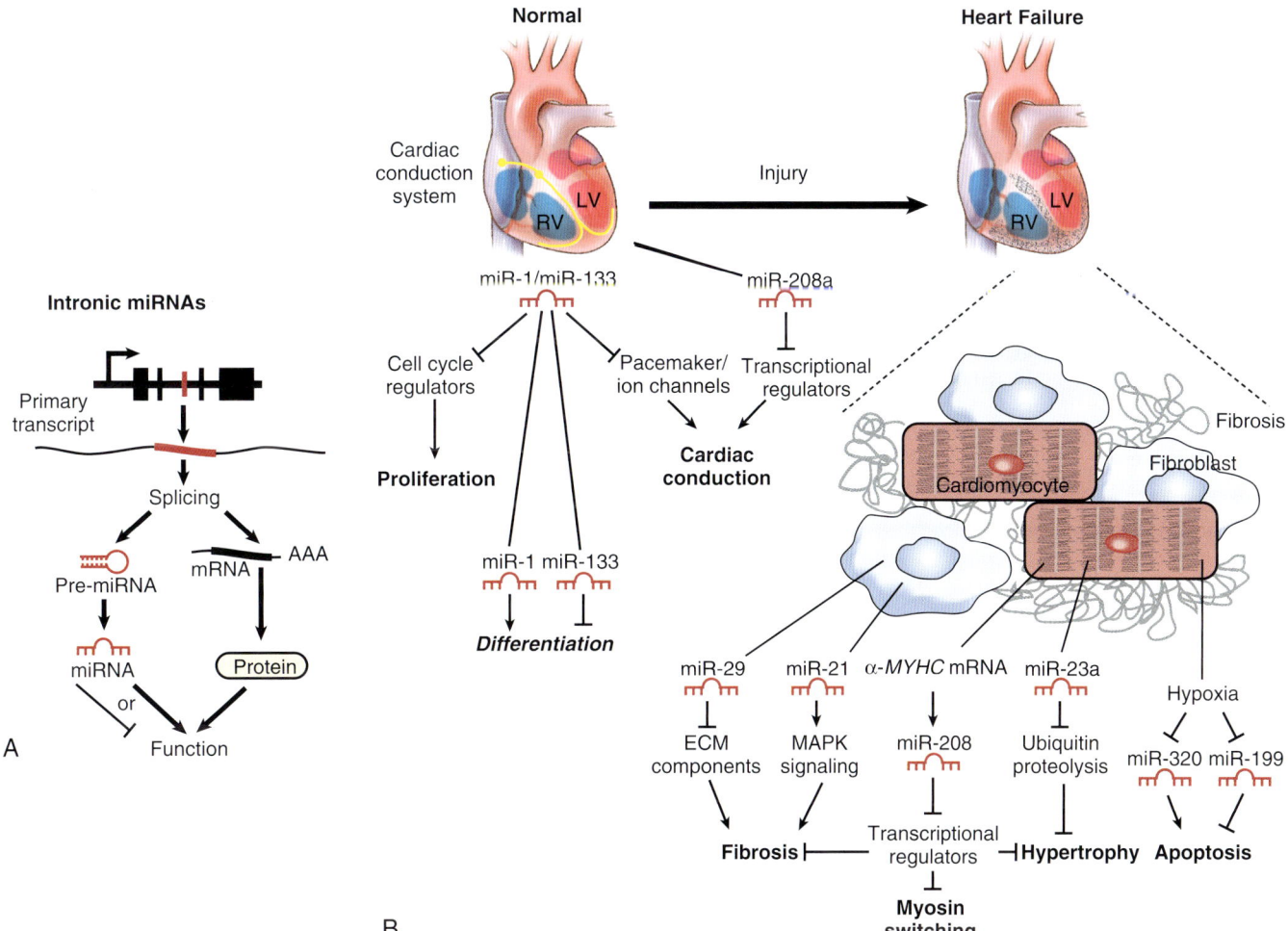

FIGURE 47.13 MicroRNAs (miRNAs) and the heart. **A,** The potential modes of miRNA-based regulation of gene expression are illustrated. Intronic microRNAs are encoded within an intron of a host gene. Messenger RNA splicing generates a protein coding transcript and a microRNA stem-loop. A common mechanism of miRNA function involves the modest repression of several mRNAs in a common biologic process by a single miRNA, most commonly through transcriptional silencing, or through enhanced mRNA degradation. Intronic miRNAs often regulate similar processes to that of the protein encoded by the host gene. *AAA,* Polyadenylated tail of the transcript; pre-miRNA, precursor miRNA. **B,** Functional role of miRNAs in the normal and failing heart. A normal heart and a hypertrophic/failing heart are shown in schematic form, depicting miRNAs that contribute to normal function or pathologic remodeling. All *arrows* denote the normal action of each component or process. The miRNAs miR-1 and miR-133 are involved in the development of a normal heart **(left)** by regulating proliferation, differentiation, and cardiac conduction. After cardiac injury **(right),** various miRNAs contribute to pathologic remodeling and the progression to heart failure: miR-29 blocks fibrosis by inhibiting the expression of extracellular matrix (ECM) components, whereas miR-21 promotes fibrosis; miR-208 controls myosin isoform switching, cardiac hypertrophy, and fibrosis; and miR-23a promotes cardiac hypertrophy by inhibiting ubiquitin proteolysis, which itself inhibits hypertrophy. Hypoxia results in the repression of miR-320 and miR-199, which promote and block apoptosis, respectively. (Modified from Small EM, Olson EN. Pervasive roles of microRNAs in cardiovascular biology. *Nature.* 2011;469:336.)

Experimental studies have shown that microRNAs have a profound effect on cardiac remodeling. MicroRNAs are noncoding RNAs that pair with specific "target" mRNAs and negatively regulate their expression through translational repression or mRNA degradation (gene silencing). The binding specificity of microRNAs depends on complementary base pairing of the approximately 6 nucleotide (nt) region at the 5′ end of the microRNA with the 3′ untranslated region (UTR) of the corresponding mRNA target. As shown in Figure 47.13A, binding of microRNAs to their cognate target mRNAs typically leads to decreased expression of target genes. Individual microRNAs modulate the expression of collections of mRNA targets that often have related functions, thereby governing complex biologic processes. Recent studies have suggested that microRNAs contribute to adverse or pathologic remodeling in experimental HF models.[57] As shown in Figure 47.13B, microRNAs regulate key components of the remodeling process, including cardiac myocyte biology, cell fate, ECM remodeling, and neurohormonal activation. Given that microRNAs are coordinately upregulated in response to stress signals, and that microRNAs regulate the expression levels of gene networks that determine the "heart failure phenotype," it is tempting to speculate that microRNAs, acting singly or in combination, may be responsible for modulating the transition from adaptive to pathologic cardiac remodeling. Moreover, it is possible that certain microRNAs may themselves become therapeutic targets using chemically modified oligonucleotides to target specific microRNAs and disrupt the binding between a specific microRNA and a specific mRNA target[57] Long noncoding RNAs are mechanistically more complex than microRNAs and likely modulate the genome at multiple different levels. For example, lncRNAs may interact with RNAs, proteins, and DNA and can either activate or silence the interaction with other molecules through conformational switching. Recent studies have shown that the profile of myocardial lncRNAs is altered in human HF, and that several lncRNAs are responsible for regulating cardiac structure and function following hemodynamic overload.[58] Inhibition of miR132, a non-coding microRNA that regulates cardiac hypertrophy and autophagy in cardiac myocytes using a synthetic locked nucleic acid antisense oligonucleotide inhibitor (antimiR-132 [CDR132L]), was shown to dose-dependently improve LV function in a large animal model of ischemic injury.[59] CDR132L has been shown to be safe in a phase I safety study in patients with NYHA class I-III HF (NCT04045405), and will be studied in a forthcoming phase II clinical trial in patients with acute myocardial infarction.

Alterations in Left Ventricular Structure

The alterations in the biology of the failing myocyte, as well as in the failing myocardium, are largely responsible for the progressive LV dilation and dysfunction that occur during cardiac remodeling. Many of the structural changes that accompany LV remodeling may contribute to worsening HF. Indeed, one of the first observations regarding the abnormal geometry of remodeled ventricle was the consistent finding that the remodeled heart was not only larger but also more spherical in shape. An important point in this context is that a change in LV shape from a prolate ellipse to a more spherical shape results in an increase in meridional wall stress of the left ventricle, thereby creating a de novo energetic burden for the failing heart. Because the load on the ventricle at end-diastole contributes importantly to the afterload on the ventricle at the onset of systole, LV dilation itself will increase mechanical energy expenditure of the ventricle, which exacerbates the underlying problems with energy utilization in the failing ventricle (Fig. 47.14).

CARDIAC ENERGETICS AND MITOCHONDRIAL BIOLOGY

Energy transfer in the cardiac myocyte occurs in three stages: uptake and metabolism, energy production through oxidative phosphorylation, and energy transfer by means of the creatine kinase (CK) shuttle. Each stage of this process can lead to contractile dysfunction of the heart. Studies in patients with end-stage cardiomyopathy have shown that myocardial ATP concentration, the total adenine nucleotide pool (ATP, ADP, and AMP), CK activity (required for synthesis of ATP), creatine phosphate (CrP) concentration, and CrP/ATP ratio are all decreased in HF. In addition, decreased levels of creatine phosphokinase have been reported, which would slow phosphocreatine shuttle, further exacerbating energy utilization in the failing heart.[60] Thus, in the failing heart, key components of the cardiac energetic system are downregulated. It is unclear at present, however, whether these energetic changes are biomarkers or drivers of LV dysfunction.

Although several mechanisms have been proposed to explain the fall in ATP content in HF, one mechanism that has received considerable attention relates to changes in substrate utilization in HF. Under normal conditions, the adult heart derives most of its energy through oxidation of fatty acids in mitochondria. The genes involved in this key energy metabolic pathway are transcriptionally regulated by members of the nuclear receptor superfamily, specifically the fatty acid–activated peroxisome proliferator–activated receptors (PPARs) and the nuclear receptor coactivator, PPAR-gamma coactivator-1α (PGC-1α). In experimental HF models, an initial decrease is seen in the oxidation of fatty acids secondary to downregulation of fatty acid–metabolizing genes, with a resultant shift toward glycolytic metabolism. Recent studies indicate that enhanced myocardial ketone use may be adaptive in HF; moreover, provisional studies in experimental models of HF and humans with HF have suggested a role for exogenous ketone therapy.[61] These observations have given rise to the suggestion that metabolic modulation may be beneficial in HF. Trimetazidine, which is a direct inhibitor of myocardial fatty acid oxidation has been approved for human use for the treatment of angina pectoris and myocardial ischemia. Clinical trials and several meta-analyses have shown that when trimetazidine is added to conventional HF therapy, it leads to improvements in NYHA functional class, LV end-systolic volume, and LV ejection fraction.[62] Trimetazidine is recommended in the ESC/HFA 2016 guidelines for the treatment of angina pectoris not responsive to beta blocker in HFrEF patients (class IIb, level of evidence A). There is no recommendation for trimetazidine in the setting of HF alone.[63]

In addition to loss of substrate, ATP generation may be impaired in the failing heart secondary to abnormalities in mitochondrial dynamics.[64] The number of mitochondria are determined through biogenic renewal and by autophagic removal (mitophagy). Studies in yeast have demonstrated that maintaining normal mitochondrial morphology and function depends on the dynamic balance of mitochondrial *fusion* and *fission* (division), collectively called "mitochondrial dynamics." The balance between mitochondrial fusion and fission determines the number, morphology, and activity of mitochondria in the heart. Fusion and fission modulate multiple mitochondrial functions, ranging from energy and ROS production to Ca^{2+} homeostasis and cell death through apoptosis programmed necrosis. Although studies in human HF are limited, data suggest that mitochondrial fusion may be reduced, which would be predicted to lead to reduced O_2 consumption and alterations in mitochondrial metabolism. Of note, abnormally small and fragmented mitochondria have been observed in end-stage DCM, myocardial hibernation, and congenital heart disease, suggesting that mitochondrial fusion/fission becomes dysregulated in cardiac disease. However, the contribution of abnormalities in mitochondrial fission/fusion in HF as a cause versus a consequence of myocardial injury remains unknown. The phase II PROGRESS-HF clinical trial, which was a randomized trial that used a mitochondrial-targeting protein (elamipretide) that enhances mitochondrial ATP synthesis and prevents mitochondrial fragmentation, did not improve LV function at 4 weeks in patients with stable HFrEF when compared with placebo.[65]

LV wall thinning also occurs as the ventricle begins to dilate and remodel. The increase in wall thinning along with the increase in afterload created by LV dilation leads to a functional "afterload mismatch" that may further contribute to a decrease in forward cardiac output. Increased LV wall stress also can lead to sustained expression of stretch-activated genes (angiotensin II, ET, TNF) and stretch activation of hypertrophic signaling pathways. Moreover, the high end-diastolic wall stress might be expected to lead to episodic hypoperfusion of the subendocardium with resultant worsening of LV function, as well as increased oxidative stress, with the resultant activation of gene families that are sensitive to free radical generation (e.g., TNF, IL-1β). Another important mechanical problem from progressive LV dilation is that the papillary muscles are pulled apart, resulting in incompetence of the mitral valve and development of "functional mitral regurgitation." In addition to the loss of forward blood flow, mitral regurgitation results in further hemodynamic volume overloading of the ventricle. Together, the mechanical burdens engendered by LV remodeling might lead to increased LV dilation, decreased forward cardiac output, and increased hemodynamic overloading (see Fig. 47.14), any of which is sufficient to contribute to worsening LV function independent of the patient's neurohormonal status.

REVERSIBILITY OF LEFT VENTRICULAR REMODELING AND RECOVERY OF LEFT VENTRICULAR FUNCTION

Clinical studies have shown that medical and device therapies that reduce HF morbidity and mortality also lead to decreased LV volume and mass and restore a more normal elliptical shape to the ventricle. These salutary changes represent the summation of a series of integrated biologic changes in cardiac myocyte size and function,

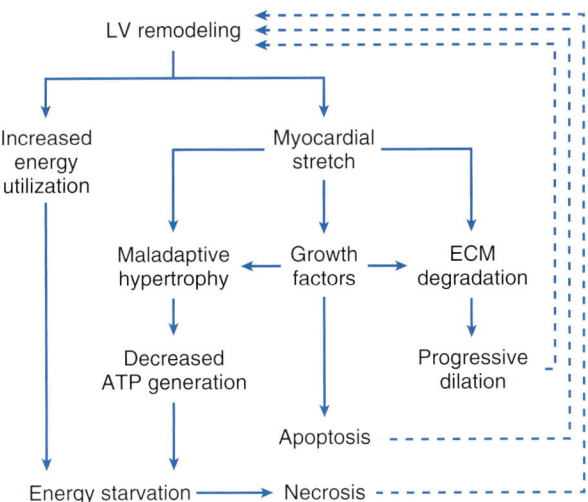

FIGURE 47.14 Self-amplifying nature of left ventricular (LV) remodeling. LV remodeling results in increased afterload on the heart, which increases energy utilization and further stimulates cardiac growth through stretch-mediated activation of growth factors. The former contributes directly to a state of energy starvation, whereas the latter contributes to further cardiac remodeling, including increased myocyte hypertrophy and further matrix remodeling. The sustained activation of growth stimuli also promotes apoptosis and myocardial fibrosis, which contribute to LV dysfunction and LV remodeling. (Modified from Katz AM. *Heart failure*. Philadelphia: Lippincott Williams & Wilkins; 2000.)

as well as modifications in LV structure and organization that are accompanied by shifts of the LV end-diastolic pressure-volume relationship toward normal. For want of better terminology, these changes are collectively referred to as "reverse LV remodeling." In the context of the present discussion, reverse LV remodeling refers to the restoration of more normal cardiac myocyte size and LV chamber geometry, resulting in a leftward shift of the end-diastolic pressure volume relationship toward normal values.[66] Importantly, reverse LV remodeling is associated with improved myocyte contractility and improved LV chamber contractility. It is important to recognize that reverse LV remodeling is associated with fewer HF hospitalizations and decreased cardiovascular mortality, and that there is a direct correlation between the extent of reverse LV remodeling and the improvement in cardiac survival.[66] Insofar as the calculation of LV ejection fraction incorporates LV end-diastolic volume in the denominator of the equation, decreases in LV end-diastolic volume are associated with a reciprocal increase in LV ejection fraction.

Although the biological basis for reverse LV remodeling and recovery of LV function is incompletely understood, several general concepts have emerged. The most prominent theme is that cardiac remodeling is a dynamic process that occurs in a bidirectional manner (i.e. forward and reverse), and that cardiac remodeling involves the coordinated regulation of multiple molecular and cellular changes that contribute to phenotypic changes in the size, shape, and function of the heart. Basic and clinical studies have consistently shown that many of the cellular and anatomic changes that occur during forward LV remodeling revert toward the normal less pathologic phenotype during reverse LV remodeling. Moreover, studies that have examined serial changes in gene expression during reverse LV remodeling have shown the normalization of gene transcription related to myocyte contractility occur before changes in genes related to the ECM, suggesting that return of myocyte function is required for reversal of the changes in LV geometry in the failing heart.[67] In addition to changes in adult cardiac myocytes during reverse LV remodeling, there are a number of important changes that occur within the myocardial ECM.[68] A second important theme, which has direct bearing on the concept of myocardial remission (discussed below), is that many of the multilevel molecular changes that occur during forward LV remodeling remain dysregulated in reverse remodeled hearts, despite improvements in structural and functional abnormalities. Transcriptional profiling of reverse remodeled hearts reveals the emergence of new sets of genes that belong to ontogenies that are not expressed in non-failing hearts.[69] Viewed together, these findings suggest that reverse LV remodeling is not simply a mirror image of the molecular and cellular pathways that become dysregulated during forward LV remodeling, but rather that reverse LV remodeling represents a coordinated multilevel process that allows the heart to adopt a new, less pathologic steady state that is associated with improved pump function and improved clinical prognosis.

Interestingly, in recognized subsets of patients, the heart undergoes reverse LV remodeling with recovery of LV function either spontaneously or after medical and device therapies or valve replacement. The recognition that LV ejection fraction improves substantially in a subset of HFrEF patients who are treated with evidenced-based medical and device therapies has led to intense interest in their outcomes and clinical management (discussed in Chapter 48).

Importantly, the subsequent clinical course of these patients is associated with fewer future HF events.[66] Recent studies have shown that, even among patients who experience complete normalization of LV function and LV structure after implementation of guideline directed medical therapies, a significant proportion of patients with a recovered LV ejection will develop recurrent LV dysfunction and recurrent HF events. The biological explanation for why some HFrecEF patients become stable clinically for prolonged periods ("myocardial remission"),[66] and why some HFrecEF patients, with similar improvements in LV structure and function "relapse" and redevelop clinical signs and symptoms of HF with recurrent LV dysfunction events is not known, but represents a significant unmet clinical need, as well as significant financial burden for health care systems that have to manage HF readmissions. One plausible explanation for this phenomenon, which is based on the consistent finding that the reverse remodeled heart retains many of the molecular features of the failing heart, is that reverse LV remodeling represents a transition to a new less pathologic steady state that allows the heart to maintain LV pump function under normal conditions, but that this adaptation has less biological and contractile reserve capacity, and is therefore more prone to redevelop LV dysfunction in response to hemodynamic, neurohormonal, or environmental stress.

FUTURE PERSPECTIVES

The clinical syndrome of HF can be considered in terms of several different clinical model systems, including cardiorenal, hemodynamic, and neurohormonal. Each of the models has strengths and weaknesses in explaining the mechanisms responsible for HF, as well as in developing effective new therapies for HF. Nonetheless, current models for explicating the mechanisms for HF are inadequate and do not adequately describe disease progression in HF. Moreover, they do not provide an adequate scaffold for understanding newer device therapies that appear to work through neurohormonally independent mechanisms. This emphasizes the importance of cardiac remodeling as a mechanism of disease progression in HF. Future therapeutic advances are likely to require a more comprehensive understanding and analysis of the pathobiology of HF, particularly cell-cell interactions during LV remodeling, as well as the complex interactions that govern the process of reverse LV remodeling. In this regard, the emerging field of systems biology, which uses network theory to describe how the interrelationships between genes, proteins, and metabolites determine functional changes at the level of the cell, tissue, and organ, may allow investigators to accelerate the pace of novel target identification, as well as improve the likelihood of success in clinical trials.

REFERENCES
Pathogenesis: Neurohormonal Mechanisms
1. Hartupee J, Mann DL. Neurohormonal activation in heart failure with reduced ejection fraction. *Nat Rev Cardiol*. 2017;14(1):30–38.
2. Notarius CF, Millar PJ, Floras JS. Muscle sympathetic activity in resting and exercising humans with and without heart failure. *Appl Physiol Nutr Metab*. 2015;40(11):1107–1115.
3. Floras JS, Ponikowski P. The sympathetic/parasympathetic imbalance in heart failure with reduced ejection fraction. *Eur Heart J*. 2015;36(30):1974-1982.
4. Anand IS, Konstam MA, Klein HU, et al. Comparison of symptomatic and functional responses to vagus nerve stimulation in ANTHEM-HF, INOVATE-HF, and NECTAR-HF. *ESC Heart Fail*. 2020;7(1):75–83.
5. Ky B, Mann DL. COVID-19 clinical trials: a primer for the cardiovascular and cardio-oncology communities. *JACC Basic Transl Sci*. 2020;5(5):501–517.

6. Hartupee J, Mann DL. Positioning of inflammatory biomarkers in the heart failure landscape. *J Cardiovasc Transl Res.* 29013;6:485-492.
7. Hafstad AD, Nabeebaccus AA, Shah AM. Novel aspects of ROS signalling in heart failure. *Basic Res Cardiol.* 2013;108(4):359.
8. Givertz MM, Anstrom KJ, Redfield MM, et al. Effects of xanthine oxidase inhibition in hyperuricemic heart failure patients: the EXACT-HF study. *Circulation.* 2015;131:1763–1771.
9. Jennings DL, Kalus JS, O'Dell KM. Aldosterone receptor antagonism in heart failure. *Pharmacotherapy.* 2005;25(8):1126–1133.
10. Zile MR, Lindenfeld J, Weaver FA, et al. Baroreflex activation therapy in patients with heart failure with reduced ejection fraction. *J Am Coll Cardiol.* 2020;76(1):1–13.
11. Lee CY, Burnett JC Jr. Natriuretic peptides and therapeutic applications. *Heart Fail Rev.* 2007;12(2):131–142.
12. Volpe M, Rubattu S, Burnett J Jr. Natriuretic peptides in cardiovascular diseases: current use and perspectives. *Eur Heart J.* 2014;35(7):419–425.
13. Chen Y, Burnett JC Jr. Biochemistry, therapeutics, and biomarker implications of neprilysin in cardiorenal disease. *Clin Chem.* 2017;63(1):108–115.
14. Volpe M, Carnovali M, Mastromarino V. The natriuretic peptides system in the pathophysiology of heart failure: from molecular basis to treatment. *Clin Sci (Lond).* 2016;130(2):57–77.
15. Armstrong PW, Pieske B, Anstrom KJ, et al. Vericiguat in patients with heart failure and reduced ejection fraction. *N Engl J Med.* 2020;382(20):1883–1893.
16. Carnicer R, Crabtree MJ, Sivakumaran V, et al. Nitric oxide synthases in heart failure. *Antioxid Redox Signal.* 2013;18(9):1078–1099.
17. Su JB. Different cross-talk sites between the renin-angiotensin and the kallikrein-kinin systems. *J Renin Angiotensin Aldosterone Syst.* 2014;15(4):319–328.
18. Yanagawa B, Nagaya N. Adrenomedullin: molecular mechanisms and its role in cardiac disease. *Amino Acids.* 2007;32(1):157–164.
19. Voors AA, Kremer D, Geven C, et al. Adrenomedullin in heart failure: pathophysiology and therapeutic application. *Eur J Heart Fail.* 2019;21(2):163–171.
20. Koguchi W, Kobayashi N, Takeshima H, et al. Cardioprotective effect of apelin-13 on cardiac performance and remodeling in end-stage heart failure. *Circ J.* 2012;76(1):137–144.
21. Ma Z, Song JJ, Martin S, et al. The Elabela-APJ axis: a promising therapeutic target for heart failure. *Heart Fail Rev.* 2020.
22. Packer M. Leptin-Aldosterone-Neprilysin axis: identification of its distinctive role in the pathogenesis of the three phenotypes of heart failure in people with obesity. *Circulation.* 2018;137(15):1614–1631.
23. Abel ED, Litwin SE, Sweeney G. Cardiac remodeling in obesity. *Physiol Rev.* 2008;88(2):389–419.
24. Adamo L, Rocha-Resende C, Prabhu SD, Mann DL. Reappraising the role of inflammation in heart failure. *Nat Rev Cardiol.* 2020;5(17):269–285.
25. Mann DL. Innate immunity and the failing heart: the cytokine hypothesis revisited. *Circ Res.* 2015;116(7):1254–1268.
26. Everett BM, Cornel J, Lainscak M, et al. Anti-Inflammatory therapy with canakinumab for the prevention of hospitalization for heart failure. *Circulation.* 2019;139:1289–1299.

Pathogenesis: Left Ventricular Remodeling

27. Hershberger RE, Morales A, Siegfried JD. Clinical and genetic issues in dilated cardiomyopathy: a review for genetics professionals. *Genet Med.* 2010;12(11):655–667.
28. Toischer K, Rokita AG, Unsold B, et al. Differential cardiac remodeling in preload versus afterload. *Circulation.* 2010;122(9):993–1003.
29. Dridi H, Kushnir A, Zalk R, et al. Intracellular calcium leak in heart failure and atrial fibrillation: a unifying mechanism and therapeutic target. *Nat Rev Cardiol.* 2020.
30. Lehnart SE, Maier LS, Hasenfuss G. Abnormalities of calcium metabolism and myocardial contractility depression in the failing heart. *Heart Fail Rev.* 2009;14(4):213–224.
31. Mohamed BA, Hartmann N, Tirilomis P, et al. Sarcoplasmic reticulum calcium leak contributes to arrhythmia but not to heart failure progression. *Sci Transl Med.* 2018;10(458):eaan0724.
32. Walweel K, Laver DR. Mechanisms of SR calcium release in healthy and failing human hearts. *Biophys Rev.* 2015;7(1):33–41.
33. Anderson DM, Makarewich CA, Anderson KM, et al. Widespread control of calcium signaling by a family of SERCA-inhibiting micropeptides. *Sci Signal.* 2016;9(457): ra119.
34. Penny WF, Hammond HK. Randomized clinical trials of gene transfer for heart failure with reduced ejection fraction. *Hum Gene Ther.* 2017;28(5):378–384.
35. Guo A, Zhang C, Wei S, Chen B, Song L-S. Emerging mechanisms of T-tubule remodelling in heart failure. *Cardiovasc Res.* 2013;98(2):204–215.
36. Aiba T, Tomaselli GF. Electrical remodeling in the failing heart. *Curr Opin Cardiol.* 2010;25(1):29–36.
37. Moreno JD, Clancy CE. Pathophysiology of the cardiac late Na current and its potential as a drug target. *J Mol Cell Cardiol.* 2012;52(3):608–619.
38. Sossalla S, Wagner S, Rasenack EC, et al. Ranolazine improves diastolic dysfunction in isolated myocardium from failing human hearts—role of late sodium current and intracellular ion accumulation. *J Mol Cell Cardiol.* 2008;45(1):32–43.
39. Lohse MJ, Engelhardt S, Eschenhagen T. What is the role of beta-adrenergic signaling in heart failure? *Circ Res.* 2003;93(10):896–906.
40. Rengo G, Pagano G, Filardi PP, et al. Prognostic value of lymphocyte G protein-coupled receptor kinase-2 protein levels in patients with heart failure. *Circ Res.* 2016;118(7):1116–1124.
41. Konstantinidis K, Whelan RS, Kitsis RN. Mechanisms of cell death in heart disease. *Arterioscler Thromb Vasc Biol.* 2012;32(7):1552–1562.
42. Zhang W, Lavine KJ, Epelman S, et al. Necrotic myocardial cells release damage-associated molecular patterns that provoke fibroblast activation in vitro and trigger myocardial inflammation and fibrosis in vivo. *J Am Heart Assoc.* 2015;4(6):e001993.
43. Del Re DP, Amgalan D, Linkermann A, et al. Fundamental mechanisms of regulated cell death and implications for heart disease. *Physiol Rev.* 2019;99(4):1765–1817.
44. Abbate A, Narula J. Role of apoptosis in adverse ventricular remodeling. *Heart Fail Clin.* 2012;8(1):79–86.
45. Haudek SB, Taffet GE, Schneider MD, Mann DL. TNF provokes cardiomyocyte apoptosis and cardiac remodeling through activation of multiple cell death pathways. *J Clin Invest.* 2007;117(9):2692–2701.
46. Nakai A, Yamaguchi O, Takeda T, et al. The role of autophagy in cardiomyocytes in the basal state and in response to hemodynamic stress. *Nat Med.* 2007;13(5):619–624.
47. Hartupee J, Szalai GD, Wang W, et al. Impaired protein quality control during left ventricular remodeling in mice with cardiac restricted overexpression of tumor necrosis factor. *Circ Heart Fail.* 2017;10(12).
48. Sciarretta S, Maejima Y, Zablocki D, Sadoshima J. The role of autophagy in the heart. *Annu Rev Physiol.* 2017.
49. Rosenberg M, Meyer FJ, Gruenig E, et al. Osteopontin predicts adverse right ventricular remodelling and dysfunction in pulmonary hypertension. *Eur J Clin Invest.* 2012;42(9):933–942.
50. Spinale FG, Zile MR. Integrating the myocardial matrix into heart failure recognition and management. *Circ Res.* 2013;113(6):725–738.
51. Zannad F, Rossignol P, Iraqi W. Extracellular matrix fibrotic markers in heart failure. *Heart Fail Rev.* 2010;15(4):319–329.
52. Kanisicak O, Khalil H, Ivey MJ, et al. Genetic lineage tracing defines myofibroblast origin and function in the injured heart. *Nat Commun.* 2016;7:12260.
53. Kakkar R, Lee RT. Intramyocardial fibroblast myocyte communication. *Circ Res.* 2010;106(1):47–57.
54. Zhang W, Chancey AL, Tzeng HP, et al. The development of myocardial fibrosis in transgenic mice with targeted overexpression of tumor necrosis factor requires mast cell-fibroblast interactions. *Circulation.* 2011;124:2106–2116.
55. Puls M, Beuthner BE, Topci R, et al. Impact of myocardial fibrosis on left ventricular remodelling, recovery, and outcome after transcatheter aortic valve implantation in different haemodynamic subtypes of severe aortic stenosis. *Eur Heart J.* 2020;41(20):1903–1914.
56. Wilcox JE, Mann DL. Beta-blockers for the treatment of heart failure with a mid-range ejection fraction: deja-vu all over again? *Eur Heart J.* 2018;39(1):36–38.
57. Small EM, Olson EN. Pervasive roles of microRNAs in cardiovascular biology. *Nature.* 2011;469(7330):336–342.
58. Thum T. Facts and updates about cardiovascular non-coding RNAs in heart failure. *ESC Heart Fail.* 2015;2(3):108–111.
59. Foinquinos A, Batkai S, Genschel C, et al. Preclinical development of a miR-132 inhibitor for heart failure treatment. *Nat Commun.* 2020;11(1):633.
60. Neubauer S. The failing heart—an engine out of fuel. *N Engl J Med.* 2007;356(11):1140–1151.
61. Selvaraj S, Kelly DP, Margulies KB. Implications of altered ketone metabolism and therapeutic ketosis in heart failure. *Circulation.* 2020;141(22):1800–1812.
62. Rosano GM, Vitale C. Metabolic modulation of cardiac metabolism in heart failure. *Card Fail Rev.* 2018;4(2):99–103.
63. Ponikowski P, Voors AA, Anker SD, et al. 2016 ESC Guidelines for the diagnosis and treatment of acute and chronic heart failure: the Task Force for the diagnosis and treatment of acute and chronic heart failure of the European Society of Cardiology (ESC) Developed with the special contribution of the Heart Failure Association (HFA) of the ESC. *Eur Heart J.* 2016;37:2129–2200.
64. Murphy E, Ardehali H, Balaban RS, et al. Mitochondrial function, biology, and role in disease: a scientific statement from the American Heart Association. *Circ Res.* 2016;118(12):1960–1991.
65. Butler J, Khan MS, Anker SD, et al. Effects of elamipretide on left ventricular function in patients with heart failure with reduced ejection fraction: the PROGRESS-HF Phase 2 trial. *J Card Fail.* 2020;26(5):429–437.

Reversibility of Heart Failure

66. Wilcox JE, Fang JC, Margulies KB, Mann DL. Heart failure with a recovered ejection fraction. *J Am Coll Cardiol.* 2020;76:719–734.
67. Weinheimer CJ, Kovacs A, Evans S, et al. Load-Dependent changes in left ventricular structure and function in a pathophysiologically relevant murine model of reversible heart failure. *Circ Heart Fail.* 2018;11(5):e004351.
68. Kim GH, Uriel N, Burkhoff D. Reverse remodelling and myocardial recovery in heart failure. *Nat Rev Cardiol.* 2018;15(2):83–96.
69. Margulies KB, Matiwala S, Cornejo C, et al. Mixed messages: transcription patterns in failing and recovering human myocardium. *Circ Res.* 2005;96:592–599.

48 Approach to the Patient with Heart Failure

JAMES L. JANUZZI JR. AND DOUGLAS L. MANN

HEART FAILURE DEFINITION AND EPIDEMIOLOGY, 933
Classification of Heart Failure, 934

THE MEDICAL HISTORY AND PHYSICAL EXAMINATION, 935
Heart Failure Symptoms and Signs, 935
The Physical Examination, 936

ROUTINE LABORATORY ASSESSMENT, 938
Chest Radiography, 938
The Electrocardiogram, 938
Measurement of Blood Chemistry and Hematologic Variables, 938

Natriuretic Peptides, 940
Other Biomarkers, 940

RISK SCORING FOR PROGNOSIS, 941

RIGHT HEART CATHETERIZATION, 942

ENDOMYOCARDIAL BIOPSY, 942

DETECTING COMORBID CONDITIONS, 942

ASSESSMENT OF QUALITY OF LIFE, 942

CARDIOPULMONARY EXERCISE TESTING, 942

USE OF IMAGING MODALITIES IN THE DIAGNOSIS AND MANAGEMENT OF PATIENTS WITH HEART FAILURE, 943
Echocardiography and Lung Ultrasound, 943
Magnetic Resonance Imaging, 943
Cardiac Computed Tomography, 943
Nuclear Imaging, 943

TIMING OF ADVANCED HEART FAILURE REFERRAL, 944

SUMMARY AND FUTURE PERSPECTIVES, 944

REFERENCES, 944

HEART FAILURE DEFINITION AND EPIDEMIOLOGY

Heart failure (HF) is a complex clinical syndrome resulting from structural and functional impairment of ventricular filling or ejection of blood. While the clinical syndrome of HF may arise due to abnormalities or disorders involving all aspects of cardiac structure and function, most patients have impairment of myocardial function, ranging from normal ventricular size and function to marked dilation and reduced function. While symptoms of HF frequently depend on the presence of elevated left or right heart filling pressures, the term "congestive" HF is no longer preferred, as many patients do not have overt congestion at the time of evaluation, and their symptoms may be due to reduction in cardiac output, for example.

The global incidence and prevalence rates of HF have reached epidemic proportions, as evidenced by the relentless increase in the number of HF hospitalizations, the growing number of HF deaths, and the spiraling costs associated with the care of HF patients. The overall prevalence of HF is increasing in part because our current therapies of cardiac disorders (such as myocardial infarction, valvular heart disease, and arrhythmias) are allowing patients to survive longer. Worldwide, HF affects nearly 23 million people. In the United States, the most recent epidemiologic data suggest that 6.2 million adult Americans have HF, and it is estimated that by 2030 the prevalence will increase 46% from current estimates.[1] Estimates of the prevalence of symptomatic HF in the general European population is similar to that in the United States, and ranges from 0.4% to 2%.[2] The prevalence of HF rises exponentially with age, and affects 4% to 8% of people over the age of 65 years (Fig. 48.1A). Although the relative incidence of HF is lower in women than men for all age groups, women constitute at least half of the cases of HF because of their longer life expectancy and the overall prevalence of HF is greater in women than men ≥80 years of age.[3] The age-adjusted incidence of HF appears greatest in black men, followed by black women, white men, and white women; the higher incidence of HF in blacks was attributed to the greater levels of atherosclerotic risk factors in this population (Fig. 48.1B).[1] In North America and Europe, the lifetime risk of developing HF is approximately one in five for a 40-year-old. Risk factors for HF include ischemic heart disease, incident or prevalent myocardial infarction, myocarditis, valvular heart disease, tachycardia, diabetes mellitus, structural heart disease related to congenital heart disease, sleep apnea, excessive drug or alcohol use, as well as obesity. A significant percentage (approximately 30% to 40%) of nonischemic HF is thought to be due to genetic factors (see Chapter 52).

In addition certain medications may increase the risk for HF, including nonsteroidal antiinflammatory medications and cancer chemotherapy.

The distribution of ejection fraction (EF) across unselected populations of HF patients is bimodal with peaks centered around 35% and 55%.[3] Approximately half of patients have HF with preserved EF (HFpEF [see Chapter 51]), while the balance have HF with reduced EF (HFrEF [see Chapter 50])[3]; HFpEF is generally defined as a left ventricular EF ≥50%, whereas HFrEF is generally defined as an EF less than 40%. Insofar as treatment strategies for treating HF are based on these two categories, these distinctions are critical and consensus is not present regarding this classification or how to consider those with HF and an EF between 40% and 50%[4]; this latter category of patients is often excluded from clinical trials, although recent HFpEF trials have included patients down to an EF of 45%.

The prevalence of HFpEF increases dramatically with age and is much more common in women than in men at any age.[1] The prevalence of HFpEF appears to be increasing, perhaps as a function of the aging population and increased recognition of the diagnosis.

An increasingly important population of patients are those with HF and "recovered" EF (HFrecEF).[5,6] Although increases in left ventricular ejection fraction (LVEF) may occur "spontaneously" in some forms of dilated cardiomyopathy (DCM), the changes generally occur in the setting of the use of guideline-directed medical and device therapy.[6] Moreover, it is usually not possible to clearly discern the "spontaneous" component to the improvement in myocardial function, because most patients are treated with guideline-directed medical therapy (GDMT). It is important to recognize that the subgroup of HFrEF patients with a recovered LVEF are clinically distinct from patients with HF with a preserved EF (HFpEF), who also have an LVEF greater than 50% along with the presence of HF signs and symptoms. Improvements in LVEF with GDMT can lead to a complete normalization of LVEF (i.e., >50%) or a partial normalization of LVEF (40% to 50%) (Fig. 48.2). Estimates of the proportion of patients with improved LVEF range widely (e.g., 10% to 40%) due to variable definitions, and the use of both observational and clinical trial datasets. Patients in this category have somewhat characteristic demographics, in that they are more likely to be younger, female, to have nonischemic HF, shorter duration of HF, and to have less remodeling of their left ventricle at the time of diagnosis. Genetic factors may play a role in recovery of EF, as certain mutations (such as those involving the titin gene) may be associated with more robust improvement in LVEF after therapy. A recent consensus statement suggested that patients

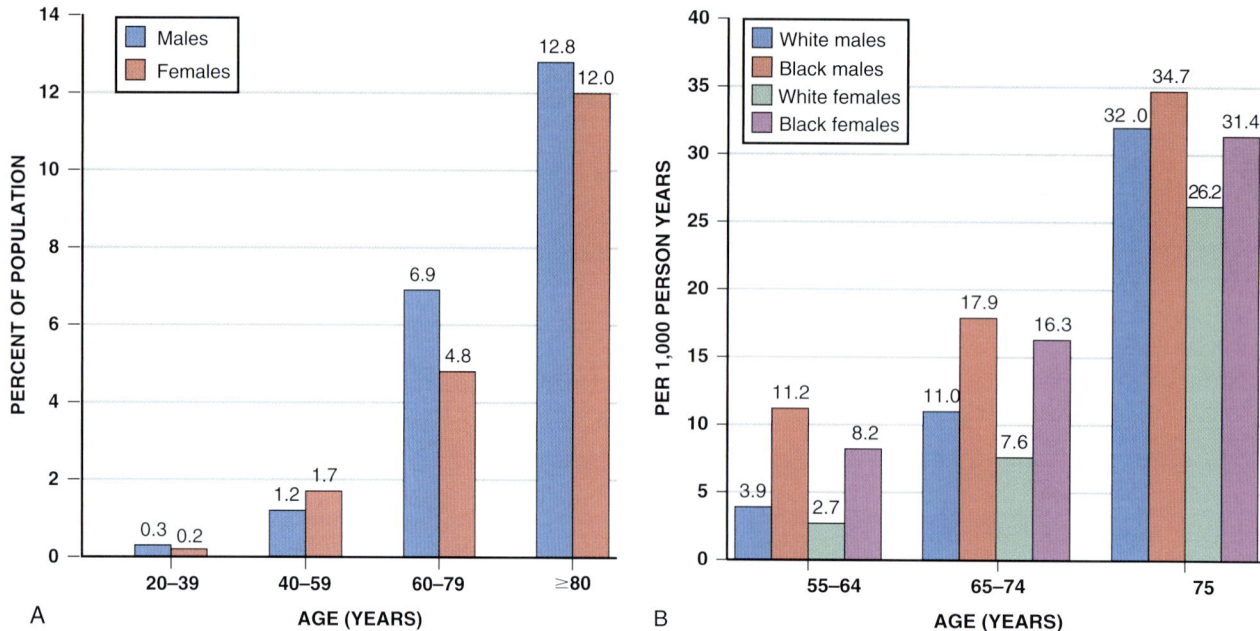

FIGURE 48.1 Prevalence and outcomes of heart failure in the United States. **A,** Prevalence of heart failure by gender and age. **B,** Prevalence of heart failure by age and racial or ethnic group. (From Virani SS, Alonso A, Benjamin EJ, et al. Heart Disease and Stroke Statistics—2020 Update: a report from the American Heart Association. *Circulation.* 2020;141[9]:e139–e596.)

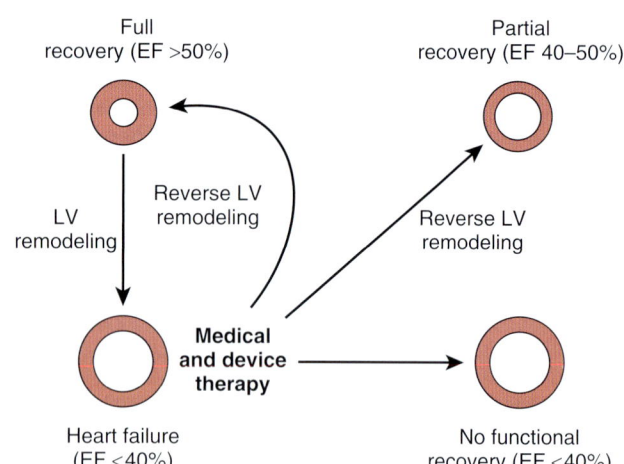

FIGURE 48.2 Changes in left ventricular (LV) ejection fraction (EF) with guideline-directed medical or device therapies (GDMT) in patients with heart failure with a reduced EF (HFrEF). HF and "recovered" EF (HFrecEF) patients treated with GDMT may have a complete recovery of left ventricular (LV) ejection fraction (EF) greater than 50%, partial recovery of LVEF (EF 40% to 50%), or no functional recovery of LVEF (EF <40%). (From Wilcox JE, Fang JC, Margulies KB, Mann DL. Heart failure with a recovered left ventricular ejection fraction. *J Am Coll Cardiol.* 2020;76[6]:719–734.)

with a recovered LVEF should be referred to as HFrecEF, to denote that they were initially HF patients with a remodeled (e.g., dilated) LV. This terminology also avoids confusing these patients with patients with HFpEF who have an LVEF greater than 50%, as well as with patients with an intermediate LVEF (40% to 50%) that may represent HFpEF patients with deteriorating LVEF.

As noted above, one of the major hurdles toward our understanding of this unique group of patients is the lack of standardization with regard to the definition of HFrecEF. A working definition of HFrecEF that is consistent with the majority of studies in the literature includes: (1) documentation of a decreased LVEF less than 40% at baseline, (2) ≥10% absolute improvement in LVEF, and (3) a second measurement of LVEF greater than 40%. These improvements in LVEF are typically accompanied by a reduction in LV volumes.[6]

Patients with HF and improved EF represent a therapeutic conundrum. Although demonstrating improvement in LVEF, many of these patients may have persistent biochemical signs of HF pathophysiology with abnormal concentrations of natriuretic peptides, and a recent study suggested that discontinuation of GDMT for HF was accompanied by an unacceptably high rate (44%) of recrudescent HFrEF.[7] Further, many patients with HF and improved EF remain at risk of adverse outcomes including return of depressed left ventricular function or hospitalization for HF. Although more studies are needed, the existing data suggest that HFrecEF patients should continue receiving GDMT despite normalization of LVEF, because of the concern for recurrence of HF, as well as the clinical observation that, among patients who experience a relapse and recurrent decline in LVEF, there is a higher likelihood of recurring myocyte injury and a diminished ability to recover LVEF the second time around.[6]

Classification of Heart Failure

Patients with HF are classified according to symptomatology and the stage of the disease. The American College of Cardiology/American Heart Association (ACC/AHA) HF staging approach (Table 48.1) emphasizes the importance of development and progression of disease,[8] whereas the New York Heart Association (NYHA) functional classification focuses more on exercise tolerance in those with established HF (see Table 48.1). While suffering from considerable subjectivity, the NYHA functional classification is widely used. Use of both systems in conjunction provides a reasonable framework for clinician communication and patient prognostication; the NYHA functional classification is also used to determine eligibility for certain therapies, such as mineralocorticoid receptor antagonists, or cardiac resynchronization therapy.

When the diagnosis of HF is suspected, the goals of the clinical assessment are to determine whether HF is present, define the underlying cause and the type of HF (HFrEF vs. HFpEF), assess the severity of HF, as well as identify comorbidities that can influence the clinical course and response to treatment. While the diagnosis of HF can be straightforward when the patient presents with a constellation of the classic signs and symptoms in the appropriate clinical setting (Tables 48.2 and 48.3), no sign or symptom alone can define the presence or severity of HF. Furthermore, detection of diagnostic physical findings of HF is imprecise, often requiring other diagnostic tools. Thus, as depicted in Figure 48.3, the clinical assessment of HF most often depends on information that is gleaned from a variety of sources including the history (both past and present), physical examination, laboratory tests, cardiac imaging, and functional studies.

TABLE 48.1 American College of Cardiology/American Heart Association (ACC/AHA) Stages of Heart Failure (HF) Compared to the New York Heart Association (NYHA) Functional Classification

	ACC/AHA STAGES OF HEART FAILURE	NYHA FUNCTIONAL CLASSIFICATION
A	At high risk for HF but without structural heart disease or symptoms of heart failure.	None
B	Structural heart disease but without signs or symptoms of heart failure.	I — No limitation of physical activity. Ordinary physical activity does not cause symptoms of heart failure.
C	Structural heart disease with prior or current symptoms of heart failure.	I — No limitation of physical activity. Ordinary physical activity does not cause symptoms of heart failure.
		II — Slight limitation of physical activity. Comfortable at rest, but ordinary physical activity results in symptoms of heart failure.
		III — Marked limitation of physical activity. Comfortable at rest, but less than ordinary activity causes symptoms of heart failure.
D	Refractory heart failure requiring specialized interventions.	IV — Unable to carry on any physical activity without symptoms of heart failure, or symptoms of heart failure at rest.

HF, Heart failure.

TABLE 48.2 Using the Medical History to Assess the Heart Failure Patient

Symptoms associated with heart failure include:
1. Fatigue
2. Shortness of breath at rest or during exercise
3. Dyspnea
4. Tachypnea
5. Cough
6. Diminished exercise capacity
7. Orthopnea
8. Paroxysmal nocturnal dyspnea
9. Nocturia
10. Weight gain/Weight loss
11. Edema (of the extremities, scrotum, or elsewhere)
12. Increasing abdominal girth or bloating
13. Abdominal pain (particularly if confined to the right upper quadrant)
14. Loss of appetite or early satiety
15. Cheyne-Stokes respirations (often reported by the family rather than the patient)
16. Somnolence or diminished mental acuity

Historical information that is helpful in determining if symptoms are due to heart failure include:
1. A past history of heart failure
2. Cardiac disease (e.g., coronary artery, valvular or congenital disease, previous myocardial infarction)
3. Risk factors for heart failure (e.g., diabetes, hypertension, obesity)
4. Systemic illnesses that can involve the heart (e.g., amyloidosis, sarcoidosis, inherited neuromuscular diseases)
5. Recent viral illness or history of HIV or Chagas disease
6. Family history of heart failure or sudden cardiac death
7. Environmental and/or medical exposure to cardiotoxic substances
8. Substance abuse
9. Noncardiac illnesses that could affect the heart indirectly (including high output states such as anemia, hyperthyroidism, arteriovenous fistulae)

THE MEDICAL HISTORY AND PHYSICAL EXAMINATION

A complete medical history and carefully focused physical examination are the foundation of the assessment in HF patients, providing important information regarding etiology of HF, identifying possible exacerbating factors, and lending pivotal data for proper management (see Chapter 13). The information obtained guides the further direction of the patient's evaluation and enables the clinician to make the most judicious use of additional tests. Further, the history helps to evaluate incongruent results that may emerge during the diagnostic process, and it can obviate the need for needless further testing.

Heart Failure Symptoms and Signs

Patients with HF may complain of a vast array of symptoms, the most common of which are listed in Table 48.2. While none of these are entirely sensitive or specific for identifying the presence of congestion (see Table 48.4), some are more reliable than others for this indication. Importantly, none are specific to HFpEF versus HFrEF. Worsening dyspnea is a cardinal symptom of HF, and is typically related to increases in cardiac filling pressures but also may represent restricted cardiac output.[9] The absence of worsening dyspnea, however, does not necessarily exclude the diagnosis of HF, because patients may accommodate symptoms by substantially modifying their lifestyle. Probing more deeply into the current level of activity may uncover a decline in exercise capacity that is not immediately apparent. Dyspnea at rest is often mentioned by patients hospitalized with HF and has a high-diagnostic sensitivity and significant prognostic ramifications in this population. However, it is also cited by patients with many other medical conditions, so that the specificity and positive predictive value of dyspnea at rest alone are low. Patients may sleep with their heads elevated to relieve dyspnea while recumbent (orthopnea); additionally, dyspnea while lying on the left side (trepopnea) may occur. Paroxysmal nocturnal dyspnea, shortness of breath developing while recumbent, is one of the most highly reliable indicators of HF. Cheyne-Stokes respiration (also referred to as periodic or cyclic respiration) is common in advanced HF and is usually associated with low cardiac output and sleep-disordered breathing (see also Chapters 50 and 89). The presence of Cheyne-Stokes respiration is generally indicative of an adverse prognosis.[10] Nocturnal cough is a frequently overlooked symptom of HF. These symptoms all typically reflect pulmonary congestion, whereas a history of weight gain, increasing abdominal girth, early satiety, and the onset of edema in dependent organs (extremities or scrotum) indicate right heart congestion; while nonspecific, right upper quadrant pain due to congestion of the liver is common in those with significant right HF, and may be incorrectly attributed to other conditions. Another cardinal symptom of HF is fatigue, generally held to be reflective of reduction in cardiac output as well as abnormal skeletal muscle metabolic responses to exercise.[11] Other causes of fatigue in HF may include major depression, anemia, renal dysfunction, endocrinologic abnormalities, as well as side effects to medications. Unintended weight loss, often leading to cachexia, may be prominent and is a major prognostic indicator.[12]

OTHER HISTORICAL INFORMATION

Information about a patient's past and current medical problems and a multigenerational family history as well as social history provides the background upon which symptoms are interpreted and a management plan is designed.

The presence of hypertension, coronary artery disease, and/or diabetes is particularly helpful because these conditions account for approximately 90% of the population attributable risk for HF in the United States.[13]

TABLE 48.3 Physical Findings of Heart Failure

1. Tachycardia
2. Extra beats or irregular rhythm
3. Narrow pulse pressure or thready pulse*
4. Pulses alternans*
5. Tachypnea
6. Cool and/or mottled extremities*
7. Elevated jugular venous pressure
8. Dullness and diminished breath sounds at one or both lung bases
9. Rales, rhonchi, and/or wheezes
10. Apical impulse displaced leftward and/or inferiorly
11. Sustained apical impulse
12. Parasternal lift
13. S3 and/or S4 (either palpable and/or audible)
14. Tricuspid or mitral regurgitant murmur
15. Hepatomegaly (often accompanied by right upper quadrant discomfort)
16. Ascites
17. Pre-sacral edema
18. Anasarca*
19. Pedal edema
20. Chronic venous stasis changes

*Indicative of more severe disease.

The medical history should also focus on what drugs are taken by the patient; notable agents associated with incident HF include cancer chemotherapy,[14] diabetes drugs (e.g., thiazolidinediones), ergot-based antimigraine drugs, appetite suppressants, certain antidepressants and antipsychotic agents (notably including clozapine), decongestants such as pseudoephedrine (due to its ability to trigger severe hypertension), as well as antiinflammatory agents such as the antimalarial drug hydroxychloroquine (uncommonly associated with an infiltrative cardiomyopathy) or nonsteroidal antiinflammatory drugs. The latter class of agents is well recognized to lead to HF through their ability to worsen renal function, trigger hypertension, and lead to fluid retention, particularly in older adults. A history of use of herbal remedies and dietary supplements should be obtained. Environmental or toxic exposures including alcohol or drug abuse should be carefully sought. A multigenerational family history should be taken for prior HF or sudden cardiac death. Information about the presence of comorbidities (as described later in the chapter) is essential in devising management plans. While most etiologies of HF are cardiac, it is worth remembering that some systemic illnesses (e.g., anemia, hyperthyroidism) can cause this syndrome without direct cardiac involvement (see Chapter 96).

The Physical Examination

The physical findings listed in Table 48.2 complement information from the medical history in defining the presence and severity of HF (see also Chapter 13). The signs of HF have been extensively described, and much as with the history of patients with HF, components of the physical exam have variable sensitivity and specificity for the diagnosis (see Table 48.4),[15] in part due to the subtlety of some physical findings as well as variability in the physical diagnostic skills of the examiner. No physical finding in HF is absolutely pathognomonic for HFpEF versus HFrEF.[15]

An evaluation for the presence and severity of HF should include consideration of the patient's general appearance, measurement of vital signs in the seated and standing position, examination of the heart and pulses, and assessment of other organs for evidence of congestion, hypoperfusion, or indications of comorbid conditions. The patient's general appearance conveys vital information. The examiner should assess the patient's body habitus and state of alertness, as well as

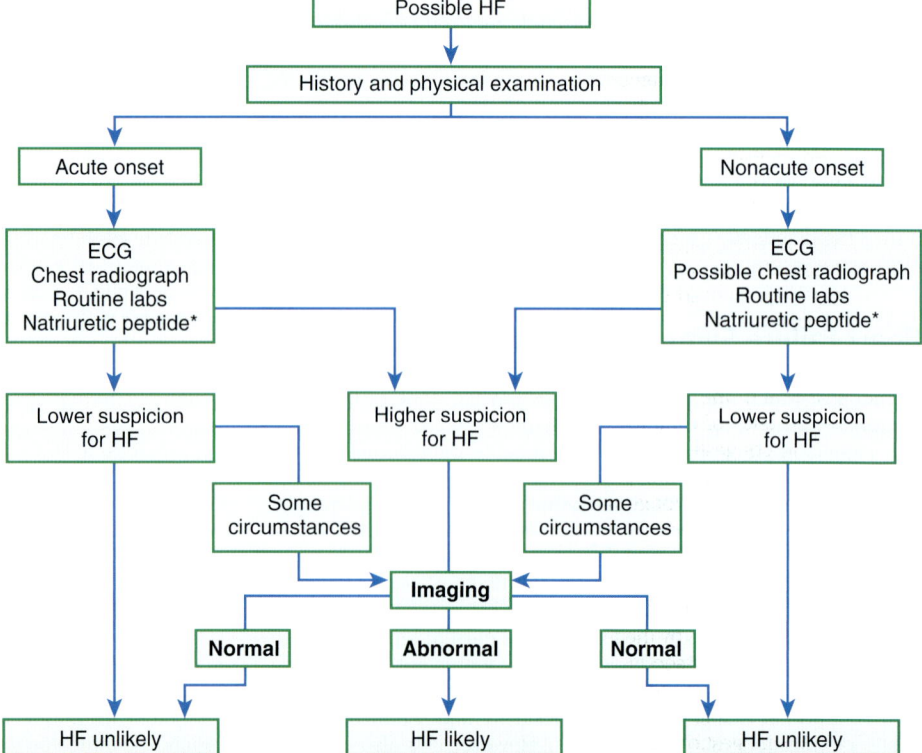

FIGURE 48.3 Flow chart for the evaluation of patients with heart failure (HF). Appropriate cut points for natriuretic peptide testing to identify or exclude HF are discussed in eTable 48.1. The diagnosis of HF is made using a combination of clinical judgment and initial and subsequent testing. Following thorough history and physical examination together with initial diagnostic testing, imaging (such as with echocardiography [ECG]) may still be necessary in ambiguous cases to definitively identify or exclude the diagnosis.

TABLE 48.4 Sensitivity and Specificity of History and Physical Exam Components for the Diagnosis of Elevated Filling Pressures in Patients with Heart Failure

H&P FINDING	FREQUENCY	SENSITIVITY	SPECIFICITY	PREDICTIVE VALUE POSITIVE	PREDICTIVE VALUE NEGATIVE	LR POSITIVE	LR NEGATIVE	OR (95% CI)
Values expressed as percentages unless otherwise indicated. LR indicates likelihood ratio; OR, odds ratio.								
Rales (≥1/3 lung fields)	26/192	15	89	69	38	1.32	1.04	1.4 (0.6, 3.4)
S3	123/192	62	32	61	33	0.92	0.85	0.8 (0.4, 1.5)
Ascites (moderate/massive)	31/192	21	92	81	40	2.44	1.15	2.8 (1.1, 7.3)
Edema (≥2+)	73/192	41	66	67	40	1.20	1.11	1.3 (0.7, 2.5)
Orthopnea (≥2 pillows)	157/192	86	25	66	51	1.15	1.80	2.1 (1, 4.4)
Hepatomegaly (>4 finger breadths)	23/191	15	93	78	39	2.13	1.09	2.3 (0.8, 6.6)
Hepatojugular reflux	147/186	83	27	65	49	1.13	1.54	1.7 (0.9, 3.5)
JVP ≥12 mm Hg	101/186	65	64	75	52	1.79	1.82	3.3 (1.8, 6.1)
JVP <8 mm Hg	18/186	4.3	81	28	33	0.23	0.85	0.2

JVP, Jugular venous pressure.

whether the patient is comfortable, short of breath, coughing, or in pain. The skin exam may show pallor or cyanosis due to under-perfusion, stigmata of alcohol abuse (such as spider angiomata or palmar erythema), erythema nodosum due to sarcoidosis, bronzing due to hemachromatosis, or easy bruising from amyloidosis; additional findings supporting amyloidosis include deltoid muscle infiltration (leading to the "shoulder pad sign"), tongue hypertrophy, and bilateral thenar wasting from carpal tunnel syndrome. The details of inspection and palpation of the heart are discussed in Chapter 13. By observing or palpating the apical impulse, the examiner can rapidly determine heart size and quality of the point of maximal impulse. In cases of severe HF, a palpable impulse corresponding to a third heart sound may be present. Cardiac auscultation (Chapter 13) is a crucial part of HF evaluation.

A characteristic holosystolic murmur of mitral insufficiency is heard in many HF patients. Tricuspid insufficiency, which is also common, can be differentiated from mitral insufficiency by the location of the murmur at the left sternal border, an increased intensity of the murmur during inspiration, and the presence of prominent "V" waves in the jugular venous waveform. Both mitral and tricuspid insufficiency murmurs may become softer as volume overload is treated, and a reduction in ventricular size (with corresponding reduction in annular diameter) improves valve coaptation and competency. Aortic stenosis is an important cause of HF because its presence greatly alters management. The presentation of aortic stenosis may be subtle, however, because the intensity of the murmur depends on blood flow across the valve and this may be reduced as HF develops. The presence of a third heart sound is a crucially important finding and suggests increased ventricular filling volume; while difficult to identify, a third heart sound is highly specific for HF, and carries a substantial prognostic meaning. A fourth heart sound usually indicates reduced ventricular compliance. In advanced HF, the third and fourth heart sounds may be superimposed, resulting in a summation gallop.

A key objective of the examination in HF patients is to detect and quantify the presence of volume retention, with or without pulmonary and/or systemic congestion. As with symptoms, evidence of congestion does not always indicate with certainty that HF is present, nor does absence of manifest congestion definitively exclude the diagnosis. Patients with HFpEF and HFrEF do not generally show significant differences in frequency or significance of the stigmata of volume overload.[16]

The most definitive method for assessing a patient's volume status by physical examination is by the measurement of jugular venous pressure (JVP), which is discussed in detail in Chapter 13. An elevated JVP has good sensitivity (70%) and specificity (79%) for elevated left-sided filling pressure (see Table 48.4).[15] The sensitivity and specificity of the JVP in detecting congestion can be considerably improved by exerting pressure on the right upper quadrant of the abdomen while assessing venous pulsations in the neck (hepatojugular reflux). Changes in JVP with therapy usually parallel changes in left-sided filling pressure. Limitations of JVP assessment include difficulties in its evaluation due to body habitus as well as significant interobserver variability in its estimation. Increase in the JVP may lag behind left heart filling pressures or may not rise at all if pulmonary artery pressure is increased to the extent that right ventricular failure or tricuspid insufficiency occur. Conversely, the JVP may be elevated without an increase in left ventricular filling pressures in patients with pulmonary arterial hypertension, in those with isolated right ventricular pressure, or when isolated severe tricuspid regurgitation is present.

While pulmonary congestion is exceedingly common in HF, physical findings indicating its presence are variable, and many are nonspecific. Dullness to percussion and diminished breath sounds at one or both lung bases suggests the presence of a pleural effusion. Bilateral pleural effusions are most common but when an effusion is present unilaterally, it is usually right sided with only approximately 10% occurring exclusively on the left side. Leakage of fluid from pulmonary capillaries into the alveoli can be manifest as rales or rhonchi, while wheezing may occur due to reactive bronchoconstriction. Pulmonary rales due to HF are usually fine in nature and extend from the base upward while those due to other causes (e.g., pulmonary fibrosis) tend to be coarser. Importantly, rales or rhonchi may be absent in congested patients with advanced HF; this may reflect compensatory increase in local lymphatic drainage. The occurrence of so-called "cardiac asthma" is due to the physical presence of fluid in the bronchial wall as well as secondary bronchospasm,[17] and can commonly result in an incorrect diagnosis of obstructive airways disease exacerbation, with consequent mis-triage and incorrect therapy with bronchodilators; such incorrect management may be associated with increased risk for mortality.[18]

Lower-extremity edema is a common finding in volume-overloaded HF patients but may commonly be the result of venous insufficiency (particularly after saphenous veins have been harvested for coronary artery bypass grafts) or as a side effect of medications (e.g., calcium channel blockers). Careful inspection of the JVP helps improve the specificity of pedal edema for HF.

Detecting reduced cardiac output and systemic hypoperfusion are key components of the examination. While patients with poor systemic perfusion usually have low systolic and narrow pulse pressures as well as weak and thready pulses, this relationship is not exact. Many patients with systolic blood pressure in the range of 80 mm Hg (or even lower) may have adequate perfusion while others with reduced cardiac output may maintain blood pressure in the normal range at the expense of tissue perfusion by greatly increasing systemic vascular resistance. Findings suggesting reduced cardiac output include poor mentation,

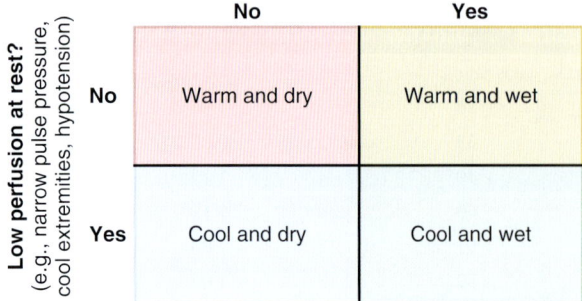

FIGURE 48.4 Schema for categorizing patients with heart failure (HF) on the basis of perfusion (warm versus cold) and presence of congestion (dry versus wet). In doing so, four categories may be identified, which have different treatment strategies. The four categories of HF identified in this schema have different treatment strategies. (Based on data from Nohria A, Tsang SW, Fang JC, et al. Clinical assessment identifies hemodynamic profiles that predict outcomes in patients admitted with heart failure. J Am Coll Cardiol. 2003;41:1797.)

reduced urine output, mottled skin, and cool extremities. Of these, cool extremities are the most broadly useful.

Assessment for systemic congestion taken together with evaluation for reduced cardiac output may be useful to categorize patients (Fig. 48.4) into "dry/warm" (uncongested with normal perfusion), "wet/warm" (congested with normal perfusion, the most common combination found in decompensated HF), "dry/cold" (uncongested but hypoperfused), and "wet/cold" (cardiogenic shock),[19] as discussed in Chapter 49. These categories are not only prognostic, but also inform treatment decision making.

ROUTINE LABORATORY ASSESSMENT

A suggested algorithm for the diagnostic evaluation of HF is presented in Figure 48.3. The laboratory testing and imaging modalities described below provide important information for the diagnosis and management of patients with suspected or proven HF.

Chest Radiography

Despite advances in other imaging technologies the chest X-ray remains a very useful component of the assessment, particularly when the clinical presentation is ambiguous. Results of chest radiography are additive to clinical variables from history and physical examination, and similarly complement the results of biomarker testing. Accordingly, chest radiography should be a routine part of the early evaluation of patients presenting with symptoms suggestive of acutely decompensated HF (see also Chapter 17).

The classical chest X-ray pattern in patients with pulmonary edema is a "butterfly" pattern of interstitial and alveolar opacities bilaterally fanning out to the periphery of the lungs. Many patients, however, present with more subtle findings, in which increased interstitial markings including Kerley B lines (thin horizontal linear opacities extending to the pleural surface caused by accumulation of fluid in the interstitial space), peri-bronchial cuffing, and evidence of prominent upper lobe vasculature (indicating pulmonary venous hypertension) are the most prominent findings. Pleural effusions and/or fluid in the right minor fissure may also be seen. In many cases, particularly in those with very advanced HF, the chest X-ray may be entirely clear, despite significant symptoms of dyspnea; the negative predictive value of chest radiography is too low to definitively exclude HF.[20]

The Electrocardiogram

The electrocardiogram (ECG) is a standard part of the initial evaluation of a patient with suspected HF, as it may provide important clues regarding incident HF, while also assisting in understanding when previously diagnosed patients experience an episode of decompensation (see also Chapter 14). In patients with HF, the ECG is infrequently normal, but may only show nonspecific findings; thus, much like the chest radiography, the positive predictive value of ECG far surpasses the negative predictive value in this setting.

Sinus tachycardia due to sympathetic nervous system activation is seen with advanced HF or during episodes of acute decompensation; beside increasing the likelihood for the diagnosis finding of elevated heart rate it is a prognostic finding in HF as well. The presence of atrial arrhythmia on the ECG as well as the ventricular response may provide clues as to the cause of HF, as well as explain why a patient may have developed decompensated symptoms; identifying atrial arrhythmia with a rapid ventricular response also provides a target for therapeutic interventions. Increased ventricular ectopy identifies a patient at risk for sudden death, particularly when the EF is very low (e.g., <30%).

The presence of increased QRS voltage may suggest left ventricular hypertrophy; in the absence of a prior history of hypertension, such a finding might be caused by valvular heart disease or by hypertrophic cardiomyopathy, particularly if bizarre repolarization patterns are noted. If right ventricular hypertrophy is present, primary or secondary pulmonary hypertension should be considered. Low QRS voltage suggests the presence of an infiltrative disease or pericardial effusion. The presence of Q waves suggests that HF may be due to ischemic heart disease, while new or reversible ST changes identify acute coronary ischemia is present even when chest pain is absent. Indeed, as acute coronary ischemia is a leading cause of acutely decompensated HF, a 12-lead ECG should be immediately obtained in this setting, to exclude acute MI.

The intervals on the ECG may provide important information regarding causes of HF, as well as yielding information with respect to treatment strategy. Prolongation of the PR interval is common in patients in this setting, and may be due to intrinsic conduction disease, but may also be seen in patients with infiltrative cardiomyopathy such as amyloidosis. With the advent of cardiac resynchronization therapy (see Chapter 58) evaluation the QRS complex has become a critical part of the clinical assessment, in that it provides important information regarding the cause of HF, as well as providing pivotal information regarding the therapeutic approach. The QT interval is often prolonged in patients with HF, and may be due to electrolyte abnormalities, myocardial disease, or from effects of commonly used drugs, such as antiarrhythmics. A lengthened QT interval may identify patients at risk for torsades de pointes and is thus an important variable to consider when utilizing therapeutic agents with effects on ventricular repolarization.

Measurement of Blood Chemistry and Hematologic Variables

Patients with new-onset HF and those with acute decompensation of chronic HF should have a panel of electrolytes, blood urea nitrogen, serum creatinine, hepatic enzymes, fasting lipid profile, thyroid stimulating hormone, transferrin saturation, uric acid, a complete blood count, and a urinalysis measured. As discussed below, the natriuretic peptides may be useful for diagnosis as well as for prognostication. A test for human immunodeficiency virus or further screening for hemachromatosis is reasonable in selected patients, while diagnostic tests for rheumatologic diseases or pheochromocytoma are reasonable when suspicion exists for these diseases. When the diagnosis of cardiac amyloidosis is entertained (see also Chapter 53), serum-free light chains may be measured to screen for the AL form of the diagnosis, however no reliable blood tests exist for diagnosis of the transthyretin form of cardiac amyloidosis, which typically requires imaging for its evaluation (see also Chapter 53).

Abnormalities of sodium are common in HF patients, particularly during periods of acute decompensation, and have substantial prognostic meaning. Studies have shown that hyponatremia (defined as serum sodium values below 135 mmol/L) may be found in up to 25% of patients with acute HF, and hyponatremia may also be seen in patients with indolently worsening HF without obvious decompensation.[21] Low-sodium concentrations in HF may be due to worsening volume retention or may be related to the use of diuretics, including thiazides. Hyponatremia is associated with impaired cognitive and neuromuscular function, and when present and persistent, low sodium is strongly prognostic for longer hospital stay, as well as a high risk for mortality.[22] Despite this fact, strategies to correct serum-sodium levels have not been shown to clearly improve the clinical course (see Chapter 50).[23] Hypernatremia, although uncommon, is also prognostic for mortality in patients with HF. Hypokalemia occurs commonly in HF patients who are treated with diuretics. Besides increasing the risk of cardiac arrhythmias, low potassium may also lead to leg cramps and muscle weakness. Conversely, hyperkalemia is less common, and most often is due to effects of medications such as angiotensin-converting enzyme inhibitors or mineralocorticoid inhibition.

Abnormalities of renal function are common in patients with HF, and occur due to renal congestion, inadequate cardiac output, or as a consequence of comorbid conditions.[24] In addition, HF therapies such as diuretics and angiotensin-converting enzyme inhibitors or angiotensin receptor blockers can increase blood urea nitrogen and creatinine. In this regard, abnormalities of renal function may have substantial effects on the ability to aggressively treat HF patients. Furthermore, abnormal renal function represents one of the more powerful prognostic variables gleaned from routine laboratory testing in HF. For these reasons, assessment of renal function should be performed as part of the initial evaluation of HF, and then periodically repeated during follow-up.

In patients hospitalized with acutely decompensated HF (see Chapter 49), registry data suggest that 60% to 70% have a reduced estimated glomerular filtration rate[25]; among such patients, the initial blood urea nitrogen and serum creatinine concentrations are both independently predictive of death.[26] Following admission, approximately 30% of patients with acute HF may also develop an increase in serum creatinine by ≥0.3 mg/dL, which is similarly prognostic for mortality.[24,25] The causes of this so-called "cardiorenal" syndrome are complex, but include the severity of right heart congestion, increased intraabdominal pressure, as well as renal hypoperfusion from inadequate cardiac output. On the other hand, worsening renal function may also occur from aggressive decongestion strategies; such decline in renal function has been linked to improved (rather than worse) prognosis, as it presumably indicates a more thorough treatment for congestion, the trigger for acute HF hospitalization.[27] Accordingly, when faced with worsening renal function, the clinician must perform a careful examination to assess volume status and tissue perfusion to decide on appropriate therapies to manage the situation. Lastly, improvement in renal function may follow therapies improving the severity of congestion, although such a finding is still associated with poor long-term prognosis.

Diabetes mellitus is common in HF patients and hyperglycemia has emerged as a possible risk factor for adverse outcome in affected patients. Because diuretics can cause gout, measuring uric acid levels can help in patient management; elevated serum uric acid levels have been noted to be prognostic, and therapies to lower their concentration are now being studied to improve HF outcomes. Abnormalities in aspartate aminotransferase, alanine aminotransferase, alkaline phosphatase, bilirubin, or lactate dehydrogenase may occur in HF patients as a consequence of either hemodynamic derangements leading to hepatic congestion, or may be due to medications, and it is important to follow levels periodically. An unexpected increase in prothrombin time in patients receiving warfarin therapy may be an early harbinger of decompensation as it may reflect impaired synthetic capacity of a congested liver. Albumin levels are an indication of the patient's nutritional status and they may be depressed due to poor appetite or impaired absorption across an engorged bowel wall; hypoalbuminemia is prognostic for mortality in acute and chronic HF.

Hematologic abnormalities are exceedingly common in HF, affecting nearly 40% of affected patients. Low hemoglobin levels have been associated with more severe HF symptoms, reduced exercise capacity and quality of life, and increased mortality.[28] While anemia may be a consequence of chronic disease in HF patients, a low hemoglobin level should trigger an evaluation to detect treatable causes, particularly iron deficiency. Increasing attention has also been given to the red cell distribution width as a prognostic variable in both acutely decompensated and chronic HF.[29] The white blood cell count and differential is helpful in detecting the presence of infection that is responsible for destabilizing a previously well-compensated patient and could provide a clue that HF is due to uncommon cause such as eosinophilic infiltration of the myocardium.

Beyond standard laboratory testing, the measurement of biomarkers has emerged over the past decade as important adjunct to the initial and subsequent evaluation of patients with suspected or proven HF. Biomarkers are now routinely used for distinguishing HF from other conditions and to establish severity of the diagnosis, and also to provide useful prognostic information in HF patients. Lastly,

TABLE 48.5 Biomarkers Used in Assessing Patients with Heart Failure

Inflammation[*,†,‡]
C-reactive protein
Tumor necrosis factor
Fas (APO-1)
Interleukins 1, 6, and 18

Oxidative stress[*,†,§]
Oxidized low-density lipoproteins
Myeloperoxidase
Urinary biopyrrins
Urinary and plasma isoprostanes
Plasma malondialdehyde

Extracellular-matrix remodeling[*,§]
Matrix metalloproteinases
Tissue inhibitors of metalloproteinases
Collagen propeptides
Propeptide procollagen type I
Plasma procollagen type III

Neurohormones[*,†,§]
Norepinephrine
Renin
Angiotensin II
Aldosterone
Arginine vasopressin
Endothelin

Myocyte injury[*,†,§]
Cardiac-specific troponins I and T
Myosin light-chain kinase I
Heart-type fatty-acid protein
Creatine kinase MB fraction

Myocyte stress[†,‡,§,¶]
B-type natriuretic peptide/N-terminal pro-B type natriuretic peptide
Midregional proadrenomedullin
ST2

New Biomarkers[†]
Chromogranin
Galectin 3
Osteoprotegerin
Adiponectin
Growth differentiation factor 15
Insulin-like growth factor binding protein 7

*Biomarkers in this category aid in elucidating the pathogenesis of heart failure.
†Biomarkers in this category provide prognostic information and enhance risk stratification.
‡Biomarkers in this category can be used to identify subjects at risk for heart failure.
§Biomarkers in this category are potential targets of therapy.
¶Biomarkers in this category are useful in the diagnosis of heart failure and in monitoring therapy.

there is considerable interest in determining the ability of biomarkers to guide therapy both in the acute and chronic settings. As shown in Table 48.5, Braunwald has proposed that HF biomarkers be divided into six distinct categories with an additional one reserved for biomarkers that have not yet been classified (see also Chapter 8 and 10).[30]

As articulated,[31] clinically useful biomarkers of HF should be easily measured with high analytical precision, should reflect important processes involved in HF presence and progression, should not recapitulate clinical information already available at the bedside, and must provide clinically useful information for caregivers to more swiftly and reliably establish/reject a diagnosis, to more accurately estimate prognosis, or to inform more successful therapeutic strategies. Only the natriuretic peptides have met these requirements, although other promising biomarkers exist for use in HF assessment.

Natriuretic Peptides

The natriuretic peptides are useful biomarkers for HF diagnosis, estimation of HF severity and prognosis, and possibly for management of HF as well. The most commonly measured natriuretic peptides are B-type natriuretic peptide (BNP) and its amino-terminal cleavage pro-peptide equivalent, NT-proBNP; these two biomarkers are released from cardiomyocytes in response to stretch, and highly precise assays exist for their detection in blood (see also Chapter 47). Given the preponderance of myocardium in the ventricles, BNP and NT-proBNP mainly reflect ventricular stretch and are synthesized in response to wall stress. Atrial natriuretic peptide (ANP) is another member of the class of natriuretic peptides and is synthesized and secreted from atrial tissue; a mid-regional pro-ANP assay is now available and appears to deliver comparable results to BNP and NT-proBNP when tested in HF patients.[32]

Due to the differences in their clearance BNP and NT-proBNP have considerably different half-lives (BNP: 20 minutes; NT-proBNP: 90 minutes), and thus they circulate with very different concentrations. Both natriuretic peptides have become an important part of the HF assessment, however much like any diagnostic test, clinicians must always remember the broad array of structural and functional reasons for BNP or NT-proBNP release to correctly interpret their values.[33] Natriuretic peptide levels tend to increase progressively with worsening NYHA functional class, and tend to be higher in HFrEF, compared to HFpEF, despite independent contributions of diastolic function to their concentrations. Patients with acute HF most often have higher values for BNP and NT-proBNP, compared to chronic stable patients, however this is by no means a universal finding, and knowledge of an individual's natriuretic peptide value when stable may be useful to better interpret a change when a change in symptoms occurs.

When using BNP or NT-proBNP, the clinician should remember that beyond left ventricular systolic and diastolic dysfunction, concentrations of both peptides are higher in patients with valvular heart disease, pulmonary hypertension, ischemic heart disease, atrial arrhythmias, and even pericardial processes such as constriction.[33] Elevation of BNP or NT-proBNP—often marked—is nearly ubiquitous in infiltrative cardiomyopathies such as cardiac amyloidosis; these elusive diagnoses should be considered in a patient with significant elevation of natriuretic peptide but without obvious congestion. Additionally, numerous relevant medical covariates with effects on natriuretic peptide values must also be kept in mind. For example, both BNP and NT-proBNP concentrations increase with age, thought to identify accumulating structural heart disease in older patients. Both natriuretic peptides are higher in patients with renal failure, partially reflective of slower clearance, but also similarly identifying heart disease in this population of patients with prevalent cardiovascular risk factors. Elevated natriuretic peptide values can also be seen in hyperdynamic states, including sepsis. Patients who have right ventricular dysfunction as a result of pulmonary embolus may have elevated natriuretic peptide concentrations. It is also important to recognize that angiotensin receptor neprilysin inhibitors (ARNIs [see Chapter 50]) may modestly increase levels of BNP, but this finding is not universal and may be transient. As NT-proBNP is not a substrate for neprilysin, its concentrations remain reflective of the clinical picture; in patients under treatment with ARNI, changes in NT-proBNP are associated with LV remodeling parameters (such as change in LVEF)[34] and strongly predict outcomes.[35,36]

Obesity is strongly linked to lower-than-expected BNP or NT-proBNP values, despite comparable or higher wall stress in heavier patients. Given the common effect on BNP, NT-proBNP, and MR-proANP, this is not likely to be a clearance effect (as each are cleared differently), rather more likely to represent suppression of natriuretic peptide gene expression or post-translational modification.

Results of BNP or NT-proBNP, although useful, should always be interpreted in the context of sound clinical judgment, integrated with results of history, physical examination, and other testing; these important biomarkers strongly supplement clinical judgment, but should not replace it. Keeping this in mind, the natriuretic peptides have been shown to be useful to identify and exclude acute HF in the emergency department, as well as more indolent HF in the outpatient setting.[37]

Pivotal data for BNP and NT-proBNP testing to diagnose acute HF came from the Breathing Not Properly and ProBNP Investigation of Dyspnea in the Emergency Department (PRIDE) studies respectively. In the Breathing Not Properly, a BNP concentration of 100 pg/mL was highly accurate for the diagnosis of acutely decompensated HF; in PRIDE, an NT-proBNP cutoff of 900 pg/mL provided comparable performance to a BNP of 100 pg/mL. Subsequently, the International Collaborative of NT-proBNP (ICON) investigators showed that age stratification improved positive predictive value of NT-proBNP in acutely dyspneic patients; as well, an NT-proBNP concentration below 300 pg/mL was useful to exclude acutely decompensated HF.[33] These data were more recently affirmed in the ICON: Re-evaluation of Acute Diagnostic Cut-Offs in the Emergency Department study, where performance of NT-proBNP to detect or exclude acute HF remained robust in a more contemporary population of patients with acute dyspnea.[38]

Knowledge of natriuretic peptide levels in the emergency department is associated with more rapid diagnosis, lower admission rate, shorter length of hospital stay, and reduced cost. As clinical uncertainty in acute dyspnea is associated with worse prognosis, it is reassuring to note that natriuretic peptide testing is particularly useful in this complex situation.

For patients with less acute presentations of dyspnea in settings other than the ED, values of BNP or NT-proBNP are most often considerably lower; when used for evaluation of the dyspneic ambulatory patient, therefore, the optimized cutoffs from emergency department studies should not be used: lower values are mandatory, and optimized for their negative predictive value to exclude (rather than identify) HF.[37] Age stratification again improves diagnostic accuracy in this setting, as older patients are expected to have generally higher concentrations of BNP or NT-proBNP in the absence of clinical HF. If a patient is found to be above such cutoffs, further diagnostic testing such as echocardiography is likely needed. Causes of falsely low BNP or NT-proBNP in the outpatient setting are comparable to those with acute dyspnea.

Natriuretic peptide levels provide useful prognostic information across all ACC/AHA stages of HF even when adjusted for important variables from history, physical examination, echocardiography, or even cardiopulmonary exercise testing (Fig. 48.5). While one natriuretic peptide measurement is prognostically meaningful, serial follow up measurements add incrementally important prognostic information. For example, in patients with acute HF, those who do not show a robust reduction in BNP or NT-proBNP by the time of hospital discharge tend to have considerably higher rates of morbidity and mortality.[39] It has thus been suggested that a BNP or NT-proBNP decrease of 30% or more by hospital discharge is desirable. Similarly, in ambulatory HF, chronically elevated or rising natriuretic peptide values identify a particularly high-risk patient population. HF therapies may lower concentrations of BNP and NT-proBNP; when this finding occurs, prognosis is improved.

Other Biomarkers

Other promising biomarkers for use in patients with HF have been identified (see Table 48.5), and some are clinically available. In general, newer biomarkers for HF have been developed to supplement the natriuretic peptides for prognostication. While most have not yet achieved the prerequisite data to justify their widespread use, a few promising biomarkers bear mention.

Concentrations of soluble ST2 (a member of the interleukin receptor family) have been shown to be strongly linked to progressive HF and death in patients across the four ACC/AHA stages of HF.[40] Originally identified in a basic science model of mechanotransduction, ST2 plays a pivotal role in the formation of fibrosis in the heart; elevated concentrations of ST2 are thus associated with progressive cardiovascular dysfunction, remodeling, and risk for death. Soluble ST2

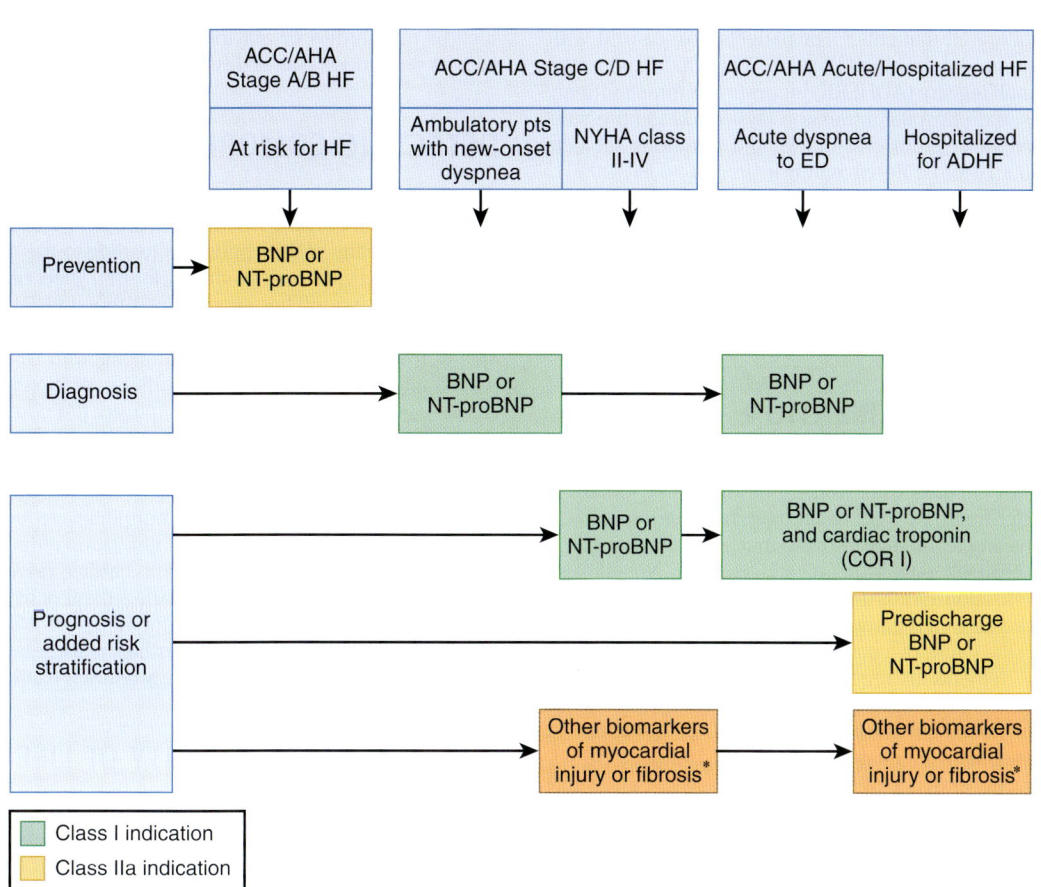

FIGURE 48.5 Indications for the use of biomarkers in heart failure. Key: *Other biomarkers of injury or fibrosis include soluble ST2 receptor, galectin-3, and high-sensitivity troponin. *ACC,* American College of Cardiology; *ADHF,* acute decompensated heart failure; *AHA,* American Heart Association; *BNP,* B-type natriuretic peptide; *COR,* Class of Recommendation; *ED,* emergency department; *HF,* heart failure; *NT-proBNP,* N-terminal pro-B-type natriuretic peptide; *NYHA,* New York Heart Association; *pts,* patients. (Modified from Yancy CW, Jessup M, Bozkurt B, et al. 2017 ACC/AHA/HFSA Focused Update of the 2013 ACCF/AHA Guideline for the Management of Heart Failure: a report of the American College of Cardiology/American Heart Association Task Force on Clinical Practice Guidelines and the Heart Failure Society of America. *J Am Coll Cardiol.* 2017;70[6]:776–803.)

concentrations are additive to natriuretic peptides for prognostication, are useful in both HFrEF and HFpEF, and are similarly dynamic to natriuretic peptides in their changes following HF therapies; in patients with both acutely decompensated and chronic HF, a chronically elevated or rising ST2 value strongly predicts adverse outcome.[41,42] Notably, among apparently normal patients in a population-based analysis, ST2 values predicted future HF, beyond other biomarkers such as BNP as well as echocardiographic parameters.[43] This implies the biochemical changes of ventricular remodeling may be detectable well before conventional biomarkers or imaging are abnormal.

The myofibrillar proteins, troponin T and I, are indicators of cardiomyocyte injury and may be elevated in HF patients in the absence of an acute coronary syndrome or even significant coronary artery disease. With the emergence of highly sensitive troponin assays, even more patients may be found to have elevated concentrations of these important predictors of risk.[44] While an elevated troponin value does not specifically identify myocardial necrosis due to coronary artery disease per se, given the importance of acute MI in the triggering of acute HF, a troponin should always be measured in this setting, although interpreted with caution. Elevated troponin concentrations in community-based normal subjects are prognostic for onset of HF (particularly if rising in serial measurement). Troponin is independently predictive of increased mortality risk across the HF spectrum.

Other novel biomarkers are emerging and may have a role in the comprehensive evaluation of the patient with HF; many of these novel markers reflect systemic stress or disarray of organs outside of the heart. For example, the mid-regional fragment of pro-adrenomedullin is a biomarker reflective of vascular and systemic stress and is powerfully prognostic for short-term adverse outcome (see also Chapter 47).[32] In a similar fashion, growth differentiation factor-15, another marker of cardiovascular stress, strongly predicts outcomes not only in established HF, but may also be prognostic for new-onset HF in apparently well subjects.[43] Lastly, novel biomarkers of renal dysfunction are emerging as strong predictors of cardiovascular risk beyond the standard measures of blood urea nitrogen or serum creatinine. Cystatin C (a ubiquitous protein found in all nucleated cells whose clearance is directly related to glomerular filtration) and β trace protein are two renal function markers whose values are tightly related to outcomes in HF, while neutrophil gelatinase-associated lipocalin, N-acetyl-β-D-glucosaminidase, and kidney injury molecule-1 are promising biomarkers of acute renal injury whose values rise well before renal function is perceived to be worsening, and impart important prognostic information in HF patients.[45]

Ultimately, for the comprehensive evaluation of HF, it seems likely that a combination or panel of biomarkers will prove to be the most useful way of assessing prognosis.

RISK SCORING FOR PROGNOSIS

During initial and subsequent evaluation of the patient with HF, the clinician should routinely assess the potential for adverse outcome. Besides biomarker testing, a number of validated methods for risk stratification in HF exist, including a variety of multivariable clinical risk scores for use in both ambulatory and hospitalized patients. One well-validated risk score (the Seattle Heart Failure model) is available in an internet-based application (www.seattleheartfailuremodel.org) and has been shown to provide robust information regarding risk of mortality in ambulatory HF patients.[46] For patients hospitalized with acute symptoms, the model developed by the Acute Decompensated Heart Failure National Registry (ADHERE) incorporates three routinely measured variables upon hospital admission (systolic blood pressure, blood urea nitrogen, and serum creatinine), and partitions subjects into categories with a 10-fold difference in risk (from 2.1% to 21.9%).[46] Importantly, clinical risk scores have not performed as well in estimating risk of hospital readmission. For this purpose, natriuretic peptide results may be of more use, particularly when measured after in-patient treatment, just prior to discharge; a lack of BNP or NT-proBNP reduction by 30% during in-patient treatment may identify those at higher risk for short-term death or rehospitalization.

RIGHT HEART CATHETERIZATION

Measurement of intracardiac pressures and hemodynamics (see also Chapter 22) as part of the diagnostic work-up or for guiding therapy is less commonly performed now than in the past, because biomarkers and noninvasive imaging techniques provide much of the information that was previously available only by heart catheterization. Nonetheless, as right heart catheterization affords unequivocal assessment of hemodynamics and filling pressures, it is particularly useful in cases where there is uncertainty about the cause of a patient's symptoms and in situations where precise measurements are required to guide therapy or decision making (e.g., selection of patients for heart transplantation). In addition, right heart catheterization is of value (and should be considered) in those with HF complicated by clinically significant hypotension, systemic hypoperfusion, dependence on inotropic infusions, or persistently severe symptoms despite adjustment of recommended therapies.

An invasive assessment with right heart catheterization is important to assess the pulmonary vascular resistance, a necessary part of the evaluation for heart transplantation. When pulmonary artery pressures are found to be elevated, response to pulmonary arterial vasodilating agents can be determined in this context, and provides important information determining whether a patient with pulmonary hypertension will be acceptable for cardiac transplantation. In addition, obtaining the pulmonary artery wedge pressure is useful for assessing volume status. The pulmonary artery wedge pressure usually estimates the left ventricular end-diastolic pressure if no obstruction to flow between the left atrium and left ventricle exists. While determination of hemodynamic variables at rest suffices in most patients, there are cases where exercise helps to reveal the presence and/or magnitude of abnormal intracardiac pressures and flow. Pulmonary hypertension, for example, can be highly dynamic and exercise measurements may be needed.

> Use of hemodynamic monitoring to guide therapy was evaluated in patients with advanced HF in the Evaluation Study of Congestive Heart Failure and Pulmonary Artery Catheterization Effectiveness (ESCAPE) trial.[47] The results did not show any clear benefit on morbidity and mortality of pulmonary artery-guided management compared to careful clinical assessment. The failure to affect postdischarge outcomes appears to be related to the fact that the hemodynamic improvements that were affected during hospitalization reverted back toward baseline within a relatively short period of time. Consequently, "tailored therapy" of HF is used less commonly now than in the past, but has a role particularly in patients with HF complicated by hypotension, systemic hypoperfusion, and end-organ dysfunction.

ENDOMYOCARDIAL BIOPSY

The role of endomyocardial biopsy for evaluating patients with HF is also discussed in Chapter 55. In general, biopsy of the myocardium is performed if a disorder with a unique prognosis or one which would benefit from a specific treatment regimen is suspected and the diagnosis cannot be made by conventional methods. The incremental diagnostic, therapeutic, and prognostic benefit offered by the information obtained from a biopsy must be weighed against the risks of the procedure. The sensitivity of endomyocardial biopsy may vary, depending on the cause of HF; for example, sensitivity is higher in more diffuse disease states such as myocarditis or amyloidosis, while more patchy disease states such as sarcoidosis may be less easily detected using biopsy.

DETECTING COMORBID CONDITIONS

The incidence of HF rises sharply from the sixth decade onward which is coincident with the time when other chronic diseases begin to manifest. In addition, many of the conditions leading to the development of HF (e.g., diabetes, hypertension, atherosclerosis) affect organs other than the heart. Thus, comorbidities are quite common in HF patients, and have a profound effect on the course of affected patients: a substantial percentage of hospitalizations suffered by patients with HF are in fact non-HF related, and not precipitated by a cardiac condition in more than half of cases.[48] Comorbidities not only complicate the course of patients with concomitant HF, but they also have a substantial impact on ability to manage patients with HF; as an example, chronic kidney disease may limit application of agents blocking the renin-angiotensin-aldosterone system. Lastly, the presence of comorbidities reduces the prognostic benefits of GDMT; for example, atrial fibrillation reduces benefit of many therapies, including beta blockers and cardiac resynchronization. With recent data suggesting aggressive management of hypertension and use of sodium-glucose co-transporter 2 inhibitors for diabetes mellitus care both may reduce HF events,[49,50] this illustrates detection and management of comorbidities is a particularly relevant exercise.

ASSESSMENT OF QUALITY OF LIFE

HF has a profound effect on quality of life, and poor health-related quality of life is a powerful predictor of adverse prognosis in HF patients. Change in health-related quality of life is now also considered an approvable endpoint for HF therapies. Determinants of poor quality of life in HF include female gender, younger age, higher body-mass index, worse symptoms, as well as the presence of depression and sleep apnea.[51] Improved quality of life has been reported following standard HF drug treatment intensification, cardiac resynchronization therapy, or in disease management programs. Given its importance, at the initial and subsequent visits, consideration should be given for quality-of-life assessment, whether through standard history or through the use of validated tools for its estimation such as the Kansas City Cardiomyopathy Questionnaire.

CARDIOPULMONARY EXERCISE TESTING

Exercise intolerance is a prime symptom of HF. Despite this fact, quantification of exercise tolerance is imprecise (see also Chapter 15); standard approaches such as the NYHA criteria or the 6-minute walk test are subjective and insensitive measures of functional capacity. Additionally, the 6-minute walk test does not reveal how close the patient may be to their maximal capacity for exercise, does not discriminate between the causes of impaired exercise capacity (e.g., cardiac, pulmonary, orthopedic) or poor motivation, and does not account for the effects of conditioning and/or age; older age may undermine accuracy of the 6-minute walk test. When more precise information is needed, cardiopulmonary exercise testing (CPX) is often used because it allows for identification of causes of exercise intolerance and quantification of exercise capacity, and delivers important physiologic information not routinely available from standard stress testing.[52]

> CPX is performed using treadmill or cycle exercise, continued to symptom limitation. Analysis of gas exchange at rest, during exercise, and in the recovery phase following exertion is performed, and measures of oxygen uptake (V_{O_2}), expiratory ventilation (V_E), and carbon dioxide output (V_{CO_2}) are generated, typically expressed as a ratio of their slope. The maximum V_{O_2} is the standard expression of capacity for endurance, based on the Fick equation, which states that V_{O_2} = cardiac output × [oxygen content$_{arterial}$ − oxygen content$_{venous}$]. Thus, V_{O_2} is a direct function of cardiac output, and indeed very strong associations are established between maximal V_{O_2}, cardiac output, and risk for death. The V_E/V_{CO_2} slope is an expression of efficiency of pulmonary CO_2 clearance

during exercise and has also been suggested to be powerfully prognostic. These variables are often used in conjunction with each other in the assessment of advanced HF.

Use of CPX is a standard part of the routine evaluation prior to heart transplantation; moderate to severely reduced maximal V_{O_2} values (e.g., <14 mL $O_2 \cdot kg^{-1} \cdot min^{-1}$) are often used as a prognostic threshold in this setting, while maximal V_{O_2} values less than 10 mL $O_2 \cdot kg^{-1} \cdot min^{-1}$ are considered severe, and particularly prognostic if the V_E/V_{CO_2} slope is ≥45.0. Many evidence-based medical and devices therapies for HF, such as certain drugs, cardiac resynchronization therapy, or exercise may result in improvement in CPX parameters, however this is not universal. For example, beta blockers have significant influence on survival, but do not significantly improve maximal V_{O_2}. Thus, as beta blockers improve prognosis across all ranges of maximal V_{O_2}, aggressive use of these agents may necessarily result in a lower optimal cut point than less than 14 mL $O_2 \cdot kg^{-1} \cdot min^{-1}$ for referral for cardiac transplantation. While CPX is most validated in HFrEF, it appears to be of prognostic value in HFpEF, although data are more limited.

USE OF IMAGING MODALITIES IN THE DIAGNOSIS AND MANAGEMENT OF PATIENTS WITH HEART FAILURE

Noninvasive cardiac imaging serves a vital role in the assessment of patients with HF and is essential for determining whether the patient should be classified as HFpEF or HFrEF (see also Chapters 16 to 20). Imaging may help confirm the diagnosis of HF by assessing the presence and severity of structural and functional changes in the heart, provide clues about the etiology of cardiac dysfunction (i.e., congenital heart disease, valvular abnormalities, pericardial disease, coronary artery disease), risk stratify patients, and possibly guide treatment strategies. Imaging modalities can also be used to help assess the efficacy of therapeutic interventions, provide ongoing prognostic information, and further guide treatment. The primary noninvasive cardiac imaging modalities used to evaluate HF patients are echocardiography (Chapter 16), magnetic resonance imaging (MRI; Chapter 19), computed tomography (CT; Chapter 20), and nuclear imaging, including single photon emission computed tomography (SPECT) and positron emission tomography (PET) techniques (Chapter 18). Imaging modalities often provide complementary data and each has the capacity to provide unique information in individual patients. While the initial evaluation of a patient with newly diagnosed HF should include a transthoracic echocardiogram, further imaging with MRI, CT, and/or nuclear techniques may be considered depending upon the need to further address questions regarding cardiac structure and function, etiology, and issues such as the potential for reversibility of systolic dysfunction with revascularization.

Echocardiography and Lung Ultrasound

Transthoracic echocardiography is an important part of the evaluation of HF,[53] can be performed without risk to the patient, does not involve radiation exposure, and can be performed at the bedside if necessary (see also Chapter 16). Increasing use of handheld echocardiography has facilitated evaluation at the point of care, such as in the emergency department setting in the context of an acute presentation.

Echocardiography is particularly well suited for evaluating the structure and function of both the myocardium and heart valves and providing information about intracardiac pressures and flows. For patients with HFrEF, LV volumes and systolic function can be assessed semi-quantitatively, or quantified using the biplane method and the modified Simpson's rule. Information about the morphology and relative sizes of the cardiac chambers may suggest specific diagnoses. For example, concentric LV hypertrophy with severe bi-atrial enlargement raises the possibility that HF is due to an infiltrative process such as amyloidosis, particularly in the absence of a prior diagnosis of hypertension; in cases such as this, strain imaging may be helpful to evaluate for the characteristic "apical sparing" seen in patients with amyloid cardiomyopathy. Diastolic function is assessed using Doppler measurements, including analyses of the mitral valve inflow pattern (early [E] and atrial [A] waveforms), tissue velocities at the mitral valve annulus, pulmonary vein flow, and the left atrial volume indexed to body surface area (see Chapter 16). Diastolic dysfunction can be further classified as grades I to III based on the above measurements, with incremental prognostic importance in HF as worsening grades of diastolic dysfunction are noted. Ratio of early mitral valve inflow to mitral valve annulus velocity determined using tissue Doppler (E/e′) is particularly helpful to determine presence and severity of diastolic dysfunction; a ratio of 15 or greater is abnormal. Pulmonary hypertension in patients without significant systolic dysfunction or pulmonary disease suggests that diastolic dysfunction may be present. Another advantage of echocardiography is the ability to noninvasively estimate right heart pressures. For example, right atrial pressures are estimated by the inferior vena cava (IVC) diameter and the relative change in diameter upon inspiration. Normal IVC diameter and inspiratory collapse of at least 50% are associated with normal RA pressures, while increased IVC diameter and smaller inspiratory changes indicate elevated RA pressure.

Lung ultrasound (LUS) has become increasingly used to evaluate patients presenting to the emergency department setting; it has been found to be useful to diagnose interstitial pulmonary edema and fluid overload through the detection of vertical reverberation artifacts, known as B-lines. Such B-lines are created at the acoustic interface between two structures with differing acoustic impedances, such as fluid-filled structures and alveolar air. Also known as "comets," in the appropriate setting, such B-lines may be highly sensitive and specific for presence of HF, particularly when incorporated with clinical judgment and other tools such as chest radiography and natriuretic peptide testing.

Magnetic Resonance Imaging

MRI provides high-quality imaging of the heart and involves no radiation, which is a significant advantage over CT (see also Chapter 19). Diagnostic images can be obtained in nearly all patients and unlike echocardiography, images can be obtained in arbitrary tomographic planes. MRI is excellent for evaluating cardiac morphology, chamber sizes, and cardiac function. Using different pulse sequences with and without gadolinium contrast, MRI can characterize myocardial tissue and assess myocardial viability. Cardiac MRI can distinguish ischemic from nonischemic cardiomyopathies based upon the pattern of delayed gadolinium enhancement from T1-weighted images: ischemic cardiomyopathies usually show characteristic sub-endocardial enhancement at the sites of prior infarctions, while nonischemic dilated cardiomyopathies most commonly have either no enhancement, mid-wall enhancement, or other patterns depending upon the cause (Fig. 48.6). Additionally, MRI is extremely useful to identify the presence of myocarditis, and may be similarly helpful in the diagnosis of specific cardiomyopathies such as infiltrative processes or left ventricular noncompaction. Use of MRI-compatible pacemakers and defibrillators has facilitated more widespread use of MRI imaging, however clinicians are advised to confirm device compatibility before imaging.

Cardiac Computed Tomography

The current role of cardiac CT in HF is mainly to help determine whether or not obstructive coronary artery disease is present via the use of CT angiography, an important application particularly for patients with lower likelihood for coronary artery disease (see also Chapter 20). Emerging applications of CT angiography may be to assist in assessment of coronary venous anatomy prior to CRT lead placement. Recent advances in CT technology have led to less radiation exposure, however cardiac CT angiography still involves administering iodinated contrast, a concern in patients who are at risk for developing nephrotoxicity.

Nuclear Imaging

A wide array of nuclear imaging techniques have been developed for the assessment of HF (see also Chapter 18). In particular, SPECT and

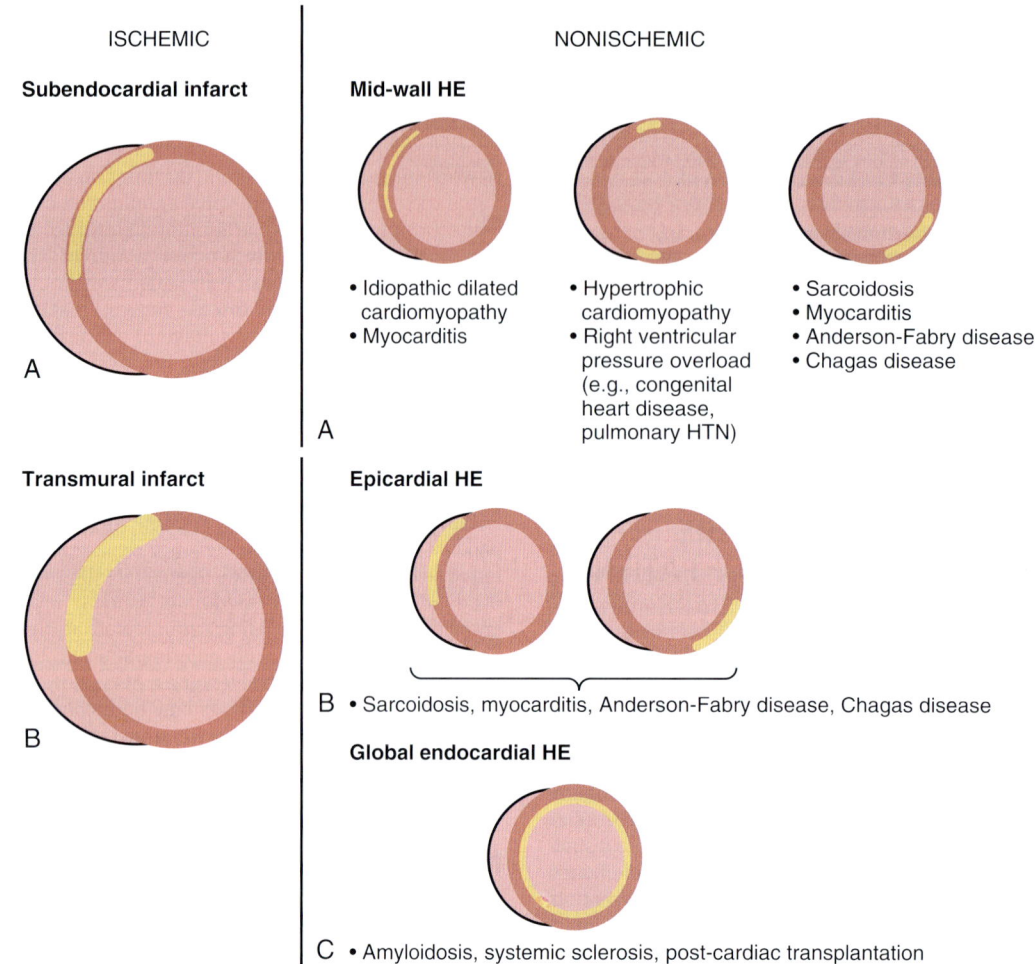

FIGURE 48.6 Patterns of hyperenhancement (HE) with magnetic resonance imaging (MRI) in various disease states. *HTN*, Hypertension. (Modified from Mahrholdt H, Wagner A, Judd RM, et al. Delayed enhancement cardiovascular magnetic resonance assessment of non-ischaemic cardiomyopathies. *Eur Heart J*. 2005;26:1461.)

PET technologies are well-suited for assessing myocardial ischemia and viability, and for evaluating myocardial function. The use of nuclear imaging to determine myocardial viability is discussed in Chapter 18. ^{18}F-fluorodeoxyglucose (^{18}F-FDG) PET scanning may be particularly helpful for diagnosis prognosis, and management of cardiac sarcoidosis[54]; a characteristic heterogeneous uptake pattern in the myocardium may be seen in patients with cardiac sarcoidosis in contrast to diffuse uptake seen in DCM and normal subjects. Following successful treatment with immunosuppressive medication, ^{18}F-FDG uptake may normalize. ^{99m}Technicium pyrophosphate (^{99m}Tc-PYP) scanning has become a major imaging modality for diagnosing transthyretin amyloidosis (see Chapter 53). Although ^{99m}Tc-PYP scans are more frequently positive in patients with transthyretin amyloidosis, they can also be modestly positive in patients with AL amyloid (see Chapter 53).[55] Lastly, cardiac scans using ^{123}I-metaiodobenzylguanidine (MIBG) may provide objective evaluation of cardiac sympathetic function; this imaging strategy may predict risk for sudden death due to arrhythmia in NYHA class II or III HFrEF when the heart-to-mediastinal ratio of ^{123}I-MIBG is low.[56]

TIMING OF ADVANCED HEART FAILURE REFERRAL

Among patients with advanced HFrEF, early identification and timely referral of select patients to a HF specialist is critical so that those with advanced disease can be considered for heart transplantation or mechanical circulatory support (see also Chapter 50). This window of opportunity is missed if referral is delayed until multiorgan failure develops, as such patients may no longer be candidates for these therapies. High-risk features include need for intravenous inotropic agents, worsening NYHA symptom severity or congestion refractory to diuretic use, rising natriuretic peptide concentrations, end-organ dysfunction, EF less than 35%, ventricular arrhythmias, recurrent hospitalizations, progressive intolerance to HF therapies, or low blood pressure/high heart rate.

SUMMARY AND FUTURE PERSPECTIVES

As treatment options for HF continue to evolve, there will be increased emphasis on more rapid, accurate, and cost-effective assessment of patients with the goal being to provide unambiguous information about the presence, severity, and cause of HF. New insights into the biology of cardiac dysfunction are likely to lead to the development of therapeutic approaches that are specific to the underlying etiology. Continued advances in the use of biomarkers and imaging techniques to diagnose, stage, and determine etiology of HF will be needed to meet these future demands. Even as these diagnostic modalities increase in their precision and accuracy, the information obtained through the history and physical examination will remain at the core of our ability to understand how to employ these tests most judiciously and to treat patients most effectively.

REFERENCES
Heart Failure Diagnosis and Epidemiology
1. Roger VL. Epidemiology of heart failure. *Circ Res*. 2013;113(6):646–659.
2. Guha K, McDonagh T. Heart failure epidemiology: European perspective. *Curr Cardiol Rev*. 2013;9(2):123–127.
3. Writing Group Members, Mozaffarian D, Benjamin EJ, et al. Executive summary: heart disease and stroke statistics—2016 update: a report from the American Heart Association. *Circulation*. 2016;133(4):447–454.

4. Kapoor JR, Kapoor R, Ju C, et al. Precipitating clinical factors, heart failure characterization, and outcomes in patients hospitalized with heart failure with reduced, borderline, and preserved ejection fraction. *JACC Heart Fail*. 2016;4(6):464–472.
5. Gulati G, Udelson JE. Heart failure with improved ejection fraction: is it possible to escape one's past? *JACC Heart Fail*. 2018;6(9):725–733.
6. Wilcox JE, Fang JC, Margulies KB, Mann DL. Heart failure with recovered left ventricular ejection fraction: JACC Scientific Expert Panel. *J Am Coll Cardiol*. 2020;76(6):719–734.
7. Halliday BP, Wassall R, Lota AS, et al. Withdrawal of pharmacological treatment for heart failure in patients with recovered dilated cardiomyopathy (TRED-HF): an open-label, pilot, randomised trial. *Lancet*. 2019;393(10166):61–73.

The Medical History and Physical Examination

8. Yancy CW, Jessup M, Bozkurt B, et al. 2013 ACCF/AHA guideline for the management of heart failure: a report of the American College of Cardiology Foundation/American Heart Association Task Force on practice guidelines. *J Am Coll Cardiol*. 2013;62(16):e147–239.
9. Solomonica A, Burger AJ, Aronson D. Hemodynamic determinants of dyspnea improvement in acute decompensated heart failure. *Circ Heart Fail*. 2012;6(1):53–60.
10. Damy T, Margarit L, Noroc A, et al. Prognostic impact of sleep-disordered breathing and its treatment with nocturnal ventilation for chronic heart failure. *Eur J Heart Fail*. 2012;14(9):1009–1019.
11. Yu DS, Chan HY, Leung DY, et al. Symptom clusters and quality of life among patients with advanced heart failure. *J Geriatr Cardiol*. 2016;13(5):408–414.
12. Rahman A, Jafry S, Jeejeebhoy K, et al. Malnutrition and cachexia in heart failure. *JPEN J Parenter Enteral Nutr*. 2016;40(4):475–486.
13. Avery CL, Loehr LR, Baggett C, et al. The population burden of heart failure attributable to modifiable risk factors: the ARIC (Atherosclerosis Risk in Communities) study. *J Am Coll Cardiol*. 2012;60(17):1640–1646.
14. Higgins AY, O'Halloran TD, Chang JD. Chemotherapy-induced cardiomyopathy. *Heart Fail Rev*. 2015;20(6):721–730.
15. Kelder JC, Cramer MJ, van Wijngaarden J, et al. The diagnostic value of physical examination and additional testing in primary care patients with suspected heart failure. *Circulation*. 2011;124(25):2865–2873.
16. Ho JE, Gona P, Pencina MJ, et al. Discriminating clinical features of heart failure with preserved vs. reduced ejection fraction in the community. *Eur Heart J*. 2012;33(14):1734–1741.
17. Buckner K. Cardiac asthma. *Immunol Allergy Clin North Am*. 2013;33(1):35–44.
18. Dharmarajan K, Strait KM, Lagu T, et al. Acute decompensated heart failure is routinely treated as a cardiopulmonary syndrome. *PLoS One*. 2013;8(10):e78222.
19. Nohria A, Tsang SW, Fang JC, et al. Clinical assessment identifies hemodynamic profiles that predict outcomes in patients admitted with heart failure. *J Am Coll Cardiol*. 2003;41(10):1797–1804.

Routine Laboratory Assessment

20. Sartini S, Frizzi J, Borselli M, et al. Which method is best for an early accurate diagnosis of acute heart failure? Comparison between lung ultrasound, chest X-ray and NT pro-BNP performance: a prospective study. *Intern Emerg Med*. 2016.
21. Urso C, Brucculeri S, Caimi G. Acid-base and electrolyte abnormalities in heart failure: pathophysiology and implications. *Heart Fail Rev*. 2015;20(4):493–503.
22. Mohammed AA, van Kimmenade RR, Richards M, et al. Hyponatremia, natriuretic peptides, and outcomes in acutely decompensated heart failure: results from the International Collaborative of NT-proBNP Study. *Circ Heart Fail*. 2010;3(3):354–361.
23. O'Connell JB, Alemayehu A. Hyponatremia, heart failure, and the role of tolvaptan. *Postgrad Med*. 2012;124(2):29–39.
24. Legrand M, Mebazaa A, Ronco C, Januzzi Jr JL. When cardiac failure, kidney dysfunction, and kidney injury intersect in acute conditions: the case of cardiorenal syndrome. *Crit Care Med*. 2014;42(9):2109–2117.
25. Damman K, Valente MA, Voors AA, et al. Renal impairment, worsening renal function, and outcome in patients with heart failure: an updated meta-analysis. *Eur Heart J*. 2014;35(7):455–469.
26. Fonarow GC, Adams Jr KF, Abraham WT, et al. Risk stratification for in-hospital mortality in acutely decompensated heart failure: classification and regression tree analysis. *J Am Med Assoc*. 2005;293(5):572–580.
27. Lala A, McNulty SE, Mentz RJ, et al. Relief and recurrence of congestion during and after hospitalization for acute heart failure: insights from diuretic optimization strategy evaluation in acute decompensated heart failure (DOSE-AHF) and cardiorenal rescue study in acute decompensated heart failure (CARESS-HF). *Circ Heart Fail*. 2015;8(4):741–748.
28. Cleland JG, Zhang J, Pellicori P, et al. Prevalence and outcomes of anemia and hematinic deficiencies in patients with chronic heart failure. *JAMA Cardiol*. 2016;1(5):539–547.
29. Huang YL, Hu ZD, Liu SJ, et al. Prognostic value of red blood cell distribution width for patients with heart failure: a systematic review and meta-analysis of cohort studies. *PLoS One*. 2014;9(8):e104861.
30. Braunwald E. Biomarkers in heart failure. *N Engl J Med*. 2008;358(20):2148–2159.

31. van Kimmenade RR, Januzzi Jr JL. Emerging biomarkers in heart failure. *Clin Chem*. 2011;58(1):127–138.
32. Shah RV, Truong QA, Gaggin HK, et al. Mid-regional pro-atrial natriuretic peptide and pro-adrenomedullin testing for the diagnostic and prognostic evaluation of patients with acute dyspnoea. *Eur Heart J*. 2012;33(17):2197–2205.
33. Ibrahim N, Januzzi JL. The potential role of natriuretic peptides and other biomarkers in heart failure diagnosis, prognosis and management. *Expert Rev Cardiovasc Ther*. 2015;13(9):1017–1030.
34. Januzzi Jr JL, Prescott MF, Butler J, et al. Association of change in N-terminal pro-B-type natriuretic peptide following Initiation of Sacubitril-Valsartan treatment with cardiac structure and function in patients with heart failure with reduced ejection fraction. *J Am Med Assoc*. 2019;1–11.
35. Januzzi Jr JL, Camacho A, Pina IL, et al. Reverse cardiac remodeling and outcome after initiation of sacubitril/valsartan. *Circ Heart Fail*. 2020;13(6):e006946.
36. Zile MR, Claggett BL, Prescott MF, et al. Prognostic implications of changes in N-terminal pro-B-type natriuretic peptide in patients with heart failure. *J Am Coll Cardiol*. 2016;68(22):2425–2436.
37. Kim HN, Januzzi Jr JL. Natriuretic peptide testing in heart failure. *Circulation*. 2011;123(18):2015–2019.
38. Januzzi Jr JL, Chen-Tournoux AA, Christenson RH, et al. N-terminal pro-B-type natriuretic peptide in the emergency department: the ICON-RELOADED study. *J Am Coll Cardiol*. 2018;71(11):1191–1200.
39. Salah K, Kok WE, Eurlings LW, et al. A novel discharge risk model for patients hospitalised for acute decompensated heart failure incorporating N-terminal pro-B-type natriuretic peptide levels: a European coLlaboration on Acute decompeNsated Heart Failure: ELAN-HF Score. *Heart*. 2014;100(2):115–125.
40. Shah RV, Januzzi Jr JL. Soluble ST2 and galectin-3 in heart failure. *Clin Lab Med*. 2014;34(1):87–97 (vi–vii).
41. Aimo A, Vergaro G, Passino C, et al. Prognostic value of soluble suppression of tumorigenicity-2 in chronic heart failure: a meta-analysis. *JACC Heart Fail*. 2017;5(4):280–286.
42. Aimo A, Vergaro G, Ripoli A, et al. Meta-analysis of soluble suppression of tumorigenicity-2 and prognosis in acute heart failure. *JACC Heart Fail*. 2017;5(4):287–296.
43. Wang TJ, Wollert KC, Larson MG, et al. Prognostic utility of novel biomarkers of cardiovascular stress: the Framingham Heart Study. *Circulation*. 2012;126(13):1596–1604.
44. Januzzi Jr JL, Filippatos G, Nieminen M, Gheorghiade M. Troponin elevation in patients with heart failure: on behalf of the third universal definition of myocardial infarction global task force: heart failure section. *Eur Heart J*. 2012;33(18):2265–2271.
45. Metra M, Cotter G, Gheorghiade M, et al. The role of the kidney in heart failure. *Eur Heart J*. 2012;33(17):2135–2142.

Risk Scoring for Prognosis

46. Alba AC, Agoritsas T, Jankowski M, et al. Risk prediction models for mortality in ambulatory patients with heart failure: a systematic review. *Circ Heart Fail*. 2013;6(5):881–889.

Right Heart Catheterization

47. Kahwash R, Leier CV, Miller L. Role of the pulmonary artery catheter in diagnosis and management of heart failure. *Cardiol Clin*. 2011;29(2):281–288.

Detecting Comorbid Conditions

48. van Deursen VM, Damman K, van der Meer P, et al. Co-morbidities in heart failure. *Heart Fail Rev*. 2012.
49. Group SR, Wright Jr JT, Williamson JD, et al. A randomized trial of intensive versus standard blood-pressure control. *N Engl J Med*. 2015;373(22):2103–2116.
50. Zinman B, Wanner C, Lachin JM, et al. Empagliflozin, cardiovascular outcomes, and mortality in type 2 diabetes. *N Engl J Med*. 2015;373(22):2117–2128.

Assessment of Quality of Life

51. Garin O, Herdman M, Vilagut G, et al. Assessing health-related quality of life in patients with heart failure: a systematic, standardized comparison of available measures. *Heart Fail Rev*. 2014;19(3):359–367.

Cardiopulmonary Exercise Testing and Imaging Modalities

52. Malhotra R, Bakken K, D'Elia E, Lewis GD. Cardiopulmonary exercise testing in heart failure. *JACC Heart Fail*. 2016;4(8):607–616.
53. Omar AM, Bansal M, Sengupta PP. Advances in echocardiographic imaging in heart failure with reduced and preserved ejection fraction. *Circ Res*. 2016;119(2):357–374.
54. Aggarwal NR, Snipelisky D, Young PM, et al. Advances in imaging for diagnosis and management of cardiac sarcoidosis. *Eur Heart J Cardiovasc Imaging*. 2015;16(9):949–958.
55. Maurer MS. Noninvasive identification of ATTRwt cardiac amyloid: the Re-emergence of nuclear Cardiology. *Am J Med*. 2015;128(12):1275–1280.
56. Travin MI. Clinical applications of myocardial innervation imaging. *Cardiol Clin*. 2016;34(1):133–147.

49 Diagnosis and Management of Acute Heart Failure

G. MICHAEL FELKER AND JOHN R. TEERLINK

EPIDEMIOLOGY, 946
Nomenclature and Definition, 946
Scope of the Problem, 946
Ejection Fraction, 946
Age, Race, and Gender, 946
Comorbidities, 947
Global Differences in Acute Heart Failure, 947

PATHOPHYSIOLOGY, 947
Congestion, 949
Myocardial Function, 949
Renal Mechanisms, 950

Vascular Mechanisms, 951
Neurohormonal and Inflammatory Mechanisms, 951

EVALUATION OF THE ACUTE HEART FAILURE PATIENT, 951
Classification, 951
Symptoms of Acute Heart Failure, 953
Physical Examination, 953
Other Diagnostic Testing, 954
Risk Stratification, 954

MANAGEMENT OF THE PATIENT WITH ACUTE HEART FAILURE, 955
Phases of Management, 955
General Approaches to Acute Heart Failure Therapy, 958
Process of Care, Outcomes, and Quality Assessment, 960
Specific Therapies, 961
Potential New Therapies, 966

FUTURE PERSPECTIVES, 972

REFERENCES, 972

Acute heart failure (AHF) is among the most common causes for hospitalization in patients older than 65 years in the developed world. Increasingly, the spectrum of worsening HF is recognized to encompass not just patients requiring acute hospitalization, but also worsening of HF in outpatient settings and in patients already hospitalized. The prevalence of HF is projected to continue to increase over time due to a convergence of several epidemiologic trends: the aging of the population, given the age-related incidence of HF; the reduction in hypertension-related mortality and the greatly improved survival after myocardial infarction (MI), resulting in more patients living with chronic heart failure (see Chapter 48); and the availability of effective therapy for prevention of sudden death (see Chapters 58 and 70) (Fig. 49.1). AHF is increasingly recognized as a distinct disorder with unique epidemiology, pathophysiology, treatments, and outcomes.

EPIDEMIOLOGY

Nomenclature and Definition

A variety of overlapping terms have been used to characterize AHF in the literature, including "acute heart failure syndromes" (AHFS), "acute decompensated heart failure" (ADHF), "acute decompensation of chronic heart failure" (ADCHF), "worsening heart failure" (WHF), and "hospitalization for heart failure" (HHF). Although none of these is universally accepted, we will use the terminology "acute heart failure" in this chapter for simplicity. Broadly speaking, AHF can be defined as the new onset or recurrence of symptoms and signs of HF requiring urgent or emergent therapy and resulting in unscheduled care or hospitalization. An important source of confusion with this proposed definition is the word "acute"—although this suggests a sudden onset of symptoms, many patients may have a more sub-acute course, with gradual worsening of symptoms that ultimately reaches a level of severity sufficient to seek unscheduled medical care.

Scope of the Problem

In the United States, HF is the primary diagnosis for more than 1 million hospitalized patients annually, and a secondary diagnosis for an additional 3 million hospitalizations.[1] Similar numbers of hospitalizations are reported in Europe.[2] The direct and indirect costs associated with HF approach 40 billion US dollars per year in the United States, and the majority of these expenditures are related to the costs of hospitalizations.[3,4] As noted earlier, the overall prevalence of chronic heart failure continues to grow. However, recent data suggest that the age-adjusted rate of HHF has begun to decrease, at least for primary heart failure events.[1] To what extent these changes are related to more effective treatments of chronic heart failure or alternatively, changes in care to create alternative care pathways for avoiding hospitalization is unknown. Changes in medical care (especially in the United States) have led to increased efforts to manage milder forms of WHF without hospitalization, utilizing outpatient diuretic clinics and observation units, although available data suggest that even these milder forms of decompensation are still associated with adverse prognosis.[5,6] Despite these potentially encouraging trends, AHF will be a major clinical and economic problem for health care systems for the foreseeable future. An important development in the understanding of the epidemiology, clinical characteristics, and outcomes of patients with AHF has been the development of large, relatively unselected registries of AHF which provide a "real-world" perspective on the epidemiology and outcomes of AHF worldwide (Table 49.1).[7]

Ejection Fraction

On the basis of available registry data, 40% to 50% of patients hospitalized have heart failure with preserved ejection fraction (HFpEF). Important epidemiologic differences exist between heart failure with reduced ejection fraction (HFrEF) and HFpEF (see Chapter 48). The in-hospital mortality of patients with HFpEF appears to be lower compared with that of patients with HFrEF, but post-discharge rehospitalization rates and long-term mortality after hospitalization are similarly high for both groups. Patients with AHF and HFpEF are more likely to be rehospitalized for and to die from non-CV causes than patients with AHF and HFrEF, reflecting their more advanced age and greater burden of comorbidity. More recently, the concept of heart failure with "mid-range ejection fraction" or "mildly reduced ejection fraction," that is, HF-mrEF, has been proposed as an additional refinement of the standard HFrEF vs HFpEF dichotomy, but specific data on AHF outcomes in this group are limited (Fig. 49.2).[8]

Age, Race, and Gender

There are significant differences in the epidemiology of AHF based on age, race, and gender. AHF disproportionately affects older people, with a mean age of 75 years in large registries. AHF affects men and women

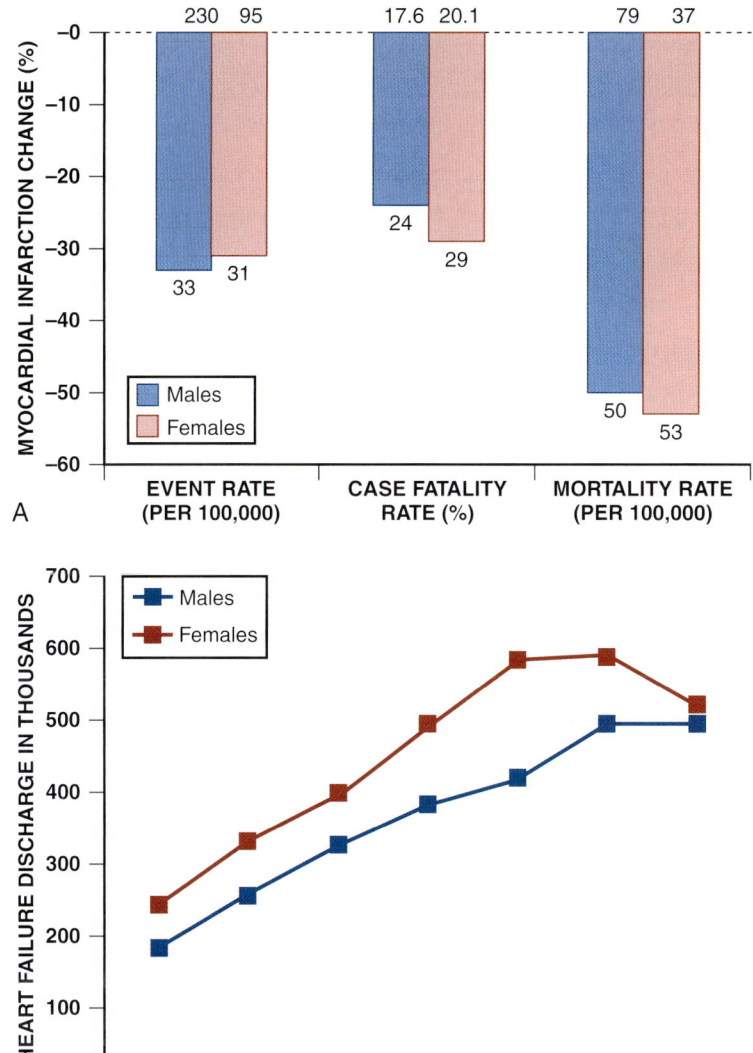

FIGURE 49.1 Reduction in myocardial infarction (MI) and increase in acute heart failure hospitalizations. **A,** Percentage change in MI rates and fatality rates in England from 2002 to 2010. **B,** Hospital discharges for heart failure by gender from 1980 to 2010. (From Braunwald E. The war against heart failure: the Lancet lecture. *Lancet.* 2015;385[9970]:812–824.)

failure, but also can complicate diagnosis and management. Hypertension is the most prevalent concurrent condition, present in approximately two-thirds of the patients (see also Chapter 26), whereas coronary artery disease (CAD) is present in about half and dyslipidemia in over one-third (see Chapters 27 and 40).[11,12] Other conditions that are the result of the vascular injury produced by these diseases, such as stroke, peripheral vascular disease, and chronic kidney disease are also very common in patients with AHF. Diabetes mellitus is present in over 40% of US patients, most likely related to increasing incidence of obesity, and ranges from 27% to 38% in Europe. The interaction between heart failure status and diabetes has been a subject of substantial interest, given the evolving data that some classes of anti-diabetic drugs, specifically the sodium-glucose co-transporter-2 (SGLT-2) inhibitors and glucagon-like peptide-1 (GLP-1) agonists, have a favorable impact on heart failure outcomes (see Chapter 50). Atrial fibrillation can both precipitate AHF and complicate its management.

Global Differences in Acute Heart Failure

Although the majority of data continues to emerge from North America and from Europe, AHF is increasingly recognized as a global issue, and important differences between regions of the world have emerged in terms of epidemiology, therapy, and outcomes.[13] Although there are a variety of country- or region-specific registries (see Table 49.1), to date most available data highlighting these differences have come from large global outcome trials. Although these studies can provide important insight into regional differences, they suffer from inherent selection bias of clinical trials and may not be truly representative of the general population. The recently reported REPORT-HF registry provides a more contemporary assessment of AHF globally (see Table 49.1).[7]

PATHOPHYSIOLOGY

The pathophysiology of AHF is complex and highly variable, with many overlapping pathogenic mechanisms that may be operative to a greater or lesser degree. This fundamental heterogeneity complicates the attempt to create a unified conceptual model. A useful framework for understanding of the pathophysiology of AHF is to consider it as the result of the interaction of underlying substrate, initiating mechanisms or triggers, and amplifying mechanisms, all of which contribute to a common set of clinical signs and symptoms (primarily related to congestion, end-organ dysfunction, or both) that define the clinical picture of AHF (Fig. 49.3). In this context, substrate refers to underlying cardiac structure and function. The underlying substrate may be one of normal ventricular function, for example patients without a prior history of HF who develop AHF because of sudden changes in ventricular function from an acute insult such as MI or acute myocarditis (see Chapter 55). Alternatively, some patients may have no prior history of HF but abnormal substrate (e.g., stage B patients with asymptomatic LV dysfunction) with a first presentation of heart failure (de novo heart failure). Finally, most patients with AHF have a substrate of chronic compensated HF who then decompensate and present with AHF (sometimes termed decompensated chronic heart failure [DCHF]).

Initiating mechanisms vary according to and interact with the underlying substrate and may be cardiac or extra-cardiac. For patients with normal substrate (normal myocardium), a substantial insult to cardiac performance (e.g., acute myocarditis) is generally required to lead to the clinical presentation of AHF. For patients with abnormal substrate at baseline (asymptomatic LV dysfunction), smaller perturbations (e.g., poorly controlled hypertension, atrial fibrillation, or ischemia) may precipitate an AHF episode. For patients with a substrate of compensated or stable chronic HF, medical or dietary nonadherence, drugs

almost equally, but there are important differences by gender. In the ADHERE registry women admitted for AHF were older than men (74 vs. 70 years), and more frequently had preserved systolic function (51% vs. 28%).[9] Differences in ethnic groups have been studied most extensively in the United States and have focused primarily on differences between African American and white patients. In the Organized Program to Initiate Lifesaving Treatment in Hospitalized Patients with Heart Failure (OPTIMIZE-HF) registry, African American patients admitted with AHF were younger (64 vs. 75 years), more likely to have left ventricular (LV) systolic dysfunction (57% vs. 51%) with a lower mean EF (35% vs. 40%), hypertensive cause for heart failure (39% vs. 19%), renal dysfunction, and diabetes compared to the non–African American group.[10] Lower crude mortality rates have been reported for African Americans compared to non–African American patients, but when adjustments are made for these differences in comorbidities and age, mortality rates are similar.

Comorbidities

Concomitant diseases are very common in patients admitted with AHF, reflective of the older population. These comorbidities not only represent diseases that are risk factors for the development of heart

TABLE 49.1 Demographics and Comorbidities of Patients Hospitalized with Acute Heart Failure from Selected Studies

	ADHERE (n = 187,565)	OPTIMIZE-HF (n = 48,612)	PERNA et al. (n = 2974)	EHFS II (n = 3580)	ATTEND (n = 4841)	DAMASCENO (n = 1006)	REPORT-HF (n = 18,102)
Region	US	US	Argentina	Europe	Japan	Africa	Global
Age (years)	75	73	68	70	73	52	67
Male (%)	48	48	59	61	58	49	61
Preserved EF (%)	53	51	26	52	47	25	45
Prior HF (%)	76	88	50	63	36	–	57
Medical History							
Coronary artery disease	57%	50%		54%	N/A		48%
Myocardial infarction	30%	N/A	22%		N/A		N/A
Hypertension	74%	71%	66%	62%	69%	56%	64%
Atrial fibrillation or flutter	31%	31*%	27%	39%	40%	18%	31%
Chronic kidney disease	30%	20%	10%	17%	N/A	8%	20%
Diabetes	44%	42%	23%	33%	34%	11%	37%
COPD/Asthma	31%	34%	15%	19%	12%	N/A	N/A

Data from ADHERE: ADHERE Scientific Advisory Committee. Acute Decompensated Heart Failure National Registry (ADHERE®) Core Module Q1 2006 Final Cumulative National Benchmark Report: Scios, Inc.; July, 2006. OPTIMIZE-HF: Gheorghiade M, Abraham WT, Albert NM, et al. Systolic blood pressure at admission, clinical characteristics, and outcomes in patients hospitalized with acute heart failure. *JAMA*. 2006;296:2217–2226. Argentina: Perna ER, Barbagelata A, Grinfeld L, et al. Overview of acute decompensated heart failure in Argentina: lessons learned from 5 registries during the last decade. *Am Heart J*. 2006;151:84–91. EHFS II: Nieminen MS, Brutsaert D, Dickstein K, et al. EuroHeart Failure Survey II (EHFS II): a survey on hospitalized acute heart failure patients: description of population. *Eur Heart J*. 2006;27:2725–2736. ATTEND: Sato N, Gheorghiade M, Kajimoto K, et al. Hyponatremia and in-hospital mortality in patients admitted for heart failure (from the ATTEND registry). *Am J Cardiol*. 2013;111:1019–25, and Dr Naoki Sato, personal communication. AFRICA: Damasceno A, Mayosi BM, Sani M, et al. The causes, treatment, and outcome of acute heart failure in 1006 Africans from 9 countries: results of the sub-Saharan Africa survey of heart failure. *Arch Intern Med*. 2012;172:1386–94. REPORT-HF: Tromp J, Bamadhaj S, Cleland JGF, et al. Post-discharge prognosis of patients admitted to hospital for heart failure by world region, and national level of income and income disparity (REPORT-HF): a cohort study. *Lancet: Global Health* 2020;8:e411–e422

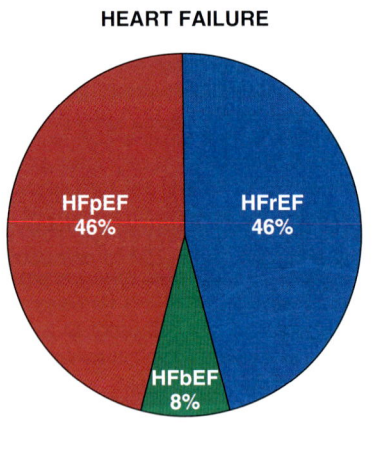
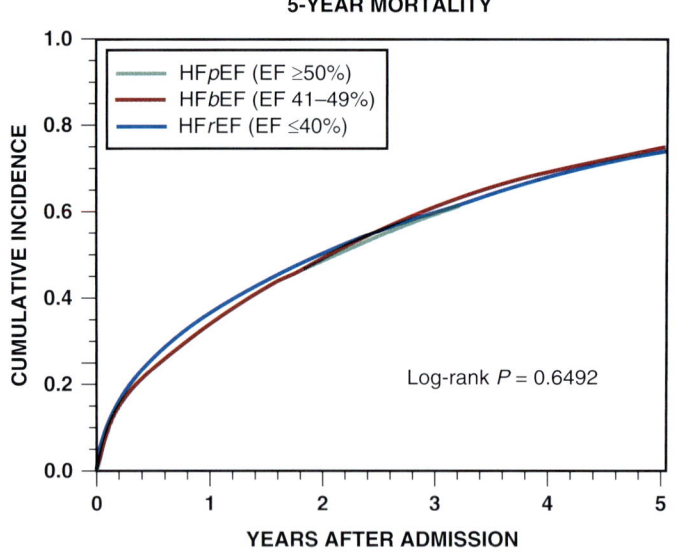

	OUTCOMES-5-YEAR EVENT RATES (%)				
	Mortality	Readmission	CV Readmission	HF Readmission	Mortality/Readmission
HFrEF	75.3	82.2	63.9	48.5	96.4
HFbEF	75.7	85.7	63.3	45.2	97.2
HFpEF	75.7	84.0	58.9	40.5	97.3

FIGURE 49.2 Outcomes after acute heart failure (AHF) hospitalization by ejection fraction. *HFbEF*, HF with borderline ejection fraction; *HFpEF*, HF with preserved ejection fraction; *HFrEF*, HF with reduced ejection fraction. (From Shah KS, Xu H, Matsouaka RA, et al. Heart failure with preserved, borderline, and reduced ejection fraction: 5-year outcomes. *JACC*. 2017;70[20]:2476–2486.)

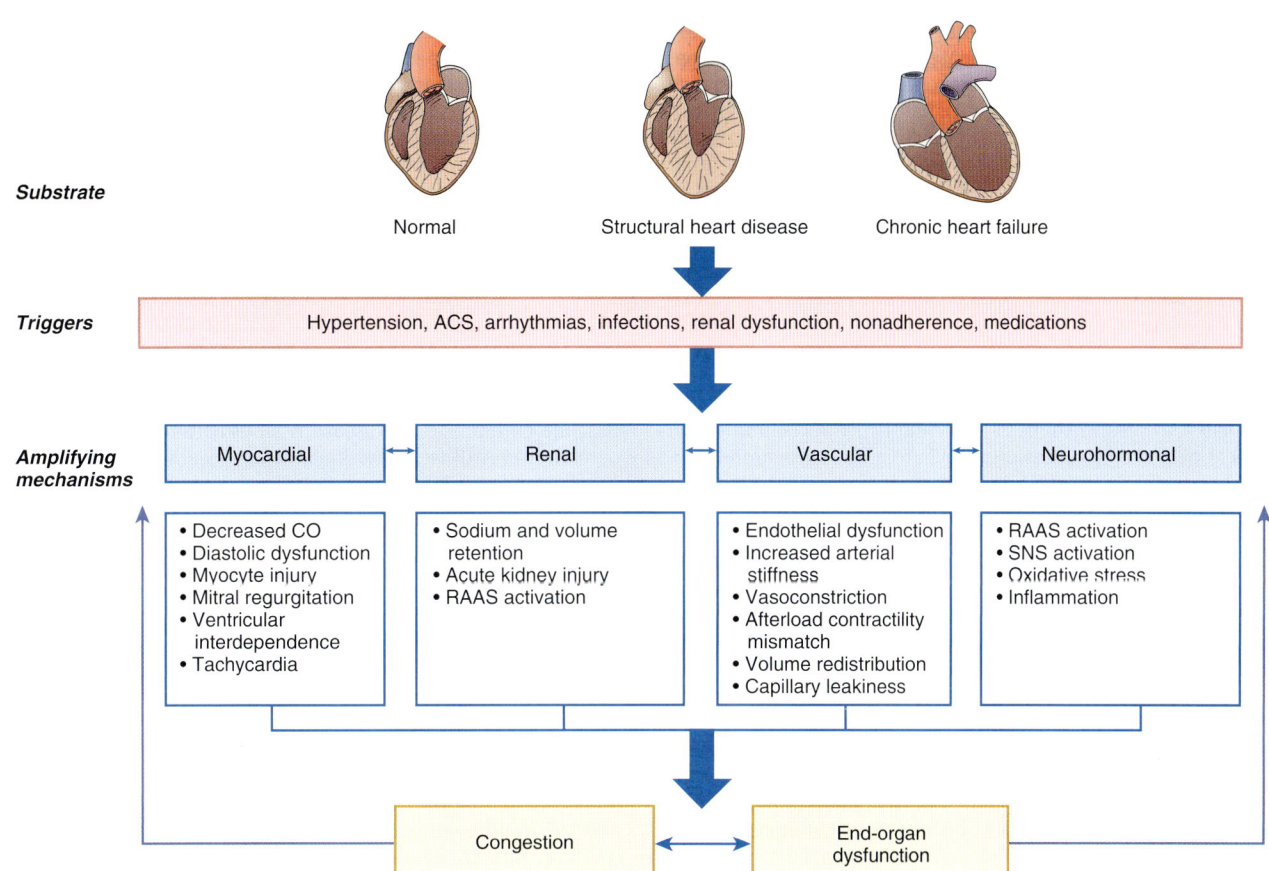

FIGURE 49.3 Schematic of the pathophysiology of acute heart failure.

such as nonsteroidal antiinflammatory agents or thiazolidinediones, and infectious processes are all common triggers for decompensation.

Regardless of the substrate or initiating factors, a variety of "amplifying mechanisms" perpetuate and contribute to the episode of decompensation. These include neurohormonal and inflammatory activation, ongoing myocardial injury with progressive myocardial dysfunction, worsening renal function, and interactions with the peripheral vasculature, all of which may contribute to the propagation and worsening of the AHF episode.

Congestion

Systemic or pulmonary congestion often due to a high ventricular diastolic pressure dominates the clinical presentation of most patients hospitalized for AHF. Congestion can be seen as a final common pathway producing clinical symptoms leading to hospitalization. An oversimplified view of AHF pathophysiology is that gradual increases in intravascular volume lead to symptoms of congestion and clinical presentation, and normalization of volume status with diuretic therapy results in restoration of homeostasis. Although some data suggest that increases in body weight often precede decompensation and hospitalization for HF, careful studies using implantable hemodynamic monitors suggest that increases in invasively measured LV filling pressures can occur without substantial changes in body weight.[14] These observations have led to increasing interest in the concept of volume redistribution and the dynamic role of the vasculature as a contributing mechanism to decompensation in heart failure (discussed in more detail in "Vascular Mechanisms" section below).

One important concept is the distinction between "clinical congestion" and "hemodynamic congestion." Although patients present with signs and symptoms of systemic congestion such as dyspnea, rales, elevated jugular venous pressure (JVP), and edema, this state is often preceded by "hemodynamic congestion," defined as high ventricular diastolic pressures without overt clinical signs. Similarly, clinical congestion may resolve with treatment but hemodynamic congestion may persist, leading to a high risk of rehospitalization. It has been postulated that hemodynamic congestion may contribute to the progression of HF because it may result in increased wall stress as well as in renin-angiotensin-aldosterone system (RAAS) and sympathetic nervous system (SNS) activation. This may trigger a variety of molecular responses in the myocardium, including myocyte loss and increased fibrosis. The natriuretic peptides (see Chapter 47), which are the intrinsic counter-regulatory hormone in heart failure, may have abnormal processing that leads to diminished biologic activity in patients with advanced heart failure.[15] In addition, elevated diastolic filling pressures may decrease coronary perfusion pressure, resulting in sub-endocardial ischemia that may further exacerbate cardiac dysfunction. Increased LV filling pressures can also lead to acute changes in ventricular architecture (more spherical shape), contributing to worsening mitral regurgitation. These mechanisms also play an important role in pathologic remodeling of the ventricle, a chronic process that may be accelerated by each episode of decompensation. Consistent with this paradigm is the well-established clinical observation that each hospitalization for AHF heralds a substantial worsening of the long-term prognosis, an effect that appears additive with recurrent hospitalizations.[16] Data from studies with implantable hemodynamic monitors have confirmed that chronically elevated filling pressures (i.e., hemodynamic congestion) are associated with increased risk of future events.[17] With the recognition of congestion as the most common aspect of AHF presentation, there has been a formal attempt to better assess and quantitate congestion in heart failure.[18]

Myocardial Function

Although a variety of extra-cardiac factors play important roles in AHF, impairments of cardiac function (systolic, diastolic, or both) remain central to our understanding of this disorder (see also Chapter 46). Changes in systolic function and decreased arterial filling can initiate a cascade of effects that are adaptive in the short term but maladaptive when elevated chronically, including stimulation of the SNS and RAAS. Activation of these neurohormonal axes leads to vasoconstriction, sodium and water retention, volume redistribution from other vascular beds, increases in diastolic filling pressures, and clinical symptoms. In patients with underlying ischemic heart disease, initial defects in systolic function may initiate a vicious cycle of decreasing coronary perfusion, increased myocardial wall stress, and progressively worsening cardiac performance. Increased LV filling pressures and changes in LV geometry can worsen functional mitral regurgitation, further decreasing cardiac output.

Importantly, abnormalities in diastolic function are present in heart failure patients regardless of EF. The impairment of the diastolic phase may be related to passive stiffness, abnormal active relaxation of the left ventricle, or both. Hypertension, tachycardia, and myocardial ischemia (even in the absence of CAD) can further impair diastolic filling. All of these mechanisms contribute to higher LV end-diastolic pressures, which are reflected back to the pulmonary capillary circulation. Diastolic dysfunction alone may be insufficient to lead to AHF, but it serves as the substrate on which other precipitating factors (such as atrial fibrillation, CAD, or hypertension) lead to decompensation. One underappreciated aspect of myocardial function in AHF relates to the interdependence of the left and right ventricles. Because of the constraints of the pericardial space, distention of either ventricle due to increased filling pressures can result in direct impingement of diastolic filling of the other ventricle. This may be particularly operative in clinical scenarios leading to abrupt failure of the right ventricle (such as pulmonary embolism or right ventricular (RV) infarction), resulting in diminished filling of the left ventricle and arterial hypotension.

The availability of increasingly sensitive assays for circulating cardiac troponins has led to evolution of our understanding of the role of myocardial injury in AHF pathophysiology. Data from both registries and clinical trial populations indicate that circulating cardiac troponins are elevated in a large proportion of patients with AHF, even in the absence of clinically overt myocardial ischemia.[19,20] In a representative analysis of data from the RELAX-AHF study using a highly sensitive assay, 90% of patients enrolled had a troponin T level above the 99th percentile upper reference limit at baseline, and troponin elevation was associated with post-discharge outcomes out to 180 days (Fig. 49.4).[21]

The precise mechanisms mediating myocardial injury in AHF are poorly defined, but increased myocardial wall stress, decreased coronary perfusion pressure, increased myocardial oxygen demand, endothelial dysfunction, activation of the neurohormonal and inflammatory pathways, platelet activation, and altered calcium handling may all contribute to myocyte injury even in the absence of epicardial CAD.[19] Specific therapeutic interventions that may increase myocardial oxygen demand (such as positive inotropic agents) or decrease coronary artery perfusion pressure (such as some vasodilators) may exacerbate myocardial injury and further contribute to the cycle of decompensation. Whether avoidance of myocardial injury is a specific target for therapy in AHF remains a subject of active investigation.

Renal Mechanisms

The kidney plays two fundamental roles relative to the pathophysiology of HF: it modulates loading conditions of the heart by controlling intravascular volume and is responsible for neurohormonal outputs (i.e., the RAAS system). Abnormalities of renal function are extremely common in patients with AHF and may be underestimated by creatinine alone.[22] Baseline chronic kidney disease is an established risk factor for poor outcomes in AHF (see Risk Stratification section later), but our understanding of the implications of changes in renal function during AHF treatment has continued to evolve.[23] The term "cardio-renal syndrome" has been increasingly used to describe pathologic interactions between the cardiac and renal axes in the setting of heart failure. Although specific definitions and nomenclature have varied, in the context of AHF the cardio-renal syndrome describes the clinical situation of worsening measures of renal function in the setting of persistent congestion. This clinical scenario has been associated with poor outcomes in a variety of observational studies. Multiple studies have investigated the pathophysiology and risk factors for this phenomenon, which is related to an intricate interplay of patient characteristics (age), comorbidities (baseline renal function as assessed by glomerular filtration rate [GFR], diabetes mellitus, hypertension), neurohormonal activation (especially of RAAS and SNS), and hemodynamic factors (central venous congestion, and less frequently arterial underfilling with renal hypoperfusion), as well as other factors such as activation of inflammatory cascades and oxidative stress.[24] Although often assumed to be related to low cardiac output and renal blood flow, careful hemodynamic studies have repeatedly confirmed that the strongest predictor of worsening renal function in heart failure patients relates to elevated central venous pressure (CVP), which is reflected back to the renal veins and leads directly to changes in GFR.[25] Importantly, recent data have emphasized the importance of evaluating changes in renal function in the context of the overall clinical picture. Worsening renal function in the setting of ongoing clinical improvement is generally reflective of successful decongestion and does not portend a poor prognosis (Fig. 49.5).[26] Although there has been substantial interest in the utility of newer biomarkers to identify episodes of frank kidney injury prior to changes in markers of renal function, the clinical utility of these markers remains uncertain. A detailed

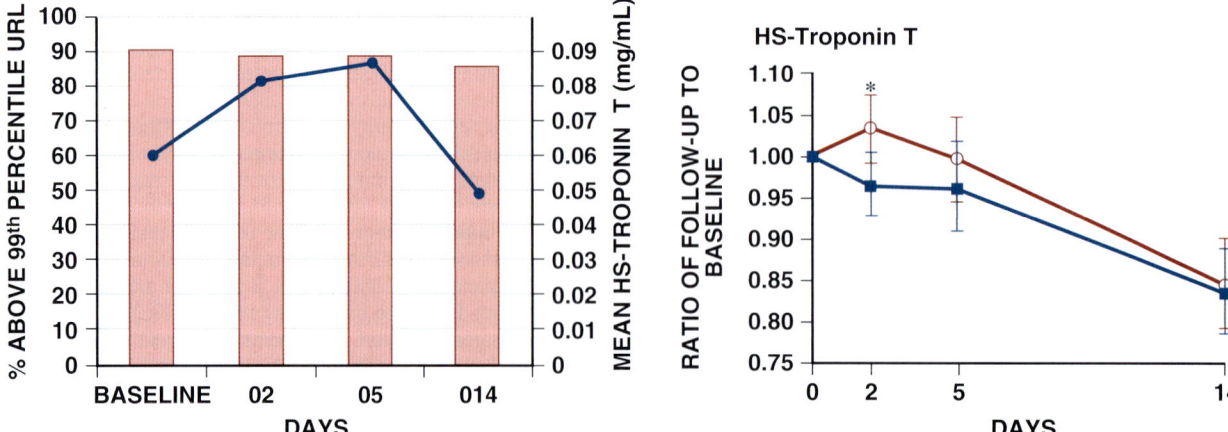

FIGURE 49.4 Incidence of elevated (above the 99th percentile upper reference limit) high-sensitivity troponin T in the RELAX-AHF study and effect of serelaxin therapy on troponin levels. (From Felker GM, Mentz FJ, Teerlink JR, et al. Serial high sensitivity cardiac troponin T measurement in acute heart failure: insights from the RELAX-AHF study. *Eur J Heart Fail*. 2015;17:1262–1270; and Metra M, Cotter G, Davison BA, et al. Effect of serelaxin on cardiac, renal, and hepatic biomarkers in the relaxin in acute heart failure (RELAX-AHF) development program: correlation with outcomes. *J Am Coll Cardiol*. 2013;61:196–206.)

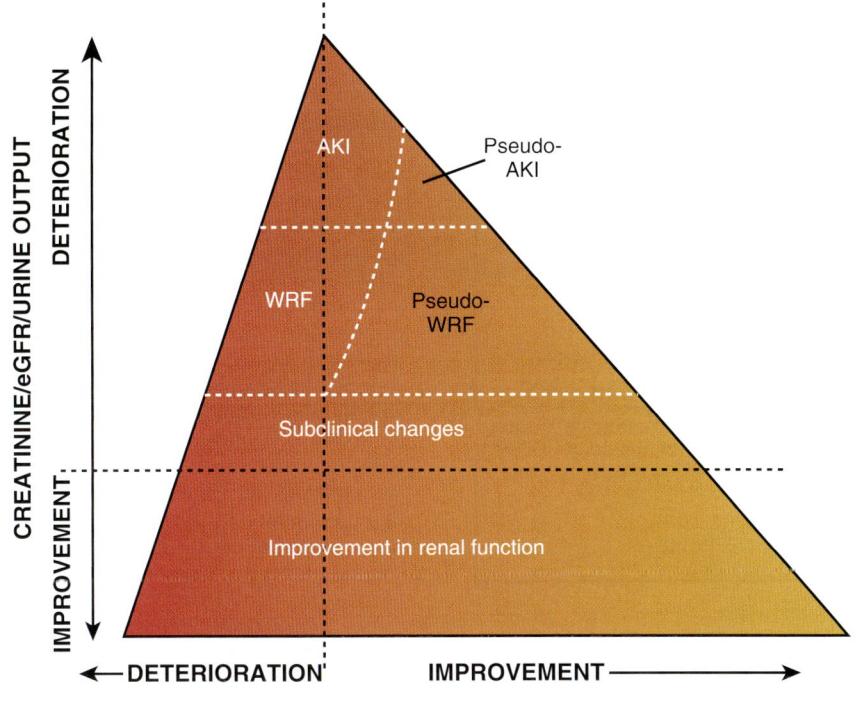

FIGURE 49.5 Schematic of changes in renal function within different clinical context in acute heart failure. AKI, acute kidney injury; WRF, worsened renal function. (From Damman K, Testani JM. The kidney in heart failure: an update. *Eur Heart J.* 2015;36:1437–1444.)

classification system for understanding the interplay between cardiac performance and renal function has been proposed and provides a framework for understanding the complex pathophysiology underlying the cardio-renal syndrome.[24]

Vascular Mechanisms

While abnormalities in cardiac function are central to the pathogenesis of AHF, there is increasing appreciation for the importance of the peripheral vasculature in this disorder. Abnormalities of endothelial function related to nitric oxide dependent regulation of vascular tone are well described in heart failure.[27] Arterial stiffness, which is related to but distinct from blood pressure, increases cardiac loading conditions and is associated with incident heart failure and worse outcomes. Peripheral vasoconstriction in the setting of AHF redistributes blood centrally, increasing pulmonary venous congestion and edema. As noted earlier, elevated CVP reduces renal function, resulting in greater fluid retention, which further elevates venous pressures. Peripheral arterial vasoconstriction increases afterload, LV filling pressures, and post-capillary pulmonary venous pressures, resulting in worsening of pulmonary edema and dyspnea. This increased afterload causes greater ventricular wall stress and increased myocardial ischemia and cardiac arrhythmias. Abnormal vascular compliance also predisposes these patients to marked blood pressure liability with relatively minor changes in intravascular volume, causing precipitous increases in afterload and ultimately in LV filling pressures resulting in pulmonary congestion. The effects of this vascular abnormality are amplified by LV diastolic dysfunction.

The clinical observation that vasodilator treatment can improve dyspnea in many acutely hypertensive patients without significant diuresis has led to the concept that afterload-contractility mismatch can lead to increased diastolic filling pressures in the setting of minimal total body volume changes. Similarly, the recognition of the large capacitance of the venous (in particular the splanchnic circulation) system has led to increased interest in volume shifts from the "venous reservoir" into the effective circulatory volume as a potentially important and under-recognized mechanism in AHF.[28] These shifts can be mediated by SNS activation, and this has been proposed as a potential explanation between the apparent disconnect between changes in filling pressures and changes in body weight during chronic hemodynamic monitoring. Whether fluid shifts involving this venous reservoir can be modulated therapeutically is a subject of active investigation.[29]

Neurohormonal and Inflammatory Mechanisms

Although elevations of circulating neurohormones are well-documented in patients with AHF, the precise role of neurohormonal activation in the pathophysiology of AHF remains to be fully delineated. Increased plasma concentrations of norepinephrine, plasma renin activity, aldosterone, and endothelin-1 (ET-1) have all been reported in patients with AHF—all of these axes are associated with vasoconstriction and volume retention, which could contribute to myocardial ischemia and congestion, thus exacerbating cardiac decompensation. Inflammatory activation and oxidative stress may also play a role. Pro-inflammatory cytokines such as tumor necrosis factor-alpha and interleukin-6 are elevated in patients with AHF and have direct negative inotropic effects on the myocardium as well as increasing capillary permeability and inducing endothelial dysfunction.[30,31] In addition to direct effects, this activation stimulates the release of other factors, such as the potent pro-coagulant tissue factor and ET-1, which can lead to further myocardial suppression, disruption of the pulmonary alveolar capillary barrier, and increased platelet aggregation and coagulation (potentially worsening ischemia).

EVALUATION OF THE ACUTE HEART FAILURE PATIENT

The initial evaluation of the patient with AHF focuses on the following critical aspects: (1) establishing a definitive diagnosis of AHF as rapidly and efficiently as possible; (2) emergent treatment for potentially life-threatening conditions (e.g., shock, respiratory failure); (3) identifying and addressing any relevant clinical triggers or other condition requiring specific treatment (e.g., acute coronary syndrome [ACS], acute pulmonary embolism, etc.); (4) risk stratification in order to triage patient to appropriate level of care (e.g., intensive care unit [ICU], telemetry unit, observation unit); and (5) defining the clinical profile of the patient (based on blood pressure, volume status, and renal function) in order to rapidly implement the most appropriate therapy. A proposed flow diagram for the initial evaluation of patients with suspected AHF is shown in Figure 49.6.[32]

Classification

The inherent heterogeneity of AHF makes the development of a comprehensive classification scheme difficult, and no single classification system has garnered universal acceptance. There are several relevant domains to consider in classifying patients with AHF (Fig. 49.7). These include underlying **substrate** (i.e., whether there is a prior history of structural heart disease or a background of chronic HF), **severity** (from mild symptoms to cardiogenic shock), **acuity** (gradual onset vs. sudden/acute onset), and **triggers** (which may be readily apparent or unknown). Each of these concepts is discussed briefly below.

Substrate
New-onset or de novo heart failure makes up about 20% of hospitalizations for AHF.[12] These patients may have no prior history of cardiovascular disease or risk factors (e.g., acute myocarditis), but more commonly, they have a background of risk factors for HF (stage A heart failure according to the

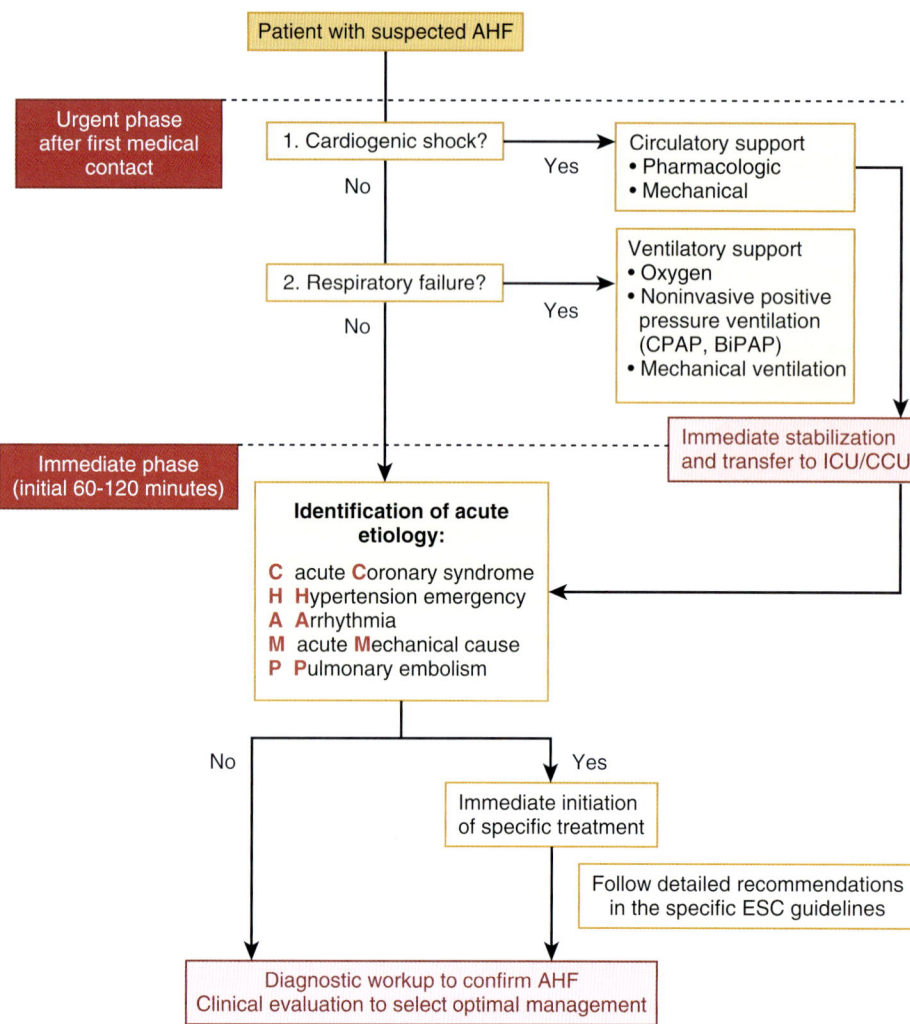

FIGURE 49.6 Algorithm for initial stabilization and management of patients with acute heart failure. (From Ponikowski P, Voors AA, Anker SD, et al. 2016 ESC Guidelines for the diagnosis and treatment of acute and chronic heart failure: the Task Force for the diagnosis and treatment of acute and chronic heart failure of the European Society of Cardiology (ESC) developed with the special contribution of the Heart Failure Association (HFA) of the ESC. *Eur Heart J.* 2016 Jul 14;37[27]:2129–2200.)

American College of Cardiology/American Heart Association [ACC/AHA] guidelines) or preexisting structural heart disease (stage B heart failure according to the ACC/AHA guidelines) (see also Chapters 48 and 50). Many of these patients with de novo heart failure develop AHF in the setting of ACS. The majority of AHF patients have a history of preexisting chronic heart failure. These patients often have a less dramatic clinical presentation because the chronic nature of the disorder has allowed for recruitment of compensatory mechanisms and remodeling (e.g., increased pulmonary lymphatic capacity). Additionally, these patients are typically already being treated with neurohormonal antagonists and loop diuretics, such that neurohormonal activation may be less profound but diuretic resistance may be more common. In patients with AHF with a background of chronic HF, these patients can be further sub-classified by ejection fraction (i.e., HFrEF, HFmrEF, HFpEF) or by cause (i.e., ischemic, nonischemic, etc.) although these factors less often impact acute management of the AHF episode.

Severity

Patients with AHF may range from modestly decompensated patients who require intensification of oral diuretics in the outpatient setting to patients with frank cardiogenic shock. Severity of presentation may be disconnected from severity of background HF. Patients with mild hypertensive heart disease may present in profound respiratory distress requiring intubation, whereas patients with very advanced chronic heart failure may present with more subtle symptoms such as fatigue and early satiety. The most severe presentations of cardiogenic shock have signs and symptoms of organ hypoperfusion despite adequate preload. Systolic blood pressure (SBP) is often (although not always) decreased, and evidence of frank or impending end-organ dysfunction (renal, hepatic, CNS) is common. Cardiogenic shock is relatively uncommon (4% of AHFS presentations in EuroHeart Failure Survey II [EHFS II]) in broad community registries but more common in tertiary care settings.

Acuity

The time course of worsening symptoms is a key component of the history for many forms of acute cardiovascular disease and AHF is no exception. Patients may develop symptoms very suddenly (over minutes) or very gradually (over weeks or longer). As noted above, the acuity of symptoms may not be aligned with the severity of heart failure and the long-term prognosis but has clear implications for the immediacy of therapy needed for stabilization. The fact that many patients may have slowly developing symptoms over days to weeks presents the possibility that early intervention with intensified therapy may prevent some hospitalizations.[33]

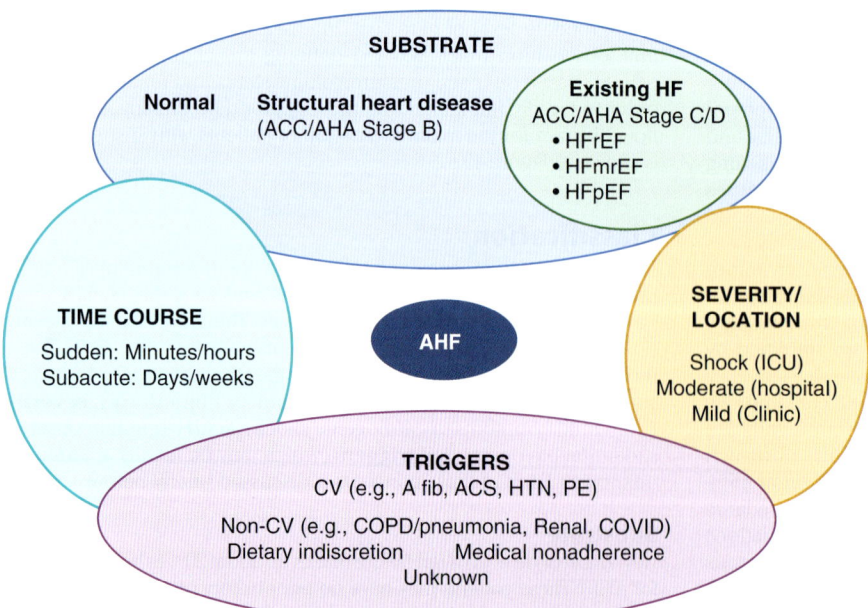

FIGURE 49.7 Systematic approach to classification of patients with acute heart failure.

Triggers

AHF may be triggered by very clear precipitants or alternatively the reason for decompensation may be obscure. In the OPTIMIZE-HF registry, 61% of enrolled subjects had an identifiable clinical precipitant, with pulmonary processes (15%), myocardial ischemia (15%), and arrhythmias (14%) being the most common.[34] More than one precipitant was identified in a substantial minority of the study population. Of the identified triggers, worsening renal function was associated with the highest in-hospital mortality (8%), whereas nonadherence to diet or medication or uncontrolled hypertension had a much better prognosis (<2% in-hospital mortality for each). Infection with the novel coronavirus Sars-CoV-2 is a rapidly evolving trigger of AHF that is discussed in detail elsewhere (see Chapter 94). In patients with a background of HFpEF, acute hypertension is a common trigger for decompensation, and may overlap with the syndrome of hypertensive emergency. Acute hypertension may be triggered by a high sympathetic tone related to dyspnea and accompanying anxiety (reactive hypertension) or acute hypertension with accompanying changes in afterload may be a trigger for decompensation. Both of these mechanisms may be operative in a given patient, and cause and effect relationships may be difficult to discern. Frank pulmonary edema with evident rales and florid congestion on chest x-ray is much more common in this group of patients than in those with more gradual onset of symptoms, likely related to difference in LV compliance, acuity of pressure changes, and pulmonary lymphatic capacity. Although often strikingly ill at the time of initial presentation with hypoxemia and the possible need for noninvasive ventilation (NIV) or even intubation, this group tends to respond well to therapy and have lower in-hospital mortality.[12]

Symptoms of Acute Heart Failure

The most common reasons for patients to seek medical care for AHF are symptoms related to congestion. A list of the most common presenting symptoms is provided in Table 49.2. Dyspnea is the most common symptom and is present in over 90% of patients presenting with AHF. The duration and time course of symptom onset can vary markedly as noted above. The sensation of dyspnea is a complex phenomenon that is influenced by multiple physiologic, psychological, and social factors, and can vary dramatically between patients.[35] Patients may also present with symptoms related to systemic venous congestion, including peripheral edema, weight gain, early satiety, and increasing abdominal girth. Importantly, atypical symptoms can predominate, especially in older patients, where fatigue, depression, altered mental status, and sleep disruptions may be the primary complaints. Bendopnea, or the sensation of dyspnea on bending over, is a commonly reported symptom that has recently been validated experimentally.[36]

Physical Examination

Despite advances in diagnostics technology, biomarkers, and imaging, heart failure remains a clinical diagnosis and the physical examination continues to play a fundamental role (see Chapters 13 and 48). A useful framework in the bedside evaluation of patients with AHF is that developed by Stevenson and colleagues, which focuses on the adequacy of perfusion ("cold" vs. "warm") and congestion at rest ("wet" vs. "dry").[37] While this framework does not completely encompass the heterogeneity of AHF, it does focus the evaluation on two critical aspects that will significantly influence both prognosis and choice of treatments.

Assessing blood pressure is a critical part in the evaluation of patients with AHF; hypotension is one of the strongest predictors of poor outcomes and helps to define appropriate therapeutic interventions. SBP is typically normal or elevated in patients with AHF, with almost 50% presenting with SBP greater than 140 mm Hg. The combination of underlying hypertension and the marked increase in sympathetic stimulation that accompanies AHF can result in elevations of SBP consistent with hypertensive urgencies or emergencies (12% of patients had an SBP over 180 mm Hg on admission). Patients with very low SBP are uncommon, with only 2% of patients in ADHERE presenting with an SBP less than 90 mm Hg. Although blood pressure is generally related to cardiac output and the state of organ perfusion, it is important to recognize that hypotension and hypoperfusion are not synonymous. Patients with systemic hypoperfusion may present with normal blood pressure, and similarly patients with advanced forms of heart failure may have chronically low blood pressure not associated with acute hypoperfusion. Pulse pressure (the difference between systolic and diastolic blood pressure) is a useful measure that is an indirect marker of cardiac output. A low pulse pressure is a marker of a low cardiac output and confers an increased risk in patients admitted with AHF. A high pulse pressure may alert the physician to a high output state including the possibility of unrecognized thyrotoxicosis, aortic regurgitation, or anemia.

The JVP is a barometer of systemic venous hypertension and is the single most useful physical examination finding in the assessment of patients with AHF. The accurate assessment of the JVP is highly dependent on examiner skill. The JVP reflects the right atrial pressure, which typically (although not always) is an indirect measure of LV filling pressures. JVP may not reflect LV filling pressures in isolated RV failure (e.g., from pulmonary hypertension or RV infarct), and significant tricuspid regurgitation can complicate the assessment of the JVP because the large "CV wave" of tricuspid regurgitation can lead to its overestimation.

Rales or inspiratory crackles are the most common physical examination finding and have been noted in 66% to 87% of patients admitted for AHF. However, rales are often not heard in patients with a background of chronic heart failure and pulmonary venous hypertension, due to increased lymphatic drainage, reinforcing the important clinical pearl that the absence of rales does not necessarily imply normal LV filling pressures. Cool extremities with palpable peripheral pulses suggest decreased peripheral perfusion consistent with a marginal cardiac index, marked vasoconstriction, or both. Of note, the temperature should be assessed at the lower leg as opposed to the foot, and this assessment is relative to the temperature of the examiner's hands.

TABLE 49.2 Common Presenting Symptoms and Signs of Decompensated Heart Failure

SYMPTOMS	SIGNS
Predominantly related to volume overload	
Dyspnea (exertional, paroxysmal nocturnal dyspnea, orthopnea, or at rest); cough; wheezing	Rales, pleural effusion
Foot and leg discomfort	Peripheral edema (legs, sacral)
Abdominal discomfort/bloating; early satiety or anorexia	Ascites/increased abdominal girth; right upper quadrant pain or discomfort; hepatomegaly/splenomegaly; scleral icterus
	Increased weight
	Elevated jugular venous pressure, abdominojugular reflux
	Increasing S_3, accentuated P_2
Predominantly related to Hypoperfusion	
Fatigue	Cool extremities
Altered mental status, daytime drowsiness, confusion, or difficulty concentrating	Pallor, dusky skin discoloration, Hypotension
Dizziness, pre-syncope, or syncope	Pulse pressure (narrow)/proportional pulse pressure (low)
	Pulsus alternans
Other signs and symptoms of AHF	
Depression	Orthostatic hypotension (hypovolemia)
Sleep disturbances	S_4
Palpitations	Systolic and diastolic cardiac murmurs

AHF, Acute heart failure.

Peripheral edema is present in up to 65% of patients admitted with AHF and is less common in patients presenting with predominantly low-output heart failure or cardiogenic shock. As with rales, the presence of edema has a reasonable positive predictive value for AHF but a low sensitivity, so its absence does not exclude that diagnosis. Edema due to AHF is usually dependent, symmetric, and pitting. It is estimated that a minimum of 4 liters of extracellular fluid is accumulated to produce clinically detectable edema.

Other Diagnostic Testing
Biomarkers
The natriuretic peptides are a family of important counter-regulatory hormones in HF with vasodilatory and other effects (see Chapters 47 and 48). In the context of AHF, both brain natriuretic peptide (BNP) and N-terminal pro-BNP (NT-proBNP) have been shown to play an important role in the differential diagnosis of patients presenting in the emergency department with dyspnea, and are now Class I recommendations in clinical guidelines.[38] In diagnostic testing, natriuretic peptides have greater negative predictive value (i.e., the ability to rule out heart failure as a cause of dyspnea) than positive predictive value (i.e., the ability to definitively identify a diagnosis of heart failure as the cause of dyspnea). As with all biomarker testing, false-positives (e.g., due to MI or pulmonary embolism) and false-negatives (primarily due to obesity, which results in lower natriuretic peptide levels for a given degree of heart failure) may occur. Although natriuretic peptide levels tend to be lower in patients with HFpEF than those with reduced systolic function, natriuretic peptide testing cannot reliably distinguish HFpEF from HFrEF in an individual patient. As noted previously, measurement of cardiac troponin is frequently elevated in patients presenting with AHF, and elevated levels are associated with worse in-hospital and post-discharge outcomes. Assessment of cardiac troponin in patients with AHF is now a Class I recommendation in clinical guidelines and serves to both establish prognosis as well as inform the likelihood of concurrent ACS. It is important to note that elevation of troponin in the context of a typical AHF hospitalization without clinical evidence of ACS is not synonymous with a Type II MI based on the updated fourth universal MI definition.[39]

Other Laboratory Testing
Assessment of renal function is a critical component in the management of patients with AHF. Estimated glomerular filtration rates (eGFRs) should be calculated because serum creatinine may underestimate the degree of renal dysfunction, especially in older adults. Blood urea nitrogen (BUN) is more directly related to the severity of AHF than creatinine, as it integrates both renal function and neurohormonal activation in AHF. A wide variety of other biomarkers, including ST2, galectin 3, and GDF15, have been evaluated in patients with AHF, but none are currently recommended for routine use in patients with AHF.[10] In patients in whom the diagnosis of AHF is uncertain, testing to establish alternative causes (e.g., D-dimer to evaluate for pulmonary embolism or procalcitonin to evaluate for evidence of infection) may be useful.

Chest Radiography, Electrocardiogram, and Echocardiogram
Chest radiography is commonly performed at the time of presentation in patients with dyspnea and is a fundamental test in the evaluation of patients with suspected AHF. In the ADHERE registry, 90% of patients underwent chest radiography during hospitalization and there was evidence of congestion in over 80% of these patients. In patients with a background of chronic heart failure and/or slow onset of symptoms, evidence of congestion on chest x-ray may be subtle and frank pulmonary edema is often absent despite substantially elevated filling pressures.

The electrocardiogram (ECG) is another standard diagnostic test that is appropriate in all patients presenting with AHF (see Chapter 14). Careful attention for ECG changes suggestive of ischemia is of importance because troponin elevation is common in AHF regardless of cause. Arrhythmias are also a common trigger for AHF, and atrial fibrillation is present in 20% to 30%.

Utilization of echocardiography (see Chapter 16) is very high in patients with AHF—over 80% of patients in EHFS II had an echocardiogram performed during the index hospitalization.[12] An echocardiogram is generally the single most useful test in evaluating the cause in the patient with AHF. Echocardiography can assess global systolic and diastolic function, regional wall motion abnormalities, valvular function, hemodynamics including estimates of filling pressures and cardiac output, and pericardial disease. The tissue Doppler ratio of peak early diastolic trans-mitral blood flow velocity (E) to the peak early diastolic mitral annular tissue velocity (E_a) ($E:E_a$ ratio) has been shown to be additive to BNP measures in diagnosing AHF patients presenting with dyspnea. An $E:E_a$ ratio of greater than 15 predicts a pulmonary capillary wedge pressure (PCWP) greater than 15 mm Hg and has been demonstrated to be accurate in the emergency room and intensive care settings.

Risk Stratification
Risk stratification can serve as important clinical tools by helping to identify those patients at both ends of the spectrum of risk; patients who are at very high risk may be observed more closely or treated more intensively, whereas patients at low risk may avoid hospitalization altogether or need less rigorous follow-up and monitoring. A variety of predictive models have been developed in AHF, which can generally be divided into two groups: those focused on in-hospital mortality, and those focused on post-discharge events (death or rehospitalization). Commonly used predictive models are summarized in Table 49.3. Although individual models differ, several variables occur repeatedly in risk models in a variety of settings: older age, lower blood pressure, higher heart rate, higher BUN and creatinine, and hyponatremia. In

TABLE 49.3 Selected Risk Prediction Models in Acute Heart Failure

	POPULATION	SAMPLE SIZE	ENDPOINTS	C-INDEX	KEY PREDICTORS
ADHERE[140]	US registry	65275	In-hospital mortality	n/a	↑BUN, ↑Cr, ↓SBP, ↑age
OPTIMIZE in hospital[141]	US registry	48612	In-hospital mortality	0.75	↑age, ↑HR, ↓SBP, ↑Cr, ↓Na
OPTIMIZE post discharge[142]	US registry	4402	60–90-day outcomes	0.72	↑age, ↑Cr, reactive airway dz, liver dz, ↓SBP, ↓Na, depression
PROTECT[143]	Global RCT	2015	In-hospital outcomes	0.67	↑BUN, ↑RR, ↓SBP, ↑HR, ↓albumin
EFFECT[144]	Canadian population data	4031	30-day and 1-year mortality	0.80	↑age, SBP, ↑RR, ↑BUN, ↓Na
OPTIME-CHF[145]	Global RCT	949	60-day mortality	0.77	↑age, ↑BUN, ↓Na, ↓Hb
ESCAPE[146]	US RCT	423	6-month mortality	0.76	↑BNP, ↑age, ↑BUN, Na, mechanical ventilation, ↑diuretic dose

BNP, Brain natriuretic peptide; *BUN*, blood urea nitrogen; *Cr*, creatinine; *Hb*, hemoglobin; *HR*, heart rate; *RCT*, randomized controlled trial; *RR*, respiratory rate; *SBP*, systolic blood pressure settings where natriuretic peptides are available, they are also powerful predictors of long-term risk, although they may be stronger predictors at hospital discharge than on admission.

MANAGEMENT OF THE PATIENT WITH ACUTE HEART FAILURE

Phases of Management

The management of AHF patients may be considered in the context of four phases of treatment with distinct goals. Optimal therapy requires a high level of coordination between the in-hospital and post-discharge caregivers and care plan. Different treatment strategies and a detailed description of various therapies will be presented later.

Phase I: Urgent/Emergent Care

The initial goals in the management of a patient presenting with AHF are to expeditiously establish the diagnosis (as discussed above), treat life-threatening abnormalities, initiate therapies to provide symptom relief, and identify the cause and precipitating triggers for the episode of AHF.

Initial therapies may follow the algorithm in Fig. 49.8. In patients with hypoxemia ($SaO_2 < 90\%$), oxygen administration is recommended. Although oxygen saturation on presentation is inversely related to short-term mortality, inhaled oxygen ($F_iO_2 \geq 0.4$) may cause detrimental hemodynamic effects (such hyperoxia-induced vasoconstriction) in patients with systolic dysfunction,[41] therefore it is not routinely recommended for patients without hypoxemia.[42] In patients with obstructive pulmonary disease, high concentrations of inhaled oxygen should not be used to avoid the risk of respiratory depression and worsening hypercarbia. Early clinical studies and meta-analyses suggest that in patients with cardiogenic pulmonary edema, treatment with continuous positive airway pressure (CPAP) or noninvasive intermittent positive pressure ventilation (NIPPV) improves symptoms and physiologic variables, and reduces the need for invasive ventilation and mortality.[43] The Three Interventions in Cardiogenic Pulmonary Oedema (3CPO) trial enrolled 1069 patients with pulmonary edema who were randomized to standard oxygen therapy, CPAP, or NIPPV.[44]

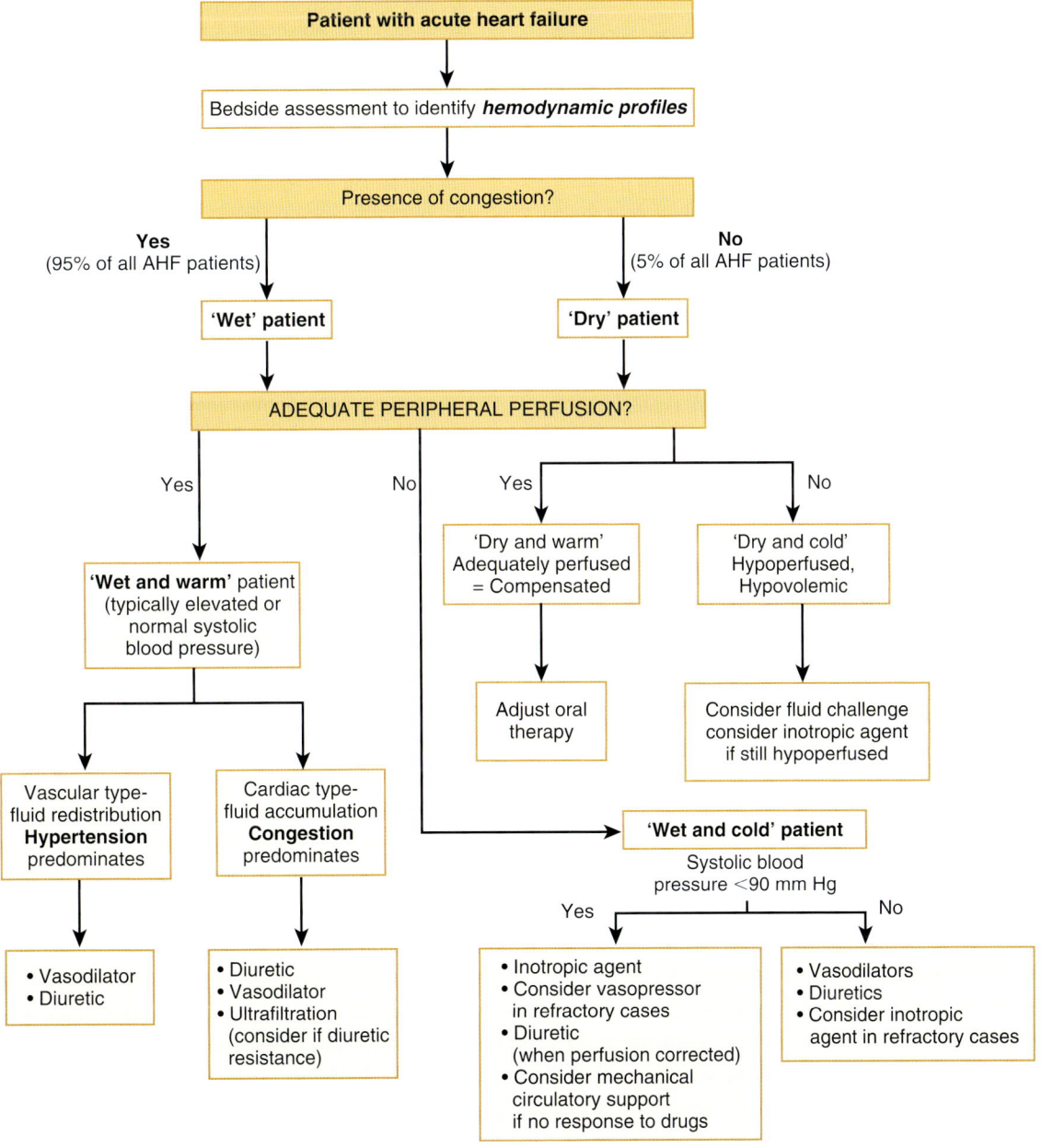

FIGURE 49.8 Algorithm for management of patients admitted with acute heart failure (AHF) based on degree of congestion and perfusion. (From Ponikowski P, Voors AA, Anker SD, et al. 2016 ESC Guidelines for the diagnosis and treatment of acute and chronic heart failure: the Task Force for the diagnosis and treatment of acute and chronic heart failure of the European Society of Cardiology (ESC) developed with the special contribution of the Heart Failure Association (HFA) of the ESC. *Eur Heart J.* 2016;37:2129–2200.)

NIV with CPAP or NIPPV was associated with greater improvement in patient-reported dyspnea, heart rate, acidosis, and hypercapnea after 1 hour of therapy, although it was not associated with a 7-day mortality benefit nor a decreased need for intubation when compared with standard oxygen therapy. Contraindications to the use of NIV include immediate need for endotracheal intubation (inability to protect the airways, life-threatening hypoxia) and lack of patient cooperation (altered sensorium, unconsciousness, anxiety, inability to tolerate mask). Caution should be used in patients with cardiogenic shock, RV failure, and severe obstructive airway disease. Potential side effects and complications include anxiety, claustrophobia, dry mucous membranes, worsening RV failure, hypercapnea, pneumothorax, and aspiration. Mechanical ventilation with endotracheal intubation is required in about 4% to 5% of all patients.[12,45] Morphine use has been associated with increased likelihood of mechanical ventilation, ICU admission, prolonged hospital stay, and mortality in some retrospective analyses.

Intravenous loop diuretics are the most frequently administered pharmacologic therapy for AHF; over 75% of patients in the emergency department receive intravenous diuretics, with a mean door to first intravenous administration time of 2.2 hours in ADHERE.[45] Whereas some patients with volume redistribution rather than hypervolemia may derive benefit from vasodilators alone, symptomatic patients with objective evidence of congestion consistent with pulmonary or systemic venous hypertension or edema should generally receive urgent diuretic therapy for relief of symptoms related to congestion. Initial therapy is typically a bolus injection with a dose between 1 and 2.5 times the patient's oral loop diuretic dose for patients on chronic diuretic therapy (see section on Diuretics below).[46] In the absence of hypotension, vasodilators may have a role in the initial therapy of patients with pulmonary edema and poor oxygenation. A treatment strategy of early initiation of intravenous nitrate therapy in patients with severe cardiogenic pulmonary edema has been shown to reduce the need for mechanical ventilation and the frequency of MI.[47]

Although low-risk patients may potentially be discharged with careful follow-up, the vast majority of patients who present to the emergency department with AHF are hospitalized.[48] Although fewer than 5% of heart failure patients are initially treated in an emergency department observation unit, these specialized care centers may be effective in decreasing hospitalizations, ICU and critical care unit (CCU) admissions, and related health care costs while maintaining the quality of patient care.[49] In general, hospitalization is recommended for patients with evidence of significant decompensated heart failure, including hypotension, worsening renal function, or altered mentation; significant hypoxemia, hemodynamically significant arrhythmia (most commonly atrial fibrillation either with rapid ventricular response or new onset); and ACS. Hospitalization should be considered in patients with worsened congestion, even in the absence of dyspnea and often reflected by significant weight gain (≥5 kg), other signs or symptoms of pulmonary or systemic congestion, newly diagnosed heart failure, complications of heart failure therapy (such as electrolyte disturbances, frequent implantable cardioverter-defibrillator [ICD] firings), or other associated comorbid conditions.[50]

SPECIFIC CLINICAL PRESENTATIONS
Atrial Fibrillation with Rapid Ventricular Response
Atrial fibrillation (see Chapter 66) with rapid ventricular response is the most common tachyarrhythmia requiring treatment in patients with AHF. It may be difficult to determine with certainty whether the atrial fibrillation was a trigger for AHF or a result of decompensation. Although the ventricular response frequently decreases in parallel with the relief of dyspnea, and consequent decreased sympathetic drive, additional therapy may be required. Immediate cardioversion is generally not indicated except in the unstable patient, as cardioversion while the patient remains significantly decompensated is associated with a high rate of recurrent atrial fibrillation. In patients with systolic dysfunction, intravenous digoxin (in the absence of an accessory pathway), cautious use of beta blocker therapy, or amiodarone may be used. Diltiazem and other agents that suppress ventricular function should be avoided in patients with significant systolic dysfunction but may be effective in patients with preserved function.

Right Ventricular Heart Failure
The most common cause of RV HF in AHF is left-sided failure. Isolated RV HF is relatively rare and is generally due to acute RV infarction, acute pulmonary embolism, or severe pulmonary hypertension. Isolated RV HF caused by an acute RV infarction is best treated with early reperfusion, whereas hemodynamically significant pulmonary embolism may be treated with thrombolytics. Hemodynamic stabilization by optimizing CVPs via carefully monitored fluid loading (target CVP approximately 10 to 12 mm Hg) and increasing RV systolic function with intravenous inotropic support under invasive hemodynamic guidance may also be necessary.[51] Selective pulmonary artery vasodilation by inhaled (nitric oxide, prostacyclin analogs) or intravenous (prostacyclin analogs, sildenafil) agents may improve RV function through decreased afterload. If the patient is mechanically ventilated, normoxia and hypocarbia should be goals using moderate tidal volumes (approximately 8 mL/kg) and as low a PEEP as possible (<12 cm H_2O) to maintain moderate plateau pressures.

Acute Coronary Syndromes (see Chapters 37 and 39)
ACS may be the underlying trigger in patients presenting with AHF, but as noted above, the diagnosis is confounded by the high prevalence of elevated troponins in AHF itself. These patients may present with chest discomfort, electrocardiographic changes consistent with ischemia, and elevated serum troponin. Aggressive therapy for ACS should be rapidly instituted. In the absence of cardiogenic shock, inodilators should be avoided in both patients with ACS and significant asymptomatic coronary disease because experimental data have shown that they can cause necrosis of ischemic and/or hibernating myocardium.

Cardiogenic Shock (see Chapter 38)
Cardiogenic shock is characterized by marked hypotension (SBP <80 mm Hg) lasting more than 30 minutes, associated with severe reduction of cardiac index (usually <1.8 L/min/m^2) in spite of adequate LV filling pressure (PCWP >18 mm Hg), resulting in organ hypoperfusion. Cardiogenic shock is an unusual presentation of AHF, occurring in less than 4% of the patients in EHFS II,[12] most of whom had a MI. Mechanical complications of acute myocardial infarction (AMI) such as mitral regurgitation, cardiac rupture with ventricular septal defect or tamponade, and isolated RV infarct may also be causes in this setting. Intravenous inotropes or even vasoconstrictors may be required in these patients, with mechanical circulatory support, such as intra-aortic balloon pump (IABP) or other forms of temporary mechanical support, including ECMO, may be required as a bridge to heart transplant or other mechanical intervention. A variety of evolving approaches to providing hemodynamic support are now available, which may permit temporary stabilization until decisions about the appropriateness of other therapies (such as durable mechanical support or transplantation) can be made (see Chapters 59 and 60).

Phase II: Hospital Care
The goals for the management of a patient with AHF during the hospitalization phase are to complete the diagnostic and acute therapeutic processes that were initiated at the time of initial presentation, to optimize the patient's hemodynamic profile, volume status, and clinical symptoms, and to initiate or optimize chronic heart failure therapy. Monitoring of daily weights, fluid intake and output, and vital signs, including orthostatic blood pressure, as well as a daily assessment of symptoms and signs is crucial. Laboratory monitoring should include daily analysis of electrolytes and renal function. Diagnostic evaluations should include an echocardiogram, if not recently performed. Evaluation for myocardial ischemia may be needed if there is suspicion of ischemia as a trigger of decompensation. Dietary sodium restriction (2 g daily) and fluid restriction (2 liters daily) may be useful to help treat congestion, although the utility of sodium and fluid restriction in this setting has increasingly been called into question.[52] The increased risk of venous thromboembolism in heart failure is exacerbated by the decreased mobility of hospitalized patients with AHF and venous thromboembolism prophylaxis is indicated in all patients unless there is a clear contraindication.

It should be recognized that AHF hospitalization represents an opportunity to review and optimize chronic heart failure therapy. Although changes in renal function may necessitate dose adjustment or temporary discontinuation of RAAS inhibitors (angiotensin-converting enzyme [ACE] inhibitors, angiotensin receptor blocker

[ARB], angiotensin receptor neprilysin inhibitor [ARNI], and/or mineralocorticoid receptor antagonists), in general discontinuation of guideline directed medical therapy should be avoided where possible. Patients admitted on beta blockers have a lower occurrence of ventricular arrhythmias, a shorter length of stay, and reduced 6-month mortality compared to those not receiving them. Patients who had beta blockers withdrawn had significantly lower outpatient use of beta blockers and higher in-hospital mortality, short-term mortality, and combined short-term rehospitalization and mortality, even after adjustments for potential confounders.[53] Therefore, patients should continue beta blocker therapy during the admission for AHF, unless significant hypotension or cardiogenic shock are present. Identification of other untreated targets (e.g., revascularization, consideration of cardiac resynchronization therapy [CRT] in appropriate candidates, etc.) should be performed during the hospitalization. Recent data from the PIONEER trial suggest that hospitalization is an ideal time to transition to sacubitril-valsartan therapy in appropriate patients rather than defer this to the outpatient setting.[54] The hospitalization phase of AHF management is also an opportunity to provide education and behavioral therapies to patients. Patients should receive specific and clear education about heart failure, including indications for specific drugs, outpatient monitoring of fluid status through daily weights, self adjustment of diuretics, exercise programs, and nutritional counseling, as well as possible consultation with physical and occupational therapy. Comorbidities should be aggressively addressed as these often complicate heart failure management. The hospitalization is also a possible opportunity to enroll the patient in appropriate heart failure disease management programs.

The Cardio-Renal Syndrome in Hospitalized Patients

The *cardio-renal syndrome* (see Chapter 101) represents a significant therapeutic challenge in patients with AHF. Cardio-renal syndrome is often described as the clinical state where the volume overload of heart failure is resistant or refractory to treatment due to progressive renal insufficiency. A commonly used practical definition is an increase in serum creatinine of greater than 0.3 mg/dL (or 25% decreases in GFR) despite evidence of persistent clinical or hemodynamic congestion. Using this definition, the cardio-renal syndrome occurs in approximately 25% to 35% of the patients admitted with AHF, associated with longer lengths of stay and higher post-discharge mortality.[23] This definition of the cardio-renal syndrome emphasizes the importance of persistent congestion, as multiple studies have suggested that changes in renal function during successful decongestion therapy are usually transient and may not be associated with adverse outcomes.[26,55]

Although the diagnosis of the cardio-renal syndrome may be straightforward, the clinical management is a major challenge. Because absolute serum creatinine concentrations can be misleading, eGFR should be calculated in patients with AHF. As noted above, arterial under-filling due to over-diuresis or low cardiac output does not appear to be the most frequent primary cause of worsening renal function, although hypotension can be an important factor.[56] Progressive deterioration of renal function (BUN >80 mg/dL and creatinine >3.0 mg/dL) or hyperkalemia may necessitate discontinuation of RAAS inhibitors, although use of other vasodilators should be considered, either intravenous (i.e., nitroglycerin or nitroprusside) or oral (isosorbide dinitrate and hydralazine). Increasing doses of diuretics are typically required, although diuretic resistance may be profound. The degree of diuretic resistance, sometimes quantified as diuretic efficiency, is known to be associated with increased length of stay and adverse prognosis.[57] Urine sodium measurements may provide a useful guide to initial diuretic response.[58] Although ultrafiltration is often considered in this scenario, clinical trial data have not supported the efficacy or safety of this approach.[59]

In-Hospital Worsening Heart Failure

Traditional assessments of the inpatient course of patients with AHF have generally lacked granularity and focused primarily on in-hospital mortality. However, there has been increasing emphasis from both a clinical and research perspective on difference in the clinical "trajectory" of patients during inpatient AHF treatment. It is apparent that different patients may have markedly different clinical courses during inpatient therapy for AHF, from relatively uncomplicated courses marked by steady improvement in heart failure status, to those characterized by progressive deterioration in clinical status (Fig. 49.9).[5] Fundamentally, the concept of in-hospital WHF encompasses clinical worsening (as manifest by worsening signs and/or symptoms of heart failure) that necessitates a significant intensification of therapy. Both terminology and specific definitions of WHF have varied between studies, leading to widely varying estimates of prevalence from 5% to 42%. In general, the development of WHF during inpatient AHF therapy is associated with both longer length of inpatient stay (by approximately 5 days in a recent pooled analysis) and adverse post-discharge outcomes (approximately 50% to 100% increase in 30 or 60 day death or HF rehospitalization).[60] As expected, different severity of WHF implies different risk, with WHF treated with increased diuretics alone associated with less increase in baseline risk than WHF requiring IV inotropes or mechanical circulatory or respiratory support. Although there has been substantial interest from researchers and regulators in the concept of WHF as a clinical trial endpoint in recent AHF studies, to date no interventions have provided definitive evidence that they are able to impact this clinical endpoint.

Phase III: Pre-Discharge Planning

The pre-discharge phase focuses on the goals of evaluating readiness for discharge, optimizing chronic oral therapy, minimizing the side effects of treatments, and ultimately preventing early readmission and improving symptoms and survival. Although there may be pressures to rapidly discharge patients, careful optimization of medical regimen prior to discharge may reduce the risk of subsequent readmissions and improve long-term outcomes.[61] Despite the fact that most patients present with congestion, many patients are discharged without significant weight loss. Available data demonstrate that persistent clinical congestion at discharge was associated with a high risk for rehospitalization.[62] Similarly, elevations of discharge BNP level have been shown to be

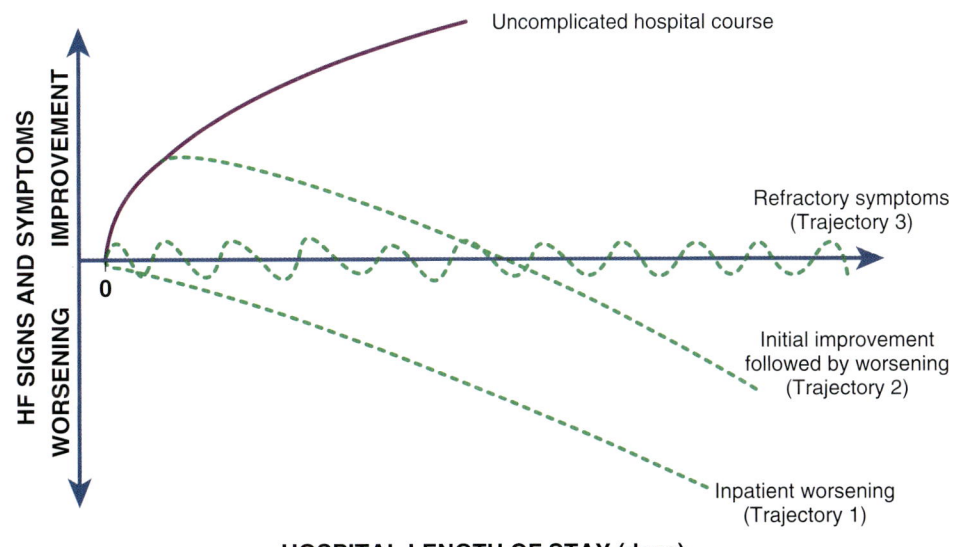

FIGURE 49.9 Various clinical trajectories of patients with acute heart failure during inpatient management. (From Butler J, Gheorghiade M, Kelkar A, et al. In-hospital worsening heart failure. *Eur J Heart Fail*. 2015;17:1104–1113.)

associated with risk for rehospitalization post-discharge.[63] Evaluation of functional capacity with simple maneuvers such as climbing one flight of stairs or walking down the corridor may be a simple and valuable tool to use prior to discharge.

Pharmacologic therapies known to improve long-term outcomes in chronic heart failure, such as beta blockers, ACE inhibitors or ARBs, ARNIs, and mineralocorticoid receptor antagonists, should be initiated as soon as reasonable during the hospitalization and prior to discharge in hemodynamically stable, appropriate patients. In patients already treated chronically with these agents prior to this episode of AHF, they should generally be continued during hospitalization. Clinical practice guidelines provide general criteria for considerations of hospital discharge, although substantial clinical judgment is still required (Table 49.4).[64]

Phase IV: Post-Discharge Management

Early recurrence of signs and symptoms of HF suggestive of worsening volume overload and/or neurohormonal activation are likely to contribute to the high rates of readmission that are observed in AHF.[65] Prompt interventions may therefore allow intervention to prevent the progression of volume overload and new admissions. At least some rehospitalizations for heart failure appear to be preventable.[66] A series of studies have also investigated the benefits of post-discharge support, especially patient-centered discharge instructions, transition coaches, follow-up telephone calls, and early physician follow-up, although results of these studies have been mixed in terms of impact on outcomes.[67,68] A follow-up appointment is optimally scheduled within approximately 7 to 10 days post-discharge, but closer follow-up (in less than a week) should be considered for patients with high-risk features.

General Approaches to Acute Heart Failure Therapy
Targeting Congestion

Treatment strategies for AHF have been largely empiric and limited by an incomplete understanding of its epidemiology and pathophysiology, as well as the relatively blunt nature of the available therapeutic tools.

TABLE 49.4 Considerations Prior to Discharge after Acute Heart Failure Hospitalization

Recommended for all heart failure patients
• Exacerbating factors addressed
• Near-optimal volume status observed
• Transition from intravenous to oral diuretic successfully completed
• Patient and family education completed, including clear discharge instructions
• LVEF documented
• Smoking cessation counseling initiated
• Near-optimal pharmacologic therapy achieved, including ACE inhibitor and beta blocker (for patients with reduced LVEF), or intolerance documented
• Follow-up clinic visit scheduled, usually for 7–10 days
Should be considered for patients with advanced heart failure or recurrent admissions for heart failure
• Oral medication regimen stable for 24 hr
• No intravenous vasodilator or inotropic agent for 24 hr
• Ambulation before discharge to assess functional capacity after therapy
• Plans for post-discharge management (scale present in home, visiting nurse or telephone follow up generally no longer than 3 days after discharge)
• Referral for disease management, if available

ACE, Angiotensin-converting enzyme; *LVEF*, left ventricular ejection fraction. Adapted from Heart Failure Society of America; Lindenfeld J, Albert NM, et al. HFSA 2010 comprehensive heart failure practice guideline. *J Card Failure.* 2010;16(6):e1–e194.

The current general approach focuses on the successful treatment of clinical and hemodynamic congestion, while limiting untoward effects on myocardial or end-organ function, identifying addressable triggers, and optimizing proven long-term therapies. This approach incorporates information from three main aspects of the patient's clinical presentation: blood pressure, volume status, and renal function.

Blood Pressure

Blood pressure reflects the interaction between vascular tone and myocardial pump function and is one of the most important prognostic indicators in AHF (see above). Most patients present with elevated blood pressures and consequently will benefit from and safely tolerate vasodilator therapy. Vasodilators may decrease preload by reversing venous vasoconstriction and the related central volume redistribution from the peripheral and splanchnic venous systems, and reduce afterload by decreasing arterial vasoconstriction with a resultant improvement in cardiac and renal function. Vasodilators are the primary therapy for AHF with pulmonary edema, and for non-hypotensive patients with low cardiac output (poor peripheral or central perfusion with SBPs above 85 to 100 mm Hg). A systematic review of clinical studies supported the ability of vasodilators to improve short-term symptoms and appear safe to administer, but revealed no data suggesting an impact on mortality.[69] However, in an international registry of 4953 patients admitted for AHF (ALARM-HF; 75% admitted to ICU/CCU care settings), analysis of a propensity-based matched cohort of 1007 matched pairs demonstrated improved in-hospital survival in patients treated with vasodilators and diuretics compared to patients only treated with diuretics with 7.8% compared to 11.0% in-hospital mortality, respectively ($P = 0.016$).[70] Interestingly, this difference in survival was particularly evident in patients with SBP less than 120 mm Hg (Fig. 49.10). The selection of agent depends on the clinical situation, local practice, and availability (see section on Specific Therapies below).

Hypotension (SBP below 85 to 90 mm Hg) or signs of peripheral hypoperfusion are poor prognostic signs in patients with AHF. Treating the potentially reversible, underlying causes, such as ACS, pulmonary embolus, and (rarely) hypovolemia, is essential. Hypovolemic hypotension, usually related to over-diuresis, is unusual in patients presenting with symptomatic AHF, and unappreciated volume overload may be present, especially in obese patients in whom neck veins and ascites are difficult to assess. If there is clear evidence of hypovolemia, carefully monitored "fluid challenges" may be attempted, although rapid intravenous fluid boluses can precipitate congestive symptoms. Asymptomatic hypotension, as an isolated finding in the absence of congestion and poor peripheral or central perfusion, does not require emergent treatment. Inotropic therapy may be indicated for persistent symptomatic hypotension or evidence of hypoperfusion in the setting of advanced systolic dysfunction. An analysis of 954 propensity-matched pairs of patients from the ALARM-HF registry suggested that IV catecholamine use was associated with 1.5-fold increase in in-hospital mortality for dopamine or dobutamine use and a greater than 2.5-fold increase for norepinephrine or epinephrine use.[70] Specific inotropic agents vary by country and local clinical practice (see section on specific agents below). In most patients, invasive pulmonary artery catheter monitoring is not necessary, because the measures of urine output, blood pressure, and end-organ function may be clinically evaluated. The use of vasoconstrictors, such as high-dose dopamine, phenylephrine, epinephrine, and norepinephrine, should generally be avoided unless absolutely necessary for refractory symptomatic hypotension or hypoperfusion. Rarely, over dosage of afterload-reducing agents can precipitate admissions for AHF with a clinical presentation similar to cardiogenic shock or "pseudo-sepsis," in which case careful administration of vasoconstrictors may be indicated.

Volume Status

Most patients with AHF have evidence of volume overload and for patients in whom this is the dominant presenting feature, such as those with significant peripheral edema or ascites, intravenous diuretics remain the foundation of AHF therapy. Patients with clinically evident congestion typically have 4 to 5 liters of excess volume and amounts greater than 10 liters are not uncommon. The choice of diuretic regimen is influenced by the amount and rapidity of the desired fluid removal and the renal function (see below). Diuresis addresses the underlying abnormality and frequently improves symptoms and signs of elevated filling pressures. However, intravenous vasodilator therapy may provide more rapid relief in highly symptomatic patients with evidence of pulmonary congestion. In fact, many patients with hypertensive AHF may require minimal diuretics. Surprisingly, in a study of 131,430 admissions for heart failure, 11% of the patients received a median of 1 liter of intravenous fluids, predominantly normal saline, during the first 2 days of hospitalization. Patients receiving intravenous fluids had increased rates of subsequent critical care admission, intubation, renal replacement therapy, and hospital death compared with those who received only diuretics.[71] Thus, careful attention to volume status is critical, as patients' symptoms of congestion may resolve despite persistent hemodynamic congestion (i.e., elevated filling pressures). Hospital discharge before hemodynamic congestion is fully treated appears to be a common cause of rehospitalization.[72]

Renal Function

Renal function (see Chapter 101) is the third main aspect of a contemporary approach to treatment of the patient with AHF. Treatment of AHF in the presence of normal renal function is generally uncomplicated. Diuretics may be given in standard doses, although renal function, electrolytes, and volume status must be carefully monitored. However, approximately two-thirds of patients present with at least moderate renal insufficiency.[22] This may be from preexisting kidney disease or may be a manifestation of WHF. Abnormal renal function is typically associated with some degree of diuretic resistance, and higher doses of diuretics or other strategies may be needed (see section on Diuretics below). The important clinical problem of worsening renal function during AHF therapy, the cardio-renal syndrome, is discussed above.

Invasive Hemodynamic Strategy

Invasive hemodynamic management with pulmonary artery catheterization (PAC) may be a useful strategy in the management of some patients with AHF. PAC is an invasive procedure that provides detailed hemodynamic data, including direct assessment of filling pressures and cardiac output, and calculation of pulmonary and systemic vascular resistance. Potential risks of PAC include bleeding, infection, arrhythmias, and rare catastrophic events, such as pulmonary artery rupture or infarction. The use of PAC in the routine management of AHF has been a subject of controversy. The Evaluation Study of Congestive Heart Failure and Pulmonary Artery Catheterization Effectiveness (ESCAPE) was a randomized controlled trial of 433 patients with severe symptomatic heart failure despite recommended therapies randomized to receive therapy guided by clinical assessment and PAC or by clinical assessment alone.[73] In ESCAPE, use of PAC did not significantly affect the days alive and out of hospital during the first 6 months (133 vs. 135 days), mortality (43 vs. 38 deaths), or the number of days hospitalized (8.7 vs. 8.3 days) compared to clinical assessment alone. Based on the results of the ESCAPE trial, the use of PAC in AHF management has declined—in EHFS II, only 5% of patients had a PAC during AHF hospitalization. Importantly, the

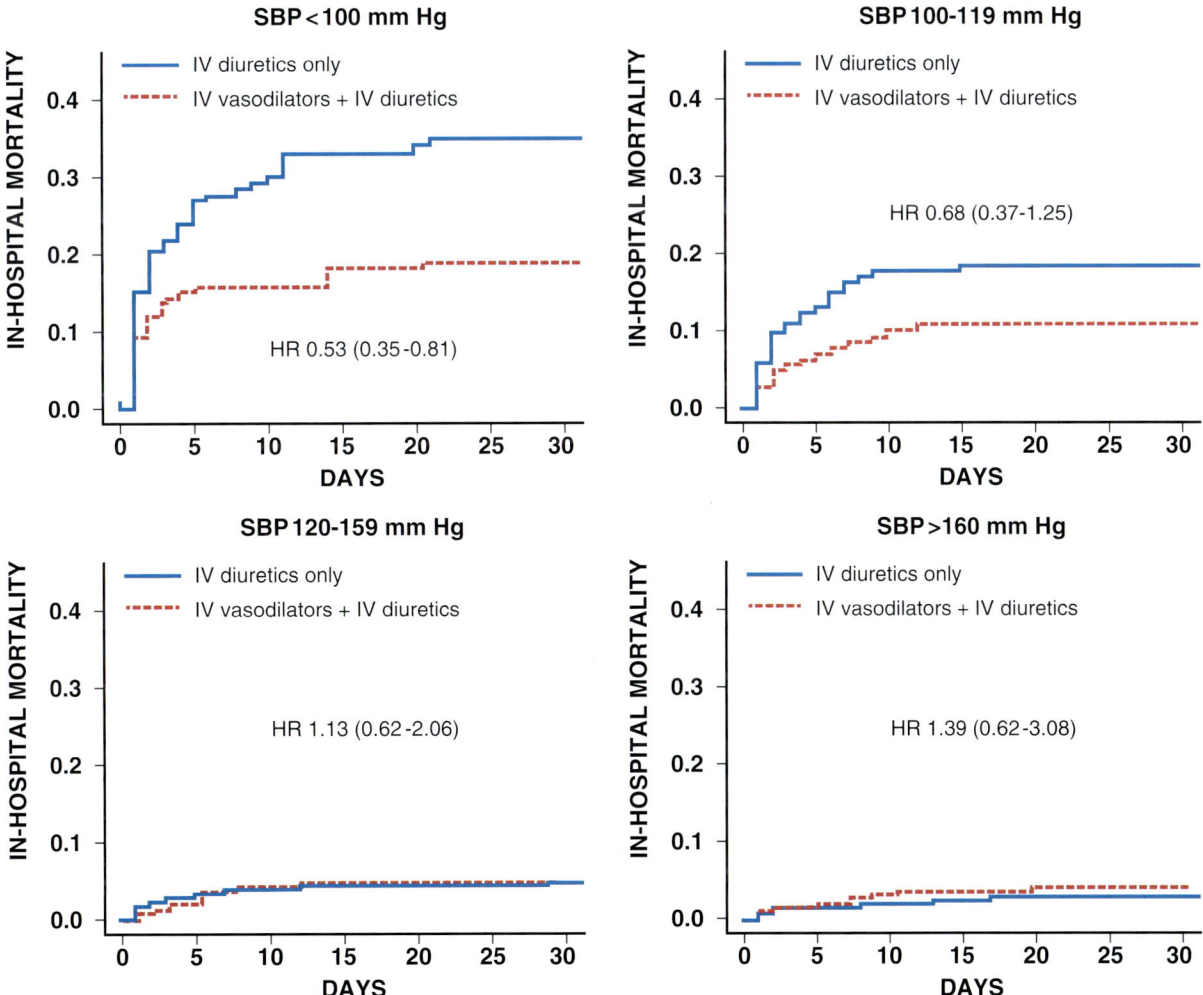

FIGURE 49.10 Effects of IV vasodilators on in-hospital mortality of patients with various levels of systolic blood pressure (SBP). SBP ranged from less than 100 to ≥160 mm Hg. The number of patients is 318, 334, 668, and 694 for SBP less than 100, 100–119, 120–159, and ≥160 mm Hg, respectively. *HR*, Hazard ratio. Value in parenthesis is the 95% confidence interval. (From Mebazaa A, Parissis J, Porcher R, et al. Short-term survival by treatment among patients hospitalized with acute heart failure: the global ALARM-HF registry using propensity scoring methods. *Intensive Care Med.* 2011;37:290–301.)

ESCAPE study excluded patients in whom the treating clinician did not have equipoise about the need for invasive hemodynamic measurement. Invasive hemodynamic assessment with PAC may still play an important role in selected patients, especially those with shock or other severe hemodynamic compromise, with oliguria or anuria, or with unclear hemodynamics and poor response to therapy. In patients with advanced heart failure in whom PAC is used to tailor therapy, an LV filling pressure as approximated by PCWP of less than 16 mm Hg, right atrial pressure less than 8 mm Hg, and a systemic vascular resistance between 1000 and 1200 dynes sec cm^{-5} are useful targets.

Process of Care, Outcomes, and Quality Assessment

The first point of contact at the admitting hospital for most patients (80%) is the emergency department.[74] Many patients with AHF may be effectively managed in and safely discharged from the emergency department and specific algorithms for care and criteria for discharge are evolving.[75] Once the patient with AHF is hospitalized, there appear to be substantial geographic differences in process of care and hospital course worldwide. In the U.S. ADHERE registry, 23% of patients were admitted to an ICU setting, whereas a substantially higher proportion (51%) had an ICU stay in a similar European registry (EHFS II). Median length of stay is also markedly different across geographic regions, with length of stay in the United States of approximately 4 days. Median length of stay is approximately twice as long in Europe (median of 9 days in EHFS II), and even higher in Japan (21 days in ATTEND registry). These differences in length of stay do not appear to be fully explained by differences in case mix or severity of illness. The longer length of stay outside the United States is generally associated with lower rates of short-term rehospitalization, although a cause-and-effect relationship is not fully established. A focus on reducing length of stay in the United States appears to have been accompanied by an increase in post-discharge events, both mortality and (in particular) rehospitalization.[76] In contrast in the U.S. Veterans Affairs hospitals, heart failure hospitalizations have increased slightly while 30-day mortality has decreased significantly.[77] In general, the natural history of AHF is characterized by relatively low in-hospital mortality but a high rate of recurrent post-discharge events (Table 49.5). Inpatient mortality in AHF ranges between 3% and 7%, with the notable exception of patients in cardiogenic shock, who have a markedly increased in-hospital mortality (40% in EHFS II).[12] Although in-hospital mortality is low, hospitalization for AHF portends a substantial worsening of the clinical course in many patients. In the EVEREST study, despite careful attention to evidence-based care in the context of a large clinical trial, 26% of enrolled patients had died in a median follow-up period of 9.9 months. Of all deaths, 41.0% were due to HF, 26.0% due to sudden cardiac death, 2.6% due to AMI, 2.2% due to stroke, and 13.2% due to non-cardiovascular causes.[78]

The Rehospitalization Problem

The high rates of rehospitalization after discharge from a heart failure hospitalization have become a major focus of clinicians, policy makers, and payers. Claims data using the U.S. Medicare sample suggest a striking rate of rehospitalization in older patients, with a 30-day rehospitalization rate of 27%, although rates are substantially lower in younger non-Medicare cohorts.[79,80] Rates of rehospitalization within 6 months approach 50% in many cohorts, in particular older adults. Of note, approximately half of the rehospitalizations are not heart failure related, which underscores the total burden of comorbidity in heart failure patients as well as the challenges in affecting this event rate with heart failure-focused interventions. In the EVEREST, careful

TABLE 49.5 Outcomes in Acute Heart Failure Patients from Selected Trials and Registries

STUDY	PATIENTS (N)	RE-HOSPITALIZATION	MORTALITY IN-HOSPITAL	MORTALITY POST-DISCHARGE
Trials				
ASCEND-HF	7,141	6% at 30 days		13% at 6 mo
EVEREST	4,133	12% at 30 days	3%	26% at 9.9 mo
RELAX-AHF	1,161	9% at 60 days		9% at 6 mo
RELAX-AHF-2	6,545	19% Hosp for HF or RF at 6 mo		12% at 6 mo
TRUE-HF	2,157	7% HF Hosp at 30 days		21% CV death at 15 mo
Registries				
Lee (Canada)	4,031	N/A	8.7%	10.6% 30 days
				31% 1 year
ADHERE (US)	187,565	N/A	3.8%	N/A
OPTIMIZE-HF (US)	41,267	30% at 60–90 days	3.8%	8.0% at 60–90 days
Tavazzi (Italy)	2,807	38.1% at 6 months	7.3%	12.8% at 6 months
EHFS II (EU)	3,580	N/A	6.7%	N/A
ATTEND (Japan)	4,837	N/A	6.3%	N/A
Damasceno (sub-Saharan Africa)	1,006	9% at 60 days (all cause)	4.2%	18% at 6 months

Data from O'Connor CM, Starling RC, Hernandez AF, et al. Effect of nesiritide in patients with acute decompensated heart failure. *N Engl J Med.* 2011;365:32–43. Konstam MA, Gheorghiade M, Burnett Jr JC, et al. Effects of oral tolvaptan in patients hospitalized for worsening heart failure: the EVEREST outcome trial. *JAMA.* 2007;297:1319–1331. Teerlink JR, Cotter G, Davison BA, et al. Serelaxin, recombinant human relaxin-2, for treatment of acute heart failure (RELAX-AHF): a randomised, placebo-controlled trial. *Lancet.* 2013;381:29–39. Teerlink MM, Cotter G, Davison BA, et al. Effects of serelaxin in patients with acute heart failure. *N Engl J Med.* 2019;381:716–726. Packer M, O'Connor C, McMurray JJV, et al. Effect of ularitide on cardiovascular mortality in acute heart failure. *N Engl J Med.* 2017;376:1956–1964. Lee DS, Austin PC, Rouleau JL, et al. Predicting mortality among patients hospitalized for heart failure: derivation and validation of a clinical model. *JAMA.* 2003;290:2581–2587. ADHERE Scientific Advisory Committee Acute Decompensated Heart Failure National Registry (ADHERE®) Core Module Q1 2006 Final Cumulative National Benchmark Report: Scios, Inc.; July, 2006. Gheorghiade M, Abraham WT, Albert NM, et al. Systolic blood pressure at admission, clinical characteristics, and outcomes in patients hospitalized with acute heart failure. *JAMA.* 2006;296:2217–2226. Tavazzi L, Maggioni AP, Lucci D, et al. Nationwide survey on acute heart failure in cardiology ward services in Italy. *Eur Heart J.* 2006;27:1207–1215. Nieminen MS, Brutsaert D, Dickstein K, et al. EuroHeart Failure Survey II (EHFS II): a survey on hospitalized acute heart failure patients: description of population. *Eur Heart J.* 2006;27:2725–2736. Sato N, Gheorghiade M, Kajimoto K, et al. Hyponatremia and in-hospital mortality in patients admitted for heart failure (from the ATTEND registry). *Am J Cardiol.* 2013;111:1019–1025. Damasceno A, Mayosi BM, Sani M, et al. The causes, treatment, and outcome of acute heart failure in 1006 Africans from 9 countries: results of the sub-Saharan Africa survey of heart failure. *Arch Int Med.* 2012;172:1386–1394.

adjudication of post-discharge hospitalizations showed that 46% were for heart failure, 15% for other cardiovascular causes, and 39% were for non-cardiovascular causes.[78] These rehospitalizations represent a major driver of health expenditures, accounting for over 39 billion US dollars spent on heart failure care per year in the United States.[4] Although controversial, reducing rehospitalization rates for heart failure has been identified as a major focus of quality improvement and cost containment by payers such as the US Centers for Medicare and Medicaid Services. As a result, a variety of interventions and initiatives related to inpatient management, discharge planning, and transitions of care have been implemented in an attempt to decrease rehospitalization rates for heart failure, although the nature, implementation, and effectiveness of these practices have varied widely across health systems.[81] Despite these significant efforts, recent evidence suggests only a minor impact on rehospitalizations.[82] There is also uncertainty about what proportion of rehospitalizations are avoidable, although a systematic review suggests that a quarter or more may be preventable.[66] To date, only improved utilization of proven evidence-based therapies (such as beta blockers and ACE inhibitors) during acute hospitalization has been shown to improve post-discharge outcomes.[61] Hospital discharge before congestion is adequately treated appears to be a common cause of early readmission.[72] Early post-discharge follow-up has also been associated with lower rehospitalization rates in retrospective registry data.[68] A variety of other interventions centered on telemedicine, disease monitoring, and disease management remain under active investigation.

Specific Therapies
Diuretics

Loop diuretics are the primary pharmacologic treatment for volume overload in patients with AHF, and typically result in rapid symptom relief in most patients.[83] (Diuretics are discussed in detail in Chapter 50.) Loop diuretics (furosemide, torsemide, bumetanide, and ethacrynic acid; Table 49.6) can lead to excretion of up to 25% of the filtered sodium and intravenous administration avoids variable bioavailability and allows for rapid onset of action (typically within 30 to 60 minutes). Preliminary data suggest that genetic variants modulate the response to furosemide in patients with decompensated HF.[84] Based on the results of the DOSE study described below, initial doses of approximately 2.5 times the outpatient dose should be considered for patients on chronic oral diuretic therapy, with underlying renal dysfunction, or with severe volume overload. Given the steep dose-response curve of these agents, titration should be rapid with doubling of the dose until an effective response is noted. If there is significant volume overload (>5 to 10 liters) or diuretic resistance, a continuous intravenous infusion can be considered. Despite their ubiquitous use in AHF, loop diuretics have generally not been tested in rigorously controlled clinical trials. Loop diuretics may lead to neurohormonal activation and electrolyte repletion, and have been associated in observational studies with both increased risk of worsening renal function and decreased survival, although a recent analysis suggested no relationship between diuretic exposure and 30-day all-cause death or HF hospitalization.[85] The DOSE trial was a randomized, double-blind study that prospectively compared diuretic strategies in AHF.[86] Using a 2 × 2 factorial design, 308 patients were randomized to treatment with IV furosemide using either twice-daily bolus dosing or a continuous infusion and to either a low (equivalent to the numerical value of the oral outpatient dose given IV) or high (2.5 times the oral dose given IV) dose strategy. There was no significant difference in either of the co-primary endpoints of global assessment of symptoms or change in creatinine at 72 hours with administration by bolus compared to infusion or with the low- versus high-dose strategy. The high-dose strategy was associated with greater relief of dyspnea and net fluid loss at 72 hours, although more patients in the high-dose group had a transient increase in creatinine greater than 0.3 mg/dL, which resolved by the time

TABLE 49.6 Therapeutic Approaches for Volume Management in Acute Heart Failure

SEVERITY OF VOLUME OVERLOAD	DIURETIC	DOSE (MG)	COMMENTS
Moderate	Furosemide, or	20–40 mg or up to 2.5 times oral dose	Intravenous administration preferable in symptomatic patients
	Bumetanide, or	0.5–1.0	Titrate dose according to clinical response
	Torsemide	10–20	Monitor Na+, K+, creatinine, BP
Severe	Furosemide, or	40–160 or 2.5 times oral dose 5–40 mg/hr infusion	Intravenously
	Bumetanide, or	1–4 / 0.5–2 mg/hr infusion (max 2–4 mg/hr, limit 2–4 hr)	Bumetanide and torsemide have higher oral bioavailability than furosemide, but intravenous administration preferable in AHF
	Torsemide	20–100/ 5–20 mg/hr	
	Ultrafiltration	200–500 mL/hr	Adjust ultrafiltration rate to clinical response, monitor for hypotension; consider hematocrit sensor
Refractory to loop diuretics	Add HCTZ, or	25–50 twice daily	Combination with loop diuretic may be better than very high dose of loop diuretics alone
	Metolazone, or	2.5–10 once daily	Metolazone more potent if creatinine clearance <30 mL/min
	Chlorothiazide, or	250–500 mg IV 500–1000 mg po	
	Spironolactone	25–50 once daily	Spironolactone best choice if patient not in renal failure and normal or low serum K+, although may not be very potent
In case of alkalosis	Acetazolamide	0.5	Intravenously
Refractory to loop diuretic and thiazides	Add dopamine (renal vasodilation), or dobutamine or milrinone (inotropic agent)		
	Ultrafiltration, or hemodialysis if co-existing renal failure		

of hospital discharge (Table e49.1). The significance of this finding is unclear; although there were no apparent differences in hospital length of stay or days alive out of the hospital, the study was not powered for long-term clinical outcomes. Overall, there were no differences in results between the continuous infusion and intermittent bolus strategies in the clinical trial setting of DOSE, suggesting that whichever approach is most likely to reliably produce the desired diuresis in the particular local clinical practice should be used.

In the setting of diuretic resistance, administration of a thiazide-like diuretic that blocks the distal tubule can provide significant augmentation of the diuretic effect.[87] Intravenous chlorothiazide (500 to 1000 mg) or oral metolazone (2.5 to 10 mg) given prior to the loop diuretic are effective agents, although care must be taken to monitor for hypotension, worsening renal function, and electrolyte abnormalities, which may be profound. Nonsteroidal anti-inflammatory drugs can greatly reduce the efficacy of diuretics by reducing renal synthesis of vasodilatory prostaglandins, and these agents should be avoided. If hypokalemia is a persistent problem with replacement requirements, administration of a potassium-sparing diuretic, such as spironolactone or eplerenone, should be considered, and may also provide synergistic diuretic effects, especially at higher doses,[88] as well as long-term beneficial effects on outcomes.

Vasodilators

In the absence of hypotension, vasodilators can be used as first-line therapy in combination with diuretics in the management of AHF patients to improve congestive symptoms (Table 49.7).[89] As noted above, in the ALARM-HF registry using propensity-matching techniques, patients admitted with AHF and treated with diuretics and vasodilators had significantly better in-hospital survival compared to patients treated with diuretics alone or those treated with inotropes,[70] while another more recent analysis of 11,078 patients admitted for AHF demonstrated no mortality benefit at 7, 30, or 365 days[90] consistent with the findings of a systematic review.[69] After extensive review of these and other data, the U.K. National Institute for Health and Care Excellence found no evidence to support the routine use of vasodilators in patients with AHF.[91] However, in practice vasodilators appear to provide symptom relief in these patients. Vasodilators can be classified as: (1) predominantly venous dilators, with consequent reduction in preload; (2) arterial dilators, leading to a decrease in afterload; and (3) balanced vasodilators, with combined action on both the venous and the arterial system. Currently available vasodilators include the organic nitrates (nitroglycerin and isosorbide dinitrate), sodium nitroprusside (SNP), and nesiritide. All of these drugs act by activating soluble guanylate cyclase (sGC) in the smooth muscle cells, leading to higher intracellular concentrations of cGMP and consequent vessel relaxation (see Chapter 47). They should be used with caution in patients who are preload or after-load dependent (e.g., severe diastolic dysfunction, aortic stenosis, and CAD), because they may cause severe hypotension. BP should be monitored frequently and the drug discontinued if symptomatic hypotension develops.

Nitrates

Organic nitrates are one of the oldest therapies for AHF. These agents are potent venodilators, producing rapid decreases in pulmonary venous and ventricular filling pressures and improvement in pulmonary

TABLE 49.7 Intravenous Vasoactive Agents for the Treatment of Acute Heart Failure

INTRAVENOUS MEDICATION	INITIAL DOSE	EFFECTIVE DOSE RANGE*	COMMENTS
Vasodilators			
Nitroglycerin; glyceryl trinitrate	20 μg/min	40–400 μg/min	Hypotension, headache; Tolerance with continuous use after 24 hr
Isosorbide dinitrate	1 mg/hr	2–10 mg/hr	Hypotension, headache; Tolerance with continuous use within 24 hr
Nitroprusside	0.3 μg/kg/min	0.3–5 μg/kg/min (usually <4 μg/kg/min)	Caution in patients with active myocardial ischemia; Hypotension; cyanide side effects (nausea, dysphoria); thiocyanate toxicity; light sensitive
Nesiritide[†]	2 μg/kg bolus with 0.010–0.030 μg/kg/min infusion[‡]	0.010–0.030 μg/kg/min	Up-titration: 1 μg/kg bolus, then increase infusion rate by 0.005 μg/kg/min no more frequently than every 3 hr, up to a maximum of 0.03 μg/kg/min
			Hypotension, headache (less than with organic nitrates)
Inotropes			
Dobutamine	1–2 μg/kg/min	2–20 μg/kg/min	For inotropy and vasodilation; Hypotension, tachycardia, arrhythmias; ?mortality
Dopamine	1–2 μg/kg/min	2–4 μg/kg/min	For inotropy and vasodilation; Hypotension, tachycardia, arrhythmias; ?mortality
	4–5 μg/kg/min	5–20 μg/kg/min	For inotropy and vasoconstriction; Tachycardia, arrhythmias; ?mortality
Milrinone	25–75 μg/kg bolus over 10–20 min[‡] followed by infusion	0.10–0.75 μg/kg/min	For vasodilation and inotropy; Hypotension, tachycardia, arrhythmias; Renal excretion; ?mortality
Enoximone[†]	0.25–0.75 mg/kg	1.25–7.5 μg/kg/min	For vasodilation and inotropy; Hypotension, tachycardia, arrhythmias; ?mortality
Levosimendan[†]	12-24 μg/kg bolus over 10 min* followed by infusion	0.5–2.0 μg/kg/min	For vasodilation and inotropy; active metabolite present for approximately 84 hr; Hypotension, tachycardia, arrhythmias; ?mortality
Epinephrine		0.05–0.5 μg/kg/min	For vasoconstriction and inotropy; Tachycardia, arrhythmias, end-organ hypoperfusion; ?mortality
Norepinephrine		0.2–1.0 μg/kg/min	For vasoconstriction and inotropy; Tachycardia, arrhythmias, end-organ hypoperfusion; ?mortality

Use higher dose range for chronic diuretic use, renal insufficiency, and severe volume overload. Diuretic naïve patients should receive lower doses, initially.
*In general, titration of medication is accomplished by doubling of dose with careful monitoring for adverse effects.
†Not approved for use in all countries.
‡Some clinicians do not administer a bolus dose, so as to decrease the risk of hypotension. Bolus not recommended in patients with hypotension.

congestion, dyspnea, and myocardial oxygen demand at low doses. At slightly higher doses and in the presence of vasoconstriction, nitrates are also arteriolar vasodilators, reducing afterload and increasing cardiac output. Nitrates are relatively selective for epicardial, compared to intramyocardial, coronary arteries, resulting in increased coronary blood flow and making them useful for patients with concomitant active myocardial ischemia. The starting dose of nitroglycerin is usually 20 μg/min with rapid up-titration occurring every 5 to 15 minutes in either 20 μg/min increments or doubling of the dose. The dose may initially be titrated to the goal of immediate symptom relief, but a blood pressure reduction of at least 10 mm Hg in mean arterial pressure with a SBP greater than 100 mm Hg may be preferable. The nitrate dose may need to be reduced if SBP is 90 to 100 mm Hg and will often need to be discontinued with SBP less than 90 mm Hg. Intravenous nitrate use appears to be more common in Europe than in the United States (38% in EHFS-II but only 9% in ADHERE).[12,45] Organic nitrates may also be administered orally, sublingually, or by spray, allowing for convenient emergent treatment prior to establishing intravenous access.

> There is limited clinical trial experience with organic nitrates. Early administration of high-dose intravenous nitrates is beneficial in improving arterial oxygenation and potentially preventing some consequences of AHF (MI, need for mechanical ventilation), compared to furosemide alone[47] or NIV,[92] although these studies were small and not blinded. In a study designed to evaluate nesiritide in patients with dyspnea at rest from decompensated heart failure, nitroglycerin treatment in 143 patients demonstrated nonsignificant, mild decreases in PCWP and no significant improvement in patient-assessed dyspnea within 3 hours, but the dose was remarkably low (42 μg/min).[93] In a small, single-site sub-study[94] where nitroglycerin was aggressively up-titrated to a mean dose of 155 μg/min by 3 hours, there were significant decreases in PCWP (4- to 6-mm Hg decrease from baseline) from 1 to 12 hours, but no difference at 24 hours. The major limitation of organic nitrates is the tolerance that typically develops within 24 hours. Headache is the most common adverse effect (20% within 24 hours[93]). Symptomatic hypotension (5%) may also be noted, but generally resolves when nitrate therapy is discontinued. Given the risk of severe hypotension with potentially catastrophic consequences, the recent use of phosphodiesterase 5 inhibitors (sildenafil, tadalafil, vardenafil, etc.) should be ruled out prior to administration of nitrates.

Sodium Nitroprusside

SNP induces a balanced reduction in afterload and preload that is exquisitely titratable, due to a very short half-life (seconds to a few minutes) and is particularly effective in the setting of markedly elevated afterload (e.g., hypertensive AHF) and moderate-severe mitral regurgitation. Intravenous administration is usually monitored with an indwelling arterial line, although automated blood pressure cuffs are now used in many centers. Titration of the SNP dose to rapidly improve symptoms and/or to achieve an SBP of 90 to 100 mm Hg are typical goals, and invasive pulmonary artery catheters may assist in meeting other hemodynamic goals. Tapering the dose of nitroprusside prior to discontinuation is advised to avoid the possibility of "rebound hypertension." Physician discomfort with the cyanide metabolites and the historical institutional requirements for invasive arterial monitoring has limited the use of this highly effective therapy to fewer than 1% of patients with AHF in Europe and the United States.[12,45]

> Nitroprusside, a pro-drug that is rapidly metabolized to nitric oxide and cyanide, has no inherent arrhythmogenic properties, may improve myocardial oxygen demand by reducing afterload and wall stress, creates no significant electrolyte disturbances, and is rarely toxic. Despite its potency, severe hypotension is unusual and rapidly resolves. However, significant vasodilation of the intra-myocardial vasculature has been noted, possibly producing a coronary steal phenomenon, and consequently, nitroprusside is not recommended for patients with active myocardial ischemia. The most common complaints with nitroprusside are related to the cyanide metabolite, including nausea, abdominal discomfort, dissociative feelings, and dysphoria. Cyanide rarely accumulates in patients, but impaired hepatic function and doses of greater than 250 μg/min for over 48 hours increase this risk. The thiocyanate metabolite can accumulate in patients with moderate to severe renal insufficiency when exposed to prolonged infusions of high doses (usually >400 μg/min) over days and is usually not relevant in the treatment of AHF. Cyanide levels may be measured, but rarely return in a timely fashion to be useful.
>
> There are no randomized studies of nitroprusside in patients with AHF, although multiple studies demonstrated dramatic reduction in PCWP (15 mm Hg) and marked increases in cardiac output, associated with increases in diuresis, natriuresis, and decreased neurohormonal activation. In a contemporary analysis of 175 consecutive patients admitted for AHF, intravenous SNP was associated with greater hemodynamic improvement and lower rates of inotropic support or worsening renal function during hospitalization and with lower rates of all-cause mortality after discharge, despite a worse hemodynamic profile at baseline.[95]

NESIRITIDE

Nesiritide (recombinant human B-type natriuretic peptide) is identical to endogenous BNP and causes potent vasodilation in the venous and arterial vasculatures, resulting in significant reductions in venous and ventricular filling pressures and mild increases in cardiac output. As with other vasodilators, nesiritide may reduce diuretic requirements, but in clinical studies, there is limited evidence for a significant direct "natriuretic" effect. Nesiritide may be used for treatment of patients with acutely decompensated congestive heart failure who have dyspnea at rest or with minimal activity, but it should not be administered for the indication of replacing diuretics, enhancing diuresis, protecting renal function, or improving survival. An optional bolus of 2 μg/kg followed by a 0.01 μg/kg/min infusion is the recommended starting dose for nesiritide. There is limited clinical trial experience with up-titration of the drug, but for patients who remain symptomatic with evidence of volume overload and sufficient blood pressure, up-titration may be considered. Nesiritide has clear effects on hemodynamics and has limited need for frequent dose adjustments and an absence of tolerance, but its high cost and lack of clear clinical benefit beyond other less expensive and more readily titratable agents have limited its use. The Vasodilation in the Management of Acute CHF (VMAC) trial randomized 489 patients with decompensated CHF and dyspnea at rest to placebo, nitroglycerin, or nesiritide.[93] After 3 hours, patients receiving nesiritide had a significantly greater decrease in PCWP compared to both nitroglycerin and placebo, and improvement in dyspnea compared to placebo (no difference from nitroglycerin). A pooled analysis of the randomized, controlled clinical trial data suggested that nesiritide may be associated with an increased risk of worsening renal function as well as increased mortality. To address these issues, the ASCEND-HF trial randomized 7141 patients with AHF to nesiritide or placebo for 24 to 168 hours.[96] At 30 days, there was no difference between patients receiving nesiritide and those receiving placebo with regard to the composite endpoint of death or rehospitalization for heart failure. The clinical effects on dyspnea were relatively modest and have generally not been felt to be clinically important compared to placebo. Use of nesiritide had no impact on worsening renal function but was associated with an increase in the rate of hypotension. Another small study (ROSE-AHF) enrolled 360 patients admitted for AHF to specifically assess the effect of low-dose nesiritide on congestion and renal function.[97] In this study, nesiritide had no beneficial effect on urine output or cystatin-C, nor on any of the other secondary endpoints reflective of decongestion, renal function, or clinical outcomes, although it was associated with more symptomatic hypotension.

Nesiritide exerts its activity via guanylyl cyclase-linked natriuretic peptide receptors (NPR A and B) causing cGMP-mediated vasodilation. Hypotension, at times prolonged (over 2 hours[93]) despite the relatively short (18 minute) half-life of the peptide, is more common in patients with volume depletion and consequently, nesiritide use should be limited to those with congestive signs and symptoms. Headache also occurs, although less frequent than with nitroglycerin. Other actions of nesiritide include neurohormonal antagonism with reduction in vasopressin, aldosterone, and sympathetic tone, and alteration of intra-renal hemodynamics and glomerular filtration. Nesiritide did not improve urine output or renal function in AHF patients with worsening creatinine.[97]

Inotropes and Inodilators

The inotropic drugs and inodilators (inotropic drugs with vasodilatory properties) increase cardiac output through cyclic adenosine monophosphate (cAMP)-mediated inotropy and reduce PCWP through vasodilation (see Table 49.7).[98] However, retrospective data from both registries and trials of AHF patients suggest that even the short-term use (hours to few days) of IV inotropes (except for digoxin) is associated with significant side effects such as hypotension, atrial or ventricular arrhythmias, and an increase in in-hospital[70] and possibly long-term mortality.[99] Patients with CAD may be at higher risk of adverse events due to reduced coronary perfusion and increased myocardial oxygen requirements with possible myocardial ischemia and injury. Therefore, these agents are reserved for use in selected situations of hypoperfusion when other interventions are inappropriate or have failed. The use of these drugs should be limited to patients with reduced EF, who present with low SBP (<90 mm Hg) or low measured cardiac output in the presence of signs of congestion and organ hypoperfusion such as decreased mentation or reduced urine output.[32,50] Despite these recommendations, inotropes are still frequently used in patients with HFpEF in some regions. Inotropic agents for AHF should be used with close hemodynamic and telemetry monitoring and should be stopped as soon as adequate organ perfusion is restored. All of these agents may increase conduction through the atrioventricular node, causing a rapid ventricular response in patients presenting with atrial fibrillation. Additionally, IV inotropes may be used in cardiogenic shock as a temporary therapy to prevent hemodynamic collapse or as a life-sustaining bridge to more definitive therapy for those patients awaiting mechanical circulatory support, ventricular assist devices, or cardiac transplantation. In North American and European registries, approximately 15% and 25% of patients were treated with inotropic agents, although given the minimal supportive clinical evidence, there is marked local variability in the use of these drugs.[100]

Dobutamine

Dobutamine is the most commonly used positive inotrope in Europe and the United States, despite evidence that it increases mortality.[101,102] Dobutamine at doses of 1 to 2 μg/kg/min may improve renal perfusion in patients with cardiogenic shock, although higher doses (5 to 10 μg/kg/min) may be necessary for more profound hypoperfusion. Tachyphylaxis may occur with infusions of over 24 to 48 hours, partially due to receptor desensitization. In general, dobutamine (or dopamine) is the preferred inotrope in patients with significant hypotension and in the setting of significant renal dysfunction, given the renal excretion of milrinone. Concomitant beta blocker therapy will result in competitive antagonism of the effects of dobutamine and higher doses of dobutamine (10 to 20 μg/kg/min) may be required to obtain the desired hemodynamic effects. The lowest effective dose of dobutamine should be used in the context of continuous blood pressure and rhythm monitoring. Dobutamine should be gradually weaned off and clinical status re-evaluated with each dose adjustment. Temporary adjustments to afterload-reducing agents or diuretics may assist in weaning.

As an agonist of both beta$_1$ and beta$_2$ adrenergic receptors (see Chapter 38) with variable effects on the alpha receptors, dobutamine has multiple actions. Beta-receptor stimulation results in increased inotropy and chronotropy through increases in intracellular cAMP and calcium, as well as via direct activation of voltage sensitive calcium channels. At low doses, stimulation of beta$_2$ and alpha receptors causes vasodilation, resulting in decreased aortic impedance and systemic vascular resistance with reduction in afterload and indirect increases in cardiac output. At higher doses, vasoconstriction can ensue with decreased venous capacitance and increased right atrial pressure. Adverse effects of dobutamine include tachycardia, increasing ventricular response to atrial fibrillation, increased atrial and ventricular arrhythmias, myocardial ischemia, and possibly cardiomyocyte necrosis via direct toxic effects and induction of apoptosis.[103]

While the hemodynamic and other effects of dobutamine have been studied, there is only one placebo-controlled, randomized trial in patients with AHF. Although there are some methodologic concerns, the CAlcium Sensitizer or Inotrope or NOne in low output heart failure (CASINO) study demonstrated significantly increased mortality with dobutamine compared to placebo, consistent with the results of other studies of this class of agents.[101]

Dopamine

In both the United States and Europe, dopamine is used as often as dobutamine, presumably as a vasoconstrictor and for its putative effects on renal vasodilation. As a precursor to the synthesis of norepinephrine, an agonist of both adrenergic and dopaminergic receptors, and an inhibitor of norepinephrine uptake, dopamine has complex effects that vary significantly with dose. Initiation of dopamine therapy causes a rapid release of norepinephrine that can precipitate tachycardia, as well as atrial and ventricular arrhythmias. In addition, intermediate to high doses can cause significant vasoconstriction, precipitating heart failure and poor perfusion. Dopamine should be gradually weaned from these doses down to 3 to 5 μg/kg/min and then discontinued to avoid potential hypotensive effects of low-dose dopamine.

Low-dose dopamine (≤2 μg/kg/min) has been proposed to cause specific dilation of renal, splanchnic, and cerebral arteries, potentially increasing renal blood flow in a selective manner, as well as promoting natriuresis through direct distal tubular effects. The DAD-HF study of 60 patients admitted for AHF suggested that a combination of low-dose furosemide and low-dose dopamine resulted in comparable urine output and dyspnea relief, but improved renal function profile and potassium homeostasis compared to high-dose furosemide.[104] However, the DAD-HF II study of 161 patients found no beneficial effect of the addition of low-dose dopamine to furosemide.[105] In the ROSE-AHF study of 360 patients hospitalized with AHF, low-dose dopamine did not increase urine volume during 72 hours, did not improve cystatin C concentrations, but did reduce hypotension and increased tachycardia compared to placebo.[97] Therefore, there does not appear to be an indication for low-dose dopamine therapy to improve renal function.

Intermediate-dose dopamine (2 to 10 μg/kg/min) results in enhanced norepinephrine release, stimulating cardiac receptors with an increase in inotropy and mild stimulation of peripheral vasoconstricting receptors. Because the positive inotropic effect is largely dependent upon myocardial catecholamine stores, which are often depleted in patients with advanced heart failure, dopamine is a poor inotrope in patients with severe systolic dysfunction.

High-dose dopamine (10 to 20 μg/kg/min) causes peripheral and pulmonary artery vasoconstriction, mediated by direct agonist effects on alpha$_1$ adrenergic receptors. These doses pose a significant risk of precipitating limb and end-organ ischemia and should be used cautiously.

Epinephrine

Epinephrine is a full beta-receptor agonist and a potent inotropic agent with balanced vasodilator and vasoconstrictor effects. The direct effect of epinephrine on increasing inotropy independent of myocardial catecholamine stores makes epinephrine a useful agent in the treatment of transplant patients with denervated hearts.

Phosphodiesterase Inhibitors

cAMP is a ubiquitous signaling molecule that increases inotropy, chronotropy, and lusitropy in cardiomyocytes and causes vasorelaxation in vascular smooth muscle (see Chapter 46). Phosphodiesterase IIIa is compartmentalized in the cardiac and vascular smooth muscle, where it terminates the signaling activity of cAMP by degrading it to AMP. Many specific inhibitors of PDE IIIa, such as milrinone and enoximone, have been developed to provide organ-specific improvements in hemodynamics through increasing myocardial and vascular smooth muscle cell cAMP concentrations. In theory, subcellular localization may provide the possibility to stimulate inotropy without increasing heart rate with low doses of highly specific phosphodiesterase inhibitors (PDEI). The independence of the mechanism from adrenergic receptors bypasses receptor down-regulation, desensitization, and antagonism by beta blockers. Although studies have shown improved hemodynamic efficacy with PDEI compared to dobutamine in patients on beta blocker therapy, such limitations of dobutamine's effects are not typically clinically relevant. In addition, this mechanism allows for synergistic effects with beta receptor agonists, such as dobutamine. Such combination therapy may be useful in patients with markedly reduced LV systolic function. PDEI cause significant peripheral and pulmonary vasodilation, reducing afterload and preload, while increasing inotropy. These effects make them well suited for patients with LV dysfunction and pulmonary hypertension or post-transplant patients.

Milrinone is the most commonly used PDEI, but only 3% of patients in ADHERE[45] and less than 1% in EHFS II[12] received it. Milrinone therapy may be initiated with a 25 to 75 μg/kg bolus over 10 to 20 min, although in clinical practice the bolus dose is usually omitted. Infusions are typically started at 0.10 to 0.25 μg/kg/min and may be up-titrated to hemodynamic effect. Given the elimination half-life of 2.5 hours and the pharmacodynamic half-life of over 6 hours, effects from up-titration are delayed by at least 15 minutes after dosage adjustment. Also due to these pharmacodynamics, patients who have had prolonged administration of milrinone may have delayed deterioration, so they should be observed for at least 48 hours after cessation. Milrinone is renally excreted, necessitating dose adjustment in the presence of renal dysfunction or substitution with dobutamine. Milrinone has many side effects, including hypotension and atrial and ventricular arrhythmias. In OPTIME-CHF (Outcomes of a Prospective Trial of Intravenous Milrinone for Exacerbations of Chronic Heart Failure),[106] 951 patients admitted with exacerbation of systolic heart failure not requiring intravenous inotropic support were randomized to milrinone or placebo infusion. There was no difference in the primary endpoint of days hospitalized for cardiovascular causes with 60 days, but significant increases in sustained hypotension and new atrial arrhythmias were noted in the milrinone-treated patients. In addition, a post-hoc sub-group analysis demonstrated increased mortality in patients with an ischemic cause of heart failure who received milrinone.[99] This study reinforces the caution that must be exercised in selecting these agents for the treatment of patients with AHF.

ENOXIMONE
Enoximone is also a PDE IIIa inhibitor that is available in Europe. Dosing is essentially 10 times that of milrinone, with a bolus dose of 0.25 to 0.75 mg/kg bolus over 10 to 20 minutes, followed by an infusion of 1.25 μg/kg/min. It is extensively metabolized by the liver into renally cleared active metabolites, so doses should be reduced in the setting of either renal or hepatic insufficiency. Otherwise, the above comments apply to this PDEI as well.

Levosimendan
Levosimendan is a novel agent that increases myocardial contractility and produces peripheral vasodilation, through cardiac myofilament calcium sensitization by calcium-dependent (systolic) troponin C binding and activation of vascular smooth muscle potassium channels, respectively. Levosimendan also has some PDEI activity, which some contend is responsible for its inotropic activity in patients.[107] Levosimendan was administered to almost 4% of patients in EHFS II[12] and is available in over 40 countries (although not in the United States), where it is used in patients with reduced LV systolic function and hypoperfusion in the absence of severe hypotension. Although it may be given with a bolus of 12 to 24 μg/kg over 10 minutes, many clinicians directly initiate a continuous infusion at a rate of 0.05 to 0.10 μg/kg/min, which may be up-titrated to 0.2 μg/kg/min. In clinical trials, levosimendan has been shown to significantly increase cardiac output, reduce PCWP and afterload, and improve dyspnea. The potent vasodilating effects of levosimendan can cause significant hypotension, the risk of which may be reduced by maintaining filling pressures.[98] Levosimendan has an active, acetylated metabolite with a half-life of over 80 hours, allowing it to have hemodynamic effects days after discontinuation of the infusion.

Initial clinical studies demonstrated reduced arrhythmias and improved survival with levosimendan compared to placebo and dobutamine. REVIVE-II (Randomized multicenter evaluation of intravenous levosimendan efficacy versus placebo in the short term treatment of decompensated heart failure), a recent study of 600 patients, demonstrated significant improvement in the clinical status, serial BNP, and hospital length of stay with levosimendan treatment compared to standard care, but there were also more episodes of hypotension, atrial fibrillation, and ventricular ectopy, as well as a nonsignificant increase in early deaths at 14 or 90 days.[108] SURVIVE (Survival of patients with AHF in need of intravenous inotropic support trial) randomized 1327 patients with systolic dysfunction, evidence of low cardiac output, and dyspnea at rest despite diuretics and vasodilators to either levosimendan or dobutamine. An early reduction in mortality was not sustained through 180 days, but levosimendan was associated with a greater incidence of atrial fibrillation and lower incidence of WHF compared to dobutamine.[109]

Vasopressors
These agents should be reserved for patients with marked hypotension in whom central organ hypoperfusion is evident. Vasopressors will redistribute cardiac output centrally at the expense of peripheral perfusion and increased afterload. *Norepinephrine* is a potent agonist of the beta$_1$ and the alpha$_1$ receptors, but is a weaker agonist of beta$_2$ receptors, resulting in marked vasoconstriction. In general, it is the preferred vasopressor for cardiogenic shock.[32] In the SOAP II trial, 1679 patients with shock were randomized to either dopamine or norepinephrine with a nonstatistical difference increase in mortality with dopamine associated with a significant increase in arrhythmic events.[110] In a subgroup analysis including the 280 patients with cardiogenic shock, norepinephrine had improved survival compared to dopamine. *Phenylephrine* is a selective alpha$_1$ receptor agonist with potent direct arterial vasoconstrictor effects. This agent may be used in case of severe hypotension, particularly when the hypotension is related to systemic vasodilation, rather than to a decrease in cardiac output. As noted above, *dopamine* may also be used for its vasoconstrictor properties. All of these agents may induce end-organ hypoperfusion and tissue necrosis.

OTHER PHARMACOLOGIC THERAPIES
Digoxin
Digoxin rapidly improves hemodynamics without increasing heart rate or decreasing BP and may be considered in patients with a low BP due to a low cardiac output.[111] Digoxin may be used intravenously with an initial bolus of 0.5 mg IV. It should be given slowly because a rapid administration may cause systemic vasoconstriction. The initial bolus should be followed by an oral or IV dose of 0.25 mg at least 12 hours after the initial dose. In patients who continue to have signs and symptoms of HF, digoxin therapy should be continued in addition to other therapies, with a dose resulting in a trough serum concentration of less than 1 ng/mL. Ischemia, hypokalemia, and hypomagnesemia may increase the likelihood of developing digitalis intoxication, even at the therapeutic doses. Digoxin should not be used in patients with moderate to severe renal impairment, ongoing ischemia, or advanced AV block.

Arginine Vasopressin Antagonists
Arginine vasopressin (AVP), also known as antidiuretic hormone, is the main regulator of plasma osmolality. Vasopressin levels are inappropriately high in both acute and chronic HF and are thought to have a major role in the pathophysiology of HF. In particular, vasopressin appears to be the major contributor to the development of the hyponatremia observed in patients with HF. In patients with AHF, volume overload, and persistent hyponatremia at risk for or having active cognitive symptoms, therapy with a vasopressin antagonist for short-term improvement in serum sodium concentration may be considered. Currently available vasopressin antagonists are tolvaptan (an oral, selective V2 receptor antagonist) and conivaptan (a V1$_a$/V2 receptor antagonist for IV use). Although both agents have been approved for the treatment of clinically significant hypervolemic and euvolemic hyponatremia, they have not been shown to improve long-term outcomes in heart failure and are not currently approved for this indication. The Efficacy of Vasopressin Antagonism in Heart Failure Outcome Study with Tolvaptan (EVEREST) was an international trial that evaluated more than 4000 patients admitted with AHF and reduced EF. Tolvaptan added to standard therapy for AHF modestly improved signs and symptoms during hospitalization and modestly reduced body weight without affecting renal function, HR, or BP, but post-discharge survival and readmission rate were not affected by chronic post-discharge therapy with tolvaptan.[112,113] A recent small double blind study of short-term (48 hours) therapy with tolvaptan vs placebo in AHF, the TACTICS study, did not show a clinically important benefit of tolvaptan therapy in this setting.[114] In patients with AHF, the addition of conivaptan to standard therapy increased urine output without a significant improvement in signs or symptoms or decrease in body weight.[115]

Calcium Channel Blockers
Calcium channel blockers (CCBs) without significant myocardial depressant effects, such as nicardipine and clevidipine, may be potentially useful in patients with AHF presenting with severe hypertension refractory to other therapies. In a pilot study of 104 patients with hypertensive AHF who exhibited pulmonary congestion, clevidipine rapidly provided significant blood pressure control associated with improvement in dyspnea compared to standard of care.[116]

Other Nonpharmacologic Therapies
Ultrafiltration

Peripheral ultrafiltration is an available modality to remove sodium and water in hospitalized patients with HF. The theoretical advantage of ultrafiltration is the removal of isotonic fluid, resulting in greater and more reliable salt removal, potentially without the neurohormonal activation seen with diuretics.[83] Potential limitations of ultrafiltration include the need for large-bore venous access, systemic anticoagulation, and increased complexity of nursing care related to management of the device. Although theoretically attractive, the appropriate use of ultrafiltration in AHF remains uncertain.

The Ultrafiltration Versus Intravenous Diuretics for Patients Hospitalized for Acute Decompensated Heart Failure (UNLOAD) trial randomized 200 patients with AHF to veno-venous ultrafiltration or standard of care within 24 hours of initial presentation. Patients receiving ultrafiltration demonstrated a greater reduction in body weight at 48 hours, but no improvements in dyspnea and/or renal function.[117] Intriguingly, there was a reduction in post-discharge events at 90 days with ultrafiltration, although the number of events was small. Other recent studies have raised questions about the optimal use of ultrafiltration in heart failure. In an observational study of 63 patients with persistent congestion refractory to hemodynamically guided intensive medical therapy, slow continuous ultrafiltration resulted in improved hemodynamics, yet was associated with high incidence of subsequent transition to renal replacement therapy and high in-hospital mortality.[118] The Cardiorenal Rescue Study in Acute Decompensated Heart Failure (CARRESS) randomized 188 patients with AHF, worsened renal function, and persistent congestion to a strategy of stepped pharmacologic care (intravenous diuretics dosed by the investigator to maintain urine output of 3 to 5 L/day plus intravenous vasodilators or inotropes if needed to achieve target urine output) or ultrafiltration (fluid removal rate 200 mL/hr).[59] Ultrafiltration resulted in similar weight loss (approximately 12 pounds), but resulted in an increase in creatinine levels, compared to standard care, and was associated with more serious adverse events, especially kidney failure, bleeding complications, and intravenous catheter-related complications.

CARRESS enrolled a high-risk population with a composite rate of death or rehospitalization at 60 days of over 50%. The AVOID-HF study (Aquapheresis Versus Intravenous Diuretics and Hospitalizations for Heart Failure, NCT01474200) was designed as an 810-patient trial that was terminated early after 224 patients were enrolled. Although underpowered, there were trends suggesting longer time to first HF event and fewer HF and cardiovascular events in the adjustable ultrafiltration group compared to those randomized to adjustable intravenous loop diuretics.[119] There was no difference in renal function, but more patients assigned to ultrafiltration experienced adverse events.

HYPERTONIC SALINE

Administration of hypertonic saline (HSS; 3%) along with high-dose furosemide and sodium and fluid restriction may be associated with greater diuretic and clinical response. The SMAC-HF study randomized 1771 patients hospitalized for AHF to a single-blind strategy of hypertonic saline solution (150 mL 3% NS) plus furosemide 250 mg intravenous bolus twice daily and sodium restriction to 120 mmol/day versus furosemide 250 mg intravenous bolus twice daily and sodium restriction to 80 mmol/day; both groups received a fluid intake of 1000 mL/day.[120] After discharge, the HSS group continued with 120 mmol Na/day; the second group continued with 80 mmol Na/day. There was a shorter length of stay, increased creatinine clearance at discharge, reduced readmission rate, and improved survival for patients in the hypertonic saline group. These hypothesis-generating data are intriguing, but they are limited by the unblinded study design and the potential confounding by post-discharge management. Larger, prospective, blinded trials are needed to further evaluate this therapeutic approach prior to adoption for clinical practice.

Potential New Therapies

Most of the large clinical trials of new therapies for AHF have been negative in terms of efficacy and/or safety (Table 49.8). A variety of potential explanations have been proposed including lack of drug efficacy, patient selection, timing of therapy, and endpoints.[121] Nonetheless, given the diverse pathophysiology of AHF, it may be unrealistic to expect that

TABLE 49.8 Selected Clinical Trials for Acute Heart Failure

TRIAL	TREATMENT ARMS	POPULATION	RESULTS
VMAC (2002) N = 489	Nesiritide (Nes; 0.01–0.03 μg/kg/min with optional 2 μg/kg bolus; from 24 hr up to 7 days) vs Placebo (Pla; only during first 3 hr) vs Nitroglycerin (NTG; from 24 hr up to 7 days)	Dyspnea at rest ≥2 signs of HF within 72 hours CXR with pulmonary edema	Change in PCWP, at 3 h (1°): −5.8 mm Hg Nes, −3.8 mm Hg NTG, −2 mm Hg Placebo (p < 0.001); at 24: −8.2 mm Hg Nes, −6.3 mm Hg NTG (p < 0.04). Self-evaluation of dyspnea at 3 h, Likert (1°): Nes vs Pla, p = 0.03; Nes vs NTG, p = 0.56; a 24 h: NTG vs Nes, p = 0.13. Self-evaluation of global clinical status, at 3 hr: Nes vs Pla, p = 0.07; Nes vs NTG, p = 0.33; at 24 hr: NTG vs Nes, p = 0.08.
OPTIME-HF (2002) N = 951	Milrinone (0.5 μg/kg/min, titratable to 0.75) vs Placebo, for 48–72 hr	Presenting within 48 hr Known systolic HF LEVF ≤40%	Days with CV hospitalization or dead in 60 days (1°): Milrinone, 12.3 vs Pla 12.5 (p = 0.71) Failure of therapy due to AE within 48 hr: Milrinone 20.6% vs Pla 9.2% (p < 0.001). Excess sustained hypotension (p = 0.004), new atrial fibrillation/flutter (p < 0.001), VT/VF (p = 0.06).
ESCAPE (2005) N = 433	Pulmonary artery catheter (PAC)-guided therapy vs clinical assessment (CA)-guided therapy	LVEF ≤30% SBP ≤125 mm Hg ≥1 sign and ≥1 symptom of HF 3 months HF symptoms despite ACEi and diuretics	Days alive out of hospital during 6 months (1°): PAC, 133 days vs CA, 135 (HR 1.00; 95% CI 0.82–1.21; p = 0.99). Greater number of adverse events in PAC group
VERITAS (2007) N = 1435	Tezosentan (Tezo; 5 mg/hr for 30 min, followed by 1 mg/hr for 24–72 hr) vs Placebo	Presenting within 24 hr Persistent dyspnea Respiratory rate ≥24 bpm At least two of: elevated BNP/NT-proBNP, clinical pulmonary edema, CXR with congestion, LV systolic dysfunction	Change in dyspnea AUC, 24 hr (1°): VERITAS-1, Tezo −562 vs Pla −550 mm * h (p = 0.80); VERITAS-2, Tezo −367 vs Pla −342 (p = 0.60). Death or worsening HF, 7 days: VERITAS-1 + 2, Tezo 26.3% vs. Pla 26.4 (p = 0.95)

TABLE 49.8 Selected Clinical Trials for Acute Heart Failure—cont'd

TRIAL	TREATMENT ARMS	POPULATION	RESULTS
SURVIVE (2007) N = 1327	Levosimendan (Levo; loading 12 µg/kg, followed 0.1–0.2 µg/kg/min; for 24 hr) vs Dobutamine (Dob; 5 µg/kg/min, titratable up to 40 µg/kg/min; for at least 24 hr)	LVEF ≤30% Requiring IV inotropic support At least one of following: dyspnea at rest, oliguria, PCWP ≥18 mm Hg or CI ≤V2.2 L/min/m²	All-cause mortality, 180 days (1°): Levo, 26% vs. Dob 28% (HR 0.91; 95% CI 0.74–1.13; p = 0.40) Change in BNP from baseline to 24 hr: Levo, −631 vs. Dob, −397, p < 0.001. No change in dyspnea at 24 hr, days alive out of hospital at 180 days, all-cause mortality at 31 days, CV mortality at 180 days.
EVEREST (2007) N = 4133	Tolvaptan (Tol; 30 mg po qd) vs Placebo, for at least 60 days	Randomized within 48 hr NYHA III–IV symptoms LVEF ≤40% Signs of volume expansion	Composite of changes in global clinical status and body weight, 7 days (1°): p < 0.001, for Tol superiority; no difference in clinical status; Change in body weight, 1 day: Tol, −1.76 kg vs. Pla, −0.97; p < 0.001. All-cause mortality (1°): Tol, 25.9% vs Pla 26.3% (HR 0.98, 95% CI 0.87–1.11, superiority p = 0.68; non-inferiority p < 0.001) CV death or HF hospitalization (1°): Tol, 42.0% vs. Pla 40.2% (HR 1.04, 95% CI 0.95–1.14, superiority p = 0.55)
UNLOAD (2007) N = 200	Ultrafiltration (UF; fluid removal titrated by investigator up to 500 mL/hr) vs Diuretic (titrated by investigator, at least twice daily oral dose), for 48 hr	Randomized within 24 hr ≥2 signs of congestion	Weight loss, 48 hr (1°): UF, −5.0 kg vs Diuretics, −3.1, p = 0.001 Dyspnea score, 48 hr (1°): UF, 6.4 vs Diuretics, 6.1; p = 0.35 HF rehospitalization, 90 days: UF, 0.22 vs Diuretics, 046, p = 0.022; Days rehospitalized: UF, 1.4 days vs Diuretics, 3.8; p = 0.022; Unscheduled HF visits: UF, 21% pts vs Diuretics, 44%, p = 0.009.
3CPO (2008) N = 1069	Noninvasive positive pressure ventilation (NIPPV) vs continuous positive airway pressure (CPAP) vs oxygen therapy (O_2)	Clinical diagnosis of Cardiogenic pulmonary edema CXR with pulmonary edema Respiratory rate >20 bpm Arterial pH <7.35	All-cause mortality, 7 days (1°): NIPPV + CPAP 9.5% vs O_2 9.8% (OR 0.97, 95% CI 0.63–1.48; p = 0.87) Composite death or intubation, 7 days (1°): NIPPV + CPAP, 11.1% vs O_2 11.7% (OR 0.94, 95% CI 0.59–1.51; p = 0.81) NIPPV + CPAP better than O_2: Change in arterial pH, 1 hr (p < 0.001); Dyspnea score, 1 hr (p = 0.008)
PROTECT (2010) N = 2033	Rolofylline 30 mg vs. placebo for up to 3 days	Randomized within 24 hr, Persistent dyspnea at rest or with minimal activity, estimated CrCl 20–80 mL/min, BNP ≥500 pg/mL or NT-proBNP ≥2000 pg/mL, IV loop diuretic therapy	Clinical composite (1°): OR for rolofylline 0.92, 95% CI 0.78–1.09, p = 0.35
DOSE (2011) N = 308	Low vs. high dose furosemide Continuous vs intermittent intravenous bolus 1:1:1:1 2×2 factorial design	Randomized within 24 hr, ≥1 sign and ≥1 symptom of HF, history of chronic HF treated with furosemide 80–240 mg/day (or equivalent) for at least 1 month	Global assessment of symptoms (1°): 4236 ± 1440 AUC bolus vs. 4373 ± 1404 AUC cont inf, P = 0.47; 4171 ± 1436 AUC low dose vs 4430 ± 1401 AUC high dose, P = 0.06 Mean change in SCr (1°): 0.05 mg/dL bolus vs. 0.07 mg/dL continuous, P = 0.45; 0.04 mg/dL low dose vs. 0.08 mg/dL high dose, P = 0.21.
ASCEND-HF (2011) N = 7141	Nesiritide (Nes) 0.01 µg/kg/min with optional 2 µg/kg bolus (from 24 hr up to 7 days) vs. Placebo (Pla)	Hospitalized for ADHF, dyspnea at rest or with minimal activity, ≥1 sign and ≥1 objective measure of ADHF, randomized within 24 hr of first IV treatment for ADHF	Self-reported dyspnea moderately or markedly better At 6 hr: 42.1% Pla vs 44.5% Nes, P = 0.03* At 24 hr: 66.1% Pla vs 68.2% Nes, P = 0.007* (*did not meet prespecified US regulatory requirement of significance) Death or rehospitalization for HF at 30 days: 10.1% Pla vs 9.4% Nes (HR 0.93, 95% CI 0.8–1.08, P = 0.31)

Continued

TABLE 49.8 Selected Clinical Trials for Acute Heart Failure—cont'd

TRIAL	TREATMENT ARMS	POPULATION	RESULTS
CARRESS-HF (2012) $N = 188$	Ultrafiltration (UF) vs stepped pharmacologic care (Pharm)	Develop cardiorenal syndrome before (within 6 weeks) or after (within 7 days from admission) hospitalization.	Change in creatinine level: UF, +0.23 mg/dL vs Pharm, -0.04 ± 0.53 mg/dL in the pharmacologic-therapy group vs in the ultrafiltration group, P = 0.003. Weight loss: 5.5 ± 5.1 kg [12.1 ± 11.3 lb] in the pharmacologic-therapy group vs. 5.7 ± 3.9 kg [12.6 ± 8.5 lb] in the ultrafiltration group, P = 0.58. Serious adverse events: 72% in the ultrafiltration group vs. 57% in the pharmacologic-therapy group, P = 0.03
RELAX-AHF (2013) $N = 1161$	Serelaxin (Ser) 30 µg/kg/day vs. Placebo (Pla) for 48 hr	Patients with dyspnea at rest or on minimal exertion, congestion on chest x-ray, BNP ≥350 ng/L (or NT-proBNP ≥1400 ng/L), eGFR 30–75 mL/min/1.73 m², and SBP > 125 mmHg	Change in dyspnea by VAS AUC to day 5 (1°): 19% improvement by Ser compared to placebo by VAS AUC (448 mm *h, 95% CI 120–775), p = 0.007. Proportion of patients with moderately or markedly improved dyspnea by Likert scale at all 3 early timepoints (6, 12, 24 hr; 1°): Ser 27% vs. Pla 26%, P = 0.70. Days alive out of hospital up to day 60: Ser 48.3 vs. Pla 47.7, p = 0.37. 180-day mortality: Pla 65 deaths vs. Ser 42, HR 0.63 (95% CI 0.43–0.93), P = 0.02
REVIVE-2 (2013) $N = 600$	Levosimendan (Levo; loading 12 µg/kg, followed by 0.1–0.2 µg/kg/min; for 24 h) vs Placebo	Dyspneic at rest. LVEF ≤35%	Clinical composite endpoint, 5 d (1°): Levo superior, p = 0.015. More frequent hypotension and cardiac arrhythmias, during the infusion period; numerically higher risk of death, 90 d (REVIVE 1&2: Levo, 49 deaths/350 pts; vs Placebo, 40/ 350, P = 0.29)
ROSE (2013) $N = 360$	Dopamine (2 µg/kg/min; n = 122). Nesiritide (0.005 µg/kg/min without bolus; n = 119). Pooled placebo group (n = 119)	Acute heart failure. Renal dysfunction (eGFR 15–60 mL/min/1.73 m²). Randomized within 24 hr of admission	Compared to placebo: Dopamine: No significant effect on 72-hr cumulative urine volume or on the change in cystatin C level; Increased tachycardia. Nesiritide: No significant effect on 72-hr cumulative urine volume or on the change in cystatin C level
DAD-HF II (2014) $N = 161$	8-hr continuous infusions of: (a) high-dose furosemide (HDF, n = 50, 20 mg/hr), (b) low-dose furosemide and low-dose dopamine (LDFD, n = 56, 5 mg/hr and 5 µg kg⁻¹ min⁻¹, respectively), or (c) low-dose furosemide (LDF, n = 55, furosemide 5 mg/hr).	Dyspnea on minimal exertion or rest dyspnea. Oxygen saturation <90% on admission arterial blood gas. One or more of the following: (a) signs of congestion, (b) interstitial congestion or pleural effusion on chest x-ray, and (c) elevated serum B-type natriuretic peptide levels	No significant differences in 60-day and one-year all-cause mortality and hospitalization for HF, dyspnea relief (Borg index), worsening renal function, and length of stay
AVOID-HF (2016) $N = 224$ (810 planned)	Adjustable ultrafiltration (AUF; N = 110). Adjustable intravenous loop diuretics (ALD; N = 114).	Chronic daily oral loop diuretics. Fluid overload. Received ≤2 iv loop diuretic doses. Randomized within 24 hr of admission to hospital	Estimated days to first HF event for the AUF (62) and ALD (34) group (p = 0.106). At 30 days, compared with the ALD group, the AUF group had fewer HF and cardiovascular events. Renal function changes were similar. More AUF patients with adverse events.
ATOMIC-AHF (2016) $N = 606$	3 sequential cohorts (approximately 200 patients per cohort): Cohort 1: Omecamtiv mecarbil (OM, target plasma concentration 115 ng/mL) vs. Placebo. Cohort 2: OM (target plasma concentration, 230 ng/mL) vs. Placebo. Cohort 3: OM (target plasma concentration 310 ng/mL) vs Placebo	LVEF ≤40%. Dyspnea at rest or with minimal exertion. Elevated natriuretic peptides. Randomized within 24 hr of initial IV diuretic.	Dyspnea relief: No significant difference compared to placebo (3 OM dose groups and pooled placebo: placebo, 41%; OM cohort 1, 42%; cohort 2, 47%; cohort 3, 51%; p 0.33); Increased dyspnea relief in Cohort 3 at 48 hr (placebo, 37% vs.OM, 51%; p = 0.034) and through 5 days (p 0.038). Plasma concentration-related increases in LV systolic ejection time (p < 0.0001) and decreases in end-systolic dimension (p < 0.05).

TABLE 49.8 Selected Clinical Trials for Acute Heart Failure—cont'd

TRIAL	TREATMENT ARMS	POPULATION	RESULTS
ATHENA-HF (2017) $N = 360$	(a) Placebo or 25 mg spironolactone (b) High-dose spironolactone (100 mg) daily for 96 hr	AHF with at least one sign and one symptom of HF NT-proBNP ≥1000 pg/mL or BNP ≥250 pg/mL within 24 hr Potassium ≤5.0 mEq/liter eGFR ≥30 mL/min/1.73m² SBP >90 mm Hg	1° endpoint, Change in NT-proBNP at 96 hr: NS (p = 0.57) All 2° endpoints and day 30 all-cause mortality or heart failure hospitalization: NS
BLAST-AHF (2017) $N = 621$	(a) Placebo (N = 183) (b) TRV027 1 mg/hr (N = 128) (c) TRV027 5 mg/hr (N = 182) (d) TRV027 25 mg/hr (N = 125)	History of heart failure (HF) Elevated natriuretic peptides ≥2 physical HF signs SBP ≥120 mm Hg and ≤200 mm Hg eGFR (sMDRD) 20–75 mL/min/1.73m² Excluded if use of ARBs 7 days prior, IV inotropes or vasopressors within 2 hr prior, or IV nitrates within 1 hr prior to randomization	1° endpoint (comprised of multiple outcomes, analyzed as a composite z-score), including (1) time from baseline to death through day 30, (2) time from baseline to heart failure rehospitalization through day 30, (3) the first assessment timepoint following worsening heart failure through day 5, (4) change in dyspnea visual analog scale (VAS) score calculated as the area under the curve (AUC) representing the change from baseline over time from baseline through day 5, and (5) length of initial hospital stay (in days) from baseline: No difference in any group.
TACTICS (2017) $N = 257$	(a) Placebo (N = 128) (b) Tolvaptan (N = 129)	AHF within 24 hr of presentation Elevated natriuretic peptides + 1 additional sign or symptom of congestion Serum sodium ≤140 mmol/L	Dyspnea relief by Likert scale was similar between tolvaptan and placebo at 8 hr (25% moderately or markedly improved for tolvaptan vs 28% placebo, p = 0.59) and at 24 hr (50% tolvaptan vs 47% placebo, p = 0.80). The proportion defined as responders at 24 hr (primary study endpoint) was 16% for tolvaptan and 20% for placebo (p = 0.32). Tolvaptan resulted in greater weight loss and net fluid loss compared to placebo, but tolvaptan-treated patients were more likely to experience worsening renal function during treatment.
SECRET of CHF (2017) $N = 250$	(a) Placebo (N = 128) (b) Tolvaptan 30 mg/day (N = 122)	AHF within 36 hr Active dyspnea Any of the following: (1) eGFR <60 mL/min/1.73 m²; (2) hyponatremia; or (3) diuretic resistance (urine output ≤125 mL/hr following intravenous furosemide ≥40 mg)	1° endpoint, 8- and 16-hr dyspnea reduction: NS (p = 0.46; p = 0.78) 2° endpoint: significantly greater weight reduction with tolvaptan (Day 1: −2.4 ± 2.1 kg vs. −0.9 ± 1.8 kg; p < 0.001). 2° endpoint: dyspnea reduction was greater with tolvaptan at Day 3 (p = 0.01).
TRUE-AHF (2017) $N = 2157$	(a) Placebo (N = 1069) (b) Ularitide (N = 1088)	Men or women, aged 18–85 years Unplanned hospitalization or ED visit for acutely decompensated heart failure Dyspnea at rest, worsened within the past week Evidence of heart failure on chest X-ray BNP >500 pg/mL or NT-pro BNP >2000 pg/mL Persistence of dyspnea at rest despite ≥40 mg of IV furosemide (or equivalent) Systolic BP ≥116 mm Hg and ≤180 mm Hg Start of study drug infusion within 12 hr after initial clinical assessment	1° endpoints, Cardiovascular death: Ularitide 235 deaths, Placebo 225; HR = 1.03 (96% CI:0.85–1.25); p = 0.75 1° endpoints, Hierarchical clinical composite at 48 hr: p = 0.82 2° endpoints, Intensive care LOS during first 120 hr, Hospital length of stay during first 30 days, Episodes of in-hospital WHF during first 120 hr, Proportion with WHF during first 120 hr, Rehospitalization for HF within 30 days of hospital discharge, Duration (hours) of IV therapy for HF during index admission, All-cause mortality or CV hospitalization at 6 months: All NS; Change in NT-proBNP at 48 hr: 47% decrease with ularitide (p < 0.001); Change in serum creatinine during first 72 hr: Increased with ularitide (p = 0.005) Adverse events: Hypotension: Placebo, 10.1% vs. Ularitide, 22.4%. No difference in renal events.

Continued

TABLE 49.8 Selected Clinical Trials for Acute Heart Failure—cont'd

TRIAL	TREATMENT ARMS	POPULATION	RESULTS
RELAX-AHF-2 (2019) N = 6545	(a) Placebo (n = 3271) (b) Serelaxin 30 μg/kg/d (n = 3274)	Presented within 16 hr prior to randomization for AHF Dyspnea at rest or with minimal exertion, Pulmonary congestion on chest radiograph, BNP ≥500 pg/mL or NT-proBNP ≥2000 pg/mL, SBP ≥125 mm Hg, eGFR ≥25 and ≤75 mL/min/1.73 m², Received at least 40 mg furosemide (or its equivalent) at any time between presentation and the start of screening.	1° endpoint, Cardiovascular death through day 180: Serelaxin, 285 (8.7%) patients vs Placebo, 290 (8.9%); hazard ratio, 0.98; 95% CI, 0.83–1.15; P = 0.77) 1° endpoint, Worsening heart failure through Day 5: Serelaxin, 227 (6.9%) patients vs. Placebo, 252 (7.7%); hazard ratio, 0.89; 95% CI, 0.75–1.07; P = 0.19) 2° endpoints: No significant difference in All-cause death at 180 days, Length of index hospital stay, or Cardiovascular death or rehospitalization for heart failure or renal failure at 180 days.
RELAX-AHF-EU (2019) N = 2666 (3183 planned)	(a) Standard-of-Care (SoC; n = 894) (b) Serelaxin 30 μg/kg/day + SoC (n = 1756)	Presented within 16 hr prior to randomization for AHF Dyspnea, Pulmonary congestion on chest radiograph, BNP ≥500 pg/mL or NT-proBNP ≥2000 pg/mL), SBP ≥125 mm Hg, eGFR ≥25 and ≤75 mL/min/1.73m² Received at least 40 mg furosemide (or its equivalent) at any time between presentation and the start of screening.	Prospective, randomized, open-label, blinded-endpoint (PROBE) trial 1° endpoint, adjudicated Worsening heart failure/all-cause death through Day 5: significantly reduced in the serelaxin+SoC vs. SoC group (5.0% vs. 6.9%; hazard ratio 0.71; 95% confidence interval 0.51–0.98; P = 0.0172) (absolute risk reduction 1.9%, number needed to treat 53)
GALACTIC (2019) N = 788	(a) Usual care (n = 402) (b) Early intensive and sustained vasodilation therapy throughout the hospitalization (n = 386)	Hospitalized for AHF Dyspnea (NYHA III/IV) BNP ≥500 ng/L or NT-proBNP ≥2000ng/L. SBP ≥100 mm Hg Planned treatment in a general ward	Prospective, randomized, open-label blinded end-point (PROBE) trial 1° endpoint, composite of all-cause mortality or rehospitalization for AHF at 180 days: Vasodilators, 117 patients (30.6%; 55 deaths [14.4%]) vs Usual Care, 111 patients (27.8%; 61 deaths [15.3%]) (absolute difference for the primary end point, 2.8% [95% CI, −3.7%–9.3%]; adjusted hazard ratio, 1.07 [95% CI, 0.83–1.39]; P = .59)

ACEi, Angiotensin-converting enzyme (ACE) inhibitor; *AUC*, area under the curve; *HF*, heart failure; *LOS*, length of stay; *NTG*, nitroglycerin; *PAC*, premature atrial complex; *PCWP*, pulmonary capillary wedge pressure; *VAS*, visual analogue scale; *VMAC*, vasodilation in the management of acute CHF; *WHF*, worsening heart failure.

Data from VMAC Investigators. Intravenous nesiritide vs nitroglycerin for treatment of decompensated congestive heart failure: a randomized controlled trial. *JAMA.* 2002;287:1531–40. Cuffe MS, Califf RM, Adams KF, et al. Short-term intravenous milrinone for acute exacerbation of chronic heart failure: a randomized controlled trial. *JAMA.* 2002;287:1541–1547. Binanay C, Califf RM, Hasselblad V, et al. Evaluation study of congestive heart failure and pulmonary artery catheterization effectiveness: the ESCAPE trial. *JAMA.* 2005;294:1625–1633. McMurray JJ, Teerlink JR, Cotter G, et al. Effects of tezosentan on symptoms and clinical outcomes in patients with acute heart failure: the VERITAS randomized controlled trials. *JAMA.* 2007;298:2009–2019. Mebazaa A, Nieminen MS, Packer M, et al. Levosimendan vs dobutamine for patients with acute decompensated heart failure: the SURVIVE Randomized Trial. *JAMA.* 2007;297:1883–1891. Gheorghiade M, Konstam MA, Burnett JC, et al. Short-term clinical effects of tolvaptan, an oral vasopressin antagonist, in patients hospitalized for heart failure: the EVEREST Clinical Status TRIALS. *JAMA.* 2007;297:1332–1343. Konstam MA, Gheorghiade M, Burnett JC Jr, et al. Effects of oral tolvaptan in patients hospitalized for worsening heart failure: the EVEREST Outcome Trial. *JAMA.* 2007;297:1319–1331. Costanzo MR, Guglin ME, Saltzberg MT, et al. Ultrafiltration versus intravenous diuretics for patients hospitalized for acute decompensated heart failure. *J Am Coll Cardiol.* 2007;49:675–683. Gray A, Goodacre S, Newby DE, et al. Noninvasive ventilation in acute cardiogenic pulmonary edema. *N Engl J Med.* 2008;359:142–151. Giamouzis G, Butler J, Starling RC, et al. Impact of dopamine infusion on renal function in hospitalized heart failure patients: results of the Dopamine in Acute Decompensated Heart Failure (DAD-HF) Trial. *J Card Fail.* 2010;16:922–930. Massie BM, O'Connor CM, Metra M, et al. Rolofylline, an adenosine A1-receptor antagonist, in acute heart failure. *N Engl J Med.* 2010;363:1419–28. Felker GM, Lee KL, Bull DA, et al. Diuretic strategies in patients with acute decompensated heart failure. *N Engl J Med.* 2011;364:797–805. O'Connor CM, Starling RC, Hernandez AF, et al. Effect of nesiritide in patients with acute decompensated heart failure. *N Engl J Med.* 2011;365:32–43. Bart BA, Goldsmith SR, Lee KL, et al. Ultrafiltration in decompensated heart failure with cardiorenal syndrome. *N Engl J Med.* 2012;367:2296–2304. Teerlink JR, Cotter G, Davison BA, et al. Serelaxin, recombinant human relaxin-2, for treatment of acute heart failure (RELAX-AHF): a randomised, placebo-controlled trial. *Lancet.* 2013;381:29–39. Packer M, Colucci WS, Fisher L, et al. Effect of levosimendan on the short-term clinical course of patients with acutely decompensated heart failure. *JACC Heart Fail.* 2013;1:103–111. Chen HH, Anstrom KJ, Givertz MM, et al. Low-dose dopamine or low-dose nesiritide in acute heart failure with renal dysfunction: the ROSE acute heart failure randomized trial. *JAMA.* 2013;310:2533–2543. Triposkiadis FK, Butler J, Karayannis G, et al. Efficacy and safety of high dose versus low dose furosemide with or without dopamine infusion: the Dopamine in Acute Decompensated Heart Failure II (DAD-HF II) trial. *Int J Cardiol.* 2014;172:115–121. Costanzo MR, Negoianu D, Jaski BE, et al. Aquapheresis versus intravenous diuretics and hospitalizations for Heart Failure. *JACC Heart Fail.* 2016;4:95–105. Teerlink JR, Felker GM, McMurray JJ, et al. Acute treatment with omecamtiv mecarbil to increase contractility in acute heart failure: the ATOMIC-AHF Study. *J Am Coll Cardiol.* 2016;67:1444–1455. Felker GM, Mentz RJ, Cole R, et al. Efficacy and safety of tolvaptan in patients hospitalized with acute heart failure. *J Am Coll Cardiol.* 2016; (epub ahead of print).

a single drug would exert beneficial effects in all patients with AHF. There remain areas of significant unmet need in the treatment of AHF, including vasodilators with proven clinical benefits, agents that improve myocardial performance without significant adverse effects, and agents that improve or protect renal function. There are a number of interesting compounds that are undergoing development and/or clinical evaluation.

Vasodilating Agents

A variety of novel molecules with vasodilator properties are in development as therapeutics for AHF.[89]

Serelaxin

Relaxin was first identified as a major hormone of pregnancy with powerful systemic and renal vascular effects, as well as beneficial effects on cardiac preconditioning and ischemia, inflammation, fibrosis, and apoptosis. Serelaxin (recombinant human relaxin-2) demonstrated encouraging effects in a dose-finding pilot study of 234 patients with AHF.[122] The Phase III RELAX-AHF (Efficacy and Safety of Relaxin for the Treatment of Acute Heart Failure) trial enrolled 1161 patients within 16 hours of presentation who had dyspnea, congestion, mild-to-moderate renal insufficiency, and SBP greater than 125 mm Hg and randomized them to standard of care with a 48-hour infusion of either serelaxin (30 μg/kg/day) or placebo.[123] The trial demonstrated efficacy of serelaxin in improving dyspnea as quantified by the area under the curve of the change from baseline dyspnea visual analog scale over 5 days, which was associated with improvements in signs of congestion, decreased in-hospital WHF, shorter length of stay, and both cardiovascular and all-cause mortality at 180 days. There were no significant changes in the dyspnea score as assessed by the 7-level Likert scale over the first 24 hours nor any endpoint related to HF rehospitalizations. Serelaxin treatment was also associated with improved markers of end-organ damage or dysfunction, including cardiac, renal, and hepatic markers.[124] There were no serious adverse events of hypotension or other safety signals in the serelaxin-treated patients. Mechanistic studies have confirmed serelaxin's beneficial effects on hemodynamics[125] and renal function.[126] The RELAX-AHF-2 trial, enrolling over 6600 patients admitted for AHF, evaluated the effects of serelaxin compared to placebo on WHF through 5 days and 180-day cardiovascular mortality and showed no significant benefit (Fig. 49.11).[127]

Natriuretic Peptides

Multiple different natriuretic peptides continue to be developed and investigated for the treatment of AHF, including naturally occurring and alternatively spliced peptides and chimeric designer peptides. Urodilatin, a modified version of pro-ANP, is a 32-amino-acid hormone, synthesized and secreted from the distal tubules of the kidney that regulates renal sodium absorption and water homeostasis via binding to NPR1 receptors and increasing intracellular cGMP levels. *Ularitide*, a synthetically produced urodilatin, has demonstrated beneficial effects on hemodynamics and symptom relief in two studies of patients with AHF.[128] The TRUE-AHF trial (NCT01661634) enrolled 2157 patients with symptomatic AHF and randomized them to a 48-hour infusion of either ularitide (15 ng/kg/min) or placebo. Ularitide did not significantly improve either primary endpoint of the clinical composite endpoint through 5 days or cardiovascular mortality during the course of the study. Ularitide had no beneficial effect on any secondary endpoint without evidence of end-organ protection and increased creatinine associated with a doubling of hypotension (see Fig. 49.11).[129]

NEUROHORMONAL ANTAGONISTS

Direct renin inhibitors (DRIs) block the first enzymatic step in the RAAS cascade, leading to a profound suppression of this neurohormonal system (see Chapters 47 and 50). Given the role of RAAS in the pathogenesis and complications of HF, as well as the improved survival associated with its inhibition, further blockade of this system may confer additional survival benefits. *Aliskiren* is the first oral DRI on the market and currently approved for the treatment of hypertension. The ASTRONAUT trial enrolled 1639 hemodynamically stable patients a median 5 days after admission for AHF with EF less than 40%, elevated natriuretic peptides, and signs or symptoms of fluid overload who were randomized to daily oral aliskiren or placebo.[130] Aliskiren treatment was associated with higher rates of hyperkalemia, hypotension, and renal impairment/renal failure compared to placebo after a median follow-up of 11.3 months, but there was no difference in cardiovascular death or heart failure rehospitalization at 6 or 12 months. *Endothelin receptor antagonists* block the actions of ET-1, the most powerful endogenous vasoconstrictor that is produced by the vascular endothelial cells. It exerts its effects by binding to two receptors, ET_A and ET_B, located on the vascular smooth muscle cells, resulting in significant systemic arterial vasoconstriction. *Tezosentan*, a nonselective ET_{A-B} antagonist, has been shown to improve hemodynamics in patients with AHF. The Value of Endothelin Receptor Inhibition with Tezosentan in Acute Heart Failure Study (VERITAS) studied more than 1400 patients admitted with AHF in a large, international trial. The addition of IV tezosentan to standard therapy did not improve symptoms nor decrease WHF or mortality at 7 days after randomization.[131] Another approach to neurohormonal antagonism in AHF included the *angiotensin II type I receptor beta-arrestin-biased ligand, TRV027*, which increases signaling of the beta-arrestin mediated pathways stimulating inotropy while simultaneously antagonizing the classic G-protein angiotensin II signaling pathways. The BLAST-AHF study enrolled 621 patients admitted with AHF in a dose-ranging study of a 48 to 96 hour infusion of TRV027 compared to placebo.[132] TRV027 did not confer any benefit over placebo at any dose with regards to the primary composite endpoint or any of the individual components, although there were no significant safety issues.

SOLUBLE GUANYLATE CYCLASE ACTIVATORS AND STIMULATORS

Cinaciguat is the first compound in a new class of vasodilators. Their mechanism of action is similar to that of organic nitrates (and their end product NO) because both classes of drugs activate the sGC in smooth muscle cells, thus leading to the synthesis of cGMP and subsequent

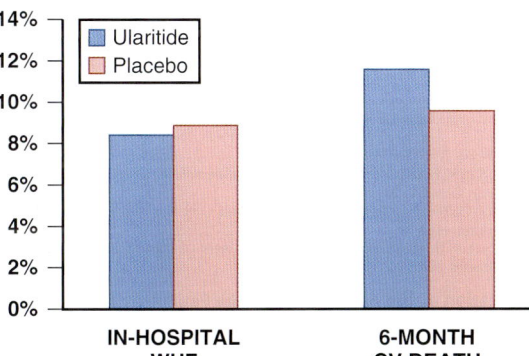
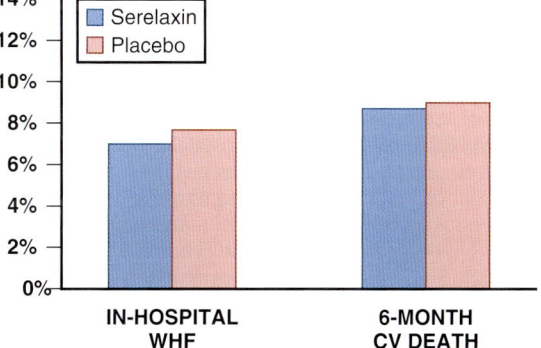

FIGURE 49.11 Overview of study population and primary results from TRUE-HF (ularitide) and RELAX-AHF-2 (serelaxin) randomized clinical trials. (Adapted from Metra M, Teerlink JR, Cotter G, et al. Effects of serelaxin in patients with acute heart failure. *N Engl J Med.* 2019;381:716–726; Packer M, O'Connor C, McMurray JJV, et al. Effect of ularitide on cardiovascular mortality in acute heart failure. *N Engl J Med.* 2017;376:1956–1964.)

vasodilation. Cinaciguat has been shown to improve hemodynamics in patients with AHF; however, at high doses, it has been associated with significant hypotension, which resulted in the termination of early clinical studies.[133] *Vericiguat* is an oral sGC stimulator that has been studied in patients enrolled in studies within 4 weeks of a WHF event. In the SOCRATES-Reduced study of 456 patients, vericiguat did not significantly improve log transformed NT-proBNP concentrations compared to placebo, but there was a suggestion of a dose response.[134]

INOTROPIC AGENTS
Cardiac Myosin Activators

Cardiac myosin activators represent a new mechanistic class of agents designed to increase myocardial contractility. These agents increase the transition rate from the weakly bound to the strongly bound state necessary for initiation of a force-generating power stroke. Unlike current inotropes, they increase the systolic ejection time without altering the rate of LV pressure development, resulting in increased stroke volume and cardiac output without increases in intracellular cAMP or calcium. *Omecamtiv mecarbil* is the first agent of this class to undergo testing in man. In both healthy volunteers and patients with chronic stable HFrEF, administration of omecamtiv mecarbil produced dose-dependent increases in systolic ejection time, fractional shortening, stroke volume, and ejection fraction and was well-tolerated over a broad range of plasma concentrations.[135] In a phase IIb dose-finding study of 606 patients with AHF (ATOMIC-AHF; NCT01300013), intravenous omecamtiv mecarbil did not meet the primary endpoint of dyspnea improvement compared to the pooled placebo, but it was generally well-tolerated, increased systolic ejection time, and improved dyspnea in the high-dose group.[136]

Istaroxime

Istaroxime, the prototype of a new class of drugs, exerts its actions on the myocyte in two ways: (1) via stimulation of the membrane-bound Na-K/ATPase, and (2) by enhancing the activity of the sarcoendoplasmic reticulum Ca/ATPase type 2a (SERCA-2a). These distinct mechanisms, respectively, result in increased cytosolic calcium accumulation during systole, with positive inotropic effects, and in rapid sequestration of cytosolic calcium into the sarcoplasmic reticulum during diastole, leading to an enhanced lusitropic effect. The HORIZON-HF study evaluated 120 patients admitted with AHF and decreased EF. The addition of istaroxime to standard therapy lowered PCWP and HR and increased SBP. The higher infusion dose increased cardiac index and reduced LVED volume. There were no changes in neurohormones, renal function, or troponin I levels during the short 6-hour infusion.[137,138]

RENOPROTECTIVE AGENTS

Therapeutics to prevent or treat acute kidney injury and maintain or improve renal function in the setting of AHF are an important unmet need. *Adenosine A$_1$ receptor antagonists* have been developed to increase renal blood flow and enhance diuresis without activating the tubuloglomerular feedback. *Rolofylline* is a highly selective adenosine A$_1$ receptor antagonist that has been studied in patients with HF. Despite the positive trends seen in the PROTECT-Pilot study, the Phase III PROTECT trial failed to show any clinical benefit, including renal protection,[139] and was associated with more seizure and stroke events when compared to placebo. Given these results, it is doubtful that these agents will undergo further evaluation in AHF.

FUTURE PERSPECTIVES

AHF remains one of the most challenging cardiovascular problems with unacceptably high post-discharge rehospitalization and mortality rates. The development of new therapies has been a persistent challenge over recent decades and most patients are still treated primarily with intravenous loop diuretics. Current management consists primarily of treating the manifestations of the syndrome rather than central pathophysiologic derangements. Improvement in understanding of underlying pathophysiology and better targeting of treatments to specific patient groups most likely to benefit will potentially provide greater success in developing efficacious new therapies for AHF. Given the heterogeneity of the AHF population, it is unlikely that a "one-therapy-fits-all" approach will lead to an improvement in outcomes.

At the same time that new therapies are sought, continued efforts to improve and standardize the use of "best practices" in terms of process of care, transitions of care, and post-discharge follow-up will potentially allow us to better use currently available therapies to improve outcomes from this highly morbid condition.

REFERENCES
Epidemiology

1. Jackson SL, Tong X, King RJ, et al. National burden of heart failure events in the United States, 2006 to 2014. *Circ Heart Fail.* 2018;11:e004873.
2. Ponikowski P, Anker SD, AlHabib KF, et al. Heart failure: preventing disease and death worldwide. *ESC Heart Failure.* 2014;1:4–25.
3. Heidenreich PA, Albert NM, Allen LA, et al. Forecasting the impact of heart failure in the United States: a policy statement from the American Heart Association. *Circ Heart Fail.* 2013;6:606–619.
4. Voigt J, John MS, Taylor A, et al. A reevaluation of the costs of heart failure and its implications for allocation of health resources in the United States. *Clin Cardiol.* 2014;37:312–321.
5. Butler J, Gheorghiade M, Kelkar A, et al. In-hospital worsening heart failure. *Eur J Heart Failure.* 2015;17:1104–1113.
6. Okumura N, Jhund PS, Gong J, et al. Importance of clinical worsening of heart failure treated in the outpatient setting: evidence from the Prospective Comparison of ARNI with ACEI to Determine Impact on Global Mortality and Morbidity in Heart Failure trial (PARADIGM-HF). *Circulation.* 2016;133:2254–2262.
7. Filippatos G, Angermann CE, Cleland JGF, et al. Global differences in characteristics, precipitants, and initial management of patients presenting with acute heart failure. *JAMA Cardiol.* 2020;5:401–410.
8. Kapoor JR, Kapoor R, Ju C, et al. Precipitating clinical factors, heart failure characterization, and outcomes in patients hospitalized with heart failure with reduced, borderline, and preserved ejection fraction. *JACC (J Am Coll Cardiol): Heart Fail.* 2016;4:464–472.
9. Galvao M, Kalman J, Demarco T, et al. Gender differences in in-hospital management and outcomes in patients with decompensated heart failure: analysis from the acute decompensated heart failure national registry (ADHERE). *J Card Fail.* 2006;12:100–107.
10. Yancy CW, Abraham WT, Albert NM, et al. Quality of care of and outcomes for African Americans Hospitalized with heart failure: findings from the OPTIMIZE-HF (Organized Program to Initiate Lifesaving Treatment in Hospitalized Patients with Heart Failure) registry. *J Am Coll Cardiol.* 2008;51:1675–1684.
11. Adams Jr KF, Fonarow GC, Emerman CL, et al. Characteristics and outcomes of patients hospitalized for heart failure in the united States: rationale, design, and preliminary observations from the first 100,000 cases in the Acute Decompensated Heart Failure National Registry (ADHERE). *Am Heart J.* 2005;149:209–216.
12. Nieminen MS, Brutsaert D, Dickstein K, et al. EuroHeart Failure Survey II (EHFS II): a survey on hospitalized acute heart failure patients: description of population. *Eur Heart J.* 2006;27:2725–2736.
13. Metra M, Mentz RJ, Hernandez AF, et al. Geographic differences in patients in a global acute heart failure clinical trial (from the ASCEND-HF trial). *Am J Cardiol.* 2016;117:1771–1778.

Pathophysiology

14. Zile MR, Bennett TD, S. John Sutton M, et al. Transition from chronic compensated to acute decompensated heart failure: pathophysiological insights obtained from continuous monitoring of intracardiac pressures. *Circulation.* 2008;118:1433–1441.
15. Dries DL, Ky B, Wu AHB, et al. Simultaneous assessment of unprocessed ProBNP1-108 in addition to processed BNP32 improves identification of high-risk ambulatory patients with heart failure. *Circ Heart Fail.* 2010;3:220–227.
16. Solomon SD, Dobson J, Pocock S, et al. Influence of nonfatal hospitalization for heart failure on subsequent mortality in patients with chronic heart failure. *Circulation.* 2007;116:1482–1487.
17. Stevenson LW, Zile M, Bennett TD, et al. Chronic ambulatory intracardiac pressures and future heart failure events. *Circ Heart Fail.* 2010;3:580–587.
18. Gheorghiade M, Follath F, Ponikowski P, et al. Assessing and grading congestion in acute heart failure: a scientific statement from the acute heart failure committee of the heart failure association of the European Society of Cardiology and Endorsed by the European Society of Intensive Care Medicine. *Eur J Heart Fail.* 2010;12:423–433.
19. Januzzi JL, Filippatos G, Nieminen M, Gheorghiade M. Troponin elevation in patients with heart failure: on behalf of the third universal definition of myocardial infarction global Task force: heart failure section. *Eur Heart J.* 2012;33:2265–2271.
20. Kociol RD, Pang PS, Gheorghiade M, et al. Troponin elevation in heart failure prevalence, mechanisms, and clinical implications. *J Am Coll Cardiol.* 2010;56:1071–1078.
21. Felker GM, Mentz RJ, Teerlink JR, et al. Serial high sensitivity cardiac troponin T measurement in acute heart failure: insights from the RELAX-AHF study. *Eur J Heart Fail.* 2015;17:1262–1270.
22. Heywood JT, Fonarow GC, Costanzo MR, et al. High prevalence of renal dysfunction and its impact on outcome in 118,465 patients hospitalized with acute decompensated heart failure: a report from the ADHERE database. *J Cardiac Fail.* 2007;13:422–430.
23. Damman K, Testani JM. The kidney in heart failure: an update. *Eur Heart J.* 2015;36:1437–1444.
24. Ronco C, Cicoira M, McCullough PA. Cardiorenal syndrome type 1: pathophysiological crosstalk leading to combined heart and kidney dysfunction in the setting of acutely decompensated heart failure. *J Am Coll Cardiol.* 2012;60:1031–1042.
25. Mullens W, Abrahams Z, Francis GS, et al. Importance of venous congestion for worsening of renal function in advanced decompensated heart failure. *J Am Coll Cardiol.* 2009;53:589–596.
26. Metra M, Davison B, Bettari L, et al. Is worsening renal function an ominous prognostic sign in patients with acute heart failure? The role of congestion and its interaction with renal function. *Circ Heart Fail.* 2012;5:54–62.
27. Marti CN, Gheorghiade M, Kalogeropoulos AP, et al. Endothelial dysfunction, arterial stiffness, and heart failure. *J Am Coll Cardiol.* 2012;60:1455–1469.
28. Fallick C, Sobotka PA, Dunlap ME. Sympathetically mediated changes in capacitance. *Circ Heart Fail.* 2011;4:669–675.
29. Fudim M, Boortz-Marx RL, Ganesh A, et al. *Splanchnic Nerve Block for Chronic Heart Failure.* JACC Heart *failure*; 2020.
30. Milo-Cotter O, Cotter-Davison B, Lombardi C, et al. Neurohormonal activation in acute heart failure: results from VERITAS. *Cardiology.* 2011;119:96–105.
31. Bozkurt B, Mann DL, Deswal A. Biomarkers of inflammation in heart failure. *Heart Failure Reviews.* 2010;15:331–341.

Evaluation of the Acute Heart Failure Patient

32. Ponikowski P, Voors AA, Anker SD, et al. ESC Guidelines for the diagnosis and treatment of acute and chronic heart failure: the task force for the diagnosis and treatment of acute and chronic heart failure of the European Society of Cardiology (ESC) developed with the special contribution of the Heart Failure Association (HFA) of the ESC. *Eur Heart J.* 2016;37:2129–2200.
33. Greene SJ, Mentz RJ, Felker GM. Outpatient worsening heart failure as a target for therapy: a review. *JAMA Cardiol.* 2018;3:252–259.

34. Fonarow GC, Abraham WT, Albert NM, et al. Factors identified as precipitating hospital admissions for heart failure and clinical outcomes: findings from OPTIMIZE-HF. *Arch Intern Med.* 2008;168:847–854.
35. Pang PS, Cleland JG, Teerlink JR, et al. A proposal to standardize dyspnoea measurement in clinical trials of acute heart failure syndromes: the need for a uniform approach. *Eur Heart J.* 2008;29:816–824.
36. Thibodeau JT, Turer AT, Gualano SK, et al. Characterization of a novel symptom of advanced heart failure: bendopnea. *JACC Heart Fail.* 2014;2:24–31.
37. Nohria A, Tsang SW, Fang JC, et al. Clinical assessment identifies hemodynamic profiles that predict outcomes in patients admitted with heart failure. *J Am Coll Cardiol.* 2003;41:1797–1804.
38. Maisel AS, Krishnaswamy P, Nowak RM, et al. Rapid measurement of B-Type natriuretic peptide in the emergency diagnosis of heart failure. *N Engl J Med.* 2002;347:161–167.
39. Thygesen K, Alpert JS, Jaffe AS, et al. Fourth universal definition of myocardial infarction (2018). *J Am Coll Cardiol.* 2018;72:2231–2264.

Management of the Patient with Acute Heart Failure

40. Chow SL, Maisel AS, Anand I, et al. Role of biomarkers for the prevention, assessment, and management of heart failure: a scientific statement from the American Heart Association. *Circulation.* 2017;135:e1054–e1091.
41. Park JH, Balmain S, Berry C, et al. Potentially detrimental cardiovascular effects of oxygen in patients with chronic left ventricular systolic dysfunction. *Heart.* 2010;96:533–538.
42. Sepehrvand N, Ezekowitz JA. Oxygen therapy in patients with acute heart failure: friend or foe? *JACC Heart Fail.* 2016;4:783–790.
43. Vital FM, Saconato H, Ladeira MT, et al. Non-invasive positive pressure ventilation (CPAP or bilevel NPPV) for cardiogenic pulmonary edema. *Cochrane Database Syst Rev.* 2008:CD005351.
44. Gray A, Goodacre S, Newby DE, et al. Noninvasive ventilation in acute cardiogenic pulmonary edema. *N Engl J Med.* 2008;359:142–151.
45. ADHERE Scientific Advisory Committee. *Acute Decompensated Heart Failure National Registry (ADHERE®) Core Module Q1 2006 Final Cumulative National Benchmark Report.* Scios, Inc.; 2006.
46. Ellison DH, Felker GM. Diuretic treatment in heart failure. *N Engl J Med.* 2018;378:684–685.
47. Cotter G, Metzkor E, Kaluski E, et al. Randomised trial of high-dose isosorbide dinitrate plus low-dose furosemide versus high-dose furosemide plus low-dose isosorbide dinitrate in severe pulmonary oedema. *Lancet.* 1998;351:389–393.
48. Weintraub NL, Collins SP, Pang PS, et al. Acute heart failure syndromes: emergency department presentation, treatment, and disposition: current approaches and future aims: a scientific statement from the American Heart Association. *Circulation.* 2010;122:1975–1996.
49. Collins SP, Pang PS, Fonarow GC, et al. Is hospital admission for heart failure really necessary?: the role of the emergency department and observation unit in preventing hospitalization and rehospitalization. *J Am Coll Cardiol.* 2013;61:121–126.
50. Yancy CW, Jessup M, Bozkurt B, et al. 2013 ACCF/AHA guideline for the management of heart failure: a report of the American College of Cardiology Foundation/American Heart Association Task force on practice guidelines. *J Am Coll Cardiol.* 2013;62:e147–e239.
51. Green EM, Givertz MM. Management of acute right ventricular failure in the intensive care unit. *Curr Heart Fail Rep.* 2012;9:228–235.
52. Aliti G, Rabelo ER, Clausell N, et al. Aggressive fluid and sodium restriction in acute decompensated heart failure: a randomized clinical trial. *JAMA Intern Med.* 2013;173:1058–1064.
53. Prins KW, Neill JM, Tyler JO, et al. Effects of beta-blocker withdrawal in acute decompensated heart failure: a systematic review and meta-analysis. *JACC Heart Fail.* 2015;3:647–653.
54. Velazquez EJ, Morrow DA, DeVore AD, et al. Angiotensin-neprilysin inhibition in acute decompensated heart failure. *N Engl J Med.* 2019;380:539–548.
55. Testani JM, Chen J, McCauley BD, et al. Potential effects of aggressive decongestion during the treatment of decompensated heart failure on renal function and survival. *Circulation.* 2010;122:265–272.
56. Dupont M, Mullens W, Finucan M, et al. Determinants of dynamic changes in serum creatinine in acute decompensated heart failure: the importance of blood pressure reduction during treatment. *Eur J Heart Fail.* 2013;15:433–440.
57. Testani JM, Brisco MA, Turner JM, et al. Loop diuretic efficiency: a metric of diuretic responsiveness with prognostic importance in acute decompensated heart failure. *Circ Heart Fail.* 2014;7:261–270.
58. Felker GM, Ellison DH, Mullens W, et al. Diuretic therapy for patients with heart failure. JACC state-of-the-art review. *J Am Coll Cardiol.* 2020;75:1178–1195.
59. Bart BA, Goldsmith SR, Lee KL, et al. Ultrafiltration in decompensated heart failure with cardiorenal syndrome. *N Engl J Med.* 2012;367:2296–2304.
60. Davison BA, Metra M, Cotter G, et al. Worsening heart failure following admission for acute heart failure: a pooled analysis of the protect and RELAX-AHF studies. *JACC Heart Fail.* 2015;3:395–403.
61. Fonarow GC, Abraham WT, Albert NM, et al. Association between performance measures and clinical outcomes for patients hospitalized with heart failure. *J Am Med Assoc.* 2007;297:61–70.
62. Ambrosy AP, Pang PS, Khan S, et al. Clinical course and predictive value of congestion during hospitalization in patients admitted for worsening signs and symptoms of heart failure with reduced ejection fraction: findings from the EVEREST trial. *Eur Heart J.* 2013;34:835–843.
63. Kociol RD, Horton JR, Fonarow GC, et al. Admission, discharge, or change in B-type natriuretic peptide and long-term outcomes: data from Organized Program to Initiate Lifesaving Treatment in Hospitalized Patients with Heart Failure (OPTIMIZE-HF) linked to Medicare claims. *Circ Heart Fail.* 2011;4:628–636.
64. Yancy CW, Jessup M, Bozkurt B, et al. 2013 ACCF/AHA guideline for the management of heart failure: a report of the American College of Cardiology foundation/American heart association Task force on practice guidelines. *J Am Coll Cardiol.* 2013;62:e147–e239.
65. Gheorghiade M, Vaduganathan M, Fonarow GC, et al. Rehospitalization for heart failure: problems and perspectives. *J Am Coll Cardiol.* 2013;61:391–403.
66. van Walraven C, Bennett C, Jennings A, et al. Proportion of hospital readmissions deemed avoidable: a systematic review. *CMAJ (Can Med Assoc J).* 2011;183:E391–E402.
67. Hansen LO, Young RS, Hinami K, et al. Interventions to reduce 30-day rehospitalization: a systematic review. *Ann Intern Med.* 2011;155:520–528.
68. Hernandez AF, Greiner MA, Fonarow GC, et al. Relationship between early physician follow-up and 30-day readmission among Medicare beneficiaries hospitalized for heart failure. *J Am Med Assoc.* 2010;303:1716–1722.
69. Alexander P, Alkhawam L, Curry J, et al. Lack of evidence for intravenous vasodilators in ED patients with acute heart failure: a systematic review. *Am J Emerg Med.* 2015;33:133–141.
70. Mebazaa A, Parissis J, Porcher R, et al. Short-term survival by treatment among patients hospitalized with acute heart failure: the global ALARM-HF registry using propensity scoring methods. *Intensive Care Med.* 2011;37:290–301.
71. Bikdeli B, Strait KM, Dharmarajan K, et al. Intravenous fluids in acute decompensated heart failure. *JACC Heart Fail.* 2015;3:127–133.
72. Blair JE, Khan S, Konstam MA, et al. Weight changes after hospitalization for worsening heart failure and subsequent re-hospitalization and mortality in the EVEREST trial. *Eur Heart J.* 2009;30:1666–1673.
73. Binanay C, Califf RM, Hasselblad V, et al. Evaluation study of congestive heart failure and pulmonary artery catheterization effectiveness: the ESCAPE trial. *J Am Med Assoc.* 2005;294:1625–1633.
74. Collins S, Storrow AB, Albert NM, et al. Early management of patients with acute heart failure: state of the art and future directions. A consensus document from the Society for Academic Emergency Medicine/Heart Failure Society of America Acute Heart Failure working group. *J Cardiac Fail.* 2015;21:27–43.
75. Miro O, Levy PD, Mockel M, et al. Disposition of emergency department patients diagnosed with acute heart failure: an international emergency medicine perspective. *Eur J Emerg Med.* 2017;24:2–12.
76. Bueno H, Ross JS, Wang Y, et al. Trends in length of stay and short-term outcomes among Medicare patients hospitalized for heart failure, 1993-2006. *J Am Med Assoc.* 2010;303:2141–2147.
77. Heidenreich PA, Sahay A, Kapoor JR, et al. Divergent trends in survival and readmission following a hospitalization for heart failure in the Veterans Affairs health care system 2002 to 2006. *J Am Coll Cardiol.* 2010;56:362–368.
78. O'Connor CM, Miller AB, Blair JE, et al. Causes of death and rehospitalization in patients hospitalized with worsening heart failure and reduced left ventricular ejection fraction: results from Efficacy of Vasopressin Antagonism in Heart Failure Outcome Study with Tolvaptan (EVEREST) program. *Am Heart J.* 2010;159:841–849.e1.
79. Allen LA, Tomic KES, Smith DM, et al. Rates and predictors of 30-day readmission among commercially insured and medicaid-enrolled patients hospitalized with systolic heart failure/clinical perspective. *Circ Heart Fail.* 2012;5:672–679.
80. Jencks SF, Williams MV, Coleman EA. Rehospitalizations among patients in the medicare fee-for-service program. *N Engl J Med.* 2009;360:1418–1428.
81. Bradley EH, Curry L, Horwitz LI, et al. Contemporary evidence about hospital strategies for reducing 30-day readmissions: a national study. *J Am Coll Cardiol.* 2012;60:607–614.
82. Bergethon KE, Ju C, DeVore AD, et al. Trends in 30-day readmission rates for patients hospitalized with heart failure: findings from the get with the guidelines-heart failure registry. *Circ Heart Fail.* 2016;9. https://doi.org/10.1161/CIRCHEARTFAILURE.115.002594.
83. Felker GM, Mentz RJ. Diuretics and ultrafiltration in acute decompensated heart failure. *J Am Coll Cardiol.* 2012;59:2145–2153.
84. de Denus S, Rouleau JL, Mann DL, et al. A pharmacogenetic investigation of intravenous furosemide in decompensated heart failure: a meta-analysis of three clinical trials. *Pharmacogenomics J.* 2017;17:192–200.
85. Mecklai A, Subacius H, Konstam MA, et al. In-hospital diuretic agent use and post-discharge clinical outcomes in patients hospitalized for worsening heart failure: insights from the EVEREST trial. *JACC Heart Fail.* 2016;4:580–588.
86. Felker GM, Lee KL, Bull DA, et al. Diuretic strategies in patients with acute decompensated heart failure. *N Engl J Med.* 2011;364:797–805.
87. Jentzer JC, DeWald TA, Hernandez AF. Combination of loop diuretics with thiazide-type diuretics in heart failure. *J Am Coll Cardiol.* 2010;56:1527–1534.
88. Bansal S, Lindenfeld J, Schrier RW. Sodium retention in heart failure and Cirrhosis. *Circ Heart Fail.* 2009;2:370–376.
89. Singh A, Laribi S, Teerlink JR, Mebazaa A. Agents with vasodilator properties in acute heart failure. *Eur Heart J.* 2017;8:317–325.
90. Ho EC, Parker JD, Austin PC, Tu JV, et al. Impact of nitrate use on survival in acute heart failure: a propensity-matched analysis. *J Am Heart Assoc.* 2016;5(2):e002531.
91. National Clinical Guideline Centre. *Acute Heart Failure: Diagnosing and Managing Acute Heart Failure in adults. NICE Clinical Guideline 187 Methods, Evidence and Recommendations.* National Institute for Health and Care Excellence; 2014.
92. Sharon A, Shpirer I, Kaluski E, et al. High-dose intravenous isosorbide-dinitrate is safer and better than Bi-PAP ventilation combined with conventional treatment for severe pulmonary edema. *J Am Coll Cardiol.* 2000;36:832–837.
93. Investigators VMAC. Intravenous nesiritide vs nitroglycerin for treatment of decompensated congestive heart failure: a randomized controlled trial. *J Am Med Assoc.* 2002;287:1531–1540.
94. Elkayam U, Akhter MW, Singh H, et al. Comparison of effects on left ventricular filling pressure of intravenous nesiritide and high-dose nitroglycerin in patients with decompensated heart failure. *Am J Cardiol.* 2004;93:237–240.
95. Mullens W, Abrahams Z, Francis GS, et al. Sodium nitroprusside for advanced low-output heart failure. *J Am Coll Cardiol.* 2008;52:200–207.
96. O'Connor CM, Starling RC, Hernandez AF, et al. Effect of nesiritide in patients with acute decompensated heart failure. *New Engl J Med.* 2011;365:32–43.
97. Chen HH, Anstrom KJ, Givertz MM, et al. Low-dose dopamine or low-dose nesiritide in acute heart failure with renal dysfunction: the ROSE acute heart failure randomized trial. *J Am Med Assoc.* 2013;310:2533–2543.
98. Hasenfuss G, Teerlink JR. Cardiac inotropes: current agents and future directions. *Eur Heart J.* 2011;32:1838–1845.
99. Felker GM, Benza RL, Chandler AB, et al. Heart failure etiology and response to milrinone in decompensated heart failure: results from the OPTIME-CHF study. *J Am Coll Cardiol.* 2003;41:997–1003.
100. Partovian C, Gleim SR, Mody PS, et al. Hospital patterns of use of positive inotropic agents in patients with heart failure. *J Am Coll Cardiol.* 2012;60:1402–1409.
101. Coletta AP, Cleland JG, Freemantle N, Clark AL. Clinical trials update from the European Society of Cardiology heart failure meeting: SHAPE, BRING-UP 2 VAS, COLA II, FOSIDIAL, BETACAR, CASINO and meta-analysis of cardiac resynchronisation therapy. *Eur J Heart Fail.* 2004;6:673–676.
102. Follath F, Cleland JG, Just H, et al. Efficacy and safety of intravenous levosimendan compared with dobutamine in severe low-output heart failure (the LIDO study): a randomised double-blind trial. *Lancet.* 2002;360:196–202.
103. Adamopoulos S, Parissis JT, Iliodromitis EK, et al. Effects of levosimendan versus dobutamine on inflammatory and apoptotic pathways in acutely decompensated chronic heart failure. *Am J Cardiol.* 2006;98:102–106.
104. Giamouzis G, Butler J, Starling RC, et al. Impact of dopamine infusion on renal function in hospitalized heart failure patients: results of the Dopamine in Acute Decompensated Heart Failure (DAD-HF) Trial. *J Cardiac Fail.* 2010;16:922–930.
105. Triposkiadis FK, Butler J, Karayannis G, et al. Efficacy and safety of high dose versus low dose furosemide with or without dopamine infusion: the Dopamine in Acute Decompensated Heart Failure II (DAD-HF II) trial. *Int J Cardiol.* 2014;172:115–121.
106. Cuffe MS, Califf RM, Adams Jr KF, et al. Short-term intravenous milrinone for acute exacerbation of chronic heart failure: a randomized controlled trial. *J Am Med Assoc.* 2002;287:1541–1547.
107. Orstavik O, Ata SH, Riise J, et al. Inhibition of phosphodiesterase-3 by levosimendan is sufficient to account for its inotropic effect in failing human heart. *Br J Pharmacol.* 2014;171:5169–5181.
108. Packer M, Colucci WS, Fisher L, et al. Effect of levosimendan on the short-term clinical course of patients with acutely decompensated heart failure. *JACC Heart Fail.* 2013;1:103–111.
109. Mebazaa A, Nieminen MS, Packer M, et al. Levosimendan vs dobutamine for patients with acute decompensated heart failure: the SURVIVE Randomized Trial. *J Am Med Assoc.* 2007;297:1883–1891.
110. De Backer D, Biston P, Devriendt J, et al. Comparison of dopamine and norepinephrine in the treatment of shock. *N Engl J Med.* 2010;362:779–789.
111. Gheorghiade M, Braunwald E. Reconsidering the role for digoxin in the management of acute heart failure syndromes. *J Am Med Assoc.* 2009;302:2146–2147.
112. Gheorghiade M, Konstam MA, Burnett Jr JC, et al. Short-term clinical effects of tolvaptan, an oral vasopressin antagonist, in patients hospitalized for heart failure: the EVEREST Clinical Status Trials. *J Am Med Assoc.* 2007;297:1332–1343.

113. Konstam MA, Gheorghiade M, Burnett Jr JC, et al. Effects of oral tolvaptan in patients hospitalized for worsening heart failure: the EVEREST Outcome Trial. *J Am Med Assoc.* 2007;297:1319–1331.
114. Felker GM, Mentz RJ, Cole R, et al. Efficacy and safety of tolvaptan in patients hospitalized with acute heart failure. *J Am Coll Cardiol.* 2016;69(11):1399–1406.
115. Goldsmith SR, Elkayam U, Haught WH, et al. Efficacy and safety of the vasopressin V1A/V2-receptor antagonist conivaptan in acute decompensated heart failure: a dose-ranging pilot study. *J Cardiac Fail.* 2008;14:641–647.
116. Peacock WF, Chandra A, Char D, et al. Clevidipine in acute heart failure: results of the a study of blood pressure control in acute heart failure-A pilot study (PRONTO). *Am Heart J.* 2014;167:529–536.
117. Costanzo MR, Guglin ME, Saltzberg MT, et al. Ultrafiltration versus intravenous diuretics for patients hospitalized for acute decompensated heart failure. *J Am Coll Cardiol.* 2007;49:675–683.
118. Patarroyo M, Wehbe E, Hanna M, et al. Cardiorenal outcomes after slow continuous ultrafiltration therapy in refractory patients with advanced decompensated heart failure. *J Am Coll Cardiol.* 2012;60:1906–1912.
119. Costanzo MR, Negoianu D, Jaski BE, et al. Aquapheresis versus intravenous diuretics and hospitalizations for heart failure. *JACC Heart failure.* 2016;4:95–105.
120. Paterna S, Fasullo S, Parrinello G, et al. Short-term effects of hypertonic saline solution in acute heart failure and long-term effects of a moderate sodium restriction in patients with compensated heart failure with New York Heart Association Class III (Class C) (SMAC-HF Study). *Am J Med Sci.* 2011;342:27–37.
121. Felker GM, Pang PS, Adams KF, et al. Clinical trials of pharmacological therapies in acute heart failure syndromes: lessons learned and directions forward. *Circ Heart Fail.* 2010;3:314–325.
122. Teerlink JR, Metra M, Felker GM, et al. Relaxin for the treatment of patients with acute heart failure (Pre-RELAX-AHF): a multicentre, randomised, placebo-controlled, parallel-group, dose-finding phase IIb study. *Lancet.* 2009;373:1429–1439.
123. Teerlink JR, Cotter G, Davison BA, et al. Serelaxin, recombinant human relaxin-2, for treatment of acute heart failure (RELAX-AHF): a randomised, placebo-controlled trial. *Lancet.* 2013;381:29–39.
124. Metra M, Cotter G, Davison BA, et al. Effect of serelaxin on cardiac, renal, and hepatic biomarkers in the Relaxin in Acute Heart Failure (RELAX-AHF) development program: correlation with outcomes. *J Am Coll Cardiol.* 2013;61:196–206.
125. Ponikowski P, Mitrovic V, Ruda M, et al. A randomized, double-blind, placebo-controlled, multicentre study to assess haemodynamic effects of serelaxin in patients with acute heart failure. *Eur Heart J.* 2014;35:431–441.
126. Voors AA, Dahlke M, Meyer S, et al. Renal hemodynamic effects of serelaxin in patients with chronic heart failure: a randomized, placebo-controlled study. *Circ Heart Fail.* 2014;7:994–1002.
127. Metra M, Teerlink JR, Cotter G, et al. Effects of serelaxin in patients with acute heart failure. *N Engl J Med.* 2019;381:716–726.
128. Anker SD, Ponikowski P, Mitrovic V, et al. Ularitide for the treatment of acute decompensated heart failure: from preclinical to clinical studies. *Eur Heart J.* 2015;36:715–723.
129. Packer M, O'Connor C, McMurray JJV, et al. Effect of ularitide on cardiovascular mortality in acute heart failure. *N Engl J Med.* 2017;376:1956–1964.
130. Gheorghiade M, Bohm M, Greene SJ, et al. Effect of aliskiren on postdischarge mortality and heart failure readmissions among patients hospitalized for heart failure: the ASTRONAUT randomized trial. *J Am Med Assoc.* 2013;309:1125–1135.
131. McMurray JJ, Teerlink JR, Cotter G, et al. Effects of tezosentan on symptoms and clinical outcomes in patients with acute heart failure: the VERITAS randomized controlled trials. *J Am Med Assoc.* 2007;298:2009–2019.
132. Felker GM, Butler J, Collins SP, et al. Heart failure therapeutics on the basis of a biased ligand of the angiotensin-2 type 1 receptor: rationale and design of the BLAST-AHF study (Biased Ligand of the Angiotensin Receptor Study in Acute Heart Failure). *JACC Heart Fail.* 2015;3:193–201.
133. Erdmann E, Semigran MJ, Nieminen MS, et al. Cinaciguat, a soluble guanylate cyclase activator, unloads the heart but also causes hypotension in acute decompensated heart failure. *Eur Heart J.* 2013;34:57–67.
134. Gheorghiade M, Greene SJ, Butler J, et al. Effect of vericiguat, a soluble guanylate cyclase stimulator, on natriuretic peptide levels in patients with worsening chronic heart failure and reduced ejection fraction: the SOCRATES-REDUCED randomized trial. *J Am Med Assoc.* 2015;314:2251–2262.
135. Liu LC, Dorhout B, van der Meer P, et al. Omecamtiv mecarbil: a new cardiac myosin activator for the treatment of heart failure. *Expert Opin Investig Drugs.* 2016;25:117–127.
136. Teerlink JR, Felker GM, McMurray JJ, et al. Acute treatment with omecamtiv mecarbil to increase contractility in acute heart failure: the ATOMIC-AHF study. *J Am Coll Cardiol.* 2016;67:1444–1455.
137. Gheorghiade M, Blair JE, Filippatos GS, et al. Hemodynamic, echocardiographic, and neurohormonal effects of istaroxime, a novel intravenous inotropic and lusitropic agent: a randomized controlled trial in patients hospitalized with heart failure. *J Am Coll Cardiol.* 2008;51:2276–2285.
138. Shah SJ, Blair JE, Filippatos GS, et al. Effects of istaroxime on diastolic stiffness in acute heart failure syndromes: results from the hemodynamic, echocardiographic, and neurohormonal effects of istaroxime, a novel intravenous inotropic and lusitropic agent: a randomized controlled trial in patients hospitalized with heart failure (HORIZON-HF) trial. *Am Heart J.* 2009;157:1035–1041.
139. Massie BM, O'Connor CM, Metra M, et al. Rolofylline, an adenosine A1-receptor antagonist, in acute heart failure. *N Engl J Med.* 2010;363:1419–1428.
140. Fonarow GC, Adams Jr KF, Abraham WT, et al. Risk stratification for in-hospital mortality in acutely decompensated heart failure: classification and regression tree analysis. *J Am Med Assoc.* 2005;293:572–580.
141. Abraham WT, Fonarow GC, Albert NM, et al. Predictors of in-hospital mortality in patients hospitalized for heart failure: insights from the Organized Program to Initiate Lifesaving Treatment in Hospitalized Patients with Heart Failure (OPTIMIZE-HF). *J Am Coll Cardiol.* 2008;52:347–356.
142. O'Connor CM, Abraham WT, Albert NM, et al. Predictors of mortality after discharge in patients hospitalized with heart failure: an analysis from the Organized Program to Initiate Lifesaving Treatment in Hospitalized Patients with Heart Failure (OPTIMIZE-HF). *Am Heart J.* 2008;156:662–673.
143. O'Connor CM, Mentz RJ, Cotter G, et al. The PROTECT in-hospital risk model: 7-day outcome in patients hospitalized with acute heart failure and renal dysfunction. *Eur J Heart Fail.* 2012;14:605–612.
144. Lee DS, Stitt A, Austin PC, et al. Prediction of heart failure mortality in emergent care: a cohort study. *Ann Intern Med.* 2012;156:767–775.W-261,W-2.
145. Felker GM, Leimberger JD, Califf RM, et al. Risk stratification after hospitalization for decompensated heart failure. *J Cardiac Fail.* 2004;10:460–466.
146. O'Connor CM, Hasselblad V, Mehta RH, et al. Triage after hospitalization with advanced heart failure: the ESCAPE (Evaluation Study of Congestive Heart Failure and Pulmonary Artery Catheterization Effectiveness) risk model and discharge score. *J Am Coll Cardiol.* 2010;55:872–878.

50 Management of Heart Failure Patients with Reduced Ejection Fraction

DOUGLAS L. MANN

ETIOLOGY, 975

PROGNOSIS, 975
Biomarkers and Prognosis, 976
Renal Insufficiency, 978

APPROACH TO THE PATIENT, 978
Patients at High Risk for Developing Heart Failure (Stage A), 978
Management of Patients With Symptomatic and Asymptomatic Heart Failure, 979
Defining the Appropriate Strategy, 979

MANAGEMENT OF FLUID RETENTION, 981
Diuretic Classes, 982
Diuretic Treatment of Heart Failure, 985
Diuretic Resistance and Management, 988
Device-Based Therapies for Management of Fluid Status, 989

PREVENTION OF DISEASE PROGRESSION, 989
Angiotensin-Converting Enzyme Inhibitors, 989
Angiotensin Receptor Blockers, 993
Angiotensin Receptor Neprilysin Inhibitors, 993
Beta-Blockers, 994

Mineralocorticoid Receptor Antagonists, 996
Renin Inhibitors, 996
Combination of Hydralazine and Isosorbide Dinitrate, 997
I_f-Channel Inhibitor, 997
Sodium-Glucose Transporter-2 Inhibitors, 997
Soluble Guanylate Cyclase Stimulators, 998
Myosin Activators, 998

MANAGEMENT OF PATIENTS WHO REMAIN SYMPTOMATIC, 998
Cardiac Glycosides, 999
N-3 Polyunsaturated Fatty Acids, 1000

PHARMACOGENOMICS/PERSONALIZED MEDICINE, 1000

MANAGEMENT OF ATHEROSCLEROTIC DISEASE, 1000

MANAGEMENT OF VALVULAR DISEASE, 1001

SPECIAL POPULATIONS, 1001
Women, 1001
Race/Ethnicity, 1001
Elderly Persons, 1001
Patients with Cancer, 1001

ANTICOAGULATION AND ANTIPLATELET THERAPY, 1001

MANAGEMENT OF CARDIAC ARRHYTHMIAS, 1002

DEVICE THERAPY, 1002
Cardiac Resynchronization, 1002
Implantable Cardioverter-Defibrillators, 1002

SLEEP-DISORDERED BREATHING, 1002

DISEASE MANAGEMENT, 1003

PATIENTS WITH REFRACTORY END-STAGE HEART FAILURE (STAGE D), 1003

INTEGRATION OF PALLIATIVE CARE INTO HEART FAILURE CARE, 1004
Primary Palliative Care, 1004
Hospice, 1004
Treatment of Symptoms Approaching End of Life, 1004

FUTURE PERSPECTIVES, 1005

REFERENCES, 1005

The epidemiology and clinical assessment of patients with heart failure (HF) is reviewed in Chapter 48, whereas the following chapter will focus on the management of patients with a reduced ejection fraction, which is referred to as *HFrEF*. The diagnosis and management of patients with acute HF is discussed in Chapter 49, and the management of patients with an HF with a preserved ejection fraction (HFpEF) is discussed in Chapter 51.

ETIOLOGY

As shown in Table 50.1, any condition that leads to an alteration in left ventricular (LV) structure or function can predispose a patient to developing HF. Although the etiology of HF in patients with HFrEF differs from that of patient with HFpEF (see Chapter 48), there is considerable overlap between the etiologies of these two conditions. In industrialized countries, coronary artery disease (CAD) is the predominant cause in etiology in men and women and is responsible for 60% to 75% of cases of HF. Hypertension contributes to the development of HF in a significant number of patients, including most patients with CAD. Both CAD and hypertension interact to augment the risk of HF. Rheumatic heart disease remains a major cause of HF in Africa and Asia, especially in the young. Hypertension is an important cause of HF in the African and African American population. Chagas disease is still a major cause of HF in South America.[1] As developing nations undergo socioeconomic development, the epidemiology of HF is becoming similar to that of Western Europe and North America, with CAD emerging as the single most common cause of HF.

In 20% to 30% of the cases of HFrEF, the exact etiologic basis is not known. These patients are referred to as having dilated or *idiopathic* cardiomyopathy if the cause is unknown (see Chapter 52). Prior viral infection (Chapter 55) or toxin exposure (e.g., alcohol [Chapter 84] or use of chemotherapeutic agents [Chapters 56 and 57]) may also lead to a dilated cardiomyopathy. Although excessive alcohol consumption can promote cardiomyopathy, alcohol consumption per se is not associated with increased risk for HF, and alcohol may protect against the development of HF when consumed in moderation.[2] It is also becoming increasingly clear that a large number of the cases of dilated cardiomyopathy are secondary to specific genetic defects, most notably those in the cytoskeleton (see Chapter 52). Most of the forms of familial dilated cardiomyopathy are inherited in an autosomal dominant fashion. Mutations of genes encoding cytoskeletal proteins (desmin, cardiac myosin, vinculin) and nuclear membrane proteins (lamin) have been identified thus far. Dilated cardiomyopathy is also associated with Duchenne, Becker, and limb girdle muscular dystrophies (see Chapter 100). Conditions that lead to a high cardiac output (e.g., arteriovenous fistula, anemia) are seldom responsible for the development of HF in a normal heart. However, in the presence of underlying structural heart disease, these conditions often lead to overt congestive failure.

PROGNOSIS

Although several recent reports have suggested that the mortality for HF patients is improving, the overall mortality rate remains higher than for many cancers, including those involving the bladder, breast, uterus, and prostate. In the Framingham Study, the median survival was 1.7 years for men and 3.2 years for women, with only 25% of men and 38% of women surviving 5 years. European studies have confirmed a similar poor long-term prognosis (Fig. 50.1).[3] More recent data from the Framingham Study have examined long-term trends in the survival of patients with HF and shown improved survival in both men and

TABLE 50.1 Risk Factors for Cardiac Failure (Olmstead County)

RISK FACTOR	ODDS RATIO (95% CI)	P VALUE	POPULATION ATTRIBUTABLE RISK (96 = 5% CI)		
			OVERALL	WOMEN	MEN
Coronary heart disease	3.05 (2.36–3.95)	<.001	0.20 (0.16–0.24)	0.16 (0.12–0.20)	0.23 (0.16–0.30)
Hypertension	1.44 (1.18–1.76)	<.001	0.20 (0.10–0.30)	0.28 (0.14–0.42)	0.13 (0.00–0.26)
Diabetes	2.65 (1.98–3.54)	<.001	0.12 (0.09–0.15)	0.10 (0.06–0.14)	0.13 (0.08–0.18)
Obesity	2.00 (1.57–2.55)	<.001	0.12 (0.08–0.16)	0.12 (0.07–0.17)	0.13 (0.07–0.19)
Ever smoker	1.37 (1.13–1.68)	.002	0.14 (0.06–0.22)	0.08 (0.00–0.15)	0.22 (0.07–0.37)

From Dunlay SM, Weston SA, Jacobsen SJ, et al. Risk factors for heart failure: a population-based case-control study. *Am J Med*. 2009;122:1023–1028.

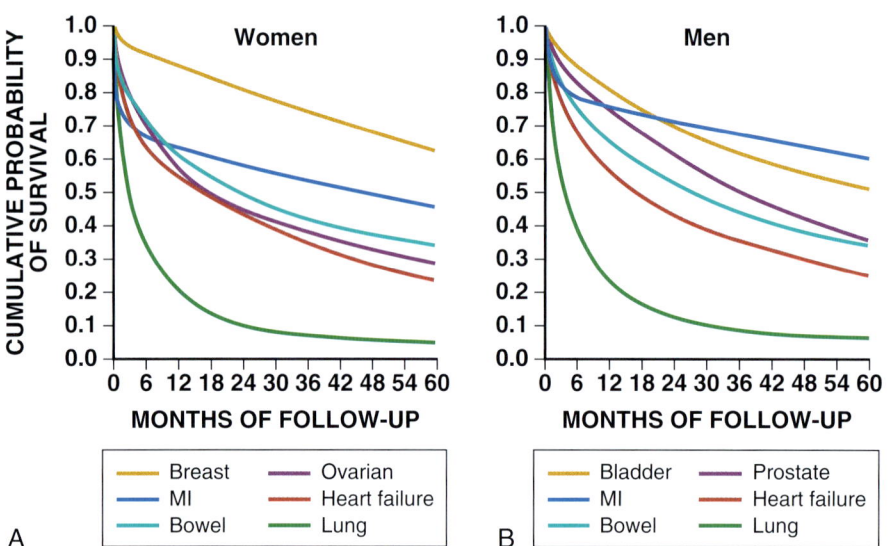

FIGURE 50.1 Survival in heart failure patients compared to cancer. Five-year survival following a first admission to any Scottish hospital in 1991 for heart failure, myocardial infarction, and the four most common sites of cancer specific to women (**A**) and men (**B**). (Modified from Stewart S, MacIntyre K, Hole DJ, et al. More "malignant" than cancer? Five-year survival following a first admission for heart failure. *Eur J Heart Fail*. 2001;3:315–322.)

women, with an overall decline in mortality of approximately 12% per decade from 1950 to 1999. Moreover, recent reports from Scotland, Sweden, and the United Kingdom also suggested that survival rates may be improving following hospital discharge.[3] Of note, the mortality of HF in epidemiologic studies is substantially higher than that reported in clinical HF trials involving drug and/or device therapies, in which the mortality figures are often deceptively low because the patients enrolled in trials are younger, are more stable clinically, and tend to be followed more closely clinically.

The role of gender and HF prognosis remains a controversial issue with respect to HF outcomes. Nonetheless, the aggregate data suggest that women with HF have a better overall prognosis than do men.[4] However, women appear to have a greater degree of functional incapacity for the same degree of LV dysfunction and also have higher prevalence of HF with a normal EF (see Chapter 51). Controversy has also arisen regarding the impact of race on outcome, with higher mortality rates being reported in blacks in some but not all studies. In the United States HF affects approximately 3% of blacks, whereas in the general population, the prevalence is about 2%.[5] Blacks with HF present at an earlier age and have more advanced LV dysfunction and a worse New York Heart Association (NYHA) class at the time of diagnosis. Although the reasons for these differences are not known, as noted above, differences in HF etiology might explain some of these observations. There may also be additional socioeconomic factors that may influence outcomes in black patients, such as geographic location and access to health care. Age is one of the stronger and most consistent predictors of adverse outcome in HF (see Special Populations below).[6]

Many other factors have been associated with increased mortality in HF patients (Table 50.2). Most of the factors listed as outcome predictors have survived, at least, univariate analysis, with many standing out independently when multifactorial analysis techniques are employed. Nonetheless, it is extraordinarily difficult to determine which prognostic variable is most important to predicting individual patient outcome in either clinical trials or, more importantly, during the day-to-day management of an individual patient. To this end several multivariate models for predicting the HF prognosis have been developed and validated. The Seattle Heart Failure Model was derived by retrospectively investigating predictors of survival among HF patients in clinical trials. The Seattle Heart Failure Model provides an accurate estimate of 1-, 2-, and 3-year survival with the use of easily obtained clinical, pharmacologic, device, and laboratory characteristics, and is accessible free of charge to all health care providers as an interactive web-based program (http://depts.washington.edu/shfm).

Biomarkers and Prognosis (see also Chapter 48)

The observation that the renin angiotensin-aldosterone, adrenergic, and inflammatory systems are activated in HF (see Chapter 47) has prompted the examination of the relationships between a variety of biochemical measurements and clinical outcomes (Table 50.3). Strong inverse correlations have been reported between survival and plasma levels of norepinephrine, renin, arginine vasopressin (AVP), aldosterone, atrial and brain natriuretic peptides (BNP and NT-proBNP), endothelin-1, and inflammatory markers such as tumor necrosis factor (TNF), soluble TNF receptors, C reactive protein, galactin-3, pentraxin-3, and soluble ST2. The GUIDE-IT trial (Guiding Evidence Based Therapy Using Biomarker Intensified Treatment in Heart Failure) was designed to prospectively study the relationship between change in natriuretic peptide concentration, cardiac remodeling, and clinical events in HFrEF patients. Although GUIDE-IT was stopped prematurely because biomarker-guided treatment was not more effective than usual care in improving outcomes, the Echocardiographic Substudy showed that lowering NT-proBNP to less than 1000 pg/mL by 12 months was associated with reverse LV remodeling and improved outcomes, regardless of the treatment strategy employed. These findings suggest the response to treatment as assessed by change in NT-proBNP is more important than the treatment strategy. Markers of oxidative stress, such as oxidized low-density lipoprotein and serum uric acid, have also been associated with worsening clinical status and impaired survival in patients with chronic HF. Cardiac troponin T and I, sensitive

TABLE 50.2 Etiology of Chronic Heart Failure

Myocardial Disease
Coronary artery disease
    Myocardial infarction*
    Myocardial ischemia*
Chronic pressure overload
    Hypertension*
    Obstructive valvular disease*
Chronic volume overload
    Regurgitant valvular disease
    Intracardiac (left-to-right) shunting
    Extracardiac shunting
Nonischemic dilated cardiomyopathy
    Familial/genetic disorders
    Infiltrative disorders*
    Toxic/drug-induced damage
    Metabolic disorder*
    Viral or other infectious agents

Disorders of Rate and Rhythm
Chronic bradyarrhythmias
Chronic tachyarrhythmias

Pulmonary Heart Disease
Cor pulmonale
Pulmonary vascular disorders
High-output states

Metabolic Disorders
Thyrotoxicosis
Nutritional disorders (beriberi)

Excessive Blood Flow Requirements
Systemic arteriovenous shunting
Chronic anemia

*Indicates conditions that can also lead to heart failure with a preserved ejection fraction.

TABLE 50.3 Prognostic Variable in Heart Failure Patients

Demographics	Exercise Testing
Gender	Metabolic assessment
Race	BP response
Age	Heart rate response
Heart Failure Etiology	6-min walk
CAD	Peak V_{O_2}
IDCM	Anaerobic threshold
Valvular heart disease	V_E/V_{CO_2}
Myocarditis	Oxygen uptake slope
Hypertrophy	**Metabolic**
Alcohol	Serum sodium
Anthracyclines	Thyroid dysfunction
Amyloidosis	Anemia
Hemachromatosis	Acidosis/alkalosis
Genetic factors	**Chest X-ray**
Comorbidities	Congestion
Diabetes	Cardiothoracic ratio
Systemic hypertension	**ECG**
Pulmonary hypertension	Rhythm (atrial fibrillation or arrhythmias)
Sleep apnea	
Obesity/cachexia (body mass)	Voltage
Renal insufficiency	QRS width
Hepatic abnormalities	QT interval
COPD	Signal-average EKG (T-wave alternans)
Clinical Assessment	
NYHA class (symptoms)	HR variability
Syncope	**Biomarkers**
Angina pectoris	NE, PRA, AVP, aldosterone
Systolic versus diastolic dysfunction	ANP, BNP, NT-proBNP, endothelin
Hemodynamics	TNF, sTNFR 1,2, galectin-3, pentraxin-3, sST2
LVEF	Cardiac troponins, hematocrit
RVEF	**Endomyocardial Biopsy**
PAP	Inflammatory states
PCWP	Degree of fibrosis
CI	Degree of cellular disarray
PAP-PCWP	Infiltrative processes
Exercise hemodynamics	

BNP, brain natriuretic peptides; *BP*, blood pressure; *CAD*, coronary artery disease; *CI*, cardiac index; *COPD*, chronic obstructive pulmonary disease; *CRP*, C-reactive protein; *ESR*, erythrocyte sedimentation rate; *HR*, hazard ratio; *IDCM*, idiopathic dilated cardiomyopathy; *IL*, interleukin; *LVEF*, left ventricular ejection fraction; *NE*, norepinephrine; *NYHA*, New York Heart Association; *PAP*, pulmonary artery pressure; *PAP-PCWP*, gradient across lung; *PCWP*, pulmonary capillary wedge pressure; *PRA*, plasma renin activity; *RVEF*, right ventricular ejection fraction; *sST2*, soluble suppression of tumorigenesis-2; *TNF*, tumor necrosis factor; V_{CO_2}, volume of exhaled carbon dioxide; *VE*, ventilation.
Modified from Young JB. The prognosis of heart failure. In: Mann DL, eds. *Heart Failure: A Companion to Braunwald's Heart Disease*. Philadelphia: Elsevier; 2004:489–506.

markers of myocyte damage, may be elevated in patients with nonischemic HF and predict adverse cardiac outcomes, as well as the development of incident HF.[7] The association between a low hemoglobin/hematocrit and adverse HF outcomes has also long been recognized, and has garnered considerable recent attention after several reports illustrated the independent prognostic value of anemia in patients with HF with either reduced or normal ejection fraction.[8]

Published estimates of the prevalence of anemia (defined as a hemoglobin concentration of <13 g/dL in men and <12 g/dL in women) in HF patients vary widely, ranging from 4% to 50% depending on the population studied and definition of anemia that is used. In general, anemia is associated with more HF symptoms, worse NYHA functional status, greater risk of HF hospitalization, and reduced survival.[9] However, it is unclear whether anemia is a cause of decreased survival, or simply a marker of more advanced disease. The underlying cause for anemia is likely multifactorial, including reduced sensitivity to erythropoietin receptors, the presence of a hematopoiesis inhibitor, and/or a defective iron supply for erythropoiesis given as possible explanations.

A standard diagnostic workup should be undertaken in anemic HF patients, recognizing that no definite etiology is identified in many of these patients. Correctable causes of anemia should be treated according to practice guidelines. The role for blood transfusions in patients with cardiovascular disease is controversial. Although a "transfusion threshold" for maintaining the hematocrit greater than 30% in patients with cardiovascular disease has been generally been accepted, this clinical practice has been based more on expert opinion rather than on direct evidence that documents the efficacy of this form of therapy. Given the risks and costs of red blood cell transfusion, the evanescent benefits of blood transfusions in patients with chronic anemia, coupled with the unclear benefit in HF patients, the routine use of blood transfusion cannot be recommended for treating the anemia that occurs in stable HF patients. Treatment of anemic HF patients with mild to moderate anemia (hemoglobin level 9.0 to 12.0 g/dL) with the erythropoietin analog darbepoetin alpha was evaluated in the RED-HF (Reduction of Events With Darbepoetin Alfa in Heart Failure) trial. There was no significant difference in the primary outcome variable of death from any cause or hospitalization for worsening HF (hazard ratio [HR] in the darbepoetin alfa group, 1.01; 95% confidence interval [CI] 0.90–1.13; $P = 0.87$), nor the secondary outcome of cardiovascular death or time to first hospitalization for worsening HF (HR in the darbepoetin alfa group 10.01, 95% CI 0.89 to 1.14; *P* = 0.2). The lack of effect of darbepoetin alfa was consistent across all prespecified subgroups. Importantly, treatment with darbepoetin alfa led to an early (within 1 month) and sustained increase in the hemoglobin level throughout the study.

Iron deficiency is a common comorbidity in patients with HFrEF, and has been associated with increased mortality and a poorer quality of life, regardless of whether there is concomitant anemia.[10] The definition of iron deficiency in HF differs from other conditions of chronic inflammation and is defined as: ferritin less than 100 μg/L or ferritin of 100 to 299 μg/L with a transferrin saturation less than 20%. Correction of iron deficiency in anemic and nonanemic patients with HFrEF (EF <30% to 45%) has been studied in several clinical trials.[11] Two of the three randomized trials conducted thus far have used intravenous ferric carboxymaltose (FCM). Studies with FCM have demonstrated an improvement in symptoms, exercise capacity, and health-related quality of life; however, the effects on major clinical events remain uncertain.[9] The one randomized clinical trial that used an oral iron polysaccharide (Oral Iron Repletion Effects On Oxygen Uptake in Heart Failure [IRONOUT], NCT02188784), did not show an improvement in peak Vo_2 by cardiopulmonary exercise testing at 16 weeks. Based on the results of the randomized trials with intravenous iron supplementation, the current ACC/AHA/HFSA guidelines recommend (class IIb, LOE B-R) that intravenous iron replacement might be reasonable in patients with NYHA class II and III HF and iron deficiency (ferritin <100 ng/mL or 100 to 300 ng/mL if transferrin saturation is <20%) to improve functional status and quality of life.[12] Although the US guidelines do not recommend any specific formulation, the European guidelines recommend treatment with IV FCM in symptomatic HF patients with iron deficiency to improve HF symptoms and quality of life (class IIa, Level of Evidence A recommendation).[9]

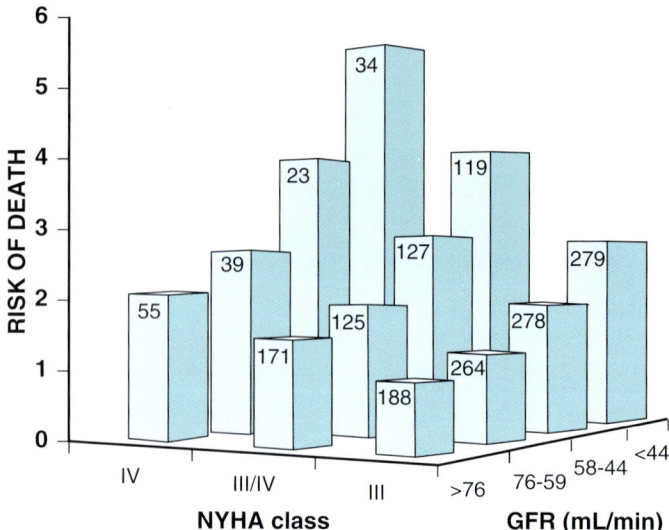

FIGURE 50.2 Effect of renal function on outcomes in heart failure patients. Three-dimensional bar graph showing risk of mortality (vertical axis) in relation to decreasing New York Heart Association (NYHA) class (horizontal axis) and decreasing quartiles of glomerular filtration rate (GFRc; diagonal axis). (From Hillege HL, Girbes AR, de Kam PJ, et al. Renal function, neurohormonal activation, and survival in patients with chronic heart failure. *Circulation*. 2000;102:203–210.)

Renal Insufficiency (see also Chapter 101)

Renal insufficiency is associated with poorer outcomes in patients with HF; however, there remains some uncertainty whether renal impairment is a simply a marker for worsening HF or whether renal impairment might be causally linked to worsening HF. Though more common in patients hospitalized for HF, at least some degree of renal impairment is still present in about half of stable HF outpatients. Patients with renal hypoperfusion or intrinsic renal disease show an impaired response to diuretics and angiotensin-converting enzymes inhibitors (ACEIs) and are at increased risk of adverse effects during treatment with digitalis. In a recent meta-analysis the majority of HF patients had some degree of renal impairment. These patients represented a high-risk group with an approximately 50% increased relative mortality risk when compared with patients who had normal renal function.[13] Similar findings were observed in the Acute Decompensated Heart Failure National Registry (ADHERE) (see Chapter 49). In the Second Prospective Randomized Study of Ibopamine on Mortality and Efficacy, impaired renal function was a stronger predictor of mortality than impaired LV function and NYHA class in patients with advanced HF (Fig. 50.2). Thus, renal insufficiency is a strong, independent predictor of adverse outcomes in HF patients. As will be discussed, below, treatment with sodium-glucose transporter-2 (SGLT2) inhibitors stabilizes renal function in patients with HFrEF.[14]

APPROACH TO THE PATIENT

HFrEF should be viewed as continuum that is comprised of four interrelated stages (see Fig. 50.3).[15] Stage A includes patients who are at high risk for developing HF, but without structural heart disease or symptoms of HF (e.g., patients with diabetes or hypertension). Stage B includes patients who have structural heart disease but without symptoms of HF (e.g., patients with a previous myocardial infarction [MI] and asymptomatic LV dysfunction). Stage C includes patients who have structural heart disease who have developed symptoms of HF (e.g., patients with a previous MI with shortness of breath and fatigue). Stage D includes patients who refractory HF requiring special interventions (e.g., patients with refractory HF who are awaiting cardiac transplantation). The clinical assessment of patients with HFrEF is discussed in detail in Chapter 48, and the diagnosis and management of patients with HFpEF is discussed in detail in Chapter 51.

Patients at High Risk for Developing Heart Failure (Stage A)

For patients at high risk of developing HFrEF, every effort should be made to prevent HF using standard practice guidelines to treat preventable conditions that are known to lead to HF, including hypertension (see Chapter 26), hyperlipidemia (see Chapter 27), and diabetes (see Chapter 31). In this regard, ACEIs are particularly useful in preventing HF in patients who have a history of atherosclerotic vascular disease, diabetes mellitus, or hypertension with associated cardiovascular risk factors.

POPULATION SCREENING

At present there is limited information available to support the screening of broad populations to detect undiagnosed HF and/or asymptomatic LV dysfunction. Although initial studies suggested that determination of BNP or NT-proBNP levels (see also Chapter 48) might be useful for screening, the positive predictive value for these tests in a low-prevalence and asymptomatic population for the purpose of detecting cardiac dysfunction varies among studies, and the possibility of false-positive results has significant cost-effectiveness implications.

Patients who are at very high risk of developing cardiomyopathy (e.g., those with a strong family history of cardiomyopathy or those receiving cardiotoxic interventions [see Chapters 56 and 57]) are appropriate targets for more aggressive screening such as 2-D echocardiography to assess LV function. St Vincent's Screening To Prevent Heart Failure (STOP-HF) showed that, in patients with known cardiovascular risk factors, screening with BNP testing followed by collaborative care between internists and cardiovascular specialists resulted in a significant reduction in LV dysfunction (odds ratio [OR], 0.55; 95% CI, 0.37 to 0.82; *P* = 0.003). Although there was no significant reduction in clinical HF events, there was a significant decrease in the incidence rates of emergency hospitalization for major cardiovascular events.[16] However, the routine periodic assessment of LV function in low-risk patients is not currently recommended. Several sophisticated clinical scoring systems have been developed to screen for HF in population-based studies, including the Framingham Criteria, which screens for HF on the basis of clinical criteria, and the National Health and Nutrition Survey (NHANES) which uses self-reporting of symptoms to identify HF patients (Table 50.4). However, as discussed in Chapter 48, additional laboratory testing is usually necessary to definitively make the diagnosis of HF when these methodologies are used.

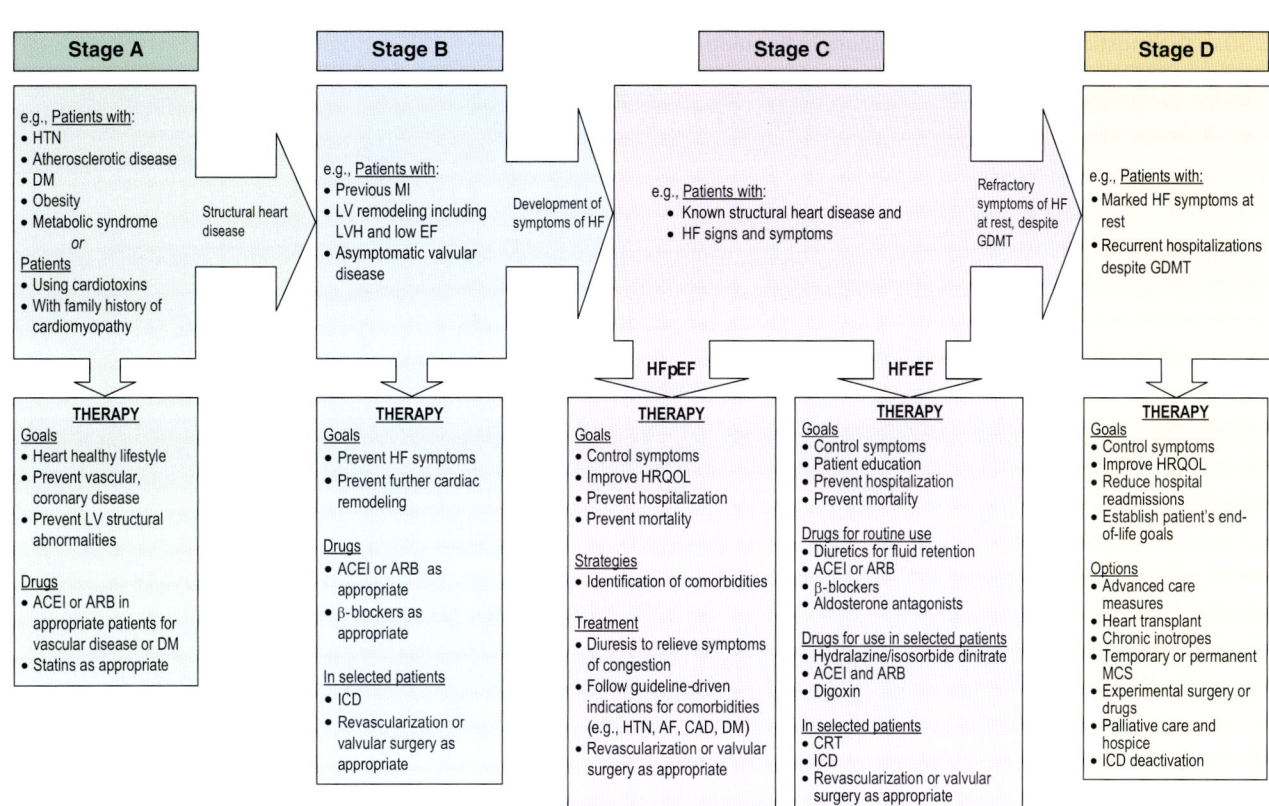

FIGURE 50.3 Stages in the development of heart failure and recommended therapy by stage. *ACEI,* Angiotensin-converting enzyme inhibitor; *AF,* atrial fibrillation; *ARB,* angiotensin-receptor blocker; *CAD,* coronary artery disease; *CRT,* cardiac resynchronization therapy; *DM,* diabetes mellitus; *EF,* ejection fraction; *GDMT,* guideline-directed medical therapy; *HF,* heart failure; *HFpEF,* heart failure with preserved ejection fraction; *HFrEF,* heart failure with reduced ejection fraction; *HRQOL,* health-related quality of life; *HTN,* hypertension; *ICD,* implantable cardioverter-defibrillator; *LV,* left ventricular; *LVH,* left ventricular hypertrophy; *MCS,* mechanical circulatory support; *MI,* myocardial infarction. (Modified from Hunt SA, Abraham WT, Chin MH, et al. 2009 focused update incorporated into the ACC/AHA 2005 Guidelines for the Diagnosis and Management of Heart Failure in Adults: a report of the American College of Cardiology Foundation/American Heart Association Task Force on Practice Guidelines: developed in collaboration with the International Society for Heart and Lung Transplantation. *Circulation.* 2009;119:e391–e479; and Yancy CW, Jessup M, Bozkurt B, et al. 2013 ACCF/AHA Guideline for the Management of Heart Failure: A Report of the American College of Cardiology Foundation/American Heart Association Task Force on Practice Guidelines. Circulation 2013;128(16):e240-327.)

Management of Patients With Symptomatic and Asymptomatic Heart Failure

Transient Left Ventricular Dysfunction

As noted in Chapter 47, the clinical syndrome of HF with reduced EF begins after an initial index event produces a decline in ejection performance of the heart. However, it is important to recognize that LV dysfunction may develop transiently in a variety of different clinical settings that may not invariably lead to the development of the clinical syndrome of HF. Figure 50.4 illustrates the important relationship between LV dysfunction (transient and sustained) and the clinical syndrome of HF (asymptomatic and symptomatic). LV dysfunction with pulmonary edema may develop acutely in patients with previously normal LV structure and function. This occurs most commonly postoperatively following cardiac surgery, or in the setting of severe brain injury, after a systemic infection, or after cessation of tachycardia. The general pathophysiologic mechanism involved is either some form of "stunning" of functional myocardium (see also Chapter 49), or activation of proinflammatory cytokines that are capable of suppressing LV function (see Chapter 47). Emotional stress can also precipitate severe, reversible LV dysfunction that is accompanied by chest pain, pulmonary edema, and cardiogenic shock in patients without coronary disease (Takotsubo syndrome [stress cardiomyopathy]). In this setting LV dysfunction is thought to occur secondary to the deleterious effects of catecholamines following heightened sympathetic stimulation.[17] Microvascular dysfunction has been suggested as an important pathogenetic determinant of myocardial ischemia in Takotsubo syndrome.[17] If LV dysfunction persists following the initial cardiac injury, patients may remain asymptomatic for a period of months to years; however, the weight of epidemiologic and clinical evidence suggests that at some point these patients will undergo the transition to overt symptomatic HF.

Defining the Appropriate Strategy (see Fig. 50.4)

The main goals of treatment are to reduce symptoms, prolong survival, improve quality of life, and prevent disease progression. As will be discussed below, the current pharmacologic device, and surgical therapeutic armamentarium for the management of patients with a reduced EF allows health care providers to achieve each of these goals in the great majority of patients. Once patients have developed structural heart disease (Stage B to D), the choice of therapy for patients with HF with a reduced EF depends on their NYHA functional classification (see Chapter 48, Table 48.1). Although this classification system is notoriously subjective, and has large interobserver variability, it has withstood the test of time and continues to be widely applied to patients with HF. For patients who have developed LV systolic dysfunction, but who remain asymptomatic (class I), the goal should be to slow disease progression by blocking neurohormonal systems that lead to cardiac remodeling (see Chapter 47). For patients who have developed symptoms (class II to IV), the primary goal should be to alleviate fluid retention, lessen disability, and reduce the risk of further disease progression and death. As will be discussed subsequently, these goals generally require a strategy that combines diuretics (to control salt and water retention) with neurohormonal interventions (to minimize cardiac remodeling).

General Measures

Identification and correction of the condition(s) responsible for the cardiac structural and/or functional abnormalities is critical (see Table 50.2), insofar as some of conditions that provoke LV structural and functional abnormalities are potentially treatable and/or reversible. Patients with HF often have multiple comorbid conditions that may interact with the syndrome of HF and or the choice of therapeutics. The 2013 ACC/AHA practice guidelines recognized the importance of comorbidities in HF, including hypertension, anemia, diabetes, arthritis, chronic kidney disease, and depression, but did not provide specific recommendations.

TABLE 50.4 Diagnostic Criteria for Heart Failure in Population-Based Studies

FRAMINGHAM CRITERIA		
MAJOR CRITERIA	**MINOR CRITERIA**	**MAJOR OR MINOR CRITERIA**
Paroxysmal nocturnal dyspnea or orthopnea	Ankle edema	Weight loss >4.5 kg in 5 days in response to treatment
Neck-vein distention	Night cough	
RALES	Dyspnea on exertion	
Cardiomegaly	Hepatomegaly	
Acute pulmonary edema	Pleural effusion	
S3 gallop	Vital capacity decreased one third from maximal capacity	
Increased venous pressure >16 cm H_2O		
Hepatojugular reflux	Tachycardia (rate >120/min)	

NHANES CRITERIA		
CATEGORIES	**CRITERIA**	**SCORE**
History	*Dyspnea:*	1
	Do you stop for breath when walking at an ordinary pace?	
	Do you stop for breath after walking for about 100 yards on flat ground?	1
	When hurrying on a hill	2
	When walking at an ordinary pace	2
Physical examination	*Heart rate:*	
	>110 beats/min	1
	91–110 beats/min	2
	Jugular venous pressure (>6 cm H_2O):	
	Alone	1
	Plus hepatomegaly or edema	2
	Rales:	
	Basilar crackles	1
	Crackles more than basilar crackles	2
Chest radiography	Upper zone flow redistribution	1
	Interstitial pulmonary edema	2
	Interstitial edema plus pleural fluid	3
	Alveolar fluid plus pleural fluid	3

The diagnosis of HF using the Framingham criteria requires the simultaneous presence of at least two major criteria or one major criterion in conjunction with two minor criteria. Minor criteria are acceptable only if they cannot be attributed to another medical condition (such as pulmonary hypertension, chronic lung disease, cirrhosis, ascites, or the nephrotic syndrome). NHANES-1 criteria: diagnosis of HF is score ≥three points.
NHANES, National Health and Nutrition Survey.
Modified from Ho KK, Pinsky JL, Kannel WB, et al. The epidemiology of heart failure: the Framingham Study. *J Am Coll Cardiol.* 1993;22:6A–13A; and Schocken DD, Arrieta MI, Leaverton PE, et al. Prevalence and mortality rate of congestive heart failure in the United States. *J Am Coll Cardiol.* 1992;20:301–306.

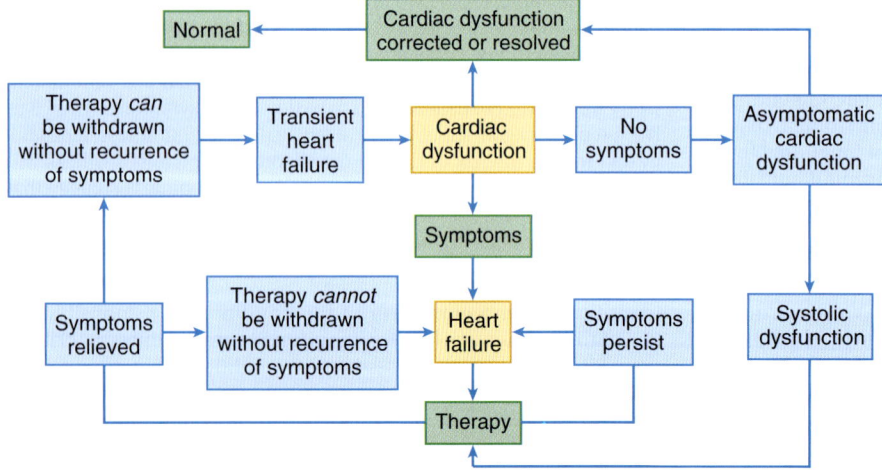

FIGURE 50.4 Relationship between cardiac dysfunction, symptomatic heart failure, and asymptomatic heart failure following appropriate treatment. (From Swedberg K, Cleland J, Dargie H, et al. Guidelines for the diagnosis and treatment of chronic heart failure: executive summary (update 2005): The Task Force for the Diagnosis and Treatment of Chronic Heart Failure of the European Society of Cardiology. *Eur Heart J.* 2005;26:1115–1140.)

However, the 2017 ACC/AHA/HFSA focused guideline update did provide specific recommendations for the treatment of hypertension, anemia, and sleep-disordered breathing.[18] In addition to searching for reversible etiologies and comorbidities that contribute to the development of HF, it is equally important to identify factors that provoke worsening HF in stable patients (Table 50.5). Among the most common causes of acute decompensation in a previously stable patient are dietary indiscretion and inappropriate reduction of HF therapy, either from patient self-discontinuation of medication, or alternatively from physician withdrawal of effective pharmacotherapy (e.g., because of concern over azotemia). HF patients should be advised to stop smoking and to limit alcohol consumption to two standard drinks per day in men or one standard drink per day in women. Patients suspected

TABLE 50.5 Factors That May Precipitate Acute Decompensation in Patients with Chronic Heart Failure

Dietary indiscretion
Inappropriate reduction in HF medications
Myocardial ischemia/infarction
Arrhythmias (tachycardia or bradycardia)
Infection
Anemia

Initiation of medications that worsen the symptoms of HF
   Calcium antagonists (verapamil, diltiazem)
   Beta-blockers
   Nonsteroidal antiinflammatory drugs
   Thiazolidinediones
   Antiarrhythmic agents (all class I agents, sotalol [class III])
   Anti-TNF antibodies

Alcohol consumption
Pregnancy
Worsening hypertension
Acute valvular insufficiency

HF, Heart failure; TNF, tumor necrosis factor.
From Mann DL. Heart Failure and Cor Pulmonale. In: Kasper DL, et al., eds. *Harrison's Principles of Internal Medicine*. 17th ed. New York: McGraw-Hill; 2007:1448.

of having an alcohol-induced cardiomyopathy should be advised to abstain from alcohol consumption indefinitely. Excessive temperature extremes and heavy physical exertion should be avoided. Certain drugs are known to make HF worse and should also be avoided. For example, nonsteroidal antiinflammatory drugs (NSAIDs), including cyclooxygenase-2 inhibitors (COX2), are not recommended in patients with chronic HF because the risk of renal failure and fluid retention is markedly increased in the setting of reduced renal function and/or ACEI use. Patients should be advised to weigh themselves on a regular basis to monitor weight gain and alert a health care provider or adjust their diuretic dose in the case of a sudden unexpected weight gain of greater than 3 to 4 pounds over a 3-day period. Although there is no documented evidence of the effects of immunization in HF patients, they are at high risk of developing pneumococcal disease and influenza. Accordingly, clinicians should consider recommending influenza and pneumococcal vaccines to their HF patient to prevent respiratory infections. It is equally important to educate the patient and family about HF, the importance of proper diet, as well the importance of compliance with the medical regimen. Supervision of outpatient care by a specially trained nurse or physician assistant and/or specialized HF clinics have all been found to be helpful, particularly in patients with advanced disease (see Disease Management below).

Activity

Although heavy physical labor is not recommended for patients with HF, routine modest exercise has been shown to be beneficial in selected patients with NYHA class I to III HFrEF. The HF-ACTION trial (Controlled Trial Investigating Outcomes of Exercise Training) was a large multicenter randomized controlled study whose primary endpoint was a composite of all-cause mortality and all-cause hospitalization. Secondary endpoints included all-cause mortality, all-cause hospitalization, and the composite of cardiovascular mortality or HF hospitalization. HF-ACTION failed to show a significant improvement in all-cause mortality or all-cause hospitalization (HR, 0.93; 95% CI 0.84 to 1.02; $p = 0.13$) in patients who received a 12-week (3 times/wk) exercise training program followed by 25 to 30 minute, 5 days/wk home-based, self-monitored exercise workouts on a treadmill or stationary bicycle. Moreover, there was no difference in all-cause mortality (HR, 0.96; 95% CI 0.79 to 1.17; $p = 0.70$). However, there was a trend towards decreased cardiovascular mortality or HF hospitalizations (HR, 0.87; 95% CI 0.74 to 0.99 $p = 0.06$) and quality of life was significantly improved in the exercise group.[19] For euvolemic patients regular isotonic exercise such as walking or riding a stationary-bicycle ergometer may be useful as an adjunct therapy, to improve clinical status after patients have undergone exercise testing to determine suitability for exercise training (ensuring that patient does not develop significant ischemia or arrhythmias). Exercise training is not recommended, however, in HFrEF patients who have had a major cardiovascular event or procedure within the last 6 weeks, in patients receiving cardiac devices that limit the ability to achieve target heart rates, and in patients with significant arrhythmia or ischemia during baseline cardiopulmonary exercise testing.

Diet

Dietary restriction of sodium (2 to 3 g daily) is recommended in all patients with the clinical syndrome of HF and preserved or depressed EF. Further restriction (<2 g daily) may be considered in moderate to severe HF. Fluid restriction is generally unnecessary unless the patient is hyponatremic (<130 mEq/L), which may develop because of activation of the renin angiotensin system, excessive secretion of AVP, or loss of salt in excess of water from prior diuretic use. Fluid restriction (<2 L/day) should be considered in hyponatremic patients (<130 mEq/L), or for those patients whose fluid retention is difficult to control despite high doses of diuretics and sodium restriction. Caloric supplementation is recommended for patients with advanced HF and unintentional weight loss or muscle wasting (cardiac cachexia); however, anabolic steroids are not recommended for these patients because of the potential problems with volume retention. The measurement of nitrogen balance, caloric intake, and prealbumin may be useful in determining appropriate nutritional supplementation. The use of dietary supplements ("nutraceuticals") should be avoided in the management of symptomatic HF because of the lack of proven benefit and the potential for significant interactions with proven HF therapeutics.

MANAGEMENT OF FLUID RETENTION

Many of the clinical manifestations of the syndrome of HF result from excessive salt and water retention that leads to an inappropriate volume expansion of the vascular and extravascular space. The use of implantable devices to monitor HF is discussed in Chapter 58. This chapter will focus on the use of diuretics in chronic HFrEF. Although both digitalis and low doses of ACEIs enhance urinary sodium excretion, few volume-overloaded HF patients can maintain proper sodium balance without the use of diuretic drugs. Indeed, attempts to substitute ACEIs for diuretics have been shown to lead to pulmonary edema and peripheral congestion. As shown in Figure 50.5, diuretic-induced negative sodium and water balance can decrease LV dilation, functional mitral insufficiency, and decrease mitral wall stress and subendocardial ischemia. In short-term clinical trials diuretic therapy has led to a reduction in jugular venous pressures, pulmonary congestion, peripheral edema, and body weight, all of which were observed within days of initiation of therapy. In intermediate-term studies, diuretics have been shown to improve cardiac function, symptoms, and exercise tolerance in HF patients.[20] To date, there have been no long-term studies of diuretic therapy in HF; thus, their effects on morbidity and mortality are not clearly known. Although retrospective analyses of clinical trials suggest that diuretic use is associated with worse clinical outcomes,[20] a meta-analysis (Cochrane Review) suggested that treatment with diuretic therapy produced a significant reduction in mortality (OR 0.24; 95% CI 0.07 to 0.83; p = 0.02) and worsening HF (OR 0.07; 95% CI 0.01 to 0.52; p = 0.01).[20] However, given the retrospective nature of this review, this analysis cannot be used as formal evidence to recommend the use diuretics to reduce HF mortality.

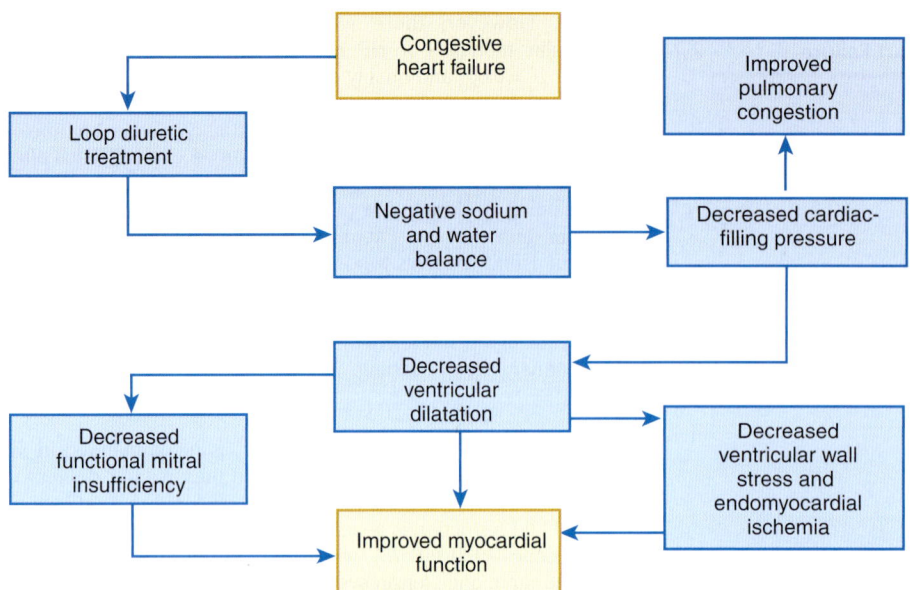

FIGURE 50.5 Potential beneficial effects of diuretics on myocardial function. Diuretic-induced negative sodium and water balance can decrease left ventricular (LV) dilation, functional mitral insufficiency, and decrease mitral wall stress and subendocardial ischemia. However, treatment with diuretics can also lead to deterioration of renal function and worsening neurohormonal activation. (Modified from Schrier RW. Use of diuretics in heart failure and cirrhosis. *Semin Nephrol.* 2011;31:503–512.)

Diuretic Classes

A number of classification schemes have been proposed for diuretics on the basis of their mechanism of action, their anatomical locus of action within the nephron, and the form of diuresis that they elicit (solute versus water diuresis). The most common classification for diuretics employs an admixture of chemical (e.g., thiazide diuretic), site of action (e.g., loop diuretics), or clinical outcomes (e.g., potassium-sparing diuretics). The loop diuretics increase sodium excretion by up to 20% to 25% of the filtered load of sodium, enhance free water clearance, and maintain their efficacy unless renal function is severely impaired. In contrast, the thiazide diuretics increase the fractional excretion of sodium to only 5% to 10% of the filtered load, tend to decrease free water clearance, and lose their effectiveness in patients with impaired renal function (creatinine clearance <40 mL/min). Consequently, the loop diuretics have emerged as the preferred diuretic agents for use in most patients with HF. Diuretics that induce a water diuresis (aquaretics) include demeclocycline, lithium, and vasopressin V2 receptor antagonists, each of which inhibits the action of AVP on the collecting duct through different mechanisms, thereby increasing free water clearance. Drugs that cause solute diuresis are subdivided into two types: osmotic diuretics, which are nonresorbable solutes that osmotically retain water and other solutes in the tubular lumen; and drugs that selectively inhibit ion transport pathways across tubular epithelia, which constitute the majority of potent, clinically useful diuretics. The classes of diuretics and individual class members are listed in Table 50.6 and their renal sites of action are depicted in Figure 50.6.

Loop Diuretics

The agents classified as loop diuretics, including furosemide, bumetanide, and torsemide, act by competing with chloride for binding to the Na^+-K^+-$2Cl^-$ symporter (NKCC2) on the apical membrane of epithelial cells in the thick ascending loop of Henle (site II, Fig. 50.6). Because furosemide, bumetanide, and torsemide are bound to plasma proteins, delivery of these drugs to the tubule by filtration is limited. However, these drugs are secreted efficiently into the tubular lumen by organic anion transporters (OAT1 and OAT2) at the basolateral membrane of proximal convoluted tubule epithelial cells and by multidrug resistance–associated protein 4 (and others) at the apical membrane or these cells.[21] Thus, the efficacy of loop diuretics is dependent upon sufficient renal plasma blood flow and proximal tubular secretion to deliver these agents to their site of action. Probenecid shifts the plasma concentration-response curve for furosemide to the right by competitively inhibiting furosemide excretion by the organic acid transport system. The bioavailability of furosemide ranges from 40% to 70% of the oral dose. In contrast the oral bioavailability of bumetanide and torsemide exceed 80%. Accordingly, these agents may be more effective in advanced HF or those with right-sided HF, albeit at considerably greater cost. Agents in a second functional class of loop diuretics typified by ethacrynic acid exhibit a slower onset of action and have delayed and only partial reversibility. Ethacrynic acid may be safely used in sulfa-allergic HF patients.

MECHANISMS OF ACTION

Loop diuretics are believed to improve symptoms of congestion by several mechanisms. First, loop diuretics reversibly bind to and reversibly inhibit the action of the Na^+-K^+-$2Cl^-$ cotransporter, thereby preventing salt transport in the thick ascending loop of Henle. Inhibition of this symporter also inhibits Ca^{++} and Mg^{++} resorption by abolishing the transepithelial potential difference that is the driving force for absorption of these cations. By inhibiting the concentration of solute within the medullary interstitium, these drugs also reduce the driving force for water resorption in the collecting duct, even in the presence of AVP (see also Chapter 47). The decreased resorption of water by the collecting duct results in the production of urine that is nearly isotonic with plasma. The increase in delivery of Na^+ and water to the distal nephron segments also markedly enhances K^+ excretion, particularly in the presence of elevated aldosterone levels.

Loop diuretics also exhibit several characteristic effects on intracardiac pressure and systemic hemodynamics. Furosemide acts as a venodilator and reduces right atrial and pulmonary capillary wedge pressure within minutes when given intravenously (0.5 to 1.0 mg/kg). Similar data, although not as extensive, have accumulated for bumetanide and torsemide. This initial improvement in hemodynamics may be secondary to the release of vasodilatory prostaglandins, insofar as studies in animals and humans have demonstrated that the venodilatory actions of furosemide are inhibited by indomethacin. There have also been reports of an acute rise in systemic vascular resistance with in response to loop diuretics, which has been attributed to transient activation of the systemic or intravascular renin-angiotensin system (RAS), which is secondary to loop diuretics directly stimulating renin secretion by macula densa cells.

The potentially deleterious rise in LV afterload reinforces the importance of initiating vasodilator therapy with diuretics in patients with acute pulmonary edema and adequate blood pressure (see Chapter 49).

Thiazide and Thiazide-Like Diuretics

The benzothiadiazides, also known as *thiazide diuretics*, were the initial class of drugs that were synthesized to block the Na^+-Cl^- transporter in the cortical portion of the ascending loop of Henle and the distal convoluted tubule (site III, Fig. 50.6). Subsequently, drugs that share similar pharmacologic properties became known as thiazide-like diuretics, even though they were technically not benzothiadiazine derivatives. Metolazone, a quinazoline sulfonamide, is a thiazide-like diuretic that is used in combination with furosemide, in patients who become resistant to diuretics (see below). Because thiazide and thiazide-like diuretics prevent maximal dilution of urine, they decrease the kidney's ability to increase free water clearance and may therefore contribute to the development of hyponatremia. Thiazides increase Ca^{2+} resorption in the distal nephron (Fig. 50.6)

TABLE 50.6 Diuretics for Treating Fluid Retention in Chronic Heart Failure

DRUG	INITIAL DAILY DOSE(S)	MAXIMUM TOTAL DAILY DOSE	DURATION OF ACTION
Loop Diuretics*			
Bumetanide	0.5–1.0 mg once or twice	10 mg	4–6 hr
Furosemide	20–40 mg once or twice	600 mg	6–8 hr
Torsemide	10–20 mg once	200 mg	12–16 hr
Ethacrynic acid	25–50 mg once or twice	200 mg	6 hr
Thiazide Diuretics**			
Chlorothiazide	250–500 mg once or twice	1000 mg	6–12 hr
Chlorthalidone	25 mg once	100 mg	24–72 hr
Hydrochlorothiazide	25 mg once or twice	200 mg	6–12 hr
Indapamide	2.5 mg once	5 mg	36 hr
Metolazone	2.5–5.0 mg once	5 mg	12–24 hr
Potassium-Sparing Diuretics			
Amiloride	5.0 mg once	20 mg	24 hr
Triamterene	50–100 mg twice	300 mg	7–9 hr
AVP Antagonists			
Satavaptan	25 mg once	50 mg once	NS
Tolvaptan	15 mg once	60 mg once	NS
Lixivaptan	25 mg once	250 mg twice	NS
Conivaptan (IV)	20 mg IV loading dose followed by	100 mg once	7–9 hr
	20 mg continuous IV infusion/day	40 mg IV	
Sequential Nephron Blockade			
Metolazone	2.5–10 mg once plus loop diuretic		
Hydrochlorothiazide	25–100 mg once or twice plus loop diuretic		
Chlorothiazide (IV)	500–1000 mg once plus loop diuretic		

*Equivalent doses: 40 mg furosemide = 1 mg bumetanide = 20 mg torsemide = 50 mg of ethacrynic acid.
**Do not use if estimated glomerular filtration is less than 30 mL/min or with cytochrome 3A4 inhibitors.
Unless indicated, all doses are for oral diuretics.
mg, Milligrams; *IV*, intravenous. *NS*, not specified.
Modified from Hunt SA, et al. ACC/AHA 2005 guideline update for the diagnosis and management of chronic heart failure in the adult: a report of the American College of Cardiology/American Heart Association Task Force on Practice Guidelines. *J Am Coll Cardiol*. 2005;46:e1–e82.

by several mechanisms, occasionally resulting in a small increase in serum Ca^{2+} levels. In contrast, Mg^{2+} resorption is diminished and hypomagnesemia may occur with prolonged use. Increased delivery of NaCl and fluid into the collecting duct directly enhances K^+ and H^+ secretion by this segment of the nephron, which may lead to clinically important hypokalemia.

MECHANISMS OF ACTION
The site of action of these drugs within the distal convoluted tubule has been identified as the Na^+-Cl^- symporter of the distal convoluted tubule. Although this cotransporter shares approximately 50% amino acid homology with the $Na^+/K^+/2Cl^-$ symporter of the ascending limb of the loop of Henle, it is insensitive to the effects of furosemide. This cotransporter (or related isoforms) is also present on cells within the vasculature and many cell types within other organs and tissues and may contribute to some of the other actions of these agents, such as their utility as antihypertensive agents. Similar to the loop diuretics, the efficacy of thiazide diuretics is dependent, at least in part, upon proximal tubular secretion to deliver these agents to their site of action. However, unlike the loop diuretics the plasma protein binding varies considerably among the thiazide diuretics; accordingly, this parameter will determine the contribution that glomerular filtration makes to tubular delivery of a specific diuretic.

Mineralocorticoid Receptor Antagonists
Mineralocorticoids (MRAs) such as aldosterone cause retention of salt and water and increase the excretion of K^+ and H^+ by binding to specific MRA receptors. Spironolactone (first-generation MRA) and eplerenone (second-generation MRA) are synthetic MRA receptors that act on the distal nephron to inhibit Na^+/K^+ exchange at the site of aldosterone action (Site IV, Fig. 50.6).

MECHANISMS OF ACTION
Spironolactone has antiandrogenic and progesterone-like effects, which may cause gynecomastia or impotence in men, and menstrual irregularities in women. To overcome these side effects, eplerenone was developed by replacing the 17 alpha-thioacetyl group of spironolactone with a carbomethoxy group. As a result of this modification, eplerenone has greater selectivity for the MRA receptor than for steroid receptors and has less sex hormone side effects than does spironolactone. Eplerenone is further distinguished from spironolactone by its shorter half-life and the fact that it does not have any active metabolites. Although spironolactone and eplerenone are both weak diuretics, clinical trials have shown that both of these agents have profound effects on cardiovascular morbidity and mortality (Fig. 50.7) by virtue of their ability to antagonize the deleterious effects of aldosterone in the cardiovascular system (see Chapter 47). Hence these agents are used in HF for their ability to antagonize the renin angiotensin aldosterone system (see below), rather than for their diuretic properties. Spironolactone (see Table 50.6) and its active metabolite, canrenone, competitively inhibit the binding of aldosterone to MRA or type I receptors in many tissues, including epithelial cells of the distal convoluted tubule and collecting duct. These cytosolic receptors are ligand-dependent transcription factors, which upon binding of the ligand (e.g., aldosterone), translocate to the nucleus where they bind to hormone response elements present in the promoter of some genes, including several involved in vascular and myocardial fibrosis, inflammation, and calcification.

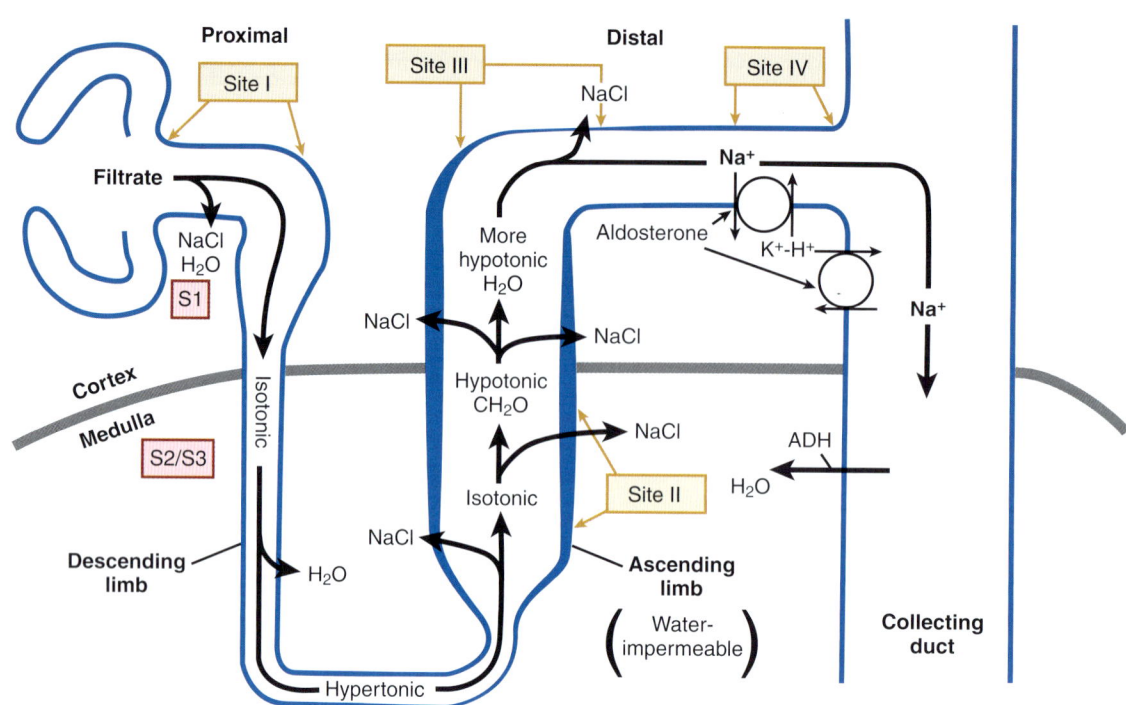

Site I (proximal convoluted tubule): carbonic anhydrase inhibitors, SGLT2 inhibitors
Site II (ascending loop of Henle): loop diuretics
Site III (distal convoluted tubule): thiazide and thiazide-like diuretics
Site IV (late distal tubule and collecting duct): potassium-sparing diuretics, MRAs
S1-S3 segments of proximal convoluted tube

FIGURE 50.6 Sites of action of diuretics in the kidney. (Modified from Wile D. Diuretics: a review. *Ann Clin Biochem.* 2012;49:419–431.)

While first- and second-generation steroid-based MRAs have been shown to reduce HF mortality rates, the broader use of these agents in HF patients has been limited by significant side effects, most notably hyperkalemia. Novel, potent, and selective "third-generation" nonsteroidal MRAs that combine the potency and efficacy of spironolactone with the selectivity of eplerenone, and have less hyperkalemia, have recently entered clinical trials. Finerenone (BAY 94-8862) is a nonsteroidal MRA that was compared to eplerenone in patients with worsening chronic HF and type 2 diabetes mellitus and/or chronic kidney disease in the phase IIb ARTS-HF (MinerAlocorticoid-Receptor antagonist Tolerability Stud) trial.[22] ARTS-HF was a randomized, double-blind, comparator-controlled multicenter trial in 1066 patients with HF (left ventricular ejection fraction [LVEF] ≤40%). The primary endpoint was the percentage of individuals with a decrease of greater than 30% in plasma NT-proBNP from baseline to Day 90. When compared with eplerenone, finerenone was well tolerated and resulted in a 30% or greater decrease in NT-proBNP levels, which was similar to the proportion of patients observed in the eplerenone-treatment group. The composite clinical endpoint of death from any cause, cardiovascular hospitalizations, or emergency presentation for worsening HF until Day 90, which was a prespecified secondary endpoint occurred less frequently in all finerenone-dose groups except for the lowest doses.

Potassium-Sparing Diuretics

Triamterene and amiloride are referred to as *potassium-sparing diuretics*. These agents share the common property of causing a mild increase in NaCl excretion, as well as having antikaluretic properties. Triamterene is a pyrazinoylguanidine derivative, whereas amiloride is a pteridine. Both drugs are organic bases that are transported into the proximal tubule, where they block Na^+ reabsorption in the late distal tubule and collecting duct (site IV, Fig. 50.7). However, since Na^+ retention occurs in more proximal nephron sites in HF, neither amiloride nor triamterene is effective in achieving a net negative Na^+ balance when given alone in HF patients. Both amiloride and triamterene appear to share a similar mechanism of action. Considerable evidence suggests that amiloride blocks Na^+ channels in the luminal membrane of the principal cells in the late distal tubule and collecting duct, perhaps by competing with Na^+ for negatively charged areas within the pore of the Na^+ channel. Blockade of Na^+ channels leads to hyperpolarization of the luminal membrane of the tubule, which reduces the electrochemical gradient that provides the driving force for K^+ secretion into the lumen. Amiloride and its congeners also inhibit Na^+/H^+ antiporters in renal epithelial cells and in many other cell types, but only at concentrations that are higher than those used clinically.

Carbonic Anhydrase Inhibitors

The zinc metalloenzyme carbonic anhydrase plays an essential role in the $NaHCO_3$ resorption and acid secretion in the proximal tubule (site I, see Fig. 50.6). Although weak diuretics, carbonic anhydrase inhibitors (see Table 50.6) such as acetazolamide, potently inhibit carbonic anhydrase, resulting in near-complete loss of $NaHCO_3$ resorption in the proximal tubule. The use of these agents in patients with HF is confined to temporary administration to correct the metabolic alkalosis that occurs as a "contraction" phenomenon in response to the administration of other diuretics. When used repeatedly, these agents can lead to metabolic acidosis as well as severe hypokalemia.

Sodium-Glucose Transporter-2 Inhibitors

The SGLT2 is a high-capacity, low-affinity transporter that is located in the S1 and S2 segments of the proximal tubule in the kidneys (Site I, Fig. 50.6). SGLT2 accounts for 90% of glucose reabsorption by the kidney, whereas the lower-capacity higher-affinity SGLT1, located in the S3 segment of the proximal tubules, accounts for the remaining 10% of glucose absorption. SGLT2 is also responsible for proximal tubular reabsorption of sodium, and the passive absorption of chloride that is driven by the resulting electrochemical gradient in the proximal tubule lumen. The increased absorption of sodium and chloride in the proximal tubule results in lower chloride concentration delivered to the macula densa, which in turn results in dilation of the afferent arteriole and increased glomerular filtration through "tubulo-glomerular feedback," which preserves renal blood flow and glomerular filtration rate.

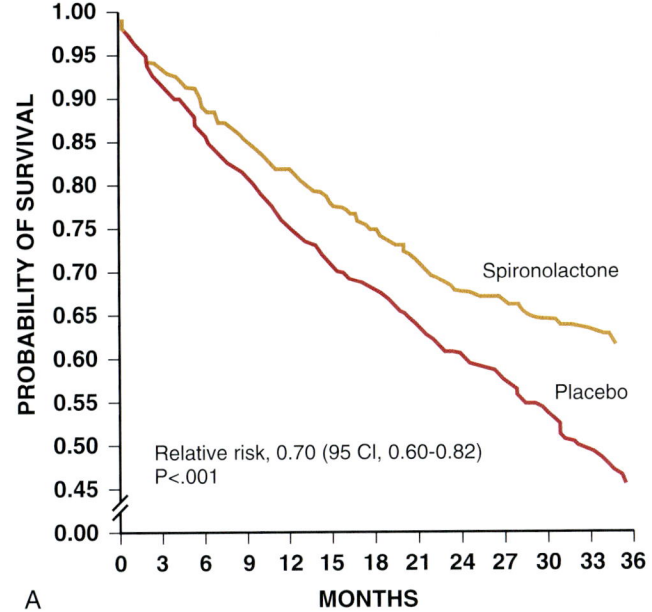

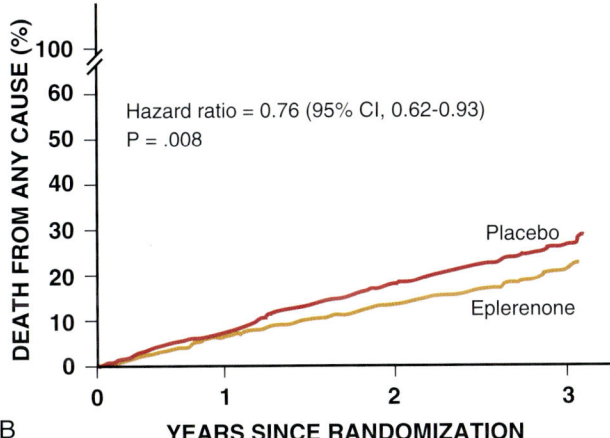

FIGURE 50.7 Kaplan-Meier analysis of the probability of survival among patients in the placebo and treatment groups in the RALES trial (**A**) with spironolactone and the EMPHASIS trial (**B**) using eplerenone. (Modified from Pitt B, Zannad F, Cody R, et al. The effect of spironolactone on morbidity and mortality in patients with severe heart failure. Randomized Aldactone Evaluation Study Investigators. *N Engl J Med.* 1999;341:709–717; and Zannad F, McMurray JJ, Krum H, et al. Eplerenone in patients with systolic heart failure and mild symptoms. *N Engl J Med.* 2011;364:11–21.)

Vasopressin Antagonists

As discussed in Chapter 47, increased circulating levels of the pituitary hormone AVP contribute to the increased systemic vascular resistance and positive water balance in HF patients. The cellular effects of AVP are mediated by interactions with three types of receptors, V_{1a}, V_{1b}, and V_2 (see Chapter 47). Selective V_{1a} antagonists block the vasoconstricting effects of AVP in peripheral vascular smooth muscle cells, whereas V_2 selective receptor antagonists inhibit recruitment of aquaporin water channels into the apical membranes of collecting duct epithelial cells, thereby reducing the ability of the collecting duct to resorb water. Combined V_{1a}/V_2 antagonists lead to a decrease in systemic vascular resistance and prevent the dilutional hyponatremia that occurs in HF patients.[24]

The AVP antagonists or "vaptans" (see Table 50.6) were developed to selectively block the V_2 receptor (e.g., tolvaptan, lixivaptan, satavaptan) or nonselectively block both the V_{1a}/V_2 receptors (e.g., conivaptan). All four AVP antagonists increase urine volume, decrease urine osmolarity, and have no effect on 24-hour sodium excretion (see also Chapter 49).[24] Long-term therapy with the V_2 selective vasopressin antagonist tolvaptan did not improve mortality but appears to be safe in patients with advanced HF.[25] Currently two vasopressin antagonists are Food and Drug Administration (FDA)-approved (conivaptan and tolvaptan) for the treatment of clinically significant hypervolemic and euvolemic hyponatremia (serum Na+ ≤125) that is symptomatic and which resisted correction with fluid restriction in patients with HF; however, neither of these agents is currently specifically approved for the treatment of HF. Use of these agents is appropriate after traditional measures to treat hyponatremia have been tried, including water restriction and maximization of medical therapies such as ACEIs or angiotensin receptor blockers (ARBs) which block or decrease angiotensin II. The use of vaptans in hospitalized HF patients is discussed in Chapter 49.

Diuretic Treatment of Heart Failure

Patients with evidence of volume overload or a history of fluid retention should be treated with a diuretic to relieve their symptoms. In symptomatic patients, diuretics should be always used in combination with neurohormonal antagonists that are known to prevent disease progression. When patients have moderate to severe symptoms or renal insufficiency, a loop diuretic is generally required. Diuretics should be initiated in low doses (see Table 50.6) and then titrated upward to relieve signs and symptoms of fluid overload. A typical starting dose of furosemide for patients with systolic HF and normal renal function is 40 mg, although doses of 80 to 160 mg are often necessary to achieve adequate diuresis. Loop diuretics have a sigmoidal dose-response curve. Importantly, in both HF and renal insufficiency, the dose response for loop diuretics shifts downward and to the right (Fig. 50.9A). Because of the steep dose-response curve and effective threshold for loop diuretics (see Fig. 50.9B), it is critical to find an adequate dose of loop diuretic that leads to a clear-cut diuretic response. One commonly employed method for finding the appropriate dose is to double the dose until the desired effect is achieved, or the maximal dose of diuretic is reached. Once patients have achieved an adequate diuresis, it is important to document their "dry weight" and make certain that patients weigh themselves daily in order to maintain their dry weight.

Although furosemide is the most commonly used loop diuretic, the oral bioavailability of furosemide is approximately 40% to 79%. Therefore, bumetanide or torsemide may be preferable because of their increased bioavailability. With the exception of torsemide, the commonly used loop diuretics are short-acting (<3 hours). For this reason, loop diuretics usually need to be given at least twice daily. Some patients may develop hypotension or azotemia during diuretic therapy. While the rapidity of diuresis should be slowed in these patients, diuretic therapy should be maintained at a lower level until the patient becomes euvolemic, insofar as persistent volume overload may compromise the effectiveness of some neurohormonal antagonists. Intravenous administration of diuretics may be necessary to relieve congestion acutely (see Fig. 50.9B and Chapter 49), and can be done safely in the outpatient setting. After a diuretic effect is achieved with short-acting loop diuretics, increasing administration frequency to twice or even three

SGLT2 inhibitors result in a 1:1 stoichiometric inhibition of sodium and glucose uptake in the proximal tubule of the kidney. This leads to contraction of the plasma volume and modest lowering of blood pressure, without activation of the sympathetic nervous system. The contraction of plasma volume may contribute to changes in markers of hemoconcentration with SGLT2 inhibitors, including increases in blood urea nitrogen and hematocrit, although the latter may also be on the basis of increased erythropoiesis. In addition, the proximal natriuresis that occurs with SGLT2 inhibition results in afferent arteriole vasoconstriction through tubulo-glomerular feedback, thereby reducing glomerular hyperfiltration (Fig. 50.8). Experimental studies showed that SGLT2 inhibitors reduced hyperfiltration and decreased inflammatory and fibrotic responses of proximal tubular cells.[23] Beyond effects on traditional cardiovascular risk factors such as HbA_{1c} and weight, SGLT2 inhibition also reduces plasma uric acid levels by 10% to 15% by increasing uricosuria via exchange of filtered glucose. Elevated uric acid levels have been implicated in worsening HF because of oxidative stress and inflammation.

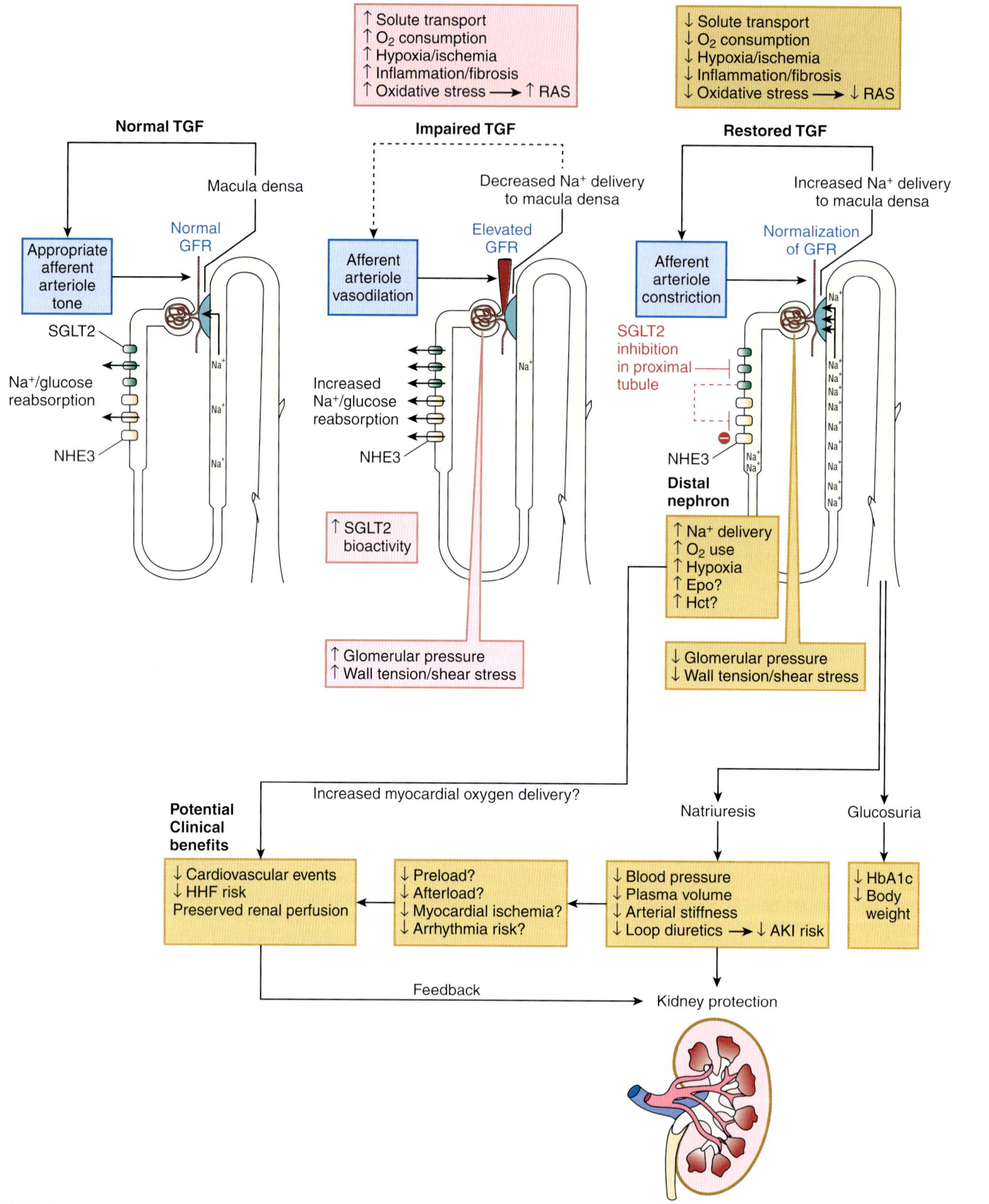

FIGURE 50.8 Selected physiologic mechanisms associated with cardiovascular and renal protection with sodium-glucose transporter-2 (SGLT2) inhibitors. Physiologic changes that occur in the setting of SGLT2 inhibitors, as well as their potential contribution to cardiovascular and renal protection, are depicted. *Red boxes* represent aberrant changes, whereas *yellow boxes* represent protective changes. *Small red circle with a white line* represents inhibition of function. *AKI*, Acute kidney injury; *Epo*, erythropoietin; *GFR*, glomerular filtration rate; *HbA1c*, glycosylated hemoglobin; *Hct*, hematocrit; *HHF*, hospitalization for heart failure; *Na+*, sodium; *NHE3*, sodium–hydrogen antiporter 3; *O2*, oxygen; *RAS*, renin-angiotensin system; *SGLT2*, sodium-glucose cotransporter-2; *TGF*, tubuloglomerular feedback. (From Cherney DZ, Odutayo A, Aronson R, et al. Sodium Glucose Cotransporter-2 Inhibition and Cardiorenal Protection. *J Am Coll Cardiol*. 2019;74[20]:2511–2524.)

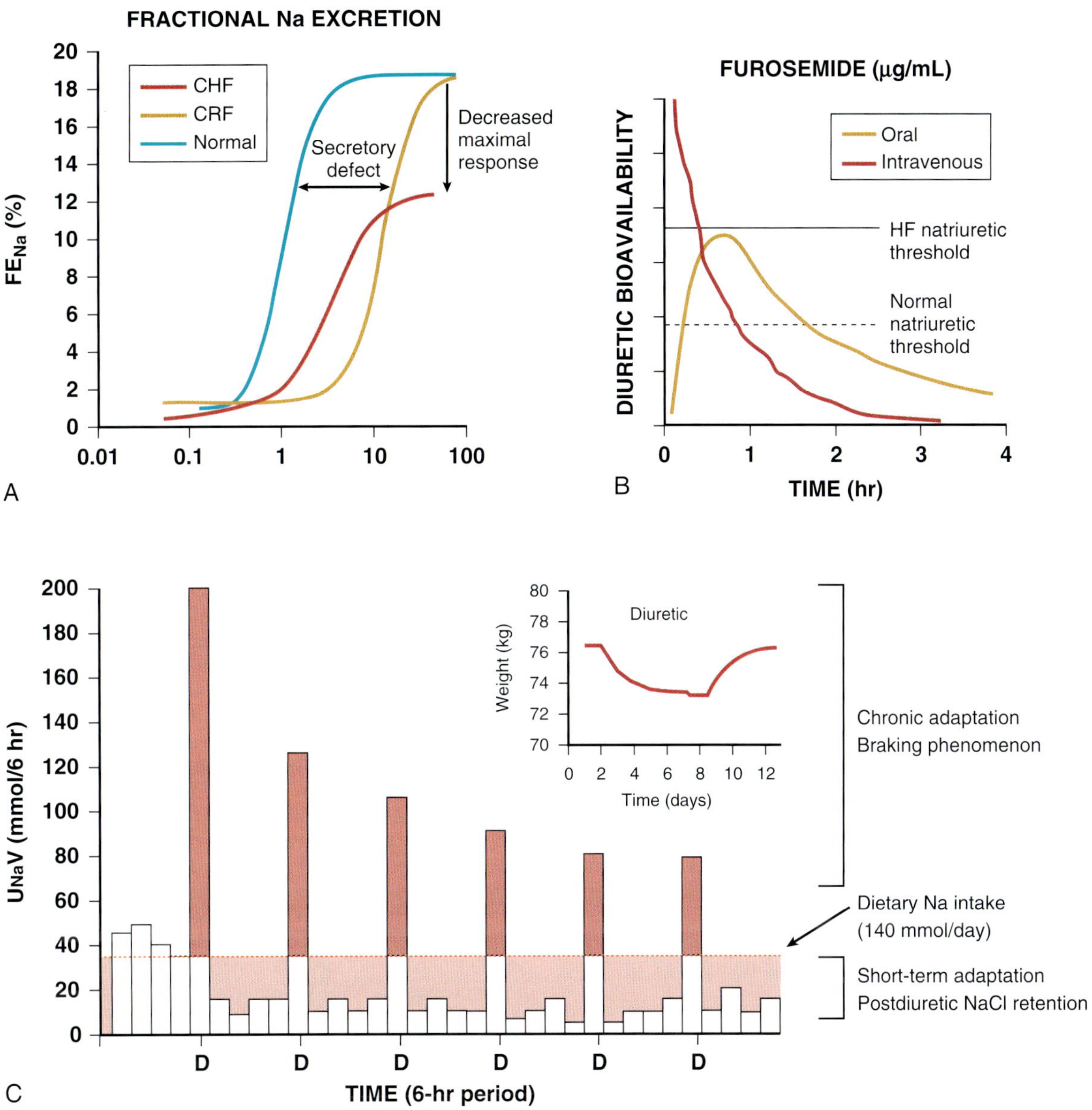

FIGURE 50.9 Pharmacokinetic and pharmacodynamic properties of loop diuretics. **A,** Dose-response curves of loop diuretics in normal patients versus patients with chronic renal failure (CRF) and chronic heart failure. **B,** Comparison of pharmacokinetics of oral versus intravenous loop diuretics (LD). **C,** An example of the braking phenomenon, whereby each additional dose of LD results in progressively less natriuresis. Each period of natriuresis is followed by a period of postdiuretic sodium retention. *ADHF*, Acute decompensated heart failure. **Inset**: effect of a diuretic on body weight, taken as an index of ECF volume. Note that steady state is reached within 6 to 8 days despite continued diuretic administration. (Modified from Ellison DH. Diuretic therapy and resistance in congestive heart failure. *Cardiology.* 2001;96:132-143.)

times per day will provide more diuresis with less physiologic perturbation than larger single doses. Once the congestion has been relieved, treatment with diuretics is continued to prevent the recurrence of salt and water retention in order to maintain the patient's ideal dry weight.

Complications of Diuretic Use

Patients with HF who are receiving diuretics should be monitored for complications of diuretics on a regular basis. The major complications of diuretic use include electrolyte and metabolic disturbances, volume depletion, as well as worsening azotemia. The interval for reassessment should be individualized based on severity of illness and underlying renal function, the use of concomitant medications such as ACEIs, ARBs and aldosterone antagonists, the past history of electrolyte imbalances, and/or need for more aggressive diuresis.

Electrolyte and Metabolic Disturbances

Diuretic use can lead to potassium depletion, which can predispose the patient to significant cardiac arrhythmias. Renal potassium losses from diuretic use can be also exacerbated by the increase in circulating levels of aldosterone observed in patients with advanced HF, as well by the marked increases in distal nephron Na^+ delivery that follow use of either loop or distal nephron diuretics. The level of dietary salt intake may also contribute to the extent of renal K^+ wasting with diuretics.

In the absence of formal guidelines with respect to the level of maintenance of serum K^+ levels in HF patients, many experienced HF clinicians have advocated that the serum K^+ should be maintained between 4.0 and 5.0 mEq/L because HF patients are often treated with pharmacologic agents that are likely to provoke proarrhythmic effects in the presence of hypokalemia (e.g., digoxin, type III antiarrhythmics, beta-agonists, or phosphodiesterase inhibitors). Hypokalemia can be prevented by increasing the oral intake of KCL. The normal daily dietary K^+ intake is approximately 40 to 80 mEq. Therefore, to increase this by 50% requires an additional 20 to 40 mEq K^+ supplementation daily. However, in the presence of alkalosis, hyperaldosteronism, or Mg^{2+} depletion, hypokalemia is quite unresponsive to increased dietary intake of KCL, and more aggressive replacement is necessary. If supplementation is necessary, oral potassium supplements in the form of KCL extended-release tablets or liquid concentrate should be used whenever possible. Intravenous potassium is potentially hazardous and should be avoided except in emergencies. Where appropriate, the use of an MRA may also prevent the development of hypokalemia.

The use of aldosterone-receptor antagonists is often associated with the development of life-threatening hyperkalemia, particularly when they are combined with ACEIs, ARBs, or angiotensin receptor-neprilysin inhibitors (ARNIs).[26] Potassium supplementation is generally stopped after the initiation of aldosterone antagonists, and patients should be counseled to avoid high potassium–containing foods. The management of acute hyperkalemia (>6.0 mEq/L) may require a short-term cessation of potassium-retaining agents and/or renin-angiotensin-aldosterone system (RAAS) inhibitors; however, RAAS inhibitors should be carefully reintroduced as soon as possible while monitoring potassium levels. Two new potassium binders, patiromer and sodium zirconium cyclosilicate, have been studied in HF patients with hyperkalemia. Patiromer is a nonabsorbed, cation-exchange polymer that contains a calcium-sorbitol counterion, and works by binding potassium in the lumen of the gastrointestinal tract, resulting in a reduction of serum-potassium levels within 7 hours of the first dose. Patiromer is FDA-approved for the treatment of hyperkalemia, but should not be used as an emergency treatment for life-threatening hyperkalemia because of its delayed onset of action. The initial clinical studies in patients with HF have shown that these therapies reduce serum potassium and prevent recurrent hyperkalemia in HF patients with chronic kidney disease who were receiving RAAS inhibitors.[27]

Diuretics may be associated with multiple other metabolic and electrolyte disturbances, including hyponatremia, hypomagnesemia, metabolic alkalosis, hyperglycemia, hyperlipidemia, and hyperuricemia. Hyponatremia is usually observed in HF patients with very high degrees of RAAS activation and/or AVP levels. Aggressive diuretic use can also lead to hyponatremia. Hyponatremia can typically be treated by more stringent water restriction. Both loop and thiazide diuretics can cause hypomagnesemia, which can aggravate muscle weakness and cardiac arrhythmias. Magnesium replacement should be administered for signs or symptoms of hypomagnesemia (arrhythmias, muscle cramps), and can be routinely given (with uncertain benefit) to all subjects receiving large doses of diuretics or requiring large amounts of K^+ replacement. The modest hyperglycemia and/or hyperlipidemia produced by thiazide diuretics is not usually clinically important, and blood glucose and lipids are usually easily controlled using standard practice guidelines. Metabolic alkalosis can generally be treated by increasing KCL supplementation, lowering diuretic doses, or transiently using acetazolamide.

Hypotension and Azotemia

The excessive use of diuretics can lead to a decreased blood pressure, decreased exercise tolerance, and increased fatigue, as well as impaired renal function. Hypotensive symptoms usually resolve after a decrease in the dose or frequency of diuretics in patients who are volume depleted. However, in most instances the use of diuretics is associated with decrease in blood pressure and/or mild azotemia that do not lead to patient symptoms. In this instance reductions in the diuretic dose are not necessary, particularly if the patient remains edematous. In some patients with advanced, chronic HF, elevated BUN and creatinine concentrations may be necessary to maintain control of congestive symptoms.

Neurohormonal Activation

Diuretics may increase the activation of endogenous neurohormonal systems in HF patients, which can lead to disease progression unless patients are receiving treatment with a concomitant neurohormonal antagonist (e.g., ACEI or beta-blocker).

Ototoxicity

Ototoxicity, which is more frequent with ethacrynic acid than the other loop diuretics, can manifest as tinnitus, hearing impairment, and deafness. Hearing impairment and deafness are usually, but not invariably, reversible. Ototoxicity occurs most frequently with rapid intravenous injections, and least frequently with oral administration.

Diuretic Resistance and Management

One of the inherent limitations of diuretics is that they achieve water loss via excretion of solute at the expense of glomerular filtration, which in turn activates a set of homeostatic mechanisms that ultimately limit their effectiveness. In normal subjects the magnitude of natriuresis following a given dose of diuretic declines over time as a result of the so-called "braking phenomenon" (see Fig. 50.9C). Studies have shown that the time-dependent decline in natriuresis for a given diuretic dose is critically dependent upon reduction of the extracellular fluid volume, which leads to an increase in solute and fluid reabsorption in the proximal tubule. In addition, contraction of the extracellular volume can lead to stimulation of efferent sympathetic nerves, which reduces urinary Na^+ excretion by reducing renal blood flow, stimulating renin (and ultimately aldosterone) release, which in turn stimulates Na^+ reabsorption along the nephron (see also Chapter 47). The magnitude of the natriuretic effect of potent loop diuretics may also decline in HF patients, particularly as HF progresses. Although the bioavailability of these diuretics is generally not decreased in HF, the potential delay in their rate of absorption may result in peak drug levels within the tubular lumen in the ascending loop of Henle that are insufficient to induce maximal natriuresis. The use of intravenous formulations may obviate this problem (see Chapter 49). However, even with intravenous dosing, a rightward shift of the dose-response curve is observed between the diuretic concentration in the tubular lumen and its natriuretic effect in HF (see Fig. 50.9A). Moreover, the maximal effect (ceiling) is lower in HF. This rightward shift has been referred to as "diuretic resistance" and is likely due to several factors in addition to the braking phenomenon described above. First, most loop diuretics (with the exception of torsemide) are short-acting drugs. Accordingly, after a period of natriuresis, the diuretic concentration in plasma and tubular fluid declines below the diuretic threshold. In this situation, renal Na^+ reabsorption is no longer inhibited and a period of antinatriuresis or postdiuretic NaCl retention ensues. If dietary NaCl intake is moderate to excessive, postdiuretic NaCl retention may overcome the initial natriuresis in patients with excessive activation of the adrenergic nervous system and RAS. This observation forms the rationale for administering short-acting diuretics several times per day to obtain consistent daily salt and water loss. Second, there is a loss of renal responsiveness to endogenous natriuretic peptides as HF advances (see Chapter 47). Third, diuretics increase solute delivery to distal segments of the nephron, causing epithelial cells to undergo both hypertrophy and hyperplasia. Although the diuretic-induced signals that initiate changes in distal nephron structure and function are not well understood, chronic loop diuretic administration increases the Na-K-ATPase activity in the distal collecting duct and cortical collecting tubule, as well as increases the number of thiazide-sensitive Na-Cl cotransporters in the distal nephron, which increases the solute resorptive capacity of the kidney as much as threefold.

In patients with HF an abrupt decline in cardiac and/or renal function or patient noncompliance with their diuretic regimen or diet may lead to diuretic resistance. Apart from these more obvious causes, it is important to query the patient with regard to the concurrent use of drugs that adversely affect renal function, such as NSAIDs and COX-2 inhibitors (see Table 50.5), and certain antibiotics (trimethoprim and gentamicin). The relative risk of increased HF hospitalization varies between individual NSAIDs; including a 1.16 (95% CI 1.07 to 1.27) increase for naproxen, a 1.18 (95% CI 1.12 to 1.23) increase for ibuprofen, a 1.19 (1.15 to 1.24) increase for diclofenac, and a 1.51 (95% 1.33 to 1.71) increase for indomethacin. The use of the COX-2 inhibitors, etoricoxib and rofecoxib, was also associated with increased risk of hospitalization.[28] The insulin-sensitizing thiazolidinediones (TZDs) have also been linked to increased fluid retention in patients with HF, although the clinical significance of this finding is not known. It has been suggested that TZDs activate proliferator-activated receptor-gamma expression in the renal collecting duct, which enhances expression of cell-surface epithelial Na^+ channels. Moreover, studies in healthy men have shown that pioglitazone stimulates plasma renin activity that may contribute to increased Na^+ retention. Rarely, drugs such as probenecid, or high plasma concentrations of some antibiotics, may compete with the organic ion transporters in the proximal tubule responsible for the transfer of most diuretics from the recirculation into the tubular lumen. The use of increasing doses of vasodilators, with or without a marked decline in intravascular volume as a result of concomitant diuretic therapy, may lower renal perfusion pressure below that necessary to maintain normal autoregulation and glomerular filtration in patients with RAS from atherosclerotic disease. Accordingly, a reduction in renal blood flow may occur despite an increase in cardiac output, thereby leading to a decrease in diuretic effectiveness.

A patient with HF may be considered to be resistant to diuretic drugs when moderate doses of a loop diuretic do not achieve the desired reduction of the extracellular fluid volume. In outpatients, a common and useful method for treating the diuretic-resistant patient is to administer two classes of diuretic concurrently. Adding a proximal tubule diuretic or a distal collecting tubule diuretic to a regimen of loop diuretics is often dramatically effective ("sequential nephron blockade"). As a general rule, when adding a second class of diuretic the dose of loop diuretic should not be altered, because the shape of the dose-response curve for loop diuretics is not affected by the addition of other diuretics, and the loop diuretic must be given at an effective dose for it to be effective. The combination of loop and distal collecting tubule diuretics has been shown to be effective through several mechanisms.[29] One is that distal collecting tubule diuretics have longer half-lives than loop diuretics and may thus prevent or attenuate postdiuretic NaCl retention. A second mechanism by which distal collecting tubule diuretics potentiate the effects of loop diuretics is by inhibiting Na^+ transport along the proximal tubule, insofar as most thiazide diuretics also inhibit carbonic anhydrase. They also inhibit NaCl transport along the distal renal tubule, which may counteract the increased solute resorptive effects of the hypertrophied and hyperplastic distal epithelial cells.

The selection of a distal collecting tubule diuretic to use as second diuretic is a matter of choice. Many clinicians choose metolazone because its half-life is longer than that of some other distal collecting tubule diuretics, and because it has been reported to remain effective even when the glomerular filtration rate is low. However, direct comparisons between metolazone and several traditional thiazides have shown little difference in natriuretic potency when they are included in a regimen with loop diuretics in HF patients.[30] Distal collecting tubule diuretics may be added in full doses (50 to 100 mg/day hydrochlorothiazide or 2.5 to 10 mg/day metolazone; see Table 50.6) when a rapid and robust response is needed. However, such an approach is likely to lead to excessive fluid and electrolyte depletion if patients are not followed up extremely closely. One reasonable approach to combination therapy is to achieve control of fluid overload by initially adding full doses of distal collecting tubule diuretic on a daily basis and then decreasing the dose of this diuretic to three times weekly to avoid excessive diuresis. An alternative strategy in hospitalized patients is to administer the same daily parenteral dose of a loop diuretic by continuous intravenous infusion, which leads to sustained natriuresis because of the continuous presence of high drug levels within the tubular lumen (see also Chapter 49), and avoids postdiuretic ("rebound") resorption of Na^+ (see Fig. 50.9C). This approach requires the use of a constant-infusion pump but permits more precise control of the natriuretic effect achieved over time, particularly in carefully monitored patients. It also diminishes the potential for a too-rapid decline in intravascular volume and hypotension as well as the risk of ototoxicity in patients given large bolus intravenous doses of a loop diuretic. A typical continuous furosemide is initiated with a 20- to 40-mg intravenous loading dose as a bolus injection, followed by a continuous infusion of 5 to 10 mg/hr for a patient who had been receiving 200 mg of oral furosemide per day in divided doses. The Diuretic Optimal Strategy Evaluation in Acute Heart Failure (DOSE) study showed that there was no significant difference in patient symptoms or renal function when patients with acute decompensated HF were treated with an IV bolus of furosemide compared to IV infusion of furosemide (see Chapter 49), suggesting that whichever approach is most likely to reliably produce the desired dieresis should be used.

Another common reason for diuretic resistance in advanced HF is the development of the cardiorenal syndrome (see also Chapters 49 and 101), which is recognized clinically as worsening renal function that limits diuresis in patients with obvious clinical volume overload.[31] In patients with advanced HF the cardiorenal syndrome is frequently present in patients who have repeated HF hospitalizations, and in whom adequate diuresis is difficult to obtain because of worsening indices of renal function. This impairment in renal function often is dismissed as "pre-renal"; however, when measured carefully, neither cardiac output nor renal perfusion pressure have been shown to be reduced in diuretic-treated patients who develop cardiorenal syndrome. Importantly, worsening indices of renal function contribute to longer hospital stays, and predict higher rates of early rehospitalization and death.[32] The mechanisms for and treatment of the cardiorenal syndrome remain poorly understood.

Device-Based Therapies for Management of Fluid Status (See also Chapter 58)

The use of mechanical methods of fluid removal, such as extracorporeal ultrafiltration (UF), may be needed to achieve adequate control of fluid retention, particularly in patients who become resistant and/or refractory to diuretic therapy. Extracorporeal UF removes salt and water isotonically by driving the patient's blood through a highly permeable filter via an extracorporeal circuit in an arteriovenous or venovenous mode. Alternative extracorporeal methods include continuous hemofiltration, continuous hemodialysis, or continuous hemodiafiltration. With slow continuous UF, the patient's intravascular fluid volume remains stable as fluid shifts from the extravascular space into the intravascular space, with the result that there is no deleterious activation of neurohormonal systems. UF has been shown to reduce right atrial and pulmonary artery wedge pressures and increase cardiac output, diuresis, and natriuresis without changes in heart rate, systolic blood pressure, renal function, electrolytes, or intravascular volume.[33]

The Relief for Acutely Fluid-Overloaded Patients With Decompensated Congestive Heart Failure (RAPID-CHF) trial, which was the first randomized controlled trial of UF for acute decompensated HF, enrolled 40 patients who were randomized to receive either usual care (diuretic) or a single 8-hour UF (using a proprietary device) in addition to usual care. The primary endpoint was weight loss 24 hours after enrollment. Fluid removal after 24 hours was approximately twofold greater in the UF group.[33] The Ultrafiltration versus IV Diuretics for Patients Hospitalized for Acute Decompensated Congestive Heart Failure (UNLOAD) compared the long-term safety and efficacy of UF therapy (using a proprietary device) to intravenous diuretics in a multicenter trial involving 200 patients, who were assessed at entry and at intervals out to 90 days. The primary endpoint was total weight loss during the first 48 hours of randomization and the change in dyspnea score during the first 48 hours of randomization. Although the two treatments were similar in their ability to relieve dyspnea, UF was associated with significantly greater fluid loss over 48 hours and a lower rate of rehospitalization during the next 90 days.[33] The use of UF in high-risk patients who are developing the cardiorenal syndrome was explored in the Cardiorenal Rescue Study in Acute Decompensated HF (CARRESS) trial, which showed that UF resulted in similar weight loss, but resulted in an increase in creatinine levels, compared to standard care, and was associated with more serious adverse events and intravenous catheter-related complications (see Chapter 49).[33]

Given the cost, need for venous access, and the nursing support necessary to implement UF, this intervention will require additional studies to determine its role in the management of volume overload in HF patients. In addition to extracorporeal methods for relieving volume overload, peritoneal dialysis can be used as a viable alternative therapy for the short-term management of refractory congestive symptoms for patients in whom vascular access cannot be obtained, or for whom appropriate extracorporeal therapies are not available.

PREVENTION OF DISEASE PROGRESSION (TABLE 50.7 AND FIG. 50.10)

Drugs that interfere with the excessive activation of renin angiotensin-aldosterone system and the adrenergic nervous system can relieve the symptoms of HFrEF patients by stabilizing and/or reversing LV remodeling (see Chapter 47). In this regard ACEIs/ARBs and beta-blockers have emerged as cornerstones of modern HF therapy for patients with a depressed EF (see Fig. 50.10).

Angiotensin-Converting Enzyme Inhibitors

There is overwhelming evidence that ACEIs should be used in symptomatic and asymptomatic patients with a reduced EF (<40%) (class I indication). ACEIs interfere with the renin angiotensin system by inhibiting the enzyme that is responsible for the conversion of angiotensin I to angiotensin II (see Chapter 47). However, because ACEIs also inhibit kininase II, they may lead to the upregulation of bradykinin, which may further enhance the effects of angiotensin suppression. ACEIs stabilize

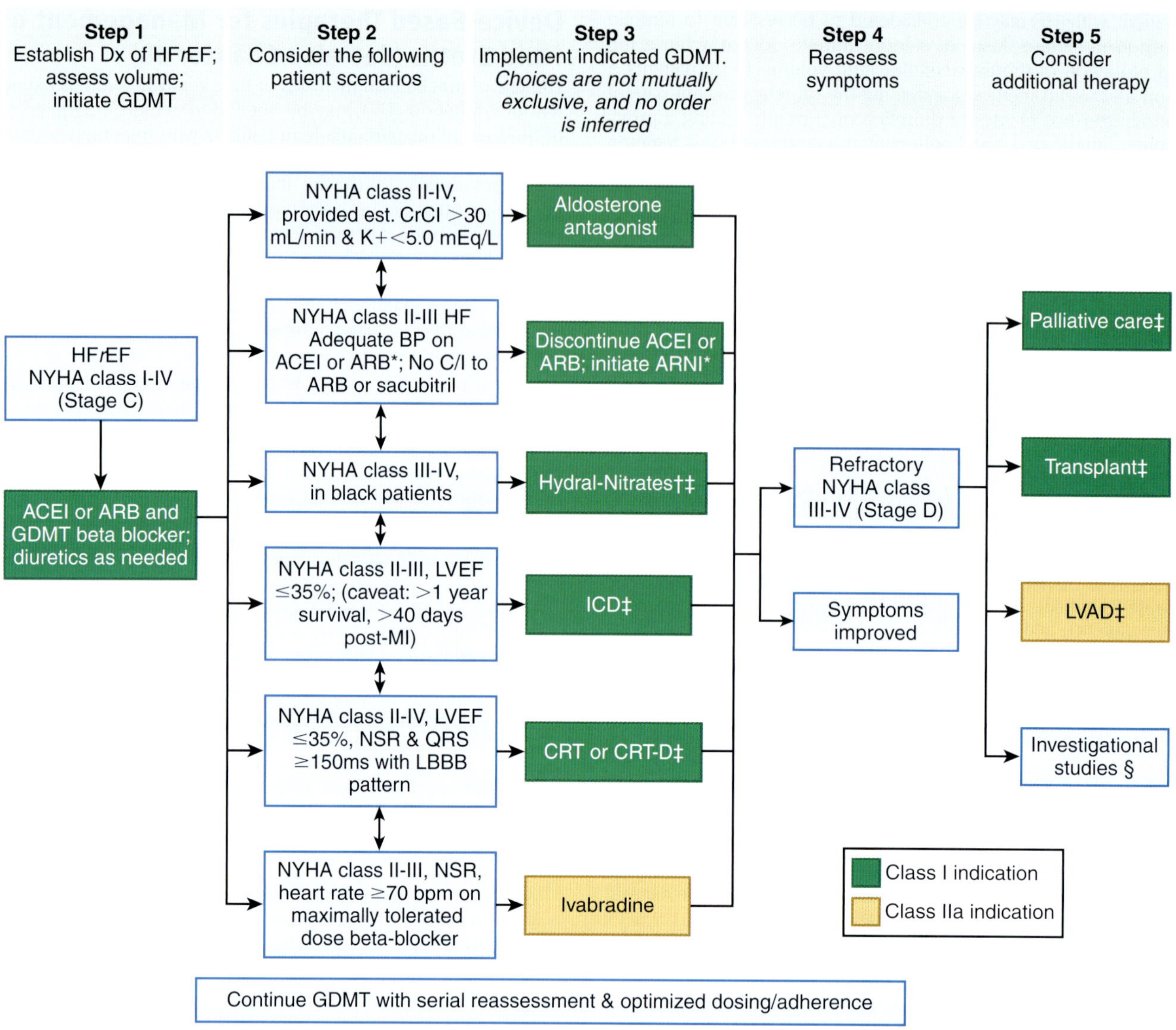

FIGURE 50.10 Treatment algorithm Stage C and D heart failure with a reduced ejection fraction. For all medical therapies, dosing should be optimized and serial assessment exercised. See text for details. (Key: *See text for important treatment directions. †**Hydral-Nitrates green box**: The combination of ISDN/HYD with ARNI has not been robustly tested. BP response should be carefully monitored. ‡See 2013 ACC/AH heart failure guidelines. §Participation in investigational studies is also appropriate for stage C, NYHA class II and III HF. *ACEI,* Angiotensin-converting enzyme inhibitor; *ARB,* angiotensin receptor blocker; *ARNI,* angiotensin receptor neprilysin inhibitor; *BP,* blood pressure; *bpm,* beats per minute; *C/I,* contraindication; *CrCl,* creatinine clearance; *CRT-D,* cardiac resynchronization therapy–device; *Dx,* diagnosis; *GDMT,* guideline-directed management and therapy; *HF,* heart failure; *HFrEF,* heart failure with reduced ejection fraction; *ICD,* implantable cardioverter-defibrillator; *ISDN/HYD,* isosorbide dinitrate hydral-nitrates; *K+,* potassium; *LBBB,* left bundle branch block; *LVAD,* left ventricular assist device; *LVEF,* left ventricular ejection fraction; *MI,* myocardial infarction; *NSR,* normal sinus rhythm; *NYHA,* New York Heart Association. (Modified from Yancy CW, Jessup M, Bozkurt B, et al. 2017 ACC/AHA/HFSA Focused Update of the 2013 ACCF/AHA Guideline for the Management of Heart Failure: A Report of the American College of Cardiology/American Heart Association Task Force on Clinical Practice Guidelines and the Heart Failure Society of America. *J Am Coll Cardiol.* 2017;70:776–803.)

LV remodeling, improve patient symptoms, prevent hospitalization, and prolong life. Because fluid retention can attenuate the effects of ACEIs, it is preferable to optimize the dose of diuretic first, before starting the ACEI. However, it may be necessary to reduce the dose of diuretic during the initiation of an ACEI, in order to prevent symptomatic hypotension. ACEIs should be initiated in low doses, followed by increments in dose if lower doses have been well tolerated. Titration is generally achieved by doubling doses every 3 to 5 days. The dose of ACEI should be increased until the doses used are similar to those that have been shown to be effective in clinical trials (see Table 50.7). Higher doses are more effective than lower doses in preventing hospitalization. For stable patients, it is acceptable to add therapy with beta-blocking agents before full target doses of either ACEIs are reached. Blood pressure (including postural changes), renal function, and potassium should be evaluated within 1 to 2 weeks after initiation of ACEIs, especially in patients with preexisting azotemia, hypotension, hyponatremia, diabetes mellitus, or in those taking potassium supplements. Abrupt withdrawal of treatment with an ACEI may lead to clinical deterioration and should, therefore, be avoided in the absence of life-threatening complications (e.g., angioedema, hyperkalemia).

The efficacy of ACEIs has been consistently demonstrated in clinical trials with patients with asymptomatic and symptomatic LV dysfunction (Fig. 50.11).[9,15] These trials recruited a broad variety of patients, including women and the elderly, as well as patients with a wide range of causes and severity of LV dysfunction. The consistency of data from the Studies on Left Ventricular Dysfunction (SOLVD) Prevention Study, Survival and Ventricular Enlargement (SAVE), and the Trandolapril Cardiac Evaluation (TRACE) has shown that asymptomatic patients with LV dysfunction will have less development of symptomatic HF and hospitalizations (Table 50.8) when treated with an ACEI. ACEIs have also consistently shown benefit for patients with symptomatic LV dysfunction. As shown in Table 50.8, all placebo-controlled chronic HF trials have demonstrated a reduction in mortality. Further, the absolute benefit is greatest in patients with the most severe HF. Indeed, the patients with NYHA class IV HF in the Cooperative North Scandinavian Enalapril Survival Study (CONSENSUS I) had a much larger effect size than the SOLVD Treatment Trial, which in turn had a larger effect size than the SOLVD Prevention Trial. Although only three placebo-controlled mortality trials

TABLE 50.7 Drugs for the Prevention and Treatment for Chronic Heart Failure

	INITIATING DOSE	MAXIMAL DOSE
Angiotensin-Converting Enzyme Inhibitors		
Captopril	6.25 mg 3 times	50 mg 3 times
Enalapril	2.5 mg twice	10 mg twice
Lisinopril	2.5–5.0 mg once	20 mg once
Ramipril	1.25–2.5 mg once	10 mg once
Fosinopril	5–10 mg once	40 mg once
Quinapril	5 mg twice	40 mg twice
Trandolapril	0.5 mg once	4 mg once
Angiotensin Receptor Blockers		
Valsartan	40 mg twice	160 mg twice
Candesartan	4–8 mg once	32 mg once
Losartan	12.5–25 mg once	50 mg once
Angiotensin Receptor Neprilysin Inhibitor		
Sacubitril/Valsartan	24 mg/26 mg 2 times daily***	97 mg/103 mg 2 times daily***
Beta-Receptor Blockers		
Carvedilol	3.125 mg twice	25 mg twice (50 mg twice if >85 kg)
Carvedilol-CR	10 mg once	80 mg once
Bisoprolol	1.25 mg twice	10 mg once
Metoprolol succinate CR	12.5–25 mg qd	target dose 200 mg qd
Mineralocorticoid Receptor Antagonists		
Spironolactone	12.5–25 mg once	25–50 mg once
Eplerenone	25 mg once	50 mg once
Other Agents		
Combination of hydralazine/isosorbide dinitrate	25 to 50 mg/10 mg 3 times	100 mg/40 mg 3 times
Fixed dose of hydralazine/isosorbide dinitrate	37.5 mg/20 mg (one tablet) 3 times	75 mg/40 mg (two tablets) 3 times
Digoxin*	0.125 mg qd	≤0.375 mg/day**
Ivabradine	5 mg twice daily	7.5 mg twice daily

*Dosing should be based on ideal body weight, age, and renal function.
**Trough level should be 0.5 to 1 ng/mL though absolute levels have not established.
***(mg sacubitril/mg valsartan).
Modified from Mann DL. Heart Failure and Cor Pulmonale, In: Kasper DL, et al., eds. *Harrison's Principles of Internal Medicine*. 17th ed. New York: McGraw-Hill; 2007:1449.

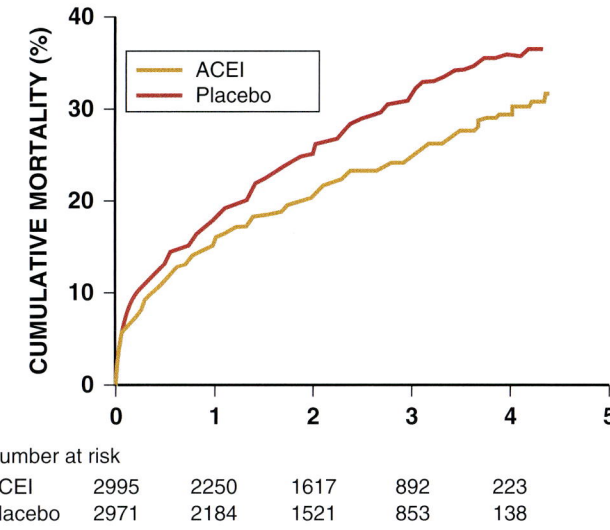

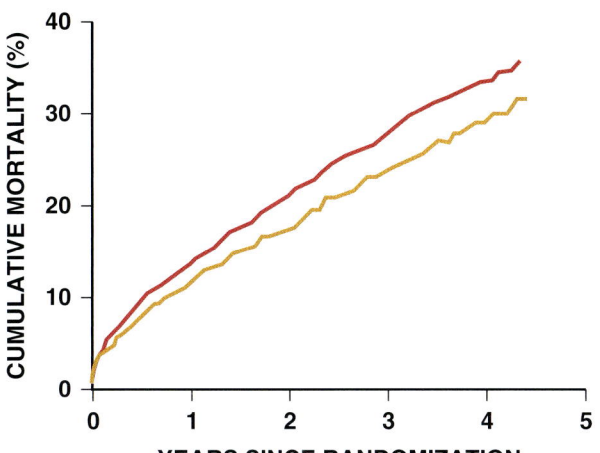

FIGURE 50.11 Meta-analysis of angiotensin-converting enzyme inhibitors (ACEI) in heart failure with reduced ejection fraction (HFrEF). **A,** Kaplan-Meier curves for mortality for patients with HF with a depressed EF treated with an ACEI following acute myocardial infarction (three trials). **B,** Kaplan-Meier curves for mortality for patients with HF with a depressed EF treated with an ACEI in five clinical trials, including post-infarction trials. The benefits of ACEI were observed early and persisted long term. (Modified from Flather MD, Yusuf S, Køber L, et al. Long-term ACE-inhibitor therapy in patients with heart failure or left-ventricular dysfunction: a systematic overview of data from individual patients. ACE-Inhibitor Myocardial Infarction Collaborative Group. *Lancet*. 2000;355:1575–1580.)

have been conducted in patients with chronic HFrEF, the aggregate data suggest that ACEIs reduce mortality in direct relation to the degree of severity of chronic HF. The Vasodilator in Heart Failure II (V-HeFT-II) trial provided evidence that ACEIs improve the natural history of HF through mechanisms other than vasodilation, inasmuch as subjects treated with enalapril had significantly lower mortality than subjects treated with the vasodilatory combination of hydralazine plus isosorbide dinitrate (which does not directly inhibit neurohormonal systems). Although enalapril is the only ACEI that has been used in placebo-controlled mortality trials in chronic HF, as shown in Table 50.8, multiple ACEIs have proven to be more or less equally effective when administered in oral form within the first week of the ischemic event in MI trials. ACEIs markedly enhance survival in patients with signs or symptoms of HF after MI. In addition to these effects on mortality, ACEIs improve the functional status of patients with HF. In contrast, ACEIs only produce small benefits in exercise capacity. Taken together, these observations support the conclusion that the effects of ACEIs on the natural history of chronic HF, post-MI LV dysfunction, or patients at high risk of developing HF represent a "class effects" of these agents. Nonetheless, it should be emphasized that patients with a low blood pressure (<90 mm Hg systolic), or impaired renal function (serum creatinine >2.5 mg/mL) were not recruited and/or represent a small proportion of patients who participated in these trials. Thus, the efficacy of these agents for these latter patient populations is less well established.

Side Effects of Angiotensin-Converting Enzyme Inhibitor Use

The majority of the adverse effects of ACEIs are related to suppression of the renin angiotensin system. The decreases in blood pressure and mild azotemia often seen during the initiation of therapy are, in general, well tolerated and do not require a decrease in the dose of the ACEI. However, if hypotension is accompanied by dizziness or if the

TABLE 50.8 Mortality Rates in Placebo-Controlled Trials Conducted in Patients with Chronic Heart Failure (EF < 40%) or Patients with Acute Myocardial Infarction or at Risk for Heart Failure

TRIAL NAME	AGENT	NYHA CLASS	NO. OF SUBJECTS ENROLLED	12-MONTH PLACEBO MORTALITY (%)	12-MONTH EFFECT SIZE (%)	P VALUE 12 MONTHS (FULL F/U)
Angiotensin-Converting Enzyme Inhibitors						
Heart Failure						
CONSENSUS-1	Enalapril	IV	253	52	↓31	0.01 (0.0003)
SOLVD-Rx	Enalapril	I-III	2569	15	↓21	0.02 (0.004)
SOLVD-Asx	Enalapril	I, II	4228	5	0	0.82 (0.30)
Post–Myocardial Infarction						
SAVE	Captopril	—	2231	12	↓18	0.11 (0.02)
AIRE	Ramipril	—	1986	20	↓22	0.01 (0.002)
TRACE	Trandolapril	—	1749	26	↓16	0.046 (0.001)
Angiotensin Receptor Blockers						
Heart Failure						
VAL-HeFT	Valsartan	II-IV	5010	9	0	NS (0.80)
CHARM-Alternative	Candesartan	II-IV	2028	NS	NS	NS (0.02)
CHARM-Added	Candesartan	II-IV	2547	NS	NS	NS (0.11)
HEAAL	Losartan	II-IV	3846	NS	NS	NS (0.24)
Post–Myocardial Infarction						
VALIANT	Valsartan	—	14,703	19.5*	NS	NA (0.98)**
Angiotensin Receptor Neprilysin Inhibitors						
PARADIGM	Sacubitril/Valsartan	II-IV	8442	NS	NS	NS ($P < 0.001$)
Mineralocorticoid Receptor Antagonists						
Heart Failure						
RALES	Spironolactone	III, IV	1663	24	↓25	NS (<0.001)
EMPHASIS	Eplerenone	II	2737	9	NS	NS (< 0.01)
Post–Myocardial Infarction						
EPHESUS	Eplerenone	I	6632	12	↓15	NS (0.005)
Beta-blockers						
Heart Failure						
CIBIS-I	Bisoprolol	III, IV	641	21	↓20***	NS (0.22)
U.S. Carvedilol	Carvedilol	II, III	1094	8	↓66***	NS (< 0.001)
ANZ—Carvedilol	Carvedilol	I,II,II	415	NS	NS	NS (> 0.1)
CIBIS-II	Bisoprolol	III, IV	2647	12	↓34***	NS (0.001)
MERIT-HF	Metoprolol CR	II-IV	3991	10	↓35***	NS (0.006)
BEST	Bucindolol	III, IV	2708	23	↓10***	NS (0.16)
COPERNICUS	Carvedilol	Severe	2289	28	↓38***	NS (0.0001)
Post–Myocardial Infarction						
CAPRICORN	Carvedilol	I	1959	NS	↓23*	NS (0.03)
BEAT	Bucindolol	I	343		↓12*	NS (0.06)

*In VALIANT the compactor group was enalapril; **Reflects differences between valsartan and enalapril; ***Effect size at the conclusion of the trial.

Note: Twelve-month mortality rates were taken from the survival curves when data were not directly available in published material.

AIRE, Acute Infarction Ramipril Efficacy; *BEAT*, bucindolol evaluation in acute myocardial infarction trial; *BEST*, Beta Blocker Evaluation of Survival Trial; *CAPRICORN*, Carvedilol Post-Infarct Survival Control in Left Ventricular Dysfunction; *CHARM*, candesartan in heart failure-assessment of reduction in mortality and morbidity; *CHF*, congestive heart failure; *CIBIS*, Cardiac Insufficiency Bisoprolol Study; *CONSENSUS*, Cooperative North Scandinavian Enalapril Survival Study; *COPERNICUS*, Carvedilol Prospective Randomized Cumulative Survival; *EPHESUS*, Eplerenone Post-Acute Myocardial Infarction Heart Failure Efficacy and Survival Study; *HEEAL*, Heart Failure Endpoint Evaluation of Angiotensin II Antagonist Losartan; *MERIT-HF*, Metoprolol CR/XL Randomized Interventional Trial in Congestive Heart Failure; *MI*, myocardial infarction; *MRAs*, mineralocorticoid receptor antagonists; *NS*, not specified; *NYHA*, New York Heart Association; *PARADIGM*, Prospective comparison of ARNI with ACEI to Determine Impact on Global Mortality and morbidity in Heart Failure trial; *RALES*, Randomized Aldactone Evaluation Study; *SAVE*, Survival and Ventricular Enlargement; *SOLVD*, Studies of Left Ventricular Dysfunction; *TRACE*, Trandolapril Cardiac Evaluation; *Val-HeFT*, Valsartan Heart Failure Trial; *VALIANT*, Valsartan in Acute Myocardial Infarction Trial.

Modified from Bristow MR, Linas S, Port DJ. Drugs in the treatment of heart failure. In: Zipes DP, et al., eds. *Braunwald's Heart Disease*. 7th ed. Philadelphia: Elsevier, 2004:573.

renal dysfunction becomes severe, it may be necessary to decrease the dose of the diuretic if significant fluid retention is not present, or alternatively decrease the dose of the ACEI if significant fluid retention is present. Potassium retention may also become problematic if the patient is receiving potassium supplements or a potassium-sparing diuretic. Potassium retention that is not responsive to these measures may require a reduction in the dose of ACEI. The side effects of ACEIs that are related to kinin potentiation include a nonproductive cough (10% to 15% of patients) and angioedema (1% of patients). In patients who cannot tolerate ACEIs because of cough or angioedema, ARBs are the next recommended line of therapy. Patients intolerant to ACEIs because of hyperkalemia or renal insufficiency are likely to experience the same side effects with ARBs. The combination of hydralazine and an oral nitrate should be considered for these latter patients (see Table 50.7).

Angiotensin Receptor Blockers

ARBs (see Table 50.7) are well tolerated in patients who are intolerant of ACEIs because of cough, skin rash, and angioedema and should, therefore, be used in symptomatic and asymptomatic patients with an EF less than 40% who are ACE intolerant for reasons other than hyperkalemia or renal insufficiency (class I indication). Although ACEIs and ARBs inhibit RAAS, they do so by a different mechanism. Whereas ACEIs block the enzyme responsible for converting angiotensin I to angiotensin II, ARBs block the effects of angiotensin II on the angiotensin type 1 receptor (see Chapter 47), the receptor subtype that is responsible for virtually all the adverse biological effects relevant to a angiotensin II on cardiac remodeling (see Chapter 47). Multiple ARBs are available to clinicians for the treatment of HFrEF. Three of these, losartan, valsartan, and candesartan, have been extensively evaluated in the setting of HFrEF (see Table 50.7). ARBs should be initiated with the starting doses shown in Table 50.7, which can be up-titrated every 3 to 5 days by doubling the dose of ARB. As with ACEIs, blood pressure, renal function, and potassium should be reassessed within 1 to 2 weeks after initiation and followed closely after changes in dose.

> In symptomatic HFrEF patients who were intolerant to ACE inhibitors the aggregate clinical data suggest that ARBs are as effective as ACEIs in reducing HF morbidity and mortality. Candesartan significantly reduced all-cause mortality, cardiovascular death, or hospital admission in the Candesartan Heart Failure: Assessment of Reduction in Mortality and Morbidity trial (CHARM-Alternative Trial).[9,15] Importantly candesartan reduced all-cause mortality, irrespective of background ACE-inhibitor or beta-blocker therapy. Similar findings were shown with valsartan in the small subgroup of patients not receiving an ACE inhibitor in the Valsartan Heart Failure Trial (Val-Heft). A direct comparison of ACEI and ARBs was assessed in the Losartan Heart Failure Survival Study (ELITE-II), which showed that although losartan did not improve survival in elderly HF patients when compared to captopril, losartan was significantly better tolerated. The question of the impact of high-dose versus low-dose ARB antagonism in ACEI-intolerant patients was evaluated in the Heart Failure Endpoint Evaluation of Angiotensin II Antagonist Losartan (HEAAL) trial.[34] During 4.7 years of follow-up, high-dose losartan (150 mg daily) was superior to low-dose losartan (50 mg daily) for the composite outcome of death or admission for heart failure (HR 0.90; 95% CI 0.82 to 0.99; (p = 0.027). Although there were more side effects with high-dose losartan, these adverse events infrequently led to discontinuation of therapy, suggesting that up-titration of ARBs may confer clinical benefit in HFrEF patients.
>
> One large trial evaluated ARB compared to ACEI in post-MI patients who developed LV dysfunction or signs of HF. The Valsartan in Acute Myocardial Infarction Trial (VALIANT) compared losartan, captopril, and the combination of the two agents on mortality in patients with MI complicated by LV systolic dysfunction, HF or both. During a follow-up period of 24.7 months, there was no significant difference in all-cause mortality in the valsartan group as compared with the captopril group (HR 1.00; 97.5 CI 0.90 to 1.11), nor was there a significant difference in all-cause mortality in the valsartan-captopril group when compared to the captopril group (HR 0.98; 97.5% CI 0.89 to 1.09; P = 0.73). Non-inferiority testing showed that valsartan was noninferior to captopril with respect to mortality (P = 0.004).[9,15] Two large HFrEF trials compared ACEI and ARB versus ACE inhibitor alone. In the CHARM-Added trial, the addition of candesartan to ACE inhibitor led to a reduction in the primary outcome of CV death or HF hospitalization (HR 0.85; 95% CI: 0.75 to 0.96).[34] However, the addition of candesartan to an ACE inhibitor resulted in an increase in the incidence of hyperkalemia increased from 0.7% to 3.4%. The addition of valsartan to an ACEI had no beneficial effect on mortality in the Valsartan Heart Failure Trial (Val-HeFT) when compared to placebo, whereas the combined endpoint of mortality and morbidity was significantly (13.2%) lower with valsartan than with placebo because of a reduction in the number of patients hospitalized for HF.[34] The interpretation of both of these trials is confounded by the observation that the dose of ACEI in the placebo may have been suboptimal.

Although one meta-analysis suggests that ARBs and ACEIs have similar effects on all-cause mortality and HF hospitalizations,[35] and although ARBs may be considered as initial therapy rather than ACEIs following MI, the ACC/AHA/HFSA guidelines recommend that ACE inhibitors remain first line therapy (class I indication) for the treatment of HFrEF, whereas ARBs were recommended for ACE-intolerant patients (class IIa indication).[9,15] The guidelines also indicate that ARBs may be considered in persistently symptomatic patients with HFrEF who are already being treated with an ACE inhibitor and a beta-blocker in whom an aldosterone antagonist is not indicated or tolerated (class IIb indication).[9]

Side Effects of Angiotensin Receptor Blocker Use

Both ACEIs and ARBs have similar effects on blood pressure, renal function, and potassium. Therefore, the problems of symptomatic hypotension, azotemia, and hyperkalemia will be similar for both of these agents. Although less frequent that with ACEIs, angioedema has also been reported in some patients who receive ARBs. In patients who are intolerant to ACEIs and ARBs, the combined use of hydralazine and isosorbide dinitrate (H-ISDN) may be considered as a therapeutic option in such patients (see Table 50.7). However, compliance with this combination has generally been poor because of the large number of tablets required and the high incidence of adverse reactions.

Angiotensin Receptor Neprilysin Inhibitors

A new therapeutic class of agents that antagonize RAAS and inhibit the neutral endopeptidase system has been developed recently. The first-in-class therapeutic agent is a molecule that combines valsartan (an AT1 receptor antagonist) with sacubitril (a neprilysin inhibitor) in a 1:1 mixture. The combination of an ARNI slows the degradation of natriuretic peptides, bradykinin and adrenomedullin, thereby enhancing diuresis, natriuresis and myocardial relaxation, as well as inhibiting renin and aldosterone secretion., while selectively blocking the AT1-receptor reduces vasoconstriction, sodium, and water retention and myocardial hypertrophy (see Chapter 47).[36] In the Prospective comparison of ARNI with ACEI to Determine Impact on Global Mortality and morbidity in Heart Failure trial (PARADIGM-HF) trial,[37] the use of fixed dose sacubitril/valsartan resulted in striking reductions in all-cause mortality, cardiovascular mortality, and HF hospitalizations when compared with the use of an ACE inhibitor (enalapril) alone in patents with mild to moderate HF (NYHA class II to IV; LVEF ≤35%) (Fig. 50.12) that was characterized by either mildly elevated natriuretic peptide levels (BNP greater than 150 pg/mL or NT-proBNP ≥ 600 pg/mL), or a prior hospitalization in the preceding 12 months and elevated natriuretic peptide levels (BNP ≥100 pg/mL or NT-proBNP ≥400 pg/mL) who were also able to tolerate both a target dose of enalapril (10 mg twice daily) and then subsequently sacubitril/valsartan (200 mg twice daily). ARNIs should be administered in low doses (sacubitril 24 mg/valsartan 26 mg twice daily) in ACEI/ARB naïve patients, or at moderate doses (sacubitril 49 mg/valsartan 51 mg twice daily) in patients who are tolerating ACEIs/ARBs. The target dose of sacubitril/valsartan in PARADIGM-HF was 97/103 mg twice daily. Although the most recent update of the ACC/AHA/HFSA guidelines do not recommend starting HFrEF patients on ARNIs (see Fig. 50.10), in patients with chronic HFrEF NYHA class II or III who are tolerating an ACE inhibitor or an ARB, ARNIs are recommended as a replacement to further reduce morbidity and mortality (class I indication).[12] Given that less than 1% of the patients in the PARADIGM-HF had NYHA class IV HF, ARNIs are not currently recommended for patients with advanced HF symptomatology.

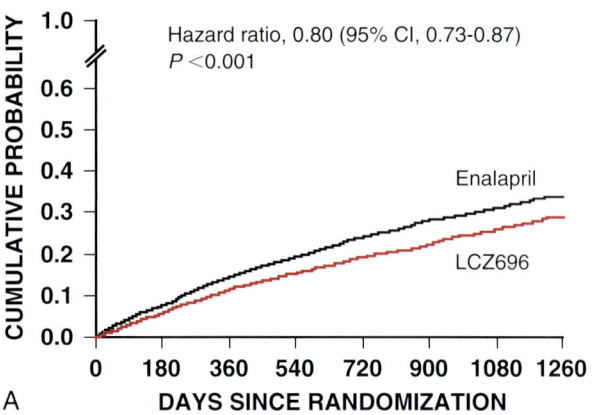
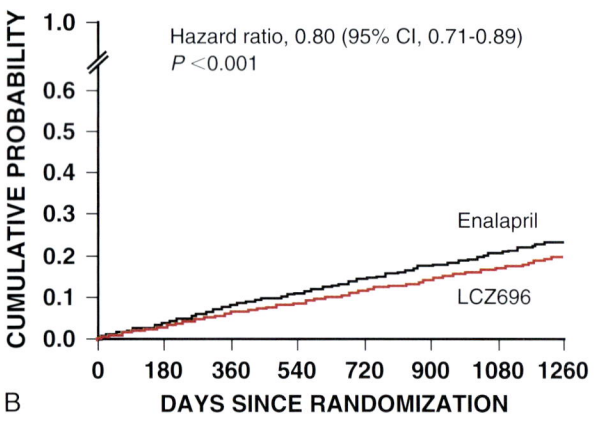
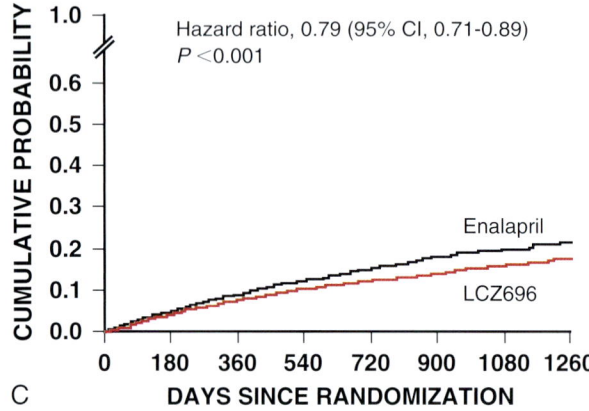

FIGURE 50.12 Kaplan-Meier analysis of outcomes in the PARADIGM trial. **A,** Death from cardiovascular causes or hospitalization for heart failure (the primary endpoint). **B,** Death from cardiovascular cause. **C,** Hospitalization for heart failure. (Modified from McMurray JJ, Packer M, Desai AS, et al. Angiotensin-neprilysin inhibition versus enalapril in heart failure. *N Engl J Med.* 2014;317:993–1004.)

The LIFE trial (NCT02816736), which compared sacubitril/valsartan with valsartan in HFrEF patients with advanced chronic HF and NYHA class IV symptoms in the previous 3 months, showed that sacubitril/valsartan was not superior to valsartan in terms of lowering NT-proBNP.[38] The use of ARNIs in acute HF is discussed in Chapter 49.

Side Effects of Angiotensin Receptor Neprilysin Inhibitors

The use of an ARNI is associated with hypotension (approximately 14%), hyperkalemia (4%), cough (11%), and a very low-frequency incidence of angioedema. Oral neprilysin inhibitors, used in combination with ACE inhibitors, can lead to angioedema; accordingly, the concomitant use of ACEIs and ARNIs is contraindicated (class III recommendation). For patients who are switching from ACEIs to sacubitril/valsartan, the ACEI should be withheld for at least 36 hours before initiating sacubitril/valsartan in order to minimize the risk of angioedema caused by overlapping ACE and neprilysin inhibition. There are additional concerns about the effects of sacubitril/valsartan on the degradation of beta-amyloid peptide in the brain, which could theoretically accelerate amyloid deposition. The optimal titration and tolerability of ARNIs, particularly with regard to blood pressure and the adjustment of concomitant HF medications, will require addition clinical experience.

Beta-Blockers

Beta-blocker therapy represents a major advance in the treatment of HF patients with a depressed EF. Beta-blockers interfere with the harmful effects of sustained activation of the central nervous system, by competitively antagonizing one or more adrenergic receptors (α_1, β_1 and β_2). Although there are a number of potential benefits to blocking all three receptors, most of the deleterious effects of sympathetic activation are mediated by the β_1 adrenergic receptor.

The functional effects of beta-blocker therapy on the failing heart are biphasic. Administration of beta-blockers may be associated with an early, short-term deterioration in cardiac function, consistent with the negative inotropic effects of withdrawing adrenergic drive. However, when given in concert with ACE inhibitors, treatment with beta-blockers is associated with decrease in LV volumes (reverse LV remodeling), favorable changes in LV shape, as well as improved LVEF. From a clinical standpoint, this initial deterioration in LV function is generally not apparent if β-blocker therapy is initiated gradually and slowly up-titrated in patients who are relatively euvolemic. In the long term when given in concert with ACEIs, beta-blockers improve patient symptoms, prevent hospitalization, and prolong life. Therefore beta-blockers are indicated for patients with symptomatic or asymptomatic HF and a depressed EF less than 40% (class I indication). Three beta-blockers have been shown to be effective in reducing the risk of death in patients with chronic HF: bisoprolol and sustained-release metoprolol succinate both competitively block the β1 receptor, and carvedilol competitively blocks the α1, β1, and β2 receptors. Analogous to the use of ACEIs, beta-blockers should be initiated in low doses (see Table 50.7), followed by gradual increments in the dose if lower doses have been well tolerated. The dose of beta-blocker should be increased until the doses used are similar to those that have been reported to be effective in clinical trials (see Table 50.7). However, unlike ACEIs, which may be up-titrated relatively rapidly, the dose titration of beta-blockers should proceed no sooner than two-week intervals, because the initiation and/or increased dosing of these agents may lead to worsening fluid retention because of the abrupt withdrawal of adrenergic support to the heart and the circulation. Therefore, it is important to optimize the dose of diuretic before starting therapy with beta-blockers. If worsening fluid retention does occur, it is likely to occur within 3 to 5 days of initiating therapy, and will be manifest as increase in body weight and/or symptoms of worsening HF. The increased fluid retention can usually be managed by increasing the dose of diuretics. Patients need not be taking high doses of ACEIs before being considered for treatment with a beta-blocker, because most patients enrolled in the beta-blocker trials were not taking high doses of ACEIs. Furthermore, in patients taking a low dose of an ACEI, the addition of a beta-blocker produces a greater improvement in symptoms and reduction in the risk of death than an increase in the dose of the ACEI. Studies have shown that beta-blockers can be safely started before discharge, even in patients hospitalized for HF, provided that the patient is stable and does not require intravenous HF therapy. Contrary to early reports, the aggregate results of clinical trials suggest that beta-blocker therapy is well tolerated by the great majority of HF patients (>85%), including patients with comorbid conditions such as diabetes mellitus, chronic obstructive lung disease, and peripheral vascular disease. Nonetheless, there is a subset of patients (10% to 15%) who remain intolerant to beta-blockers because of worsening fluid retention or symptomatic hypotension.

The first placebo-controlled multicenter trial with a beta-blocking agent was the Metoprolol in Dilated Cardiomyopathy (MDC) trial, which used the shorter-acting tartrate preparation at a target dose of 50 mg three times a day in symptomatic HF patients with idiopathic dilated cardiomyopathy. Metoprolol tartrate at an average dose of 108 mg/day reduced the prevalence of the primary endpoint of death or need for cardiac transplantation by 34%, which did not quite reach statistical significance (p = 0.058). The benefit was due entirely to a reduction by metoprolol in the morbidity component of the primary endpoint, with no favorable trends in the mortality component of the primary endpoint. A more efficacious formulation of metoprolol was subsequently developed, metoprolol (succinate) CR/XL, which has a better pharmacologic profile than metoprolol tartrate because of its controlled-release profile and longer half-life. In the Metoprolol CR/XL Randomized Intervention Trial in Congestive Heart Failure (MERIT-HF), metoprolol CR/XL provided a significant relative risk reduction of 34% reduction in mortality in subjects with mild to moderate HF and moderate to severe systolic dysfunction when compared with the placebo group (Fig. 50.13, top).[9,15] Importantly, metoprolol CR/X reduced mortality from both sudden death and progressive pump failure. Further, mortality was reduced across most demographic groups, including older versus younger subjects, nonischemic versus ischemic etiology, and lower versus higher ejection fractions.

Bisoprolol is a second-generation β_1 receptor-selective blocking agent with approximately 120-fold higher affinity for human β1 versus β2 receptors. The first trial performed with bisoprolol was the Cardiac Insufficiency Bisoprolol Study I (CIBIS-I) trial, which examined the effects of bisoprolol on mortality in subjects with symptomatic ischemic or nonischemic cardiomyopathy. CIBIS-I showed a nonsignificant (p = 0.22) 20% risk reduction for mortality at 2 years follow-up. Because the sample size for CIBIS-I was based on an unrealistically high expected event rate in the control group, a follow-up trial with more conservative effect size estimates and sample size calculations was conducted. In CIBIS-II bisoprolol reduced all-cause mortality by 32% (11.8% versus 17.3%, (p = 0.002), sudden cardiac death by 45% (3.6% versus 6.4%, (p = 0.001), HF hospitalizations by 30% (11.9% bisoprolol versus 17.6% placebo, (p < 0.001), and all-cause hospitalizations by 15% (33.6% versus 39.6%, (p = 0.002) (see Fig. 50.13, middle). The CIBIS-III trial addressed the important question of whether an initial treatment strategy using the beta-blocker bisoprolol was noninferior to a treatment strategy of using an ACEI (enalapril) first, among patients with newly diagnosed mild to moderate HF. The two strategies were compared in a blinded manner with regard to the combined primary endpoint of all-cause mortality or hospitalization, as well as with regard to each of the components of the primary endpoint individually. Although the per-protocol primary endpoint analysis of death or rehospitalization did not meet the prespecified criteria for noninferiority, the intent-to-treat analysis showed that bisoprolol was noninferior to enalapril (HR 0.94, 95% CI 0.77 to 1.16, (p = 0.019 for noninferiority). Although CIBIS-III did not provide clear-cut evidence to justify starting with a beta-blocker first, the overall safety profile of the two strategies was similar. Current guidelines continue to recommend starting with an ACEI first, followed by the addition of a beta-blocker.

Of the three beta-blockers that are approved for the treatment of HF, carvedilol has been studied most extensively (see Table 50.8). The phase III U.S. Trials Program, composed of four individual trials managed by single Steering and Data and Safety Monitoring Committee, was stopped prematurely because of a highly significant (p < 0.0001) 65% reduction in mortality with carvedilol that was observed across all four trials. This was followed by a second study, the Australia-New Zealand Heart Failure Research Collaborative Group Carvedilol Trial (ANZ-Carvedilol), which showed there was a significant improvement in LVEF (p < 0.0001) and a significant (p = 0.0015) reduction in LV end-diastolic volume index in the carvedilol-treated group at 12 months, as well as a significant relative risk reduction of 26% in the clinical composite of death or hospitalization for the carvedilol group at 19 months. Rates of hospitalization were also significantly lower for patients treated with carvedilol (48%) compared to placebo (58%). The Carvedilol Prospective Randomized Cumulative Survival (COPERNICUS) study extended these benefits to patients with more advanced HF. In COPERNICUS patients with advanced HF symptoms had to be clinically euvolemic and have an LVEF less than 25%. When compared with placebo, carvedilol reduced the mortality risk at 12 months by 38% (see Table 50.8) and the relative risk of death or HF hospitalization by 31% (see Fig. 50.13, bottom). Carvedilol has also been evaluated in a post-MI trial which enrolled patients with LV dysfunction. The Carvedilol Post-Infarct Survival Controlled Evaluation (CAPRICORN) trial was a randomized, placebo-controlled trial designed to test the long-term efficacy of carvedilol on morbidity and mortality in patients with LV dysfunction after MI who were already treated with ACEIs. Although carvedilol did not reduce the prespecified primary endpoint of mortality plus cardiovascular hospitalization, it did significantly reduce total mortality by 23% (p = 0.03), cardiovascular mortality by 25 % (p < 0.05), and nonfatal MI by 41% (p = 0.014). Finally, in the Carvedilol or Metoprolol European Trial (COMET) carvedilol (target dose 25 mg twice daily) was compared

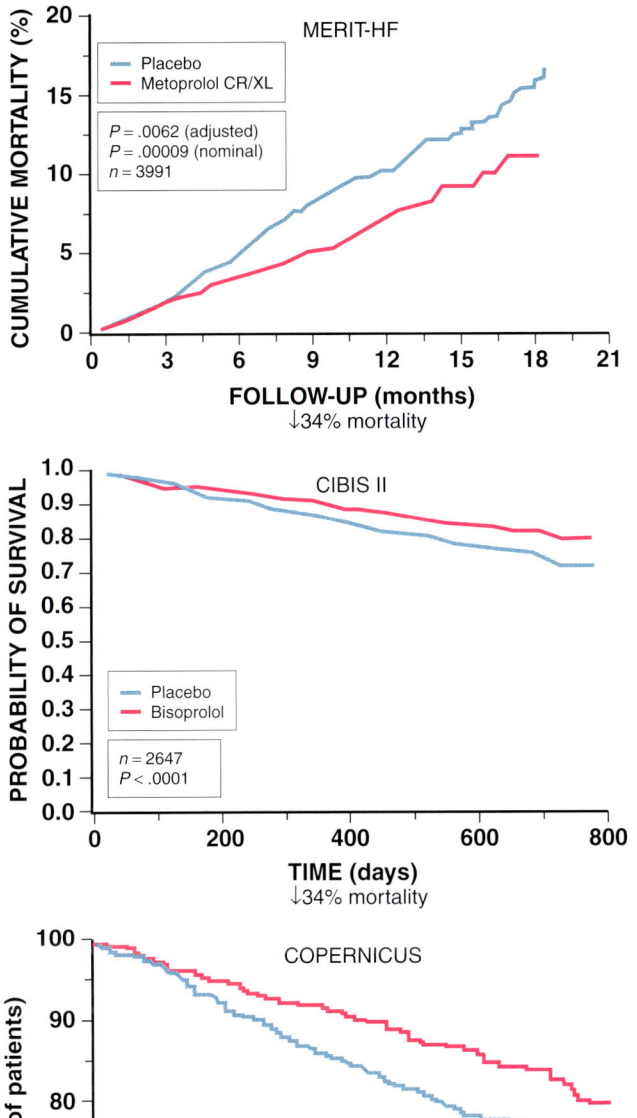

FIGURE 50.13 Kaplan-Meier analysis of the probability of survival among patients in the placebo and beta-blocker groups in the MERIT-HF **(top)**, CIBIS II **(middle)**, and COPERNICUS **(bottom)** trials. *CHF,* Chronic heart failure; *CI,* confidence interval. (Data from The Cardiac Insufficiency Bisoprolol Study II [CIBIS II]. *Lancet.* 1999;353:9–13; Metoprolol CR/XL randomized intervention trial in congestive heart failure [MERIT-HF]. *Lancet.* 1999;353:2001–2007; and Packer M, Coats AJS, Fowler MB, et al; for The Carvedilol Prospective Randomized Cumulative Survival Study Group. Effect of carvedilol on survival in severe chronic heart failure. *N Engl J Med.* 2001;344:1651–1658.)

with immediate-release metoprolol tartrate (target dose 50 mg twice daily) with respect to the primary endpoint of all-cause mortality. In COMET carvedilol was associated with a significant 33% reduction in all-cause mortality when compared with metoprolol tartrate (33.9% versus 39.5%, HR 0.83, 95% CI 0.74 to 0.93, P = 0.0017).[9,15] Based on the results of the COMET trial, short-acting metoprolol tartrate is not recommended for use in the treatment of HF. The results of the COMET trial emphasize the importance of using doses and formulations of beta-blockers that have been shown to be effective in clinical trials. There have been no trials to ascertain whether the survival benefits of carvedilol are greater than those of metoprolol (succinate) CR/XL when both drugs are used at the appropriate target doses.

Not all studies with beta-blockers have been universally successful, suggesting that the effects of beta-blockers should not necessarily be viewed broadly as a class effect. Indeed, early studies with the first generation of nonspecific β_1 and β_2 receptors without ancillary vasodilating properties (e.g., propranolol) resulted in significant worsening of HF and death. The Beta Blocker Evaluation of Survival Trial (BEST) evaluated the third-generation beta-blocking agent bucindolol, which is a completely nonselective β_1 and β_2 blocker with some α_1 receptor blockade properties. Although the BEST trial showed that there was a nonsignificant (p = .10) 10% reduction in total mortality in the bucindolol-treated group, there was a statistically significant (p = 0.01) 19% reduction in mortality in white patients. The differential response of bucindolol in white patients has been suggested to be secondary to a polymorphism (Arginine 389) in the beta$_1$-adrenergic receptor that is more prevalent in white patients. Nebivolol is a selective β1 receptor antagonist with ancillary vasodilatory properties that are mediated, at least in part, by nitric oxide (NO). In the Study of Effects of Nebivolol Intervention on Outcomes and Rehospitalization in Seniors with Heart Failure (SENIORS), nebivolol significantly reduced the composite outcome of death or cardiovascular hospitalizations (HR: 0.86; 95% CI 0.74 to 0.99; (p < 0.04), which was the primary endpoint of the trial; however, nebivolol did not reduce mortality significantly. Although approximately 35% of the patients in SENIORS had an LVEF greater than 35%; more than half of these patients had an EF ranging from 35% to 50%, and thus would not be considered as HF with a midrange LVEF or HFpEF patients. Nebivolol is not FDA approved for the treatment of HFrEF.

Side Effects of Beta-Blockers

The adverse effects of beta-blockers are generally related to the predictable complications that arise from interfering with the adrenergic nervous system. These reactions generally occur within several days of initiating therapy, and are generally responsive to adjusting concomitant medications, as described above. Treatment with a beta-blocker can be accompanied by feelings of general fatigue or weakness. In most instances, the increased fatigue spontaneously resolves within several weeks or months; however, in some patients, it may be severe enough to limit the dose of beta-blocker or require the withdrawal or reduction of treatment. Therapy with beta-blockers can lead to bradycardia and/or exacerbate heart block. Moreover, beta-blockers (particularly those that block the α_1 receptor) can lead to vasodilatory side effects. Accordingly, the dose of beta-blockers should be decreased if the heart rate decreases to less than 50 beats/min and/or second- or third-degree heart block develops, or symptomatic hypotension develops. Continuation of beta-blocker treatment during an episode of acute decompensation is safe, although dose reduction may be necessary.[39] Beta-blockers are not recommended for patients with asthma with active bronchospasm.

Mineralocorticoid Receptor Antagonists

Although classified as potassium-sparing diuretics, MRAs that block the effects of aldosterone (e.g., spironolactone) have beneficial effects that are independent of the effects of these agents on sodium balance. Although ACEI may transiently decrease aldosterone secretion, with chronic therapy there is a rapid return of aldosterone to levels similar to those before ACEI, which is referred to as *aldosterone breakthrough*.[40] The administration of an MRA is recommended for patients with NYHA class II to IV HF who have a depressed EF (≤35%), and who are receiving standard therapy including diuretics, ACEIs, and beta-blockers (class I indication) (see Fig. 50.10).[41] The dose of aldosterone antagonist should be increased until the doses used are similar to those that have been shown to be effective in clinical trials (see Table 50.7). Spironolactone should be initiated at a dose of 12.5 to 25 mg daily, and up-titrated to 50 mg daily, whereas eplerenone should be initiated as doses of 25 mg/day and increased to 50 mg daily (see Table 50.7). As noted above, potassium supplementation is generally stopped after the initiation of aldosterone antagonists, and patients should be counseled to avoid high-potassium foods. Potassium levels and renal function should be rechecked within 3 days and again at 1 week after initiation of an aldosterone antagonist. Subsequent monitoring should be dictated by the general clinical stability of renal function and fluid status but should occur at least monthly for the first 6 months.

The first evidence that MRAs could produce a major clinical benefit in HF was demonstrated by the Randomized Aldactone Evaluation Study (RALES) trial,[9,15] which evaluated spironolactone (25 mg/day initially, titrated to 50 mg/day for signs of worsening HF) versus placebo in NYHA class III or IV HF patients with a LVEF less than 35%, who were being treated with an ACEI, a loop diuretic, and, in most cases, digoxin. As shown in Figure 50.7A, spironolactone led to a 30% reduction in total mortality when compared with placebo (p = 0.001). The frequency of hospitalization for worsening HF was also 35% lower in the spironolactone group than in the placebo group. Although the mechanism for the beneficial effect of spironolactone has not been fully elucidated, prevention of extracellular matrix remodeling (see Chapter 47) and prevention of complications secondary to hypokalemia are plausible mechanisms. Although spironolactone was well tolerated in RALES, gynecomastia was reported in 10% of men who were treated with spironolactone, as compared with 1% of men in the placebo group (P < 0.001). The Eplerenone in Mild Patients Hospitalization and Survival Study in Heart Failure (EMPHASIS-HF) trial, which was performed in patients with NYHA class II HF with an EF less than 30% (or 35% if the QRS width was >130 msec), demonstrated that eplerenone (titrated to 50 mg/day) led to a significant 27% decrease in cardiovascular death or HF hospitalization (HR 0.63; 95% CI 0.54 to 0.74; P < 0.001) (see Fig. 50.7B).[9,15] There were also significant decreases in all-cause death (24%), cardiovascular death (24%), all-cause hospitalization (23%), and HF hospitalizations (43%). Importantly, the effect of eplerenone was consistent across all prespecified subgroups. In contrast to the RALES trial, which was conducted prior to the widespread adoption of beta-blockers, the background therapy for EMPHASIS-HF included ACEIs or ARBs and beta-blockers. The findings in RALES and EMPHASIS-HF are consistent with findings in randomized clinical trials in patients with acute MI and LV dysfunction. The Eplerenone Post-Acute Myocardial Infarction Heart Failure Efficacy and Survival Study (EPHESUS) evaluated the effect of eplerenone (titrated to a maximum of 50 mg/day) on morbidity and mortality among patients with acute MI complicated by LV dysfunction and HF. Treatment with eplerenone led to 15% decrease in all-cause death in the EPHESUS trial (RR 0.85; 95% CI 0.75 to 0.96; P = 0.008). Based on the results of the RALES and EMPHASIS-HF trials,[9,15] aldosterone antagonists are currently recommended for all patients with persistent NYHA class II to IV symptoms and an EF ≤35%, in addition to treatment with an ACEI (or an ARB if an ACEI is not tolerated) and a beta-blocker (class I indication).

Side Effects of Mineralocorticoid Receptor Antagonists

The major problem with the use of aldosterone antagonists is the development of life-threatening hyperkalemia, which is more prone to occur in patients who are receiving potassium supplements, or who have underlying renal insufficiency. Aldosterone antagonists are not recommended when the serum creatinine is greater than 2.5 mg/dL (or creatinine clearance is <30 mL/min) or serum potassium is greater than 5.5 mmol/L. The development of worsening renal function should lead to consideration regarding stopping aldosterone antagonists because of the potential risk of hyperkalemia. Painful gynecomastia may develop in 10% to 15% of patients who use spironolactone, in which case eplerenone may be substituted.

Renin Inhibitors

Aliskiren is an orally active direct renin inhibitor that appears to suppress RAS to a degree similar to ACE inhibitors.[42] Although the benefits of ACEIs and ARBs in HF have been clearly established, these agents provoke a compensatory increase in renin and downstream intermediaries of the renin-angiotensin-aldosterone system, which may attenuate the effects of ACEIs and ARBs ("aldosterone breakthrough"). Aliskiren is

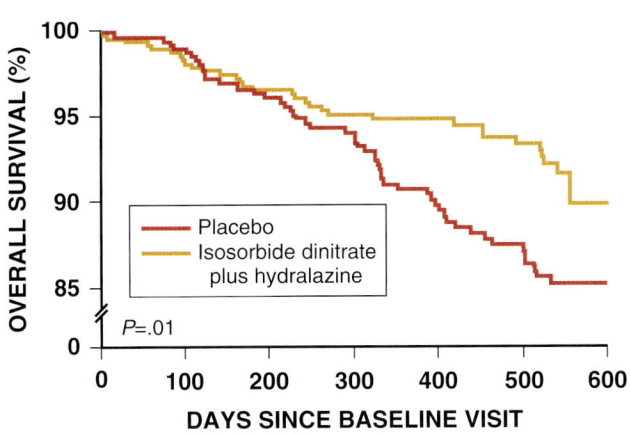

FIGURE 50.14 Kaplan-Meier analysis of the probability of survival among patients in the placebo and isosorbide dinitrate plus hydralazine treatment arms of the A-HeFT study. (Modified from Taylor AL, Ziesche S, Yancy C, et al. Combination of isosorbide dinitrate and hydralazine in blacks with heart failure. *N Engl J Med*. 2004;351:2050–2057.)

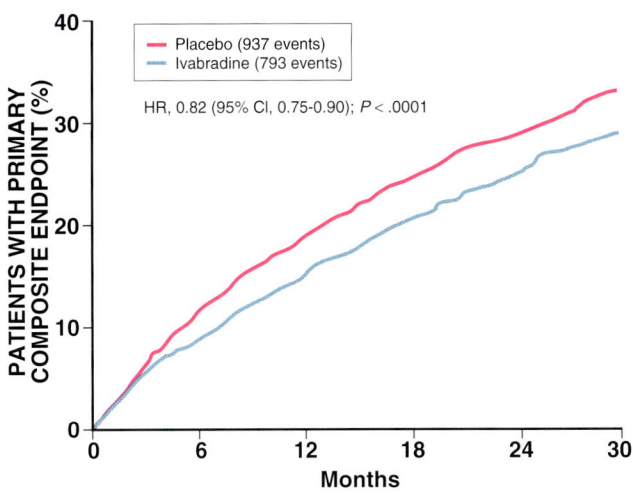

FIGURE 50.15 Kaplan-Meier cumulative event curves for the primary composite endpoint of cardiovascular death or hospitalization for worsening HF in patients treated with ivabradine compared to placebo. (Modified from Swedberg K, Komajda M, Böhm M, et al. Ivabradine and outcomes in chronic heart failure (SHIFT): a randomised placebo-controlled study. *Lancet*. 2010;376:875–885.)

a nonpeptide inhibitor that binds to the active site (S1/S3 hydrophobic binding pocket) of renin, thereby preventing the conversion of angiotensinogen to angiotensin I (see Fig. 47.3). In the Aliskiren Observation of Heart Failure Treatment (ALOFT) trial[43] treatment with aliskiren significantly (p < 0.01) decreases NT-proBNP and urinary aldosterone excretion. Based on these promising early results, several large pivotal outcomes trials were initiated to determine whether adding aliskiren to standard HF therapy would improve clinical outcomes. However, both the Aliskiren Trial on Acute Heart Failure Outcomes (ASTRONAUT)[44] and the Efficacy and Safety of Aliskiren and Aliskiren/Enalapril Combination on Morbi-mortality in Patients With Chronic Heart Failure (ATMOSPHERE)[45] clinical trials failed to improve outcomes in HFrEF patients. Aliskiren is not currently recommended as an alternative to an ACEI, ARBs, or in combination with ACEIs for the treatment of HFrEF.

Combination of Hydralazine and Isosorbide Dinitrate

Therapy with the combination of H-ISDN has been shown to reduce all-cause mortality in African Americans. There are two placebo-controlled trials (V-HeFT-I and A-HeFT) and one active-controlled (V-HeFT) randomized trial with H-ISDN in HFrEF patients. In A-HeFT, a total 1050 self-identified African American HFrEF patients with NYHA class III to IV HF who were receiving standard medical therapy for HF were randomized to placebo or fixed dose H-ISDN. The primary endpoint was a weighted composite score of all-cause mortality, first hospitalization for HF, and quality of life. The study was terminated early because of a significantly higher mortality rate (10.2% versus 6.2%, P = 0.02) in the placebo group than in the H-ISDN treatment group (Fig. 50.14). The combination of H-ISDN is recommended (class I indication) for African Americans with NYHA class III to IV HFrEF who remain symptomatic despite concomitant use of ACE inhibitors, beta blockers, and aldosterone antagonists (see Fig. 50.10).[46] There is evidence to suggest that the combination of H-ISDN is beneficial as a first line therapy in non-African Americans with HFrEF, although this has never been tested formally in a clinical trial.[15] The combination of H-ISDN is used in patients who are intolerant to ACEI/ARBs/ARNIs (class IIa recommendation).

I_f-Channel Inhibitor

Ivabradine is a heart rate-lowering agent that acts by selectively blocking the cardiac pacemaker I_f ("funny") current that controls the spontaneous diastolic depolarization of the sinoatrial node. Ivabradine blocks I_f channels in a concentration-dependent manner by entering the channel pore from the intracellular side, and thus can only block the channel when it is open. The magnitude of I_f inhibition is directly related to the frequency of channel opening and would therefore be expected to be most effective at higher heart rates. Ivabradine was shown to improve outcomes in the Systolic Heart Failure Treatment with the I_f Inhibitor Ivabradine Trial (SHIFT), which enrolled symptomatic patients with an LVEF ≤35%, who were in sinus rhythm with heart rate ≥70 beats/min and on standard medical therapy for HF (including beta-blockers). In the SHIFT trial ivabradine (up-titrated to a maximal dosage of 7.5 mg twice daily) reduced the primary composite outcome of cardiovascular death or HF hospitalization by 18% (HR 0.82, 95% CI 0.75 to 0.90, (p < 0.0001) (Fig. 50.15). The composite

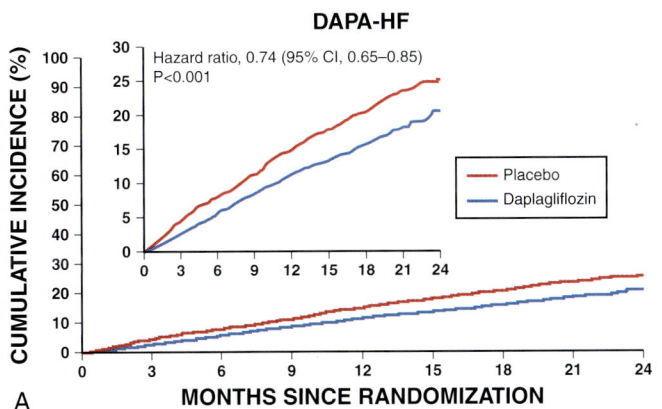
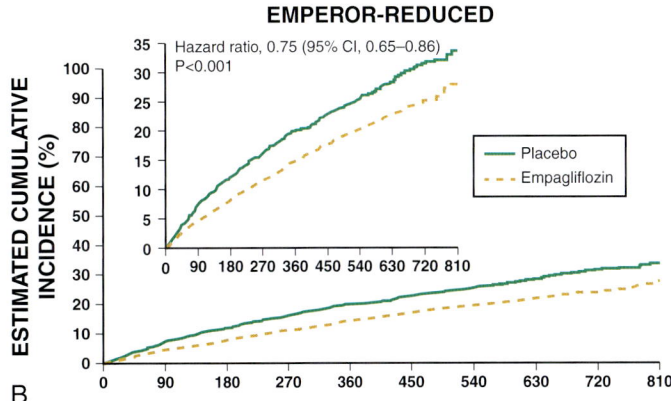

FIGURE 50.16 Kaplan-Meier Analysis of SGLT2 inhibitors in HFrEF patients. **A,** Effect of dapigflozin on worsening heart failure or cardiovascular death in NYHA class II to IV HF patients with an LVEF of ≤40 in the DAPA-HF trial. **B,** Effect of empagliflozin on CV death or hospitalization for worsening heart failure in NYHA class II to IV HF patients with an LVEF of ≤40 in the EMPEROR-Reduced trial. *HF,* Heart failure; *HfrEF,* heart failure with reduced ejection fraction; *LVEF,* left ventricular ejection fraction; *NYHA,* New York Heart Association; *SGLT2,* sodium-glucose transporter-2. (**A** from McMurray JJV, Solomon SD, Inzucchi SE, et al. Dapagliflozin in Patients with Heart Failure and Reduced Ejection Fraction. *N Engl J Med*. 2019;381[21]:1995–2008; **B** from Packer M, Anker SD, Butler J, et al. Cardiovascular and Renal Outcomes with Empagliflozin in Heart Failure. *N Engl J Med*. 2020;383[15]:1413–1424.)

endpoint was driven primarily by reducing hospital admissions for worsening HF (HR 0.74, CI 0.66 to 0.83; (p < 0.0001), insofar as there was no decrease in cardiovascular deaths (HR 0.91; 95% CI 0.80 to 1.03), (p = 0.13) or all-cause deaths.[47] Given that ivabradine lowered heart rate by approximately 10 beats/min and that only 26% of the patients in the trial were on optimal doses of beta-blockers, it is possible that titrating beta-blockers to recommended disease may have reduced the HF hospitalizations to a similar degree. Ivabradine is recommended by the ACC/AHA/HFSA guidelines (class IIa recommendation) to reduce HF hospitalization in HFrEF patients in sinus rhythm with a HR greater than 70 beats/min who are receiving guideline-directed medical therapy (GDMT).

Sodium-Glucose Transporter-2 Inhibitors

Medicines in the SGLT2 class of inhibitors include canagliflozin, dapagliflozin, and empagliflozin. The landmark EMPA-REG OUTCOME (Empagliflozin Cardiovascular Outcome Event Trial in Type 2 Diabetes Mellitus Patients) demonstrated that empagliflozin reduced death from CV causes by 38%, hospitalization for HF by 35%, and progression to end-stage kidney disease in patients with type 2 DM and established CV disease (see also Chapter 31).[48] The question of whether SGLT2 inhibitors are beneficial in HFrEF patients without diabetes has been addressed in two large clinical trials, which showed that dapagliflozin (DAPA-HF) and empagliflozin (EMPEROR-Reduced) significantly reduced worsening HF and CV death in NYHA class II to IV HF patients (Fig. 50.16).[49,50]

> In the DAPA-HF trial (Effect of Dapagliflozin on the Incidence of Worsening Heart Failure or Cardiovascular Death in Patients With Chronic Heart Failure), 4744 patients with NYHA class II, III, or IV HF and an LVEF of ≤ 40% were randomized to receive either dapagliflozin (10 mg once daily) or placebo, in addition to GDMT.[49] The primary outcome was a composite of worsening HF (hospitalization or an urgent visit resulting in intravenous therapy for HF) or cardiovascular death. After a follow-up of 18.2 months, dapagliflozin was associated with a 26% reduction in risk (HR, 0.74; 95% CI, 0.59 to 0.83; p = 0.00001) (see Fig. 50.16A). Importantly, event rates for all the components of the composite outcome favored dapagliflozin; hospitalizations for worsening HF were reduced (HR 0.70; 95% CI, 0.59 to 0.83), as well as death from CV cause (HR 0.82; 95% CI 0.69 to 0.98). The outcomes were similar in patients with and without diabetes. Moreover, this benefit was consistent across all subgroups of background therapy and combinations of background therapy analyzed, with HRs ranging from 0.57 to 0.86 and no significant randomized treatment-by-subgroup interaction. There was no difference in a composite of worsening renal function. In the EMPEROR-Reduced (Empagliflozin outcome trial in Patients with Chronic Heart Failure With Reduced Ejection Fraction) trial 3730 patients with NYHA class II, III, or IV HF and an ejection fraction of LVEF of ≤ 40% were randomized to receive empagliflozin (10 mg once daily) or placebo, in addition to standard guideline-directed medical therapy. The primary outcome was a composite of CV death or hospitalization for worsening HF. After a median follow-up of 16 months, empagliflozin was associated with 25% reduction in risk (HR 0.75; 95% CI, 0.65 to 0.86; P < 0.001) (see Fig. 50.16B).[50] The primary outcome was similar in patients with or without diabetes. In contrast to DAPA-HF, the primary endpoint in EMPEROR-Reduced was driven by decreased HF hospitalization (HR, 0.70; 95% CI, 0.58 to 0.85); whereas there was no significant difference in CV mortality (HR 0.92; 95% CI, 0.75 to 1.12). Although the reasons for the discrepancy in CV outcomes between these two trials are not known, the patients in EMPEROR-Reduced had on average more severe HF than those in DAPA-HF, raising the possibility that SGLT2 inhibitors are less effective in advanced HF. Another important difference between EMPEROR-Reduced and DAPA-HF is that a composite renal outcome was significantly reduced with the use of empagliflozin, whereas it was not with dapagliflozin. At the time of this writing, neither the ACC/AHA/HFSA guidelines nor the European HF guidelines have provided recommendations with respect to the use of SGLT2 inhibitors in HFrEF. However, the Canadian Cardiovascular Society and the Canadian Heart Failure Society recommend the use the use of SGLT2 inhibitors in patients with mild or moderate HF who have an LVEF less than 40% or less to improve symptoms and quality of life and to reduce the risk of hospitalization and cardiovascular mortality.[51]

Soluble Guanylate Cyclase Stimulators

As discussed in Chapter 47, in HF there is an imbalance between oxidative stress and NO availability (see Fig. 47.4). The decrease in NO bioavailability contributes to the development of endothelial dysfunction, as well as LV dysfunction. Vericiguat is a novel oral soluble guanylate cyclase (see Fig. 47.6) stimulator that enhances the cyclic guanosine monophosphate (GMP) production pathway, by directly stimulating soluble guanylate cyclase activity, as well as sensitizing soluble guanylate cyclase to endogenous NO.[52] In the Vericiguat Global Study in Subjects with Heart Failure with Reduced Ejection Fraction (VICTORIA) trial, 5050 patients with chronic NYHA class II to IV HF and an LVEF less than 45% were randomized to receive vericiguat (target dose, 10 mg once daily) or placebo, in addition to GDMT.[52] The primary outcome was a composite of CV death or first hospitalization for HF. At 10.8 months of follow-up there were fewer CV death and HF hospitalizations in the vericiguat group than in the placebo group (HR 0.90; 95% CI 0.82 to 0.98; P = 0.02). There was, however, no significant difference in CV death in the vericiguat group when compared with the placebo group (HR 0.93; 95% CI 0.81 to 1.06). At the time of this writing, neither the ACC/AHA/HFSA guidelines nor the European HF guidelines have provided recommendations with respect to the use of vericiguat in HFrEF patients.

Myosin Activators

Cardiac myosin activators represent a new mechanistic class of therapeutic agents designed to increase myocardial contractility without increasing intracellular concentrations of cyclic adenosine monophosphate and calcium, and without increasing myocardial oxygen consumption, thus avoiding the major toxic effects of classic inotropic agents (see Chapter 49). Omecamtiv mecarbil is a small-molecule activator of myosin that prolongs myocardial systole by increasing the fraction of sarcomeric myosin molecules that are strongly bound to actin (see Chapter 46), thereby leading to increased myocardial force generation and increased contractility. Administration of omecamtiv mecarbil in patients with HFrEF results in dose-dependent increases in systolic ejection time, fractional shortening, stroke volume, and LVEF. In the Chronic Oral Study of Myosin Activation to Increase Contractility in Heart Failure (COSMIC-HF), a phase 2 trial, 448 patients with HFrEF were randomized to receive placebo or omecamtiv mecarbil (25 mg twice daily with pharmacokinetic-guided dose selection to 50 mg twice daily) for 20 weeks. In patients who received omecamtiv mecarbil, systolic ejection time and stroke volume both increased, while diastolic filing parameters were not worsened.[53] The GALACTIC-HF (Global Approach to Lowering Adverse Cardiac Outcomes Through Improving Contractility in Heart Failure trial [NCT02929329]), which enrolled 8200 patients with HFrEF, showed that treatment with omecamtiv mecarbil significantly reduced the composite of CV death or HF hospitalization and other urgent treatment for HF compared to placebo in patients treated with standard of care (HR 0.92; 95% CI 0.86 to 0.99; (p = 0.025).

MANAGEMENT OF PATIENTS WHO REMAIN SYMPTOMATIC

As noted above an ACEI/ARB or ARNI, a beta-blocker and MRAs should be standard background therapy for patients with HFrEF. However, the addition of an ARB to the combination of ACEI or MRA is not recommended in HFrEF patients because of the risk of hyperkalemia. Moreover, the combination of ARNI with an ACEI is not recommended because of the risk of angioedema. Additional pharmacologic therapy (polypharmacy) or device therapy (see below) should be considered in patients who have persistent symptoms or progressive worsening despite optimized therapy with evidence-based medical and device therapies. Digoxin is recommended for patients with symptomatic HFrEF to reduce hospitalizations despite receiving standard therapy, including ACEIs (or ARBs), ARNIs, beta-blockers, and MRA receptor antagonists (class IIa indication).

Cardiac Glycosides

Digoxin, first described by William Withering in 1775, is by far the oldest drug in the HF armamentarium. Digoxin and digitoxin are the most frequently used cardiac glycosides. Given that digoxin is most commonly used, and is the only glycoside that has been evaluated in placebo-controlled trials, there is little reason to prescribe other cardiac glycosides for the management of patients with chronic HF. Digoxin exerts its effects by inhibiting the sodium potassium adenosine trisphosphate (Na^+-K^+ ATPase) pump in cell membranes, including the sarcolemmal Na^+-K^+ ATPase pump of cardiac myocytes (see Chapters 46 and 47). Inhibition of Na^+-K^+ ATPase pump leads to an increase in intracellular calcium and hence increased cardiac contractility, which led to the suggestion that beneficial effects of digoxin were secondary to its inotropic properties. However, the more likely mechanism of digoxin in HF patients is to sensitize Na^+-K^+ ATPase activity in vagal afferent nerves, leading to an increase in vagal tone that counterbalances the increased activation of the adrenergic system in advanced HF. Digoxin also inhibits Na^+-K^+ ATPase activity in the kidney and may therefore blunt renal tubular resorption of sodium. Therapy with digoxin is commonly initiated and maintained at a dose of 0.125 to 0.25 mg daily. For the great majority of patients the dose should be 0.125 mg daily and the serum digoxin level should be less than 1.0 ng/mL, especially in elderly patients, patients with impaired renal function, and patients with a low lean body mass. Higher doses (e.g., digoxin >0.25 mg daily) are rarely used, and not recommended for the management of HF patients in sinus rhythm or who have atrial fibrillation (AF).

Although clinicians have used cardiac glycosides to treat patients with chronic HF for well over 200 years, there is still considerable debate regarding the effectiveness of the cardiac glycosides in HF patients. Whereas small-and medium-sized trials conducted in the 1970s and 1980s yielded equivocal results, two relatively large digoxin withdrawal studies in the early 1990s, the Randomized Assessment of Digoxin and Inhibitors of Angiotensin-Converting Enzyme (RADIANCE) and the Prospective Randomized Study of Ventricular Function and Efficacy of Digoxin (PROVED), provided strong support for clinical benefit from digoxin.[15] In these studies, worsening HF and HF hospitalizations developed in more patients who were withdrawn from digoxin than in patients who were maintained on digoxin. Insofar as withdrawal studies are difficult to interpret with respect to efficacy of a given therapeutic agent, the Digoxin Investigator Group (DIG) trial was a prospective trial conducted to assess the role of digitalis in chronic HF. Although the DIG trial showed that digoxin had a neutral effect on the primary endpoint of mortality, digoxin reduced hospitalizations (including 30-day readmissions for HF),[15] and favorably affected the combined endpoints of death or hospitalization due to worsening HF. Data from the DIG trial indicated a strong trend (p = 0.06) toward a decrease in deaths secondary to progressive pump failure, which was offset by an increase in sudden and other nonpump failure cardiac deaths (p = 0.04). One of the most important findings to emerge from the DIG trial was that mortality was directly related to the digoxin serum level.[15] In men enrolled in the DIG trial, trough levels between 0.6 and 0.8 ng/mL were associated with decreased mortality, suggesting that trough levels of digitalis should be maintained between 0.5 and 1.0 ng/mL. There is also evidence that digoxin may be potentially harmful in women. In a post-hoc multivariable analysis of the DIG trial, digoxin was associated with a significantly higher risk (23%) of death from any cause among women, but not men, possibly because of the relatively lower body weights in women, who were prescribed doses of digoxin the basis of a nomogram rather than trough levels.[15] The DIG trial was conducted prior to the widespread use of β-blockers, and no large trial of digoxin in addition to contemporary GDMT with both ACE inhibitors and β-blockers has been performed.

Complications of Digoxin Use

The principal adverse effects of digoxin are (1) cardiac arrhythmias including heart block (especially in the elderly) and ectopic and reentrant cardiac rhythms, (2) neurologic complaints such as visual disturbances, disorientation, and confusion, and (3) gastrointestinal symptoms such as anorexia, nausea, and vomiting. As noted above, these side effects can generally be minimized by maintaining trough levels of 0.5 to 0.8 ng/mL. In patients with HF, overt digitalis toxicity tends to emerge at serum concentrations that are greater than 2.0 ng/mL; however, digitalis toxicity may occur with lower digoxin levels, particularly if hypokalemia or hypomagnesemia coexist. Oral potassium administration is often useful for atrial, AV junctional, or ventricular ectopic rhythms, even when the

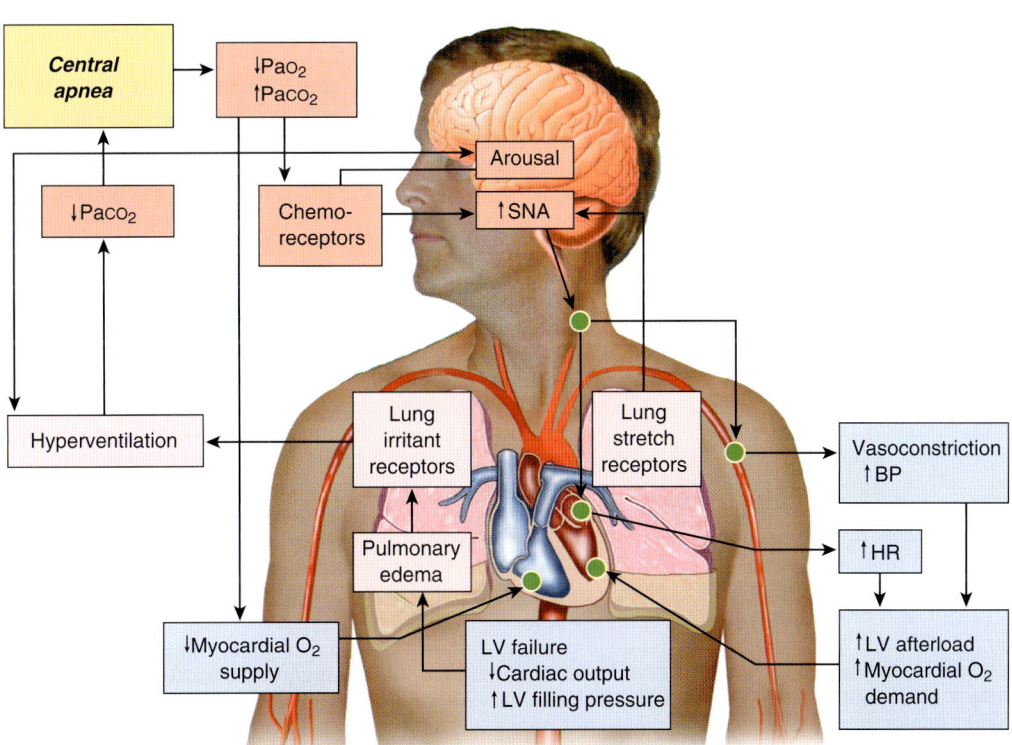

FIGURE 50.17 Pathophysiology of central sleep apnea and Cheyne-Stokes respiration in heart failure (HF). HF leads to increased left ventricular (LV) filling pressure. The resulting pulmonary congestion activates lung vagal irritant receptors, which stimulate hyperventilation and hypocapnia. Superimposed arousals cause further abrupt increases in ventilation and drive the partial pressure of carbon dioxide in arterial blood ($Paco_2$) below the threshold for ventilation, triggering a central apnea. Central sleep apneas are sustained by recurrent arousal resulting from apnea-induced hypoxia and the increased effort to breathe during the ventilatory phase because of pulmonary congestion and reduced lung compliance. Increased sympathetic activity causes increases in blood pressure (BP) and heart rate (HR) and increases myocardial oxygen (O_2) demand in the presence of reduced supply. SNA, Sympathetic nervous system activity; Pao_2, partial pressure of oxygen in arterial blood. (Redrawn from Bradley TD, Floras JS. Sleep apnea and heart failure. Part II: Central sleep apnea. Circulation. 20003;107:1822.)

serum potassium is in the normal range, unless high-grade AV block is also present. However, serum K+ levels must be monitored carefully to avoid hyperkalemia, especially in patients with renal failure or taking aldosterone receptor antagonists. Potentially life-threatening digoxin toxicity can be reversed by antidigoxin immunotherapy using purified Fab fragments. The concomitant use of quinidine, verapamil, spironolactone, flecainide, propafenone, and amiodarone can increase serum digoxin levels and may increase the risk of adverse reactions. Patients with advanced heart block should not receive digitalis unless a pacemaker is in place.

N-3 Polyunsaturated Fatty Acids

There is a large body of experimental evidence suggesting that n-3 polyunsaturated fatty acids (PUFA) have favorable effects on inflammation, including a reduction of endothelial activation and production of inflammatory cytokines, platelet aggregation, autonomic tone, blood pressure, heart rate, and LV function. The Gruppo Italiano per lo Studio della Sopravvivenza nell'Insufficienza cardiaca-Heart Failure (GISSI-HF) showed that long-term administration of 1 g/day of omega n-3 PUFA resulted in a significant reduction in both all-cause mortality (adjusted HR 0.91; 95.5% CI 0.83 to 0.99; p = 0.041) and all-cause mortality and cardiovascular admissions (adjusted HR 0.92; 99% CI 0.850 to 0.999; p = 0.009), in all the predefined subgroups, including HF patients with nonischemic cardiomyopathy.[54] The most recent ACC/AHA/HFSA and ESC guidelines endorse the use of n-3 PUFAs as adjunctive therapy (class IIa indication) for HFrEF patients who are receiving optimal evidence-based medical therapy.[9]

PHARMACOGENOMICS/PERSONALIZED MEDICINE

As discussed in Chapter 9, *pharmacogenomics* is the study of how genetic variations affect drug response, including genetic variants of enzymes that metabolize drugs, variants in drug receptors or drug transporters, as well as drug targets. These variations can result in gain or loss of therapeutic efficacy, influence optimal drug dosing of a drug, or favor alternative drug treatment. Given the tremendous heterogeneity that exists in HF patients, it is likely that genetic variations play a significant role in determining drug metabolism, disposition, and functional activity in HF patients. Recent advances in the field of pharmacogenetics suggest an analysis of underlying gene polymorphism in disease-causing pathways may one day enable clinicians to develop personalized therapeutic regimens for HF patients. Indeed, polymorphisms have been identified in the genes that appear to influence the therapeutic efficacy of ACEIs, beta-blockers, nitrates, and diuretics.

Personalized medicine seeks to use genetic information to "personalize" and improve diagnosis, prevention, and therapy. The personalized management of HF involves a large spectrum of potential applications, from diagnosis of monogenic disorders (see Chapters 52 to 54) to prevention and management strategies based on modifier genes, as well as to pharmacogenomics. However, the major challenge in applying pharmacogenomics to everyday clinical practice in patients with HFrEF is the absence of robust clinical data that supports the differential utilization of neurohormonal antagonists in the management of HFrEF patients with specific gene polymorphisms.[55] Indeed, all of the extant pharmacogenomic analyses in HFrEF have come from post-hoc, retrospective analyses of clinical trial data or from observational patient series studies, rather than prospective outcomes studies that have randomized HFrEF patients to a pharmacogenomic-guided therapy versus standard of care. The study Genetically Targeted Therapy for the Prevention of Symptomatic Atrial Fibrillation in Patients With Heart Failure (GENETIC-AF) enrolled patients with paroxysmal or persistent AF, HF, and an LVEF less than 50%.[56] Patients who had a specific genotype for the beta-1 adrenergic receptor (β1389 Arg/Arg genotype) were randomized to bucindolol or metoprolol succinate. The primary endpoint was a composite outcome of all-cause mortality or recurrent AF or atrial flutter at 24 weeks. The trial also incorporated a unique adaptive design that permitted patients to be transitioned into phase III clinical trial, if an interim analysis suggested benefit of bucindolol. At 24 weeks event rates for the bucindolol group (54%) were similar to those of the metoprolol group (53%), with a HR of 1.01 (95% CI: 0.71 to 1.42). However, when GENETIC-AF patients were divided between those with HRrEF (LVEF <40%) and those with HF with a midrange EF (HFmrEF), there was a reduction of approximately 60% in the primary endpoint of recurrent AF/flutter or all-cause mortality for patients with HFmrEF, which was not observed in patients with HFrEF.[56] The PRECISION-HF trial will evaluate the effect of bucindolol in HF patients with a β1389 Arg/Arg genotype and an LVEF ≥40% and ≤55%.

MANAGEMENT OF ATHEROSCLEROTIC DISEASE

The clinical evaluation of atherosclerotic cardiovascular heart disease in HF patients is discussed in Chapter 48. In patients with a prior MI and HF without angina, the use of ACEIs and beta-blockers has been shown to decrease the risk of reinfarction and death. Although the role of aspirin in HF patients of ischemic etiology has not been clearly established in randomized trials, and remains controversial because of the concern that aspirin may attenuate the beneficial effects of ACEI, long-term treatment with an antiplatelet agents, including aspirin (75 to 81 mg), is recommended for patients with HF due to ischemic etiology, regardless of whether they are receiving ACEIs.[57] Alternative antiplatelet agents (e.g., clopidogrel) may not interact adversely with ACEIs and may have superior effects in preventing clinical events; however, their ability to favorably affect outcomes in HF has not been demonstrated. Both beta-blockers and ivabradine (in selected patients) are effective for controlling angina in HFrEF patients.[58]

Although coronary artery bypass grafting (CABG) has not been shown to improve cardiac function or symptoms, or prevent reinfarction or death in HF patients without angina, CABG has been shown to improve symptoms and survival in patients with modestly reduced EF and angina. The Surgical Treatment for Ischemic Heart Failure (STICH) trial showed that CABG did not reduce all-cause death (HR 0.86 [95% CI 90.7 to 1.04]; $P = .12$), which was the primary endpoint of the trial; CABG did, however, reduce the composite endpoint of cardiovascular death, death from any cause, or hospitalization for cardiovascular causes (HR for CABG 0.74 [95% CI, 0.64 to 0.85]; $P < 0.001$), which was a prespecified secondary analysis. The 10-year follow-up to the original STICH trial demonstrated a significantly lower mortality in patients who underwent CABG when compared to medical therapy. The results of STICH suggest that CABG is beneficial in HF patients of ischemic etiology, who are otherwise suitable for surgery. Although the data are less robust, percutaneous coronary intervention (PCI) may be considered as an alternative to CABG in patients unsuitable for surgery. Current ACC/AHA/HFSA guidelines (class I indication) recommend revascularization with CABG or PCI for HFrEF patients on appropriate medical therapy, who have angina and suitable coronary anatomy for revascularization, especially left main stenosis (>50%) or left main equivalent disease.

MANAGEMENT OF VALVULAR DISEASE

Functional mitral regurgitation secondary to LV dysfunction and LV remodeling in HFrEF is powerful predictor of adverse clinical outcomes. Two randomized clinical trials have examined percutaneous mitral valve repair (PMVR) using the MitraClip closure device in addition to GDMT in HFrEF patients with moderate to severe mitral regurgitation. The MitraClip device for Severe Functional/ Secondary Mitral Regurgitation (MITRA-FR) did not demonstrate any improvement in the composite of death from any cause or unplanned hospitalization for HF at 12 months (OR 1.16; 95% CI, 0.73 to 1.84; $P = 0.53$), whereas the Cardiovascular Outcomes Assessment of the MitraClip Percutaneous Therapy for Heart Failure Patients with Functional Mitral Regurgitation (COAPT) trial showed a significant decrease in all hospitalizations for HF (HR 0.53; 95% CI 0.40 to 0.70; $P < 0.001$). In the COAPT trial, death from any cause (prespecified secondary outcome) within 24 months occurred in significantly fewer patients in the device group when compared to the control group (HR 0.62; 95% CI 0.46 to 0.82; $P < 0.001$). Importantly, these two trials differed with respect to patient characteristics and outcome definitions and duration of follow-up. At the time of this writing the ACC/AHA/HFSA and European Society of Cardiology have not provided guidelines for the use of PMVR in HFrEF.

SPECIAL POPULATIONS

Women (see also Chapter 91)

Although women account for a significant proportion of the growing HF epidemic, they have been poorly represented in clinical trials. Women with HF are more likely to be older (see Fig. 48.1), have a preserved ejection fraction (see Chapter 51) and nonischemic etiology for their HF. Although some studies have reported that HF outcomes are worse for women with than for men, the aggregate data suggest that women have a survival advantage when they develop HF. Although the explanation for this observation is unclear, it may be related to gender differences in etiology for HF. Nonetheless, while women appear to have a survival advantage after the diagnosis of HF, they experience increased morbidity, with worse equality of life, and have increased depression. Moreover, women are at increased risk of developing HF following acute MI.[59] Pooled analysis of several large-scale prospective clinical trials with β-blockers and ACEIs suggest that these agents provide similar survival benefits in women with reduced ejection fraction as in men.[59]

Race/Ethnicity

Epidemiologic and clinical trial data have raised awareness of potential areas of concern regarding the evaluation and treatment of HF in specific racial and ethnic groups. The efficacy of pharmacologic treatments in such subgroups is somewhat controversial, because there have been so few randomized clinical trials of HF treatment that have prespecified a subgroup analysis of outcomes stratified by race or ethnicity, that also have sufficient numbers of subjects for meaningful statistical analysis. Several retrospective analyses have highlighted that differences between African American and white populations in response to some standard HF therapies. Unfortunately, few data exist for Hispanic and Asian HF populations. Retrospective analyses from SOLVD and the V-HeFT trials suggested that African Americans do not benefit from ACEIs. In contrast, post-hoc analysis of studies with approved beta-blockers have found that African American patients benefit, although the magnitude of the effect appears to be diminished.[60] As noted above, the use of The H-ISDN was associated with a significant 43% reduction in the rate of death from any cause in the A-HeFT trial (see Fig. 50.14) and a significant 33% relative reduction in the rate of first hospitalization for HF. The mechanism for the beneficial effect of the hydralazine isosorbide regimen may be related to an improvement in NO bioavailability; however, the combination therapy group also had a small (but significant) effect on blood pressure lowering.

Elderly Persons (see also Chapter 90)

As noted at the outset, the prevalence of HF increases with age (see Fig. 48.1) and is the most common reason for hospitalization in elderly patients. Of note, the presentation of HF may differ in elderly patients with HF. Although they commonly present with the classic symptoms of dyspnea and fatigue, the elderly are more likely than younger patients to present with atypical symptoms such as altered mental status, depression, or poor executive functioning.[6] The therapeutic approach to HF with a reduced EF in the elderly should be, in principal, identical to that in younger patients with respect the choice of pharmacologic therapy. However, altered pharmacokinetic and pharmacodynamic properties of cardiovascular drugs in the elderly may require that these therapies be applied more cautiously, with reductions in drug dosages when appropriate (see also Chapter 90). Other complicating factors may include, blunting of baroreceptor function, and orthostatic dysregulation of blood pressure, which may make it difficult to use target doses of some neurohormonal antagonists. Multidisciplinary HF programs have been successful in decreasing the rate of readmission and associated morbidity in elderly patients (see below).

Patients with Cancer

Patients with cancer are particularly predisposed to the development of HF as a result of the cardiotoxic effects of many cancer chemotherapeutic agents. The management of these patients is discussed in Chapters 56 and 57.

ANTICOAGULATION AND ANTIPLATELET THERAPY

Patients with HF have an increased risk for arterial or venous thromboembolic events. In clinical HF trials the rate of stroke ranges from 1.3% to 2.4%/yr. Depressed LV function is believed to promote relative stasis of blood in dilated cardiac chambers with increased risk of thrombus formation. Thromboembolism prophylaxis in patients with HF and AF should be individualized and based on an assessment of the risk of stroke versus the risk of bleeding on an anticoagulant. In general most patients with HFrEF will have an increased risk of stroke, as assessed by a variety of risk scores (e.g., Cardiac failure, Hypertension, Age ≥75 (Doubled), Diabetes, Stroke (Doubled)-Vascular disease, Age 65 to 74 and Sex category (Female) [CHA2DS2-VASc]). A recent meta-analysis of clinical trials in patients with nonvalvular AF suggests that, when compared to warfarin, novel oral anticoagulants (NOACs) have a favorable risk-benefit profile, with significant reductions in stroke, intracranial hemorrhage, and mortality, and with similar major bleeding as for warfarin, but increased gastrointestinal bleeding.[61] Other studies have suggested comparable efficacy but fewer major bleeding events. On the basis of these studies, the ESC HF guidelines recommend NOACs, recognizing that their safety in older subjects and subjects with impaired renal function is not known.[9] Anticoagulation is also recommended for all patients with a history of systemic or pulmonary emboli, including stroke or transient ischemic attack. Patients with symptomatic or asymptomatic ischemic cardiomyopathy and documented recent large anterior MI or recent MI with documented LV thrombus should be treated with warfarin (goal INR 2.0 to 3.0) for the initial 3 months after MI unless there are contraindications. The question of whether HF patients who are in sinus rhythm should be treated with anticoagulants to reduce stroke was addressed in the Warfarin Versus Aspirin in Reduced Cardiac Ejection Fraction (WARCEF) trial, which showed that treatment with warfarin as compared with aspirin did not reduce the composite outcome of time to ischemic stroke, intracerebral hemorrhage, or death from any cause (HR 0.93; 95% CI, 0.79 to 1.10, $P = 0.40$).[62] Although treatment with warfarin was associated with a significant reduction in the rate of ischemic stroke (HR 0.52; 95% CI, 0.33 to 82; $P = 0.005$), this benefit was offset by a significant increase in the rate of major hemorrhage. Interestingly, the rates of intracerebral and intracranial hemorrhage did not differ significantly between the two treatment groups. Based on the results of the WARCEF trial, there is no compelling reason to use warfarin rather than aspirin in HF patients with a reduced LVEF who are in sinus rhythm.

MANAGEMENT OF CARDIAC ARRHYTHMIAS

AF is the most common arrhythmia in HF (see also Chapters 65 and 66), and occurs in 15% to 30% of patients. AF may lead to worsening HF symptoms (see Table 50.5), and increases the risk of thromboembolic complications, particularly stroke. The Atrial Fibrillation and Congestive Heart Failure (AF-CHF) trial tested rate control versus rhythm control in patients with chronic HFrEF (EF <35%) and a history of AF. In AF-CHF a strategy of rhythm control (pharmacologic or electrical cardioversion) was superior to a strategy of controlling ventricular rate with respect to reducing death from cardiovascular causes (HR rhythm-control group 1.06; 95% CI 0.86 to 1.30; $P = 0.59$).[63] Secondary outcomes were also similar in the rate and rhythm control groups, including death from any cause, stroke, worsening HF, and the composite of death from cardiovascular causes, stroke, or worsening HF.[63] Accordingly, a rhythm-control strategy is best suited for patients with a reversible secondary cause of AF, or in patients who are not amenable to a rate strategy. For control of heart rate in HFrEF patients with AF, beta-blockers are preferred over digoxin, insofar as digoxin does not provide rate control during exercise. Although the effectiveness of beta-blockers in HFrEF patients with coexisting AF was cast in doubt by a patient-level meta-analysis, a recent substudy of the AF-CHF trial showed that the use of beta-blockers was associated with significantly lower mortality, but no difference in CV and non-CV hospitalization in patients with HFrEF and AF. The mortality reduction was not altered by the type of AF (i.e., paroxysmal or persistent) or the proportion of time spent in AF.[64] Importantly, the combination of digoxin and a beta-blocker is more effective than a beta-blocker alone in controlling the ventricular rate at rest. When beta-adrenergic blockers cannot be used, amiodarone has been used by some physicians, but chronic use has potentially significant risks, including thyroid disease and lung toxicity (see below). The short-term intravenous administration of diltiazem or amiodarone has been used for the acute treatment of patients with AF with very rapid ventricular response; however, the negative inotropic effects of nondihydropyridine calcium channel blockers such as diltiazem and verapamil must be considered if these agents are used. The optimum control of ventricular rate in patients with HF and AF is unclear at present. Although a resting ventricular response of 60 to 80 beats/min and a ventricular response between 90 and 115 beats/min during moderate exercise has been suggested by some experts, the RACE II study (Rate Control Efficacy in Permanent Atrial Fibrillation: a Comparison between Lenient versus Strict Rate Control II) did not show a difference in a composite of clinical outcomes when a strategy of strict rate control (<80 beats/min at rest and <110 beats/min during a 6 minute walk) was compared with lenient rate control.[65] Recognizing that sustained tachycardia can lead to a cardiomyopathy, AV node ablation and cardiac resynchronization (CRT) have been suggested for control of ventricular rate (<100 to 110 beats/min) in extreme cases of a rapid ventricular response with AF.[9]

> Most antiarrhythmic agents, with the exception of amiodarone and dofetilide, have negative inotropic effects and are proarrhythmic. Amiodarone is a class III antiarrhythmic that has little or no negative inotropic and/or proarrhythmic effects and is effective against most supraventricular arrhythmias (see also Chapter 66). Amiodarone is the preferred drug for restoring and maintaining sinus rhythm and may improve the success of electrical cardioversion in patients with HF. Amiodarone increases the level of phenytoin and digoxin, and will prolong the INR in patients taking warfarin. Therefore it is often necessary to reduce the dose of these drugs by as much as 50% when initiating therapy with amiodarone. The risks of adverse events, such as hyperthyroidism, hypothyroidism, pulmonary fibrosis, and hepatitis are relatively low, particularly when lower doses of amiodarone are used (100 to 200 mg/day). Dronedarone is a novel antiarrhythmic drug that reduces the incidence of AF and atrial flutter and has electrophysiologic properties that are similar to those of amiodarone, but does not contain iodine, and thus does not cause iodine-related adverse reactions. Although dronedarone was significantly more effective than placebo in maintaining sinus rhythm in several studies, the ANDROMEDA trial (European Trial of Dronedarone in Moderate to Severe Congestive Heart Failure) had to be terminated prematurely because of a twofold increase in mortality (HR 2.13; 95% CI 1.07 to 4.25; $P = .167$) in the dronedarone-treated HF patients.[66] The excess mortality was predominantly related to worsening of HF. As a result of this study dronedarone is contraindicated in patients with class IV HF, or those with class II or III HF who have had a recent HF decompensation. Because of the risk of proarrhythmic effects of antiarrhythmic agents in patients with LV dysfunction, it is preferable to treat ventricular arrhythmias with implantable cardioverter-defibrillators (ICDs), either alone or in combination with amiodarone (see also Chapter 69).

Two randomized clinical trials in HFrEF patients have demonstrated a reduction in all-cause mortality and hospitalizations with catheter ablation for AF. The AATAC (Ablation versus Amiodarone for Treatment of Atrial Fibrillation in Patients With Congestive Heart Failure and an Implanted ICD/CRTD) trial showed that catheter ablation of AF was superior to amiodarone in terms of achieving freedom from AF at long-term follow-up (primary endpoint) and reducing unplanned hospitalization and mortality (secondary endpoint RR 0.55; 95% CI 0.39 to 0.76).[67] The CASTLE-AF (Catheter Ablation versus Standard Conventional Treatment in Patients with Left Ventricular Dysfunction and Atrial Fibrillation) trial showed that catheter ablation reduced death from any cause or hospitalization for worsening HF (primary endpoint) in NYHA class II to IV HFrEF patients (HR 0.62; 95% CI 0.43 to 0.87; $P = 0.007$) with symptomatic paroxysmal or persistent AF.[68]

DEVICE THERAPY

Cardiac Resynchronization

CRT is discussed in detail in Chapters 58 and 69. When CRT is added to optimal medical therapy in patients in sinus rhythm there is a significant decrease in patient mortality and hospitalization, a reversal of LV remodeling, as well as improved quality of life and exercise capacity (see Chapter 58).[9,46] CRT should be considered for patients in NYHA class II to IV HF with a depressed EF less than 30% to 35% and a wide QRS who are on GDMT, and may be considered in select patients with NYHA class I HF with a wide QRS. For eligible patients, consideration should be given for implantation of CRT with an ICD (CRT-ICD).

Implantable Cardioverter-Defibrillators

ICDs are discussed in detail in Chapters 58, 69, and 70. Briefly, the prophylactic implantation of ICDs in patients with mild to moderate HF (NYHA class II to III) has been shown to reduce the incidence of sudden cardiac death in patients with ischemic or nonischemic cardiomyopathy (see Chapters 58 and 69). Accordingly, implantation of an ICD should be considered for patients in NYHA class II to III HF with a depressed EF less than 30% to 35%, who are on are on GDMT, and who have a reasonable expectation of survival with a good functional status for more than 1 year (class I indication}. CRT-ICD should be considered for NYHA class IV patients.

SLEEP-DISORDERED BREATHING

The general topic of sleep disorders in cardiovascular disease is discussed in detail Chapter 89. HF patients with a reduced EF (<40%) commonly exhibit sleep-disordered breathing: approximately 40% of patients exhibit central sleep apneas (CSA), commonly referred to as Cheyne-Stokes breathing (see also Chapter 48); whereas another 10% exhibit obstructive sleep apneas (OSA). CSA associated with Cheyne-Stokes respiration is a form of periodic breathing in which central apneas and hypopneas alternate with periods of hyperventilation that have a waxing-waning pattern of tidal volume. Risk factors for the development of CSA in an HF patient include male gender, age older than 60 years, the presence of AF, and hypocapnia.[69] Figure 50.17 illustrates the proposed mechanisms that underlie periodic oscillations in ventilation in HF, including heightened sensitivity to arterial partial pressure and long circulation time. The main clinical significance of CSA in HF is its association with increased mortality. Whether this is simply because Cheyne-Stokes respiration with central sleep apnea is a reflection of advanced disease with poor LV function, or whether its presence constitutes a separate and additive adverse influence on outcomes is not clear. This statement notwithstanding, multivariate analyses suggest that central sleep apnea remains an independent risk factor for death or cardiac transplantation, even after controlling for potentially confounding risk factors. The potential mechanism(s) for adverse outcomes in HF patients with CSA may be attributed to marked neurohumoral activation (especially norepinephrine). Studies have suggested that Cheyne-Stokes respirations can resolve with proper treatment of HF. However, if the patient continues to have symptoms related to sleep-disordered breathing for the treatment of nocturnal hypoxemia in OSA, despite optimization of HF therapies, a comprehensive overnight sleep study-polysomnography is indicated.

Although current guidelines recommend that continuous positive airway pressure (CPAP) may be reasonable to improve sleep quality and daytime sleepiness in patients with OSA,[12] there is no consensus as to how CSA should be treated. Insofar as CSA is to some extent a manifestation of advanced HF, the first consideration is to optimize drug therapy, including aggressive diuresis to lower cardiac-filling pressure, along with the use of ACEIs/ARBs, ARNIs, beta-blockers and MRAs, which may lessen the severity of CSA. In some cases, however, metabolic alkalosis arising from diuretic use may predispose to CSA by narrowing the difference between the circulating $Paco_2$ level and the $Paco_2$ threshold that is necessary for apnea to develop. The use of nocturnal oxygen and devices that provide CPAP has been reported to alleviate CSA, abolish apnea-related hypoxia, decrease nocturnal norepinephrine levels, as well as producing symptomatic and functional improvement in HF patients when used in the short term (up to 1 month). However, the effects of supplemental oxygen on cardiovascular endpoints over more prolonged periods have not been assessed. Although there is no direct evidence that treatment of sleep-disturbed breathing prevents the development of HF, treatment with CPAP has been shown to improve LV structure and function in patients with either obstructive or central sleep apnea disturbed-breathing syndrome.[69] Despite these objective measurements of improvement with CPAP, this treatment modality did not lead to a prolongation of life in the Canadian Continuous Positive Airway Pressure for Patients with Central Sleep Apnea and Heart Failure (CANPAP) trial,[69] which was discontinued early after concerns about the early divergence of transplantation-free survival favoring the control group. There was no difference in the primary endpoint of death or transplantation (p = 0.54), nor was there a significant difference in the frequency of hospitalization between groups (0.56 vs. 0.61 hospitalizations per patient year, (p = 0.45). However, a post-hoc analysis of the CANPAP study suggested that adequate suppression of CSA by CPAP was associated with improved heart transplant–free survival.[69] The role of adaptive servo-ventilation (ASV), which alleviates CSA by delivering servo-controlled inspiratory pressure support on top of expiratory positive airway pressure, was evaluated in the SERVE-HF trial (Treatment of Sleep-Disordered Breathing with Predominant Central Sleep Apnea by Adaptive Servo Ventilation in Patients with Heart Failure).[70] In patients with HFrEF (LVEF ≤ 45%) who predominately had CSA, ASV had no effect on the primary endpoint, which was a time-to-event analysis of the first event of death from any cause, lifesaving cardiovascular intervention (cardiac transplantation, implantation of a ventricular assist device, resuscitation after sudden cardiac arrest, or appropriate lifesaving shock), or unplanned hospitalization for worsening HF. However, all-cause mortality (HR 1.28 [95% CI, 1.06 to 1.55]; P = 0.01) and cardiovascular mortality (HR 1.34 [95% CI, 1.09 to 1.65]; p = 0.006) were significantly higher in the ASV group than in the control group. Therefore, ASV is not recommended in patients with NYHA class II to IV HFrEF and predominately CSA (Level III: harm[12]). Thus, the data remain unclear whether elimination of apnea will lead to improved clinical outcomes. Other therapies that have been proposed for sleep-disordered breathing in HF include nocturnal oxygen, CO_2 administration (by adding dead space), theophylline, and acetazolamide and diaphragmatic pacing; these have not yet been systematically studied in outcome-based prospective randomized trials (see Chapter 89).

DISEASE MANAGEMENT

Despite the compelling scientific evidence that ACEIs/ARBs, beta-blockers, and aldosterone antagonists reduce hospitalizations and mortality in patients with HF, these life-prolonging therapies continue to be underutilized outside of the highly artificial environment of clinical trials. Indeed, numerous studies in a variety of different clinical settings have documented that a significant proportion of patients with HF are not receiving treatment with guideline-recommended, evidence-based therapies. The failure to deliver optimal medical care to HF patients is almost certainly multifactorial, as it is with other complex chronic conditions that have substantial morbidity and mortality. Further, the elderly nature of many HF patients, who often have a myriad of comorbidities, also presents special challenges to health care providers. Optimal HF care includes a trained network of healthcare providers involved in the delivery of HF management and interventions, including nurses, case managers, physicians, pharmacists, case workers, dietitians, physical therapists, psychologists, and information systems specialists; a method for communicating this knowledge to the patient, including patient education, education of caregivers and family members, medication management, peer support, or some form of post-acute care; and a method of ensuring that the patient has received and understood the knowledge; a system for encouraging adherence to the recommended regimen and monitoring patient compliance (Fig. 50.18). Numerous studies have shown that many of the challenges to delivering optimal care to HF patients can be met through an integrated specialized HF clinic approach that uses nurse and physician extenders to deliver and ensure the implementation of care. Technology-driven strategies that employ low-cost telemonitoring also appear promising in terms of improving HF management and outcomes (see also Chapter 58)[71]; however, the optimum approach to noninvasive remote monitoring is uncertain and the data from randomized clinical trials have been inconsistent, and so these strategies are not recommended by current practice guidelines.

A disease management approach to HF has been shown to reduce hospitalizations and increase the percentage of patients receiving ideal, guideline-recommended therapy. Recent studies demonstrate that disease management programs need not be confined to the outpatient setting and that hospital-based disease management systems can also improve medical care and education of hospitalized HF patients and accelerate use of evidence-based, guideline-recommended therapies by administering them before hospital discharge.[41] Although disease management strategies can lead to improved survival, it is not clear that these strategies are necessarily more cost effective. Accordingly, the biggest challenge to disease management programs will be to determine how to support the additional personnel required in this model of care.

PATIENTS WITH REFRACTORY END-STAGE HEART FAILURE (STAGE D)

Most patients with HFrEF respond well to evidenced-based pharmacologic and nonpharmacologic treatments and enjoy a good quality of life with a meaningful prolongation of life. However, for reasons that are not clear, some patients do not improve or will experience a rapid recurrence of symptoms despite optimal medical and device therapies. These individuals represent the most advanced stage of HF (stage D) and should be considered for specialized treatment strategies, such as mechanical circulatory support (see Chapter 59), continuous intravenous positive inotropic therapy, or referral for cardiac transplantation (see Chapter 60). However, before a patient is considered to have refractory HF, physicians should identify any contributing conditions (see Table 50.5) and ensure that all conventional medical strategies have been optimally employed. When no further therapies are appropriate, the focus of disease management should shift to palliation of symptoms.

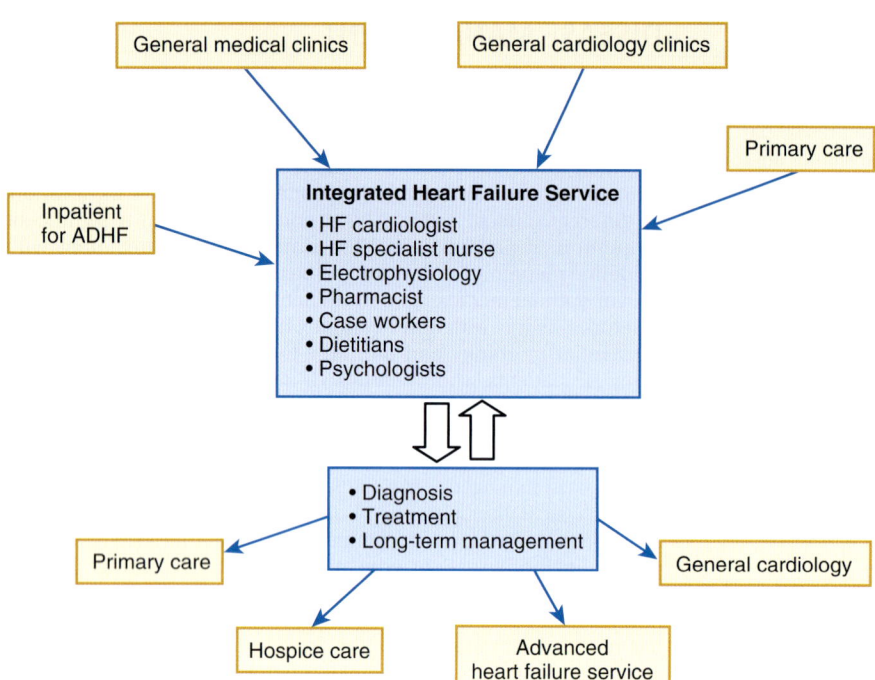

FIGURE 50.18 Integrated disease management program in heart failure. (Modified from McDonagh TA. Lessons from the management of chronic heart failure. *Heart.* 2005;91[suppl 2]:ii24–ii27.)

INTEGRATION OF PALLIATIVE CARE INTO HEART FAILURE CARE

Ideally, patients should continue to be cared for by a team of health care providers with whom they have established a longitudinal relationship, and who apply palliative care principles (Table 50.9). Palliative care is designed to improve quality of life for patients and their families through anticipation of declining health status and major events, clarification of goals of care, relief of physical symptoms, provision of psychosocial and spiritual support, coordination of care, and assistance with bereavement (Fig. 50.19).[72] The high prevalence, morbidity, and lethality of HF creates a substantial need for palliative care at the end of life. However, many providers of cardiovascular care do not distinguish between palliative care and hospice, nor do they understand the indications for these services. Palliative approaches to care should be integrated throughout the care of patients with cardiovascular disease, with intensification during major events and approaching the end of life.

Primary Palliative Care

All clinicians caring for patients with advanced cardiovascular disease play a role in the provision of supportive and palliative interventions. This role is vital insofar as (1) many of the therapies that improve symptoms and quality of life derive from treatment of the underlying cardiovascular disease; (2) prognosis and complex decisions are often best understood by the cardiovascular specialist; (3) integrated care is often preferable to further fragmentation through another consult team; and (4) there are not enough palliative care specialists to provide such services to everyone in need. Provision of supportive care by the usual care team has been designated as "primary" palliative care, to distinguish it from "secondary" or "subspecialty" palliative care.[73] Clinicians supervising inpatient or longitudinal care for patients with cardiovascular disease should regard expertise in providing palliative care as integral to their professional competence.

Hospice

The term *hospice* is used to describe a specific model of palliative care that is offered to patients who are at the end of life with a terminal disease when curative or life-prolonging therapy is no longer a focus of treatment. Historically, hospice was developed for patients with cancer, but it is increasingly used for patients with cardiovascular disease, with 14.7% of admissions to US hospices in 2014 having a primary diagnosis of heart disease. In the United States, referral is guided by the Centers for Medicare and Medicaid Services (CMS) hospice eligibility guidelines, which require that a physician estimate that life expectancy is 6 months or less.[74] While the 6-month time period is rarely reached, patients who survive beyond it can usually continue to receive hospice benefits if the prognosis remains poor.

Treatment of Symptoms Approaching End of Life

Progressive symptoms are the most common reason for reductions in health status among patients with HF. Indeed, symptom burden at the end of life is often greater than for patients with advanced lung or pancreatic cancer.[75] Accordingly, the design of the cardiovascular regimen and general palliative approaches are critical near the end of life. The best treatment to relieve late-stage cardiac symptoms is often continuation of the regimen that was initiated to decrease progression from earlier stages of disease. The primary treatment of symptomatic congestion remains diuretic therapy. Supplementation with oral, sublingual, or topical nitrates can temporarily help redistribute volume when adequate diuresis cannot be achieved. If symptoms relate to diuretic resistance or hypotension, decrease or discontinuation of neurohormonal antagonists may improve comfort by enhancing diuretic response and

TABLE 50.9 Key Messages for Managing Patients with Cardiovascular Disease Nearing End of Life

1. Worsening disease should trigger preparation with patients and families, but without specifically answering the question of how much time remains, which is usually bounded by wide uncertainty.
2. "What-if" conversations should be standard prior to any major intervention in the setting of advanced cardiac disease or other serious medical conditions, including frailty.
3. Difficult discussions now will simplify difficult decisions in the future.
4. Shared decisions include a broad spectrum of potential interventions beyond those relating to resuscitation preferences.
5. Deactivation of the defibrillation function of ICDs should be explained and offered regularly to patients with poor prognosis and must be done before transition to hospice.
6. Palliative care specialist consultation may be particularly helpful to facilitate decision making within challenging family dynamics and to improve relief of refractory symptoms.
7. Clinicians with existing relationships should shoulder the primary responsibility for presenting an end-of-life plan consistent with values and goals expressed by patient and family.
8. The transition separating "Do Everything" from hospice may be bridged through a phase of "Quality Survival" during which time patients increasingly weigh the benefits, risks, and burdens of initiating or continuing life-sustaining treatments.
9. Revision of the medical regimen for symptom relief and quality of life may involve discontinuation of some recommended therapies and addition of therapies not usually recommended.
10. The end-of-life plan should honor patient preference for site of death as feasible, with agreement upon a "Plan B" if that becomes unsupportable.

From Allen LA, Stevenson LW. Management of patients with cardiovascular disease approaching end of life. In: Zipes DP, Libby P, Bonow RO, et al., eds. *Braunwald's Heart Disease.* 11th ed. Elsevier; 2019:590.

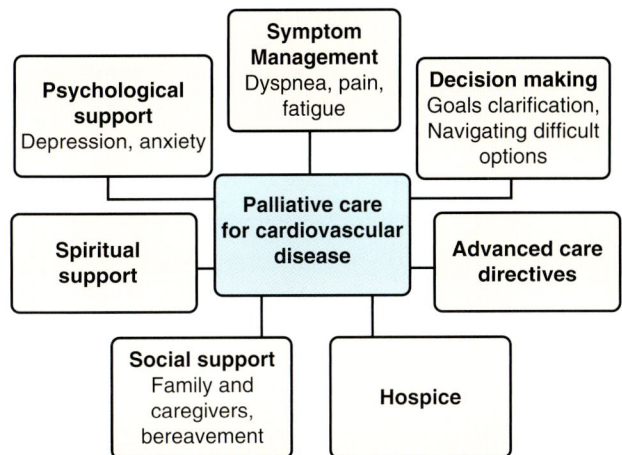

FIGURE 50.19 Components of palliative care for end-stage heart failure. (From Allen LA, Stevenson LW. Management of patients with cardiovascular disease approaching end of life. In: Zipes DP, Libby P, Bonow RO, et al., eds. *Braunwald's Heart Disease*. 11th ed. Elsevier; 2019:590.)

increasing systemic blood pressure. Although discontinuation of these agents is associated with worsening HF over time in stable patients, it is unlikely to worsen cardiac function or symptoms in the final days of life. Caution is required in certain situations; for example, withdrawal of beta-blockers may worsen symptom burden in patients with frequent angina or tachyarrhythmias. Relaxation of chronic sodium and fluid restriction often worsens symptoms of congestion; but favorite foods and beverages can be a major factor in quality of life and social interaction for some patients at a time when few other shared pleasures remain.

FUTURE PERSPECTIVES

As discussed in the foregoing chapter treatment with ACEIs/ARBs, beta-blockers, MRAs, and cardiac devices has substantially improved quality and quantity of life for patients with HFrEF. Moreover, recent success with the use of ARNIs and SGLT2 inhibitors has opened up the possibility of combining traditional neurohormonal approaches with additional drugs, whose mode of action is not completely understood. Ongoing approaches with small molecules that modulate contractility and gene therapy, accompanied by growing appreciation of the role of pharmacogenomics (see Chapter 7), will undoubtedly lead to further advances in the field.

REFERENCES

Etiology and Prognosis

1. Bocchi EA. Heart failure in South America. *Curr Cardiol Rev*. 2013;9(2):147–156.
2. Walsh CR, Larson MG, et al. Alcohol consumption and risk for congestive heart failure in the Framingham Heart Study. *Ann Intern Med*. 2002;136(3):181–191.
3. McMurray JJ, Adamopoulos S, Anker SD, et al. ESC guidelines for the diagnosis and treatment of acute and chronic heart failure 2012: the task force for the diagnosis and treatment of acute and chronic heart failure 2012 of the European Society of Cardiology. Developed in collaboration with the Heart Failure Association (HFA) of the ESC. *Eur Heart J*. 2012;33:1787–1847.
4. Go AS, Mozaffarian D, Roger VL, et al. Heart disease and stroke statistics—2013 update: a report from the American Heart Association. *Circulation*. 2013;127(1):e6–e245.
5. Yancy CW. Heart failure in African Americans. *Am J Cardiol*. 2005;96(7B):3i–12i.
6. Thomas S, Rich MW. Epidemiology, pathophysiology, and prognosis of heart failure in the elderly. *Heart Fail Clin*. 2007;3(4):381–387.
7. Jaffe AS, Miller WL. Meta-analyses and interpretation of troponin values in heart failure. *JACC Heart Fail*. 2018;6(3):198–200.
8. von HS, Anker MS, Jankowska EA, et al. Anemia in chronic heart failure: can we treat? What to treat? *Heart Fail Rev*. 2012;17(2):203–210.
9. Ponikowski P, Voors AA, Anker SD, et al. 2016 ESC Guidelines for the diagnosis and treatment of acute and chronic heart failure: the task force for the diagnosis and treatment of acute and chronic heart failure of the European Society of Cardiology (ESC)Developed with the special contribution of the Heart Failure Association (HFA) of the ESC. *Eur Heart J*. 2016;37:2129–2200.
10. Fitzsimons S, Doughty RN. Iron deficiency in patients with heart failure. *Eur Heart J Cardiovasc Pharmacother*. 2015;1(1):58–64.
11. von Haehling S, Ebner N, Evertz R, et al. Iron deficiency in heart failure. An Overview. 2019;7(1):36–46.

Approach to the Patient and Management

12. Yancy CW, Jessup M, Bozkurt B, et al. 2017 ACC/AHA/HFSA focused update of the 2013 ACCF/AHA guideline for the management of heart failure: a report of the American College of Cardiology/American Heart Association Task force on clinical practice guidelines and the Heart Failure Society of America. *Circulation*. 2017;136(6):e137–e161.
13. Cole RT, Masoumi A, Triposkiadis F, et al. Renal dysfunction in heart failure. *Med Clin North Am*. 2012;96(5):955–974.
14. Kelly RB. Microtubules, membrane traffic, and cell organization. *Cell*. 1990;61:5–7.
15. Yancy CW, Jessup M, Bozkurt B, et al. 2013 ACCF/AHA guideline for the management of heart failure: a report of the American College of Cardiology Foundation/American Heart Association Task Force on Practice Guidelines. *Circulation*. 2013;128:e240–e327.
16. Ledwidge M, Gallagher J, Conlon C, et al. Natriuretic peptide-based screening and collaborative care for heart failure: the STOP-HF randomized trial. *J Am Med Assoc*. 2013;310(1):66–74.
17. Dias A, Nunez Gil IJ, Santoro F, et al. Takotsubo syndrome: state-of-the-art review by an expert panel - part 1. *Cardiovasc Revasc Med*. 2019;20(1):70–79.
18. Yancy CW, Jessup M, Bozkurt B, et al. 2017 ACC/AHA/HFSA focused update of the 2013 ACCF/AHA guideline for the management of heart failure: a report of the American College of Cardiology/American Heart Association Task Force on Clinical Practice Guidelines and the Heart Failure Society of America. *J Am Coll Cardiol*. 2017;70(6):776–803.
19. O'Connor CM, Whellan DJ, Lee KL, et al. Efficacy and safety of exercise training in patients with chronic heart failure: HF-ACTION randomized controlled trial. *J Am Med Assoc*. 2009;301(14):1439–1450.
20. Faris RF, Flather M, Purcell H, et al. Diuretics for heart failure. *Cochrane Database Syst Rev*. 2012;2:CD003838.
21. Ellison DH, Felker GM. Diuretic treatment in heart failure. *N Engl J Med*. 2017;377(20):1964–1975.
22. Filippatos G, Anker SD, Bohm M, et al. A randomized controlled study of finerenone vs. eplerenone in patients with worsening chronic heart failure and diabetes mellitus and/or chronic kidney disease. *Eur Heart J*. 2016;37(27):2105–2114.
23. Cherney DZ, Odutayo A, Aronson R, et al. Sodium glucose cotransporter-2 inhibition and cardiorenal protection. *J Amer Coll Cardiol*. 2019;74(20):2511–2524.
24. Finley JJ, Konstam MA, Udelson JE. Arginine vasopressin antagonists for the treatment of heart failure and hyponatremia. *Circulation*. 2008;118(4):410–421.
25. Konstam MA, Gheorghiade M, Burnett Jr JC, et al. Effects of oral tolvaptan in patients hospitalized for worsening heart failure: the EVEREST Outcome Trial. *J Am Med Assoc*. 2007;297(12):1319–1331.
26. Juurlink DN, Mamdani MM, Lee DS, et al. Rates of hyperkalemia after publication of the randomized Aldactone evaluation study. *N Engl J Med*. 2004;351(6):543–551.
27. Pitt B, Bakris GL, Bushinsky DA, et al. Effect of patiromer on reducing serum potassium and preventing recurrent hyperkalaemia in patients with heart failure and chronic kidney disease on RAAS inhibitors. *Eur J Heart Fail*. 2015;17(10):1057–1065.
28. Arfe A, Scotti L, Varas-Lorenzo C, et al. Non-steroidal anti-inflammatory drugs and risk of heart failure in four European countries: nested case-control study. *BMJ*. 2016;354:i4857.
29. Wile D. Diuretics: a review. *Ann Clin Biochem*. 2012;49(Pt 5):419–431.
30. Ellison DH. Diuretic therapy and resistance in congestive heart failure. *Cardiology*. 2001;96(3–4):132–143.
31. Stevenson LW, Nohria A, Mielniczuk L. Torrent or torment from the tubules? challenge of the cardiorenal connections. *J Am Coll Cardiol*. 2005;45(12):2004–2007.
32. Schefold JC, Filippatos G, Hasenfuss G, et al. Heart failure and kidney dysfunction: epidemiology, mechanisms and management. *Nat Rev Nephrol*. 2016;12(10):610–623.
33. Mentz RJ, Kjeldsen K, Rossi GP, et al. Decongestion in acute heart failure. *Eur J Heart Fail*. 2014;16(5):471–482.
34. Leong DP, McMurray JJV, Joseph PG, Yusuf S. From ACE inhibitors/ARBs to ARNIs in coronary artery disease and heart failure (Part 2/5). *J Am Coll Cardiol*. 2019;74(5):683–698.
35. Lee VC, Rhew DC, Dylan M, et al. Meta-analysis: angiotensin-receptor blockers in chronic heart failure and high-risk acute myocardial infarction. *Ann Intern Med*. 2004;141(9):693–704.
36. Braunwald E. The path to an angiotensin receptor antagonist-neprilysin inhibitor in the treatment of heart failure. *J Am Coll Cardiol*. 2015;65(10):1029–1041.
37. Rubio DM, Schoenbaum EE, Lee LS, et al. Defining translational research: implications for training. *Acad Med*. 2010;85(3):470–475.
38. Mann DL, Greene SJ, Givertz MM, et al. Sacubitril/valsartan in advanced heart failure with reduced ejection fraction: rationale and design of the LIFE trial. *JACC Heart Fail*. 2020.
39. Jondeau G, Neuder Y, Eicher JC, et al. B-CONVINCED: beta-blocker CONtinuation Vs. INterruption in patients with Congestive heart failure hospitalized for a decompensation episode. *Eur Heart J*. 2009;30(18):2186–2192.
40. Schrier RW. Aldosterone "escape" vs "breakthrough". *Nat Rev Nephrol*. 2010;6(2):61.
41. Jessup M, Abraham WT, Casey DE, et al. 2009 focused update: ACCF/AHA guidelines for the diagnosis and management of heart failure in adults: a report of the American College of Cardiology Foundation/American Heart Association Task Force on Practice Guidelines: developed in collaboration with the International Society for Heart and Lung Transplantation. *Circulation*. 2009;119(14):1977–2016.
42. Seed A, Gardner R, McMurray J, et al. Neurohumoral effects of the new orally active renin inhibitor, aliskiren, in chronic heart failure. *Eur J Heart Fail*. 2007;9(11):1120–1127.
43. Cleland JG, Abdellah AT, Khaleva O, et al. Clinical trials update from the European Society of Cardiology Congress 2007: 3CPO, ALOFT, PROSPECT and statins for heart failure. *Eur J Heart Fail*. 2007;9(10):1070–1073.
44. Gheorghiade M, Bohm M, Greene SJ, et al. Effect of aliskiren on postdischarge mortality and heart failure readmissions among patients hospitalized for heart failure: the ASTRONAUT randomized trial. *J Am Med Assoc*. 2013;309(11):1125–1135.
45. McMurray JJ, Krum H, Abraham WT, et al. Aliskiren, enalapril, or aliskiren and enalapril in heart failure. *N Engl J Med*. 2016;374(16):1521–1532.
46. Yancy CW, Jessup M, Bozkurt B, et al. 2016 ACC/AHA/HFSA focused update on new pharmacological therapy for heart failure: an update of the 2013 ACCF/AHA guideline for the management of heart failure: a report of the American College of Cardiology/American Heart Association Task Force on Clinical Practice Guidelines and the Heart Failure Society of America. *J Am Coll Cardiol*. 2016.
47. Swedberg K, Komajda M, Bohm M, et al. Ivabradine and outcomes in chronic heart failure (SHIFT): a randomised placebo-controlled study. *Lancet*. 2010;376(9744):875–885.
48. Zinman B, Wanner C, Lachin JM, et al. Empagliflozin, cardiovascular outcomes, and mortality in type 2 diabetes. *N Engl J Med*. 2015;373(22):2117–2128.
49. McMurray JJV, Solomon SD, Inzucchi SE, et al. Dapagliflozin in patients with heart failure and reduced ejection fraction. *N Engl J Med*. 2019.
50. Packer M, Anker SD, Butler J, et al. Cardiovascular and renal outcomes with empagliflozin in heart failure. *N Engl J Med*. 2020.
51. O'Meara E, McDonald M, Chan M, et al. CCS/CHFS heart failure guidelines: clinical trial update on functional mitral regurgitation, SGLT2 inhibitors, ARNI in HFpEF, and Tafamidis in Amyloidosis. *Can J Cardiol*. 2020;36(2):159–169.
52. Armstrong PW, Pieske B, Anstrom KJ, et al. Vericiguat in patients with heart failure and reduced ejection fraction. *N Engl J Med*. 2020;382(20):1883–1893.
53. Teerlink JR, Felker GM, McMurray JJ, et al. Chronic Oral Study of Myosin Activation to Increase Contractility In Heart Failure (COSMIC-HF): a phase 2, pharmacokinetic, randomised, placebo-controlled trial. *Lancet*. 2016;388(10062):2895–2903.
54. GISSI-HF Investigators. Effect of n-3 polyunsaturated fatty acids in patients with chronic heart failure (the GISSI-HF trial): a randomised, double-blind, placebo-controlled trial. *Lancet*. 2008;372:1223–1230.
55. Krittanawong C, Namath A, Lanfear DE, Tang WH. Practical pharmacogenomic approaches to heart failure therapeutics. *Curr Treat Options Cardiovasc Med*. 2016;18(10):60.
56. Piccini JP, Abraham WT, Dufton C, et al. Bucindolol for the maintenance of sinus rhythm in a genotype-defined HF population: the GENETIC-AF trial. *JACC Heart Fail*. 2019;7(7):586–598.

57. Lindenfeld J, Albert NM, Boehmer JP, et al. HFSA 2010 comprehensive heart failure practice guideline. *J Card Fail.* 2010;16(6):e1–194.
58. Borer JS, Swedberg K, Komajda M, et al. Efficacy profile of ivabradine in patients with heart failure plus angina pectoris. *Cardiology.* 2017;136(2):138–144.
59. Dunlay SM, Roger VL. Gender differences in the pathophysiology, clinical presentation, and outcomes of ischemic heart failure. *Curr Heart Fail Rep.* 2012;9(4):267–276.
60. Lanfear DE, Hrobowski TN, Peterson EL, et al. Association of beta-blocker exposure with outcomes in heart failure differs between African American and white patients. *Circ Heart Fail.* 2012;5(2):202–208.
61. Ruff CT, Giugliano RP, Braunwald E, et al. Comparison of the efficacy and safety of new oral anticoagulants with warfarin in patients with atrial fibrillation: a meta-analysis of randomised trials. *Lancet.* 2014;383(9921):955–962.
62. Homma S, Thompson JL, Pullicino PM, et al. Warfarin and aspirin in patients with heart failure and sinus rhythm. *N Engl J Med.* 2012;366(20):1859–1869.
63. Roy D, Talajic M, Nattel S, et al. Rhythm control versus rate control for atrial fibrillation and heart failure. *N Engl J Med.* 2008;358(25):2667–2677.
64. Cadrin-Tourigny J, Shohoudi A, Roy D, et al. Decreased mortality with beta-blockers in patients with heart failure and coexisting atrial fibrillation: an AF-CHF substudy. *JACC Heart Fail.* 2017;5(2):99–106.
65. Van Gelder IC, Groenveld HF, Crijns HJ, et al. Lenient versus strict rate control in patients with atrial fibrillation. *N Engl J Med.* 2010;362(15):1363–1373.
66. Kober L, Torp-Pedersen C, McMurray JJ, et al. Increased mortality after dronedarone therapy for severe heart failure. *N Engl J Med.* 2008;358(25):2678–2687.
67. Di Biase L, Mohanty P, Mohanty S, et al. Ablation versus amiodarone for treatment of persistent atrial fibrillation in patients with congestive heart failure and an implanted device: results from the AATAC multicenter randomized trial. *Circulation.* 2016;133(17):1637–1644.
68. Marrouche NF, Brachmann J, Andresen D, et al. Catheter ablation for atrial fibrillation with heart failure. *N Engl J Med.* 2018;378(5):417–427.
69. Sharma B, McSharry D, Malhotra A. Sleep disordered breathing in patients with heart failure: pathophysiology and management. *Curr Treat Options Cardiovasc Med.* 2011;13(6):506–516.
70. Cowie MR, Woehrle H, Wegscheider K, et al. Adaptive servo-ventilation for central sleep apnea in systolic heart failure. *N Engl J Med.* 2015;373(12):1095–1105.

Disease Management, Patients with End-Stage Heart Failure and Palliative Care

71. Maric B, Kaan A, Ignaszewski A, Lear SA. A systematic review of telemonitoring technologies in heart failure. *Eur J Heart Fail.* 2009;11(5):506–517.
72. Braun LT, Grady KL, Kutner JS, et al. Palliative care and cardiovascular disease and stroke: a policy statement from the American Heart Association/American Stroke Association. *Circulation.* 2016;134(11):e198–e225.
73. World Palliative Care Alliance; WHO. *Global Atlas of Palliative Care at the End of Life. 2014.* Worldwide Palliative Care Alliance; 2014.
74. CMS Services. Medicare benefit policy manual: coverage of hospice services under hospital insurance. In: CMS Services, ed. *Centers for Medicare and Medicaid Services Rev.* 246th ed. Centers for Medicare and Medicaid Services; 2018.
75. Bekelman DB, Rumsfeld JS, Havranek EP, et al. Symptom burden, depression, and spiritual well-being: a comparison of heart failure and advanced cancer patients. *J Gen Intern Med.* 2009;24(5):592–598.

51 Heart Failure with Preserved and Mildly Reduced Ejection Fraction

CAROLYN S.P. LAM, SANJIV J. SHAH, AND SCOTT D. SOLOMON

EPIDEMIOLOGY, 1007
Prevalence, 1007
Incidence, 1008
Risk Factors, 1008
Atrial Fibrillation, 1008
Prognosis, 1008
Quality of Life, 1010

DIAGNOSIS, 1010

PATHOPHYSIOLOGY, 1017

Pathophysiology of HFpEF and HFmrEF, 1017

TREATMENT OF HFPEF AND HFMREF, 1020
General Considerations, 1021
Empiric Therapy of HFpEF and HFmrEF, 1023
Specific Pharmacologic Treatment, 1024
Device Therapy in HFpEF and HFmrEF, 1026

Lifestyle Modification and Exercise Training, 1028
Unsuccessful and Potentially Harmful Treatments in HFpEF, 1028
Emerging Concepts in the Treatment of HFpEF and HFmrEF, 1028
Ongoing Clinical Trials in HFpEF, 1028

REFERENCES, 1028

The pathophysiologic definition of heart failure (HF)—the "inability of the heart to pump blood to the body at a rate commensurate with its needs, or to do so only at the cost of high filling pressures"[1]—is based on the presence of hemodynamic congestion that results in a clinical syndrome characterized by breathlessness, fatigue, and edema but importantly makes no assumption regarding underlying left ventricular (LV) ejection fraction (EF). Yet with the advent of major randomized clinical trials in HF that included an upper LVEF exclusion criterion, the diagnosis of HF became intertwined with ejection fraction. The focus on patients with reduced LVEF has been understandable given their higher mortality rates and the benefit observed in trials of neurohormonal agents. Isolated case reports and small case series in the 1980s served as reminders that HF could occur in the absence of overt reduction in LVEF.[2-4] However, this syndrome received little attention until the more widespread use of noninvasive assessment of LVEF provided robust epidemiologic evidence of the scope of HF in the absence of reduced LVEF. Collectively, these early epidemiologic data showed that approximately half of patients with HF did not have a markedly reduced LVEF and that these patients had a significantly increased risk of death and hospitalization compared with the general population.[5,6]

Although the term HFpEF is nearly universally used currently, there remains debate what LVEF cutoff should be used to define it and indeed what to name this broad syndrome. Whereas some have used the term to define HF with EF above the range generally considered reduced (40% or less), a nomenclature that was first used to distinguish the component of the CHARM program in which patients had HF and LVEF >40%, the most recent guidelines suggest that "HFpEF" be defined using an LVEF cutoff of ≥50%,[7-9] (instead of >40% in CHARM-Preserved). The 2016 European Society of Cardiology HF Guidelines adopted the term "HF with mid-range EF" to refer to patients with LVEF 40% to 50%, while the 2013 American College of Cardiology/American Heart Association HF Guidelines used "borderline" to describe this group. Importantly, this new nomenclature led to an upsurge of publications related to this previously neglected subgroup of HF.[10] More recently, "HF with mid-range EF" has been renamed as "HF with mildly reduced EF."[11,12] Accordingly, this chapter discusses the epidemiology, pathophysiology, diagnosis, and therapy of patients with HFpEF and HF with mildly reduced ejection fraction (HFmrEF). Of note, most epidemiologic and pathophysiologic studies in patients with HF and EF >40% have focused on the subgroup with HFpEF (EF ≥50%), although several completed and ongoing clinical trials have included both types of patients.

EPIDEMIOLOGY

Estimates of the prevalence and incidence of HFpEF and HFmrEF depend on the definition used, method of ascertainment, and population studied. As HF is a clinical syndrome, its ascertainment in epidemiologic studies is challenging, typically relying on hospitalization diagnostic codes with or without additional adjudication using well-accepted clinical criteria such as the Framingham criteria.[13] Furthermore, the determination of LVEF is not always available at the time of HF presentation or using standardized state-of-the-art methods (including echocardiography).

Prevalence

Multiple community-based cohorts have reported on the prevalence of HFpEF in diverse populations across the United States and Europe. Together, these studies showed that approximately half the HF population have LVEF >50%. Although the overall prevalence of HF in the community increases with age, the prevalence of HFpEF is higher in women than in men at any given age, although men are more represented at lower ejection fractions.[14]

Estimating temporal trends in the prevalence of HFpEF is challenged by changes in diagnostic criteria and measurement techniques. Early epidemiologic studies did not include echocardiography, but increased awareness, availability, and routine use of both (more advanced) echocardiography and natriuretic peptides may have contributed to a reported increase in the prevalence of HFpEF and HFmrEF in recent years. Nonetheless, large studies of hospitalized HF in the United States consistently show that the proportion of hospitalized HFpEF has increased over time relative to hospitalized HF with reduced EF (HFrEF).[5] Among 110,621 patients hospitalized for HF in 275 U.S. hospitals in Get With the Guidelines-Heart Failure, from 2005 to 2010, the proportion of patients with LVEF ≥40% increased from 48% to 53%, with a projected increase to 65% by 2020.[15,16] The latter study also provided estimates of the proportion of patients with LVEF in the 40% to 50% range, which averaged ~15% and did not change over time. Conversely, the proportion with LVEF ≥50% increased from 33% in 2005 to 39% in 2010, while the proportion with LVEF <40%, decreased from 52% to 47% over the same time frame. Similar observations have been reported in Japan.[17,18] *In summary, the prevalence of HFpEF and HFmrEF is high and increasing over time relative to HFrEF, a phenomenon related to aging of the population,*[19] *making these the predominant forms of HF in aging societies.*

TABLE 51.1 Risk Factors for Heart Failure

HFpEF	sHR* (95% CI)	P
Age, per 10 years	1.90 (1.74-2.07)	<0.0001
Male sex	0.93 (0.78-1.11)	0.43
Systolic BP, per 20 mm Hg	1.14 (1.05-1.24)	0.003
Body mass index, per 4 kg/m²	1.28 (1.21-1.37)	<0.0001
Antihypertensive treatment	1.42 (1.18-1.71)	0.0002
Previous myocardial infarction	1.48 (1.12-1.96)	0.006
HFrEF	**sHR* (95% CI)**	**P**
Age, per 10 years	1.66 (1.52-1.80)	<0.0001
Male sex	1.84 (1.55-2.19)	<0.0001
Systolic BP, per 20 mm Hg	1.20 (1.10-1.30)	<0.0001
Body mass index, per 4 kg/m²	1.19 (1.11-1.28)	<0.0001
Antihypertensive treatment	1.35 (1.13-1.63)	0.001
Diabetes mellitus	1.83 (1.48-2.26)	<0.0001
Current smoker	1.41 (1.14-1.75)	0.0015
Previous myocardial infarction	2.60 (2.08-3.25)	<0.0001
ECG LV hypertrophy	2.12 (1.55-2.90)	<0.0001
Left bundle branch block	3.17 (2.11-4.78)	<0.0001

BP, Blood pressure; *CI*, confidence interval; *sHR*, sub-distribution hazard ratio; *LV*, left ventricular.

Adapted from Ho JE, et al. Predictors of new-onset heart failure: differences in preserved versus reduced ejection fraction. Circ Heart Fail. 2013;6(2):279-286.

Incidence

The reported incidence of HFpEF and HFmrEF in community-based studies has varied, from a 12-year cumulative HF incidence of 4.2% in the Prevention of Renal and Vascular End-Stage Disease (PREVEND) study (36.9% HF with EF >45%) to 13.7% (53.3% HF with EF >45%) in the Cardiovascular Health Study (CHS), with the incidence rate related to the baseline age of the population (lower incidence in younger cohorts).[20,21] The age- and sex-adjusted incidence of HF declined from 3.2 to 2.2 cases per 1000 person-years from 2000 to 2010 in Olmstead County, Minnesota; with a smaller reduction for HFpEF than HFrEF, and more pronounced reduction in women than in men.[22] As a result, HFpEF constituted an increasing proportion of incident HF cases over time (from 47.8% in 2000-2003 to 56.9% in 2004-2007 and 52.3% in 2008-2010).[22]

Risk Factors

Although population-based longitudinal studies have established the well-known clinical risk factors for incident HF, few have taken into account different HF types. In the Framingham Heart Study (FHS),[23] an examination of predictors of 8-year risk of HF patients with LVEF >45% versus those with LVEF ≤45% showed that predictors of all incident HF included older age, male sex, hypertension, higher body mass index (BMI), increasing heart rate, coronary artery disease (CAD), diabetes mellitus, smoking, valve disease, lower HDL cholesterol, atrial fibrillation, and the presence of LV hypertrophy or left bundle branch block. Specifically in those with higher LVEF, risk factors included higher BMI, smoking, and a history of atrial fibrillation. In contrast male sex, hypertension, higher heart rate, prior cardiovascular disease, higher cholesterol level, LV hypertrophy, and left bundle branch block were associated with higher risk of HFrEF. However, older age was associated with a higher risk of HFpEF and HFmrEF whereas male sex and prior myocardial infarction were associated with higher risk of HFrEF (Table 51.1).[23] Of note, the cumulative incidences of HFpEF and HFmrEF in men and women were similar; whereas the cumulative incidence of HFrEF in men was markedly higher than in women.

Pooling individual level data from FHS, PREVEND, and CHS,[20] independent predictors of incident HF with EF >45% included older age, higher systolic blood pressure, increased BMI, antihypertensive treatment, and previous myocardial infarction. After adjusting for other clinical risk factors, sex was not an independent predictor in the model specific for HF with EF >45%. Instead, male sex was independently associated with significantly higher risk for HFrEF. Left bundle branch block, previous myocardial infarction, smoking, and LV hypertrophy were more strongly associated with HFrEF, whereas older age was more strongly associated with HF with EF >45% (see Table 51.1).[20] In summary, aging is a potent risk factor for heart failure with LVEF >40%. Although women predominate among patients with HFpEF and the prevalence of HFpEF is higher in women than men at any age, this may be related to aging rather than to an intrinsically higher risk of HFpEF in women versus men, because women outlive men on average (Fig. 51.1).

Atrial Fibrillation

Atrial fibrillation is the most common arrhythmia in patients with HFpEF and HFmrEF, with a prevalence of 20% to 40% at the time of presentation, and occurring in two-thirds of these patients at some point during their course.[24,25] Both atrial fibrillation and HF are age-related conditions that frequently coexist, and share common clinical manifestations (e.g., breathlessness and effort intolerance).[26,27] Furthermore, atrial fibrillation is a potent and independent prognostic factor in patients with HFpEF and HFmrEF.[28-30] In addition, atrial fibrillation can complicate the diagnosis of HF because atrial fibrillation alone increases natriuretic peptides, even in the absence of overt HF.

Prognosis
Mortality

Estimates of mortality in HFpEF and HFmrEF have differed depending on baseline status of the study population (especially hospitalized versus outpatient status), study design (epidemiologic study versus clinical trial), LVEF cutoff level used, and various selection biases (use of natriuretic peptide level for the diagnosis, missing LVEF data, participation bias). In general, mortality rates reported in unselected observational studies are higher than in clinical trial populations, and those in cohorts of hospitalized, acute decompensated HF is higher than in outpatient cohorts of chronic HF.

Epidemiologic reports showed that the high 5-year mortality rates in hospitalized HFpEF were comparable or only slightly lower compared with that in HFrEF (Fig. 51.2),[5,6] with estimates ranging from 53% to 74% and no change over the past decade.[22] The Meta-Analysis Global Group in Chronic Heart Failure (MAGGIC) meta-analysis, inclusive of data from clinical trials, reported that patients with HFpEF had lower risk of death from any cause compared with those with HFrEF independent of age, sex, and etiology.[31] The death rate was 12.1 (95% CI: 11.7, 12.6) per 100 patient-years in HFpEF and 14.1 (95% CI: 13.8, 14.4) per 100 patient-years in HFrEF, with an adjusted hazard ratio (HR) of 0.68 (95% CI: 0.64, 0.71) for HFpEF versus HFrEF (Fig. 51.2, *bottom left panel*); death rates were lower in randomized trials alone, and the lower risk in HFpEF than HFrEF was more prominent in ambulatory versus hospitalized patients.[31] More recently, a prospective multicenter longitudinal study in Singapore and New Zealand, specifically designed to compare outcomes among HF types, found that over 2 years, all-cause death rates were 7.5 (95% CI: 6.0 to 9.3) per 100 patient-years in HFpEF and 10.9 (95% CI: 9.6 to 12.4) per 100 patient-years in HFrEF, thus confirming a lower risk of death in HFpEF (adjusted HR 0.62; 95% CI: 0.46 to 0.85) compared with HFrEF (Fig. 51.2, *right panel*).[32]

Beyond all-cause mortality rates, cause of death differs in HFpEF and HFmrEF compared with HFrEF. As expected with older age and greater prevalence of age-related comorbidities in those with higher LVEF, the proportion of deaths from noncardiovascular causes is generally higher in HFpEF and HFmrEF than in HFrEF, accounting for 32% to 49% of deaths in HFpEF in observational studies[33,34] and 28% to 30% in clinical trials. Importantly, cardiovascular causes still comprise the predominant cause of death even in HF patients with LVEF above 40%.[35]

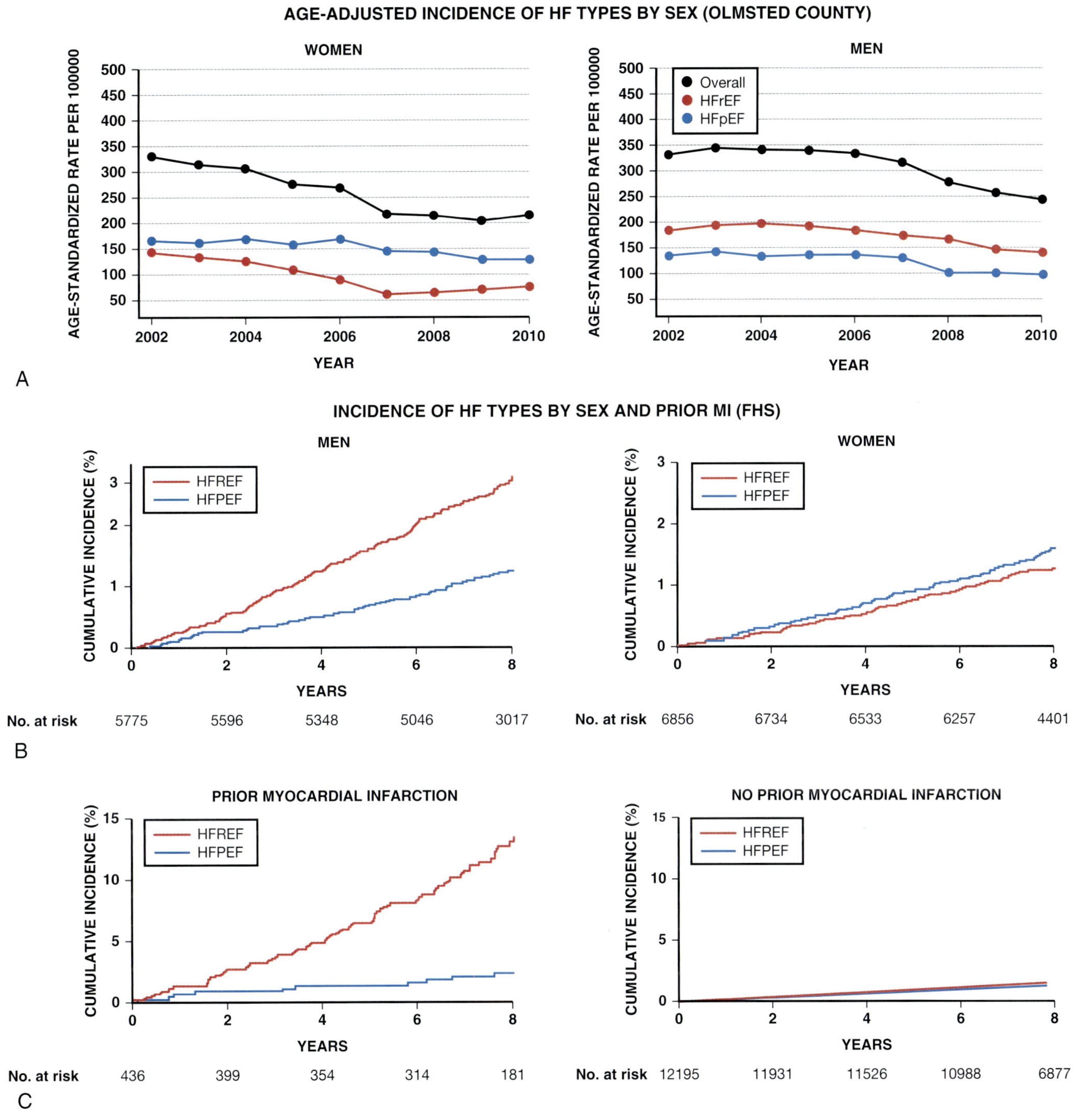

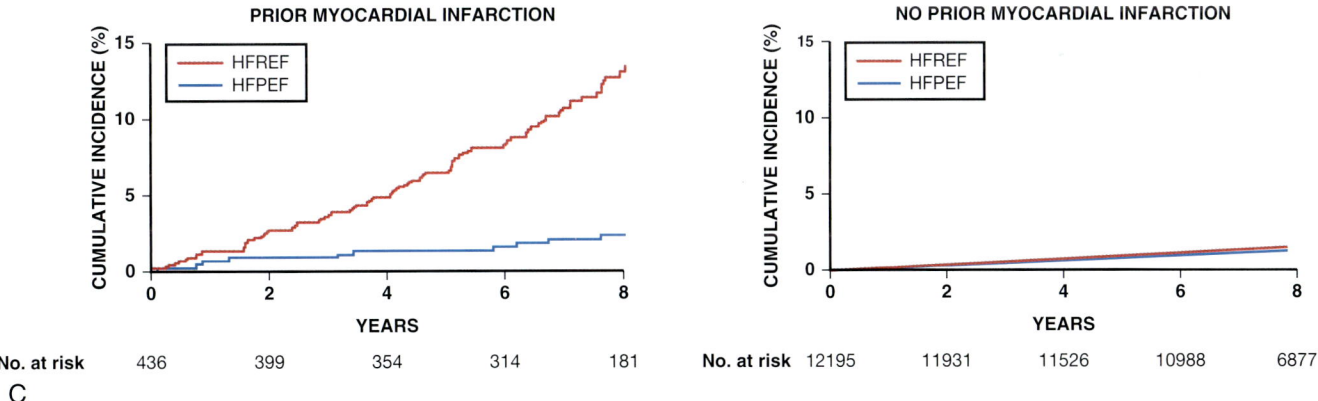

FIGURE 51.1 Prevalence and incidence of HF types by sex. A, Age-adjusted incidence of HF types by sex. **B,** Incidence of HF types by sex. **C,** Incidence of HF types by prior myocardial infarction (from Framingham Heart Study). (**A** adapted from Gerber Y, et al. A contemporary appraisal of the heart failure epidemic in Olmsted County, Minnesota, 2000 to 2010. JAMA Intern Med. 2015;175(6):996-1004. **B, C** modified from Ho JE, et al. Predictors of new-onset heart failure: differences in preserved versus reduced ejection fraction. Circ Heart Fail. 2013;6[2]:279-286.)

Among cardiovascular causes of death, sudden death accounted for up to 43% of cardiovascular mortality (~25% to 30% of total deaths) in clinical trials that included patients with HF and LVEF >40%, with HF deaths accounting for another 20% to 30% of cardiovascular deaths.[34]

Hospitalization

In contrast to lower death rates compared with HFrEF, the high hospitalization rates in HFpEF and HFmrEF are similar, if not even higher, than in HFrEF.[22,36] Following a new diagnosis of HFpEF, patients were hospitalized an average of 1.39 times per year in Olmsted County, Minnesota,[22] with hospitalizations for noncardiovascular causes being more common (0.88 per person-year) than cardiovascular hospitalizations (0.46 per person-year). Although total hospitalization rates were similar across the spectrum of LVEF, noncardiovascular hospitalizations were higher in those with HFpEF, whereas cardiovascular hospitalizations were lower, when compared with HFrEF.

Importantly, recurrent hospitalizations are common in HFpEF and HFmrEF and contribute to a high total hospitalization burden.[37] Compared with epidemiologic studies, the proportion of cardiovascular hospitalizations in HFpEF clinical trials was higher: 56% of hospitalizations in the Irbesartan in Heart Failure and Preserved Ejection

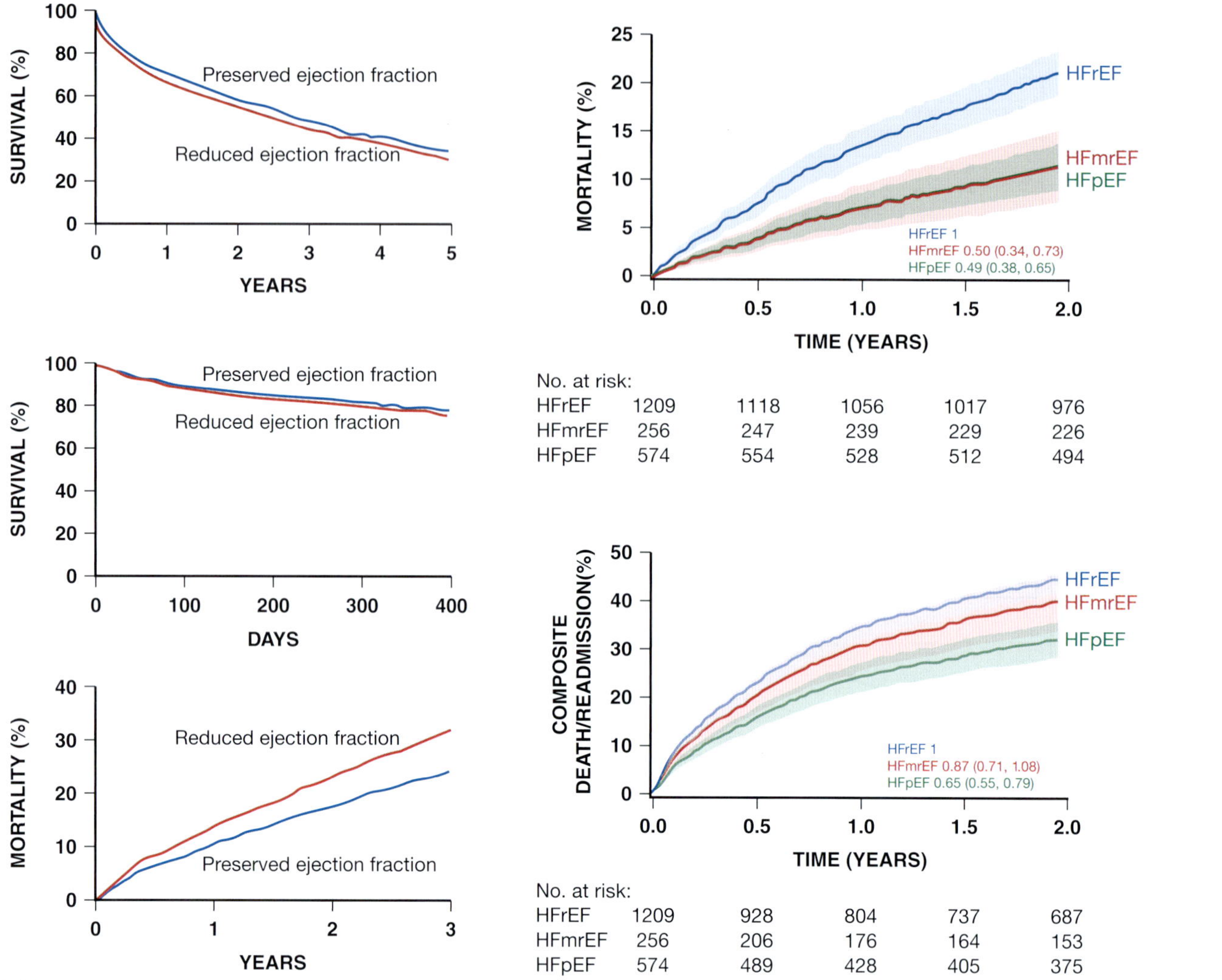

FIGURE 51.2 Survival among patients with heart failure in two epidemiologic studies, an individual patient-level meta-analysis (inclusive of clinical trials), and a prospective dual nation multicenter observational study. (From Owan TE, et al. N Engl J Med. 2006;355:251-259; Bhatia RS, et al, N Engl J Med. 2006;355:260–269; MAGGIC, Eur Heart J. 2012;33:1750-1757; Lam CSP, et al Eur Heart J. 2018;39[20]:1770-1780.)

Fraction (I-PRESERVE) trial[38] and 55% of hospitalizations in CHARM-Preserved.[37] Of note, a prior HF hospitalization heralds a higher risk of death or rehospitalization, with the highest risk close to the time postdischarge and declining over time.[38-40]

Quality of Life

Beyond mortality and hospitalizations, patients with HFpEF also have significantly reduced quality of life, similar to that in HFrEF. Health-related quality of life is often measured in HFpEF clinical trials using either the Kansas City Cardiomyopathy Questionnaire (KCCQ) or the Minnesota Living with Heart Failure Questionnaire (MLHFQ). In the Treatment of Preserved Cardiac Function Heart Failure With an Aldosterone Antagonist (TOPCAT) trial, 43% of participants at baseline had either very low or low KCCQ scores (0 to 50), indicating poor quality of life.[41] In PARAGON-HF, mean KCCQ-overall summary score at randomization was 71, with lowest mean KCCQ score in the symptom stability domain.[42] Low KCCQ scores correlated with worse New York Heart Association functional class, higher NT-proBNP concentration, and more signs and symptoms of HF.

Prior studies have also shown that KCCQ is a valid and reliable measure of health status in HFpEF, has comparable performance in patients with HFpEF and HFrEF,[43] and may be used in serial evaluations to reflect risk of subsequent death and cardiovascular hospitalization in HFpEF and HFrEF.[44,45] Compared with patients with HFrEF in the Prospective Comparison of ARNI with an ACE-Inhibitor to Determine Impact on Global Mortality and Morbidity in Heart Failure (PARADIGM-HF) trial, those with HFpEF in PARAGON-HF had lower mean scores in nearly all domains, as well as lower mean scores in most physical and social activities (except for intimate or sexual relationships).[42]

DIAGNOSIS

The diagnosis of HFpEF and HFmrEF relies on (1) a clinical diagnosis of HF and (2) evidence of a preserved or only mildly reduced LVEF (LVEF >40%). The former is corroborated by typical signs and symptoms of HF, which are similar across the spectrum of LVEF, including evidence of elevated cardiac filling pressures on physical examination (elevated jugular venous pressure), as well as supportive testing including biomarkers (elevated natriuretic peptides), echocardiography (increased E/e' ratio, dilated inferior vena cava, or left atrial [LA] enlargement), or invasive hemodynamic testing (elevated pulmonary capillary wedge pressure [PCWP]). The specific LVEF cutoff for HFpEF has been debated and has been different in different contexts, with recent guidelines suggesting that HFpEF should be defined as LVEF ≥50% and HFmrEF defined as LVEF between 40% and 49%.[9] Nevertheless, many clinicians and trials have used the term HFpEF to refer to patients with HF and LVEF as low as 40%.

In patients hospitalized with HF or in outpatients with overt HF and signs of fluid overload (including chest radiographic evidence of pulmonary vascular congestion or pulmonary edema), the diagnosis is

TABLE 51.2 Noncardiac Etiologies That Can Mimic the HFpEF Syndrome

Obesity
Chronic lung disease
Chronic kidney disease with minimal cardiac structural or functional abnormalities
Primary cirrhosis
Extrinsic compression of the LA, LV, or IVC
IVC obstruction
Lymphedema
Anemia

often straightforward. However, the diagnosis can be challenging in patients with dyspnea and exercise intolerance who do not have overt signs of elevated filling pressures and natriuretic peptide levels below typical thresholds used to make the diagnosis of HF, which occurs commonly in some patients (up to 30% to 40%, especially in patients who are obese).[46] In these patients, provocative testing (e.g., exercise) can be useful to make the diagnosis by echocardiography (elevated E/e′ ratio at peak exercise) or invasive hemodynamic testing (PCWP ≥25 mm Hg with passive leg raise or during exercise).[47] It is important to proceed with invasive hemodynamic testing (with or without exercise) in any patient with suspected HFpEF or HFmrEF in whom the diagnosis is in question because signs and symptoms of HF can be nonspecific and many of the comorbidities that coexist with HFpEF and HFmrEF can mimic the HF syndrome.

Echocardiographic evidence of LV diastolic dysfunction is challenging and should not be used as the sole criteria for the diagnosis of HFpEF for several reasons: (1) diastolic function on echocardiography may be uninterpretable, equivocal, or misinterpreted; (2) many older patients without the HF syndrome have evidence of diastolic dysfunction; (3) while echocardiography is useful for the diagnosis of impaired relaxation, E/e′ ratio (an estimate of LV filling pressures) is often in the indeterminate range (8 to 15), and echocardiography has not proven useful for the assessment of LV chamber compliance in the clinical setting. Thus, while the presence of diastolic dysfunction in the appropriate clinical context is supportive, the absence of significant diastolic dysfunction should not be used to exclude the diagnosis of HFpEF, and further testing with exercise stress or invasive hemodynamics should be considered.

The diagnosis of HFpEF and HFmrEF relies on the exclusion of noncardiac causes of dyspnea, exercise tolerance, or fluid overload. For example, a patient with severe chronic obstructive pulmonary disease on oxygen would likely have symptoms of dyspnea and exercise intolerance and may have signs of central venous congestion due to cor pulmonale with right ventricular hypertrophy. Although the patient has symptoms of "heart failure," the diagnosis is COPD and not HF. Thus, in each patient with suspected HFpEF and HFmrEF, it is important to consider alternate etiologies (Table 51.2).

HFpEF Diagnostic Scores

Two scoring systems have been developed to assist in the diagnosis of HFpEF in patients with dyspnea in whom the diagnosis is in question: the H_2FPEF[48] score and the HFA-PEFF score[49] (Fig. 51.3). Both of these scores offer simple approaches to the diagnosis of HFpEF, and although not specifically designed for HFmrEF, may be helpful in the diagnosis of HFmrEF as well. The H_2FPEF score was systematically derived and validated at a single center (Mayo Clinic, Rochester, MN).[48] HFpEF was diagnosed in patients with PCWP ≥15 mm Hg at rest or ≥25 mm Hg during exercise. The final diagnostic model included the following weighted components: BMI >30 g/m² (2 points), 2 or more antihypertensive medications (1 point), atrial fibrillation (3 points), echocardiographic pulmonary artery (PA) systolic pressure >35 mm Hg (1 point), age >60 years (1 point), and echocardiographic E/e′ >9 (1 point). The overall score AUC was 0.84 and the score was found to be superior to other consensus criteria developed for the diagnosis of HFpEF. The score was then validated in a separate test, where it was found to perform well (AUC, 0.89). The authors developed a nomogram that provides the likelihood of the HFpEF diagnosis based on the calculated score in an individual patient (Fig. 51.3A). Given the ease of use of the H_2FPEF score, it may be particularly helpful in the primary care setting where at-risk patients with dyspnea could be screened using the score to help establish the diagnosis.

The HFA-PEFF score was developed by a group of experts convened by the European Society of Cardiology Heart Failure Association.[49] The "PEFF" mnemonic stands for Pre-test assessment; Echocardiography and natriuretic peptide score; Functional testing; and Final etiology. The recommended pretest assessment involves evaluation of HF symptoms and signs, clinical comorbidities typically associated with HFpEF, laboratory tests, electrocardiography, and echocardiography (Fig. 51.3B). The HFA-PEFF score is based on functional and morphologic echocardiographic criteria, and natriuretic peptide criteria. Components of the functional domain include echocardiographic tissue Doppler e′ velocities, E/e′ ratio, tricuspid regurgitation velocity, and LV global longitudinal strain. Components of the morphologic domain include LA volume index, LV mass index, relative wall thickness, and LV wall thickness. Each domain included major criteria (2 points) or minor criteria (1 point) (Fig. 51.3B). A score of ≥5 points is diagnostic of HFpEF, whereas a score of <2 points excludes HFpEF. In both the H_2FPEF and HFA-PEFF scores have been further assessed for external validation and although not perfect, appear to be clinically useful for making the diagnosis of HFpEF.

KEY TESTS FOR THE EVALUATION OF HFpEF AND HFmrEF

Biomarkers

Natriuretic peptides (NPs; B-type natriuretic peptide [BNP] and N-terminal pro-BNP [NT-proBNP]) are the most widely studied and used diagnostic and prognostic biomarkers in HFpEF and HFmrEF. NPs are secreted by both the ventricular and atrial myocardium in response to increased wall stress, which is directly related to chamber size and inversely related to wall thickness. NP levels are consistently on average higher in patients with HFrEF compared with patients with higher LVEF most likely due to the increased ventricular dilation in lower LVEF patients.[50] In patients with HFrEF, LV dilation is common and wall thickness is frequently normal, whereas in HFpEF, LV volumes are normal or small, and wall thickness can be increased. Thus, for any given rise in LV diastolic pressure elevation, patients with HFpEF or HFmrEF often have lower NP levels compared with HFrEF, and these syndromes have been considered states of relative NP deficiency, which may contribute to the clinical syndrome, including hypertension and fluid retention.

Although an elevated NP level can be helpful to diagnose HF in patients with LVEF >40%, other causes of elevated NP levels such as atrial fibrillation, pulmonary arterial hypertension, primary RV failure, acute pulmonary embolism, and chronic kidney disease must be considered in the differential diagnosis. NP levels should not be used to exclude the diagnosis of HF in patients with intermediate to high pretest probability because 30% to 40% of patients with HFpEF have NP levels below typical diagnostic thresholds, NP levels are lower in HFpEF and HFmrEF than in HFrEF, and morbid obesity is associated with lower NP levels due to NP clearance receptors on adipocytes and lower NP production in obese patients. In these patients, further diagnostic testing should be performed. In patients with prevalent HFpEF and HFmrEF, elevated NP levels are a useful prognostic marker.

High-sensitivity troponin (hsTnT) is also useful in the evaluation of patients with HFpEF and HFmrEF, and elevation in hsTnT can signify a more "myocardial" phenotype of HFpEF, can alert the clinician to the potential presence of an infiltrative cardiomyopathy such as cardiac amyloidosis, and may reflect impaired subendocardial perfusion due to coronary microvascular dysfunction, particularly if measured during or immediately after exercise testing. Moreover, elevated levels portend a worse prognosis.[51,52] In the future, proteomic or metabolomic analysis of the blood may provide additional insight into better diagnostic tests and sub-phenotyping in HFpEF and HFmrEF.

Echocardiography (see Chapter 16)

Comprehensive echocardiography, including Doppler and tissue Doppler imaging, along with speckle-tracking echocardiography for the assessment of cardiac mechanics, should be performed on all patients with suspected or known HFpEF and HFmrEF. Conventional echocardiography provides important diagnostic and etiologic clues in these patients. Importantly, echocardiography is essential to rule out other causes of a patient's signs and symptoms, including other forms of heart disease. Although not all patients with HFpEF or HFmrEF have LV hypertrophy, the majority have concentric LV remodeling, defined by a relative wall thickness (2 × posterior wall thickness/LV end-diastolic dimension) >0.42.[53] Assessment of LV mass index in relation to relative

	Clinical Variable	Values	Points
H₂	**H**eavy	Body mass index > 30 kg/m²	2
	Hypertensive	2 or more antihypertensive medicines	1
F	Atrial **f**ibrillation	Paroxysmal or persistent	3
P	**P**ulmonary hypertension	Doppler echocardiographic estimated pulmonary artery systolic pressure > 35 mmHg	1
E	**E**lder	Age > 60 years	1
F	**F**illing pressure	Doppler echocardiographic E/e' > 9	1
		H₂FPEF score	Sum (0–9)

Total points	0	1	2	3	4	5	6	7	8	9
Probability of HFpEF			0.2	0.3	0.4	0.5	0.6	0.7	0.8	0.9	0.95

A

	Functional	Morphological	Biomarker (SR)	Biomarker (AF)
Major	Septal e' < 7 cm/s or lateral e' < 10 cm/s or Average E/e' ≥ 15 or TR velocity > 2.8 m/s (PASP > 35 mm Hg)	LAVI > 34 mL/m² or LVMI ≥ 149/122 g/m² (m/w) and RWT > 0,42	NT-proBNP > 220 pg/mL or BNP > 80 pg/mL	NT-proBNP > 660 pg/mL or BNP > 240 pg/mL
Minor	Average E/e' 9–14 or GLS < 16%	LAVI 29–34 mL/m² or LVMI > 115/95 g/m² (m/w) or RWT > 0,42 or LV wall thickness ≥ 12 mm	NT-proBNP 125–220 pg/mL or BNP 35–80 pg/mL	NT-proBNP 365–660 pg/mL or BNP 105–240 pg/mL

Major criteria : 2 points	≥ 5 points: HFpEF
Minor criteria : 1 point	2–4 points: Diastolic stress test or invasive hemodynamic measurements

B

FIGURE 51.3 HFpEF scores. A, Description of the H₂FPEF score and point allocations for each clinical characteristic (*top*), with associated probability of having heart failure with preserved ejection fraction (HFpEF) based on the total score as estimated from the model (*bottom*). **B,** Calculating and interpreting the HFA-PEFF score. Echocardiographic and natriuretic peptide heart failure with preserved ejection fraction workup and scoring system (diagnostic workup). (**A** from Reddy YNV, et al. A simple, evidence-based approach to help guide diagnosis of heart failure with preserved ejection fraction. Circulation. 2018;138[9]:861-870. **B** from Pieske B, et al. How to diagnose heart failure with preserved ejection fraction: the HFA-PEFF diagnostic algorithm: a consensus recommendation from the Heart Failure Association [HFA] of the European Society of Cardiology [ESC]. Eur Heart J. 2019;40(40):3297-3317.)

wall thickness can also be helpful because it can be used to categorize LV geometry (normal, concentric remodeling, concentric hypertrophy, or eccentric hypertrophy), which can provide clues to the etiology (Fig. 51.4A). LA volume is also very useful for the diagnosis because it provides insight into chronic LA pressure overload. Although maximal LA volume index to body surface area ≥34 mL/m² is the guideline-based cutoff for LA enlargement, it can be challenging to use because of the high prevalence of obesity in these patients, which results in lower values. For these reasons, it is important to examine the LA in relation to the other chambers of the heart. An LA that is as large or larger than the LV implies that the LA is not emptying properly to adequately fill the LV, which is common in HFpEF. Therefore, LA minimal volume or LA reservoir strain (see later) may be better tools to help diagnose and manage these patients. It is important to note that other conditions can result in LV hypertrophy and/or LA enlargement in the setting of a preserved LVEF. These include athlete's heart, high output states (e.g., cirrhosis), and atrial fibrillation, underscoring the importance of comprehensive echocardiographic assessment in these patients.

Conventional echocardiography is also useful for the assessment of load on the right heart in patients with HFpEF and HFmrEF. Elevated

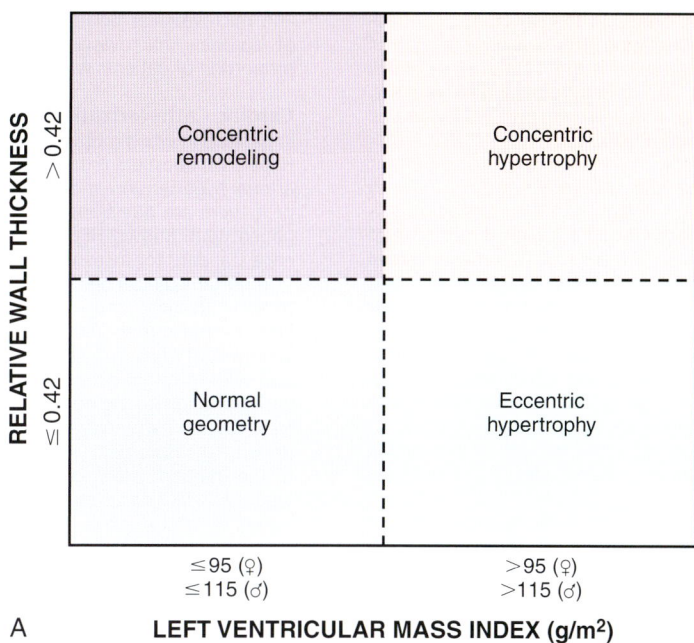
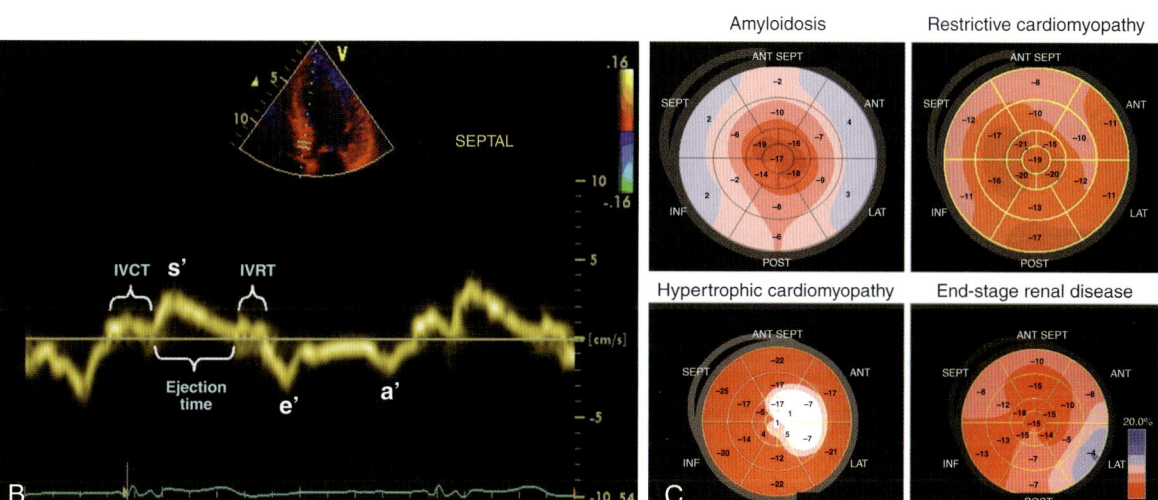

FIGURE 51.4 A, Hypertrophy subtypes: comparison of relative wall thickness (RWT). Patients with normal LV mass can have either concentric remodeling (normal LV mass with increased RWT >0.42) or normal geometry (RWT ≤0.42) and normal LV mass. Patients with increased LV mass can have either concentric (RWT >0.42) or eccentric (RWT ≤0.42) hypertrophy. These LV mass measurements are based on linear measurements. **B,** Tissue Doppler imaging can be used to determine the extent of myocardial involvement in HFpEF. Reductions in systolic (s'), early diastolic (e'), and late diastolic (a') velocities, prolongation of isovolumic contraction time (IVCT) and isovolumic relaxation time (IVRT), and reduction in ejection time are all signs of a sick myocardium. **C,** LV global longitudinal strain bullseye maps. The strain maps show particular patterns suggestive of amyloidosis (*upper left*), restrictive cardiomyopathy (*upper right*), apical hypertrophic cardiomyopathy (*lower left*), and end-stage renal disease with a pattern suggestive of Fabry disease (*lower right*). *ANT,* Anterior; *ANT SEPT,* anteroseptal; *INF,* inferior; *LAT,* lateral; *POST,* posterolateral; *SEPT,* septal. (**A** from Lang RM, et al. Recommendations for cardiac chamber quantification by echocardiography in adults: an update from the American Society of Echocardiography and the European Association of Cardiovascular Imaging. Eur Heart J Cardiovasc Imaging. 2015;16[3]:233-270; **B** from Shah SJ. 20th Annual Feigenbaum lecture: echocardiography for precision medicine-digital biopsy to deconstruct biology. J Am Soc Echocardiogr. 2019;32[11]:1379-1395e1372; **C** from Marwick TH, et al. Myocardial strain in the assessment of patients with heart failure: a review. JAMA Cardiol. 2019;4[3]:287-294.)

pulmonary artery systolic pressure (>40 mm Hg) especially when coupled with LA enlargement or dysfunction, is common in HFpEF, and this elevation is considered secondary to left sided heart disease. As HFpEF worsens, RV enlargement and dysfunction often occur in response to chronic elevation in LA and pulmonary venous pressures. Thus, it is important to examine and quantify the right heart on echocardiography in all patients with HFpEF with indices such as RV fractional area change (normal >35%), tricuspid annular plane systolic excursion (normal >1.6 cm), and RV s' velocity (normal >10 cm/sec). The ratio of tricuspid regurgitation velocity (in m/sec) to RV outflow tract velocity time integral (in cm) >0.18 is indicative of elevated total pulmonary resistance and should prompt evaluation of the possibility of pulmonary vascular disease. Assessment of septal flattening during systole and diastole provides insight into RV pressure and volume overload, respectively. Notching of the RV outflow tract pulse wave Doppler velocity profile is a sign that pulmonary vascular resistance (PVR) is elevated due to interruption of the normal forward RV outflow by the reflected wave from the stiff distal pulmonary vasculature. Finally, assessment of inferior vena cava size and collapsibility, along with hepatic vein flow, can provide valuable information on estimated right atrial pressure and etiologies such as severe tricuspid regurgitation, constrictive pericarditis, and restrictive cardiomyopathy. Assessment of the RV and right atrium on echocardiography is also important for differentiating heart failure from pulmonary arterial hypertension.[54]

Measures of Diastolic Function and Strain. Tissue Doppler imaging (TDI) can be helpful in the assessment of patients with suspected HFpEF or HFmrEF (Fig. 51.4B). The early diastolic (e') velocity is a marker of LV relaxation and is usually reduced in patients with heart failure regardless of LVEF. However, TDI provides additional clues for the diagnosis and management of HFpEF; thus, clinicians should examine the s' and a' velocities along with the ejection time and the isovolumic contraction and relaxation times on the TDI tracing. The s' velocity (a marker of longitudinal motion of the myocardium) is often reduced in HFpEF patients, especially in patients with CAD or infiltrative cardiomyopathy. A reduced a' velocity is reflective of impaired LA contraction and/or reduced LV end-diastolic chamber compliance.

Speckle-tracking echocardiography has emerged as an important diagnostic and prognostic tool in patients with HFpEF and HFmrEF and has provided insights into the pathophysiology.[55] Similar to s' velocity, a reduced absolute LV global longitudinal strain (GLS) value is indicative of reduced longitudinal fiber LV function (a marker of LV subendocardial function, which is often affected by risk factors that lead to HFpEF) even in the setting of a preserved LVEF and is often present in patients with HFpEF.[56] Although values of GLS can vary based on type of echocardiography machine and software used, an absolute GLS value of >18% is considered normal, 16% to 18% borderline, and <16% abnormal (Fig. 51.4C). Polar bullseye maps of the LV longitudinal strain pattern are also useful for determining the potential etiology of HFpEF (Fig. 51.4C) because it can help differentiate patients who have diffuse myocardial fibrosis from those who have cardiac amyloidosis, who would generally have an apical sparing pattern.

Strain measures of the left atrium and right ventricle can also be performed. LA longitudinal strain consists of three components (reservoir, conduit, and booster strains). LA reservoir strain is indicative of the ability of the LA to fill during ventricular systole; when reduced, it is associated with poor prognosis and reflects increased LA pressure and/or reduced compliance of the LA.[57] LA conduit strain reflects the ability of the LA to empty properly during passive filling of the LV in early diastole, and LA booster strain is indicative of the ability of the LA contractile function. When LA strain indices are abnormal out of proportion to the extent of LV dysfunction, a primary LA myopathy as a cause of HFpEF should be considered. Reduced RV free wall strain is often present in HFpEF and is also associated with adverse events; it can be reduced in the setting of elevated pulmonary vascular resistance or a primary myocardial process that is affecting both the LV and the RV and resulting in HFpEF.

Most compensated patients with HFpEF do not have symptoms at rest but become very symptomatic with exertion. Thus, exercise echocardiography can be very useful in the evaluation of HFpEF patients.[58] Despite the routine use of exercise testing in other cardiovascular conditions (especially CAD), exercise testing is still underutilized in the diagnosis and management of HFpEF. Exercise echocardiography can provide an assessment of ischemia (i.e., wall motion abnormalities), LV filling pressures (e.g., E/e' and PA systolic pressure), and can rule out dynamic valvular disease (such as exercise-induced mitral regurgitation). In HFpEF patients, bicycle stress echocardiography is typically easier for patients compared with treadmill testing because HFpEF patients are often older, frail, and debilitated.

Cardiac Magnetic Resonance Imaging (see Chapter 19)

Although echocardiography can provide a wealth of information to assist with the diagnosis and management of HFpEF and HFmrEF, acoustic windows can be challenging in many HFpEF patients because of the high prevalence of obesity and concomitant lung disease. Furthermore, echocardiography is limited in its ability to provide tissue characterization and assessment of extracardiac structures. For these reasons, cardiac magnetic resonance (CMR) imaging can be a very useful diagnostic test in HFpEF and HFmrEF.[59]

CMR is the reference standard for assessment of cardiac structure and global systolic function given its high temporal resolution. Furthermore, late gadolinium enhancement provides assessment of myocardial scar, which may be due to myocardial infarction, myocarditis, or specific cardiomyopathies depending on its distribution. However, some patients with HFpEF and HFmrEF have diffuse myocardial fibrosis which cannot be easily detected on conventional CMR imaging with contrast; instead, T1 mapping with quantitation of the extracellular volume content can be used and when elevated (typically >25%) is indicative of either diffuse myocardial fibrosis or extracellular deposition of proteins as is seen in cardiac amyloidosis. T2 mapping is also useful for the diagnosis of myocardial edema, which can be present in cases of myocarditis. In addition, T2* imaging can be useful for the quantitation of myocardial iron content when the diagnosis of hemochromatosis is under consideration. CMR imaging is also useful to detect thickening and/or enhancement of the pericardium. Dynamic deep breathing cine images can also detect evidence of diastolic septal bounce which reflects ventricular interdependence and can be seen in the setting of constrictive pericarditis. Finally, vasodilator perfusion CMR imaging can be used to detect coronary macrovascular and microvascular perfusion defects, the latter of which is indicative of coronary microvascular dysfunction and is present in a large proportion of patients with HFpEF.[60]

Cardiac Catheterization (see Chapter 22)

In patients in whom noninvasive tests are equivocal and the diagnosis of HFpEF is in question, if there is need to differentiate between pulmonary arterial hypertension and HFpEF (i.e., pulmonary venous hypertension), or if there are questions about the physiology or volume status of a patient with known HFpEF, cardiac catheterization remains the reference standard for assessment of invasive hemodynamics.

Important clinical decisions are made on the basis of invasive hemodynamic testing; thus, proper and careful technique is essential. Pressure tracings should be scrutinized not only for the correct measurement of pressure values but also for the clues provided by the pressure waveforms. In general, pressure measurements should be made at end-expiration during normal, free breathing without asking the patient to perform breath hold maneuvers. Respiratory variation in intracardiac pressure measurements is often exaggerated in HFpEF patients because of the frequent presence of concomitant morbid obesity and chronic lung disease. Right atrial pressure and PCWP tracings should be measured mid-A wave or at the base of the A wave in patients in sinus rhythm and at the base of the V wave in patients with atrial arrhythmias in the absence of A waves.

Tall A waves in the RA pressure tracing are indicative of preserved RA contractile function and a stiff RV. Tall V waves in the RA pressure tracing can be seen in severe tricuspid regurgitation or in the presence of a stiff RA. A rapid X and Y descent can be seen in patients with the HFpEF clinical syndrome who have a restrictive cardiomyopathy (which can be isolated to the RV) or constrictive pericarditis. A rise in RA pressure during inspiration (Kussmaul's sign) can be seen in patients with HFpEF who have a stiff RV, constrictive pericarditis, or significant tricuspid regurgitation. A high RV nadir pressure can be indicative of significant volume overload, and an exaggerated A wave in the RV pressure tracing can be seen in patients with a stiff RV. A dip-and-plateau (square root sign) morphology of the RV pressure tracing can be seen in restrictive cardiomyopathy or constrictive pericarditis.

Patients with HFpEF and HFmrEF often have elevated PA pressures, which is most commonly due to pulmonary venous hypertension. PA pulse pressure (PA systolic minus PA diastolic pressure) is often elevated in HFpEF and HFmrEF due to proximal PA stiffening. A high PA systolic pressure can also occur because of the reflected wave from the distal pulmonary pressures (often due to a high PCWP), which causes augmentation of the PA pressure waveform in systole. High PA systolic and PA pulse pressures can lead to high mean PA pressures causing the pulmonary vascular resistance (PVR) to be elevated in HFpEF patients. Elevated PVR (>3 Wood units) primarily due to PA systolic pressure elevation can be differentiated from PVR elevation due to concomitant pulmonary arteriopathy and venopathy by examining the diastolic pressure gradient (DPG; PA diastolic pressure minus PCWP) which will be elevated (>5 to 7 mm Hg) in these cases. The ratio of pulmonary to systemic vascular resistance can also be helpful in HFpEF patients; a high ratio is suggestive of the presence of intrinsic pulmonary vascular disease.

By definition, PCWP should be elevated at rest (≥15 mm Hg) or with passive leg raise or exercise (≥ 25 mm Hg) in patients with HFpEF and HFmrEF. Tall V waves in the PCWP tracing are also often seen either at rest, during exercise, or during intravenous fluid challenge in HFmrEF and HFpEF and typically reflects a stiff LA more commonly than severe mitral regurgitation. Although PCWP and LV end-diastolic pressure (LVEDP) are often thought of as interchangeable, there can be important differences in the PCWP and LVEDP values, which, in turn, can provide insight into cardiovascular physiology.[61] PCWP is an integrated measure of the burden of LA stiffness (and indirectly the LV stiffness) on the pulmonary circulation, while the LVEDP only provides information on LV compliance. Thus, if PCWP can be measured accurately, it is the best measure to use for the calculation of PVR because poor LA compliance (with resultant accentuated LA pressure waves) is what the pulmonary circulation "sees" and what overloads it, not the LVEDP.

Assessment of cardiac output and stroke volume are important to rule out high-output HF, which has specific etiologies and differs from typical HFpEF. Either thermodilution or Fick cardiac output can be used, but the latter can suffer from assumptions made of oxygen consumption, and direct measurement of oxygen consumption is preferred when available. A low stroke volume in the setting of HFpEF is an important sign and should be interrogated further to determine the cause. Restrictive cardiomyopathy, LA failure due to atrial fibrillation or LA myopathy, valvular heart disease, pulmonary vascular disease, and RV failure are all potential causes of a low stroke volume in the setting of elevated cardiac filling pressures.

Dynamic "perturbation" during invasive hemodynamic testing can be very helpful in patients with HFpEF and can be done with passive leg raise, exercise, fluid challenge, and administration of systemic vasodilators. In patients with unexplained dyspnea, a passive leg raise alone can be helpful for making the diagnosis of HFpEF.[62] As mentioned earlier, exercise can be used in equivocal cases, and exercise invasive hemodynamic testing is considered to be the gold standard test for diagnosis. V waves in the PCWP tracing often become exaggerated during exercise because the LA is unable to handle the extra load that occurs due to splanchnic vasoconstriction leading to a large volume shift of blood from the splanchnic circulation and liver to the stiff left heart. Assessment of the relative rise in mean PA pressure and PCWP during exercise can also be helpful. In patients with passive pulmonary venous hypertension, the mean PA pressure and PCWP will rise in parallel with increasing cardiac output during exercise whereas the mean PA pressure will rise more rapidly compared with PCWP in the setting of intrinsic pulmonary vascular disease (Fig. 51.5). A fluid challenge (10 cc/kg of warmed normal saline over a few minutes) can be safely administered to patients with HFpEF who have an RA pressure ≤12 mm Hg. Exaggerated rise in PCWP is indicative of HFpEF; exaggerated rise in PA pressure relative to PCWP is indicative of pulmonary vascular disease; and lack of augmentation (or reduced) cardiac output after fluid challenge can be seen in the setting of constrictive pericarditis, RV failure, or LA dysfunction. In patients with elevated PVR, administration of a systemic vasodilator such as intravenous nitroprusside can be helpful to differentiate pulmonary venous hypertension from intrinsic pulmonary vascular disease. If nitroprusside administration results in reduction in SVR, PCWP, and mean PA pressure, the pulmonary hypertension is likely due to pulmonary venous hypertension. However, if there is a reduction in SVR and PCWP and yet the mean PA pressure remains elevated (in which case the PVR and DPG will also remain elevated), intrinsic pulmonary vascular disease is likely present.

Coronary evaluation is also helpful in patients with suspected HFpEF or HFmrEF. Although most often first examined noninvasively with nuclear or echocardiographic stress testing (or via coronary computed tomography), invasive coronary angiography is helpful when the diagnosis of CAD or ischemia is uncertain. Coronary vasodilator testing with assessment of coronary flow reserve (CFR) and the index of microvascular resistance (IMR) are also helpful in determining whether or not coronary microvascular dysfunction are present.[63] CFR is defined as the ratio of hyperemic coronary flow (in response to adenosine, for example) to resting coronary flow, and can be measured using invasive coronary flow testing, positron emission tomography (PET), CMR, or transthoracic Doppler echocardiography. The cutoff for defining coronary microvascular dysfunction varies by type of study but is generally defined as CFR <2.0 to 2.5. A reduced CFR can be due to intrinsic coronary microvascular dysfunction but can also be present in patients with epicardial CAD, extrinsic compression of the coronary microvasculature (e.g., due to interstitial myocardial fibrosis), coronary microvascular capillary rarefaction (due to severely diseased coronary microvasculature), or elevated cardiac filling pressures. IMR, which is more specific to the coronary microvasculature, may be less susceptible to hemodynamic factors but currently can be measured only with invasive coronary flow techniques. An IMR ≥23 is abnormal and indicative of coronary microvascular dysfunction. The combination of a reduced CFR and elevated IMR is most specific for coronary microvascular dysfunction and has been associated with a poor prognosis in HFpEF patients.

Endomyocardial Biopsy
Although not routinely indicated, endomyocardial biopsy can be safely performed during right heart catheterization in patients in whom there is a suspicion for infiltrative or toxic cardiomyopathies. In a single-center study of 108 patients with HFpEF who underwent endomyocardial biopsy, myocardial fibrosis and cardiomyocyte hypertrophy were very common (93% and 88%, respectively) but were mild in the majority of cases. In particular, myocardial fibrosis was absent in 7%, mild or patchy in 66%, moderate in 17%, and severe in only 10% of patients. Of the 108 patients examined, 15 (14%) of the patients were found to have cardiac amyloidosis, 50% in whom the diagnosis was unsuspected.[64] Although there was no evidence of overt inflammation in the biopsy samples, evidence of monocyte infiltration was common in HFpEF, with twofold higher CD68+ cells/mm^2 compared with controls. Figure 51.6 displays representative histologic findings of myocardial biopsy specimens in HFpEF patients.

Cardiopulmonary Exercise Testing
Cardiopulmonary exercise testing (CPET) is the reference standard test for assessment of exercise intolerance and dyspnea. CPET is especially useful to distinguish heart failure from other causes of dyspnea, including lung disease, anemia, obesity, or deconditioning. In patients in whom the diagnosis of HFpEF has been established, CPET can be useful to pinpoint the source of exercise intolerance, as shown in Table 51.3, and can be used to classify HF into sub-phenotypes based on differential combination of CPET abnormalities.[65] Nevertheless, CPET cannot diagnose all cases of HFpEF. Reduced peak oxygen consumption is reflective of inadequate augmentation of cardiac output and/or peripheral skeletal muscle extraction during exercise, both of which are frequently present in HFpEF. However, some patients, particularly those with early, milder forms of HFpEF, have an isolated problem of elevated LV filling pressures during exercise, and can still augment cardiac output appropriately.[66] Thus, additional testing, such as diastolic stress echocardiography or invasive exercise hemodynamics may be necessary to rule in or rule out heart failure in such patients.

Extracardiac Considerations
Aorta. Increased central aortic stiffness is common in HFpEF and HFmrEF and may be a major driver of its pathogenesis. Reflected waves from a stiff systemic vasculature result in augmentation of aortic pressure, which in turn creates increased load on the LV during ventricular systole and increases systolic LV wall stress.[67] Increased aortic stiffening can also reduce the ability of the aorta to act as a buffer to the pulsatile flow resulting in barotrauma to organs such as the kidney and brain. A variety of techniques are available for the measurement of aortic stiffness, including systemic pulse pressure (systolic minus diastolic blood pressure), arterial tonometry (for measurement of aortic augmentation index and pulse wave velocity), and imaging techniques such as echocardiography and CMR, which can be used to calculate pulse wave velocity.
Lungs. Systematic evaluation of pulmonary function, including chest radiography, pulmonary function tests (PFTs), and computed

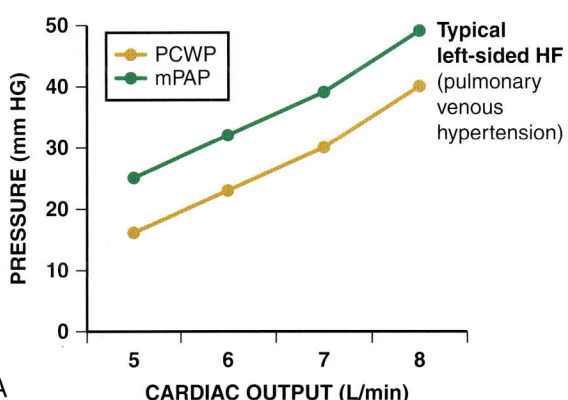
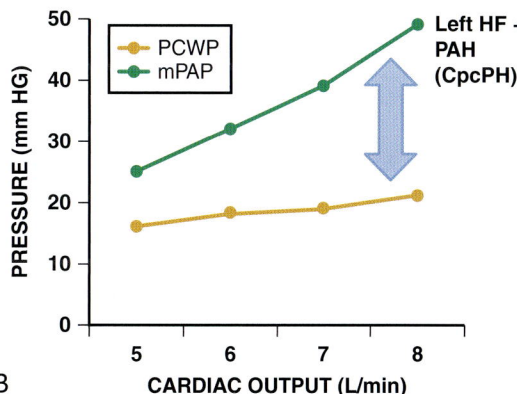

FIGURE 51.5 A, In patients with HFpEF or HFmrEF who develop isolated pulmonary venous hypertension due to left heart disease, the PCWP and mean PA pressure (mPAP) will go up in parallel as cardiac output increases with exercise. **B,** In patients with HFpEF or HFmrEF who develop combined post- and precapillary pulmonary hypertension (CpcPH), mPAP will rise more steeply than the rise in PCWP as cardiac output increases with exercise.

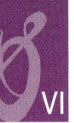

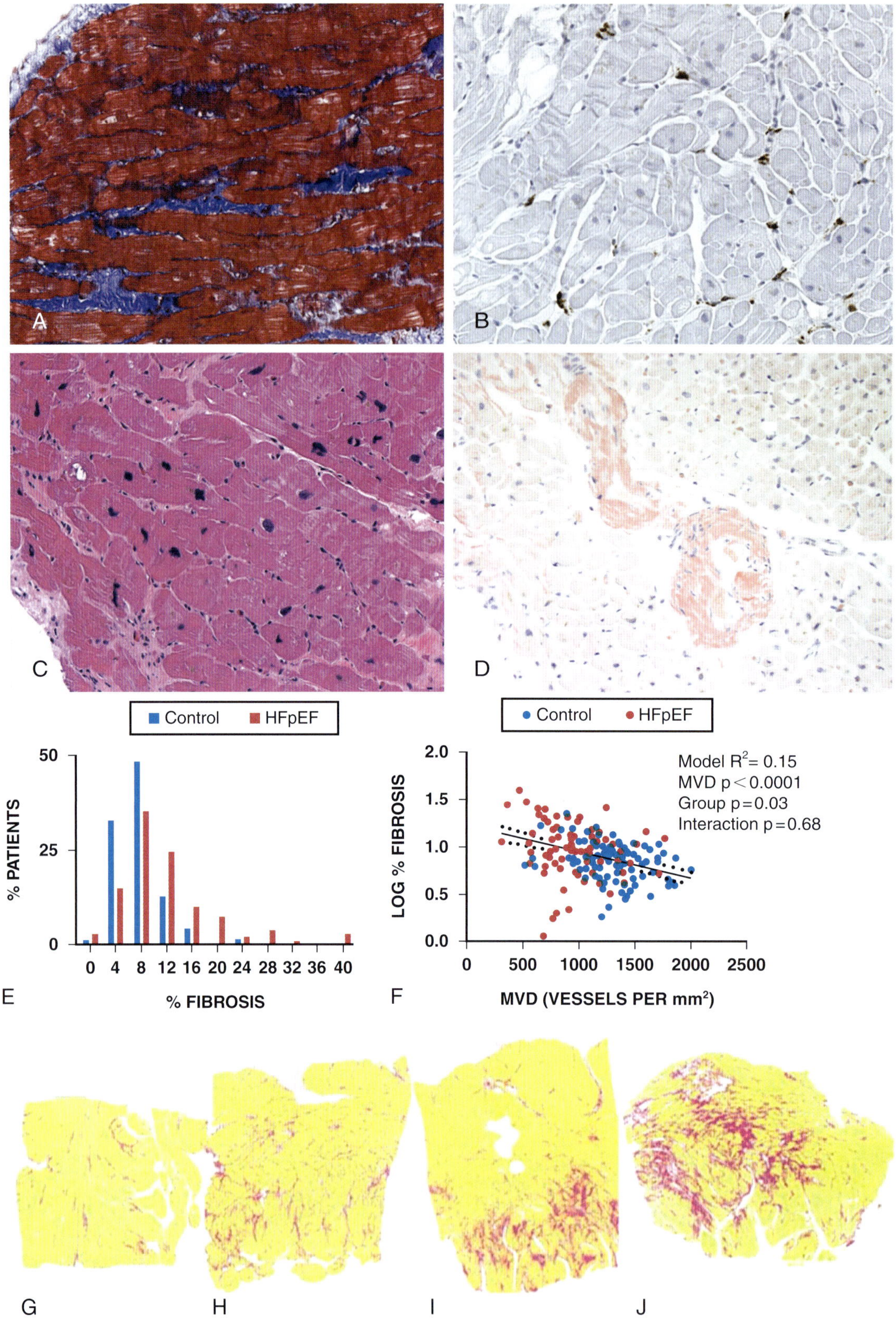

FIGURE 51.6 **A-D,** Endomyocardial biopsy in HFpEF. **A,** Interstitial fibrosis (blue) on Masson's trichrome stain. **B,** CD68+ cells (brown) on immunohistochemistry. **C,** Myocyte hypertrophy on hematoxylin and eosin stain. **D,** Cardiac amyloidosis on Congo Red stain. **E-J,** Cardiac fibrosis in HFpEF and control. **E,** The frequency distribution for percent area fibrosis is shifted upward in HFpEF. **F,** Log-transformed percent area fibrosis increases similarly with decreasing MVD in HFpEF and controls, but it remains higher in HFpEF than in control at any level of MVD. **G-J,** representative examples of SAB stained left ventricular sections with algorithm-defined fibrosis (red), myocardium (yellow), and space (white) from HFpEF patients with 3% **(G)**, 7% **(H)**, 10% **(I)**, and 21% **(J)** fibrosis. *HFpEF,* heart failure with preserved ejection fraction; *MVD,* microvascular density; *SAB,* sulfated Alcian blue. (**A-D** adapted from Hahn V, et al. Endomyocardial biopsy characterization of heart failure with preserved ejection fraction and prevalence of cardiac amyloidosis. JACC Heart Fail. 2020;8[9]:712-724; **E-J** adapted from Mohammed S, et al. Coronary microvascular rarefaction and myocardial fibrosis in heart failure with preserved ejection fraction. Circulation. 2015;131[6]:550-559.)

TABLE 51.3 Cardiopulmonary Exercise Testing in HFpEF and HFmrEF

CPET PARAMETER	INTERPRETATION
RER <1.05	Submaximal test limited by noncardiopulmonary factor
Peak V_{O_2} < 80% predicted	Indicative of impaired exercise capacity
Discrepancy between unindexed peak V_{O_2} and indexed peak V_{O_2}	In patients with obesity-induced limitation of exercise capacity, unindexed peak V_{O_2} (percent predicted) will be relatively preserved but once indexed to body weight will be much more abnormal
Peak V_E/maximum voluntary V_E <70%	Evaluate for intrinsic pulmonary disease
Reduced O_2 pulse	Look for low stroke volume as a potential cause
Blunted heart rate response	Medication-induced (e.g., beta blocker) versus chronotropic incompetence
Elevated V_E/V_{CO_2}	Can be a sign of elevated PA pressure and PVR; and does not require a maximal test; also a prognostic sign in HFpEF
Exercise oscillatory breathing	Indicative of a worse prognosis in HFpEF

tomography (CT) of the chest is important in patients suspected with HFpEF and HFmrEF to exclude a pulmonary cause of symptoms. Chronic lung diseases, particularly chronic obstructive pulmonary disease (COPD), are often present in patients with HFpEF and HFmrEF and can contribute to its pathogenesis. In patients with COPD with hyperinflation, a chronically underfilled left heart can lead to reduced stroke volume and cardiac output, which triggers neurohormonal activation and can lead to systemic hypertension, which can eventually cause HF. Patients with COPD and chronic bronchitis appear to share risk factors with HFpEF and HFmrEF such as obesity. In patients with either COPD or interstitial lung disease, pulmonary hypertension can result in RV dysfunction, which can further exacerbate HFpEF and right heart failure. Even in the absence of chronic lung disease, HFpEF and HFmrEF patients may have abnormal PFT findings, including reduced forced vital capacity (especially in the setting of obesity) and reduced diffuse capacity of carbon monoxide (COPD) due to pulmonary venous congestion, interstitial edema, alveolar edema, and pulmonary vascular disease.

Central and obstructive sleep apnea (CSA and OSA, respectively) are also common in HFpEF and HFmrEF. CSA can occur in decompensated HF regardless of underlying EF, and increased laryngeal edema and obesity can result in OSA. Thus, overnight polysomnography can be useful in the assessment of HFpEF but should be performed after adequate diuresis to ensure that fluid overload alone is not the cause of either CSA or OSA.[68]

Kidney. Impaired renal function is important in the pathogenesis of HFpEF, often coexists with HFpEF, and can be a major cause of fluid retention. However, because of the crude nature of clinical assessment of renal function (which is reliant on creatinine for estimation of glomerular filtration rate [GFR]), assessment of renal function in HFpEF is often inaccurate and misleading. In patients with overt fluid overload, the serum creatinine level can be hemodiluted, resulting in false reassurance of "normal" renal function. Conversely, diuresis in HFpEF is often halted due to elevation in serum creatinine despite its beneficial effects because clinicians fail to understand the concept of hemoconcentration during diuresis.[69] Several studies have shown that hemoconcentration during diuresis, despite being associated with rising serum creatinine, is associated with improved outcomes in the setting of HF.

Skeletal Muscle. Several studies have demonstrated the concept of sarcopenic obesity in HFpEF.[70] As in other chronic diseases, there is loss of skeletal muscle and increased intramuscular adiposity. Furthermore, there is a transition between type I to type II muscle fibers in HFpEF, which results in impaired exercise tolerance in HFpEF.[71] Patients with HFpEF also have systemic microvascular dysfunction, which, when present in the skeletal muscles, results in decreased oxygen extraction, which has been shown to account for 50% of the reduction in peak V_{O_2} in HFpEF patients. CPET is therefore a useful tool for the assessment of skeletal muscle dysfunction in HFpEF (based on measurement of arteriovenous O_2 difference). Magnetic resonance spectroscopy can also be utilized to directly examine skeletal muscle energetics and skeletal muscle composition, though such techniques are currently primarily used in the research setting.

Liver. In patients with signs and symptoms of HFpEF, clinical evaluation of the liver is important to exclude primary cirrhosis with high-output heart failure. Nonalcoholic fatty liver disease (NAFLD) is common in morbidly obese patients and is associated with worse LV longitudinal strain, diastolic dysfunction, and higher stroke volume in the general population, all of which can contribute to a HFpEF phenotype.[72] Conversely, severe HFpEF with right heart failure can result in passive congestion of the liver, ultimately leading to cirrhosis. Therefore, liver function tests (particularly bilirubin and alkaline phosphatase as markers of liver congestion) and radiologic assessment of the liver by ultrasound, CT, or MRI can be useful in teasing out the role of the liver in patients with HFpEF.

Adipose Tissue. Increased visceral adiposity is a major contributor to HFpEF pathophysiology and is not always apparent by simply examining the BMI in HFpEF patients.[73] Certain subgroups of patients, especially those of South Asian descent, can have lower BMI but high visceral adiposity. Excessive epicardial adipose tissue may be particularly relevant to the pathophysiology of HFpEF patients.[47,74] Multiple methods for evaluating the presence and extent of visceral adiposity are available, including waist-hip circumference ratio, dual-energy X-ray absorptiometry (DEXA) scanning, and CT or MRI of the chest and abdomen. Several biomarkers, including increased triglyceride/HDL ratio, hyperglycemia with insulin resistance, increased plasminogen activator inhibitor-1 (PAI-1), and reduced vitamin D levels are also indicative of increased visceral adiposity.

PATHOPHYSIOLOGY

Pathophysiology of HFpEF and HFmrEF

From a hemodynamic perspective, the cardinal abnormality in HFpEF patients is LV end-diastolic pressure elevation (with resultant LA pressure elevation) at rest or with exertion. Patients with HFpEF have marked elevation in PCWP with minimal exertion. How and why cardiac pressure elevation occurs in HFpEF has been a matter of intense investigation over the past 25 years. In HFrEF, the primary cardiac insult results in myocardial injury (e.g., myocardial infarction, genetic cardiomyopathy, toxins [including chemotherapy], pathogens [e.g., viruses], or other causes), leading to progressive ventricular dysfunction, ventricular dilatation, and elevated filling pressure. Similar mechanisms may be in part responsible for the clinical syndrome in HFmrEF, especially in patients whose LVEF is reduced because of ischemic heart disease. The mechanisms of myocardial dysfunction in HFpEF, where LVEF is normal, remains unclear.

Once HFpEF is clinically overt, a variety of potential pathophysiologic abnormalities can be present (Fig. 51.7).[75] Although the presence of abnormal myocardial relaxation and reduced LV chamber compliance are common in HFpEF and previously thought to be the major pathophysiologic abnormality in HFpEF, it is likely that HFpEF represents a systemic syndrome with multiple cardiac and extracardiac pathophysiologic mechanisms beyond diastolic dysfunction. From a cardiac perspective, LV systolic dysfunction is often impaired despite a preserved LVEF. Longitudinal fiber LV systolic dysfunction (i.e., abnormal LV global longitudinal strain and reduced TDI s' velocities) are often present in HFpEF[57]; furthermore, patients with HFpEF often have impaired LV contractile reserve. LA dysfunction is common in HFpEF, and some patients may have a primary LA myopathy out of proportion to LV dysfunction. Worse LA reservoir function (i.e., impaired ability of the LA to expand during LV systole) promotes chronic increases in pulmonary venous pressure, which can lead to pulmonary hypertension and right-sided heart failure. Atrial dilation in response to the HFpEF syndrome often leads to mitral and tricuspid annular dilation with resultant mitral and tricuspid regurgitation, both of which can exacerbate the HFpEF syndrome. Additional potential mechanisms in HFpEF include abnormal ventricular-arterial coupling and chronotropic incompetence.

Systemic and coronary endothelial dysfunction are common in HFpEF. CFR is reduced in up to 75% of HFpEF patients,[60] and evidence of coronary microvascular disease is present in the majority of HFpEF

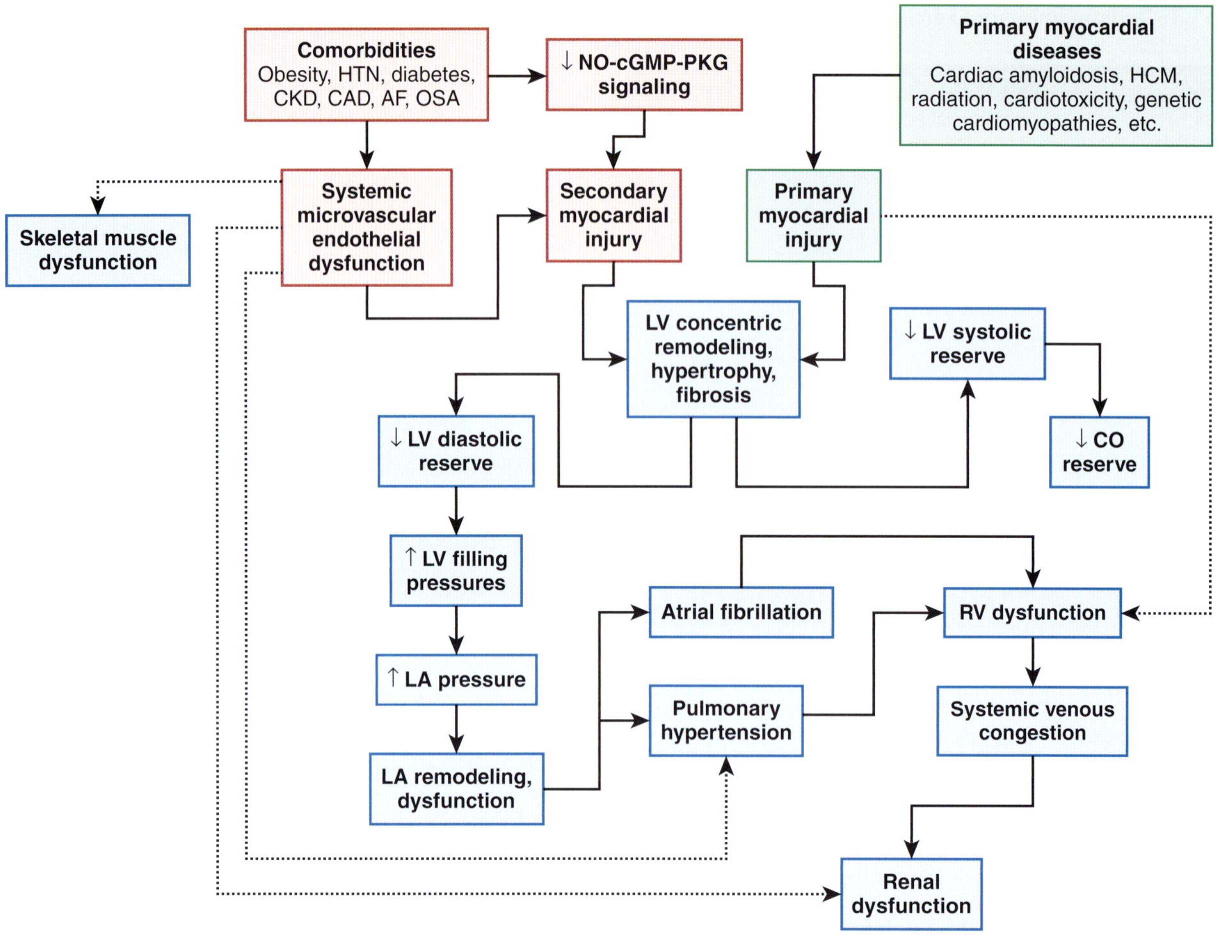

FIGURE 51.7 Etiologic and pathophysiologic model of HFpEF. Etiologic and pathophysiologic model of heart failure with preserved ejection fraction. HFpEF can result from primary or secondary myocardial injury, with the latter being more typical of the syndrome. Comorbidities are thought to lead to systemic inflammation, which is associated with systemic endothelial dysfunction and decreased NO-cGMP-PKG signaling that result in secondary myocardial injury. Other diseases such as cardiac amyloidosis and HCM result in primary myocardial injury. Regardless of the cause, LV concentric remodeling and hypertrophy ensues, which results in a cascade of LV dysfunction, LA dysfunction, and RV dysfunction, ultimately leading to pulmonary and systemic venous congestion. Systemic endothelial dysfunction also likely contributes to skeletal muscle dysfunction and renal dysfunction, both of which are present in the vast majority of HFpEF patients. *AF*, Atrial fibrillation; *CKD*, chronic kidney disease; *CAD*, coronary artery disease; *cGMP*, cyclic guanosine monophosphate; *CO*, cardiac output; *HCM*, hypertrophic cardiomyopathy; *HTN*, hypertension; *LA*, left atrial; *LV*, left ventricular; *NO*, nitric oxide; *OSA*, obstructive sleep apnea; *PKG*, protein kinase G; *RV*, right ventricular. (From Shah SJ. Innovative clinical trial designs for precision medicine in heart failure with preserved ejection fraction. J Cardiovasc Transl Res. 2017;10[3]:322-336.)

patients on autopsy[76] (Fig. 51.8). Reduced CFR is associated with systemic endothelial dysfunction and worse cardiac structure and function in HFpEF and may be a key factor underlying the poor systolic and diastolic reserve present in the setting of HFpEF. In addition, coronary microvascular dysfunction can involve the RV, resulting in impaired RV function independent of RV dysfunction due to increased RV afterload. Systemic endothelial dysfunction can lead to pulmonary, renal, and skeletal muscle dysfunction in HFpEF, all of which likely lead to and exacerbate the HFpEF syndrome.

Less is known about the underlying pathophysiology of HFmrEF due to a general lack of detailed studies in this HF subtype. Because of the mildly reduced LVEF, HFmrEF share some pathophysiologic similarities with patients with HFrEF. Longitudinal systolic dysfunction (i.e., abnormal LV global longitudinal strain) and impaired contractile reserve are more exaggerated in HFmrEF compared with HFpEF. Nevertheless, HFmrEF patients share many of the same comorbidities as HFpEF and may therefore also share some pathophysiologic similarities such as systemic and coronary endothelial dysfunction, abnormal ventricular-arterial coupling, and chronotropic incompetence.

Molecular Mechanisms Underlying HFpEF And HFmrEF

Several molecular mechanisms have been investigated in preclinical studies of HFpEF.[77] Comorbidity-induced systemic inflammation and endothelial dysfunction, cyclic guanosine monophosphate (cGMP)-protein kinase G (PKG) deficiency, interstitial myocardial fibrosis related to hypertension and diabetes, abnormal cardiomyocyte calcium handling, lipotoxicity, metabolic defects in fuel utilization and efficiency, and loss of cytoprotective signaling are some of the molecular mechanisms thought to be present in common forms of HFpEF, as shown in Figure 51.9.[75] Less is known about the molecular mechanisms of HFmrEF due to the lack of basic science studies of this HF phenotype.

The comorbidity-inflammation-endothelial dysfunction paradigm has garnered recent attention in HFpEF because patients with HFpEF often have multiple comorbidities such as hypertension, obesity, diabetes, chronic kidney disease, CAD, and COPD, and markers of systemic inflammation are more potent risk factors for incident HFpEF compared with incident HFrEF. Comorbidities are thought to result in systemic inflammation leading to endothelial dysfunction in multiple organs throughout the body. Inflammation-induced endothelial dysfunction affects the myocardium, lungs, skeletal muscle, and kidneys leading to diverse HFpEF phenotypes with variable amounts of myocardial remodeling and dysfunction, pulmonary hypertension, renal sodium retention, and deficient skeletal muscle oxygen extraction during exercise. In the heart, inflammation-induced coronary endothelial dysfunction can result in coronary microvascular dysfunction with subendocardial ischemia, particularly during exertion. Endothelial inflammation also causes increased reactive oxygen species, reduced nitric oxide bioavailability, and production of peroxynitrite, resulting in reduced soluble guanylate cyclase activity, lower cGMP content, and reduced PKG. Decreased PKG has protean manifestations germane to HFpEF: increased cardiomyocyte hypertrophy, increased cardiomyocyte stiffness (due to changes in titin phosphorylation), pulmonary vasoconstriction, impaired renal and skeletal muscle function, and increased adiposity. Inflammation also results in increased endothelial expression of adhesion molecules, which attract infiltrating leukocytes that secrete transforming growth factor β

(TGF-β), which converts fibroblasts to myofibroblasts thereby enhancing interstitial collagen deposition and promoting interstitial myocardial fibrosis.[78,79]

Systemic inflammation also leads to the activation of monocytes and macrophages, which release pro-fibrotic cytokines including interleukin-10 and TGF-β, thereby promoting interstitial fibrosis in multiple organs, including the heart.[80] Importantly, collagen cross-linking tends to be higher in HFpEF with increased profibrotic potential in HFpEF compared with HFrEF.[78] Measurement of circulating markers of fibrosis in HFpEF and HFmrEF patients have shown that collagen synthesis is increased, and collagen degradation is decreased. Both mineralocorticoid antagonists and sacubitril/valsartan appear to reverse these processes resulting in a less pro-fibrotic profile in HFpEF and HFmrEF patients treated with these drugs.[78,81]

Although endothelium-derived NO is reduced in HFpEF, inducible NO synthase (iNOS), which is activated by systemic inflammation, may be upregulated and could be a pathogenic factor leading to HFpEF. In a recent study that utilized a novel 2-hit mouse model of HFpEF leading to hypertension and obesity, NOS was upregulated, which resulted in nitrosative stress of the endonuclease inositol-requiring protein 1α (IRE1α), leading to defective splicing of an unfolded protein response effector (the spliced form of X-box-binding protein 1 [XBP1s]). XBP1s, in turn, was reduced in both the rodent HFpEF model and also in myocardial samples from patients with HFpEF. Defective splicing of XBP1s leads

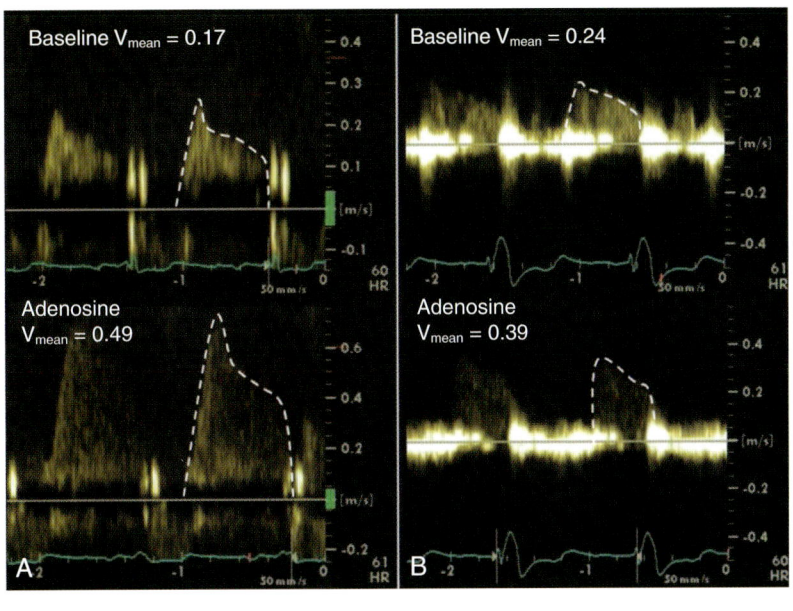

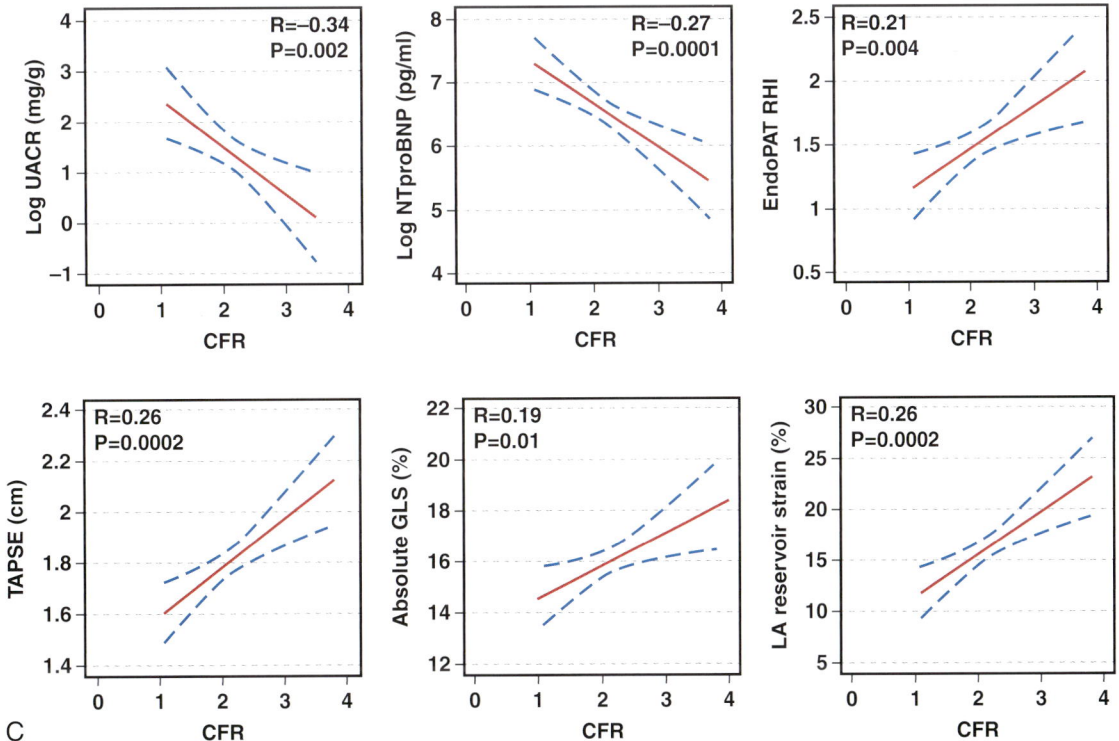

FIGURE 51.8 Coronary microvascular dysfunction in HFpEF and HFmrEF. **A** and **B**, Examples of transthoracic coronary Doppler echocardiography tracings at rest and with adenosine in a HFpEF patient without coronary microvascular dysfunction (**A**) versus a HFpEF patient with coronary microvascular dysfunction (**B**). The patient without coronary microvascular dysfunction had a normal coronary flow reserve (2.88), whereas the patient with coronary microvascular dysfunction had a reduced coronary flow reserve (1.63). **C**, Correlations between coronary flow reserve (CFR) and biomarkers, systemic endothelial function, and echocardiographic parameters in the PROMIS-HFpEF study. *EndoPAT*, endothelial peripheral artery tonometry; *GLS*, left ventricular global longitudinal strain; *LA*, left atrial; *NTproBNP*, N-terminal pro-B-type natriuretic peptide; *RHI*, reactive hyperemia index, a marker of systemic endothelial function; *TAPSE*, tricuspid annular plane systolic excursion; *UACR*, urinary albumin-to-creatinine ratio.

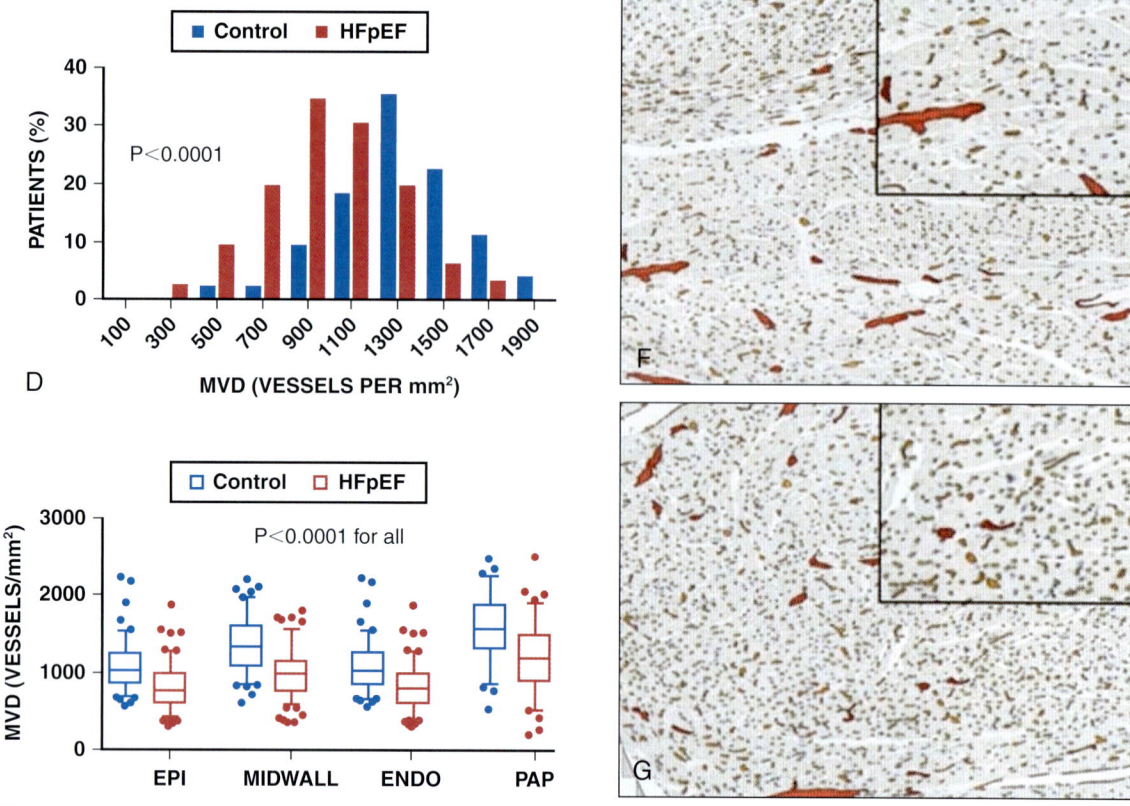

FIGURE 51.8 cont'd D-G, Coronary microvascular density (MVD) in HFpEF and control. **D,** The frequency distribution for total MVD is shifted downward in HFpEF. **E,** Tukey box plots (*box,* median, 75th, and 25th percentiles; *whiskers,* highest value within 75th percentile plus 1.5 × IQR and lowest value within the 25th percentile minus 1.5 × IQR; symbols show outliers if present) of regional MVD demonstrate similar reduction in MVD across the subepicardial (*Epi*), midmyocardial (*Midwall*), subendocardial (*Endo*), and papillary muscle (*Pap*) in HFpEF. Representative examples of antiplatelet endothelial cell adhesion molecule-1/ anti-CD31 stained left ventricular sections with algorithm-defined capillaries (*yellow*), precapillary arterioles (*orange*), and larger intramyocardial arteries (*red*) illustrate **(F)** the lower MVD in HFpEF in comparison with **(G)** control subjects. *CD31,* cluster of differentiation 31; *HFpEF,* heart failure with preserved ejection fraction; *IQR,* interquartile range. (**A-C** adapted from Shah SJ, et al. Prevalence and correlates of coronary microvascular dysfunction in heart failure with preserved ejection fraction: PROMIS-HFpEF. Eur Heart J. 2018;39[37]:3439-3450; **D-G** from Mohammed S, et al. Coronary microvascular rarefaction and myocardial fibrosis in heart failure with preserved ejection fraction. Circulation. 2015;131[6]:550-559.)

to increased levels of unfolded proteins within the cardiomyocytes, which are thought to interfere with normal cardiomyocyte function.[82]

Multiple mechanisms present in HFpEF can result in stiffening of titin, the major molecular spring within the cardiomyocyte, thereby leading to increased passive stiffness of cardiomyocytes (with resultant increased LV chamber stiffness). As stated earlier, reduced PKG leads to abnormal phosphorylation of key sites within titin and increases in its stiffness. Other mechanisms of increased stiffness of titin include cardiomyocyte stretch induced ERK-2 signaling, sympathetically mediated PKA stimulation, reactive oxygen species-induced CaMKII abnormalities, and endothelin- and angiotensin-II-mediated increases in PKCα.[75]

Abnormal calcium homeostasis in cardiomyocytes has long been known to be associated with abnormalities in systolic and diastolic function and are likely impaired in HFpEF and HFmrEF patients. T-tubule disruption, increased calcium entry into cardiomyocytes due to enhanced late inward sodium current, defective ryanodine receptor functioning, reduced SERCA2a activity, and abnormal myofilament calcium handling are all potential mechanisms underlying defective cardiomyocyte calcium homeostasis and could represent therapeutic targets in HFpEF and HFmrEF.[75]

Strategies for Phenotypic Subtyping of HFpEF

Because of the heterogeneous nature of the HFpEF syndrome, multiple potential mechanisms, and widespread endothelial dysfunction that can variably affect multiple organs with varying severity, several potential HFpEF sub-phenotypes exist.[83] For these reasons, the creation of a rationale, unified classification system for HFpEF has been challenging. Nevertheless, several ways of classifying HFpEF are available and can assist with clinical management of HFpEF (Table 51.4): (1) clinical subtypes (based on etiologic and echocardiographic features); (2) dominant HFpEF pathophysiology; (3) clinical presentation (exercise-induced LA pressure elevation, overt volume overload, or pulmonary hypertension/RV failure); and (4) extent of cardiac (vs. extracardiac) involvement. While these HFpEF sub-phenotypes are not necessarily mutually exclusive and may represent different stages of the disease they are nevertheless helpful in the clinical setting and also may explain why HFpEF clinical trials have met with little success. For example, a HFpEF patient with exercise-induced LA pressure elevation with minimal signs of overt fluid overload and a HFpEF patient with significant RV enlargement/dysfunction and pulmonary hypertension may both have elevated natriuretic peptides and LA enlargement and therefore meet inclusion of contemporary HFpEF clinical trials. However, the management of these two types of patients would likely differ dramatically in the clinical setting. The first patient may benefit from structured exercise training whereas the second patient may benefit from implantable hemodynamic monitoring to guide diuresis. Besides pathophysiologic and etiologic sub-phenotypes of HFpEF, it is now also recognized that there are important geographical differences in HFpEF, likely related to different underlying risk factors and genetic backgrounds.[84]

TREATMENT OF HFPEF AND HFMREF

The treatment of HF with a LVEF of 40% or less (HFrEF) has been informed by an abundance of large clinical outcomes trials that have tested several classes of pharmacologic and device therapies and afforded clinicians a full armamentarium of treatments designed to reduce morbidity and mortality (see also Chapter 50). In contrast, there have been limited large clinical outcomes trials to inform therapeutic approaches in patients with HF and LVEF >40%, and treatment of these patients has been mostly empiric. While many of the basic principles of HF management are similar regardless of LVEF, several therapies that have proven beneficial in HFrEF have shown no or limited benefit in patients with HF and higher LVEF (>55% to 60%). Moreover, the treatment of HFpEF and HFmrEF is complicated by the added complexity

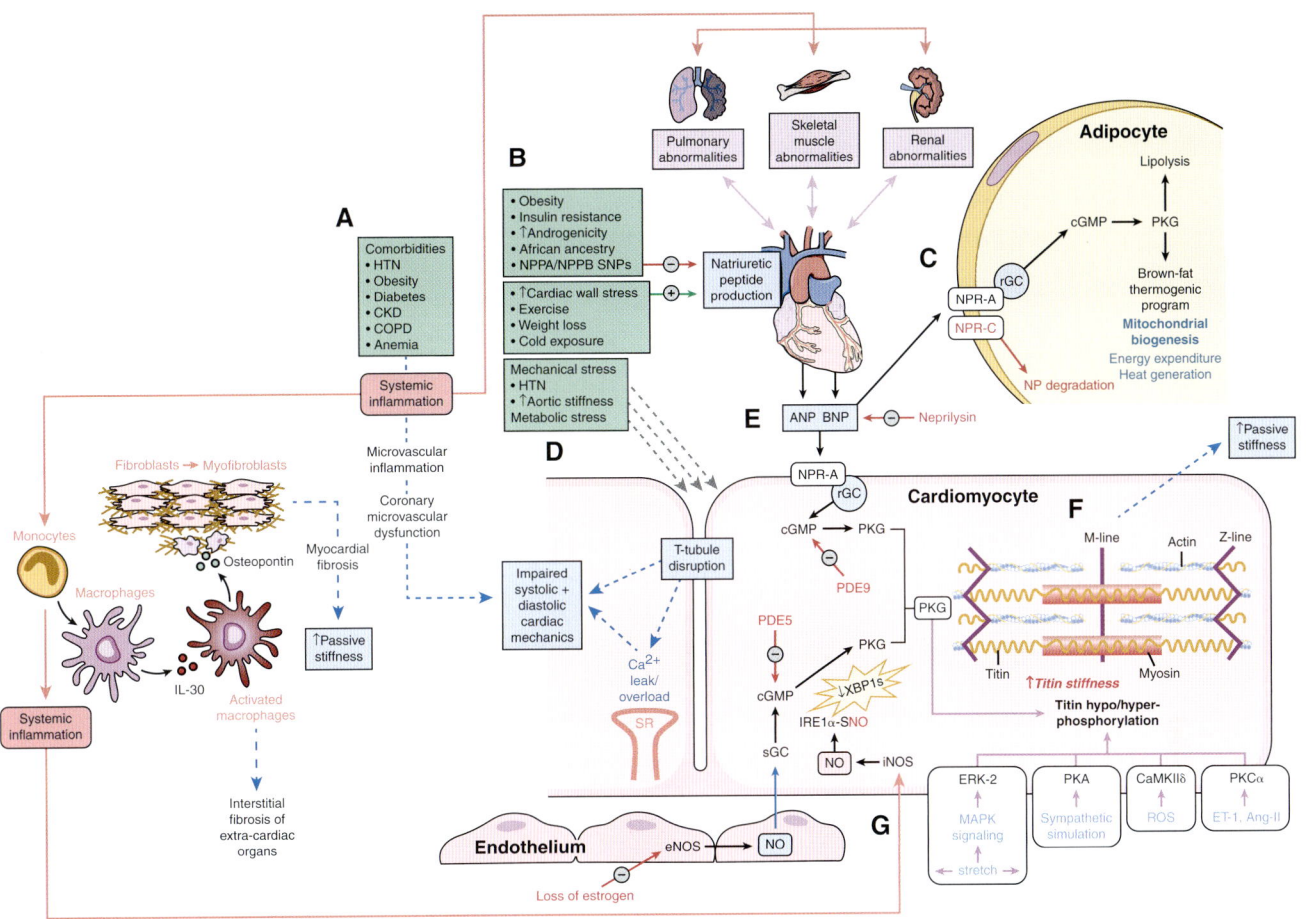

FIGURE 51.9 Proposed molecular mechanisms underlying HFpEF. **A,** Comorbidities are common in HFpEF and are thought to lead to systemic inflammation, which results in microvascular inflammation, widespread endothelial dysfunction (in multiple organs), and coronary microvascular dysfunction, leading to abnormal systolic and diastolic cardiac mechanics and poor cardiac reserve. Systemic inflammation also leads to the activation of monocytes and macrophages, which release profibrotic cytokines, including IL-10 and transforming growth factor-β, thereby promoting interstitial organ fibrosis, which in the heart increases passive myocardial stiffness. **B,** Several factors promote a relative natriuretic peptide (NP) deficiency state in HFpEF, including obesity, sedentary lifestyle, African ancestry, insulin resistance, increased androgenicity in women, genetic variation in the *NPPA* and *NPPB* genes, and a lower amount of wall stress (compared with heart failure with reduced ejection fraction). **C,** NPs are active in adipose tissue, where the relative ratio of the NP receptor A (*NPRA*) to NP receptor C (*RC*) is important in dictating whether beneficial NP effects are possible. With increased NPRA, there is increased cGMP and protein kinase G (*PKG*) production, leading to lipolysis and the brown-fat thermogenic program. With increased NPRC, these beneficial effects are minimized because there is increased NP breakdown. **D,** Mechanical and metabolic stressors on the cardiomyocyte lead to T-tubule disruption and abnormal calcium handling within the cardiomyocyte, which leads to intracellular calcium overload and inefficient myocardial contraction and relaxation. **E,** NPs act through a receptor guanylate cyclase (rGC) pathway that results in the creation of cGMP and stimulation of PKG, which has a variety of beneficial effects in the heart and multiple other organs. There is also an intracellular, soluble guanylate cyclase that is stimulated by nitric oxide (*NO*), which also leads to increased cGMP and activation of PKG. Phosphodiesterase (*PDE*) 5 results in the breakdown of the NO-based cGMP pool, whereas PDE9 results in the breakdown of the NP-based cGMP pool. **F,** Multiple mechanisms present in HFpEF can result in stiffening of titin, the major molecular spring within the cardiomyocyte, thereby leading to increased cardiomyocyte (and subsequently cardiac chamber) passive stiffness. Because of insufficient NPs and NO, PKG is reduced in HFpEF, which leads to hypophosphorylation of key sites within titin and increases its stiffness. Extracellular signal–regulated kinase 2 (ERK-2; stimulated by increased cardiomyocyte stretch), protein kinase A (*PKA*; stimulated by sympathetic stimulation), calmodulin-dependent protein kinase II (*CaMKII*; stimulated by reactive oxygen species [ROS]), and protein kinase Cα (PKCα; stimulated by endothelin-1 [ET-1] and angiotensin-II) all can have deleterious prostiffening effects on titin. **G,** Although endothelium-derived NO is reduced in HFpEF, inducible NO synthase (*iNOS*), which is activated by systemic inflammation, is upregulated and could be a pathogenic factor leading to HFpEF. In a recent study that used a novel two-hit mouse model of HFpEF (Nω-nitro-l-arginine methyl ester, which induces hypertension (HTN)]+high-fat diet [obesity]), iNOS was upregulated, which resulted in S-nitrosylation (nitrosative stress) of the endonuclease inositol-requiring protein 1α (*IRE1α*), leading to defective splicing of an unfolded protein response effector (the spliced form of X-box-binding protein 1 [*XBP1s*]). XBP1s, in turn, was reduced in both the rodent HFpEF model and in myocardial samples from patients with HFpEF, leading to increased levels of unfolded proteins within the cardiomyocytes, which are thought to interfere in normal cardiomyocyte function. *ANP,* atrial NP; *BNP,* brain NP; *CKD,* chronic kidney disease; *COPD,* chronic obstructive pulmonary disease; *eNOS,* endothelial NO synthase; *IL,* interleukin; *MAPK,* mitogen-activated protein kinase; *SNO,* S-nitrosylation; *SNP,* single nucleotide polymorphism. (From Shah SJ, et al. Research priorities for heart failure with preserved ejection fraction: National Heart, Lung, and Blood Institute Working Group Summary. Circulation. 2020;141[12]:1001-1026.)

of diagnosis in a syndrome in which signs and symptoms overlap with other diseases, and in which clear evidence of cardiac abnormalities are often lacking, a problem that has also confounded the testing of therapies in clinical trials.

General Considerations
Exclusion of Other Causes of Signs/Symptoms

Once the diagnosis of HFpEF or HFmrEF is clear, it is important to recognize that several potential etiologies can result in signs and symptoms of HF, a preserved or mildly reduced LVEF, and elevated cardiac filling pressures (Table 51.5). Because the signs and symptoms associated with HFpEF and HFmrEF are relatively nonspecific, it is necessary that other diseases that can mimic these be considered and ruled out.

Ischemic heart disease resulting in anginal equivalent of shortness of breath can be mistaken for HF. Hypertensive crisis can present with signs and symptoms of HF that can be alleviated with blood pressure control. Both obstructive and interstitial forms of lung disease, as well as pulmonary venoocclusive disease, can mimic the shortness of breath in HF, and elevation in pulmonary pressures can lead to right-sided symptoms and signs, including early satiety, pleural effusions, and edema. All of these conditions have pathophysiologic features that are distinct from HF and can be treated by specific therapies.

Additionally, several distinct disease entities that can present with HF and in which ejection fraction can be relatively preserved should be ruled out, including amyloid heart disease, hypertrophic cardiomyopathy, and constrictive pericarditis (see also Chapters 53, 54, and 86). There are several clinical clues that should alert the clinician to the

TABLE 51.4 Classification Schemes for HFpEF

CLASSIFICATION SCHEME	CATEGORIES OF HFPEF	DESCRIPTION
Clinical classification	"Garden-variety" HFpEF	Hypertension, diabetes, obesity, and/or chronic kidney disease
	CAD-HFpEF	Typically multivessel CAD with prior coronary revascularization
	Right heart failure–HFpEF	Predominant right-sided HF with or without pulmonary hypertension
	Atrial fibrillation–predominant HFpEF	Atrial arrhythmias dominate the clinical presentation
	HCM-like HFpEF	These patients do not have genetic forms of HCM, but their clinical course and echocardiography features are typical of HCM
	High-output HFpEF	Typically due to liver disease and severe anemia
	Valvular HFpEF	Multiple moderate valvular lesions
	Rare causes of HFpEF	For example, infiltrative cardiomyopathies, cardiotoxicities, and genetic cardiomyopathies
Presentation phenotypes	Exercise-induced increase in LA pressure	These patients typically are very breathless with exertion but do not have overt signs of volume overload and typically do not have a history of HF hospitalization
	Volume overload	Signs and symptoms of volume overload: typically have a history of HF hospitalization
	RV failure + pulmonary hypertension	Right heart failure predominates the clinical picture: often pulmonary hypertension is present and systemic blood pressure is reduced
Myocardial phenotypes	Type 1: HCM	Typical genetic forms of HCM
	Type 2: infiltrative	Cardiac amyloidosis and other forms of infiltrative or restrictive cardiomyopathies
	Type 3: non-HTN. non-LVH	No history of hypertension and LV wall thickness <1.2 cm
	Type 4: HTN	Typical, "garden-variety" form of HFpEF with history of HTN
Latent class analysis	A: younger males with CAD, lower LVEF	Based on latent class analysis of the I-PRESERVE and CHARM-Preserved trials. The authors used latent class analysis of 11 clinical features (age, gender, BMI, atrial fibrillation. CAD, diabetes, hyperlipidemia, valvular disease, alcohol use, cGFR, and hematocrit) to find six distinct groups of HFpEF in IPRESERVE and validated these findings in CHARM-Preserved
	B: younger females with lowest NT-proBNP	
	C: obesity, hyperlipidemia, diabetes mellitus, anemia, and renal insufficiency	
	D: obese females	
	E: older males with CAD, lowest LVEF	
	F: female predominance, advanced age, lower BMI, atrial fibrillation, CKD, highest NT-proBNP	
Phenomapping	Pheno-group 1: BNP deficiency syndrome	Based on model-based clustering of 67 continuous variables (phenotypes): physical characteristics, vital signs, ECG data laboratory data, and echocardiography parameters
	Pheno-group 2: obesity–cardiometabolic phenotype	
	Pheno-group 3: RV failure + cardiorenal phenotype	

BMI, Body mass index; *CAD*, coronary artery disease; *CKD*, chronic kidney disease; *HCM*, hypertrophic cardiomyopathy; *HTN*, hypertension; *LVH*, left ventricular hypertrophy; *LVEF*, left ventricular ejection fraction; *NTproBNP*, N-terminal pro-B-type natriuretic peptide; *RV*, right ventricular.
Data from Shah SJ. Precision medicine for heart failure with preserved ejection fraction: an overview. *J Cardiovasc Transl Res.* 2017;10(3):233–244.

TABLE 51.5 Differential Diagnosis of HFpEF

ETIOLOGY	DIAGNOSTIC TOOLS	TREATMENT
Cardiac amyloidosis	Monoclonal proteins, radionuclide scintigraphy, biopsy	Tafamidis (for transthyretin amyloidosis) or chemotherapy (for light-chain amyloidosis); avoid neurohormonal antagonists
Hypertrophic cardiomyopathy	Echocardiography, cardiac MRI	Beta blockers, calcium channel blockers, or septal reduction therapies (for obstructive cardiomyopathy); avoid vasodilators
Cardiac sarcoidosis	Cardiac MRI, FDG-PET, biopsy	Immunosuppressive agents
Constrictive pericarditis	Echocardiography, cardiac MRI or CT imaging, invasive hemodynamic measurements	Pericardiectomy
Valvular heart disease	Echocardiography, invasive hemodynamic measurements with ventriculography	Surgical or percutaneous valve interventions
Coronary artery disease	Invasive coronary angiography, stress imaging[†] or CT imaging	Revascularization, aspirin, statins, beta blockers, and nitrates
High-output heart failure	Evaluate for arteriovenous shunts and liver disease	Treatments directed at the cause of high cardiac output (such as fistula ligation for shunts, liver transplantation for cirrhosis)
Myocarditis	Cardiac MRI, endomyocardial biopsy	Immunosuppressive agents for some types (such as giant cell myocarditis or eosinophilic myocarditis)
Toxins	Assessment of clinical history, blood testing, endomyocardial biopsy	Removal of offending toxin (such as alcohol, cocaine, chemotherapy or radiation therapy, or heavy metals)

possibility of an atypical cause of the syndrome (Table 51.6). While these diseases can overlap with HFpEF and HFmrEF, the specific underlying etiology and pathophysiology are distinct, and targeted treatment options are either available or emerging.

Pathophysiologic Considerations of Therapy

The pathophysiology of HF, regardless of LVEF, is characterized by insufficient cardiac output to meet the body's metabolic needs, elevation in cardiac filling pressures, or both. Despite normal or mildly reduced LVEF, stroke volume (and hence cardiac output) can be low in patients with HFpEF and HFmrEF because of relatively small LV volume and LA failure, resulting in an inability to augment stroke volume during exertion, or to do so only by elevating filling pressure. Thus, while cardiac output may be sufficient at rest, during exertion it may be insufficient, resulting in symptoms. Unlike HFrEF where augmentation of stroke volume can potentially be of value, in HF with higher LVEF, it is not clear that increases in contractile function would be of benefit, as LVEF is already relatively high, even though patients with HFpEF do often have evidence of LV systolic dysfunction and impaired contractile reserve. One situation in which inadequate cardiac output might contribute to a patients' symptoms in HFpEF and HFmrEF is *chronotropic incompetence*, in which patients lack the ability to adequately increase heart rate in the setting of exertion.[85] In cases of true chronotropic incompetence, in which the contribution of medications such as beta blockers or calcium channel blockers has been ruled out, pacemaker therapy may have a role in ensuring adequate cardiac output (see later and Chapters 68 and 69).

LV diastolic dysfunction is present in the majority of patients with HFpEF and HFmrEF, and likely contributes to the pathophysiology of the syndrome. While several lusitropic therapies have been tested in patients with HFpEF and HFmrEF, few therapies other than blood pressure management (see later) have been shown to specifically improve diastolic function.

Mortality Reduction in HFpEF and HFmrEF

The overall goals of HF therapy are to reduce mortality, reduce hospitalization, and improve symptoms and functional capacity. Although mortality is increased in patients with HFpEF and HFmrEF compared with the general population, the absolute incidence of mortality in HF declines as LVEF rises, as does the proportion of deaths attributed to noncardiovascular causes. It has therefore been more difficult to demonstrate mortality benefit in HFpEF and HFmrEF than in HFrEF, both because of the lower event rates, and because therapies that are predominantly aimed at the cardiovascular system will be less able to modify noncardiovascular mortality.[86] Thus, reducing mortality in patients with HFpEF and HFmrEF requires focusing on factors that contribute to known risk factors for death, including treatment of both cardiac and noncardiac comorbidities that increase that risk. Beyond mortality reduction it is important to recognize that reduction in hospitalization and improvement in symptoms and functional capacity are critical patient-centered goals in the management of HFpEF and HFmrEF.

Empiric Therapy of HFpEF and HFmrEF

Decongestive Therapy with Diuretics

As in all patients with HF, those with HFpEF and HFmrEF typically have some degree of volume overload. Many will have evidence of elevated intracardiac filling pressures, both at rest and during exertion, which contributes to shortness of breath, orthopnea, paroxysmal nocturnal dyspnea, and right-sided symptoms such as lower extremity edema and early satiety. Thus, decongestive therapy with diuretics remains empiric cornerstone therapy for patients with HFpEF and HFmrEF. While diuretic therapy has not been specifically tested in HFpEF and HFmrEF in rigorous clinical trials, there is sufficient empiric evidence and overall collective experience, in addition to evidence from strategy trials using intracardiac monitoring (see later) that most clinicians agree that these patients require and benefit from diuretic therapy. Both the choice of type of diuretic (e.g., loop diuretic versus thiazide diuretic) and the frequency of use are empiric. As with other forms of HF, loop diuretics tend to be more potent than thiazide diuretics, but there are limited data to inform which diuretics are best. Combining loop and thiazide diuretics can be useful in patients in whom volume management is more challenging, or who become refractory to treatment, and empiric use of variable dose and frequency based on careful monitoring of a patient's weight is a commonly utilized strategy. Likewise, combinations of thiazide and potassium sparing diuretics are commonly used empirically in HFpEF and play a role both in decongestion and treatment of hypertension. Mineralocorticoid receptor antagonists (MRAs) are weak diuretics, although their potential benefits in HFpEF may go beyond their diuretic properties (see later), and in the setting of chronic loop diuretic therapy, sodium resorption in other areas of the nephron are heightened; thus, the addition of an MRA to loop diuretic therapy can result in augmented diuresis. As is the case in HFrEF, overdiuresis and volume depletion can predispose patients, especially elderly patients, to hypotension and renal dysfunction, and caution should be taken to avoid overdiuresis in vulnerable patients.

Blood Pressure Management

Although the general principles of blood pressure management (see also Chapter 26) apply to patients with HFpEF and HFmrEF, there

TABLE 51.6 Clues to Atypical Causes of HFpEF

CLUE TO ATYPICAL CAUSE OF HFPEF	NOTES/RATIONALES
HFpEF in a younger patient (age <55 years), especially if conventional HFpEF risk factors are lacking	Patients with common forms of HFpEF are often older and frequently have multiple comorbidities; if these are absent there may be an atypical cause of HFpEF.
Low BP, or LV hypertrophy without hypertension	Hypertension is very common in HFpEF; LV hypertrophy without hypertension is an indicator of an atypical cause of HFpEF.
Definite HFpEF (e.g., documented elevated LV filling pressures, prior HF hospitalization) but low H_2FPEF score	The H_2FPEF score combines common HFpEF risk factors with Doppler echocardiographic evidence of elevated LV filling pressures; if the score is low but definite HF is present, an atypical cause of HFpEF should be excluded.
Kussmaul's sign: ↑JVP with inspiration	Kussmaul's sign can be a sign of constrictive pericarditis, restrictive cardiomyopathy, severe tricuspid regurgitation, or a primary RV cardiomyopathy.
Persistent, low-level troponin elevation	Persistent low-level troponin elevation can be a sign of infiltrative cardiomyopathy such as cardiac amyloidosis.
Low prealbumin (= transthyretin)	Transthyretin (also known as prealbumin) can be measured clinically. A reduced transthyretin level may be indicative of increased propensity for transthyretin cardiac amyloidosis (but is not diagnostic of this disorder, so further testing must be completed).
Restrictive cardiomyopathy	On echocardiography, look for a "sparkling" myocardium, severely reduced tissue Doppler s' and e' velocities, preserved radial function and reduced longitudinal function, and hepatic vein systolic flow reversal during inspiration. On invasive hemodynamics look for concordant LV and RV pressure tracings during respiration.
Constrictive pericarditis	On echocardiography, look for a diastolic septal bounce, preserved e' velocity, septal e' velocity equal to or greater than lateral e' velocity, respiratory variation in mitral inflow, preserved longitudinal function and reduced radial function, and systolic flow reversal during expiration. On invasive hemodynamics, look for discordant LV and RV pressure tracings during respiration.

may be an additional rationale for lowering blood pressure in these patients. Blood pressure lowering has been shown to improve measures of diastolic function.[87] Although not specifically conducted in patients with HF, several trials of intensive versus standard blood pressure treatment, including HYVET[88] and SPRINT,[89] demonstrated reduction in HF hospitalizations in patients assigned to more intensive blood pressure lowering arms, suggesting that blood pressure reduction may be useful as a means to reduce HF hospitalizations in at-risk patients. Although most of the neurohormonal modulators that have been tested rigorously in HFpEF and HFmrEF are antihypertensive agents, post hoc analyses have suggested that the potential beneficial effects of therapy appeared to be independent of blood pressure reduction,[90] suggesting that the benefits of these agents extend beyond blood pressure lowering.

Atrial Fibrillation
Atrial fibrillation is extremely common in patients with HFpEF and HFmrEF (see earlier), and even patients who have never experienced atrial fibrillation are at markedly increased risk of developing atrial fibrillation. Atrial fibrillation can worsen HF in these patients by reducing the LA contribution to cardiac output and by reducing diastolic filling time when heart rates are rapid. Stroke volume is typically reduced even in patients with atrial fibrillation who have controlled heart rates due to reduced filling and emptying of the LA. Patients with HFpEF who are compensated are more likely to decompensate when they go into atrial fibrillation.[91]

The principles of treatment of atrial fibrillation in patients with HFpEF and HFmrEF are similar to the treatment of atrial fibrillation in general (see Chapter 66), including both rate control and anticoagulation. Beta blockers can be helpful in prevention of atrial fibrillation in those who are in sinus rhythm but have been in atrial fibrillation in the past although the experience in HFpEF and HFmrEF is largely anecdotal. One outstanding question in the treatment of atrial fibrillation in patients with HFpEF and HFmrEF is whether rhythm control rather than just rate control would reduce hospitalizations for HF, and, if so, which rhythm control strategies would be best. Most practitioners agree that patients with HFpEF and HFmrEF who are symptomatic despite empiric therapy and remain in atrial fibrillation deserve a trial of restoration of sinus rhythm, either through electrical or chemical cardioversion or an ablation procedure, although there are no randomized data to support this recommendation. The benefit observed in randomized trials of atrial fibrillation ablation in HFrEF raises the possibility that ablation might be a viable strategy in HFpEF and HFmrEF as well, although there are no rigorous clinical trials. The use of prophylactic rhythm control in patients with paroxysmal atrial fibrillation is also unclear, although beta blockade is often used in these patients empirically. Whether other antiarrhythmic drugs or ablation would reduce the incidence of atrial fibrillation–related hospitalization in these patients remains unknown. Unless contraindicated, anticoagulation with warfarin or a direct-acting oral anticoagulant should be utilized in patients with HFpEF and HFmrEF because of the high risk of thromboembolism in patients with concomitant atrial fibrillation and HF.

Management of Other Comorbidities
Comorbidities such as hypertension, obesity, diabetes, CAD, chronic kidney disease, chronic lung disease, sleep apnea, and anemia are extremely common in patients with HFpEF and HFmrEF. Generally, these comorbidities should be managed according to established guidelines in patients with HFpEF and HFmrEF. Maintaining euvolemia is important in patients with concomitant chronic lung disease and obstructive sleep apnea because elevated pulmonary venous pressure will exacerbate hypoxemia in patients with parenchymal lung disease, and oropharyngeal edema can exacerbate obstructive sleep apnea. Obesity is a very frequent comorbidity in HFpEF, and even when BMI is <30 kg/m², significant visceral adiposity is often present in HFpEF. Obesity is also a major determinant of NYHA class and exercise intolerance in HFpEF. Thus, treatment of obesity should be part of the therapeutic plan in HFpEF patients. Lifestyle modifications (see later) can be useful in improving several comorbidities commonly present in patients with HFpEF and HFmrEF.

Specific Pharmacologic Treatment
Calcium Channel Blockers and Beta Blockers
Both nondihydropyridine calcium channel blockers and beta blockers, which have previously been thought to improve myocardial diastolic properties, have been neutral in small trials in HFpEF and HFmrEF. There are virtually no data to support a role for calcium channel blockers in either HFpEF or HFmrEF beyond blood pressure lowering. The SENIORS trial tested the selective beta blocker nebivolol in patients with HF and showed a modest overall reduction in all-cause mortality or cardiovascular hospitalization.[92] That there was no heterogeneity in the treatment response based on ejection fraction has led some to conclude that this beta blocker might be beneficial in patients with HF and higher LVEF, although only 15% of patients in the trial had LVEF >50%. Carvedilol was tested in 245 patients in the J-DHF trial followed for 3.2 years and was not associated with greater reduction in cardiovascular death or HF hospitalization, although the trial was markedly underpowered. Others have suggested that beta blockade might be detrimental in patients with HFpEF,[93] although the data to support harm are likely confounded. The role of beta blockers for rate reduction in patients with atrial fibrillation, or in prevention of atrial fibrillation, is well established, and these benefits likely extend to patients with HFpEF or HFmrEF. Because beta blockers can lower blood pressure, they might limit the use of therapies that also affect blood pressure and for which more data exist. Nevertheless, the proportion of patients with HFpEF and HFmrEF taking beta blockers for hypertension is high, approaching 80% in recent clinical trials. In patients with reduced cardiac output at rest or during exertion, withdrawal of nondihydropyridine calcium channel blockers or beta blockers may be warranted, particularly in those patients with lack of augmentation of stroke volume during exercise. In these patients, improving chronotropic responsiveness may help augment cardiac output during exertion, thereby potentially improving symptoms.

Renin-Angiotensin-Aldosterone System Inhibitors
Neurohormonal modulators, particularly renin-angiotensin-aldosterone (RAAS) inhibitors have been the cornerstone of treatment of HFrEF but have proven less effective in large clinical trials of HFpEF. The postulated effects of RAAS inhibition in HFpEF and HFmrEF include lowering blood pressure, improvement of diastolic function, and reduction of myocardial fibrosis. Overall, there is less activation of the renin-angiotensin system in HF with higher ejection fraction, which might account for the limited therapeutic success of these agents.

Angiotensin Converting Enzyme Inhibitors
The initial CONSENSUS trial compared enalapril versus placebo in NYHA Class IV HF irrespective of ejection fraction, although the majority likely had HFrEF because cardiomegaly was an entry requirement. The ACE inhibitor perindopril was compared with placebo in patients with HF and LVEF >45% in the PEP-CHF trial,[94] an 850-patient trial in which event rates were lower than expected and in which many patients withdrew from therapy after a year (with a high frequency of crossover to ACE inhibitor therapy in the placebo arm). Overall, the hazard ratio for the primary endpoint, a composite of all-cause mortality and unplanned HF hospitalization, was 0.92 (95% CI 0.70 to 1.21), although at 1 year, before a substantial number of dropouts from the ACE inhibitor arm, there was nominal reduction in both the primary endpoint and HF hospitalization, as well as improvement in functional class and 6-minute walk test distance.

Angiotensin Receptor Blockers
Two large outcomes trials with angiotensin receptor blockers have been performed in patients with HF and LVEF >40%: CHARM-Preserved,[95] which compared candesartan to placebo in patients with HF and LVEF >40%, and I-PRESERVE,[96] which compared irbesartan to placebo in patients with HF and LVEF >45%. CHARM-Preserved was a component of the larger CHARM program that enrolled patients with HF across the ejection fraction spectrum; entry criteria for the entire program were similar regardless of ejection fraction. CHARM-Preserved enrolled 3023 patients with HF and LVEF >40%, and the hazard ratio for the primary endpoint of time to first HF hospitalization or cardiovascular

TABLE 51.7 Comparison of HFpEF Trials: Design and Inclusion Criteria

	CHARM-P	PEP-CHF	I-PRESERVE	TOPCAT	PARAGON-HF	EMPEROR-PRESERVED	DELIVER-HF
N	3023	850	4128	3445	4800	5988	6200
Treatment arms	Candesartan vs. placebo	Perindopril vs. placebo	Irbesartan vs. placebo	Spironolactone vs. placebo	Sacubitril/valsartan vs. valsartan	Empagliflozin vs. placebo	Dapagliflozin vs. placebo
Key inclusion criteria	NYHA Class II to IV, prior CV hospitalization	Clinical diagnosis of DHF with ≥ signs/symptoms of HF, ≥2 of the following: LAE/LVH/Impaired LV filling/AFib	NYHA Class II to IV + any corroborating evidence (e.g., HF sign), LVH or LAE considered optional corroborating evidence, HFH required unless in NYHA Class III to IV	≥1 HF symptom + ≥1 HF sign, elevated NP or HFH	NYHA Class II to IV, Elevated NT-proBNP (adjusted for atrial fibrillation and higher if no recent HF hospitalization), structural heart disease (LAE or LVH)	NYHA Class II to IV, elevated NT-proBNP.	NYHA Class II to IV, elevated NT-proBNP (adjusted for atrial fibrillation), structural heart disease (LAE or LVH)
Endpoint	First of either CVD or HFH	First of either all-cause death of HFH	First of either all-cause death or CVH	First of either CVD, HFH, or RSD	CVD and TOTAL HFH (first and recurrent).	CVD or hospitalization for HF	CVD or hospitalization for HF either in the full population or in patients with LVEF <60%

death was 0.89 (95% CI 0.77 to 1.03), $P = 0.12$. This result was stronger in several prespecified and post hoc analyses, including an analysis adjusting for baseline covariates, and in analyses using total number of hospitalization events rather than time to first event.[37] There was no observed effect on mortality. In contrast, the I-PRESERVE trial did not show a benefit comparing irbesartan to placebo in patients with HF and an LVEF above 45%. The primary outcome of all-cause death or cardiovascular hospitalization was similar between treatment groups (HR 0.95, 95% CI 0.86 to 1.05; $P = 0.35$). Each of these trials had slightly different inclusion and exclusion criteria (Table 51.7). More contemporary clinical trials in this population have shown that the majority of patients with HFpEF are treated with ACE inhibitors or angiotensin receptor blockers despite lack of a specific indication for these therapies, suggesting that in the majority of patients being treated, these agents are being used for comorbidities such as hypertension, chronic kidney disease, or diabetes.

Mineralocorticoid Receptor Antagonists

Mineralocorticoid receptor antagonists (MRAs) are potassium-sparing diuretics that have been used as a diuretic and for treatment of hypertension for several decades. Their benefit in HF was first shown in severe HFrEF (see also Chapter 50). Aldosterone is a known contributor to fibrosis in the heart, vasculature, and kidneys, and MRA receptor activation has been implicated in disorders of blood vessels, including hypertension and endothelial dysfunction, and abnormalities of cardiac structure, including myocardial hypertrophy. Moreover, experimental evidence supported a potential role for MRAs in reducing myocardial fibrosis,[97] improving diastolic function,[98] and endothelial vasomotor function.

These data provided the rationale for the TOPCAT trial,[99] which compared spironolactone to placebo in 3445 patients with HFpEF. The entry criteria for TOPCAT required signs and symptoms of HF with either elevation in natriuretic peptides or a history of HF hospitalization within the past year, and only patients with potassium <5.0 mmol/L, serum creatinine <2.5 mg/dL, and estimated glomerular filtration rate ≥30 mL/min/1.73 m² were included. The primary endpoint of the trial was a composite of cardiovascular death, HF hospitalization or aborted cardiac arrest, and the overall results showed an 11% nonsignificant risk reduction (HR 0.89, 95% CI 0.77 to 1.04, $P = 0.14$).[100] The trial enrolled patients from several countries around the world, and following unblinding, it became apparent that patients enrolled in the United States, Canada, Argentina, and Brazil had a nearly fivefold higher event rate than in patients enrolled in Russia and the Republic of Georgia, raising the possibility that patients enrolled in these regions may not have had HF.[101] The treatment effect of spironolactone was similarly attenuated in these regions. These revelations and subsequent metabolite data showing that a high proportion of sampled patients in Russia and the Republic of Georgia were not taking study drug[102] raised the possibility that in the right patients in whom the therapy was being taken, spironolactone would have shown benefit (Fig. 51.10A).

These data have been used to support incorporation of spironolactone, a generic and inexpensive therapy generic, into several guidelines for potential use in HFpEF (currently listed in the AHA/ACC/HFSA guidelines as a class IIb indication). Because spironolactone is readily available, but can elevate serum potassium, the decision to use it in patients with HFpEF and HFmrEF should be based on individual benefit-risk determination. For example, patients in TOPCAT with evidence of chronic kidney disease demonstrated a reduced benefit-risk ratio compared with those with better renal function,[103] whereas patients with HF with LVEF 45% to 60% appeared to benefit the most from spironolactone in TOPCAT.[104] Based on available data, unless otherwise contraindicated, an MRA should be added to loop diuretic therapy instead of potassium supplementation in patients with HFpEF and HFmrEF. When using an MRA in HFpEF or HFmrEF, potassium and renal function should be closely monitored 1 week and 1 month after initiating MRA therapy, and on a regular basis thereafter. Recently an FDA advisory voted in support of an indication for spironolactone in HFpEF.

Angiotensin Receptor Neprilysin Inhibition

Sacubitril/valsartan in a crystalline compound composed of the angiotensin receptor blocker valsartan and sacubitril, a prodrug neprilysin inhibitor. Neprilysin breaks down several vasoactive peptides, including the biologically active natriuretic factors, ANP, BNP, and CNP; adrenomedullin; endothelin; and angiotensin II; pairing both a neprilysin inhibitor with a renin-angiotensin system (RAS) inhibitor simultaneously blocks the RAS and augments the endogenous vasoactive peptide system.[105] Sacubitril/valsartan reduced cardiovascular mortality, HF hospitalization and all-cause mortality in 8399 patients with HFrEF in the PARADIGM-HF trial.[106] In a phase II trial in patients with HF and LVEF of 45% or greater, sacubitril/valsartan reduced NT-proBNP, a natriuretic peptide marker that is not directly affected by a neprilysin inhibitor, improved NYHA class, and reduced LA size compared with valsartan.[107] Based on these findings, the PARAGON-HF trial tested sacubitril/valsartan compared with valsartan in 4822 patients with NYHA Class II to IV HF, and LVEF ≥45%.[108] In contrast to prior HFpEF trials, patients were required to have elevation in natriuretic peptides and evidence of structural heart disease (see Table 51.7). Moreover, the primary endpoint of PARAGON-HF was a composite of cardiovascular death and total (first and recurrent) HF hospitalizations utilizing a novel recurrent events analysis (see also Chapter 4). PARAGON-HF showed a 13% reduction in total HF hospitalizations and cardiovascular death (rate ratio 0.87, 95% CI 0.75 to 1.01, $P = 0.059$), which just missed statistical significance. Nevertheless, several secondary endpoints, including measures of functional status, quality of life, and renal function were strongly suggestive of a true benefit. Moreover, there was evidence of substantial heterogeneity, with a treatment effect that was most pronounced in patients with LVEF that was at or below the median of 57%, and in women, with women appearing to derive greater benefit than men to a higher ejection fraction[109] (Fig. 51.10B). These findings have led to an FDA expanded approval for the use of sacubitril/valsartan in patients with chronic HF, noting that benefit was most evident in those with ejection fraction below normal.

Device Therapy in HFpEF and HFmrEF
Diagnostic Devices

A number of therapeutic and diagnostic devices have been tested, or are currently being tested, in HFpEF and HFmrEF. Several diagnostic devices have been developed to aid physicians in remote management of patients with HF (see Chapter 58). The CardioMEMS heart sensor is an implantable hemodynamic monitor that is inserted into a pulmonary artery and transmits pulmonary pressures to healthcare providers. In the CHAMPION trial,[110] the CardioMEMS sensor was tested in conjunction with a protocol-driven algorithm by which physicians utilized device information to make therapeutic changes. Patients were randomized to either an algorithm-based strategy based on utilizing remote data from the device, or standard medical therapy. Patients in the device-strategy arm demonstrated a significant decrease in pulmonary artery diastolic and systolic pressures, as well as a 52% decrease in HF-related events, an increase in days alive out of hospital and improvement in quality of life. The benefit observed was similar in patients across the spectrum of ejection fraction, suggesting that careful assessment of hemodynamic variables and application of therapeutic algorithms based on these assessments could improve outcomes in patients with HF regardless of ejection fraction. These devices are likely most helpful in HFpEF and HFmrEF patients

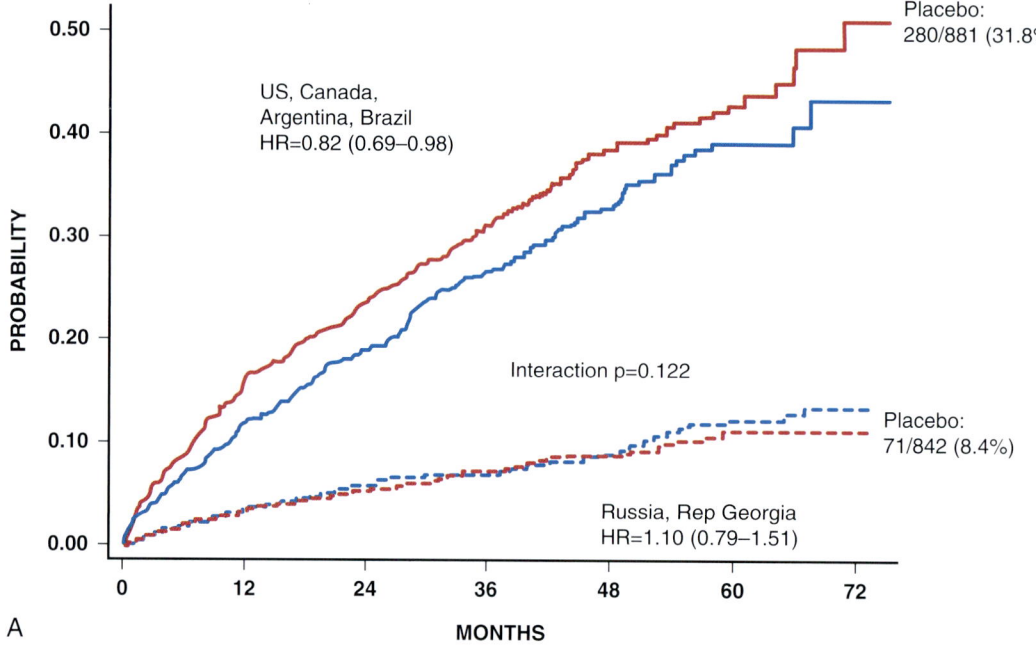

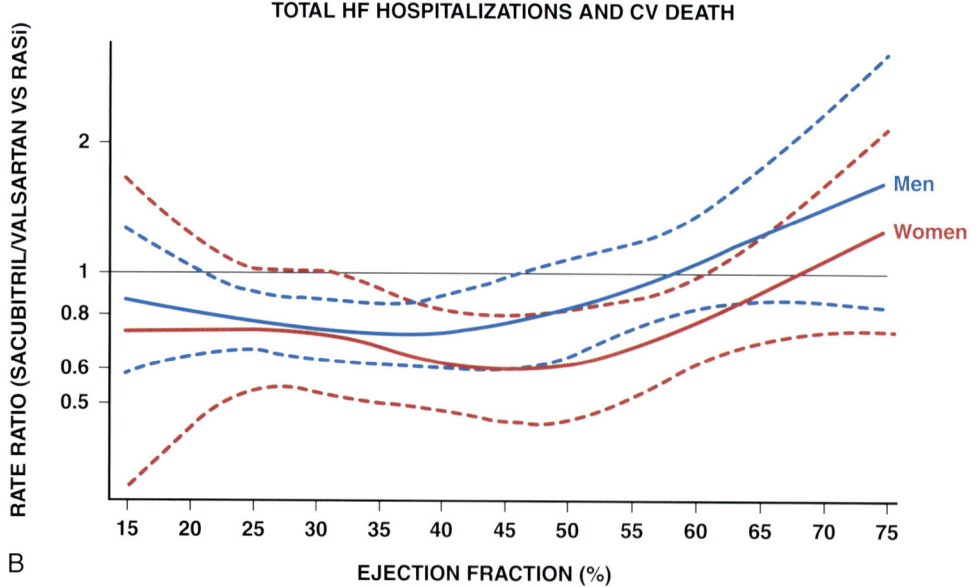

FIGURE 51.10 Phase III randomized controlled trials in HFpEF and HFmrEF. HFpEF and HFmrEF. **A,** Treatment effect comparing spironolactone and placebo in both the Americas region (United States, Canada, Argentina, Brazil) and in Russia and Republic of Georgia in the TOPCAT trial. The event rate in Russia and Republic of Georgia was approximately fivefold lower than in the Americas. **B,** Treatment effect for sacubitril/valsartan across the spectrum of heart failure from both the PARADIGM-HF and PARAGON-HF trials. The treatment benefit of sacubitril/valsartan declines as ejection fraction rises into the normal range in both men and women, with women deriving greater benefit to a higher ejection fraction than men.

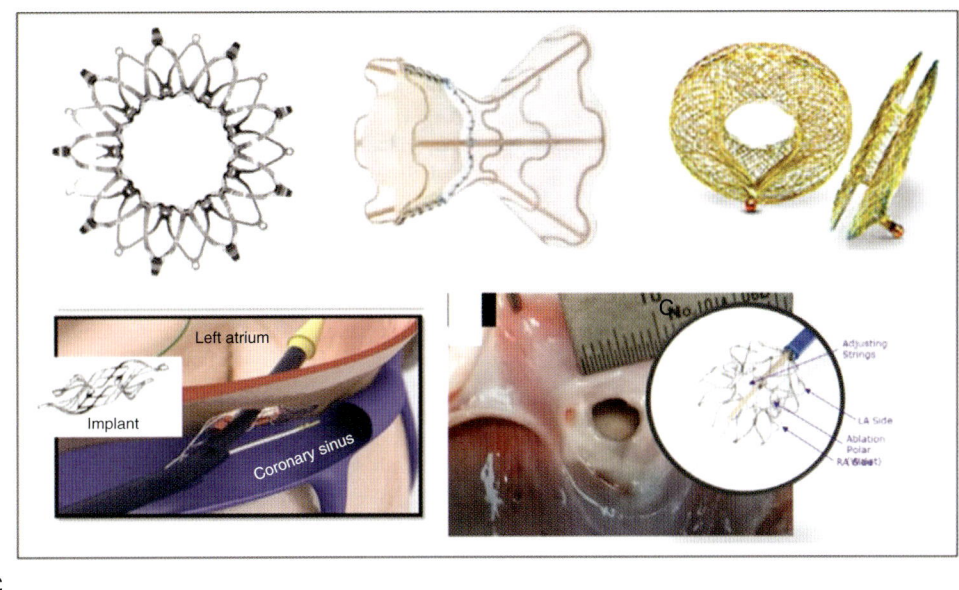

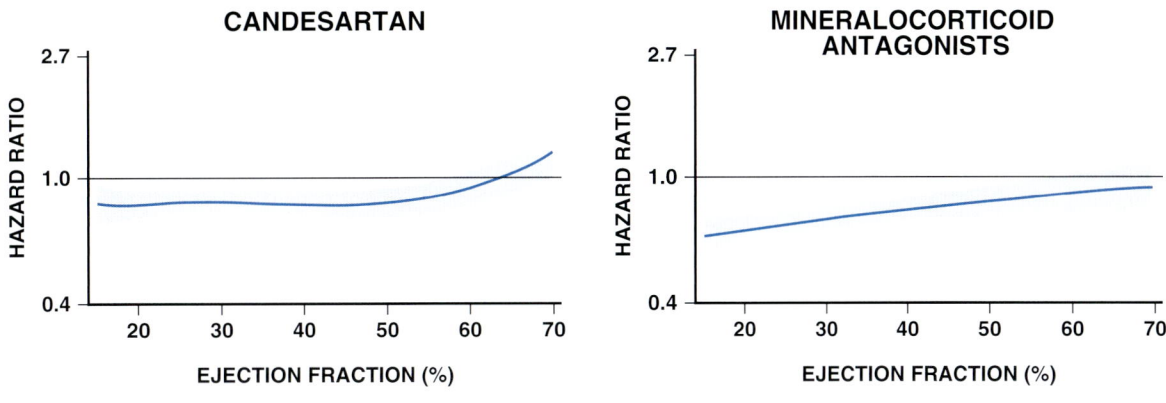

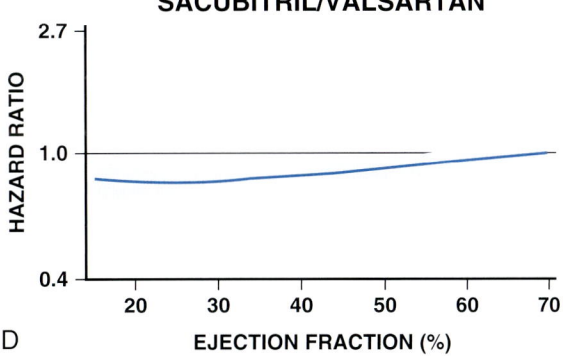

FIGURE 51.10 cont'd C, Interatrial shunt devices designed to lower left atrial pressure in heart failure. **D,** Treatment effect of the ARB candesartan, the MRA spironolactone, and sacubitril/valsartan across the spectrum of ejection fraction showing evidence of benefit for all three therapies in the reduced and mildly reduced ejection fractions. (**A** from Pfeffer MA, et al. Regional variation in patients and outcomes in the Treatment of Preserved Cardiac Function Heart Failure With an Aldosterone Antagonist (TOPCAT) trial. Circulation. 2015;131[1]:34-42. **B** from Solomon SD, et al. Sacubitril/valsartan across the spectrum of ejection fraction in heart failure. Circulation. 141[5]:352-361. **C** from Griffin JM, et al. Impact of interatrial shunts on invasive hemodynamics and exercise tolerance in patients with heart failure. J Am Heart Assoc. 2020;9[17]:e016760. **D** from Dewan P, et al. Interactions between left ventricular ejection fraction, sex and effect of neurohumoral modulators in heart failure. Eur J Heart Fail. 2020;22[5]:898-901.)

who experience frequent hospitalizations and can be helpful in keeping these patients out of the hospital. Many of these patients have the cardiorenal syndrome; implantable hemodynamic monitoring can be helpful to carefully guide diuresis in order to maintain euvolemia without exacerbating renal dysfunction. Several other diagnostic devices, including those that monitor heart rate and rhythm, impedance, respiration and other parameters are currently being tested in HFpEF and HFmrEF.

Therapeutic Devices

As elevation of LA pressures represents the pathophysiologic sine qua non of HF, another strategy that has been explored the placement of a shunt device between the left and right atria to lower LA pressures both at rest and on exertion. Interatrial shunt devices have been tested in preliminary trials (Fig. 51.10C), which have suggested that this approach is both safe and might improve hemodynamics;[111,112] pivotal data will be forthcoming from ongoing trials.

Neither ICDs nor CRT devices are currently recommended for patients with LVEF above 40%, although some patients with HFpEF and HFmrEF are at risk for sudden death, and dyssynchrony may contribute to worsening hemodynamics in patients with HF regardless of LVEF.[113] Patients with chronotropic incompetence who satisfy other requirements for standard pacemaker placement may benefit from pacemaker therapy. In addition, in patients with HFpEF and HFmrEF who already have pacemakers for other reasons and evidence of low resting cardiac output or inadequate stroke volume increase with exercise, raising the basal pacemaker rate or increasing the rate responsiveness of the pacemaker may improve symptoms and exercise tolerance.

Lifestyle Modification and Exercise Training

Both diet and lifestyle modification may have a role in the treatment of HFpEF and HFmrEF, although neither have been rigorously studied. As with HFrEF, sodium and fluid restriction may be useful in HFpEF, especially in patients with evidence of fluid overload. While strategies meant to treat obesity, including bariatric surgery, have been shown to have a variety of beneficial cardiovascular effects (see also Chapter 30), whether obesity reversal would improve outcomes in HFpEF is unknown. Pharmacologic treatment of obesity is currently being tested in clinical trials in HFpEF and HFmrEF.

In contrast to most pharmacologic intervention trials for HFpEF, exercise-based interventions have consistently demonstrated clinically meaningful improvements in objectively measured exercise capacity (peak oxygen uptake, total exercise time, and 6-minute walk distance), symptoms, and quality of life.[114] The benefits have been ascribed to the effect of exercise on a number of factors that influence exercise tolerance, including general metabolic benefits and effects on skeletal muscle.[115,116] While the majority of exercise trials have tested aerobic (endurance) training, others have incorporated strength training or high-intensity interval training. One of the major factors influencing the success of exercise programs is adherence, which has been only modest in trials.[117] In a randomized trial of patients with obesity and HFpEF, in which both caloric restriction and aerobic exercise were tested in a factorial design, the combination of approaches led to improved exercise capacity, quality of life in conjunction with greater weight loss and improvement in inflammatory biomarkers.[118] A recent multi-center trial of high-intensity interval training versus moderate continuous training versus guideline-based physical activity advice (control) in HFpEF patients showed that the two types of exercise training resulted in some improvement in peak V_{O_2} at 3 months (although not meeting the prespecified minimal clinically important difference of 2.5 mL/kg/min) compared with control during which time exercise training was done in a supervised setting.[119] However, after the initial 3 months, these improvements were attenuated during telehealth exercise over the next 9 months. Results for high intensity interval training and moderate continuous training were similar. Overall, these data suggest that exercise training can be useful to improve exercise tolerance and quality of life in patients with HFpEF and HFmrEF and should be recommended with a specific exercise program prescription in all patients.

Unsuccessful and Potentially Harmful Treatments in HFpEF

Numerous treatments have been tested unsuccessfully in HFpEF. Phosphodiesterase type 5 (PDE5) inhibitors have shown benefit and are currently approved for treatment of pulmonary arterial hypertension, but in several randomized trials in HFpEF, including in HFpEF with known elevation in pulmonary pressures, PDE5 inhibitors failed to show hemodynamic benefits.[120,121] Vericiguat, a soluble guanylate cyclase inhibitor, has been tested in two phase II trials in HFpEF and failed to show hemodynamic benefits or improvement in quality of life.[122,123] Neither organic[124] nor inorganic nitrates[125] have proven beneficial in HFpEF thus far, and isosorbide mononitrate was associated with lower activity levels compared with placebo in HFpEF in the NEAT trial.[124] Ivabradine, a pure heart rate reducing agent, was tested in the EDIFY trial in 179 patients with HFpEF,[126] and failed to show improvement of E/e', 6-minute walk test distance, or NT-proBNP at 6 months.

Emerging Concepts in the Treatment of HFpEF and HFmrEF

Emerging data suggest that patients with HF and LVEF that is above the range generally considered "reduced" but below normal (which overlaps with the HFmrEF category) may be phenotypically intermediate between HFrEF and HFpEF but may respond to therapies that have been proven beneficial in patients with HFrEF. Post hoc analyses from both the CHARM-Preserved and TOPCAT trials suggest greater treatment benefit with either candesartan or spironolactone in patients with LVEFs at the lower end of the spectrum of LVEF enrolled in those trials (Fig. 51.10D), and with treatment responses similar to what was seen in patients with HFrEF for the same therapies.[127] In a prespecified analysis, the PARAGON-HF trial also found significant therapeutic heterogeneity based on LVEF with patients in the lower end of the ejection fraction spectrum studied (LVEF <57%) demonstrating greater benefit from sacubitril/valsartan compared with valsartan.[108] These data collectively suggest that HF patients with mildly reduced ejection fraction may benefit from therapies that benefit HFrEF patients, and this concept is reflected in the recent FDA approval for sacubitril/valsartan.

Ongoing Clinical Trials in HFpEF

Several pharmacologic therapies are currently being tested in large outcomes trials in patients with HF and LVEF >40%. SGLT-2 inhibitors have been shown to reduce morbidity and cardiovascular mortality in HFrEF. In the EMPEROR-Preserved trial empagliflozin compared with placebo reduced first heart failure hospitalization or cardiovascular death in patients with HFpEF. These results were driven by reduction in heart failure hospitalization and the benefit declined with increasing ejection fraction.[128] The DELIVER trial (testing data dapagliflozin compared with placebo) will report in early 2022. Recently, two trials demonstrated marked reduction in HF hospitalization in patients with diabetes and recent hospitalization for HF with the SGLT-1/2 inhibitor sotagliflozin, including in patients with LVEF >40%.[129] Because SGLT-2 inhibitors have been shown to have similar overall effects in patients with and without diabetes in HFrEF, these data are encouraging for the role of these agents in HFpEF and HFmrEF. Another large outcomes trial in HFpEF and HFmrEF is testing the nonsteroidal MRA finerenone, which may have potential advantages over steroidal MRAs such as spironolactone. Spironolactone is also currently being tested in two additional large outcomes trials in HFpEF (SPIRRIT and SPIRIT trials) in an effort to validate the findings in TOPCAT-Americas. Numerous additional trials are currently underway in HFpEF, with the hope that novel treatments beyond diuretics and neurohormonal therapies will begin to demonstrate beneficial results in these patients.

REFERENCES

1. Braunwald E. *Heart Disease: A Textbook of Cardiovascular Medicine*. 4th ed. Philadelphia: Saunders; 1992.
2. Dougherty AH, Naccarelli GV, Gray EL, Hicks CH, Goldstein RA. Congestive heart failure with normal systolic function. *Am J Cardiol*. 1984;54(7):778–782.
3. Topol EJ, Traill TA, Fortuin NJ. Hypertensive hypertrophic cardiomyopathy of the elderly. *N Engl J Med*. 1985;312(5):277–283.
4. Soufer R, Wohlgelernter D, Vita NA, et al. Intact systolic left ventricular function in clinical congestive heart failure. *Am J Cardiol*. 1985;55(8):1032–1036.
5. Owan TE, Hodge DO, Herges RM, et al. Trends in prevalence and outcome of heart failure with preserved ejection fraction. *N Engl J Med*. 2006;355(3):251–259.
6. Bhatia RS, Tu JV, Lee DS, et al. Outcome of heart failure with preserved ejection fraction in a population-based study. *N Engl J Med*. 2006;355(3):260–269.
7. Yancy CW, Jessup M, Bozkurt B, et al. 2017 ACC/AHA/HFSA focused update of the 2013 ACCF/AHA guideline for the management of heart failure: a report of the American College of Cardiology/American Heart Association task force on clinical practice guidelines and the Heart Failure Society of America. *Circulation*. 2017;136(6):e137–e161.
8. Yancy CW, Jessup M, Bozkurt B, et al. 2013 ACCF/AHA guideline for the management of heart failure: executive summary: a report of the American College of Cardiology Foundation/American Heart Association Task Force on practice guidelines. *Circulation*. 2013;128(16):1810–1852.
9. Ponikowski P, Voors AA, Anker SD, et al. 2016 ESC Guidelines for the diagnosis and treatment of acute and chronic heart failure: the task force for the diagnosis and treatment of acute and chronic heart failure of the European Society of Cardiology (ESC) developed with the special contribution of the Heart Failure Association (HFA) of the ESC. *Eur Heart J*. 2016;37(27):2129–2200.
10. Nauta JF, Hummel YM, van Melle JP, et al. What have we learned about heart failure with midrange ejection fraction one year after its introduction? *Eur Heart J*. 2017;19(12):1569–1573.
11. Bozkurt B, Coats A, Tsutsui H. Universal definition and classification of heart failure. *J Card Fail*. 2021.
12. Lam CSP, Voors AA, Piotr P, et al. Time to rename the middle child of heart failure: heart failure with mildly reduced ejection fraction. *Eur Heart J*. 2020;41(25):2353–2355.
13. McKee PA, Castelli WP, McNamara PM, Kannel WB. The natural history of congestive heart failure: the Framingham study. *N Engl J Med*. 1971;285(26):1441–1446.
14. Ceia F, Fonseca C, Mota T, et al. Prevalence of chronic heart failure in southwestern Europe: the EPICA study. *Eur J Heart Fail*. 2002;4(4):531–539.

15. Steinberg BA, Zhao X, Heidenreich PA, et al. Trends in patients hospitalized with heart failure and preserved left ventricular ejection fraction: prevalence, therapies, and outcomes. *Circulation.* 2012;126(1):65–75.
16. Oktay AA, Rich JD, Shah SJ. The emerging epidemic of heart failure with preserved ejection fraction. *Curr Heart Fail Rep.* 2013;10(4):401–410.
17. Nochioka K, Shiba N, Kohno H, et al. Both high and low body mass indexes are prognostic risks in Japanese patients with chronic heart failure: implications from the CHART study. *J Card Fail.* 2010;16(11):880–887.
18. Shiba N, Nochioka K, Miura M, et al. Trend of westernization of etiology and clinical characteristics of heart failure patients in Japan: first report from the CHART-2 study. *Circ J.* 2011;75(4):823–833.
19. Dunlay SM, Roger VL. Understanding the epidemic of heart failure: past, present, and future. *Curr Heart Fail Rep.* 2014;11(4):404–415.
20. Ho JE, Enserro D, Brouwers FP, et al. Predicting heart failure with preserved and reduced ejection fraction: the International Collaboration on Heart Failure Subtypes. *Circ Heart Fail.* 2016;9(6). https://doi.org/10.1161/CIRCHEARTFAILURE.115.003116.
21. Dunlay SM, Roger VL, Redfield MM. Epidemiology of heart failure with preserved ejection fraction. *Nat Rev Cardiol.* 2017;14(10):591–602.
22. Gerber Y, Weston SA, Redfield MM, et al. A contemporary appraisal of the heart failure epidemic in Olmsted County, Minnesota, 2000 to 2010. *JAMA Intern Med.* 2015;175(6):996–1004.
23. Ho JE, Lyass A, Lee DS, et al. Predictors of new-onset heart failure: differences in preserved versus reduced ejection fraction. *Circ Heart Fail.* 2013;6(2):279–286.
24. Santhanakrishnan R, Wang N, Larson MG, et al. Atrial fibrillation begets heart failure and vice versa: temporal associations and differences in preserved versus reduced ejection fraction. *Circulation.* 2016;133(5):484–492.
25. Zakeri R, Chamberlain AM, Roger VL, Redfield MM. Temporal relationship and prognostic significance of atrial fibrillation in heart failure patients with preserved ejection fraction: a community-based study. *Circulation.* 2013;128(10):1085–1093.
26. Kotecha D, Lam CS, Van Veldhuisen DJ, et al. Heart failure with preserved ejection fraction and atrial fibrillation: vicious twins. *J Am Coll Cardiol.* 2016;68(20):2217–2228.
27. Lam CS, Rienstra M, Tay WT, et al. Atrial fibrillation in heart failure with preserved ejection fraction: association with exercise capacity, left ventricular filling pressures, natriuretic peptides, and left atrial volume. *JACC Heart Fail.* 2017;5(2):92–98.
28. Kotecha D, Chudasama R, Lane DA, et al. Atrial fibrillation and heart failure due to reduced versus preserved ejection fraction: a systematic review and meta-analysis of death and adverse outcomes. *Int J Cardiol.* 2016;203:660–666.
29. Linssen GC, Rienstra M, Jaarsma T, et al. Clinical and prognostic effects of atrial fibrillation in heart failure patients with reduced and preserved left ventricular ejection fraction. *Eur J Heart Fail.* 2011;13(10):1111–1120.
30. Olsson LG, Swedberg K, Ducharme A, et al. Atrial fibrillation and risk of clinical events in chronic heart failure with and without left ventricular systolic dysfunction: results from the Candesartan in Heart failure-Assessment of Reduction in Mortality and morbidity (CHARM) program. *J Am Coll Cardiol.* 2006;47(10):1997–2004.
31. Meta-analysis Global Group in Chronic Heart Failure (MAGGIC). The survival of patients with heart failure with preserved or reduced left ventricular ejection fraction: an individual patient data meta-analysis. *Eur Heart J.* 2012;33(14):1750–1757.
32. Lam CSP, Gamble GD, Ling LH, et al. Mortality associated with heart failure with preserved vs. reduced ejection fraction in a prospective international multi-ethnic cohort study. *Eur Heart J.* 2018;39(20):1770–1780.
33. Aschauer S, Zotter-Tufaro C, Duca F, et al. Modes of death in patients with heart failure and preserved ejection fraction. *Int J Cardiol.* 2017;228:422–426.
34. Vaduganathan M, Patel RB, Michel A, et al. Mode of death in heart failure with preserved ejection fraction. *J Am Coll Cardiol.* 2017;69(5):556–569.
35. Solomon SD, Anavekar N, Skali H, et al. Influence of ejection fraction on cardiovascular outcomes in a broad spectrum of heart failure patients. *Circulation.* 2005;112(24):3738–3744.
36. Nichols GA, Reynolds K, Kimes TM, et al. Comparison of risk of re-hospitalization, all-cause mortality, and medical care resource utilization in patients with heart failure and preserved versus reduced ejection fraction. *Am J Cardiol.* 2015;116(7):1088–1092.
37. Rogers JK, Pocock SJ, McMurray JJ, et al. Analysing recurrent hospitalizations in heart failure: a review of statistical methodology, with application to CHARM-Preserved. *Eur J Heart Fail.* 2014;16(1):33–40.
38. Carson PE, Anand IS, Win S, et al. The hospitalization burden and post-hospitalization mortality risk in heart failure with preserved ejection fraction: results from the I-PRESERVE trial (Irbesartan in Heart Failure and Preserved Ejection Fraction). *JACC Heart Fail.* 2015;3(6):429–441.
39. Bello NA, Claggett B, Desai AS, et al. Influence of previous heart failure hospitalization on cardiovascular events in patients with reduced and preserved ejection fraction. *Circ Heart Fail.* 2014;7(4):590–595.
40. Vaduganathan M, Claggett BL, Desai AS, et al. Prior heart failure hospitalization, clinical outcomes, and response to sacubitril/valsartan compared with valsartan in HFpEF. *J Am Coll Cardiol.* 2020;75(3):245–254.
41. Lewis EF, Kim HY, Claggett B, et al. Impact of spironolactone on longitudinal changes in health-related quality of life in the treatment of preserved cardiac function heart failure with an aldosterone antagonist trial. *Circ Heart Fail.* 2016;9(3):e001937.
42. Chandra A, Vaduganathan M, Lewis EF, et al. Health-related quality of life in heart failure with preserved ejection fraction: the PARAGON-HF trial. *JACC Heart Fail.* 2019;7(10):862–874.
43. Joseph SM, Novak E, Arnold SV, et al. Comparable performance of the Kansas City Cardiomyopathy Questionnaire in patients with heart failure with preserved and reduced ejection fraction. *Circ Heart Fail.* 2013;6(6):1139–1146.
44. Pokharel Y, Khariton Y, Tang Y, et al. Association of serial Kansas City Cardiomyopathy Questionnaire assessments with death and hospitalization in patients with heart failure with preserved and reduced ejection fraction: a secondary analysis of 2 randomized clinical trials. *JAMA Cardiol.* 2017;2(12):1315–1321.
45. Butler J, Hamo CE, Udelson JE, et al. Exploring new endpoints for patients with heart failure with preserved ejection fraction. *Circ Heart Fail.* 2016;9(11).
46. Anjan VY, Loftus TM, Burke MA, et al. Prevalence, clinical phenotype, and outcomes associated with normal B-type natriuretic peptide levels in heart failure with preserved ejection fraction. *Am J Cardiol.* 2012;110(6):870–876.
47. Obokata M, Reddy YNV, Pislaru SV, et al. Evidence supporting the existence of a distinct obese phenotype of heart failure with preserved ejection fraction. *Circulation.* 2017;136(1):6–19.
48. Reddy YNV, Carter RE, Obokata M, et al. A simple, evidence-based approach to help guide diagnosis of heart failure with preserved ejection fraction. *Circulation.* 2018;138(9):861–870.
49. Pieske B, Tschope C, de Boer RA, et al. How to diagnose heart failure with preserved ejection fraction: the HFA-PEFF diagnostic algorithm: a consensus recommendation from the Heart Failure Association (HFA) of the European Society of Cardiology (ESC). *Eur Heart J.* 2019;40(40):3297–3317.
50. Iwanaga Y, Nishi I, Furuichi S, et al. B-type natriuretic peptide strongly reflects diastolic wall stress in patients with chronic heart failure: comparison between systolic and diastolic heart failure. *J Am Coll Cardiol.* 2006;47(4):742–748.
51. Fudim M, Ambrosy AP, Sun JL, et al. High-sensitivity troponin I in hospitalized and ambulatory patients with heart failure with preserved ejection fraction: insights from the Heart Failure Clinical Research Network. *J Am Heart Assoc.* 2018;7(24):e010364.
52. Obokata M, Reddy YNV, Melenovsky V, et al. Myocardial injury and cardiac reserve in patients with heart failure and preserved ejection fraction. *J Am Coll Cardiol.* 2018;72(1):29–40.
53. Katz DH, Beussink L, Sauer AJ, et al. Prevalence, clinical characteristics, and outcomes associated with eccentric versus concentric left ventricular hypertrophy in heart failure with preserved ejection fraction. *Am J Cardiol.* 2013;112(8):1158–1164.
54. McLaughlin VV, Shah SJ, Souza R, Humbert M. Management of pulmonary arterial hypertension. *J Am Coll Cardiol.* 2015;65(18):1976–1997.
55. Marwick TH, Shah SJ, Thomas JD. Myocardial strain in the assessment of patients with heart failure: a review. *JAMA Cardiol.* 2019;4(3):287–294.
56. Kraigher-Krainer E, Shah AM, Gupta DK, et al. Impaired systolic function by strain imaging in heart failure with preserved ejection fraction. *J Am Coll Cardiol.* 2014;63(5):447–456.
57. Freed BH, Daruwalla V, Cheng JY, et al. Prognostic utility and clinical significance of cardiac mechanics in heart failure with preserved ejection fraction: importance of left atrial strain. *Circ Cardiovasc Imaging.* 2016;9(3).
58. Obokata M, Kane GC, Reddy YN, et al. Role of diastolic stress testing in the evaluation for heart failure with preserved ejection fraction: a simultaneous invasive-echocardiographic study. *Circulation.* 2017;135(9):825–838.
59. Barison A, Aimo A, Todiere G, et al. Cardiovascular magnetic resonance for the diagnosis and management of heart failure with preserved ejection fraction. *Heart Fail Rev.* 2020.
60. Shah SJ, Lam CSP, Svedlund S, et al. Prevalence and correlates of coronary microvascular dysfunction in heart failure with preserved ejection fraction: PROMIS-HFpEF. *Eur Heart J.* 2018;39(37):3439–3450.
61. Reddy YNV, Nishimura RA. Not all secondary mitral regurgitation is the same-potential phenotypes and implications for mitral repair. *JAMA Cardiol.* 2020.
62. Borlaug BA, Nishimura RA, Sorajja P, et al. Exercise hemodynamics enhance diagnosis of early heart failure with preserved ejection fraction. *Circ Heart Fail.* 2010;3(5):588–595.
63. Dryer K, Gajjar M, Narang N, et al. Coronary microvascular dysfunction in patients with heart failure with preserved ejection fraction. *Am J Physiol Heart Circ Physiol.* 2018;314(5):H1033–H1042.
64. Hahn VS, Yanek LR, Vaishnav J, et al. Endomyocardial biopsy characterization of heart failure with preserved ejection fraction and prevalence of cardiac amyloidosis. *JACC Heart Fail.* 2020;8(9):712–724.
65. Houstis NE, Eisman AS, Pappagianopoulos PP, et al. Exercise intolerance in heart failure with preserved ejection fraction: diagnosing and ranking its causes using personalized O_2 pathway analysis. *Circulation.* 2018;137(2):148–161.
66. Reddy YNV, Olson TP, Obokata M, et al. Hemodynamic correlates and diagnostic role of cardiopulmonary exercise testing in heart failure with preserved ejection fraction. *JACC Heart Fail.* 2018;6(8):665–675.
67. Chirinos JA. Deep phenotyping of systemic arterial hemodynamics in HFpEF (Part 2): clinical and therapeutic considerations. *J Cardiovasc Transl Res.* 2017;10(3):261–274.
68. Sanderson JE, Fang F, Lu M, et al. Obstructive sleep apnoea, intermittent hypoxia and heart failure with a preserved ejection fraction. *Heart.* 2021;107(3):190–194.
69. Griffin M, Rao VS, Fleming J, et al. Effect on survival of concurrent hemoconcentration and increase in creatinine during treatment of acute decompensated heart failure. *Am J Cardiol.* 2019;124(11):1707–1711.
70. Kitzman DW, Haykowsky MJ, Tomczak CR. Making the case for skeletal muscle myopathy and its contribution to exercise intolerance in heart failure with preserved ejection fraction. *Circ Heart Fail.* 2017;10(7).
71. Kitzman DW, Nicklas B, Kraus WE, et al. Skeletal muscle abnormalities and exercise intolerance in older patients with heart failure and preserved ejection fraction. *Am J Physiol Heart Circ Physiol.* 2014;306(9):H1364–H1370.
72. VanWagner LB, Wilcox JE, Colangelo LA, et al. Association of nonalcoholic fatty liver disease with subclinical myocardial remodeling and dysfunction: a population-based study. *Hepatology.* 2015;62(3):773–783.
73. Kitzman DW, Shah SJ. The HFpEF obesity phenotype: the elephant in the room. *J Am Coll Cardiol.* 2016;68(2):200–203.
74. Packer M. Epicardial adipose tissue may mediate deleterious effects of obesity and inflammation on the myocardium. *J Am Coll Cardiol.* 2018;71(20):2360–2372.
75. Shah SJ, Borlaug BA, Kitzman DW, et al. Research priorities for heart failure with preserved ejection fraction: National Heart, Lung, and Blood Institute working group summary. *Circulation.* 2020;141(12):1001–1026.
76. Mohammed SF, Hussain S, Mirzoyev SA, et al. Coronary microvascular rarefaction and myocardial fibrosis in heart failure with preserved ejection fraction. *Circulation.* 2015;131(6):550–559.
77. Mishra S, Kass DA. Cellular and molecular pathobiology of heart failure with preserved ejection fraction. *Nat Rev Cardiol.* 2021.
78. Shah SJ, Kitzman DW, Borlaug BA, et al. Phenotype-specific treatment of heart failure with preserved ejection fraction: a multiorgan roadmap. *Circulation.* 2016;134(1):73–90.
79. Paulus WJ, Tschope C. A novel paradigm for heart failure with preserved ejection fraction: comorbidities drive myocardial dysfunction and remodeling through coronary microvascular endothelial inflammation. *J Am Coll Cardiol.* 2013;62(4):263–271.
80. DeBerge M, Shah SJ, Wilsbacher L, Thorp EB. Macrophages in heart failure with reduced versus preserved ejection fraction. *Trends Mol Med.* 2019;25(4):328–340.
81. Cunningham JW, Claggett BL, O'Meara E, et al. Effect of sacubitril/valsartan on biomarkers of extracellular matrix regulation in patients with HFpEF. *J Am Coll Cardiol.* 2020;76(5):503–514.
82. Schiattarella GG, Altamirano F, Tong D, et al. Nitrosative stress drives heart failure with preserved ejection fraction. *Nature.* 2019;568(7752):351–356.
83. Shah SJ. Precision medicine for heart failure with preserved ejection fraction: an overview. *J Cardiovasc Transl Res.* 2017;10(3):233–244.
84. Tromp J, Ferreira JP, Janwanishstaporn S, et al. Heart failure around the world. *Eur J Heart Fail.* 2019;21(10):1187–1196.
85. Phan TT, Shivu GN, Abozguia K, et al. Impaired heart rate recovery and chronotropic incompetence in patients with heart failure with preserved ejection fraction. *Circ Heart Fail.* 2010;3(1):29–34.
86. Wolsk E, Claggett B, Køber L, et al. Contribution of cardiac and extra-cardiac disease burden to risk of cardiovascular outcomes varies by ejection fraction in heart failure. *Eur J Heart Fail.* 2017;20(3):504–510.
87. Solomon SD, Janardhanan R, Verma A, et al. Effect of angiotensin receptor blockade and antihypertensive drugs on diastolic function in patients with hypertension and diastolic dysfunction: a randomised trial. *Lancet.* 2007;369(9579):2079–2087.
88. Beckett NS, Peters R, Fletcher AE, et al. Treatment of hypertension in patients 80 years of age or older. *New Engl J Med.* 2008;358(18):1887–1898.
89. Group SR, Wright Jr JT, Williamson JD, et al. A randomized trial of intensive versus standard blood-pressure control. *N Engl J Med.* 2015;373(22):2103–2116.
90. Selvaraj S, Claggett B, Shah SJ, et al. Systolic blood pressure and cardiovascular outcomes in heart failure with preserved ejection fraction: an analysis of the TOPCAT trial. *Eur J Heart Fail.* 2017;20(3):483–490.
91. Cikes M, Claggett B, Shah AM, et al. Atrial fibrillation in heart failure with preserved ejection fraction. *JACC Heart Failure.* 2018;6(8):689–697.
92. van Veldhuisen DJ, Cohen-Solal A, Böhm M, et al. Beta-blockade with nebivolol in elderly heart failure patients with impaired and preserved left ventricular ejection fraction. *J Am Coll Cardiol.* 2009;53(23):2150–2158.

93. Silverman DN, Plante TB, Infeld M, et al. Association of β-blocker use with heart failure hospitalizations and cardiovascular disease mortality among patients with heart failure with a preserved ejection fraction. *JAMA Network Open*. 2019;2(12):e1916598.
94. Cleland JG, Tendera M, Adamus J, et al. The perindopril in elderly people with chronic heart failure (PEP-CHF) study. *Eur Heart J*. 2006;27(19):2338–2345.
95. Pfeffer MA, Swedberg K, Granger CB, et al. Effects of candesartan on mortality and morbidity in patients with chronic heart failure: the CHARM-Overall programme. *Lancet*. 2003;362(9386):759–766.
96. Massie BM, Carson PE, McMurray JJ, et al. Irbesartan in patients with heart failure and preserved ejection fraction. *New Engl J Med*. 2008;359(23):2456–2467.
97. Suzuki G, Morita H, Mishima T, et al. Effects of long-term monotherapy with eplerenone, a novel aldosterone blocker, on progression of left ventricular dysfunction and remodeling in dogs with heart failure. *Circulation*. 2002;106(23):2967–2972.
98. Bauersachs J, Heck M, Fraccarollo D, et al. Addition of spironolactone to angiotensin-converting enzyme inhibition in heart failure improves endothelial vasomotor dysfunction. *J Am Coll Cardiol*. 2002;39(2):351–358.
99. Desai AS, Lewis EF, Li R, et al. Rationale and design of the treatment of preserved cardiac function heart failure with an aldosterone antagonist trial: a randomized, controlled study of spironolactone in patients with symptomatic heart failure and preserved ejection fraction. *Am Heart J*. 2011;162(6):966–972.e910.
100. Pitt B, Pfeffer MA, Assmann SF, et al. Spironolactone for heart failure with preserved ejection fraction. *New Engl J Med*. 2014;370(15):1383–1392.
101. Pfeffer MA, Claggett B, Assmann SF, et al. Regional variation in patients and outcomes in the Treatment of Preserved Cardiac Function Heart Failure With an Aldosterone Antagonist (TOPCAT) trial. *Circulation*. 2015;131(1):34–42.
102. de Denus S, O'Meara E, Desai AS, et al. Spironolactone metabolites in TOPCAT — new insights into regional variation. *New Engl J Med*. 2017;376(17):1690–1692.
103. Beldhuis IE, Myhre PL, Claggett B, et al. Efficacy and safety of spironolactone in patients with HFpEF and chronic kidney disease. *JACC Heart Failure*. 2019;7(1):25–32.
104. Solomon SD, Claggett B, Lewis EF, et al. Influence of ejection fraction on outcomes and efficacy of spironolactone in patients with heart failure with preserved ejection fraction. *Eur Heart J*. 2016;37(5):455–462.
105. Vardeny O, Miller R, Solomon SD. Combined neprilysin and renin-angiotensin system inhibition for the treatment of heart failure. *JACC Heart Failure*. 2014;2(6):663–670.
106. McMurray JJV, Packer M, Desai AS, et al. Angiotensin–neprilysin inhibition versus enalapril in heart failure. *New Engl J Med*. 2014;371(11):993–1004.
107. Solomon SD, Zile M, Pieske B, et al. The angiotensin receptor neprilysin inhibitor LCZ696 in heart failure with preserved ejection fraction: a phase 2 double-blind randomised controlled trial. *Lancet*. 2012;380(9851):1387–1395.
108. Solomon SD, McMurray JJV, Anand IS, et al. Angiotensin–neprilysin inhibition in heart failure with preserved ejection fraction. *New Engl J Med*. 2019;381(17):1609–1620.
109. Solomon SD, Vaduganathan M, Claggett B L, et al. Sacubitril/valsartan across the spectrum of ejection fraction in heart failure. *Circulation*. 2020;141(5):352–361.
110. Abraham WT, Adamson PB, Bourge RC, et al. Wireless pulmonary artery haemodynamic monitoring in chronic heart failure: a randomised controlled trial. *Lancet*. 2011;377(9766):658–666.
111. Hasenfuß G, Hayward C, Burkhoff D, et al. A transcatheter intracardiac shunt device for heart failure with preserved ejection fraction (REDUCE LAP-HF): a multicentre, open-label, single-arm, phase 1 trial. *Lancet*. 2016;387(10025):1298–1304.
112. Feldman T, Mauri L, Kahwash R, et al. Transcatheter interatrial shunt device for the treatment of heart failure with preserved ejection fraction (REDUCE LAP-HF I [Reduce Elevated Left Atrial Pressure in Patients with Heart Failure]): a phase 2, randomized, sham-controlled trial. *Circulation*. 2018;137(4):364–375.
113. Santos ABS, Kraigher-Krainer E, Bello N, et al. Left ventricular dyssynchrony in patients with heart failure and preserved ejection fraction. *Eur Heart J*. 2013;35(1):42–47.
114. Pandey A, Parashar A, Kumbhani DJ, et al. Exercise training in patients with heart failure and preserved ejection fraction. *Circ Heart Fail*. 2015;8(1):33–40.
115. Dhakal BP, Malhotra R, Murphy RM, et al. Mechanisms of exercise intolerance in heart failure with preserved ejection fraction. *Circ Heart Fail*. 2015;8(2):286–294.
116. Pandey A, Khera R, Park B, et al. Relative impairments in hemodynamic exercise reserve parameters in heart failure with preserved ejection fraction. *JACC Heart Fail*. 2018;6(2):117–126.
117. Fleg JL, Cooper LS, Borlaug BA, et al. Exercise training as therapy for heart failure. *Circ Heart Fail*. 2015;8(1):209–220.
118. Kitzman DW, Brubaker P, Morgan T, et al. Effect of caloric restriction or aerobic exercise training on peak oxygen consumption and quality of life in obese older patients with heart failure with preserved ejection fraction. *J Am Med Assoc*. 2016;315(1):36.
119. Mueller S, Winzer EB, Duvinage A, et al. Effect of high-intensity interval training, moderate continuous training, or guideline-based physical activity advice on peak oxygen consumption in patients with heart failure with preserved ejection fraction: a randomized clinical trial. *J Am Med Assoc*. 2021;325(6):542–551.
120. Hoendermis ES, Liu LCY, Hummel YM, et al. Effects of sildenafil on invasive haemodynamics and exercise capacity in heart failure patients with preserved ejection fraction and pulmonary hypertension: a randomized controlled trial. *Eur Heart J*. 2015;36(38):2565–2573.
121. Redfield MM, Chen HH, Borlaug BA, et al. Effect of phosphodiesterase-5 inhibition on exercise capacity and clinical status in heart failure with preserved ejection fraction. *J Am Med Assoc*. 2013;309(12):1268.
122. Armstrong PW, Lam CSP, Anstrom KJ, et al. Effect of vericiguat vs placebo on quality of life in patients with heart failure and preserved ejection fraction. *J Am Med Assoc*. 2020;324(15):1512.
123. Pieske B, Maggioni AP, Lam CSP, et al. Vericiguat in patients with worsening chronic heart failure and preserved ejection fraction: results of the SOluble guanylate Cyclase stimulatoR in heArT failurE patientS with PRESERVED EF (SOCRATES-PRESERVED) study. *Eur Heart J*. 2017;38(15):1119–1127.
124. Redfield MM, Anstrom KJ, Levine JA, et al. Isosorbide mononitrate in heart failure with preserved ejection fraction. *New Engl J Med*. 2015;373(24):2314–2324.
125. Borlaug BA, Anstrom KJ, Lewis GD, et al. Effect of inorganic nitrite vs placebo on exercise capacity among patients with heart failure with preserved ejection fraction. *J Am Med Assoc*. 2018;320(17):1764.
126. Komajda M, Isnard R, Cohen-Solal A, et al. Effect of ivabradine in patients with heart failure with preserved ejection fraction: the EDIFY randomized placebo-controlled trial. *Eur J Heart Fail*. 2017;19(11):1495–1503.
127. Dewan P, Jackson A, Lam CSP, et al. Interactions between left ventricular ejection fraction, sex and effect of neurohumoral modulators in heart failure. *Eur J Heart Fail*. 2020;22(5):898–901.
128. Anker SD, Butler J, Filippatos G, et al; EMPEROR-Preserved Trial Investigators. Empagliflozin in heart failure with a preserved ejection fraction. *N Engl J Med*. Aug 27, 2021. https://doi.org/10.1056/NEJMoa2107038.
129. Bhatt DL, Szarek M, Steg PG, et al. Sotagliflozin in patients with diabetes and recent worsening heart failure. *N Engl J Med*. 2021;384(2):117–128.

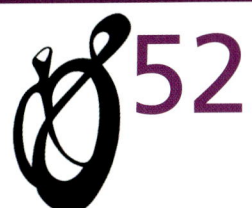

52. The Dilated, Restrictive, and Infiltrative Cardiomyopathies

RAY E. HERSHBERGER

THE DILATED CARDIOMYOPATHIES, 1032
Genetics of Dilated Cardiomyopathy, 1035
Genetics of Familial Dilated Cardiomyopathy, 1035
Approach to Clinical Genetic Evaluation, 1037
Therapy for Dilated Cardiomyopathy, 1039
Arrhythmogenic Right Ventricular Cardiomyopathy, 1039
Alcoholic and Diabetic Cardiomyopathies, 1041
Left Ventricular Noncompaction, 1041

Tachycardia-Induced Cardiomyopathy, 1041
Peripartum Cardiomyopathy, 1042
Takotsubo Cardiomyopathy, 1042

RESTRICTIVE AND INFILTRATIVE CARDIOMYOPATHIES, 1043
Approach to Identifying a Cause of Restrictive Cardiomyopathy, 1043
Sarcoid Cardiomyopathy, 1044
Fabry Disease, 1046

Gaucher Disease and Glycogen Storage Diseases, 1047
Hemochromatosis, 1048
Endomyocardial Disease, 1048
Carcinoid Heart Disease, 1048
Löffler (Eosinophilic) Endocarditis, 1049
Endomyocardial Fibrosis, 1049

FUTURE PERSPECTIVES, 1049

REFERENCES, 1049

There remains no satisfying universal definition of cardiomyopathy. Even though it is now agreed that myocardial disease secondary to atherosclerotic coronary artery disease (CAD), valvular disease, congenital heart disease, and systemic hypertension should not be classified as a cardiomyopathy, opinion differs as to whether the condition should be defined on the basis of morphology and whether molecular disturbances such as the channelopathies should be included. An American Heart Association definition[1] described cardiomyopathies as "a heterogeneous group of diseases of the myocardium associated with mechanical and/or electrical dysfunction that usually (but not invariably) exhibit inappropriate ventricular hypertrophy or dilation and are due to a variety of causes and frequently are genetic. Cardiomyopathies either are confined to the heart or are part of a generalized systemic disorder often leading to cardiovascular death or progressive heart failure–related disability." This classification included patients with predominantly electrical dysfunction of the heart, a group not included in a European Working Group definition.[2] Both U.S. and European experts, however, have recognized the growing importance of genetics in patients with cardiomyopathy since these position papers were released.

The ability to combine genetic information with phenotypic information regarding both left ventricular (LV) and right ventricular (RV) structure and function forms the basis of cardiovascular genetic medicine (Fig. 52.1). Clinical genetic testing enhances the care of patients who present with symptoms as well as family members of these patients through proper cascade risk assessment. Despite the expansion of ClinVar, a publicly accessible database of clinically relevant variants, the field still lacks a comprehensive variant- coupled with phenotype-specific database. Nevertheless, as genomic information proliferates, coupled with useful and accurate phenotype information in large, publicly accessible databases, such information will both help predict the natural history and guide therapy.

Clinical genetic testing made feasible by next-generation sequencing over the past decade has rapidly expanded with many commercially available options that are commonly supported by US insurers with appropriate documentation and pre-test genetic counseling. Although this brings opportunities to define a cardiomyopathy by assigning a specific genetic etiology, it also brings new challenges: knowing which tests to order, how to conduct pretest counseling and obtain consent, and how to interpret genetic test results. Table 52.1[3-5] presents an overview of the classification of cardiomyopathies based on key phenotype information. Phenotype information includes key cardiac morphology, physiology, and cellular and molecular pathology data, supported by details of the patient's environment relevant to the specific disease in question.[6]

Despite rapid expansion of genetic knowledge, clinical, or phenotype, information continues to drive the interpretation of genetic information.[4,5] This can be expressed as a phenotype-first (vs. genotype-first) approach to genetic medicine. In short, for the cardiomyopathies, we still rely on phenotype information to identify an individual with a clinical abnormality that fits into one of the conventional categories (dilated cardiomyopathy [DCM], arrhythmogenic right ventricular cardiomyopathy [ARVC], hypertrophic cardiomyopathy [HCM], restrictive cardiomyopathy [RCM]), and we then interpret specific variants in genes having been curated for their relevance by phenotype. It is abundantly clear that nearly all that we think we understand about cardiomyopathy genetics has been gained from a phenotype-first approach. This will remain in the mainstream for the foreseeable future, because when a genotype-first approach is used, we observe differences, sometimes quite dramatic, in variants considered to be highly likely to be pathogenic in individuals who have no evidence of the phenotype of interest, as has recently been shown in a remarkably reduced estimated penetrance of truncating variants in ARVC genes.[7] Thus, phenotype assessment still relies on the most complete and comprehensive information regarding LV and RV chamber size and function, at times also informed by the presence and character of conduction system disease and arrhythmias, as well as cellular and subcellular function. Numerous genes have had rare variants reported in association with one or more of the genetic cardiomyopathies (Fig. 52.2). This observation itself argues that a phenotype-first approach will need to continue until greater mechanistic insights are available to explain how variants in the same gene, perhaps influenced by an individual's specific genetic, epigenetic, or environmental background, or from alternative disease models (e.g., an oligemic model[8]), cause divergent phenotypes.

The enormous progress made to understand the genetic basis of cardiomyopathy has only led to new questions yet to be addressed. Perhaps most important is that of environmental influence on a genetic background predisposing to cardiomyopathy. Hypertension has been postulated as the most prevalent environmental aspect to hasten the emergence of cardiomyopathy. But it is now also clear that given an appropriate genetic background, established myocardial toxins such as alcohol[9] or drugs used to treat cancer[10] can facilitate the development of DCM. The interplay of genetics with environment to influence disease onset and presentation remains as a major incompletely understood aspect of cardiomyopathy.

Moreover, the prevailing and prototypical genetic paradigm has been mendelian for the cardiomyopathies, that is, where one highly penetrant variant in a well-established gene explains the specific cardiomyopathy phenotype in all affected members of a multi-generational pedigree. This view, rightfully so, has been based on the

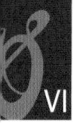

FIGURE 52.1 Interaction of genome and phenome. The *arrow* depicts the bimodal interaction between genes and the environment, or the genome and phenome. The goal of human genetic studies has always been to understand genomic variation and its impact on phenotypes, and vice versa. Our ultimate understandings are limited by the depth and integrity of data of both types, and then how well each data type is integrated and leveraged with the other for the greatest insight into health and disease.

very large pedigrees that provided the basis to find the first genes that underlie the cardiomyopathies. While this continues to be the nearly universal paradigm for HCM and the long QT syndrome, a growing body of data, still preliminary, suggests that ARVC and DCM have genetic complexity beyond mendelian in a substantial number of probands and families.[8,11,12]

Finally, although this chapter focuses primarily on nonsyndromic cardiomyopathies, there are multiple syndromes in which a cardiomyopathy develops in concert with multiorgan system involvement. HCM (see Chapter 54) is also mentioned briefly herein because of its significant genetic overlap with DCM (see Fig. 52.2), as is amyloid cardiomyopathy (see Chapter 53) due to its phenotypic presentation as a RCM.

THE DILATED CARDIOMYOPATHIES

DCM is characterized by an enlarged left ventricle with systolic dysfunction that is not caused by ischemic or valvular heart disease. At the outset the DCM nomenclature can be confusing because the DCM term can be applied regardless of etiology, that is, ischemic, valvular, or other causes based only on LV enlargement and reduced function. Thus, a clear grasp of this nomenclature is foundational to navigating the clinical and genetic literature around DCM.[13] Due to the prevalence of ischemic cardiomyopathy, the most common clinical and clinical research approach is to sort DCM into ischemic or nonischemic categories. However, the latter category, having systolic dysfunction and LV enlargement, can include virtually any etiology (except ischemic), including genetic cause. In this category resides those patients diagnosed with "idiopathic" DCM, where other clinically identifiable causes have been excluded. When multiple individuals are identified in a family meeting idiopathic DCM criteria, such families are assigned a *familial* DCM diagnosis.[13] These DCM families provided the initial substrate for the discovery of the first DCM genes. For clinical practice, though, most DCM rigorously classified as idiopathic presents as sporadic, not familial, DCM, even after the clinical screening of first-degree family members. The question, not yet resolved, remains as to whether nonfamilial DCM results principally from underlying rare variant genetic cause. A nearly completed NIH study[12,14] may provide clarity to this fundamental question. A related question applicable to all of the cardiomyopathies is whether cause stems largely from one single highly penetrant rare variant, or is the amalgamation of genetics, both rare, with a possibly substantial oligogenic overlay for some conditions, and common, along with possible epigenetic and environmental impacts.

When investigating a patient with DCM, a full history, including risk factors for CAD, should be acquired.[13] Unless the patient is questioned in detail, the duration of symptoms may be significantly underestimated. Angina may occur, even in the absence of epicardial coronary disease, but symptoms suggestive of angina should raise the possibility of CAD. Patients should be questioned carefully about alcohol consumption (see Chapter 84), both present and past. If a spouse is available, that person's input may be of great value because underreporting of heavy alcohol intake is common. A history to elicit exposure to cardiotoxic drugs, such as anthracyclines or others commonly given for cancer treatment, is also important, although the clinician should be aware that other much less commonly used drugs such as chloroquine or hydroxychloroquine can also underlie cardiomyopathy. Other well-established myocardial toxins, even if rare, such as heavy metal exposure from ingestion or inhalation, should also be ruled out. Finally, a history directed to finding subtle signs of neuromuscular disease is always indicated, as key proteins of several genes causing cardiomyopathy are also expressed in skeletal muscle.[13]

A family history is essential for all patients with any type of cardiomyopathy. Known diagnoses of cardiomyopathy should be elicited in all first-, second-, and third-degree relatives, as well as any family members who have had history of heart failure or sudden cardiac death. Relevant procedures include family members who have had coronary bypass operations, which implies ischemic etiology. If possible to exclude ischemic etiology, a family history of devices such as pacemakers, implantable cardioverter-defibrillators (ICDs), or ventricular assist devices, or a history of heart transplant, should raise concern for shared genetic risk between family members. Patients will commonly have little medically informed family history information available unless prompted to obtain this either before or following the initial medical interview. Notably, symptoms suggestive of heart failure but also of sudden cardiac death are commonly conflated and reported as the relevant family member having had a "heart attack." Relevant medical records can be invaluable, especially of such close relatives who have recently died of cardiovascular cause.

Findings on clinical examination may reflect the biventricular dysfunction that may present in DCM (see Chapters 13 and 48), although DCM also commonly presents with predominant LV involvement. Electrocardiography frequently reveals LV hypertrophy, nonspecific ST-T wave changes, or bundle branch block (see Chapter 48). Conduction system disease has specific gene associations (e.g., *LMNA* cardiomyopathy). Pathologic Q waves may be present, although their presence should also raise the possibility of advanced atherosclerotic heart disease. In advanced cases with extensive fibrosis, low-voltage limb leads may be seen.

Echocardiography (see also Chapter 16) reveals LV systolic dysfunction (Fig. 52.3) that may also show biventricular dysfunction in at least one third of cases,[15] all of which can range from mild to severe. LV wall thickness is almost always within the normal range, but the LV mass is invariably increased. Most commonly, global LV hypokinesis is present, but regional wall motion abnormalities may also be seen, particularly septal dyskinesis in those with left bundle branch block. Disproportionate thinning of a dyskinetic wall should raise the possibility of CAD rather than primary cardiomyopathy. Mitral and tricuspid regurgitation is frequently present and may be severe, even when the clinical examination does not reveal a loud murmur. Other than impaired leaflet coaptation, the mitral and tricuspid valves appear to be structurally normal, and valvular structural abnormalities suggest primary valvular disease rather than cardiomyopathy. Diastolic function in DCM ranges from normal to restrictive (see also Chapter 51). A restrictive pattern is most commonly seen in patients with volume overload in "decompensated" heart failure and often improves with initiation of diuretic or vasodilator therapy.

Coronary angiography (see Chapter 21) should be considered in all patients who have risk factors for CAD, most importantly cigarette smoking or a prominent family history of early-onset CAD observed in familial hypercholesterolemia, or in those who are of an age where CAD is commonly observed regardless of added risk factors, conventionally above 40 years in males and above 45 years in females. Alternatively, computed tomography (CT) coronary angiography (see Chapter 20) may be used, although it does not allow hemodynamic study, which may be useful in some patients. Because CAD is common, the functional significance of any obstructive coronary lesions found should be carefully evaluated insofar as their presence may be coincidental to DCM.

Cardiac magnetic resonance imaging (CMR) (see also Chapter 19) has become foundational for the evaluation of a patient who presents with a recently diagnosed cardiomyopathy. A pattern of nontransmural delayed gadolinium enhancement in a noncoronary distribution in a dilated left ventricle suggests a nonischemic cause. Certain conditions, such as sarcoidosis, may have a rather typical appearance. CMR is able to evaluate the extent of myocardial fibrosis in DCM and may provide information complementary to that obtained with cardiac biopsy. Unless a specific condition is suspected, cardiac biopsy is often unrewarding in the evaluation of DCM, but it may occasionally provide an

TABLE 52.1 Classification of the Cardiomyopathies by Phenome and Genome

TYPE	PHENOME				GENOME	
	MORPHOLOGY	PHYSIOLOGY	PATHOLOGY	SYSTEMIC CONDITIONS, CLINICAL FEATURES, RISK FACTORS	NONSYNDROMIC, USUALLY SINGLE GENE	SYNDROMIC
Dilated (DCM)	Dilation of LV and RV with minimal or no wall thickening	Reduced contractility is the primary defect; variable degree of diastolic dysfunction	Myocyte hypertrophy; scattered fibrosis	Hypertension; alcohol; thyrotoxicosis, myxedema; persistent tachycardia; toxins (e.g., chemotherapy, especially anthracyclines); radiation	Diverse gene ontology (see Fig. 52.2, Fig. 52.6) with >30 genes implicated	Diverse array of associated conditions, especially muscular dystrophies: Emery-Dreifuss muscular dystrophy, limb-girdle muscular dystrophy, Duchenne/Becker muscular dystrophy; Laing distal myopathy; Barth syndrome; Kearns-Sayre syndrome; others[3-5]
Restrictive (RCM)	Usually normal chamber sizes; minimal to moderate wall thickening	Contractility normal or near-normal with a marked increase in end-diastolic filling pressure	Specific to type, diagnosis: amyloid, iron, glycogen storage disease, others	Endomyocardial fibrosis, amyloid, sarcoid, scleroderma, Churg-Strauss syndrome, cystinosis, lymphoma, pseudoxanthoma elasticum, hypereosinophilic syndrome, carcinoid	If not associated with systemic genetic disease, genetic cause usually from sarcomeric gene rare variants	Gaucher disease, hemochromatosis, Fabry disease, familial amyloidosis; mucopolysaccharidoses; Noonan syndrome
Hypertrophic (HCM)	Usually normal or reduced internal chamber dimension; wall thickening pronounced, especially septal hypertrophy	Systolic function increased or normal	Myocyte hypertrophy, classically with disarray	Severe hypertension can confound clinical, morphologic diagnosis	Rare variants of genes encoding sarcomeric proteins (see Chapter 54)	Noonan syndrome, LEOPARD syndrome, Danon syndrome, Fabry disease, Wolff-Parkinson-White syndrome, Friedreich ataxia, MERRF, MELAS (see Chapter 100)
Arrhythmogenic right ventricular cardiomyopathy (ARVC)	Scattered fibrofatty infiltration, classically of RV but also of LV; dilation of RV or LV, or both, is common but not universal	Ventricular arrhythmias (VT, VF) early or late, reduced contractility with progressive disease; can mimic DCM	Islands of fatty replacement; fibrosis	Palmoplantar keratoderma, wooly hair in Naxos syndrome	Rare variants of genes encoding proteins of desmosome (see Fig. 52.2; Fig. 52.6)	Naxos syndrome
Inflammatory	Normal or dilated without hypertrophy	Reduced systolic function	Inflammatory infiltrates	Hypereosinophilic syndrome (see text), acute myocarditis (see Chapter 55)		
Ischemic	Normal or dilated without hypertrophy	Reduced systolic function	Areas of infarcted myocardium	Hypercholesterolemia, hypertension, diabetes, cigarette smoking, family history	Familial hypercholesterolemia; other heritable lipid disorders	Familial hypercholesterolemia
Infectious	Normal or dilated without hypertrophy	Reduced systolic function	Specific to infection	Viral (especially acute myocarditis); protozoal (e.g., Chagas disease); bacterial, direct infection (e.g., Lyme disease) or from acute cellular toxicity as result of systemic toxins (e.g., Streptococcus, gram-negative, others) (see Chapter 55)	Genetic predisposition to infection and/or variable response to infective agent	

LV, Left ventricle; MELAS, mitochondrial encephalopathy, lactic acidosis, and strokelike symptoms; MERRF, myoclonic epilepsy associated with ragged-red fibers; RV, right ventricle; VF, ventricular fibrillation; VT, ventricular tachycardia.

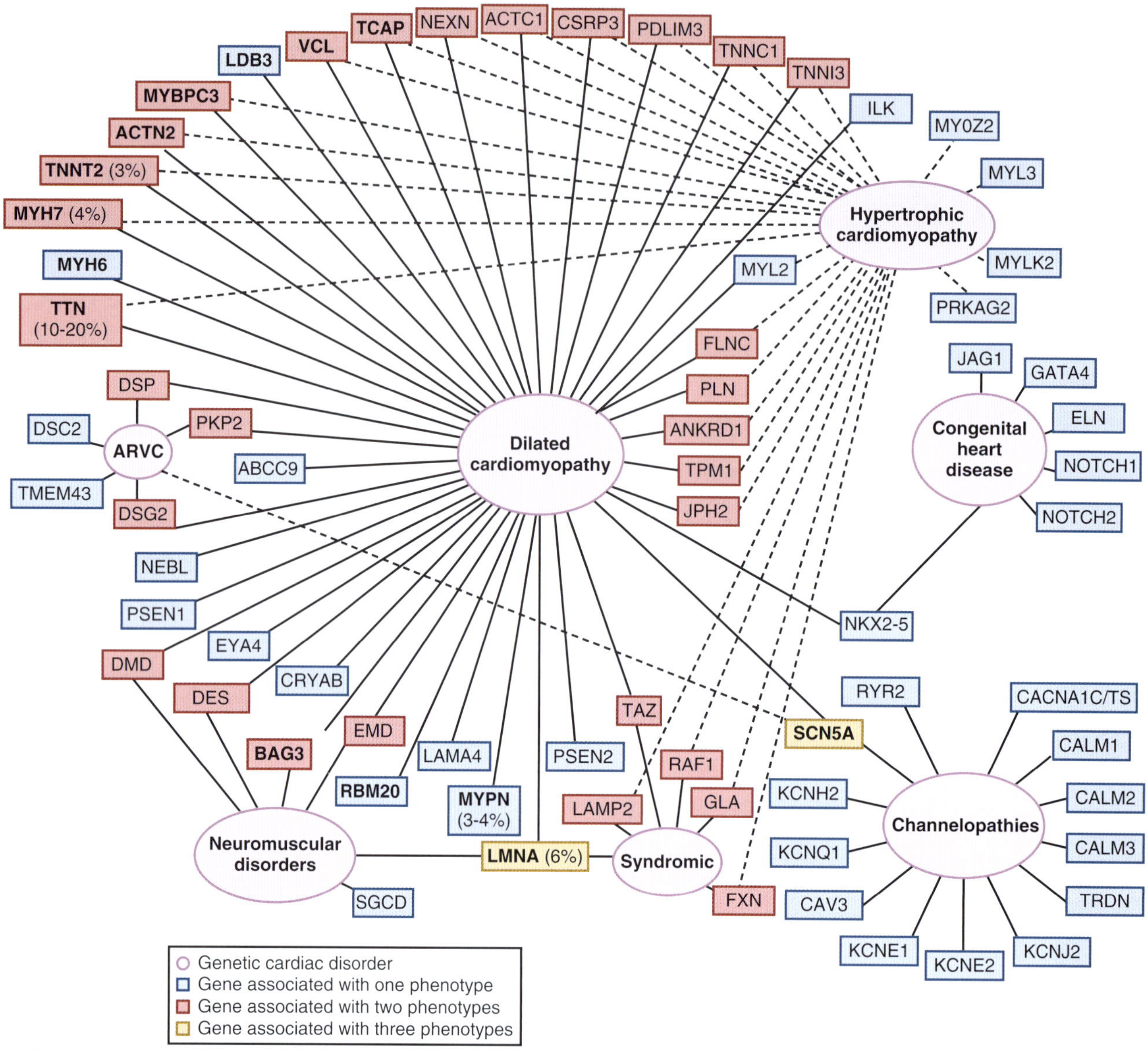

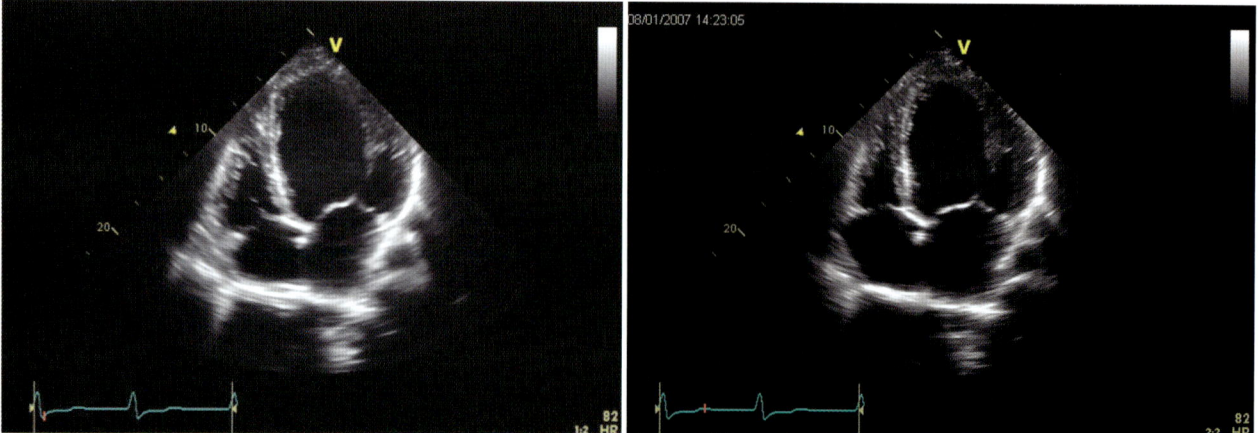

FIGURE 52.2 Relationships of genes implicated in causing cardiovascular and related phenotypes. The gene relationships for several cardiovascular phenotypes are shown, with the principal focus on dilated cardiomyopathy (DCM) genetics. Common cardiac phenotypes are shown in the *purple ovals*, and lines connect each phenotype to the gene or genes (shown in a box) of which rare variants have been implicated in causing the phenotype. The gene boxes are color-coded according to the number of phenotypes with which they are associated: *blue* indicates one phenotype, *red* indicates two phenotypes, and *yellow* indicates three phenotypes (as shown in the lower left corner of the figure). For a gene causing 3% or more of familial DCM cases, the frequency is included with its name. Hypertrophic cardiomyopathy (HCM) gene associations are indicated by *dotted lines*. Well-established HCM genes include two sarcomere genes (*MYH7* and *MYBPC3*) that together account for 80% of HCM cases for which a genetic cause can be identified. Three other sarcomere genes (*TNNT2*, *TNNI3*, and *TPM1*) account for an additional 15% of such cases. The other numerous genes implicated have caused only one or a few reported cases. The evidence in support of rare variants in the genes shown and their relevance for the specified cardiomyopathy varies considerably.

FIGURE 52.3 Echocardiogram in a patient with dilated cardiomyopathy. The end-diastolic frame (**left**) and end-systolic frame (**right**) in a 40-year-old man with severe dilated cardiomyopathy (DCM; ejection fraction <20%) are shown. Note the globular left ventricular (LV) shape, typical of advanced DCM. Despite the severe reduction in LV ejection fraction, he had only mild symptoms, attributable, in part, to preservation of stroke volume because of the marked increase in LV end-diastolic volume.

unexpected diagnosis. Multimodality imaging has become the norm for most cases of DCM.[16]

Once a diagnosis has been established in a patient meeting rigorous clinical criteria for idiopathic DCM, a full genetic evaluation should be initiated.

Genetics of Dilated Cardiomyopathy

In a significant proportion of patients with DCM, no obvious cause can be found even with a comprehensive clinical evaluation; these patients are assigned a diagnosis of *idiopathic DCM*. Family-based studies from the 1990s have shown that if clinical screening with an electrocardiogram (ECG) and/or echocardiogram is conducted in the first-degree family members of patients with DCM, evidence of DCM will be found in 10% to 20% or more,[17] thereby establishing a diagnosis of *familial DCM*. Familial DCM is now known to have a genetic basis of diverse ontology (see Fig. 52.2).[11] Despite the discovery of many genes, plausible genetic cause can only be identified in 25% to 30% of familial cases, with lower sensitivity in sporadic cases of DCM, as more stringent analytical approaches have become the norm.[12] In the largest series to date of 1040 individuals with DCM, with presumed mostly sporadic disease and assuming a mendelian paradigm, sensitivity of testing was approximately 15% when the enrichment of rare variants was assessed compared to population controls.[18] Truncating variants in the giant scaffolding protein titin (*TTN*) have been shown to be the most common, associated with 10% to 20% of cases of DCM depending upon cohort studied (Fig. 52.4).[18–20] Penetrance issues are also highly relevant for *TTN*, also illustrated by genetics-first approaches, with evidence suggesting a marked reduction in penetrance in individuals of African ancestry compared to European ancestry.[21] The proportion of rare variants thought to be causative of DCM attributed to any specific gene is much smaller, usually ranging from less than 1% to 3%. Even though familial DCM is now considered to have a genetic basis due to the observed heritability, the issue of whether sporadic DCM (that is, where no evidence of familial DCM is apparent after clinical screening of relatives) has a genetic basis has not been resolved. While some sporadic cases will show pathogenic or likely pathogenic variants, many will only harbor a rare variant of unknown significance or no variants in any known DCM genes.[12]

Patients with DCM typically have an asymptomatic phase for many years before symptomatic heart failure, an arrhythmia, or an embolic event develops later in the course of the disease (Fig. 52.5).[22] Occasionally, asymptomatic but clinically detectable DCM is discovered serendipitously during routine or preprocedural medical screening, usually prompted by subtle abnormalities on an ECG that prompt an echocardiogram. The time span needed for clinical disease to develop illustrates the remarkable ability of the myocardium to maintain normal—or close to normal—cardiac output and filling pressure for years despite clinically detectable asymptomatic DCM. This principle underlies the observation that the family history is much less sensitive than clinical screening by echocardiography in detecting DCM among family members of an individual with a new diagnosis of idiopathic DCM. This also emphasizes the necessity of clinical screening of all first-degree family members when a new diagnosis of any cardiomyopathy has been made.

Genetics of Familial Dilated Cardiomyopathy

The genes shown to cause familial DCM are classified by subcellular location (gene ontology). As shown in Figure 52.2, most of the implicated genes encode sarcomere, Z-disc, or cytoskeleton proteins. The broad representation of other genes encoding a wide variety of proteins demonstrates the diverse pathways that can lead to a final phenotype of DCM.[11] Presumably, other yet unknown pathways may also be relevant in the pathogenesis of DCM. More than 30 genes have been identified to cause DCM (referred to as locus heterogeneity) of diverse subcellular localization (Fig. 52.6). The diverse subcellular locations of genes implicated in DCM differentiate this form of cardiomyopathy from HCM (see also Chapter 54) and ARVC, which are caused by variants in genes encoding sarcomeric or desmosomal proteins, respectively (see Fig. 52.2). In addition to locus heterogeneity, the molecular genetics of DCM is also characterized by

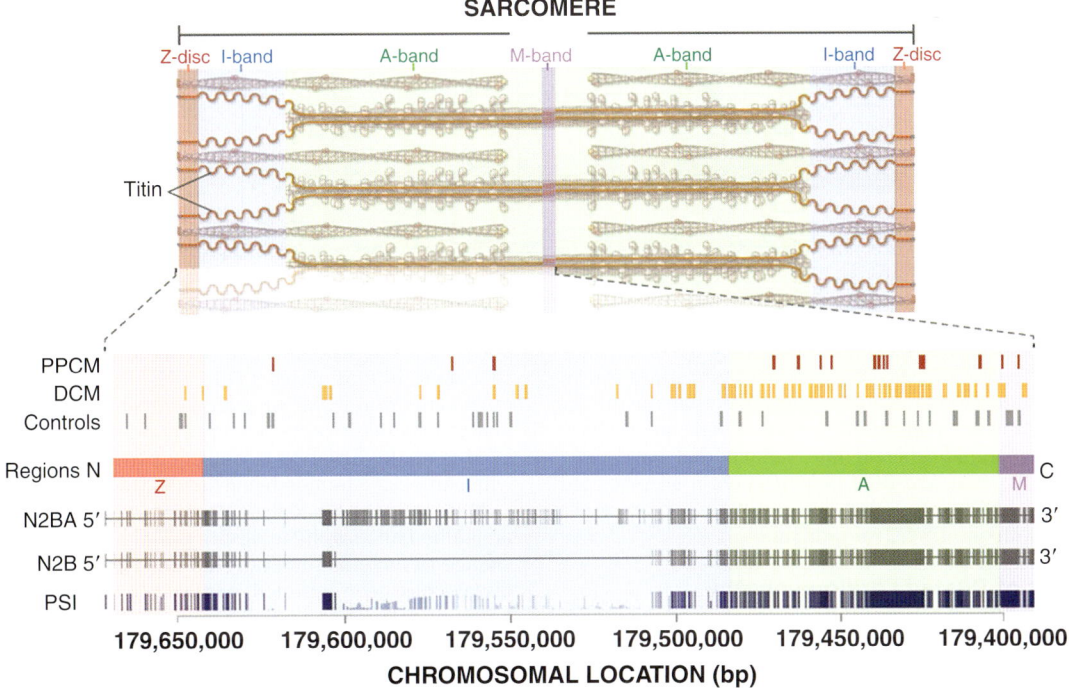

FIGURE 52.4 The giant protein titin and its involvement in dilated cardiomyopathy (DCM). Titin, the largest protein in the body, which is made up of more than 35,000 amino acids, is encoded by *TTN*, which acts as a scaffolding protein for sarcomere assembly. The large size of *TTN* made investigation extremely challenging prior to the development of next-generation sequencing strategies. Recent work has implicated truncating variants of *TTN* in 15% to 25% of familial DCM patients and 10% to 15% of nonfamilial DCM patients. Truncating variants include nonsense, frameshift, splice site, or other variants that cause the protein to be truncated. The upper part of the diagram shows the protein structure, with sarcomeric regions labeled (Z-disc and I, A, and M bands). The lower portion shows the locations of truncating variants in peripartum cardiomyopathy (PPCM), DCM, or controls. The exons of the primary two cardiovascular transcripts expressed (N2BA, N2B) are shown, along with their proportions spliced in (PSI). (From Ware JS, Li J, Mazaika E, et al. Shared genetic predisposition in peripartum and dilated cardiomyopathies. *N Engl J Med*. 2016;374:233–241.)

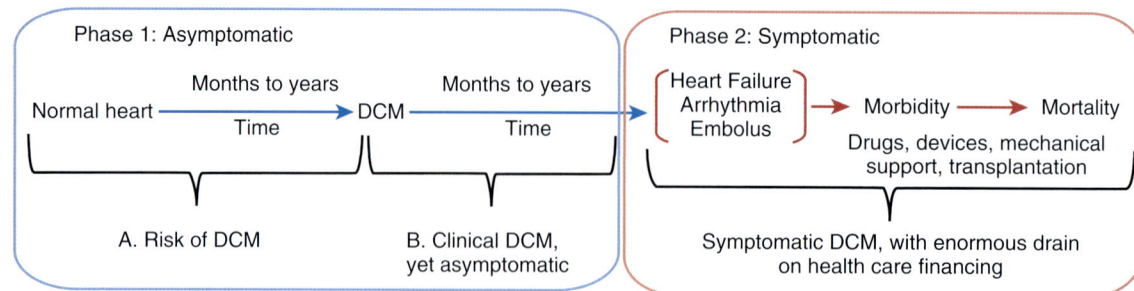

FIGURE 52.5 Asymptomatic and symptomatic phases of dilated cardiomyopathy (DCM). Phase 1 includes two periods, both asymptomatic. In the first period (1A), individuals who harbor one or more rare DCM variants have a risk of developing DCM over time. During this phase, genetic information identifies the individuals who would benefit from periodic clinical screening to detect early clinical disease. In phase 1B, DCM is present but asymptomatic, at times for years, and may evade detection unless periodic clinical cardiovascular imaging efforts detect it. Once disease has been detected, medical therapy can be initiated in an effort to prevent progression to phase 2. In phase 2, disease becomes late-stage and symptomatic with heart failure, arrhythmia, or embolus, the presenting features of DCM. (From Morales A, Hershberger RE. The rationale and timing of molecular genetic testing for dilated cardiomyopathy. *Can J Cardiol*. 2015;31:1309–1312.)

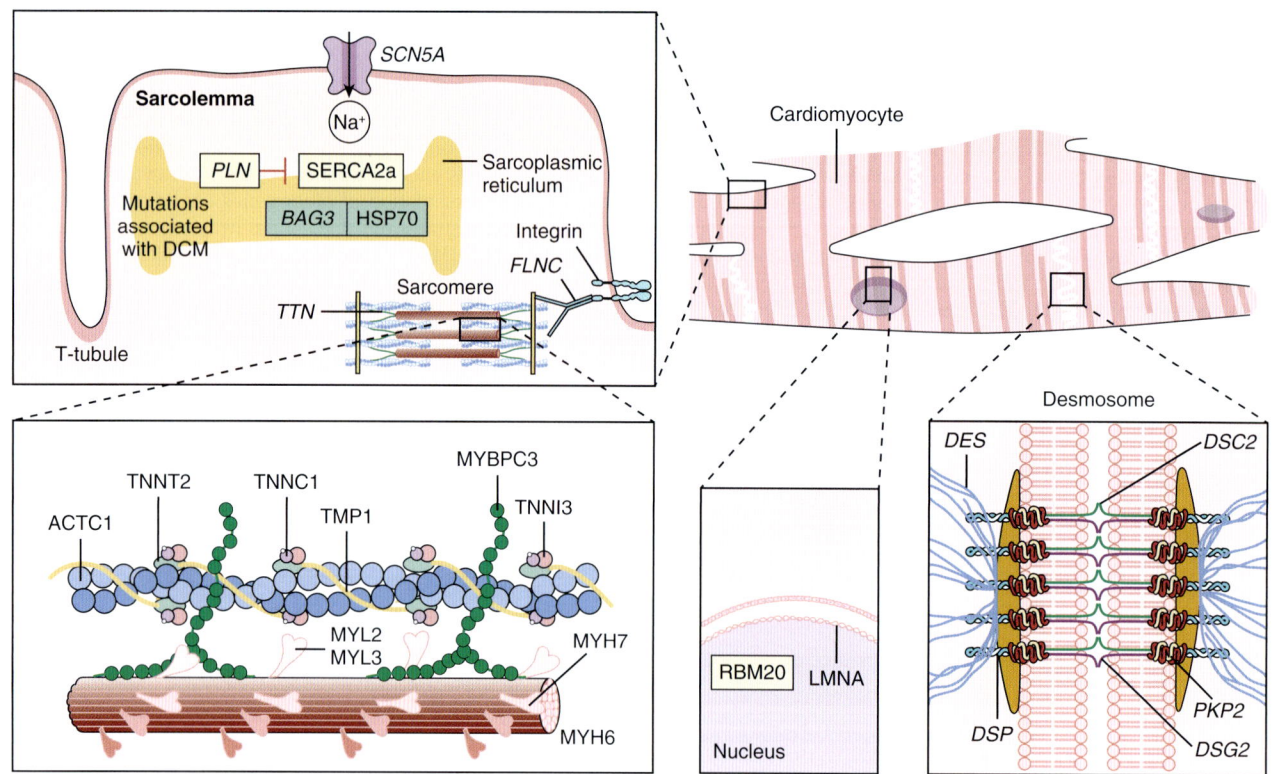

FIGURE 52.6 Subcellular localization of key cardiomyopathy proteins (see text for abbreviations). (Adapted from Schultheiss H-P, Fairweather D, Caforio ALP, et al. Dilated cardiomyopathy. *Nat Rev Dis Primers*. 2019;5:32. https://doi.org/10.1038/s41572-019-0084-1.)

allelic heterogeneity; that is, rare variants commonly occur at many locations in a DCM gene, and many rare variant sites in genes shown to cause both DCM and HCM are specific to that cardiomyopathy. So-called overlap phenotypes particularly for sarcomeric genes have occasionally been reported, wherein rare variants that have been shown to cause DCM, HCM, and RCM may be seen in an extended pedigree. One family has been reported showing all three phenotypes (HCM, RCM, DCM) with one *TNNT2* rare variant.[23]

Clinical Genetics of Dilated Cardiomyopathy

DCM is characterized by a relatively unitary final phenotype[11] of "generic" DCM. That is, for almost all genes implicated in DCM, there are no unique or distinguishing clinical features that have been associated with specific gene rare variants. The only general variation in phenotype commonly recognized[17,24] is "DCM with prominent conduction system disease," which has been observed in lamin A/C (*LMNA*) DCM and some cases of sodium channel (*SCN5A*) or desmin (*DES*) DCM. Occasionally, a clinically mild muscular dystrophy phenotype can be identified in patients with *LMNA* cardiomyopathy and a new diagnosis of DCM. However, if the muscular dystrophy is prominent, in most cases it will have been identified in a neuromuscular clinic with DCM being an incidental finding at the time of evaluation. Regardless of the setting, when a new diagnosis of idiopathic DCM is made, vigilance in detecting syndromic disease is essential, with particular attention being directed to neuromuscular phenotypes.

Most cases of familial DCM are transmitted via autosomal dominant inheritance, with the offspring of a mutation carrier having a 50% chance of inheriting the rare variant (Fig. 52.7). Autosomal recessive disease has been reported, particularly in consanguineous families. X-linked DCM resulting from rare variants in the gene for Duchenne muscular dystrophy (*DMD*) in patients without any findings of muscular dystrophy has been reported both in males and in carrier females, although the prevalence of DMD-DCM in cohorts of patients with idiopathic DCM has not been studied systematically. Mitochondrial DCM has also been reported, particularly in the setting of syndromic disease.[11]

Familial DCM is characterized by age-dependent penetrance, which means that an individual harboring a DCM-causing allele will manifest

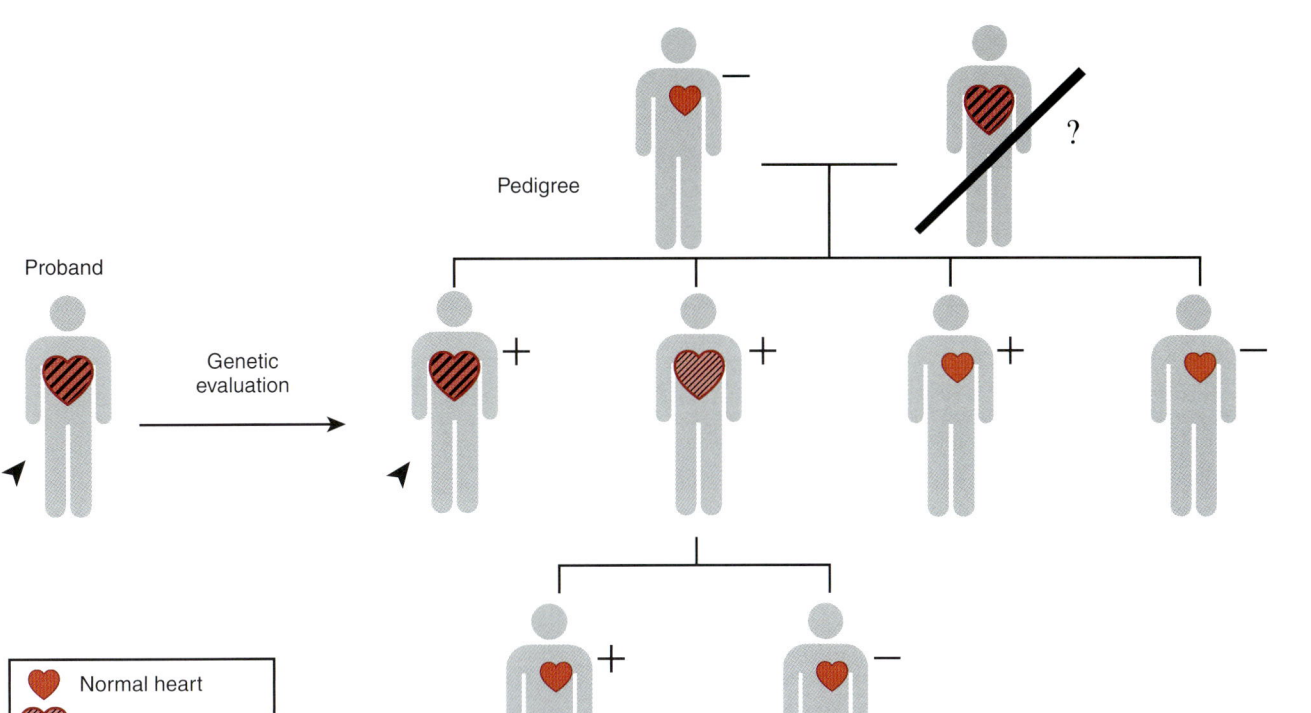

FIGURE 52.7 Genetic evaluation for cardiomyopathy. The goal of a genetic evaluation is to assess genetic risk of the proband and the proband's at-risk family members. The proband is the first patient identified with the trait or disease of interest, here depicted as an individual with dilated cardiomyopathy (DCM) and shown as an enlarged heart. The at-risk relatives can be shown by a pedigree, or a graphical depiction of the family relationships. A genetic evaluation includes a comprehensive family history for three generations or more and genetic and family counseling for all patients and families. In this example, the proband's mother died with a known diagnosis of DCM, but neither a genetic evaluation nor family screening was undertaken. With a new diagnosis of cardiomyopathy, clinical screening of first-degree relatives is indicated. In this example, the proband's three siblings are clinically evaluated. One is found to have asymptomatic DCM; the other two do not have clinical evidence of DCM. Because DCM has been found in one sibling, the sibling's children also have undergone clinical cardiovascular screening. A genetic evaluation is also indicated. In most cases, genetic testing should be undertaken for the one clearly affected person in a family to facilitate family screening and management. In this case, the proband is sequenced first, and a pathogenic rare variant is identified. This permits sequencing of the at-risk family members. The affected sibling is a mutation carrier, as is one unaffected sibling, who will be advised to have ongoing surveillance with clinical screening for early-onset DCM so that treatment can be initiated prior to the development of symptomatic DCM. One sibling is shown to not carry the mutation, so that individual can be released from clinical surveillance. The affected sibling's offspring can now also undergo genetic testing to assess risk. The one who is a mutation carrier will need clinical surveillance for development of DCM, with early intervention to attempt to prevent symptomatic disease. In this pedigree, the negative genetic testing result of the unaffected individual in the first generation indicates that the rare variant, inherited by multiple individuals in the second generation, was transmitted from the affected individual in the first generation. The finding that three affected family members all carried the same rare variant builds the evidence that the variant indeed is the pathogenic variant in this family. The *solid diagonal line* in the first generation represents a deceased individual.

evidence of the DCM phenotype with increasing age.[17,24] Most genetic DCM cases become evident in the fourth to seventh decades, although DCM occurring in adolescence, childhood, or infancy is not uncommon. Variations in the age at onset of DCM are common across families with rare variants in the same DCM gene, at times marked, and even in family members of an extended pedigree with the same rare variant (see Fig. 52.7). Penetrance in familial DCM is commonly incomplete; that is, an individual with a disease-causing allele may not manifest any aspect of the disease phenotype (see Fig. 52.7). Also, expression is variable in that the clinical features and the phenotype can vary significantly between individuals in the same family or between families with the same rare variant. Both incomplete penetrance and variable expressivity confound the assessment of familial DCM in family pedigrees. This is particularly relevant for a newly discovered or novel candidate rare variant in a family because full segregation of the candidate rare variant with the disease phenotype in one or more extended families is one of the most helpful approaches for determining the pathogenicity of such variants.

Incomplete penetrance and variable expressivity at times result in marked phenotypic variability within and between families with DCM, even with the same rare variant. The explanation for this phenomenon is not clear. Both environmental and genetic factors have been postulated and range from intrinsic (e.g., hypertension) and extrinsic phenomic components (e.g., toxins, viruses, adverse or favorable drug exposure) to a combination of various genomic variants resulting in a different genetic milieu (e.g., a second rare variant in a different disease gene, risk alleles in the same or other relevant DCM pathways, variability in epigenetics or gene expression, and others).

Allelic heterogeneity, in which rare variants in one gene can give rise to different and distinct phenotypes seemingly unrelated to one another (see Fig. 52.2), is also observed with some DCM genes, and knowledge of these allelic variants can be critical when considering a genetic diagnosis of DCM. One of the most remarkable examples is *LMNA*, which encodes the proteins lamin A and lamin C, key components of the inner nuclear membrane. For example, mutations in *LMNA* cause a distinctive DCM phenotype in which conduction system disease and arrhythmia occur before the onset of DCM. Mutant lamin proteins also cause a variety of syndromic diseases spanning striated muscle, adipose, nerve, and vascular tissues. These phenotypes, collectively termed the *laminopathies*, include skeletal myopathies (autosomal dominant Emery-Dreifuss muscular dystrophy, limb-girdle muscular dystrophy type 1B, and others [see Chapter 100]), lipodystrophy syndromes, peripheral neuropathy, and accelerated aging syndromes, most notably Hutchinson-Gilford progeria.

Approach to Clinical Genetic Evaluation

With a new cardiomyopathy diagnosis a genetic evaluation should be initiated.[4,5] A genetic evaluation precedes genetic testing, and at times may not require genetic testing. Genetic testing (Fig. 52.8) is always

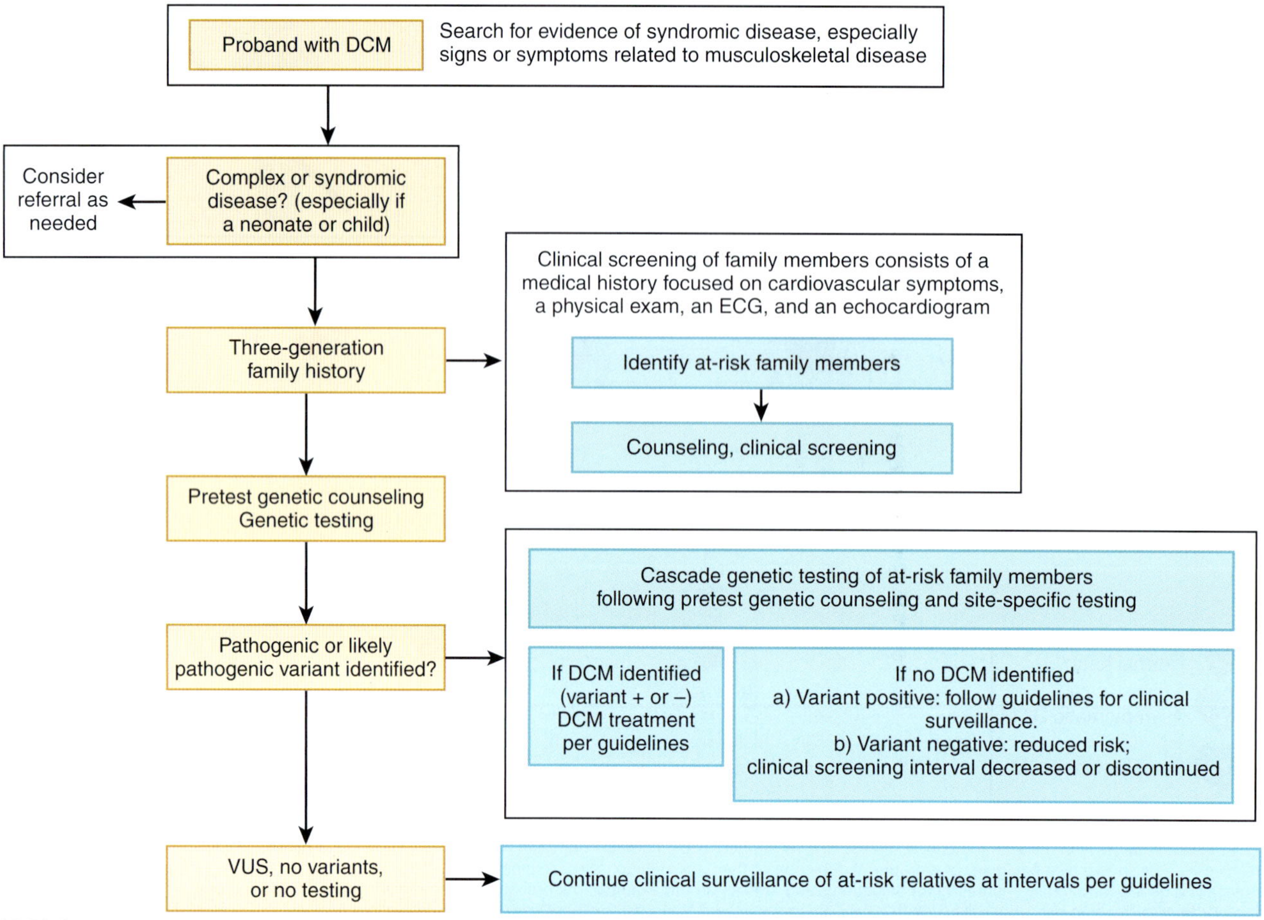

FIGURE 52.8 Flow diagram of clinical genetic testing. The conceptual approach to clinical genetic testing of a proband, the individual first identified in the family of interest, and the proband's at-risk family members, is shown. VUS, variant of unknown significance. Please see Fig. 52.7 for how this could be implemented into a multigenerational family.

TABLE 52.2 Genetic Cardiomyopathy Guidelines*

1	Family history of at least three generations
2	Clinical screening for first-degree relatives
3	Referral for genetic evaluation as needed
4	Genetic testing for DCM, HCM, ARVC, or RCM
5	Genetic counseling for patients and families
6	Cardiovascular evaluation for secondary findings
7 and 8	Therapies based on phenotype are recommended
9	Consider ICD** use before usual criteria are met

ARVC, Arrhythmogenic right ventricular cardiomyopathy; *DCM*, dilated cardiomyopathy; *HCM*, hypertrophic cardiomyopathy; *RCM*, restrictive cardiomyopathy.
*See text for expanded explanation. From the Heart Failure Society of America[4] and the American College of Genetics and Genomics.[5]
**ICD, Implantable cardioverter-defibrillator.

recommended to be performed as a component of a genetic evaluation.[4,5] Components of a genetic evaluation for a new diagnosis of cardiomyopathy include five key tasks (Table 52.2). This first two are fundamental and will help define the nature and extent of the cardiomyopathy observed in a patient and include (1) a comprehensive family history for at least three generations, and (2) the clinical screening of all first-degree relatives for cardiomyopathy (see Fig. 52.7). Evidence of cardiomyopathy in closely related family members defines familial cardiomyopathy, and this clinical determination is strong evidence for genetic etiology. This information may also aid in the interpretation and inferences drawn from genetic test results. If local evaluative expertise is not available, (3) a referral for expert evaluation is recommended, especially for complex clinical or genetic cases, or infants or children where syndromic and metabolic disease should be considered and excluded. Then (4) genetic testing (see Fig. 52.8) and (5) genetic counseling should be provided for DCM, ARVC, HCM, and RCM, all of which have been shown to have a genetic basis.[4,5]

The sixth item (see Table 52.2) provides guidance for cardiovascular specialists who are sent individuals who have secondary (sometimes referred to as incidental) genetic findings in genes known to cause cardiovascular disease, such as the cardiomyopathies. In most cases these variants have been observed in clinical exome testing or expanded medically relevant gene panels. In short, a search for the relevant phenotypic features of the condition should be undertaken,[4,5] understanding that penetrance in a "genetics-first" approach rather than a "phenotype-first" approach may give dramatically different penetrance estimates (e.g., for ARVC variants[7]), as noted above. The remaining items (see Table 52.2) reflect current medical or device interventions, including a recommendation for early ICD use as may be indicated by a specific genetic diagnosis that incurs substantial risk of sudden cardiac death before LV systolic dysfunction reaches an ejection fraction less than 35%.

Guidelines for evaluation and clinical genetic testing for DCM, applicable to all cardiomyopathies with a possible genetic cause (see Fig. 52.8), include a comprehensive three- to four-generation search of the family history for any evidence of any type of cardiomyopathy, muscular dystrophy, or other evidence of syndromic disease that may have a cardiomyopathy component. However, as noted earlier, even if it is obtained by a skilled genetics professional, the family history may well be negative because DCM is commonly asymptomatic in family members. Accordingly, cardiovascular clinical screening of all first-degree relatives is essential; history taking, a physical examination, an ECG, and echocardiography should be acquired at a minimum. If evidence of DCM is identified in a relative, screening of that relative's first-degree relatives is indicated (i.e., stepwise or cascade clinical screening).

Genetic testing, within the context of genetic counseling, is indicated with any evidence of familial disease because identification of a disease-associated rare variant (in one or more clearly affected family members) can permit molecular genetic testing of other at-risk family members with preclinical disease and thereby aid in their risk stratification. Those who test negative for the family's disease-associated rare variant should have a significantly reduced risk for the development of DCM; those harboring the family DCM rare variant should undergo enhanced clinical screening to detect early DCM, with the rationale that early drug intervention, for example with an angiotensin-converting enzyme (ACE) inhibitor or a beta blocker, may delay or prevent progression of the disease.

Genetic Testing

Genetic testing (see Fig. 52.8) is now conducted by next-generation sequencing in panels of genes ranging from 50 to 80 or more. In the United States, most insurers pay for genetic testing with appropriate genetic counseling and diagnosis coding. Genetic testing should always be conducted within the context of genetic counseling, the goals of which are to review the genetic inheritance patterns and clinically relevant facts regarding idiopathic and familial DCM and ensure that a comprehensive family history has been completed and properly interpreted, including identification of at-risk relatives. Counseling is also essential to provide information regarding the risks, benefits, and limitations of clinical genetic testing, including the possible consequences of uncertain or inconclusive results or the discovery of heritable disease and its potential psychological implications. These processes are time-consuming and require specialized knowledge; guidelines suggest that referral of patients to individuals or centers with experience should be considered if local resources for completion of the process are not available.

Post-test counseling is indicated regardless of finding a pathogenic or likely pathogenic variant in a relevant cardiomyopathy gene, because the sensitivity of genetic testing, that is, the likelihood that a relevant rare variant will be found, ranges from 20% to 25% for DCM, and 25% to 50% for ARVC and HCM. Sensitivity of testing for RCM is 10%. If testing does not return a pathogenic or likely pathogenic variant, at-risk first-degree family members are counseled to continue with clinical surveillance. If a pathogenic or likely pathogenic variant is identified in the proband, then testing of any other family members who already show evidence of cardiomyopathy builds the case that the identified variant is indeed relevant for disease (see Fig. 52.7). Other at-risk family members who do not yet show a phenotype can be tested to aid in their risk stratification. Those who test negative for the family's disease-associated rare variant should have a significantly reduced risk for the development of cardiomyopathy; those harboring the family rare variant should undergo enhanced clinical screening to detect early disease. The rationale for this for DCM and ARVC is that early drug intervention, for example with an ACE inhibitor, a beta blocker, or an ICD, may delay or prevent progression of the disease or sudden death.

The recommendation for genetic testing recognizes that with the greater number of genes being tested in pan-cardiomyopathy panels, a greater number of variants of uncertain significance may be encountered.[4,5,22] Clinicians ordering clinical genetic testing must understand this concept and be prepared to deal with this reality as the results become available. The emergence of next-generation sequencing of panels of genes has fueled an extremely active period for reevaluation of testing strategies, including approaches to interpreting large numbers of variants. All of this will require careful, comprehensive translational research to understand the optimal testing strategies, including the accumulation of large databases of disease-associated variants.

Therapy for Dilated Cardiomyopathy

Therapy for DCM is similar to that for all types of heart failure with a reduced ejection fraction and is discussed in detail in Chapter 50. Attention should be paid to treatment of atrial arrhythmias (see Tachycardia-Induced Cardiomyopathy, later). In selected patients, cardiac resynchronization therapy should be considered (see Chapter 58), and/or referral for a ventricular assist device or cardiac transplantation may be also needed (see also Chapters 59 and 60).

Arrhythmogenic Right Ventricular Cardiomyopathy

ARVC is now considered a genetically determined cardiomyopathy that has been historically characterized by lethal arrhythmias in relatively young adults and with fibrofatty replacement of the myocardium, especially of the right ventricle. The ARVC nomenclature is preserved to reflect the current medical literature.[25] Some have proposed to change the nomenclature to the simpler "arrhythmogenic cardiomyopathy" while enlarging the "arrhythmic" phenotypes[26] well beyond the conventional task force-specific ARVC category,[25] but issues have been noted with this approach[27] including an effort to take into account the arrhythmias that occur in cardiomyopathies beyond ARVC. A recognized misnomer in the ARVC term is that biventricular involvement occurs in up to 50% of cases and a small proportion of cases affect predominantly the left ventricle. Nevertheless, the current approach works well: the applied task force criteria provide a reasonable sensitivity to a specific gene ontology, that is, genes encoding proteins of the desmosome (see Fig. 52.6). The disorder is classically conceptualized as having three stages: an early subclinical phase in which imaging studies are negative but during which sudden cardiac death can still occur; next, a phase in which (usually) RV abnormalities are obvious without any clinical manifestation of RV dysfunction but with the development of a symptomatic ventricular arrhythmia; and, finally, progressive fibrofatty replacement and infiltration of the myocardium leading to severe RV dilation and aneurysm formation and associated right-sided heart failure. LV dilation and failure may also arise at this stage or may occur later (sometimes referred to as phase 4).[28] Exercise is a key facilitator of arrhythmias at all stages of disease.[25,26,28]

The electrical manifestations of ARVC reflect the pathologic disturbance. In the early stage, slow conduction and electrical uncoupling may lead to a fatal arrhythmia. As the disease progresses, fibrofatty infiltration results in inhomogeneous activation and a further delay in conduction. The predominant site of cardiac involvement, known as the triangle of dysplasia, was believed to involve the RV outflow tract, an area below the tricuspid valve, and the RV apex. However, recent data suggest that the RV apex is only involved in advanced disease and that an area involving the basal inferior and anterior right ventricle and the posterolateral left ventricle may be most commonly involved.[29] Patients with ARVC exhibit a typical monomorphic ventricular tachycardia (VT) characterized by left bundle branch block morphology with a superior axis[30] and typical T wave inversions extending to V_3 or beyond. A classic "epsilon wave" in the right precordial leads is a specific but insensitive finding (Fig. 52.9).

Genomic Cause of Arrhythmogenic Right Ventricular Cardiomyopathy

Unlike genetic DCM, which has extensive locus heterogeneity, ARVC is driven by rare variants in genes encoding proteins that are key for cell-to-cell adhesion.[28] Extensive work over the past decade has implicated genes encoding the desmosome, one of three key components of the intercalated disc, the end-to-end connection between ventricular myocytes,[28,31] in the pathogenesis of ARVC. In addition to desmosomes, the intercalated disc includes gap junctions mediating small-molecule communications. Mechanical coupling is mediated through the desmosome and adherens junctions (see Chapter 46), and disruptions of desmosomal proteins have been associated with ARVC. The classic hallmark of ARVC, fibrofatty replacement, is now understood to be related to aberrant Wnt signaling of desmosomal proteins, as well as direct plakoglobin signaling, which transforms myocytes into adipocytes with disease progression.[28,31]

MOLECULAR GENETICS
When a genetic cause can be identified, rare variants in the genes encoding plakophilin 2 (*PKP2*), desmoglein 2 (*DSG2*), and desmoplakin (*DSP*) account for most genetic causes of ARVC (see Fig. 52.2).

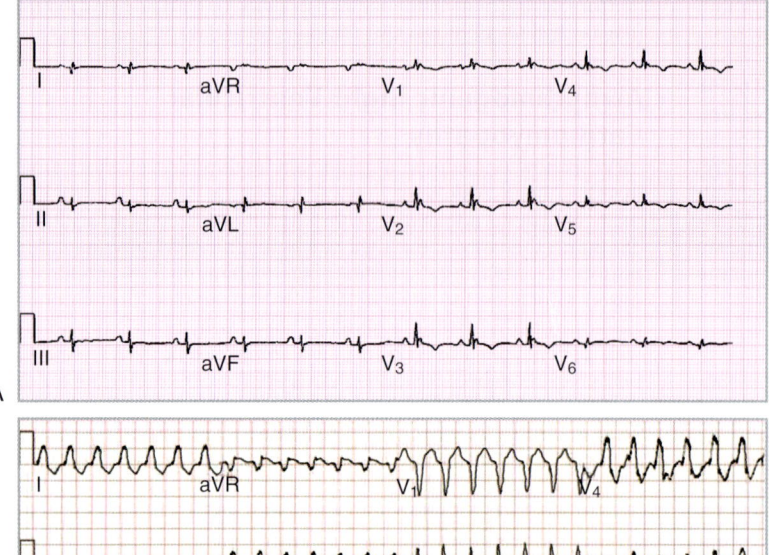
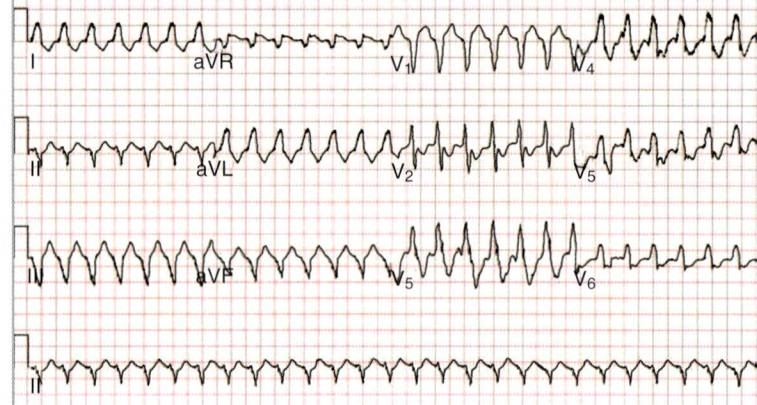

FIGURE 52.9 Arrhythmogenic right ventricular cardiomyopathy (ARVC). **A,** Electrocardiogram (ECG) of a patient with ARVC. A typical ECG shows inverted T waves in the anterior precordial leads and an "epsilon potential" early during ventricular repolarization representing a "late potential" caused by delayed depolarization of an area of the right ventricle. **B,** Ventricular tachycardia in a patient with ARVC. There are left bundle branch block morphologic findings with a leftward axis. (From Hauer RN, Cox MGPJ, Groeneweg JA. Impact of new electrocardiographic criteria in arrhythmogenic cardiomyopathy. *Front Physiol.* 2012;3:352.)

Rare variants in other genes encoding the desmosomal proteins (desmocollin [*DSC2*], junction plakoglobin [*JUP*]) or affecting desmosomal physiology (e.g., transmembrane protein [*TMEM*]) also cause ARVC (see Fig. 52.6). The ClinGen gene-validity curation for ARVC has found these six genes to have definitive evidence.[32] The degree of locus heterogeneity is similar for HCM and ARVC, in which five or fewer genes contribute to most of the identifiable genetic causes. However, as for DCM and HCM, the genes implicated in ARVC show extensive allelic heterogeneity.

CLINICAL GENETICS
The autosomal recessive syndromic *Naxos disease*, so named because it was discovered on the Greek island of Naxos, is manifested as ARVC cosegregating with palmoplantar keratoderma and wooly hair. Molecular genetic analysis has shown a homozygous two–base pair frameshift deletion of *JUP*, which encodes plakoglobin. This observation first implicated the desmosome in ARVC and prompted the molecular genetic discovery of other desmosomal proteins. Other rare variants in *JUP* have also been associated with cutaneous disease or wooly hair phenotypes, although cardiovascular phenotypes have not been identified in most of these allelic variants.[31] A second autosomal recessive syndromic disease, *Carvajal syndrome*, resembles Naxos disease in that individuals have palmoplantar keratoderma and wooly hair, but individuals with Carvajal syndrome manifest DCM, not ARVC. Carvajal syndrome is caused by a frameshift rare variant in *DSP*, which encodes desmoplakin.[31] Other rare variants in *DSP* have been identified with only ARVC or with only skin or hair manifestations. Even though reduced penetrance and variable expressivity are commonly observed in all genetic cardiomyopathies, these features may be particularly prominent in ARVC, recently highlighted in a genetics first study where penetrance was estimated to be only 6%,[7] in part because of the difficulty of assessing the phenotype and also because the arrhythmia component may be the only feature of the disease in some individuals long before structural changes can be identified. ARVC has also been noted to have highly variable penetrance, in part attributed to an oligogenic basis in some.[27]

Diagnosis
The more advanced the disease, the easier the diagnosis, but recognition of earlier stages, which may be manifested as aborted sudden death without detectable structural abnormalities, can be difficult. In addition, with increasing use of CMR for the diagnosis of cardiac pathology, a trend toward overdiagnosis of ARVC is now being recognized (see also Chapter 19). Although, in experienced hands, CMR is a useful tool for both diagnosis and evaluation of the extent of structural abnormalities in ARVC, early disease may not be apparent despite ventricular arrhythmia,[33] and overdiagnosis of the disease by less-experienced CMR readers has been recognized. Endomyocardial biopsy for ARVC is one of the diagnostic criteria but is rarely undertaken because of the potential for higher complication rates and for false-negative findings.[33] The diagnosis of ARVC currently rests primarily on the combination of clinical, electrocardiographic, and genetic findings, which are divided into major and minor diagnostic criteria as proposed in a 2010 consensus statement.

Approach to Clinical Genetic Evaluation, Including
Clinical Genetic Testing
The general approach to genetic evaluation reviewed above for DCM is fully relevant for ARVC. Current studies estimate that a plausible genetic cause can be identified in approximately half of ARVC cases.[4,34,35] The impact of multiple rare variants in desmosomal genes has been emphasized, as well as the impact of the revised task force clinical criteria, which has increased the sensitivity of molecular genetic testing.[35] A study of 439 index patients and their 562 family members showed an earlier onset of disease in those who were positive for the rare variant, although clinical characteristics were similar for both groups with disease onset.[36] Genetic testing is indicated for ARVC so that cascade testing of at-risk family members can be accomplished. This is particularly relevant for ARVC insofar as arrhythmias, especially sudden cardiac death, can occur before other phenotypic features become evident. Pan-cardiomyopathy testing, especially for a phenotype of prominent VT, ventricular fibrillation, or sudden cardiac death with biventricular dilation and systolic dysfunction of unknown cause otherwise consistent with DCM, may also yield rare variants in the genes associated with ARVC. Even though conventional recommendations currently discourage the use of genetic testing for the diagnosis of ARVC, molecular genetic testing will probably be used more frequently in the near future to assist in making the diagnosis, especially as genetic testing proliferates and is used more commonly for all cardiomyopathies regardless of phenotype.

Differential Diagnosis
The differential diagnosis of ARVC in the early stages (before the onset of visible structural abnormalities) includes idiopathic and RV outflow tract VTs. The morphology of the classic ARVC-related VT differs from these entities, and in the presence of precordial T wave inversion during sinus rhythm, ARVC should be the initial diagnosis. Cardiac sarcoidosis may occasionally mimic ARVC morphologically and be indistinguishable, even with multiple imaging modalities. Cardiac biopsy in patients with sarcoidosis often fails to show the pathognomonic granulomas but may reveal extensive fibrosis, which may also be confused with ARVC.

Treatment
Currently, the mainstay of therapy for ARVC is suppression and prevention of ventricular arrhythmias and the risk for sudden cardiac death, and prevention of disease progression. A systematic review estimated arrhythmic events at approximately 10% per year, with predictors being male gender, syncope, T wave inversions in V_3 to V_6,

RV dysfunction, prior VT or ventricular fibrillation, and exercise.[37] Intense physical exertion is associated with an earlier onset of symptoms and an increased risk of sustained VT, and therefore patients with a diagnosis of ARVC are advised not to participate in athletic activity.[38] The classic monomorphic VT in ARVC with predominant RV involvement is generally well tolerated, even at a rapid rate, possibly because of preserved LV function in most patients. Nevertheless, VT of a different morphology may occur and sudden death is not uncommon. Antiarrhythmic drugs may suppress a symptomatic arrhythmia but have not been shown to prevent sudden death. Beta-blocking agents may suppress catecholamine-triggered arrhythmia and slow progression of ventricular dysfunction and have been recommended as potentially valuable in all patients with ARVC.[38] An ICD is recommended in patients with aborted sudden death, syncope, or decreased LV function and may be considered in other patients. Catheter ablation has not been shown to reduce sudden death but is valuable in a patient with an ICD and frequent arrhythmias or in occasional patients with very well-tolerated single-morphology VT. Ablation appears to be most successful when lesions are made in both the epicardial and endocardial surfaces of the heart; it should be performed only at centers experienced in the technique, either as a combined procedure or with epicardial ablation reserved for recurrence after endocardial ablation.[39] Heart failure may occur in advanced ARVC and is treated with standard drugs. Because a history of vigorous sustained exercise among carriers of a pathogenic ARVC desmosome rare variant is associated with an earlier onset of symptoms and a higher prevalence of VT or ventricular fibrillation,[40] there is a task force recommendation that persons with definite or suspected ARVC should not compete in most competitive sports.

Alcoholic and Diabetic Cardiomyopathies

Excessive alcohol intake is cardiotoxic and may be manifested as DCM, and is discussed in detail in Chapter 84.[41] The importance of obtaining as accurate an alcohol history as possible in assessing patients with DCM cannot be overstated. The existence of a specific diabetic cardiomyopathy independent of the effect of diabetes on the vasculature is debated, both in terms of its existence and in the form that it takes. Abnormalities initially in diastolic and then systolic function are prevalent in diabetic patients, but their clinical relevance to the development of overt disease is unclear.[42] Nevertheless, data do support good glycemic control as a preventative against the development of heart failure (see Chapter 31).[43] The addition of SGLT2 inhibitors to the management of diabetic patients with heart failure with reduced ejection fraction is discussed in Chapter 50.

Left Ventricular Noncompaction

In 2006 LVNC was included as a genetic cardiomyopathy in an AHA scientific statement.[1] In 2008, the European Society of Cardiology questioned whether LVNC should be classified as a cardiomyopathy or "merely a congenital or acquired morphologic trait that is shared by many phenotypically distinct cardiomyopathies."[2] Most authorities have suggested that evidence to classify LV noncompaction (LVNC) as a distinct cardiomyopathy is insufficient,[4,44-49] and rather consider LVNC as a morphologic trait that is shared by many cardiomyopathies as well as by other conditions, such as the channelopathies and congenital heart disease. A pattern of LVNC can emerge with intense exercise or pregnancy and resolve with diminished exercise or in the postpartum period, thus suggesting a paradigm of remodeling and reverse remodeling as seen in other conditions affecting LV size or function. Underlying this debate is the lack of adverse outcomes of LVNC itself, as published accounts of adverse events stem from a defined cardiomyopathy or arrhythmia phenotype. Mounting evidence has increased to favor a variant phenotype rather than one inherently pathologic.[46,48] LVNC does not have its own gene ontology but intersects with those of DCM, HCM, and ARVC (see Fig. 52.6).

Defining the LVNC phenotype has been confounded by various echocardiographic or CMR approaches that have led to an estimate of its frequency in a population-based study of as high as 23%; furthermore, the concordance of three different echocardiographic diagnostic schemata was congruent in only 30% of cases.[45] These diagnostic criteria have been summarized and include four that are echocardiographic-based and two that are cardiac CMR-based. If LVNC is identified in concert with another cardiomyopathy (DCM, HCM, RCM) the approach to the primary cardiomyopathy will drive the genetic evaluation process, as outlined earlier. It is not clear that any specific management is indicated for LVNC independent of some other cardiovascular diagnosis or complication.

Tachycardia-Induced Cardiomyopathy

Tachycardia for a prolonged period can result in diastolic and systolic ventricular dysfunction, even in the absence of other cardiac diseases. This condition is known as tachycardia-induced cardiomyopathy.[50] It is a diagnosis that can be made only retrospectively when correction of an arrhythmia is associated with improved ventricular function. However, it should be considered in any patient with tachycardia and LV systolic dysfunction who is not in sinus rhythm. The cardiomyopathy may be manifested either as an isolated condition or in association with preexisting cardiac disease. Thus a patient with mild DCM in whom atrial fibrillation develops may have a tendency for the development of decompensated heart failure, not only because of the loss of atrial function but also because the rapid, irregular rate of atrial fibrillation leads to further systolic dysfunction. Hyperthyroidism should be ruled out because it may cause both tachycardia and, rarely, an independent DCM. The "purest" form of tachycardia-induced cardiomyopathy is probably that caused by incessant or extremely frequent atrial tachycardia or permanent reciprocating junctional tachycardia, often in a child or young patient with systolic dysfunction.[51] However, almost any arrhythmia can cause tachycardia-induced cardiomyopathy, including very frequent premature ventricular contractions (PVCs) or recurrent nonsustained VT.[52] Incessant atrial tachycardia causing tachycardia-induced cardiomyopathy may be mistaken for sinus tachycardia. If a previous ECG is available, comparison may be helpful, with specific attention being paid to subtle differences in P-wave morphology.

The duration of the arrhythmia, more than the heart rate, is probably a critical factor in tachycardia-induced cardiomyopathy. Among 30 patients with incessant atrial tachycardia and tachycardia-induced cardiomyopathy, the mean duration of symptoms was 6 years. The mean ventricular response was just 117 beats/min, and rate control (primarily by ablation) was associated with normalization of the ejection fraction in all but one patient.[51] A decreased ejection fraction in the presence of atrial fibrillation may occasionally improve after the restoration of sinus rhythm. If the ventricular rate is well controlled, improvement of LV systolic function in atrial fibrillation with a reduced ejection fraction is uncommon, but it is important to assess ventricular rate control with 24-hour monitoring to confirm control during both exercise and rest. Most patients with PVC-associated tachycardia-induced cardiomyopathy have more than 20,000 PVCs over a 24-hour period, but the condition has also been described with a lesser frequency of arrhythmia.[39] Catheter ablation of PVCs, if possible, is generally associated with improvement in ventricular function in these patients.

Most cases of tachycardia-induced cardiomyopathy improve within 3 to 6 months after correction of the arrhythmia, but occasionally patients have been seen with late improvement, up to 1 year. Because the rapid, irregular ventricular response to atrial fibrillation is associated with marked beat-to-beat variation in the ejection fraction, the most accurate way to determine whether an improvement in systolic function has really occurred is to evaluate the ejection fraction early after restoration of sinus rhythm and then compare it with a reevaluation 3 to 6 months later.

Following restoration of sinus rhythm, subtle abnormalities in LV function may remain, such as mild LV dilation despite normalization of the ejection fraction, and recurrence of arrhythmia can be associated with deterioration of LV function.[53] In an animal model, tachycardia was associated with diastolic dysfunction often before a decrease in systolic function. Tachycardia-induced LV diastolic dysfunction may occur in humans in the presence of a normal ejection fraction. Although poorly studied, it may be responsible for the symptoms of heart failure in some patients with arrhythmia and a preserved LV ejection fraction.[54] Few data on improvement in diastolic dysfunction following correction of arrhythmia are available.

Peripartum Cardiomyopathy

Peripartum cardiomyopathy (PPCM) has been defined as DCM that occurs in a temporal relationship to pregnancy (see also Chapter 92). While PPCM has traditionally been considered etiologically separate from DCM, evidence now clearly indicates that at least a portion of PPCM cases results from genetic risk, at least in part, from genes known to cause DCM. Definitive evidence of this was recently shown,[20] where 172 women with PPCM underwent sequencing for DCM genes, with *TTN* truncating variants (TTNtvs) identified in 26 of the 172 (15%). A similar frequency of TTN truncating mutations in cohorts of patients with DCM is suggestive that at least a portion of PPCM may be DCM occurring during pregnancy. Two earlier studies also observed that in some proportion of cases a rare variant genetic cause, similar to that of DCM, was at play,[55,56] where rare variants in DCM genes were present in 6 of 19 women who had sequence information available.[55] In a second earlier study, among 90 families with DCM, 6% were found to have at least one member with PPCM, and genetic screening of relatives of three patients with PPCM who failed to show complete recovery revealed undiagnosed DCM in all three families.[56] From these studies comes the recommendation that in DCM occurring during or following pregnancy, the same guidelines for DCM presented earlier should be followed, namely, obtaining a comprehensive family history, performing clinical screening of first-degree relatives, and conducting genetic testing.

However, it can also be argued that of the many additional women who harbor TTNtvs only a small fraction develop PPCM, and the additional risk factors, whether genetic, epigenetic, or endogenous environmental factors, may well be at play.[57] Extensive prior studies have implicated risk for DCM during pregnancy that range from autoimmune conditions or nutritional deficiencies to inflammation of the myocardium. Animal models of vascular-hormonal features known to be associated with PPCM, focused primarily on elevated prolactin and its physiology and downstream signaling in late pregnancy and the peripartum period, have contributed to this vascular hypothesis. Bromocriptine, now considered experimental only, had been earlier advocated for treatment based on data from uncontrolled studies, but more recent randomized (without a control group) studies have shown no convincing benefit, and the significant adverse effects of bromocriptine await a properly randomized and controlled trial to show benefit.[57]

Clinical Features

The U.S. incidence is estimated to be between 1 in 1000 and 1 in 4000 live births, with a major risk factor that of African ancestry; significantly higher incidence has been reported in countries with predominant African ancestry. Preeclampsia, older age, and multiple-fetus pregnancies are also risk factors. In patients with PPCM, symptoms and signs of heart failure develop during late pregnancy or after delivery, similar to those of any patient with heart failure caused by LV systolic dysfunction. Most diagnoses are made in the 4 months following delivery; prepartum diagnoses are most commonly made in the last month of pregnancy. However, the disorder has also been described in early pregnancy (pregnancy-associated cardiomyopathy). Because symptoms similar to those of heart failure (dyspnea, fatigue, and edema) may occur in normal pregnancy, it is possible that a proportion of cases have a delayed diagnosis. Furthermore, because spontaneous resolution of LV dysfunction is known to occur, mild cases in the peripartum period may be overlooked. Given the rarity of the disease, it is not possible to precisely determine the incidence of PPCM in subsequent pregnancies of patients who have had a previous episode. However, recurrence appears to be related to the degree of recovery from the initial episode; PPCM seems less likely to recur in women who enter a second pregnancy with a normal ejection fraction than in those with a persistent reduction in the ejection fraction.[58]

In approximately 50% of patients with PPCM who are given standard medical therapy, the LV ejection fraction returns to normal, although the patients may still be at risk for recurrent PPCM. The remainder are often stabilized with medical therapy; however, a proportion of patients may experience progressive heart failure. Following delivery, treatment of PPCM is the same as for other causes of systolic dysfunction. However, if heart failure occurs during pregnancy, ACE inhibitors or angiotensin-receptor blockers are contraindicated because of the risk for fetotoxic effects. Diuretics should be used with caution, and metoprolol should be used rather than carvedilol. Eplerenone should be avoided, but spironolactone can be used cautiously later in pregnancy. Heart transplantation has been performed in patients with severe PPCM. In the United States, approximately 5% of all women undergoing cardiac transplantation have PPCM as their primary indication; it represents the fourth most common cause in women. Post-transplantation outcomes of PPCM are similar to those for other indications.

Takotsubo Cardiomyopathy (see also Chapters 37 and 38)

Takotsubo cardiomyopathy (TC) (referred to as Takotsubo syndrome [TTS] in Europe)[59,60] or stress-induced cardiomyopathy, is an acute, reversible condition first recognized in the 1990s, now with an updated uniform definition (Table 52.3). It is estimated that in 2012, about 5500 patients were admitted to U.S. hospitals with TC, with an even greater number developing the condition while they were in the hospital secondary to a comorbid condition or stress. In an International Takotsubo Registry of 1750 patients, 89.8% were women, the vast majority postmenopausal.[61] Chest pain was the predominant symptom in 76%, dyspnea in 47%, and syncope in 7.7%. A preceding physical trigger occurred in 36% and an emotional trigger in 28%, and troponin values were elevated in 87%, with ST elevation shown on the ECG in almost half of the patients. While men can be affected, women are 10-fold more likely to show TC overall, and women older than 55 years are five times more likely to experience TC compared to those less than 55 years.[59] Of those younger than 50 years, men were more commonly affected with more antecedent neurologic or psychiatric disorders compared to older individuals.[62]

A complete explanation for the pathophysiology of TC remains elusive, but activation of the sympathetic nervous system appears central, with an identifying emotional or physiologic stimulus preceding onset in most cases. Multi-vessel epicardial coronary artery spasm has been postulated as the pathophysiologic pathway due to the generalized myocardial contractile abnormalities that do not follow a specific coronary artery territory, as observed in acute coronary obstruction in atherosclerotic disease. Abnormalities of coronary microcirculation have also been postulated. Familial clustering has only rarely been observed, and genetics, if at play, may be from common variants that facilitate adrenergic signaling or its downstream amplification.

The diagnosis of TC, and in particular, differentiating it from an acute coronary syndrome in the emergency room, has been aided by an algorithm developed by an international Takotsubo task force (Table 52.4).

> The LV contractile abnormalities in TC are prominent, and although they involve the LV apex (resulting in the synonym of "apical ballooning syndrome") in more than 80% of patients, regional wall motion abnormalities may be limited to the midventricular wall or other LV walls in a minority of patients. Compensatory hyperdynamic contraction of the basal LV segments with associated apical LV dyskinesis may result in acute LV outflow tract obstruction because of systolic anterior motion of the mitral valve with an associated outflow tract gradient and hypotension. Although the long-term prognosis is good, an in-hospital mortality rate of 4.1% has been reported, primarily because of irreversible cardiogenic shock, LV rupture, or embolization of LV thrombi. Malignant ventricular arrhythmia, particularly torsades de pointes associated with Takotsubo-related QT prolongation, may occur, as (rarely) may complete heart block.[63]

TABLE 52.3 International Takotsubo Diagnostic Criteria (InterTAK Diagnostic Criteria)

1. Patients show transient* left ventricular dysfunction (hypokinesia, akinesia, or dyskinesia) presenting as apical ballooning or midventricular, basal, or focal wall motion abnormalities. Right ventricular involvement can be present. Besides these regional wall motion patterns, transitions between all types can exist. The regional wall motion abnormality usually extends beyond a single epicardial vascular distribution; however, rare cases can exist where the regional wall motion abnormality is present in the subtended myocardial territory of a single coronary artery (focal TTS).**
2. An emotional, physical, or combined trigger can precede the takotsubo syndrome event, but this is not obligatory.
3. Neurologic disorders (e.g., subarachnoid hemorrhage, stroke/transient ischemic attack, or seizures) as well as pheochromocytoma may serve as triggers for takotsubo syndrome.
4. New electrocardiogram (ECG) abnormalities are present (ST-segment elevation, ST-segment depression, T wave inversion, and QTc prolongation); however, rare cases exist without any ECG changes.
5. Levels of cardiac biomarkers (troponin and creatine kinase) are moderately elevated in most cases; significant elevation of brain natriuretic peptide is common.
6. Significant coronary artery disease is not a contradiction in takotsubo syndrome.
7. Patients have no evidence of infectious myocarditis.**
8. Postmenopausal women are predominantly affected.

*Wall motion abnormalities may remain for a prolonged period of time or documentation of recovery may not be possible. For example, death before evidence of recovery is captured.
**Cardiac magnetic resonance imaging is recommended to exclude infectious myocarditis and diagnosis confirmation of takotsubo syndrome.
From Ghadri JR, Wittstein IS, Prasad A, et al. International Expert Consensus Document on Takotsubo Syndrome (Part I): Clinical Characteristics, Diagnostic Criteria, and Pathophysiology. *Eur Heart J.* 2018;39:2032–2046.

TABLE 52.4 An InterTAK Clinical Score to Differentiate Takotsubo Syndrome from Acute Coronary Syndrome

Female sex 25 points
Emotional stress 24 points
Physical stress 13 points
No ST-segment depression (except aVR) (12 points)
Psychiatric disorders 11 points
Neurologic disorders 9 points
QTc prolongation 6 points

≤70 points, low/intermediate probability of TTS; >70 points, high probability

From Ghadri JR, Cammann VL, Jurisic S, et al. A novel clinical score (InterTAK Diagnostic Score) to differentiate takotsubo syndrome from acute coronary syndrome: results from the International Takotsubo Registry. *Eur J Heart Fail.* 2017;19:1036–1042.

RESTRICTIVE AND INFILTRATIVE CARDIOMYOPATHIES

The RCMs are a heterogeneous group of diseases characterized by a nondilated left ventricle, often with a normal or near-normal LV ejection fraction. The predominant manifestation is diastolic dysfunction as a result of myocardial disease, and although severe hypertensive disease, aortic stenosis, and some cases of HCM may feature restrictive pathophysiology, these conditions are not classified as RCMs. Some infiltrative cardiac diseases such as amyloidosis (see Chapter 53) produce an RCM, whereas others, such as sarcoidosis, have an infiltrative component but appear as RCM or DCM. Thus, just as DCM is a morphologic condition that encompasses several causes of cardiomyopathy, the terms *restrictive cardiomyopathy* and *infiltrative cardiomyopathy* are pathophysiologic and anatomic definitions of cardiomyopathies that have overlaps with several well-defined conditions.

Approach to Identifying a Cause of Restrictive Cardiomyopathy

Because RCM is not always an isolated cardiac disease but may arise secondary to other acquired or genetic diseases, the diagnostic approach is challenging for the cardiovascular specialist (see Table 52.1). Endomyocardial biopsy may be more relevant for the diagnosis of a specific cause in patients with RCM than in those with DCM or HCM insofar as RCM may be caused by an infiltrative cardiac process without systemic involvement or with subclinical involvement of other organs.[64] However, CMR imaging with T1, T2, and extracellular volume mapping has increased the diagnostic yield and thus reduced the need for endomyocardial biopsy. When a cause cannot be identified, the condition is known as *idiopathic RCM*. Unlike with DCM, *familial RCM* is distinctly uncommon. Regardless of whether a cause can be found, a comprehensive family history should always be obtained as should clinical screening of first-degree relatives. As noted above, genetic testing is now indicated for any case of RCM where the etiology is uncertain or unknown, even when the family history is negative (see Fig. 52.8).

Clinical and Molecular Genetics of Restrictive Cardiomyopathy

The clinical genetic features of familial RCM are similar to those of DCM in that reduced penetrance and a variable age at onset are commonly observed. Genes with rare variants implicated in the cause of idiopathic and nonsyndromic RCM are in most cases ones that encode sarcomeric proteins.[65,66] Although some locus heterogeneity is apparent, it is much less so than with DCM. Because cardiac hemodynamic findings commonly exhibit restrictive physiology in HCM, the genetic similarity of HCM and RCM suggests that in these cases the RCM phenotype at times may be viewed as a "minimally hypertrophic" HCM phenotype with prominent restrictive physiology. As noted earlier, at times "overlap" or "crossover"

Therapy

TC is a self-limited disorder, usually with rapid resolution of symptoms and LV dysfunction. Classification has been recommended into lower-risk and higher-risk categories, with the latter based on an LV ejection fraction of less than 45%, hypotension and an outflow tract gradient of greater than 40 mm Hg, and/or the presence of an arrhythmia. Use of an ACE inhibitor or a beta blocker, or both, is recommended in the higher-risk groups. Because of the occasional association with acute QT prolongation, care should be taken to avoid using QT-prolonging medications, such as macrolide antibiotics or certain antiarrhythmic agents. In patients with hypotension associated with TC, pressors should be used with caution because LV outflow tract obstruction may be precipitated. Occasionally, thrombus formation may occur in the dyskinetic segment, and anticoagulation is routinely used for this indication. In most cases resolution is complete or nearly complete within days to weeks, although the major adverse events, including cardiogenic shock or death, mandate observation of the acute phase of TC in an intensive care unit (ICU) setting. Major adverse events occur in approximately 5% of individuals, with younger males most at risk. The recurrence risk has been estimated at 5%, usually within the first year. Overall mortality of TC has been estimated to follow that of coronary disease, even though most patients have no demonstrable atherosclerotic plaque. The use of ACE inhibitors long term have been shown to reduce recurrence. In contrast, prophylactic use of beta blockers has not been shown to reduce recurrence, even though attempting to minimize a catecholamine-induced trigger provides a rationale for their use. Likewise, for depression or other psychiatric disorders, treatment has been postulated to possibly reduce recurrence, but evidence is lacking largely due to the difficulty of conducting controlled trials when the recurrence rate is low. Even though a visualized thrombus mandates anticoagulation, long-term anticoagulation has not been recommended.

phenotypes of RCM and HCM have been observed in families with rare variants in sarcomeric genes that demonstrate this principle.[65,66]

Clinical Features of Idiopathic Restrictive Cardiomyopathy

Idiopathic RCM has been described in individuals from infancy to late adulthood; it usually carries a poor prognosis, especially in children.[67] The disease is rare, and the largest adult series contains only 91 cases seen over a 17-year period.[68] In one series of 32 unrelated patients with end-stage disease, RCM was considered to be genetically determined either by the identification of pathogenic rare variants (60%) or by evidence of familial disease without a known pathogenic rare variant (in an additional 5 patients), for a total of 75%.[69] Symptoms of idiopathic RCM are nonspecific and reflect the presence of heart failure. Dyspnea is an initial complaint in most patients; edema occurs in approximately half; and palpitations, fatigue, and orthopnea are reported by 22% to 33%. Physical examination is usually consistent with biventricular heart failure, with jugular venous distention noted in most patients but ascites and significant edema being found in advanced cases. Atrial fibrillation is common, and a third heart sound is heard in one in four patients; murmurs are not a feature. Assuming that amyloidosis has been excluded, the ECG has normal voltage, with only a minority of patients showing intraventricular conduction delay.

Echocardiography reveals a typical pattern of biatrial enlargement and nondilated ventricles with a normal or near normal LV ejection fraction and LV wall thickness (Fig. 52.10). At *cardiac catheterization* RV and LV filling pressures are elevated with a dip-and-plateau tracing often seen; unlike in constrictive pericarditis, however, equalization of diastolic pressures is uncommon. Careful evaluation of simultaneously recorded LV and RV pressures during respiration demonstrates concordant changes in systolic pressures in RCM, rather than a discordance (inspiratory increase in RV systolic pressure with a simultaneous decrease in LV pressure) seen in constrictive pericarditis.[70] Endomyocardial biopsy demonstrates nonspecific findings such as myocyte hypertrophy, interstitial fibrosis, and, not uncommonly, endocardial fibrosis. The survival rate is reduced in comparison with that of an age- and sex-matched population; the observed survival rate from the time of diagnosis is 64% at 5 years and 37% at 10 years.[71] Most deaths are associated with cardiac causes, either suddenly or secondary to heart failure, although a third die of noncardiac causes related to progressive age.

The differential diagnosis of idiopathic RCM includes the infiltrative cardiomyopathies, such as amyloidosis, or constrictive pericarditis.[72] Unlike idiopathic RCM, amyloidosis is associated with increased LV wall thickness and subtle abnormalities in LV systolic function, with specific findings on cardiac biopsy; it can also be heritable with variants in *TTR* (see also Chapter 53). Constrictive pericarditis is more difficult to differentiate from RCM because most of the clinical features overlap between the two disorders. A thickened pericardium noted on echocardiography, CT, or CMR in a patient with heart failure and a preserved ejection fraction without wall thickening suggests constrictive pericarditis; however, it bears emphasis that 18% of patients with constrictive pericarditis have normal pericardial thickness.[70] Advanced echocardiographic or CMR-imaging techniques may be of help in distinguishing constrictive pericarditis from RCM (see also Chapters 16 and 19), but endomyocardial biopsy may be required unless an alternative diagnosis is clear. Treatment of idiopathic RCM is generally limited to medical treatment emphasizing judicious use of diuretics, but in selected advanced cases, cardiac transplantation has been performed with similar outcomes as in those with nonrestrictive cardiomyopathy.[68]

Sarcoid Cardiomyopathy

Sarcoidosis is a multisystem disorder of unknown cause characterized histologically by noncaseating granulomas. In the United States the disease is most commonly seen in the black population and is more common in women than in men. Sarcoid has a higher incidence in Scandinavia and Japan. Cardiac involvement takes the form of ventricular dysfunction, heart block, and/or ventricular arrhythmias. Despite

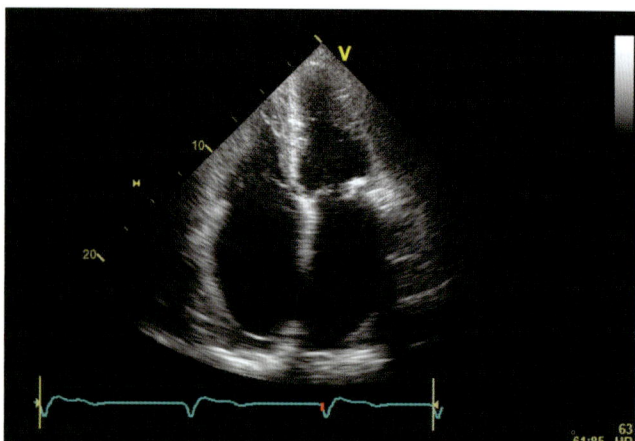

FIGURE 52.10 Echocardiogram showing restrictive cardiomyopathy. An apical four-chamber view is shown in an 80-year-old man with long-standing restrictive cardiomyopathy (RCM). The left ventricular (LV) ejection fraction was normal, with evidence of severe diastolic dysfunction on echocardiography and cardiac catheterization. Note the massive biatrial enlargement and normal LV wall thickness.

frequently being described as an RCM, sarcoid heart disease can also present as a DCM, occasionally with aneurysm formation. Although most patients with sarcoid cardiomyopathy also have evidence of noncardiac disease, particularly lung disease, clinically isolated cardiac sarcoidosis is increasingly being recognized as a cause of heart block and ventricular arrhythmias. Sudden death, presumably from heart block or a ventricular arrhythmia, may be the first manifestation either of sarcoidosis itself or of heart disease in a patient with known pulmonary or systemic sarcoid. The prevalence of cardiac involvement in patients with pulmonary sarcoidosis was previously thought to be no more than 5%, but autopsy studies indicate a much higher prevalence, and recent cardiac imaging studies have demonstrated abnormalities in at least 25% of patients with pulmonary sarcoidosis.[73]

Pathology

The pathology of sarcoid heart disease raises puzzling questions about the cause of the systolic dysfunction, which can be severe. Noncaseating granulomas, the hallmark of the disease, are patchily distributed even in severe disease and thus may not alone account for the severe systolic dysfunction. Granulomatous lesions are associated with edema and inflammation, and widespread myocardial fibrosis is seen late in the disease (Fig. 52.11). The patchy nature of granulomatous infiltration and the sometimes extensive fibrosis render cardiac biopsy a low-yield procedure for detecting diagnostic histology in cardiac sarcoidosis, and finding granulomas may be difficult even at autopsy, because end-stage disease is characterized predominantly by fibrosis.[74] Occasionally, the right ventricle may be severely and predominantly involved. Recently several cases of meeting criteria for ARVC with a typical appearance on multimodality imaging have been described that are later found to show noncaseating granulomas and other signs consistent with sarcoidosis.[75,76] RV function can be impaired in patients with severe pulmonary sarcoidosis and pulmonary hypertension, even in the absence of direct sarcoid involvement of the heart.

Clinical Features

The most common noncardiac site of sarcoid involvement is the lungs, with approximately half of patients having overt parenchymal disease and the remainder having isolated bilateral hilar lymphadenopathy. Other findings, in decreasing order of frequency, are hepatic and gastrointestinal involvement, ocular sarcoidosis, and neurologic sarcoidosis. Skin involvement in sarcoidosis is not uncommon, and lesions appear to have a predilection for scars and tattoos. In patients with established extracardiac sarcoid, LV systolic dysfunction is most commonly due to associated cardiac sarcoidosis.

The most common clinical feature of cardiac sarcoidosis is biventricular heart failure. Mitral regurgitation, often caused by papillary muscle involvement in addition to LV dilation, may be severe.

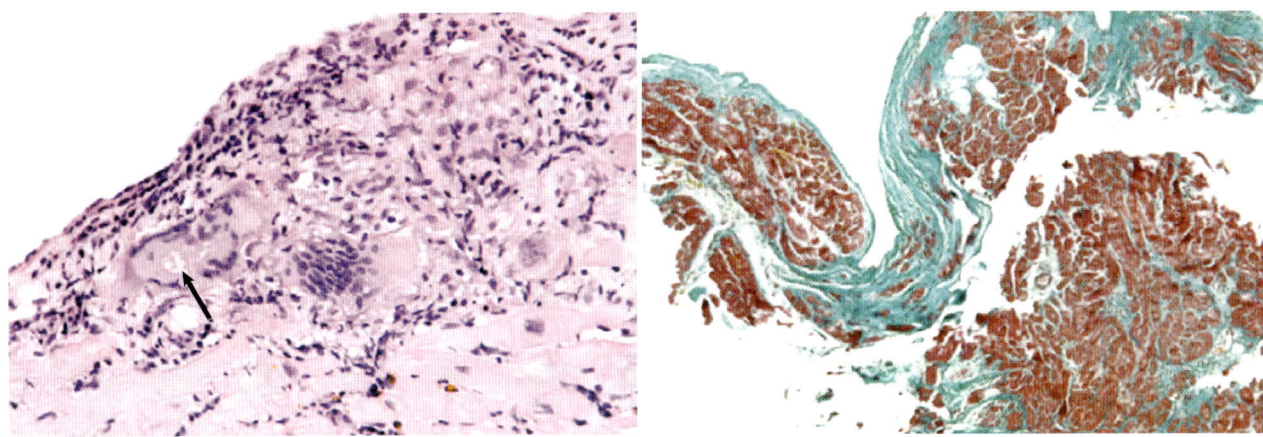

FIGURE 52.11 Myocardial biopsy for sarcoid cardiomyopathy. The **left panel** shows an initial biopsy specimen (hematoxylin-eosin staining) with an inflammatory noncaseating granuloma typical of sarcoid. The *arrow* points to an "asteroid body" in the cytoplasm of the giant cell; this is a common finding in various granulomatous diseases. The **right panel** shows a follow-up biopsy specimen (Masson trichrome stain, initial magnification 100×) in the same patient. No granulomas are present, and there is now extensive interstitial fibrosis (*green-staining area*). This demonstrates how granulomas may be missed on biopsy, particularly in advanced sarcoid cardiomyopathy, when fibrosis is extensive. (From Leone O, Veinot JP, Angelini A, et al. 2011 consensus statement on endomyocardial biopsy from the Association for European Cardiovascular Pathology and the Society for Cardiovascular Pathology. *Cardiovasc Pathol*. 2012;21:245.)

Sarcoid granulomas have a predilection for the cardiac conduction system, and high-degree atrioventricular (AV) block may occur, either as an initial manifestation of cardiac sarcoidosis or later in the disease (Fig. 52.12). Both atrial and ventricular arrhythmias are common, the latter arising from either ventricle. Once causes such as Lyme disease have been ruled out, complete heart block in a young patient suggests sarcoidosis, especially if ventricular arrhythmias are present, and imaging should be pursued in all such cases. Sudden cardiac death is almost always associated with grossly visible scarring and fibrosis at autopsy. A rare manifestation of cardiac sarcoidosis is acute sarcoid myocarditis, characterized by high-degree AV block, malignant ventricular arrhythmia, and heart failure. It may be difficult to distinguish this from giant cell myocarditis unless systemic features of sarcoid are also present.

Diagnosis

Laboratory testing for sarcoidosis is generally unrewarding. An elevated sedimentation rate may be present but is nonspecific, as is a finding of elevated immunoglobulins. Hypercalcemia (believed to be due to activation of vitamin D by macrophages in sarcoid granulomas), although uncommon, is a useful clue. Although elevation of serum ACE may be helpful for diagnosis, there is a wide range in the normal population because of a polymorphism in the *ACE* gene. Normal ACE levels may be seen in patients with untreated sarcoidosis, and serial ACE levels do not appear to correlate with treatment response.

CMR with gadolinium enhancement (see also Chapter 19) is a sensitive test for detecting cardiac abnormalities (Fig. 52.13). Delayed gadolinium enhancement may be found in either a coronary or noncoronary distribution, is usually nontransmural, and has a predilection for the basal and/or midventricular septum.[73] The finding of myocardial late gadolinium enhancement by CMR in a patient with proven extracardiac sarcoidosis is a marker for subsequent major cardiac events, including sudden death, and the risk of major events is proportional to the amount of late gadolinium enhancement.[77] In the acute stage, T2-weighted imaging may show myocardial edema, which is characterized by focal areas of thickening and increased signal intensity on T2-weighted and early gadolinium-enhanced images.[78]

^{18}F-fluorodeoxyglucose (FDG) positron emission tomography (PET) scanning (see also Chapter 18, Figs. 18.2, 18.36, 18.37, and 18.39) is complementary to CMR in patients with sarcoidosis; it reveals areas of inflammation in active disease, permits serial evaluation of response to therapy, and is becoming an important tool for the diagnosis and management of cardiac disease.[79] An example of a combined PET-CT scan in a patient with cardiac amyloidosis is shown in Figure 52.14.

TISSUE BIOPSY

A positive cardiac biopsy showing noncaseating granulomas is diagnostic of cardiac sarcoidosis if giant cell myocarditis is ruled out. However, the patchy nature of the granulomatous infiltration results in a low yield of positive biopsies. Targeted biopsy of another organ, such as enlarged hilar lymph nodes, may give a higher yield, or alternatively, biopsy of an area of definite abnormality seen on PET or CMR may be valuable. Although the 2006 recommendations of the Japanese Society of Sarcoidosis and of the Granulomatous Disorders suggest diagnosis by a combination of major and minor criteria, including myocardial biopsy, PET-CT and CMR are more sensitive and are playing an increasing role.

Treatment

No randomized clinical trials of the treatment of cardiac sarcoidosis have been completed, although the design of a Canadian study where patients will be randomized to prednisone or prednisone plus methotrexate has been published.[80] Standard heart failure therapy should be instituted if heart failure is present, but in addition, steroid therapy is often given, particularly in patients with newly diagnosed sarcoidosis and systolic dysfunction. Steroids are frequently effective in noncardiac sarcoidosis, and nonrandomized data suggest a benefit in patients with cardiac sarcoid complicated by heart failure, particularly early in the disease when irreversible fibrosis has not yet developed. Prednisone is generally initiated in doses between 1 mg/kg and 40 mg daily and tapered gradually over a period of several months with careful monitoring.[81] Methotrexate is often used as a second agent if steroid therapy is unsuccessful,[82] and several recent case reports have shown promising responses to anti-tumor necrosis factor (anti-TNF) monoclonal antibodies.

Management of arrhythmia often requires a pacemaker and/or ICD. On the assumption that high-degree AV block in systemic sarcoidosis is a marker of associated myocardial sarcoidosis, use of a pacemaker-ICD has been recommended for any patient with sarcoidosis who requires pacing. Prophylactic use of an ICD based on a reduced ejection fraction, similar to other patients with heart failure with a depressed ejection fraction, is also appropriate (see also Chapter 58), but the role of an ICD in a patient with sarcoidosis and mild cardiac disease but no high-degree AV block or frequent ventricular arrhythmia is less clear.[83] The 2014 Heart Rhythm Society Consensus Recommendations for ICD implantation in patients with cardiac sarcoidosis are a useful guide, and suggest incorporation of advanced imaging and possible electrophysiologic study in such patients.[84] A recent meta-analysis of 585 patients from 10 studies showed substantial benefit of ICD placement, with 39% receiving appropriate therapy over a mean follow-up period of 25 months.[85] Cardiac transplantation may be undertaken in patients with severe cardiac sarcoidosis after careful evaluation for noncardiac involvement. Less than 0.2% of transplants in the United States are performed for cardiac sarcoidosis; outcomes are at least equivalent to those of other cardiac transplant patients.[85]

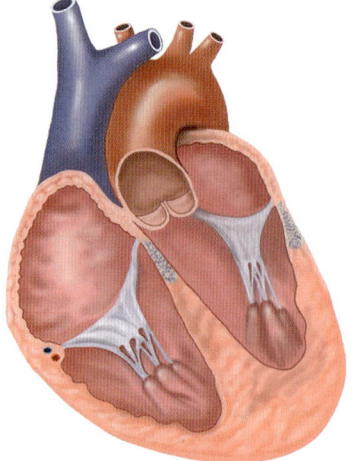
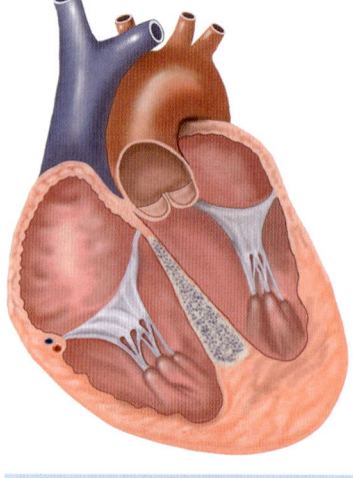
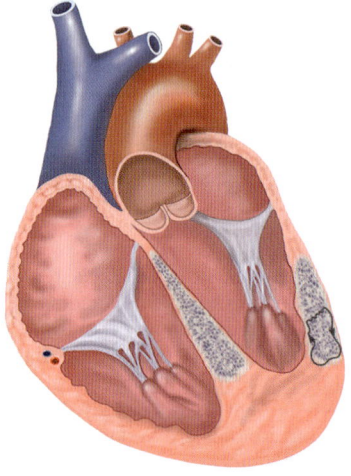
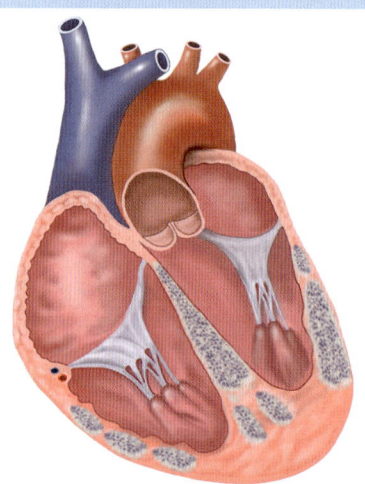

Small patches of basal involvement, usually clinically silent

Large area of septal involvement, often clinically manifest as heart block

Re-entrant circuit involving area of granuloma/fibrosis leading to VT

Extensive areas of LV and RV involvement, often clinically manifest as heart failure +/− heart block +/− VT

FIGURE 52.12 Illustrative examples of the extent of cardiac sarcoid pathologic changes in relation to clinical manifestations of the disease. (From Birnie DH, Nery PB, Ha AC, Beanlands RSB. Cardiac sarcoidosis. *J Am Coll Cardiol.* 2016;68:411–421.)

Fabry Disease

Fabry disease is caused by progressive lysosomal accumulation of neutral glycosphingolipids, primarily globotriaosylceramide; it results from deficiency of the enzyme alpha-galactosidase A, which is encoded by *GLA* on the X chromosome.[86] As an X-linked condition, most disease occurs in males with transmission by female carriers, although significant disease in later years can also be seen in women.[86–88] The disease phenotype encompasses diverse signs and symptoms with the following major manifestations: angiokeratomas, acroparesthesias, anhidrosis, ocular changes, and eventually cardiovascular, cerebrovascular, and renal disease, all largely related to the central pathophysiology of small-vessel vascular disease from the deposition of glycosphingolipid and consequent vascular insufficiency. The hallmark of the classic early-onset disease in males in childhood is episodic crises of severe pain in the extremities (acroparesthesias), characterized by burning pain in the distal end of the extremities, triggered by a variety of stressors, and resulting in ischemia of peripheral nerves from small-vessel disease. Angiokeratomas, red and purple punctate dermal lesions involving the lower midsection, buttocks, thighs, and upper part of the legs, may be one of the earliest signs of the disease and accumulate progressively with age. Anhidrosis is also an early finding in most cases. A survey of the phenotypic characteristics derived from a Fabry registry[87] showed that the age at onset and phenotypic variability were related to the degree of alpha-galactosidase A deficiency, with less than 1% of the activity associated with the earliest and most aggressive disease.[86–88]

Most morbid and mortal manifestations of Fabry disease are related to cardiovascular, cerebrovascular, and renal disease and occur in men in midlife who have had the classic phenotype and onset in early life, although the age at onset of advanced disease is variable and in some cases it may occur in the second and third decades. Cerebrovascular issues related to small-vessel disease include transient ischemic attacks and thrombosis resulting in stroke in up to a quarter of patients in a variety of locations, most commonly the posterior circulation. Cardiovascular involvement is not usually clinically apparent until the third or fourth decade, but eventually some manifestation of cardiovascular disease occurs in most patients. The most common finding is LV hypertrophy on echocardiography, although the degree of hypertrophy is mild in many cases in the third decade but is progressive with age. Worsening LV hypertrophy is associated with angina that occurs consequent to small-vessel disease, and epicardial coronary disease is uncommon. Findings on the ECG initially include a short PR interval and LV hypertrophy, with later evidence of heart block. Nonspecific intraventricular conduction delays are also seen. Bradycardia is common and a few patients will require pacemakers. Nonspecific ST-T changes are also common. Echocardiographic features range from mild to severe LV hypertrophy, the latter being more common in older patients, and mild to significant diastolic dysfunction. In most cases systolic function is normal, although heart failure has been reported with advanced disease. Palpitations and arrhythmia also occur.

Atypical phenotypes of Fabry disease have been categorized as cardiac or renal variants. Although most classic Fabry disease

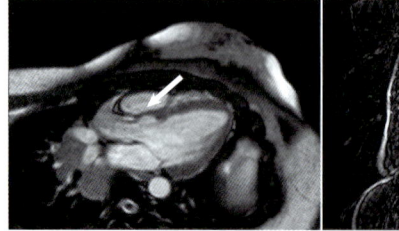
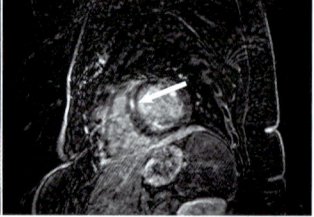

FIGURE 52.13 Cardiac MRI in a patient with sarcoidosis. Heart failure developed late in pregnancy and was initially diagnosed as peripartum cardiomyopathy (PPCM). Echocardiography revealed a reduced ejection fraction with the basal septal thinning typical of sarcoidosis. The appearance was confirmed on MRI (**left panel**, *arrow*). Delayed gadolinium uptake showed midmyocardial gadolinium uptake (**right panel**, *arrow*) consistent with sarcoidosis, which was subsequently confirmed on a biopsy specimen.

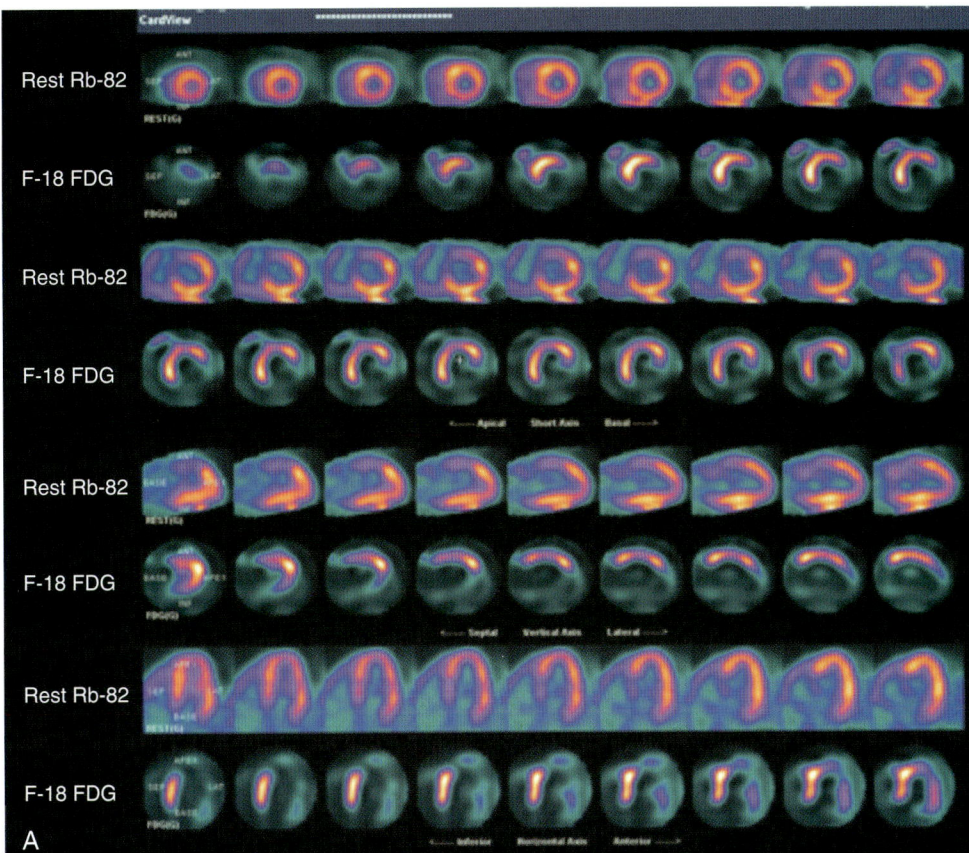

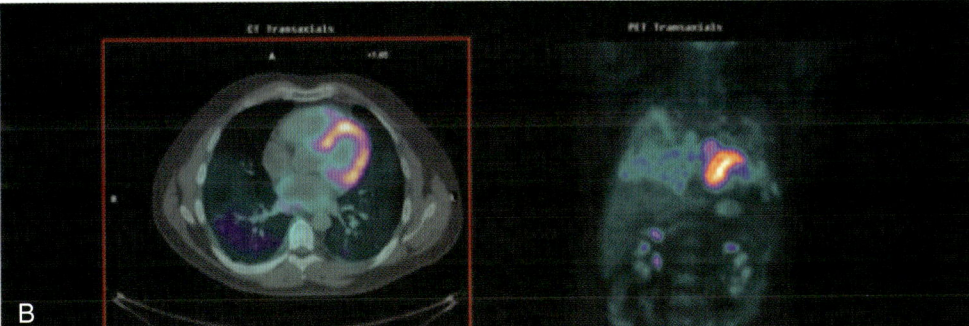

FIGURE 52.14 Positron emission tomography (PET) scan in a patient with sarcoidosis. A combined resting PET scan using rubidium-82 and ¹⁸F-FDG (a glucose analogue) is shown for a 53-year-old man with a history of pulmonary sarcoidosis who had palpitations and atrial flutter. **A,** From the top, each pair of images represents the rubidium-82 scan and, underneath it, the corresponding ¹⁸F-FDG image. The scans show a basal and midanteroseptal perfusion defect with intense FDG uptake in these regions suggestive of myocardial inflammation. Normal myocardium does not exhibit any FDG uptake because it is using free fatty acids. **B,** Combined CT-PET images in the same patient demonstrating the intense cardiac uptake. (Courtesy of Dr. Sharmila Dorbala, Brigham and Women's Hospital, Boston. From Dubrey SW, Falk RH. Diagnosis and management of cardiac sarcoidosis. *Prog Cardiovasc Dis.* 2010;52:336.)

is syndromic, as noted earlier, and in the vast majority of cases a diagnosis of Fabry disease will be established before referral for cardiovascular or renal consultation, occasionally patients will be referred to cardiovascular or renal specialists for organ-specific disease before the diagnosis of Fabry disease is made. The atypical cardiac variant phenotype has few or none of the classic signs and symptoms but rather may be manifested as unexplained LV hypertrophy in the sixth to eighth decades, at times accompanied by cardiomyopathy, mitral insufficiency, and mild proteinuria but minimal or no renal dysfunction. Because of its protean manifestations, the frequency of Fabry disease in patients who have unexplained LV hypertrophy consistent with a diagnosis of HCM has been investigated. In a study of 1386 patients at 13 European centers that included men and women older than 35 and 40 years, respectively, all with diagnoses of HCM, systematic screening for Fabry disease was performed by searching for *GLA* rare variants, and when identified, it was confirmed by alpha-galactosidase A levels.[89] Seven individuals (0.5%) were identified, four of the seven being women 45 to 72 years of age, all with significant LV hypertrophy (ranging from 15 to 22 mm). Only three had other signs of Fabry disease, most commonly angiokeratomas. Exclusion of rare variants in other genes encoding sarcomeric proteins known to cause HCM was not reported in this study, but comprehensive molecular (panel) testing for HCM would now identify sarcomeric variants, as well as *GLA* variants. Fabry disease has also been found in unexplained cardiomyopathy cases with gadolinium uptake where all other usual genetic causes have been excluded.[90]

The diagnosis of Fabry disease rests on showing reduced alpha-galactosidase A activity and molecular genetic testing for rare variants in *GLA*. An endomyocardial biopsy alpha-galactosidase A specimen showing inclusions in vascular endothelial cytoplasm on light or electron microscopy can also lead to the diagnosis. Because the cardiovascular findings in adults with Fabry disease usually include LV hypertrophy, in many cases a diagnosis of HCM is considered. Genetic testing with gene panels now includes *GLA* to ensure that atypical cases of Fabry disease will not be missed.

Importantly, treatment of Fabry disease is available as intravenous enzyme replacement therapy (ERT), which can arrest the deposition of globotriaosylceramide and in some cases reverse the disease phenotype, ameliorate symptoms, and restore organ function. For this reason, the diagnosis of Fabry disease is important, even though rarely encountered by most physicians.

Another commercially approved treatment for Fabry disease in an oral chaperone therapy called migalastat is a pharmacologic chaperone that reversibly binds to the active site of the alpha-galactosidase and stabilizes the protein, which allows it to be trafficked from the endoplasmic reticulum into the lysosome where it exerts its action. Migalastat is only approved for use in Fabry disease patients who have GLA variants that result in abnormally folded, less stable forms of the alpha-galactosidase A, so-called amenable variants. Newer approaches, including periodic administration of mRNA encoding human α-Gal A, are now in preclinical studies,[91] which if successful could expand therapeutic options.

Gaucher Disease and Glycogen Storage Diseases

Gaucher disease is an autosomal recessive glycogen storage disease that results from deficient beta-glucocerebrosidase enzyme activity caused by homozygous or compound heterozygous rare variants in *GBA*.[92] The clinical spectrum of disease varies greatly and ranges from a lethal acute perinatal form and a subacute juvenile form, both of which share major central nervous system disease, to a mostly asymptomatic adult form; all forms share splenomegaly, hepatomegaly, cytopenia, and pulmonary disease because of deposition of glucosylceramide in reticuloendothelial cells, including peripheral blood leukocytes. Cardiac involvement is uncommon to rare but has been reported in patients with allelic variants, with mitral and aortic valve calcification leading to valvular insufficiency and stenosis in the setting of corneal opacification and splenomegaly. Recurrent pericarditis resulting in constriction, as well as DCM with systolic dysfunction, has also been reported. ERT is now available, and in most cases will stabilize or reverse the disease process, thus accentuating the relevance of identifying Gaucher disease.

Hemochromatosis

Hemochromatosis is a disease caused by iron overload in which iron infiltrates major organs, especially the liver, heart, thyroid, gonads, skin, and pancreatic islet cells, to give the characteristic clinical findings of advanced disease that include cirrhosis, cardiomyopathy, diabetes, and endocrine disease. Hemochromatosis is categorized as hereditary (or primary) when arising from genetic disease or as secondary when caused by increased absorption associated with the thalassemias, sickle cell disease, or the sideroblastic anemias, or when related to excess blood transfusions for myelodysplasia or aplastic anemia. The content and distribution of iron are tightly regulated because of its toxicity and the inability of the body to excrete iron. Recent progress has been made in further understanding the molecular mechanisms of iron adsorption, use, storage, and recycling.[93]

HFE (hemochromatosis gene)-associated hereditary hemochromatosis is an autosomal recessive disease that in almost all cases results from the homozygous rare variant Cys282Tyr, although 3% to 8% of cases are compound heterozygotes for Cys282Tyr and His63Asp. The carrier frequency of the Cys282Tyr variant ranges as high as 11% in individuals of European descent, although the disease is twice as likely to develop in women and penetrance varies even with Cys282Tyr homozygotes.[94] A recent study with homozygous His63Asp showed only hypertension with minimal cardiac hypertrophy but without other adverse events.[95] The onset of clinical disease from iron overload is insidious, and signs and symptoms are insensitive and nonspecific. Screening tests include serum ferritin and percent transferrin saturation, with the accepted level being 200 ng/mL in women and 300 ng/mL in men or 45% in women and 50% in men. If both tests are negative, iron overload is effectively excluded. With elevated transferrin saturation, molecular genetic testing for *HFE* is indicated. With elevated transferrin saturation and ferritin levels higher than 1000, iron removal, usually by phlebotomy, is indicated, and evaluation of liver and cardiac function is indicated.

The cardiovascular findings of hemochromatosis, regardless of cause, are similar and may bring the patient to medical attention before diagnosis because of other organ system involvement in a minority of cases, so clinicians always need to consider hemochromatosis in the differential diagnosis of a nondilated cardiomyopathy with mild to moderate systolic dysfunction. Cardiovascular dysfunction begins with a restrictive nondilated phenotype that with advancing disease progresses to systolic dysfunction, mild to moderate LV dilation consistent with DCM, and then advanced disease and eventual heart failure.[96] In most cases, arrhythmias and conduction system disease accompany the progressive myocardial dysfunction and include AV and bundle branch blocks and bradyarrhythmias and tachyarrhythmias, some of which may result in syncope and sudden cardiac death. CMR has evolved to become a sensitive noninvasive diagnostic modality. A definitive tissue-based diagnosis of iron overload causing cardiac dysfunction can also be made by endomyocardial biopsy, which may be particularly useful if other testing is inconclusive or the degree of cardiovascular involvement by hemochromatosis is confounded by other cardiovascular disease (e.g., coronary disease). Definitive treatment is centered on iron removal, usually by phlebotomy in *HFE*-associated hereditary hemochromatosis, and as iron stores are depleted, cardiac function will improve in most cases, sometimes to a dramatic degree. Cardiac transplantation can be avoided in most patients with timely diagnosis and phlebotomy.

Endomyocardial Disease

The endomyocardial diseases, another cause of RCM, are unified by the finding of endocardial fibrosis. Several conditions share the pathologic end phenotype of fibrosis of the endocardium, but no unifying hypothesis for this pathology has emerged, and each condition may have its own distinctive cause. *Endomyocardial fibrosis* (EMF), a disease first described in Uganda in 1948 (initially termed tropical endocardial disease or endocardial fibroelastosis [EFE]), may well be the most common cause of RCM worldwide.[97] Although only rarely observed in North America, related conditions that pathologically resemble EMF include Löffler endocarditis, usually observed in adults, or the distinctly different onset of neonatal endocardial fibroelastosis associated with hypoplastic left-heart syndrome and other congenital heart disease or in utero mumps infection. EFE, recently recapitulated in a model system,[98] can be differentiated from EMF by its epidemiology and more diffuse involvement of the left ventricle, whereas endocardial fibrosis more involves the RV and LV apices and subvalvular apparatus. Neonatal EFE has been observed in a few families, and a genetic cause has been considered, and the X-linked *Barth syndrome* (see OMIM 302060) is categorized as a DCM with associated EFE, a proximal skeletal myop-athy, and growth retardation.

Carcinoid Heart Disease

Carcinoid heart disease is a rare condition that occurs as part of carcinoid syndrome, a systemic disorder mediated by elevated circulating levels of vasoactive substances, including serotonin (5-hydroxytryptamine [5-HT]), 5-hydroxytryptophan, histamine, bradykinin, tachykinins, and prostaglandins produced by a rare metastatic neuroendocrine malig-nancy, carcinoid.[99] *Carcinoid syndrome* is characterized by a triad of symptoms—flushing, diarrhea, and bronchospasm—that occur in association with hepatic metastases. The metastases produce high levels of these vasoactive substances, particularly 5-HT, which reaches the systemic circulation via the hepatic vein. High levels in the right side of the heart cause progressive fibrotic endocardial plaque.[100] Inactivation in the lung to hydroxyindoleacetic acid (5-HIAA) generally protects the left-sided heart structures, but these structures may become involved if levels are very high or if a patent foramen ovale allows right-to-left shunting.[101] Carcinoid heart disease has also very rarely been described in association with nonmetastatic ovarian cancer.

The characteristic pathologic features of carcinoid heart disease are right-sided valve thickening and retraction resulting from myofibroblast proliferation along with deposition of collagen and smooth muscle cells. Tricuspid annular and subvalvar involvement and pulmonary root constriction also occur, thereby adding to the valvular dysfunction. Very rarely the heart is involved directly by carcinoid metastases.[99] Physical examination reveals evidence of RV volume and pressure overload with murmurs of tricuspid and pulmonary regurgitation and stenosis. In the late stage of the disease, peripheral edema and ascites with low cardiac output occur, although the valvular disease may be hemodynamically severe before significant clinical deterioration takes place. Symptoms of right-sided heart failure in the setting of known carcinoid syndrome are highly suggestive of carcinoid heart disease, but cardiac involvement may occasionally be the initial feature of carcinoid syndrome. Chest radiography and electrocardiography are generally unrevealing in carcinoid heart disease. Elevation of urinary 5-HIAA levels is highly specific and moderately sensitive for the diagnosis of carcinoid syndrome, and the echocardiographic and CMR features of thickened immobile tricuspid and pulmonary valves with combined stenosis and regurgitant lesions are highly suggestive of carcinoid heart disease.[102]

Untreated patients with carcinoid syndrome have a median survival time of 3 to 4 years, and the presence of carcinoid heart disease shortens this to less than 1 year.[99] Therapy is not generally curative and includes debulking the hepatic metastases by embolization or partial hepatic resection and by the use of octreotide, a somatostatin analogue that binds to somatostatin receptors on the surface of carcinoid tumor cells and inhibits the secretion of vasoactive substances. Newer treatment includes radiation therapy delivered by peptide receptor-linked radiotherapy.[103] Although the development and progression of carcinoid heart disease are associated with increasing 5-HIAA levels,[104,105] a decrease in 5-HIAA levels afterward does not appear to cause a change in the cardiac valvular lesions, and they may even progress. Valve replacement in carcinoid heart disease can be performed successfully[101] but carries unique challenges, such as the development of an *acute carcinoid crisis* characterized by profound hypotension, severe flushing bronchoconstriction, and arrhythmias. Thus a surgical and anesthetic team knowledgeable about the condition and working with an endocrinologist, both intraoperatively and perioperatively, is of critical importance. Once advanced carcinoid valve disease is recognized on echocardiography, surgery is recommended even in the absence of significant right-sided heart dysfunction; patients who have undergone surgery are believed to be likely to have a more favorable outcome.[99]

Löffler (Eosinophilic) Endocarditis

Löffler endocarditis occurs within the spectrum of the hypereosinophilic conditions in which increased numbers of eosinophils invade and damage tissues in a variety of organs, including the endocardium and myocardium, by releasing highly active biologic substances. The cause of the eosinophilia in Löffler endocarditis includes known and idiopathic causes, such as a broad spectrum of helminthic or other parasitic infections, malignancy including carcinoma or eosinophilic leukemia, and allergy including drug reactions, all of which may have associated hypereosinophilia, as well as idiopathic hypereosinophilia syndrome. Hypereosinophilia has been defined as either a chronic absolute eosinophil count higher than 1500 cells/mL for at least 1 month, although hypereosinophilia persisting for 6 months or longer is common, or pathologic evidence of hypereosinophilic tissue invasion. One family has been reported with autosomal dominant transmission linked to 5q31-q33, and more recently, hypereosinophilia syndrome in the setting of myeloproliferative disease has responded to tyrosine kinase inhibitors, but a unifying genetic or environmental hypothesis is not yet available.

Hypereosinophilic syndromes affecting the heart, although rare, when present cause considerable morbidity and mortality. Some cases of myocardial hypereosinophilic disease may be identified at endomyocardial biopsy during evaluation for idiopathic RCM, and in such situations a thorough evaluation for an underlying cause should be completed. Regardless of cause, eosinophilic-mediated cardiac disease has been categorized into three stages: acute, intermediate, and fibrotic. In the acute phase, usually characterized by few or no signs or symptoms, eosinophils invade the myocardium, degranulate, and aided by lymphocytes, cause intense myocardial inflammation and eventually myocardial necrosis. Even though findings on echocardiography may be normal during this phase, contrast-enhanced CMR can detect disease,[106,107] and myocardial biomarkers may be elevated to variable degrees. In the second stage, thrombus favoring the apices covers the affected endocardium. Symptoms include chest pain or dyspnea. Other evidence of disease includes mitral or tricuspid valvular regurgitation, cardiomegaly, and heart failure. Embolism of endocardial thrombus to the brain or other organs is common and may be the initial feature of the disease. The ECG may show T wave inversions, and imaging studies will reveal mural thrombus in affected areas, at times so extensive that large portions of the myocardial chamber are obliterated with clot. The third fibrotic phase progresses with diffuse scarring that results in endocardial fibrosis and RCM. The scar process commonly involves the mitral and tricuspid subvalvular structures; it impairs their mobility and leads to valvular regurgitation. Valve leaflet scarring can also occur. If disease can be identified in the first stage, therapy is focused on treatment of the underlying condition. Corticosteroids and cytolytic therapies have been used with some response. The fibrotic stage needs to be addressed surgically by valve release, repair, or replacement and by resection of the endocardial scar to mitigate the restrictive nature of the endocardial fibrosis.

Endomyocardial Fibrosis

EMF, an unusual disease in North America but common in Africa, is characterized by fibrosis of the LV and RV apical endocardium causing an RCM.[97] First reported in Uganda, it has been found in tropical regions of Africa, the south Asian subcontinent, and Brazil, although it is also found in subtropical Africa and some cases occur rarely in moderate climates, including North America. A population prevalence of approximately 20% in rural Mozambique has been reported,[108] with more males affected than females (23% vs. 17%). In addition, family clustering was identified in this study, although whether this was related to environmental exposure common to the family units selected for study, to a genetic predisposition, or to both was not addressed. A bimodal peak in age has been noted in several studies, with onset in the first decade and a second peak occurring in the second to fourth decades of life.

The cause of EMF remains unknown, but its pathology resembles that of other conditions in North America that are more commonly encountered, such as eosinophilic cardiomyopathy or hypereosinophilic syndrome, discussed earlier. However, elevated eosinophil counts in peripheral blood or cardiac tissue from endomyocardial biopsy have seldom been observed in EMF. Although one or more infectious agents could be causal, no consistent unifying infectious cause has been established. Environmental exposure to cerium, a rare element present in affected areas, has also been considered. Family-based disease has been observed in several reports, but whether familial predisposition is related to environmental or genetic causes, or to both, remains unknown.

In most cases heart failure symptoms from left or right restrictive physiology predominate the clinical findings and include dyspnea on exertion, paroxysmal nocturnal dyspnea, and edema. Ascites, at times a prominent feature, is common to all the endomyocardial diseases. Cardiovascular imaging shows restrictive filling with apical fibrosis that commonly involves the mitral and tricuspid subvalvular apparatus, accompanied by atrial enlargement. As noted earlier, successful surgical resection of the endocardial fibrosis with valve repair or replacement can have a dramatic effect on symptoms and survival, although the operation itself is associated with a significant risk for morbidity and mortality.

FUTURE PERSPECTIVES

Enormous progress has recently been made in understanding the genetic basis of cardiomyopathy, accelerated in large part by large panel and genome-wide next-generation sequencing strategies. The genomic information reviewed herein, limited in most cases by numbers of well-phenotyped individuals with rare variant surveys of only a few known genes, will give way to comprehensive genome-wide strategies to identify and understand rare and common variants relevant to disease susceptibility and cause, including structural and other nonprotein coding genomic variants, in much larger populations. This will enable a more comprehensive and insightful understanding of the genomic basis of human disease. Our present rudimentary understandings of "mendelian genetics," likely an oversimplified concept of "single-gene" genetics for many of the cases of DCM and ARVC, in the next few years will evolve into greater insight to the complexity that likely underlies the cardiomyopathies.

REFERENCES
The Dilated Cardiomyopathies
1. Maron BJ, Towbin JA, Thiene G, et al. Contemporary definitions and classification of the cardiomyopathies: an American Heart Association scientific statement from the council on clinical cardiology, heart failure and transplantation committee; quality of care and outcomes research and functional genomics and translational biology interdisciplinary working groups; and council on epidemiology and prevention. *Circulation.* 2006;113:1807–1816.
2. Elliott P, Andersson B, Arbustini E, et al. Classification of the cardiomyopathies: a position statement from the European Society of Cardiology working group on myocardial and pericardial diseases. *Eur Heart J.* 2008;29:270–276.
3. Hershberger RE, Cowan J, Morales A, Siegfried JD. Progress with genetic cardiomyopathies: screening, counseling, and testing in dilated, hypertrophic, and arrhythmogenic right ventricular dysplasia/cardiomyopathy. *Circ Heart Fail.* 2009;2:253–261.
4. Hershberger RE, Givertz M, Ho CY, et al. Genetic evaluation of cardiomyopathy—a heart failure society of America practice guideline. *J Card Fail.* 2018;24(5):281–302.
5. Hershberger RE, Givertz MM, Ho CY, et al. Genetic evaluation of cardiomyopathy: a clinical practice resource of the American College of Medical Genetics and Genomics (ACMG). *Genet Med.* 2018;20:899–909.
6. Piran S, Liu P, Morales A, Hershberger RE. Where genome meets phenome: rationale for integrating genetic and protein biomarkers in the diagnosis and management of dilated cardiomyopathy and heart failure. *J Am Coll Cardiol.* 2012;60:283–289.
7. Carruth ED, Young W, Beer D, et al. Prevalence and electronic health record-based phenotype of loss-of-function genetic variants in arrhythmogenic right ventricular cardiomyopathy-associated genes. *Circ Genom Precis Med.* 2019;12:e002579.

8. Cowan JR, Kinnamon DD, Morales A, et al. Multigenic disease and bilineal inheritance in dilated cardiomyopathy is illustrated in nonsegregating LMNA pedigrees. *Circ Genom Precis Med*. 2018;11:e002038.
9. Ware JS, Amor-Salamanca A, Tayal U, et al. Genetic etiology for alcohol-induced cardiac toxicity. *J Am Coll Cardiol*. 2018;71:2293–2302.
10. Garcia-Pavia P, Kim Y, Restrepo-Cordoba MA, et al. Genetic variants associated with cancer therapy-induced cardiomyopathy. *Circulation*. 2019;140:31–41.
11. Hershberger RE, Hedges DJ, Morales A. Dilated cardiomyopathy: the complexity of a diverse genetic architecture. *Nat Rev Cardiol*. 2013;10:531–547.
12. Morales A, Kinnamon DD, Jordan E, et al. Variant interpretation for dilated cardiomyopathy: refinement of the American College of Medical Genetics and Genomics/ClinGen guidelines for the DCM precision medicine study. *Circ Genom Precis Med*. 2020;13:e002480.
13. Hershberger RE, Morales A, Siegfried JD. Clinical and genetic issues in dilated cardiomyopathy: a review for genetics professionals. *Genet Med*. 2010;12:655–667.
14. Kinnamon DD, Morales A, Bowen DJ, et al. Toward genetics-driven early intervention in dilated cardiomyopathy: design and implementation of the DCM precision medicine study. *Circ Cardiovasc Genet*. 2017;10:e001826.
15. Gulati A, Ismail TF, Jabbour A, et al. The prevalence and prognostic significance of right ventricular systolic dysfunction in nonischemic dilated cardiomyopathy. *Circulation*. 2013;128:1623–1633.
16. Donal E, Delgado V, Bucciarelli-Ducci C, et al. Multimodality imaging in the diagnosis, risk stratification, and management of patients with dilated cardiomyopathies: an expert consensus document from the European Association of Cardiovascular Imaging. *Eur Heart J Cardiovasc Imaging*. 2019;20:1075–1093.
17. Burkett EL, Hershberger RE. Clinical and genetic issues in familial dilated cardiomyopathy. *J Am Coll Cardiol*. 2005;45:969–981.
18. Mazzarotto F, Tayal U, Buchan RJ, et al. Reevaluating the genetic contribution of monogenic dilated cardiomyopathy. *Circulation*. 2020;141:387–398.
19. Herman DS, Lam L, Taylor MR, et al. Truncations of titin causing dilated cardiomyopathy. *N Engl J Med*. 2012;366:619–628.
20. Ware JS, Li J, Mazaika E, et al. Shared genetic predisposition in peripartum and dilated cardiomyopathies. *N Engl J Med*. 2016;374:233–241.
21. Haggerty CM, Damrauer SM, Levin MG, et al. Genomics-first evaluation of heart disease associated with titin-truncating variants. *Circulation*. 2019;140:42–54.
22. Morales A, Hershberger RE. The rationale and timing of molecular genetic testing for dilated cardiomyopathy. *Can J Cardiol*. 2015;31:1309–1312.
23. Menon S, Michels V, Pellikka P, et al. Cardiac troponin T mutation in familial cardiomyopathy with variable remodeling and restrictive physiology. *Clin Genet*. 2008;74:445–454.
24. Hershberger RE, Siegfried JD. State of the Art Review. Update 2011: clinical and genetic issues in familial dilated cardiomyopathy. *J Am Coll Cardiol*. 2011;57:1641–1649.
25. James CA, Calkins H. Arrhythmogenic right ventricular cardiomyopathy: progress toward personalized management. *Annu Rev Med*. 2019;70:1–18.
26. Towbin JA, McKenna WJ, Abrams DJ, et al. 2019 HRS expert consensus statement on evaluation, risk stratification, and management of arrhythmogenic cardiomyopathy. *Heart Rhythm*. 2019;16:e301–e372.
27. Elliott PM, Anastasakis A, Asimaki A, et al. Definition and treatment of arrhythmogenic cardiomyopathy: an updated expert panel report. *Eur J Heart Fail*. 2019;21:955–964.
28. Corrado D, Basso C, Judge DP. Arrhythmogenic cardiomyopathy. *Circ Res*. 2017;121:784–802.
29. Te Riele AS, James CA, Philips B, et al. Mutation-positive arrhythmogenic right ventricular dysplasia/cardiomyopathy: the triangle of dysplasia displaced. *J Cardiovasc Electrophysiol*. 2013;24:1311–1320.
30. Hauer RN, Cox MG, Groeneweg JA. Impact of new electrocardiographic criteria in arrhythmogenic cardiomyopathy. *Front Physiol*. 2012;3:352.
31. Swope D, Li J, Radice GL. Beyond cell adhesion: the role of armadillo proteins in the heart. *Cell Signal*. 2013;25:93–100.
32. ClinGen Cardiovascular Domain Working Group.
33. te Riele AS, James CA, Rastegar N, et al. Yield of serial evaluation in at-risk family members of patients with ARVD/C. *J Am Coll Cardiol*. 2014;64:293–301.
34. den Haan AD, Tan BY, Zikusoka MN, et al. Comprehensive desmosome mutation analysis in North Americans with arrhythmogenic right ventricular dysplasia/cardiomyopathy. *Circ Cardiovasc Genet*. 2009;2:428–435.
35. Quarta G, Muir A, Pantazis A, et al. Familial evaluation in arrhythmogenic right ventricular cardiomyopathy: impact of genetics and revised task force criteria. *Circulation*. 2011;123:2701–2709.
36. Groeneweg JA, Bhonsale A, James CA, et al. Clinical presentation, long-term follow-up, and outcomes of 1001 arrhythmogenic right ventricular dysplasia/cardiomyopathy patients and family members. *Circ Cardiovasc Genet*. 2015;8:437–446.
37. Bosman LP, Sammani A, James CA, et al. Predicting arrhythmic risk in arrhythmogenic right ventricular cardiomyopathy: a systematic review and meta-analysis. *Heart Rhythm*. 2018;15:1097–1107.
38. Corrado D, Wichter T, Link MS, et al. Treatment of arrhythmogenic right ventricular cardiomyopathy/dysplasia: an international task force consensus statement. *Circulation*. 2015;132:441–453.
39. Santangeli P, Zado ES, Supple GE, et al. Long-term outcome with catheter ablation of ventricular tachycardia in patients with arrhythmogenic right ventricular cardiomyopathy. *Circ Arrhythm Electrophysiol*. 2015;8:1413–1421.
40. James CA, Bhonsale A, Tichnell C, et al. Exercise increases age-related penetrance and arrhythmic risk in arrhythmogenic right ventricular dysplasia/cardiomyopathy-associated desmosomal mutation carriers. *J Am Coll Cardiol*. 2013;62:1290–1297.
41. Guzzo-Merello G, Segovia J, Dominguez F, et al. Natural history and prognostic factors in alcoholic cardiomyopathy. *JACC Heart Fail*. 2015;3:78–86.
42. Jia G, Hill MA, Sowers JR. Diabetic cardiomyopathy: an update of mechanisms contributing to this clinical entity. *Circ Res*. 2018;122:624–638.
43. Fitchett D, Zinman B, Wanner C, et al. Heart failure outcomes with empagliflozin in patients with type 2 diabetes at high cardiovascular risk: results of the EMPA-REG OUTCOME(R) trial. *Eur Heart J*. 2016;37:1526–1534.
44. Sen-Chowdhry S, McKenna WJ. Left ventricular noncompaction and cardiomyopathy: cause, contributor, or epiphenomenon? *Curr Opin Cardiol*. 2008;23:171–175.
45. Kohli SK, Pantazis AA, Shah JS, et al. Diagnosis of left-ventricular non-compaction in patients with left-ventricular systolic dysfunction: time for a reappraisal of diagnostic criteria? *Eur Heart J*. 2008;29:89–95.
46. Arbustini E, Weidemann F, Hall JL. Left ventricular noncompaction: a distinct cardiomyopathy or a trait shared by different cardiac diseases? *J Am Coll Cardiol*. 2014;64:1840–1850.
47. Anderson RH, Jensen B, Mohun TJ, et al. Key questions relating to left ventricular noncompaction cardiomyopathy: is the emperor still wearing any clothes? *Can J Cardiol*. 2017;33:747–757.
48. Hershberger RE, Morales A, Cowan J. Is left ventricular noncompaction a trait, phenotype, or disease? The evidence points to phenotype. *Circ Cardiovasc Genet*. 2017;10.
49. Ross SB, Jones K, Blanch B, et al. A systematic review and meta-analysis of the prevalence of left ventricular non-compaction in adults. *Eur Heart J*. 2020;41:1428–1436.
50. Gopinathannair R, Etheridge SP, Marchlinski FE, et al. Arrhythmia-induced cardiomyopathies: mechanisms, recognition, and management. *J Am Coll Cardiol*. 2015;66:1714–1728.
51. Medi C, Kalman JM, Haqqani H, et al. Tachycardia-mediated cardiomyopathy secondary to focal atrial tachycardia: long-term outcome after catheter ablation. *J Am Coll Cardiol*. 2009;53:1791–1797.
52. Hasdemir C, Ulucan C, Yavuzgil O, et al. Tachycardia-induced cardiomyopathy in patients with idiopathic ventricular arrhythmias: the incidence, clinical and electrophysiologic characteristics, and the predictors. *J Cardiovasc Electrophysiol*. 2011;22:663–668.
53. Dandamudi G, Rampurwala AY, Mahenthiran J, et al. Persistent left ventricular dilatation in tachycardia-induced cardiomyopathy patients after appropriate treatment and normalization of ejection fraction. *Heart Rhythm*. 2008;5:1111–1114.
54. Selby DE, Palmer BM, LeWinter MM, Meyer M. Tachycardia-induced diastolic dysfunction and resting tone in myocardium from patients with a normal ejection fraction. *J Am Coll Cardiol*. 2011;58:147–154.
55. Morales A, Painter T, Li R, et al. Rare variant mutations in pregnancy-associated or peripartum cardiomyopathy. *Circulation*. 2010;121:2176–2182.
56. van Spaendonck-Zwarts KY, van Tintelen JP, van Veldhuisen DJ, et al. Peripartum cardiomyopathy as a part of familial dilated cardiomyopathy. *Circulation*. 2010;121:2169–2175.
57. Davis MB, Arany Z, McNamara DM, et al. Peripartum cardiomyopathy: JACC state-of-the-art review. *J Am Coll Cardiol*. 2020;75:207–221.
58. Elkayam U, Tummala PP, Rao K, et al. Maternal and fetal outcomes of subsequent pregnancies in women with peripartum cardiomyopathy. *N Engl J Med*. 2001;344:1567–1571.
59. Ghadri JR, Wittstein IS, Prasad A, et al. International expert consensus document on takotsubo syndrome (Part I): clinical characteristics, diagnostic criteria, and pathophysiology. *Eur Heart J*. 2018;39:2032–2046.
60. Ghadri JR, Wittstein IS, Prasad A, et al. International expert consensus document on takotsubo syndrome (Part II): diagnostic workup, outcome, and management. *Eur Heart J*. 2018;39:2047–2062.
61. Templin C, Ghadri JR, Diekmann J, et al. Clinical features and outcomes of takotsubo (stress) cardiomyopathy. *N Engl J Med*. 2015;373:929–938.
62. Cammann VL, Szawan KA, Stahli BE, et al. Age-related variations in takotsubo syndrome. *J Am Coll Cardiol*. 2020;75:1869–1877.
63. Syed FF, Asirvatham SJ, Francis J. Arrhythmia occurrence with takotsubo cardiomyopathy: a literature review. *Europace*. 2011;13:780–788.

Restrictive Cardiomyopathies

64. Stollberger C, Finsterer J. Extracardiac medical and neuromuscular implications in restrictive cardiomyopathy. *Clin Cardiol*. 2007;30:375–380.
65. Kaski JP, Syrris P, Burch M, et al. Idiopathic restrictive cardiomyopathy in children is caused by mutations in cardiac sarcomere protein genes. *Heart*. 2008;94:1478–1484.
66. Caleshu C, Sakhuja R, Nussbaum RL, et al. Furthering the link between the sarcomere and primary cardiomyopathies: restrictive cardiomyopathy associated with multiple mutations in genes previously associated with hypertrophic or dilated cardiomyopathy. *Am J Med Genet*. 2011;155A:2229–2235.
67. Webber SA, Lipshultz SE, Sleeper LA, et al. Outcomes of restrictive cardiomyopathy in childhood and the influence of phenotype: a report from the Pediatric Cardiomyopathy Registry. *Circulation*. 2012;126:1237–1244.
68. Depasquale EC, Nasir K, Jacoby DL. Outcomes of adults with restrictive cardiomyopathy after heart transplantation. *J Heart Lung Transplant*. 2012;31:1269–1275.
69. Gallego-Delgado M, Delgado JF, Brossa-Loidi V, et al. Idiopathic restrictive cardiomyopathy is primarily a genetic disease. *J Am Coll Cardiol*. 2016;67:3021–3023.
70. Talreja DR, Edwards WD, Danielson GK, et al. Constrictive pericarditis in 26 patients with histologically normal pericardial thickness. *Circulation*. 2003;108:1852–1857.
71. Ammash NM, Seward JB, Bailey KR, et al. Clinical profile and outcome of idiopathic restrictive cardiomyopathy. *Circulation*. 2000;101:2490–2496.
72. Pereira NL, Grogan M, Dec GW. Spectrum of restrictive and infiltrative cardiomyopathies: Part 1 of a 2-part series. *J Am Coll Cardiol*. 2018;71:1130–1148.
73. Patel MR, Cawley PJ, Heitner JF, et al. Detection of myocardial damage in patients with sarcoidosis. *Circulation*. 2009;120:1969–1977.
74. Bagwan IN, Hooper LV, Sheppard MN. Cardiac sarcoidosis and sudden death. The heart may look normal or mimic other cardiomyopathies. *Virchows Arch*. 2011;458:671–678.
75. Vasaiwala SC, Finn C, Delpriore J, et al. Prospective study of cardiac sarcoid mimicking arrhythmogenic right ventricular dysplasia. *J Cardiovasc Electrophysiol*. 2009;20:473–476.
76. Kerkar A, Hazard F, Caleshu C, et al. Pathological overlap of arrhythmogenic right ventricular cardiomyopathy and cardiac sarcoidosis. *Circ Genom Precis Med*. 2019;12:452–454.
77. Murtagh G, Laffin LJ, Beshai JF, et al. Prognosis of myocardial damage in sarcoidosis patients with preserved left ventricular ejection fraction: risk stratification using cardiovascular magnetic resonance. *Circ Cardiovasc Imaging*. 2016;9:e003738.
78. Gupta A, Singh Gulati G, Seth S, Sharma S. Cardiac MRI in restrictive cardiomyopathy. *Clin Radiol*. 2012;67:95–105.
79. Ramirez R, Trivieri M, Fayad ZA, et al. Advanced imaging in cardiac sarcoidosis. *J Nucl Med*. 2019;60:892–898.
80. Birnie D, Beanlands RSB, Nery P, et al. Cardiac sarcoidosis multi-center randomized controlled trial (CHASM CS- RCT). *Am Heart J*. 2020;220:246–252.
81. Sadek MM, Yung D, Birnie DH, et al. Corticosteroid therapy for cardiac sarcoidosis: a systematic review. *Can J Cardiol*. 2013;29:1034–1041.
82. Cremers JP, Drent M, Bast A, et al. Multinational evidence-based World Association of Sarcoidosis and Other Granulomatous Disorders recommendations for the use of methotrexate in sarcoidosis: integrating systematic literature research and expert opinion of sarcoidologists worldwide. *Curr Opin Pulm Med*. 2013;19:545–561.
83. Birnie DH, Nery PB, Ha AC, Beanlands RS. Cardiac sarcoidosis. *J Am Coll Cardiol*. 2016;68:411–421.
84. Perkel D, Czer LS, Morrissey RP, et al. Heart transplantation for end-stage heart failure due to cardiac sarcoidosis. *Transplant Proc*. 2013;45:2384–2386.
85. Halawa A, Jain R, Turagam MK, et al. Outcome of implantable cardioverter defibrillator in cardiac sarcoidosis: a systematic review and meta-analysis. *J Interv Card Electrophysiol*. 2020.
86. Mehta A, Hughes DA. Fabry Disease. 1993.
87. Eng CM, Fletcher J, Wilcox WR, et al. Fabry disease: baseline medical characteristics of a cohort of 1765 males and females in the Fabry Registry. *J Inherit Metab Dis*. 2007;30:184–192.
88. Wilcox WR, Oliveira JP, Hopkin RJ, et al. Females with Fabry disease frequently have major organ involvement: lessons from the Fabry Registry. *Mol Genet Metab*. 2008;93:112–128.
89. Elliott P, Baker R, Pasquale F, et al. Prevalence of Anderson-Fabry disease in patients with hypertrophic cardiomyopathy: the European Anderson-Fabry Disease survey. *Heart*. 2011;97:1957–1960.
90. Moonen A, Lal S, Ingles J, et al. Prevalence of Anderson-Fabry disease in a cohort with unexplained late gadolinium enhancement on cardiac MRI. *Int J Cardiol*. 2020;304:122–124.
91. Zhu X, Yin L, Theisen M, et al. Systemic mRNA therapy for the treatment of Fabry disease: preclinical studies in wild-type mice, fabry mouse model, and wild-type non-human primates. *Am J Hum Genet*. 2019;104:625–637.
92. Pastores GM, Hughes DA. Gaucher Disease. 1993.
93. Fleming RE, Ponka P. Iron overload in human disease. *N Engl J Med*. 2012;366:348–359.

94. Barton JC, Edwards CQ. HFE Hemochromatosis. *GeneReviews(R)*; 2000. Apr 3 [Updated 2018 Dec 6].
95. Selvaraj S, Seidelmann S, Silvestre OM, et al. HFE H63D polymorphism and the risk for systemic hypertension, myocardial remodeling, and adverse cardiovascular events in the ARIC study. *Hypertension*. 2019;73:68–74.
96. Murphy CJ, Oudit GY. Iron-overload cardiomyopathy: pathophysiology, diagnosis, and treatment. *J Card Fail*. 2010;16:888–900.
97. Mocumbi AO, Stothard JR, Correia-de-Sa P, Yacoub M. Endomyocardial fibrosis: an update after 70 years. *Curr Cardiol Rep*. 2019;21:148.
98. Friehs I, Illigens B, Melnychenko I, et al. An animal model of endocardial fibroelastosis. *J Surg Res*. 2012.
99. Davar J, Connolly HM, Caplin ME, et al. Diagnosing and managing carcinoid heart disease in patients with neuroendocrine tumors: an expert statement. *J Am Coll Cardiol*. 2017;69:1288–1304.
100. Bhattacharyya S, Davar J, Dreyfus G, Caplin ME. Carcinoid heart disease. *Circulation*. 2007;116:2860–2865.
101. Castillo JG, Silvay G, Solis J. Current concepts in diagnosis and perioperative management of carcinoid heart disease. *Semin CardioThorac Vasc Anesth*. 2012.
102. Agha AM, Lopez-Mattei J, Donisan T, et al. Multimodality imaging in carcinoid heart disease. *Open Heart*. 2019;6:e001060.
103. Davis LM, Nicou N, Martin W, et al. Timing of peptide receptor radiotargeted therapy in relation to cardiac valve surgery for carcinoid heart disease in patients with neuroendocrine metastases and cardiac syndrome. A single-centre study from a centre of excellence. *Nucl Med Commun*. 2020;41:575–581.
104. Bhattacharyya S, Toumpanakis C, Chilkunda D, et al. Risk factors for the development and progression of carcinoid heart disease. *Am J Cardiol*. 2011;107:1221–1226.
105. Buchanan-Hughes A, Pashley A, Feuilly M, et al. Carcinoid heart disease: prognostic value of 5-hydroxyindoleacetic acid levels and impact on survival—a systematic literature review. *Neuroendocrinology*. 2021;111:1–15.
106. Debl K, Djavidani B, Buchner S, et al. Time course of eosinophilic myocarditis visualized by CMR. *J Cardiovasc Magn Reson*. 2008;10:21.
107. Qureshi N, Amin F, Chatterjee D, et al. MR imaging of endomyocardial fibrosis (EMF). *Int J Cardiol*. 2011;149:e36–e37.
108. Mocumbi AO, Ferreira MB, Sidi D, Yacoub MH. A population study of endomyocardial fibrosis in a rural area of Mozambique. *N Engl J Med*. 2008;359:43–49.

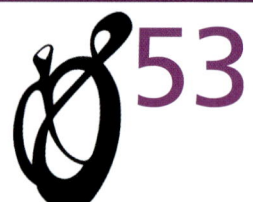

53 Cardiac Amyloidosis

FREDERICK L. RUBERG AND MATHEW S. MAURER

EPIDEMIOLOGY, 1052
Light Chain Amyloidosis, 1052
Transthyretin Amyloidosis, 1052

PATHOPHYSIOLOGY, 1053

CLINICAL FEATURES AND PROGNOSIS, 1054

Prognosis, 1054

DIAGNOSIS, 1055

CLINICAL MANAGEMENT, 1058
Supportive Non–Disease-Modifying Therapies, 1058
Disease-Targeted Therapeutics, 1058

CONCLUSION, 1060

REFERENCES, 1060

The systemic amyloidoses are a group of diseases characterized by the extracellular deposition of insoluble, misfolded fibrillar proteins in the form of β-pleated sheets, resulting in organ dysfunction. First applied to human disease by Rudolph Virchow in 1854, amyloid derives its name from the Latin amylum or starch, because amyloid was initially and erroneously thought to be composed of cellulose owing to a positive iodine-staining reaction. Amyloid deposits evaluated by electron microscopy demonstrated that amyloid fibrils are nonbranching protein structures, 80 to 100 Angstroms in width and of variable length. They are resistant to proteolysis. Amyloid fibrils avidly bind to the histologic stain Congo red imparting a hyaline pink appearance under light microscopy, while under polarized light, fibrils reflect a characteristic apple-green birefringence.[1] Precursor protein identification is essential to define the type of amyloidosis, inform prognosis, and guide therapy. The taxonomy is defined by abbreviating the type with an A (for amyloid) followed by a protein abbreviation.[2] The two most common types of amyloidosis that affect the heart are light chain (AL) amyloidosis and transthyretin (ATTR) amyloidosis. ATTR amyloidosis is further subclassified by the sequence of the *TTR* gene, which resides on chromosome 18. Hereditary or variant transthyretin amyloidosis (hATTR or ATTRv) results from single nucleotide polymorphisms of the *TTR* gene and are inherited in an autosomal dominant fashion. In ATTRv, amino acid substitution results in a destabilization and misfolding process that leads to amyloidogenesis. Historical nomenclature places a one- or three-letter abbreviation for the normal amino acid at the position of substitution in the protein followed by the substituted amino acid (e.g., ATTR Val122Ile signifies isoleucine replacing valine at position 122 in the TTR amino acid sequence). More contemporary nomenclature includes the 20-amino acid signal peptide sequence in the count of residues such that pVal142Ile (or pV142I) refers to the same variant as Val122Ile. In contrast, wild-type transthyretin amyloidosis (ATTRwt) is a sporadic disease characterized by a normal *TTR* genetic sequence, with unclear causes of TTR misfolding. Secondary amyloidosis (AA), composed of serum amyloid A protein, can result from intense and persistent systemic inflammation but rarely affects the heart. Finally, uncommon genetic variants also known to affect the heart include atrial natriuretic peptide (ANP), apolipoprotein A1 (ApoA1), fibrinogen (Afib), and gelsolin (Agel). This chapter will focus attention on AL and ATTR amyloidosis, by far the most relevant types for the practicing clinician.

EPIDEMIOLOGY

Light Chain Amyloidosis

Epidemiologic studies suggest that AL amyloidosis is a rare disease with an annual incidence of approximately 1 per 100,000 individuals, accounting for approximately 5000 new annual cases in the United States. Cardiac involvement can be demonstrated in up to 70% of cases of AL amyloidosis. Although AL amyloidosis can affect individuals from the fourth decade of life onward, the prevalence of AL amyloidosis increases with age, with a median age of diagnosis at 63 years, and slight male predominance (between 55% and 65%). The current estimated prevalence is 40 to 58 cases per million persons. AL amyloidosis is related to, but distinct from, multiple myeloma and monoclonal gammopathy of unknown significance (MGUS) (other clonal plasma cell disorders). Among patients with MGUS, only a small percentage will develop AL amyloidosis (1% overall, relative risk 8.8). Although most patients with AL amyloidosis do not have multiple myeloma, up to 10% to 15% of patients with multiple myeloma have coexisting AL amyloidosis.[3]

Transthyretin Amyloidosis

The epidemiology ATTR amyloidosis varies by type (ATTRwt and ATTRv) and by specific variant, but conclusive data regarding population incidence and prevalence are lacking. Autopsy studies have demonstrated that up to 25% of decedents older than age 85 years have demonstrable myocardial TTR amyloid deposits, with a prevalence that increases with age, male sex, and is associated with a clinical diagnosis of heart failure.[4] Contemporary imaging suggests that of older (>60 year) patients hospitalized with heart failure and preserved ejection fraction with an increased left ventricular wall thickness, between 10% and 15% of patients may have ATTRwt amyloidosis. Other studies of older individuals with severe aortic stenosis demonstrate similar prevalence and male predilection for ATTRwt amyloidosis.[5] Larger-scale epidemiology studies designed to assess the prevalence of ATTRwt amyloidosis are presently underway.

In contrast to ATTRwt, hATTR or ATTRv is caused by a genetic mutation in the TTR gene. The TTR gene is composed of 4 exons (127 amino acids) in which more than 100 mutations have been described that can cause hereditary amyloidosis. Linked to a genetic founder, each variant is endemic to a particular geographic region or follows population migration patterns. Disease expression manifests as a polyneuropathy or cardiomyopathy (previously termed familial amyloidogenic polyneuropathy [FAP] or cardiomyopathy [FAC]). Phenotypic penetrance varies widely by mutation and increases with age (Table 53.1). The most common variant observed outside of the United States is pVal50Met (Val30Met), endemic to Portugal, northern Sweden, Japan, and Brazil. This variant causes predominantly a polyneuropathy phenotype, but at a later age of onset causes amyloid cardiomyopathy. The pThr80Ala (Thr60Ala) variant first identified in a northern region of the Republic of Ireland, causes both cardiomyopathy and polyneuropathy. Prevalence can approach 1% in endemic areas but is very uncommon elsewhere in the world. By far the most common *TTR* variant is pVal142Ile (Val122Ile), which has been reproducibly identified in approximately 3.5% of self-identified Black persons in the United States.[6] As a cause of ATTR cardiomyopathy, this allele frequency translates into more than 1.6 million persons in the United States as carriers and therefore at risk

TABLE 53.1 Comparison of the Most Common Types of Cardiac Amyloidosis

FEATURES	AL	ATTR					
PRECURSOR PROTEIN	LIGHT CHAIN—KAPPA OR LAMBDA	VARIANT TTR					
		CARDIOGENIC			NEUROPATHIC/MIXED		
SPECIFIC MUTATION		VAL122ILE (pV142I)	LEU111MET (pL131M)	ILE68LEU (pI88L)	THR60ALA (pT80A)	VAL30MET (pV50M)	WILD-TYPE TTR
Average age (range)	63 (30–80)	72 (47–90)	48 (35–60)	71 (40–80)	66 (41–82)	Early onset (30–50) Endemic, neuropathic Late onset (>50)— nonendemic, mixed phenotype	75 (50->100)
Gender (% male)	55%–60%	70%	64%	78%	60%	50%	90%
Race/ethnicity	Not specific	Black/Afro-Caribbean	Danish	Italian	Irish	Portuguese, Swedish, Japanese	Not specific
Cardiac involvement (%)	~70%	100%	100%	96%	100%	More common in late onset	100%
Fat pad biopsy	70%–80%*	<50%	<50%	<50%	<50%	<50%	<20%
Primary referral route	Hematology, cardiology, nephrology, dermatology	Cardiology	Cardiology	Cardiology	Neurology and cardiology	Neurology and cardiology	Cardiology
Extracardiac manifestations	Nephrotic syndrome/renal failure; Autonomic dysfunction; Purpura; Macroglossia; Carpal tunnel syndrome	Autonomic dysfunction; Carpal tunnel; Lumbar spinal stenosis	Carpal tunnel syndrome	Polyneuropathy (rare); Carpal tunnel syndrome	Polyneuropathy; Autonomic dysfunction; Carpal tunnel syndrome	Polyneuropathy; Autonomic dysfunction; GI motility disorder; Carpal tunnel syndrome	Carpal tunnel syndrome; Lumbar spinal stenosis; Biceps Tendon Rupture
Median survival/stage	1: Not reached (at 12 years); 2: 9.4 years; 3: 4.3 years; 3b: 1 year	1: 54 months; 2: 28.8 months; 3: 17.7 months	NR	Median overall survival of 36 months	1: 77 months; 2: 54 months; 3: 21 months	Survival usually >10 years and improved with liver transplant and tafamidis	1: 75 months; 2: 46 months; 3: 20 months

AL, light chain amyloidosis; ATTR, transthyretin amyloidosis; NAC, National Amyloidosis Centre, London, UK; NR, not reported.
*Dependent on extent of amyloid.

for ATTR cardiomyopathy. In addition, individuals of Hispanic/Latino ancestry may also harbor this mutation which increases the risk of developing heart failure nearly 50%. Unfortunately, among the vast majority of allele carriers with heart failure, the diagnosis is delayed or missed.[7] That stated, the phenotypic penetrance of ATTR cardiomyopathy is unclear and depends upon the age of ascertainment, with increasing penetrance with advancing age. Other TTR variants seen worldwide that predominantly result in ATTR cardiac amyloidosis include pIle88Leu (Ile68Leu, Italy) and pLeu131Met (Leu111Met, Denmark).[8]

PATHOPHYSIOLOGY

In AL amyloidosis, a dysregulated plasma cell clone produces kappa or lambda immunoglobulin light chain fragments that have a propensity to misfold, aggregate, and deposit in the myocardial interstitium. Lambda light chain amyloidosis is more common than kappa, and organ systems affected include the heart, kidneys, liver, nervous system (including autonomic nervous system), gastrointestinal tract, and soft tissues. The titer of light chain does not predict the site of target organ deposition. Cardiac AL amyloidosis is viewed as a "toxic-infiltrative" cardiomyopathy involving two mechanisms: (1) interstitial and/or perivascular amyloid fibril deposition leading to disruption of tissue architecture, microvascular dysfunction with angina/ischemia, and inhibition of contractile/relaxation functions and (2) direct toxicity to cardiomyocytes through, in part, p38 mitogen-activated protein kinase (MAPK) signaling. Interstitial deposition results in a restrictive cardiomyopathy and heart failure, and direct cellular toxicity is thought to occur through induction of reactive oxygen species and apoptosis in cardiomyocytes.[3]

Transthyretin, also known as prealbumin, is a tetrameric protein consisting of four identical subunits, synthesized in the liver, but also by the choroid plexus and retinal pigmented epithelial cells. TTR derives its name from its function as a circulating transporter of thyroid hormone and retinol (vitamin A). In hATTR, amino acid substitutions alter the properties of the protein favoring tetramer dissociation which is the rate-limiting step in amyloid fibril formation. Monomers then misfold and aggregate into amyloid fibrils that deposit in body tissues with specific organ tropism. Precisely why native (i.e., genetically normal), wild-type TTR becomes kinetically unstable and aggregates is unclear, but the process definitively occurs with advancing age (typically older than 60 years). Disease expression may also be influenced by age-related degradation in cellular systems that manage misfolded proteins. ATTR amyloidosis results in progressive myocardial deposition (infiltrating between myocytes) and restrictive cardiomyopathy and/or a small fiber, length-dependent peripheral and autonomic neuropathy. Tissue tropism or organ system involvement in ATTR amyloidosis is incompletely understood; however, there is developing evidence that the amyloid fibril composition may play a role. Amyloid deposits composed of TTR fragments (type A fibrils) are associated with later-onset disease with cardiac involvement in ATTRv and with ATTRwt, whereas full-length TTR fibrils (type B fibrils) in amyloid deposits correlate with earlier-onset disease without a strong cardiac phenotype.[9]

CLINICAL FEATURES AND PROGNOSIS

There are various impediments that hinder the recognition of cardiac amyloidosis by the cardiovascular clinician. First, the disease is generally perceived to be rare and presents with clinical and imaging features associated with more common conditions. Second, cardiac amyloidosis was, until recently, an untreatable disease with extremely poor prognosis lending credence to therapeutic nihilism. Third and finally, the diagnostic approach required endomyocardial biopsy, a procedure not appropriate in a scenario of low-pretest likelihood or for widespread screening. Recent discoveries in epidemiology, advancements in diagnostic imaging, and the development of novel therapeutics have rendered each of these conceptions invalid. Nevertheless, significant delays in disease recognition persist. Among patients with ATTR amyloidosis, data demonstrate increasing frequency of hospitalizations and visits for heart failure without disease recognition in the 3 years preceding ultimate diagnosis.[10]

Although differing by precursor protein, the final common pathophysiologic pathway of cardiac amyloidosis is one of myocardial infiltration and progressive impairment in diastolic and systolic function that elicits symptoms of congestive heart failure. Left ventricular ejection fraction (LVEF) is preserved in early stages of the disease, while longitudinal contraction is impaired. Progressive infiltration and/or direct myocyte toxicity subsequently results in decrement in global left and right ventricular systolic function. Signs of heart failure in more advanced disease become predominantly right-sided, with lower extremity edema, ascites, and hepatic enlargement. For this reason, the disease, particularly in early stages, is misrecognized for more common wall-thickening processes such as hypertensive remodeling or hypertrophic cardiomyopathy (HCM). The electrocardiogram (ECG) classically demonstrates a low-voltage pattern in approximately 50% of patients with AL cardiac amyloidosis, while inferior or anterior pseudoinfarcts are seen in greater than 70% of AL cases. Low voltage is seen in only 25% to 40% of patients with ATTR, while up to 15% can show evidence of left ventricular hypertrophy. Conduction disease progressing to heart block is more commonly a feature of ATTR amyloidosis. Atrial dysrhythmias, particular atrial fibrillation (AF) and flutter, are seen in up to 40% to 60% of patients with wtATTR amyloidosis at diagnosis and in up to 90% over time. The risk of intracardiac thrombus is increased in all patients with cardiac amyloidosis, even those in sinus rhythm, with stroke or systemic embolization occurring in some patients. Although a low-voltage pattern itself can be attributable to other causes (pericardial effusion, lung hyper-expansion), integration of increased wall thickness seen by echocardiography in the setting of a low-voltage pattern (the mass to voltage ratio), increases diagnostic accuracy.

One strategy to increase recognition involves identification of other, noncardiac features of AL or ATTR amyloidosis in the context of heart failure. Clinical features of AL amyloidosis are myriad and follow organ system infiltration including renal (proteinuria, often nephrotic range), soft tissue (macroglossia, carpal tunnel syndrome), gastrointestinal (bleeding), or neurologic (peripheral or autonomic neuropathy). Periorbital ecchymosis resulting from capillary fragility is considered a pathognomonic feature of AL amyloidosis and is not seen in ATTR amyloidosis. Hereditary ATTR amyloidosis presents as a small fiber, length-dependent peripheral neuropathy manifesting as paresthesis, pain, or sensory loss on the hands and feet. However, autonomic neuropathy, most commonly manifesting as abnormal sweating, orthostatic hypotension, gastrointestinal dysmotility, and erectile dysfunction, can also be observed in AL or ATTR. As noted previously, different TTR variants present with either cardiomyopathy or neuropathy symptoms, or both. For example, the pVal50Met variant causes predominantly neuropathy in early-onset disease (third or fourth decade) but cardiomyopathy and neuropathy in later onset (sixth or seventh decade of life). The pThr80Ala variant causes either cardiomyopathy or neuropathy, or both, with onset in the fifth decade. The common variant pVal142Ile affects individuals of West African origin generally in the seventh decade of life, but nearly exclusively causes cardiomyopathy. Rare ATTRv manifestations resulting from leptomeningeal involvement include hydrocephalus and vitreous opacities. Wild-type ATTR was previously held to be principally a cardiac-restricted disease, although soft tissue deposition manifesting as carpal tunnel syndrome, lumbar spinal stenosis (ligamentum flavum thickening), and spontaneous tendon ruptures (biceps in particular) is now widely recognized. It is held that the orthopedic/soft tissue manifestations of ATTRwt amyloidosis precede the cardiac, often by many years. The presence of neuropathy in ATTRwt is often difficult to disentangle for other age-associated neuropathies or comorbidities (including diabetes mellitus or alcohol intake).

Prognosis

The prognosis of AL cardiac amyloidosis varies greatly depending upon two important contingencies: the stage of disease upon diagnosis and, importantly, the response to chemotherapy directed against the affected plasma cell clone. Prognosis is assessed by a combination of biomarker risk assessment models and cardiac imaging. Biomarker testing (Mayo or Boston University scoring systems) involves measurement of brain natriuretic peptides (NT-pro-BNP or BNP), cardiac troponin I or T, and direct measurement of lambda and kappa light chain.[11,12] Patients are classified into stages depending upon the values of these biomarkers. Recent data demonstrate that median survival for stage 2 patients (with either troponin or BNP above threshold) is approximately 9.5 years, whereas for those with advanced disease (stage 3b), median survival remains approximately 1 year. Imaging studies demonstrate that poor prognosis is also associated with lower echocardiographic stroke volume, increasing impairment global longitudinal strain, increasingly severe cardiac magnetic resonance imaging (CMR) late gadolinium enhancement (LGE), and increasing CMR extracellular volume fraction (ECV).[13] Each of these imaging features is a marker of more advanced disease and is strongly associated with cardiac biomarkers. Hematologic response status and change in cardiac biomarkers with treatment also predict prognosis. The attainment of a complete hematologic response is the goal of all therapy and is strongly associated with improved survival. A reduction in BNP or NT-pro BNP of greater than 30% from baseline is also indicative of a cardiac response and is associated with improved prognosis.

The prognosis of ATTR amyloidosis differs between hereditary and wild-type genotype. Similar to AL amyloidosis, staging systems using cardiac biomarkers and renal function have been developed to inform prognosis. Despite the larger population of affected patients as compared with AL, data limited to case series estimate median survival in ATTRwt amyloidosis to be approximately 3.5 years and for ATTRv amyloidosis pVal142Ile to be approximately 2.5 years from diagnosis. However, as in AL, prognosis depends upon stage of disease at diagnosis. Using a combination of NT-proBNP and troponin T (Mayo system) or NT-proBNP and estimated glomerular filtration rate (eGFR, National Amyloidosis Centre system), data demonstrate that for ATTRwt median survival following diagnosis ranges from 5 to 7 years for stage 1 (early stage) to 2 to 3 years for stage 3 (advanced stage).[14,15] It is important to emphasize that the natural history studies currently available do not account for contemporary TTR-specific therapies which can extend survival. Like AL, imaging also informs prognosis with increasing CMR LGE and ECV and worsening global longitudinal strain associated with impaired survival.

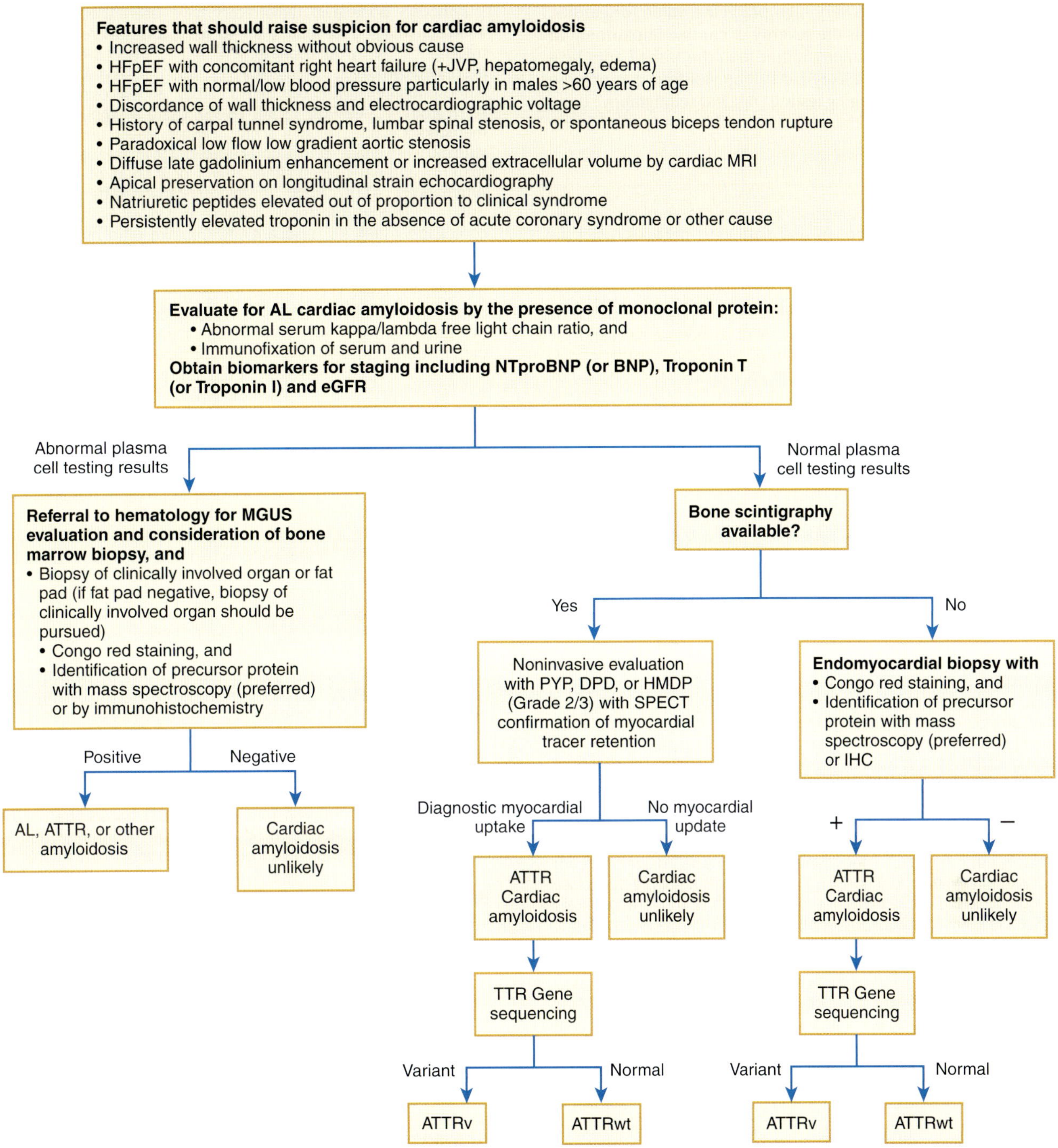

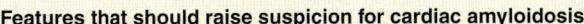

FIGURE 53.1 Algorithm for cardiac amyloidosis diagnosis. Accurate diagnosis of cardiac amyloidosis can be made by tissue biopsy or by noninvasive methods (bone-seeking nuclear tracers) following exclusion of monoclonal protein. Note appropriate testing for monoclonal protein involves serum-free light chain assay and serum and urine immunofixation electrophoresis (not serum protein electrophoresis). Nuclear imaging with bone-seeking radiotracers (PYP, DPD, or HMDP) can be performed concurrent to monoclonal protein assessment to afford additional information. *DPD*, ^{99m}Tc-3,3-diphosphono-1,2-propanedicarboxylic acid; *HMDP*, ^{99m}Tc-hydhydroxyl-methylene-diphosphonate; *MGUS*, monoclonal gammpopathy of unknown significance; *PYP*, ^{99m}Tc-pyrophosphate.

DIAGNOSIS

The critical step to enable a diagnosis of cardiac amyloidosis is clinical suspicion forged, in part, by attention to associated signs/symptoms and reassessment of changes in clinical features previously attributed to other processes. Examples of the latter point include intolerance to beta blockade (a feature of restrictive filling), intolerance to angiotensin-converting enzyme (ACE) inhibitors, angiotensin receptor blockers (ARBs), or angiotensin receptor/neprilysin inhibitors (ARNIs), or a reduced requirement for antihypertensives. Heightened awareness in specific affected populations is also essential, such as severe aortic stenosis, particularly the low-flow, low-gradient phenotype. In addition, several "red flag" features have been proposed including extreme left ventricle (LV) wall thickening (>15 mm), discordant ECG voltage as predicted from wall thickness, orthopedic/soft tissue manifestations, and characteristic patterns on imaging testing.[16] A clinical algorithm to guide the approach toward accurate diagnosis of cardiac amyloidosis can be found in Figure 53.1.

Diagnosis of amyloidosis classically requires tissue biopsy with Congo red (or Thioflavin) staining and precursor protein identification by immunohistochemistry and/or mass spectrometry. In the case of AL amyloidosis, a tissue biopsy is required to establish the diagnosis. Establishment of cardiac amyloidosis, however, does not require an endomyocardial biopsy, as supportive evidence from imaging and biomarker testing afford a very high predictive value for cardiac involvement.[17] Furthermore, it is the severity of cardiac impairment in AL that defines treatment regimens, rather than the binary adjudication of cardiac involvement. Unlike AL, ATTR amyloidosis can now be accurately diagnosed with imaging testing (nuclear scintigraphy) combined with testing for light chain amyloidosis, when performed in the proper clinical context.

BIOMARKERS

Persistent and unexplained elevation in cardiac biomarkers, including the aforementioned troponins and natriuretic peptides, are hallmark features of cardiac amyloidosis but are nonspecific. Although candidates have been proposed, there are no specific biomarkers yet reported that can definitively identify cardiac amyloidosis. In AL, abnormal increase in either lambda (more common) or kappa free light chain with abnormal ratio, and/or identification of a monoclonal band on immunofixation electrophoresis is indicative of a plasma cell dyscrasia. In the proper context, these findings can increase suspicion for AL but are not diagnostic. Furthermore, it is common in the setting of chronic kidney disease to observe a kappa predominance with abnormal free light chain ratio, confusing interpretation. In addition, MGUS incidence increases with age and plasma cell testing abnormalities can be seen in up to 40% to 50% of patients with ATTR amyloidosis.[18] Thus hematologic consultation is indispensable in unclear scenarios. A serum protein electrophoresis (SPEP) is insensitive for identifying AL amyloidosis and should not be obtained without subsequent immunofixation. Emerging data suggest that lower prealbumin (TTR) concentration may identify patients with ATTRv amyloidosis and can inform prognosis in ATTRwt. Similarly, the TTR ligand retinol-binding protein 4 (RBP4), also appears to identify ATTRv pVal142Ile amyloidosis, although its capacity to predict prognosis has not been well explored.[19]

IMAGING

Cardiac imaging plays an essential role in the diagnostic pathway for cardiac amyloidosis identification (Table 53.2). Recently published multisocietal consensus recommendations for the acquisition, analysis, and reporting of imaging in cardiac amyloidosis have conferred important standardization.[20,21] Echocardiography is indispensable (see also Chapter 16). Findings include increased biventricular thickening (above the upper limit of normal for age and sex but often ≥12 mm for the LV), dilated atria, interatrial septal thickening, valvular thickening, evidence of right ventricular thickening, pericardial effusion, dilated inferior vena cava, diastolic dysfunction, and increased left atrial pressures (see also Fig. 16.31). Global measures of systolic function are generally preserved in early to midstage disease; however, segmental variation in systolic function is evident early. Global longitudinal strain is often reduced and in specific, basal segments often are hypokinetic relative to apical segments. This distinctive pattern is described as "apical sparing" (Fig. 53.2) and can be quantified with longitudinal systolic strain deformational imaging with an approximate apical/basal ratio of greater than 2 or apical/basal+mid strain greater than 0.7 (relative apical sparing). Increased LVEF/global longitudinal strain ratio greater than 4 is also suggestive of amyloid cardiomyopathy.[22] Echocardiographic features, although raising suspicion of amyloid cardiomyopathy, are not in themselves diagnostic. Another echocardiographic parameter that has utility in identifying cardiac amyloidosis and predicting clinical outcomes is the myocardial contraction fraction (MCF, ratio of LV stroke volume to myocardial wall volume).

CMR imaging (see Chapter 19) with LGE affords the capacity to visualize the extracellular space expansion that results from amyloid fibril deposition.[23] As in echocardiography, AL and ATTR patterns overlap; thus, although useful for adjudication of amyloid from nonamyloid, the specific type cannot be reliably identified. Cardiac amyloidosis demonstrates diffuse enhancement throughout the myocardial segments, either in a global subendocardial or transmural pattern, often with atrial involvement. The inability to suppress ("null") the myocardium in cine-inversion recovery (Look-Locker) sequences is a common feature. LGE CMR is approximately 85% to 90% sensitive and specific for identification of amyloid cardiomyopathy in patients with clinically suspected disease. As extracellular amyloid fibril deposition increases, the interstitial space between myocytes expands. Parametric T1 mapping demonstrates increased native (noncontrast) T1 and ECV is typically greater than 0.40. One distinct advantage of CMR over other imaging modalities is its capacity to differentiate other diseases that may mimic the amyloid cardiomyopathy phenotype (e.g., HCM, Fabry disease).

Although bone avid radiotracers have been used for myocardial infarction imaging for more than 40 years, it is now recognized that the tracers ^{99m}Tc-pyrophosphate (PYP), ^{99m}Tc-3,3-diphosphono-1,2-propanedicarboxylic acid (DPD), and ^{99m}Tc-hydroxyl-methylene-diphosphonate (HMDP) can detect cardiac amyloidosis and differentiate ATTR from AL (see Figs. 18.34, 18.35). Using a simple semiquantitative methodology (the Perugini score), cardiac tracer uptake is compared with rib with grade 0 (no uptake) to grade 3 (cardiac uptake greater than rib) and determined either after 1 or 3 hours of tracer incubation. Alternatively, ATTR cardiac amyloidosis can be differentiated from AL using ^{99m}Tc PYP (the tracer available in United States) by a heart to contralateral lung (H/CL) quantitative uptake ratio of greater than 1.5 from a region of interest drawn over the heart and contralateral chest after a 1 hour of tracer incubation. Single-photon emission computed tomography (SPECT) is required to confirm myocardial (and not blood pool) tracer uptake. A large international collaboration using a cohort of biopsy-proven AL and ATTR cardiac amyloidosis patients demonstrated that nuclear tracers provided 100% specificity when grade 2 or 3 uptake was seen in the absence of a monoclonal protein by serum or urine in individuals with heart failure and typical echocardiographic or CMR features of amyloidosis.[24] In addition, a multicenter study validated these results with ^{99m}Tc-PYP and additionally showed H/CL ratio greater than 1.6 conferred worse survival.[25] It is essential that lab testing excludes evidence of a monoclonal gammopathy in conjunction with nuclear imaging to properly interpret the testing results. For these reasons, ATTR cardiac amyloidosis can now be diagnosed using bone avid tracers and blood testing without the need for confirmatory cardiac tissue biopsy when properly applied. It is appropriate to note that there remains some disagreement in the optimal timing of imaging following tracer injection. That stated, with the adoption, awareness, and growing availability of this imaging technique, recognition of ATTR amyloidosis has increased. Nuclear techniques have noted ATTR amyloidosis in 16% of patients with aortic stenosis undergoing transcatheter aortic valve replacement and 5% of patients with presumed HCM, with 26% of those referred for HCM older than 80 years of age having cardiac amyloidosis. Although nuclear techniques hold great promise as a means to screen for ATTR amyloidosis when applied in the proper clinical context, endomyocardial biopsy remains necessary in cases of demonstrated monoclonal gammopathy or in cases of equivocal tracer uptake and high clinical suspicion. Although not widely available, positron emission tomography (PET) tracers specific for amyloid deposits (florbetapir, florbetaben, 11C-Pittsburgh-B) also identify cardiac amyloidosis and may prove clinically useful in the future.

BIOPSY

Endomyocardial biopsy remains the "gold standard" for diagnosis of cardiac amyloidosis and is considered 100% sensitive and specific if biopsy specimens are collected from multiple sites (four or more are recommended). Definitive typing for the precursor protein must be determined by immunohistochemistry or via the more preferred, laser dissection with tandem mass spectrometry (LC MS/MS) analysis. Endomyocardial biopsy carries a small but notable risk of perforation, tamponade, or access site complications and as such is reserved for confirmatory testing in suspected cases wherein imaging testing is inconclusive (or isolated AL cardiac amyloidosis). Abdominal fat aspirate with Congo red staining can be helpful; however, sensitivity for ATTRwt is low (only approximately 20%) and a negative result should not dissuade continued evaluation.[26] Biopsies of other sites (e.g., gastrointestinal), have widely reported sensitivities/specificities, and as with fat aspirate, a negative result should not dissuade further testing in scenarios of high clinical suspicion.

GENOTYPING

Genotyping of *TTR* is a final critical step in the ATTR amyloidosis diagnostic algorithm because it has implications for treatment as well as raises the possibility of gene inheritance for first-degree relatives. One approach proposed as means to achieve amyloidosis screening involves widespread genotyping. Such an approach can accurately identify known variants associated with ATTR amyloidosis, although it is important to note that clinical penetrance is unclear and varies with age and family history. This has been most widely explored for the pVal142Ile genotype. Although data clearly demonstrate that the inheritance of the pVal142Ile allele increases the risk of heart failure,[7] evidence from other studies suggest that the allele does not necessarily result in imaging evidence of ATTR amyloidosis.[27] Furthermore, a genotyping-only approach will fail to identify ATTRwt, the most common type of cardiac amyloidosis. Although rare, the possibility of non-*TTR* variants including gelsolin, AApoA1, A2, and AFib (fibrinogen) should be considered in the presence of defined cardiac amyloidosis and a strong family history with normal *TTR* gene sequence.

TABLE 53.2 Comparison of Diagnostic Imaging Modalities in Cardiac Amyloidosis

FEATURE	ECHOCARDIOGRAPHY	MRI	BONE SCINTIGRAPHY
Clinical clues	Pericardial or pleural effusions, thick right ventricle, small LV cavity, intra-atrial septal thickening, and impaired global longitudinal strain characteristically with sparing of the apex	Elevated native T1, increased extracellular volume fraction, late gadolinium enhancement in any pattern, abnormal gadolinium kinetics	Diagnostic for transthyretin amyloid cardiomyopathy (ATTR-CM) if normal light chain assays and grade 2/3 cardiac uptake with confirmation of myocardial retention by SPECT False positives due to AL cardiac amyloidosis, previous myocardial infarction, diffuse myocardial scarring, overlying previous rib fracture, blood pool, hydroxychloroquine toxicity, and unusual forms of cardiac amyloidosis (ApoA1)
Relative cost	$	$$	$
Specialized expertise required for interpretation	No	Yes	No
Exposure to ionizing radiation	No	No	Yes
Cardiac devices affect image quality	No	Yes	No
Can identify nonamyloid causes of LV thickening	Yes (valvular disease, HCM, diastolic function) though amyloid CM may also be present	Yes (infiltrative disease, HCM)	No
Distinguish AL and ATTR	No	No	Yes*
Markers of worse prognosis	Lower stroke volume, greater regional variation in global longitudinal strain, worse global longitudinal strain, lower MCF, low EF (late phase)	Late gadolinium enhancement, higher extracellular volume fraction, higher native T1	H/CL ratio ≥1.6 at 1 hr

AL, Amyloidogenic light chain; *ApoA1*, apolipoprotein A1; *EF*, ejection fraction; *H/CL*, heart to contralateral lung; *HCM*, hypertrophic cardiomyopathy; *LV*, left ventricle; *MCF*, myocardial contraction fraction; *SPECT*, Single-photon emission computed tomography.
*In the context of normal serum and urine immunofixation electrophoresis and serum kappa/lambda ratio.

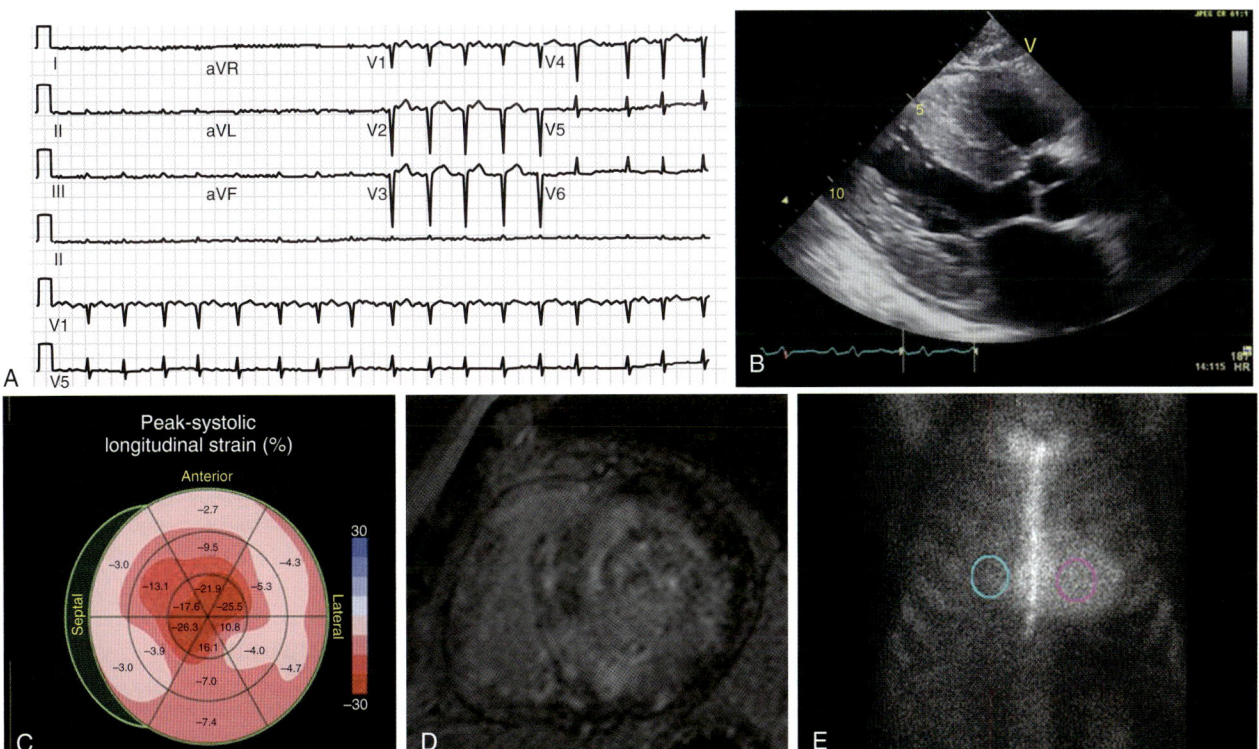

FIGURE 53.2 Electrocardiographic and imaging findings in cardiac amyloidosis. A 77-year-old male with dyspnea and palpitations presents for evaluation. **A,** Electrocardiogram (ECG) demonstrates atrial fibrillation, with low voltage in the limb leads and a pseudoinfarct pattern in the anterior leads. **B,** Still-frame image from parasternal long-axis echocardiogram illustrating severely increased wall thickness (19 mm) discordant from ECG low-voltage findings. **C,** Echocardiographic global longitudinal strain polar map showing apical-sparing pattern. **D,** Cardiac MR with phase-sensitive inversion recovery late gadolinium enhancement (PSIR-LGE) imaging demonstrating diffuse subendocardial and transmural enhancement. **E,** Planar Tc^{99m} pyrophosphate (PYP) image showing grade 3 tracer uptake, confirmed by single-photon emission computed tomography (SPECT), with a heart to contralateral chest ratio of 1.7. Endomyocardial biopsy confirmed ATTRwt amyloidosis.

CLINICAL MANAGEMENT

Supportive Non–Disease-Modifying Therapies

In contrast to other etiologies of heart failure, the evidence basis underlying clinical management in cardiac amyloidosis, although increasing, remains sparse. As such, management strategies are largely drawn from smaller, nonrandomized, observational case series. That being stated, aforementioned consensus recommendations for imaging and a recently reported AHA Scientific Statement distilled available evidence into coherent recommendations to guide clinical management.[28] In general, the approach to a patient with cardiac amyloidosis involves treatment of the underlying cause (chemotherapy for AL, TTR-directed therapies for ATTR) and concurrent management of heart failure, arrhythmia, and concomitant symptoms. As such, the general principles underlying non–disease-modifying therapy for cardiac amyloidosis include symptom management, maintenance of euvolemia, avoidance of polypharmacy (particularly in elderly patients), avoidance of medications that may cause symptomatic hypotension, implantation of electrical devices (pacemakers, defibrillators), and consideration of advanced circulatory support/transplant for refractory heart failure in a minority of patients.

MANAGEMENT OF HEART FAILURE

Maintenance of euvolemia and optimization of perfusion in patients with cardiac amyloidosis can be a distinct challenge. Perturbations of filling hemodynamics from diastolic dysfunction with impairment of stroke volume (restriction), renal dysfunction from intrinsic renal disease, poor perfusion, or the cardiorenal syndrome, and in some individuals, concurrent autonomic dysfunction from amyloid neuropathy renders a very narrow range of tolerable circulating volume. Bioavailable loop diuretics and aldosterone antagonists are the preferred first-line agents with frequent dose adjustments to address changes in volume status that may result from concomitant chemotherapies for AL amyloidosis, such as steroids. Patients with orthostasis from poor vascular tone owing to impaired autonomic function may require the alpha-agonist midodrine to maintain adequate systolic blood pressure.

Evidence-based therapies that have proven beneficial in other causes of heart failure including ACE inhibitors, ARBs, ARNIs, and beta blockers are generally poorly tolerated in patients with advanced cardiac amyloidosis owing to fixed stroke volume and impaired hemodynamic compensatory mechanisms. Lower doses are often useful to manage hypertension or AF heart rate in earlier stage patients. Non-dihydropyridine calcium channel blockers (CCBs) are generally contraindicated in cardiac amyloidosis because they can bind amyloid fibrils (demonstrated in AL only), and worsen heart failure through heart-rate slowing, negative inotropy, and potentiation of conduction block. Interestingly, the affinity of TTR amyloid fibrils for various bone-seeking radiotracers is thought to be calcium related, thereby suggesting a potential mechanism for increased binding of CCBs to amyloid fibrils. Dihydropyridine CCBs may be useful as adjunctive agents for blood pressure management, particularly in the context of renal dysfunction, although potentiation of lower-extremity edema may limit application. Although an in vitro study demonstrated that isolated AL amyloid fibrils bind digoxin with high affinity, digoxin has been recently reconsidered if used cautiously as adjunctive management in AF rate control.[29]

ARRHYTHMIA MANAGEMENT

Atrial dysrhythmias, particularly AF and atrial flutter, are extremely common in ATTR amyloidosis and less commonly seen in AL amyloidosis. Management involves anticoagulation to prevent thromboembolism and rate control, and if exacerbating symptoms of heart failure, rhythm control is also appropriate. As with maintenance of euvolemia, heart rate control can also be challenging to optimize because both tachycardia and bradycardia are poorly tolerated, resulting from restrictive hemodynamics. Maintaining sinus rhythm and the atrial contribution to ventricular filling in cardiac amyloidosis may be less important because many patients have significantly reduced atrial mechanical function, reducing the atrial contribution to ventricular filling. Regularization and slowing of heart rate likely provide equal or greater benefit. The stroke risk among patients with AF and cardiac amyloidosis is exceedingly high because of blood stasis and elevated pressures, and atrial amyloid deposition may potentiate thrombosis. Left atrial appendage thrombosis has been observed in the context of normal sinus rhythm and after therapeutic anticoagulation, underscoring the imperative to perform transesophageal echocardiography prior to attempts at restoration of sinus rhythm by cardioversion.[30] Heparins, vitamin K antagonists, or direct-acting oral anticoagulants are all effective in reducing thromboembolic risk and should be considered as indefinite therapy with minimal interruption. As specified in recent American College of Cardiology/American Heart Association/Heart Rhythm Society (ACC/AHA/HRS) recommendations, agents that may be used for rhythm control include amiodarone (most commonly) and dofetilide.[29] Data supporting the use of catheter ablation in cardiac amyloidosis are limited. In early-stage patients, cavotricuspid isthmus ablation may help to maintain sinus rhythm in the setting of atrial flutter, while pulmonary venous isolation procedures are generally less effective at controlling AF than in nonamyloid populations.

In ATTR in particular, deposits of amyloid fibrils infiltrate the conduction system, with a significant percentage of patients requiring permanent pacing. Pacing following AV junctional ablation for refractory AF management can also be considered. Biventricular pacing can be considered for patients with preexisting reduced LVEF. The routine use of automatic implantable cardioverter-defibrillators (ICDs) in patients with cardiac amyloidosis is debatable as sudden cardiac death related to ventricular tachycardia (VT) or ventricular fibrillation (VF) is relatively uncommon and mortality typically results from pulseless electrical activity. If anticipated survival is less than 1 year, then practice guidelines do not recommend ICD placement for the primary prevention of sudden cardiac death.[29] Device implantation for primary prevention is debatable, although ICD placement after aborted sudden death or sustained VT/VF is less controversial provided survival is expected to exceed 1 year.

ADVANCED CIRCULATORY SUPPORT AND ORGAN TRANSPLANTATION

Selected patients with advanced heart failure may qualify for orthotopic heart transplantation (OHT) and/or mechanical circulatory support (MCS) after careful assessment for the extent of systemic involvement. Acceptable outcomes have been reported in small series of carefully selected patients with AL that underwent OHT followed by treatment for AL (typically stem cell transplant–based regimens but more recently targeted anti-plasma cell therapy alone). Similarly, outcomes after OHT in ATTR patients with wild-type or cardiac-restricted variant disease (typically pVal142Ile) do not differ from those transplanted for other nonamyloid indications. Patients with ATTRv can be treated with OHT followed by TTR-specific pharmacotherapies to slow allograft TTR deposition. MCS with left ventricular assist devices (LVADs) or total artificial heart has been reported as a bridge to transplant in a small number of highly selected patients, but outcomes are worse in part because of small ventricular chamber size leading to suction events and, in the case of LVAD, concomitant right heart failure.

The majority of circulating TTR protein (95%) is produced by the liver. Orthotopic liver transplantation (OLT) replaces amyloidogenic mutant TTR with wild-type TTR and theoretically arrests amyloid formation. Prior to contemporary pharmaceutical therapies, OLT was the only available TTR-specific treatment for ATTRv amyloidosis. The treatment is largely effective among patients without demonstrable cardiac involvement; however, among those with cardiac amyloidosis, there is still a risk of progressive cardiac deposition after isolated OLT owing to continued wild-type TTR deposition upon the template of previous amyloid deposits. Combined OHT and OLT was formerly a strategy in ATTRv disease with a neuropathic *TTR* variant but has been largely rendered obsolete by contemporary therapies.[28]

Disease-Targeted Therapeutics
Light Chain Amyloidosis

The ultimate goal of chemotherapy for AL amyloidosis is elimination of the plasma cell clone that produces the amyloidogenic light chain. Arresting amyloid production reverses disease progression, preserves organ function, and enhances survival. Chemotherapeutics are drawn from the armamentarium of agents developed for multiple myeloma. The objective is attainment of a complete hematologic response (CR) defined as normalization of the involved free light chain and light chain ratio, elimination of a monoclonal band by immunofixation electrophoresis, and normalization of the bone marrow plasma cell population. Degrees of hematologic response are defined by the proportion of light chain reduction from complete, very good partial,

TABLE 53.3 Therapies for Amyloidogenic Transthyretin Amyloidosis

DRUG NAME	MECHANISM OF ACTION	INDICATION	ROUTE	DOSE	COMMON, SERIOUS OR POTENTIAL SIDE EFFECTS	CONCOMITANT THERAPY	MONITORING	COST
Patisiran	Silencer	Neuropathy	IV	0.3 mg/kg q3 weeks up to 30 mg	Infusion-related reactions Vitamin A deficiency	With IV infusion: • IV steroids • Acetaminophen • IV H1 blocker • IV H2 blocker • Daily vitamin A supplements	None	$450,000 annual list price $345,000 average effective net annual price
Inotersen	Silencer	Neuropathy	SQ	284 mg weekly	Thrombocytopenia/ glomerulonephritis, requiring testing before treatment and monitoring during therapy Infusion-site reactions, fever Vitamin A deficiency	Daily vitamin A supplements	Weekly platelet counts. Every 2 weeks measures of serum creatinine, eGFR urinalysis, and urine protein to creatinine ratio	$450,000 annual list price $345,000 average effective net annual price
Tafamidis meglumine	Stabilizer	Neuropathy/ Cardio-myopathy	Oral	20 mg once a day 80 mg once a day	Side effects were less common than with placebo in cardiomyopathy	None	None	€100,000 per year $225,000 per year
Tafamidis free salt	Stabilizer	Cardio-myopathy	Oral	61 mg once a day	Unknown	None	None	$225,000 per year
Diflunisal	Stabilizer	Neuropathy/ Cardio-myopathy	Oral	250 mg PO twice a day	Related to NSAID properties: • Bleeding • Hypertension • Fluid retention • Renal dysfunction	Proton pump inhibitor	Monitor renal function, platelet count, hemoglobin 1–2 weeks after initiation and then every 3 months	$300-500 per year

eGFR, Estimated glomerular filtration rate; *hATTR*, Hereditary transthyretin amyloidosis; *NSAID*, nonsteroidal antiinflammatory drug.

partial, and no response. As noted earlier, the biomarker scoring systems developed for prognosis are also used to follow response to treatment. First-line strategies vary by institutional experience and must be individualized to a particular patient. In appropriately selected patients managed at highly specialized referral centers with extensive experience, high-dose melphalan-based chemotherapy coupled with autologous stem cell transplant (HDM/SCT) can be applied as a means to rapidly reduce the light chain concentration. In such centers, a complete or very good partial response can be induced in approximately 60% of patients with a peritransplant mortality less than 2% while durable, long-term complete response (>15 years) can be achieved.[31] Eligibility for HDM/SCT is defined by various clinical parameters including (but not limited to) LVEF, pulmonary function, blood pressure, and performance status.[32] For those not eligible for HDM/SCT, contemporary advances in chemotherapy offer many alternative and highly effective options. Regimens include combinations of drugs such as proteasome inhibitors, immune modulators, and most recently, monoclonal antibodies. In specific, a monoclonal antibody targeting the CD38-receptor (daratumumab), developed for the treatment of patients with relapsed multiple myeloma, has produced a rapid and profound hematologic response with minimal toxicity.[33] This agent, which can be delivered subcutaneously, results in robust hematologic and organ responses with an acceptable safety profile.[34] Daratumumab is the first and only agent specifically approved by FDA for AL amyloidosis and is now considered first line therapy in combination with cytoxan, bortizimib, and dexamthasone.

Transthyretin Amyloidosis

There are numerous pharmacologic strategies developed to ameliorate ATTR amyloidosis, including TTR silencing or knockdown, TTR stabilization, and TTR amyloid fibril disruption/extraction (Table 53.3). Presently, there are three U.S. Food and Drug Administration (FDA)-approved therapies for ATTR amyloidosis including the TTR silencers patisiran and inotersen, and the TTR stabilizer tafamidis, with additional novel agents in clinical trials. In addition, the FDA-approved nonsteroidal antiinflammatory drug (NSAID) diflunisal has been repurposed for ATTR amyloidosis treatment and demonstrated efficacy in smaller, nonrandomized, retrospective studies.

TTR Stabilizers

As a therapeutic class, TTR stabilizers are orally available small molecules that bind to TTR and inhibit its dissociation and subsequent amyloid fibril formation. Tafamidis is a benzoxazole derivative lacking NSAID activity specifically engineered to bind to the thyroxine-binding sites of TTR with high affinity and selectivity, stabilizing the tetramer and slowing dissociation and subsequent aggregation. The efficacy of tafamidis in ATTR cardiac amyloidosis was demonstrated in the phase III clinical study Amyloid Transthyretin

Amyloidosis Cardiomyopathy Trial (ATTR-ACT), where treatment resulted in lower all-cause mortality and reduction in cardiovascular hospitalizations.[35] Treatment also resulted in a lower rate of decline in distance for the 6-minute walk test and in the Kansas City Cardiomyopathy Questionnaire (KCCQ-OS) as compared with controls. Tafamidis was approved in May of 2019 as the only therapeutic approved for ATTRwt cardiac amyloidosis. Given its extremely high initial cost, the cost-effectiveness of the therapy was deemed poor despite the efficacy.[36]

Diflunisal is an NSAID that, like tafamidis, binds to the TTR tetramer at the thyroxine-binding site, kinetically stabilizing it from dissociation. Used off-label in a phase III study of patients with ATTRv amyloidosis, diflunisal at a reduced dose of 250 mg twice daily improved symptoms of amyloid polyneuropathy.[37] Retrospective studies have demonstrated the safety of diflunisal in selected patients with eGFR greater than 45 mL/min and efficacy as determined by improved echocardiographic markers of decline with increased survival in treated patients. Diflunisal has emerged as a cost-effective alternative therapy in selected patients with careful monitoring of volume status and renal function.[4] An additional stabilizer with a separate molecular TTR-binding site (acoramidis, or AG10) is currently in a phase III clinical trial with promising preliminary results from smaller phase II studies.[38]

TTR Silencers

TTR protein silencers hold great promise to halt or even reverse ATTR cardiac amyloidosis by significantly reducing circulating TTR. Patisiran is a small interfering RNA (siRNA) delivered intravenously that specifically targets hepatic TTR messenger RNA (mRNA) to elicit degradation and subsequent inhibition of TTR protein translation. Administered every 3 weeks, the drug reduces circulating TTR protein levels by approximately 90%. Patisiran must be co-administered with corticosteroids and histamine receptor blockers to blunt immune/histamine response. Efficacy of patisiran in ATTRv amyloidosis with polyneuropathy was demonstrated in the phase III APOLLO trial, where patients randomized to active drug experienced improved neuropathy (as measured by the modified neuropathy impairment score, mNIS+7) and quality of life.[39] More than 50% of patients in APOLLO had cardiac amyloid involvement, and in a cardiac subgroup analysis with wall thickness greater than 13 mm, patisiran resulted in significant improvements in NT-proBNP, LV wall thickness, global longitudinal strain, and gait speed compared with placebo.[40] Patisiran was approved by the FDA for ATTRv amyloidosis and polyneuropathy, with or without cardiomyopathy. Patisiran and another RNA interfering therapeutic, vutrisiran (delivered subcutaneously every 3 months) are presently being evaluated in phase III trials of cardiac amyloidosis patients that includes those with ATTRwt.

The 2'-O-methoxyethyl–modified antisense oligonucleotide inotersen is a short synthetic RNA that binds and inhibits translation of target hepatic *TTR* mRNA, thereby suppressing expression. Efficacy of inotersen in ATTRv amyloidosis in ameliorating clinically assessed polyneuropathy and quality of life was demonstrated in the NEURO-TTR study.[41] Inotersen received FDA approval for ATTRv amyloid polyneuropathy with or without cardiomyopathy (as in patisiran). Both agents were deemed not cost-effective in cost-effective analyses based on current U.S. prices.[42] Given observed toxicities of thrombocytopenia and glomerulonephritis (both 3%), inotersen was approved with a Risk Evaluation and Mitigation Strategy (REMS) that includes weekly monitoring of platelet counts and every 2-week monitoring of renal function and urinary protein. A small, open-label study of inotersen in patients with ATTR cardiomyopathy demonstrated stabilization of LV wall thickness, mass, global longitudinal strain, and functional capacity.[43] Ongoing clinical trials of inotersen and the related ligand-conjugated antisense oligonucleotide (LICA, trial CADRIO-TTRansform) in ATTR cardiac amyloidosis, including ATTRwt, are ongoing. A promising, early-stage report of a clustered regularly interspaced short palindromic repeats and associated Cas9 endonuclease (CRISPR-Cas9) based therapeutic (NTLA-2001) affords the potential for permanent silencing of TTR expression.[44]

CONCLUSION

The diagnostic and therapeutic landscape for cardiac amyloidosis has dramatically changed over the recent past. A disease that formerly was conceived as uncommon and untreatable is now increasingly recognized with available therapies that dramatically extend survival and mitigate symptoms. Advances in noninvasive diagnosis coupled with concurrent demonstration of efficacy and approval of specific therapies has shifted cardiac amyloidosis from a rarely encountered and untreatable "zebra," to a condition that cardiovascular clinicians should consider in daily practice.

REFERENCES

Etiologies

1. Sipe JD, Cohen AS. Review: history of the amyloid fibril. *J Struct Biol*. 2000;130:88–98.
2. Wechalekar AD, Gillmore JD, Hawkins PN. Systemic amyloidosis. *Lancet*. 2016;387:2641–2654.
3. Merlini G, Dispenzieri A, Sanchorawala V, et al. Systemic immunoglobulin light chain amyloidosis. *Nat Rev Dis Primers*. 2018;4:38.
4. Ruberg FL, Grogan M, Hanna M, et al. Transthyretin amyloid cardiomyopathy: JACC state-of-the-art review. *J Am Coll Cardiol*. 2019;73:2872–2891.
5. Castano A, Narotsky DL, Hamid N, et al. Unveiling transthyretin cardiac amyloidosis and its predictors among elderly patients with severe aortic stenosis undergoing transcatheter aortic valve replacement. *Eur Heart J*. 2017;38:2879–2887.
6. Buxbaum JN, Ruberg FL. Transthyretin V122I (pV142I)* cardiac amyloidosis: an age-dependent autosomal dominant cardiomyopathy too common to be overlooked as a cause of significant heart disease in elderly African Americans. *Genet Med*. 2017;19:733–742.
7. Damrauer SM, Chaudhary K, Cho JH, et al. Association of the V122I hereditary transthyretin amyloidosis genetic variant with heart failure among individuals of African or Hispanic/Latino ancestry. *J Am Med Assoc*. 2019;322:2191–2202.
8. Maurer MS, Hanna M, Grogan M, et al. Genotype and phenotype of transthyretin cardiac amyloidosis: THAOS (transthyretin amyloid outcome survey). *J Am Coll Cardiol*. 2016;68:161–172.
9. Suhr OB, Lundgren E, Westermark P. One mutation, two distinct disease variants: unravelling the impact of transthyretin amyloid fibril composition. *J Intern Med*. 2017;281:337–347.
10. Lane T, Fontana M, Martinez-Naharro A, et al. Natural history, quality of life, and outcome in cardiac transthyretin amyloidosis. *Circulation*. 2019;140:16–26.

Diagnosis

11. Kumar S, Dispenzieri A, Lacy MQ, et al. Revised prognostic staging system for light chain amyloidosis incorporating cardiac biomarkers and serum free light chain measurements. *J Clin Oncol*. 2012;30:989–995.
12. Lilleness B, Ruberg FL, Mussinelli R, et al. Development and validation of a survival staging system incorporating BNP in patients with light chain amyloidosis. *Blood*. 2019;133:215–223.
13. Falk RH, Quarta CC, Dorbala S. How to image cardiac amyloidosis. *Circ Cardiovasc Imaging*. 2014;7:552–562.
14. Gillmore JD, Damy T, Fontana M, et al. A new staging system for cardiac transthyretin amyloidosis. *Eur Heart J*. 2018;39:2799–2806.
15. Grogan M, Scott CG, Kyle RA, et al. Natural history of wild-type transthyretin cardiac amyloidosis and risk stratification using a novel staging system. *J Am Coll Cardiol*. 2016;68:1014–1020.
16. Witteles RM, Bokhari S, Damy T, et al. Screening for transthyretin amyloid cardiomyopathy in everyday practice. *JACC Heart Failure*. 2019;7:709–716.
17. Aljama MA, Sidiqi MH, Dispenzieri A, et al. Comparison of different techniques to identify cardiac involvement in immunoglobulin light chain (AL) amyloidosis. *Blood Adv*. 2019;3:1226–1229.
18. Phull P, Sanchorawala V, Connors LH, et al. Monoclonal gammopathy of undetermined significance in systemic transthyretin amyloidosis (ATTR). *Amyloid*. 2018;25:62–67.
19. Arvanitis M, Simon S, Chan G, et al. Retinol binding protein 4 (RBP4) concentration identifies V122I transthyretin cardiac amyloidosis. *Amyloid*. 2017;24:120–121.
20. Dorbala S, Ando Y, Bokhari S, et al. ASNC/AHA/ASE/EANM/HFSA/ISA/SCMR/SNMMI expert consensus recommendations for multimodality imaging in cardiac amyloidosis: Part 1 of 2-evidence base and standardized methods of imaging. *J Card Fail*. 2019;25:e1–e39.
21. Dorbala S, Ando Y, Bokhari S, et al. ASNC/AHA/ASE/EANM/HFSA/ISA/SCMR/SNMMI expert consensus recommendations for multimodality imaging in cardiac amyloidosis: Part 2 of 2-diagnostic criteria and appropriate utilization. *J Card Fail*. 2019;25:854–865.
22. Pagourelias ED, Mirea O, Duchenne J, et al. Echo parameters for differential diagnosis in cardiac amyloidosis: a head-to-head Comparison of deformation and nondeformation parameters. *Circ Cardiovasc Imaging*. 2017;10:e005588.
23. Martinez-Naharro A, Baksi AJ, Hawkins PN, Fontana M. Diagnostic imaging of cardiac amyloidosis. *Nat Rev Cardiol*. 2020;17:413–426.
24. Gillmore JD, Maurer MS, Falk RH, et al. Nonbiopsy diagnosis of cardiac transthyretin amyloidosis. *Circulation*. 2016;133. 2404-2012.
25. Castano A, Haq M, Narotsky DL, et al. Multicenter study of planar technetium 99m pyrophosphate cardiac imaging: predicting survival for patients with ATTR cardiac amyloidosis. *JAMA Cardiol*. 2016;1:880–889.
26. Quarta CC, Gonzalez-Lopez E, Gilbertson JA, et al. Diagnostic sensitivity of abdominal fat aspiration in cardiac amyloidosis. *Eur Heart J*. 2017;38:1905–1908.
27. Quarta CC, Buxbaum JN, Shah AM, et al. The amyloidogenic V122I transthyretin variant in elderly black Americans. *N Engl J Med*. 2015;372:21–29.

Management

28. Kittleson MM, Maurer MS, Ambardekar AV, et al. Cardiac amyloidosis: evolving diagnosis and management: a scientific statement from the American heart association. *Circulation*. 2020;142:e7–e22.
29. Towbin JA, McKenna WJ, Abrams DJ, et al. 2019 HRS expert consensus statement on evaluation, risk stratification, and management of arrhythmogenic cardiomyopathy. *Heart Rhythm*. 2019;16:e301–e372.
30. El-Am EA, Dispenzieri A, Melduni RM, et al. Direct current cardioversion of atrial arrhythmias in adults with cardiac amyloidosis. *J Am Coll Cardiol*. 2019;73:589–597.
31. Muchtar E, Gertz MA, Kumar SK, et al. Improved outcomes for newly diagnosed AL amyloidosis over the years 2000–2014: cracking the glass ceiling of early death. *Blood*. 2017;129:2111–2119.
32. Varga C, Comenzo RL. High-dose melphalan and stem cell transplantation in systemic AL amyloidosis in the era of novel anti-plasma cell therapy: a comprehensive review. *Bone Marrow Transplant*. 2019;54:508–518.
33. Sanchorawala V, Sarosiek S, Schulman A, et al. Safety, tolerability, and response rates of daratumumab in relapsed AL amyloidosis: results of a phase 2 study. *Blood*. 2020;135:1541–1547.

34. Palladini G, Kastritis E, Maurer MS, et al. Daratumumab plus CyBorD for patients with newly diagnosed AL amyloidosis: safety run-in results of ANDROMEDA. *Blood*. 2020;136:71–80.
35. Maurer MS, Schwartz JH, Gundapaneni B, et al. Tafamidis treatment for patients with transthyretin amyloid cardiomyopathy. *N Engl J Med*. 2018;379:1007–1016.
36. Kazi DS, Bellows BK, Baron SJ, et al. Cost-effectiveness of tafamidis therapy for transthyretin amyloid cardiomyopathy. *Circulation*. 2020;141:1214–1224.
37. Berk JL, Suhr OB, Obici L, et al. Repurposing diflunisal for familial amyloid polyneuropathy a randomized clinical trial. *J Am Med Assoc*. 2013;310:2658–2667.
38. Judge DP, Falk RH, Maurer MS, et al. Transthyretin stabilization by AG10 in symptomatic transthyretin amyloid cardiomyopathy. *J Am Coll Cardiol*. 2019.
39. Adams D, Gonzalez-Duarte A, O'Riordan WD, et al. Patisiran, an RNAi therapeutic, for hereditary transthyretin amyloidosis. *N Engl J Med*. 2018;379:11–21.
40. Scott D, Solomon DA, Kristen A, et al. Effects of patisiran, an RNA interference therapeutic, on cardiac parameters in patients with hereditary transthyretin-mediated amyloidosis: an analysis of the APOLLO study. *Circulation*. 2019;139(4):431–443.
41. Benson MD, Waddington-Cruz M, Berk JL, et al. Inotersen treatment for patients with hereditary transthyretin amyloidosis. *N Eng J Med*. 2018;379:22–31.
42. Inotersen and Patisiran for Hereditary Transthyretin Amyloidosis. *Effectiveness and Value Evidence Report*. Institute for Clinical and Economic Review (ICER); 2018.
43. Dasgupta NR, Benson MD. Treatment of ATTR cardiomyopathy with a TTR specific antisense oligonucleotide, inotersen. *Amyloid*. 2019;26:20–21.
44. Gillmore JD, Gane E, Taubel J, et al. CRISPR-Cas9 in vivo gene editing for transthyretin amyloidosis. *N Engl J Med* 2021;385:493–502.

54 Hypertrophic Cardiomyopathy

CAROLYN Y. HO AND STEVE R. OMMEN

DIAGNOSIS, MORPHOLOGY, AND ETIOLOGY OF HYPERTROPHIC CARDIOMYOPATHY, 1062
Diagnosis and Morphology, 1062
Etiology and Genetic Basis of Hypertrophic Cardiomyopathy, 1063

PATHOPHYSIOLOGY, 1063

NATURAL HISTORY, 1066

GENETIC TESTING AND FAMILY MANAGEMENT, 1066
Genetic Testing, 1066
Family Management, 1067

CLINICAL MANAGEMENT, 1069
Sudden Cardiac Death Risk Stratification, 1069
Management of Symptoms, 1070

PATIENTS WITH OBSTRUCTIVE HYPERTROPHIC CARDIOMYOPATHY, 1071

PATIENTS WITH NONOBSTRUCTIVE HYPERTROPHIC CARDIOMYOPATHY, 1072
Management of Atrial Fibrillation, 1072
Exercise and Sports Participation, 1072

CLINICAL TRIALS AND EMERGING THERAPIES, 1073

SUMMARY, 1075

REFERENCES, 1075

Hypertrophic cardiomyopathy (HCM) is a primary disorder of the myocardium. It is defined by the presence of unexplained left ventricular hypertrophy (LVH), occurring in the absence of identifiable factors that may account for increased left ventricular wall thickness, including pressure overload and infiltrative or storage disorders. Classically, myocyte hypertrophy, disarray, and myocardial fibrosis are present histologically. The prevalence has been estimated to be 1 in 500 in the general population. Familial disease is well characterized, and pathogenic variants in the genes encoding the cardiac sarcomere are the most common etiology of HCM. Pathogenic sarcomeric variants are present in more than 60% of patients with a family history of HCM, but are also seen in individuals with sporadic disease. However, the cause of disease cannot be easily identified in many patients. Additionally, there is substantial heterogeneity in cardiac morphology and disease course, ranging from low symptom burden and relatively normal longevity to marked functional limitations, advanced heart failure, and sudden cardiac death. Clinical management requires assessment of the individual patient's pathophysiology and symptoms, as well as systematic evaluation of family members. This chapter describes the diagnosis, natural history, and management of HCM.

DIAGNOSIS, MORPHOLOGY, AND ETIOLOGY OF HYPERTROPHIC CARDIOMYOPATHY

Diagnosis and Morphology

Hypertrophic cardiomyopathy (HCM) is a highly complex disorder with a myriad of effects on the heart. Historically and currently the diagnosis of HCM has relied solely on the most overt feature: left ventricular hypertrophy that has developed in the absence of an obvious cause. In many ways this remains a diagnosis of exclusion. A maximum left ventricular wall thickness of ≥15 mm has been the standard threshold to diagnose disease in adults, although a threshold of ≥13 mm is recommended if there is a family history of HCM or if the individual in question carries a disease-causing (pathogenic) sarcomeric gene variant.[1] Standards for diagnosing pediatric-onset HCM have been more variable but typically require a left ventricular wall thickness at least two standard deviations greater than the body surface area–corrected population mean (z score ≥2.5).[2,3]

At the histopathologic level, HCM is characterized by myocyte hypertrophy, disarray, and fibrosis (Fig. 54.1). These intrinsic tissue abnormalities, particularly myocyte hypertrophy and myocardial fibrosis, likely contribute to clinical manifestations of heart failure (systolic and diastolic) and to the genesis of arrhythmias (ventricular and atrial). Notably, these histologic changes are not uniformly distributed and affect deeper layers of the myocardium; therefore endocardial biopsy is generally not useful in yielding a tissue diagnosis of HCM.

The location and degree of hypertrophy are variable, and ventricular volumes are typically small. Although asymmetric septal hypertrophy resulting in reversed septal curvature is the classic and most common morphologic subtype of HCM, hypertrophy can involve any left ventricular (LV) segment and may be focal or concentric (Fig. 54.2). Apical HCM is a well-described morphologic variant in which hypertrophy involves the distal LV, below the level of the papillary muscles. As such, apical HCM is not associated with left ventricular outflow tract obstruction (LVOTO). Apical HCM was first reported in Japan[4] and is more prevalent in individuals of Japanese versus European descent (13% to 25% vs. 1% to 2%).[5] Although early studies suggested a more benign prognosis for apical HCM, a broad spectrum of clinical outcomes has been described.[6]

Septal morphology and location of hypertrophy are moderately predictive of genetic background. Patients with classic reversed septal curvature are most likely to have pathogenic sarcomeric gene variants whereas patients with a sigmoidal septum (discrete upper septal thickening) or apical hypertrophy are least likely to have sarcomeric disease.[7,8] This latter pattern of hypertrophic remodeling is relatively common in older adults with hypertension and thus nonspecific. However, even within families with HCM who share the same underlying pathogenic sarcomeric variant, both the degree and morphology of hypertrophy are often varied.[9]

The differential diagnosis for HCM includes other conditions that may also result in increased left ventricular wall thickness, including syndromic, metabolic, storage, or infiltrative disorders (e.g., Noonan syndrome/RASopathies, Fabry disease, Pompe disease, cardiac amyloidosis, mitochondrial disease) and compensatory or secondary hypertrophic heart disease attributed to pressure overload (hypertension) or intense athletic training. These disorders are genocopies—phenotypically similar but genetically different—that mimic HCM as they share a common feature of cardiac hypertrophy. However, they are distinct from HCM and have different underlying pathobiology and natural history (Table 54.1). For HCM to be diagnosed with confidence, these conditions should be excluded. Age of presentation can be informative. Family history should be carefully ascertained to determine if disease is genetic, and if so, the pattern of inheritance can provide valuable information. Clinical features and physical examination should focus on identifying key extracardiac features, such as bilateral carpal tunnel

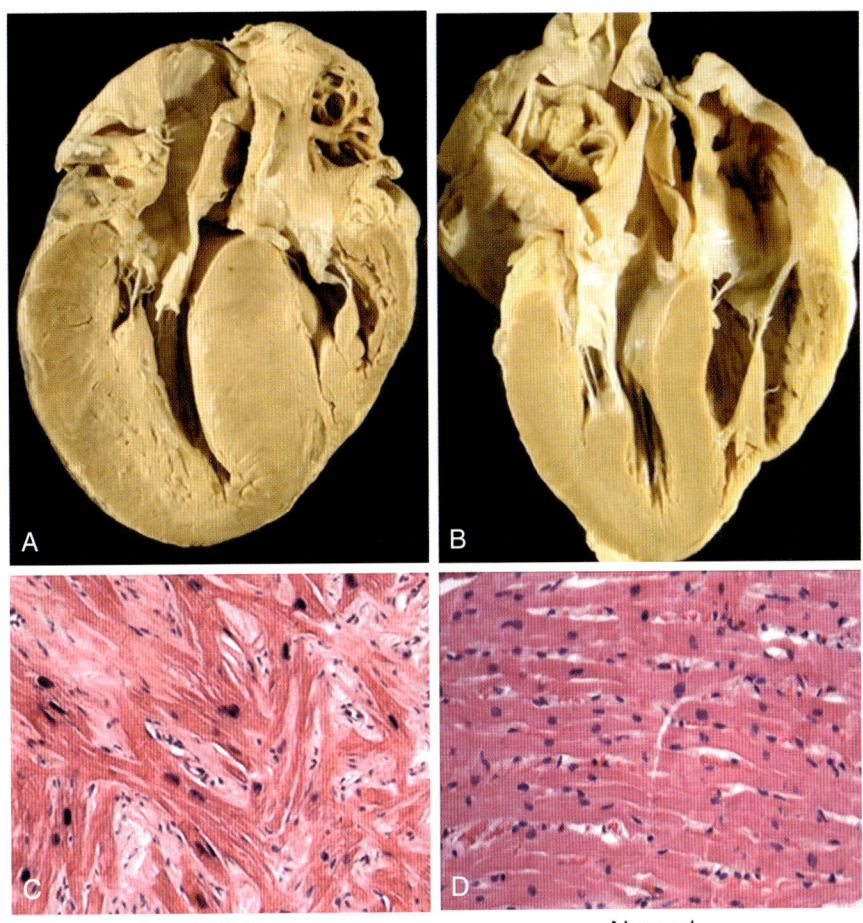

FIGURE 54.1 Gross and microscopic appearance of hypertrophic cardiomyopathy (HCM). **A** and **C**, HCM characterized by left ventricular hypertrophy, myocyte disarray, and myocardial fibrosis. **B** and **D**, Normal heart.

syndrome, biceps tendon rupture, skin changes (suggesting amyloidosis, particularly transthyretin [ATTR] amyloidosis), plasma cell dyscrasias (suggesting light chain [AL] amyloidosis), skin, neurologic and renal involvement (suggesting Fabry disease), and syndromic features (suggesting Noonan syndrome and mitochondrial disease). Cardiac magnetic resonance imaging (CMR) can help characterize myocardial tissue composition, identifying evidence of fibrosis or other infiltrative processes; however, biopsy (myocardial or of another affected site) is sometimes warranted to obtain a tissue diagnosis. Genetic testing can also provide key information to differentiate HCM from genocopies that also result in increased LV wall thickness (see Genetic Testing section later).

Etiology and Genetic Basis of Hypertrophic Cardiomyopathy

HCM was the first genetic cardiomyopathy to be characterized at the molecular level. Seminal genetic studies performed on families with HCM in the 1980s to 1990s established that HCM is a disease of the sarcomere—most frequently caused by pathogenic variation in genes encoding cardiac-specific sarcomeric proteins (Table 54.2), particularly myosin binding protein C (*MYBPC3*), myosin heavy chain (*MYH7*), troponin T (*TNNT2*), troponin I (*TNNI3*), myosin light chains (*MYL2* and *MYL3*), alpha-tropomyosin (*TPM1*), and actin (*ACTC*).[10–13] Sarcomeric variants are found in approximately 30% of HCM patients with apparently sporadic disease and over 60% of patients with a family history of HCM[14] or among those diagnosed in childhood. Variants in *MYBPC3* and *MYH7* are most common; collectively responsible for over 80% of sarcomeric HCM (caused by pathogenic sarcomeric variants identified by genetic testing) (Fig. 54.3). The population prevalence of HCM is approximately 1:500,[1] making it the most common monogenic heart disease. The cause of HCM in patients who do not carry sarcomere variants (non-sarcomeric HCM) remains largely unknown but likely reflects more complex interactions between genetic background and environment.

The sarcomere (Fig. 54.4) is the fundamental unit of contraction of all muscle cells. Cardiac sarcomeric proteins are organized into thick (myosin heavy and light chains, myosin binding protein C) and thin (actin, the troponin complex, and α-tropomyosin) filaments that interdigitate with muscle fiber shortening and lengthening. Excitation-contraction coupling relies on highly coordinated alterations in protein confirmation and calcium flux to drive thick and thin filament interaction and cardiac contraction and relaxation.[15] Membrane depolarization by the action potential elicits calcium influx through L-type calcium channels on the cardiomyocyte membrane. Ryanodine receptors on the sarcoplasmic reticulum (SR) are then activated to trigger calcium-induced calcium release. With the resultant increase in intracellular Ca^{2+} concentration, calcium binds to troponin C, leading to conformational changes in troponins I and T that release steric hindrance of tropomyosin from actin, permitting actin-myosin cross-bridge formation. Adenosine triphosphate (ATP) is then hydrolyzed to allow actin-myosin detachment and reuptake of calcium into the SR through the sarcoplasmic reticulum calcium-ATPase (SERCA) to complete the heart's chemomechanical cycle.

The exact mechanisms by which sarcomeric gene variants lead to the complex phenotype of HCM are not completely understood and likely involve multiple underlying pathways. Most pathogenic variants that cause HCM appear to act in a dominant negative or poison peptide fashion whereby mutant proteins are incorporated into the sarcomere and alter contractile performance.[16,17] *MYBPC3* is an exception in that the majority of pathogenic variants in *MYBPC3* result in premature termination codons and haploinsufficiency appears to be the predominant mechanism of disease.[18–20] Animal and basic science models have identified increased force generation, increased calcium sensitivity, impaired and disordered relaxation, and abnormal myocardial energetics, including increased energy consumption, as fundamental abnormalities associated with sarcomeric variants and HCM.[18,21–25]

Some of these fundamental findings have been corroborated by investigating individuals who carry pathogenic sarcomeric gene variants but have not yet developed a clinically overt phenotype of HCM. Studying these at-risk preclinical or subclinical variant carriers allows interrogation of the early manifestations of sarcomeric variants without confounding effects created by pathophysiologic abnormalities that accompany cardiac remodeling and disease development. Abnormalities in myocardial structure, function, and biochemistry are identifiable prior to the development of LVH. Decreased LV cavity size,[26] impaired LV relaxation, increased LV ejection fraction (LVEF),[27,28] altered myocardial energetics,[22,29] electrocardiographic abnormalities,[30] increased mitral valve leaflet length,[31,32] and evidence of a profibrotic state[33,34] can be identified in sarcomeric variant carriers when left ventricular wall thickness is normal. These findings also emphasize that although LVH is the most obvious manifestation, it is not an absolute marker of HCM. Further investigation is needed to characterize the entire spectrum of disease.

PATHOPHYSIOLOGY

The clinical manifestations of HCM can be tied to a complex interplay of cellular abnormalities, impaired myocardial function, and anatomic changes that alter hemodynamics, and may predispose to

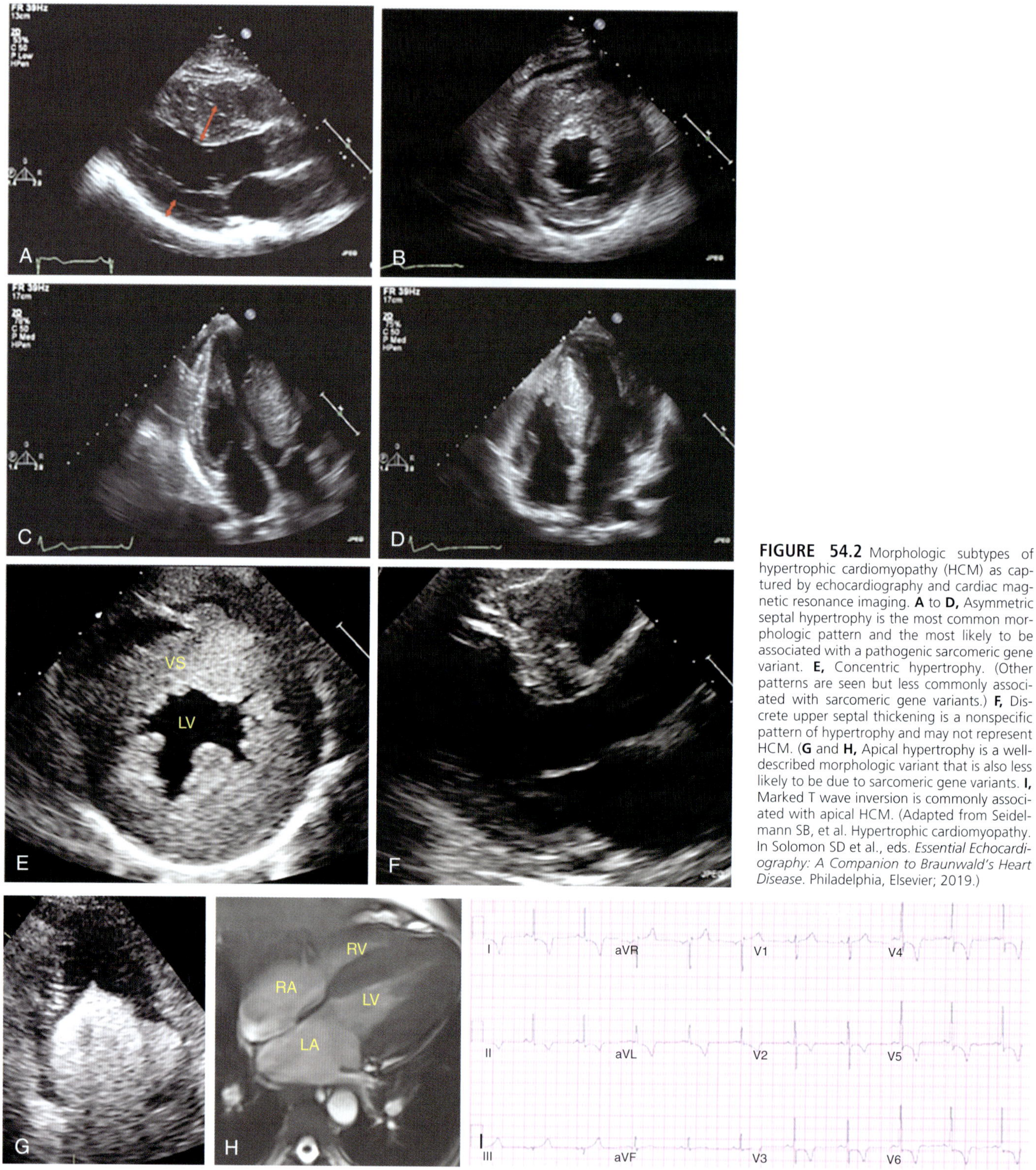

FIGURE 54.2 Morphologic subtypes of hypertrophic cardiomyopathy (HCM) as captured by echocardiography and cardiac magnetic resonance imaging. **A** to **D,** Asymmetric septal hypertrophy is the most common morphologic pattern and the most likely to be associated with a pathogenic sarcomeric gene variant. **E,** Concentric hypertrophy. (Other patterns are seen but less commonly associated with sarcomeric gene variants.) **F,** Discrete upper septal thickening is a nonspecific pattern of hypertrophy and may not represent HCM. (**G** and **H,** Apical hypertrophy is a well-described morphologic variant that is also less likely to be due to sarcomeric gene variants. **I,** Marked T wave inversion is commonly associated with apical HCM. (Adapted from Seidelmann SB, et al. Hypertrophic cardiomyopathy. In Solomon SD et al., eds. *Essential Echocardiography: A Companion to Braunwald's Heart Disease*. Philadelphia, Elsevier; 2019.)

development of arrhythmias. At the cellular level, abnormal calcium handling and altered interaction between actin-myosin has been identified, leading to abnormal contraction and relaxation. Coupled with the inherent stiffness of the hypertrophied left ventricle, some degree of diastolic dysfunction is present in nearly all patients with HCM.[35–37] Early diastolic tissue Doppler velocities are reduced in most patients with HCM, and abnormalities can be identified before the development of overt LVH in individuals who carry pathogenic sarcomeric variants.[38,39] Because the capillary network is less dense in HCM, subendocardial ischemia is readily manifest and can further worsen diastolic function. Delayed relaxation impacts the entire left ventricle at the macroscopic and myofilament level and also has carry-over effects on systolic function. However, contractile function has been more difficult to characterize. Animal, tissue, and cellular models of HCM have generally, but not universally, suggested increased contractility. There is some evidence suggesting that individuals who carry pathogenic sarcomeric variants but have not yet developed HCM (preclinical HCM) have preserved or slightly increased systolic strain by echo.[27,40] However, echocardiographic and CMR-derived systolic strain are abnormal in most patients with clinically overt HCM, potentially as a result of developing

TABLE 54.1 Genocopies of Hypertrophic Cardiomyopathy and Differentiating Features

ETIOLOGIES	TYPICAL AGE AT PRESENTATION	SYSTEMIC FEATURES	DIAGNOSTIC CONSIDERATIONS
RASopathies Glycogen storage diseases, other metabolic or mitochondrial diseases	Infants (0–12 months) and toddlers	Dysmorphic features Failure to thrive Metabolic acidosis	Geneticist assessment and genetic testing Newborn metabolic screening and additional metabolic assessment
RASopathies Mitochondrial diseases	Early childhood	Dysmorphic features Delayed or abnormal cognitive development Visual or hearing impairment	Biochemical screening Genetic testing
Friedrich ataxia Danon disease Mitochondrial disease	School age and adolescence	Skeletal muscle weakness or movement disorder	Biochemical screening Neuromuscular assessment Genetic testing
Friedrich ataxia Glycogen storage disorder (e.g., Fabry disease) Infiltrative disorders (e.g., light chain (AL) or transthyretin (ATTR) cardiac amyloidosis)	Late adolescence and adulthood	Movement disorder Peripheral or autonomic neuropathy Renal dysfunction Skin involvement Plasma cell dyscrasia Bilateral carpal tunnel syndrome, biceps tendon rupture	Biochemical screening Neuromuscular assessment Genetic testing Biopsy

Adapted from Ommen SR, Mital S, Burke MA, et al. AHA/ACC guideline for the diagnosis and treatment of patients with hypertrophic cardiomyopathy: a report of the American College of Cardiology/American Heart Association Joint Committee on Clinical Practice Guidelines. *J Am Coll Cardiol.* 2020;76(25):e159–e240.

TABLE 54.2 Major Genes Associated with Hypertrophic Cardiomyopathy and Genocopies

CORE SARCOMERIC GENES	PROTEIN ENCODED	% HCM ATTRIBUTABLE[4]
MYBPC3	Cardiac myosin-binding protein C	~50%
MYH7	Cardiac β myosin heavy chain	30%–35%
TNNI3	Cardiac troponin I	~5%
TNNT2	Cardiac troponin T	~5%
TPM1	α-tropomyosin	<3%
MYL2	Myosin regulatory light chain	<3%
MYL3	Myosin essential light chain	<3%
ACTC1	α-cardiac actin	~1%
Other HCM-Associated Genes		
CSRP3	Muscle LIM protein	<1%
TNNC1	Cardiac troponin C	<1%
ACTN2	α-actinin	<1%
JPH2	Junctophilin-2	Rare
Genocopies		
Storage Diseases		
LAMP2 (Danon disease)	Lysosome-associated membrane protein 2 (X chromosome)	
PRKAG2 (Glycogen storage disease)	Protein Kinase AMP-Activated Non-Catalytic Subunit Gamma 2	
GLA (Fabry disease)	α-galactosidase (X chromosome)	
Infiltrative Disease		
TTR (familial amyloidosis)	Transthyretin	
Noonan syndrome/RASopathies		
PTPN11 (Noonan syndrome)	Protein tyrosine phosphatase non-receptor type 11	
RAF1	Raf-1 Proto-Oncogene	

HCM, Hypertrophic cardiomyopathy.

myocardial abnormalities (fibrosis, disarray, hypertrophy) that accompany clinically overt disease. Moreover, calculated LVEF may not be a reliable measure of overall systolic function in HCM as the small LV cavity size associated with HCM is in the denominator of the formula and may artificially elevate ejection fraction. Accordingly, patients with HCM are considered to have significantly impaired systolic function if the ejection fraction less than 50%.

The most clinically apparent, and treatable, pathophysiologic mechanism in HCM is that of LVOTO.[41–43] Obstruction is present at rest or with physiologic provocation in up to two-thirds of patients with HCM and occurs as the hypertrophied septum redirects flow across, rather than along the mitral valve, which causes systolic anterior motion (SAM), further narrowing the outflow tract. The mitral valve itself is often elongated and positioned more anteriorly, which amplifies this effect.[44,45] The anterior mitral leaflet, rather than closing normally, is pushed further into the outflow tract, narrowing the latter and interfering with coaptation. Together, this results in increased LV systolic pressure and obstruction to outflow, particularly in late systole, increased myocardial oxygen demand, and posteriorly directed mitral regurgitation (Fig. 54.5). Patients are considered to have obstructive physiology if they have maximum instantaneous gradients across the outflow tract of at least 30 mm Hg. Resting or provoked gradients exceeding 40 to 50 mm Hg are considered capable of causing limiting symptoms. Patients with effort-related symptoms and resting LVOT gradients less than 40 mm Hg should have provocative maneuvers included with noninvasive evaluation. Bedside maneuvers such as Valsalva or squat-to-stand can be helpful in identifying latent outflow obstruction.[46] Provocation with exercise (e.g., exercise echocardiography) is a highly relevant and physiologic method to assess effort intolerance and should be considered in patients with symptoms whose resting gradients are not sufficiently high to account for their symptoms.[47,48] Symptom management is discussed under "Clinical Management," later.

Atrial fibrillation (AF) is a common arrhythmia in patients with HCM and is associated with decreased quality of life and a relatively high risk for systemic thromboembolism.[49–51] The loss of atrial contribution to LV filling, and the compromised diastolic filling period with rapid heart rates can result in decreased LV preload and thereby increased LVOT gradient. Aggressive rate control or restoration of sinus rhythm, both in combination with oral anticoagulation are felt to be important for patients with HCM (see Clinical Management, Management of Atrial Fibrillation, later).

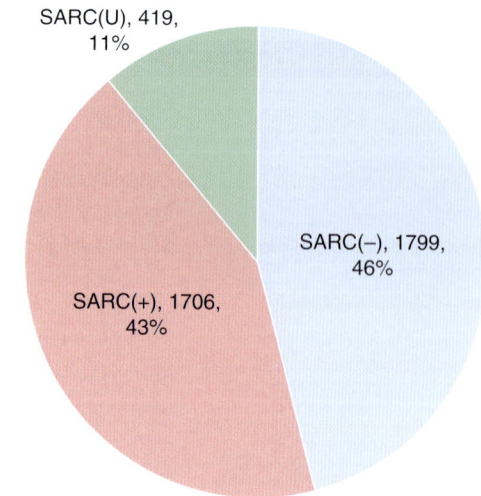
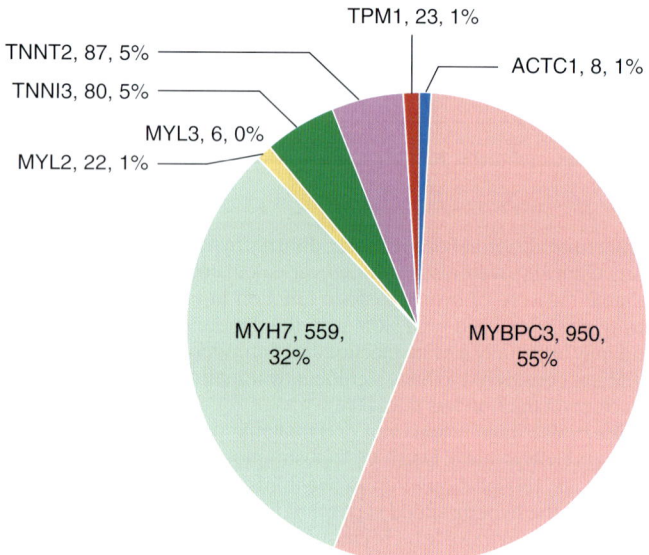

FIGURE 54.3 Top, Prevalence of sarcomeric versus nonsarcomeric hypertrophic cardiomyopathy (HCM). Examining 3924 HCM probands who had genetic testing and are cared for at high-volume HCM centers participating in the multicenter Sarcomeric Human Cardiomyopathy Registry (SHaRe),[49] 43% had pathogenic or likely pathogenic sarcomeric variants (SARC(+)), 46% did not have clinically significant variants identified (SARC(−)), and 11% had sarcomeric variants of unknown significance (SARC(U)). **Bottom,** Distribution of sarcomeric genes in HCM. Focusing on patients with sarcomeric HCM, myosin heavy chain and myosin binding protein C are most commonly implicated, collectively accounting for over 80% of HCM with an identified genetic etiology. *MYH7,* Myosin heavy chain; *MYBPC3,* myosin binding protein C; *MYL2/MYL3,* myosin essential and regulatory light chain; *TNNI3,* troponin I; *TNNT2,* troponin T; *TPM1,* alpha-tropomyosin; *ACTC1,* actin.

Ventricular arrhythmias are also an important cause for concern in HCM.[52] Sudden cardiac arrest occurs in just less than 1% of patients with HCM each year necessitating periodic risk assessment to identify patients with features that suggest higher risk and who may benefit from implantable cardioverter-defibrillator (ICD) placement (see Clinical Management, Sudden Cardiac Death Risk Stratification later). Nonfatal ventricular arrhythmias can also be problematic for some patients. This is often felt to result from intramyocardial scar and/or apical LV aneurysm.

NATURAL HISTORY

Natural history has been difficult to study and accurately characterize because disease course is highly variable. Many patients experience relatively normal longevity and modest symptom burden, whereas many others experience adverse clinical outcomes including heart failure, arrhythmias, and sudden cardiac death. Several large, multicenter HCM registries have recently been developed to better characterize clinical outcomes and their predictors.[49,53-55] Overall morbidity in HCM is dominated by heart failure and atrial fibrillation. Similarly, mortality is driven by complications of heart failure and noncardiac death, both of which are more common than lethal arrhythmias. Genotype is associated with clinical outcomes. Patients with sarcomeric HCM are diagnosed at an earlier age and had a greater burden and earlier onset of HCM-related complications than patients with nonsarcomeric HCM.[49,56-58] Sex also impacts the clinical course in HCM. Females are typically diagnosed at an older age and typically have more symptomatic heart failure and higher mortality.[59,60]

The lifetime cumulative burden of HCM was shown to be greatest in patients diagnosed earlier in life, and those with sarcomere mutations.[49] While the incidence of malignant ventricular arrhythmias and risk for sudden cardiac death decline with age, the risk for heart failure and atrial fibrillation increases. The majority of these HCM-related complications occur later in life, becoming most prevalent by middle to late adulthood, even in patients diagnosed before age 40 years (Fig. 54.6). These observations underscore the need for lifelong surveillance and for developing effective strategies to attenuate progressive disease burden.

Approximately 8% of patients with HCM experience more advanced cardiac remodeling marked by a decrease in LV systolic function.[61] Because HCM is characteristically associated with increased LVEF, an LVEF of 50% or less is abnormal and has traditionally defined HCM with LV systolic dysfunction (HCM-LVSD). Risk predictors for incident development of systolic dysfunction included the presence of pathogenic sarcomeric variants, particularly in thin filament genes, increased left ventricular wall thickness, left ventricular dilation, and borderline low ejection fraction (50% to 59%). The natural history of HCM-LVSD is variable; however, the majority of patients experience adverse events. Approximately one-third of patients died or required cardiac transplantation or durable mechanical support within a decade of developing systolic dysfunction.[61] Risk predictors of poor prognosis for patients with HCM-LVSD are multiple pathogenic/likely pathogenic sarcomeric variants, atrial fibrillation, and LVEF less than 35%.[61] Management is discussed later under "Clinical Management."

GENETIC TESTING AND FAMILY MANAGEMENT

Genetic Testing

The goals of genetic testing are to provide a definitive diagnosis in patients with known or suspected HCM and to guide management of at-risk or undiagnosed relatives.[62] There are two major types of genetic testing: diagnostic and predictive/variant confirmation testing in families. *Diagnostic genetic testing* is performed on an individual with unexplained LVH or a clinical diagnosis of HCM, typically using multigene panels specifically tailored for HCM that include at least the core sarcomeric genes (*MYH7, MYBPC3, TNNT2, TNNC1, TNNI3, TPM1, MYL2, MYL3, ACTC1*), as well as genes associated with other conditions that result in increased LV wall thickness, including glycogen storage disease and lysosome storage diseases (*LAMP2, PRKAG2, GLA* [Fabry disease], *GAA* [Pompe disease]), metabolic and mitochondrial disease, hereditary amyloidosis (*TTR*), and other genetic syndromes such as Noonan syndrome (involving genes in the Ras/MAP kinase pathway) (see Table 54.2). As such, diagnostic genetic testing can clarify diagnosis and identify the underlying disease process, including differentiating HCM from these genocopies. Accurately making these distinctions will critically impact clinical management.

One of the greatest challenges for genetic testing is determining whether an identified sequence variant is the cause of disease. In contrast to typical laboratory testing, genetic testing is probabilistic and classifies variants along a continuum that reflects the estimated likelihood that a variant is disease causing, based on current evidence. The American College of Medical Genetics and Genomics and the Association for Molecular Pathology developed guidelines for variant interpretation, proposing five tiers of classification: pathogenic, likely pathogenic, uncertain significance, likely benign, and benign, drawing upon a variety of evidence, including population, functional, computational, and segregation data to determine classification.[63] Variants classified as pathogenic and likely pathogenic are generally considered

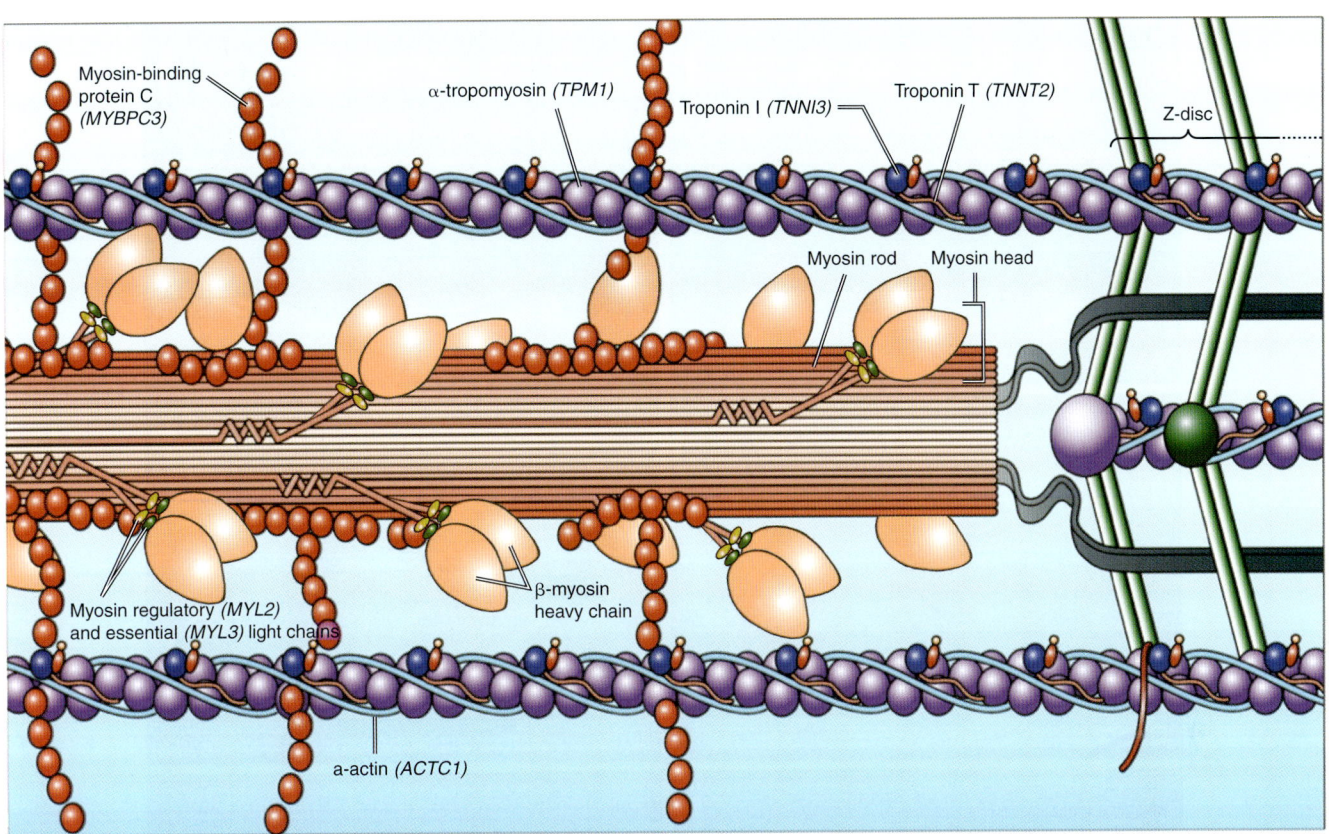

FIGURE 54.4 Cardiac sarcomere. The sarcomere is the fundamental unit of contraction for cardiac myocytes. Pathogenic variants in the genes that encode the different elements of the sarcomere are the most common genetic cause of hypertrophic cardiomyopathy. (Adapted from Seidelmann SB, et al. Hypertrophic cardiomyopathy. In Solomon SD et al., eds. *Essential Echocardiography: A Companion to Braunwald's Heart Disease*. Philadelphia, Elsevier; 2019.)

"positive" genetic testing results, meaning there is reasonable to high confidence that they are the genetic etiology of disease. These results may be considered for clinical decision making, including predictive genetic testing. A classification of a variant of uncertain significance (VUS) is an indeterminate result that does not provide a definitive genetic etiology and should not be used for clinical decision making or predicting risk in unaffected relatives. Negative results should be considered cautiously because this does not imply that genetic disease is excluded but rather indicates that a causative variant was not identified with available technology and knowledge. Clinical evaluation of at-risk healthy relatives is often still advisable. Additional genetic testing may be considered in the future if there are important advances in knowledge and technology. Furthermore, variants of uncertain significance should be reassessed periodically to determine if new data have emerged that allows reclassification into a more definitive category.

Family Management

Because HCM is often genetic, management extends beyond the individual patient to also include their family. The goals of family screening are to provide timely cardiac evaluation and initiate early treatment that may help mitigate adverse outcomes, particularly sudden death and symptomatic heart failure. The initial step is to obtain a multigenerational family history, ideally in pedigree format, to capture family structure, medical diagnoses and events, and ages and causes of death. This type of structured review assists in determining if familial disease is present, establish the inheritance pattern, and identify relatives at risk for developing disease. If familial disease is confirmed or cannot be excluded, clinical screening is performed to identify affected relatives and to follow currently unaffected relatives who are at risk for developing clinical disease.

The systematic process of evaluating relatives at risk for a genetic condition is termed cascade testing and may incorporate both clinical screening and genetic testing (Figs. 54.7 and 54.8). If genetic etiology has not been established in the family or if relatives do not wish to pursue genetic testing, the family evaluation relies on clinical screening (physical examination, electrocardiogram, echocardiogram) for first-degree relatives of an individual with HCM. If HCM is diagnosed in relatives during screening, their first-degree relatives are evaluated, and so forth. Due to the variable penetrance and expressivity of HCM, symptoms or signs may not develop until early or middle adulthood; thus longitudinal clinical screening is recommended for at-risk relatives.

The overall strategy for family screening is summarized in Figure 54.8. Initiation and repetition of clinical screening (echocardiography and ECG) varies by age. For adult and adolescent first-degree relatives of patients with HCM, screening is recommended to commence at the time of diagnosis in the proband and repeated at regular intervals (late childhood through adolescence every 1 to 2 years, and every 5 years through adulthood). For younger children, clinical screening can commence at any time but no later than the onset of puberty. Earlier initiation of screening can be considered if there is a family history of early-onset HCM, a particularly malignant history of HCM-related adverse outcomes, and/or heightened parental concern. For children and adolescents, once clinical screening is initiated, the repeat surveillance interval is every 1 to 2 years.[3]

If a definitively pathogenic variant is identified by diagnostic genetic testing on an affected family member, focused *predictive or variant confirmation genetic testing* can be offered to relatives to determine whether the variant has been inherited in other relatives. Relatives found to carry the pathogenic variant are at risk of developing disease. They should undergo serial clinical evaluation and be informed of the risk of transmission to offspring (see Figs. 54.7 and 54.8). However, the penetrance (the likelihood that an individual who carries a variant develops disease) of pathogenic variants is variable and cannot be predicted prospectively. In addition to not being able to accurately predict when or if HCM will develop, we currently are not able to predict how severe manifestations will be (expressivity). Therefore, broad longitudinal clinical follow-up of all at-risk relatives is currently recommended. In contrast, relatives who have negative predictive genetic testing and do not carry their family's pathogenic variant can generally be reassured that they neither they nor their children are at increased risk for developing HCM. They can be dismissed from longitudinal screening, although they should undergo prompt

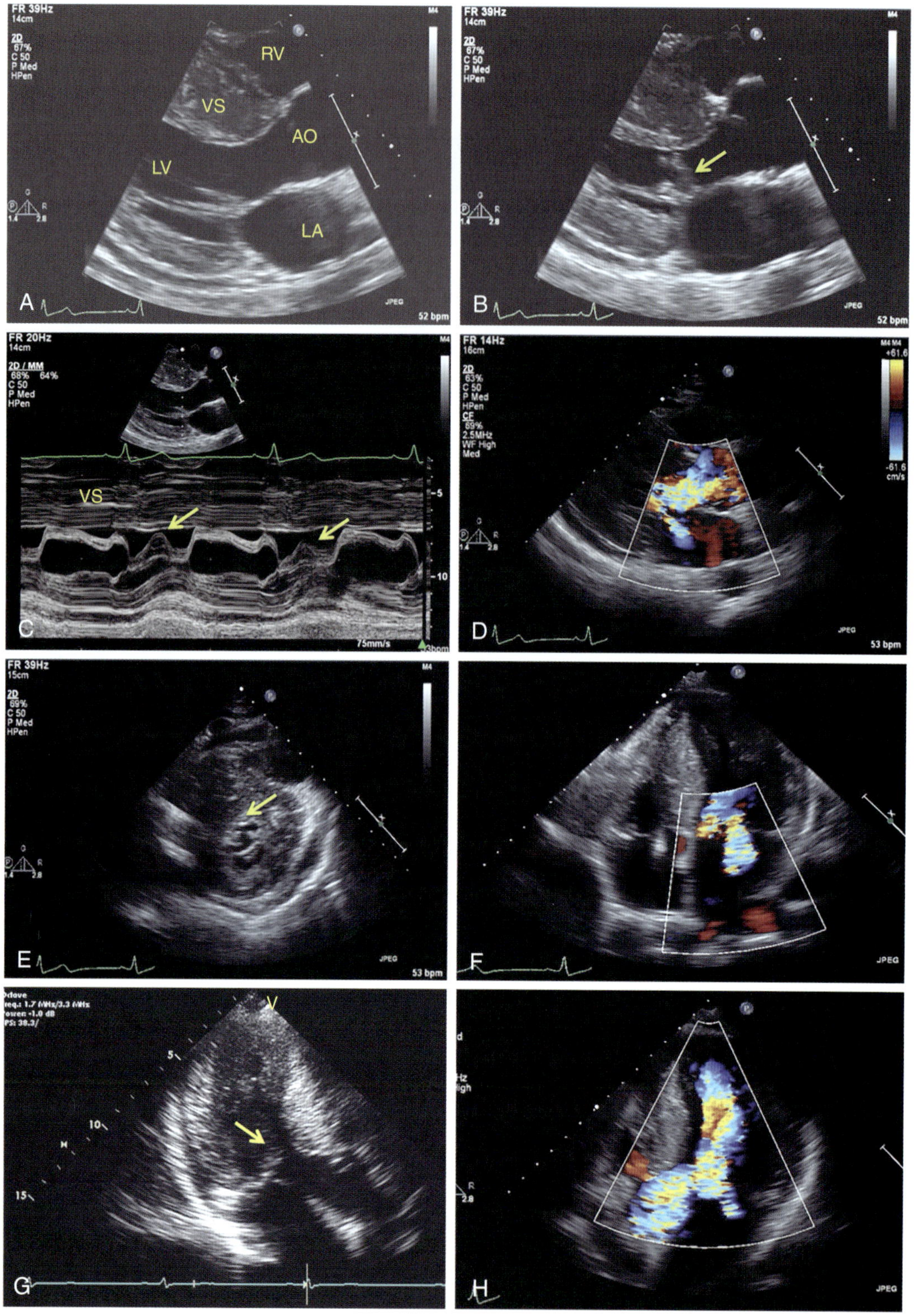

FIGURE 54.5 Systolic anterior motion of the mitral valve and left ventricular outflow tract obstruction. Still-frame images illustrate typical systolic anterior motion (SAM), showing the anterior mitral leaflet as it makes septal contact, producing mechanical impedance to LV outflow and mitral regurgitation. **A,** Parasternal long axis view in diastole. **B,** Parasternal long axis view in midsystole showing typical SAM in which the anterior mitral leaflet bends acutely (*arrows*), becoming almost perpendicular to the LV outflow tract in systole, resulting in focal septal contact and obstruction to flow. **C,** M-mode depiction of mitral valve motion demonstrating anterior motion of the mitral valve and septal contact in midsystole (*arrows*). The degree and duration of SAM-septal contact relates directly to the magnitude of the outflow gradient. **D,** Parasternal long axis image in midsystole with color Doppler demonstrating turbulent flow in the LV outflow tract due to systolic anterior motion and posteriorly directed mitral regurgitation. **E,** Parasternal short axis image in midsystole showing that the typical anterior motion of the mitral valve occurs in the center of the anterior mitral valve leaflet (*arrow* demonstrates septal contact). **F,** Apical four-chamber view in midsystole with color Doppler demonstrating turbulent flow in the LV outflow tract and mitral regurgitation. **G** and **H,** Apical three- and five-chamber view in midsystole demonstrating elongated mitral leaflets, particularly the anterior leaflet (AML), producing LV outflow obstruction from SAM (*arrow*) as shown by the accompanying color Doppler image. *AO,* Aorta; *LA,* left atrium; *LV,* left ventricle; *RV,* right ventricle; *VS,* ventricular septum. (From Seidelmann SB, et al. Hypertrophic cardiomyopathy. In: Solomon SD et al., eds. *Essential Echocardiography: A Companion to Braunwald's Heart Disease*. Philadelphia, Elsevier; 2019.)

evaluation in response to clinical changes. In cases where diagnostic genetic testing is not performed or a causal variant is not identified (diagnostic genetic testing was negative or identified variants were not definitively pathogenic), predictive genetic testing for healthy, at risk relatives is not an option and serial clinical evaluation is the default strategy, typically starting with first-degree relatives of affected individuals and expanding as new diagnoses are made.

Predictive genetic testing can also be used for reproductive planning either with prenatal testing (using amniocentesis or chorionic villus sampling) during an ongoing pregnancy to determine whether

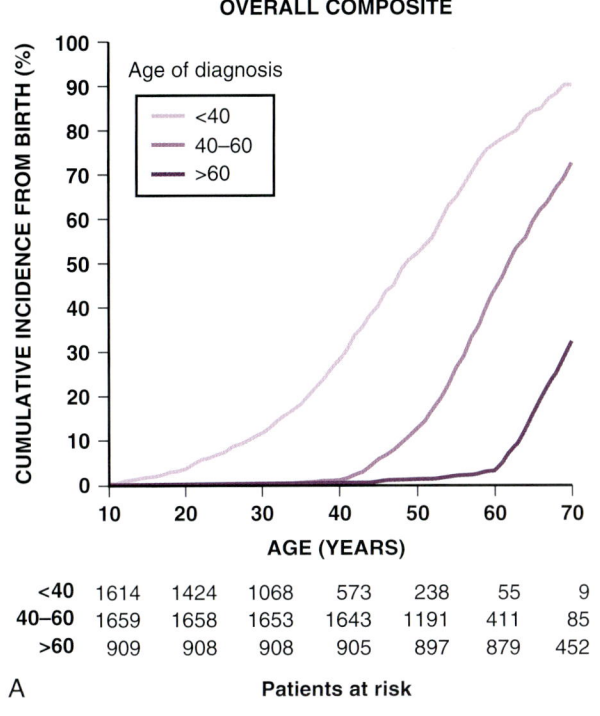
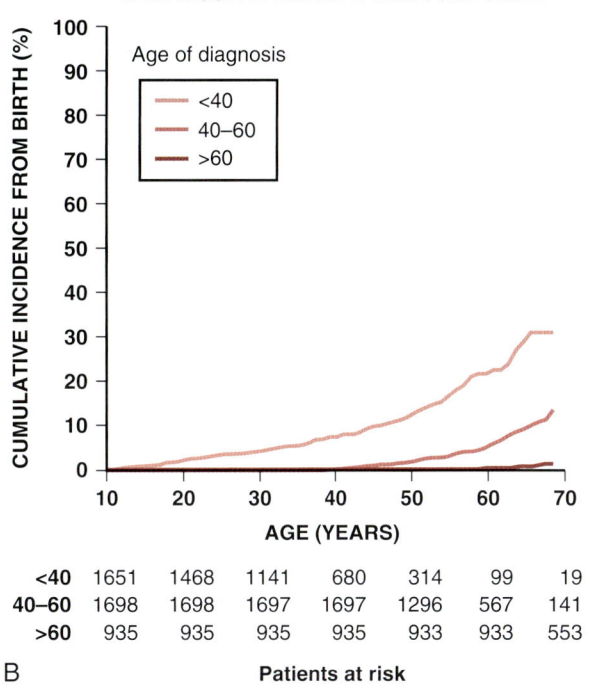
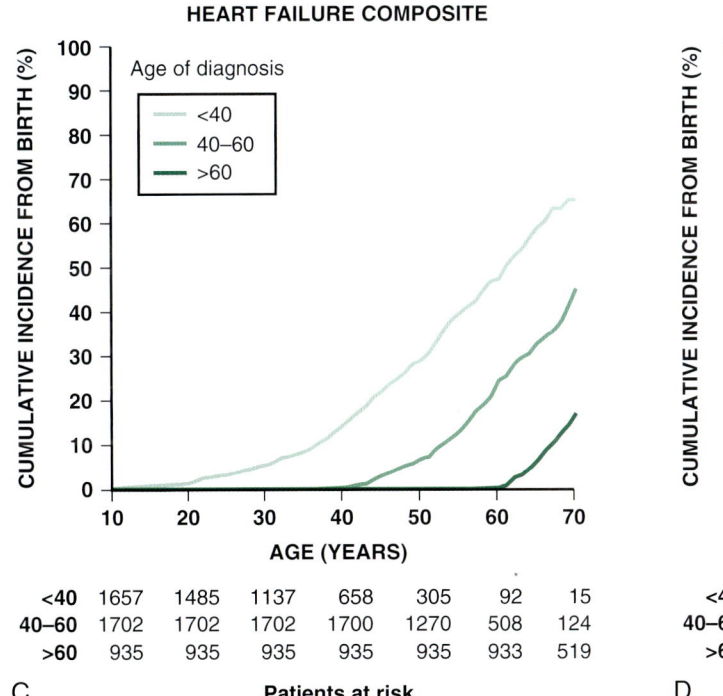
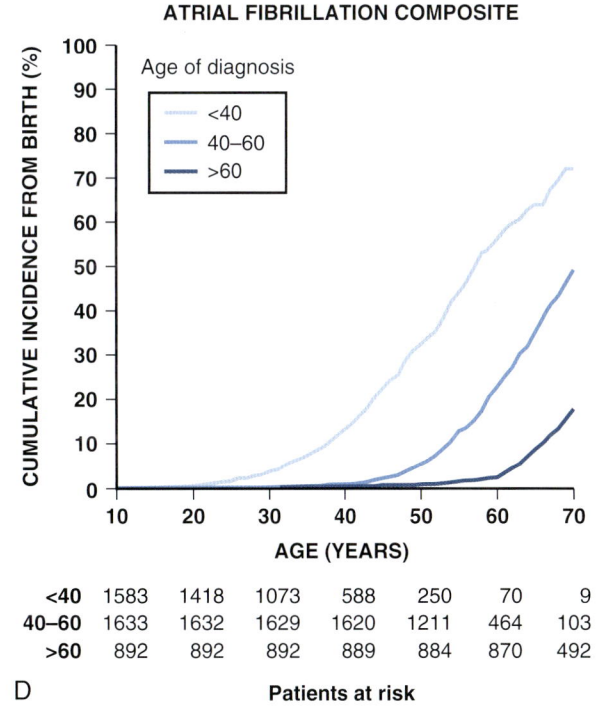

FIGURE 54.6 Age at diagnosis is associated with the lifetime cumulative burden of events. These curves depict the cumulative incidence of events from birth for outcomes of interest, stratified by age at diagnosis <40, 40 to 60, and >60 years. Earlier age at diagnosis is associated with a higher burden of adverse events. **A,** Overall composite outcome (first occurrence of all-cause mortality, sudden cardiac death, resuscitated cardiac arrest, appropriate implantable cardioverter-defibrillator therapy, cardiac transplantation, LV assist device implantation, New York Heart Association class III/IV symptoms, atrial fibrillation). **B,** Ventricular arrhythmia composite (first occurrence of sudden cardiac death, resuscitated cardiac arrest, or appropriate implantable cardioverter-defibrillator therapy). **C,** Heart failure composite (first occurrence of cardiac transplantation, LV assist device implantation, LVEF <35%, or New York Heart Association class III/IV symptoms). **D,** Atrial fibrillation. (From Ho CY, Day SM, Ashley EA, et al. Genotype and lifetime burden of disease in hypertrophic cardiomyopathy: insights from the sarcomeric human cardiomyopathy registry (SHaRe). *Circulation.* 2018;138:1387–1398.)

or not the fetus inherited the causal variant or through preimplantation genetic diagnosis (PGD). With PGD, genetic testing is performed on a single cell from embryos created using in vitro fertilization. Only embryos without evidence for the family's pathogenic variant are used for implantation, with a goal of achieving pregnancy without transmitting the genetic susceptibility for HCM.

CLINICAL MANAGEMENT

Sudden Cardiac Death Risk Stratification

The approach to the patient with HCM involves advice about family screening/surveillance (discussed earlier), risk stratification for SCD, and management of symptoms. As mentioned earlier, SCD occurs in

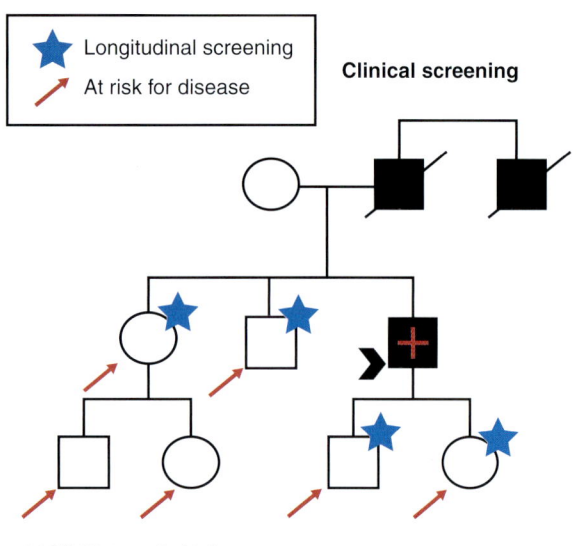

FIGURE 54.7 Family screening strategies using **(A)** clinical evaluation or **(B)** genetic testing. **A,** Clinical screening: All family members are at risk for developing hypertrophic cardiomyopathy (HCM) (*red arrows*). Guidelines recommend that all first-degree relatives (*blue stars*) of an affected individual undergo serial, longitudinal clinical screening to monitor for disease development. If found to have HCM (or develop HCM during follow-up), their first-degree relatives should be screened; a process referred to as *cascade screening*. The frequency of longitudinal screening varies by age and clinical status and is outlined in the 2020 ACC/AHA and 2014 ESC guidelines.[1,3] **B,** Predictive genetic testing is recommended for all members of families in whom a pathogenic variant has been identified. This allow unambiguous identification of relatives who are and are not at risk for developing HCM. With these results, family screening can evolve from broad, longitudinal screening of all potentially at-risk relatives (**A**) to focused longitudinal screening of relatives who are definitively at risk for disease by virtue of having inherited the family's pathogenic variant (*red plus signs and arrows* in **B**). Relatives who have not inherited the family's pathogenic variant (*red minus sign*) and their children are not at risk of developing HCM. Longitudinal follow-up is not required unless there is a clinical change in these patients. *Black arrowheads* indicate family proband. *Squares* indicate males and *circles* indicate females. *Solid black squares* indicate relatives diagnosed with HCM, and *open circles and squares* denote clinically unaffected relatives. (Adapted from Ahluwalia M, Ho CY. Heart 2021;107:183–189.)

just less than 1% of patients with HCM each year, and the appropriate utilization of ICDs has resulted in significantly improved outcomes. Patients who have previously experienced cardiac arrest or sustained ventricular arrhythmias have class 1 indications for ICD placement as secondary prevention.[1,3] Risk assessment and advice regarding primary-prevention ICDs remains a blend of science and clinical judgement (Fig. 54.9). Several clinical features have been associated with SCD, but the importance of the risk factors varies with age (i.e., some risk markers carry more weight in children than adults, and vice versa), and the overall risk appears to diminish with advanced age.[64-66] Although there are numerous exceptions, generally, the more severe the phenotypic expression of HCM, the higher the risk for SCD. Massive LV wall thickness (either as a binary variable or as a continuous variable), syncope felt to be arrhythmogenic, family history of SCD, overt systolic dysfunction, LV apical aneurysm, nonsustained ventricular tachycardia (NSVT), and extensive intramyocardial scarring (as assessed with CMR) have all been identified as being associated with SCD. Severe LVOTO has also been shown to be associated with SCD, but the effect size is modest and given the inherently dynamic nature of obstruction, this metric can be problematic to use in practice. Left atrial size, as a surrogate for phenotypic severity, has also been incorporated into risk calculators.[67] These tools can be useful to help patients with one or more of the SCD risk markers understand the magnitude of that risk.

In adult patients, the risk markers that appear to carry the most significance are massive hypertrophy (wall thickness approaching or exceeding 30 mm), family history of SCD in first-degree relatives younger than the age of 40 to 50 (or potentially multiple second-degree relatives), arrhythmogenic syncope, LV systolic dysfunction, and LV apical aneurysm. NSVT appears to be more important for younger patients or when the runs of NSVT are frequent, longer, and/or faster.[3,68] Extensive late gadolinium enhancement (LGE) on CMR indicates scarring in the LV wall which has also been shown to be associated with adverse outcomes including heart failure and ventricular arrhythmias.[69]

For children with HCM, massive hypertrophy (defined as z score approaching 20), arrhythmogenic syncope, and NSVT appear to be the most prominent risk predictors of SCD.[64] There are discordant data regarding family history of SCD, but a family event may be most useful if the event occurred in very young family members, or if it has occurred in multiple family members. Systolic dysfunction, apical aneurysm, and extensive LGE have not widely studied in children with HCM, but if present would seem important to consider as representing a particularly severe phenotype. The decision to proceed with ICD placement in children also must consider the complexity of placement, the need to account for somatic growth, and the greater number of years a device will be present.[70]

Management of Symptoms

Apart from SCD risk stratification, management of patients with HCM has traditionally focused on symptom management. Although clinical trial evidence is relatively scant, no pharmacologic agent has been shown to improve survival, and no invasive therapy has been shown to alter mortality in asymptomatic patients. This means that asymptomatic patients do not require initiation of therapy. Advice on health lifestyle, family evaluation, and management of other health concerns

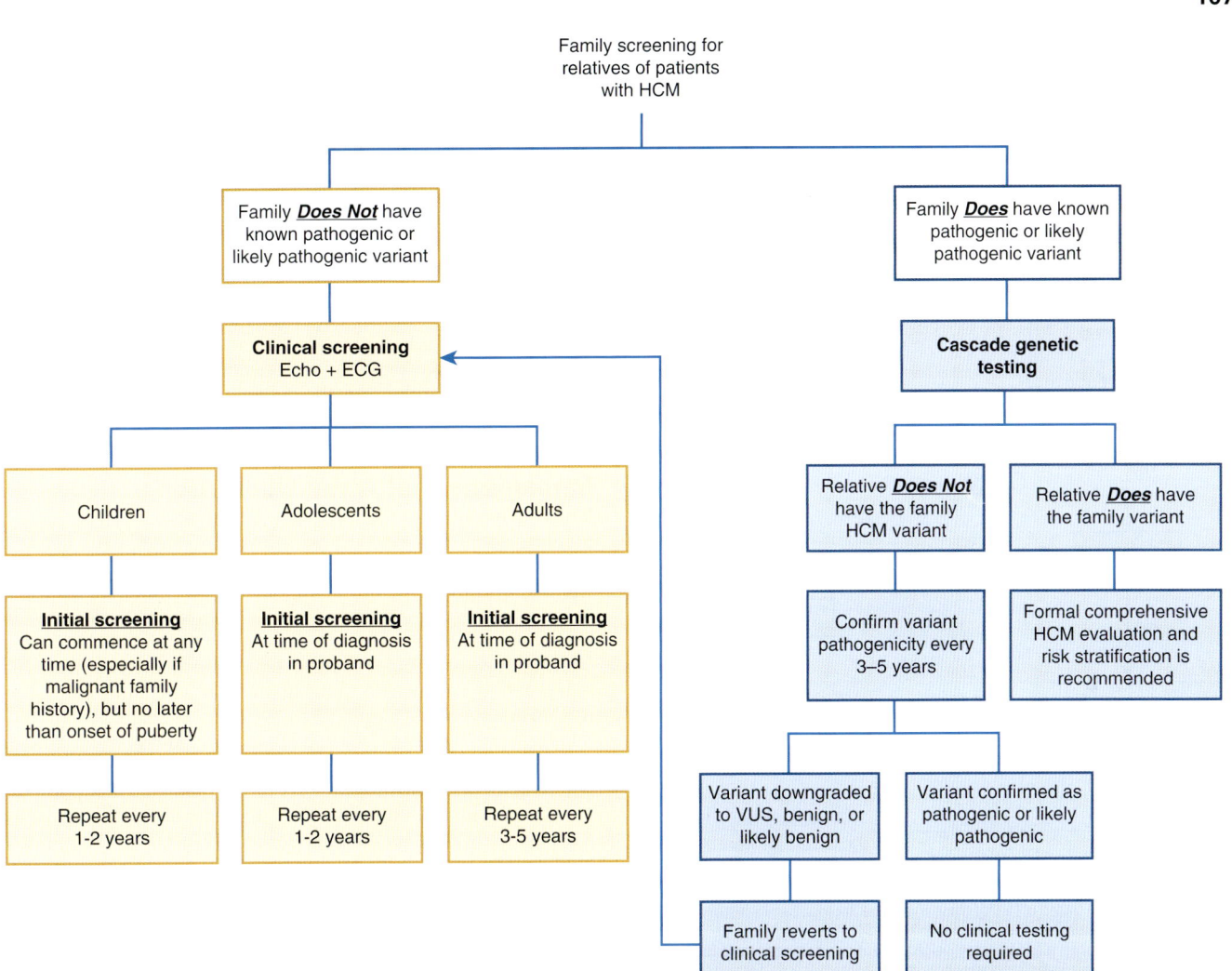

FIGURE 54.8 Strategy for family screening. Current recommendations suggest that clinical screening be repeated every 1 to 2 years during late childhood to early adulthood and every 5 years throughout adulthood. (From Ahluwalia M, Ho CY. Cardiovascular genetics: the role of genetic testing in diagnosis and management of patients with hypertrophic cardiomyopathy. Heart. 2021;107[3]:183–189.)

are the focus for these patients. For patients who have exertional dyspnea, angina, or syncope/presyncope, it is useful to base treatment on whether the symptoms are driven by obstructive physiology, nonobstructive disease, arrhythmia, or other processes (Fig. 54.10).

PATIENTS WITH OBSTRUCTIVE HYPERTROPHIC CARDIOMYOPATHY

Dyspnea, chest pain/pressure, and/or presyncope that vary from day to day are the hallmark symptoms attributable to LVOTO. Because gradient is highly dependent on loading conditions, anything that causes systemic vasodilation (e.g., ambient temperature, postprandial state, alcohol consumption) or volume depletion may exacerbate symptoms. Symptoms are most dramatically promoted by physical effort as systemic vascular resistance drops and contractility is augmented. Patients are rarely symptomatic at rest unless there is another disease state (e.g., sepsis) that alters loading conditions dramatically. Although randomized clinical trials have not been performed, the general approach for symptomatic patients with obstructive physiology is to optimize volume status (encourage vigorous hydration), eliminate or reduce any vasodilator therapies, and empirically start beta blockers, verapamil, or diltiazem because these agents have negative chronotropic effects which help maximize preload by increasing the diastolic filling interval, and negative inotropic effects.[3] Therapeutic efficacy is guided by the symptomatic response of the patient, not changes in gradient. If patients remain symptomatic after maximizing one of these agents, then switching to one of the other agents is the usual next step in care. Persistent symptoms beyond this prompts consideration of advanced options including disopyramide (added to one of the other agents).[71] Novel agents that directly target the enhanced actin-myosin interaction of HCM are in trials at this time (see Clinical Trials and Emerging Therapy, later).[72]

Although medical therapies are used to target myocardial function and/or loading conditions to indirectly improve obstruction, septal reduction therapy (surgical septal myectomy or alcohol septal ablation) directly addresses the anatomic cause of obstruction. Septal myectomy has evolved since its introduction over 60 years ago.[73] Performed via an aortotomy, muscle resection is now extended and involves a larger surface area of the septum down to the level of the papillary muscles. Some operators also include plication or other manipulation of the anterior mitral leaflet, particularly if mitral regurgitation or mitral valve pathology is thought to contribute importantly to pathophysiology.[74–76] Successful myectomy normalizes the flow pattern in the ventricle such that the mitral valve can coapt normally and outflow tract gradient is substantially reduced or abolished (Fig. 54.11). Muscle does not "regrow" at the myectomy site; therefore results are durable (recurrent or residual obstruction likely results from inadequate initial resection). In experienced centers, operative (30-day) mortality is less than 1% with a 90% to 95% success rate.[77,78]

Septal ablation is a percutaneous procedure during which alcohol is infused into the septal perforator artery that supplies the obstructive hypertrophied septum. This results in a scar which causes retraction of the septum as the myocardium remodels post infarct (Fig. 54.12).

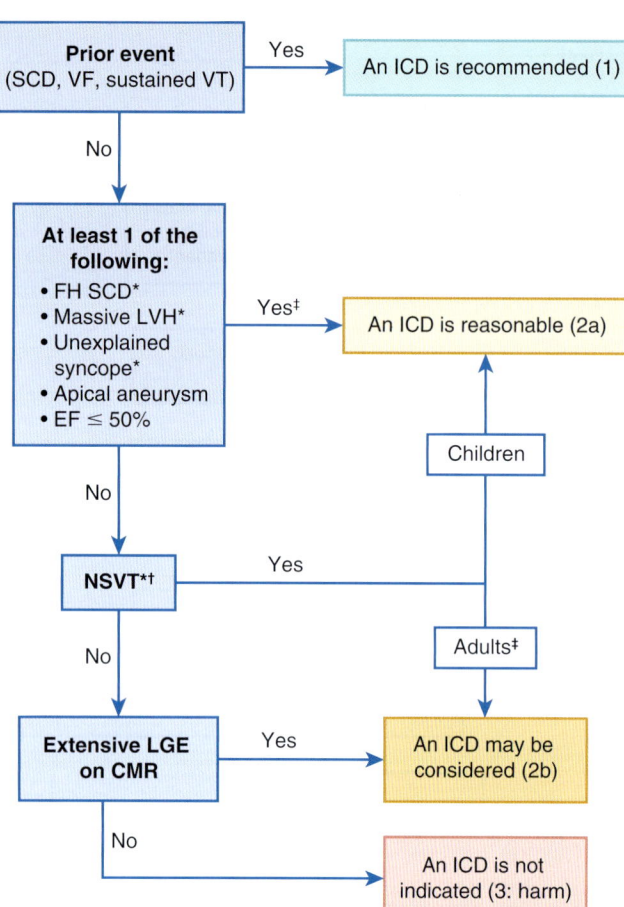

FIGURE 54.9 Patient selection for ICD placement. *ICD decisions in pediatric patients with HCM are based on ≥1 of these major risk factors: family history of HCM SCD, NSVT on ambulatory monitor, massive LVH, and unexplained syncope. †It would seem most appropriate to place greater weight on frequent, longer, and faster runs of NSVT. ‡In patients >16 years of age, 5-year risk estimates can be considered to fully inform patients during shared decision-making discussions. *CMR,* Cardiovascular magnetic resonance; *EF,* ejection fraction; *FH,* family history; *HCM,* hypertrophic cardiomyopathy; *ICD,* implantable cardioverter-defibrillator; *LGE,* late gadolinium enhancement; *LVH,* left ventricular hypertrophy; *NSVT,* nonsustained ventricular tachycardia; *SCD,* sudden cardiac death; *VF,* ventricular fibrillation; *VT,* ventricular tachycardia. (Adapted from Ommen SR, Mital S, Burke MA, et al. AHA/ACC guideline for the diagnosis and treatment of patients with hypertrophic cardiomyopathy: a report of the American College of Cardiology/American Heart Association Joint Committee on Clinical Practice Guidelines. J Am Coll Cardiol. 2020;76[25]:e159–e240.)

Patients who respond to ablation have similar symptomatic improvements as patients treated with septal myectomy, and long-term survival is similar.[79,80] However, there is a higher need for reintervention following ablation, and higher rate of heart block requiring permanent pacemaker placement. Clinical decision making to determine whether to pursue myectomy versus ablation can be complex and considers factors including access to experienced operators, a comprehensive discussion of the benefits and risks of both procedures, and patient-specific features that may make one option more appropriate, including septal morphology and suitable coronary artery anatomy. Patients who have other cardiovascular disease requiring surgical intervention are usually treated with surgical myectomy. Younger patients, patients with more severe LVH (>18 mm), and patients with severe resting gradients (>100 mm Hg) appear to have better outcomes with surgery.[81] Patients who are frail or have significant comorbidity that makes a surgical approach riskier are better candidates for septal ablation.

PATIENTS WITH NONOBSTRUCTIVE HYPERTROPHIC CARDIOMYOPATHY

Patients who do not have obstructive physiology can also have symptoms of angina or dyspnea. The former is likely due to subendocardial ischemia, and the latter falls into a spectrum of heart failure with preserved ejection fraction. Empiric treatment also uses beta blockers, verapamil, or diltiazem as first agents. Diuretics are used for patients with persistent dyspnea and/or signs of congestion. Nonobstructive patients with preserved systolic function (i.e., LVEF >50%) and severe symptoms that do not respond to these therapies are often considered for advanced heart failure options (medical therapy and advanced therapies) in accordance with the heart failure guidelines (see Fig. 54.10).[82] Cardiac transplantation is typically pursued as mechanical circulatory support has not been widely successful, particularly if LV cavity size is small.

As described previously under Natural History, specific to patients with HCM, systolic dysfunction is believed to be present when LVEF falls below 50% (as compared with ejection fraction <40%) with most other forms of cardiomyopathy guideline-directed management for systolic heart failure should be applied when appropriate.[3]

Management of Atrial Fibrillation

It has been estimated that up to half of patients with HCM may experience atrial fibrillation, with prevalence increasing with age.[49] Similar to other patients, this may be asymptomatic. However, patients with HCM, particularly those with obstructive physiology, are prone to develop symptoms when preload is decreased. The onset of atrial fibrillation can substantially reduce preload through loss of atrial contribution to LV filling, and as heart rates increase, the diastolic filling period is truncated. Slowing the heart rate and restoring sinus rhythm are important targets for therapy. Beta blockers, verapamil, and diltiazem can be helpful for rate control, and amiodarone, dofetilide, sotalol, and disopyramide have all be used for rhythm control.[3] The potential for proarrhythmia needs consideration in HCM, particularly in patients who do not have an ICD. Catheter ablation is considered a reasonable option for patients whose AF is not well controlled with medications. Similarly, for patients with HCM and AF who are referred for surgical myectomy, intraoperative AF ablation techniques can be added.

The risk of thromboembolism in patients with HCM and AF is higher than in patients without structural heart disease.[83] As such, risk-scoring systems (e.g., CHADs2VASc) are not used in patients with HCM, but rather oral anticoagulation is considered appropriate in all patients with both HCM and AF. Direct oral anticoagulants or warfarin are considered as viable options in patients with HCM. As with other patients with AF lasting more than 24 hours, the recommendation for oral anticoagulation is clear. For AF episodes less than 24 hours, the choice to initiate anticoagulation would need to be individualized accounting for bleeding risk, total AF burden, and other risk factors for thromboembolism.

Exercise and Sports Participation

The benefits of a healthy lifestyle that includes regular light to moderate physical activity appear to extend to patients with HCM.[84,85] The challenge is that among competitive athletes who have had cardiac arrest, HCM is overrepresented as an underlying diagnosis. This fact led to a generalized exclusion of individuals with HCM from participation in competitive athletics regardless of their clinical status.[86] The increasing societal interest in higher-intensity exercise led to renewed studies to determine for patients with HCM if there was a safe intensity level. These investigations, starting from the population of patients with HCM rather than from patients with cardiac arrest, have not shown increased adverse event rates with increasing effort intensity or participation in sports.[87,88] Taken together, these seemingly disparate results likely reflect that the highest level of physical activity (competitive sports) does represent a level of increased risk for cardiac arrest, but that the incremental relative risk of participation compared with nonparticipation is so small that the most recent studies are underpowered to detect that risk. From a practical standpoint, each person with HCM who is interested in higher-intensity training must be informed of this risk, the inability to accurately estimate the risk, and determine his or her own level of tolerance for the unknown risk.[3]

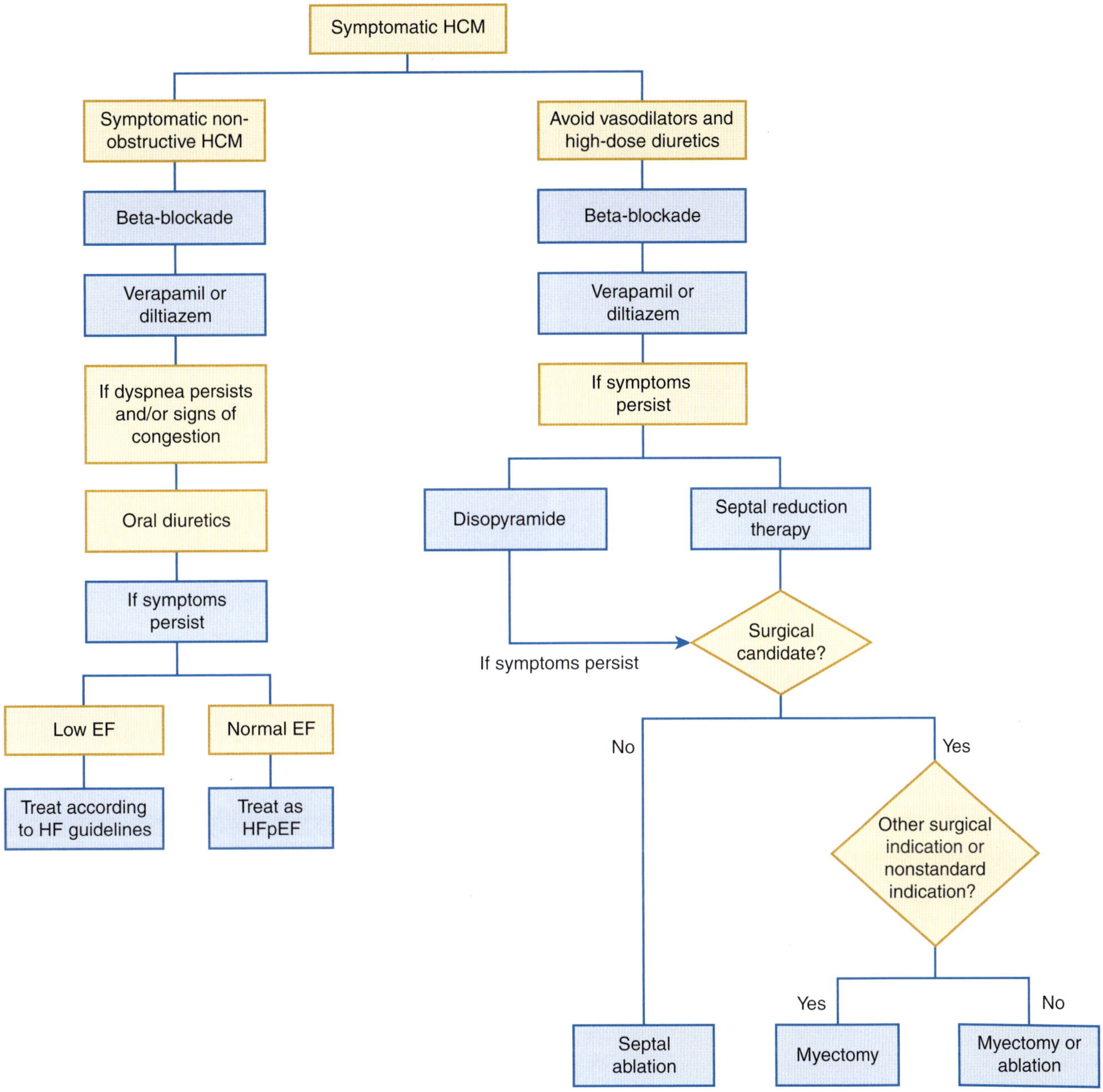

FIGURE 54.10 Management of symptoms in patients with hypertrophic cardiomyopathy.

CLINICAL TRIALS AND EMERGING THERAPIES

Owing to its relative rarity and heterogeneous disease expression, very few robust, prospective, appropriately controlled trials have been performed in HCM. To date, fewer than 100 trials have been published, the vast majority studying fewer than 50 patients and lacking randomization, blinding, or comparison with placebo.[89,90] Historically and currently, treatment has relied on off-label use of available medications (beta blockers, L-type calcium channel blockers, and disopyramide) to mitigate symptoms by leveraging nonspecific pharmacologic properties. These limitations have been well recognized and, in concert with growing understanding of underlying disease pathways, there has been renewed interest in developing more mechanistically driven therapies. However, small trials of potentially promising therapeutic targets in obstructive and nonobstructive HCM have failed to demonstrate efficacy. These include attempts to modulate myocardial energetics using perhexiline and trimetazidine,[91,92] to inhibit the late-sodium channel using ranolazine and eleclazine,[93,94] and to decrease fibrosis using spironolactone, valsartan, and losartan.[95–98]

Newer treatments and concepts in development include disease-modifying and prevention strategies, targeting sarcomeric variant carriers prior to development of clinically overt HCM, myosin inhibitors, and gene-based therapies. No treatments have been proven to alter the natural history of disease or to be beneficial for either sarcomeric variant carriers with normal LV wall thickness or for asymptomatic patients with HCM. However, with improved understanding of how sarcomere variants cause HCM, treatments are being pursued attempting to target early, disease-initiating pathways. The goal of these therapies would be to attenuate disease progression and, ultimately, disease emergence. Studies in mouse models of sarcomeric HCM have demonstrated that treatment with agents, including diltiazem, losartan, and mavacamten (see later), was able to attenuate disease development if given early in life, prior to the development of diagnostic features of disease.[99–101] Pilot efforts at translation to human disease are being attempted, but further investigation and experience are required.[102,103]

Novel, oral selective allosteric inhibitors of cardiac myosin ATPase have recently been developed to address fundamental abnormalities associated with HCM, namely increased contractile force. The first such agent, mavacamten, reduces actin-myosin cross-bridge formation, thereby reducing myocardial contractility and improving myocardial energetics.[104] Animal studies demonstrated that mavacamten reduces

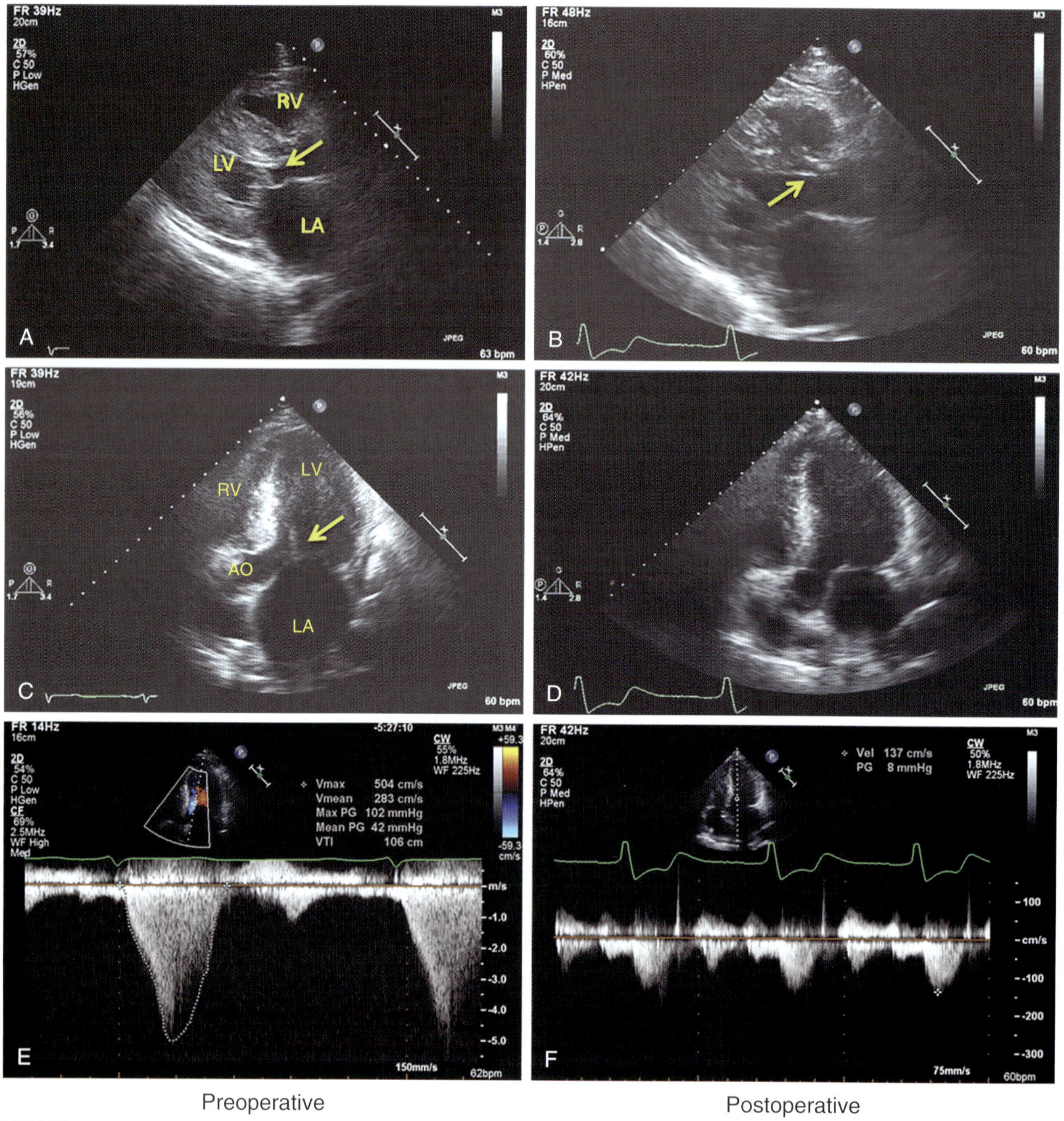

FIGURE 54.11 Surgical myectomy to manage symptomatic obstructive hypertrophic cardiomyopathy (HCM). **A,** Preoperative: Parasternal long axis view shows marked hypertrophy of the septum and systolic anterior motion of the mitral valve (SAM) (*arrow*). **B,** Postoperative: Parasternal long axis view shows a myectomy "trough" (*arrow*) representative of the portion of the upper septum that was resected, resulting in an increase of the cross-sectional area of the LV outflow tract, ultimately, eliminating SAM and LVOT obstruction. **C,** Preoperative: Apical five-chamber view showing hypertrophy of the ventricular septum and SAM (*arrow*). **D,** Postoperative: Apical five-chamber view showing resection of the basal ventricular septum and resolution of SAM. **E,** Preoperative: Apical five-chamber view with continuous wave Doppler showing a peak velocity of 5.0 m/sec. **F,** Postoperative: Apical five-chamber view with continuous wave Doppler showing a reduction in peak velocity to 1.4 m/sec post resection. *AO,* Aorta; *LA,* left atrium; *LV,* Left ventricle; *RV,* right ventricle; *VS,* ventricular septum. (From Seidelmann SB, et al. Hypertrophic cardiomyopathy. In: Solomon SD, et al., eds. *Essential Echocardiography: A Companion to Braunwald's Heart Disease.* Philadelphia, Elsevier; 2019.)

myocardial contraction in a dose-dependent manner and relieves left ventricular outflow obstruction.[101,105] A phase III clinical trial of mavacamten versus placebo in patients with symptomatic obstructive HCM demonstrated that treatment with mavacamten significantly improved exercise capacity, LVOT obstruction, symptoms, and health status.[72] Substantial reduction in outflow tract gradients were achieved with only modest reduction in LVEF; however, careful dose titration and monitoring are required given that the mechanism of action is to decrease contractility. Furthermore, although initial experience with myosin inhibitors targeted patients with obstructive HCM and focused on reducing contractility and obstruction, there is also potential mechanistic rationale that myosin inhibitors may improve relaxation abnormalities and impaired myocardial energetics associated with disease.[104,106] A phase II study of mavacamten versus placebo in patients with symptomatic nonobstructive HCM demonstrated that treatment with mavacamten was associated with a significant reduction in N-terminal propeptide of B-type natriuretic peptide.[107] Although this initial experience has been promising, further investigation is needed to determine long-term safety and benefit over standard therapy.

Gene-based therapy is also emerging as a potential strategy, including genome editing, exon skipping, allele-specific silencing, spliceosome-mediated RNA trans-splicing, and gene replacement.[108,109] The therapeutic goal is to replace, remove, or mitigate the effect of the germline genetic defect. Technologies are being developed and tested

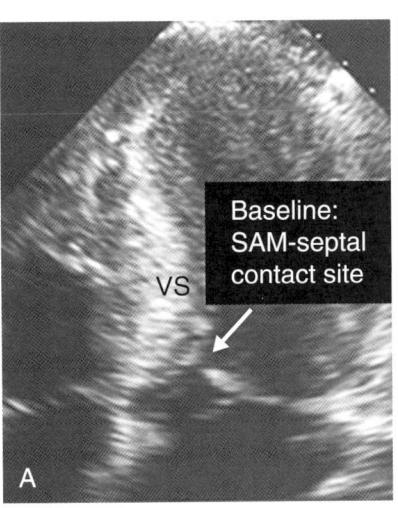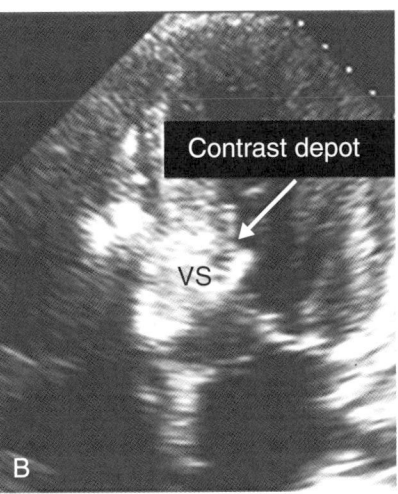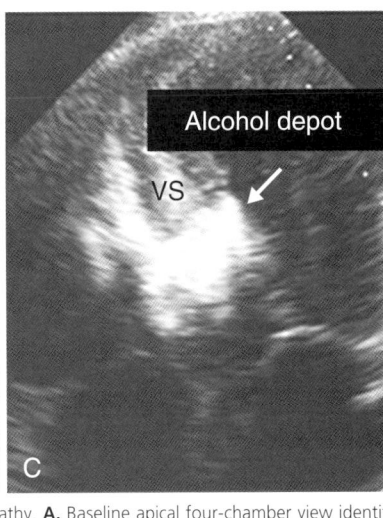

FIGURE 54.12 Alcohol septal ablation for management of symptomatic obstructive hypertrophic cardiomyopathy. **A,** Baseline apical four-chamber view identifies the area of maximal systolic anterior motion (SAM)-septal contact to target for ablation (*arrow*). **B,** Intracoronary injection of echocardiographic contrast is used to verify that the identified septal perforator branch supplies the target area of the ventricular septum, at the site of maximal SAM-septal contact. The region supplied by the injected septal branch is highlighted by the contrast agent manifest as an echogenic signal created by the accumulation of contrast within the myocardium (*arrow*). Contrast defines the site of potential ablation and determines if infarction size will be too large or involve unintended structures such as the right ventricle. **C,** After defining the site of potential ablation, alcohol is injected into the selected septal perforator branch, targeting the region of the septum that is highlighted by intracoronary contrast and seen as an intensely echobright signal from the alcohol collection within the myocardium (*arrow*). (From Seidelmann SB, et al. Hypertrophic cardiomyopathy. In: Solomon SD, et al., eds. *Essential Echocardiography: A Companion to Braunwald's Heart Disease*. Philadelphia, Elsevier; 2019.)

in animal and human-induced pluripotent stem cell models of HCM. Genetic variants resulting in haploinsufficiency as the mechanism of disease, such as most HCM caused by *MYBPC3* variants, may be most amenable to gene therapy.

SUMMARY

HCM is a primary myocardial disorder defined by otherwise unexplained left ventricular hypertrophy. As an intriguing and complex clinical entity and the first cardiomyopathy to be explained at the molecular genetic level, HCM has been the focus of intense clinical and basic science investigation for decades. Optimal clinical management requires thoughtful assessment of an individual patient's pathophysiology, as well as systematic care of their family. Further studies to better understand the relationships between genotype, phenotype, and outcomes over a lifetime are critical to improve risk stratification and to guide patient management. These insights will also support development of targeted therapies intended to modify disease progression and prevent adverse sequelae.

REFERENCES

1. Elliott PM, Anastasakis A, Borger MA, et al. 2014 ESC guidelines on diagnosis and management of hypertrophic cardiomyopathy: the task force for the diagnosis and management of hypertrophic cardiomyopathy of the European Society of Cardiology (ESC). *Eur Heart J.* 2014;35:2733–2779.
2. Norrish G, Field E, McLeod K, et al. Clinical presentation and survival of childhood hypertrophic cardiomyopathy: a retrospective study in United Kingdom. *Eur Heart J.* 2019;40:986–993.
3. Ommen SR, Mital S, Burke MA, et al. 2020 AHA/ACC guideline for the diagnosis and treatment of patients with hypertrophic cardiomyopathy: a report of the American College of Cardiology/American Heart Association Joint Committee on Clinical Practice Guidelines. *J Am Coll Cardiol.* 2020;76:e159–e240.
4. Yamaguchi H, Ishimura T, Nishiyama S, et al. Hypertrophic nonobstructive cardiomyopathy with giant negative T waves (apical hypertrophy): ventriculographic and echocardiographic features in 30 patients. *Am J Cardiol.* 1979;44:401–412.
5. Kitaoka H, Doi Y, Casey SA, et al. Comparison of prevalence of apical hypertrophic cardiomyopathy in Japan and the United States. *Am J Cardiol.* 2003;92:1183–1186.
6. Hughes RK, Knott KD, Malcolmson J, et al. Apical hypertrophic cardiomyopathy: the variant less known. *J Am Heart Assoc.* 2020;9:e015294.
7. Bos JM, Will ML, Gersh BJ, et al. Characterization of a phenotype-based genetic test prediction score for unrelated patients with hypertrophic cardiomyopathy. *Mayo Clin Proc.* 2014;89:727–737.
8. Gruner C, Ivanov J, Care M, et al. Toronto hypertrophic cardiomyopathy genotype score for prediction of a positive genotype in hypertrophic cardiomyopathy. *Circ Cardiovasc Genet.* 2013;6:19–26.
9. Arad M, Penas-Lado M, Monserrat L, et al. Gene mutations in apical hypertrophic cardiomyopathy. *Circulation.* 2005;112:2805–2811.
10. Geisterfer-Lowrance AA, Kass S, Tanigawa G, et al. A molecular basis for familial hypertrophic cardiomyopathy: a beta cardiac myosin heavy chain gene missense mutation. *Cell.* 1990;62:999–1006.
11. Georgakopoulos D, Christe ME, Giewat M, et al. The pathogenesis of familial hypertrophic cardiomyopathy: early and evolving effects from an alpha-cardiac myosin heavy chain missense mutation [see comments]. *Nat Med.* 1999;5:327–330.
12. Seidman CE, Seidman JG. Identifying sarcomere gene mutations in hypertrophic cardiomyopathy: a personal history. *Circ Res.* 2011;108:743–750.
13. Watkins H, McKenna WJ, Thierfelder L, et al. Mutations in the genes for cardiac troponin T and alpha-tropomyosin in hypertrophic cardiomyopathy. *N Engl J Med.* 1995;332:1058–1064.
14. Alfares AA, Kelly MA, McDermott G, et al. Results of clinical genetic testing of 2,912 probands with hypertrophic cardiomyopathy: expanded panels offer limited additional sensitivity. *Genet Med.* 2015;17:880–888.
15. Eisner DA, Caldwell JL, Kistamas K, Trafford AW. Calcium and excitation-contraction coupling in the heart. *Circ Res.* 2017;121:181–195.
16. Bottinelli R, Coviello DA, Redwood CS, et al. A mutant tropomyosin that causes hypertrophic cardiomyopathy is expressed in vivo and associated with an increased calcium sensitivity. *Circ Res.* 1998;82:106–115.
17. Cuda G, Fananapazir L, Epstein ND, Sellers JR. The in vitro motility activity of beta-cardiac myosin depends on the nature of the beta-myosin heavy chain gene mutation in hypertrophic cardiomyopathy. *J Muscle Res Cell Motil.* 1997;18:275–283.
18. van Dijk SJ, Dooijes D, dos Remedios C, et al. Cardiac myosin-binding protein C mutations and hypertrophic cardiomyopathy: haploinsufficiency, deranged phosphorylation, and cardiomyocyte dysfunction. *Circulation.* 2009;119:1473–1483.
19. Helms AS, Tang VT, O'Leary TS, et al. Effects of MYBPC3 loss-of-function mutations preceding hypertrophic cardiomyopathy. *JCI Insight.* 2020;5.
20. Helms AS, Thompson AD, Glazier AA, et al. Spatial and functional distribution of MYBPC3 pathogenic variants and clinical outcomes in patients with hypertrophic cardiomyopathy. *Circ Cardiovasc Genet.* 2020;13(5):396–405.
21. Sequeira V, Wijnker PJ, Nijenkamp LL, et al. Perturbed length-dependent activation in human hypertrophic cardiomyopathy with missense sarcomeric gene mutations. *Circ Res.* 2013;112:1491–1505.
22. Witjas-Paalberends ER, Guclu A, Germans T, et al. Gene-specific increase in the energetic cost of contraction in hypertrophic cardiomyopathy caused by thick filament mutations. *Cardiovasc Res.* 2014;103:248–257.
23. Marian AJ, Braunwald E. Hypertrophic cardiomyopathy: genetics, pathogenesis, clinical manifestations, diagnosis, and therapy. *Circ Res.* 2017;121:749–770.
24. Alamo L, Ware JS, Pinto A, et al. Effects of myosin variants on interacting-heads motif explain distinct hypertrophic and dilated cardiomyopathy phenotypes. *eLife.* 2017;6.
25. Toepfer CN, Garfinkel AC, Venturini G, et al. Myosin sequestration regulates sarcomere function, cardiomyocyte energetics, and metabolism, informing the pathogenesis of hypertrophic cardiomyopathy. *Circulation.* 2020;141:828–842.
26. Ho CY, Day SM, Colan SD, et al. The burden of early phenotypes and the influence of wall thickness in hypertrophic cardiomyopathy mutation carriers: findings from the HCMNet study. *JAMA Cardiol.* 2017;2:419–428.
27. Ho CY, Carlsen C, Thune JJ, et al. Echocardiographic strain imaging to assess early and late consequences of sarcomere mutations in hypertrophic cardiomyopathy. *Circ Cardiovasc Genet.* 2009;2:314–321.
28. Ho CY, Cirino AL, Lakdawala NK, et al. Evolution of hypertrophic cardiomyopathy in sarcomere mutation carriers. *Heart.* 2016.
29. Crilley JG, Boehm EA, Blair E, et al. Hypertrophic cardiomyopathy due to sarcomeric gene mutations is characterized by impaired energy metabolism irrespective of the degree of hypertrophy. *J Am Coll Cardiol.* 2003;41:1776–1782.
30. Lakdawala NK, Thune JJ, Maron BJ, et al. Electrocardiographic features of sarcomere mutation carriers with and without clinically overt hypertrophic cardiomyopathy. *Am J Cardiol.* 2011;108:1606–1613.
31. Captur G, Lopes LR, Mohun TJ, et al. Prediction of sarcomere mutations in subclinical hypertrophic cardiomyopathy. *Circ Cardiovasc Imaging.* 2014;7:863–871.
32. Groarke JD, Galazka PZ, Cirino AL, et al. Intrinsic mitral valve alterations in hypertrophic cardiomyopathy sarcomere mutation carriers. *Eur Heart J Cardiovascular Imaging.* 2018;19:1109–1116.
33. Ho CY, Lopez B, Coelho-Filho OR, et al. Myocardial fibrosis as an early manifestation of hypertrophic cardiomyopathy. *N Engl J Med.* 2010;363:552–563.
34. Ho CY, Abbasi SA, Neilan TG, et al. T1 measurements identify extracellular volume expansion in hypertrophic cardiomyopathy sarcomere mutation carriers with and without left ventricular hypertrophy. *Circ Cardiovasc Imaging.* 2013;6:415–422.
35. Paulus WJ, Lorell BH, Craig WE, et al. Comparison of the effects of nitroprusside and nifedipine on diastolic properties in patients with hypertrophic cardiomyopathy: altered left ventricular loading or improved muscle inactivation? *J Am Coll Cardiol.* 1983;2:879–886.
36. Soullier C, Obert P, Doucende G, et al. Exercise response in hypertrophic cardiomyopathy: blunted left ventricular deformational and twisting reserve with altered systolic-diastolic coupling. *Circ Cardiovasc Imaging.* 2012;5:324–332.

37. Villemain O, Correia M, Khraiche D, et al. Myocardial stiffness assessment using Shear wave imaging in pediatric hypertrophic cardiomyopathy. *JACC Cardiovasc Imaging*. 2018;11:779–781.
38. Ho CY, Sweitzer NK, McDonough B, et al. Assessment of diastolic function with Doppler tissue imaging to predict genotype in preclinical hypertrophic cardiomyopathy. *Circulation*. 2002;105:2992–2997.
39. Nagueh SF, McFalls J, Meyer D, et al. Tissue doppler imaging predicts the development of hypertrophic cardiomyopathy in subjects with subclinical disease. *Circulation*. 2003;108: 395–398.
40. Williams LK, Misurka J, Ho CY, et al. Multilayer myocardial mechanics in genotype-positive left ventricular hypertrophy-negative patients with hypertrophic cardiomyopathy. *Am J Cardiol*. 2018;122:1754–1760.
41. Maron MS, Olivotto I, Betocchi S, et al. Effect of left ventricular outflow tract obstruction on clinical outcome in hypertrophic cardiomyopathy. *N Engl J Med*. 2003;348:295–303.
42. Maron MS, Olivotto I, Zenovich AG, et al. Hypertrophic cardiomyopathy is predominantly a disease of left ventricular outflow tract obstruction. *Circulation*. 2006;114:2232–2239.
43. Sorajja P, Nishimura RA, Gersh BJ, et al. Outcome of mildly symptomatic or asymptomatic obstructive hypertrophic cardiomyopathy: a long-term follow-up study. *J Am Coll Cardiol*. 2009;54:234–241.
44. Numata S, Yaku H, Doi K, et al. Excess anterior mitral leaflet in a patient with hypertrophic obstructive cardiomyopathy and systolic anterior motion. *Circulation*. 2015;131:1605–1607.
45. Sherrid MV, Gunsburg DZ, Moldenhauer S, Pearle G. Systolic anterior motion begins at low left ventricular outflow tract velocity in obstructive hypertrophic cardiomyopathy. *J Am Coll Cardiol*. 2000;36:1344–1354.
46. Ayoub C, Geske JB, Larsen CM, et al. Comparison of valsalva maneuver, amyl nitrite, and exercise echocardiography to demonstrate latent left ventricular outflow obstruction in hypertrophic cardiomyopathy. *Am J Cardiol*. 2017;120:2265–2271.
47. Joshi S, Patel UK, Yao SS, et al. Standing and exercise doppler echocardiography in obstructive hypertrophic cardiomyopathy: the range of gradients with upright activity. *J Am Soc Echocardiogr*. 2011;24:75–82.
48. Reant P, Dufour M, Peyrou J, et al. Upright treadmill vs. semi-supine bicycle exercise echocardiography to provoke obstruction in symptomatic hypertrophic cardiomyopathy: a pilot study. *Eur Heart J Cardiovasc Imaging*. 2018;19:31–38.
49. Ho CY, Day SM, Ashley EA, et al. Genotype and lifetime burden of disease in hypertrophic cardiomyopathy: insights from the Sarcomeric Human Cardiomyopathy Registry (SHaRe). *Circulation*. 2018;138:1387–1398.
50. Olivotto I, Cecchi F, Casey SA, et al. Impact of atrial fibrillation on the clinical course of hypertrophic cardiomyopathy. *Circulation*. 2001;104:2517–2524.
51. Rowin EJ, Orfanos A, Estes NAM, et al. Occurrence and natural history of clinically silent episodes of atrial fibrillation in hypertrophic cardiomyopathy. *Am J Cardiol*. 2017;119:1862–1865.
52. Link MS, Bockstall K, Weinstock J, et al. Ventricular tachyarrhythmias in patients with hypertrophic cardiomyopathy and defibrillators: triggers, treatment, and implications. *J Cardiovasc Electrophysiol*. 2017;28:531–537.
53. Elliott P, Charron P, Blanes JR, et al. European cardiomyopathy pilot registry: EURObservational Research Programme of the European society of Cardiology. *Eur Heart J*. 2016;37:164–173.
54. Charron P, Elliott PM, Gimeno JR, et al. The Cardiomyopathy Registry of the EURObservational Research Programme of the European Society of Cardiology: baseline data and contemporary management of adult patients with cardiomyopathies. *Eur Heart J*. 2018;39:1784–1793.
55. Neubauer S, Kolm P, Ho CY, et al. Distinct subgroups in hypertrophic cardiomyopathy in the NHLBI HCM registry. *J Am Coll Cardiol*. 2019;74:2333–2345.
56. Sedaghat-Hamedani F, Kayvanpour E, Tugrul OF, et al. Clinical outcomes associated with sarcomere mutations in hypertrophic cardiomyopathy: a meta-analysis on 7675 individuals. *Clin Res Cardiol*. 2018;107:30–41.
57. Ingles J, Burns C, Bagnall RD, et al. Nonfamilial hypertrophic cardiomyopathy: prevalence, natural history, and clinical implications. *Cir Cardiovasc Genet*. 2017;10.
58. Li Q, Gruner C, Chan RH, et al. Genotype-positive status in patients with hypertrophic cardiomyopathy is associated with higher rates of heart failure events. *Cir Cardiovasc Genet*. 2014;7:416–422.
59. Olivotto I, Maron MS, Adabag AS, et al. Gender-related differences in the clinical presentation and outcome of hypertrophic cardiomyopathy. *J Am Coll Cardiol*. 2005;46:480–487.
60. Geske JB, Ong KC, Siontis KC, et al. Women with hypertrophic cardiomyopathy have worse survival. *Eur Heart J*. 2017;38:3434–3440.
61. Marstrand P, Han L, Day SM, et al. Hypertrophic cardiomyopathy with left ventricular systolic dysfunction: insights from the SHaRe registry. *Circulation*. 2020;141:1371–1383.
62. Cirino AL, Harris S, Lakdawala NK, et al. Role of genetic testing in inherited cardiovascular disease: a review. *JAMA Cardiol*. 2017;2:1153–1160.
63. Richards S, Aziz N, Bale S, et al. Standards and guidelines for the interpretation of sequence variants: a joint consensus recommendation of the American College of Medical Genetics and Genomics and the Association for Molecular Pathology. *Genet Med*. 2015;17:405–424.
64. Miron A, Lafreniere-Roula M, Steve Fan CP, et al. A validated model for sudden cardiac death risk prediction in pediatric hypertrophic cardiomyopathy. *Circulation*. 2020;142:217–229.
65. Norrish G, Cantarutti N, Pissaridou E, et al. Risk factors for sudden cardiac death in childhood hypertrophic cardiomyopathy: a systematic review and meta-analysis. *Eur J Prev Cardiol*. 2017;24:1220–1230.
66. Rowin EJ, Sridharan A, Madias C, et al. Prediction and prevention of sudden death in young patients (<20 years) with hypertrophic cardiomyopathy. *Am J Cardiol*. 2020;128:75–83.
67. O'Mahony C, Jichi F, Pavlou M, et al. A novel clinical risk prediction model for sudden cardiac death in hypertrophic cardiomyopathy (HCM risk-SCD). *Eur Heart J*. 2014;35:2010–2020.
68. Monserrat L, Elliott PM, Gimeno JR, et al. Non-sustained ventricular tachycardia in hypertrophic cardiomyopathy: an independent marker of sudden death risk in young patients. *J Am Coll Cardiol*. 2003;42:873–879.
69. Weng Z, Yao J, Chan RH, et al. Prognostic Value of LGE-CMR in HCM: a meta-analysis. *JACC Cardiovasc Imaging*. 2016;9:1392–1402.
70. Maron BJ, Spirito P, Ackerman MJ, et al. Prevention of sudden cardiac death with implantable cardioverter-defibrillators in children and adolescents with hypertrophic cardiomyopathy. *J Am Coll Cardiol*. 2013;61:1527–1535.
71. Sherrid MV, Barac I, McKenna WJ, et al. Multicenter study of the efficacy and safety of disopyramide in obstructive hypertrophic cardiomyopathy. *J Am Coll Cardiol*. 2005;45:1251–1258.
72. Olivotto I, Oreziak A, Barriales-Villa R, et al. Mavacamten for treatment of symptomatic obstructive hypertrophic cardiomyopathy (EXPLORER-HCM): a randomised, double-blind, placebo-controlled, phase 3 trial. *Lancet*. 2020.
73. Nguyen A, Schaff HV. Surgical myectomy: subaortic, midventricular, and apical. *Cardiol Clin*. 2019;37:95–104.
74. Balaram SK, Ross RE, Sherrid MV, et al. Role of mitral valve plication in the surgical management of hypertrophic cardiomyopathy. *Ann Thorac Surg*. 2012;94:1990–1997; discussion 1997-8.
75. Hong JH, Schaff HV, Nishimura RA, et al. Mitral regurgitation in patients with hypertrophic obstructive cardiomyopathy: implications for concomitant valve procedures. *J Am Coll Cardiol*. 2016;68:1497–1504.
76. Schoendube FA, Klues HG, Reith S, et al. Long-term clinical and echocardiographic follow-up after surgical correction of hypertrophic obstructive cardiomyopathy with extended myectomy and reconstruction of the subvalvular mitral apparatus. *Circulation*. 1995;92:II122–I127.
77. McLeod CJ, Ommen SR, Ackerman MJ, et al. Surgical septal myectomy decreases the risk for appropriate implantable cardioverter defibrillator discharge in obstructive hypertrophic cardiomyopathy. *Eur Heart J*. 2007;28:2583–2588.
78. Ommen SR, Maron BJ, Olivotto I, et al. Long-term effects of surgical septal myectomy on survival in patients with obstructive hypertrophic cardiomyopathy. *J Am Coll Cardiol*. 2005;46:470–476.
79. Batzner A, Pfeiffer B, Neugebauer A, et al. Survival after alcohol septal ablation in patients with hypertrophic obstructive cardiomyopathy. *J Am Coll Cardiol*. 2018;72:3087–3094.
80. Nguyen A, Schaff HV, Hang D, et al. Surgical myectomy versus alcohol septal ablation for obstructive hypertrophic cardiomyopathy: a propensity score-matched cohort. *J Thorac Cardiovasc Surg*. 2019;157:306–315 e3.
81. Sorajja P, Binder J, Nishimura RA, et al. Predictors of an optimal clinical outcome with alcohol septal ablation for obstructive hypertrophic cardiomyopathy. *Catheter Cardiovasc Interv*. 2013;81:E58–E67.
82. Yancy CW, Jessup M, Bozkurt B, et al. 2017 ACC/AHA/HFSA focused update of the 2013 ACCF/AHA guideline for the management of heart failure: a report of the American College of Cardiology/American Heart Association Task Force on Clinical Practice Guidelines and the Heart Failure Society of America. *Circulation*. 2017;136:e137–e161.
83. Guttmann OP, Rahman MS, O'Mahony C, et al. Atrial fibrillation and thromboembolism in patients with hypertrophic cardiomyopathy: systematic review. *Heart*. 2014;100:465–472.
84. Saberi S, Wheeler M, Bragg-Gresham J, et al. Effect of moderate-intensity exercise training on peak oxygen consumption in patients with hypertrophic cardiomyopathy: a randomized clinical trial. *J Am Med Assoc*. 2017;317:1349–1357.
85. Piercy KL, Troiano RP, Ballard RM, et al. The physical activity guidelines for Americans. *J Am Med Assoc*. 2018;320:2020–2028.
86. Maron BJ, Levine BD, Washington RL, et al. Eligibility and disqualification recommendations for competitive athletes with cardiovascular abnormalities: task force 2: preparticipation screening for cardiovascular disease in competitive athletes: a scientific statement from the American Heart Association and American College of Cardiology. *Circulation*. 2015;132:e267–e272.
87. Harmon KG, Asif IM, Klossner D, Drezner JA. Incidence of sudden cardiac death in National Collegiate Athletic Association athletes. *Circulation*. 2011;123:1594–1600.
88. Ullal AJ, Abdelfattah RS, Ashley EA, Froelicher VF. Hypertrophic cardiomyopathy as a cause of sudden cardiac death in the young: a meta-analysis. *Am J Med*. 2016;129:486–496 e2.
89. Ammirati E, Contri R, Coppini R, et al. Pharmacological treatment of hypertrophic cardiomyopathy: current practice and novel perspectives. *Eur J Heart Fail*. 2016;18:1106–1118.
90. Wong TC, Martinez M. Novel pharmacotherapy for hypertrophic cardiomyopathy. *Cardiol Clin*. 2019;37:113–117.
91. Abozguia K, Elliott P, McKenna W, et al. Metabolic modulator perhexiline corrects energy deficiency and improves exercise capacity in symptomatic hypertrophic cardiomyopathy. *Circulation*. 2010;122:1562–1569.
92. Coats CJ, Pavlou M, Watkinson OT, et al. Effect of trimetazidine dihydrochloride therapy on exercise capacity in patients with nonobstructive hypertrophic cardiomyopathy: a randomized clinical trial. *JAMA Cardiol*. 2019;4:230–235.
93. Olivotto I, Camici PG, Merlini PA, et al. Efficacy of ranolazine in patients with symptomatic hypertrophic cardiomyopathy: the RESTYLE-HCM randomized, double-blind, placebo-controlled study. *Circ Heart Fail*. 2018;11:e004124.
94. Olivotto I, Hellawell JL, Farzaneh-Far R, et al. Novel approach targeting the complex pathophysiology of hypertrophic cardiomyopathy: the impact of late sodium current inhibition on exercise capacity in subjects with symptomatic hypertrophic cardiomyopathy (LIBERTY-HCM) trial. *Circ Heart Fail*. 2016;9:e002764.
95. Kawano H, Toda G, Nakamizo R, et al. Valsartan decreases type I collagen synthesis in patients with hypertrophic cardiomyopathy. *Circ J*. 2005;69:1244–1248.
96. Penicka M, Gregor P, Kerekes R, et al. The effects of candesartan on left ventricular hypertrophy and function in nonobstructive hypertrophic cardiomyopathy: a pilot, randomized study. *J Mol Diagn*. 2009;11:35–41.
97. Axelsson A, Iversen K, Vejlstrup N, et al. Efficacy and safety of the angiotensin II receptor blocker losartan for hypertrophic cardiomyopathy: the INHERIT randomised, double-blind, placebo-controlled trial. *Lancet Diabetes Endocrinol*. 2015;3:123–131.
98. Maron MS, Chan RH, Kapur NK, et al. Effect of spironolactone on myocardial fibrosis and other clinical variables in patients with hypertrophic cardiomyopathy. *Am J Med*. 2018;131:837–841.
99. Semsarian C, Ahmad I, Giewat M, et al. The L-type calcium channel inhibitor diltiazem prevents cardiomyopathy in a mouse model. *J Clin Invest*. 2002;109:1013–1020.
100. Teekakirikul P, Eminaga S, Toka O, et al. Cardiac fibrosis in mice with hypertrophic cardiomyopathy is mediated by non-myocyte proliferation and requires Tgf-beta. *J Clin Invest*. 2010;120:3520–3529.
101. Green EM, Wakimoto H, Anderson RL, et al. A small-molecule inhibitor of sarcomere contractility suppresses hypertrophic cardiomyopathy in mice. *Science*. 2016;351:617–621.
102. Ho CY, Lakdawala NK, Cirino AL, et al. Diltiazem treatment for pre-clinical hypertrophic cardiomyopathy sarcomere mutation carriers: a pilot randomized trial to modify disease expression. *JACC Heart Fail*. 2015;3:180–188.
103. Ho CY, McMurray JJV, Cirino AL, et al. The Design of The Valsartan for Attenuating Disease Evolution in Early Sarcomeric Hypertrophic Cardiomyopathy (VANISH) trial. *Am Heart J*. 2017;187:145–155.
104. Kawas RF, Anderson RL, Ingle SRB, et al. A small-molecule modulator of cardiac myosin acts on multiple stages of the myosin chemomechanical cycle. *J Biol Chem*. 2017;292:16571–16577.
105. Stern JA, Markova S, Ueda Y, et al. A small molecule inhibitor of sarcomere contractility acutely relieves left ventricular outflow tract obstruction in feline hypertrophic cardiomyopathy. *PloS One*. 2016;11:e0168407.
106. Mamidi R, Li J, Doh CY, et al. Impact of the myosin modulator mavacamten on force generation and cross-bridge behavior in a murine model of hypercontractility. *J Am Heart Assoc*. 2018;7:e009627.
107. Ho CY, Mealiffe ME, Bach RG, et al. Evaluation of mavacamten in symptomatic patients with nonobstructive hypertrophic cardiomyopathy. *J Am Coll Cardiol*. 2020;75:2649–2660.
108. Prondzynski M, Mearini G, Carrier L. Gene therapy strategies in the treatment of hypertrophic cardiomyopathy. *Pflugers Arch*. 2019;471:807–815.
109. Ma H, Marti-Gutierrez N, Park SW, et al. Correction of a pathogenic gene mutation in human embryos. *Nature*. 2017;548:413–419.

55 Myocarditis

LESLIE T. COOPER JR. AND KIRK U. KNOWLTON

OVERVIEW AND DEFINITION, 1077
EPIDEMIOLOGY, 1077
SPECIFIC ETIOLOGIC AGENTS, 1078
Viruses, 1078
Bacteria, 1081
Protozoa, 1081
Helminths, 1083
Physical Agents, Including Adverse Drug Effects, 1083

PATHOGENESIS OF VIRAL MYOCARDITIS, 1083
Viral Infection, 1083
Innate Immunity, 1085
Acquired Immunity, 1085
Cardiac Remodeling, 1086
CLINICAL SYNDROMES, 1086
DIAGNOSTIC APPROACHES, 1086
Laboratory Testing, 1087

Cardiac Imaging, 1087
Endomyocardial Biopsy, 1088
PROGNOSIS, 1088
TREATMENT, 1088
FUTURE PERSPECTIVES, 1089
REFERENCES, 1089

OVERVIEW AND DEFINITION

In its broadest sense, *myocarditis* refers to any inflammation of the myocardium. Inflammation can be found after any form of injury to the heart, including ischemic damage, mechanical trauma, and genetic cardiomyopathies. More specifically, however, *classic myocarditis* refers to inflammation of the heart muscle occurring as a result of exposure to either discrete external antigens, such as viruses, bacteria, parasites, toxins, or drugs, or internal triggers, such as autoimmune activation against self-antigens. Although viral infection remains the most commonly identified cause of myocarditis, drug hypersensitivity and toxic drug reactions, other infections, and peripartum cardiomyopathy also can lead to myocarditis.

The pathogenesis of myocarditis is a classic paradigm of cardiac injury followed by immunologic response from the host resulting in cardiac inflammation. The relative incidence of viral causes is continually evolving as new diagnostic tools based on molecular epidemiology become available. Indeed, more than 20 viruses have been associated with myocarditis, and the most frequent are currently parvovirus B19 (B19V) and human herpesvirus 6.[1] Enteroviruses such as coxsackievirus B continue to be commonly identified pathogens, and strains of enterovirus remain widely used in mouse models of the disease.[2] If the host immune response is overwhelming or inappropriate, the inflammation may destroy the heart tissue acutely or may linger, producing cardiac remodeling that leads to dilated cardiomyopathy (DCM), heart failure, or death. Fortunately for most patients, clinical myocarditis often is self-limited if proper support and follow-up care are available. In many cases the virus is cleared successfully, and the immune response is downmodulated. In some patients, however, an autoimmune reaction to endogenous antigens lingers beyond this phase and can cause persistent cardiac dysfunction. Sometimes viral genomes persist in the heart with or without acute inflammation.[3] Viral genomes commonly are detected in endomyocardial biopsy (EMB) specimens from patients with DCM and may signal a disease-related infection. As discussed in this chapter, with new insights into the understanding of the pathophysiology of myocarditis and new therapies for this condition, the outlook for affected patients is continuing to improve.

EPIDEMIOLOGY

As estimated in the 2019 Global Burden of Disease study the prevalence of myocarditis in 2019 was 712,780 (612,466 to 817,245, 95% uncertainty interval [UI]) or a prevalence rate of 9.21 per 100,000 (7.92 to 10.56, 95% UI).[4] This rate increased from 8.04 (6.85 to 9.19, 95% UI) in 1990. Disability from myocarditis is largely due to heart failure.

The age standardized, global disability-adjusted life years (DALYs) rate per 100,000 due to myocarditis in 2019 was 977,238 (803,762 to 1,126,804, 95% UI). There were an estimated 32,449 (23,164 to 37,087, 95% UI) deaths or 0.42 (0.30 to 0.48, 95% UI) deaths per 100,000 due to myocarditis.[4]

The death rate from myocarditis is higher in the first year of life than between ages 1 and 14 years for both males and females. After age 15 years, DALYs, number of deaths, and death rate due to myocarditis are higher in males than females.[4]

The rates of myocarditis vary by region with higher rates seen in parts of Southeast Asia, East Asia, Oceania, Central Europe, Eastern Europe, and Central Asia (Table 55.1). Myocarditis can be difficult to distinguish from other forms of cardiomyopathy in areas that rely on clinical presentation and echocardiography for diagnosis, suggesting imprecision in diagnosis within the larger category of cardiomyopathy. Myocarditis is responsible for sudden cardiovascular death in approximately 2% of infants, 5% of children, and 5% to 14% of young athletes.[4-6]

Myocarditis is responsible for a substantial minority of DCM cases (see also Chapters 48 and 52). In a review of DCM case series from 1978 to 1995 in which EMB was performed, the incidence of biopsy-proven myocarditis varied widely, ranging from 0.5% to 67%, with an average of 10.3%. Data from the U.S. Pediatric Cardiomyopathy Registry, in which 46% (222/485) of children with an identified cause of DCM had myocarditis, are illustrative of recent reports. As in most DCM case series, only a minority of children in this series, 34% of 1426, had a specific cause of DCM identified.[7] The differing histologic criteria used to define myocarditis are responsible for some of the variation in the reported prevalence of myocarditis. The standard Dallas criteria define idiopathic myocarditis as an inflammatory infiltrate of the myocardium with necrosis and/or degeneration of adjacent myocytes not typical of the ischemic damage associated with coronary artery disease (Fig. 55.1A and Table 55.2).[8] These criteria have been criticized because of interreader variability in interpretation, lack of prognostic value, and low sensitivity due in part to sampling error. Specific immunohistochemical stains that detect cellular antigens, such as anti-CD3 (T lymphocytes), anti-CD68 (macrophages), and class I and II human leukocyte antigens (see Fig. 55.1B), may have greater sensitivity for small infiltrates than that of hematoxylin-eosin stain. Markers of complement activity such as C4d also are commonly found in native cardiomyopathic hearts. Newer immunohistochemical stains have a greater predictive value for cardiovascular events than the Dallas criteria.[9]

The presence of viral genomes in heart tissue may indicate an active infectious myocarditis. In the posttransplantation setting, the presence of viral genomes in myocardial biopsy material predicts future rejection episodes and graft loss in children.[10] Viruses for which testing is commonly done in the setting of suspected myocarditis are B19V, adenovirus, cytomegalovirus, enterovirus, Epstein-Barr virus, hepatitis

C virus, herpes simplex viruses 1, 2, and 6, and influenza viruses A and B. New diagnostic criteria that rely on higher B19V copy numbers or evidence of active viral replication have been proposed.[2] For epidemiologic studies in which universal EMB is not feasible, diagnostic classifications that rely on clinical syndromes, biomarkers, and/or imaging abnormalities have been used (Table 55.3).[11]

SPECIFIC ETIOLOGIC AGENTS

In most cases, myocarditis is triggered by an inciting event, such as infection or exposure to a drug or toxin that activates the immune response. A subset of cases is due to primary immunologic abnormalities in the affected patient. Advanced techniques in virology, immunology, and molecular biology have demonstrated that there are many potential causes of myocarditis. Almost any infectious agent has been associated with myocarditis. In clinical practice, however, it is often difficult to identify a specific etiologic agent.

Viruses

Viral infection has been implicated as one of the most common infectious causes of myocarditis (Table 55.4). The earliest evidence of virus infection and its association with myocarditis and pericarditis was acquired during outbreaks of influenza, poliomyelitis, measles, and mumps, and in cases of pleurodynia associated with enterovirus infection.[12] Modern virologic and molecular techniques have demonstrated that adenoviruses, enteroviruses, and parvovirus are among the most commonly identified infectious agents in myocarditis. Although SARS-CoV-2 viral genomes and proteins have been identified in the heart tissue, the presence of SARS-CoV-2 viral genomes in the heart is generally not accompanied by a classic lymphocytic myocarditis (see also Chapter 94).

The precise incidence of myocarditis caused by these infectious agents varies geographically and temporally (Fig. 55.2). Nevertheless, in meta-analyses, polymerase chain reaction (PCR) studies in patients with clinically suspected myocarditis or cardiomyopathy who subsequently underwent heart biopsy demonstrated that virus could be identified 3.8 times more frequently in patients with myocarditis than in control subjects. Additional evidence indicates that persistence of the viral genome in patients with cardiomyopathy is associated

TABLE 55.1 Deaths from Myocarditis by Geographic Regions (Global Burden of Disease Study 2019)

GEOGRAPHIC REGION	DEATHS PER 100,000	95% UNCERTAINTY INDEX
Southeast Asia, East Asia, and Oceania	0.76	0.46–0.93
Central Europe, Eastern Europe, and Central Asia	0.79	0.57–0.93
High-income regions*	0.29	0.18–0.30
Latin America and Caribbean	0.22	0.18–0.35
North Africa and Middle East	0.36	0.26–0.65
South Asia	0.21	0.15–0.29
Sub-Saharan Africa	0.20	0.13–0.33

*High income regions are defined as Southern Latin America, Western Europe, High Income North America, Australasia, and High Income Asia Pacific.
From Roth GA, Mensah GA, Johnson CO, et al. Global burden of cardiovascular diseases and risk factors, 1990 to 2019: update from the global burden of disease 2019. *J Am Coll Cardiol*. 2020;76:2982–3021. Epublished DOI: 10.1016/j.jacc.2020.11.010.

TABLE 55.2 Endomyocardial Biopsy Diagnosis of Myocarditis: The Dallas Criteria

Definition

Idiopathic *myocarditis*: "an inflammatory infiltrate of the myocardium with necrosis and/or degeneration of adjacent myocytes not typical of the ischemic damage associated with coronary artery disease"

Classification

First biopsy
- Myocarditis with or without fibrosis
- Borderline myocarditis (repeat biopsy may be indicated)
- No myocarditis

Subsequent biopsy
- Ongoing (persistent) myocarditis with or without fibrosis
- Resolving (healing) myocarditis with or without fibrosis
- Resolved (healed) myocarditis with or without fibrosis

	DESCRIPTORS	
	INFLAMMATORY INFILTRATE	FIBROSIS
Distribution	Focal, confluent, diffuse	Endocardial, interstitial
Extent	Mild, moderate, severe	Mild, moderate, severe
Type	Lymphocytic, eosinophilic, granulomatous, giant cell, neutrophilic, mixed	Perivascular, replacement

Modified from Leone O, Veinot JP, Angelini A, et al. 2011 consensus statement on endomyocardial biopsy from the Association for European Cardiovascular Pathology and the Society for Cardiovascular Pathology. *Cardiovasc Pathol*. 2012;21:245.

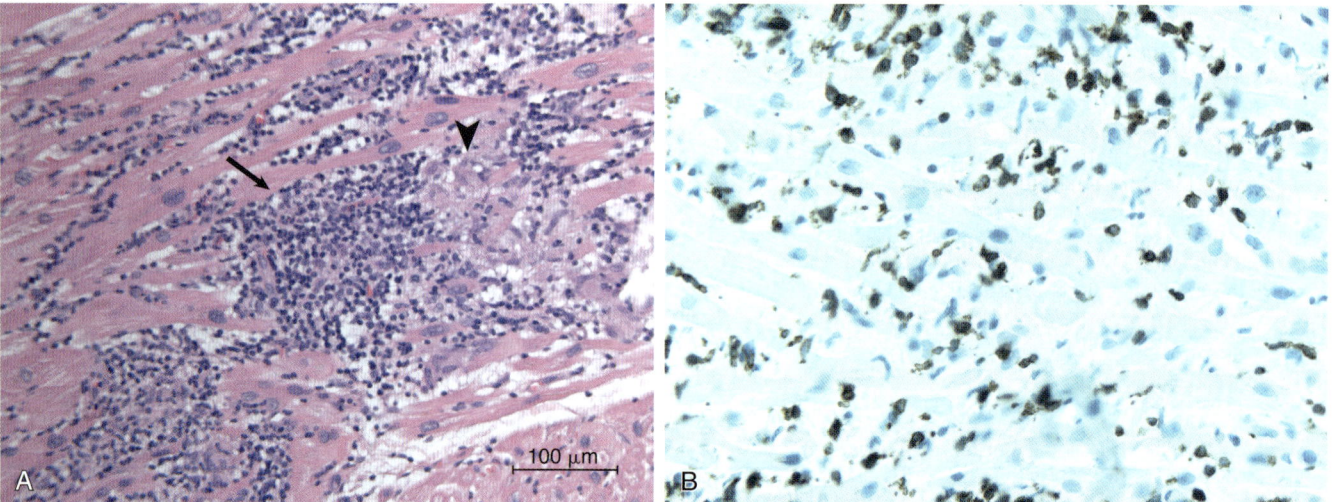

FIGURE 55.1 **A,** Acute myocarditis with widespread lymphocytic and histiocytic infiltrate *(arrow)* and associated myocyte damage *(arrowhead)*. **B,** CD3 immunostaining of T lymphocytes in a patient with acute myocarditis. (Courtesy of Dylan Miller, MD. From Cooper LT. Myocarditis. *N Engl J Med*. 2009;360:1526.)

TABLE 55.3 Three-Tiered Clinical Classification for Diagnosis of Myocarditis by Level of Diagnostic Certainty

DIAGNOSTIC CATEGORY	CRITERIA	HISTOLOGIC CONFIRMATION	BIOMARKER, ECG, OR IMAGING ABNORMALITIES CONSISTENT WITH MYOCARDITIS	TREATMENT NEEDED
Possible subclinical acute myocarditis	In the clinical context of possible myocardial injury *without* cardiovascular symptoms but with at least one of the following: Biomarkers of cardiac injury raised ECG findings suggestive of cardiac injury Abnormal cardiac function on echocardiogram or CMR	Absent	Required	Not known
Probable acute myocarditis	In clinical context of possible myocardial injury *with* cardiovascular symptoms and at least one of the following: Biomarkers of cardiac injury raised ECG findings suggestive of cardiac injury Abnormal cardiac function on echocardiogram or CMR	Absent	Required	Per clinical syndrome
Definite myocarditis	Histologic or immunohistologic evidence of myocarditis	Present	Not required	Tailored to specific cause

CMR, Cardiac magnetic resonance imaging; *ECG*, electrocardiogram.
Modified from Sagar S, Liu PP, Cooper LT, Jr. Myocarditis. *Lancet*. 2012;379:738.

TABLE 55.4 Causes of Myocarditis

VIRUSES AND VIRAL DISORDERS	BACTERIA AND BACTERIAL DISORDERS	CARDIOTOXINS	HYPERSENSITIVITY MEDIATORS AND FACTORS
Adenovirus*	*Chlamydia*	Anthracycline drugs*	Cephalosporins
B19V	Cholera	Arsenic	Clozapine
Coxsackievirus B*	Leptospirosis	Carbon monoxide	Diuretics
Cytomegalovirus*	Lyme disease	Catecholamines	Hypereosinophilia
Epstein-Barr virus	*Mycoplasma*	Chagas disease	Insect bites
Hepatitis C virus	*Neisseria*	Cocaine*	Kawasaki disease
Herpes simplex virus	Relapsing fever	Copper	Lithium
HIV*	*Salmonella*	Ethanol*	Sarcoidosis
Influenza virus	Spirochete	Heavy metals	Snake bites
Mumps	*Staphylococcus*	Lead	Sulfonamides
Poliovirus	*Streptococcus*	Leishmaniasis	Systemic disorders
Rabies	Syphilis	Malaria	Tetanus toxoid
Rubella	Tetanus	Mercury	Tetracycline
SARS-CoV-2	Tuberculosis	Protozoa	Wegener granulomatosis
Varicella-zoster virus			
Yellow fever			

*Frequent cause of myocarditis.
HIV, Human immunodeficiency virus.
Modified from Elamm C, Fairweather D, Cooper LT. Pathogenesis and diagnosis of myocarditis. *Heart J*. 2012;98:835.

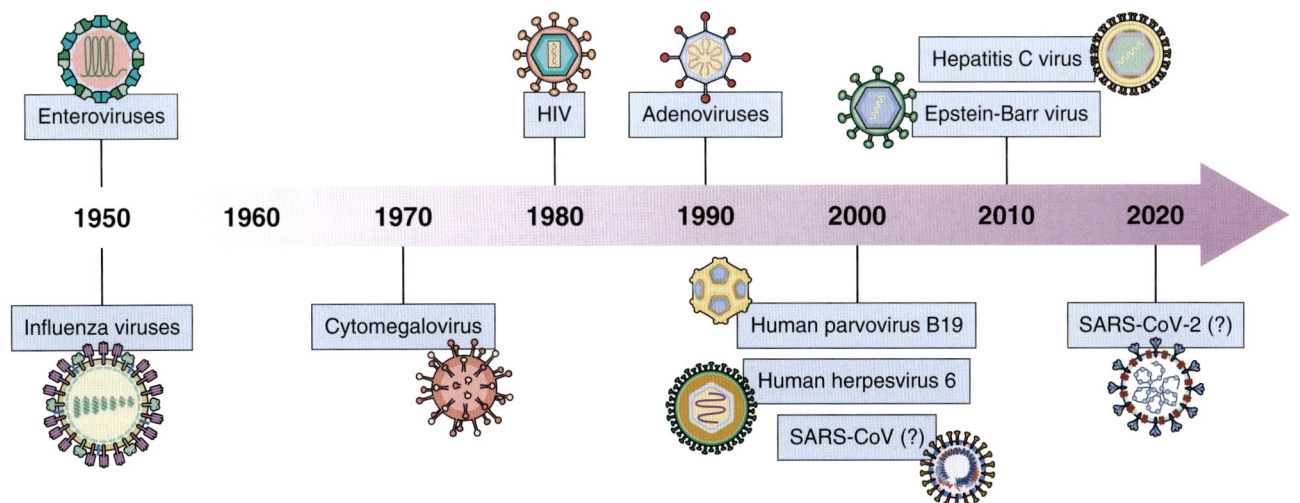

FIGURE 55.2 Prominent viruses associated with inflammatory cardiomyopathy over time. Over the years, the number of recognized viruses associated with inflammatory cardiomyopathy has grown. This evolution is partly influenced by the intentional detection of a broader repertoire of viruses over time as well as by the occurrence of novel viruses or virus genotypes in the heart. The association between severe acute respiratory syndrome coronavirus (SARS-CoV) and SARS-CoV-2 and inflammatory cardiomyopathy is not yet clear. "(?)" denotes unclear, needing further investigation; HIV, human immunodeficiency virus. (Adapted from Tschope C, Ammirati E, Bozkurt B, et al. Myocarditis and inflammatory cardiomyopathy: current evidence and future directions. *Nat Rev Cardiol*. 2020;Oct 12:1–25. https://doi.org/10.1038/s41569-020-00435-x.)

with increased ventricular dysfunction and worse outcome during follow-up.

Enteroviruses, Including Coxsackieviruses. Coxsackievirus is a member of the Enterovirus genus, Picornaviridae family. It is a nonenveloped lytic virus. Its capsid proteins harbor a single, positive-strand RNA genome of 7.4 Kb. Throughout the history of studies that address the causes of myocarditis, enteroviruses such as coxsackievirus B3 or echovirus are commonly identified in a subset of patients at a higher frequency than in control subjects. Using molecular techniques such as PCR and in situ hybridization, the enterovirus genome has been identified in the heart of 15% to 30% of patients with myocarditis and 7% to 30% of specimens with DCM, although the incidence in different studies varies considerably. Coxsackievirus infection meets the criteria of Koch's postulates as a cause of myocarditis in humans: It can be regularly found in the lesions of the disease; it has been isolated in pure culture from patients with myocarditis; and when inoculated into a mouse it can recapitulate the disease, after which the virus can be recovered from the heart of the infected mouse.

Coxsackievirus is a close relative of the poliovirus and rhinovirus, viruses that have been studied extensively. Although the disease phenotypes are different, the many similarities in viral replication cycles have facilitated an understanding of the mechanisms by which coxsackievirus can cause disease. Coxsackievirus typically enters the host through the gastrointestinal or respiratory system. It uses the coxsackievirus-adenovirus receptor (CAR), a transmembrane adhesion protein, as its primary receptor for cell entry. It can cause a broad range of clinical syndromes, including meningitis, skin rashes, acute respiratory illness, skeletal myositis, and myocarditis. Most recently, evaluation of patients with myocarditis has demonstrated a decrease in the prevalence of enteroviruses in the myocardium. This is particularly evident in Western Europe. The reason for this decrease is not clear but may be related to a herd immunity that occurs after a period of prolonged exposure to the virus. The lower incidence may also be confounded by seasonal outbreaks of enterovirus infections, thereby making the exact incidence dependent on the outbreaks.

Adenovirus. Adenoviruses are nonenveloped DNA viruses that also use CAR (adenovirus types 2 and 5), as well as integrins, as receptors for entry into the target cell. The adenovirus capsid harbors a double-stranded DNA genome. Adenoviruses commonly infect mucosal surfaces. The adenovirus genome is consistently identified in a subset of patients with myocarditis. The incidence in myocarditis patients has been recorded to be as high as 23% and as low as less than 2%.[13] Although mechanisms of adenoviral infection have been studied in considerable detail in cell culture and other diseases, it has been challenging to study adenovirus-mediated myocarditis, in the face of difficulties identifying an appropriate mouse model using the same adenoviruses that affect humans.

Parvovirus. The role of parvovirus B19 (B19V) of the genus Erythrovirus in the pathogenesis of myocarditis has been identified as a potentially important contributor to myocarditis because of the high prevalence of B19V DNA in hearts of patients with myocarditis. Parvovirus is a nonenveloped, nonlytic virus with a single-strand, positive-strand DNA genome of approximately 5.6 Kb. Humans are the only known host for B19V, making it challenging to study in animal models, but examples of myocarditis in mice stimulated with the capsid protein VP1 or antibodies against VP1 have been reported.[14] Its primary receptor is globoside, also known as group P antigen. This antigen is found primarily on erythroid progenitors, erythroblasts, and megakaryocytes. It also has been shown to be expressed on endothelial cells. This finding may be important for its role in the pathogenesis of myocarditis. The infection is thought generally to be spread by the respiratory route. The incidence of infection in the general population is also high, with evidence of B19V infection demonstrated in approximately 50% of children at age 15 years, and detectable IgG directed against B19V found in as many as 80% of older adult patients. With PCR studies, the PVB genome has been identified in 11% to 56% of patients with myocarditis and in 10% to 51% of patients with DCM.[14]

In keeping with the high prevalence of B19V in the general population, the pathogenic role of B19V continues to be clarified. In one study, B19V was assessed by immunohistochemistry and PCR assay. The investigators found that B19V was detectable by immunohistologic analysis in 65% of patients with myocarditis, 35% of patients with DCM, and 8% of noninflamed control hearts. The viral load was assessed by genome copy numbers in the samples that were positive for B19V on immunohistologic analysis. The viral load was significantly higher in patients with acute myocarditis, followed by those with DCM, and it was lowest in the patients with normal hearts without inflammation. In addition, viral RNA replicative intermediates were detected only in patients with inflamed hearts. It has also been determined that evidence of viral transcription is associated with an anomalous host myocardial transcriptome.[15,16] These findings indicate that the amount of B19V viral DNA is associated with the disease phenotype. Of importance, the virus was found in endothelial cells and not myocardial cells. Other studies have suggested a bystander role for B19V in adult myocarditis, with persistence of low-level B19V titers a frequent finding, but unrelated to ongoing myocardial injury. Additional experimentation is needed to determine mechanisms by which B19V could contribute to myocarditis and cardiomyopathy.

Human Immunodeficiency Virus. The improved survival rate of patients with human immunodeficiency virus (HIV) infection has affected the incidence of heart disease in this population (see also Chapter 85). Myocarditis with lymphocytic infiltration has been reported in 40% to 52% of patients who die of acquired immunodeficiency syndrome (AIDS). The incidence of myocardial disease, however, appears to have decreased with increased antiretroviral therapy.

Hepatitis C Virus. Hepatitis C virus infection appears to be mainly associated with cardiomyopathy in Asian countries such as Japan. A low incidence of hepatitis C virus antibodies (4.4%) was identified in patients who were studied in the Myocarditis Treatment Trial. This occurrence rate was nevertheless higher than that (1.8%) in the general U.S. population. Perhaps the higher incidence of hepatitis C virus infection in DCM is related to the overall higher incidence of this infection in Asia. Myocardial biopsy samples from patients with cardiomyopathy have demonstrated the presence of the hepatitis C viral genome, and a rise in serum antibody titers has been documented in patients so affected. The phenotype associated with hepatitis C virus also has been reported to include hypertrophic cardiomyopathy, suggesting that hepatitis C may have a direct effect on growth and hypertrophy of the myocardial cells. Symptomatic myocarditis generally is observed in the first to third weeks of illness. It has been reported that heart function can return to normal with clearance of the virus.

Influenza Virus. Influenza A virus infection is a well-recognized cause of myocarditis, and this association should be kept in mind during periodic outbreaks of influenza A. The exact incidence of myocarditis with influenza A outbreaks is not known, but it generally is considered to be in the 5% range. During pandemics such as the 2009 H1N1 pandemic, myocarditis was reported in 5% to 15% of cases as diagnosed by changes on the electrocardiogram (ECG) and the presence of cardiac symptoms. Some cases manifested with fulminant myocarditis. Histopathologic examination usually demonstrates the presence of the inflammatory infiltrate that is typical of myocarditis (see also Chapter 94).

Coronavirus. As the world has turned its attention to the COVID-19 pandemic, it became clear during the early stages of the disease that patients who were admitted to the hospital for COVID-19 had a 20% to 35% incidence of myocardial injury manifested by an increase in troponin and type B natriuretic factor. It was also clear that the extent of myocardial injury correlated directly with a worsening prognosis of intubation and death. It was assumed initially that this myocardial injury was secondary to a classical form of myocarditis precipitated by infection of cardiac cells by SARS-CoV-2. Case reports from some of the most severely affected areas supported that hypothesis. However, diagnoses were often made by clinical findings and evidence of myocarditis on cardiac magnetic resonance (cMR) imaging. Subsequent reports of myocarditis have been varied, which may be related to definitions that used to define myocarditis.[17] An autopsy report from a young person with sudden death found to have COVID-19 demonstrated that SARS-CoV-2 could be identified within isolated, but adjacent myocytes. Correlative experiments in human IPS-derived cardiomyocytes (hiPS-CMs) demonstrate that hiPS-CMs can be infected by SARS-CoV-2 and that cell fusion can be mediated by proteolytically activated SPIKE protein.[18] The pathogenesis of cardiac injury in COVID-19 is complex with mechanisms that include viral mediated injury, microvascular dysfunction/thrombosis, cytokines, and type II myocardial infarctions. The histological features seen at autopsy include increased macrophages and cytokine elevation. Classic lymphocytic myocarditis is relatively uncommon in COVID-19 patients.[19,20] Additional research will be needed to clearly define mechanisms of cardiac injury following SARS-CoV2 infection. The cause of injury is likely multifactorial with evidence of inflammation as manifest by macrophage infiltration and less commonly a typical lymphocytic myocarditis.

Attention has turned to whether myocarditis or cardiac injury might be identified by cardiac MR after patients recover from COVID-19. Myocarditis identified by MR after SARS-CoV-2 infection varies widely, from

0.6% in young athletes to 32% in older patients with elevated troponin.[21] COVID-19 in children and young adults <21 years of age was associated with a multisystem inflammatory syndrome (MIS-C). A total of 36/99 (36%) of the patients were diagnosed with Kawasaki disease or atypical (or incomplete) Kawasaki disease, whereas 52/99 (53%) had clinical evidence of myocarditis (see also Chapter 94).[17] COVID vaccines have been highly successful at reducing the risk of illness and hospitalization from SARS-CoV-2 infection. A small increase in the rate of myocarditis and pericarditis has been observed following mRNA vaccines. The rate of myocarditis and pericarditis has been reported as 1.0 per 100,000 and 1.8 per 100,000, respectively. None of the patients that had myocarditis or pericarditis died following vaccination. Additional studies are needed to confirm these findings. In addition, the incidence and severity of vaccine-associated myocarditis and pericarditis is much less than the devastating effects of COVID-19 infection.[21a]

Bacteria

Nonviral pathogens such as bacteria and parasites can affect the heart and, in some cases, activate an immune reaction in the heart. Virtually any bacterial agent can cause myocardial dysfunction, but it does not necessarily mean that the bacterium has infected the myocardium. In the case of sepsis or other severe bacterial infections, the myocardial dysfunction generally is attributed to activation of inflammatory mediators (see Chapter 47). Of note, however, bloodstream infection by virtually any bacterial infection can result in metastatic foci in the myocardium. This finding is most commonly associated with bacterial endocarditis. Some bacterial infections are well known to have specific effects on the heart that can be mediated by direct infection or activation of inflammatory mechanisms. The most common of these include diphtheria, rheumatic heart disease, and streptococcal infections.

Corynebacterium Infection. Myocardial involvement with *Corynebacterium diphtheriae* is a serious complication and is the most common cause of death in diphtheria. In up to one half of fatal cases, evidence of cardiac involvement can be found. Studies from the last decade indicate that there is evidence of myocardial involvement in 22% to 28% of patients. The overall incidence has decreased in developed countries because of vaccination, but recently there have been a growing number of unprotected individuals in developed countries as well. This may be related to vaccine avoidance. *C. diphtheriae* produces an exotoxin that severely damages the myocardium and the cardiac conduction system. Cardiac damage is due to the liberation of this exotoxin, which inhibits protein synthesis by interfering with host translational mechanisms. The toxin appears to have an affinity for the cardiac conduction system. Both antitoxin therapy and antibiotics are important in the treatment of diphtheria.

Streptococcal Infection. The most commonly detected cardiac complication after beta-hemolytic streptococcal infection is acute rheumatic fever, which is followed by rheumatic valve disease in approximately 60% of affected patients. Rarely, involvement of the heart by the streptococcus may produce a nonrheumatic myocarditis distinct from acute rheumatic carditis (see also Chapter 97). This clinical entity is characterized by the presence of an interstitial infiltrate composed of mononuclear cells with occasional polymorphonuclear leukocytes, which may be focal or diffuse. In contrast with rheumatic heart disease, streptococcal myocarditis usually occurs coincident with the acute infection or within a few days of the pharyngitis. Electrocardiographic abnormalities, including ST elevation and prolongation of the PR and QT intervals, are common. Rare sequelae may include sudden death, conduction disturbances, and arrhythmias.

Tuberculosis. Involvement of the myocardium by Mycobacterium tuberculosis (not tuberculous pericarditis) is rare. Tuberculous involvement of the myocardium occurs by means of hematogenous or lymphatic spread or may arise directly from contiguous structures and may cause nodular, miliary, or diffuse infiltrative disease. On occasion, it may lead to arrhythmias, including atrial fibrillation and ventricular tachycardia, complete atrioventricular block, heart failure, left ventricular aneurysms, and sudden death.

Whipple Disease. Although overt involvement is rare, intestinal lipodystrophy, or Whipple disease, is not uncommonly associated with cardiac involvement. Periodic acid–Schiff–positive macrophages can be found in the myocardium, pericardium, coronary arteries, and heart valves of patients with this disorder. Electron microscopy has demonstrated rod-shaped structures in the myocardium similar to those found in the small intestine, representing the causative agent of the disease, Tropheryma whipplei, a gram-negative bacillus related to the actinomycetes. An inflammatory infiltrate and foci of fibrosis also may be present. The valvular fibrosis may be severe enough to result in aortic regurgitation and mitral stenosis. Although it usually is asymptomatic, nonspecific electrocardiographic changes are most common; systolic murmurs, pericarditis, complete heart block, and even overt congestive heart failure may occur. Antibiotic therapy appears to be effective in treatment of the basic disease, but relapses can occur, often more than 2 years after the initial diagnosis.

Lyme Carditis. Lyme disease is caused by a tick-borne spirochete (*Borrelia burgdorferi*). It usually begins during the summer months with a characteristic rash (erythema chronicum migrans), followed by acute neurologic, joint, or cardiac involvement, usually with few long-term sequelae. Early studies indicated that up to 10% of untreated patients with Lyme disease demonstrated evidence of transient cardiac involvement, the most common manifestation being atrioventricular block of variable degree. With the early use of antibiotics, however, Lyme carditis is now considered to be a rare manifestation.[22] Of patients with Lyme disease reported to the Centers for Disease Control (CDC), only 1.1% were identified as having Lyme carditis.[23] Syncope due to complete heart block is frequent with cardiac involvement because of the commonly associated depression of ventricular escape rhythms. Diffuse ST-segment and T wave abnormalities are transient and usually asymptomatic. An abnormal gallium scan is compatible with cardiac involvement, and the demonstration of spirochetes in myocardial biopsy specimens of patients with Lyme carditis suggests a direct cardiac effect. Patients with second-degree or complete heart block should be hospitalized and undergo continuous electrocardiographic monitoring. Temporary transvenous pacing may be required for a week or longer in patients with a high-grade block. It is thought that antibiotics can prevent subsequent complications and may shorten the duration of the disease; therefore, they are used routinely in patients with Lyme carditis. Intravenous antibiotics are suggested, although oral antibiotics can be used when only mild cardiac involvement is present. Corticosteroids may reduce myocardial inflammation and edema, which in turn can shorten the duration of the heart block. It is thought that treatment of the early manifestations of the disease will prevent development of late complications.

Protozoa

Chagas disease is one of the major causes of nonischemic cardiomyopathy throughout the world, although the incidence is changing. In a remarkable tale of discovery at the beginning of the 20th century, Carlos Chagas almost single-handedly identified the parasite, *Trypanosoma cruzi*, which causes the entity now known as Chagas disease. He also elucidated the relatively complex life cycle of the parasite in poor, rural areas of Brazil. The parasite resides in and replicates in an infected host such as an armadillo or a domestic cat. The parasite then infects triatomine insects, including the hematophagous reduviid bug that feeds on the blood of infected vertebrate carriers. The triatomine acts as the vector of infection when it bites a human, depositing the parasite in its feces in the area of the bite wound, conjunctiva, or other mucous membranes. Transmission can also occur through blood transfusions, organ transplantation, consumption of food or beverages that have been contaminated by the vector or vector feces, as well as *in utero* from mother to fetus. Once within the now-infected individual, the parasite replicates and infects target organs such as the heart. Parasitic infection of cardiac myocytes and activation of the associated immune function damage the heart and other organs and lead to the clinical manifestations of Chagas disease; Fig. 55.3 shows the life cycle.[24]

Chagas disease is endemic in poor, rural areas of Central and South America. The distribution of Chagas disease is changing to include more urban and traditionally nonendemic areas because of migration of infected individuals from the rural to urban areas. Vector control initiatives in the endemic areas and aggressive screening of the blood supply has reduced the overall incidence of Chagas disease. In the 1980s, 17.4 million people were infected in 18 endemic countries.[25] By 2010, it was estimated that the number of infected persons had dropped to nearly 5.7 million. In 1990, it was

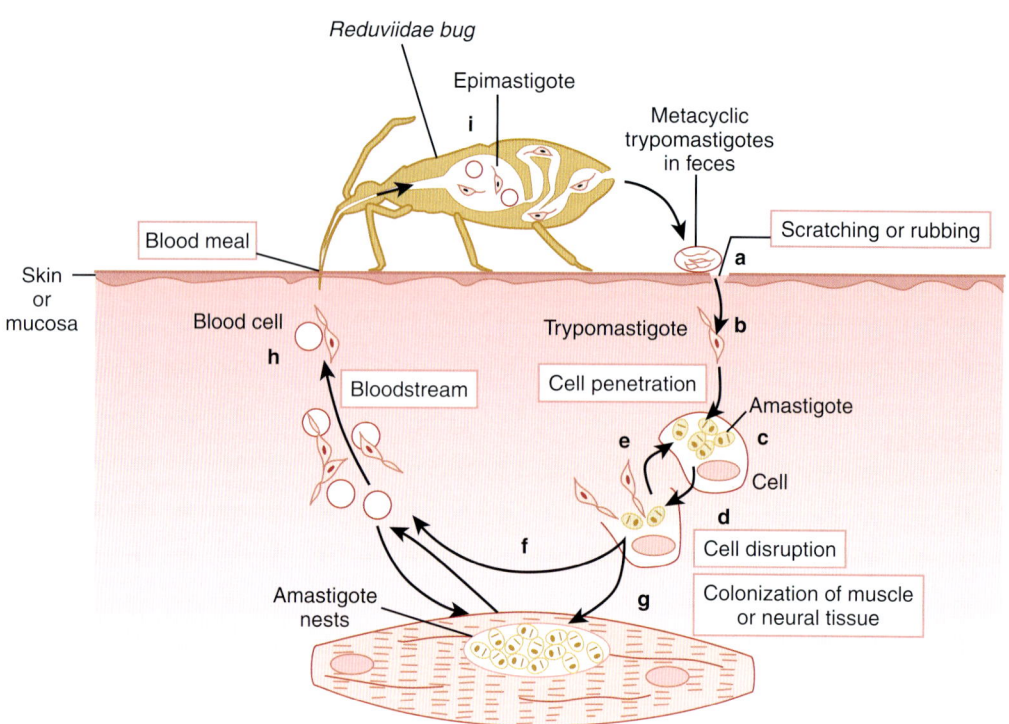

FIGURE 55.3 The life cycle of *Trypanosoma cruzi*. Reduviidae bugs transmit *T. cruzi*. While partaking of a blood meal (a), the insect defecates on the host's skin, releasing the infective trypomastigote form of the parasite. The trypomastigotes penetrate the host's skin or mucous membrane through abrasions caused by scratching or rubbing the bitten area (b). Trypomastigotes can infect host cardiac, skeletal, smooth muscle, or neural cells, subsequently giving rise to the round amastigote form that can replicate intracellularly (c). Amastigotes can give rise to trypomastigotes that can lyse cells (d). Amastigotes and trypomastigotes released from dying cells can propagate the infection or reenter the circulation (e-g). Insects can pick up the parasite when consuming a blood meal (h); it develops into the epimastigote form that replicates in the insect gut (i). (From Macedo AM, Oliveira RP, Pena SDJ. Chagas' disease: role of parasite genetic variation in pathogenesis. Expert Rev Mol Med. 2002;4:1.)

estimated that 700,000 new cases were diagnosed each year. In 2010, that number had decreased to 29,925. Similarly, the number of annual deaths from Chagas disease has decreased, from 50,000 per year in 1990 to approximately 12,500 per year.[26] However, at the same time that Chagas disease is decreasing worldwide, the incidence in the developed world is increasing because of immigration from endemic areas. It is currently estimated that 240,000 to 350,000 people in the United States are infected with *T. cruzi*.[26] This has important implications in relation to blood transfusion and organ donation, because the infectious agent can be transferred from donor to recipient; this is a particularly important consideration in the immunocompromised transplant recipient.

Symptoms from *T. cruzi* infection typically begin 1 to 2 weeks after a bite from an infected triatomine, or can occur up to a few months after transfusion of infected blood. The parasite load can affect the severity of clinical presentation. The initial acute phase of the disease begins 1 to 2 weeks after infection and lasts for up to 4 to 8 weeks. In the acute phase, the most sensitive diagnostic test is the identification of *T. cruzi* genetic material in the blood using PCR assay. During the acute phase of parasite infection, most affected patients are either asymptomatic or have a mild, subacute febrile illness. Other potential manifestations include adenopathy, hepatomegaly, myocarditis, and meningoencephalitis. Cardiovascular abnormalities during the acute phase might include nonspecific ECG changes, first-degree atrioventricular block, and cardiomegaly on chest x-ray examination. Death occurs from myocarditis or meningoencephalitis in less than 5% to 10% of symptomatic patients. In up to 90% of patients, the symptoms of disease resolve spontaneously, even without therapeutic intervention. Of these, approximately 60% to 70% develop an intermediate form of the disease that is characterized by the absence of signs or symptoms of cardiac or gastrointestinal involvement. Although these patients will remain seropositive throughout life, there are no other laboratory findings of Chagas disease. The prognosis is excellent for this form of the disease.

The other 30% to 40% of patients will develop manifestations of the chronic Chagas disease 5 to 15 years after the acute phases of the disease. Cardiac involvement in the chronic form of Chagas is characterized by myocardial fibrosis, destruction of the conduction system, ventricular dilation, thinning of the apex of the heart, and formation of a thrombus in the apex of the heart. These changes lead to DCM, symptomatic heart failure, arrhythmias, atrioventricular and bundle branch block, and possible thromboembolism. The Latin American guidelines for the diagnosis and treatment of cardiovascular involvement in Chagas disease define 5 different stages of Chagas heart disease based on the presence or absence of ECG changes, LV dysfunction, and development of symptoms of heart failure.[27] Gastrointestinal disturbances also can be a prominent part of the presentation. Congenital transmission of the parasite to a fetus from the mother is another important mechanism of transmission of the parasite. Conversely, the parasite can be passed from the mother to the infant at the time of birth. *T. cruzi* also has been shown to infect the placenta and subsequently infect the fetus in utero. Congenital transmission occurs in 1% to 5% of pregnancies when the mother has chronic Chagas disease. Congenital transmission of this disease results in spontaneous abortion, premature birth, or infection of organs in the fetus.[26]

Benznidazole and nifurtimox, which both inhibit *T. cruzi* DNA replication, and are effective against the trypomastigote and amastigote forms of the parasite, are currently the only treatments for treating Chagas disease. Benznidazole is considered to be the first line of therapy because of its better tolerability; however, both drugs produce significant side effects. Current treatment recommendations are based on the phase of the disease and age of the patient. The cure rates for treating congenital cases (96%) and children in the acute (76%) early chronic phase (62%) are well established. However, the cure rates for adults with chronic disease are less well established.[28] Treatment with benznidazole is recommended for children in acute and congenital cases, reactivations, and in the chronic indeterminate phase. The therapy of adult patients with intermediate or established Chagas cardiomyopathy remains controversial. The BENEFIT trial was a prospective study of 2854 patients with Chagas cardiomyopathy randomized to receive benznidazole or placebo for up to 80 days. The primary outcome variable was a clinical composite of death, resuscitated cardiac arrest, sustained ventricular tachycardia, insertion of a pacemaker or implantable cardioverter-defibrillator, cardiac transplantation, new heart failure, stroke, or other thromboembolic event. BENEFIT showed that although benznidazole significantly reduced the detection of parasite in the serum, it had no effect on the primary outcome (adjusted HR, 0.92; 95% CI, 0.81 to 1.06; p = 0.26).[29] Current guidelines recommend that adults ≤50 years of age in the indeterminate phase with minimal cardiac involvement should be offered treatment.[28] However, there is insufficient evidence supporting effectiveness of treatment in older adults and adults with cardiomyopathy. Nonetheless, given that it is not currently possible to predict which asymptomatic adult patients > 50 years of age will progress to the chronic form of the disease, it may be reasonable to also consider therapy for this group of patients on a case-by-case basis, because treatment remains the best way to prevent morbidity and mortality in Chagas disease.[28]

Helminths

Infection by a wide variety of helminth parasites, commonly *Trichinella* and *Echinococcus*, can result in myocardial injury ultimately progressing to cardiomyopathy.

Physical Agents, Including Adverse Drug Effects

A wide variety of substances other than infectious agents can act on the heart and damage the myocardium. In some cases, the damage is acute, transient, and associated with evidence of an inflammatory myocardial infiltrate with myocyte necrosis (e.g., with the arsenicals and lithium). Other agents that damage the myocardium can lead to chronic changes with resulting histologic evidence of fibrosis and a clinical picture of a dilated or restrictive cardiomyopathy. Numerous chemicals and drugs (both industrial and therapeutic) can lead to cardiac damage and dysfunction. Several other physical agents (e.g., radiation, excessive heat, hypothermia) also can contribute directly to myocardial damage.

Drugs. Drug-induced hypersensitivity syndrome may involve the heart and be associated with myocarditis. The syndrome usually emerges within 8 weeks of the initiation of a new drug but can occur at any time after drug consumption. Common agents include antiepileptics, antimicrobials, allopurinol, and sulfa-based drugs. Dobutamine, often used for hemodynamic support in patients with failing hearts, may be associated with eosinophilic myocarditis, and the drug should be stopped when eosinophilia appears or when an unexpected decline in left ventricular function is noted. Presenting characteristics may include a rash (unless the patient is immunologically compromised), fever, and multiorgan dysfunction (including hepatitis, nephritis, and myocarditis). Diffuse myocardial involvement may result in systemic hypotension and thromboembolic events. CMR imaging and measurement of cardiac biomarkers may help identify patients with cardiac involvement. EMB may demonstrate eosinophils, histiocytes, lymphocytes, myocardial necrosis, and occasionally granuloma and vasculitis. Myocardial involvement is patchy, so a definitive diagnosis is made only when the biopsy findings are positive. Corticosteroids and drug withdrawal usually resolve this syndrome; however, some patients may display a prolonged and relapsing course.

Clozapine is an effective antipsychotic medication that is used to treat severe, refractory schizophrenia. Myocarditis is a rarely reported side effect of clozapine therapy, with the initial incidence reported at between 0.01% and 0.001%. More recent observations, however, have found an incidence of myocarditis in 1% to 10% of patients. Perhaps the increased incidence is related to an increased awareness of the risk. Myocarditis can develop at any time during treatment but occurs most frequently within the first 4 days to 22 weeks after initiation of clozapine. The peak incidence is at around 19 to 21 days. Clozapine-related myocarditis probably is the result of a hypersensitivity reaction. It may be accompanied by eosinophilia, with eosinophilic infiltration seen in myocardial biopsy material. Clozapine also is a potent anticholinergic compound, and high levels associated with altered metabolism from CYP450 enzymes also could contribute to the cardiac effects. With clear evidence of myocarditis in a patient taking this drug, immediate discontinuation is indicated.[30]

Vaccination for smallpox among uniformed service members has been demonstrated to be associated with myopericarditis. In a prospective assessment of myocarditis following smallpox vaccination, clinical myopericarditis and subclinical myocarditis were noted at an incidence of 463 and 2868 per 100,000 subjects, respectively (in a healthy cohort the incidence was 2.2 clinical myopericarditis patients per 100,000). There were no cases of clinical myopericarditis or subclinical myocarditis in a control group that received trivalent influenza vaccination.[31]

As new chemotherapeutic agents are developed to target specific pathways in the heart, it is becoming increasingly apparent that cancer chemotherapy can induce cardiomyopathy that may be associated with myocarditis (**see** also Chapters 56 and 57). Antibodies against programmed cell death-1 (PD-1) (nivolumab, pembrolizumab, cemiplimab), T-lymphocyte-associated protein-4 (CTLA-4) (ipilimumab), and programmed cell death ligand 1 (PD-L1) (atezolizumab, avelumab, durvalumab)—termed "immune checkpoint inhibitors" (ICIs)—have revolutionized cancer treatment by increasing native immune activation and enhancing tumor antigen expression. As an unwanted consequence of immune activation, self-antigens (once regulated by checkpoint receptors) are recognized as foreign and result in autoimmunity including myocarditis in 0.3% to 1.0%. Fulminant myocarditis has been treated with high-dose corticosteroids and sometimes alemtuzumab or abatacept, T cell inhibitors.[32]

PATHOGENESIS OF VIRAL MYOCARDITIS

Much of the current understanding of the pathogenesis of myocarditis is derived from mouse models of enteroviral infection, particularly coxsackievirus B3, and rodent models of autoimmune myocarditis. The principles derived from these models have been applied to human myocarditis of different causes.[2] The description of the pathogenesis draws from cellular animal and human data. The pathogenesis of viral myocarditis can be divided into three major components: viral infection and replication, immunologic response (innate and adaptive immune response), and, ultimately, a phase of chronic cardiac remodeling (Fig. 55.4). MicroRNAs have also been shown to have a role in myocarditis.

Viral Infection

Viruses enter the host through a variety of locations, including the gastrointestinal system and respiratory system. The virus may undergo initial replication in the host in organs such as the liver, spleen, and pancreas. Ultimately, the virus reaches the heart via dissemination through the blood or lymphatic vessels. The steps include attachment of the virus to its receptor, entry of the virus into the cell, replication of the virus within the affected cell in the heart, and for lytic viruses, exit of the virus from the cell to allow infection of other cardiac cells. In the case of coxsackievirus, the virus infects the cardiac myocyte. In addition, however, other viruses may infect other cells in the heart, such as B19V that has been demonstrated to infect the cardiac endothelial cell and is not found in the cardiac myocyte.[16]

Initially, the virus binds to a viral receptor, ultimately resulting in internalization of the virus. This process includes entry of the viral capsid proteins and the viral genome. In the case of coxsackieviruses and adenoviruses, the receptor is a transmembrane molecule, CAR, named for these two viruses, which are known to use it as a receptor.[33] Genetic deletion of CAR in the cardiac myocyte markedly inhibits infection of the heart and development of myocarditis.[34] In addition to CAR, coxsackievirus infection can be facilitated by interaction with the decay-accelerating factor (DAF), or CD55. CAR acts as a receptor in both human and mouse cells. CAR is a tight junction protein in noncardiac cells and is expressed at high levels in the intercalated disc of myocardial cells. Entry of the virus through the receptor activates a signaling complex that includes p56[lck], Abl, and Fyn kinase.[33]

On entry of the enterovirus into the cell, the positive, single-strand RNA is released from the icosahedral capsid and translated using host translational mechanisms. The viral RNA is translated as a single, monocistronic polyprotein, which is cleaved into its separate peptides by the viral proteases 2A and 3C; through an autocatalytic cleavage process, VP0 is cleaved into VP2 and VP4. This results in generation of capsid and nonstructural proteins, including an RNA-dependent RNA polymerase that is required for replication of the viral genome. The other nonstructural proteins also are required for replication of the positive-strand RNA through a negative-strand intermediate. Once the numbers of viral capsid proteins have been amplified and the positive-strand RNA has replicated, the positive-strand RNA is encapsidated into the newly formed viral capsid proteins VP1, VP2, VP3, and VP4. The encapsidated coxsackievirus RNA is released from the myocardial cell through a process of cell lysis and disruption of the sarcolemmal membrane.

Several mechanisms are recognized to affect membrane integrity, thus affecting in turn release of the replicated virus. Muscle cells rely on the subsarcolemmal protein dystrophin and the associated proteins in the dystrophin-glycoprotein complex to maintain the integrity of the sarcolemmal membrane. Hereditary absence of dystrophin in Duchenne muscular dystrophy, for example, causes cardiac and skeletal muscle dysfunction (see Chapter 100). In enterovirus-induced murine myocarditis, it has been demonstrated that one of the nonstructural proteins, protease 2A, is able to directly cleave dystrophin, thus disrupting the dystrophin-glycoprotein complex. This decreases the sarcolemmal

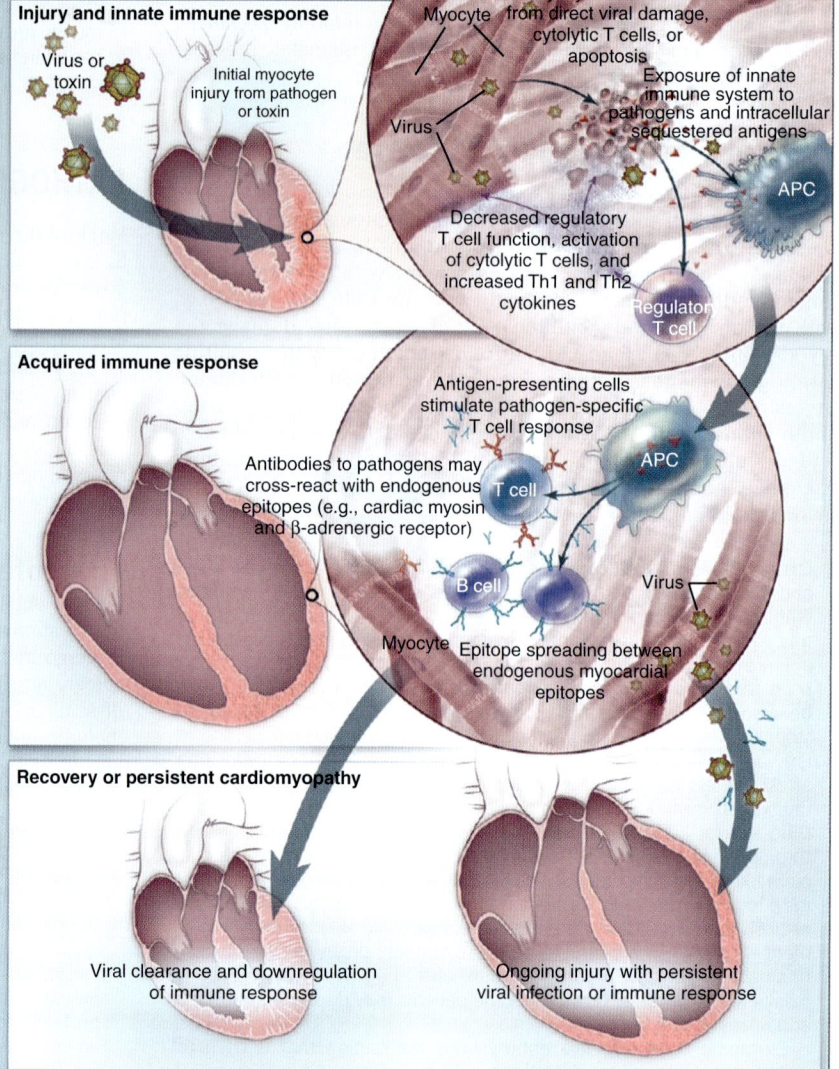

FIGURE 55.4 Pathogenesis of myocarditis. The current understanding of the cellular and molecular pathogenesis of postviral and autoimmune myocarditis is based solely on animal models. In these models, the progression from acute injury to chronic dilated cardiomyopathy may be simplified into a three-stage process. Acute injury leads to cardiac damage, exposure of intracellular antigens such as cardiac myosin, and activation of the innate immune system. Over weeks, specific immunity that is mediated by T lymphocytes and antibodies directed against pathogens and similar endogenous heart epitopes causes robust inflammation. In most patients, the pathogen is cleared and the immune reaction is downregulated, with few sequelae. In other patients, however, the virus is not cleared, and it causes continued myocyte damage; heart-specific inflammation may persist because of mistaken recognition of endogenous heart antigens as pathogenic entities. *APC,* antigen-presenting cell. (From Cooper LT. Myocarditis. *N Engl J Med.* 2009;360:1526.)

membrane integrity and facilitates the release of the virus from the myocardial cell. When dystrophin is not present in the mouse heart, as occurs in Duchenne muscular dystrophy, coxsackievirus is released more efficiently from the myocyte to infect adjacent cells.[35] However, when a dystrophin protein is expressed that cannot be cleaved by protease 2A, viral replication and the extent of myocardial damage is decreased.[35] Proteases 2A and 3C can cleave other host proteins that are involved in the maintenance of membrane integrity, initiation of translation of host proteins, regulation of apoptosis, innate immune response, and serum response factor.[3]

As genetic profiles have been assessed in patients, especially children with myocarditis, there is a growing body of literature that supports the concept that abnormalities in the cytoskeletal proteins occur more frequently in patients with myocarditis than in control populations. One study demonstrates that, in patients with acute myocarditis, there is an increase in the percentage who have homozygous or compound heterozygous variants in genes that have been associated with DCM. Interestingly, they found that potentially pathogenic variants occurred in the genes DSP, PKP2, and TNNI3 that code for the cytoskeletal and contractile proteins desmoplakin, plakophilin-2, and troponin I type 3. In addition, there were alterations in BAG3, which encodes BCL2-associated athanogene 3, which is an important mediator of apoptosis. Other genes that were abnormal in acute myocarditis included SCN5A, which encodes the sarcolemmal sodium channel, voltage-gated type V alpha subunit, which has been associated with the dystrophin-glycoprotein complex. Finally, RYR2, which encodes the ryanodine receptor 2, was mutated.[36] Additional evidence for an interaction between myocarditis and cytoskeletal abnormalities has been demonstrated in other case reports including one in monozygotic twins with a desmoplakin gene variant.[37] Desmoplakin cardiomyopathy has been shown to have an inflammatory component as well.[38]

Generally, the activation of the innate and adaptive, antigen-specific immune response eliminates or greatly reduces the replication of the virus within the host cell. In some cases, however, the virus can persist within the myocardium. In keeping with the presence of the enteroviral genome in a subset of patients with DCM, it is thought that persistence of the enteroviral genome could contribute to the ongoing remodeling that occurs with DCM. The feasibility of this concept has been shown in a mouse model, in which low-level, cardiac-specific expression of a replication-defective enteroviral genome can cause cardiomyopathy. However, the proportion of patients in whom the enteroviral genome can be identified with reverse transcriptase PCR (rtPCR) or in situ hybridization techniques generally is less than 10%. The early phases of enteroviral infection and intramyocardial innate immunity can now be studied in human-induced pluripotent stem cells that are differentiated to cardiac myocytes.[39]

Other types of viruses also have been detected in cardiac biopsy specimens from patients with DCM. These viruses include B19V, herpesvirus, cytomegalovirus, hepatitis C virus, and others. Distinguishing whether the presence of a viral genome in each patient is causative or an incidental finding in cardiomyopathy has not been trivial. For example, the B19V viral genome can be detected in a high percentage of patients independent of whether they have cardiomyopathy. It has been demonstrated that only 15.9% of patients that have evidence of

B19V DNA on EMB have evidence of B19V mRNA. Interestingly, there is a significant difference in expression profiling in the biopsies that show transcriptionally active B19V, suggesting that transcriptional activity of the B19V may have a role in the pathogenesis.[16]

Innate Immunity

Innate immunity is effective during the earliest stages of virus infection. It is an antigen-independent defense mechanism that protects the host from a broad range of microbial pathogens. Innate immunity is initiated in the first days of enteroviral infection and is the major immune mechanism responsible for inhibiting viral infection and replication during the first 4 to 5 days after infection (Fig. 55.5). In addition to innate immune mechanisms in noncardiac organs, important innate immune responses also are activated in the cardiac myocyte.[40] One of the classic and best-characterized examples of innate immunity is the activation of interferon (IFN) signaling that occurs with viral infection. The two broad classes of IFNs use different receptors: Type I IFNs bind to the IFN-α receptor and include IFN-α and IFN-β, whereas IFN-γ is the sole type II IFN member. Both types I and II IFNs are effective at limiting viral replication when added to infected cells or when administered to a coxsackievirus-infected mouse.[40] The absence of type I IFN receptors or IFN-β in mice is associated with a marked increase in mortality rates but has less effect on early viral replication in the heart. In a phase II clinical trial, it has been demonstrated that administration of IFN-β to virus-positive patients with symptoms of heart failure caused significant clearance or reduction of the virus load and improvement in the New York Heart Association (NYHA) functional class and quality of life. In enterovirus-positive patients, IFN-β may improve survival rates.[41]

Acquired Immunity

Acquired immunity becomes a prominent manifestation of viral myocarditis beginning approximately 4 to 5 days after the viral infection, although the peak and pattern of activation are variable. The acquired immune response is an antigen-specific response that is directed to a single antigen and is mediated by T and B cells. T cells are targeted to infected cells and attempt to limit infection by destroying the host cell through secretion of cytokines or perforins. These can contribute to the death of the infected cell through necrotic and/or apoptotic mechanisms. Thus, although T cell–mediated immune mechanisms are important for controlling and limiting viral replication, they also can have detrimental effects on the infected organ by stimulating cell death mechanisms in the infected host. Appropriately limiting the T cell and B cell immune mechanisms could limit damage to the heart, but such inhibition needs to be balanced by the need to inhibit viral replication.[42]

The acquired immune process is initiated when the variable region of the T cell receptor binds to peptides with specific amino acid sequences that are recognized as foreign to the host. When CD4+ T cells interact with antigen-presenting cells such as dendritic cells, the CD4+ cells can differentiate into different effector cell subsets, such as the classic Th1 and Th2 cell subtypes, namely Th17 and T regulatory (Treg) cells. Cytokines in the cellular microenvironment can control how the cells differentiate. The precise cellular signaling cascades and pattern

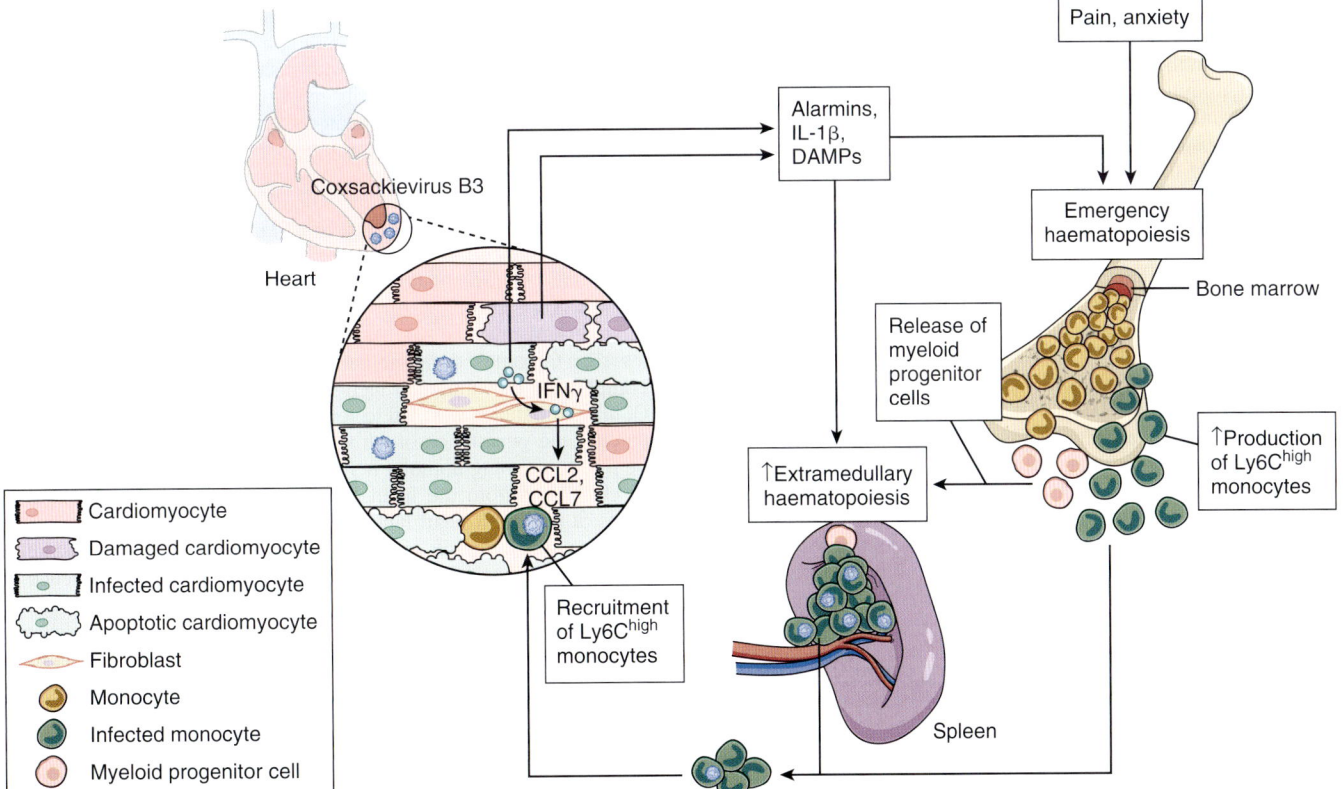

FIGURE 55.5 Cardiosplenic axis in coxsackievirus B3-induced myocarditis. In the heart, coxsackievirus B3 infection of cardiomyocytes leads to cell damage and death and the release of IL-1β and damage-associated molecular patterns (DAMPs), which trigger the recruitment and activation of cells from the innate immune system. Pain, anxiety, and the release of danger signals into the systemic circulation trigger emergency hematopoiesis in the bone marrow, leading to medullary monocytopoiesis as well as release of myeloid progenitor cells into the circulation. Myeloid progenitor cells then migrate to the spleen, where extramedullary monocytopoiesis takes place to replenish the pool of proinflammatory Ly6C^{high} monocytes, which can be rapidly mobilized to the damaged heart. In the heart, interferon γ (IFNγ) released by infected cardiomyocytes boosts the production by fibroblasts of the pro-inflammatory C-C motif chemokines CCL2 and CCL7, which promote the homing of Ly6C^{high} monocytes to the heart. Given that the spleen is a target organ of coxsackievirus B3 and monocytes target cells of coxsackievirus B3, the recruited Ly6C^{high} monocytes might be infected with coxsackievirus B3 and thereby transport the virus into the heart, further contributing to the viral infection. Activation of the innate immune system in the heart is beneficial for its antiviral effects but excessive or persistent activation can lead to exaggerated and/or chronic inflammation that triggers myocardial destruction and remodeling, culminating in cardiac dysfunction. (Adapted from Tschope, C, Ammirati E, Bozkurt B, et al. Myocarditis and inflammatory cardiomyopathy: current evidence and future directions. Nat Rev Cardiol. 2020;Oct 12:1–25. https://doi.org/10.1038/s41569-020-00435-x.)

of cytokine production that are associated with differentiation of these distinct T cell subtypes has been reviewed elsewhere.[42,43] Appropriate regulation of effector T cells is needed to control infections and at the same time avoid inappropriate immunologic destruction of host tissue such as myocardial cells. Activation of T cells also leads to B cell activation, which results in secretion of antigen-specific antibodies directed against the invading pathogen. After initial activation, the immune cells undergo clonal expansion to attack the source of antigen, which could include a viral coat protein or, in some cases, proteins in the cardiac myocyte such as myosin. There is evidence that cross reaction with the host may occur because of "molecular mimicry" between the virus and the host. Treg cells have important functions for the suppression of Th1-cell and Th2-cell immune responses and were previously identified as T-helper cells. They are characterized by the expression of the forkhead transcription factor, Foxp3, and are defined as $CD4^+CD25^+Foxp3^+$. The classic model held that commitment of $CD4^+$ cells to the different effector lineages involved stable programs of gene expression and that once differentiated, they maintained that effector phenotype even as changes in the microenvironment occurred. This model, however, has evolved, because of evidence that $CD4^+$ T cells have an element of plasticity in that they can alter their functional programs and in this way change the balance between Treg cells and cytokine-producing T cells and the type of cytokines that they produce.[42] This plasticity may be important as new therapeutic strategies are developed. The activation of T cells is highly dependent on an interaction with the innate immune-signaling cascade. For example, signaling through the T cell receptor uses p56lck. It is interesting that p56lck also has been shown to bind to the CAR-DAF receptor complex and that it is involved in viral entry. When p56lck is genetically deleted from the mouse, typical myocarditis is almost eliminated, with no significant mortality rates after infection.[44]

Alterations in any of the pathogenic mechanisms just described could, theoretically, affect the susceptibility to viral infection. For example, alterations in the mechanism of viral entry and replication, innate or acquired immune-signaling mechanisms, or the integrity of the sarcolemmal membrane could affect the susceptibility to develop myocarditis on exposure to a given virus. Nutrition is also likely to influence the susceptibility to viral infection. It is thought that a deficiency of selenium can increase the risk of myocarditis, as has been described in the Keshan province in China. When selenium deficiency was prevented, the incidence of myocarditis and DCM decreased. Furthermore, selenium deficiency in mice also increased the susceptibility to enteroviral myocarditis. The number of mechanisms known to affect the susceptibility to myocarditis in humans is far from complete.

Cardiac Remodeling

Remodeling of the heart after cardiac injury (see also Chapter 47) can significantly affect cardiac structure and function, and the degree of such remodeling may mean the difference between appropriate healing and the development of DCM. The virus can directly enter the endothelial cells and myocytes and effect changes that lead to direct cell death or hypertrophy. The virus also can modify the myocyte cytoskeleton, as mentioned earlier, leading to DCM. The inflammatory process outlined earlier for both innate and acquired immunity can lead to cytokine release and activation of matrix metalloproteinases that digest the interstitial collagen and elastin framework of the heart (see Chapter 47).

CLINICAL SYNDROMES

Myocarditis has a wide-ranging array of potential clinical presentations, a feature that contributes to the difficulties in diagnosis and classification. The clinical picture may be one of asymptomatic electrocardiographic or echocardiographic abnormalities or may include signs and symptoms of chest pain, cardiac dysfunction, arrhythmias or heart failure, and/or hemodynamic collapse. Transient electrocardiographic or echocardiographic abnormalities have been observed frequently during community viral outbreaks or influenza epidemics, but most patients remain asymptomatic from a cardiac standpoint and have few long-term sequelae. Chest pain from myocarditis may resemble typical angina and be accompanied by ECG changes, including ST-segment elevation. Coronary vasospasm, demonstrated using intra-coronary acetylcholine infusion, is one cause for chest pain in patients with clinical signs of myocarditis in the absence of significant coronary atherosclerosis. Chest pain also may mimic that in pericarditis, suggesting epicardial inflammation with adjacent pericardial involvement. The outcome of myopericarditis generally is good, with only two sudden deaths reported from four published case series ($N = 128$).

Myocarditis typically has a bimodal distribution in terms of age in the population, with the acute or fulminant presentation more commonly seen in young children and teenagers. By contrast, the presenting symptoms are more subtle and insidious, often with DCM and heart failure, in the older adult population. The difference in presentation probably is related to the maturity of the immune system, whereby the young tend to mount an exuberant response to the initial exposure of a provocative antigen. By contrast, older persons would have developed a greater degree of tolerance and show a chronic inflammatory response only to the chronic presence of a foreign antigen or with a dysregulated immune system that predisposes to autoimmunity. Myocarditis probably is responsible for 10% to 50% of new-onset cases of idiopathic DCM, a rate that varies depending on the criteria used for diagnosis. Viral myocarditis has been associated with heart failure from both systolic and isolated diastolic dysfunction.[45]

The presentation of myocarditis varies by cause. For example, B19V frequently causes chest pain from endothelial dysfunction, whereas ventricular arrhythmias and heart block are more common in giant cell myocarditis (GCM).[45] Associated physical examination findings point to specific causes for myocarditis. Enlarged lymph nodes with hilar adenopathy on the chest radiograph may suggest systemic sarcoidosis. A pruritic, maculopapular rash with an elevated eosinophil count suggests a hypersensitivity reaction to a drug or toxin. Patients who present with DCM complicated by sustained or symptomatic ventricular tachycardia or high-grade heart block are at high risk for having GCM or cardiac sarcoidosis. A study of 72 young Finnish patients with initially unexplained atrioventricular block revealed that 25% had either cardiac sarcoidosis (19%) or GCM (6%). Of these 18 patients, 7 (39%) experienced sustained ventricular tachycardia or cardiac death or required transplantation over an average follow-up period of 48 months (Fig. 55.6).[46] A prospective study of 12 patients with biopsy-proven GCM revealed that 25% of patients with a cardiomyopathy of less than 6 months' duration that failed to respond to usual care or was complicated by ventricular tachycardia or high-grade heart block had GCM.[47] In patients who fail to recover from an acute episode of myocarditis, the persistence of left ventricular dysfunction can sometimes be due to ongoing immune activation or chronic myocarditis. Failure to clear virus from the heart has been postulated to underlie some cases of persistent heart failure. Recognition of endogenous proteins, such as cardiac myosin, as "foreign" may contribute to ongoing inflammation even after successful viral clearance.[4,48] In clinical practice, the distinction between a noninflammatory DCM and a chronic inflammatory DCM with or without viral infection requires EMB. As discussed below, the lack of positive large-scale trial data supporting either immunosuppression or antiviral therapy currently limits the application of EMB in this setting.

DIAGNOSTIC APPROACHES

The diagnosis of myocarditis traditionally has required a histologic diagnosis according to the classic Dallas criteria. However, because of low sensitivity due to the patchy nature of the inflammatory infiltrates in the myocardium and the reluctance of clinicians to perform an invasive diagnostic procedure, myocarditis is severely underdiagnosed. Because the incidence of the disease is likely to be much higher than is appreciated, a high level of clinical suspicion, together with hybrid clinical and laboratory criteria and new imaging modalities, may help

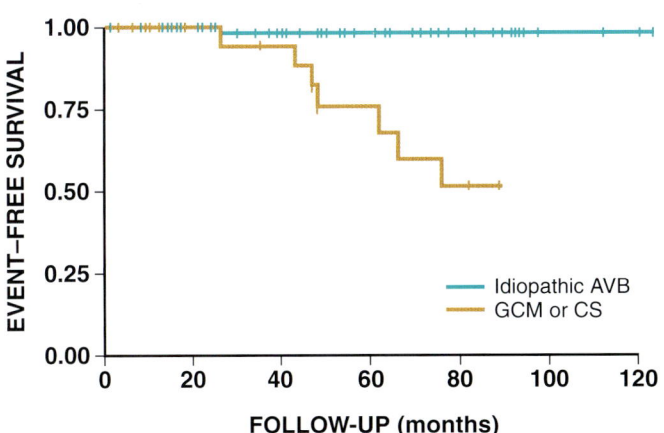

FIGURE 55.6 Kaplan-Meier curves for survival free of major adverse cardiac events (cardiac death, cardiac transplantation, ventricular fibrillation, or treated sustained ventricular tachycardia) in patients with pacemaker implantation for atrioventricular block (AVB) that remained idiopathic or AVB due to cardiac sarcoidosis (CS) or giant cell myocarditis (GCM). (From Kandolin R, Lehtonen J, Kupari M. Cardiac sarcoidosis and giant cell myocarditis as causes of atrioventricular block in young and middle-aged adults. *Circ Arrhythm Electrophysiol.* 2011;4:303.)

secure the diagnosis without necessarily resorting to biopsy in all cases (see Table 55.3).[2] Although clinical and imaging criteria have been used to estimate the myocarditis prevalence in various cohorts without EMB confirmation, such criteria probably sacrifice diagnostic specificity.

Laboratory Testing

The role of cardiac injury biomarkers in screening for myocarditis in patients with acute viral illness has been investigated in accordance with the hypothesis that a diagnosis of heart damage in this setting may indicate a greater risk of arrhythmias or cardiomyopathy. In this regard, elevated cardiac troponin values help to confirm cases of suspected myocarditis. Whereas older studies suggested that the sensitivity of troponins for myocarditis was low, more recent studies using more sensitive assays in less chronic disease support the value of troponin. For example, troponin levels predicted the severity of myocarditis and short-term prognosis in a case series of 65 children with recent-onset myocarditis. Fulminant myocarditis was associated with higher levels of cardiac troponins I and T (cTnI and cTnT) than acute myocarditis, and a higher cardiac troponin level was associated with a lower left ventricular ejection fraction.[49] In a case series of adults hospitalized with acute or fulminant myocarditis, creatine kinase–MB concentrations of greater than 29.5 ng/mL predicted in-hospital death with a sensitivity of 83% and a specificity of 73%. A growing literature also supports a role for TnI as an autoantigen as well as a biomarker for diagnosis.[50]

Renko and associates prospectively measured cTnI levels in 1009 children to determine the incidence of myocarditis in children hospitalized for an acute infection. TnI levels exceeded the screening limit (0.06 μg/L) in only six children, none of whom had electrocardiographic or echocardiographic abnormalities. Thus, the incidence of acute myocarditis during childhood viral infections appears to be low, so routine TnI screening for asymptomatic myocarditis in unselected children without cardiac symptoms probably is not indicated.[51] The rate of asymptomatic increases in troponin after smallpox vaccination is as high as 28.7 per 1000.[32] The risk of acute cardiomyopathy appears low in the first year after smallpox vaccination, but the longer-term significance of a troponin rise in this setting is not known.

A variety of other biomarkers have demonstrated prognostic value in acute myocarditis. In children with fulminant myocarditis, higher serum creatinine, lactate, and aspartate transaminase (AST) levels are associated with increased in-hospital mortality rates.[52] N-terminal pro–B type (brain) natriuretic peptide (NT-pro-BNP) is predictably elevated in children with acute DCM due to myocarditis and generally declines rapidly in children who recover left ventricular function.[53] In adults, higher interleukin-10 and soluble Fas concentrations are associated with an increased risk of death. Anti–heart antibodies have been reported to predict an increased risk of death or need for transplantation. However, few anti–heart antibody tests are standardized or available in clinical laboratories. Nonspecific biomarkers of inflammation, such as the leukocyte count, C-reactive protein, and erythrocyte sedimentation rate, have low specificity. Circulating viral antibody titers do not correlate with tissue viral genomes and are rarely of diagnostic use in clinical practice.[54]

Pathognomonic ECG findings are lacking in acute myocarditis, but nonspecific repolarization changes and sinus tachycardia are common (see also Chapter 14). PR-segment depression and diffuse ST-segment elevation may accompany a clinical presentation of myopericarditis. The presence of a QRS width greater than 120 milliseconds in duration and Q waves is associated with a great risk of cardiac death or need for heart transplantation.[55]

Cardiac Imaging

An assessment of left ventricular function by means of cardiac imaging (see also Chapters 16 to 19) is essential in all cases of suspected myocarditis. Echocardiography is an excellent choice for imaging, although there are no specific echocardiographic features of myocarditis. In patients who have an acute cardiomyopathy, the most common pattern is a dilated, spherical ventricle with reduced systolic function. Patients with heart failure due to fulminant myocarditis typically present with small cardiac chambers and mild and reversible ventricular hypertrophy from inflammation. Right ventricular dysfunction is less common and heralds a poor prognosis. Of interest, segmental wall motion abnormalities often are present early and may mimic the regional changes seen in a myocardial infarction. A pericardial effusion usually signifies myopericarditis.

CMR (see Chapter 19) has become the primary noninvasive imaging modality for assessment of myocardial inflammation in patients with suspected myocarditis. Certain patterns of signal abnormality on CMR are strongly suggestive of acute myocarditis.[56] Myocardial necrosis can be detected by late gadolinium enhancement (LGE). The T1-weighted, myocardial-delayed enhancement technique can quantitate regions of damage and possibly predict the risk of cardiovascular death and ventricular arrhythmias after myocarditis.[57] T2-weighted imaging can be used to detect myocardial edema. However, the T2-weighted, short tau inversion recovery (STIR) and T1-weighted-delayed postcontrast signal abnormalities seen in acute myocarditis usually decrease with time. The sensitivity and specificity of CMR in suspected myocarditis more than 14 days after symptom onset were poor (sensitivity, 63%; specificity, 40%).[58] Thus, CMR performs best in the setting of acute cardiomyopathy or chest pain with elevated troponin. Both T1- and T2-weighted sequences should be used, to optimize the sensitivity and specificity.[59] An anteroseptal pattern of delayed enhancement is associated with greater risk of MACE as is an increase in DGE on follow-up CMR 6 months after presentation. A decrease in LGE on follow-up CMR is associated with a low risk of MACE.[57] Because of the absence of large-scale multicenter data with CMR in myocarditis, current recommendations with respect to the CMR diagnosis of myocarditis are based on expert opinion, rather than rigorous data of pulse sequences that have been evaluated against myocardial biopsy in clearly defined clinical subsets of patients. The "Lake Louise Criteria" is a consensus document that provides suggested CMR criteria for diagnosing myocardial inflammation in patients with suspected myocarditis. The diagnostic accuracy of the Lake Louise Criteria ranges from 68% to 78%, depending on the number of tissue markers used in CMR studies.[60]

Although most nuclear imaging techniques are ancillary in the evaluation of suspected myocarditis, positron emission tomography (PET) imaging remains useful for diagnosing cardiac sarcoidosis.[61] Isiguzo and colleagues recently showed a significant association of metabolism-perfusion mismatch by rubidium-fluorodeoxyglucose (FDG) PET with clinically active disease in cardiac sarcoidosis patients.[62] Case control series suggest that patients with cardiomyopathy or ventricular arrhythmias due to cardiac sarcoidosis may benefit from steroid therapy.

Endomyocardial Biopsy

EMB remains essential for the diagnosis of specific forms of myocarditis.[63] The rate of major complications with EMB is less than 1 in 1000 when the procedure is done by experienced operators. In children with suspected myocarditis, EMB demonstrating myocarditis can identify responders to medical treatment. Because myocarditis may only involve regions of one ventricle, several large-volume cardiac centers are routinely performing left as well as right ventricular biopsy. In these centers, the safety of left ventricular biopsy is equivalent to that of right ventricular biopsy, and the diagnostic yield is greater.[64,65]

The clinical scenarios in which EMB is most useful are suspected GCM and fulminant lymphocytic myocarditis in the setting of an acute cardiomyopathy (Fig. 55.7).[66,67] GCM should be considered in acute DCM that fails to respond to usual care or is complicated by high-grade heart block or sustained ventricular tachycardia. The use of immunosuppressive therapy that includes cyclosporine probably increases the transplant-free survival rate in patients with GCM whose symptoms are of less than 6 months' duration.[47,68] Histologically, GCM is defined by a diffuse or multifocal inflammatory infiltrate of lymphocytes and multinucleated giant cells in the absence of granuloma. In contrast with cardiac sarcoidosis, in which the giant cells are located within the granuloma, the giant cells often are located at the edges of the inflammation, where myocyte damage is present. Eosinophils are significantly more common in GCM, whereas fibrosis is significantly more common in cardiac sarcoidosis. Immunohistochemistry may be beneficial in differentiating GCM from cardiac sarcoidosis.

PROGNOSIS

The prognosis for patients with acute myocarditis varies in relation to the clinical scenario and degree of left ventricular dysfunction at presentation.[69] Patients who present with myopericarditis or chest pain suggestive of an acute coronary syndrome usually do well if their left ventricular function is normal or near normal.[70] However, approximately 15% of patients with myopericarditis may develop recurrent myopericarditis. In acute DCM, the risk of death or need for cardiac transplantation is increased in those myocarditis patients with lower left ventricular function, lower right ventricular function, and higher pulmonary artery pressures. In children, the time course of left ventricular functional recovery extends to at least 8 years, and the overall risk of death or requirement for transplantation approaches 30% (Fig. 55.8).[71,72] In patients with a recent onset of DCM who were bridged to recovery with a left ventricular assist device, myocardial inflammation was present but fibrosis was less evident.[73] There is a risk of late heart failure due to diastolic dysfunction years after the apparent resolution of acute myocarditis.[45]

In chronic DCM, the presence of inflammatory cells on EMB may define a subset of patients who will improve with a short course of immunosuppression. Some investigators have demonstrated that the presence of active myocarditis defined by immunohistology, but not conventional Dallas criteria, predicts the risk of death or need for transplantation. The presence of viral genomes on EMB may portend a poor outcome. Older clinical data for enteroviruses in acute cardiomyopathy were mostly consistent with this conclusion, but in recent years, the impact of viral genomes on the outcome has been questioned. Possibly the variable findings with respect to viral genomes may be due to a changing spectrum of viruses, from enteroviruses to B19V and human herpesvirus 6. In addition, genetic background differences in study populations, and possibly unmeasured environmental toxins or nutritional deficiencies, may account for differences in study outcomes. Studies that have evaluated the impact of CMR imaging–associated delayed gadolinium enhancement on the cardiovascular risk following acute myocarditis generally support an association between delayed gadolinium enhancement and subsequent arrhythmic events.[59]

TREATMENT

The first-line therapy for all patients with myocarditis and heart failure is supportive care (see Chapter 50). A small proportion of patients will require hemodynamic support that ranges from vasopressors (see Chapter 49) to intraaortic balloon pump and ventricular assist devices (see Chapter 59) (Fig. 55.9). Guidelines for myocarditis management have been published by the American Heart Association (AHA),[74] Japanese Circulatory Society, and European Society of Cardiology (ESC) working group on myocarditis and pericarditis.[63] In patients who present with an acute DCM and a syndrome of heart failure, the current American College of Cardiology (ACC)/AHA guidelines for heart failure care should be followed.[45] Clinical experience suggests that standard pharmacotherapy is effective in myocarditis, although trials of heart failure management in myocarditis have not been done.

Routine treatment of mild to moderately severe acute myocarditis with immunosuppressive drugs is not recommended for adults.

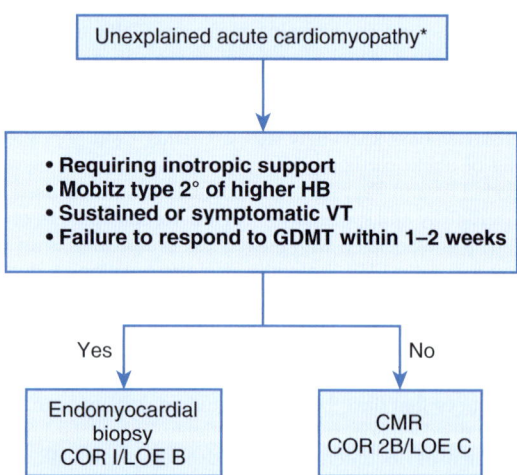

FIGURE 55.7 Algorithm for the evaluation of suspected myocarditis in the setting of unexplained acute cardiomyopathy. Unexplained acute cardiomyopathy will usually present as a dilated cardiomyopathy. However, patients with fulminant myocarditis may have normal end-diastolic diameter with mildly increased left ventricular wall thickness. It is also important to exclude ischemic, hemodynamic (valvular, hypertensive), metabolic, and toxic causes of acute cardiomyopathy, as indicated clinically. *CMR*, Cardiac magnetic resonance imaging; *COR*, class of recommendation; *LOE*, level of evidence. (From Bozkurt B, Colvin M, Cook J, et al; American Heart Association Committee on Heart Failure and Transplantation of the Council on Clinical Cardiology; Council on Cardiovascular Disease in the Young; Council on Cardiovascular and Stroke Nursing; Council on Epidemiology and Prevention; and Council on Quality of Care and Outcomes Research. Current Diagnostic and Treatment Strategies for Specific Dilated Cardiomyopathies: A Scientific Statement From the American Heart Association. *Circulation.* 2016;134:e579-e646.)

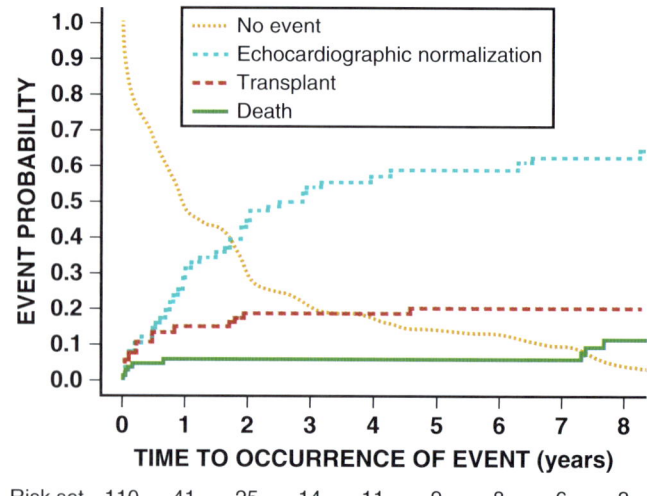

FIGURE 55.8 Crude cumulative incidence rates of echocardiographic normalization, cardiac transplantation, and death among children with biopsy-confirmed myocarditis. (From Foerster SR, Canter CE, Cinar A, et al. Ventricular remodeling and survival are more favorable for myocarditis than for idiopathic dilated cardiomyopathy in childhood: an outcomes study from the Pediatric Cardiomyopathy Registry. *Circ Heart Fail.* 2010;3:689.)

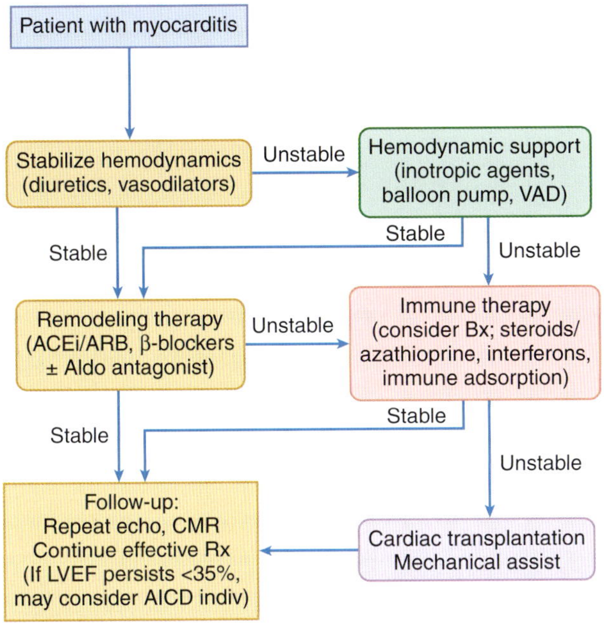

FIGURE 55.9 Treatment algorithms for patients with myocarditis, depending on hemodynamic stability and response to general supportive and remodeling treatment regimen at each step. All patients require aggressive support and appropriate follow-up. Immune therapy at present is still indicated mainly to support those who have failed to improve spontaneously. *ACEi*, Angiotensin-converting enzyme inhibitor; *AICD*, automatic implantable cardioverter-defibrillator; *Aldo*, aldosterone; *ARB*, angiotensin receptor blocker; *Bx*, biopsy; *CMR*, cardiac magnetic resonance; *echo*, echocardiography; *indiv*, based on individual assessment of risk versus benefit; *LVEF*, left ventricular ejection fraction; *VAD*, ventricular assist device.

These data are based on the U.S. Myocarditis Treatment Trial, in which immunosuppression with prednisone and either azathioprine or cyclosporine effected similar changes in the left ventricular ejection fraction and transplant-free survival rates compared with placebo. Significant exceptions are recognized, including those of patients with GCM, cardiac sarcoidosis, eosinophilic myocarditis, and myocarditis associated with inflammatory connective tissue disorders. Also, the data from case-controlled series regarding the use of intravenous immunoglobulin (IVIG) and immunosuppressive drugs are neutral to favorable in the pediatric literature. Treatment of viral infection may be helpful in the management of posttransplantation viral heart disease in children.[10] However, in adult patients with chronic DCM and viral genomes detected by PCR in heart biopsy tissues, one trial series suggests that 6 mIU of IFN-β three times per week improves enteroviral or adenoviral heart infection.[41] There may be a role for a short course of immunosuppression in patients with chronic DCM who fail to respond to guideline-based heart failure management. In the Tailored Immunosuppression in Inflammatory Cardiomyopathy (TIMIC) trial, 85 patients with chronic inflammatory cardiomyopathy without persistent viral infection were randomly assigned to receive either prednisone and azathioprine or placebo. Immunosuppressive treatment was associated with an increase in the left ventricular ejection fraction from 26% to 46% and an improved quality of life, whereas none of the patients in the placebo arm improved their left ventricular ejection fraction.[75] Larger, multicenter trials are needed to assess whether immunosuppression will affect clinically meaningful end points such as the risk of death or admission to hospital in this population.

Patients with ventricular arrhythmias or heart block due to acute myocarditis should be hospitalized for electrocardiographic monitoring. Arrhythmias usually resolve after several weeks. The ACC/AHA/ESC guidelines for the management of arrhythmias recommended that acute arrhythmia emergencies be managed conventionally in the setting of myocarditis. Generally, the indications for an implantable cardiac defibrillator (ICD) are the same as with nonischemic DCM. In the setting of GCM or cardiac sarcoidosis, the high rate of ventricular arrhythmias may warrant early consideration for an ICD. In patients with suspected lymphocytic myocarditis and nonsustained ventricular tachycardia, a temporary external defibrillator vest may be used while it is determined whether the arrhythmias will persist after the acute inflammatory phase.

Mechanical circulatory support (see also Chapter 59) or extracorporeal membrane oxygenation may allow a bridge to transplantation or recovery in patients with cardiogenic shock despite optimal medical care. In those patients who recover, the time to recovery in acute myocarditis varies, ranging from a few weeks to a few months. Transplantation also is an effective therapy for patients with myocarditis who have refractory heart failure despite optimal medical therapy and mechanical circulatory support. Survival rates after transplantation for myocarditis are similar to survival rates for other causes of cardiac transplantation. However, the risk of graft loss may be greater in children who undergo transplantation.

FUTURE PERSPECTIVES

One of the major gaps in the management of myocarditis is the lack of a sensitive and specific noninvasive test. In this regard, diagnostic techniques are evolving to identify novel blood-based biomarkers reflecting cardiac inflammation through microarray and proteomic analysis of tissues from both laboratory models and patient samples.[3] Moreover, with improved understanding of pathophysiologic mechanisms, new therapies also are being developed and evaluated in clinical trials. These new treatments, including cell-based therapies that selectively inhibit T cell responses, induce apoptosis of activated T cells, and increase Treg cells, will be evaluated in planned clinical trials. Such prospective investigations should be designed specifically to establish efficacy in women. Translational studies focused on genomic markers in biopsy samples and peripheral blood should help refine risk assessments and target therapies to the populations at highest need.

REFERENCES

Definition and Epidemiology

1. Schultheiss HP, Kuhl U, Cooper LT. The management of myocarditis. *Eur Heart J.* 2011;32:2616–2625.
2. Heymans S, Eriksson U, Lehtonen J, Cooper LT. The quest for new approaches in myocarditis and inflammatory cardiomyopathy. *J Am Coll Cardiol.* 2016;68:2348–2364.
3. Fung G, Luo H, Qiu Y, et al. Myocarditis. *Circulation Res.* 2016;118:496–514.
4. Mensah GA, Roth GA, Fuster V. The global burden of cardiovascular diseases and risk factors. *J Am Coll Cardiol.* 2019;74:2529–2532.
5. Maron BJ, Udelson JE, Bonow RO, et al. Eligibility and disqualification recommendations for competitive athletes with cardiovascular abnormalities: Task Force 3: hypertrophic cardiomyopathy, arrhythmogenic right ventricular cardiomyopathy and other cardiomyopathies, and myocarditis. *Circulation.* 2015;132.
6. Harmon KG, Asif IM, Maleszewski JJ, et al. Incidence and etiology of sudden cardiac arrest and death in high school athletes in the United States. *Mayo Clin Proc.* 2016;91:1493–1502.
7. Towbin JA, Lowe AM, Colan SD, et al. Incidence, causes, and outcomes of dilated cardiomyopathy in children. *J Am Med Assoc.* 2006;296:1867.
8. Leone O, Veinot JP, Angelini A, et al. 2011 consensus statement on endomyocardial biopsy from the association for European Cardiovascular Pathology and the Society for Cardiovascular Pathology. *Cardiovasc Pathol.* 2012;21:245–274.
9. She RC, Hammond EH. Utility of immunofluorescence and electron microscopy in endomyocardial biopsies from patients with unexplained heart failure. *Cardiovasc Pathol.* 2010;19:e99–e105.
10. Moulik M, Breinholt JP, Dreyer WJ, et al. Viral endomyocardial infection is an independent predictor and potentially treatable risk factor for graft loss and coronary vasculopathy in pediatric cardiac transplant recipients. *J Am Coll Cardiol.* 2010;56:582–592.
11. Nunes MCP, Beaton A, Acquatella H, et al. Chagas cardiomyopathy: an update of current clinical knowledge and management: a scientific statement from the American Heart Association. *Circulation.* 2018;138.

Specific Etiologic Agents

12. Knowlton KU, Anderson JL, Savoia MC, Oxman MN. Myocarditis and pericarditis. *Mandell, Douglas, and Bennett's Principles and Practice of Infectious Diseases.* 9th ed. Philadelphia: Elsevier; 2019:1151–1164.
13. Manga P, McCutcheon K, Tsabedze N, et al. HIV and nonischemic heart disease. *J Am Coll Cardiol.* 2017;69:83–91.
14. Verdonschot J, Hazebroek M, Merken J, et al. Relevance of cardiac parvovirus B19 in myocarditis and dilated cardiomyopathy: review of the literature. *Eur J Heart Fail.* 2016;18:1430–1441.
15. Ammirati E, Frigerio M, Adler ED, et al. Management of acute myocarditis and chronic inflammatory cardiomyopathy: an expert consensus document. *Circ Heart Fail.* 2020;13:e007405.
16. Kuhl U, Lassner D, Dorner A, et al. A distinct subgroup of cardiomyopathy patients characterized by transcriptionally active cardiotropic erythrovirus and altered cardiac gene expression. *Basic Res Cardiol.* 2013;108.
17. Knowlton KU. Pathogenesis of SARS-CoV-2 induced cardiac injury from the perspective of the virus. *J Mol Cell Cardiol.* 2020;147:12–17.
18. Jay S, David P, Chanakha N, et al. SARS-CoV-2 direct cardiac damage through spike-mediated cardiomyocyte fusion. *Nat Res.* 2020.
19. Basso C, Leone O, Rizzo S, et al. Pathological features of COVID-19-associated myocardial injury: a multicentre cardiovascular pathology study. *Eur Heart J.* 2020;41:3827–3835.
20. Halushka MK, Vander Heide RS. Myocarditis is rare in COVID-19 autopsies: cardiovascular findings across 277 postmortem examinations. *Cardiovasc Pathol.* 2020;50:107300.

21. Martinez MW, Tucker AM, Bloom OJ, et al. Prevalence of inflammatory heart disease among professional athletes with prior COVID-19 infection who received systematic return-to-play cardiac screening. *JAMA Cardiol.* 2021;6(7):745–752.
21a. Diaz GA, Parsons GT, Gering SK, et al. Myocarditis and pericarditis after vaccination for COVID-19. *JAMA.* Published online August 4, 2021. doi:10.1001/jama.2021.13443.
22. Krause PJ, Bockenstedt LK. Lyme disease and the heart. *Circulation.* 2013;127.
23. Forrester JD, Meiman J, Mullins J, et al. Notes from the field: update on Lyme carditis, groups at high risk, and frequency of associated sudden cardiac death—United States. *MMWR Morb Mortal Wkly Rep.* 2014;63:982–983.
24. Lidani KCF, Andrade FA, Bavia L, et al. Chagas disease: from discovery to a worldwide health problem. *Front Public Health.* 2019;7:166.
25. Moncayo Á, Silveira AC. Current epidemiological trends for Chagas disease in Latin America and future challenges in epidemiology, surveillance and health policy. *Mem Inst Oswaldo Cruz.* 2009;104:17–30.
26. Bern C, Messenger LA, Whitman JD, Maguire JH. Chagas disease in the United States: a public health approach. *Clin Microbiol Rev.* 2019;33.
27. Santos E, Menezes Falcao L. Chagas cardiomyopathy and heart failure: from epidemiology to treatment. *Rev Port Cardiol.* 2020;39:279–289.
28. Meymandi S, Hernandez S, Park S, et al. Treatment of Chagas disease in the United States. *Curr Treat Options Infect Dis.* 2018;10:373–388.
29. Morillo CA, Marin-Neto JA, Avezum A, et al. Randomized trial of benznidazole for chronic Chagas' cardiomyopathy. *N Engl J Med.* 2015;373:1295–1306.
30. De Berardis D, Serroni N, Campanella D, et al. Update on the adverse effects of clozapine: focus on myocarditis. *Curr Drug Safety.* 2012;7:55–62.
31. Engler RJM, Nelson MR, Collins Jr LC, et al. A prospective study of the incidence of myocarditis/pericarditis and new onset cardiac symptoms following smallpox and influenza vaccination. *PloS One.* 2015;10:e0118283–e.
32. Bonaca MP, Olenchock BA, Salem J-E, et al. Myocarditis in the setting of cancer therapeutics: proposed case definitions for emerging clinical syndromes in Cardio-Oncology. *Circulation.* 2019;140:80–91.

Pathogenesis

33. Coyne CB, Bergelson JM. Virus-induced Abl and Fyn kinase signals permit coxsackievirus entry through Epithelial tight junctions. *Cell.* 2006;124:119–131.
34. Shi Y, Chen C, Lisewski U, et al. Cardiac deletion of the coxsackievirus-adenovirus receptor Abolishes coxsackievirus B3 infection and prevents myocarditis in vivo. *J Am Coll Cardiol.* 2009;53:1219–1226.
35. Lim B-K, Peter AK, Xiong J, et al. Inhibition of Coxsackievirus-associated dystrophin cleavage prevents cardiomyopathy. *J Clini Invest.* 2013;123:5146–5151.
36. Belkaya S, Kontorovich AR, Byun M, et al. Autosomal recessive cardiomyopathy presenting as acute myocarditis. *J Am Coll Cardiol.* 2017;69:1653–1665.
37. Kissopoulou A, Fernlund E, Holmgren C, et al. Monozygotic twins with myocarditis and a novel likely pathogenic desmoplakin gene variant. *ESC Heart Fail.* 2020;7:1210–1216.
38. Smith ED, Lakdawala NK, Papoutsidakis N, et al. Desmoplakin cardiomyopathy, a fibrotic and inflammatory form of cardiomyopathy distinct from typical dilated or Arrhythmogenic right ventricular cardiomyopathy. *Circulation.* 2020;141:1872–1884.
39. Bouin A, Gretteau P-A, Wehbe M, et al. Enterovirus persistence in cardiac cells of patients with idiopathic dilated cardiomyopathy is linked to 5′ terminal genomic RNA-deleted viral populations with viral-encoded proteinase activities. *Circulation.* 2019;139:2326–2338.
40. Yajima T, Knowlton KU. Viral myocarditis. *Circulation.* 2009;119:2615–2624.
41. Schultheiss H-P, Piper C, Sowade O, et al. Betaferon in chronic viral cardiomyopathy (BICC) trial: effects of interferon-β treatment in patients with chronic viral cardiomyopathy. *Clini Res Cardiol.* 2016;105:763–773.
42. Zhou L, Chong MMW, Littman DR. Plasticity of CD4+ T cell lineage differentiation. *Immunity.* 2009;30:646–655.
43. Huber SA. Viral myocarditis and dilated cardiomyopathy: etiology and pathogenesis. *Curr Pharm Des.* 2016;22:408–426.
44. Liu P, Aitken K, Kong Y-Y, et al. The tyrosine kinase p56lck is essential in coxsackievirus B3-mediated heart disease. *Nat Med.* 2000;6:429–434.
45. Kociol RD, Cooper LT, Fang JC, et al. Recognition and initial management of fulminant myocarditis. *Circulation.* 2020;141.
46. Kandolin R, Lehtonen J, Kupari M. Cardiac sarcoidosis and giant cell myocarditis as causes of atrioventricular block in young and middle-aged adults. *Circ Arrhythm Electrophysiol.* 2011;4:303–309.
47. Kandolin R, Lehtonen J, Salmenkivi K, et al. Diagnosis, treatment, and outcome of giant-cell myocarditis in the era of combined immunosuppression. *Circ Heart Fail.* 2013;6:15–22.
48. Ammirati E, Veronese G, Brambatti M, et al. Fulminant versus acute nonfulminant myocarditis in patients with left ventricular systolic dysfunction. *J Am Coll Cardiol.* 2019;74:299–311.

Diagnostic Approaches

49. Al-Biltagi M, Issa M, Hagar HA, et al. Circulating cardiac troponins levels and cardiac dysfunction in children with acute and fulminant viral myocarditis. *Acta Paediatr.* 2010;99:1510–1516.
50. Kaya Z, Katus HA, Rose NR. Cardiac troponins and autoimmunity: their role in the pathogenesis of myocarditis and of heart failure. *Clini Immunol (Orlando, Fla).* 2010;134:80–88.
51. Renko M, Leskinen M, Kontiokari T, et al. Cardiac troponin-I as a screening tool for myocarditis in children hospitalized for viral infection. *Acta Paediatr.* 2009.
52. Younis A, Matetzky S, Mulla W, et al. Epidemiology characteristics and outcome of patients with clinically diagnosed acute myocarditis. *Am J Med.* 2020;133:492–499.
53. Mlczoch E, Darbandi-Mesri F, Luckner D, et al. NT-pro BNP in acute childhood myocarditis. *J Pediatr.* 2012;160:178–179.
54. Mahfoud F, Gartner B, Kindermann M, et al. Virus serology in patients with suspected myocarditis: utility or futility? *Eur Heart J.* 2011;32:897–903.
55. Ukena C, Mahfoud F, Kindermann I, et al. Prognostic electrocardiographic parameters in patients with suspected myocarditis. *Eur Heart Fail.* 2011;13:398–405.
56. Gräni C, Eichhorn C, Bière L, et al. Prognostic value of cardiac magnetic resonance tissue characterization in risk stratifying patients with suspected myocarditis. *J Am Coll Cardiol.* 2017;70:1964–1976.
57. Aquaro GD, Ghebru Habtemicael Y, Camastra G, et al. Prognostic value of repeating cardiac magnetic resonance in patients with acute myocarditis. *J Am Coll Cardiol.* 2019;74:2439–2448.
58. Lurz P, Luecke C, Eitel I, et al. Comprehensive cardiac magnetic resonance imaging in patients with suspected myocarditis. *J Am Coll Cardiol.* 2016;67:1800–1811.
59. Ferreira VM, Schulz-Menger J, Holmvang G, et al. Cardiovascular magnetic resonance in non-ischemic myocardial inflammation. *J Am Coll Cardiol.* 2018;72:3158–3176.
60. Friedrich MG, Sechtem U, Schulz-Menger J, et al. Cardiovascular magnetic resonance in myocarditis: A JACC White Paper. *J Am Coll Cardiol.* 2009;53:1475–1487.
61. Blankstein R, Osborne M, Naya M, et al. Cardiac positron emission tomography enhances prognostic assessments of patients with suspected cardiac sarcoidosis. *J Am Coll Cardiol.* 2014;63:329–336.
62. Isiguzo M, Brunken R, Tchou P, et al. Metabolism-perfusion imaging to predict disease activity in cardiac sarcoidosis. *Sarcoidosis Vasc Diffuse Lung Dis.* 2011;28:50–55.
63. Caforio ALP, Pankuweit S, Arbustini E, et al. Current state of knowledge on aetiology, diagnosis, management, and therapy of myocarditis: a position statement of the European Society of Cardiology Working Group on Myocardial and Pericardial Diseases. *Eur Heart J.* 2013;34:2636–2648.
64. Yilmaz A, Kindermann I, Kindermann M, et al. Comparative evaluation of left and right ventricular endomyocardial biopsy. *Circulation.* 2010;122:900–909.
65. Chimenti C, Frustaci A. Contribution and risks of left ventricular endomyocardial biopsy in patients with cardiomyopathies. *Circulation.* 2013;128:1531–1541.
66. Cooper LT, Baughman KL, Feldman AM, et al. The role of endomyocardial biopsy in the management of cardiovascular disease. *Circulation.* 2007;116:2216–2233.
67. Bennett MK, Gilotra NA, Harrington C, et al. Evaluation of the role of endomyocardial biopsy in 851 patients with unexplained heart failure from 2000–2009. *Circ Heart Fail.* 2013;6:676–684.
68. Maleszewski JJ, Orellana VM, Hodge DO, et al. Long-term risk of recurrence, morbidity and mortality in giant cell myocarditis. *Am J Cardiol.* 2015;115:1733–1738.

Prognosis and Treatment

69. Gilotra NA, Bennett MK, Shpigel A, et al. Outcomes and predictors of recovery in acute-onset cardiomyopathy: a single-center experience of patients undergoing endomyocardial biopsy for new heart failure. *Am Heart J.* 2016;179:116–126.
70. Imazio M, Brucato A, Barbieri A, et al. Good prognosis for pericarditis with and without myocardial involvement. *Circulation.* 2013;128:42–49.
71. Foerster SR, Canter CE, Cinar A, et al. Ventricular remodeling and survival are more favorable for myocarditis than for idiopathic dilated cardiomyopathy in childhood. *Circ Heart Fail.* 2010;3:689–697.
72. Alvarez JA, Orav EJ, Wilkinson JD, et al. Competing risks for death and cardiac transplantation in children with dilated cardiomyopathy: results from the pediatric cardiomyopathy registry. *Circulation.* 2011;124:814–823.
73. Boehmer JP, Starling RC, Cooper LT, et al. Left ventricular assist device support and myocardial recovery in recent onset cardiomyopathy. *J Cardiac Fail.* 2012;18:755–761.
74. Bozkurt B, Colvin M, Cook J, et al. Current diagnostic and treatment strategies for specific dilated cardiomyopathies: a scientific statement from the American Heart Association. *Circulation.* 2016;134.
75. Seferović PM, Polovina M, Bauersachs J, et al. Heart failure in cardiomyopathies: a position paper from the heart failure association of the European Society of Cardiology. *Eur J Heart Fail.* 2019;21:553–576.

56 Cardio-Oncology: Managing Cardiotoxic Effects of Cancer Therapies

BONNIE KY

EPIDEMIOLOGY, CLINICAL MANIFESTATIONS, AND PATHOPHYSIOLOGY OF CANCER THERAPY CARDIOTOXICITY, 1091
Traditional Chemotherapeutic Agents, 1091
Additional Cancer Therapies, 1094

IMMUNOTHERAPY, 1094
Immune Checkpoint Inhibitors, 1094
Chimeric Antigen Receptor T Cell Therapies, 1094

TARGETED THERAPY, 1095
ErbB Antagonists (Trastuzumab, Pertuzumab), 1095
Tyrosine Kinase Inhibitors and Monoclonal Antibodies, 1095

HORMONAL THERAPY, 1096
Androgen Deprivation Therapies, 1096
Selective Estrogen Receptor Modulators and Aromatase Inhibitors, 1096

RADIATION THERAPY, 1097
STEM CELL TRANSPLANTATION, 1097
MECHANISTIC OVERLAP BETWEEN CARDIOVASCULAR DISEASE AND CANCER, 1097
FUTURE PERSPECTIVES, 1097
REFERENCES, 1098

Cardiovascular (CV) disease and cancer are highly prevalent and two major causes of mortality worldwide, resulting in a substantial public health burden. Global estimates suggest 422 million prevalent cases of CV disease.[1] Each year, there are an estimated 17 million incident cases of cancer.[2] CV disease accounts for an estimated 17.9 million deaths and cancer 9.6 million deaths worldwide each year.[3] The overlap in the epidemiology of these two diseases, as well as the shared biologic mechanisms of both CV disease and cancer have led to the birth and maturation of the field of cardio-oncology.

Cardio-oncology is a multidisciplinary field that encompasses the following broad clinical areas: (1) the care of patients with pre-existing CV risk factors or disease who develop cancer; (2) cancer patients and survivors who are at greater propensity for the development of CV risk factors or disease secondary to cancer or cancer therapy; and (3) patients with active or a prior history of cancer who subsequently develop overt CV risk factors or disease. Incident CV disease related to cancer therapy is often termed *cardiotoxicity*. The diseases encompassed by the term include not only heart failure (HF) (see Chapters 49–51), cardiomyopathy (CM), and left ventricular (LV) dysfunction (often referred to as cancer therapeutics related cardiac dysfunction, or CTRCD), but also a broad range of CV disease states, including hypertension (HTN) (see Chapter 26), coronary disease and myocardial ischemia (see Chapters 37, 38, 40), arrhythmia (see Chapters 65–68), pulmonary HTN (see Chapter 88), pericardial disease (see Chapter 86), valvular disease (see Chapters 72–76), myocarditis (see Chapter 55), peripheral arterial disease (PAD; see Chapter 43), and venous and arterial thrombosis.

Both the incidence and significance of cardiotoxicity with cancer therapy are believed to be growing. There are several potential reasons for this. First, survival rates among cancer patients are increasing, potentially related to early detection and more effective treatment regimens, and as a result, the observed "late effects" of cancer therapies are becoming more evident. Second, cancer therapies are rapidly evolving, and while many conventional chemotherapies are still being used, new drug development has led to the development of "targeted" strategies, many of which can also affect fundamental signaling pathways that are necessary for cardiomyocyte and endothelial cell function and homeostasis. This chapter reviews the epidemiology, clinical manifestations, and pathophysiology of CV disease with commonly used chemotherapeutic agents, targeted therapies, immune therapies, hormonal therapy, and radiation therapy (RT) (Table 56.1, Fig. 56.1). Care of the CV patient prior to, during, and after therapy and strategies to mitigate cardiotoxicity are discussed in Chapter 57.

EPIDEMIOLOGY, CLINICAL MANIFESTATIONS, AND PATHOPHYSIOLOGY OF CANCER THERAPY CARDIOTOXICITY

Traditional Chemotherapeutic Agents
Anthracyclines
The American College of Cardiology and American Heart Association HF Guidelines classify exposure to cardiotoxic therapies, such as anthracyclines, as stage A HF.[4] Reports of the incidence of anthracycline-associated cardiotoxicity have varied widely in the literature, in part, secondary to the variability in the definition of CV outcomes across retrospective analyses and the lack of systematic and rigorously ascertained longitudinal follow-up data, particularly in adults. Historically, cardiotoxicity has been classified as acute, subacute, or chronic although recent studies have substantially challenged this paradigm.

A study of 2625 patients treated with anthracyclines, primarily for breast cancer and hematologic disease, followed over a median of 5.2 years (interquartile range [IQR] 2.6 to 8.0) with serial echocardiography monitoring noted an overall incidence of cardiotoxicity of 9%.[5] Cardiotoxicity was defined as a decrease in the LV ejection fraction (LVEF) of more than 10% from baseline to less than an absolute value of 50%. In 98% of cases, cardiotoxicity was detected within the first year after chemotherapy had been completed, with a median time between the last dose of anthracyclines and the development of cardiotoxicity of 3.5 months (IQR, 3 to 6). In five patients, cardiotoxicity was detected after 5.5 years. The LVEF at the completion of chemotherapy and the cumulative anthracycline dose were independently associated with cardiotoxicity risk. A very small number of patients were hospitalized; the majority were managed as outpatients. HF therapy was initiated in all patients who developed cardiotoxicity, and 82% of the patients recovered their LVEF, either fully or partially. Data from a carefully phenotyped, prospective observational cohort study of breast cancer patients treated with standard dosages of anthracyclines, doxorubicin 240 mg/m^2, also support the observation that modest declines in quantitative LVEF, on the order of 3% to 4%, occur and are detectable during the 1 to 2 years after the initiation of anthracycline chemotherapy.[6] Altogether, these findings suggest that declines in cardiac function, which may be subclinical, can occur relatively early after chemotherapy completion; these data also challenge the notion of irreversible LVEF declines.

Anthracyclines are a mainstay of therapy in childhood cancers. Cardiotoxicity, when carefully evaluated, is also observed in patients early after exposure to anthracyclines. In clinical trial participants

TABLE 56.1 Cardiotoxic Effects of Cancer Therapies

AGENT	REPORTED CARDIOTOXIC EFFECTS	COMMENTS
Anthracyclines		
Doxorubicin, daunorubicin, epirubicin, idarubicin, mitoxantrone	Cardiac arrhythmias, CM, HF	Risk factors include cumulative dose, although genetic variation may confer increased risk at lower dosages; conventional CV risk factors and disease; age; gender; additional cardiotoxic therapies, including RT or trastuzumab
Anti-Microtubule Therapies—Taxanes (See Supplement)		
Paclitaxel, docetaxel	Arrhythmia, myocardial ischemia	May exacerbate risk of anthracycline cardiotoxicity secondary to pharmacokinetic effects
Alkylating and Alkylating-Like Agents (See Supplement)		
Cyclophosphamide	Myopericarditis, arrhythmias	Rare; CV complications reported primarily at high dosages; emerging data in the transplant setting may suggest increased CV risk.
Cisplatin, carboplatin, oxaliplatin	Vasculotoxicity, including endothelial dysfunction, arterial vasospasm, HTN	Small studies suggest acute vasculotoxic effects; relationship to long-term events unknown.
Antimetabolites (See Supplement)		
5-Fluorouracil, capecitabine	Coronary vasospasm, myocardial ischemia, infarction, arrhythmias, ECG changes, sudden death	May be related to endothelial injury, vasoconstriction, and vasospasm; typically managed with nitrates and calcium channel blockers
Monoclonal Antibody Tyrosine Kinase Inhibitors		
Bevacizumab	HTN, CM, HF, thrombosis	Low risk of CM or HF
Trastuzumab	CM, HF	Increased risk of CM and HF with anthracyclines; HTN, obesity, and borderline normal baseline LVEF are also established risk factors; many LVEF declines are reversible, but as noted in clinical trial data, in approximately 20% of patients, reversibility is not seen
Pertuzumab	CM, HF	Risk of CM and HF remains incompletely defined, but thus far, it has been modest
Proteasome Inhibitors		
Bortezomib and carfilzomib	CM, HF, edema, HTN, acute coronary syndrome, pulmonary hypertension, arrhythmia	Bortezomib is a reversible proteasome inhibitor; carfilzomib is an irreversible proteasome inhibitor; cardiotoxicity rates greater
Small-Molecule Tyrosine Kinase Inhibitors		
Sunitinib	HTN, CM, HF, ischemia, thrombosis	Risk of HTN that tends to occur early; relationship between afterload and CM risk remains to be determined
Sorafenib	HTN, CM, ischemia, thrombosis	Risk of HTN; also associated with ischemia
Imatinib	Edema, pericardial effusion	Very low risk of CM
Nilotinib	Peripheral vascular disease, ischemic heart disease, QT prolongation, cardiometabolic effects	Multi-targeted oral tyrosine kinase inhibitor; cardiometabolic effects include hyperglycemia and hyperlipidemia
Ponatinib	Peripheral vascular disease, ischemic heart disease, HTN, HF	Multi-targeted oral tyrosine kinase inhibitor
Dasatinib	Pulmonary HTN, pericardial effusion	Cardiopulmonary status should be evaluated prior to and during therapy
Ibrutinib	HTN, atrial fibrillation, ventricular arrhythmias, HF, bleeding	Bruton's tyrosine kinase inhibitor
Immune-Modulating Agents		
Immune checkpoint inhibitors	Myocarditis	Myocarditis is very rare but can be fulminant; worse with combination therapy; typically occurs earlier in course of therapy but can occur at any time
CAR T cell therapy	Cytokine release syndrome associated adverse CV events (hypotension, arrhythmia)	Treatment for cytokine release syndrome includes tocilizumab
Androgen-Deprivation Therapy		
Leuprolide, goserelin, triptorelin, degarelix, flutamide, bicalutamide	Metabolic syndrome, ischemia, coronary artery disease, HTN	Mixed data regarding an increased risk of adverse CV events with mechanisms of CV disease unclear; patients with pre-existing CV disease may be at a more substantially increased risk
Estrogen-Receptor Modulators		
Tamoxifen	Thrombosis	Favorable effects on lipids
Aromatase inhibitors (anastrozole, letrozole, exemestane)	Hypercholesterolemia, HTN, HF, combined endpoint of dysrhythmia, valvular disease, and pericarditis	Studies evaluated aromatase inhibitors in comparison to tamoxifen and demonstrated worse CV effects
Radiation Therapy	Valvular disease, pericardial disease, vascular disease, ischemia, coronary artery disease, CM, HF	Major CV events tend to occur late, although early abnormalities in cardiac function and perfusion are observed; mean heart dose associated with mortality

CM, Cardiomyopathy; *CV*, cardiovascular; *ECG*, electrocardiogram; *HF*, heart failure; *HTN*, hypertension; *RT*, radiation therapy.

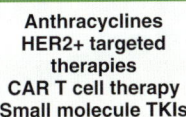

FIGURE 56.1 Cardiotoxicities of common cancer therapies. This figure demonstrates commonly used cancer therapies and the associated potential cardiovascular risk factors and diseases. *CAR*, Chimeric antigen receptor; *HER2*, human epidermal growth factor receptor 2; *LV*, left ventricular; *TKI*, tyrosine kinase inhibitor; *VEGF*, vascular endothelial growth factor (Adapted from Harries I, Liang K, Williams M, et al. Magnetic resonance imaging to detect cardiovascular effects of cancer therapy. JACC Cardio Oncl. 2020;2(2):270–292.)

younger than 30 years of age receiving frontline treatment for acute myelogenous leukemia, the cumulative incidence of cardiotoxicity, as defined by National Cancer Institute Common Terminology Criteria for Adverse Events (version 3.0) grade 2 or worse LV systolic dysfunction, was 12%.[7] The standard induction and intensification treatment protocol included daunorubicin and mitoxantrone. In this study, 25% of the cardiotoxicity events were infection associated and 70% of these occurred early, with a median time to cardiotoxicity of 4.3 months (IQR, 3.1 to 5.9) after chemotherapy initiation. Both 5-year event free and overall survival were significantly worsened in patients who suffered from cardiotoxicity. These findings not only indicate an early cardiotoxicity onset, but also suggest treatment-related cardiotoxicity in children results in worse overall outcomes.

Clinical risk factors for anthracycline-induced cardiotoxicity include age of exposure, traditional, modifiable CV risk factors (HTN, diabetes, obesity, and hyperlipidemia), prior chest RT, anthracycline dose, genetic factors, and pre-existing CV disease. In adult survivors of childhood cancer, the prevalence of CM is 4.7% to 10.7%, and increases with age, with an adjusted odds of CM development 2.7 (95% CI 1.1 to 6.9) fold greater compared to patients not exposed to anthracyclines.[8] More recent studies also suggest that the association between anthracycline dose and HF is modified by age of treatment, with a greater relative risk (RR) of CV disease among those who received high-dose anthracycline chemotherapy (≥ 250 mg/m^2) at ≤ 13 years of age, as compared to children older than 13 years.[9] Here, children that were ≤ 13 years at diagnosis had a RR of 2.4 to 4.0 fold of any CV disease compared to those older than 13 years. In addition to modifiable CV risk factors and age at anthracycline exposure, concomitant treatment exposures such as RT (>15 Gy) are associated with an increased risk of CV disease. In 1820 adult survivors of childhood cancer treated with anthracyclines, chest-directed RT, or both, there was a high prevalence of subclinical dysfunction in those with an LVEF $\geq 50\%$, with abnormal GLS in 28% and diastolic dysfunction in 8.7%,[10] greatest in those who received both anthracyclines and RT.

While multiple studies document a dose-dependent relationship between anthracycline exposure and risk of HF and CM, it is recognized that anthracycline cardiotoxicity can occur at any dose. Older retrospective analyses suggest an incidence of HF, as defined by clinical signs and symptoms, of 1.7% at a cumulative dose of 300 mg/m^2, 4.7% at 400 mg/m^2, 15.7% at 500 mg/m^2, and 48% at 650 mg/m^2.[5] It is notable that standard errors for many of these estimates are large, given the small sample sizes. Moreover, with respect to dose, emerging data suggest that the equivalency ratios for mitoxantrone relative to doxorubicin is 10.5 (95% CI 6.2 to 19.1), much greater than previously published (0.6 (95% CI 0.4 to 1.0) for daunorubicin, 0.8 (95% CI 0.5 to 2.8) for epirubicin).[11] Data from childhood cancer survivors also indicate that genetic variations in single-nucleotide polymorphisms modify the association between the anthracycline dose and CM risk and confer an increased risk of cardiotoxicity at lower dosages.[12] The genetic determinants of anthracycline cardiotoxicity is an active area of research, with ongoing studies in candidate genes and genome-wide association studies.

Several basic mechanisms have been proposed to explain anthracycline-induced cardiotoxicity. The first is formation of reactive oxygen species (ROS) and increased oxidative stress via redox cycling of the quinone moiety of doxorubicin, formation of anthracycline-iron complexes, and topoisomerase-2β (Top2β) inhibition (Fig. 56.2).[13] Furthermore, anthracyclines have been shown to cause impaired calcium signaling and intracellular sequestration affecting myocardial relaxation, a decrease in cardiac progenitor cells, and alterations in neuregulin (NRG)/ErbB signaling.[13,14] Recent data also suggest a role for phosphoinositide 3-kinase γ (PI3Kγ) in the pathophysiology of anthracycline cardiotoxicity, perhaps related to the release of mitochondrial DNA by injured organelles and contained autolysosomes.[15] The most widely cited and unifying mechanism is the formation of ROS, leading to oxidative stress and subsequent injury to cardiac myocytes and endothelial cells.[13,14] The quinone moiety of the anthracycline enters cells and undergoes redox cycling, generating free radicals via both an enzymatic pathway involving the mitochondrial respiratory chain and also via a nonenzymatic pathway involving direct interactions between anthracyclines and intracellular iron. Toxic hydroxyl radicals from anthracycline-iron complexes act as cytotoxic messengers. This results in impaired mitochondrial function, cellular membrane damage, and cytotoxicity. Nitric oxide synthase (NOS) also contributes to the generation of anthracycline-mediated reactive nitrogen species, worsening nitrosative stress. The formation of ROS may occur via the isozyme Top2, and, more specifically, Top2β, in cardiomyocytes.[13] Mice lacking Top2β are protected from anthracycline-induced DNA damage, cardiomyocyte death, and declines in cardiac function. These findings need to be validated. Interestingly, dexrazoxane, an iron chelator and cardioprotectant, binds to Top2β and results in Top2β degradation.

Data derived from in vitro and in vivo animal models support the hypothesis that anthracyclines also affect the population of cardiac progenitor cells. Anthracycline chemotherapy may also render cardiomyocytes more susceptible to alterations in NRG-1 and ErbB signaling and downstream pro-survival pathways.[13,14] In vitro studies have demonstrated an inhibitory effect of doxorubicin on hypoxia-inducible factor (HIF) and downstream pathways. Anthracyclines also result in impaired diastolic relaxation via calpain-dependent titin proteolysis. More recent studies have used human induced pluripotent stem cell–derived cardiomyocytes (hiPSC-CMs) to model the predilection to anthracycline cardiotoxicity in patients, and corroborated decreased cell viability, impaired mitochondrial and metabolic function, impaired calcium handling, decreased antioxidant pathway activity, and increased ROS production as mechanisms of toxicity.[16]

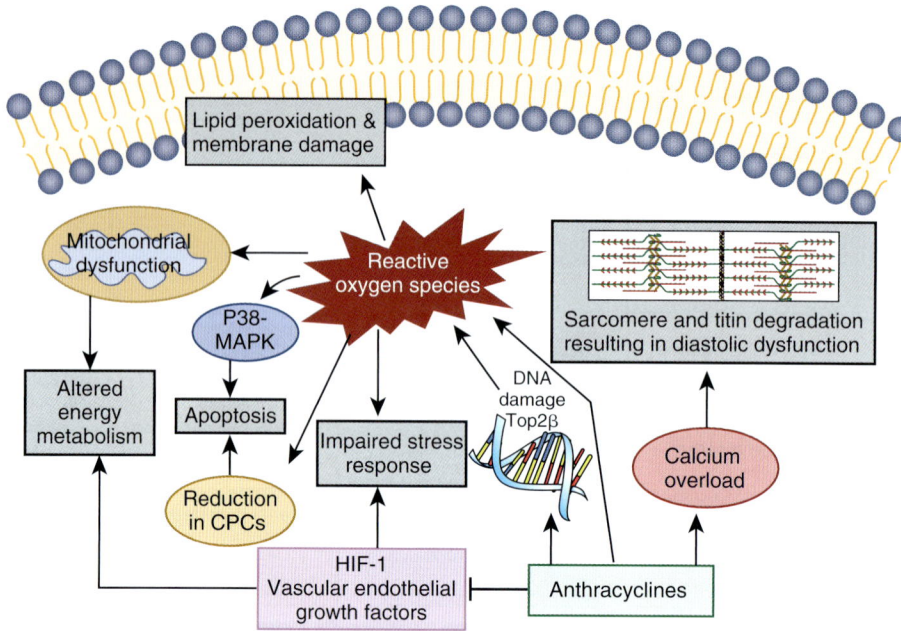

FIGURE 56.2 Proposed mechanisms of anthracycline cardiotoxicity. Using anthracyclines results in the generation of reactive oxygen species (ROS), potentially via topoisomerase 2β inhibition, as well as calcium overload, reduction in cardiac progenitor cells (CPCs), and hypoxia-inducible factor (HIF) inhibition.

Several other traditional chemotherapeutic agents, including taxanes, alkylating and alkylating-like agents, and antimetabolites can also lead to cardiotoxicity.

Additional Cancer Therapies
Proteasome Inhibitors

Proteasome inhibitors, including bortezomib and carfilzomib, are used in the treatment of relapsed or refractory and newly diagnosed cases of multiple myeloma. Bortezomib is a reversible nonselective inhibitor of proteasomes that blocks chymotrypsin-like activity at the 26S proteasome; carfilzomib is an irreversible selective inhibitor of proteasomes that blocks chymotrypsin activity of the 20S proteasome.

The reported incidence of all-grade and grade 3 and higher adverse CV events with these proteasome inhibitors from a meta-analysis of Phase 1 to 3 clinical trials was 18.1% and 8.2%, respectively.[17] HF (4.1%) and HTN (12.2%) were the most common adverse CV events, followed by arrhythmias (2.4%) and ischemia (1.8%). In a multi-center, longitudinal prospective cohort study of 95 patients, the rates of adverse CV events were much greater, occurring in 50.7% in patients receiving carfilzomib and 16.7% receiving bortezomib.[18] Most occurred during carfilzomib therapy; HF and HTN were similarly noted as most common, with grade 3 and 4 HF and HTN events occurring in 20% and 23%, respectively. Arrhythmia, acute coronary syndrome, and pulmonary HTN were also noted. In case series, both HF with preserved and reduced ejection fraction have been reported. Predictors of adverse CV events with carfilzomib include a history of HF, baseline diastolic dysfunction, higher doses of carfilzomib, and abnormal NT-proBNP levels at baseline or during therapy. It is postulated that proteasome inhibitors alter protein homeostasis[19] and reduce phosphorylation of AMPKalpha and downstream autophagy related proteins, such as Raptor.[20]

IMMUNOTHERAPY
Immune Checkpoint Inhibitors

Immune checkpoint inhibitors have become the standard of care in the treatment of a variety of solid and liquid tumors, revolutionizing cancer care, replacing cytotoxic therapies for many malignancies. These monoclonal antibodies, which target cytotoxic T lymphocyte–associated antigen 4 (CTLA-4) and the programmed death receptor (PD-1) and its ligand PD-L1, are associated with a risk of immune-related adverse events. In a retrospective analysis of 448 patients with advanced melanoma treated in Phase I-III trials, 94.9% of treated patients experienced adverse events over a median follow-up of 13.2 months, with 55.4% being grade 3 to 4. Dermatologic, gastrointestinal, endocrine, hepatic, and pulmonary adverse events are most common. Myocarditis, however, occurs much less frequently, on the order of 0.06% to 1%,[21,22] but is notable given its potential morbidity and mortality.

The data related to immunotherapy cardiotoxicity are still emerging. Many published studies are derived from retrospective cohort studies or case series. These suggest that myocarditis typically occurs early, at a median time of 34 to 65 days, but over a broad range as there are also published reports of late myocarditis. Additional clinical manifestations include dyspnea, palpitations, and HF. Biomarkers, including troponin and natriuretic peptides have been studied as diagnostic and prognostic tools, as have imaging markers including global longitudinal strain, with associations with adverse cardiac events in small studies.[23–25]

Combination therapies have been noted to be associated with an approximate twofold increased risk of myocarditis compared to monotherapy. Myositis has also been reported to be common in patients who develop myocarditis. The relevance of other autoimmune diseases or CV disease or risk factors in the development of myocarditis remains incompletely defined. Other toxicities have been reported with immunotherapy, including arrhythmias, pericardial effusions, and CM. Whether these are completely distinct entities from myocarditis is not clear. Moreover, these are emerging data regarding potential associations with accelerated atherosclerosis.

Chimeric Antigen Receptor T Cell Therapies

Chimeric antigen receptor (CAR) T cells targeting CD19 are a newer class of therapies that have shown to be highly effective in the treatment of refractory and relapsing hematologic malignancies, including pediatric acute lymphoblastic leukemia and adult large B-cell lymphoma.[26] Toxicities associated with CAR T cell therapy include cytokine release syndrome, a multi-organ system toxicity that occurs with widespread release of inflammatory cytokines and chemokines, including interleukin (IL)-2, soluble IL-2Ra, interferon gamma, IL-6, soluble IL-6R, and granulocyte-macrophage colony-stimulating factor. Adverse CV events most commonly occur with cytokine release syndrome, and include hypotension, arrhythmia, HF, and potentially cardiac death. Treatment for cytokine release syndrome includes tocilizumab.

TARGETED THERAPY

The treatment of a number of malignant neoplasms has changed dramatically with the advent of targeted therapies. As opposed to traditional chemotherapeutics which target basic cellular processes present in most cells, these therapies target pathways that are dysregulated in cancerous cells. It was hoped that this approach would reduce toxicities typical of conventional chemotherapeutics and be more effective at treating the cancer. However, concerns about cardiotoxicity have surfaced for several agents, likely given the mechanistic commonalities to both CV disease and cancer.

ErbB Antagonists (Trastuzumab, Pertuzumab)

Trastuzumab is a humanized monoclonal antibody that binds subdomain IV of human epidermal growth factor receptor 2 (HER2)/neu, also known as ErbB2. Trastuzumab exerts its antitumor effects by blocking HER2 cleavage, resulting in antibody-dependent, cell-mediated cytotoxicity and inhibition of ligand-independent, HER2-mediated signaling affecting the following downstream pathways: PI3K, serine/threonine-specific protein kinase Akt, mitogen-activated protein kinase (MAPK), extracellular-signal–regulated kinase 1/2 (ERK1/2), and the mechanistic target of rapamycin (mTOR).[13] Trastuzumab also exerts antiangiogenic effects. First approved by the Food and Drug Administration (FDA) in 1998 for metastatic disease, it received indications for early-stage HER2+ breast cancer in 2007.

Phase III clinical trials with trastuzumab suggest that the risk of severe HF is low, on the order of 1.7% to 4.1%, but the risk of LVEF declines is greater, on the order of 7.1% to 18.6%.[5,27] Compared to retrospective and prospective cohort studies, these rates are lower. This may be secondary to the lack of generalizability of the clinical trial population given stringent exclusion/inclusion criteria. Retrospective analyses from various large data sources, including the Surveillance, Epidemiology, and End Results (SEER) Program, the Cancer Research Network, and the Canadian health care system databases, indicate a higher incidence of HF and CM.[5] SEER analyses suggested an HF incidence of 41.9% at 3 years following combination therapy with anthracyclines and trastuzumab; however, these data are also subject to limitations including potential misclassification. In the Cancer Research Network, there was a 20.1% incidence of HF and/or CM with combination therapy. Ontario Cancer Registry data suggested an estimated cumulative 5-year incidence of HF of 5.2% with trastuzumab regimens, with a HF risk that was greatest in the first 1.5 years of cancer therapy.[28] In this analysis, patients treated with sequential anthracyclines and trastuzumab therapy had a cumulative incidence of 6.6% for major cardiac events at 3 years. The adjusted risk of major cardiac events was higher with sequential therapy (HR 3.96, 95% CI 3.01 to 5.22) and trastuzumab without anthracyclines (HR 1.76, 95% CI 1.19 to 2.60) compared with other chemotherapy. There are clear data that indicate the risk of HF and CM with trastuzumab therapy is increased in the setting of sequential anthracycline and trastuzumab exposure. Additional risk factors for trastuzumab cardiotoxicity include obesity, a lower baseline LVEF, HTN, or diabetes; non-Caucasian race; and older age.

Importantly, LVEF declines with trastuzumab are largely reversible and typically occur during therapy. As a consequence, trastuzumab-associated cardiotoxicity was initially termed type II dysfunction, to distinguish it from anthracycline-associated cardiotoxicity, termed type I dysfunction.[5] This classification has largely fallen out of favor secondary to its oversimplification and because of the lack of strong evidence that the biologic underpinnings and clinical manifestations of anthracycline and trastuzumab cardiotoxicity are fundamentally distinct without overlap. Moreover, the reversibility of LVEF declines with trastuzumab is not universally observed. In the HERceptin Adjuvant (HERA) Trial, a phase III randomized trial of trastuzumab, approximately 20% to 30% of patients did not demonstrate LVEF recovery, and some patients suffered a subsequent decline in LVEF even after an initial recovery was noted. Conversely, as noted above, LVEF recovery is observed with anthracyclines.[29] There are also data to suggest that there are longer-term consequences and a risk of late HF with trastuzumab.[30]

Dose delays and interruptions have also been shown to be associated with worse overall survival rates, emphasizing the importance of safe cancer therapy delivery. The clinical determinants of LV recovery, as defined by an improvement in LVEF, have not been rigorously defined with trastuzumab, but observations suggest that temporary cessation of therapy and/or institution of cardiac medications (e.g., angiotensin-converting enzyme [ACE] inhibitors and beta blockers) are associated with recovery. Very small studies have also suggested that trastuzumab can be continued in the setting of modest LVEF declines, of 40% of greater.[31] Longitudinal data defining the changes in cardiac size and function over time suggest that measures of LV size (primarily end-systolic volumes), contractility (longitudinal and circumferential strain), and ventricular-arterial coupling (afterload) are independently associated with LVEF decline and recovery.[6]

It is widely speculated that the cardiac dysfunction observed with trastuzumab is a direct consequence of ErbB2 inhibition in cardiomyocytes, but this remains to be definitively proven.[13,14] Basic studies have been limited, in part, by the lack of robust systems to directly study the in vitro and in vivo effects of trastuzumab. The NRG/ErbB system functions as a paracrine and juxtacrine system between microvascular endothelial cells and cardiomyocytes. NRG-1 is expressed in vascular endothelial cells, and ErbB2 and ErbB4 are expressed in cardiomyocytes and endothelial cells. Recombinant NRG-1β activates ErbB2 and ErbB4 receptor phosphorylation in cardiomyocytes in vitro. Important downstream mediators, as noted above, include PI3K/Akt, MAPK/ERK, steroid receptor activator (Src)/focal adhesion kinase, and NOS. All of these pathways are fundamental for cardiac homeostasis, cell survival, mitochondrial function, cell growth, and focal adhesion formation. Mice with a cardiac-specific deletion of ErbB2 develop dilated CM and demonstrate exaggerated systolic dysfunction after pressure overload compared with wild-type mice. ErbB2 and ErbB4 expression is preserved during compensated hypertrophy, but it declines in the early stages of systolic dysfunction in mice subjected to pressure overload. Overall, these findings suggest that perturbations in ErbB receptor signaling are important in the maintenance of cardiac function. Data also suggest that disruption of ErbB2 signaling results in endothelial dysfunction and an altered vascular phenotype, potentially contributing to the cardiomyopathic phenotype.

There are a number of newer ErbB antagonists, including pertuzumab, ado-trastuzumab Emtansine (T-DM1), and tucatinib. Pertuzumab is a humanized monoclonal antibody that binds HER2 at subdomain II of the HER2 extracellular domain; it is administered in conjunction with trastuzumab for high-risk and metastatic HER2+ breast cancer.[32] Pertuzumab also stimulates antibody-dependent, cell-mediated cytotoxicity, and prevents dimerization to other ligand-activated HER receptors, especially HER3. Although the CV effects are still being elucidated, Phase III trial data have not demonstrated a substantial cardiotoxic signal with pertuzumab and trastuzumab, T-DM1, or tucatinib that is greater than trastuzumab alone.[32] However, the external validity of these findings remains a question, as the epidemiology of LVEF declines and recovery have not completely been defined in the non-clinical trial setting.

Tyrosine Kinase Inhibitors and Monoclonal Antibodies

Many of the targeted cancer therapeutics inhibit the activity of tyrosine kinases (TKs). TKs attach phosphate groups to tyrosine residues of other proteins, thereby changing the activity, subcellular localization, and rate of degradation of the proteins. In the normal cell, these wild-type (i.e., normal) TKs play many roles in regulating basic cellular functions. However, in leukemias and cancers, the gene encoding the causal (or contributory) TKs is amplified (leading to overexpression) or mutated, leading to a constitutively activated state that drives proliferation of the cancerous clonal cells or blocks their normal death.

Vascular Endothelial Growth Factor Signaling Pathway Inhibitors

Vascular endothelial growth factor receptor (VEGFR) signaling pathway inhibitors are used in the treatment of metastatic renal cell cancers; gastrointestinal stromal tumors; and thyroid, hepatocellular, and colon cancers. Bevacizumab is a humanized recombinant anti-VEGF antibody. The CV risks associated with bevacizumab include HTN, a low incidence of HF (1.6%, but with a RR of 4.7 compared with placebo), and arterial thromboembolic events (7.1% with bevacizumab versus 2.5% with chemotherapy alone).

Sorafenib, sunitinib, axitinib, pazopanib, lenvatinib, cabozantinib, and vandetanib are other small-molecule tyrosine kinase inhibitors (TKIs) that inhibit multiple TKs, in addition to the VEGFR signaling pathway.[13,33] These antiangiogenic TKIs have been associated with HTN, CM and HF, cardiac ischemia, and arterial thrombotic events. Of these agents, we focus on describing the epidemiology and basic mechanisms of sunitinib, because it is one of the most well studied agents to date. This discussion is relevant to other TKIs that have primarily off-target effects on VEGFR and PDGFR.

> Sunitinib results in HTN, as well as declines in LVEF. In phase III trials and subsequent clinical experience, the incidence of HTN ranges from 5% to 47% and the incidence of significant LVEF declines is estimated to be on the order of 10%.[14] HTN secondary to sunitinib tends to occur early, with the median time to HTN (defined as a systolic blood pressure of ≥140 mm Hg or diastolic blood pressure of ≥90 mm Hg) occurring within 1 to 20 days of the first two cycles of sunitinib therapy. The incidence of systolic HTN in one pooled analysis was 58% by the end of cycle 1 and 80% by the end of cycle 2. Increases in blood pressure tend to be greater in those with a history of HTN. Additional single center retrospective data suggest that average systolic blood pressure increases of 8.5 mm Hg and diastolic blood pressure increases of 6.7 mm Hg occur with any TKI therapy, greatest with axitinib.[34]
>
> Prospective observational data suggest that the rate of LV dysfunction in the metastatic renal cell cancer population, as defined by declines in LVEF, is on the order of 9.7%. Most of these events occur early after the initiation of therapy, primarily within the first 3 months. LVEF declines have also been observed to be reversible and manageable, although predictors of recovery remain to be defined. The mechanisms of sunitinib cardiotoxicity are believed to be secondary to the inhibition of signaling pathways critical to CV homeostasis, energy compromise, and increased afterload.[14]

Bcr-Abl Targeted Therapies

Imatinib, the first targeted small-molecule TK inhibitor of the fusion protein Bcr-Abl, which arises from the chromosomal translocation that creates the Philadelphia chromosome, revolutionized the treatment of chronic myeloid leukemia.[35] However, clinically, imatinib may be associated with a very low incidence of HF, with admittedly conflicting data. Newer generation Bcr-Abl TKIs have raised more substantive concerns. Dasatinib, with more potent activity than imatinib against Bcr-Abl, has been associated with significant pulmonary HTN that is observed to be largely reversible with cessation of the drug. This finding prompted the FDA to recommend that patients be evaluated for cardiopulmonary disease prior to and during dasatinib treatment. Nilotinib and ponatinib have both been associated with PVD and ischemic heart disease. Moreover, nilotinib has been associated with cardiometabolic effects, including hyperglycemia and hyperlipidemia, and QT prolongation. The incidence of PVD has been reported to be 1.3% to 6.2%, and the incidence of combined CV events, including ischemic heart disease, cerebrovascular disease, and PVD, is on the order of 10% to 15.9%.[35] Ponatinib has been associated with HTN, ischemic events, and HF, potentially related to VEGFR1-3 inhibition. In the Ponatinib Ph-Positive Acute Lymphoblastic Leukemia and CML Evaluation (PACE) trial, 6% of patients experienced CV events, 3% experienced cerebrovascular events, and 4% experienced PAD at 12 months.[36] At a median follow-up of 24 months, the cumulative incidences increased to 10%, 7%, and 7%, respectively. The biologic mechanisms of cardiotoxicity remain unknown, but again are likely related to their multi-targeted kinase inhibition. Comprehensively deciphering the mechanisms of these kinase inhibitors remains challenging given their nonselectivity; as they typically affect more than 30 different kinases. Ibrutinib is a small molecule Bruton's TKI that is used in the treatment of chronic lymphocytic leukemia, Waldenstrom macroglobulinemia, mantle cell lymphoma, marginal zone lymphoma, and chronic graft versus host disease. CV toxicities include HTN, atrial fibrillation and supraventricular arrhythmias, ventricular arrhythmias, HF, and bleeding. One pharmacovigilance database study indicated an elevated reporting odds ratio (ROR) for each of these, that occurred soon after the first dose.[37] For HTN, the ROR was 1.7 (95% CI 1.5 to 1.9); supraventricular arrhythmias (largely atrial fibrillation) 23.1 (95% CI 21.6 to 24.7); ventricular arrhythmias 4.7 (95% CI 3.7 to 5.9); HF 3.5 (95% CI 3.1 to 3.8); and central nervous system bleeding 3.7 (3.4 to 4.1). These were each associated with an increased risk of death, except HTN.

HORMONAL THERAPY

Androgen Deprivation Therapies

In prostate cancer, androgen deprivation therapy (ADT) is used to reduce levels of androgens in the circulation and decrease prostate cell growth. ADT includes gonadotropin-releasing hormone (GnRH) agonists, such as leuprolide, goserelin, and triptorelin; GnRH antagonists (Degarelix); and antiandrogens, such as flutamide and bicalutamide. These therapies have adverse cardiometabolic effects, and low testosterone is also implicated in metabolic syndrome. Studies suggest that they result in increased body weight (particularly visceral adiposity), decreased insulin sensitivity, and dyslipidemia (increased low-density lipoprotein [LDL] and triglycerides). Changes in body composition occur early, within the first few months of therapy. Multiple cohort studies indicate an increased risk of CV events in men with prostate cancer. Moreover, treatment with ADT has also been associated with adverse CV events, including coronary disease, myocardial infarction, HF, sudden cardiac death, or death due to CV disease. Not all studies corroborate this effect, however, including a meta-analyses of 4141 patients from 8 randomized trials. It may also be that these effects are worsened in patients with preexisting CV disease, and new CV events have been reported within the first 6 months of initiation of therapy.[38] CV risk in patients treated with ADT may vary according to severity of comorbidities, with ADT reported as having a greater and worse impact on CV survival in patients who have greater baseline CV risk and worse overall comorbidities.

Selective Estrogen Receptor Modulators and Aromatase Inhibitors

Tamoxifen is a selective estrogen receptor modulator widely used in adjuvant therapy for estrogen receptor–positive breast cancer. Data regarding the cardioprotective effect of tamoxifen have been conflicting. Tamoxifen does exert a favorable effect on lipids, with a reduction in total cholesterol and LDL levels. Some studies demonstrate a potential effect on decreasing the ischemic heart disease incidence, with a RR of 0.76 (95% CI, 0.60 to 0.95; $P = 0.02$), although other studies demonstrate no significant effect.[39] An increased risk of thromboembolic events, however, is well established; they occur largely during the first 2 years of exposure and in older women. A meta-analysis from the Early Breast Cancer Trialists' Collaborative Group confirmed a significant, but small, increased risk in venous thromboembolism with tamoxifen.

Aromatase inhibitors (e.g., anastrozole, letrozole, exemestane) block the conversion of androgens to estrogen. The two major classes that are currently in use differ according to their ability to bind reversibly versus irreversibly to aromatase. Data regarding the potential CV effects of aromatase inhibitors have been conflicting, but it is hypothesized that these agents inhibit the beneficial effects of estrogen related to the regulation of lipids, coagulation, antioxidant systems, and nitric oxide production. Aromatase inhibitors are associated with worse hypercholesterolemia and HTN, and a longer duration of exposure is reportedly associated with an increased risk of CV disease. Pooled data analyses from multiple large cohort studies suggest that there is a modestly increased risk of CV disease, as defined by myocardial infarction, angina, or HF with aromatase inhibitors compared with tamoxifen (odds ratio [OR], 1.26; 95% CI, 1.10 to 1.43; p < 0.001).[40] Another large retrospective analysis determined that compared with tamoxifen, aromatase inhibitors were not associated with an increased risk of CV ischemia or stroke, or HF/CM, but were associated with a combined outcome of dysrhythmia, valvular dysfunction, and pericarditis.[41] A population-based, retrospective cohort study suggested that in 23,525 women newly diagnosed with breast cancer, of which 17,922 initiated treatment with an aromatase inhibitor (n = 8139) or tamoxifen (n = 9783), aromatase inhibitors were associated with an increased risk of HF (incidence rate, 5.4 versus 1.8 per 1000 person-years; HR 1.86 95% CI 1.14 to 3.03) and CV mortality (incidence rate, 9.5 versus 4.7 per 1000 person-years; HR 1.50, 95% CI 1.11 to 2.04) compared with tamoxifen.[42]

RADIATION THERAPY

RT has been critical for improved cancer control and survival rates. Despite these gains, incidental irradiation to cardiac structures results in an increased risk of CV morbidity and mortality.[43] The clinical manifestations of RT cardiotoxicity include coronary disease, CM and HF, valvular disease, arrhythmia, and pericardial disease. Increasing data suggest that early subclinical changes, including cardiac perfusion defects and longitudinal strain abnormalities, can occur earlier, within 6 months of RT, even with the use of current techniques.

In a meta-analysis of over 23,000 women with breast cancer, there was an excess of deaths not resulting from breast cancer as early as 5 years following RT, principally due to CV disease and lung cancer. Subsequent studies support these results. In one study of women treated from 1954 to 1984 evaluated approximately 28 years after cancer therapy, RT was associated with a 1.76-fold increased risk of cardiac mortality and a 1.33-fold increased risk of vascular mortality. Patients with left-sided disease had a 1.56-fold increased risk of cardiac mortality compared with right-sided disease. Moreover, a study of women treated for breast cancer between 1958 and 2001 suggested that major CV events increased by 7.4% for each Gy increase in mean heart dose.[44]

Studies in lymphoma survivors corroborate an association between RT dose to the heart and a progressive risk of CV disease, with a CV complications risk three- to five-fold greater than the general population. Relative to healthy age-matched controls, the standard incidence ratio was 3.19 for coronary artery bypass surgery, 1.55 for revascularization, 9.19 for valve surgery, 12.91 for pericardial stripping or pericardiocentesis, and 1.9 for defibrillator or pacemaker placement.

Most recently, data from the lung cancer population have also suggested an increased CV risk. In RTOG 0617, a randomized trial of standard versus high-dose RT in locally advanced lung cancer, high-dose RT was associated with a 38% increased risk of all-cause mortality,[45] and RT dose to the heart specifically was associated with worse overall survival. A single-center retrospective analysis of 748 non-small cell lung cancer patients treated with RT (median age 65 years, IQR 57 to 73 years), of whom 35.8% had pre-existing coronary disease, noted that coronary disease, HF, or cardiac death occurred in 10.3%.[46]

In addition to the RT dose delivered (total and mean heart dose), which is a critical determinant of the development of cardiac disease, additional risk factors include the radiation field, younger age, higher number of fractions, concomitant chemotherapy (anthracyclines), CV risk factors (diabetes, tobacco use, obesity, HTN, hypercholesterolemia), and CV disease.

Irradiation also results in valvular disease with leaflet thickening, fibrosis, and calcification. Left-sided valves are more commonly affected, particularly the aortic valve, followed by the mitral and tricuspid valves. Fibrosis and calcification of the aortic root, aortic valve annulus, aortic valve leaflets, aortic-mitral intervalvular fibrosa, mitral valve annulus, and the base and mid portions of the mitral valve leaflets typically occur. Sparing of the mitral valve tips and commissures has been noted as a distinguishing feature. Regurgitation is more common than stenosis, with the exception of the aortic valve. The reported incidence of significant valve disease is 1% at 10 years, 5% at 15 years, and 6% at 20 years, with the incidence increasing significantly after 20 years and related to dose. The pathophysiology of radiation-induced heart disease may be related to an increase in TGF-β and osteogenic factors, including bone morphogenetic protein 2, osteopontin, and alkaline phosphatase.

RT is also associated with the development of HF and CM. Diffuse myocardial fibrosis and microvascular and macrovascular injury result in systolic and diastolic dysfunction, and can manifest as a restrictive CM phenotype. RT has also been associated with an increased risk of HF with preserved ejection fraction. On a microvascular level, irradiation results in endothelial cell loss and dysfunction, increased inflammation, and decreased capillary density. On a macrovascular level, there is proximal (ostial) involvement of coronary arteries, and lesions can be fibrous, fibrocalcific, fibrofatty, and laden with cholesterol and lipid. Irradiation also results in autonomic dysfunction, defined by an elevated resting heart rate and abnormal heart rate recovery. Finally, radiation-induced pericardial disease can occur acutely, as pericarditis and pericardial effusions. Pericardial thickening and constrictive pericarditis have also been noted, and can be delayed several weeks to years after RT.

STEM CELL TRANSPLANTATION

Advances in hematopoietic stem cell transplantation (HCT) for hematologic malignancies have led to improvements in transplant outcomes resulting in a growing survivor population. However, CV disease is a competing risk and a major cause of morbidity and mortality in this population. Compared with the general population, there is a markedly increased rate of CV death, HF/CM, and ischemic heart disease, with incidence rate differences on the order of 3.6 (1.7 to 5.5), 8.8 (5.7 to 11.8), and 3.3 (0.7 to 5.9), respectively.[47] These effects are worsened in younger survivors less than 60 years of age. Moreover, there is a significantly increased hazard of CV death (HR 2.3, 95% CI 1.1 to 48) and HF/CM (HR 1.9, 95% 1.1 to 3.3). Highly prevalent, modifiable CV risk factors in the HCT survivor population contribute significantly to CV disease. The burden of modifiable CV risk factors after HCT in this population is substantial. At 1-year post transplant, HCT survivors (median age 44 years) have a cumulative incidence of HTN of 28.4%; dyslipidemia 33.6%, diabetes 10.8%, and multiple CV risk factors 16.1%.[47] These numbers increase substantially over time, and at 10 years, 37.7% suffer from HTN, 46.7% from dyslipidemia, 18.1% diabetes, and 31.4% multiple CV risk factors.

MECHANISTIC OVERLAP BETWEEN CARDIOVASCULAR DISEASE AND CANCER

An emerging area in the field of cardio-oncology research that links both cancer-associated mutations and CV disease is clonal hematopoiesis.

FUTURE PERSPECTIVES

The field of cardio-oncology continues to evolve. The need for the dedicated CV care of cancer patients will continue to grow as both cancer and CV disease remain highly prevalent; as there is a growing population of survivors; and as newer cancer therapies affect fundamental CV signaling pathways, resulting in both subclinical and overt cardiotoxic effects. With this growth comes a call to: (1) advance our understanding of the basic pathophysiologic mechanisms; (2) translate these findings to improve upon cancer therapeutics and cardioprotective strategies; (3) understand the epidemiology and natural history of cardiotoxicity and CV remodeling with cancer therapies; (4) develop robust mechanisms to identify high-risk CV patients; and (5) personalize the delivery of therapy to maximize its oncologic effectiveness and minimize its cardiotoxic potential. There is a great need for continued clinical and research education and expertise and collaborative efforts among cardiologists, oncologists, industry partners, patient advocates, and the National Institutes of Health and FDA, as well as analogous global organizations, so that a framework can be built to address gaps in knowledge and personalize care through evidence-based medicine.[48]

REFERENCES

Epidemiology, Clinical Manifestations, and Pathophysiology of Cancer Therapy Cardiotoxicity

1. Roth GA, Johnson C, Abajobir A, et al. Global, regional, and national burden of cardiovascular diseases for 10 causes, 1990 to 2015. *J Am Coll Cardiol*. 2017;70(1):1–25.
2. American Cancer Society. *Global Cancer Facts & Figures*. 4th ed. Atlanta: American Cancer Society; 2018.
3. Roth GA, Abate D, Abate KH, et al. Global, regional, and national age-sex-specific mortality for 282 causes of death in 195 countries and territories, 1980–2017: a systematic analysis for the Global Burden of Disease Study 2017. *Lancet*. 2018;392(10159):1736–1788.

Traditional Chemotherapeutic Agents

4. Yancy CW, Jessup M, Bozkurt B, et al. 2013 ACCF/AHA guideline for the management of heart failure: a report of the American College of Cardiology Foundation/American Heart Association Task Force on practice guidelines. *Circulation*. 2013;128(16):e240–e327.
5. Bloom MW, Hamo CE, Cardinale D, et al. Cancer therapy-related cardiac dysfunction and heart failure: Part 1: definitions, pathophysiology, risk factors, and imaging. *Circ Heart Fail*. 2016;9(1):e002661.
6. Narayan HK, Finkelman B, French B, et al. Detailed echocardiographic phenotyping in breast cancer patients: associations with ejection fraction decline, recovery, and heart failure symptoms over 3 years of follow-up. *Circulation*. 2017;135(15):1397–1412.
7. Getz KD, Sung L, Ky B, et al. Occurrence of treatment-related cardiotoxicity and its impact on outcomes among children treated in the AAML0531 clinical trial: a report from the Children's Oncology Group. *J Clin Oncol*. 2019;37(1):12–21.
8. Mulrooney DA, Armstrong GT, Huang S, et al. Cardiac outcomes in adult survivors of childhood cancer exposed to cardiotoxic therapy: a cross-sectional study. *Ann Intern Med*. 2016;164(2):93–101.
9. Bates JE, Howell RM, Liu Q, et al. Therapy-related cardiac risk in childhood cancer survivors: an analysis of the childhood cancer survivor study. *J Clin Oncol*. 2019;37(13):1090–1101.
10. Armstrong GT, Joshi VM, Ness KK, et al. Comprehensive echocardiographic detection of treatment-related cardiac dysfunction in adult survivors of childhood cancer: results from the St. Jude lifetime cohort study. *J Am Coll Cardiol*. 2015;65(23):2511–2522.
11. Feijen EAM, Leisenring WM, Stratton KL, et al. Derivation of anthracycline and anthraquinone equivalence ratios to doxorubicin for late-onset cardiotoxicity. *JAMA Oncol*. 2019;5(6):864–871.
12. Zamorano JL, Lancellotti P, Rodriguez Muñoz D, et al. 2016 ESC Position Paper on cancer treatments and cardiovascular toxicity developed under the auspices of the ESC Committee for Practice guidelines: the task force for cancer treatments and cardiovascular toxicity of the European Society of Cardiology (ESC). *Eur Heart J*. 2016;37(36):2768–2801.
13. Ky B, Vejpongsa P, Yeh ET, et al. Emerging paradigms in cardiomyopathies associated with cancer therapies. *Circ Res*. 2013;113(6):754–764.
14. Hahn VS, Lenihan DJ, Ky B. Cancer therapy-induced cardiotoxicity: basic mechanisms and potential cardioprotective therapies. *J Am Heart Assoc*. 2014;3(2):e000665.
15. Li M, Sala V, De Santis MC, et al. Phosphoinositide 3-kinase gamma inhibition protects from anthracycline cardiotoxicity and reduces tumor growth. *Circulation*. 2018;138(7):696–711.
16. Burridge PW, Li YF, Matsa E, et al. Human induced pluripotent stem cell-derived cardiomyocytes recapitulate the predilection of breast cancer patients to doxorubicin-induced cardiotoxicity. *Nat Med*. 2016;22(5):547–556.

Additional Cancer Therapies

17. Waxman AJ, Clasen S, Hwang WT, et al. Carfilzomib-associated cardiovascular adverse events: a systematic review and meta-analysis. *JAMA Oncol*. 2018;4(3):e174519.
18. Cornell RF, Ky B, Weiss BM, et al. Prospective study of cardiac events during proteasome inhibitor therapy for relapsed multiple myeloma. *J Clin Oncol*. 2019;37(22):1946–1955.
19. Willis MS, Patterson C. Proteotoxicity and cardiac dysfunction–Alzheimer's disease of the heart? *N Engl J Med*. 2013;368(5):455–464.
20. Efentakis P, Kremastiotis G, Varela A, et al. Molecular mechanisms of carfilzomib-induced cardiotoxicity in mice and the emerging cardioprotective role of metformin. *Blood*. 2019;133(7):710–723.

Immunotherapy

21. Johnson DB, Balko JM, Compton ML, et al. Fulminant myocarditis with combination immune checkpoint blockade. *N Engl J Med*. 2016;375(18):1749–1755.
22. Mahmood SS, Fradley MG, Cohen JV, et al. Myocarditis in patients treated with immune checkpoint inhibitors. *J Am Coll Cardiol*. 2018;71(16):1755–1764.
23. Awadalla M, Mahmood SS, Groarke JD, et al. Global longitudinal strain and cardiac events in patients with immune checkpoint inhibitor-related myocarditis. *J Am Coll Cardiol*. 2020;75(5):467–478.
24. Zhang L, Awadalla M, Mahmood SS, et al. Cardiovascular magnetic resonance in immune checkpoint inhibitor-associated myocarditis. *Eur Heart J*. 2020;41(18):1733–1743.
25. Chitturi KR, Xu J, Araujo-Gutierrez R, et al. Immune checkpoint inhibitor-related adverse cardiovascular events in patients with lung cancer. *JACC (J Am Coll Cardiol): CardioOncol*. 2019;1(2):182–192.
26. Ghosh AK, Chen DH, Guha A, et al. CAR T cell therapy–related cardiovascular outcomes and management. *JACC (J Am Coll Cardiol): CardioOncol*. 2020;2(1):97–109.

Targeted Therapies

27. Advani PP, Ballman KV, Dockter TJ, et al. Long-term cardiac safety analysis of NCCTG N9831 (Alliance) adjuvant trastuzumab trial. *J Clin Oncol*. 2016;34(6):581–587.
28. Goldhar HA, Yan AT, Ko DT, et al. The temporal risk of heart failure associated with adjuvant trastuzumab in breast cancer patients: a population study. *J Natl Cancer Inst*. 2016;108(1).
29. Cardinale D, Colombo A, Bacchiani G, et al. Early detection of anthracycline cardiotoxicity and improvement with heart failure therapy. *Circulation*. 2015;131(22):1981–1988.
30. Banke A, Fosbøl EL, Ewertz M, et al. Long-term risk of heart failure in breast cancer patients after adjuvant chemotherapy with or without trastuzumab. *JACC Heart Fail*. 2019;7(3):217–224.
31. Leong DP, Cosman T, Alhussein MM, et al. Safety of continuing trastuzumab despite mild cardiotoxicity. *JACC (J Am Coll Cardiol): CardioOncol*. 2019;1(1):1–10.
32. Jerusalem G, Lancellotti P, Kim SB. HER2+ breast cancer treatment and cardiotoxicity: monitoring and management. *Breast Cancer Res Treat*. 2019;177(2):237–250. https://doi.org/10.1007/s10549-019-05303-y.
33. Haas NB, Manola J, Ky B, et al. Effects of adjuvant sorafenib and sunitinib on cardiac function in renal cell carcinoma patients without overt metastases: results from ASSURE, ECOG 2805. *Clin Cancer Res*. 2015;21(18):4048–4054.
34. Waliany S, Sainani KL, Park LS, et al. Increase in blood pressure associated with tyrosine kinase inhibitors targeting vascular endothelial growth factor. *JACC (J Am Coll Cardiol): CardioOncology*. 2019;1(1):24–36.
35. Moslehi JJ, Deininger M. Tyrosine kinase inhibitor-associated cardiovascular toxicity in chronic myeloid leukemia. *J Clin Oncol*. 2015;33(35):4210–4218.
36. Cortes JE, Kim DW, Pinilla-Ibarz J, et al. A phase 2 trial of ponatinib in Philadelphia chromosome-positive leukemias. *N Engl J Med*. 2013;369(19):1783–1796.
37. Salem JE, Manouchehri A, Bretagne M, et al. Cardiovascular toxicities associated with ibrutinib. *J Am Coll Cardiol*. 2019;74(13):1667–1678.

Hormonal Therapy

38. O'Farrell S, Garmo H, Holmberg L, et al. Risk and timing of cardiovascular disease after androgen-deprivation therapy in men with prostate cancer. *J Clin Oncol*. 2015;33(11):1243–1251.
39. Davies C, Pan H, Godwin J, et al. Long-term effects of continuing adjuvant tamoxifen to 10 years versus stopping at 5 years after diagnosis of oestrogen receptor-positive breast cancer: ATLAS, a randomised trial. *Lancet*. 2013;381(9869):805–816.
40. Amir E, Seruga B, Niraula S, et al. Toxicity of adjuvant endocrine therapy in postmenopausal breast cancer patients: a systematic review and meta-analysis. *J Natl Cancer Inst*. 2011;103(17):1299–1309.
41. Haque R, Shi J, Schottinger JE, et al. Cardiovascular disease after aromatase inhibitor use. *JAMA Oncol*. 2016;2(12):1590–1597.
42. Khosrow-Khavar F, Filion KB, Bouganim N, et al. Aromatase inhibitors and the risk of cardiovascular outcomes in women with breast cancer: a population-based cohort study. *Circulation*. 2020;141(7):549–559.

Radiation Therapy

43. Early Breast Cancer Trialists' Collaborative G, Darby S, McGale P, et al. Effect of radiotherapy after breast-conserving surgery on 10-year recurrence and 15-year breast cancer death: meta-analysis of individual patient data for 10,801 women in 17 randomised trials. *Lancet*. 2011;378(9804):1707–1716.
44. Darby SC, Ewertz M, McGale P, et al. Risk of ischemic heart disease in women after radiotherapy for breast cancer. *N Engl J Med*. 2013;368(11):987–998.
45. Bradley JD, Paulus R, Komaki R, et al. Standard-dose versus high-dose conformal radiotherapy with concurrent and consolidation carboplatin plus paclitaxel with or without cetuximab for patients with stage IIIA or IIIB non-small-cell lung cancer (RTOG 0617): a randomised, two-by-two factorial phase 3 study. *Lancet Oncol*. 2015;16(2):187–199.
46. Atkins KM, Rawal B, Chaunzwa TL, et al. Cardiac radiation dose, cardiac disease, and mortality in patients with lung cancer. *J Am Coll Cardiol*. 2019;73(23):2976–2987.

Stem Cell Transplantation

47. Armenian SH, Ryan TD, Khouri MG. Cardiac dysfunction and heart failure in hematopoietic cell transplantation survivors: emerging paradigms in pathophysiology, screening, and prevention. *Heart Fail Clin*. 2017;13(2):337–345.

Future Directions

48. Minasian LM, Dimond E, Davis M, et al. The evolving design of NIH-funded cardio-oncology studies to address cancer treatment-related cardiovascular toxicity. *JACC (J Am Coll Cardiol): CardioOncol*. 2019;1(1):105–113.

57 Cardio-Oncology: Approach to the Patient

JOERG HERRMANN

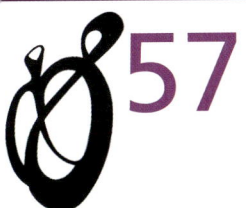

APPROACH TO THE CANCER PATIENT AT RISK OF OR WITH CARDIOVASCULAR DISEASES BEFORE CANCER THERAPY, 1099
Cardiomyopathy/Heart Failure Considerations, 1099
Vascular Disease Considerations, 1100
Arrhythmia Considerations, 1101

APPROACH TO THE CANCER PATIENT AT RISK OF OR WITH CARDIOVASCULAR DISEASES DURING CANCER THERAPY, 1103

Cardiomyopathy/Heart Failure Management, 1103
Vascular Disease Management, 1104
Arrhythmia Management, 1104

APPROACH TO THE CANCER PATIENT AT RISK OF OR WITH CARDIOVASCULAR DISEASES AFTER CANCER THERAPY, 1104
Cardiomyopathy/Heart Failure in Cancer Survivorship, 1104

Vascular Disease in Cancer Survivorship, 1105
Arrhythmias in Cancer Survivorship, 1105

CARDIO-ONCOLOGY CARE TEAM AND CLINICS, 1105

FUTURE PERSPECTIVES, 1105

REFERENCES, 1106

Never in history have there been more cancer survivors than presently, and thus, never have the chances been greater for a cardiologist to treat a patient with a cancer diagnosis. The latter conclusion holds true even more so in view of the general aging of the population and the fact that aging is a risk factor for both cancer and cardiovascular diseases (CVD).[1,2] The same applies to obesity, and a sedentary lifestyle and smoking add to the list of factors that increase the risk not only for CVD but also cancer. Thus, the cancer patient of today often presents with cardiovascular (CV) risk factors and diseases that require optimal management, in particular as they can complicate cancer care. Furthermore, cancer therapy can cause CVD, as outlined in **Chapter 56**, with significant implications for morbidity and mortality. Indeed, cancer patients with CVD, either present before or developing during cancer therapy, have worse overall survival, emphasizing the call for the optimal management of both.[3] This call extends to all cardiologists, who need to have a basic understanding of how to approach CVD in the cancer patient, as well as those who specialize in this area that has become known as cardio-oncology.

One intuitive and practical approach to the cancer patient with CVD can be summarized under the acronym SCI-FI (CV **S**ubject, Oncology **C**ontext, Cardio-Oncology **I**nteraction, and **F**ollow-up on **I**ntervention, Fig. 57.1). It begins with the CV issue in question, then takes the oncology/hematology context into consideration, and finally integrates these entities. The three CVD groups to be attentive to in particular are cardiomyopathy/heart failure (HF), vascular disease, and arrhythmias. These compose most of the referrals and can lead to fatal outcomes if not recognized and managed appropriately. Last but not least, the specific management aspects of these CVD vary by stage of presentation in the continuum of cancer care: before, during, or after cancer therapy (Fig. 57.2). This chapter will follow this framework.

APPROACH TO THE CANCER PATIENT AT RISK OF OR WITH CARDIOVASCULAR DISEASES BEFORE CANCER THERAPY

Patients who were diagnosed with cancer and are about to undergo oncological or hematological treatment are referred for a cardiology consultation most commonly out of concern that the presence or risk of CVD could pose a threat to the completion of cancer therapy and the patient. A comprehensive understanding of CVD, as well as cancer, its treatment, and how it affects the CV system is needed to address such referrals. A conceptual model that provides a useful foundation and can almost universally be applied is the multiple-hit model (Fig. 57.3).[4] The key concept is that injuries from cancer therapies add to any pre-existing impairment of CV function decreasing the CV reserve to the point of its exhaustion and eventually the clinical appearance of disease states. Very pertinent questions for any patient who is to undergo cancer therapy with concerns for CVD are: how much of the CV reserve is left, what is the margin for toxicities, and what is to be expected? Aligned with this basic concept, applicable consensus documents and guidelines are in general agreement that all cancer patients who are about to start any (potentially) cardiotoxic therapy should have a baseline assessment of cardiac function, with echocardiography as the preferred imaging modality, an assessment of any potential CVD and CV risk factors, and optimal control of any of the CV abnormalities identified.[5]

Cardiomyopathy/Heart Failure Considerations

Cardiotoxicity has historically received the greatest interest and over the years has been defined by many different criteria (see also Chapter 56). Moreso, two subtypes had been proposed on the basis of the cardiotoxicity reversibility pattern (irreversible cardiac injury, or type 1, and reversible cardiac dysfunction, or type 2), and the 2014 American Society of Echocardiography (ASE)/European Association of Cardiovascular Imaging (EACI) consensus document assigned all (potentially) cardiotoxic medication to one of these two groups.[5] This model even set the tone for pre-, on-, and posttreatment evaluations. However, recent data have challenged this concept and indicate that breast cancer patients who experienced trastuzumab cardiotoxicity have an impaired CV function even years later.[6] Furthermore, improvement in cardiac function may be seen even in patients with anthracycline cardiotoxicity.[7,8] Alternative classification systems have been proposed, and in the general approach to cancer patients at risk of cardiac dysfunction it might be useful to consider the mechanisms that can account for the decrease in cardiac function: (1) directly harmful effects on the myocardium, (2) indirectly harmful effects on the myocardium, for example, via progression of coronary artery disease (CAD), ischemia, metabolic derangement, and (3) mediated by inflammation (Table 57.1).[9] Such an approach directs to optimal treatment strategies, for example, neurohormonal blockade in case of cardiomyopathy versus improvement in coronary blood flow in case of CAD or coronary vasospasm versus antiinflammatory in case of myocarditis.

Radiation-induced heart disease involves every structure of the heart and can lead to restrictive cardiomyopathy, constrictive pericarditis, valvular heart disease, and conduction and autonomic function

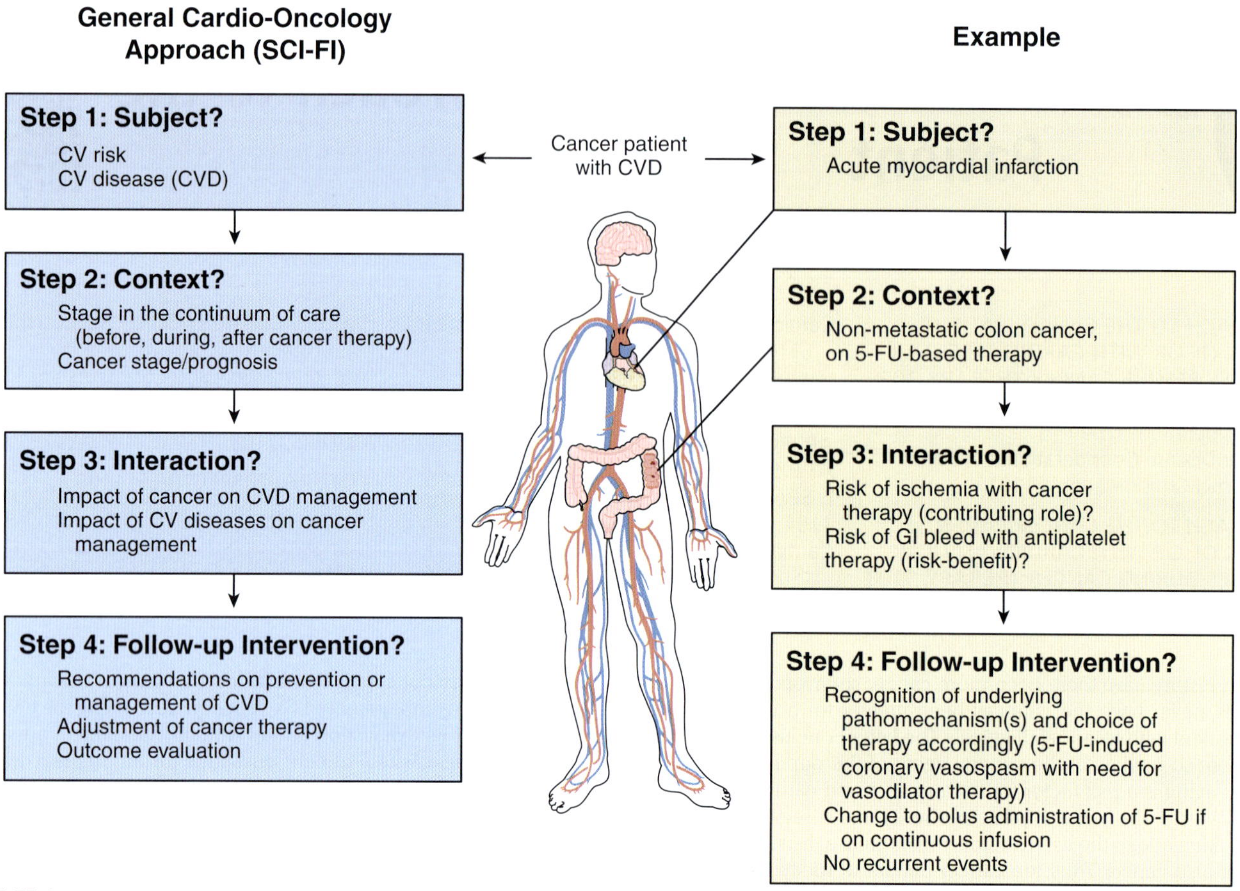

FIGURE 57.1 Approach to the cancer patient at risk of or with cardiovascular disease (CVD). The basic approach starts with defining the CVD problem in the context of the patient's malignancy and its treatment. This interplay is evaluated further to reach a conclusion on the management of both CVD and the malignancy. Follow-up assessment allows for the adjustment of recommendations and the successful management of the patient. *5-FU*, 5-fluorouracil; *GI*, gastrointestinal.

abnormalities (see also Chapter 56).[10,11] Every patient undergoing chest and/or neck radiation therapy should therefore be carefully counseled. Patients with a history of CAD and myocardial infarction (MI) in particular should be informed about the risks and benefits of undergoing chest radiation therapy. An increased risk of acute coronary events was seen in particular in this subgroup of women who underwent radiation therapy for breast cancer.[12] The risk of these events is not immediate but within the timeline of years. Time to onset of cardiomyopathy is usually beyond 10 years and classically presents as restrictive cardiomyopathy and HF with preserved ejection fraction.[13] Reduction of dose exposure is the best preventive strategy and several techniques are available. Anti-inflammatory and antioxidant therapies including statins and angiotensin converting enzyme (ACE) inhibitors are theoretically attractive but have not been proven beneficial in clinical practice.

Vascular Disease Considerations

In addition to the historically well-known increased risk of venous thromboembolism (VTE), cancer patients can present with typical and atypical chest pain episodes, MI, transient ischemic attack, stroke, claudication, critical limb ischemia, and Raynaud's.[14] Based on pathophysiology, one may propose three main vascular toxicity types: acute thrombosis, acute vasospasm, and accelerated atherosclerosis (Table 57.2).[15]

The risk of venous thrombosis in cancer patients relates not to a single but several factors (patient-, cancer-, and treatment-related). These are captured in risk prediction models such as the most widely used Khorana risk score.[16] Based on data indicating a 60% reduction in VTE and/or VTE-related deaths, practice guidelines of various societies suggest the use of direct oral anticoagulants (DOACs) as primary thromboprophylaxis in ambulatory cancer patients who are about to start chemotherapy and have a Khorana score ≥2, if there are no drug-drug interactions and no high-risk scenario for bleeding.[16]

Low-molecular-weight heparin (LMWH) remains an option for outpatient thromboprophylaxis in high-risk patients. For patients with multiple myeloma receiving "IMiD"-based combination therapy, current guidelines recommend aspirin 81 to 325 mg daily if none or only one individual/myeloma risk factor, otherwise LMWH equivalent to 40 mg enoxaparin daily or full-dose warfarin. In hospitalized patients with major surgery or acute medical illness, thromboprophylaxis with heparin or LMWH is recommended per standard recommendations with consideration for 4 weeks extension in high-risk postoperative patients in the setting of abdominal and pelvic surgery for malignancy.

Regarding arterial thromboembolic events (ATEs), the highest risk period is within 1 month before and after cancer diagnosis, thereafter declining by persisting for at least 12 months.[17,18] Advanced (stage 3 and 4) cancers and those of the gastrointestinal tract and the lung pose the highest malignancy-related risk categories for ATEs, similar to VTE.[18] A therapy-related risk of ATEs is seen in particular with vascular endothelial growth factor (VEGF) inhibitors and platinum drugs.

Acute vasospasm should be anticipated for patients to be started on 5-fluorouracil (5-FU), capecitabine, paclitaxel, cisplatin, bleomycin, VEGF inhibitors such as sorafenib, and Bcr-Abl inhibitors such as dasatinib.[15] Risk factors for 5-FU cardiotoxicity have variably been described but likely a history of cardiac disease (in particular ischemic heart disease [IHD]) and especially MI is relevant. Furthermore, smoking is likely of significance for peripheral vasoconstriction.[19] Accelerated atherosclerosis in cancer patients is most commonly associated with radiation therapy but has received attention with the use of Bcr-Abl inhibitors such as nilotinib and ponatinib in recent years; it may also be seen with VEGF inhibitors and cisplatin.[15]

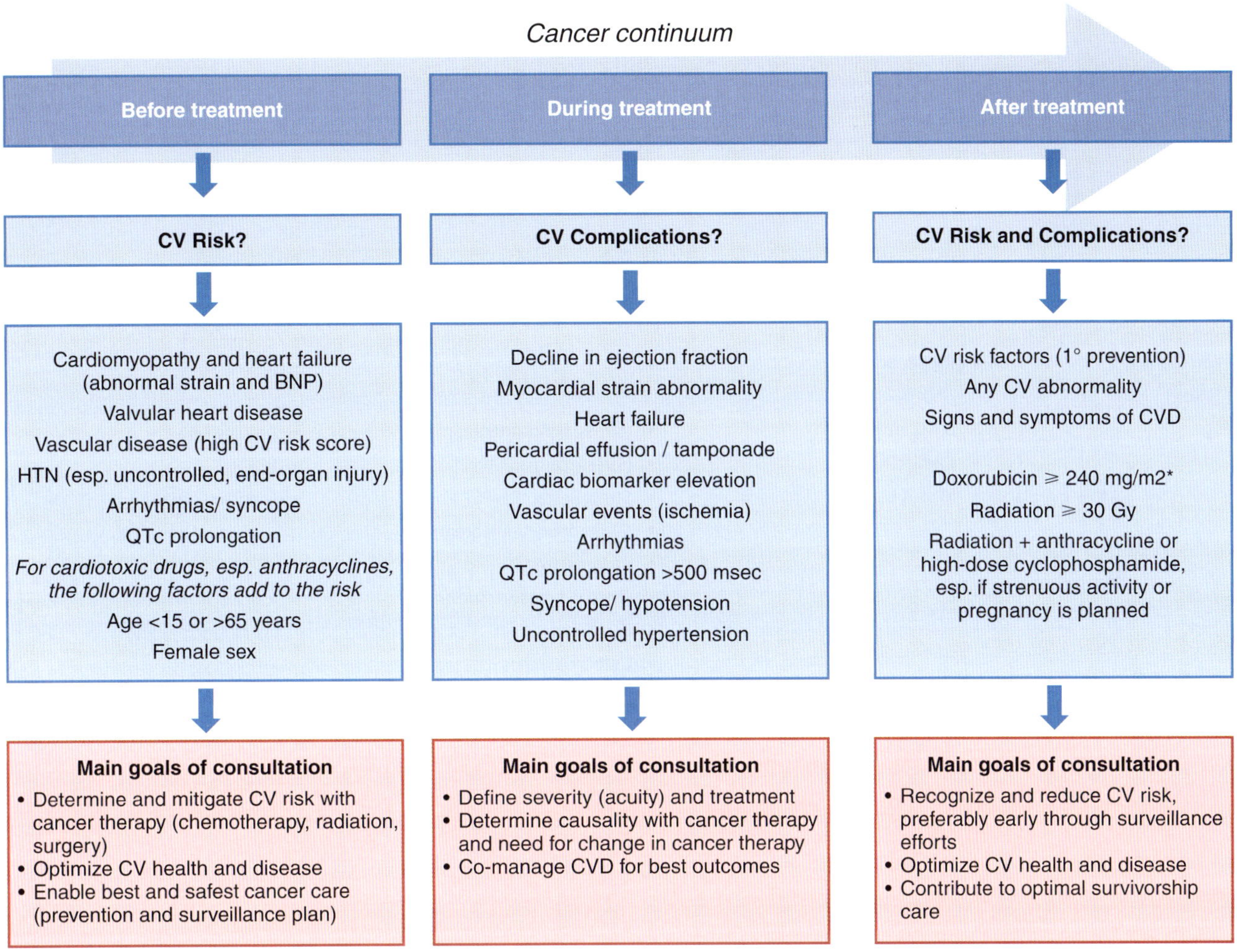

FIGURE 57.2 Cardiovascular disease management aspects across the cancer continuum. The needs of cancer patients vary based on their stand relative to treatment and so do the goals of the cardio-oncology consultation. Orienting oneself to this grid serves well in a practice that aims to cover the vast scope of cardiology and oncology/hematology.

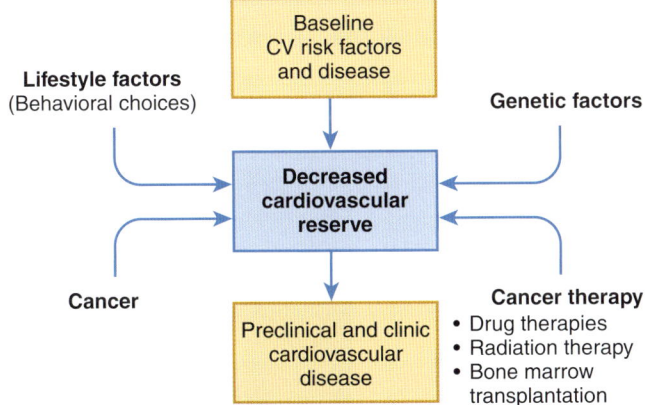

FIGURE 57.3 Multiple-hit model for cardio-oncology. In most cancer patients a number of factors (or "hits") lead to the clinical emergence of cardiovascular disease (CVD). Many patients already have cardiovascular risk factors or (subclinical) CVD that lower the reserve to tolerate additional stressors such as cancer and cancer therapy. Lifestyle factors and genetics further influence the equation.

Arrhythmia Considerations

Patients with cancer who have electrocardiogram (ECG) abnormalities, impaired exercise capacity, or CVD at baseline should be assumed to be more susceptible to cancer therapy-induced arrhythmias, as are those undergoing treatment regimens with known cardiotoxicity potential. Therefore, as a general rule, comorbidities that could represent a possible arrhythmogenic substrate should be identified and treated aggressively before and during cancer therapy. Early identification and appropriate management of cardiac ischemia, dysfunction, and remodeling is also likely to be the best strategy to modulate the arrhythmogenic substrate and improve outcomes in patients with cancer therapy-induced arrhythmias. These recommendations hold true for QTc prolongation and related ventricular arrhythmias.[9]

Crizotinib, dasatinib, lapatinib, nilotinib, pazopanib, sorafenib, sunitinib, vandetanib, and vemurafenib should be administered with caution in patients with pre-existing QTc prolongation or QTc-prolongation-related risk factors. As illustrated for several tyrosine kinase inhibitors (TKIs), such as vandetanib, electrolytes should be corrected before initiation of cancer therapy (goal value for serum K^+ levels ≥ 4 mEq/L and for magnesium and calcium within normal limits) and monitored along with ECGs, as outlined above (at baseline, at 2 to 4 weeks, at 8 to 12 weeks, and every 3 months thereafter). The common cutoffs for the QTc interval are 450 msec before and 500 msec during therapy (the one exception being nilotinib 480 msec). Full-dose therapy can be given if the QTc is less than 450 msec, half-dose if between 450 and upper limit, no dose if above the upper limit.[9]

The other common reason for referral is atrial fibrillation (AF), more commonly pre-existing though some cancer populations and therapeutics have been recognized as being more predisposed. The impact in terms of morbidity and mortality is the same and the approach to these patients should be the same as in the general population.[9]

TABLE 57.1 Overview of the Three Principal Presentations of Cardiotoxicity with Cancer Therapy

	CATEGORIES OF CANCER THERAPY-RELATED CARDIOTOXICITIES		
	Direct Impairing Effect on the Myocardium	Indirect Impairing Effect on the Myocardium	Impairing Effect Owing to Myocarditis
Risk with Cancer Therapy			
Doxorubicin	+	+	+ (toxic or reactive)
Cyclophosphamide	+	+	+ (toxic or reactive)
5-Fluorouracil	+	+	NR
HER2 inhibitors	+	Inconclusive findings	NR
VEGF inhibitors	+ (TKIs)	+	NR
Immune checkpoint inhibitors	Inconclusive findings	+	+ (immune-mediated)
Radiation therapy	+ (at high dose)	+	+ (toxic or reactive)
Diagnosis			
Imaging	• Echocardiogram • Cardiac MRI • MUGA scan	• (Stress) echocardiogram • (Stress) cardiac MRI • Stress Sestamibi–PET • CT coronary angiogram • Vasoreactivity studies	• Cardiac MRI • PET • Echocardiogram
Biomarkers	• Cardiac troponins • Natriuretic peptides (especially chronically)	• Thyroid function studies • Cytokines • Catecholamines	• Cardiac troponins • Natriuretic peptides
Management			
Treatment	• Stop cancer therapy • Beta-blocker (carvedilol and nebivolol) • ACE inhibitor • ARB • Spironolactone	• Stop cancer therapy • Therapy directed to the underlying cause (e.g., correction of myocardial ischemia or valve disease)	• Stop cancer therapy • For ICI: anti-inflammatory or immunosuppressive therapy, supportive care (e.g., ECMO)
Prevention	• Screening for comorbidities • For anthracyclines: cardiovascular medications (as above) • Exercise	• Screening for predisposing conditions • For radiation therapy: dose reduction, for example by shielding, positioning or proton beam • Dose and type of administration of cancer therapeutics	• Screening for comorbidities (efficacy not proven) • Early detection with biomarkers and/or ECG changes (heart blocks, ventricular arrhythmias including ectopy and tachycardia, atrial fibrillation)

ACE, Angiotensin converting enzyme; *ARB*, angiotensin receptor blocker; *CT*, computed tomography; *ECMO*, extracorporeal membrane oxygenation; *ICI*, immune checkpoint inhibitor; *MRI*, magnetic resonance imaging; *MUGA*, multigated acquisition scan; *NR*, not reported; *PET*, positron emission tomography; *TKI*, tyrosine kinase inhibitors; *VEGF*, vascular endothelial growth factor.
From Herrmann J. Adverse cardiac effects of cancer therapies: cardiotoxicity and arrhythmia. *Nat Rev Cardiol.* 2020;17:474–502.

TABLE 57.2 Overview of the Three Principal Presentations of Arterial Vascular Toxicity with Cancer Therapy

PRESENTATION	ACUTE VASOSPASM	ACUTE THROMBOSIS	ACCELERATED ATHEROSCLEROSIS

Onset after cancer therapy	Days to weeks	Weeks to months	Months to years
Reversibility	Very likely	Likely	Very unlikely
Examples of cancer therapeutics	5-fluorouracil, capecitabine, platinum drugs, VEGF inhibitors	Platinum drugs, bleomycin, vinca alkaloids, VEGF inhibitors, ICIs	Nilotinib, ponatinib, cisplatin, VEGF inhibitors
Treatment	Nitrates, calcium-channel blocker (CCB)	Thrombectomy with/without PTCA, stent, DAPT, statin therapy	Revascularization, aspirin, statin, amlodipine, ACE-inhibitor, exercise
On-therapy screening	Signs and symptoms	Signs and symptoms	Signs and symptoms
Prevention	Vasoreactivity studies, ECG (ST-segment elevation monitoring)	vWF levels, circulating endothelial cell and/or endothelial progenitor cell levels	Ankle–brachial index, cardiac stress test, coronary CT angiography

ACE, angiotensin-converting enzyme; *ASCDV*, atherosclerotic cardiovascular disease; *CCB*, calcium channel blockers; *CT*, computed tomography; *CVD*, cardiovascular disease; *DAPT*, dual antiplatelet therapy; *ECG*, electrocardiogram; *ICI*, immune checkpoint inhibitor; *PTCA*, percutaneous transluminal coronary angioplasty; *VEGF*, vascular endothelial growth factor; *vWF*, von Willebrand factor.
From Herrmann J. Vascular toxic effects of cancer therapies. *Nat Rev Cardiol.* 2020;17:503–522.

APPROACH TO THE CANCER PATIENT AT RISK OF OR WITH CARDIOVASCULAR DISEASES DURING CANCER THERAPY

Patients are referred for a cardiology evaluation during active cancer treatment most commonly to seek guidance on how a noted CVD issue could be managed, its causal relationship with cancer therapy, and its overall impact on the patient's cancer treatment plan. Such management decisions and judgment calls are among the most challenging given the unique characteristics and comorbidities of patients with active cancer, demanding a broader knowledge and experience with their trajectory. Standard practice guidelines written for the general population may need to be modified, although for the most part these should be followed and translate into better clinical outcomes. Pertinent societal recommendations and considerations for cancer patients with CVD presentations are covered elsewhere.[9,15] The 2020 European Society of Medicine Oncology (ESMO) recommendations for management of cardiac disease in cancer patients are outlined.[20]

Cardiomyopathy/Heart Failure Management

Cardiotoxicity is commonly used as an umbrella term for any cardiac abnormality encountered with cancer therapy. The first step is therefore to define the abnormality, its causes, and implications. Of the advocated cardiac surveillance parameters, left ventricular ejection fraction (LVEF) is most commonly reported and reacted to. That being said, various consensus documents have forwarded different definitions of cardiotoxicity, and the consensus definition that emerges is a drop of greater than 10% to below the lower limit of normal, which is set at 53% in the ASE/EACI consensus and at 50% in the ESMO consensus.[5,20] The cutoff to stop cancer therapy is not universally defined but most would agree with an LVEF of 40% as originally outlined for trastuzumab therapy for cessation of therapy and as outlined in the most recent ESMO document.[20] Cancer therapy of any type is to be discontinued in any patient who develops HF. These patients as well as those with an EF less than 50% should receive neurohormonal therapy in accordance with the American Heart Association (AHA)/American College of Cardiology (ACC) HF guidelines (Chapter 50).[21] For global longitudinal strain (GLS), a 15% relative change (confirmed within 2 to 3 weeks upon repeat assessment) is considered to represent subclinical left ventricular dysfunction and is predictive of a more evident future decline in LVEF. At present, however, there is no clear guidance how to react to such changes.[5] The same holds true for cTn elevations, though it has been used as a trigger to start ACE inhibitor therapy. For both parameters, the main merit is in the high negative predictive value.

As outlined above, it is important not to default to the assumption that a decline in cardiac function is always due to the cancer therapy, and even when it is, that is always due to a direct (toxic) effect on the cardiomyocytes. Some cancer therapeutics affect the vasculature more so than the myocardium and a decline in cardiac function is seen because of a reduction in blood supply. This would be even more so in the case in patients with CAD and other CVD conditions. The pre-therapy evaluation therefore serves a very important role as does an evaluation for any additional contributing factor during therapy should complications arise. Very important in view of the increasing use and the potential fatal implications is the recognition of ICI myocarditis (Fig. 57.4).

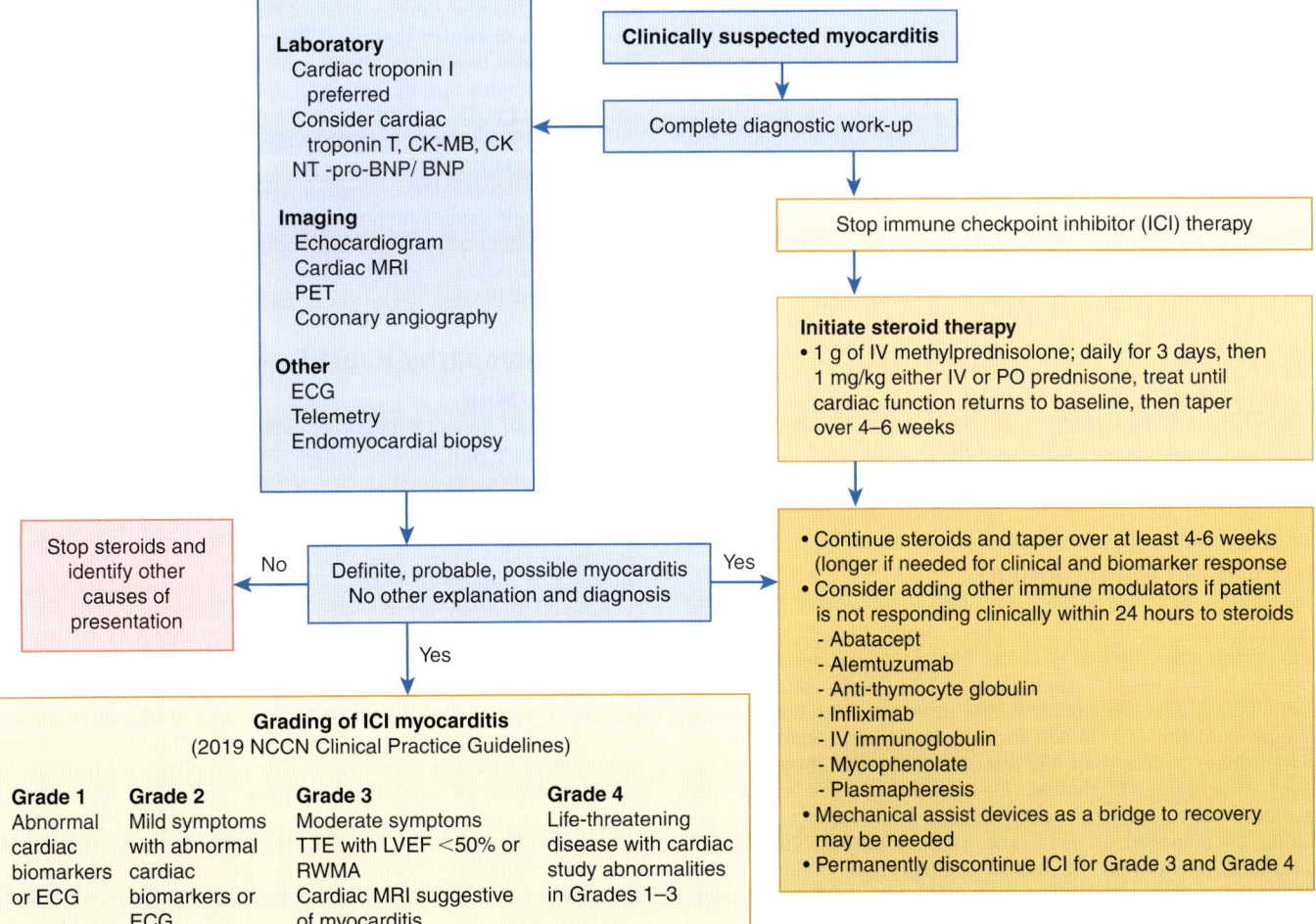

FIGURE 57.4 Outline of the approach to immune checkpoint inhibitor (ICI) myocarditis. Some patients on ICI therapy may undergo routine, serial (e.g., every 4 weeks) testing with biomarkers (cardiac troponin and natriuretic peptides) and electrocardiograms (ECG), while others present with symptoms that raise concerns for myocarditis. The work-up includes cardiac imaging studies, coronary angiography, and endomyocardial biopsy as prompted clinically. ICI therapy is to be stopped and steroids are to be started already at this stage. Once a diagnosis of myocarditis is substantiated, steroids are continued with additional immunosuppressive therapies as needed. Depending on the grade/severity of myocarditis, ICI is not to be resumed. *CK*, creatine kinase; *BNP*, brain natriuretic peptide; *ECG*, electrocardiogram; *LVEF*, left ventricular ejection fraction; *MRI*, magnetic resonance imaging; *PET*, positron emission tomography; *TTE*, transthoracic echocardiogram; *RWMA*, regional wall motion abnormalities.

Vascular Disease Management

Management of VTE in cancer patients is challenging because of their predisposition to both thrombosis and bleeding. Recurrence of VTE despite anticoagulation (so-called anticoagulation failure) is seen in 15% of patients on warfarin (rate of 2.5% per month).[22] LMWH has superior efficacy in this regard at similar major bleeding rates than warfarin. Compared with LMWH, DOACs have similar (edoxaban) or improved (rivaroxaban, apixaban) efficacy rates but higher bleeding rates, especially gastrointestinal (GI) bleeding rates.[23] Patients with mucosal tumors (GI/GU malignancy) should receive anticoagulation other than with DOACs. Treatment should continue for as long as the cancer disease process is deemed active, and at a minimum for 3 to 6 months.

As outlined above, cancer patients are also at risk of ATEs,[17] and presentations range from unstable angina to MI with and without arrhythmias (polymorphic ventricular tachycardia [VT] or heart block) in the coronary circulation, from transient ischemic attack to stroke in the carotid/cerebral circulation, and bowel ischemia, acute renal failure, and critical limb ischemia in the peripheral circulation. Treatment is in agreement with current practice guidelines and is outlined in Chapters 43 and 45. Antiplatelet therapy is a key element and based on current ACC/AHA guidelines, dual antiplatelet therapy (DAPT) should be continued for 1 year in patients with ACS, thereafter guided by risk calculators such as the DAPT score (see also Chapters 37 and 40).[24] These, however, do not take malignancy into consideration. Similar to VTE recommendations, one might argue for the continuation of DAPT as long as active cancer is present; however, there are no data for such a recommendation yet. Moreover, all of these interventions need to be balanced with the bleeding risk. In this context thrombocytopenia is an important factor to consider and the Society for Cardiovascular Angiography and Interventions (SCAI) recommendations for platelet cutoffs are as following: for surgical interventions platelet counts greater than 50K are recommended, for percutaneous coronary intervention (PCI) with DAPT platelet counts greater than 30K, and for angiography platelet counts greater than 10K.[25]

While acute coronary vasospasm, especially if profound and prolonged, can lead to MI, VT/ventricular fibrillation to the point of sudden cardiac death (SCD), and cardiac dysfunction, even Takotsubo's, HF, and cardiogenic shock, the typical presentation is angina with concomitant ST-segment elevation on ECG, resolving promptly with vasodilator therapy. In case of 5-FU, the presentation can be so typical that treatment with vasodilator therapy is both diagnostic and therapeutic. For patients experiencing acute vasospasm, vasodilators such as nitrates and calcium channel blockers (CCBs) are mainstay therapy and have been used even in combination.

Arrhythmia Management

QTc prolongation noted on surveillance ECGs should prompt the adjustment of therapy. For most drugs, therapy should be held if the QTc interval exceeds 500 msec and resumed at a reduced dose upon resolution of QTc prolongation. With nilotinib, any QTc greater than 480 msec requires cessation of therapy until the QTc is 450 to 480 msec (then resume therapy at half dose) or less than 450 msec (then resume therapy at full dose). Any grade 4 (that is, life-threatening) QTc event also precludes any further cancer therapy. Ventricular arrhythmias should be managed as usual according to clinical guidelines.[26] Important to address in cancer patients on multiple other medications are drug-drug interactions and electrolyte abnormalities (goal value for serum K^+ levels ≥ 4 mEq/L and for calcium and magnesium within normal limits).

The principles and goals of the management of AF in patients with cancer are generally the same as those in the general population, albeit with some important nuances. The first is a more lenient heart rate goal (<115 beats/min [bpm]) with the use of beta-blockers, CCBs, and digoxin. The second is the potential for drug-drug interactions, especially with antiarrhythmic drugs, which are indicated if patients remain symptomatic.

Anticoagulation in patients with cancer can be problematic in general and especially in patients receiving ibrutinib because of a predisposition to bleeding.[27] Ibrutinib has a unique antiplatelet effect, inhibiting mainly von Willebrand factor (vWF) and collagen-mediated platelet activation (in addition to fibrinogen-activated platelet activation).[28] Importantly, these activation pathways are distinct from those inhibited by aspirin (cyclooxygenase) and thienopyridines adenosine diphosphate ((ADP) receptor), and combination therapy would lead to a profoundly additive effect and bleeding risk; therefore, this strategy is not recommended. Anticoagulation strategies in cancer patients are outlined above.

APPROACH TO THE CANCER PATIENT AT RISK OF OR WITH CARDIOVASCULAR DISEASES AFTER CANCER THERAPY

Patients who have completed their cancer therapy and are cured of their disease (survivors) remain at risk of secondary malignancies as well as long-term consequences and complications of their malignancy and its treatment. These patients are referred to see a cardiologist to discuss long-term risk and preventive strategies. Often though, cardiologists may encounter these patients presenting with CVD, which can be due to (a) the continuum of vascular disease that was present even before the cancer treatment, and/or (b) the new development of vascular disease during or after completion of cancer therapy. Whereas the first scenario requires follow-up and treatment in keeping with published guidelines, the second scenario has to take into account the uniqueness of the cancer therapy the patient has received. Some cancer therapeutics affect the CV system only for the time of therapy, and especially if any impact is ruled out at the time, any newly developing CVD years later is very difficult to causally link to it. The situation is different with cancer therapies that have a prolonged effect and late onset. Cultivating an understanding of the most likely clinical course and potential contributing mechanisms is again the most recommendable approach.

Cardiomyopathy/Heart Failure in Cancer Survivorship

The profound impact cancer therapies can have on the CV system has been very well illustrated in cardiopulmonary exercise studies outlining a drop in peak VO_2.[29] A sharp decline in exercise capacity is seen after cancer therapy, which, however, may not become evident at the time. It may, and likely will with additional risk factors, progress to the symptomatic stage. This matches conceptually the progression through the AHA HF stages. Patients after exposure to cardiotoxic therapy are considered to be in Stage A HF just like patients with hypertension, diabetes, and other well-known risk predisposition. How to best follow these patients and when to act and in which format is not well defined. Serial echocardiographic studies over the first 3 years after cancer therapy indicate that the main negative deflection in LVEF is occurring in the first year after start of cancer therapy.[30] This provides the rationale for current American Society of Clinical Oncology (ASCO) and National Comprehensive Cancer Network (NCCN) follow-up recommendations (see below). However, several studies do outline a cumulative increase in HF presentations over time and not only in patients after anthracycline-based therapy, but also in patients after trastuzumab treatment and especially after the combination of these agents.[31,32] Reportedly, breast cancer patients who underwent chemotherapy also have an increased risk of late (10+ years) CV mortality. The sequence and causal link of reduction of cardiac function, HF, and mortality in these patients is yet to be proven though, as is the mantra of early detection and intervention.[33] Following radiation therapy, an increase in HF rates is seen after 15 years in breast cancer patients and an exponential increase in CV events follow the same timeline in lymphoma patients after chest radiation.[34] The effects of anthracycline exposure and radiation therapy are additive. While anthracycline therapy in adults leads to a dilative cardiomyopathy and HF with reduced LVEF, radiation therapy classically leads to a restrictive cardiomyopathy and HF with preserved LVEF. As HF can be the final common pathway of the various elements in the spectrum of radiation-induced heart disease, all contributing factors need to be evaluated, including ischemic and structural heart disease. Otherwise, treatment recommendations follow the ACC/AHA HF guidelines for the various stages of HF. Exercise is to be encouraged and cardio-oncology rehabilitation programs have emerged.[35]

Vascular Disease in Cancer Survivorship

Cancer patients have a sixfold higher risk of VTE recurrence with an annual rate as high as 30% in the absence of anticoagulation and as high as 20% even within the initial 6 months on anticoagulation therapy. The rate of VTE recurrence differs significantly by cancer type, stage of disease, and progression over time; specific risk factors include brain, lung, pancreatic, or ovarian cancer; myeloproliferative or myelodysplastic disorders; stage IV cancer; cancer stage progression; or leg paresis.[22] The original and modified Ottawa prediction scores were developed to risk stratify for recurrent VTE; among the variables included in the score, female gender and lung cancer increase the risk, whereas breast cancer and stage I (/II) decrease the risk.[36] If outlined risk factors are present, it is likely best to continue anticoagulation (premature discontinuation of anticoagulation should be avoided). Importantly, the risk for VTE remains increased in cancer survivors, especially in childhood cancer survivors who face a 25-fold higher risk than their non-diseased siblings.[37,38]

> In terms of VTE, most cancer therapies do not pose a long-term risk though exceptions need to be recognized. The first is cisplatin, and its circulating levels can remain detectable for decades after completion of cancer therapy. The second is Bcr-Abl TKIs, especially nilotinib and ponatinib, though ischemic events may not relate to thrombosis (alone); the same holds true for radiation therapy.[12] Proactive screening for thrombosis is usually not done; the evaluation is driven by signs and symptoms. In these patients it remains important to consider embolic thrombotic events (VTE with patent foramen oval, marantic endocarditis, AF, atrial or ventricular thrombus) as well as plaque rupture or erosion with subsequent in situ thrombosis. Treatment is directed toward the underlying etiology and per guidelines with options including anticoagulation, fibrinolysis, antiplatelet therapy, and revascularization.[39,40] Preventive efforts are mainly secondary prevention efforts and are directed toward improving endothelial health and reducing the risk of thrombus formation. For the long-term (>1 year past event) use of DAPT, the presumed anti-ischemic benefit must be weighed against the bleeding risk. Calculators to estimate these risks are available but need to be validated in cancer patients and the long-term dynamics of thrombotic risk in these patients remain to be defined.[24,41]

For many years after completion of therapy, cancer patients can experience an altered vasoreactivity profile, which can present as typical and atypical angina, microvascular angina, cardiac syndrome X, and Raynaud's. CCBs are usually first-line therapy for patients with Raynaud's, especially slow-release/long-acting dihydropyridine CCB such as nifedipine XL. They may also be more effective than nitrates in cases of microcirculatory involvement (microvascular angina).

Accelerated atherosclerosis is the leading entity in terms of vascular risk after completion of cancer therapy. The risk is particularly high in patients who received Bcr-Abl inhibitors or radiation therapy, and also after allogenic bone marrow transplantation. These patients may benefit from preemptive screening of vascular territories most likely to be involved, including ankle-brachial index (ABI), carotid ultrasound and noninvasive coronary imaging, and stress tests. Following chest radiation therapy, consensus guidelines recommend a cardiac stress test every 5 years in patients with defined high-risk features. As the increase in risk with the combination of radiation therapy and CV risk factors is profound, regular screening for these is recommended.[11] For patients who present with accelerated atherosclerosis (progressive arterial occlusive disease), treatment is in keeping with societal guidelines.

Arrhythmias in Cancer Survivorship

Arrhythmias in cancer survivors are most commonly expected after radiation therapy to the chest and therapies that exerted a lasting negative effect on cardiac function. This includes patients who sustained a MI as a consequence of cancer therapy with subsequent scar formation. Patients after anthracycline therapy may have such poor heart function that they are at risk of malignant arrhythmias and SCD. Indeed, current literature is supportive of the fact that among patients with a LVEF less than 35% and meeting qualifications for an ICD/cardiac resynchronization therapy-defibrillator (CRT-D) the risk of VT and ventricular fibrillation and the benefit from device therapy is the same for anthracycline and dilated/ischemic cardiomyopathy. Device therapy should therefore not be withheld for cancer survivors. AF can be seen in those with cardiomyopathy or valvular heart disease, especially after radiation therapy. Management follows standard guidelines. Heart block can be seen after radiation therapy. Sinus tachycardia is by far the most common rhythm abnormality in cancer patients, even as a reflection of autonomic dysfunction, after radiation as well as after anthracycline therapy.

CARDIO-ONCOLOGY CARE TEAM AND CLINICS

Cardio-oncology allows for further specialization and dedicated care of cancer patients with CVD. A multidisciplinary team is at the core of the cardio-oncology clinic and expands to a larger network that includes general practitioners and other subspecialties as patients are undergoing long-term comprehensive care (Fig. 57.5). Three milestones can be distinguished toward establishing a cardio-onco-hematology clinic (vision, institutional support and organization, and implementation and operation). The structure and scope of the cardio-onco-hematology clinic needs to be individualized for the specific practice environment it is to successfully operate in and will require reevaluation and re-adjustment based on outcome measures and developments in the field.[42] The overreaching goal of the clinic and the outlined approach in this chapter is to enable cancer patients to receive the best possible cancer therapy at the lowest pos-sible CV risk.

FUTURE PERSPECTIVES

It is the expectation that in the years to come the demands for cardio-oncology will grow and with it the need for education (including core knowledge and competencies), best practice recommendations (including practice guidelines and quality metrics), and research (providing the much-needed evidence base). These currently ongoing developments will refine the approach to the cancer patient at risk of or with evident CVD or CV toxicity. In addition, emerging trends will shape the cardio-oncology practice including ongoing advances in cancer therapies, artificial intelligence innovations, and changing health care environments such as those imposed by viral pandemics.

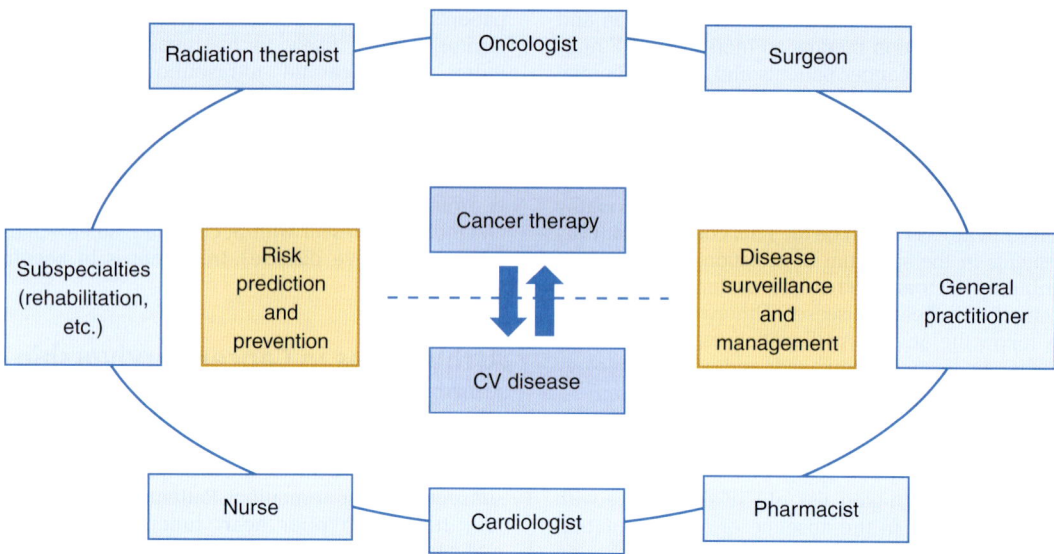

FIGURE 57.5 The cardio-oncology network. The cardio-oncology approach is multidisciplinary in nature. It requires the expertise and interaction of multiple providers to most optimally follow and treat the cancer patient through their continuum of care.

REFERENCES

Approach to the Cancer Patient at Risk of or with Cardiovascular Diseases Before Cancer Therapy

1. Herrmann J. Adverse cardiac effects of cancer therapies: cardiotoxicity and arrhythmia. *Nat Rev Cardiol.* 2020;17(8):474–502.
2. Herrmann J. Vascular toxic effects of cancer therapies. *Nat Rev Cardiol.* 2020;17(8):503–522.
3. Youn JC, et al. Cardiovascular disease burden in adult patients with cancer: an 11-year nationwide population-based cohort study. *Int J Cardiol.* 2020;317:167–173.
4. Jones LW, et al. Early breast cancer therapy and cardiovascular injury. *J Am Coll Cardiol.* 2007;50(15):1435–1441.
5. Plana JC, et al. Expert consensus for multimodality imaging evaluation of adult patients during and after cancer therapy: a report from the American Society of Echocardiography and the European Association of Cardiovascular Imaging. *J Am Soc Echocardiogr.* 2014;27(9):911–939.
6. Yu AF, et al. Long-term cardiopulmonary consequences of treatment-induced cardiotoxicity in survivors of ERBB2-positive breast cancer. *JAMA Cardiol.* 2020.
7. Cardinale D, et al. Early detection of anthracycline cardiotoxicity and improvement with heart failure therapy. *Circulation.* 2015;131(22):1981–1988.
8. Mazur M, et al. Burden of cardiac arrhythmias in patients with anthracycline-related cardiomyopathy. *JACC Clin Electrophysiol.* 2017;3(2):139–150.
9. Herrmann J. Adverse cardiac effects of cancer therapies: cardiotoxicity and arrhythmia. *Nat Rev Cardiol.* 2020.
10. Lancellotti P, et al. Expert consensus for multi-modality imaging evaluation of cardiovascular complications of radiotherapy in adults: a report from the European Association of Cardiovascular Imaging and the American Society of Echocardiography. *J Am Soc Echocardiogr.* 2013;26(9):1013–1032.
11. Iliescu C, et al. SCAI expert consensus statement: evaluation, management, and special considerations of cardio-oncology patients in the cardiac catheterization laboratory (Endorsed by the Cardiological Society of India, and Sociedad Latino Americana De Cardiologia Intervencionista). *Catheter Cardiovasc Interv.* 2016;87(5):895–899.
12. Darby SC, et al. Risk of ischemic heart disease in women after radiotherapy for breast cancer. *N Engl J Med.* 2013;368(11):987–998.
13. Saiki H, et al. Risk of heart failure with preserved ejection fraction in older women after contemporary radiotherapy for breast cancer. *Circulation.* 2017;135(15):1388–1396.
14. Herrmann J, et al. Vascular toxicities of cancer therapies: the old and the new—an evolving avenue. *Circulation.* 2016;133(13):1272–1289.
15. Herrmann J. Vascular toxic effects of cancer therapies. *Nat Rev Cardiol.* 2020.
16. Key NS, et al. Venous thromboembolism prophylaxis and treatment in patients with cancer: ASCO clinical practice guideline update. *J Clin Oncol.* 2020;38(5):496–520.
17. Oren O, Herrmann J. Arterial events in cancer patients-the case of acute coronary thrombosis. *J Thorac Dis.* 2018;10(suppl 35):S4367–S4385.
18. Navi BB, et al. Risk of arterial thromboembolism in patients with cancer. *J Am Coll Cardiol.* 2017;70(8):926–938.
19. Wigley FM, Flavahan NA. Raynaud's phenomenon. *N Engl J Med.* 2016;375(6):556–565.

Approach to the Cancer Patient at Risk of or with Cardiovascular Diseases During Cancer Therapy

20. Curigliano G, et al. Management of cardiac disease in cancer patients throughout oncological treatment: ESMO consensus recommendations. *Ann Oncol.* 2020;31(2):171–190.
21. Yancy CW, et al. ACC/AHA/HFSA focused update of the 2013 ACCF/AHA guideline for the management of heart failure: a report of the American College of Cardiology/American Heart Association task force on clinical practice guidelines and the Heart Failure Society of America. *J Am Coll Cardiol.* 2017.
22. Chee CE, et al. Predictors of venous thromboembolism recurrence and bleeding among active cancer patients: a population-based cohort study. *Blood.* 2014;123(25):3972–3978.
23. Li A, et al. Direct oral anticoagulant (DOAC) versus low-molecular-weight heparin (LMWH) for treatment of cancer associated thrombosis (CAT): a systematic review and meta-analysis. *Thromb Res.* 2019;173:158–163.
24. Yeh RW, et al. Development and validation of a prediction rule for benefit and harm of dual antiplatelet therapy beyond 1 year after percutaneous coronary intervention. *J Am Med Assoc.* 2016;315(16):1735–1749.
25. Iliescu CA, et al. SCAI expert consensus statement: evaluation, management, and special considerations of cardio-oncology patients in the cardiac catheterization laboratory (endorsed by the Cardiological Society of India, and Sociedad Latino Americana De Cardiologia Intervencionista). *Catheter Cardiovasc Interv.* 2016;87(5):E202–E223.
26. Al-Khatib SM, et al. AHA/ACC/HRS guideline for management of patients with ventricular arrhythmias and the prevention of sudden cardiac death: a report of the American College of Cardiology/American Heart Association task force on clinical practice guidelines and the Heart Rhythm Society. *J Am Coll Cardiol.* 2018;72(14):e91–e220.
27. Aguilar C. Ibrutinib-related bleeding: pathogenesis, clinical implications and management. *Blood Coagul Fibrinolysis.* 2018;29(6):481–487.
28. Shatzel JJ, et al. Ibrutinib-associated bleeding: pathogenesis, management and risk reduction strategies. *J Thromb Haemost.* 2017;15(5):835–847.

Approach to the Cancer Patient at Risk of or with Cardiovascular Diseases After Cancer Therapy

29. Koelwyn GJ, et al. Running on empty: cardiovascular reserve capacity and late effects of therapy in cancer survivorship. *J Clin Oncol.* 2012;30(36):4458–4461.
30. Narayan HK, et al. Detailed echocardiographic phenotyping in breast cancer patients: associations with ejection fraction decline, recovery, and heart failure symptoms over 3 years of follow-up. *Circulation.* 2017;135(15):1397–1412.
31. Chen J, et al. Incidence of heart failure or cardiomyopathy after adjuvant trastuzumab therapy for breast cancer. *J Am Coll Cardiol.* 2012;60(24):2504–2512.
32. Bowles EJ, et al. Risk of heart failure in breast cancer patients after anthracycline and trastuzumab treatment: a retrospective cohort study. *J Natl Cancer Inst.* 2012;104(17):1293–1305.
33. Bradshaw PT, et al. Cardiovascular disease mortality among breast cancer survivors. *Epidemiology.* 2016;27(1):6–13.
34. Lee CK, Aeppli D, Nierengarten ME. The need for long-term surveillance for patients treated with curative radiotherapy for Hodgkin's disease: University of Minnesota experience. *Int J Radiat Oncol Biol Phys.* 2000;48(1):169–179.
35. Gilchrist SC, et al. Cardio-oncology rehabilitation to manage cardiovascular outcomes in cancer patients and survivors: a scientific statement from the American Heart Association. *Circulation.* 2019;139(21):e997–e1012.
36. Delluc A, et al. Accuracy of the Ottawa score in risk stratification of recurrent venous thromboembolism in patients with cancer-associated venous thromboembolism: a systematic review and meta-analysis. *Haematologica.* 2020;105(5):1436–1442.
37. Madenci AL, et al. Long-term risk of venous thromboembolism in survivors of childhood cancer: a report from the childhood cancer survivor study. *J Clin Oncol.* 2018;JCO2018784595.
38. Faber J, et al. Burden of cardiovascular risk factors and cardiovascular disease in childhood cancer survivors: data from the German CVSS-study. *Eur Heart J.* 2018;39(17):1555–1562.
39. O'Gara PT, et al. ACCF/AHA guideline for the management of ST-elevation myocardial infarction: a report of the American College of Cardiology Foundation/American Heart Association task force on practice guidelines. *J Am Coll Cardiol.* 2013;61(4):e78–e140.
40. Amsterdam EA, et al. AHA/ACC guideline for the management of patients with non-ST-elevation acute coronary syndromes: a report of the American College of Cardiology/American Heart Association task force on practice guidelines. *J Am Coll Cardiol.* 2014;64(24):e139–e228.
41. Costa F, et al. Derivation and validation of the predicting bleeding complications in patients undergoing stent implantation and subsequent dual antiplatelet therapy (PRECISE-DAPT) score: a pooled analysis of individual-patient datasets from clinical trials. *Lancet.* 2017;389(10073):1025–1034.
42. Herrmann J, Loprinzi C, Ruddy K. Building a cardio-onco-hematology program. *Curr Oncol Rep.* 2018;20(10):81.

58 Devices for Monitoring and Managing Heart Failure

JOANN LINDENFELD AND MICHAEL R. ZILE

VENTRICULAR DYSSYNCHRONY: THE TARGET OF CARDIAC RESYNCHRONIZATION THERAPY, 1107
Randomized Controlled Trials of Cardiac Resynchronization Therapy in New York Heart Association Class III and IV HFrEF Patients, 1107
Randomized Controlled Trials of Cardiac Resynchronization Therapy in NYHA Class I and II Patients, 1110
Indications for Cardiac Resynchronization Therapy in Patients with Heart Failure, 1111
Limitations of Cardiac Resynchronization Therapy, 1111

SUDDEN CARDIAC DEATH IN CHRONIC HEART FAILURE, 1111
Randomized Controlled Trials of Implantable-Cardioverter Defibrillators for Primary Prevention of SCD in HFrEF, 1111

GUIDELINES FOR CARDIAC RESYNCHRONIZATION AND IMPLANTABLE CARDIOVERTER-DEFIBRILLATORS IN HEART FAILURE WITH A REDUCED EJECTION FRACTION, 1113

NEW IMPLANTABLE THERAPEUTIC DEVICES FOR HEART FAILURE, 1113
Central Sleep Apnea, 1114
Transcatheter Mitral Valve Repair Secondary (Functional) Mitral Regurgitation, 1114

Cardiac Contractility Modulation, 1114
Baroreflex Activation Therapy, 1114

IMPLANTABLE DEVICES TO MONITOR HEART FAILURE, 1114
Device-Based Heart Failure Diagnostics, 1114
Ventricular Filling Pressures as a Target for Monitoring, 1116
Implantable Hemodynamic Monitors, 1116

INTERPLAY BETWEEN DRUGS AND DEVICES, 1117

CONCLUSIONS, 1117

REFERENCES, 1118

While implantable cardioverter defibrillators (ICDs) were first approved by the U.S. Food and Drug Administration (FDA) for the secondary prevention of sudden cardiac death (SCD) in 1985, the advent of device-based therapy for the management of heart failure (HF) did not begin until 2001 when the FDA approved cardiac resynchronization therapy (CRT) to reduce the symptoms of moderate to severe HF. In 2003, the Center for Medicaid Services (CMS) issued the first coverage decision for the use of ICDs for the primary prevention of SCD in patients with HF and reduced ejection fraction (HFrEF) post–myocardial infarction (post-MI) followed later by more expansive coverage to include nonischemic HFrEF patients. After a hiatus of nearly two decades, several new therapeutic devices that target central sleep apnea (CSA), secondary mitral regurgitation (SMR), abnormal myocardial contractility, and autonomic imbalance have been approved by the FDA for the treatment of patients with HF. Devices have also been developed to monitor and transmit physiologic data that provide important information about the events preceding HF exacerbations, allowing testing of treatment strategies based on remotely monitored data to avert HF exacerbations, reduce HF hospitalizations (HFHs), and reduce mortality. This chapter reviews the use of CRT, ICDs, and newer approved devices for management of HF and discusses the ability of monitoring devices to provide data to improve symptoms and reduce HF exacerbations. Medical management of HF is discussed in Chapters 48 to 51.

VENTRICULAR DYSSYNCHRONY: THE TARGET OF CARDIAC RESYNCHRONIZATION THERAPY

Intraventricular conduction abnormalities are common in patients with chronic HF and are associated with increased morbidity and mortality.[1] Conduction delay resulting in a QRS duration greater than 120 msec on the surface electrocardiogram has been termed electrical dyssynchrony. The difference in the timing of mechanical contraction or relaxation between different segments of the left ventricle that results from electrical dyssynchrony has been termed mechanical dyssynchrony and can result in suboptimal ventricular filling, a reduction in left ventricular (LV) contractility, greater degree and prolonged duration of mitral regurgitation (MR), and paradoxical septal wall motion.[2] Using this definition of a QRS duration of greater than 120 milliseconds, about one-third of patients with HFrEF have ventricular dyssynchrony.[2] CRT improves ventricular dyssynchrony with implantation of pacing leads to pace both the right and left ventricles. Optimal placement of two leads, one on the right ventricular septum and a second in the coronary sinus at the site of latest LV activation allows for simultaneous or near simultaneous activation of both ventricles and improves inter- and intra-ventricular synchrony. Early studies demonstrated a benefit of CRT in patients with HFrEF and ventricular dyssynchrony on hemodynamics, functional outcomes and quality of life (QoL) leading to the initial indications for this therapy.[3] These results led to large-scale randomized controlled trials (RCTs) confirming the beneficial effects of CRT on functional status and demonstrating an important morbidity and mortality benefit.

Randomized Controlled Trials of Cardiac Resynchronization Therapy in New York Heart Association Class III and IV HFrEF Patients (Table 58.1)

The following RCTs are considered among the most important studies of CRT in the severe HFrEF patient population: the Multisite Stimulation in Cardiomyopathy (MUSTIC) study,[4] the Multicenter InSync Randomized Clinical Evaluation (MIRACLE) trial,[5] the MIRACLE ICD trial,[6] the CONTAK CD trial,[7] the Comparison of Medical Therapy, Pacing and Defibrillation in Heart Failure (COMPANION),[8] and the Cardiac Resynchronization in Heart Failure (CARE HF) trial.[9] To understand and compare the size and design, clinical benefits, baseline medical therapy, and limitations of CRT with or without an ICD, these studies are described in Table 58.1 with specific comments in the text that follows.

Multisite Stimulation in Cardiomyopathy (MUSTIC) Trial. The MUSTIC trial was a single-blind randomized controlled crossover study of CRT that enrolled 67 patients with enrollment criteria outlined in Table 58.1.[4] The CRT device was implanted in all patients and after a run-in period, patients were randomized to either VVI pacing at a fixed rate of 40 beats/min ("inactive pacing") or atrio-biventricular pacing ("active pacing") for 12 weeks followed by a crossover to the alternate treatment assignment. Forty-eight patients completed the study. The primary endpoint of peak exercise oxygen consumption (V_{O_2}) improved with CRT vs. no CRT as did all the secondary endpoints. The blinded crossover design of this trial suggested substantial improvements in

TABLE 58.1 Pivotal Trials for Cardiac Resynchronization Therapy

TRIAL (YEAR PUBLISHED)	N	INCLUSION CRITERIA	STUDY DESIGN	MEAN FOLLOW-UP	PRIMARY ENDPOINT	SECONDARY ENDPOINTS	MEDICAL THERAPY*
MUSTIC (2001)	67	• QRS >150 msec • NYHA Classes III and IV • LVEF <35% • Sinus rhythm	Single-blind, crossover RCT CRT on vs. CRT off	24 wk	CRT on vs. CRT off 6MHWD (active vs. inactive pacing) 399 ± 100 m vs. 326 ± 134 m ($p \leq 0.001$)	CRT on vs. CRT off QoL 29.6 ± 21.3 vs. 43.2 ± 22.8 ($p < 0.001$) V_{O_2} 16.2 ± 4.7 vs. 15 ± 4.9 mL/kg/min ($p < 0.029$)	ACEI/ARB 96% BB 28% MRA 22% Diuretics† 94% Digoxin 48%
MIRACLE (2002)	453	• QRS ≥130 msec • NYHA III, IV • LVEF ≤35%	Double-blind prospective RCT CRT on vs. CRT off	6 mo	CRT on vs. CRT off 6MWHD +39 vs. +10 M ($p = 0.001$) QoL −18 vs. −9 points ($p < 0.001$) NYHA Improved ($p < 0.001$)	CRT on vs. CRT off Measures of exercise performance (V_{O_2}) and total exercise time, LVEF, area of MR jet, QRS duration—all improved ($p < 0.001$)	ACEI/ARB 93% BB 62% MRA NR Diuretics† 94% Digoxin 78%
MIRACLE-ICD (2003)	369	• QRS ≥130 msec • NYHA Classes III, IV • LVEF ≤35% • Indication for secondary prevention • ICD or history of inducible sustained ventricular tachycardia	Double-blind, prospective RCT CRT-ICD implanted in all with CRT off in control group	6 mo	CRT on vs. off 6MWHD +55 CI = 44–79] vs. +53 m [CI = 43–75] ($p = 0.36$) QoL −17.5 [CI = −21 to −14] vs. −11.0 [CI = −16 to −7] m ($p = 0.02$) NYHA Improved ($p = 0.007$)	CRT on vs. off No significant differences in changes in left ventricular size or function, overall HF status, survival, and rates of hospitalization	ACEI/ARB 93% BB 62% MRA NR Diuretics† 93%
CONTAK CD (2003)	490	• QRS ≥120 msec • NYHA Classes II–IV • LVEF ≤35% • Indication for primary prevention ICD	Single-blind, prospective RCT parallel-controlled CRT-ICD implanted with CRT off in control group	6 mo	CRT vs. no CRT Progression of HF, defined as ACM, hospitalization for HF, and VT/VF requiring device intervention 15% reduction in HF progression with CRT vs. no CRT ($p = 0.35$)	CRT vs. no CRT V_{O_2} 0.8 mL/kg/min vs. 0.0 mL/kg/min ($p = 0.03$) 6MHWD 35 m vs. 15 m ($p = 0.043$) QoL ($p = NS$)	ACEI/ARB 81% BB 45% MRA NR Diuretics† 92% Digoxin 72%
COMPANION (2004)	1520	• QRS ≥120 msec • NYHA Classes III–IV • LVEF ≤35%	Prospective RCT Randomized 1:2:2 to OPT (optimal medical therapy) vs. CRT-D (CRT+ICD) vs. CRT-P (CRT alone)	NR	Time to ACM or hospitalization for any cause CRT-P vs. OPT (HR= 0.81; $p = 0.014$) CRT-D vs. OPT (HR, 0.80; $P = 0.01$)	ACM CRT-P vs. OPT (reduced by 24%, $p = 0.059$) CRT-D vs. OPT (reduced 36%, $p = 0.003$) 6MWD OPT vs. CRT-P vs. CRT-I 1 ± 93 vs. 40 ± 96 ($p < 0.001$) vs. 46 ± 98 ($p < 0.001$) QoL OPT vs. CRT-P vs. CRT-D −12 ± 23 vs. −25 ± 26 ($p < 0.001$) vs. −26 ±28 ($p < 0.001$)	ACEI/ARB 89% BB 68% MRA 53% Loop diuretics 94%
CARE HF (2005)	813	• QRS ≥150 msec or 120–150 msec with echocardiographic dyssynchrony • NYHA Classes III–IV • LVEF ≤35%	Unblinded, prospective RCT CRT vs. no CRT	29.4 mo	CRT vs. no CRT Time to ACM or unplanned cardiovascular hospitalization HR = 0.63; 95% CI = 0.51–0.77; $P < 0.001$	CRT vs. no CRT ACM (HR= 0.64; 95% CI 0.48–0.85; $P < 0.002$) QoL difference (mean ± SD) at 90 −10 (−8 to −12) ($p < 0.001$)	ACEI/ARB 95% BB 70% MRA 54% Loop diuretics 44% Digoxin 40%

TABLE 58.1 Pivotal Trials for Cardiac Resynchronization Therapy—cont'd

TRIAL (YEAR PUBLISHED)	N	INCLUSION CRITERIA	STUDY DESIGN	MEAN FOLLOW-UP	PRIMARY ENDPOINT	SECONDARY ENDPOINTS	MEDICAL THERAPY*
REVERSE (2008)	610	• QRS ≥120 msec • NYHA Classes I-II • LVEF ≤40%	Double-blind, prospective RCT CRT on vs. off	12 mo	CRT on vs. off Clinical composite response (improved, unchanged or worsened) CRT on vs. off 16% vs. 21% worsened (p = 0.19)	CRT on vs. off LVESVI –18.4 ± 29.5 vs. –1.3 ± 23.4 mL/m² (p < 0.0001)	ACE/ARB 96% BB 96% MRA NR Diuretics NR
MADIT-CRT (2009)	1820	• QRS ≥130 msec • NYHA Classes I-II • LVEF ≤30% • Candidate for primary prevention ICD	Unblinded, prospective double-blind CRT-ICD vs. ICD	2.4 yr	CRT-ICD vs. ICD ACM or HF event CRT-ICD 17.2% vs. ICD 25.3% (HR = 0.66, CI = 0.52-0.84, p = 0.001)	CRT-ICD vs. ICD ACM 6.8% vs. 7.3% (p = 0.99) HF events CRT-ICD 13.9% vs. 22.8% (p < 0.001)	ACEI 77% ARB 21% BB 93% MRA 32% Diuretics† 76%
RAFT (2010)	1798	• QRS ≥120 msec or ≥200 msec if paced • NYHA Classes II-III • LVEF ≤30%	Double-blind, prospective RCT ICD-CRT vs. ICD alone	40 mo	ICD-CRT vs. ICD ACM or HFH HR 0.75, CI 0.64-0.87 (p < 0.0001)	ICD-CRT vs. ICD ACM HR 0.75, CI 0.62-0.91 (p < 0.0001) AE double in ICD-CRT compared with ICD at 30 days	ACEI/ARB 96% BB 90% MRA 42% Diuretics† 85% Digoxin 34%
ECHO-CRT (2012)	809	• QRS ≤130 msec • NYHA Classes III-IV • LVEF ≤30% and echo evidence of LV dyssynchrony	Prospective RCT CRT vs. control	19.4 mo	CRT vs. control ACM or first HFH HR 1.20, CI = 0.92-1.57, p = 0.15	CRT vs. control ACM HR 1.81, CI, 1.11-2.93 (p = 0.02)	ACEI/ARB 95% BB 96% MRA 61% Diuretics 86%
BLOCK-HF (2013)	691	• Indications for pacing with AV block • NYHA Classes I-III • LVEF ≤50% • Patients with standard indication for CRT excluded	Prospective RCT CRT vs. RV pacing	37 mo	CRT vs. RV pacing Time to ACM or urgent HF visit or a 15% increase in LVESVI HR, 0.74; CI, 0.60-0.90	CRT vs. RV pacing ACM + urgent HF care HR 0.73, CI 0.56-0.94 ACM + HFH HR 0.77, CI 0.58-1.00 ACM HR 0.83, CI 0.59-1.17 HFH HR 0.68 (049-0.94)	NR

*All medical therapy for CRT group.
†All diuretic types.

ACEI, Angiotensin converting enzyme inhibitors; ACM, all-cause mortality; AE, adverse events; ARB, angiotensin receptor blockers; BB, beta blockers; CI, confidence intervals; HF, heart failure; HFH, heart failure hospitalization; HR, hazard ratio; LVEF, left ventricular ejection fraction; MRA, mineralocorticoid receptor antagonists; NR, not reported; NYHA, New York Heart Association Classification; QoL, quality of life (Minnesota Living with Heart Failure for all studies); RCT, randomized controlled trial; RV, right ventricular; 6MHWD, 6-minute hall walk distance; Vo₂, peak exercise oxygen consumption.

functional capacity and QoL with CRT that were dependent on ongoing pacing.

Multicenter InSync Randomized Clinical Evaluation (MIRACLE). MIRACLE was the first prospective RCT designed to evaluate the benefits of CRT in patients with the inclusion criteria outlined in Table 58.1.[5] Patients assigned to CRT experienced an improvement in each of the primary endpoints at 6 months: 6MHWD, NYHA functional class, and QoL. The trial also provided evidence of substantial LV reverse remodeling with CRT as outlined in Table 58.1. The results of this trial led to FDA approval of the InSync system in 2001, the first approved CRT system in the United States.

Multicenter Insync–Implantable Cardioverter-Defibrillator Randomized Clinical Evaluation. MIRACLE ICD was a prospective RCT designed to evaluate the benefits of an implantable cardiac defibrillator (ICD) + CRT vs. ICD alone.[6] The inclusion criteria and primary endpoints were the same as in MIRACLE with the additional requirement that subjects have an indication for a secondary prevention ICD or have a history of inducible sustained ventricular tachycardia. With CRT, the improvements in QoL and (NYHA) classification were similar to those in MIRACLE but there was no difference in 6MHWD. However, Vo_2 and total exercise time were improved. The ventricular remodeling benefits seen with CRT in MIRACLE were not reproduced in MIRACLE ICD. The combined CRT-ICD device used in this study was approved by the FDA in June 2002 for use in NYHA Class III and IV HFrEF patients with ventricular dyssynchrony and an ICD indication.

CONTAK CD. CONTAK CD was similar to MIRACLE ICD except NYHA Class II patients were enrolled.[7] Both the study design (crossover) and primary endpoint (Vo_2) were changed during the study to a parallel design and a composite HF progression endpoint. The 15% reduction in HF progression was not significant but Vo_2 and 6MWHD were improved. Significant reductions in ventricular dimensions and improvement in left ventricular ejection fraction (LVEF) similar to those seen in MIRACLE were demonstrated with CRT.

Comparison of Medical Therapy, Pacing, and Defibrillation in Heart Failure (COMPANION). COMPANION randomized patients to optimal medical therapy (OPT), CRT-P (CRT alone), and CRT-D (CRT+ICD) and was the first reported large RCT to include mortality in the primary endpoint.[8] COMPANION confirmed the results of earlier CRT trials in improving symptoms, exercise tolerance, and QoL for HF patients with electrical dyssynchrony. COMPANION was also the first large RCT to demonstrate the impact of CRT-D in reducing all-cause mortality (ACM) and suggested incremental benefit from combined ICD and CRT therapies.

Mean systolic blood pressure was significantly higher in both the CRT-P and CRT-D groups compared to the OPT group at 3, 6, and 12 months (Fig. 58.1). This improvement in systolic blood pressure following CRT may allow uptitration of guideline-directed medical therapy (GDMT), further improving morbidity and mortality.

Cardiac Resynchronization in Heart Failure Trial. The CARE-HF trial convincingly demonstrated the benefits of CRT+ medical therapy vs. medical therapy alone on morbidity and mortality in patients with NYHA Class III or IV HF and ventricular dyssynchrony[9] (Fig. 58.2). CRT also led to a significant reduction in MR area by echocardiography and significant myocardial reverse remodeling and reduced N-terminal pro B-type natriuretic peptide (NT-proBNP) at 18 months. These benefits were achieved irrespective of the use of beta blockers, mineralocorticoid receptor antagonists (MRAs), or digoxin. In addition, the mean systolic blood pressure was 5.8 mm Hg (CI, 3.5 to 8.2, p = 0.001) higher in the CRT group than in the control group at 3 months; this difference was maintained at 18 months, confirming the blood pressure improvements in COMPANION.

Randomized Controlled Trials of Cardiac Resynchronization Therapy in NYHA Class I and II Patients (Table 58.1)

CRT studies described earlier in this chapter focused specifically on patients with HFrEF and NYHA Classes III and IV. These studies also provided preliminary data that informed the design of studies that allowed expanded indications to patients with an LVEF between 30% and 35% and NYHA Class I and II HFrEF patients.

The echo data from MIRACLE-ICD suggested a significant improvement in LV remodeling with CRT even in the small cohort of NYHA Class II patients enrolled similar to that seen in the more symptomatic patients in CARE-HF.[10] This finding led to three important trials with CRT in patients with mild HF including the Resynchronization Reverses Remodeling in Systolic Left Ventricular Dysfunction (REVERSE) trial,[11] Multicenter Automatic Defibrillator Implantation Trial with Cardiac Resynchronization Therapy (MADIT-CRT),[12] and Resynchronization/defibrillation for Ambulatory Heart Failure Trial (RAFT).[13]

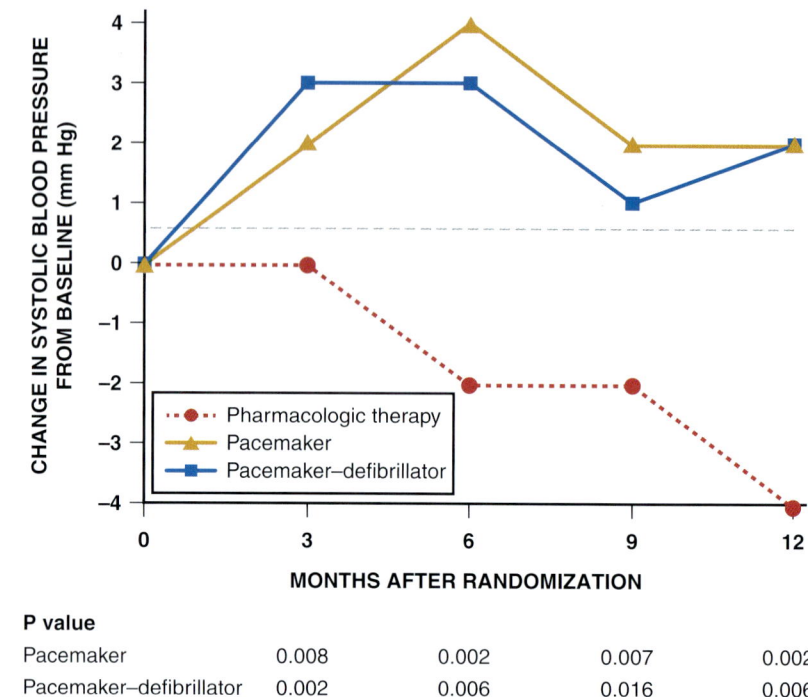

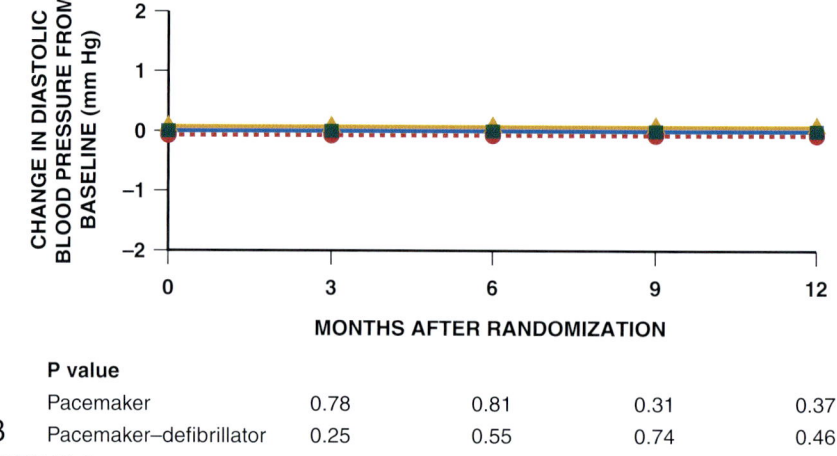

FIGURE 58.1 Median change from baseline in systolic **(A)** and diastolic **(B)** blood pressure at 3, 6, 9, and 12 months in the COMPANION trial. P values are for the comparison with optimal pharmacologic therapy. (Modified from Bristow MR, et al. Cardiac-resynchronization therapy with or without an implantable defibrillator in advanced chronic heart failure. N Engl J Med. 2004;350:2140-2150.)

Resynchronization Reverses Remodeling in Systolic Left Ventricular Dysfunction Trial. The primary endpoint (an HF composite) in REVERSE was not significantly changed but the CRT-on vs. CRT-off group had a greater improvement in measures of LV remodeling.[11] As noted in CARE-HF, the benefits of CRT on remodeling were present irrespective of the presence or dose of beta blockers. Despite the negative primary endpoint, this trial suggested a benefit of CRT on ventricular remodeling in mildly symptomatic HFrEF patients.

Multicenter Automatic Defibrillator Implantation Trial With Cardiac Resynchronization Therapy. The MADIT-CRT trial was an unblinded RCT designed to determine if CRT + primary prevention ICD vs. primary prevention ICD alone reduced the risk of ACM and nonfatal HF events in HFrEF patients with NYHA Class I (ischemic etiology) and NYHA Class II (ischemic or nonischemic etiology) symptoms.[12] The significant reduction in the primary endpoint was due to a reduction in HF events in both the ischemic and nonischemic groups. A subsequent analysis demonstrated that the benefit of CRT was seen only in those with a left bundle branch block (LBBB).[14] A larger benefit of CRT was noted for women (HR = 0.37, CI 0.22 to 0.62) than men (HR = 0.76, CI 0.59 to 0.97, p = 0.01 for interaction) and in patients with a QRS of 150 milliseconds or longer. The MADIT-CRT trial led the FDA to expand the indication for CRT to NYHA Class II or ischemic Class I patients, with LVEF less than 30%, QRS duration longer than 130 milliseconds, and LBBB. MADIT-CRT also demonstrated substantial improvement in ventricular size and function in patients randomized to CRT, with the outcomes benefit directly related to the degree of reverse remodeling.[15]

Initially the RAFT trial included patients in NYHA Class II and III but when the CARE HF trial showed a reduction in mortality for NYHA Class III patients, the protocol was revised to include only patients in Class II.[13] The RAFT trial was the first to show a mortality benefit of combined CRT-ICD over an ICD alone, and a mortality reduction with the addition of CRT in patients in NYHA Class II HF. *The results of REVERSE, MADIT-CRT, and RAFT resulted in the FDA expanding the indication CRT to include patients with mildly symptomatic HF.*

Cardiac Resynchronization Therapy in Patients With Narrow QRS Complex and Mechanical Dyssynchrony. Patients with HFrEF and a

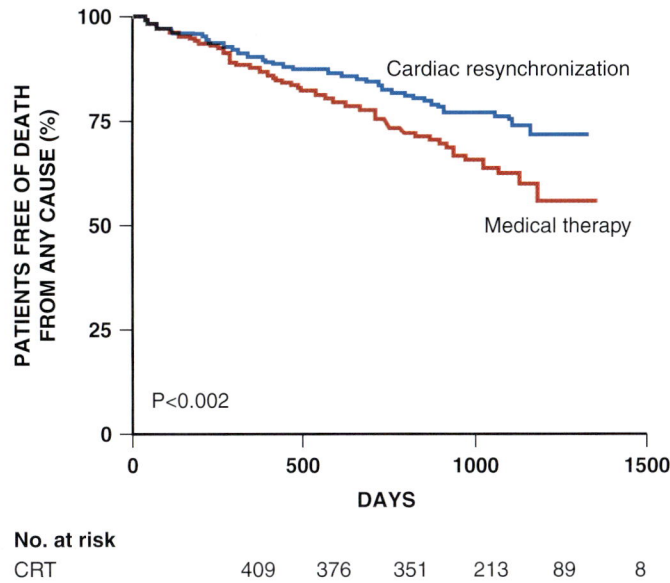

FIGURE 58.2 Kaplan-Meier estimates of survival in patients randomized to cardiac resynchronization therapy (CRT) compared to conventional medical therapy in the CARE-HF trial. (Modified from Cleland JGF, et al. The effect of cardiac resynchronization on morbidity and mortality in heart failure. *N Engl J Med*. 2005;352:1539-1549.)

narrow QRS complex may demonstrate mechanical dyssynchrony using imaging techniques such as echocardiography. Small trials suggested a benefit in these patients but a larger trial, Echocardiography Guided Cardiac Resynchronization Therapy (EchoCRT), did not confirm these benefits.[16] The primary endpoint was not significant, but the secondary endpoint of ACM was higher in the CRT group than in the control group (Table 58.3), demonstrating the potential for harm in using CRT in narrow-QRS patients. Thus CRT is considered contraindicated in these patients.

Patients Requiring Right Ventricular pacing. Early studies of CRT specifically excluded patients with high degrees of atrioventricular block to avoid the confounding effects of right ventricular (RV) pacing with its potential to cause ventricular dyssynchrony.[3] To determine whether CRT might reduce mortality, morbidity, and adverse LV remodeling in patients requiring RV pacing, the Biventricular vs. Right Ventricular Pacing in Heart Failure Patients with Atrioventricular Block (BLOCK HF) study was designed.[17] Patients with standard guideline indications for CRT were excluded. Patients received a CRT and ICD (ICD if the patient had an indication for ICD therapy) and were assigned to standard RV pacing or CRT. Patients randomly assigned to CRT had a significantly lower incidence of the primary outcome than did those assigned to RV pacing (Table 58.2) This led to a guideline recommendation to consider CRT in patients with and LVEF of ≤50% who require RV pacing.

Indications for Cardiac Resynchronization Therapy in Patients with Heart Failure

Although electrical and mechanical dyssynchrony often coexist, CRT guideline recommendations are based on electrical dyssynchrony alone. This recommendation is due to the volume of clinical trial data using QRS duration as an enrollment criterion and the results of the Predictors of Response to CRT (PROSPECT) study.[18] The PROSPECT trial was designed to find echocardiographic or tissue Doppler measures of dyssynchrony that predicted a positive response to CRT by improvement in a clinical composite score or a ≥15% reduction in left ventricular end-systolic volume (LVESV) at 6 months in patients with standard CRT indications. No single measure had adequate sensitivity or specificity to improve patient selection for CRT beyond the current QRS guidelines.

Limitations of Cardiac Resynchronization Therapy

While, overall, RCTs have shown that HFrEF patients derive substantial benefits from CRT, some patients are "nonresponders" and do not have reductions in symptoms or HF hospitalizations and do not achieve LV reverse remodeling. Factors reported to contribute to the nonresponder rate include suboptimal LV lead placement, suboptimal atrioventricular (AV) and ventricular-ventricular (VV) timing, ventricular scar, and HF disease progression.[3] Factors associated with a particularly beneficial (super) response include LBBB, longer QRS duration, female sex, lack of prior myocardial infarction, and smaller left atrial volume.[19] Patients may have a wide range of responses to CRT (or any medical or device therapy) as outlined in Fig. 58.3. Super responders show a large benefit—some as "super" as normalization of ventricular function. Some patients (nonprogressors) do not show a measurable benefit of CRT, but also do not have the predicted worsening HF over time as do nonresponders. Negative responders are those who have clinical worsening of their disease after CRT implantation. A number of advances in CRT pacing are being developed to address the nonresponder rate, including biomarker-guided selection, optimal AV and VV timing, and the use of epicardial and endocardial LV pacing leads.[3]

CRT has been standard therapy for HFrEF for nearly two decades but there are a number of clinical situations for which more data would be valuable. Perhaps the most important of these is the benefit of CRT in patients with atrial fibrillation (AF). Patients with AF were excluded from most of the pivotal trials of CRT but the prevalence of AF is as high as 40% in some HFrEF studies. Because of the lack of strong clinical trial data, the recommendations for CRT in patients with persistent AF with or without AV nodal ablation and RV pacing are weaker than those for similar patients with sinus rhythm. In patients with AF, adequate rate control or AV ablation to allow consistent pacing is important to achieve a response.[20] Another gap in knowledge for CRT is in patients with HF and preserved or mid-range ejection fraction in whom mechanical and electrical dyssynchrony may be present, but no large studies have yet addressed the benefits of CRT in these patients.[21]

SUDDEN CARDIAC DEATH IN CHRONIC HEART FAILURE

Sudden cardiac death (SCD) is a leading cause of mortality in patients with HFrEF and occurs at a rate severalfold higher than in the general population (see also Chapter 70). Given this high rate of SCD, the use of prophylactic ICDs was hypothesized to reduce total mortality in HFrEF. A series of studies performed more than two decades ago have provided proof of this hypothesis.

Randomized Controlled Trials of Implantable-Cardioverter Defibrillators for Primary Prevention of SCD in HFrEF

The most important trials establishing a role for ICDs as primary prevention of mortality in HFrEF patients are the Multicenter Automatic Defibrillator Implantation II Trial (MADIT II),[22] Prophylactic Defibrillator Implantation in Patients with Nonischemic Dilated Cardiomyopathy (DEFINITE),[23] and the Sudden Cardiac Death–Heart Failure Trial (SCD-HeFT).[24] A more recent study, the Danish Study to Assess the Efficacy of ICDs in Patients with Non-ischemic Systolic Heart Failure on Mortality (DANISH) trial, has raised questions regarding the efficacy of prophylactic ICD use in nonischemic HF patients.[25] To allow comparison of these studies their size and design, clinical benefits, baseline medical therapy, and limitations are outlined in Table 58.2, with specific comments in the text that follows.

Multicenter Automatic Defibrillator Implantation II Trial. MADIT II was designed and powered to assess the survival benefit of ICDs in post-MI patients with reduced EF (<30%).[22] The trial was stopped early because of a marked benefit of ICD therapy. Survival benefits of ICD therapy were present in all age groups and NYHA classes.
Prophylactic Defibrillator Implantation in Patients With Nonischemic Dilated Cardiomyopathy Trial. The DEFINITE trial was the first RCT evaluating an ICD for primary prevention of ACM in patients with nonischemic cardiomyopathy.[23] At the time the trial was conducted there were inadequate data regarding the benefit of an ICD

in nonischemic HF patients and previous observations had suggested that prophylactic amiodarone might reduce the risk of SCD in these patients. Although the primary endpoint of ACM was not reduced with an ICD, a post hoc analysis suggested a highly significant reduction in SCD with an ICD. This result was based on SCD in 3 patients in the ICD group and 14 in the control group. The mortality in DEFINITE was lower than in MADIT II, perhaps in part, due to the higher use of angiotensin-converting enzyme inhibitors (ACEIs) and beta blockers. The study was underpowered for ACM but did suggest a strong trend toward a survival advantage based on the expected reduction in SCD for patients receiving an ICD.

Sudden Cardiac Death: Heart Failure Trial. The results of the SCD-HeFT trial have had a substantial impact on current practice guidelines for ICDs.[24] SCD-HeFT randomized patients to three arms—comparing an ICD to amiodarone and placebo in patients with both ischemic and nonischemic causes of HFrEF (Fig. 58.4). Similar degrees of benefit on ACM with an ICD were noted in patients with ischemic and nonischemic HFrEF, confirming the findings of MADIT II and DEFINITE. The neutral results on ACM with amiodarone effectively ended its routine use for primary prevention of SCD in HFrEF. The SCD-HeFT trial provided the most robust evidence to date supporting the prophylactic use of an ICD in patients with NYHA Class II and III HFrEF irrespective of etiology.

Danish Study to Assess the Efficacy of ICDs in Patients with NonIschemic Systolic Heart Failure on Mortality. With improvements in medical therapy that reduce both SCD and death from progressive HF the value of primary prevention ICDs in patients with nonischemic HF has been questioned. The DANISH trial randomized patients with non-ischemic HFrEF to usual clinical care vs. usual care plus an ICD. Fifty-eight percent of patients in each group received CRT.[25] There was no benefit of primary prevention ICD implantation on ACM in this patient group. However, the secondary endpoint of SCD was significantly reduced in patients in the ICD group. While the results questioned the use of prophylactic ICDs in a nonischemic HFrEF population who had appropriate CRT use, the substantial reduction in SCD, overall, and the decrease in ACM in younger patients have left considerable uncertainty about ICD use in patients with nonischemic HFrEF.

Using older trials for guideline recommendations is increasingly problematic as new medical therapies continue to reduce the risk of both progressive HF death and SCD in HFrEF, potentially reducing the

TABLE 58.2 Pivotal Trials for ICDs for Primary Prevention of SCD

TRIAL (YEAR PUBLISHED)	N	INCLUSION CRITERIA	STUDY DESIGN	% ISCHEMIC	MEAN FOLLOW-UP	PRIMARY ENDPOINT	MORTALITY/YEAR	MEDICAL THERAPY*
MADIT II (2002)	1232	• LVEF ≤30% • Prior MI • ≥1 month post-MI	RCT 3:2 ICD + medical therapy vs. medical therapy	100%	20 mo	ICD + MT vs. MT ACM HR = 0.69 (95% CI, 0.51-0.93; P = 0.016)	ICD 8.5% Control 11.9%	ACEI 68% ARB NR BB 70% MRA NR Dig 57% Diuretics† 72%
DEFINITE (2004)	458	• Nonischemic • LVEF <36% • PVCs or NSVT	RCT ICD + MT vs. MT	0%	29 mo	ICD + MT vs. MT ACMHR = 0.65 (95% CI, 0.40-1.06; P = 0.08) Post hoc analysis of SCD HR = 0.20 (95% CI, 0.06-0.71; P = 0.006) (no. of events = 17)	ICD 3.9% Control 7.0%	ACEI 84% ARB 14% BB 86% MRA NR Dig 42% Diuretics† 87%
SCD-HeFT (2005)	2521	• LVEF ≤35% • NYHA Classes II-II • >3 mo post-HF onset	RCT ICD + MT vs. amiodarone + MT vs. MT	52%	45.5 mo	ACM ICD vs. MT HR = 0.77 (97.5% CI, 0.62-0.96, p = 0.007) Amiodarone + MT vs. MT HR = 0.77 (97.5% CI, 0.86-1.3, P = 0.53)	ICD 5.8% Control 7.6%	ACEI/ARB 94% BB 69% MRA 20%‡+ Dig 67% Loop diuretics 82%
DANISH (2016)	1116	• LVEF ≤35% • NYHA Classes II-II (or IV if CRT planned) • NT-proBNP >200 pg/mL • Nonischemic	RCT ICD + MT vs. MT	0%	67.6 mo	ICD + MT vs. MT ACM HR = 0.87 (95% CI, 0.68-1.12; P = 0.28) Other endpoints CV death HR = 0.77 (95% CI, 0.57-1.05; P = 0.10) SCD HR = 0.50 (95% CI, 0.31-0.82; P = 0.005)	ICD 4.4% Control 5.0%	ACEI/ARB 96% BB 92% MRA 59% Dig NR Loop diuretics NR CRT 58%

*All medical therapy for CRT group.
†All diuretic types.
‡potassium-sparing diuretics (unknown % of MRA)

Abbreviations as for Table 58.1. *ACM*, All-cause mortality; *ACMHR*, all-cause mortality hazard ratio; *ARB*, angiotensin receptor blockers; *BB*, beta blockers; *CRT*, cardiac resynchronization therapy; *CV*, cardiovascular; *HR*, hazard ratio; *ICD*, implantable cardiac defibrillator; *LVEF*, left ventricular ejection fraction; *MI*, myocardial infarction; *MRA*, mineralocorticoid receptor antagonists; *MT*, medical therapy; *NR*, not reported; *NSVT*, nonsustained ventricular tachycardia; *NYHA*, New York Heart Association; *PVCs*, premature ventricular contractions; *RCT*, randomized controlled trial; *SCD*, sudden cardiac death.

absolute benefit of ICDs.[26] While the absolute rate of both SCD and progressive HF increase as NYHA symptom class worsens, the relative risk of SCD is higher in less symptomatic patients. Thus, by improving symptom class, improved medical therapy for HFrEF may shift the relative percentage of deaths to more SCD increasing the potential benefit of ICDs.[3] Indeed recent meta-analyses support the efficacy of ICD use for nonischemic cardiomyopathy, despite the results of the DANISH trial.[27] Furthermore, in a recent analysis of the Prospective Comparison of ARNI (Angiotensin Receptor–Neprilysin Inhibitor) with ACEI (Angiotensin-Converting–Enzyme Inhibitor) to Determine Impact on Global Mortality and Morbidity in HF Trial (PARADIGM-HF), ICD use was associated with lower rates of SCD, regardless of HFrEF etiology.[28] Thus it is unlikely that current guideline recommendations for ICDs will change, despite the results of the DANISH trial.

GUIDELINES FOR CARDIAC RESYNCHRONIZATION AND IMPLANTABLE CARDIOVERTER-DEFIBRILLATORS IN HEART FAILURE WITH A REDUCED EJECTION FRACTION

The American College of Cardiology, American Heart Association, and Heart Rhythm Society (ACC/AHA/HRS) 2012 guidelines for device-based therapy of cardiac rhythm abnormalities,[29] and 2017 guidelines for management of patients with ventricular arrhythmias and the prevention of sudden cardiac death,[30] and the 2017 AHA/ACC/HFSA Heart Failure Guidelines[31] provide the most recent recommendations for CRT and ICD therapies. The only Class I recommendation for CRT is for patients with LVEF ≤35%, LBBB with QRS duration of ≥150 msec, sinus rhythm, NYHA Class II, III, or ambulatory Class IV, and receiving GDMT. The only Class I indication for primary prevention ICD is for patients with HFrEF at least 40 days post-MI with LVEF <35%, NYHA Class II or II, and receiving GDMT. There are a number of Class II recommendations.[29-31]

NEW IMPLANTABLE THERAPEUTIC DEVICES FOR HEART FAILURE (TABLE 58.3)

Abnormal myocardial contractility often leads to HF resulting in a number of secondary manifestations including neurohormonal activation, autonomic imbalance, arrhythmias, ventricular dyssynchrony, myocardial remodeling, secondary mitral regurgitation (SMR), and sleep disordered breathing. These manifestations generally become more common and more severe as HF progresses. Device therapy has been instrumental in filling gaps in treatment for some of these manifestations that were only partially addressed or not addressed at all with medical therapy. For example, CRT improves myocardial dyssynchrony still present after GDMT and ICDs treat the ventricular arrhythmias that still occur despite GDMT in HFrEF patients. More recently, devices have been developed to reduce episodes of central sleep

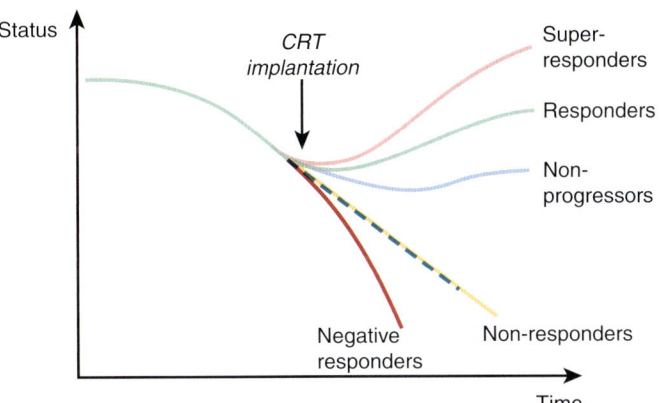

FIGURE 58.3 Possible clinical courses after CRT implantation. Responders show a measurable effect, whereas superresponders show excellent response up to normalization after CRT implantation. Nonprogressors do not show a benefit of CRT, but also do not follow their predicted natural course of deterioration as a result of chronic heart failure (*dashed line*) like nonresponders. Negative responders demonstrate clinical worsening of their disease after CRT implantation. *CRT,* cardiac resynchronization therapy. (From Steffel J, Ruschitzka F. Superresponse to cardiac resynchronization therapy. Circulation. 2014;130:87-90.)

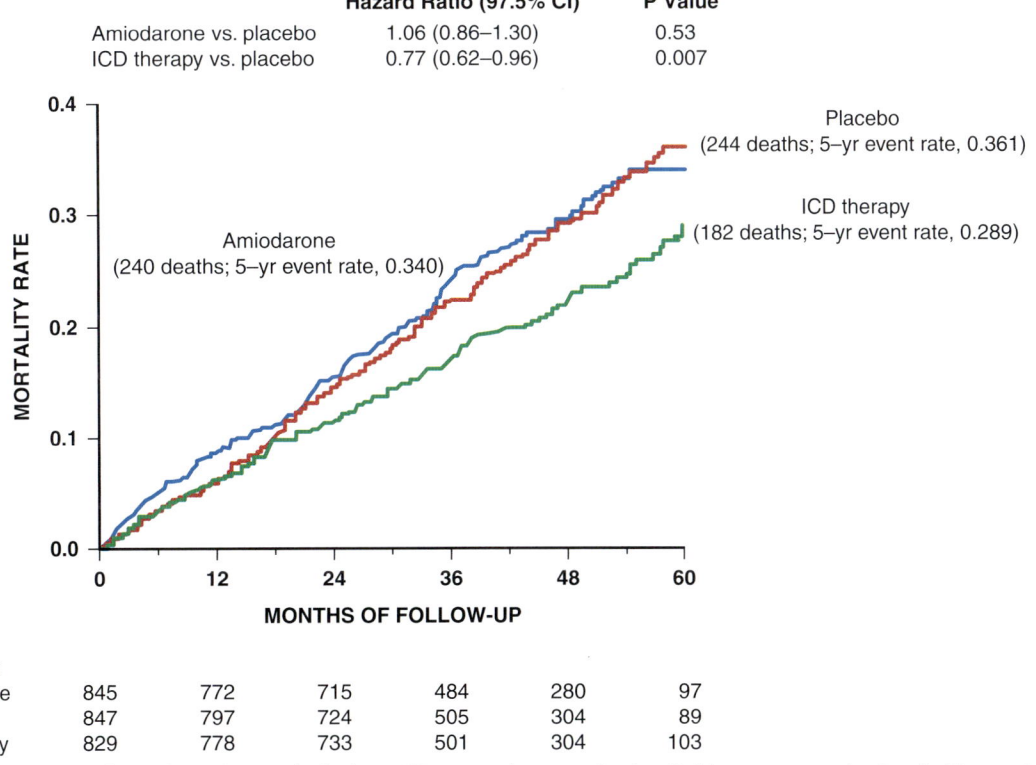

FIGURE 58.4 Kaplan-Meier estimates of survival in patients randomized to an ICD compared to conventional medical therapy or conventional medical therapy plus amiodarone in the SCD-HeFT trial. (Modified from Bardy GH, et al. Amiodarone or an implantable cardioverter-defibrillator for congestive heart failure. *N Engl J Med.* 2005;352:225-237.)

apnea, reduce SMR, improve myocardial contractility, and restore autonomic imbalance in HFrEF patients. The pivotal clinical trials for new approved therapeutic devices for HFrEF include the Remede System Pivotal Study,[32] the Cardiovascular Outcomes Assessment of the MitraClip Percutaneous Therapy for Heart Failure Patients with Functional Mitral Regurgitation (COAPT) trial,[33] the Evaluate Safety and Efficacy of the OPTIMIZER System in Subjects with Moderate-to Severe Heart Failure (FIX-HF-5C),[34] and the BAROSTIM NEO-Baroreceptor Activation Therapy for Heart Failure (BEAT-HF) trial.[35]

Central Sleep Apnea

Both obstructive sleep apnea and CSA are common even in optimally medically managed patients with HFrEF and are associated with worse symptoms and increased mortality.[36] The Remede system was designed to avert episodes of CSA by direct stimulation of the phrenic nerve via a transvenous lead in either the left pericardiophrenic or right brachiocephalic vein connected to a pulse generator. The device is programmed to deliver stimulation during sleep, thereby preventing episodes of CSA. The Remede System Pivotal Study enrolled 151 subjects, 96 of whom had NYHA Class I-IV HF.[32] At 6 months, the device "on" group was more likely to have a ≥50% reduction in Apnea-Hypopnea Index (AHI) from baseline (51% vs. 11%). The Remede system (Respicardia, Minnetonka, MN) was FDA approved in 2017 for the treatment of moderate to severe CSA in adult patients. The device does not have a specific guideline indication for HF and it remains uncertain if CSA should be routinely treated in patients with HFrEF because of concern generated by the Adaptive Servo-Ventilation for Central Sleep Apnea in Systolic HF (SERVE-HF) trial.[37] The SERVE-HF trial randomized 1625 subjects with HFrEF and predominantly CSA to adaptive servo-ventilation (ASV) or control. ASV had no significant effect on the primary endpoint, time to the first event of death from any cause, lifesaving cardiovascular intervention, or unplanned hospitalization for worsening HF, but all-cause and cardiovascular mortality were both increased with ASV. The increase in mortality was due to an increase in cardiovascular death without a preceding hospitalization for worsening HF.[38] Thus additional data are necessary to determine if the excess mortality seen in SERVE-HF in patients with HFrEF and CSA was due to the treatment modality (ASV) or the reduction in CSA.

Transcatheter Mitral Valve Repair Secondary (Functional) Mitral Regurgitation

SMR is associated with a poor prognosis in patients with HFrEF.[39] Two recent trials, Cardiovascular Outcomes Assessment of the MitraClip Percutaneous Therapy for HF Patients with Functional Mitral Regurgitation (COAPT)[33] and Percutaneous Repair with the MitraClip Device for Severe Functional/Secondary Mitral Regurgitation (MITRA-FR)[40] evaluated the role of transcatheter edge to edge repair (TEER) of the mitral valve in patients with HFrEF and moderately severe to severe SMR and demonstrated markedly differently results, with COAPT demonstrating a large benefit on HFH and ACM and MITRA-FR demonstrating no benefit. (See also Chapter 78.) The explanation for these disparate results remains a source of considerable discussion. However, in 2019, the FDA approved the MitraClip (Abbott, Menlo Park, CA) device for repair of moderately severe to severe SMR in patients with symptomatic HF and an LVEF of 20% to 50% despite optimally titrated (GDMT based on the results of the COAPT trial). The 2020 ACC/AHA Valvular Heart Disease Guidelines have a new IIa recommendation for TEER of the mitral valve in patients with chronic severe secondary MR related to LV systolic dysfunction and symptomatic HF who meet the inclusion criteria of the COAPT trial.[41]

Cardiac Contractility Modulation

Myocardial contractility is impaired in patients with HFrEF despite optimal GDMT. Cardiac contractility modulation (CCM) uses the Optimizer Smart System (Impulse Dynamics, Stuttgart, Germany), which includes an implantable pulse generator (IPG), one atrial and two ventricular leads, a programmer, and a transcutaneous charger.[42] The IPG stimulates the ventricular myocardium with high-voltage, nonexcitatory (does not stimulate contraction) impulses to improve myocardial contractility.[42] The precise molecular mechanism by which CCM improves contractility is uncertain but does appear to be associated with improved myocardial calcium handling.[42] The FIX-HF-5C trial combined patients from a similar previous trial (FIX-HF-5) and 160 new subjects with an LVEF ≥25% and ≤45%, NYHA Class III or IV symptoms, QRS duration <130 msec, and normal sinus rhythm with[34,43] (Table 58.3). The difference in peak VO2 favored the CCM group, as did all the secondary endpoints (Table 58.3). The FDA approved the Optimizer Smart System) in with the indications outlined in Table 58.3. There are no current guideline recommendations for CCM.

Baroreflex Activation Therapy

HF is associated with autonomic imbalance—enhanced activation of the sympathetic nervous system and decreased parasympathetic activity—that results in increased heart rate and blood pressure, myocardial remodeling, decreased diuresis and enhanced renin secretion as well as increased morbidity and mortality.[44] Baroreflex activation therapy (BAT) is designed to restore this autonomic imbalance by inhibiting the sympathetic system and activating the parasympathetic system by electrically stimulating the baroreceptors in the carotid sinus.

The BAROSTIM NEO system (CVRx, Inc., Minneapolis, MN), consists of a pulse generator and a carotid sinus lead implanted surgically to deliver BAT. In a randomized, open-label phase II trial of 146 subjects with NYHA Class III and an LVEF of ≤35% comparing GDMT alone to GDMT + BAT, each of the three primary endpoints—6MHWD, QoL, and NT-pro BNP—was improved in the BAT group.[45] The benefits were most prominent in the subgroup of patients without CRT.[46] Thus CRT was an exclusion in the subsequent phase III BEAT-HF trial. Initial results demonstrated significant improvements in QoL and 6MHW distance but not NT pro-BNP at 6 months.[35] However, patients with an NT-proBNP <1600 pg/mL benefitted significantly from BAT. Thus, an additional cohort of patients enrolled concurrently, with the same inclusion criteria, and a requirement for an NT-proBNP <1600 pg/mL were analyzed. Combining this cohort with the subjects in the early cohort with NT-proBNP <1600 pg/mL (n = 246 patients) resulted in a highly statistically significant benefit of BAT for all three endpoints (Table 58.3). These beneficial changes occurred despite a disproportionately increased use of ACEI/ARB, beta blockers, and MRAs during the 6-month study period in the GDMT alone group.[35] Based on the totality of data, BAT was approved by the FDA on August 16, 2019. The BEAT-HF trial was the first trial designed under the FDA expedited access pathway for premarket approval of devices and has a planned postmarket phase (now fully enrolled) to expand the indication to reduction of HF hospitalizations and cardiovascular mortality.[47]

IMPLANTABLE DEVICES TO MONITOR HEART FAILURE

Device-Based Heart Failure Diagnostics

Despite advances in medical and device therapy for HFrEF, HFH and mortality remain high. In addition, no therapies have been developed for HFpEF that have been shown to definitely reduce HFH and mortality.[48] The cost of care for HF in the United States is expected to double by 2030, with HFH accounting for 80% of the costs, thus there is intense interest in reducing HFH to both reduce societal costs of HF and improve QoL for patients.[48] Studies using changes in heart rate, blood pressure, body weight, and symptoms or any combination of these parameters to predict an HF exacerbation and guide therapies that prevent HFH have had inconsistent success. There are several potential reasons for these disappointing results. Some of these metrics are relatively insensitive in predicting an HF exacerbation, some become abnormal only late in the course of HF decompensation, and some are difficult to assess in a continuous and remote fashion.[49] These issues led to the search for physiologic parameters that might be more sensitive and specific in predicting HFH. Many implantable CRT, ICD, and pacemaker devices can now record and transmit individual

TABLE 58.3 Pivotal Trials of New Therapeutic Devices for Heart Failure

TRIAL (YEAR PUBLISHED)	N	THERAPEUTIC TARGET	INCLUSION CRITERIA	STUDY DESIGN	PRIMARY ENDPOINT	FDA APPROVAL DATE AND INDICATION	MEDICAL THERAPY[†]
Remede System Pivotal Study (2016)	151 (96 with HF)	Central sleep apnea	AHI of ≥ 20 central sleep apnea events per hour with central sleep apneas ≥ 50% of all apneas	RCT Neurostimulation vs. no neurostimulation	% of patients with a reduction in AHI of ≥50% from baseline to 6 mo Neurostimulation vs. no neurostimulation 51 vs. 11% (CI = 25-54, $p < 0.001$)	10.6.2017 Remede System Indicated for the treatment of moderate to severe central sleep apnea in adult patients	NR
COAPT (2018)	614	Secondary mitral regurgitation	• LVEF 20%-50% • 3-4 + MR • NYHA Class II-IVa • LVESD ≤70 mm	RCT MitraClip + optimal GDMT vs. optimal GDMT alone	Freedom from all HFH for 24 mo HR = 0.53 (95% CI = 0.40-0.70, $p < 0.001$)	3.14.2019 MitraClip NT and NTR/XTR Delivery System: for the treatment of symptomatic, moderate-to-severe secondary MR in patients with LVEF 20%-50% and LVESD ≤70 mm	ACEI/ARB/ARNI 72% BB 91% MRA 51% Diuretics 89%
FIX-HF-5C (2018)	160*	Myocardial contractility	• LVEF 25%-45% • NYHA Classes III-IV • NSR • QRS<130 msec • No CRT indication	RCT Cardiac contractility modulation (CCM) vs. control	CCM vs. control Peak V_{O_2} +0.84 mL O_2/kg/min (0.12-1.55) (posterior probability of 0.989) Secondary endpoint of 6MHWD and QoL also improved	3.21.2019 Optimizer Smart system: to improve 6MHWD, QoL, and functional status of NYHA Class III HF patients who remain symptomatic despite GDMT, are in normal sinus rhythm, and not indicated for CRT and have an LVEF of 25%-45%	NR
BEAT-HF (2020)	408	Autonomic imbalance	• LVEF ≤35% • NYHA Class III or II (if recent III) • QRS<130 msec • No CRT indication	RCT Baroreflex activation therapy (BAT) vs. control	BAT vs. control All three of following must be significant: QoL −14.1 (95% CI = −19 to −9, $p < 0.001$) 6MHWD +60 m (95% CI = 40-80 m, $p < 0.001$) NT-proBNP −25% (95% CI = −38 to −9, $p = 0.004$)	8.16.2019 BAROSTIM NEO system: For the improvement of symptoms of HF-QoL, 6MHWD, and functional status (NYHA) for patients who are in NYHA Class III or Class II (if recent Class III) have an LVEF ≤35%, an NT-proBNP < 1600 pg/mL, and no indication for CRT	ACEI/ARB/ARNI 88% BB 95% MRA 48% Diuretics 85%

*30% borrowing from FIX-HF-5.
[†]All diuretic types.

ACEI, Angiotensin converting enzyme inhibitors; ARB, angiotensin receptor blockers; BB, beta blockers; HF, heart failure; CCM, cardiac contractility modulation; GDMT, guideline-directed medical therapy; HFH, heart failure hospitalization; HR, hazard ratio; LVEF, left ventricular ejection fraction; LVESD, left ventricular end systolic diameter; MRA, mineralocorticoid receptor antagonists; NT-proBNP, brain natriuretic peptide; NYHA, New York Heart Association; QoL, quality of life; RCT, randomized controlled trial.

physiologic parameters including atrial and ventricular heart rate and rhythm, patient activity level, heart rate variability, and intrathoracic impedance, a measure of lung water. Some devices also record measurements of respiratory activity such as rapid shallow breathing, respiratory rate, and tidal volume as well as the presence and intensity of third and fourth heart sounds.[50] Some of these metrics, alone or combined in a predictive model, change in the days to weeks prior to an HFH and predict the likelihood of an impending HFH allowing time for an intervention to reverse the decompensation and prevent an HFH.[49-51] In addition to monitoring individual device-based HF diagnostic parameters, algorithms based on combined parameters can stratify patients into subgroups of high risk, medium risk, and low risk for HFH.[50] These metrics can be measured remotely and be transmitted to secure networks for monitoring by providers. Several of these multisensor, multiparameter, integrated, diagnostic risk scores have been validated and approved by the FDA including HeartLogic (Boston Scientific) and TriageHF (Medtronic). However, to date, randomized trials in which providers use individual monitoring parameters or algorithms combining multiple parameters to guide therapy have not consistently led to a reduction in HFH or mortality.[52-54]

Ventricular Filling Pressures as a Target for Monitoring

Data using an implantable right ventricular pressure monitor that provides an estimate of diastolic pulmonary artery pressure (PAP) has shown that one of the earliest and most consistent changes prior to an HF exacerbation is an increase in estimated diastolic PAP that closely reflects the increase in pulmonary capillary wedge pressure (PCWP).[55] Estimated diastolic PAP most often rises gradually, generally preceding symptoms and HFH by days to weeks[55] (Fig. 58.5A). While these changes in PAP are generally small, they are accurately measured by implantable devices, are similar in patients with HFrEF and HFpEF, and are not consistently associated with changes in body weight.[55] Algorithms based on multisensors have demonstrated a similar timeline prior to an HF exacerbation (Fig. 58.5B).[50] Both high baseline estimated diastolic PAP and an increase in estimated diastolic PAP are associated with increased HFH and increased mortality.[56] These data stimulated the development of implantable devices to directly measure PAP and the design of a large RCT using direct PAP monitoring.

Implantable Hemodynamic Monitors

The CardioMEMS Heart Sensor Allows Monitoring of Pressure to Improve Outcomes in NYHA Class III Heart Failure Patients (CHAMPION) trial evaluated the use of the CardioMEMS heart sensor—a device implanted in a small pulmonary artery that records high-fidelity pulmonary artery pressures that are downloaded and transmitted intermittently. The CHAMPION trial randomized HF patients with the implanted device, regardless of LVEF, to two groups: one in which clinicians were able to view PAP and respond according to a suggested algorithm or to standard of care alone without access to PAP.[57] The CHAMPION trial differed from prior studies of implantable hemodynamic monitors in that specific pressure targets and treatment algorithms were suggested by protocol to ensure adequate testing of the hypothesis. The primary endpoint of the trial was the rate of HFH over 6 months, and long-term outcomes were also prospectively evaluated. Over a 6-month period, significantly fewer HFH occurred in the treatment group (83) than in the control group (120). During the entire single-blinded follow-up averaging 15 months, the treatment group had a 37% RRR in HF hospitalizations compared with the control group

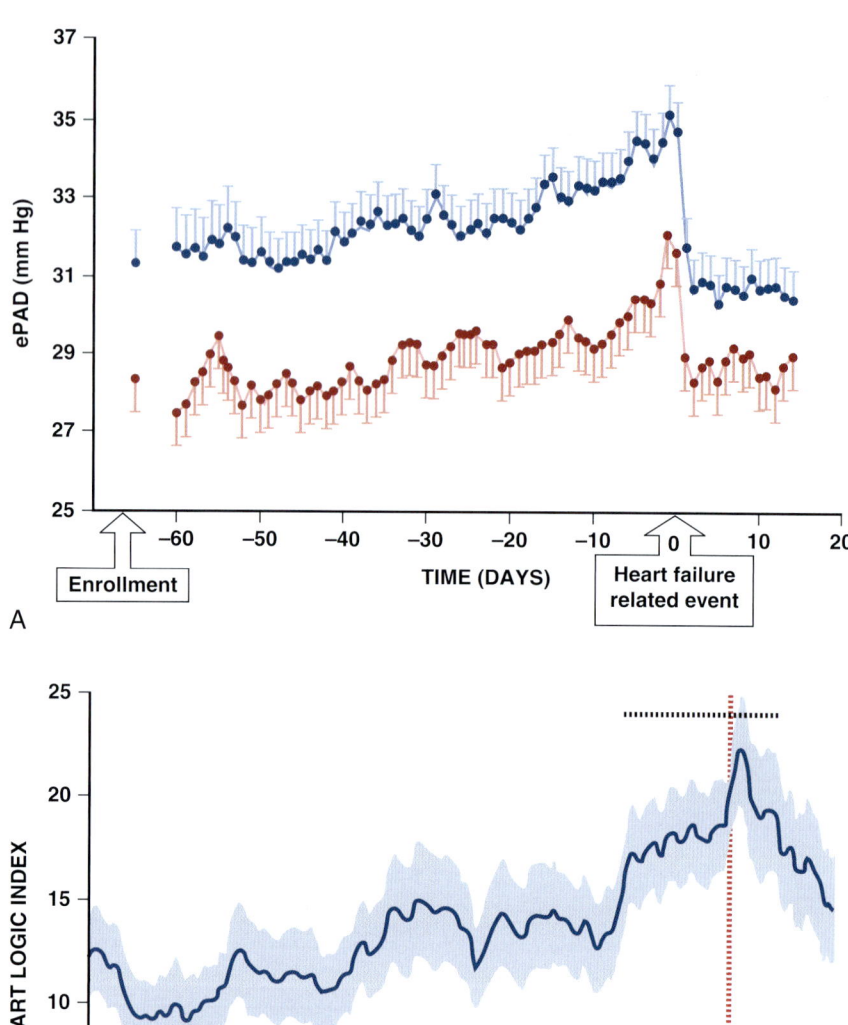

FIGURE 58.5 A, Daily median implantable hemodynamic monitor (IHM)-derived pressures (ePAD) in patients who experienced a heart failure related event (HFRE). Trends in daily median estimated pulmonary artery diastolic pressures (ePAD) are shown beginning 60 days before a hypervolemic HFRE and continuing for 14 days after the event. Systolic HF patients are represented by blue circles and diastolic HF patients by red circles. **B,** Temporal profile of HeartLogic index trends in patients with and without heart failure events. Data are displayed as mean ± SEM. The shaded regions represent the SEM. HeartLogic index in patients with usable HFE (*blue line*) aligned by the date of the HFE (*vertical line*) at day 0; HeartLogic index in patients without HFE (*black line*) aligned by the last available HeartLogic index date for each patient (day 30). (**A** from Zile MR, et al. Transition from chronic compensated to acute decompensated heart failure: pathophysiological insights obtained from continuous monitoring of intracardiac pressures. *Circulation.* 2008;118:1433-1441; **B** from Boehmer JP, et al. A multisensor algorithm predicts heart failure events in patients with implanted devices: results from the MultiSENSE study. *JACC Heart Fail.* 2017;5:216-225.)

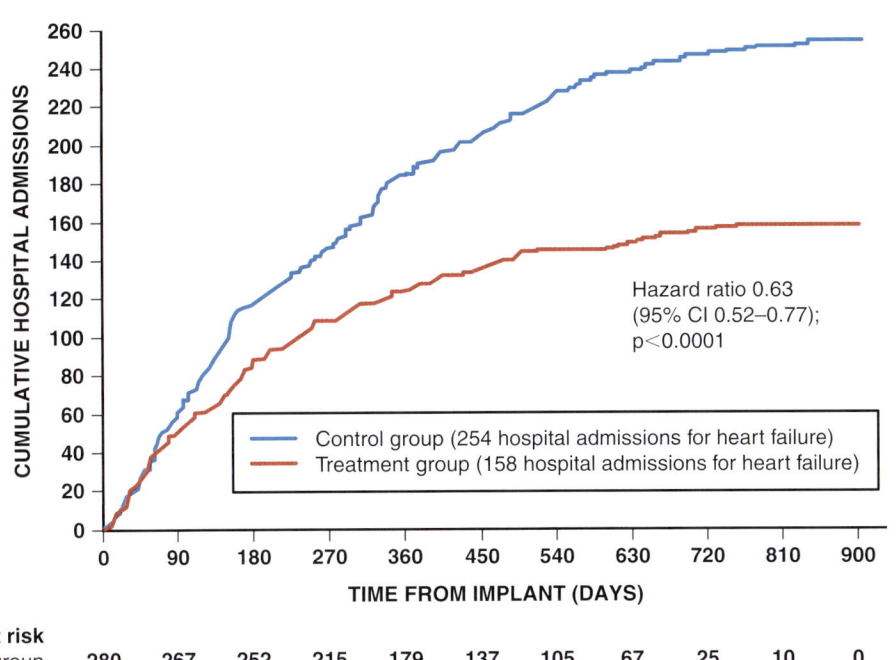

FIGURE 58.6 Primary (6-month) and extended results of the CHAMPION trial for the primary endpoint of heart failure (HF) hospitalization rate. (Modified from Abraham WT, et al. Wireless pulmonary artery haemodynamic monitoring in chronic heart failure: a randomised controlled trial. *Lancet.* 2011;377:658-666.)

($p < 0.001$) (Fig. 58.6). Twice as many medication changes occurred in the actively monitored group and two-thirds of these changes were increases in medication doses while one-third were decreases.[58] The majority of pressure-based medication changes (≈75%), as expected, were diuretics. All four prespecified secondary endpoints were met favoring the treatment group, including PAP reduction, proportion of patients hospitalized for HF, days alive and out of the hospital for HF, and QoL score. Importantly, all results mentioned above were statistically significant in both the HFrEF and HFpEF patients; in fact, the highest reduction in HFH (52%) occurred in the HFpEF subgroup, which composed 22% of the patients studied.

The results of the CHAMPION trial led to FDA approval of the first implantable hemodynamic monitoring system in 2014, for use in HFrEF and HFpEF patients with NYHA Class III symptoms and a history of HF hospitalization within the previous year. The CHAMPION trial confirmed previous data that higher baseline estimated diastolic PAP predicts mortality and increases in PAP from baseline in PAP are also associated with increased mortality.[55]

Building on the results of this trial, the Hemodynamic-GUIDEd Management of Heart Failure (GUIDE-HF) Trial was designed. GUIDE-HF is a multicenter, trial consisting of a fully enrolled, double-blind, randomized arm ($n = 1000$) and a larger unblinded, unrandomized arm that is still enrolling.[59] In the randomized arm, patients with both NYHA Class II to IV, HFrEF or HFpEF and either or both a previous HFH or elevated BNP or NT-proBNP level underwent device implantation and then were randomized 1:1 to either PAP-guided therapy vs. no PAP guided therapy (control) for 12 months. The primary endpoint is ACM + HFH and is scheduled to be reported in 2021. Other implantable hemodynamic monitors are currently in development. Current AHA/ACC/HFSA guidelines do not include a recommendation for PAP monitoring.

INTERPLAY BETWEEN DRUGS AND DEVICES

As new medical and device therapies for HF are developed it will be important to refine and standardize definitions of response in order to initiate or continue therapies in likely "responders" (see Fig. 58.3). As HFrEF is generally a progressive disease, nonprogression may be a favorable response in some patients.[19] Further, it will be necessary to understand the interplay and potential synergies of drugs and devices. For example, CRT raises the systolic blood pressure, creating opportunity to either maintain or further uptitrate medical therapies that were limited by hypotension pre-CRT[8,9,60] (see Fig. 58.1). In the MADIT-CRT trial the greater degree of myocardial remodeling in the CRT group the more likely it was for patients to remain on either an ACEI or angiotensin receptor blocker (ARB) and/or to reduce diuretic doses or avoid diuretics entirely.[61] The ability to continue ACEI/ARBs and/or avoid diuretic escalation with CRT were both associated with a lower risk of ACM + HFH.[61] Furthermore, in a study of 650 patients who were on maximally tolerated GDMT prior to CRT, post-CRT uptitration of ACEI/ARB and beta blockers was possible in 45% and 57%, respectively.[62] Successful uptitration of either therapy was associated with a large reduction in ACM + HFH, a finding confirmed in another large observational trial.[63] It is, however, possible that the ability to uptitrate medical therapy following CRT is a marker of a group with better outcomes rather than the result of uptitration of medical therapy.

There is also an intriguing possibility that medical therapy may enhance the response to device therapies. A retrospective analysis of the COMPANION trial suggested that the relative benefit of CRT was larger with the addition of each of three classes of neurohormonal antagonists (ACEI/ARB, beta blockers, and MRA).[60] A similar result was suggested from a recent analysis of a CRT registry.[64] Further studies are required to determine whether this is a synergistic effect of CRT and medical therapies or if the ability to add or uptitrate medical therapy is a marker for patients who are more responsive to CRT.

Finally, it is important to remember that devices must be monitored to ensure proper functioning. CRT becomes less beneficial and perhaps ineffective as the percentage of pacing falls below 95%.[65] Patients with HFrEF may develop indications for device therapies over time so that candidacy for devices should be reconsidered at intervals, especially if HF worsens. LBBB appears in about 2.4% of HFrEF patients per year[1] and moderately severe or severe MR in about 3% to 4% per year in HFrEF patients on maximally tolerated GDMT.[36] The development of LBBB and/or significant SMR provides opportunities for CRT and TMVr, respectively, and should be considered in any HFrEF patient, especially in those who have progression of HF.

CONCLUSIONS

Implantable devices for monitoring and managing HF, particularly HFrEF, have become an integral part of standard therapy. Recently, several therapeutic devices have been developed and approved to address important pathophysiologic mechanisms often incompletely addressed by medical therapy. Additional data will inform the most beneficial use of these devices and their potential synergies with medical therapy.

REFERENCES

Dyssynchrony

1. Kristensen SL, Castagno D, Shen L, et al. Prevalence and incidence of intraventricular conduction delays and outcomes in patients with heart failure and reduced ejection fraction: insights from PARADIGM-HF and ATMOSPHERE [published online ahead of print, 2020 Jul 28]. *Eur J Heart Fail.* 2020.
2. Kirk JA, Kass DA. Cellular and molecular aspects of dyssynchrony and resynchronization. *Card Electrophysiol Clin.* 2015:585–597.
3. Hussein AA, Wilkoff BL. Cardiac implantable electronic device therapy in heart failure. *Circ Res.* 2019;124:1584–1597.

Randomized Controlled Trials of Cardiac Resynchronization Therapy

4. Cazeau S, Leclercq C, Lavergne T, et al. Effects of multisite biventricular pacing in patients with heart failure and intraventricular conduction delay. *N Engl J Med.* 2001;344(12):873–880.
5. Abraham WT, Fisher WG, Smith AL, MIRACLE Study Group, et al. Multicenter InSync randomized clinical evaluation. Cardiac resynchronization in chronic heart failure. *N Engl J Med.* 2002;346:1845–1853.
6. Young JB, Abraham WT, Smith AL, et al. Combined cardiac resynchronization and implantable cardioversion defibrillation in advanced chronic heart failure: the MIRACLE ICD Trial. *J Am Med Assoc.* 2003;289:2685–2694.
7. Higgins SL, Hummel JD, Niazi IK, et al. Cardiac resynchronization therapy for the treatment of heart failure in patients with intraventricular conduction delay and malignant ventricular tachyarrhythmias. *J Am Coll Cardiol.* 2003;42:1454–1459.
8. Bristow MR, Saxon LA, Boehmer J, et al. Cardiac-resynchronization therapy with or without an implantable defibrillator in advanced chronic heart failure. *N Engl J Med.* 2004;350:2140–2150.
9. Cleland JG, Daubert JC, Erdmann E, et al. The effect of cardiac resynchronization on morbidity and mortality in heart failure. *N Engl J Med.* 2005;352:1539–1549.
10. Abraham WT, Young JB, León AR, et al. Effects of cardiac resynchronization on disease progression in patients with left ventricular systolic dysfunction, an indication for an implantable cardioverter-defibrillator, and mildly symptomatic chronic heart failure. *Circulation.* 2004;110:2864–2868.
11. Linde C, Abraham WT, Gold MR, et al. Randomized trial of cardiac resynchronization in mildly symptomatic heart failure patients and in asymptomatic patients with left ventricular dysfunction and previous heart failure symptoms. *J Am Coll Cardiol.* 2008;52:1834–1843.
12. Moss AJ, Hall WJ, Cannom DS, et al. Cardiac-resynchronization therapy for the prevention of heart-failure events. *N Engl J Med.* 2009;361:1329–1338.
13. Tang AS, Wells GA, Talajic M, et al. Cardiac-resynchronization therapy for mild-to-moderate heart failure. *N Engl J Med.* 2010;363:2385–2395.
14. Zareba W, Klein H, Cygankiewicz I, et al. Effectiveness of cardiac resynchronization therapy by QRS morphology in the Multicenter Automatic Defibrillator Implantation Trial-Cardiac Resynchronization Therapy (MADIT-CRT). *Circulation.* 2011;123:1061–1072.
15. Solomon SD, Foster E, Bourgoun M, et al. Effect of cardiac resynchronization therapy on reverse remodeling and relation to outcome: multicenter automatic defibrillator implantation trial: cardiac resynchronization therapy. *Circulation.* 2010;122:985–992.
16. Ruschitzka F, Abraham WT, Singh JP, et al. Cardiac-resynchronization therapy in heart failure with a narrow QRS complex. *N Engl J Med.* 2013;369:1395–1405.
17. Curtis AB, Worley SJ, Adamson PB, Biventricular vs. Right Ventricular Pacing in Heart Failure Patients with Atrioventricular Block (BLOCK HF) Trial Investigators, et al. Biventricular pacing for atrioventricular block and systolic dysfunction. *N Engl J Med.* 2013;368:1585–1593.
18. Chung ES, Leon AR, Tavazzi L, et al. Results of the predictors of response to CRT (PROSPECT) trial. *Circulation.* 2008;117:2608–2616.
19. Steffel J, Ruschitzka F. Superresponse to cardiac resynchronization therapy. *Circulation.* 2014;130(1):87–90.
20. Ruwald MH, Mittal S, Ruwald AC, et al. Association between frequency of atrial and ventricular ectopic beats and biventricular pacing percentage and outcomes in patients with cardiac resynchronization therapy. *J Am Coll Cardiol.* 2014;64:971–981.
21. Friedman DJ, Emerek K, Kisslo J, et al. Left bundle-branch block is associated with asimilar dyssynchronous phenotype in heart failure patients with normal and reduced ejection fractions. *Am Heart J.* 2020;231:45–55.

Primary Prevention of Sudden Cardiac Death

22. Moss AJ, Zareba W, Hall WJ, et al. Prophylactic implantation of a defibrillator in patients with myocardial infarction and reduced ejection fraction. *N Engl J Med.* 2002;346:877–883.
23. Kadish A, Dyer A, Daubert JP, et al. Prophylactic defibrillator implantation in patients with nonischemic dilated cardiomyopathy. *N Engl J Med.* 2004;350:2151–2158.
24. Bardy GH, Lee KL, Mark DB, Sudden Cardiac Death in Heart Failure Trial (SCD-HeFT) Investigators, et al. Amiodarone or an implantable cardioverter-defibrillator for congestive heart failure. *N Engl J Med.* 2005;352:225–237.
25. Køber L, Thune JJ, Nielsen JC, DANISH Investigators, et al. Defibrillator implantation in patients with nonischemic systolic heart failure. *N Engl J Med.* 2016;375:1221–1230.
26. Shen L, Jhund PS, Petrie MC, et al. Declining risk of sudden death in heart failure. *N Engl J Med.* 2017;377:41–51.
27. Shun-Shin MJ, Zheng SL, Cole GD, et al. Implantable cardioverter defibrillators for primary prevention of death in left ventricular dysfunction with and without ischaemic heart disease: a meta-analysis of 8567 patients in the 11 trials. *Eur Heart J.* 2017;38:1738–1746.
28. Rohde LE, Chatterjee NA, Vaduganathan M, et al. Sacubitril/valsartan and sudden cardiac death according to implantable cardioverter-defibrillator use and heart failure cause: a PARADIGM-HF analysis. *JACC Heart Fail.* 2020;8:844–855.

Guidelines

29. Tracy CM, Epstein AE, Darbar D, et al. 2012 ACCF/AHA/HRS focused update of the 2008 guidelines for device-based therapy of cardiac rhythm abnormalities: a report of the American College of Cardiology Foundation/American Heart Association Task Force on Practice Guidelines and the Heart Rhythm Society [corrected]. *Circulation.* 2012;126:1784–1800.
30. Al-Khatib SM, Stevenson WG, Ackerman MJ, et al. 2017 AHA/ACC/HRS guideline for management of patients with ventricular arrhythmias and the prevention of sudden cardiac death: executive summary: a report of the American College of Cardiology/American Heart Association Task Force on Clinical Practice Guidelines and the Heart Rhythm Society. *Heart Rhythm.* 2018;15:e190–e252.
31. Yancy CW, Jessup M, Bozkurt B, et al. 2017 ACC/AHA/HFSA focused update of the 2013 ACCF/AHA guideline for the management of heart failure: a report of the American College of Cardiology/American Heart Association Task Force on Clinical Practice Guidelines and the Heart Failure Society of America. *Circulation.* 2017;136(6):e137–e161.

New Therapeutic Devices for Heart Failure

32. Costanzo MR, Ponikowski P, Javaheri S, et al. Transvenous neurostimulation for central sleep apnoea: a randomised controlled trial. *Lancet.* 2016;388:974–982.
33. Stone GW, Lindenfeld J, Abraham WT, et al. Transcatheter mitral-valve repair in patients with heart failure. *N Engl J Med.* 2018;379:2307–2318.
34. Abraham WT, Kuck KH, Goldsmith RL, et al. A randomized controlled trial to evaluate the safety and efficacy of cardiac contractility modulation. *JACC Heart Fail.* 2018;6(10):874–883.
35. Zile MR, Lindenfeld J, Weaver FA, et al. Baroreflex activation therapy in patients with heart failure with reduced ejection fraction. *J Am Coll Cardiol.* 2020;76(1):1–13.
36. Coats AJS. Monitoring for sleep-disordered breathing in heart failure. *Eur Heart J Suppl.* 2019;21(suppl M):M36–M39.
37. Cowie MR, Woehrle H, Wegscheider K, et al. Adaptive servo–ventilation for central sleep apnea in systolic heart failure. *N Engl J Med.* 2015;373:1095–1105.
38. Eulenburg C, Wegscheider K, Woehrle H, et al. Mechanisms underlying increased mortality risk in patients with heart failure and reduced ejection fraction randomly assigned to adaptive servoventilation in the SERVE-HF study: results of a secondary multistate modelling analysis. *Lancet Respir Med.* 2016;4:873–881.
39. Nasser R, Van Assche L, Vorlat A, et al. Evolution of functional mitral regurgitation and prognosis in medically managed heart failure patients with reduced ejection fraction. *JACC Heart Fail.* 2017;5:652–659.
40. Obadia JF, Messika-Zeitoun D, Leurent G, et al. Percutaneous repair or medical treatment for secondary mitral regurgitation. *N Engl J Med.* 2018;379(24):2297–2306.
41. Otto CM, Nishimura RA, Bonow RO, et al. 2020 ACC/AHA guideline for the management of patients with valvular heart disease: a report of the American College of Cardiology/American Heart Association Joint Committee on Clinical Practice Guidelines. *J Am Coll Cardiol.* 2020;80:S0735–S1097.
42. Campbell CM, Kahwash R, Abraham WT. Optimizer Smart in the treatment of moderate-to-severe chronic heart failure. *Future Cardiol.* 2020;16:13–25.
43. Wiegn P, Chan R, Jost C, et al. Safety, Performance, and efficacy of cardiac contractility modulation delivered by the 2-lead optimizer Smart system: the FIX-HF-5C2 Study. *Circ Heart Fail.* 2020;13.
44. Sobowale CO, Hori Y, Ajijola OA. Neuromodulation therapy in heart failure: combined use of drugs and devices. *J Innov Card Rhythm Manag.* 2020;11(7):4151–4159.
45. Abraham WT, Zile MR, Weaver FA, et al. Baroreflex activation therapy for the treatment of heart failure with a reduced ejection fraction. *JACC Heart Fail.* 2015;3(6):487–496.
46. Zile MR, Abraham WT, Weaver FA, et al. Baroreflex activation therapy for the treatment of heart failure with a reduced ejection fraction: safety and efficacy in patients with and without cardiac resynchronization therapy. *Eur J Heart Fail.* 2015;17:1066–1074.
47. Zile MR, Abraham WT, Lindenfeld J, et al. First granted example of novel FDA trial design under expedited access pathway for premarket approval: BeAT-HF. *Am Heart J.* 2018;204:139–150.

Implantable Devices to Monitor Heart Failure

48. Jackson SL, Tong X, King RJ, et al. National burden of heart failure events in the United States, 2006 to 2014. *Circ Heart Fail.* 2018;11(12):e004873.
49. Abraham WT, Perl L. Implantable hemodynamic monitoring for heart failure patients. *J Am Coll Cardiol.* 2017;70:389–398.
50. Boehmer JP, Hariharan R, Devecchi FG, et al. A multisensor algorithm predicts heart failure events in patients with implanted devices: results from the MultiSENSE study. *JACC Heart Fail.* 2017;5:216–225.
51. Ali O, Hajduczok AG, Boehmer JP. Remote physiologic monitoring for heart failure. *Curr Cardiol Rep.* 2020;22:68.
52. Heist EK, Herre JM, Binkley PF, et al. Analysis of different device-based intrathoracic impedance vectors for detection of heart failure events (from the Detect Fluid Early from Intrathoracic Impedance Monitoring study). *Am J Cardiol.* 2014;114:1249–1256.
53. Morgan JM, Kitt S, Gill J, et al. Remote management of heart failure using implantable electronic devices. *Eur Heart J.* 2017;38(30):2352–2360.
54. Hindricks G, Taborsky M, Glikson M, et al. Implant-based multiparameter telemonitoring of patients with heart failure (IN-TIME): a randomised controlled trial. *Lancet.* 2014;384:583–590.
55. Zile MR, Bennett TD, St John Sutton M, et al. Transition from chronic compensated to acute decompensated heart failure: pathophysiological insights obtained from continuous monitoring of intracardiac pressures. *Circulation.* 2008;118:1433–1441.
56. Zile MR, Bennett TD, El Hajj S, et al. Intracardiac pressures measured using an implantable hemodynamic monitor: relationship to mortality in patients with chronic heart failure. *Circ Heart Fail.* 2017;10:1–9.
57. Abraham WT, Adamson PB, Bourge RC, et al. Wireless pulmonary artery haemodynamic monitoring in chronic heart failure: a randomised controlled trial. *Lancet.* 2011;377:658–666.
58. Costanzo MR, Stevenson LW, Adamson PB, et al. Interventions linked to decreased heart failure hospitalizations during ambulatory pulmonary artery pressure monitoring. *JACC Heart Fail.* 2016;4:333–344.
59. Lindenfeld J, Abraham WT, Maisel A, et al. Hemodynamic-GUIDEd management of Heart Failure (GUIDE-HF). *Am Heart J.* 2019;214:18–27.

Interplay Between Drugs and Devices

60. Bristow MR, Saxon LA, Feldman AM, et al. Lessons learned and insights gained in the design, analysis, and outcomes of the COMPANION trial. *JACC Heart Fail.* 2016;4:521–535.
61. Penn J, Goldenberg I, McNitt S, et al. Changes in drug utilization and outcome with cardiac resynchronization therapy: a MADIT-CRT substudy. *J Card Fail.* 2015l;21:541–547.
62. Martens P, Verbrugge FH, Nijst P, et al. Feasibility and association of neurohumoral blocker up-titration after cardiac resynchronization therapy. *J Card Fail.* 2017;23:597–605.
63. Witt CT, Kronborg MB, Nohr EA, et al. Optimization of heart failure medication after cardiac resynchronization therapy and the impact on long-term survival. *Eur Heart J Cardiovasc Pharmacother.* 2015;1:182–188.
64. Schmidt S, Hürlimann D, Starck CT, et al. Treatment with higher dosages of heart failure medication is associated with improved outcome following cardiac resynchronization therapy. *Eur Heart J.* 2014;35:1051–1060.
65. Ruwald MH, Mittal S, Ruwald AC, et al. Association between frequency of atrial and ventricular ectopic beats and biventricular pacing percentage and outcomes in patients with cardiac resynchronization therapy. *J Am Coll Cardiol.* 2014;64(10):971–981.

59 Mechanical Circulatory Support

KEITH D. AARONSON AND FRANCIS D. PAGANI

INDICATIONS, STRATEGIES, AND DEVICE SELECTION, 1119
Bridge to Recovery, 1119
Bridge to Transplantation, 1120
Destination Therapy, 1120

DESIGN OF VENTRICULAR ASSIST DEVICES, 1122

PATIENT SELECTION, COMORBIDITY, AND TIMING OF INTERVENTION, 1122

Renal Function, 1122
Pulmonary Function and Pulmonary Hypertension, 1123
Hepatic Function, 1123
Right Ventricular Function, 1124
Coagulation, 1124
Other Medical Considerations, 1124

PATIENT OUTCOMES, 1124
Temporary Mechanical Circulatory Support, 1124

Devices Intended for Long-Term Mechanical Circulatory Support, 1127

INTERAGENCY REGISTRY OF MECHANICALLY ASSISTED CIRCULATORY SUPPORT, 1129

FUTURE PERSPECTIVES, 1130

REFERENCES, 1131

Mechanical circulatory support (MCS) devices are mechanical pumps designed to assist or replace the function of the left and/or right ventricle(s) of the heart. Important features that characterize MCS devices include: (1) location of the pumping chamber; (2) ventricle(s) supported by the pump; (3) pumping mechanism; and (4) intended use and duration of support (Table 59.1). Typically, temporary MCS devices, used for days or weeks of support, are *extracorporeal* (or *paracorporeal*) pumps (pump located outside the body), whereas durable devices, used for months to years of support, are implantable (*intracorporeal*) systems.

INDICATIONS, STRATEGIES, AND DEVICE SELECTION

MCS devices are indicated to provide hemodynamic support to patients with cardiogenic shock or symptomatic advanced heart failure (HF) refractory to guideline-directed medical care. The goal of MCS therapy is to provide hemodynamic support to the patient in one of three clinical scenarios: (1) patients with severe but potentially reversible heart dysfunction until native heart function sufficiently recovers to have the MCS device successfully withdrawn for anticipated long-term survival without MCS (i.e., bridge to recovery, BTR); (2) patients with severe and irreversible heart dysfunction who are failing medical therapy, to allow sufficient time for allocation and transplantation of a donor heart (i.e., bridge to heart transplantation, BTT); or (3) patients with severe and irreversible heart dysfunction who are failing medical therapy but not eligible for heart transplantation, for permanent support (i.e., destination therapy [DT]). Candid discussion with each patient about which ventricular assist device (VAD) treatment strategy is being used is both legally and morally essential, allays unreasonable expectations, and improves patient satisfaction. However, that discussion should include the understanding that recipients often move between strategies as their clinical circumstances evolve. The decision to initiate MCS must include an analysis of the intended use and clinical setting, patient variables and conditions, the type of MCS devices available for the selected indication, medical society guidelines for use of the device, and financial considerations.

Bridge to Recovery

BTR refers to the use of MCS devices in patients with acute cardiogenic shock or acute decompensated HF that is refractory to guideline-directed medical therapy. In these clinical scenarios, there is a reasonable expectation that the myocardial injury is reversible and that myocardial function will recover during a short period of temporary MCS; this is generally the default strategy when applying temporary MCS. The use of MCS for BTR is the most common application of MCS in the United States.[1] Examples of reversible forms of myocardial injury are acute myocardial infarction (AMI), acute myocarditis, and postcardiotomy cardiogenic shock resulting from ischemic myocardial stunning. Several types of MCS devices can provide temporary circulatory support in these circumstances, including intra-aortic balloon pumps (IABP) (Fig. 59.1), surgically or percutaneously placed extracorporeal/paracorporeal VADs (Figs. 59.2 to 59.4), and systems for extracorporeal life support (ECLS; Fig. 59.5) (or extracorporeal membrane oxygenation [ECMO]), which can provide both cardiac and pulmonary support. Typically, temporary MCS devices such as the IABP, Impella VAD (Abiomed, Inc., Danvers, MA), or TandemHeart VAD (TandemLife, Inc., Pittsburgh, PA) are placed percutaneously to enable rapid initiation of cardiac support and subsequent ease of removal when cardiac function recovers. Some types of extracorporeal VAD systems (i.e., CentriMag VAD; Abbott Labs, Chicago, IL) require major operative procedures with sternotomy or less-invasive thoracotomy incisions for access and placement of the outflow and inflow cannulas, and more frequently are initiated in the operating room for postcardiotomy HF following failure to wean from cardiopulmonary bypass (CPB; see Fig. 59.2).

The assumption that myocardial injury is reversible may not be accurate, and this may be especially so when the patient presents with significant hemodynamic compromise and significant organ injury. Temporary MCS may be instituted with the expectation of clinical improvement, but the subsequent recognition that myocardial recovery has not occurred and is unlikely to occur despite an extended period of hemodynamic support requires strategic adjustment. In such situations, temporary MCS can be continued as a bridge to placement of a durable, implantable VAD or total artificial heart (TAH; *bridge to bridge* [BTB] application), or continued as a bridge to heart transplantation.[2] The use of temporary MCS devices in this way is not an approved indication for these devices but occasionally may be appropriate because of the inherent difficulties in accurately assessing the potential for myocardial recovery in all clinical settings. Historically, durable, implantable VADs have been the most common form of MCS to provide BTT support. However, recent changes to the United States heart transplant allocation system have given greater relative priority to patients supported with temporary MCS devices, including ECMO, compared to durable, implantable VADs.[2] As a result, there has been a significant change in clinical practice patterns with more patients being bridged to heart transplantation with temporary MCS devices, particularly with IABP counterpulsation support.[2]

As a rule, patients should be excluded from consideration for temporary MCS if myocardial recovery is unlikely and the option of heart transplantation or implantation of a long-term, durable VAD is not feasible. In these clinical scenarios, MCS should not be instituted and is considered futile.

Bridge to Transplantation

The second indication for MCS applies to patients presenting with cardiogenic shock or decompensated advanced HF refractory to guideline directed medical management in whom myocardial function is unlikely to recover (e.g., longstanding ischemic, valvular, or idiopathic cardiomyopathy; severe AMI or myocarditis), and who are considered eligible for heart transplantation. Durable, implantable MCS devices designed for long-term use (months to years) permit untethered patient mobility and discharge from the hospital and are appropriate devices for BTT indication (Figs. 59.6 to 59.8). A major operative procedure, including CPB, is generally required for placement in most patients, although newer, smaller device designs permit less-invasive implant techniques without CPB.[3] These devices are ideally placed in patients with significant symptoms of HF who are either receiving intravenous (IV) inotropes or who are not on inotropes but have limiting symptoms at rest or with minimal activity, and in whom hemodynamics are stable and end-organ function is preserved or slowly deteriorating. Select patients with acutely unstable hemodynamics and compromised organ function may be better served by a bridge to decision (BTD) strategy consisting of temporary MCS, followed by placement of a durable MCS device only for those who respond with improvements in hemodynamics and organ function. Although durable, implantable MCS devices (VADs) are most frequently used in situations of chronic irreversible cardiac dysfunction, recovery of myocardial function may also occur to such a degree to permit removal of the durable MCS device.[4,5] Patients thought to have irreversible dysfunction, but who demonstrate sufficient recovery of cardiac function to permit explant of durable, implantable VADs, are most commonly young patients with short durations of HF and with a nonischemic cause of the HF.[4,5]

Recently, clinical trials evaluating newer durable, implantable MCS devices (left ventricular assist devices [LVADs]) have developed alternative terminology for durable, implantable MCS device use and have used the terms "short-term" support to refer to clinical situations where patients are receiving durable VADs as BTT therapy or BTR and "long-term" support to refer to clinical situations where patients are receiving durable VADs as BTT or DT.[6,7] Although confusing to use the term "short-term support" to refer to an indication for temporary and durable devices, the important message is that the ultimate indication for durable VAD implantation in a significant proportion of patients is unknown at the time of implant and patients may transition to either heart transplantation or DT depending on the clinical course following device implantation. Importantly, the initial intent—BTT or DT—does not appear to have a significant impact on long-term survival with durable VAD therapy.[7]

Destination Therapy

The feasibility of durable, implantable MCS devices to provide long-term support demonstrated through the BTT experience prompted further expansion of indications for durable, implantable MCS devices as a permanent alternative to heart transplantation. DT is the application of durable, implanted MCS in patients with chronic refractory symptoms of advanced HF that result from irreversible forms of either nonischemic or ischemic cardiomyopathy and who are ineligible for heart transplantation. Use of durable, implantable devices that permit

TABLE 59.1 Terminology Describing Characteristics of Mechanical Circulatory Support Devices

Pump Location
Extracorporeal: Pump located outside the body
Paracorporeal: Pump located outside but adjacent to the body
Intracorporeal: Pump implanted within the body
Orthotopic: In the normal position of the heart (TAH)

Ventricle Supported
LV support (LVAD)
RV support (RVAD)
Biventricular support (BiVAD)
Biventricular replacement (TAH)

Intended Use
Short-term: Days to weeks (BTR indication)
1. Patient remains hospitalized
2. Patient tethered to pump
Long-term: Months to years (BTT or DT indication)
1. Patient discharged with untethered, "hands-free" mobility

Pump Mechanism[6,7]
Pulsatile flow, volume displacement with:
1. Pneumatic actuation, *or*
2. Electrical actuation
Continuous-flow rotary pump with *axial design* (flow of blood is along axis of symmetry of pump) *and*
1. Bearing support of impeller (mechanical pivot), *or*
2. Magnetic or hydrodynamic levitation of impeller (bearingless design)
Continuous-flow rotary pump with *centrifugal design* (flow of blood from center to periphery of pump) *and*
1. Bearing support of impeller, *or*
2. Magnetic or hydrodynamic levitation of impeller (bearingless design)

BiVAD, Biventricular assist device; *BTR*, bridge to recovery; *BTT*, bridge to transplantation; *DT*, destination therapy; *LVAD*, left ventricular assist device; *RVAD*, right ventricular assist device; *TAH*, total artificial heart.

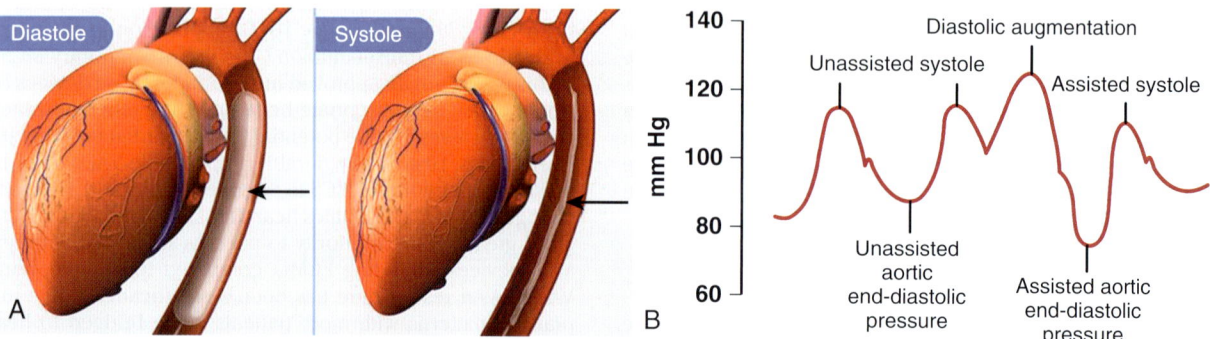

FIGURE 59.1 A, Intra-aortic balloon pump (IABP) positioned in descending aorta and inflated during diastole (increasing diastolic blood pressure and coronary perfusion) and deflated during systole (reducing ventricular afterload). **B,** Aortic pressure tracing during IABP support. Balloon counterpulsation is occurring after every other heartbeat (1:2 counterpulsation). With correct timing, balloon inflation begins immediately after aortic valve closure, signaled by the dicrotic notch of the arterial waveform. Compared with unassisted ejection, the pump augments diastolic blood flow by increasing peak aortic pressure during diastole. Balloon deflation before systole decreases ventricular afterload, with lower aortic end-diastolic pressure and lower peak systolic pressure.

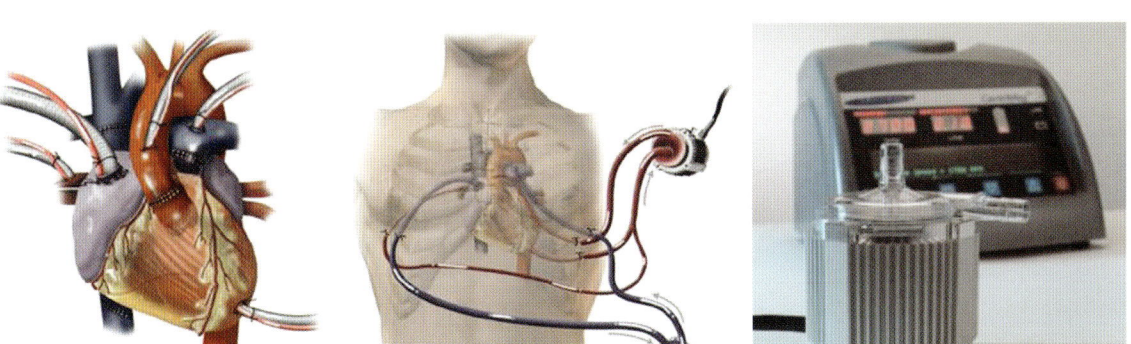

FIGURE 59.2 Temporary extracorporeal mechanical circulatory support: CentriMag Ventricular Assist System (Abbott Labs, Chicago, IL). **A,** Surgically implanted cannula for biventricular support configuration. *Left ventricular support*: A cannula is positioned in the right superior pulmonary vein (cannula depicted on the far left of the picture) and drains blood from the left atrium and pumps it back to the aorta. (Alternative cannula configuration includes a cannula inserted into the left ventricular apex (far bottom right of the figure) draining the left ventricle and returning blood to the cannula positioned in the ascending aorta). *Right ventricular support*: A cannula positioned in the right atrial appendage (second from left) drains blood from the right atrium and pumps it to the main pulmonary artery (cannula in the upper right corner of the figure). **B,** Cannula connected to external blood pumps (extracorporeal pumps) supporting right and left ventricles. **C,** The CentriMag is a continuous-flow rotary pump with centrifugal design and full magnetic levitation of the internal rotor.

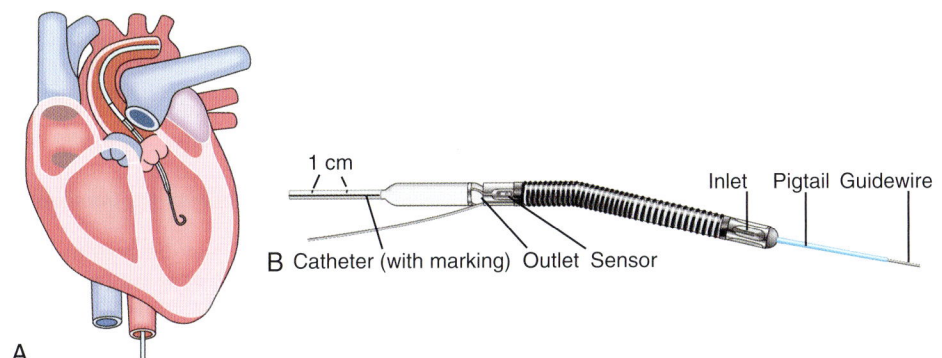

FIGURE 59.3 Temporary mechanical circulatory support: Impella (Abiomed, Inc., Danvers, MA). **A,** The Impella is a continuous-flow, microaxial pump designed to propel blood from the left ventricle into the ascending aorta, in series with the left ventricle. The tip is positioned within the left ventricle, and blood is pumped from the left ventricle into the ascending aorta. **B,** The tip of the catheter is a flexible pigtail loop that stabilizes the device within the left ventricle. The catheter connects to a cannula that contains the pump inlet and outlet areas, motor housing, and pump-pressure monitor. The proximal end of the catheter is connected to the external pump. (From Thunberg CA, Gaitan BD, Arabia FA, et al. Ventricular assist devices today and tomorrow. *J Cardiothorac Vasc Anesth*. 2010;24:656.)

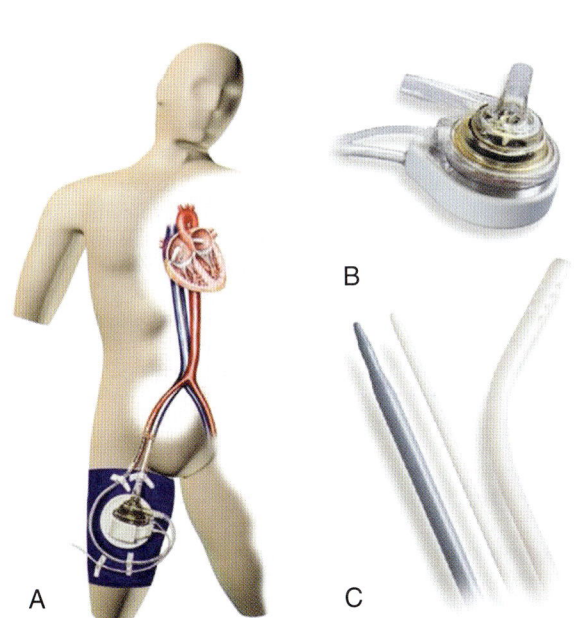

FIGURE 59.4 Temporary mechanical circulatory support: TandemHeart percutaneous ventricular assist device (pVAD) (TandemLife, Inc., Pittsburgh, PA). **A,** The TandemHeart pVAD has four components: a centrifugal pump with hydrodynamic levitation of the internal rotor positioned on the right thigh **(B)**, a 21F transseptal cannula **(C)**, a femoral arterial cannula, and a control console.

untethered "hands-free" patient mobility at home is appropriate in this clinical situation. A major operative procedure is required for placement of these implantable pumps, which, as in the setting of BTT, are ideally used in patients with significant symptoms of advanced HF with stable hemodynamics and without manifestations of significant organ injury, irreversible frailty, or cachexia. The benefits of MCS for DT, in terms of survival, function, and quality of life, for the treatment of chronic advanced HF were first established in a prospective, randomized trial known as REMATCH (Randomized Evaluation of Mechanical Assistance in the Treatment of Congestive Heart Failure).[8] REMATCH evaluated the use of a durable, implantable LVAD compared with optimal medical management (OMM) for refractory chronic advanced HF. LVAD therapy halved (relative risk [RR], 0.52; 95% confidence interval [CI] 0.34 to 0.78) the mortality seen in the control population (92% at 2 years) treated with OMM. Despite serious adverse events (e.g., stroke, infection, bleeding, and device malfunction) attributable to MCS, LVAD recipients experienced a better quality of life than those in the OMM group.

Patients evaluated for DT must meet specific criteria for reimbursement from CMS that include: (1) ineligibility for heart transplantation; (2) significant functional limitations consistent with New York Heart Association (NYHA) Class IIIB or IV symptoms for 45 of the preceding 60 days, despite the use of maximally tolerated doses of drugs outlined in guidelines for HF treatment; (3) left ventricular ejection fraction (LVEF) less than 25%; and (4) a peak exercise oxygen consumption (peak VO_2) of 14 mL/kg/min or less, unless the patient is dependent on IV inotropes for 14 days or IABP for 7 days.[9] Although the current reimbursement framework requires determination of DT or BTT status, it is often not possible when assessing VAD candidacy to accurately determine future transplant eligibility. Many patients present with hemodynamic compromise, significant pulmonary hypertension, organ injury, cachexia, or debilitation, all of which represent relative contraindications to heart transplantation but may be reversible with a period of MCS.

The terms *bridge to candidacy* (BTC) and *bridge to decision* reflect the unknown efficacy of MCS therapy to reverse the clinical conditions that represent relative barriers to heart transplantation. In a similar vein, patients receiving MCS for BTT indication may experience significant

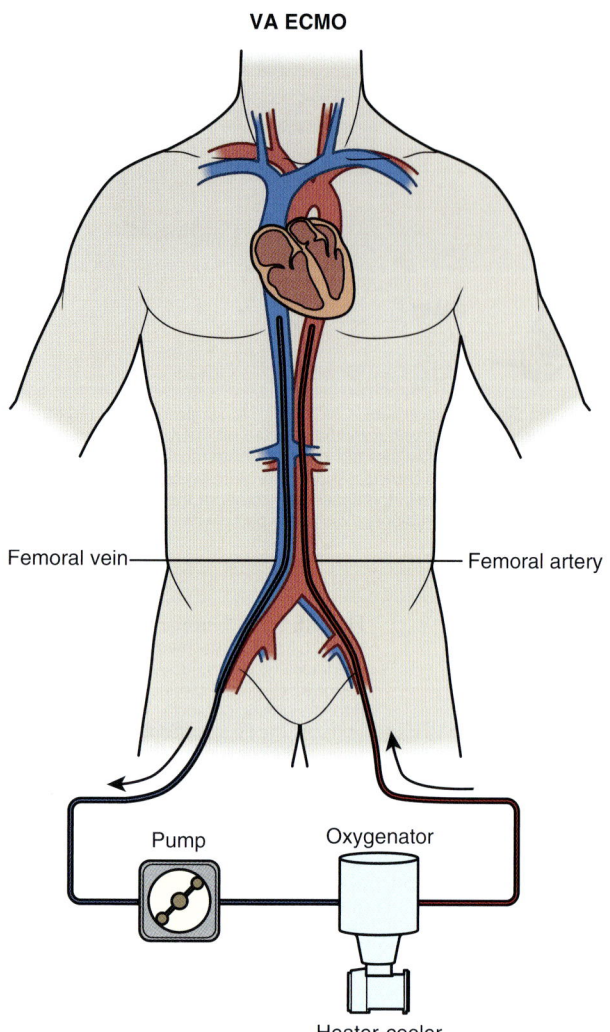

FIGURE 59.5 Extracorporeal life support (ECLS) or extracorporeal membrane oxygenation (ECMO) circuit. The ECMO circuit is used to establish rapid initiation of mechanical circulatory support. The circuit consists of a pump (typically a centrifugal pump system), oxygenator, and heater-cooler element. A typical configuration for emergent application of ECMO is percutaneous placement of cannulas in the femoral vein and femoral artery.

complications after implantation of an MCS device that could adversely affect transplantation candidate status. Recent clinical trials investigating new devices for durable VAD therapy have attempted to reframe VAD candidacy without reference to transplant candidacy by using patient characteristics and physiologic parameters to define an indication for "long-term support."[6,7,10] In the future, this unifying indication of long-term support with coverage determination likely will encompass MCS therapy with durable devices for long-term support independent of transplant eligibility.

DESIGN OF VENTRICULAR ASSIST DEVICES

An MCS pump or pumps may be positioned extracorporeally (outside the body) (see Figs. 59.1 through 59.5) or intracorporeally (contained within the body) (see Figs. 59.6 through 59.9) as a biventricular assist device (BiVAD), a right ventricular assist device (RVAD), or more often as an LVAD. The pump's flow characteristic further classifies pump type as *pulsatile flow* or *continuous flow*. The older generation, pulsatile flow, volume displacement pumps, such as the HeartMate XVE and Novacor LVAS, were large, had limited durability, and are now of only historical interest.[11] Newer-generation continuous-flow pumps are smaller, capable of a similar degree of pumping support (6 to 10 liters per minute [L/min]), more durable, and functionally dependent on both preload and afterload. These include the HeartMate 3 (HM3) (see Fig. 59.6), the HeartMate II (HMII) (see Fig. 59.7), and HeartWare ventricular assist device (HVAD) (see Fig. 59.8).[6,7,10,12–16] The improvements in design attributes of the newest continuous-flow pump (HM3) with centrifugal design, including complete magnetic levitation of the internal rotor, decreased mechanical wear, operation at low flow, and improved potential for hemocompatibility were recently studied in the MOMENTUM 3 (Multi-center Study of MagLev Technology in Patients Undergoing MCS Therapy with HeartMate 3) clinical trial.[6,7,10,16]

PATIENT SELECTION, COMORBIDITY, AND TIMING OF INTERVENTION

Appropriately timing the initiation of MCS is crucial to obtaining satisfactory patient outcomes. There are no absolute hemodynamic criteria to meet to initiate MCS for any indication. Generally, patients presenting with acute forms of myocardial injury exhibit recognizable changes in hemodynamics. A cardiac index less than 1.8 to 2.2 L/min/m^2, systolic blood pressure less than 90 mm Hg, pulmonary capillary wedge pressure (PCWP) greater than 20 mm Hg, and evidence of poor tissue perfusion, reflected by oliguria, rising serum creatinine, arterial lactate, and liver transaminases, mental status changes, or cool extremities, despite the use of guideline directed medical therapy, constitute general indications for initiation of MCS.[17–19] Patient history and overall clinical setting also need to be considered in the decision. When the patient's clinical status reaches this degree of hemodynamic compromise, the risk of death is substantial, exceeding more than 50% at 30 days, despite the availability of OMM, invasive circulatory monitoring, thrombolysis, and IABP support.[17–19]

More subtle indications to initiate MCS may be present, particularly in patients with chronic advanced HF who are being evaluated for BTT or DT. These indications include resting tachycardia, progressive organ dysfunction, and persistent significant HF symptoms resulting in limited functional capacity and poor quality of life despite guideline directed medical therapy, with or without inotrope use.[20,21] In chronic HF patients who had previously maintained good end-organ function and functional performance despite substantially compromised hemodynamics, deterioration in end-organ function or progressive decline in functional performance may occur in the absence of any significant change in hemodynamic parameters.[22] Ambulatory patients with NYHA Class IIIB or IV symptoms who do not tolerate guideline directed medical therapy for advanced HF, or who experience renal insufficiency or hypotension with optimal dosages of angiotensin-converting enzyme (ACE) inhibitors or beta blockers, may need evaluation for MCS therapy.[22] Patients who require inotrope therapy or who do not tolerate inotrope therapy as a result of refractory ventricular arrhythmias, or those who have life-threatening coronary anatomy and unstable angina not amenable to revascularization and are at risk of imminent death (hours, days, or weeks), may be considered for MCS without necessarily meeting hemodynamic criteria.

Renal Function

Renal dysfunction has consistently been one of the greatest risks for morbidity and mortality with the use of MCS.[23] Renal dysfunction may be secondary to decreased perfusion of the kidney in cardiogenic shock or advanced HF, but elevated central venous pressure is the hemodynamic abnormality most closely associated with worsening renal function during in-hospital diuresis. Kidney dysfunction may result from intrarenal hemodynamic derangements reflecting overactivity of the renin-angiotensin-aldosterone (RAAS) and sympathetic nervous systems in advanced HF as well as from the effects of guideline directed medical therapy blocking these systems (although renal deterioration resulting from the latter should generally not limit their use) and immune-mediated nephrotoxicity or complications of noncardiac comorbidity. In patients with shock or advanced HF, it is difficult to assess the reversibility of renal dysfunction. Acute onset of renal failure requiring renal replacement therapy is not necessarily a contraindication to initiate short-term MCS but may be a greater obstacle to successful long-term support with implantable devices for BTT and in particular, DT. In the setting of cardiogenic shock with acute renal failure, establishing normal hemodynamics with MCS may resolve the renal failure in a relatively short period. However, a preimplant creatinine clearance of less than 30 mL/min/m^2 is associated with a 22% 3-month mortality in recipients of a continuous-flow LVAD, and this constitutes a relative contraindication to durable LVAD implantation at most centers.[23] Thus the degree and duration of cardiogenic shock, along with the patient's baseline renal function, must be considered in estimating the probability of recovery of renal function.

Pulmonary Function and Pulmonary Hypertension (see Chapter 88)

HF may be associated with a restrictive pattern on pulmonary function testing. However, this often improves with removal of interstitial fluid and pleural effusions after placement of an MCS device and resolution of lung congestion. Patients with a long history of smoking or a history of other intrinsic lung disease with significant abnormalities on pulmonary function testing—for example, less than 50% of predicted normal value for forced vital capacity (FVC), forced expiratory volume at 1 second (FEV$_1$), or diffusion capacity for carbon monoxide (DLco)—should undergo high-resolution computed tomography (CT). Patients with low oxygen saturation (<92%) on room air also require evaluation with echocardiography to rule out a right-to-left shunt from an atrial septal defect or patent foramen ovale. If results are negative, spiral (helical) CT or radionuclide scanning (in patients without pulmonary abnormalities on chest radiography) is warranted to rule out thromboembolic disease. Patients with severe pulmonary disease and HF patients with chronically elevated pulmonary venous pressures may have an elevated pulmonary vascular resistance (PVR) that is fixed (not responsive to pulmonary artery vasodilators). High fixed PVR (thresholds vary from 3 to 6 Wood units) represents a contraindication to heart transplantation and consequently to use of LVAD for BTT indication. Moderate elevations in PVR can be encountered in patients with cardiogenic shock and especially in those with long-established HF and does not preclude successful use of LVAD, if lowering of PVR (reversibility) is achieved with inotropes or pulmonary vasodilators. PVR frequently declines a few months after LVAD implantation, so patients deemed not transplantable because of elevated PVR at the time of implant may later become eligible. Perioperative hypoxia secondary to significant underlying lung disease also may contribute to pulmonary vasoconstriction, leading to right ventricular (RV) failure after institution of VAD support. Sleep apnea is present in a significant number of patients with HF, which may contribute to pulmonary hypertension.

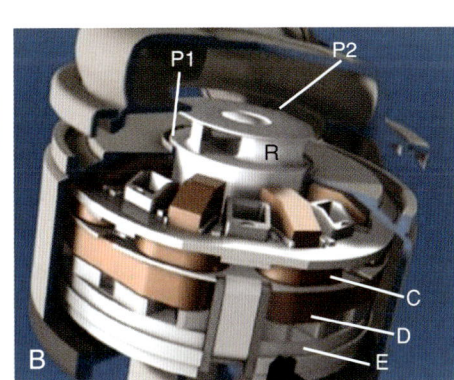

FIGURE 59.6 Implantable durable left ventricular assist device—HeartMate 3 (HM3, Abbott Labs, Chicago, IL). **A,** The HM3 left ventricular assist device (LVAD) is a continuous-flow rotary pump with centrifugal design and complete magnetic levitation of the internal rotor. The blood pump is positioned within the pericardial space, with its integral inflow conduit in the left ventricle and outflow graft (*not shown*) attached to the ascending aorta. The percutaneous power cable is tunneled through the abdominal wall and is attached to the system controller that receives power from two lithium-ion batteries. The implanted components include the inflow cannula, pump housing, motor, control electronics, outflow graft and bend relief, and percutaneous driveline. The HM3 uses a centrifugal flow pump that has a capacity to pump blood up to 10 L/min. Left ventricular (LV) blood is drawn into the inflow cannula along a central axis and is expelled at right angles by and between the impeller blades of a rotor rotating about the central axis. Blood is angularly accelerated and travels around a volute before it is diffused to a desired pressure and flow rate by being directed tangentially into the outflow graft. The pump rotor is fully supported by magnetic levitation, obviating mechanical or fluid bearings and essentially eliminating mechanical wear as a reliability factor. Both drive (i.e., rotation) and levitation of the rotor is accomplished using a single stator comprising iron pole pieces, a back-iron, copper coils, and position sensors. Measuring the position of a permanent magnet in the rotor and controlling the current in the drive and levitation coils enables active control of the radial position and rotational speed of the rotor. Because the permanent magnet is attracted to the iron pole pieces, the rotor passively resists excursion in the axial direction, whether translating or tilting. The electronics and software necessary to control motor drive and levitation are integrated into the lower housing with the stator; these components plus the rotor comprise the motor. **B,** Cross section of an implantable durable continuous-flow rotary pump with centrifugal design and complete magnetic levitation of the internal rotor. The rotor (*R*) is magnetically levitated by electromagnetic coils (*C*) and rotated by motor drive coils (*D*). The levitated rotor produces wide recirculation passages radially (*P1*) and axially (*P2*). A second axial passage beneath the rotor is hidden in this view. Motor electronics (*E*) are incorporated into the implantable pump. (From Heatley G, Sood P, Goldstein D, et al. Clinical trial design and rationale of the Multicenter Study of MagLev Technology in Patients Undergoing Mechanical Circulatory Support Therapy with HeartMate 3 (MOMENTUM 3) investigational device exemption clinical study protocol. *J Heart Lung Transplant*. 2016;35:528.)

Hepatic Function

Preoperative total bilirubin level (in the absence of Gilbert syndrome) and transaminase levels more than three times normal are independent risk factors for RV failure and reduced survival following LVAD implantation. The cause of the hyperbilirubinemia may be multifactorial, including congestive hepatopathy, cirrhosis, or a combination of causative disorders. Abnormal liver function often is associated with abnormal coagulation factors, as well as low serum albumin. Attempts should be made to normalize all indices of liver function and the cause(s) of any abnormalities preoperatively. The presence of portal hypertension with liver cirrhosis is a contraindication to initiating MCS support. A history of significant alcohol use should be ruled out in

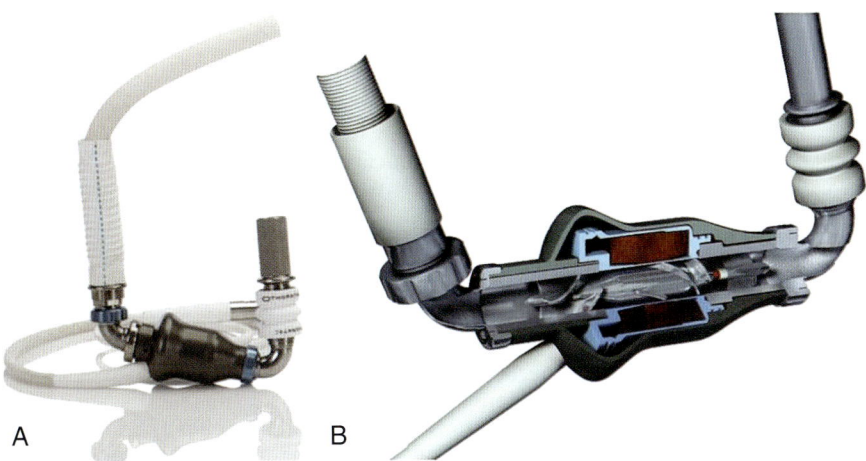

FIGURE 59.7 Implantable durable left ventricular assist device—HeartMate II (HMII; Abbott Labs, Chicago, IL). **A,** The HMII left ventricular assist device (LVAD) is a continuous-flow rotary pump with axial design and mechanical support of the internal rotor. The device is positioned outside the pericardial space in a preperitoneal pump pocket. The inlet cannula is inserted into the apex of the left ventricle, and the outflow graft is attached to the ascending aorta. **B,** Internal view of the HMII device demonstrating blood flow path with internal rotor containing a magnet suspended by mechanical pivots (stators) and external wiring (coils), creating a rotating magnetic field that spins the rotor (and internal magnet).

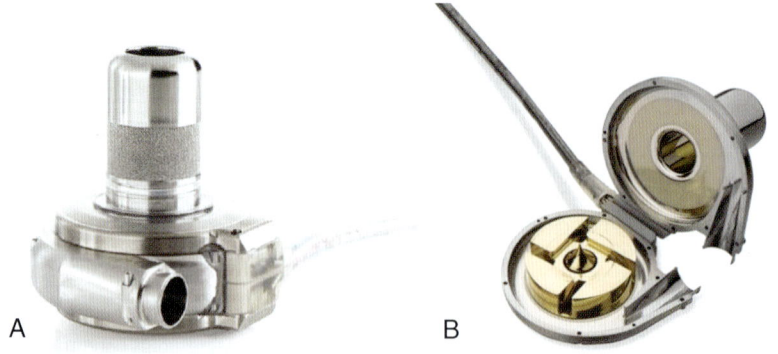

FIGURE 59.8 Implantable durable left ventricular assist device (LVAD)—HeartWare ventricular assist device (HVAD; Medtronic, Inc., Minneapolis, MN). **A,** The HVAD LVAD is a continuous-flow rotary pump with centrifugal design and hydrodynamic and magnetic levitation of the internal rotor. The pump is positioned within the pericardial space with the integrated inlet cannula positioned within the apex of the left ventricle and the outflow graft (*not shown*) sewn to the ascending aorta. The percutaneous driveline traverses the skin and attaches to an external controller and power source (batteries). **B,** Internal view of the pump demonstrating internal rotor that is levitated by magnets (passive magnetic field) positioned in the impeller and central post. Hydrodynamic forces generated by the top surface of the impeller stabilize impeller position.

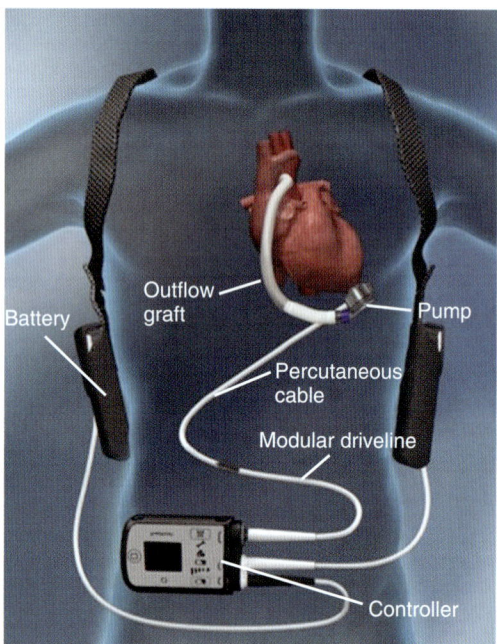

FIGURE 59.9 Typical configuration for a wearable durable left ventricular assist device (LVAD). The pump is attached to the apex of the left ventricle, and the outflow graft is attached to the ascending aorta. The power supply for implantable pumps is delivered through a percutaneous lead (also referred to as driveline) that traverses the skin and connects the external power system (batteries or stationary power unit) with the internal pump. The external components of an implantable system generally consist of a power source (i.e., batteries or an alternating-current [AC] power unit) and a small, portable computer (controller) that controls device speed and monitors device function.

all potential candidates for MCS therapy, especially those with abnormal liver function. Patients also should be tested for previous infection with hepatitis A, B, and C viruses. Ultrasound visualization of the liver is a good screening test in patients with significant hepatomegaly to rule out infiltrative disease, mass, or other pathologic condition that may warrant biopsy. Decrease in hepatic congestion and recovery of synthetic function can occur with institution of MCS.

Right Ventricular Function

Patients with advanced HF frequently have coexisting RV failure, a major contributor to morbidity and mortality after initiation of MCS.[24-26] RV failure is most commonly a result of LV failure. Compared to patients with HF resulting from coronary artery disease, patients with a nonischemic cause are more likely to develop significant RV failure and have a three- to fourfold greater risk of requiring both LV and RV support. Patients who require BiVAD support have significantly higher preoperative creatinine and total bilirubin levels and a greater need for mechanical ventilation before MCS device insertion than patients requiring LVAD support only. The need for BiVAD support is associated with substantially worse survival with both short-term and long-term MCS devices because of a greater degree of compromised preoperative organ function.[24] RV failure is a prominent factor leading to renal dysfunction after LVAD implantation, because significantly elevated right atrial (RA) pressures lead to changes in glomerular filtration from cortical to medullary nephrons, with secondary reduction in urine output and resistance to diuretic therapy. Preoperative optimization of RV function with a goal RA pressure ideally at 10 to 12 mm Hg is important in reducing the need for postoperative RV support. The higher the left atrial (LA) pressure or PCWP at device implantation, the greater is the benefit to the right ventricle and pulmonary artery pressure when the left ventricle is totally unloaded and LA pressure falls. Postoperative recovery of RV function, however, may lag for several days, because total decompression of the left ventricle allows a significant shift of the interventricular septum toward the left ventricle, with further distention and dysfunction of the RV.[25-30]

Coagulation (see Chapter 95)

Coagulopathy is a significant risk factor and a common abnormality noted in patients with refractory HF. An abnormal international normalized ratio (INR) in the absence of warfarin use is of added concern because it may reflect chronically high RA pressures, leading to hepatic congestion and, ultimately, to hepatic fibrosis and cirrhosis. Prolonged abnormal INR and low platelet count combined with use of anticoagulation or antiplatelet therapy are associated with significant perioperative bleeding, requiring multiple transfusions, leading to increased PVR, RV failure, decline in renal function, hemodynamic instability, and multiple-organ failure. In addition, patients with severe HF typically have a nutritional basis for abnormal coagulation because of depletion of several specific coagulation factors, such as factor VII. The minimum preoperative screen for coagulation abnormalities should include INR, platelet count, and in view of the high likelihood of previous heparin exposure, a heparin-induced thrombocytopenia (HIT) assay. The presence or development of HIT is associated with a high risk of bleeding, as well as thrombosis of MCS devices.

Other Medical Considerations

Other important medical considerations in instituting MCS include the presence or absence of significant aortic, mitral, or tricuspid valve disease, coronary artery disease, and atrial and ventricular arrhythmias, as well as intracardiac shunts.

PATIENT OUTCOMES

Temporary Mechanical Circulatory Support

Temporary MCS is indicated in patients with cardiogenic shock refractory to medical therapy when *rapidly achieved* augmentation of cardiac output and reduction of ventricular filling pressures are required to sustain life.[1] When used in the setting of medically refractory myocarditis or Takotsubo cardiomyopathy, temporary MCS may provide time for spontaneous recovery and discontinuation of MCS. When cardiogenic shock complicates longstanding HF, temporary MCS can provide the time needed for patients, family members, and physicians to make critical decisions about long-term MCS and heart transplantation. Patients with HF severe enough to warrant long-term MCS but with reversible clinical characteristics (e.g., coagulopathy from hepatic congestion, acute renal failure from low cardiac output and high RA pressure, hypoalbuminemia resulting from cardiac cachexia and bowel edema) that put them at high risk for perioperative death with a long-term device may benefit from temporary MCS, if their risk profile could be substantially improved with temporary MCS to the extent that they would become good candidates for a durable MCS device. The clinical evaluation of temporary MCS devices for treatment of cardiogenic shock generally has not involved randomized clinical trials but rather has relied on the use of prospective, single-arm observation studies to validate device design, safety, and efficacy. Table 59.2 summarizes extracorporeal assist devices and their characteristics.

Intra-Aortic Balloon Pump (see Chapter 38)

The IABP pump remains the most commonly used MCS device (see Fig. 59.1). The IABP consists of a balloon catheter and a pump console to control the timing of balloon inflation and deflation. The catheter is a double-lumen, 7.5- to 8.0-French (F) catheter with a polyethylene balloon attached at its distal end, with one lumen of the catheter attached to the pump and used to inflate the balloon with gas. Helium is used because its low viscosity facilitates rapid transfer in and out of the balloon, and because it absorbs very rapidly in blood if the balloon ruptures. Timing of balloon inflation and deflation is based on electrocardiogram (ECG) or pressure triggers. The balloon inflates with the onset of diastole, which roughly corresponds with electrophysiologic repolarization or the middle of the T wave on the surface ECG, or just after the dicrotic notch on the aortic pressure tracing. Following diastole, the balloon rapidly deflates at the onset of LV systole, which is timed electrocardiographically to the peak of the R wave on the surface ECG. The IABP increases diastolic blood pressure, decreases afterload, decreases myocardial oxygen consumption, increases coronary artery perfusion, and modestly enhances cardiac output. The IABP provides modest ventricular unloading but does increase mean arterial pressure and coronary blood flow. Patients must have some level of LV function and electrical stability for an IABP to be effective because any increase in cardiac output depends on the work of the heart itself. Optimal hemodynamic effect from the IABP depends on several factors, including the balloon's position in the aorta, the blood displacement volume, the balloon diameter in relation to aortic diameter, the timing of balloon inflation in diastole and deflation in systole, and the patient's own heart rate, blood pressure, and vascular resistance.

The efficacy of IABP counterpulsation was recently evaluated in the SHOCK II clinical trial (Randomized Clinical Study of Intra-aortic Balloon Pump Use in Cardiogenic Shock Complicating Acute Myocardial Infarction), a randomized, prospective, open-label, multicenter trial comparing IABP therapy with best available medical therapy for treatment of acute myocardial infarction (AMI) complicated by cardiogenic shock.[31] All patients were expected to undergo early revascularization (by means of percutaneous coronary intervention or bypass surgery). At 30 days, 119 patients in the IABP group (39.7%) and 123 patients in the control group (41.3%) had died (RR with IABP, 0.96; 95% CI 0.79 to 1.17; $P = 0.69$). No significant differences were found in secondary endpoints or in process-of-care measures, including the time to hemodynamic stabilization, the length of stay in the intensive care unit,

TABLE 59.2 Temporary Mechanical Circulatory Support Devices*

DEVICE	PUMP MECHANISM	PUMP ENERGY SOURCE	METHOD OF PLACEMENT	VENTRICLE SUPPORTED	DEGREE OF SUPPORT[†]
Intra-aortic balloon pump (IABP) (several manufacturers)	Counterpulsation	Pneumatic	Percutaneous placement via femoral artery or operative placement in ascending aorta or axillary artery	Principal effect: reduction of left ventricular (LV) afterload and increase in coronary perfusion	Partial-support device
Extracorporeal life support (ECLS) (several manufacturers depending on pump selected)	Continuous-flow rotary pump with centrifugal design	Variable; depends on pump used for ECLS circuit (most frequently a continuous-flow rotary pump with centrifugal design)	Percutaneous or operative placement	Venous-arterial configuration. Partial unloading of right and left ventricles by reduction in preload with oxygenation of blood	Full-support device (4–6 L/min)
CentriMag VAD (Abbott Labs, Chicago, IL)	Continuous-flow rotary pump with centrifugal design (magnetic levitation; no bearing)	Electric motor	Operative placement	Right, left, or biventricular support	Full-support device (4–6 L/min)
TandemHeart pVAD (TandemLife, Inc., Pittsburgh, PA)	Continuous-flow rotary pump with centrifugal design (hydrodynamic support of impeller)	Electric motor	Percutaneous placement. Requires transseptal placement of cannula for left atrial drainage. Arterial return to femoral artery	LV support[‡]	Partial-support device (2–4 L/min)
Impella 2.5, CP, 5.0, or RP (Abiomed Inc., Danvers, MA)	Continuous-flow rotary pump with microaxial design (bearing support of impeller)	Electric motor	Percutaneous via femoral artery (Impella 2.5, CP, or 5.0) or operative placement via aorta or axillary artery depending on device size (Impella 5.0, CP). Placement across aortic valve (Impella 5.0, CP). Inflow from left ventricle and outflow in ascending aorta	LV support or right ventricular (RV) support (Impella RP)[‡]	Partial-support device. 1–3 L/min for Impella 2.5 or full-support device. 3.5–4 L/min for Impella CP. 5 L/min for Impella 5.0

*The table includes representative mechanical circulatory support devices and is not meant to be an exhaustive listing of all devices currently available in the United States or internationally.
[†]Values of cardiac support represent approximate ranges and capabilities of the device.
[‡]Impella RP designed specifically for right ventricular support. Provides 4 liters or greater of flow.

serum lactate levels, dose and duration of catecholamine therapy, and renal function. The use of IABP counterpulsation did not significantly reduce 30-day mortality in patients with AMI complicated by cardiogenic shock for whom an early revascularization strategy was planned. There have not been adequately powered randomized clinical trials of IABP therapy to assess for a mortality benefit in cardiogenic shock occurring outside the context of an AMI.

IABP placement via the left axillary artery is increasingly being used for advanced HF patients who require short-term hemodynamic support as a bridge to transplantation. In part, this is the result of the October 2018 revision to the UNOS Heart Allocation Policy that prioritizes heart donor allocation to patients receiving temporary MCS over those receiving durable MCS. Moreover, in patients for whom the degree of hemodynamic support afforded by an IABP is adequate for successful bridging, major surgery and the associated prolonged recovery is avoided, as is the forced immobility and resulting further deconditioning associated with transfemoral insertion. In the largest single center published experience, 133 of 195 patients (68%) receiving an axillary IABP were successfully bridged to transplant (120 patients) or durable implanted LVAD (13 patients).[32] Sixteen patients died while on IABP and 18 needed additional circulatory support. Forty-nine percent (49%) needed bedside repositioning of the IABP, 37% required fluoroscopic exchange or repositioning, and IABP removal occurred in 14%. Unique complications of axillary IABP are folding of the balloon within the aorta or entry of the catheter tip into a branch of the abdominal aorta (Fig. 59.10). Kinking of the balloon may occur without eliciting system alarms so serial surveillance x-rays to confirm positioning are essential. Other complications included bacteremia requiring antibiotic treatment (9.2%), left arm ischemia (3.5%), mesenteric ischemia (3%), and stroke (2.6%). A fully ambulatory counterpulsation device intended for more prolonged hemodynamic support in the outpatient setting, potentially in less advanced HF patients, is under investigation (Fig. 59.11).[33]

Extracorporeal Life Support and Extracorporeal Membrane Oxygenation

ECMO provides cardiopulmonary support for patients whose heart and/or lungs can no longer provide adequate physiologic support (see Fig. 59.5).[34,35] ECMO can be configured for respiratory support (venovenous [VV-ECMO]) or for respiratory and circulatory support (venoarterial [VA-ECMO]). In cases of biventricular failure, VA-ECMO is the MCS device of choice for patients in cardiogenic shock and impaired oxygenation, because it provides full cardiopulmonary support. ECMO may be placed at the bedside without fluoroscopic guidance. ECMO is similar to a CPB circuit used in cardiac surgery with some modifications. VA-ECMO involves a circuit composed of a continuous-flow centrifugal pump for blood propulsion (most commonly) and a membrane oxygenator for gas exchange. A venous cannula drains deoxygenated blood into a membrane oxygenator for gas exchange, and oxygenated blood is subsequently infused into the patient through an arterial cannula. VA-ECMO provides systemic circulatory support with flow capabilities approximating 4 to 6 L/min depending on cannula size. Because of the increase in systemic afterload, however, VA-ECMO alone may not significantly reduce ventricular wall stress and may result in LV distension in cases where residual LV function is inadequate to eject against the increase in systemic afterload.[36] This may result in high myocardial oxygen demand (secondary to high filling pressures and volume). This may have negative consequences on myocardial recovery unless the LV is unloaded by concomitant IABP, an LV vent, atrial septostomy, or use of a percutaneous LV-to-aorta VAD. Inadequate LV unloading may also result in pulmonary hemorrhage.

Numerous large clinical series have reported successful use of ECLS for cardiac and respiratory support in adult, pediatric, and neonatal patients.[34,35,37–41] Reports of contemporary survival outcomes are significantly impacted by adult or pediatric application, cause of the cardiac

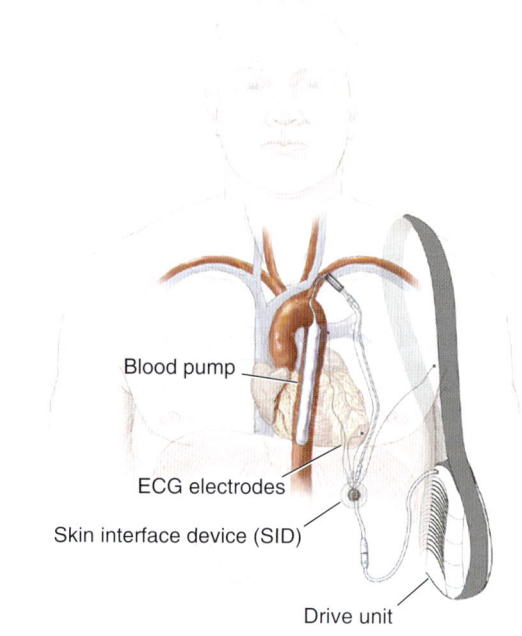

FIGURE 59.11 The iVAS is an external heart assist device that has several components. The intravascular component is a 50-cc displacement pump (similar to an intra-aortic balloon) placed in the descending aorta. The skin interface device (SID) is an electromechanical and pneumatic conduit with a chimney that allows for shuttling of air between the pump and external driver and communication of the captured electrocardiogram (ECG) signals that are transmitted to the driver from 3 subcutaneous electrodes. The SID is placed onto the lower chest cage and connects a driver to an external driveline. An external and wearable drive unit provides compressed ambient air to inflate and deflate the pump. (From Jeevanandam V, Song T, Onsager D, et al. The first-in-human experience with a minimally invasive, ambulatory, counterpulsation heart assist system for advanced congestive heart failure. *J Heart Lung Transplant*. 2018;37(1):1–6.)

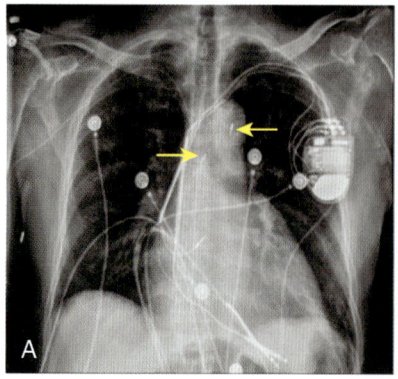 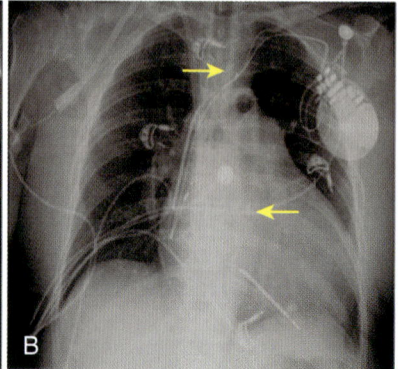 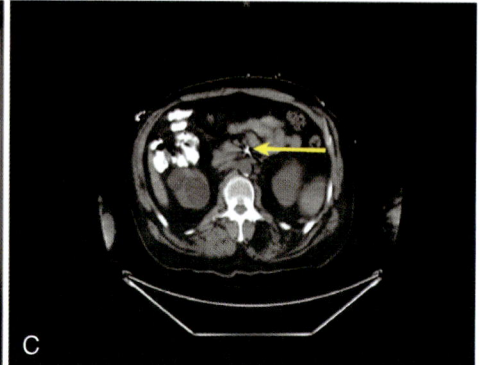

FIGURE 59.10 Images depicting complications unique to axillary intra-aortic balloon pumps (IABP). **A**, Chest radiograph of IABP folded into the aortic arch with the distal marker at the aortic knob and the proximal marker in the ascending aorta (*arrows*). **B**, Chest radiograph of IABP partially folded into the ascending aorta. The distal marker is pulled up into the thoracic aorta whereas the proximal marker remains close to ideal position (*arrows*). **C**, Abdominal computed tomography of the metallic tip of the IABP projecting into a branch of the abdominal aorta (*arrow*). (From Bhimaraj A, Agrawal T, Duran A, et al. Percutaneous left axillary artery placement of intra-aortic balloon pump in advanced heart failure patients. *JACC Heart Fail*. 2020;8(4):313–323.)

and/or respiratory failure, and heterogeneity of the patient population and mode of presentation.[34,35,37–41]

Left Atrium to Aorta Assist Device
The TandemHeart percutaneous ventricular assist device (pVAD) is a paracorporeal device inserted as a LA–aorta assist device that pumps blood from the left atrium to the femoral artery through a transseptal positioned LA cannula, thereby entirely bypassing the LV (see Fig. 59.4). The TandemHeart system includes a 21F transseptal cannula, a centrifugal pump, a femoral arterial cannula, and a control console. The TandemHeart is approved by FDA to incorporate an oxygenator to the circuit, allowing for concomitant LV unloading and oxygenation. The centrifugal blood pump contains a hydrodynamic bearing that supports a spinning impeller. The impeller is powered by a brushless direct-current (DC) electromagnetic motor, rotating between 3000 and 7500 rpm. The external console controls the pump and provides battery backup in case of power failure. A continuous infusion of heparinized saline flows into the lower chamber of the pump, which provides lubrication and cooling, and prevents thrombus formation. The redirection of blood from the left atrium reduces LV preload, LV workload, filling pressures, wall stress, and myocardial oxygen demand. The increase in arterial blood pressure and cardiac output supports systemic perfusion.[36] The flow through the TandemHeart is additive to LV output through the aortic valve (parallel circulation). However, the contribution from the native heart is typically reduced as MCS support is increased due to changes in LV loading conditions (i.e., decrease in preload and increase in afterload). Coronary flow is driven by the perfusion pressure (diastolic pressure–RA pressure). With a parallel circulation, the aorta is perfused and pressured by both the left ventricle and the TandemHeart. Not infrequently, LV contraction (native heart output) may be negligible, and systemic perfusion is pump dependent, with a flat mean arterial pressure curve. This situation can result in stasis of blood within the aortic root, resulting in thrombus formation and stroke.

In a randomized comparison of the IABP with the TandemHeart, the TandemHeart provided more effective improvement in cardiac power index as well as other hemodynamic and metabolic variables compared to the IABP.[42,43] Moreover, complications, such as severe bleeding and limb ischemia, were encountered more frequently after Tandem-Heart VAD support. Thirty-day mortality rates were similar between the groups, but the study was underpowered to compare mortality between groups.

Left Ventricle to Aorta Assist Device
The Impella is a continuous flow microaxial pump designed to pump blood from the LV into the ascending aorta, in series with the LV (see Fig. 59.3). Several versions of the pump are available, including the Impella 2.5, Impella CP, Impella CP with SmartAssist, Impella 5.0, Impella LD, and Impella 5.5 with SmartAssist. The pumps are U.S. FDA-approved to treat patients with cardiogenic shock. A pump specifically designed to support the right ventricle, the Impella RP is U.S. FDA-approved to treat right HF or decompensation following left VAD implantation, myocardial infarction, heart transplant, or postcardiotomy failure to wean from CPB. The SmartAssist technology uses optical sensors to assess aortic pressure. The devices for LV assist are designed to be placed via the femoral artery, either percutaneously (Impella 2.5 and CP) or with a surgical cutdown (Impella 5.0 and 5.5). Alternate access sites such as the subclavian artery have also been described. The Impella pumps blood from the LV into the ascending aorta, thereby unloading the LV and increasing forward flow. It reduces myocardial oxygen consumption, increases coronary perfusion, improves mean arterial pressure, and reduces PCWP.[36] The Impella 2.5 provides a greater increase in cardiac output than the IABP but less than the TandemHeart device. The more powerful Impella CP and 5.0 devices are comparable to the TandemHeart device in terms of support. Similar to the TandemHeart, adequate RV function or concomitant RVAD is necessary to maintain LV preload and hemodynamic support during biventricular failure or unstable ventricular arrhythmias.

In a prospective, randomized clinical trial comparing the Impella 2.5 to the IABP, cardiac index was significantly increased in patients with the Impella 2.5 compared with patients supported with an IABP.[44] Overall mortality rates at 30 days were similar in both groups, but the study was not adequately powered to assess for a mortality difference.[44]

Despite the absence of suitably powered randomized clinical trials demonstrating a mortality benefit over IABP therapy (which itself has no proven mortality benefit), the use of temporary MCS devices in patients with cardiogenic shock is likely to continue. In comparison with an IABP, these devices provide a much larger increment in cardiac output and superior LV unloading.[44,45]

Devices Intended for Long-Term Mechanical Circulatory Support
The introduction of continuous-flow technology into clinical practice was a milestone in the field of MCS therapy and led to significant improvements in survival and reduction of serious major adverse events, especially in the area of device malfunction. Compared with pulsatile-flow devices, continuous-flow technology provides functionally equivalent hemodynamic support improvement of kidney and liver function. Long-term survival with continuous-flow technology is significantly better with half the rate of stroke and infection and one-third the rate of device malfunction compared to pulsatile-flow technology. Table 59.3 summarizes the characteristics of durable MCS devices intended for long-term use.

Durable Implantable Left Ventricular Assist Devices
HeartMate 3
The HM3 is FDA-approved for both short-term (BTR or BTT indication) and long-term (BTT, BTC, or DT indication) support of patients with advanced HF (see Fig. 59.6). The HM3 recently completed clinical evaluation in the MOMENTUM 3 clinical trial. MOMENTUM 3 was a multicenter randomized clinical trial evaluating the HM3 to the HMII pump.[6,10] The final analysis included 1028 enrolled patients: 516 in the HM3 group and 512 in the HMII group. In the final analysis of the primary endpoint, 397 patients (76.9%) in the HM3 group, as compared with 332 (64.8%) in the HMII group, remained alive and free of disabling stroke or reoperation to replace or remove a malfunctioning device at 2 years (RR, 0.84; 95% CI, 0.78 to 0.91; P < 0.001 for superiority). There was no difference in deaths alone. Pump replacement was less common in the HM3 group than in the HMII group (12 patients [2.3%] vs. 57 patients [11.3%]; RR, 0.21; 95% CI, 0.11 to 0.38; P < 0.001). The numbers of events per patient-year for stroke of any severity, major bleeding, and gastrointestinal hemorrhage were lower in the HM3 group than in the HMII group (Table 59.4).

HeartMate II
The HMII (see Fig. 59.7) is intended for long-term support of patients with advanced HF and is the most evaluated MCS device to date, with more than 20,000 implantations worldwide. Patient outcomes after implantation of the HMII have been extensively evaluated in five major scientific reports on its use for BTT and DT indications within the context of pre- and post-approval clinical trials (see Table 59.4).[12,44–47]

HeartWare Ventricular Assist Device
[NOTE: On June 3, 2021, worldwide sales and distribution of the HVAD was discontinued by the manufacturer. This was in response to a study showing poorer survival at 1 year with the HVAD than with the HM3, with a hazard ratio ~ 3.[49a] At the time of this publication, previously implanted patients continue to be supported by this device, and it is recommended that the HVAD not be prophylactically exchanged for an alternative LVAD.[49b]]

The HVAD has undergone clinical evaluation in the United States for BTT indication in a prospective, nonrandomized clinical trial, AD-VANCE (see Table 59.4).[50,51] The unique feature of ADVANCE was the use of a contemporaneous, observational control arm derived from registrants entered into Interagency Registry for Mechanically Assisted Circulatory Support (INTERMACS). The primary outcome in ADVANCE was success defined as survival on the originally implanted device, transplantation, or explantation for ventricular recovery at

TABLE 59.3 Long-term Durable Mechanical Circulatory Support Devices*

DEVICE	PUMP MECHANISM	PUMP ENERGY SOURCE	METHOD OF PLACEMENT	VENTRICLE SUPPORTED	INDICATION
HeartMate 3 (Abbott Labs, Chicago, IL)	Continuous-flow rotary pump with centrifugal design and magnetic levitation of internal impeller	Electric motor. Power to pump delivered via percutaneous lead with external power source and computer controller	Operative	Left ventricle. Implantable pump with intrapericardial placement	Approved for "Short-term" and "Long-term" support (intended for BTT, BTC, or DT indication)
HeartMate II (Abbott Labs, Chicago, IL)	Continuous flow rotary pump with axial design with mechanical pivot support of internal impeller	Electric motor. Power to pump delivered via percutaneous lead with external power source and computer controller	Operative	Left ventricle. Implantable pump requiring preperitoneal pocket	BTT, DT
HVAD (Medtronic, Minneapolis, MN)	Continuous-flow rotary pump with centrifugal design with magnetic and hydrodynamic levitation of internal impeller	Electric motor. Power to pump delivered via percutaneous lead with external power source and computer controller	Operative	Left ventricle. Implantable pump with intrapericardial placement. No preperitoneal pocket required	BTT, DT
SynCardia TAH-t (SynCardia Systems, Tucson, AZ)	Pulsatile, volume displacement (50-cc and 70-cc displacement devices)	Pneumatic. Patient tethered to portable drive unit	Operative	Biventricular support. Orthotopic placement with removal of both ventricles	BTT DT†

*The table includes representative mechanical circulatory support devices and is not meant to be an exhaustive list of all devices currently available in the United States or internationally.
†Currently under clinical evaluation for DT indication.
BTC, Bridge to candidacy; BTT, Bridge to transplantation; DT, destination therapy.

TABLE 59.4 Clinical Trials of Durable, Implantable Continuous-Flow Rotary Devices for Mechanical Circulatory Support in United States

CLINICAL TRIAL	PATIENTS (n)	FOLLOW-UP DURATION	STUDY DEVICE SURVIVAL (6 MONTHS/1 YEAR/2 YEARS)	COMPARATOR GROUP (PATIENTS, DEVICE USED)	TRIAL DESIGN	COMPARATOR GROUP SURVIVAL (6 MONTHS/1 YEAR/2 YEARS)
HeartMate II Pivotal BTT trial[12]	133	Median duration of support: 126 days	75%/68%/—	None	Observational Single arm	N/A
HeartMate II Pivotal BTT trial and CAP[46]	281	Median duration of support: 155 days	82%/73%/72% (18 months)	None	Observational Single arm	N/A
HVAD Pivotal BTT trial[50]	140	Duration of follow-up: 89.1 patient-years	94%/86%/—	499 Commercially implanted devices for BTT (INTERMACS)	Observational Contemporaneous control group	90%/85%/—
HVAD Pivotal BTT trial and CAP[51]	332	—	91%/84%/—	None	Observational Single arm	N/A
HeartMate II Post-approval BTT study[49]	169	Median duration of support: 386 days	90%/85%/—	169 HeartMate XVE or Thoratec pVAD or IVAD (INTERMACS)	Observational Contemporaneous control group	79%/70%/—
HeartMate II Pivotal DT trial—original cohort[47]	134	Median duration of support: 1.7 years	—/68%/58%	66 HeartMate XVE	Randomized clinical trial	—/55%/24%
HeartMate II Pivotal DT trial—CAP[48]	281	Median duration of support: 1.7 years	—/73%/63%	None	Observational Single arm	N/A
HVAD DT Pivotal Trial[52]	297	Complete follow-up to 24 months	(—/—/60%)	148 HeartMate II	Randomized	(—/—/68%)
HeartMate 3 Pivotal trial[6]	516	Complete follow-up to 24 months	90%/86.6%/79%	512 HeartMate II	Randomized clinical trial	89%/84%/77%

CAP, Continued access protocol; N/A, not applicable.

180 days and was evaluated for both noninferiority and superiority. A total of 140 patients received the investigational pump, and 499 patients received a commercially available pump (the HMII in at least 95% of cases) implanted contemporaneously. Success was achieved in 90.7% of patients on the investigational pump and in 90.1% of controls, establishing the noninferiority of the investigational pump ($P < 0.001$; 15% noninferiority margin). At 6 months, median 6-minute walk distance increased by 128.5 meters, and both disease-specific and global quality-of-life scores improved significantly. The HVAD was approved for use in the United States for the BTT indication in 2012. The HVAD underwent clinical evaluation in the United States for DT indication in the ENDURANCE and ENDURANCE Supplemental Trials (A Clinical Trial to Evaluate the HeartWare Ventricular Assist System).[52,53] In the ENDURANCE trial, 297 participants were assigned to the HVAD and 148 participants assigned to the control device, the HMII. The primary endpoint, defined as survival at 2 years free from disabling stroke or device removal for malfunction or failure, was achieved in 164 patients in the HVAD group and 85 patients in the HMII group.[52] The analysis of the primary endpoint showed noninferiority of the HVAD relative to the HMII device (estimated success rates, 55.4% and 59.1%, respectively, calculated by the Weibull model; absolute difference, 3.7 percentage points; 95% upper confidence limit, 12.56 percentage points; $P = 0.01$ for noninferiority). More patients in the HMII group than in the study group had device malfunction or device failure requiring replacement (16.2% vs. 8.8%), and more patients in the HVAD group had strokes (29.7% vs. 12.1%). Quality of life and functional capacity improved to a similar degree in the two groups. Due to the high rate of stroke in the HVAD device in ENDURANCE, a supplemental clinical trial was performed to investigate the effect of an improved blood pressure control management algorithm on incidence of stroke associated with HVAD support.[53] The primary endpoint for the trial was the 12-month incidence of transient ischemic attack or stroke with residual deficit 24 weeks post-event. The ENDURANCE Supplemental trial demonstrated that an enhanced blood pressure protocol significantly reduced mean arterial blood pressure. However, the primary endpoint was not achieved (14.7% with HVAD vs. 12.1% with the HMII, noninferiority [margin 6%] $P = 0.14$). However, a post-hoc analysis of a secondary composite endpoint, consisting of freedom from death, disabling stroke, or need for device replacement or urgent transplantation, demonstrated superiority of HVAD (76.1%) versus the HMII (66.9%) ($P = 0.04$). The incidence of stroke in HVAD subjects was reduced 24.2% in ENDURANCE Supplemental compared with ENDURANCE ($P = 0.10$), and hemorrhagic cerebrovascular accident was reduced by 50.5% ($P = 0.02$).

Total Artificial Heart
SynCardia Total Artificial Heart–Temporary
Another option for MCS is the TAH. The 70-mL stroke volume version of the SynCardia CardioWest Total Artificial Heart–Temporary (TAH-t; Fig. 59.12) was evaluated in a large, prospective, nonrandomized trial conducted in five centers for BTT indication in 81 patients at risk for imminent death from irreversible biventricular cardiac failure.[54] The study cohort was compared with a nonrandomized, observational control cohort of 35 patients. The primary study endpoints included the rates of survival to heart transplantation and survival after transplantation. The rate of survival to transplantation was 79% (95% CI 68% to 87%). Of the 35 patients in the control cohort who met the same entry criteria but did not receive the TAH-t, 16 (46%) survived to transplantation ($P < 0.001$). Overall, the 1-year survival rate among the patients who received the TAH was 70%, compared with 31% among the controls ($P < 0.001$). After transplantation, 1-year and 5-year survival rates among patients who had received the TAH were 86% and 64%.[54] The SynCardia TAH-t was approved by the FDA for BTT in 2007. The TAH-t is currently being evaluated in the United States for DT indication. A smaller version of the device (50-cc ventricle) is also available.

INTERAGENCY REGISTRY OF MECHANICALLY ASSISTED CIRCULATORY SUPPORT

An important milestone in the advance of MCS therapy has been the development of the INTERMACS. INTERMACS is a national registry

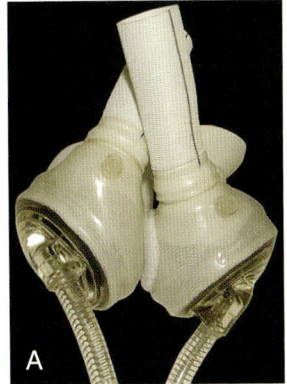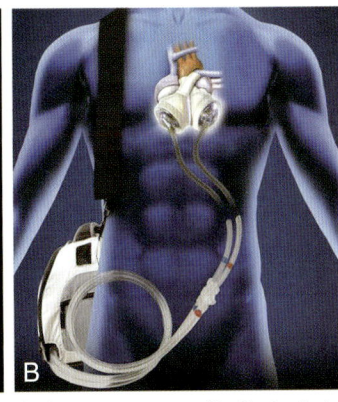

FIGURE 59.12 SynCardia Total Artificial Heart-Temporary (SynCardia Systems, Tucson, Arizona). **A,** The TAH-t consists of a right and left prosthetic ventricle. The prosthetic ventricles, made of biocompatible polyurethane, have a capacity of 70 mL. A 50-cc prosthetic ventricle is also available for use in patients with small body habitus. The ventricles are pneumatically driven with four flexible polyurethane diaphragms positioned between the blood surface and the air sac. When compressed air is forced into the air sacs simultaneously, compression is affected onto the blood sac and ejection occurs in simulation of cardiac systole. Cardiac ejection in the TAH-t thus occurs in parallel from the left and right sides. As the air sac is deflated, the blood sac is filled passively from the atrial connection. Two mechanical valves are situated along the prosthetic ventricle to provide unidirectional inflow and outflow. The prosthetic ventricles are connected by quick-connect silicone cuffs to two atrial connectors on the cuffs (not shown), and two connectors on the end of the grafts are sewn to the aorta and pulmonary artery. The compressed air is delivered by an external console (not shown) through two separate air tubes connected to the right and left prosthetic ventricles. The console has two independent controllers that allow redundancy for emergency backup. Compressed air cylinders inside the console can be used to mobilize the patient. **B,** Portable drive unit to permit hospital discharge and improve patient mobility is also available.

currently administered by The Society of Thoracic Surgeons, and is the largest available data repository for the study of durable MCS outcomes.[55] INTERMACS was formerly a collaboration between National Heart, Lung and Blood Institute (NHLBI), FDA, Centers for Medicare and Medicaid Services (CMS), device manufacturers, and the professional community and began prospective patient enrollment and data collection in June 2006. In March 2009, CMS and the U.S. Department of Health and Human Services mandated that all U.S. hospitals approved for use of MCS for DT enter MCS patient data into INTERMACS for all non-investigative MCS devices approved by FDA. Although mandated data entry was discontinued by CMS in October 2013, the number of DT implants entered annually into INTERMACS has increased. Since the inception of INTERMACS, the ongoing evolution of strategies for device application and the types of available devices has continued to refine the landscape of MCS. A major limitation of INTERMACS is the inability to enter patient information on investigative devices currently in evaluation in the United States, which represents a barrier for capture of all patients receiving durable, implantable MCS therapy. To date, data on more than 22,000 patients receiving durable MCS therapy have been reported to INTERMACS.[55] The overall survival rate for all patients undergoing primary implantation of a durable MCS device is approximately 82% at 1 year and 72% at 2 years (Fig. 59.13).[55] A competing outcomes analysis demonstrates that at 5 years, 23% of patients remain alive on support, 34% have undergone heart transplantation, 39% have died, and 4% underwent device explantation for myocardial recovery.[55]

One of the most important contributions to the MCS field has been the development of a subjective classification system based on severity of illness, termed "INTERMACS Patient Profiles," which range from Profile 1 (critical cardiogenic shock) to Profile 7 (advanced NYHA Class III HF) (Table 59.5).[56] This classification system has added enhanced resolution of patient outcomes in the advanced stages of HF or cardiogenic shock beyond that offered by the NYHA classification system. INTERMACS patient profiles are associated with short-term survival following LVAD implantation and are used to inform appropriate timing of intervention with durable, implantable MCS devices. Patients undergoing implantation of an MCS device who have critical cardiogenic shock (INTERMACS Patient Profile 1) have worse long-term outcomes than patients with more stable forms of advanced HF (INTERMACS Patient Profile levels 2 through 7).[57] Patients with significant organ dysfunction at MCS device implantation, accompanied

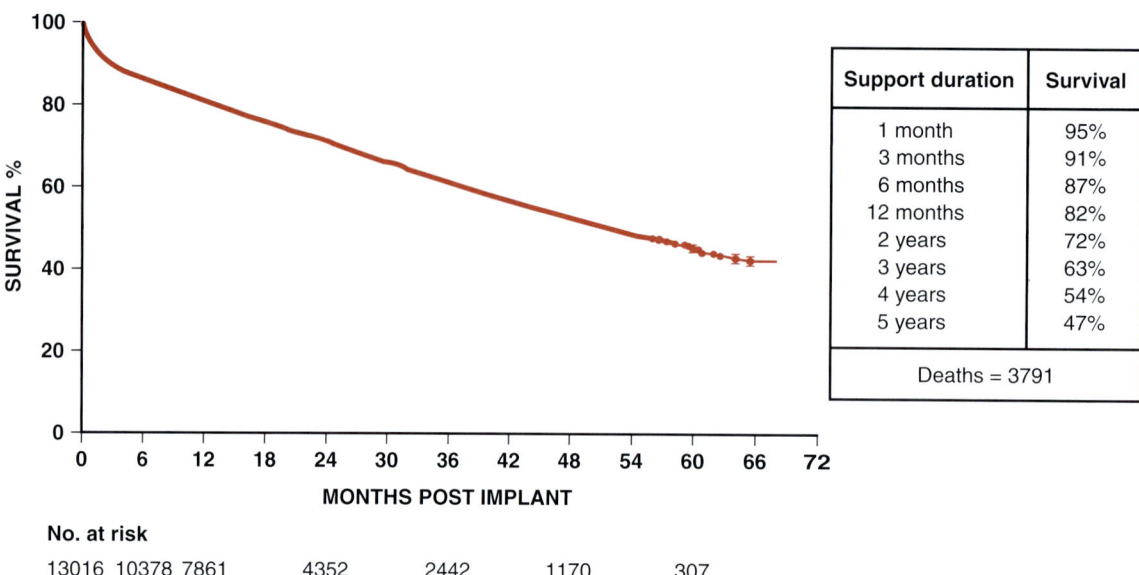

FIGURE 59.13 Actuarial survival after implantation of primary continuous-flow left ventricular assist devices without concomitant right ventricular assist device (RVAD) support. The *curve* displays the Kaplan-Meier survival estimates over time. (Data from Teuteberg JJ, Cleveland JC Jr, Cowger J, et al. The Society of Thoracic Surgeons Intermacs 2019 Annual Report: The changing landscape of devices and indications. *Ann Thorac Surg.* 2020;109:649–660.)

TABLE 59.5 INTERMACS Patient Profiles

PROFILE	DEFINITION	DESCRIPTION
1	"Crashing and burning"	Life-threatening hypotension and rapidly escalating inotropic pressor support, with critical organ hypoperfusion confirmed by worsening acidosis and lactate levels.
2	"Inotrope dependent and worsening"	Shows signs of continuing deterioration in nutrition, renal function, fluid retention, or other major status indicator *or* refractory volume overload, ± evidence of impaired perfusion, with inotropic infusion intolerance due to tachyarrhythmias, clinical ischemia, or other.
3	"Stable on inotropes"	Clinically stable on mild-moderate doses of IV inotropes (or has a temporary MCSD) after repeated failures to wean without symptomatic hypotension, worsening symptoms, or progressive organ dysfunction. May be either at home or in the hospital.
4	"Frequent flyer/resting symptoms"	At home on oral therapy but frequently has symptoms of congestion at rest or with ADLs. May have orthopnea, SOB during ADLs, GI symptoms, disabling ascites, or severe lower extremity edema.
5	"Exercise intolerant"	Comfortable at rest but unable to engage in any activity, living predominantly within the house or housebound. No congestive symptoms, but may have chronically elevated volume status, frequently with renal dysfunction, and may be characterized as exercise intolerant.
6	"Walking wounded"	Comfortable at rest without evidence of fluid overload, but able to do some mild activity. ADLs are comfortable and minor activities outside the home can be performed, but fatigue results within a few minutes of any meaningful physical exertion. Occasional episodes of worsening symptoms; likely to have had a hospitalization for heart failure within the past year.
7	"Advanced NYHA Class III"	Clinically stable with a reasonable level of comfortable activity, despite history of previous decompensation that is not recent. Usually able to walk more than a block. Any decompensation requiring IV diuretics or hospitalization within the previous month should make this person a Patient Profile 6 or lower.

ADLs, Activities of daily living; *GI,* gastrointestinal; *IV,* intravenous; *MCSD,* mechanical circulatory support device; *NYHA,* New York Heart Association; *SOB,* shortness of breath.
From Stevenson LW, Pagani FD, Young JB, et al. INTERMACS profiles of advanced heart failure: the current picture. *J Heart Lung Transplant.* 2009;28:535–541.

by a greater degree of hemodynamic compromise, are significantly more likely to require BiVAD support and are at higher risk for major adverse events and at significantly higher risk for death during use of MCS devices.

FUTURE PERSPECTIVES

Recent rapid technological advancements and successful clinical application of MCS have provided a major impetus to extending the use of this modality. Important initiatives that will contribute significantly to future directions in MCS therapy include (1) introduction of new MCS devices that focus on miniaturization and biventricular support applications; (2) implementation of partial-support MCS devices and management paradigms to enhance long-term myocardial recovery; (3) design of fully implantable MCS devices, with elimination of the percutaneous lead and introduction of wireless energy transfer; (4) specific developments in the field of pediatric MCS, including appropriately designed MCS devices, clinical trials, and national registry development; (5) evaluation of MCS therapy in patients with less advanced HF; and (6) harmonization of the global MCS experience through international registry initiatives.

The percutaneous lead has been a significant source of morbidity and adversely influences quality of life for patients on MCS support.[58] The introduction of wireless energy transfer will allow MCS systems to receive energy transcutaneously without the need for the percutaneous lead.[59] The entire MCS system will be implantable, with an internal power source providing short periods of support, allowing the patient to pursue activities that are restricted with current technology, such as swimming and bathing. The incorporation of this type of technology, if successful, can be expected to increase patient satisfaction and quality of life significantly.

Important developments in the pediatric field include the PumpKIN Trial (Pumps in Kids, Infants and Neonates).[60] PumpKIN is an NHLBI initiative to investigate the use of several novel pump designs and ECLS systems for pediatric MCS application. The trial is investigating an implantable pump design based on the Jarvik 2000 VAD.[61] The initiative is a collaboration between industry, clinical centers, and the New England Research Institutes (NERI), designated as the data-coordinating center for the trial.

Widespread interest in MCS therapies has resulted in global adoption and clinical application of this technology. An understanding of international outcomes based on uniform definitions of outcomes and adverse events is essential to the sustainability of MCS therapy and to foster efficient device development and clinical evaluation. IMACS is an international registry collaboration supported by the International Society of Heart and Lung Transplantation and INTERMACS that was initiated to achieve international cooperation on reporting of MCS outcomes.[62] Efforts to create uniform registration and reporting requirements worldwide constitute an important initiative of the FDA to facilitate clinical device evaluation in the United States.[63]

REFERENCES

Indications and Device Selection

1. Rihal CS, Naidu SS, Givertz MM, et al. 2015 SCAI/ACC/HFSA/STS clinical expert consensus statement on the use of percutaneous mechanical circulatory support devices in cardiovascular care: endorsed by the American Heart Association, the Cardiological Society of India, and Sociedad Latino Americana de Cardiologia Intervencion; Affirmation of Value by the Canadian Association of Interventional Cardiology-Association Canadienne de Cardiologie d'intervention. *J Am Coll Cardiol*. 2015;65:e7–e26.
2. Hanff TC, Harhay MO, Kimmel SE, et al. Trends in mechanical support use as a bridge to adult heart transplant under new allocation rules. *JAMA Cardiol*. 2020:e200667.
3. McGee Jr E, Danter M, Strueber M, et al. Evaluation of a lateral thoracotomy implant approach for a centrifugal-flow left ventricular assist device: the lateral clinical trial. *J Heart Lung Transplant*. 2019;38:344–351.
4. Wever-Pinzon O, Drakos SG, McKellar SH, et al. Cardiac recovery during long-term left ventricular assist device support. *J Am Coll Cardiol*. 2016;68:1540–1553.
5. Topkara VK, Garan AR, Fine B, et al. Myocardial recovery in patients receiving contemporary left ventricular assist devices: results from the Interagency Registry for Mechanically Assisted Circulatory Support (INTERMACS). *Circ Heart Fail*. 2016;9(7). https://doi.org/10.1161/CIRCHEARTFAILURE.116.003157 e003157.
6. Mehra MR, Uriel N, Naka Y, et al. A fully magnetically levitated left ventricular assist device—final report. *N Engl J Med*. 2019;380:1618–1627.
7. Goldstein DJ, Naka Y, Horstmanshof D, et al. Association of clinical outcomes with left ventricular assist device use by bridge to transplant or destination therapy intent: the multicenter study of Maglev Technology in Patients Undergoing Mechanical Circulatory Support Therapy with Heartmate 3 (MOMENTUM 3) randomized clinical trial. *JAMA Cardiol*. 2020;5:411–419.
8. Rose EA, Gelijns AC, Moskowitz AJ, et al. Long-term mechanical left ventricular assistance for end-stage heart failure. *N Engl J Med*. 2001;345:1435.
9. Centers for Medicare & Medicaid Services. Decision Memo for ventricular assist devices as destination therapy (CAG-00119R). Assessed June 1, 2020 https://www.cms.gov/medicare-coverage-database/details/nca-decision-memo.aspx?NCAId=268.
10. Heatley G, Sood P, Goldstein D, MOMENTUM 3 Investigators, et al. Clinical trial design and rationale of the multicenter study of Maglev Technology in Patients Undergoing Mechanical Circulatory Support Therapy with Heartmate 3 (MOMENTUM 3) investigational device exemption clinical study protocol. *J Heart Lung Transplant*. 2016;35:528–536.

Design of Ventricular Assist Devices

11. Frazier OH, Rose EA, Oz MC, et al. Multicenter clinical evaluation of the HeartMate vented electric left ventricular assist system in patients awaiting heart transplantation. *J Thorac Cardiovasc Surg*. 2001;122:1186.
12. Miller LW, Pagani FD, Russell SD, et al. Use of a continuous-flow device in patients awaiting heart transplantation. *N Engl J Med*. 2007;357:885.
13. Pagani FD. Continuous flow rotary left ventricular assist devices with "3rd generation" design. *Semin Thorac Cardiovasc Surg*. 2008;20:255.
14. Moazami N, Fukamachi K, Kobayashi M, et al. Axial and centrifugal continuous flow rotary pumps: a translation from pump mechanics to clinical practice. *J Heart Lung Transplant*. 2013;32:1.
15. Netuka I, Sood P, Pya Y, et al. Fully magnetically levitated left ventricular assist system for treating advanced heart failure: a multicenter study. *J Am Coll Cardiol*. 2015;66:2579–2589.
16. Mehra MR, Naka Y, Uriel N, et al. A fully magnetically levitated circulatory pump for advanced heart failure. *N Engl J Med*. 2017;376:440–450.

Patient Selection, Comorbidities, and Timing of Intervention

17. Reynolds HR, Hochman JS. Cardiogenic shock: current concepts and improving outcomes. *Circulation*. 2008;117:686–697.
18. Hochman JS, Sleeper LA, Webb JG, et al. Early revascularization in acute myocardial infarction complicated by cardiogenic shock. *N Engl J Med*. 1999;341:625.
19. Vahdatpour C, Collins D, Goldberg S. Cardiogenic shock. *J Am Heart Assoc*. 2019;8(8):e011991.
20. Yancy CW, Jessup M, Januzzi JL. 2017 ACC expert consensus decision pathway for optimization of heart failure treatment: answers to 10 pivotal issues about heart failure with reduced ejection fraction. *J Am Coll Cardiol*. 2018;71:201–230.
21. Yancy CW, Jessup M, Bozkurt B, et al. 2017 ACC/AHA/HFSA focused Update of the 2013 ACCF/AHA guideline for the management of heart failure: a report of the American College of Cardiology/American Heart Association Task Force on clinical practice guidelines and the Heart Failure Society of America. *Circulation*. 2017;136:e137–e161.
22. Guglin M, Zucker MJ, Borlaug BA. Evaluation for heart transplantation and LVAD implantation. *J Am Coll Cardiol*. 2020;75:1471–1487.
23. Kirklin JK, Naftel DC, Kormos RL, et al. Quantifying the effect of cardiorenal syndrome on mortality after left ventricular assist device implant. *J Heart Lung Transplant*. 2013;32:1205–1213.
24. Kormos RL, Teuteberg JJ, Pagani FD, et al. Right ventricular failure in patients with the HeartMate II continuous-flow left ventricular assist device: incidence, risk factors, and effect on outcomes. *J Thorac Cardiovasc Surg*. 2010;139:1316.
25. Kiernan MS, Grandin EW, Brinkley Jr M, et al. Early right ventricular assist device use in patients undergoing continuous-flow left ventricular assist device implantation: incidence and risk factors from the Interagency registry for mechanically assisted circulatory support. *Circ Heart Fail*. 2017;10(10):e003863.
26. Cleveland JC, Naftel DC, Reece TB, et al. Survival after biventricular assist device implantation: an analysis of the Interagency registry for mechanically assisted circulatory support database. *J Heart Lung Transplant*. 2011;30:862.
27. Kukucka M, Potapov E, Stepanenko A, et al. Acute impact of left ventricular unloading by left ventricular assist device on the right ventricle geometry and function: effect of nitric oxide inhalation. *J Thorac Cardiovasc Surg*. 2011;141:1009.
28. Santamore WP, Gray LA. Left ventricular contributions to right ventricular systolic function during LVAD support. *Ann Thorac Surg*. 1996;61:350.
29. Pavie A, Leger P. Physiology of univentricular versus biventricular support. *Ann Thorac Surg*. 1996;61:347.
30. Mandarino WA, Winowich S, Gorcsan J, et al. Right ventricular performance and left ventricular assist device filling. *Ann Thorac Surg*. 1997;63:1044.

Patient Outcomes

31. Thiele H, Zeymer U, Neumann FJ, et al. Intraaortic balloon support for myocardial infarction with cardiogenic shock. *N Engl J Med*. 2012;367:1287.
32. Bhimaraj A, Agrawal T, Duran A, et al. Percutaneous left axillary artery placement of intra-aortic balloon pump in advanced heart failure patients. *JACC Heart Fail*. 2020;8(4):313–323.
33. Jeevanandam V, Song T, Onsager D, et al. The first-in-human experience with a minimally invasive, ambulatory, counterpulsation heart assist system for advanced congestive heart failure. *J Heart Lung Transplant*. 2018;37(1):1–6.
34. Rao P, Khalpey Z, Smith R, et al. Venoarterial extracorporeal membrane oxygenation for cardiogenic shock and cardiac arrest. *Circ Heart Fail*. 2018;11(9):e004905.
35. Guglin M, Zucker MJ, Bazan VM, et al. Venoarterial ECMO for adults: JACC scientific expert panel. *J Am Coll Cardiol*. 2019;73:698–716.
36. Burkhoff D, Sayer G, Doshi D, Uriel N. Hemodynamics of mechanical circulatory support. *J Am Coll Cardiol*. 2015;66:2663–2674.
37. Squiers JJ, Lima B, DiMaio JM. Contemporary extracorporeal membrane oxygenation therapy in adults: fundamental principles and systematic review of the evidence. *J Thorac Cardiovasc Surg*. 2016;152(1):20–32.
38. Rastan AJ, Dege A, Mohr M, et al. Early and late outcomes of 517 consecutive adult patients treated with extracorporeal membrane oxygenation for refractory postcardiotomy cardiogenic shock. *J Thorac Cardiovasc Surg*. 2010;139:302–311.e1.
39. Bartlett RH, Roloff DW, Custer JR, et al. Extracorporeal life support: the University of Michigan experience. *J Am Med Assoc*. 2000;283:904.
40. Aubin H, Petrov G, Dalyanoglu H, et al. A supra-institutional network for remote extracorporeal life support: a retrospective cohort study. *JACC Heart Fail*. 2016;4:698–708.
41. Eckman PM, Katz JN, El Banayosy A, et al. Veno-arterial extracorporeal membrane oxygenation for cardiogenic shock: an introduction for the busy clinician. *Circulation*. 2019;140:2019–2037.
42. Thiele H, Sick P, Boudriot E, et al. Randomized comparison of intra-aortic balloon support with a percutaneous left ventricular assist device in patients with revascularized acute myocardial infarction complicated by cardiogenic shock. *Eur Heart J*. 2005;26:1276.
43. Burkhoff D, Cohen H, Brunckhorst C, et al. TandemHeart Investigators Group. A randomized multicenter clinical study to evaluate the safety and efficacy of the TandemHeart percutaneous ventricular assist device versus conventional therapy with intraaortic balloon pumping for treatment of cardiogenic shock. *Am Heart J*. 2006;152.469.e1-469.e4698.
44. Seyfarth M, Sibbing D, Bauer I, et al. A randomized clinical trial to evaluate the safety and efficacy of a percutaneous left ventricular assist device versus intra-aortic balloon pumping for treatment of cardiogenic shock caused by myocardial infarction. *J Am Coll Cardiol*. 2008;52:1584.
45. Werdan K, Gielen S, Ebelt H, Hochman JS. Mechanical circulatory support in cardiogenic shock. *Eur Heart J*. 2014;35:156–167.
46. Pagani FD, Miller LW, Russell SD, et al. Extended mechanical circulatory support with a continuous flow rotary left ventricular assist device. *J Am Coll Cardiol*. 2009;54:312.
47. Slaughter MS, Rogers JG, Milano CA, et al. Advanced heart failure treated with continuous-flow left ventricular assist device. *N Engl J Med*. 2009;361:2241.
48. Park SJ, Tector A, Piccioni W, et al. Left ventricular assist devices as destination therapy: a new look at survival. *J Thorac Cardiovasc Surg*. 2005;129(9):2005; erratum 129:1464.
49. Starling RC, Naka Y, Boyle AJ, et al. Results of the post–U.S. Food and Drug Administration–approval study with a continuous flow left ventricular assist device as a bridge to heart transplantation: a prospective study using the INTERMACS (Interagency Registry for Mechanically Assisted Circulatory Support). *J Am Coll Cardiol*. 2011;57:1890.

49a. Pagani FD, Cantor R, Cowger J, et al. Concordance of treatment effect: an analysis of The Society of Thoracic Surgeons Intermacs Database [published online ahead of print, 2021 Jun 1]. *Ann Thorac Surg*. 2021; S0003-4975(21)00929-2. https://doi.org/10.1016/j.athoracsur.2021.05.017.

49b. Medtronic Recalls HVAD Pump Implant Kits Due to Delayed or Failed Restart After the Pump is Stopped. U.S. Food and Drug Administration Website. https://www.fda.gov/medical-devices/medical-device-recalls/medtronic-recalls-hvad-pump-implant-kits-due-delayed-or-failed-restart-after-pump-stopped. Accessed July 7, 2021.

50. Aaronson KD, Slaughter MS, Miller LW, et al. Use of an intrapericardial, continuous-flow, centrifugal pump in patients awaiting heart transplantation. *Circulation*. 2012;125:3191.
51. Slaughter MS, Pagani FD, McGee EC, et al. HeartWare ventricular assist system for bridge to transplant: combined results of the bridge to transplant and continued access protocol trial. *J Heart Lung Transplant*. 2013;32:675.
52. Rogers JG, Pagani FD, Tatooles AJ, et al. Intrapericardial left ventricular assist device for advanced heart failure. *N Engl J Med*. 2017;376:451–460.
53. Milano CA, Rogers JG, Tatooles AJ, et al. HVAD: the ENDURANCE supplemental trial. *JACC Heart Fail*. 2018;6:792–802.
54. Copeland JG, Smith RG, Arabia FA, et al. Cardiac replacement with a total artificial heart as a bridge to transplantation. *N Engl J Med*. 2004;351:859.

Interagency Registry of Mechanically Assisted Circulatory Support

55. Teuteberg JJ, Cleveland Jr JC, Cowger J, et al. The Society of Thoracic Surgeons INTERMACS 2019 annual report: the changing landscape of devices and indications. *Ann Thorac Surg*. 2020;109:649–660.
56. Stevenson LW, Pagani FD, Young JB, et al. INTERMACS profiles of advanced heart failure: the current picture. *J Heart Lung Transplant*. 2009;28:535–541.
57. Kormos RL, Cowger J, Pagani FD, et al. The Society of Thoracic Surgeons Intermacs database annual report: evolving indications, outcomes, and scientific partnerships. *J Heart Lung Transplant*. 2019;38:114–126.

Future Perspectives

58. Goldstein DJ, Naftel D, Holman W, et al. Continuous-flow devices and percutaneous site infections: clinical outcomes. *J Heart Lung Transplant*. 2012;31:1151.
59. Pya Y, Maly J, Bekbossynova M, et al. First human use of a wireless coplanar energy transfer coupled with a continuous-flow left ventricular assist device. *J Heart Lung Transplant*. 2019;38:339–343.
60. Baldwin JT, Borovetz HS, Duncan BW, et al. The national, heart, lung, and blood institute pediatric circulatory support program: a summary of the 5-year experience. *Circulation*. 2011;123:1233.
61. Adachi I. Current status and future perspectives of the PumpKIN trial. *Transl Pediatr*. 2018;7:162–168.
62. Kirklin JK, Mehra MR. The dawn of the ISHLT Mechanical Assisted Circulatory Support (IMACS) registry: fulfilling our mission. *J Heart Lung Transplant*. 2012;31:115.
63. US Food and Drug Administration Center for Devices and Radiological Health. Japan–U.S. "Harmonization by doing" HBD Pilot Program initiative; 2010. http://www.fda.gov/MedicalDevices/DeviceRegulationandGuidance/InternationalInformation/ucm053067.htm.

60 Cardiac Transplantation

RANDALL C. STARLING

HISTORICAL ASPECTS, 1132

EPIDEMIOLOGY OF HEART TRANSPLANTATION, 1132

EVALUATION OF THE POTENTIAL RECIPIENT, 1132
Medical Issues, 1132
Psychosocial Evaluation, 1134
Substance Abuse, 1134

DONOR ALLOCATION SYSTEM, 1134

THE CARDIAC DONOR, 1134
Donor Evaluation, 1134
Hepatitis C and Drug Overdose Cause of Death, 1135

Donation After Circulatory Determined Death Donors, 1135

SURGICAL CONSIDERATIONS, 1136

IMMUNOSUPPRESSION, 1136

REJECTION, 1137
Cellular Rejection, 1137
Antibody-Mediated Rejection, 1137

OUTCOMES AFTER HEART TRANSPLANTATION, 1138
Surveillance for Rejection and Coronary Artery Vasculopathy, 1138
Survival, 1138
Functional Outcomes, 1139

INFECTION, 1139

MEDICAL COMPLICATIONS AND COMORBID CONDITIONS, 1140
Malignancy, 1140
Diabetes, 1140
Hypertension, 1140
Renal Insufficiency, 1140
Hyperlipidemia, 1141
Cardiac Allograft Vasculopathy, 1141

FUTURE PERSPECTIVES, 1142

ACKNOWLEDGMENTS, 1143

REFERENCES, 1143

HISTORICAL ASPECTS

Cardiac transplantation in humans began over 50 years ago in Cape Town, South Africa.[1] After rapid initial growth in the United States, transplantation stopped because of poor outcomes. The initial 1-year survival was only approximately 20%, and most centers ceased cardiac transplantation programs. In 1984 with the approval of cyclosporine, there was a proliferation of heart transplant centers in the United States as the survival improved significantly. Currently, there are over 140 active heart transplant centers in the United States. The valiant efforts of pioneering heart surgeons, cardiologists, pathologists, and immunologists have all contributed to the ongoing improvements in the technical and management aspects of cardiac transplantation now achieving outstanding short- and long-term outcomes.

EPIDEMIOLOGY OF HEART TRANSPLANTATION

Heart transplantation is performed internationally, as well as at over 140 centers in the United States. The International Society of Heart and Lung Transplantation (ISHLT; https://ishlt.org/research-data/registries/ttx-registry) maintains an international registry that contains in excess of 140,000 heart transplants, reported from 390 international centers. The Scientific Registry of Transplant Recipients (https://www.srtr.org/transplant-centers/?organ=heart) is a USA-based registry of heart transplant recipients and provides program specific outcomes. The United Network of Organ Sharing (UNOS; https://unos.org/) also provides extensive information for heart transplant centers and outcomes. In 2019 a record number of 3552 heart transplants were performed in the United States, representing a 4.2% increase over the 3408 transplants performed in 2018. Over the past decade the number of heart transplants has continuously grown; in 2010 2332 heart transplants were performed compared with 3552 heart transplants in 2019, representing a 34% increase in 9 years in heart transplant volume. There were 669 heart transplants performed in Europe in 2019 (https://www.eurotransplant.org/organs/heart/).

The tremendous growth in transplant volume has been attributed to successful treatment of hepatitis C and expansion of the donor pool.[2] Secondly, the opiate crisis in the United States and Europe has increased the numbers of suitable donors secondary to drug overdoses.[3,4] Based on early and emerging outcomes data, the results are equivalent using these donors. Combined heart-lung, heart-liver, and heart-kidney transplantation can be performed with excellent results, but the numbers are very limited.

EVALUATION OF THE POTENTIAL RECIPIENT

Medical Issues

The benchmark for the consideration of cardiac transplantation is marked reduction in functional capacity despite implementation of all conventional therapies (see also Chapters 50 and 59). The advanced heart failure specialist must consider and exhaust all treatment options before recommending transplantation. Figure 60.1 summarizes the details of testing and evaluation for patients undergoing an evaluation for cardiac transplantation. The convention is to measure exercise capacity objectively with cardiopulmonary exercise testing or a 6-minute walk test. A peak oxygen consumption ($\dot{V}o_2$) less than 50% of age and gender predicted is considered a marked functional limitation. In general, a peak $\dot{V}o_2$ of less than 10 mL-kg-minute is considered as an indication for cardiac transplantation, and a peak $\dot{V}o_2$ less than 14 mL/kg/min is considered a poor prognosis. A 6-minute walk of less than 300 m is considered a marked impairment. Additional testing is required for a full review of all organ systems, with a goal to ensure there are no life-threatening comorbidities and or conditions that would complicate the ability to survive heart transplant surgery or limit life span for noncardiac reasons. Most malignancies in remission and/or with a disease-free interval for 5 years or longer will not preclude cardiac transplantation. Concomitant severe renal, pulmonary, or hepatic disease may indicate a need for the consideration of dual organ transplantation. The details of full evaluation for heart transplantation in the patient with advanced heart failure are described in detail in a recent American College of Cardiology report.[5] Figure 60.2 provides an algorithm for the consideration of heart transplantation and left ventricular assist device (LVAD) (see also Chapter 59). Evaluation of the pulmonary artery pressures and pulmonary vascular resistance (PVR) is essential. Patients with World Health Organization (WHO) group 2 pulmonary artery hypertension (see also Chapter 88) generally respond well to diuresis and pharmacologic or mechanical unloading with acceptable PVR. Patients with elevation of the PVR and transpulmonic gradient refractory to treatment may require consideration of heart and lung transplantation. Many patients listed for cardiac transplantation will require support with LVAD while awaiting a donor heart. In the United States, almost

Evaluation of the Heart Transplant Candidate

- Clinical history and physical examination
- Laboratory evaluation: Complete blood count, basic metabolic panel, liver function tests, urinalysis, coagulation studies, thyroid evaluation, urine drug screen, alcohol level, HIV testing, hepatitis testing, tuberculosis screening, CMV IgG and IgM, RPR/VDRL, panel reactive antibodies, ABO and Rh blood type, lipids, hemoglobin A1c
- Chest x-ray, pulmonary function testing
- ECG
- Right and left heart catheterization
- Cardiopulmonary exercise testing
- Age-appropriate malignancy screening
- Psychosocial evaluation (including substance abuse history, mental health, and social support)
- Financial screening

FIGURE 60.1 Evaluation of the heart transplant candidate. (From Guglin M, Zucker MJ, Borlaug BA, et al. ACC Heart Failure and Transplant Member Section and Leadership Council. Evaluation for Heart Transplantation and LVAD Implantation: JACC Council perspectives. *J Am Coll Cardiol.* 2020;75:1471–1487.)

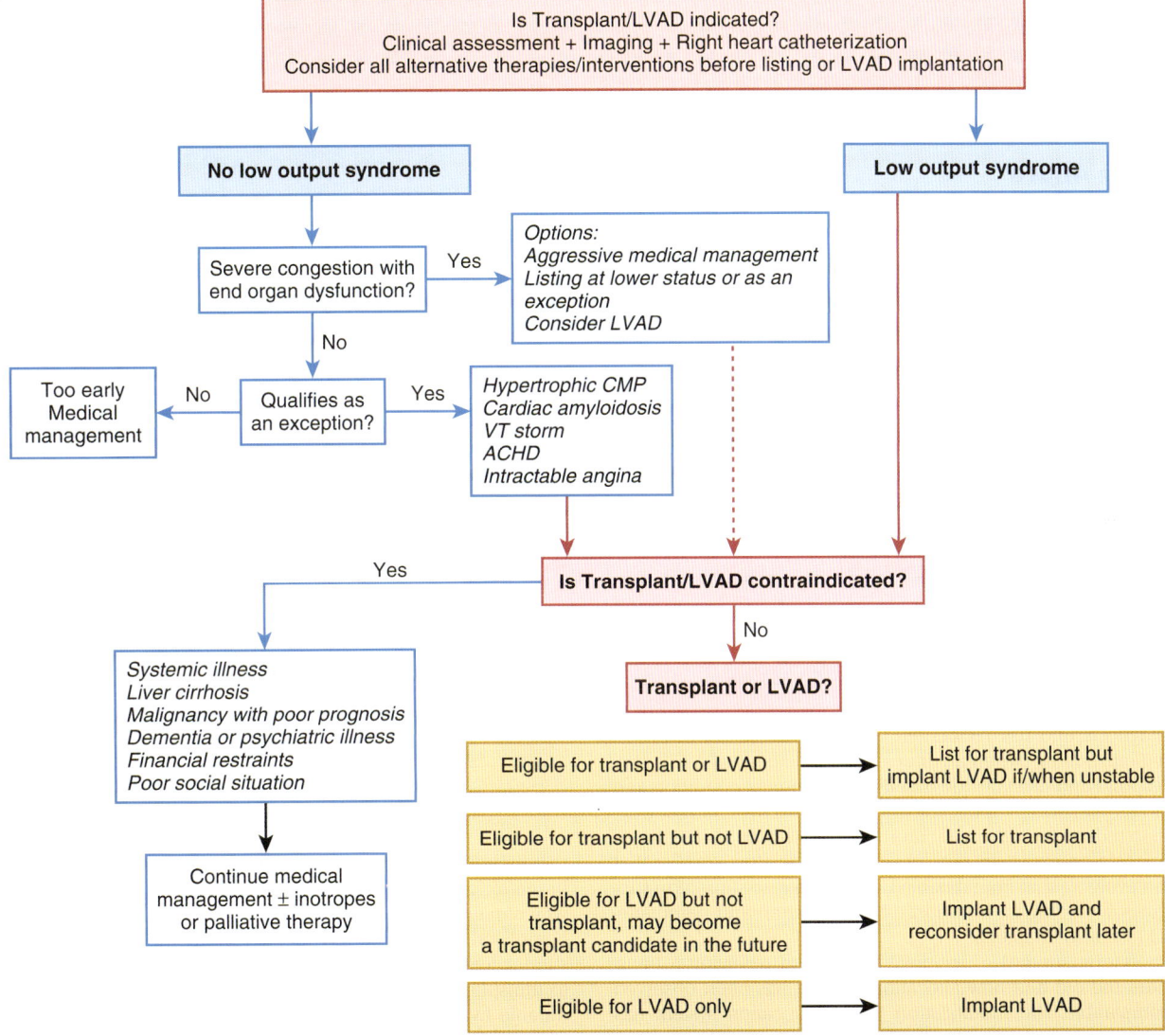

FIGURE 60.2 Algorithm for choosing cardiac transplantation or left ventricular assist device (LVAD) in patients with advanced heart failure. The evaluation process within the advanced heart failure center consists of three main parts: identification of indications for heart transplantation and/or LVAD implantation, ruling out contraindications, and deciding on the strategy: proceed with listing, proceed with LVAD placement, continue management, or administer palliative care. In the latter two scenarios, the patient may be sent back to the referring center or co-managed by both teams. *ACHD*, Adult congenital heart disease; *CMP*, cardiomyopathy; *VT*, ventricular tachycardia. (From Guglin M, Zucker MJ, Borlaug BA, et al. Evaluation for heart transplantation and LVAD implantation. *J Am Coll Cardiol.* 2020;75[12]:1471–1487.)

half of those transplanted are on LVAD historically. Transplant outcomes are essentially equivalent with LVAD support when compared with those not supported with LVAD. A decision to support with LVAD prior to transplant is made by the local transplant team and relates to waiting time, severity of illness, and decisions related to best strategy to achieve a successful heart transplant.

Age is a variable that generates robust discussion. There is a "U-" shaped relationship historically regarding mortality post heart transplant, with increased mortality in those younger than 18 years of age and those older than 65 years of age. There are numerous isolated reports of excellent survival in recipients older than age 65 to 70 years from individual centers. The registry data clearly demonstrate reduced survival that increases by decade of age older than 60 years. Individual centers generally have established algorithms for patient treatment with LVAD and heart transplantation related to recipient age. Some centers have adopted an approach of using donors that would be otherwise discarded (e.g., donor age older than 55 years) as "extended donors" for potential recipients that exceed local established upper limits of age. The ethics of transplantation and allocation of a "scarce" resource is often discussed when evaluating which patient groups will be most likely to have successful outcomes with heart transplantation.

Psychosocial Evaluation

The Stanford Integrated Psychosocial Assessment for Transplantation (SIPAT) is used by most U.S. heart transplant centers to quantify a candidate's psychosocial milieu and determine compliance and social support.[6] It has been well established that lack of a support structure and noncompliance portend poor outcomes after cardiac transplantation. The SIPAT is an objective tool that quantifies and scores each candidate and has been linked to survival post transplantation. The ISHLT has published guidelines for the psychosocial evaluation of adult heart transplant recipients.[7] The psychosocial evaluation is an integral and essential component of a heart transplant evaluation. The social worker is an active, important member of every heart transplant team.

Substance Abuse

Most U.S. programs will not consider an active user of a tobacco product for transplant and require cessation for a minimum of 6 months before listing for transplant. Substance abuse is considered a contraindication to heart transplantation. A patient with an active opiate addiction will not be considered for heart transplantation and will be referred to an addiction specialist for recommendations for recovery. The use of cannabis is generally considered a contraindication, but there are statewide variations. Most heart failure centers will offer LVAD to patients with advanced heart failure and active addiction; hence providing a lifesaving device to enable the patient an opportunity to embark upon a recovery program with the hope for potential transplant listing in the future.

DONOR ALLOCATION SYSTEM

Allocation of donor hearts in the United States is based upon a new algorithm developed by the United Network for Organ Sharing that was implemented October 2018. In contrast to the prior donor allocation system which categorized patients as status 1A, 1B, and 2, there are now six categories that were designated, based upon severity of illness, diagnosis, and risk factors felt to be associated with wait list mortality (Table 60.1).[8] When an offer is made, the center has 30 minutes to respond and must decide based upon recipient condition and donor variables to accept or decline the donor offer. The changes were designed to reduce the waiting list mortality and reduce waiting times, while maintaining excellent outcomes. Early indicators suggest that there is an evolving shift from durable LVAD support to short-term support devices, including an intra-aortic balloon pump and percutaneous LVAD (see also Chapter 59).

The short-term survival of recipients listed and receiving a transplant under the old and new allocation systems has been observed to be comparable. The modification to the allocation system has resulted in several changes to the clinical management of patients undergoing heart transplantation. The implications of these practice changes should be closely monitored to ensure, at minimum, equivalent outcomes. The impact of the revised allocation system has shown a marked increase in the use of the intra-aortic balloon pump pretransplant with the Scientific Registry for Transplant Recipients (SRTR) registry report demonstrating an increase from 7.6% to 28.3% after the allocation revision. There is variability across UNOS regions in the proportion of patients undergoing heart transplantation at the most urgent listing statuses,[1–3] ranging from 29% in region six (Pacific Northwest) to 63% in region eight (Central Plains). Clinicians may

TABLE 60.1 Adult Heart Allocation Criteria for Medical Urgency Status

Tier		
1.	i.	VA ECMO (up to 7 days)
	ii.	Nondischargeable BIVAD
	iii.	Mechanical circulatory support with life-threatening ventricular arrhythmia
2.	i.	Intra-aortic balloon pump (up to 14 days)
	ii.	Acute percutaneous endovascular circulatory support (up to 14 days of support)
	iii.	Ventricular tachycardia/ventricular fibrillation; mechanical circulatory support not required
	iv.	Mechanical circulatory support with device malfunction/device failure
	v.	Total artificial heart
	vi.	Dischargeable BIVAD or RVAD
3.	i.	LVAD for up to 30 days
	ii.	Multiple inotropes of single high-dose inotrope with continuous hemodynamic monitoring
	iii.	Mechanical circulatory support with device infection
	iv.	Mechanical circulatory support with thromboembolism
	v.	Mechanical circulatory support with device-related complications other than infection, thromboembolism, device
4.	i.	Diagnosis of congenital heart disease (CHO) with:
		a. Unrepaired/incompletely repaired complex CHO, usually with cyanosis
		b. Repaired CHD with two ventricles
		c. Single ventricle repaired with Fontan or modifications
	ii.	Diagnosis of ischemic heart disease with intractable angina
	iii.	Diagnosis of hypertrophic cardiomyopathy
	iv.	Diagnosis of restrictive cardiomyopathy
	v.	Stable LVAD patient after 30 days
	vi.	Inotropes without hemodynamic monitoring
	vii.	Diagnosis of amyloidosis
	viii.	Retransplant
5.	i.	Approved combined organ-transplants: heart-lung, heart-liver, heart-kidney
6.	i.	All remaining active candidates
7.	i.	Inactive/not transplantable

BIVAD, biventricular assist device; *LVAD*, left ventricular assist device; *RVAD*, right ventricular assist device; *VA ECMO*, venoarterial extracorporeal membrane oxygenation.

recommend placement of a balloon pump or extracorporeal membrane oxygenation to sustain life and hence expedite transplantation, which might potentially expose patients to higher daily risks of device complications. In some geographic regions, waiting times appear to be shorter for those in urgent need. The use of durable LVAD as bridge to transplant (BTT) has declined. Meanwhile, among patients with a durable LVAD listed for transplant, transplantation rates are low, and these patients are listed as status 4. When a specified device-related complication occurs, it may permit escalation to status 2 or 3, hence hopefully facilitating a shorter waiting time.

THE CARDIAC DONOR

Donor Evaluation

In light of an inadequate number and increasing organ demand, efficacious donor management and selection are crucial in maintaining excellent transplant volumes and outcomes. Obviously, it is critical

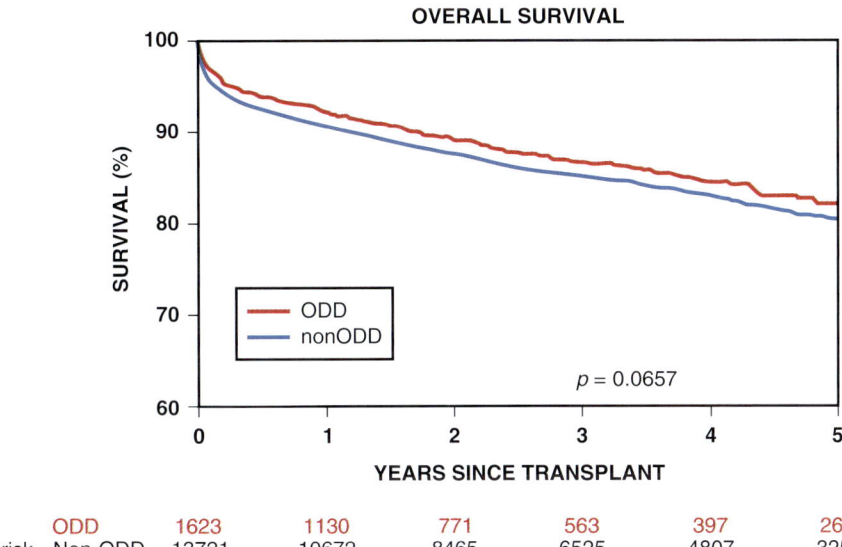

FIGURE 60.3 Impact of the opioid epidemic on heart transplantation. **A,** National average percentage of cardiac transplants from overdose-death donors (ODD) compared with overdose deaths involving opioids per 100,000 population. **B,** Kaplan-Meier analysis for survival on the basis of ODD status. *blue line*, Non-ODD; *No.*, number; *Red line*, ODD. (From Phillips KG, Ranganath NK, Malas J, et al. Impact of the opioid epidemic on heart transplantation: donor characteristics and organ discard. *Ann Thorac Surg.* 2019;108[4]:1133–1139.)

to obtain a complete medical history for the donor, including any relevant cardiovascular disorders before brain death. All donors are screened for communicable diseases, including viral disorders such as hepatitis and HIV infection. Specific information that is relevant for the assessment of cardiac donor suitability also includes the presence or absence of thoracic trauma, disseminated cancer, donor hemodynamic stability, pressor and inotropic requirements, duration of cardiac arrest, and need for cardiopulmonary resuscitation. In some cardiac donors, hemodynamic deterioration may be caused by brain death. Cardiac echocardiography is required on all donors, and coronary arteriography is required to evaluate the presence of coronary artery disease in donors older than 45 to 50 years, depending on other risk factors.

The acceptable cold ischemia time for cardiac transplantation is approximately 4 to 5 hours; systems of ex vivo heart perfusion of human heart donors are under investigation.[9] Prolonged ischemic time has been shown to be a significant risk factor for death after cardiac transplantation, especially when it is coupled with other risk factors, such as older donor age. Donors up to the age of 60 to 65 years are currently considered, depending on transport distance and other donor risk factors. The final decision to accept a heart for transplantation is made at the time of harvesting, after direct examination of the heart for coronary calcification, as well as left ventricular hypertrophy or dilation. Many regions have instituted a process of systematically reviewing donor turndown events to reduce variability and increase confidence in expanded criteria for donors. These outcome reviews have resulted in improved donor organ utilization and transplant volumes.[10]

Hepatitis C and Drug Overdose Cause of Death

Over the past 5 years it has become more common to accept donor organs that are hepatitis C–positive donors or donors when the cause of death is related to overdose. As shown in Figure 60.3A the percent of overdose-death donors was 1.1% in 2000 and rose to 14.2% in 2017.[11]

Registry data indicate that survival with overdose-death donors is equivalent to non–overdose-death donors (see Fig. 60.3B). The advent of antiviral agents now permits use of use of hepatitis C–positive donors and subsequent cure if seroconversion occurs.[2] Prolonged follow-up will provide important information as to the suitability of these donor organs. An early report suggests that hepatitis C–positive donor recipients may experience a higher frequency of acute allograft rejection.[12] Although this report was in a limited cohort of 22 viremic recipients, it will be imperative to track the outcomes of these patients carefully. Any systemic viral infection that involves the endothelium could, in theory, accelerate coronary vascular disease. At present this expanded donor pool will save lives at minimum with excellent short-term survival.

Donation After Circulatory Determined Death Donors

This form of organ donation is now beginning to advance in the United States in efforts to expand the donor pool. Donation after circulatory determined death (DCD) involves donors with devastating brain injury who depend on life support but do not meet the legal criteria for brain death. After the withdrawal of life support, death is declared on the basis of cardiac arrest and organ harvest ensues thereafter. If widely adopted, DCD has the estimated potential to increase overall heart transplant volume by more than 20%. A report from the United Kingdom over a 5-year period from 2015 to 2020 at a single transplant center demonstrated a 48% increase in transplantation with similar 30-day and 1-year survival between DCD and standard donors.[13] The history, techniques, and role for the future is explained in detail regarding the potential to expand the donor pool.[14]

SURGICAL CONSIDERATIONS

The two most common surgical approaches for the implantation of the donor heart are the biatrial and the bicaval anastomoses. The bicaval anastomosis technique was introduced with the intention to reduce right atrial size, to minimize distortion of the recipient heart, to preserve atrial conduction pathways, and to decrease tricuspid regurgitation. This alternative procedure entails five anastomoses: left atrium, pulmonary artery, aorta, inferior vena cava, and superior vena cava. Although no prospective trial has been conducted to establish the superiority of either technique, the bicaval technique is now being done most often in the United States, primarily because it appears to decrease the need for permanent pacemakers in transplant recipients.[15] Most important, the number of patients coming to transplantation with ventricular assist devices in place has steadily increased, so that transplant procedures are riskier and result in more device-related complications. Each prior sternotomy increases risk; it is now commonplace for the heart transplant recipient to have undergone one or more prior sternotomies, and this should not be considered as a contraindication.

The most common reason for failure to wean a heart transplant recipient from cardiopulmonary bypass is right-sided heart failure, evidenced by a low cardiac output despite a rising central venous pressure. The right side of the heart can be seen in the surgical field to dilate and to contract poorly. Intraoperative transesophageal echocardiography shows a dilated, poorly contracting right ventricle and an underfilled, vigorously contracting left ventricle. Right ventricular function may be enhanced with inotropes and pulmonary vasodilators, but the prognostic importance of preoperative PVR becomes obvious in these first few hours after surgery.[16] A most important and essential element of assessing suitability for cardiac transplantation is to measure the PVR. Often a challenge with vasodilator therapy and adjunctive measures to improve left heart function and reduce pulmonary capillary wedge pressure are necessary to determine reversibility of WHO group 2 pulmonary hypertension. Patients receiving LVAD as BTT with pulmonary hypertension often normalize after unloading with LVAD, and serial measures with right heart catheterization are often required to document reversal.

IMMUNOSUPPRESSION

Immunosuppressive regimens begin with the simultaneous use of three classes of drugs: glucocorticoids, calcineurin inhibitors (CNIs), and antiproliferative agents.[17] In the immediate postoperative period, immunosuppressive agents are given parenterally with a quick transition to oral formulations. In a subset of patients, transplant teams use a variety of drugs for "induction therapy" to rapidly enhance immune tolerance. This practice was based upon the prior experiences in renal transplantation. Over the past 30 years there has been a vast experience with different agents.[18] Globally, transplant centers are divided, and approximately half use induction therapy.[19] The arguments in favor of induction are to minimize the risk of rejection and to minimize steroid use. The downsides include infection, malignancy, and the potential for mortality as a consequence. The two most commonly used agents are basiliximab and T cell cytolytic agents. Basiliximab is a chimeric mouse-human monoclonal antibody to the α chain (CD25) of the interleukin-2 (IL-2) receptor of T cells. Antithymocyte globulins (ATGs) are the T cell cytolytic agents. A large registry analysis compared recipients receiving no induction versus basiliximab or ATGs.[20] Survival was equivalent with no induction or ATGs and reduced with basiliximab. More deaths attributable to malignancy were seen in the ATG group. Another common practice is to delay the introduction of a CNI early after transplant, to avoid the potential associated nephrotoxicity. A "renal sparing" approach without a CNI and use of an induction agent in theory may prevent early post-transplant acute kidney injury.

The mainstay of chronic immunotherapy is corticosteroids. Steroids are given intravenously (IV) preoperatively and postoperatively and are rapidly converted to oral therapy. There is tremendous variability regarding steroid dosing, and most centers aim to remove steroids after the first year if it is feasible. Corticosteroids are nonspecific antiinflammatory agents that work primarily by lymphocyte depletion. Side effects are common and include cushingoid appearance, fluid retention, hypertension, dyslipidemia, weight gain with central obesity, gastrointestinal bleeding, pancreatitis, cataract formation, hyperglycemia, and osteoporosis with avascular necrosis of bone. Bone densitometry monitoring and treatment with vitamin D and calcium supplements are often necessary.

The advent of the CNI cyclosporine, approved for use in the United States in 1984, was a pivotal landmark that changed heart transplantation in the United States. The introduction of cyclosporine, the first in class CNI led to improved survival, fewer infections, and the ability to minimize steroid use. There are two CNIs, cyclosporine and tacrolimus, commonly in use. Nephrotoxicity and hypertension are common adverse events. Tacrolimus was subsequently developed with the hope for superior efficacy and fewer adverse events. Their primary mechanism of action involves binding to specific proteins (cyclophilin or FK-binding protein) to form complexes that block the action of calcineurin, a key participant in T cell activation. They suppress the immune system by blocking T cell proliferation through the inhibition of its key signaling phosphatase calcineurin, thus called CNIs. The CNIs serve to block the signal transduction pathways responsible for T cell and B cell activation.

Tacrolimus is the CNI currently used and may be administered IV, orally, or sublingually. Tacrolimus is given twice a day, and the dosing is based upon monitoring 12-hour trough levels. Target trough levels tend to decrease after the first year. The most common patient-centered adverse events are tremor and hypertension. Acute nephrotoxicity, usually reversible, can be seen and is potentiated by the concurrent use of nonsteroid antiinflammatory agents, which should be strictly avoided. Chronic nephrotoxicity is a late consequence of CNI use and may be definitively diagnosed only by renal biopsy and pathology. Hirsutism, gingival hyperplasia, hyperlipidemia, and neuropathy may also occur.

Antiproliferative agents work to either directly or indirectly inhibit the expansion of activated T cell and B cell clones after antigen presentation. Historically, azathioprine was the first agent used in this class and served as the mainstay of immunosuppression with steroids before the routine use of cyclosporine. Mycophenolate mofetil (MMF) has replaced azathioprine as the first-line antiproliferative agent based upon clinical trials demonstrating superiority and a reduction in rejection with hemodynamic compromise.[21] MMF is hydrolyzed to mycophenolic acid, which inhibits de novo purine synthesis. Both azathioprine and MMF cause leukopenia as their major adverse effect; the use of MMF can be limited by diarrhea and nausea and may be associated with a form of colitis. MMF is given IV or orally twice a day. There is an enteric coated, long-acting once-a-day form of the drug. There is also concern that viral infections, primarily cytomegalovirus (CMV), may be more prevalent in the presence of MMF.

Mammalian target of rapamycin (mTOR) are immunosuppressive drugs that inhibit the mTOR, which is a serine/threonine-specific protein kinase. Rapamycin inhibits cellular proliferation and cell cycle progression, and it was discovered to have immunosuppressive properties in the 1980s. Sirolimus (often called rapamycin) and everolimus are two mTOR inhibitors that block activation of T cells after autocrine stimulation by IL-2. They also are known to inhibit proliferation of endothelial cells and fibroblasts. Originally, it was hoped that mTOR inhibitors might have unique characteristics to reduce the scourge of cardiac transplantation, cardiac allograft vasculopathy (CAV). A clinical trial published in 2003 provided optimism for the role of this class of immunosuppressive drugs, showing a reduction in CAV.[22] Their action is complementary to that of CNIs, and both sirolimus and everolimus have been used as maintenance immunosuppression, as alternatives to standard immunosuppression, and as rescue drugs for rejection. The mTOR inhibitors have been shown to slow progression of CAV in patients with established disease and to reduce development of de novo CAV.[23,24] The use of sirolimus as a primary immunosuppressive agent has been observed to reduce CAV and improve survival, but definitive data from randomized clinical trials do not exist.[25] The drugs inhibit the proliferation of fibroblasts and may theoretically cause delayed wound healing although this was not observed with everolimus in the randomized trial with de novo use. Finally, reduced

TABLE 60.2 ISHLT Standardized Cardiac Biopsy Grading Compared with an Earlier System

2004 SYSTEM		1990 SYSTEM	
GRADE 0 R	NO REJECTION	GRADE 0	NO REJECTION
Grade 1 R, mild	Interstitial and/or perivascular infiltrate with up to one focus of myocyte damage	Grade 1, mild	
		A—focal	Focal perivascular and/or interstitial infiltrate without myocyte damage
		B—diffuse	Diffuse infiltrate without myocyte damage
Grade 2 R, moderate	Two or more foci of infiltrate with associated myocyte damage	Grade 2, moderate (focal)	One focus of infiltrate with associated myocyte damage
Grade 3 R, severe	Diffuse infiltrate with multifocal myocyte damage ± edema, ± hemorrhage, ± vasculitis	Grade 3, moderate	
		A—focal	Multifocal infiltrate with myocyte damage
		B—diffuse	Diffuse infiltrate with myocyte damage
		Grade 4, severe	Diffuse, polymorphous infiltrate with extensive myocyte damage ± hemorrhage ± vasculitis

ISHLT, International Society of Heart and Lung Transplantation.
Modified from Stewart S, Winters GL, Fishbein MC, et al. Revision of the 1990 working formulation for the standardization of nomenclature in the diagnosis of heart rejection. J Heart Lung Transplant. 2005;24:1710.

occurrence of CMV viremia and infection has been observed with everolimus-based regimens and forms the basis for use in some recipients with recurrent CMV disease. Despite the accumulated efficacy data with everolimus, it has not been approved by the FDA for the indication of cardiac transplantation and its use is "off label" in the United States. The main concern of the FDA was related to worse renal outcomes observed in the two large, randomized trials performed in the United States.[22,26–28] The withdrawal of CNI and replacement with mTOR should be considered with caution and careful observation if implemented.

REJECTION

Rejection, which once limited the effectiveness of cardiac transplantation, has become a much less common occurrence in the current era. Rejection has been primarily an asymptomatic diagnosis based upon surveillance endomyocardial biopsy and pathologic examination of the specimens. Although heart biopsy has been considered the "gold standard," it is well established that there may be significant variability between pathologists with concordance studies showing up to 25% of biopsies receiving different pathologic grades. This has created variability among centers and the requirement for external pathology panels is a necessity in clinical trials. Over the past decade, noninvasive and laboratory-based assays have become available, challenging the need for routine, frequent surveillance endomyocardial biopsies.

From the beginning, rejection has referred to the infiltration of lymphocytes within the myocardium. The intensity of the lymphocytic infiltration and the degree of myocyte injury and necrosis determines the pathologic grade of rejection. Heart biopsies are graded by a standardized international grading system developed by the International Society for Heart and Lung Transplantation shown in Table 60.2.[29] Rejection is subdivided as cellular and antibody mediated.

Cellular Rejection

Cellular rejection has been the basis of surveillance endomyocardial biopsy justification. Early reports indicated up to 50% of patient demonstrating moderate forms of rejection in the first 6 months; currently the rates observed have decreased to approximately 10%. Factors contributing to the reduced rates are related to improved donor-recipient matching with improvements in organ matching based upon "virtual" crossmatching and improvements in immunosuppressive regimens. Virtual crossmatch uses solid phase assays to detect anti-HLA antibodies in the recipient and allows exclusion of donors with unacceptable HLA antigens. The previous mandate for a negative prospective crossmatch has been largely eliminated based upon the use of virtual crossmatches and high concordance with final crossmatches when lymphoid tissue from the donor becomes available.

In most cases of cellular rejection diagnosed from a surveillance endomyocardial biopsy, the patient is asymptomatic and will have no evidence of cardiac allograft dysfunction. This explains why imaging of the functioning allograft with echo is insensitive to detect cellular rejection, which most often is a pathologic diagnosis without changes in heart function or physiology. Most often, cellular rejection is treated by steroid augmentation or adjustment of baseline immunosuppressive medications. Heart biopsies that are triggered by patient symptoms, or a decline in graft function that demonstrates moderate to severe cellular rejection require hospitalization, IV steroids, and other adjunctive therapies often including antithymocyte globulin. Some patients will require hemodynamic monitoring or inotropic or mechanical support; fortunately for most patients, graft dysfunction from cellular rejection is reversible with treatment and full recovery is expected. Numerous other techniques, including cardiac MRI (see also Chapter 19), have been studied, with varying degrees of effectiveness, but none have replaced the endomyocardial biopsy.[30]

The advent of gene expression profiling assays has proliferated over the past decade and become mainstream to monitor the cardiac allograft. A commercially available test, the AlloMap, is based upon a validated 11 gene panel to diagnosis cellular rejection. The panel of 11 informative genes and 9 controlled genes detects changes in gene expression associated with acute rejection and provides an actionable score. The usefulness of this test was studied in a multicenter study over a decade ago; however, the uptake of the blood test to replace endomyocardial biopsy has been gradual.[31] Most recently an ancillary blood test measuring donor-derived cell-free DNA has been developed, envisioned to be combined with gene expression profiling to monitor the cardiac allograft.[32]

Antibody-Mediated Rejection

Antibody-mediated rejection (AMR) was formally defined based on the 2005 ISHLT publication revising the pathologic standards for rejection. Prior to this formulation, it was recognized that heart transplant recipients would present with graft dysfunction and hemodynamic compromise and only mild cellular rejection present on heart biopsy. Eventually, it was observed that most of these patients had developed donor-specific antibodies to HLA loci. Subsequently with the advent of staining for complement, the observation of complement deposition in the heart biopsies of patients with hemodynamic compromise led to the terminology of "humoral rejection with hemodynamic compromise." Hence the terminology of AMR was formally defined and subsequently refined in 2011.[33] AMR remains a challenge; there is variability in monitoring, and currently there is not a validated noninvasive or blood test. Most often, HLA antibody in the form of donor-specific assays are present, but it is also known that non-HLA antibody may be implicated in AMR. Heart biopsy and the presence of complement with adjunctive histologic criteria are the basis of the pathologic diagnosis. The treatment is less standardized but most often includes cytolytic agents, antibody depletion, and specific therapies directed at B cell lymphocytes.[34] AMR can present early or late post transplant, and the most vulnerable patients are those with positive crossmatch, elevated preformed antibody levels, and demographically multiparous female recipients. AMR is often associated with graft dysfunction and hemodynamic compromise. Treatment may require prolonged antibody depletion with plasmapheresis, and protocols with photopheresis have been described.

Recently a tissue-based molecular diagnostic system has been developed aimed to increase the accuracy of both T cell–mediated cellular rejection and AMR.[35] RNA is extracted from endomyocardial biopsy specimens, and analyses are performed to detect rejection-associated transcripts associated with known profiles from renal transplant T cell–mediated and AMR. The hope is that this modality will provide a new tool to improve the accuracy of diagnosis and calibration of histology interpretations.

OUTCOMES AFTER HEART TRANSPLANTATION

Surveillance for Rejection and Coronary Artery Vasculopathy

The conventions for performing heart biopsy and coronary angiography were established decades ago by the original U.S. heart transplant programs. Endomyocardial biopsies were performed 12 to 15 times the first year post transplant and gradually reduced in frequency after year 1. Many programs continued surveillance heart biopsies twice a year indefinitely. Much variation exists throughout the United States now, with some programs stopping endomyocardial biopsy after the first year and using laboratory and imaging techniques and only a clinical event-driven approach to heart biopsy. The majority of U.S. programs perform routine surveillance heart biopsies at minimum for the first year post transplant. As was discussed, the endomyocardial biopsy is the only technique that can diagnose both cellular and AMR. AMR can be diagnosed by light microscopy on the basis of histology and either immunohistochemistry or immunofluorescence. The limitation of the gene expression profiling assay (AlloMap) is that it is validated only for cellular rejection. Most heart transplant programs follow their recipients long term and continue routine testing and clinic visits designed to diagnose asymptomatic rejection or coronary disease before a clinical manifestation occurs.

The convention for surveillance coronary angiography is yearly for the lifetime of the transplant recipient. Coronary artery vasculopathy (CAV) is common and can occur within the first year after transplant or much later after the first decade. Monitoring techniques have included coronary angiography, intravascular ultrasound (IVUS), and coronary optical coherence tomography. The latter two procedures are primarily investigational, although IVUS is used in conjunction with percutaneous coronary interventions (PCIs) routinely. Based on evidence obtained from clinical trials, it was felt that IVUS determined findings of coronary changes even without the concurrent demonstration of angiographic disease were important and predictive of the development of angiographic disease. Insurers typically will not reimburse for IVUS studies, and its use for surveillance has waned recently. Many patients with high-grade, epicardial coronary obstructions may be asymptomatic when referred for surveillance cardiac cath. Most patients are treated with drug-eluting stents, even if asymptomatic. The dogma has been that denervated heart transplant recipients do not always exhibit typical angina. Most noninvasive techniques have been studied for CAV surveillance; however, they lack the necessary sensitivity and specificity to replace the routine use of coronary angiography. Perhaps the most promising noninvasive strategy for coronary surveillance is the use of PET imaging.[36] At present, coronary angiography yearly or less frequently and supplemented with yearly noninvasive stress imaging is the basis for CAV surveillance. It is believed that aspirin and statin use should be routine in heart transplant recipients even without elevation of low-density lipoprotein (LDL). Lipid abnormalities should be aggressively treated.

Survival

Patients with stage D heart failure are estimated to have a mortality of 50% at 6 months and nearly 100% at 1 year. These projections are based on reported mortality for patients deemed to be inotrope dependent. When listing a patient for transplant, most often the decision is based upon reduced quality of life and poor functional capacity. Advances in medical and device therapies for heart failure have markedly reduced mortality; hence a patient listed for transplant may have an estimated 1-year mortality of 20% to 30% or less depending on the clinical situation. Acknowledging the potential "survival benefit" is important when recommending cardiac transplantation. From a long-term perspective the survival advantage for transplantation becomes very clear when looking at survival projections at 10 years and beyond. Thus two common situations exist; the hospitalized patient in extremis related to an acute event or chronic decompensation and the "walking wounded" patient with chronic heart failure being managed as an outpatient with poor quality of life and reduced exercise tolerance. LVADs have played a role in the management of patients in both scenarios and provided both improved survival and quality of life while waiting for a donor heart; it is referred to as the "bridge to transplant" strategy for LVAD therapy (see also Chapter 59).

The major source of information for heart transplantation survival is based upon the ISHLT registry that contains data on over 146,000 transplants. The registry is updated yearly and provides detailed information related to demographics, era, and immunosuppression. The 2019 registry report shows survival related to era of transplantation: the median survival from 1992 to 2001 was 10.5 years and increased to 12.5 years in the era 2002 to 2009 (Fig. 60.4).[37] Survival, activity, and outcome metrics for all U.S. heart transplant programs can be viewed in detail on the Health Resources and Services Administration (HRSA) website *The Scientific Registry for Transplant Recipients* (https://srtr.transplant.hrsa.gov/).[38] Many successful U.S. heart transplant programs report 1-year survival greater than 90% and 3-year survival greater than 85%. There are over 140 active heart transplant programs in the United States, with volumes varying from fewer than 10 to more than 100 transplants each year. Data from the SRTR show the common causes of mortality in the first 5 years after transplant (Fig. 60.5), including graft failure, infection, coronary artery disease, and malignancy. A feared and fortunately uncommon complication is primary graft failure (PGF). PGF typically occurs in the early post-transplant period and can manifest as profound allograft dysfunction and cardiogenic shock without evidence of acute rejection or any specific etiology. PGF is felt to be related to ischemic time, age of the donor, preservation, and surgical factors that are poorly understood. Patients require support often with extracorporeal membrane oxygenation, and many will fully recover; however, the 30-day mortality rate is 30%.[39] Numerous factors related to the donor including age, mechanism of brain death, and gender may all influence early and late outcomes.[40] Over the past decade the donor pool has been expanded by using organs that in the past would have been discarded, yet outstanding outcomes have been maintained or improved.

As noted earlier, the allocation system for heart donors changed in October 2018. The changes were designed to reduce the waiting list mortality and reduce waiting times, while maintaining excellent outcomes. Early indicators suggest that there is an evolving shift from durable LVAD support to short-term support devices, including an intra-aortic balloon pump and percutaneous LVAD. The argument has been made that LVAD will provide equivalent survival to transplantation and lengthen the overall life span for an individual, acknowledging the median survival post heart transplant is limited to approximately 12 years. Contemporary data (Fig. 60.6) suggest that the 1- and 5-year survival for heart transplant (with or without BTT LVAD support) is superior when compared with outcomes of patients receiving a chronic or destination (DT) LVAD.[40] Overall 1-year survival was 87.7% in those wait-listed for heart transplant compared with 76.4% in the DT LVAD group, whereas the 5-year

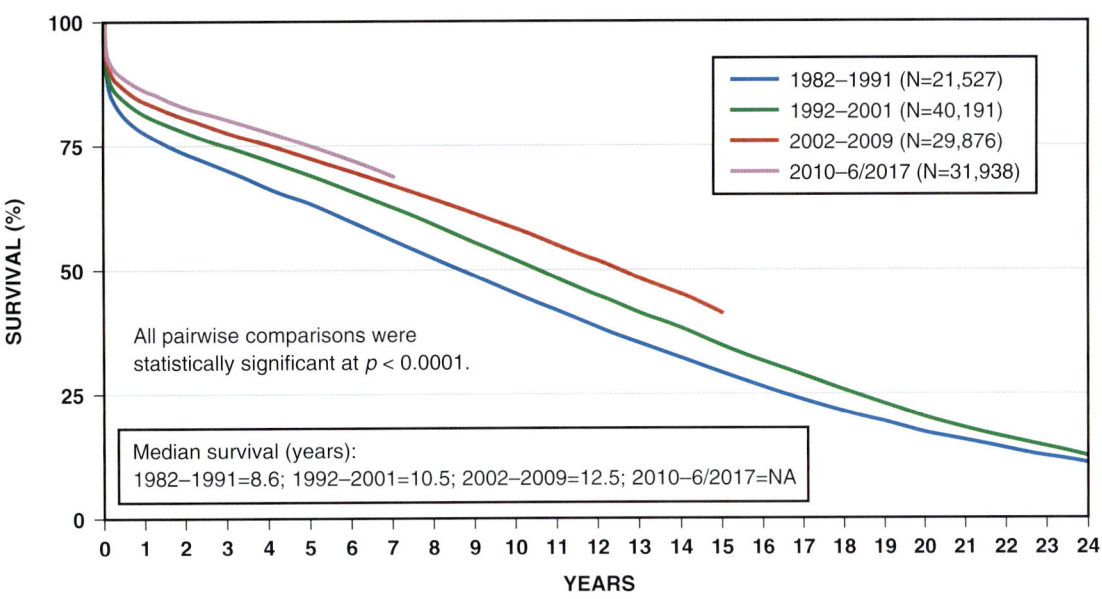

FIGURE 60.4 Kaplan-Meier survival estimates for adult heart transplant patients by era. (From Khush KK, Cherikh WS, Chambers DC, et al. International Society for Heart and Lung Transplantation. The International Thoracic Organ Transplant Registry of the International Society for Heart and Lung Transplantation: Thirty-sixth adult heart transplantation report—2019; focus theme: Donor and recipient size match. *J Heart Lung Transplant*. 2019;38[10]:1056–1066. doi: 10.1016/j.healun.2019.08.004. Epub 2019 Aug 10. Erratum in: *J Heart Lung Transplant*. 2020;39:91. https://ishltregistries.org/registries/slides.asp?yearToDisplay=2020.)

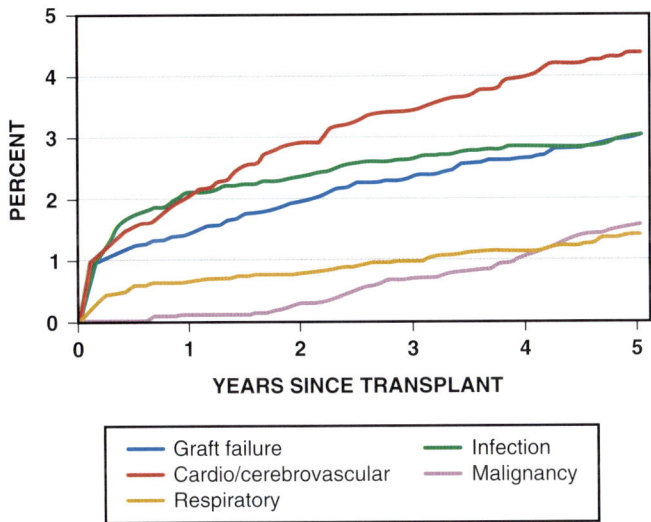

FIGURE 60.5 Five-year cumulative incidence of death by cause among adult heart transplant recipients, 2012–2013. Primary causes of death are as reported on the Organ Procurement Transplant Network Transplant Recipient Registration and Follow-up Forms. Other causes of death include hemorrhage, trauma, nonadherence, unspecified other, unknown, etc. Cumulative incidence is estimated using Kaplan-Meier competing risk methods. (From https://srtr.transplant.hrsa.gov/annual_reports/2018/Heart.aspx)

report showed that peak $\dot{V}O_2$ of less than or equal to 60% and VE/$\dot{V}CO_2$ greater than or equal to 34 with exercise were associated with a high hazard for CAV in heart transplant recipients at 1 year after transplant.[42] Cardiac rehabilitation is routinely recommended for all heart transplant recipients to optimize their recovery potential.[43] The Karnofsky Index, which is routinely reported after cardiac transplantation, provides an objective measure of functional capacity. Most heart transplant recipients reach near-normal function based on their Karnofsky grade, and over 90% are physically fit to return to most all occupations with excellent cardiopulmonary function. A typical heart transplant recipient should expect to regain full activity and be able to return to usual social and employment activities within 6 to 12 months after transplantation.

INFECTION

A successful result after cardiac transplantation is a balance between preventing rejection and overzealous use of immunosuppression. The incidence of rejection has decreased, but opportunistic infection remains an important risk due to immunosuppression. Infections cause approximately 20% of deaths within the first year after transplantation and continue to be a common contributing factor in morbidity and mortality throughout the recipient's life. The most common infections are bacterial and viral, specifically CMV. The recipient and the donor are assessed for prior CMV infection with IgG antibody titers.[44] The highest risk for CMV infection is from a CMV-positive donor in a negative CMV recipient. Standard prophylaxis for CMV infection with valganciclovir for 3 to 6 months post transplant reduces the burden of disease. Routinely patients are monitored for CMV DNA, which may become seropositive in the absence of a clinical infection. The spectrum of disease may vary from asymptomatic viremia to a serious, tissue-invasive infection, for example CMV pneumonitis. The use of an mTOR inhibitor (everolimus) may be considered in a high-risk patient with recurrent CMV infection concurrent with the elimination of mycophenolic acid mofetil to mitigate the risk of future active CMV infection. Mortality is highest for fungal infections, followed by protozoal, bacterial, and viral infections. Aspergillosis and candidiasis are the most common fungal infections after heart transplantation. *Pneumocystis jirovecii* and herpes simplex virus infections and oral candidiasis, require prophylactic regimens to be used during the first 6 to 12 months after transplantation. Prophylactic IV ganciclovir or oral valganciclovir generally is given for variable periods

survival was 72.1% in the heart transplant group versus 36.1% in the DT LVAD group.[41] The improvement in survival was primarily related to whether or not the patient underwent heart transplantation. Given that there may have been medical reasons why certain patients were deemed DT versus BTT, a randomized clinical trial to definitively address is required. The clinical data that are available suggest that clinical outcomes with cardiac transplantation are superior to those of DT LVAD therapy.[40]

Functional Outcomes

Cardiac transplantation dramatically improves quality of life and functional capacity. The improvement is referenced based upon the pretransplant degree of impairment. A normal heart transplant recipient's exercise capacity is below that of an age-matched control, normal individual but much improved compared with pretransplant. A recent

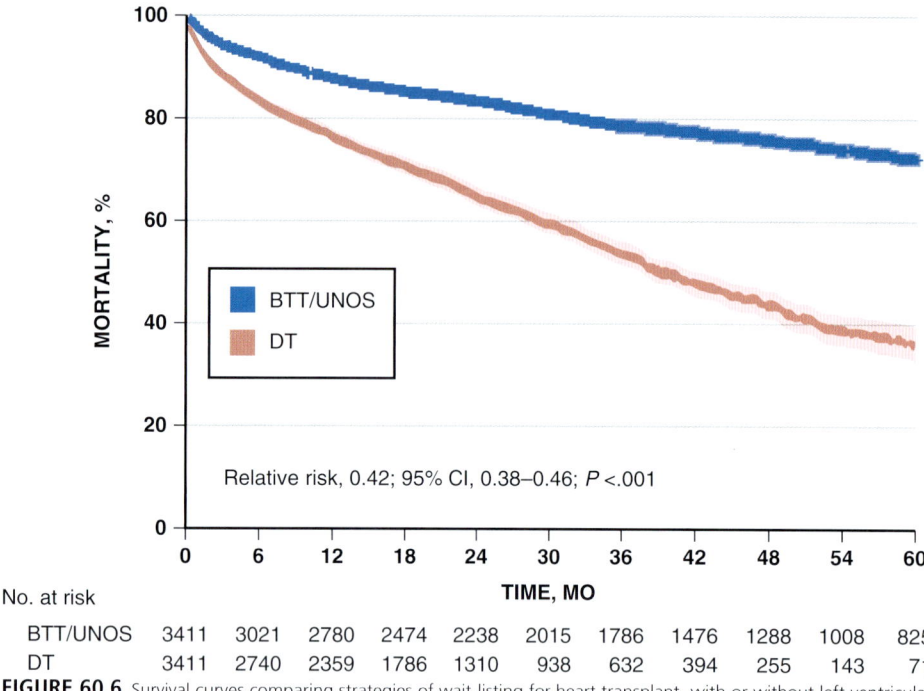

FIGURE 60.6 Survival curves comparing strategies of wait-listing for heart transplant, with or without left ventricular assist device (LVAD) when compared with LVAD destination therapy (DT). The strategy of wait-listing for heart transplant (with or without LVAD) was associated with a superior outcome at 5 years (relative risk [RR], 0.42; 95% CI, 0.38–0.46) after adjusting for select clinical factors. These survival curves accounted for waiting-list mortality with or without bridge to transplant (BTT) LVAD. (From Lala A, Rowland JC, Ferket BC, et al. Strategies of wait-listing for heart transplant vs durable mechanical circulatory support alone for patients with advanced heart failure. *JAMA Cardiol*. 2020;5:652–659.)

in CMV-seronegative recipients of a transplant from a CMV-positive donor. Patients who undergo transplantation with infected LVAD represent a unique and high-risk group for infectious complications post heart transplantation. Surgical management with irrigation and infection control at the time of transplant and prolonged postoperative antibiotics are necessary.

MEDICAL COMPLICATIONS AND COMORBID CONDITIONS

The complications that follow heart transplantation reflect, in part, the premorbid status of a majority of transplant recipients, who have vascular disease and other significant medical conditions.[45] After 5 years, more than 90% of recipients have hypertension, at least 80% have hyperlipidemia, and more than 30% have diabetes, as shown in Table 60.3. Each year after transplantation, clinically significant CAV—which is the major limitation to long life after transplantation—will develop in a larger number of patients. By 5 years, almost 30% of recipients will have CAV, and at least half will be so afflicted at 10 years. It is the most common reason why retransplant is undertaken in the United States (Fig. 60.7). Likewise, progressive renal insufficiency is an insidious problem that is only recently being addressed by substitution protocols to limit the administration of CNIs. Safety and efficacy remain devoid of evidence for the use of mTOR inhibitors as a replacement for CNIs.

Malignancy

Patients are generally considered for transplantation if they have at least a 5-year disease-free interval regarding a preexisting malignancy such as breast, lung, or colon cancer. Malignancy after cardiac transplant is related to a number of risk factors, including age, race, cigarette use, and others (Table 60.4). Most U.S. transplant centers require a cigarette-free interval of a minimum of 6 months before permitting active listing for transplant. More than 10% of adult heart transplant recipients may develop de novo malignancy between years 1 and 5 after transplantation, which is accompanied by increased mortality.[46] Lymphoma and lung cancer are the most common malignancies, with reduced 5-year survival rates of 32% and 21%, respectively, after the time of diagnosis.[47] A dialogue between the transplant cardiologist and the treating oncologist is necessary (see also Chapters 56 and 57) both to discuss the advantage of immunosuppression reduction, as well as monitoring for cardiotoxicity with specific agents with known cardiotoxicity, such as anthracyclines, immune checkpoint inhibitors, and tyrosine kinase inhibitors. Sirolimus, which is uncommonly used as a chronic maintenance immunosuppressive drug, has been associated with reduced occurrences of malignancies in a single center study.[48] Specific to transplant is a malignancy known as post-transplant lymphoproliferative disorder (PTLD). There are known risk factors for PTLD, including an Epstein-Barr virus (EBV)-negative recipient of an EBV+ donor and the use of induction immunotherapy, and others risks that are less well established.[49] Specific treatment often includes immunosuppression reduction, rituximab, and close follow-up monitoring. Skin malignancies are common in all solid organ recipients, and prophylaxis includes limiting exposure to ultraviolet light and liberal use of sunscreen and barrier protection.

Diabetes

Patients in whom new-onset diabetes mellitus develops after transplantation are at increased risk for morbidity and mortality. Accumulating evidence suggests that long-term outcomes, including patient survival and graft survival, may be adversely affected. Much of the diabetes that occurs is attributed to the high-dose corticosteroids used early after transplant surgery, but it is now appreciated that the CNIs play an important role as well. Impaired B cell function appears to be the primary mechanism of CNI-induced new-onset diabetes.

The risk factors for the development of diabetes after transplantation include obesity, increased age, family history of diabetes, abnormal glucose tolerance, and African American or Hispanic descent. Changing trends in the demographics of transplant patients, such as increased age and increased body mass index (BMI), suggest that these patients may now be at a greater risk for new-onset diabetes than in the past. Increased BMI increases risk of insulin resistance, and corticosteroids can cause glucose intolerance, insulin resistance, and frank hyperglycemia. African Americans are more likely to develop new-onset diabetes mellitus regardless of the immunosuppression used but are particularly susceptible after treatment with tacrolimus.

Hypertension

Hypertension is prevalent in heart transplant recipients and associated with the use of CNIs.[50] The control of hypertension and achieving a target blood pressure can be challenging and often require multiple agents (see also Chapter 26). Calcium channel blockers and ACE inhibitors are commonly used. Long-term use of CNIs may lead to the development of chronic kidney disease and refractory hypertension. It is recommended to aggressively treat all cardiac risk factors, including optimal blood pressure control in heart transplant recipients.

Renal Insufficiency

The development of chronic kidney disease is a concern and potentially avoidable after cardiac transplant. A major contributor to the risk of renal disease is CNI nephrotoxicity. The cumulative incidence of chronic renal failure (defined as a glomerular filtration rate of 29 mL/min per 1.73 m^2 of body-surface area or less or the development of end-stage renal disease [ESRD]) 5 years after cardiac transplant is

TABLE 60.3 Cumulative Post–Heart Transplant Morbidity Rates for Adult Patients

OUTCOME	WITHIN 5 YEARS (%)	TOTAL NO. OF PATIENTS WITH KNOWN RESPONSE	WITHIN 10 YEARS	TOTAL NO. OF PATIENTS WITH KNOWN RESPONSE
Hypertension	92	13,023	Not available	Not available
Renal dysfunction	52	15,769	68%	5428
Abnormal creatinine <2.5 mg/dL	33		39%	
Creatinine >2.5 mg/dL	15		20%	
Chronic dialysis	2.9		6.0%	
Renal transplantation	1.1		3.6%	
Hyperlipidemia	88	14,372	Not available	Not available
Diabetes	38	15,458	Not available	Not available
Cardiac allograft vasculopathy	30	11,511	50%	3146

Cumulative prevalence in survivors at 5 and 10 years after transplantation (January 1995 to June 2013).
Adapted from Lund LH, Edwards LB, Kucheryavaya AY, et al. The registry of the International Society for Heart and Lung Transplantation: thirty-first official adult heart transplant report—2014; focus theme: retransplantation. *J Heart Lung Transplant*. 2014;33:996–1008.

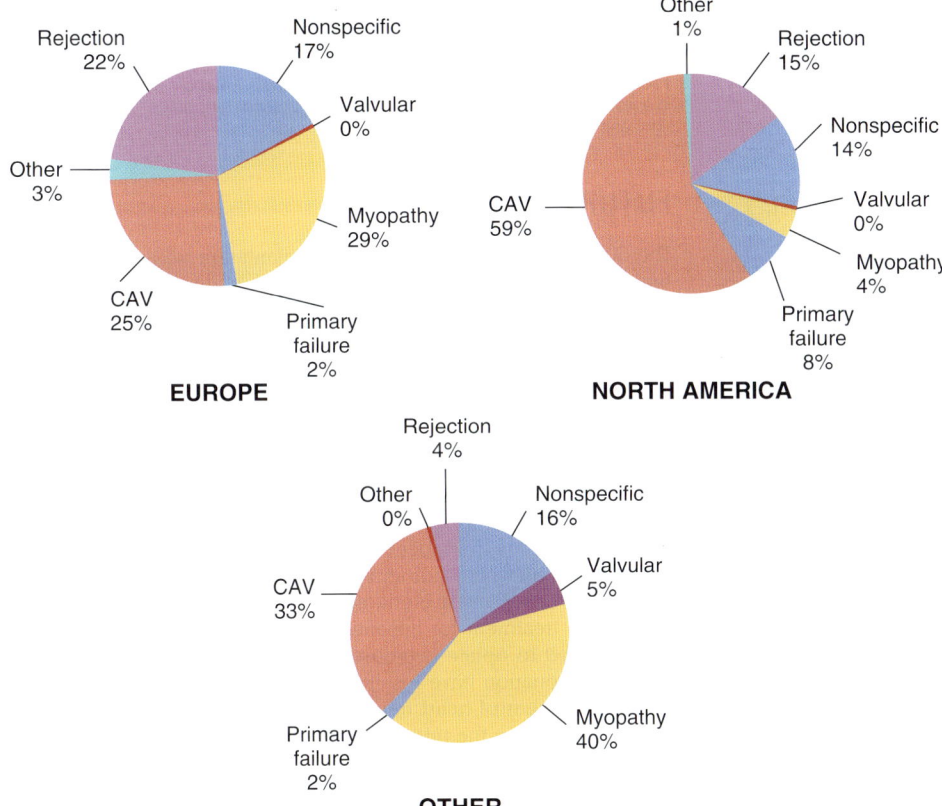

FIGURE 60.7 Indication for retransplantation by geographic location for adult heart retransplantation (2006–June 2013). *CAV*, Coronary allograft vasculopathy. (From Lund LH, Edwards LB, Kucheryavaya AY, et al. The registry of the International Society for Heart and Lung Transplantation: thirty-first official adult heart transplant report—2014; focus theme: retransplantation. *J Heart Lung Transplant*. 2014;33[10]:996–1008.)

10.9%.[51] Known contributing risk factors include age, gender, diabetes mellitus, hypertension, and hepatitis C infection. The high mortality associated with ESRD post heart transplant can be significantly mitigated with renal transplantation (see also Chapter 101).

Hyperlipidemia

Hyperlipidemia is common after transplantation, as it is in the general population. The concern has been that many studies have demonstrated an association of hyperlipidemia with the development of CAV and cerebrovascular and peripheral vascular disease, with the attendant morbidity and mortality of these vascular disorders. Typically, total cholesterol, LDL cholesterol, and triglycerides increase by 3 months after transplantation and then generally fall somewhat after the first year. A number of drugs commonly used after transplantation contribute to the hyperlipidemia observed. Corticosteroids may lead to insulin resistance, increased free fatty acid synthesis, and increased very-LDL production. Cyclosporine increases serum LDL cholesterol and binds to the LDL receptor, decreasing its availability to absorb cholesterol from the bloodstream; tacrolimus probably causes less hyperlipidemia. Sirolimus and MMF also have unfavorable effects on lipids. Sirolimus in escalating doses has been shown to result in prominent elevation of triglyceride levels.

Lipid-lowering therapy with any statin, or HMG-CoA reductase inhibitor, was strongly associated with a marked improvement in 1-year survival in the Heart Transplant Lipid registry. In heart transplant recipients, pravastatin and simvastatin have been associated with outcome benefits in survival, severity of rejection, incidence of CAV, and even malignancies.[52]

Cardiac Allograft Vasculopathy

The development of coronary artery vasculopathy (CAV) is a well-known limitation of cardiac transplantation. CAV may occur in young or older recipients, and its prevalence increases with older donor age. CAV remains the most prominent long-term complication of heart transplantation, with an annual incidence rate of 5% to 10%. CAV is detected angiographically in up to 20% of transplant hearts at 1 year and in 40% to 50% at 5 years. CAV occurring early is predominantly an immune-mediated phenomena with myointimal proliferative lesions characterized by intense cellular infiltration. CAV occurring after the first decade and beyond is similar in its pathologic characteristics as native coronary artery disease. There is evidence to implicate donor-specific antibody production, and AMR with accelerated CAV. CAV angiographically is graded by the ISHLT grading system (Table 60.5) and characterized by diffuse disease and the distal obliteration or "pruning" of the coronary arteries (Fig. 60.8).[53] ISHLT CAV grade 3 represents the most extensive degree of coronary disease based upon angiographic assessment. A single center experience has observed worsening severity of CAV was associated with progressively worse long-term survival. Among patients with CAV, long-term survival in those with CAV amenable to PCI was greater than that in those with severe CAV not treatable with PCI.[54] There is evidence that statin therapy improves outcomes for heart transplant recipients, and statin use is advised in all patients irrespective of lipid levels. The

TABLE 60.4 Multivariable Risk Model for First Invasive Malignancy

LATE PHASE VARIABLE	RELATIVE RISK	P-VALUE
Older age (60 vs. 45 years)	2.1	<0.0001
Black male recipient	1.4	0.04
History of cigarette use	1.2	0.05
History of invasive malignancy	1.6	0.02
Earlier date of transplant (1995 vs. 2005)	2.1	<0.0001

TABLE 60.5 Recommended Nomenclature for Cardiac Allograft Vasculopathy

ISHLT CAV_0	(Not significant): No detectable angiographic lesion
ISHLT CAV_1	(Mild): Angiographic left main (LM) <50%, or primary vessel with maximum lesion of <70%, or any branch stenosis <70% (including diffuse narrowing) without allograft dysfunction
ISHLT CAV_2	(Moderate): Angiographic LM <50%; a single primary vessel >70%, or isolated branch stenosis >70% in branches of 2 systems, without allograft dysfunction
ISHLT CAV_3	(Severe): Angiographic LM >50%, or two or more primary vessels >70% stenosis, or isolated branch stenosis >70% in all 3 systems; or ISHLT CAV_1 or CAV_2 with allograft dysfunction (defined as LVEF <45% usually in the presence of regional wall motion abnormalities) or evidence of significant restrictive physiology (which is common but not specific; see text for definitions)

Definitions

a. A primary vessel denotes the proximal and middle 33% of the left anterior descending artery, the left circumflex, the ramus and the dominant or co-dominant right coronary artery with the posterior descending and posterolateral branches.

b. A secondary branch vessel includes the distal 33% of the primary vessels or any segment within a large septal perforator, diagonals and obtuse marginal branches or any portion of a nondominant right coronary artery.

c. Restrictive cardiac allograft physiology is defined as symptomatic heart failure with echocardiographic E to A velocity ratio >2 (>1.5 in children), shortened isovolumetric relaxation time (<60 msec), shortened deceleration time (<150 msec), or restrictive hemodynamic values (right atrial pressure >12 mm Hg, pulmonary capillary wedge pressure >25 mm Hg, cardiac index <2 $L/min/m^2$).

CAV, Coronary artery vasculopathy; ISHLT, International Society of Heart and Lung Transplantation; LVEF, left ventricular ejection fraction.
From Mehra MR, Crespo-Leiro MG, Dipchand A, et al. International Society for Heart and Lung Transplantation working formulation of a standardized nomenclature for cardiac allograft vasculopathy—2010. J Heart Lung Transplant. 2010;29(7):717–727.

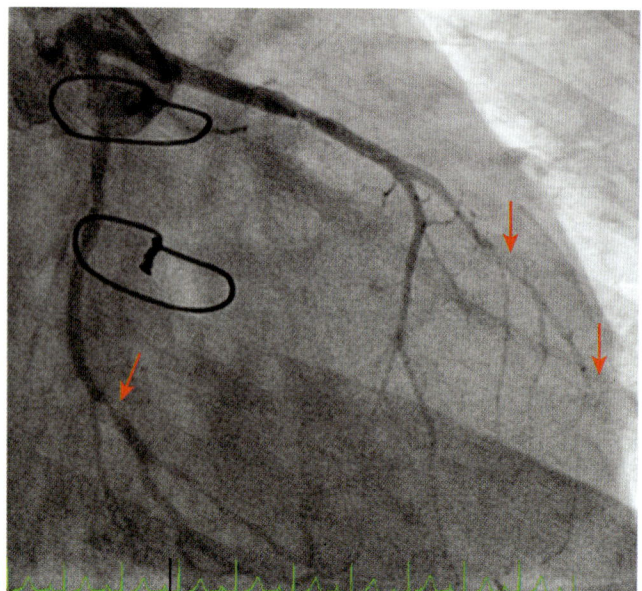

FIGURE 60.8 Coronary artery angiogram showing coronary artery vasculopathy in a heart transplant patient. Arrows indicate distal obliteration or "pruning" of the right and left coronary arteries.

use of low-dose aspirin (81 mg) is also recommended substantiated by isolated reports demonstrating improved survival with aspirin use.[55] Ultimately the only treatment for extensive CAV may be retransplantation. Patients with extensive CAV and no other risk factors experience improved long-term survival with retransplantation; however, medical management in the absence of systolic dysfunction should be considered.[56,57] Lack of donor organs creates an ethical discussion when considering the option of retransplantation. The option of using an mTOR inhibitor (everolimus, sirolimus) as part of the immunosuppressive regimen in patients with established CAV has been advocated.[58] The strategy for heart transplant recipients for the longitudinal surveillance, and follow-up of established CAV varies widely across centers. Although yearly coronary angiography was the initial standard, followed by the use of IVUS in conjunction with angiography, more centers now are using various noninvasive testing protocols. CAV remains an area in dire need of continued research to establish best practices for primary and secondary prevention.

FUTURE PERSPECTIVES

The 50th anniversary of cardiac transplantation was recently celebrated and provided the opportunity to reflect upon the tremendous progress that has occurred over the past 5 decades. Successful transplantation requires excellence in multiple facets including organ harvesting and preservation, surgical implantation, immunosuppression, and post-transplant surveillance, and multi-disciplinary care. Clearly over the past 2 decades a shift has occurred with greater care pre- and post-transplant provided by cardiologists. Importantly, the discipline of transplant cardiology emerged in 2010 with the opportunity for board certification in the United States. Organ preservation systems have been developed for longer ischemic times with good organ function. Surgical techniques have been refined. The standard approach to monitor for rejection with histology is now moving toward molecular diagnostics and fewer invasive endomyocardial biopsies. The emergence of effective treatment for hepatitis C and the knowledge that donor death related to opiate overdose is not a contraindication to heart transplant donation have resulted in an expanding donor pool and a greater number of heart transplants. The challenges that will need to be addressed in the future include personalizing, minimizing, and improving immunosuppression and overall protocols. The prospect of immune tolerance does not appear to be a near-term reality; hence we must continue to immunosuppress our patients. Our goal must be to determine the least amount of immunosuppression necessary to avoid the adverse impact of immunotherapy while maintaining graft survival. Mechanical circulatory support has also advanced tremendously over the past 25 years (see Chapter 59) but still cannot match the outcomes with cardiac transplantation. CAV remains a devastating problem limiting the long-term success of cardiac transplantation and should remain an active area of research to advance the field. The mechanisms of early coronary vasculopathy are certainly primarily immune mediated and will be overcome only if we understand and develop treatments to prevent and/or mitigate. Evidence is required to improve outcomes, which is challenging in heart transplantation with limited patient numbers.[59] Risk factor modification is imperative in this patient population at high risk for vascular complications. The future may find that sodium-glucose cotransporter inhibitors have an important role to mitigate adverse events, but well-designed randomized clinical trials must be conducted to advance our knowledge. For now, cardiac transplantation unquestionably remains the best treatment option for eligible potential recipients with stage D, advanced heart failure.

ACKNOWLEDGMENTS

The author gratefully acknowledges Drs. Mariell Jessup, Pavan Alturi, and Michael A. Acker, whose chapter on this topic in the prior edition of *Braunwald's Heart Disease: A Textbook of Cardiovascular Medicine* served as the partial basis for the current chapter.

This chapter is dedicated in memory of the late David O. Taylor, MD, and the advanced heart failure and cardiac transplant medicine fellows that have trained at the Cleveland Clinic.

REFERENCES

History, Epidemiology and Evaluation of the Recipient

1. Stehlik J, Kobashigawa J, Hunt SA, et al. Honoring 50 years of clinical heart transplantation in *Circulation*: in-depth State-of-the-Art review. *Circulation*. 2018;137(1):71–87.
2. Woolley AE, Singh SK, Goldberg HJ, et al. Heart and lung transplants from HCV-infected donors to uninfected recipients. *N Engl J Med*. 2019;380(17):1606–1617.
3. Vaduganathan M, Machado SR, DeFilippis EM, et al. Organ donation and drug intoxication-related deaths in the United States. *N Engl J Med*. 2019;380(6):597–599.
4. Mehra MR, Jarcho JA, Cherikh W, et al. The drug-Intoxication epidemic and solid-organ transplantation. *N Engl J Med*. 2018;378(20):1943–1945.
5. Guglin M, Zucker MJ, Borlaug BA, et al. Evaluation for heart transplantation and LVAD implantation: JACC Council perspectives. *J Am Coll Cardiol*. 2020;75(12):1471–1487.

Donor and Surgery Considerations, Allocation, Immunosuppression

6. Maldonado JR, Sher Y, Lolak S, et al. The Stanford Integrated psychosocial assessment for transplantation: a prospective study of medical and psychosocial outcomes. *Psychosom Med*. 2015;77(9):1018–1030.
7. Dew MA, DiMartini AF, Dobbels F, et al. The 2018 ISHLT/APM/AST/ICCAC/STSW recommendations for the psychosocial evaluation of adult cardiothoracic transplant candidates and candidates for long-term mechanical circulatory support. *J Heart Lung Transplant*. 2018;37(7):803–823.
8. Truby LK, Rogers JG. Advanced heart failure: epidemiology, diagnosis, and therapeutic approaches. *JACC Heart Fail*. 2020;8(7):523–536.
9. Ardehali A, Esmailian F, Deng M, et al. Ex-vivo perfusion of donor hearts for human heart transplantation (PROCEED II): a prospective, open-label, multicentre, randomised non-inferiority trial. *Lancet*. 2015;385:2577–2584.
10. Smith JW, O'Brien KD, Dardas T, et al. Systematic donor selection review process improves cardiac transplant volumes and outcomes. *J Thorac Cardiovasc Surg*. 2016;151:238–243.
11. Phillips KG, Ranganath NK, Malas J, et al. Impact of the opioid epidemic on heart transplantation: donor characteristics and organ discard. *Ann Thorac Surg*. 2019;108(4):1133–1139.
12. Gidea CG, Narula N, Reyentovich A, et al. Increased early acute cellular rejection events in hepatitis C-positive heart transplantation. *J Heart Lung Transplant*. 2020;S1053–2498(20)31624-7.
13. Messer S, Cernic S, Page A, et al. 5-Year single Centre early experience of heart transplantation from Donation After Circulatory Determined death (DCD) donors. *J Heart Lung Trans*. 2020;S1053–2498(20):31765-4.
14. Rajab TK, Jaggers J, Campbell DN. Heart transplantation following donation after cardiac death: history, current techniques, and future. *J Thorac Cardiovasc Surg*. 2020;S0022-5223(20)30529-8.
15. Davies RR, Russo MJ, Morgan JA, et al. Standard versus bicaval techniques for orthotopic heart transplantation: an analysis of the United Network for Organ Sharing database. *J Thorac Cardiovasc Surg*. 2010:700–708, 8 e1–2.
16. Bermudez CA, Rame JE. Reversible but risky: pulmonary hypertension in advanced heart failure is the Achilles' heel of cardiac transplantation. *J Thorac Cardiovasc Surg*. 2015;150:1362–1363.
17. Soderlund C, Radegran G. Immunosuppressive therapies after heart transplantation—the balance between under- and over-immunosuppression. *Transplant Rev (Orlando)*. 2015;29:181–189.
18. Whitson BA, Kilic A, Lehman A, et al. Impact of induction immunosuppression on survival in heart transplant recipients: a contemporary analysis of agents. *Clin Transplant*. 2015;29:9–17.
19. Khush KK, Potena L, Cherikh WS, et al. The international thoracic organ transplant registry of the international Society for heart and lung transplantation: 37th adult heart transplantation report-2020; focus on deceased donor characteristics. *J Heart Lung Transplant*. 2020;S1053–2498(20):31660-0.
20. Nozohoor S, Stehlik J, Lund LH, et al. Induction immunosuppression strategies and long-term outcomes after heart transplantation. *Clin Transplant*. 2020;34:e13871.
21. Kobashigawa JA, Meiser BM. Review of major clinical trials with mycophenolate mofetil in cardiac transplantation. *Transplantation*. 2005;80(suppl 2):S235–S243.
22. Eisen HJ, Tuzcu EM, Dorent R, et al. Everolimus for the prevention of allograft rejection and vasculopathy in cardiac-transplant recipients. *N Engl J Med*. 2003;349(9):847–858.
23. Topilsky Y, Hasin T, Raichlin E, et al. Sirolimus as primary immunosuppression attenuates allograft vasculopathy with improved late survival and decreased cardiac events after cardiac transplantation. *Circulation*. 2012;125(5):708–720.
24. Kobashigawa JA, Pauly DF, Starling RC, et al. Cardiac allograft vasculopathy by intravascular ultrasound in heart transplant patients: substudy from the everolimus versus mycophenolate mofetil randomized, multicenter trial. *JACC Heart Fail*. 2013;1(5):389–399.
25. Asleh R, Briasoulis A, Kremers WK, et al. Long-term sirolimus for primary immunosuppression in heart transplant recipients. *J Am Coll Cardiol*. 2018;71(6):636–650.
26. Eisen HJ. CAVEAT mTOR: You've heard about the benefits of using mTOR inhibitors, here are some of the risks. *Am J Transplant*. 2020;21:449–450.
27. Tsay AJ, Eisen HJ. mTOR inhibitors vs calcineurin inhibitors: a Catch-22-preventing nephrotoxicity or acute allograft rejection after heart transplantation. *Am J Transplant*. 2019;19(11):2967–2968.
28. Eisen HJ, Kobashigawa J, Starling RC, et al. Everolimus versus mycophenolate mofetil in heart transplantation: a randomized, multicenter trial. *Am J Transplant*. 2013;13(5):1203–1216.

Rejection, Outcomes, Infection

29. Stewart S, Winters GL, Fishbein MC, et al. Revision of the 1990 working formulation for the standardization of nomenclature in the diagnosis of heart rejection. *J Heart Lung Transplant*. 2005;24(11):1710–1720.
30. Estep JD, Shah DJ, Nagueh SF, et al. The role of multimodality cardiac imaging in the transplanted heart. *JACC Cardiovasc Imaging*. 2009;2(9):1126–1140.
31. Pham MX, Teuteberg JJ, Kfoury AG, et al. Gene-expression profiling for rejection surveillance after cardiac transplantation. *N Engl J Med*. 2010;362(20):1890–1900.
32. Khush KK, Patel J, Pinney S, et al. Noninvasive detection of graft injury after heart transplant using donor-derived cell-free DNA: a prospective multicenter study. *Am J Transplant*. 2019;19(10):2889–2899.
33. Berry GJ, Angelini A, Burke MM, et al. The ISHLT working formulation for pathologic diagnosis of antibody-mediated rejection in heart transplantation: evolution and current status (2005–2011). *J Heart Lung Transplant*. 2011;30(6):601–611.
34. Colvin MM, Cook JL, Chang P, et al. Antibody-mediated rejection in cardiac transplantation: emerging knowledge in diagnosis and management: a scientific statement from the American Heart Association. *Circulation*. 2015;131(18):1608–1639.
35. Halloran PF, Potena L, Van Huyen JD, et al. Building a tissue-based molecular diagnostic system in heart transplant rejection: the heart Molecular Microscope Diagnostic (MMDx) System. *J Heart Lung Transplant*. 2017;36(11):1192–1200.
36. Chih S, Chong AY, Erthal F, et al. PET assessment of epicardial intimal disease and Microvascular dysfunction in cardiac allograft vasculopathy. *J Am Coll Cardiol*. 2018;71(13):1444–1456.
37. ISHLT registry. www. https://ishltregistries.org/registries/slides.asp.
38. Scientific registry of transplant recipients. https://www.srtr.org/transplant-centers/?organ=heart&recipientType=adult&query=.
39. Kittleson MM, Kobashigawa JA. Cardiac transplantation: current outcomes and contemporary controversies. *JACC Heart Fail*. 2017;5(12):857–868.
40. Khush KK, Potena L, Cherikh WS, et al. The international thoracic organ transplant registry of the international society for heart and lung transplantation: 37th adult heart transplantation report-2020; focus on deceased donor characteristics. *J Heart Lung Transplant*. 2020;39(10):1003–1015.
41. Lala A, Rowland JC, Ferket BS, et al. Strategies of wait-listing for heart transplant vs durable mechanical circulatory support alone for patients with advanced heart failure. *JAMA Cardiol*. 2020;5(6):652–659.
42. Mingxi DY, Liebo MJ, Lundgren S, et al. Impaired exercise tolerance early after heart transplantation is associated with development of cardiac allograft vasculopathy. *Transplantation*. 2020;104(10):2196–2203.
43. Kobashigawa JA, Leaf DA, Lee N, et al. A controlled trial of exercise rehabilitation after heart transplantation. *N Engl J Med*. 1999;340(4):272–277.
44. Kotton CN, Kumar D, Caliendo AM, et al. The Third international Consensus guidelines on the management of cytomegalovirus in solid-organ transplantation. *Transplantation*. 2018;102(6):900–931.

Medical Complications, Comorbidities, and Future Perspective

45. Singh TP, Milliren CE, Almond CS, Graham D. Survival benefit from transplantation in patients listed for heart transplantation in the United States. *J Am Coll Cardiol*. 2014;63:1169–1178.
46. Youn JC, Stehlik J, Wilk AR, et al. Temporal trends of de novo malignancy development after heart transplantation. *J Am Coll Cardiol*. 2018;71(1):40–49.
47. Higgins RS, Brown RN, Chang PP, et al. A multi-institutional study of malignancies after heart transplantation and a comparison with the general United States population. *J Heart Lung Transplant*. 2014;33(5):478–485.
48. Asleh R, Clavell AL, Pereira NL, et al. Incidence of malignancies in patients treated with sirolimus following heart transplantation. *J Am Coll Cardiol*. 2019;73(21):2676–2688.
49. Dierickx D, Habermann TM. Post-transplantation lymphoproliferative disorders in adults. *N Engl J Med*. 2018;378(6):549–562.
50. Campbell PT, Krim SR. Hypertension in cardiac transplant recipients: tackling a new face of an old foe. *Curr Opin Cardiol*. 2020;35(4):368–375.
51. Ojo AO, Held PJ, Port FK, et al. Chronic renal failure after transplantation of a nonrenal organ. *N Engl J Med*. 2003;349(10):931–940.
52. Frohlich GM, Rufibach K, Enseleit F, et al. Statins and the risk of cancer after heart transplantation. *Circulation*. 2012;126:440–447.
53. Mehra MR, Crespo-Leiro MG, Dipchand A, et al. International Society for Heart and Lung Transplantation working formulation of a standardized nomenclature for cardiac allograft vasculopathy-2010. *J Heart Lung Transplant*. 2010;29(7):717–727. Erratum in: J Heart Lung Transplant. 2011 Mar;30(3):360. PMID: 20620917.
54. Agarwal S, Parashar A, Kapadia SR, et al. Long-term mortality after cardiac allograft vasculopathy: implications of percutaneous intervention. *JACC Heart Fail*. 2014;2(3):281–288.
55. Kim M, Bergmark BA, Zelniker TA, et al. Early aspirin use and the development of cardiac allograft vasculopathy. *J Heart Lung Transplant*. 2017;36(12):1344–1349.
56. Goldraich LA, Stehlik J, Kucheryavaya AY, et al. Retransplant and medical therapy for cardiac allograft vasculopathy: international Society for heart and lung transplantation registry analysis. *Am J Transplant*. 2016;16(1):301–309.
57. Barghash MH, Pinney SP. Heart retransplantation: Candidacy, outcomes, and management. *Curr Transplant Rep*. 2020;7(1):12–17.
58. Asleh R, Alnsasra H, Lerman A, et al. Effects of mTOR inhibitor-related proteinuria on progression of cardiac allograft vasculopathy and outcomes among heart transplant recipients. *Am J Transplant*. 2021;21:626–635.
59. Shah MR, Starling RC, Schwartz Longacre L, et al. Heart transplantation research in the next decade–a goal to achieving evidence-based outcomes: National Heart, Lung, and Blood Institute Working Group. *J Am Coll Cardiol*. 2012;59(14):1263–1269.

第七部分　心律失常

吴灵敏　姚焰　导读

心脏最核心的功能是泵血功能，实现机械泵血功能的前提是有正常的心电活动。心律失常是心脏电活动异常的外在表现，其发生机制是电冲动的形成异常和（或）传导异常。心血管内科一直被誉为内科学的皇冠，而心律失常则是皇冠上最耀眼的那颗明珠。心律失常发病率、致死致残率高，其诊断、风险评估和治疗一直是公认的难点和痛点。随着我国人口老龄化的加剧，从事各学科的医务工作者均应掌握一定的心律失常基础知识以指导临床实践。

心律失常种类繁多，按照临床表现可分为快速性心律失常和缓慢性心律失常。快速性心律失常主要涵盖窦性心动过速、房性期前收缩、房性心动过速、心房扑动、心房颤动、室性期前收缩、室性心动过速（室速）、心室扑动和心室颤动（室颤）等；缓慢性心律失常则主要包括病态窦房结综合征、房间传导阻滞、房室传导阻滞、束支传导阻滞等。Braunwald 教授曾预言心力衰竭和心房颤动是本世纪心脏病学面临的最大挑战，然而，心房颤动仅仅是众多心律失常中的一种而已。

近半个世纪来，心律失常领域的进展层出不穷，已经取得了丰硕的成果。实际上，现代医学能够根治的疾病殊为有限，而在快速性心律失常治疗领域，导管消融手术的出现和成熟，使得大部分心律失常的根治成为现实。随着导管消融技术领域的持续进步，既往被认为是禁区的顽固性器质性室速/室颤领域，也出现了骄人的成绩。对于致命性的恶性室性心律失常，植入式心脏复律除颤器作为生命的最后保障，挽救了无数的生命。缓慢性心律失常领域，起搏器植入作为一项近乎根治性疗效的治疗策略，已经发展至更加符合生理的希浦系统起搏阶段，并且该技术为我国学者所原创。此外，心脏神经节改良消融技术在心律失常治疗领域已展现出诱人的前景，我国学者也是该领域的主要原创者之一。简言之，在诸多医学亚专科当中，心律失常领域属于较早的进入了微创、根治的先进行列，并且我国学者勇立潮头，在推动学科的发展中发挥了重要的作用。

《Braunwald 心脏病学》第 61～71 章为心律失常部分，其撰写高屋建瓴、气势恢宏，全面阐述了各种心律失常的发病机制、诊断和鉴别诊断、风险分层和治疗等领域的基础知识和最新进展。其中，第 61 章对心律失常的诊断和评估进行了总的概述；第 62 章详细论述了心律失常的发病机制；第 63 章结合最新的遗传学研究成果，全面介绍了心律失常相关遗传学知识；第 64 章系统概述了快速性心律失常的治疗进展；第 65 章梳理了各种类型室上性心动过速的定义、流行病学、临床特征和治疗策略；第 66 章针对心房颤动的临床特征、机制和管理进行了深入浅出的论述；第 67 章对各种室性心律失常的管理进行了阐述；第 68～69 章介绍了各种缓慢性心律失常和传导阻滞，并论述了起搏器和除颤器植入的基础知识和最近进展；第 70 章全面介绍了心搏骤停和心脏性猝死的相关知识，包括定义、流行病学、病因等，重点介绍了防治策略尤其是公共安全防治措施等；第 71 章对低血压和晕厥进行了概述，并重点关注了心脏神经改良消融技术的应用价值。

故书不厌百回读，熟读深思子自知。掌握坚实的基础知识，是正确临床实践和推动医学科学发展的前提条件。尤其对于临床实践而言，世界上没有两个完全一样的患者，个体化是临床诊疗的最高准则，从理论到实践的反复轮回是必要的保证。千秋邈矣独留我，百战归来再读书。希望本书能为读者提供一份有益的思想启迪和现实帮助。

PART VII ARRHYTHMIAS, SUDDEN DEATH, AND SYNCOPE

61 Approach to the Patient with Cardiac Arrhythmias

ANNE B. CURTIS AND GORDON F. TOMASELLI

GENERAL APPROACH TO THE HISTORY AND PHYSICAL EXAM, 1145
History, 1145
Physical Examination, 1146

SIGNS AND SYMPTOMS, 1146
Palpitations, 1146
Syncope, Presyncope, and Altered Level of Consciousness, 1147
Sudden Cardiac Arrest and Aborted Sudden Cardiac Death, 1148

CLINICAL AND LABORATORY TESTING, 1148
Resting Electrocardiogram, 1148
Cardiac Imaging, 1149
Stress Electrocardiography, 1149
Long-term Electrocardiogram Recording: Holter Monitoring, Event Recording, and Insertable Loop Recorders, 1151

HEAD UP TILT, 1155
Invasive Electrophysiologic Testing, 1156
Complications of Electrophysiologic Studies, 1159

REFERENCES, 1161

The evaluation of patients with suspected cardiac arrhythmias is highly individualized and must include a comprehensive assessment of the patient. Evaluation of the patient begins with a careful history and physical examination and should usually progress from the simplest to the most complex diagnostic test, from the least invasive and safest to the most invasive and risky, and from the least expensive out-of-hospital evaluations to those that require hospitalization and sophisticated, costly, and potentially risky procedures. However, two key features—the history and the electrocardiogram (ECG)—are pivotal in directing the diagnostic evaluation and treatment. The physical examination is focused on determining whether there is cardiopulmonary disease that is associated with specific cardiac arrhythmias. The absence of significant cardiopulmonary disease often, but not always, suggests a benign cause of a cardiac rhythm disturbance. The judicious use of noninvasive diagnostic tests is an important element in the evaluation of patients with arrhythmias, and the most important is the ECG, particularly if recorded at the time of symptoms.

An evidence-based approach to the history and physical examination for patients with suspected cardiovascular (CV) disease is presented in Chapter 13. This chapter focuses on features most germane to the patient with cardiac rhythm disturbances. However, it is essential to understand that the general medical condition of the patient may profoundly influence the presentation of any cardiac arrhythmia. This chapter discusses the approach to and diagnostic evaluation of the patient with a suspected arrhythmia, keeping in mind that arrhythmia management has two goals: addressing the patient's symptoms as well as whatever risks the arrhythmia poses to the individual.

GENERAL APPROACH TO THE HISTORY AND PHYSICAL EXAM

History

Patients with cardiac arrhythmias exhibit a wide spectrum of clinical presentations, ranging from asymptomatic incidental ECG abnormalities to survival from sudden cardiac arrest (SCA). The presenting features may vary with circumstances, and arrhythmias are common in the setting of CV and medical diseases, leading to overlap of symptoms and signs. The history is key to directing the evaluation of patients. In general, the more severe the presenting symptoms, the more aggressive are the evaluation and treatment. The presence of structural heart disease and prior myocardial infarction (MI) often dictates a change in the approach to the management of syncope or a presumed cardiac arrhythmia.

In assessing a patient with a known or suspected arrhythmia, several key pieces of information should be obtained that can help determine a diagnosis or guide further diagnostic testing. The mode of onset of an episode can provide clues about the type of arrhythmia or preferred treatment option. For example, palpitations that occur in the setting of exercise, fright, or anger are often caused by catecholamine-sensitive automatic or triggered tachycardias that may respond to adrenergic blocking agents. Palpitations that occur at rest or that awaken the patient can be caused by enhanced vagal tone; an example of such an arrhythmia is atrial fibrillation (AF). Lightheadedness or syncope occurring in the setting of a tightly fitting collar or turning the head suggests carotid sinus hypersensitivity. The triggering event may help establish the presence of an inherited ion channel abnormality such as the long-QT syndrome (LQTS) (see Chapter 63). The mode of termination of episodes can also be helpful: palpitations that are reliably terminated by breath-holding or by Valsalva or other vagal maneuvers probably involve the atrioventricular (AV) node as an integral part of a tachycardia circuit. On occasion, focal atrial tachycardia (AT) or ventricular tachycardia (VT) can be terminated with vagal maneuvers, as can VT originating in the right ventricular outflow tract. Patients should be asked about the frequency and duration of episodes and the severity of symptoms. These features help guide how aggressively and quickly the physician needs to pursue a diagnostic or therapeutic plan (a patient with daily episodes associated with near-syncope or severe dyspnea warrants a more expeditious evaluation than does one with infrequent episodes of mild palpitations and no other symptoms). Patients should be encouraged to report their heart rate during an episode (either rapid or slow, regular or irregular) by counting the pulse directly or by using a blood pressure or heart rate monitor, wearable, or smart phone application. Devices recording an ECG waveform provide the most reliable data.

A careful drug and dietary history should also be sought; some nasal decongestants can provoke tachycardia episodes, whereas beta-adrenergic receptor-blocking eye drops for the treatment of glaucoma can drain into tear ducts, be absorbed systemically, and precipitate syncope secondary to bradycardia. Dietary supplements, particularly those containing stimulants, can cause arrhythmias. A growing list of drugs can directly or indirectly affect ventricular repolarization and produce or exacerbate long-QT interval–related tachyarrhythmias (see Chapter 9). The patient should be questioned about the presence of systemic

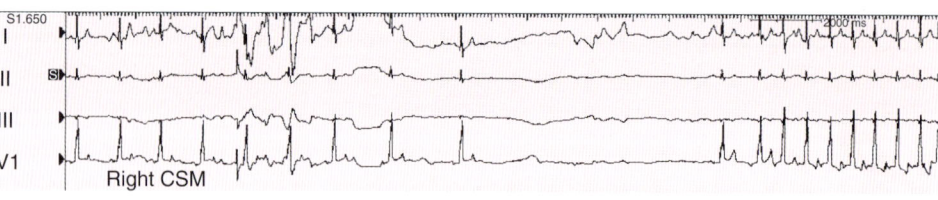

FIGURE 61.1 Right carotid sinus massage (CSM) produces sinus arrest and a 7.2-second pause in a patient with episodic dizziness. (Image courtesy Dr. Joseph Marine.)

illnesses that may be associated with arrhythmias, such as chronic obstructive pulmonary disease, thyrotoxicosis (see Chapter 94), pericarditis (Chapter 86), and chronic heart failure (Chapters 49 and 50), as well as previous chest injury, surgery, radiation therapy, or chemotherapy.

A family history of a significant cardiac arrhythmia may not directly inform the prognosis of a patient, but it should alert the practitioner to the possibility of a heritable trait such as a channelopathy (Chapter 63), cardiomyopathy (Chapters 52 and 54) or neuromuscular disease (Chapter 100) that may increase susceptibility to development of an arrhythmia.

Physical Examination

In the absence of symptoms, the physical examination is focused on determining whether CV or general medical disease is present. The lack of significant cardiopulmonary disease often, but not always, suggests benignity of a rhythm disturbance. Conversely, palpitations, syncope, or near-syncope in the setting of significant heart or lung disease have a more ominous prognosis. In addition, the physical examination may reveal the presence of a persistent arrhythmia such as AF. The detailed approach to the CV physical examination is outlined in Chapter 13 and may suggest the presence of structural heart disease (and thus generally a clinically more serious situation with a worse overall prognosis), even in the absence of an arrhythmia episode. For example, a laterally displaced or dyskinetic apical impulse, a regurgitant or stenotic murmur, or a third heart sound in an older adult can denote significant myocardial or valvular dysfunction or damage.

The general physical examination is also important and can identify medical conditions associated with cardiac manifestations and arrhythmias. Inspection of the skin may reveal erythema chronicum migrans, the rash associated with Lyme disease; hair loss and exophthalmos may reflect the presence of thyroid disease; and ptosis, cataracts, and skeletal muscle wasting or myotonia may indicate the presence of neuromuscular disease (see Chapter 100). Even facial features may suggest an associated rhythm disorder (e.g., cataracts and early balding with myotonic dystrophy, micrognathia, and low-set ears in Andersen-Tawil syndrome).

If tachycardia is present, the priorities are evaluation of the heart rate and blood pressure, and to obtain a 12-lead ECG if the patient is hemodynamically stable. If it is not possible to obtain an ECG, several clues on the physical examination can help to make a diagnosis. The presence of regular cannon A waves in the jugular venous pulse would be consistent with 1:1 retrograde ventriculoatrial activation, as in tachycardias such as atrioventricular reentrant tachycardia (AVRT), atrioventricular nodal reentrant tachycardia (AVNRT), and some junctional tachycardias and VTs. In contrast, patients may have physical examination features of AV dissociation, such as intermittent "cannon" A waves, indicative of right atrial contraction against a closed tricuspid valve, variable intensity of the first heart sound, and variable peak systolic blood pressure, consistent with arrhythmias, including VT and nonparoxysmal AV junctional tachycardia, without retrograde capture of the atria (see Chapter 13).

The Valsalva maneuver and carotid sinus massage (CSM) during the physical examination can be useful to interrupt arrhythmias sensitive to autonomic tone or identify the patient with a hypersensitive carotid sinus reflex. CSM is performed with the patient supine and comfortable and the head turned slightly away from the side being stimulated. The examiner first needs to listen carefully over both carotid arteries to be certain that no bruit is present. The area of the carotid sinus, at the artery's bifurcation, is palpated lightly at the angle of the jaw until a good pulse is felt. Even this minimal amount of pressure can induce a hypersensitive response in susceptible individuals. If no initial effect is noted, a side-to-side or rotating motion of the fingers over the site is performed for up to 5 seconds. Lack of effect on the ECG after 5 seconds of pressure adequate to cause mild discomfort is considered a negative response. Because responses to carotid massage may differ on the two sides, the maneuver can be repeated on the opposite side; however, both sides should never be stimulated simultaneously. Findings may not be readily reproducible, even within minutes of a prior attempt. Gentle massage is usually sufficient to terminate a sensitive tachycardia or produce significant periods of sinus arrest or AV block in susceptible patients. The most definitive responses to CSM are tachycardia termination, as may be observed in AVRT, AVNRT, sinus node reentry, adenosine-sensitive AT, and idiopathic right ventricular outflow tract tachycardia. CSM can gradually slow a sinus tachycardia without termination and decrease the ventricular response to AT, atrial flutter, and AF without termination, allowing examination of atrial activity. CSM transiently terminates the permanent form of AV junctional reciprocating tachycardia, which then restarts when carotid massage ceases. CSM generally does not affect reentrant ventricular or junctional tachycardias (Fig. 61.1). During wide-QRS tachycardias with a 1:1 relationship between the P waves and QRS complexes, vagal influence can terminate or slow a supraventricular tachycardia (SVT) that depends on the AV node for perpetuation; on the other hand, vagal effects on the AV node can transiently block retrograde conduction and thus establish the diagnosis of VT by demonstrating AV dissociation (Fig. 61.2). Because the effect of either of these physical maneuvers typically lasts only seconds, clinicians must be ready to observe or record any changes in rhythm on an ECG when the maneuver is performed.

SIGNS AND SYMPTOMS

Palpitations

Palpitations are the awareness of the heartbeat that may be caused by a rapid heart rate, irregularities in heart rhythm, or an increase in the force of cardiac contraction, as occurs with a post–extrasystolic beat; however, this perception can also exist in the setting of a completely normal cardiac rhythm. Patients who complain of palpitations describe the sensation of an unpleasant awareness of a forceful, irregular, or rapid beating of the heart. Many patients are acutely aware of any cardiac irregularity, whereas others are oblivious, even to long runs of a rapid VT or AF with a rapid ventricular rate. The latter is particularly noteworthy because if untreated, it may be associated with stroke or may produce a tachycardia-induced cardiomyopathy. Patients may use terms such as a "pounding" or "flipping" sensation in the chest; a fullness or pounding in the throat, neck, or chest; or a pause in the heartbeat, or "skipped beat." The skip often results from the pause after a premature ventricular complex (PVC) or the resetting of sinus rhythm after a premature atrial complex (PAC). Usually, the premature beat, particularly if it is a ventricular extrasystole, occurs too early to permit sufficient ventricular filling to cause a sensation when the ventricle contracts. The ventricular systole that ends the compensatory pause is often responsible for the actual palpitation, the result of a more forceful contraction from prolonged ventricular filling or increased motion of the heart in the chest.

Anxiety over such symptoms is usually the complaint that brings the patient to the physician's attention. Premature atrial or ventricular complexes constitute the most common causes of palpitations. If the premature complexes are frequent, or particularly if a sustained tachycardia is present, patients are more likely to have additional symptoms, such as lightheadedness, syncope or near-syncope, chest discomfort, fatigue, or shortness of breath. The context and symptoms associated

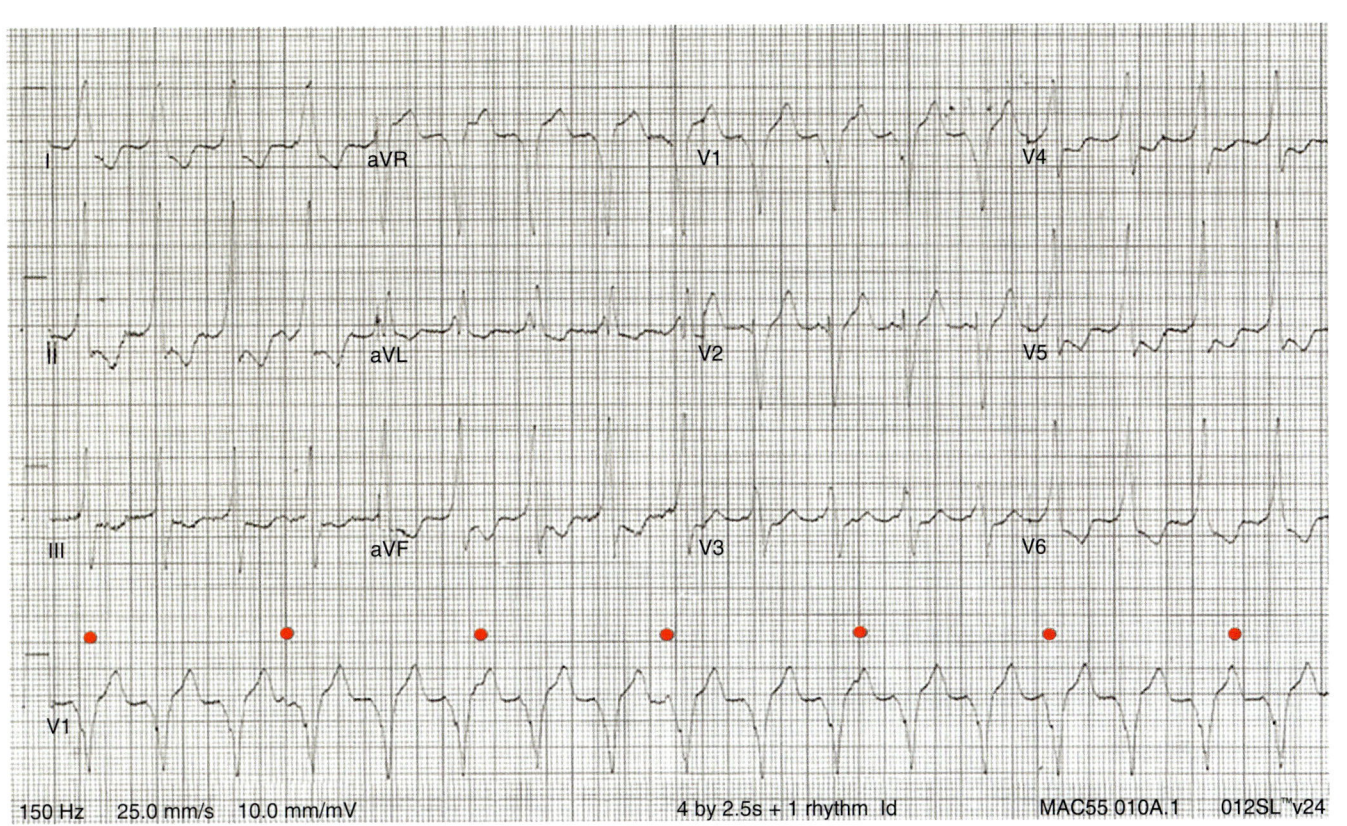

FIGURE 61.2 Wide complex tachycardia with AV dissociation establishing the diagnosis of ventricular tachycardia. P waves are dissociated from the QRS complexes and are indicated by the red dots; the sinus rate is approximately 40 beats/min.

with palpitations can be diagnostically and prognostically informative. Low-risk features include isolated palpitations not induced by exercise, the absence of structural heart disease or symptoms such as syncope or chest pain, no family history of sudden cardiac death (SCD), and a normal 12-lead ECG. Associated symptoms, such as syncope or chest pain, the presence of structural heart disease or a documented arrhythmia, and family history of SCD may be associated with a more ominous cause of palpitations.[1]

The differential diagnosis of palpitations is broad. The age of the patient and the presence of associated CV problems influence the nature of the symptoms. For example, an SVT at a rate of 180 beats/min can provoke chest pain in a patient with coronary artery disease (CAD) or syncope in a patient with aortic stenosis but may result in mild breathlessness in an otherwise healthy young person. The onset and offset of palpitations can suggest the etiology of the arrhythmia. A sudden, abrupt onset, "like a light switch turning on," is consistent with a paroxysmal tachycardia such as AVNRT (see Chapter 65), whereas gradual speeding and slowing are more consistent with atrial or sinus tachycardia. However, even tachycardias that start abruptly can begin and end with extra beats appearing to have a more gradual onset and offset. Termination by Valsalva maneuver or CSM suggests a tachycardia incorporating nodal tissue in the reentrant pathway, such as sinus node reentry, AVRT, or AVNRT (see Chapters 62 and 65).

The rate of an untreated tachycardia often narrows diagnostic possibilities, and patients should be taught to count their radial or carotid pulse rate, noting whether it is regular or irregular. Ventricular rates of 150 beats/min should always suggest the diagnosis of atrial flutter with 2:1 AV block (see Chapter 65), whereas most SVTs, such as those caused by AVNRT or AVRT, usually occur at rates exceeding 150 beats/min. The rates of VTs overlap with those of SVTs. Patients with bradyarrhythmias may have symptoms of low cardiac output, including fatigue, weakness, dizziness, dyspnea, and syncope (see Chapter 68). Palpitations can result from an increased force of contraction associated with longer ventricular filling times and may be prominent symptoms in bradycardias.

Syncope, Presyncope, and Altered Level of Consciousness

Syncope, commonly referred to as "fainting" or "passing out," is a transient, self-limited loss of consciousness and posture resulting from a drop in blood pressure with cerebral hypoperfusion and should always prompt a search for a cause (see Chapter 71). It is important to distinguish syncope from other causes of transient loss of consciousness, such as seizures, metabolic disorders (hypoglycemia, hypoxia [e.g., airline decompression]), intoxication, cataplexy, and pseudosyncope. The etiologies of true syncope are varied with similarly diverse prognoses. The unheralded loss of consciousness in any patient, even if benign from the cardiac perspective, can be dangerous depending on the circumstances (e.g., while driving a vehicle, or standing at the top of a flight of stairs). However, because syncope can be a harbinger of SCD, it is important to identify cardiac from more benign causes of syncope.[2-4] When caused by a cardiac arrhythmia, the onset of syncope is rapid and the duration is usually brief, with or without a preceding aura, and it is not typically followed by a postictal confusional state. It can be associated with bodily injury if the patient falls while unconscious. Palpitations preceding a syncope may support an arrhythmic cause of syncope but are often absent if the loss of consciousness is rapid. Seizure activity is uncommon and occurs mostly after prolonged asystole or a rapid ventricular arrhythmia. Therefore, the seizure does not begin with or anticipate the syncope, whereas in epileptic seizures, convulsive movements start within seconds of the onset of syncope. Tongue biting or incontinence is also uncommon in cardiac syncope. In summary, syncope with early seizure activity is frequently caused by epilepsy, whereas later seizure activity is more likely caused by a cardiac arrhythmia with cerebral hypoperfusion.

The history of syncope should be elicited and interpreted carefully, because older people who have fallen might deny loss of consciousness during the event because of retrograde amnesia. Common arrhythmic causes of syncope include bradyarrhythmias caused by sinus node dysfunction or AV block and tachyarrhythmias, most often ventricular, but on occasion supraventricular. Bradycardia can follow tachycardia in patients with the bradycardia-tachycardia syndrome, and treatment of both may be necessary. Of the reflex syncopes—neurocardiogenic, carotid hypersensitivity, and situational—neurocardiogenic is the most common. It should be differentiated from syncope caused by orthostasis, which may be seen in autonomic failure (e.g., due to diabetes).[5] Vasodepressor and cardioinhibitory syncope usually unfold more slowly and can be preceded by manifestations of autonomic hyperactivity such as nausea, abdominal cramping, diarrhea, sweating, or yawning. In fact, palpitations are common in this setting. On recovery, the patient may be bradycardic, pale, sweaty, and fatigued, unlike the patient recovering from a Stokes-Adams attack or an episode of VT, who may be flushed and may have a sinus tachycardia, usually without persistent mental confusion. Palpitations and presyncope on standing can be symptoms of postural orthostatic tachycardia syndrome (POTS).[6] Drug-induced (orthostatic hypotension, bradyarrhythmia) and nonarrhythmic cardiac causes of syncope such as aortic stenosis, hypertrophic cardiomyopathy, pulmonary stenosis, pulmonary hypertension, and acute MI can be excluded by the history, physical examination, ECG, echocardiography, and other laboratory tests. Noncardiac causes of syncope, such as hypoglycemia, transient ischemic attack, and psychogenic causes, can often be excluded by a careful history (see Chapter 71).

Sudden Cardiac Arrest and Aborted Sudden Cardiac Death

SCD is common, although estimates of the incidence are confounded by inadequate case identification and secular trends that have influenced both the rates and the etiologies of sudden death (see Chapter 70).[7] SCD caused by cardiac arrhythmias is most often the result of VT or ventricular fibrillation (VF); however, it can result from profound bradycardia, as might be observed in complete heart block or asystole. A variety of noncardiac conditions may be associated with life-threatening arrhythmias, including neurologic diseases (stroke, intracranial hemorrhage, epilepsy, neuromuscular disease, and Parkinson disease), diabetes, obesity, cirrhosis, anorexia, and bulimia. In well-adjudicated cases, coronary heart disease (CHD) is the most common finding in SCD and can be the first and last manifestation. Up to 80% of cases of SCD occur in patients with some form of structural heart disease, such as CHD, cardiomyopathy, or congenital heart disease. Other cardiac causes of SCD, referred to as "autopsy negative," include primary electrical diseases such as LQTS, Brugada syndrome, catecholaminergic polymorphic ventricular tachycardia (CPVT), idiopathic ventricular fibrillation (IVF), and under some circumstances, Wolff-Parkinson-White (WPW) syndrome (see Chapters 63 and 65). The remaining sudden deaths are usually not cardiac in etiology.

For the purposes of evaluation, SCA should be considered as SCD that someone has survived. It is essential that patients who have SCA undergo a comprehensive evaluation to identify the cause and proper treatment. A history of cardiac disease is critically important in directing the evaluation and management, as is a family history of SCD or significant cardiac arrhythmias. The circumstances at the time of SCA are often informative. Cardiac symptoms that predate the SCD suggest preexisting structural heart disease. A variety of precipitating factors can provide clues to the etiology of SCA. Exercise, emotional upset, or stress may precipitate cardiac arrest in the setting of a variety of structural heart diseases, arrhythmogenic cardiomyopathy (arrhythmogenic right ventricular cardiomyopathy/dysplasia, ARVC/D), and primary electrical diseases such as LQTS (types 1 and 2) and CPVT. SCD in LQTS3 or Brugada syndrome is more likely to occur at rest or with sleep. Fever is a common precipitant of the characteristic ECG abnormality (Fig. 61.3) and arrhythmias in Brugada syndrome.

Medications and recreational drugs can increase the risk of lethal arrhythmias; patients should be asked about the use of antiarrhythmic drugs, stimulants, decongestants, psychotropics, antibiotics, alcohol, amphetamines, cocaine, and supplements, especially those used for weight loss and energy enhancement. Patients with LQTS and Brugada syndrome should be cautioned about the use of medications that may increase risk of arrhythmias. Drugs that should be avoided are listed on https://www.crediblemeds.org/and http://www.brugadadrugs.org/, respectively. Structural heart diseases, such as dilated (DCM) or hypertrophic (HCM) cardiomyopathy (HCM SCD risk calculator https://doc-2do.com/hcm/webHCM.html) are associated with delayed ventricular repolarization, an acquired form of LQTS, and the same drugs can produce life-threatening arrhythmias in these patients.

The presence of a family history of serious ventricular arrhythmias, premature sudden death, stillbirths, sudden infant death syndrome (SIDS), unexplained motor vehicle and other accidents, and relatives with permanent pacemakers or implantable cardioverter-defibrillators (ICDs) may be relevant and will influence the evaluation of presumed heritable arrhythmias. If available, biologic materials from related decedents may be suitable for genetic testing or a molecular autopsy in suspected cases of heritable causes of SCD.

CLINICAL AND LABORATORY TESTING

The history, physical examination, and ECG are of paramount importance in the evaluation of patients with a suspected arrhythmia. A number of other studies, alone or in combination, may assist in the diagnosis and management of patients with cardiac arrhythmias.

Resting Electrocardiogram

The judicious use of noninvasive diagnostic tests is an important element in the evaluation of patients with arrhythmias, and there is no test more important than the ECG (see Chapter 14). Uncommon but

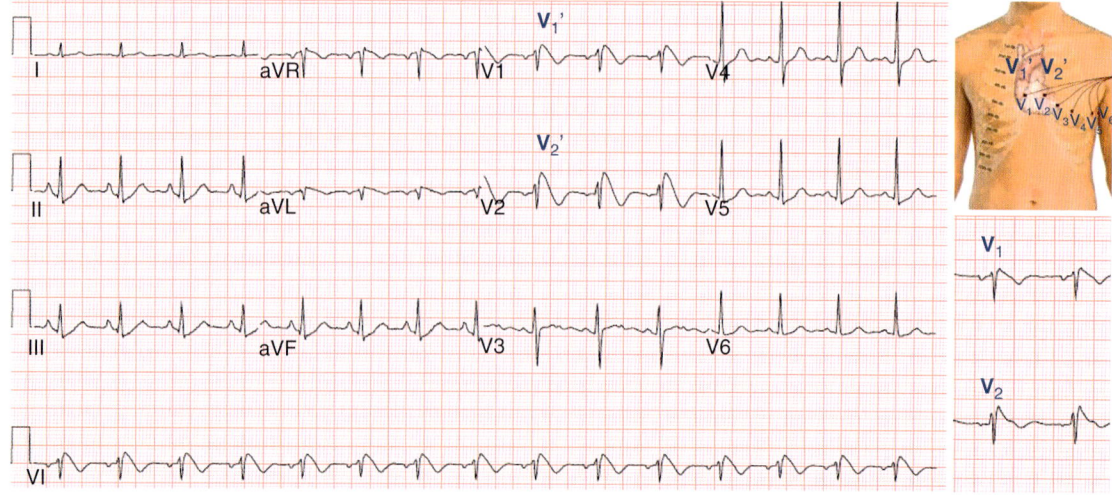

FIGURE 61.3 12-Lead electrocardiogram from a patient with Brugada syndrome with V_1' and V_2' recorded in the second intercostal space, as shown on the torso. *Inset*, Appearance of leads V1 and V2 in the standard positions in this patient.

diagnostically important signatures of electrophysiologic disturbances may be unearthed on the resting ECG, such as delta waves in WPW syndrome, prolongation or shortening of the QT interval, right precordial ST-segment abnormalities characteristic of Brugada syndrome, and epsilon waves in ARVC/D (Fig. 61.4).

During an arrhythmia, the ECG is the primary tool for diagnosis; an electrophysiologic study (EPS), in which intracardiac electrode catheters are used to record activity from several regions of the heart at one time, is more definitive but infrequently available immediately. A 12-lead ECG in addition to a long continuous recording with the use of a lead that shows distinct P waves is often helpful for closer analysis; typically, this is one of the inferior leads (II, III, and aVF), V_1, or aVR. The ECG obtained during an arrhythmia may be diagnostic by itself and obviate the need for further diagnostic testing.

Fig. 61.5 depicts an algorithm for the diagnosis of specific tachyarrhythmias from the 12-lead ECG (see Chapters 65 and 67). A major branch point in the differential diagnosis concerns the QRS duration: wide-QRS (>0.12 second) tachycardias are often VTs, and narrow-QRS (≤0.12 second) tachycardias are almost always SVTs, but there is some overlap (Table 61.1). Next, the most important questions to answer, regardless of QRS width, concern the characteristics of P waves. If P waves are not clearly visible on the regular ECG, atrial activity can occasionally be discerned by placing the right and left arm leads in various anterior chest positions (so-called Lewis leads), by recording atrial electrograms using intracardiac right atrial recordings (via permanent or temporary transvenous pacing leads), or by using esophageal electrodes or an echocardiogram. The last three methods are not readily available in most clinical situations and consume valuable time when dealing with a sick patient. A long rhythm strip can usually be obtained and can yield important clues by revealing P waves if perturbations occur during the arrhythmia (e.g., changes in rate, premature complexes, sudden termination, and the effect of physical maneuvers, as noted earlier). In a stable patient, if P waves are not clearly visible, the administration of adenosine by rapid intravenous bolus (6 mg followed by 12 mg if no response to the first dose) while running a rhythm strip may cause transient AV block and either terminate the tachycardia or allow discernment of P waves and diagnosis of the arrhythmia (Fig. 61.6).

Each arrhythmia should be approached in a systematic manner to answer several key questions; as suggested earlier, many of these questions relate to P wave characteristics and underscore the importance of assessing the ECG carefully for them. If P waves are visible, are the atrial and ventricular rates identical? Are the P-P and R-R intervals regular or irregular? If irregular, is it a consistent, repeating irregularity? Is there a P wave related to each QRS complex? Does the P wave seem to precede (long RP interval) or follow (short RP interval) the QRS complex (Fig. 61.7)? Are the resultant RP and PR intervals constant? Are all P waves and QRS complexes identical? Is the P wave vector normal or abnormal? Are P, PR, QRS, and QT durations normal? Once these questions have been addressed, the clinician needs to assess the significance of the arrhythmia in view of the clinical setting. Should it be treated, and if so, how? For SVTs with a normal QRS complex, a branching decision tree such as that shown in Fig. 61.5 may be useful.

The Ladder Diagram: A ladder diagram, derived from the ECG, is used to depict depolarization and conduction schematically to aid in understanding the rhythm (Fig. 61.8). Because the ECG and therefore the ladder diagram represent electrical activity as a function of time along the x-axis, conduction is indicated by the lines of the ladder diagram sloping in a left-to-right direction. Activity originating in an ectopic site such as the ventricle is indicated by lines emanating from that tier. Sinus nodal discharge and conduction and, under certain circumstances, AV junctional discharge and conduction can only be inferred; their activity is not directly recorded on the ECG.

Cardiac Imaging

The prognostic implications of a cardiac arrhythmia depend on context, most importantly the presence of structural heart disease. The presence of structural heart disease may be apparent from the history and physical examination, chest radiograph, and ECG itself. Cardiac imaging plays an important role in the detection and characterization of myocardial structural abnormalities that can render the heart more susceptible to arrhythmias. Ventricular tachyarrhythmias, for instance, occur more frequently in patients with ventricular systolic dysfunction and chamber dilation, in HCM, and in the setting of infiltrative diseases such as sarcoidosis. Supraventricular arrhythmias may be associated with particular congenital conditions, including AV reentry in the setting of Ebstein anomaly (see Chapter 82). Echocardiography (Chapter 16) is frequently employed to screen for disorders of cardiac structure and function. Increasingly, magnetic resonance imaging (MRI) of the myocardium (Chapter 19) is being used to screen for scar burden, fibrofatty infiltration of the myocardium as seen in ARVC, and other structural changes that affect arrhythmia susceptibility. Both contrast-enhanced MRI and 18F-fluorodeoxyglucose positron emission tomography with computed tomographic transmission (18F-FDG PET/CT) have been used in the diagnosis, management, and response to treatment of cardiac sarcoidosis (Fig. 61.9) (see Chapter 18).

Stress Electrocardiography

Exercise electrocardiographic stress testing may be particularly useful in the evaluation of patients who experience symptoms with exertion (Chapter 15). Exercise stress testing is important in determining the

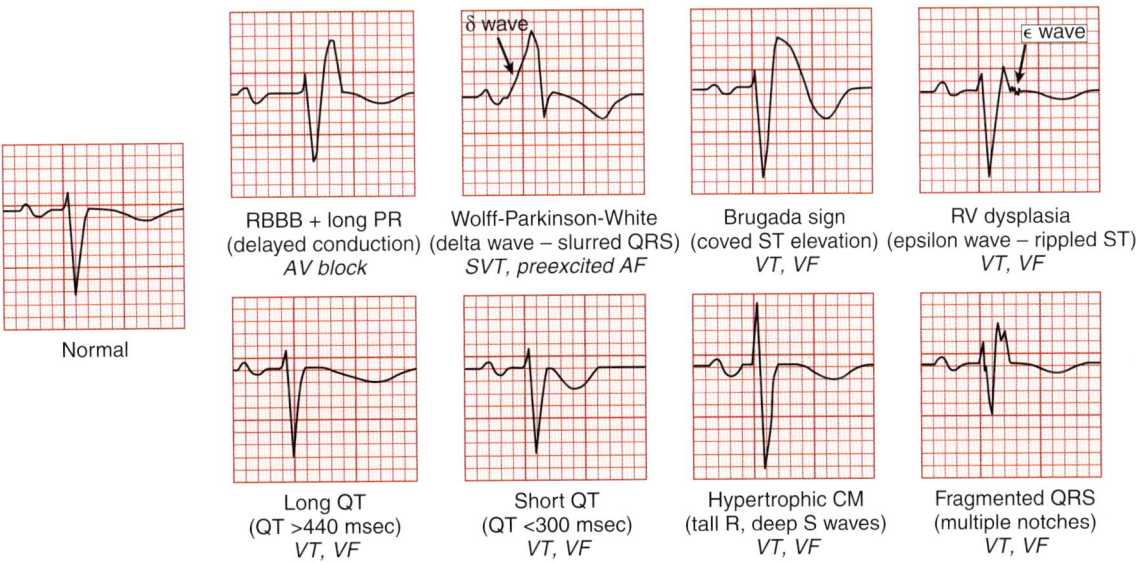

FIGURE 61.4 Resting QRS abnormalities that suggest potential for arrhythmia. Lead V1 is shown in each example; a normal complex is presented at *left* for reference. *CM,* Cardiomyopathy; *RBBB,* right bundle branch block; *RV,* right ventricular.

presence of myocardial demand ischemia and other arrhythmic substrates, such as alterations in repolarization and the dynamic behavior of the QT interval (see Chapter 63). Microscopic alterations in the T wave (T wave alternans, see below) at low heart rates may identify patients at risk for ventricular arrhythmias. Altered heart rate recovery may indicate autonomic dysfunction associated with heightened arrhythmic risk. A persistent elevation in heart rate after the end of exercise (delay in return to baseline) is associated with a worse CV prognosis, as is a rapid resting heart rate.

It is important to recognize that not all arrhythmias induced by exercise have an ominous prognosis. Approximately one third of individuals without heart disease will have ventricular ectopy associated with exercise. Typically, this manifests as occasional uniform PVCs, more likely to occur at faster heart rates, and not reproducible from one test to the next. Three to six beats of nonsustained VT can occur in normal subjects, especially elderly persons, and its occurrence neither implicates ischemia or other forms of heart disease nor predicts increased CV morbidity or mortality. However, multiform PVCs and VT are an infrequent response to exercise in healthy individuals; thus, the development of more complex ventricular arrhythmias during exercise testing should prompt a search for underlying structural heart disease.[8,9] Ventricular ectopy occurs in about half of patients with CAD, generally appearing more reproducibly and at lower heart rates (<130 beats/min) than in healthy individuals and often in the early recovery period. Frequent PVCs (>10 per minute), polymorphic PVCs, and VT are more likely to occur in patients with CAD. PVCs at rest can be suppressed by exercise in patients with CAD; therefore, this observation does not necessarily imply a benign prognosis or absence of underlying structural heart disease.

Patients who have symptoms consistent with an arrhythmia induced by exercise (e.g., syncope, sustained palpitations) should be considered for stress testing. Stress testing may be indicated to provoke supraventricular and ventricular arrhythmias, to determine the relationship of the arrhythmia to activity, to aid in choosing antiarrhythmic therapy

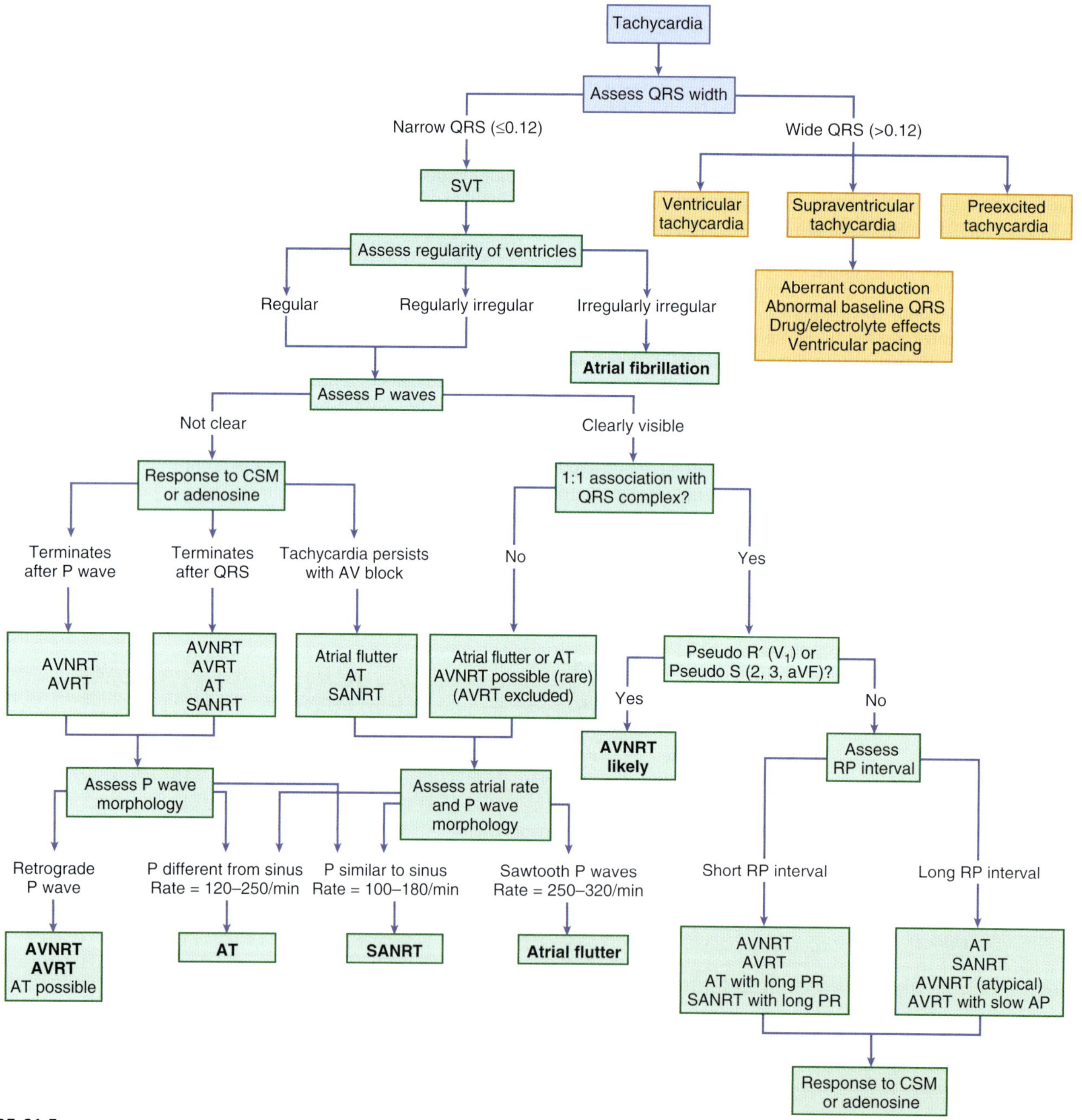

FIGURE 61.5 Stepwise approach to diagnosis of the type of tachycardia based on a 12-lead electrocardiogram during the episode. The initial step is to determine whether the tachycardia has a wide or narrow QRS complex. For wide-complex tachycardia, see Table 61.1; the remainder of the algorithm is helpful in diagnosis of the type of narrow-complex tachycardia. *AP,* Accessory pathway; *AT,* atrial tachycardia; *AVNRT,* atrioventricular nodal reentrant tachycardia; *AVRT,* atrioventricular reciprocating tachycardia; *CSM,* carotid sinus massage; *SANRT,* sinoatrial nodal reentry tachycardia.

TABLE 61.1 Electrocardiographic Distinctions for Diagnosis of Wide–QRS Complex Tachycardia

FAVOR SUPRAVENTRICULAR TACHYCARDIA	FAVOR VENTRICULAR TACHYCARDIA
Initiation with a premature P wave	Initiation with a premature QRS complex
Tachycardia complexes identical to those in resting rhythm	Tachycardia beats identical to PVCs during sinus rhythm
"Long-short" sequence preceding initiation	"Short-long" sequence preceding initiation
Changes in the P-P interval preceding changes in the R-R interval	Changes in the R-R interval preceding changes in the P-P interval
QRS contours consistent with aberrant conduction (V_1, V_6)	QRS contours inconsistent with aberrant conduction (V_1, V_6)
Slowing or termination with vagal maneuvers	AV dissociation or other non-1:1 AV relationship
Onset of the QRS to its peak (positive or negative) <50 msec	Onset of the QRS to its peak (positive or negative) ≥50 msec
	Fusion beats, capture beats
QRS duration ≤0.14 sec	QRS duration >0.14 sec
Normal QRS axis (0–+90 degrees)	Left-axis deviation (especially –90–180 degrees)
	Concordant R-wave progression pattern
	Contralateral bundle branch block pattern from the resting rhythm
	Initial R, q, or r >40 msec or notched Q in aVR
	Absence of an "rS" complex in any precordial lead

AV, Atrioventricular; PVC, premature ventricular complexes.

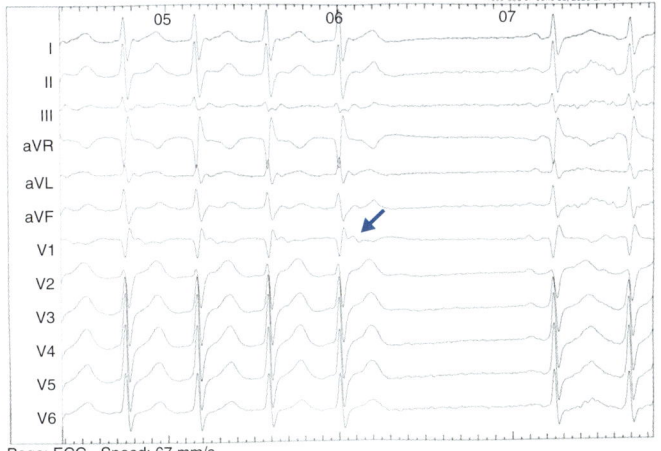

FIGURE 61.6 Supraventricular tachycardia, typical AV reentry tachycardia terminated by 6 mg of IV adenosine. The tachycardia terminates with a retrograde P wave *(arrow)*. After the pause, the temporal relationship of the P wave to the QRS changes indicating conversion to sinus rhythm.

and uncovering proarrhythmic responses, and to provide some insight into the mechanism of the tachycardia.

Exercise testing has diagnostic or prognostic value in patients with primary electrical abnormalities such as LQTS, CPVT, and Brugada syndrome (see Chapter 63). Since the QT interval can be normal in up to one quarter of patients with genetically proven LQTS, exercise testing can stress repolarizing reserves and can be useful to expose ECG abnormalities in these patients. An abnormal response of the QT interval to the heart rate acceleration produced by standing is seen in patients with LQTS compared with normal patients. Exercise testing can unmask polymorphic PVCs and VT in patients with CPVT (Fig. 61.10).[10] In patients with Brugada syndrome, significant ST-segment elevation with coving of the ST segment during the recovery phase predicts arrhythmic events during follow-up.[11]

Long-Term Electrocardiogram Recording: Holter Monitoring, Event Recording, and Insertable Loop Recorders

The fundamental diagnostic principle in managing patients with an undocumented cardiac rhythm disturbance is to record the ECG during a symptomatic episode and establish a causal relation between the arrhythmia and symptoms. As importantly, recording normal sinus rhythm during a patient's typical symptomatic episode effectively excludes cardiac arrhythmia as a cause. In patients not suspected of having a life-threatening arrhythmia, Holter monitoring and event recording, continuously or intermittently, record the ECG over longer periods, enhancing the possibility of observing the cardiac rhythm during symptoms. The type and duration of ECG monitoring depend on the frequency of symptoms. Most continuous recording systems are equipped with patient-triggered recording to enable correlation of the ECG with symptoms. Continuous recording systems do not require patient recognition of an arrhythmia but some do allow for patient-activated ECG data transmission.

In Hospital Electrocardiographic Recording

ECG monitoring systems are used in increasing proportions of inpatients regardless of history or suspicion of arrhythmias. These systems can provide valuable information about rhythm abnormalities, including mode of onset and termination, and allow prompt acquisition of a full 12-lead ECG for more detail. Telemetry can disclose intermittent heart block in a patient with presyncope that may warrant consideration of pacemaker implantation or reveal nonsustained VT in a patient with previous MI and left ventricular dysfunction and prompt an EPS for further assessment of risk. Although telemetry is helpful in many cases, it can be misleading: artifacts can simulate VT or VF, heart block, or asystole. Careful scrutiny is necessary to avoid unnecessary tests and procedures in patients with these artefactual arrhythmias (Fig. 61.11).

Ambulatory Electrocardiographic (Holter) Recording

Continuous electrocardiographic recorders include the traditional Holter monitor and digitally record three or more electrocardiographic channels for 24 to 48 hours. Computers scan the recording, with human oversight, to provide a report with snapshot recordings of symptomatic events and other important findings such as asymptomatic arrhythmias or ST-segment changes. Holter monitoring is most useful in patients with frequent (daily or more often) symptoms. From 25% to 50% of patients experience a symptom during a 24-hour recording; in 2% to 15% the complaint is caused by an arrhythmia (Fig. 61.12). The ability to correlate symptoms temporally with abnormalities on the ECG is one of the strengths of this technique. This section addresses the requirement for maintenance of clinical competence in ambulatory electrocardiography.

Significant rhythm disturbances are uncommon in healthy young persons. Sinus bradycardia with heart rates of 35 to 40 beats/min, sinus arrhythmia with pauses exceeding 3 seconds, sinoatrial exit block, type I (Wenckebach) second-degree AV block (often during sleep), wandering atrial pacemaker, junctional escape complexes, and PACs and PVCs can be observed and are not necessarily abnormal. Frequent and complex atrial and ventricular rhythm disturbances are less frequently observed, however, and type II second-degree AV conduction disturbances (see Chapter 68) are not recorded in normal patients. Elderly patients have a higher prevalence of arrhythmias, some of which may be responsible for neurologic symptoms (Fig. 61.13, see Chapter 90).

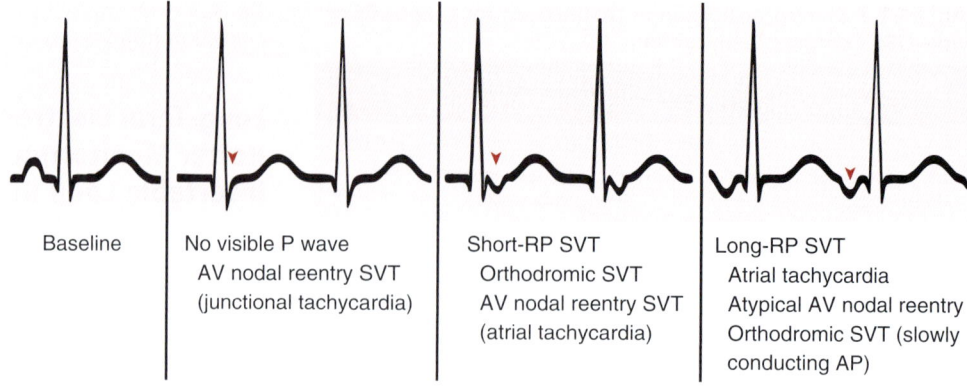

FIGURE 61.7 Differential diagnosis of types of supraventricular tachycardia based on timing of atrial activity (RP and PR intervals). **Left,** Normal beat. The types of tachycardia are listed below the representative electrocardiographic patterns that they can produce, as categorized by P wave position relative to the QRS complex. An *arrowhead* shows the location of the P wave in each example. Diagnoses in parentheses are rare causes of the noted findings. *AP,* Accessory pathway.

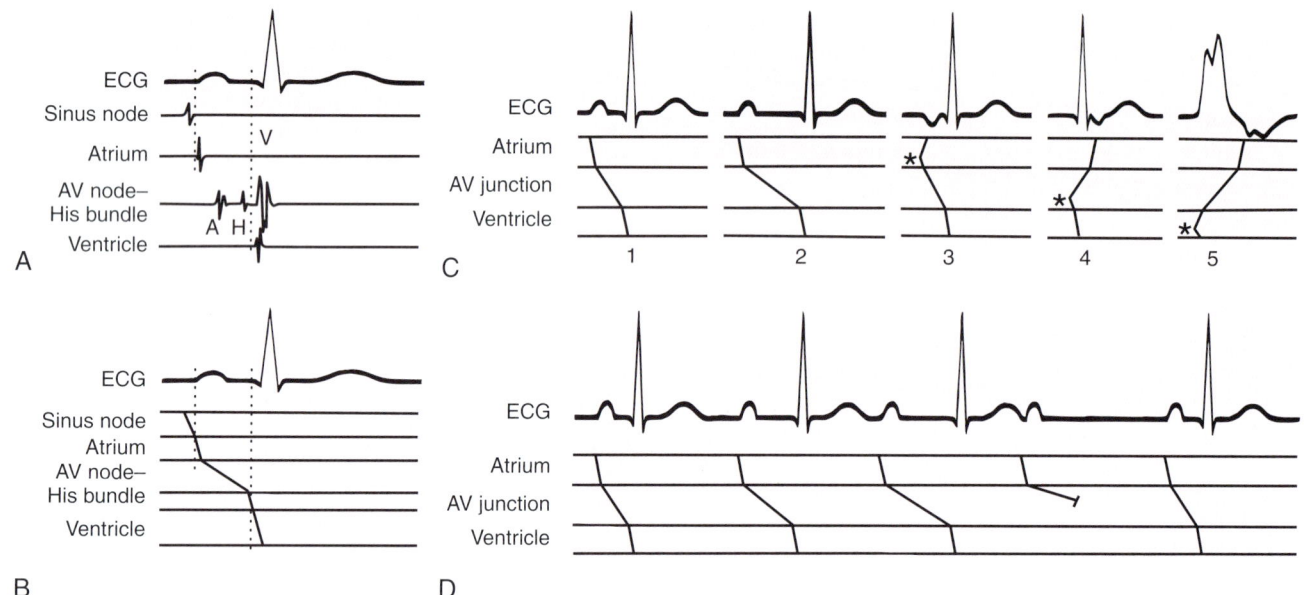

FIGURE 61.8 Intracardiac signals and ladder diagrams. **A,** A single beat is shown with accompanying intracardiac signals from the sinus node, right atrium, atrioventricular (AV) nodal and His bundle regions, and right ventricle. **B,** The same beat is shown with the accompanying ladder diagram below. Cardiac regions have been divided into tiers separated by horizontal lines. Vertical *dotted lines* denote onset of the P wave and QRS complexes. The relatively steep lines indicate rapid conduction through the atrium, His bundle, and ventricular muscle and more gently sloping lines the slower conduction in the sinus and AV nodes. **C,** Different situations with accompanying explanatory ladder diagrams. Beat 1 is normal, as in **B**; beat 2 shows first-degree AV delay, with the more gradual slope than normal in the AV nodal tier signifying very slow conduction in this region. In beat 3 an atrial premature complex is shown (starting in the atrial tier at the *asterisk*) and is producing an inverted P wave on the ECG. In beat 4 an ectopic impulse arises in the His bundle *(asterisk)* and propagates to the ventricle, as well as retrogradely through the AV node to the atrium. In beat 5 a ventricular ectopic complex *(asterisk)* conducts retrogradely through the His bundle and AV node and eventually to the atrium. **D,** Wenckebach AV cycle (type I second-degree block). As the PR interval progressively increases from left to right in the figure, the slope of the line in the AV nodal region flattens until it fails to propagate at all after the fourth P wave (small line perpendicular to the sloping AV nodal conduction line), after which the cycle repeats. *A,* Atrial recording; *H,* His recording; *V,* ventricular recording.

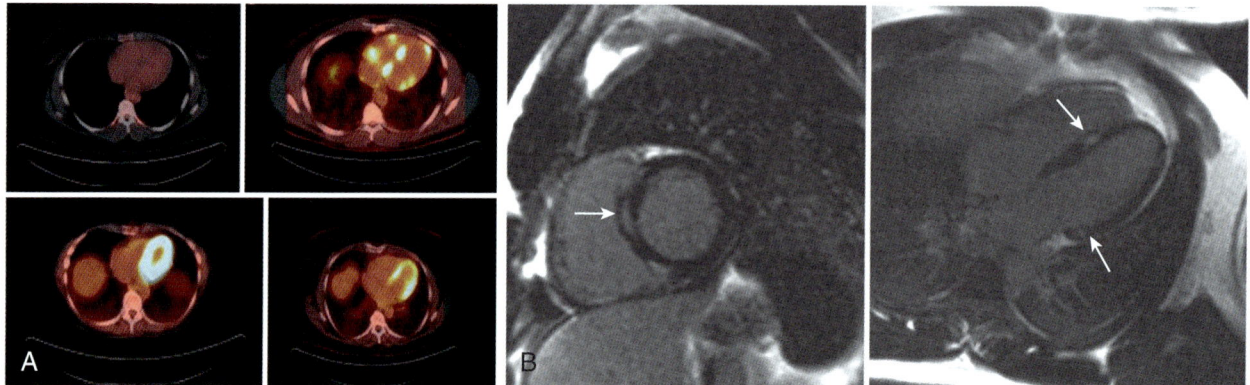

FIGURE 61.9 Sarcoidosis **A,** Four images show the pattern of 18F-fluorodeoxyglucose uptake on positron emission tomography (PET) scan. **B,** Two cardiac magnetic resonance images show evidence of delayed gadolinium enhancement in the midwall of the left ventricle *(arrows).* (Modified from Hamzeh N, Steckman DA, Sauer WH, et al. Pathophysiology and clinical management of cardiac sarcoidosis. *Nat Rev Cardiol.* 2015;12:278.)

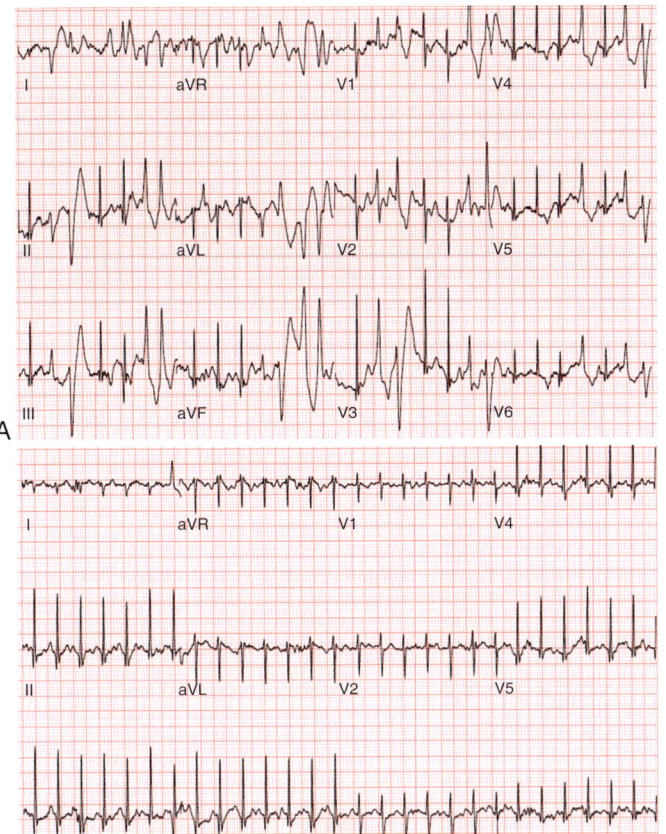

FIGURE 61.10 Exercise-induced polymorphic premature ventricular complexes and ventricular tachycardia (VT) in a young woman with dizziness; palpitations caused by a ryanodine receptor (RyR2) mutation producing catecholaminergic polymorphic VT (CPVT). **A,** ECG at peak exercise before treatment. **B,** ECG while receiving treatment with nadolol and flecainide.

a pacemaker stimulus is detected, facilitating diagnosis of potential pacemaker malfunction. On occasion, artifacts on the ECG can mimic bradycardias or tachycardias and lead to erroneous therapy. Finally, most systems can also provide heart rate variability and QT data (see below). Use of these systems for detection of myocardial ischemia (ST-segment analysis) has yielded mixed results for both specificity and sensitivity.

Event Recording

In many patients, the 24- or 48-hour snapshot provided by the Holter recording is insufficient to document the cause of the patient's symptoms. Event recorders are indicated when symptoms occur less frequently (e.g., several episodes per month), and because the monitors are typically patient activated, and well-suited for correlating symptoms with rhythm disturbances. These devices come in various forms and are kept by the patient for an extended time, often up to 30 days. Event recorders can be continuous with auto-triggered or patient-activated recording. Discontinuous transtelephonic monitoring systems without looping memory require patient activation. When being worn by the patient, digital recordings can be made during symptomatic episodes and can be transmitted to a receiving station by telephone at the patient's convenience (see Fig. 61.13). Some of these recorders store more than 30 seconds of the ECG before the patient activates the recording. These loop recorders record continuously, but only a small window of time is present in memory at any moment. When the patient presses the event button, the current window is frozen while the device continues recording for another 30 to 60 seconds, depending on how it is configured. Event recorders are highly effective in documenting infrequent events, but the quality of the recordings is more subject to motion artifact than with Holter monitors, and usually only one channel can be recorded. With most systems, the device automatically begins recording the rhythm when the heart rate increases or decreases outside preset parameters. Some systems incorporate cell phone technology that automatically notifies a central monitoring facility when certain conditions are met (e.g., extreme bradycardia or tachycardia). This can significantly shorten the time between occurrence and effective treatment of serious arrhythmias.

The use of wearables for cardiac monitoring has enabled detection of abnormalities in heart rate and rhythm on a much broader basis than physician-prescribed monitoring.[13] Fitness bands and other wearables may have accelerometers that detect movement during exercise and other daily activities and correlate it with heart rate. There are a number of other devices that are accurate and easy to use, including smartphones and watches that use camera-based plethysmography to assess heart rate and rhythm. Algorithms have been developed to detect irregularity of the heart rate and notify a patient of "possible AF." Although heart rate measurements tend to be fairly accurate, subsequent cardiac monitoring to confirm AF in patients alerted to a possible arrhythmia has shown confirmation of AF in less than half of the patients.[14] Both iPhones and Android phones have applications for real-time ECG monitoring. They are useful for on-demand arrhythmia diagnosis and monitoring arrhythmia burden and are being used as a phenotyping platform in population studies.[15-17] A small, lightweight device is available that has two electrodes on which the fingers of the left and right hands are placed to record a lead I ECG rhythm strip for 30 seconds. More recently, a third electrode has been added that allows for all six limb leads to be recorded. These rhythm strips can be uploaded to the cloud and downloaded to a physician's office for subsequent verification of the rhythm. The latest versions of smartwatches can also record a single-lead rhythm strip by opening an app and placing the fingers of the hand opposite to the watch on the crown of the watch for 30 seconds.

Most currently available pacemakers and ICDs can provide Holter-like data when premature beats or tachycardia episodes occur and can store electrograms of these events from the implanted leads (Fig. 61.14). Dual-chamber devices can record atrial and ventricular high-rate episodes that can be correlated with the electrograms during such events (see Chapter 69). The device can then

It is worth repeating that the long-term prognosis of even frequent and complex PVCs in asymptomatic healthy patients is very good, without an increased risk of mortality. However, frequent PVCs (>15% of the total) have been shown to produce a cardiomyopathy and heart failure in some people, which can be reversed following elimination of the PVCs. Most patients with ischemic heart disease, particularly after MI (see Chapters 37 to 39), exhibit PVCs when they are monitored for 24 hours. The frequency of PVCs progressively increases during the first several weeks and then decreases at about 6 months after infarction. Frequent and complex PVCs are associated with a two- to five-fold increased risk for cardiac or sudden death in patients after MI, but treating these PVCs may not improve the prognosis. Recent data indicate that ablation of PVCs after MI may improve previously depressed ventricular function.[12]

Long-term recording of the ECG has also exposed potentially serious arrhythmias and complex ventricular ectopy in patients with left ventricular hypertrophy, as well as in those with hypertrophic, dilated, and ischemic cardiomyopathy; in those with mitral valve prolapse (see Chapter 76); in those with otherwise unexplained syncope (Chapter 71) or transient vague cerebrovascular symptoms or stroke; and in those with conduction disturbances, sinus node dysfunction, bradycardia-tachycardia syndrome, WPW syndrome (Chapter 65), and pacemaker malfunction (Chapter 69). It has been shown that asymptomatic AF occurs far more often than symptomatic episodes in patients with AF.

Variations of Holter recording have been used for particular applications. Some monitoring systems are able to reconstruct a full 12-lead ECG from a seven-electrode recording system. This is especially useful in trying to document the ECG morphology of VT before an ablation procedure or a consistent morphology of PVCs that may arise from an ablatable focus of VT or VF. Most Holter recording and analysis systems can place a clearly recognizable deflection on the recording when be interrogated and the electrograms printed for analysis. Many implanted device systems incorporate remote monitoring so that if symptoms develop, the information can be transmitted via the Internet to the physician's office, thus enabling more prompt diagnosis and treatment than if the patient had to schedule an outpatient visit. For serious rhythm disturbances, such as sustained VT, this information can lead to timely changes in therapy; in other cases, such as incidentally discovered AF, therapeutic implications (e.g., initiation of anticoagulation) are less clear. Implantable monitors or insertable loop recorders (ILRs) are typically used for the evaluation of suspected serious arrhythmias that occur infrequently and cannot be provoked at diagnostic EPS. An ILR, a single-lead ECG monitoring device placed subcutaneously at approximately the level of the anterior second rib, monitors the cardiac rhythm for as long as 24 to 36 months. Both P waves and QRS complexes can be recorded by an ILR. These devices have both auto-triggered and patient-activated arrhythmia-recording capabilities. Use of such devices has been successful in recording tachyarrhythmias and, more often, bradyarrhythmias. The devices can be configured to store patient-activated episodes, automatically activated recordings (heart rate outside preset parameters), or a combination of these. ECG recordings can be sent to an analyzing center transtelephonically and then to physicians via the Internet. Interrogation of ILRs can also be performed remotely over a landline telephone. Technologic advances have resulted in further reduction in size and ease of implantation of ILRs, which has led to increased clinical deployment of these devices. ILRs have primarily been used in the evaluation of syncope, but their use is increasing in monitoring arrhythmia density, especially AF.[18]

ELECTROCARDIOGRAM DYNAMICS/ANALYTICS

Various methods for evaluating components of the ECG and heart rate have been developed, mainly for the purpose of enhancing SCD risk stratification of patients. Few of them are used routinely today because of suboptimal sensitivity and specificity. **Heart rate variability** is used to evaluate vagal and sympathetic influences on the sinus node (inferring that the same activity is also occurring in the ventricles) and to identify patients at risk for a CV event or death. R-R variability predicts all-cause mortality after MI, as does left ventricular ejection fraction or nonsustained VT.[19,20] Similar results have been obtained in patients with dilated cardiomyopathy (see Chapters 50 and 52).

Heart rate turbulence is a measure of reflex vagal control of the heart. Abnormal heart rate turbulence is a strong independent predictor of mortality in patients with CAD and dilated cardiomyopathy. **QRS and QT dispersion and T wave abnormalities** are a reflection of heterogeneity in refractoriness and conduction velocity, which is a hallmark of reentrant arrhythmias. Dispersion indices usually measure the maximum difference (shortest to longest) in the intervals of interest. Abnormally high QRS and QT dispersion

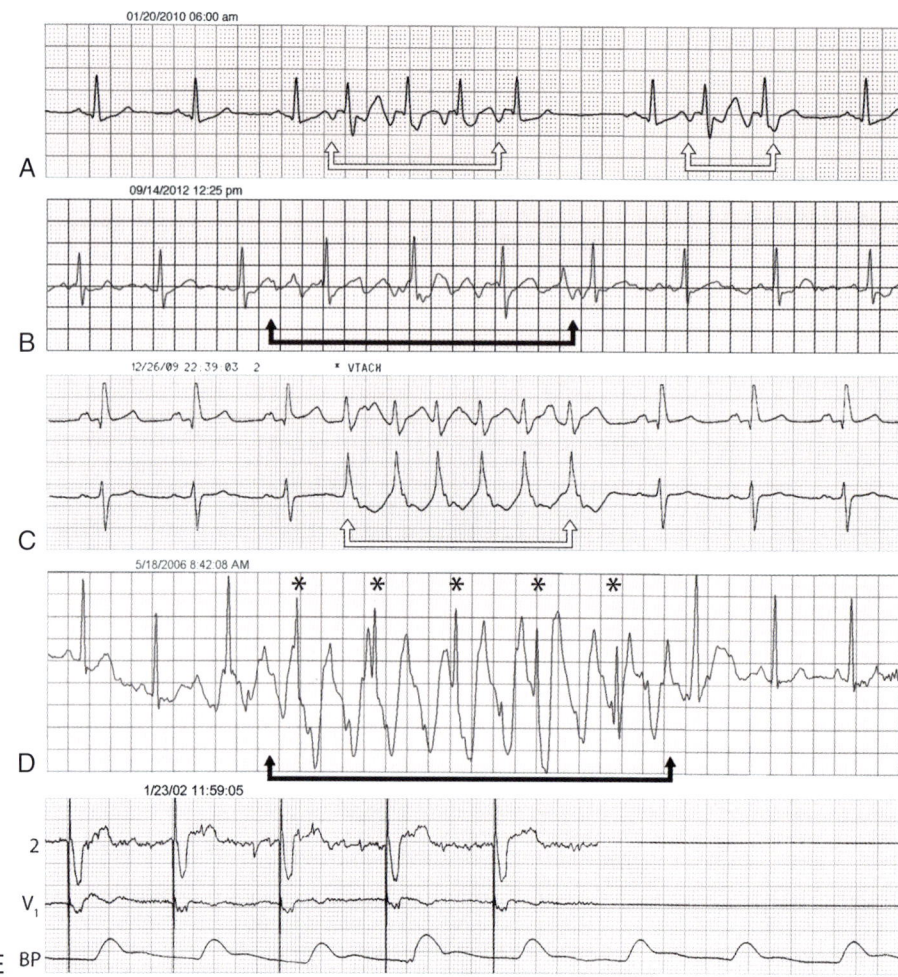

FIGURE 61.11 Electrocardiographic events and artifacts. **A,** Sinus rhythm punctuated by short episodes of atrial tachycardia with a more rapid rate (between the *white arrows*). **B,** Pseudo–atrial arrhythmia. Sinus rhythm is present throughout (no variation in the R-R interval) despite the appearance of an artifact that mimics short episode of atrial flutter or fibrillation (between the *black arrows*). **C,** Nonsustained VT (between the *white arrows*) with wide rapid QRS complexes not preceded by a P wave and seen in two monitor leads. **D,** Pseudo-VT. Despite the appearance of VT (between the *black arrows*), sinus rhythm is present throughout (including complexes indicated by *asterisks*). **E,** Pseudo–pacemaker failure. After the first five paced complexes, the ECG is flat in *both* monitor leads, thus suggesting failure of pacemaker output; however, the pulse contour on the blood pressure (BP) tracing indicates that the heart is still contracting and the pacemaker is still working whereas the ECG monitor is not.

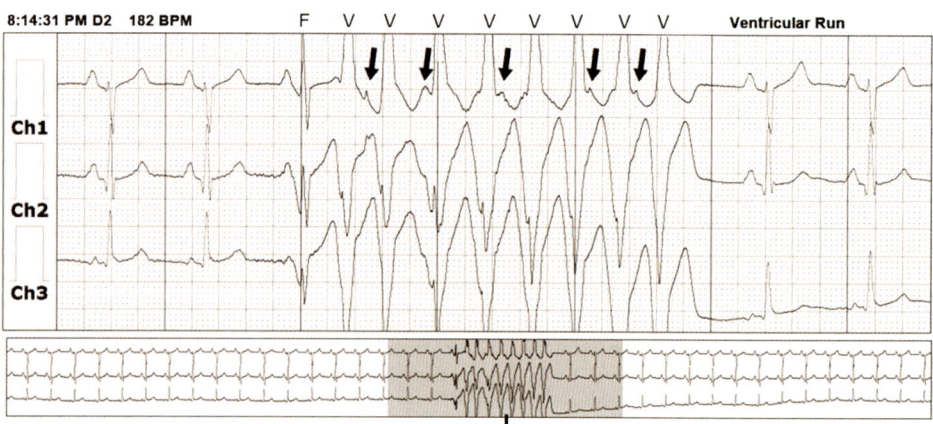

FIGURE 61.12 Long-term electrocardiographic recording in a patient with palpitations. A three-channel monitor shows sinus rhythm followed by nine wide QRS complexes of VT (labeled "V"); the complex that precedes these is a fusion between the normal complex and wide ("F"). *Arrows* indicate retrograde P waves during tachycardia. The presence of fewer P waves than QRS complexes and a fusion complex at the outset confirm the diagnosis of VT (which correlated with the patient's palpitations).

have been correlated with risk for overall mortality and arrhythmic death in patients with various disorders. **Signal-averaged electrocardiography and late potentials** Signal averaging is a method that improves the signal-to-noise ratio when signals are recurrent and noise is random. Signal averaging can detect late ventricular potentials of 1 to 25 μV that correspond to the delayed and fragmented conduction in the ventricles recorded with direct mapping techniques in patients with VT. In specific situations, it can be helpful, as in a patient suspected of having ARVC. **T wave alternans** is beat-to-beat alternation in the amplitude or morphology of the ECG recording of ventricular repolarization, the ST segment, and the T wave. It has been found in conditions favoring the development of ventricular tachyarrhythmias, such as ischemia and LQTS, and in patients with ventricular arrhythmias. A positive T wave alternans test result has been associated with a worse arrhythmic prognosis in various disorders, including ischemic heart disease and nonischemic cardiomyopathy. **Body surface mapping** is used to provide a complete picture of the effects of currents from the heart on the body surface. The potential distributions are represented by contour lines of equal potential, and each distribution is displayed instant by instant throughout activation, recovery, or both. **Electrocardiographic imaging** is a method for recording cardiac electrical activity at the skin surface and spatially integrating it with imaging data (currently, cardiac CT scanning). Using complex mathematical processing of electrical data collected from 224 electrodes on the skin surface, this technique can plot or project atrial and ventricular electrical activity on an epicardial "shell" of the patient's own heart and thereby follow the course of activation or repolarization during sinus rhythm or an arrhythmia.[21]

HEAD UP TILT

Tilt-table testing (TTT) is useful in the evaluation of patients without structural heart disease and recurrent syncope in whom there is a suspicion that exaggerated vagal tone producing cardioinhibitory and/or vasodepressor responses may play a causal role. In patients with structural heart disease, TTT may be indicated in those with syncope in whom other causes (e.g., asystole, tachyarrhythmias) have been excluded. TTT has been suggested as a useful tool in the diagnosis of and therapy for recurrent idiopathic vertigo, chronic fatigue syndrome, recurrent transient ischemic attacks, and repeated falls of unknown etiology in elderly patients without much evidence. Importantly, TTT is relatively contraindicated in the presence of severe CAD with proximal coronary stenoses, known severe cerebrovascular disease, severe mitral stenosis, and obstruction to left ventricular outflow (e.g., aortic stenosis).

Patients are placed on a tilt table in the supine position and tilted upright to a maximum of 60 to 80 degrees for 20 to 45 minutes or longer if necessary. Isoproterenol, administered as a bolus or infusion, may provoke syncope in patients whose initial upright TTT result shows no abnormalities or, after a few minutes of tilt, may shorten the time needed to produce a positive response on the test. An initial intravenous isoproterenol dose of 1 μg/min can be increased in 0.5-μg/min steps until symptoms occur or a maximum of 4 μg/min is given. Isoproterenol induces a vasodepressor response in upright susceptible patients (decrease in heart rate and blood pressure along with near-syncope or syncope). Tilt-table test (TTT) results are positive in two-thirds to three-fourths of patients susceptible to neurally mediated syncope. They are reproducible in approximately 80% of patients but have a 10% to 15% false-positive response rate. A positive test result is more meaningful when it reproduces symptoms that have occurred spontaneously.

The physiologic response to TTT is incompletely understood; however, redistribution of blood volume and increased ventricular contractility occur consistently. Exaggerated activation of a central reflex in response to TTT produces a stereotypic response of an initial increase in heart rate, followed by drop in blood pressure and then a reduction in heart rate characteristic of neurally-mediated hypotension. Positive responses can be divided into cardioinhibitory, vasodepressor, and mixed categories. In patients with orthostatic hypotension and autonomic insufficiency, blood pressure will drop with only a minimal increase in heart rate. Patients with neurocardiogenic syncope or near syncope have been treated with beta blockers, disopyramide, theophylline, selective serotonin reuptake inhibitors, midodrine, fludrocortisone, salt loading, tilt-training, and thigh-high support stockings, alone or in combination. However, none of these treatments is reliably effective in most patients.

POTS is another aberrant variant of a neurocardiogenic reflex characterized

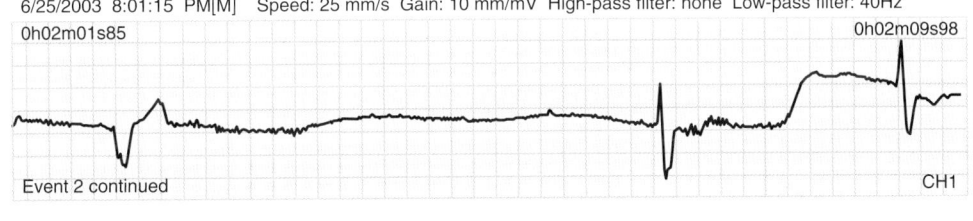
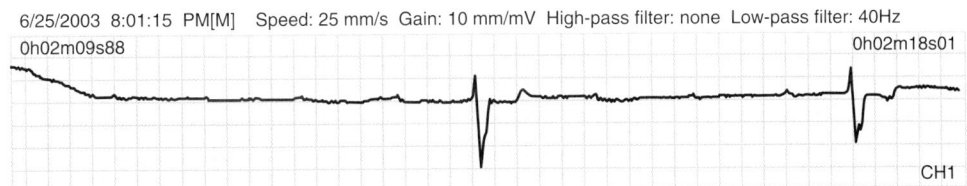

FIGURE 61.13 Continuous electrocardiographic recording from a patient-activated event monitor during an episode of lightheadedness. Sinus rhythm at 75 beats/min with sudden AV block is present with pauses of longer than 4 seconds, and in the *bottom strip* there is an effective heart rate of approximately 8 beats/min.

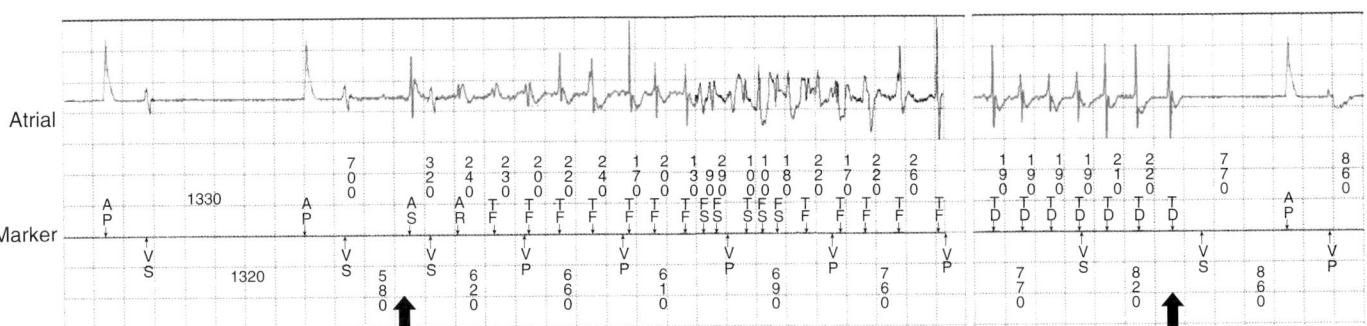

FIGURE 61.14 Recordings from a pacemaker log showing an episode of atrial fibrillation (AF) at its onset *(left arrow)* and termination *(right arrow)*, more than four days later. Two atrial paced complexes (AP) are followed by an episode of AF characterized by rapid erratic deflections. When the episode ends, atrial pacing resumes. The patient was unaware of the episode, but when discovered at a routine office follow-up visit, this information prompted initiation of anticoagulation in light of an elevated stroke risk and newly discovered AF.

by the inability to tolerate the upright posture and a dramatic increase (>30 beats/min) in heart rate (>120 beats/min) within 10 minutes of assuming an upright posture. A wide array of symptoms complicates the diagnosis of POTS, which is often confused with anxiety disorder, inappropriate sinus tachycardia, chronic fatigue syndrome, and fibromyalgia.[22,23] Data from an international registry suggest that endurance and strength-training programs may be useful in managing POTS.[24]

Invasive Electrophysiologic Testing

The EPS is central to the understanding and treatment of many cardiac arrhythmias. The indications for EPS fall into several broad categories: to define the mechanism of an arrhythmia, to deliver catheter-based ablative treatment, and to determine the etiology of symptoms that may be caused by an arrhythmia (e.g., syncope, palpitations). An invasive EPS involves introducing multipolar electrode catheters into the venous or arterial system and positioning them at various intracardiac sites or percutaneously into the pericardium to record or stimulate cardiac electrical activity. The positioning of these catheters is guided by complementary imaging modalities including fluoroscopy, intracardiac echocardiography (ICE) and electroanatomic mapping (EAM), often using MRI and CT to merge cardiac images with the EAM information. This section addresses the requirement for maintenance of clinical competence in electrophysiological procedures including electrophysiological studies, catheter ablation, and cardiac rhythm device implantation and management.

The components of the EPS are baseline measurements of conduction under resting and stressed (rate or pharmacologic) conditions and maneuvers, both pacing and pharmacologic, to induce arrhythmias. Assessment of AV conduction at rest is done by positioning electrodes along the septal leaflet of the tricuspid valve and measuring the atrial-His interval (an estimate of AV nodal conduction time; normally, 60 to 125 milliseconds) and the His-ventricular (H-V) interval (a measure of infranodal conduction; normally, 35 to 55 milliseconds). The heart is stimulated from portions of the atria or ventricles and from the region of the His bundle, bundle branches, accessory pathways, and other structures. EP studies are performed *diagnostically* to provide information about the type of clinical rhythm disturbance and insight into its electrophysiologic mechanism. EPS are used *therapeutically* to terminate a tachycardia by electrical stimulation or electroshock, to evaluate the effects of therapy by determining whether a particular intervention modifies or prevents electrical induction of a tachycardia or whether an electrical device properly senses and terminates an induced tachyarrhythmia, and to ablate myocardium involved in the tachycardia and prevent further episodes. EPS have also been used prognostically to identify patients at risk for SCD. The study can be helpful in patients with AV block, intraventricular conduction disturbance, sinus node dysfunction, tachycardia, and unexplained syncope or palpitations (see Chapter 71).

An EPS is usually effective at initiating VT and SVT when these tachyarrhythmias have occurred spontaneously. Particularly for VT, programmed stimulation is used in a systematic attempt to induce the arrhythmia. Short bursts of fixed rate ventricular pacing (e.g., eight beats at 100 to 150 beats/min, corresponding to a pacing cycle length of 600 to 400 msec) are followed by single ventricular extrastimuli at varying coupling intervals, and eventually two or three extrastimuli are added. The ability to induce an arrhythmia using such stimulation techniques before an intervention (e.g., drug therapy or catheter or surgical ablation) allows one to assess the efficacy of treatment afterward by using the same stimulation techniques and demonstrating noninducibility. However, false-negative responses (not finding a particular electrical abnormality known to be present) and false-positive responses (induction of a nonclinical arrhythmia) may complicate interpretation of the results because many lack reproducibility. Altered autonomic tone in a supine patient undergoing EPS, hemodynamic or ischemic influences, changing anatomy (e.g., new infarction) after the study, day-to-day variability, and the use of an artificial trigger (electrical stimulation) to induce the arrhythmia are several of many factors that can explain the occasional disparity between test results and spontaneous occurrence of arrhythmia. Overall, the diagnostic validity and reproducibility of these studies are good, and they are safe when performed by skilled clinical electrophysiologists.

ATRIOVENTRICULAR BLOCK

In patients with AV block, the site of block usually dictates the clinical course of the patient and whether a pacemaker is needed (see Chapter 68). In general, the site of AV block can be determined from analysis of the surface ECG. When the site of block cannot be determined from such an analysis and when knowing the site of block is imperative for management of the patient, an invasive EPS is indicated. Candidates include symptomatic patients in whom His-Purkinje block is suspected but not established, patients with second- or third-degree AV block, for whom information about the site of block or its mechanism may help direct therapy or assess prognosis, and patients suspected of having concealed His bundle extrasystoles. Patients with block in the His-Purkinje system become symptomatic because of periods of bradycardia or asystole and require pacemaker implantation more often than do patients who have AV nodal block. Type I (Wenckebach) AV block in older patients can have clinical implications similar to those for type II AV block. However, the results of EPS for evaluating the conduction system must be interpreted with caution. In rare cases, the process of recording conduction intervals alters their values. For example, catheter pressure on the AV node or His bundle can cause prolongation of the atrial-His or H-V interval and could lead to erroneous diagnosis and therapy. Finally, patients with AV block treated with a pacemaker who continue to be symptomatic and in whom a causal ventricular tachyarrhythmia is suspected are also candidates for EPS.

INTRAVENTRICULAR CONDUCTION DISTURBANCE

For patients with an intraventricular conduction disturbance, an EPS provides information about the duration of the H-V interval, which can be prolonged with a normal PR interval, or normal with a prolonged PR interval. A prolonged H-V interval (>55 msec) is associated with a greater likelihood of the development of a complete AV block (but typically the rate of progression is slow, 2% to 3% annually) and for having structural heart disease and a higher mortality.[25] The finding of very long H-V intervals (>80 to 90 msec) identifies patients at increased risk for the development of AV block. The H-V interval has high specificity (approximately 80%) but low sensitivity (66%) for predicting the development of complete AV block. During an EPS, atrial pacing is used to uncover abnormal His-Purkinje conduction. A positive response is provocation of distal His block during 1:1 AV nodal conduction at rates of 135 beats/min or less. Again, sensitivity is low but specificity is high. Drug infusion, such as with procainamide or ajmaline (not available in the United States), sometimes exposes abnormal His-Purkinje conduction (Fig. 61.15). An EPS is indicated in patients with an intraventricular conduction disturbance with symptoms (syncope or presyncope) that appear to be related to a bradyarrhythmia when no other cause of symptoms is identified, including with prolonged ECG monitoring. However, for many of these patients, ventricular tachyarrhythmias rather than AV block can be the cause of their symptoms, with obvious therapeutic implications. Consequently, programmed stimulation to see if ventricular tachyarrhythmias can be provoked is a standard part of the evaluation of such patients with EPS.

SINUS NODE DYSFUNCTION

Demonstration of slow sinus rates, sinus exit block, or sinus pauses on an ECG temporally related to symptoms suggests a causal relationship and usually obviates the need for further diagnostic studies (see Chapters 65 and 68). Carotid sinus pressure that results in several seconds of complete asystole or AV block and reproduces the patient's usual symptoms exposes the presence of a hypersensitive carotid sinus reflex. CSM must be done cautiously; rarely, it can precipitate a stroke. Neurohumoral agents, adenosine, or stress testing can be used to evaluate the effects of autonomic tone on sinus node automaticity and sinoatrial conduction time (SACT).

Sinus Node Recovery Time

Sinus node recovery time (SNRT) is a technique that can be useful for evaluating sinus node function. Atrial pacing is initiated at a fixed rate faster than the sinus rate for 30 to 60 seconds, after which is it abruptly terminated. The interval between the last paced high right atrial response and the first spontaneous (sinus) high right atrial response after termination of pacing is measured to determine SNRT. Because the spontaneous sinus rate influences SNRT, the value is corrected by subtracting the spontaneous sinus node cycle length (before pacing) from the SNRT (Fig. 61.16). This value, the corrected SNRT (CSNRT), is generally shorter than 525 milliseconds. A prolonged CSNRT has been found in patients suspected of having sinus node dysfunction. After cessation of pacing, the first return sinus cycle can be normal but can be followed by secondary pauses (a strong indicator of sinus node dysfunction). It is important to evaluate AV node and His-Purkinje function in patients with sinus node dysfunction because many also exhibit impaired AV conduction.

Sinoatrial Conduction Time

SACT can be estimated by simple pacing techniques based on the assumptions that (1) conduction times into and out of the sinus node are equal, (2) no depression of sinus node automaticity occurs, and (3) the pacemaker site does not shift after premature stimulation. These assumptions can be erroneous, particularly in patients with sinus node dysfunction. The sensitivity of the SACT and SNRT tests is only approximately 50% for each test alone and 65% when combined. The specificity, combined, is approximately 88%, with a low predictive value. Thus, if these test results are abnormal, the likelihood of the patient having sinus node dysfunction is great. However, normal results do not exclude the possibility of sinus node disease. Candidates for invasive EPS to evaluate sinus node function are symptomatic patients in whom sinus node dysfunction is suspected but has not yet been established as a cause of the symptoms. In patients with suspected clinical sinus node dysfunction, EPS is also important in excluding other causes of symptoms (e.g., tachyarrhythmias).

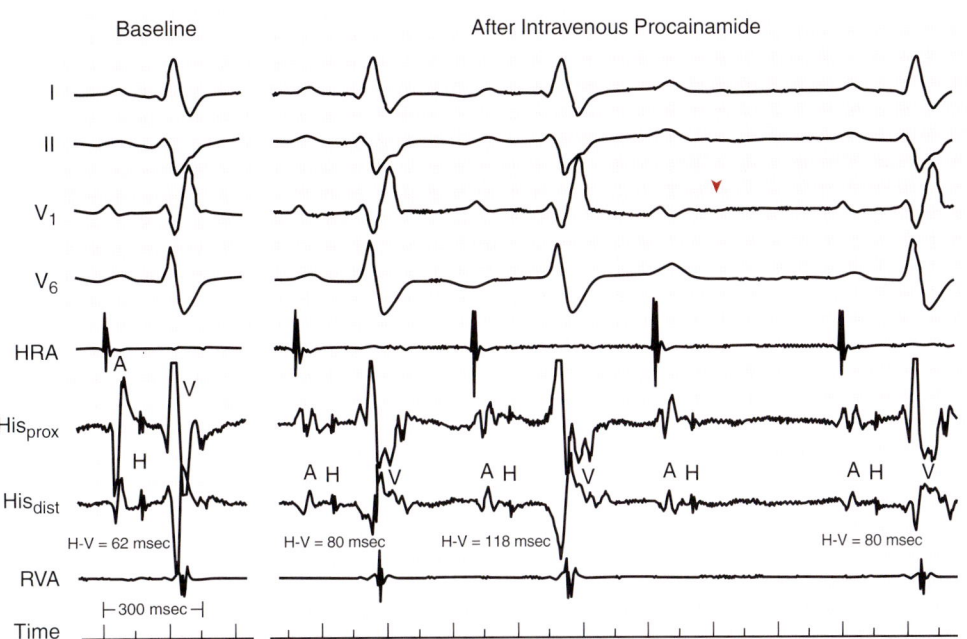

FIGURE 61.15 Testing the His-Purkinje system. A 43-year-old woman with sarcoidosis underwent EPS after a syncopal episode. Surface leads I, II, V$_1$, and V$_6$ are shown, with intracardiac recordings from catheters in the high right atrium (*HRA*), the proximal (*His$_{prox}$*), and distal (*His$_{dist}$*) electrode pairs of a catheter at the AV junction to record the His potential, and right ventricular apex (*RVA*). During baseline recording, the H-V interval is only slightly prolonged (62 msec). After infusion of intravenous procainamide, the H-V interval is longer and infra-His Wenckebach block is present. *Arrowhead* denotes the missing QRS complex caused by infra-His block. *A*, Atrial electrogram; *H*, His potential; *V*, ventricular electrogram.

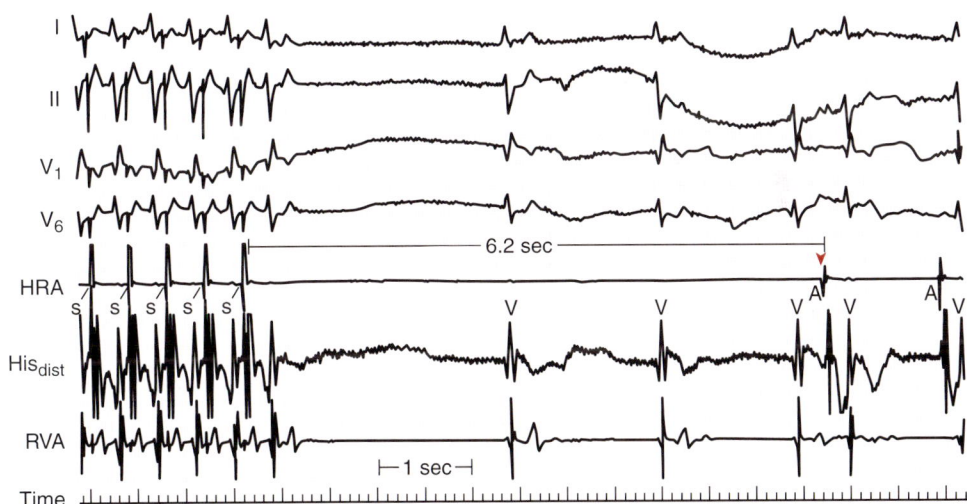

FIGURE 61.16 Abnormal sinus node function. The recording format is similar to that in Fig. 61.15. The last five complexes of a 1-minute burst of atrial pacing (*S*) at a cycle length of 400 msec are shown, after which pacing is stopped. The sinus node does not spontaneously discharge (sinus node recovery time (SNRT)) until 6.2 seconds later (*arrowhead*). Three junctional escape beats occurred before this time. *His$_{dist}$*, Distal electrode pair; *HRA*, high right atrium; *RVA*, right ventricular apex.

TACHYCARDIA

In patients with tachycardias, an EPS can be used to diagnose the arrhythmia, to determine and deliver therapy, to establish the anatomic sites involved in the tachycardia, to identify patients at high risk for the development of serious arrhythmias, and to gain insight into the mechanisms responsible for the arrhythmia (see Chapters 65 and 67). The study can differentiate aberrant supraventricular conduction from ventricular tachyarrhythmias when standard electrocardiographic criteria are equivocal. An SVT is recognized electrophysiologically by an H-V interval equaling or exceeding that recorded during a normal sinus rhythm (Fig. 61.17). In contrast, during VT, the H-V interval is shorter than normal, or the His deflection cannot be recorded clearly because of superimposition of the larger ventricular electrogram. Only two situations exist in which a consistently short H-V interval occurs: during retrograde activation of the His bundle from activation originating in the ventricle (i.e., PVC, ventricular pacing, or VT) and during AV conduction over an accessory pathway (preexcitation syndrome). Atrial pacing at rates exceeding the tachycardia rate can demonstrate the ventricular origin of a wide-QRS tachycardia by producing fusion and capture beats and normalization of the H-V interval. The only VT that exhibits an H-V interval equal to or slightly exceeding the normal sinus H-V interval is bundle branch reentry, but His activation will be in the retrograde direction.

An EPS should be considered for the following circumstances: (1) in patients who have symptomatic, recurrent, or drug-resistant supraventricular or ventricular tachyarrhythmias to help select optimal therapy; (2) in patients with tachyarrhythmias occurring too infrequently to permit adequate diagnostic or therapeutic assessment; (3) for differentiation of SVT and aberrant conduction from VT; (4) whenever nonpharmacologic therapy, such as the use of electrical devices, catheter ablation, or surgery, is contemplated; (5) in patients surviving an episode of cardiac arrest occurring more than 48 hours after acute MI or without evidence of an acute Q wave MI in an effort to establish a mechanism; and (6) for assessment of the risk for sustained VT in

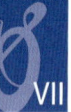

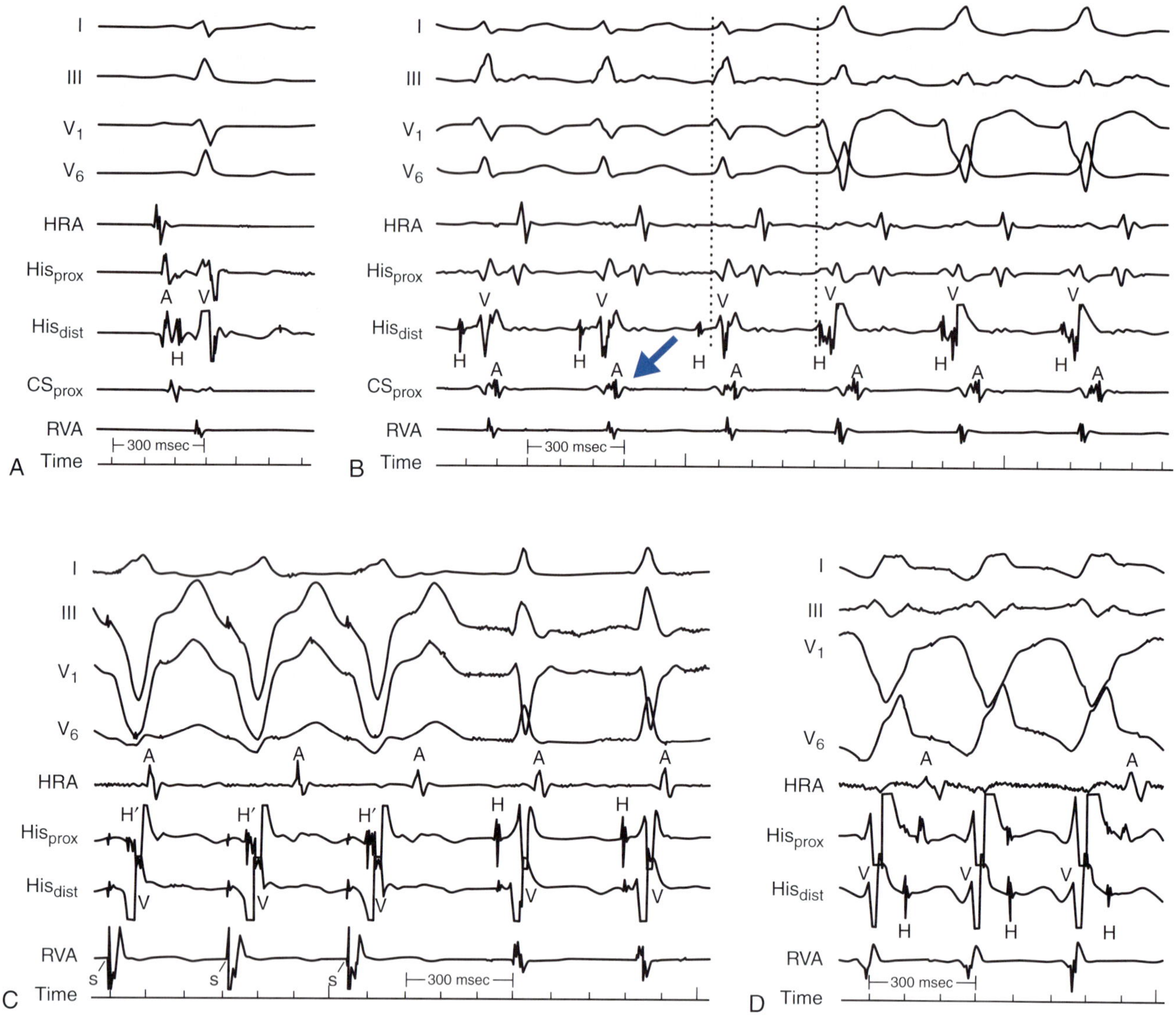

FIGURE 61.17 Bundle of His recordings in a format similar to that in Figs. 61.14 and 61.15. **A,** Baseline sinus rhythm with normal AV conduction. **B,** Orthodromic supraventricular tachycardia (SVT) with retrograde conduction over a left-sided accessory pathway throughout the tracing (earliest atrial activation in CS$_{prox}$, *arrow*). The first three beats have a narrow QRS complex with a normal H-V interval; the last three QRS complexes represent a fusion of conduction over the AV node–His bundle and a slowly conducting right-sided accessory pathway (left bundle aberrant conduction is a clue). The His potential occurs after onset of the wide QRS complex *(dashed lines)*. **C,** Three paced ventricular beats are shown with a retrograde His potential (H′), followed by initiation of AV node reentrant SVT (atrial depolarization near the end of the QRS complex, as seen in the HRA tracing). **D,** VT with delayed activation of the His potential and complete retrograde AV node block (dissociated atrial complexes). *CS$_{prox}$*, Proximal coronary sinus; *His$_{dist}$*, distal electrode pair; *His$_{prox}$*, proximal electrode pair; *HRA,* high right atrium; *RVA,* right ventricular apex.

patients with a previous MI, ejection fraction of 0.3 to 0.4, no evidence of heart failure, and nonsustained VT on an ECG. In general, EPS is not indicated in patients with LQTS and torsades de pointes.

The process of initiation and termination of SVT or VT with programmed electrical stimulation to establish precise diagnoses and help select sites for catheter ablation is the most common application of EPS in patients with tachycardia. Noninvasive stimulation from an implanted pacemaker or defibrillator can be used to test the effects of drug therapy given in an attempt to decrease the frequency of arrhythmias, as well as to test the ICD's ability to detect and treat VT that has been slowed or otherwise altered by drug effect.

UNEXPLAINED SYNCOPE

The three common arrhythmic causes of syncope are sinus node dysfunction, AV block, and tachyarrhythmias. Of the three, tachyarrhythmias are most reliably evaluated in the electrophysiology laboratory, followed by sinus node abnormalities and His-Purkinje block. Patients with a single episode of syncope and no evidence of structural heart disease, as well as those with a nondiagnostic EPS, have a low incidence of sudden death and an 80% remission rate over the ensuing 10 years. In those with recurrent syncope, the test is falsely negative in 20%, usually because of failure to find an AV block or sinus node dysfunction. Conversely, in many patients with structural heart disease, several abnormalities may be present that could account for syncope and can be diagnosed at EPS. Deciding which among these abnormalities is responsible for syncope and therefore requires therapy, and of what type, can be difficult (Fig. 61.18). Mortality and the incidence of SCD are determined mainly by the presence of underlying heart disease (see Chapter 70).

Syncopal patients considered for an EPS are those whose spells remain undiagnosed despite general, neurologic, and noninvasive cardiac evaluation, particularly if the patient has structural heart disease. The diagnostic yield is approximately 70% in that group but only 12% in patients without structural heart disease. Therapy for a putative cause found during EPS prevents recurrence of syncope in approximately 80% of patients. Among arrhythmic causes of syncope, intermittent conduction disturbances are the most difficult to diagnose. EPS are poor in establishing this diagnosis despite an array of provocative tests that can be used. When tachyarrhythmias have been thoroughly sought and excluded and clinical suspicion for intermittent heart block is high (e.g., bundle branch block or long H-V interval), empiric permanent pacing may be justified.

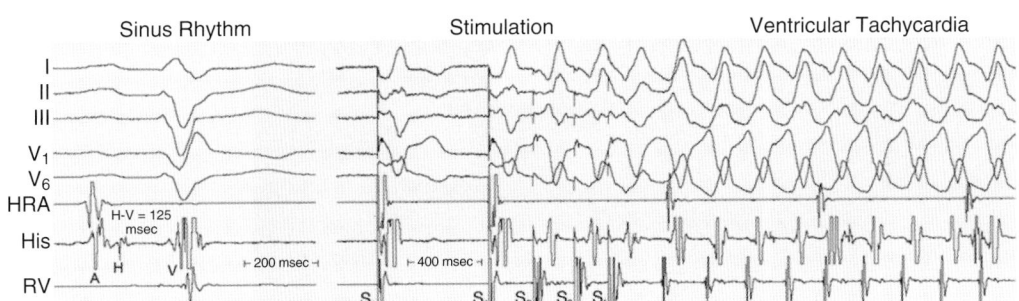

FIGURE 61.18 Surface ECG and intracardiac recordings in a patient with prior myocardial infarction and syncope. The format is similar to previous figures. In **left panel**, a sinus rhythm complex shows a right bundle branch block and left axis deviation, with a very prolonged H-V interval of 125 milliseconds (normal, 35 to 55); thus heart block could have caused syncope. However, in **right panel,** ventricular stimulation with three extrastimuli (S2, S3, S4) induces sustained VT, another potential cause of syncope (note the different time scales in the two panels).

PALPITATIONS

An EPS is indicated in patients with palpitations who have had a pulse documented by medical personnel to be inappropriately rapid or slow without an electrocardiographic recording and in those suspected of having clinically significant arrhythmias without electrocardiographic documentation. In patients with syncope or palpitations, the sensitivity of EPS may be low but can be increased at the expense of specificity. For example, more aggressive pacing techniques (e.g., use of three or four premature stimuli), administration of drugs (e.g., isoproterenol), or left ventricular pacing can increase the likelihood of induction of ventricular arrhythmias by precipitating nonclinical ventricular tachyarrhythmias, such as nonsustained polymorphic VT or VF. Similarly, aggressive techniques during atrial pacing can induce nonspecific episodes of atrial flutter (AF). A diagnostic dilemma arises when the patient's clinical, symptom-producing arrhythmia is one of these nonspecific arrhythmias that can be produced in a normal patient who has no arrhythmia. In most patients, these arrhythmias are regarded as *nonclinical* (i.e., nonspecific responses to intense stimulation). In other patients, such as those with hypertrophic or dilated nonischemic cardiomyopathy, they may be clinically relevant arrhythmias. However, induction of sustained SVT (e.g., AVNRT, AVRT) or monomorphic VT is almost never an artifact of stimulation, no matter how intense. Initiation of these arrhythmias in patients who have not had known spontaneous episodes of these tachycardias is uncommon and provides important information; for example, the induced tachyarrhythmia may be clinically significant and responsible for the patient's symptoms. In addition, inducible SVT episodes can have important implications for patients with ICDs that may deliver inappropriate therapy for such arrhythmias. In general, other abnormalities, such as prolonged sinus pauses after overdrive atrial pacing or His-Purkinje block, are not induced in patients who do not or may not spontaneously experience these abnormalities.

Complications of Electrophysiologic Studies

The risks associated with undergoing only an EPS are small. Myocardial perforation with cardiac tamponade, pseudoaneurysms at arterial access sites, and provocation of nonclinical arrhythmias can occur, each with less than a 1/500 incidence; the addition of therapeutic maneuvers (e.g., ablation) to the procedure increases the incidence of complications. In many centers, diagnostic EPS and even ablation procedures are performed on an outpatient basis (i.e., same-day discharge). With the increasing use of extensive ablation in the left atrium to treat AF, an increase in systemic thromboembolic complications has been observed, as have pericardial effusion and tamponade, valve damage, and phrenic nerve injury (see Chapter 66).[26-29] In addition pericardial approaches (subxyphoid and anterior) to epicardial VT ablation can rarely be associated with pericardial bleeding, RV puncture, and very rarely the need for cardiac surgery.[30]

DIRECT CARDIAC MAPPING: RECORDING POTENTIALS DIRECTLY FROM THE HEART

Cardiac mapping is a method whereby potentials recorded directly from the heart are spatially depicted as a function of time in an integrated manner. The location of recording electrodes (e.g., epicardial, intramural, or endocardial) and the recording mode used (unipolar vs. bipolar), as well as the method of display (isopotential, isochronal, unipolar, or bipolar voltage maps), depend on the problem under consideration. Direct cardiac mapping by catheter electrodes or less frequently at cardiac surgery can be used to identify and localize the areas responsible for rhythm disturbances in patients with supraventricular and ventricular tachyarrhythmias for catheter or surgical ablation, isolation, or resection. Conditions amenable to this approach include accessory pathways associated with WPW syndrome, the slow or fast pathways in AVNRT, AV node–His bundle ablation, sites of origin of focal AT and VTs, isolated pathways essential for the maintenance of reentrant ATs or VTs, and various substrates responsible for episodes of AF (see Chapter 66). Mapping can also be used to delineate the anatomic course of the His bundle and phrenic nerve to avoid injury during catheter ablation or open heart surgery for repair of congenital heart disease.

Specialized mapping systems use computers to log not only the activation times and electrogram amplitude (voltage) at various points in the heart, but also the physical locations from which they were obtained. The mapping information acquired in this way can be displayed on a screen to show relative activation times in a color-coded sequence. Using such systems, dozens or even hundreds of sites can be sampled relatively quickly, thereby leading to a clear picture of cardiac activation and potential target sites for ablation (Figs. 61.19 and 61.20). These systems can also record the signal amplitude at each site sampled to allow differentiation of normal from scarred myocardium, which can help in planning ablation strategies (Fig. 61.21). Other mapping systems can acquire data from several thousand points simultaneously by using a multipolar electrode array. This may be useful for hemodynamically unstable tachycardias or those that terminate spontaneously within seconds, which precludes detailed point-to-point mapping.

Pace mapping is a technique in which pacing is performed at putative sites from which arrhythmias arise (a focus) or exit (reentrant circuit). The greater the degree of "match" in QRS complexes (for VT) or intracardiac activation sequences (for ATs), the more likely that the paced site may be an appropriate site for ablation. Software has been developed to calculate the fidelity of match of the paced complexes to the target arrhythmia; ideally, this should approach 100% (see Chapter 64 , and Figs. 64.17 and 64.19). Other algorithms have been developed to analyze propagation patterns during complex arrhythmias such as AF by recording signals from multielectrode "basket" catheters in the atrium (Fig. 61.22). This has resolved many cases of an apparently chaotic rhythm to one in which erratic patterns of propagation emanate from a stable rapid source (either rotor or focus). Ablation at these source sites can eliminate AF in some cases. Lastly, although computerized mapping systems acquire activation time and voltage at given sites in the heart, these features have been displayed separately. Current mapping systems have the ability to integrate previous imaging studies (CT, MRI) into the procedure for additional anatomic reference and to derive anatomic information by moving a catheter throughout a cardiac chamber to develop a contour of its inner surface, on which activation or voltage data can be plotted.

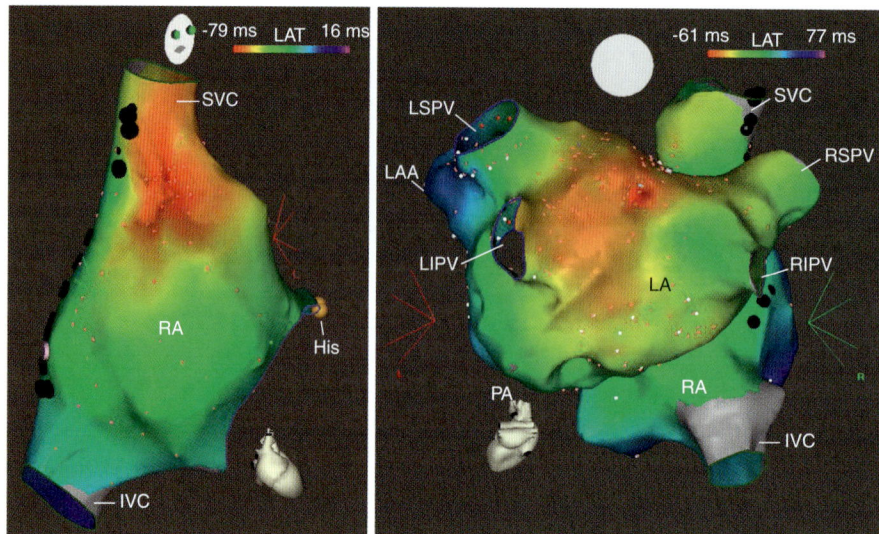

FIGURE 61.19 Electroanatomic maps of focal atrial tachycardias. **Left,** A focal right atrial tachycardia is shown from a right lateral view. A color-coded time scale of activation is shown at the top right; *red* indicates earliest activation and *purple,* latest. This atrial tachycardia arose in the anterolateral right atrium *(RA),* slightly anterior to where the sinus node resides; ablation here eliminated tachycardia while leaving sinus node function unaffected. **Right,** Activation map of a left atrial focal tachycardia with a posterior view of both RA and left atrium *(LA).* The tachycardia arose from the region of the *small red spot* at top center of the LA, with all other areas activated centrifugally. Ablation at this site eliminated the tachycardia. *SVC,* Superior vena cava; *IVC,* inferior vena cava; *His,* His bundle area *(orange dots); LIPV,* left inferior pulmonary vein *(PV); LSPV,* left superior PV; *RIPV,* right inferior PV; *RSPV,* right superior PV.

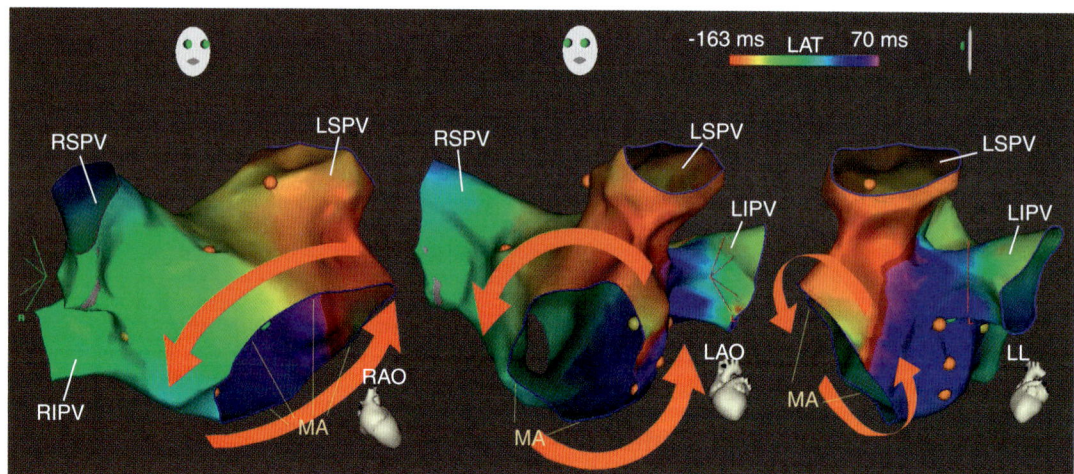

FIGURE 61.20 Electroanatomic activation map of "perimitral" reentrant atrial flutter. Three views of the left atrium are shown: right anterior oblique *(RAO),* left anterior oblique *(LAO),* and left lateral *(LL).* The wave front propagates around the mitral annulus *(MA)* in a "counterclockwise" direction as indicated by *orange arrows*; in this complete circuit, early activation *(red)* abuts late activation *(purple)* at the lateral mitral annulus. The cycle length of the tachycardia was 235 msec, almost completely described by the points shown in the figure (from −163 to +70 msec, a total of 233 msec; time scale at *top*). Abbreviations as in Fig. 61.19.

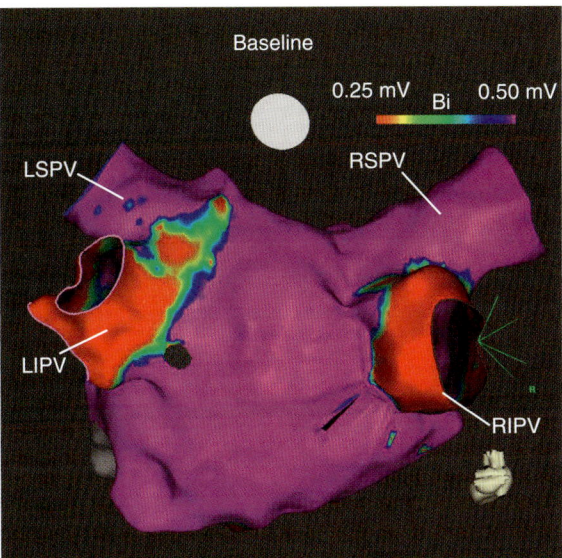
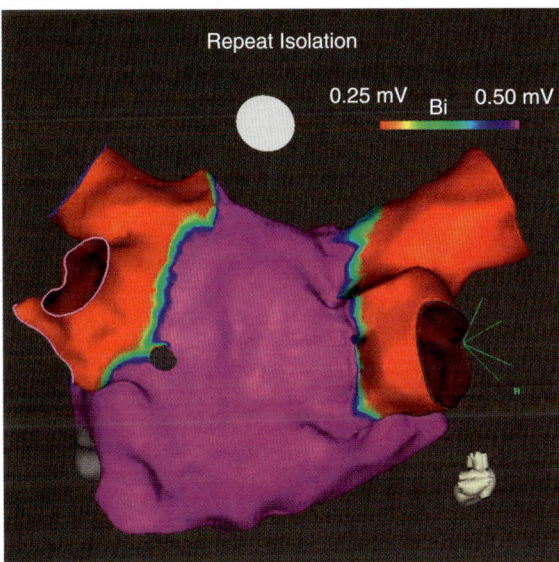

FIGURE 61.21 Electroanatomic left atrial voltage maps during sinus rhythm in a patient with recurrent atrial fibrillation after prior pulmonary vein (PV) isolation. **Top,** Posterior view of the left atrium at baseline, showing low voltage *(red,* tantamount to electrical isolation) in the left *(LIPV)* and right *(RIPV)* inferior PVs, but high residual voltage *(purple)* in the left *(LSPV)* and right *(RSPV)* superior PVs. **Bottom,** After repeat ablation around the PVs, the superior veins now have no residual voltage *(red)*; all four PVs are now isolated. The patient has had no recurrence of symptoms. Voltage scales are shown at *top right* of each panel.

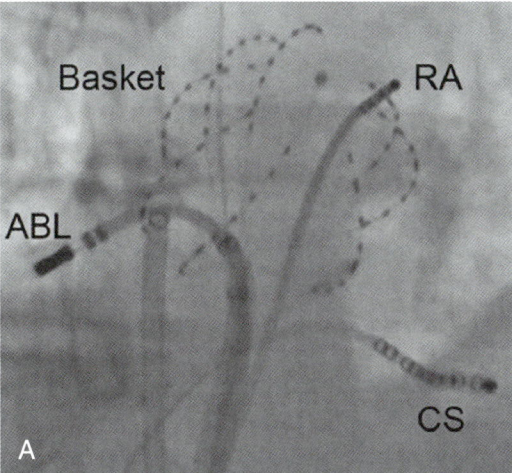
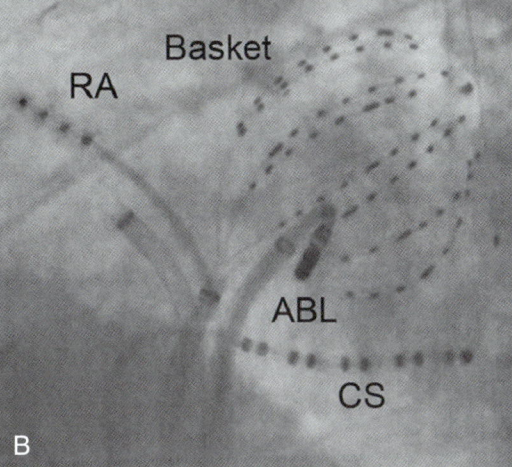

FIGURE 61.22 Basket catheter for mapping atrial fibrillation. Right **(A)** and left **(B)** anterior oblique fluoroscopic views of an eight-spline, eight electrodes per spline (64 total electrodes) "basket" catheter in the left atrium; other catheters are right atrial *(RA)*, coronary sinus *(CS)*, and an ablation catheter *(ABL)* in the right inferior pulmonary vein.

REFERENCES

Signs and Symptoms

1. Giada F, Raviele A. Clinical approach to patients with palpitations. *Card Electrophysiol Clin.* 2018;10:387–396.
2. Goldberger ZD, Petek BJ, Brignole M, et al. ACC/AHA/HRS versus ESC guidelines for the diagnosis and management of syncope: JACC guideline comparison. *J Am Coll Cardiol.* 2019;74:2410–2423.
3. Puppala VK, Akkaya M, Dickinson O, et al. Risk stratification of patients presenting with transient loss of consciousness. *Cardiol Clin.* 2015;33:387–396.
4. Albassam OT, Redelmeier RJ, Shadowitz S, et al. Did this patient have cardiac syncope?: the rational clinical examination systematic review. *J Am Med Assoc.* 2019;321:2448–2457.
5. Novak P. Autonomic disorders. *Am J Med.* 2019;132:420–436.
6. Bryarly M, Phillips LT, Fu Q, et al. Postural orthostatic tachycardia syndrome: JACC focus seminar. *J Am Coll Cardiol.* 2019;73:1207–1228.
7. Wong CX, Brown A, Lau DH, et al. Epidemiology of sudden cardiac death: global and regional perspectives. *Heart Lung Circ.* 2019;28:6–14.
8. Jeserich M, Merkely B, Olschewski M, et al. Patients with exercise-associated ventricular ectopy present evidence of myocarditis. *J Cardiovasc Magn Reson.* 2015;17:100.

Clinical and Laboratory Testing

9. Kim J, Kwon M, Chang J, et al. Meta-analysis of prognostic implications of exercise-induced ventricular premature complexes in the general population. *Am J Cardiol.* 2016;118:725–732.
10. Skinner JR, Winbo A, Abrams D, et al. Channelopathies that lead to sudden cardiac death: clinical and genetic aspects. *Heart Lung Circ.* 2019;28:22–30.
11. Subramanian M, Prabhu MA, Harikrishnan MS, et al. The utility of exercise testing in risk stratification of asymptomatic patients with type 1 brugada pattern. *J Cardiovasc Electrophysiol.* 2017;28:677–683.
12. Marcus GM. Evaluation and management of premature ventricular complexes. *Circulation.* 2020;141:1404–1418.
13. Sana F, Isselbacher EM, Singh JP, et al. Wearable devices for ambulatory cardiac monitoring: JACC state-of-the-art review. *J Am Coll Cardiol.* 2020;75:1582–1592.
14. Perez MV, Mahaffey KW, Hedlin H, et al. Large-scale assessment of a smartwatch to identify atrial fibrillation. *N Engl J Med.* 2019;381:1909–1917.
15. Wasserlauf J, You C, Patel R, et al. Smartwatch performance for the detection and quantification of atrial fibrillation. *Circ Arrhythm Electrophysiol.* 2019;12:e006834.
16. Turakhia MP, Desai M, Hedlin H, et al. Rationale and design of a large-scale, app-based study to identify cardiac arrhythmias using a smartwatch: the apple heart study. *Am Heart J.* 2019;207:66–75.
17. Godin R, Yeung C, Baranchuk A, et al. Screening for atrial fibrillation using a mobile, single-lead electrocardiogram in Canadian primary care clinics. *Can J Cardiol.* 2019;35:840–845.
18. Giancaterino S, Lupercio F, Nishimura M, et al. Current and future use of insertable cardiac monitors. *JACC Clin Electrophysiol.* 2018;4:1383–1396.
19. Melillo P, Izzo R, Orrico A, et al. Automatic prediction of cardiovascular and cerebrovascular events using heart rate variability analysis. *PloS One.* 2015;10:e0118504.
20. Al-Zaiti SS, Pietrasik G, Carey MG, et al. The role of heart rate variability, heart rate turbulence, and deceleration capacity in predicting cause-specific mortality in chronic heart failure. *J Electrocardiol.* 2019;52:70–74.
21. Rudy Y. Noninvasive ECG imaging (ECGI): mapping the arrhythmic substrate of the human heart. *Int J Cardiol.* 2017;237:13–14.

22. Sheldon RS, Grubb 2nd BP, Olshansky B, et al. 2015 heart rhythm society expert consensus statement on the diagnosis and treatment of postural tachycardia syndrome, inappropriate sinus tachycardia, and vasovagal syncope. *Heart Rhythm*. 2015;12:e41–e63.
23. Raj SR, Guzman JC, Harvey P, et al. Canadian cardiovascular society position statement on postural orthostatic tachycardia syndrome (POTS) and related disorders of chronic orthostatic intolerance. *Can J Cardiol*. 2020;36:357–372.
24. George SA, Bivens TB, Howden EJ, et al. The international pots registry: evaluating the efficacy of an exercise training intervention in a community setting. *Heart Rhythm*. 2016;13:943–950.

Invasive EP Testing

25. Boule S, Ouadah A, Langlois C, et al. Predictors of advanced his-purkinje conduction disturbances in patients with unexplained syncope and bundle branch block. *Can J Cardiol*. 2014;30:606–611.
26. Voskoboinik A, Sparks PB, Morton JB, et al. Low rates of major complications for radiofrequency ablation of atrial fibrillation maintained over 14 years: a single centre experience of 2750 consecutive cases. *Heart Lung Circ*. 2018;27:976–983.
27. Peichl P, Wichterle D, Pavlu L, et al. Complications of catheter ablation of ventricular tachycardia: a single-center experience. *Circ Arrhythm Electrophysiol*. 2014;7:684–690.
28. Dukkipati SR, Choudry S, Koruth JS, et al. Catheter ablation of ventricular tachycardia in structurally normal hearts: indications, strategies, and outcomes-part i. *J Am Coll Cardiol*. 2017;70:2909–2923.
29. Shivkumar K. Catheter ablation of ventricular arrhythmias. *N Engl J Med*. 2019;380:1555–1564.
30. Keramati AR, DeMazumder D, Misra S, et al. Anterior pericardial access to facilitate electrophysiology study and catheter ablation of ventricular arrhythmias: a single tertiary center experience. *J Cardiovasc Electrophysiol*. 2017;28:1189–1195.

Guidelines

31. Crawford MH, Bernstein SJ, Deedwania PC, et al. ACC/AHA guidelines for ambulatory electrocardiography. A report of the American College of Cardiology/American Heart Association task force on practice guidelines (committee to revise the guidelines for ambulatory electrocardiography). Developed in collaboration with the North American Society for Pacing and Electrophysiology. *J Am Coll Cardiol*. 1999;34:912–948.
32. Kadish AH, Buxton AE, Kennedy HL, et al. ACC/AHA clinical competence statement on electrocardiography and ambulatory electrocardiography: a report of the ACC/AHA/ACP-ASIM task force on clinical competence (ACC/AHA Committee to develop a clinical competence statement on electrocardiography and ambulatory electrocardiography) endorsed by the International Society for Holter and Noninvasive Electrocardiology. *Circulation*. 2001;104:3169–3178.
33. Zipes DP, Calkins H, Daubert JP, et al. 2015 ACC/AHA/HRS advanced training statement on clinical cardiac electrophysiology (a revision of the ACC/AHA 2006 update of the clinical competence statement on invasive electrophysiology studies, catheter ablation, and cardioversion). *J Am Coll Cardiol*. 2015;66:2767–2802.
34. Zipes DP, DiMarco JP, Gillette PC, et al. Guidelines for clinical intracardiac electrophysiological and catheter ablation procedures. A report of the American College of Cardiology/American Heart Association task force on practice guidelines (committee on clinical intracardiac electrophysiologic and catheter ablation procedures), developed in collaboration with the North American Society of Pacing and Electrophysiology. *J Am Coll Cardiol*. 1995;26:555–573.
35. Shen WK, Sheldon RS, Benditt DG, et al. 2017 ACC/AHA/HRS guideline for the evaluation and management of patients with syncope: a report of the American College of Cardiology/American Heart Association task force on clinical practice guidelines and the Heart Rhythm Society. *J Am Coll Cardiol*. 2017;70:e39–e110.
36. Aliot EM, Stevenson WG, Almendral-Garrote JM, et al. EHRA/HRS expert consensus on catheter ablation of ventricular arrhythmias: developed in a partnership with the European Heart Rhythm Association (EHRA), a registered branch of the European Society of Cardiology (ESC), and the Heart Rhythm Society (HRS); in collaboration with the American College of cardiology (ACC) and the American Heart Association (AHA). *Heart Rhythm*. 2009;6:886–933.

62 Mechanisms of Cardiac Arrhythmias
STANLEY NATTEL AND GORDON F. TOMASELLI

FOUNDATIONS OF CARDIAC ELECTROPHYSIOLOGY, 1163
The Functions of the Cardiac Electrical System, 1163
The Cardiac Action Potential, 1163
Physiology of Ion Channels, 1163
Phases of the Cardiac Action Potential, 1166
Normal Automaticity, 1170
Molecular Structure of Key Cardiac Ion Channels and Transporters, 1171
Gap Junction Channels and Intercalated Discs, 1173

STRUCTURE AND FUNCTION OF THE CARDIAC ELECTRICAL NETWORK, 1175
Sinoatrial Node, 1175
Atrioventricular Junctional Area and Intraventricular Conduction System, 1175
Bundle of His (Penetrating Portion of Atrioventricular Bundle), 1176
Innervation of Atrioventricular Node, His Bundle, and Ventricular Myocardium, 1177

Arrhythmias and the Autonomic Nervous System, 1178
MECHANISMS OF ARRHYTHMOGENESIS, 1179
Disorders of Impulse Formation, 1179
Disorders of Impulse Conduction, 1183
Specific Arrhythmias Illustrating Mechanistic Principles, 1186

REFERENCES, 1189

FOUNDATIONS OF CARDIAC ELECTROPHYSIOLOGY

The Functions of the Cardiac Electrical System

While this might come as a surprise to some electrophysiologists, the role of the electrical system of the heart is not to generate nice-looking action potentials (APs) and conduction patterns. Its role is to subserve and control the mechanical function of the heart appropriately. The key elements of this function are illustrated in Figure 62.1A. The electrical system must initiate contraction at a rate and rhythm that is appropriate to the body's moment-to-moment needs for blood supply to various organs. Appropriate timing of the contraction of different parts of each cardiac chamber (atria and ventricles) needs to be ensured, as does the relative timing of the atria versus the ventricles. The atria serve a primer-pump role and need to contract before the ventricles with an appropriate delay to allow optimal ventricular filling (which is a key determinant of cardiac contractility via the Frank-Starling principle). Finally, excessively rapid and excessively slow rates must be prevented, as these can have disastrous effects on cardiac function.

As illustrated by the schematic diagram of the relationship between heart rate and cardiac output in Figure 62.1B, cardiac output is more or less a linear function of the heart rate between about 50 and 150 beats/min (consistent with the relationship cardiac output = heart rate × stroke volume, as long as stroke volume is fairly constant). At heart rates below or above this range, cardiac output can fall precipitously. The key properties underlying the functions listed in Figure 62.1A are automaticity, conduction, electromechanical coupling, and refractoriness. The central cellular characteristic that underlies these properties and cardiac electrical function is the cardiac action potential.

The Cardiac Action Potential

The cardiac action potential (AP) is illustrated in Figure 62.2. The AP is a graph of the voltage difference between the inside of a cardiac cell and the outside of the cell (as seen from the inside, for example by a fine-tipped electrode placed inside the cell), as a function of time. Cardiac cells normally have a negative intracellular resting potential, which for most of the heart (working atrial and ventricular muscle, specialized His-Purkinje conducting system) is about –80 to –90 mV. The exceptions are the sinoatrial (SA) and central atrioventricular (AV) node regions, which have resting potentials between about –50 and –65 mV. The cardiac AP is by convention divided into four phases, the AP-upstroke (phase 0), which depolarizes the cell from its negative resting potential to a potential positive to 0 mV; the initial rapid repolarization phase (phase 1); the so-called plateau (phase 2) in which the AP voltage changes relatively slowly; and the final (phase 3) rapid repolarization phase, which brings the cell back to its resting potential (referred to as phase 4).

During phase 0, there is a rapid inrush of positively charged Na$^+$ ions that mediate depolarization and carry a large inward current (the direction of current is by convention defined by the movement of positive ions), which provides the energy for electrical conduction. Phase 1 sets the voltage level for the subsequent critical phase 2. Phase 2 is the portion of the AP during which Ca^{2+} enters the cell and causes a large secondary release of Ca^{2+} from the sarcoplasmic reticulum (SR), the main cellular Ca^{2+}-storage organelle. The SR Ca^{2+}-release rapidly increases free intracellular [Ca^{2+}], which causes cellular contraction and mediates electromechanical coupling. Finally, phase 3 (carried by a rapid egress of K$^+$) brings the cell back to its negative resting potential. Because the cell cannot be activated by normal means at voltages positive to –60 mV, from when the cell reaches –60 mV during phase 0 until the time that it repolarizes to –60 mV during phase 3 the cell cannot be fired and is "refractory" to activation. Thus, the timing of phase 3 sets the refractory period (RP). The mechanisms by which the crucial AP properties are set depend critically on the function of ion channels, which is discussed in detail below.

Physiology of Ion Channels

Electrical signaling in the heart involves the passage of ions through ionic channels. The sodium, potassium, calcium, and chloride (Na$^+$, K$^+$, Ca^{2+}, and Cl$^-$) ions are the major charge carriers, and their movement across the cell membrane through channel pores creates a flow of current that generates excitation and signals in cardiac myocytes (Table 62.1).

When a semipermeable membrane allows an ion to cross, and the concentration of the ion is different on the two sides of the membrane, a small number of ions will move across the membrane and create an electrical field. For example, consider the case of K$^+$ and the cardiac cell membrane. The concentration of K$^+$ is maintained (by a complex set of pumps and transporters) at about 150 mM inside the cardiac cell and is about 4 mM outside. Cardiac cell membranes are highly permeable to K$^+$ at rest, largely because of a specific ion channel, the inward-rectifier K$^+$ channel (carrying the current I_{K1}). K$^+$ tends to leave the cell, down its chemical gradient. However, each K$^+$ ion that leaves the cell (unaccompanied by a negative ion, because the cell membrane is largely impermeable to them at rest) leaves the interior of the cell with a slightly negative charge relative to the outside. Equilibrium is created when the chemical force tending to push K+ out of the cell is balanced by an equal and opposite electrical force created by the net intracellular negative charge tending to pull the K+ back into the cell. The voltage at which these forces balance is called the "equilibrium potential." In the case of K+, the equilibrium potential is given by the Nernst equation (E = RT/F·ln([K+$_o$]/[K+$_i$]), where R is the universal gas constant, T = absolute temperature, F = Faraday's constant, and [K+$_o$], [K+$_i$] = extracellular and intracellular K+ concentration, respectively. This value, designated "E_K," for K+ equilibrium potential, is about −95 mV. Thus, at rest the high permeability to K+ results in a resting potential of about −90 mV (see Fig. 62.2), close to the K+ equilibrium potential.

As shown in Figure 62.2, membrane voltages during a cardiac AP vary over the range of approximately −90 to +30 mV. Each phase of the cardiac AP is characterized by its dominant ionic permeabilities (shown in green in Fig. 62.2), which determine the direction in which the transmembrane potential moves during that phase. Phase 0 happens when there is a rapid increase in membrane permeability to Na+, and K+ permeability falls, making Na+ the dominant conductance. At the peak of phase 0 (the "overshoot"), the cell moves close to the Na+ equilibrium potential, which is quite positive because in contrast to K+, Na+ is more concentrated outside the cell than inside and the Na+ chemical force makes it move into the cell, making the interior more positive. Phase 1 is carried by a transient, rapid exit of K+ from the cell. Because the calculated reversal potential of a cardiac Ca2+ channel is +64 mV (assuming P_K/P_{Ca} = 1/3000, Ca_i = 100 nM, and Ca_o = 2 mM), passive Ca2+ flux is into the cell. During phase 2, the transmembrane potential is governed by balanced permeabilities to Ca2+ and K+, while during phase 3 a rapid increase in K+ permeability offsets the decreasing Ca2+ conductance and repolarizes the cell. In some cardiac cells (notably His-Purkinje cells) a late Na+ current (I_{NaL}) contributes inward current during the phase 2 plateau.

The changes in ionic permeabilities during the AP are determined by the opening and closing of ion channels. The opening of ion channels allows selected ions to flow passively down the electrochemical activity gradient at a very high rate (>10^6 ions per second). The high transfer rates and restriction to "downhill" fluxes not stoichiometrically coupled to the hydrolysis of energy-rich phosphates distinguish ion channel mechanisms from other ion-transporting structures (pumps and exchangers), such as the sarcolemmal Na+,K+–adenosine triphosphatase (Na+,K+–ATPase, which largely maintains the physiological Na+ and K+ concentrations inside the cell), sarcoendoplasmic reticulum (SR) Ca2+-ATPase (SERCA, the SR Ca2+-uptake mechanism), or the Na+/Ca2+ exchanger (NCX, which removes from the cell interior the extra Ca2+ that has entered during phase 2). Ion channels may be induced to open or close (gated) by extracellular and intracellular receptor-ligands, changes in transmembrane voltage ("voltage-gated"), or mechanical stress (see Table 62.1). The most important ion channels in generating the AP are voltage-gated. Ion currents and gating of single ion channels can best be studied by means of the "patch-clamp" technique, in which a glass microelectrode tip is attached to the cell membrane (to record single channel opening), and in some cases a small patch of membrane is torn away to allow electrical continuity between the inside of the cell and the contents of the microelectrode (to measure transmembrane currents). The microelectrode is filled with an electrically conducting fluid that is connected to an amplifier that measures the potential difference between the microelectrode and a reference electrode, generally located in the extracellular fluid.

The *permeability ratio* is commonly used to define a channel's ionic selectivity, defined as the ratio of the permeability of one ion type to that of the main permeant ion type. Permeability ratios of voltage-gated K+ and Na+ channels for other monovalent and divalent (e.g., Ca2+)

Functions of the Cardiac Electrical System

- To initiate rhythmic contraction at a rate appropriate to the needs of the body.
- To ensure appropriate timing of contraction for each cardiac chamber.
- To prevent heart rates that are excessively slow or rapid for the body's needs.

A

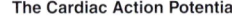

B

FIGURE 62.1 A, Functions of the cardiac electrical system. **B,** Plot of the cardiac output as a function of heart rate.

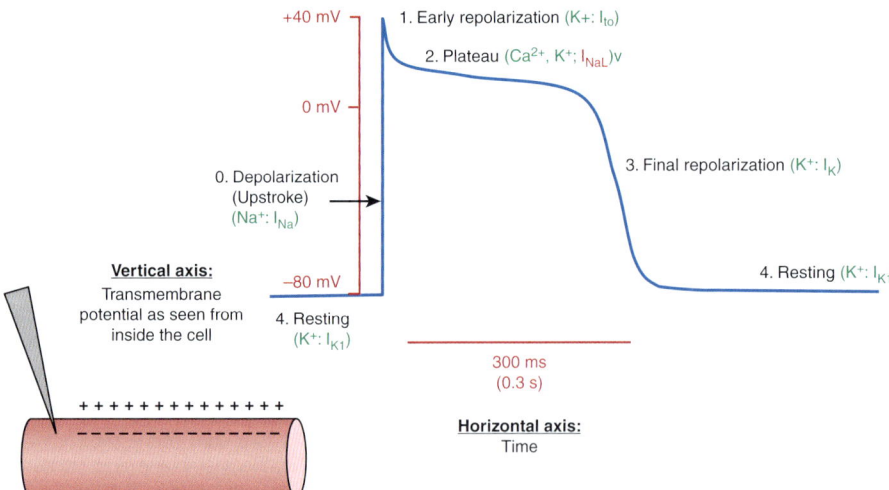

FIGURE 62.2 A representative ventricular action potential, with phases numbered 0 to 4. The major ionic currents active during each phase are shown in green type. The late Na current I_{NaL} is augmented in some forms of heritable and acquired heart disease. The drawing at lower left of the figure depicts cardiac muscle impaled with an electrode. The resting membrane potential of the inside of the cell is negative with respect to the outside.

TABLE 62.1 Synopsis of Transsarcolemmal Ionic Currents in Mammalian Cardiac Myocytes

CURRENT	SUBUNIT	FUNCTIONAL PROPERTIES
A. Sodium Currents		
I_{Na}	Nav1.5, Nav1.1, Nav1.3, Nav1.6, Nav1.8 (alpha subunits)	TTX-resistant (Nav1.5, Nav1.8) and TTX-sensitive (Nav1.1, Nav1.3, Nav1.6) voltage-gated currents; Nav1.5 is the major cardiac isoform; neuronal Na$^+$ channel isoforms contribute to SA node pacemaking and ventricular repolarization
B. Calcium Currents		
$I_{Ca,L}$	Cav1.2 (alpha subunit)	L-type (*l*ong lasting, *l*arge conductance) Ca^{2+} currents through voltage-gated Ca^{2+} (Cav) channels blocked by dihydropyridine antagonists (e.g., nifedipine), phenylalkylamines (e.g., verapamil), benzodiazepines (e.g., diltiazem), and various divalent ions (e.g., Cd^{2+}); activated by dihydropyridine agonists (e.g., Bay K 8644); responsible for phase 0 depolarization and propagation in SA and AV nodal tissue and contributing to the plateau of atrial, His-Purkinje, and ventricular cells; main trigger of Ca^{2+} release from the sarcoplasmic reticulum (Ca^{2+}-induced Ca^{2+} release); the noninactivating or "window" component underlies EADs
$I_{Ca,T}$	Cav3.1/alpha$_{1G}$ (alpha subunit)	T-type (*t*ransient current, *t*iny conductance) Ca^{2+} currents through Cav channels blocked by mibefradil and efonidipine but insensitive to dihydropyridines; may contribute an inward current to the later phase of phase 4 depolarization in pacemaker cells and action potential propagation in AV nodal cells; role in triggering Ca^{2+}-induced Ca^{2+} release uncertain
I_f	HCN4 (alpha subunit)	Hyperpolarization-activated "funny" current carried by Na$^+$ and K$^+$ in SA and AV nodal cells and His-Purkinje cells; involved in generating phase 4 depolarization; increases the rate of impulse initiation in pacemaker cells
C. Potassium Currents		
I_{K1}	Kir2.1 (alpha subunit)	K$^+$ current through inwardly rectifying K$^+$ (Kir) channels, voltage-dependent block by Ba^{2+} at micromolar concentrations; responsible for maintaining resting the membrane potential in atrial, His-Purkinje, and ventricular cells; channel activity is a function of both membrane potential and [K$^+$]$_o$; inward rectification appears to result from depolarization-induced internal block by Mg^{2+} and neutral or positively charged amino acid residues in the cytoplasmic channel pore
$I_{K,G}$ ($I_{K,ACh}$, $I_{K,Ade}$)	Kir3.1/Kir3.4 (alpha subunit)	Inwardly rectifying K$^+$ current activated by muscarinic (M$_2$) and purinergic (type 1) receptor stimulation via GTP regulatory (G) protein signal transduction; expressed in SA and AV nodal cells and atrial cells, where it causes hyperpolarization and action potential shortening; activation causes negative chronotropic and dromotropic effects
I_{Ks}	KvLQT1, Kv7.1 (alpha subunit)/minK (beta subunit)	K$^+$ current carried by a voltage-gated K$^+$ (Kv) channel (delayed rectifier K$^+$ channel); plays a major role in determining phase 3 of the action potential
I_{Kr}	hERG, Kv11.1 (alpha subunit)/MiRP1 (beta subunit)	Rapidly activating component of delayed rectifier K$^+$ current; I_{Kr} specifically blocked by dofetilide and sotalol in a reverse use–dependent manner; inward rectification of I_{Kr} results from depolarization-induced fast inactivation; plays a major role in determining the APD
I_{Kur}	Kv1.5 (alpha subunit)	K$^+$ current through a Kv channel with ultrarapid activation but ultraslow inactivation kinetics; expressed in atrial myocytes; determines the APD
$I_{K,Ca}$	SK1-3 (alpha subunit)	K$^+$ current through small-conductance Ca^{2+}-activated channels; blocked by apamin and expressed in human atrial and ventricular myocytes; determines the APD; upregulated in failing cardiomyocytes
I_{to} (I_{to1}, I_A)	Kv4.3 (alpha subunit)/KChIP2 (beta subunit)	Transient outward K$^+$ current through voltage-gated (Kv) channels; exhibits fast activation and inactivation and recovery kinetics; blocked by 4-aminopyridine in a reverse use–dependent manner; contributes to the time course of phase 1 repolarization; transmural differences in I_{to} properties contribute to regional differences in early repolarization
D. Chloride Currents		
$I_{Cl,Ca}$ (I_{to2})	?	4-Aminopyridine–resistant transient outward current carried by Cl$^-$ ions; activated by an increase in intracellular calcium level; blocked by stilbene derivatives (SITS, DIDS); contributes to the time course of phase 1 repolarization; may underlie spontaneous transient inward currents under conditions of Ca^{2+} overload; molecular correlate uncertain
$I_{Cl,cAMP}$	?	Time-independent chloride current regulated by the cAMP/adenylate cyclase pathway; slightly depolarizes resting membrane potential and significantly shortens the APD; antagonizes action potential prolongation associated with beta-adrenergic stimulation of $I_{Ca,L}$
$I_{Cl,swell}$ or $I_{Cl,vol}$	?	Outwardly rectifying, swelling-activated Cl$^-$ current; inhibited by 9-anthracene carboxylic acid; activation causes resting membrane depolarization and action potential shortening
$I_{K,ATP}$	Kir6.2 (alpha subunit)/SUR	Time-independent K$^+$ current through Kir channels activated by a fall in intracellular ATP concentration; inhibited by sulfonylurea drugs, such as glibenclamide; activated by pinacidil, nicorandil, cromakalim; causes shortening of the APD during myocardial ischemia or hypoxia
$I_{Cir,swell}$	?	Inwardly rectifying, swelling-activated cation current; permeable to Na$^+$ and K$^+$; inhibited by Gd^{3+}; depolarizes resting membrane potential and prolongs terminal (phase 3) repolarization
E. Electrogenic Pumps and Exchangers		
$I_{Na/Ca}$	NCX1.1	Current carried by Na$^+$/Ca^{2+} exchanger; causes net Na$^+$ outward current and Ca^{2+} inward current (reverse mode) or net Na$^+$ inward and Ca^{2+} outward current (3 Na$^+$ for 1 Ca^{2+}); direction of Na$^+$ flux depends on membrane potential and intracellular and extracellular concentrations of Na$^+$ and Ca^{2+}; Ca^{2+} influx mediated by $I_{Na/Ca}$ can trigger SR Ca^{2+} release; underlies I_{ti} (transient inward current) under conditions of intracellular Ca^{2+} overload

Continued

TABLE 62.1 Synopsis of Transsarcolemmal Ionic Currents in Mammalian Cardiac Myocytes—cont'd

CURRENT	SUBUNIT	FUNCTIONAL PROPERTIES
$I_{Na/K}$	Alpha subunit/beta subunit	Na^+ outward current generated by Na^+,K^+-ATPase (stoichiometry: 3 Na^+ leave and 2 K^+ enter); inhibited by digitalis
I_{ti}	?	Transient inward current activated by Ca^{2+} waves; I_{ti} possibly reflects 3 Ca^{2+}-dependent components: I_{NCX}, $I_{Cl,Ca}$, and a *TRPM4* (transient receptor potential cation channel, member 4 gene)–mediated current
F. Electroneutral Ion-Exchanging Proteins		
Ca^{2+}-ATPase	SERCA2	Extrudes cytosolic calcium
Na/H	Cardiac myocytes express isoform NHE1	Exchanges intracellular H^+ for extracellular Na^+; specifically inhibited by the benzoylguanidine derivatives HOE 694 and HOE 642; inhibition causes intracellular acidification
Cl^--HCO_3^-		Exchanges intracellular HCO_3^- for external Cl^-; inhibited by SITS
Na^+-K^+-$2Cl^-$	Na-K-Cl NKCC1	Cotransporter blocked by amiloride

APD, Action potential duration; *AV*, atrioventricular; *DIDS*, 4,4′-diisothiocyanatostilbene-2,2′-disulfonic acid; *EADs*, early afterdepolarizations; *GTP*, guanosine triphosphate; *SA*, sinoatrial; *SITS*, 4-acetamido-4′-isothiocyanatostilbene-2,2′-disulfonic acid; *TTX*, tetrodotoxin.

cations (cations are positively charged ions, so called because they are attracted to a "cathode" or negative electrode) versus their permeant ion are usually less than 1:10. Voltage-gated Ca^{2+} channels exhibit a more than 1000-fold discrimination against Na^+ and K^+ ions (e.g., P_K/P_{Ca} = 1/3000) and all of these are impermeable to anions (negatively charged ions like Cl^-, attracted to an "anode").

Because ions are charged, net ionic flux through an open channel is determined by both the concentration and the electrical gradients across the membrane (electrodiffusion). As discussed above, the potential at which the passive flux of ions resulting from the chemical driving force is exactly balanced by the electrical driving force is called the *equilibrium* or *reversal potential* of the channel. In a channel that is perfectly selective for one ion species, the reversal potential equals the thermodynamic equilibrium potential of that ion, E_S, which is given by an equation of the form:

$$E_S = (RT/zF) \ln ([S_o] / [S_i])$$

where $[S_i]$ and $[S_o]$ are the intracellular and extracellular concentrations of the permeant ion, respectively, z is the valence of the ion, R is the gas constant, F is the Faraday constant, T is the absolute temperature (kelvin), and ln is the natural logarithm (the Nernst equation is this equation applied to K^+). If the current through an open channel is carried by more than one permeant ion, the reversal potential becomes a weighted mean of all the equilibrium potentials.

ION FLUX THROUGH VOLTAGE-GATED CHANNELS

The activation of voltage-dependent cardiac channels generally increases with membrane depolarization. Channels do not have a sharp voltage threshold for opening. Rather, the dependence of channel activation on membrane potential is a continuous function of voltage and follows a sigmoidal curve (Fig. 62.3A, *blue curve*). The potential at which activation is half-maximal and the steepness of the activation curve govern channel permeability changes in response to changes in membrane potential. Some channels (like Na^+, L-type Ca^{2+} and transient-outward K^+ channels) also show inactivation, with a voltage dependence qualitatively similar to activation but generally occurring at more negative voltages (Fig. 62.3A, *gold curve*). Both channel activation and inactivation are time-dependent, with a change in voltage causing a progressive change in gating toward the steady-state values shown in Figure 62.3A. The time constant of a gating process indicates the time required to get to about 63% of steady state, and ranges from about 1 msec (msec, 1/1000 second) for Na^+ channel activation to about 5 to 10 msec for L-type Ca^{2+} channels to 100 msec for delayed-rectifier K^+ channels. Inactivation is generally about an order of magnitude slower than activation.

Activation occurs rapidly on membrane depolarization, causing channel opening. Inactivation proceeds with a slight delay because of its slower kinetics, allowing for a substantial number of channels to open and carry current before inactivation occurs. If membrane depolarization persists, the channel remains inactivated and cannot reopen. Inactivation curves of the various cardiac voltage-gated ion channels differ in their voltage dependence. For example, sustained membrane depolarization to −50 mV (as may occur in acutely ischemic myocardium) causes almost complete inactivation of the Na^+ channel, whereas the L-type Ca^{2+} channel (see Voltage-Gated Ca^{2+} Channels) exhibits little inactivation at this membrane potential. Activation and inactivation curves can overlap over a voltage range with finite steady-state conductance (hatched area in Fig. 62.3A), in which case a steady-state noninactivating inward current can flow, potentially causing spontaneous depolarization. L-type Ca^{2+} channel and Na^+ channel window currents have been implicated in the genesis of triggered activity arising from early afterdepolarizations (EADs).[1]

Channels recover from inactivation and then enter the closed state, from which they can be reactivated and open again (Fig. 62.3B). Rates of recovery from inactivation vary among the different types of voltage-dependent channels and usually follow monoexponential or multiexponential time courses, with time constants ranging from a few milliseconds for Na^+ current to several seconds for some subtypes of K^+ currents.

PRINCIPLES OF IONIC CURRENT MODULATION

The whole-cell current amplitude I is the product of the number of functional channels in the membrane available for opening (N), the probability that a channel will open (P_o), and the single-channel current amplitude (i) (Fig. 62.3C), or $I = N \cdot P_o \cdot i$. Changes in total current therefore result from alterations in N, P_o, i, or any combination of these factors. Changes in the number of available channels in the cell membrane result from up- or down-regulation of the expression of ion channel–encoding genes. The magnitude of the single-channel current amplitude depends in part on the ionic concentration gradient across the membrane. Changes in channel activation (i.e., P_o) can result from phosphorylation or dephosphorylation of the channel protein, or from gene mutations that alter channel gating or conductivity properties.

Phases of the Cardiac Action Potential

As discussed above, the cardiac AP consists of five phases: *phase 0*, upstroke or rapid depolarization; *phase 1*, early rapid repolarization; *phase 2*, plateau; *phase 3*, final rapid repolarization; and *phase 4*, resting membrane potential and diastolic depolarization (see Fig. 62.2). These phases are the result of passive ion fluxes moving down their electrochemical gradients established by active ion pumps and exchange mechanisms. Each ion moves primarily through its own ion-specific channel. Different regions in the heart have different AP morphologies. However, two specific regions have quite distinct APs from the rest of the heart: the SA and AV nodes. Unlike the APs shown in Figure 62.2, these areas have APs with much less negative resting potentials and much slower phase-0 upstrokes (Fig. 62.4), often referred to as "slow-response APs." The following discussion explains the detailed electrogenesis of each of these phases and how it can be altered.

RESTING MEMBRANE POTENTIAL

The intracellular potential during electrical quiescence in diastole is −50 to −95 mV, depending on the type of cell (Table 62.2 and Figure 62.4).

Outward potassium current through open, inwardly rectifying K^+ channels (I_{K1}) under normal conditions determines the resting membrane potential in atrial and ventricular myocytes, as well as in the specialized conducting cells of the His-Purkinje system. Slow-response tissues have a less negative resting potential because they have much

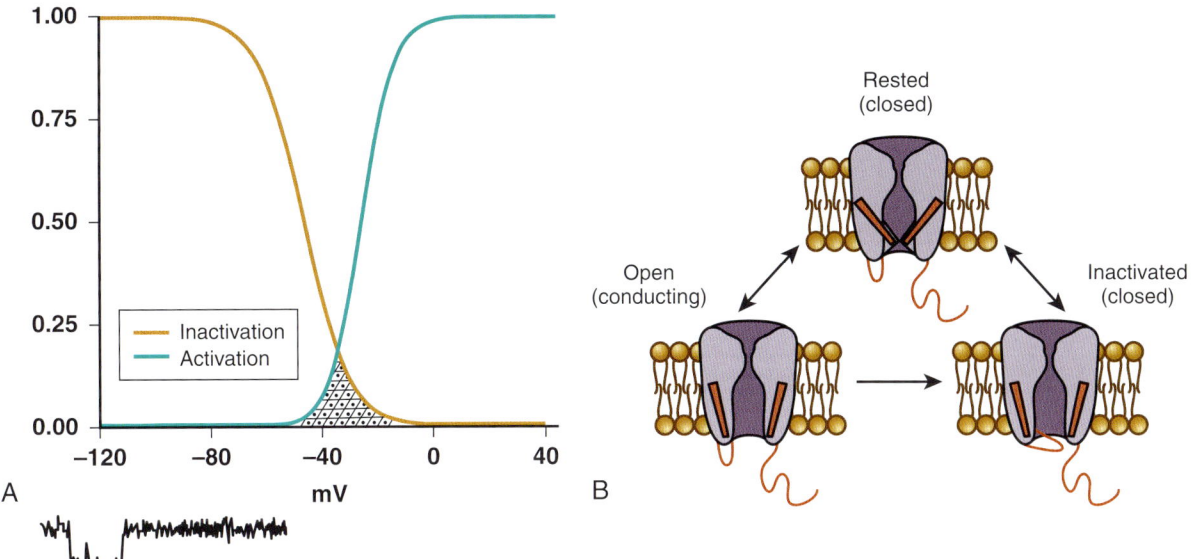

FIGURE 62.3 **A,** Curves that describe the voltage dependence of channel opening or the transition from the rested, closed to the open, conducting state (activation curve, *teal*) and channel availability (inactivation, *gold*). The inactivation or availability curve describes the voltage dependence of the occupancy of the inactivated state, and channels may transition to the inactivated state by way of the open or the rested, closed state. Generally, an inactivated channel must first return to the closed state to be available to open again. The crosshatched area indicates voltages at which there is steady-state opening of the channels because there is finite activation and inactivation is incomplete. In this overlap region, steady-state "window current" flows and can cause excessive action-potential depolarization and/or arrhythmogenic afterdepolarizations. **B,** Principal conformations of voltage-dependent channels. The position of the activation gate changes with the transition from closed to open, and the transition to the inactivated state is determined by the position of the inactivation gate. **C,** Single-channel current recordings showing the opening of sodium (Na) channels in response to a step change in voltage. The *middle tracing* reflects the activity of two channels, each with a single-channel amplitude of 1.4 pA.

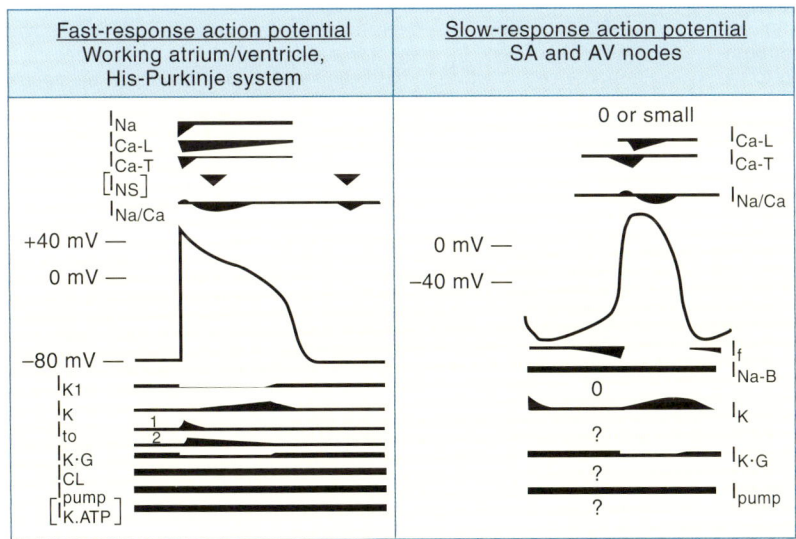

FIGURE 62.4 Currents and channels involved in generating resting membrane and action potentials. The time course of a stylized action potential of atrial and ventricular cells is shown on the **left** and that of sinoatrial (SA) node cells is on the **right**. Above and below are the various channels and pumps that contribute the currents underlying the electrical events. (See Table 62.1 for identification of the symbols and description of the channels or currents.) Where possible, the approximate time courses of the currents associated with the channels or pumps are shown symbolically, without trying to represent their magnitudes relative to each other. I_K incorporates at least two currents, I_{Kr} and I_{Ks}. There appears to be an ultrarapid component as well, designated I_{Kur}. The *heavy bars* for I_{Cl}, I_{pump}, and $I_{K,ATP}$ indicate only the presence of these channels or pump, without implying magnitude of currents, because the magnitude would vary with physiologic and pathophysiologic conditions. The channels identified by *brackets* (I_{NS} and $I_{K,ATP}$) are active only under pathologic conditions. I_{NS} may represent a swelling-activated cation current. For the SA node cells, I_{NS} and I_{K1} are small or absent. Question marks indicate that experimental evidence is not yet available to determine the presence of these channels in SA node cell membranes. Although it is likely that other ionic current mechanisms exist, they are not shown here because their roles in electrogenesis are not sufficiently well defined.

lower I_{K1} channel-density in their membranes than other parts of the heart.

The intracellular ion concentrations that govern the AP are set by a group of ion pumps and exchangers that transport ions more slowly than open ion channels, but are active continuously throughout the cardiac cycle. The most important pump in establishing the transmembrane ionic distribution gradient is the Na-K pump, which pumps Na⁺ out of the cell and simultaneously pumps K⁺ into the cell against their respective chemical gradients, keeping the intracellular K⁺ concentration high and the intracellular Na⁺ concentration low. The Na-K pump is "electrogenic": each cycle of the pump carries 3 Na⁺ ions out for every 2 K⁺ ions pumped in, leaving a net negative intracellular charge. The rate of Na⁺-K⁺ pumping must increase as the heart rate increases to maintain the same ionic gradients, because the cell gains a small amount of Na⁺ and loses a small amount of K⁺ with each depolarization. Rapid cardiac activation makes the resting potential more negative because of the electrogenic properties of the activated Na-K pump. The energy for the Na-K pump is generated by its catalytic activity that breaks high-energy phosphate bonds in adenosine triphosphate (ATP), so it is often called the "Na⁺,K⁺-ATPase." Excess inhibition of Na⁺,K⁺-ATPase function (e.g.,

TABLE 62.2 Properties of Transmembrane Potentials in Heart Cells

PROPERTY	SA NODAL CELL	ATRIAL MYOCYTE	AV NODAL CELL	HIS PURKINJE CELL	VENTRICULAR MYOCYTE
Resting potential (mV)	−50 to −60	−80 to −90	−60 to −70	−90 to −95	−80 to −90
Action Potential Features					
Amplitude (mV)	60–70	110–120	70–80	120	110–120
Overshoot (mV)	0–10	30	5–15	30	30
Duration (msec)	100–300	100–300	100–300	300–500	200–300
V̇max (V/sec)	1–10	100–200	5–15	500–700	100–200
Propagation velocity (m/sec)	<0.05	0.3–0.4	0.1	2–3	0.3–0.4
Fiber diameter (μm)	5–10	10–15	1–10	100	10–15

AV, Atrioventricular; *SA,* sinoatrial; *V̇max,* maximal rise of membrane potential.
Modified from Sperelakis N. Origin of the cardiac resting potential. In: Berne RM et al., eds. *Handbook of Physiology: The Cardiovascular System.* Bethesda, MD: American Physiological Society; 1979:190.

by digitalis glycoside toxicity) can cause substantial cardiac-cell depolarization and seriously impair cardiac electrical function, leading to conduction block and arrhythmias.

The resting potential can be made more negative by interventions that increase the K^+ permeability; for example, both adenosine and acetylcholine (ACh) activate a G-protein coupled K^+ channel ($I_{K,G}$, Table 62.1) and increase resting K^+ conductance. In fast-response tissues, the normal resting K^+ conductance is high and $I_{K,G}$ activation produces small changes in resting potential. However, in SA and AV nodes, with very limited baseline K^+ conductance, $I_{K,G}$ activation substantially increases resting K^+ conductance and can have a major hyperpolarizing effect that slows automaticity and conduction.

PHASE 0: UPSTROKE (RAPID DEPOLARIZATION)

Cardiac activation normally proceeds from the SA node pacemaker and is conducted throughout the heart. Electrical changes in the AP follow a relatively fixed time and voltage relationship that differs according to specific cell types (Fig. 62.5). The AP can also be initiated by an electrical stimulus, as is induced by an artificial pacemaker. Normally, the AP morphology is independent of the size of the depolarizing stimulus, provided that the pulse exceeds a threshold value. Small, subthreshold depolarizing stimuli depolarize the membrane in proportion to the strength of the stimulus, but fail to elicit an AP. When the stimulus is sufficiently intense to depolarize membrane potential to a threshold value in the range of about −70 to −65 mV (for normal fast-response tissues), an "all-or-none" response results.

The upstroke of the cardiac AP in fast-response tissues results from a rapid increase in membrane conductance for Na^+. Rapid depolarization opens Na^+ channels before they have a chance to close via inactivation. When the depolarization is sufficiently rapid, Na^+ channel opening allows Na^+ ions to enter the cell, depolarizing it rapidly and causing more channels to open, producing further depolarization in a self-sustaining process (the "all-or-none" phase 0 depolarization). This process stops when Na^+ channels inactivate to a significant degree (within 1 to 2 msec), allowing the membrane to reach a voltage of about +40 mV, near the Na^+ equilibrium potential (+60 mV).

The rate at which depolarization occurs during phase 0, that is, the maximum rate of change in voltage over time, is indicated by the expression dV/dt_{max} or $\dot{V}max$ (see Table 62.2). $\dot{V}max$ (dV/dt_{max}) is an indicator of the rate and magnitude of phase 0 Na^+ entry into the cell, which is a determinant of tissue conduction velocity (CV). Depolarization must be rapid in order to initiate a fast-response AP. A slow depolarization allows Na^+ channels to inactivate, reducing the maximal conductance they can achieve when activated from that depolarized potential. Thus, clinical processes like hyperkalemia, which slowly depolarize the cell (by reducing the transmembrane K^+ concentration gradient and consequently the K^+ equilibrium potential) result in reduced phase 0 Na^+ current and can produce important conduction slowing.

In cardiac Purkinje fibers, the SA node region, and to a lesser extent, ventricular muscle, different populations of Na^+ channels exist. By far the most common is the tetrodotoxin (TTX)-resistant Nav1.5 isoform (encoded by the *SCN5A* gene). The Nav1.8 TTX-resistant isoform (*SCN10a*) contributes little to peak I_{Na}, but plays an important role in the late Na^+ current (I_{NaL}) that contributes importantly to the prolongation of AP-duration (APD) with cardiac disease or ion-channel mutations. TTX-sensitive Na^+ channels may also participate in I_{NaL}, although the precise contribution remains to be better defined.[2]

Normal fast-response APs have phase 0 dV/dt_{max} values of the order of 200 to 1000 mV/msec. Slow-response APs in the SA and AV nodes have much slower upstrokes (of the order of 4 to 20 mV/msec) because of the slower activation of Ca^{2+} channels compared to Na^+ channels (see Figs. 62.4 and 62.5). The slow phase 0 upstroke is associated with much slower conduction in slow versus fast response tissues. Slow conduction through the AV node is responsible for creating a delay between atrial and ventricular activation, helping to ensure optimal efficiency of the atrial "primer pump" function to optimize ventricular filling just before ventricular contraction. Under certain circumstances, diseased working myocardial cells can have slow-response type cells (see Fig. 62.5F).

The threshold for activation of $I_{Ca,L}$ is about −30 to −40 mV. In fibers of the fast-response type, $I_{Ca,L}$ is normally activated during phase 0 caused by the fast I_{Na}. Current flows through both fast and slow channels during the latter part of the AP upstroke. However, $I_{Ca,L}$ is much smaller than the peak I_{Na} and therefore contributes little to the AP until the fast I_{Na} is inactivated after completion of phase 0. Thus, $I_{Ca,L}$ affects mainly the plateau of APs recorded in atrial and ventricular muscle and His-Purkinje fibers. $I_{Ca,L}$ may play a prominent role in depolarized fast-response cells in which I_{Na} has been inactivated, if conditions are appropriate for slow-channel activation. Although T-type Cav channels have not been directly recorded in human myocardium, the corresponding genes have been cloned from human hearts, and experimental evidence in animals has suggested that these channels might play an important role in determining SA node automaticity and AV nodal conduction.[3]

PHASE 1: EARLY RAPID REPOLARIZATION

Following phase 0, the membrane repolarizes rapidly and transiently to almost 0 mV (early notch), partly because of inactivation of I_{Na} and concomitant activation of several outward currents. The most important of these in the human heart is the 4-aminopyridine–sensitive transient outward K^+ current, commonly termed I_{to} (or I_{to1}), which is activated rapidly by depolarization and then rapidly inactivates. Both the density and the recovery of I_{to} from inactivation exhibit transmural gradients in the left and right ventricular (RV) free wall, with the density decreasing and reactivation becoming progressively prolonged from epicardium to endocardium. Transmural differences in the expression of KChIP2, the auxiliary subunit that forms the I_{to} channel in working atrial and ventricular muscle along with Kv4.3 pore-forming alpha subunits, contributes to the transmural gradient in I_{to} properties and densities.[4] This gradient gives rise to regional differences in AP shape, with increasingly slower phase 1 restitution kinetics and diminution of the notch along the transmural axis. These regional differences create transmural voltage gradients, thereby increasing dispersion of repolarization and allowing for arrhythmogenic transmural current flow, contributing to arrhythmogenesis in Brugada syndrome (see Chapters 63 and 67). Downregulation of I_{to} is at least partially responsible for slowing of phase 1 repolarization in failing human cardiomyocytes.

Studies have demonstrated that these changes in the phase 1 notch of the cardiac AP cause a reduction in the kinetics and peak amplitude of the AP–evoked intracellular Ca^{2+} transient because of failed recruitment and synchronization of SR Ca^{2+} release through $I_{Ca,L}$. Thus, modulation of I_{to} appears to play a physiologic role in controlling cardiac excitation-contraction coupling. It remains to be determined whether transmural differences in phase 1 repolarization translate into similar differences in regional contractility that are important for overall contractile function.

The 4-aminopyridine–resistant, Ca^{2+}-activated chloride current $I_{Cl,Ca}$ (or I_{to2}) might also contribute to outward current during phase 1 repolarization.[1] This current is activated by the AP–evoked intracellular Ca^{2+} transient. Other chloride currents may also play a role in early repolarization, such as the cyclic adenosine monophosphate (cAMP)- or swelling-activated chloride conductances $I_{Cl,cAMP}$ and $I_{Cl,swell}$.

PHASE 2: PLATEAU

During the plateau phase, which may last several hundred milliseconds, membrane conductance of all ions falls to rather low values. Accordingly, smaller changes in current are needed to produce changes in transmembrane potential than near the resting potential. This phenomenon makes the plateau a vulnerable time for the generation of arrhythmogenic afterdepolarizations (see discussion of EADs below). The plateau is maintained by competition between the outward current carried by K+ and the inward current carried by Ca^{2+} moving through $I_{Ca,L}$ and Na+ being exchanged for internal Ca^{2+} by the NCX. After depolarization, I_{K1} conductance falls to low levels during the plateau as a result of inward rectification, despite the large electrochemical driving force on K+ ions.

The plateau is a critical time for Ca^{2+} entry through activated L-type Ca^{2+} channels. The entry of Ca^{2+}, principally during the plateau, triggers a much larger secondary release of Ca^{2+} from SR stores and is an essential component of cardiac excitation-contraction coupling (see Chapter 46).

Several potassium currents are open during the plateau phase, including the rapid (I_{Kr}) and slow (I_{Ks}) components of the delayed rectifier current I_K (see Voltage-Gated K+ Channels). "Delayed rectification" refers to the time-dependent opening of the I_K channel. In addition, I_{Kr} shows a phenomenon called "inward rectification," which involves a decrease in channel opening at more positive potentials. Inward rectification is a prominent feature of the background I_{K1} channel, whose conductance drops dramatically at positive potentials to prevent wasteful excess loss of K+ and allow efficient phase 0 depolarization. I_{Kr} also shows prominent inward rectification, due to extremely rapid inactivation that occurs during depolarization. This fast inactivation mechanism is sensitive to changes in extracellular K+, with the degree of inactivation being accentuated at low extracellular K+ concentrations, explaining how hypokalemia can prolong APD (by decreasing I_{Kr}).

I_{Ks} also contributes to plateau duration. Mutations in the KvLQT1 subunit, which in combination with the I_{Ks} ancillary (beta) subunit (KCNE1, encoding a protein also called minK) carries I_{Ks}, are associated with abnormally prolonged ventricular repolarization (long-QT syndrome [LQTS] type 1; see Chapters 63 and 67). Although I_{Ks} activates slowly compared to the APD, it is only slowly inactivated. Therefore, increases in heart rate cause I_{Ks} activation to accumulate, contributing to APD abbreviation at higher heart rates.

In conditions of reduced intracellular ATP concentration (e.g., hypoxia, acute ischemia), K+ efflux through activated I_{KATP} channels reduces APD and increases K+ concentration in the extracellular space, which in turn decreases the K driving force, I_{K1} amplitude, and cell resting potential. Other ionic mechanisms that control plateau duration include $I_{Ca,L}$ inactivation and steady-state (window-current) components of both I_{Na} and $I_{Ca,L}$.

PHASE 3: FINAL RAPID REPOLARIZATION

Repolarization of the terminal portion of the AP proceeds rapidly largely because of changes in two currents: time-dependent inactivation of $I_{Ca,L}$, with a decrease in the inward movement of positive charges, and activation of repolarizing K+ currents, particularly I_{Kr} and I_{Ks}, which increase the movement of positive charges out of the cell. As the cell repolarizes, the transmembrane potential moves to voltages at which the inward rectification of I_{K1} is removed, so I_{K1} contributes substantially to the terminal part of phase 4. A small-conductance Ca^{2+}-activated K+ current, I_{KCa}, expressed in human atrial myocytes, may also contribute to phase 3 repolarization.[5]

Loss-of-function mutations in the human ether-a-go-go–related or hERG gene (KCNH2), which encodes the pore-forming (α) subunit of I_{Kr}, delay phase 3 repolarization and predispose to the development arrhythmias associated with LQTS. A wide range of non-cardiac drugs, such as erythromycin, many antipsychotics, antimalarial/antiinflammatory drugs like hydroxychloroquine, and antifungal drugs such as ketoconazole, inhibit I_{Kr} and can cause acquired forms of LQTS (see Chapters 63 and 67). A decrease in I_{K1} function, as occurs in heart failure or mutations in the associated KCNJ2 gene, prolong APD and reduce resting membrane potential.

PHASE 4: DIASTOLIC DEPOLARIZATION

Normally, the membrane potential of atrial and ventricular muscle cells remains steady throughout diastole. In specialized conducting cells of the His-Purkinje system and in the SA and AV nodes, the resting membrane potential does not remain constant in diastole but gradually depolarizes (see Figs. 62.4 and 62.5). The property possessed by spontaneously automatic cells is called spontaneous phase 4 diastolic depolarization. When spontaneous phase 4 depolarization reaches a

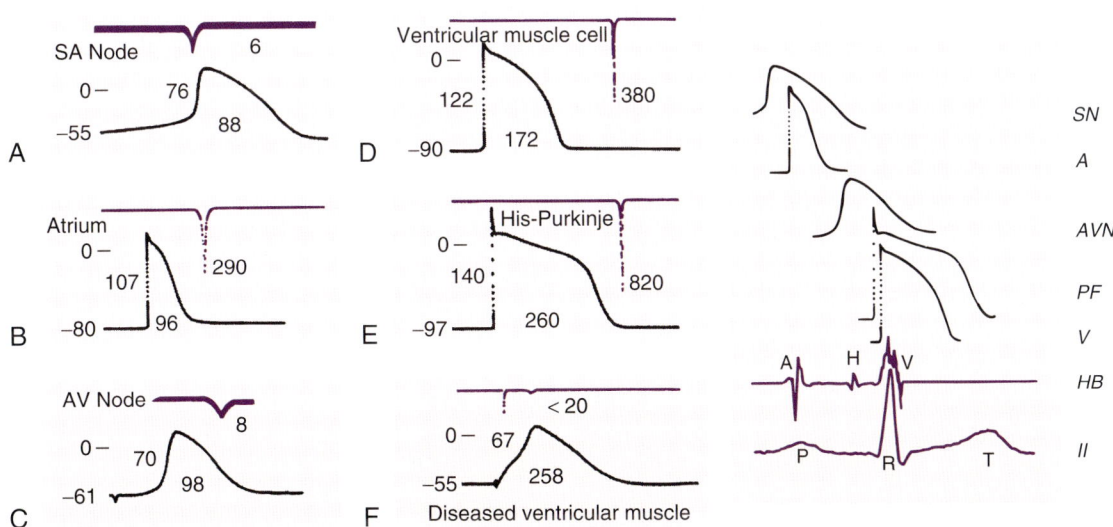

FIGURE 62.5 Action potentials recorded from different tissues in the heart **(left)** remounted along with a His bundle recording and scalar electrocardiogram from a patient **(right)** to illustrate the timing during a single cardiac cycle. **A** to **F**, Top tracing is dV/dt of phase 0, and the second tracing is the action potential. For each panel, the numbers (from left to right) indicate maximum diastolic potential (mV), action potential amplitude (mV), action potential duration at 90% of repolarization (milliseconds), and rate of depolarization of phase 0 (V/sec). Zero potential is indicated by the *short horizontal line* next to the zero on the upper left of each action potential. **A**, Rabbit sinoatrial node. **B**, Canine atrial muscle. **C**, Rabbit AV node. **D**, Canine ventricular muscle. **E**, Canine Purkinje fiber. **F**, Diseased human ventricle. Note that the action potentials recorded in **A**, **C**, and **F** have reduced resting membrane potentials and amplitudes relative to the other action potentials. In the right panel, *A*, Atrial muscle potential; *AVN*, atrioventricular nodal potential; *HB*, His bundle recording; *II*, lead II; *PF*, Purkinje fiber potential; *SN*, sinus nodal potential; *V*, ventricular muscle potential. Horizontal calibration on the left: 50 milliseconds for **A** and **C**, 100 milliseconds for **B**, **D**, **E**, and **F**; 200 milliseconds on the right. Vertical calibration on the left: 50 mV; horizontal calibration on the right: 200 milliseconds. (Modified from Gilmour RF Jr, Zipes DP. Basic electrophysiology of the slow inward current. In: Antman E, Stone PH, eds. *Calcium blocking agents in the treatment of cardiovascular disorders.* Mount Kisco, NY: Futura; 1983:1–37.)

voltage at which a sufficient number of phase 0 inward current channels (Na+ channels in His-Purkinje system, Ca2+ channels in SA and AV nodes) open, spontaneous cell-firing occurs. The voltage at which an AP is generated is called the "threshold potential." The time from the maximum (most negative) diastolic potential (MDP) at the end of phase 3 to the arrival at threshold potential determines the "intrinsic" spontaneous cycle length of the tissue. The intrinsic rate of SA node automaticity normally exceeds the intrinsic rate of other potentially automatic pacemaker sites; thus the SA mode maintains dominance of the cardiac rhythm. The SA node is heavily innervated by the parasympathetic and sympathetic nervous systems. Parasympathetic activation slows SA node automaticity and sympathetic activation accelerates it. This dual control allows for very fine regulation of SA node rate in relation to the body's needs, with heart rate being the most important single determinant of cardiac output (see Fig. 62.1). Enhanced or abnormal automaticity at other sites (as well as other arrhythmia mechanisms, see below) can cause them to discharge at rates faster than the SA node and usurp control of cardiac rhythm for one or many cycles (see Chapter 65). The intrinsic pacemaking ability of other tissues produces important "escape" rhythms should the sinus node fail or should conduction between the atria and ventricles be blocked because of disease in the AV node or specialized His-Purkinje ventricular conducting system.

Normal Automaticity

Two models of contributors to SA node pacemaking have been proposed.[3] In the "membrane clock" model, HCN channels (see Cardiac Pacemaker Channels and Table 62.1) are activated by repolarization from the plateau to normal diastolic membrane potentials. HCN channels carry a current called I_f ("funny current"), often called the "pacemaker current," with the unusual feature of time-dependent activation at negative potentials (unlike all other voltage-dependent cardiac channels). During the diastolic interval between consecutive APs, the probability of HCN channels being open increases. Open HCN channels conduct both Na+ and K+, but at these negative membrane potentials at which the driving force for Na+ is high and for K+ is low, Na+ entry predominates. The inward Na+ current through HCN channels depolarizes pacemaker cells to threshold, repetitively triggering APs to generate a periodically firing pacemaker.[1,3]

In the "Ca2+ clock" model, periodic increases in [Ca2+]i serve as an internal generator of rhythmic signals that are transformed into changes in membrane voltage via modulation of calcium-sensitive ion channels and transporters in the cell membrane. This concept is illustrated in Figure 62.6, in which simultaneous [Ca2+]i and voltage measurements in isolated SA node myocytes are used as an example. Local submembrane increases in [Ca2+]i (denoted by the white arrows in Fig. 62.6B) occurring during the latter part of the spontaneous diastolic depolarization (transmembrane APs are shown in blue) precede the rapid upstroke of the AP. SR Ca2+-release activates the Na+/Ca2+ exchange inward (i.e., depolarizing) current (I_{NCX}), which then results in membrane depolarization, which activates membrane L-type Ca2+ channels to initiate the AP phase-0 upstroke. Thus, the NCX plays an essential role in converting the driver intracellular Ca2+ signals into membrane (i.e., voltage) signals. Once an AP has been initiated, two highly interacting, concurrent series of events proceed (Fig. 62.6C). In a surface membrane delimited series of events, depolarization-induced activation of I_K leads to membrane repolarization, which is followed by slow diastolic depolarization via a number of inward currents, particularly I_f and I_{CaT} (see Table 62.1). In a second, parallel cycle of events, AP-induced SR Ca2+ release is followed by Ca2+ reuptake into the SR, giving rise to spontaneous Ca2+-release and subsequent inward I_{NCX}.

In reality, the calcium and membrane clock systems function together, to ensure that the important SA node pacemaking function is protected by system redundancy, somewhat like dual computers producing a fail-safe system controlling key aircraft guidance functions.

The rate of SA node discharge is regulated by autonomic and other influences. Alterations in the slope of diastolic depolarization, MDP, or threshold potential can alter the discharge rate. For example, if the slope of diastolic depolarization steepens, the discharge rate increases (e.g., Fig. 62.6A, dashed line). The molecular mechanisms that mediate acceleration of the SA node discharge rate in response to adrenergic stimulation are complex. Adrenergic stimulation increases inward HCN current, mainly by virtue of cyclic AMP shifting the HCN channel activation curve to more depolarized

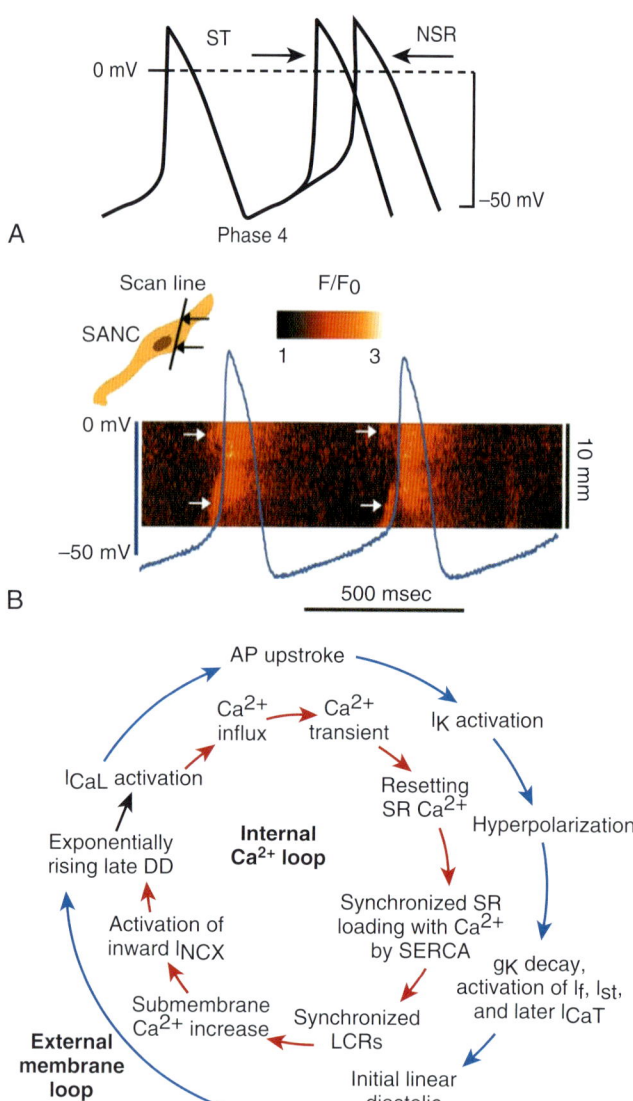

FIGURE 62.6 A, Sympathetic stimulation of heart rate in the sinoatrial node (SAN). Simulated SAN action potentials during baseline (NSR) and sympathetic stimulation (ST [sinus tachycardia]). Sympathetic stimulation increases the rate of diastolic depolarization (not shown) and shifts the maximum diastolic potential to a less negative value, thereby accelerating action potential firing. **B and C,** Spontaneous sarcoplasmic reticulum (SR) Ca2+-release events trigger membrane excitation in SAN myocytes. **B,** Confocal line scan images of Ca2+ signals measured in spontaneously beating rabbit sinoatrial node cells (SANC) with simultaneous recording (blue lines) of transmembrane action potentials; the orientation of the scan line is shown in the inset. Arrows in the confocal image show the local Ca2+ release in the submembrane space during late diastolic depolarization that precedes the rapid upstroke of the action potential. **C,** Model of sinoatrial node cell pacemaking, as suggested by Maltsev and coworkers. I_{NCX}, Na+/Ca2+ exchange current; DD, diastolic depolarization; LCR, local Ca2+ release; SERCA, sarcoendoplasmic reticulum Ca2+-ATPase. (B and C from Maltsev VA, Vinogradovad TM, Lakatta EG. The emergence of a general theory of the initiation and strength of the heartbeat. J Pharmacol Sci. 2006;100:338.)

potentials.[1] In addition, cAMP-activation of protein kinase A (PKA) increases phosphorylation of key Ca2+-handling proteins like the cardiac ryanodine-receptor (RyR2), phospholamban (see Chapter 46), SERCA, and voltage-gated Ca2+ channels. Phosphorylation of these proteins increases the rate of spontaneous SR Ca2+ release and SR Ca2+ uptake via synergistic activation of these proteins. ACh shifts the MDP to more negative values, moving it further away from threshold and slowing the spontaneous firing rate.

PASSIVE MEMBRANE ELECTRICAL PROPERTIES

In addition to the active electrical properties that govern APs, cardiac electrical function is also determined by passive electrical properties. When a cell membrane depolarizes, the Na+ that rushes in changes the

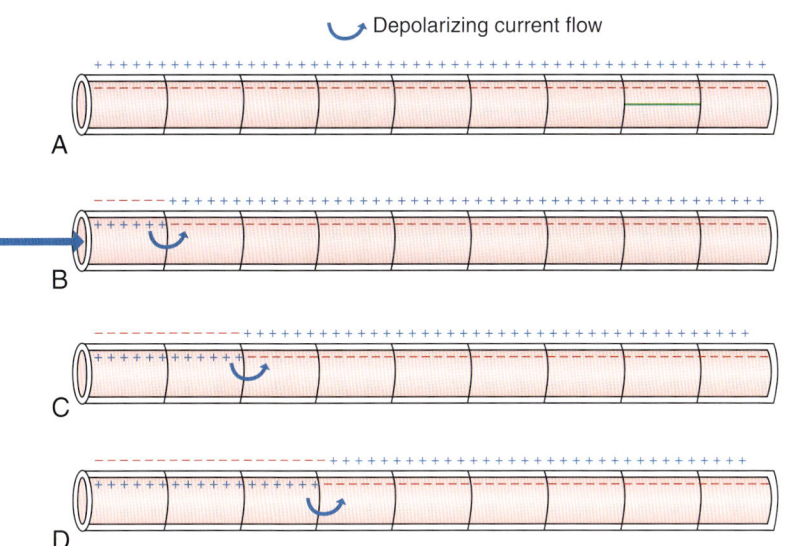

FIGURE 62.7 Schematic of an electrical impulse traversing a cardiac fiber bundle. The bundle is comprised of electrically coupled cardiomyocytes simulating a continuous cable. **A**, A resting bundle, with a negative *(inside)* transmembrane potential. **B**, Activation of the bundle from the left; the first cardiomyocyte in the bundle is depolarized, initiating an action potential and cell-to-cell current flow *(curved arrow)* and causing progressive depolarization of cells in the fiber (**C** and **D**).

local transmembrane potential quite strongly. Figure 62.7 illustrates how an electrical impulse travels along a cardiac fiber bundle composed of multiple cardiac cells (cardiomyocytes). Cardiomyocytes are electrically coupled to each other by low-resistance "gap junctions" (see below), making a bundle of cardiac fibers behave like a continuous cable. Panel A represents the resting bundle, with cardiomyocytes having a transmembrane potential of −80 mV due to more negative charges on the internal side of the membrane. Panel B illustrates what happens when an impulse arrives from an activated cell to the left, depolarizing the first cardiomyocyte in the bundle. The cell membrane, depolarized to threshold, undergoes phase 0 and changes rapidly from being relatively negative internally (−80 mV transmembrane potential) to becoming positive (+40 mV). A flow of electrical current (by definition, movement of positive ions) ensues as illustrated by the curved arrow in B, depolarizes adjacent membrane to threshold and causes cellular activation, as shown in C. The impulse then spreads further as shown in D, and eventually makes its way to the end of the bundle. One major determinant of impulse spread is how fast depolarizing current flow spreads from the activated region to the region that is not yet activated. When a depolarizing current is passed across an electrical resistor (like the lipid cell membrane), the voltage change produced depends on the resistance (by virtue of Ohm's law, E = IR, where E = voltage change, I = current, R = resistance). Thus, membrane resistance is an important factor governing conduction speed in the heart. The resting fast-response cardiac cell membrane has a relatively low resistance because of the high K^+ conductance through I_{K1}; rapid conduction therefore requires a very large current flow (ensured by large phase 0 Na^+ current). Slow-channel tissue has a much higher resistance because of lack of I_{K1}, allowing the relatively small I_{CaL} to produce conduction, albeit much more slowly than in fast-response tissue. Membrane resistance is a very important "passive" membrane property, as opposed to active membrane functions mediated by ion channels.

Molecular Structure of Key Cardiac Ion Channels and Transporters

The changes in membrane permeability that mediate the phases of the cardiac AP are largely produced by the time- and voltage-dependent function of cardiac ion channels, the building blocks of biologic electricity in the heart, brain, skeletal muscle, and other excitable tissues. Specialized transmembrane glycoproteins form ion channels: ion-selective pores in cell membranes that open and close *(gating)* in response to an appropriate biologic signal. The ion channels most centrally involved in controlling cardiac AP gate in response to changes in transmembrane voltage ("voltage-gated channels"). Other physiologically important channels respond to chemical ligands such as ACh, ATP, and Ca^{2+}. Electrophysiologic studies have detailed the functional properties of Na^+, Ca^{2+}, and K^+ currents in cardiomyocytes, and molecular cloning has revealed a large number of pore-forming (α) and auxiliary (β, γ, and δ) subunits that form ion channels. Mutations in the genes encoding cardiac ion channel subunits are responsible for many forms of inherited cardiac arrhythmias (see Chapter 63). The expression and functional properties of myocardial ion channels also change in a number of acquired disease states, and these alterations can predispose to cardiac arrhythmias.[6]

VOLTAGE-GATED NA+ CHANNELS

Voltage-gated Na^+ (Nav) channel pore-forming (α) subunits have four homologous domains (I to IV), each of which contains six-transmembrane–spanning regions (designated S1 to S6), and these four domains come together to form the Na^+-permeable pore (Fig. 62.8A).[7] Among the multiple Nav α subunits, Nav1.5 (which is encoded by the *SCN5A* gene) is the most strongly expressed in mammalian myocardium. The name of the voltage-gated sodium channel protein consists of the chemical symbol of the principal permeating ion (Na^+) and v, which indicates its principal physiologic regulator (voltage). The number following v indicates the gene subfamily (Nav1), and the number following the decimal point identifies the specific channel isoform (e.g., Nav1.1). An identical nomenclature applies to voltage-gated calcium and potassium channels. Mutations in *SCN5A*, which are associated with LQT3 syndrome, disrupt Nav channel inactivation and thereby give rise to a sustained inward Na^+ current during the plateau phase of the AP and to APD prolongation. Mutations in *SCN5A* are also linked to Brugada syndrome. Brugada syndrome mutations result in reduced I_{Na} amplitude, which leads to slowing of the phase 0 AP upstroke, reduced AP amplitude, and altered phase 1 early repolarization.

Nav1.5 pore-forming α subunits coassemble with one to two auxiliary Nav β subunits to form functional cell-surface Na^+ channels in cardiomyocytes.[8] Nav β subunits appear to play an important role in anchoring ion channel proteins to the cell membrane. Subpopulations of Nav1.5 channels are present in different subcellular regions, such as the intercalated disc and T-tubular membranes. As with many other ion channels, Nav1.5 channels are part of macromolecular complexes including both channel and regulatory proteins.[8,9]

VOLTAGE-GATED Ca²⁺ CHANNELS

As with Nav channels, cardiac voltage-gated Ca^{2+} (Cav) channels are assemblies of a pore-forming $α_1$ subunits and auxiliary Cav β or Cav $α_2$–δ subunits (see Fig. 62.8C). Among the various α subunits, Cav1.2, also known as $α_{1C}$ encoded by the *CACNA1C* gene, is the prominent Cav $α_1$ subunit expressed in mammalian myocardium. Cav1.2 channels exhibit many of the time- and voltage-dependent properties and pharmacologic sensitivities of cardiac L-type Ca^{2+} currents (see Table 62.1). Cav1.3 channel subunits may also form L-type Ca^{2+} channels, particularly in the SA node and atria. Accessory subunits modulate the functional properties of Cav channels.[10]

Cav3.1/$α_1$ G alpha subunits form a Ca^{2+}-selective channel with time- and voltage-dependent characteristics and pharmacologic sensitivities that resemble those of the low-voltage activated T-type Ca^{2+} channel. Disruption of the gene encoding Cav3.1 subunits *(CACNA1G)* in mice slows the sinus node rate and AV conduction, and reduces the heart-rate response to adrenergic stimulation, consistent with a role in SA and AV node function.[11]

VOLTAGE-GATED K+ CHANNELS

Voltage-gated K^+ channels (Kv) are the most diverse family of voltage-dependent channels in the heart. Kv channels are composed of four separate pore-forming (α) subunits, each containing six-membrane–spanning domains (S_1 through S_6)[12] (see Fig. 62.8B). Kvα subunits expressed in the human heart include members of the Kv1, Kv4, hERG

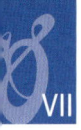

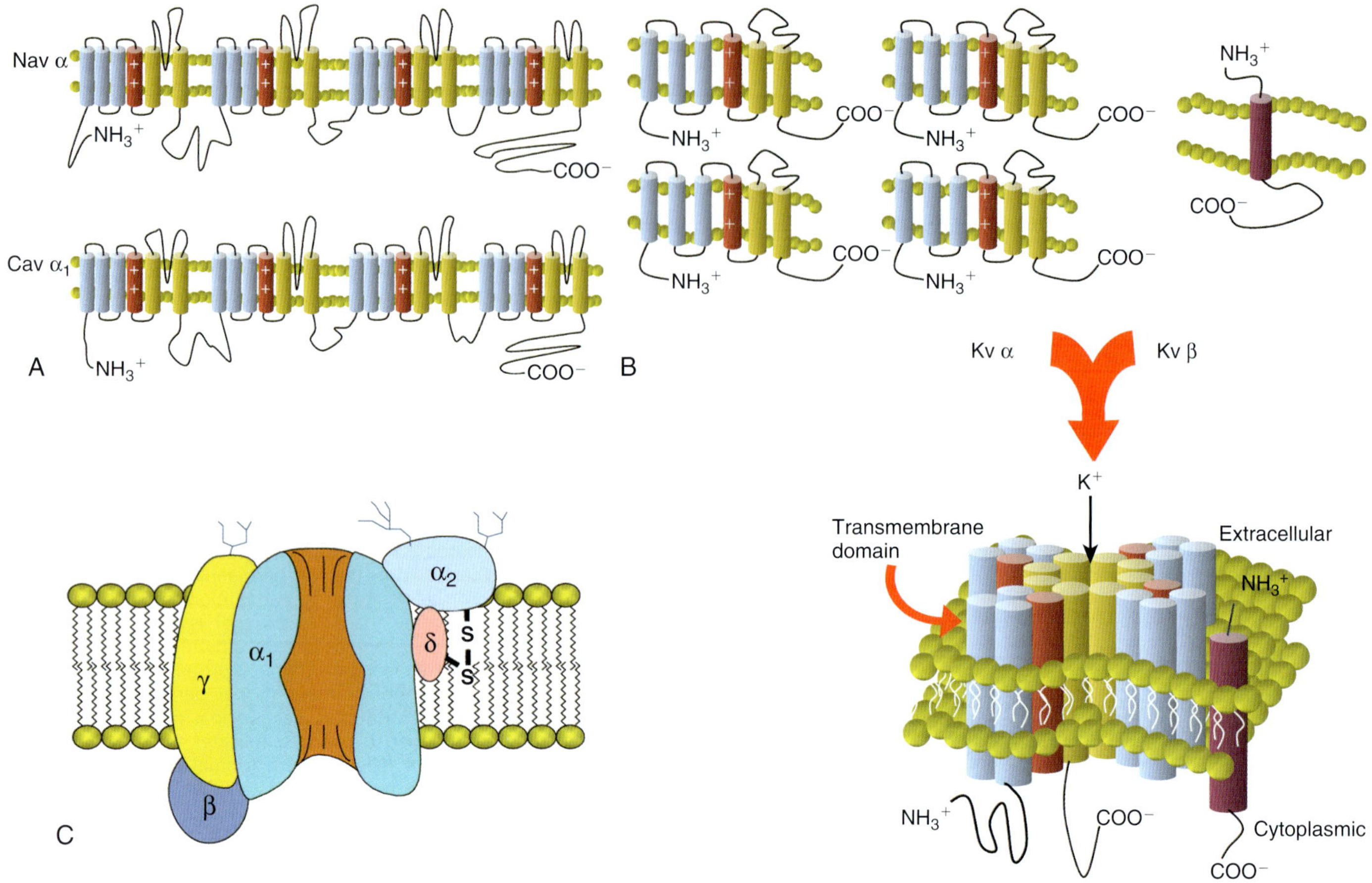

FIGURE 62.8 Transmembrane topology and schematic of the structure of ion channels. **A,** Voltage-gated Na$^+$ and Ca^{2+} channels are composed of a single tetramer consisting of four covalently linked repeats of the six-transmembrane–spanning motifs. **B,** Voltage-gated K$^+$ channels are composed of four separate subunits, each containing a single six-transmembrane–spanning motif. Inwardly rectifying K$^+$ channels are formed by inward rectifier K$^+$ channel pore-forming (alpha) subunits (Kir). In contrast to voltage-gated K$^+$ channel alpha subunits, the Kir alpha subunits have only two (not six) transmembrane domains. **C,** All ion channels are multisubunit proteins, as exemplified by the schematic subunit structure of L-type Ca channels.

(Kv7), and KvLQT (Kv11) subfamilies. In addition, Kv channel α subunit proteins interact with Kv channel accessory subunits, including minK, KChIP2, and MiRP1 (see Table 62.1), to form functional cell surface channels with distinct time- and voltage-dependent properties. Co-assembly of the Kv4.3 α subunits and the accessory subunit KChIP2 gives rise to the cardiac transient outward Kv channel I_{to} (see Phase 1: Early Rapid Repolarization). hERG α subunits, possibly together with MiRP1 accessory subunits, form functional cardiac I_{Kr} channels. Mutations in the gene encoding hERG *(KCNH2)* have been shown to underlie congenital LQT2 syndrome. These LQT2 mutations are loss-of-function mutations that lead to reduced functional I_{Kr} channel expression or to alterations in channel processing or trafficking (see Chapter 63).

KvLQT1 α subunits associate with minK (encoded by *KCNE1*) accessory subunits to form channels that carry slowly activating, noninactivating K$^+$ currents, identified with I_{Ks} in human myocardium. Mutations in the gene encoding KvLQT1 α subunits, *KCNQ1*, are linked to LQT1 syndrome. Mutations in the minK-encoding gene *KCNE1* are associated with LQT5 syndrome. These mutations are all loss-of-function mutations that reduce expression of functional I_{Ks} channels in the cell membrane.

Kv1.5 α subunits contribute to K$^+$-selective channels with time- and voltage-dependent characteristics that underlie the rapidly activating and slowly inactivating I_{Kur} in human atrial myocytes.[13] I_{Kur} is downregulated in the atria of patients with chronic AF.

Small-conductance, Ca^{2+}-sensitive K$^+$ channels are tetrameric assemblies of SK α subunits (encoded by *KCNN1-3*) and underlie a Ca^{2+}-activated K$^+$ current, I_{KCa}, in human cardiomyocytes.[5] Common variants in *KCNN3* discovered in genome-wide analyses have been associated with AF.[14]

INWARDLY RECTIFYING CARDIAC K$^+$ CHANNELS

Kir channels in cardiac myocytes, as in other cells, conduct inward current at membrane potentials negative to E_K (see earlier, Physiology of Ion Channels) and smaller outward currents (due to inward rectification) at membrane potentials positive to E_K. The current through Kir channels is a function of both the membrane potential and the extracellular K$^+$ concentration ($[K^+]_o$) and is the major determinant of the resting membrane potential in working myocardium and the specialized ventricular conducting system. When $[K^+]_o$ increases, the E_K moves to more positive values and the cell depolarizes.

Inward rectification reduces the permeability of K$^+$ channels at depolarized voltages to prevent too much K$^+$ leaving the cell. Mechanisms include channel block by binding of magnesium and positively charged organic ions to the channel (for I_{K1}) and extremely rapid inactivation (for I_{Kr}).[15] In contrast to Kv α subunits, Kir α subunits have only two (not six) transmembrane domains. The α subunits Kir2.1 and Kir2.2 encoded by *KCNJ2* and *KCNJ3*, respectively, are the main subunits underlying the I_{K1} inwardly rectifying current in cardiomyocytes.

The K$^+$-selective sarcolemmal $I_{K,ATP}$ channel is formed by the association of pore-forming Kir6 α subunits and sulfonylurea receptor (SUR) subunits. In cardiomyocytes, Kir6.2 α subunits (encoded by *KCNJ11*) assemble with SUR1 and SUR2 subunits encoded by *ABCC8* and *ABCC9*, respectively, to carry $I_{K,ATP}$. Different anatomic regions of the heart may express $I_{K,ATP}$ comprised of differing channel and SUR subunits. $I_{K,ATP}$ channels play a pivotal role in myocardial ischemia and preconditioning, by reducing APD and myocardial metabolic demands when cellular ATP content goes down. Opening of cardiac sarcolemmal $I_{K,ATP}$ channels underlies ST-segment elevation during acute myocardial ischemia. $I_{K,ATP}$ is an important regulator of the function of multiple tissues. For example, in blood vessels, $I_{K.ATP}$ leads to vasodilation and in the pancreas, $I_{K.ATP}$ inhibits insulin secretion. Drugs like nicorandil and diazoxide open ATP-sensitive K+ channels, whereas sulfonylurea compounds (e.g., glibenclamide) inhibit $I_{K.ATP}$. In addition to the sarcolemmal $I_{K.ATP}$ channel an ATP-sensitive potassium conductance in mitochondria (mitoK[ATP]) is involved in cardioprotection and arrhythmias. The molecular composition of this channel is uncertain but likely involves another type of inwardly rectifying K+ channel.[16]

The ACh-activated K+ channel $I_{K.ACh}$ is a heteromultimer of two inwardly rectifying potassium channel subunits, Kir3.1 and Kir3.4.[12,15] Stimulation of $I_{K.ACh}$ by vagally secreted ACh hyperpolarizes SA and AV node cells, decreases the slope of spontaneous depolarization in the SA node, slowing heart rate, and slows conduction in the AV node. Adenosine, through type 1 purinergic receptor–mediated G-protein activation, opens the $I_{K.ACh}$ channel (in this context carrying a current referred to as $I_{K.Ado}$) in atrial, SA node, and AV node cells. Adenosine and vagal-enhancement maneuvers are useful for the acute termination of arrhythmias involving the AV node as part of the reentry circuit, such as atrioventricular reentrant (AVRT) and atrioventricular nodal reentrant tachycardias (AVNRT) (see later, Mechanisms of Arrhythmogenesis).

CARDIAC PACEMAKER CHANNELS

The I_f pacemaker current prominently contributes to diastolic depolarization in all tissues with spontaneous automaticity. I_f activates slowly at negative potentials and deactivates rapidly with depolarization, carrying a mixed monovalent cation (Na+ and K+) current. I_f is highly regulated; beta-adrenergic stimulation increases the probability of channel opening by shifting the channel's activation curve to more positive potentials, accelerating diastolic depolarization. The HCN channels underlying I_f are topologically similar to voltage-dependent K+ channels and related to cyclic nucleotide–gated channels in photoreceptors in the retina. Of the four known HCN pore-forming α subunits, HCN4 is the most highly expressed in the mammalian myocardium. Mutations in the human HCN4 gene have been linked to familial sinus bradycardia and inappropriate sinus tachycardia.[17] I_f-blocking drugs have been approved for the treatment of angina and are under investigation for the treatment of various forms of heart failure and arrhythmias.[18]

ELECTROGENIC TRANSPORTERS
Na+/Ca2+ Exchanger

The NCX is an ion transporter that exchanges three Na+ ions for one Ca2+ and is very strongly expressed in the mammalian heart. With each cycle, NCX exchanges three positive charges (Na+ ions) for every Ca2+ ion (two positive charges) that it handles, producing a net current in the direction of Na+ movement (its function is therefore "electrogenic"). NCX almost always functions to extrude Ca2+, resulting in a net inward current. The cardiac NCX is a transmembrane glycoprotein proposed to have nine-transmembrane repeats based on hydropathy analysis (Fig. 62.9A,B). The intracellular loop contains domains that bind Ca2+ (CBD 1 and 2) and the endogenous NCX inhibitory domain, XIP.

Ion exchange through NCX can occur in either direction. With each heartbeat, the phase-2 entry of Ca2+ triggers a large cytosolic Ca2+ release from SR stores through the release-channel RyR2. Intracellular [Ca2+] then increases from the resting level of less than 100 nM to approximately 1 μM. Outward Ca2+ flux through the NCX (in exchange for Na+, generating an inward current) along with Ca2+ reuptake into the SR by the SR Ca2+-ATPase (SERCA) remove cytosolic Ca2+ during diastole, restoring diastolic [Ca2+] to its resting level. NCX current is time-independent and largely reflects changes in intracellular [Ca2+] during the AP. Thus, NCX can contribute to determining the transmembrane voltage. At depolarized potentials, reverse-mode Na+/Ca2+ exchange (Ca2+ influx, net outward current) can occur; however, the role of reverse-mode exchange in initiating SR Ca2+ release and contraction is uncertain.

NCX current is an important component of the inward current that underlies delayed afterdepolarizations (DADs). DADs are spontaneous membrane depolarizations after complete repolarization of the AP. They generally result from spontaneous diastolic SR Ca2+ release events under pathologic conditions. The cytosolic Ca2+ transient resulting from Ca2+ release causes Ca2+ to be extruded via NCX in exchange for extracellular Na+ release, producing a depolarizing inward current. When the resulting membrane depolarization reaches threshold it initiates an ectopic AP; repeated DADs can cause or trigger tachyarrhythmias.[19]

Na+,K+-ATPase

Also called the Na+ pump, Na+,K+-ATPase maintains the high intracellular K+ and low intracellular Na+ concentration of cardiomyocytes. The Na+ pump belongs to the widely distributed class of P-type ATPases cation transporters. The P-type designation refers to the formation of a phosphorylated aspartyl intermediate during the catalytic cycle. The Na+,K+-ATPase hydrolyzes a molecule of ATP to transport two K+ into the cell and three Na+ out and thus is electrogenic, generating a time-independent hyperpolarizing outward current. The Na+,K+-ATPase is oligomeric, consisting of α and β subunits and a tissue-specific regulator protein called phospholemman (PLM). PLM belongs to a family of single-membrane–spanning proteins called FXYD proteins, which share a characteristic 35-amino acid sequence including a PFXYD (proline-phenylalanine-X-tyrosine-aspartic acid) sequence in their extracellular domain. PLM (FXYD1) is expressed in heart and skeletal muscle, which binds to and inhibits Na+,K+-ATPase, acting as an important endogenous regulator.[20]

Na+,K+-ATPase isoforms are diverse and exhibit tissue-specific distributions. The structural diversity of the Na+,K+-ATPase comes from variations in α and β genes, splice variants of the α subunits and promiscuity of subunit associations. The α subunit is catalytic and binds digitalis glycosides in the extracellular linker between the first and second membrane-spanning region (Fig. 62.9C and D).

Gap Junction Channels and Intercalated Discs

Another family of ion channel proteins critical to cardiac electrophysiology forms gap junctional channels. These dodecameric channels are found in the intercalated discs between adjacent cells (Fig. 62.10A,B). Three types of specialized junctions make up each intercalated disc. The macula adherens (or "desmosome") and the fascia adherens form areas of strong adhesion between cells that provide linkage for the transfer of mechanical energy from one cell to the next. The *nexus*, also called the tight or gap junction (Fig. 62.10C–E), is a region of functional intercellular contact in the intercalated disc. Membranes at these junctions are separated by only about 10 to 20 Å and are connected by hexagonally packed subunit bridges (or "gap junction channels"). These specialized channels provide biochemical and low-resistance electrical coupling between adjacent cells, by establishing aqueous pores that directly link their cytoplasm. Gap junctions allow the movement of ions (e.g., Na+, Cl−, K+, Ca2+) and small molecules (e.g., cAMP, cGMP, inositol 1,4,5-triphosphate [IP_3]) between adjacent cells, thereby linking their interiors.

Gap junctions permit a multicellular structure such as the heart to function electrically as an orderly, synchronized, interconnected unit. Gap junctions are mostly located at cell ends. Thus, the anatomic and biophysical properties of cardiac muscle bundles vary according to the direction in which they are measured, a property called "anisotropy." CV is generally two to three times faster longitudinally, in the direction of the long axis of the fiber, than it is transversely, perpendicular to this long axis. Resistivity (the inverse of permeability) is lower longitudinally than transversely. Cardiac conduction is discontinuous because of resistive discontinuities created by the gap junctions. The *safety factor for conduction*, the energy for normal conduction relative to the minimum energy that propagates, determines the success of AP propagation. Interestingly, the *safety factor for propagation* is greater transversely than horizontally. Conduction delay or block thus occurs more easily in the longitudinal direction than it does transversely.

Gap junctions also provide "biochemical coupling," which permits cell-to-cell movement of ATP (or other high-energy phosphates), cyclic nucleotides, and IP_3, the activator of the IP_3-sensitive SR Ca2+-release channel. Diffusion of second-messenger substances through gap junctional channels enables coordinated responses of the myocardial syncytium to physiologic stimuli.[21]

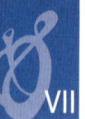

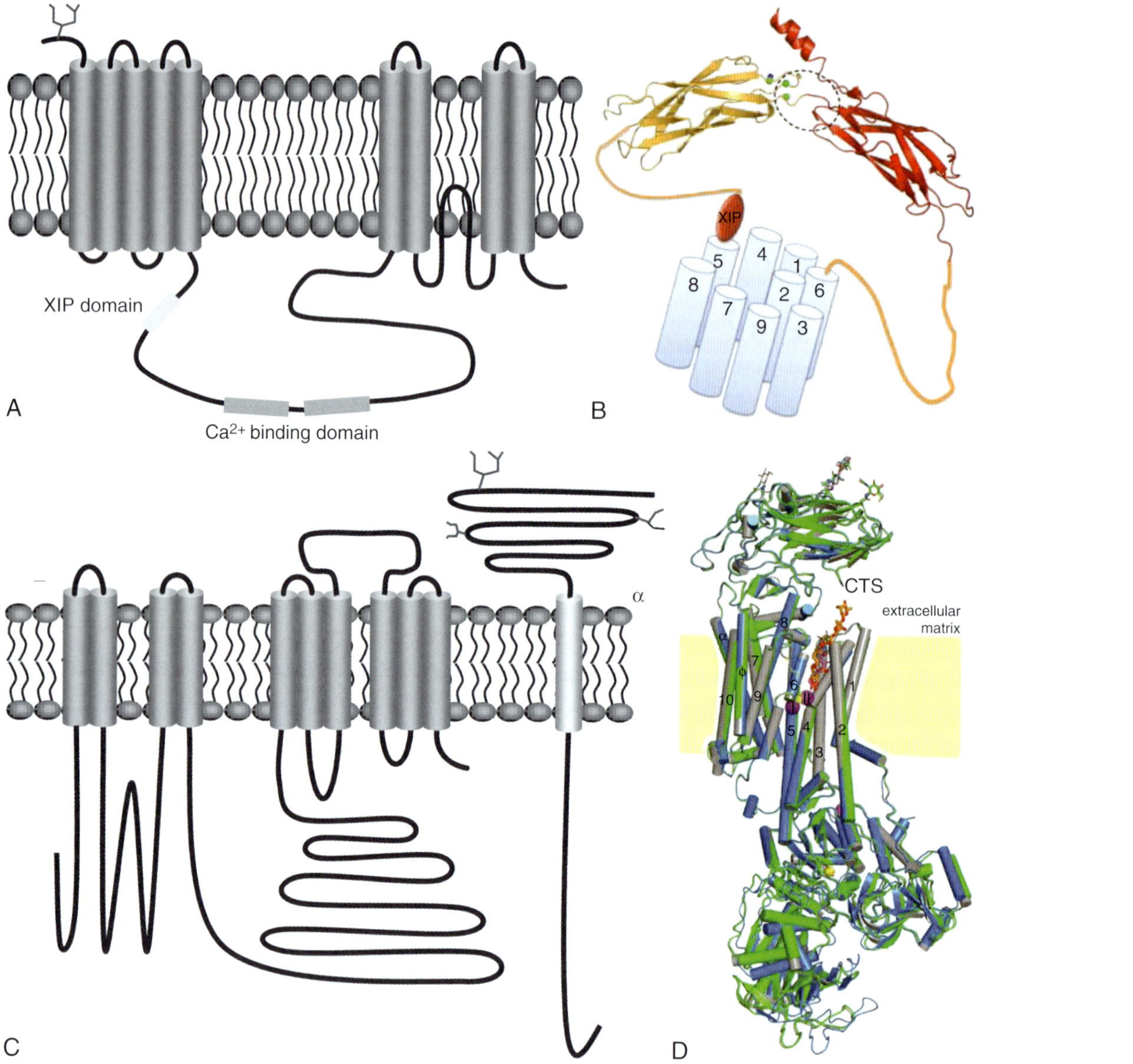

FIGURE 62.9 Transmembrane topology and predicted structures of Na+/Ca2+ exchanger (NCX) and the Na+,K+-ATPase (Na pump). **A,** Predicted topology of NCX, the cytoplasmic segment includes an autoinhibitory domain (XIP) and two Ca2+-binding domains. **B,** Predicted structure; the cytoplasmic surface is on top. **C,** Topologic structure of the α and β subunits of Na+,K+-ATPase. **D,** Overlapping structures of the Na pump bound to three different cardiotonic steroids. *CTS,* Cardiotonic steroid. (**B** from Khaninshvilli D. The SLC8 gene family of sodium-calcium exchangers (NCX)—structure, function, and regulation in health and disease. *Mol Aspects Med.* 2013;34:220–235. **D** from Laursen M, Gregersen JL, Yatime L, et al. Structures and characterization of digoxin- and bufalin-bound Na+,K+-ATPase compared with the ouabain-bound complex. *Proc Natl Acad Sci U S A.* 2015;112:1755–1760.)

Gap junction function is dynamic. When the intracellular calcium level rises, as in myocardial infarction (MI), gap junctions close to seal off injured from noninjured cells. Acidosis increases, and alkalosis decreases, gap junctional resistance. Increased gap junctional resistance slows the rate of AP propagation, leading to conduction delay or block. The small number of transverse gap junctions means that inactivation of gap junctions impairs transverse conduction to a greater degree than longitudinal, resulting in increased anisotropy.

Connexins are the proteins that form the intercellular channels of gap junctions. Six connexin proteins assemble to form a *"connexon,"* a hemichannel that connects to a complementary connexon hemichannel in an adjacent cell to create a permeable channel connecting the cells. Each connexon is formed by six integral membrane connexin subunits, which surround an aqueous pore and thereby create a low-resistance connection (Fig. 62.10A). *Connexin 43,* a 43-kDa polypeptide, is the most abundant cardiac connexin in heart cells, with connexins 40 and 45 being found in smaller amounts. Ventricular muscle expresses connexins 43 and 45, whereas atrial muscle and the specialized conduction system express connexins 43, 45, and 40.

The various connexin types form gap junctional channels with characteristic unitary conductances, voltage sensitivities, and permeabilities. Tissue-specific connexin expression and the spatial distribution of gap junctions contribute to distinct conduction properties of cardiac tissues. The functional diversity of cardiac gap junctions is further enhanced by the ability of different connexin isoforms to form hybrid gap junctional channels with unique electrophysiologic properties (Fig. 62.10B). These channel chimeras appear to have a major function in controlling impulse transmission at the SA node–atrium border, the atrium–AV node transitional zone, and the Purkinje-myocyte border.[1,22]

Alterations in the distribution and function of cardiac gap junctions are associated with increased susceptibility to arrhythmias. Conduction slowing and arrhythmogenesis have been associated with redistribution of connexin 43 (Cx43) gap junctions from the end of cardiomyocytes to the lateral borders and with decreased phosphorylation of Cx43 in a dog model of nonischemic dilated cardiomyopathy (Fig. 62.10C–E). Adult mice genetically engineered to lack cardiac Cx43 exhibited increased susceptibility to the induction

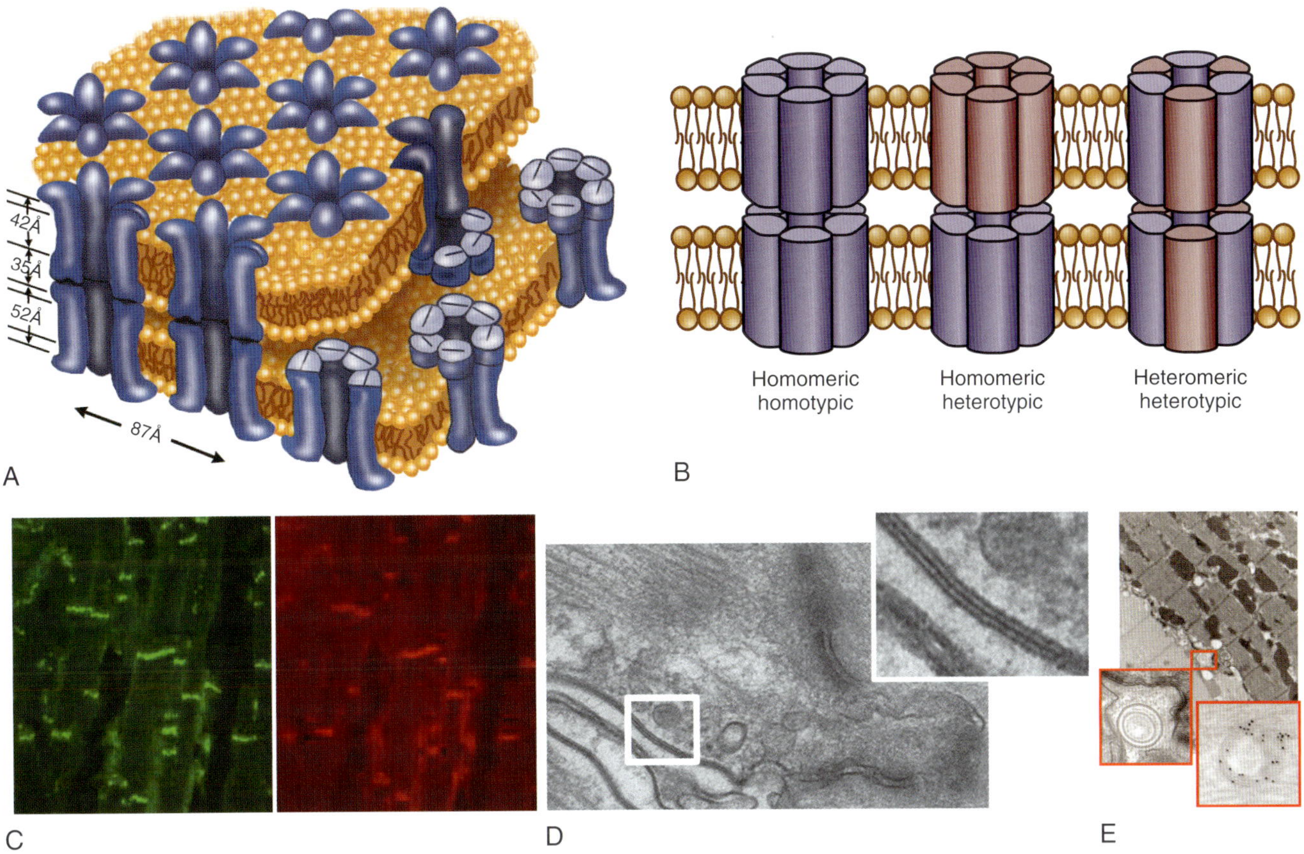

FIGURE 62.10 A, Model of the structure of a gap junction based on the results of x-ray diffraction studies. Individual channels are composed of paired hexamers in the membranes of adjacent cells and adjoin in the extracellular gap to form an aqueous pore that provides continuity of the cytoplasm of the two cells; Å, ångstroms. **B,** Mixing of connexin subunits to form gap junction channels may occur at interfaces between tissue types in the heart. Homomeric, homotypic channels contain a single connexin isoform; homomeric, heterotypic channels are composed of connexons (hemichannels) comprising a single connexin isoform; and heteromeric, heterotypic channels are made from connexons containing more than one connexin isoform. **C,** Connexin 43 (Cx43) is concentrated at the intercalated discs at cell ends in ventricular myocardium *(green)* and colocalizes with junctional proteins such as N-cadherin *(red)*. **D,** Electron microscopic view of an intercalated from normal ventricular myocardium reveals a pentalaminar membrane *(inset)* characteristic of gap junctions. **E,** Remodeling of gap junctions in the failing heart. Immunoreactive Cx43 is increased along lateral cell borders, and annular gap junctions that label with anti-Cx43 immunogold antibodies *(insets)* can be observed. (**A** from Saffitz JE. Cell-to-cell communication in the heart. *Cardiol Rev.* 1995;3:86; **C** and **E** modified from Hesketh GA, Shah MH, Halperin VL, et al. Ultrastructure and regulation of lateralized connexin43 in the failing heart. *Circ Res.* 2010;106:1153–1163.)

of fatal tachyarrhythmias. Side-to-side electrical coupling between cardiomyocytes is reduced following acute MI, exaggerating anisotropy and facilitating reentrant activity. Lastly, mutations in the atrial-specific connexin 40 gene have been associated with AF.[23] Normal electrical coupling of cardiomyocytes through gap junctions depends on cell-to-cell mechanical coupling through adhesion junctions. Defects in cell-cell adhesion prevent normal localization of connexins in gap junctions, potentially causing lethal tachyarrhythmias. Mutations in *desmoplakin,* a protein that links desmosomal adhesion molecules to *desmin,* a filament protein of the cardiomyocyte cytoskeleton, and *plakoglobin,* a protein that connects N-cadherins to actin and desmosomal cadherins to desmin, produce autosomal recessive variants of arrhythmogenic RV cardiomyopathy (ARVC), Carvajal disease, and Naxos disease, respectively (see Chapter 52).[24] Notably, restoring plakoglobin (*JUP* gene) levels in a mouse model of Naxos disease caused by a truncation of plakoglobin prevented cardiac dysfunction, consistent with a loss of function defect of the truncated protein. Loss of N-cadherin expression in mouse hearts decreases Cx43 expression in gap junctions, impairs and promotes arrhythmias.

STRUCTURE AND FUNCTION OF THE CARDIAC ELECTRICAL NETWORK

Sinoatrial Node

The SA node is a spindle-shaped structure composed of a fibrous tissue matrix containing closely packed cells. In man, it is 10 to 20 mm long and 2 to 3 mm wide, narrowing caudally toward the inferior vena cava (IVC). The SA node is superficial, lying less than 1 mm from the epicardial surface, laterally in the right atrial sulcus terminalis at the junction of the superior vena cava (SVC) and right atrium. The proximity to the right phrenic nerve is an important consideration when catheter ablation or modification of the sinoatrial node (SAN) is contemplated (Fig. 62.11). The artery supplying the SAN branches from the right (55% to 60% of the time) or the left (40% to 45%) circumflex coronary artery and approaches the node around the junction of the SVC and right atrium.

Atrioventricular Junctional Area and Intraventricular Conduction System
Atrioventricular Node

Based on histology and immunolabeling, the normal AV junctional area is composed of multiple distinct structures, including transitional tissue, inferior nodal extension (INE), compact portion, penetrating bundle, His bundle, atrial and ventricular muscle, central fibrous body, tendon of Todaro, and valves (Fig. 62.12A).[26] The properties of AV node cells are diverse, with the compact AV node populated by relatively depolarized cells displaying slow response APs and cells more like working atrium in other sections.[27]

At the level of the AV junction, the tract of nodal tissue is divided into two major components, the INE and the penetrating bundle.[26,28]

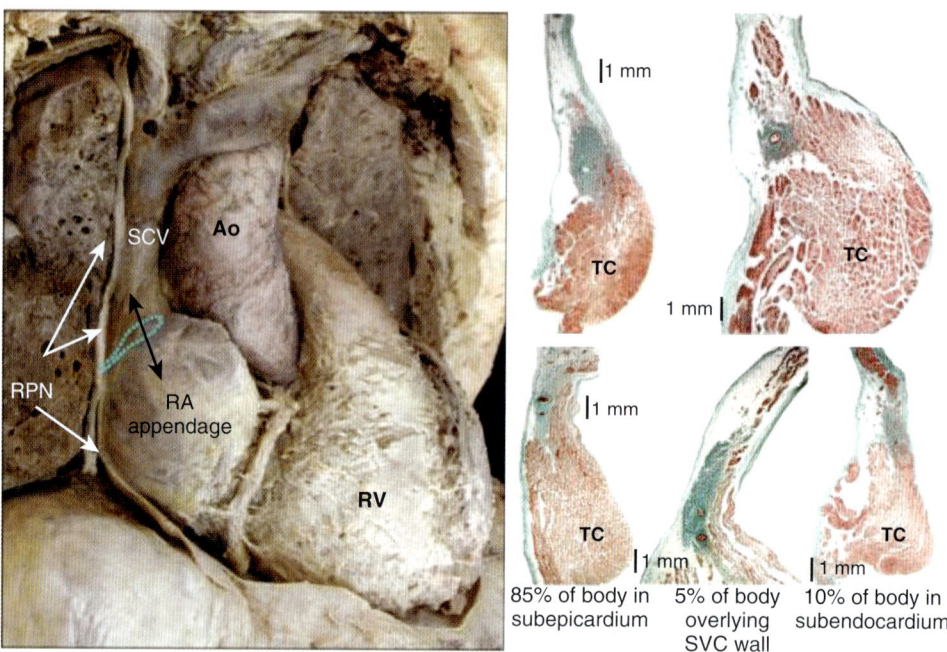

FIGURE 62.11 **Left,** Anterior view of the heart in a cadaver that has been dissected to show the course of the right phrenic nerve *(RPN)* relative to the right atrium *(RA).* The anticipated location of the sinus node outlined with the *dots.* The *double-headed arrow* represents the sectioning plane used for making the cross sections through the sinus node and the terminal crest *(TC)* shown in the histologic sections. *Ao,* Aorta; *RV,* right ventricle; *SCV,* superior caval vein. The histologic sections in the two **upper right panels** show variations in sizes of the sinus node cross section and the TC. With this stain (Masson trichrome), the node is recognizable by its fibrous matrix *(green)* and its artery. Two **lower right panels** show variations in nodal location relative to the epicardial and endocardial surfaces and to the SCV. *SVC,* Superior vena cava. (From Ho SY, Sanchez-Quintana D. Anatomy and pathology of the sinus node. *J Interv Card Electrophysiol.* 2016;46:3–8.)

The INE is located between the coronary sinus and the tricuspid valve, and the end of the INE is covered by transitional tissue (Fig. 62.12D). The small myocytes in the INE are dispersed among connective tissue and do not express connexin 43, whereas myocytes in the transitional zone do express Cx43; however, unlike the Cx43-positive atrial myocytes in the working myocardium, they are loosely packed between collagen septa (Fig. 62.12B, C). The INE is continuous with the penetrating bundle, which penetrates the fibrous tissue separating the atria and ventricles and emerges in the ventricles as the bundle of His. Both structures are covered by connective tissue and are therefore enclosed. Myocytes in the *penetrating bundle* express Cx43 and are dispersed among connective tissue. A tract of Cx43-positive nodal tissue projects into the Cx43-negative INE.

The compact portion of the AV node (Fig. 62.12A) is a superficial structure lying just beneath the right atrial endocardium, anterior to the ostium of the coronary sinus, and directly above the insertion of the septal leaflet of the tricuspid valve. It is at the apex of a triangle formed by the tricuspid annulus and the *tendon of Todaro* (Fig. 62.12), which originates in the central fibrous body and passes posteriorly through the atrial septum to continue with the Eustachian valve. The term *triangle of Koch,* however, has to be used with caution because histologic studies of anatomically normal adult hearts have demonstrated that the tendon of Todaro, which forms one side of the triangle of Koch, is absent in about two thirds of hearts. The compact node is located at the junction where the Cx43-negative nodal tissue meets the Cx43-positive nodal tissue (see Fig. 62.12B–D).

In 85% to 90% of human hearts, the arterial supply to the AV node is derived from a branch of the right coronary artery that originates at the posterior intersection of the AV and interventricular grooves (crux). A branch of the circumflex coronary artery provides the arterial supply to the AV node in the remaining hearts.

During normal anterograde AV conduction, the AP propagates from the SAN through atrial working myocardium (while the involvement of specialized internodal conduction pathways has been suggested, their existence remains controversial) and enters the tract of nodal tissue at two points (see Fig. 62.12D). The first point is at the end of the INE (next to the penetrating bundle) via transitional tissue. This conduction pathway most likely corresponds to the fastpathway route. Second, the AP enters near the atrial origin of the INE. This conduction pathway probably constitutes the slow-pathway route. The AP cannot enter nodal tissue at other tissue points, because of separation by a vein and connective tissue. From the two entry points, the APs propagating anterogradely and retrogradely along the INE usually annihilate each other, whereas the APs entering the nodal tract via the transitional zone propagate into the compact node and then reach the His bundle to enter the left and right bundle branches.

Transmembrane APs recorded from cardiomyocytes in situ at various locations within the nodal tract exhibit distinct shapes and time courses. Cells from the compact AV node are depolarized and have much slower phase 0 upstrokes due to the relatively small underlying Ca^{2+} current.[27] This smaller rate of depolarization, along with more limited electrical coupling, results in slowing of conduction across the compact portion and penetrating bundle (CV <10 cm/sec versus 35 cm/sec in atrial working myocardium), thereby giving rise to the AV conduction delay. APs from extranodal atrial tissue and the His bundle have more negative diastolic potentials and faster upstrokes than myocytes in the transitional zone and penetrating bundle.

Bundle of His (Penetrating Portion of Atrioventricular Bundle)

This structure is the continuation of the penetrating bundle on the ventricular side of the AV junction before it divides to form the left and right bundles. Myocytes in the His bundle are small and Cx43 positive (see Fig. 62.12). Large, well-formed fasciculoventricular connections between the penetrating portion of the AV bundle and the ventricular septal crest are occasionally found in adult hearts, possibly underlying preexcitation. Branches from the anterior and posterior descending coronary arteries supply the upper muscular interventricular septum with blood, which makes the conduction system at this site more impervious to ischemic damage unless the ischemia is extensive.

Bundle Branches (Branching Portion of Atrioventricular Bundle)

The bundle branches begin at the superior margin of the muscular interventricular septum, immediately beneath the membranous septum, with cells of the left bundle branch (LBB) cascading downward as a continuous sheet onto the septum beneath the noncoronary aortic cusp (Fig. 62.13A). The AV bundle may then give off other discrete bundle tracts. Sometimes these constitute a true bifascicular system with an anterosuperior branch and an inferoposterior system, constituting (when damaged) the anatomical basis of electrocardiographic left anterior and left posterior hemiblock respectively. In other cases, the AV bundle may give rise to a group of central fibers, and in still others, the offshoots appear as a network without clear division into a fascicular system (Fig. 62.13B,C). The right bundle branch continues intramyocardially as an unbranched extension of the AV bundle down the right side of the interventricular septum to the apex of the right ventricle

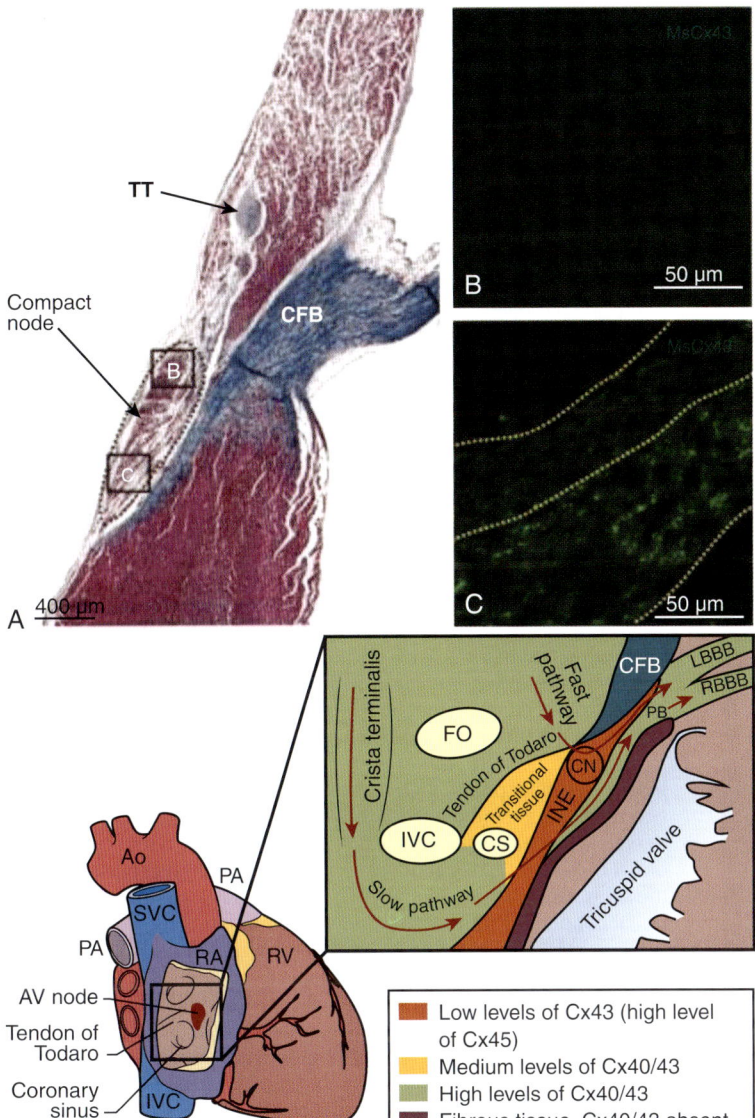

Purkinje fibers penetrate only the inner third of the endocardium, whereas in pigs, they almost reach to the epicardium. These differences influence changes produced by myocardial ischemia, because Purkinje fibers are more resistant to ischemia than ordinary myocardial fibers. Purkinje myocytes are found in the His bundle and bundle branches, and cover most of the endocardium of both ventricles (see Fig. 62.13B); they align to form multicellular bundles in longitudinal strands separated by collagen. Although conduction of cardiac impulses is their principal function, large free-running Purkinje fibers composed of many Purkinje cells, often called *false tendons*, are capable of contraction. APs propagate within the thin Purkinje fiber bundles from the base to the apex before activating surrounding myocytes. Purkinje myocytes have less well-developed transverse tubules, which reduces membrane capacitance and thus accelerates AP propagation. Purkinje fiber coupling relies on connexins 40 and 45. The molecular identity of the connexin type at the Purkinje fiber–myocyte junction (PMJ) is unclear. Purkinje cells have markedly longer repolarization times than surrounding myocytes (see Fig. 62.5E) and may be preferential sites of afterdepolarization generation.

Innervation of Atrioventricular Node, His Bundle, and Ventricular Myocardium

Pathways of Innervation

The AV node and His bundle region are richly innervated by cholinergic and adrenergic fibers with densities exceeding the ventricular myocardium.[1] Innervation density is variable in the AV junctional area. For example, the INE has a higher density of cholinergic and adrenergic nerves than working atrial myocardium; the opposite is true for the compact node. Ganglia, nerve fibers, and nerve nets lie close to the AV node.

In general, autonomic neural input to the heart exhibits some degree of "sidedness," with the right sympathetic and vagal nerves affecting the SA node more than the AV node and the left sympathetic and vagal nerves affecting the AV node more than the SA node. The distribution of neural input to the SA and AV nodes is complex because of substantial overlapping innervation. Despite the overlap, specific branches of the vagal and sympathetic nerves can be shown to innervate certain regions preferentially. Stimulation of the right stellate ganglion produces sinus tachycardia with less effect on AV nodal conduction, whereas stimulation of the left stellate ganglion generally shifts the sinus pacemaker to an ectopic site and consistently shortens AV nodal conduction time and refractoriness. Left stellate stimulation produces variable and usually smaller degrees of SAN acceleration. Stimulation of the right cervical vagus nerve primarily slows the SA nodal discharge rate, whereas stimulation of the left vagus primarily prolongs AV nodal conduction time and refractoriness. Neither sympathetic nor vagal stimulation affects normal conduction in the His bundle. The negative dromotropic response of the heart to vagal stimulation is mediated by the activation of $I_{K,ACh}$, which hyperpolarizes AV nodal cells, making them harder to activate.

FIGURE 62.12 **A**, Masson's trichrome–stained section through the compact node of the rabbit heart (*red*, myocytes; *blue*, connective tissue). The compact node is enclosed with a *dashed line*. **B** and **C**, High-magnification images of boxed regions in **A** (**B** is the compact node; **C** is the lower nodal bundle) showing Cx43 expression (immunofluorescence, *bright-green* punctate spots). **C**, *Dotted yellow lines* divide tissue into Cx43-negative (*top*) and Cx43-positive (*bottom*) regions. (Modified from Dobrzynski H, Nikolski VP, Sambelashvili AT, et al. Site of origin and molecular substrate of atrioventricular junctional rhythm in the rabbit heart. *Circ Res*. 2003;93:1102–1110.) *CFB*, Central fibrous body; *TT*, tendon of Todaro. **D**, Color-coded map of the distribution of connexins (Cx) in the atrioventricular (AV) junction. *Ao*, Aorta; *CN*, compact AV node; *CS*, coronary sinus; *FO*, foramen ovale; *INE*, inferior nodal extension; *IVC*, inferior vena cava; *LBBB*, left bundle branch block; *PA*, pulmonary artery; *PB*, penetrating bundle; *RA*, right atrium; *RBBB*, right bundle branch block; *RV*, right ventricle. (From Temple IP, Inada S, Dobrzynski H, et al. Connexins and the atrioventricular node. *Heart Rhythm*. 2010;10:297.)

and base of the anterior papillary muscle. In some human hearts, the His bundle traverses the right interventricular crest and gives rise to a right-sided narrow stem origin of the LBB. The anatomy of the LBB system can be variable and may not conform to a constant bifascicular division. However, the concept of a trifascicular system remains useful to both electrocardiographers and clinicians (see Chapter 14).

Terminal Purkinje Fibers

The Purkinje fibers connect with the ends of the bundle branches to form interweaving networks on the endocardial surface of both ventricles and transmit the cardiac impulse almost simultaneously to the right and left ventricular endocardium. Purkinje fibers tend to be less concentrated at the base of the ventricle and at the papillary muscle tips. They penetrate the myocardium transmurally from the endocardium for varying distances, depending on the species. In humans,

Most efferent sympathetic impulses reach the canine ventricles over the ansae subclavia, branches from the stellate ganglia. Sympathetic nerves then synapse primarily in the caudal cervical ganglia and form individual cardiac nerves that innervate relatively localized parts of the ventricles. The major route to the heart is the recurrent cardiac nerve on the right side and the ventrolateral cardiac nerve on the left. In general, the right sympathetic chain shortens refractoriness primarily of the anterior portion of the ventricles, and the left affects primarily the posterior surface of the ventricles, although overlapping areas of distribution occur. Asymmetrical sympathetic activation may be associated with arrhythmogenesis and stellate ganglion block is sometimes used to treat certain refractory ventricular arrhythmia syndromes.

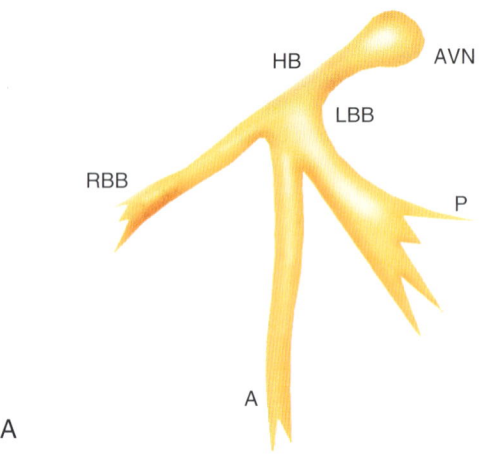

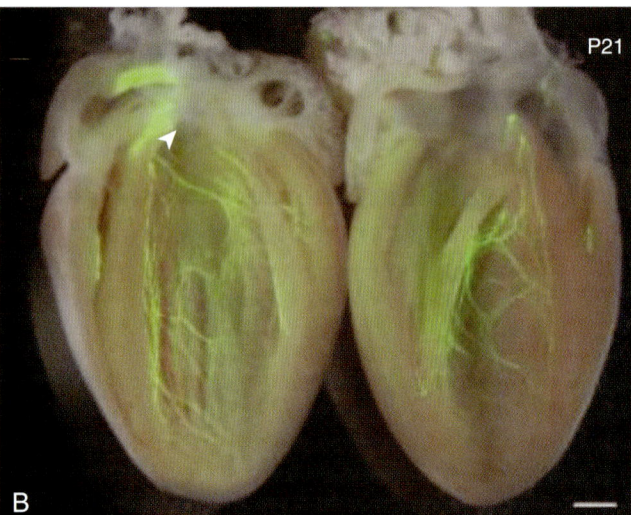

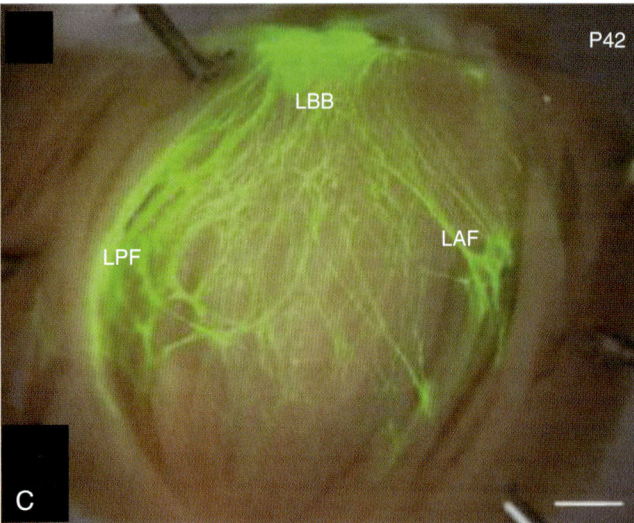

FIGURE 62.13 A, Schematic representation of the trifascicular bundle branch conduction system. **B** and **C,** Whole mount of murine hearts expressing contactin-2 eGFP reporter gene (Cntn2EGFP) demonstrate the presence of Cntn2 throughout the cardiac conduction system. The hearts are from mice **(B)** 21 days (P21) and **(C)** 42 days (P42) postpartum. There is robust expression of Cntn2 within the atrioventricular node *(AVN) (arrowhead)* His bundle *(HB),* bundle branches, and Purkinje network. Scale bars = 500 μm. *LAF,* Left anterior fascicle; *LBB,* left bundle branch; *LPF,* left posterior fascicle; *RBB,* right bundle branch. (**A** modified from Rosenbaum MB et al. *The Hemiblocks.* Oldsmar, FL: Tampa Tracings; 1970, cover illustration; **B** and **C** from Maass K, Shekhar A, Lu J, et al. Isolation and characterization of embryonic stem cell–derived cardiac Purkinje cells. *Stem Cells.* 2015;33:1102–1112.)

The intraventricular route of sympathetic nerves generally follows the coronary arteries. Afferent and efferent sympathetic nerves travel in the superficial layers of the epicardium and dive to innervate the endocardium. Vagal fibers travel intramurally or subendocardially and travel to the epicardium at the AV groove (Fig. 62.14A). Sympathetic nerve density in the left ventricle is higher in the epicardial than endocardium, which at least in part results from transmural gradients in cytokines during cardiac development that influence sympathetic nerve growth (Fig. 62.14B).[1,29]

Effects of Vagal Stimulation

The principal effects of vagus nerve activation are due to opening of $I_{K,ACh}$ channels. In addition, vagal discharge modulates cardiac sympathetic activity at prejunctional and postjunctional sites by regulating the amount of norepinephrine released and by inhibiting cAMP-induced phosphorylation of cardiac proteins, including ion channels and calcium pumps. Tonic vagal stimulation thus produces a greater absolute reduction in the SAN rate in the presence of tonic background sympathetic stimulation, a sympathetic-parasympathetic interaction termed *accentuated antagonism.* In contrast, changes in AV conduction during concomitant sympathetic and vagal stimulation are essentially the algebraic sum of the individual AV conduction responses to tonic vagal and sympathetic stimulation alone. Cardiac responses to brief vagal bursts begin and dissipate quickly; in contrast, cardiac responses to sympathetic stimulation commence and dissipate more slowly. Periodic *vagal bursting,* as may occur each time that a systolic pressure wave arrives at the baroreceptor regions in the aortic and carotid sinuses, induces phasic changes in sinus cycle length and can entrain the sinus node to discharge faster or slower at periods identical to those of the vagal burst. In a similar phasic manner, vagal bursts prolong AV nodal conduction time and are influenced by background levels of sympathetic tone. Because the peak vagal effects on sinus rate and AV nodal conduction occur at different times in the cardiac cycle, a brief vagal burst can slow the sinus rate without affecting AV nodal conduction or can prolong AV nodal conduction time and not slow the sinus rate.

Effects of Sympathetic Stimulation

Nonuniform distribution of sympathetic nerves—and thus norepinephrine levels—may produce nonuniform electrophysiologic effects during sympathetic activation because the ventricular content of norepinephrine is greater at the base than at the apex of the heart. In humans, both direct and reflex sympathetic stimulation increases regional differences in cardiac repolarization. The dispersion of repolarization is significantly enhanced in patients with ischemic cardiomyopathy.[1] Afferent vagal activity is higher in the posterior ventricular myocardium, which may account for the vagomimetic effects of inferior MI.

The vagi exert very small effects on ventricular tissue; decreased contractility and prolonged refractoriness are demonstrable under careful experimental observation. In addition, the vagus can exert indirect effects by modulating sympathetic influences.

Beyond the beat-to-beat regulation of rate and contractile force, sympathetic input to the heart, through both translational and posttranslational modifications, exerts long-term regulation of adrenergic receptor sensitivity and ion channels. These long-term changes in autonomic responsiveness and cardiac electrical properties appear to be mediated, at least in part, by highly localized signaling cascades involving neurally released molecules such as NPY.[1] In addition, adrenergic neurotransmitters (both released in the heart and in circulating forms) have major neurohumoral effects and promote cellular and structural remodeling that contribute to heart failure and arrhythmias.

Arrhythmias and the Autonomic Nervous System

Alterations in vagal and sympathetic innervation (autonomic remodeling) can influence the development of arrhythmias and contribute to sudden cardiac death (SCD) from ventricular tachyarrhythmias.[30] Damage to nerves extrinsic to the heart, such as the stellate ganglia,

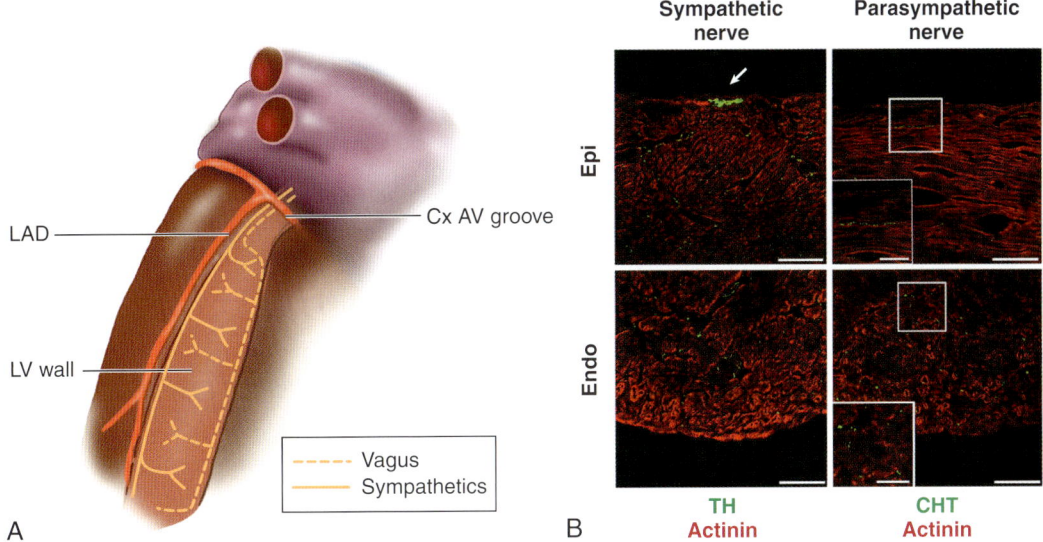

FIGURE 62.14 A, Intraventricular route of the sympathetic and vagal nerves to the left ventricle (*LV*); *LAD*, left anterior descending artery. **B,** Distribution of sympathetic and parasympathetic nerves in the mammalian heart. Immunofluorescence staining for the sympathetic and parasympathetic nerve markers tyrosine hydroxylase (*TH*) and choline transporter (*CHT*) is shown in the LV of a rat heart (*green*, nerves; *red*, alpha-actinin, a cardiomyocyte marker). TH-positive nerves are more abundant in the subepicardial (Epi) layer than in the subendocardial (Endo) layer. *Arrow* indicates sympathetic nerves at the epicardial surface. No CHT-positive nerves are present at the epicardial surface, and CHT-positive nerves are more abundant in the subendocardial layer. Higher magnification views of the boxed regions are shown in the *insets*. Scale bars = 100 μm. (**A** from Ito M, Zipes DP. Efferent sympathetic and vagal innervation of the canine right ventricle. *Circulation.* 1994;90:1459. By permission of the American Heart Association; **B** from Kanazawa H, Ieda M, Kimura K, et al. Heart failure causes cholinergic transdifferentiation of cardiac sympathetic nerves via gp130-signaling cytokines in rodents. *J Clin Invest.* 2010;120:408.)

and to intrinsic cardiac nerves from diseases that may affect primarily nerves, such as viral infections, or from diseases that secondarily cause cardiac damage may produce cardioneuropathy. Although the mechanisms by which altered sympathetic innervation modulates cardiac electrical properties are largely unknown, spatially heterogeneous sympathetic hyperinnervation could result in enhanced dispersion of myocardial excitability and refractoriness through patchy adrenergic stimulation of ionic currents, including $I_{Ca,L}$, I_{Ks}, and I_{Cl} (see Table 62.1). Sympathetic hypoinnervation has been shown to increase the sensitivity of adrenergic receptors to activation by circulating catecholamines (*denervation supersensitivity*).

Numerous studies have suggested an important role of altered cardiac sympathetic innervation in arrhythmogenesis. Nerve growth factor (NGF) infusion into the left stellate ganglion in dogs with chronic MI causes spatially heterogeneous sympathetic cardiac hyperinnervation (nerve sprouting) and dramatically increases the incidence of SCD from ventricular tachyarrhythmias. Malignant ventricular arrhythmias are preceded by increased neuronal discharge. Explanted human hearts from transplant recipients with a history of arrhythmias exhibit greater and more heterogeneous expression of sympathetic nerve fibers versus patients without arrhythmias. In a canine model of heart failure with dyssynchronous ventricular contraction, cardiac resynchronization therapy (CRT) restored sympathovagal balance and reduced arrhythmogenic afterdepolarizations. In patients with congestive heart failure, sympathetic neural tone is upregulated, leading to adverse myocardial effects, including depletion of cardiac norepinephrine content, adverse cellular remodeling, tissue fibrosis and lethal arrhythmias, and arrhythmogenesis.[31] Neurotransmitter switching and transdifferentiation from catecholaminergic into cholinergic neurons occurs in the chronically failing heart.

The junctions between PVs and the left atrium are highly innervated. Sympathetic and parasympathetic nerves are colocalized and concentrated in "ganglionated plexuses" around the PVs. Selective ablation of ganglionated plexuses, as well as regional ablation targeting anatomic areas containing ganglionated plexuses, has been shown to prevent paroxysmal AF in some but not all clinical and experimental studies.[32] Mutations in genes encoding cardiac ion channel subunits also affect channel function in the central and peripheral autonomic nervous system and thereby result in abnormal firing properties of affected neurons.[1] This observation may partially explain the clinical finding that SCD in some variants of LQTS (see Chapters 63 and 67)

is typically preceded by sympathetic arousal. Also, the antiarrhythmic efficacy of surgical left cardiac sympathetic denervation has previously been demonstrated in young patients with catecholaminergic polymorphic ventricular tachycardia (CPVT, see later). Thus the cardiac sympathetic nervous system provides a potentially useful target for treating patients at risk for clinical arrhythmias.[29] Overall, while there are some established indications for targeted autonomic-nerve manipulation in cardiac arrhythmias, the clear indications are limited and this is still an evolving area.

MECHANISMS OF ARRHYTHMOGENESIS

The mechanisms responsible for cardiac arrhythmias are generally divided into disorders of impulse formation, disorders of impulse conduction, or combinations of both (Table 62.3). In many cases, currently available diagnostic tools do not permit unequivocal determination of the electrophysiologic mechanisms responsible for many clinical arrhythmias. It is clinically difficult to separate microanatomic reentry from automaticity, and often one is left with the consideration that a particular arrhythmia is "most consistent with" or "best explained by" one or the other electrophysiologic mechanism. Some tachyarrhythmias can be started by one mechanism and perpetuated by another. This is particularly true of reentrant arrhythmias, which often require an initiating premature activation resulting from some type of abnormal impulse generation. Entrainment and the response to the creation of critical lines of block by ablation (e.g., for AV reentrant arrhythmias, atrial flutter, critical conduction channels for ventricular tachyarrhythmias) can identify arrhythmias caused by macroreentry (see later and Chapter 65).

Disorders of Impulse Formation

Disorders of impulse formation are characterized by an inappropriate discharge rate of the normal pacemaker, the SA node (e.g., sinus rates too fast or too slow for physiologic needs of patient), or discharge of an ectopic pacemaker that then controls the atrial or ventricular rhythm, either as an escape rhythm or accelerated automaticity. Pacemaker discharges from ectopic sites, often called *latent* or *subsidiary* pacemakers, can occur in fibers located in several parts of the atria, coronary sinus and PVs, AV valves, portions of the AV junction, and His-Purkinje system. Usually kept from reaching the level of threshold potential because of overdrive suppression by the more rapidly firing sinus node, ectopic pacemaker activity at one of these latent sites manifests when the SAN rate slows or block occurs between the SA node and the ectopic pacemaker site, permitting *escape* of the latent pacemaker at the latter's normal discharge rate. A clinical example would be sinus bradycardia to a rate of 45 beats/min that permits an AV junctional escape complex to occur at a rate of 50 beats/min.

The discharge rate of a latent pacemaker can accelerate inappropriately and usurp control of cardiac rhythm from the SA node, as may occur with a premature ventricular complex (PVC) or a burst of ventricular tachycardia (VT). Such disorders of impulse formation can be caused by alteration in a *normal* pacemaker mechanism (e.g., phase 4 diastolic depolarization that is physiologically normal for SA node or for ectopic site such as a Purkinje fiber, but occurs inappropriately fast or slow) or by a physiologically *abnormal* pacemaker mechanism.

A patient with persistent sinus tachycardia at rest or sinus bradycardia during exertion exhibits inappropriate SAN rates, but the underlying ionic mechanisms responsible can still be basically normal, with changes in the kinetics or magnitude of relevant currents underlying the abnormal rate. Conversely, when a patient experiences VT during acute MI, myocardial ischemia and infarction can depolarize normally non-automatic myocardial cells to membrane potentials at which inactivation of K^+-currents and activation of I_{CaL} cause automatic discharge.

Abnormal Automaticity

The mechanisms responsible for normal automaticity are described earlier (Phase 4: Diastolic Depolarization). Abnormal automaticity can arise from cells that have reduced maximum diastolic potentials, often at membrane potentials positive to −50 mV, in the activation range of both I_K and I_{CaL}. Automaticity at membrane potentials more negative than −70 mV may be caused by I_f. Electrotonic effects from surrounding normally polarized or more depolarized myocardium influence the development of automaticity.

Partial depolarization and failure to reach normal maximal diastolic potential can induce automatic discharges in most if not all cardiac fibers. Although this type of spontaneous automatic activity has been found in human atrial and ventricular fibers, its relationship to the genesis of clinical arrhythmias has not been established. Abnormal automaticity in Purkinje cells can be caused by spontaneous, submembrane Ca^{2+} elevations through activation of calcium-sensitive membrane conductances, similar to processes identified in SA node myocytes. Rhythms resulting from abnormal automaticity may be slow atrial, junctional, or ventricular escape rhythms; certain types of atrial tachycardias (ATs) (e.g., those produced by digitalis or perhaps those coming from PVs); accelerated junctional (nonparoxysmal junctional tachycardia) and idioventricular rhythms (see Chapters 65 and 67).

Triggered Activity

Triggered activity is initiated by *afterdepolarizations*, which are depolarizing oscillations in membrane voltage induced by one or more preceding APs. Thus, triggered activity is related to *the consequences of a preceding impulse or series of impulses*, without which electrical quiescence occurs (Figs. 62.15 and 62.16). This triggering activity is not caused by an automatic self-generating mechanism, and the term "triggered automaticity" is therefore contradictory. Afterdepolarizations can occur before or after full repolarization of the fiber, termed *early afterdepolarizations* when they arise before full repolarization of the AP (Fig. 62.15C) or *delayed afterdepolarizations* (see Fig. 62.15B) when they occur after completion of repolarization (phase 4), at more negative membrane potentials than EADs. Not all afterdepolarizations reach the threshold potential, but those that do can trigger another afterdepolarization and thus self-perpetuate.

Delayed Afterdepolarizations

DADs and triggered activity have been demonstrated in Purkinje fibers, atrial and ventricular muscle cells in a wide range of experimental and clinical contexts (see Fig. 62.16). When fibers in the rabbit, canine, simian, and human mitral valves and in the canine tricuspid valve and coronary sinus are superfused with norepinephrine, they exhibit the capability for sustained, triggered rhythmic activity that may correspond to some forms of clinical tachyarrhythmia.

In vivo, atrial and ventricular arrhythmias caused by triggered activity have been reported in experimental models and in humans. Clinical arrhythmias likely due to DADs include some arrhythmias precipitated by digitalis, spontaneous atrial ectopic beats, and some cases of AF

TABLE 62.3 Mechanisms of Arrhythmias

DISORDER	EXPERIMENTAL EXAMPLES	CLINICAL EXAMPLES
Disorders of Impulse Formation		
Automaticity		
Normal automaticity	Normal in vivo or in vitro in SA nodal, AV nodal, and Purkinje cells	Sinus tachycardia or bradycardia inappropriate for the clinical situation; possibly ventricular parasystole
Abnormal automaticity	Depolarization-induced automaticity in Purkinje myocytes	Accelerated ventricular rhythms after myocardial infarction
Triggered Activity		
EADs	Drugs (sotalol, N-acetylprocainamide, terfenadine, erythromycin), cesium, barium, low $[K^+]_o$	Acquired LQTS and associated ventricular arrhythmias
DADs	Gain-of-function mutations in the gene encoding RyR2	Catecholaminergic polymorphic ventricular tachycardia; atrial ectopic beats
Disorders of Impulse Conduction		
Block and Reentry		
Bidirectional or unidirectional without reentry	SA, AV, bundle branch, Purkinje muscle	Sinoatrial, AV, bundle branch block
Unidirectional block with reentry	AV node, Purkinje-muscle junction, infarcted myocardium	Reciprocating tachycardia in Wolff-Parkinson-White syndrome, AV nodal reentry tachycardia, ventricular tachycardia caused by bundle branch reentry
Combined Disorders		
Interactions between automatic foci	Depolarizing or hyperpolarizing subthreshold stimuli speed or slow the automatic discharge rate	Modulated parasystole
Interactions between automaticity and conduction	Deceleration-dependent block, overdrive suppression of conduction, entrance and exit block	Similar to experimental

AV, Atrioventricular; *DADs*, delayed afterdepolarizations; *EADs*, early afterdepolarizations; *LQTS*, long-QT syndrome; *SA*, sinoatrial.

arising from DADs in PVs and arrhythmias caused by certain congenital arrhythmia syndromes (e.g., CPVT). The accelerated idioventricular rhythm and VTs 1 day after experimental canine MI may be caused by DADs, and certain specific VTs, such as those arising in the RV outflow tract, may be caused by DADs, whereas other data suggest that EADs are responsible.

Major Role of Intracellular Ca^{2+}-Handling Abnormalities in Delayed Afterdepolarization Generation

It is well-recognized that DADs result from the activation of a calcium-sensitive inward current elicited by spontaneous increases in intracellular free calcium concentration due to aberrant diastolic Ca^{2+} release (see Fig. 62.16). Acquired or inherited abnormalities in the properties and/or function of the SR RyR2 calcium-release channels or SR calcium-binding proteins underlie spontaneous calcium-release events.

As discussed above, rapid mobilization of Ca^{2+} from the SR into the cytosol is mediated by the synchronous opening of RyRs. The cardiac RyR is composed of four equivalent subunits (homotetramer), each encoded by the *RYR2* gene. During cardiac systole, the small influx of calcium ions through L-type Cav channels triggers a massive release of Ca^{2+} from the SR via synchronous opening of RyR2 channels, a process called Ca^{2+}-induced Ca^{2+} release (see Chapter 46). During diastole, RyR2 channels close and Ca^{2+} is recycled into the SR via calcium pumps, thereby refilling SR Ca^{2+} stores for the next release cycle. The duration and amplitude of Ca^{2+} efflux from the SR are therefore tightly controlled by the gating of RyR2 channels. RyR2 interacts with a number of accessory proteins to form a macromolecular Ca^{2+}-release complex. Proteins interact with RyR2 at multiple sites within the cytosolic domains of RyR2 and in the SR (e.g., calsequestrin, the major calcium-binding protein in the SR lumen). Among the cytosolic ligands, FKBP-12.6 (calstabin 2) has been implicated in stabilizing the closed state of the RyR2 channel and thus preventing diastolic Ca^{2+} leakage.[1]

Mutations in the human *RYR2* gene and in *CASQ2*, which encodes calsequestrin, have been linked to CPVT. Experimental studies have revealed that the *RYR2* and *CASQ2* mutations that underlie CPVT increase the sensitivity of the RyR2 channel to luminal Ca^{2+} activation.

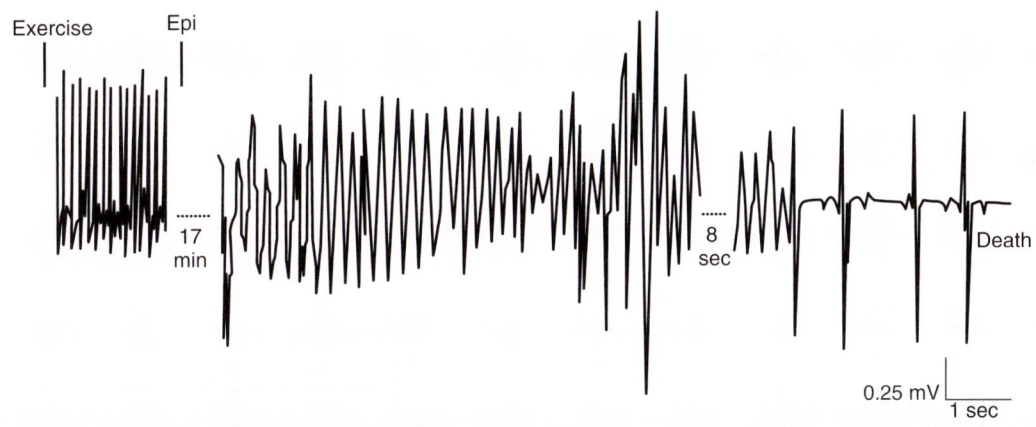

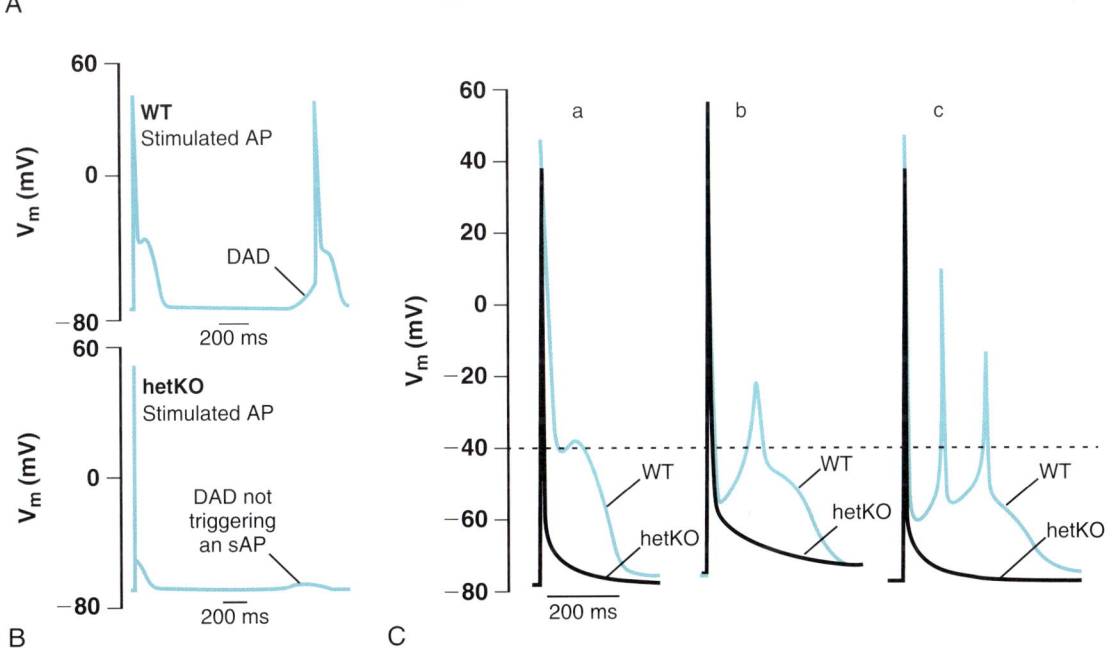

FIGURE 62.15 A, Electrocardiogram after exercise and administration of epinephrine in a mouse heterozygous for a loss-of-function mutation in the gene encoding ankyrin-B (AnkB$^{-/+}$). Polymorphic ventricular tachycardia (torsades de pointes) occurred within about 17 minutes of epinephrine administration, followed by marked bradycardia and death 2 minutes after the arrhythmia. **B,** Impaired translation of delayed afterdepolarizations (DADs) into spontaneous action potentials (APs) in heterozygous knockout of Na$^+$/Ca^{2+} exchanger (hetKO) versus wild-type (WT) exposed to isoproterenol and an arrhythmogenic pacing protocol. The first AP is initiated by current injection. The second AP in the **upper panel** is triggered by a DAD in the WT; it fails to generate an AP in the hetKO. **C,** Early afterdepolarizations (EADs) in WT and heterozygous knockout of Na$^+$/Ca^{2+} exchanger. The EAD shape varied between low-amplitude, slow-transient membrane fluctuations (a), spike-like depolarizations (b), and steep upstrokes (c). (**A** from Mohler PJ, Schott JJ, Gramolini AO, et al. Ankyrin-B mutation causes type 4 long-QT cardiac arrhythmia and sudden cardiac death. *Nature*. 2003;421:634; **B** and **C** from American Heart Association; Bögeholz N, Pauls P, Bauer BK, et al. Suppression of early and late afterdepolarizations by heterozygous knockout of the Na$^+$/Ca^{2+} exchanger in a murine model. *Circ Arrhythm Electrophysiol.* 2015;8:1210.)

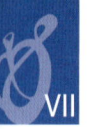

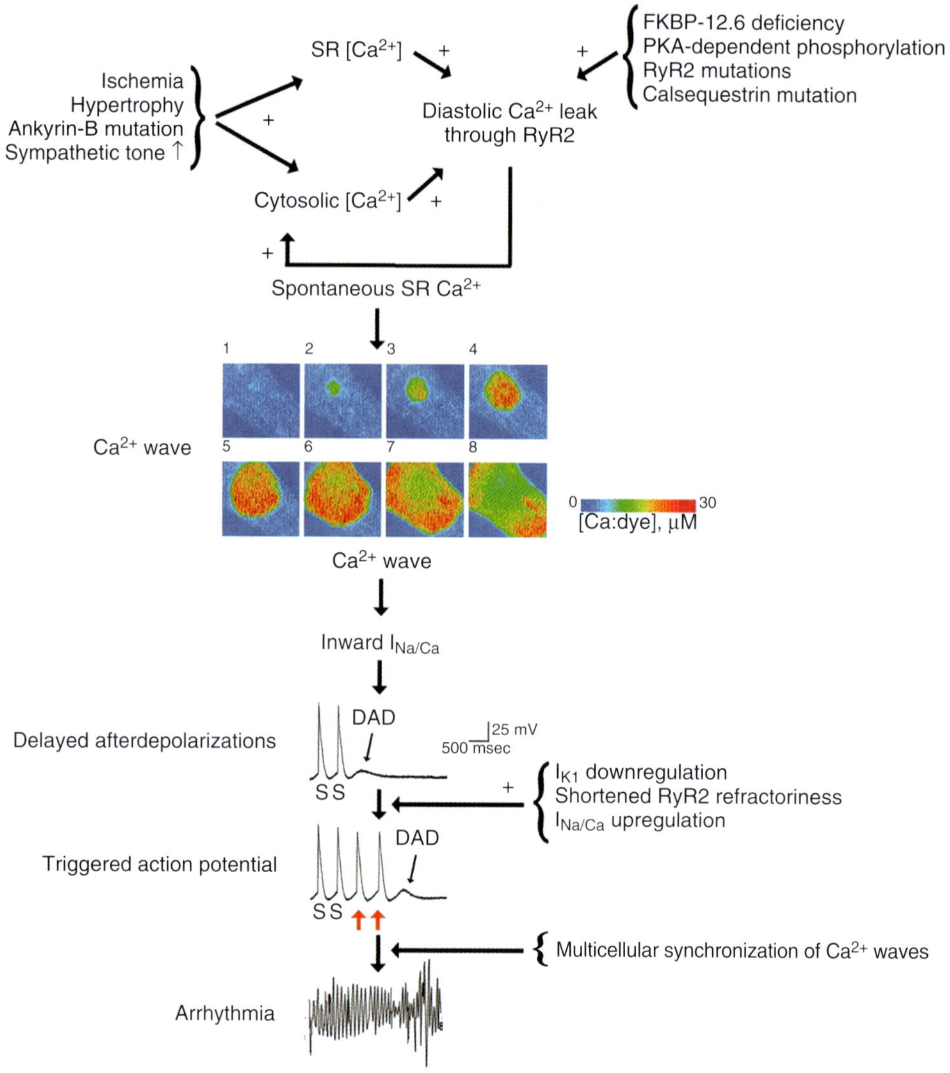

FIGURE 62.16 Proposed sequence of events leading to delayed afterdepolarizations (DADs) and triggered tachyarrhythmia. **Top panel,** Congenital (e.g., gain-of-function mutations in the *RYR2* or *CASQ2* genes) or acquired (e.g., ischemia, hypertrophy, increased sympathetic tone, heart failure) factors will cause a diastolic Ca²⁺ leak through RyR2 that results in localized and transient increases in [Ca²⁺]$_i$ in cardiomyocytes. **Middle panel,** Representative series of images showing changes in [Ca²⁺]$_i$ during a Ca²⁺ wave in a single cardiomyocyte loaded with a Ca²⁺-sensitive fluorescent dye. Images were obtained at 117-msec intervals. Focally elevated Ca²⁺ (*frame 2*) diffuses to the adjacent junctional sarcoplasmic reticulum (SR), where it initiates more Ca²⁺ release events that result in a propagating Ca²⁺ wave (*frames 3 to 8*). **Bottom panel,** The Ca²⁺ wave, through activation of inward I$_{Na/Ca}$, will depolarize the cardiomyocyte (DAD). If of sufficient magnitude to overcome the source-sink mismatch, the DAD will depolarize the cardiomyocyte above threshold and result in a single or repetitive premature activations (*red arrows*), which can trigger an arrhythmia. Downregulation of the inwardly rectifying potassium current (I$_{K1}$), upregulation of I$_{Na/Ca}$, and shortened Ca²⁺ signaling refractoriness because of ryanodine receptor phosphorylation and/or oxidation can promote the generation of DAD-triggered action potentials. S, Stimulus. (Modified from Rubart M, Zipes DP. Mechanisms of sudden cardiac death. *J Clin Invest.* 2005;115:2305. With permission from the Journal of Clinical Investigation.)

Thus, increased catecholamine release due to adrenergic stimulation (e.g., from emotional or physical stress), which increases SR Ca²⁺ stores and phosphorylates RyR2 (increasing its Ca²⁺ sensitivity further), enhances the propensity for spontaneous, diastolic SR Ca²⁺ release and DAD-triggered arrhythmias (accounting for the "C" in CPVT). The regulatory protein FKBP-12.6 appears to inhibit RyR2 sensitivity and Ca²⁺ release. Reduced FKBP-12.6 binding caused by PKA–mediated RyR2 hyperphosphorylation has been implicated in cardiac arrhythmogenesis associated with heart failure. Polymorphic VT, as well as inducible AF, develop in FKBP-12.6–deficient mice on adrenergic stimulation. Treatment with the 1,4-benzothiazepine derivatives JTV519 and S107, which restore FKBP-12.6 affinity for RyR2, has been shown to suppress CPVT in FKBP-12.6–deficient mice, although these agents also have other potential antiarrhythmic actions.[1] Purkinje myocytes isolated from mice heterozygous for a CPVT-causing mutation in *RyR2* are more susceptible to arrhythmogenic Ca²⁺-handling abnormalities than nonmutant cardiomyocytes, and Purkinje cells appear to be more prone to developing arrhythmogenic afterdepolarizations than working ventricular myocytes.[33]

The IP$_3$ receptor (IP3R) is another Ca²⁺-release channel in cardiomyocytes that is activated by binding of the second messenger IP$_3$ and cytosolic Ca²⁺. The IP3R exists as a homotetramer or heterotetramer, each subunit encoded by the *ITPR1, ITPR2,* or *ITPR3* gene. The type 2 IP3R is the predominant subtype in atrial myocytes, where they are located near RyR2 channels at the SR Ca²⁺-release sites and contribute to altered excitation-contraction coupling and arrhythmogenesis in the atria. In Purkinje myocytes, type 1 IP3Rs colocalize with type 3 RyR in the subsarcolemmal space to form a functional dyad that regulates electrical excitability. IP$_3$-dependent Ca signaling has been implicated in cardiac arrhythmias due to ischemia and reperfusion injury, inflammation, and cardiac failure. IP3Rs are upregulated in heart failure and AF.[1] In atrial and Purkinje myocytes, IP$_3$ causes spontaneous [Ca²⁺]$_i$ transients, Ca²⁺ waves, and Ca²⁺ alternans and facilitates the generation of afterdepolarizations. Recent work suggests that perinuclear IP$_3$R upregulation in AF may enhance nuclear Ca²⁺ load and contribute the gene-reprograming associated with AF-related remodeling.[34]

The cascade of events linking cellular Ca²⁺-handling abnormalities to cardiac arrhythmias is illustrated in Figure 62.16. Ca²⁺ leak via RyR2 during diastole gives rise to localized increases in cytosolic calcium concentrations in single cardiomyocytes. Since RyR2 release occurs in response to a critical level of Ca²⁺, RyR2 leak may occur because of increased RyR2 sensitivity or increased Ca²⁺ load. When large enough, the focally elevated Ca²⁺ resulting from RyR2 release causes a propagating Ca²⁺ wave that depolarizes the cardiomyocyte membrane and triggers a DAD through activation of the inward Na⁺/Ca²⁺exchange current (I$_{Na/Ca}$) which handles the increased Ca²⁺. Calmodulin kinase type-II (CaMKII) is a key player in promoting DADs, via phosphorylation of multiple membrane proteins, in particular RyR2 which, when CaMKII-phosphorylated shows enhanced sensitivity to Ca²⁺. CaMKII inhibition suppresses arrhythmogenic DADs and may provide a strategy for new therapeutic development.[35,36] Because intracellular Na⁺ is exchanged for Ca²⁺, drugs that reduce I$_{Na}$ suppress Na⁺ load and, indirectly, Ca²⁺ load, NCX current, and DADs. DADs likely play a causative role in arrhythmogenesis in the failing heart, where enhanced CaMKII activity, upregulation of I$_{Na/Ca}$, and downregulation of the inward rectifier K⁺ current I$_{K1}$, facilitate DAD generation.[37]

Short coupling intervals and pacing at rates more rapid than the triggered activity rate (*overdrive pacing*) increase the amplitude and shorten the cycle length of DADs after cessation of pacing (*overdrive acceleration*), because they enhance cellular Ca²⁺ loading. The clinical implication is that tachyarrhythmias caused by DAD-triggered activity may not be suppressed easily or indeed may be precipitated by rapid rates, either spontaneously, as with sinus tachycardia, or induced by pacing. Because a single premature stimulus can theoretically both initiate and terminate triggered activity, differentiation from reentry (see later) becomes difficult.

Early Afterdepolarizations

Various interventions can cause EADs, with most of them delaying repolarization. The sentinel finding in clinically identifiable EAD-associated syndromes is thus prolongation of the electrocardiographic QT interval, the macroscopic manifestation of cellular APD prolongation. EADs almost certainly play a central role in the tachyarrhythmias seen in the acquired and congenital forms of LQTS (see Fig. 62.15 and Chapters 63 and 67).

Long-QT Syndrome

Patients with heritable LQTS have an abnormally prolonged ventricular APD and are at increased risk of SCD from ventricular tachyarrhythmias (see Chapters 63 and 67). When the AP is excessively prolonged, the membrane potential remains at levels that allow recovery of enough steady-state Ca^{2+} (particularly during phase 2) or Na^+ (during phase 3) current to depolarize the cell, producing an EAD. It appears that, because of their longer APD and unique Ca^{2+} handling properties, Purkinje cells are particularly sensitive to EAD-inducing interventions.[33,38] Purkinje cell EADs raise to threshold adjacent ventricular muscle cells that have already repolarized, producing an unstimulated extrasystole. This activation can initiate tachyarrhythmias either by the induction of unstable transmural reentry or via repetitive rapid EADs inducing repetitive ventricular beats in rapid succession. Transmural variation in APD can produce substantial repolarization gradients, particularly under EAD-promoting conditions, creating favorable conditions for reentry in which functional conduction block within the ventricular wall plays an important role.

While DADs and EADs clearly have different features and occur under different conditions, both centrally involve cell Ca^{2+} homeostasis and abnormal Ca^{2+} dynamics are central to both. APD is a major determinant of Ca^{2+} entry; EAD-associated APD prolongation increases Ca^{2+} influx through L-type Ca^{2+} channels and produces Ca^{2+} loading in the SR, thus increasing the likelihood of DAD generation. Thus, EADs and DADs may occur together with common initiating conditions.[39]

Genetically modified mice have been used extensively to model congenital arrhythmogenic disorders, including LQTS. While for some LQTS forms the ionic derangements show similar physiology in mice and men (e.g., I_{Na} inactivation deficiencies responsible for LQT3), for others (particularly delayed-rectifier K^+ channel abnormalities), the mouse APD does not share the same determinants with human. The ability to generate patient-specific human iPSCs offers a new paradigm for modeling human disease. These have been used extensively to model and study mechanisms of LQTS.[40] For example, a Medline search with the term "iPSC cardiomyocytes long QT syndrome" identified 169 papers (as of April 2021). Cardiomyocytes differentiated from iPSC cells of LQTS patients recapitulate the disease phenotype in vitro, including marked APD prolongation and increased susceptibility to spontaneous or pharmacologically induced triggered activity. Large-scale production of human iPSC–derived cardiomyocytes has made it possible to generate sufficient numbers of uniform cardiac monolayers and higher-order three-dimensional models that can be used for the study of arrhythmia mechanisms in vitro.[41] Collectively, pluripotent stem cell technology now offers a unique platform to evaluate patient-specific arrhythmia mechanisms, to evaluate and optimize patient therapy and for high-throughput screens for drug proarrhythmic effects.[42]

Experimental observations have also suggested an important role of transmural or longitudinal heterogeneity of repolarization. Marked transmural dispersion of repolarization can create a vulnerable window for the development of reentry. Direct experimental evidence of the existence of transmural dispersion in the AP has been provided for the human heart. Normal hearts showed midmyocardial islands of cells that had distinctly long APDs with steep local APD gradients. In contrast, failing hearts were observed to have significantly reduced transmural repolarization gradients and to lack islands of cells with delayed repolarization. The ionic mechanisms underlying transmural dispersion of repolarization in the human heart likely include spatial variations in expression of the transient outward potassium current I_{to} and the delayed rectifier potassium current I_{Ks} (see Table 62.1).[1,43]

Sympathetic stimulation can increase EAD amplitude to provoke ventricular tachyarrhythmias. Beta-adrenergic stimulation produces a balanced increase in inward (especially $I_{Ca,L}$) and outward (I_{Ks}) currents. In LQT1, the I_{Ks} alpha subunit is defective and adrenergic stimulation causes an unopposed increase in depolarizing current, potentially producing important APD prolongation and EADs. LQT1 patients are particularly prone to adrenergic provocation of ventricular arrhythmias and tend to respond well to beta-adrenoceptor blockers.

Acquired LQTS and torsades de pointes from class III antiarrhythmic drugs like quinidine, sotalol, or dofetilide and a host of non-cardiac agents like cisapride, erythromycin, moxifloxacin, and psychoactive drugs, likely mediated by EADs (see Chapters 9 and 64).[44] Almost all of these drugs block I_{Kr}- the hERG alpha-subunit that has a large inner vestibule which easily accommodates many drugs that have HERG-block as an off-target effect.[45] Screening for hERG block and potential QT - prolongation are thus now an important part of the preclinical toxicology screen for most new drugs.[46] The problem is compounded by the idiosyncratic nature of the proarrhythmic effect, related in large measure to genetically determined "repolarization reserve." In addition, drugs may additively prolong APD and provoke EADs/torsades de pointes. In addition, drug interactions at the level of hepatic metabolism or (less commonly) renal excretion may increase the concentration of an at-risk compound.[47]

Disorders of Impulse Conduction

Conduction delay and block can result in bradyarrhythmias or tachyarrhythmias. Bradyarrhythmias occur when the propagating impulse is blocked and is followed by asystole or a slower escape rhythm; tachyarrhythmias occur when the delay and block produce reentrant excitation (see later, Reentry). Various factors involving both active and passive membrane properties determine the CV and successful propagation of an impulse. These factors include the stimulating efficacy of the propagating impulse, which is related to the amplitude and rate of rise of phase 0 (an indicator of the size of the activating phase 0 inward current); the excitability of the tissue to which the impulse is conducted; and the geometry of the tissue.

DECELERATION-DEPENDENT BLOCK

Diastolic depolarization has been suggested as a cause of conduction block at slow rates, so-called bradycardia- or deceleration-dependent block (see Chapter 68). However, excitability and the speed of impulse propagation *increase* as the membrane depolarizes until approximately −70 mV despite a reduction in AP amplitude *(supernormal conduction).* This type of block has also been referred to as "phase 4 block," but experiments in Purkinje fiber bundles have demonstrated that diastolic (phase 4) depolarization is not a necessary condition for the occurrence of deceleration-dependent block. Evidently, depolarization-induced inactivation of fast Na^+ channels is offset by other factors, such as a reduction in the difference between membrane potential and threshold potential and an increase in membrane excitability.

TACHYCARDIA-DEPENDENT BLOCK

More often, impulses are blocked at rapid rates or short cycle lengths as a result of incomplete recovery of refractoriness (postrepolarization refractoriness) caused by incomplete time- or voltage-dependent recovery of excitability. For example, such incomplete recovery is the usual mechanism responsible for a nonconducted premature P wave or one that conducts with a functional bundle branch block.

DECREMENTAL CONDUCTION

"Decremental conduction" refers to the phenomenon whereby an impulse with a low safety factor loses activation effectiveness as it spreads anterogradely. This property is most typically seen in the AV node, in relation to the relatively small amplitude of phase 0 Ca^{2+}

FIGURE 62.17 Reentry and entrainment. **A** to **E**, Criteria for entrainment exemplified in a case of postinfarction ventricular tachycardia (VT). **A**, *left,* Two leads of the ECG of a VT and intracardiac recordings from a mapping catheter (Map) at a left ventricular site critical for VT continuation, as well as from the right ventricular apex (RV). Note the diastolic potential *(red arrowhead)* during VT. Recordings are similarly arranged in all subsequent panels. **A**, *right,* RV pacing in the setting of sinus rhythm. **B**, RV pacing at a cycle length (CL) slightly shorter than VT produces a QRS complex that is a blend between fully VT and fully paced ("fusion") complexes. All recordings are accelerated to the paced CL, and after pacing ceases, the same VT resumes. Each fused QRS complex is identical, and the last beat is entrained, but surface fusion is absent. **C** and **D**, The same phenomena, but at shorter-paced CLs. Note that the fused QRS complex appears to be more similar to pacing than to VT as the pacing CL shortens. **B** to **D**, Progressive degrees of fusion on ECG. Map recording of **B, C,** and **D** also shows a progression of fusion, with both the morphology and timing of a portion of the electrogram changing with faster pacing. **E**, Finally, an even shorter-paced CL results in a sudden change in both map electrogram (block in small diastolic potential, *red arrowhead)* and surface ECG, which is now fully paced. When pacing ceases, VT has been interrupted. **F**, Diagrammatic representation of the reentrant circuit during spontaneous atrial flutter (AFL) and transient entrainment of the AFL. **Left,** Reentrant circuit during spontaneous type I AFL; *f* = circulating wavefront of the AFL. **Center,** Introduction of the first pacing impulse (X) during rapid pacing from a high atrial site during AFL. The *black arrowhead* indicates entry of the pacing impulse into the reentrant circuit, where it is conducted orthodromically (Ortho) and antidromically (Anti). The antidromic wavefront of the pacing impulse (X) collides with the previous beat, in this case the circulating wavefront of the spontaneous AFL *(f),* which results in an atrial fusion beat and, in effect, terminates the AFL. However, the orthodromic wavefront from the pacing impulse (X) continues the tachycardia and resets it to the pacing rate. **Right,** Introduction of the next pacing impulse (X + 1) during rapid pacing from the same high atrial site. The *black arrowhead* again indicates entry of the pacing impulse into the reentrant circuit, where it is conducted orthodromically and antidromically. Once again, the antidromic wavefront from the pacing impulse (X + 1) collides with the orthodromic wavefront of the previous beat. In this case, it is the orthodromic wavefront of the previous paced beat (X), and an atrial fusion beat results. The orthodromic wavefront from the pacing impulse (X + 1) continues the tachycardia and resets it to the pacing rate. In all three parts, *arrows* indicate the direction of spread of the impulses; the *serpentine line* indicates slow conduction through a presumed area of slow conduction *(stippled region)* in the reentrant circuit. (**A** to **E** from Zipes DP. A century of cardiac arrhythmia: in search of Jason's golden fleece. *J Am Coll Cardiol.* 1999;34:959; **F** from Waldo AL. Atrial flutter: entrainment characteristics. *J Cardiovasc Electrophysiol.* 1997;8:337.)

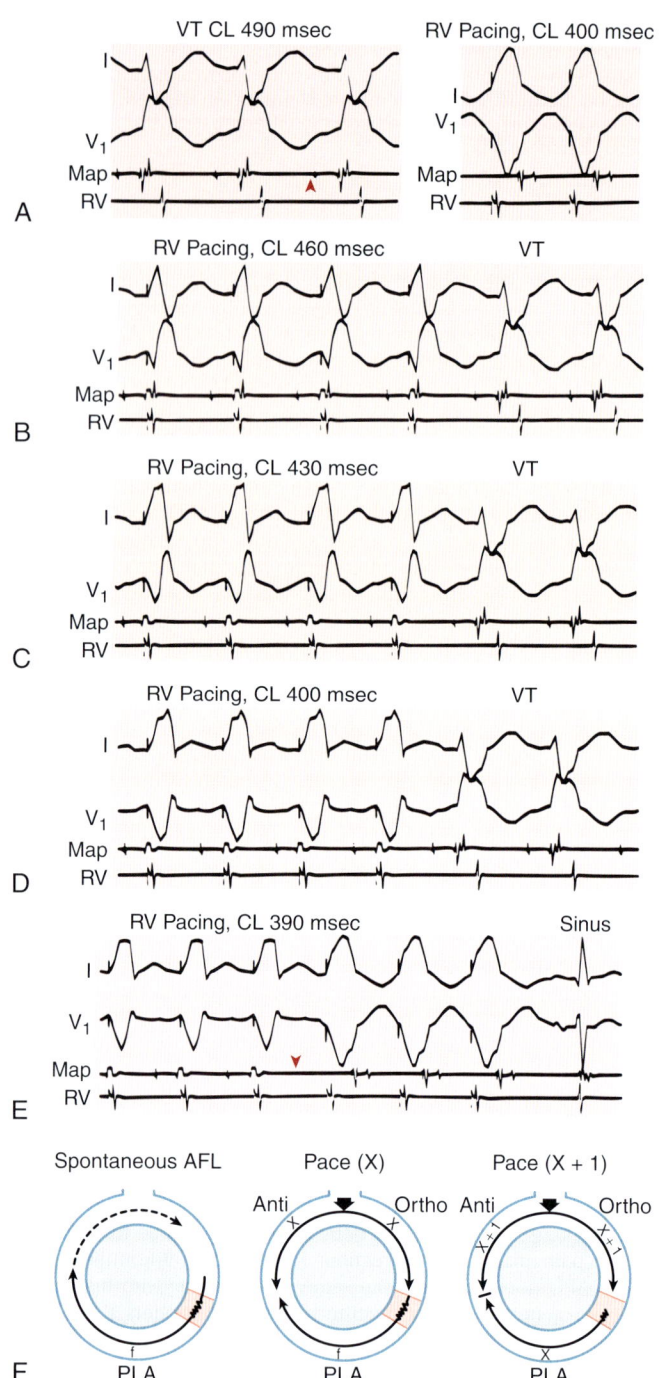

current in slow channel tissue, especially at fast rates and in the presence of disease. It is also a feature of diseased tissue with conduction impairment due to cell death, fibrosis, and/or reduced phase 0 activating current. Decremental conduction is associated with increased risk of conduction block.

REENTRY
During the normal cardiac cycle, activation begins in the SAN pacemaker and continues until the entire heart has been activated. The cardiac impulse stops propagating when all fibers have been discharged and are completely refractory. During this absolute RP, the cardiac impulse has "no place to go." Activation is then reinitiated by the next sinus impulse. If, however, a group of fibers not activated during the initial wave of depolarization recovers excitability in time to be reactivated before the impulse dies out, the fibers may serve as a link to reexcite areas that were just discharged and have now recovered from the initial depolarization. Such a process has been given various names—reentry, reentrant excitation, circus movement, reciprocal or echo beat, and reciprocating tachycardia—and all have approximately the same meaning.

ENTRAINMENT
Entraining a tachycardia (i.e., increasing the rate of the tachycardia through capture of the reentry circuit by pacing),[48] with resumption of the intrinsic rate of the tachycardia when pacing is stopped, is a clinically accessible way to establish the presence of reentry (Fig. 62.17A). Entrainment represents capture or continuous resetting of the tachycardia by the pacing-induced activation. Each pacing stimulus creates a wavefront that travels in an anterograde direction (orthodromic) and resets the tachycardia to the pacing rate. A wavefront propagating retrogradely in the opposite direction (antidromic) collides with the orthodromic wavefront of the previous beat. In the clinical example shown in Figure 62.17, as the RV pacing rate is increased, the paced QRS morphology (Fig. 62.17B–D) changes, the result of more of the tachycardia circuit being captured by the anterograde activation wave, yet when pacing is stopped, the tachycardia is still present; this is referred to as *progressive fusion.* These wavefront interactions create electrocardiographic and electrophysiologic features that can be explained only by reentry. Therefore, the demonstration of entrainment can be used to prove the reentrant mechanism of a clinical tachycardia and form the basis for localizing the pathway traveled by the tachycardia wavefront. Such localization can be useful to guide ablation therapy.

Anatomic Reentry
Anatomic reentry inspired the first conceptual models of reentry.[48] In anatomic reentry, there is a discrete anatomical barrier separating alternate conduction pathways, and allowing reentry to be initiated and maintained. A conceptual model presented as a schematic of the occurrence of anatomic reentry with the required conditions is shown in Figure 62.18. In many individuals, the AV node behaves as if there are two functionally independent pathways with common connections at top and bottom, but longitudinally dissociated in between. Typically, the pathway with the faster conduction has a longer RP. Both pathways have RPs much shorter than the SAN cycle

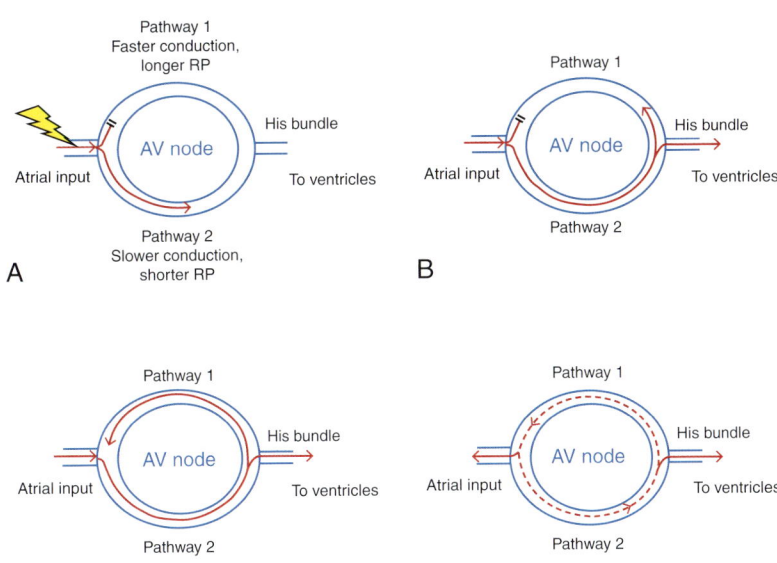

FIGURE 62.18 Schematic of reentry in the AV node (AVN). Differences in conduction and refractoriness in the fast (1) and slow (2) pathways permit reentry to occur. **A**, Activation of the AVN from the atrium with block in the fast, longer refractory period pathway with conduction down the slow pathway. **B**, Activation of the His bundle and ventricle from the slow pathway with the activation wave retrogradely activating the fast pathway. **C**, Atrial activation from the AVN over the fast pathway with a short time from ventricular (QRS) to atrial (retrograde P) activation. **D**, Typical AV node reentry tachycardia circuit.

length, so a premature beat is required in order to engage the AV node during the RP of either pathway. Figure 62.18A illustrates a premature beat arriving during the RP of the fast pathway (here designated Pathway 1) but after the shorter-RP pathway (Pathway 2) has recovered excitability. The impulse then travels antegradely down Pathway 2 to the His bundle entrance, conducting via the His bundle to the ventricles (Fig. 62.18B). If the distal end of Pathway 1 has now had time to recover, the impulse will propagate retrogradely up Pathway 1 (Fig 62.18C). If the circuit time (the time to leave each point in the circuit and get back to the initial point of reference) is longer than the RP of Pathway 2, it will now be reexcited in the antegrade direction and the process can continue indefinitely (Fig 62.18D) if the conditions are right. The key determinants are: (1) alternative conducting pathways separated longitudinally but with connections at each end; (2) different RPs of the alternate pathways allowing for block of a premature beat in one pathway; and (3) a circuit time longer than the longest RO in the pathway.

A realistic example of AV nodal reentry using different pathways is illustrated in Figure 62.19. Because the two pathways have different electrophysiologic properties (e.g., shorter RP and slower conduction in one pathway versus a longer RP and faster conduction in the other), the impulse is first blocked anterogradely in the fast pathway with the longer RP and then propagates slowly in the adjacent slow pathway, whose RP is shorter (Fig. 62.19A). If conduction in this alternative route is sufficiently slow, the propagating impulse finds tissue that has recovered from refractoriness throughout its circuit, exciting tissue beyond the blocked pathway and returning in the reverse direction along the pathway initially blocked, to reexcite tissue proximal to the site of block (Fig. 62.19B). A clinical arrhythmia caused by anatomic reentry is most likely to have a monomorphic morphology on ECG. For anatomic reentry to occur, the time for conduction within the depressed but unblocked area and for excitation of the distal segments must exceed the RP of the initially blocked pathway and the tissue proximal to the site of block.

CONDITIONS FOR ANATOMIC REENTRY

The length of the pathway is fixed and determined by the anatomy. Conditions that depress CV or abbreviate the RP promote the development of reentry in this model, whereas prolonging refractoriness and speeding CV hinder it. The maintenance of anatomic reentry requires the existence of an "excitable gap," a region ahead of the reentrant wavefront that has recovered excitability and is available for re-excitation. Conceptually, the distance traveled by the impulse in one RP is the minimum distance that can support reentry with anatomical reentry. This distance, termed the reentrant wavelength (λ) is equal to the minimum circuit time (the RP) multiplied by the mean CV. The actual length of the pathway minus λ gives the length of the excitable gap.

In reentrant circuits with an excitable gap, CV determines the revolution time of the impulse around the circuit and therefore the rate of the tachycardia. Prolongation of refractoriness does not influence the revolution time around the circuit or the rate of the tachycardia, with the rare exception when the revolution exactly equals the RP and makes the impulse propagate in relatively refractory tissue. Anatomic reentry occurs in patients with Wolff-Parkinson-White (WPW) syndrome (Fig. 62.20), in AV nodal reentry, in some atrial flutters, and in some VTs.

Functional Reentry

Functional reentry lacks confining anatomic boundaries and can occur in contiguous fibers that exhibit functionally different electrophysiologic properties caused by local differences in transmembrane AP, APD, or other determinants of excitability. Dispersion of excitability, refractoriness, or both, as well as anisotropic distributions of intercellular resistance, permit initiation and maintenance of reentry. Functional heterogeneities in the electrophysiologic properties of the myocardium have been shown to contribute to the generation and maintenance of tachycardia and fibrillation. These heterogeneities can be fixed, as in the case of spatial redistribution of gap junctions in the failing heart or infarct border zone, or with spatial gradients in the magnitude of the background K^+ current I_{K1}. They can also change dynamically, as in an acutely ischemic myocardium or in the presence of dynamic autonomic tone changes that influence RP in a spatially heterogeneous way (e.g., vagal AF).

An important concept in understanding functional reentry is that of a spiral wave rotor.[49] The development of functional block along a line of tissue causes the impulse to circulate around the initial zone of block. The pattern of propagation is often represented as a circle or ellipse, but its shape depends on underlying tissue properties, anisotropy, and heterogeneity. A schematic of such a system is shown in Figure 62.21A. The reentrant wavefront (shown by a solid red curve) has a curvature that is greatest near the center of the wave, and gradually decreases at portions of the front progressively further from the core. Behind the propagating wavefront, there is a zone of refractory tissue that ends at the dashed red curve, with the tissue inside the dashed border having recovered excitability. Where the curvature is relatively flat (see brown box and insert), the propagating wavefront stimulates a region of tissue in front of it that is about the same size as the wavefront. As the curvature increases (black box), the emanating wavefront has to activate much larger regions of tissue relative to the source wavefront. At the center of the spiral is a zone where the curvature is so great that the source-sink mismatch causes failure of activation. This zone creates a "core" of excitable but non-excited tissue. If the properties of the tissue are such that the recirculating "rotor" can continue uninterrupted, the resulting stable rotor will cause a sustained tachycardia. An example of such a reentrant wave in simulated 2-dimensional tissue is shown in Figure 62.21B. If there are multiple unsynchronized rotors, or a single rotor with a variable tissue response with irregular propagation patterns, fibrillation results. Fibrillatory activity can be maintained by highly unstable rotors, providing their rate of formation is greater or equal to their rate of destruction.

The detection of rotors in tissue can be facilitated by the use of "phase mapping," which defines the activation at each point in space relative to the phase in an activation cycle in which it occurs.[49] At the inner tip of the activation wavefront, there is a location at which all phases meet, called a "phase singularity" (PS). Identifying and following the PS trajectory over time is useful to keep track

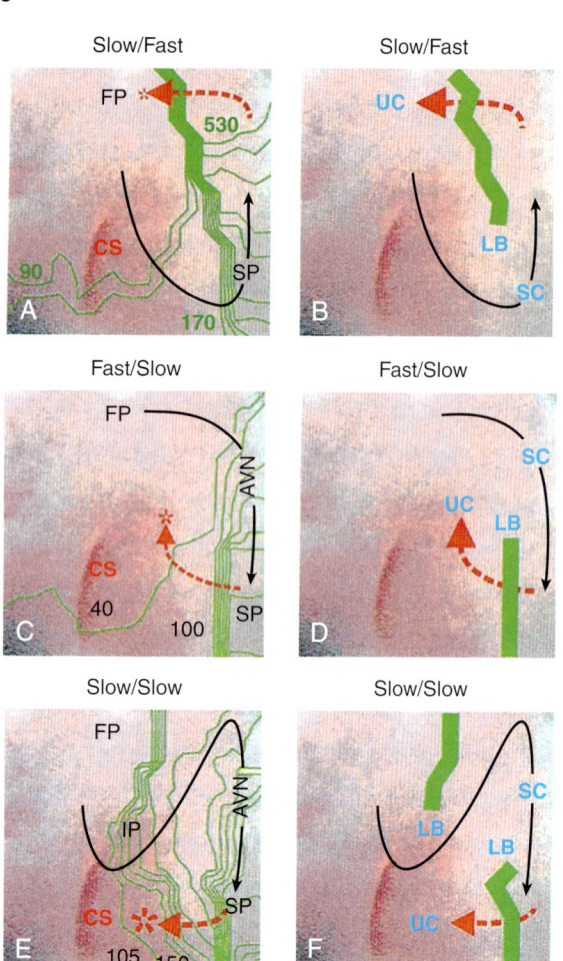

FIGURE 62.19 Reentrant circuits of different types of atrioventricular nodal reentrant tachycardia (AVNRT). Pictures of the optical activation maps of A_2 stimuli obtained from three different experiments at A_2 coupling intervals of 190, 220, and 190 milliseconds, respectively, were merged with the pictures of the mapping area to show the initiation of echo beats in **A** (Slow/Fast), **C** (Fast/Slow), and **E** (Slow/Slow) circuits. The numbers on the maps indicate the activation times in reference to the A_2 stimulus. The *black arrow* indicates anterograde conduction, and the *asterisk* and the *dashed red arrow* represent the site of earliest retrograde atrial activation. The corresponding locations of the lines of block (LB, *green*), slow anterograde conduction (SC, *black arrow*), and unidirectional conduction (UC, *red*) are shown in **B, D,** and **F,** respectively. *CS,* Coronary sinus; *FP,* fast pathway; *IP,* intermediate pathway; *SP,* slow pathway. (From Wu J, Zipes DP. Mechanisms underlying atrioventricular nodal conduction and the reentrant circuit of atrioventricular nodal reentrant tachycardia using optical mapping. J Cardiovasc Electrophysiol. 2002;13:831.)

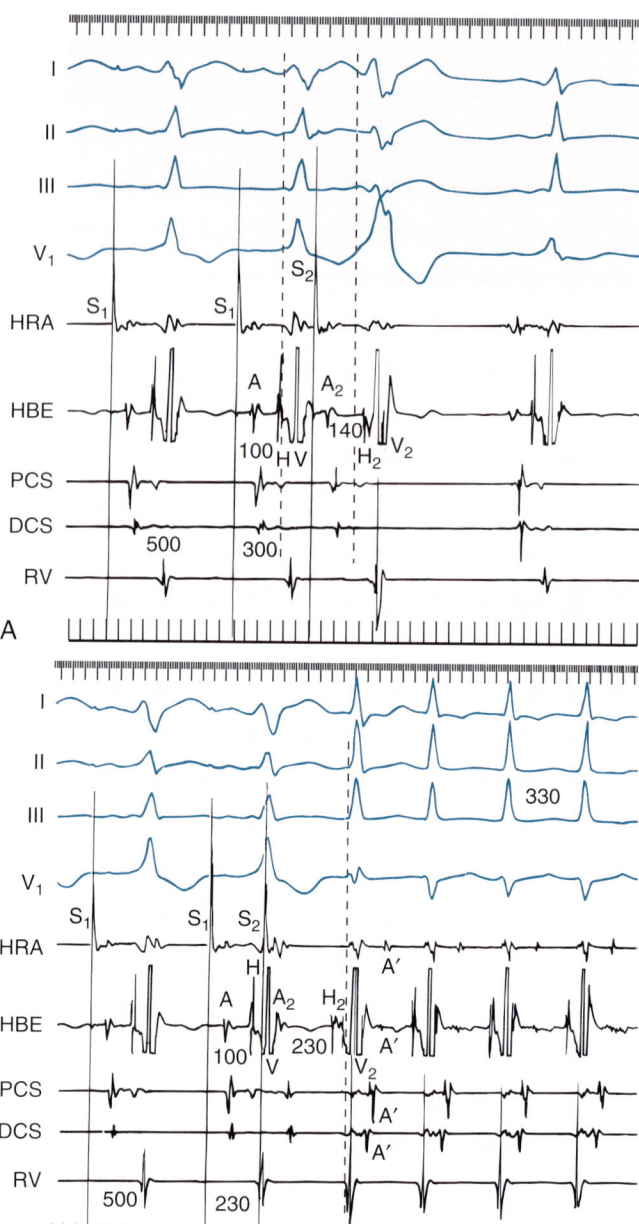

FIGURE 62.20 A, Wolff-Parkinson-White syndrome. Following high right atrial pacing at a cycle length of 500 milliseconds (S_1–S_1), premature stimulation at a coupling interval of 300 milliseconds (S_1–S_2) produces physiologic delay in AV nodal conduction, which results in an increase in the A-H interval from 100 to 140 milliseconds but no delay in the AV interval. Consequently, activation of the His bundle follows activation of the QRS complex *(second interrupted line),* and the QRS complex becomes more anomalous in appearance because of increased ventricular activation over the accessory pathway. **B,** Induction of reciprocating AV tachycardia. Premature stimulation at a coupling interval of 230 milliseconds prolongs the A_2–H_2 interval to 230 milliseconds and results in anterograde block in the accessory pathway and normalization of the QRS complex (a slight functional aberrancy in the nature of incomplete right bundle branch block occurs). Note that H_2 precedes onset of the QRS complex *(interrupted line).* Following V_2, the atria are excited retrogradely (A′) beginning in the distal coronary sinus, followed by atrial activation in leads recording from the proximal coronary sinus, His bundle, and high right atrium. A supraventricular tachycardia is initiated at a cycle length of 330 milliseconds. I, II, III, and V_1 indicate scalar electrocardiographic leads. A, H–V, atrial, His bundle, and ventricular activation during the drive train; A_2, H_2, V_2, atrial, His bundle, and ventricular activation during the premature stimulus; *DCS,* distal coronary sinus electrogram; *HBE,* His bundle electrogram; *HRA,* high right atrium; *PCS,* proximal coronary sinus electrogram; *RV,* right ventricular electrogram. Timelines are in 50- and 10-millisecond intervals. S_1, Stimulus of the drive train; S_2, premature stimulus. (From Zipes DP, Mahomed Y, King RD, et al. Wolff-Parkinson-White syndrome: cryosurgical treatment. Indiana Med. 1986;89:432.)

of complex, often short-lived rotors. Sophisticated mapping studies have revealed reentrant rotors in a wide range of experimental and clinical arrhythmias, including VT and atrial and ventricular fibrillation.[50]

Specific Arrhythmias Illustrating Mechanistic Principles

Other chapters in this book deal with various forms of specific arrhythmias including supraventricular and VTs, flutter, and fibrillation (see Chapters 65 and 67). We will discuss a variety of arrhythmias here focused on their mechanistic properties to illustrate the basic principles of electrophysiology and arrhythmogenesis discussed in the present chapter.

Atrial Flutter
Reentry is the most likely cause of the usual form of atrial flutter, with the reentrant circuit being confined to the right atrium in typical atrial flutter, where it usually travels counterclockwise in a caudocranial direction in the interatrial septum and in a craniocaudal direction in the right atrial free wall. An area of slow conduction is present in the posterolateral to posteromedial inferior area of the right atrium, along with a central area of block that can include an anatomic (IVC) and functional component. This area of slow

conduction is rather constant and represents the site of successful ablation of typical atrial flutter. Ablation results are consistent with a macroreentry circuit.

Different reentrant circuits exist in patients with other types of atrial flutter, such as those that occur after surgery or ablation or that are associated with an atrial septal defect (see Chapter 82).

Atrial Fibrillation

Spatiotemporal Organization and Focal Discharge

AF is characterized by rapid irregular atrial activity. The classical theory is that of multiple disorganized reentrant waves, encapsulated by Moe's "multiple-wavelet hypothesis," but a variety of competing theories and ideas of AF pathophysiology have emerged (see Chapter 66).[49,51] While atrial activation during AF appears to be random, there is in fact an underlying organization, likely related to both discrete determining electrophysiological characteristics and non-random sources. The activity of underlying sources may be reflected in dominant frequencies of activation in spectral analyses of recordings of atrial electrical activity. The notion that a single or small number of underlying focal or rotor sources underlie AF and may be susceptible to targeted ablation is a very attractive idea. There is extensive evidence that the PVs are particularly prone to host both focal and reentrant sources, and PV ablation is the single most effective procedure for AF management.[52] The localization of sources in other regions, which seem to be increasingly important as AF becomes more persistent and enduring, has proved difficult and is the object of extensive ongoing technological, scientific, and clinical investigation.[53]

Several experimental models have been used to study the structural and basic electrophysiologic properties of PVs that are thought to play a role in initiation and maintenance of AF. Morphologic studies have demonstrated the presence of complex anatomic structures and phenotypically different cardiomyocytes in PVs.[1,54] Electrophysiologic studies have shown that both reentrant and nonreentrant mechanisms (automaticity and triggered activity) may underlie initiation of AF from the PVs.

ION CHANNEL ABNORMALITIES IN ATRIAL FIBRILLATION
Monogenic (Familial) Atrial Fibrillation

Although familial forms of AF are relatively rare, identification of mutations in AF kindreds has provided valuable insight into the molecular pathways underlying the arrhythmia. Most mutations linked to familial AF have been located in genes that encode sodium or potassium channel subunits. Functional analyses of these mutations have revealed either gain-of-function or loss-of-function effects. Mutations in genes encoding pore-forming alpha or auxiliary beta subunits of the delayed rectifier potassium channel and the voltage-gated sodium channel (I_{Ks} and I_{Na}, respectively; see Table 62.1) have been reported in familial AF. The mechanisms by which these mutations cause AF are not fully understood. Gain-of-function mutations in I_{Ks} give rise to increased repolarizing currents, which then shorten the APD and atrial refractoriness, thereby facilitating fibrillatory activity. An augmented inward sodium current can increase excitability and promote triggered activity. Conversely, a reduced inward sodium current might promote reentry by favoring block and the initiation of reentry. Other potassium channel mutations in the *KCNJ2* and *KCNA5* genes, which encode the inward rectifier and ultrarapid delayed rectifier potassium current, respectively, have been associated with AF (see Table 62.1). Finally, mutations in the *GJA5* gene, which encodes the gap junction channel subunit connexin 40, have been linked to familial AF. Abnormal intercellular electrical coupling can produce conduction heterogeneity, localized block, and facilitated reentry.

Polygenic Factors in Atrial Fibrillation

A significant portion of AF risk is heritable. Genome-wide association studies (GWAS) have identified variations in multiple genomic regions that are associated with lone AF. These regions encode ion channels (e.g., calcium-activated potassium channel gene *KCNN3*, HCN channel gene *HCN4*), transcription factors related to cardiopulmonary development (e.g., homeodomain transcription factor PRRX1), and cell-signaling molecules (e.g., CAV1, a cellular membrane protein involved in signal transduction). The mechanistic links between these genetic variations and susceptibility to AF remain to be determined.[55] Only a small percentage of the AF risk can be attributed to known gene polymorphisms; a more expansive approach combining GWAS, whole blood epigenome-wide association, and transcriptome-wide association reveals almost 2000 genes linked to AF and accounts for about three times as much (about 10% vs. 3%) of the AF risk.[56] Nevertheless, there are still major risk determinants outside present genetically identified factors. With the rapid technologic development of genetic approaches and the creation of ever-larger merged databases, the identification of genetic factors underlying AF will certainly progress; however, since genetics account for only a portion of AF risk and disease factors like hypertension, heart disease, diabetes, and toxins (cigarette smoke, environmental pollution, etc.) are also major determinants there will likely be a limit to how much insight into AF risk genetic studies can provide.

A number of studies have probed the primary role of abnormalities in ion channel expression or related properties in causing AF. In human tissue studies, diastolic Ca^{2+} leak and associated triggered activity in right atrial appendage myocytes are associated with paroxysmal and persistent AF, as well as post-operative AF.[57] Conduction abnormalities are frequently found in AF patients and are likely related to reentry-promoting tissue fibrosis[58,59] and disturbances in connexin expression and/or function.[21,58]

Remodeling of the Atria

Remodeling of atrial structure and/or electrical function occurs as a result of risk factors, heart disease, and AF itself, and appears to be a key determinant of AF occurrence, persistence, and resistance to therapy. Prolonged rapid atrial rates cause electrophysiologic alterations in the atria, including shortening and loss of the physiologic rate adaptation of refractoriness and a decrease in CV. The ionic mechanisms underlying shortening of the RP and slowing of conduction includes downregulation of L-type Ca^{2+} and Na^+ currents, upregulation of I_{K1}, and disturbances in connexin expression and distribution.[57] In addition, remodeling of autonomic innervation and function appears to play an important role in both triggering and maintaining AF.[60] Rapid rates and a variety of underlying conditions promote the development of atrial fibrosis, which favors AF progression. Finally, there is extensive emerging evidence that inflammatory signaling plays a central role in AF pathophysiology, contributing to the ion channel/transporter and structural changes that underlie the AF substrate.[61,62]

Sinus Node Reentry

The SA node shares with the AV node electrophysiologic features like the potential for dissociation of conduction; that is, an impulse can be conducted in some nodal fibers but not in others, permitting reentry to occur (see Chapter 65). The reentrant circuit can be located entirely within the SA node or may involve both the SA node and atrium. Supraventricular tachycardias caused by sinus node reentry are generally less symptomatic than other SVTs because of slower rates. Ablation of the SA node may occasionally be necessary for refractory tachycardia.

Atrial Reentry

Reentry within the atrium, unrelated to the SA node, can be a cause of SVT in humans. Distinguishing AT caused by automaticity or afterdepolarizations from AT sustained by reentry over small areas (i.e., microanatomic reentry) is difficult.

Atrioventricular Nodal Reentry

The mechanisms underlying AV node reentry are discussed in detail above. For further information, see Chapter 65.

Preexcitation Syndrome

Preexcitation results from fibers that bypass the AV node and allow for more rapid communication between atria and ventricles than is normally permitted by the AV node. These connections can produce the substrate for anatomical reentry involving the atria, AV node, ventricles, and bypass tract, generally referred to as "*atrioventricular reciprocating tachycardia*" (AVRT). In most patients who have reciprocating tachycardias associated with WPW syndrome, the accessory pathway conducts more rapidly than the normal AV node but takes a longer time to recover excitability; that is, the anterograde RP of the accessory pathway exceeds that of the AV node. Consequently, a premature

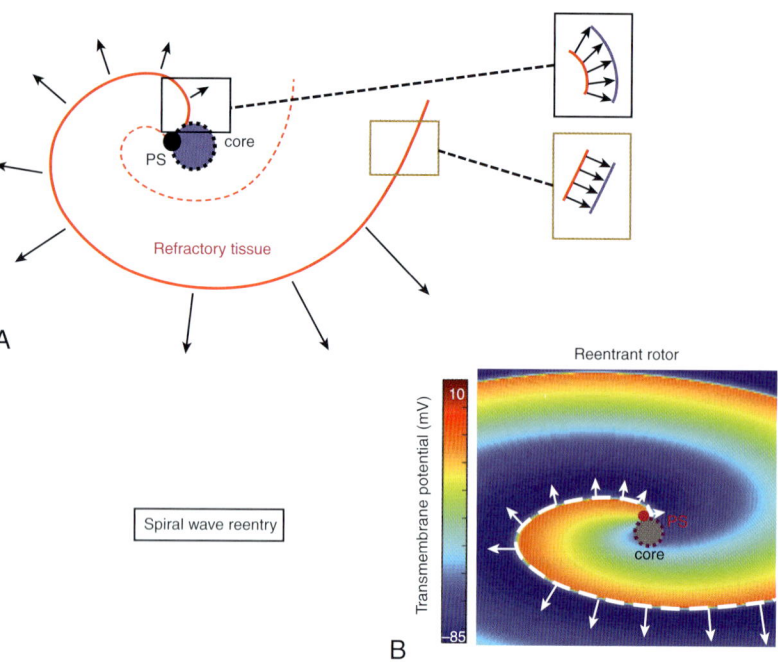

FIGURE 62.21 Spiral wave reentry due to functional block generating a rotor. **A,** Reentrant wavefront (*solid red curve*) with greatest curvature near the center of the wave. Tissue behind the wavefront is refractory (ending at the *dashed red curve*), with the tissue inside the dashed border having recovered excitability. The core is characterized by a high degree of curvature causing inexcitability due to source-sink mismatch. **B,** An example of a reentrant wave in simulated 2-dimensional tissue.

atrial complex that occurs sufficiently early is blocked anterogradely in the accessory pathway and continues to the ventricle over the normal AV node and His bundle. After the ventricles have been excited, the impulse is able to enter the accessory pathway retrogradely and return to the atrium. A continuous conduction loop of this type establishes the circuit for the tachycardia. The usual (orthodromic) activation wave during such a reciprocating tachycardia in a patient with an accessory pathway occurs anterogradely over the normal AV node–His-Purkinje system and retrogradely over the accessory pathway, which results in a normal-duration QRS complex (see Fig. 62.20). Occasionally, the activation wave travels in a reverse (antidromic) direction to the ventricles over the accessory pathway and to the atria retrogradely up the AV node. Two accessory pathways can form the circuit in some patients with antidromic AVRT. In some patients, the accessory pathway may be capable of only retrograde conduction ("concealed"), but the circuit and mechanism of AVRT remain the same. Less frequently, the accessory pathway can conduct only anterogradely. The pathway can be localized by ECG analysis. Developmental studies in mice have demonstrated that myocardium-specific inactivation of T-box 2 (Tbx2), a transcription factor essential for AV canal patterning, leads to the formation of fast-conducting accessory pathways, malformation of the annulus fibrosus, and ventricular preexcitation in mice.[63]

Ventricular Tachycardia Caused by Reentry

Reentry in the ventricle, both anatomic and functional, as a cause of sustained VT has been supported by many animal and clinical studies (see Chapter 67). Reentry in ventricular muscle, with or without contributions from specialized tissue, is responsible for many or most VTs in patients with ischemic heart disease. The area of microreentry appears to be small, and less often a macroreentry circuit is found around the infarct scar. Surviving myocardial tissue separated by connective tissue provides serpentine routes of activation traversing infarcted areas that can establish reentry pathways. Bundle branch reentry, macroreentry using the specialized conduction system, can cause sustained VT, particularly in patients with dilated cardiomyopathy.

Both figure-of-eight and single-circle reentrant loops have been described as circulating around an area of functional block or as conducting slowly across an apparent area of block created by anisotropy. When intramural myocardium survives, it can form part of the reentrant loop. Structural discontinuities that separate muscle bundles—as a result of the naturally occurring myocardial fiber orientation and anisotropic conduction, as well as collagen matrices formed from the fibrosis after MI—establish the basis for slowed conduction and fragmented electrograms, which can lead to reentry. After MI, the surviving epicardial border zone undergoes substantial electrical remodeling, including reduced CV and increased anisotropy associated with the occurrence of reentrant circuits and VT. Slowing of conduction arises from alterations in the spatial distribution and electrophysiologic properties of connexin 43 gap junctions, as well as from reduced voltage-gated sodium current. It has been speculated that myocyte depolarization secondary to electrotonic coupling to adjacent myofibroblasts (which typically have a much more depolarized potential) plays a role in electrical dysfunction in postinfarction border-zone myocardium. While sophisticated studies using advanced microscopy techniques suggest that such coupling is possible,[64] their actual role in clinically relevant arrhythmogenesis and potential for therapeutic targeting are still uncertain. During acute ischemia, various factors, including elevated $[K^+]_o$ and reduced pH, combine to create depressed APs in ischemic cells that impede conduction and can lead to reentry. A great deal of effort has gone into defining the ionic basis of these changes; however, efforts to apply this knowledge to provide viable clinical therapeutics have largely failed and interest has shifted to primary prevention against the atherosclerosis leading to MI and prevention of myocardial damage by rapid reperfusion of acutely ischemic tissue via interventional procedures.

Brugada Syndrome

Brugada syndrome is a congenital sudden death syndrome involving characteristic electrocardiographic abnormalities. These typically include ST-segment elevation (unrelated to ischemia, electrolyte abnormalities, or structural heart disease) in the right precordial (V_1 to V_3) leads of the ECG, often but not always accompanied by an apparent right bundle branch block (see Fig. 61.3). Early repolarization in localized myocardial regions is often a central factor, although conduction abnormalities have also been observed, and the relative role of repolarization versus depolarization abnormalities remains controversial. The hereditary nature of the syndrome is well established; however, a wide variety of genes and ion-channel abnormalities have been associated and it is apparent that simple mendelian transmission does not explain the phenotypic expression in many cases.[65] The single most common genetic abnormalities in Brugada syndrome are loss-of-function mutations in *SCN5A* (Table 62.1), which encodes the pore-forming cardiac sodium channel alpha subunit Nav1.5, and mutations in *SCN1B*, *SCN2B*, and *SCN3B*, which encode the function-modifying sodium channel beta subunits (see Chapter 63). However, mutations in the α and β subunits of the Ca^{2+} channel and several potassium channel genes have been found in some patients with Brugada syndrome, as have mutations in the glycerol-3-phosphate dehydrogenase 1–like (*GPD1L*) and other genes that encode proteins that regulate the functional expression of the Na$^+$ current I_{Na}. Brugada syndrome–associated gene defects cause a reduction or loss of sodium or calcium current in combination with altered functional properties of voltage-gated sodium channels.[65] While the apparent localization of Brugada syndrome substrates points to the potential applicability of catheter ablation, results to date have been mixed and improvement is needed before ablation becomes an effective and widely applicable therapy.[66]

Catecholaminergic Polymorphic Ventricular Tachycardia

CPVT is an inherited arrhythmogenic syndrome characterized by stress-induced, adrenergically mediated polymorphic VT occurring in structurally normal hearts. The common mechanism underlying RyR2-associated CPVT is spontaneous diastolic Ca^{2+} leak from the SR via RyR2, leading to intracellular Ca^{2+} waves and triggered activity. While RyR2 mutations are responsible for about 95% of cases, CPVT can also occur because of mutations in genes encoding calsequestrin, calmodulin, and triadin, all proteins that interact with RyR2 and regulate its function.[67] Beta-adrenergic tone resulting from stimulation by catecholamines has a central role in modulating RyR2 function, both by increasing RyR2-sensitivity to Ca^{2+} by enhancing PKA and CaMKII-mediated phosphorylation, and by increasing SR Ca^{2+}-loading through increased $I_{Ca,L}$ and SERCA activity, effects that largely account for the "C" in CPVT. Thus, beta-adrenergic receptor blockade is the mainstay of CPVT therapy. For patients that are not adequately controlled by beta-blockers, flecainide is a safe and largely effective therapy,[68] acting by directly inhibiting RyR2 Ca^{2+}-release and/or by inhibiting I_{Na} to decrease cellular excitability and cellular Ca^{2+}-loading through the reduced phase-0 Na^+-influx and subsequent exchange for extracellular Ca^{2+} via NCX.

Arrhythmogenic Right Ventricular Cardiomyopathy

ARVC is an inherited myopathy characterized by sustained monomorphic VT and sudden death (see Chapter 52). At least 16 genes have been associated with ARVC-causing mutations.[69] The majority are mutations in genes encoding proteins of the cardiac desmosome, a component of the intercalated disc essential for mechanical coupling between cardiomyocytes. Mutations in the desmosomal proteins, intercalated disk proteins, nuclear envelope proteins, along with desmin, titin, phospholamban, channel proteins, and growth factors have been identified in patients with ARVC. Approximately 20% to 45% of the pathogenic mutations linked to ARVC are in the gene encoding plakophilin 2 (*PKP2*), which interacts with other cytoskeletal proteins to stabilize the desmosome. Loss of *PKP2* expression reduces the voltage-gated sodium current and connexin 43 expression at the intercalated disc and thus results in slowed AP propagation. Shared phenotypic, genetic, and functional features suggest pathogenic links between ARVC and Brugada syndrome.[69] The pathophysiology of ARVC illustrates the interrelatedness of tissue mechanical integrity and cardiac bioelectricity, as well as the critical role of the intercalated disk in electrophysiological function.

Ventricular Fibrillation: Fibrillation Initiation and Maintenance

Previous experimental and simulation investigations point to reentry as the central mechanism underlying VF (see Chapter 67). While the reentry underlying VF was classically thought to be randomly maintained by wandering wavelets of activation, more recent investigations have suggested underlying spatiotemporal organization and pointed to the role of spiral-wave reentry in maintaining VF. Important roles have been identified for both focal activity in initiating reentry and rotor sources maintaining VF.[70] These have been translated into promising ablation approaches for patients with recurrent VF episodes.[71]

The hallmark of cardiac fibrillation is ongoing wave break (or wave splitting). Wave break is caused by conduction block occurring at a specific site along the wavefront while the remaining portions of the front continue to propagate. This localized block, wave break, causes splitting of a primary spiral wavefront into two daughter wavelets. The daughter wavefronts can collide and annihilate each other, or can form independent reentry-supporting spiral-wave generators.[49,70] Two hypotheses exist regarding the genesis of wave breaks during fibrillation. The "mother rotor" hypothesis states that VF is maintained by a single, stationary, intramural stable reentrant circuit (i.e., the mother rotor) in a dominant domain, which has the shortest RP from which activations propagate into the more slowly activating domains with longer RPs. In this case, the fastest activating (i.e., dominating) rotor rather than ongoing wave break is the engine driving cardiac fibrillation, and wave break occurs only secondarily. High-resolution electrical mapping has suggested that fast activation during VF is driven by Purkinje fibers. Spatial heterogeneity in the magnitude of ionic currents has been implicated in the generation of spatial gradients in activation rates and in maintaining rotor stability in the fastest activating regions. For example, the magnitude of the inward rectifying K^+ current I_{K1} (see Table 62.1) is a critical determinant of rotor frequency and sustainability.[49]

The involvement of rotors in cardiac fibrillation does not require the presence of a single or small number of dominant rotors. As long as the destruction and creation rate of rotors are such that a critical number of rotor generators are present at all times, fibrillation will sustain itself indefinitely. A major determinant of the dynamically induced component of heterogeneity leading to reentry has been identified as electrical restitution, or variation of the AP duration and CV with the diastolic interval. For example, it has been proposed that the breakup of periodic waves is precipitated by APD alternans sufficiently large to cause conduction block along the spiral wavefront. Simulations have shown that a reentrant rotor becomes unstable and breaks down into multiple rotors when the slope of the restitution curve for the APD versus the diastolic interval is greater than 1. At the cellular level, the steepness of the APD restitution curve and intracellular calcium level ($[Ca^{2+}]_i$) dynamics cause the APD and $[Ca^{2+}]_i$ transient to alternate. Given the bidirectional coupling between changes in $[Ca^{2+}]_i$ and membrane potential—for example, the membrane potential determines the activity of L-type Ca channels, and conversely, the $[Ca^{2+}]_i$ transient amplitude strongly modulates the APD through its effects on Ca^{2+}-sensitive currents (e.g., $I_{Na/Ca}$ and I_{Ca}) during the AP plateau—an alternation in $[Ca^{2+}]_i$ transient amplitude causes a secondary alternation in the APD. Recent work has shown that AF-induced Ca^{2+}-handling remodeling promotes aberrant RyR2 Ca^{2+}-releases associated with enhanced Ca^{2+} and APD alternans, leading to a vulnerability spatially discordant alternans that initiates and stabilizes AF.[72] Manipulations that alter cellular Ca^{2+}-handling in a way that decreases alternans might provide novel approaches to prevent fibrillation.

REFERENCES

1. Tomaselli GF, Rubart M, Zipes DP. Mechanisms of cardiac arrhythmias. In: Zipes DP, Libby P, Bonow RO, Mann DL, Tomaselli GF, eds. *Braunwald's Heart Disease, a Textbook of Cardiovascular Medicine*. 11th ed. Philadelphia, PA: Elsevier; 2016.
2. Bengel P, Ahmad S, Tirilomis P, et al. Contribution of the neuronal sodium channel Nav1.8 to sodium- and calcium-dependent cellular proarrhythmia. *J Mol Cell Cardiol*. 2020;144:35–46.
3. Carmeliet E. Pacemaking in cardiac tissue. From Ik2 to a coupled-clock system. *Physiol Rep*. 2019;7:e13862.
4. Yang KC, Nerbonne JM. Mechanisms contributing to myocardial potassium channel diversity, regulation and remodeling. *Trends Cardiovasc Med*. 2016;26:209–218.
5. Shamsaldeen YA, Culliford L, Clout M, et al. Role of SK channel activation in determining the action potential configuration in freshly isolated human atrial myocytes from the SKArF study. *Biochem Biophys Res Commun*. 2019;512:684–690.
6. Rahm AK, Lugenbiel P, Schweizer PA, et al. Role of ion channels in heart failure and channelopathies. *Biophys Rev*. 2018;10:1097–1106.
7. Jiang D, Shi H, Tonggu L, et al. Structure of the cardiac sodium channel. *Cell*. 2020;180:122–134 e110.
8. Ahern CA, Payandeh J, Bosmans F, et al. The hitchhiker's guide to the voltage-gated sodium channel galaxy. *J Gen Physiol*. 2016;147:1–24.
9. Balse E, Eichel C. The cardiac sodium channel and its protein partners. *Handb Exp Pharmacol*. 2018;246:73–99.
10. Briot J, Tetreault MP, Bourdin B, et al. Inherited ventricular arrhythmias: the role of the multi-subunit structure of the l-type calcium channel complex. *Adv Exp Med Biol*. 2017;966:55–64.
11. Li Y, Zhang X, Zhang C, et al. Increasing t-type calcium channel activity by beta-adrenergic stimulation contributes to beta-adrenergic regulation of heart rates. *J Physiol*. 2018;596:1137–1151.
12. Nerbonne JM. Molecular basis of functional myocardial potassium channel diversity. *Card Electrophysiol Clin*. 2016;8:257–273.
13. Jeevaratnam K, Chadda KR, Huang CL, et al. Cardiac potassium channels: physiological insights for targeted therapy. *J Cardiovasc Pharmacol Ther*. 2018;23:119–129.
14. Tucker NR, Clauss S, Ellinor PT. Common variation in atrial fibrillation: navigating the path from genetic association to mechanism. *Cardiovasc Res*. 2016;109:493–501.
15. Grandi E, Sanguinetti MC, Bartos DC, et al. Potassium channels in the heart: structure, function and regulation. *J Physiol*. 2017;595:2209–2228.
16. Papanicolaou KN, Ashok D, Liu T, et al. Global knockout of ROMK potassium channel worsens cardiac ischemia-reperfusion injury but cardiomyocyte-specific knockout does not: implications for the identity of mitoKATP. *J Mol Cell Cardiol*. 2020;139:176–189.
17. Baruscotti M, Bucchi A, Milanesi R, et al. A gain-of-function mutation in the cardiac pacemaker HCN_4 channel increasing cAMP sensitivity is associated with familial inappropriate sinus tachycardia. *Eur Heart J*. 2017;38:280–288.
18. Ide T, Ohtani K, Higo T, et al. Ivabradine for the treatment of cardiovascular diseases. *Circ J*. 2019;83:252–260.
19. Kistamas K, Veress R, Horvath B, et al. Calcium handling defects and cardiac arrhythmia syndromes. *Front Pharmacol*. 2020;11:72.
20. Himes RD, Smolin N, Kukol A, et al. L30A mutation of phospholemman mimics effects of cardiac glycosides in isolated cardiomyocytes. *Biochemistry*. 2016;55:6196–6204.
21. Delmar M, Laird DW, Naus CC, et al. Connexins and disease. *Cold Spring Harb Perspect Biol*. 2018;10.
22. Hoagland DT, Santos W, Poelzing S, et al. The role of the gap junction perinexus in cardiac conduction: potential as a novel anti-arrhythmic drug target. *Prog Biophys Mol Biol*. 2019;144:41–50.
23. Noureldin M, Chen H, Bai D. Functional characterization of novel atrial fibrillation-linked GJA5 (Cx40) mutants. *Int J Mol Sci*. 2018;19.
24. Vimalanathan AK, Ehler E, Gehmlich K. Genetics of and pathogenic mechanisms in arrhythmogenic right ventricular cardiomyopathy. *Biophys Rev*. 2018;10:973–982.
25. Eckhardt LL, Kalscheur MM. Replacing hardware with "viralware". *J Am Coll Cardiol*. 2019;73:1688–1690.
26. Markowitz SM, Lerman BB. A contemporary view of atrioventricular nodal physiology. *J Interv Card Electrophysiol*. 2018;52:271–279.
27. Billette J, Tadros R. An integrated overview of AV node physiology. *Pacing Clin Electrophysiol*. 2019;42:805–820.
28. George SA, Faye NR, Murillo-Berlioz A, et al. At the atrioventricular crossroads: dual pathway electrophysiology in the atrioventricular node and its underlying heterogeneities. *Arrhythm Electrophysiol Rev*. 2017;6:179–185.
29. Fukuda K, Kanazawa H, Aizawa Y, et al. Cardiac innervation and sudden cardiac death. *Circ Res*. 2015;116:2005–2019.

30. Manolis AA, Manolis TA, Apostolopoulos EJ, et al. The role of the autonomic nervous system in cardiac arrhythmias: the neuro-cardiac axis, more foe than friend? *Trends Cardiovasc Med.* 2020.
31. Bencivenga L, Liccardo D, Napolitano C, et al. Beta-adrenergic receptor signaling and heart failure: from bench to bedside. *Heart Fail Clin.* 2019;15:409–419.
32. Stavrakis S, Kulkarni K, Singh JP, et al. Autonomic modulation of cardiac arrhythmias: methods to assess treatment and outcomes. *JACC Clin Electrophysiol.* 2020;6:467–483.
33. Boyden PA, Dun W, Robinson RB. Cardiac Purkinje fibers and arrhythmias; the GK Moe award Lecture 2015. *Heart Rhythm.* 2016;13:1172–1181.
34. Qi XY, Vahdahi Hassani F, Hoffmann D, et al. Inositol trisphosphater receptors and nuclear calcium in atrial fibrillation. *Circ Res.* 2021;128:619–635.
35. Nassal D, Gratz D, Hund TJ. Challenges and opportunities for therapeutic targeting of calmodulin kinase II in heart. *Front Pharmacol.* 2020;11:35.
36. Sufu-Shimizu Y, Okuda S, Kato T, et al. Stabilizing cardiac ryanodine receptor prevents the development of cardiac dysfunction and lethal arrhythmia in ca(2+)/calmodulin-dependent protein kinase IIδc transgenic mice. *Biochem Biophys Res Commun.* 2020;524:431–438.
37. Hegyi B, Morotti S, Liu C, et al. Enhanced depolarization drive in failing rabbit ventricular myocytes: calcium-dependent and beta-adrenergic effects on late sodium, l-type calcium, and sodium-calcium exchange currents. *Circ Arrhythm Electrophysiol.* 2019;12:e007061.
38. Iyer V, Roman-Campos D, Sampson KJ, et al. Purkinje cells as sources of arrhythmias in long QT syndrome type 3. *Sci Rep.* 2015;5:13287.
39. Koleske M, Bonilla I, Thomas J, et al. Tetrodotoxin-sensitive Na_vs contribute to early and delayed afterdepolarizations in long QT arrhythmia models. *J Gen Physiol.* 2018;150:991–1002.
40. Sala L, Gnecchi M, Schwartz PJ. Long QT syndrome modelling with cardiomyocytes derived from human-induced pluripotent stem cells. *Arrhythm Electrophysiol Rev.* 2019;8:105–110.
41. van Gorp PRR, Trines SA, Pijnappels DA, et al. Multicellular in vitro models of cardiac arrhythmias: focus on atrial fibrillation. *Front Cardiovasc Med.* 2020;7:43.
42. da Rocha AM, Campbell K, Mironov S, et al. hiPSC-CM monolayer maturation state determines drug responsiveness in high throughput pro-arrhythmia screen. *Sci Rep.* 2017;7:13834.
43. Priori SG, Napolitano C. J-wave syndromes: electrocardiographic and clinical aspects. *Card Electrophysiol Clin.* 2018;10:355–369.
44. Woosley RL, Black K, Heise CW, et al. CredibleMeds.org: what does it offer? *Trends Cardiovasc Med.* 2018;28:94–99.
45. Butler A, Helliwell MV, Zhang Y, et al. An update on the structure of hERG. *Front Pharmacol.* 2019;10:1572.
46. Wallis R, Benson C, Darpo B, et al. CiPA challenges and opportunities from a non-clinical, clinical and regulatory perspectives. An overview of the safety pharmacology scientific discussion. *J Pharmacol Toxicol Methods.* 2018;93:15–25.
47. Etchegoyen CV, Keller GA, Mrad S, et al. Drug-induced QT interval prolongation in the intensive care unit. *Curr Clin Pharmacol.* 2017;12:210–222.
48. Aguilar M, Nattel S. The pioneering work of George Mines on cardiac arrhythmias: groundbreaking ideas that remain influential in contemporary cardiac electrophysiology. *J Physiol.* 2016;594:2377–2386.
49. Nattel S, Xiong F, Aguilar M. Demystifying rotors and their place in clinical translation of atrial fibrillation mechanisms. *Nat Rev Cardiol.* 2017;14:509–520.
50. Hansen BJ, Zhao J, Li N, et al. Human atrial fibrillation drivers resolved with integrated functional and structural imaging to benefit clinical mapping. *JACC Clin Electrophysiol.* 2018;4:1501–1515.
51. Dharmaprani D, Schopp M, Kuklik P, et al. Renewal theory as a universal quantitative framework to characterize phase singularity regeneration in mammalian cardiac fibrillation. *Circ Arrhythm Electrophysiol.* 2019;12:e007569.
52. Terricabras M, Verma A. Is pulmonary vein isolation enough for persistent atrial fibrillation? *J Cardiovasc Electrophysiol.* 2020.
53. Hyman MC, Marchlinski FE. Persistent atrial fibrillation: when the pulmonary veins are no longer the answer. *J Cardiovasc Electrophysiol.* 2020;31:1861–1863.
54. Bond RC, Choisy SC, Bryant SM, et al. Ion currents, action potentials, and noradrenergic responses in rat pulmonary vein and left atrial cardiomyocytes. *Physiol Rep.* 2020;8:e14432.
55. Choi SH, Jurgens SJ, Weng LC, et al. Monogenic and polygenic contributions to atrial fibrillation risk: results from a national biobank. *Circ Res.* 2020;126:200–209.
56. Wang B, Lunetta KL, Dupuis J, et al. Integrative omics approach to identifying genes associated with atrial fibrillation. *Circ Res.* 2020;126:350–360.
57. Nattel S, Heijman J, Zhou L, et al. Molecular basis of atrial fibrillation pathophysiology and therapy: a translational perspective. *Circ Res.* 2020;127:51–72.
58. Callegari S, Macchi E, Monaco R, et al. A clinico-pathological "bird's-eye" view of left atrial myocardial fibrosis in 121 patients with persistent atrial fibrillation: developing architecture and main cellular players. *Circ Arrhythm Electrophysiol.* 2020.
59. Nattel S. Molecular and cellular mechanisms of atrial fibrosis in atrial fibrillation. *JACC Clin Electrophysiol.* 2017;3:425–435.
60. Gussak G, Pfenniger A, Wren L, et al. Region-specific parasympathetic nerve remodeling in the left atrium contributes to creation of a vulnerable substrate for atrial fibrillation. *JCI Insight.* 2019;4.
61. Hiram R, Xiong F, Naud P, et al. The inflammation-resolution promoting molecule resolvin-d1 prevents atrial proarrhythmic remodeling in experimental right heart disease. *Cardiovasc Res.* 2021;117:1776–1789.
62. Yao C, Veleva T, Scott Jr L, et al. Enhanced cardiomyocyte nlrp3 inflammasome signaling promotes atrial fibrillation. *Circulation.* 2018;138:2227–2242.
63. Meyers JD, Jay PY, Rentschler S. Reprogramming the conduction system: onward toward a biological pacemaker. *Trends Cardiovasc Med.* 2016;26:14–20.
64. Schultz F, Swiatlowska P, Alvarez-Laviada A, et al. Cardiomyocyte-myofibroblast contact dynamism is modulated by connexin-43. *FASEB J.* 2019;33:10453–10468.
65. Cerrone M. Controversies in Brugada syndrome. *Trends Cardiovasc Med.* 2018;28:284–292.
66. Rizzo A, de Asmundis C, Brugada P, et al. Ablation for the treatment of Brugada syndrome: current status and future prospects. *Expert Rev Med Devices.* 2020;17:123–130.
67. Wleklinski MJ, Kannankeril PJ, Knollmann BC. Molecular and tissue mechanisms of catecholaminergic polymorphic ventricular tachycardia. *J Physiol.* 2020;598:2817–2834.
68. Wang G, Zhao N, Zhong S, et al. Safety and efficacy of flecainide for patients with catecholaminergic polymorphic ventricular tachycardia: a systematic review and meta-analysis. *Medicine (Baltim).* 2019;98:e16961.
69. Gandjbakhch E, Redheuil A, Pousset F, et al. Clinical diagnosis, imaging, and genetics of arrhythmogenic right ventricular cardiomyopathy/dysplasia: JACC state-of-the-art review. *J Am Coll Cardiol.* 2018;72:784–804.
70. Aras KK, Kay MW, Efimov IR. Ventricular fibrillation: rotors or foci? Both! *Circ Arrhythm Electrophysiol.* 2017;10.
71. Singh P, Noheria A. Ablation approaches for ventricular fibrillation. *Curr Treat Options Cardiovasc Med.* 2018;20:21.
72. Liu T, Xiong F, Qi XY, et al. Altered calcium handling produces reentry-promoting action potential alternans in atrial fibrillation-remodeled hearts. *JCI Insight.* 2020;5.

63 Genetics of Cardiac Arrhythmias

JOHN R. GIUDICESSI, DAVID J. TESTER, AND MICHAEL J. ACKERMAN

THE QT-OPATHIES, 1191
Long QT Syndrome, 1191
Triadin Knockout Syndrome, 1195
Timothy Syndrome, 1196
Cardiac-Only Timothy Syndrome, 1197
Short QT Syndrome, 1197
Drug-Induced Torsade de Pointes, 1197

THE OTHER CHANNELOPATHIES, 1199
Andersen-Tawil Syndrome, 1199
Ankyrin-B Syndrome, 1199

Brugada Syndrome, 1200
Catecholaminergic Polymorphic Ventricular Tachycardia, 1201
Calcium Release Channel Deficiency Syndrome, 1203
Early Repolarization Syndrome, 1204
Familial Atrial Fibrillation, 1204
Idiopathic Ventricular Fibrillation, 1205
Multifocal Ectopic Purkinje-Related Premature Contractions, 1205

Progressive Cardiac Conduction Disease, 1205
Sick Sinus Syndrome, 1206

CONCLUSIONS, 1206

FUTURE PERSPECTIVES, 1206

REFERENCES, 1207

Cardiac arrhythmias encompass a large and heterogenous group of electrical abnormalities of the heart with or without underlying structural heart disease. Cardiac arrhythmias can be innocuous, can predispose to the development of potentially lethal stroke or embolus, or can present emergently with a life-threatening condition that may result in sudden cardiac death (SCD), one of the most common causes of death in the developed countries. In the United States, for example, an estimated 300,000 to 400,000 individuals die suddenly each year, with the vast majority involving the elderly; 80% are caused by ventricular fibrillation (VF) in the context of ischemic heart disease. In comparison, SCD in the young is relatively uncommon, with an incidence between 1.3 and 8.5 per 100,000 patient-years.[1] However, tragically, thousands of otherwise healthy individuals under the age of 40 years die suddenly each year without warning signs. Most SCD in the young can be attributed to structural cardiovascular anomalies identifiable at autopsy. However, 30% to 50% of sudden death in the young remains unexplained following a complete autopsy and medicolegal investigation (see Chapter 70).

Potentially lethal and inheritable arrhythmia syndromes—classified under "the cardiac channelopathies" including congenital long QT syndrome (LQTS), Brugada syndrome (BrS), catecholaminergic polymorphic ventricular tachycardia (CPVT), and related disorders—involve electrical disturbances with the propensity to cause fatal arrhythmias in the setting of a structurally normal heart. These often unassuming electrical abnormalities have the capacity to cause the heart of an unsuspecting individual to develop a potentially lethal arrhythmia, leading to a sudden and early demise of an otherwise healthy individual. In fact, it is now recognized that nearly a third of autopsy-negative sudden unexplained death (SUD) in the young and approximately 10% of sudden infant death syndrome (SIDS) stem from these inherited cardiac channelopathies.[1]

Through molecular advances in the field of cardiovascular genetics, the underlying bases responsible for many inherited cardiac arrhythmia syndromes have been identified, while other underlying genetic substrates are on the cusp of discovery. Over the past two decades, a set of themes including extreme genetic heterogeneity, reduced/incomplete penetrance, and variable expressivity have proven to be central themes among the cardiac channelopathies. However, for some disorders, important genotype-phenotype correlations have been recognized and have provided diagnostic, prognostic, and therapeutic impact.

Given the potentially devastating impact that these disorders can have on a family and their communities, we sought to illustrate the clinical description, genetic basis, and the genotype-phenotype correlations associated with these inherited arrhythmia syndromes.

Specifically, this chapter will discuss cardiac channelopathies, focusing on the subset of QT-opathies [LQTS including calmodulinopathic LQTS, triadin knockout (TKO) syndrome, Timothy syndrome (TS), cardiac-only Timothy syndrome (COTS), short QT syndrome (SQTS), and drug-induced torsade de pointes (DI-TdP)] and other channelopathies [Andersen-Tawil syndrome (ATS), ankyrin-B syndrome (ABS), BrS, CPVT, early repolarization syndrome (ERS), familial atrial fibrillation (FAF), idiopathic ventricular fibrillation (IVF), multifocal ectopic Purkinje-related premature contractions (MEPPC), progressive cardiac conduction defect (PCCD), and sick sinus syndrome (SSS)].

THE QT-OPATHIES

Long QT Syndrome

Clinical Description and Manifestations of Long QT Syndrome

Congenital LQTS comprises a distinct group of cardiac channelopathies characterized by delayed repolarization of the myocardium resulting in heart rate-corrected QT prolongation (QTc >480 msec as the 50th percentile among individuals with genetically confirmed LQTS; Fig. 63.1A) and an increased risk of syncope, seizures, and SCD in the setting of a structurally normal heart. The incidence of LQTS may exceed 1 in 2500 persons. However, individuals with LQTS may not manifest QT prolongation on a resting 12-lead surface electrocardiogram (ECG). This repolarization abnormality almost always is without consequence; however, it is rarely triggered by exertion, swimming, emotion, auditory stimuli such as an alarm clock, or the postpartum period, which can cause the heart to become electrically unstable and develop a life-threatening and sometimes lethal arrhythmia, torsade de pointes (TdP) (see Chapter 70). Though the cardiac rhythm often returns to normal spontaneously, resulting in only transient syncope, 5% of untreated and unassuming LQTS individuals succumb to a fatal arrhythmia as their sentinel event. However, it is estimated that nearly half of individuals experiencing SCD, stemming from this very treatable arrhythmogenic disorder, may have exhibited prior warning signs (i.e., exertional syncope, family history of premature sudden death) that went unrecognized. LQTS may explain approximately 20% of autopsy-negative SUD in the young and 10% of SIDS.[1]

GENETIC BASIS FOR LONG QT SYNDROME

LQTS is a genetically heterogeneous disorder of cardiac repolarization inherited predominantly in an autosomal dominant pattern (formerly referred to as Romano-Ward syndrome). It is rarely inherited in a recessive pattern as illustrated by Jervell and Lange-Nielsen Syndrome (JLNS),

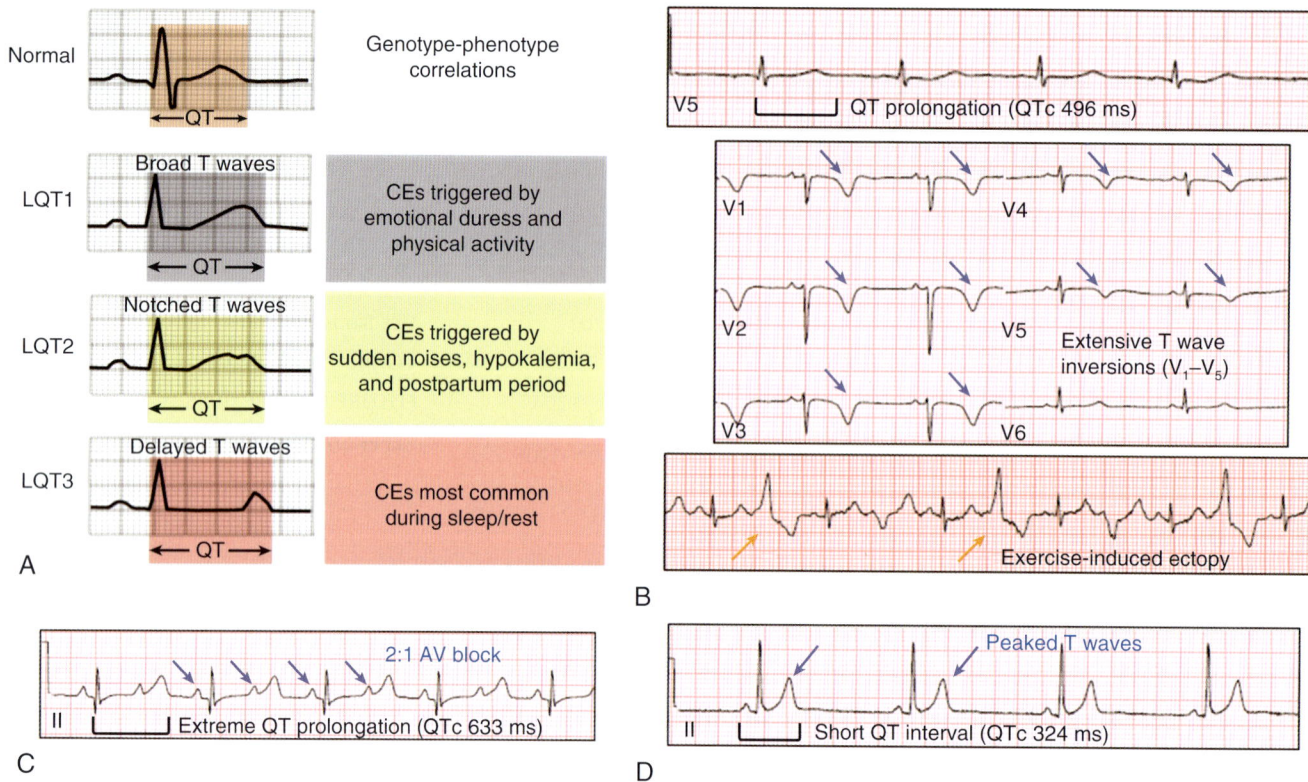

FIGURE 63.1 Notable electrocardiographic findings in the QT-opathies. **A,** Canonical (i.e., LQT1-3) long QT syndrome genotype-specific electrocardiogram patterns and clinically relevant genotype-phenotype correlations. **B,** QTc prolongation (top panel, *black bracket*), extensive precordial T wave inversions (middle panel, *blue arrows*), and exercise-induced ventricular ectopy (bottom panel, *orange arrows*) observed in a triadin knockout syndrome patient homozygous for p.D18fs*13-TRDN. **C,** Rhythm strip from a Timothy syndrome patient harboring p.G406R-CACNA1C that displays extreme QTc prolongation (*black bracket*) and 2:1 atrioventricular block (*blue arrows*). **D,** Rhythm strip from a patient with short QT syndrome displaying characteristic QTc shortening (*black bracket*) and peaked T waves (*blue arrows*). *AV,* Atrioventricular; *CEs,* cardiac events; *QTc,* heart rate-corrected QT interval.

characterized by extreme QTc prolongation, high risk of SCD, and sensorineural hearing loss. Spontaneous/sporadic germline mutations can account for nearly 5% to 10% of LQTS. To date, hundreds of mutations have now been identified in LQTS-susceptibility genes responsible for a nonsyndromic "classical" LQTS phenotype. In addition, three extremely rare, multisystem disorders (ATS formerly referred to as LQT7; ABS formerly referred to as LQT4; and TS formerly referred to as LQT8) associated with marked QTc prolongation and an array of extra-cardiac manifestations have also been described and are detailed in the later sections of this chapter.

Approximately 75% of patients with a clinically robust diagnosis of LQTS host either loss-of-function or gain-of-function pathogenic/likely pathogenic variants in one of these three major/canonical LQTS genes—*KCNQ1*-encoded I_{Ks} ($K_v 7.1$) potassium channel (LQT1, approximately 35%, loss-of-function); *KCNH2*-encoded I_{Kr} ($K_v 11.1$) potassium channel (LQT2, approximately 30%, loss-of-function); and *SCN5A*-encoded I_{Na} ($Na_v 1.5$) sodium channel (LQT3, approximately 10%, gain-of-function)—which are responsible for the inscription of the cardiac action potential (Fig. 63.2). Approximately 5% to 10% of patients have multiple mutations and such patients present at a younger age and with greater expressivity.[1]

Following the discovery of the canonical LQTS-susceptibility genes in 1995 and 1996, rapid advances in deoxyribonucleic acid (DNA) sequencing technology has facilitated the discovery of new disease-susceptibility genes in scenarios (i.e., singletons and small pedigrees) not feasible with classical linkage analysis.[2] As a result, the last two decades have seen a rapid explosion in the number of new disease-susceptibility genes, which includes the 14 minor LQTS-susceptibility genes that may underlie an additional 5% to 10% of LQTS cases.

However, many of the minor LQTS-susceptibility genes (e.g., *AKAP9, ANK2, CAV3, KCNE1, KCNE2, SCN4B,* and *SNTA1*) were discovered using hypothesis-driven, candidate-based analysis of

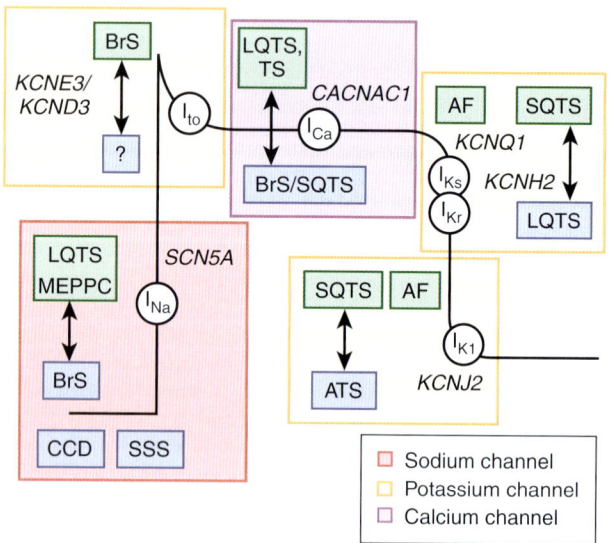

FIGURE 63.2 Cardiac action potential disorders. Illustrated are the key ion currents (*white circles*) along the ventricular cardiomyocyte's action potential that are associated with potentially lethal cardiac arrhythmia disorders. Disorders resulting in gain-of-function mutations are shown in *green rectangles* and those with loss-of-function mutations shown in *blue rectangles*. For example, while gain-of-function mutations in the *SCN5A* encoding cardiac sodium channel responsible for INa, lead to LQTS, loss-of-function *SCN5A* mutations result in BrS, CCD, and SSS. *AF,* Atrial fibrillation; *ATS,* Andersen-Tawil syndrome; *BrS,* Brugada syndrome; *CCD,* cardiac conduction disease; *LQTS,* long QT syndrome; *MEPPC,* multifocal ectopic Purkinje-related premature contractions; *SSS,* sick sinus syndrome; *SQTS,* short QT syndrome; *TS,* Timothy syndrome.

biologically plausible genes rather than unbiased approaches (linkage analysis, next-generation sequencing-based trio/pedigree analysis, etc.).[2,3] Furthermore, many putative disease-causative variants used to establish these minor LQTS disease-gene associations (GDAs) were discovered before the true background rate of rare and presumably innocuous amino acid-altering variants was illuminated by large-scale sequencing projects such as the Genome Aggregation Database (gnomAD).[4] Therefore, it comes as little surprise that some putative LQTS-causative nonsynonymous variants are observed at frequencies in public exomes/genomes that far exceed the anticipated contribution of the minor LQTS-susceptibility gene in which it resides (i.e., 1:250,000 or 0.0004% for a ≤ 1% contributor) or in some cases the estimated prevalence of LQTS as a whole (i.e., 1:2500 or 0.04%).[3,5]

As a result, the strength of many minor LQTS GDAs is rightfully in question. To this end, the Clinical Genome Resource (ClinGen) Clini-cal Domain Channelopathy Working Group recently released a semi-quantitative, evidence-based assessment of the GDA strength for the 17 putative LQTS-susceptibility genes.[6,7] However, the canonical LQTS-susceptibility genes (*KCNQ1*/LQT1, *KCNH2*/LQT2, and *SCN5A*/LQT3) and redundant genes (*CALM1-3*) responsible for calmodulinopathic LQTS received "definitive" evidence designations, and the majority of the remaining LQTS-susceptibility genes received a "limited" or "disputed" evidence designation.[6,7] As a result, the majority (9/17; 53%) of alleged LQTS-susceptibility genes have now been demoted to so-called gene of uncertain significance (GUS) status.[6]

Unfortunately, owing to the limited number of sentinel variants used to establish initial GDAs, nearly all novel, nonsynonymous variants identified in a minor LQTS-GUS are destined to receive, at best, an ambiguous variant of uncertain significance (VUS) designation in accordance with the current American College of Medical Genetics and Genomics (ACMG) guidelines.[8,9] Therefore, the continued inclusion of GUS on gene panels likely elevates the signal-to-noise ratio associated with LQTS genetic testing as well as the risk of genetic testing misinterpretation, and subsequent diagnostic miscues.[8,9]

However, in light of (1) the increasing contribution of common genetic variants (oligogenic/polygenic basis) to the genetic architecture of LQTS, particularly in the approximately 10% to 20% of individuals that remain genotype-negative,[10,11] (2) clear role of rare and common variants in some GUS, most notably the *KCNE1*-encoded MiRP1 β-subunit,[8,12–14] in low penetrant and acquired/drug-induced forms of LQTS, and (3) potential that new evidence could elevate the ClinGen designation of a minor LQTS GUS, it is difficult to argue for the blanket removal of all limited- and disputed-evidence genes from commercial LQTS genetic testing panels at this time.

As minor LQTS GUS are likely to remain on LQTS genetic testing panels for the foreseeable future, ordering health care professionals should prioritize clinically actionable (ACMG pathogenic/likely pathogenic) variants identified in ClinGen definitive (*KCNQ1, KCNH2, SCN5A,* and *CALM1-3*), strong (*TRDN*), and moderate (*CACNA1C*) evidence genes and approach any variant (ACMG pathogenic, likely pathogenic, or VUS) identified in a ClinGen limited/disputed evidence gene with caution, as detailed in Figure 63.3. Importantly, if any doubt exists in regards to the clinical implications of variants labeled, currently or previously, as pathogenic/likely pathogenic in a GUS or VUS in definitive, strong, or moderate-evidence LQTS-susceptibility genes, strong consideration should be given to referring the patient to a dedicated Cardiovascular Genomics Clinic with the suitable infrastructure and expertise needed to carefully interpret, continually reappraise, and if needed act on these genetic findings (see Fig. 63.3).[2]

Phenotypic Correlates for the Three Canonical Long QT Syndrome Genotypes

Specific genotype/phenotype associations in LQTS have emerged, suggesting relatively gene-specific triggers, ECG patterns, and response to therapy (see Fig. 63.1A). Swimming and exertion-induced cardiac events are strongly associated with mutations in *KCNQ1* (LQT1), whereas auditory triggers and events occurring during the postpartum period most often occur in patients with LQT2. While exertion- or emotional stress-induced events are most common in LQT1, events occurring during periods of sleep/rest are most common in LQT3. In a study of 721 LQT1 and 634 LQT2 genetically confirmed patients from the U.S. portion of the international LQTS registry, a multivariate analysis was used to assess the independent contribution of clinical and mutation-specific factors in the occurrence of a first triggered event associated with exercise, arousal, or sleep/rest.[1] Among the 221 symptomatic LQT1 patients, their first cardiac event was most often associated with exercise (55%) followed by sleep/rest (21%), arousal (14%), and non-specific (10%) triggers, whereas the 204 symptomatic LQT2 patients most often had their first event associated with either arousal triggers (44%) or nonexercise/nonarousal triggers (43%), and only 13% of the symptomatic LQT2 patients had an exercise-induced triggered first event. For LQT2 patients, the rate of arousal-triggered events was similar between male and female children, whereas there was a significantly higher rate of arousal-triggered events in women than men (26% vs. 6%, at age 40 years) following the onset of adolescence. Characteristic gene-suggestive ECG patterns have been described previously. LQT1 is associated with a broad-based T wave, LQT2 with a low amplitude notched or biphasic T wave, and LQT3 with a long isoelectric segment followed by a narrow-based T wave (see Fig. 63.1A).

However, exceptions to these relatively gene-specific T wave patterns exist, and due caution must be exercised with making a pre-genetic test prediction of the particular LQTS subtype involved, as the most common clinical mimicker of the LQT3-looking ECG is seen among patients with LQT1. This is key because the underlying genetic basis heavily influences the response to standard LQTS pharmacotherapy where beta blockers are extremely protective in LQT1 patients and moderately protective in patients with LQT2 and LQT3. Additionally, targeting the pathologic, LQT3-associated late sodium current with agents such as mexiletine, flecainide, or ranolazine represents a gene-specific therapeutic option for LQT3. Attenuation in repolarization with clinically apparent shortening in the QTc has been demonstrated with such a strategy and recently, a reduction in LQT3-triggered events using this strategy has been demonstrated. While the generalization that beta-blocker efficacy is genotype-type dependent has been well accepted, the effectiveness of beta-blocker therapy may be largely trigger-specific, rather than dependent on genotype. For both LQT1 and LQT2 patients, beta-blockade was associated with a pronounced 71% (LQT2 patients) to 78% (LQT1 patients) reduction in the risk for exercise-triggered cardiac events, but had no statistically significant effect on the apparent risk for arousal- or sleep/rest-triggered events.[1] However, it should be noted that many symptomatic LQT1 and LQT2 patients experience a subsequent cardiac event associated with a different trigger. For example, an LQT2 patient first presenting with an arousal event or event during sleep may present subsequently with an exercise-triggered event. Therefore, beta-blocker therapy remains first-line therapy even for patients experiencing a non-exercise-associated first event.

In addition, intra-genotype risk stratification has been realized for the two most common subtypes of LQTS based on mutation type, mutation location, and cellular function. Patients with LQT1 secondary to $K_v7.1$ missense mutations localizing to the transmembrane-spanning domains clinically have a twofold greater risk of a LQT1-triggered cardiac event than LQT1 patients with mutations localizing to the C-terminal region. In addition, missense mutations localizing to the so-called cytoplasmic loops (C-loops) within the transmembrane-spanning domains, an area of the protein involved in adrenergic channel regulation, are associated with the highest rate of both exercise- and arousal-triggered events, but were not associated with an increase rate of sleep/rest associated events.[1] C-loop $K_v7.1$ missense mutations were consistently associated with a sixfold increase in risk for exercise-triggered events compared to non-missense mutations, and a nearly threefold increase compared to N- and C-terminal missense mutations.[1]

Patients with mutations resulting in a greater degree of $K_v7.1$ loss-of-function at the cellular in vitro level (dominant negative) have a twofold greater clinical risk compared to mutations that damaged the biology of the $K_v7.1$ channel less severely (haploinsufficiency). Adding to the traditional clinical risk factors, molecular location and cellular function are independent risk factors used in the evaluation of patients with LQTS.

Akin to molecular risk stratification in LQT1, patients with LQT2 secondary to $K_v11.1$ pore-region mutations have a longer QTc, a more severe clinical manifestation of the disorder, and experience significantly more arrhythmia-related cardiac events occurring at a younger age than those LQT2 patients with non-pore mutations in $K_v11.1$.[1] Similarly, in a Japanese cohort of LQT2 patients, those with

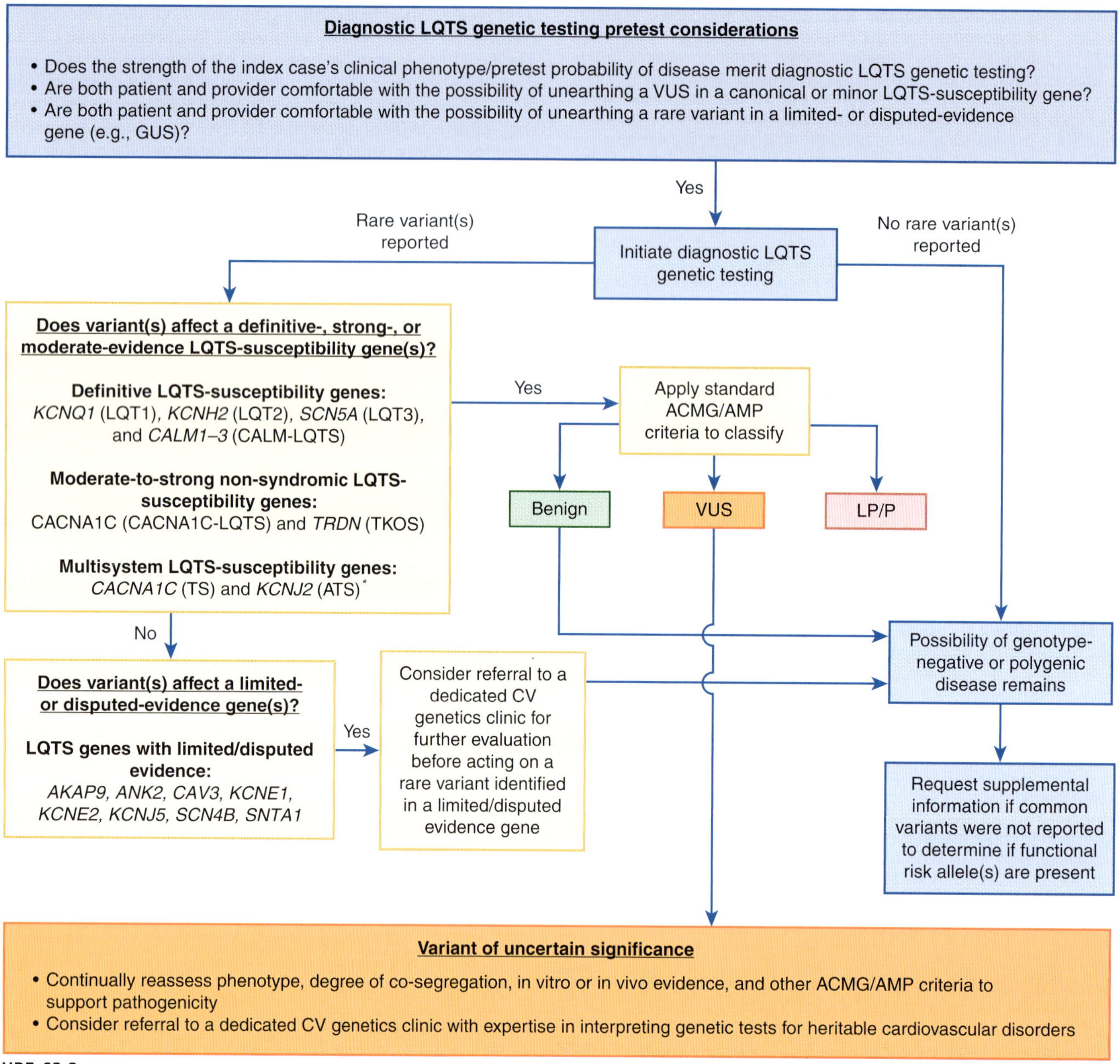

FIGURE 63.3 A rational approach to long QT syndrome genetic testing initiation and interpretation. *Blue boxes* denote basic considerations pertaining to the initiation of long QT syndrome genetic testing. *Light yellow boxes* denote a tiered approach to the assessment of rare variants in long QT syndrome-susceptibility genes with variable gene-disease association evidence strength. *Orange boxes* denote basic considerations pertaining to the identification of rare variants of uncertain significance in self-sufficient long QT syndrome-susceptibility genes that currently lack sufficient evidence to classify as either benign or pathogenic/likely pathogenic. *Due to the lack of a true QT prolongation phenotype, the authors recommend against the routine inclusion of *KCNJ2* on diagnostic LQTS testing panels. *ACMG*, American College of Medical Genetics and Genomics; *AMP*, Association for Molecular Pathology; *LP*, likely pathogenic; *LQTS*, long QT syndrome; *P*, pathogenic; *TKOS*, triadin knockout syndrome; *TS*, Timothy syndrome; *GUS*, gene of uncertain significance; *VUS*, variant of uncertain significance. (Adapted from Giudicessi JR, et al. *Trends Cardiovasc Med.* 2018;28[7]:453–464.)

pore mutations had a longer QTc, though not significant among probands, non-probands with pore mutations experienced their first cardiac event at an earlier age than those with a non-pore mutation. Most recently, additional information has been gleaned suggesting that LQT2 patients with mutations involving the transmembrane pore region had the greatest risk for cardiac events, those with frame-shift/nonsense mutations in any region had an intermediate risk, and those with missense mutations in the C-terminus had the lowest risk for cardiac events. Interestingly, LQT2 patients with mutations in the pore-loop region of the $K_v11.1$ channel have a greater than twofold increased risk for arousal-triggered events, and LQT2 patients with non-pore loop TM region mutations have a nearly sevenfold increase in the risk for exercise-triggered cardiac events compared with patients with N-terminal/C-terminal mutations.[1]

Incomplete penetrance and variable expressivity are clinical hallmark features of LQTS, and it has been long thought that co-inheritance of a true disease-causing mutation and either a common or rare channel genetic variant may determine the expressed severity of the disorder. For example, the co-existence of the common *K897T-KCNH2* polymorphism and the *A1116V-KCNH2* mutation (on opposite alleles) led to a more severe clinical course in a single Italian LQTS family. The *A1116V* mutation by itself produced a sub-clinical phenotype of mild QT prolongation and an asymptomatic course, while the proband hosting both variants had clinically overt disease consisting of a diagnostic QT prolongation, presyncopal episodes, and cardiac arrest. Besides cardiac ion channels, single nucleotide polymorphisms (SNPs) of non-ion channel genes like *NOS1AP* (the gene encoding the nitric oxide synthase 1 adapter protein), *ADRA2C* (alpha-2C adrenergic receptor), and *ADRB1* (beta-1 adrenergic receptor) can modify disease severity in LQTS.[1]

There is compelling evidence for a strong disease modifying effect of a 3′ untranslated region (3′UTR) *KCNQ1* allele-specific haplotype in LQT1 mutation positive pedigrees; the magnitude of the effect on the QTc and symptomology go well beyond any other currently described genetic modifiers.[1] The *KCNQ1* gene encodes a single K_v7.1 ion channel alpha subunit that assemble to create a pore-forming K_v7.1 tetrameric channel. Therefore, if a patient had a heterozygous *KCNQ1* mutation (i.e., one normal *KCNQ1* gene allele and one mutant allele), one would expect that if both the normal and mutant gene alleles were expressed in equal amounts, then 1/16 of the K_v7.1 channels would be a normal homomeric tetramer and 1/16 of the K_v7.1 channels would be a mutant homomeric tetramer. The remaining channels would be hybrids containing both normal and mutant alpha-subunits. If expression of the normal *KCNQ1* gene allele was somehow suppressed, then there would be relatively more *KCNQ1* mutant alpha-subunits translated and ultimately assembled to provide more dysfunctional K_v7.1 channels, thus leading to a more severe manifestation of the disorder. The opposite would be true if the mutation containing the *KCNQ1* allele was suppressed.

Most genes have a 3′ UTR that generates an mRNA transcript containing regions of cis-regulatory binding sites for small noncoding microRNAs (miRNAs) that bind to the transcript and ultimately inhibit that gene's expression. Naturally occurring genetic variation within these 3′UTRs (miR-SNPs) can either abolish existing or creating new miRNA binding sites. SNPs in the *KCNQ1* 3′UTR create a "suppressive" haplotype by generating new miRNA binding sites that suppress the expression of the *KCNQ1* allele in which they reside. Inheritance of the "suppressive" haplotype residing on the normal "healthy" allele produced a more severe LQT1 phenotype, whereas the inheritance of the "suppressive" haplotype residing on the same allele as the *KCNQ1* mutation gave a less severe LQT1 phenotype (shorter QTc and fewer symptoms).[1] This intriguing discovery both explains a significant component of reduced penetrance and variable expressivity that is a common feature of arrhythmia syndromes, and also represents a paradigm shift in our thinking about disease-modifying genetic-drivers of mendelian disorders (as one of the most important genetic determinants of disease severity in LQT1 appears to be the 3′UTR *KCNQ1* haplotype on the allele inherited from the unaffected "non-LQTS" parent).

In line with the concept that common variants within noncoding regions of the human genome may impact the penetrance and expressivity (a.k.a. clinical variability) of rare LQTS pathogenic/likely pathogenic variants, recent studies have demonstrated that an aggregate polygenic risk score (PRS) comprised of common variants that influence QTc duration at the level of population[15–17] can explain 2% to 15% of the clinical variability observed among LQTS patients.[10,18] Although the clinical utility of these PRSs in the management of genotype-positive LQTS patients remains unclear, they do provide intriguing and potentially clinically relevant insights into the genetic architecture of the 10% to 20% of LQTS patients that remain genotype-negative for monogenic LQTS.

Of note, the recent rare disease genome-wide association study (GWAS) by Lahrouchi et al.[10] provided compelling evidence, by way of a 68 SNP/common variant–weighted PRS, that genotype-negative LQTS likely represents a polygenic subtype that arises secondary to the accumulation of multiple QTc-prolonging common genetic variants. Interestingly, in comparison to patients with canonical LQTS (i.e., LQT1-LQT3), these genotype-negative patients had longer aggregate QTc intervals and a similar rate of event-free survival.[10] These observations are in line with those from other genetic heart diseases considered, at least initially, to be predominantly mendelian/monogenic such as familial hypercholesterolemia and BrS.[19]

LQTS, like many cardiovascular disorders, appears to have a more complex genetic architecture than anticipated initially that likely includes monogenic, oligogenic, and polygenic subtypes (Fig. 63.4).[2] As our understanding of the genetic architecture underlying LQTS continues to grow, it appears increasingly likely that commercial gene panel-based LQTS genetic tests in use today require an overhaul to better accommodate assessment of the 10% to 20% of patients that have oligogenic/polygenic subtypes, and the genetic background that influences the penetrance and expressivity of canonical LQTS-causative variants.

Calmodulinopathic Long QT Syndrome

In the early 2010s, three independent, unbiased exome sequencing studies implicated heterozygous sporadic/de novo pathogenic variants in the biologically redundant *CALM1*, *CALM2*, and *CALM3* genes that collectively encode calmodulin (an ubiquitously expressed and essential calcium-handling protein) in infants/young children with extreme QT prolongation (i.e., >600 msec) and adrenergic-triggered life-threatening ventricular arrhythmias.[20] Subsequently, pathogenic variants in *CALM1-3* have also been identified in patients with CPVT, IVF, and CPVT/LQTS overlap phenotypes. However, recent data from the multicenter International Calmodulinopathy Registry indicate that LQTS (49%) and CPVT (28%) phenotypes predominate.[20]

From a pathophysiological perspective, it is interesting to note that all LQTS-causative *CALM1-3* mutations described to date localize within or proximal to calcium-coordinating residues of the C-terminal lobe (C-lobe) of calmodulin and impart a marked reduction in calcium-binding affinity.[20,21] Although calmodulin is known to regulate a number of cardiac ion channels, the predominant effect of LQTS pathogenic/likely pathogenic *CALM1-3* variants appears to be loss of calcium-dependent inactivation (CDI) of the L-type calcium channel (LTCC) resulting in unrestrained calcium influx (i.e., LTCC/I_{CaL} gain-of-function).[21] In contrast, CPVT pathogenic/likely pathogenic variants in *CALM1-3* localized at the N-terminal (N-lobe) and C-lobe increase RyR2-binding affinity/single channel open probability and spontaneous calcium release from the sarcoplasmic reticulum rather than calcium-binding affinity.[21]

Unfortunately, the calmodulinopathies (such as CALM-LQTS and CALM-CPVT) are frequently refractory to conventional LQTS- and CPVT-directed therapies (beta-blockers).[20] At present, it is not known whether the varying levels of neurodevelopmental delay observed in a minority of patients with a calmodulinopathy (17%) are secondary to anoxic brain injury in the setting of recurrent cardiac arrhythmias or are related to developmental effects of perturbed calcium-handling in the central nervous system.[20] Regardless, a combination of pharmacologic, sympathectomy, and device-related therapies is typically required and even then is often inadequate. As such, the calmodulinopathies represent an important target for gene-therapy and other targeted precision medicine approaches.

Triadin Knockout Syndrome

In 2015, Altmann et al. described a rare autosomal recessive form of LQTS characterized by transient/consistent QT prolongation with extensive precordial ($V_1–V_4$) T wave inversions (see Fig. 63.1B), severe and often refractory exercise-induced ventricular arrhythmias during childhood. In addition, they described mild-to-moderate proximal skeletal myopathy secondarily due to either homozygous (p.D18fs*13-TRDN and p.K147fs0*-TRDN) or compound heterozygous (p.N9fs*5-TRDN and p.K147fs*0-TRDN) frame-shift/null pathogenic/likely pathogenic variants in *TRDN*-encoded triadin (a key structural component of the cardiac release unit [CRU]).[21,22] Interestingly, some of the same TRDN null variants (p.D18fs*13-TRDN and p.N9fs*5-TRDN) were implicated previously in recessively inherited CPVT,[21] suggesting that Triadin knockout syndrome (TKOS) may represent a unique clinical entity with clinical characteristics of both LQTS and CPVT.

To this end, a recent study from the International TKOS Registry attempted to clarify the phenotype observed in individuals with homozygous/compound heterozygous TRDN null variants.[23] Whereas the mean QTc observed in TKOS patients was 472 ± 34 msec, exercise-induced ectopy was observed in 89%.[23] Furthermore, 90% of TKOS patients experienced SCA/SCD, and 74% suffered breakthrough cardiac events despite a myriad of medical, surgical (sympathectomy), and device therapy highlighting the malignant nature of the distinct TKOS clinical phenotype.[23]

Like calmodulinopathies, TKOS is primarily a disorder of calcium-handling. Although the TKOS patient-specific human induced pluripotent stem cell-derived cardiomyocytes (iPSC-CM) have yet to be characterized, insights gleaned from ventricular arrhythmia-prone *TRDN* null mice suggest that complete ablation of triadin, as would be expected in TKOS patients, disrupts the approximation of the

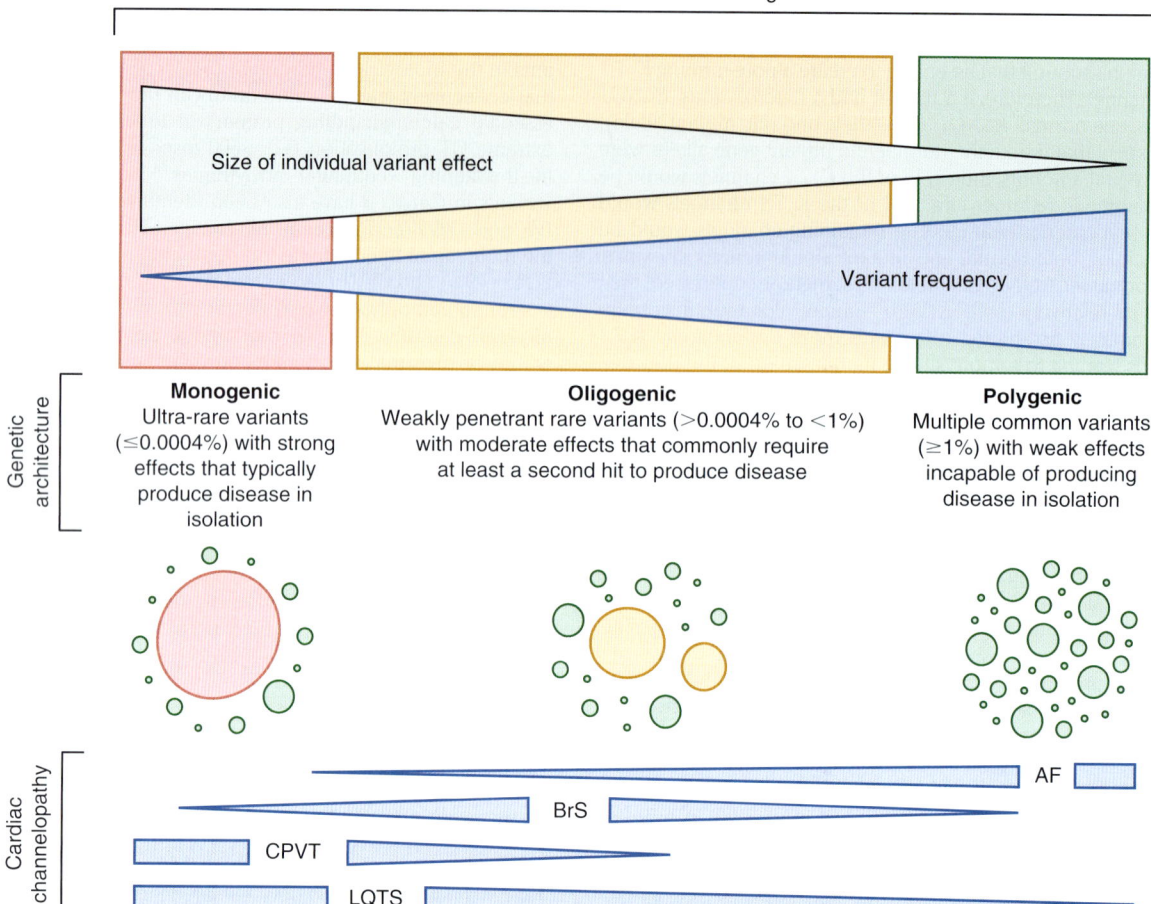

FIGURE 63.4 The spectrum of genetic variation underlying the heritable component of select cardiac channelopathies. At the severe (*red*) end of the spectrum are ultra-rare disease-causative pathogenic variants with strong effects on gene function that typically result in monogenic disorders. In the middle of the spectrum (*yellow*) are weakly penetrant and comparably more common rare variants with moderate effects on gene function that rarely produce disease in isolation, but in the presence of one or more second hits result in so-called oligogenic disease. At the benign (*green*) end of the spectrum are common variants with weak effects on gene function, largely discovered through large genome-wide association studies, that are incapable of producing disease in isolation, but may confer disease risk when multiple risk-associated common variants are present within the genome of an individual exposed to environmental risk factors, resulting in so-called polygenic disease. In recognition that the genetic architecture of most cardiac channelopathies is variable, *blue triangles* denote the spectrum of genetic variation shown to contribute to genetic basis of select cardiac channelopathies. *AF*, Atrial fibrillation; *BrS*, Brugada syndrome; *CPVT*, catecholaminergic polymorphic ventricular tachycardia; *LQTS*, long QT syndrome. (Adapted from Giudicessi JR, Ackerman MJ. *Transl Res*. 2013;161[1]:1–14.)

T-tubule and junctional sarcoplasmic reticulum within the cardiac dyad and reduces the expression of key proteins such as RyR2, calsequestrin2, and junctin reducing the co-localization of the LTCC/RyR2 and RyR2/Calsequestrin2 in the CRU.[21] The resulting remodeling of the CRU leads to reduced sarcoplasmic reticulum calcium release and impaired LTCC CDI that ultimately leads to calcium overload in the sarcoplasmic reticulum.[21] These molecular events likely contribute to an underlying proarrhythmic electrophysiological substrate capable of triggering delayed afterdepolarization- and/or early afterdepolarization-mediated ventricular arrhythmias. This explains the distinct and particularly malignant clinical phenotype, with elements of LQTS and CPVT, observed in TKOS patients.[21,23]

Timothy Syndrome
Clinical Description and Manifestations of Timothy Syndrome

Timothy syndrome (TS) is an extremely rare (<30 patients described worldwide) multisystem, highly lethal arrhythmia disorder, associated with both cardiac and extracardiac abnormalities. The typical cardiac manifestation of TS includes fetal bradycardia, extreme prolongation of the QT interval (QTc >500 msec) often with macroscopic T wave alternans and 2:1 atrioventricular block at birth (see Fig. 63.1C). These abnormalities often coincide with congenital heart defects or cardiomyopathies. Extracardiac abnormalities often consist of simple syndactyly (webbing of the toes and fingers), dysmorphic facial features, abnormal dentition, immune deficiency, severe hypoglycemia, and developmental delay (including autism). Currently, most TS patients die before reaching puberty. While the majority of TS has been described as sporadic/de novo occurrences, few cases with somatic mosaicism associated with a less severe phenotype have recently been described. For example, the *CACNA1C* mutation may be present in the patient's skeletal muscle, but could only be present in traces or even completely absent in other cell types of the human body (i.e., absent in heart, blood lymphocytes), where the patient may present with simple syndactyly.

GENETIC BASIS FOR TIMOTHY SYNDROME

In 2004, Splawski et al. identified the molecular basis for this highly lethal arrhythmia and named it *Timothy syndrome* (TS) after Katherine Timothy, Drs. Keating's and Splawski's study coordinator who meticulously phenotyped these cases.[1] Remarkably, in all 13 unrelated patients where DNA was available, Splawski identified the same recurrent sporadic de novo missense mutation, p.G406R-CACNA1C, in the alternatively spliced exon 8A of the *CACNA1C*-encoded cardiac LTCC (Ca$_v$1.2), which is important for excitation-contraction coupling in the heart and mediates an inward depolarizing current in cardiomyocytes (Fig. 63.2) similar to the cardiac sodium channel Na$_v$1.5. Through alternative splicing, the human L-type Ca channel consists of two mutually exclusive isoforms: one containing exon 8A and the other with exon 8. A year later, they described two cases of atypical TS with similar features of TS yet without syndactyly. As with other TS cases, these two atypical cases were identified as having sporadic de novo *CACNA1C* mutations in exon 8. One case hosted a mutation analogous to the classic TS mutation, *p.G406R-CACNA1C*, whereas the other case hosted a *p.G402R-CACNA1C* missense mutation. All three mutations confer gain-of-function to the LTCC/Ca$_v$1.2 channels through impaired channel inactivation and reside very near the end of the S6 transmembrane segment of domain 1 in the beginning of the intracellular loop between domain I and II of the Ca$_v$1.2 alpha subunit.

In 2011, Gillis et al. identified a novel *CACNA1C* mutation, *p.A1473G-CACNA1C*, in a single patient with a prolonged QT interval, dysmorphic facial features, syndactyly, and joint contractures consistent with TS.[1] In 2015, Boczek et al. identified a novel *CACNA1C* mutation, *p.I1166T-CACNA1C*, in a patient exhibiting a TS phenotype with QT prolongation, patent ductus arteriosus, seizures, facial dysmorphism, joint hypermobility, hypotonia, hand anomalies, intellectual impairment, and tooth decay.[24] Patch-clamp analysis of *p.I1166T-CACNA1C* demonstrated a novel electrophysiological phenotype distinct from the loss of inactivation seen with the previously established TS mutations. Instead, p.I1166T-CACNA1C electrophysiological studies illustrated a loss of current density and a gain-of-function shift in activation, leading to an increase in window current.[24] Interestingly, both p.I1166T-CACNA1C's and p.A1473G-CACNA1C's topological position (a few amino acids away from the S6 transmembrane segment of the domain III and IV, respectively) in the channel architecture is very similar to the position of the three original TS mutations (S6 segment of domain I).

Cardiac-Only Timothy Syndrome

In 2015, Boczek et al. used exome sequencing to identify a novel *CACNA1C* mutation p.R518C-CACNA1C that was most likely responsible for the observed phenotype in a large pedigree with concomitant LQTS, hypertrophic cardiomyopathy (HCM), congenital heart defects, and sudden cardiac death.[25] None of the patients had extracardiac phenotypes, such as those observed with TS. A subsequent *CACNA1C* exon 12 specific analysis in 5 additional unrelated index cases with a similar phenotype of LQTS and a personal/family history of HCM identified 2 additional pedigrees with mutations at the same amino acid position; either p.R518C-CACNA1C or p.R518H-CACNA1C. Patch-clamp studies on both revealed a complex Ca$_v$1.2 electrophysiological phenotype consisting of loss of current density and inactivation in combination with increased window and late current. All three pedigrees hosting p.R518C-CACNA1C/p.R518H-CACNA1C presented with this unique and atypical phenotypic sequela consistent with cardiac-only Timothy syndrome (COTS).[25]

The spectrum of QT-opathies associated with LTCC/Ca$_v$1.2 gain-of-function currently encompasses nonsyndromic LQTS (i.e., CACNA1C-LQTS/LQT8), COTS, and TS.[21] The electrophysiological mechanisms and clinical phenotypes that differentiate this spectrum of LTCC/Ca$_v$1.2-mediated disorders are detailed in Figure 63.5 and are the focus of several recent comprehensive reviews.[21,26]

Short QT Syndrome
Clinical Description and Manifestations of Short QT Syndrome

Short QT syndrome (SQTS), first described in 2000 by Gussak et al., is associated with a short QT-interval (usually ≤320 msec) on a 12-lead ECG (Fig. 63.1D), paroxysmal atrial fibrillation (AF), syncope, and an increased risk for SCD. Giustetto et al. analyzed the clinical presentation of 53 patients with SQTS from 29 families (the largest cohort studied to date). They found that 62% of the patients were symptomatic, with cardiac arrest being the most common symptom (31% of patients) and frequently the first manifestation of the disorder. A fourth of the patients had a history of syncope, and nearly 30% had a family history of SCD. Symptoms including syncope or cardiac arrest most often occurred during periods of rest or sleep. Nearly one-third presented with AF. SCD was observed during infancy, suggesting the potential role for SQTS as a rare pathogenic basis for some cases of SIDS.[1]

GENETIC BASIS FOR SHORT QT SYNDROME
SQTS is most often inherited in an autosomal dominant manner; however, some de novo sporadic cases have been described. To date, mutations in six genes have been implicated in the pathogenesis of SQTS, including gain-of-function mutations in the potassium channel encoding genes *KCNH2* (SQT1), *KCNQ1* (SQT2), and *KCNJ2* (SQT3) and loss-of-function mutations in *CACNA1C* (SQT4), *CACNB2b* (SQT5), and *CACNA2D1* (SQT6) encoding for LTCC alpha, beta, and delta subunits, respectively (Fig. 63.2).[1] However, despite the identification of these SQTS-susceptibility genes, the proportion of SQTS expected to be SQT1-6 genotype positive and that awaiting genetic elucidation are unknown. It is estimated that over 75% of SQTS remains elusive genetically.

Genotype-Phenotype Correlates in Short QT Syndrome

While there are insufficient data to clearly define genotype-phenotype correlations in SQTS (probably fewer than 60 cases have been described in the literature to date), gene-specific ECG patterns are beginning to emerge. The typical ECG pattern consists of a QT-interval of ≤320 msec (QTc ≤340 msec) and tall, peaked T waves in the precordial leads with either a short ST segment present or no ST-segment at all. The T waves tend to be symmetrical in SQT1 but asymmetrical in SQT2-4. In SQT2, inverted T waves can be observed. In SQT5, a BrS-like ST elevation in the right precordial lead could be observed as well.[1]

Owing to the prematurely small sample size, a recent report revealed that SQTS patients with *KCNH2* mutations have a shorter QT and a greater response to hydroquinidine therapy than patients with a non-KCNH2 mediated SQTS.[1] Based on a clinical variable analysis of 65 mutation-positive SQTS patients among 132 SQTS cases previously reported in the literature, Harrell et al. indicated that patients with *KCNH2*-mediated SQTS (SQT1) exhibit a later age of onset of manifestation, whereas patients with *KCNQ1*-mediated SQTS (SQT2) have a higher prevalence of bradyarrhythmias and AF.[27]

Drug-Induced Torsade de Pointes (see Chapter 9)
Clinical Description and Manifestations of Drug-Induced Torsade de Pointes

Drug-induced long QT syndrome (DI-LQTS) and torsades de pointes is a multifactorial clinical entity that tends to surface in the setting of multiple modifiable (electrolyte abnormalities such as hypokalemia, co-administration of multiple QT-prolonging drugs, drug accumulation due to renal/hepatic impairment or inhibition of cytochrome P450 metabolism) and non-modifiable (female sex, underlying genetic disposition, structural heart disease, and diabetes) risk factors (see Chapters 9 and 64). The estimated incidence of DI-LQTS/DI-TdP is drug-dependent, while class III anti-arrhythmic agents range between 1% and 8% depending on the drug and dose. DI-TdP and subsequent sudden death are rare events; however, the list of potential "QT-liability" or "torsadegenic" drugs is extensive and includes both anti-arrhythmic drugs (quinidine, sotalol and dofetilide) and many noncardiac medications (antipsychotics, methadone, antimicrobials, antihistamines, and the gastrointestinal stimulant cisapride [see https://www.crediblemeds.org for a comprehensive list]).[1]

hERG/K$_v$11.1 Channel Blockade and Cardiac Repolarization Reserve

In addition to their intended function/mechanism of action, the vast majority of drugs associated with DI-LQTS and DI-TdP also cause unwanted, intracellular drug-induced blockade of the rapidly activating component of phase 3 delayed rectifier K$^+$ current (I_{Kr}) conducted by *KCNH2*-encoded hERG/K$_v$11.1 K$^+$ channels. In effect, QT-prolonging drugs create a "LQT2-like" phenotype through reduced repolarization efficiency, lengthening and exaggerated spatial dispersion of the cardiac action potential. However, I_{Kr} drug blockade alone does not appear sufficient to provide the potentially lethal TdP substrate. One particular thesis centers on the observation that cardiac repolarization relies on the interaction of several ion currents that provide some level of redundancy in order to protect against extreme QT prolongation by "QT-liability" drugs. This so-called repolarization reserve may be reduced through anomalies in the repolarization machinery as a result of common or rare genetic variants in critical ion channels that produce a subclinical loss

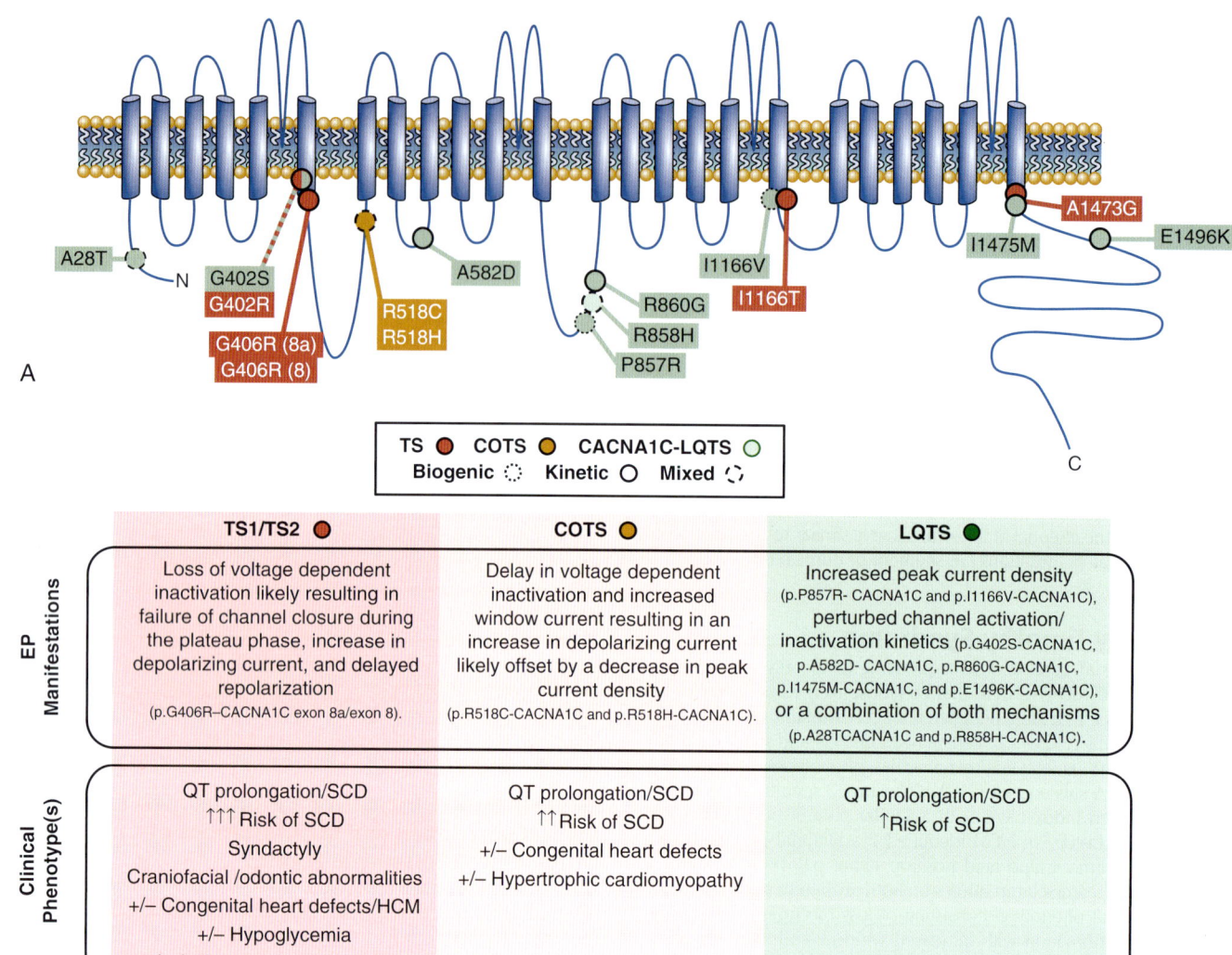

FIGURE 63.5 Electrophysiological and clinical manifestations of putative LQTS-causative gain-of-function CACNA1C mutations. **A,** The location of Timothy syndrome (TS; *red circles*)-, cardiac-only Timothy syndrome (COTS; *orange circles*)-, and LQTS (CACNA1C-LQTS; *green circles*)-causative CACNA1C pathogenic variants are depicted on the Cav1.2 linear protein topology. Biogenic (*small dashed outline*), biophysical/kinetic (*solid outline*), and mixed (*large dashed outline*) electrophysiologic manifestations of individual CACNA1C pathogenic variants are indicated by the contrasting circle outlines. **B,** Summary of the electrophysiological and clinical manifestations of TS, COTS, and LQTS. *EP,* Electrophysiologic; *HCM,* hypertrophic cardiomyopathy; *SCD,* sudden cardiac death. (Adapted from Giudicessi JR, et al. Circ Arrhythm Electrophysiol. 2016;9[7]:e002480.)

of the repolarizing I_{Ks} and I_{Kr} currents.[1] Prior studies have demonstrated that (1) 10% to 15% of patients with DI-TdP host rare ion channel mutations,[1] and (2) weighted-effect PRSs, designed to measure the aggregate effect of QTc-influencing common genetic variants identified previously in the general population[9,17] can identify those at greatest risk of developing an exaggerated QTc response/TdP following exposure to known QT prolonging drugs.[28] As a result, these studies provide further credence to the concept that multiple genetic and environmental hits to the "repolarization reserve" are involved in the pathogenesis of DI-LQTS/DI-TdP.

Furthermore, emerging evidence suggests that drug-induced blockade of hERG/K$_v$11.1 channels is not the only mechanism involved in the pathogenesis of DI-LQTS/DI-TdP. Over the last several years, inhibition of phosphoinositide 3-kinase (PI3K) signaling and its downstream effect on multiple depolarizing and repolarizing currents [primarily reduced I_{Kr} and increased late/sustained Na$^+$ (I_{NaL}) currents] has emerged as another important mechanism underling DI-LQTS/DI-TdP risk.[28] Interestingly, drugs such as dofetilide, sotalol, and azithromycin that also inhibit PI3K and increase I_{NaL} current appear to be more torsadogenic than those that only cause hERG/K$_v$11.1 blockade. Therefore, in vitro markers of DI-LQTS risk, most notably the hERG/K$_v$11.1 half-maximal inhibitory concentration (IC$_{50}$), which is used currently for pre-clinical drug screening, may underestimate the true DI-LQTS/DI-TdP liability of some pharmacologic agents.[28]

Common Ion Channel Polymorphisms and DI-TdP Risk
(see Chapter 9).

Among the common polymorphisms of the *KCNH2*-encoding I_{Kr} potassium channel, the p.K897T-KCNH2 and p.R1047L-KCNH2 polymorphisms have gained the most attention. Paavonen et al. observed that p.T897-KCNH2 channels exhibit slower activation kinetics with a higher degree of inactivation, an alteration expected to decrease channel function and perhaps alter drug sensitivity since several commonly used drugs inhibiting I_{Kr} channel function bind preferentially to the inactivated state of the channel. This finding reveals that p.T897T-KCNH2 may genetically "reduce repolarization reserve" and facilitate a pro-arrhythmic response that may be enhanced in the setting of I_{Kr} channel blocking drugs. In fact, p.K897T-KCNH2 appears to affect the QTc response to ibutilide in a gender-specific manner. In one study, among 105 AF patients treated with dofetilide, p.R1047L-KCNH2 was over-represented among those patients who developed DI-TdP. Besides these common potassium channel alpha-subunit polymorphisms, three common polymorphisms (p.D85N-KCNE1, p.T8A-KCNE2, and p.Q9E-KCNE2) involving auxiliary beta subunits have been implicated in drug-induced arrhythmia susceptibility.[1]

Of note, there is particularly strong epidemiological (DI-LQTS odds ratio of 9.0 [3.5 to 22.9]) and functional (decreased I_{Ks} and I_{Kr} secondary to altered activation/inactivation kinetics) evidence to support a role for p.D85N-KCNE1, a common variant observed in approximately 1% of individuals of European-descent, in DI-LQTS/DI-TdP risk.[29] In addition, p.D85N-KCNE1 may cause transient QTc prolongation in isolation[8,14] and influence QTc duration in both the general population[8] and congenital LQTS patients.[10] Nevertheless, owing to its common nature, some commercial genetic testing companies continue to relegate reporting of p.D85N-KCNE1 and other clinically relevant common variants (p.K897T-KCNH2, p.S1103Y-SCN5A, etc.) to supplemental reports that must be requested by the ordering health care professional.[8]

In addition to common genetic variants that affect the KVLQT1/K_v7.1 (I_{Ks}) and hERG/K_v11.1 (I_{Kr}) potassium channels, common variants in the SCN5A-encoded Na_v1.5 cardiac sodium channel that increase late sodium current may also serve as potentially pro-arrhythmic genetic substrate in patients exposed to QT-prolonging drugs. Of note, the p.S1103Y-SCN5A common variant observed in approximately 8% to 10% of individuals of African descent has been associated with baseline QT prolongation and a small persistent risk of arrhythmia/SCD across the age spectrum (DI-LQTS odds ratio of 8.7 [3.2 to 23.9]).[8] Interestingly, in heterologous expression systems the very subtle biophysical alterations imparted by p.S1103Y-SCN5A do not appear to alter action potential duration (APD). However, in the setting of a "second hit" such as hERG/K_v11.1 block or intracellular acidosis, the modest increase in late sodium current generated by p.S1103Y-SCN5A significantly prolongs the APD in in vitro and in silico models.[8]

Recent GWAS have associated common variants of the NOS1AP-encoded nitric oxide synthase 1 adapter protein (NOS1AP) with QT interval duration. NOS1AP is a regulator of the neuronal nitric oxide synthase (nNOS), which regulates intracellular calcium levels and myocyte contraction through its effect on the LTCCs. Common SNPs in NOS1AP are associated with drug-induced QT prolongation and ventricular arrhythmia.[1] This association was most pronounced among those patients using amiodarone, one of the most common antiarrhythmic drugs. It has been hypothesized that individuals hosting genetic variants in NOS1AP that suppress the gene's expression may in turn result in increased LTCC currents and subsequently QT prolongation and such individuals may be at increased arrhythmogenic risk while on amiodarone.[1] However, although QT prolongation is observed routinely with amiodarone, DI-TdP attributed to amiodarone is exceedingly rare.

Additionally, genetic variation or individual differences in drug elimination or metabolism may contribute to individual risk for drug DI-TdP. For example, patients with genetically mediated reduction in CYP3A enzymatic activity could be vulnerable to DI-TdP in the setting of I_{Kr} blockers that depend on the cytochrome P450 enzyme CYP3A for its metabolism.[1]

THE OTHER CHANNELOPATHIES

Andersen-Tawil Syndrome

Clinical Description and Manifestations of Andersen-Tawil Syndrome

ATS, first described in 1971 in a case report by Andersen and later described by Tawil in 1994, is now recognized as a rare (≤1:1,000,000) autosomal-dominant cardiac channelopathy characterized clinically by the triad of periodic paralysis, frequent ventricular ectopy/arrhythmia (Fig. 63.6A), and variable developmental abnormalities.[1]

Initially, ATS was classified erroneously as a multisystem form of LQTS (and called LQT7) due to the inclusion of prominent U-waves that result in substantial prolongation of the QT-U interval (see Fig. 63.6A).[2] However, once the U-waves are excluded properly, the QTc values of ATS patients are typically within the normal range (i.e., <440 msec).[2] Furthermore, the burden and nature of the electrocardiographic abnormalities (mostly ventricular bigeminy, polymorphic VT, and in rare circumstances bi-directional VT) observed in ATS is reminiscent of the electrocardiographic hallmarks of CPVT and can lead to misdiagnosis. However, the presence of these findings at rest as well as the variable presence of micrognathia, low-set ears, widely spaced eyes, and clinodactyly helps differentiate ATS from CPVT. Correctly distinguishing between true ATS and CPVT is critical as the treatment strategies are quite different.

Of note, despite an often-alarming burden of ventricular ectopy, the long-term prognosis in ATS has generally been considered favorable. However, in the largest multicenter registry of ATS patients assembled to date, Mazzanti et al. demonstrated recently that the rate of SCA/SCD in ATS (9.3%)[30] was much higher than reported previously (2.7%) and similar to the lifetime SCA/SCD observed in other cardiac channelopathies such as LQTS (~13%). As such, the natural history of ATS could be more malignant than anticipated previously and the efficacy of conventional pharmacotherapies in terms of SCA/SCD prevention (i.e., nadolol plus flecainide, amiodarone) remains currently in question.[30]

GENETIC BASIS FOR ANDERSEN-TAWIL SYNDROME

To date, more than 40 unique mutations in KCNJ2 have been described as causative for ATS1. Mutations in KCNJ2 account for approximately two-thirds of ATS, while the molecular basis of the residual third of ATS cases remains genetically and mechanistically elusive. However, the prevalence of KCNJ2 mutations may be as high as 75% to 80% for patients with at least two ATS phenotypic features (i.e., typical ATS).[1] Most ATS-associated mutations in KCNJ2 are inherited in an autosomal dominant inheritance pattern, however as much as one-third of mutations in KCNJ2 could be sporadic de novo occurrences. In addition, somatic mosaicism has also been described in at least one KCNJ2-associated ATS family. Localized to chromosome 17q23, KCNJ2 encodes for Kir2.1, a two-membrane spanning repeat potassium channel alpha subunit expressed in brain, skeletal muscle, and heart that is critically responsible for the inward rectifying cardiac I_{K1} current (Fig. 63.2). In the heart, I_{K1} plays an important role in setting the heart's resting membrane potential, buffering extracellular potassium, and modulating the action potential waveform. Most KCNJ2 mutations described in ATS are missense mutations that cause a loss-of-function of I_{K1} either through a dominant negative effect on Kir2.1 subunit assembly or through haploinsufficiency as a result of protein trafficking defects.[1]

Phenotypic Correlates in KCNJ2-Mediated Andersen-Tawil Syndrome (ATS1)

Genotype-specific electrocardiographic features of ATS are beginning to emerge. Zhang et al. examined ECG T-U morphology and found that 91% of KCNJ2 mutation positive ATS1 patients had characteristic T-U-wave patterns (including prolonged terminal T wave down-slope, a wide T-U junction, and biphasic and enlarged U-waves) compared to none of the 61 unaffected family members or 29 genotype-negative ATS patients. In a subsequent study, 88% of KCNJ2 mutation positive ATS patients had an abnormal U-wave. Additionally, while the U-wave is markedly abnormal in ATS1, it is typically normal in LQTS. Consequently, this KCNJ2 gene-specific T-U morphology can be very useful in differentiating ATS1 patients from KCNJ2 mutation-negative ATS and LQT1-3 patients. This could facilitate a cost-effective approach towards genetic testing of the appropriate disorder. Interestingly, topological location of KCNJ2 mutations may influence the phenotypic expression of ATS features. The vast majority (approximately 90%) of KCNJ2 mutations reside either in the N- or C-terminus of this two-transmembrane single pore channel. C-terminal mutations appear to be more often associated with typical ATS (>2 ATS features), dysmorphism, and periodic paralysis. Meanwhile, N-terminal mutations were more often observed in atypical ATS (only 1 ATS feature, predominately a cardiac phenotype only) cases.[1]

Ankyrin-B Syndrome

The ANK2 gene encodes for ankyrin B protein, a member of large family of proteins that anchor various integral membrane proteins to the spectrin-based cytoskeleton. Specifically, ankyrin B is involved in anchoring the Na/K-ATPase, Na/Ca exchanger, and InsP3 receptor to specialized microdomains in the cardiomyocyte transverse tubules. In murine models, ANK2 haploinsufficiency results in altered calcium handling and a complex cardiac phenotype consisting of atrial arrhythmias, sinus bradycardia, modest heart rate-corrected QT interval prolongation, catecholamine-induced ventricular arrhythmias, and a propensity for SCD.[31] In humans, loss-of-function variants in *ANK2* were shown to cause a dominantly inherited cardiac arrhythmia with an increased risk for SCD in the setting of overt QTc prolongation. As a result, *ANK2* was subsequently assigned the label of type 4 LQTS (LQT4). However, subsequent studies have demonstrated that baseline QTc prolongation is inconsistently observed in ankyrin B syndrome (ABS). Similar to ATS, this initial discrepancy appears to have been caused partly by the erroneous inclusion of prominent U-waves/sinusoidal T-U abnormalities in QTc calculations. As a result, the QT-U interval may appear markedly prolonged in ABS, but true QTc values typically reside in the normal-to-borderline range as commonly reported. As a result, this disorder has been renamed SSS with bradycardia or the ABS.[1]

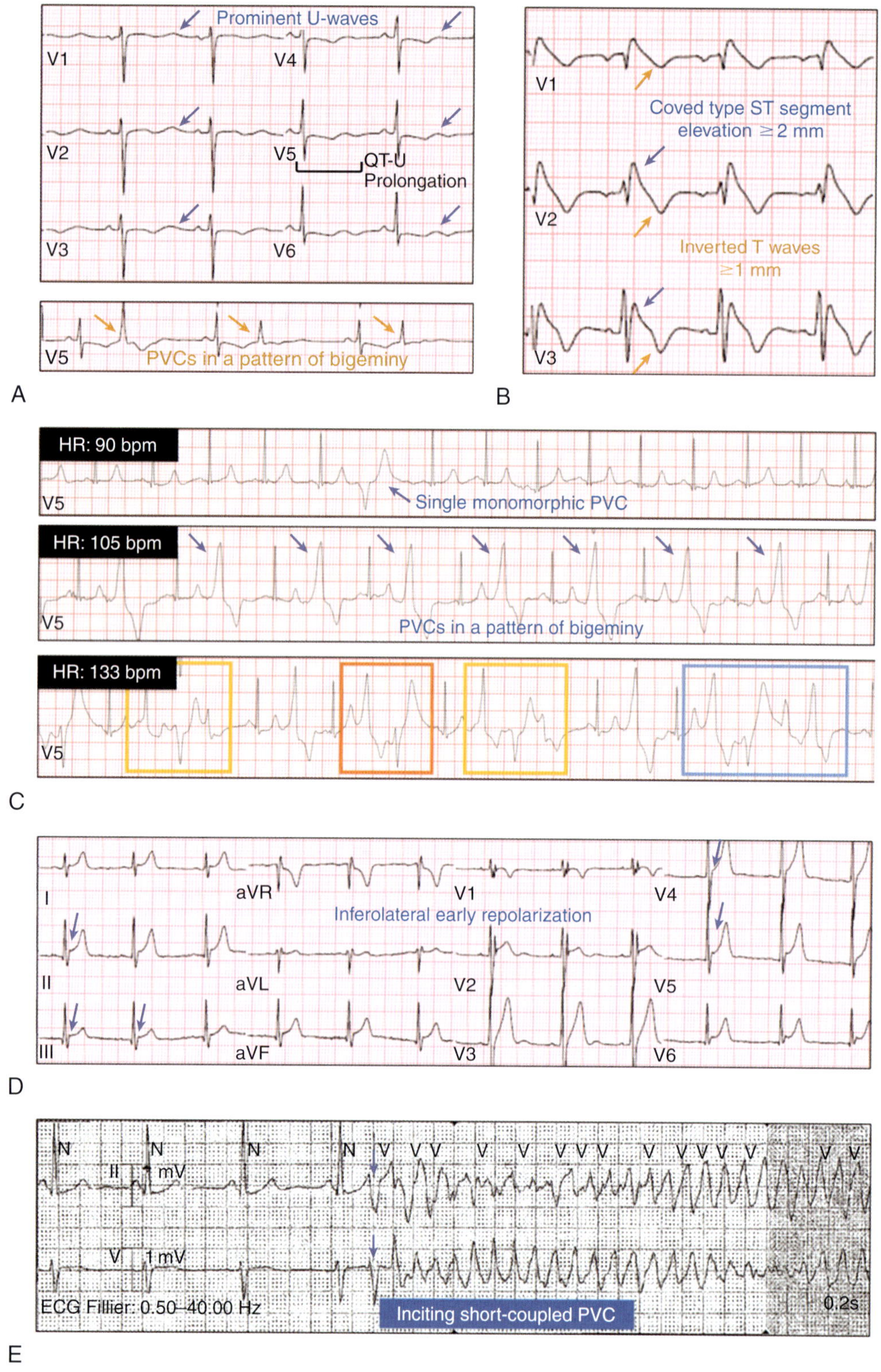

Of note, the first human *ANK2* mutation (p.E1425G-ANK2) was identified in a large multi-generational French kindred presenting with "atypical LQTS" displaying a phenotype of prolonged QT-interval, severe sinus bradycardia, polyphasic T waves and AF.[1] Following this sentinel discovery, significant loss-of-function ankyrin B variants of differing degrees of functionality have now been identified in patients with a wide array of arrhythmia including bradycardia, sinus node dysfunction (SND), delayed cardiac conduction/conduction block, IVF, AF, DI-LQTS, exercise-induced VT, and even BrS and CPVT phenotypes.

However, it is important to note that 2% to 4% of ostensibly healthy white and 8% to 10% of black subjects (including the most common "black" specific variant p.L1622I-ANK2) also host rare variants in *ANK2*, making it difficult to distinguish ABS-causative variants from background genetic noise (i.e., VUS). Furthermore, the majority of alleged ABS-causative loss-of-function variants, including p.E1424G-ANK2, used to establish the initial GDA between *ANK2* and ABS have now been observed with perplexingly high frequency in public exomes/genomes (i.e., >100 individuals). This revealed that the genetic basis of ABS may be substantially more complex than initially anticipated.[5]

Brugada Syndrome
Clinical Description and Manifestations of Brugada Syndrome

Brugada syndrome (BrS) is a heritable arrhythmia syndrome characterized clinically by spontaneous or

FIGURE 63.6 Select electrocardiographic findings in the non-QT-opathies. **A,** Prominent U-waves (*blue arrows*), QT-U interval prolongation (*black bracket*), and frequent ventricular ectopy (*orange arrows*) in a p.R82W-KCNJ2–positive Andersen-Tawil syndrome patient. After exclusion of the U-wave in the top panel, the patient's QT interval (443 msec) is within normal limits. **B,** A spontaneous type 1 Brugada syndrome pattern (coved/downsloping ST elevation ≥2 mm [*blue arrows*] with T wave inversions ≥1 mm [*orange arrows*] in the right precordial leads) in a genotype-negative patient with Brugada syndrome and easily inducible ventricular fibrillation from the right ventricular outflow tract on electrophysiology study. **C,** The progression of exercise-induced ventricular ectopy in a p.N98S-CALM1-positive catecholaminergic polymorphic ventricular tachycardia patient. During the early stages of exercise (*top panel*), occasional premature ventricular contractions (*blue arrow*) are observed. With increasing workloads (*middle panel*), more complex patterns of ventricular ectopy, most notable premature ventricular contractions in a pattern of bigeminy (*blue arrows*), is observed. At peak exercise (*bottom panel*), untreated or sub-optimally treated patients' manifest findings such as bi-directional couplets (*orange box*) and triplets (*gold boxes*) and bidirectional ventricular tachycardia (nonsustained in this case; *blue box*). **D,** Early repolarization in the inferior and lateral leads observed in a genotype-negative patient who presented with a sentinel cardiac arrest and has suffered appropriate implantable cardioverter defibrillator shocks. **E,** Telemetry rhythm strip demonstrating so-called short coupled torsades de pointes (premature ventricular contraction with a coupling interval of approximately 300 msec is indicated by *blue arrows*) in a genotype-negative patient who presented with a sentinel out-of-hospital cardiac arrest.

class I antiarrhythmic-provoked coved type ST-segment elevation (≥2 mm) followed by a negative T wave in ≥1 mm right precordial leads (V_1 or V_2, often referred to as a type 1 Brugada ECG pattern; Fig. 63.6B) on ECG and an increased risk of SCD during rest, sleep, or febrile episodes.[1] Although initially thought to disproportionately affect males with structurally normal hearts, recent imaging,[32,33] post-mortem necropsy, and concomitant electroanatomic mapping/targeted endomyocardial biopsy[34] studies have provided evidence that BrS is defined by electroanatomic and structural abnormalities involving the right ventricular outflow tract (RVOT) epicardium. As a result, BrS is best classified as a focal epicardial arrhythmogenic cardiomyopathy rather than a true cardiac channelopathy.

GENETIC BASIS OF BRUGADA SYNDROME

Classically, BrS is considered a mendelian/monogenic disorder inherited in an autosomal dominant fashion. However, many BrS cases arise sporadically, and marked incomplete penetrance and variable expressivity is a hallmark of the disorder. Therefore, the use of unbiased gene-discovery techniques (i.e., linkage analysis and trio/pedigree-based exome sequencing) to identify monogenic causes of BrS have largely proven unsuccessful.

At present, loss-of-function pathogenic/likely pathogenic variants in the *SCN5A*-encoded $Na_v1.5$ cardiac sodium channel underlie approximately 20% to 30% of BrS cases and constitute Brugada syndrome type 1 (BrS1). Interestingly, the yield of mutation detection may be significantly higher among familial forms than in sporadic cases. In one study, *SCN5A* mutations were identified in 38% of familial BrS cases compared to none in 27 sporadic cases (p = 0.001). The majority of the mutations were missense (66%), followed by frameshift (13%), nonsense, (11%), splice-site (7%), and in-frame deletions/insertions (3%) mutations. Approximately 3% of the genotype-positive patients host multiple putative pathogenic *SCN5A* mutations. Similar to the genotype-phenotype observations in LQTS, patients hosting multiple *SCN5A* mutations tend to be younger at diagnosis (29.7 ± 16 years) than those having a single mutation (39.2 ± 14.4 years).[1] Similar to LQT3, there is no particular mutational "hotspot", as nearly 80% of the BrS related *SCN5A* mutations occur as "private" single family mutations.

However, nearly 10% of the 438 unrelated putative disease-causative *SCN5A* variant-positive patients hosted one of the following four mutations: p.E1784K-SCN5A (14 patients), p.F861Wfs*90-SCN5A (11 patients), p.D356N-SCN5A (8 patients), and p.G1408R-SCN5A (7 patients). Interestingly, the most common occurring BrS1 mutation (p.E1784K-SCN5A) has also been reported as the most commonly seen LQT3-associated *SCN5A* mutation, illustrating how the same exact DNA alteration in a given gene can lead to two distinct cardiac arrhythmia syndromes. This is most likely a result of other environmental or genetic modifying factors. In fact, p.E1784K-SCN5A represents the quintessential example of a cardiac sodium channel mutation with the capacity to provide for a mixed clinical phenotype of LQT3, BrS, and conduction disorders.[1]

Besides ultra-rare pathogenic/likely pathogenic variants, common genetic variants in *SCN5A* (and other genes) also contribute a substantive role in the pathogenesis of BrS. In particular, a rare disease GWAS identified and validated the association of three genetic loci [*SCN5A* (rs11708996) *SCN10A* (rs10428132) on chromosome 3 and *HEY2* (rs9388451) on chromosome 6] in BrS patients of European descent. Interestingly, the likelihood of manifesting a type 1 BrS ECG pattern rose substantially as individuals accumulated risk alleles within these genetic loci (two risk alleles conferred an odds ratio of 1.9 whereas greater than four risk alleles conferred an odds ratio of 21.5). Importantly, this simple "PRS" has now been validated independently in Japanese and Taiwanese cohorts.[19,35] However, approximately 1.5% of individuals of European-descent possess greater than 4 risk alleles in the aforementioned BrS-associated genetic loci identified by Bezzina et al.[19] Therefore, it is highly unlikely that these common genetic loci are sufficient to cause BrS, a disorder with an estimated prevalence less than 1:5000 (0.02%).[19,36]

In addition to putative BrS-causative *SCN5A* rare variants and the polygenic cocktail of common variants in *SCN5A*, *SCN10A*, and *HEY2*, alleged BrS-causative variants have now been described in greater than 20 additional BrS-susceptibility genes. Mechanistically, many of the "minor" BrS-susceptibility genes encode components of the Na_v1.5 macromolecular complex and have been shown to perturb Na_v1.5 trafficking in vitro (*GPD1L*, *RANGRF* [aka *MOG1*], *PKP2*, *SLMAP*, and the more recently described *RRAD*)[1,37] or gating/conduction (*SCN1B*, *SCN2B*, and *SCN3B*) and decrease I_{Na} in a manner analogous to BrS-causative variants in *SCN5A*. The vast majority of the remaining minor BrS-susceptibility genes encode pore-forming α- and accessory β-subunits that impart either a loss-of-function to the depolarizing L-type calcium current ($I_{Ca,L}$; *CACNA1C*, *CACNA2D1*, and *CACNB2*) or a gain-of-function to repolarizing transient outward (I_{to}; *KCND3*, *KCNE3*, and *KCNE5*) and ATP-sensitive potassium (I_{KATP}; *ABCC9* and *KCNJ8*) currents.[1]

However, with the notable exception of the p.A280V-GPD1L variant in the *GPD1L*-encoded glycerol-3-phosphate dehydrogenase 1-like protein (discovered using linkage analysis)[1] and the recently described p.R211H-RRAD variant in *RRAD*-encoded Ras-Related Associated with Diabetes GTPase discovered by exome sequencing,[37] the remaining minor BrS-susceptibility genes were largely discovered using hypothesis-driven candidate gene approaches. Unfortunately, the only BrS-susceptibility gene where rare variants are statistically over-represented in BrS cases versus controls is *SCN5A*.[38]

In this context, it is surprising that *SCN5A* is the only BrS-susceptibility gene to receive a ClinGen "definitive" evidence designation.[39] Although some of the more recently described BrS-susceptibility genes (*RRAD*, *SEMA3A*) were not assessed, the 20 BrS-susceptibility genes that were evaluated by the ClinGen Channelopathy Working Group all received "disputed" evidence designations demoting them to ambiguous GUS status.[39] As a result, extreme caution should be used when interpreting any rare variant identified in alleged minor BrS-susceptibility gene and the identification of such a variant should **never** be used as the sole means of diagnosing a BrS.[40,41] Ultimately, the (1) the probable demise of most alleged minor BrS-susceptibility genes,[39] (2) large number of BrS cases that remain genetically elusive, and (3) low penetrance and variable expressivity associated with many BrS-causative *SCN5A* pathogenic variants determines whether the majority of BrS is a genetically heterogeneous monogenic disorder or an admixture of monogenic, oligogenic/polygenic, and nongenetic etiologies that through developmental- and/or immune-mediated mechanisms result in a shared final common pathway of epicardial RVOT inflammation, fibrosis, and conduction disorders (Fig. 63.7).

Phenotypic Correlates of *SCN5A*-Mediated Brugada Syndrome

As the majority of BrS cases remain elusive genetically, genotype-phenotype correlations in BrS have not been analyzed to the same degree as in LQTS. *SCN5A* mutations are associated with a higher incidence of conduction abnormalities in BrS patients, and the presence of a long PQ interval may be indicative of *SCN5A*-mediated BrS1. In fact, Crotti et al., reported that compared to a less than 10% yield for a positive *SCN5A* genetic test for those with a PQ less than 200 msec, the yield was almost 40% among those with a PQ interval ≥200 msec. Interestingly, young BrS males (<20 years, 83%) had a significantly higher *SCN5A* pathogenic/likely pathogenic variant detection rate than males aged 20 to 40 years (21%) and those over 40 years (11%, $P < 0.0001$). In addition, BrS1, patients with non-sense, frameshift, and premature truncation causing mutations exhibit a more severe phenotype. Unlike LQTS genetic testing where the triad of diagnostic, prognostic, and therapeutic impact has been fulfilled, BrS genetic testing is currently limited by its lower yield (25% for BrS versus 75% for LQTS) and relative absence of a therapeutic contribution from knowing the genotype.[1] As a result, the clinical utility of BrS genetic testing is limited largely to *SCN5A*-specific genetic testing in order to facilitate the cascade screening of potentially at-risk relatives.[42–44]

Catecholaminergic Polymorphic Ventricular Tachycardia

Clinical Description and Manifestations of Catecholaminergic Polymorphic Ventricular Tachycardia

Catecholaminergic polymorphic ventricular tachycardia (CPVT) is a heritable arrhythmia syndrome that affects an estimated 1 in 10,000 individuals, and manifests clinically with exercise-induced syncope or sudden death in individuals with otherwise structurally normal hearts. Similar to LQT1, swimming is a potentially lethal arrhythmia-precipitating trigger in CPVT. In fact, both LQT1 and CPVT have been shown to underlie several cases of unexplained drowning or near-drowning in the young healthy swimmer. However, aside from

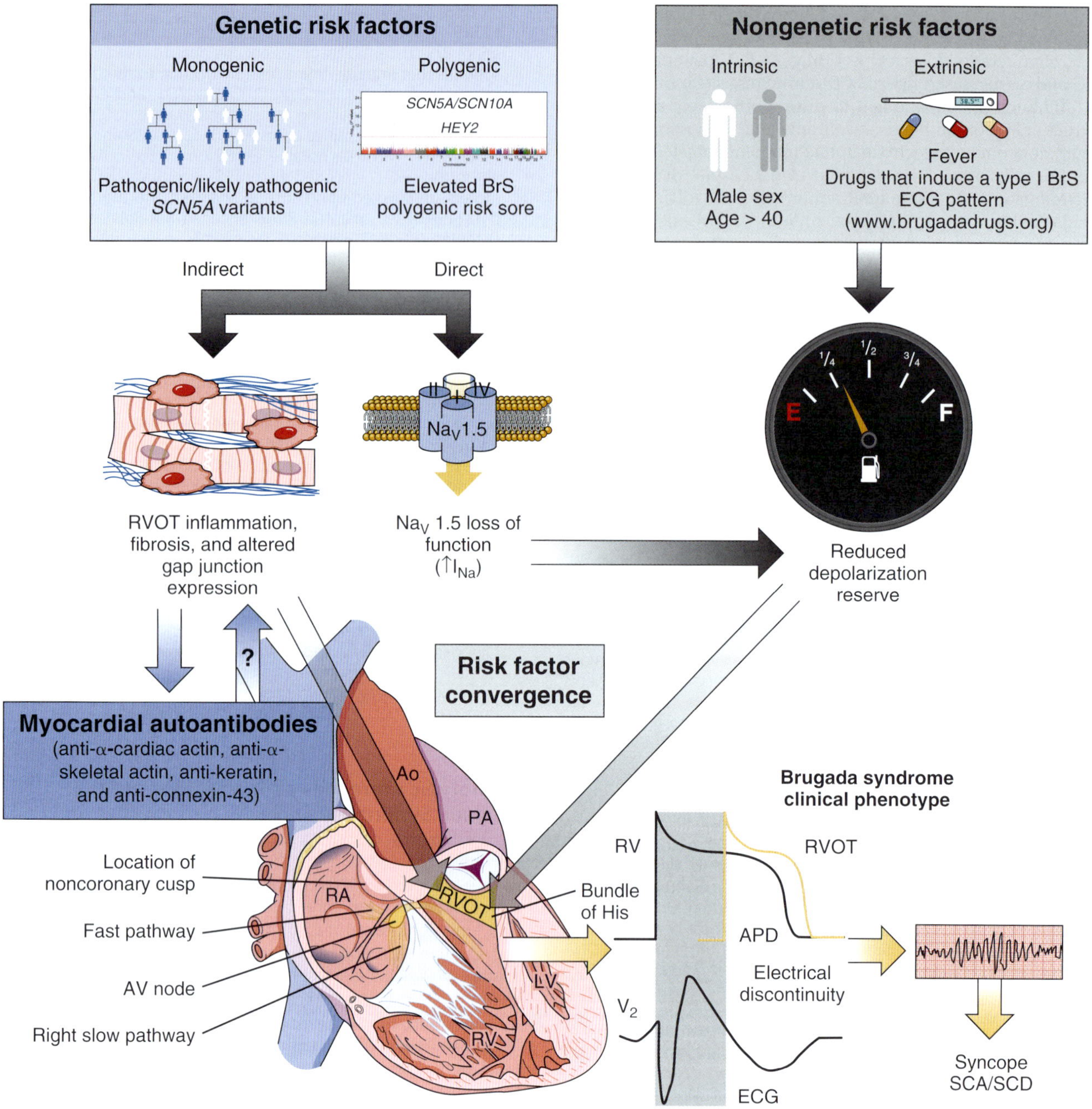

FIGURE 63.7 The evolving genetic architecture and pathophysiology of Brugada syndrome. The contribution of genetic (*blue box*) and nongenetic (*gray box*) risk factors to Brugada syndrome pathogenesis. *Black arrows* denote the potential myocardial and electrophysiological effect(s) of known genetic and nongenetic risk factors. *Blue arrows* demonstrate the recent identification of myocardial autoantibodies sensitive and specific for Brugada syndrome, as well as their potential role in disease pathogenesis. *Gray arrows* demonstrate the convergence of myocardial and electrophysiological effects in the right ventricular outflow tract resulting in a localized delay in depolarization/conduction. *Yellow arrows* demonstrate how electrical discontinuity between the right ventricular (*black tracing*) and right ventricular outflow tract (*yellow tracing*) are capable of generating the classic electrocardiogram findings observed in Brugada syndrome as well as an increased risk of syncope and/or sudden cardiac arrest/death secondary to sustained ventricular arrhythmias. *AP*, Action potential; *BrS*, Brugada syndrome; *ECG*, electrocardiogram; I_{Na}, RV, right ventricle; *RVOT*, right ventricular outflow tract; *SCA*, sudden cardiac arrest; *SCD*, sudden cardiac death.

nonspecific findings such as bradycardia and subtle U-waves, the resting 12-lead ECG in CPVT is completely normal. As a result, the use of exercise stress testing (EST), or catecholamine provocation testing (CPT), is needed to unearth the adrenergically induced ventricular ectopy/arrhythmias (Fig. 63.6C), including the pathognomonic finding of bidirectional VT (Fig. 63.6C), that serve as the electrocardiographic hallmarks of CPVT.[1]

Clinically, a presentation of exercise-induced syncope or cardiac arrest in the setting of a QTc less than 460 msec should always prompt first consideration of CPVT rather than so-called "concealed" or "normal QT interval" LQT1. Furthermore, exercise-induced premature ventricular complexes occurring in a pattern of bigeminy is a far more likely observation than the more specific but less sensitive finding of bidirectional VT. Unfortunately, failure to perform an EST/CPT or the misinterpretation of appropriately obtained EST/CPT results represents a common reason for a delayed or missed CPVT diagnosis.[45] As a result, the 2017 ACC/AHA/HRS guidelines have called for the inclusion of an EST (or CPT for those unable to exercise) in the primary evaluation of all patients presenting with arrhythmic symptoms occurring during exertion or emotion.[42] However, as over a quarter of CPVT patients in the Pediatric and Congenital Electrophysiology Society multicenter CPVT registry that experienced a prior SCA did so during non-exertional wakeful activities (i.e., rest and playing a musical instrument),[46] the argument could be made to extend the inclusion of an EST/CPT in the work-up of all unexplained SCA survivors.

Once thought to manifest only during childhood, recent studies have suggested that the age of first presentation can range from infancy to 40 years of age. CPVT's potential lethality is illustrated by mortality rates of 30% to 50% by 35 years of age and the presence of a positive family history of young (<40 years) SCD for more than a third of CPVT individuals and in as many as 60% of families hosting RyR2 mutations. Moreover, approximately 15% of autopsy negative SUD in the young and some cases of SIDS have been attributed to CPVT.[1]

GENETIC BASIS OF CATECHOLAMINERGIC POLYMORPHIC VENTRICULAR TACHYCARDIA

Perturbations in key components of intracellular calcium-induced calcium release from the sarcoplasmic reticulum serve as the pathogenic basis for CPVT (see Chapter 62). Inherited in an autosomal dominant fashion, mutations in the *RYR2*-encoded cardiac ryanodine receptor/calcium release channel represent the most common genetic subtype of CPVT (CPVT1), accounting for 60% of clinically "strong" cases of CPVT (Fig. 63.8). Gain-of-function mutations in RyR2 produce leaky calcium release channels leading to excessive calcium release, particularly during sympathetic stimulation that can precipitate calcium overload, delayed depolarizations (DADs), and ventricular arrhythmias. Again, most unrelated CPVT families are identified with their own unique *RYR2* mutation and about 5% of unrelated mutation-positive patients host multiple putative pathogenic mutations.

RYR2 is one of the largest genes in the human genome with 105 exons that transcribe/translate one of the largest cardiac ion channel proteins comprising 4967 amino acid residues. While there appears to be no specific mutation "hot-spots," there are three regional "hot-spots" or "domains" where unique mutations reside (see Fig. 63.8). Greater than 90% of *RYR2* mutations discovered to date represent missense mutations; however, as much as 5% of unrelated CPVT patients host large gene rearrangements consistent with large whole exon deletions, similar to findings with LQTS. While to date genotype-phenotype correlations are very limited, a recent publication revealed that family members hosting C-terminal (ion channel-forming domain) RyR2 mutations may have a higher burden of nonsustained ventricular tachycardia (NSVT) than those hosting N-terminal or central domain RyR2 localizing mutations.[1]

Strikingly, nearly a third of "possible/atypical" LQTS (QTc <480 msec) cases with exertion-induced syncope have also been identified as *RYR2* mutation positive. In fact, it has been reported that nearly 30% of patients with CPVT have been misdiagnosed as "LQTS with normal QT-intervals" or "concealed LQTS," indicating the critical importance of properly distinguishing between CPVT and LQTS at the clinical level, as risk assessments and treatment strategies of these unique disorders may vary. Similarly, loss-of-function variants in the *KCNJ2*-encoded $K_{ir}2.1$ potassium channel (the same gene/mechanism that causes ATS) have also been observed in patients diagnosed with CPVT who experience exercise-induced bi-directional VT. Although a distinct electrophysiological phenotype (protein kinase A-dependent I_{k1} reduction) has been elucidated for the type 3 CPVT (CPVT3)-causative *KCNJ2* variant (p.Val227Phe-KCNJ2),[1] it is unclear if ATS and CPVT3 represent a disease continuum or separate entities differentiated by distinct electrophysiological/pathophysiological mechanisms.

In addition to *KCNJ2*, pathogenic/likely pathogenic variants in three additional genes (*CASQ2*-encoded calequestrin-2, *TRDN*-encoded triadin, and *CALM1*- and *CALM3*-encoded calmodulin) also have been implicated in the pathogenesis of CPVT. Whereas *CASQ2* and *TRDN* were associated with autosomal recessive forms of CPVT, *CALM1*/*CALM3*, like *RYR2* and *KCNJ2*, is associated with an autosomal dominant form. However, the recent realization that some CASQ2-CPVT-causative variants are capable of generating a CPVT phenotype in heterozygous individuals has re-defined the heritability of this minor CPVT subtype (i.e., both an autosomal dominant and recessive disorder).[47]

Calcium Release Channel Deficiency Syndrome

In early 2020, Tester et al. described two seemingly unrelated, multigenerational Amish families with multiple recessively inherited and exercise-associated youthful SUDs. Interestingly, exome sequencing and subsequent analysis using an autosomal recessive model failed to identify any homozygous or compound heterozygous nonsynonymous variants within a candidate gene(s).[48] However, copy number variant analysis identified a homozygous tandem duplication involving the 5′ untranslated/promoter regions and the first four exons of *RYR2* in all affected individuals (i.e., youthful SCA/SCD) with available genetic material. Unlike CPVT1, patients with this new disorder termed "calcium release channel deficiency syndrome" or CRC deficiency syndrome display relatively nonspecific ECG findings (i.e., intermittent QTc prolongation with U-waves) and modest or no ventricular ectopy during EST/CPT or prolonged ambulatory Holter monitoring.[48]

Mechanistically, CRC deficiency syndrome patient-specific

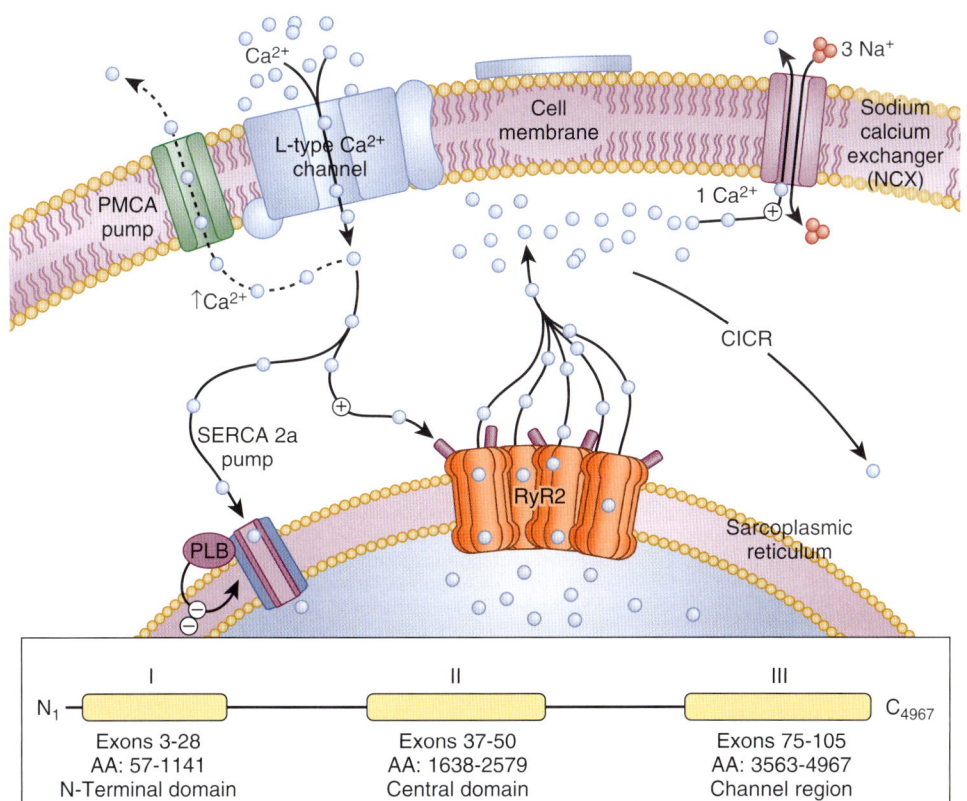

FIGURE 63.8 Catecholaminergic polymorphic ventricular tachycardia: a disorder of intracellular calcium handling. Perturbations in key components of the calcium-induced calcium release (CICR) mechanism responsible for cardiac excitation-contraction coupling is the pathogenic basis for CPVT. At the center of this mechanism is the *RYR2*-encoded cardiac ryanodine receptor/calcium release channel located in sarcoplasmic reticulum membrane. Mutations in RyR2 are clustered and distributed in three "hot-spot" regions of this 4967 amino acid (AA) protein; Domain I or N-terminal Domain (AA 57-1141), Domain II or the Central Domain (AA 1638-2579), and Domain III or Channel Region (AA 3563-4967).

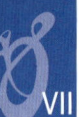

iPSC-CM display a profound reduction in the transcription and translation of RyR2, and loss of calcium responsiveness to isoproterenol and caffeine. Therefore, unlike the RyR2 gain-of-function (i.e., hyperactive/hyperreactive "leaky" channels) observed in CPVT1, CRC deficiency syndrome appears to result in RyR2 loss-of-function that nearly ablates calcium-induced calcium release in response to catecholamine infusion.[49]

Interestingly, RyR2 loss-of-function variants (e.g., p.A4860G-RYR, and p.S4938F-RYR2) have also been observed in patients with so-called short-coupled TdP/PVC-triggered VF and unremarkable ESTs diagnosed with either atypical CPVT or IVF.[50] As such, these studies provide compelling evidence that genetic defects in RyR2 likely increase SCA/SCD risk through a variety of electrophysiologic mechanisms, which may have both risk-stratification and management implications in the future.

Early Repolarization Syndrome
Clinical Description and Manifestations of Early Repolarization Syndrome

The early repolarization (ER) pattern is characterized by the elevation (≥ 1 mm above baseline) of the QRS-ST junction (the so-called J-point) manifesting as either QRS slurring (at the transition of the QRS to the ST-segment) or notching (a positive deflection inscribed on terminal S wave), ST-segment elevation with upper concavity and prominent T waves in ≥ 2 contiguous leads (Fig. 63.6D). The prevalence of the ER pattern in the general population has been reported to range from less than 1% to 13%, depending on age, sex, race, and the criteria for J-point elevation. This electrocardiographic phenomenon has long been considered an innocuous variant among healthy individuals. However, Haissaguerre et al. have noted that J-point elevation (≥ 1 mm above baseline) on inferolateral ECG leads was over represented significantly (31%) and was greater in magnitude among 206 case subjects who experienced cardiac arrest due to IVF compared to 412 (5%, $p < 0.001$) age, sex, race, and level of physical activity matched controls. Those patients with ER were more often males and have a personal history of syncope or cardiac arrest during sleep than those without ER pattern. Other studies have observed an over representation of J-point elevation in IVF patients compared to controls, with the same male predominance among those with ER.[1]

In a community-based general population of 10,864 middle-aged (30 to 59 years of age, 52% male) Finnish subjects, Tikkanen et al. identified 630 subjects overall (5.8%) with J-point elevation of at least 0.1 mV; J-point elevation. This overall prevalence of ER pattern was reduced to only 0.33% when considering a J-point elevation of ≥ 0.2 mV. Following a 30-year follow-up with the end point being cardiac death, Tikkanen et al. noted that compared to subjects without a J-point elevation, subjects with ER (J-point ≥ 0.1 mV) in the inferior leads had both an increased risk of cardiac death (adjusted relative risk [ARR] = 1.28, 95% confidence interval [CI] = 1.04 to 1.59; $P = 0.03$) and arrhythmias (ARR = 1.43, 95% CI = 1.06 to 1.94, p = 0.03) and this risk was further elevated (cardiac death, ARR = 2.98, 95% CI = 1.85 to 4.92, p < 0.001; arrhythmia, ARR = 2.92; 95% CI = 1.45 to 5.89, p < 0.001) with increasing elevation (≥ 0.2 mV) of the J-point. However, ER pattern localizing to only the lateral leads did not show a statistically significant association with increased risk for arrhythmic cardiac death.[1] Obviously, the vexing clinical conundrum with respect to this Inferolateral Early Repolarization syndrome is distinguishing the potentially lethal ERS from the all too often observed juvenile ER pattern seen in healthy individuals, particularly athletes.

GENETIC BASIS FOR EARLY REPOLARIZATION SYNDROME

The inclination for a genetic basis for ERS stems from Haissaguerre's observation that 16% of their IVF patients with an ER pattern had a family history of unexplained sudden death. The first gene to be implicated in ERS was described by Haissaguere et al., who reported finding a rare, functionally uncharacterized, missense mutation (p.S422L-KCNJ8) in the KCNJ8-encoding pore-forming subunit Kir6.1 of the ATP-sensitive potassium channel in a 14-year-old female with IVF. Since then, this same mutation has been described now in additional cases of BrS and ERS and has been shown to have a gain-of-function in

electrophysiological phenotype. However despite its abnormal in vitro functional phenotype, it is now appreciated that p.S422L-KCNJ8 is far more common than once thought, thus questioning its pathophysiological role. In fact, since its implication in disease, p.S422L-KCNJ8 is now known to have heterozygous frequency of 0.5% (168/33,363) among European Caucasians in the exome aggregation consortium (ExAC) and as high as 4% among the Ashkenazi Jewish population. Thus, these findings reveal that this variant may be a functional common variant that contributes to disease phenotype rather than a monogenic disease-causative pathogenic mutation.[1] In addition, gain-of-function variants in ABBC9, a component of the hetero-octameric $K_{ir}6.1$ ATP-sensitive potassium channels, and the KCND3-encoded $K_v4.3$ voltage-gated potassium channel as well as loss-of-function variants in the LTCC (CACNA1C, CACNB2b, and CACNA2D1) and $Na_v1.5$ (SCN5A and SCN10A) macromolecular complex constituents have been linked to ERS.[36] However, not all of these genetic variants have been characterized functionally, while p.S422L-KCNJ8 could appear to be over-represented in public exomes/genomes.

As such, no definitive evidence exists to show that ERS has a mendelian/monogenic (i.e., single gene) basis. Although initial ER pattern GWAS studies were inconclusive, a recent larger GWAS study identified a statistical association between a locus in KCND3 and an ER pattern (not ERS).[51] In light of the clinical similarities between the so-called J-wave syndromes (i.e., ERS and BrS) and the emerging polygenic genetic architecture of BrS, it stands to reason that the bulk of ERS may also have a oligogenic/polygenic basis driven by relatively common functional risk alleles such as p.S422L-KCNJ8.

Familial Atrial Fibrillation (see Chapter 66)
Clinical Description and Manifestations of Familial Atrial Fibrillation

AF is the most common cardiac arrhythmia with a prevalence of about 1% in the general population and 6% in people over the age of 65 years. Most often AF is associated with underlying cardiac pathology, including cardiomyopathy, valvular disease, hypertension, and atherosclerotic cardiovascular disease and is responsible for over a third of cardioembolic episodes. However, AF can present even at an early age without any identifiable cardiac anomalies and is termed lone AF, accounting for 2% to 16% of all AF cases. Further, approximately one-third of lone AF patients have a family history of AF suggesting familial forms of the disease.[1]

GENETIC BASIS FOR FAMILIAL ATRIAL FIBRILLATION

While the majority of FAF remains genetically elusive, several genetic loci and causative genes have been described in recent decades. In 1996, Brugada et al. identified three families with autosomal dominant arterial fibrillation (AF). The age of onset ranged from in utero to 45 years. Genetic linkage analysis of these families revealed a novel locus for AF on chromosome 10 (10q22). In 2003, a second locus at 6q14-16, again associated with autosomal dominant inheritance, was identified. To date, the underlying causative genes for both loci remain unknown.

However, in 2003 an AF-associated locus on chromosome 11 in a large four-generation family and subsequent identification of a SQTS-like gain-of-function variant, p.S140G-KCNQ1, in $K_v7.1$ (I_{Ks}) was identified, thus providing a causal link between a cardiac potassium ion channel mutation and FAF for the first time. Interestingly, a second de novo mutation involving KCNQ1 was identified in a patient with a severe form of AF and SQTS presenting in utero.[1]

Following these discoveries, gain-of-function variants a number of genes encoding potassium channel α- [KCNH2 ($K_v11.1$), KCNJ2 ($K_{ir}2.1$), KCND3 (I_{to}), and KCNJ8 ($K_{ir}6.1$)] and accessory β-subunits (KCNE1, KCNE2, KCNE3, KCNE4, and KCNE5) have been linked to familial AF. In addition, loss-of-function variants in genes encoding potassium channel α-subunits [KCNJ5 (I_{KACh}), KCNA5 (I_{Kur}), and hyperpolarization-activated cyclic nucleotide gated channel 4 (HCN4) (I_f)] have also been described.[52]

Besides these potassium channels, $Na_v1.5$ has also been implicated in lone and familial AF. In fact, AF is a fairly common arrhythmia among patients with loss-of-function sodium cardiac channelopathies (up to 15% to 20% of BrS cases developing AF). In 2008, a novel SCN5A mutation (p.M1875T-SCN5A) in a family characterized with juvenile onset of atrial arrhythmias that progressed to AF in the absence of structural heart disease or ventricular arrhythmias was described. Functional studies of this mutant channel produced an increased peak current density and a depolarizing shift of activation (gain-of-function). *SCN5A* channel mutations have been identified in approximately 3% of AF cases.[1] Moreover, putative AF-causative variants have also been described in Na$_v$1.5 accessory β-subunits (*SCN1B*, *SCN2B*, *SCN3B*, *SCN4B*, and *SCN1Bb*) as well as the *SCN10A*-encoded Na$_v$1.8 sodium channel through a modulatory effect on late sodium current.[52]

In addition, non-ion channel genes have been implicated in familial and lone AF. Hodgson-Zingman et al. identified a frameshift mutation in the *NPPA* gene in a large pedigree with FAF. *NPPA* encodes for the atrial natriuretic peptide which modulates ionic currents in myocardial cells and may shorten atrial conduction time. The clinical phenotype of neonatal onset of AF, with an autosomal recessive inheritance pattern, was recently linked to a mutation in *NUP155*, which encodes for a member of the nucleoporins family of proteins. Gollob et al. identified 4 heterozygote *GJA5* missense mutations in 4 of 15 patients with early onset idiopathic AF. Most interestingly, three of the four mutations were shown to be in cardiac tissue only (somatic) and not germline in origin. *GJA5* encodes for the cardiac gap-junction protein connexin 40 that is predominantly expressed in atrial myocytes and mediates the finely orchestrated electrical activation of the atria. Yang et al. have identified either *GATA4* (*p.S70T-GATA4* and *p.S160T-GATA4*), or *GATA5* (*p.G184V-GATA5*, *p.K218T-GATA5* and *p.A266P-GATA5*) missense mutations in 5/130 (3.8%) unrelated Han Chinese individuals with familial AF.[1] *GATA4* and *GATA5* belong to a family of cardiac transcription factors critical for cardiogenesis.

Importantly, the overall fraction of AF cases that have a mendelian/monogenic (i.e., single gene) basis is exceedingly small and the clinical utility of genetic testing in familial/lone AF-susceptibility is limited. Rather, as demonstrated by recent AF GWAS, the heritable component for the vast majority of AF patients is likely polygenic in nature and arises secondary to the contribution of a number of relatively common variants residing in genes that encode ion channel macromolecular complexes (e.g., *CAV1*, *KCNN3*, *KCND3*), structural proteins (i.e., *NEBL*, *TTN*, *SYNE2*), transcription factors (e.g., *PITX2*, *TBX5*, *ZFHX3*), and those with a myriad of other functions.[52] Although recent GWAS meta-analyses have demonstrated that the collective contribution of AF-associated loci explain approximately 11% of AF heritability,[53] the translation of these findings into clinically meaningful PRSs capable of enhancing AF risk prediction independent of or in concert with traditional risk factors has been slow.[54]

Idiopathic Ventricular Fibrillation
Clinical Description and Manifestations of Idiopathic Ventricular Fibrillation

VF is a major cause of SCD and often is the "final common arrhythmic pathway" for all the aforementioned channelopathies. In the absence of an identifiable cardiac (structural and genetic), respiratory, metabolic, or toxicological cause, resuscitated cardiac arrest victims in which VF is documented are termed "idiopathic"' ventricular fibrillation (IVF).[43] In essence, like SIDS, IVF is a diagnosis of exclusion and can stem from several underlying mechanisms. It accounts for as much as 10% of sudden deaths, especially in the young. About 30% of IVF-labeled individuals will have recurrent episodes of VF. In 20% of such cases, there is a family history of sudden death or IVF, suggesting a hereditary component in some cases. Unfortunately, the vast majority of IVF patients are diagnosed only after experiencing a sentinel out-of-hospital cardiac arrest.

GENETIC BASIS FOR IDIOPATHIC VENTRICULAR FIBRILLATION
At present, pathogenic/likely pathogenic variants in *CALM1-3*-encoded calmodulin, the *IRX3*-encoded Iroquois homeobox gene family transcription factor, *RYR2*-encoded RyR2 calcium release channel, and a promoter haplotype in the *DPP6* gene locus on chromosome 7q36 have been found to be linked to IVF.[1,55] However, many patients with IVF-causative variants in these genes have documented evidence of short-coupled TdP/PVC-triggered VT/VF (Fig. 63.6e), which is often considered to be synonymous with IVF but could represent a distinct clinical entity/phenotype.

Despite the identification of these IVF-susceptibility genes, the current ACC/AHA and EHRA/HRS guideline-endorsed role for genetic testing in individuals with IVF is to provide further evidence of a specific underlying SCD-predisposing genetic heart disease (i.e., a cardiomyopathy in a pre-cardiomyopathic electrical state or cardiac channelopathy) when there is reasonable clinical suspicion.[42] However, given the likelihood of unearthing ≥ 1 ambiguous VUS in a strong evidence channelopathy- or cardiomyopathy-susceptibility gene, the 2013 HRS/EHRA guidelines discouraged the use of large gene panels as seen in pan-arrhythmia, pan-cardiac, and exome-based genetic testing in individuals with a diagnosis of IVF.

Even with this guidance, several referral centers have published their experience with genetic testing in IVF, most using large commercial gene panels (i.e., pan-arrhythmia or pan-cardiac genetic testing) and/or exome sequencing.[29,56-58] Of note, within the slate of SCD-predisposing channelopathy- and cardiomyopathy-susceptibility genes tested variably in each study, the yield of ambiguous VUS (range 15% to 26%) far exceeded that of clinically-actionable pathogenic/likely pathogenic variants (range 2% to 17%).[29,56-58] As such, the decision to pursue any form of genetic testing in IVF should not be taken lightly and should be performed in a dedicated cardiovascular genetics clinic.

Multifocal Ectopic Purkinje-Related Premature Contractions

In addition to AF, LQTS, BrS, and progressive cardiac conduction disease (PCCD), pathogenic/likely pathogenic genetic variants in the *SCN5A*-encoded Na$_v$1.5 cardiac sodium channel have been linked to MEPPC. This rare condition results in a high burden of narrow complex, polymorphic ventricular ectopy of fascicular/Purkinje origin, increased risk of sudden death, and in some cases, a reversible and likely PVC-mediated dilated cardiomyopathy.[59,60]

Initially, MEPPC was thought to arise secondary to a specific gain-of-function variant (*p.R222Q-SCN5A*) observed in several unrelated families. However, additional variants within (*p.G213N-SCN5A*, *p.R225P-SCN5A*, and *p.L828F-SCN5A*) or in close proximity (*p.I141V-SCN5A* and *p.M1851V-SCN5A*) to the S4 transmembrane segments that play a critical role in Na$_v$1.5 voltage-sensing have been observed in patients with a MEPPC-like phenotype with time.[60] Furthermore, it appears that some LQT3-causative variants (voltage-sensing domain variants such as *p.N1325S-SCN5A* and *p.R1623Q-SCN5A*) are capable of causing a LQT3-MEPPC overlap syndrome consisting of QTc prolongation and frequent narrow complex PVCs/short-coupled ventricular arrhythmias that is associated with a higher risk of VF (SCA and appropriate ICD shocks) when present.[61]

Mechanistically, the majority of MEPPC-causative *SCN5A* variants result in the generation of increased "window current" that arise secondary to hyperpolarizing shifts in Nav1.5 voltage-dependent activation and inactivation.[59,62] Interestingly, despite possessing *SCN5A* variants that cause a LQT3-like Na$_v$1.5 gain-of-function, patients with MEPPC have normal QTc values suggesting that cardiac APD is not prolonged globally. Recent evidence from a *p.R222Q-SCN5A* knock-in murine cardiomyocyte/Purkinje cell model suggest that this phenomenon is due to the generation of an APD-shortening outward gating-pore current conducted through alternative cation permeation pathways adjacent to the S4 transmembrane.[63,64] Therefore, the absence of QTc prolongation in MEPPC may be explained by the offsetting effects of increased Na$_v$1.5 window current amplitude (APD-prolonging) and the generation of a distinct outward gating-pore current (APD-shortening) on cardiac repolarization.

Progressive Cardiac Conduction Disease
Clinical Description and Manifestations of Progressive Cardiac Conduction Defect

Cardiac conduction disease (CCD) causes a potentially life-threatening alteration in normal impulse propagation through the cardiac conduction system. CCD can be a result of several physiologic mechanisms, acquired or congenital, in the presence or absence of structural heart disease. PCCD, also known as Lev-Lenègre disease, is one of the most common cardiac conduction disturbances in the absence of structural heart disease and is characterized by progressive (age-related) impairment of impulse propagation through the His-Purkinje system, with right or left bundle branch block and widening of the QRS complex. This leads to a complete AV block, syncope, and occasionally sudden death.

GENETIC BASIS FOR PROGRESSIVE CARDIAC CONDUCTION DISEASE

In 1999, Schott et al. further expanded the spectrum of loss-of-function SCN5A disease with the inclusion of familial PCCD. They identified a splice-site SCN5A mutation (c.3963+2 T>C) associated with an autosomal dominant inheritance pattern in a large French family. Since then, investigators have identified over 30 PCCD-associated mutations in SCN5A. In addition to SCN5A, mutations in SCN1B can cause BrS with conduction disease. These mutations present with a loss-of-function phenotype through reduced current density and enhanced slow inactivation of the channel. As with most loss-of-function SCN5A-mediated disorders, the phenotypic expression of PCCD can be complex and is often present with a concomitant BrS or BrS-like phenotype. In fact, PCCD is the prevailing phenotype in BrS-associated SCN5A pathogenic/likely pathogenic variant carriers, where the penetrance of conduction defects can be as high as 76%.[1]

In 2009, Meregalli et al. demonstrated that SCN5A variant type can have a profound effect on the severity of PCCD and BrS. Studying 147 individuals hosting one of 32 different SCN5A variants, Meregalli found that patients with either a premature truncation mutation (i.e., nonsense or frameshift) or a severe loss-of-function missense mutation (>90% reduction in peak I_{Na}) had a significantly longer PR interval compared with those patients with missense variants having less impairment to the sodium current (≤90% reduction). Furthermore, these patients had significantly more episodes of syncope than those with an "active" variant.[1] These findings suggest that those mutations with a more deleterious loss of sodium current produce a more severe phenotype of syncope and conduction defect, providing the first evidence for intragenotype risk stratification associated with SCN5A loss-of-function disease.

Gain-of-function variants (p.E7K-TRPM4, p.R164W-TRPM4, p.A432T-TRPM4, and p.G844D-TRPM4) in the TRPM4-encoded transient receptor potential melastatin type 4 ion channel have been identified as a cause of autosomal dominant isolated cardiac conduction disorder and progressive familial heart block. This is possible by classical linkage analysis and subsequent mutational analysis of TRPM4 in four different large multigenerational pedigrees. As such, the calcium-activated nonselective cation channel contributes importantly to the cardiac conduction system.[1]

Sick Sinus Syndrome

Clinical Description and Manifestations of Sick Sinus Syndrome

SND or "sick sinus syndrome" (SSS) manifesting as inappropriate sinus bradycardia, sinus arrest, atrial standstill, tachycardia-bradycardia syndrome, or chronotropic incompetence is the leading diagnosis for pacemaker implantation (see Chapter 68). SSS commonly occurs in the elderly (1 in 600 cardiac patients >65 years of age) with acquired cardiac conditions including cardiomyopathy, congestive heart failure, ischemic heart disease, or metabolic diseases. However, there are no identifiable cardiac anomalies or conditions underlying sinus node dysfunction ("idiopathic SND"), which can occur at any age including in utero in a significant number of cases. Additionally, familial forms of idiopathic SND consistent with autosomal dominant inheritance with reduced penetrance and recessive forms with complete penetrance have been reported.[1]

GENETIC BASIS OF SICK SINUS SYNDROME

Mutational analysis of small cohorts and case reports of patients with idiopathic SSS have so far implicated four genes: SCN5A, HCN4, ANK2, and MYH6. To date, 15 putative SSS-causative variants have been reported in SCN5A. These variants either produced nonfunctional sodium channels through loss of expression or channels with mild to severe loss-of-function through altered biophysical properties of the channel. In 2003, based on prior observations of arrhythmias and conduction disturbances, SCN5A was identified as a gene for congenital SSS diagnosed in the first decade of life. Compound heterozygote variants (p.T220I-SCN5A + p.R1623X- SCN5A, p.P1298L-SCN5A + p.G1408R-SCN5A, and p.delF1617- SCN5A + p.R1632H-SCN5A) implicated SCN5A in autosomal recessive SSS.[1] Moreover, many of the SCN5A positive patients displayed a mixed phenotype consisting of SSS, BrS and/or CCD. The expressivity of the mixture can be highly variable within affected families, and the environmental and/or genetic modifiers responsible for this phenomenon are poorly understood. A patient with SSS, CCD, and recurrent VT was described with an p.L1821fsX10-SCN5A frameshift variant that exhibited a 90% reduction in current density (consistent with BrS/SSS/CCD), and an increase in late sodium current (consistent with LQT3) for those channels that are expressed. The absence of symptoms in a number of other family members highlights the incomplete or low penetrance of this SCN5A-mediated disorder.

Two loss-of-function variants in HCN4, have been identified in idiopathic SND. The HCN4 gene encodes the so-called I_f "funny" or pacemaker current and plays a key role in the automaticity of the sinus node. In one study, a frameshift variant (p.P544fsX30-HCN4) was identified in a patient with idiopathic SND. In another study, a patient with idiopathic SND had a missense variant (p.D553N-HCN4) that resulted in abnormal trafficking of the pacemaker channel. Interestingly, while the frameshift mutation identified in a 66-year-old woman produced a mild phenotype associated with sinus rhythm during exercise, the p.D553N-HCN4 missense mutation identified in a 43-year-old woman was associated with severe bradycardia, recurrent syncope, QT prolongation, and polymorphic ventricular tachycardia (TdP), suggesting the potential for lethality in HCN4-mediated disease.[1] Further studies (larger cohorts) are required to determine if the preliminary 10% to 15% yield for defective HCN4-encoded pacemaker channels in idiopathic SND (derived from the two small cohorts) is durable.

Genetic dysfunction in ANK2-encoded ankyrin B has been reported in two large families with high penetrant and severe SND. Ankyrin B is essential for normal membrane organization of ion channels and transporters in the cardiomyocytes within the SA node and is required for proper physiological cardiac pacing. Dysfunction of ankyrin B-based trafficking pathway causes abnormal electrical activity in the SA node and SND. Like the Na_v1.5 sodium channel, variants in ANK2 have been associated with a variety of cardiac dysfunctions.

In a GWAS in the Icelandic population including 792 individuals with SSS and 37,592 controls, a rare missense variant (c.2161C>T, p.R721W-MYH6) in MYH6-encoded alpha heavy chain 6 subunit of cardiac myosin was significantly associated with SSS. Moreover, the lifetime risk of being diagnosed with SSS was only 6% for non-carriers of c.2161C>T compared to 50% for carriers of the MYH6 variant. Ishikawa et al. identified a 3 bp in-frame deletion resulting in a single amino acid deletion (p.delE933-MYH6) in a genotype-negative proband with SSS. The mutant slowed down action potential propagation when heterologously expressed in HL-1 atrial myocytes. Moreover, morpholino knockdown of MYH6 in zebrafish led to a reduced heart rate that could be restored when co-expressed with wild-type MYH6, but not when co-expressed with dE933-MYH6.[1]

CONCLUSIONS

This novel discipline of genetic cardiology has grown substantially over the past two decades. The pathogenic insights into the molecular underpinnings for nearly all these syndromes have matured through the entire continuum of research from discovery, translation, incorporation into routine clinical practice. This bench-to-bedside maturation now requires the learned interpretation of the available genetic tests for these syndromes with a clear understanding of the diagnostic, prognostic, and therapeutic implications associated with genetic testing of these channelopathies.

FUTURE PERSPECTIVES

As illustrated by LQTS, genetic testing in the cardiac channelopathies has the potential to substantially impact the diagnosis, risk-stratification, and clinical management of patients with these potentially lethal but highly treatable genetic heart disorders. However, the full promise of precision genomic medicine is far from being completely realized. As such, over the next decade, well-designed and adequately powered studies as well as educational efforts are needed to:

1. Better define the genetic architecture of the cardiac channelopathies (Fig. 63.4), particularly in regards to the role of limited- and disputed-evidence disease-susceptibility genes (also known as GUSs), the ability of common genetic variants/PRSs to explain genotype-negative disease, and the marked incomplete penetrance and variable expressivity observed in these putative mendelian/monogenic disorders.

2. Enhance our ability to distinguish pathogenic/likely pathogenic variants from rare and likely innocuous background genetic noise in definitive/strong evidence cardiac channelopathy-susceptibility genes.
3. Strengthen the genetics/genomics literacy of all cardiovascular health care providers and improve access to dedicated cardiovascular genetics clinics/cardiovascular-specific genetic counseling.
4. Use our ever-expanding understanding of the genetic and electrophysiological basis of cardiac channelopathies to develop new and targeted therapies, particularly for disorders (e.g., TS, TKOS, CASQ2-CPVT/CPVT2) that are often refractory to available medical, surgical, and device therapies.

These efforts will allow cardiovascular health care providers to fully capitalize on the promise of precision genomic medicine and deliver genetics- and genomics-guided care to an increasing number of patients with monogenic- and polygenic-driven cardiac arrhythmias.

REFERENCES

QT-opathies

1. Tester DJAM. Genetics of cardiac arrhythmias. In: Zipes D, Mann DL, Libby P, Bonow RO, Tomaselli GF, eds. *Braunwald's Heart Disease: A Textbook of Cardiovascular Medicine*. Elsevier; 2019:604–618.
2. Giudicessi JR, Wilde AAM, Ackerman MJ. The genetic architecture of long QT syndrome: a critical reappraisal. *Trends Cardiovasc Med*. 2018;28(7):453–464.
3. Giudicessi JR, et al. Variant frequency and clinical phenotype call into question the nature of minor, nonsyndromic long-QT syndrome-susceptibility gene-disease associations. *Circulation*. 2020;141(6):495–497.
4. Karczewski KJ, et al. The mutational constraint spectrum quantified from variation in 141,456 humans. *Nature*. 2020;581(7809):434–443.
5. Giudicessi JR, Ackerman MJ. Established loss-of-function variants in ANK2-encoded ankyrin-B rarely cause a concerning cardiac phenotype in humans. *Circ Genom Precis Med*. 2020;13(2):e002851.
6. Adler A, et al. An international, multicentered, evidence-based reappraisal of genes reported to cause congenital long QT syndrome. *Circulation*. 2020;141(6):418–428.
7. Strande NT, et al. Evaluating the clinical validity of gene-disease associations: an evidence-based framework developed by the clinical genome Resource. *Am J Hum Genet*. 2017;100(6):895–906.
8. Giudicessi JR, et al. Classification and reporting of potentially proarrhythmic common genetic variation in long QT syndrome genetic testing. *Circulation*. 2018;137(6):619–630.
9. Giudicessi JR, Kullo IJ, Ackerman MJ. Precision cardiovascular medicine: state of genetic testing. *Mayo Clin Proc*. 2017;92(4):642–662.
10. Lahrouchi N, et al. Transethnic genome-wide association study provides insights in the genetic architecture and heritability of long QT syndrome. *Circulation*. 2020;142(4):324–338.
11. Turkowski KL, et al. The QTc-polygenic risk score (QTc-PRS) and its contribution to type 1, type 2, and type 3 long QT syndrome in probands and genotype-positive family members. *Circ Genom Precis Med*. 2020.
12. Roberts JD, et al. An international multicenter evaluation of type 5 long QT syndrome: a low penetrant primary arrhythmic condition. *Circulation*. 2020;141(6):429–439.
13. Garmany R, et al. Clinical and functional reappraisal of alleged type 5 long QT syndrome: causative genetic variants in the KCNE1-encoded minK beta-subunit. *Heart Rhythm*. 2020;17(6):937–944.
14. Lane CM, et al. Long QT syndrome type 5-Lite: defining the clinical phenotype associated with the potentially proarrhythmic p.Asp85Asn-KCNE1 common genetic variant. *Heart Rhythm*. 2018;15(8):1223–1230.
15. Pfeufer A, et al. Common variants at ten loci modulate the QT interval duration in the QTSCD Study. *Nat Genet*. 2009;41(4):407–414.
16. Newton-Cheh C, et al. Common variants at ten loci influence QT interval duration in the QTGEN Study. *Nat Genet*. 2009;41(4):399–406.
17. Arking DE, et al. Genetic association study of QT interval highlights role for calcium signaling pathways in myocardial repolarization. *Nat Genet*. 2014;46(8):826–836.
18. Turkowski KL, et al. Corrected QT interval-polygenic risk score and its contribution to type 1, type 2, and type 3 long-QT syndrome in probands and genotype-positive family members. *Circ Genom Precis Med*. 2020;13(4):e002922.
19. Bezzina CR, et al. Common variants at SCN5A-SCN10A and HEY2 are associated with Brugada syndrome, a rare disease with high risk of sudden cardiac death. *Nat Genet*. 2013;45(9):1044–1049.
20. Crotti L, et al. Calmodulin mutations and life-threatening cardiac arrhythmias: insights from the International Calmodulinopathy Registry. *Eur Heart J*. 2019;40(35):2964–2975.
21. Giudicessi JR, Ackerman MJ. Calcium revisited: new insights into the molecular basis of long-QT syndrome. *Circ Arrhythm Electrophysiol*. 2016;9(7).
22. Altmann HM, et al. Homozygous/compound heterozygous triadin mutations associated with autosomal-recessive long-QT syndrome and pediatric sudden cardiac arrest: elucidation of the triadin knockout syndrome. *Circulation*. 2015;131(23):2051–2060.
23. Clemens DJ, et al. International triadin knockout syndrome registry. *Circ Genom Precis Med*. 2019;12(2):e002419.
24. Boczek NJ, et al. Novel Timothy syndrome mutation leading to increase in CACNA1C window current. *Heart Rhythm*. 2015;12:211–219.
25. Boczek NJ, et al. Identification and functional characterization of a novel CACNA1C-mediated cardiac disorder characterized by prolonged QT intervals with hypertrophic cardiomyopathy, congenital heart defects, and sudden cardiac death. *Circulation*. 2015;8(5):1122–1132.
26. Landstrom AP, Dobrev D, Wehrens XHT. Calcium signaling and cardiac arrhythmias. *Circ Res*. 2017;120(12):1969–1993.
27. Harrell DT, et al. Genotype-dependent differences in age of manifestation and arrhythmia complications in short QT syndrome. *Int J Cardiol*. 2015;190:393–402.
28. Giudicessi JR, Ackerman MJ, Camilleri M. Cardiovascular safety of prokinetic agents: a focus on drug-induced arrhythmias. *Neuro Gastroenterol Motil*. 2018;30(6):e13302.
29. Giudicessi JR, Ackerman MJ. Role of genetic heart disease in sentinel sudden cardiac arrest survivors across the age spectrum. *Int J Cardiol*. 2018;270:214–220.

Other Channelopathies

30. Mazzanti A, et al. Natural history and risk stratification in andersen-tawil syndrome type 1. *J Am Coll Cardiol*. 2020;75(15):1772–1784.
31. Koenig SN, Mohler PJ. The evolving role of ankyrin-B in cardiovascular disease. *Heart Rhythm*. 2017;14(12):1884–1889.
32. Bastiaenen R, et al. Late gadolinium enhancement in Brugada syndrome: a marker for subtle underlying cardiomyopathy? *Heart Rhythm*. 2017;14(4):583–589.
33. Gray B, et al. Relations between right ventricular morphology and clinical, electrical and genetic parameters in Brugada Syndrome. *PloS One*. 2018;13(4):e0195594.
34. Pieroni M, et al. Electroanatomic and pathologic right ventricular outflow tract abnormalities in patients with Brugada syndrome. *J Am Coll Cardiol*. 2018;72(22):2747–2757.
35. Juang JJ, et al. Validation and disease risk assessment of previously reported genome-wide genetic variants associated with Brugada syndrome: SADS-TW BrS registry. *Circ Genom Precis Med*. 2020.
36. Antzelevitch C, et al. J-Wave syndromes expert consensus conference report: emerging concepts and gaps in knowledge. *Heart Rhythm*. 2016;13(10):e295–324.
37. Belbachir N, et al. RRAD mutation causes electrical and cytoskeletal defects in cardiomyocytes derived from a familial case of Brugada syndrome. *Eur Heart J*. 2019;40(37):3081–3094.
38. Le Scouarnec S, et al. Testing the burden of rare variation in arrhythmia-susceptibility genes provides new insights into molecular diagnosis for Brugada syndrome. *Hum Mol Genet*. 2015;24(10):2757–2763.
39. Hosseini SM, et al. Reappraisal of reported genes for sudden arrhythmic death. *Circulation*. 2018;138(12):1195–1205.
40. Behr ER, et al. Role of common and rare variants in SCN10A: results from the Brugada syndrome QRS locus gene discovery collaborative study. *Cardiovasc Res*. 2015;106(3):520–9.
41. Le Scouarnec S, et al. Testing the burden of rare variation in arrhythmia-susceptibility genes provides new insights into molecular diagnosis for Brugada syndrome. *Hum Mol Genet*. 2015;24(10):2757–63.
42. Al-Khatib SM, et al. 2017 AHA/ACC/HRS guideline for management of patients with ventricular arrhythmias and the prevention of sudden cardiac death: a report of the American College of Cardiology/American Heart Association task force on clinical practice guidelines and the Heart Rhythm Society. *Circulation*. 2018;138(13):e272–e391.
43. Priori SG, et al. HRS/EHRA/APHRS expert consensus statement on the diagnosis and management of patients with inherited primary arrhythmia syndromes: document endorsed by HRS, EHRA, and APHRS in May 2013 and by ACCF, AHA, PACES, and AEPC in June 2013. *Heart Rhythm*. 2013;10(12):1932–1963.
44. Priori SG, et al. 2015 ESC guidelines for the management of patients with ventricular arrhythmias and the prevention of sudden cardiac death: the task force for the management of patients with ventricular arrhythmias and the prevention of sudden cardiac death of the European Cociety of Cardiology (ESC). Endorsed by: Association for European Paediatric and Congenital Cardiology (AEPC). *Eur Heart J*. 2015;36(41):2793–2867.
45. Giudicessi JR, Ackerman MJ. Exercise testing oversights underlie missed and delayed diagnosis of catecholaminergic polymorphic ventricular tachycardia in young sudden cardiac arrest survivors. *Heart Rhythm*. 2019;16(8):1232–1239.
46. Roston TM, et al. The clinical and genetic spectrum of catecholaminergic polymorphic ventricular tachycardia: findings from an international multicentre registry. *Europace*. 2018;20(3):541–547.
47. Ng K, et al. An international multi-center evaluation of inheritance patterns, arrhythmic risks, and underlying mechanisms of CASQ2- catecholaminergic polymorphic ventricular tachycardia. *Circulation*. 2020;142(10):932–947.
48. Tester DJ, et al. Identification of a novel homozygous multi-exon duplication in RYR2 among children with exertion-related unexplained sudden deaths in the Amish community. *JAMA Cardiol*. 2020;5(3):13–18.
49. Tester DJ, et al. Molecular characterization of the calcium release channel deficiency syndrome. *JCI Insight*. 2020;5(15).
50. Fujii Y, et al. A type 2 ryanodine receptor variant associated with reduced Ca(2+) release and short-coupled torsades de pointes ventricular arrhythmia. *Heart Rhythm*. 2017;14(1):98–107.
51. Teumer A, et al. KCND3 potassium channel gene variant confers susceptibility to electrocardiographic early repolarization pattern. *JCI Insight*. 2019;4(23).
52. Feghaly J, et al. Genetics of atrial fibrillation. *J Am Heart Assoc*. 2018;7(20):e009884.
53. Nielsen JB, et al. Biobank-driven genomic discovery yields new insight into atrial fibrillation biology. *Nat Genet*. 2018;50(9):1234–1239.
54. Weng LC, et al. Genetic predisposition, clinical risk factor burden, and lifetime risk of atrial fibrillation. *Circulation*. 2018;137(10):1027–1038.
55. Koizumi A, et al. Genetic defects in a His-Purkinje system transcription factor, IRX3, cause lethal cardiac arrhythmias. *Eur Heart J*. 2016;37(18):1469–1475.
56. Leinonen JT, et al. The genetics underlying idiopathic ventricular fibrillation: a special role for catecholaminergic polymorphic ventricular tachycardia? *Int J Cardiol*. 2018;250:139–145.
57. Mellor G, et al. Genetic testing in the evaluation of unexplained cardiac arrest: from the CASPER (cardiac arrest survivors with preserved ejection fraction registry). *Circ Cardiovasc Genet*. 2017;10(3).
58. Visser M, et al. Next-generation sequencing of a large gene panel in patients initially diagnosed with idiopathic ventricular fibrillation. *Heart Rhythm*. 2017;14(7):1035–1040.
59. Laurent G, et al. Multifocal ectopic Purkinje-related premature contractions: a new SCN5A-related cardiac channelopathy. *J Am Coll Cardiol*. 2012;60(2):144–156.
60. Wilde AAM, Amin AS. Clinical spectrum of SCN5A mutations: long QT syndrome, Brugada syndrome, and cardiomyopathy. *JACC Clin Electrophysiol*. 2018;4(5):569–579.
61. Barake W, et al. Purkinje system hyperexcitability and ventricular arrhythmia risk in type 3 long QT syndrome. *Heart Rhythm*. 2020;17(10):1768–1776.
62. Ter Bekke RMA, et al. Beauty and the beat: a complicated case of multifocal ectopic Purkinje-related premature contractions. *HeartRhythm Case Rep*. 2018;4(9):429–433.
63. Daniel LL, et al. SCN5A variant R222Q generated abnormal changes in cardiac sodium current and action potentials in murine myocytes and Purkinje cells. *Heart Rhythm*. 2019;16(11):1676–1685.
64. Moreau A, et al. Gating pore currents are defects in common with two Nav1.5 mutations in patients with mixed arrhythmias and dilated cardiomyopathy. *J Gen Physiol*. 2015;145(2):93–106.

64 Therapy for Cardiac Arrhythmias

JOHN M. MILLER AND KENNETH A. ELLENBOGEN

PHARMACOLOGIC THERAPY, 1208
General Considerations Regarding Antiarrhythmic Drugs, 1208
Antiarrhythmic Agents, 1213

ELECTROTHERAPY FOR CARDIAC ARRHYTHMIAS, 1227

Direct-Current Electrical Cardioversion, 1227
Implantable Electrical Devices for Treatment of Cardiac Arrhythmias, 1229
Ablation Therapy for Cardiac Arrhythmias, 1229

SURGICAL THERAPY FOR TACHYARRHYTHMIAS, 1241
Supraventricular Tachycardias, 1241
Ventricular Tachycardia, 1242

REFERENCES, 1243

It is estimated that almost a third of people will have a problematic tachyarrhythmia, most often atrial fibrillation (AF), at some point during a normal life span. Thus, most clinicians will need to manage their patients' rhythm problems, or those treatments may impact or may be impacted by treatment of the patient's other disorders. Treatment of patients with tachyarrhythmias has evolved dramatically over the last 40 years and has become more complex and specialized. A few, relatively ineffective antiarrhythmic drugs (AADs) were the only therapeutic option until the late 1960s, when surgical therapy to cure (not just suppress) tachyarrhythmias was developed. This mode in turn was replaced by catheter ablation for better control or even cure of many types of supraventricular tachycardias (SVTs) and ventricular tachycardias (VTs) in the absence of structural heart disease starting in the 1980s. The implantable cardioverter-defibrillator (ICD) was introduced in the early 1980s and has become standard therapy for patients with serious ventricular arrhythmias in the presence of structural heart disease. Some patients require a combination of treatments, such as an ICD and AADs or surgery and an ICD; drug therapy can also affect ICD function, positively or negatively. Drug therapy for arrhythmias, at one time the only option, has largely been replaced as the mainstay of therapy by ablation or implanted devices. In most patients, however, tachyarrhythmias are initially treated with AADs, and thus these agents continue to have a significant role in management of patients with a variety of arrhythmias.

PHARMACOLOGIC THERAPY

The principles of clinical pharmacokinetics and pharmacodynamics are discussed in Chapter 9.

General Considerations Regarding Antiarrhythmic Drugs

Most of the AADs currently available can be classified according to whether they exert blocking actions predominantly on sodium (Na^+), potassium (K^+), or calcium (Ca^{2+}) channels and/or what receptors they block (Table 64.1). The commonly used classification (Vaughan Williams) is still a useful framework for categorizing drug action but is limited because it is based on the electrophysiologic effects exerted by an arbitrary concentration of the drug, generally on a laboratory preparation of normal cardiac tissue.

In practice, the actions of these drugs are complex and depend on tissue type, degree of acute or chronic damage, heart rate, membrane potential, ionic composition of the extracellular milieu, autonomic influences (see Chapter 102), genetics (see Chapter 63), age (Chapter 90), and other factors (see Table 64.1). Many drugs exert more than one type of electrophysiologic effect or operate indirectly, such as by altering hemodynamics, myocardial metabolism, or autonomic neural transmission. Therefore, it is more appropriate to think of classes of action rather than classes of drugs, although the major classification schemes categorize drugs by their predominant action. Some drugs have active metabolites that exert effects different from those of the parent compound. Not all drugs in the same class have identical effects (e.g., amiodarone, sotalol, and ibutilide). Whereas all class III agents are dramatically different, some drugs in different classes have overlapping actions (e.g., class IA and class IC drugs). Thus, in vitro studies on healthy myocardium usually establish the idealized properties of AADs rather than their actual antiarrhythmic properties in vivo. Since many AADs affect ventricular repolarization and thus have the potential for producing lethal ventricular arrhythmias, development and approval of new agents is uncommon (no new agents in the United States since dronedarone in 2009).[1]

Despite its limitations, the Vaughan Williams classification is widely known and provides a useful communication shorthand, but the reader is cautioned that drug actions are more complex than those depicted by the classification. A more realistic but not widely used framework regarding AADs is provided by the "Sicilian Gambit." This approach to drug classification is an attempt to identify the mechanisms of a particular arrhythmia, to determine the vulnerable parameter of the arrhythmia most susceptible to modification, to define the target most likely to affect the vulnerable parameter, and then to select a drug that will modify the target (Table 64.2; also see Table 64.1).[2] More recently, a modified Vaughan Williams classification has been proposed that takes into account additional drug targets, including effects on connexins, molecules underlying longer-term signaling processes, and mechanically sensitive ion channels (Fig. 64.1).[3] This revised classification, incorporating advances in both basic and clinical sciences, also emphasizes that most AADs affect multiple targets and can be used to facilitate decisions about drug choices in specific clinical settings. Classes 0-VII have been described; currently available agents are limited to Classes 0-IV and several unclassified drugs.

Drug Classification
Class 0
This class includes drugs that block the HCN channel mediated pacemaker current (I_f). Inhibition of the I_f channel (or "funny" current) reduces the depolarization rate of the sinus node pacemaker cells and reduces heart rate.

According to the Vaughan Williams classification, class I drugs predominantly block the voltage gated fast sodium channel (I_{Na}). These in turn are divided into four subgroups, classes IA, IB, IC and ID. Some also block potassium channels at pharmacologically relevant concentrations.

Class IA
This class includes drugs that reduce $\dot{V}_{max}$ (rate of rise in action potential upstroke [phase 0]) and prolong the action potential duration (APD; see Chapter 62)—quinidine, procainamide, and disopyramide. The kinetics of onset and offset of class IA drugs blocking the Na^+

TABLE 64.1 Actions of Drugs Used in Treatment of Arrhythmias

DRUG	FAST	NA* MED	SLOW	CA	K_R	K_S	HCN	α	β	M_2	P	NA-K ATPASE	LV FUNCTION	SINUS RATE	EXTRACARDIAC
Quinidine		●A			◉			○	○			—		↑	◉
Procainamide		●I			◉							↓		—	◉
Disopyramide		●A			◉				○			↓		var	●
Ajmaline		●A										—		—↓	○
Lidocaine	○											—		—↓	○
Mexiletine	○											—		—	○
Phenytoin	○											—		—	◉
Flecainide			●A		○							↓		—	○
Propafenone		●A			○				◉			↓		↓	○
Propranolol	○								●			↓		↓	○
Nadolol									●			↓		↓	○
Amiodarone	○		◉	●	◉			◉	◉			—		↓	●
Dronedarone	○		◉	●	◉			◉	◉			—		↓	○
Sotalol					◉				●			↓		↓	○
Ibutilide	activator				○							—		↓	○
Dofetilide					●							—		—	○
Verapamil	○			●					◉			↓		↓	○
Diltiazem				◉								↓		↓	○
Adenosine											□	—		↓	◉
Digoxin										○		●	↑	↓	◉
Atropine										●		—		↑	◉
Ranolazine	○				○							—		—	○
Ivabradine							●						○	↓	○

*Fast, med (medium), and slow refer to kinetics of recovery from sodium (Na) channel blockade.
Relative potency of blockade or extracardiac side effect: ○, low; ◉, moderate; ●, high; □, agonist; A, activated state blocker; I = inactivated state blocker.
—, minimal effect; ↑, increase; ↓, decrease; var, variable effects.
Ca, calcium channel; HCN, hyperpolarization-activated cyclic nucleotide-gated channel; K_R, Rapid component of delayed rectifier K+ current; K_s, slow component of delayed rectifier K+ current; LV, left ventricular; M_2, muscarinic receptor subtype 2; Na, sodium channel; NaK- ATPase, sodium pump; P, A, purinergic receptor;.
Modified from Schwartz PJ, Zaza A. Haemodynamic effects of a new multifactorial antihypertensive drug. Eur Heart J. 1992;13:26.

channel is of intermediate rapidity (<5 seconds) when compared with class IB and class IC agents.

Class IB
This class of drugs does not reduce $\dot{V}_{max}$ and shortens the APD—mexiletine, phenytoin, and lidocaine. The kinetics of onset and offset of these drugs in blocking the sodium channel is rapid (<500 milliseconds).

Class IC
This class of drugs, including flecainide and propafenone, can reduce $\dot{V}_{max}$, slow conduction velocity, and prolong refractoriness minimally. These drugs have slow onset and offset kinetics (10 to 20 seconds).

Class ID
This class of drugs includes ranolazine, which preferentially inhibits the late Na+ current affecting APD and recovery and increases refractoriness and repolarization reserve. Class ID drugs cause a reduction in early afterdepolarization-induced triggered activity.

Class II
These drugs block beta-adrenergic receptors and include propranolol, metoprolol, nadolol, carvedilol, nebivolol, and timolol.

Class III
This class of drugs predominantly blocks potassium channels (e.g., I_{Kr}) and prolongs repolarization. Included are sotalol, amiodarone, dronedarone, and ibutilide. Although these drugs are all classified as class III, they differ significantly in their effects on additional ion channels. For example, amiodarone is a nonselective K+ channel blocker while the other agents primarily block I_{Kr}.

Class IV
This class of drugs predominantly blocks the L-type or slow calcium channel ($I_{Ca,L}$)—verapamil, diltiazem, nifedipine, and others (felodipine blocks $I_{Ca,T}$).

Antiarrhythmic agents appear to cross the cell membrane and interact with receptors in the membrane channels when the channels are in the resting, activated, or inactivated state (see Table 64.1 and Chapter 62), and each of these interactions is characterized by different association and dissociation rate constants of a drug from its receptor. Such interactions depend on voltage and time. Transitions among resting, activated, and inactivated states are time- and voltage-dependent. When the drug is bound (associated) to a receptor site at or close to the channel pore (the drug may not actually "plug" the channel), the channel cannot conduct, even in the activated state.

USE DEPENDENCE
Some drugs exert greater inhibitory effects on the upstroke of the action potential at more rapid rates of stimulation and after longer periods of stimulation, a characteristic called *use dependence*. Drugs with this property depress $\dot{V}_{max}$ to a greater extent after the channel has been "used" (i.e., after action potential depolarization rather than after a rest period). Agents with class IB action exhibit rapid binding and unbinding from their receptor site on the channel protein, or exhibit

TABLE 64.2 Classification of Drug Actions on Arrhythmias Based on Modification of Vulnerable Parameter

MECHANISM	ARRHYTHMIA	VULNERABLE PARAMETER (EFFECT)	DRUGS (EFFECT)
Automaticity			
Enhanced normal	Inappropriate sinus tachycardia	Phase 4 β-adrenergic induced rate acceleration and I_f block	β-Adrenergic blocking agents and I_f blockers
Abnormal	Atrial tachycardia	Maximum diastolic potential (hyperpolarization)	M_2 agonist
		Phase 4 depolarization (decrease)	Ca^{2+} or Na^+ channel blocking agents
			M_2 agonist
	Accelerated idioventricular rhythms	Phase 4 depolarization (decrease)	Ca^{2+} or Na^+ channel blocking agents
Triggered Activity			
EAD	Torsades de pointes	Action potential duration (shorten)	β-adrenergic agonists; vagolytic agents (increase rate)
		EAD (suppress)	Ca^{2+} channel blocking agents; Mg^{2+}; β-adrenergic blocking agents; ranolazine
DAD	Digitalis-induced arrhythmias	Calcium overload (unload)	Ca^{2+} channel blocking agents
		DAD (suppress)	Na^+ channel blocking agents
	RV outflow tract ventricular tachycardia	Calcium overload (unload)	β-adrenergic blocking agents
		DAD (suppress)	Ca^{2+} channel blocking agents; adenosine
Reentry—Na^+ Channel Dependent			
Long excitable gap	Typical atrial flutter	Conduction and excitability (depress)	Type IA, IC Na^+ channel blocking agents
	Circus movement tachycardia in WPW	Conduction and excitability (depress)	Type IA, IC Na^+ channel blocking agents
	Sustained uniform ventricular tachycardia	Conduction and excitability (depress)	Na^+ channel blocking agents
Short excitable gap	Atypical atrial flutter	Refractory period (prolong)	K^+ channel blocking agents
	Atrial fibrillation	Refractory period (prolong)	K^+ channel blocking agents
	Circus movement tachycardia in WPW	Refractory period (prolong)	Amiodarone, sotalol
	Polymorphic and uniform ventricular tachycardia	Refractory period (prolong)	Type IA Na^+ channel blocking agents
	Bundle branch reentry	Refractory period (prolong)	Type IA Na^+ channel blocking agents; amiodarone
	Ventricular fibrillation	Refractory period (prolong)	
Reentry—Ca^{2+} Channel Dependent			
	AV nodal reentrant tachycardia	Conduction and excitability (depress)	Ca^{2+} channel blocking agents
	Circus movement tachycardia in WPW	Conduction and excitability (depress)	Ca^{2+} channel blocking agents
	Verapamil-sensitive ventricular tachycardia	Conduction and excitability (depress)	Ca^{2+} channel blocking agents

AV, Atrioventricular; *DAD*, delayed afterdepolarization; *EAD*, early afterdepolarization; *RV*, right ventricular; *WPW*, Wolff-Parkinson-White syndrome.
Modified from Task Force of the Working Group on Arrhythmias of the European Society of Cardiology. The Sicilian gambit: a new approach to the classification of antiarrhythmic drugs based on their actions on arrhythmogenic mechanisms. *Circulation.* 1991;84:1831. Copyright 1991, American Heart Association.

use-dependent block of the fast channel at fast rates. Class IC drugs have slow kinetics, and class IA drugs are intermediate. With increased time spent in diastole (slower rate), a greater proportion of receptors unbind drug, and the drug exerts less effect. The clinical consequence is that these drugs with slower kinetics have greater electrophysiologic effects at more rapid heart rates. For example, a class IC drug would cause more Na^+ channel blockade at more rapid heart rates, and this translates into greater QRS widening with faster heart rates. Unhealthy cells with reduced (i.e., abnormal) membrane potentials recover more slowly from drug actions than do healthier cells with more negative (i.e., normal) membrane potentials. This is referred to as *voltage dependence of block*.

REVERSE USE DEPENDENCE
Some drugs exert greater effects at slow rates than at fast rates, a property known as *reverse use dependence*. This is particularly true for drugs that lengthen repolarization; in the ventricle the QT interval becomes more prolonged at slow rather than at fast rates. This effect is not an ideal antiarrhythmic property, because prolongation of refractoriness should be increased at fast rates to interrupt or prevent a tachycardia and should be minimal at slow rates to avoid precipitation of torsades de pointes (TdP).

MECHANISMS OF ARRHYTHMIA SUPPRESSION
Given that enhanced automaticity, triggered activity, or reentry can cause cardiac arrhythmias (see Chapter 62), **mechanisms** by which AADs suppress arrhythmias in general can only be postulated (see Table 64.2) as some arrhythmias may encompass multiple mechanisms. AADs can slow the spontaneous discharge frequency of an automatic pacemaker by depressing the slope of diastolic depolarization, shifting the threshold voltage toward zero, or hyperpolarizing the resting membrane potential. In general, most AADs at therapeutic concentrations depress the automatic firing rate of spontaneously discharging ectopic sites while minimally affecting the discharge rate of the normal sinus node. Other agents act directly on the sinus node to slow heart rate, whereas drugs that exert vagolytic effects, such as disopyramide and quinidine, can increase the sinus rate. Drugs that suppress early (early afterdepolarization [EAD]) or delayed (delayed afterdepolarization [DAD]) afterdepolarizations can eliminate triggered arrhythmias based on these mechanisms.

Reentry depends critically on the interrelationships between refractoriness and conduction velocity, the presence of unidirectional block in one of the pathways, and other factors that influence refractoriness and conduction, such as excitability (see Chapter 62). An antiarrhythmic agent can stop ongoing reentry that is already present or

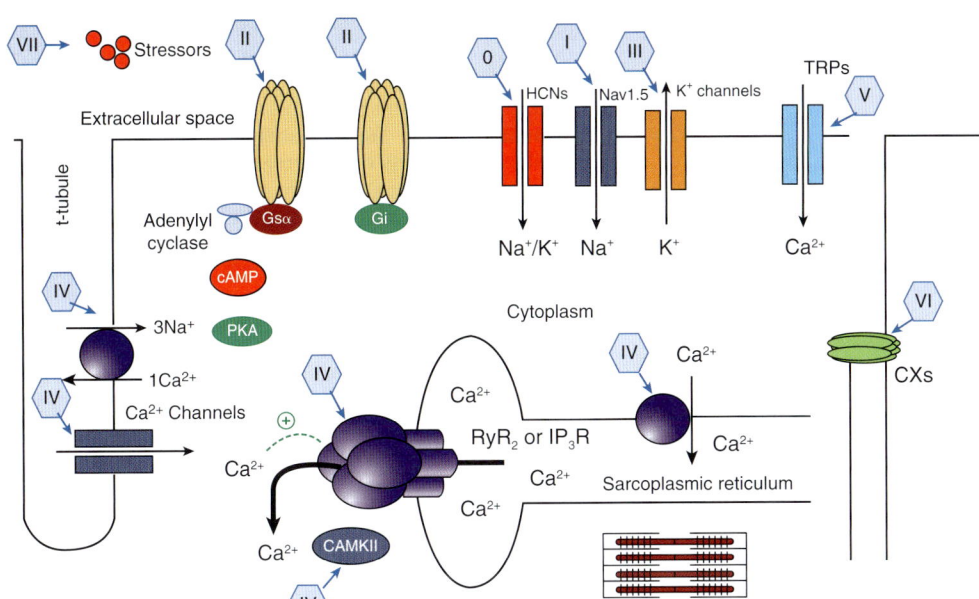
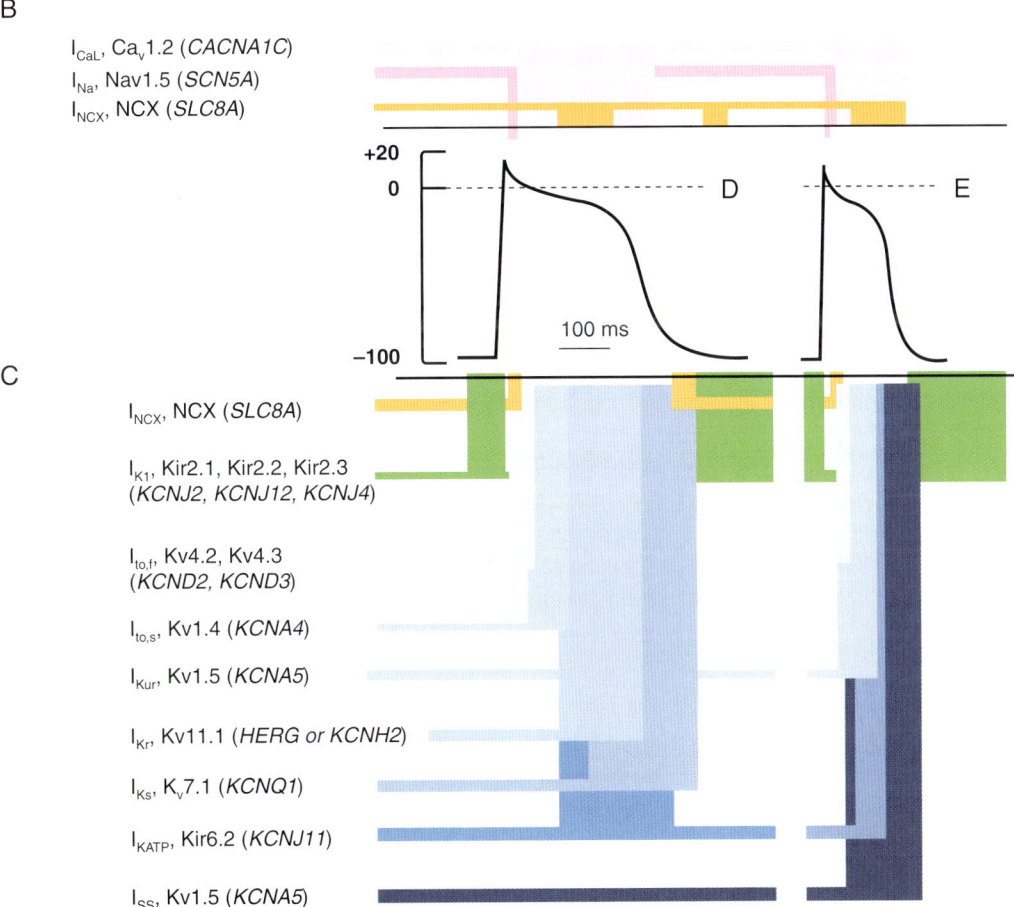

FIGURE 64.1 A, Surface and intracellular membrane ion channels, ion exchangers, transporters, and ionic pumps involved in cardiomyocyte electrophysiological excitation and activation; Roman numerals in blue hexagons refer to classes (0, HCN channel blockers; I, voltage-gated sodium channel blockers; II, autonomic inhibitors/activators; III, potassium channel blockers/openers; IV, calcium handling modulators; V, mechanosensitive channel blockers; VI, gap junction channel blockers; VII, upstream target modulators). **B** to **E**, Activation and inactivation of ion channels, currents, underlying proteins, and encoding genes and their contributions to (**B**) inward depolarizing and (**C**) outward repolarizing currents inscribing cardiac action potentials (APs). Ventricular (**D**) and atrial (**E**) APs comprise rapid depolarizing (phase 0), early repolarizing (phase 1), brief (atrial) or prolonged (ventricular) phase 2 plateaus (phase 2), phase 3 repolarization, and phase 4 electric diastole. In these, inward Na^+ or Ca^{2+} currents drive phase 0 depolarization and Ca^{2+} current maintains the phase 2 plateau (**B**), and a range of outward K^+ currents (**C**) drive phase 1 and phase 3 repolarization. Phase 4 resting potential restoration is accompanied by a refractory period required for Na^+ channel recovery. The resulting wave of electric activity and refractoriness is propagated through successive sino-atrial node, atrial, atrioventricular, Purkinje, and endocardial and epicardial ventricular cardiomyocytes. CaMKII indicates calcium/calmodulin kinase II; Cx, connexin; Gi, inhibitory G protein; Gs, stimulatory G-protein; HCN, hyperpolarization-activated cyclic nucleotide-gated channel; Nav1.5, cardiac Na^+ channel protein; PKA, protein kinase A; RyR2, cardiac ryanodine receptor type 2; TRP, transient receptor potential channel. (Adapted from Lei M, Wu L, Terrar DA, et al. Modernized classification of cardiac antiarrhythmic drugs. *Circulation*. 2018;138:1879–1896 with permission. Copyright (c) 2018, American Heart Association.)

can prevent it from starting if the drug depresses or, alternately, improves conduction. For example, improving conduction can (1) eliminate unidirectional block so that reentry cannot begin or (2) facilitate conduction in the reentrant loop so that the returning wavefront reenters too quickly, encounters cells that are still refractory, and is extinguished. A drug that depresses conduction can transform unidirectional block into bidirectional block and thus terminate reentry or prevent it from starting by creating an area of complete block in the reentrant pathway. Conversely, a drug that slows conduction without producing block or significantly lengthening refractoriness can actually promote reentry. Lastly, most AADs share the ability to prolong refractoriness relative to their effects on APD; that is, the ratio of the effective refractory period (ERP) to APD exceeds 1.0. If a drug prolongs the refractoriness of fibers in the reentrant pathway, the pathway may not recover excitability in time to be depolarized by the reentering impulse, and reentrant propagation ceases. Different types of reentry influence the effectiveness of a drug.

In considering the properties of a drug, it is important to define carefully the situation or model from which conclusions are drawn. Electrophysiologic, hemodynamic, autonomic, pharmacokinetic, and adverse effects can all differ in normal individuals compared with patients, in normal versus abnormal tissue, in cardiac muscle compared with specialized conduction fibers, and in atrial versus ventricular muscle.

DRUG METABOLITES

Drug metabolites can add to or alter the effects of the parent compound by exerting similar actions, competing with the parent compound, or mediating drug toxicity. Quinidine has at least four active metabolites, but none with a potency exceeding that of the parent drug, and none implicated in causing TdP. About 50% of procainamide is metabolized to N-acetylprocainamide (NAPA), which prolongs repolarization and is a less effective sodium channel blocker but competes with procainamide for renal excretion and can increase the parent drug's elimination half-life. A lidocaine metabolite can compete with the parent drug for sodium channels and partially antagonize its blocking effect.

PHARMACOGENETICS

Genetically determined metabolic pathways account for many of the differences in patients' responses to some drugs (see Chapter 9).[4]

The superfamily of cytochrome P-450 (CYP450) enzymes metabolize propafenone, hydroxylate several beta blockers, and biotransform flecainide. The CYP4502D6 exhibits extensive genetic and functional heterogeneity. Lack of this enzyme (in approximately 7% of white patients and 5% of Blacks) reduces metabolism of the parent compound and thereby leads to increased plasma concentrations of the parent drug and reduced concentrations of metabolites. Propafenone is metabolized by CYP450 to a compound with slightly less antiarrhythmic and beta-adrenergic blocking effects, as well as fewer central nervous system (CNS) side effects. Thus, poor metabolizers may experience more heart rate slowing and neurotoxicity than extensive metabolizers do.

Drugs such as rifampin, phenobarbital, and phenytoin induce the synthesis of larger amounts of various CYP450 isoforms, which leads to lower concentrations of the parent drugs because of extensive metabolism, whereas erythromycin, clarithromycin, fluoxetine, and grapefruit juice inhibit enzyme activity, which leads to accumulation of the parent compound. Therefore, clinicians caring for patients who take AADs should be sensitive to the effects of non-cardiac medications and supplements on AAD metabolism and elimination and drug-drug interactions. Over-the-counter (OTC) drugs such as proton pump inhibitors can promote hypokalemia and hypomagnesemia and interact with a simple antibiotic such as ceftriaxone to cause TdP.[5,6] Many astute clinicians use, and refer their patients to, websites such as Crediblemeds.org, where updated information on drug interactions of this type is available. A list of drugs that prolong the QT interval can also be found at www.sads.org.

Clinical Use

In treating cardiac rhythm disorders, most drugs are given on a daily basis (in one to three doses) to prevent episodes from occurring or, in some cases of AF, to control the ventricular rate. Efficacy can be judged in various ways, depending on the clinical circumstances. Symptom reduction (in the case of benign arrhythmias, such as most premature ventricular complexes [PVCs]) and electrocardiographic monitoring (long-term or event; see Chapter 61) are useful; electrophysiologic study (EPS) has been used in the past, with suppression of electrical induction of arrhythmia being the goal, but is rarely used for this purpose currently. Interrogation of implanted devices can also provide an indicator of the success of drug therapy by providing PVC counts and burden of atrial arrhythmias.

In some patients, tachycardia episodes are infrequent enough (months between occurrences) and symptoms mild enough that reactive drug administration is more reasonable than chronic daily dosing. The patient takes a medication only after an episode has started, in the hope that the tachycardia can be terminated and a visit to a physician's office or emergency department avoided. This "pill in the pocket" strategy has worked well for some patients with AF, who have been given one of various medications orally in a monitored setting to ensure safety as well as efficacy before allowing self-medication at home or elsewhere.

Adverse Effects

AADs produce one group of adverse effects related to excessive dosage and plasma concentrations that result in both non-cardiac (e.g., neurologic defects) and cardiac (e.g., heart failure, some arrhythmias) toxicity. Another group of side effects unrelated to plasma concentrations is termed *idiosyncratic*; examples include amiodarone-induced pulmonary fibrosis and some arrhythmias, such as quinidine-induced TdP, which can occur in individuals with a forme fruste of long-QT syndrome (i.e., marked prolongation of normal QT interval in the presence of certain medications; see Chapters 9 and 63). Genetic variants can underlie susceptibility to idiosyncratic reactions.

The U.S. Food and Drug Administration (FDA) has recently determined that the risk of adverse events during pregnancy and lactation (previously categorized as A, B, C, D, and X; see Table 64.3) should be modified (the Pregnancy and Lactation Labeling rule of 2015). The old classification scheme was confusing and did not accurately differentiate the risks to the fetus. This rule applies to all new prescription drugs after June 2015 and is being phased in gradually for drugs approved between 2001 and 2015. This process is underway but until completed, adverse event risk in this setting is characterized using the previous classification.[7] We have attempted to summarize some information about AAD safety during pregnancy in Table 64.4.

Proarrhythmia

Drug-induced or drug-exacerbated cardiac arrhythmias (proarrhythmia) constitute a major clinical problem.[1,8] Proarrhythmia can manifest as an increase in frequency of a preexisting arrhythmia, sustaining of a previously non-sustained arrhythmia (even making it incessant), or development of arrhythmias that the patient has not previously experienced. Electrophysiologic mechanisms are probably related to prolongation of repolarization or an increase in transmural dispersion, development of EADs with resultant TdP, and alterations in reentry pathways to initiate or sustain tachyarrhythmias. Proarrhythmic events can occur in as many as 5% to 10% of patients receiving antiarrhythmic agents; heart failure increases this risk. Reduced left ventricular function, treatment with digitalis and diuretics, bradycardia and a longer pretreatment QT interval identify patients who experience AAD-induced ventricular fibrillation (VF). The more commonly known proarrhythmic events occur within several days of

TABLE 64.3 Antiarrhythmic Drug Use During Pregnancy

Considered Safe
Adenosine (C)
Propranolol (C)
Metoprolol (C)
Lidocaine (B)
Digoxin* (C)
Sotalol (B)
Verapamil (C)
Limited Data; Recommend Use With Caution
Adenosine (C)
Propranolol (C)
Metoprolol (C)
Carvedilol (C)
Propafenone (C)
Flecainide* (C)
Propafenone (C)
Sotalol* (B)
Diltiazem (C)
Verapamil (C)
Ivabradine (D)
Contraindicated
Amiodarone (D)
Dronedarone (X)

A, No demonstrated risk to the fetus based on well-controlled human studies; *B*, No demonstrated risk to the fetus based on animal studies; *C*, Animal studies have demonstrated fetal adverse events, but no human study data; *D*, Demonstrated high human fetal risk, and X: demonstrated high risk for human fetal abnormalities and should not be used.
*Digoxin, flecainide, and sotalol have been used to treat fetal arrhythmias during pregnancy.
Adapted from Regitz-Zagrosek V, Ross-Hesselink JW, Bauersachs J, et al. 2018 ESC guidelines for the management of cardiovascular diseases during pregnancy. *Eur Heart J*. 2018;39:3165–3241.

beginning drug therapy or changing dosage and are represented by such developments as incessant VT and long-QT–related TdP. In the Cardiac Arrhythmia Suppression Trial (CAST), however, researchers found that encainide and flecainide reduced spontaneous ventricular arrhythmias but were associated with a total mortality of 7.7%, versus 3.0% in the placebo group. Deaths were equally distributed throughout the treatment period, indicating that another type of proarrhythmic response can occur sometime after the beginning of drug therapy. Such late proarrhythmic effects may be related to drug-induced exacerbation of the regional myocardial conduction delay caused by ischemia and to heterogeneous drug concentrations that can promote reentry. In the future, a candidate antiarrhythmic compound's potential for proarrhythmia may be modeled computationally and tested in stem cells.

The availability of catheter ablation (see later) and implantable devices (pacemakers and ICDs; see Chapter 69) to treat a wide variety of arrhythmias has largely relegated drug therapy to a secondary role in the treatment of serious arrhythmias. Drugs are still useful to prevent or to decrease the frequency of recurrences in patients who have relatively infrequent episodes of benign tachycardias, as well as in those who have had incomplete success with catheter ablation procedures and in patients with an ICD, to decrease the frequency of shocks because of supraventricular or ventricular arrhythmias.

Antiarrhythmic Agents
Class IA Agents
Quinidine

Quinidine and quinine are isomeric alkaloids isolated from cinchona bark. Although quinidine shares the antimalarial, antipyretic, and vagolytic actions of quinine, only quinidine has direct cellular electrophysiologic effects. It blocks several channels, including the rapid inward sodium channel (I_{Na}), I_{Kr}, I_{to}, and to a lesser extent the slow inward calcium channel, I_{Ks}, and the adenosine triphosphate (ATP)–sensitive potassium current (K_{ATP}). Quinidine causes alpha-adrenergic and cholinergic blockade. The ultimate biologic effect of the drug in a given patient depends on heart rate, drug concentration, and which channels are more prominently affected. Because of decreased demand for quinidine, manufacturing had ceased for a time, with little remaining supply in many countries, but recent renewed demand for its use in patients with Brugada syndrome and idiopathic VF have resulted in quinidine becoming more readily available.

ELECTROPHYSIOLOGIC ACTIONS
Quinidine exerts little effect on automaticity of the normal sinus node but suppresses automaticity in normal Purkinje fibers (Tables 64.1, 64.2). In patients with sinus node dysfunction, quinidine can further depress sinus node automaticity. Quinidine lengthens the QT interval in part via formation of EADs in experimental preparations and in humans, which appears to be responsible for TdP. Because of its significant anticholinergic effect and the reflex sympathetic stimulation resulting from alpha-adrenergic blockade, which causes peripheral vasodilation, quinidine can cause a reflex increase in the sinus node discharge rate and improve atrioventricular (AV) nodal conduction. Quinidine prolongs repolarization, an effect that is more prominent at slow heart rates (reverse use dependence) because of block of I_{Kr} (as well as enhancing the late inward Na$^+$ current at low concentrations). Faster rates result in more block of sodium channels and less unblocking because a smaller percentage of time is spent in the rested state (use dependence). Isoproterenol can modulate the effects of quinidine on reentrant circuits in humans. Quinidine at higher doses inhibits the late inward Na$^+$ current. As noted, quinidine blocks the transient outward current I_{to}, which probably explains its efficacy in suppressing ventricular arrhythmias in Brugada syndrome and patients with idiopathic VF (see Chapter 63).

HEMODYNAMIC EFFECTS
Quinidine induces vasodilation by blocking alpha-adrenergic receptors and can cause significant hypotension. It does not cause significant direct myocardial depression.

PHARMACOKINETICS
Plasma quinidine concentrations peak at approximately 1.5 to 3 hours after an oral dose of a quinidine gluconate preparation (see Table 64.4). Approximately 80% of plasma quinidine is protein bound, especially to α_1-acid glycoprotein. Both the liver and the kidneys remove quinidine; dose adjustments may be made to achieve appropriate serum concentrations. Its elimination half-life is 8 to 9 hours after oral administration.

DOSAGE AND ADMINISTRATION. The usual oral dose of quinidine sulfate for an adult is 300 to 600 mg four times daily, which results in a steady-state level within about 24 hours (see Table 64.4). A loading dose of 600 to 800 mg produces an earlier effective concentration. Oral doses of the gluconate are about 30% higher than those of the sulfate form. Important interactions with other drugs occur.

INDICATIONS. Quinidine is a versatile AAD that was used previously to treat premature supraventricular and ventricular complexes and sustained tachyarrhythmias. However, because of its side effect profile and potential for causing TdP, as well as its limited usefulness in preventing VT and VF in most applications, its use has decreased greatly. In recent years, however, interest has increased in quinidine for treating primary (idiopathic) VF, ventricular arrhythmias in patients with Brugada syndrome (see Chapter 63),[9] and short-QT syndrome. Quinidine crosses the placenta so it can be used to treat fetal arrhythmias.

ADVERSE EFFECTS. The most common adverse effects of chronic oral quinidine therapy are gastrointestinal (GI) and include nausea, vomiting, diarrhea, abdominal pain, and anorexia (milder with the gluconate form). CNS toxicity includes tinnitus, hearing loss, visual disturbances, confusion, delirium, and psychosis (cinchonism). Allergic reactions include rash, fever, immune-mediated thrombocytopenia, hemolytic anemia, and rarely, anaphylaxis. Side effects may preclude long-term administration of quinidine in 30% to 40% of patients.

Quinidine can slow cardiac conduction, sometimes to the point of block, which is manifested as prolongation of the QRS duration or as sinoatrial (SA) or AV nodal conduction disturbances. Quinidine can produce syncope in 0.5% to 2.0% of patients, most often the result of a self-terminating episode of TdP. Quinidine prolongs the QT interval in most patients (not dose related), regardless of whether ventricular arrhythmias occur, but significant QT prolongation (QT interval of 500 to 600 milliseconds) is often a characteristic of patients with quinidine-related syncope, who may have a genetic predisposition underlying such a response (see Chapter 9). Many of these patients are also receiving digitalis or diuretics or have hypokalemia; women are more susceptible than men. Importantly, syncope is unrelated to plasma concentrations of quinidine or the duration of therapy, although most episodes occur within the first 2 to 4 days of therapy initiation, often after conversion of AF to sinus rhythm. This proarrhythmic effect during initiation of treatment is reproducible and because of this, the drug should not be taken on an intermittent basis. Therapy of proarrhythmia requires immediate discontinuation of use of the drug; magnesium given intravenously (2 g over 1 to 2 minutes, followed by an infusion of 3 to 20 mg/min) is the initial drug treatment of choice. Atrial or ventricular pacing can be used to suppress the ventricular tachyarrhythmia, perhaps by suppressing EADs. When pacing is not available, isoproterenol can be given with caution. The arrhythmia gradually dissipates as quinidine is cleared and the QT interval returns to baseline. Affected patients should not use quinidine thereafter and also should avoid other drugs that prolong the QT interval (see Crediblemeds.org).

Drugs that induce hepatic enzyme production, such as phenobarbital and phenytoin, can shorten the duration of action of quinidine by increasing its rate of elimination. Quinidine can increase plasma concentrations of flecainide by inhibiting the CYP450 enzyme system. Quinidine can elevate serum digoxin concentrations by decreasing its clearance and volume of distribution and the affinity of tissue receptors.

Procainamide

ELECTROPHYSIOLOGIC ACTIONS
The cardiac actions of procainamide on automaticity, conduction, excitability, and membrane responsiveness resemble those of quinidine (see

TABLE 64.4 Dosage and Other Information for Clinical Use of Common Antiarrhythmic Agents

DRUG	INTRAVENOUS (MG) LOADING	INTRAVENOUS (MG) MAINTENANCE	ORAL (MG) LOADING	ORAL (MG) MAINTENANCE	TIME TO PEAK PLASMA CONCENTRATION (ORAL) (HR)	EFFECTIVE SERUM OR PLASMA CONCENTRATION (MCG/ML)	HALF-LIFE (HR)	BIOAVAILABILITY (%)	MAJOR ROUTE OF ELIMINATION	PREGNANCY CLASS
Quinidine	6–10 mg/kg at 0.3–0.5 mg/kg/min	—	800–1000	300–600 q6h	1.5–3.0	3–6	5–9	60–80	Liver > kidneys	C
Procainamide	6–13 mg/kg at 0.2–0.5 mg/kg/min	2–6 mg/min	500–1000	250–1000 q4–6h	1	4–10	3–5	70–85	Kidneys > liver	C
Disopyramide	1–2 mg/kg over 15–45 min*	1 mg/kg/hr*	N/A	100–300 q6-8h	1–2	2–5	4–10	80–90	Kidneys	C
Lidocaine	1–2 mg/kg at 20–50 mg/min	1–4 mg/min	N/A	N/A	N/A	1–5	1–2	N/A	Liver	B
Mexiletine	500 mg*	0.5–1.0 g/24 hr*	400–600	150–300 q8-12h	2–4	0.75–2.0	10–17	80–90	Liver	C
Phenytoin	100 mg q5min for ≤1000 mg	N/A	1000	100–400 q12-24h	8–12	10–20	18–36	50–70	Liver	D
Flecainide	2 mg/kg*	100–200 q12h*	N/A	50–200 q12h	3–4	0.2–1.0	20	95	Kidneys	C
Propafenone	1–2 mg/kg*	N/A	600–900	150–300 q8-12h	1–3	0.5–2.0	2–10 (extensive metabolizers); 10–32 (poor metabolizers)	3–25	Liver	C
Propranolol	0.25–0.5 mg q5min to ≤0.20 mg/kg	N/A	N/A	10–200 q6-8h	4	0.02–0.2	3–6	35–65	Liver	C
Amiodarone	15 mg/min for 10 min; 1 mg/min for 6 hr; 0.5 mg/min thereafter	0.5 mg/min	400 to 800 mg/day for 7–14 days	200–600 qd	Variable	0.5–1.5	56 days	25	Liver	D
Dronedarone	N/A	N/A	N/A	400 mg q12h	3–4	0.3–0.6	13–19	70–90	Liver	X
Sotalol	60–112.5 mg over 1 h	75–112.5 mg over 5 h	N/A	80–160 q12h	2.5–4	2.5	10–20	90–100	Kidneys	B
Ibutilide	1 mg over 10 min	N/A	N/A	N/A	N/A	N/A	2–12		Kidneys	C
Dofetilide		N/A	N/A	0.125–0.5 q12h			7–13	90	Kidneys	C
Verapamil	5–10 mg over 1–2 min	0.005 mg/kg/min	N/A	80–120 q6-8h	1–2	0.10–0.15	3–8	20–35	Liver, kidneys	C
Adenosine	6–18 mg (rapidly)	N/A	N/A	N/A	N/A	N/A	Seconds	100	Blood cells	C
Digoxin	0.5–1.0 mg	0.125–0.25 mg	0.5–1.0	0.125–0.25 qd	2–6	0.0008–0.002	36–48	60–80	Kidneys	C
Ranolazine	N/A	N/A	N/A	500–1000 bid	4–6	N/A	7	60–75	Kidneys > liver	C
Ivabradine	N/A	N/A	N/A	2.5–7.5 mg bid	1	N/A	6	40%	Gut and liver	D

Pill in the Pocket Approach

1. Chronic oral beta blocker therapy or diltiazem or verapamil
2. If NOT on chronic beta blocker therapy, rapid acting beta blockers such as metoprolol 25–50 mg, propranolol 20–80 mg, diltiazem 30–90 mg or verapamil 30–60 mg at least 30 min prior to antiarrhythmic drug therapy
3. Flecainide as single dose of 200–300 mg; 200 mg if weight <70 kg

OR

Propafenone as single dose of 450–600 mg; 450 mg if weight <70 kg

Recommended that the first dose of a class IC agent or first trial of pill in the pocket consideration should be given to have it administered under monitored therapy

*Intravenous use investigational or unavailable in United States.
N/A, not applicable; q4–6h, every 4 to 6 hours; qd, every day; bid, twice daily.
Results presented may vary according to doses, disease state, and IV or oral administration.
Pregnancy Class: A, controlled studies show no fetal risk; B, no controlled studies, but no evidence of fetal risk; fetal harm unlikely; C, fetal risk cannot be excluded; drug should be used only if potential benefits outweigh potential risk;

Tables 64.1, 64.2). Procainamide predominantly blocks the inactivated state of I_{Na}. It also blocks I_{Kr}, I_{K1}, and $I_{K,ATP}$. Like quinidine, procainamide usually prolongs the ERP more than it prolongs the APD and thus may prevent reentry. Procainamide exerts the least anticholinergic effects among type IA drugs. High levels of NAPA, such as in patients with renal disease, can produce EADs, triggered activity, and TdP. Because of decreased demand, availability of intravenous (IV) and oral procainamide is greatly limited.

HEMODYNAMIC EFFECTS

Procainamide can depress myocardial contractility in high concentrations. It does not produce alpha blockade but can result in peripheral vasodilation, possibly through antisympathetic effects on the brain or spinal cord, which can impair cardiovascular reflexes (e.g., provoking orthostatic symptoms).

PHARMACOKINETICS

Oral administration produces a peak plasma concentration in approximately 1 hour. Approximately 80% of oral procainamide is bioavailable; the overall elimination half-life of procainamide is 3 to 5 hours, with 50% to 60% of the drug eliminated by the kidneys and 10% to 30% metabolized by the liver (see Table 64.4). The drug is acetylated to NAPA, which is excreted almost exclusively by the kidneys. As renal function decreases and in patients with heart failure, NAPA levels increase and, because of the risk for serious cardiotoxicity, need to be carefully monitored in these situations. NAPA has an elimination half-life of 7 to 8 hours, but the half-life exceeds 10 hours if high doses of procainamide are used. Increased age, congestive heart failure, and reduced creatinine clearance lower the clearance of procainamide and necessitate a reduced dosage.

DOSAGE AND ADMINISTRATION. Procainamide can be given by the oral, IV, or intramuscular (IM) route to achieve plasma concentrations in the range of 4 to 10 μg/mL and produce an antiarrhythmic effect (see Table 64.4). Several IV regimens have been used to administer procainamide, but usually doses of 10 to 15 mg/kg are used at a rate of up to 50 mg/min until the arrhythmia has been controlled, hypotension results, or the QRS complex is prolonged more than 50%. With this method, the plasma concentration falls rapidly during the first 15 minutes after the loading dose, with parallel effects on refractoriness and conduction. A constant-rate IV infusion of procainamide can be given at a dosage of 2 to 6 mg/min, depending on the patient's response.

Oral administration of procainamide requires a 3- to 4-hour dosing interval at a total daily dose of 2 to 6 g, with a steady-state concentration being reached within 1 day. When a loading dose is used, it should be twice the maintenance dose. Frequent dosing is required because of its short elimination half-life in normal persons. For the extended-release forms of procainamide, dosing is at 6- to 12-hour intervals. Procainamide by IM injection is almost 100% bioavailable.

INDICATIONS. Procainamide is used to treat both supraventricular and ventricular arrhythmias in a manner comparable to that of quinidine. Although both drugs have similar electrophysiologic actions, either drug can effectively suppress a supraventricular or ventricular arrhythmia that is resistant to the other drug. Procainamide can be used to convert recent-onset AF to sinus rhythm. As with quinidine, prior treatment with beta or calcium channel blockers is recommended to prevent acceleration of the ventricular response during atrial flutter or fibrillation after procainamide therapy. Procainamide can block conduction in the accessory pathway of patients with Wolff-Parkinson-White (WPW) syndrome and can be used in patients with AF and a rapid ventricular response related to conduction over the accessory pathway. It can produce His-Purkinje block and is sometimes administered during an EPS to stress the His-Purkinje system and evaluate the need for a pacemaker (see Fig. 61.15). However, it should be used with caution in patients with evidence of His-Purkinje disease (bundle branch block) for whom a ventricular pacemaker is not readily available.

Procainamide is more effective than lidocaine in acutely terminating sustained VT. IV procainamide is recommended along with IV amiodarone and IV sotalol in the Advanced Cardiac Life Support (ACLS) Guidelines for the treatment of stable wide QRS tachycardia presumed to be VT. Most consistently, procainamide slows the VT rate, a change correlated with the increase in QRS duration. The drug also has diagnostic applications when given intravenously (10 mg/kg over 5 to 10 minutes). In patients with suspected Brugada syndrome who have a normal resting electrocardiogram (ECG), drug infusion can result in the characteristic "Brugada sign," whereas in patients with WPW syndrome, the drug can cause sudden loss of preexcitation.

ADVERSE EFFECTS. Noncardiac adverse effects from administration of procainamide include rash, myalgia, digital vasculitis, and Raynaud phenomenon. Fever and agranulocytosis may be the result of hypersensitivity reactions, and a complete blood count should be assessed at regular intervals. GI side effects are less frequent than with quinidine, and adverse CNS side effects are less frequent than with lidocaine. Toxic concentrations of procainamide can diminish myocardial performance and promote hypotension. Various conduction disturbances or ventricular tachyarrhythmias can occur, similar to those produced by quinidine. NAPA can cause QT prolongation and TdP. In the absence of sinus node disease, procainamide does not adversely affect sinus node function. In patients with sinus node dysfunction, however, procainamide can prolong sinus node recovery time and worsen symptoms in some patients with bradycardia-tachycardia syndrome.

Arthralgia, fever, pleuropericarditis, hepatomegaly, and hemorrhagic pericardial effusion with tamponade have been described in a systemic lupus erythematosus (SLE)-like syndrome related to procainamide administration. The syndrome occurs more frequently and earlier in patients who are slow acetylators of procainamide and is genetically influenced (see Chapter 9). Acetylation of procainamide to form NAPA appears to block the SLE-inducing effect. In 60% to 70% of patients receiving long-term procainamide therapy, anti-nuclear antibodies (ANAs) develop, with clinical symptoms occurring in 20% to 30%; this is reversible when procainamide is stopped. Positive serologic test results are not necessarily a reason to discontinue drug therapy; however, the development of symptoms with a positive anti-DNA antibody generally indicates that drug therapy should be discontinued. Corticosteroid administration in these patients may eliminate the symptoms. In this syndrome, in contrast to naturally occurring SLE, the brain and kidneys are typically spared, and there is no predilection for women.

Disopyramide

Disopyramide has been approved in the United States for oral administration to treat patients with ventricular and supraventricular arrhythmias.

ELECTROPHYSIOLOGIC ACTIONS

Disopyramide produces electrophysiologic effects similar to those of quinidine and procainamide, causing use-dependent block of I_{Na} and non–use-dependent block of I_{Kr} (see Tables 64.1, 64.2). Disopyramide is a muscarinic blocker and can increase the sinus node discharge rate and shorten AV nodal conduction time and refractoriness when the nodes are under cholinergic (vagal) influence. It exerts greater anticholinergic effects than quinidine and does not appear to affect alpha or beta adrenoceptors. The drug prolongs atrial and ventricular refractory periods, but its effect on AV nodal conduction and refractoriness is not consistent. Disopyramide prolongs His-Purkinje conduction time, but infra-His block rarely occurs. It can be administered safely to patients who have first-degree AV delay and narrow QRS complexes.

HEMODYNAMIC EFFECTS

Disopyramide suppresses ventricular systolic performance and is a mild arterial vasodilator. The drug should generally be avoided in patients with reduced left ventricular systolic function because they tolerate its negative inotropic effects poorly.

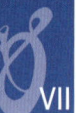

PHARMACOKINETICS

Oral disopyramide is 80% to 90% absorbed, with a mean elimination half-life of 8 to 9 hours in healthy volunteers but almost 10 hours in patients with heart failure (see Table 64.4). Renal insufficiency prolongs its elimination time. Thus, in patients with renal, hepatic, or cardiac insufficiency, loading and maintenance doses need to be reduced. Peak blood levels after oral administration occur in 1 to 2 hours. Approximately 50% of an oral dose is excreted unchanged in urine, with 30% occurring as the mono-*N*-dealkylated metabolite. The metabolites appear to exert less effect than the parent compound. As with other class IA antiarrhythmic drugs, macrolide antibiotics inhibit its metabolism.

DOSAGE AND ADMINISTRATION. Doses are generally 100 to 300 mg orally every 6 hours, with a range of 400 to 1200 mg/day (see Table 64.4). A controlled-release preparation can be given as 200 to 300 mg every 12 hours.

INDICATIONS. Disopyramide appears to be comparable to quinidine and procainamide in reducing the frequency of PVCs and effectively preventing recurrence of VT in selected patients. Disopyramide has been combined with other drugs, such as mexiletine, to treat patients who do not respond or respond only partially to one drug.

Although rarely used for this, disopyramide helps prevent recurrence of AF after successful cardioversion as effectively as quinidine and may terminate atrial flutter. In treating patients with AF, particularly atrial flutter, the ventricular rate must be controlled before disopyramide is administered, or the combination of a decrease in atrial rate with vagolytic effects on the AV node can result in 1:1 AV conduction during atrial flutter (see Chapter 66). It has been used in patients with hypertrophic cardiomyopathy for both AF therapy and its negative inotropic effect.

ADVERSE EFFECTS. Three types of adverse effects follow disopyramide administration. The most common effects are related to the drug's potent parasympatholytic properties and include urinary hesitancy or retention, constipation, blurred vision, closed-angle glaucoma, and dry mouth. Symptoms are less with the sustained-release form. Second, disopyramide can produce ventricular tachyarrhythmias frequently associated with QT prolongation and TdP. Cross-sensitization to both quinidine and disopyramide occurs in some patients, and TdP can develop while receiving either drug. When drug-induced torsades de pointes (DI-TdP) occurs, agents that prolong the QT interval should be used cautiously or not at all. Lastly, disopyramide can reduce contractility of the normal ventricle, but the depression of ventricular function is much more pronounced in patients with preexisting ventricular failure. Rarely, cardiovascular collapse can result.

Ajmaline

Ajmaline, a rauwolfia derivative, has been used extensively to treat patients with ventricular and supraventricular arrhythmias in Europe and Asia but is not available in the United States.

ELECTROPHYSIOLOGIC ACTIONS

As with other class IA drugs, ajmaline produces use-dependent block of INa; it also weakly blocks IKr. The drug has mild anticholinergic activity (see Tables 64.1, 64.2).

HEMODYNAMIC EFFECTS

Ajmaline mildly suppresses ventricular systolic performance but does not affect peripheral resistance. It also inhibits platelet activity more potently than aspirin does.

PHARMACOKINETICS, DOSAGE, AND ADMINISTRATION

Ajmaline is well absorbed with a mean elimination half-life of 13 minutes in most patients, thus making it poorly suited to long-term oral use. The dose for termination of acute arrhythmia is generally 50 mg intravenously infused over 1 to 2 minutes.

INDICATIONS

Although it is useful for terminating SVTs by IV infusion, other medications have largely supplanted ajmaline for this purpose and its use has evolved to that of a diagnostic tool. When administered intravenously at doses of 50 mg over a 3-minute period, or 10 mg/min, to a total dose of 1 mg/kg, ajmaline can have the following effects: (1) delta wave disappearance in patients with WPW syndrome (indicating an accessory pathway anterograde ERP longer than 250 milliseconds); (2) ST-T abnormalities and interventricular conduction block in patients with occult Chagasic cardiomyopathy; (3) heart block in patients with bundle branch block and syncope, but in whom no rhythm disturbance had been discovered; and (4) right precordial ST elevation in patients with suspected Brugada syndrome in whom findings on the resting ECG are normal. It is in this last setting that ajmaline is used most frequently.

ADVERSE EFFECTS

Ajmaline can produce mild anticholinergic side effects, as well as mild depression of left ventricular systolic function, and can worsen AV conduction in patients with His-Purkinje disease. Rare occurrences of TdP have been reported. Ajmaline can increase the defibrillation threshold.

Class IB Agents
Lidocaine

ELECTROPHYSIOLOGIC ACTIONS

Lidocaine blocks I_{Na}, predominantly in the open or inactivated state. It has rapid onset and offset kinetics and does not affect normal sinus node automaticity in usual doses but does depress other normal and abnormal forms of automaticity, as well as EADs and DADs in Purkinje fibers in vitro (see Tables 64.1, 64.2). Lidocaine has only a modest depressant effect on $\dot{V}_{max}$; however, faster rates of stimulation, acidosis, increased extracellular K^+ concentration, and reduced membrane potential (changes that can result from ischemia) increase the ability of lidocaine to block I_{Na}. Lidocaine can convert areas of unidirectional block into bidirectional block during ischemia and inhibit the development of VF by preventing fragmentation of organized large wavefronts into heterogeneous wavelets.

Except in very high concentrations, lidocaine does not affect slow-Ca channel–dependent action potentials despite its moderate suppression of the Ca current. Lidocaine has minimal effect on atrial fibers and does not affect conduction in accessory pathways. Depressed automaticity or conduction can develop in patients with preexisting sinus node dysfunction, abnormal His-Purkinje conduction, or junctional or ventricular escape rhythms. Part of lidocaine's effects may involve inhibition of cardiac sympathetic nerve activity.

HEMODYNAMIC EFFECTS

Clinically significant adverse hemodynamic effects are rarely noted with lidocaine at the usual drug concentrations unless left ventricular function is severely impaired.

PHARMACOKINETICS

Lidocaine is used only parenterally because oral administration results in extensive first-pass hepatic metabolism and unpredictably low plasma levels, as well as excessive metabolites that can produce toxicity (see Table 64.4). Hepatic metabolism of lidocaine depends on hepatic blood flow; severe hepatic disease or reduced hepatic blood flow, as in heart failure or shock, can greatly decrease the rate of lidocaine metabolism. Beta-adrenoceptor blockers can decrease hepatic blood flow and increase the serum concentration of lidocaine. Prolonged infusion can reduce lidocaine clearance. Its elimination half-life averages 1 to 2 hours in normal individuals, longer than 4 hours in patients after uncomplicated myocardial infarction (MI), longer than 10 hours in patients after MI complicated by heart failure, and even longer in the presence of cardiogenic shock. Maintenance doses should be reduced by one third to one half in patients with low cardiac output.

DOSAGE AND ADMINISTRATION. Although lidocaine can be given intramuscularly, the IV route is most often used, with an initial bolus of 1 to 2 mg/kg body weight at a rate of 20 to 50 mg/min and a second injection of half the initial dose 20 to 40 minutes later to maintain the therapeutic concentration (see Table 64.4).

If the initial bolus of lidocaine is ineffective, up to two more boluses of 1 mg/kg may be administered at 5-minute intervals. Patients who require more than one bolus to achieve a therapeutic effect generally need a higher maintenance dose to sustain these higher concentrations, with infusion rates in the range of 1 to 4 mg/min to produce steady-state plasma levels of 1 to 5 mg/mL in patients with uncomplicated MI. These rates must be reduced during heart failure or shock because of the concomitant reduced hepatic blood flow. Higher doses and concentrations are unlikely to provide additional benefit but do increase the risk for toxicity.

INDICATIONS. Lidocaine has moderate efficacy against ventricular arrhythmias of diverse causes; it is generally ineffective against supraventricular arrhythmias and rarely terminates monomorphic VT. Although once used in an attempt to prevent VF in the first 2 days after acute MI, its efficacy was marginal, and because it can produce side effects such use is now not recommended.

ADVERSE EFFECTS. The most frequently reported adverse effects of lidocaine are dose-related manifestations of CNS toxicity: dizziness, paresthesias, confusion, delirium, stupor, coma, and seizures. Occasional sinus node depression and His-Purkinje block have been reported. Rarely, lidocaine can cause malignant hyperthermia.

Mexiletine

Mexiletine, a local anesthetic congener of lidocaine with anticonvulsant properties, is used for the oral treatment of patients with symptomatic ventricular arrhythmias. It is rarely used as a single agent for the treatment of ventricular arrhythmias.

ELECTROPHYSIOLOGIC ACTIONS

Mexiletine is similar to lidocaine in many of its electrophysiologic actions. In vitro, mexiletine shortens the APD and ERP of Purkinje fibers and, to a lesser extent, ventricular muscle. It depresses the V_{max} of phase 0 by blocking I_{Na}, especially at faster rates, and depresses the automaticity of Purkinje fibers but not that of the normal sinus node. Its onset and offset kinetics are rapid. Hypoxia or ischemia can increase its effects (see Tables 64.1, 64.2).

Mexiletine can result in severe bradycardia and abnormal sinus node recovery time in patients with sinus node disease, but not in those with a normal sinus node. It does not affect AV nodal conduction and can depress His-Purkinje conduction, but not greatly, unless conduction was abnormal initially. Mexiletine does not appear to affect human atrial muscle. It does not affect the QT interval. It has been used in treating a variety of other disorders, including erythromelalgia (red, painful extremities) in children and myotonia.

HEMODYNAMIC EFFECTS

Mexiletine exerts no major hemodynamic effects on ventricular contractile performance or peripheral resistance.

PHARMACOKINETICS

Mexiletine is rapidly and almost completely absorbed after oral ingestion by volunteers, with peak plasma concentrations being attained in 2 to 4 hours (see Table 64.4). Its elimination half-life is approximately 10 hours in healthy individuals but 17 hours in post-MI patients. Therapeutic plasma levels of 0.5 to 2 mcg/mL are maintained by oral doses of 200 to 300 mg every 6 to 8 hours. Absorption with less than a 10% first-pass hepatic effect occurs in the upper part of the small intestine and is delayed and incomplete in patients receiving narcotics or antacids. Approximately 70% of the drug is protein bound; the apparent volume of distribution is large because of extensive tissue uptake. Normally, mexiletine is eliminated metabolically by the liver, with less than 10% being excreted unchanged in urine. Doses should be reduced in patients with cirrhosis or left ventricular failure. Renal clearance of mexiletine decreases as urinary pH increases. Its known metabolites exert no electrophysiologic effects. Metabolism can be increased by phenytoin, phenobarbital, and rifampin and can be reduced by cimetidine.

DOSAGE AND ADMINISTRATION. The recommended starting dose is 200 mg orally every 8 hours when rapid arrhythmia control is not essential (see Table 64.4). Doses may be increased or decreased by 50 to 100 mg every 2 to 3 days and are better tolerated when given with food. The total daily dose should generally not exceed 1200 mg. In some patients, administration every 12 hours can be effective.

INDICATIONS. Mexiletine is a moderately effective antiarrhythmic agent for the treatment of acute and chronic ventricular tachyarrhythmias, but not SVTs. Success rates vary from 6% to 60% and can be increased in some patients if mexiletine is combined with other drugs such as procainamide, beta blockers, quinidine, disopyramide, propafenone, or amiodarone. Most studies show no clear superiority of mexiletine over other class I agents. Mexiletine may be very useful in children with congenital heart disease and serious ventricular arrhythmias. In treating patients with a long QT interval, mexiletine may be safer than drugs that increase the QT interval further, such as quinidine. Limited experience in treating subsets of patients with long-QT syndrome (LQT3, which is related to the *SCN5A* gene for the cardiac sodium channel) suggests a beneficial role (see Chapter 63). Mexiletine has also been used to treat myotonia in patients with neuromuscular diseases such as myotonic dystrophy. Involvement of the conduction system in these diseases can predispose these patients to advanced life-threatening heart rate slowing, mandating mexiletine be used with caution or backup pacing in this situation (Chapter 100).

ADVERSE EFFECTS. Up to 40% of patients may require a change in dose or discontinuation of mexiletine therapy as a result of adverse effects, including tremor, dysarthria, dizziness, paresthesia, diplopia, nystagmus, confusion, nausea, vomiting, and dyspepsia. Cardiovascular side effects are rare but include hypotension, bradycardia, and exacerbation of arrhythmia. The adverse effects of mexiletine appear to be dose related, and toxic effects can occur at plasma concentrations that are sub-therapeutic or only slightly higher than therapeutic levels. Therefore, its effective use requires careful titration of dose and monitoring for adverse effects and possibly plasma concentration. Lidocaine use as an AAD should be avoided in patients receiving mexiletine.

Phenytoin

Phenytoin was used originally to treat seizure disorders. Its value as an AAD is limited to rare cases of digitalis-toxic atrial and ventricular tachyarrhythmias (for which more rapid and effective control can be achieved with digitalis-specific antibodies) and occasional cases of ventricular arrhythmias when used in combination with other agents (see Tables 64.1, 64.2, 64.4).

Class IC Agents
Flecainide

Flecainide is approved by the FDA to treat patients with life-threatening ventricular arrhythmias, as well as various supraventricular arrhythmias.

ELECTROPHYSIOLOGIC ACTIONS

Flecainide exhibits marked use-dependent depressant effects on the rapid sodium channel by decreasing V_{max} and has slow onset and offset kinetics (see Tables 64.1, 64.2). Drug dissociation from the sodium channel is slow, with time constants of 10 to 30 seconds (versus 4 to 8 seconds for quinidine and <1 second for lidocaine). Thus, marked drug effects can occur at physiologic heart rates. Flecainide shortens the duration of the Purkinje fiber action potential but prolongs it in ventricular muscle, actions that, depending on the circumstances, could enhance or reduce electrical heterogeneity and create or suppress arrhythmias. Flecainide profoundly slows conduction in all cardiac fibers and, in high concentrations, inhibits the slow Ca^{2+} channel (see Chapter 62). Conduction time in the atria, ventricles, AV node, and His-Purkinje system is prolonged. Minimal increases in atrial or ventricular refractoriness or in the QT interval result. Anterograde and retrograde refractoriness in accessory pathways can increase significantly in a use-dependent manner. Sinus node function remains unchanged in normal individuals but may be depressed in patients with sinus node dysfunction. Flecainide can facilitate or inhibit reentry and may transform AF to flutter. Pacing and defibrillation thresholds are characteristically slightly to significantly increased.

HEMODYNAMIC EFFECTS

Flecainide depresses cardiac performance, particularly in patients with compromised ventricular systolic function, and should be used cautiously or not at all in those with moderate or severe ventricular systolic dysfunction.

PHARMACOKINETICS

Flecainide is at least 90% absorbed, with peak plasma concentrations achieved in 3 to 4 hours. Its elimination half-life in patients with ventricular arrhythmias is 20 hours, with 85% of the drug excreted unchanged or as an inactive metabolite in urine (see Table 64.4). Its two major metabolites have less potency than the parent drug. Elimination is slower in patients with renal disease and heart failure, and doses should be reduced in these situations. Therapeutic plasma concentrations range from 0.2 to 1.0 mcg/mL. Approximately 40% of the drug is protein bound. Increases in serum concentrations of digoxin (15% to 25%) and propranolol (30%) result during co-administration with flecainide. Propranolol, quinidine, and amiodarone may increase flecainide serum concentrations. Five to 7 days of dosing may be required to reach a steady-state concentration in some patients.

DOSAGE AND ADMINISTRATION. The starting dose is 100 mg every 12 hours, increased in increments of 50 mg twice daily, no sooner than every 3 to 4 days, until efficacy is achieved or an adverse effect is noted, or to a maximum of 400 mg/day (see Table 64.4). Cardiac rhythm and QRS duration should be monitored after changes in dose.

INDICATIONS. Flecainide is indicated for the treatment of life-threatening ventricular tachyarrhythmias, SVTs, and paroxysmal AF. Encouraging experimental and early clinical data support its use for catecholaminergic polymorphic VT (see Chapter 63). The dosage is adjusted to achieve the desired effect, but the serum concentration should not exceed 1.0 μg/mL. Flecainide is particularly effective in suppressing PVCs and short runs of non-sustained VT. As with other class I AADs, no data from controlled studies indicate that the drug favorably affects survival or sudden cardiac death, and data from CAST indicate increased mortality in patients with coronary artery disease (CAD). Flecainide produces a use-dependent prolongation of VT cycle length, which can improve hemodynamic tolerance. Flecainide is also useful for various SVTs, such as atrial tachycardia (AT), atrial flutter, and AF (including oral loading to terminate episodes acutely). Flecainide and propafenone may both be used in combination with beta or calcium channel blockers as a "pill in the pocket" approach to terminate AF as an outpatient (Table 64.4). When flecainide toxicity occurs, isoproterenol can reverse some of its electrophysiologic effects. It is important to slow the ventricular rate before treatment of AF with flecainide (e.g., with beta blockers or verapamil or diltiazem) to avoid the 1:1 AV conduction of slowed atrial flutter that may result from the effect of flecainide on fibrillation. Flecainide has been used to treat fetal arrhythmias and arrhythmias in children. Flecainide administration can produce ST elevation in lead V_1, characteristic of Brugada syndrome, in susceptible patients (see Chapter 63) and has been used as a diagnostic tool in persons suspected of having this disorder.

ADVERSE EFFECTS. Proarrhythmic effects are some of the most important adverse effects of flecainide. Its marked slowing of conduction precludes its use in patients with second-degree AV block without a pacemaker and warrants cautious administration in patients with intraventricular conduction disorders. Worsening of existing ventricular arrhythmias or the onset of new ventricular arrhythmias can occur in 5% to 30% of patients, especially in those with preexisting sustained VT, cardiac decompensation, and higher doses of the drug. Failure of the flecainide-related arrhythmia to respond to therapy, including electrical cardioversion-defibrillation, may result in mortality as high as 10% in patients in whom proarrhythmic events develop. Negative inotropic effects can precipitate or worsen heart failure episodes. Patients with sinus node dysfunction may experience sinus arrest, and an increase in the pacing and defibrillation thresholds may develop in those with pacemakers and ICDs, respectively. In CAST, patients treated with flecainide had higher mortality or nonfatal cardiac arrest compared to the placebo group, possibly related to an interaction between the drug and myocardial ischemia. Exercise can amplify the conduction slowing in the ventricle produced by flecainide and in some cases can precipitate a proarrhythmic response. Therefore, exercise testing has been recommended to screen for proarrhythmia (as well as occult ischemia) before and periodically during treatment. CNS complaints, including confusion and irritability, represent the most frequent noncardiac adverse effects. The safety of flecainide during pregnancy has not been determined, although as noted previously, it is occasionally used to treat fetal arrhythmias. It is concentrated in breast milk to a level 2.5- to 4-fold higher than in plasma. High doses of class IC agents can result in a markedly prolonged QRS duration, bundle branch block and wide and bizarre QRS morphologies during tachycardia.

Propafenone

Propafenone has been approved by the FDA for the treatment of patients with life-threatening ventricular tachyarrhythmias, as well as AF.

ELECTROPHYSIOLOGIC ACTIONS

Propafenone blocks the fast sodium current in a use-dependent manner in Purkinje fibers and to a lesser degree in ventricular muscle (see Tables 64.1, 64.2). Its use-dependent effects contribute to its ability to terminate AF. Its dissociation constant from the receptor is slow, similar to that of flecainide. Effects are greater in ischemic than in normal tissue and with reduced membrane potentials. Propafenone decreases excitability and suppresses spontaneous automaticity and triggered activity. The drug is a weak blocker of I_{Kr} and beta-adrenergic receptors. Although ventricular refractoriness increases, slowing of conduction is the major effect. Propafenone has several active metabolites that exert electrophysiologic effects. It depresses sinus node automaticity, and the A-H, H-V, PR, and QRS intervals increase, as do the refractory periods of all tissues. The QT interval increases only as a function of increased QRS duration.

HEMODYNAMIC EFFECTS

Propafenone and 5-hydroxypropafenone exhibit negative inotropic properties at high concentrations. In patients with left ventricular ejection fraction (EF) exceeding 40%, the negative inotropic effects are well tolerated, but patients with preexisting left ventricular dysfunction and congestive heart failure may exhibit worsening of their symptoms.

PHARMACOKINETICS

With more than 95% of the drug absorbed, the maximum plasma concentration of propafenone is achieved in 1 to 3 hours (see Table 64.4). Systemic bioavailability is dose dependent and ranges from 3% to 40% because of variable presystemic clearance. Bioavailability increases as the dose increases, and the plasma concentration is therefore not linearly related to dose. A threefold increase in dosage (300 to 900 mg/day) results in a 10-fold increase in plasma concentration, presumably because of saturation of hepatic metabolic mechanisms. Propafenone is 97% bound to alpha$_1$-acid glycoprotein, with an elimination half-life of 5 to 8 hours. Maximum therapeutic effects occur at serum concentrations of 0.2 to 1.5 μg/mL. The marked interpatient variability in pharmacokinetics and pharmacodynamics may be the result of genetically determined differences in metabolism (see Chapter 9). Approximately 7% of the white population are poor metabolizers and have an elimination half-life of 15 to 20 hours for the parent compound. The (+)-enantiomer provides nonspecific beta-adrenergic receptor blockade with 2.5% to 5% of the potency of propranolol, but because plasma propafenone concentrations may be 50 or more times higher than propranolol levels, these beta-blocking properties may be relevant. Poor metabolizers have a greater beta receptor–blocking effect than extensive metabolizers.

DOSAGE AND ADMINISTRATION

Most patients respond to oral propafenone doses of 150 to 300 mg every 8 hours, not to exceed 1200 mg/day (see Table 64.4). Doses are similar for patients of both metabolizing phenotypes. A sustained-release form is available for the treatment of AF; dosing is 225 to 425 mg twice daily. Concomitant food administration increases its bioavailability, as does hepatic dysfunction. No good correlation between the plasma propafenone concentration and suppression of arrhythmia has been shown. Doses should not be increased more often than every 3 to 4 days. Propafenone increases plasma concentrations of warfarin, digoxin, and metoprolol.

INDICATIONS. Propafenone is indicated for the treatment of paroxysmal SVT, AF, and life-threatening ventricular tachyarrhythmias, and effectively suppresses spontaneous PVCs and nonsustained and sustained VT. Acute termination of AF episodes occurred with a single 600-mg oral dose of propafenone in 76% of patients given the drug (twice the rate of those given placebo). It has been used effectively in the pediatric age group. Propafenone increases the pacing threshold but minimally affects the defibrillation threshold. The beta blocking effect contributes to a reduction in the sinus rate during exercise.

ADVERSE EFFECTS. Minor noncardiac effects occur in approximately 15% of patients, with dizziness, disturbances in taste, and blurred vision being the most common and GI side effects next. Exacerbation of bronchospastic lung disease can occur because of mild beta-blocking effects. Cardiovascular side effects develop in 10% to 15% of patients, including AV block, sinus node depression, and worsening of heart failure. Proarrhythmic responses, which occur more often in patients with a history of sustained VT and decreased EF, appear less often than with flecainide. Applicability of data from CAST about flecainide to propafenone is not clear but limiting the use of propafenone in a manner similar to that of other class IC drugs seems prudent; however, its beta-blocking actions may make it different. The safety of propafenone administration during pregnancy has not been established (class C).

Class II Agents
Beta Adrenoceptor–Blocking Agents

Although many beta adrenoceptor–blocking drugs have been approved for use in the United States, metoprolol, carvedilol, atenolol, propranolol, and esmolol have been most widely used to treat supraventricular and ventricular arrhythmias. Acebutolol, nadolol, timolol, betaxolol, pindolol, and bisoprolol have been used less extensively for the treatment of arrhythmias. Metoprolol, atenolol, carvedilol, timolol, and propranolol decrease overall mortality and sudden death after MI (see Chapter 70). It is generally thought that beta blockers possess class effects, and that when titrated to the proper dose, all can be used effectively to treat cardiac arrhythmias, hypertension, or other disorders. However, differences in pharmacokinetic or pharmacodynamic properties that confer safety, reduce adverse effects, or affect dosing intervals or drug interactions influence the choice of agent. For example, nadolol may be particularly effective in patients with long-QT syndrome (see Chapter 63). Also, some beta blockers, such as sotalol, pindolol, and carvedilol, exert unique actions in addition to beta receptor blockade.

Beta receptors can be separated into those that affect predominantly the heart (β_1) and those that affect predominantly blood vessels and the bronchi (β_2). In low doses, selective beta blockers can block β_1 receptors more than they block β_2 receptors and might be preferable for the treatment of patients with pulmonary or peripheral vascular disease. In high doses, the "selective" β_1 blockers also block β_2 receptors. Carvedilol also exerts alpha-blocking effects and is used primarily in patients with heart failure (see Chapters 49 and 50). It is a relatively poor agent for rate control in AF because of the alpha-blocking–induced hypotension that accompanies doses large enough to block the AV node adequately.

Some beta blockers exert intrinsic sympathomimetic activity; that is, they slightly activate the beta receptor. These drugs appear to be as efficacious as beta blockers without intrinsic sympathomimetic actions and may cause less slowing of the heart rate at rest and less prolongation of AV nodal conduction time. They have been shown to induce less depression of left ventricular function than do beta blockers without intrinsic sympathomimetic activity. Beta blockers without intrinsic sympathomimetic activity have been shown to reduce mortality in patients after MI, with nonselective agents possibly conferring slightly greater benefit (see Chapters 37 and 38).

The following discussion focuses on the use of propranolol as a prototypic antiarrhythmic agent but is generally applicable to other beta blockers.

ELECTROPHYSIOLOGIC ACTIONS

Beta blockers exert an electrophysiologic action by competitively inhibiting binding of catecholamines at beta adrenoceptor sites (see Tables 64.1, 64.2). Thus, beta blockers exert their major effects in cells most actively stimulated by adrenergic actions. At a beta-blocking concentration, propranolol slows spontaneous auto-maticity in the sinus node or in Purkinje fibers that are being stimulated by adrenergic tone and produces an I_f block (see Chapter 62). Beta blockers also block the $I_{Ca,L}$ stimulated by beta agonists. In the absence of adrenergic stimulation, only high concentrations of propranolol slow normal automaticity in Purkinje fibers, probably by a direct membrane (ion channel blocking) action.

Concentrations that cause beta receptor blockade, but no local anesthetic effects, do not alter the normal resting membrane potential, maximum diastolic potential amplitude, V_{max}, repolarization, or refractoriness of atrial, Purkinje, or ventricular muscle cells in the absence of catecholamine stimulation. However, in the presence of isoproterenol, a relatively pure beta receptor stimulator, beta blockers reverse isoproterenol's accelerating effects on repolarization. Propranolol reduces the amplitude of digitalis-induced DADs and suppresses triggered activity in Purkinje fibers.

Propranolol slows the sinus discharge rate in humans by 10% to 20%, although severe bradycardia occasionally results if the heart is particularly dependent on sympathetic tone or if sinus node dysfunction is present. The PR interval lengthens, as do AV nodal conduction time and AV nodal effective and functional refractory periods (at a constant heart rate), but refractoriness and conduction in the normal His-Purkinje system remain unchanged, even after high doses of propranolol. Beta blockers do not affect conduction or repolarization in normal ventricular muscle, as evidenced by their lack of effect on the QRS complex and QT interval, respectively.

Because administration of beta blockers that do not have direct membrane action prevents many arrhythmias resulting from activation of the autonomic nervous system, it is thought that the beta-blocking action is responsible for their antiarrhythmic effects. Nevertheless, the possible importance of the direct membrane effect of some of these drugs cannot be discounted totally, because beta blockers with direct membrane actions can affect the transmembrane potentials of diseased cardiac fibers at much lower concentrations than are needed to affect normal fibers directly. However, indirect actions on the arrhythmogenic effects of ischemia are probably the most important.

HEMODYNAMIC EFFECTS

Beta blockers exert negative inotropic effects and can precipitate or worsen heart failure. However, beta blockers clearly improve survival in patients with heart failure (see Chapter 50). By blocking β receptors, these drugs may allow unopposed alpha-adrenergic effects to produce peripheral vasoconstriction and exacerbate coronary artery spasm or pain from peripheral vascular disease in some patients.

Pharmacokinetics

Although various types of beta blockers exert similar pharmacologic effects, their pharmacokinetics differ substantially. Propranolol is almost 100% absorbed, but the effects of first-pass hepatic metabolism reduce its bioavailability to approximately 30% and produce significant interpatient variability in plasma concentration with a given dose (see Table 64.4). Reduced hepatic blood flow, as in patients with heart failure, decreases the hepatic extraction of propranolol; in these patients, propranolol may further decrease its own elimination rate by reducing cardiac output and hepatic blood flow. Beta blockers eliminated by the kidneys tend to have longer half-lives and exhibit less interpatient variability in drug concentration than do beta blockers metabolized by the liver.

DOSAGE AND ADMINISTRATION. The appropriate dose of propranolol is best determined by a measure of the patient's physiologic response, such as changes in resting heart rate or prevention of exercise-induced sinus tachycardia, because wide individual differences exist between the observed physiologic effect and plasma concentration. For example, IV dosing is best achieved by titration of the dose to clinical effect, beginning with doses of 0.25 to 0.50 mg, increasing to 1.0 mg if necessary, and administering doses every 5 minutes until either a desired effect or toxicity is produced or a total of 0.15 to 0.20 mg/kg has been given. In many cases, the short-acting effects of esmolol are preferred. Orally, propranolol is given in four divided doses, usually ranging from 40 to 160 mg/day up to no more than 640 mg/day (see Table 64.4). Some beta blockers, such as carvedilol and pindolol, need to be given twice daily; many are also available as once-daily long-acting preparations. In general, if one agent in adequate doses does not produce the desired effect, other beta blockers will also be ineffective. Conversely, if one agent produces the desired physiologic effect but a side effect develops, another beta blocker can often be substituted successfully.

INDICATIONS. Arrhythmias associated with thyrotoxicosis or pheochromocytoma and arrhythmias largely related to excessive cardiac adrenergic stimulation, such as those initiated by exercise or emotion, often respond to beta-blocker therapy. Beta-blocking drugs do not usually convert chronic atrial flutter or AF to normal sinus rhythm but may do so if the arrhythmia is of recent onset and in patients who have recently undergone cardiac surgery. The atrial rate during atrial flutter or fibrillation is not changed, but the ventricular response decreases because beta blockade prolongs AV nodal conduction time and refractoriness. Esmolol can be used intravenously for rapid control of the heart rate. For reentrant SVTs using the AV node as one of the reentrant pathways, such as AV nodal reentrant tachycardia (AVNRT) and orthodromic reciprocating tachycardia in WPW syndrome or inappropriate sinus tachycardia, or for AT, beta blockers can slow or terminate the tachycardia and can be used prophylactically to prevent a recurrence (see Chapters 65 and 66). Combining beta blockers with digitalis, quinidine, or various other agents can be effective when the beta blocker as a single agent fails.

Beta blockers can be effective for digitalis-induced arrhythmias such as AT, nonparoxysmal AV junctional tachycardia, PVCs, or VT. If a significant degree of AV block is present during digitalis-induced arrhythmia, lidocaine or phenytoin may be preferable to propranolol. Beta blockers can also be useful to treat ventricular arrhythmias associated with prolonged–QT interval syndrome (see Chapter 63) and with mitral valve prolapse (see Chapter 76). For patients with ischemic heart disease, beta blockers do not generally prevent the episodes of recurrent monomorphic VT that occur in the absence of acute ischemia. It is well accepted that several beta blockers reduce the incidence of both total and sudden death after MI (see Chapters 37 and 38). The mechanism of this reduction in mortality is not entirely clear and may be related to reduction of the extent of ischemic damage, autonomic effects, a direct antiarrhythmic effect, or combinations of these factors. Beta blockers may have been protective against proarrhythmic responses in CAST.

ADVERSE EFFECTS. Adverse cardiovascular effects from beta blockers include unacceptable hypotension, bradycardia, and congestive heart failure. The bradycardia can be caused by sinus slowing or AV block. Sudden withdrawal of propranolol in patients with angina pectoris can precipitate or worsen angina and cardiac arrhythmias and cause acute MI, possibly as a result of the heightened sensitivity to beta agonists caused by previous beta blockade (receptor upregulation). Heightened sensitivity may begin several days after cessation of beta-blocker therapy and can last 5 or 6 days. Other adverse effects of beta blockers include worsening of asthma or chronic obstructive pulmonary disease, intermittent claudication, Raynaud phenomenon, mental depression, increased risk for hypoglycemia in insulin-dependent diabetic patients, easy fatigability, disturbingly vivid dreams or insomnia, and impaired sexual function. Many of these side effects were noted less frequently with the use of β_1-selective agents, but even so-called cardioselective beta blockers can exacerbate asthma or diabetic control in individual patients.

Class III Agents
Amiodarone

Amiodarone is an iodinated benzofuran derivative approved by the FDA for the treatment of patients with life-threatening ventricular tachyarrhythmias when other drugs are ineffective or not tolerated.

ELECTROPHYSIOLOGIC ACTIONS

With long-term oral administration, amiodarone prolongs the APD and refractoriness of all cardiac fibers without affecting resting membrane potential (see Tables 64.1, 64.2 and Chapter 62). When acute effects are evaluated, amiodarone and its metabolite desethylamiodarone prolong the APD of ventricular muscle but shorten the APD of Purkinje fibers. It depresses V_{max} in ventricular muscle in a rate- or use-dependent manner by blocking inactivated sodium channels, an effect that is accentuated by depolarized and reduced by hyperpolarized membrane potentials. Amiodarone depresses conduction at fast rates more than at slow rates (use dependence). It does not prolong repolarization more at slow than at fast rates (i.e., does not demonstrate reverse use dependence) but does exert time-dependent effects on refractoriness, which may in part explain its high antiarrhythmic efficacy and low incidence of TdP.

Desethylamiodarone has relatively greater effects on fast-channel tissue, which probably contributes to its antiarrhythmic efficacy. The delay in building up adequate concentrations of this metabolite may in part explain the delay in amiodarone's antiarrhythmic action.

Amiodarone noncompetitively antagonizes alpha and beta receptors and blocks conversion of thyroxine (T_4) to triiodothyronine (T_3), which may account for some of its electrophysiologic effects. Amiodarone exhibits slow channel–blocking effects; with oral administration, it slows the sinus rate by 20% to 30% and prolongs the QT interval, at times changing the contour of the T wave and producing U waves.

The ERP of all cardiac tissues is prolonged. The H-V interval increases, and the QRS duration lengthens, especially at fast rates. Amiodarone given intravenously modestly prolongs the refractory period of atrial and ventricular muscle. The PR interval and AV nodal conduction time lengthen. The duration of the QRS complex lengthens at increased rates but less than after oral amiodarone. Thus the increase in prolongation of conduction time (except for AV node), duration of repolarization, and refractoriness is much less after IV administration than after the oral route. Considering these actions, it is clear that amiodarone has class I (blocks I_{Na}), class II (antiadrenergic), and class IV (blocks $I_{Ca,L}$) actions in addition to its class III effects (blocks I_K). Amiodarone's actions approximate those of a theoretically ideal drug that exhibits use-dependent Na^+ channel blockade with fast diastolic recovery from block and use-dependent prolongation of the APD. It does not increase and may decrease QT dispersion. Catecholamines can partially reverse some of the effects of amiodarone.

HEMODYNAMIC EFFECTS

Amiodarone is a peripheral and coronary vasodilator. When administered intravenously (150 mg over 10 minutes, then a 1-mg/min infusion), amiodarone decreases the heart rate, systemic vascular resistance, and left ventricular dP/dt. Oral doses of amiodarone sufficient to control cardiac arrhythmias do not depress the left ventricular EF, even in patients with reduced EF. However, because of the antiadrenergic actions of amiodarone, it should be given cautiously, particularly intravenously, to patients with marginal cardiac compensation.

PHARMACOKINETICS

Amiodarone is slowly, variably, and incompletely absorbed, with a systemic bioavailability of 25% to 65% (see Table 64.4). Plasma concentrations peak 3 to 6 hours after a single oral dose. There is a minimal first-pass effect, indicating minimal hepatic extraction. Elimination is by hepatic excretion into bile with some enterohepatic recirculation. Extensive hepatic metabolism occurs, with desethylamiodarone being a major metabolite. Both accumulate extensively in the liver, lung, fat, "blue" skin, and other tissues. The concentration in myocardium is 10 to 50 times that found in plasma. Plasma clearance of amiodarone is low, and renal excretion is negligible. Doses do not need to be reduced in patients with renal disease. Amiodarone and desethylamiodarone are not dialyzable. The volume of distribution is large but variable, with an average of 60 L/kg. Amiodarone is highly protein bound (96%), crosses the placenta (10% to 50%), and is found in breast milk.

The onset of action after IV administration generally occurs within 1 to 2 hours. After oral administration, the onset of action may require 2 to 3 days, often 1 to 3 weeks, and on occasion even longer. Loading doses reduce this time interval. Plasma concentrations relate well to oral doses during chronic treatment and average approximately 0.5 mg/L (0.5 μg/mL) for each 100 mg/day at doses between 100 and 600 mg/day. Amiodarone's elimination half-life is multiphasic, with an initial 50% reduction in plasma concentration 3 to 10 days after cessation of drug ingestion (probably representing elimination from well-perfused tissues), followed by a terminal half-life of 26 to 107 days (mean, 53 days), with most patients in the 40- to 55-day range. To achieve a steady-state concentration without a loading dose takes about 265 days. Interpatient variability in these pharmacokinetic parameters mandates close monitoring of the patient. Therapeutic serum concentrations range from 0.5 to 1.5 μg/mL. Greater suppression of arrhythmias may occur with up to 3.5 μg/mL, but the risk for side effects increases.

DOSAGE AND ADMINISTRATION. There is no standard dosing schedule for amiodarone applicable to all patients. One recommended approach is to treat with 800 to 1200 mg/day for 1 to 3 weeks, 400 to 800 mg/day for 1 to 2 weeks, and finally after 2 to 3 months of treatment, a maintenance dose of 200 mg per day (see Table 64.4). Maintenance drug can be given once or twice daily and should be titrated to the lowest effective dose to minimize the occurrence of side effects; in general, the earlier during drug loading that arrhythmia control is achieved, the lower the maintenance dose can be. Doses as low as 100 mg every other day can be effective in some patients. Regimens must be individualized for a given patient and clinical situation. To achieve more rapid loading and effect in emergencies, amiodarone can be administered intravenously at initial doses of 15 mg/min for 10 minutes, followed by 1 mg/min for 6 hours and then 0.5 mg/min for the remaining 18 hours and the next several days as necessary. Supplemental infusions of 150 mg over a 10-minute period can be used for breakthrough VT or VF. Intravenous infusions can be continued safely for 2 to 3 weeks. IV amiodarone is generally well tolerated, even in patients with left ventricular dysfunction. Patients with depressed EF should receive IV amiodarone with great caution because of hypotension. High-dose oral loading (800 to 2000 mg/day to maintain trough serum concentrations of 2 to 3 µg/mL) may suppress ventricular arrhythmias in 5 to 7 days.

INDICATIONS. Amiodarone has been used to suppress a wide spectrum of supraventricular and ventricular tachyarrhythmias in utero, in adults, and in children, including AV node and AV reentry, junctional tachycardia, atrial flutter and fibrillation, VT and VF associated with CAD, and hypertrophic cardiomyopathy. Success rates vary widely, depending on the population of patients, arrhythmia, underlying heart disease, length of follow-up, definition and determination of success, and other factors. In general, however, the efficacy of amiodarone equals or exceeds that of all other AADs and may be in the range of 60% to 80% for most supraventricular tachyarrhythmias and 40% to 60% for ventricular tachyarrhythmias. IV amiodarone is recommended in the 2015 ACLS algorithm for treatment of a shockable rhythm during the cardiac arrest VF/pulseless VT/cardiac arrest asystole/pulseless electrical activity (PEA) algorithm. Amiodarone may be useful in improving outcomes in patients with ventricular tachyarrhythmia during and after resuscitation from cardiac arrest. Amiodarone given before open heart surgery, as well as postoperatively, has been shown to decrease the incidence of postoperative AF. Amiodarone is superior to class I AADs and sotalol in maintaining sinus rhythm in patients with recurrent AF.

Patients who have an ICD receive fewer shocks if they are treated with amiodarone than if treated with conventional drugs. Amiodarone has little effect on the pacing threshold but typically increases the electrical defibrillation threshold modestly and slows the rate of VT (sometimes below the ICD's detection rate).

Several prospective, randomized controlled trials and meta-analyses have demonstrated improved survival with amiodarone therapy versus placebo. However, amiodarone has been shown to result in inferior survival compared with ICD therapy, and in the SCD-HeFT population (New York Heart Association [NYHA] class II or III heart failure; EF, 35%), survival of amiodarone-treated patients was no different than for the placebo group. The drug may still be used adjunctively in ICD-treated patients to decrease the frequency of shocks from VT and VF episodes or to control supraventricular tachyarrhythmias that elicit device therapy (see Chapter 65). As noted, the drug can slow the ventricular rate during spontaneous VT episodes beneath the detection rate of the device; careful patient assessment and, occasionally, device reprogramming and testing are necessary. It also can be used to slow the ventricular rate during AF and atrial flutter.

Because of the serious nature of the arrhythmias being treated, the unusual pharmacokinetics of the drug, and its adverse effects, consideration should be given to starting amiodarone therapy with the patient hospitalized and monitored for at least several days. Combining other AADs with amiodarone may improve efficacy in some patients.

ADVERSE EFFECTS. Adverse effects are reported by about 75% of patients treated with amiodarone for 5 years, and these effects compel stopping the drug in 18% to 37%. The most frequent side effects requiring drug discontinuation involve pulmonary and GI complaints or abnormal test results. Most adverse effects are reversible with dose reduction or cessation of treatment. Adverse effects are more common when therapy is continued in the long term and at higher doses. Of the non-cardiac adverse reactions, pulmonary toxicity is the most serious[10]; in one study, it occurred in 33 of 573 patients between 6 days and 60 months of treatment, with three deaths. The mechanism is unclear but may involve a hypersensitivity reaction, widespread phospholipidosis, or both. Dyspnea and nonproductive cough are the most common symptoms, along with fine crackles on examination, hypoxia, abnormal gallium scan results, reduced carbon monoxide diffusion capacity (D_{LCO}), and radiographic evidence of pulmonary infiltrates. Amiodarone must be immediately discontinued if such pulmonary changes occur. Corticosteroids can be tried, but no controlled studies have been done to support their use. Up to 10% mortality results in patients with pulmonary inflammatory changes, often in those with unrecognized pulmonary involvement that is attributed to other causes and is thus allowed to progress. Chest radiography and pulmonary function testing, including D_{LCO}, is recommended at baseline and then yearly chest radiographs are recommended. At maintenance doses lower than 200 mg/day, pulmonary toxicity is uncommon but can still occur. Advanced age, high maintenance doses, and reduced predrug D_{LCO} are risk factors for the development of pulmonary toxicity. An unchanged D_{LCO} on therapy may be a negative predictor of pulmonary toxicity.

Although asymptomatic elevations in liver enzyme levels are found in most patients, amiodarone is not stopped unless values exceed two or three times the upper limit of normal in a patient with initially normal values. Cirrhosis occurs infrequently but may be fatal.[11] Neurologic dysfunction, photosensitivity (perhaps minimized by sunscreens), bluish skin discoloration, GI disturbances, and hyperthyroidism (1% to 2%) or hypothyroidism (2% to 4%) can occur. Because amiodarone appears to inhibit the peripheral conversion of T_4 to T_3, chemical changes result and are characterized by a slight increase in T_4, reverse T_3, and thyroid-stimulating hormone (TSH) and a slight decrease in T_3 levels. The reverse T_3 concentration has been used as an index of drug effect. During hypothyroidism the TSH level increases greatly, whereas the level of T_3 increases in hyperthyroidism. Thyroid function tests should be performed approximately every 3 months for the first year while amiodarone is being taken and once or twice yearly thereafter, or sooner if symptoms develop that are consistent with thyroid dysfunction. Corneal microdeposits occur in almost 100% of adults receiving the drug longer than 6 months. More serious ocular reactions, including optic neuritis and atrophy with visual loss, have been reported but are rare, and causation by amiodarone has not been firmly established.[12] Among the most common side effects limiting long-term drug use are neurologic, and these side effects are both dose and duration related as well as idiosyncratic. Lowering the dose of amiodarone frequently decreases the severity of the side effect. A wide variety of neurologic toxicities have been described including tremor, ataxia, peripheral neuropathy, and rarely myopathy and encephalopathy. Some general guidelines for monitoring outpatients taking amiodarone are seen in Table 64.5.

Cardiac side effects include symptomatic bradycardias in approximately 2% of patients; and the rare development of TdP in 1% to 2%. Despite QT prolongation, amiodarone causes TdP rarely presumably due to the inhibition of multiple K channels and L-type Ca channels.

In general, the lowest possible maintenance dose of amiodarone that is still effective should be used to avoid significant adverse effects. Many supraventricular arrhythmias can be managed successfully with daily dosages of 200 mg or less, whereas ventricular arrhythmias generally require higher doses. Adverse effects are less common at dosages of 200 mg/day or less but can still occur. Monitoring of patients on this agent at any dose is critical.[13]

TABLE 64.5 Recommended Follow-up for Amiodarone

ECG at routine clinic follow ups, and at least every 12 months
Liver function tests at baseline and every 6 months or if patient presents with clinical features of liver disease
Thyroid function test (thyroid stimulating hormone) at baseline and every 4–6 months or if patient presents with clinical features suggestive of thyroid disease
Chest radiography at baseline and every year or for new and changing symptoms
Pulmonary function tests at baseline (including D_{LCO}) and if symptoms develop, especially in patients with underlying lung disease or abnormalities on chest radiography
Skin examination at routine follow-up every 6–12 months
Neurologic examination at routine follow-up. Note side effects are dose- and duration-related. Reduced dose should ameliorate symptoms.
Ophthalmologic examination at baseline if there is visual impairment and yearly or for any change in vision
Be aware of numerous drug interactions and drugs contraindicated with concomitant use of amiodarone, especially drugs that prolong QT interval or interact with amiodarone metabolism

Important interactions with other drugs occur, and when given concomitantly with amiodarone, the doses of warfarin, digoxin, and other AADs should be reduced by one third to one half and the patient observed closely. Drugs with synergistic actions, such as beta blockers or calcium channel blockers, must be given cautiously. The safety of amiodarone during pregnancy is controversial but categorized currently as class D. It should be used in pregnant patients only if no alternatives exist but should be avoided during breastfeeding.

Dronedarone

Dronedarone is approved by the FDA to facilitate maintenance of sinus rhythm in patients with atrial flutter and AF.

ELECTROPHYSIOLOGIC ACTIONS

As with amiodarone, dronedarone alters the activity of multiple cardiac ion channels (see Tables 64.1, 64.2). It is a more potent blocker of I_{Na} than amiodarone and exhibits similar effects on the L-type calcium current. Blockade of both I_{Kr} and I_{Ks} by dronedarone is also similar to that by amiodarone, whereas its effect on atrial $I_{K,Ach}$ and antiadrenergic effects (via noncompetitive binding) are significantly more potent than for amiodarone. Sinus node function is depressed to a minor degree. Pacing and defibrillation thresholds are slightly increased.

HEMODYNAMIC EFFECTS

Dronedarone has minimal effect on cardiac performance except in patients with compromised ventricular systolic function and should not be used in those with clinical signs of heart failure.

PHARMACOKINETICS

Dronedarone is 70% to 90% absorbed after oral administration, with peak plasma concentrations achieved in 3 to 4 hours; absorption is enhanced by food (see Table 64.4). Unlike the very long half-life of amiodarone, the elimination half-life of dronedarone is 13 to 19 hours, with 85% of the drug being excreted unchanged in feces and the remainder in urine. Dronedarone is metabolized by and slightly inhibits the activity of CYP3A4 (as well as CYP2D6) and should not be used in conjunction with other agents that strongly inhibit these enzyme systems. There is minimal warfarin interaction, but dronedarone increases serum levels of dabigatran.

DOSAGE AND ADMINISTRATION. The standard recommended dose of dronedarone is 400 mg every 12 hours with food (see Table 64.4). No parenteral form is currently available.

INDICATIONS. Dronedarone is indicated to facilitate cardioversion of atrial flutter or AF or to maintain sinus rhythm after restoration of sinus rhythm. It is slightly less effective than amiodarone and type IC drugs in this regard.[14] In the ANDROMEDA (Antiarrhythmic Trial with Dronedarone in Moderate-to-Severe Congestive Heart Failure Evaluating Morbidity Decrease) study, dronedarone-treated patients had a mortality rate more than twice that of the placebo group (8.1% vs. 3.8%). Similarly, in the PALLAS (Permanent Atrial Fibrillation Outcome Study Using Dronedarone on Top of Standard Therapy) trial, patients with permanent AF who were taking dronedarone had a greater than twofold higher risk for death, stroke, systemic embolism, or MI than did control patients. Thus, the medication should not be used in patients with current or recent episodes of clinical heart failure or those with permanent AF (as a rate control agent). Patients taking dronedarone should be evaluated periodically to ensure that permanent AF or heart failure has not developed.[15]

ADVERSE EFFECTS. A transient, predictable increase in serum creatinine, without adversely affecting actual glomerular filtration or other measures of renal function, occurs with standard dosing and is not a reason to alter the dose or to discontinue use of dronedarone. As noted, patients with NYHA class III or IV heart failure, as well as those with permanent AF, should not be given the drug because these patients have higher mortality. Patients with severe liver dysfunction should not generally receive dronedarone. The QT interval is predictably prolonged, but proarrhythmic effects from this or other mechanisms are rare (although sinus bradycardia is sometimes seen). Rash, photosensitivity, nausea, diarrhea, dyspepsia, headache, and asthenia have occurred in treated patients at higher frequency than in controls.

Absence of the iodine appears to account for the lower prevalence of lung and thyroid toxicity in dronedarone-treated patients than in those taking amiodarone. Dronedarone should not be used during pregnancy (category X, evidence or risk of fetal harm) and is possibly unsafe during breastfeeding.

Sotalol

Sotalol is a nonspecific beta adrenoceptor blocker without intrinsic sympathomimetic activity that prolongs repolarization. It is approved by the FDA to treat patients with life-threatening ventricular tachyarrhythmias and those with AF.[16]

ELECTROPHYSIOLOGIC ACTIONS

Both the *d*- and *l*-isomers have similar effects on prolonging repolarization, whereas the *l*-isomer is responsible for almost all the beta-blocking activity (see Tables 64.1, 64.2). Sotalol does not block alpha adrenoceptors and does not block I_{Na} (no membranestabilizing effects) but does prolong atrial and ventricular repolarization times by reducing I_{Kr}, thus prolonging the plateau of the action potential. Action potential prolongation is greater at slower rates (reverse use dependence). Resting membrane potential, action potential amplitude, and V_{max} are not significantly altered. Sotalol prolongs atrial and ventricular refractoriness, A-H and QT intervals, and sinus cycle length (see Chapter 65).

HEMODYNAMICS

Sotalol exerts a negative inotropic effect only through its beta-blocking action. Although it can slightly increase the strength of contraction by prolonging repolarization, which occurs maximally at slow heart rates, the negative inotropic effects predominate. In patients with reduced cardiac function, sotalol can decrease the cardiac index, increase filling pressure, and precipitate overt heart failure. Therefore, it must be used cautiously in patients with marginal cardiac compensation but is well tolerated in those with normal cardiac function.

PHARMACOKINETICS

Sotalol is completely absorbed and not metabolized, thus making it 90% to 100% bioavailable. It is not bound to plasma proteins, is excreted unchanged primarily by the kidneys, and has an elimination half-life of 10 to 15 hours (see Table 64.4). Peak plasma concentrations occur 2.5 to 4 hours after oral ingestion. Over the dose range of 160 to 640 mg, sotalol displays dose proportionality with plasma concentration (usually in the range of 2.5 μg/mL). The dose must be reduced in patients with renal disease. The beta-blocking effect is half-maximal at 80 mg/day and maximal at 320 mg/day.

DOSAGE. The typical oral dose is 80 to 160 mg every 12 hours, with 2 to 3 days between dose adjustments to attain a steady-state concentration and to monitor the ECG for arrhythmias and QT prolongation (see Table 64.4). Doses exceeding 320 mg/day can be used in patients when the potential benefits outweigh the risk for proarrhythmia. Because of its ability to prolong significantly the QT interval in some patients and cause TdP or provoke severe bradycardia, consideration should be given to inpatient initiation of the drug, especially in those with AF (in whom conversion to sinus bradycardia may cause syncope and/or further QT prolongation at slow rates), as well as in women (with longer baseline QT intervals). Intravenous sotalol has been approved for use in the United States; loading doses of 60 to 112.5 mg (depending on creatinine clearance) can be given over 1 hour, monitoring the QTc interval.

INDICATIONS. Approved by the FDA to treat patients with ventricular tachyarrhythmias and AF, sotalol is also useful to prevent recurrence of a wide variety of SVTs, including atrial flutter, AT, AV node reentry, and AV reentry (see Chapter 65). It slows the ventricular response to atrial tachyarrhythmias, but rarely causes conversion to sinus rhythm. Sotalol appears to be more effective than conventional AADs and may be comparable to amiodarone in the treatment of patients with ventricular tachyarrhythmias, as well as in prevention of recurrences of AF after cardioversion. Sotalol has been used successfully to decrease the incidence of AF after cardiac surgery. It may be effective in fetal and pediatric patients and young adults with congenital heart disease. Unlike most other AADs, sotalol may decrease the frequency of ICD discharges and reduce the defibrillation threshold but typically does not slow VT rates.

ADVERSE EFFECTS. Proarrhythmia is the most serious adverse effect. Overall, new or worsened ventricular tachyarrhythmias occur in approximately 4% of patients taking sotalol; this response is the result of TdP in approximately 2.5% but increases to 4% in patients with a history of sustained VT and is dose related (only 1.6% at 320 mg/day but 4.4% at 480 mg/day). This proarrhythmic effect was probably the cause of excess mortality in patients given *d*-sotalol (the enantiomer lacking a beta-blocking effect) after acute MI in the SWORD (Survival With Oral *d*-Sotalol) trial. Other adverse effects typically seen with other beta blockers also apply to sotalol. Sotalol should be used with caution or not at all in combination with other drugs that prolong the QT interval. However, such combinations have occasionally been used successfully.

Ibutilide

Ibutilide is an agent released for acute termination of episodes of atrial flutter and AF (see Chapter 66). Ibutilide also blocks accessory pathway conduction.

ELECTROPHYSIOLOGIC ACTIONS

As with other class III agents, ibutilide prolongs repolarization (see Tables 64.1, 64.2). Although similar to other class III agents that block outward potassium currents, such as I_{Kr}, ibut-ilide is unique in that it also activates a slow inward sodium current. IV ibutilide has minimal effects on AV conduction or QRS duration, but the QT interval is characteristically prolonged. Ibutilide has no significant effect on hemodynamics.

PHARMACOKINETICS

Ibutilide is administered intravenously and has a large volume of distribution (see Table 64.4). Clearance is predominantly renal, with a drug half-life averaging 6 hours, but with considerable interpatient variability. Protein binding is approximately 40%. One of the drug's metabolites has weak class III effects.

DOSAGE AND ADMINISTRATION. Ibutilide is given as an IV infusion of 1 mg over 10 minutes (see Table 64.4). It should not be given in the presence of a QTc interval longer than 440 milliseconds or other drugs that prolong the QT interval or in patients with uncorrected hypokalemia, hypomagnesemia, or bradycardia. A second 1-mg dose may be given after the first dose is finished if the arrhythmia persists. Patients must have continuous electrocardiographic monitoring throughout the dosing period and for up to 4 hours thereafter because of the risk for ventricular arrhythmias. Pretreatment with IV magnesium may decrease the risk for ventricular arrhythmias and enhance efficacy in treating some atrial arrhythmias. Up to 60% of patients with AF and 70% of those with atrial flutter convert to sinus rhythm after 2 mg of ibutilide has been administered.[17]

INDICATIONS. Ibutilide is indicated for termination of an established episode of atrial flutter or AF. It should not be used in patients with frequent short paroxysms of AF because it merely terminates episodes and is not useful for long-term prevention. Patients whose condition is hemodynamically unstable should proceed to direct-current (DC) cardioversion. Ibutilide has been used safely and effectively in patients who were already taking amiodarone or propafenone, but should be used with caution in these patients. Ibutilide has been administered at transthoracic electrical cardioversion to increase the likelihood of termination of AF. In one study, all 50 patients given ibutilide before attempted electrical cardioversion achieved sinus rhythm, whereas only 34 of 50 who did not receive the drug converted to sinus rhythm. Of note, all 16 patients who did not respond to electrical cardioversion without ibutilide were successfully electrically cardioverted to sinus rhythm when a second attempt was made after ibutilide pretreatment.

Ibutilide prolongs accessory pathway refractoriness and can temporarily slow the ventricular rate during preexcited AF. The drug can rarely terminate episodes of organized AT, as well as sustained, uniform-morphology VT.

ADVERSE EFFECTS. The most significant adverse effect of ibutilide is QT prolongation–related TdP, which occurs in approximately 2% of patients given the drug (twice as often in women as in men). This effect develops within the first 4 hours of dosing or until the QTc has returned to baseline, after which the risk is negligible. Thus, patients must undergo electrocardiographic monitoring for up to 4 hours after dosing (or longer, until QTc returns to baseline). This requirement makes using ibutilide in emergency departments or private offices problematic. The safety of ibutilide during pregnancy has not been well studied, and its use in pregnant women should be restricted to those in whom no safer alternative exists.

Dofetilide

Dofetilide is approved for the acute conversion of AF to sinus rhythm, as well as for chronic suppression of recurrent AF.

ELECTROPHYSIOLOGIC ACTIONS

The sole electrophysiologic effect of dofetilide is block of the rapid component of the delayed rectifier potassium current (I_{Kr}), important in repolarization (see Tables 64.1, 64.2). This effect is more prominent in the atria than in the ventricles—30% increase in the atrial refractory period versus 20% in the ventricle. The effect of dofetilide on I_{Kr} is prolongation of refractoriness without slowing conduction, which is believed to be largely responsible for its antiarrhythmic effect. It is also responsible for prolongation of the QT interval on the ECG, which averages 11% but can be much greater. This effect on the QT interval is dose dependent and linear. No other important electrocardiographic changes are observed with the drug. It has no significant hemodynamic effects. Dofetilide is more effective than quinidine at converting AF to sinus rhythm. Its long-term efficacy is similar to that of other agents.[18]

PHARMACOKINETICS

Oral dofetilide is absorbed well, and more than 90% is bioavailable. Its mean elimination half-life is 7 to 13 hours, with 50% to 60% excreted unchanged in urine (see Table 64.4). The remainder of the drug undergoes hepatic metabolism to inert compounds. Significant drug-drug interactions have been reported in patients taking dofetilide; cimetidine, verapamil, ketoconazole, and trimethoprim, alone or in combination with sulfamethoxazole, cause a significant elevation in the dofetilide serum concentration and should not be used with this drug.

DOSAGE AND ADMINISTRATION. Dofetilide is available only as an oral preparation. Dosing is from 0.125 to 0.5 mg twice daily and must be initiated in a hospital setting with continuous electrocardiographic monitoring to ensure that excessive QT prolongation and TdP do not develop (see Table 64.4). Physicians must be specially certified to prescribe the drug. Its dosage must be decreased in the presence of impaired renal function or an increase in the QT interval of more than 15%, or 500 milliseconds. Dofetilide should not be given to patients with a creatinine clearance lower than 20 mL/min or a baseline QTc interval longer than 440 milliseconds.

INDICATIONS. Oral dofetilide is indicated for prevention of episodes of supraventricular tachyarrhythmias, particularly atrial flutter and fibrillation. The role of dofetilide in the treatment of ventricular arrhythmias is less clear; it has been shown to decrease the defibrillation threshold in patients with an ICD, as well as decrease the frequency of ICD therapies for ventricular arrhythmias.

ADVERSE EFFECTS. The most significant adverse effect of dofetilide is QT interval prolongation–related TdP, which occurs in 2% to 4% of patients. Risk is highest in patients with a baseline prolonged QT interval, in those who are hypokalemic, in those taking some other agent that prolongs repolarization, and after conversion from AF to sinus rhythm. Because the risk for TdP is highest at drug initiation, it should be used continuously and not as intermittent outpatient dosing. The drug is otherwise well tolerated, with few side effects. Its use in pregnancy has not been studied extensively, and it should probably be avoided in pregnant women if possible.

Class IV Agents

Calcium Channel Antagonists: Verapamil and Diltiazem

Verapamil, a synthetic papaverine derivative, is the prototype of a class of drugs that block the slow calcium channel and reduce $I_{Ca,L}$ in cardiac muscle (see Chapter 46). Diltiazem has electrophysiologic actions similar to those of verapamil. Nifedipine and other dihydropyridine agents exhibit minimal electrophysiologic effects at clinically used doses; these drugs are not discussed here.

ELECTROPHYSIOLOGIC ACTIONS

By blocking $I_{Ca,L}$ in all cardiac fibers, verapamil reduces the plateau height of the action potential, slightly shortens muscle action potential at pharmacologic concentrations, and slightly prolongs Purkinje fiber action potential (see Tables 64.1, 64.2). It does not appreciably affect the action potential amplitude, V_{max} of phase 0, or resting membrane voltage in cells that have fast-response characteristics related to I_{Na} (e.g., atrial and ventricular muscle, His-Purkinje system). Verapamil suppresses slow responses elicited by various experimental methods, as well as sustained triggered activity and EADs and DADs. Verapamil and diltiazem suppress electrical activity in the normal sinus and AV nodes. Verapamil depresses the slope of diastolic depolarization in sinus node cells, V_{max} of phase 0, and maximum diastolic potential and prolongs conduction time and refractory periods of the AV node. The AV node–blocking effects of verapamil and diltiazem are more apparent at faster rates of stimulation (use dependence) and in depolarized fibers (voltage dependence). Verapamil slows activation of the slow channel and delays its recovery from inactivation.

Verapamil does exert some local anesthetic activity because the d-isomer of the clinically used racemic mixture exerts slight blocking effects on I_{Na}. The l-isomer blocks the slow inward current carried by calcium, as well as other ions, traveling through the slow channel. Verapamil does not affect calcium-activated adenosine triphosphatase (ATPase), nor does it block beta receptors, but it may block alpha receptors and potentiate vagal effects on the AV node. Verapamil can also cause other effects that indirectly alter cardiac electrophysiology, such as decreasing platelet adhesiveness or reducing the extent of myocardial ischemia.

In humans, verapamil prolongs conduction time through the AV node (the A-H interval) and lengthens AV nodal anterograde and retrograde refractory periods without affecting the P wave or QRS duration or the H-V interval. The spontaneous sinus rate may decrease slightly, an effect only partially reversed by atropine. More often, the sinus rate does not change significantly because verapamil causes peripheral vasodilation, transient hypotension, and reflex sympathetic stimulation, which mitigates any direct slowing effect that verapamil exerts on the sinus node. If verapamil is given to a patient who is also receiving a beta blocker, the sinus node discharge rate may slow because reflex sympathetic stimulation is blocked. Verapamil does not exert a significant direct effect on atrial or ventricular refractoriness or on the anterograde or retrograde properties of accessory pathways. However, reflex sympathetic stimulation after IV verapamil administration may increase the ventricular response over the accessory pathway during AF in patients with WPW syndrome, sometimes dangerously so.

HEMODYNAMIC EFFECTS

Because verapamil interferes with excitation-contraction coupling, it inhibits vascular smooth muscle contraction and causes marked vasodilation in coronary and other peripheral vascular beds. The reflex sympathetic effects of verapamil may reduce its marked negative inotropic action on isolated cardiac muscle, but the direct myocardial depressant effects of verapamil may predominate when the drug is given in high doses. In patients with well-preserved left ventricular function, combined therapy with propranolol and verapamil appears to be well tolerated, but in some cases, beta blockade can accentuate the hemodynamic depressant effects produced by oral verapamil. Patients with reduced left ventricular function may not tolerate the combined blockade of beta receptors and calcium channels; thus, in these patients, verapamil and a beta blocker should be used in combination either cautiously or not at all. Verapamil reduces myocardial oxygen demand while decreasing coronary vascular resistance. Such changes may be indirectly antiarrhythmic.

Peak alterations in hemodynamic variables occur 3 to 5 minutes after completion of a verapamil injection, with the major effects dissipating within 10 minutes. Systemic resistance and mean arterial pressure decrease, as does left ventricular dP/dt_{max}, and left ventricular end-diastolic pressure increases. Heart rate, cardiac index, and mean pulmonary artery pressure do not change significantly in individuals with normal resting left ventricular systolic function. Thus the afterload reduction produced by verapamil significantly counterbalances its negative inotropic action, so the cardiac index may not be reduced. In addition, when verapamil slows the ventricular rate in a patient with tachycardia, hemodynamics may also improve. Nevertheless, caution should be exercised in giving verapamil to patients with myocardial depression or those receiving beta blockers or disopyramide because hemodynamic deterioration may progress in some patients.

PHARMACOKINETICS

After single oral doses of verapamil, measurable prolongation of AV nodal conduction time occurs in 30 minutes and lasts 4 to 6 hours (see Table 64.4). After IV administration, AV nodal conduction delay occurs within 1 to 2 minutes and A-H interval prolongation is still detectable after 6 hours. After oral administration, absorption is almost complete, but its overall bioavailability of 20% to 35% suggests substantial first-pass metabolism in the liver, particularly of the l-isomer. Verapamil's elimination half-life is 3 to 8 hours, with up to 70% of the drug excreted by the kidneys. Norverapamil is a major metabolite that may contribute to the electrophysiologic actions of verapamil. Serum protein binding is approximately 90%. With diltiazem, the percentage of heart rate reduction in AF is related to its plasma concentration.

DOSAGE AND ADMINISTRATION. For acute termination of SVT or rapid achievement of ventricular rate control during AF, the most common IV dose of verapamil is up to 10 mg infused over 1 to 2 minutes while cardiac rhythm and blood pressure are monitored (see Table 64.4). A second injection of an equal dose may be given 30 minutes later. The initial effect achieved with the first bolus injection, such as slowing of the ventricular response during AF, can be maintained by continuous infusion of the drug at a rate of 0.005 mg/kg/min. The oral dose is 240 to 480 mg/day in divided doses. Diltiazem is given intravenously at a dose of 0.25 mg/kg as a bolus over 2 minutes, with a second dose in 15 minutes if necessary. Because it is generally better tolerated (less hypotension) with long-term administration, such as for control of the ventricular rate during AF, diltiazem is preferred over verapamil in this setting. Significant hypotension resulting from IV diltiazem can be countered by volume expansion or judicious use of a pure vasoconstrictor agent such as phenylephrine. Orally, doses must be adjusted to the patient's needs, with a 120- to 360-mg range. Various long-acting preparations (once daily) are available for verapamil and diltiazem.

INDICATIONS. After simple vagal maneuvers have been tried and adenosine has been given, IV verapamil or diltiazem is the next treatment of choice for termination of sustained AV node reentry or orthodromic AV reciprocating tachycardia associated with an accessory pathway (see Chapter 65). Verapamil is as effective as adenosine for termination of these arrhythmias. Assuming that the patient is stable, verapamil should definitely be tried before termination is attempted by digitalis administration, pacing, electrical DC cardioversion, or acute blood pressure elevation with vasopressors. Verapamil and diltiazem terminate 60% to 90% or more episodes of paroxysmal SVT within several minutes. Verapamil may also be of use in some fetal SVTs. Although IV verapamil has been given along with IV propranolol, this combination should be used only with great caution because of combined adverse hemodynamic effects.

Verapamil and diltiazem decrease the ventricular response over the AV node during AF or atrial flutter, possibly converting a small number of episodes to sinus rhythm, particularly if the atrial flutter or AF is of recent onset. AF can occur in some patients with atrial flutter after verapamil administration. As noted earlier, in patients with preexcited ventricular complexes during AF associated with WPW syndrome, IV verapamil may accelerate the ventricular response; therefore, the IV route is contraindicated in this situation. Verapamil can terminate some ATs. Even though verapamil can often terminate an idiopathic left septal VT, hemodynamic collapse can occur if IV verapamil is given to patients with the more common forms of VT because these generally occur in the setting of decreased left ventricular systolic function. A general rule for avoiding complications, however, is not to administer verapamil intravenously to any patient with wide-QRS tachycardia unless one is certain of the nature of the tachycardia and its probable response to verapamil.

Orally, verapamil or diltiazem can prevent the recurrence of AV node reentrant and orthodromic AV reciprocating tachycardias associated with an accessory pathway, as well as help maintain a decreased ventricular response during atrial flutter or AF in patients without an accessory pathway. Verapamil has not generally been effective in treating patients who have recurrent ventricular tachyarrhythmias, although it may suppress some forms of VT, such as left septal VT (noted earlier). It can also be useful in patients with ventricular arrhythmias related to coronary artery spasm. Calcium channel blockers have not been shown to reduce mortality or to prevent sudden cardiac death in patients after acute MI, except for diltiazem in those with non–ST-segment elevation infarctions (see Chapter 39).

ADVERSE EFFECTS. Verapamil must be used cautiously in patients with significant hemodynamic impairment or in those receiving beta blockers, as noted earlier. Hypotension, bradycardia, AV block, and asystole are more likely to occur when the drug is given to patients who are already receiving beta-blocking agents. Hemodynamic collapse has been noted in infants, and verapamil should be used cautiously in children younger than 1 year. Verapamil should also be used with caution in patients with sinus node abnormalities because marked depression of sinus node function or asystole can result in some of these patients. IV isoproterenol, calcium, glucagon, dopamine, or atropine, which may be only partially effective, or temporary pacing may be necessary to counteract some of the adverse effects of verapamil. Isoproterenol may be more effective for the treatment of bradyarrhythmias, and calcium may be used for the treatment of hemodynamic dysfunction secondary to verapamil. AV node depression is common in overdoses. Contraindications to the use of verapamil and diltiazem include the presence of advanced heart failure, second- or third-degree AV block without a pacemaker in place, AF and anterograde conduction over an accessory pathway, significant sinus node dysfunction, most VTs, cardiogenic shock, and other hypotensive states. Although these drugs should probably not be used in patients with overt heart failure, if it is caused by one of the supraventricular tachyarrhythmias noted earlier, verapamil or diltiazem may restore sinus rhythm or significantly decrease the ventricular rate and thereby lead to hemodynamic improvement. Also, verapamil can decrease the excretion of digoxin by approximately 30%. Hepatotoxicity may occur on occasion. Verapamil crosses the placental barrier; its use in pregnancy has been associated with impaired uterine contraction, fetal bradycardia, and possibly fetal digital defects. It should therefore be used only if no effective alternatives exist.

Other Antiarrhythmic Agents
Adenosine

Adenosine is an endogenous nucleoside present throughout the body and has been approved by the FDA to treat patients with SVTs.

ELECTROPHYSIOLOGIC ACTIONS

Adenosine interacts with G-protein coupled A_1 receptors present on the extracellular surface of cardiac cells and activates K^+ channels ($I_{K,Ach}$, $I_{K,Ado}$) in a manner similar to that produced by acetylcholine (see Tables 64.1, 64.2). The increase in K^+ conductance shortens the atrial APD, hyperpolarizes the membrane potential, and decreases atrial contractility. Similar changes occur in the sinus and AV nodes. In contrast to these direct effects mediated through the gua-nine nucleotide regulatory proteins G_i and G_o, adenosine antagonizes catecholamine-stimulated adenylate cyclase to decrease accumulation of cyclic adenosine monophosphate (AMP) and to decrease $I_{Ca,L}$ and the pacemaker current I_f in sinus node cells along with a decrease in V_{max}. Shifts in the pacemaker site within the sinus node and sinus exit block may occur. Adenosine slows the sinus rate in humans, followed within seconds by a reflex increase in the sinus rate. In the AV node, adenosine produces transient prolongation of the A-H interval, often with transient first-, second-, or third-degree AV node block lasting up to a few seconds. The delay in AV nodal conduction is rate dependent. His-Purkinje conduction is not generally affected directly. Adenosine does not affect conduction in normal accessory pathways. Conduction may be blocked in unusual accessory pathways that have long conduction times or decremental conduction properties. Patients with heart transplants exhibit a supersensitive response to adenosine.

PHARMACOKINETICS

Adenosine is removed from the extracellular space by washout, enzymatically by degradation to inosine, by phosphorylation to AMP, or by reuptake into cells through a nucleoside transport system (see Table 64.4). The vascular endothelium and erythrocytes contain these elimination systems, which result in very rapid clearance of adenosine from the circulation. Its elimination half-life is 1 to 6 seconds. Most of adenosine's effects are produced during its first passage through the circulation. Important drug interactions occur; methylxanthines are competitive antagonists, and therapeutic concentrations of theophylline totally block the exogenous effects of adenosine. Dipyridamole is a nucleoside transport blocker that blocks reuptake of adenosine, thus delaying its clearance from the circulation or interstitial space and potentiating its effect. Smaller adenosine doses should be used in patients receiving dipyridamole and in heart transplant patients where denervation makes the sinus and AV node supersensitive.

DOSAGE AND ADMINISTRATION. To terminate tachycardia, a bolus of adenosine is rapidly injected intravenously at doses of 6 to 12 mg, followed by a flush (see Table 64.4). Pediatric (<50 kg) dosing should be 0.05 to 0.3 mg/kg. When it is injected into a central vein and in patients after heart transplantation or those receiving dipyridamole, the initial dose should be reduced to 3 mg. Transient sinus slowing or AV node block results but lasts less than 5 seconds. Doses higher than 18 mg are unlikely to revert a tachycardia and should not be used.

INDICATIONS. Adenosine has become the drug of first choice to terminate an SVT acutely, such as AV node or AV reentry (see Chapter 65), and is useful in pediatric patients. Adenosine can produce AV nodal block or terminate ATs and sinus node reentry. It results in only transient AV block during atrial flutter or fibrillation and is thus useful only for diagnosis, not therapy. Adenosine terminates a group of VTs whose maintenance depends on adrenergic drive, which is most often located in the right ventricular outflow tract but can be found at other sites as well; however, idiopathic left septal VT rarely responds. When properly administered, adenosine usually causes transient hypotension, chest discomfort, and dyspnea; if tachycardia persists in the absence of these effects, the drug may not have been given correctly. Adenosine has less potential than verapamil for producing prolonged hypotension, should tachycardia persist after injection.

Doses as low as 2.5 mg terminate some tachycardias; doses of 12 mg or less terminate 92% of SVTs, usually within 30 seconds. Successful termination rates with adenosine are comparable to those achieved with verapamil. Because of its effectiveness and extremely short duration of action, adenosine is preferable to verapamil in most cases, particularly in patients who have previously received IV beta adrenoceptor blockers, in those with poorly compensated heart failure or severe hypotension, and in neonates. Verapamil might be chosen first in patients receiving drugs such as theophylline (which is known to interfere with adenosine's actions or metabolism), in patients with active bronchoconstriction, and in those with inadequate venous access.

Adenosine may be useful to help differentiate among causes of wide-QRS tachycardias because it terminates many SVTs with aberrancy or reveals the underlying atrial mechanism and does not block conduction over an accessory pathway or terminate most VTs. In rare cases, however, adenosine terminates some VTs, characteristically those of right ventricular outflow tract origin as noted earlier, and therefore tachycardia termination is not completely diagnostic of an SVT. This agent may predispose to the development of AF and might transiently increase the ventricular response in patients with AF conducting over an accessory pathway. Adenosine may also be useful in differentiating conduction over the AV node from that over an accessory pathway during ablative procedures designed to interrupt the accessory pathway. However, this distinction is not absolute because adenosine can block conduction in slowly conducting accessory pathways and does not always produce block in the AV node.

ADVERSE EFFECTS. Transient side effects occur in almost 40% of patients with SVT given adenosine and usually consist of flushing, dyspnea, and chest pressure. These symptoms are fleeting, lasting less than 1 minute, and are well tolerated. PVCs, transient sinus bradycardia, sinus arrest, and AV block are common when an SVT is terminated abruptly. AF is occasionally observed (12% in one study) with adenosine administration, perhaps because of the drug's effect in shortening atrial refractoriness. Induction of AF can be problematic in patients with WPW syndrome and rapid AV conduction over the accessory pathway.

Digoxin

Cardiac actions of digitalis glycosides have been recognized for several centuries. In adults, digoxin is used mainly for control of the ventricular rate during AF, whereas its use in pediatrics is in a broader range of arrhythmias. Use of digoxin has decreased because of the availability of agents with greater and more reliable efficacy and a wider therapeutic to toxic drug concentration range. Its use is generally discouraged in adults.

ELECTROPHYSIOLOGIC ACTIONS

Digoxin acts mainly through the autonomic nervous system, in particular by enhancing both central and peripheral vagal tone. These actions are confined largely to slowing of the sinus node discharge rate, shortening of atrial refractoriness, and prolongation of AV nodal refractoriness (see Tables 64.1, 64.2). Electrophysiologic effects on the His-Purkinje system and ventricular muscle are minimal, except with toxic concentrations. In studies of denervated hearts, digoxin has relatively little effect on the AV node and causes a mild increase in atrial refractoriness.

The sinus rate and P wave duration are minimally changed in most patients taking digoxin. The sinus rate may decrease in patients with heart failure whose left ventricular performance is improved by the drug; individuals with significant underlying sinus node disease also have slower sinus rates or even sinus arrest. Similarly, the PR interval is generally unchanged, except in patients with underlying AV node disease. The QRS and QT intervals are unaffected. The characteristic ST and T wave abnormalities seen with use of digoxin do not represent toxicity.

PHARMACOKINETICS

IV digoxin yields some electrophysiologic effect within minutes, with a peak effect occurring after 1.5 to 3 hours (see Table 64.4). After oral dosing, the peak effect occurs in 4 to 6 hours. The extent of digoxin absorption after oral administration varies according to the preparation; tablet forms are 60% to 75% absorbed, whereas encapsulated gel forms are almost completely absorbed. Ingestion of cholestyramine or an antacid preparation at the same time as digoxin ingestion decreases its absorption. The serum half-life of digoxin is 36 to 48 hours, and the drug is excreted unchanged by the kidneys.

DOSAGE AND ADMINISTRATION. In acute loading doses of 0.5 to 1.0 mg, digoxin can be given orally or intravenously (see Table 64.4). Chronic daily oral dosing should be adjusted on the basis of clinical indications and the extent of renal dysfunction. Most patients require 0.125 to 0.25 mg/day as a single dose. However, some patients undergoing renal dialysis need as little as 0.125 mg every other day, whereas young patients may require as much as 0.5 mg/day. Serum digoxin levels may be used to monitor compliance with therapy, as well as to determine whether digitalis toxicity is the cause of new symptoms compatible with the diagnosis. However, routine monitoring of digoxin levels is not warranted in patients whose ventricular rate is controlled during AF and who have no symptoms of toxicity.

INDICATIONS. Digoxin can be used intravenously to slow the ventricular rate during AF and atrial flutter; it was formerly used in an attempt to convert SVTs to sinus rhythm, but its onset of action is much slower and its success rate less than that of adenosine, verapamil, or beta blockers. Thus, it is now rarely used in this fashion. Digoxin is more often used orally to control the ventricular rate in permanent ("chronic") AF. When a patient with AF is at rest and vagal tone predominates, the ventricular rate can be maintained between 60 and 100 beats/min in 40% to 60% of cases. However, when the patient begins to exercise, the decrease in vagal tone and increase in adrenergic tone combine to diminish the beneficial effects of digoxin on AV nodal conduction. Patients can experience a marked increase in ventricular rate with even mild exertion. Digoxin is therefore rarely used as a single agent to control the ventricular rate in AF. The drug has little ability to prevent episodes of paroxysmal AF or to control the ventricular rate during episodes and may even provoke episodes in patients with so-called vagal AF. Furthermore, digoxin is not more effective than placebo in terminating episodes of acute- or recent-onset AF.

ADVERSE EFFECTS. The use of digoxin has decreased because of is its potential for serious adverse effects, the narrow window between therapeutic and toxic concentrations and extensive drug-drug interactions. Digitalis toxicity produces various symptoms and signs, including headache, nausea and vomiting, altered color perception, halo vision, and generalized malaise. Less common but more serious than these are digitalis-related arrhythmias, which include bradycardias related to a greatly enhanced vagal effect (e.g., sinus bradycardia or arrest, AV node block) and tachyarrhythmias that may be caused by DAD-mediated triggered activity (e.g., junctional, and fascicular or VT). Worsening renal function, advanced age, hypokalemia, chronic lung disease, hypothyroidism, and amyloidosis increase a patient's sensitivity to digitalis-related arrhythmias. The diagnosis of toxicity can be confirmed by determination of the serum digoxin level. Therapy for most bradycardias consists of withdrawal of digoxin; atropine or temporary pacing may be needed in symptomatic patients. Phenytoin can be used to control atrial tachyarrhythmias, whereas lidocaine has been successful in treating infranodal tachycardias. Life-threatening arrhythmias can be treated with digoxin-specific antibody fragments. Electrical DC cardioversion should be performed only when absolutely necessary in a digitalis-toxic patient because life-threatening VT or VF can result and can be difficult to control. Some data incriminate digoxin in increasing mortality in patients with AF.[19]

Ranolazine

Ranolazine, approved by the FDA for the treatment of chronic angina, has significant electrophysiologic properties. It has been shown to decrease the incidence of AF, SVT, and ventricular arrhythmias relative to controls in trials of the drug's antianginal effects.

ELECTROPHYSIOLOGIC ACTIONS

Ranolazine blocks I_{Kr}, as well as the late Na current; at higher concentrations, the L-type Ca current is mildly affected (see Tables 64.1, 64.2). The drug prolongs atrial and ventricular refractoriness and induces postrepolarization refractoriness; the P wave, PR interval, and QRS are unaffected, but the QT interval is mildly prolonged. Unlike other I_{Kr}-blocking drugs, ranolazine does not induce EADs. Its effects are more pronounced on atrial than on ventricular myocardium, and the drug shows promise for the treatment of AF, particularly when combined with dronedarone.[20]

HEMODYNAMIC EFFECTS

Ranolazine has no important hemodynamic effects; it does not appear to produce meaningful changes in contractility or vascular resistance.

PHARMACOKINETICS

Absorption of oral ranolazine is mediated in part by the P-glycoprotein system, modulators of which may increase or decrease drug exposure. About 75% of a dose is bioavailable, with peak levels reached in 2 to 5 hours (see Table 64.4). Absorption is not affected by food. Its half-life is approximately 7 hours; hepatic metabolism to minimally or wholly inactive products occurs via the CYP3A and, to a lesser extent, the CYP2D6 pathways. Approximately 75% of the drug is excreted in urine, the remainder in feces.

DOSAGE AND ADMINISTRATION. The typical oral dose of ranolazine is 500 mg twice daily, to a maximum of 1000 mg twice daily. The dose should be decreased in the setting of moderate liver disease. It should not be used in conjunction with strong inhibitors of CYP3A, which could increase the drug's serum concentration threefold.

ADVERSE EFFECTS. The most widely known potential adverse effect of ranolazine is QTc prolongation, which averages 6 to 15 milliseconds (sometimes more in patients with severe liver failure), because of inhibition of I_{Kr}. Despite this effect on the QT interval, TdP is rare, probably in part because of only modest QT prolongation combined with the drug's inhibition of the late inward Na current, which mitigates the QT effect. As noted, ranolazine does not cause EADs or increases in transmural dispersion of refractoriness, which are believed to be prerequisites for torsades. Ranolazine produces a mild elevation in measured serum creatinine (0.1 mg/dL) without changing the actual glomerular filtration rate. The drug is pregnancy category C; its concentration in breast milk is unknown.

Ivabradine

Ivabradine is approved by the FDA for reducing the risk of hospitalization for worsening heart failure in patients with stable, symptomatic heart failure and a reduced EF in sinus rhythm with a resting heart rate ≥70 beats/min and taking maximally tolerated doses of beta blockers. Ivabradine has been used to treat inappropriate sinus tachycardia.

ELECTROPHYSIOLOGIC ACTIONS

Ivabradine blocks the pacemaker or "funny" current (I_f), the current responsible for generating spontaneous depolarization in the sinus node. The funny current is a mixed Na+-K+ inward current activated by hyperpolarization. Ivabradine blocks the intracellular portion of the transmembrane ion pore and inhibits cation movement with a high degree of selectivity leading to a reduction in the slope of diastolic depolarization. Ivabradine causes a dose-dependent reduction in heart rate. It has been used to treat inappropriate sinus tachycardia, especially when beta blockers and calcium channel blockers have failed or are poorly tolerated. Little long-term data exists on its efficacy.[21]

HEMODYNAMIC EFFECTS
There are no hemodynamic effects or alterations of cardiac contractility caused by ivabradine.

PHARMACOKINETICS
The drug undergoes extensive first-pass hepatic metabolism and is metabolized by CYP3A4. The dose needs to be adjusted for severe hepatic or renal impairment. The pharmacokinetics properties appear to be linear with respect to dosing.

DOSAGE AND ADMINISTRATION. Ivabradine is typically started at a dose of 5 mg twice per day (2.5 mg bid if the resting heart rate is <60 beats/min) and may be increased to 7.5 mg twice daily to increase its effects. The dosage may be lowered if excessive bradycardia is encountered. The dose is typically titrated after 2 weeks.

SIDE EFFECTS. The drug may cause excessive sinus slowing or AV nodal block, and caution should be exercised when given to patients with sinus bradycardia or first-degree AV block. The most common non-cardiac side effect is visual disturbances, specifically transient flashes of brightness in the visual field. When ivabradine is used in combination with other QT prolonging drugs it may increase the risk of TdP. There may be an increased incidence of AF with this agent. Ivabradine is contraindicated in pregnant mothers due to possible fetal toxicity.

Antiarrhythmic Effects of Nonantiarrhythmic Drugs
Several medications commonly used for other indications also have some degree of antiarrhythmic effect. In some cases, physicians can use these drugs for their standard indications and achieve additional, although often small, amounts of benefit in treating the patient's rhythm disturbance. These drugs include angiotensin-converting enzyme (ACE) inhibitors and angiotensin receptor–blocking agents; aldosterone antagonists such as eplerenone, statins, and omega-3 fatty acids (prevention of sudden death); and these same classes of drugs with the addition of non-dihydropyridine calcium channel blockers and ranolazine (less AF and perhaps VF). The mechanisms whereby these drugs exert their attenuating effect on arrhythmias is not clear in most cases, and they should not be relied on as the sole form of antiarrhythmic therapy. In patients who have arrhythmias, as well as another disorder that requires drug therapy (hypertension, heart failure), one of these medications may be preferable to agents that treat the primary disorder but do not possess antiarrhythmic effects. There are a number of drugs used for other indications that have been considered for repurposed use in the treatment of arrhythmias. Prominent are drugs used to treat neurological disorders such gabapentins, flunarizine, and riluzole which have ion channel blocking effects and vanoxerine a dopamine reuptake inhibitor. It is imperative to remember that all drugs that have effects on electrical properties of the heart can also produce proarrhythmic effects.

New Antiarrhythmic Agents

VERNAKALANT
Vernakalant is a mixed potassium and sodium channel blocker used intravenously for conversion of AF to sinus rhythm. The drug, currently available in Europe, is a use-dependent inhibitor of I_{Na} and blocks the atrial-specific potassium current I_{Kur} as well as $I_{K.ACh}$ and I_{to}. Vernakalant prolongs atrial APD and refractoriness. The safety for IV conversion of AF (initial dose of 3 mg/kg over 10 minutes followed by 2 mg/kg over 15 minutes for persistent arrhythmia) have been demonstrated in the Atrial Arrhythmia Conversion Trials 1 and 3 (ACT1, ACT3). The drug was well tolerated in these studies, with minimal side effects and no TdP episodes. Transient hypotension and bradycardia were observed in 5% to 10% of patients.

ELECTROTHERAPY FOR CARDIAC ARRHYTHMIAS

Direct-Current Electrical Cardioversion
Cardioversion is a general term used to indicate the termination of an arrhythmia, usually a tachyarrhythmia, by various means, including electrical, pharmacologic, or manual/surgical. *Electrical cardioversion* refers to the delivery of an electrical shock to the heart to terminate a tachycardia, flutter, or fibrillation and includes the technique of both synchronous cardioversion (see below) and defibrillation. It offers obvious advantages over drug therapy because under conditions optimal for close supervision and monitoring, a precisely regulated "dose" of electricity can restore sinus rhythm immediately and safely. The distinction between supraventricular and ventricular tachyarrhythmias, crucial to the proper medical management of arrhythmias, becomes less significant, and the time-consuming titration of drugs with potential side effects is obviated.

MECHANISMS
Electrical cardioversion is most effective in terminating tachycardias related to reentry, such as atrial flutter and many cases of AF, AV node reentry, reciprocating tachycardias associated with WPW syndrome, most forms of VT, ventricular flutter, and VF. The electrical shock, by depolarizing all excitable myocardium and possibly by prolonging refractoriness, interrupts reentrant circuits and establishes electrical homogeneity, which terminates reentry. The mechanism by which a shock successfully terminates VF has not been completely explained. If the precipitating factors are no longer present, interruption of the tachyarrhythmia for only the brief time produced by the shock may prevent its return for long periods, even though the anatomic and electrophysiologic substrates required for the tachycardia are still present.

Tachycardias thought to be caused by disorders of impulse formation (automaticity) include parasystole, some forms of AT, junctional tachycardia (with or without digitalis toxicity), accelerated idioventricular rhythm, and relatively uncommon forms of VT (see Chapters 62 and 67). An attempt to cardiovert these tachycardias electrically is not indicated in most cases because they typically recur within seconds after the shock, and release of endogenous catecholamines consequent to the shock can perpetuate the arrhythmia. It has not been established whether cardioversion can terminate tachycardias caused by enhanced automaticity or triggered activity.

Technique
Synchronous cardioversion refers to a specific technique of delivering an electrical shock, usually of lower energy and timed to the QRS complex ("R wave"), to avoid the vulnerable period of the T wave. Before elective synchronous cardioversion, careful physical examination should be performed, including palpation of limb pulses and inspection of the chest wall and airway. A 12-lead ECG is usually obtained before and after cardioversion, as well as a rhythm strip during the shock delivery. The patient, who should be informed completely about what to expect, is in a fasting state and respiratory function and electrolyte values should be normal, with no evidence of drug toxicity. Withholding of digitalis for several days before elective cardioversion in patients without clinical evidence of digitalis toxicity is not necessary, although patients in whom digitalis toxicity is suspected should not be electrically cardioverted until this situation has been corrected. Administration of maintenance AADs 1 to 2 days before planned electrical cardioversion of patients with AF can revert some patients to sinus rhythm, help prevent recurrence of AF once sinus rhythm is restored, and assist in determining the patient's tolerance of the drug for long-term use.[14] There is also evidence that statin drugs, as well as ACE inhibitors and angiotensin receptor blockers, may help prevent recurrence of AF, especially in patients with ventricular dysfunction.[22]

Self-adhesive patches applied in the standard apicoanterior or anteroposterior paddle positions have transthoracic impedances similar to those of paddles and are useful in elective synchronous cardioversions or other situations in which time is available for their application. Patches 12 to 13 cm in diameter can be used to deliver maximum current to the heart, but the benefits of these patches versus patches 8 to 9 cm in diameter have not been clearly established. Larger

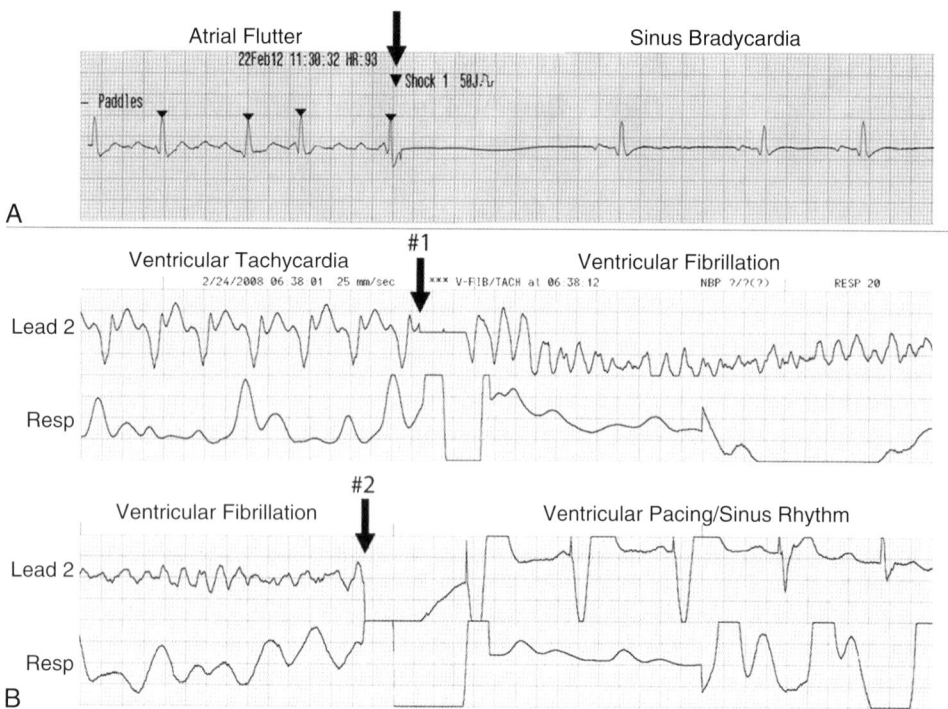

FIGURE 64.2 Cardioversions. **A,** Synchronized shock (note the synchronization mark in the apex of the QRS complex, *arrowhead*) during atrial flutter is followed by sinus bradycardia. **B** *(top),* Shock (*#1*) is delivered during ventricular tachycardia but asynchronously (on the T wave); this results in ventricular fibrillation, which is then treated with a second, asynchronous shock (*#2*) that results in sinus rhythm with tracked ventricular pacing. *Resp,* Respirations.

During elective cardioversion, a short-acting barbiturate such as methohexital, a sedative such as propofol, or an amnesic such as diazepam or midazolam can be used. A physician skilled in airway management should be in attendance; an IV route should be established; and pulse oximetry, the ECG, and blood pressure should be monitored. All equipment necessary for emergency resuscitation should be immediately accessible. Before cardioversion, 100% oxygen may be administered for 5 to 15 minutes by nasal cannula or facemask and is continued throughout the procedure. Manual ventilation of the patient may be necessary to avoid hypoxia during periods of deepest sedation. Adequate sedation of the patient undergoing even urgent cardioversion is essential.

In up to 5% of patients with AF, sinus rhythm cannot be restored by external countershock despite all the preceding measures, including ibutilide pretreatment and biphasic shocks. It is important to distinguish between inability to *attain* sinus rhythm, indicating failure of the shock to convert the arrhythmia, and inability to *maintain* sinus rhythm after transient termination of fibrillation; the latter condition (early re-initiation of AF) does not respond to higher-energy shocks because fibrillation has already been terminated but quickly recurs. Pretreatment with an AAD may help maintain sinus rhythm after subsequent shocks. Patients in whom AF simply cannot be terminated with an external shock tend to be very obese or have severe obstructive lung disease. In such patients, internal cardioversion can be performed with the use of specially configured catheters that have multiple large electrodes covering several centimeters of the distal portion of the catheter for distributing the shock energy. Internal shocks of 2 to 15 J can terminate AF in more than 90% of patients whose arrhythmia was refractory to transthoracic shock. Esophageal cardioversion has also been reported. Rarely, simultaneous shocks from two defibrillators have been reported to terminate refractory AF or VF.

Indications

As a general rule, any non-sinus tachycardia that produces hypotension, congestive heart failure, mental status changes, or angina and does not respond promptly to medical management should be terminated electrically. Very rapid ventricular rates in patients with AF and WPW syndrome are often best treated by electrical cardioversion. In almost all cases, the patient's hemodynamic status improves after cardioversion. Rarely, a patient may experience hypotension, reduced cardiac output, or congestive heart failure after the shock. This problem may be related to complications of the cardioversion, such as embolic events, myocardial depression resulting from the anesthetic agent or the shock itself, hypoxia, lack of restoration of left atrial contraction despite return of electrical atrial systole, or post-shock arrhythmias. DC countershock of digitalis-induced tachyarrhythmias is contraindicated (see earlier).

Favorable candidates for electrical cardioversion of AF include patients who (1) have symptomatic AF of less than 12 months' duration, (2) continue to have AF after the precipitating cause has been removed (e.g., after treatment of thyrotoxicosis), (3) have a rapid ventricular rate that is difficult to slow, or (4) have symptoms of decreased cardiac output (e.g., fatigue, lightheadedness, dyspnea) attributable to lack of atrial contraction's contribution to ventricular filling. In patients who have indications for chronic anticoagulants to prevent stroke, the hope of avoiding these medications by restoring sinus rhythm is not a reason to attempt cardioversion, because these patients are still at

patches may distribute the intracardiac current over a wider area and reduce the possibility of shock-induced myocardial injury.

A synchronized shock (i.e., one delivered during the QRS complex; Fig. 64.2) is used for all cardioversions except for very rapid ventricular tachyarrhythmias, such as ventricular flutter or VF. For defibrillation of the latter, energies greater than those for synchronous cardioversion are required, and synchronization is not necessary because there is no vulnerable period of the T wave to avoid. Although generally minimal, shock-related myocardial damage increases directly with increases in applied energy, and thus the minimum effective shock should be used. Therefore, shocks are "titrated" when the clinical situation permits. Except for AF, shocks in the range of 25 to 50 joules (J) successfully terminate most SVTs and should be tried initially. If the shock is unsuccessful, a second shock of higher energy can be delivered. The starting level to terminate AF with older monophasic machines should be no less than 100 J, but with newer biphasic systems, a shock as low as 25 J may succeed. Delivered energy can be increased in stepwise fashion; up to 360 J can be used safely. It is critical to remember to resynchronize the defibrillator to the QRS complex after an unsuccessful shock before delivery of another shock to avoid initiation of VF (machines typically revert to the asynchronous mode after each shock). Anteroposterior patches may have a higher efficacy rate by placing more of the atrial mass in the shock vector than is the case with apicoanterior patches. If a shock of 360 J fails to convert the rhythm, 1 or 2 additional shocks at the same energy may still succeed by decreasing chest wall impedance; reversing patch polarity can occasionally help as well. Administration of ibutilide has been shown to facilitate electrical cardioversion of AF to sinus rhythm. Intracardiac or transesophageal defibrillation can be tried if all attempts at external cardioversion fail. For patients with stable VT, starting levels in the range of 25 to 50 J can be used. If there is some urgency to terminate the tachyarrhythmia, the clinician can begin with higher energies. To terminate VF, a biphasic 100 to 200 J shock (200 to 360 J with monophasic machines) is generally used, although much lower energies (<50 J) terminate VF when the shock is delivered soon after onset of the arrhythmia, for example, using previously placed adhesive patches in the electrophysiology laboratory.

increased risk for thromboembolic events. Several large trials have shown that maintenance of sinus rhythm confers no survival advantage over rate control and anticoagulation; thus, not all patients with newly discovered AF warrant an attempt at restoration of sinus rhythm. Treatment must be determined individually (see Chapter 66). In a recently published study, early cardioversion was not superior at restoring sinus rhythm at 4 weeks compared to a wait-and-see approach with delayed cardioversion.[23]

Unfavorable candidates include patients with (1) digitalis toxicity, (2) no symptoms and a well-controlled ventricular rate without therapy, (3) sinus node dysfunction and various unstable supraventricular tachyarrhythmias or bradyarrhythmias—often bradycardia-tachycardia syndrome—in whom AF finally develops and is maintained, which in essence represents a cure for sick sinus syndrome, (4) little or no symptomatic improvement with normal sinus rhythm, (5) prompt reversion to AF after cardioversion despite drug therapy, (6) a large (>5 cm) left atrium and longstanding AF, (7) episodes of AF that revert spontaneously to sinus rhythm, (8) no mechanical atrial systole after the return of electrical atrial systole, (9) AF and advanced heart block, (10) cardiac surgery planned in the near future, and (11) AAD intolerance. AF is more likely to recur after cardioversion in patients who have significant chronic obstructive lung disease, congestive heart failure, mitral valve disease (particularly mitral regurgitation), AF present longer than 1 year, and an enlarged left atrium (echocardiographic diameter >5.5 cm).

In patients with atrial flutter, slowing the ventricular rate by administration of beta or calcium channel blockers or terminating the flutter with an antiarrhythmic agent may be difficult, and electrical cardioversion is often the initial treatment of choice. For patients with other types of SVT, electrical cardioversion may be used when (1) vagal maneuvers or simple medical management (e.g., IV adenosine and verapamil) has failed to terminate the tachycardia and (2) the clinical setting dictates prompt restoration of sinus rhythm because of hemodynamic decompensation or other clinical consequences of the tachycardia. Similarly, in patients with VT, the hemodynamic and electrophysiologic consequences of the arrhythmias determine the need for and urgency of DC cardioversion. Electrical countershock is the initial treatment of choice for ventricular flutter or VF. Speed is essential (see Chapter 70).

If reversion of the arrhythmia to sinus rhythm does not occur after the first shock, a higher energy level should be tried. When transient ventricular arrhythmias result after an unsuccessful shock, a bolus of lidocaine can be given before delivery of a shock at the next energy level. If sinus rhythm returns only transiently and is promptly supplanted by the tachycardia, a repeated shock can be tried, depending on the tachyarrhythmia being treated and its consequences. Administration of an AAD intravenously may be useful before delivery of the next cardioversion shock (e.g., ibutilide for resistant AF). After cardioversion, the patient should be monitored, at least until full consciousness has been restored and preferably for 1 hour or more thereafter, depending on the duration of recovery from the particular form of sedation or anesthesia used. If ibutilide has been given, the ECG should be monitored for up to 4 hours because TdP can develop in the first few hours after administration.

Results
Electrical cardioversion restores sinus rhythm in up to 95% of patients, depending on the type of tachyarrhythmia. However, sinus rhythm remains after 12 months in less than one third to one half of patients with longstanding persistent AF. Thus, maintenance of sinus rhythm, once established, is the difficult problem, not immediate termination of the tachyarrhythmia. The likelihood of maintaining sinus rhythm depends on the particular arrhythmia, the presence of underlying heart disease, and the response to AAD therapy. Atrial size often decreases after termination of AF and restoration of sinus rhythm, and functional capacity improves.

Complications
Arrhythmias induced by electrical cardioversion are generally caused by inadequate synchronization, with the shock occurring during the ST segment or T wave (see Fig. 64.2). On occasion, even a properly synchronized shock can produce VF. Post-shock arrhythmias are usually transient and do not require therapy. Asystole is rare and typically lasts no more than a few seconds before a sinus or junctional rhythm ensues; most defibrillators are also capable of transcutaneous pacing if needed. Embolic episodes are reported to occur in 1% to 3% of patients converted from AF to sinus rhythm. Prior therapeutic anticoagulation with warfarin (international normalized ratio [INR], 2.0 to 3.0) or newer agents such as dabigatran, rivaroxaban, apixaban or edoxaban, should be used consistently for at least 3 weeks by patients who have no contraindication to such therapy and have had AF for longer than 2 days or of indeterminate duration. It is important to note that 3 weeks of therapeutic anticoagulation is not the same as simply administering warfarin for 3 weeks, because the warfarin dose may not achieve a therapeutic INR. However, the newer agents confer almost immediate anticoagulation, such that 3 weeks of treatment equals 3 weeks of anticoagulation. Anticoagulation for at least 4 weeks afterward is recommended because restoration of atrial mechanical function lags behind that of electrical systolic function, and thrombi can still form due to delayed mechanical recovery, although the atria are electrocardiographically in sinus rhythm. Exclusion of left atrial thrombi by transesophageal echocardiography immediately before cardioversion may not always preclude embolism days or weeks after cardioversion of AF. Atrial thrombi can be present in patients with non–fibrillation-related atrial tachyarrhythmias, such as atrial flutter and AT in patients with congenital heart disease. The same precardioversion and postcardioversion anticoagulation recommendations apply to these patients as to those with AF. Although DC shock has been demonstrated in animals to cause myocardial injury, studies in humans have indicated that elevations in myocardial enzymes after cardioversion are not common. ST-segment elevation, sometimes dramatic, can occur immediately after elective DC cardioversion and can last for up to 1 to 2 minutes, although cardiac enzymes and myocardial scintigraphy may be unremarkable. ST elevation lasting longer than 2 minutes usually indicates myocardial injury unrelated to the shock. A decrease in serum K^+ and Mg^{2+} levels can occur after cardioversion of VT.

Cardioversion of VT can also be achieved by a chest thump. Its mechanism of termination is probably related to a mechanically induced PVC that interrupts a tachycardia circuit and may be related to commotio cordis. The thump cannot be timed accurately and is probably effective only when delivered during a nonrefractory part of the cardiac cycle. The thump can alter a VT and possibly induce ventricular flutter or VF if it occurs during the vulnerable period of the T wave. Because there may be a slightly greater likelihood of converting a stable VT to VF than of terminating VT to sinus rhythm, chest thump cardioversion should not be attempted unless a defibrillator is unavailable.

Implantable Electrical Devices for Treatment of Cardiac Arrhythmias
Implantable devices that monitor the cardiac rhythm and can deliver competing pacing stimuli and low- and high-energy shocks have been used effectively in selected patients (see Chapter 69).

Ablation Therapy for Cardiac Arrhythmias
The purpose of catheter ablation is to destroy myocardial tissue by delivery of energy, generally electrical energy or cryoenergy, through electrodes on a catheter placed next to an area of the myocardium integrally related to onset or maintenance of the arrhythmia. For tachycardias with an apparent focal origin (e.g., automatic, triggered activity, microreentry), the focus itself (<5 mm in diameter) is targeted. In macroreentrant AT and VT, inexcitable scar tissue typically separates strands of surviving myocardium, and wavefronts propagate around these scars. The target for ablation is a narrow portion of myocardium between inexcitable areas (e.g., scar, valve annulus; Fig. 64.3). The first catheter ablation procedures were performed with DC shocks, but this energy source has been supplanted by radiofrequency (RF) energy, which is delivered from an external generator and destroys tissue by controlled heat production.

Lasers and microwave energy sources have been used, but not frequently; cryothermal catheter ablation has been approved for use in humans. When a target tissue has been identified by EPS, the tip of the ablation catheter is maneuvered into apposition with this tissue. After stable catheter position and recordings have been ensured, RF energy is delivered between the catheter tip and an indifferent electrode, usually an electrocautery-type grounding pad on the skin of the patient's thigh. Because energies in the RF portion of the electromagnetic spectrum are poorly conducted by cardiac tissue, RF energy instead causes resistive heating in the cells close to the tip of the catheter (i.e., these cells transduce the electrical energy into thermal energy). When tissue temperature exceeds 50°C, irreversible cellular damage and tissue death occur. An expanding front of conducted heat emanates from the region of resistive heating while RF delivery continues over the next 30 seconds and results in the production of a homogeneous, roughly hemispheric lesion of coagulative necrosis 3 to 5 mm in diameter (Fig. 64.4A). RF-induced heating of tissue that has inherent automaticity (e.g., His bundle, foci of automatic tachycardias) results in initial acceleration of a rhythm, whereas RF delivery during a reentrant arrhythmia typically causes slowing and termination of the arrhythmia. In most cases, RF delivery is painless, although ablation of atrial or right ventricular tissue can be uncomfortable for some patients.

Cooled-Tip Radiofrequency Ablation

In some situations, the catheter can be delivered to the correct location, but conventional RF energy delivery cannot eliminate the tachycardia. In some of these cases the amount of damage—depth or breadth—caused by standard RF energy is inadequate. With the use of standard RF energy, power delivery is usually regulated to maintain a preset catheter tip temperature (typically, 55°C to 70°C). Tip temperatures higher than 90°C are associated with coagulation of blood elements on the electrode, which precludes further energy delivery and could also cause this material to become detached and embolize. Cooling of the catheter tip by internal circulation of liquid or continuous fluid infusion through small holes in the tip electrode can prevent excessive heating of the tip and allow delivery of higher power, thus producing a larger lesion (see Fig. 64.4B) and potentially enhancing efficacy.[24] Cooled-tip ablation has been used to good advantage in cases in which standard (4-mm tip) catheter ablation has failed, as well as for primary therapy for atrial flutter and fibrillation and VT associated with structural heart disease, in which additional damage to already-diseased areas is not harmful and may be required to achieve the desired result.

Catheter-delivered cryoablation causes tissue damage by freezing cellular structures. Nitrous oxide is delivered to the tip of the catheter, where it is allowed to internally boil and cool the tip electrode, after which the gas is circulated back to the delivery console. Catheter tip temperature can be regulated, with cooling to as low as −80°C. Cooling to 0°C causes reversible loss of function and can be used as a diagnostic test (i.e., termination of a tachycardia when the catheter is in contact with a group of cells critical to its perpetuation, or determining its effect on normal conduction when close to the AV node). The catheter tip can then be cooled more deeply to produce permanent damage and thus cure of the arrhythmia. Cryoablation has been used for pulmonary vein isolation to treat paroxysmal AF by situating a collapsed balloon at the end of a catheter near a pulmonary vein ostium and inflating the balloon with nitrous oxide at −80°C. During cryoballoon occlusion of the vein for 3 to 4 minutes at a time, pulmonary vein isolation can usually be effected with one or two applications.[25] Real-time recordings can be done simultaneously to monitor conduction. Cryoablation appears to cause less endocardial damage than RF energy does and may thus engender less risk for thromboemboli after ablation, as well as less chance of esophageal injury with ablation of AF (although it is not eliminated). However, balloon cryotherapy to isolate right pulmonary veins for the treatment of AF has resulted in phrenic nerve injury, and care must be taken to establish the location of the phrenic nerve. Larger balloon sizes, with more proximal zones of cryoablation, and monitoring

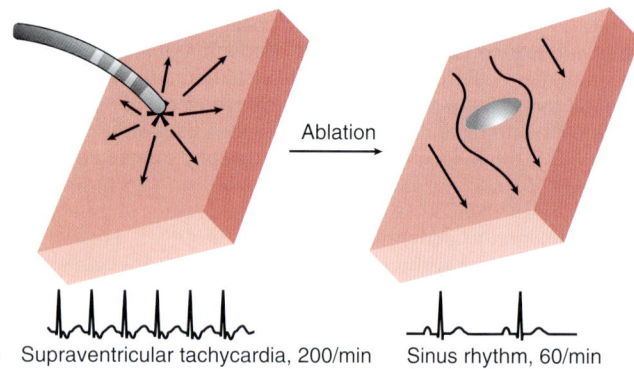
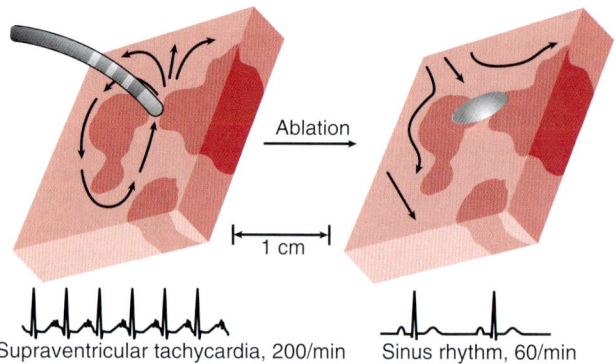

FIGURE 64.3 Strategies for catheter ablation. **A,** Focal tachycardia. *Left,* SVT is caused by an atrial focus, with activation emanating in all directions. *Right,* Ablation of the focus eliminates the arrhythmia with minimal disruption of normal activation. **B,** Macroreentrant SVT in setting of previous atrial damage resulting in scar formation. *Left,* During SVT, a wavefront circulates around a scarred area and through a narrow isthmus between this and another area of scar. *Right,* Ablation at this critical site prevents further reentry.

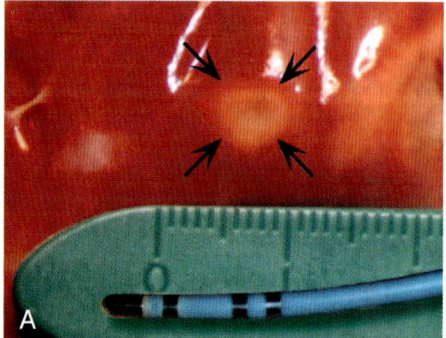
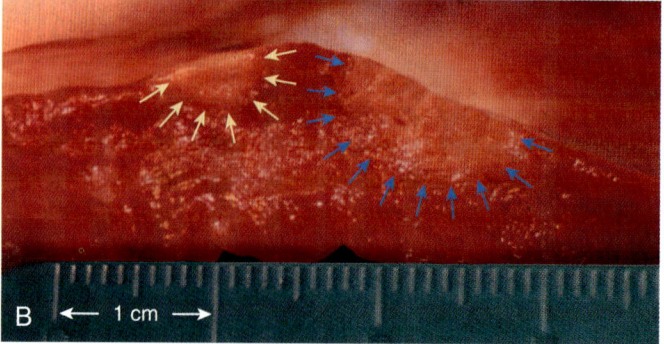

FIGURE 64.4 Radiofrequency lesion in human ventricular myocardium (explanted heart at transplantation). **A,** Energy was applied for 30 seconds at the location denoted by arrows, with the tip of the catheter shown. The lesion is 5 mm in diameter and has a well-demarcated border. A central depression in the lesion results from partial desiccation of tissue. **B,** Extent of radiofrequency lesions (cut surface of specimen in **A**). The lesion outlined by *yellow arrows* was made with a standard electrode (15 W for 30 sec); the lesion outlined by *blue arrows* was made with an irrigated catheter, cooling the tip to allow more power delivery (50 W for 30 sec). The lesion made by the irrigated catheter is more than twice the diameter and 12 times the volume of the standard catheter lesion.

diaphragmatic contraction during transvenous phrenic nerve pacing, have markedly decreased the risk of phrenic damage.

OTHER FORMS OF ABLATION

Laser energy has been used for pulmonary vein isolation and in VT; the wavelengths used cannot penetrate blood and thus the energy must be delivered through a water-filled balloon that is in direct contact with tissue, or blood must be flushed from the endocardial target tissue with saline. Laser energy can be very effective in these applications but the equipment is expensive and remains cumbersome. Pulsed field ablation, in which high energy current is delivered through a variety of electrode designs, can result in irreversible electroporation of target cardiac tissue. This promising technique appears to be capable of causing very focused myocardial damage, destroying heart muscle relatively selectively while almost entirely sparing vascular, esophageal and nerve tissue.[26]

Radiofrequency Catheter Ablation of Accessory Pathways

Location of Pathways

The safety, efficacy, and cost-effectiveness of RF catheter ablation of an accessory AV pathway have made ablation the treatment of choice in most adult and many pediatric patients who have AV reentrant tachycardia (AVRT) or atrial flutter or fibrillation associated with a rapid ventricular response over the accessory pathway (see Chapter 65). When RF energy is delivered to an immature heart, the lesion size can increase as the heart grows; however, this has not been shown to cause problems later in life.

An EPS is performed initially to determine that the accessory pathway is part of the tachycardia circuit or capable of rapid AV conduction during AF and to localize the accessory pathway (the optimal site for ablation). Pathways can exist in the right or left free wall or the septum of the heart (Fig. 64.5). Septal accessory pathways are further classified as superoparaseptal, midseptal, and posterior paraseptal. Pathways classified as posterior paraseptal are posterior to the central fibrous body within the so-called pyramidal space, which is bounded by the posterosuperior process of the left ventricle and the inferomedial aspects of both atria and is behind (posterior to) the true atrial septum. Superoparaseptal pathways are found near the His bundle, and an accessory pathway activation potential as well as a His bundle potential can be recorded simultaneously from a catheter placed at the His bundle region. Midseptal pathways are close to the AV node and can usually be ablated from a right-sided approach; rarely, a left atrial approach is needed. Right posterior paraseptal pathways insert along the tricuspid ring in the vicinity of the coronary sinus ostium, whereas left posterior paraseptal pathways are further into the coronary sinus and may be located at a subepicardial site around the proximal coronary sinus, within a middle cardiac vein or coronary sinus diverticulum, or subendocardially along the ventricular aspect of the mitral annulus.

Pathways at all locations and in all age groups can be ablated successfully. Multiple pathways are present in about 5% of patients. Occasional pathways with epicardial locations may be more easily approached from within the coronary sinus. Rarely, pathways can connect an atrial appendage with adjacent ventricular epicardium, 2 cm or more from the AV groove.

ABLATION SITE

The optimal ablation site can be found by direct recordings of the accessory pathway (Fig. 64.6), although deflections that mimic accessory pathway potentials can be recorded at other sites. The ventricular insertion site can be determined by finding the site of the earliest onset of the ventricular electrogram in relation to the onset of the delta wave. Other helpful guidelines include unfiltered unipolar recordings that register a QS wave and an accessory pathway signal during preexcitation. A major ventricular potential synchronous with onset of the delta wave can be a target site in left-sided preexcitation, whereas earlier ventricular excitation in relation to the delta wave can be found for right-sided preexcitation. The atrial insertion site of manifest or concealed pathways (i.e., delta wave present or absent, respectively) can be found by locating the site showing the earliest atrial activation during retrograde conduction over

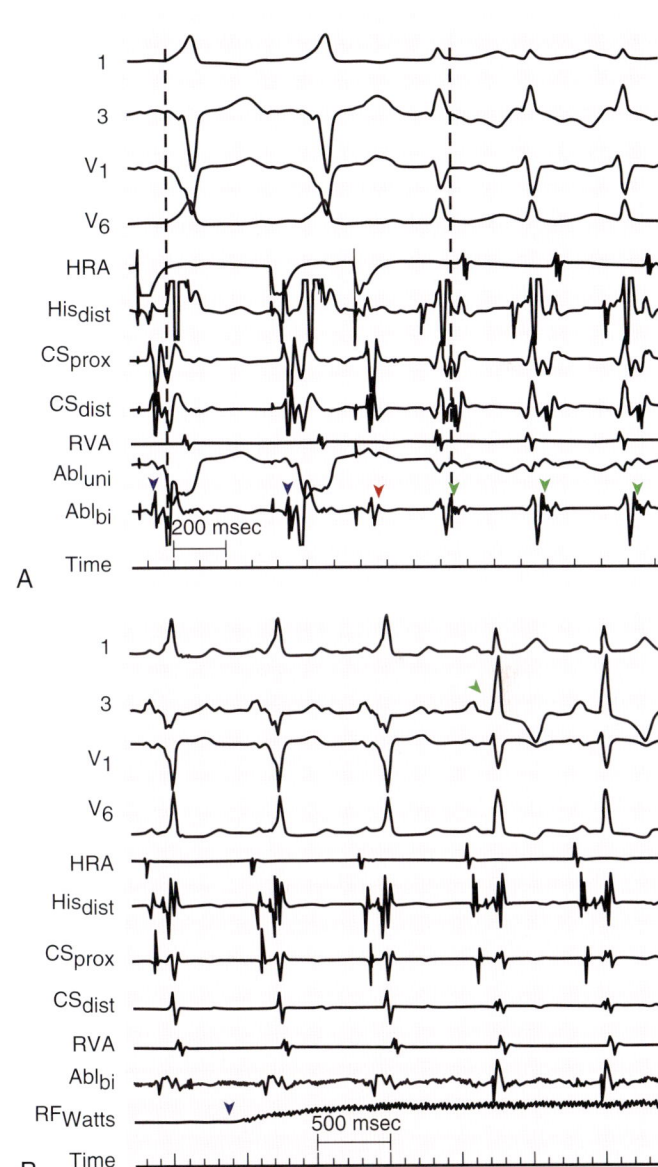

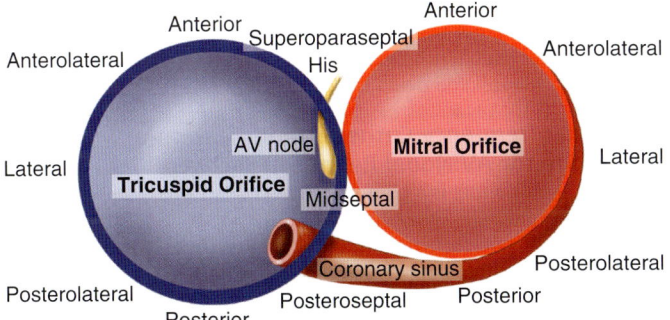

FIGURE 64.5 Locations of accessory pathways by anatomic region. The tricuspid and mitral valve annuli are depicted in a left anterior oblique view. Locations of the coronary sinus, atrioventricular node, and bundle of His are shown. Accessory pathways may connect the atrial to the ventricular myocardium in any of the regions shown.

FIGURE 64.6 Wolff-Parkinson-White syndrome. Surface ECG leads 1, 3, V_1, and V_6 are shown, with intracardiac recordings from high right atrium (HRA), distal His (His_{dist}) bundle region, proximal (CS_{prox}) and distal (CS_{dist}) coronary sinus, right ventricular apex (RVA), and unipolar (Abl_{uni}) and bipolar (Abl_{bi}) tip electrodes of the ablation catheter. RF power in watts (RF_{Watts}) is also shown. **A,** Two beats of atrial pacing are conducted over the accessory pathway (blue arrowheads in the Abl_{bi} recording from the site of the accessory pathway) and resulted in a delta wave on the ECG. A premature atrial stimulus (center) encounters accessory pathway refractoriness (red arrowhead) and instead is conducted over the AV node and bundle of His and resulted in a narrow QRS complex and started an episode of AVRT. After each narrow QRS complex is an atrial deflection, the earliest portion of which is recorded at the ablation site (green arrowheads). **B,** Ablation of this pathway by delivery of RF energy from the ablation catheter tip. The blue arrowhead denotes the onset of delivery of RF energy; two QRS complexes later, the delta wave is abruptly lost (green arrowhead in lead 3) because of elimination of conduction over the accessory pathway.

the pathway. Reproducible mechanical inhibition of accessory pathway conduction during catheter manipulation and subthreshold stimulation has also been used to determine the optimal site. Accidental catheter trauma should be avoided, however, because it can hide the target for prolonged periods. Right free wall and superoparaseptal pathways are particularly susceptible to catheter trauma.

Left-sided accessory pathways typically cross the mitral annulus obliquely. Consequently, the earliest site of retrograde atrial activation and the earliest site of anterograde ventricular activation are not directly across the AV groove from each other (i.e., ventricular insertion closer to coronary sinus ostium). Identification of the earliest site of atrial activation is usually performed during orthodromic AVRT or relatively rapid ventricular pacing so that retrograde conduction using the AV node does not confuse assessment of the location of the earliest atrial activation.

Successful ablation sites should exhibit anatomic/fluoroscopic stability and consistent electrical characteristics. During sinus rhythm, local ventricular activation at the successful ablation site precedes onset of the delta wave on the ECG by 10 to 35 milliseconds; during orthodromic AVRT, the interval between onset of ventricular activation in any lead and local atrial activation is usually 70 to 90 milliseconds (see Fig. 64.6). When temperature-measuring ablation catheters are used, a stable rise in catheter tip temperature is a helpful indicator of catheter stability and adequate contact between the electrode and tissue. In such a case, tip temperature generally exceeds 50°C. The retrograde transaortic and transseptal approaches have been used with equal success to ablate accessory pathways located along the mitral annulus. Routine performance of an EPS weeks after the ablation procedure is not generally indicated but may be considered in patients who have a recurrent delta wave or symptoms of tachycardia. Catheter-delivered cryoablation can be useful in patients with septal accessory pathways (located near AV node or His bundle). With use of this system, the catheter tip and adjacent tissue can be reversibly cooled to test a potential site. If accessory pathway conduction fails while normal AV conduction is preserved, deeper cooling can be performed at the site to complete the ablation. If, however, normal AV conduction is worsened, permanent damage is almost always averted by allowing the catheter tip to rewarm quickly.

Atriofascicular accessory pathways have connections consisting of a proximal, AV node–like portion on the atrial side of the annulus, which is responsible for conduction delay and decremental conduction properties, and a long distal segment crossing the annulus and extending along the endocardial surface of the right ventricular free wall, which has electrophysiologic properties similar to those of the right bundle branch. The distal end of the right atriofascicular accessory pathway can insert into the apical region of the right ventricular free wall, close to the distal right bundle branch, or can actually fuse with the latter. Right atriofascicular accessory pathways might represent a duplication of the AV conduction system and can be localized for ablation by recording potentials from the rapidly conducting distal component, which crosses the tricuspid annulus (analogous to the His bundle) and extends to the apical region of the right ventricular free wall. Ablation at such a site on the annulus is usually successful; these pathways are very sensitive to catheter trauma, and the operator must use great care to avoid such trauma (that may eliminate pathway conduction for minutes or hours).

Indications

Ablation of accessory pathways is indicated in patients who have symptomatic AVRT that is drug resistant or who are drug intolerant or do not desire long-term drug therapy. It is also indicated in patients who have AF or other atrial tachyarrhythmias and a rapid ventricular response, by means of an accessory pathway when the tachycardia is drug resistant, or in those who are drug intolerant or do not desire long-term drug therapy. Other potential candidates with an accessory pathway include the following: (1) patients with AVRT or AF with rapid ventricular rates identified during an EPS for another arrhythmia; (2) asymptomatic patients with ventricular preexcitation whose livelihood, profession, important activities, insurability, or mental well-being and the public safety would be affected by spontaneous tachyarrhythmias or by the presence of the electrocardiographic abnormality; (3) patients with AF and a controlled ventricular response by means of the accessory pathway; and (4) patients with asymptomatic preexcitation and a family history of sudden cardiac death. Controversy remains whether all patients with accessory pathways (even those without symptoms) need treatment; however, ablation has such a high success rate and low complication rate that in most centers, patients who need any form of therapy are referred for catheter ablation.

Results

Currently, in the hands of an experienced operator, the success rate for accessory pathway ablation is greater than 95% (slightly less for right free wall pathways, in which stable catheter-tissue contact is more problematic), with a 2% recurrence rate after an apparently successful procedure. There is a 1% to 2% complication rate, including bleeding, vascular damage, myocardial perforation with cardiac tamponade, valve damage, stroke, and MI. Heart block occurs in less than 3% of septal pathways. Procedure-related death is very rare.

Radiofrequency Catheter Modification of AV Node for AV Nodal Reentrant Tachycardias

AV node reentry is a common cause of SVT episodes (see Chapters 62 and 65). Although controversy still exists about the exact nature of the tachycardia circuit, abundant evidence has indicated that two pathways in the region of the AV node participate, one with relatively fast conduction but long refractoriness and the other with shorter refractoriness but slower conduction. Premature atrial complexes can encounter refractoriness in the fast pathway, conduct over the slow pathway, and reenter the fast pathway retrogradely, thereby initiating AV nodal reentrant SVT (Fig. 64.7). Although this is the most common manifestation of

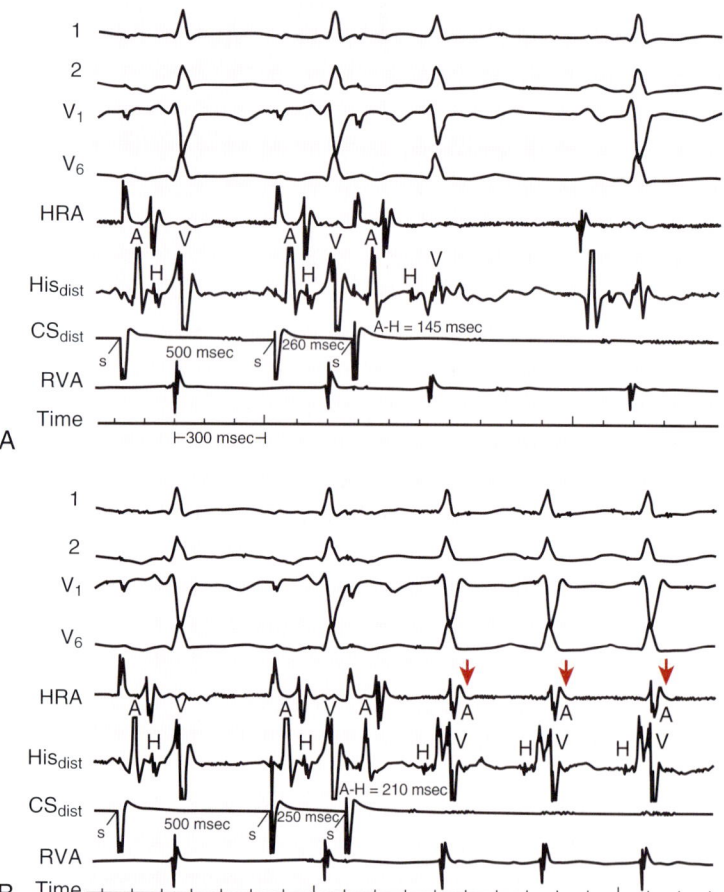

FIGURE 64.7 Atrioventricular node reentry. **A,** Two atrial paced complexes from the coronary sinus (CS) are followed by an atrial premature stimulus at a coupling interval of 260 milliseconds and resulted in an A-H interval of 145 milliseconds. **B,** The same atrial drive train is followed by an atrial extrastimulus 10 milliseconds earlier than before (250 milliseconds). This resulted in a marked increase in the A–H interval to 210 milliseconds, after which atrioventricular (AV) nodal reentrant tachycardia ensues because the extrastimulus encounters block in a "fast" AV node pathway, conducts down a "slow" pathway, and then conducts back up the fast pathway in a repeating fashion. *Red arrowheads* denote atrial electrograms coincident with QRS complexes, characteristic of the most common type of AV node reentry. Recording was done as in the previous figure.

AV node reentry, some patients have what appears to be propagation in the opposite direction in this circuit (anterograde fast, retrograde slow), as well as a "slow-slow" variant. Other, much less common types have been described. Two or more of these variants can exist in the same patient (Fig. 64.8).

FAST PATHWAY ABLATION

Ablation can be performed to eliminate conduction in the fast pathway or the slow pathway. Currently, fast pathway ablation is rarely performed because it is associated with a prolonged PR interval, a higher recurrence rate (10% to 15%), and a slightly higher risk for complete AV block (2% to 5%) than with slow pathway ablation. One uncommon situation in which fast pathway ablation may be preferred is for patients who have a greatly prolonged PR interval at rest and no evidence of anterograde fast pathway conduction. In such patients, ablation of the anterograde slow pathway may produce complete AV block, whereas retrograde fast pathway ablation can eliminate SVT without altering AV conduction.

SLOW PATHWAY ABLATION

The slow pathway can be located by mapping along the posteromedial tricuspid annulus close to the coronary sinus os. Electrographic recordings are obtained with an atrial-to-ventricular electrogram ratio of less than 0.5 and either a multicomponent atrial electrogram or a recording consistent with a possible slow pathway potential. In the anatomic approach, target sites are selected fluoroscopically. A single RF application eliminates slow pathway conduction in many cases, but in others, serial RF applications may be needed, starting at the most posterior site (near the coronary sinus os) and progressing along the tricuspid annulus more anteriorly. An accelerated junctional rhythm usually occurs when RF energy is applied at a site that will result in successful elimination of SVT (Fig. 64.9). The success rate is equivalent with the anatomic and electrographic mapping approaches, and most often, combinations of both are used and yield success rates of greater than 95%, with less than a 1% chance of complete heart block.[27] Catheter-delivered cryoablation has been used for the treatment of AVNRT with excellent results and is considered by some to be safer than RF (less chance of permanent AV block) but in most series has a somewhat higher rate of SVT recurrence after apparent successful ablation.

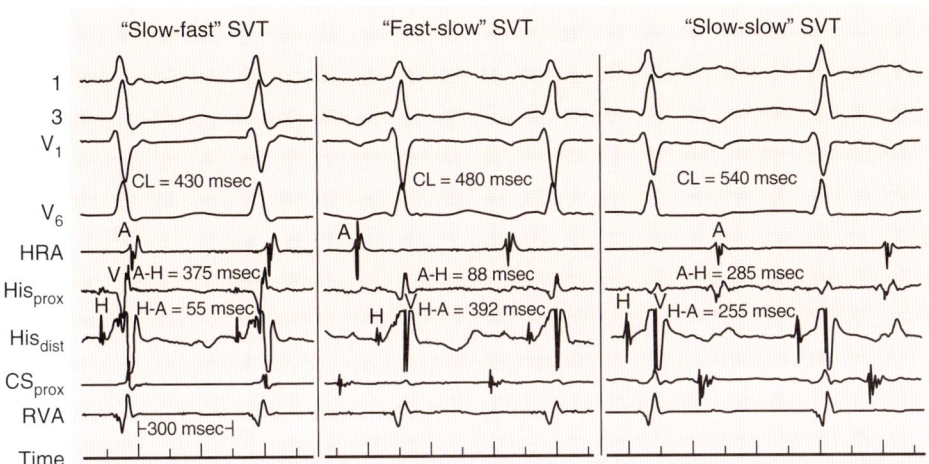

FIGURE 64.8 Three variants of atrioventricular (AV) node reentrant supraventricular tachycardia (SVT) in the same patient. **Left,** Most common type of AV node SVT (anterograde slow pathway, retrograde fast). Atrial activation is coincident with ventricular activation. **Center,** "Atypical" AV node reentry with anterograde fast pathway conduction and retrograde conduction over a slow pathway. **Right,** A rare variety is shown that consists of anterograde conduction over a slow pathway and retrograde conduction over a second slow pathway. Note the similar atrial activation sequences in the last two (coronary sinus before the right atrium), as distinct from that of slow-fast AV node reentry (coronary sinus and right atrial activation almost simultaneous). Note also the different P-QRS relationships, from simultaneous activation (left, short RP interval) to P in front of the QRS (middle, long RP interval) and P midway in the cardiac cycle (right). Recording was done as in previous figures. CL, Cycle length.

Patients in whom slow pathway conduction is completely eliminated almost never have recurrent SVT episodes. Approximately 40% of patients can have evidence of residual slow pathway function after successful elimination of sustained AVNRT, usually manifested as persistent dual AV node physiology and single AV node echoes during atrial extrastimulation. The surest endpoint for slow pathway ablation is elimination of sustained AVNRT, with and without an infusion of isoproterenol or epinephrine.

AVNRT recurs in approximately 5% of patients after slow pathway ablation; repeat ablation is almost always successful. In some patients the ERP of the fast pathway decreases after slow pathway ablation, possibly because of eliminating electrotonic interaction between the two pathways. Atypical forms of reentry can result after ablation, as can apparent parasympathetic denervation, and result in inappropriate sinus tachycardia. This usually resolves within 3 months after ablation.

At present, the slow pathway approach is the preferred method for ablation of typical AVNRT. Ablation of the slow pathway is also a safe and effective means for the treatment of atypical forms of AVNRT. In patients with AVNRT undergoing slow pathway ablation, junctional ectopy during application of the RF energy is a sensitive but nonspecific marker of successful ablation; it occurs in longer bursts at effective than at ineffective target sites. Ventriculoatrial conduction should be expected during the junctional ectopy, and poor ventriculoatrial conduction or actual block may herald subsequent anterograde AV block. Junctional ectopic rhythm is caused by heating of the AV node and does not occur with cryoablation.

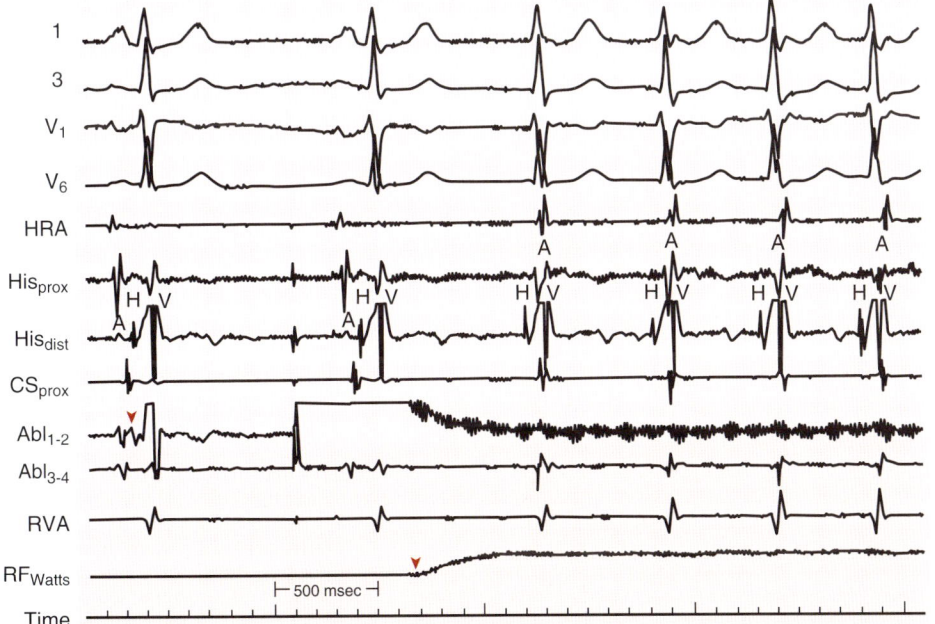

FIGURE 64.9 Atrioventricular node slow pathway modification for cure of atrioventricular (AV) node reentrant supraventricular tachycardia. The ablation recording (*arrowhead* in Abl$_{1-2}$) shows a slurred deflection between the atrial and ventricular electrogram components; this may represent the AV node slow pathway deflection (but it is not the bundle of His deflection, which is instead recorded from a separate catheter 15 mm away). Shortly after the onset of radiofrequency delivery (*arrowhead* in RF$_{Watts}$), an accelerated junctional rhythm begins and gradually speeds up further. Retrograde conduction is present during the junctional rhythm. Abl$_{3-4}$, Proximal electrode recording from ablation catheter.

Indications
RF catheter ablation for AVNRT can be considered in patients with recurrent, symptomatic, sustained AVNRT that is drug resistant or who are drug intolerant or do not desire long-term drug treatment. The procedure can also be considered for patients with sustained AVNRT identified during EPS or catheter ablation of another arrhythmia, or when EPS reveals dual–AV node pathway physiology and atrial echoes but without AVNRT in patients with suspected AVNRT clinically.

Results
Most centers currently use slow pathway ablation, which results in a procedural success rate of 98%, a recurrence rate of less than 5%, and an incidence of heart block requiring permanent pacing of 1% or less. Late development of heart block (months to years later) is rare.

Junctional Tachycardia
Junctional tachycardia, often called ectopic junctional tachycardia (although if the location is junctional, by definition it is ectopic) is a rare form of SVT in which the ECG resembles that in AVNRT but is distinct in that (1) the mechanism is automatic, not reentrant, and (2) the atrium is clearly not involved in the tachycardia. This disorder is most often observed in young healthy individuals, in women more often than in men, and is usually catecholamine dependent. Ablation must be carried out close to the His bundle, and the risk for heart block requiring pacemaker insertion exceeds 5%.

Radiofrequency Catheter Ablation of Arrhythmias Related to the Sinus Node
Inappropriate sinus tachycardia is a syndrome characterized by high sinus rates with exercise and at rest. Patients complain of palpitations at all times of day that correlate with inappropriately high sinus rates. They may not respond well to beta-blocker therapy because of lack of desired effect or occurrence of side effects. Ivabradine, which blocks I_f (principal pacemaker current in sinus node) is indicated for treatment of heart failure but has been used with some success in patients with inappropriate sinus tachycardia.[28] When the sinus node area is to be ablated because of drug-refractory symptoms, it can be identified anatomically and electrophysiologically, and ablative lesions are usually placed between the superior vena cava and crista terminalis at sites of early atrial activation. Intracardiac echocardiography can help in defining the anatomy and in positioning the ablation catheter. Isoproterenol may be helpful in "forcing" the site of impulse formation to cells with the most rapid discharge rate. Care must be taken to apply RF energy at the most cephalad sites first; initial ablation performed farther down the crista terminalis does not alter the atrial rate at the time but can damage any subsidiary pacemaker regions that may be needed after the sinus node has eventually been ablated.

Indications
Patients with *persistent* inappropriate sinus tachycardia should be considered for ablation only after clear failure of medical therapy, because the results of ablation are often less than completely satisfactory. Whenever ablation is performed in the region of the sinus node, the patient should be apprised of the chance of needing a pacemaker after the procedure. Phrenic nerve damage and superior vena caval stenosis are also possibilities.

Results
Although a good technical result may be obtained at the time of the procedure for inappropriate sinus tachycardia, symptoms often persist because of recurrence of rapid sinus rates (at or near preablation rates) or for nonarrhythmic reasons. In some, after the atrial rate decreases, an inappropriately rapid junctional rhythm (80 to 90/min) is present; this may indicate an overall increased sensitivity of cells with pacemaker capacity to catecholamines in these patients. Multiple ablation sessions are needed in some patients, and approximately 20% eventually undergo pacemaker implantation; however, not all these patients have relief of symptoms, including palpitations, despite a normal heart rate.

Radiofrequency Catheter Ablation of Atrial Tachycardia
ATs are a heterogeneous group of disorders; causative factors include rapid discharge of a focus (focal tachycardia) and reentry. The former can occur in anyone, regardless of the presence of structural abnormalities of the atria, whereas reentrant ATs almost always occur in the setting of structurally damaged atria. Symptoms vary from none, with relatively infrequent or slow ATs in patients without heart disease, to syncope (rapid AT with compromised cardiac function) or heart failure (incessant AT over weeks or months). All forms of AT are amenable to catheter ablation (see Chapter 65).

FOCAL ATRIAL TACHYCARDIA
In focal ATs (automatic or triggered foci or microreentry), activation mapping is used to determine the source of the AT by recording the earliest onset of local activation. These tachycardias can behave capriciously and can be practically noninducible during EPS despite the patient complaining of multiple daily episodes before the EPS. Approximately 10% of patients can have multiple atrial foci. Sites tend to cluster near the pulmonary veins in the left atrium and the mouths of the atrial appendages and along the right atrial crista terminalis (Figs. 64.10A, 64.11, and 64.12). Activation times at these sites typically occur only 15 to 40 milliseconds before onset of the P wave on the ECG. Care must be taken to avoid inadvertent damage to the phrenic nerve (see Fig. 64.12); its location can be determined by pacing at high current at a candidate site of ablation while observing for diaphragmatic contraction. Ablation should not be performed at a site at which this is seen, if at all possible.

REENTRANT ATRIAL TACHYCARDIA
As noted, these ATs usually occur in the setting of structural heart disease, especially after previous surgery involving an atrial incision (repair of congenital heart disease such as an atrial septal defect, Mustard or Senning repair of transposed great vessels, or one of a variety of Fontan repairs for tricuspid atresia and other disorders), or previous atrial ablation (e.g., for AF). The region of slow conduction is typically related to an end of an atriotomy or previous ablation scar, the location of

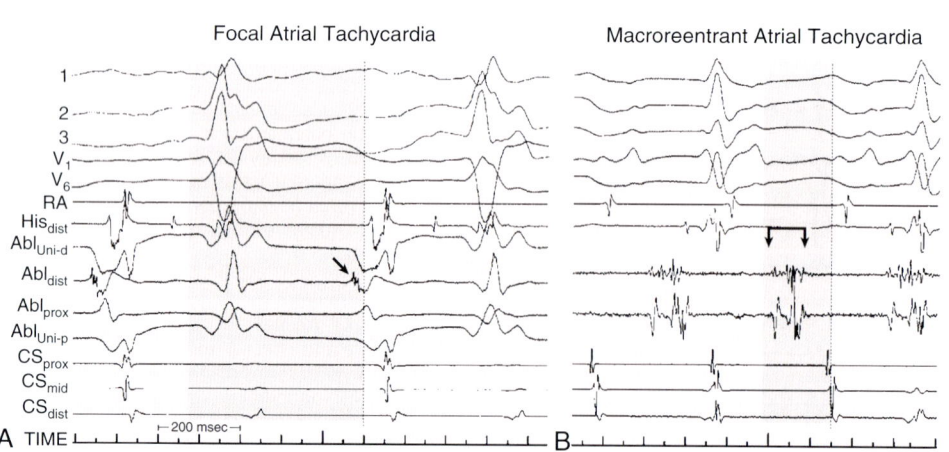

FIGURE 64.10 Atrial tachycardia. In both panels the interval from the end of one P wave to the beginning of the next (atrial diastole) is in *gray*. A *dashed line* denotes onset of the P wave during tachycardia. **A,** Focal atrial tachycardia (AT) arising in the right atrium. Two tachycardia complexes are shown; the earliest site found (Abl$_{dist}$, at which ablation eliminated the tachycardia) is shown as a multicomponent recording that starts only approximately 40 milliseconds before onset of the P wave. The unipolar recording (Abl$_{Uni-d}$) has a deep negative deflection (indicating propagation away from the electrode). The activation sequence of recordings is very different from that during sinus rhythm, in which the right atrial (RA) recording is at the onset of the P wave. **B,** Macroreentrant AT in a patient who had undergone repair of an atrial septal defect years earlier. The ablation catheter is in the posterior right atrium, where a fragmented signal (between *arrows*) is recorded that almost fills atrial diastole. Ablation at this site terminated the tachycardia.

which varies from patient to patient. Therefore, preprocedural review of operative and ablation procedure reports and careful electrophysiologic mapping are essential. Because reentry within a complete circuit is occurring, activation can be recorded throughout the entire cardiac cycle. The ablation strategy is to identify regions with mid-diastolic atrial activation during tachycardia (see Fig. 64.10B) that can be proved by pacing techniques to be integral to the tachycardia. Such sites are attractive ablation targets because they are composed of relatively few cells—thus electrical silence on the surface ECG in atrial diastole—and so are more easily eliminated by the small amount of damage effected by a typical application of RF energy. Focal ablation of these sites can then be performed, but often tachycardia can still be initiated (usually at a slower rate) or recurs after the procedure. Because these sites are typically located at a relatively narrow zone between the ends of previous scars, surgical incisions, or ablation lines and another nonconducting barrier (e.g., another scar, caval orifice, valve annulus), a line of ablative lesions is generally made from the end of the scar to the nearest electrical barrier; thus reentry can be prevented. This technique is analogous to that used in curing atrial flutter (see later). Because these patients frequently have extensive atrial disease with islands of scar that could serve as barriers for additional ATs, specialized mapping techniques may be needed to locate these regions and preemptively connect them with ablative lesions to prevent future AT episodes.

Indications
Catheter ablation for ATs should be considered in patients who have recurrent episodes of symptomatic sustained ATs that are drug resistant, or who are drug intolerant or do not desire long-term drug treatment.

Results
Success rates for ablation of focal AT range from 80% to 95%, largely depending on the ability to induce episodes at EPS. When episodes can be initiated with pacing, isoproterenol, or other means, the AT can usually be ablated. Reentrant ATs, although more readily induced by an EPS, are often more difficult to eliminate completely; initial success rates are high (90%), but recurrences are seen in up to 20% of patients and necessitate drug therapy or another ablation procedure. Complications, which occur in 1% to 2% of patients, include phrenic nerve damage, cardiac tamponade, and heart block (with rare perinodal ATs).

Radiofrequency Catheter Ablation of Atrial Flutter
Atrial flutter can be defined electrocardiographically (most typically, negative sawtooth waves in leads II, III, and aVF at a rate of approximately 300 beats/min) or electrophysiologically (rapid, organized macroreentrant AT, the circuit for which is anatomically determined). Understanding of the reentrant pathway in all forms of atrial flutter is essential for development of an ablation strategy (see Chapter 65).

Reentry in the right atrium, with the left atrium passively activated, constitutes the mechanism of the typical electrocardiographic variety of atrial flutter, with caudocranial activation along the right atrial septum and craniocaudal activation of the right atrial free wall (Fig. 64.13A). Ablating tissue in a line between any two anatomic barriers that transects a portion of the circuit necessary for perpetuation of reentry can be curative. Typically, this is across the isthmus of atrial tissue between the inferior vena caval orifice and the tricuspid annulus (the cavotricuspid isthmus), a relatively narrow point in the circuit. Locations for RF delivery can be guided anatomically or electrophysiologically. Less frequently, the direction of wavefront propagation in this large right atrial circuit is reversed ("clockwise" flutter proceeding cephalad up the right atrial free wall and caudad down the septum, with upright flutter waves in the inferior leads; Fig. 64.13A, left panel). These two arrhythmias constitute cavotricuspid isthmus–dependent flutter, that can be ablated by cavotricuspid isthmus interruption, and are distinct from other rapid atrial arrhythmias that may have a similar appearance on the ECG but use different (and often multiple) circuits in other parts of the right or left atrium. Ablation can be more difficult in these cases, which often occur in the setting of advanced lung disease or previous cardiac surgery or ablation. A common theme in these complex reentrant arrhythmias is the presence of an anatomically determined zone of

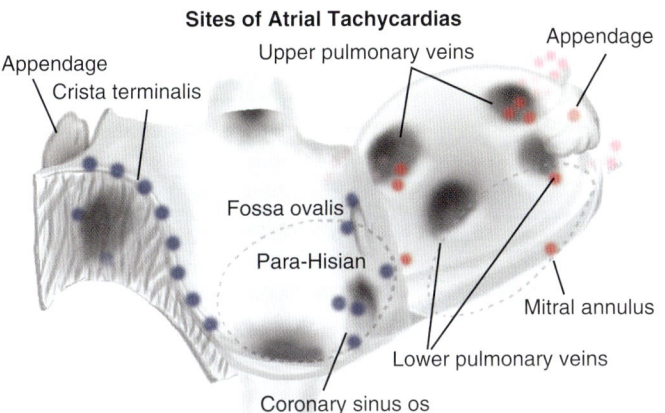

FIGURE 64.11 Locations of origins of focal atrial tachycardias. The atria are viewed from the front with the right atrial free wall retracted to show the interior. Structures are labeled as shown; right atrial foci appear in shades of *blue*, left atrial foci in shades of *red*.

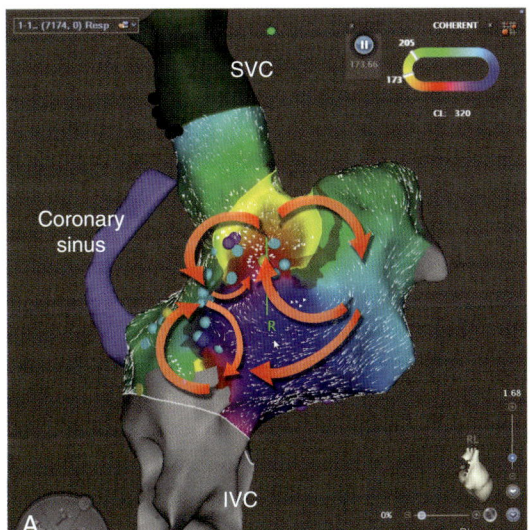 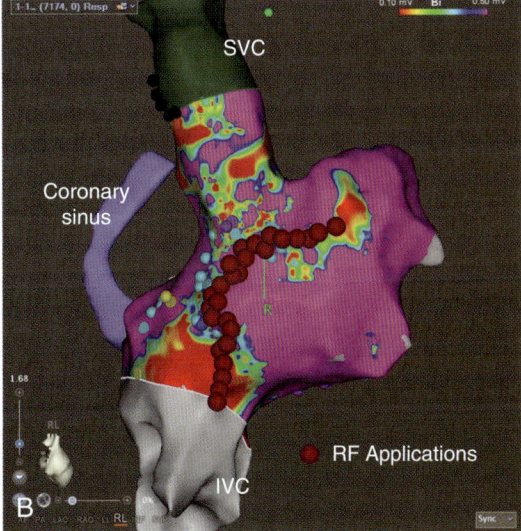

FIGURE 64.12 Reentrant atrial tachycardia. **A,** Electroanatomic activation map of the right atrium is shown in a patient with a previous right atrial incision for closure of an atrial septal defect. *Orange arrows* depict a complex double loop of reentry around presumed scars with a common diastolic pathway between scars. *Small white arrows* depict the vectoral direction of activation during tachycardia. The *color bar* shows progression of activation times during AT (from *red* through *green*, *blue*, and *purple*). The tachycardia cycle length (320 msec) is entirely represented in the range of colors. **B,** *Red dots* denote ablation sites connecting scars (transecting diastolic pathway) and connecting one scar to the *IVC* to preclude reentry around all barriers. *SVC,* superior vena cava; *IVC,* inferior vena cava.

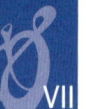

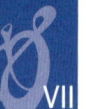

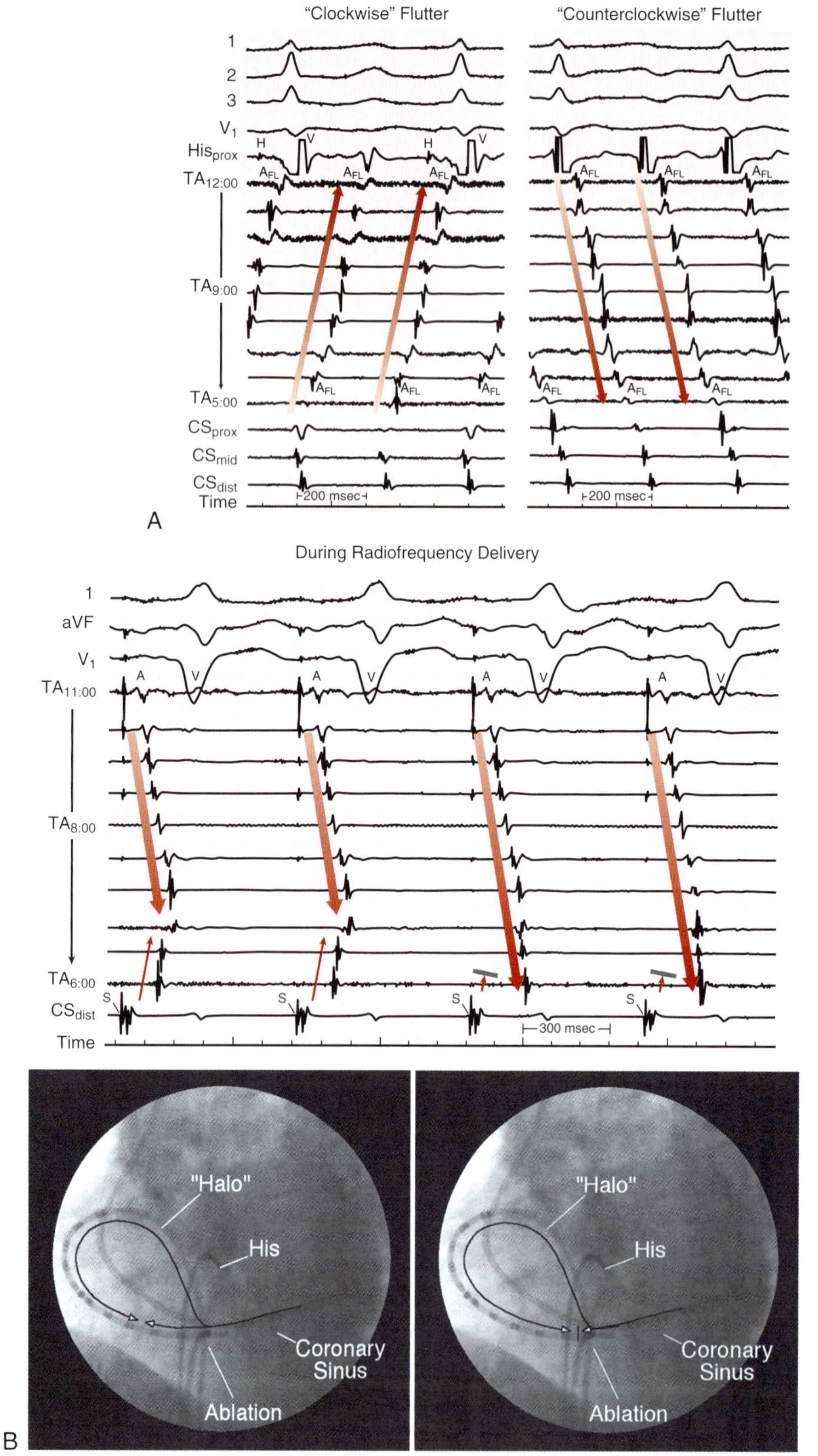

FIGURE 64.13 **A,** Two forms of atrial flutter in the same patient are shown. A halo catheter with 10 electrode pairs is situated on the atrial side of the tricuspid annulus *(TA)*, with recording sites displayed from the top of the annulus (12:00) to the inferomedial aspect (5:00), as shown in the fluoroscopic views in **B.** *Left,* the wavefront of atrial activation proceeds in a clockwise fashion *(arrows)* along the annulus. *Right,* the direction of propagation is the reverse. **B,** Ablation of the isthmus of atrial tissue between the tricuspid annulus and the inferior vena caval orifice for cure of atrial flutter. Recordings are displayed from the multipolar catheter around much of the circumference of the tricuspid annulus (see the left anterior oblique fluoroscopic images). Ablation of this isthmus is performed during coronary sinus pacing. In the two beats on the **left,** atrial conduction proceeds in two directions around the tricuspid annulus, as indicated by arrows and recorded along the halo catheter. In the two beats on the **right,** ablation has interrupted conduction in the floor of the right atrium, thereby eliminating one path for transmission along the tricuspid annulus. The halo catheter now records conduction, proceeding all the way around the annulus. This finding demonstrates a unidirectional block in the isthmus; block in the other direction may be demonstrated by pacing from one of the halo electrodes and observing a similar lack of isthmus conduction. The bundle of His recording in **A** *(right panel)* is lost because of catheter movement.

inexcitability around which an electrical wavefront can circulate. Specialized mapping tools and skills are necessary to achieve successful ablation in these cases.

In patients with AF, an AAD can slow intra-atrial conduction to such an extent that atrial flutter results and fibrillation is no longer observed. In some of these patients, ablation of atrial flutter and continued AAD therapy can prevent recurrences of these atrial arrhythmias.

The endpoint of atrial flutter ablation procedures was initially termination of atrial flutter with RF application, accompanied by noninducibility of the arrhythmia. However, with use of these criteria, up to 30% of patients had recurrent flutter because of lack of complete and permanent conduction block in the cavotricuspid isthmus. Thus, the current endpoint of ablation has changed to ensuring a line of bidirectional block is present in this region, usually by pacing from opposite sides of the isthmus (see Fig. 64.13B). With use of these criteria, recurrence rates have fallen to less than 5%.

Indications

Candidates for RF catheter ablation include patients with recurrent episodes of atrial flutter that are drug resistant, those who are drug intolerant, and those who do not desire long-term drug therapy. Many patients who undergo AF ablation (see Chapter 66) also have episodes of flutter during the procedure that can be treated by ablation of the cavotricuspid isthmus at the same setting.

Results

Regardless of circuit location, atrial flutter can be ablated successfully in more than 90% of cases, although patients with complex right or left atrial flutter require more extensive and complex procedures. Recurrence rates are less than 5% except in patients with extensive atrial disease, in whom new circuits can develop over time as new areas of conduction delay and block form. Complications are rare and include inadvertent heart block and phrenic nerve paralysis.

Ablation and Modification of Atrioventricular Conduction for Atrial Tachyarrhythmias

In some patients who have rapid ventricular rates despite optimal drug therapy during complex atrial tachyarrhythmias that are less amenable to ablation, RF ablation can be used to eliminate or modify AV conduction and control the ventricular rates.

To achieve this, a catheter is placed across the tricuspid valve and positioned to record a small His bundle electrogram associated with a large atrial electrogram. RF energy is applied until complete AV block has been achieved and is continued for an additional 30 to 60 seconds (Fig. 64.14). If no change in AV conduction is observed after 15 seconds of RF ablation despite good contact, the catheter is repositioned and the attempt repeated. In occasional patients, attempts at RF ablation via this right-sided approach fail to achieve heart block. These patients can undergo an attempt from

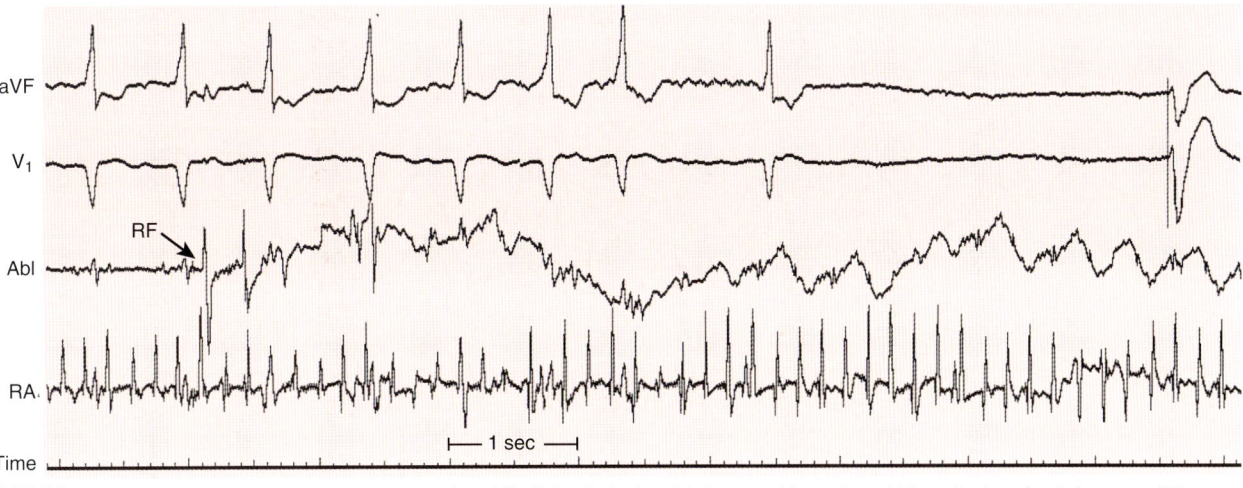

FIGURE 64.14 Atrioventricular nodal ablation for rate control of atrial fibrillation (AF). The ECG shows rapidly conducted AF; application of radiofrequency (RF) energy (arrow) results in complete AV block within seconds, followed by a ventricular paced complex.

the left ventricle with a catheter positioned along the interventricular septum, just beneath the aortic valve, to record a large His bundle electrogram. Success rates currently approach 100%, with AV conduction recurring in less than 5% of cases. Improved left ventricular function can result from control of the ventricular rate during AF and withdrawal of rate-controlling medications that have negative inotropic action. Permanent right, His bundle or biventricular pacing is typically required after ablation. With continuing advances in direct ablation of complex atrial arrhythmias, AV nodal ablation is less often used currently except in elderly patients. Whereas in some cases the AV junction can be modified to slow the ventricular rate without producing complete AV block by ablation in the region of the slow pathway (as described with AV node modification for AV node reentry), this strategy has been almost entirely abandoned due to poor predictability of long-term outcome despite good acute results.

Indications

Ablation and modification of AV conduction can be considered in the following cases: (1) patients with symptomatic atrial tachyarrhythmias who have inadequately controlled ventricular rates, unless primary ablation of the atrial tachyarrhythmia is possible (especially when a permanent pacemaker is already present for treatment of bradycardia-tachycardia syndrome); (2) similar patients when drugs are not tolerated or patients do not choose to take them, even though the ventricular rate can be controlled; (3) patients with symptomatic, nonparoxysmal junctional tachycardia that is drug resistant or in whom drugs are not tolerated or are not desired; (4) patients resuscitated from sudden cardiac death related to atrial flutter or AF with a rapid ventricular response in the absence of an accessory pathway; and (5) patients with a dual-chamber pacemaker and pacemaker-mediated tachycardia that cannot be treated effectively by drugs or reprogramming of the pacemaker. The last three situations are rarely encountered.

Results

As previously noted, successful interruption of AV conduction can be achieved in almost all cases; recurrent conduction is observed in less than 5%. Significant complications occur in 1% to 2%. In early studies, up to 4% of patients had an episode of sudden death after AV junction ablation despite adequate pacemaker function, presumably because of relative bradycardia after long periods of rapid ventricular rates serving as the setting for repolarization-related ventricular arrhythmias. Since then, backup pacing rates are set to 80 to 90/min for the first 1 to 3 months after ablation in most cases, which has almost entirely eliminated this problem. Improvements in quality-of-life indices, as well as in cost-effectiveness, have been demonstrated for this procedure.

Radiofrequency Catheter Ablation of Atrial Fibrillation

See Chapters 65 and 66.

Radiofrequency Catheter Ablation of Ventricular Arrhythmias (see Chapter 67)

In general, the success rate for ablation of VTs is lower than that for AV node reentry or AV reentry because of the heterogeneity of substrates and presentations. In the ideal case, induction of the VT must be reproducible, with uniform QRS morphology from beat to beat, and VT must be sustained and hemodynamically stable so that the patient can tolerate the VT long enough during the procedure to undergo the extensive mapping necessary to localize optimal ablation target sites. These conditions are often not met. Patients with several electrocardiographically distinct, uniform morphologies of VT can still be candidates for ablation, because in many cases a common reentrant pathway is shared by two or more VT morphologies. Also, the target for ablation must be fairly circumscribed and preferably endocardially situated, although catheter mapping and ablation from the epicardial surface after percutaneous pericardial access is performed in many centers. Very rapid VT, polymorphic VT, and infrequent, nonsustained VT can be addressed with catheter ablation using different strategies.

LOCATION AND ABLATION

RF catheter ablation of VT can be divided into idiopathic VT, which occurs in patients with essentially structurally normal hearts and includes patients with isolated PVCs; VT that occurs in various disease settings but without CAD; and VT in patients with CAD and usually previous MI. In the first group, VTs/PVCs can arise in either ventricle. Right VTs most frequently originate in the outflow tract and have a characteristic left bundle branch block–like, inferior axis morphology (see Chapter 67); less often, VTs/PVCs arise in the inflow tract or free wall. Initiation of tachycardia can often be facilitated by catecholamines. Most left VTs in structurally normal hearts are septal in origin and have a characteristic QRS configuration (i.e., right bundle branch block, superior axis). Other VTs/PVCs also occur and arise from different areas of the left ventricle, including the left ventricular outflow region and the aortic sinuses of Valsalva, and are similar in electrocardiographic appearance and clinical behavior to those arising in the right ventricular outflow tract. VTs in abnormal hearts without CAD can be the result of either intramyocardial or bundle branch reentry, most often observed in patients with dilated cardiomyopathy, or as a focal process. Epicardial foci and circuits are more common in this than in other groups. In patients with bundle branch reentry, ablation of the right bundle branch eliminates the tachycardia. VT can occur in patients with right ventricular dysplasia (see Chapter 63), sarcoidosis, Chagas disease, hypertrophic cardiomyopathy (see Chapters 52 to 54), and a host of other noncoronary disease states.

Activation mapping and pace mapping are effective in patients with idiopathic VTs/PVCs to locate the site of origin of the VT. In *activation mapping* the timing of endocardial electrograms sampled by the mapping catheter as it is moved around the chamber is compared with the onset of the surface QRS complex. Sites that are activated 20 to 40 milliseconds before onset of the surface QRS are near the origin of the arrhythmia. In idiopathic VT/PVCs, ablation at a site at which the unipolar

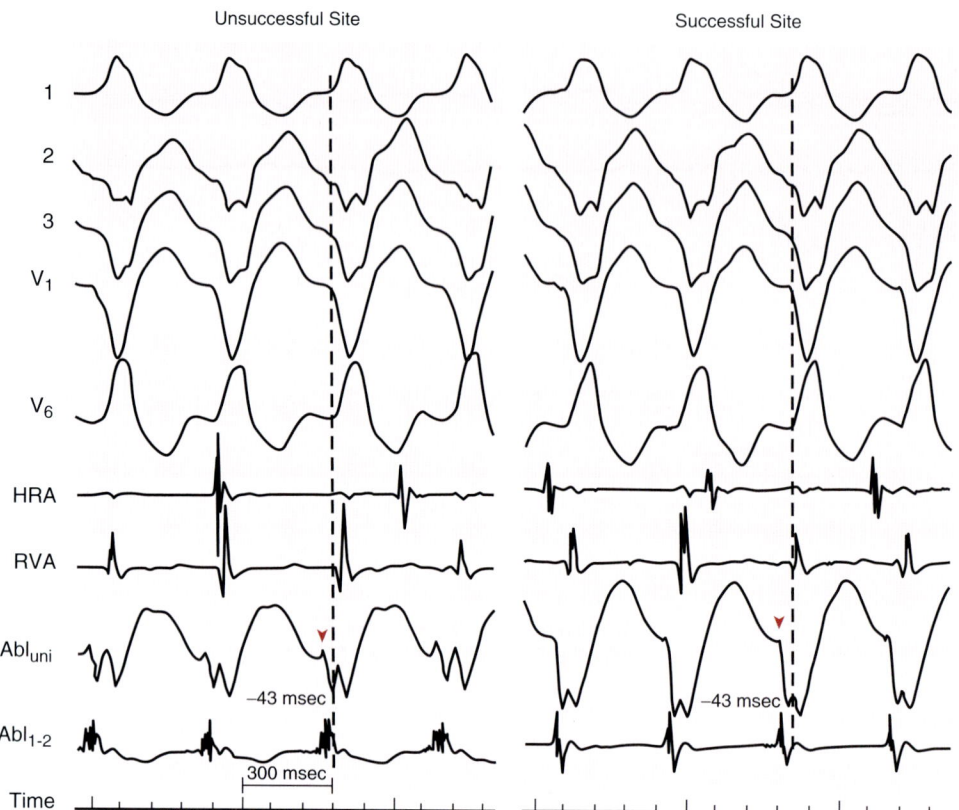

FIGURE 64.15 Recordings from unsuccessful and successful ablation sites in a patient with idiopathic ventricular tachycardia arising in the inferior right ventricular wall. In the recordings from the unsuccessful ablation site, the unipolar signal *(arrowhead)* has a small r wave, which indicates that a portion of the wavefront from the focus of tachycardia is approaching the site from elsewhere. At the successful site, the unipolar recording has a QS configuration, thus indicating that all depolarization is emanating from this site. In each site the bipolar recording (Abl$_{1-2}$) occurs an identical 43 milliseconds before onset of the QRS *(dashed lines)*.

electrogram shows a QS complex may yield greater success than if an rS potential is observed (Fig. 64.15). *Pace mapping* involves stimulation of various ventricular sites to produce a QRS contour that duplicates the QRS contour of the spontaneous VT or PVC, thus establishing the apparent site of origin of the arrhythmia (Fig. 64.16). This technique is limited by several methodologic problems but may be useful when the arrhythmia cannot be initiated and when a 12-lead ECG has been obtained during spontaneous episodes. Presystolic Purkinje potentials, as well as very-low-amplitude mid-diastolic signals, can be recorded during VT from sites at which ablation cures VT in most patients with left ventricular VTs that have a right bundle branch block superior axis; this VT characteristically terminates with IV verapamil and is the only significant idiopathic VT with a reentrant basis. Localization of optimal ablation sites for VT in patients with CAD and previous MI can be more challenging than in patients with structurally normal hearts because of the altered anatomy and electrophysiology. Pace mapping has a lower sensitivity and specificity than for idiopathic VT. Furthermore, reentry circuits can sometimes be large and resistant to the relatively small lesions produced by RF catheter ablation in scarred endocardium.

In scar-based VT (e.g., after MI, cardiomyopathies), finding a protected region of diastolic activation used as a critical part of the reentrant circuit is desirable because ablation at this site has a good chance of eliminating the tachycardia (Fig. 64.17). As a result of the extensive derangement in electrophysiology caused by the previous damage (e.g., infarct, myopathy), many areas of the ventricle may have diastolic activation but may not be relevant to perpetuation of the VT. These "bystander sites" make activation mapping more difficult. Pacing techniques such as entrainment can be used to test whether a site is actually part of a circuit or is a bystander. *Entrainment* involves pacing for several complexes during a tachycardia at a rate slightly faster than the VT rate; after pacing is stopped and the same tachycardia resumes, the timing of the first complex relative to the last paced beat is an indicator of how close the pacing site is to a part of the VT circuit (Fig. 64.18). During entrainment, part of the ventricle is activated by the paced wavefront and part by the VT wavefront being forced to exit earlier than it normally would, thereby resulting in a fusion complex on the ECG. Pacing from within a critical portion of the circuit itself produces an exact QRS match with the VT; fusion occurs only within the circuit and is "concealed" (not evident on the surface ECG). Sites with a low-amplitude, isolated, mid-diastolic potential that cannot be dissociated from the tachycardia by pacing perturbations, at which entrainment with concealed fusion can be demonstrated, are highly likely to be successful ablation sites.

In a significant proportion of patients with VT and structural heart disease, activation mapping and entrainment cannot be performed because of poor hemodynamic tolerance of the arrhythmia or inability to initiate sustained tachycardia during an EPS. In these situations, additional methods can be used that are categorized as *substrate mapping*, in which areas of low electrical voltage or from which very delayed potentials are recorded during sinus rhythm, or at which pacing closely replicates a known VT 12-lead ECG morphology (pace mapping) are targeted for ablation without needing any mapping during VT (Fig. 64.19). Other strategies include searching for and eliminating possible conduction channels within scar tissue, homogenization of scar tissue, or surrounding the arrhythmogenic zone with RF applications to isolate this "core." These methods, usually requiring very extensive ablation in diseased areas, have yielded very good results in many cases. In other patients, hemodynamic support in the form of catecholamine infusion, intra-aortic balloon counterpulsation, or a percutaneous temporary ventricular assist device or extracorporeal membrane oxygenation has been used to facilitate activation mapping during VT.

In patients without structural heart disease, only a single VT is usually present, and catheter ablation of that VT is most often curative. In patients with extensive structural heart disease, multiple VTs are usually present. Most of these patients already have, or soon will have, an ICD; ablation can be used to decrease the frequency of ICD therapies but is generally not intended to cure the patient of all ventricular arrhythmias. Catheter ablation of a single VT in such patients may be only palliative and may not eliminate the need for further AAD or device therapy, but can improve quality of life by decreasing ICD shocks. The genesis of multiple tachycardia morphologies is not clear, although in some cases they are merely different manifestations of one circuit (e.g., different directions of wavefront propagation or exit to the ventricle as a whole), and ablation of one may prevent recurrence of others. The presence of multiple VT morphologies contributes to the difficulties in mapping and ablation of VT in these patients, because pacing techniques used to validate recordings at potential sites of ablation may result in a change in morphology to another VT that may not arise in the same region.

After ablation of VT, ventricular stimulation is repeated to assess efficacy. In some cases, rapid polymorphic VT or VF can be initiated. The clinical significance of these arrhythmias is unclear, but some evidence has suggested that they have a low likelihood of spontaneous occurrence during follow-up.

As noted earlier, most cases of polymorphic VT and VF are not currently amenable to standard ablation methods because of hemodynamic instability and beat-to-beat changes in activation sequence. However, some cases appear to have a focal source (similar to the focal sources of AF), and if the focus can be identified and ablated, further arrhythmia episodes can be prevented. In such cases, repeated episodes of arrhythmia have constant electrocardiographic features of the initiating beat or beats, thus suggesting a consistent source, which may be in either ventricle. The electrogram at sites of successful ablation often has very sharp presystolic potentials reminiscent of Purkinje potentials, with a 50- to 100-millisecond delay until onset of the QRS (Fig. 64.20).[29] In some cases of VF, "rotors" (sites of rapid circulation within a small region)

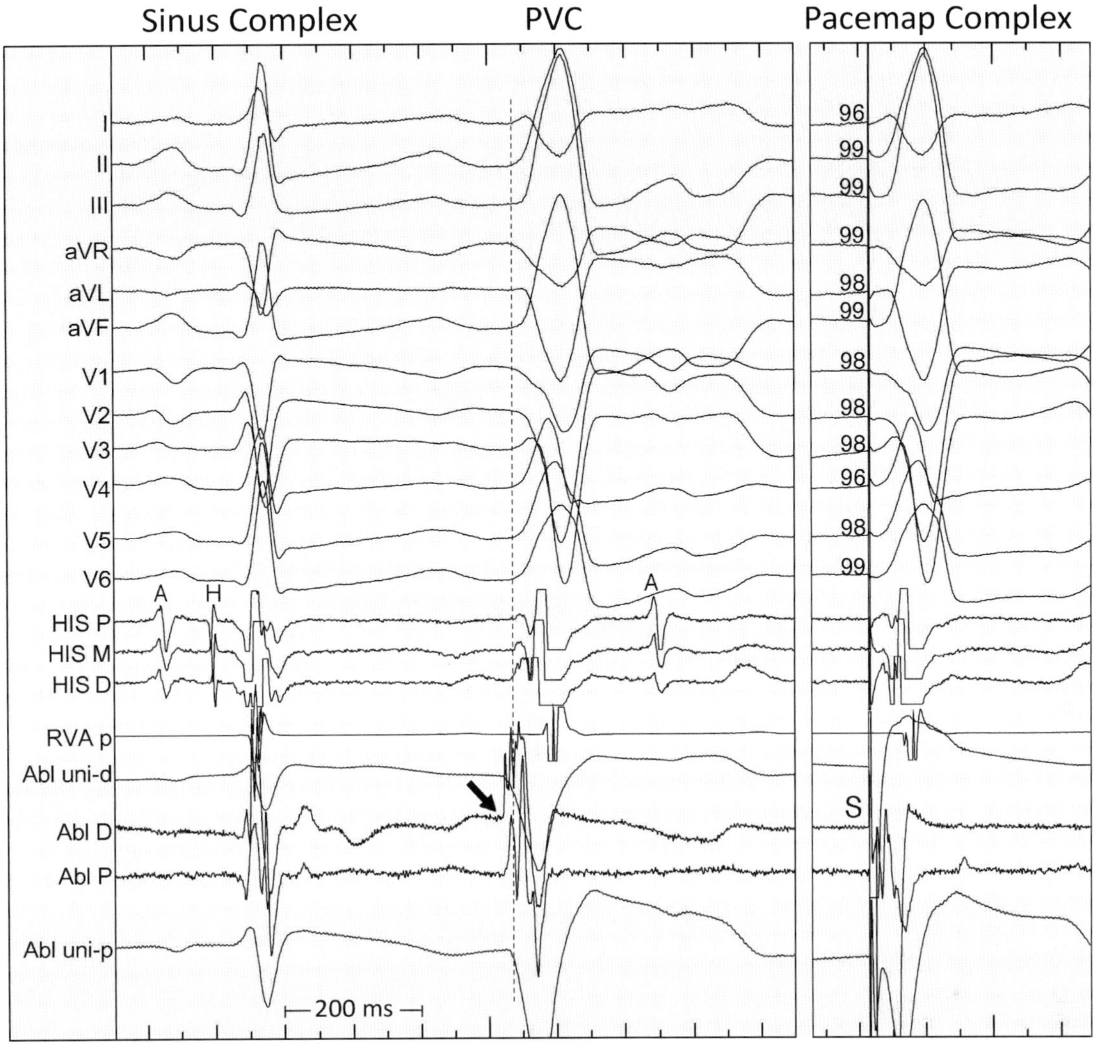

FIGURE 64.16 Premature ventricular complex (PVC) and pace mapping. All 12 surface ECG leads are shown, along with intracardiac recordings in sinus rhythm, a spontaneous PVC, and pacing (S) at the site of Abl D (distal recordings of ablation catheter). The Abl D recording shows a sharp deflection (arrow) occurring about 25 milliseconds before onset of the QRS (dashed line). In the **right panel,** pacing is performed from this site. This produces an identical QRS complex in each lead, with a short stimulus–QRS interval; numbers indicate percentage of "match" between PVC and paced QRS complexes using an algorithm in the recording system. Ablation at this site eliminated VT in 2 seconds. *uni,* Unipolar recording; *A,* atrial electrogram; *H,* His electrogram.

have been reported, ablation of which has prevented recurrences (similar to the case with AF). This work is promising but preliminary.

Indications

Patients considered for RF catheter ablation of VT in the absence of structural heart disease are those with symptomatic, sustained monomorphic VT when the tachycardia is drug resistant, when the patient is drug intolerant, or when the patient does not desire long-term drug therapy. Patients with structural heart disease who are candidates for ablation include those with bundle branch reentrant VT and those with sustained monomorphic VT and an ICD who are receiving multiple shocks not manageable by reprogramming or concomitant drug therapy. In some patients (usually without structural heart disease, but also in patients with diseased ventricles), nonsustained VT or even severely symptomatic PVCs warrant RF catheter ablation. In some of these patients, in whom the ventricular ectopy occurs frequently, significant left ventricular systolic dysfunction has occurred (presumably similar to tachycardia-related cardiomyopathy). After successful ablation, ventricular function may improve significantly or even normalize.

Results

In patients with structurally normal hearts, the success rate of VT or PVC ablation is approximately 85%.[30] In patients with postinfarction VT, more than 70% no longer have recurrences of VT after the ablation procedure despite inducibility of rapid VT or VF; only approximately 30% of patients will have no inducible ventricular arrhythmia of any type and no spontaneous recurrences. As noted earlier, most of these patients already have, or will have, an ICD as backup. Significant complications occur in up to 3%, including vascular damage, heart block, worsening of heart failure, cardiac tamponade, stroke, and valve damage. Death is rare but can occur in patients with severe CAD and/or systolic dysfunction.

NEW MAPPING AND ABLATION TECHNOLOGIES
Multielectrode Mapping Systems

Some of the limitations of ablation are related to inadequate mapping. These problems include having only isolated premature complexes during the EPS instead of sustained tachycardias (in idiopathic AT and VT), nonsustained episodes of VT, poor hemodynamic tolerance of VT, and multiple VT morphologies. Standard mapping techniques sample single sites sequentially and are poorly suited to these situations. New mapping systems are available that enable sampling of many sites simultaneously and incorporate sophisticated computer algorithms for analysis and display of global maps. These mapping systems use various technologies ranging from multiple electrodes situated on each of several splines of a basket catheter, to the use of low-intensity electrical or magnetic fields to localize the tip of the catheter in the heart and record and plot activation times on a contour map of the chamber, to the use of complex mathematics to compute "virtual" electrograms recorded from a mesh electrode situated in the middle of a chamber cavity or on the body surface. Some of these systems are capable of generating activation maps of an entire chamber by using only one

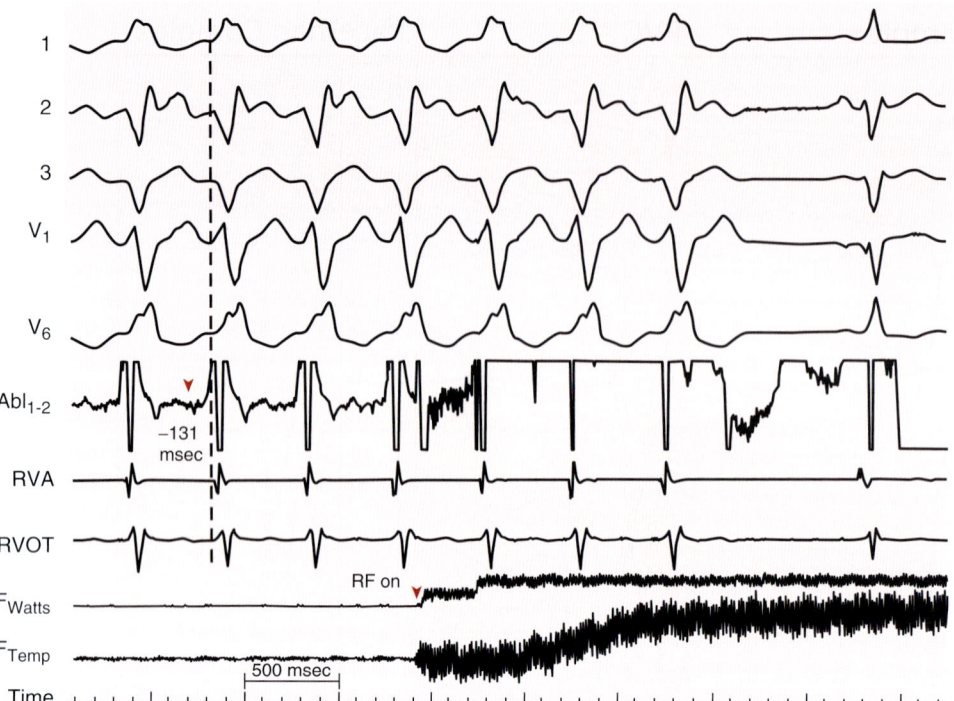

cardiac complex, an obvious advantage in patients with only rare premature complexes, nonsustained arrhythmias, or poor hemodynamic tolerance of sustained arrhythmias.

Epicardial Catheter Mapping

Although most VTs can be ablated from the endocardium, occasional cases are resistant to this therapy. In many of these cases, epicardial ablation may be successful. It is often needed in VT attributable to cardiomyopathy but less frequently in postinfarction patients and those without structural heart disease.

For gaining access to the pericardial space for epicardial mapping and ablation, a long spinal anesthesia needle is introduced from a subxiphoid approach under fluoroscopic guidance. As the pericardium is approached, a small amount of radiocontrast agent is injected. If the tip of the needle is still outside the pericardium, the dye stays where it is injected; when the pericardial space has been entered, the dye disperses and outlines the heart. A guidewire is introduced through the needle and a standard vascular introducer sheath exchanged over the wire. The pericardial space is then accessible for a mapping/ablation catheter, and standard mapping techniques can then

FIGURE 64.17 Radiofrequency ablation of postinfarction ventricular tachycardia. The electrogram in the ablation recording (Abl$_{1-2}$, *arrowhead*) precedes onset of the QRS *(dashed line)* by 131 msec. Ablation here (RF on) results in slight deceleration of VT before termination in 1.3 seconds. Temperature monitored from the catheter tip had just peaked (≈70°C) at the time that VT terminated.

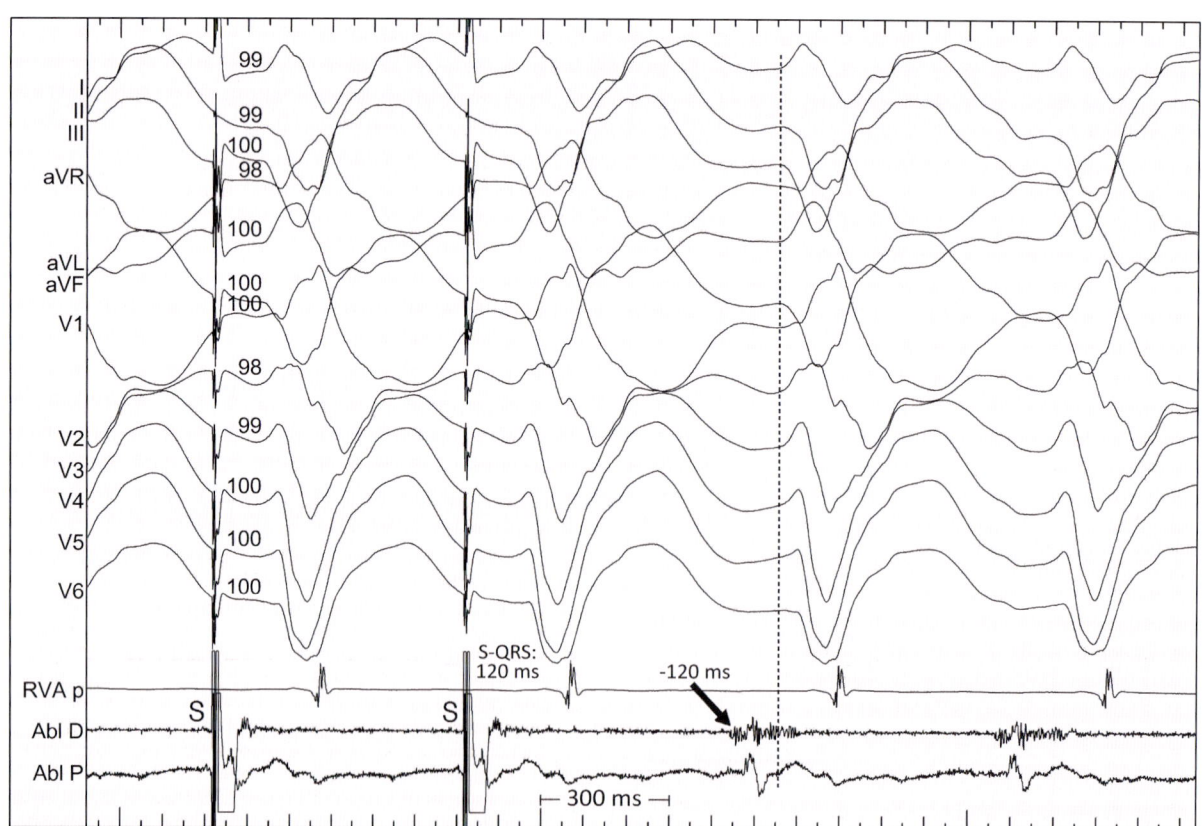

FIGURE 64.18 Concealed" entrainment of postinfarction ventricular tachycardia. The two complexes on the *left* are pacing during VT, with a stimulus (S)-QRS interval 120 milliseconds; after pacing ends, VT resumes. The electrogram *(arrow)* in Abl D (distal electrode pair of the ablation catheter) is 120 milliseconds before QRS onset *(dotted line)*. The paced and VT QRS complexes are almost identical (numbers above paced complexes indicate algorithmic "match" assessed by recording system). Ablation at this site quickly terminated VT. *RVA p*, Right ventricular apex; *Abl P*, recording from proximal electrodes on ablation catheter.

be applied. When a site is selected for possible ablation, coronary arteriography is usually warranted to avoid delivery of RF energy near a coronary artery. This is less important in cases of postinfarction VT because the VT substrate is typically in a region of previous transmural infarction. For left ventricular sites, high-output pacing should be performed to assess proximity to the left phrenic nerve; if captured, another ablation site may be sought at which phrenic capture is absent, or a balloon can be placed in the pericardial space (or air or fluid instilled) to physically displace and thus protect the nerve from damage during ablation. Treatment of ventricular arrhythmias in some right ventricular pathologies, such as arrhythmogenic right ventricular cardiomyopathy and Brugada syndrome, often require epicardial mapping and ablation. Epicardial mapping can be used for patients who have previously undergone cardiac surgery, although adhesions may obliterate portions of the pericardial space; on occasion, a small subxiphoid incision is needed for better access and visualization of the space. The most frequent complication of epicardial mapping is pericarditis related to the ablation; cardiac tamponade is rare.

Chemical Ablation

Chemical ablation of an area of myocardium can be used for treatment of VT refractory to drug and standard catheter ablation. Using this specialized technique, an angioplasty catheter is maneuvered into an arterial (or venous) branch in the region of the VT (determined by mapping). After verifying the correct vessel by injecting iced saline into it and observing transient slowing or termination of VT, the angioplasty balloon is inflated (to prevent spillage of alcohol) and 100% ethanol is injected into the vessel. This generally terminates VT and kills the cells responsible for its continuation. Recurrences of tachycardia several days after apparently successful ablation are possible. Excessive myocardial necrosis is the major complication, and alcohol ablation should be considered only when other ablative approaches fail or cannot be done.

Several other mapping/imaging techniques have been developed recently, including integration of a previously obtained computed tomography or magnetic resonance study into computerized mapping systems and use of intracardiac ultrasound to construct a facsimile of the intracardiac anatomy in any chamber during ablation procedures, to guide placement of anatomic ablation and reduce fluoroscopic exposure. Other techniques include use of algorithms to select complex fractionated atrial electrograms for ablation in patients with AF and algorithms to assess the fidelity of pace maps with native tachycardia complexes. Cryoablation, high-frequency focused ultrasound, laser energy, and delivery of RF energy between two catheters on opposite sides of a ventricular wall, or through a needle electrode inserted into myocardium, have had some success in select patients.

Non-Invasive Radioablation

Recently, external radiation has been used to treat VT refractory to medication and catheter ablation strategies.[31] With this method, once a target area in the ventricles has been precisely designated, one of a variety of sources of radiation is focused at these specific coordinates from different angles in order to minimize collateral damage to skin and normal tissue near the ablation target. This technique requires expertise coordinated among many disciplines (electrophysiology, nuclear medicine, radiation physics) and is not widely available; preliminary results are promising.

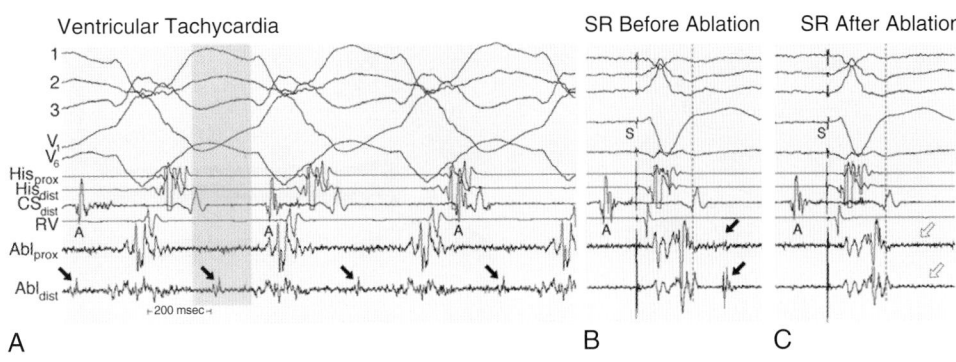

FIGURE 64.19 Mid-diastolic potentials during ventricular tachycardia correlating with late potentials in sinus rhythm (SR). **A,** Ventricular tachycardia (VT); diastole (from the end of one QRS complex to the beginning of the next) is shaded in gray. In the Abl$_{dist}$ recording, a small, sharp signal is seen in mid-diastole that corresponds to a protected corridor of propagation. **B,** After termination of VT with pacing, recording at the same location shows a delayed ("late") potential in SR that tracked ventricular pacing (black arrows; the dashed line denotes the end of the QRS complex). **C,** Ablation here eliminated the late potential (clear arrows), as well as inducible VT. A, Atrial recording; S, stimulus artifact.

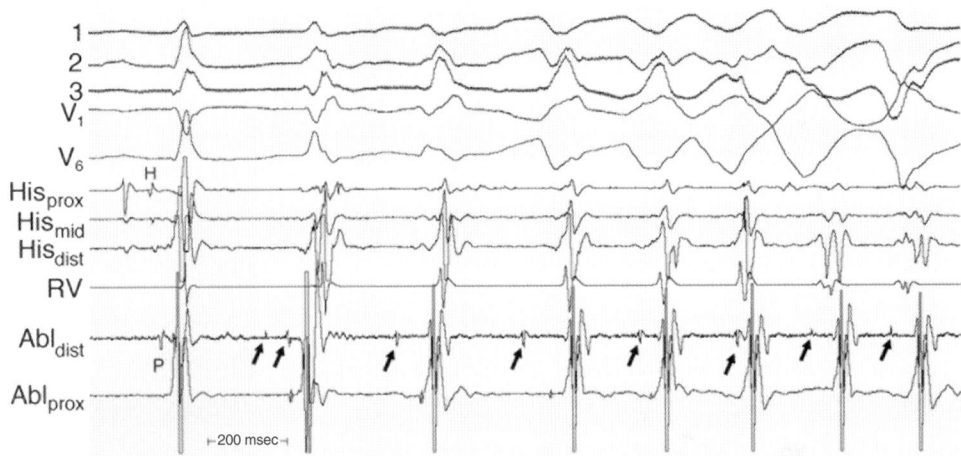

FIGURE 64.20 "Focal ventricular fibrillation." Recordings are shown from a patient with multiple episodes of VF in a day. A sinus rhythm complex, during which a Purkinje potential (P) is recorded from the ablation (Abl) electrode, is followed by a premature complex from this site that is preceded by sharp Purkinje spikes (arrows) that continue to precede subsequent complexes of polymorphic ventricular tachycardia that degenerated to ventricular fibrillation (VF). Ablation at this site eliminated recurrent episodes of VF.

SURGICAL THERAPY FOR TACHYARRHYTHMIAS

The objectives of a surgical approach to treatment of a tachycardia are to excise, isolate, or interrupt tissue in the heart critical for initiation, maintenance, or propagation of the tachycardia while preserving or even improving myocardial function. In addition to a direct surgical approach to the arrhythmia, indirect approaches such as aneurysmectomy, coronary artery bypass grafting, and relief of valvular regurgitation or stenosis can be useful in select patients by improving cardiac hemodynamics and myocardial blood supply. *Cardiac sympathectomy* (stellate ganglionectomy) alters adrenergic influences on the heart and has been effective in some patients, particularly those who have recurrent VT with long-QT syndrome despite beta blockade, and catecholaminergic polymorphic VT.

Supraventricular Tachycardias

Surgical procedures exist for patients (adults and children) with AT, atrial flutter and fibrillation, AV node reentry, and AV reentry (Fig. 64.21). RF catheter ablation adequately treats most of these patients and thus has replaced direct surgical intervention, except for the occasional patient in whom RF catheter ablation fails or who is

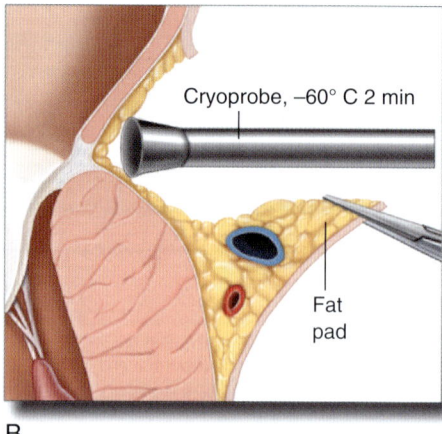

FIGURE 64.21 Schematic diagram showing the two approaches for surgical interruption of an accessory pathway. **A,** Left atrioventricular groove and its vascular contents the coronary sinus (CS) and circumflex coronary artery (CA). Multiple accessory pathways (AP) course through the fat pad. **B,** Approach for epicardial dissection. **C,** Endocardial dissection. Both approaches clear out the fat pad and interrupt any accessory pathways. (From Zipes DP. Cardiac electrophysiology: promises and contributions. *J Am Coll Cardiol*. 1989;13:1329. Reprinted by permission of the American College of Cardiology.)

undergoing concomitant cardiovascular surgery. In some cases, a prior attempt at RF catheter ablation complicates surgery by obliterating the normal tissue planes that exist in the AV groove or by rendering tissues friable. On occasion, patients with ATs have multiple foci that require surgical intervention. Several surgical procedures have been developed to treat AF and are reviewed in Chapter 66.

Ventricular Tachycardia

In contrast to patients with supraventricular arrhythmias, candidates for surgical therapy for ventricular arrhythmias often have severe left ventricular dysfunction, generally the result of CAD. The cause of the underlying heart disease influences the type of surgery performed. Candidates are patients with drug-resistant, symptomatic, recurrent ventricular tachyarrhythmias who ideally have a segmental wall motion abnormality (scar or aneurysm) with preserved residual left ventricular function, have not benefited from previous attempts at catheter ablation, or are not candidates for catheter ablation because of hemodynamic instability during VT or the presence of left ventricular thrombi (precluding endocardial catheter ablation).

Idiopathic Ventricular Tachycardia/Premature Ventricular Complexes and Nonischemic Cardiomyopathy

Patients with VT or PVCs in the absence of structural heart disease or with nonischemic cardiomyopathy who have undergone unsuccessful drug and catheter ablation therapy for their arrhythmias are candidates for surgical therapy.

The procedure is usually performed through a limited thoracotomy, exposing only the area of the ventricles believed responsible for the arrhythmia. In idiopathic VT/PVC cases, this is often at the basal aspect of the anterior left ventricle, an area where epicardial catheter ablation is difficult because of thick epicardial fat and proximity to major coronary arteries. After exposing the area of the ventricular epicardial surface of interest, mapping is done to confirm the source of the arrhythmia, after which cryoablation is usually performed (Fig. 64.22). This typically results in cessation of the arrhythmia. Extensive ablation is often needed in patients with nonischemic cardiomyopathy, in whom epicardial and intramural scarring in the basal left and right ventricles is a common substrate for ventricular arrhythmias.

Ischemic Heart Disease

In almost all patients who have VT associated with ischemic heart disease, the arrhythmia, regardless of its configuration on the surface ECG, arises in the left ventricle or on the left ventricular side of the interventricular

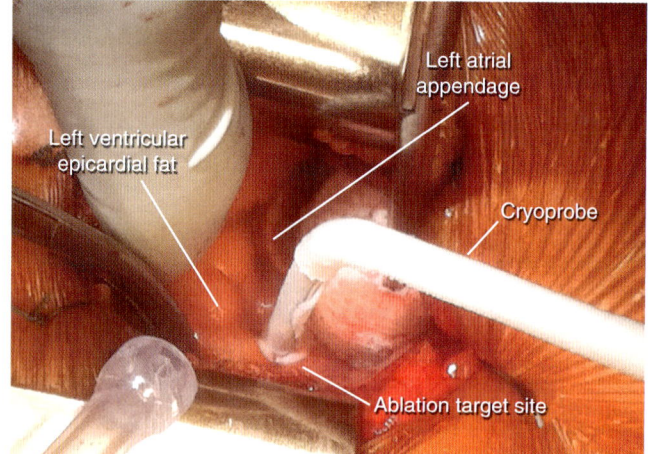

FIGURE 64.22 Epicardial cryoablation for treatment of symptomatic, drug-refractory premature ventricular complexes (PVCs) that could not be ablated from an endo- or epicardial catheter approach. The left ventricular base is exposed through a limited left thoracotomy; after mapping to pinpoint the sites of origin of PVCs, a cryoprobe is used to freeze the area.

septum. The electrocardiographic contour of the VT can change from a right bundle branch block to a left bundle branch block pattern without a change in the site of earliest diastolic activation, thus suggesting that the location of the circuit within the left ventricle remains the same, often near the septum, but that its exit pathway is altered.

Indirect surgical approaches, including coronary artery revascularization, and ventricular aneurysm or infarct resection with or without coronary artery bypass grafting, have been successful in no more than 20% to 30% of VT cases. Coronary artery bypass grafting as a primary therapeutic approach has generally been successful only in patients who experience rapid VT because of severe ischemia, as well as in patients with ischemia-related VF, but it can sometimes be useful in patients with coronary disease resuscitated from sudden death who have no inducible arrhythmias at EPS. These patients generally show a clear relationship between episodes of ventricular arrhythmia and immediately antecedent severe ischemia and have no evidence of infarction or minimal wall motion abnormalities but have preserved overall left ventricular function. Patients with sustained monomorphic VT or only polymorphic VT rarely have their arrhythmias affected by coronary bypass surgery, although it can reduce the frequency of the arrhythmic episodes in some patients and prevent new ischemic events. Percutaneous (temporary) stellate ganglion blockade, or left or bilateral cardiac sympathectomy, has been shown to be effective in controlling refractory VT and VF in many cases.

SURGICAL TECHNIQUES

In general, two types of direct surgical procedures are used, resection and ablation (Fig. 64.23). The first direct surgical approach to VT was encircling endocardial ventriculotomy, which entails performing a transmural ventriculotomy to isolate areas of endocardial fibrosis that were recognized visually; this procedure is rarely used now. Another procedure, subendocardial resection, is based on data indicating that arrhythmias after MI arise mostly at the subendocardial borders between normal and infarcted tissue. Subendocardial resection involves peeling off a 1- to 3-mm-thick layer of endocardium, often near the rim of an aneurysm, that has been demonstrated by mapping procedures to contain sites of mid-diastolic activation recorded during VT. Tachycardias arising from near the base of the papillary muscles are treated with a cryoprobe cooled to −70°C. Cryoablation can also be used to isolate areas of the ventricle that cannot be resected and is often combined with resection. Lasers have also been used with good success, but the equipment is expensive and cumbersome.

For ventricular tachyarrhythmias, operative mortality ranges from 5% to 10%, related to poor LV function and comorbidities extant prior to surgery. Success, defined as the absence of recurrence of spontaneous ventricular arrhythmias, is achieved in 59% to 98% of patients. In experienced centers, operative mortality can be as low as 5% in stable patients undergoing elective procedures, with 85% to 95% of survivors being free of inducible or spontaneous ventricular tachyarrhythmias. Long-term recurrence rates range from 2% to 15% and correlate with results of the patient's postoperative electrophysiologic stimulation study. Operative survival is strongly influenced by the degree of left ventricular dysfunction.

ELECTROPHYSIOLOGIC STUDIES
Preoperative Electrophysiologic Study

In patients for whom direct surgical therapy for VT is planned, a preoperative EPS is usually warranted. This study involves initiation of the VT and electrophysiologic mapping to localize the area to be resected, as is done with catheter ablation. Preoperative catheter mapping is contraindicated in patients with known left ventricular thrombi that might be dislodged by the mapping catheter.

Intraoperative Ventricular Mapping

Electrophysiologic mapping is also performed at surgery, with the surgeon using a handheld probe or an electrode array coupled with computer techniques that instantaneously provide an overall activation map, cycle by cycle. The sequence of activation during VT can be plotted and the area of earliest activation determined. Resection or ablation of tissue from which these recordings are made usually cures the VT, thus indicating that they represent a critical portion of the reentrant circuit. When the earliest recordable endocardial electrical activity occurs less than 30 milliseconds before onset of the QRS complex, the critical portions of the circuit may be in the interventricular septum or near the epicardium of the free wall. In some patients, intramural mapping using a plunge needle electrode can be useful. Most centers have used a strategy of "sequential" subendocardial resection in which VT is initiated, mapped, and ablated (resected or cryoablated) while the heart is warm and beating, and stimulation is repeated immediately. If VT can still be initiated, mapping and resection are also repeated until VT can no longer be initiated. Reentry around an inferior scar, with a critical diastolic pathway confined to an isthmus of ventricular muscle between the scar and mitral valve annulus, can be cured by cryoablation of this isthmus. Cure rates in this situation exceed 93%, although risk of late exacerbation of heart failure remains a concern.

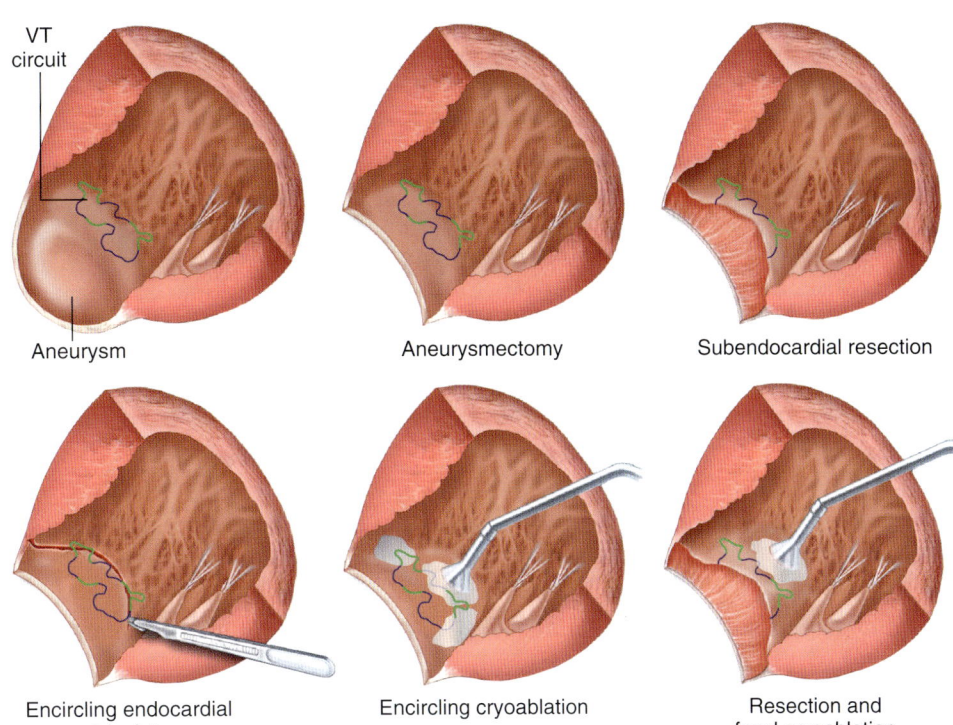

FIGURE 64.23 Schematic diagram showing surgical procedures for the treatment of postinfarction ventricular tachycardia with a left ventricular aneurysm. A damaged left ventricle is depicted as opened along the lateral wall and showing the septum and papillary muscles. The tachycardia circuit *(upper left)* takes a meandering course near the point where the aneurysm meets normal myocardium and at times is superficial *(purple lines)* and at other times is coursing deeper *(green lines)*. Simple aneurysmectomy that leaves a portion of the aneurysm for suturing often misses the circuit and thus does not cure the arrhythmia. By subendocardial resection, a layer of endocardium and subjacent tissue is removed, including at least some of the tachycardia circuit. Such resection results in elimination of the tachycardia. Encircling endocardial ventriculotomy attempts to isolate the circuit electrically without removal of tissue, but it probably actually works by incising portions of the circuit. Cryoablation can be used to encircle the infarct zone, alone or in combination with resection of damaged tissue too deep in the wall to be resected safely.

REFERENCES
Pharmacologic Therapy

1. Lester RM, Olbertz J. Early drug development: assessment of proarrhythmic risk and cardiovascular safety. *Expert Rev Clin Pharmacol.* 2016;9:1611–1618.
2. Rosen MR, Janse MJ. Concept of the vulnerable parameter: the Sicilian Gambit revisited. *J Cardiovasc Pharmacol.* 2010;55:428–437.
3. Lei M, Wu L, Terrar DA, et al. Modernized classification of cardiac antiarrhythmic drugs. *Circulation.* 2018;138:1879–1896.
4. Zaiou M, El Amri H. Cardiovascular pharmacogenetics: a promise for genomically-guided therapy and personalized medicine. *Clin Genet.* 2017;91:355–370.
5. Tomaselli Muensterman E, Tisdale JE. Predictive analytics for identification of patients at risk for QT interval prolongation: a systematic review. *Pharmacotherapy.* 2018;38:813–821.
6. Lorberbaum T, Sampson KJ, Woosley RL, et al. An integrative data science pipeline to identify novel drug interactions that prolong the QT interval. *Drug Saf.* 2016;39:433–441.
7. Wright JM, Page RL, Field ME. Antiarrhythmic drugs in pregnancy. *Expert Rev Cardiovasc Ther.* 2015;13:1433–1444.
8. Li Z, Ridder BJ, Han X, et al. Assessment of an in silico mechanistic model for proarrhythmia risk prediction under the CiPA initiative. *Clin Pharmacol Ther.* 2019;105:466–475.
9. Brodie OT, Michowitz Y, Belhassen B. Pharmacological therapy in Brugada syndrome. *Arrhythm Electrophysiol Rev.* 2018;7:135–142.
10. Mankikian J, Favelle O, Guillon A, et al. Initial characteristics and outcome of hospitalized patients with amiodarone pulmonary toxicity. *Respir Med.* 2014;108:638–646.
11. Hussain N, Bhattacharyya A, Prueksaritanond S. Amiodarone-induced cirrhosis of liver: what predicts mortality? *ISRN Cardiol.* 2013;617943.
12. Wang AG, Cheng HC. Amiodarone-associated optic neuropathy: clinical review. *Neuro Ophthalmol.* 2017;41:55–58.
13. Epstein AE, Olshansky B, Naccarelli GV, et al. Practical management guide for clinicians who treat patients with amiodarone. *Am J Med.* 2016;129:468–475.
14. Valembois L, Audureau E, Takeda A, et al. Antiarrhythmics for maintaining sinus rhythm after cardioversion of atrial fibrillation. *Cochrane Database Syst Rev.* 2019;9:CD005049.
15. De Vecchis R, Ariano C. Effects of dronedarone on all-cause mortality and on cardiovascular events in patients treated for atrial fibrillation: a meta-analysis of RCTs. *Minerva Cardioangiol.* 2019;67:163–171.
16. Kpaeyeh JA, Wharton JM. Sotalol. *Card Electrophysiol Clin.* 2016;8:437–452.
17. Vinson DR, Lugovskaya N, Warton EM, et al. Ibutilide effectiveness and safety in the cardioversion of atrial fibrillation and flutter in the community emergency department. *Ann Emerg Med.* 2018;71:96–108.e2.

18. Naksuk N, Sugrue AM, Padmanabhan D, et al. Potentially modifiable factors of dofetilide-associated risk of torsades de pointes among hospitalized patients with atrial fibrillation. *J Interv Card Electrophysiol.* 2019;54:189–196.
19. Erath JW, Vamos M, Hohnloser SH. Effects of digitalis on mortality in a large cohort of implantable cardioverter defibrillator recipients: results of a long-term follow-up study in 1020 patients. *Eur Heart J Cardiovasc Pharmacother.* 2016;2:168–174.
20. Guerra F, Romandini A, Barbarossa A, et al. Ranolazine for rhythm control in atrial fibrillation: a systematic review and meta-analysis. *Int J Cardiol.* 2017;227:284–291.
21. Koruth JS, Lala A, Pinney S, et al. The clinical use of ivabradine. *J Am Coll Cardiol.* 2017;70:1777–1784.
22. Sanders P, Elliott AD, Linz D. Upstream targets to treat atrial fibrillation. *J Am Coll Cardiol.* 2017;70:2906–2908.

Electrotherapy

23. Pluymaekers N, Dudink E, Luermans J, et al. Early or delayed cardioversion in recent-onset atrial fibrillation. *N Engl J Med.* 2019;380:1499–1508.
24. Houmsse M, Daoud EG. Biophysics and clinical utility of irrigated-tip radiofrequency catheter ablation. *Expert Rev Med Devices.* 2012;9:59–70.
25. Andrade JG, Dubuc M, Guerra PG, et al. The biophysics and biomechanics of cryoballoon ablation. *Pacing Clin Electrophysiol.* 2012;35:1162–1168.
26. Reddy VY, Neuzil P, Koruth JS, et al. Pulsed field ablation for pulmonary vein isolation in atrial fibrillation. *J Am Coll Cardiol.* 2019;74:315–326.
27. Katritsis DG, Zografos T, Siontis KC, et al. Endpoints for successful slow pathway catheter ablation in typical and atypical atrioventricular nodal re-entrant tachycardia: a contemporary, multicenter study. *JACC Clin Electrophysiol.* 2019;5:113–119.
28. Reissmann B, Fink T, Schluter M, et al. Catheter ablation for inappropriate sinus tachycardia: clinical outcomes of sinus node ablation. *HeartRhythm Case Rep.* 2020;6:81–85.
29. Cheniti G, Vlachos K, Meo M, et al. Mapping and ablation of idiopathic ventricular fibrillation. *Front Cardiovasc Med.* 2018;5:123.
30. Marchlinski FE, Haffajee CI, Beshai JF, et al. Long-term success of irrigated radiofrequency catheter ablation of sustained ventricular tachycardia: post-approval THERMOCOOL VT trial. *J Am Coll Cardiol.* 2016;67:674–683.
31. Cuculich PS, Schill MR, Kashani R, et al. Noninvasive cardiac radiation for ablation of ventricular tachycardia. *N Engl J Med.* 2017;377:2325–2336.

65 Supraventricular Tachycardias

JONATHAN M. KALMAN AND PRASHANTHAN SANDERS

DEFINITIONS, 1245
ASSESSMENT OF THE PATIENT WITH PALPITATIONS, 1245
SUPRAVENTRICULAR ARRHYTHMIA TYPES, 1246
Atrial Premature Complexes or Ectopic Beats, 1246

Atrial Tachycardias, 1247
Focal Atrial Tachycardia, 1247
Inappropriate Sinus Tachycardia, 1251
Atrial Flutter or Macroreentrant Atrial Tachycardia, 1252
Paroxysmal Supraventricular Tachycardia, 1257

DIFFERENTIAL DIAGNOSIS OF WIDE COMPLEX TACHYCARDIA, 1270
REFERENCES, 1270

DEFINITIONS

The 2015 American College of Cardiology/American Heart Association/Heart Rhythm Society (ACC/AHA/HRS) guidelines[1] defined supraventricular tachycardia (SVT) as:

An umbrella term used to describe tachycardias (atrial and/or ventricular rates in excess of 100 bpm at rest), the mechanism of which involves tissue from the His bundle or above. These SVTs include inappropriate sinus tachycardia, atrial tachycardia (including focal and multifocal AT), macroreentrant AT (including typical atrial flutter), junctional tachycardia, atrioventricular nodal reentrant tachycardia (AVNRT), and various forms of accessory pathway-mediated reentrant tachycardias (AVRT).

They further define paroxysmal SVT (PSVT) as: "A clinical syndrome characterized by the presence of a regular and rapid tachycardia of abrupt onset and termination. These features are characteristic of AVNRT or AVRT, and, less frequently, AT. PSVT represents a subset of SVT."

ASSESSMENT OF THE PATIENT WITH PALPITATIONS

When a patient complains of palpitations, this can reflect a broad range of differing symptoms that will frequently point to the correct diagnosis. For example, some patients may simply develop a subjective awareness of their heartbeat, which is often described as a slow forceful beating. Frequently these symptoms will be most obvious at night and will often be reported while lying on the left-hand side presumably as the cardiac apex is felt more clearly against the chest wall.

Symptoms of ectopic beats are most usually reported as a skipped beat associated with a strange sensation in the throat or an impulse to cough. This may be repetitive, and patients can often describe the frequency of these (every third beat, etc.). The symptoms may occasionally be associated with transient light-headedness and shortness of breath, although these are usually mild and momentary. If repetitive, the symptoms may be described as lasting for hours and it is important to ascertain whether this is a continuous rapid arrhythmia lasting for hours or alternately intermittent symptoms coming and going over hours. Many patients with ectopic beats, including high-burden ectopy, are completely asymptomatic, and the reason for this symptom variance remains unclear.

Symptomatic sinus tachycardia produces regular palpitations with heart rate generally in the range of 120 to 130 bpm, although it can be much faster depending on the underlying cause. Onset of symptoms in inappropriate sinus tachycardia (IAST) may be gradual or sudden as patients may become aware of sinus tachycardia only when a particular heart rate is reached. Termination is gradual usually over many minutes, and episodes can last for hours. Patients may feel breathless on minor exertion, mildly light-headed, and fatigued. Symptoms can overlap with those of SVT.

SVT is usually described as sudden in onset with rapid racing (often too fast to count) with a sensation that the heart is trying to beat out of the chest. The episodes may be triggered by sudden movements such as sudden running for the bus or by bending and standing up. Episodes may last continuously from minutes to hours and terminate suddenly. They may respond to vagal maneuvers. SVT may be associated with transient light-headedness at onset, which is occasionally severe and resulting in presyncope, although syncope is unusual. Accompanying symptoms include anxiety as a secondary phenomenon, although some patients (particularly women) have been given an erroneous diagnosis of panic attacks or primary anxiety disorder. Patients may also become breathless and develop chest discomfort during prolonged episodes. Polyuria may be reported during and early after SVT episodes due to release of atrial natriuretic peptide at these elevated rates. Symptoms are generally more severe in older age-groups, although rate is also an important determinant of symptom severity. Recurrent short bursts (seconds to minutes) of rapid palpitations with normal rhythm interspersed suggests an automatic focal AT. Prolonged irregularly irregular racing points to atrial fibrillation (AF). Sudden syncope is rarely associated with SVT and when arrhythmic in origin generally suggests ventricular tachycardia (VT) or a significant pause as a result of sinus arrest or atrioventricular (AV) block.

The physical examination may be helpful in demonstrating findings associated with valvular pathology, cardiac failure, or thyrotoxicosis or when an incessant or persistent arrhythmia is present. Investigations include a 12-lead electrocardiogram (ECG) in sinus rhythm. This will determine whether preexcitation is present and identify P wave abnormalities and bundle branch block patterns.

Routine blood tests include biochemistry and thyroid function tests. When patients present to an emergency department with tachyarrhythmias, troponin will often be elevated. In this setting, this is a nonspecific response frequently secondary to the tachycardia and not necessarily indicative of obstructive coronary artery disease.[2] An echocardiogram is usually performed to evaluate ventricular function and atrial size and to rule out significant valvular pathology.

Most important is documentation of the tachycardia. This may involve finding ambulance traces or emergency department ECGs. For patients without documented arrhythmias, a range of monitoring strategies are available and may be chosen according to symptom frequency and patient preference. When symptoms occur daily, simple 24-hour Holter monitoring will obtain the diagnosis. Documentation of onset and termination of the arrhythmia may add important diagnostic information. For example, an IAST may have gradual increase in rate over 30 seconds to several minutes, whereas a focal AT usually has sudden onset with a "warm-up" over several beats. For less frequent episodic events, a range of wearable technologies or devices used with a smart phone are now available and this has greatly facilitated documentation of the arrhythmia (see Chapter 61). Alternative approaches include more prolonged monitoring of up to 30 days with a variety of different devices of variable patient tolerability. An implanted loop recorder may be considered in the unusual event that documentation cannot be obtained with simpler monitoring approaches. Finally, in patients with classic symptoms of sudden onset and offset tachycardia highly suggestive of SVT, documentation is not essential and an initial approach of a diagnostic electrophysiologic study (EPS) with a view to catheter ablation may be considered.

SUPRAVENTRICULAR ARRHYTHMIA TYPES

Atrial Premature Complexes or Ectopic Beats

Atrial premature complexes are very common in the general population. In an unselected population over the age of 50, the average frequency was approximately 1 or 2 per hour and increased with each decade of life.[3] Increase in atrial ectopy occurred not only in relation to advancing age but also in association with other cardiovascular disease. Regular physical exercise was protective. Transient increase in atrial ectopics may occur in response to intercurrent illness, in stress and anxiety, and in response to alcohol and caffeine.

Usually ectopic beats are asymptomatic but may be associated with a range of sensations, including a heightened awareness of the heart beating, the sensation that the heart has given an extra beat or missed a beat, a fluttering sensation in the chest or throat, and occasionally a momentary feeling of faintness or dizziness.

A diagnosis is generally made with ECG monitoring with documentation that symptoms occur corresponding with atrial ectopic events.

Although in the vast majority of patients atrial premature complexes are benign, the seminal paper by Haissaguerre et al. described the triggering of AF by focal atrial ectopics originating from sleeves of myocardium within the pulmonary veins.[4] Subsequent studies showed that patients with both paroxysmal and persistent forms of AF demonstrate an increased atrial ectopic burden when compared with a control population. Furthermore, increased premature atrial complex (PAC) burden is associated with incident AF risk both in the general population and in patients with cryptogenic stroke. Longitudinal studies have described an association between excess PACs (>30/hour or runs of nonsustained AT >20 beats) and the outcomes of incident AF, stroke, and death. In 15-year follow-up, patients with excess PACS and a CHADs-VASc score of 2 or greater demonstrated an annual stroke risk comparable to that of patients with AF.[5] A number of opinions have suggested that atrial ectopy and AF may be markers of an underlying atrial myopathy that is the primary determinant of stroke risk and adverse outcomes.[6,7] Isolated case reports have indicated that frequent PACs (20% to 40% daily burden) also may be associated with development of a reversible cardiomyopathy.[8]

Despite the association of frequent atrial ectopy with potential for adverse events, to date there is no evidence that treatment of isolated atrial ectopy reduces risk or improves long-term outcomes. Therefore, the only indication for treatment of PACs is when they are sufficiently symptomatic. The vast majority of patients with atrial ectopics will not require any treatment other than reassurance. In those with severe symptoms, treatment would initially involve a beta blocker or calcium channel antagonist. Occasionally it might be appropriate to prescribe an antiarrhythmic medication such as flecainide. In highly symptomatic patients unresponsive to or intolerant of medication, catheter ablation may be considered when the ectopic burden is high and the atrial ectopic is unifocal in origin.

The appearance of an atrial ectopic on an ECG is characterized by an early atrial beat with a P wave morphology different from that of the sinus beat. However, the P wave is frequently inscribed within the preceding T wave and the morphology therefore unclear (Fig. 65.1). An atrial ectopic may be conducted normally, with prolongation of the PR interval and possibly aberrancy or widening of the QRS but also may be nonconducted. A nonconducted or blocked atrial ectopic is one of the most common causes of an unexpected pause on an ECG (Fig. 65.1A,

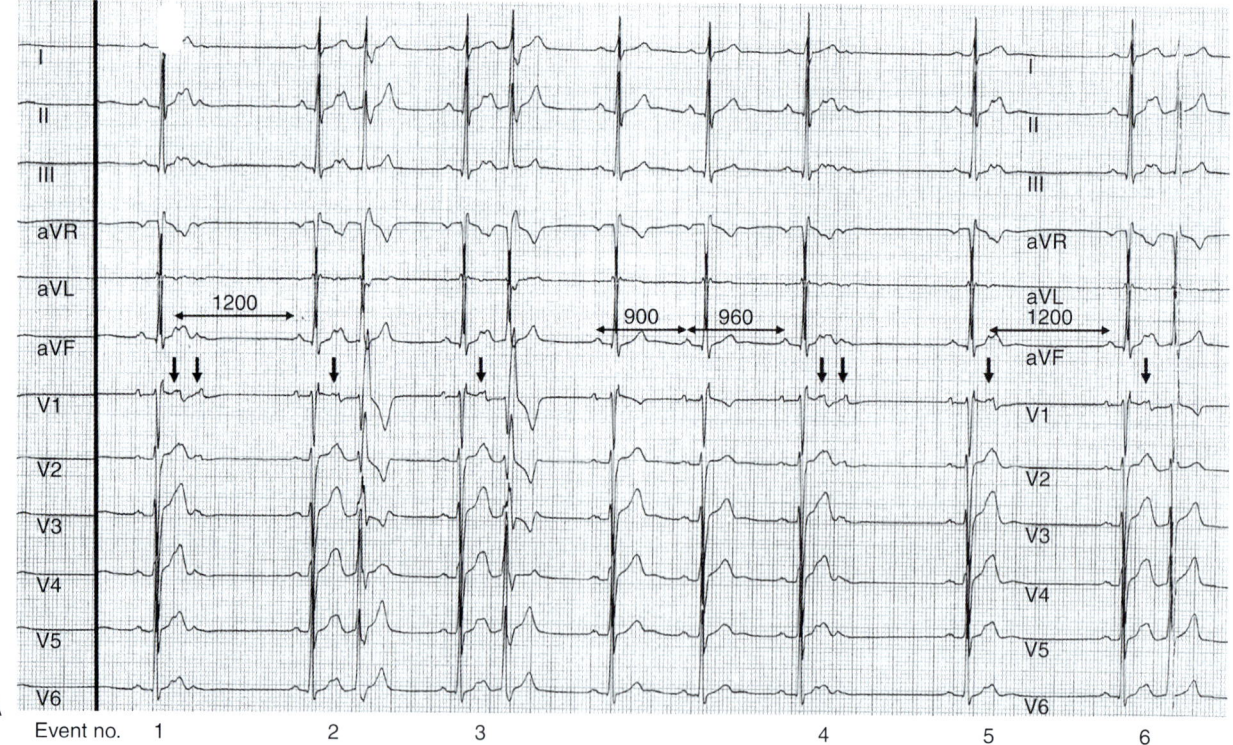

FIGURE 65.1 A, Continuous 12-lead ECG with frequent atrial ectopics. Events 1 and 4 demonstrate 2 atrial ectopic beats in quick succession; the first is inscribed within the initial component of the T wave and the P wave morphology is obscured. The second occurs immediately after the T wave, and the morphology is very different from the sinus morphology. This is particularly evident in lead III and V₁. Neither of these two ectopics in event 1 or 4 are conducted, creating the appearance of an unexpected sinus pause. Similarly, event 5 has a single ectopic beat inscribed within the T wave, which is nonconducted and also creates an apparently unexpected pause. Close inspection of the T wave immediately before the pause clearly demonstrates the mechanism. The pause duration from ectopic to next sinus beat (1200 msec) is longer than a single sinus interval (900 msec). This longer interval includes the conduction time into the node, depolarization and reset of the node possibly with overdrive suppression, and then conduction out from the node (sinoatrial conduction time). Note that in event 1 the pause from first ectopic to the following sinus beat is also 1200 msec, indicating that the second ectopic beat has not resulted in further sinus node reset. This is presumably because the perinodal region was refractory as a result of the immediately preceding ectopic. In events 2, 3, and 6, the ectopic is conducted with a prolonged PR interval as the early ectopic is conducted to the AV node while still relatively refractory and therefore decremental or slow conduction occurs. The QRS complex in these conducted beats demonstrates right bundle branch block aberrancy. The long preceding interval produced by the pause is followed by a short interval, which renders the right bundle branch refractory at that moment. Note that the right bundle branch has a longer refractory period than that of the left bundle branch.

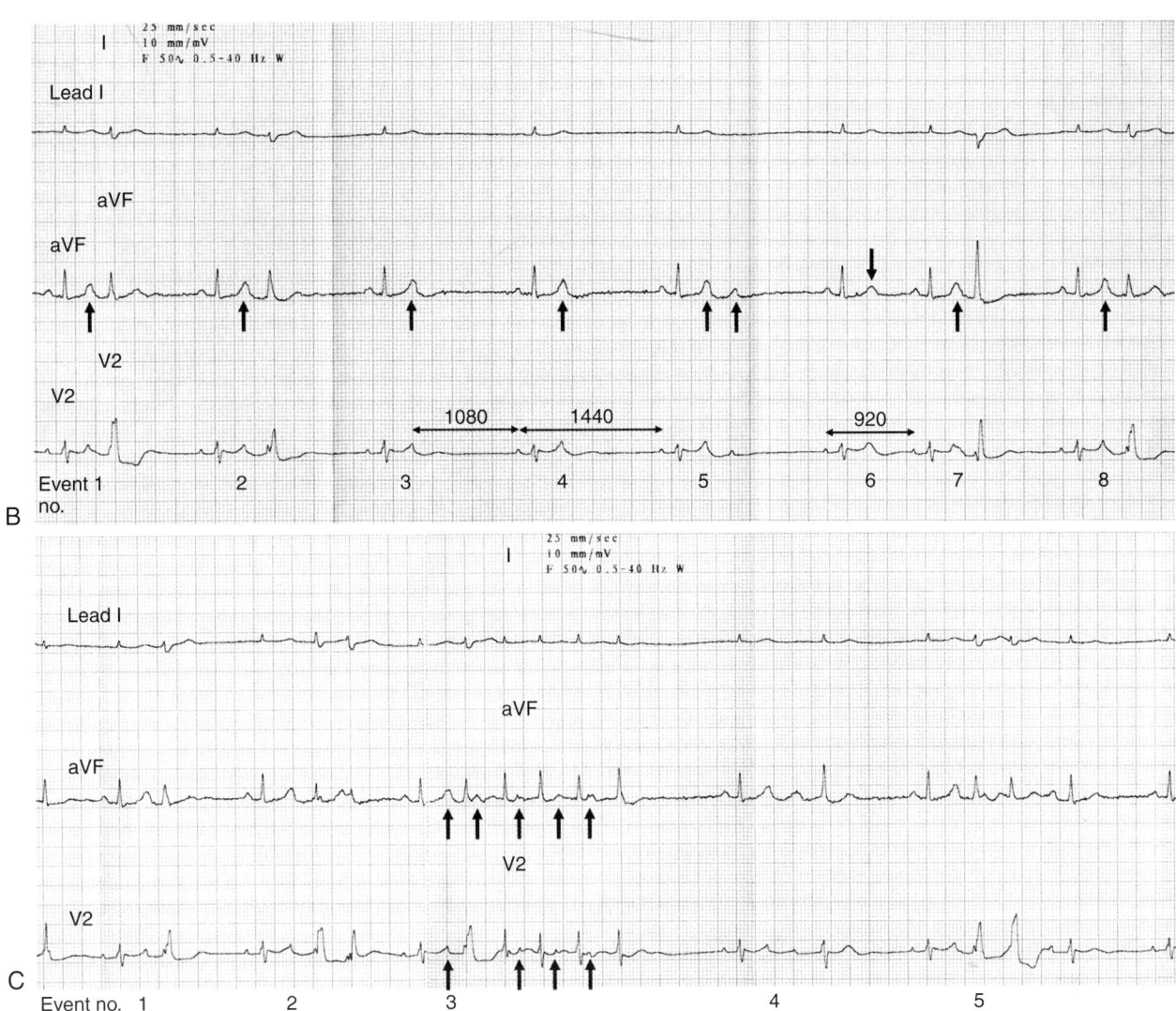

FIGURE 65.1–cont'd B, Continuous 3-lead rhythm strip with high burden of atrial ectopics. In events 1, 2, 7, and 8, the ectopic beat is conducted with a long PR interval and right bundle branch aberrancy. In events 3, 4, and 5 there is a nonconducted atrial ectopic beat occurring within the T wave, creating a pause. The bigeminal pattern of atrial ectopy therefore creates the impression of a marked sinus bradycardia with apparent sinus interval of 1440 msec. In event 5, a second atrial premature beat occurs immediately after the T wave and the visible morphology indicates that this is different from the sinus morphology (best appreciated in aVF). Event 6 is the only normal T wave appearance because there is no inscribed atrial ectopic (*downward pointing arrow*). The sinus interval following the absence of an atrial premature beat is 920 msec rather than the apparent interval of 1440 msec. The interval between the nonconducted atrial premature beat and the following sinus beat (1080 msec) is longer than the sinus interval of 920 msec. **C,** Continuous three-lead ECG in event 1, an atrial premature beat that conducts with a long PR interval and right bundle branch block (RBBB) aberrancy. In events 2, 3, 4, and 5 there are short (variable duration) runs of nonsustained atrial tachycardia. Again we see conduction with a long PR interval and some beats showing RBBB aberrancy. In event 3 the P wave preceding each QRS complex can be clearly seen when examining both aVF and V$_2$ (*arrows*). This constellation of arrhythmias is frequently observed on monitoring in patients with paroxysmal atrial fibrillation.

B). Nonconducted ectopics in a bigeminal pattern may create the appearance of marked sinus bradycardia (see Fig. 65.1B). Frequent atrial ectopics accompanied by recurrent bursts of nonsustained AT indicates a very active focal trigger or triggers and is a pattern commonly seen in patients who also demonstrate paroxysms of AF (Fig. 65.1C). This is usually because of activity originating in the pulmonary vein sleeves.

Atrial Tachycardias

The term *atrial tachycardia* encompasses a range of different tachycardias that originate in the atria and do not require the participation of the AV node for maintenance of the arrhythmia.[9] These tachycardias have differing arrhythmia mechanisms and are often related to anatomic structures.[9,10] Broadly AT can be considered to be in one of two major categories: focal or macroreentry. Focal AT has been defined as atrial activation starting rhythmically at a small area (focus) from which it spreads out centrifugally.[11] Impulses occur with a given periodicity separated by a quiescent interval recorded on the surface ECG as an isoelectric period. The main tenet of this definition is that, in contrast to activation seen in macroreentrant AT (also termed *atrial flutter* [AFL]), atrial activity originates from a focal location. In macroreentry, activation occurs around a large central obstacle, such as an anatomic structure or region of scarring; electrical activity can be recorded throughout the *entire* atrial cycle length. These include typical AFL and other well-characterized macroreentrant circuits in the right and left atrium, which are also frequently referred to as types of "atypical AFL." More recently a third category of AT has been described although not routinely included in all classifications. These have been termed "small circuit" or "localized" reentry (see later).[12]

Focal Atrial Tachycardia

Focal AT is a form of SVT characterized by regular, organized atrial activity with discrete P waves and typically an isoelectric segment between P waves (Fig. 65.2, *left*). However, when focal AT rate is particularly rapid, an isoelectric interval may not be apparent (Fig. 65.2, *right*). Focal AT may display some irregularity particularly at onset ("warm-up") and termination ("cool-down"),[1] usually occurring over several beats. Atrial mapping reveals a focal point of origin. Mechanisms of focal AT include abnormal or enhanced automaticity (abnormal impulse initiation in an individual or cluster of myocytes),

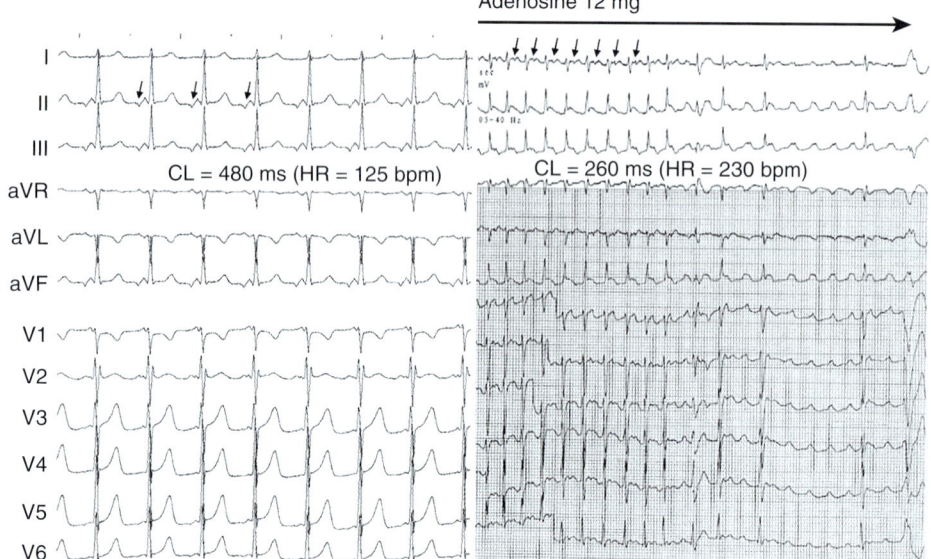

FIGURE 65.2 Focal atrial tachycardia. *Left,* Heart rate is 125 bpm and there is a P wave easily visible before each QRS preceded by a clear isoelectric interval. The P wave morphology is unusual, most notably in the inferior leads, where the pattern demonstrates a biphasic negative-positive appearance incompatible with a sinus origin. This patient (a 22-year-old woman) had an incessant tachycardia originating in the left septal region. This tachycardia falls into the group of long RP tachycardia. *Right,* Rapid tachycardia (heart rate 230 bpm) treated with adenosine. During 1:1 conduction to the ventricle, the P wave appears within the initial part of the T wave, which is deformed (arrows on lead I). This is therefore a short R-P tachycardia. The rapid rate coupled with delayed atrioventricular (AV) conduction at this rate is responsible for the position of the P wave within the preceding T wave. After administration of adenosine, AV conduction is blocked but the tachycardia continues uninterrupted. At this rapid rate, there appears to be almost continuous undulation (V_1 and inferior leads) resembling macroreentry. This was a focal atrial tachycardia originating in the left superior pulmonary vein. *CL,* cycle length

triggered activity (abnormal impulse initiation due to oscillations of membrane potential, termed early or delayed after-depolarizations) and reentry (when myocardial regions activated later in propagation reexcite regions that have already recovered excitability).[13] In practice, there is considerable overlap in electrophysiologic properties, and it is not always possible to be certain of the underlying mechanism during a clinical EPS. For example, tachycardias due either to reentry or to triggered activity may be initiated and terminated with programmed electrical stimulation during an EPS. Tachycardias due to enhanced automaticity and triggered activity may initiate in response to isoprenaline infusion or adrenergic stimulation and may demonstrate multiple spontaneous onsets and terminations (Fig. 65.3). The arrhythmia may also demonstrate cycle length variability (see Fig. 65.3). Finally, focal AT due to either microreentry or triggered activity may be terminated with adenosine.[10]

Epidemiology. Focal AT is the least common mechanism of PSVT, accounting for approximately 10% to 20% of patients with PSVT.[14] Focal AT has a slight preponderance in women, although this has not been a consistent finding in all studies. AT can occur across the age spectrum but gradually increases in prevalence with age and peaking between the age of 40 and 60 years.[15] Automatic AT tends to be more common in younger populations, whereas focal AT due to microreentry is more common in older populations, although many exceptions to this generalization occur. Older patients are more likely to have right-sided AT and multiple ATs.[16] The majority of patients with focal AT do not have underlying structural heart disease or atrial abnormalities, but focal AT may also occur in this context.

Clinical Features. Focal AT is usually manifested by atrial rates between 130 and 250 bpm but may be as low as 100 bpm or as high as 300 bpm[9] (see Fig. 65.2). In general, younger patients tend to have faster AT, with rates up to 340 bpm observed in infants. The P wave morphology is usually different from that of sinus rhythm (see Fig. 65.2), but foci arising from the region of the crista terminalis (particularly the superior crista) may have morphology consistent with a sinus origin (Fig. 65.4). The properties of the atrial focus may be similar to that of the sinus node in that they are responsive to changes in activity and autonomic tone, with the rate varying according to activity. In incessant tachycardias, rates during sleep may be up to 40 bpm less than those during waking hours.

Patients experience a variety of symptoms, including palpitations, dizziness, chest pain, dyspnea, fatigue, and presyncope.[9] Syncope is unusual unless tachycardia rates are extremely rapid or there is associated underlying structural heart disease.

Tachycardia-mediated cardiomyopathy (TMC) has been reported to occur in a small percentage of patients with incessant ATs. In a large series of patients with focal AT, the incidence of TMC was 10%. TMC occurred exclusively in the context of incessant or very frequent (almost incessant) paroxysmal tachycardia. Patients with TMC were younger, were more frequently male, and had slower tachycardias (mean rate 117 bpm). Incessant tachycardias arise from specific anatomic locations, including the right atrial (RA) and left atrial (LA) appendages (Fig. 65.5) and from the pulmonary venous ostia. Importantly, after successful ablation, left ventricular (LV) function normalizes in virtually all patients.

Embolic events and stroke have rarely been reported in patients with AT, and treatment with anticoagulation is generally not indicated.[1,13] Spontaneous remission of focal AT has been reported in both adults and children after cessation of medical therapy. In fact, the AT disappeared in 55% of patients under the age of 25, compared with just 14% of patients aged 26 or older.

Diagnosis and Differential Diagnosis
Detection of AT is usually straightforward. Most patients can be diagnosed by a routine ECG during sustained tachycardia (see Fig. 65.2). However, those with self-reverting paroxysmal AT may require monitoring for diagnosis. If symptoms are frequent, this may require a 24-hour Holter monitor and, if infrequent, various wearable monitoring technologies are available to facilitate ECG documentation if only on a single lead. It should be noted that brief (3 to 10 beats) nonsustained AT is a common finding on routine Holter recordings and is seldom associated with symptoms. Occasionally the ECG differentiation of focal AT from other forms of SVT or from macroreentrant AT may be more challenging.

Inappropriate Sinus Tachycardia versus AT
Differentiating AT from IAST on the ECG alone can at times be difficult, particularly for tachycardias originating at the superior crista terminalis. Although the P wave in AT usually has a morphology different from that of the sinus P wave (see Fig. 65.2), in which case the diagnosis will be clear, when AT arises from the superior crista terminalis these differences may be subtle (see Fig. 65.4). AT usually demonstrates an abrupt onset and termination or may warm up and cool down over 3 or 4 beats. In contrast, IAST gradually increases in rate over approximately 30 seconds to several minutes. In addition, demonstration that onset occurs with a tightly coupled P wave, particularly located in the preceding T wave, is virtually diagnostic of AT (see Fig. 65.3).

AT versus AVNRT/AVRT
The most important differentiating factor on ECG between AT and AVNRT and AVRT is the R-P relationship. Both typical AVNRT and AVRT have a short R-P interval that does not vary (the former superimposed on the QRS and the latter in the ST segment), and the P wave morphology usually cannot be clearly discerned. Although most commonly associated with a long R-P interval, AT can occur with either a short R-P interval or a long R-P interval depending on the tachycardia rate and the speed of AV nodal conduction. It can therefore mimic either AVNRT or AVRT. The ability to demonstrate "unlinking" or variability of the R to P relationship invariably indicates AT. In AT

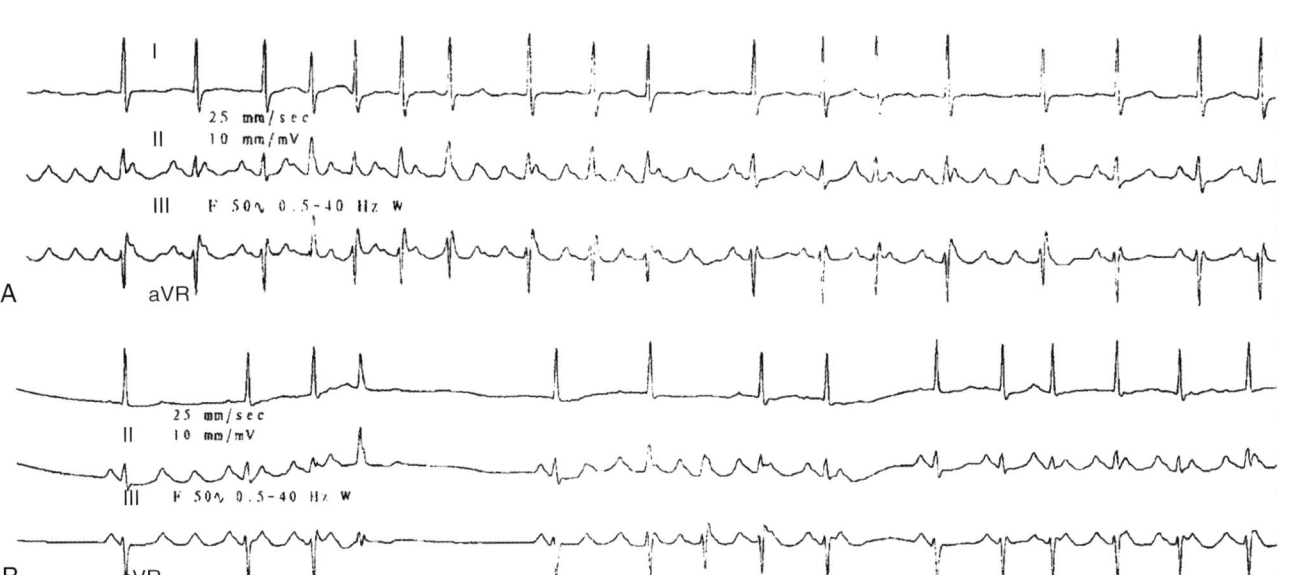

FIGURE 65.3 A, This rhythm strip resembles atrial flutter with continuous P wave undulation. However, on closer inspection, there is marked cycle length variability indicating that this is not macroreentry but rather likely to be focal. **B,** Spontaneous initiations and terminations of the arrhythmia confirming a focal mechanism related either to abnormal automaticity or triggered automaticity. This pattern is incompatible with a reentrant arrhythmia.

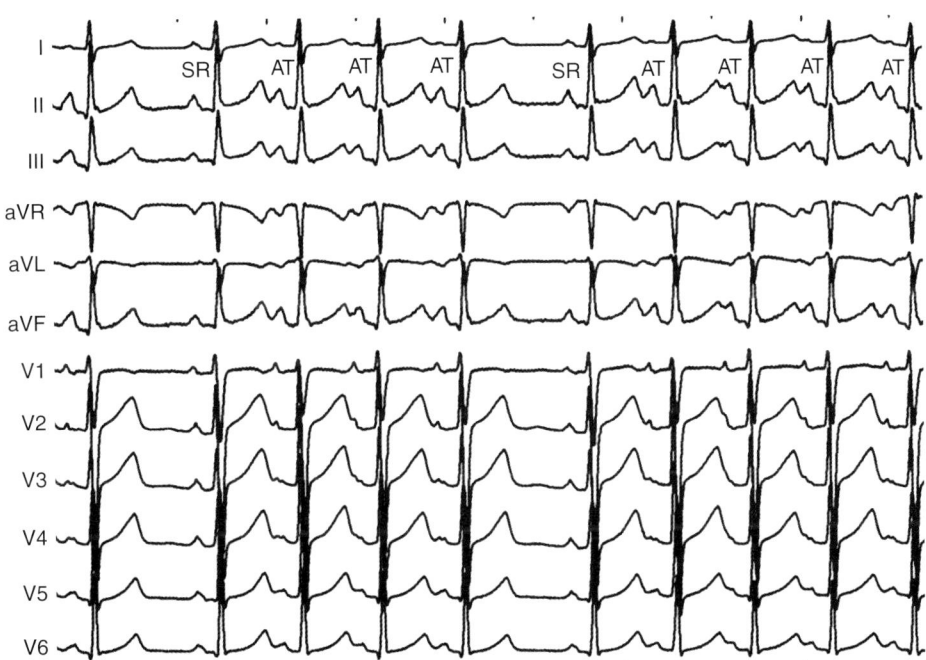

FIGURE 65.4 Continuous 12-lead ECG indicating short bursts of atrial tachycardia from the region of the superior crista terminalis. Note that the P wave morphology of the tachycardia beats (atrial tachycardia [AT]) is very similar to the morphology of the sinus beats (SR).

the R-P relationship is incidental and hence possibly variable. In AVRT and AVNRT this relationship will be constant because it is integral to the tachycardia mechanism. Another clue to the diagnosis is the presence of an inferior P wave axis. This excludes AVRT or AVNRT because it suggests an origin high in the atrium. A superiorly directed P wave vector may indicate AVRT or AVNRT or an AT focus originating from the coronary sinus ostium or annular structures. Of note, atypical AVNRT and a concealed accessory pathway with slow retrograde conduction may have long R-P intervals but have constant R-P intervals and a superior P wave axis. Automatic AT may also manifest with recurrent self-limiting bursts of tachycardia that can exhibit warm-up and cool-down phases.

Focal AT versus Macroreentrant AT

In most cases of focal AT it is possible to observe a discrete P wave with an intervening isoelectric interval (see Fig. 65.2A). However, when the atrial rate is very rapid and, if atrial conduction slowing is present, there may be no isoelectric baseline and the appearance may mimic that of macroreentrant AT (see Fig. 65.2, right). Conversely, although macroreentrant AT (including typical AFL) frequently demonstrates a continuous undulation without an isoelectric period on the ECG, patterns resembling focal AT (with an isoelectric period) also have been described. Variation in the tachycardia rate with spontaneous termination and then reinitiation is diagnostic of a focal AT, usually the result of enhanced automaticity or triggered activity (see Fig. 65.3). Spontaneous bursts of tachycardia do not occur with macroreentrant tachycardias.

The rate of the tachycardia does not help discriminate between focal and macroreentrant AT as the rate ranges of both focal AT and macroreentrant AT are too wide to be reliably used for determination of arrhythmia mechanism. The rate range of focal AT is usually between 130 and 250 bpm but may be as low as 100 bpm or as high as 300 bpm. Similarly, although macroreentrant atrial arrhythmias usually have a rate between 240 and 310 bpm, conduction delays within the circuit either due to atrial pathology or use of conduction slowing antiarrhythmics can slow the rate to less than 150 bpm.

Focal AT versus Multifocal AT versus AF

True multifocal AT is a relatively uncommon arrhythmia that occurs in the context of underlying conditions, including pulmonary disease, pulmonary hypertension, coronary disease, and valvular heart disease. However, bursts of focal AT may masquerade as multifocal AT because of the variable P wave appearance when there are varying degrees of fusion with the preceding T wave or QRS complex. Indeed, during rapid focal AT it may be quite difficult to discern a clear P wave morphology because the majority of beats are at least partially obscured by the T waves and QRS complexes unless higher grades of AV conduction block are present (Fig. 65.6). Similarly, when focal AT is fast, it has some P wave interval irregularity in cycle length, and there is varying AV conduction, the trace may superficially resemble AF, particularly if there is only a single monitor lead. A careful appraisal of the trace will generally indicate a P wave fused with the T wave visible before most conducted beats (see Fig. 65.6).

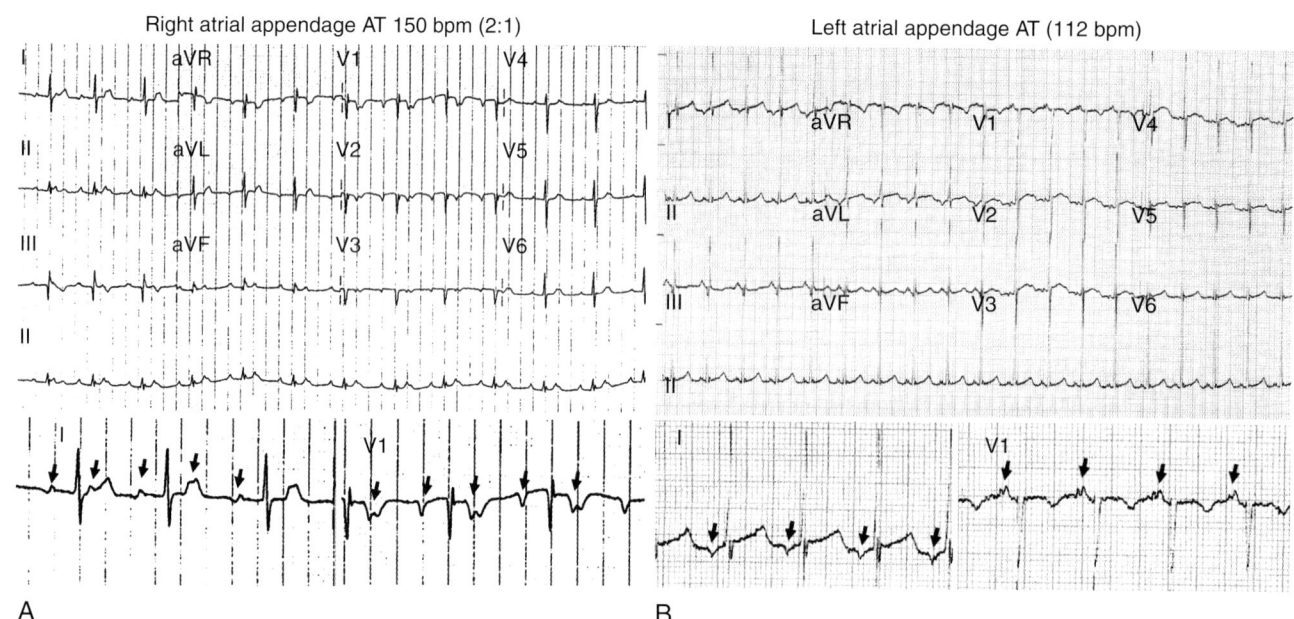

FIGURE 65.5 A, A 12-lead ECG of an incessant tachycardia originating in the right atrial appendage. The atrial rate is 150 bpm, and there is 2:1 conduction to the ventricle. The P wave is deeply inverted from V_1 to V_3 consistent with an origin in the right atrial appendage (anterior location), and lead I has an unusual biphasic negative-positive appearance inconsistent with a sinus origin. **B,** A 12-lead ECG of an incessant tachycardia originating in the left atrial appendage. The P wave morphology is characteristic, showing a broad upright and notched appearance in V_1, a similar pattern in inferior leads (especially well seen in aVF) and a deeply inverted pattern in lead I (characteristic for a left appendage origin). The incessant tachycardia at 112 bpm did not produce symptomatic palpitations, but the patient presented with heart failure due to tachycardia-mediated cardiomyopathy that was reversed after successful ablation.

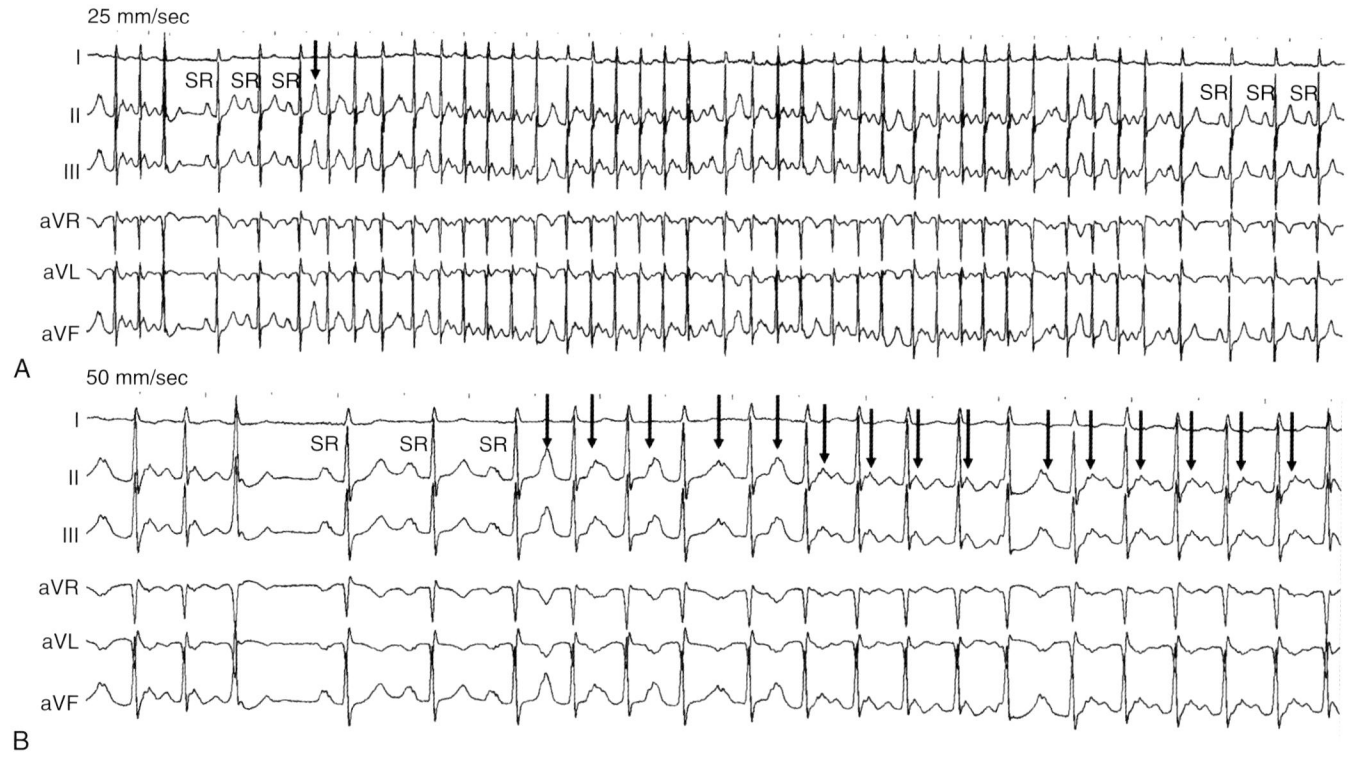

FIGURE 65.6 A, Continuous ECG at a sweep speed of 25 mm/sec; on the left there is termination of an arrhythmia followed by 3 sinus beats (SR) before onset of a rapid irregular tachycardia with a P wave on the peak of the T wave (*arrow*). At first glance this trace suggests atrial fibrillation. The arrhythmia terminates spontaneously on the right of the trace. **B,** The tachycardia initiation is shown at a faster sweep speed (50 mm/sec). It is now possible to see the P wave deforming the T wave and the tail end of the QRS throughout the burst of tachycardia ruling out atrial fibrillation. Because the P wave shows variable fusion with the T wave it is possible to think there is variation in morphology that would suggest a multifocal atrial tachycardia. In fact this was a single-focus atrial tachycardia arising in the left atrial roof.

Anatomic Distribution

Focal ATs do not occur randomly throughout the atria but rather have a characteristic anatomic distribution (Fig. 65.7). In the right atrium they tend to cluster around the crista terminalis,[17] coronary sinus ostium (CS os), para-Hisian or perinodal region, tricuspid annulus (TA), and RA appendage. In the left atrium, the majority originate from the pulmonary veins, with the mitral annulus, LA appendage, and left septum being less common. More recently, focal AT has been described originating from the noncoronary cusp of the aortic valve.[18] The specific reasons for this anatomic distribution remain speculative. For example, the crista terminalis is an area of marked anisotropy with poor transverse but rapid linear

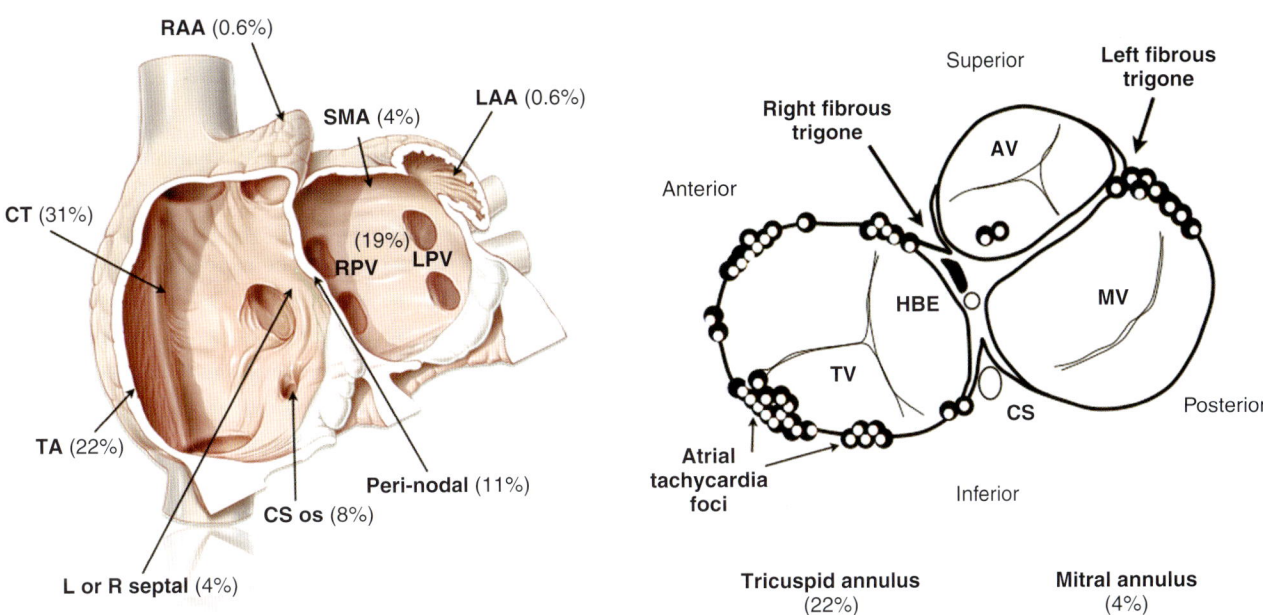

FIGURE 65.7 Anatomic distribution of focal atrial tachycardias. Approximately 75% of atrial tachycardias originate in the right atrium, with the most common locations being the crista terminalis (CT), the tricuspid annulus (TA), the coronary sinus ostium (CS os), and the perinodal region. In the left atrium, the most common location is the ostium of the pulmonary veins and the superior mitral annulus (SMA). Less common locations include the left atrial (LAA) and right atrial appendages (RAA). Tachycardias originating near the midline can sometimes be safely and successfully ablated from within the noncoronary cusp. (From Kistler PM, et al. P-Wave morphology in focal atrial tachycardia: development of an algorithm to predict the anatomic site of origin. J Am Coll Cardiol 2006;48:1010-1017.)

conduction, creating a potential substrate for reentry. In addition, the sinus node complex is located along the crista terminalis, and the presence of automatic tissue with anisotropy may favor abnormal automaticity.

In the context of this classic anatomic distribution, the P wave morphology can provide a reliable and relatively specific guide as to the likely anatomic site of focal AT origin and a number of different P wave algorithms have been proposed.[19] The important caveat is that no significant structural atrial disease is present and the patient has not had prior catheter ablation, because either of these factors may fundamentally change the shape of the P wave. In general, an upright P wave in V_1 suggests LA origin whereas a negative P wave in V1 suggests RA origin.

Sinus Node Reentry

Although the sinus node reentry arrhythmia remains as a separate entity in recent guidelines documents,[1,13] there has been some debate as to whether tachycardias due to reentry within the sinus node truly exist.[11] Sinus node reentry is clinically defined as a tachycardia that can be induced and terminated with programmed stimulation and has a P wave morphology identical or similar to that of the sinus P wave. It is now well recognized that the sinus node is not a discrete structure but rather a diffuse pacemaker complex located along the long axis of the crista terminalis. AT has been described arising from sites along the length of this structure, and it may be best to define these simply as crista terminalis AT.[11]

Management of Focal AT

Acute Management of Focal AT. Initial management of a focal AT in the emergency department might involve administration of adenosine as for other mechanisms of SVT (6 to 12 mg intravenously). For focal AT, the arrhythmia may either terminate, transiently slow, and then return to the pre-adenosine rate or continue with AV block and unmasked P waves (see Fig. 65.2). If unsuccessful, intravenous beta blockers or calcium channel blockers (verapamil or diltiazem) may be effective in hemodynamically stable patients. If ineffective, antiarrhythmic agents such as flecainide, ibutilide, or amiodarone may be considered. Alternatively, if drug treatment is unsuccessful or the patient is hemodynamically unstable, synchronized DC cardioversion may be used. This would be inappropriate for automatic forms of tachycardia with recurrent bursts of tachycardia separated by 1 or more sinus beats. Similarly, for incessant automatic tachycardias, there is a high probability of recurrence of the arrhythmia after cardioversion.

Chronic Management. Catheter ablation is recommended as a first-line therapy in patients with symptomatic focal AT as an alternative to pharmacologic therapy (class 1).[1,13] Catheter ablation for the most part involves the use of a three-dimensional mapping system to identify the earliest site of atrial activation (Fig. 65.8). Mapping will generally indicate a site from which there is centrifugal spread of activation away from that site. Contemporary ablation series indicate a high procedural success rate in excess of 85% with a very low risk of major complications. The caveat is that for some automatic or triggered forms of focal AT, on occasion all attempts at inducing the arrhythmia may be unsuccessful rendering mapping and ablation impossible on that day.

When catheter ablation is not preferred or not appropriate, pharmacologic management may be considered. However, there are no long-term, randomized, placebo-controlled studies on the use of antiarrhythmic therapy in focal AT. The available studies are observational, with small numbers and mostly conducted over a decade ago. There is widespread agreement that antiarrhythmic agents have low efficacy in the treatment of focal AT.

When drug therapy is preferred, beta blockers or non-dihydropyridine calcium channel blockers (verapamil or diltiazem) may be considered. In patients without structural or ischemic heart disease, propafenone or flecainide also may be considered. Less commonly, agents such as sotalol, amiodarone, or ivabradine have been used.

Inappropriate Sinus Tachycardia

IAST is defined as an elevated heart rate of greater than 100 bpm at rest or on minimal exertion out of keeping with the level of activity or stress.[20,21] The mean 24-hour heart rate is above 90 bpm. The diagnosis can be made when there are accompanying symptoms attributable to the elevated heart rate such as palpitations, breathlessness on minor activity, light-headedness, chest pain, and fatigue. The impact on quality of life can be substantial and is frequently associated with significant psychosocial distress.[20,21] Overwhelmingly the condition manifests in young women. Other than the symptoms that may be debilitating, IAST does not have adverse prognostic significance and reports of tachycardia-induced cardiomyopathy are extremely rare. It is important to rule out secondary causes as a critical part of the initial evaluation before the diagnosis may be considered. A broad range of secondary causes of sinus tachycardia, including anxiety, anemia,

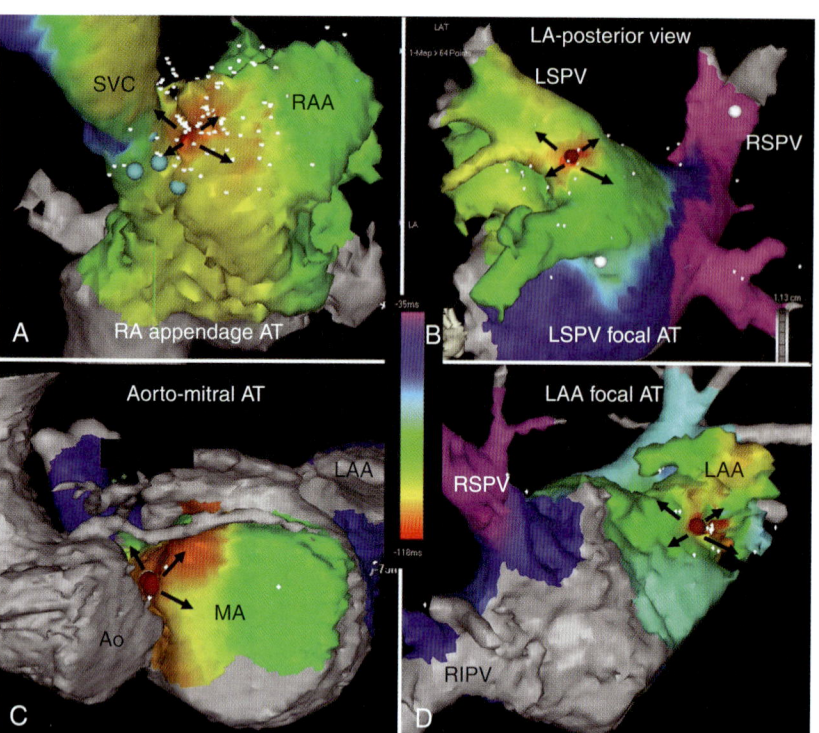

FIGURE 65.8 Three-dimensional electroanatomic maps of focal atrial tachycardia originating from four different anatomic locations. The earliest site of activation is represented by *red*, with *yellow, green, light blue, dark blue*, and *purple* representing progressively later activation. The *black arrows* indicate centrifugal spread away from the site of focal origin where ablation was successful in eliminating the tachycardia. **A,** Origin at the superior base of the right atrial appendage (RAA). **B,** Origin from the posterior inferior ostium of the left superior pulmonary vein. **C,** Origin from the aortomitral continuity. **D,** Origin from the anterior base of the left atrial appendage (LAA). *Ao,* Aortic root; *LA,* left atrium; *LSPV,* left superior pulmonary vein; *MA,* mitral annulus; *RIPV,* right inferior pulmonary vein; *RSPV,* right superior pulmonary vein; *SVC,* superior vena cava.

Atrial Flutter or Macroreentrant Atrial Tachycardia

Epidemiology

Data indicate that AFL is one of the most common cardiac arrhythmias in humans, with an estimated prevalence of 190,000 people in the United States in 2005. Similar to predictions for AF (Chapter 66), its prevalence is expected to increase to 440,000 by 2050 owing to the increasing aging of the population.[22] AFL often occurs in the context of structural heart disease (e.g., valvular, ischemic heart disease, cardiomyopathy) but may also manifest during an acute disease process (e.g., sepsis, myocardial infarction).

Relationship Between Atrial flutter and Atrial Fibrillation. AFL and AF have been described as two sides of the same coin.[23,24] The two arrhythmias frequently coexist clinically with documented AF in up to 75% of AFL patients. In both animal and human studies, the onset of AFL is usually preceded by a transitional period of AF. When AFL terminates it is also generally via transitional AF (Fig. 65.9). It appears that AF provides both the necessary trigger and electrophysiologic preconditions to initiate and sustain AFL. Furthermore, existing atrial remodeling, which underlies the development of AF, also promotes maintenance of AFL and development of sinus node dysfunction. In addition, antiarrhythmic agents such as flecainide, propafenone, and amiodarone, which slow atrial conduction, promote the conversion of AF to AFL. These agents slow both atrial and ventricular conduction. The atrial rate may slow to 200 to 230 bpm, potentially facilitating 1:1 AV conduction. At these rates, class 1C agents may result in slowed ventricular conduction with the appearance of a very-wide-complex tachycardia resembling VT (Fig. 65.10). It is for this reason that guidelines recommend addition of an AV nodal blocking drug when treating AF with a class 1C agent. An example of AFL with an atrial rate slowed to 230 bpm with amiodarone therapy is shown in Fig. 65.11A. The three panels of Fig. 65.11 show 1:1 conduction resembling a rapid SVT in panel A, the classic 2:1 conduction of typical flutter in panel B, and variable Wenckebach conduction in panel C.

The risk of developing AF late after a flutter ablation is high and increases with both intensity of monitoring and duration of follow-up. In some studies the likelihood of detecting AF during 2 years of follow-up reaches 50%.[25] Risk factors for developing AF after ablation of AFL include previously documented AF, impaired LV function, ischemic and other structural heart disease, and LA enlargement.

Symptoms in patients with AFL resemble those of AF, with palpitations, breathlessness, and reduction in exercise tolerance. A minority of patients with AFL may be minimally symptomatic. In the setting of 1:1 flutter, patients may experience presyncope or syncope. In addition, in the presence of persistent rapid ventricular response rates of 2:1 flutter, patients may develop a decline in LV ejection fraction due to development of a TCM. This is usually fully reversible within approximately 3 months of resumption of sinus rhythm.

Patients with AFL (whether or not AF has also been documented) are considered to have a similar thromboembolic risk to patients with AF. Therefore, recommendation regarding anticoagulation of patients with AFL reflect those for AF both in long-term management and at the time of reversion (pharmacologic, electrical, or with catheter ablation).[1,13]

Classification of Atrial Flutter

The terms *atrial flutter* and *atrial macroreentry* continue to be used interchangeably, with the use of the historical term *atrial flutter* remaining predominant. A suggested AFL classification is shown in Table 65.1, with broad division into those that are dependent on the cavo-tricuspid isthmus (CTI-dependent or typical AFL) and those that are not ("atypical" or non-CTI dependent) (Fig. 65.12). These arrhythmias classically involve reentry around a central obstacle (which may be an anatomic structure or a region of scarring) and the presence of slow conduction to facilitate perpetuation of the arrhythmia.

volume depletion, thyrotoxicosis, fever, pulmonary embolus, cardiac failure, sepsis, stimulants, and drug withdrawal must first be excluded. The heart rate in IAST is not necessarily persistently elevated, and considerable fluctuation is often present. Resting heart rates are frequently in the normal range, and diurnal variation is generally preserved. However, significant rate increases occur with minor activity and positional changes and at other times may be unexplained.[20] Heart rate increases generally occur gradually over 30 seconds to several minutes in contrast to onset of focal AT, which demonstrates sudden onset with a tightly coupled initiating beat and perhaps "warm-up" phenomenon over 2 to 3 beats. The P wave morphology of IAST reflects an origin in the region of the superior crista terminalis in the right atrium with a biphasic positive-negative appearance in V_1 and upright P waves in inferior leads and lead I. This resembles the morphology of a focal AT originating in the same anatomic region. The differential diagnosis also includes both postural orthostatic tachycardia syndrome (POTS) and physical deconditioning, which may have many overlapping features.

The mechanism of IAST is not well understood, and both intrinsic (sinus node hyperactivity) and extrinsic (related to dysautonomia or neurohormonal dysregulation) mechanisms have been suggested. A number of recent reports have described the development of inappropriate sinus tachycardia with elevated mean heart rates and reduced heart rate variability as a manifestation of post COVID-19 syndrome.[21a]

Treatment requires effective communication, support, and reassurance, which may improve outcomes. Lifestyle interventions such as exercise training and volume expansion may be helpful. Ivabradine, a selective blocker of the pacemaker current (I_f) has been found to be safe and effective in several small trials.[1,13] Addition of beta blockade to ivabradine therapy or the use of beta blockers alone may also be useful. However, beta blockers may increase postural dizziness and fatigue. Sinus node modification (catheter ablation) and surgical ablation are not recommended as a part of routine care for patients with IAST. Although these may have early effect and most patients have recurrent symptoms and even with complete surgical removal of the sinus pacemaker complex, fast rates are often generated from the junctional region and left atrium.

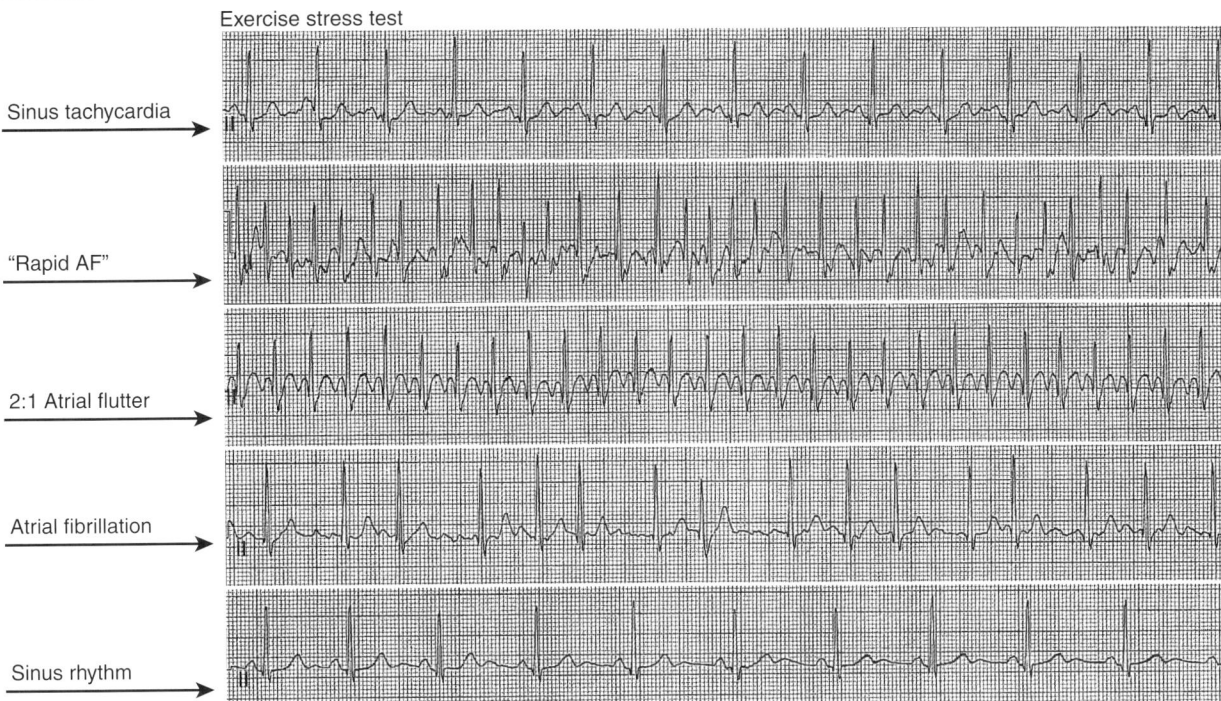

FIGURE 65.9 Exercise stress test indicating progressively: sinus tachycardia, followed by onset of atrial fibrillation (AF) with rapid ventricular response rate, followed by organization into atrial flutter with 2:1 conduction, followed by degeneration back to AF during the recovery phase, and finally termination to sinus rhythm. The example highlights the fact that AF acts as the critical initiator of atrial flutter, establishing regions of functional block and the critical unidirectional block in the flutter circuit required for initiation of the arrhythmia.

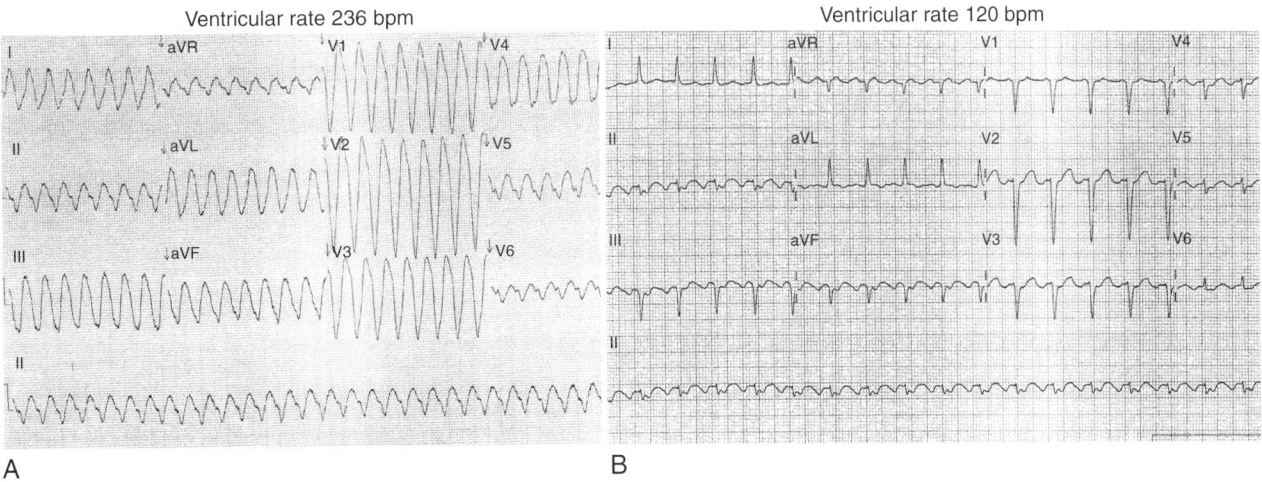

FIGURE 65.10 A patient treated with flecainide for atrial fibrillation presents with a wide-complex tachycardia at 236 bpm (**A**) and profound hemodynamic compromise. The patient spontaneously reverted to atrial flutter (AF) with 2:1 conduction with a ventricular rate almost exactly half that of the wide-complex tachycardia **B,** This provides strong evidence that the initial presenting arrhythmia was AF with 1:1 conduction to the ventricle. The profound use-dependent conduction slowing effect of flecainide in the ventricle is responsible for the extremely broad QRS complexes at this rate. This is a potentially life-threatening arrhythmia because of the risk of degeneration into sine wave ventricular tachycardia and asystole. Flecainide was discontinued, and the patient underwent ablation of the atrial flutter.

The term *atypical AFL* denotes a heterogeneous group of macroreentrant circuits that may occur in either atrium or involve both chambers and a range of anatomic boundaries (see Fig. 65.12). These circuits do not involve the CTI. Broadly, atypical AFL may occur in the context of previous atrial surgery (congenital, valvular heart disease, Maze procedures), after catheter ablation for AF (the ablation areas creating scar around which reentry occurs), cardiac transplantation, or in the absence of previous atrial surgery.

Cavo-Tricuspid Isthmus Dependent Flutter. The circuit of (typical) CTI-dependent flutter has been extensively described.[26] Typical flutter is as a macroreentrant circuit within the right atrium. It can be considered to be a broad activation wavefront rotating between the tricuspid annulus (TA) anteriorly and the crista terminalis-eustachian ridge/inferior vena cava (IVC) posteriorly (Fig. 65.12A). More recently, it is recognized that the posterior barrier may be a line of block running between the superior and IVCs.[26] The CTI is the narrowest anatomic segment of the circuit. In the most common form (approximately 90%) the circuit rotates in a counterclockwise direction when viewed in the frontal plane. In 10%, rotation is clockwise. Numerous variations of this classic circuit have been described,[26] with the most common being lower loop reentry (Fig. 65.12B) where the activation wavefront crosses the posterior line of block. Other less common variations include upper loop reentry and intra-isthmus reentry.

The ECG of typical counterclockwise AFL is characterized by the classic inferior lead flutter wave appearance ("saw-tooth" pattern) demonstrating an initial gradual downsloping segment followed by a deeply inverted component with a terminal positive component (Fig. 65.13A).

TABLE 65.1 Classification of Supraventricular Tachycardias

Atrial arrhythmias
Atrial premature beats
Sinus tachycardias
• Physiologic sinus tachycardia
• Inappropriate sinus tachycardia
• Postural orthostatic tachycardia syndrome (POTS)
• Sinus node reentry (a subset of focal AT)
Focal AT
Multifocal AT
Atrial flutter or macroreentrant atrial tachycardia (MRAT)
• Cavo-tricuspid isthmus-dependent flutter
• Typical atrial flutter—counterclockwise
• Typical atrial flutter—clockwise
• Lower loop reentry
• Intra-isthmus reentry
• Non–cavo-tricuspid isthmus-dependent macroreentry (atypical flutter)
• Right atrial atypical flutter
• Left atrial atypical flutter
Small circuit/localized atrial tachycardia
AV junctional tachycardias
Atrioventricular nodal reentrant tachycardia (AVNRT)
• Typical
• Atypical
Nonreentrant junctional tachycardia
• JET (junctional ectopic or focal junctional tachycardia)
• Other nonreentrant variants
Atrioventricular reentrant tachycardia (AVRT)
• Orthodromic (including PJRT)
• Antidromic (with retrograde conduction through the AVN or, rarely, over another pathway; includes atriofascicular pathways)
Preexcited atrial fibrillation

AT, Atrial tachycardia; *AVN*, atrioventricular node; *JET*, junctional ectopic tachycardia; *PJRT*, permanent junctional reciprocating tachycardia.

In the precordial leads, V_1 classically demonstrates an initial isoelectric component followed by an upright component. With progression across the precordial leads, the initial component becomes inverted and the second component isoelectric such that V_5 and V_6 demonstrate an inverted flutter wave. Lead I is low amplitude/isoelectric and aVL usually upright (see Fig. 65.13A). Unusual flutter wave morphologies may be seen with counterclockwise AFL and a left AFL may occasionally mimic the counterclockwise AFL appearance.[27]

It has long been recognized that typical flutter has a characteristic rate of 300 bpm. With 2:1 conduction, this equates to a ventricular rate of 150 bpm. Both the stereotypical morphology and cycle length reflect the RA anatomy that defines the circuit. However, multiple factors can significantly slow this rate and it is not unusual to see atrial rates as slow as 200 bpm for typical flutter in certain circumstances. Marked RA enlargement, atrial remodeling with significant conduction slowing, and antiarrhythmic agents which slow atrial conduction are associated with slower flutter rates.

In clockwise AFL, although the anatomic boundaries are identical to those of counterclockwise AFL, the wavefront is reversed and there is more variability in the ECG appearance. Nevertheless, characteristic features appear in the inferior leads where a broad and notched upright component is preceded by an inverted segment. V_1 is characterized by a broad negative and usually notched deflection with transition to an upright deflection in V_6 (Fig. 65.13B).

Non Cavo-Tricuspid Isthmus–Dependent Flutter (Atypical Atrial Flutter). Atypical AFL encompasses a range of macroreentrant atrial arrhythmias that are not dependent on the CTI. They have markedly varied ECG characteristics (Fig. 65.13C), and the flutter wave morphology is generally not particularly useful for determining the circuit location, although some broad generalizations can be made. Atypical flutter may occur primarily in the right or the left atrium. When the V_1 flutter wave is deeply inverted, this is highly likely to represent a right atrial circuit. Conversely, when the V_1 flutter wave is upright, this generally indicates an LA circuit. However, many variations exist and these findings lack sensitivity and specificity. Occasionally, atypical flutter may present ECG characteristics suggesting an isthmus-dependent mechanism. Similarly, the atrial rate in atypical flutter has wide limits (120 to 300 bpm) depending on the underlying circuit and pathology).

AFL is classically described as showing a continuously undulating appearance of the flutter wave on the 12-lead ECG, reflecting continuous atrial activation. This distinguishes macroreentry from focal AT, which typically demonstrates discrete P waves separated by an isoelectric interval. Although this is generally true of CTI-dependent flutter, in patients with atypical flutter, extensive atrial scarring may result in extremely low-amplitude flutter morphology and the appearance of either discrete P waves or very-low-amplitude P waves. Conversely, when focal AT is very rapid (e.g., >250 bpm), the P waves may appear to show continuous undulation.

The pathology underlying atypical flutter is highly variable, and these circuits may occur in the context of (1) prior corrective atrial surgery (congenital heart disease [CHD], valvular heart disease, after a Maze procedure or cardiac transplantation),[28] (2) previous AF ablation, (3) advanced atrial disease associated with atrial enlargement (these patients frequently have underlying pathologies such as heart failure [systolic or diastolic] or unoperated valvular heart disease such as severe mitral regurgitation[29]), or (4) in patients with normal atrial size and without an obvious underlying pathologic condition. In these patients, spontaneous scarring of unknown cause may be found at the time of atrial mapping. These circuits have particularly been described in the RA free wall.[30]

The circuits involved in atypical (non–isthmus dependent) AFL are highly variable and involve a range of anatomic boundaries. These might be anatomic structures, surgical scars, or regions of low voltage and slowed conduction. Stereotypical anatomic locations associated with certain underlying pathologic conditions or procedures have been defined. These include surgical repair of complex CHD such as Mustard or Senning repair, Fontan repair, or simpler atrial surgeries such as atrial septal defect (ASD) repair (Fig. 65.12E). Mitral valve surgery (repair or replacement) has been associated with a high late incidence of both typical and atypical flutter.[31] In patients with prior atrial surgery, circuits particularly involve atriotomy scars and it is important to review operative reports to ascertain the nature of atrial access incisions. The circuits associated with different access incisions vary accordingly. In patients with prior LA ablation, circuits may be around the pulmonary veins (roof dependent) or around the mitral annulus (mitral isthmus dependent). Frequently both circuits may occur in an individual patient (Fig. 65.14). Dual-loop or figure-of-8 reentry has been described when there are two simultaneous circuits. This may occur in either the left atrium (Fig. 65.15) or the right atrium (Fig. 65.16) and is not uncommon in the context of prior AF ablation or prior atrial surgery.[29,30]

Small Circuit Reentry. As noted earlier, a third category of AT termed *small circuit reentry* has been increasing recognized in the era of high-density three-dimensional mapping. These reentrant circuits occur in a localized region with a diameter of 1 to 2 cm; the hallmark is that the entire circuit can be recorded on a single catheter with a high density of electrodes in this specific region (Fig. 65.17). These circuits generally occur in the context of advanced atrial remodeling, and although they have been recognized across a range of pathologies they are most commonly observed in patients with a history of persistent AF, atrial enlargement, and prior AF ablation. It is important to recognize that these circuits are not necessarily due to proarrhythmia created by prior ablation but rather reflect regions of advanced atrial remodeling with markedly slowed conduction, which is a necessary prerequisite to stabilize these small circuits.[12,32]

Treatment

Acute Management. For patients who are hemodynamically unstable, synchronized cardioversion is indicated. For hemodynamically stable patients, DC cardioversion is also preferred if trained personnel are available. Alternatively, intravenous ibutilide or oral dofetilide may be trialed. These should be administered in hospital with careful monitoring for the potential risk of ventricular proarrhythmia. This risk is increased in patients with impaired LV function.

For patients with implanted dual-chamber devices (pacemaker or defibrillator) attempts at high-rate atrial overdrive pacing may be considered if appropriate expertise is available.

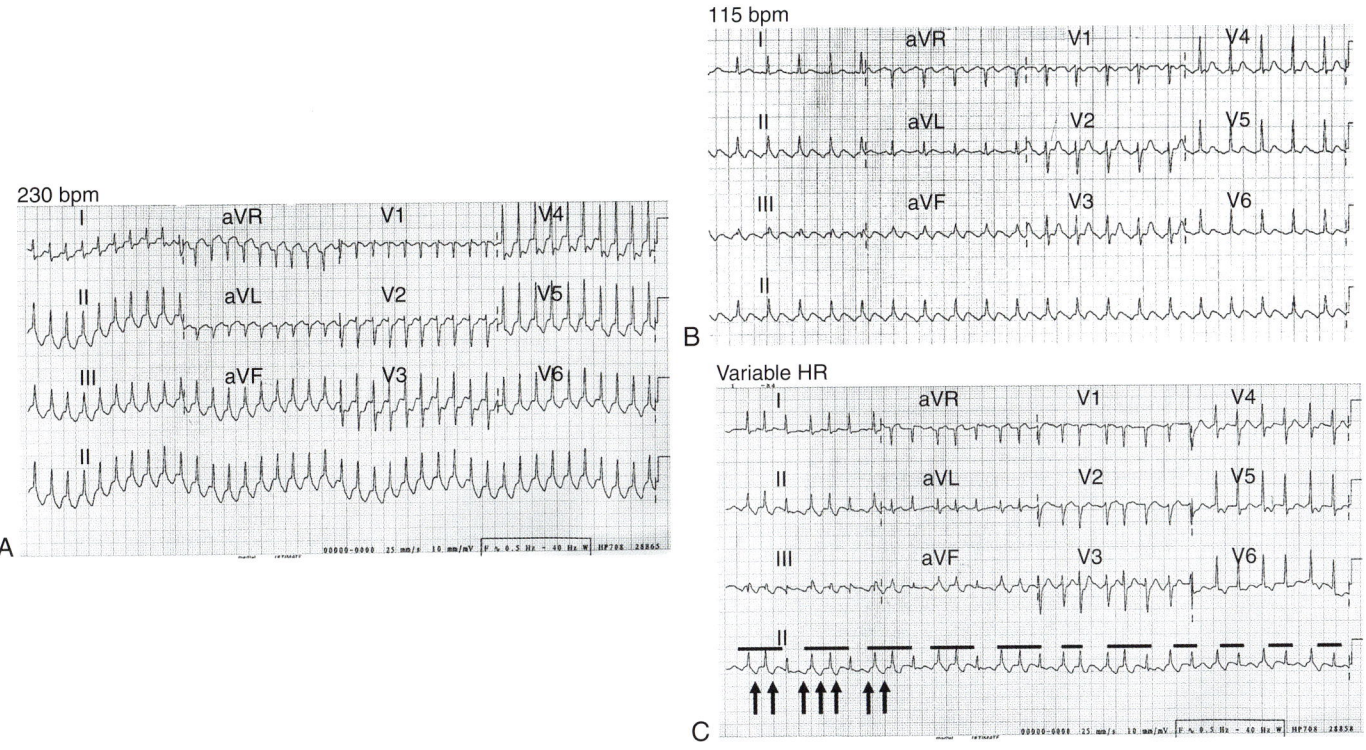

FIGURE 65.11 A, Atrial flutter (AF) with 1:1 conduction. Atrial rate is slowed due to amiodarone facilitating 1:1 atrioventricular nodal conduction with a narrow QRS. **B,** Typical AF with 2:1 conduction. **C,** Typical AF with variable Wenckebach-type conduction. The *horizontal lines* highlight the grouped beating of Wenckebach conduction. The *arrows* indicate the flutter waves.

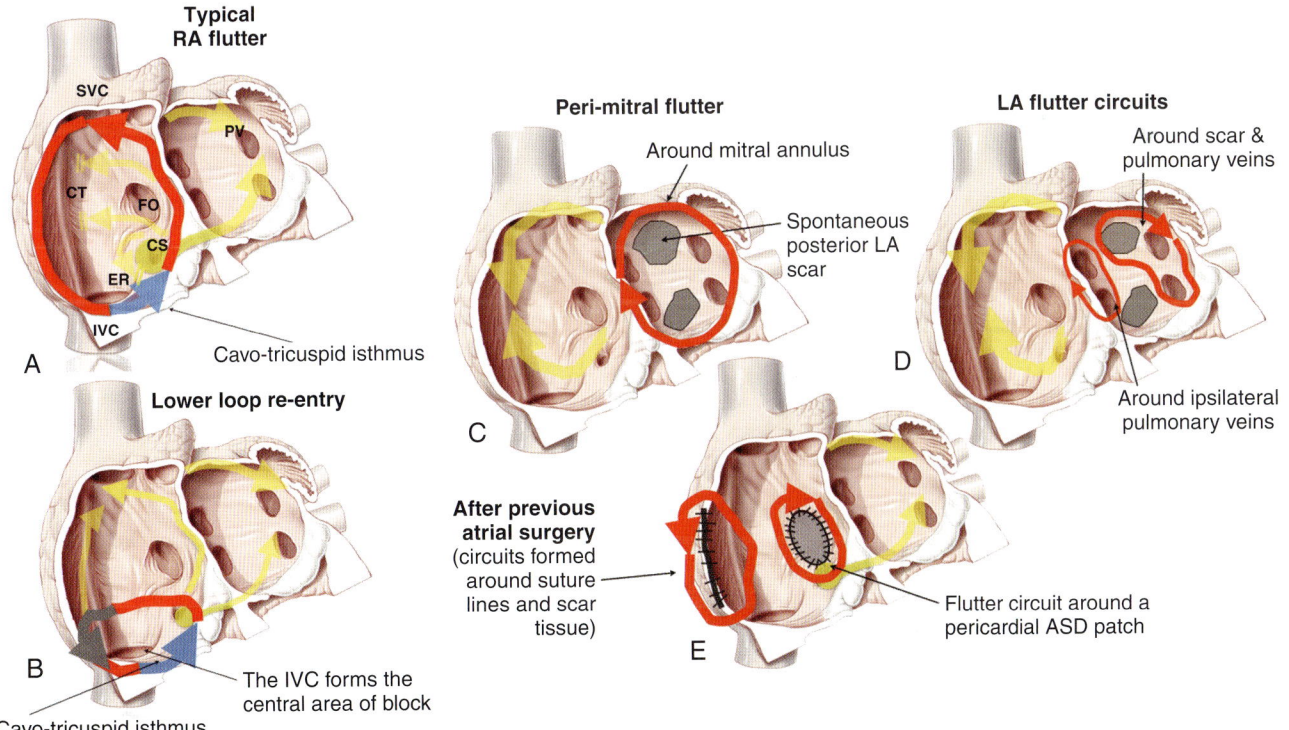

FIGURE 65.12 Examples of different types of atrial macroreentry or atrial flutter (AF). **A,** Typical counterclockwise AF confined within the right atrium. *Blue arrow* indicates conduction through the cavo-tricuspid isthmus and the *red arrow* completion of the circuit around the right atrium. The wavefront is constrained between the tricuspid annulus anteriorly (cutaway in this image), the posterior line of block formed by the crista terminalis (CT), and the continuation into the eustachian ridge (ER). The left atrium and the posterior right atrium are passively activated (*yellow arrows*) and do not form part of the circuit. **B,** Lower loop reentry with the circuit cutting across the posterior line of block to complete the circuit (*gray arrow*). **C,** Perimitral valve flutter with a region of posterior spontaneous scarring. **D,** Examples of other left atrial macroreentrant circuit with one around the left-sided pulmonary veins and an area of scarring in the posterior left atrium. The other is around the right-sided pulmonary veins. This may occur in an atrium with significant remodeling and conduction slowing or may occur as a result of prior ablation. **E,** Circuits after prior atrial surgery. Most macroreentrant circuits late after atrial septal defect (ASD) repair are typical cavo-tricuspid isthmus–dependent flutter or occur around the atrial incision in the free wall. Circuits around a septal patch are less common. In the current era, most ASDs are closed with a percutaneously placed closure device. *CS,* Coronary sinus ostium; *FO,* fossa ovalis; *IVC,* inferior vena cava; *PV,* pulmonary veins; *SVC,* superior vena cava. (From Lee G, et al. Catheter ablation of atrial arrhythmias: state of the art. Lancet 2012;380(9852):1509-1519.)

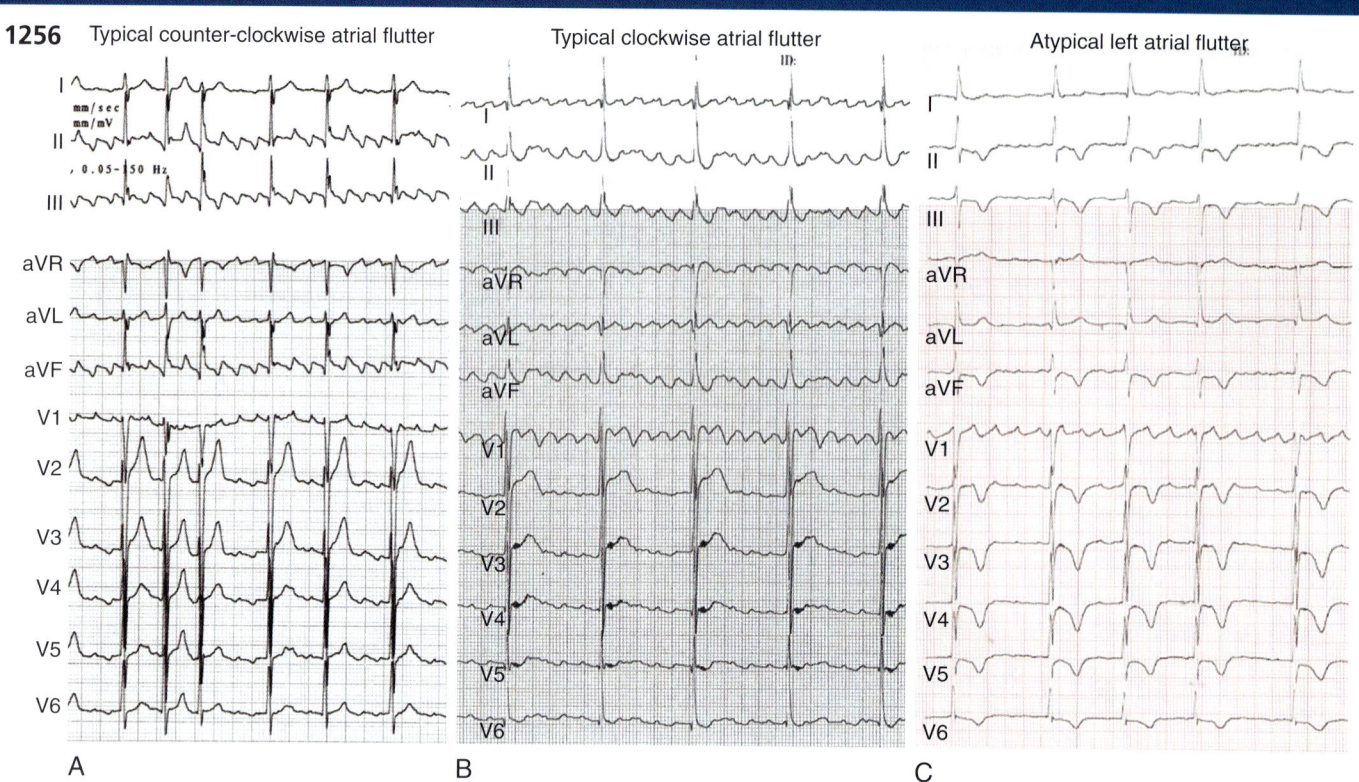

FIGURE 65.13 Variants of atrial flutter. **A,** ECG of typical counterclockwise atrial flutter (AFL). **B,** ECG of typical clockwise AFL. **C,** ECG of an atypical left AFL.

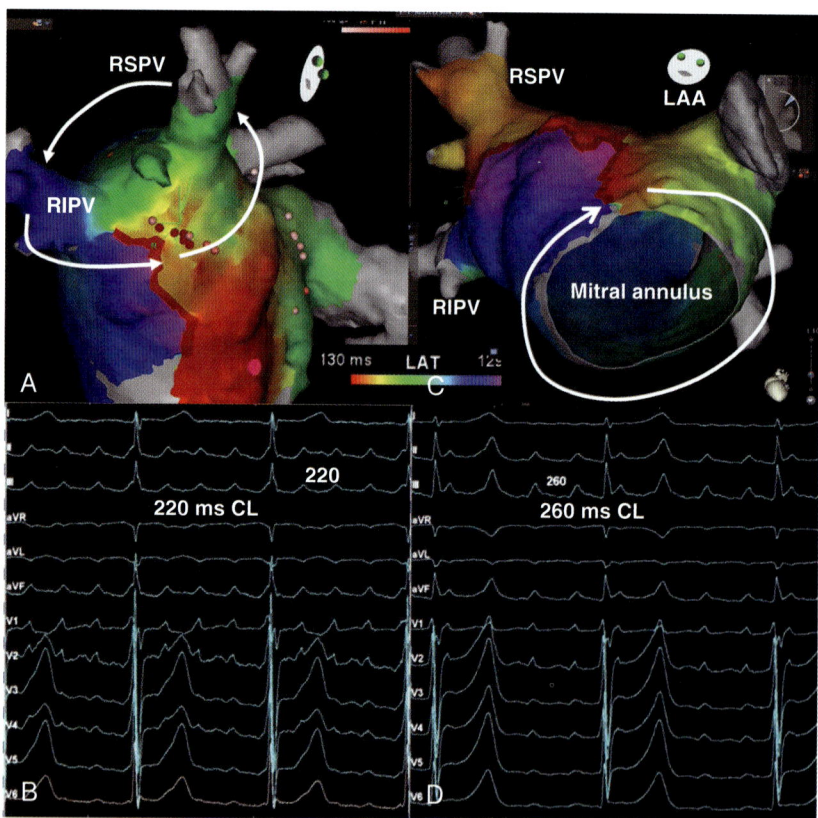

FIGURE 65.14 Patient with a prior history of persistent atrial flutter and previous catheter ablation. Three-dimensional color-coded activation maps and corresponding ECGs are shown. Activation timing is earliest in *red* through *yellow, green, light blue,* and *dark blue,* with the latest area activated in *purple*. The *deep red line* where purple meets red is the region of "head meets tail" of a reentrant circuit. **A,** Circuit rotating around the right-sided pulmonary veins in a counterclockwise direction is shown. This is considered a "roof-dependent" flutter. **B,** The corresponding ECG indicates an atypical flutter with upright morphology in V₁ and precordial leads and also upright in inferior leads and a cycle length of 220 msec. An ablation line was created across the atrial roof between the right superior (RSPV) and left superior (LSPV) pulmonary veins. **C,** A remap indicated that the circuit had changed and was now rotating around the mitral annulus in a counterclockwise direction. This may be termed a *mitral isthmus-dependent flutter*. The absence of change in the flutter wave morphology reflects the poor sensitivity and specificity of the flutter morphology for localization of atypical flutter circuits. This is particularly the case in the context of structural heart disease and prior ablation. **D,** With completion of the ablation line there was a sudden increase in cycle length to 260 msec without any apparent change in the flutter wave morphology.

Rate control with oral or intravenous beta blockers or non-dihydropyridine calcium channel blockers (verapamil or diltiazem) may be used for rate control. Class 1C agents should not be used in patients with AFL because of the risk of slowing atrial rate and facilitating 1:1 AV conduction with concomitant profound conduction slowing in the ventricle (see Fig. 65.10).

Chronic Therapy. Catheter ablation now represents the cornerstone management strategy in patients with AFL. It may be considered after a first episode or in patients with recurrent or persistent episodes. It is particularly indicated in patients who develop TMC. These recommendations apply to both CTI-dependent (typical) AFL and non–isthmus-dependent (atypical) flutters.

In CTI-dependent flutter, ablation is across the CTI from the annulus to the eustachian ridge at the anterior margin of the IVC. The end point is the demonstration of bidirectional conduction block across this line using standard electrophysiology mapping techniques. The acute success rate is in excess of 97%, and the recurrence rate is now approximately 5% to 10%.[1,13] The procedural risk of serious adverse events is under 1%.[33]

In patients with atypical flutter or non–CTI-dependent flutter, the success rate is much more variable and depends on the nature of the underlying cardiac disease. For example, in patients with simple forms of scar-related flutter such as after ASD repair or mitral valve repair, success rates are similarly high, approaching 90%.[30,34] However, the requirement for multiple procedures is more common than for CTI-dependent flutter (>20% to 30%) because the frequent presence of multiple circuits and the late incidence of AF is high (>30% at 2 years). In patients with more advanced forms of surgically repaired CHD such as Fontan repair for univentricular physiology or Mustard/Senning repair for D-transposition of the great arteries (D-TGA), acute success rates are lower, the need for multiple procedures is higher, and long-term recurrences are common.[28,35] Patients generally have multiple different circuits due to the extensive atrial surgery performed and the underlying anatomic abnormalities. Nevertheless, ablation can represent an effective palliative procedure as part of a more

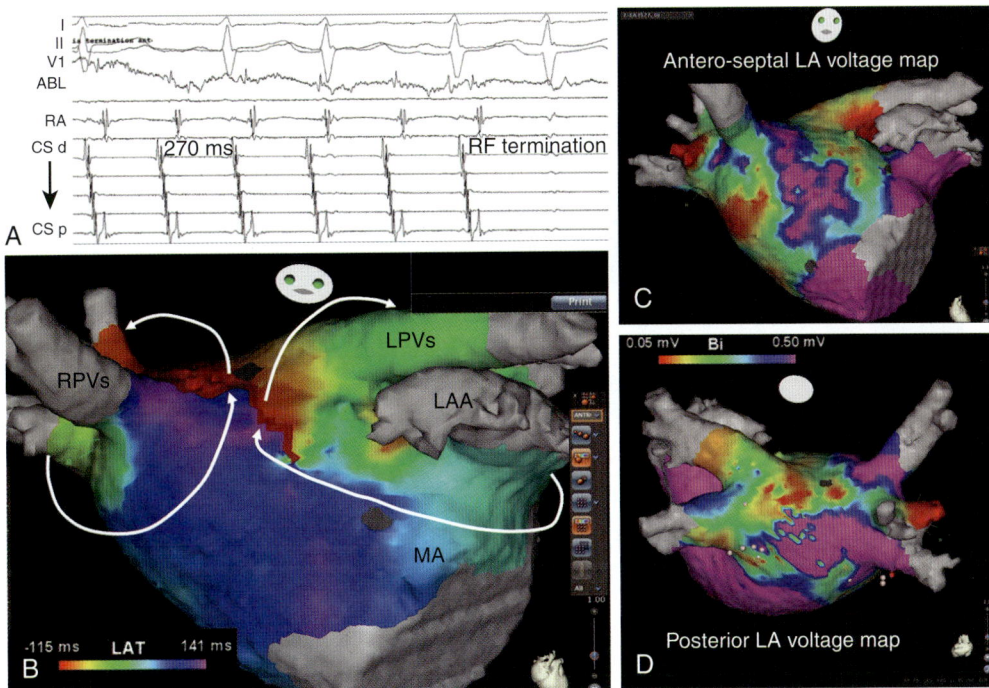

FIGURE 65.15 Example of dual-loop reentry in a patient with prior persistent atrial fibrillation (AF), advanced atrial remodeling, and prior AF ablation. **A,** Demonstration of ECG recordings and simultaneous intracardiac recordings from the ablation catheter (ABL), the right atrium (RA), and the coronary sinus (CS, distal to proximal) during a radiofrequency application that terminated the flutter. **B,** Electroanatomic color-coded activation map with colors superimposed on the left atrial CT scan, with the earliest activation indicated in *red* through *yellow, green, light blue, dark blue,* and *purple*. The *deep red line* where purple meets red is the region of "head meets tail" of both simultaneous reentrant circuits. The simultaneous circuits are indicated by the *white arrows* with one rotating around the right pulmonary veins (RPVs) and the other around the left pulmonary veins (LPVs) and the left atrial appendage (LAA). Both circuits are "roof-dependent." Linear ablation through the LA roof from the superior RPV to the superior LPV terminated the flutter as shown in **A**. **C** and **D,** The nature of advanced remodeling in this atrium. The colors in these images indicate atrial voltage with normal amplitudes represented by *purple* and *blue;* and abnormally low voltages by *red* and *yellow*. There are extensive low-voltage regions, indicative of fibrosis and associated with slow conduction in this atrium both anteriorly and septally (**C**) and posteriorly (**D**).

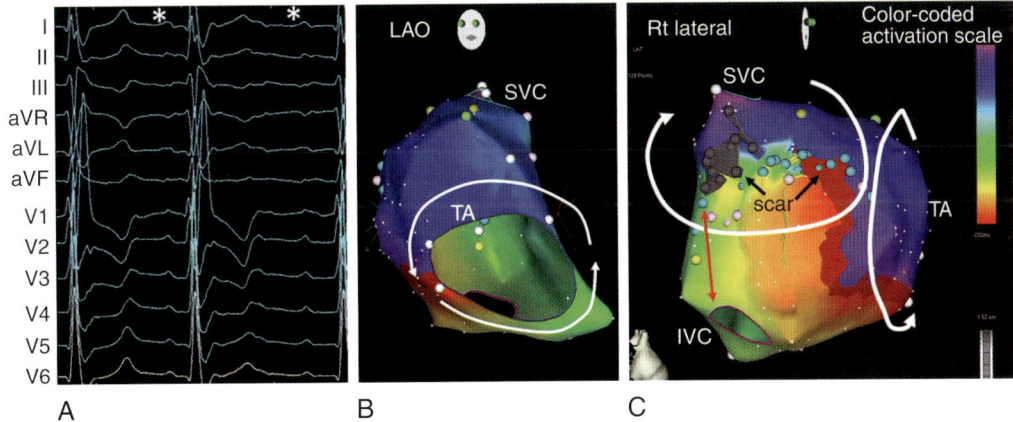

FIGURE 65.16 Dual-loop reentry in a 52-year-old man with prior atrial septal defect (ASD) repair. **A,** The flutter wave morphology *(asterisks)* is very unusual across all ECG leads. **B,** The three-dimensional electroanatomic map with a counterclockwise circuit around the tricuspid annulus (TA) in the right atrium in the left anterior oblique (LAO) view. Progression of activation is according to the color code at *right*. The activation is characteristic of typical counterclockwise atrial flutter, but the ECG is inconsistent with this. **C,** The right lateral view of the right atrium demonstrates that there are two simultaneous loops of activation. One is around the TA, but the other is around the region of the superior vena cava and an area of scar (*gray patch* and *blue dots* arrowed). This is presumed to be the region of the atriotomy scar required for access to repair the ASD. This latter circuit alone would be termed *upper loop reentry*. Ablation in the cavo-tricuspid isthmus interrupted the circuit around the TA without any change in the cycle length due to the ongoing upper loop circuit. Ablation from the scar to the inferior vena cava (*red double-headed arrow*) terminated this second circuit.

general strategy that includes careful attention to structural and hemodynamic issues.[36]

A common form of atypical flutter in the era of AF ablation is due to circuits occurring after AF ablation procedures. These may occur in up to 20% of patients and are more common in those who have undergone persistent AF ablation, particularly when extensive or linear ablation has been performed or in those with more advanced atrial remodeling. Patients may have multiple circuits and the need for multiple procedures is common.[37,38] Nevertheless, when control can be achieved, the long-term freedom from AF is high.

For patients in whom catheter ablation is contraindicated (e.g., advanced age, comorbidities, patient preference) or is not feasible (e.g., presence of mechanical valves, multiple unstable circuits, previously failed) a number of antiarrhythmic agents may be considered for maintenance of sinus rhythm. These include sotalol, dofetilide, or amiodarone depending on efficacy, tolerability, and nature of comorbidities (e.g., amiodarone preferred in the presence of significant LV dysfunction).

For patients in whom a rhythm control strategy is unsuccessful or not preferred, a rate control strategy may be adopted. This might be with a beta blocker or a non-dihydropyridine calcium channel blocker (verapamil or diltiazem). If drug therapy is unsuccessful or poorly tolerated and ventricular response rates remain high, pacing (usually biventricular or His bundle pacing) followed by AV node ablation may be considered.

Due to the frequent coexistence of AF and AFL, anticoagulant management of patients with AFL generally follows the same recommendations as for AF both at the time of reversion and during chronic management, in which decisions should be dictated by the $CHADS_2$-VA_2Sc score rather than apparent rhythm control.[1,13]

Paroxysmal Supraventricular Tachycardia

ECG Characteristics and ECG Classification of PSVT

SVT is most classically a regular narrow-complex tachycardia with a wide rate range from just in excess of 100 bpm to over 250 bpm in some patients (Fig. 65.18). In some patients bundle branch aberrancy may be present during tachycardia. This is more commonly right bundle aberrancy due to the longer refractory period of the right bundle compared with the left bundle (Fig 65.18A). Occasionally, patients with SVT may have a preexisting bundle branch block even in sinus rhythm, resulting in a wide complex tachycardia that nevertheless has a typical bundle branch block appearance (Fig. 65.19). In cases of aberrancy, the differential diagnosis may include some forms of VT such as a fascicular VT (Fig. 65.20).

The ECG of PSVT can be classified according to the VA relationship (Fig. 65.21). When there are more atrial than ventricular complexes

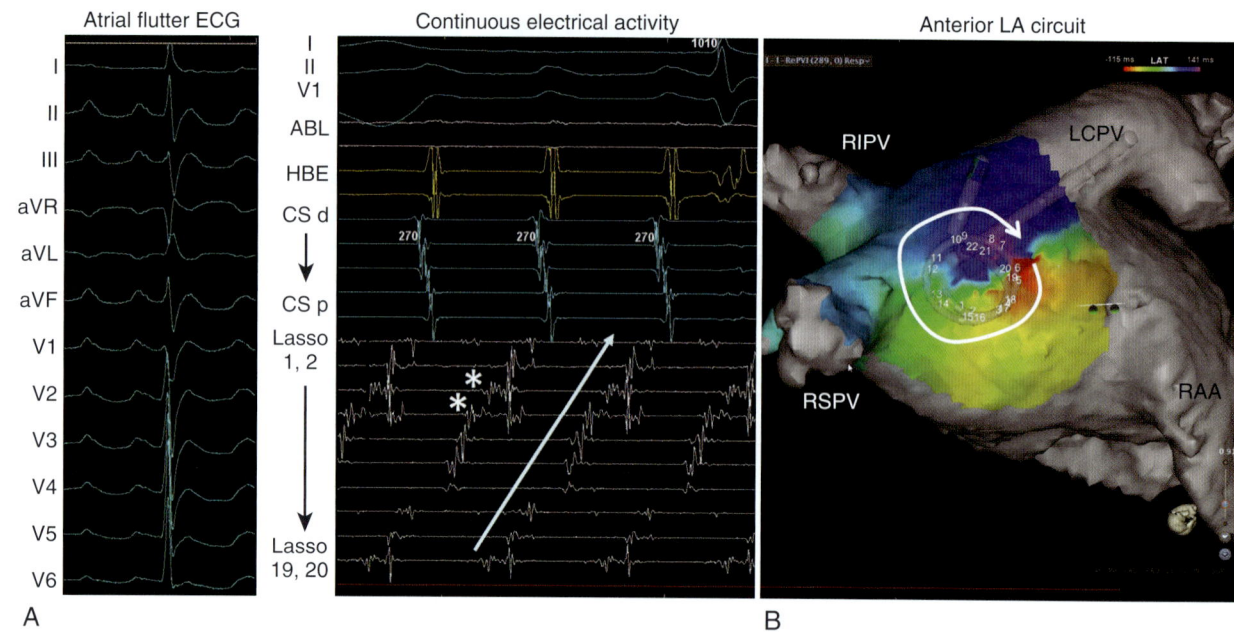

FIGURE 65.17 Atypical atrial flutter due to small circuit reentry in a patient with a history of persistent atrial fibrillation. **A,** Flutter wave morphology, which is upright in V_1 (indicating a probable left atrial origin) and upright in inferior leads (indicating a probable superior origin). The signals in the *middle panel* recorded by a lasso catheter in the anterior left atrium show activation spanning the entire cycle length. The *asterisks* indicate long fractionated multicomponent electrograms that span almost half the tachycardia cycle length and indicate a region of markedly slowed conduction necessary to maintain these small reentrant circuits. These signals reflect advanced atrial remodeling. **B,** An anatomic view of the left atrium viewed from superior aspect. The lasso catheter is shown in the anterior LA roof. The activation sequence goes from *red* through *yellow, green, light blue, dark blue,* and *purple.* Where purple meets red is the "head meets tail" location of the reentrant circuit (*arrow*). This circuit was interrupted by ablation at the site of the fractionated electrograms.

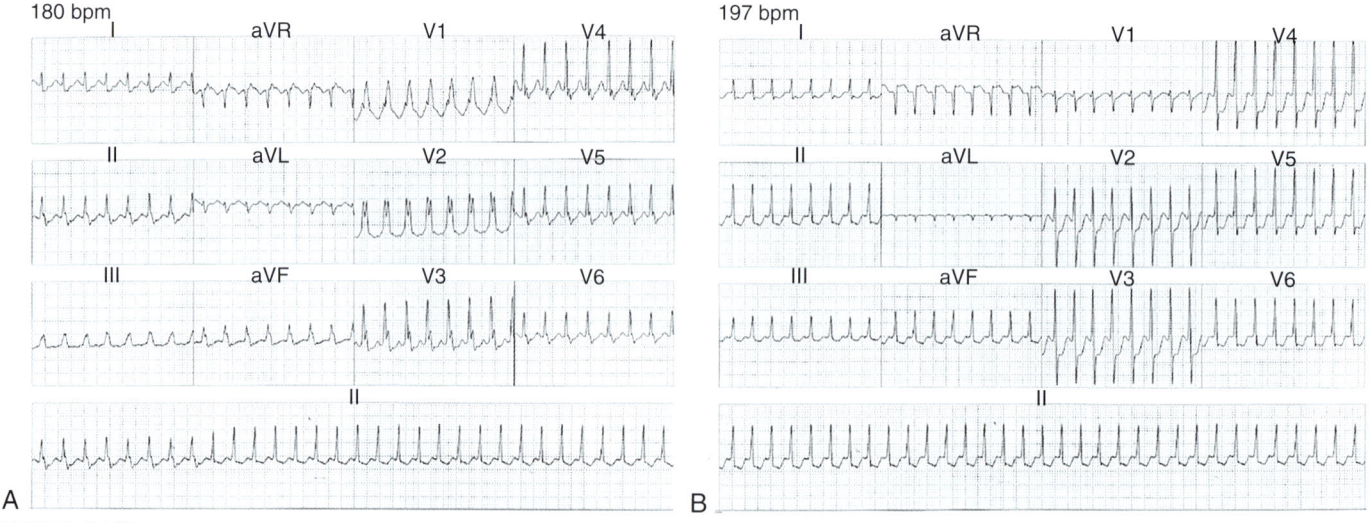

FIGURE 65.18 A, Initial ECG demonstrates characteristic appearance of a regular tachycardia, which is relatively narrow but displays a typical right bundle branch block (RBBB) morphology at a heart rate of 180 bpm. The RBBB occurs at initiation when a "long-short" onset sequence finds the right bundle refractory. The RBBB persists due to transseptal concealed conduction (linking). Activation over the left bundle then crosses the septum and invades the right bundle retrogradely maintaining the block to antegrade conduction. **B,** Minutes later, the bundle branch block normalized spontaneously. Two possible mechanisms for this spontaneous resolution are either "accommodation," in which the antegrade refractory period of the right bundle gradually shortens or, alternatively, distal migration of the site of collision between antegrade activation of the RBBB and transseptal retrograde penetration. This resolution despite the higher heart rate confirms that the block was functional. Note also the widespread ST segment depression, which usually does not imply the presence of myocardial ischemia.

the possibilities include focal AT (see Fig. 65.5), AV node reentry with block (Fig. 65.22) or AFL (see Fig. 65.11B,C). When there are fewer atrial than ventricular complexes during a narrow-complex tachycardia, the differential diagnosis includes only quite rare entities, including junctional ectopic tachycardia (JET), a concealed nodofascicular pathway and high septal fascicular VT (see Fig. 65.21). Most commonly, when the atrial and ventricular complexes occur 1:1, the tachycardia can be further defined in terms of whether the P wave falls in the first half of the R-R interval (short RP tachycardia) or the second half of the R-R interval (long RP tachycardia). Short RP tachycardias can be further divided into those in which the P wave falls largely within the QRS when it may not be visible (RP <70 msec) or after the QRS within the T wave (RP >70 msec) (see Fig. 65.21).

Clinical Presentation

As described in the introduction, PSVT may be viewed as a subset of SVT and involves a classic clinical picture characterized by sudden onset and termination of rapid palpitations documented as a regular narrow-complex tachycardia. This clinical picture implies the presence of AVNRT, AVRT, or less frequently AT.

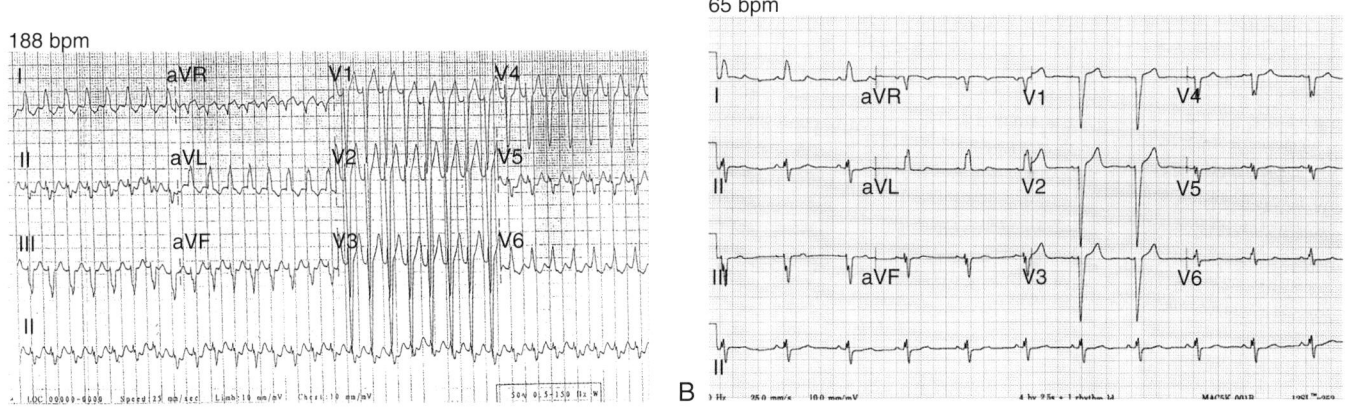

FIGURE 65.19 A, Left bundle branch block and left axis tachycardia at 188 bpm. The appearance is of a typical left bundle with a deep S wave in right precordial leads and in inferior leads and loss of the septal Q wave in the lateral precordial leads. **B,** In sinus rhythm at 65 bpm the identical QRS morphology is present indicating that the ECG is highly likely to represent SVT. The rhythm was proven to be atrioventricular nodal reentrant tachycardia.

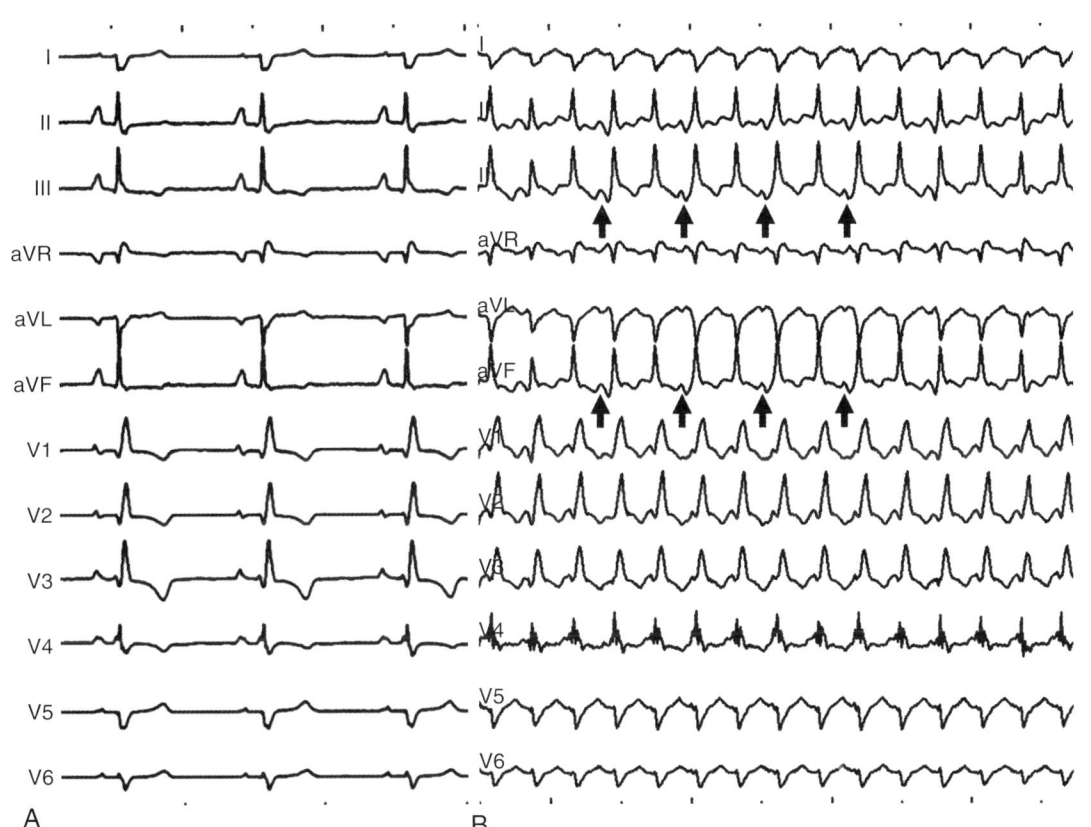

FIGURE 65.20 A, Sinus rhythm ECG demonstrating a right bundle branch block pattern with right axis deviation due to presence of a left posterior hemiblock. **B,** Tachycardia with the identical QRS morphology suggests that this is likely to be a supraventricular tachycardia. However, there is VA dissociation (P waves indicated by the *solid arrows* seen best in lead III and aVF. The mechanism of the arrhythmia was a form of bundle branch reentry with the antegrade limb being the left posterior hemifascicle (hence the same morphology as sinus rhythm) and the retrograde limb being the right bundle, which had slow conduction. *VA,* ventriculoatrial.

rapid rates.[10] In adults with PSVT, asymptomatic episodes are quite uncommon. AF may develop in up to 12% of patients diagnosed with PSVT during follow-up.

Episodes of PSVT are usually initiated by atrial or ventricular ectopic beats or couplets. Patients frequently describe classic triggers such as sudden movements, bending over, or exercise, although a wide range of triggers with variable frequency have been reported.

A description of multiple stop-start episodes in succession usually indicates a focal AT, whereas a single prolonged episode is more common with AVRT or AVNRT. Adults with a long history of episodes that began in childhood and teenage years are more likely to have AVNRT or AVRT rather than AT.

Patients with PSVT may have been diagnosed and treated as having anxiety and panic attacks, a misdiagnosis more commonly observed in women.[10]

Typically, rapid palpitations may be accompanied by lightheadedness, chest discomfort, and dyspnea, but the severity of these symptoms varies considerably. Very rapid and more prolonged episodes particularly in older patients are more likely to be associated with severe symptoms. Conversely, younger patients will frequently have no symptoms other than an awareness of rapid palpitations. Intense light-headedness or occasionally presyncope may be reported at onset of the tachycardia and may be perceived immediately before awareness of rapid palpitations. However, syncope is rare in SVT. Patients will often describe fatigue, which may persist for 24 hours after an event. Polyuria is occasionally described as a feature and is presumed to be the result of atrial natriuretic peptide release at

Epidemiology. AV node reentry (AVNRT) is the most common documented mechanism of PSVT in patients undergoing catheter ablation.[15] After the age of 20, AVNRT accounts for the largest number of ablations in each age group. There is a consistent 2:1 female-to-male predominance observed in multiple series. AVRT is the most common mechanism of SVT in the first decade of life, accounting for 55% to 60% of PSVT cases.[15] Thereafter there is a progressive decline that continues through each decade of life such that beyond 60 years of age AVRT represents under 10% of SVT cases. In contrast, the prevalence of AT is low in the first decades of life (<10%), slowly increasing with age to represent over 20% of cases beyond age 60.

AVNRT: Anatomy, Physiology and ECG Characteristics.

The AVNRT circuit most probably involves the compact AV node, perinodal transitional inputs to the node, which may be left or right sided (fast and slow pathways), and the perinodal atrial region. However, it must be emphasized that the precise anatomic location of the entire circuit is unknown. The critical components of the circuit are located within the anatomic triangle of Koch bounded anteriorly by the TA, posteriorly by the tendon of Todaro, superiorly by the membranous septum and the penetrating bundle of His, and inferiorly by the ostium of the coronary sinus. At the apex of the triangle is the compact node. The fast AV nodal pathway approaches the compact node at the superior aspect of the triangle, and the slow pathway approaches the node from the inferior aspect of the triangle and the CS os region. In addition, there are both anterior and posterior inputs to the AV node from the left side of the septum, which may participate in tachycardia. A proposed schema for the different forms of AVNRT from the work of Katritsis and Becker is shown in Fig. 65.23.[39] The theoretical possibilities include a right-sided circuit, a left-sided circuit, simultaneous right and left circuits, and figure-of-8 reentry.

Typical AVNRT

The typical form of AVNRT involves antegrade conduction over the slow pathway and retrograde activation via the fast pathway. Retrograde activation to the atrium via the fast pathway occurs synchronously with antegrade activation over the His Purkinje system to the ventricle resulting in simultaneous atrial and ventricular activation. In approximately 50% of cases, the P wave is not visible because it is occurs completely within the QRS. In 45% of cases, the final component of the P wave occurs at the tail end of the QRS, producing a pseudo right bundle appearance in V_1 and a pseudo S wave pattern in the inferior leads (Fig. 65.22A). This appearance has been reported to indicate typical AVNRT with an accuracy of 100%.[40] Occasionally the tachycardia exhibits 2:1 conduction to the ventricle (Fig. 65.22B). This generally occurs early after onset of the arrhythmia and is characterized by the appearance of a P wave exactly in the middle of two consecutive QRS complexes (Fig. 65.22B). The usual site of block is within or below the bundle of His (Fig. 65.22C), and

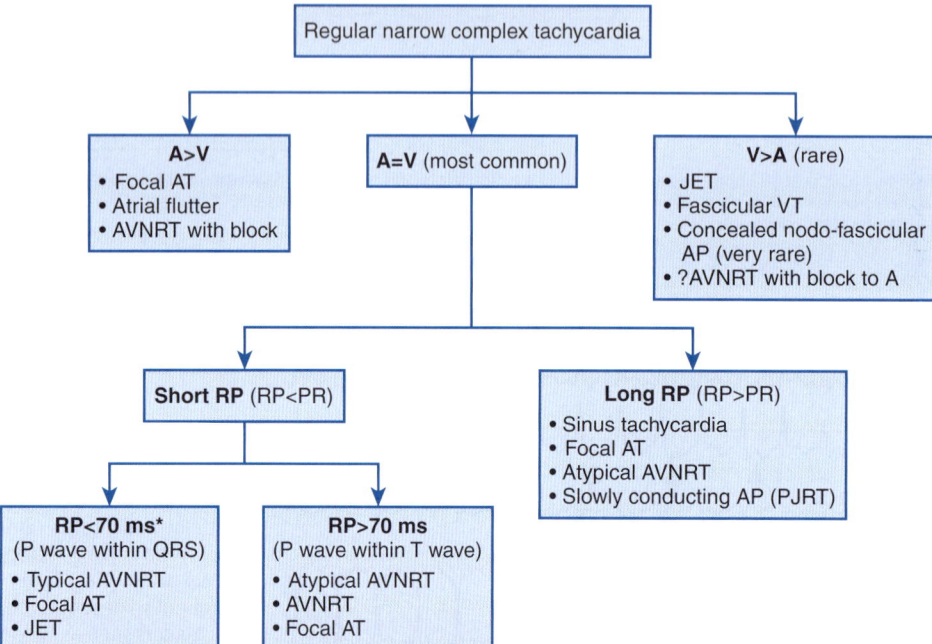

FIGURE 65.21 Algorithm for evaluation of narrow-complex tachycardia. The P wave is either not visible or visible as a pseudo R prime in V_1. The interval of 70 msec is derived from the VA time on the His bundle electrogram during electrophysiologic study. When using the onset of the surface QRS to onset of the visible P wave the intervals used are less than 90 msec and greater than 90 msec. *A,* Atrium; *AP,* accessory pathway; *AT,* atrial tachycardia; *AVNRT,* atrioventricular nodal reentrant tachycardia; *JET,* junctional ectopic tachycardia; *PJRT,* permanent junctional reciprocating tachycardia; *V,* ventricle; *VT,* ventricular tachycardia. (Modified from Brugada J, et al. 2019 ESC guidelines for the management of patients with supraventricular tachycardia the task force for the management of patients with supraventricular tachycardia of the European Society of Cardiology (ESC): developed in collaboration with the Association for European Paediatric and Congenital Cardiology (AEPC). Eur Heart J 2020;41:655-720.)

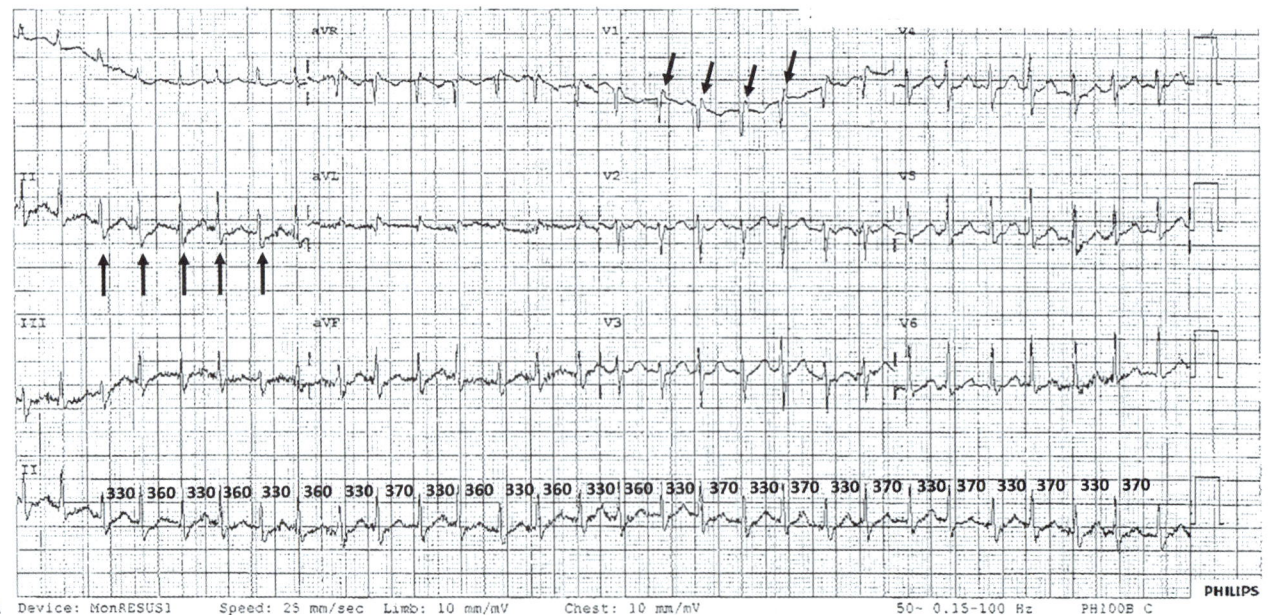

FIGURE 65.22 A, 1:1 atrioventricular nodal reentrant tachycardia (AVNRT). Note the presence of the pseudo R prime in V_1 (*downward arrows*) and the pseudo S wave in inferior leads (*upward arrows*) due to the retrograde P wave. Note also the presence of cycle length alternans varying between 330 and 360/370 msec on alternate beats. This suggests the presence of two antegrade slow pathways. Despite this cycle length alternans, the position of the retrograde P wave remains fixed at the same location in the final component of the QRS as indicated by the *arrows*. This fixed VA time despite cycle length variation rules out focal atrial tachycardia and confirms the presence of typical AVNRT. *VA,* ventriculoatrial.

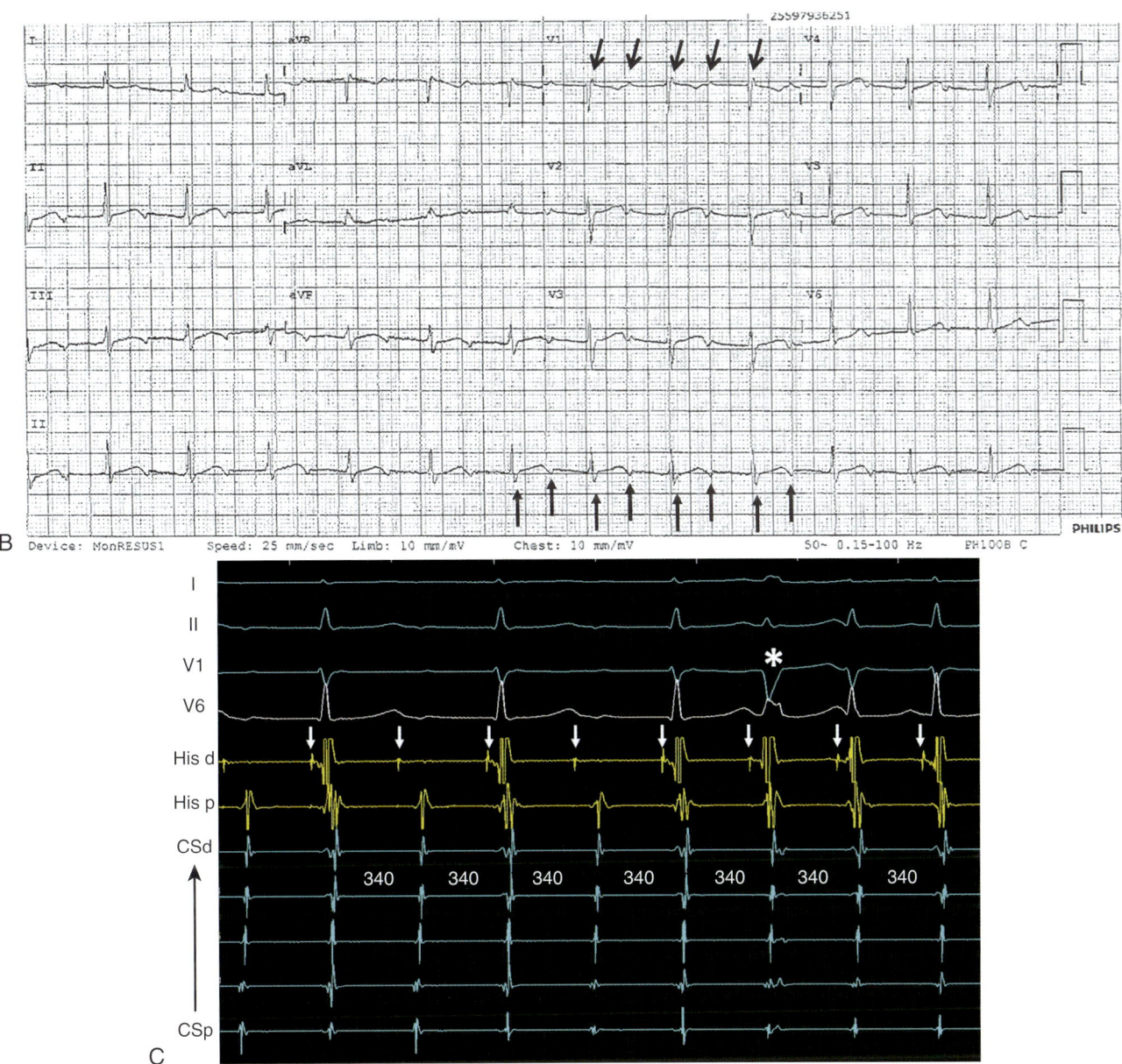

FIGURE 65.22—cont'd **B,** 2:1 AVNRT in the same patient; note that there is a P wave (inverted in inferior leads; upright in V$_1$) precisely located in the middle between two QRS complexes. In V$_1$ there is a pseudo R prime at the tail end of the QRS (pseudo partial RBBB) and indicated by the *downward arrows,* which corresponds to the final component of the P wave. This can be readily appreciated by viewing the identical appearance of the P wave located between the two QRS complexes. Similarly, in inferior leads, the pseudo S wave appearance (*upward arrows*) is due to the P wave occurring in the final component of the QRS. Again, this can be appreciated by noting the P wave located between the QRS complexes that has the identical morphology to the pseudo S wave. **C,** Four ECG leads and intracardiac recordings from a His bundle catheter (distal and proximal) and from a coronary sinus catheter (CS) with recordings displayed from proximal at the *bottom* to distal at the *top*. The panel shows 2:1 AVNRT, which changes to 1:1 spontaneously during an electrophysiology study and ablation procedure. The cycle length is 340 msec (176 bpm). On the *left* of the panel, every other His spike (*white arrows*) is not followed by a QRS complex. Thus, there is 2:1 "infra-Hisian" block. This is not pathologic but rather reflects functional block. On the *right* of the screen, the tachycardia spontaneously goes 1:1, with the first beat showing only left bundle aberrancy (*asterisk*) before the tachycardia then becomes 1:1 with narrow complexes (final 2 beats).

although block occurring in a lower final common AV nodal pathway above the His bundle has previously been proposed, definitive evidence for this is lacking.[40] Several ECG features may allow differentiation of *typical* AVNRT from a focal AT:

1. When onset of the tachycardia is recorded, an early atrial ectopic that blocks in the fast pathway (due to the relatively longer refractory period of the fast pathway) conducts down the slow pathway with a long PR interval is highly suggestive of AVNRT. Activity then travels retrogradely via the fast pathway, which has now recovered excitability, and the tachycardia is initiated. Onset of focal AT is also generally with a tightly coupled atrial premature beat, but it will not necessarily be conducted with a long PR interval over a slow pathway.
2. When cycle length variability occurs during the tachycardia, the presence of a fixed ventriculoatrial (VA) relationship (reflecting fast pathway conduction) provides strong evidence in favor of AVNRT rather than AT, in which this relationship is incidental (see Fig. 65.22A).
3. When termination of the tachycardia is documented, spontaneous termination with a P wave as the final event also provides strong evidence against AT and therefore in favor of AVNRT.

Atypical AVNRT

Atypical AVNRT may be fast-slow or slow-slow, the latter indicating the presence of more than one slow pathway. Fast-slow AVNRT is a long RP tachycardia usually with a PR interval of less than 200 msec (Fig. 65.24).[40] In fast-slow AVNRT the distance from the atrium to His recording (the AH interval) is shorter than the subsequent HA interval. The inferior leads characteristically show inverted P waves due to the

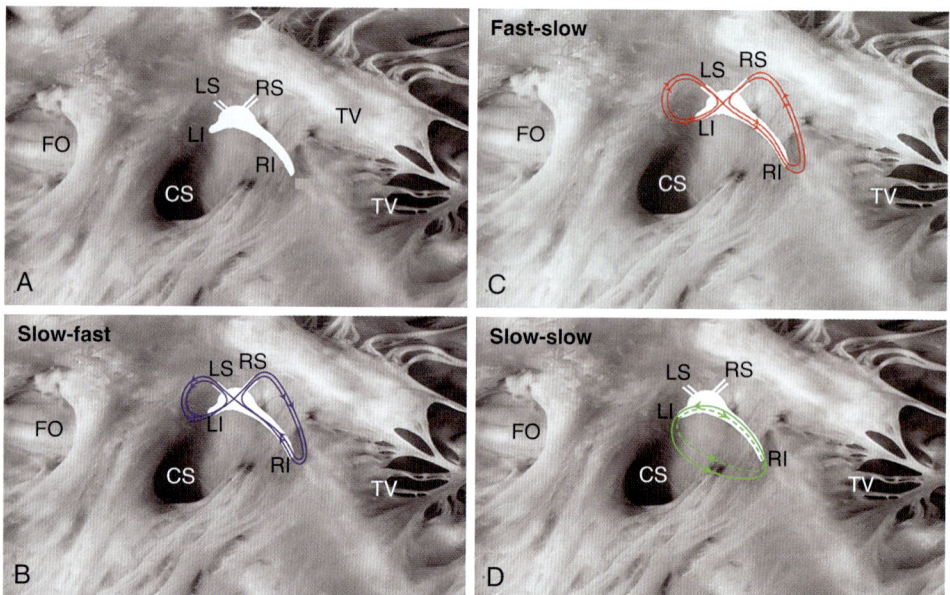

retrograde slow pathway exit that is frequently in the vicinity of the CS os. Slow-slow AVNRT is diagnosed when the VA interval is >70 msec, but the AH interval is longer than the HA interval.

Treatment of AVNRT

ACUTE MANAGEMENT. Patients should be educated in vagal maneuvers to be performed in the supine position with leg elevation.[41] When performed under instruction in the emergency department this may be effective in 40% to 50% of patients.

In patients who fail vagal maneuvers, adenosine 6 to 12 mg intravenous bolus is the treatment of choice. Care must be taken to warn the patient that they may feel chest tightness and a transient sense of impending doom. In patients who fail adenosine reversion, intravenous verapamil or diltiazem or alternatively an intravenous beta blocker (metoprolol or esmolol) may be considered.

DC cardioversion is appropriate in hemodynamically unstable patients or when all other measures fail but is rarely required.

FIGURE 65.23 A proposed schema for the different forms of atrioventricular nodal reentry tachycardia (AVNRT). The theoretical possibilities include a right-sided circuit, a left-sided circuit, simultaneous right and left circuits, and figure-of-8 reentry. **A,** Schema of the anatomy of the atrioventricular nodal region showing the coronary sinus ostium (CS), the tricuspid valve (TV), and the fossa ovalis (FO). The compact node is shown with right inferior (RI), left inferior (LI), right superior (RS), and left superior (LS) inputs to the node. **B,** Slow-fast typical AVNRT circuits. The most common form approaches the node from the RI input and exits from the RS input. A small region of perinodal atrium completes the circuit. The circuit also may be localized to the left-sided inputs. **C,** Fast-slow AVNRT with activation in the reverse direction with input to the node over the RS or LS and exits from wither the RI or LI pathways. **D,** Slow-slow AVNRT uses the two inferior inputs to the node as entrance and exit. As in all forms of AVNRT, perinodal atrium completes the circuit. (From Katritsis DG, Becker A. The atrioventricular nodal reentrant tachycardia circuit: a proposal. Heart Rhythm 2007;4:1354-1360.)

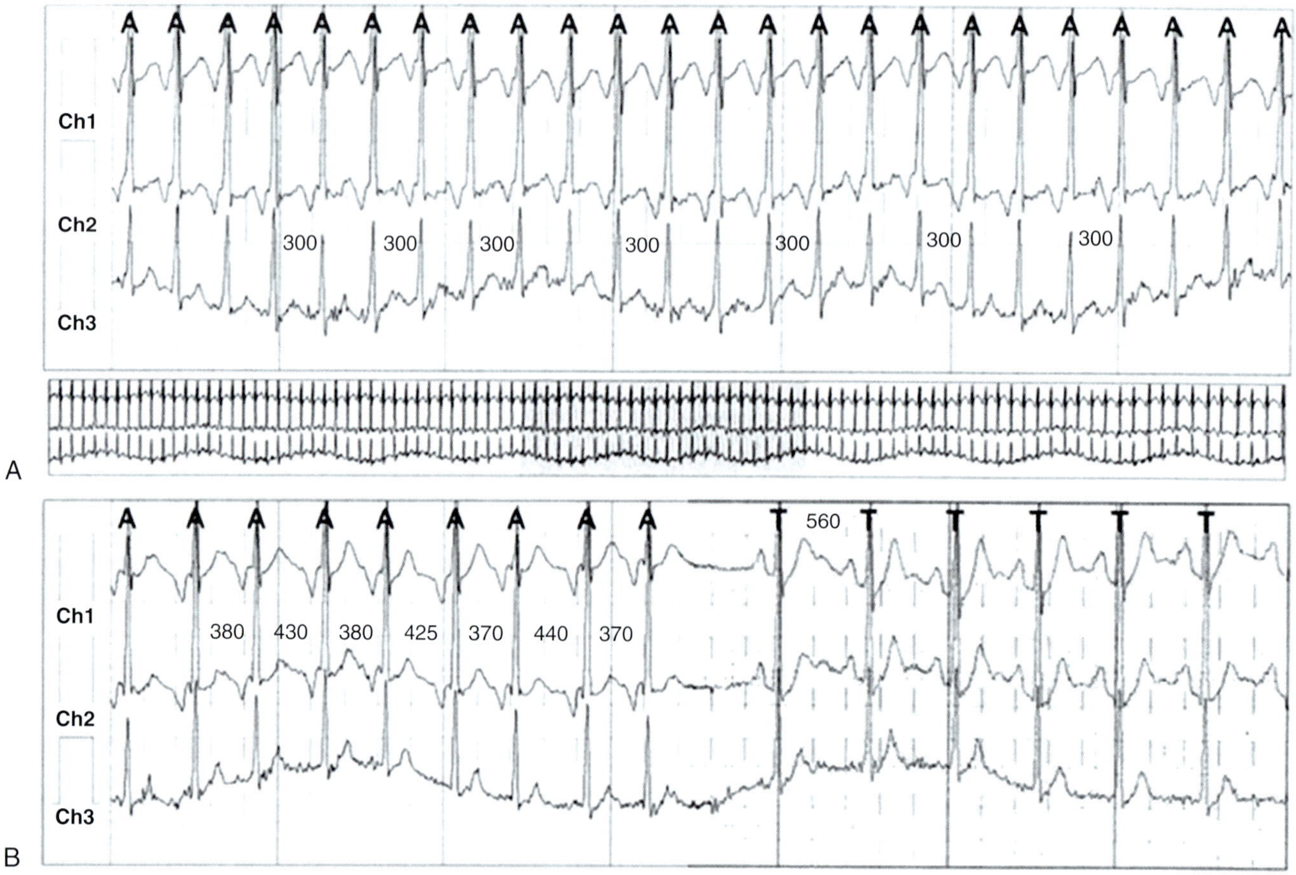

FIGURE 65.24 Holter monitor trace of a long R-P tachycardia with inverted P waves in Ch1 and Ch2 indicative of a superiorly directed axis. The differential diagnosis includes focal atrial tachycardia, atypical atrioventricular nodal reentrant tachycardia (AVNRT), or permanent junctional reciprocating tachycardia (slowly conducting retrograde pathway). **A,** The tachycardia cycle length is relatively fixed at approximately 300 msec (200 bpm). **B,** Immediately before termination the tachycardia cycle length has prolonged and is varying by up to 70 msec (cycle length approximately 400 msec equivalent to heart rate of 150 bpm). Note that even with marked variability the PR interval remains fixed (150 msec), indicating that the variation is in the VA interval. This "unhooking of the VA" favors a diagnosis of focal atrial tachycardia but does not on its own eliminate the other two diagnoses as variable retrograde conduction over a slow atrioventricular nodal pathway or a slowly conducting accessory pathway could produce a similar pattern. Termination with the last complex being ventricular (QRS) is also consistent with all three diagnoses. Indeed, at electrophysiologic study the arrhythmia was proven to be atypical fast-slow AVNRT with variable conduction in the retrograde slow pathway. VA, ventriculoatrial

CHRONIC MANAGEMENT. Patients with infrequent episodes associated with mild symptoms and that are responsive to vagal maneuvers may elect no treatment.

However, for more frequent episodes, unpredictable episodes, or episodes with severe symptoms, the treatment of choice is catheter ablation targeting the slow pathway region.[1,13] Numerous observational trials have documented both the efficacy and safety of catheter ablation for AVNRT. In addition, a recent randomized trial comparing catheter ablation versus antiarrhythmics confirmed the superiority of ablation and the relative long-term inefficacy of medical therapy. At 5 years of follow up none of the ablation patients had a recurrence necessitating hospital presentation compared with over 75% in the medical arm by 2 years.[42] Large series have confirmed the efficacy and safety of catheter ablation for both typical and atypical forms of AVNRT.[43] Long-term success rates in excess of 95% are generally reported. In addition, large contemporary series have reported an incidence of AV block between 0.1% and 0.4% and no mortality.[42,44,45] In the pediatric age group there is a preference toward using cryoablation because some studies have suggested a lower rate of inadvertent AV block, but the recurrence rate is higher.[46,47] However, in the adult population no consistent benefit has been demonstrated with cryoablation.[48] Catheter ablation has been shown to improve quality of life and reduce ongoing costs.

In patients who prefer medical therapy, the first-line long-term treatment options are either a nondihydropyridine calcium channel blocker (verapamil or diltiazem) or a beta blocker. These may reduce the frequency and duration of events but rarely abolish the tachycardia. In addition, 20% to 50% of patients will discontinue therapy for reasons including inefficacy or intolerance.[40]

Junctional Ectopic Tachycardia (Nonreentrant Junctional Tachycardia). JET is a rare arrhythmia that occurs in several specific clinical contexts:

1. It may occur early after surgical repair of CHD with an incidence of 1% to 5%.[49,50]
2. As a congenital arrhythmia presenting in the first 6 months of life, in which it has been associated with a high morbidity and mortality.[51] In this age group the arrhythmia is more likely to be incessant and has higher rates.
3. In the pediatric age group beyond the age of 6 months. For management, a wide range of antiarrhythmic medications have been trialed and the majority of patients require combination therapy.[52] Complete suppression of the arrhythmia is rare; more frequently the rate and frequency of episodes is decreased. In up to 20% of cases, antiarrhythmics are completely ineffective. The agent with highest reported efficacy is amiodarone. Catheter ablation is playing an increasing role using either radiofrequency or cryoablation approaches. In the largest study published to date, these modalities had comparable acute efficacy (82% to 85%) and recurrence rates (13% to 14%). Inadvertent permanent third-degree AV block occurred in 3 of 17 (18%) patients who underwent radiofrequency ablation and in none of the cryoablation patients.[53]
4. Rarely, this arrhythmia may manifest in adults.[54] In a small ablation series of JET in adults (mean age 58), recurrence rates (37%), requirement for multiple procedures, and risk of AV block (20%) were high.

The ECG characteristics of JET are those of a narrow-complex tachycardia resembling typical AVNRT with a P wave at the terminal end of the QRS (Fig. 65.25) or with VA dissociation when conduction block is present between the junctional focus and the surrounding atrium. On monitoring, the arrhythmia demonstrates multiple spontaneous (not ectopic induced) onsets and terminations and rates may occur in excess of 250 bpm.

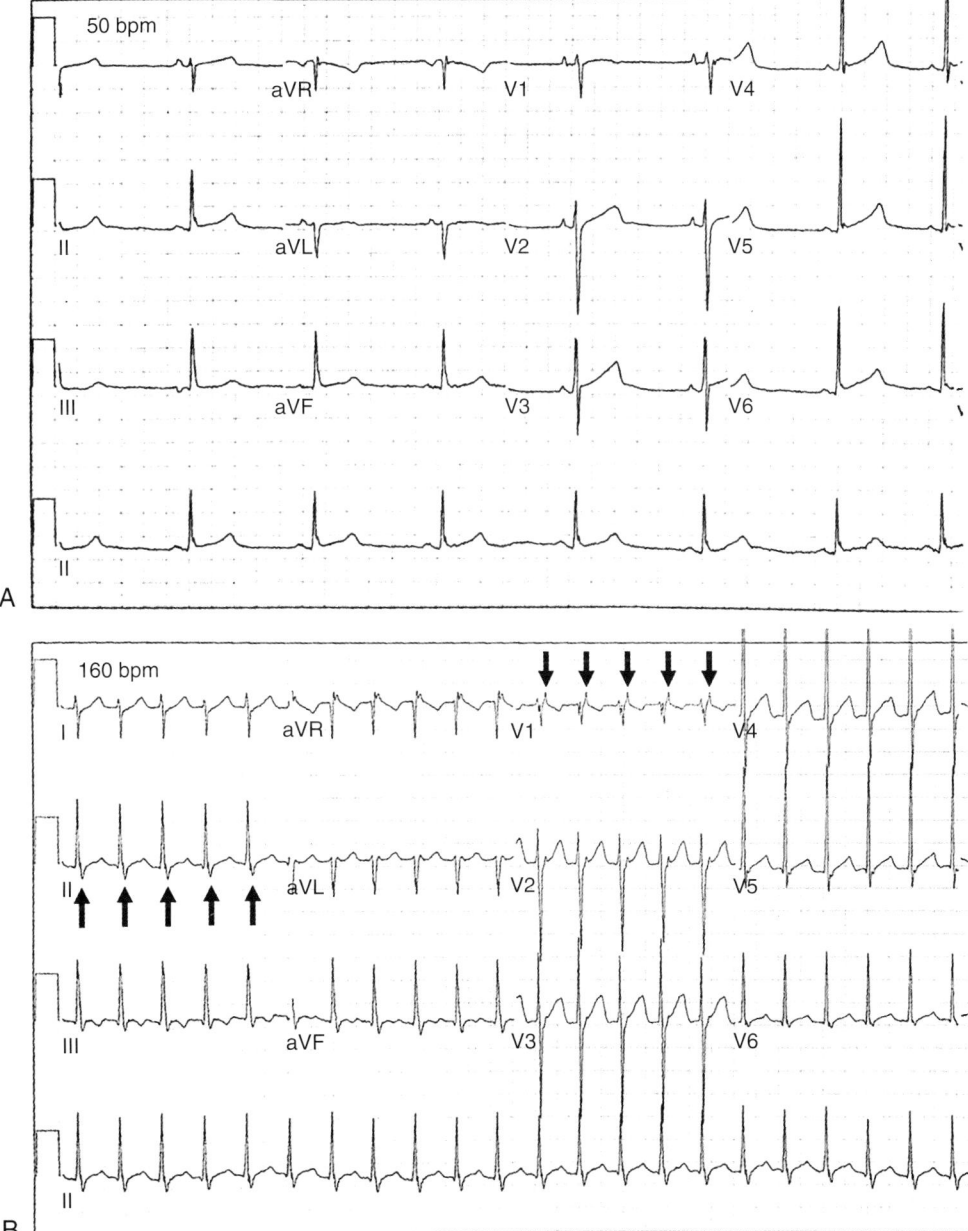

FIGURE 65.25 ECGs recorded in a 12-yr-old boy with incessant tachycardia refractory to medical therapy. **A,** Sinus rhythm at 50 bpm. **B,** Junctional tachycardia at 160 bpm (on Holter monitoring rates would frequently reach 240 bpm during minor activity). Note the presence of the P wave visible after the tail end of the QRS in V_1 as a sharp pseudo R prime (*downward arrows*) and in the inferior leads as a sharp pseudo S wave (*upward arrows* in lead II). On a snapshot ECG, the arrhythmia is indistinguishable from typical atrioventricular reentrant tachycardia. Holter monitoring revealed repeated onsets and terminations with a junctional beat (no preceding P wave).

Tachycardias due to an Accessory Pathway

Accessory Pathway Epidemiology

The prevalence of a Wolff-Parkinson-White (WPW) pattern on a sinus rhythm ECG in the general population has been estimated at between 0.15% and 0.25%. Although not classically considered to be an inherited disorder, the prevalence does increase significantly among first-degree relatives of patients with WPW to 0.55%.[55] However, in many patients, WPW is intermittent and not all with the ECG pattern will develop tachyarrhythmias.

Accessory pathways may occur in the context of the *PRKAG2* gene variant cardiac glycogenosis, which causes a syndrome characterized by cardiomyopathy with increased ventricular wall thickness, conduction disease and AV block, and ventricular preexcitation.[56]

Accessory pathways are classically recognized in patients with Ebstein anomaly, occurring in approximately 25% of this population.[57] They occur in relation to the tricuspid valve malformation and are therefore invariably right sided; frequently there may be multiple pathways, the majority of which are manifest (Fig. 65.26). It is important to recognize that in addition to AVRT, patients with Ebstein anomaly may sustain a wide range of arrhythmias, including typical and atypical AFL, focal AT, AF, and ventricular arrhythmias.

Accessory Pathway Anatomic Considerations. The musculature of the atrium and ventricles is normally separated by the electrically inert fibrous skeleton of the heart, with the only connection being the bundle of His. This electrical conducting bundle penetrates through the central fibrous body of the heart and then divides into the bundle branch system, which directs the impulse to the right and left ventricles. An accessory pathway represents a congenital persistence of bridging AV working myocardium in the form of a muscle bundle. Another form of accessory pathway involves a muscular bridge from the sleeve of myocardium investing the coronary sinus and its branches and the epicardial myocardium of the left ventricle most usually in the posteroseptal region.

Anatomically, accessory pathways are most commonly located along the mitral annulus and termed *left free wall pathways* (60%); approximately 25% are in the septal region of the tricuspid or mitral annulus, and a minority (15%) are on the right free wall.[10]

Concealed vs. Manifest Accessory Pathways. An accessory pathway may conduct in the antegrade direction (termed *manifest* due to the characteristic ECG appearance), the retrograde direction, or both. When an accessory pathway conducts only in the retrograde direction it is termed *concealed* and the surface ECG is normal. On occasion, manifest accessory pathways conduct in the antegrade direction only (these represent only approximately 10% of all accessory pathways).

The WPW ECG

The sinus rhythm 12-lead ECG of WPW classically exhibits a short PR interval (rapid conduction over the accessory pathway) and a slurred QRS onset (delta wave) (Fig. 65.27). The QRS complex represents a fusion beat between conduction over the accessory pathway and conduction over the AV node. The normal AV node has slow and decremental conduction that accounts for the normal PR interval. *Decrement* refers to the fact that conduction in the AV node slows further for an abnormally fast input such as an AT or AF. In contrast, an accessory pathway generally has rapid antegrade conduction such that there is a very short PR interval and the P wave is followed immediately by the QRS without an isoelectric interval.

Because initial ventricular activation occurs via the accessory pathway inserting directly into ventricular myocardium, the initial appearance of the QRS is a slurred onset and the beginnings of a wide QRS (due to relatively slow ventricular conduction). However, shortly after this onset, activation over the AV node is complete and the remainder of ventricular activation then occurs rapidly over the His-Purkinje fibers. This creates an inflection point in the QRS between the slow delta wave due to ventricular myocardial conduction and the subsequent rapid His-Purkinje upstroke (Fig. 65.28 and Fig. 65.29). The extent of ventricular preexcitation depends on a number of factors, including the anatomic location of the pathway and the relative speed of conduction over the accessory pathway compared with the node. For example, a left lateral accessory pathway may demonstrate minimal preexcitation because by the time atrial activation has spread from the sinus node in the high right atrium over to a left lateral location, antegrade conduction though the AV node may have already occurred. In

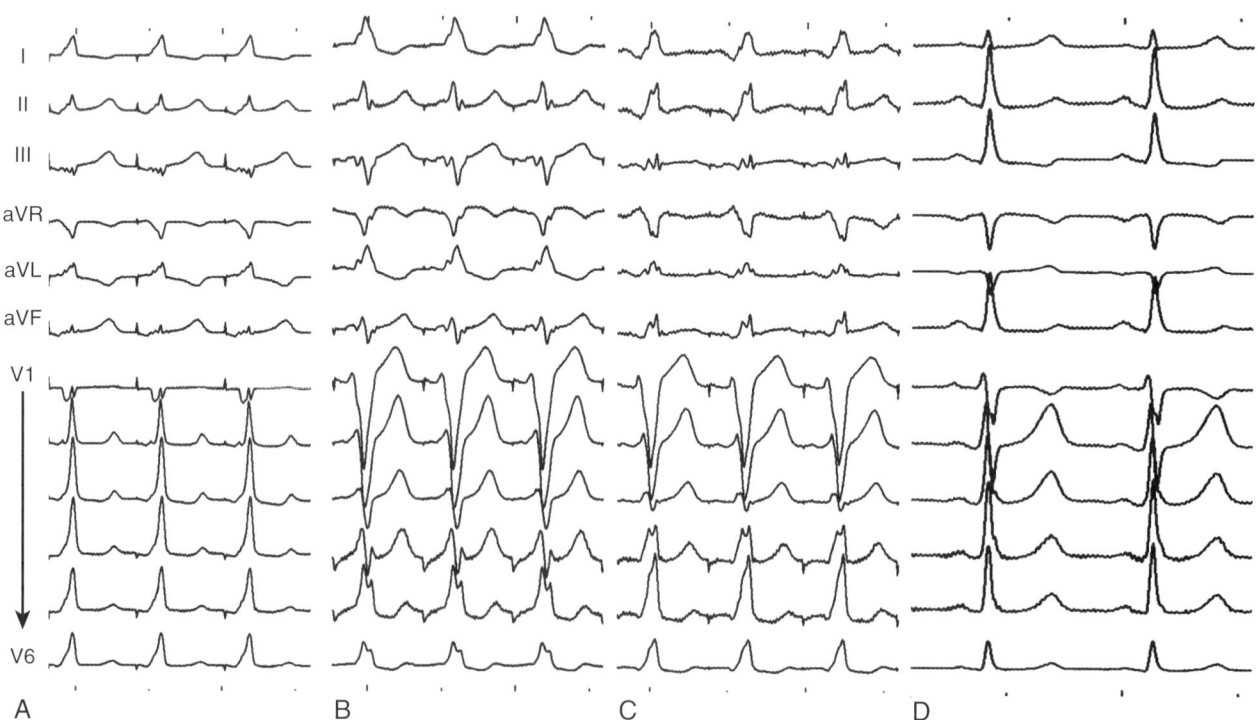

FIGURE 65.26 Patient with Ebstein anomaly and three accessory pathways around the tricuspid annulus. The ECGs were performed during an electrophysiologic study, and pacing is from the atrium near the accessory pathway insertion site in order to maximize the preexcitation. **A,** An accessory pathway located in a midseptal location. The precordial transition is between V_1 and V_2 localizing the pathway to the septum. Leads II and III are isoelectric with a small positive delta wave in lead II. This pattern is consistent with a midseptal location (deeply negative delta waves would suggest a posteroseptal location and steeply positive delta wave in the inferior leads would suggest an anteroseptal location). **B,** A second accessory pathway with a precordial transition occurs after V_3, putting this pathway on the right free wall. The pathway was right lateral. **C,** A third right-sided accessory pathway with another differing delta wave vector. The precordial transition after V_3 indicating right free wall and a more inferiorly directed delta wave axis (upright in lead II and aVF). The pathway was right anterolateral. **D,** After catheter ablation of all three pathways, the QRS morphology normalized.

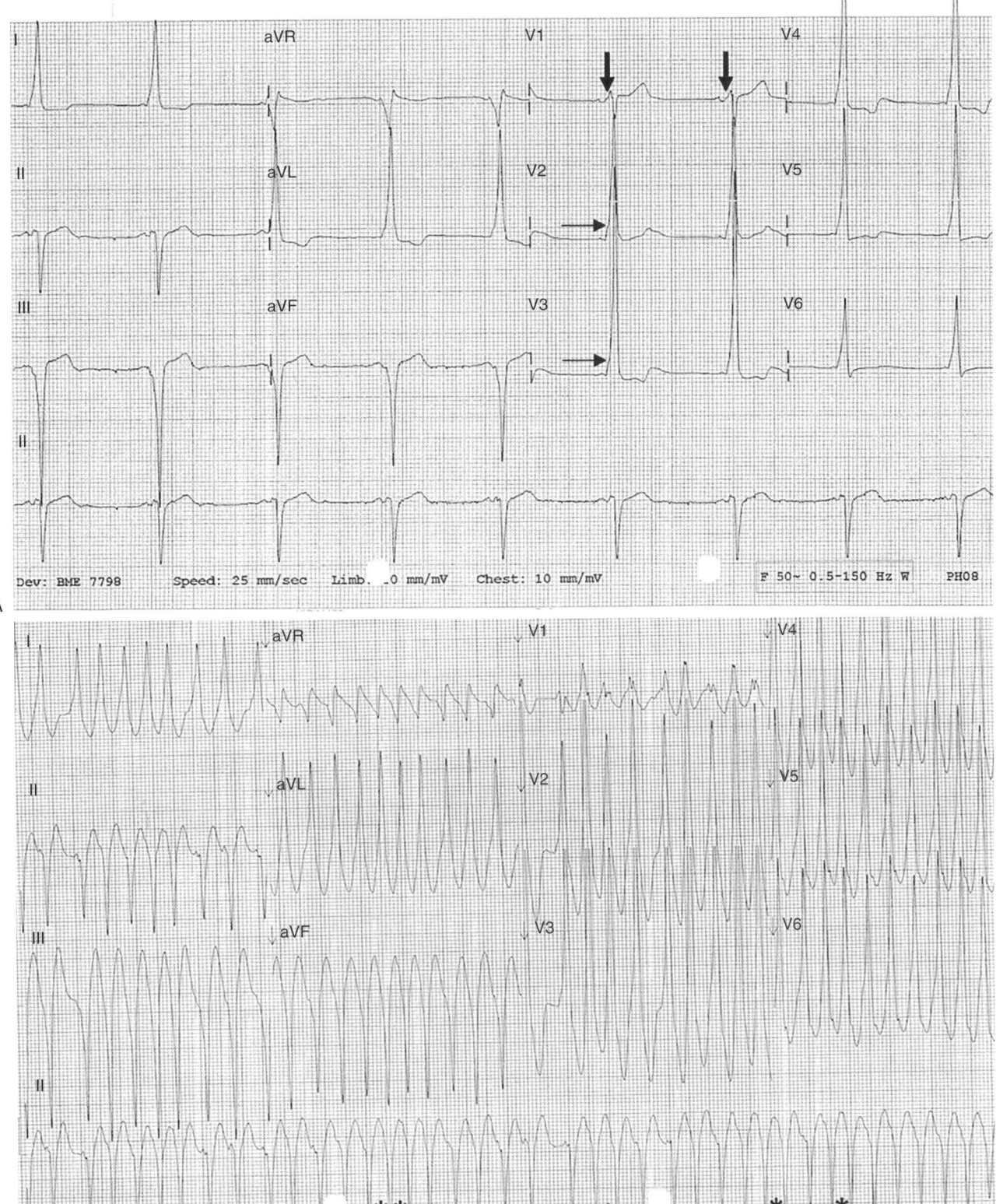

FIGURE 65.27 A, Sinus rhythm ECG showing a short PR interval and delta wave classic for Wolf-Parkinson-White syndrome (WPW). The delta wave vector is upright in V_1 (*downward arrows*) and across the precordium and negative in the inferior leads, consistent with a left posterior accessory pathway location. The inflection point between slow ventricular myocardial activation from the delta wave insertion into ventricular myocardium and rapid activation over the His-Purkinje tissue once slower conduction over the atrioventricular node has occurred is well seen in V_2 and V_3 (*horizontal arrows*). **B,** Preexcited atrial fibrillation, the hallmark of which is an irregularly irregular wide-complex tachycardia that appears largely monomorphic (some variability may occur due to capture and fusion). The delta wave morphology is upright in V_1 during maximal preexcitation. There are some very short R-R intervals of 200 msec or less (*asterisks*) equivalent to a heart rate of over 300 bpm. In general, a shortest preexcited R-R interval of less than 250 msec is a risk factor for progression to ventricular fibrillation and sudden death.

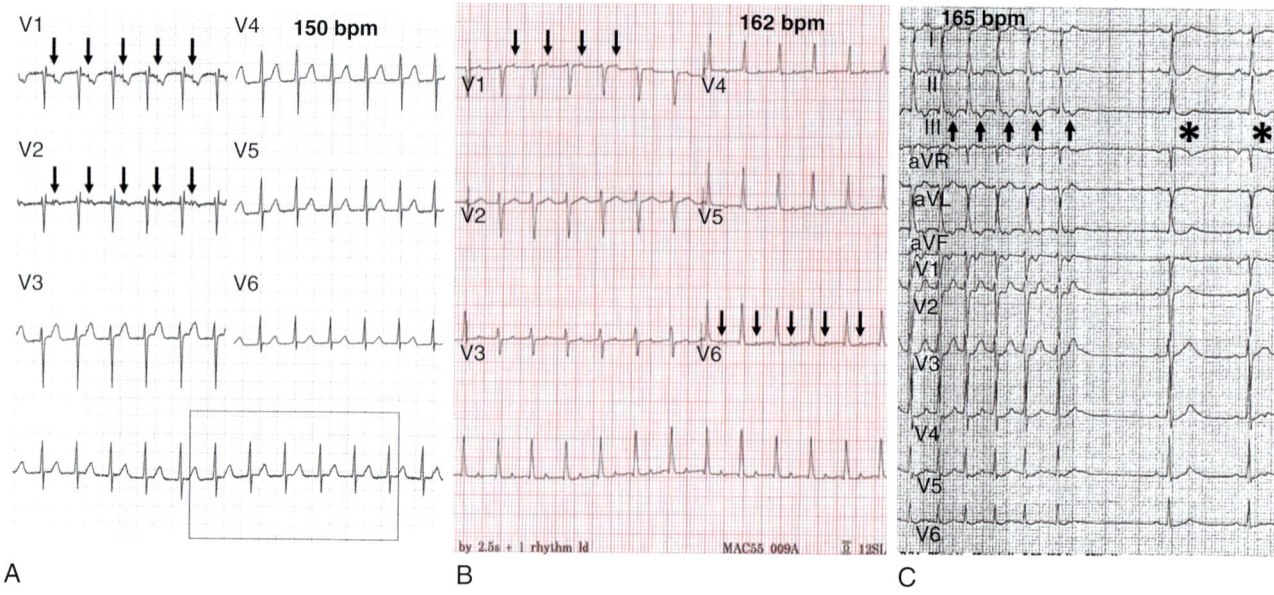

FIGURE 65.28 A, Precordial leads showing atrioventricular reentrant tachycardia (AVRT) with the retrograde P wave clearly observed deforming the T wave in V1 and in V2 (*arrows*). The patient had a concealed anteroseptal accessory pathway. **B,** Precordial leads of atrial tachycardia originating from the anteroseptal tricuspid annulus. (The P wave morphology cannot be clearly identified within the T wave). The P wave occupies the same position deforming the T wave as in the AVRT example in panel A. However, the arrhythmia is a focal atrial tachycardia. At this heart rate, there is slow conduction over the AV node to the ventricle such that the P wave is inscribed within the preceding T wave (*arrows*). The arrhythmia is independent of AV nodal conduction, and the position of the P wave is therefore incidental. Nevertheless, on the ECG alone, the two mechanisms cannot be distinguished. **C,** On the left of this continuous 12-lead trace is a regular narrow-complex tachycardia at 165 bpm with the retrograde P wave observed within the T wave (*upward arrows*). There is spontaneous termination with the final activation being the retrograde P wave. This essentially rules out an atrial tachycardia as it would be highly unlikely for the tachycardia to terminate at the precise moment when there was coincidental AV block. This implies antegrade block in the AV node, which must form part of the circuit being either AVRT or atypical atrioventricular nodal reentrant tachycardia. In this case, the arrhythmia was AVRT due to a concealed right posteroseptal accessory pathway. Note that the final 2 sinus beats are not preexcited. The *asterisks* highlight the absence of the retrograde P waves during sinus rhythm.

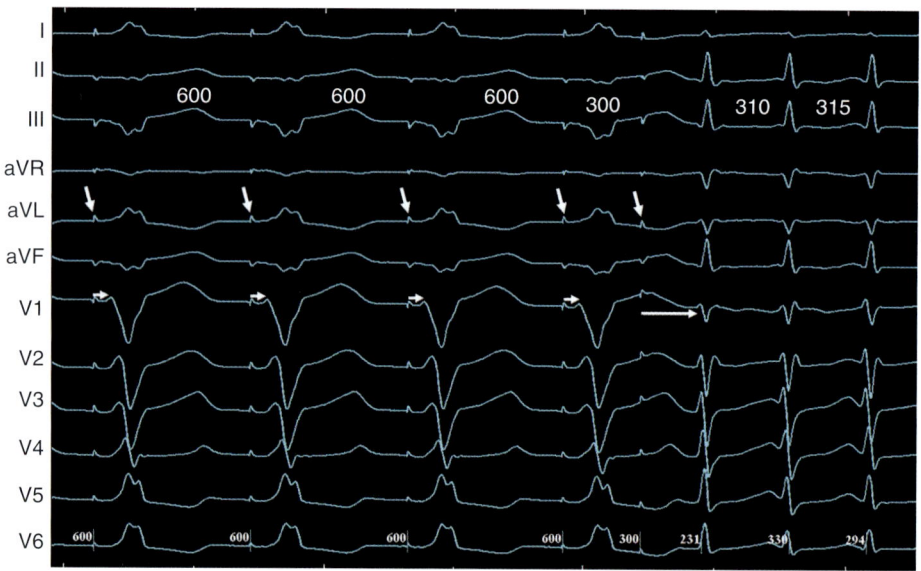

FIGURE 65.29 Continuous 12-lead ECG during atrial programmed stimulation at electrophysiology study. The patient has a right free wall accessory pathway (late precordial transition at V4). An atrial pacing drive train is being delivered at cycle length of 600 msec (pacing artefact—*downward arrows*). There is a short PR interval, and the QRS morphology is maximally preexcited due to pacing close to the accessory pathway location. An atrial extra-stimulus is introduced at a coupling interval of 300 msec. There is antegrade block in the accessory pathway with a much longer PR interval due to antegrade conduction over the AV node. The QRS of this beat is narrow because preexcitation is no longer present, and all activation occurred over the AV node and His-Purkinje system. Tachycardia is initiated as the accessory pathway–recovered excitability in the retrograde direction setting up the reentrant loop. In this case, the retrograde P waves during these initial tachycardia beats (cycle length 310/315 msec) cannot be clearly detected.

Accessory Pathway Localization. A variety of ECG algorithms to predict the likely anatomic location of the accessory pathway are based on the delta wave vector.[10] Broadly, a positive delta wave in V1 indicates a left-sided accessory pathway (see Fig. 65.28), a negative delta wave in V1 with early precordial transition to upright in V2 usually indicates a right septal accessory pathway (see Fig. 65.29), and later transition of the precordial delta wave at or after V3 most usually a right free wall accessory pathway (see Fig. 65.27). The pattern in the limb leads aids with localization to relatively more superior or inferior sites or more septal or lateral sites. These algorithms are most specific when there is significant or maximal preexcitation, which can be achieved during EPS by pacing close to the accessory pathway site.[58]

Arrhythmias Associated with Accessory Pathways

ORTHODROMIC AVRT. The most common form of tachycardia associated with an accessory pathway is orthodromic AVRT. In patients with a manifest pathway, this accounts for 90% to 95% of AVRT episodes. This circuit involves antegrade conduction over the AV node and His-Purkinje system and is therefore classically a regular narrow-complex tachycardia. Retrograde conduction occurs over the accessory pathway after ventricular activation. Therefore, the retrograde P wave occurs after ventricular activation and generally creates a visible sharp deflection deforming the T wave most usually best seen in V1 (see Fig. 65.28). Note that this location of the P wave is not specific to AVRT and may also occur in AT (see Fig. 65.28B) and in atypical AVNRT.

contrast, right free wall pathways, being very close to the AV node, may demonstrate marked preexcitation in sinus rhythm due to the proximity of the accessory pathway to sinus node activation (see Fig. 65.29). An accessory pathway with slow conduction such as an atriofascicular pathway may show no preexcitation because AV nodal conduction is more rapid.

In sinus rhythm, although the accessory pathway conducts more rapidly than the AV node, the refractory period of the accessory pathway (time taken to recover excitability) is usually longer than AV nodal refractory period. This is particularly true in sinus rhythm when the cycle length is long compared with that in tachycardia. Thus, a tight-coupled atrial premature complex can find the accessory pathway refractory but conduct slowly antegradely down the AV node (see Fig. 65.29). Conduction time down the node and His-Purkinje and across the ventricle allows recovery of accessory pathway excitability in the retrograde direction and AV reentry is initiated. When block in the accessory pathway occurs with antegrade conduction over the AV node, preexcitation is lost and the QRS normalizes because all ventricular activation is over the His-Purkinje system.

ANTIDROMIC AVRT. Antidromic AVRT is a regular wide-complex arrhythmia in which antegrade conduction occurs over the accessory pathway (fully preexcited), with retrograde activation occurring over the AV node or over a second accessory pathway present in 30% to 60% of patients with spontaneous antidromic AVRT[13] (Fig. 65.30). The P wave is inscribed within the broad QRS and is usually not visible. It accounts for only approximately 5% of AVRT episodes.

PREEXCITED TACHYCARDIA. In preexcited tachycardia, the arrhythmia originates in the atrium and is conducted passively to the ventricle over the accessory pathway, which acts as a bystander. Examples of this include AT (Fig. 65.31) or AV node reentry with passive conduction over the accessory pathway. A rapidly conducting accessory pathway does not exhibit any decremental conduction in response to a rapid input such as an AT or AF. The development of AF in the presence of an accessory pathway with a short antegrade refractory period (<250 msec) and a shortest R-R interval during AF of less than 250 msec can result in ventricular response rates of up to 300 bpm with the potential to trigger ventricular fibrillation (VF) and sudden death. The characteristic ECG is a wide-complex tachycardia (maximal preexcitation) with an irregularly irregular ventricular rhythm (see Fig. 65.28B and Fig. 65.29B).

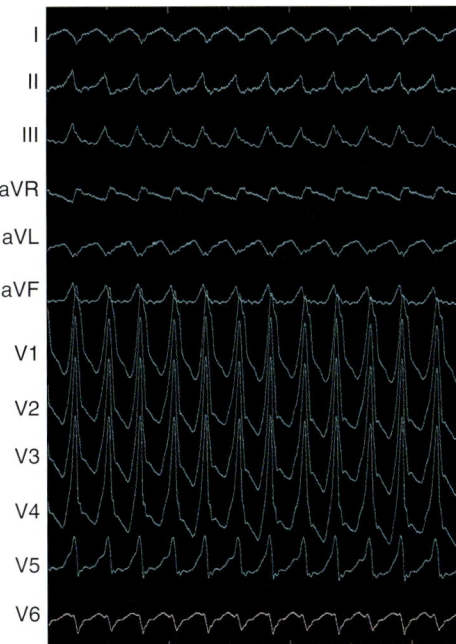

FIGURE 65.30 Antidromic tachycardia recorded during a catheter ablation procedure. The tachycardia is a regular monomorphic wide-complex tachycardia with antegrade conduction over the accessory pathway and retrograde conduction over the atrioventricular node. All ventricular myocardium is depolarized from the accessory pathway insertion point with slow conduction over ventricular myocardium producing maximal preexcitation. The delta wave vector is markedly upright in V_1 (left-sided), upright in inferior leads (anteriorly located) and negative in leads I and aVL (far left lateral) consistent with a left anterolateral pathway. The arrhythmia was proven at electrophysiologic study to be antidromic tachycardia, but the differential diagnosis of this wide-complex regular tachyarrhythmia includes ventricular tachycardia and other forms of preexcited tachycardia.

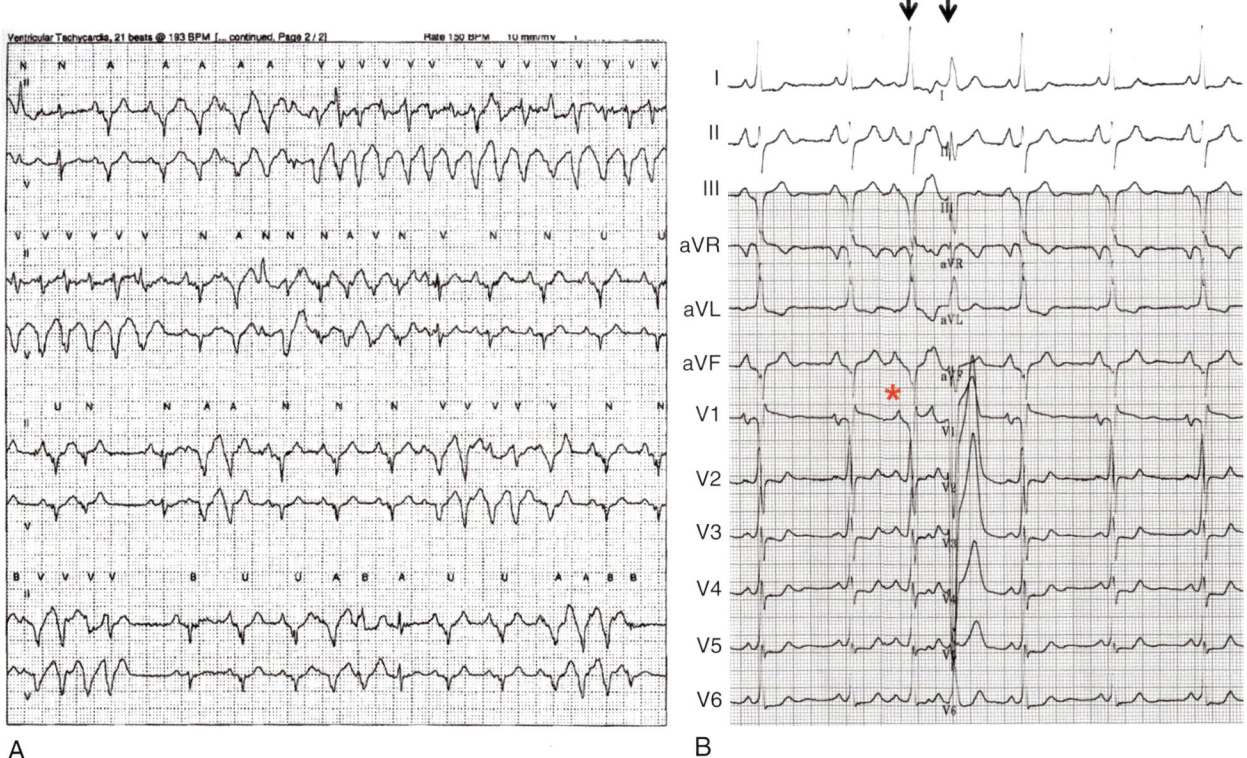

FIGURE 65.31 A 57-year-old man with recurrent palpitations and presyncope. **A,** Holter monitor trace showing bursts of wide-complex tachycardia. Analysis of the sinus beats suggests the presence of preexcitation. There are bursts of atrial tachycardia with increasing preexcitation. **B,** Continuous 12-lead ECG showing sinus rhythm with an atrial couplet from the atrial tachycardia focus. The first 2 sinus beats are preexcited with a pattern consistent with a right posteroseptal accessory pathway (precordial transition between V_1 and V_2; superiorly directed delta wave axis). There are then two atrial ectopics (*downward arrows*) with an increase in QRS duration due to increasing preexcitation. This occurs due to the decremental conduction properties of the AV node, whereas the accessory pathway demonstrates no such decrement. The atrial ectopic focus P wave is upright in V_1 and upright in inferior leads and was successfully ablated at the ostium of the left superior pulmonary vein.

Treatment of AVRT

As with any regular narrow-complex SVT, initial management may include vagal maneuvers best performed in the supine position with leg elevation.[41]

In patients who fail vagal maneuvers, adenosine 6- to 12-mg intravenous bolus is the treatment of choice but must be used with caution in AVRT due to the potential for induction of AF with rapid antegrade conduction over the accessory pathway. Electrical cardioversion must be available. In patients who fail adenosine reversion, drugs that act on the AV nodal limb of the circuit, including intravenous verapamil or diltiazem or a beta blocker (metoprolol or esmolol), may be considered. Alternatively, drugs acting on the accessory pathway such as ibutilide, procainamide, or a class 1C agent (flecainide or propafenone) may be used. In antidromic tachycardia, drugs active on the accessory pathway are preferred because when multiple accessory pathways are present they may form both limbs of the circuit. DC cardioversion is appropriate in hemodynamically unstable patients or when antiarrhythmic medications fail.

ACUTE TREATMENT OF PREEXCITED AF. Acute treatment of preexcited AF when the patient is hemodynamically unstable is DC cardioversion. When hemodynamically stable, drugs acting on the accessory pathway such as ibutilide, procainamide, or a class 1C agent (flecainide or propafenone) may be used. Amiodarone should be avoided because enhanced AV nodal conduction and VF have been described in a number of reports. Similarly, AV nodal–blocking drugs should not be used because they may also contribute to a risk of VF.

CHRONIC THERAPY IN AVRT. Catheter ablation is the treatment of choice for patients with symptoms associated with recurrent AVRT or who have sustained preexcited AF.[1,13]

Contemporary ablation success rates are in the vicinity of 95%, and complications rates are under 1% in experienced centers. In a large series of 11,601 accessory pathway catheter ablations performed between 1998 and 2011 there was a zero mortality.[59]

Beta blockers or non-dihydropyridine calcium channel blockers (verapamil or diltiazem) should be considered for concealed accessory pathway AVRT (no preexcitation on sinus rhythm ECG) when ablation is not preferred or is unsuccessful. Class 1C agents (propafenone or flecainide) may be considered for AVRT with a manifest or concealed accessory pathway when ablation is not preferred or has been unsuccessful and when no other contraindications are present (ischemic heart disease, impaired LV function etc.).[13]

ASYMPTOMATIC WPW. When WPW is found incidentally on a routine ECG or an ECG performed for a nonarrhythmic indication, it raises the question as to whether the patient is at risk of sudden death and what the most appropriate approach is. This remains a controversial area of electrophysiology. Of patients with asymptomatic WPW, 80% will go through life without arrhythmic events. In the 20% who do develop arrhythmias, the most common is AVRT in 80%. Preexcited AF may develop in 20% to 30%, with the small associated risk of sudden death estimated at 2.4 per 100 person-years in patients with asymptomatic WPW.[13] The risk estimates associated with asymptomatic preexcitation vary widely and depend on the population being considered. Preexcitation has been estimated to cause sudden death in only 3.6 per 10 million person-years in the general population.[60]

There are advocates for invasive testing and ablation if the accessory pathway has a short effective refractory period (ERP),[13,61] whereas others point out that the risk of an adverse outcome is so low that intervention is not warranted as a routine approach.[60,62,63] This exceedingly low risk must be balanced against the small procedural risk and the possibility of accessory pathway recurrence after an initially successful ablation. Nevertheless, the 2019 European Society of Cardiology guidelines provide a Class 1 recommendation of catheter ablation in asymptomatic patients who have an accessory pathway with high-risk properties at EPS. To emphasize the controversy, however, the 2015 ACC/AHA/HRS guidelines provide a class 2A recommendation for diagnostic EPS with a view to catheter ablation of high-risk pathways or alternatively an identical 2A recommendation for observation without further evaluation or treatment.[1] This decision in general involves a detailed discussion and must take into account patient preferences. Patients in high-risk occupations (e.g., pilots) may require catheter ablation to allow maintenance of licensing. Low-risk features of WPW include intermittent loss of preexcitation on ECG, Holter monitoring, or exercise stress test. High-risk features include the presence of multiple accessory pathways, a short antegrade refractory period of the accessory pathway, young age (the risk of sudden cardiac death associated with WPW is highest in the first two decades of life), and symptomatic AVRT episodes. In addition, because children may not describe classic symptoms associated with SVT, the threshold for electrophysiologic evaluation will be considerably lower.

Unusual Forms of Accessory Pathway. Permanent junctional reciprocating tachycardia (PJRT) is an unusual type of long RP SVT that occurs predominantly in infants and children.[64] The arrhythmia is due to a concealed accessory pathway with slow, decremental retrograde conduction. The accessory pathway is most commonly located in the right posteroseptal region but has also been described in the left posteroseptal area, the right free wall, and the left free wall. The tachycardia is incessant in over 50% of patients and not uncommonly results in a TMC. This is generally fully reversible on resumption of persistent sinus rhythm. In a recent large multicenter series of 194 patients with PJRT, the median age at diagnosis was 3.2 months, with the majority being diagnosed before age 1. However, there were patients diagnosed throughout childhood years and into early teenage years. The tachycardia manifests as a long RP rhythm with spontaneous initiation classically heralded by a slight shortening of the sinus cycle length (Fig. 65.32). Medical therapy is frequently ineffective, and the majority of patients will eventually undergo catheter ablation with a success rate in excess of 90% and low complication rate.[64]

Atriofascicular Pathways and Variants. The original description by Mahaim was of an anatomic connection between the AV node and the right ventricle.[65] Subsequent work describing the electrophysiologic properties of pathways with antegrade only and decremental conduction assumed that this was associated with these previously characterized anatomic connections. However, surgical mapping demonstrated that the majority of these pathways consisted of an accessory AV node and His-Purkinje system with origin from the right atrium with a distal insertion either into the distal right bundle branch (atriofascicular) or into right ventricular myocardium (AV). The most common anatomic location for these atrio-connections is at the anterior lateral TA, but they also may occur at other sites around the tricuspid ring. Because of the antegrade decremental properties of the pathway, patients will usually not have any evidence of preexcitation on a resting 12-lead ECG or minimal preexcitation only because activation occurs first over the AV node (Fig. 65.33A). Tachycardia is an antidromic arrhythmia with antegrade conduction over the pathway and retrograde conduction over the right bundle followed by bundle of His and then AV node (Fig. 65.33B). Less commonly, retrograde conduction occurs over a second accessory pathway. During tachycardia, due to the insertion near the RV apex, the QRS morphology is classically of left bundle branch appearance with a late precordial transition and a superior axis. Atriofascicular pathways have been described in association with Ebstein anomaly, in which accessory pathway conduction can mask the underlying right bundle branch block (Fig. 65.33C). Catheter ablation is the treatment of choice in patients with an atriofascicular pathway. After proving the presence of an atriofascicular pathway responsible for tachycardia, mapping is performed along the lateral tricuspid ring looking for a typical M potential. This is the equivalent of the His bundle potential being a sharp deflection located between the atrial and ventricular signals. Ablation can be technically challenging because of the common difficulty of stabilizing the ablation catheter on the TA, but success can be achieved in over 90% of cases.

Manifest antegrade only nodofascicular and nodoventricular pathways do occur but are rare. The pathway extends from the AV node to the right bundle or RV myocardium. The clinical characteristics appear very similar to those of an atriofascicular pathway (no preexcitation at baseline, with a tachycardia demonstrating left bundle branch block morphology. The distinction is made during a detailed EPS and, in the majority, ablation can be successfully achieved in the slow pathway region.

Rarely a nodofascicular pathway may be concealed, demonstrating retrograde conduction only. These very rare pathways are associated with a narrow-complex tachycardia with antegrade conduction over the AV node and His-Purkinje system and retrograde conduction over the concealed nodofascicular pathway. These pathways are most frequently right sided. The retrograde P wave may be concealed within the QRS,

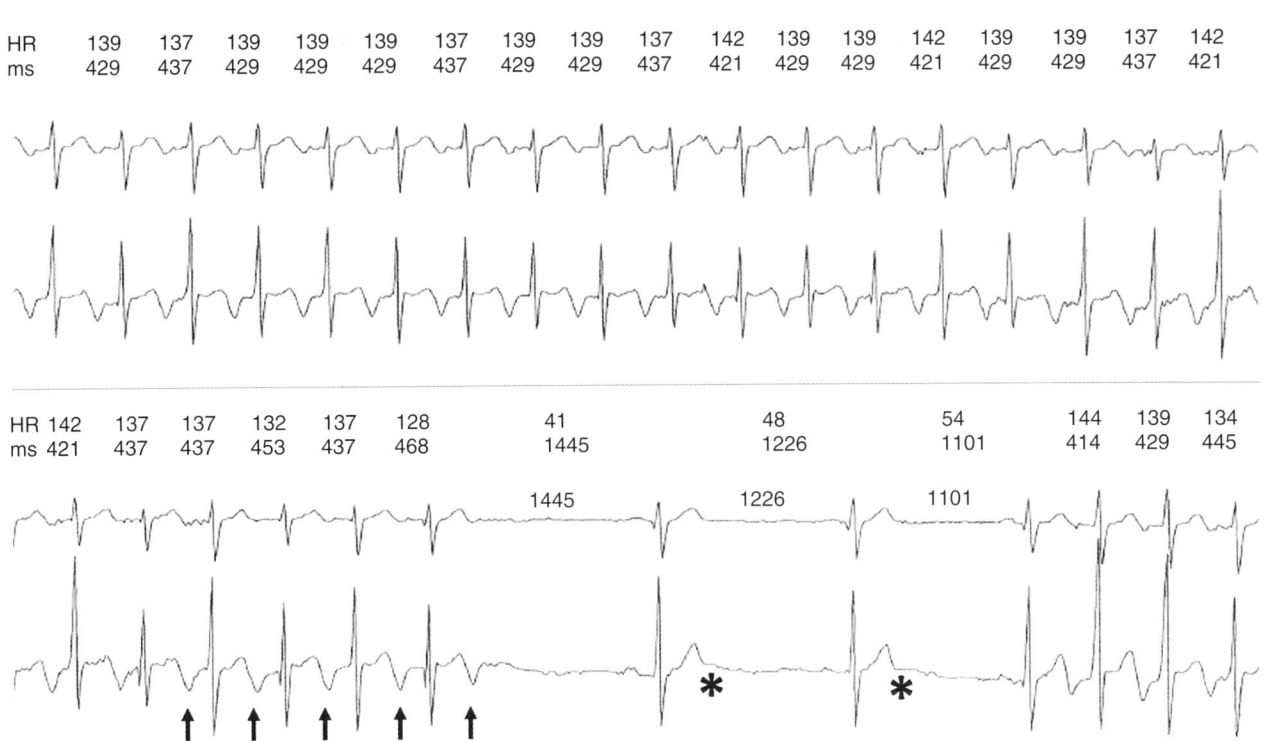

FIGURE 65.32 Holter monitor trace showing a spontaneous termination and then reinitiation of a long-RP tachycardia. Note the inverted P waves closer to the following QRS (*upward arrows*). There is spontaneous termination with the last recording being a retrograde P wave (*final upward arrow*). This effectively rules out an atrial tachycardia. Note that there are then 3 sinus beats (*asterisks* indicating absence of a retrograde P wave) before the tachycardia then reinitiates spontaneously. This spontaneous reinitiation is proceeded by a shortening of the sinus cycle length. This sinus cycle length shortening classically proceeds tachycardia onset in permanent junctional reciprocating tachycardia. This mechanism was confirmed at electrophysiology study.

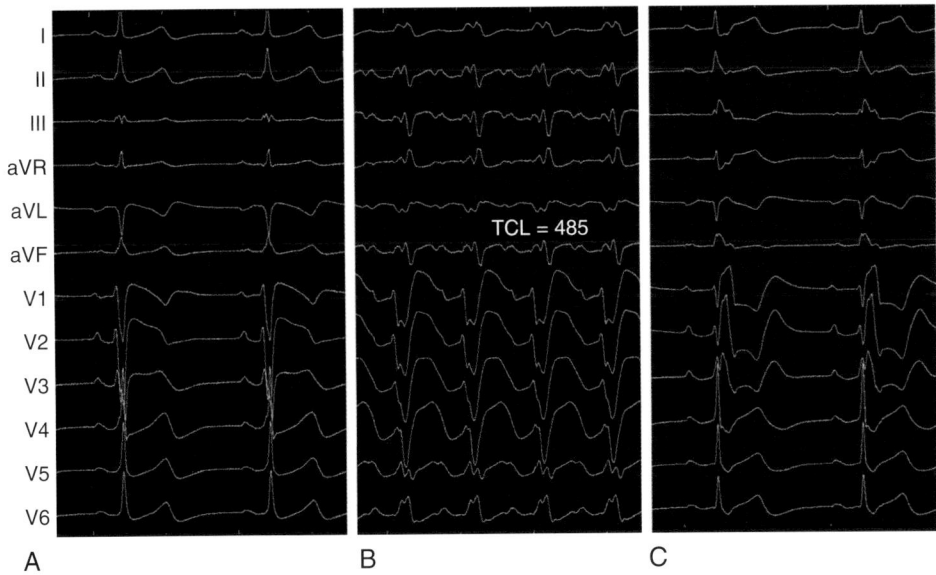

FIGURE 65.33 Recordings made during electrophysiology study and ablation procedure for patient with Ebstein anomaly and atriofascicular pathway. The pathway represents an accessory atrioventricular (AV) node, His-Purkinje system originating on the lateral tricuspid annulus and inserting into the apical region of the right bundle branch. The pathway conducts in the antegrade direction only and shows decremental properties. **A,** Baseline sinus rhythm ECG. The PR interval is normal, and there is only a hint of slurring in the initial portion of the QRS seen particularly in V_4-V_6. **B,** During antidromic preexcited tachycardia (rate 125 bpm) the QRS is broad with an LBBB morphology, late precordial transition after V_4 and a superiorly directed axis. This pattern is characteristic of tachycardia due to antegrade conduction over an atriofascicular pathway with retrograde conduction over the AV node. **C,** After successful ablation of the atriofascicular pathway the underlying first-degree AV block and right bundle branch block pattern characteristic of Ebstein anomaly is now manifest. Before ablation, this pattern had been obscured by the presence of an accessory atriofascicular pathway.

thereby mimicking typical AVNRT, or there may be retrograde block to the atrium in which case there will be VA dissociation during the narrow-complex tachycardia.[66,67]

Supraventricular Tachycardia in Adults Late after Surgical Repair of Congenital Heart Disease. Supraventricular arrhythmias are particularly common in adults late after repair of CHD. The most common mechanism is macroreentrant AT (atypical flutter) due to circuits around scars and prosthetic material. They are most common in patients with more complex forms of CHD such as Fontan repair for single ventricular physiology or Mustard or Senning repair for D-TGA.[68] However, these circuits are also common in less complex forms of CHD such as tetralogy of Fallot and simple forms such as ostium secundum ASD. In patients with complex CHD, the combination of atrial enlargement, atrial surgical scarring, and extensive remodeling often results in the presence of multiple different tachycardia circuits (Fig. 65.34).

Patients with CHD may also develop focal AT or either AVNRT or AVRT.

It is important to be aware that atrial arrhythmias in patients with complex CHD can be life-threatening. Patients often have little hemodynamic reserve, and rapid arrhythmias can lead to cardiac arrest. An arrhythmia that causes stable symptoms with 2:1 conduction may cause hemodynamic collapse if 1:1 conduction develops. This is a significant risk due to the relatively long cycle length of the arrhythmia in many cases.

Medical therapy is commonly with beta blockers for rate control. The threshold for amiodarone use in this population is relatively low because most other antiarrhythmics such as sotalol and class 1C drugs are contraindicated. Bradyarrhythmias are also common and pacing may be required. Catheter ablation is a therapeutic option to control recurrent arrhythmias. In view of extensive atrial scarring, the

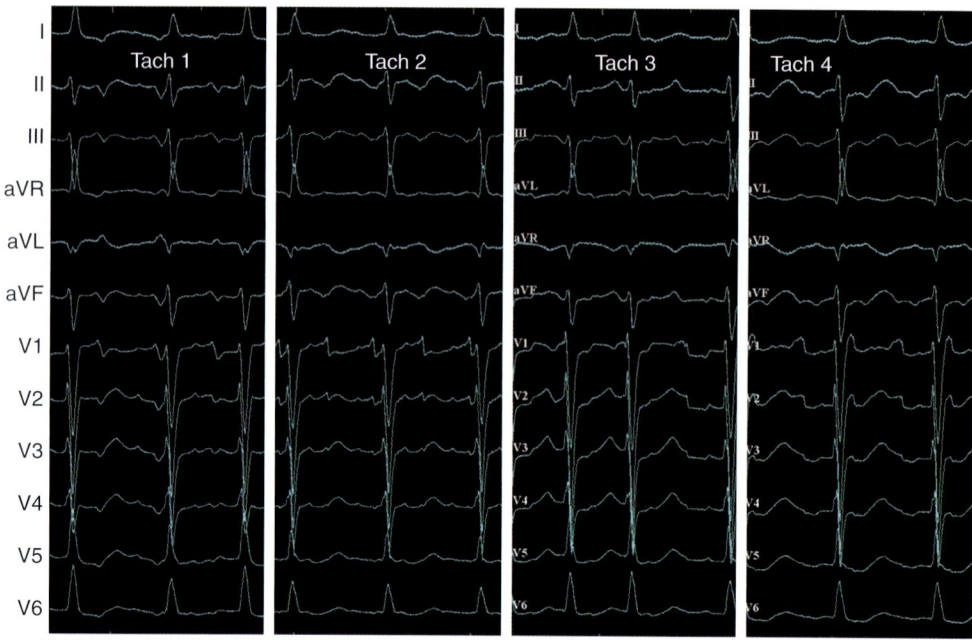

FIGURE 65.34 A 37-year-old man with prior atriopulmonary Fontan due to single ventricular physiology. Four different tachycardia morphologies recorded during an electrophysiology study. These patients frequently have profound right atrial enlargement together with extensive surgical scarring and atrial remodeling, which together create the possibility for numerous different circuits.

QRS (initial RS interval shorter in SVT with aberrancy), (5) chest lead concordance, with negative or positive being highly specific for VT but relatively insensitive; (6) QRS axis (e.g., northwest axis rarely seen in SVT with aberrancy), (7) when available, comparison with the baseline ECG may provide important clues; (8) onsets, terminations, and transitions may provide diagnostic information. For example, transition from wide to narrow complex or the reverse at a similar rate is highly suggestive of SVT with aberrancy; and (9) beyond the ECG alone, the clinical context can provide critically important information. Knowledge of a prior myocardial infarct with persistent scar would point strongly toward VT. Alternatively, a history of paroxysmal AF treated with a class 1C agent such as flecainide suggests atrial flutter with ventricular conduction slowing.

TABLE 65.2 Regular Wide-Complex Tachycardia

Ventricular tachycardia
Fascicular tachycardia

SVT with bundle branch aberrancy
    Rate-related
    Preexisting
    Antiarrhythmic induced (e.g., flecainide)
    Metabolic derangement (e.g., hyperkalemia)

Accessory pathway related
    Antidromic tachycardia
    Preexcited tachycardia (atrial tachycardia or AVNRT with bystander accessory pathway)

Rapid ventricular pacing

AVNRT, Atrioventricular nodal reentrant tachycardia; *SVT,* supraventricular tachycardia.

procedure is generally not curative but excellent palliative results can be obtained. Management of adults late after surgical repair of CHD should be undertaken only in specialist units where CHD physicians and electrophysiologists experienced in complex arrhythmia ablation work closely together.

Patients with atrial arrhythmias and CHD generally warrant anticoagulation with an oral anticoagulant.

DIFFERENTIAL DIAGNOSIS OF WIDE COMPLEX TACHYCARDIA

The differential diagnosis of wide-complex tachycardia is considered in Table 65.2. The differentiation of VT from supraventricular tachyarrhythmias associated with broad QRS complexes can be a diagnostic challenge with important clinical implications. A range of different stepwise, points-based, and single criteria methods have been devised that largely are focused on the same key criteria.[69] These have included (1) the AV relationship and specifically whether AV dissociation is present, (2) morphologic QRS criteria asking the question of whether this is a typical left or right bundle branch block pattern; (3) QRS duration (broader in VT), (4) activation velocity of the initial and terminal components of the

REFERENCES
General Considerations

1. Page RL, Joglar JA, Caldwell MA, et al. ACC/AHA/HRS guideline for the management of adult patients with supraventricular tachycardia: a report of the American College of Cardiology/American Heart Association task force on clinical practice guidelines and the Heart Rhythm Society. *J Am Coll Cardiol.* 2016;67:e27–e115.
2. Murer M, Cuculi F, Toggweiler S, et al. Elevated high-sensitivity troponin does not indicate the presence of coronary artery disease in patients presenting with supraventricular tachycardia. *Cardiol J.* 2017;24:642–648.
3. Conen D, Adam M, Roche F, et al. Premature atrial contractions in the general population: frequency and risk factors. *Circulation.* 2012;126:2302–2308.
4. Haissaguerre M, Jais P, Shah DC, et al. Spontaneous initiation of atrial fibrillation by ectopic beats originating in the pulmonary veins. *N Engl J Med.* 1998;339:659–666.
5. Larsen BS, Kumarathurai P, Falkenberg J, et al. Excessive atrial ectopy and short atrial runs increase the risk of stroke beyond incident atrial fibrillation. *J Am Coll Cardiol.* 2015;66:232–241.
6. Marcus GM, Dewland TA. Premature atrial contractions: a wolf in sheep's clothing? *J Am Coll Cardiol.* 2015;66:242–244.
7. Sajeev JK, Koshy AN, Dewey H, et al. Association between excessive premature atrial complexes and cryptogenic stroke: results of a case-control study. *BMJ Open.* 2019;9:e029164.
8. Liuba I, Schaller RD, Frankel DS. Premature atrial complex-induced cardiomyopathy: case report and literature review. *Heart Rhythm Case Rep.* 2020;6:191–193.
9. Roberts-Thomson KC, Kistler PM, Kalman JM. Atrial tachycardia: mechanisms, diagnosis, and management. *Curr Probl Cardiol.* 2005;30:529–573.
10. Olgin JE, Zipes DP. Supraventricular arrhythmias. In: Zipes DP, et al., ed. *Braunwald's Heart Disease, a Textbook of Cardiovascular Medicine.* 11th ed. Philadelphia, PA: Elsevier; 2016.
11. Saoudi N, Cosio F, Waldo A, et al. A classification of atrial flutter and regular atrial tachycardia according to electrophysiological mechanisms and anatomical bases; a statement from a joint expert group from the working group of arrhythmias of the European Society of Cardiology and the North American Society of Pacing and Electrophysiology. *Eur Heart J.* 2001;22:1162–1182.
12. Frontera A, Takigawa M, Haissaguerre M, et al. High-density characterization of a localized reentry circuit occurred after AF ablation. *Pacing Clin Electrophysiol.* 2019;42:111–112.
13. Brugada J, Katritsis DG, Arbelo E, et al. 2019 ESC guidelines for the management of patients with supraventricular tachycardia: the task force for the management of patients with supraventricular tachycardia of the European Society of Cardiology (ESC). *Eur Heart J.* 2020;41:655–720.
14. Poutiainen AM, Koistinen MJ, Airaksinen KE, et al. Prevalence and natural course of ectopic atrial tachycardia. *Eur Heart J.* 1999;20:694–700.
15. Porter MJ, Morton JB, Denman R, et al. Influence of age and gender on the mechanism of supraventricular tachycardia. *Heart Rhythm.* 2004;1:393–396.
16. Hillock RJ, Kalman JM, Roberts-Thomson KC, et al. Multiple focal atrial tachycardias in a healthy adult population: characterization and description of successful radiofrequency ablation. *Heart Rhythm.* 2007;4:435–438.

Supraventricular Arrhythmic Types

17. Morris GM, Segan L, Wong G, et al. Atrial tachycardia arising from the crista terminalis, detailed electrophysiological features and long-term ablation outcomes. *JACC Clin Electrophysiol.* 2019;5:448–458.
18. Beukema RJ, Smit JJ, Adiyaman A, et al. Ablation of focal atrial tachycardia from the non-coronary aortic cusp: case series and review of the literature. *Europace.* 2015;17:953–961.
19. Kistler PM, Roberts-Thomson KC, Haqqani HM, et al. P-wave morphology in focal atrial tachycardia: development of an algorithm to predict the anatomic site of origin. *J Am Coll Cardiol.* 2006;48:1010–1017.
20. Olshansky B, Sullivan RM. Inappropriate sinus tachycardia. *Europace.* 2019;21:194–207.
21. Sheldon RS, Grubb 2nd BP, Olshansky B, et al. 2015 Heart Rhythm Society expert consensus statement on the diagnosis and treatment of postural tachycardia syndrome, inappropriate sinus tachycardia, and vasovagal syncope. *Heart Rhythm.* 2015;12:e41–63.
21a. Arano Llach J, Bazan V, Llados G, et al. Inappropriate sinus tachycardia in post-Covid-19 syndrome. *Europace.* 2021;23(suppl 3):euab116.114.
22. Benjamin EJ, Muntner P, Alonso A, et al. Heart disease and stroke statistics-2019 update: a report from the American Heart Association. *Circulation.* 2019;139:e56–e528.

23. Kumar S, Michaud GF. Atrial fibrillation: mechanisms, clinical features and management. In: Zipes DP, et al., ed. *Cardiac Electrophysiology: From Cell to Bedside*. 7th ed. Philadelphia, PA: Elsevier; 2018.
24. Waldo AL. Atrial fibrillation and atrial flutter: two sides of the same coin!. *Int J Cardiol*. 2017;240:251–252.
25. Maskoun W, Pino MI, Ayoub K, et al. Incidence of atrial fibrillation after atrial flutter ablation. *JACC Clin Electrophysiol*. 2016;2:682–690.
26. Pathik B, Lee G, Sacher F, et al. New insights into an old arrhythmia: high-resolution mapping demonstrates conduction and substrate variability in right atrial macro-re-entrant tachycardia. *JACC Clin Electrophysiol*. 2017;3:971–986.
27. Medi C, Kalman JM. Prediction of the atrial flutter circuit location from the surface electrocardiogram. *Europace*. 2008;10:786–796.
28. Moore BM, Anderson R, Nisbet AM, et al. Ablation of atrial arrhythmias after the atriopulmonary Fontan procedure: mechanisms of arrhythmia and outcomes. *JACC Clin Electrophysiol*. 2018;4:1338–1346.
29. Derval N, Takigawa M, Frontera A, et al. Characterization of complex atrial tachycardia in patients with previous atrial interventions using high-resolution mapping. *JACC Clin Electrophysiol*. 2020;6:815–826.

Management Strategies

30. Markowitz SM, Thomas G, Liu CF, et al. Atrial tachycardias and atypical atrial flutters: mechanisms and approaches to ablation. *Arrhythm Electrophysiol Rev*. 2019;8:131–137.
31. Enriquez A, Santangeli P, Zado ES, et al. Postoperative atrial tachycardias after mitral valve surgery: mechanisms and outcomes of catheter ablation. *Heart Rhythm*. 2017;14:520–526.
32. Luther V, Sikkel M, Bennett N, et al. Visualizing localized reentry with ultra-high density mapping in iatrogenic atrial tachycardia: beware pseudo-reentry. *Circ Arrhythm Electrophysiol*. 2017;10.
33. Holmqvist F, Kesek M, Englund A, et al. A decade of catheter ablation of cardiac arrhythmias in Sweden: ablation practices and outcomes. *Eur Heart J*. 2019;40:820–830.
34. Wang H, Wang C, Chen J, et al. Long-term outcome of catheter ablation for atrial tachyarrhythmias in patients with atrial septal defect. *J Interv Card Electrophysiol*. 2019;54:217–224.
35. Anguera I, Dallaglio P, Macias R, et al. Long-term outcome after ablation of right atrial tachyarrhythmias after the surgical repair of congenital and acquired heart disease. *Am J Cardiol*. 2015;115:1705–1713.
36. Saul JP, Kanter RJ, Writing Commitee, et al. PACES/HRS expert consensus statement on the use of catheter ablation in children and patients with congenital heart disease: developed in partnership with the Pediatric and Congenital Electrophysiology Society (PACES) and the Heart Rhythm Society (HRS). Endorsed by the governing bodies of PACES, HRS, the American Academy of Pediatrics (AAP), the American Heart Association (AHA), and the Association for European Pediatric and Congenital Cardiology (AEPC). *Heart Rhythm*. 2016;13:e251–e289.
37. Gopinathannair R, Mar PL, Afzal MR, et al. Atrial tachycardias after surgical atrial fibrillation ablation: clinical characteristics, electrophysiological mechanisms, and ablation outcomes from a large, multicenter study. *JACC Clin Electrophysiol*. 2017;3:865–874.
38. Gucuk Ipek E, Marine J, Yang E, et al. Predictors and incidence of atrial flutter after catheter ablation of atrial fibrillation. *Am J Cardiol*. 2019;124:1690–1696.
39. Katritsis DG, Becker A. The atrioventricular nodal reentrant tachycardia circuit: a proposal. *Heart Rhythm*. 2007;4:1354–1360.
40. Katritsis DG, Josephson ME. Classification, electrophysiological features and therapy of atrioventricular nodal reentrant tachycardia. *Arrhythm Electrophysiol Rev*. 2016;5:130–135.
41. Appelboam A, Reuben A, Mann C, et al. Postural modification to the standard Valsalva manoeuvre for emergency treatment of supraventricular tachycardias (revert): a randomised controlled trial. *Lancet*. 2015;386:1747–1753.
42. Katritsis DG, Zografos T, Katritsis GD, et al. Catheter ablation vs. Antiarrhythmic drug therapy in patients with symptomatic atrioventricular nodal re-entrant tachycardia: a randomized, controlled trial. *Europace*. 2017;19:602–606.
43. Feldman A, Voskoboinik A, Kumar S, et al. Predictors of acute and long-term success of slow pathway ablation for atrioventricular nodal reentrant tachycardia: a single center series of 1,419 consecutive patients. *Pacing Clin Electrophysiol*. 2011;34:927–933.
44. Chrispin J, Misra S, Marine JE, et al. Current management and clinical outcomes for catheter ablation of atrioventricular nodal re-entrant tachycardia. *Europace*. 2018;20:e51–e59.
45. Katritsis DG, Zografos T, Siontis KC, et al. Endpoints for successful slow pathway catheter ablation in typical and atypical atrioventricular nodal re-entrant tachycardia: a contemporary, multicenter study. *JACC Clin Electrophysiol*. 2019;5:113–119.
46. Insulander P, Bastani H, Braunschweig F, et al. Cryoablation of atrioventricular nodal re-entrant tachycardia: 7-year follow-up in 515 patients-confirmed safety but very late recurrences occur. *Europace*. 2017;19:1038–1042.
47. Karacan M, Celik N, Akdeniz C, et al. Long-term outcomes following cryoablation of atrioventricular nodal reentrant tachycardia in children. *Pacing Clin Electrophysiol*. 2018;41:255–260.
48. Chan NY, Mok NS, Yuen HC, et al. Cryoablation with an 8-mm tip catheter in the treatment of atrioventricular nodal re-entrant tachycardia: results from a randomized controlled trial (cryoablate). *Europace*. 2019;21:662–669.
49. Makhoul M, Oster M, Fischbach P, et al. Junctional ectopic tachycardia after congenital heart surgery in the current surgical era. *Pediatr Cardiol*. 2013;34:370–374.
50. El Amrousy DM, Elshmaa NS, El-Kashlan M, et al. Efficacy of prophylactic dexmedetomidine in preventing postoperative junctional ectopic tachycardia after pediatric cardiac surgery. *J Am Heart Assoc*. 2017;6:e004780.
51. Kylat RI, Samson RA. Junctional ectopic tachycardia in infants and children. *J Arrhythm*. 2020;36:59–66.
52. Ergul Y, Ozturk E, Ozgur S, et al. Ivabradine is an effective antiarrhythmic therapy for congenital junctional ectopic tachycardia-induced cardiomyopathy during infancy: case studies. *Pacing Clin Electrophysiol*. 2018;41:1372–1377.
53. Collins KK, Van Hare GF, Kertesz NJ, et al. Pediatric nonpost-operative junctional ectopic tachycardia medical management and interventional therapies. *J Am Coll Cardiol*. 2009;53:690–697.
54. Dar T, Turagam MK, Yarlagadda B, et al. Outcomes of junctional ectopic tachycardia ablation in adult population-a multicenter experience. *J Interv Card Electrophysiol*. 2020.
55. Vidaillet Jr HJ, Pressley JC, Henke E, et al. Familial occurrence of accessory atrioventricular pathways (preexcitation syndrome). *N Engl J Med*. 1987;317:65–69.
56. Lopez-Sainz A, Dominguez F, Lopes LR, et al. Clinical features and natural history of PRKAG2 variant cardiac glycogenosis. *J Am Coll Cardiol*. 2020;76:186–197.
57. Wei W, Zhan X, Xue Y, et al. Features of accessory pathways in adult Ebstein's anomaly. *Europace*. 2014;16:1619–1625.
58. Pambrun T, El Bouazzaoui R, Combes N, et al. Maximal pre-excitation based algorithm for localization of manifest accessory pathways in adults. *JACC Clin Electrophysiol*. 2018;4:1052–1061.
59. Garg J, Shah N, Krishnamoorthy P, et al. Catheter ablation of accessory pathway: 14-year trends in utilization and complications in adults in the United States. *Int J Cardiol*. 2017;248:196–200.
60. Obeyesekere MN, Klein GJ. Application of the 2015 ACC/AHA/HRS guidelines for risk stratification for sudden death in adult patients with asymptomatic pre-excitation. *J Cardiovasc Electrophysiol*. 2017;28:841–848.
61. Pappone C, Santinelli V. Electrophysiology testing and catheter ablation are helpful when evaluating asymptomatic patients with Wolff-Parkinson-White pattern: the pro perspective. *Card Electrophysiol Clin*. 2015;7:371–376.
62. Obeyesekere MN, Klein GJ. Preventing sudden death in asymptomatic Wolf-Parkinson-White patients. *JACC Clin Electrophysiol*. 2018;4:445–447.
63. Skanes AC, Obeyesekere M, Klein GJ. Electrophysiology testing and catheter ablation are helpful when evaluating asymptomatic patients with Wolff-Parkinson-White pattern: the con perspective. *Card Electrophysiol Clin*. 2015;7:377–383.
64. Kang KT, Potts JE, Radbill AE, et al. Permanent junctional reciprocating tachycardia in children: a multicenter experience. *Heart Rhythm*. 2014;11:1426–1432.
65. Hoffmayer KS, Han FT, Singh D, et al. Variants of accessory pathways. *Pacing Clin Electrophysiol*. 2020;43:21–29.
66. Soares Correa F, Lokhandwala Y, Cruz Filho F, et al. Part II: clinical presentation, electrophysiologic characteristics, and when and how to ablate atriofascicular pathways and long and short decrementally conducting accessory pathways. *J Cardiovasc Electrophysiol*. 2019;30:3079–3096.
67. Anderson RH, Sanchez-Quintana D, Mori S, et al. Unusual variants of pre-excitation: from anatomy to ablation: Part I—Understanding the anatomy of the variants of ventricular pre-excitation. *J Cardiovasc Electrophysiol*. 2019;30:2170–2180.
68. Khairy P, Van Hare GF, Balaji S, et al. PACES/HRS expert consensus statement on the recognition and management of arrhythmias in adult congenital heart disease: developed in partnership between the Pediatric And Congenital Electrophysiology Society (PACES) and the Heart Rhythm Society (HRS). Endorsed by the governing bodies of PACES, HRS, the American College of Cardiology (ACC), the American Heart Association (AHA), the European Heart Rhythm Association (EHRA), the Canadian Heart Rhythm Society (CHRS), and the International Society for Adult Congenital Heart Disease (ISACHD). *Can J Cardiol*. 2014;30:e1–e63.
69. Kashou AH, Noseworthy PA, DeSimone CV, et al. Wide complex tachycardia differentiation: a reappraisal of the state-of-the-art. *J Am Heart Assoc*. 2020;9:e016598.

66 Atrial Fibrillation: Clinical Features, Mechanisms, and Management

HUGH CALKINS, GORDON F. TOMASELLI, AND FRED MORADY

ELECTROCARDIOGRAPHIC FEATURES, 1272
CLASSIFICATION OF ATRIAL FIBRILLATION, 1272
EPIDEMIOLOGY OF ATRIAL FIBRILLATION, 1272
MECHANISMS OF ATRIAL FIBRILLATION, 1273
GENETIC FACTORS, 1274
CAUSES OF ATRIAL FIBRILLATION, 1274
CLINICAL FEATURES, 1274
DIAGNOSTIC EVALUATION, 1275
PREVENTION OF THROMBOEMBOLIC COMPLICATIONS, 1275
Risk Stratification, 1275

Aspirin, 1276
Warfarin, 1276
Direct-Acting Oral Anticoagulants, 1276
Low-Molecular-Weight Heparin, 1277
Excision or Closure of the Left Atrial Appendage, 1277
ACUTE MANAGEMENT OF ATRIAL FIBRILLATION, 1277
LONG-TERM MANAGEMENT OF ATRIAL FIBRILLATION, 1279
Pharmacologic Rate Control Versus Rhythm Control, 1279
Pharmacologic Rate Control, 1279
Pharmacologic Rhythm Control, 1279
Rhythm Control with Agents Other Than Antiarrhythmic Drugs, 1280

NONPHARMACOLOGIC MANAGEMENT OF ATRIAL FIBRILLATION, 1280
Risk Factor Modification, 1280
Pacing to Prevent Atrial Fibrillation, 1280
Catheter Ablation of Atrial Fibrillation, 1280
Ablation of the Atrioventricular Node, 1283
SPECIFIC CLINICAL SYNDROMES, 1284
Postoperative Atrial Fibrillation, 1284
Wolff-Parkinson-White Syndrome, 1284
Congestive Heart Failure, 1284
Hypertrophic Cardiomyopathy, 1285
Pregnancy, 1285
FUTURE PERSPECTIVES, 1285
REFERENCES, 1285

ELECTROCARDIOGRAPHIC FEATURES

Atrial fibrillation (AF) is a supraventricular arrhythmia characterized electrocardiographically by low-amplitude baseline oscillations (fibrillatory or f waves from the fibrillating atria) and an irregularly irregular ventricular rhythm. The f waves, 300 to 600 beats/min, are variable in amplitude, shape, and timing. Atrial flutter waves have a rate of 250 to 350 beats/min and are constant in timing and morphology (Fig. 66.1). In lead V_1, f waves sometimes appear uniform and can mimic flutter waves (Fig. 66.2). In some patients, f waves are very small and not perceptible on the electrocardiogram, and the diagnosis of AF is based on the irregularly irregular ventricular rhythm (Fig. 66.3).

The ventricular rate during untreated AF typically is 100 to 160 beats/min. Patients with the Wolff-Parkinson-White (WPW) syndrome can experience ventricular rates during AF exceeding 250 beats/min because of conduction over the accessory pathway (see Chapter 65). The ventricular rate during AF can appear more regular when the rate is extremely rapid (>170 beats/min) (Fig. 66.4), when a junctional tachycardia independently controls the ventricles, when there is high-degree atrioventricular (AV) block with a regular escape rhythm (Fig. 66.5), or when the QRS complexes all are paced. In these cases the diagnosis of AF is based on the presence of f waves. Infrequently, a junctional tachycardia can exhibit Wenckebach exit block (often during digitalis toxicity) and cause a regularly irregular ventricular rate.

CLASSIFICATION OF ATRIAL FIBRILLATION

Atrial fibrillation that terminates spontaneously within 7 days is termed *paroxysmal*, and AF present continuously for more than 7 days is called *persistent*. AF that persists for longer than 1 year is termed *longstanding persistent*. The term *permanent AF* is used when the patient and clinician jointly decide to abandon further attempts at restoring and/or maintaining sinus rhythm.[1] This "acceptance of AF" represents a therapeutic attitude rather than a pathophysiologic characteristic of the AF and should not be taken literally. Some patients with paroxysmal AF occasionally can have episodes that are persistent and vice versa. The predominant form of AF determines how it should be categorized.

A confounding factor in the classification of AF is cardioversion and antiarrhythmic drug (AAD) therapy. For example, if a patient undergoes transthoracic cardioversion 24 hours after AF onset, it is unknown whether the AF would have persisted for more than 7 days. Furthermore, AAD therapy can change persistent AF into paroxysmal AF. The classification of AF should not be altered on the basis of the effects of electrical cardioversion or AAD therapy.

Lone atrial fibrillation refers to AF that occurs in patients younger than 60 years who do not have hypertension or any evidence of structural heart disease. This designation is a historical descriptor that has been variably applied to different low-risk subsets of AF patients. Because the definitions have not been consistent, and the potentially confusing definitions of this term, this designation should be abandoned.

Paroxysmal AF also can be classified clinically on the basis of the autonomic setting in which it most often occurs. Approximately 25% of patients with paroxysmal AF have *vagotonic* AF, in which AF is initiated in the setting of high vagal tone, typically in the evening when the patient is relaxing or during sleep. Drugs exerting a vagotonic effect (e.g., digitalis) can aggravate vagotonic AF, and drugs with a vagolytic effect (e.g., disopyramide) may be particularly appropriate for prophylactic therapy. Adrenergic AF occurs in approximately 10% to 15% of patients with paroxysmal AF in the setting of high sympathetic tone, as during strenuous exertion. In patients with adrenergic AF, beta blockers not only provide rate control but may prevent episodes of AF. Most patients have a mixed or random form of paroxysmal AF, with no consistent pattern of onset. In some, alcohol can be a precipitant.[2,3]

EPIDEMIOLOGY OF ATRIAL FIBRILLATION

Atrial fibrillation is the most common arrhythmia treated in clinical practice and the most common arrhythmia for which patients are hospitalized; approximately 33% of arrhythmia-related hospitalizations are for AF. In 2010 the prevalence of AF was estimated to be between 2.1 and 6.1 million persons. This is predicted to increase to 12.1 million persons by 2030.[4] AF is associated with approximately a fivefold increase in the risk of cerebrovascular accident (stroke), a twofold increase in the risk of all-cause mortality, and a twofold increase in cognitive dysfunction.[4] AF also is associated with the development of heart failure and has been linked to sudden death.

The incidence of AF is related to age and sex, ranging from 0.1% per year before age 40 to more than 1.5% per year in women and more than 2% per year in men older than 80. Advanced age, congestive heart failure, male sex, tall stature, a family history of AF at less than 50 years of age, left atrial enlargement, and hypertension are independent risk factors for the development of AF, as are obesity and obstructive sleep apnea. AF is less common in African Americans.[1]

MECHANISMS OF ATRIAL FIBRILLATION

The mechanisms responsible for AF are complex and incompletely understood. The three main mechanistic concepts that have emerged over time consist of multiple reentrant wavelets, rapidly discharging autonomic foci, and a single reentrant circuit with fibrillatory conduction. Considerable progress has been made in defining the mechanisms underlying initiation, perpetuation, and progression of AF.[5-8] A key breakthrough that had an immediate therapeutic impact was the recognition that in many patients, AF is triggered and/or maintained by rapidly firing foci in the pulmonary veins.[7] It is now well accepted the focal firing is the key mechanism underlying initiation and perpetuation of paroxysmal AF. In contrast, the mechanisms that underlie maintenance of persistent AF appear far more complex. In persistent AF, changes in the atrial substrate, including interstitial fibrosis that

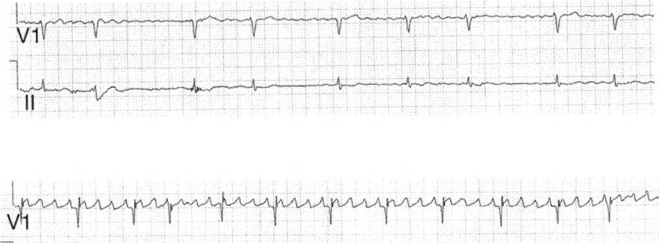

FIGURE 66.1 Comparison between the f waves of AF **(top panel)** and the flutter waves of atrial flutter **(bottom panel).** Note that f waves are variable in rate, shape, and amplitude, whereas flutter waves are constant in rate and morphology. Shown are leads V_1 and II.

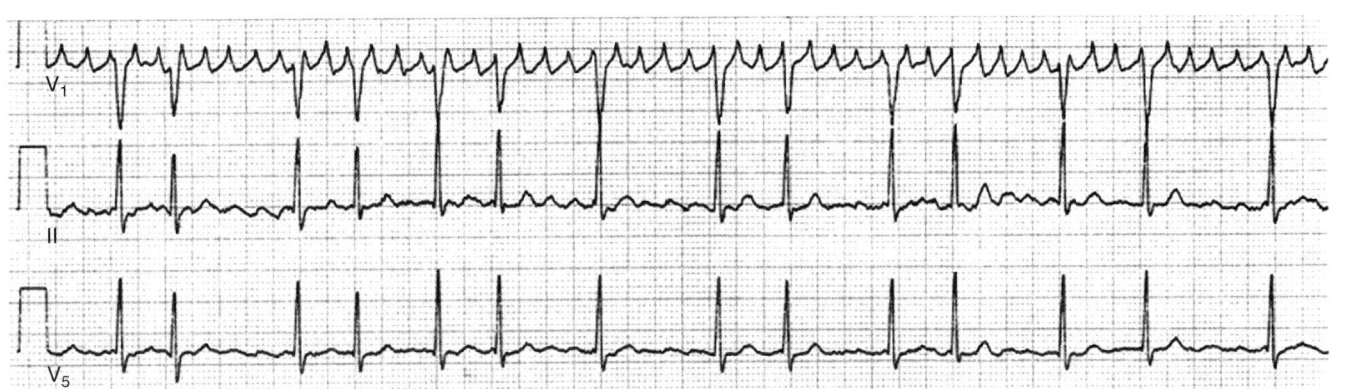

FIGURE 66.2 An example of AF with prominent f waves in V_1 that mimic atrial flutter waves. Note that typical f waves are present in leads II and V_5, establishing the diagnosis of AF.

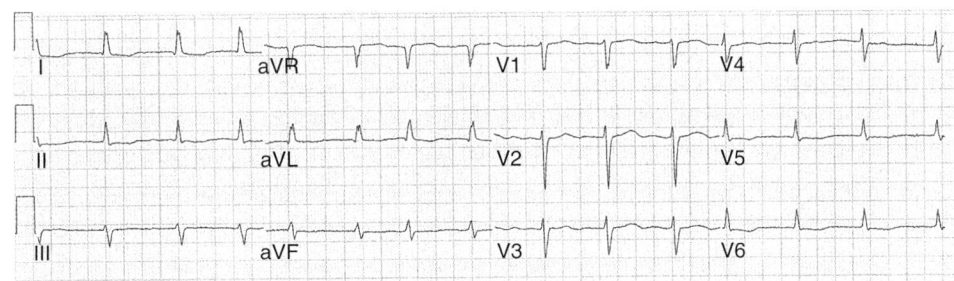

FIGURE 66.3 A 12-lead electrocardiogram of AF in which f waves are not discernible. The irregularly irregular ventricular rate indicates that this is AF.

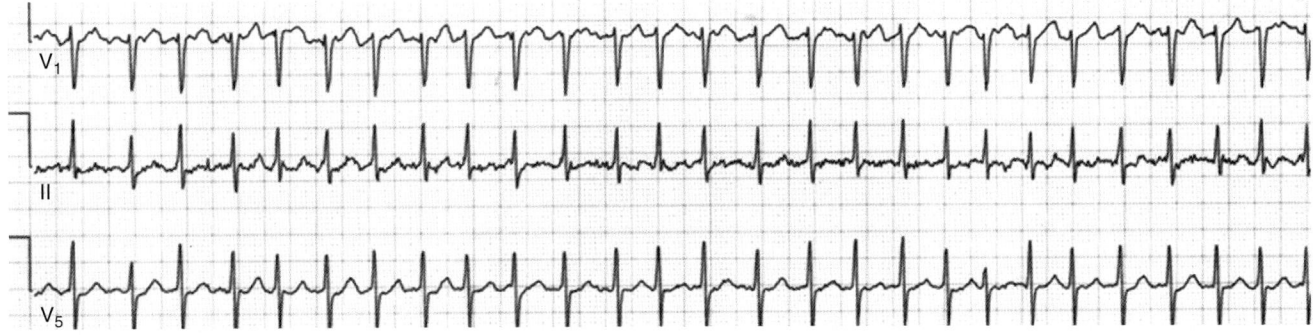

FIGURE 66.4 A recording of AF with a rapid ventricular rate of 160 beats/min. Shown are leads V_1, II, and V_5. On quick review, there may appear to be a regular rate consistent with paroxysmal supraventricular tachycardia. On closer inspection, it is clear that the rate is irregularly irregular.

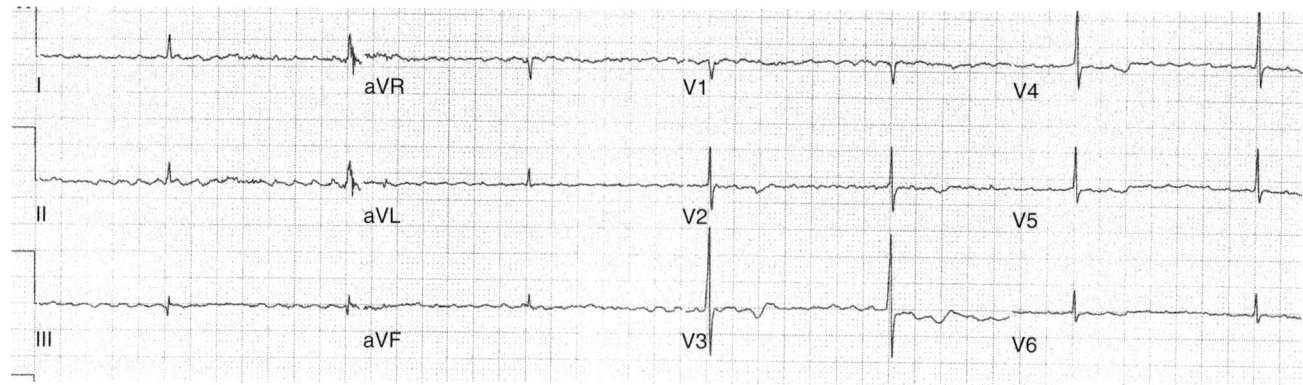

FIGURE 66.5 A 12-lead electrocardiogram of AF and a regular junctional rhythm at a rate of 43 beats/min. There is either underlying third-degree AV block or second-degree AV block with extremely slow atrioventricular conduction allowing a junctional escape rhythm to become manifest.

contributes to slow, discontinuous, and anisotropic conduction, may give rise to wandering or stationary reentry. It is for this reason that the outcomes of AF ablation targeted at the pulmonary veins (PVs) alone results in lower efficacy than in patients with paroxysmal AF.

GENETIC FACTORS

It is now well established that susceptibility to AF is heritable.[9,10] Individuals who have a first-degree relative with AF have a 40% increased risk of developing AF. In the last decade, considerable progress has been made in identifying the genetic determinants of AF. Population-based studies have been used to identify many AF risk loci. A recent study tested the association between AF genetic susceptibility and recurrence of AF after AF ablation using a polygenic risk score. A higher AF genetic susceptibility was associated with younger age and fewer clinical risk factors, but not AF recurrence.[10] Although progress has been made, studies continue to better define the link between genetic factors and AF and how these genetic factors impact the response to therapy.

CAUSES OF ATRIAL FIBRILLATION

The majority of patients with AF have hypertension (usually with left ventricular hypertrophy; Chapter 26) or some other form of structural heart disease. In addition to hypertensive heart disease, the most common cardiac abnormalities associated with AF are ischemic heart disease (Chapters 37 to 40), mitral valve disease (Chapters 75 and 76), hypertrophic cardiomyopathy (Chapter 54), and dilated cardiomyopathy (Chapter 52). Less common causes of AF are restrictive cardiomyopathies such as amyloidosis (Chapter 53), constrictive pericarditis (Chapter 86), and cardiac tumors (see Chapter 98). Severe pulmonary hypertension often is associated with AF (Chapter 88).

Obstructive sleep apnea and obesity are associated with each other, and both independently increase the risk of AF (see Chapter 89).[11] The possible mechanisms of AF in patients with sleep apnea include hypoxia, surges in autonomic tone, and hypertension. Available data suggest that atrial dilation and an increase in local and systemic inflammatory factors are responsible for the relationship between obesity and AF. Obesity is associated with increased deposits of epicardial fat (see Chapter 30). A growing body of data has demonstrated that epicardial fat is strongly associated with the presence, severity, and recurrence of AF in many clinical settings. The most likely arrhythmogenic mechanisms by which epicardial fat predisposes to AF include adipocyte infiltration, profibrotic effects, proinflammatory effects.[12] The LEGACY study demonstrated that sustained weight loss and exercise can reduce the AF burden.[13]

AF is sometimes caused by tachycardia. Patients with tachycardia-induced AF most often have AV nodal reentrant tachycardia or a tachycardia related to WPW syndrome that degenerates into AF. AF in a patient with a history of rapid and regular palpitations before the onset of irregular palpitations or with a WPW electrocardiographic pattern suggest that the patient may have tachycardia-induced AF. Treatment of the tachycardia that triggers the AF often (but not always) prevents recurrences of AF.

CLINICAL FEATURES

The symptoms of AF range from none to severe and functionally disabling. The most common symptoms are palpitations, fatigue, dyspnea, effort intolerance, and lightheadedness. Polyuria can occur because of release of atrial natriuretic peptide. Many patients with symptomatic paroxysmal AF also have asymptomatic episodes, and some patients with persistent AF have symptoms only intermittently, making it difficult to assess accurately the frequency and duration of AF on the basis of symptoms.

An estimated 25% of patients with AF are asymptomatic, more often elderly patients and patients with persistent AF. Such patients sometimes are erroneously classified as being "asymptomatic" despite having symptoms of fatigue or effort intolerance. Because fatigue is a nonspecific symptom, it may not be clear that the cause is persistent AF. Many elderly patients incorrectly assume that their effort intolerance is attributable to aging. A "diagnostic cardioversion" may be helpful by maintaining sinus rhythm for at least a few days to determine whether a patient feels better in sinus rhythm. This strategy is especially valuable in a patient under the age of 80 years who presents for a routine physical examination and is found to be in AF. Rather than quickly declaring the patient "asymptomatic," many experienced clinicians will restore sinus rhythm with a cardioversion to evaluate symptomatic improvement. This strategy also is useful in patients with newly diagnosed persistent AF as the longer a patient is in continuous AF, the more difficult it is to restore and maintain sinus rhythm. This approach can provide a basis to pursue a rhythm-control versus rate-control strategy.

Syncope, an uncommon symptom of AF, can be caused by a long sinus pause on termination of AF in a patient with the sick sinus syndrome. Syncope also can occur during AF with a rapid ventricular rate because of neurocardiogenic (vasodepressor) syncope triggered by the tachycardia or because of a severe drop in blood pressure caused by a reduction in cardiac output.

Asymptomatic or minimally symptomatic AF patients are not prompted to seek medical care and can present with a thromboembolic complication such as stroke or the insidious onset of heart failure symptoms, eventually presenting in florid congestive heart failure caused by tachycardia-induced cardiomyopathy.

The hallmark of AF on physical examination is an irregularly irregular pulse. Short R-R intervals during AF do not allow adequate time for left ventricular diastolic filling, resulting in a low stroke volume and the absence of palpable peripheral pulse. This results in a "pulse deficit," during which the peripheral pulse is not as rapid as the apical rate. Other manifestations of AF on the physical examination are irregular jugular venous pulsations and variable intensity of the first heart sound.

DIAGNOSTIC EVALUATION

The history should be directed at determination of the type and severity of symptoms, the first onset of AF, whether the AF is paroxysmal or persistent, the triggers of AF, whether the episodes are random or occur at particular times (e.g., during sleep), and the frequency and duration of episodes. When it is unclear from the history, 2 to 4 weeks of continuous or autotrigger ambulatory monitoring, or by mobile cardiac outpatient telemetry, is useful to determine whether AF is paroxysmal or persistent and to quantitate the AF burden in patients with paroxysmal AF. The history also should be directed at identification of potentially correctable causes (e.g., hyperthyroidism, excessive alcohol intake), structural heart disease, and comorbidities.

In a patient who describes irregular or rapid palpitations suggestive of paroxysmal AF, ambulatory monitoring is useful to document whether AF is responsible for the symptoms. If the symptoms occur on a daily basis, a 24-hour Holter recording is appropriate. However, extended monitoring for 2 to 4 weeks with an event monitor or continuous rhythm monitor or by mobile cardiac outpatient telemetry is appropriate for patients whose symptoms are sporadic (see Chapter 61).[14] Another option is an insertable monitor, which is placed subcutaneously and has a battery life of approximately 3 years.[15] A recent trial demonstrated that among patients with a cryptogenic stroke and no AF seen on a 24-hour Holter monitor, AF was detected in 8.9% of patients who had an implantable cardiac monitor within 6 months.[15] One of the most important benefits of a continuous monitor over weeks to years is that the burden of AF can be precisely defined.

Laboratory testing should include thyroid, liver, and renal function blood tests. Echocardiography always is appropriate to evaluate atrial size and left ventricular function and to look for left ventricular hypertrophy, congenital heart disease (see Chapter 82), and valvular heart disease (Chapters 72 to 77). Chest radiography is appropriate if the history or physical examination is suggestive of pulmonary disease (Chapter 17). A stress test is appropriate for evaluation of ischemic heart disease in at-risk patients (Chapter 15).

PREVENTION OF THROMBOEMBOLIC COMPLICATIONS

Risk Stratification

The most important therapeutic goal in AF patients is to prevent thromboembolic complications, especially stroke.[16,17] Anticoagulants (warfarin or one of the direct oral anticoagulants) are far more effective than antiplatelet agents (e.g., aspirin or clopidogrel) for prevention of thromboembolic complications.[16,17] However, because of the risk of hemorrhage from anticoagulants, their use should be limited to patients whose risk of thromboembolic complications is greater than the risk of hemorrhage. Therefore, it is useful to risk stratify patients with AF to identify appropriate candidates for anticoagulation.

The strongest predictors of ischemic stroke and systemic thromboembolism are a history of stroke or transient ischemic episode and mitral stenosis. When patients with AF and a prior ischemic stroke are treated with aspirin, the risk of another stroke is very high, in the range of 10% to 12% per year. At the other end of the risk spectrum are younger patients with AF and no comorbidities whose cumulative 15-year risk of stroke is in the range of 1% to 2%. Aside from prior stroke, the best-established risk factors for stroke in patients with nonvalvular AF are diabetes (relative risk [RR], 1.7), hypertension (RR, 1.6), heart failure (RR, 1.4), and age 70 or older (RR, 1.4 per decade).[1,17,18]

Renal failure also is an independent risk factor for stroke in patients with AF.[19] The RR of a thromboembolic event in the absence of anticoagulation was 1.4 in patients with non–end-stage chronic kidney disease and 1.8 in patients requiring hemodialysis or a renal transplant. The predictive strength of chronic kidney disease for a thromboembolic event appears to be equivalent to that of heart failure and advanced age. Therefore, it may be appropriate to take into account chronic kidney disease when evaluating the risk profile of a patient with AF.

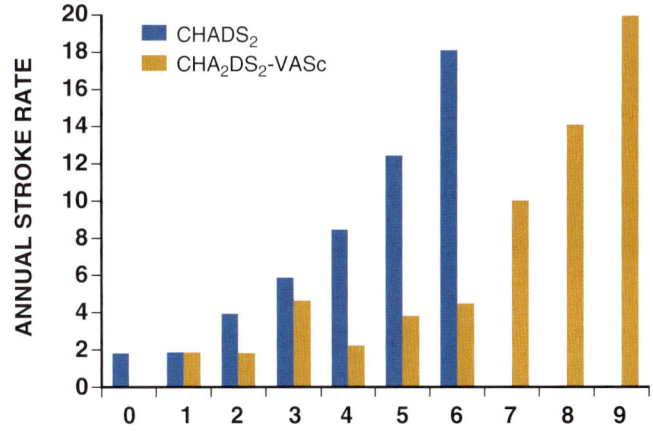

FIGURE 66.6 The annual risk of stroke (percent risk/year) based on the CHADS$_2$ and CHA$_2$DS$_2$-VASc scores. (From Lip GY. Implications of the CHA(2)DS(2)-VASc and HAS-BLED Scores for thromboprophylaxis in atrial fibrillation. Am J Med 2011;124:111-114.)

At present the CHA$_2$DS$_2$-VASc score is recommended for estimation of stroke risk (cardiac failure, hypertension, age >75 years; diabetes, stroke, or transient ischemic attack (TIA), age 65 to 74 years, vascular disease, female sex category).[18,20] Each risk factor counts as 1 point, with the exception of prior stroke or transient ischemic events and age $\geq$ 75 years, which count for 2 points. Correction for the inclusion of female sex is accomplished in the updated 2019 AF Guidelines by specifying a higher CHA$_2$DS$_2$-VASc score in women than in men (i.e., $\geq$3 in women and $\geq$ 2 in men to achieve a class I recommendation for anticoagulation) for each anticoagulation cutoff.[18] When considering the CHA$_2$DS$_2$-VASc score, it is important to recognize that there are risk factors for stroke that are not included in the CHA$_2$DS$_2$-VASc score. These include left atrial size, mitral annular calcification, and AF burden.

The clinical value of the CHA$_2$DS$_2$-VASc score lies in its simplicity and predictive value. There is a direct relationship between the CHA$_2$DS$_2$-VASc score and the annual risk of stroke in the absence of aspirin or anticoagulant therapy. The annual risk of stroke is zero or close to zero when the CHA$_2$DS$_2$-VASc score is 0, compared with approximately 3% when the CHA$_2$DS$_2$-VASc score is 3 (Fig. 66.6).[17] Other risk scores that incorporate other metrics include biomarkers that have been developed and calibrated and may improve risk benefit assessment in AF patients that are candidates for anticoagulation.[21]

The AF burden in persistent AF is 100% and always higher than in patients with paroxysmal AF. It may seem reasonable to assume that the risk of stroke is higher in patients with persistent AF. This recently has been confirmed by several studies, which reported a higher stroke risk in patients with persistent than paroxysmal AF.[17,22] Despite the results of these recent studies, neither the CHA$_2$DS$_2$-VASc score nor the current United States and European AF management guidelines have incorporated AF burden as a risk factor for stroke or into anticoagulation recommendations.[18,23]

Pacemakers and implantable cardioverter-defibrillators (ICDs) that incorporate an atrial lead are capable of detecting short episodes of asymptomatic AF that are subclinical. Subclinical atrial tachyarrhythmias were independently associated with a 2.5-fold increase in the risk of stroke. Long-term intracardiac monitoring in patients with recently implanted pacemakers or ICDs has detected subclinical AF (SCAF) in up to 50% of patients. In a multicenter prospective study, electrocardiographic monitors were implanted in patients $\geq$ 65 years of age with left atrium (LA) enlargement or elevated pro-BNP but no history of AF with either CHA$_2$DS$_2$-VASc $\geq$ 2, sleep apnea or body mass index (BMI) >30 kg/m^2. About half of the patients had a history of stroke or TIA. SCAF (>5 minutes duration) was detected in 40% of patients who suffered a stroke or TIA and 30% of those who did not over 16 months of follow-up.[24] SCAF is common in older adults and more frequently detected due to the widespread use of implanted electrocardiographic monitoring devices. However, whether anticoagulation lowers stroke risk in this subset of AF patients currently is unknown; SCAF may be a risk marker, not a cause of stroke. The 2019 AHA/ACC/HRS AF Guidelines provides a class I level of evidence (LOE) B recommendation that the presence of recorded atrial high rate episodes on an implanted device should prompt further evaluation to document clinically relevant AF to guide treatment decisions.[18] It is important to recognize that not all mode switch events that are classified as AF by an implanted device are truly AF. In the absence of data from clinical trials, most clinicians today would advise anticoagulation for patients with device-detected AF who have episodes of at least 5 hours in duration and have an elevated stroke risk profile.

An important consideration in patients treated with an oral anticoagulant is the risk of bleeding. Several risk-scoring systems have been developed to assess a patient's susceptibility to hemorrhagic complications. The scoring system with the best balance of simplicity and accuracy is the HAS-BLED score.[25] The components of this score are hypertension, abnormal renal or liver function, stroke, bleeding history or predisposition, labile international normalized ratio (INR), older adults (>75 years), and concomitant drug (antiplatelet agent or nonsteroidal anti-inflammatory drug) or alcohol use. Each of these components is 1 point. As the score increases from 0 to the maximum of 9, there is a stepwise increase in the risk of bleeding in patients treated with warfarin. While these scores may be helpful in identifying patients at elevated breeding risk, their clinical utility was deemed insufficient to be included as a formal recommendation in the 2014 ACC/AHA/HRS AF Guidelines.[1,18]

The 2019 AHA/ACC/HRS AF Guidelines give a class I LOE A recommendation for anticoagulation of men with a CHA_2DS_2-VASc score of 2 or higher and women with a CHA_2DS_2-VASc score of 3 or higher.[18] For men with a CHA_2DS_2-VASc score of 1 and women with a CHA_2DS_2-VASc score of 2, anticoagulation should be considered (class IIa, LOE A). While the CHA_2DS_2-VASc score provides a valuable guideline for anticoagulation, other factors should be considered, including patient preference. Some patients may prefer to accept an increased risk of stroke instead of long-term anticoagulation. Other patients with a low CHA_2DS_2-VASc score of 0 to 1 may prefer to take an anticoagulant to protect against even the small risk of a stroke.

Aspirin

Aspirin is not effective for preventing thromboembolic complications in patients with AF. In a meta-analysis of five randomized clinical trials, aspirin did not significantly reduce the risk of stroke compared with placebo in patients with AF.[26] In a large cohort study of patients with nonvalvular AF, aspirin had no therapeutic efficacy for preventing strokes.[1] In several network meta-analyses, the variable and modest reduction in stroke risk with aspirin is not greater than that expected for reduction of risk for vascular stroke. It is notable that a major update of the 2019 ACC/AHA/HRS AF Guidelines, as compared with the 2014 AHA/ACC/HRS AF Guidelines, is that aspirin is no longer recommended for stroke prevention in AF patients.[1,18] In patients with a low CHA_2DS_2-VASc score, the recommended options for stroke prevention are now an anticoagulant versus no therapy.

Warfarin

A meta-analysis of the major randomized clinical trials that compared warfarin with placebo for prevention of thromboembolism in patients with AF demonstrated that warfarin reduced the risk of all strokes (ischemic and hemorrhagic) by approximately 60%.[26,27] The target INR should be 2.0 to 3.0. This range of INRs provides the best balance between stroke prevention and hemorrhagic complications. In clinical practice, maintenance of the INR in therapeutic range has been challenging, and a large proportion of patients often have an INR of less than 2.0. A large prospective study of community-based practices demonstrated that the mean time in therapeutic range (TTR) in patients treated with warfarin was only 66% and that the TTR was less than 60% in 34% of patients.[28] Even in clinical trials there are significant lapses in maintaining warfarin TTR. Maintaining the INR at a level of 2.0 or higher is important because even a relatively small decrease in INR from 2.0 to 1.7 more than doubles the risk of stroke.

The annual risk of a major hemorrhagic complication during anticoagulation with warfarin is in the range of 1% to 2%, and a strong predictor of major bleeding events is an INR greater than 3.0. For example, the risk of intracranial bleeding is approximately twice as high at an INR of 4.0 than 3.0. This emphasizes the importance of maintaining the INR in the range of 2.0 to 3.0.

Some studies have indicated that advanced age can be a risk factor for intracranial hemorrhage in patients with AF treated with warfarin. However, the available data indicate that warfarin and the direct-acting oral anticoagulants (DOACs) have a favorable risk-to-benefit ratio even in patients older than 75.[29]

Direct-Acting Oral Anticoagulants

Direct thrombin inhibitors and factor Xa inhibitors have several advantages over vitamin K antagonists such as warfarin: (1) a fixed dosing regimen that eliminates the need for monitoring the INR, (2) rapid onset and offset, (3) equal or greater efficacy for stroke prevention, (4) a lower risk of intracranial hemorrhage, (5) no interactions with dietary factors such as alcohol or vitamin-K containing foods, and (6) far fewer drug interactions.[30]

Dabigatran, an oral direct thrombin inhibitor, and rivaroxaban, apixaban, and edoxaban, which are factor Xa inhibitors, are approved by the U.S. Food and Drug Administration (FDA) for prevention of stroke/embolism in patients with nonvalvular AF. Randomized clinical trials demonstrated that each of these four DOACs is noninferior or superior to warfarin in efficacy and safety in patients with nonvalvular AF who had risk factors for stroke.[30] One of the most serious risks of anticoagulation is intracranial hemorrhage. The trials, which were performed for FDA approval of each of these NOACs, revealed that the risk of intracranial hemorrhage is about 50% lower with DOACs compared with warfarin.

Because of these major advantages, the 2019 ACC/AHA/HRS AF Guidelines recommend the use of DOACs over warfarin for prevention of thromboembolic complications in patients with AF.[18]

DOACs also have some disadvantages compared with warfarin: higher cost, more gastrointestinal side effects in the case of dabigatran, twice-daily dosing for dabigatran and apixaban, the absence of a readily available laboratory test to verify compliance, and restricted use in patients with prosthetic valves. Furthermore, use of these agents requires great care in patients with severe renal disease. The pharmacokinetics of apixaban suggest it could be used in severe renal disease and recent studies have demonstrated safety/efficacy,[31] but randomized controlled trials are needed.

Until recently another limitation of DOACs was that there were no specific reversal agents. However, reversal agents now are available for all DOACs.[30,32-34] The first reversal agent to receive FDA approval, both for uncontrolled bleeding and the need for urgent surgery, was idarucizumab, an antibody fragment that reverses the anticoagulant effects of dabigatran within minutes.[30,34] Since that time andexanet alfa has been approved for acute major bleeding in patients taking a factor Xa inhibitor.[32] A limitation of andexanet alfa is high cost compared with a prothrombin concentrate.

When a reversal agent is not available or not desired, administration of prothrombin complex concentrate can reverse the anticoagulant effect of the DOACs.

Older studies demonstrated the frequent underutilization of warfarin in patients with AF and risk factors for stroke. The inconvenience and potential risks of warfarin likely contributed to its underutilization. However, the underutilization of and low adherence to oral anticoagulant use in patients with AF has continued to be the case even with the advent of DOACs.[35]

The major professional societies have incorporated recommendations regarding the use of the factor Xa- and direct thrombin-inhibitors into their most recent guidelines for the management of AF.[18,23] As noted above, the ACC/AHA/HRS AF guidelines recommend DOACs over warfarin for prevention of stroke and systemic embolism in patients with nonvalvular paroxysmal or persistent AF and risk factors for stroke. This recommendation is limited to patients without valvular AF. Valvular AF is defined as AF in patients with a prosthetic valve or with moderate to severe mitral stenosis. Based on recent data, the 2019 ACC/AHA/HRS AF Guidelines provide a 2B recommendation for reduced-dose DOAC therapy in patients with moderate to severe kidney disease.[18] These guidelines also state that dabigatran, rivaroxaban, and edoxaban are not recommended in patients with end-stage kidney disease or patients on dialysis. Recent studies indicate the apixaban may be safe to use in such patients.[31]

The results of a large number of clinical trials have indicated that the DOACs are as effective as warfarin for prevention of thromboembolic complications associated with cardioversion.[36] This is the case regardless of whether or not a transesophageal echocardiogram is performed before cardioversion to look for left atrial thrombus.

The onset of action of the DOACs is approximately 1.5 to 2 hours after a dose. Their half-life is approximately 12 hours. The rapid onset of action and washout eliminates the need for bridging therapy with heparin when treatment with one of the DOACs is interrupted for a surgical or invasive medical procedure. Recent data indicate that the risk of major periprocedural complications does not differ significantly between patients who undergo radiofrequency catheter ablation of AF during uninterrupted therapy with warfarin and patients anticoagulated with an uninterrupted DOAC.[30,37]

Low-Molecular-Weight Heparin

Low-molecular-weight heparin (LMWH) has a longer half-life than unfractionated heparin and a predictable antithrombotic effect that is attained with a fixed dosage administered subcutaneously twice daily. Because LMWH can be self-injected outside the hospital, it is a practical alternative to unfractionated heparin for initiation of anticoagulation with warfarin in patients with AF. Bridging therapy with LMWH should be continued until the INR is 2.0 or higher.

Because of its high cost, LMWH rarely is used in clinical practice as a substitute for long-term conventional anticoagulation. In the past, LMWH typically was used as a temporary bridge to therapeutic anticoagulation when therapy with warfarin was initiated or in high-risk patients for a few days before and after a medical or dental procedure when anticoagulation with warfarin was been suspended. In contemporary practice, the use of DOACs has greatly limited the need for LMWH in patients with nonvalvular AF.

Excision or Closure of the Left Atrial Appendage

Approximately 90% of left atrial thrombi form in the left atrial appendage (LAA), and therefore successful excision or closure of the LAA should greatly reduce the risk of thromboembolic complications in patients with AF. Surgical techniques consist of either excision or closure by suturing or stapling. The efficacy of these techniques is variable and probably dependent on both the technique and the operator. Transesophageal echocardiography (TEE) should be performed after surgical closure of the LAA to confirm successful closure before discontinuation of anticoagulation.

In recent years, several percutaneous LAA occlusion and ligation devices have been developed as alternatives to surgical closure techniques. These devices have their greatest utility in high-risk AF patients who cannot tolerate or who refuse to take an oral anticoagulant.

The only percutaneous occlusion device approved by the FDA specifically for stroke prevention as an alternative to warfarin is the WATCHMAN (Boston Scientific, Marlborough, Massachusetts).[38] This nitinol plug covered with fenestrated fabric became widely available for clinical use after FDA approval in 2015 (Fig. 66.7). After implantation of the WATCHMAN using femoral vein access and transseptal catheterization, anticoagulation with warfarin is recommended for at least 45 days, at which time anticoagulation can be discontinued if there is no TEE evidence of peridevice flow.[39] Since initial release of this device, considerable evidence has demonstrated that DOACs can be used instead of warfarin.[40,41]

Another device used in the United States for LAA occlusion is the LARIAT (Sentreheart, Redwood City, California). This device has FDA

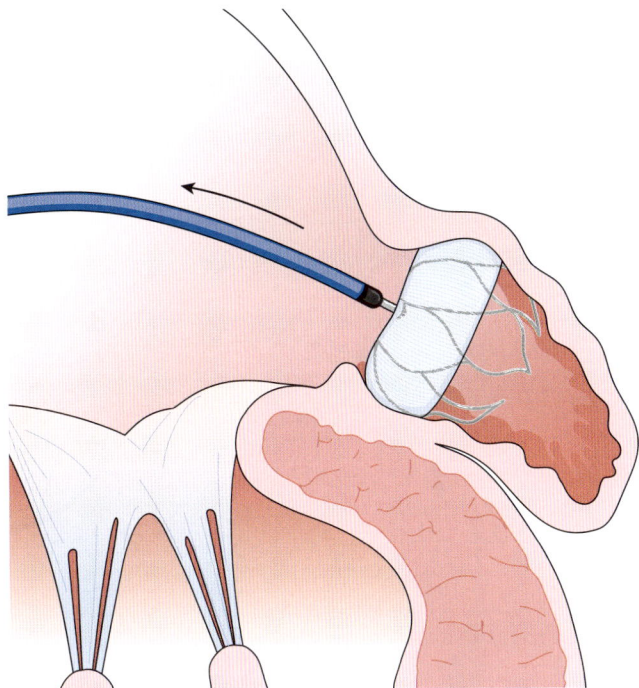

FIGURE 66.7 WATCHMAN device positioned in the left atrial appendage. The delivery sheath is removed once the device is well seated.

approval for soft tissue approximation (not stroke prevention) and has been used off-label in clinical practice in the United States and elsewhere for LAA occlusion. A guidewire with a magnetic tip is inserted into the left atrium after transseptal catheterization and is positioned at the tip of the LAA. It functions as a rail for an epicardial snare. Entry into the pericardial space is attained using a percutaneous approach. A snare with a pretied suture is inserted into the pericardial space and guided toward the LAA (Fig. 66.8). The pretied suture then is tightened to occlude the LAA. In a large multicenter registry, complete LAA closure was achieved in 94% of 712 patients. There was one procedure-related death, and cardiac perforation occurred in 3.4% of patients, with open heart surgery required to repair the perforation in 1.4% of patients.[42] Clinical trial data establishing the efficacy of the LARIAT for stroke prevention are lacking. At present, this device is being used in the AMAZE clinical trial, which is seeking to determine whether PV isolation plus appendage ligation with the LARIAT device is superior to PV isolation alone in patients with persistent AF. The study has completed enrollment and the results should be available in 2021. Percutaneous or surgical LAA occlusion are considered class IIa and IIb recommendations, respectively, in situations where anticoagulation is contraindicated or the patient is undergoing cardiac surgery.

ACUTE MANAGEMENT OF ATRIAL FIBRILLATION

Patients who present to the emergency department because of AF often have a rapid ventricular rate, and control of the ventricular rate is most rapidly achieved with intravenous diltiazem or esmolol. If the patient is hemodynamically unstable, immediate transthoracic cardioversion may be appropriate. Cardioversion should ideally be preceded by TEE to rule out a left atrial thrombus if the AF has been present for longer than 48 hours or if the duration is unclear and the patient is not already anticoagulated. However, if the patient has marked hemodynamic compromise, immediate cardioversion without a TEE is advised.

If the patient is hemodynamically stable, the decision to restore sinus rhythm by cardioversion is based on several factors, including symptoms, prior AF episodes, age, left atrial size, and current AAD therapy. For example, in an elderly patient whose symptoms resolve once

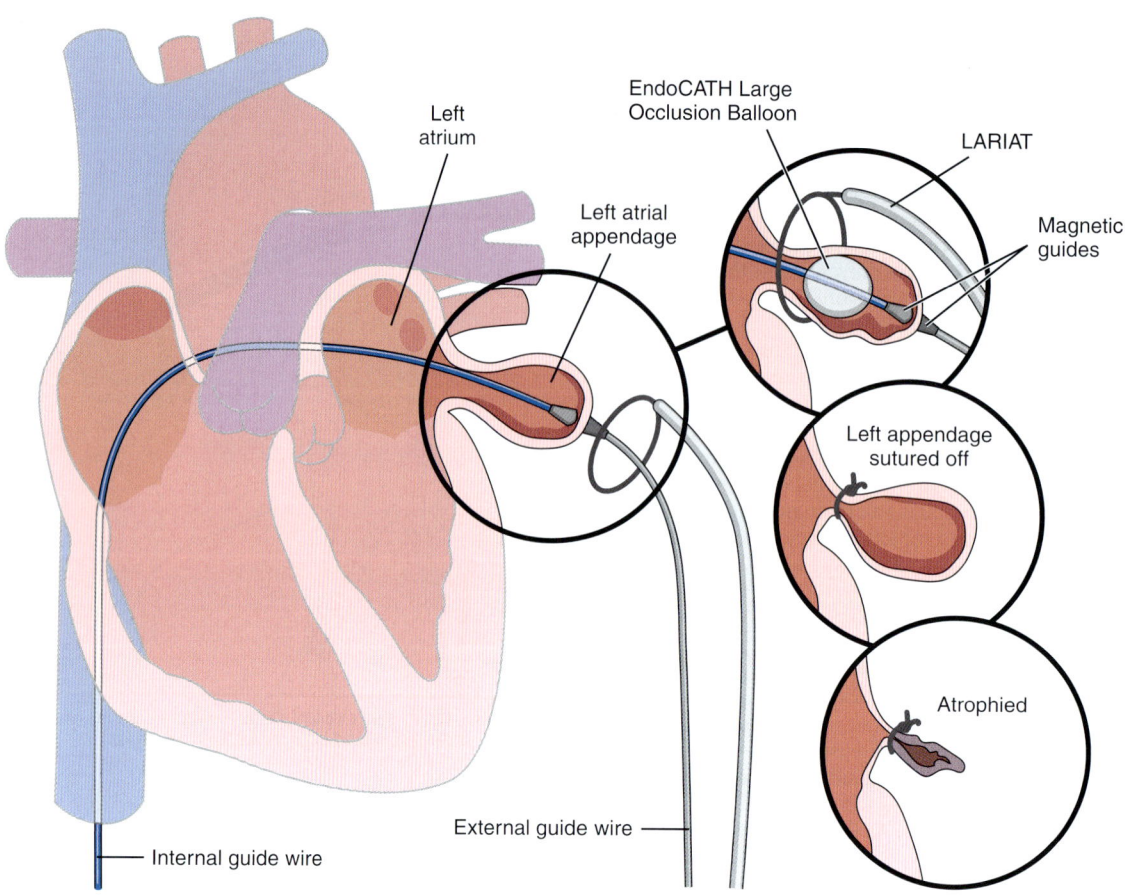

FIGURE 66.8 Steps involved in deploying the LARIAT catheter for occlusion of the left atrial appendage.

the ventricular rate is controlled and who already has had early recurrences of AF despite rhythm-control drug therapy, further attempts at cardioversion usually are not appropriate. On the other hand, cardioversion usually is appropriate for patients with symptomatic AF who present with a first episode of AF or who have had long intervals of sinus rhythm between prior episodes.

If cardioversion is decided upon for a hemodynamically stable patient who presents with AF that does not appear to be self-limited, two management decisions must be made: early versus delayed cardioversion and pharmacologic versus electrical cardioversion.

The advantages of early cardioversion are rapid relief of symptoms, avoidance of the need for TEE or therapeutic anticoagulation for 3 to 4 weeks before cardioversion if cardioversion is performed within 48 hours of AF onset, and possibly a lower risk of early AF recurrence because of less atrial remodeling (see Chapter 64). A reason to defer cardioversion is the unavailability of TEE in a patient who has not been anticoagulated with AF of unclear duration or duration more than 48 hours. Other reasons include a left atrial thrombus by TEE (see Chapter 16), a suspicion (based on prior AF episodes) that AF will convert spontaneously within a few days, or in rare cases, a correctable cause of AF such as hyperthyroidism.

When cardioversion is performed early in the course of an episode of AF, there is the option of either pharmacologic or electrical cardioversion. Pharmacologic cardioversion has the advantage of not requiring general anesthesia or deep sedation. In addition, the probability of an immediate recurrence of AF is lower with pharmacologic cardioversion than with electrical cardioversion. However, pharmacologic cardioversion is associated with the risk of adverse drug effects and is not as effective as electrical cardioversion. Pharmacologic cardioversion is unlikely to be effective if the duration of AF is longer than 7 days.

Drugs that can be administered intravenously for cardioversion of AF consist of ibutilide, procainamide, and amiodarone. For AF episodes fewer than 2 to 3 days in duration, efficacy is approximately 60% to 70% for ibutilide, 40% to 50% for amiodarone, and 30% to 40% for procainamide. To minimize the risk of QT prolongation and polymorphic ventricular tachycardia (torsades de pointes; see Chapter 67), the use of ibutilide should be limited to patients with an ejection fraction greater than 35%.

Acute pharmacologic cardioversion of AF also can be attempted with oral drugs in patients without structural heart disease. The most common oral agents for acute conversion of AF are propafenone (300 to 600 mg) and flecainide (100 to 200 mg). When flecainide is used, patients generally take a beta blocker on AF onset and then take the flecainide one or more hours later. It is recommended that these drugs be administered under surveillance upon first use, as patients may have a pronounced postconversion pause. If no adverse drug effects are observed, the patient may then be an appropriate candidate for episodic, self-administered AAD therapy on an outpatient basis (the "pill-in-the-pocket" approach).

The efficacy of transthoracic cardioversion exceeds 95%. Biphasic waveform shocks convert AF more effectively than monophasic waveform shocks and allow the use of lower energy shocks, resulting in less skin irritation. An appropriate first-shock strength using a biphasic waveform is 150 to 200 J, followed by higher output shocks if needed. If a 360-J biphasic shock is unsuccessful, ibutilide should be infused before another shock is delivered because it lowers the defibrillation energy requirement and improves the success rate of transthoracic cardioversion.

Transthoracic cardioversion can fail to restore sinus rhythm. An increase in shock strength, an infusion of ibutilide, or repeat CV with greater pressure applied to the defibrillation patches, often results in successful repeat cardioversion. The second type of failure is an immediate recurrence of AF within a few seconds of successful conversion to sinus rhythm. This occurs in approximately 25% of AF episodes less than 24 hours in duration and 10% of episodes more than 24 hours in duration. For this type of cardioversion failure, an increase in shock strength is of no value. If the patient has not been receiving an oral rhythm-control agent, infusion of ibutilide may be helpful to prevent an immediate recurrence of AF.

Regardless of whether cardioversion is performed pharmacologically or electrically, *therapeutic* anticoagulation is necessary for 3 weeks or more before cardioversion to prevent thromboembolic complications if the AF has been ongoing for more than 48 hours. If the time of onset of AF is unclear, for the sake of safety, the AF duration should be assumed to be more than 48 hours. These patients should be therapeutically anticoagulated for 4 weeks after cardioversion to prevent thromboembolic complications that may occur because of atrial stunning. If the patient's stroke risk profile is elevated, anticoagulation should be continued indefinitely. If the duration of AF is known to be less than 48 hours, cardioversion can be performed without anticoagulation. However, if the patient's stroke risk profile is elevated and long-term anticoagulation is advised, immediate initiation of anticoagulation with a DOAC is recommended.[42]

When AF duration exceeds 48 hours or is unclear, an alternative to 3 weeks of therapeutic anticoagulation before cardioversion is anticoagulation with heparin and a TEE to check for a left atrial thrombus. If no thrombi are seen, the patient can be cardioverted safely but still requires 4 weeks of therapeutic anticoagulation after cardioversion to prevent thromboembolism related to atrial stunning. The major clinical benefit of the TEE-guided approach over the conventional approach is that sinus rhythm is restored several weeks sooner. Compared with the conventional approach, the TEE approach has not been found to reduce the risk of stroke or major bleeding or to affect the proportion of patients still in sinus rhythm at 8 weeks after cardioversion.[18]

LONG-TERM MANAGEMENT OF ATRIAL FIBRILLATION

Pharmacologic Rate Control Versus Rhythm Control

Several randomized studies have compared a rate-control strategy with a rhythm-control strategy in patients with AF. Overall, these studies have demonstrated a significantly lower rate of rehospitalization with a rate-control strategy but no significant differences in other major outcomes, such as all-cause mortality, strokes, bleeding events, worsening heart failure, or quality of life.[43]

The results of these randomized studies should not be applied systematically to all patients with AF. It is important to note that many patients in the rhythm-control arms of these studies continued to have AF, and that the possible beneficial effects of sinus rhythm over AF could have been negated by adverse effects of the AADs. Furthermore, most patients enrolled in these studies were elderly and had few AF symptoms, and the duration of follow-up was several years. It remains uncertain what the implications are of decades of continuous AF in terms of the risks of stroke, heart failure, dementia, and death.

The decision to pursue a rhythm-control strategy versus a rate-control strategy should be individualized based on several factors. These include the nature, frequency, and severity of symptoms; the length of time that AF has been present continuously in patients with persistent AF; left atrial size; comorbidities; the response to prior cardioversions; age; the side effects and efficacy of the AADs already used to treat the patient; patient age and activity level; and the patient's preference.

The duration of continuous AF is a predictor of the ability to restore and maintain sinus rhythm. The chance of successful AF rhythm control is higher in patients with paroxysmal or early persistent AF (<6 months) than for patients who have been in continuous AF for one or more years. This is an important consideration when faced with asymptomatic or minimally symptomatic patients with newly diagnosed persistent AF. It is well established that the presence of AF is associated with a higher risk of stroke risk, heart failure risk, cognitive dysfunction, and mortality. Recent studies indicate that the stroke risk is higher in a patient with continuous AF than paroxysmal AF.[17,22] While no study has shown that restoration of sinus rhythm with AF ablation impacts any of these complications of AF, it may. Of particular note is the CABANA trial.[44] This prospective randomized clinical trial randomized 2204 patients with AF to catheter ablation or medical therapy. The primary endpoint was a composite of death, disabling stroke, serious bleeding, or cardiac arrest. No difference in the primary endpoint was present after a median follow-up of 48.5 months. But the secondary endpoint of death or cardiovascular hospitalizations was significantly lower in the ablation arm than in the medical therapy arm (51.7% vs. 58.1%, p = 0.001). For this reason, the 2017 HRS/EHRA/ECAS Consensus Document on AF ablation provides a class IIb recommendation for catheter ablation of AF in patients who are asymptomatic.[8]

Pharmacologic Rate Control

An excessively rapid ventricular rate during AF often results in uncomfortable symptoms and decreased effort tolerance and can cause a tachycardia-induced cardiomyopathy if it is sustained for several weeks to months. Optimal heart rates during AF vary with age and should be similar to the heart rates that a patient would have at a particular degree of exertion during sinus rhythm. Heart rate control must be assessed both at rest and during exertion. The 2014 and 2019 ACC/AHA/HRS AF Guidelines advise that the optimal metric for rate control is a resting heart rate <80 beats/min.[1,18] Based on a single European clinical trial, a more lenient rate control metric of <110 beats/min is provided with a class IIb recommendation.[1,18] Assessment of the degree of heart rate control can be obtained with a 24-hour Holter monitor. A 12-lead ECG provides an indication of the resting ventricular rate but fails to provide information on the ventricular rate during a patient's daily activities.

Oral agents available for long-term heart rate control in patients with AF are digitalis, beta blockers, calcium channel antagonists, and amiodarone[1] (see Chapter 64). The first-line agents for rate control are beta blockers and the calcium channel antagonists verapamil and diltiazem. A combination is often used to improve efficacy or to limit side effects by allowing the use of smaller dosages of the individual drugs. In patients with sinus node dysfunction and tachycardia-bradycardia syndrome, the use of a beta blocker with intrinsic sympathomimetic activity (pindolol, acebutolol) may provide rate control without aggravating sinus bradycardia.

Digitalis may adequately control the rate at rest but often does not provide adequate rate control during exertion as it works mainly by increasing vagal tone. Digitalis is no longer recommended for rate control except in patients with heart failure because digitalis has been shown to increase the risk of all-cause mortality, particularly among patients with AF. The 2014 and 2019 AHA/ACC/HRS Guidelines recommend digoxin for rate control only in patients with heart failure.[1,18]

Amiodarone is much less frequently used for rate control than the other negative dromotropic agents because of the risk of organ toxicity associated with long-term therapy. Amiodarone can be an appropriate choice for rate control if the other agents are not tolerated or are ineffective. For example, amiodarone would be an appropriate choice for a patient with persistent AF, heart failure, and reactive airway disease who cannot tolerate either a calcium channel antagonist or a beta blocker and who has a rapid ventricular rate despite treatment with digitalis. Amiodarone as a rate-control medication is provided with a class IIb recommendation in the 2014 ACC/AHA/HRS AF Guidelines.[1,18]

Pharmacologic Rhythm Control

The results of studies on the efficacy of AADs for suppression of AF suggest that all the available drugs except amiodarone have similar efficacy and are associated with a 40% to 60% reduction in the odds of recurrent AF during 1 year of treatment (see Chapter 64). The one drug that stands out as having higher efficacy than the others is amiodarone. In studies that directly compared amiodarone with sotalol or class I drugs, amiodarone was 60% to 70% more effective in suppressing AF. However, because of the risk of organ toxicity, amiodarone is not appropriate first-line drug therapy for most patients with AF. The 2014 and

2019 AHA/ACC/HRS AF Guidelines recommend that amiodarone be used as first-line antiarrhythmic medication only in patients with heart failure.[1,18] In all other subsets of patients, amiodarone should only be used after a less toxic AAD has proven ineffective or poorly tolerated. Because the efficacy of rhythm-control agents other than amiodarone is in the same general range, the selection of a particular AAD to prevent AF often is dictated by the issues of safety and side effects.

Ventricular proarrhythmia from class Ia agents (quinidine, procainamide, disopyramide) and class III agents (sotalol, dofetilide, dronedarone, amiodarone) is manifested as QT prolongation and polymorphic ventricular tachycardia (torsades de pointes). Risk factors for this type of proarrhythmia include female sex, left ventricular dysfunction, hypokalemia, and concomitant use of another QT-prolonging drug. The risk of torsades de pointes appears to be much lower with dronedarone and amiodarone than with the other class III drugs. The ventricular proarrhythmia from class Ic agents (flecainide and propafenone) manifests as monomorphic ventricular tachycardia, sometimes associated with widening of the QRS complex during sinus rhythm, but not QT prolongation. They also increase the propensity for ventricular fibrillation in the setting of myocardial ischemia or infarction (see Chapters 9 and 64). For this reason, class Ic agents are not recommended in patients with established coronary artery disease (CAD).[1,18]

Adverse drug events or side effects resulting in discontinuation of drug therapy are fairly common with rhythm-control drugs, with discontinuation rates reported to be as high as 40%.[45]

The best options for drug therapy to suppress AF depend on the patient's comorbidities. In patients with AF in the setting of a structurally normal heart, flecainide, propafenone, sotalol, dofetilide, and dronedarone are all reasonable first-line drugs. Amiodarone can be considered if the first-line agents are ineffective or not tolerated, especially if AF ablation is not preferred by the patient. As noted above, in patients with CAD, class Ic drugs have been found to increase the risk of death, and the safest first-line options are dofetilide, sotalol, or dronedarone, with amiodarone reserved for use as a second-line agent. In patients with heart failure, several AADs have been associated with increased mortality, and the only two drugs known to have a neutral effect on survival are amiodarone and dofetilide (see Chapter 64).

Dronedarone should not be used as a rate-control agent in patients with persistent AF. At the time of FDA approval, it was not known that dronedarone increased mortality in New York Heart Association (NYHA) Class IV heart failure or patients with a recent episode of decompensated heart failure. After a higher mortality risk was demonstrated in a subsequent randomized clinical trial,[46] dronedarone was labeled as being contraindicated when used as a rate-control agent and also in patients with decompensated heart failure.

Rhythm Control with Agents Other Than Antiarrhythmic Drugs

Experimental studies have indicated that angiotensin-converting enzyme (ACE) inhibitors and angiotensin receptor blockers (ARBs) have favorable effects on electrical and structural remodeling (see Chapters 62 and 64). This explains why some studies have shown that ACE inhibitors and ARBs prevent AF. However, other studies have demonstrated that these agents do not prevent AF. At present, there is insufficient evidence to support the use of ACE inhibitors and ARBs for the sole purpose of preventing AF. Available data also do not support the use of statins or omega-3 polyunsaturated fatty acids (PUFAs) for the prevention of AF.[18]

NONPHARMACOLOGIC MANAGEMENT OF ATRIAL FIBRILLATION

Risk Factor Modification

An important development in AF management in the past decade has been the recognition of the importance of risk factor management in the treatment of patients with AF.[11] Historically, the three pillars of AF management have been stroke prevention, rate control, and rhythm control. There is now is strong evidence that risk factor management should be considered the fourth pillar of AF management. The modifiable AF risk factors consist of obesity, hypertension, diabetes, sleep apnea, CAD, heart failure, lack of cardiovascular fitness, and tobacco and alcohol use.

An overview of risk factor management in patients with AF is provided in this chapter. More detailed information is provided in the recently published AHA Scientific Statement on Lifestyle and Risk Factor Modification for Reduction in Atrial Fibrillation.[47]

Obesity is closely linked to the development of AF. The risk of developing AF increases 29% with every 5-point increase in BMI. The scientific basis for this link between obesity and AF has been studied extensively in animal models. Several clinical studies have demonstrated that weight loss combined with comprehensive risk factor management reduces AF and also improves the efficacy of catheter ablation.[11,47,48] This has also been shown recently to be a cost-effective treatment strategy.[49]

Hypertension is a modifiable risk factor for AF. Hypertension causes ventricular hypertrophy and atrial enlargement, as well as activation of the renin-angiotensin system.[1,50] One small study enrolling 76 patients with severe resistant hypertension, demonstrated that renal denervation was associated with a significant reduction in both BP and AF burden at 12 months' follow-up.[51] There also is a strong association between diabetes and AF, probably because of fibrotic changes in the atria and downregulation of connexin-43 and associated abnormalities of conduction in the atrium.[52]

Cigarette smoking augments the risk of AF by causing an increase in sympathetic tone, inflammation, endothelial dysfunction, atrial fibrosis, and oxidative stress. Alcohol use has also been linked to development of AF.[2,3] This link results from direct cellular effects of alcohol on atrial myocytes with acute oxidative stress and also from activation of the sympathetic nervous system. A recent study demonstrated that abstinence from alcohol results in a reduction in AF burden.[2]

Physical inactivity is another modifiable AF risk factor. Physical activity has been demonstrated to reduce the incidence of cardiovascular disease. Sedentary lifestyles have also been shown to be other risk factors for AF, particularly obesity. Cardiovascular fitness has been found to reduce the AF burden independent of weight loss.

Another modifiable risk factor to consider is sleep apnea. Sleep apnea is common among AF patients. A number of studies have shown that sleep apnea increases the risk of new-onset AF. Treatment of sleep apnea has been shown to reduce the probability of recurrent AF after cardioversion and AF catheter ablation.

Based on the growing body of literature linking AF development to the presence of modifiable risk factors, especially obesity, the AHA/ACC/HRS 2019 AF Guideline provides a class I LOE B recommendation that overweight and obese patients with AF should lose weight as part of a risk factor modification program.[18] The goal of weight loss ideally should be a BMI of ≤ 27 kg/m^2.

Pacing to Prevent Atrial Fibrillation

Multiple studies have been performed to determine whether various atrial pacing strategies can prevent or terminate AF. Overall, there has been no convincing evidence that any atrial pacing strategy is effective in preventing or terminating episodes of AF, and therefore atrial pacing is not indicated for prevention of AF in patients without bradycardia or AV block.

Catheter Ablation of Atrial Fibrillation

Catheter ablation reliably and permanently eliminates several types of arrhythmias, such as AV nodal reentrant tachycardia (AVNRT) and accessory pathway–mediated tachycardias (see Chapters 64 and 65). Success rates greater than 95% are attainable when the arrhythmia substrate is well defined, localized, and temporally stable. In contrast, the arrhythmia substrate of AF is not completely understood, is usually widespread, is variable between patients, and is often progressive. Furthermore, several factors that promote AF cannot be addressed simply by catheter ablation, including comorbidities (e.g., hypertension, obesity, obstructive sleep apnea), structural remodeling of the atria, systemic inflammatory factors, and genetic factors (see Chapter 7). Therefore, whereas late recurrences of AVNRT or accessory pathway conduction are very rare, AF can recur after an initially successful ablation procedure. For this reason, AF ablation should not be considered a "cure" for AF but rather a palliative measure to keep the patient in sinus rhythm for as long as possible.[8] This section of the chapter provides an overview of the techniques and outcomes of catheter ablation of AF.

Catheter Ablation Technique and Outcomes of AF Ablation

Cox and colleagues developed and demonstrated the efficacy of surgical AF ablation in the early 1990s. Although a large number of investigators attempted to replicate the surgical maze procedure with catheter ablation techniques, these clinical trials reported limited success. A major step forward occurred in 1998 when Haissaguerre et al. identified the PVs as the most common site of focal triggers that initiate AF.[7] After an initial approach of focal RF ablation within the PVs, it was quickly recognized that electrical isolation of the PVs is the optimal technique for eliminating triggers and drivers arising in the PVs. This is true for ablation of paroxysmal and persistent AF. Electrical isolation of the PVs can be achieved by focal PV ostial ablation, circumferential ostial ablation, or circumferential ablation in the antral areas of the PVs, 1 to 2 cm from the ostium. Circumferential antral isolation of the PVs results in 1 year of freedom from AF of between 60% and 80% in patients with paroxysmal AF, 40% to 60% in patients with persistent AF, and 20% to 40% in patients with longstanding persistent AF.[8] Because of the lower success rate of antral PV isolation in patients with the persistent forms of AF, a number of strategies have been developed to improve outcomes in this cohort of patients. These techniques include linear ablation to isolate the left atrial posterior wall, linear ablation in other regions of the left atrium and right atrium, ablation of complex fractionated electrograms, ablation of nonpulmonary vein triggers, isolation of the LAA, focal impulse and rotor modulation ablation, ablation of atrial scar identified by MRI or voltage mapping, and electrical isolation of the superior vena cava. Despite single-center cohort studies that reported promising results, none of the adjunctive approaches has been shown to be superior in efficacy compared with the others when subjected to a prospective, randomized clinical trial.[8,53] This remains an active area of clinical investigation and a number of prospective randomized clinical trials are underway.

The efficacy of AF ablation is closely linked with how success is defined and the intensity of ECG monitoring postablation.[54,55] In general, the more monitoring performed, the lower the success rate. The CIRCA-DoSE trial recently examined this relationship closely.[54] In this trial, 346 patients with paroxysmal AF were randomized to catheter ablation with the cryoballoon or with RF energy. An implantable rhythm monitor was implanted at least 1 month before ablation in all patients. The success of AF ablation was approximately 55% at 1 year if the definition of success was defined as freedom from a 30 second or longer episode of an atrial arrhythmia after the 3-month blanking period. The success rate increased to approximately 80% if the definition of success was freedom from a symptomatic atrial arrhythmia. Importantly, AF burden was reduced by approximately 98%. The outcomes of AF ablation were similar in the cryoballoon and RF arms of the study. These results have been reproduced in a more recent trial.[55]

The two most common ablation energy sources are radiofrequency energy and cryoenergy. Radiofrequency energy applied on a point-by-point basis was the first method that became widely adapted for AF ablation. In contemporary practice, radiofrequency ablation typically is performed in association with a three-dimensional electroanatomic mapping system as a nonfluoroscopic navigation guide and to create a visual record of the sites that already have been ablated (Fig. 66.9). To improve anatomic accuracy, the electroanatomic map of the left atrium can be merged with a computed tomography scan or magnetic resonance image of the left atrium and PVs or with an ultrasound image generated by intracardiac echocardiography. An important determinant of lesion depth and durability is *contact force*, and the newest

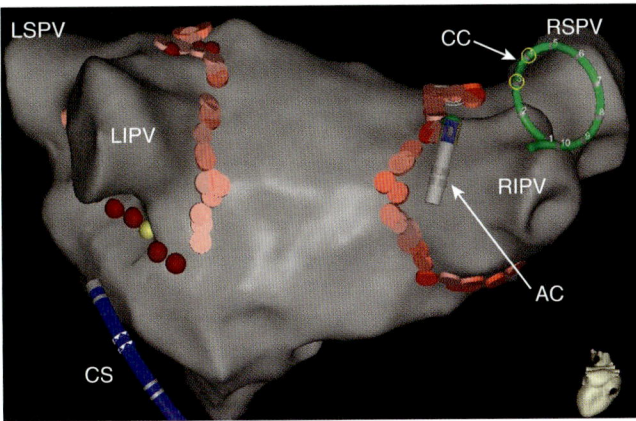

FIGURE 66.9 An electroanatomic map of the left atrium. Icons representing the distal portion of the ablation catheter *(AC)*, circular catheter *(CC)* in the right superior pulmonary vein *(RSPV)*, and a catheter positioned within the coronary sinus *(CS)* are visualized in real time. Circumferential antral ablation was performed around the left and right pulmonary veins. Each one of the *pink, red,* and *yellow* tags represents a site at which radiofrequency energy was delivered. *LIPV,* Left inferior pulmonary vein; *LSPV,* left superior pulmonary vein; *RIPV,* right inferior pulmonary vein.

generation of RF ablation catheters provides the operator with immediate feedback on contact force.

In 2010 a cryoballoon catheter designed to isolate PVs became widely available for use in the United States. In contrast to point-by-point RF ablation around the PVs, the cryoballoon was designed to fit into the antrum of a PV and to create a circumferential ablation lesion using cryoenergy. Cryoenergy is delivered through the entire distal half of the second-generation cryoballoon catheter currently in clinical use. Complete occlusion of the PV by the inflated balloon is essential for reliable PV isolation (Fig. 66.10). Various strategies are used to deliver the cryoenergy, ranging from one or two applications of 3 to 4 minutes to applications of variable duration based on specific freezing parameters[56] (Fig. 66.11).

Avoidance of entry of the cryoballoon into the luminal portion of a PV is important to avoid PV stenosis. The most commonly used cryoballoon catheter has a 28-mm diameter when the balloon is fully inflated. The relatively large size of the balloon typically allows occlusion of a PV from the antrum. A multielectrode catheter inserted through a central lumen of the cryoballoon catheter often allows recording of PV potentials during an application of cryoenergy. The endpoint of the cryoballoon ablation procedure is electrical isolation of all PVs. Disappearance or dissociation of PV potentials within the first minute of a cryoenergy application is a strong independent predictor of durable PV isolation (Fig. 66.12). Other independent predictors are a temperature recorded by a thermocouple proximal to the balloon of at least –40°C within 60 seconds of an application of cryoenergy and an interval thaw time to 0°C of >10 seconds upon completion of a cryoenergy application. In addition to the cryoballoon, a visually-guided laser balloon (VGLB) system now also is available for clinical use.[57] A randomized clinical trial demonstrated that the VGLB was noninferior to radiofrequency catheter ablation in regards to efficacy.[58]

There have been a number of head-to-head comparisons of the safety and efficacy of radiofrequency ablation versus cryoballoon ablation.[54,59] These studies have reported remarkably similar outcomes. The cryoballoon procedures are generally shorter, require more fluoroscopy, and have a higher risk of phrenic nerve injury and a lower risk of pericardial tamponade.[55] The tool an operator chooses is largely based on his or her own personal training and experience. Some operators have great skill with point-by-point RF ablation and rarely if ever use the cryoballoon system. Other operators use the cryoballoon system for 100% of first-time ablation procedures and reserve the RF approach for complete isolation of PVs that cannot be successfully isolated with the cryoballoon catheter, for repeat ablation procedures, and also in patients in whom the operator wishes to ablate sites outside the PVs. RF ablation also may be needed to ablate typical or atypical atrial flutter.

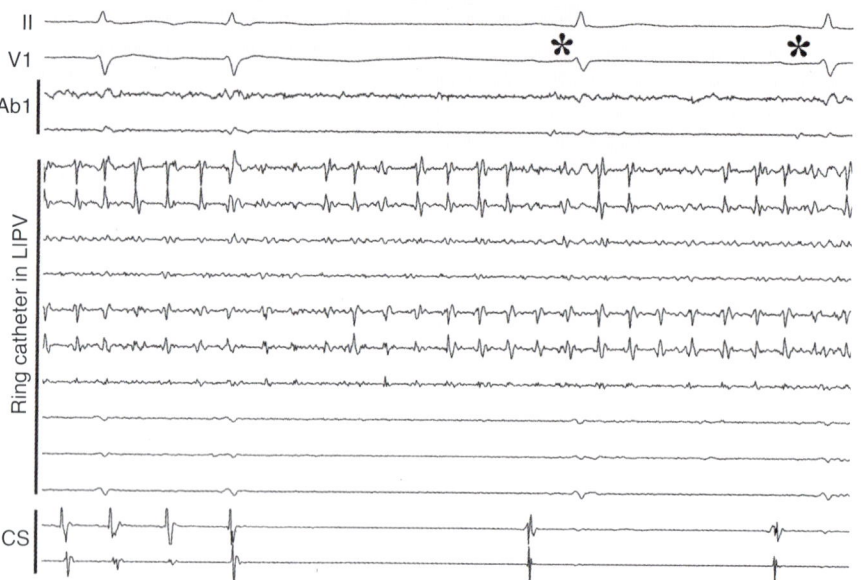

FIGURE 66.10 A tachycardia with a cycle length of 80 milliseconds arising in a left inferior pulmonary vein (LIPV) during AF. AF converted to sinus rhythm *(asterisks)* during radiofrequency ablation when the LIPV was electrically isolated. The pulmonary vein tachycardia persisted inside the vein. Conversion to sinus rhythm on electrical isolation of the LIPV is strong evidence that the tachycardia arising in the muscle sleeve of this pulmonary vein was the driver of AF in this patient. Shown are leads II and V₁, the electrograms recorded by the ablation catheter *(Abl)*, by a ring catheter in the LIPV, and in the coronary sinus *(CS)*.

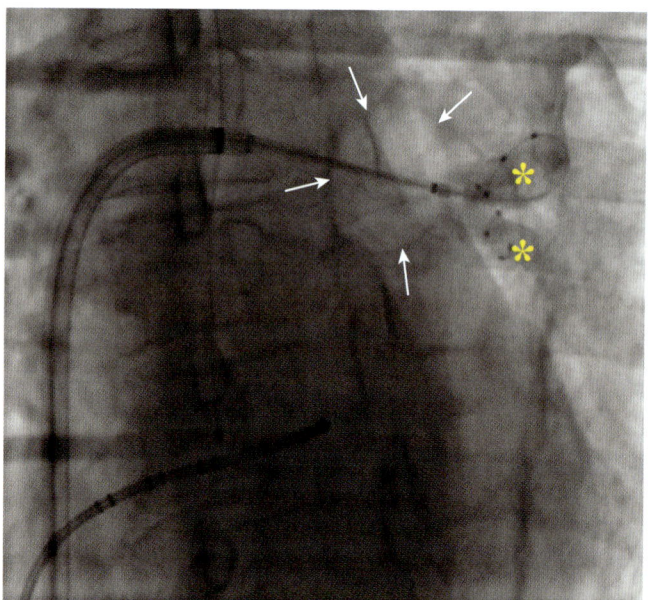

FIGURE 66.11 A right anterior oblique fluoroscopic image of the heart showing a cryoballoon catheter positioned in the antrum of the left inferior pulmonary vein. The 28-mm balloon *(arrows)* is inflated, and there is no leakage of contrast injected through the lumen of the cryoballoon catheter into the vein *(asterisks)*. This indicates complete occlusion of the vein, a necessary requirement for durable pulmonary vein isolation. A diagnostic ring catheter is positioned within the vein.

When performed by experienced operators, catheter ablation of AF has a major complication rate of 1% to 3%.[8] The potential complications include stroke (0.5%), cardiac tamponade (0.5% to 1.5%), phrenic nerve injury (0.2%), femoral vein-related complications (1%), pulmonary vein stenosis (0.5%), and death (0.1%).

The most feared complication of AF ablation is an atrial esophageal fistula. The risk of esophageal perforation is reported to be in the range of 0.01% to 0.02%.[60] Despite its rarity, this complication is of great concern because it often is lethal. Patients typically present 3 to 14 days after ablation with one of more of the following: dysphagia, odynophagia, fever, leukocytosis, bacteremia, and stroke. Computed tomography of the chest with intravenous contrast is the diagnostic test of choice. The presence of contrast in the esophagus or air in the mediastinum or cardiac chambers is indicative of an esophageal perforation or fistula formation. Instrumentation of the esophagus should be avoided.

Monitoring of the position of the esophagus and intraluminal esophageal temperature monitoring have been used to prevent esophageal injury during ablation along the posterior wall. Although these maneuvers may reduce the risk, they clearly do not prevent all cases of esophageal injury, since 90% of patients with an esophageal perforation had undergone monitoring of the esophageal position or temperature.[60] There is evidence that limiting the power of RF energy applications to 20 to 25 watts for less than 30 seconds when ablating along the posterior left atrial wall and the use of periprocedural proton pump inhibitors reduce the risk of esophageal injury.[61]

Based on the results of a recent global survey, 72% of patients with an esophageal perforation had evidence of an atrial-esophageal fistula, and mortality among these patients was 79%. In contrast, among the 28% of patients with an esophageal perforation who did not have an atrial-esophageal fistula, mortality was 13%.[60] This highlights the importance of early diagnosis and treatment of esophageal perforations. Early surgical intervention is appropriate regardless of whether an atrial-esophageal fistula is present.

Most published series have reported a small or zero mortality risk.[8,44] However, two recent studies examined the mortality of AF ablation in large claims databases. One study examined the major complication rate and mortality among 190,398 patients in the Nationwide Inpatient Sample.[62] The complication rate was 7.21% and the mortality rate was 0.24%. The complication and mortality rates were more than twice that of patients undergoing ablation for supraventricular tachycardia (SVT). The complication rate was about 30% lower but the in-hospital mortality rate was only 13% of that of patients undergoing ablation for VT.[62] A lower operator- and center-procedure-volume were associated with a higher complication rate. A second recent study reported a similar mortality rate of 0.46%, half of which occurred during an early readmission following the index procedure.[63] These studies serve as a sober reminder that AF ablation can be risky and that both operator experience and center procedure volume are important factors that influence risk.

Indications for Ablation and Selection of Patients

The indications for catheter ablation of AF reflect the safety and efficacy of the procedure.[8,18,23] Various documents have been published that provide specific indications for AF ablation. The most widely recognized management guidelines are the 2014 and 2019 AHA/ACC/HRS AF Guidelines, the 2016 ESC AF Guidelines, and the 2017 HRS/EHRA/ECAS Consensus Document on AF Ablation. The 2017 HRS/EHRA/ECAS Consensus Document provides the most detailed recommendations.[8] In this section, the appropriate indications for catheter ablation of AF are reviewed.

Several principles should be considered when selecting patients who are appropriate candidates for AF ablation. First, the only proven benefit of AF ablation is an improvement in quality of life. While cohort studies have provided evidence suggesting that AF ablation may reduce stroke risk, heart failure risk, cognitive dysfunction risk, and mortality, none of these benefits have been conclusively proven in randomized clinical trials. As noted earlier, the CABANA trial randomized 2204 patients to ablation or medical therapy. No difference was seen in the composite primary endpoint of death, disabling stroke, serious

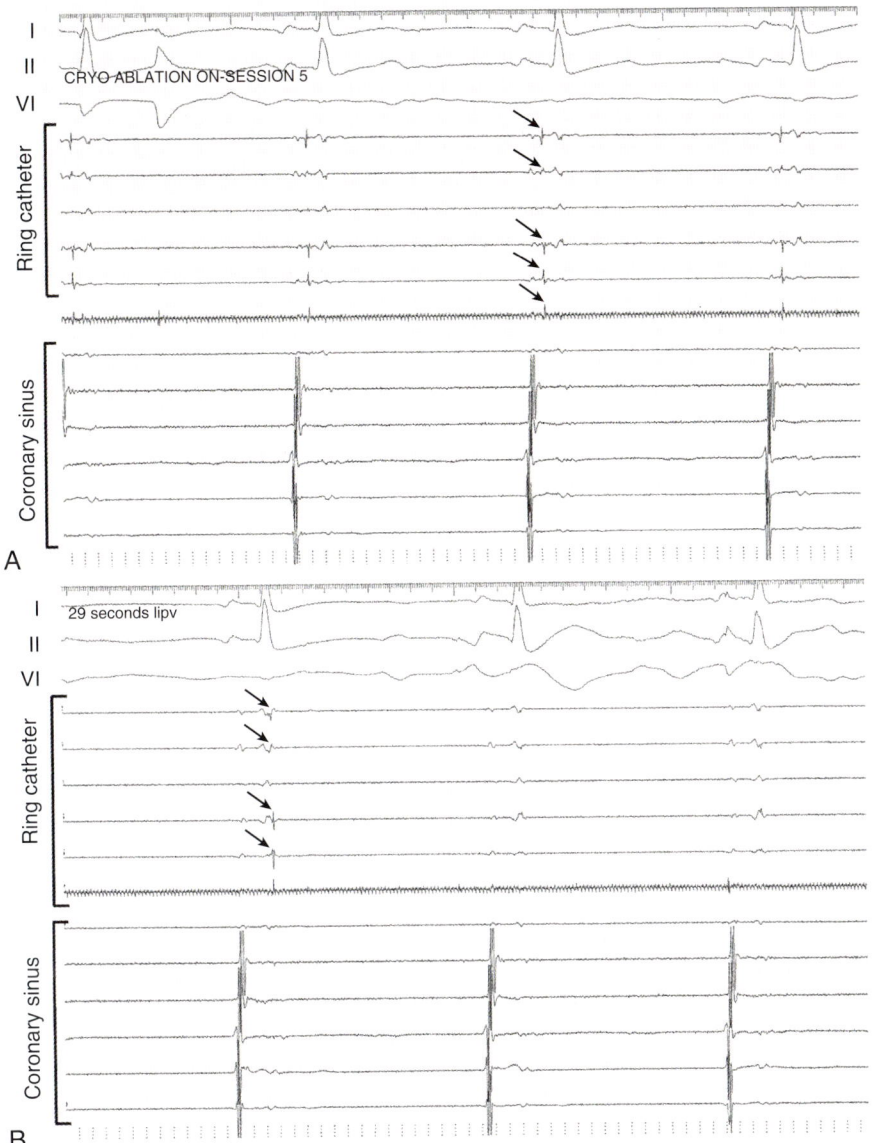

FIGURE 66.12 **A,** Pulmonary vein potentials *(arrows)* recorded from within the left inferior pulmonary vein at the onset of an application of cryoenergy during sinus rhythm at a rate of 54 beats/min. **B,** At 29 seconds into an application of cryoenergy, there is a conduction delay in the pulmonary vein potentials *(arrows)* followed by their complete disappearance, indicating isolation of the left inferior pulmonary vein *(lipv)*. The application of cryoenergy was continued for a total of 4 minutes.

bleeding, or cardiac arrest.[44] It is notable, however, that a secondary treatment analysis revealed that catheter ablation was associated with a lower mortality than medical therapy. The CASTLE AF study is also important to consider. This trial randomized 363 patients with AF heart failure, each of whom had an ICD, to catheter ablation or medical therapy. After a median follow-up of 37.8 months, the primary composite endpoint of death from any cause or hospitalization for worsening heart failure was lower in the ablation arm.[64]

Because of the absence of strong data demonstrating a survival benefit of AF ablation in the absence of heart failure, this procedure is most commonly performed to improve quality of life in patients with symptomatic AF. Other factors to consider when recommending catheter ablation include the type of AF (paroxysmal, persistent, or longstanding persistent), duration of continuous AF, severity of symptoms and quality of life, age, left atrial size, response to rate- and rhythm-control medications, response to cardioversion, and patient preference.

The optimal patients for AF ablation, for which the guidelines provide a class I indication, are patients with symptomatic paroxysmal AF who have not responded well to least one antiarrhythmic medication.[8,18,23] Because of patient preference, ablation sometimes is performed as first-line treatment, in preference to an antiarrhythmic medication. Catheter ablation in medication-naïve patients is a class II indication. Similarly, the recommendation for AF ablation in patients with persistent or longstanding persistent AF is weaker than for patients with paroxysmal AF. This reflects the fact that most trials have primarily enrolled patients with paroxysmal AF and because outcomes after catheter ablation are less satisfactory in patients with the persistent forms of AF.

Surgical Ablation of Atrial Fibrillation

The maze procedure was developed and first reported by Cox et al. in 1987.[1,8] The operation initially required a sternotomy and cardiopulmonary bypass and consisted of multiple atrial incisions to create lines of block and compartmentalize the left atrium and right atrium. In addition, the left and right atrial appendages were excised. Although this procedure had a high success rate, it was technically challenging and the risks were considerable. For this reason, this "cut-and-sew" approach is rarely if ever still performed.

The current iteration of the procedure is the Cox maze 4.[8] This procedure has a similar lesion set, but various tools are used to create the lines of block instead of surgical incisions. These tools include a bipolar clamp RF ablation tool to electrically isolate the PVs. Cryoablation energy delivered with a handheld probe is used to create linear lesions. A bipolar RF clamp is used to electrically isolate the LAA. AF ablation using this open-chest approach is performed in conjunction with open-chest heart surgical procedures such as mitral valve repair or replacement or coronary artery bypass grafting.

Stand-alone surgical AF ablation is performed using a minimally invasive approach referred to as the "mini maze." This procedure involves recreating the maze lesion set using a thorascopic approach with ablation tools specifically designed for percutaneous use.

A single randomized clinical trial[65] and a review of cohort studies[66] have indicated that surgical ablation has greater efficacy than catheter ablation but that it is associated with a higher rate of complications including the need for a permanent pacemaker.[65,66] In many centers this procedure is reserved for AF patients who are poor candidates for catheter ablation, often due to the presence of longstanding persistent AF with severe left atrial dilation, or inefficacy of catheter ablation procedures.

An evolving surgical ablation strategy is a hybrid AF ablation approach in which cardiac surgeons and electrophysiologists participate. Hybrid AF ablation can be performed sequentially during a single ablation session. Some centers prefer a staged approach in which the surgical portion of the procedure is performed first followed by catheter ablation at a separate session, usually several weeks later. The choice of a single combined procedure versus a staged procedure is largely based on operator preference.

Ablation of the Atrioventricular Node

Radiofrequency catheter ablation of the AV node results in complete AV nodal block and substitutes a regular, paced rhythm for an irregular and rapid native rhythm. It is a useful strategy in patients who are symptomatic from AF because of a rapid ventricular rate that cannot be adequately controlled pharmacologically by medications and who either are not good candidates for AF ablation or have already undergone unsuccessful attempts at ablation. AV node ablation also can be helpful in patients with heart failure and AF to maximize the benefits of cardiac resynchronization therapy (CRT) if there already is not 100% ventricular pacing.

In patients with AF and an uncontrolled ventricular rate, AV node ablation improves the left ventricular ejection fraction (EF) if there is a tachycardia-induced cardiomyopathy. AV node ablation also has been shown to improve symptoms, quality of life, and functional capacity and to reduce the use of health care resources.[67-69]

The disadvantages of AV node ablation are that it creates a lifelong need for ventricular pacing and does not restore AV synchrony. Although symptoms and functional capacity typically improve after AV node ablation in patients with AF and an uncontrolled ventricular rate, some patients may not feel as well as during sinus rhythm.

Atrioventricular node ablation is a technically simple procedure with an acute and long-term success rate of 98% or higher and a very low risk of complications. In patients with persistent AF, a ventricular pacemaker is implanted. A dual-chamber pacemaker is appropriate if the AF is paroxysmal. Most patients have a good clinical outcome with right ventricular pacing, but in patients with left ventricular dysfunction, biventricular pacing for CRT is appropriate.[67,69] In some cases, rate-responsive pacing may improve exercise capacity after AV node ablation.[70] In patients with an ischemic or nonischemic cardiomyopathy and EF of 30% to 35% or lower, an ICD may be appropriate for primary prevention of sudden death. However, a pacemaker without the ICD often is adequate for patients with a borderline EF (30% to 35%) and a rapid ventricular rate because the EF typically improves after the ventricular rate has been controlled by AV node ablation. In patients without a bundle branch block, His bundle pacing is optimal because it avoids the dyssynchrony associated with right ventricular pacing and eliminates the need for a lead in the coronary sinus that is required for biventricular pacing.[71,72]

SPECIFIC CLINICAL SYNDROMES

Postoperative Atrial Fibrillation

Atrial fibrillation is common after open heart surgery, occurring in 25% to 40% of patients who undergo coronary artery bypass graft (CABG) surgery or valve replacement. AF in this setting is associated with a twofold increase in the risk of postoperative stroke and is the most common reason for prolonged hospitalization. The incidence of AF peaks on the second postoperative day. The pathogenesis of postoperative AF is multifactorial and probably involves various combinations of adrenergic activation, inflammation, atrial ischemia, electrolyte disturbances, and genetic factors.[73] Several risk factors for AF after open heart surgery have been identified, including age over 70 years, history of prior AF, male sex, left ventricular dysfunction, left atrial enlargement, chronic lung disease, diabetes, and obesity.

The incidence of AF after open heart surgery can be significantly reduced by prophylactic treatment with amiodarone,[74] sotalol, or beta blockers.[75] Hypomagnesemia is common after open heart surgery and can heighten the risk of AF. Magnesium administration has been reported to decrease the risk of postoperative AF. Right atrial or biatrial pacing using temporary electrodes has been reported to reduce the risk of postoperative AF.[76]

A number of other interventions have been assessed for their efficacy in reducing the incidence of AF after cardiac surgery, typically not in large randomized clinical trials. The use of colchicine,[77] statins,[78] and steroids[79] to address postoperative inflammation have produced variable results in reducing AF burden. These agents should be used with caution since the impact on postoperative AF may not be a class effect[80] and other adverse effects have been reported.[79] Omega-3 PUFAs also have an anti-inflammatory effect, but randomized studies on their efficacy for preventing postoperative AF have reported conflicting results.[81]

Another approach to the prevention of AF after cardiac surgery is injection of botulinum toxin into the four major epicardial fat pads at operation. This causes temporary autonomic blockade and has been shown to reduce the incidence of AF after CABG to less than 10% and reduced the AF burden for up three years after surgery.[82]

Patients who develop postoperative AF can be managed using a rate- or rhythm-control strategy. In a randomized comparison of rate- and rhythm-control strategies in patients with AF after cardiac surgery, there were no significant differences between the two strategies in the number of days of hospitalization, mortality, or adverse events.[83] The decision regarding which type of strategy to employ in these patients should be based on the severity of symptoms, hemodynamic effects of the AF, and the patient-specific risk of side effects or adverse reactions to the various rate- and rhythm-control drugs.

AF that occurs after cardiac surgery often resolves within 3 months. In a randomized comparison of rate control versus rhythm control in patients with new-onset AF after cardiac surgery, approximately 95% of patients in both groups were in sinus rhythm at 60 days and had not experienced AF during the prior 30 days.[83] Treatment with an oral anticoagulant should be continued after discharge. Because new-onset AF after cardiac surgery often does not recur after 60 to 90 days, rhythm-control medications can be discontinued at that time, and if there is no subsequent evidence of symptomatic or asymptomatic AF, as confirmed by monitoring (e.g., 3- to 4-week autotrigger event monitor), anticoagulation can be safely discontinued unless needed for another indication.

New-onset AF occurs postoperatively in less than 5% of patients undergoing major noncardiac surgery. Some of the possible mechanisms of postoperative AF after cardiac surgery (e.g., sympathetic activation, electrolyte abnormalities, hypoxia) most likely also play a role in AF after noncardiac surgery. Beta blockers have been shown to significantly reduce the risk of AF after major noncardiac surgery,[84] but one must be vigilant for the development of bradycardia and hypotension.[85]

Wolff-Parkinson-White Syndrome

Patients with the WPW syndrome and an accessory pathway with a short refractory period can experience a very rapid ventricular rate during AF (see Chapters 64 and 65). Ventricular rates greater than 250 to 300 beats/min can result in loss of consciousness or precipitate ventricular fibrillation and a cardiac arrest. Patients with WPW syndrome who present in AF with a rapid ventricular rate should undergo transthoracic cardioversion if there is hemodynamic instability. If the patient is hemodynamically stable, intravenous procainamide or ibutilide can be used for pharmacologic cardioversion. Procainamide may be preferable to ibutilide because it blocks accessory pathway conduction and slows the ventricular rate before AF has converted to sinus rhythm. Digitalis and calcium channel antagonists are contraindicated in patients with WPW syndrome and AF. These agents selectively block conduction in the AV node and can result in acceleration of conduction through the accessory pathway.

The preferred therapy for patients with WPW syndrome and AF with a rapid ventricular rate is catheter ablation of the accessory pathway. When performed by experienced operators, the efficacy of catheter ablation is 95% or higher for most types of accessory pathways, and the risk of a major complication is very low. AF typically no longer recurs after successful accessory pathway ablation, probably because AF in the WPW syndrome often is induced by AV reciprocating tachycardia that degenerates into AF.

Congestive Heart Failure

Atrial fibrillation is a common arrhythmia in patients with heart failure, with a prevalence ranging from 10% in patients with NYHA functional Class I up to 50% in Class IV patients (see Chapters 48 and 49). AF may be the cause of heart failure in patients who present with a nonischemic cardiomyopathy and AF with a rapid ventricular rate. It now is recognized that AF can cause left ventricular dysfunction and heart failure even when the ventricular rate is not rapid. In patients with structural heart disease and preexisting left ventricular dysfunction, AF often worsens the heart failure. The deleterious hemodynamic effects of AF are mediated by a rapid and/or irregular ventricular rate and loss of AV synchrony.

The most appropriate rate-control drugs in patients with systolic heart failure are beta blockers and digitalis. If necessary, amiodarone also can be used for rate control. In patients with diastolic heart failure, nondihydropyridine calcium antagonists can be used safely for rate control. Amiodarone and dofetilide are the only two rhythm-control drugs that are not associated with an increased risk of death in patients with heart failure. AV node ablation is appropriate for patients when the ventricular rate during AF is not adequately controlled by drug therapy. Because left ventricular dysfunction and heart failure can be aggravated by right ventricular pacing, biventricular pacing should be instituted after AV node ablation. The decision to implant a biventricular pacemaker versus a biventricular ICD is based on clinical judgment. If it seems likely that the EF will remain less than 30% to 35% after optimal heart rate control, a biventricular ICD is appropriate for primary prevention of sudden cardiac death. It may take 2 to 3 months to evaluate the response of the LVEF to restoration of sinus rhythm. The decision on an ICD can be safely deferred by use of a wearable defibrillator pending reevaluation of the LVEF.

In patients with heart failure who undergo CRT, AF often results in intrinsic and/or fused QRS complexes even when the rate is considered to be adequately controlled. This can limit the extent of biventricular capture, which undermines the maximum therapeutic effect of CRT. If this is the case in a patient with heart failure and AF, AV node ablation is appropriate to maximize the benefit of CRT by allowing 100% biventricular capture.

A large number of trials have been performed to evaluate the safety and efficacy of AF catheter ablation in patients with heart failure.[8,64,86] Meta-analysis of these trials concluded that catheter ablation of AF in patients with heart failure was associated with a greater improvement in LVEF, greater increase in 6-minute walk distance, improved quality of life, and a significantly reduced mortality. Another more recent meta-analysis concluded that AF ablation reduces the risk of death, stroke, and hospitalization compared with medical therapy in heart failure patients.[87] The CASTLE AF trial randomized 363 heart failure patients, each of whom had an ICD in place, to AF catheter ablation or medical therapy. After a median follow-up of 37.8 months, the primary composite endpoint of death from any cause or hospitalization for worsening heart failure was lower in the ablation arm.[64] While these studies strongly suggest that AF ablation should be considered in patients with heart failure, it is important to recognize that these trials were limited by small numbers of highly selected patients. It is for this reason that the 2019 AHA/ACC/HRS AF Guidelines provides only a class IIb recommendation for AF ablation in patients with heart failure.[18]

As in other patients with AF, the decision to pursue a rate-control or a rhythm-control strategy in patients with heart failure should be individualized. But it is important to recognize that sinus rhythm is the best type of rate control. It is also important to recognize that AF can cause or aggravate left ventricular dysfunction and heart failure despite adequate heart rate control. Because of this, a reasonable approach is to first use a rhythm-control strategy in patients with newly diagnosed AF associated with heart failure. Amiodarone or dofetilide can be used to help maintain sinus rhythm after sinus rhythm is restored by cardioversion. If a patient does not want to be on these AADs long term or if these AADs do not prevent early recurrences of AF, catheter ablation of the AF or rate-control alone should be considered.

A rate-control strategy is appropriate for patients who do not respond adequately to amiodarone or dofetilide and either are not suitable candidates for catheter ablation of the AF or have had an unsuccessful outcome from ablation.

Hypertrophic Cardiomyopathy (see Chapter 54)

Atrial fibrillation occurs in approximately 25% of patients with hypertrophic cardiomyopathy (HCM) and can cause severe hemodynamic impairment because of an inadequate diastolic filling time and loss of atrial-ventricular synchrony. Because of a high risk of thromboembolic complications, anticoagulation is indicated in AF patients with HCM, independent of the CHA_2DS_2-VASc score.[1,18]

Severe left ventricular hypertrophy increases the risk of drug-induced torsade de pointes as a complication of AAD therapy. Catheter ablation of AF also is an option. A large number of studies have reported that catheter ablation in AF is associated with an acceptable efficacy and safety profile.[8]

Pregnancy (see Chapter 92)

The prevalence of AF during pregnancy is very low, approximately 60/100,000 pregnancies. When it occurs, there often is underlying congenital or valvular heart disease, thyrotoxicosis, or electrolyte abnormalities. Pregnancy is associated with a hypercoagulable state, but there are no data indicating that pregnancy increases the risk of thromboembolic complications related to AF. In women with paroxysmal AF before pregnancy, the frequency of episodes may or may not increase during pregnancy.

The decision to anticoagulate a pregnant woman with AF should be made using the same criteria as in nonpregnant women. If anticoagulation is deemed necessary, warfarin (not a DOAC) is recommended from the second trimester until 1 month before the due date, and subcutaneous LMWH is recommended during the first trimester and during the final month of pregnancy.

Transthoracic cardioversion is considered safe at all stages of pregnancy. The recommended pharmacologic agents for acute management of AF consist of intravenous metoprolol for rate control and flecainide or sotalol for conversion to sinus rhythm. If ongoing therapy is deemed necessary, the recommended rate-control drug is digoxin. If ineffective, a beta blocker can be used, but only after the first trimester. If there is no structural heart disease, flecainide and sotalol are recommended for long-term rhythm control.[88] In the patient with structural heart disease, amiodarone is recommended for rhythm control.

FUTURE PERSPECTIVES

The past few years have witnessed significant progress in the field of catheter ablation of AF, but there is room for further improvement and limited data on the durability of rhythm control.[89] The failure to create permanent pulmonary vein isolation often accounts for recurrences of AF after both radiofrequency catheter ablation and cryoballoon ablation. The development of new ablation tools that improve the ability to safely create transmural lesions could reduce the need for redo ablation procedures. At present, several studies are underway to determine whether electroporation, also known as pulse field ablation, may be a more effective and safer energy source than either RF or cryoablation. Early data suggest that this energy source results in a high rate of permanent PV isolation and also reduces the risk of injury to surrounding structures such as the phrenic nerve and esophagus.[90,91]

AF is a progressive condition that results in atrial remodeling. In patients with persistent AF, a better understanding of AF mechanisms could result in more efficient and successful ablation strategies. The best chance for treating AF is early in the course of the disease. New trials are underway to examine the outcomes of early AF ablation even if episodes of paroxysmal or persistent AF are infrequent.

Perhaps most pressing, as the population ages, the incidence of chronic disease and AF will continue to rise. This will create a public health challenge that is linked to other preventable diseases that share modifiable risk factors. This underscores the need for primordial prevention strategies that delay the onset of AF by minimizing risk factors and behaviors and optimizing the management of predisposing diseases.[92]

REFERENCES

Epidemiology

1. Morady F, Zipes DP. Atrial fibrillation: clinical features, mechanisms, and management. In: Zipes DP, et al., ed. *Braunwald's heart disease, a textbook of cardiovascular medicine*. 11 ed. Philadelphia, PA: Elsevier; 2016.
2. Voskoboinik A, Kalman JM, De Silva A, et al. Alcohol abstinence in drinkers with atrial fibrillation. *N Engl J Med*. 2020;382:20–28.

3. Johansson C, Lind MM, Eriksson M, et al. Alcohol consumption and risk of incident atrial fibrillation: a population-based cohort study. *Eur J Intern Med*. 2020;76:50–57.
4. Benjamin EJ, Virani SS, Callaway CW, et al. Heart disease and stroke statistics-2018 update: a report from the American Heart Association. *Circulation*. 2018;137:e67–e492.

Mechanisms

5. Nattel S. Molecular and cellular mechanisms of atrial fibrosis in atrial fibrillation. *JACC Clin Electrophysiol*. 2017;3:425–435.
6. Lee S, Sahadevan J, Khrestian CM, et al. Characterization of foci and breakthrough sites during persistent and long-standing persistent atrial fibrillation in patients: studies using high-density (510-512 electrodes) biatrial epicardial mapping. *J Am Heart Assoc*. 2017;6:e005274.
7. Haissaguerre M, Jais P, Shah DC, et al. Spontaneous initiation of atrial fibrillation by ectopic beats originating in the pulmonary veins. *N Engl J Med*. 1998;339:659–666.
8. Calkins H, Hindricks G, Cappato R, et al. HRS/EHRA/ECAS/APHRS/SOLAECE expert consensus statement on catheter and surgical ablation of atrial fibrillation. *Europace*. 2017;20:e1–e160. 2018.
9. Shoemaker MB, Husser D, Roselli C, et al. Genetic susceptibility for atrial fibrillation in patients undergoing atrial fibrillation ablation. *Circ Arrhythm Electrophysiol*. 2020;13:e007676.
10. Roselli C, Chaffin MD, Weng LC, et al. Multi-ethnic genome-wide association study for atrial fibrillation. *Nat Genet*. 2018;50:1225–1233.
11. Miller JD, Aronis KN, Chrispin J, et al. Obesity, exercise, obstructive sleep apnea, and modifiable atherosclerotic cardiovascular disease risk factors in atrial fibrillation. *J Am Coll Cardiol*. 2015;66:2899–2906.
12. Wong CX, Ganesan AN, Selvanayagam JB. Epicardial fat and atrial fibrillation: current evidence, potential mechanisms, clinical implications, and future directions. *Eur Heart J*. 2017;38:1294–1302.
13. Pathak RK, Middeldorp ME, Meredith M, et al. Long-term effect of goal-directed weight management in an atrial fibrillation cohort: A long-term follow-up study (legacy). *J Am Coll Cardiol*. 2015;65:2159–2169.
14. Tung CE, Su D, Turakhia MP, et al. Diagnostic yield of extended cardiac patch monitoring in patients with stroke or tia. *Front Neurol*. 2014;5:266.
15. Brachmann J, Morillo CA, Sanna T, et al. Uncovering atrial fibrillation beyond short-term monitoring in cryptogenic stroke patients: Three-year results from the cryptogenic stroke and underlying atrial fibrillation trial. *Circ Arrhythm Electrophysiol*. 2016;9:e003333.

Management

16. Sun Q, Chang S, Lu S, et al. The efficacy and safety of 3 types of interventions for stroke prevention in patients with cardiovascular and cerebrovascular diseases: a network meta-analysis. *Clin Ther*. 2017;39:1291. 1312 e1298.
17. Link MS, Giugliano RP, Ruff CT, et al. Stroke and mortality risk in patients with various patterns of atrial fibrillation: results from the ENGAGE AF-TIMI 48 trial (effective anticoagulation with factor Xa next generation in atrial fibrillation-thrombolysis in myocardial infarction 48). *Circ Arrhythm Electrophysiol*. 2017;10:e004267.
18. January CT, Wann LS, Calkins H, et al. AHA/ACC/HRS focused update of the 2014 AHA/ACC/HRS guideline for the management of patients with atrial fibrillation: a report of the American College of Cardiology/American Heart Association task force on clinical practice guidelines and the heart rhythm society. *J Am Coll Cardiol*. 2019;74:104–132. 2019.
19. Bonde AN, Lip GY, Kamper AL, et al. Renal function and the risk of stroke and bleeding in patients with atrial fibrillation: an observational cohort study. *Stroke*. 2016;47:2707–2713.
20. Freedman B, Camm J, Calkins H, et al. Screening for atrial fibrillation: a report of the af-screen international collaboration. *Circulation*. 2017;135:1851–1867.
21. Berg DD, Ruff CT, Jarolim P, et al. Performance of the abc scores for assessing the risk of stroke or systemic embolism and bleeding in patients with atrial fibrillation in engage af-timi 48. *Circulation*. 2019;139:760–771.
22. Takabayashi K, Hamatani Y, Yamashita Y, et al. Incidence of stroke or systemic embolism in paroxysmal versus sustained atrial fibrillation: the Fushimi atrial fibrillation registry. *Stroke*. 2015;46:3354–3361.
23. Kirchhof P, Benussi S, Kotecha D, et al. 2016 ESC guidelines for the management of atrial fibrillation developed in collaboration with EACTS. *Eur Heart J*. 2016;37:2893–2962.
24. Healey JS, Alings M, Ha A, et al. Subclinical atrial fibrillation in older patients. *Circulation*. 2017;136:1276–1283.
25. Proietti M, Rivera-Caravaca JM, Esteve-Pastor MA, et al. Predicting bleeding events in anticoagulated patients with atrial fibrillation: a comparison between the HAS-BLED and GARFIELD-AF bleeding scores. *J Am Heart Assoc*. 2018;7:e009766.
26. Assiri A, Al-Majzoub O, Kanaan AO, et al. Mixed treatment comparison meta-analysis of aspirin, warfarin, and new anticoagulants for stroke prevention in patients with nonvalvular atrial fibrillation. *Clin Ther*. 2013;35:967–984 e962.
27. Tereshchenko LG, Henrikson CA, Cigarroa J, et al. Comparative effectiveness of interventions for stroke prevention in atrial fibrillation: a network meta-analysis. *J Am Heart Assoc*. 2016;5:e003206.
28. Pokorney SD, Simon DN, Thomas L, et al. Patients' time in therapeutic range on warfarin among us patients with atrial fibrillation: results from orbit-af registry. *Am Heart J*. 2015;170:141–148. 148 e141.
29. Shah SJ, Singer DE, Fang MC, et al. Net clinical benefit of oral anticoagulation among older adults with atrial fibrillation. *Circ Cardiovasc Qual Outcomes*. 2019;12:e006212.
30. Steffel J, Verhamme P, Potpara TS, et al. The 2018 European heart rhythm association practical guide on the use of non-vitamin k antagonist oral anticoagulants in patients with atrial fibrillation. *Eur Heart J*. 2018;39:1330–1393.
31. Stanifer JW, Pokorney SD, Chertow GM, et al. Apixaban versus warfarin in patients with atrial fibrillation and advanced chronic kidney disease. *Circulation*. 2020;141:1384–1392.
32. Connolly SJ, Crowther M, Eikelboom JW, et al. Full study report of andexanet alfa for bleeding associated with factor Xa inhibitors. *N Engl J Med*. 2019;380:1326–1335.
33. Tomaselli GF, Mahaffey KW, Cuker A, et al. acc expert consensus decision pathway on management of bleeding in patients on oral anticoagulants: a report of the American College of Cardiology solution set oversight committee. *J Am Coll Cardiol*. 2020;76:594–622.
34. Pollack CV Jr, Reilly PA, Eikelboom J, et al. Idarucizumab for dabigatran reversal. *N Engl J Med*. 2015;373:511–520.
35. Ozaki AF, Choi AS, Le QT, et al. Real-world adherence and persistence to direct oral anticoagulants in patients with atrial fibrillation: a systematic review and meta-analysis. *Circ Cardiovasc Qual Outcomes*. 2020;13:e005969.
36. Gibson CM, Basto AN, Howard ML. Direct oral anticoagulants in cardioversion: a review of current evidence. *Ann Pharmacother*. 2018;52:277–284.
37. Cardoso R, Willems S, Gerstenfeld EP, et al. Uninterrupted anticoagulation with non-vitamin K antagonist oral anticoagulants in atrial fibrillation catheter ablation: lessons learned from randomized trials. *Clin Cardiol*. 2019;42:198–205.
38. Freeman JV, Varosy P, Price MJ, et al. The ncdr left atrial appendage occlusion registry. *J Am Coll Cardiol*. 2020;75:1503–1518.
39. Brouwer TF, Whang W, Kuroki K, et al. Net clinical benefit of left atrial appendage closure versus warfarin in patients with atrial fibrillation: a pooled analysis of the randomized protect-af and prevail studies. *J Am Heart Assoc*. 2019;8:e013525.
40. Boersma LV, Ince H, Kische S, et al. Evaluating real-world clinical outcomes in atrial fibrillation patients receiving the watchman left atrial appendage closure technology: final 2-year outcome data of the Evolution trial focusing on history of stroke and hemorrhage. *Circ Arrhythm Electrophysiol*. 2019;12:e006841.
41. Sondergaard L, Wong YH, Reddy VY, et al. Propensity-matched comparison of oral anticoagulation versus antiplatelet therapy after left atrial appendage closure with watchman. *JACC Cardiovasc Interv*. 2019;12:1055–1063.
42. Lakkireddy D, Afzal MR, Lee RJ, et al. Short and long-term outcomes of percutaneous left atrial appendage suture ligation: results from a us multicenter evaluation. *Heart Rhythm*. 2016;13:1030–1036.
43. Sethi NJ, Feinberg J, Nielsen EE, et al. The effects of rhythm control strategies versus rate control strategies for atrial fibrillation and atrial flutter: a systematic review with meta-analysis and trial sequential analysis. *PLoS One*. 2017;12:e0186856.

Ablation

44. Packer DL, Mark DB, Robb RA, et al. Effect of catheter ablation vs antiarrhythmic drug therapy on mortality, stroke, bleeding, and cardiac arrest among patients with atrial fibrillation: the cabana randomized clinical trial. *JAMA*. 2019;321:1261–1274.
45. Allen LaPointe NM, Dai D, Thomas L, et al. Antiarrhythmic drug use in patients <65 years with atrial fibrillation and without structural heart disease. *Am J Cardiol*. 2015;115:316–322.
46. Boriani G, Blomstrom-Lundqvist C, Hohnloser SH, et al. Safety and efficacy of dronedarone from clinical trials to real-world evidence: implications for its use in atrial fibrillation. *Europace*. 2019;21:1764–1775.
47. Chung MK, Eckhardt LL, Chen LY, et al. Lifestyle and risk factor modification for reduction of atrial fibrillation: a scientific statement from the American Heart Association. *Circulation*. 2020;141:e750–e772.
48. Middeldorp ME, Pathak RK, Meredith M, et al. PREVEntion and regReSsive effect of weight-loss and risk factor modification on atrial fibrillation: the REVERSE-AF study. *Europace*. 2018;20:1929–1935.
49. Pathak RK, Evans M, Middeldorp ME, et al. Cost-effectiveness and clinical effectiveness of the risk factor management clinic in atrial fibrillation: the CENT study. *JACC Clin Electrophysiol*. 2017;3:436–447.
50. Cipollini F, Arcangeli E, Seghieri G. Left atrial dimension is related to blood pressure variability in newly diagnosed untreated hypertensive patients. *Hypertens Res*. 2016;39:583–587.
51. Romanov A, Pokushalov E, Ponomarev D, et al. Pulmonary vein isolation with concomitant renal artery denervation is associated with reduction in both arterial blood pressure and atrial fibrillation burden: data from implantable cardiac monitor. *Cardiovasc Ther*. 2017;35. https://doi.org/10.1111/1755-5922.12264.
52. Fatemi O, Yuriditsky E, Tsioufis C, et al. Impact of intensive glycemic control on the incidence of atrial fibrillation and associated cardiovascular outcomes in patients with type 2 diabetes mellitus (from the action to control cardiovascular risk in diabetes study). *Am J Cardiol*. 2014;114:1217–1222.
53. Verma A, Jiang CY, Betts TR, et al. Approaches to catheter ablation for persistent atrial fibrillation. *N Engl J Med*. 2015;372:1812–1822.
54. Andrade JG, Champagne J, Dubuc M, et al. Cryoballoon or radiofrequency ablation for atrial fibrillation assessed by continuous monitoring: a randomized clinical trial. *Circulation*. 2019;140:1779–1788.
55. Duytschaever M, De Pooter J, Demolder A, et al. Long-term impact of catheter ablation on arrhythmia burden in low-risk patients with paroxysmal atrial fibrillation: the close to cure study. *Heart Rhythm*. 2020;17:535–543.
56. Aryana A, Braegelmann KM, Lim HW, et al. Cryoballoon ablation dosing: from the bench to the bedside and back. *Heart Rhythm*. 2020;17:1185–1192.
57. Tohoku S, Bordignon S, Chen S, et al. From point by point to single shot: evolution of visually guided pulmonary vein isolation using the third-generation laser balloon catheter. *J Cardiovasc Electrophysiol*. Apr 22 2020.
58. Dukkipati SR, Cuoco F, Kutinsky I, et al. Pulmonary vein isolation using the visually guided laser balloon: A prospective, multicenter, and randomized comparison to standard radiofrequency ablation. *J Am Coll Cardiol*. 2015;66:1350–1360.
59. Kuck KH, Furnkranz A, Chun KR, et al. Cryoballoon or radiofrequency ablation for symptomatic paroxysmal atrial fibrillation: reintervention, rehospitalization, and quality-of-life outcomes in the fire and ice trial. *Eur Heart J*. 2016;37:2858–2865.
60. Barbhaiya CR, Kumar S, Guo Y, et al. Global survey of esophageal injury in atrial fibrillation ablation: characteristics and outcomes of esophageal perforation and fistula. *JACC Clin Electrophysiol*. 2016;2:143–150.
61. Kapur S, Barbhaiya C, Deneke T, et al. Esophageal injury and atrioesophageal fistula caused by ablation for atrial fibrillation. *Circulation*. 2017;136:1247–1255.
62. Hosseini SM, Rozen G, Saleh A, et al. Catheter ablation for cardiac arrhythmias: utilization and in-hospital complications, 2000 to 2013. *JACC Clin Electrophysiol*. 2017;3:1240–1248.
63. Cheng EP, Liu CF, Yeo I, et al. Risk of mortality following catheter ablation of atrial fibrillation. *J Am Coll Cardiol*. 2019;74:2254–2264.
64. Marrouche NF, Brachmann J, Andresen D, et al. Catheter ablation for atrial fibrillation with heart failure. *N Engl J Med*. 2018;378:417–427.
65. Boersma LV, Castella M, van Boven W, et al. Atrial fibrillation catheter ablation versus surgical ablation treatment (fast): a 2-center randomized clinical trial. *Circulation*. 2012;125:23–30.
66. Kearney K, Stephenson R, Phan K, et al. A systematic review of surgical ablation versus catheter ablation for atrial fibrillation. *Ann Cardiothorac Surg*. 2014;3:15–29.
67. Mittal S, Musat DL, Hoskins MH, et al. Clinical outcomes after ablation of the AV junction in patients with atrial fibrillation: impact of cardiac resynchronization therapy. *J Am Heart Assoc*. 2017;6:e007270.
68. Garcia B, Clementy N, Benhenda N, et al. Mortality after atrioventricular nodal radiofrequency catheter ablation with permanent ventricular pacing in atrial fibrillation: outcomes from a controlled nonrandomized study. *Circ Arrhythm Electrophysiol Jul*. 2016;9:e003993.
69. Brignole M, Pokushalov E, Pentimalli F, et al. A randomized controlled trial of atrioventricular junction ablation and cardiac resynchronization therapy in patients with permanent atrial fibrillation and narrow qrs. *Eur Heart J*. 2018;39:3999–4008.
70. Palmisano P, Aspromonte V, Ammendola E, et al. Effect of fixed-rate vs. rate-responsive pacing on exercise capacity in patients with permanent, refractory atrial fibrillation and left ventricular dysfunction treated with atrioventricular junction ablation and biventricular pacing (responsible): a prospective, multicentre, randomized, single-blind study. *Europace*. 2017;19:414–420.
71. Vijayaraman P, Subzposh FA, Naperkowski A. Atrioventricular node ablation and His bundle pacing. *Europace*. 2017;19:iv10–iv16.
72. Huang W, Su L, Wu S, et al. Benefits of permanent His bundle pacing combined with atrioventricular node ablation in atrial fibrillation patients with heart failure with both preserved and reduced left ventricular ejection fraction. *J Am Heart Assoc*. 2017;6:e005309.

Postoperative Atrial Fibrillation

73. Dobrev D, Aguilar M, Heijman J, et al. Postoperative atrial fibrillation: mechanisms, manifestations and management. *Nat Rev Cardiol*. 2019;16:417–436.
74. Atreya AR, Priya A, Pack QR, et al. Use and outcomes associated with perioperative amiodarone in cardiac surgery. *J Am Heart Assoc*. 2019;8:e009892.
75. Blessberger H, Lewis SR, Pritchard MW, et al. Perioperative beta-blockers for preventing surgery-related mortality and morbidity in adults undergoing cardiac surgery. *Cochrane Database Syst Rev*. 2019;9:CD013435.
76. Ruan Y, Robinson NB, Naik A, et al. Effect of atrial pacing on post-operative atrial fibrillation following coronary artery bypass grafting: pairwise and network meta-analyses. *Int J Cardiol*. 2020;302:103–107.

77. Lee JZ, Singh N, Howe CL, et al. Colchicine for prevention of post-operative atrial fibrillation: a meta-analysis. *JACC Clin Electrophysiol*. 2016;2:78–85.
78. Zhen-Han L, Rui S, Dan C, et al. Perioperative statin administration with decreased risk of postoperative atrial fibrillation, but not acute kidney injury or myocardial infarction: a meta-analysis. *Sci Rep*. 2017;7:10091.
79. Dvirnik N, Belley-Cote EP, Hanif H, et al. Steroids in cardiac surgery: a systematic review and meta-analysis. *Br J Anaesth*. 2018;120:657–667.
80. Yuan X, Du J, Liu Q, et al. Defining the role of perioperative statin treatment in patients after cardiac surgery: a meta-analysis and systematic review of 20 randomized controlled trials. *Int J Cardiol*. 2017;228:958–966.
81. Wang H, Chen J, Zhao L. N-3 polyunsaturated fatty acids for prevention of postoperative atrial fibrillation: updated meta-analysis and systematic review. *J Interv Card Electrophysiol*. 2018;51:105–115.
82. Romanov A, Pokushalov E, Ponomarev D, et al. Long-term suppression of atrial fibrillation by botulinum toxin injection into epicardial fat pads in patients undergoing cardiac surgery: three-year follow-up of a randomized study. *Heart Rhythm*. 2019;16:172–177.
83. Gillinov AM, Bagiella E, Moskowitz AJ, et al. Rate control versus rhythm control for atrial fibrillation after cardiac surgery. *N Engl J Med*. 2016;374:1911–1921.
84. Bessissow A, Khan J, Devereaux PJ, et al. Postoperative atrial fibrillation in non-cardiac and cardiac surgery: an overview. *J Thromb Haemost*. 2015;13(suppl 1):S304–312.
85. Blessberger H, Lewis SR, Pritchard MW, et al. Perioperative beta-blockers for preventing surgery-related mortality and morbidity in adults undergoing non-cardiac surgery. *Cochrane Database Syst Rev*. 2019;9:CD013438.

Perspectives

86. Ganesan AN, Nandal S, Luker J, et al. Catheter ablation of atrial fibrillation in patients with concomitant left ventricular impairment: a systematic review of efficacy and effect on ejection fraction. *Heart Lung Circ*. 2015;24:270–280.
87. Saglietto A, De Ponti R, Di Biase L, et al. Impact of atrial fibrillation catheter ablation on mortality, stroke, and heart failure hospitalizations: a meta-analysis. *J Cardiovasc Electrophysiol*. 2020;31:1040–1047.
88. Wright JM, Page RL, Field ME. Antiarrhythmic drugs in pregnancy. *Expert Rev Cardiovasc Ther*. 2015;13:1433–1444.
89. Gaita F, Scaglione M, Battaglia A, et al. Very long-term outcome following transcatheter ablation of atrial fibrillation. Are results maintained after 10 years of follow up? *Europace*. 2018;20:443–450.
90. Koruth JS, Kuroki K, Kawamura I, et al. Pulsed field ablation versus radiofrequency ablation: esophageal injury in a novel porcine model. *Circ Arrhythm Electrophysiol*. 2020;13:e008303.
91. Bradley CJ, Haines DE. Pulsed field ablation for pulmonary vein isolation in the treatment of atrial fibrillation. *J Cardiovasc Electrophysiol*. 2020;31(8):2136–2147.
92. Kornej J, Borschel CS, Benjamin EJ, et al. Epidemiology of atrial fibrillation in the 21st century: novel methods and new insights. *Circ Res*. 2020;127:4–20.

67 Ventricular Arrhythmias

WILLIAM G. STEVENSON AND KATJA ZEPPENFELD

PREMATURE VENTRICULAR COMPLEXES, NONSUSTAINED VENTRICULAR TACHYCARDIAS, COUPLETS, 1288
Electrocardiographic Recognition, 1288
Clinical Features, 1289
Management, 1289

ACCELERATED IDIOVENTRICULAR RHYTHM, 1292
Electrocardiographic Recognition, 1292
Management, 1292

SUSTAINED VENTRICULAR TACHYCARDIA, 1292

Monomorphic Ventricular Tachycardia, 1292
Mechanisms and Clinical Correlations, 1294
Clinical Features, 1295
Evaluation and Long-Term Management, 1296
Specific Ventricular Tachycardias, 1297
Nonischemic Dilated Cardiomyopathy, 1299
Arrhythmogenic Right Ventricular Cardiomyopathy, 1299
Congenital Heart Disease, 1302
Hypertrophic Cardiomyopathy, 1302
Inflammatory Heart Disease, 1302
Idiopathic Ventricular Tachycardias, 1303

Polymorphic Ventricular Tachycardia, 1304
Specific Disorders with Polymorphic Ventricular Tachycardias, 1304
J Wave Syndromes: Brugada and Early Repolarization Syndromes, 1308

VENTRICULAR FIBRILLATION, 1309
Electrocardiographic Recognition, 1309
Clinical Features, 1310
Management, 1310

VENTRICULAR FLUTTER, 1310

REFERENCES, 1310

Ventricular arrhythmias originate in the ventricular myocardium or His-Purkinje system. These include premature ventricular complexes (PVCs), nonsustained and sustained ventricular tachycardias (VT), and ventricular fibrillation (VF). They can occur in all forms of structural heart disease that involve the ventricles and can be the initial presentation of disease. Sustained arrhythmias are an important cause of sudden death. Some genetic abnormalities of cardiac ion channels can cause sudden death from ventricular arrhythmias despite the absence of structural heart disease. Ventricular arrhythmias that occur in the absence of structural heart disease and a defined ion channel abnormality are referred to as idiopathic and are usually benign. Evaluation and management are guided by symptoms, underlying heart disease, and the risk of arrhythmic sudden death. Because of the differences in prognosis and treatment, proper diagnosis is critical.

PREMATURE VENTRICULAR COMPLEXES, NONSUSTAINED VENTRICULAR TACHYCARDIAS, COUPLETS

Electrocardiographic Recognition

PVCs are due to abnormal impulse formation (automaticity, triggered activity) or reentry (Chapter 62) in the ventricular myocardium or Purkinje system, producing a depolarization wavefront that propagates through the ventricles independent of activation from the atrium and AV node. The mechanism cannot usually be determined with certainty. A PVC is characterized by the premature occurrence of an abnormal QRS complex that usually has a duration exceeding 120 msec. The corresponding T wave is typically broad and in the opposite direction of the major QRS deflection. It is typically not preceded by a P-wave. Premature atrial or junctional beats that conduct with bundle branch block can mimic PVCs.

The timing of the PVC and its interaction with the conduction system determine the effect on rhythm (Fig. 67.1). Often the PVC excitation wavefront propagates retrogradely in the His Purkinje system. It may block in the conduction system or collide in the AV node with the sinus impulse. In either case it fails to reach the atrium and has no effect on sinus node automaticity. The next sinus beat is on time, resulting in a compensatory pause with the R – R interval from the sinus beat preceding the PVC to the one following the PVC equal to twice the sinus cycle length. If the PVC conducts to the atrium, the retrograde P-wave is usually visible at the end of its QRS. The retrograde P-wave can then reset the sinus node, advancing its next spontaneous depolarization and producing an incomplete compensatory pause (see Fig. 67.1C), which is more commonly associated with premature atrial beats. PVCs can also fall between sinus beats without disturbing AV conduction and without producing a pause, defined as interpolated PVCs (see Fig. 67.1D). If PVCs are relatively late in the cardiac cycle the PVC activation wavefront may collide with a sinus wavefront that has already reached the ventricles, producing fusion beats.

The QRS morphology of the PVC reflects its origin within the ventricles. The wide QRS is due to the initial activation of the ventricles by wavefronts propagating through ventricular myocardium or part of the Purkinje system rather than simultaneously through right and left bundle branches. The ventricular activation sequence is largely determined by the site of initial ventricular activation and hence the QRS morphology is an indication of the location of the ventricular arrhythmia origin (Fig. 67.2). Those that have a dominant S wave in V1 are termed left bundle branch block (LBBB)—like and generally originate in the right ventricular (RV) or interventricular septum. Those with a dominant R wave in V1 are termed right bundle branch block (RBBB)—like and generally originate in the left ventricle (LV) in the morphologically normal heart. Analysis of the frontal plane axis and precordial lead patterns further refine prediction of the likely origin. Initial depolarization of the inferior wall produces a superior frontal plane axis, and depolarization of the anterior wall produces an inferiorly directed frontal plane axis. Exceptions occur and predicting the arrhythmia origin from the QRS morphology is less reliable when structural heart disease with scar that changes ventricular activation is present.

PVCs with a single QRS morphology are referred to as unifocal (see Fig. 67.1E, beats 3, 5, 7). The presence of PVCs with different QRS morphologies (see Fig. 67.1D) is referred to as multifocal or multiform and usually indicates more than one PVC focus, although variable conduction away from a single focus is also a possible cause. Frequent multifocal PVCs are more often associated with structural heart disease.

PVCs may occur in repetitive patterns. Every conducted sinus beat followed by a PVC is bigeminy (Fig. 67.2, sites 1, 3, and 4 and Fig. 67.3B). Every two sinus beats followed by a PVC is trigeminy (see Fig. 67.2, site 6). The coupling interval between the sinus beat and PVC may be fixed or variable. A fixed coupling interval is consistent with reentry or triggered activity as the mechanism (Chapter 62). Variable coupling with a common interval between PVCs suggests abnormal automaticity from a parasystolic focus that is relatively protected from ventricular activation from conducted sinus beats.

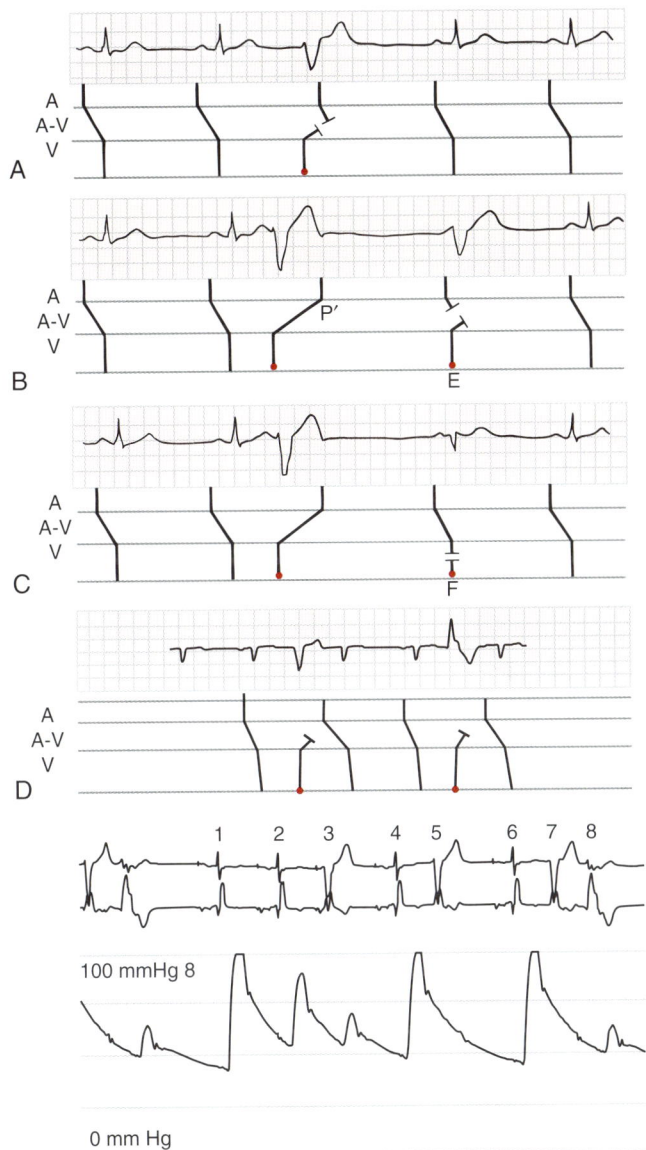

FIGURE 67.1 Premature ventricular complexes (PVCs). **A,** Late PVC results in a compensatory pause. **B,** Slower sinus rate and slightly earlier PVC result in retrograde atrial excitation (P'). The sinus node is reset, followed by a noncompensatory pause. Before the sinus-initiated P wave that follows the retrograde P wave can conduct to the ventricle, a ventricular escape beat (E) occurs. **C,** A PVC with a noncompensatory pause similar to B except that a ventricular fusion beat (F) results after the PVC because of a slightly faster sinus rate. **D,** Interpolated multifocal PVCs are followed by slightly prolonged PR interval of the sinus-initiated beat due to concealed conduction from the PVC into the AV node. **E,** Hemodynamic effect of PVCs. The ECG shows PVCs (beats 3, 5, 7, and 8). The femoral arterial tracing shows a small or absent pressure contour following the PVCs, producing an effective heart rate slower than 30 beats/min.

heart failure during long-term follow-up. PVCs are identified on a standard ECG in fewer than 1% of individuals younger than 20 years of age, increasing with age to more than 2% of those older than 50 years.[1] On ambulatory monitoring PVCs increase with age and cardiovascular risk factors including hypertension and smoking.[2] Of 1139 subjects older than 65 years who had normal LV systolic function and no heart failure, the median PVC frequency at baseline was 0.01% (approximately 10 PVCs per day).[3] The 15-year risk of heart failure increased from 19.3% for those with 0.01% PVCs/day to 30.8% for those who had 1% (approximately 1000 PVCs) per day at baseline.

Couplets and nonsustained VTs are less common than PVCs but are often present in patients who have frequent PVCs and increase with underlying disease severity. Runs of VT that are polymorphic, faster than 220 beats/min, or that start near the peak of the T-wave of the preceding sinus beat (see Figs. 67.4 and 67.5B) raise concern for risk of rapid sustained arrhythmias causing syncope or sudden death.[4]

During exercise testing 7 or more PVCs/minute occur at some stage (before, during exertion, or during recovery) in fewer than 10% of patients without a history of heart disease. PVCs may emerge during exertion, then suppress with elevation of sinus rate and reemerge in recovery as the sinus rate slows. Nonsustained VT occurs in fewer than 5%, is typically 5 beats in duration or shorter, and slower than 200 beats/minute. Benign idiopathic arrhythmias often originate from the right ventricular outflow tract (see Fig. 67.5A). Exercise-induced arrhythmias can also be associated with underlying structural heart disease, or be a manifestation of rare genetic arrhythmia syndromes, particularly catecholaminergic polymorphic VT (see Fig. 67.5C) or early arrhythmogenic RV cardiomyopathy. Exercise-induced PVCs and non-sustained VT (NSVT) have been associated with increased mortality during long-term follow-up in some studies, but generally not after adjusting for associated disease and ventricular dysfunction. In competitive athletes without evidence of heart disease, 7% have PVCs during exercise testing, usually fewer than 10, and these were associated with a benign prognosis in one study.[5]

PVCs can be produced by direct mechanical, electrical, or chemical stimulation of the myocardium and are often noted during acute coronary syndromes (see Fig. 67.4C,D), myocarditis,[6] hypoxia, and electrolyte abnormalities, particularly hypokalemia. Management is directed at correcting the underlying illness.

PVCs are commonly asymptomatic. Symptoms include palpitations, lightheadedness, weakness, and fatigue. They are often responsive to sympathetic stimulation, increasing with emotion or exertion. Palpitations are often perceived as a "thump" or strong beat from the sinus beat terminating a longer period of ventricular filling after the PVC (see Fig. 67.1E). When a PVC conducts retrogradely to the atrium, the atria contract against a closed tricuspid valve. These atrial pressure waves may elicit a vagal reflex sensation, similar to pacemaker syndrome.

Physical examination reveals pauses that are often compensatory and do not disturb the expected cadence of the pulse. Although the stroke volume of the PVC is often insufficient to produce a palpable pulse, premature heart sounds are commonly audible. Frequent PVCs may effectively produce bradycardia (see Fig. 67.1E). Cannon A waves may be present in the venous pulse when the atria contract during ventricular systole of the PVC.

Two consecutive PVCs are referred to as a PVC couplet (Fig. 67.4C). Three consecutive beats is a triplet. Nonsustained VT is defined as a run of consecutive ventricular beats persisting for 3 beats to 30 seconds (Fig. 67.5A). VT is also characterized by its QRS morphology. Monomorphic VT has the same QRS morphology from beat to beat (see Fig. 67.5A), consistent with a single origin for each beat. Polymorphic VT (see Figs. 67.4B and D and 67.5B) has a continually changing QRS morphology. The initial beats of a run of monomorphic VT may have a variable QRS morphology.

Clinical Features

PVCs occur in apparently healthy individuals but can also be a marker for underlying disease. PVC frequency is associated with mortality and

Management

The importance of PVCs depends on the clinical setting. Initial evaluation focuses on determining whether PVCs are an indication of underlying structural or electrical heart disease (Table 67.1). Symptoms of syncope, near syncope, anginal chest pain, and dyspnea warrant careful evaluation and can be due to episodes of ventricular tachycardia or other underlying heart disease. Physical examination focuses on signs of underlying heart disease. A 12-lead ECG of the arrhythmia should be obtained whenever possible to confirm the diagnosis and assess its likely origin, which is often a clue to underlying heart disease. Any ECG abnormality warrants further investigation including assessment of biventricular function for cardiomyopathies, and assessment for coronary artery disease in those at risk. Consideration of genetic ion channel abnormalities is also important (see Table 67.1).

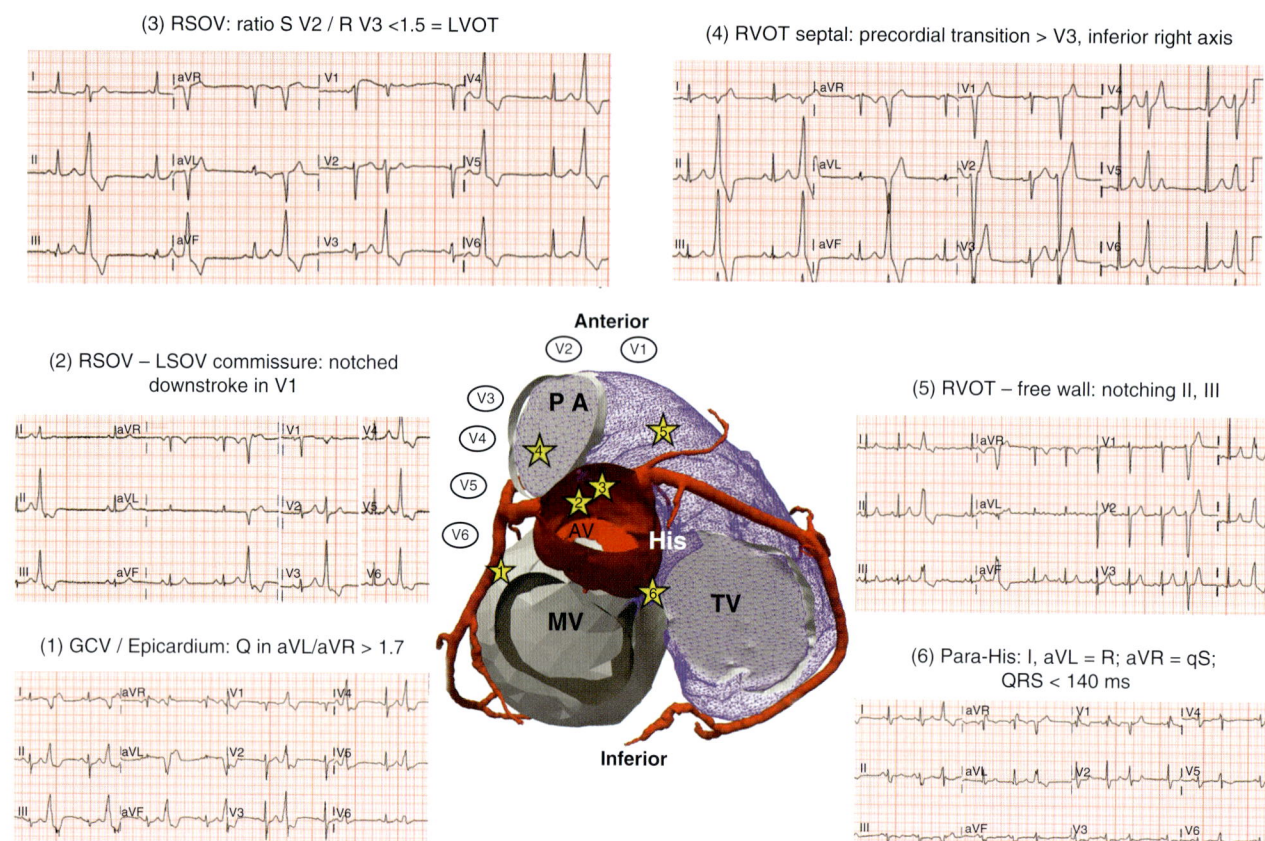

FIGURE 67.2 Premature ventricular complexes (PVCs) from the outflow tracts and tricuspid annulus. At the center, the heart is viewed from the base. Sites are indicated by stars with numbers corresponding to the ECG. Depolarization at the RVOT (sites 4, 5) and LVOT/Aorta (sites 2, 3) generates inferiorly directed ventricular activation producing dominant monophasic R waves in II, III, aVF. The RVOT and pulmonary artery sites are anterior to the aorta such that depolarization of the RVOT (sites 4 and 5) produces activation that moves away from the anterior chest wall, producing a qS or minimal initial r in V1, V2. Activation at the LVOT produces initial activation toward V1/V2 such that r/S ratio increases as the PVC originates from progressively more posterior sites (LSOV, GCV). The leftward aspect of the RVOT is left of the aorta, such that PVCs from this location can have a right inferior axis (site 4), whereas PVCs from the aortic valve ring (sites 2, 3) have a left inferior axis, as do PVCs from the rightward aspect of the RVOT and tricuspid annulus. Sites on the tricuspid annulus and those adjacent to the His bundle are lower than the RVOT, and have a more horizontal frontal plane axis. Distinguishing ECG features of these locations are noted. *GCV*, Great cardiac vein; *His*, His bundle; *LSOV*, left sinus of Valsalva; *LVOT*, left ventricular outflow tract; *MV*, mitral valve; *PA*, pulmonary artery; *RSOV*, right sinus of Valsalva; *RVOT*, right ventricular outflow tract; *TA*, tricuspid annulus; *TV*, tricuspid valve.

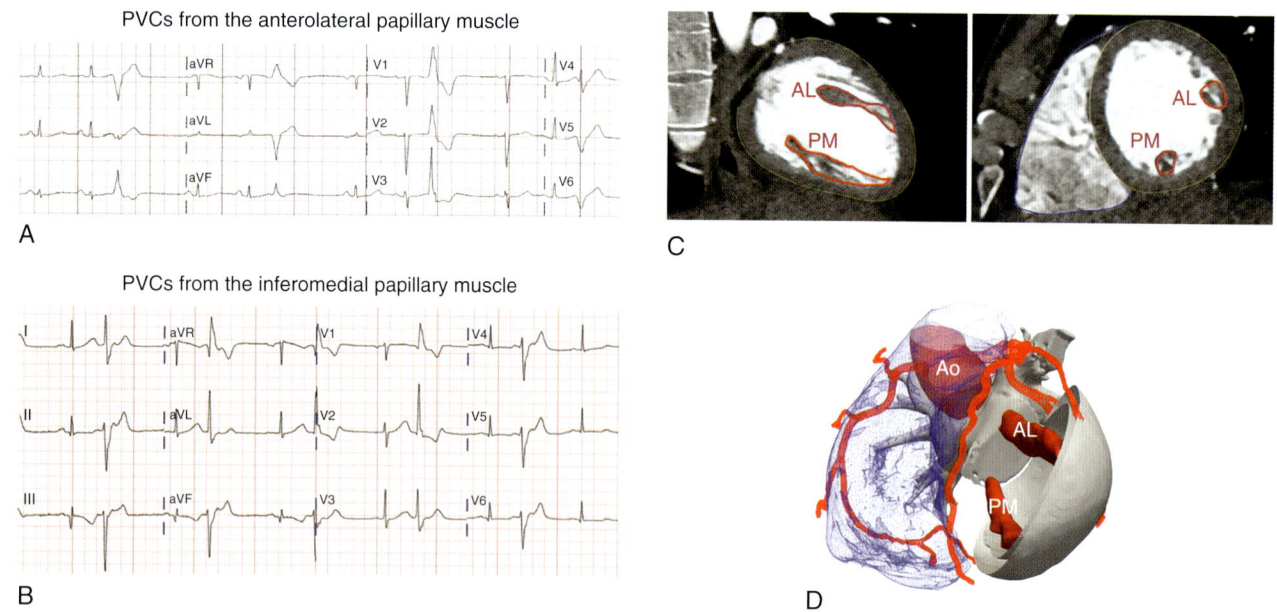

FIGURE 67.3 Premature ventricular complexes (PVCs) from the anterior lateral **(A)** and inferior medial **(B)** LV papillary muscles. The LV papillary muscles are mid-cavity structures and produce a right bundle branch block like-configuration with an rS configuration in leads V3, V4 and inferiorly directed axis (anterolateral) or superiorly directed axis (inferomedial papillary muscle). **C,** MR images of the LV with the papillary muscles in long axis *(left)* and short axis *(right)* views. **D,** Left anterior oblique view of the 3-dimensional reconstruction of the LV *(gray)* with overlying RV *(blue)*, aorta *(Ao)*, and coronary arteries *(red)*. The papillary muscles are shown in red. *AL*, Anterolateral papillary muscle; *PM*, posteromedial papillary muscle.

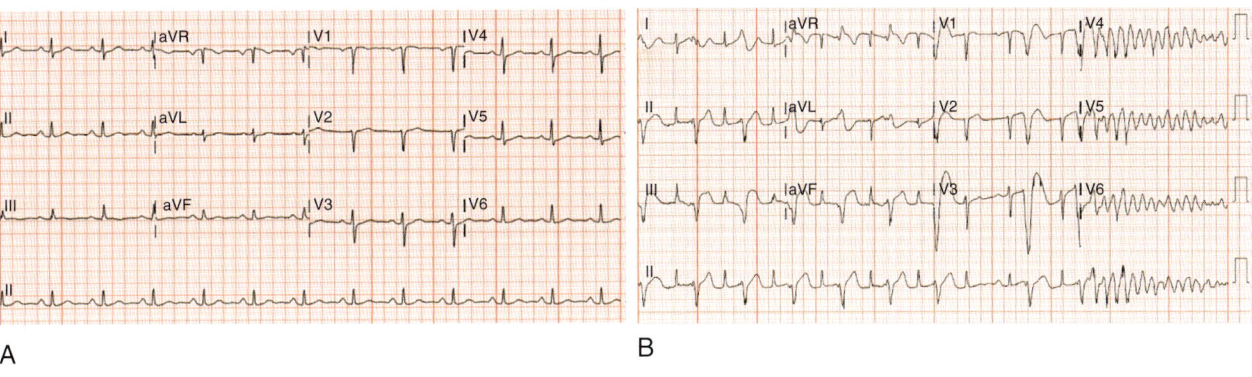
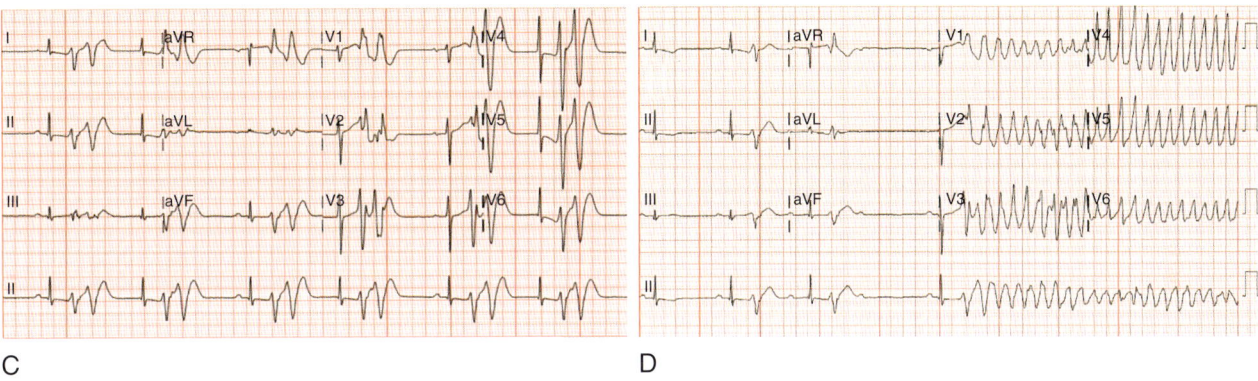

FIGURE 67.4 Polymorphic ventricular tachycardias (VTs). 12—lead ECG and continuous lead II are shown. **A** and **B,** ECGs from a patient with idiopathic VF. **A,** Normal ECG with normal repolarization, QT. **B,** Ventricular bigeminy with short coupled premature ventricular complexes interrupting the T-wave of the preceding sinus beat initiate polymorphic VT degenerating to ventricular fibrillation. **C** and **D,** During acute myocardial ischemia ventricular couplets with close coupling to the preceding sinus beat. **D,** Closely coupled PVCs are present and initiate polymorphic VT.

Idiopathic Premature Ventricular Complexes/NSVT with No Structural or Electrical Heart Disease

Idiopathic PVCs most often originate from a single site in the right or left ventricular outflow tracts, along the valve annuli, or from a papillary muscle (see Figs. 67.2 and 67.3). Multifocal PVCs are more often associated with underlying structural heart disease. In the absence of associated structural or electrical disease PVCs are benign. Some patients with idiopathic PVCs also have nonsustained or sustained VT from the same focus. Very rarely closely coupled PVCs that start near the peak of the T wave of the preceding sinus beat initiate rapid polymorphic VT/VF that causes cardiac arrest (see Fig. 67.4B).

Asymptomatic PVCs do not require therapy unless they are occurring with sufficient frequency to depress ventricular function. Symptoms often wax and wane over long periods of time and may resolve in over a third of patients.[7] Mild symptoms are often sufficiently managed by reassurance. Removal of provocative factors, such as caffeine, is reasonable. If treatment is required, chronic administration of a beta-blocker is a reasonable first therapy, particularly if PVCs are increased with activity or emotion. Efficacy is relatively low, but symptoms can be improved despite lack of a major impact on PVC frequency. Nondihydropyridine calcium channel blockers, verapamil or diltiazem, are sometimes effective. Class IC antiarrhythmic drugs flecainide and propafenone can also be effective. Amiodarone can be effective but is avoided due to long-term toxicities.

Catheter ablation should be considered when therapy is warranted and beta-blockers are ineffective or not desired, particularly when a single dominant PVC morphology is identified.[1] The likelihood of successful ablation depends on whether the PVCs are present at the time of the procedure to allow localization of its origin, and whether the focus is accessible. Success rates are greatest for the RV outflow tract, lower for papillary muscles and those that arise from the basal LV septum. A randomized trial found that catheter ablation effectively reduced RV outflow tract PVCs in 81% of patients and was more effective than chronic metoprolol or propafenone therapy.[8] Serious complications are uncommon but femoral bleeding, pseudoaneurysm, cardiac perforation, tamponade, coronary injury, and heart block can occur.

Premature Ventricular Complexes in Structural Heart Disease

In the absence of evidence that PVCs are depressing ventricular function, suppression of PVCs with antiarrhythmic medications has not generally been shown to improve outcomes. Treatment with the Class IC drug flecainide and the Class III drug D-sotalol increased mortality in post-infarct patients, possibly due to proarrhythmic effects.[1] PVCs that are symptomatic or sufficiently frequent to contribute to ventricular dysfunction warrant consideration of therapy. In patients with depressed ventricular function, amiodarone is a therapeutic option, but long-term toxicities are an important consideration (see Chapters 9 and 64). Catheter ablation can be considered if a dominant PVC morphology is present that can be targeted for ablation. During acute myocardial infarction, routine attempts to suppress PVCs with antiarrhythmic medications do not improve outcome and are not warranted. PVCs that trigger recurrent episodes of VF (see Fig. 67.4B) may respond to quinidine.[9]

Premature Ventricular Complex Induced Cardiomyopathy

Very frequent PVCs can cause reversible depression of ventricular function.[10-12] The mechanism is uncertain. Patients may be asymptomatic, or have fatigue, exertional limitation, or heart failure. Most have more than 15% PVCs as assessed from at least 24 hours of ambulatory recording, but PVC frequency during any 24-hour period can vary substantially and ventricular dysfunction has been seen in patients with

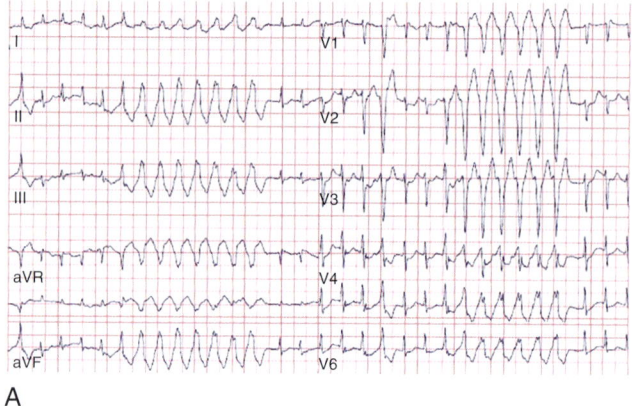
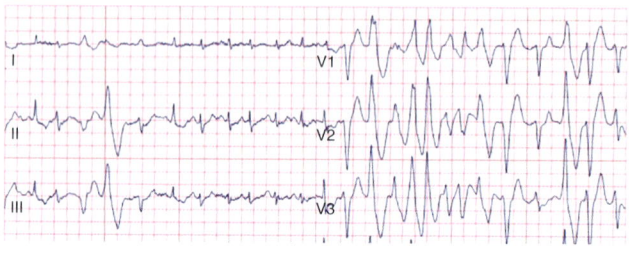
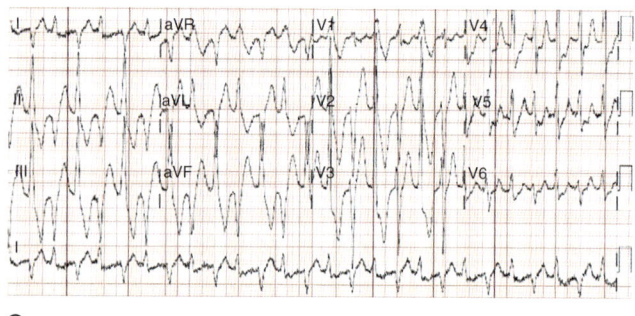

FIGURE 67.5 Exercise induced ventricular tachycardias. **A,** Nonsustained monomorphic ventricular tachycardias (VT) occurring in repetitive bursts. VT has a left bundle branch block configuration in V1 with transition after V3 and monophasic R waves in II, III, aVF consistent with origin in the RVOT. **B,** Polymorphic VT. **C,** Bidirectional ventricular tachycardia during exercise in a patient with catecholaminergic polymorphic VT.

only 5% PVCs during a single monitoring period. Multiday ECG monitoring may provide a better assessment of PVC burden.

When depressed ventricular function is encountered in a patient with frequent PVCs there are four major possibilities: (1) cardiac contractility may be normal, but the frequent PVCs are impairing measurement of ventricular function; (2) PVCs are depressing cardiac contractility; (3) an underlying cardiomyopathic process is present and causing the PVCs; and (4) An underlying cardiomyopathy is present and the PVCs are further depressing ventricular function. Sinus QRS duration greater than 130 msec, a PVC burden less than 17%, substantial LV dilation, multifocal PVCs, and areas of late gadolinium enhancement on MR imaging suggest underlying cardiomyopathy.[13] If PVCs are suspected to cause or contribute to cardiomyopathy, suppression of PVCs and reassessment of ventricular function is warranted. Beta-adrenergic blockers and amiodarone are the major pharmacologic options. Catheter ablation is recommended if there is a dominant PVC morphology that can be targeted and antiarrhythmic drug therapy is ineffective, not tolerated, or not preferred for long-term therapy.[1,14]

Patients who have frequent PVCs but normal ventricular function at presentation have a low risk of developing ventricular dysfunction. In a cohort of 100 subjects with greater than 5% PVCs/24 hours and normal LV ejection fraction followed for more than 4 years, PVCs spontaneously decreased to less than 1% in 44%, although they increased again in 9%.[7] Only 4% of patients developed LV ejection fraction less than 50%, all of whom had persistently frequent PVCs. Patients with very frequent PVCs and normal ventricular function warrant follow-up. Optimal risk assessment and surveillance is not defined but annual ambulatory recording and echocardiogram is reasonable for subjects with more than 15% to 20% PVCs.

In patients for whom cardiac resynchronization pacing has improved ventricular function, frequent PVCs can interfere with pacing and impair cardiac function, which may improve following PVC suppression.

ACCELERATED IDIOVENTRICULAR RHYTHM

Electrocardiographic Recognition

The ventricular rate is typically 60 to 100 beats/minute, often only slightly exceeding the sinus rate, producing interference AV dissociation (Fig. 67.6). Conduction of sinus beats to the ventricle producing fusion beats and capture beats is common. The mechanism is likely automaticity. This arrhythmia is usually seen in patients with structural heart disease, particularly during reperfusion of acute myocardial infarction and in myocarditis. It lasts for seconds to minutes and does not usually have an important hemodynamic effect.

Management

Suppressive therapy is rarely necessary but may be needed if loss of AV synchrony and acceleration of heart rate produces symptoms or a fall in blood pressure in a compromised patient. Accelerating the atrial rate with administration of atropine or atrial pacing can suppress the rhythm.

SUSTAINED VENTRICULAR TACHYCARDIA

Ventricular tachycardia can be due to reentry, triggered activity, or automaticity. The management and prognosis depend on the specific type of VT and underlying heart disease.

Monomorphic Ventricular Tachycardia
Electrocardiographic Recognition

Monomorphic VT is a wide QRS tachycardia that has the same QRS configuration from beat to beat indicating a stable ventricular depolarization sequence for each beat (Fig. 67.7). The QRS duration typically exceeds 120 msec, but is occasionally shorter for VTs originating in the septum or that utilize a portion of the Purkinje system. It is usually regular, but 20 msec variation in cycle length is not uncommon, and occasionally marked cycle length variation is encountered in the presence of antiarrhythmic medications, or at the onset and prior to spontaneous termination. Rates can range from slower than 100/min to faster than 270/min.

Monomorphic VT has to be distinguished from other causes of uniform wide QRS tachycardias including supraventricular tachycardia with bundle branch block aberrancy, supraventricular tachycardias conducted to the ventricles over an accessory pathway (preexcited tachycardias) (see Chapter 65), and rapid cardiac pacing if a pacemaker or implanted defibrillator is present. Rapid pacing is usually evident from pacing artifacts prior to the QRS. The rate will be at or below the maximum programmed pacing rate and the QRS morphology is the same as that during pacing at slow rates. Interrogation of the pacing device may be needed for confirmation. Preexcited tachycardias are uncommon, can be indistinguishable from monomorphic VT, and should be managed as monomorphic VT when the diagnosis is not certain.

TABLE 67.1 Etiologic Considerations

MONOMORPHIC VT	CARDIAC STRUCTURE	SINUS ECG	FH/GENETICS	VT FEATURES	USUAL INITIAL MANAGEMENT
Coronary disease	Old infarction	Abnormal	CAD+	Multiple morphologies	ICD
NICM	Fibrosis, often in the basal LV	Usually abnormal	40%—LMNA, TTN, PLM, desmosomal	Multiple morphologies	ICD
Post-viral	Fibrosis after healing			Lateral subepicardial LV origin most common	ICD
ARVC	RV fibrosis starts epicardial, LV involvement in some	Abnormal, PVCs	>60% desmosomal mutations	LBBB, multiple morphologies	ICD
Sarcoidosis	LV, RV fibrosis. + FDG PET if active inflammation	AV conduction impairment common, PVCs		RBBB or LBBB, endocardial and epicardial	ICD
Repaired TOF, VSD	Ventricular fibrosis, patch material	RBBB common		LBBB	Dependent on biventricular function
Idiopathic outflow VT	Normal	Normal, PVCs		Single monomorphic VT, PVCs often present	Beta-blocker
Idiopathic LV fascicular reentrant VT	Normal	Normal		Single RBBB monomorphic VT	Beta-blocker, verapamil
Polymorphic VT/VF					
Coronary disease	Acute ischemia	Abnormal	CAD+	Variable initiation	Reperfusion, CAD management
LV failure/hypertrophy from any cause	LVH, fibrosis, dilation	Abnormal			ICD
Acquired LQTS	Normal or any disease	QTc usually >0.48 sec, but can be short	Occasional	Pause dependent PMVT/torsade de pointes	Mg, removal of inciting factors
Idiopathic VF	Normal	Normal or early repolarization	Occasional	PMVT	ICD, quinidine, ablation
Congenital LQTS	Normal	QT prolongation, but variable	Mutations in ion channel genes	PMVT/torsade de pointes	Beta-blocker
Catecholaminergic polymorphic VT	Normal	Normal, PVCs on exertion	Mutation in RyR2, Calsequestrin	Exertion, stress induced polymorphic PVCs, VT	Beta-blocker, flecainide
Brugada syndrome	Normal	Normal or ST elevation V1—2	20%–30% SCN5A, others	Nocturnal cardiac arrest	ICD
Early repolarization	Normal, small epicardial scars?	J-point elevation	Occasional	PMVT/VF	ICD quinidine
Short QT syndrome	Normal	QTc <0.34 – 0.36s	Yes	AF, PMVT	ICD, quinidine

AF, atrial fibrillation; *ARVC*, arrhythmogenic right ventricular cardiomyopathy; *CAD*, coronary artery disease; *FDG PET*, fluorodeoxyglucose positron emission tomography; *FH*, family history; *ICD*, implantable cardioverter defibrillator; *LBBB*, left bundle branch block; *LMNA*, Lamin A/C; *LQTS*, long QT syndrome; *LVH*, left ventricular hypertrophy; *NCIM*, nonischemic cardiomyopathy; *NICM*, non-ischemic cardiomyopathy; *PMVT*, polymorphic ventricular tachycardia; *PVC*, premature ventricular contraction; *RBBB*, right bundle branch block; *RyR2*, type 2 ryanodine receptor; *SCN5A*, cardiac sodium channel gene; *TOF*, tetraology of Fallot; *TTN*, titin; *PLM*, phospholamban; *VSD*, ventricular septal defect.

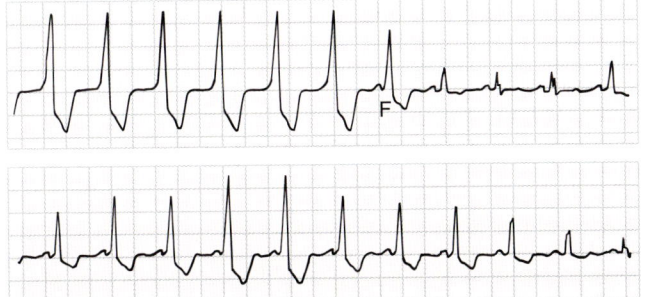

FIGURE 67.6 Accelerated idioventricular rhythm. In this continuous monitor lead recording, an accelerated idioventricular rhythm competes with the sinus rhythm. Wide QRS complexes at a rate of 110 beats/min fuse (F) with the sinus rhythm, which takes control briefly, generates the narrow QRS complexes, and then yields once again to the accelerated idioventricular rhythm as the P waves move "in and out" of the QRS complex. This example of isorhythmic AV dissociation may be caused by hemodynamic modulation of the sinus rate via the autonomic nervous system.

Ventricular Tachycardias Versus Supraventricular Tachycardia with Aberrancy

Sustained monomorphic VT is usually regular. The atrium is not involved in the tachycardia. The presence of dissociation between ventricular and atrial activity strongly favors VT over supraventricular tachycardia, the exception being junctional ectopic tachycardia with aberrancy, which is rare in adults, and some rare forms of AV nodal reentry (Chapter 65). Although P waves are often difficult to perceive, AV dissociation may be evident as subtle deflections superimposed on QRS and ST-T waves (Fig. 67.8). AV dissociation may be evident from the presence of fusion beats or capture beats. Vagotonic maneuvers or administration of adenosine may increase AV block exposing a supraventricular arrhythmia with aberration, or if 1:1 VA conduction is present in VT, may cause transient VA dissociation, confirming VT. It is important to recognize that a 1:1 relation between atrium and ventricle does not exclude VT because retrograde VA conduction may occur such that each QRS is followed by a retrograde p-wave. In many cases P-waves are difficult to discern and the relation between P-waves and QRS complexes cannot be determined with certainty.

Comparison of the QRS morphology during tachycardia with that during sinus rhythm can be helpful. The same wide QRS morphology during sinus rhythm and the tachycardia suggests supraventricular tachycardia with aberrancy; this can also occur, however, in patients with bundle branch reentry VT (see below). A number of QRS morphology criteria help distinguish VT from SVT with aberrancy (see

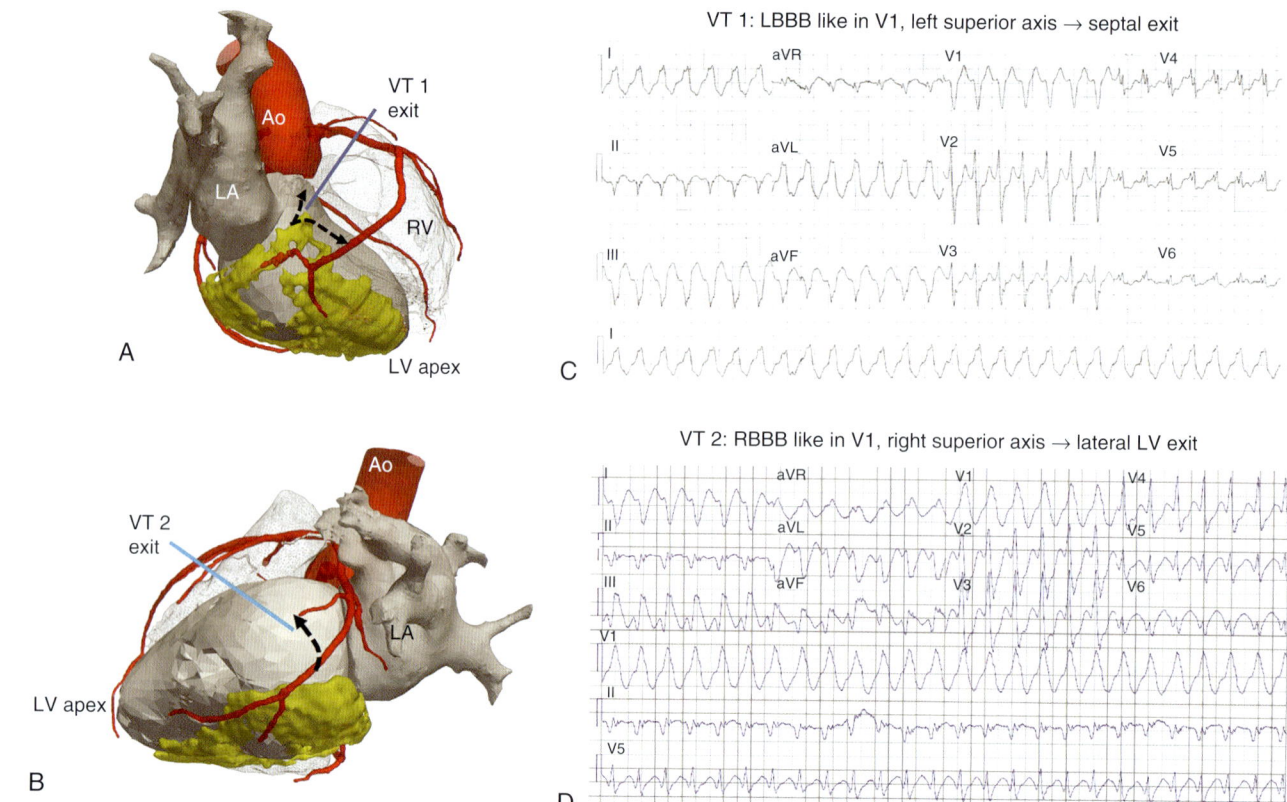

FIGURE 67.7 Sustained monomorphic ventricular tachycardias (VTs) from a patient with prior inferior myocardial infarction. Reconstructed images from segmented magnetic resonance and multidetector computed tomography imaging that shows the coronary arteries (**A,** right inferior projection; **B,** left lateral projection) demonstrate a large area of late gadolinium enhancement (LGE) in the LV consistent with a large inferior wall infarction (*yellow*). Two different VTs originated from this infarct. **C** and **D** show the 12-lead ECGs with a continuous lead I (**C**) or V1, II and V5 (**D**) at bottom. The VT morphologies are defined by the locations of the reentry circuit exits (black arrows) along the infarct margins. **C,** VT is LBBB-like in V1, consistent with a septal exit from a reentry circuit; with a superiorly directed axis, consistent with its location in the inferior LV. **D,** VT is RBBB-like in V1 with a dominant R, and axis directed rightward, consistent with activation preceding from a reentry circuit exit in the lateral wall scar margin. *Ao,* Aorta; *LA,* left atrium; *LV,* left ventricle; *LBBB,* left bundle branch block; *RV,* right ventricle.

Fig. 67.8). None are completely reliable, particularly in advanced heart disease, where the sinus rhythm QRS can be very abnormal. In structurally normal hearts, VTs that arise from the Purkinje system are more likely to fail to meet QRS criteria for VT.

Mechanisms and Clinical Correlations
Scar—Related Ventricular Tachycardia

The majority of sustained monomorphic VT associated with structural heart disease are due to reentry (Fig. 67.9) through regions of myocardial scar, consisting of fibrosis and surviving myocyte bundles. Diminished coupling between myocyte bundles and complex anatomic arrangement of the bundles contributes to slow conduction and facilitates conduction block needed for reentry. The slow conduction occurs during propagation through the scar, which is typically a small mass of myocardium that does not contribute to the surface ECG. The QRS is inscribed when the VT wavefront reaches the border of the scar and propagates across the ventricles. The QRS configuration reflects the "exit" of the reentry circuit from the scar (see Fig. 67.7). Hence the location of the scar can often be inferred from the VT QRS morphology, which is then an indication of the infarct or scar location. Cardiac imaging will often show the area of scar as a region of late gadolinium enhancement, absence of perfusion, or abnormal wall motion. Small areas of scar, however, particularly in the RV may escape detection with imaging. In the electrophysiology laboratory scars are evident as areas of low electrogram voltage due to replacement of myocardium by fibrosis (see Fig. 67.9A) and abnormal electrograms.

Scars causing VT are often able to support more than one reentry circuit. Hence, patients may have more than one QRS morphology of monomorphic VT (see Fig. 67.7). This is often seen when attempts to terminate VT by rapid pacing from an ICD initiates a new morphology of VT. Scar is a persistent electrophysiologic substrate such that episodes of VT may recur with variable frequency extending over years, often despite antiarrhythmic drug therapy.

Bundle Branch Reentry and Other Purkinje System—Related Ventricular Tachycardias

In the presence of disease of the Purkinje system and surrounding myocardium VT can be due to reentry circuits that utilize the bundle branches or fascicles. The VT has a QRS morphology consistent with activation of the ventricles from the Purkinje system, resembling bundle branch block. These VTs are uncommon, occurring in fewer than 10% of patients with recurrent VT referred for catheter ablation, but are important to recognize because they can mimic supraventricular tachycardia with aberrancy and most are well treated with ablation.

Bundle branch reentry is the most common form (Fig. 67.10). The circulating wavefront usually propagates down the right bundle branch, through the septum and up the left bundle branch to complete the circuit. VT has a typical LBBB configuration. Rarely the circuit revolves in the reverse direction giving rise to an RBBB configuration. The VT is often rapid, faster than 200/min. It is associated with disease of the Purkinje system and often with severe LV dysfunction. Most patients have an interventricular conduction delay or even a pattern of complete LBBB during sinus rhythm, despite the ability of the left bundle to sustain repetitive retrograde conduction during VT. Catheter ablation of the right bundle branch is curative, but anterograde His Purkinje conduction is often poor, warranting back-up bradycardia pacing. Most patients have other, scar-related VTs that warrant an ICD.

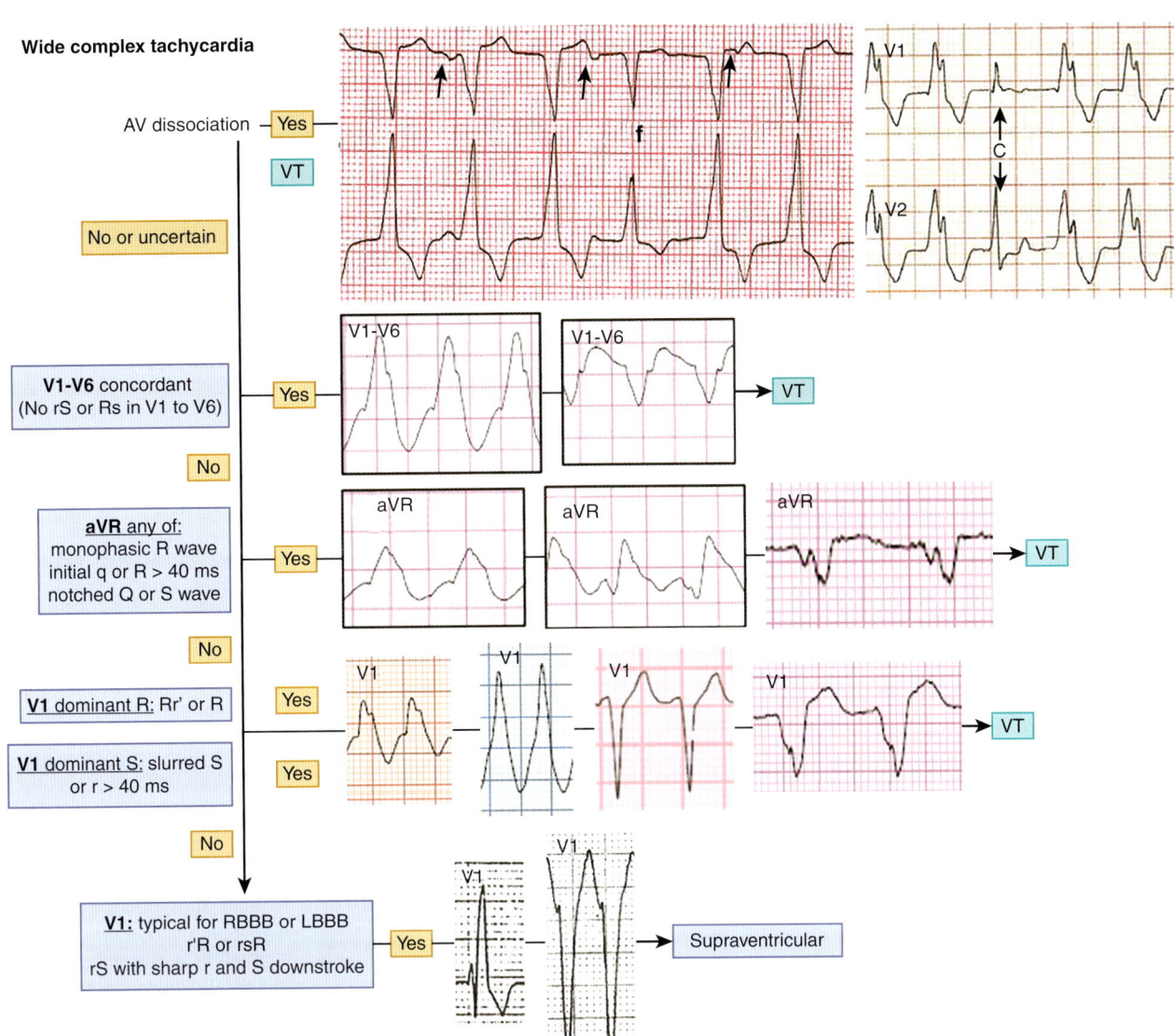

FIGURE 67.8 Flow diagram for distinguishing VT from SVT with aberrancy. Top ECG panels show AV dissociation *(arrows)* with a fusion beat (f) and capture beat (C). *LBBB,* Left bundle branch block; *RBBB,* right bundle branch block. (From Kindwall KE, Brown J, Josephson ME. Electrocardiographic criteria for ventricular tachycardia in wide complex left bundle branch block morphology tachycardias. *Am J Cardiol.* 1988;61:1279; Wellens HJ, Bär FW, Lie KI. The value of the electrocardiogram in the differential diagnosis of a tachycardia with a widened QRS complex. *Am J Med.* 1978;64:27; Brugada P, Brugada J, Mont L, et al. A new approach to the differential diagnosis of a regular tachycardia with a wide QRS complex. *Circulation.* 1991;83:1649; and Vereckei A, Duray G, Szénási G, et al. New algorithm using only lead aVR for differential diagnosis of wide QRS complex tachycardia. *Heart Rhythm.* 2008;5:89.)

The Purkinje system is also involved in idiopathic LV fascicular tachycardia that is due to reentry involving a portion of the LV Purkinje fascicles for part of the circuit (Fig. 67.11).

Automaticity in the Purkinje system can give rise to fascicular origin tachycardias that have a QRS morphology similar to supraventricular tachycardias with aberrancy.

Purkinje fibers can also be involved in rare malignant arrhythmias.[15] PVCs originating from the RV or LV Purkinje network can initiate rapid polymorphic VT in idiopathic VF. Multifocal ectopic Purkinje-related PVCs due to an *SCN5A* mutation can present with dilated cardiomyopathy that is responsive to arrhythmia suppression with quinidine or flecainide.[16]

Focal Origin Ventricular Tachycardias

VT can originate from a small focus of triggered activity or reentry. The mechanism can usually not be established with certainty. These are most often encountered in patients who do not have structural heart disease, often associated with PVCs of the same QRS morphology. Common locations of origin are in the outflow tracts (see Fig. 67.2), including sleeves of myocardium that extend along the aorta or pulmonary artery, along valve annuli and in the papillary muscles. The Purkinje system also gives rise to some focal tachycardias, particularly from the septum, papillary muscles, and occasionally in infarcts. Focal VTs tend to be enhanced by beta-adrenergic stimulation. The QRS morphology is an excellent guide to their location. Beta-blockers can be helpful and catheter ablation is usually an option when therapy is warranted.

Clinical Features

The clinical presentation of monomorphic VT varies depending on the rate and duration of the arrhythmia, underlying cardiac function, and autonomic adaptations in response to the arrhythmia. Patients may present with palpitations, dyspnea, chest pain, or may be asymptomatic. Rapid VT, faster than 200 beats/min, usually causes hypotension that may present as syncope, or cardiac arrest. VT can degenerate to VF, which may then be the initial rhythm detected by emergency medical responders; this is rare in patients without structural heart disease. Hemodynamic stability during the arrhythmia does not exclude VT.

Acute Management of Sustained Monomorphic Ventricular Tachycardia

Acute management of ongoing VT (Fig. 67.12) follows Advanced Cardiac Life Support guidelines. The patient should be immediately connected to an external defibrillator with ECG monitoring as hypotension

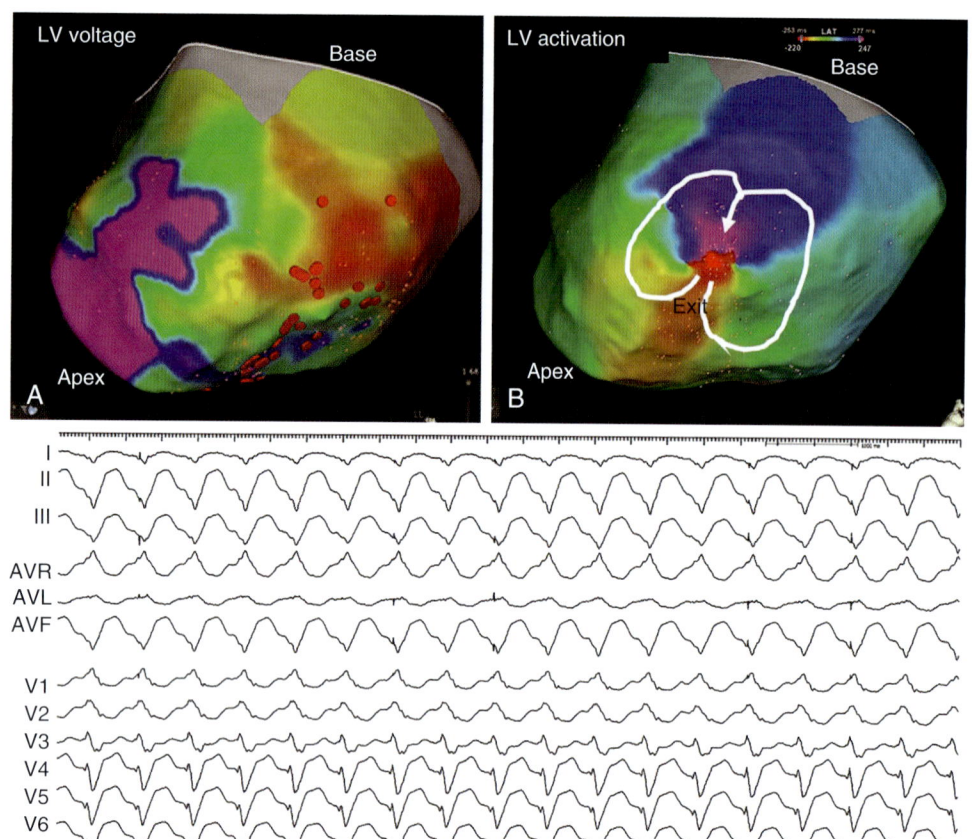

FIGURE 67.9 Nonischemic dilated cardiomyopathy with subepicardial scar-related ventricular tachycardias (VT). **A** and **B**, Maps of the epicardial LV viewed from the lateral aspect of the LV. **A**, Voltage map shows an extensive region of low voltage (*red, yellow, green, blue*) over the lateral LV from base to near the apex. **B** and **C** show one of the inducible VTs. In **B**, the activation emerges at the mid-lateral LV (*red*, and propagates clockwise and counterclockwise around the region, returning to the very low voltage region forming a figure-of-eight type of reentry circuit. **C**, ECG of the VT shows an RBBB-like superior rightward axis consistent with the reentry circuit exit in the inferolateral left ventricle. Dissociated atrial pacing spikes are also seen, indicating AV dissociation. The red dots in **A** are ablation sites for this VT, as well as others that were induced. *RBBB*, Right bundle branch block.

or degeneration to VF can occur at any time and may be precipitated by drug administration for attempted termination. QRS synchronous electrical cardioversion should be performed in case of impaired consciousness, hypotension, or pulmonary edema, after sedation if possible if the patient is conscious. For hemodynamically stable wide QRS tachycardia a 12-lead ECG should be obtained. If the diagnosis is uncertain, an intravenous bolus of adenosine may be administered during ECG monitoring, as this may transiently interrupt AV or VA conduction, clarifying the diagnosis. For acute pharmacologic termination, intravenous procainamide was more effective for termination than amiodarone in one trial.[17] Both are vasodilators that induce hypotension in up to 30% of patients. Procainamide should not be given to patients with end-stage renal disease due to the risks of accumulation of its metabolite n-acetylprocainamide that can cause QT prolongation and polymorphic VT. Intravenous lidocaine is less effective than amiodarone. Intravenous sotalol is available, but experience is limited.

If the patient is known to have an idiopathic VT without structural heart disease, acute management is dependent on the specific VT. Intravenous administration of beta-blockers can often terminate these VTs. If the diagnosis of idiopathic left ventricular fascicular reentrant tachycardia is certain, intravenous verapamil or diltiazem will usually terminate the arrhythmia. Administration of calcium channel blockers is contraindicated for acute management of other sustained VTs due to the risk of inducing hemodynamic instability.

Reversible conditions contributing to the initiation and perpetuation of VT should be sought and corrected including factors that increase sympathetic tone, often related to other acute illness, hypokalemia, hypoxia, and acidosis. Assessment for evidence of acute MI from ECG and cardiac biomarkers is appropriate, but acute MI is rarely a cause of sustained monomorphic VT. Elevations in cardiac enzymes are more likely to indicate injury secondary to hypotension and ischemia from the VT. Subsequent management is determined by the underlying heart disease and frequency of VT.

Electrical Storm

Sustained monomorphic VT usually occurs as an isolated episode. VT that occurs 3 or more times within 24 hours has been defined as an "electrical storm" and is associated with difficult to control VT and increased mortality.[18,19] Ongoing electrical storm with VT that recurs frequently after cardioversion or is incessant despite termination attempts is a life-threatening emergency. Precipitating factors, most commonly elevated sympathetic tone, should be addressed. Very wide sinusoidal tachycardia (see below) should prompt immediate consideration and treatment for hyperkalemia. Intravenous amiodarone and measures to reduce sympathetic tone should be initiated. The nonselective beta-blocker propranolol was more effective than metoprolol in one study, suggesting a role for potent nonselective beta-blockade.[20] Sedation escalating to general anesthesia is often effective. Other means of reducing cardiac sympathetic stimulation include percutaneous stellate ganglion block and high thoracic epidural anesthesia.[21] Patients with electrical storm from monomorphic VT often have a history of VT, have an ICD and are already receiving antiarrhythmic drugs. Assessment of appropriate ICD function and possible proarrhythmic effects from antiarrhythmic medications should be considered. If initial measures are ineffective, emergent catheter ablation should be considered.[1,14,22]

Evaluation and Long-Term Management

After the initial presentation of sustained VT, underlying heart disease should be characterized (see Table 67.1) and consideration given to therapy to reduce the risk of arrhythmia recurrence and sudden death. Most patients will be found to have an area of ventricular scar as the cause, most commonly prior myocardial infarction. The sinus rhythm ECG often suggests the possible underlying disease, with evidence of prior myocardial infarction, or abnormalities suggesting a cardiomyopathic process. An assessment of left and right ventricular function with echocardiography or cardiac MR imaging should be obtained. Evidence of scar or ventricular dysfunction that is not due to coronary artery disease warrants further investigation. Approximately 40% of nonischemic cardiomyopathies are genetic in origin and their detection has prognostic and family screening implications. Arrhythmogenic right ventricular cardiomyopathy (ARVC) and cardiac sarcoidosis (see below) are especially important considerations for patients with RV origin VTs. Other important causes include prior myocarditis, and ventricular scars from prior cardiac surgery, such as repaired tetralogy of

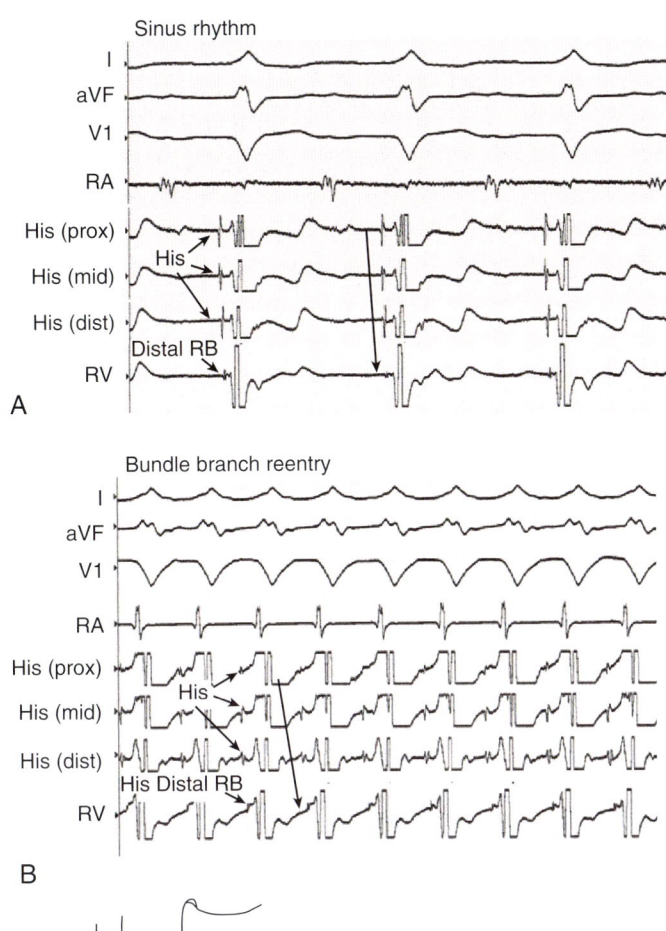

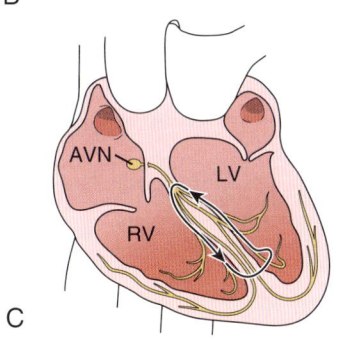

FIGURE 67.10 Surface and intracardiac recordings in a patient with inducible bundle branch reentry ventricular tachycardias. Catheter recording sites are labeled on the left. The His catheter is somewhat distal in its recording position, and the RV catheter is positioned in the right ventricle to record a distal right bundle potential. **A,** His bundle recordings and distal right bundle branch recording (on the RV catheter) during sinus rhythm. Notice that the right bundle potential (RB) is normally activated after the His bundle. **B,** Bundle branch reentry induced with the S_1-S_2. The distal His bundle and right bundle are activated anterogradely, and the H-V interval during bundle branch reentry is slightly longer than in sinus rhythm **(A). C,** Schematic of the reentry circuit. The circulating wavefront propagates down the right bundle branch, through the septum and up the left bundle branch to complete the circuit. *prox,* Proximal; *dist,* distal; *RA,* right atrium; *RV,* right ventricle.

Fallot. In the absence of structural heart disease VT is referred to as idiopathic.

Long-Term Therapy

Patients with scar-related sustained monomorphic VT are at risk for cardiac arrest from VT recurrence, which varies with the type and severity of the underlying disease. Placement of an ICD that will terminate VT should it recur is usually warranted provided the patient has a reasonable expectation for survival with acceptable quality of life for the next year and desires the protection of the ICD. ICDs reduce arrhythmic death in patients with depressed ventricular function who have had sustained hypotensive or syncopal VT that is not related to a reversible cause (secondary prevention), and also in patients who are at increased risk for a first episode of sustained VT (primary prevention of sudden death).[1,23]

ICDs terminate VT by antitachycardia pacing (ATP) or delivery of a cardioversion shock if ATP is not effective (Fig. 67.13), but do not prevent VT occurrences. Of patients who receive an ICD for primary or secondary prevention, 20% to 70% will have spontaneous VT terminated by the device within 3 years depending on the type of disease and presentation. The significance of the recurrences varies. Some are asymptomatic, terminated promptly by ATP, and infrequent such that additional therapy is not required. Others are symptomatic with syncope, or patients remain conscious and experience painful ICD shocks for VT termination. ICD shocks often cause post-traumatic stress disorder and even "mild" recurrences with palpitations and tachycardia termination by pacing may elicit substantial anxiety. VT recurrences are also associated with increased mortality over the following months for several potential reasons.[24] VT may be a marker for more severe disease and disease progression. VT episodes and ICD shocks may elicit detrimental increases in sympathetic tone and lead to implementation or escalation of therapies that have toxicities and potential adverse effects. Following a VT recurrence potential precipitating factors should be sought and addressed. The recurrence may be an indication of deteriorating cardiac function and warrant an assessment of heart failure therapies. Antiarrhythmic drug therapy or catheter ablation to prevent or reduce VT recurrences is often needed (Table 67.2).[25] Early catheter ablation after initial presentation does reduce future VT recurrences but has not been shown to reduce mortality and does expose patients who would not recur to procedure risks.[14,26] The risks and efficacy of catheter ablation varies with the underlying heart disease. Treatment is therefore individualized.

Idiopathic VT in the absence of structural heart disease rarely causes sudden death and an ICD is not usually warranted. Beta-adrenergic blockers or catheter ablation are often effective.

Specific Ventricular Tachycardias
Ischemic Cardiomyopathy

Sustained monomorphic VT may present any time after myocardial infarction, but often more than 10 years after the acute infarction. Remodeling of the infarct scar with fibrosis that promotes slow conduction is likely a factor in the late emergence of scar-related reentrant VT. Most patients have LV ejection fraction of less than 40%. Wide complex tachycardia, syncope, and cardiac arrest are common presentations. Multiple QRS morphologies of VT are common due to multiple potential reentry circuits within the infarct scar (see Fig. 67.7). The QRS morphology reflects the infarct scar location and its border zone with healthy myocardium. Inferior wall infarcts often give rise to VTs that have a superiorly directed frontal plane axis. Anteroseptal infarcts often give rise to LBBB-like VTs when the exit is on the septum and RBBB-like VTs when the VT exit is at the lateral infarct border. Myocardial ischemia is not required, and when present is more often secondary to hemodynamic consequences of VT, rather than primary. Myocardial revascularization does not adequately reduce the risk of recurrent VT.

An episode of sustained VT late after myocardial infarction usually warrants placement of an ICD (Chapters 69 and 70).[1] Recurrent VT terminated by the ICD is detected in up to 70% of patients over the following 2 to 3 years.[14,26] ICDs are also recommended for infarct survivors who are at risk for a first episode of VT based on LV ejection fraction of 35% or less with symptoms of heart failure or less than 30% even in the absence of symptoms provided that they are: (1) at least 40 days from acute infarction and (2) are more than 90 days from a revascularization procedure. These criteria were adopted after trials showed a mortality benefit in those groups. ICDs are also recommended for those with inducible sustained VT at electrophysiology study. ICDs have been shown to reduce mortality in both secondary and primary prevention patients.[1] This benefit, however, is limited for patients with serious comorbidities that limit survival and an ICD should not be implanted

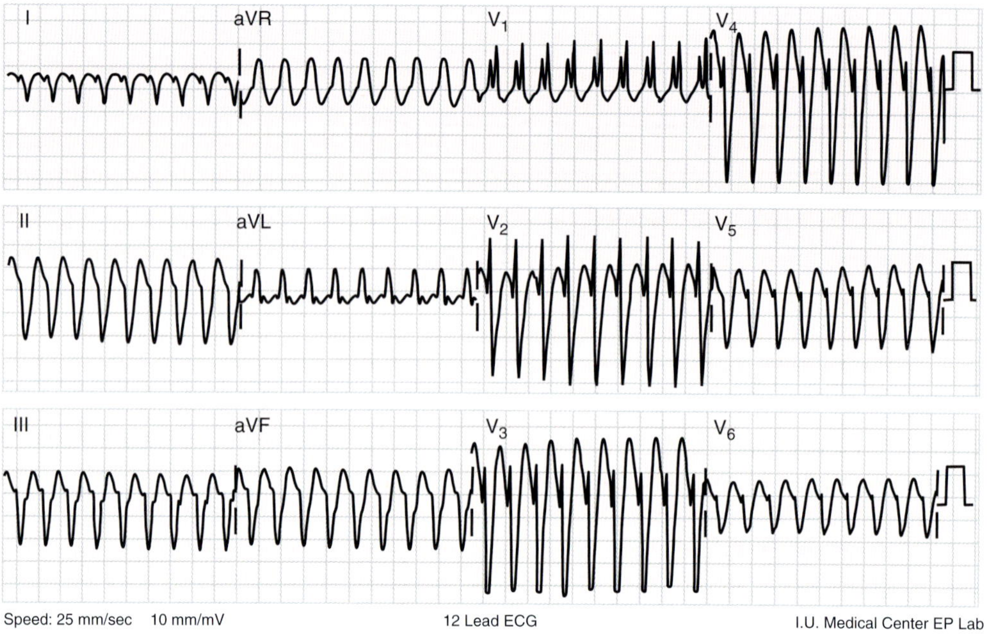

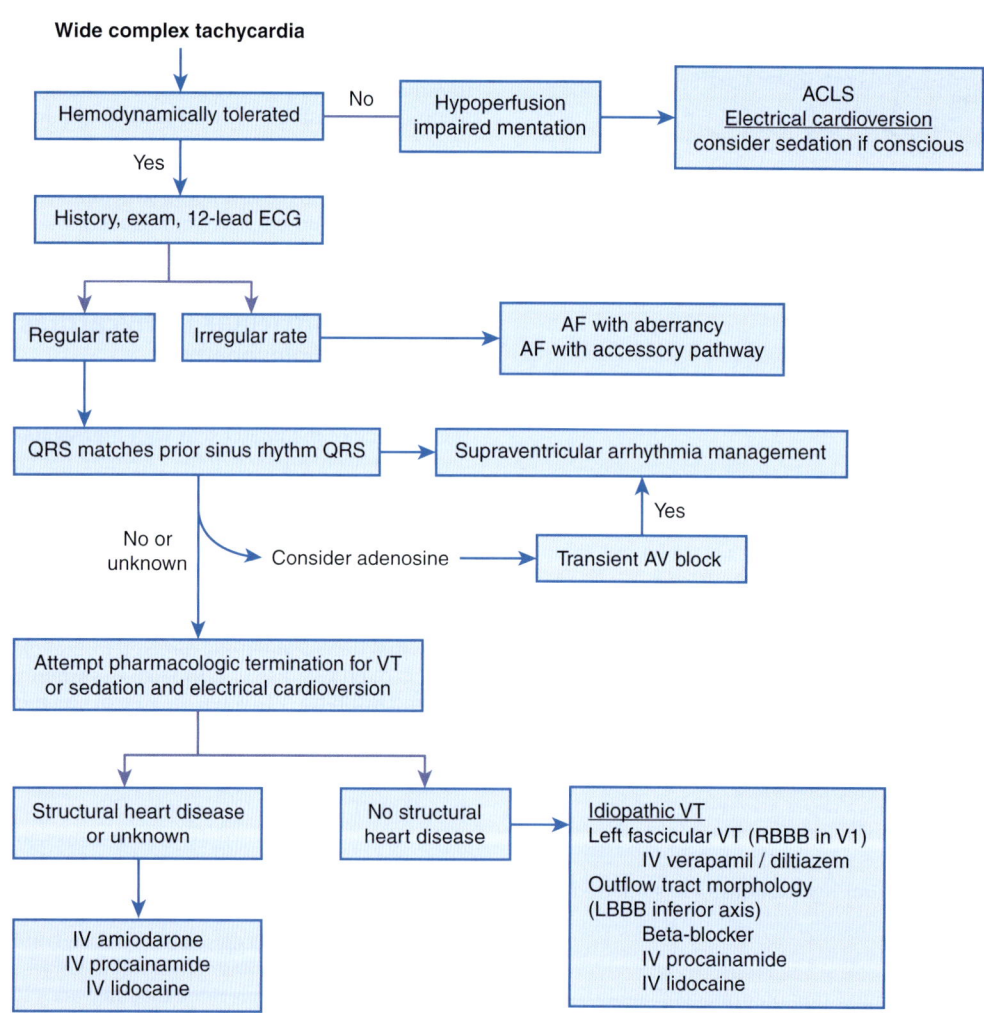

FIGURE 67.11 Left fascicular reentrant ventricular tachycardias. This tachycardia is characterized by a right bundle branch block contour with relatively narrow QRS, typically less than 150 msec. In this instance the axis was superior rightward, consistent with exit from a reentry circuit involving the posterior fascicles of the left bundle branch.

FIGURE 67.12 Management of the patient with a wide QRS tachycardia.

if the patient does not have a reasonable expectation for survival with acceptable quality of life over the following year.[23]

Over a third of patients will have recurrent VT which often warrants treatment with medications or catheter ablation to reduce recurrences (see Table 67.2). Amiodarone is more effective than sotalol for VT prevention, but long-term toxicities are of concern.[27] If VT recurs despite amiodarone, outcomes with catheter ablation are more favorable than escalating drug therapy by increasing amiodarone dose or adding mexiletine to amiodarone.[25] During the catheter ablation the infarct containing the VT substrate is usually identifiable as a region of low voltage, abnormal

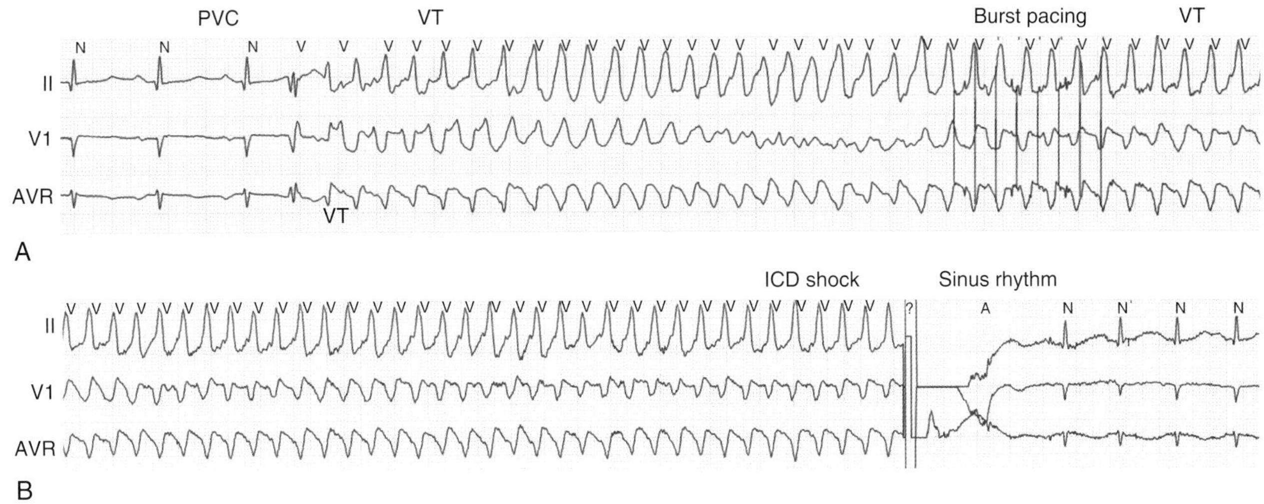

FIGURE 67.13 ICD treatment of ventricular tachycardias (VT). **A,** Initiation of sustained polymorphic VT by a premature ventricular complex is followed by burst pacing from an implanted defibrillation, which fails to terminate the VT, although the QRS becomes more organized. **B,** VT continues and the ICD delivers a shock that converts the rhythm to sinus.

electrograms that can be targeted for ablation without necessarily needing to induce VT.[14] Catheter ablation abolishes VT in about 50% of patients, and reduces the frequency of recurrences in an additional 20% to 30%.[25,28] Procedure-related mortality is 1% to 3% with patients who have severe ventricular dysfunction and comorbidities at greatest risk.[14] Complications occur in 5% to 8%, most commonly femoral bleeding, but stroke, tamponade, and vascular injury can occur. Recurrent VT after catheter ablation is a marker for increased long-term mortality.[28]

Nonischemic Dilated Cardiomyopathy

Areas of late gadolinium enhancement consistent with ventricular scar are detected by cardiac MR imaging in approximately a third of patients with nonischemic dilated cardiomyopathy (NICM) and are associated with increased risk of sudden death. A genetic mutation is identifiable in approximately 40% of patients and is associated with worse long-term mortality, occurrence of VT, and sudden death than those without an identifiable genetic cause of cardiomyopathy.[29] Sustained monomorphic VT occurs in approximately 2% to 3% of patients per year, and polymorphic VT/VF occurs with similar frequency.[29] Sustained monomorphic VT is most commonly due to reentry in regions of scar often near the base of the heart (Figs. 67.9 and 67.14).[30]

Presentation and management are similar to that for VT in ischemic heart disease.[1] An ICD is usually warranted and is also recommended for patients who have had syncope that could be due to VT. Primary prevention ICDs are also recommended for patients who have LV ejection fraction of 35% or less despite medical therapy for ventricular dysfunction and for patients with high-risk genetic cardiomyopathies, including many with lamin A/C mutations.[1,31,32] The benefit of ICDs is greater in patients younger than 60 years of age and is limited in older patients who have other diseases likely to limit survival.

Recurrent episodes of VT requiring suppressive therapy are treated with antiarrhythmic drug therapy or catheter ablation. Catheter ablation is less often successful in NICM compared to coronary disease.[33,34] The VT substrate can be intramural and epicardial (see Fig. 67.9) and more difficult to approach with catheter ablation. Percutaneous pericardial access is more often required to address subepicardial substrate and is associated with a greater risk of bleeding compared to endocardial ablation.[35] Heart block from ablation of VT originating from the basal septum can occur and warrants biventricular pacing.[36]

Arrhythmogenic Right Ventricular Cardiomyopathy

ARVC is an inherited disorder characterized by fibrofatty replacement of the right ventricular free wall that typically extends from the tricuspid annulus and RV outflow region toward the apex creating the substrate for PVCs and sustained monomorphic VT and less commonly polymorphic VT/VF. Other regions of the RV and LV can also be involved. Approximately half of the patients have an identifiable mutation involving a desmosomal protein, most commonly plakophilin-2, desmoplakin, and desmoglein, followed by other desmosomal and non-desmosomal proteins. Inheritance is autosomal dominant for most. Approximately half of patients have a family history of sudden death. LV involvement is not uncommon and may predominate, which has led to use of the term arrhythmogenic cardiomyopathy (AMC). Patients present with palpitations, syncope, or cardiac arrest most commonly in their third or fourth decade. Penetrance is quite variable. Prolonged chronic exercise increases the disease expression and progression and athletes are likely to present earlier than less active individuals. A common presentation is sustained monomorphic VT with an LBBB configuration in V1 (Fig. 67.15). The distinction of ARVC, which has a risk of sudden death from idiopathic VT, which is benign, is extremely important and can be difficult. Task force criteria have been developed for establishing the diagnosis.[37] Both ARVC and idiopathic VT can cause RVOT origin VTs that have an LBBB inferior axis VT. LBBB VT with a superior axis or multiple VTs favors ARVC. The sinus rhythm ECG is normal in idiopathic VT, but commonly shows T wave inversions in V1 to V3 or beyond, which is abnormal in individuals older than 14 years of age (see Fig. 67.15B). A prolonged terminal activation duration (nadir of the S wave to QRS offset >55 msec in V1), or less commonly epsilon waves are found in ARVC. Early in the course of ARVC cardiac imaging may be normal, but more commonly echocardiography shows some degree of RV enlargement. Cardiac MRI may show RV enlargement and areas of late gadolinium enhancement in ARVC. Electrophysiology study can be helpful. Multiple morphologies of inducible VT and isoproterenol induced multiple morphologies of PVCs are common in ARVC and rare in idiopathic VT. RV epicardial and endocardial mapping reveals areas of low amplitude abnormal electrograms in ARVC that are rare in idiopathic VT.[38] Cardiac sarcoid can be indistinguishable from ARVC, sometimes only identified at heart transplantation. AV conduction delay, evidence of septal scar, and evidence of extracardiac sarcoidosis favor sarcoid as the diagnosis (see Fig. 67.15D).

Arrhythmias are commonly provoked by exertion. Chronic therapy with a beta-blocker is recommended.[1] An ICD is recommended for those who have had sustained arrhythmias, syncope, or RV or LV dysfunction with ejection fraction of 35% or less, and is considered for patients with less severe manifestations of disease because the initial symptomatic event can be sudden death. With avoidance of exercise unaffected gene carriers appear to have an excellent outcome without therapy. If VT recurrences require suppression, sotalol, amiodarone, and

TABLE 67.2 Clinical Trials on Treatment to Reduce Ventricular Tachycardia Recurrences in Patients with ICDs

STUDY	PATIENT INCLUSION	ENDPOINTS	TREATMENT ARMS	KEY RESULTS
Antiarrhythmic Drug Trials				
RAID (Zareba 2018)	ICD for primary or secondary prevention. 54% CAD. N = 1012	Death + VT/VF	Ranolazine / Placebo	No difference in primary outcome
OPTIC (Connolly 2006)	VT or VF receiving an ICD. 80% prior MI. N = 412	ICD shock for any reason	Randomized to BB, sotalol, or amiodarone + BB	Annual rate of VT treated with ATP or shocks: Amiodarone + BB most effective 13% vs. 39% for sotalol and 45% for BB. Adverse thyroid and pulmonary effects more common with amiodarone
ALPHEE (Kowey 2011)	ICD and VT/VF. 75% CAD	Sudden death or appropriate ICD therapy	Amiodarone / Placebo	Amiodarone improved primary endpoint: 45.3% vs. 61.5%
(Pacifico 1999)	ICD for VT/VF. 70% CAD	Death or ICD shock	Sotalol / Placebo	Improved freedom from death or ICD shock in sotalol group (66% vs. 46% at 1 year)
CASCADE substudy (Dolack 1994)	VF out of hospital, CAD, ICD. N = 88	ICD shocks	Amiodarone / Other AADs	Improved 2 years free survival without ICD shocks for amiodarone vs. other AADs; 77% vs. 42%
Kettering 2002	ICD	VT/VF recurrence	Sotalol / Metoprolol	VT/VF recurred in 63% of pts with no difference between groups
QUIDAM (Andorin 2017)	Brugada syndrome	Appropriate ICD shock	Hydroquinidine / Placebo / 18 months crossover. 50 patients total	2 VF events during placebo treatment. No VF during hydroquinidine treatment, but stopped for side effects in 26%
Catheter Ablation Trials				
VANISH (Sapp 2016)	CAD with SMVT despite AAD therapy. N = 259	Death, VT Storm or ICD shock	CA / Escalation of AAD	CA Improved outcome overall (59.1% vs. 68.5%); In subanalysis CA similar to switching from sotalol to amiodarone; CA superior to escalating amiodarone
SMS (Kuch 2017)	Unstable VT or cardiac arrest. CAD. LVEF ≤40%. N = 111	Time to first recurrence VT/VF	CA before ICD implant / ICD implant with no CA	No difference with recurrent VT in 49% vs. 52.4% at 2 years
VTACH (Kuch 2010)	Hemodynamically tolerated SMVT. CAD. LVEF ≤50%. N = 107	Time to first recurrence VT/VF	CA / No CA	CA prolonged time to recurrent VT to 18.6 months vs. 5.6 months
BERLIN VT (Willems 2020)	SMVT, CAD. LVEF 30%–50%. N = 159	Death or unplanned hospitalization	CA / No CA	Terminated for futility. Trends for CA to reduce VT but with more hospitalizations
SMASH-VT (Reddy 2017)	ICD for unstable VT/VF syncope. CAD. N = 128	Survival free from appropriate ICD therapy	CA / No CA	CA reduced ICD therapy to 12% vs. 33%
CALYPSO (AL-Khatib)	CAD with SMVT despite AAD	Feasibility	Ablation / AAD	27 enrolled of 243 screened

AAD, Antiarrhythmic drug; *ATP,* antitachycardia pacing; *BB,* beta blocker; *CA,* catheter ablation; *ICD,* implantable cardioverter defibrillator; *SMVT,* sustained monomorphic VT.

Zareba W, Daubert JP, Beck CA, et al. Ranolazine in high-risk patients with implanted cardioverter-defibrillators: the RAID Trial. *J Am Coll Cardiol.* 2018;72:636–645.

Connolly SJ, Dorian P, Roberts RS, et al. Comparison of beta-blockers, amiodarone plus beta-blockers, or sotalol for prevention of shocks from implantable cardioverter defibrillators: the OPTIC Study: a randomized trial. *JAMA.* 2006;295:165–171.

Kowey PR, Crijns HJ, Aliot EM, et al. Efficacy and safety of celivarone, with amiodarone as calibrator, in patients with an implantable cardioverter-defibrillator for prevention of implantable cardioverter-defibrillator interventions or death: the ALPHEE study. *Circulation.* 2011;124:2649–2660.

Continued

Pacifico A, Hohnloser SH, Williams JH, et al. Prevention of implantable-defibrillator shocks by treatment with sotalol. d,l-Sotalol Implantable Cardioverter-Defibrillator Study Group. *N Engl J Med.* 1999;340:1855–1862.

Dolack GL. Clinical predictors of implantable cardioverter-defibrillator shocks (results of the CASCADE trial). Cardiac Arrest in Seattle, Conventional versus Amiodarone Drug Evaluation. *Am J Cardiol.* 1994;73:237–241.

Kettering K, Mewis C, Dornberger V, et al. Efficacy of metoprolol and sotalol in the prevention of recurrences of sustained ventricular tachyarrhythmias in patients with an implantable cardioverter defibrillator. *Pacing Clin Electrophysiol.* 2002;25:1571–1576.

Andorin A, Gourraud JB, Mansourati J, et al. The QUIDAM study: Hydroquinidine therapy for the management of Brugada syndrome patients at high arrhythmic risk. *Heart Rhythm.* 2017;14:1147–1154.

Sapp JL, Wells GA, Parkash R, et al. Ventricular tachycardia ablation versus escalation of antiarrhythmic drugs. *N Engl J Med.* 2016;375:111–121.

Kuck KH, Tilz RR, Deneke T, et al. Impact of substrate modification by catheter ablation on implantable cardioverter-defibrillator interventions in patients with unstable ventricular arrhythmias and coronary artery disease: results from the multicenter randomized controlled SMS (Substrate Modification Study). *Circ Arrhythm Electrophysiol.* 2017;10:e004422.

Kuck KH, Schaumann A, Eckardt L, et al. Catheter ablation of stable ventricular tachycardia before defibrillator implantation in patients with coronary heart disease (VTACH): a multicentre randomised controlled trial. *Lancet.* 2010;375:31–40.

Willems S, Tilz RR, Steven D, et al. Preventive or deferred ablation of ventricular tachycardia in patients with ischemic cardiomyopathy and implantable defibrillator (BERLIN VT): a multicenter randomized trial. *Circulation.* 2020;141:1057–1067.

Reddy VY, Reynolds MR, Neuzil P, et al. Prophylactic catheter ablation for the prevention of defibrillator therapy. *N Engl J Med.* 2007;357:2657–2665.

Al-Khatib SM, Daubert JP, Anstrom KJ, et al. Catheter ablation for ventricular tachycardia in patients with an implantable cardioverter defibrillator (CALYPSO) pilot trial. *J Cardiovasc Electrophysiol.* 2015;26:151–157.

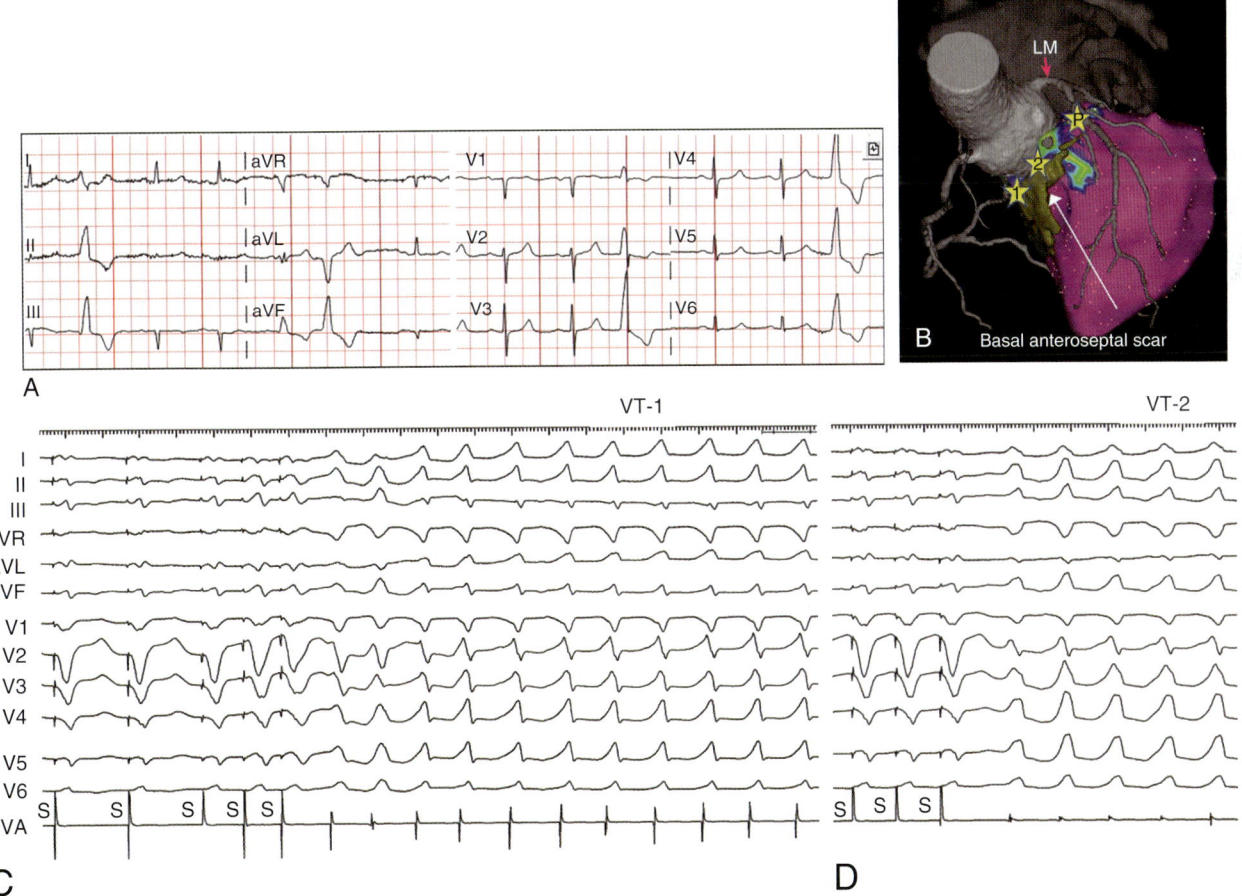

FIGURE 67.14 Arrhythmias in a patient with genetic cardiomyopathy due to a titin (*TTN*) mutation. Frequent PVCs were recognized as a young adult. Several decades later the patient presented with syncope due to ventricular tachycardias (VT) and LV ejection fraction of approximately 40%. **A,** Resting ECG shows sinus rhythm with unifocal PVCs that have an RBBB inferior right axis configuration and dominant R waves from V3 to V6 consistent with activation from a focus at the aortic mitral continuity area (site *P* in **B**). **B,** The voltage map of the LV merged with CT scan and the segmented magnetic resonance–derived scar (in *yellow*) is viewed from the superior aspect. An area of low voltage (*red, green*) consistent with scar is present at the basal LV septum. Purple is greater than 1.5 mV. Ablation areas for the PVCs (site *P*) and VTs (sites *1* and *2*) are shown (*stars*). **C,** During programmed stimulation two extrastimuli following a pacing train at 150 beats/min (*S*) induced sustained monomorphic VT that has a left bundle branch block configuration in V1, dominant R in V2 and axis of + 30 degrees, consistent with activation from site 1 at the LV basal septum. **D,** A burst of rapid pacing was performed during VT-1 (last three stimuli shown) converted VT-1 to VT-2 that has an axis of + 60 degrees, consistent with an exit at site 2. Multiple monomorphic VTs are common in scar-related VT.

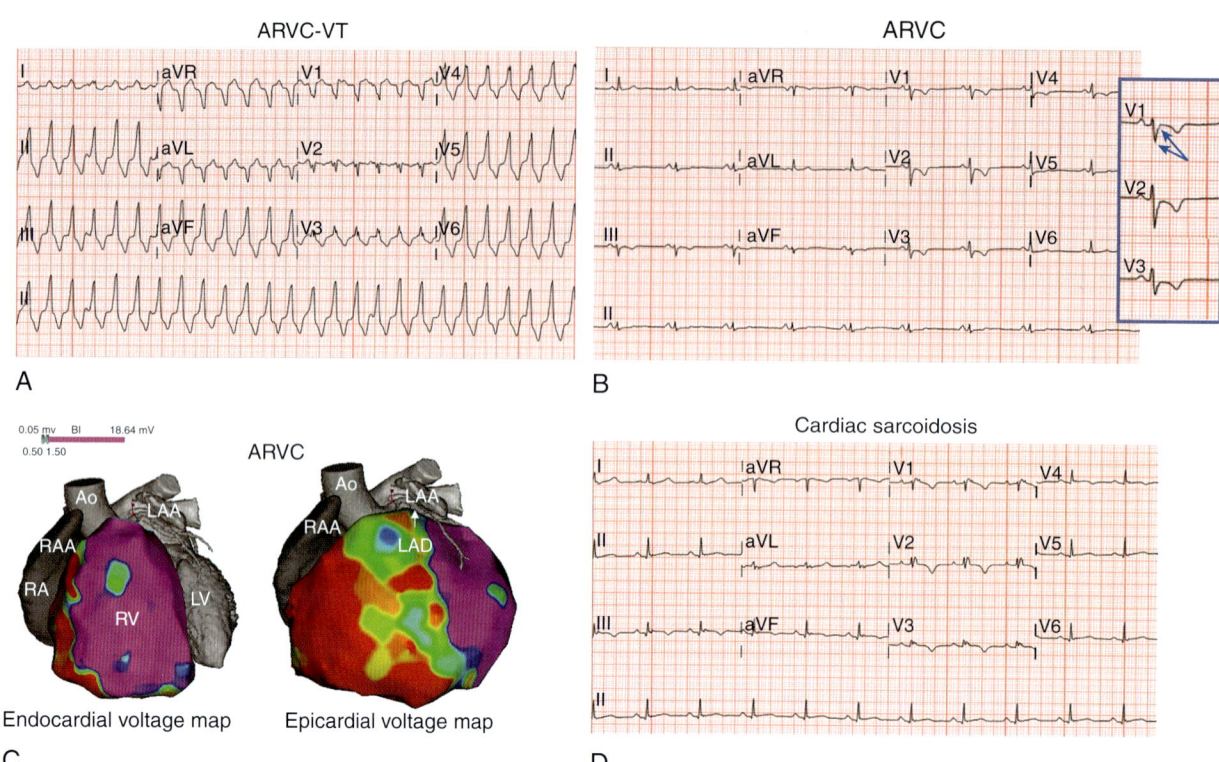

FIGURE 67.15 Arrhythmogenic RV cardiomyopathy (ARVC) (**A** to **C**) can be mimicked by sarcoidosis (**D**). **A,** sustained monomorphic VT has a left bundle branch block–like configuration in V1 and inferior axis consistent with an RVOT origin. **B,** Following conversion to sinus rhythm the ECG shows T wave inversions in V1 to V4 with a delayed S nadir to J point in V1 of greater than 50 msec consistent with an RV abnormality (arrows in enlargement at right). **C** and **D** Bipolar voltage maps viewed from an anterior projection. The endocardial bipolar voltage map (left) shows a small area of low voltage (red) along the tricuspid annulus. The epicardial voltage map (right) shows extensive low voltage (red, yellow, green) over the entire free wall of the RV. **D,** A 12-lead ECG from a patient with sarcoidosis involving the RV. T wave inversions in V1–V3 can occur in ARVC or sarcoidosis. PR interval prolongation (>0.2 s) favors sarcoidosis over ARVC.

flecainide have been used. Catheter ablation, which often requires an epicardial approach, reduces episodes.[14]

Congenital Heart Disease

The incidence of serious ventricular arrhythmias in the population of adults with congenital heart disease (CHD) is relatively low (<0.1% per year).[39,40] Approximately 10% of deaths, however, are sudden. The risk varies with the specific lesion and increases with severity of heart disease. In patients with progressive failure of the systemic or subpulmonary ventricle polymorphic VT and VF can occur independent of surgical scars. In contrast, sustained monomorphic VT is usually due to reentry facilitated by scar areas that are often associated with prior surgical repair, most commonly in tetralogy of Fallot (Fig. 67.16).[41–43] The substrate for these often-fast VTs has been well characterized. Areas of dense fibrosis owing to surgical incisions, patch material, and the valve annuli form regions of conduction block that define reentry circuit borders and create anatomically defined isthmuses with slow conduction that allow macroreentrant VTs. These isthmuses can be identified during stable rhythm and be ablated with very low rates of VT recurrence if conduction block in the isthmus can be achieved. Catheter ablation is generally considered an adjunct to an ICD, but has been used as an alternative to an ICD in selected patients.[41] VT may be associated with pulmonary regurgitation and RV enlargement late after repair such that percutaneous or surgical pulmonary valve replacement is warranted. It is important to consider ablation for VT prior to or combined with these procedures as placement of a valved conduit does not abolish VT and may prevent future access to the isthmus causing VT.

Hypertrophic Cardiomyopathy

Sudden death occurs at a rate of 1% per year in patients with genetic hypertrophic cardiomyopathy (Chapter 54).[1] Polymorphic VT (PMVT) and VF are the most common rhythms identified at sudden death. These can be precipitated by rapid rates during sinus tachycardia or atrial fibrillation. Ventricular myocyte disarray, interstitial fibrosis, and susceptibility to myocardial ischemia are likely arrhythmogenic factors. Sustained monomorphic VT is uncommon but can occur due to scar-related reentry, most commonly in patients who have a fibrotic apical aneurysm, which occurs in fewer than 5% of patients.[44,45] An ICD is recommended for survivors of cardiac arrest or sustained VT, or who have had recent unexplained syncope or other markers of sudden death risk (Chapter 70). Nonsustained VT occurs in 20% to 30% of patients on ambulatory monitoring and its relation to risk of sudden death remains controversial, although it is associated with increased risk of spontaneous VT in patients who have received an ICD.[46] Symptomatic PVCs and recurrent VT may respond to therapy with beta-blockers or amiodarone. Catheter ablation can be successful for scar-related sustained monomorphic VT.

Inflammatory Heart Disease
Cardiac Sarcoidosis

Sarcoidosis is characterized by noncaseating granulomas that can involve any organ.[47] Cardiac involvement can cause atrial and ventricular arrhythmias, heart block, and heart failure. VT is the presenting event in one-third of patients.[48] The granulomas heal, leaving areas of fibrosis that can be the substrate for scar-related reentrant sustained monomorphic VT that persists after active inflammation resolves. Purkinje-related arrhythmias also occur. Ventricular scar can occur anywhere in the left or right ventricles. When involvement is confined to the right ventricle the clinical findings can be indistinguishable from arrhythmogenic RV cardiomyopathy.

Cardiac sarcoidosis should be suspected for any patient presenting with ventricular arrhythmias associated with areas of unexplained ventricular scar, but establishing the diagnosis is often difficult. Biopsy of involved noncardiac tissue should be obtained if identified. If involvement is confined to the heart, cardiac biopsy is an option but is unrevealing in the majority of cases due to the often patchy nature of cardiac involvement. Cardiac positron emission tomography with fluorodeoxyglucose (FDG-PET) after a carbohydrate-free diet is helpful

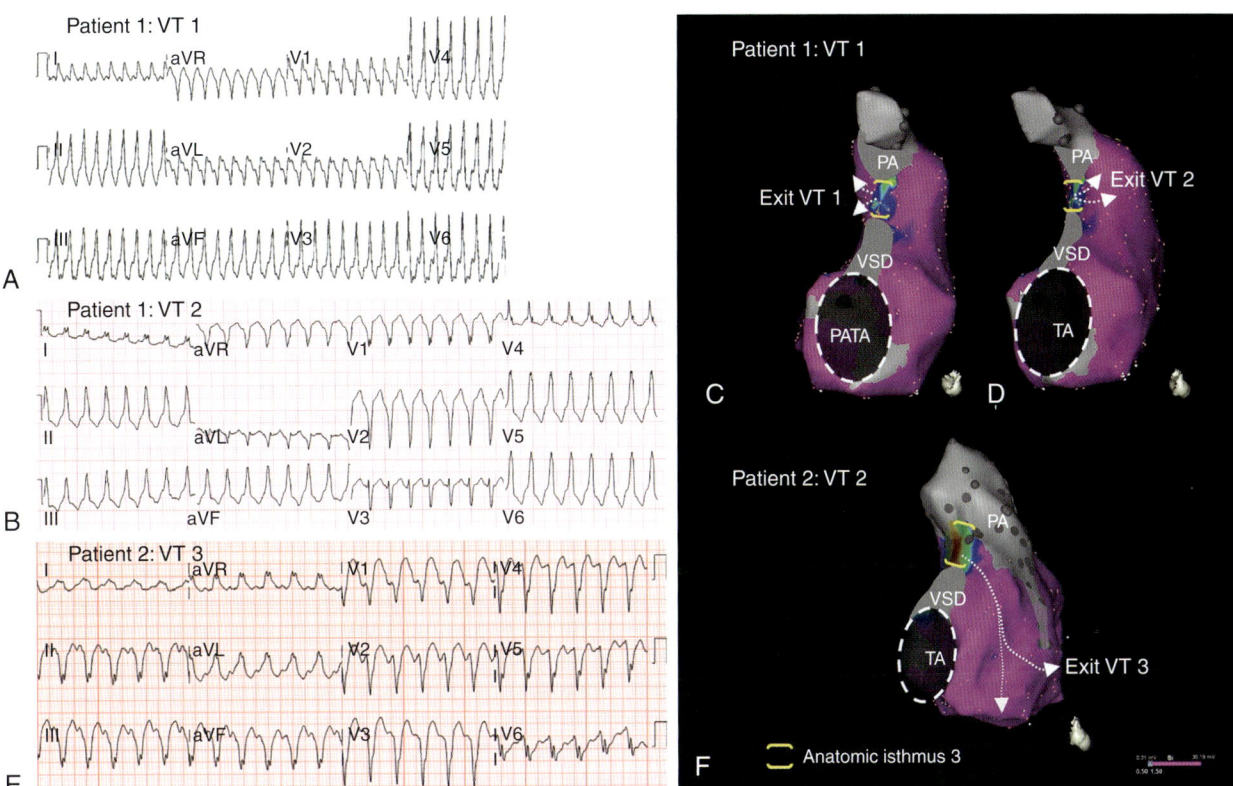

FIGURE 67.16 Tetralogy of Fallot. Ventricular tachycardia (VT) morphology depends on the location of the exit from anatomically defined isthmuses and the extension of surgical incisions. ECGs of VT (**A** and **B**) and RV voltage maps viewed from the posterior projection (**C** and **D**) from patient 1. **A**, VT1 has an RBBB-like V1 with inferior axis due to a leftward exit from the infundibular RVOT isthmus between the pulmonary artery (PA) and VSD patch (**C**). **B**, VT2 has an LBBB configuration with inferior axis, due to exit from the rightward side of the same isthmus as for VT1 (**D**). **E** and **F**, VT from patient 2 has an LBBB, superior axis configuration. This VT also uses an infundibular isthmus, but there is extensive free wall RV scar, so the apparent exit is in the inferior RV, producing the superior axis. This anatomic isthmus bordered by the PA and the VSD patch is the most common isthmus causing VT in repaired tetralogy of Fallot. (From Brouwer C, Kapel GFL, Jongbloed MRM, et al. Noninvasive identification of ventricular tachycardia-related anatomical isthmuses in repaired tetralogy of Fallot: what is the role of the 12-lead ventricular tachycardia electrocardiogram. *JACC Clin Electrophysiol.* 2018;4:1308–1318.)

in revealing active inflammation that supports the diagnosis (Chapter 18). Cardiac MR imaging may show a nonspecific pattern of fibrosis in a distribution that does not follow coronary anatomy (Chapter 19). Management is as for VT in NICM. Sustained VT or syncope warrants placement of an ICD.[1] Sustained VT is usually, but not always, associated with depressed ventricular function. ICDs are also considered for primary prevention of sudden death, particularly if there is evidence of depressed LV function, scar on cardiac MR imaging, or inducible VT at electrophysiologic testing. Immunosuppressive therapy may prevent or slow active disease progression and may improve AV block and PVCs but is unlikely to prevent recurrences of sustained VT once the fibrotic substrate is present. Recurrent episodes of VT are treated with antiarrhythmic drug therapy or catheter ablation. Catheter ablation is often challenging due to the varied scar locations and potential disease progression and recurrence rates exceed 50%.[34]

Myocarditis
Acute myocarditis from viral, autoimmune disease, or toxins can cause arrhythmias and sudden death. Active inflammation associated with myocarditis can cause multifocal PVCs, nonsustained VT, accelerated idioventricular rhythms, and polymorphic VT/VF.[6] In a series of patients with lymphocytic myocarditis, PVCs and nonsustained VT often originated from the inferior LV giving rise to RBBB superior axis QRS morphologies. With healing, myocarditis may leave areas of scar detectable as late gadolinium enhancement on MR imaging that can be a persistent substrate for reentrant sustained monomorphic VT and PVCs. Some patients presenting with PVCs and depressed ventricular function show cardiac inflammation on FDG-PET consistent with myocarditis as a cause of PVCs that sometimes resolves over time.[49,50]

Chagas Disease
Chagas disease is due to infection with the parasite *Trypanosoma cruzi* that is endemic to Latin America, where it is estimated that 6 million people are infected.[51] As a consequence of migration it is occasionally encountered outside the Western Hemisphere, and in the United States alone an estimated 300,000 people are infected. The acute infection is often unrecognized, but occasionally causes severe myocarditis. The disease then enters a chronic phase with seropositivity and no evidence of heart disease. Over years to decades 20% to 30% of patients develop cardiac disease of varying severity that appears to be due to persistent cardiac inflammation with a low level of parasite present. RBBB, left anterior hemiblock, and PVCs can be early manifestations followed over years by ventricular dysfunction, often with aneurysms, and VT. Sudden death can be the first clinical manifestation of disease and can be from ventricular arrhythmias or heart block. Sustained monomorphic VT is due to scar-related reentry, most commonly from the inferolateral left ventricle giving rise to VT that has an RBBB right axis QRS configuration.

Idiopathic Ventricular Tachycardias
Idiopathic VT is defined as monomorphic VT in patients who do not have structural heart disease Most have a single origin that is indicated by the QRS morphology. PVCs from the same focus are often present. The presence of more than one morphology of monomorphic VT, or VT with different morphologies of PVCs increases concern for underlying heart disease. The prognosis of idiopathic VT is good. The arrhythmia may be controlled by beta-blockers, verapamil or diltiazem as well as antiarrhythmic drugs such as flecainide and propafenone. Most originate from locations amenable to catheter ablation.

Outflow Tract Arrhythmias
The right and left ventricular outflow regions are the most common locations for idiopathic VT as well as PVCs (see Fig. 67.2). These most frequently arise in tissue along the pulmonary or aortic valve rings.

This tissue can extend above the valve ring giving rise to supravalvular foci that require ablation from within the pulmonary artery or aorta. The initiating mechanism is likely triggered activity. VT can be paroxysmal or exercise induced. It may occur as repetitive monomorphic VT with bursts of tachycardia separated by a variable number of sinus beats (see Fig. 67.5A). The QRS morphology of the VT has an inferiorly directed frontal plane axis, with tall monophasic R waves in leads II, III, AVF.[52]

For many patients these arrhythmias are provoked by exertion, stress, isoproterenol infusion, or rapid pacing. Termination with vagal maneuvers can occur. Suppression can often be achieved with beta-blockers or verapamil or diltiazem. Flecainide and propafenone have also been used for chronic therapy. When drug therapy is ineffective, not tolerated, or not desired by the patient, catheter ablation is a useful option. Efficacy varies for specific origins and generally exceeds 80%. Failure of ablation is often due to inability to initiate the arrhythmia to allow mapping in the electrophysiology laboratory, or origin from an inaccessible location that may be deep in the interventricular septum or subepicardial adjacent to a coronary artery where ablation is not performed. Serious complications are uncommon, but can include cardiac perforation, coronary injury, and femoral access site bleeding.

Annular Arrhythmias
Ventricular arrhythmias that arise adjacent to the tricuspid or mitral annuli have clinical characteristics similar to outflow tract arrhythmias with characteristic QRS morphologies that suggest the origin (see Fig. 67.2). Most are amenable to ablation. For those that originate close to the His bundle ablation has a risk of heart block.

Crux Arrhythmias
The crux of the heart encompasses the tissue in the inferior portion of the septum extending from the basal inferior septum near the coronary sinus apically and inferiorly.[53] The QRS shows a left superior frontal plane axis with QS complexes in II, III, and an LBBB or RBBB morphology, often with a prominent R in V2. The focus can be subepicardial, and approachable from within the middle cardiac vein or pericardial space for ablation but can also be protected by overlying posterior descending coronary artery and epicardial fat making ablation difficult.

Papillary Muscle Arrhythmias
PVCs, nonsustained VT, and occasionally sustained VT can originate from a focal source within the papillary muscles of the left or right ventricle. From the left ventricular papillary muscles the QRS has an RBBB configuration with either superior axis and S waves in V4 to V6 (posteromedial papillary muscle origin) or inferior rightward axis (anterolateral papillary muscle origin).[54] These arrhythmias can be associated with mitral valve prolapse. Most are benign, but very frequent arrhythmias may depress ventricular function and rare cases of papillary muscle PVC-induced VF occur. The presence of mitral annular disjunction (Chapter 76) and myocardial fibrosis in the adjacent LV wall has been associated with more severe arrhythmias.[55] The papillary muscles can also be sources for arrhythmias in cardiomyopathies and coronary artery disease.

Left Fascicular Reentrant Tachycardia
Left fascicular reentrant tachycardia, also known as verapamil-sensitive fascicular tachycardia is due to reentry involving one or more of the left ventricular fascicles and adjacent ventricular tissue in the septum or papillary muscles.[14] Patients are most commonly young adults. There is a male predominance. Tachycardia is sustained, often exercise induced, and hemodynamically tolerated. The most common form involves the LV posterior fascicle giving rise to an RBBB – like tachycardia with a superior left axis (see Fig. 67.11). Less common forms have a right inferior axis, or rarely, a narrow QRS. It can often be terminated by intravenous administration of verapamil, while intravenous administration of class I agents such as procainamide slow the tachycardia without termination. Chronic oral verapamil and beta-blockers have variable efficacy for preventing episodes. Catheter ablation of the common form is highly effective.

Polymorphic Ventricular Tachycardia
Electrocardiographic and Clinical Features
Polymorphic VT is characterized by a continually changing QRS morphology that indicates the changing ventricular activation sequence (Figs. 67.5, 67.17, and 67.18). Torsade de pointes is a specific type of polymorphic VT that has a waxing and waning QRS amplitude and is often associated with QT prolongation prior to initiation (see Fig. 67.17). The tachycardia is unstable and either terminates spontaneously or degenerates to VF. The distinction of where polymorphic VT ends and VF begins is often not clear. Polymorphic VT presents with light-headedness, syncope, or cardiac arrest. Polymorphic VT can be associated with myocardial ischemia (see Fig. 67.4D), left ventricular hypertrophy, or scar, but also occurs in structurally normal hearts in a number of genetic sudden death syndromes (long QT, short QT, early repolarization [ER], Brugada, catecholaminergic polymorphic VT) as well as digoxin toxicity. The mechanism may be reentry with continually changing reentry paths and has been associated with marked dispersion of ventricular repolarization. In CPVT and digoxin toxicity it is likely due to multiple competing foci of triggered activity. Unlike sustained monomorphic VT it is less likely to be associated with areas of ventricular scar, although scar is occasionally the arrhythmia substrate.[30]

Management
Sustained episodes causing hemodynamic collapse require immediate cardioversion. Following cardioversion further treatment is guided by the likely cause. Possible myocardial ischemia versus prolonged ventricular repolarization as causes should be immediately considered. In patients with coronary artery disease and electrocardiographic evidence of ischemia or ongoing infarction, emergent coronary angiography is often warranted. For torsade de pointes associated with QT prolongation intravenous administration of magnesium sulfate and removal of precipitating factors are first steps.

Specific Disorders with Polymorphic Ventricular Tachycardias
Acute Myocardial Infarction and Ischemia
Polymorphic VT degenerating to VF associated with acute ischemia or infarction is a common cause of out of hospital sudden death in Western societies. Evidence of acute infarction is found in approximately half of out of hospital VF survivors. Polymorphic VT degenerating to VF occurs within the first 24 to 48 hours in up to 10% of patients under care for acute type I myocardial infarction and may occur before, during, or after reperfusion.[1] It also occurs in up to 8% of non-ST elevation infarctions (see Fig. 67.4D). It is associated with a larger infarct territory, worse ventricular function, current smoking, and in some studies, the presence additional comorbidities. The electrocardiographic characteristics of the onset are variable. It may initiate with early or late coupled PVCs, during tachycardia or bradycardia, and with or without a preceding long R to R cycle (pause). With prompt defibrillation it is usually an isolated event. Recurrent episodes suggest ongoing ischemia warranting angiography for consideration of further intervention. Rarely recurrent episodes are due to automaticity from damaged cells in the infarct border region.[22] Amiodarone or quinidine suppress the arrhythmia in some.[9] Episodes usually resolve within days, but catheter ablation is occasionally required.

PMVT/VF during hospitalization for acute myocardial infarction is associated with greater in-hospital mortality, likely related to larger infarct size and comorbidities.[56] Mortality is greater for those with arrhythmia that occurs more than 48 hours after infarction. Although PMVT/VF within the first 48 hours of infarction is associated with greater in-hospital mortality, it is not associated with increased risk of sudden death over the following 5 years for those surviving to hospital discharge, and is not an indication for an ICD.[56]

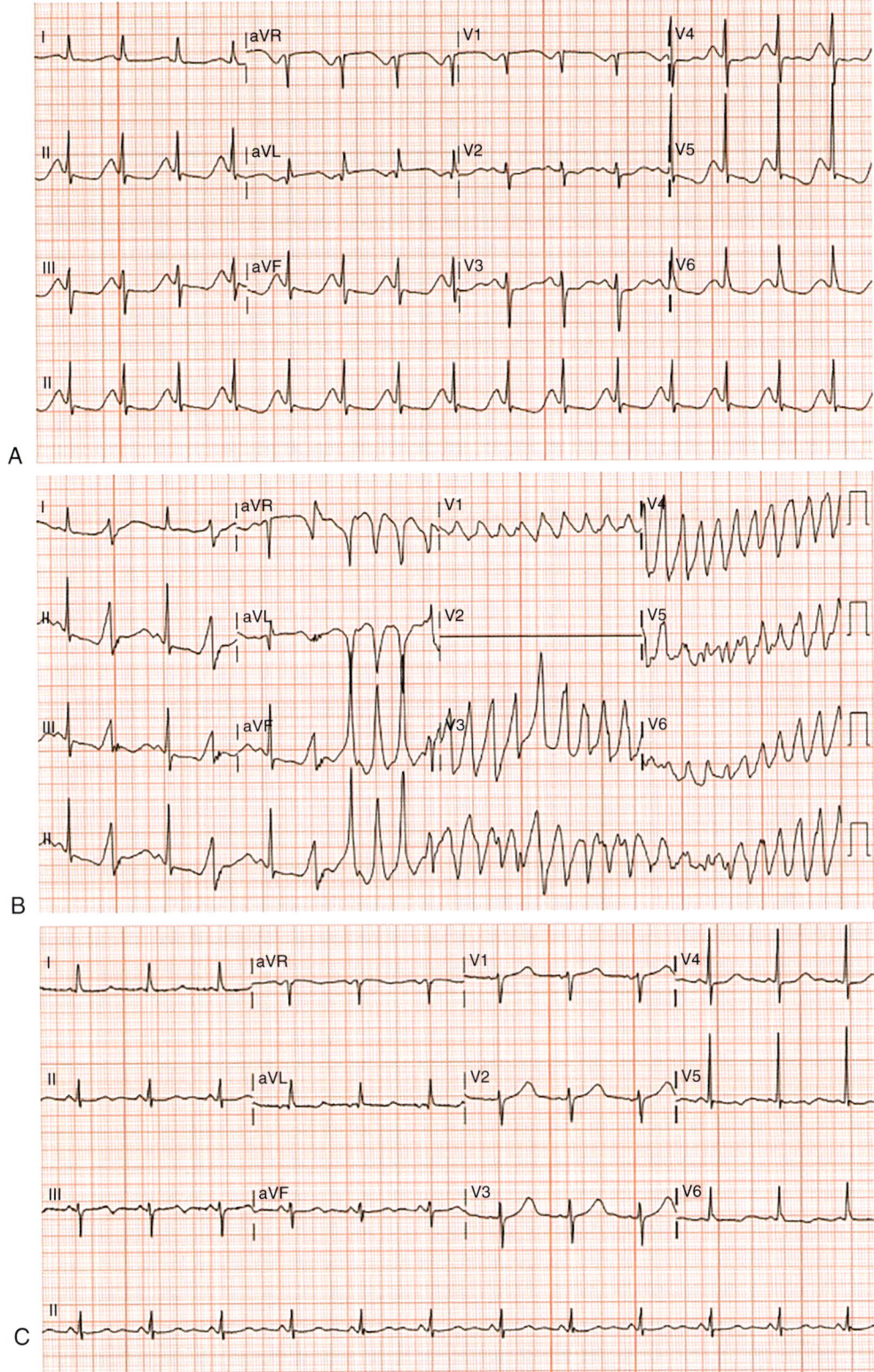

FIGURE 67.17 Long QT syndrome. **A-C** Long QT syndrome type 1. **A,** During hypokalemia there is marked QT prolongation with broad-based T waves. **B,** PVCs with initiation of the polymorphic VT torsade de pointes. **C,** After restoration of potassium, QT interval has shortened markedly. **D-F** Long QT syndrome 2.

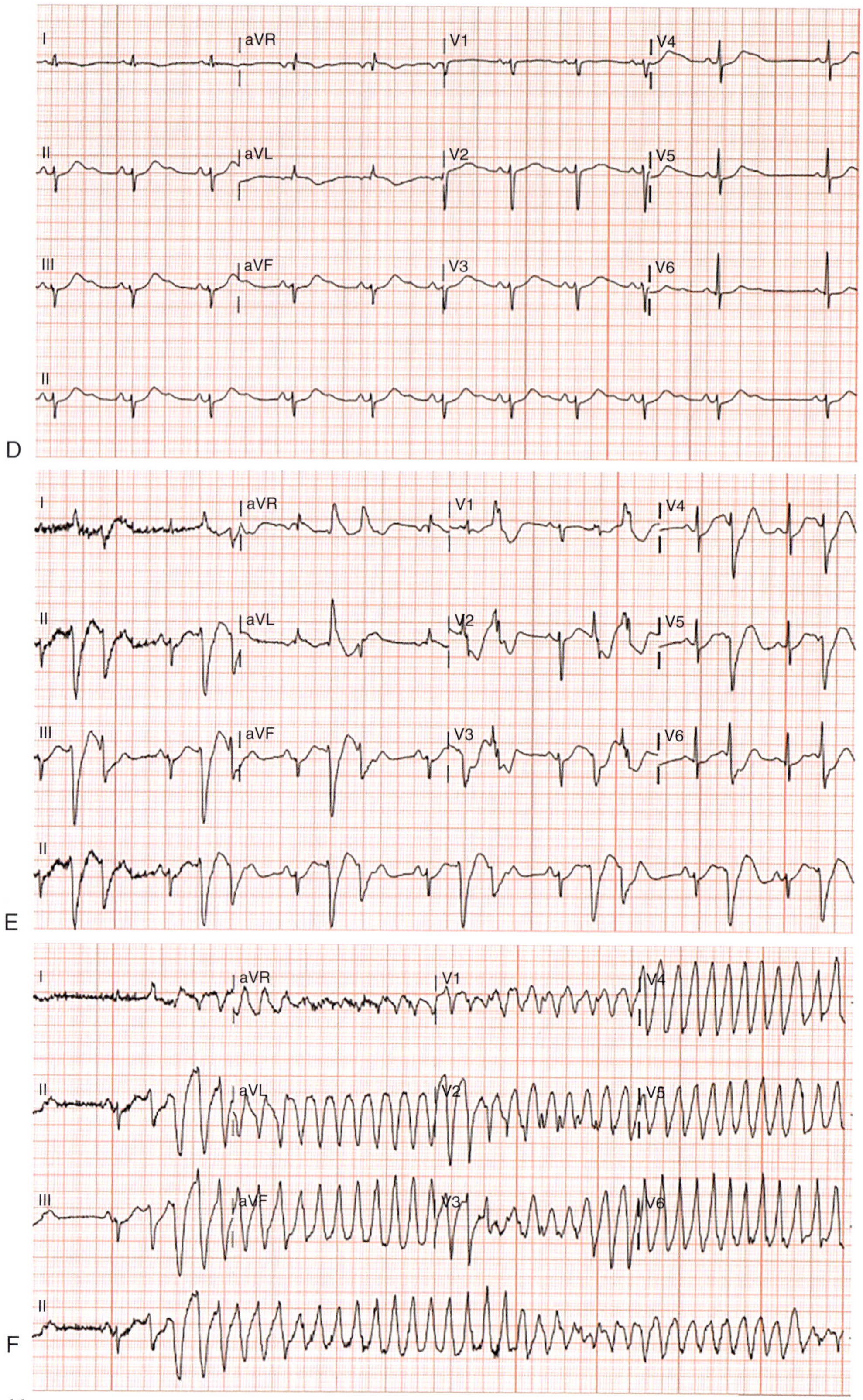

FIGURE 67.17—Cont'd **D,** QT prolongation with notched T-waves. **E,** PVCs and couplets. **F,** A pause initiates torsade de pointes.

Acquired Long QT Syndrome and Torsade de Pointes

The polymorphic VT torsade de pointes associated with QT interval prolongation is due to prolonged repolarization that allows recovery of time-dependent inward currents with creation of early afterdepolarizations that cause PVCs as well as repolarization heterogeneity facilitating reentry. Episodes are usually initiated by heart rate slowing or a PVC-induced pause. PVCs and runs of nonsustained VT are common. Sustained episodes may degenerate to VF. Prior to VT, the QTc interval is typically prolonged greater than 0.48 sec. Following defibrillation, the QT may be shorter in response to tachycardia and catecholamine administration, obfuscating the initial cause.

Any cause of QT prolongation can cause torsade de pointes. Drugs that block the repolarizing potassium current IKr are the most common offenders (dofetilide, ibutilide, sotalol, quinidine). Amiodarone also

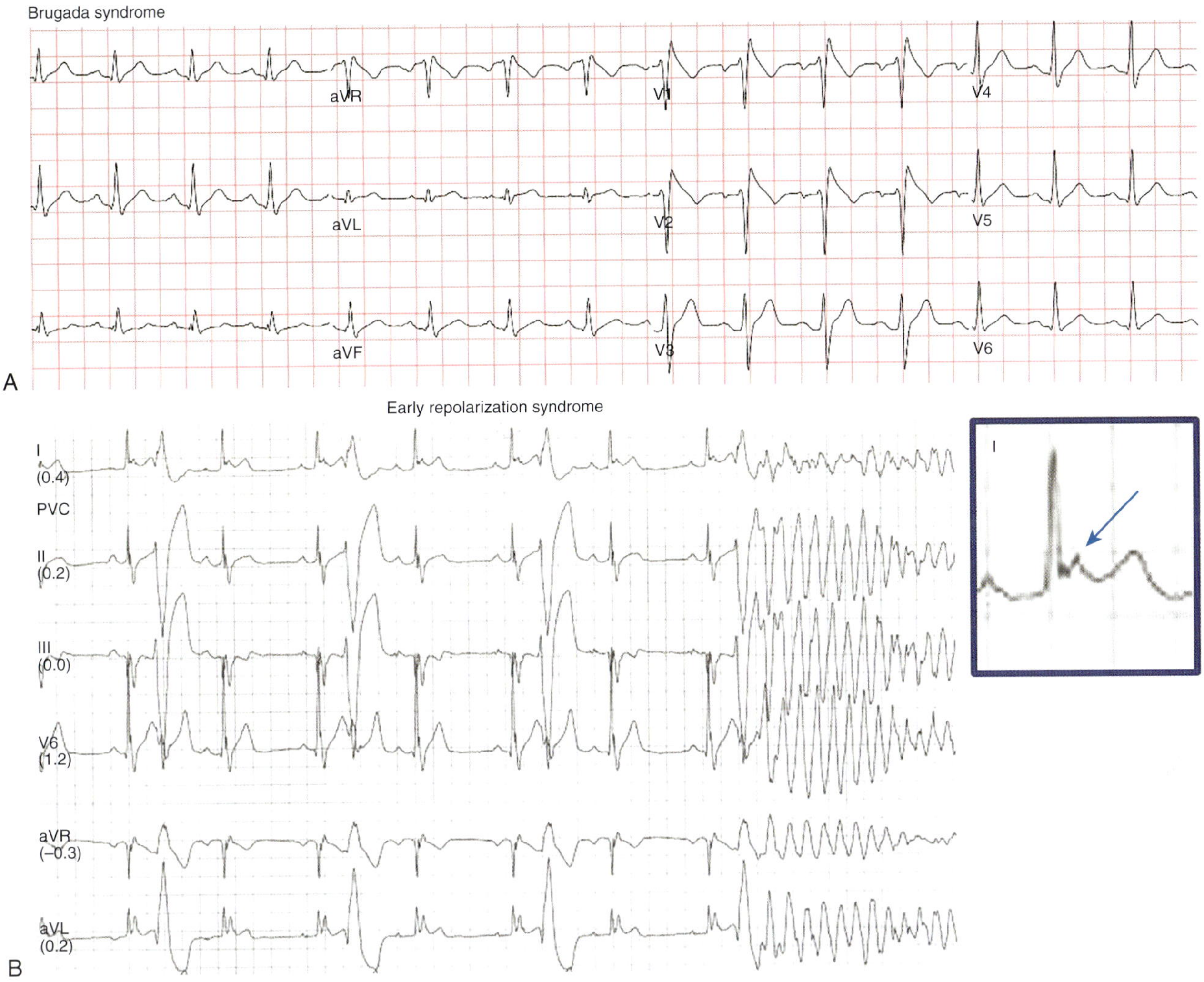

FIGURE 67.18 A, Type 1 ECG pattern of Brugada syndrome with J-point elevation greater than 2 mm in V1, V2. **B,** Early repolarization syndrome. Marked J-point elevation is present in lead I (arrow in *inset*); trigeminal short-coupled PVCs are present, interrupting the T wave of the preceding sinus beat, followed by initiation of polymorphic VT.

prolongs the QT interval, but rarely causes torsade de pointes. Many non-antiarrhythmic drugs also have IKr blocking capability (including a number of psychiatric and antibiotic medications). An updated list is maintained at www.crediblemeds.org. Bradycardia and hypokalemia are also important causes. Women are more susceptible than men, likely due to their sex-related longer QTc. In many cases a combination of factors is responsible. With genetic testing some patients are found to have inherited long QT syndrome.[57] Various combinations of single nucleotide polymorphisms that influence repolarization are genetic factors in determining risk, and have yet to be clarified sufficiently for clinical applications.[58] Drug interactions that increase concentrations of an offending agent or metabolite are also important causes.

Sustained episodes require immediate defibrillation. Recurrent episodes can usually be suppressed by 1 to 2 g of magnesium sulfate administered by rapid intravenous infusion and repeated as needed to suppress PVCs and NSVT. Bradycardia should be corrected by isoproterenol infusion or implementation of pacing at a rate that suppresses PVCs and nonsustained PMVT. Provocative drugs should be stopped and electrolyte abnormalities corrected. Shortening of the QT interval may lag excretion of the drug by several days. Patients who have had torsade de pointes should be viewed as having a susceptibility that warrants avoidance of all medications that can prolong the QT interval.

Inherited Long QT syndrome

The inherited long QT syndrome (LQTS) is due to genetic mutations that impair ventricular repolarization and prolong the QT interval (Chapter 63).[1,59] The incidence is approximately 1 in 2500. Most are autosomal dominant with variable penetrance. Although many individuals remain asymptomatic, others present with palpitations, syncope, or cardiac arrest due to torsade de pointes that can degenerate to VF (see Fig. 67.17). Episodes can present in childhood and may be misdiagnosed as seizures or benign syncope. A family history of sudden death may be present. The QTc interval is prolonged greater than 0.48 in most symptomatic individuals but can vary over time (see Fig. 67.17A, C) and can be normal on any individual ECG. Risk increases with the degree of QTc prolongation. Some phenotype correlations with genotype are described including classic triggers for arrhythmia episodes and sex differences in risk and timing of presentation and efficacy of therapies (Chapter 63).

Type 1 (LQTS1) causes over a third of congenital LQTS. It is due to a mutation that decreases the repolarizing current IKs. Episodes of syncope are classically triggered by exertion, including swimming, or emotional stress. The ECG typically shows broad symmetric T-wave (see Fig. 67.17A). Chronic therapy with beta-adrenergic blockers is highly effective in preventing episodes.

Type 2 (LQTS2) is due to a mutation that decreases the repolarizing current IKr, which is the same current that is most commonly blocked by agents causing acquired LQTS. Episodes of arrhythmia are classically provoked by emotional stress or surprise, such as sudden noises and are pause dependent. The risk is increased for women during the 9-month post-partum period. The ECG classically shows notched or humped appearing T waves (see Fig. 67.17D), similar to those often observed in acquired LQTS. Chronic therapy with beta-adrenergic blockers is protective.

Type 3 (LQTS3) is due to a mutation in *SCN5A* that increases inward Na current (INa). Episodes of arrhythmia or sudden death tend to occur during sleep and slow heart rates. The ECG typically shows a flat ST segment with a peaked T-wave. Therapy with beta-blockers is recommended. The sodium channel blocker mexiletine significantly shortens the QT interval in some individuals.

Many other mutations have been described that can cause LQTS, including ones with noncardiac features (Timothy Syndrome, Andersen-Tawil Syndrome) and a recessive form accompanied by congenital deafness (Jervell Lange-Nielsen Syndrome) (see Chapter 63).

Management

Management of recurrent acute episodes of polymorphic VT includes intravenous administration of magnesium sulfate and overdrive pacing to shorten the QT interval. Long term, avoidance of QT prolonging medications is critical. Asymptomatic individuals with mild QTc prolongation may not warrant additional therapy.[60] Chronic beta-blocker therapy with propranolol or nadolol is often sufficient, particularly for type 1 and 2 LQTS; metoprolol is less effective.[1] ICDs are considered in patients who have had cardiac arrest or who continue to have symptoms despite therapy. Specific therapeutic strategies for the type of LQTS are emerging, including potassium supplementation for type 2 and sodium channel blockers for type 3 LQTS. Surgical cardiac sympathectomy is an option when these therapies fail. When a proband is discovered, cascade genetic screening for other affected family members is important.

Inherited Short QT Syndrome

The short QT syndrome is characterized by polymorphic VT and atrial fibrillation in patients with a structurally normal heart and a QTc ≤340 to 360 milliseconds.[61] It is rare and caused by mutations that result in gain of function in repolarizing potassium channels (IKr and IKs) or loss of function in the L-type calcium current channel. Patients present with atrial fibrillation or palpitations, syncope, or cardiac arrest from polymorphic VT. Cardiac arrest is the initial manifestation in up to 40% of patients. Symptoms may occur at rest, with routine activity, or with exertion. A family history of sudden death is common. Most patients present with arrhythmias before 40 years of age. There is a male predominance. An ICD is recommended for patients who have had symptomatic arrhythmias. Quinidine may be helpful in diminishing episodes of VT.

J Wave Syndromes: Brugada and Early Repolarization Syndromes

Brugada Syndrome

Brugada syndrome (BrS) is characterized by transient or persistent coved type ST-segment elevation in at least one right pre-cordial ECG lead (see Fig. 67.18A).[62] BrS is associated with syncope and sudden death due to ventricular arrhythmias (see Chapter 63). Approximately 25% to 30% of affected patients have a mutation in the *SCN5A* gene. *SCN5A* mutations may also produce other phenotypes including AV conduction delay, sinus node dysfunction, and atrial fibrillation, features that can occur in BrS, or may occur isolated or in combinations in other family members.[63] Phenotypic manifestations can also overlap with ARVC.[62] Arrhythmic sudden death due to polymorphic VT/VF is the first manifestation in 4% of BrS patients, usually occurring at rest or during sleep. The average age at presentation is 40 years. There is approximately an 8 to 1 male dominance. The arrhythmia mechanisms are debated. There is evidence for both, abnormalities of repolarization with heterogeneously shortened action potentials, as well as abnormal conduction in regions of fibrosis in the subepicardial free wall of the RVOT tract. Rapid monomorphic VT (average cycle length of 298 ± 45 milliseconds) occurs in up to 4.2% of patients with BrS who have received an ICD and is the arrhythmia detected in 31% of those that have an appropriate ICD therapy.[64]

A type-1 ECG—consisting of a coved ST elevation ≥2 mm followed by a descending negative T wave in at least one right precordial lead, with the electrodes positioned in the 2nd, 3rd, or 4th intercostal space that is present either spontaneously or after provocative drug test with intravenous administration of sodium-channel blockers—is required for diagnosis of BrS. The ECG pattern can vary markedly and be normal at times. Enhanced vagal tone, fever, and several drugs (particularly sodium channel blocking antiarrhythmic and psychotropic drugs) can unmask the BrS pattern in some subjects who otherwise have a normal ECG. The type-2 and type-3 ECGs, defined by a saddleback pattern with broad R' followed by ST elevation ≥2 mm (type-2) or less than 2 mm (type 3) in the anterior precordial leads are not diagnostic and not, by themselves, associated with increased risk for sudden cardiac death (SCD).

The absolute risk of developing VF among asymptomatic patients with a type-1 ECG is lower than initially estimated and the majority of patients are likely to remain asymptomatic. Risk stratification in asymptomatic patients remains controversial and challenging.

Management

The ICD is the only established therapy to protect against SCD and is recommended for patients with a history of cardiac arrest or syncope consistent with an arrhythmia who have a type-1 ECG. In asymptomatic patients, the prognostic value of inducible PMVT at electrophysiology study and a family history of sudden death are less well defined. Lifestyle changes, including avoidance of drugs and intoxicating amounts of alcohol and immediate treatment of fever are important.

For patients with recurrent arrhythmias hydroquinidine or quinidine can reduce or prevent recurrences, but long-term treatment is hampered by side effects. Catheter ablation targeting areas of abnormal electrocardiograms in the subepicardial RVOT can normalize the ECG and prevent PMVT recurrences.[15]

Early Repolarization and J Wave Syndromes

Early repolarization (ER) *syndrome* is diagnosed in (1) a patient with an ER pattern who has been resuscitated from otherwise unexplained VF; or (2) in an SCD victim with a negative autopsy and a previous ECG with the ER pattern. An ER *pattern* is defined as a J-point elevation (or a J-wave producing slurring of the terminal QRS) ≥1 mm in at least 2 contiguous inferior and/or lateral leads of the 12-lead ECG and a QRS duration less than 120 milliseconds in leads without J waves (see Fig. 67.18B). The prevalence of ER varies between 1% and 24% in the general population and is particularly common in young men, athletes, and African Americans. Although the absolute arrhythmia risk is estimated to be very low (0.07%), ER patterns have been associated with VF initiated by Purkinje or myocardial triggers and sudden cardiac death. The ER pattern has also been associated with an increased incidence of ventricular arrhythmias during myocardial ischemia and in dilated or hypertrophic cardiomyopathies. The pathophysiology is uncertain.[15,62] Heterogeneity of the transmural voltage gradient across the ventricular wall due to abnormal rapid repolarization or delayed depolarization have been suggested. In contrast to BrS, the abnormal areas may more commonly involve the inferior aspects of the ventricles. Some have been associated with areas of subepicardial fibrosis over the inferior RV or LV that may facilitate reentry, similar to BrS.

There is currently no reliable risk stratification strategy to identify the small subset of patients at high risk among the large number of individuals with an ER pattern. Suspected arrhythmogenic syncope, in particular with a dynamic and high J wave amplitude recorded immediately after the event, J waves greater than 2.0 mm in inferior leads with horizontal/descending ST segment (≤0.1 mV 100 msec after J-point), J waves in several leads, a family history of SCD or ERS, and coexistence of other ECG abnormalities (LQT, short QT, Brugada) appear to be associated with a higher risk.

Management

An ICD is recommended for patients resuscitated from VT or VF or who have had syncope attributable to VT. Oral quinidine therapy can suppress recurrent episodes. Ablation of areas with delayed abnormal fractionated electrograms involving particularly the RV epicardium appears to reduce VF recurrence in highly symptomatic patients and can abolish the ER pattern.[15] In patients with VF storm administration of isoproterenol or quinidine can often suppress the arrhythmia. Ablation targeting the abnormal epicardial substrate or PVC triggers (Figs. 67.4B and 67.18B) can be lifesaving.

Catecholaminergic Polymorphic Ventricular Tachycardias

Catecholaminergic polymorphic VT (CPVT) is a rare disorder characterized by exercise- or stress-induced ventricular arrhythmias including PVCs, bidirectional VT (see Fig. 67.5C), and polymorphic VT/VF (see Chapter 63). These arrhythmias are due to abnormal calcium handling with increased intracellular calcium during sympathetic stimulation causing delayed afterdepolarizations and triggered activity. Mutations in the gene coding for the cardiac ryanodine receptor (*RYR2*) cause an autosomal dominant form. Mutations in the genes coding for calsequestrin, calmodulin, Kir2.1, and triadin cause very rare forms. Patients typically present in childhood with palpitations, syncope, or cardiac arrest during exertion or stress, although a quarter of patients have events during wakeful activity at rest.[65] The resting 12-lead ECG is normal. Exercise stress testing should be performed in suspected cases.[66] Monomorphic PVCs consistent with an outflow-tract origin in ≈60% typically occur at HR of ≈100 bpm, progressing to bigeminy, polymorphic PVCs, and VT or VF at higher rates. Bidirectional VT, although not common, is considered pathognomonic in young individuals without structural heart disease. Bidirectional VT is also seen in digoxin toxicity, myocarditis, and Anderson-Tawil syndrome.

Chronic therapy with beta-adrenergic blockers and limiting exercise are first-line treatments.[1] The addition of flecainide, propafenone, or verapamil suppresses arrhythmias in some patients. Those who continue to have symptoms often benefit from cardiac surgical left sympathectomy. Implantable defibrillators are avoided if possible. Shocks from the device, including inappropriate shocks for supraventricular tachycardia, can elicit sympathetic activation and VT storms.[67]

VENTRICULAR FIBRILLATION

Electrocardiographic Recognition

VF is a terminal arrhythmia followed by death or severe brain injury from lack of perfusion if not corrected within 3 to 5 minutes. It is characterized by irregular undulations of varying contour and amplitude without distinct QRS complexes (Fig. 67.19C).

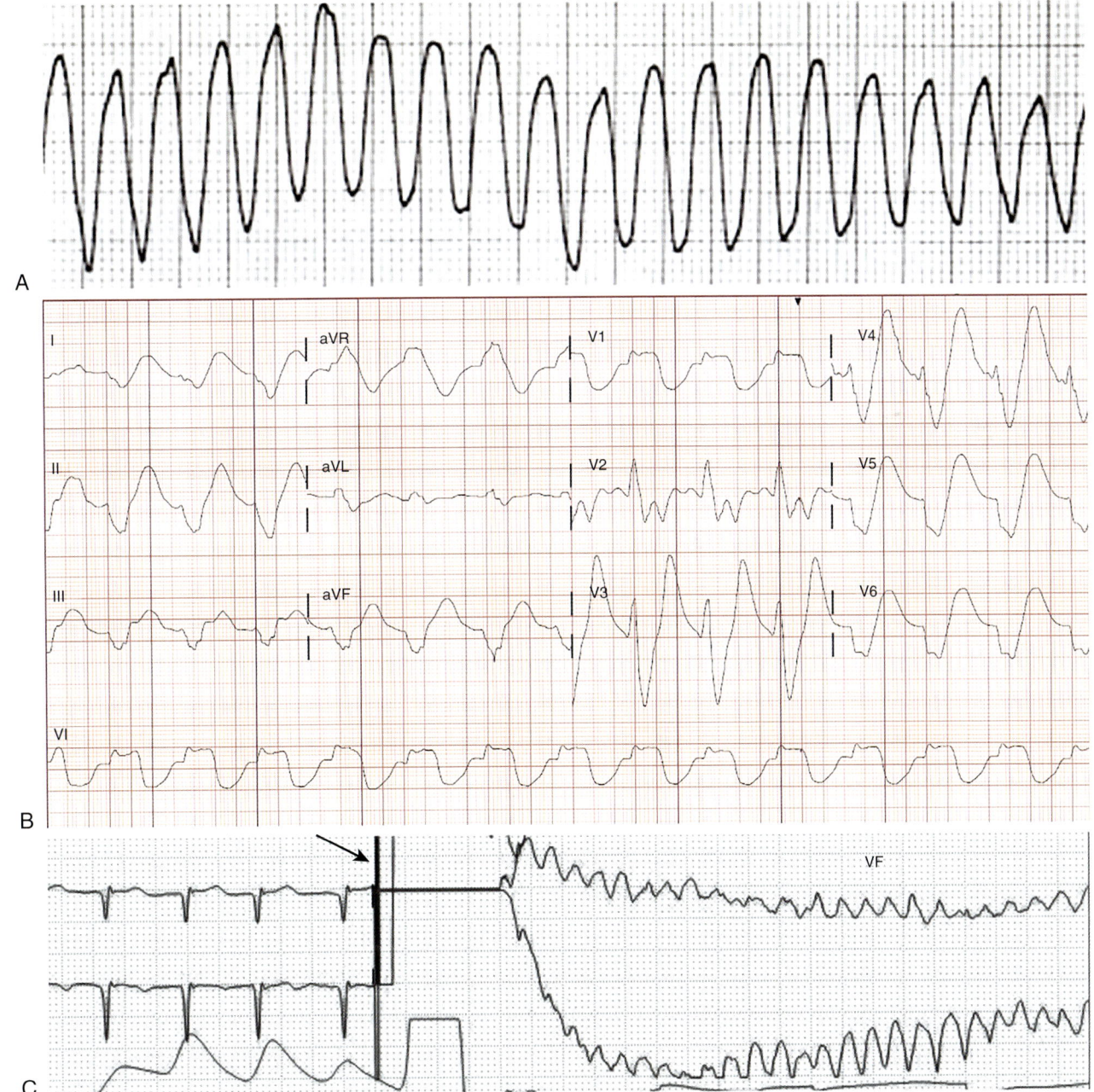

FIGURE 67.19 **A,** Rapid ventricular flutter. **B,** Slow sinusoidal rhythm with markedly wide QRS complexes due to severe hyperkalemia. **C,** Initiation of ventricular fibrillation by an external cardioversion shock *(arrow)* that fell during the T wave.

Clinical Features

VF and rapid ventricular flutter are most commonly encountered in coronary artery disease with ongoing myocardial ischemia and can follow from polymorphic VT or monomorphic VT of any cause. In structurally normal hearts VF can be elicited by electrical shock (see Fig. 67.19C) or a precordial impact that causes cardiac depolarization during the T-wave (commotio cordis). It can also be caused by very rapid ventricular rates during atrial fibrillation in patients with an accessory pathway in the Wolff-Parkinson-White syndrome or by early PVCs or unusually rapid idiopathic VT to cause idiopathic VF. There is no coordinated cardiac contraction, no detectable blood pressure, and absence of heart sounds. Eventually electrical activity of the heart ceases.

Management

Management should follow basic life support and advanced cardiac life support guidelines. Asynchronous DC cardioversion using 200 J to 400 J is mandatory therapy for VF, ventricular flutter, and pulseless VT. Cardiopulmonary resuscitation is performed until cardioversion can be performed and resumed immediately after each shock. If the first shock is ineffective subsequent shocks should be delivered at maximum defibrillator output. A bolus of intravenous amiodarone of 300 mg can be administered if initial shocks are unsuccessful while cardiopulmonary resuscitation is continued. Recurrent fibrillation is common after an initially successful shock. Close monitoring should be continued with immediate ability to defibrillate again as further evaluation seeks to identify and treat the underlying cause.

VENTRICULAR FLUTTER

Ventricular flutter (see Fig. 67.19A) is a sinusoidal tachycardia during which it is not possible to separate the QRS from the ST-T wave with certainty. Rapid ventricular flutter has rates faster than 280 beats/minute and can be a rapid monomorphic VT for which the etiologies are the same as for slower monomorphic VT, but can also occur during acute myocardial infarction or severe metabolic derangements. It usually produces hemodynamic collapse and degenerates to VF. Immediate electrical cardioversion or defibrillation is required. Correct synchronization of the defibrillator shock to the QRS, rather than T-wave, is not possible and an asynchronous shock should be used, always being prepared to apply a following shock for VF.

Relatively slow ventricular flutter is a wide QRS tachycardia due to slow conduction through the myocardium that can be due to hyperkalemia, drug toxicity, particularly cardiac sodium channel blocking drugs, severe global ischemia, and severe metabolic derangements (see Fig. 67.19B). It is usually associated with hypotension or hemodynamic collapse warranting cardioversion. For suspected hyperkalemia administration of intravenous calcium followed separately by sodium bicarbonate is warranted, followed by measures to lower serum potassium. Toxicity from a sodium channel blocking antiarrhythmic drug including flecainide, propafenone, and procainamide may respond to administration of hypertonic saline, which can be in the form of sodium bicarbonate.[68] Tachycardia increases sodium channel blockade by these drugs. Measures to slow the underlying sinus rate are helpful.

REFERENCES

1. Al-Khatib SM, Stevenson WG, Ackerman MJ, et al. 2017 AHA/ACC/HRS guideline for management of patients with ventricular arrhythmias and the prevention of sudden cardiac death: a report of the American college of cardiology/American heart association task force on clinical practice guidelines and the heart rhythm society. *Circulation*. 2018;138:e272–e391.
2. Kerola T, Dewland TA, Vittinghoff E, et al. Modifiable predictors of ventricular ectopy in the community. *J Am Heart Assoc*. 2018;7:e010078.
3. Dukes JW, Dewland TA, Vittinghoff E, et al. Ventricular ectopy as a predictor of heart failure and death. *J Am Coll Cardiol*. 2015;66:101–109.
4. Kim YR, Nam GB, Kwon CH, et al. Second coupling interval of nonsustained ventricular tachycardia to distinguish malignant from benign outflow tract ventricular tachycardias. *Heart Rhythm*. 2014;11:2222–2230.
5. Verdile L, Maron BJ, Pelliccia A, et al. Clinical significance of exercise-induced ventricular tachyarrhythmias in trained athletes without cardiovascular abnormalities. *Heart Rhythm*. 2015;12:78–85.
6. Peretto G, Sala S, Rizzo S, et al. Ventricular arrhythmias in myocarditis: characterization and relationships with myocardial inflammation. *J Am Coll Cardiol*. 2020;75:1046–1057.
7. Lee AKY, Andrade J, Hawkins NM, et al. Outcomes of untreated frequent premature ventricular complexes with normal left ventricular function. *Heart*. 2019;105:1408–1413.
8. Ling Z, Liu Z, Su L, et al. Radiofrequency ablation versus antiarrhythmic medication for treatment of ventricular premature beats from the right ventricular outflow tract: prospective randomized study. *Circ Arrhythm Electrophysiol*. 2014;7:237–243.
9. Viskin S, Chorin E, Viskin D, et al. Quinidine-responsive polymorphic ventricular tachycardia in patients with coronary heart disease. *Circulation*. 2019;139:2304–2314.
10. Latchamsetty R, Bogun F. Premature ventricular complex-induced cardiomyopathy. *JACC Clin Electrophysiol*. 2019;5:537–550.
11. Huizar JF, Ellenbogen KA, Tan AY, et al. Arrhythmia-induced cardiomyopathy: JACC state-of-the-art review. *J Am Coll Cardiol*. 2019;73:2328–2344.
12. Berruezo A, Penela D, Jauregui B, et al. Mortality and morbidity reduction after frequent premature ventricular complexes ablation in patients with left ventricular systolic dysfunction. *Europace*. 2019;21:1079–1087.
13. Penela D, Fernandez-Armenta J, Aguinaga L, et al. Clinical recognition of pure premature ventricular complex-induced cardiomyopathy at presentation. *Heart Rhythm*. 2017;14:1864–1870.
14. Cronin EM, Bogun FM, Maury P, et al. 2019 HRS/EHRA/APHRS/LAHRS expert consensus statement on catheter ablation of ventricular arrhythmias. *Heart Rhythm*. 2020;17:e2–e154.
15. Nademanee K, Haissaguerre M, Hocini M, et al. Mapping and ablation of ventricular fibrillation associated with early repolarization syndrome. *Circulation*. 2019;140:1477–1490.
16. Doisne N, Waldmann V, Redheuil A, et al. A novel gain-of-function mutation in SCN5A responsible for multifocal ectopic Purkinje-related premature contractions. *Hum Mutat*. 2020;41:850–859.
17. Ortiz M, Martin A, Arribas F, et al. Randomized comparison of intravenous procainamide vs. intravenous amiodarone for the acute treatment of tolerated wide QRS tachycardia: the PROCAMIO study. *Eur Heart J*. 2017;38:1329–1335.
18. Vergara P, Tzou WS, Tung R, et al. Predictive score for identifying survival and recurrence risk profiles in patients undergoing ventricular tachycardia ablation: the I-VT score. *Circ Arrhythm Electrophysiol*. 2018;11:e006730.
19. Vergara P, Tung R, Vaseghi M, et al. Successful ventricular tachycardia ablation in patients with electrical storm reduces recurrences and improves survival. *Heart Rhythm*. 2018;15:48–55.
20. Chatzidou S, Kontogiannis C, Tsilimigras DI, et al. Propranolol versus metoprolol for treatment of electrical storm in patients with implantable cardioverter-defibrillator. *J Am Coll Cardiol*. 2018;71:1897–1906.
21. Meng L, Tseng CH, Shivkumar K, et al. Efficacy of stellate ganglion blockade in managing electrical storm: a systematic review. *JACC Clin Electrophysiol*. 2017;3:942–949.
22. Komatsu Y, Hocini M, Nogami A, et al. Catheter ablation of refractory ventricular fibrillation storm after myocardial infarction. *Circulation*. 2019;139:2315–2325.
23. Beggs SAS, Gardner RS, McMurray JJV. Who benefits from a defibrillator-balancing the risk of sudden versus non-sudden death. *Curr Heart Fail Rep*. 2018;15:376–389.
24. Almehmadi F, Porta-Sanchez A, Ha ACT, et al. Mortality implications of appropriate implantable cardioverter defibrillator therapy in secondary prevention patients: contrasting mortality in primary prevention patients from a prospective population-based registry. *J Am Heart Assoc*. 2017;6.
25. Sapp JL, Wells GA, Parkash R, et al. Ventricular tachycardia ablation versus escalation of antiarrhythmic drugs. *N Engl J Med*. 2016;375:111–121.
26. Willems S, Tilz RR, Steven D, et al. Preventive or deferred ablation of ventricular tachycardia in patients with ischemic cardiomyopathy and implantable defibrillator (BERLIN VT): a multicenter randomized trial. *Circulation*. 2020;141:1057–1067.
27. Kheiri B, Barbarawi M, Zayed Y, et al. Antiarrhythmic drugs or catheter ablation in the management of ventricular tachyarrhythmias in patients with implantable cardioverter-defibrillators: a systematic review and meta-analysis of randomized controlled trials. *Circ Arrhythm Electrophysiol*. 2019;12:e007600.
28. Tung R, Vaseghi M, Frankel DS, et al. Freedom from recurrent ventricular tachycardia after catheter ablation is associated with improved survival in patients with structural heart disease: an International VT Ablation Center Collaborative Group study. *Heart Rhythm*. 2015;12:1997–2007.
29. Gigli M, Merlo M, Graw SL, et al. Genetic risk of arrhythmic phenotypes in patients with dilated cardiomyopathy. *J Am Coll Cardiol*. 2019;74:1480–1490.
30. Piers SR, Everaerts K, van der Geest RJ, et al. Myocardial scar predicts monomorphic ventricular tachycardia but not polymorphic ventricular tachycardia or ventricular fibrillation in nonischemic dilated cardiomyopathy. *Heart Rhythm*. 2015;12:2106–2114.
31. El Moheb M, Nicolas J, Khamis AM, et al. Implantable cardiac defibrillators for people with non-ischaemic cardiomyopathy. *Cochrane Database Syst Rev*. 2018;12:CD012738.
32. Wahbi K, Ben Yaou R, Gandjbakhch E, et al. Development and validation of a new risk prediction score for life-threatening ventricular tachyarrhythmias in laminopathies. *Circulation*. 2019;140:293–302.
33. Zeppenfeld K. Ventricular tachycardia ablation in nonischemic cardiomyopathy. *JACC Clin Electrophysiol*. 2018;4:1123–1140.
34. Vaseghi M, Hu TY, Tung R, et al. Outcomes of catheter ablation of ventricular tachycardia based on etiology in nonischemic heart disease: an international ventricular tachycardia ablation center collaborative study. *JACC Clin Electrophysiol*. 2018;4:1141–1150.
35. Aryana A, Tung R, d'Avila A. Percutaneous epicardial approach to catheter ablation of cardiac arrhythmias. *JACC Clin Electrophysiol*. 2020;6:1–20.
36. Nakamura T, Narui R, Zheng Q, et al. Atrioventricular block during catheter ablation for ventricular arrhythmias. *JACC Clin Electrophysiol*. 2019;5:104–112.
37. Bosman LP, Cadrin-Tourigny J, Bourfiss M, et al. Diagnosing arrhythmogenic right ventricular cardiomyopathy by 2010 Task Force Criteria: clinical performance and simplified practical implementation. *Europace*. 2020;22:787–796.
38. Venlet J, Piers SR, Jongbloed JD, et al. Isolated subepicardial right ventricular outflow tract scar in athletes with ventricular tachycardia. *J Am Coll Cardiol*. 2017;69:497–507.
39. Koyak Z, de Groot JR, Bouma BJ, et al. Sudden cardiac death in adult congenital heart disease: can the unpredictable be foreseen? *Europace*. 2017;19(3):401–406.
40. Wu MH, Lu CW, Chen HC, et al. Adult congenital heart disease in a nationwide population 2000-2014: epidemiological trends, arrhythmia, and standardized mortality ratio. *J Am Heart Assoc*. 2018;7.
41. Kapel GF, Reichlin T, Wijnmaalen AP, et al. Re-entry using anatomically determined isthmuses: a curable ventricular tachycardia in repaired congenital heart disease. *Circ Arrhythm Electrophysiol*. 2015;8:102–109.
42. Brouwer C, Kapel GFL, Jongbloed MRM, et al. Noninvasive identification of ventricular tachycardia-related anatomical isthmuses in repaired tetralogy of Fallot: what is the role of the 12-lead ventricular tachycardia electrocardiogram. *JACC Clin Electrophysiol*. 2018;4:1308–1318.
43. Kapel GF, Sacher F, Dekkers OM, et al. Arrhythmogenic anatomical isthmuses identified by electroanatomical mapping are the substrate for ventricular tachycardia in repaired tetralogy of Fallot. *Eur Heart J*. 2017;38:268–276.
44. Rowin EJ, Maron BJ, Chokshi A, et al. Left ventricular apical aneurysm in hypertrophic cardiomyopathy as a risk factor for sudden death at any age. *Pacing Clin Electrophysiol*. 2018.
45. Igarashi M, Nogami A, Kurosaki K, et al. Radiofrequency catheter ablation of ventricular tachycardia in patients with hypertrophic cardiomyopathy and apical aneurysm. *JACC Clin Electrophysiol*. 2018;4:339–350.
46. Wang W, Lian Z, Rowin EJ, et al. Prognostic implications of nonsustained ventricular tachycardia in high-risk patients with hypertrophic cardiomyopathy. *Circ Arrhythm Electrophysiol*. 2017;10.

47. Birnie DH, Sauer WH, Bogun F, et al. HRS expert consensus statement on the diagnosis and management of arrhythmias associated with cardiac sarcoidosis. *Heart Rhythm.* 2014;11:1305–1323.
48. Kandolin R, Lehtonen J, Airaksinen J, et al. Cardiac sarcoidosis: epidemiology, characteristics, and outcome over 25 years in a nationwide study. *Circulation.* 2015;131:624–632.
49. Ammirati E, Cipriani M, Moro C, et al. Clinical presentation and outcome in a contemporary cohort of patients with acute myocarditis: multicenter Lombardy registry. *Circulation.* 2018;138:1088–1099.
50. Lakkireddy D, Turagam MK, Yarlagadda B, et al. Myocarditis causing premature ventricular contractions: insights from the MAVERIC registry. *Circ Arrhythm Electrophysiol.* 2019;12:e007520.
51. Nunes MCP, Beaton A, Acquatella H, et al. Chagas cardiomyopathy: an update of current clinical knowledge and management: a scientific statement from the American Heart Association. *Circulation.* 2018;138:e169–e209.
52. Anderson RD, Kumar S, Parameswaran R, et al. Differentiating right- and left-sided outflow tract ventricular arrhythmias: classical ECG signatures and prediction algorithms. *Circ Arrhythm Electrophysiol.* 2019;12:e007392.
53. Kawamura M, Gerstenfeld EP, Vedantham V, et al. Idiopathic ventricular arrhythmia originating from the cardiac crux or inferior septum: epicardial idiopathic ventricular arrhythmia. *Circ Arrhythm Electrophysiol.* 2014;7:1152–1158.
54. Al'Aref SJ, Ip JE, Markowitz SM, et al. Differentiation of papillary muscle from fascicular and mitral annular ventricular arrhythmias in patients with and without structural heart disease. *Circ Arrhythm Electrophysiol.* 2015;8:616–624.
55. Dejgaard LA, Skjolsvik ET, Lie OH, et al. The mitral annulus disjunction arrhythmic syndrome. *J Am Coll Cardiol.* 2018;72:1600–1609.
56. Bougouin W, Marijon E, Puymirat E, et al. Incidence of sudden cardiac death after ventricular fibrillation complicating acute myocardial infarction: a 5-year cause-of-death analysis of the FAST-MI 2005 registry. *Eur Heart J.* 2014;35:116–122.
57. Itoh H, Crotti L, Aiba T, et al. The genetics underlying acquired long QT syndrome: impact for genetic screening. *Eur Heart J.* 2016;37:1456–1464.
58. Strauss DG, Vicente J, Johannesen L, et al. Common genetic variant risk score is associated with drug-induced QT prolongation and torsade de pointes risk: a pilot study. *Circulation.* 2017;135:1300–1310.
59. Mazzanti A, Maragna R, Vacanti G, et al. Interplay between genetic substrate, QTc duration, and arrhythmia risk in patients with long QT syndrome. *J Am Coll Cardiol.* 2018;71:1663–1671.
60. MacIntyre CJ, Rohatgi RK, Sugrue AM, et al. Intentional nontherapy in long QT syndrome. *Heart Rhythm.* 2020;17:1147–1150.
61. El-Battrawy I, Besler J, Liebe V, et al. Long-term follow-up of patients with short QT syndrome: clinical profile and outcome. *J Am Heart Assoc.* 2018;7:e010073.
62. Antzelevitch C, Yan GX, Ackerman MJ, et al. J-Wave syndromes expert consensus conference report: emerging concepts and gaps in knowledge. *Europace.* 2017;19:665–694.
63. Wilde AAM, Amin AS. Clinical spectrum of SCN5A mutations: long QT syndrome, Brugada syndrome, and cardiomyopathy. *JACC Clin Electrophysiol.* 2018;4:569–579.
64. Rodriguez-Manero M, Sacher F, de Asmundis C, et al. Monomorphic ventricular tachycardia in patients with Brugada syndrome: a multicenter retrospective study. *Heart Rhythm.* 2016;13:669–682.
65. Roston TM, Yuchi Z, Kannankeril PJ, et al. The clinical and genetic spectrum of catecholaminergic polymorphic ventricular tachycardia: findings from an international multicentre registry. *Europace.* 2018;20:541–547.
66. Giudicessi JR, Ackerman MJ. Exercise testing oversights underlie missed and delayed diagnosis of catecholaminergic polymorphic ventricular tachycardia in young sudden cardiac arrest survivors. *Heart Rhythm.* 2019;16:1232–1239.
67. Roston TM, Jones K, Hawkins NM, et al. Implantable cardioverter-defibrillator use in catecholaminergic polymorphic ventricular tachycardia: a systematic review. *Heart Rhythm.* 2018;15:1791–1799.
68. Brumfield E, Bernard KR, Kabrhel C. Life-threatening flecainide overdose treated with intralipid and extracorporeal membrane oxygenation. *Am J Emerg Med.* 2015;33:1840.e3–1845.

68 Bradyarrhythmias and Atrioventricular Block

KRISTEN K. PATTON AND JEFFREY E. OLGIN

BRADYARRHYTHMIAS, 1312
Sinus Bradycardia, 1312
Sinus Arrhythmia, 1312
Sick Sinus Syndrome, 1313

ATRIOVENTRICULAR BLOCK (HEART BLOCK), 1315

First-Degree Atrioventricular Block, 1315
Second-Degree Atrioventricular Block, 1315
High-Grade Atrioventricular Block, 1317
Third-Degree (Complete) Atrioventricular Block, 1317

ATRIOVENTRICULAR DISSOCIATION, 1319
Autonomic/Neurally Mediated Bradycardia, 1320

REFERENCES, 1320

BRADYARRHYTHMIAS

Based on large population studies of healthy individuals, the lower limit of normal resting heart rate is defined as 50 beats/min.[1,2] Frequently, bradyarrhythmias are physiologic, as in well-conditioned athletes with low resting heart rates or in type I atrioventricular (AV) block during sleep. In other cases, bradyarrhythmias can be pathologic. Similar to tachyarrhythmias, bradyarrhythmias can be categorized on the basis of the level of disturbance in the hierarchy of the normal impulse generation and conduction system (from sinus node to AV node to His-Purkinje system) (see Chapter 65 and Table 65.1).

Sinus Bradycardia

Electrocardiographic Recognition

Sinus bradycardia is diagnosed in an adult when the sinus node discharges at a rate less than 50 beats/min (Fig. 68.1A). P waves have a normal contour, and are usually upright in leads I, II, and aVF, and occur before each QRS complex, usually with a constant PR interval longer than 120 msec. Sinus arrhythmia often coexists.

Clinical Features

Sinus bradycardia can result from excessive vagal or decreased sympathetic tone, as an effect of medications, or from anatomic changes in the sinus node. In most cases, symptomatic sinus bradycardia is caused or worsened by the effects of medication. Asymptomatic sinus bradycardia frequently occurs in healthy young adults, particularly well-trained athletes, and decreases in prevalence with advancing age. During sleep, the normal heart rate can fall to 35 to 40 beats/min, especially in adolescents and young adults, with marked sinus arrhythmia sometimes producing pauses of 2 seconds or longer. Eye surgery, coronary arteriography, meningitis, intracranial tumors, increased intracranial pressure, cervical and mediastinal tumors, and certain disease states (e.g., severe hypoxia, myxedema, hypothermia, fibrodegenerative changes, convalescence from some infections, gram-negative sepsis, mental depression) can produce sinus bradycardia. Sinus bradycardia also occurs during vomiting or vasovagal syncope[3,4] (see Chapter 71) and can be produced by carotid sinus stimulation or by the administration of parasympathomimetic drugs, lithium, amiodarone, beta adrenoceptor–blocking drugs, clonidine, propafenone, ivabradine (a specific I_f pacemaker current blocker; see Chapter 62), or calcium antagonists. Conjunctival instillation of beta blockers for glaucoma can produce sinus or AV nodal abnormalities, especially in elderly patients.

In most cases, sinus bradycardia is a benign arrhythmia that can actually be beneficial by producing a longer period of diastole and increasing ventricular filling time, especially in heart failure patients. Conversely, it can be associated with syncope caused by an abnormal autonomic reflex (cardioinhibitory; see Chapter 71). Sinus bradycardia occurs in 10% to 15% of patients with acute myocardial infarction (MI) and may be even more prevalent when patients are seen in the early hours of infarction. Unless it is accompanied by hemodynamic decompensation or arrhythmias, sinus bradycardia is generally associated with a more favorable outcome after MI than sinus tachycardia. It is usually transient and occurs more commonly during inferior than during anterior MI; sinus bradycardia has also been noted during reperfusion with thrombolytic agents (see Chapter 38). Bradycardia that follows resuscitation from cardiac arrest is associated with a poor prognosis.

Management

Treatment of sinus bradycardia is not usually necessary unless cardiac output is inadequate or arrhythmias result from the slow rate. Atropine (0.5 mg intravenously as an initial dose, repeated if necessary) is generally acutely effective; lower doses, particularly given subcutaneously or intramuscularly, can exert an initial parasympathomimetic effect, possibly by a central action. For recurrent symptomatic episodes, temporary or permanent pacing may be needed (see Chapters 64 and 69). Although theophylline and terbutaline can be used to increase the sinus rate, as a general rule, no drugs are available that increase the heart rate reliably and safely during long periods without undesirable side effects.

Sinus Arrhythmia

Sinus arrhythmia is characterized by a phasic variation in sinus cycle length during which the maximum sinus cycle length minus the minimum sinus cycle length exceeds 120 msec or the maximum sinus cycle length minus the minimum sinus cycle length divided by the minimum sinus cycle length exceeds 10% (Fig. 68.1B). It is the most frequent form of arrhythmia and is physiologically normal. P wave morphology does not usually vary, and the PR interval exceeds 120 msec and remains unchanged because the focus of discharge remains relatively fixed within the sinus node. On occasion, the pacemaker focus can wander within the sinus node, or its exit to the atrium may change and produce P waves of a slightly different contour (although not retrograde) and a slightly changing PR interval that exceeds 120 msec.

> Sinus arrhythmia usually occurs in the young, especially those with slower heart rates or with enhanced vagal tone, for example, following the administration of digitalis or morphine, or due to athletic training. The prevalence of sinus arrhythmia decreases with age or with autonomic dysfunction, such as in diabetic neuropathy. Sinus arrhythmia appears in two basic forms. In the respiratory form, the P-P interval cyclically shortens during inspiration, primarily as a result of reflex inhibition of vagal tone, and slows during expiration; breath-holding eliminates the variation in cycle length (see Chapter 61). Nonrespiratory sinus arrhythmia is characterized by a phasic variation in the P-P interval unrelated to the respiratory cycle and can be the result of digitalis intoxication. Loss of sinus rhythm variability is a risk factor for sudden cardiac death (see Chapter 70).

Symptoms produced by sinus arrhythmia are uncommon, but on occasion, if the pauses are excessively long, palpitations or dizziness can result. Marked sinus arrhythmia can produce a sinus pause sufficiently long to cause syncope if it is not accompanied by an escape rhythm. Treatment is usually unnecessary. Increasing the heart rate by exercise or drugs generally abolishes sinus arrhythmia. Symptomatic individuals may experience relief from palpitations with sedatives, tranquilizers, atropine, ephedrine, or isoproterenol administration, as for the treatment of sinus bradycardia.

VENTRICULOPHASIC SINUS ARRHYTHMIA

The most common example of ventriculophasic sinus arrhythmia occurs during complete AV block and a slow ventricular rate, when P-P cycles that contain a QRS complex are shorter than P-P cycles without a QRS complex. Similar lengthening can be present in the P-P cycle that follows a premature ventricular complex (PVC) with a compensatory pause. Alterations in the P-P interval are probably caused by the influence of the autonomic nervous system responding to changes in ventricular stroke volume.

SINUS PAUSE OR SINUS ARREST

Sinus pause or sinus arrest is recognized by a pause in the sinus rhythm. The P-P interval delimiting the pause does not equal a multiple of the basic P-P interval. Differentiation of sinus arrest, which is thought to be caused by slowing or cessation of spontaneous sinus node automaticity, and therefore is a disorder of impulse formation, from sinoatrial (SA) exit block in patients with sinus arrhythmia can be difficult without direct recordings of sinus node discharge. Failure of sinus nodal discharge results in the absence of atrial depolarization and can also result in ventricular asystole if escape beats initiated by latent pacemakers do not occur. Involvement of the sinus node by acute MI, degenerative fibrotic changes, digitalis toxicity, stroke, or excessive vagal tone can produce sinus arrest. Transient sinus arrest (especially while sleeping) may have no clinical significance by itself if latent pacemakers promptly escape to prevent ventricular asystole or the genesis of other arrhythmias precipitated by slow rates. Sinus arrest and AV block have been demonstrated in many patients with sleep apnea (see Chapter 89).

Treatment is as outlined earlier for sinus bradycardia. In patients who have a chronic form of sinus node disease characterized by marked sinus bradycardia or sinus arrest, permanent pacing is often necessary. However, as a general rule, chronic pacing for sinus bradycardia is indicated only in symptomatic patients.

SINOATRIAL EXIT BLOCK

SA exit block is an arrhythmia that is recognized electrocardiographically by a pause resulting from absence of the normally expected P wave. The duration of the pause is a multiple of the basic P-P interval. SA exit block is caused by a conduction disturbance during which an impulse formed within the sinus node fails to depolarize the atria or does so with delay. An interval without P waves that equals approximately two, three, or four times the normal P-P cycle characterizes type II second-degree SA exit block. During type I (Wenckebach) second-degree SA exit block, the P-P interval progressively shortens before the pause, and the duration of the pause is less than two P-P cycles. (See Chapter 14 for further discussion of Wenckebach intervals.) First-degree SA exit block cannot be recognized on the electrocardiogram (ECG) because SA nodal discharge is not recorded. Third-degree SA exit block can be manifested as a complete absence of P waves and is difficult to diagnose with certainty without sinus node electrograms.

Excessive vagal stimulation, acute myocarditis, MI, or fibrosis involving the atrium, as well as drugs such as quinidine, procainamide, flecainide, and digitalis, can produce SA exit block. SA exit block is usually transient. It may be of no clinical importance except to prompt a search for the underlying cause. On occasion, syncope can result if the SA block is prolonged and unaccompanied by an escape rhythm. SA exit block can occur in well-trained athletes. Therapy for patients who have symptomatic SA exit block is as outlined earlier for sinus bradycardia.

Sick Sinus Syndrome
Electrocardiographic Recognition

Sick sinus syndrome is a term applied to a syndrome encompassing several sinus nodal abnormalities, including (1) persistent spontaneous sinus bradycardia inappropriate for the physiologic circumstance, (2) sinus arrest or exit block (Fig. 68.2), (3) combinations of SA and AV conduction disturbances, and often, (4) alternation of paroxysms of rapid regular or irregular atrial tachyarrhythmias and periods of slow atrial and ventricular rates (bradycardia-tachycardia syndrome; Fig. 68.3). More than one of these conditions can be seen in the same patient on different occasions, and their mechanisms are often causally interrelated and combined with an abnormal state of AV conduction or automaticity.

Patients with sinus node disease can be categorized as having intrinsic

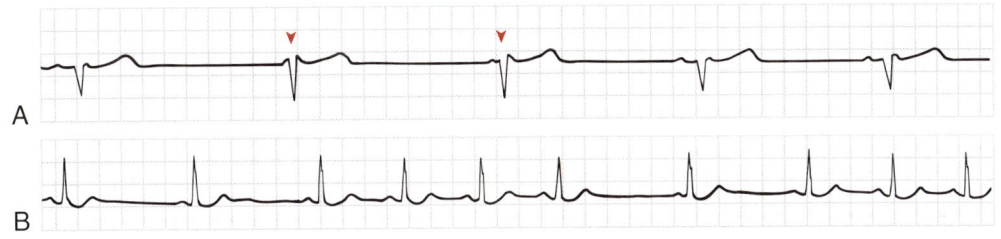

FIGURE 68.1 **A,** Sinus bradycardia at a rate of 40 to 48 beats/min. The second and third QRS complexes *(arrowheads)* represent junctional escape beats. Note the P waves at the onset of the QRS complex. **B,** Nonrespiratory sinus arrhythmia occurring as a consequence of digitalis toxicity. Monitor leads were used.

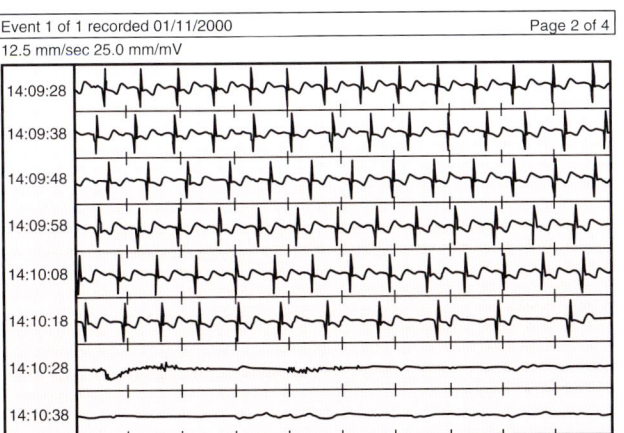
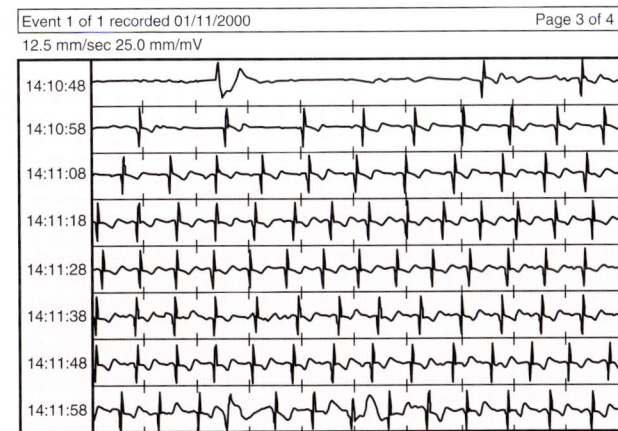

FIGURE 68.2 Continuous recording from an implanted loop recorder in a patient with syncope. The tracing shows paroxysmal sinus node arrest and a sinus pause of nearly 30 seconds. The preceding sinus cycle length appears to lengthen just before the pause, which suggests an autonomic component of the pause. There is also a single ventricular escape complex at 14:10:48.

disease unrelated to autonomic abnormalities or as exhibiting combinations of intrinsic and autonomic abnormalities. Symptomatic patients with sinus pauses or SA exit block frequently show abnormal responses on electrophysiologic testing and can have a relatively high incidence of atrial fibrillation. In children, sinus node dysfunction most frequently occurs in those with congenital or acquired heart disease, particularly after corrective cardiac surgery. Sick sinus syndrome can occur in the absence of other cardiac abnormalities. The course of the disease is frequently intermittent and unpredictable because it is influenced by the severity of the underlying heart disease. Excessive physical training can heighten vagal tone and produce syncope related to sinus bradycardia or AV conduction abnormalities in otherwise normal individuals.

The anatomic basis of sick sinus syndrome can involve total or subtotal destruction of the sinus node, areas of nodal-atrial discontinuity, inflammatory or degenerative changes in the nerves and ganglia surrounding the node, and pathologic changes in the atrial wall. Fibrosis and fatty infiltration occur, and the sclerodegenerative processes generally involve the sinus node and the AV node or the bundle of His and its branches or distal subdivisions. Occlusion of the sinus node artery can cause sinus node dysfunction.

Chronotropic Incompetence

Chronotropic incompetence (CI) is diagnosed when the heart rate does not increase appropriately in the setting of increased physiologic demand (Fig. 68.4). Although many studies use a definition of failure to obtain 80% or 85% of either maximal expected heart rate, or of inadequate heart rate reserve (the difference between resting heart rate and age predicted maximal heart rate),[2] the variance in individual heart rate range can require meticulous clinical assessment. If required, a reliable technique using ventilatory expired gas analysis during exercise to calculate the chronotropic index allows for an objective calculation of the relationship between metabolic reserve and heart rate reserve adjusted for age and functional capacity (see Chapter 15).[5]

The normal heart rate increase with exercise and rapid decline with cessation of activity results from an exquisite balance of inputs from the sympathetic and parasympathetic nervous system to the sinus node. Increase in heart rate due to physiologic demand is the principal determinant of rate of oxygen consumption (Vo_2) and exercise capacity. The fourfold increase in Vo_2 during exercise is largely due to a 2.2-fold increase in heart rate. Genome-wide association studies have confirmed heritability of heart rate increase with exercise and heart rate recovery. Candidate genes are related to the central nervous system, cardiac development, and cardiac ion channels.[6] Aging alone can confer CI; the age-related decline in heart rate response to exercise is inevitable even in healthy older athletes.

Symptomatic CI is common, and frequently associated with SA node disease, atrial fibrillation, coronary artery disease (CAD), and heart failure.[7] Symptoms are grounded in intolerance of exertion, and often include dyspnea, lightheadedness, and overall limited exercise capacity. Interestingly, beta-blocker therapy is not universally associated with CI in either the CAD or heart failure populations. Similar to sinus bradycardia treatment is based on symptoms. Despite the clear association between CI and mortality, the evidence supporting atrial-based rate responsive pacing therapy and improvement in mortality risk is scant, but promising.

Tachycardia-Bradycardia Syndrome

Tachycardia-bradycardia syndrome (TBS) occurs when a patient has tachyarrhythmias and bradyarrhythmias closely associated in time. That can occur when a tachyarrhythmia, typically atrial fibrillation or atrial flutter terminates, with a resultant excessive post-conversion pause (Fig. 68.5). TBS can also occur during atrial fibrillation when periods of atrial fibrillation with rapid ventricular rates alternate with periods of excessive bradycardia (due to high-grade AV block) during atrial fibrillation. While TBS can occur without medication, it typically occurs as a result of treatment with beta blockers or calcium channel blockers.

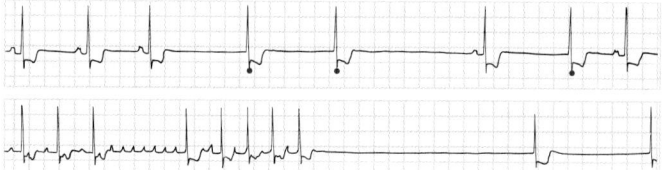

FIGURE 68.3 Sick sinus syndrome with bradycardia-tachycardia in a continuous monitor lead recording. **Top,** Intermittent sinus arrest is apparent with junctional escape beats at irregular intervals *(red circles)*. **Bottom,** A short episode of atrial flutter is followed by almost 5 seconds of asystole before a junctional escape rhythm resumes. The patient became presyncopal at this point.

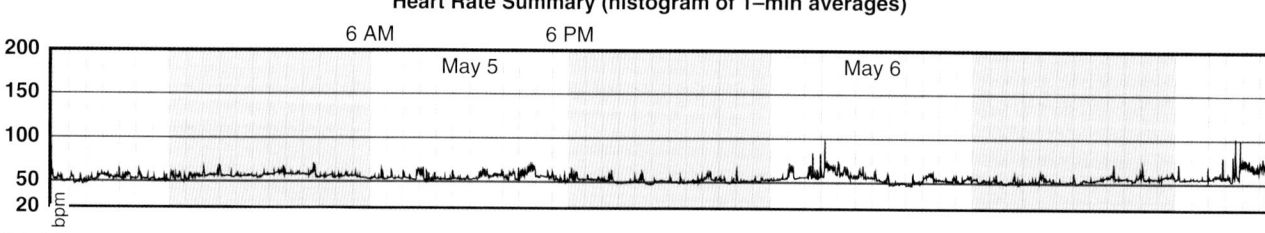

FIGURE 68.4 Three-day monitor revealing markedly suppressed heart rate histogram curve, showing a heart rate range between 55 and 91 beats/min, with an average of 45 beats/min. Correlation of symptoms and rate remain essential.

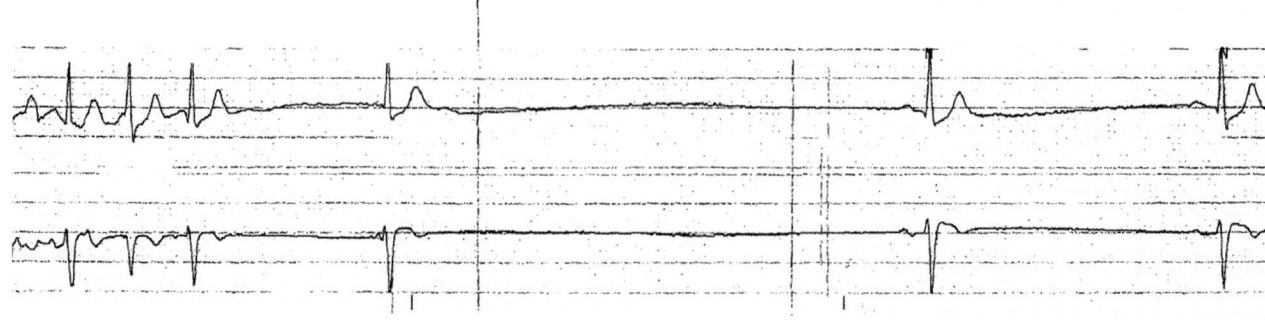

FIGURE 68.5 Telemetry monitor example of atrial fibrillation with rapid ventricular response with termination followed by a sinus pause with a junctional escape beat, and a second, longer sinus pause.

Management

For patients with sick sinus syndrome, treatment depends on the basic rhythm problem but usually involves permanent pacemaker implantation when symptoms are manifest (see Chapter 69). Pacing for bradycardia, combined with drug therapy to treat the tachycardia, is required in those with bradycardia-tachycardia syndrome.

ATRIOVENTRICULAR BLOCK (HEART BLOCK)

Heart block is a disturbance of impulse conduction that can be permanent or transient, depending on the anatomic or functional impairment. It must be distinguished from *interference*, a normal phenomenon that is a disturbance of impulse conduction caused by physiologic refractoriness resulting from inexcitability secondary to a preceding impulse. Interference or block can occur at any site where impulses are conducted, but they are recognized most often between the sinus node and atrium (SA block), between the atria and ventricles (AV block), within the atria (intra-atrial block), or within the ventricles (intraventricular block). SA exit block was discussed earlier (see Sinus Bradycardia). AV block exists if the atrial impulse is conducted with delay or is not conducted at all to the ventricle when the AV junction is not physiologically refractory. During AV block, the site of block can be in the AV node, His bundle, or bundle branches. In some cases of bundle branch block (BBB), the impulse may only be delayed and not completely blocked in the bundle branch, yet the resulting QRS complex may be indistinguishable from a QRS complex generated by a complete BBB.

AV block is classified by severity into three categories. During first-degree heart block, conduction time is prolonged but all impulses are conducted. Second-degree heart block occurs in two forms, Mobitz type I (Wenckebach) and type II. Type I heart block is characterized by progressive lengthening of the conduction time until an impulse is not conducted. Type II heart block denotes an occasional or repetitive sudden block of conduction of an impulse, without prior measurable lengthening of conduction time. When no impulses are conducted, complete or third-degree block is present. The degree of block may depend in part on the direction of impulse propagation. For unknown reasons, retrograde conduction can still occur in the presence of advanced anterograde AV block. The reverse can also occur. Some electrocardiographers use the term *advanced* or *high-grade heart block* to indicate blockage of two or more consecutive impulses.

First-Degree Atrioventricular Block

During first-degree AV block, every atrial impulse is conducted to the ventricles and a regular ventricular rate is produced, but the PR interval exceeds 0.20 second in adults. PR intervals as long as 1.0 second have been noted and can at times exceed the P-P interval, a phenomenon known as *skipped P waves*. Clinically important PR interval prolongation can result from a conduction delay in the AV node (A-H interval), in the His-Purkinje system (H-V interval), or at both sites. Equally delayed conduction over both bundle branches can infrequently produce PR prolongation without significant QRS complex widening. On occasion, intra-atrial conduction delay can result in PR prolongation. If the QRS complex on the ECG is normal in contour and duration, the AV delay almost always resides in the AV node and rarely within the His bundle itself. If the QRS complex shows a BBB pattern, the conduction delay may be within the AV node or the His-Purkinje system (Fig. 68.6). In the latter case, a His bundle electrogram is necessary to localize the site of conduction delay. Acceleration of the atrial rate or enhancement of vagal tone by carotid massage can cause first-degree AV nodal block to progress to type I second-degree AV block. Conversely, type I second-degree AV nodal block can revert to a first-degree block with deceleration of the sinus rate.

Second-Degree Atrioventricular Block

Blocking of some atrial impulses conducted to the ventricle at a time when physiologic interference is not involved defines second-degree AV block (Figs. 68.7 to 68.9). The nonconducted

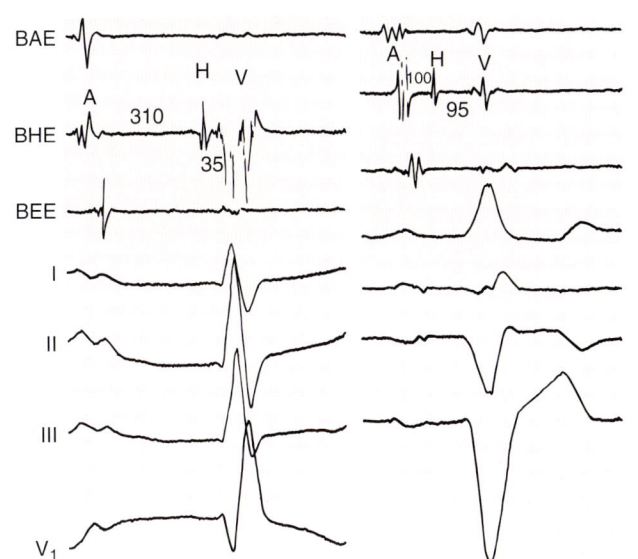

FIGURE 68.6 First-degree atrioventricular (AV) block. One complex during sinus rhythm is shown. **Left,** The PR interval measured 370 msec (PA = 25 msec; A-H = 310 msec; H-V = 39 msec) during a right bundle branch block. Conduction delay in the AV node causes the first-degree AV block. **Right,** The PR interval is 230 msec (PA = 39 msec; A-H = 100 msec; H-V = 95 msec) during a left bundle branch block. The conduction delay in the His-Purkinje system is causing the first-degree AV block. *BAE,* Bipolar atrial electrogram; *BEE,* bipolar esophageal electrogram; *BHE,* bipolar His electrogram.

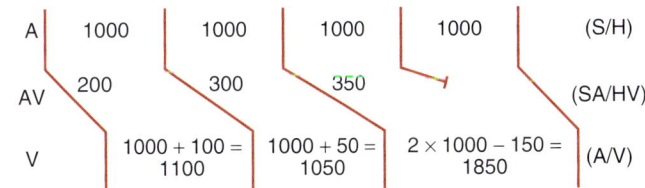

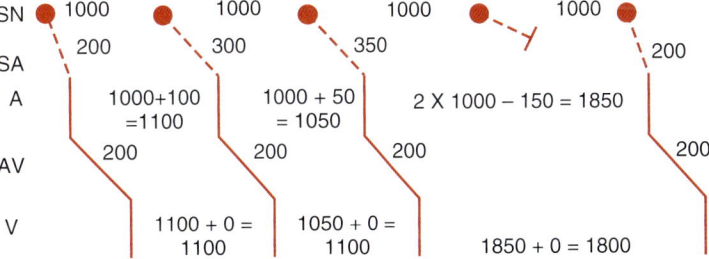

FIGURE 68.7 A, Ladder diagram of typical 4:3 atrioventricular Wenckebach cycle. P waves (A tier) occur at a cycle length of 1000 msec. The PR interval (AV tier) is 200 msec for the first beat and generates a ventricular response (V tier). The PR interval increases by 100 msec in the next complex, which results in an R-R interval of 1100 msec (1000 + 100). The increment in the PR interval is only 50 msec for the third cycle, and the PR interval becomes 350 msec. The R-R interval shortens to 1050 msec (1000 + 50). The next P wave is blocked, and an R-R interval is created that is less than twice the P-P interval by an amount equal to the increments in the PR interval. Thus the Wenckebach features explained in the text can be found in this diagram. If the increment in the PR interval of the last conducted complex increased rather than decreased (e.g., 150 msec rather than 50 msec), the last R-R interval before the block would increase (1150 msec) rather than decrease and thus become an example of an atypical Wenckebach cycle (see Fig. 68.8). **B,** If this were a Wenckebach exit block from the sinus node to the atrium, the sinus node cycle length (S) would be 1000 msec, and the SA interval would increase from 200 to 300 to 350 msec and culminate in a block. These events would not be apparent on a scalar electrocardiogram (ECG). However, the P-P interval on the ECG would shorten from 1100 to 1050 msec, and finally, there would be a pause of 1850 msec (A). If this rhythm were a junctional rhythm arising from the His bundle and conducting to the ventricle, the junctional rhythm cycle length would be 1000 msec (H) and the H-V interval would progressively lengthen from 200 to 300 to 350 msec, whereas the R-R interval would decrease from 1100 to 1050 msec and then increase to 1850 msec (V). The only clue to the Wenckebach exit block would be the changes in cycle length in the ventricular rhythm.

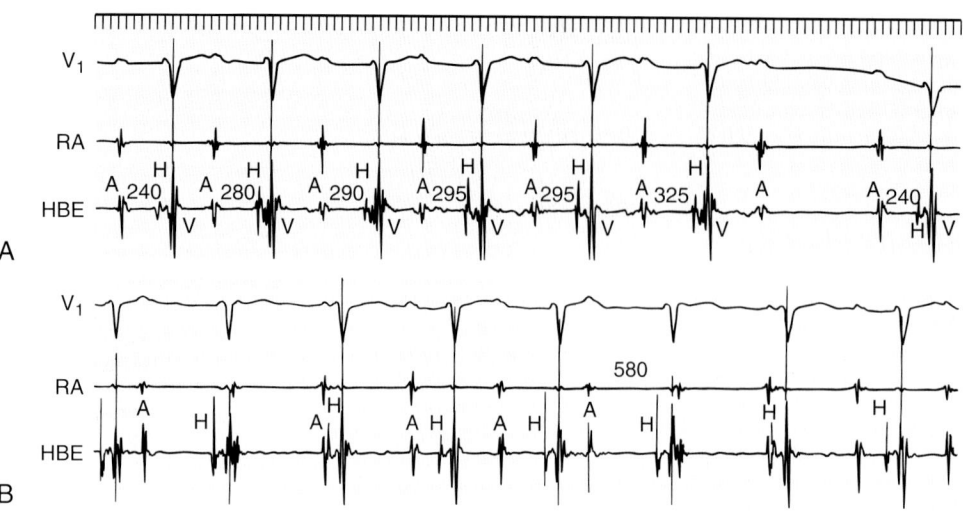

FIGURE 68.8 **A,** Type I (Wenckebach) atrioventricular (AV) nodal block. During spontaneous sinus rhythm, progressive PR prolongation occurs and culminates in a nonconducted P wave. From the His bundle recording (HBE), it is apparent that the conduction delay and subsequent block occur within the AV node (prolongation of the AH interval). Because the increment in conduction delay does not consistently decrease, the R-R intervals do not reflect the classic Wenckebach structure. **B,** Recorded 5 minutes after the intravenous administration of atropine, 0.5 mg. Atropine has had its predominant effect on sinus and junctional automaticity by this time, with little improvement in AV conduction. Consequently, more P waves are blocked and AV dissociation is present, caused by a combination of AV block and an enhanced junctional discharge rate. When atropine finally improved AV conduction (not shown), 1:1 AV conduction occurred. *RA,* Right atrium.

block in the His-Purkinje system in a patient with a BBB can closely resemble an AV nodal Wenckebach block, the site of Wenchekbach block most commonly occurs in the AV node (Fig. 68.9B).[8]

Certain features of type I second-degree block deserve special emphasis because when actual conduction times are not apparent on the ECG—for example, during SA, junctional, or ventricular exit block (see Fig. 68.7)—a type I conduction disturbance can be difficult to recognize. During a typical type I block, the increment in conduction time is greatest in the second beat of the Wenckebach group, and the absolute increase in conduction time decreases progressively over subsequent beats. These two features serve to establish the characteristics of classic Wenckebach group beats: (1) the interval between successive beats progressively decreases, although the conduction time increases (but by a decreasing function); (2) the duration of the pause produced by the nonconducted impulse is less than twice the interval preceding the blocked impulse (which is usually the shortest interval); and (3) the cycle that follows the nonconducted beat (beginning the Wenckebach group) is longer than the cycle preceding the blocked impulse. Although much emphasis has been placed on this characteristic grouping of cycles, primarily to be able to diagnose a Wenckebach exit block, this typical grouping occurs in fewer than 50% of patients with a type I Wenckebach AV nodal block.

Differences in these cycle-length patterns can result from changes in sinus pacemaker rate (e.g., sinus arrhythmia), neurogenic control of conduction, and in the increment of conduction delay. For example, if the PR increment in the last cycle increases, the R-R cycle of the last conducted beat can lengthen rather than shorten. In addition, because the last conducted beat is often at a critical state of conduction, it can become blocked and produce a 5:3 or 3:1 conduction ratio instead of a 5:4 or 3:2 ratio. During a 3:2 Wenckebach structure, the duration of the cycle that follows the nonconducted beat will be the same as the duration of the cycle that precedes the nonconducted beat.

Although it has been suggested that type I and type II AV block are different manifestations of the same electrophysiologic mechanism that differ only quantitatively in the size of the increments, clinical separation of second-degree AV block into types I and II serves a useful function, and in most cases the differentiation can be made easily and reliably from the surface ECG. Type II AV block often antedates the development of Adams-Stokes syncope[3] and complete AV block, whereas type I AV block with a normal QRS complex is generally more benign and does not progress to more advanced forms of AV conduction disturbance. In older people, type I AV block with or without BBB has been associated with a clinical picture similar to that seen in type II AV block.

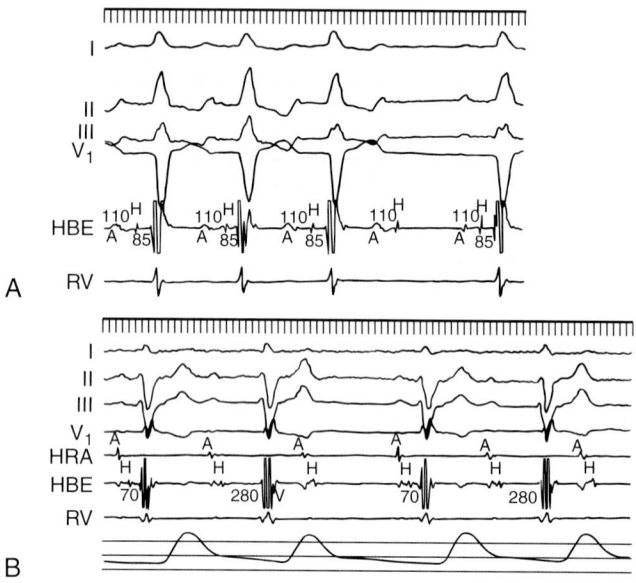

FIGURE 68.9 Type II atrioventricular (AV) block. **A,** The sudden development of His-Purkinje block is apparent. The A-H and H-V intervals remain constant, as does the PR interval. A left bundle branch block is present. **B,** Wenckebach AV block in the His-Purkinje system. The QRS complex exhibits a right bundle branch block morphology. However, note that the second QRS complex in the 3:2 conduction exhibits a slightly different contour from the first QRS complex, particularly in leads III and V$_1$. This finding is the clue that the Wenckebach AV block might be in the His-Purkinje system. The H-V interval increases from 70 to 280 msec, and then a block distal to the His bundle results. *HBE,* His bundle electrogram; *HRA,* high right atrium; *RV,* right ventricle.

In a patient with an acute MI, type I AV block usually accompanies inferior infarction (perhaps more often if a right ventricular infarction also occurs), is transient, and does not require temporary pacing, whereas type II AV block occurs in the setting of acute anterior MI, can require temporary or permanent pacing, and is associated with high mortality, generally as a result of pump failure. A high degree of AV block can occur in patients with acute inferior MI and is associated with more myocardial damage and a higher mortality rate than in those without AV block.

Although type I conduction disturbance is ubiquitous and can occur in any cardiac tissue in vivo as well as in vitro, the site of block for the usual forms of second-degree AV block can generally be determined from the surface ECG with sufficient reliability to permit clinical decisions without an invasive electrophysiologic study (EPS). Type I AV block with a normal QRS complex almost always takes place at the level of the AV node, proximal to the His bundle. An exception is the uncommon patient with type I intrahisian block. Type II AV block, particularly in association with a BBB, is localized to the His-Purkinje system. Type I AV block in a patient with a BBB can be caused by a

P wave can be intermittent or frequent, can occur at regular or irregular intervals, and may be preceded by fixed or lengthening PR intervals. A distinguishing feature is that conducted P waves relate to the QRS complex with recurring PR intervals; that is, the association of P with QRS is not random. Electrocardiographically, typical type I second-degree AV block is characterized by progressive PR prolongation culminating in a nonconducted P wave (Figs. 68.8 and 68.9B), whereas in type II second-degree AV block, the PR interval remains constant before the blocked P wave (Fig. 68.9A). In both cases, the AV block is intermittent and generally repetitive. Frequently, the eponyms Mobitz type I and Mobitz type II are applied to the two types of block, whereas Wenckebach block refers to type I block only. Although Wenckebach block in the AV node or in the His-Purkinje system. Type II AV block in a patient with a normal QRS complex can be caused by an intrahisian AV block, but the block is likely to be a type I AV nodal block, which exhibits small increments in AV conduction time.

DIFFERENTIATION OF TYPE I FROM TYPE II SECOND-DEGREE ATRIOVENTRICULAR BLOCK

The preceding generalizations encompass most patients with second-degree AV block. However, certain caveats must be heeded to avoid misdiagnosis because of subtle electrocardiographic changes or exceptions.

1. 2:1 AV block can be a form of type I or type II AV block (Fig. 68.10). If the QRS complex is narrow, the block is more likely to be type I and located in the AV node, and one should search for transition of the 2:1 block to a 3:2 block, during which the PR interval lengthens in the second cardiac cycle. If BBB is present, the block can be located in the AV node or His-Purkinje system.
2. AV block can occur simultaneously at two or more levels and cause difficulty in distinguishing between types I and II.
3. If the atrial rate varies, it can alter conduction times and cause type I AV block to stimulate type II block or change type II AV block into type I. For example, if the shortest atrial cycle length that has just achieved 1:1 AV nodal conduction at a constant PR interval is decreased by only 10 or 20 msec, the P wave of the shortened cycle can block conduction at the level of the AV node without an apparent increase in the antecedent PR interval. An apparent type II AV block in the His-Purkinje system can be converted to type I in the His-Purkinje system in some patients by increasing the atrial rate.
4. Concealed premature His depolarizations can create electrocardiographic patterns that simulate type I or II AV block.
5. Abrupt transient alterations in autonomic tone can cause sudden block of one or more P waves without altering the PR interval of the conducted P wave before or after the block. Thus, an apparent type II AV block would be produced at the AV node. Clinically, a burst of vagal tone usually lengthens the P-P interval, as well as produces AV block.
6. The response of the AV block to autonomic changes, either spontaneous or induced, to distinguish type I from type II AV block can be misleading. Although vagal stimulation generally increases and vagolytic agents decrease the extent of type I AV block, such conclusions are based on the assumption that the intervention acts primarily on the AV node and fail to consider rate changes. For example, atropine can minimally improve conduction in the AV node and greatly increase the sinus rate, which results in an increase in AV nodal conduction time and the degree of AV block as a result of the faster atrial rate (see Fig. 68.8B). Conversely, if an increase in vagal tone minimally prolongs AV conduction time but greatly slows the heart rate, the net effect on type I AV block may be to improve conduction. In general, however, carotid sinus massage improves and atropine worsens AV conduction in patients with His-Purkinje block, whereas the opposite results are to be expected in patients with AV nodal block. Similarly, exercise or isoproterenol is likely to increase the sinus rate and improve AV nodal block but worsen His-Purkinje block. These interventions can help differentiate the site of block without invasive study, although damaged His-Purkinje tissue may be variably influenced by changes in autonomic tone.
7. During type I AV block with high ratios of conducted beats, the increment in PR interval can be quite small and can suggest type II AV block if only the last few PR intervals before the blocked P wave are measured. Comparing the PR interval of the first beat in the long Wenckebach cycle with that of the beats immediately preceding the blocked P wave readily reveals the increment in AV conduction time.
8. The classic AV Wenckebach structure depends on a stable atrial rate and a maximal increment in AV conduction time for the second PR interval of the Wenckebach cycle along with a progressive decrease in PR lengthening in subsequent beats. Unstable or unusual alterations in the increment of AV conduction time or in the atrial rate, often seen with long Wenckebach cycles, result in atypical forms of type I AV block in which the last R-R interval can lengthen because the PR increment increases; such alterations are common.
9. Finally, the PR interval on the ECG consists of conduction through the atrium, AV node, and His-Purkinje system. An increment in H-V conduction, for example, can be masked on the ECG by a reduction in the A-H interval, and the resulting PR interval will not reflect the entire increment in His-Purkinje conduction time. Very long PR intervals (200 msec) are more likely to result from AV nodal conduction delay (and block), with or without concomitant His-Purkinje conduction delay, although an H-V interval of 390 msec is possible. The above discussion highlights the importance of measuring all intervals in an AV block series.

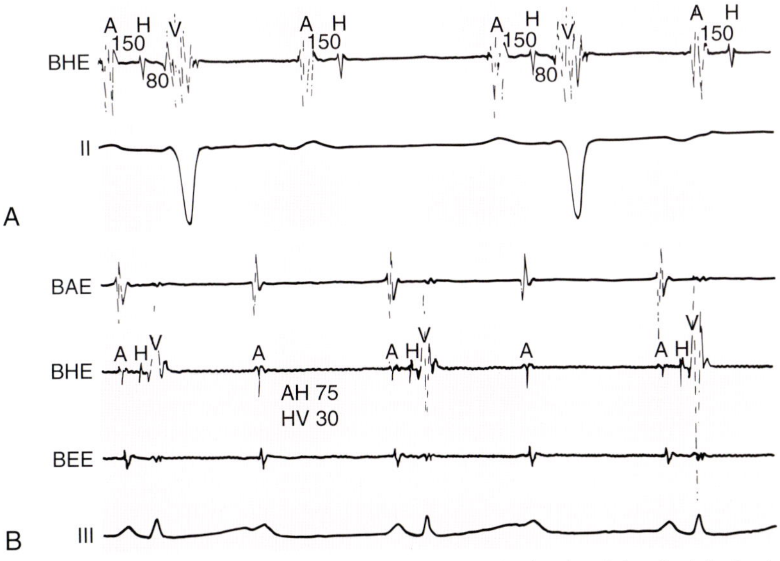

First-degree and type I second-degree AV block can occur in normal healthy children, and Wenckebach AV block can be a normal phenomenon in well-trained athletes, as noted earlier, probably related to an increase in resting vagal tone. On occasion, progressive worsening of the Wenckebach AV conduction disorder can result, and the athlete becomes symptomatic and needs to decondition. In patients who have chronic second-degree AV nodal block (proximal to the His bundle) without structural heart disease, the course is generally benign (except in older age groups), whereas in those with structural heart disease, the prognosis is poor and related to the type and severity of the underlying heart disease.

High-Grade Atrioventricular Block

High-grade, or "advanced," AV block is differentiated from complete AV block by an intermittent relationship between atrial and ventricular activity, yet conduction that is more impaired than in second-degree AV block. Some studies define high-grade AV block as Mobitz type II second-degree or third-degree AV block. The ventricular rhythm will not be regular since the diagnosis of high-grade AV block requires demonstration of intermittent AV conduction. Commonly, two or more consecutive non-conducted P waves are noted on ECG (Fig. 68.11). Etiologies include acute coronary syndromes, rheumatic heart disease, autoimmune disorders, myocarditis, and infiltrative cardiomyopathies.[8] The clinical presentation, symptoms, and outcomes are indistinguishable from third-degree AV block.

Third-Degree (Complete) Atrioventricular Block

Third-degree or complete AV block occurs when no atrial activity is conducted to the ventricles and therefore the atria and ventricles are controlled by independent pacemakers. Thus, complete AV block is one type of complete AV dissociation. The atrial pacemaker can be sinus or ectopic

FIGURE 68.10 2:1 atrioventricular (AV) block proximal and distal to the His bundle deflection in two different patients. **A,** 2:1 AV block seen on the scalar electrocardiogram occurs distal to the His bundle recording site in a patient with a right bundle branch block and anterior hemiblock. The A-H interval (150 msec) and H-V interval (80 msec) are both prolonged. **B,** 2:1 AV block proximal to the bundle of His in a patient with a normal QRS complex. The A-H interval (75 msec) and the H-V interval (30 msec) remain constant and normal. *BAE,* Bipolar atrial electrogram; *BEE,* bipolar esophageal electrogram; *BHE,* bipolar His electrogram.

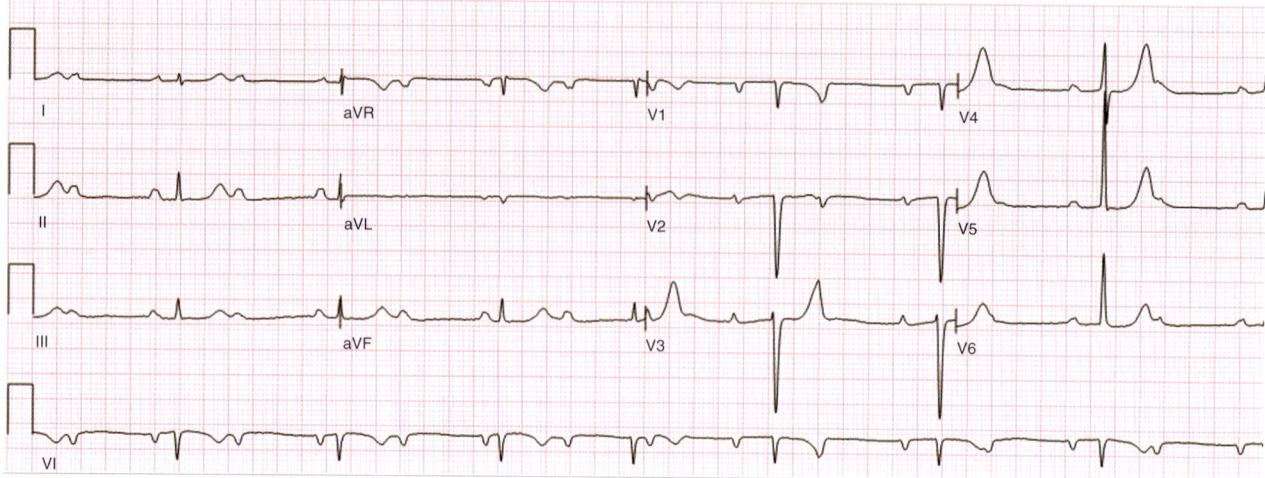

FIGURE 68.11 Electrocardiogram showing high-grade heart block. Sinus rate is 82 beats/min. The RR intervals are variable, indicating intermittent conduction and not complete heart block (QRS #4 and #5 have shorter preceding RR intervals compared with the others).

(tachycardia, flutter, or fibrillation) or can result from an AV junctional focus occurring above the level of block with retrograde atrial conduction. The ventricular focus is usually located just below the region of the block, which can be above or below the His bundle bifurcation. Sites of ventricular pacemaker activity that are in or closer to the His bundle appear to be more stable and can produce a faster escape rate than those located more distally in the ventricular conduction system. The ventricular rate in acquired complete heart block is less than 40 beats/min but can be faster with congenital complete AV block. The ventricular rhythm, usually regular, can vary in response to PVCs, a shift in the pacemaker site, an irregularly discharging pacemaker focus, or autonomic influences.[8]

Complete AV block can result from a block at the level of the AV node (usually congenital; Fig. 68.12), within the bundle of His, or distal to the His in the Purkinje system (usually acquired).[8] Block proximal to the His bundle generally exhibits normal QRS complexes and rates of 40 to 60 beats/min because the escape focus that controls the ventricle arises in or near the His bundle. In complete AV nodal block, the P wave is not followed by a His deflection, but each ventricular complex is preceded by a His deflection (Fig. 68.12). His bundle recording can be useful to differentiate AV nodal from intrahisian block because the intrahisian may carry a more serious prognosis than the AV nodal block. Intrahisian block is recognized infrequently without invasive studies. In patients with AV nodal block, atropine generally speeds both the atrial and the ventricular rate. Exercise can reduce the extent of AV nodal block. Acquired complete AV block occurs most often distal to the bundle of His because of trifascicular conduction disturbance. Each P wave is followed by a His deflection, and the ventricular escape complexes are not preceded by a His deflection. The QRS complex is abnormal, and the ventricular rate is generally less than 40 beats/min. A hereditary form of conduction block caused by degeneration of the His bundle and bundle branches has been linked to the *SCN5A* gene, which is also responsible for LQT3 (see Chapter 63).

Paroxysmal AV block in some cases can be caused by exaggerated responsiveness of the AV node to vagotonic reflexes.[9] Surgery, electrolyte disturbances, myoendocarditis, tumors, Chagas disease, rheumatoid nodules, calcific aortic stenosis, myxedema, polymyositis, infiltrative processes (e.g., amyloidosis, sarcoidosis, scleroderma), and an almost endless assortment of common and unusual conditions can produce complete AV block. In adults, rapid rates may be followed by block (called *tachycardia-dependent* AV block), which is thought to result from phase 3 block (block caused by incomplete action potential recovery), postrepolarization refractoriness, and concealed conduction in the AV node. Less common than tachycardia-dependent AV block, *pause-dependent paroxysmal* AV block can also occur; it results in AV block after a pause or during relative bradycardia and thus can be difficult to distinguish from vagal AV block. This form of AV block is often referred to as a *phase 4 block* because it is thought that

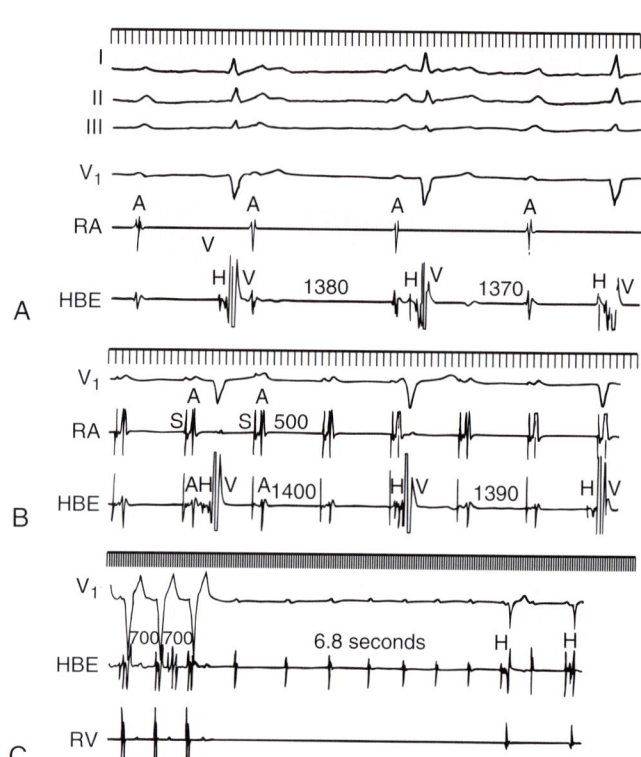

FIGURE 68.12 Congenital third-degree atrioventricular (AV) block. **A,** Complete AV nodal block is apparent. No P wave is followed by a His bundle potential, whereas each ventricular depolarization is preceded by a His bundle potential. **B,** Atrial pacing (cycle length of 500 msec) fails to alter the cycle length of the junctional rhythm. Still, no P wave is followed by a His bundle potential. **C,** After 30 seconds of ventricular pacing (cycle length of 700 msec), suppression of the junctional focus results for almost 7 seconds (overdrive suppression of automaticity). *HBE,* His bundle electrogram; *RA,* right atrium; *RV,* right ventricle.

spontaneous depolarizations during the resting phase of the action potential result in an inability to depolarize, although other mechanisms may also play a role.

In children, the most common cause of AV block is congenital (see Chapter 82). In such circumstances, the AV block can be an isolated finding or associated with other lesions. Neonatal autoimmune disease, from maternal antibodies crossing the placenta, accounts for most cases of heart block in utero or in the immediate neonatal period but only for rare cases of congenital heart block occurring after this period. Anatomic disruption between the atrial musculature and peripheral parts of the conduction system and nodoventricular discontinuity are two common histologic findings. Children are most often asymptomatic; however, in some children, symptoms requiring pacemaker implantation develop. Mortality from congenital AV block is highest in the neonatal period, is much lower during childhood and adolescence, and increases slowly later in life. Adams-Stokes attacks can occur in patients with congenital heart block at any age. It is difficult to predict the prognosis in an individual patient. A persistent heart rate at rest of 50 beats/min or less correlates with the incidence of syncope, and extreme bradycardia can contribute to the frequency of Adams-Stokes attacks in children with congenital complete AV block. The site of block may not distinguish symptomatic children who have congenital or surgically induced complete heart block from those without symptoms. Prolonged recovery times of escape foci after rapid pacing (see Fig. 68.12C), slow heart rates on 24-hour electrocardiographic recordings, and the occurrence of paroxysmal tachycardias may be factors predisposing to the development of symptoms.

Clinical Features
Many of the signs of AV block are evident at the bedside. First-degree AV block can be recognized by a long *a* to *c* wave interval in the jugular venous pulse and by diminished intensity of the first heart sound (S_1) as the PR interval lengthens (see Chapter 13). In type I second-degree AV block, the heart rate may increase imperceptibly with gradually diminishing intensity of S_1; widening of the *a* to *c* interval, terminated by a pause; and an *a* wave not followed by a *v* wave. Intermittent ventricular pauses and *a* waves in the neck not followed by *v* waves characterize type II AV block. S_1 maintains a constant intensity. In complete AV block, the findings are the same as those in AV dissociation (see later).

Significant clinical manifestations of first- and second-degree AV block usually consist of palpitations or subjective feelings of the heart "missing a beat." Persistent 2:1 AV block can produce symptoms of chronic bradycardia. Complete AV block can be accompanied by signs and symptoms of reduced cardiac output, syncope or presyncope, angina, or palpitations from ventricular tachyarrhythmias.

Management
For patients with transient or paroxysmal AV block and presyncope or syncope, the diagnosis can be elusive. Ambulatory monitoring (Holter or external loop recorders) can be useful, but monitoring for longer periods may be necessary, with extended (>3 weeks) Holter or external loop recorders being required. Longer periods of recording require an implantable loop recorder to establish the diagnosis. In patients with presyncope or syncope, one should suspect intermittent infrahisian block in those with BBB or an intraventricular conduction defect. An EPS to evaluate AV conduction thoroughly (including infusion of isoproterenol and/or procainamide) may be warranted to make the diagnosis, particularly in those with severe symptoms (see Chapter 61).

Drugs cannot be relied on to increase the heart rate for more than several hours to several days in patients with symptomatic heart block without producing significant side effects. Therefore, temporary or permanent pacemaker insertion is indicated for patients with symptomatic bradyarrhythmias. For short-term therapy, when the block is likely to be evanescent but still requires treatment or until adequate pacing therapy can be established, vagolytic agents such as atropine are useful for patients who have AV nodal disturbances, whereas catecholamines such as isoproterenol can be used transiently to treat patients who have heart block at any site (see earlier, Sinus Bradycardia). Isoproterenol should be used with extreme caution or not at all in patients with acute MI. The use of transcutaneous or temporary transvenous pacing is preferable. For symptomatic AV block or high-grade AV block (e.g., infrahisian, type II AV block, third-degree heart block not caused by congenital AV block), permanent pacemaker placement is the treatment of choice.[2,9] There is growing evidence that some patients with AV block, especially those with preexisting left ventricle dysfunction, may benefit from biventricular pacing rather than right ventricle–only pacing to prevent the development or progression of symptoms caused by heart failure.[10]

ATRIOVENTRICULAR DISSOCIATION
As the term indicates, *dissociated* or *independent* beating of the atria and ventricles defines AV dissociation. AV dissociation is never a primary disturbance of rhythm but rather is a "symptom" of an underlying rhythm disturbance produced by one of three causes or a combination of causes that prevents the normal transmission of impulses from atrium to ventricle.

CLASSIFICATION
1. Slowing of the dominant pacemaker of the heart (usually the sinus node), which allows escape of a subsidiary or latent pacemaker. AV dissociation by default of the primary pacemaker to a subsidiary one in this manner is often a normal phenomenon. It may occur during sinus arrhythmia or sinus bradycardia and permit an independent AV junction rhythm to arise (see Fig. 68.1A).
2. Acceleration of a latent pacemaker, for example, a tachycardia in which the atria are not required and that usurps control of the ventricles. An abnormally enhanced discharge rate of a usually slower subsidiary pacemaker is pathologic and typically occurs during nonparoxysmal AV junctional tachycardia or VT without retrograde atrial capture.
3. A block, generally at the AV junction, that prevents impulses formed at a normal rate in a dominant pacemaker from reaching the ventricles and allows the ventricles to beat under the control of a subsidiary pacemaker. Junctional or ventricular escape rhythm during AV block, without retrograde atrial capture, is a common example in which block gives rise to AV dissociation. Complete AV block is not synonymous with complete AV dissociation. Patients who have complete AV block have complete AV dissociation, but patients who have complete AV dissociation may or may not have complete AV block (see Fig. 68.11).
4. A combination of causes, as when excess digitalis results in the production of nonparoxysmal AV junctional tachycardia associated with SA or AV block.

MECHANISMS
With this classification in mind, it is important to emphasize that AV dissociation is not a diagnosis but a finding and is used in a manner similar to jaundice or fever. One must state that "AV dissociation is present and is caused by..." and then give the cause. An accelerated rate of a slower, normally subsidiary pacemaker and a slower rate of a faster, normally dominant pacemaker that prevents conduction because of physiologic collision and mutual extinction of opposing wavefronts (interference) or the manifestations of AV block are the basic disturbances producing AV dissociation. The atria in all these cases beat independently from the ventricles, under control of the sinus node or ectopic atrial or AV junctional pacemakers, and can exhibit any type of supraventricular rhythm. If a single pacemaker establishes control of both the atria and the ventricles for one beat (capture) or a series of beats (e.g., sinus rhythm, AV junctional rhythm with retrograde atrial capture, ventricular tachycardia [VT] with retrograde atrial capture), AV dissociation is abolished for that period. Conversely, whenever the atria and ventricles fail to respond to a single impulse for one beat (PVC without retrograde capture of the atrium) or a series of beats (VT without retrograde atrial capture), AV dissociation exists for that period. Interruption of AV dissociation by one or a series of beats under the control of one pacemaker, anterogradely or retrogradely, indicates that the AV dissociation is incomplete. Complete or incomplete dissociation can also occur in association with all forms of AV block. Usually, when AV dissociation results from AV block, the atrial rate exceeds the ventricular rate. For example, a subsidiary pacemaker with a rate of 40 beats/min can escape in the presence of a 2:1 AV block when the atrial rate is 78 beats/min. If the AV block is bidirectional, AV dissociation results.

Electrocardiographic and Clinical Features
The ECG demonstrates the independence of P waves and QRS complexes. P wave morphology depends on the rhythm controlling the atria—sinus, atrial tachycardia, junctional, flutter, or fibrillation. During complete AV dissociation, both the QRS complex and the P waves appear to be regularly spaced without a fixed temporal relationship to each other. When the dissociation is incomplete, a QRS complex with a supraventricular contour occurs early and is preceded by a P wave at

a PR interval exceeding 0.12 second and within a conductible range. This combination indicates ventricular capture by the supraventricular focus. Similarly, a premature P wave with retrograde morphology and a conductible RP interval may indicate retrograde atrial capture by the subsidiary focus.

Physical findings include a variable intensity of the first heart sound as the PR interval changes, atrial sounds, and *a* waves in the jugular venous pulse lacking a consistent relationship to ventricular contraction. Intermittent large (cannon) *a* waves may be seen in the jugular venous pulse when atrial and ventricular contractions occur simultaneously. The second heart sound can split normally or paradoxically, depending on the manner of ventricular activation. A premature beat representing ventricular capture can interrupt a regular heart rhythm. When the ventricular rate exceeds the atrial rate, a cyclic increase in intensity of the first heart sound is produced as the PR interval shortens, climaxed by a very loud sound (bruit de canon). This intense sound is followed by a sudden reduction in intensity of the first heart sound and the appearance of giant *a* waves as the PR interval shortens and P waves "march through" the cardiac cycle.

Management
Management is directed toward the underlying heart disease and precipitating cause. The individual components producing the AV dissociation, not the AV dissociation per se, determine the specific type of therapeutic, antiarrhythmic approach.

Autonomic/Neurally Mediated Bradycardia
Since the sinus node and AV node are richly innervated by the autonomic nervous system, both sinus bradyarrhythmias (sinus pauses, sinus arrest, and sinus arrhythmia) and AV block (typically type I AV block, or intermittent complete block) can be caused by autonomic influences without any underlying conduction system disease.[3] Increases in parasympathetic (vagal) tone can be triggered by a variety of events that can result in bradyarrhythmias and include hypersensitive carotid sinus syndrome, vasovagal syncope, cough syncope, stimulation of the Bezold-Jarisch receptors during an inferior MI, autonomic dysfunction, and others (see Chapter 71).[3]

Electrocardiographic Recognition
Neurally-mediated bradyarrhythmias are characterized most frequently by ventricular asystole caused by cessation of atrial activity as a result of sinus arrest or SA exit block (see Fig. 68.2). AV block is observed less frequently, probably in part because the absence of atrial activity from sinus arrest precludes the manifestations of AV block. However, if an atrial pacemaker maintained an atrial rhythm during the episodes, a higher prevalence of AV block would probably be noted. In symptomatic patients, AV junctional or ventricular escapes generally do not occur or are present at very slow rates, suggesting that heightened vagal tone and sympathetic withdrawal can suppress subsidiary pacemakers located in the ventricles, as well as in supraventricular structures.

Clinical Features
There are generally two types of neutrally mediated responses, and frequently both occur in the same patient to varying degrees. A *cardioinhibitory* response is generally defined as ventricular asystole exceeding 3 seconds, although normal limits have not been definitively established. In fact, asystole exceeding 3 seconds during carotid sinus massage is not common but can occur in asymptomatic subjects (see Fig. 68.2). A *vasodepressor* response is usually defined as a decrease in systolic blood pressure (SBP) of 50 mm Hg or more without associated cardiac slowing or a decrease in SBP exceeding 30 mm Hg when the patient's symptoms are reproduced.

Management
Atropine acutely abolishes cardioinhibitory responses to neurally mediated bradyarrhythmias. However, symptomatic patients with a cardioinhibitory response may benefit from pacemaker implantation. Because AV block can occur with a cardioinhibitory response, some form of ventricular pacing, with or without atrial pacing, is generally required. Atropine and pacing do not prevent the SBP decrease in the vasodepressor response, which may result from inhibition of sympathetic vasoconstrictor nerves and possibly from activation of cholinergic sympathetic vasodilator fibers. Combinations of vasodepressor and cardioinhibitory responses can occur, and vasodepression can account for syncope after pacemaker implantation in some patients. Patients who have neurally mediated bradyarrhythmias that do not cause symptoms require no treatment. Drugs such as digitalis, methyldopa, clonidine, and propranolol can enhance neurally mediated bradyarrhythmias and be responsible for symptoms in some patients. Elastic support hose and sodium-retaining drugs may be helpful in patients with vasodepressor responses.

REFERENCES
1. Rijnbeek PR, van Herpen G, Bots ML, et al. Normal values of the electrocardiogram for ages 16–90 years. *J Electrocardiol*. 2014;47:914–921.
2. Kusumoto FM, Schoenfeld MH, Barrett C, et al. 2018 ACC/AHA/HRS guideline on the evaluation and management of patients with bradycardia and cardiac conduction delay: a report of the American College of Cardiology/American Heart Association task force on clinical practice guidelines and the heart rhythm society. *Circulation*. 2019;140:e382–e482.
3. Bennett MT, Leader N, Krahn AD. Recurrent syncope: differential diagnosis and management. *Heart*. 2015;101:1591–1599.
4. Goldberger ZD, Petek BJ, Brignole M, et al. ACC/AHA/HRS versus ESC guidelines for the diagnosis and management of syncope: JACC guideline comparison. *J Am Coll Cardiol*. 2019;74:2410–2423.
5. Wilkoff BL, Miller RE. Exercise testing for chronotropic assessment. *Cardiol Clin*. 1992;10:705–717.
6. van de Vegte YJ, Tegegne BS, Verweij N, et al. Genetics and the heart rate response to exercise. *Cell Mol Life Sci*. 2019;76:2391–2409.
7. Brubaker PH, Kitzman DW. Chronotropic incompetence: causes, consequences, and management. *Circulation*. 2011;123:1010–1020.
8. Barra SNC, Providencia R, Paiva L, et al. A review on advanced atrioventricular block in young or middle-aged adults. *Pacing Clin Electrophysiol*. 2012;35:1395–1405.
9. Aste M, Brignole M. Syncope and paroxysmal atrioventricular block. *J Arrhythm*. 2017;33:562–567.
10. Tanawuttiwat T, Cheng A. Which patients with AV block should receive CRT pacing? *Curr Treat Options Cardiovasc Med*. 2014;16:291.

69 Pacemakers and Implantable Cardioverter-Defibrillators

MINA K. CHUNG AND JAMES P. DAUBERT

TYPES OF DEVICES, 1321
DEVICE RADIOGRAPHY, 1321
TYPES OF PACEMAKERS, 1321
INDICATIONS FOR PACEMAKERS, 1322
CAPTURE AND SENSING, 1323
Capture and Stimulation, 1323
Electrograms and Sensing Function in Pacemakers, 1324
Hemodynamic Aspects of Pacing, 1326
PACING MODE AND TIMING CYCLES, 1326
Definitions, 1326
Common Pacing Modes, 1326
Rate Responsive Pacing, 1327
Choosing a Single- or Dual-Chamber Pacing Device, 1328
Pacemaker Troubleshooting, 1328

IMPLANTABLE CARDIOVERTER-DEFIBRILLATORS, 1331
Types of ICDs, 1331
Indications for ICDs, 1331
ICD SYSTEM SELECTION, 1333
Dual- versus Single-Chamber Transvenous ICDs, 1333
Transvenous versus Subcutaneous ICD Systems, 1334
ICD THERAPY, 1336
General Considerations, 1336
ICD TROUBLESHOOTING, 1339
Ventricular Oversensing, 1339
Shocks: Diagnosis and Management, 1339
Failure to Deliver Therapy or Delayed Therapy, 1340

ICD Lead Failure: Presentation and Management, 1341
COMPLICATIONS, 1343
Vascular Access Complications, 1343
Lead Placement Complications, 1343
Pocket Hematoma and CIED Infections, 1343
Subcutaneous ICD Complications, 1343
Leadless Pacemaker Complications, 1343
FOLLOW-UP AND MANAGEMENT, 1343
Remote Monitoring, 1343
CIED Diagnostics for Atrial Fibrillation, 1344
Device Clinic Follow-Up, 1344
Electromagnetic Interference, 1344
Common Clinical Issues in CIED Patients, 1346
REFERENCES, 1347

Cardiac implantable electrical devices (CIEDs) refer to implanted devices that deliver therapeutic electrical stimuli and include permanent pacemakers and implantable cardioverter-defibrillators (ICDs).

TYPES OF DEVICES

Electrical therapy for cardiac arrhythmias includes low-voltage (typically 1 to 5 V) pacing stimuli (pulses) and high-voltage (typically 500 to 1400 V) stimuli (shocks). Pacemakers deliver pacing pulses to treat bradycardia. ICDs deliver shocks to defibrillate ventricular fibrillation (VF) or to cardiovert ventricular tachycardia (VT). ICDs also have antibradycardia pacing functions that can deliver pacing pulses to treat bradycardia, as well as antitachycardia pacing functions that can deliver sequences of rapid pacing pulses to treat ventricular or atrial tachyarrhythmias. Cardiac resynchronization therapy (CRT) pacemakers (CRT-P) or ICDs (CRT-D) also provide electrical therapy for heart failure in the form of pacing pulses that resynchronize the ventricular contraction sequence. This chapter covers antiarrhythmic electrical therapy delivered by CIEDs. See Chapters 50 and 58 for CRT in the treatment of heart failure and devices for hemodynamic monitoring, and see Chapter 61 for devices implanted for rhythm monitoring.

DEVICE RADIOGRAPHY

Chest and occasionally abdominal radiography can help to identify the type, manufacturer, and integrity of implanted devices. Transvenous system pulse generators are typically located subcutaneously in the upper chest, though in pediatric patients, some older larger devices, or devices with leads inserted via the femoral vein or epicardially, the pulse generator may be in the abdomen. Pacemaker pulse generators are smaller than ICD devices (Figs. 69.1 and 69.2). Transvenous pacemaker leads are typically implanted with lead tips in the right ventricle and right atrium. Epicardial leads may be tunneled to the devices. ICDs are readily identified by the presence of defibrillation coils on the leads (see Fig. 69.2). For CRT, leads may be placed in a left ventricular branch of the coronary sinus (Fig. 69.3) or on the LV epicardium. Some pacing leads are now being placed at the His bundle or deep septally from the right ventricle to capture the subendocardial left bundle branch conduction system (Fig. 69.4). Subcutaneous ICDs are typically placed subcutaneously in the left chest along the axillary line with leads tunneled subcutaneously (Fig. 69.5). Leadless devices can also be visualized radiographically (Fig. 69.6B).

TYPES OF PACEMAKERS

Conventional pacemaker components include a pulse generator (PG) that contains the battery and circuitry and the lead system. The lead system consists of one to three leads that are connected to the pacemaker PG via the lead pin. The lead body includes conducting wires that are surrounded by insulating material and connected to sensing and stimulating electrodes. The tip of the leads connect to the heart via an active (screw) or passive (e.g., tine) fixation mechanisms (Fig. 69.7). Conventional single-chamber systems have one lead that usually connect to the right ventricular (RV) endocardium or in some cases to the right atrium (RA). Dual-chamber systems usually have leads that connect to the right ventricle and RA (see Fig. 69.1). Cardiac resynchronization devices have a third lead that is placed to pace the left ventricle (LV) via a lead in a branch of the coronary sinus or implanted on the LV epicardial surface (see Fig. 69.3). (See Chapter 50.) Newer pacemaker configurations include leads intended to pace the cardiac conduction system, using leads placed at the His bundle or into the interventricular septum to capture the left bundle branch (see Fig. 69.4). Leadless pacemakers are also commercially available and include self-contained devices implanted via a catheter to the right ventricle (Fig. 69.6B). These provide single chamber pacing; algorithms that are designed to detect atrial contraction may be able to provide atrial synchronous pacing as well. Investigational leadless devices include right atrial or left ventricular components.

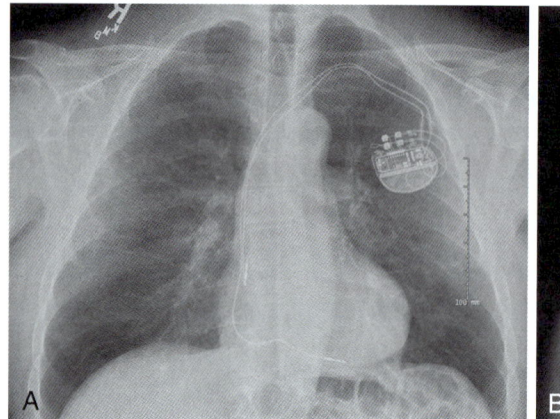
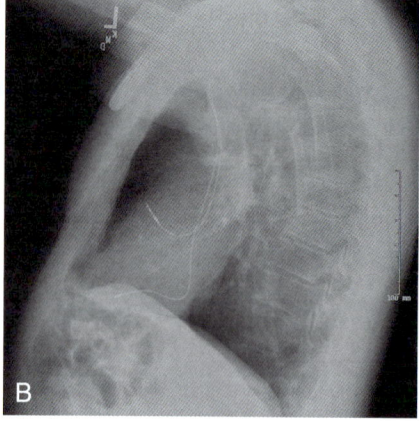

FIGURE 69.1 Chest radiograph of a dual-chamber pacemaker system. Posteroanterior (**A**) and lateral (**B**) projections demonstrate leads extending from the prepectoral pacemaker pulse generator to the right atrium and right ventricular apex.

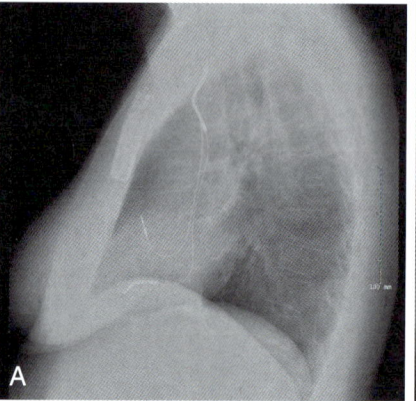
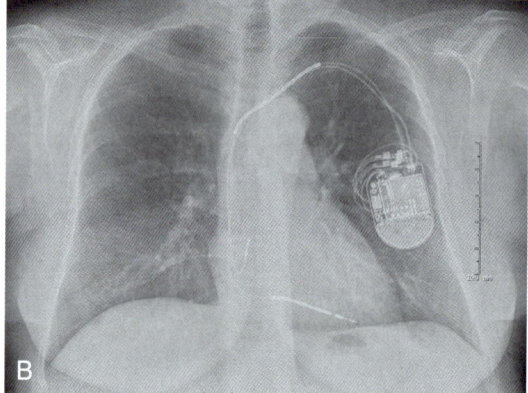

FIGURE 69.2 Chest radiograph of a dual-chamber implantable cardioverter-defibrillator (ICD) system. Lateral (**A**) and posteroanterior (**B**) projections demonstrate the ICD pulse generator in the left prepectoral region with a pacing lead extending to the right atrium and a pace/sense, dual coil defibrillation lead extending to the right ventricular apex. Defibrillation coils are evident in the brachiocephalic–superior vena cava and in the RV portions of the defibrillation lead.

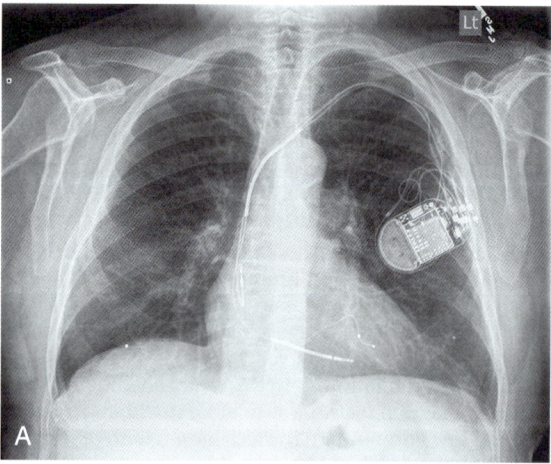
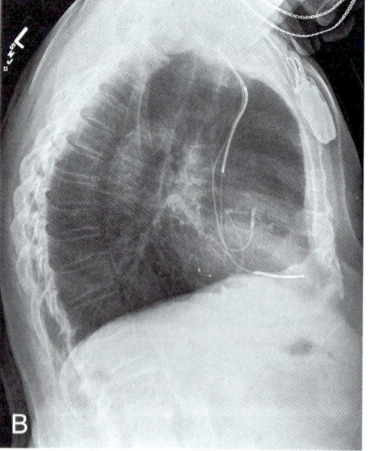

FIGURE 69.3 Chest radiograph of a cardiac resynchronization therapy defibrillator (CRT-D) system. Posteroanterior (**A**) and lateral (**B**) projections demonstrate the CRT-D ICD pulse generator in the left prepectoral region with a pacing lead extending to the right atrium, a pace/sense, dual coil defibrillation lead extending to the right ventricular apex, and a bipolar pacing lead extending to a left ventricular branch of the coronary sinus.

INDICATIONS FOR PACEMAKERS

Simply put, pacemakers are indicated for symptomatic bradycardia.[1] In the early pacemaker era such patients mainly had complete AV block with resultant intermittent asystole known as Stokes-Adams attacks.[2] In higher income countries, more pacemakers are implanted at present for symptomatic sinus node dysfunction. Patients at high risk of complete atrioventricular (AV) block due to advanced, infranodal conduction system disease may also receive a pacemaker prophylactically.[3] There is a marked age-related pacemaker indication and implantation rate with an overall prevalence of pacemakers of 500/100,000 in the U.S. Medicare population (>65) but 40/100,000 for ages 18 to 64 and 2600/100,000 for age >75.[4]

PACEMAKER LEAD AND GENERATOR DESIGN

Transvenous pacing leads are insulated wires 6 to 8F (2.0 to 2.67 mm) in diameter that carry electrical signals between a pacemaker generator, usually in the prepectoral area (superficial to the pectoralis muscle) and the endocardial surface of the heart (see Fig. 69.7). Bipolar leads have a 1 to 2 mm metallic electrode tip and a slightly larger ring electrode situated about 10 to 15 mm proximally. The electrodes are made of polished titanium and platinum alloys. Unipolar leads, now used much less commonly, though occasionally used in coronary sinus or epicardial placement, have only the tip electrode and use the metallic pacemaker generator surface as the return electrode. The tip is secured to the myocardium with passive fixation (2 to 3 mm flexible polyurethane tines that embed in trabeculated myocardium) or active fixation (via a ~1 mm screw that secures) to the endomyocardium (Fig. 69.7A). Epicardial leads are used primarily in patients with congenital heart disease, tricuspid valve replacement, endocarditis, or in the pediatric age range (Fig. 69.7C). They either screw into or are sewn onto the epicardial surface; the generator resides in the abdominal wall or pectoral region. Ventricular leads comprise RV and coronary sinus LV leads. Epicardial leads can be used on any chamber's epicardial aspect. Leads are insulated with silicone and/or polyurethane and more recently polytetrafluoroethylene. Silicone is soft and flexible but needs to be thicker, has relatively high frictional surface resistance, and is prone to abrasions. Polyurethane is stiffer, more slippery, more durable, and can be made thinner but is prone to two forms of degradation, including environmental stress cracking (ESC) and metal ion oxidation (MIO).[2] Nearly all transvenous leads have a hollow lumen for a thin malleable stylet or wire to shape or advance the lead for implantation. In cross section the lead design can be coaxial with the wire to the tip electrode in the center surrounded by insulation then the ring electrode surrounded by additional insulation or co-radial with the two different (insulated) coils wound together around the central lumen (Fig. 69.7B). Passive fixation leads are generally placed in the RV apex. Active fixation leads can be secured anywhere in the RV or in the RA. Passive fixation atrial leads have a J shape and are placed in the RA appendage, with the tines intended to secure to the trabeculated myocardium there. The connection between the lead and the generator is via a terminal pin that usually conforms to the 3.2 mm diameter IS-1 standard at present, but other size and configurations still exist.[2] Attention to these details is critical when reoperating on patients with very old leads.

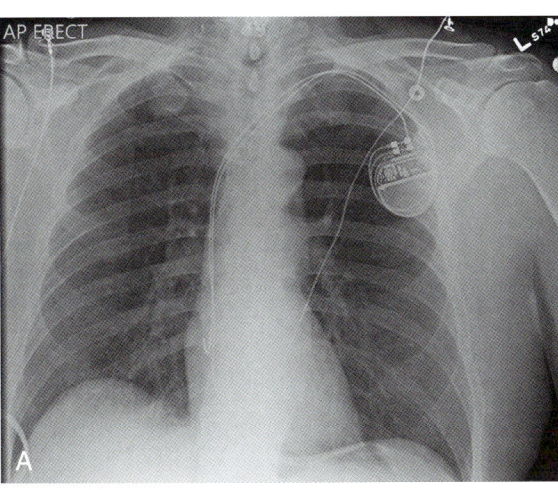
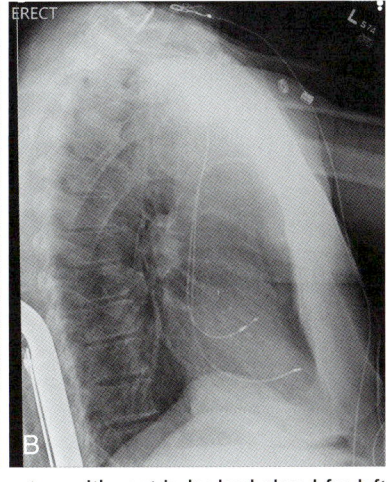

FIGURE 69.4 Chest radiograph of a dual-chamber pacemaker system with ventricular lead placed for left bundle branch pacing. Posteroanterior (**A**) and lateral (**B**) projections demonstrate pacing leads extending from the prepectoral pacemaker pulse generator to the right atrium and right ventricle with the tip inserted septally to achieve left bundle branch pacing.

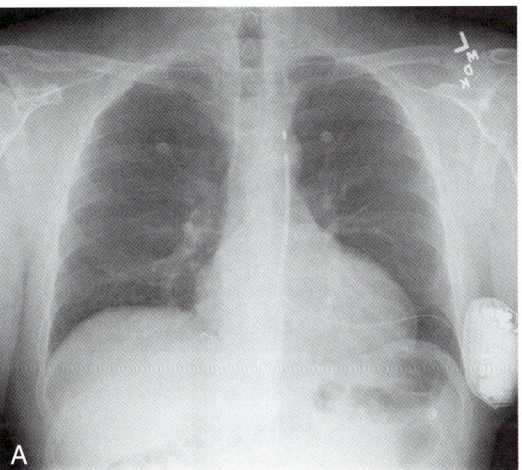
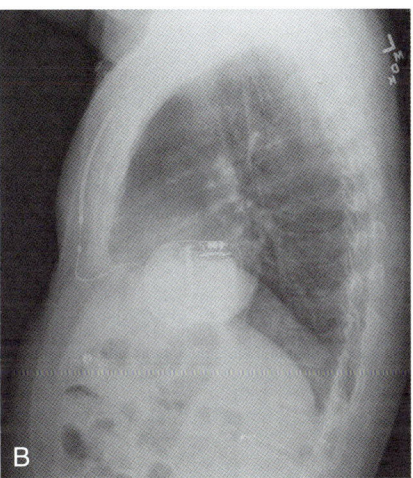

FIGURE 69.5 Chest radiograph of a subcutaneous implantable cardioverter-defibrillator (S-ICD) system. Posteroanterior (**A**) and lateral (**B**) projections demonstrate the ICD pulse generator in the left axillary region with a defibrillation lead tunneled subcutaneously to the left parasternal region.

Pacemaker generators are hermetically sealed titanium casings of varying shapes with a volume of ~10 to 15 cc housing the battery (typically lithium-iodine), sensing circuitry, activity sensors, hybrid circuit RF communication antenna, and logic boards. Glued to the generator is a clear epoxy header into which the leads are placed and secured using setscrews.

CAPTURE AND SENSING

Capture and Stimulation

Modern cardiac pacemakers perform a number of functions, but their most critical two actions remain pacing and sensing. Pacing means delivering a small (compared with a defibrillation shock) electrical stimulus of ~1 to 5 V that captures a small myocardial region adjacent to the pacing electrode yielding a propagating wavefront in the chambers of interest (i.e., the atria or ventricles).

A pacing stimulus that fails to capture is subthreshold. A stronger stimulus is required during the relative refractory period compared with electrically recovered tissue; cathodal versus anodal stimuli exhibit different characteristics, too.[5] Events leading to capture are complex when the three-dimensional structure and fiber orientation is taken into account with some stimuli leading to hyperpolarization versus depolarization occurring in adjacent regions.[2] Determinants of the threshold for a given pacing lead, above which "capture" occurs, include the stimulus strength (in voltage or current) and the pulse duration. An important relationship is Ohm's law (V = IR, where V is voltage, I is current, and R is resistance).

The strength-duration curve describes the relationship between pulse strength (usually voltage) and duration and whether capture occurs or not (Fig. 69.8). At an infinitely long pulse duration, practically estimated as about 1.5 to 2.0 msec, a minimal pulse strength (in V) eliciting capture is known as the rheobase. With shorter pulse durations, the threshold voltage (i.e., that required to capture) gradually and then abruptly increases at very short pulse durations (about 0.1 to 0.2 msec). The pulse duration at which the voltage threshold is twice the rheobase voltage is defined as the chronaxie. These concepts are important to understand threshold measurements, defining a safe margin for capture and optimizing battery longevity. Energy usage by pacing pulses are described by $J = VIt = V^2 t(1/R)$ (where J is energy, V = voltage, I = current, t = pulse duration, and R = impedance). Monophasic pulses are used for pacing, whereas biphasic ones have advantages for defibrillation. Cathodal stimulation is used in pacing, so the distal electrode is the cathode. Pacing stimuli can be unipolar, wherein the return pole is the pacemaker generator housing or bipolar with an anodal ring electrode. Under certain circumstances, capture may occur at both sites (i.e., "anodal capture"). Of note, the capacitor-generated pulse declines over the course of the stimulus from a leading to a trailing edge voltage.

As illustrated in Figure 69.8, increasing the pulse width beyond about 1 msec provides little safety margin. Similarly, increasing the voltage at very short pulse durations (0.1 to 0.15 msec) is ineffective due to the steep ascent of the curve. Examining the energy curve (see Fig. 69.8) illustrates that the optimal combination of safety margin, and efficiency usually is found near the chronaxie.[2] Thresholds can be measured manually by reducing the voltage while maintaining the pulse width constant (or vice versa). A reliable electrocardiogram (ECG) is required to avoid prolonged loss of capture in device-dependent patients and correctly interpret the results for safety and battery longevity.

Thresholds are also measured automatically by most devices, in some or all chambers, usually by assessing for an evoked response indicating tissue capture, as distinguished from electrode polarization right after the pacing pulse. The device can be programmed to adjust the pacing output to achieve a desired safety margin automatically. In some devices, capture is confirmed on a beat-to-beat basis and using a pacing output only slightly (0.125 to 0.5 V) above threshold. In other devices and/or chambers, once the threshold is measured, pacing is set at a programmable amount, often two times the threshold, and the threshold is measured one or more times a day. In the latter scenario, beat-to-beat capture, using an evoked response, is not determined. For some devices, when AV conduction is present, atrial threshold is measured automatically by ascertaining a conducted ventricular event. Alternatively, the native atrial response to a premature atrial test pulse can determine whether capture occurs. LV threshold can be measured by evaluating whether an RV event is sensed after an LV pacing test pulse.

Pacing thresholds frequently vary over time early after implantation. For active fixation leads, transient myocardial injury elicited by securing them produces an elevated threshold for minutes to hours.

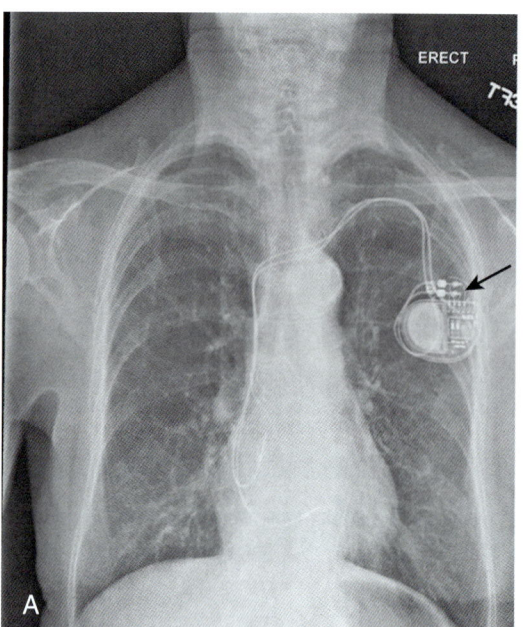
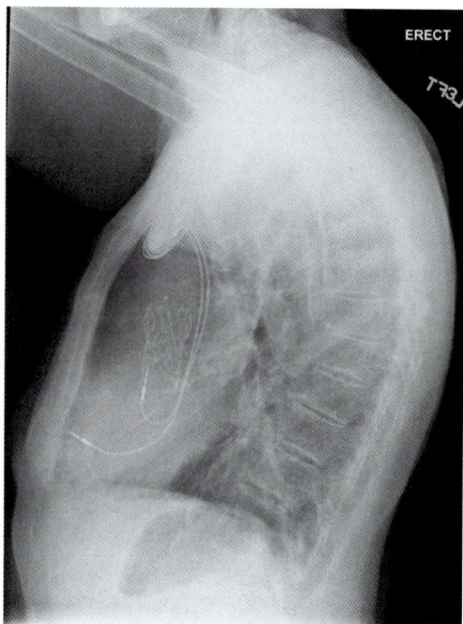
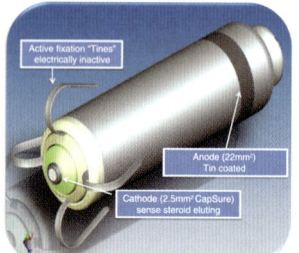
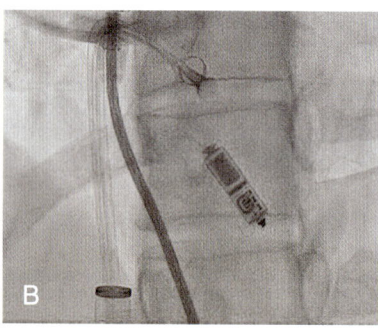
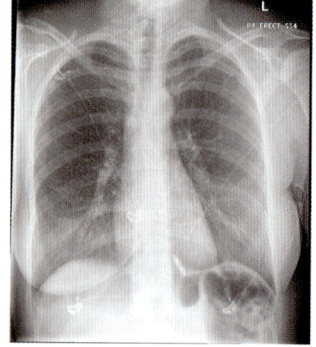
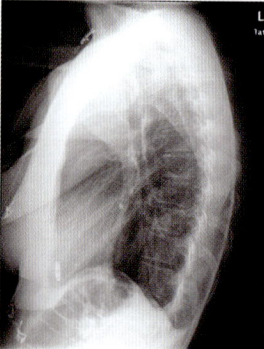

FIGURE 69.6 Transvenous and leadless pacemakers. **A,** Dual-chamber pacing system with bipolar right atrial active fixation and bipolar right ventricular active fixation leads with PA (*left*) and lateral (*right*) projections. The patient is post-TAVR, which resulted in complete heart block. Note the lead terminal pins (*arrow*) inserted into the pacemaker header and secured with set screws. Terminal pins have had several formats, but IS-1 is used predominantly for pacing leads now. **B,** Leadless cardiac pacemaker (*upper left panel*). *Lower left,* Insertion catheter has been decoupled from the leadless cardiac pacemaker after implantation and is being removed. An angiogram is usually performed through the catheter before implantation. *Right,* leadless cardiac pacemaker in PA and lateral projections in the right ventricular apex. *TAVR,* transcutaneous aortic valve replacement.

Inflammation at the electrode tissue interface leads to a subacute threshold rise resolving in about 6 weeks. However, the magnitude of this rise has been minimized with corticosteroid-eluting leads. Nevertheless, even with such leads, a fibrous capsule develops around the implanted electrode. Smaller electrodes display a higher impedance thus favorably reducing current drain (Ohm's law). However, they are more prone to threshold elevation and exit block due to the reactive fibrous cap. Electrode porosity, a fractal design in effect increasing the surface area, avoiding corrosion, and chemical composition are other important aspects of pacing electrode design.

Drugs, electrolyte perturbations, and metabolic changes also affect pacing thresholds. Severe hyperkalemia results in an elevation of pacing thresholds; significant hyperglycemia, severe hypothyroidism, and also acidosis or alkalosis can elevate thresholds. Some studies, but not all, have found that sodium channel blocking drugs (flecainide, propafenone, and others, as well as amiodarone) may elevate the pacing threshold as well. Acute ischemia and chronic infarction may also result in loss of capture.

Electrograms and Sensing Function in Pacemakers

Apart from pacemakers functioning in the asynchronous modes (VOO, DOO; see Table 69.1), pacemakers need to accurately detect underlying atrial and/or ventricular native signals in order to know whether to and when to deliver a pacing stimulus. A stable position abutting viable myocardial tissue makes this possible, but numerous challenges exist. Sensing is dependent on the electrogram (EGM) characteristics, including amplitude and frequency content, but also filtering within the device.

The EGM derives from the temporal change in the local voltage between the two electrodes (for a bipolar lead or between the tip electrode and the generator for a unipolar sensing circuit) as the activation wavefront travels toward and then away from the electrode(s).[6,7] For a unipolar lead, as the wavefront moves toward the electrode, a positive EGM is inscribed and crosses baseline when it reaches the electrode; a negative

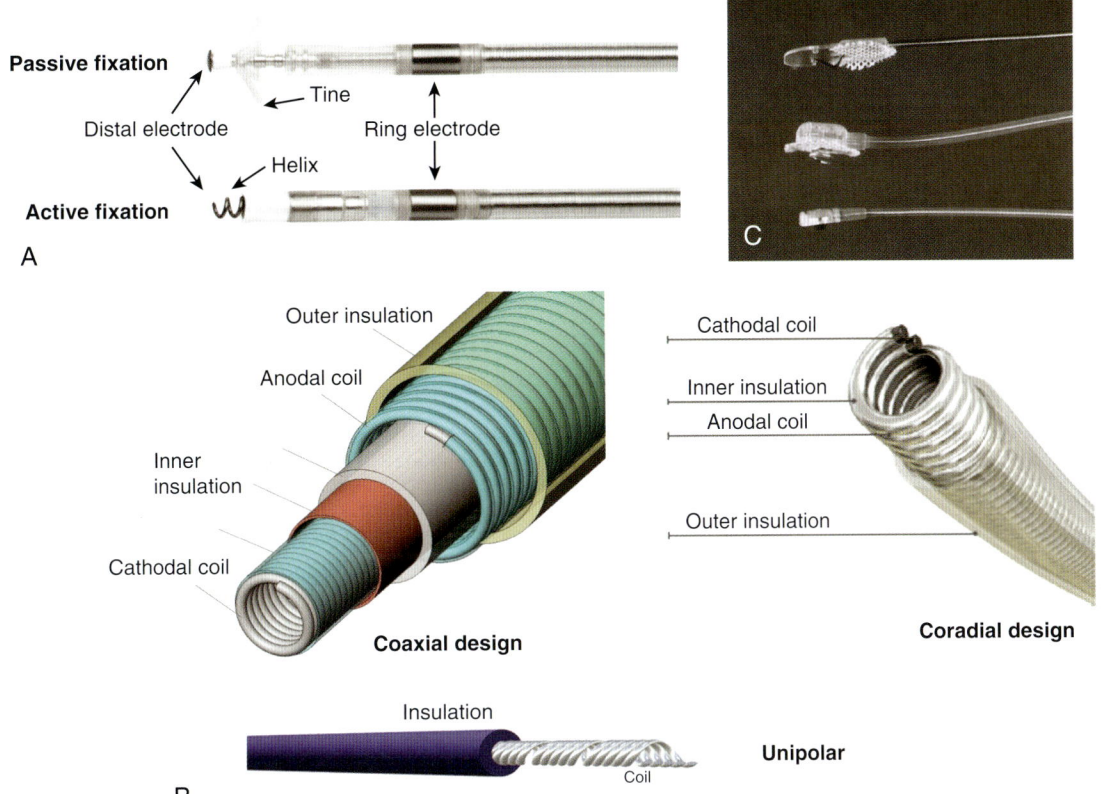

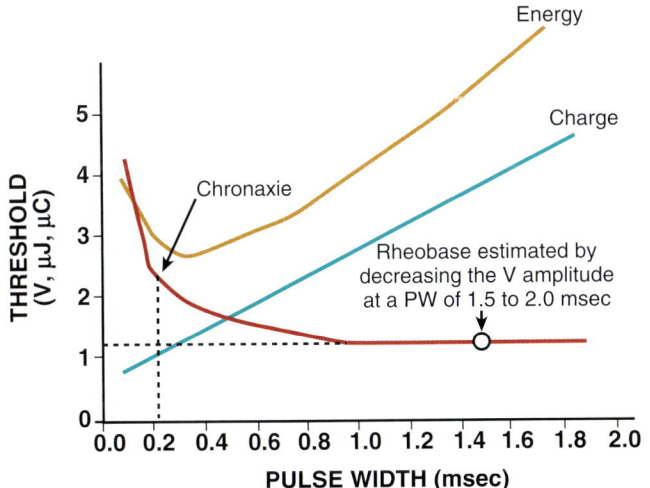

FIGURE 69.7 Pacing lead design. **A,** Lead fixation types. *Top,* Passive fixation (tined design) bipolar lead. *Bottom,* Active fixation bipolar lead with helical screw serving as distal electrode. Active fixation leads may have either extendable-retractable or fixed screws that are covered with mannitol that dissolves after several minutes in the bloodstream. **B,** Lead design types. *Left,* Coaxial leads have the distal or tip electrode (cathodal) coil on the inside with one or more layers of polyurethane or silicone insulation around the coil, the ring or proximal (anodal) electrode's coil wound around that inner insulation, and then another layer (or more) of outer insulation. *Right,* Coradial leads have the distal electrode and proximal electrode's coils individually insulated adjacent to each other and surrounded by one (or more) layers of outer insulation. *Bottom,* Unipolar leads are simple with the single electrode surrounded by insulation. **C,** Epicardial leads, which have puncture, screw-in, or sew-on fixation and contact mechanisms. They are used when endocardial leads are not feasible in certain types of congenital heart disease, young children, and after endocarditis or tricuspid valve replacement.

FIGURE 69.8 Strength-duration curve. The red curve displays the chronic, pacing threshold in volts (V), on the y-axis, from a canine at specific pulse durations (x-axis), known as the strength-duration curve. Capture occurs above and to the right of this curve. Also plotted are charge (µC), and energy (µJ) for the combination of voltage and pulse duration. Rheobase is the threshold at an infinitely long pulse width (PW) duration. Chronaxie is the pulse duration at twice the rheobase. (From Stokes K, Bornzin G. The electrode-biointerface stimulation. In Barold SS, editor: Modern Cardiac Pacing. Mount Kisco, NY: Futura; 1985, pp 33-77.)

TABLE 69.1 NASPE/BPEG Generic Code for Bradycardia Pacing

Category	POSITION			
	I	II	III	IV
	Chamber(s) paced	Chamber(s) sensed	Response to sensing	Rate modulation
	O = None	O = None	O = None	O = None
	A = Atrium	A = Atrium	T = Triggered	R = Rate modulation
	V = Ventricle	V = Ventricle	I = Inhibited	
	D = Dual (A + V)	D = Dual (A + V)	D = Dual (T + I)	
Manufacturers' designation only	S = Single (A or V)	S = Single (A or V)		

See text for explanation of use of the code.
BPEG, British Pacing and Electrophysiology Group; *NASPE,* North American Society of Pacing and Electrophysiology.
(Modified from Bernstein AD, et al. The revised NASPE/BPEG generic code for antibradycardia, adaptive-rate, and multisite pacing. Pacing Clin Electrophysiol 2002;25:260.)

signal is inscribed as the waveform moves away. With a bipolar lead the EGM is the difference between the two unipolar electrodes. Thus, the direction of the activation wavefront with respect to the bipolar pair influences the EGM size and shape, too. Bipolar leads in the ventricle sense the activation wavefront (commonly called the local R wave) but may also sense the repolarization signal (local T wave), and rarely the atrial activation event (e.g., if placed basally near the tricuspid annulus). Sensed signals vary in their timing, amplitude, and frequency content. Thus, bandpass filters are used to reduce the likelihood of sensing the wrong electrical events. Sensing of T waves can to some degree be avoided with a high pass filter above about 15 Hz (i.e., excludes lower frequencies). Local atrial and ventricular signals exhibit frequencies in the 5 to 50 Hz range, and T waves and far-field R waves exhibit frequencies in the 1 to 10 Hz range. The timing of events can also be used to exclude certain signals and thereby avoid inappropriate sensing, for example, the ventricular blanking and refractory periods and the postventricular atrial blanking and postventricular atrial refractory period. The signal from the lead undergoes amplification, filtering, and rectification and is then evaluated for whether it meets the sensing level programmed. Sensing in the atrial signals is more challenging due to the presence of large far-field ventricular signals. These far-field R waves exhibit a lower frequency range than the local atrial signal, as noted above. At implantation, P waves of about 1.5 mv or greater and R waves of 5 mv or greater are sought. Sensing thresholds for P waves thus are usually set at between 0.25 and 1.0 mv, and in the ventricle at about 2.0 mv. Setting the sensing threshold to a lower number *increases* the sensitivity reducing the chance of undersensing (but increasing the chance of oversensing). With unipolar leads, oversensing of pectoral myopotentials from the generator is a concern; in the ventricle this could lead to asystole in a pacemaker-dependent patient.

Hemodynamic Aspects of Pacing

Severe bradycardia and/or complete heart block with a junctional or ventricular escape adversely affects cardiac output. Instituting ventricular pacing at normal rates dramatically improves cardiac output by 25% to 30%. Restoring AV synchrony augments cardiac output still more by about 20%.[2] Studies in the 1980s demonstrated that chronotropic response was dominant in improving exercise capacity over AV synchrony.

Nevertheless, there are additional advantages of maintaining the AV relationship. When patients were randomized to different rate responsive modes, most preferred a mode that maintained AV synchrony (i.e., DDDR rather than VVIR).[2] Moreover, pacemaker syndrome occurs in 3% to 30% of patients who have ongoing sinus activity (i.e., not atrial fibrillation) when subjected to ventricular pacing. Its manifestations include fatigue, dyspnea, dizziness, neck pulsations, chest pain, and hypotension. It is most common when a fixed VA relationship is present, wherein the atrial contractions encounter closed AV valves. Dual-chamber as compared with single-chamber pacing leads to reduced occurrence of atrial fibrillation and of stroke and better quality of life in follow-up.[2]

For dual-chamber pacing the AV interval is of importance. Pacemaker syndrome can occur with a severely prolonged PR interval analogously to the problem with VA conduction alluded to above. On the other hand, too short of an AV interval or a marked interatrial conduction delay adversely affects performance. A hemodynamically optimal AV interval is typically about 150 msec at rest and somewhat less with exertion.[2]

The potential deleterious effects of RV pacing were initially obscured by the advantages of (1) any pacing over severe bradycardia, (2) AV sequential pacing over ventricular-only pacing, and (3) rate-responsive pacing over fixed-rate pacing. Although slightly reduced LV function occurs acutely, even in patients with normal ventricular function, RV pacing rarely exhibits clinically obvious adverse effects in the short term in such patients.[2] Elegant studies of direct His bundle stimulation clearly identified that both the contribution of atrial systole (by varying PR interval) and ventricular activation sequence (by comparing atrial-His bundle with atrial-RV) influenced ventricular function.

Clinicians became much more aware of the adverse effects of (right) ventricular stimulation on ventricular function, especially over the long term in the early 2000s. The ameliorative role of biventricular pacing (CRT) in treating LBBB-related ventricular dysfunction cemented this observation since conduction with LBBB resembles RV apical pacing. Studies comparing ventricular pacing to native ventricular activation, especially in those with LV systolic dysfunction, demonstrated significantly increased heart failure events.[2] The magnitude of the detriment with RV pacing worsened with greater QRS prolongation and worse baseline LV function.[2]

The adverse effects of RV pacing were initially attributed to the RV apex in particular. However, targeting alternative sites such as the septum actually proved somewhat elusive and led to minimal advantages.[8] Thus, algorithms emerged to limit RV pacing in dual-chamber pacemakers (as discussed later).[2] These algorithms sometimes fostered very prolonged AV intervals, however, with potential hemodynamic consequences akin to pacemaker syndrome and an increased tendency toward atrial fibrillation and pause-dependent arrhythmias.[2]

When ventricular pacing was unavoidable, as in AV block, achieving more physiologic ventricular activation has become important using either biventricular or His bundle or LBB-area pacing.[2,9,10,11]

His Bundle and Left Bundle Branch Area Pacing

Permanent His bundle pacing was reported in a small cohort in 2000. However, owing to the perceived technical difficulty, rudimentary tools, and frequently elevated thresholds, uptake was modest. The field has exploded since 2014 when a cohort study reported high procedural success rates and better outcomes than with conventional DDD pacing.[12] Dedicated sheaths and leads have eventually emerged and more improvements are expected.[9,13] His bundle capture can be selective or nonselective wherein local ventricular tissue is captured in addition to the His bundle.[14] The electrocardiography of His bundle pacing has been reviewed.[14] His bundle pacing is being used in advanced AV block but also when atrial pacing is needed with marked first-degree AV block to avoid worsening AV dyssynchrony. In addition, it has been used to correct LBBB leading to corroboration of concepts that BBB could be very proximal or even within the His bundle.[15] Elevated thresholds especially for correcting LBBB but even for His bundle capture in follow-up, and the potential for distal conduction system progression, have led to an iterative approach of targeting the LBBB, its fascicles, or the immediate region.[16]

PACING MODE AND TIMING CYCLES

Definitions

The current convention for naming pacemaker modes stems from 2001 consensus between the North American Society for Pacing and Electrophysiology (NASPE) and the British Pacing and Electrophysiology Groups (see Table 69.1). This convention specifies that five positions describe the functionality of pacemakers. The first position lists the chambers paced (A, V, or both, D). The second similarly describes the chambers sensed. The third letter specifies the device's response(s) to sensed events. Position or letter IV specifies the presence or absence of rate response. Position V specifies the location or absence of multisite pacing (i.e., biatrial or biventricular pacing with at least two stimulation sites in each case).

Timing cycles, usually in msec, characterize the function of a pacemaker in different modes. Various periods, like a clock, run sequentially or simultaneously and specify what the pacemaker will do at the end of the period or during the period if another event occurs.

Common Pacing Modes

VOO is the simplest mode (Fig. 69.9A). From the first through third letter, respectively, the mode paces only in the ventricle, does not sense the atrium or ventricle (O), and behaves asynchronously (O). There is one timing clock, the ventricular escape interval. For example, for VOO 60 bpm, the ventricular escape interval is 1000 msec (60,000 msec/min/60/min = 1000 msec). Thus every 1000 msec the pacemaker delivers a ventricular pacing pulse (even if a native ventricular beat has occurred).

VVI implies pacing in the ventricle (V) and sensing in the ventricle (V), and if a sensed event occurs, the next scheduled pacing pulse is inhibited (I) (Fig. 69.9B). The sensed event resets the ventricular escape interval. This mode adds a ventricular refractory period, during which sensed events are ignored. This prevents double counting ventricular events or local T waves and falsely inhibiting pacing.

In most pacemakers, applying a magnet converts the function from VVI to VOO. Depending upon the manufacturer, model, and

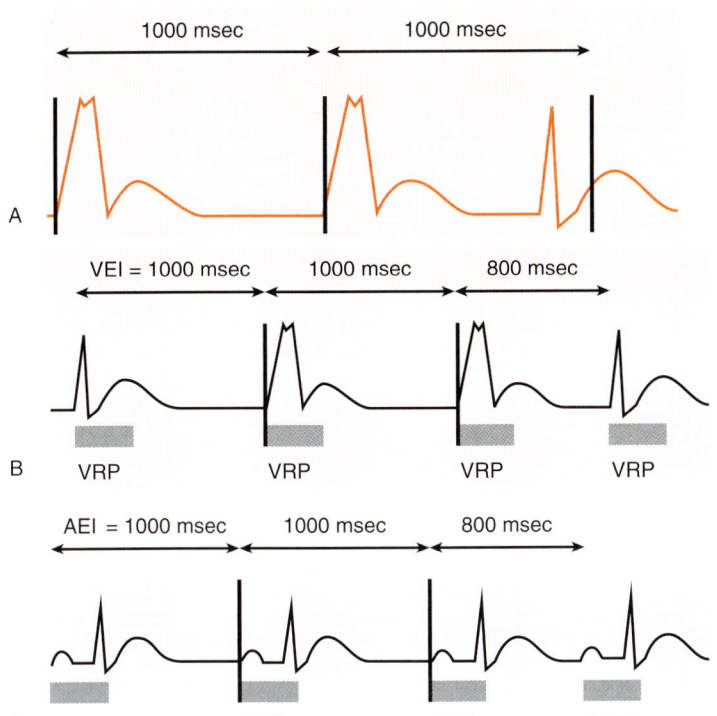

FIGURE 69.9 Single chamber modes. **A,** VOO mode. The device does not sense; it paces at a fixed rate even if intrinsic beats occur (third complex). **B,** VVI mode. The VVI timing cycle consists of a defined lower rate limit and a ventricular refractory period (VRP, gray rectangles). When the ventricular escape interval (VEI) from the ventricular sensed event of 1000 msec is completed, a paced event occurs. Because no ventricular sensed event occurs within 1000 msec after the paced event, a second ventricular paced event occurs. Because a ventricular sensed event occurs 800 msec later, a ventricular paced event does not occur. A VRP begins with any sensed or paced ventricular activity. **C,** AAI mode. The AAI timing cycle consists of a defined lower rate limit and an atrial refractory period (ARP, gray rectangles). When the atrial escape interval (AEI) from the atrial sensed event of 1000 msec is completed, a paced event occurs. Analogous to VVI mode.

programming magnet application may also change the pacing rate and/or initiate other temporary behavior (e.g., performing a pacing threshold test). The VOO mode is useful when oversensing is present as in a lead fracture or is anticipated due to electrocautery or other electromagnetic interference (EMI).

With respect to single chamber atrial pacing, AOO is analogous to VOO and AAI resembles VVI. In AAI, the device paces only in the atrium and senses in the atrium (Fig. 69.9C). In response to a sensed event, the next scheduled pacing pulse is inhibited, resetting the atrial escape interval. This mode, like VVI, has a refractory period, the atrial refractory period, during which sensed events are ignored. This prevents double counting atrial signals, or inappropriate sensing of far-field ventricular events that would falsely inhibit pacing. This mode is infrequently used due to the absence of ventricular support in the event of AV block.

Dual-chamber modes more than double the complexity. In DDD, the most commonly used one, pacing as well as sensing may occur in both the atrium and ventricle, as is evident from the first two letters (Fig. 69.10). The third letter indicates that both inhibition and triggered events occur depending upon the circumstances. DDD preserves AV synchrony where possible. Unlike VVI or AAI there is an upper rate limit in addition to a lower rate limit. The occurrence of pacing versus native activity in the atrium and in the ventricle depends on the programmed rate and AV interval compared with the native sinus rate and AV conduction characteristics. Timing can be based on either the atrium or the ventricle. The AV interval may be different for sensed atrial versus paced atrial events and may shorten with faster rates.

An atrial paced atrial event initiates a post-atrial ventricular blanking period to minimize the chance of the ventricular channel sensing the atrial pacing spike, also called crosstalk, and inappropriately inhibiting resulting in ventricular asystole in the setting of complete AV block. Since crosstalk may even occur after the 40 to 60 msec post-atrial ventricular blanking period, DDD timing features a ventricular safety pacing interval (ending at about 100 to 110 msec after the atrial pacing spike). Should ventricular sensing occur between the end of the post-atrial ventricular blanking period and the end of the ventricular safety pacing interval (due to crosstalk, a premature ventricular complex [PVC], or very rapid native conduction), the device will V pace using an abbreviated AV interval (~100 to 110 msec). If the sensing in this interval was due to crosstalk, asystole is prevented. If the sensing was due to a PVC, the abbreviated AV interval seeks to pace early enough after a PVC to avoid an R-on-T event. The post-atrial ventricular blanking tries to prevent crosstalk, while the safety pacing interval and function prevents asystole if crosstalk occurs. These blanking and safety pacing intervals don't exist after atrial sensed events. The chance for crosstalk can be reduced by using bipolar rather than unipolar atrial pacing, reducing the atrial output to an appropriate safety margin, using bipolar ventricular (rather than unipolar) sensing, decreasing the ventricular sensitivity (increasing the numerical value), and increasing the post-atrial ventricular blanking period duration.

The ventricular sensed or paced event initiates an atrial refractory period, the postventricular atrial refractory period (PVARP). PVARP seeks to prevent the atrial channel from sensing either the far-field ventricular event or retrograde atrial events initiated by the ventricular event or atrial tachyarrhythmias. As in VVI, a ventricular refractory period is present as well to prevent double counting.

The DDI mode is used much less often. Unlike DDD, it does not exhibit atrial tracking. Thus, it can be useful in the setting of atrial oversensing to avoid inappropriate ventricular pacing. Another use of DDI is when there is intermittent atrial fibrillation but suboptimal atrial sensing prevents mode switching (in DDD); tracking of the AF is avoided in DDI. Operationally, in DDI, if the sinus rate is below the lower rate limit (LRL) the device will atrial pace at the LRL and then either native ventricular conduction will occur or the device will pace the ventricle at the conclusion of the AV delay. If the sinus rate is above the LRL the device will inhibit in the atrium; if AV conduction is absent it will pace the ventricle at the LRL (at a different rate than the atrium is firing, thus losing AV synchrony).

The VDD mode is adequate for patients with intact sinus node function but with AV block. However, should sinus bradycardia below the LRL develop, the device will pace the ventricle (only, as the initial letter implies) at the LRL losing AV synchrony.

Rate Responsive Pacing

Each of the aforementioned modes can function in a rate responsive fashion as well, provided the pacemaker generator has a sensor (or sensors) for rate adaptive pacing. As discussed above, the most important mechanism for increasing cardiac output with exercise is the capacity to double or triple the heart rate since stroke volume can only be increased slightly compared with rest. Most sensors attempt to detect motion by the patient, such as walking, via an accelerometer.

Limitations to the effectiveness of a motion-based sensor include the potential for a car passenger on a bumpy road or a patient with a tremor to experience a rate increase (worse with vibration sensors), or conversely, for a rock climber or cyclist (whose torso is moving little) to undergo negligible rate augmentation (e.g., with accelerometers). Consequently, numerous modalities have been attempted to detect the need for increased rate including respiratory volume change, catecholamine-induced increased myocardial contractility, the QT interval, pH, dP/dt, central venous temperature, oxygen saturation, peak endocardial acceleration as a measure of myocardial contractility, and RV lead impedance (correlated with contractility or inotropy). Of these, accelerometers are most widely used, with minute ventilation and RV lead impedance also in use.

For the single chamber modes (VOO, VVI, AAI, AOO), which do not have an upper rate limit and only an LRL, their rate-responsive forms (VOOR, VVIR, AAIR, AOOR) now add an upper rate limit. When the patient is at rest, the device paces at the LRL. Otherwise the pacing rate

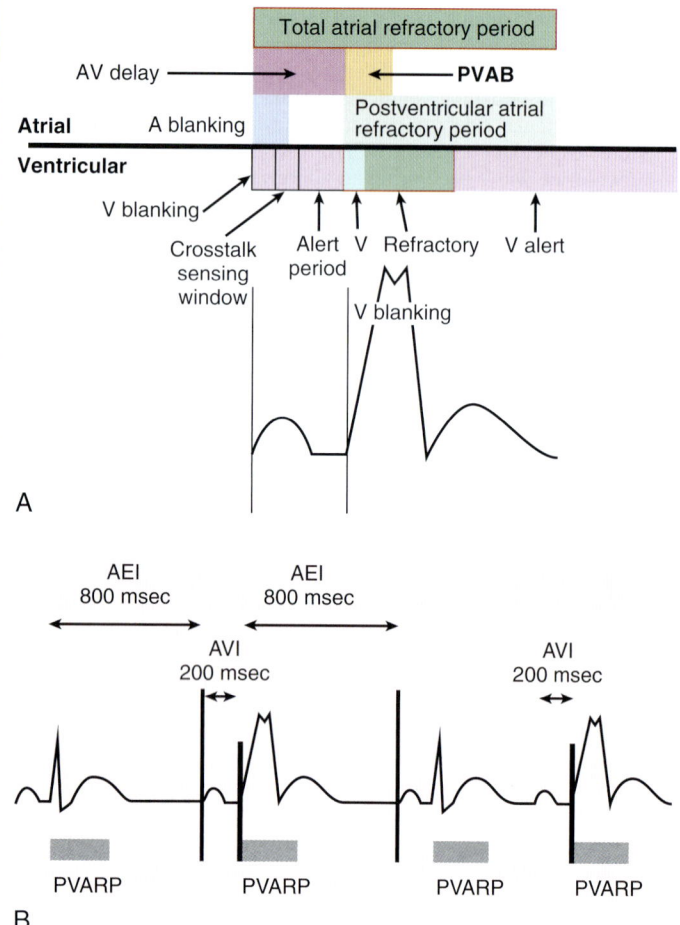

FIGURE 69.10 Basic DDD timing cycle and operation. A, The timing cycle in DDD. *Top,* Atrial channel. *Bottom,* Ventricular channel. Total atrial refractory period (TARP) is the sum of the AV delay and the postventricular atrial refractory period (PVARP). Postventricular atrial blanking (PVAB) is the time that the atrial channel is blanked after a ventricular event. "A blanking" is the atrial blanking period, representing the blanking period after an atrial event. There are two ventricular blanking periods, one after the atrial paced event, which prevents atrial paced events from being sensed on the ventricular channel, and one after the ventricular event. A ventricular sensed event in the crosstalk sensing window will result in safety pacing. There are two ventricular alert periods, one at the end of the AV delay and one after the ventricular refractory period. **B,** Operation of DDD mode. Because an intrinsic atrial event occurs and is followed by an intrinsic ventricular event within the AV interval, no ventricular pacing occurs in the first beat. In ventricular-based timing, the time from a ventricular paced or sensed event to the next atrial paced event is called the atrial escape interval (AEI), which is the lower rate limit interval minus the AV interval. Because no intrinsic atrial event occurs before the AEI times out, a paced atrial event occurs in the second beat. Since no intrinsic ventricular event occurs within the AV interval after this atrial paced event, a ventricular paced event occurs. Following this ventricular paced event an atrial paced event is delivered when the AEI times out 800 msec later to initiate the third beat. Since AV conduction follows this atrial paced event, ventricular pacing is inhibited. The fourth beat begins with an intrinsic atrial event that is not followed by an intrinsic ventricular event within the AV interval. Hence the intrinsic atrial event is "tracked" and followed by a paced ventricular event. The AV delay may vary for an atrial sensed or atrial paced event, at different rates (rate responsive AV delay), and to minimize RV pacing.

is determined by the sensor. The goal is the gradual increase in rate to match the activity and after return to rest a gradual (not immediate) decrease in rate to baseline. Sensor gain or function can be calibrated to the patient's specific physiology and activities with thresholds and response curves and other adjustments. Devices with dual sensor can use one to cross check the other or to blend the input from the two. For dual-chamber modes, already featuring an upper (tracking) rate limit, a second upper rate limit is defined for the sensor as well as the one for the maximum rate allowed in tracking the atrial rhythm.

Enhancements to the DDD Pacing Mode
Response to Atrial Tachyarrhythmias. When first devised, the DDD mode was highly problematic for patients with atrial tachyarrhythmias because atrial fibrillation would cause the device to abruptly pace at or near the upper rate limit. This problem led to the development of an ability to detect the presence of atrial fibrillation (flutter or tachycardia) and when present "mode switch" to a non-tracking mode, DDI(R) (Fig. 69.11). Practically DDI(R) functions as VVI(R) but allows ongoing surveillance of the status of the atrial arrhythmia.

To achieve mode switching, atrial events needed to be identified even within certain refractory zones such as the PVARP. A minimal atrial rate to define the arrhythmia is programmable. The device switches back to tracking (DDD or DDDR) when it confirms that the tachyarrhythmia has ended.

A related issue is nonphysiologic noise detection and response. External electromagnetic interference, such as electrocautery, could be sensed as intrinsic cardiac rhythm leading to inappropriate inhibition, and in the pacemaker-dependent patient, asystole. Noise detection and rejection algorithms can allow the device to pace asynchronously in this scenario; if noise is anticipated, the pacemaker can be programmed to an asynchronous mode (DOO, VOO, or AOO) or a magnet could be applied.

The ADI Mode to Reduce Right Ventricular Pacing
While dual-chamber pacing restores AV synchrony, it exhibits the disadvantage of a tendency to pace the right ventricle, even in the absence of complete AV block. As compared with native sinus rhythm, when the atrium is paced, intraatrial conduction is prolonged, and at faster rates AV nodal conduction may be prolonged. These two factors tend to result in ventricular pacing, unless the AV delay is set to a nonphysiologic long setting. Lengthening the AV delay also compromises the upper tracking rate. The heightened focus on the detrimental effect of RV pacing led to the development of modes or algorithms to reduce RV pacing for patients with generally intact AV conduction. Initially, these algorithms consisted of a programmable increase in AV interval. When conduction is lost, pacing occurs at a shorter, more physiologic AV interval, and periodic testing for AV conduction occurs by lengthening the AV delay. However, these proved only moderately effective at reducing RV pacing. Instead new modes that functioned essentially as single chamber atrial pacing (AAI/AAIR) but with backup ventricular pacing in the event of temporary AV block were devised. These can be described in the BPEG naming convention as ADI/ADIR (Fig. 69.12). When persistent AV block develops, the device switches to DDD/DDDR. Some variation of their function among the different manufacturers exists.[17]

Choosing a Single- or Dual-Chamber Pacing Device
Randomized trials have established that dual-chamber pacing is superior in reducing the occurrence of atrial fibrillation and possibly stroke, though a reduction in mortality has not been proven.[2] Consequently a dual-chamber device is favored except when permanent atrial fibrillation is present. The recent availability of single chamber (ventricular) leadless pacemakers has led to a greater usage of these single chamber systems in some patients who would traditionally receive a dual-chamber device. Optimal leadless pacemaker candidates include those with increased infection risk, with limited vascular access, and who are expected to have a low (ventricular) pacing burden, as well as patients with minimal benefit from dual-chamber pacing due to advanced comorbidities or reduced activity.[18] In addition, leadless devices with some atrial tracking capability have been developed, although atrial pacing is not available yet.

Pacemaker Troubleshooting
With growing complexity of pacemaker systems, many suspected pacing abnormalities are eventually deemed normal function after evaluation. Nevertheless, device dysfunction does occur and can result in serious consequence. Potential malfunction should be evaluated thoroughly via a multimodality approach harnessing all potential resources, such as telemetry, multichannel electrocardiography, the device programmer, and knowledge of the programmed parameters including active device algorithms. Moreover, it is important to take into account the patient's location and potential external environment (EMI), radiography, stored device data, and provocative investigation such as pocket manipulation or arm movement. The most frequent

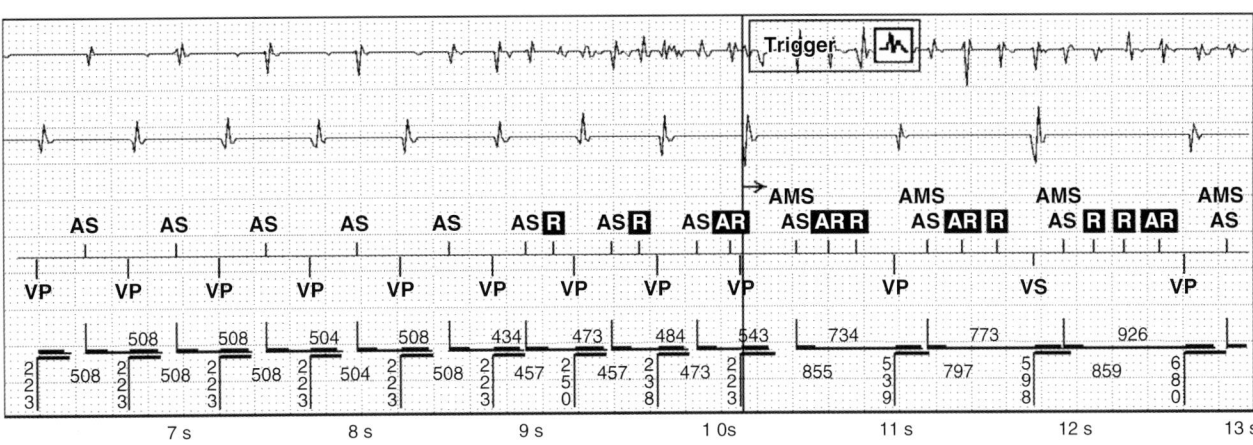

FIGURE 69.11 Mode switch. The device changes from the DDDR to the DDIR mode during an episode of atrial fibrillation. Essentially it is VVIR but it is sensing in the atrium to detect termination of the atrial arrhythmia. This mode prevents tracking an atrial arrhythmia at or near the upper rate. The top channel is the atrial electrogram. The second channel is the ventricular electrogram. The third channel is the marker channel. At the bottom the AA and VV intervals are shown horizontally and the AV intervals displayed vertically. The first five atrial events (AS) are sinus beats tracked with the programmed interval for atrial sensing (AS) and ventricular pacing (VP). Atrial fibrillation begins after the fifth atrial event with AS and AR (atrial refractory) events. Automatic mode switch (AMS) occurs when the number of rapid intervals is met. After AMS, in the DDIR mode, A events are not tracked, and the device exhibits VP or VS (ventricular sensed) events depending upon the conduction rate in atrial fibrillation and patient activity (for rate responsive pacing). When atrial fibrillation ceases, the device resumes atrial tracking (not shown).

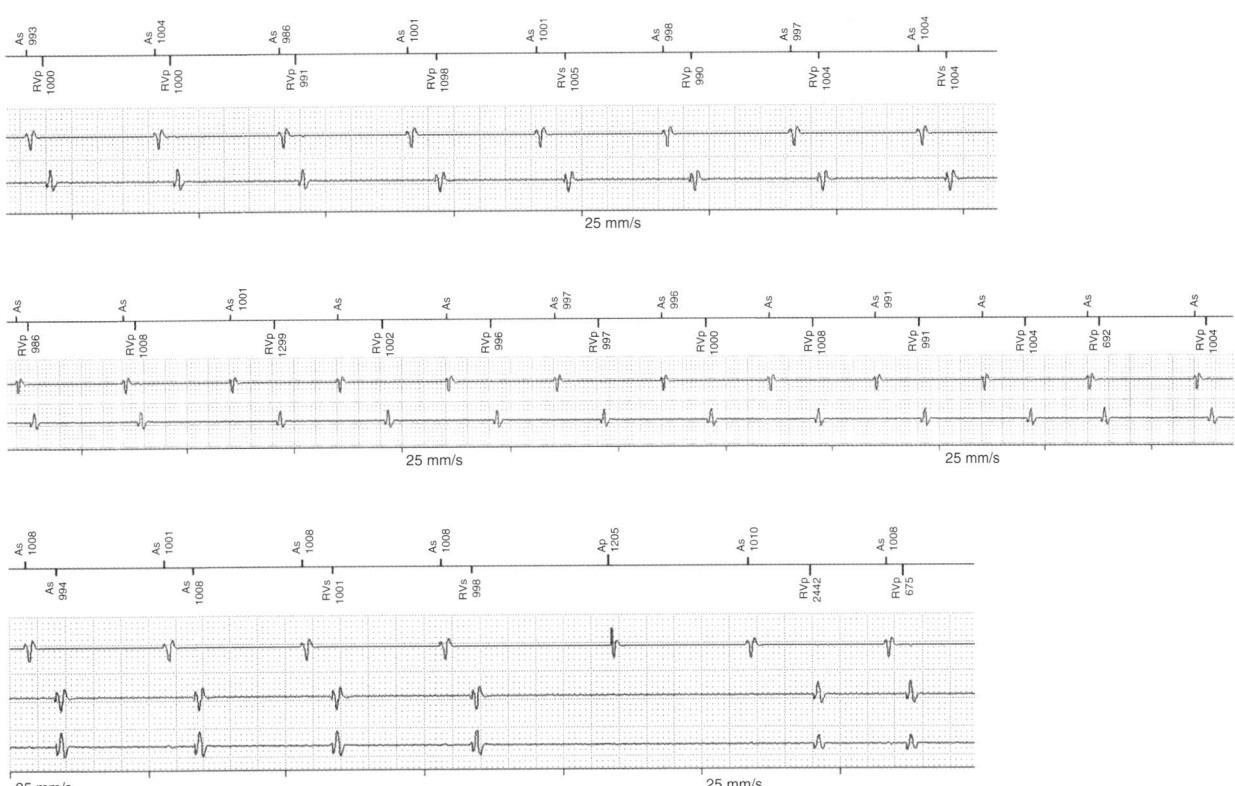

FIGURE 69.12 ADI mode or RV pacing minimization strategy. Marker channel, atrial, and ventricular electrograms from top to bottom in each panel. **Top panel,** AS-RVP (atrial sense-RV paced) occurs; the AV delay is lengthened automatically to try to allow native AV conduction and is successful in transitioning to AS-RVS (RV sensed) rhythm. **Middle panel,** AS-RVP rhythm is present; the AV delay is lengthened automatically to try to allow native AV conduction but is unsuccessful, so the AV delay shortens to the programmed interval for the DDD/DDDR mode in the last two beats. **Bottom panel,** Termination of ADI mode. AS-RVS rhythm is present but the native atrial event does not occur resulting in an AP (atrial paced event). AV conduction does not occur either, possibly due to increased vagal tone; after the next atrial event RVP occurs at the maximal allowed AV delay or maximal V-V interval depending upon the specific mode characteristics. In the last beat, there is resumption of DDD/DDDR mode with the programmed AV delay for that mode. After a programmable time interval, the device will attempt to search for native AV conduction again (as in top panel) by lengthening the AV delay (not shown).

issues are undersensing, failure to capture, failure to pace, and pacing at an unexpected rate (Table 69.2).

Failure to Capture

Especially in the acute period after implantation, pacing lead dislodgement or elevation of threshold (to a value greater than the programmed value) will cause failure to capture (Fig. 69.13). Threshold elevation sometimes is mitigated by device-automated threshold determination and programmed output alteration. Lead fracture or other failure can cause loss of capture. Lead connection issues at the generator's header are also important to consider. Pathologic capture failure must be distinguished from physiologic capture failure that occurs when a pacing impulse falls in the refractory period, sometimes due to undersensing.

Failure to Pace

The flipside of failure to capture is failure to pace. Either can result in ventricular asystole. Failure to pace usually stems from oversensing,

TABLE 69.2 Common Causes of Pacemaker Problems

Failure to Capture
Pacing output below threshold
Changes at electrode-myocardial interface
Output programmed below threshold
Lead dislodgement
Lead insulation failure or conductor fracture
Connection problem between header and lead
Functional failure to capture (undersensing or asynchronous pacing)

Failure to Pace
Corrected by magnet or programming to asynchronous mode
Oversensing of physiologic or nonphysiologic signals
Not corrected by magnet or programming to asynchronous mode
Failure in the pulse generator
Lead conductor fracture
Connection problem between header and lead

Pacing at a Rate Not Consistent with Programmed Rate
Shorter-than-expected escape interval: undersensing
Longer-than-expected escape interval: oversensing
Battery depletion

Unanticipated Rapid Pacing
Pacemaker-mediated tachycardia
Inappropriate ventricular tracking of rapid sensed atrial rates, electromagnetic interference, or myopotentials
Sensor-driven pacing unrelated to patient activity

either of physiologic signals (P, R, or T waves), of noncardiac or external noise (EMI), of lead fracture, or from a loose header connection (Fig. 69.14). Advanced battery depletion or catastrophic device failure can cause loss of output, too. A special case of failure to pace, called crosstalk, is only possible in dual-chamber devices and is discussed above.

Unexpected Pacing at or Near the Upper Rate

Several conditions are prominent causes of pacing at or near the upper rate limit. One should recall that atrial fibrillation with a rapid, natively conducted ventricular response can result in rapid rates just as in patients without pacemakers. For rate responsive devices, unexpected activation of an accelerometer sensor can occur due to vibratory movement (e.g., transportation) or hyperventilation for minute ventilation devices. In dual-chamber devices, tracking nonphysiologic atrial arrhythmias, atrial lead noise (fracture or EMI), or pacemaker-mediated tachycardia are causes of unexpectedly rapid (ventricular) pacing. Tracking an atrial tachyarrhythmia may occur if mode switch is not programmed on, if the atrial arrhythmia is below the mode switch rate, or if the atrial arrhythmia is undersensed. A special example of the latter is when every other atrial flutter beat falls in the postventricular atrial blanking period. Rapid nonphysiologic signals due to atrial lead fracture can lead to tracking near the upper rate. Similarly, external electromagnetic noise detected by the atrial lead can produce rapid ventricular pacing.

Pacemaker-mediated tachycardia (PMT), or endless loop tachycardia, originates with a ventricular impulse (especially a PVC) that conducts retrogradely to the atrium, where it is sensed and thus triggers a paced ventricular beat at the expiration of the AV delay. Subsequently, that ventricular-paced beat may again conduct retrogradely to the atrium and the "reentrant loop" continues. The ECG shows ventricular pacing at or near the upper rate limit, and retrograde P waves. PMT can be prevented by programming the PVARP to an interval longer than the observed VA conduction interval; in addition, PVARP extension can be programmed to occur for PVCs. Once begun, PMT termination algorithms function by omitting tracking for one atrial event. Applying a magnet will terminate it as well. PMT will not

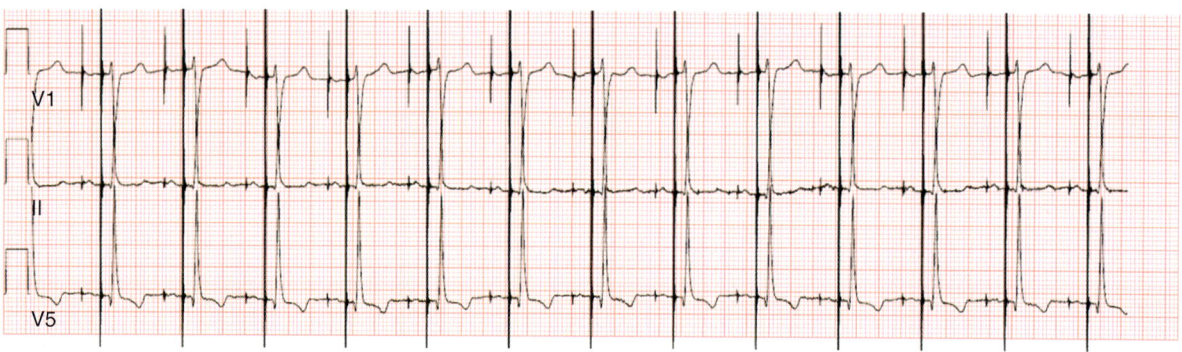

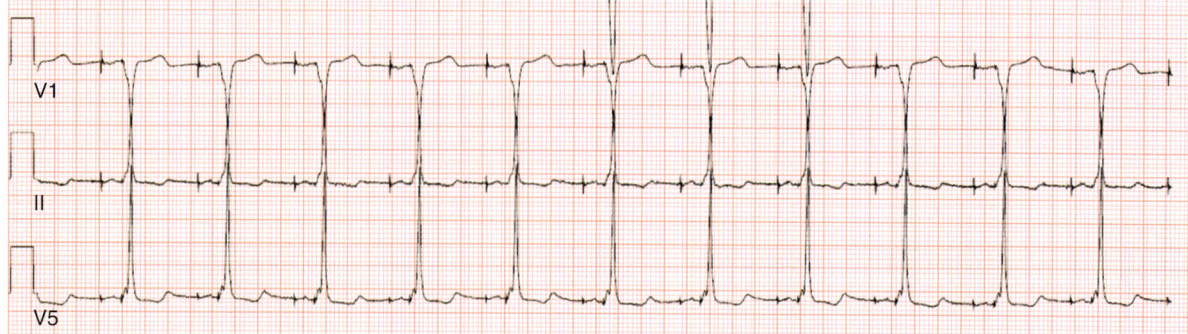

FIGURE 69.13 Failure to capture. Top panel, Unipolar atrial and ventricular pacing via epicardial temporary wires. There is atrial capture (P wave evident after first spike of each beat) but there is an isoelectric interval after the second spike followed by a native (narrow) QRS complex due to intrinsic AV conduction. The device was determined to be delivering ventricular stimuli below the capture threshold. **Bottom panel,** Atrial and ventricular capture after insertion of a permanent pacemaker (with bipolar pacing, note smaller stimulus artifact).

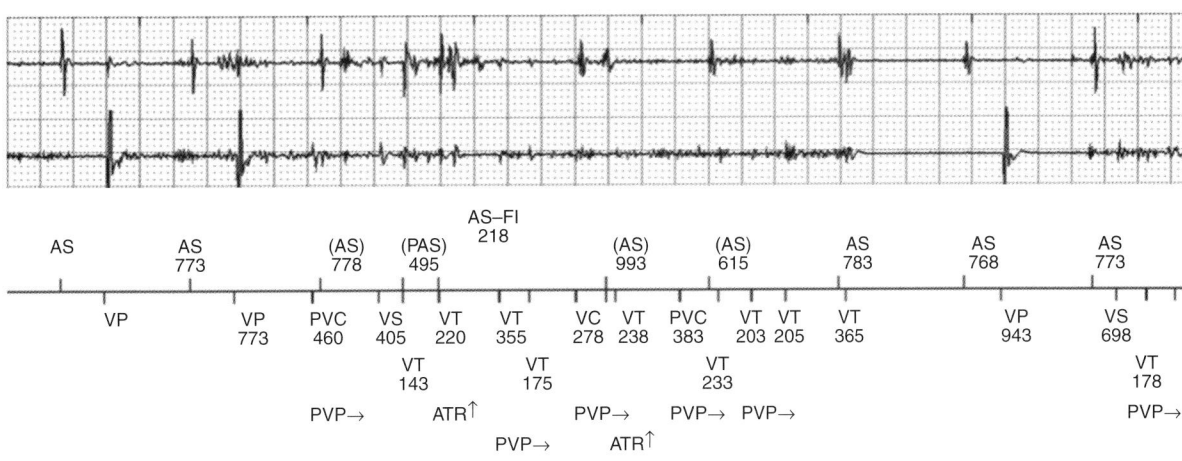

FIGURE 69.14 Failure to pace. The atrial electrogram is on top, ventricular electrogram below, and at the bottom is marker channel. AV block is present. The first two beats are atrial sensed (AS) and ventricular paced (VP). Noise is present on the atrial and ventricular electrograms due to electromagnetic interference or failure of both leads. The ventricular noise is sensed as VT inhibiting pacing output leading to a pause.

occur in the DDI mode since it is dependent upon atrial tracking, but it can occur in VDD, as well as DDD.

Non-reentrant ventricular-atrial synchrony, similar to PMT, also starts most commonly with a PVC that conducts retrogradely. However, due to timing and programming particulars, it falls in the PVARP. Atrial pacing then occurs at the LRL (or at the sensor indicated rate). However, in this scenario the atrial pacing pulse does not capture due to functional refractoriness from the preceding retrograde atrial activation. The sequence then repeats. It can be prevented by shortening the AV delay, reducing the PVARP and/or by reducing the lower rate, such as by inactivating rate-response pacing.[19]

Unexpected Drop in Pacing Rate
If the sinus rate exceeds the upper tracking rate in the setting of AV block, the pacing rate will fall. Dependent upon certain timing relationships (upper tracking rate [UTR], atrioventricular interval [AVI], PVARP), a phenomenon resembling AV Wenckebach or of 2:1 AV block can occur. Ideally, the UTR should be programmed high enough to avoid a drop in pacing rate with exercise. See Figure 69.15 for details.

Pacing-Induced Proarrhythmia
Pacing-induced proarrhythmia includes several subtypes. The simplest form is an R-on-T ventricular pacing in the VOO mode triggering VT or VF. Any form of ventricular or atrial undersensing may allow pacing to trigger an arrhythmia. Even ventricular escape pacing at a low rate can rarely trigger ventricular tachyarrhythmias. A pause in pacing due to loss of capture during a threshold test or an RV pacing-minimization algorithm can initiate VT or VF by a short-long-short sequence. A pacing lead may mechanically trigger ectopic impulses, too. Competitive atrial pacing can trigger atrial tachyarrhythmias. Some manufacturers enable programming of a noncompetitive atrial pacing interval to minimize such events.

Pseudo-Malfunction
Numerous forms of pacemaker function can appear abnormal depending upon the type and amount of ECG data available, the presence or absence of marker channels, and the type of algorithms and programming in effect. ECG records may either suggest a pacing pulse is not present or fail to disclose one (bipolar pacing, dependent on lead vector, etc.). In-person threshold tests with loss of capture or change in rate may be noted on later review of telemetry as a possible abnormality. Similarly, automatic pacing thresholds or AV search algorithms may prompt concern when seen on a monitor strip.

IMPLANTABLE CARDIOVERTER-DEFIBRILLATORS

Types of ICDs
Like implanted pacemakers, conventional ICD components include a PG that contains the battery and circuitry, and a lead system. The PG is larger than those for pacemakers, as the device must contain a larger battery and capacitors capable of generating higher voltage shocks. Transvenous ICDs incorporate fully functional antibradycardic pacing. The lead system consists of at least one lead that has one or two defibrillating coils along with pace/sense electrodes, typically placed at the RV apex (Figs. 69.2 and 69.16). Dual-chamber ICDs include a pace/sense port that is usually connected to a lead placed in the RA, thus providing along with the RV lead, dual-chamber pacing capabilities. A third port for CRT can be connected to a pacing lead placed to pace the LV via a lead in a branch of the coronary sinus or implanted on the LV epicardial surface (see Fig. 69.3). Like pacing systems, newer pacemaker configurations may include a lead intended to pace the cardiac conduction system, using a lead placed at the His bundle or deep into the interventricular septum to capture the left bundle branch. Subcutaneous ICDs are also commercially available and consist of a PG typically placed subcutaneously in the left lateral chest connected to a subcutaneously tunneled sensing and defibrillation lead (Fig. 69.5).

Indications for ICDs
ICDs are indicated for prevention of sudden death from VT/VF, either as *secondary prevention* in patients who have been resuscitated from VT/VF or *primary prevention* in patients who have not had VT/VF but are at sufficiently high risk to warrant protection with an ICD.

Secondary Prevention
ICDs are the treatment of choice for secondary prevention of VT/VF, providing patients remain at risk for recurrence of VT/VF and have sufficient life expectancy and quality of life to justify implantation. The strong consensus for secondary prevention ICDs is based on randomized trials comparing ICD implantation to medical therapy for patients who survived cardiac arrest or hemodynamically significant sustained ventricular arrhythmias (Table 69.3). The largest trial, Antiarrhythmics Versus Implantable Defibrillators (AVID),[20] randomized 1016 patients who were resuscitated from near-fatal VF, sustained VT with syncope, or sustained VT with left ventricular

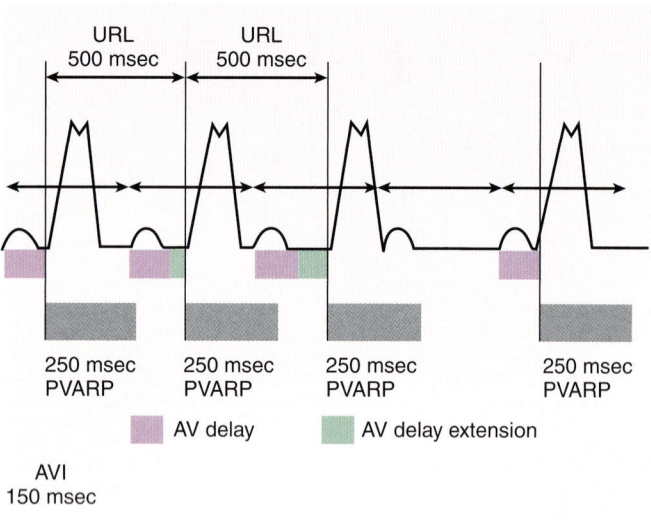

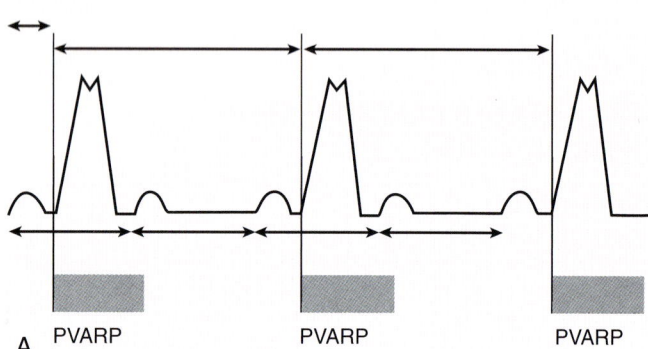

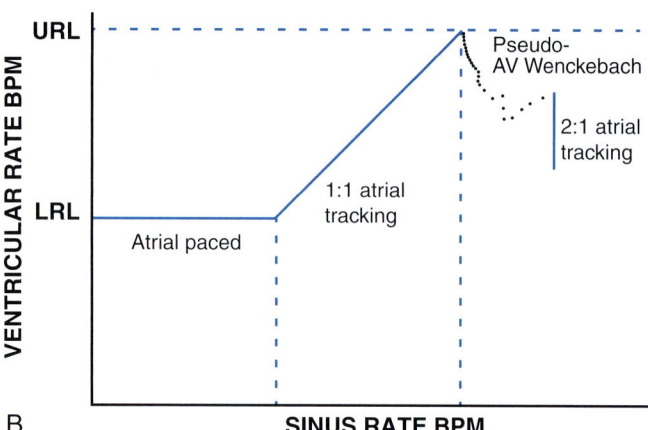

FIGURE 69.15 Upper rate limit behavior of dual-chamber pacemaker. **A,** *Top,* Pseudo-Wenckebach behavior occurs when the sinus rate exceeds the programmed maximum tracking rate but the P-P interval is longer than the total atrial refractory period (TARP, sum of atrioventricular interval [AVI] and postventricular atrial refractory period [PVARP]). *Bottom,* When the P-P interval is less than the TARP, every other P falls within the PVARP and therefore cannot be tracked. Thus the ventricular rate falls to half the atrial rate (2:1 atrial tracking). **B,** Response of DDD pacemaker (*ordinate*) as sinus rate (*abscissa*) increases. BPM, Beats per minute; LRL, programmed lower rate limit; URL, programmed upper rate limit.

ejection fraction (LVEF) of ≤40% and symptoms suggesting severe hemodynamic compromise due to an arrhythmia to ICD implantation or antiarrhythmic drugs (mostly amiodarone). Overall survival was significantly greater in the ICD group ($p < 0.02$).[20] The 2017 AHA/ACC/HRS Guideline for Management of Patients with Ventricular Arrhythmias and the Prevention of Sudden Cardiac Death[21] recommends ICD implantation in patients who survive sudden cardiac arrest due to VT/VF, hemodynamically unstable VT, stable sustained VT not due to reversible causes, or unexplained syncope with inducible sustained VT on electrophysiologic study, if meaningful

TABLE 69.3 Major ICD Trials for Secondary Prevention of Sudden Cardiac Death

TRIAL	YEAR	TOTAL N	RANDOMIZATION	MORTALITY OUTCOME WITH ICD
AVID (AVID Investigators)	1997	1016	ICD, Class III AAD (mostly amiodarone)	HR 0.62 ($p < 0.02$)
CASH (Kuck et al.)	2000	288	ICD, amiodarone, propafenone, metoprolol	HR 0.766 ($P = 0.081$)
CIDS (Connolly et al.)	2000	659	ICD, amiodarone	RRR 19.7% ($p = 0.142$)

AAD, Antiarrhythmic drug; *HR,* hazard ratio; *ICD,* implantable cardioverter-defibrillator; *RRR,* relative risk ratio.
See reference[20] for individual trials.

survival greater than 1 year is expected (Class I recommendation). An algorithm for secondary prevention of sudden cardiac death in ischemic heart disease is shown in Figure 69.17 and for nonischemic cardiomyopathy in Figure 69.18.

Primary Prevention
Several randomized clinical trials have provided indications for ICD implantation for primary prevention of sudden cardiac death (Table 69.4).[20] Clinical decisions for ICD implantation in ischemic or nonischemic cardiomyopathy are largely informed by three randomized clinical trials. The MADIT II trial of patients with ischemic cardiomyopathy and LVEF of 30% or less demonstrated significant survival benefit of an ICD[20] with survival benefit evident through 8 years of follow-up.[22] The SCD-HeFT trial of patients with LVEF of 35% or less and ischemic or nonischemic cardiomyopathy with NYHA functional Class II or III heart failure found that ICDs reduced total mortality.[20] MUSTT randomized patients with CAD and LVEF 40% or less with asymptomatic nonsustained VT to electrophysiology-guided therapy with antiarrhythmic drugs or ICD implantation versus no antiarrhythmic treatment; patients who received an ICD experienced reduced mortality.[20] However, retrospective analyses suggest that ICDs may not prolong life in identifiable subgroups with extensive comorbidities, including advanced heart failure and renal failure. Further, these trials were performed before present pharmacologic therapy and CRT for HF. A subsequent randomized controlled trial of patients with nonischemic cardiomyopathy and LVEF of 35% or less (DANISH trial) found that ICDs did not reduce total mortality in patients who received guideline-directed medical therapy (GDMT) and indicated CRT pacemakers, though sudden cardiac death mortality was reduced.[20]

Clinical trials do not support ICD implantation in low-LVEF patients within 40 days of myocardial infarction (MI) or 90 days of surgical revascularization; low-LVEF patients with recent percutaneous revascularization are not well represented in clinical trials.[20] With few exceptions,[23] ICD implantation in these patients is not indicated. Algorithms for primary prevention of sudden cardiac death in nonischemic and ischemic heart disease are shown in Figure 69.18 and Figure 69.19.

Expert consensus statements provide recommendations for ICD implantation in patients under specific circumstances not covered in clinical trials[23] and clinical scenarios not addressed by guidelines.[24] These include high-risk patients with less common diseases, including specific cardiomyopathies (e.g., hypertrophic cardiomyopathy; Chapter 54), ion channelopathies (Chapter 63), and certain forms of congenital heart disease (Chapter 82).

ICD LEADS AND GENERATORS
Defibrillation Leads
An ICD system comprises the generator and at least one defibrillation lead. Usually, the generator is implanted pectorally, and a single, transvenous defibrillation lead is implanted in the right ventricle (analogous to a ventricular pacemaker lead) (Fig. 69.20A, *left panel*). Dual-chamber

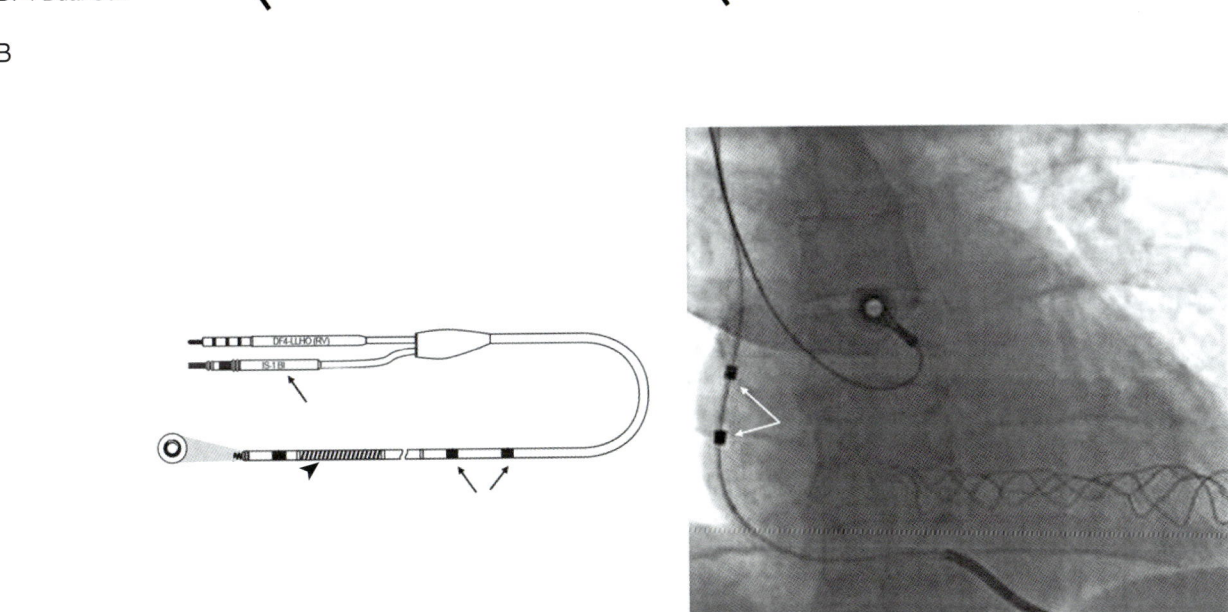

FIGURE 69.16 ICD leads. A, Cross section of transvenous ICD lead. *ETFE,* Ethyltetrafluoroethylene; *PTFE,* polytetrafluoroethylene. **B,** Dual coil lead (*arrows* to coils) with in-line modern DF4 header connection. **C,** RV lead with atrial sensing electrodes (*arrows*) and single defibrillation coil (*arrow head*).

ICDs incorporate a bipolar atrial pace-sense lead to provide dual-chamber bradycardia pacing and dual-chamber algorithms that discriminate supraventricular tachycardia (SVT) from VT. CRT-Ds incorporate an LV pacing lead (see Chapter 58). The totally subcutaneous[25] ICD system consists of a defibrillation lead implanted parallel to the sternum and tunneled to the ICD generator located near the left anterior axillary line.

ICD Generators

ICD generators include a clear-plastic header that connects to the lead(s) and a titanium can that houses high-voltage electronics, in addition to the battery and other low-voltage components found in pacemakers.

Unlike pacemakers, ICDs must deliver high-voltage shocks in addition to low-voltage pacing pulses. However, low-voltage batteries have approximately 1000 times the energy density of high-voltage capacitors. Thus, ICDs require a high-voltage transformer and charging circuit to convert electrochemical energy stored in an electrochemical cell (about 3 V) to the high voltage needed for defibrillation shocks (750 to 900 V for transvenous ICDs; 1400 V for subcutaneous ICDs). Unlike pacemaker batteries, ICD batteries must be able to deliver high current (up to 3 A) and high power (up to 10 W) to provide high-voltage electricity for shocks. The charging circuit requires 6 to 15 seconds for transvenous ICDs and 15 to 25 seconds for subcutaneous ICDs. During charging, high-voltage electricity is stored in a high-voltage capacitor. To deliver the shock, the high-voltage capacitor is disconnected from the charging circuit and connected to the shock electrodes.

ICD SYSTEM SELECTION

Dual- versus Single-Chamber Transvenous ICDs

In addition to providing dual-chamber bradycardia pacing, dual-chamber ICDs provide atrial EGMs that enhance physician interpretation of stored EGMs and permit both diagnostics for AF and dual-chamber algorithms to discriminate SVT from VT. The present

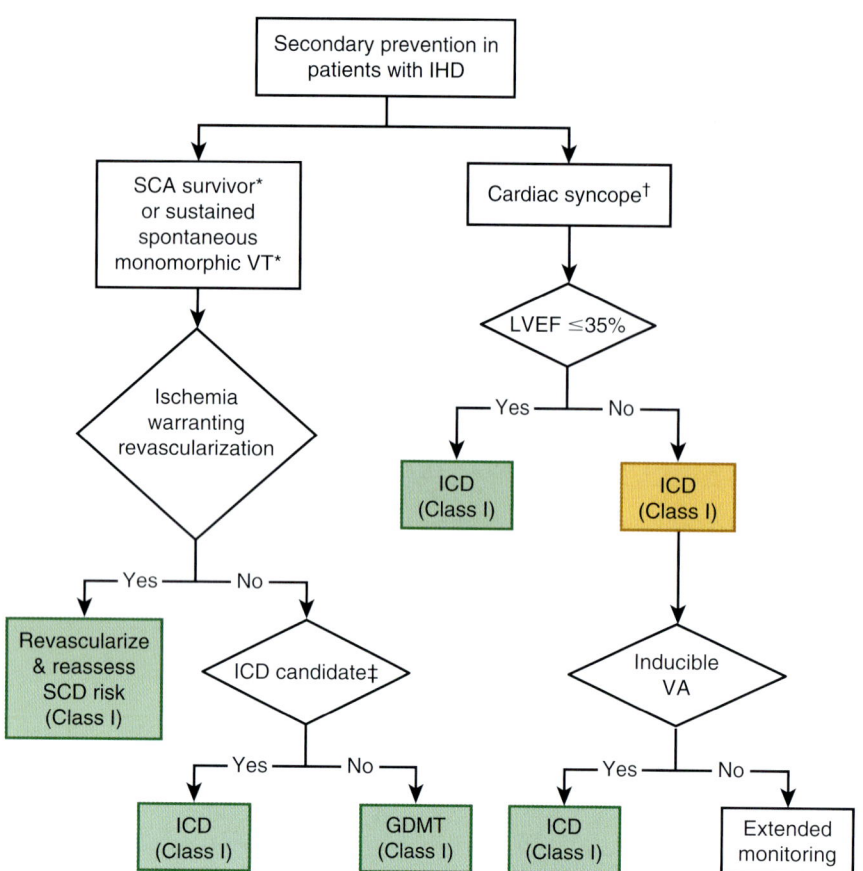

FIGURE 69.17 Secondary prevention of SCD in patients with ischemic heart disease. From 2017 AHA/ACC/HRS Guideline for Management of Patients With Ventricular Arrhythmias and the Prevention of Sudden Cardiac Death: A Report of the American College of Cardiology/American Heart Association Task Force on Clinical Practice Guidelines and the Heart Rhythm Society. Colors correspond to class of recommendation per reference 21. *Exclude reversible causes. †History consistent with an arrhythmic etiology for syncope. ‡ICD candidacy as determined by functional status, life expectancy, or patient preference. *GDMT*, guideline-directed management and therapy; *ICD*, implantable cardioverter-defibrillator; *IHD*, ischemic heart disease; *LVEF*, left ventricular ejection fraction; *SCA*, sudden cardiac arrest; *SCD*, sudden cardiac death; *VT*, ventricular tachycardia.

consensus recommends reserving dual-chamber ICDs for patients who need dual-chamber pacing or have SVT and monomorphic VT at overlapping ventricular rates.[23]

Transvenous versus Subcutaneous ICD Systems

The subcutaneous ICD[25] eliminates morbidity associated with transvenous lead insertion, lead-related complications during MRI scans, and the hazards of transvenous extraction when lead removal is required. Candidates for a subcutaneous ICD undergo screening using surface ECG electrodes to assess the risk of T wave oversensing or R wave double-counting; 7% to 10% of candidates fail screening. Despite this, inappropriate shocks caused by oversensing are more common in subcutaneous ICDs than in modern transvenous ICDs (5% to 10% versus <2% in the first year).[25-27] Subcutaneous ICDs cannot perform ATP, resynchronization, or long-term bradycardia pacing. However, future models are expected to communicate with leadless capsule pacemakers.

TRANSVENOUS DEFIBRILLATION LEADS
Dual Versus Single Coil
Dual-coil leads improved defibrillation efficacy of early ICDs but do not provide a clinically significant advantage for left pectoral implants in present ICDs.[28]

They provide better defibrillation for some right-sided implants as well as reliable atrial cardioversion and alternate EGMs for diagnostic interpretation. However, the proximal coil often adheres to the superior vena cava. If lead extraction is required, this increases procedural difficulty and may increase risk. Thus, single-coil leads usually are preferred for left pectoral implants in younger patients, but dual coils may be preferable for patients expected to have high defibrillation thresholds (e.g., patients with severe ventricular dysfunction or enlargement), although prediction of high defibrillation thresholds remains suboptimal.

Integrated Versus Dedicated Sensing Bipoles
Compared with dedicated bipolar leads, the integrated bipolar design simplifies the lead by reducing the number of conductors. However, reliable leads have been developed with both designs. Integrated bipolar EGMs have a wider field of view than dedicated bipolar EGMs and are thus more likely to oversense nonphysiologic signals or physiologic signals (such as myopotentials from the chest wall or diaphragm) that do not reflect local myocardial depolarization.[29]

ICD SENSING AND DETECTION
Sensing in ICDs is more challenging than for pacemakers given the top priority of treating lethal arrhythmias, especially VF, and thus needing to sense VF reliably. As discussed under pacemakers, simply increasing the sensitivity level (by decreasing the numerical value) poses a high risk of oversensing other signals, especially T waves. To meet both the goal of sensing potentially small and variable signals in VF along with avoiding sensing normal non–R wave signals (especially T waves), sensing is dynamically adjusted rather than using a constant level as in pacemakers (Fig. 69.21). After a sensed event, the sensitivity becomes greater until the next signal is sensed. The magnitude of the starting mV sensitivity level, after the absolute refractory period, varies on the basis of the most recent native signals but is often 50% to 75% of that value and declines, linearly, exponentially or in steps down to a programmed maximal sensitivity level, usually 0.3 to 0.5 mv. Sensing after pacing in some devices has a longer blanking period but then starts from a lower value to avoid undersensing.

The maximal sensitivity is programmable to various levels in different ICDs. In addition, some manufacturers offer other variations to enhance the ability to detect VF (such as a lower starting level or shorter initial sensing level or blanking period). Conversely, if oversensing of T waves is noted, a higher high-pass filter, longer period before sensing becomes more sensitive, or reduced maximal sensitivity are possible programming options that vary by manufacturer. One manufacturer uses a specific algorithm set that compares the differential of the filtered EGM, which magnifies the difference between R waves and T waves due to a higher slew rate (dv/dt) for R waves to allow pattern recognition of T wave oversensing that can inhibit therapy. Other algorithms try to recognize baseline noise and when noted, adjust the sensing floor to a less sensitive value to avoid myopotential oversensing. Any change in sensing function or decline in native signals can make underdetection of VF possible and consideration should be given to testing for sensing of induced VF.

Building on how a single signal is sensed, the detection of VT and VF can be described (Table 69.5 and Fig. 69.22). One or more zones of detection and therapy are programmable. Within a zone, a rate range or cycle length range is defined. In addition a duration is programmed so as not to treat a nonsustained arrhythmia. All manufacturers use some form of probabilistic detection algorithm in the VF zone, since the marked variability in signal size and coupling interval often leads to some underdetection with some intervals thus falling out of the VF zone. The number of intervals is often specified as X of

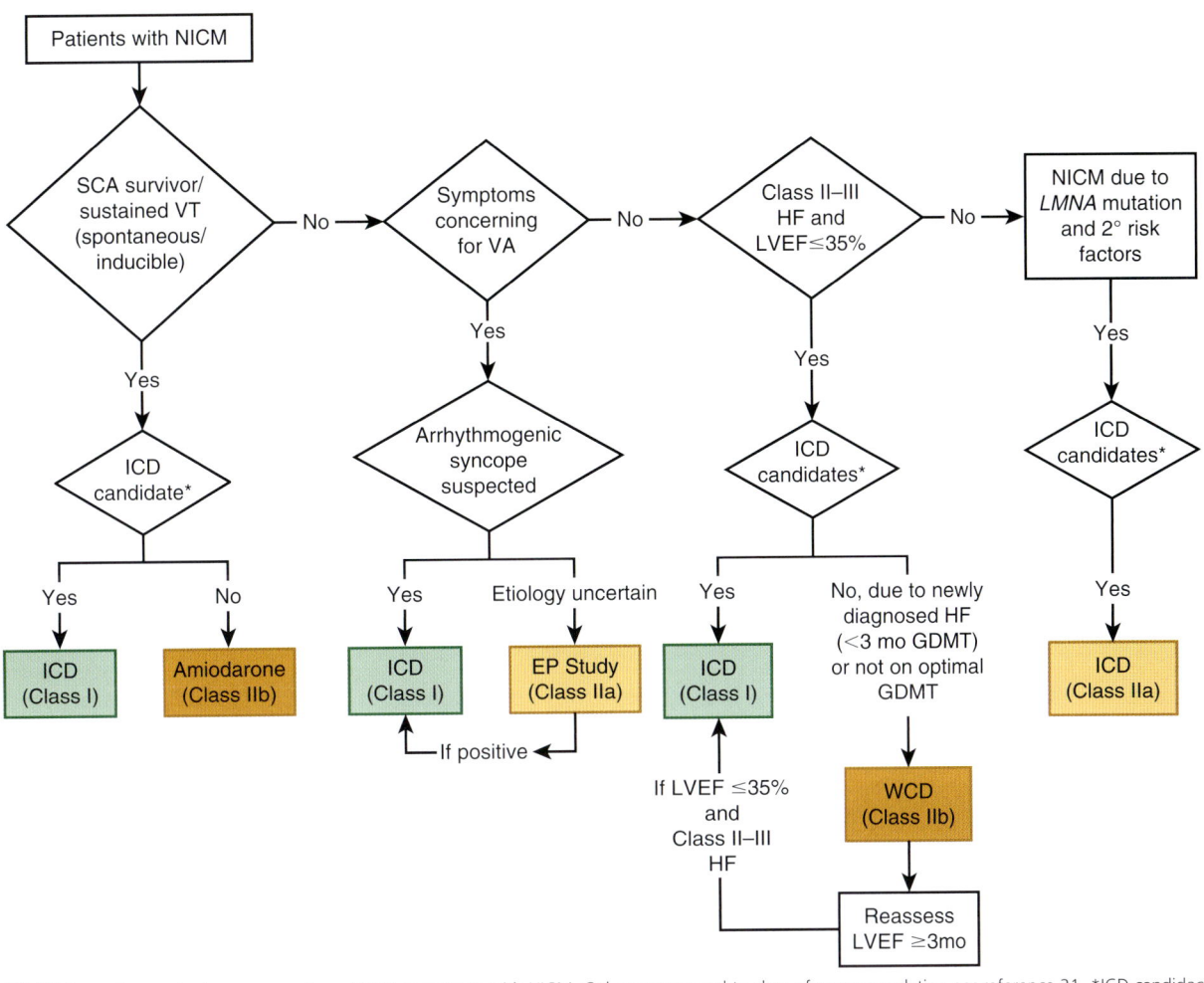

FIGURE 69.18 Secondary and primary prevention of SCD in patients with NICM. Colors correspond to class of recommendation per reference 21. *ICD candidacy as determined by functional status, life expectancy, or patient preference. 2° indicates secondary. *VA*, Ventricular arrhythmia; *WCD*, wearable cardiac defibrillator.

Y, for example 8 of 10 or 30 of 40 intervals for detection. This may or may not be programmable. One manufacturer requires a continuous string of fast beats in a VF zone; others use counters that increment or decrement if slower beats are detected. Each type of zone has its own strengths and weaknesses, requiring a sophisticated knowledge of the device and the patient's possible or likely arrhythmia characteristics. Once VT or VF detection criteria is satisfied, then therapy (ATP or charging for a shock) proceeds.

After the therapy is delivered, the device attempts to detect whether VT or VF is still present or if sinus rhythm has been restored. Because the hemodynamic state deteriorates with longer VT or especially VF, and signals may become more attenuated, redetection criteria are usually a shorter number of intervals, and shocks may be committed to avoid inappropriately aborting therapy for VF.

In addition to rate-based (plus duration) detection criteria, other measures are possible for confirming the presence of VT or VF and differentiating it from SVT, AF, or abnormal sensing. These discriminators are considered in VT zones or sometimes in the slower portion of a VF zone but not for the fastest arrhythmias so as to avoid inappropriate withholding of therapy. In single-chamber devices, available criteria include EGM morphology, sudden onset, and regularity. Morphology criteria compare a previously obtained template of either the rate sensing or shock EGM to the tachycardia under consideration for therapy. If it is deemed to differ by programmable criteria, VT is declared or vice versa. Pitfalls can include aberration, noise on the morphology channel (from exercise for example), or suboptimal template capture. Sudden onset attempts to distinguish sinus tachycardia, which develops gradually, from VT that typically occurs abruptly. Drawbacks with this criterion include a VT that starts slower than the detection rate but then gradually accelerates to the detection rate and thus falsely being declared as SVT (sinus tachycardia). Regularity or stability seeks to identify atrial fibrillation as opposed to most monomorphic VTs, which display regularity. Obviously polymorphic VT is also irregular, so this criterion should be disabled for fast arrhythmias.

In dual-chamber ICDs the atrial lead can be used to help diagnose the arrhythmia. First, atrial fibrillation can be diagnosed by rate-based criteria. Second, the rate in the ventricle and atria can be compared; if the former is faster, VT is diagnosed and treated. However, there can be undersensing in the atria due to blanking of atrial events during or after ventricular ones. VT, however, can exhibit a constant 1:1 retrograde conduction. The pattern or relationship between the A and V is used in some of these algorithms. The chamber initiating the tachycardia is a powerful diagnostic modality used in one family of devices.

Inappropriate shocks are painful, may lead to myocardial injury and hemodynamic effects, impair patient quality of life, and increase health care costs; when repetitive they may engender a posttraumatic distress syndrome. Rarely, inappropriate therapy can trigger VT or VF. Some but not all studies have identified a mortality signal associated with them. These facts led to research studies focusing on primary prevention patients comparing standard programming with novel programming using faster rate detection criteria and/or longer detection durations before therapy. These studies confirmed the benefit in reducing inappropriate therapy, the safety in doing so (lack of increase in mortality or syncope), and some found a reduction in mortality with the novel programming. Nevertheless, it is undoubtedly true that some patients may present with hemodynamically unstable or otherwise dangerous VT just below the cutoff zone, although such cases are relatively uncommon. Undersensing as well as the unintended function of some algorithms may impair VF sensing and detection that may be fatal. In programming tachycardia detection in

TABLE 69.4 Major ICD Trials for Primary Prevention of Sudden Cardiac Death

TRIAL (FIRST AUTHOR)	YEAR	N	DESIGN	POPULATION	TIMING	MORTALITY, HAZARD RATIO ICD
MADIT (Moss et al.)	1996	196	ICD versus conventional medical therapy	Prior MI; LVEF ≤35%; NSVT; inducible nonsuppressible sustained VT/VF at EPS	>3 wk post MI >2 mo post CABG >3 mo post PTCA	0.46 ($p = 0.009$)
MUSTT (Buxton et al.)	1999	704	Electrophysiology-guided therapy with antiarrhythmic drugs or ICD versus no antiarrhythmic treatment	CAD; LVEF≤40%; asymptomatic NSVT; Inducible sustained ventricular tachyarrhythmia	≥4 d post MI or revascularization	0.40 ($p < 0.001$)
MADIT II (Moss et al.)	2002	1232	3:2 ICD versus medical therapy	Prior MI LVEF ≤30%	>1 mo post MI >3 mo post revasc	0.69 ($P = 0.016$)
SCDHeFT (Bardy et al.)	2005	2521	ICD versus amiodarone versus placebo	Ischemic or nonischemic cardiomyopathy, LVEF ≤35% NYHA FC II or III		0.77 ($p = 0.007$)
DINAMIT (Hohnloser et al.)	2004	674	ICD versus no ICD	Recent MI, LVEF ≤35%; ↓HRV or average HR ≥80 bpm	6-40 d post MI	1.08 ($p = 0.66$) Arrhythmic death 0.42 ($p= 0.009$)
IRIS (Steinbeck et al.)	2009	898	ICD versus no ICD	Recent MI, LVEF ≤40%, HR ≥90 bpm or NSVT	5-31 d post MI	1.04 ($p = 0.78$) SCD 0.55 ($p = 0.049$)
CABGPatch (Bigger et al.)	1997	900	Epicardial ICD versus no ICD with CABG	CABG, LVEF ≤35%, abnormal SAECG	At time of CABG	1.07 (NS)
CAT (Bansch et al.)	2002	104	ICD versus no ICD	Nonischemic, recent onset dilated cardiomyopathy	≤9 mo	NS
DEFINITE (Kadish et al.)	2004	458	Single chamber ICD versus medical therapy	Non-ischemic dilated cardiomyopathy, LVEF <36%, and PVCs or NSVT	-	0.65 ($p = 0.08$)
AMIOVERT (Strickberger et al.)	2003	103	ICD versus amiodarone	Nonischemic dilated cardiomyopathy, LVEF ≤35%, NSVT	-	NS
COMPANION (Bristow et al.)	2004	1520	1:2:2 optimal medical therapy, CRT-P, CRT-D	Ischemic or nonischemic cardiomyopathy, NYHA FC III or IV heart failure, QRS ≥120 msec, PR150 msec	HF hospitalization in preceding 12 mo	0.64 ($p = 0.003$) CRT-D versus medical therapy
DANISH (Kober et al.)	2016	556	ICD versus usual clinical care; 58% received CRT in both groups	Nonischemic cardiomyopathy LVEF ≤35%		0.87 ($p = 0.28$); SCD 0.50 ($p = 0.005$)

See reference[20] for individual trials.
CABG, Coronary artery bypass graft surgery; *CAD*, coronary artery disease; *CRT*, cardiac resynchronization therapy; *EPS*, electrophysiologic study; *HR*, heart rate; *HRV*, heart rate variability; *ICD*, implantable cardioverter defibrillator; *LVEF*, left ventricular ejection fraction; *MI*, myocardial infarction; *NS*, nonsignificant; *NSVT*, nonsustained ventricular tachycardia; *NYHA FC*, New York Heart Association functional class; *PVCs*, premature ventricular complexes; *SAECG*, signal-averaged electrocardiogram; *SCD*, sudden cardiac death; *VF*, ventricular fibrillation; *VT*, ventricular tachycardia.

ICDs, tachyarrhythmia duration detection criteria is recommended to allow the tachycardia to continue at least 6 to 12 seconds, or 30 intervals, to reduce therapies for both primary and secondary prevention ICD patients. Discrimination algorithms to distinguish SVT from VT are also recommended to include rates faster than 200 bpm and potentially up to 230 bpm unless contraindicated, to reduce inappropriate therapies. Furthermore, activation of lead failure alerts are recommended to detect possible lead problems.[30]

ICD THERAPY

General Considerations

Modern ICDs terminate ventricular arrhythmias by antitachycardia pacing and/or by one or more shocks. Except for VF, ATP is often used first, and if unsuccessful shocks are applied (up to five to eight before therapy is ceased). ATP is used preferentially because of the adverse effects of shocks discussed above. As discussed above, zones of therapy for detection are sometimes used, allowing differentiation of the degree of aggressiveness in diagnosis (longer or shorter detection) and in therapy (none, some to extensive attempts at ATP versus shocks only). Previously, low-energy shocks were used more often, but these result in a similar degree of discomfort and may have a higher propensity at inducing atrial arrhythmias, as well as being unsuccessful for VT or VF and thus requiring more than one shock. Smaller shocks do require a shorter time for charging, but this is infrequently a substantial concern with normal, modern ICD function. In single zone configurations, commonly called a VF zone, many of the actual arrhythmias treated are rapid monomorphic VTs that are amenable to ATP.

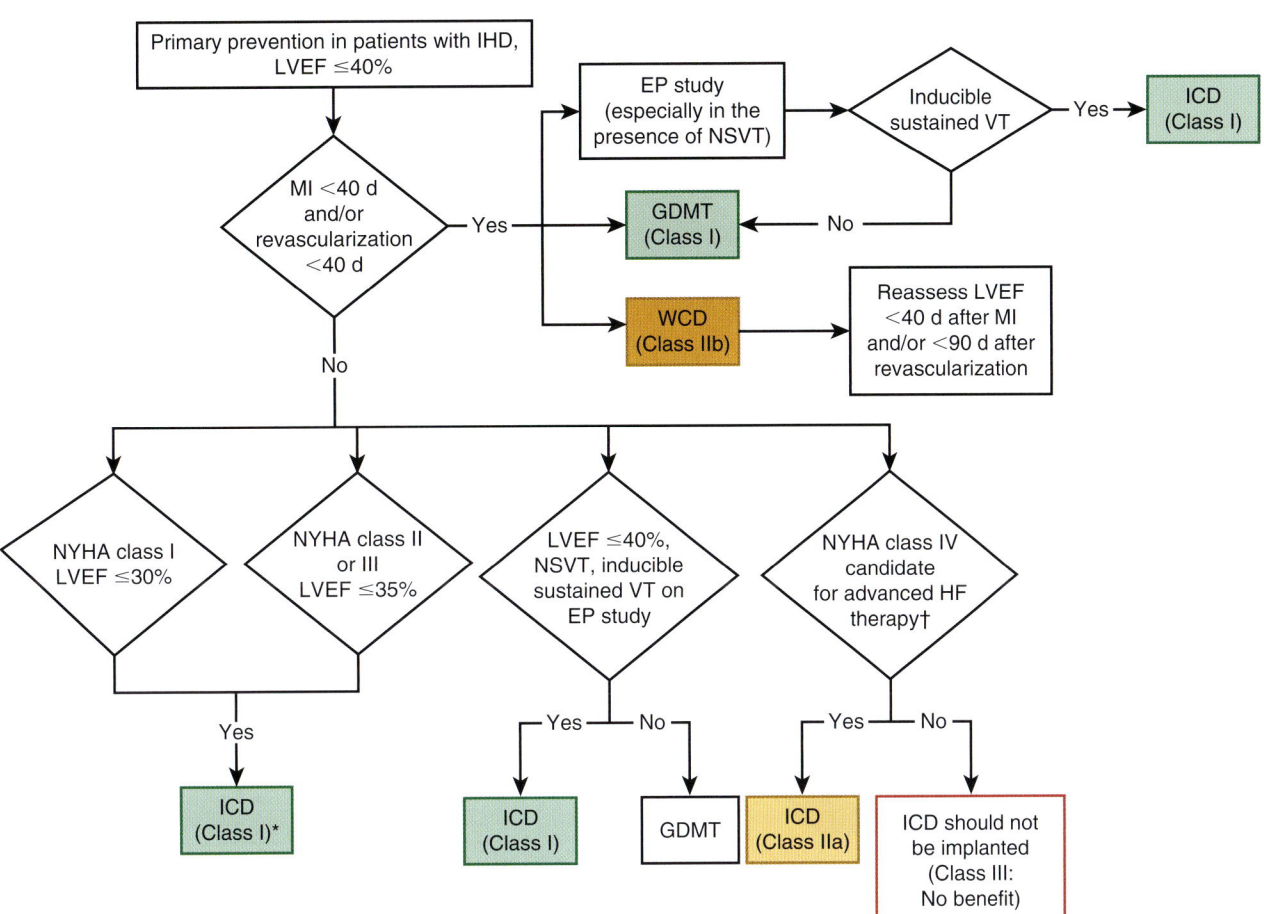

FIGURE 69.19 Primary prevention of SCD in patients with ischemic heart disease and LVEF ≤40%. Colors correspond to class of recommendation per reference 21. *Advanced HF therapy includes CRT, cardiac transplant, and LVAD. †Scenarios exist for early ICD placement in select circumstances such as patients with a pacing indication or syncope thought due to VT. These are detailed elsewhere in an HRS/ACC/AHA expert consensus statement. *MI,* myocardial infarction; *NSVT,* nonsustained ventricular tachycardia; *NYHA,* New York Heart Association. Other abbreviations are as in Fig. 69.17.

Antitachycardia Pacing

Antitachycardia pacing (ATP) differs from bradycardia pacing by the rate at which it is delivered and other aspects (Fig. 69.23). The underpinnings were established by Waldo and colleagues studying the interruption of atrial flutter using epicardial pacing wires after cardiac surgery.[2] To capture locally, at a rate even faster than the tachycardia (leading to relative refractoriness) as well as to penetrate the reentrant circuit, a higher output near the maximal pacing output is used (5 to 8 V), and a train of stimuli (usually 6 to 10) is used to progressively shorten the refractory period and allow access to the circuit. When effective, the ATP impulses enter the reentry circuit, travel in the antidromic direction, and collide with the previous impulse; meanwhile, the ATP impulse conducts in the orthodromic direction (same as during the tachycardia) but blocks due to greater refractoriness because the pacing rate is faster than the tachycardia. In addition to termination, the ATP could have no effect, accelerate the VT, or terminate and reinduce it. Thus, more than one sequence is often used, and if significant acceleration occurs, shocks are used. Two different protocols are commonly used, burst (having a constant cycle length within the train) and ramp (featuring a decrement in cycle length from beginning to end). Some studies have found ramp more effective but more prone to acceleration, and others found burst more effective. Programming more than two sequences has limited yield and delays definitive shock therapy. In single zone programming, only one ATP sequence is used.

For slower VTs, ATP is reportedly effective in 80% to 90% of events, with acceleration occurring 2% to 4% of the time. When applied to faster VTs (188 to 250 bpm), ATP has been reported to be successful for 70% to 80% of events with 2% acceleration. Prior studies had shown lower success rates and higher acceleration occurrences.[2] These success rates need to be interpreted in light of the VT duration before intervention since some VTs will self-terminate. In the MADIT-RIT study, treated VT above 200 bpm occurred half as often in the long duration arm than the conventional arm, implying self-termination occurred in many in the conventional arm, and for the episodes that persisted, the success of ATP appeared lower (58% versus 76%).[31]

In primary prevention, a single zone or two zones beginning at between 185 and 200 bpm is appropriate. A single ATP sequence is now often used to treat rapid MMVT (not VF) in single zone or in the VF zone. Current ATP programming recommendations are that for all patients with structural heart disease and ATP-capable ICDs, ATP should be active for all detection zones, including arrhythmias up to 230 bpm, with one ATP attempt, except when ATP has been documented to be ineffective or proarrhythmic.[30] Burst ATP is preferred to ramp ATP to improve termination rates of VT. For *secondary prevention* patients, when MMVT has been noted, two sequences of ATP may have added value in the fast VT zone, and two to three sequences in a slow VT zone for three-zone programming.[30]

Defibrillation and Cardioversion Shock Therapy

Although the risk of a shock inducing VF has been known since the 1700s and 1800s, the termination of VF by an electric shock was noted incidentally in the late 1800s and established in the 1930s by Wiggers and others.[32] Background work, by Gurvich in the USSR in 1939, established the supremacy of direct current (DC) shock over alternating current (AC) for terminating VF. It was appreciated in the West about 15 years later. Size constraints for implantable defibrillators led to use of a capacitor, and the high incidence of the tail end of the waveform reinducing VF led to truncation of the shock, based on work by John Schuder.

The mechanism of defibrillation has been debated since its demonstration, and theories have included transient incapacitation of the myocardium, halting the fibrillation in a critical mass of the myocardium (not necessarily the entire musculature), and termination of the reentrant rotors plus avoiding triggering new activation wavefronts leading to VF recurrence (Fig. 69.24).[33] Biphasic waveforms with a smaller or shorter second phase have supplanted monophasic waveforms due to lower defibrillation thresholds.[32,34]

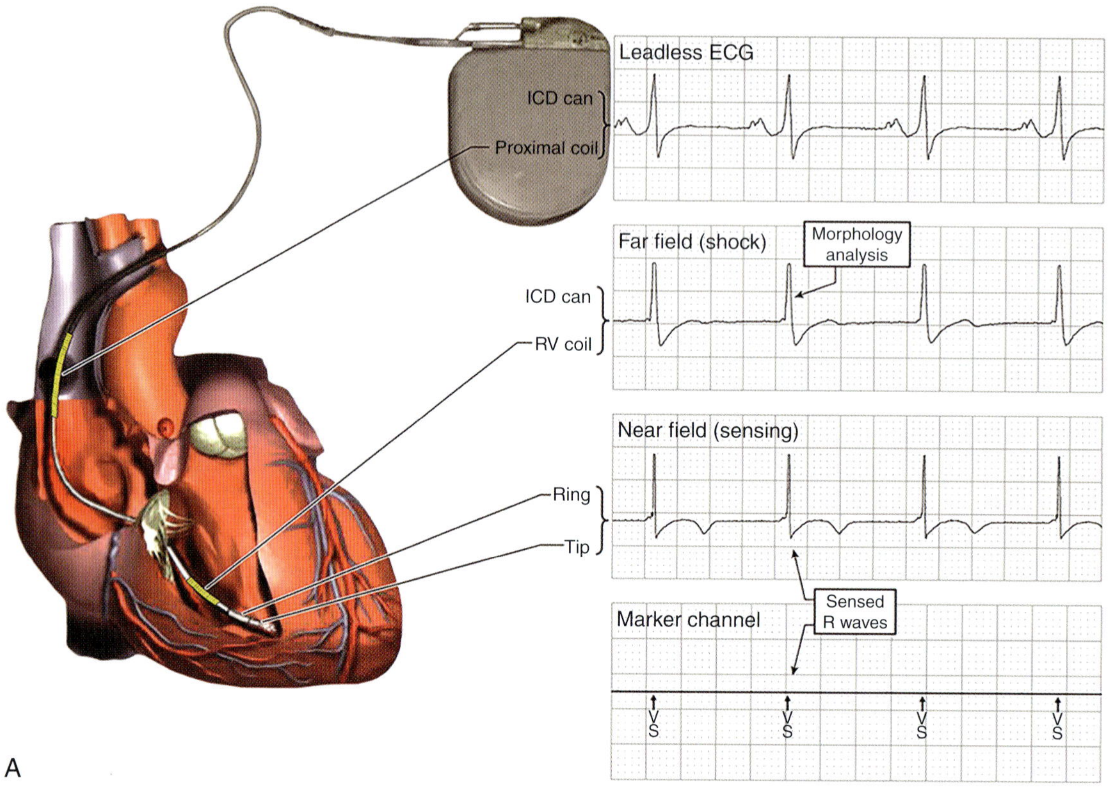

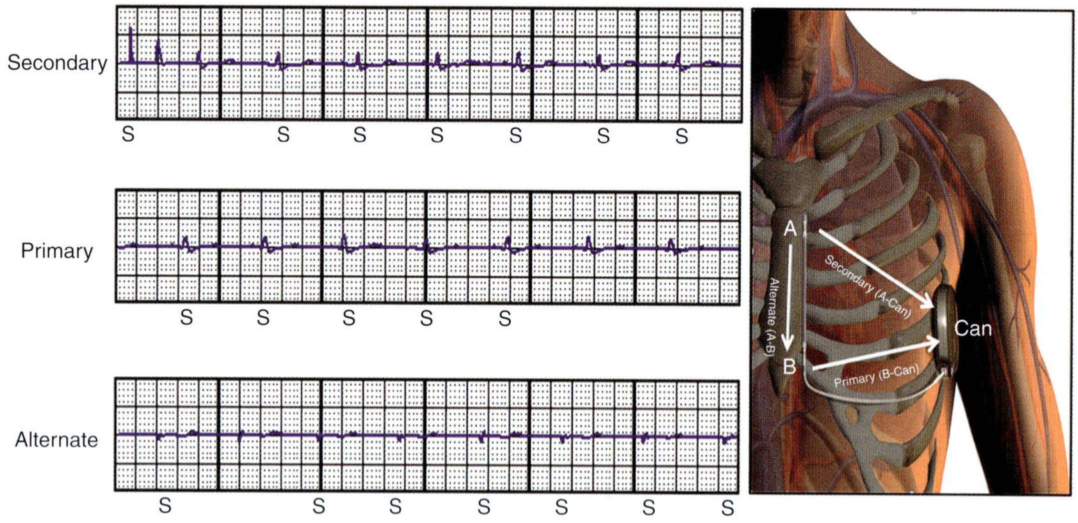

FIGURE 69.20 Implantable cardioverter-defibrillators and electrograms (EGMs). **A,** *Left,* Single-chamber ICD system, including left pectoral active can and right ventricle (RV) lead. *Right,* Telemetered EGM recorded between proximal coil and can ("leadless ECG"), high-voltage (shock) far-field EGM, and sensing near-field EGM, with annotated markers. The dual-coil lead uses true bipolar sensing between tip and ring electrodes. Marker channel denotes timing of sensed R waves from the near-field EGM (*arrows*) and ICD's classification of each ventricular event by letter symbols. "VS" denotes sensed ventricular events in the sinus rate zone. Sensing is accurate because there is a 1:1 correspondence between ventricular EGMs and markers. Morphology of shock EGMs stored during detected tachycardias is useful for distinguishing ventricular tachycardia from supraventricular tachycardia. Leadless electrocardiograms (ECGs) provide a signal with an identifiable atrial EGM with a single-chamber ICD if a dual-coil lead is used. **B,** Subcutaneous ICD records subcutaneous EGMs from one of three vectors. The amplitude of the alternate vector is smallest (as in this tracing) because it often overlies atrial tissue and the sternum. The secondary vector is prone to myopotential artifact because it usually overlies the pectoralis muscles. *S,* sensed ventricular events in the sinus rate zone. (From Swerdlow CD, Friedman P. Implantable cardioverter-defibrillator: clinical aspects. In Zipes D, Jalife J, editors: Cardiac Electrophysiology: From Cell to Bedside. 7th ed. Philadelphia: Saunders Elsevier; 2018.)

Defibrillation success rates with respect to shock size exhibit a probabilistic relationship with a sigmoidal shape, rather than a distinct threshold like myocardial capture with pacing (Fig. 69.25). Thus testing whether a given implanted lead and device would succeed in terminating VF at a given energy has proved challenging. In early decades, one or more tests involving induction and termination of VF were deemed mandatory to establish a margin of successful defibrillation. But to accurately understand the defibrillation success curve, multiple inductions are needed. Unfortunately, multiple conversions increase the risk of nonconversion, myocardial stunning, and embolization. Shortcuts with one or two inductions at levels sufficiently below the maximum output are moderately predictive of shock success for spontaneous events. An alternative or complementary approach to defibrillation threshold (DFT) testing is upper limit of vulnerability testing. As leads, devices, and waveforms have improved, the likelihood of true defibrillation incapability with a transvenous system, especially left pectoral, is low. Consequently, studies were therefore performed to assess whether not testing after implantation would have inferior or similar outcomes to a limited confirmation of defibrillation efficacy. These studies have shown similar outcomes.[35] Currently, defibrillation testing is recommended in all patients undergoing an S-ICD implant, as DFTs are higher. Defibrillation testing may be reasonable to omit in patients undergoing left pectoral transvenous ICD implantation where appropriate sensing, pacing, and impedance values and well-positioned leads are confirmed by fluoroscopy.[30] For the patient at higher risk for elevated defibrillation, such as with a right pectoral implant or patients undergoing ICD replacements, particularly with older components, testing is reasonable.

In terms of shock energy, lower energies require slightly less charge time but result in similar degree of patient discomfort, so using a maximum energy shock as the first shock is reasonable and minimizes the duration of an episode and the need for more than one (painful) shock. Particularly with evidence that for most patients testing DFTs does not improve outcomes this approach has become more common. Devices can deliver five or more shocks in a given zone for a given episode, after which point more shocks offer negligible benefit. With biphasic shocks the order of the polarity can have some bearing on success, with the RV coil being the anode for the first phase tending to be superior in some studies. For one or more of subsequent shocks, that would only be given in the event of failure of prior shocks, it is typical to try a reversed polarity sequence. Defibrillation success is also influenced by metabolic and drug effects, as well as ischemia and hemodynamic decompensation.

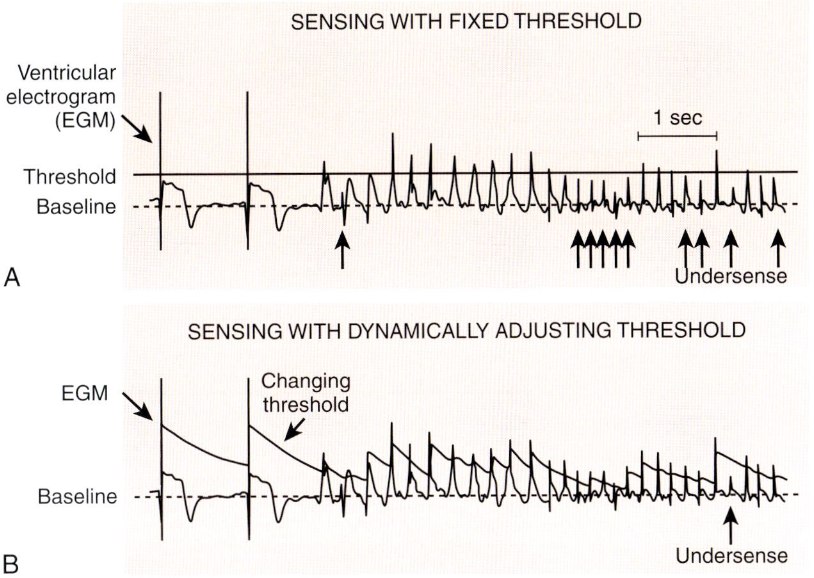

ICD TROUBLESHOOTING

Ventricular Oversensing

In early ICDs, ventricular oversensing of rapid signals usually presented as inappropriate detection of VT/VF with delivered therapy or aborted shocks. In modern ICDs with enhanced sensing features, oversensing typically presents as oversensing alerts.

Oversensing can be classified by EGM morphology, temporal pattern (cyclic versus noncyclic), source type (physiologic versus nonphysiologic), and source location (intracardiac versus extracardiac). Signals that vary with the cardiac cycle (cyclic signals) indicate an intracardiac source. Nonphysiologic sources usually are extracardiac (e.g., EMI), except for those generated by intracardiac lead failures. Physiologic signals can be intracardiac (P, R, or T waves that cause one oversensed signal per cardiac cycle) or extracardiac (myopotentials). Specific sources can generate oversensed signals with characteristic features that differ from true cardiac EGMs in frequency content and amplitude.[29]

FIGURE 69.21 Fixed versus dynamic sensing threshold in VF. **A,** Fixed sensitivity requires that the sensed potential exceed a fixed threshold. Because of the highly variable amplitude during VF, undersensing occurs (arrows). If the threshold is lowered, T wave oversensing may occur. Note that the threshold is just above the T wave amplitude during sinus rhythm, first two complexes. **B,** Dynamic adjustment of sensitivity. At the end of the blanking period after each sensed (or paced) event, the sensing threshold is set to a high value. It then decreases with time until a minimum value is reached. Undersensing is diminished while still retaining a safety margin to prevent T wave oversensing. (Modified from Olson WH. Tachyarrhythmia sensing and detection. In Singer I, editor. Implantable Cardioverter-Defibrillator. Armonk, NY: Futura; 1994, pp 71-107.)

TABLE 69.5 Strategic Programming Principles for Shock Reduction*

PRINCIPLE	RATIONALE
Sufficiently long detection time	Do not treat self-terminating VT. AF with rapid ventricular rate is less likely to exceed the rate threshold for a longer detection time.
Fast VT detection rate in primary prevention patients and secondary-prevention survivors of VF	Do not treat slower tachycardias, which are more likely to be SVT.
SVT-VT discrimination	Do not treat SVT.
ATP in all VT/VF detection zones	ATP is painless. Even in the "VF" zone, most rhythms are monomorphic VT; many can be terminated by ATP.
Maximum shock strength†	Minimize unsuccessful shocks for VT, VF, or AF with rapid ventricular rate.
Enhanced sensing features	Minimize shocks for oversensing.

*Providing AV conduction is normal and discriminator is reliable.
†Adult patients.
AF, Atrial fibrillation; *ATP,* antitachycardia pacing; *SVT,* supraventricular tachycardia; *VT,* ventricular tachycardia.

Shocks: Diagnosis and Management

Minimizing shocks requires strategic programming, use of patient alerts, and remote monitoring. Once shocks occur, diagnosis and management tools include clinical data (history, chest radiograph), ICD diagnostics (e.g., lead impedance trends), and stored EGMs (Fig. 69.26).

Approach to the Patient with Shocks

Figure 69.27 summarizes a three-step approach to the patient who presents with a shock. First, analyze stored EGMs to determine if it was delivered in response to a tachycardia or oversensing. Second, if the shock responded to a tachycardia, determine if

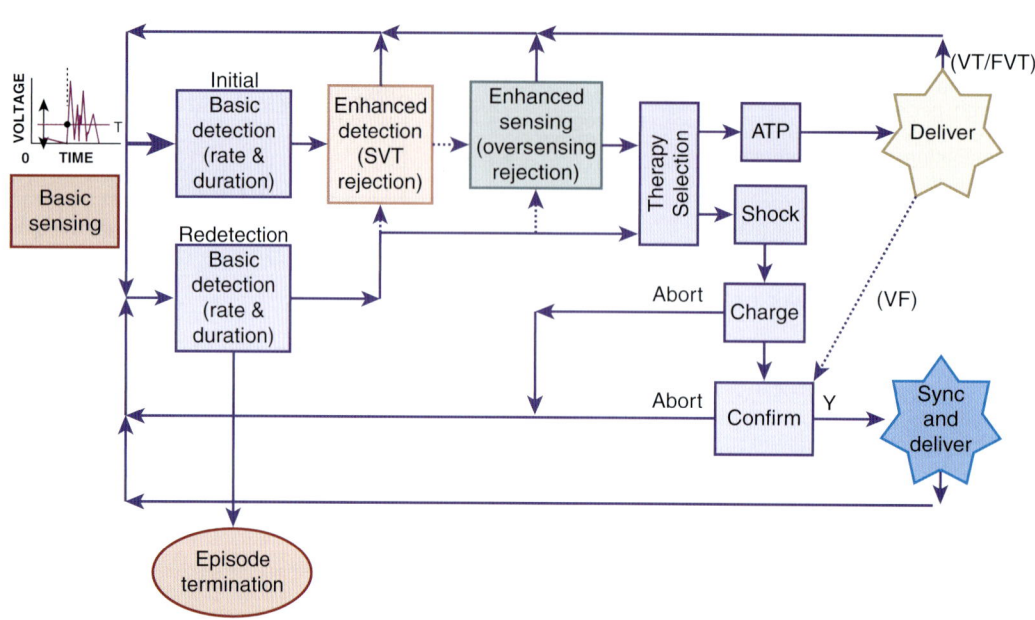

FIGURE 69.22 Overview of ICD detection algorithm. After initial basic (rate and duration) criteria are fulfilled, algorithms apply enhanced detection comprising supraventricular tachycardia–ventricular tachycardia (SVT-VT) discrimination, enhanced sensing features to detect and redetect VT, fast ventricular tachycardia (FVT), and ventricular fibrillation (VF). Enhanced sensing features may be applied either before intervals are counted or (as shown) after rate and duration are fulfilled. In the first case, oversensed signals are rejected, and only validated intervals contribute to the count. In the second case, episodes are classified specifically as oversensing events. Next, SVT-VT discriminators may classify the tachycardia as SVT; otherwise it is classified as VT/VF. When VT/VF is detected, antitachycardia pacing (ATP) is delivered immediately, but shocks require capacitor charging, which takes 6 to 15 seconds for maximum-energy. After charging is completed, ICDs perform a brief *confirmation* or *reconfirmation* process to determine if VT/VF is still present. The shock is delivered if VT/VF is reconfirmed; otherwise it is aborted. After therapy, ICDs monitor the rhythm for persistence of VT/VF or return to baseline. *Redetection* is the process by which ICDs determine whether VT/VF persists; typically it is less strict than initial detection. If VT/VF is redetected, the next programmed therapy is delivered. Simultaneously, ICDs monitor for a sufficient duration of slow intervals to fulfill the *episode termination* criterion, returning to the initial detection criteria. The VT/VF episode continues until either the ICD redetects VT or declares *episode termination*. Y, Yes. (Modified from Swerdlow C, et al. Sensing and detection with cardiac implantable electronic devices. In Ellenbogen KA, et al., editors. Clinical Cardiac Pacing, Defibrillation and Resynchronization Therapy. 5th ed. Philadelphia: Saunders; 2017.)

the rhythm is VT or SVT using established principles of ECG and EGM analysis. Third, determine whether an appropriate shock for VT/VF could have been avoided by either strategic programming (see Table 69.5) or nondevice interventions.

Because shocks for VT/VF or rapidly conducted AF are associated with increased mortality over subsequent weeks to months,[2] the clinician should not only diagnose and treat the immediate precipitant of shocks but also consider treatments to reduce delayed mortality, including reassessment for HF and ischemia.

The approach to shocks delivered for oversensing is guided by the cause of oversensing. T wave oversensing was once a common cause of inappropriate shocks in transvenous ICDs (Fig. 69.28), but its frequency has been reduced by multiple sensing enhancements and programming options.[29] However, in subcutaneous ICDs, despite electrocardiographic prescreening, it remains the most common cause of oversensing, although a new filtering algorithm has reduced these events.[26,27] Shocks for SVT may be corrected by reprogramming (rate zones or SVT-VT discriminators) and treatment with beta blockers, antiarrhythmic drugs, or ablation. Most avoidable shocks for self-terminating VT may be prevented by strategic programming.

A patient with a *single shock* can be evaluated in person or by remote monitoring within 24 to 48 hours. In contrast, *repetitive shocks* constitute an emergency (see Fig. 69.27). The cause must be determined, and VT/VF detection may be disabled using a programmer or magnet. Repetitive shocks for VT/VF may be caused by multiple unsuccessful shocks for a single episode or recurrent VT/VF after successful shock termination ("VT storm"). Multiple or inappropriate shocks for AF or SVT with rapid rates, or detection of noise, requires prompt intervention for the underlying arrhythmia or malfunction and generally require emergent reprogramming of detection criteria or disabling of detection and hospitalization.

Treatment of VT storm includes reversal of precipitating events, beta blockers, and/or pharmacologic or ablative antiarrhythmic therapy. Neuraxial interventions may also be useful.[36] Causes include acute ischemia, exacerbation of HF, metabolic abnormalities (e.g., hypokalemia, amiodarone-induced hyperthyroidism), and drug proarrhythmia or noncompliance.

Unsuccessful Shocks

Table 69.6 summarizes causes of unsuccessful shocks. If an ICD classifies a shock for VT/VF as unsuccessful, stored EGMs should be reviewed to determine if the shock truly failed to terminate VT/VF or if the ICD misclassified effective therapy as ineffective (e.g., due to immediate arrhythmia recurrence). Because defibrillation success is probabilistic, occasionally shocks fail, but failure of two maximum-output shocks is rare if the safety margin is adequate. Shocks from chronic ICD systems may fail to terminate true VT/VF because of both patient-related and ICD system–related causes. Many patient-related causes can be reversed, but system-related causes usually require operative intervention. ICD data should be reviewed for clues to system-related causes, including excessive detection or charge times, evidence of lead or connection failure, mismatch between programmed and delivered shock strength, and out-of-range high-voltage impedance, suggesting a failure in lead components of the shock circuit. In the absence of a diagnosis, defibrillation testing should be performed.

Failure to Deliver Therapy or Delayed Therapy

Delayed therapy or failure to deliver therapy can be caused by sensing problems, programmed detection parameters, or ICD system malfunction. In modern ICDs, clinically significant undersensing of VF is rare but may be caused by low-amplitude EGMs, rapidly varying EGM amplitudes (see Fig. 69.28C), drug effects, post-shock tissue changes, and device-device or intradevice interactions.[29] Rarely, enhanced

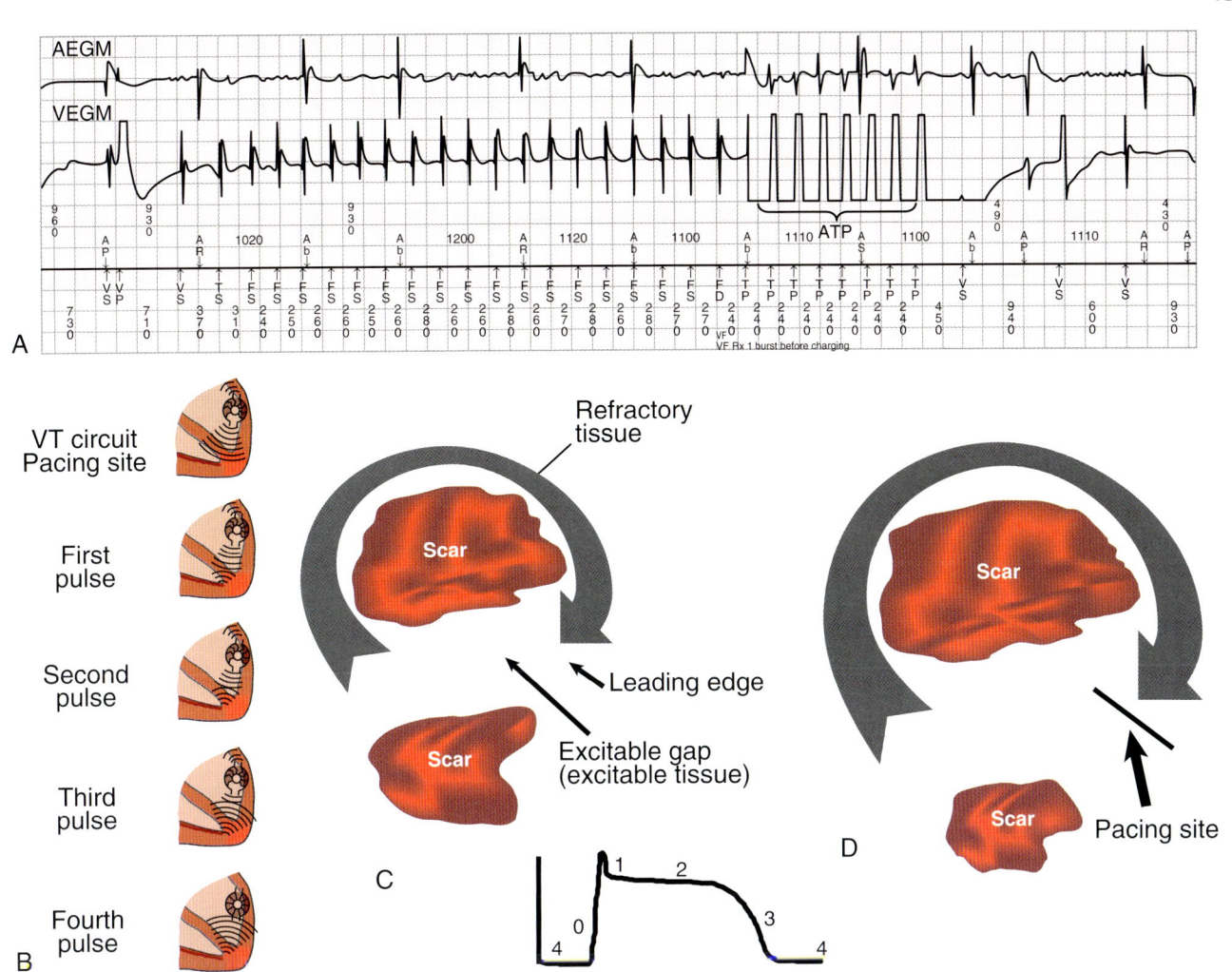

FIGURE 69.23 Antitachycardia pacing (ATP) for monomorphic ventricular tachycardia (VT). **A,** Stored atrial (AEGM) and ventricular (VEGM) electrograms and atrial and ventricular marker channels from an episode of rapid monomorphic VT (cycle length, 240 to 270 msec; rate, 220 to 250 beats/min). VT with AV dissociation begins with the second VEGM. After 18 intervals shorter than the programmed ventricular fibrillation (VF) detection interval of 320 msec, an adaptive train of eight ATP pulses is delivered at a cycle length of 240 msec, 88% of the VT cycle length, to terminate the VT. On the marker channel, VS, TS, and FS indicate intervals classified in the sinus, VT, and VF rate zones, respectively. FD, Detection of VF; TP, ATP. Note that a burst of ATP is delivered even though the intervals are in the VF zone. AP, Atrial paced events. "Ab" and "AR" indicate atrial intervals in the postventricular atrial blanking and refractory periods, respectively. **B,** Vertical panels show a conceptual model of why multiple ATP pulses are required in a train. *Top image* shows that during VT the region between the pacing lead in the right ventricular apex and the VT reentry circuit in the left ventricle is activated by the circuit. Subsequent images represent conditions after the first, second, third, and fourth ATP pulses. After each successive pulse, ATP propagates to more of the region before colliding with the VT wavefront. **C** and **D,** a conceptual model of the interaction between ATP pulses and the VT circuit. **C,** The circuit around a fixed scar is depicted by the *large curved arrow.* The head of the arrow depicts the leading edge of the wavefront, and the body of the arrow back to the tail (*gray*) represents depolarized tissue that is refractory because the wavefront has just propagated through it. The repolarized tissue between the tip and the tail of the arrow is excitable ("excitable gap"). For the head of the arrow to continue around the scar, an excitable gap must be present; if the wavefront encounters refractory tissue, it cannot proceed. **D,** A wavefront generated by an ATP pulse enters the excitable gap and terminates the VT. Tachycardias with a small excitable gap (i.e., the head of the arrow follows the tail very closely so that only a small "moving rim" of excitable tissue is in the circuit) are less likely to be terminated with ATP. (**B-D** from Hayes DL, Friedman PA, editors. Cardiac Pacing and Defibrillation: A Clinical Approach. 2nd ed. West Sussex, UK: Wiley-Blackwell; 2008.)

sensing features may classify VF as oversensing and withhold therapy. VF may be underdetected despite adequate sensing due to device inactivation or programming (sensitivity, rate, duration, SVT-VT discriminators). Lead, connector, or generator malfunction can also prevent shock delivery.

ICD Lead Failure: Presentation and Management

The serious consequences of ICD lead failure combined with reliability concerns for specific lead models have focused efforts on early diagnosis.[37] Excluding leads with known high failure rates, the overall incidence of clinical failure is about 1.3/100 lead-years.[38,2]

Clinical Presentations

Pace-sense malfunctions account for most failures. Oversensing is the most common initial electrical abnormality with either conductor fracture or insulation breach.[37] Conductor fractures usually cause a characteristic pattern of oversensing[2] (Fig. 69.29). Unlike conductor fractures, insulation breaches themselves do not generate abnormal signals. Instead, oversensing occurs because external signals enter the conductor at the breach; EGM patterns vary, reflecting the source signal. Several enhanced sensing features incorporate specific features of lead-related oversensing to alert patients and physicians and, in some cases, withhold inappropriate shocks[29,37] (see Fig. 69.28B).

Pacemakers and ICDs periodically measure DC electrical resistance ("impedance") of the pacing circuit. Usually, pacing impedance is in the normal range when oversensing occurs. Pace-sense malfunctions can also present with pacing impedance changes, loss of capture, or abrupt decrease in R wave amplitude. Pacemaker lead failures present identically to failures of ICD pace-sense components, except that oversensing causes only inhibition of pacing, not inappropriate therapy for VF.

Shock-component malfunction presents with shock-impedance changes, abnormal signals on shock EGMs, or failed defibrillation

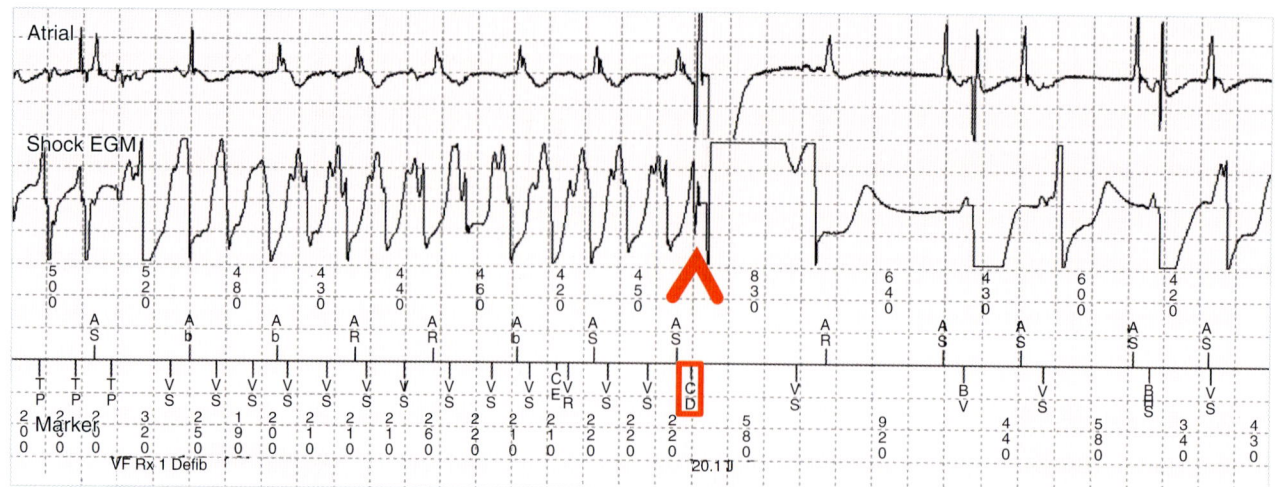

FIGURE 69.24 **Dual-chamber EGM showing polymorphic VT with AV dissociation treated with shock.** The atrial EGM, high-voltage ("shock") EGM, and dual-chamber marker channel are shown. The red arrowhead denotes shock, designated by *CD* (charge delivered) on the marker channel. After the shock, the atrial rhythm is sinus with premature atrial complexes; the ventricular rhythm is biventricular (BV) paced with premature ventricular complexes (PVCs) in the sinus rate zone (VS). The second BV beat (BV/VS) has a slightly shorter paced AV delay (110 versus 130 msec) than first BV beat because a PVC occurs during the AV delay and triggers "safety pacing," a feature that reduces crosstalk inhibition.

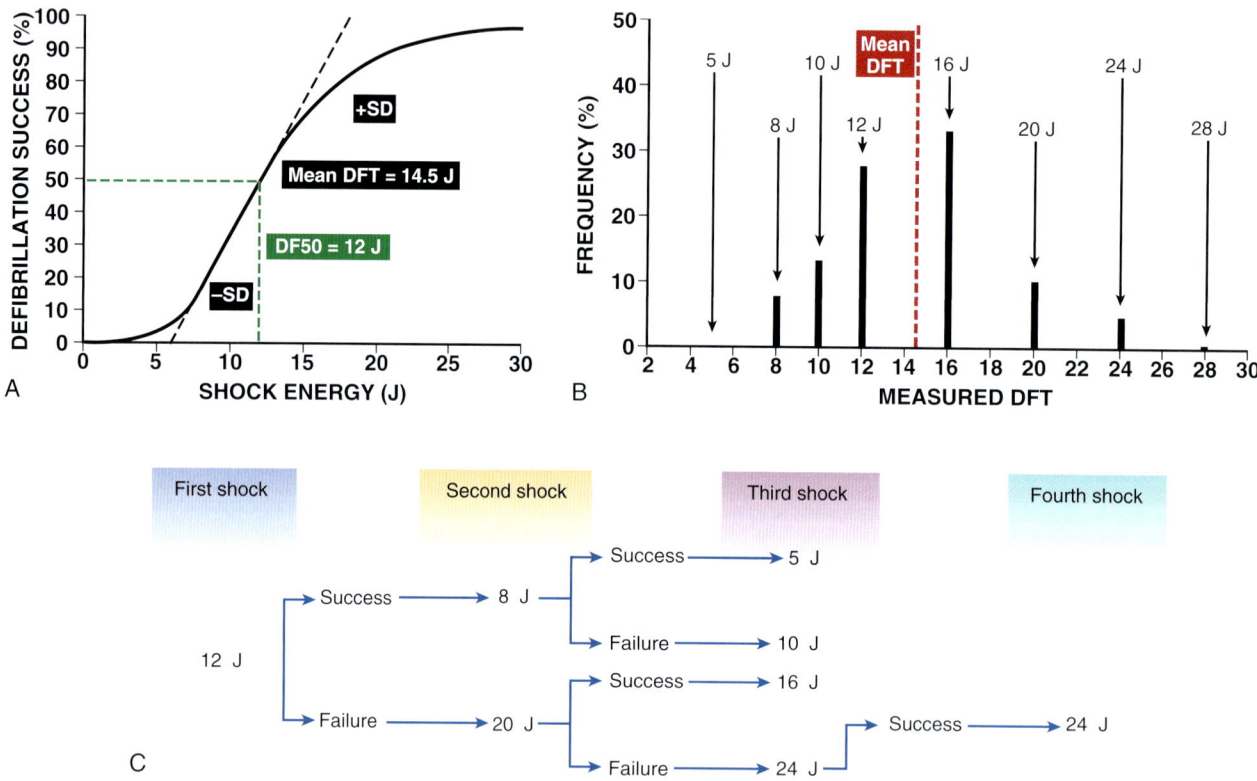

FIGURE 69.25 Relationship in an individual, simulated patient between the defibrillation probability-of-success curve and the measured defibrillation threshold (DFT) using a binary search protocol. **A,** Patient's defibrillation probability-of-success curve. **B,** Plot showing frequency of individual measured DFT values during repeated testing. **C,** Binary search sequence of three or four test shocks used to measure each DFT, starting at 12 J, the shock strength with a 50% probability of success (DF50). The process defined by the binary search protocol results in a single value, which the clinician records as the patient's "DFT." (Modified from Smits K, Virag N. Impact of defibrillation test protocol and test repetition on the probability of meeting implant criteria. Pacing Clin Electrophysiol 2011;34:1515.)

shocks. Insulation breaches that cause high-voltage short circuits may also cause ICD generator failure.

Impedance and Impedance Trends in Diagnosis of Lead Failure

Conductor fractures may cause abrupt increases in impedance; conversely, insulation breaches may cause abrupt decreases in impedance. Oversensing usually precedes impedance changes in pace-sense component failures, but impedance changes occur before or concurrently with oversensing in a minority of cases. When the cause of oversensing is in doubt, impedance abnormalities confirm the diagnosis of lead failure.

Fractures of high-voltage conductors can present as abrupt increases in shock impedance. Low shock impedance occurs in some high-voltage insulation breaches. However, diagnosing high-voltage insulation breaches by painless measurements of shock impedance is challenging because high-voltage shocks above the insulating material's dielectric breakdown voltage can cause catastrophic short circuits even if low-voltage test pulses encounter intact insulation.

Imaging

The chest x-ray film is unrevealing in most cases of lead failure, but it should be inspected for lead conductor discontinuity, kinks, or acute angles that identify stress points and twisting that suggests "twiddler's syndrome." It is important for excluding alternative causes of oversensing, such as lead dislodgement, abandoned leads, or lead fragments that cause a lead-lead interaction, and incomplete insertion of DF-1 pins into the header. Cinefluoroscopy in multiple views is more sensitive than chest radiography for identifying "inside-out" insulation breaches that cause cable conductors to protrude outside the outer insulation (externalized cables). [39,40,41]

Approach to the Patient

Figure 69.30 summarizes the approach to patients with findings suggestive of lead failure. All lead-failure diagnostics have false-positives, and the diagnosis of lead failure must be confirmed before surgical intervention to remove a failed lead.[37] Connection problems between the lead and header must be excluded. System revision involves either abandoning or extracting the failed lead and inserting a replacement lead. Usually, lead abandonment is associated with lower procedural risk, and lead extraction with fewer long-term problems. The trade-offs depend on multiple factors related to the patient, expertise of the operator/institution, specific lead model, and patient preference.[37,39,40,41]

COMPLICATIONS

Complications can be broken down temporally into acute perioperative and delayed ones. Pacemaker and ICD complications are essentially the same with the exception of shock-related issues discussed above under ICD troubleshooting. Some complications are common to all CIED devices while others are unique to transvenous, leadless, or subcutaneous-type devices. While awareness and recognition of complications should be broadly known, techniques and knowledge for the minimization and avoidance of complications, equally important, are available elsewhere.[42,43]

Vascular Access Complications

Common vascular access complications for transvenous devices include pneumothorax, hemothorax, pocket hematoma, and more rarely inadvertent arterial access.[44,45] Pneumothorax occurs in about 1% of implants, is avoidable with the cephalic vein access approach, is minimized with the extrathoracic approach, is diagnosed with chest x-ray, and if large or symptomatic, is treated with a chest tube. Venous injury or other access site bleeding, including arterial cannulation or injury can cause a pocket hematoma or hemothorax. Inadvertent placement of the lead via the subclavian vein or via a patent foramen ovale (PFO) into the left cardiac chambers can lead to stroke. The lateral view on a post-implant chest x-ray is vital to exclude this complication. Acute or subacute subclavian vein thrombosis may lead to ipsilateral upper extremity swelling; it should be managed with elevation and anticoagulation.

Lead Placement Complications

Important complications related to lead placement include cardiac perforation, dislodgement, extracardiac stimulation, and lead terminal pin to header connection problems. Cardiac perforation may present acutely or subacutely; likewise the manifestations may range from overt cardiac tamponade to pericarditis-related pain with a small effusion. Some perforations are only recognized years later having been seemingly occult, in which case the main problem is if extraction is needed for infection. Inadvertent nonmyocardial stimulation can include the right phrenic nerve from a lateral RA lead, the left phrenic nerve from an LV lead, the diaphragm itself directly from an RV lead (usually perforated but rarely at high output without perforation), and the chest wall including intercostal muscles from possible perforation. Connection issues can present with unexpected pacing observations (such as ventricle first for lead connection reversal), abnormal impedances, noise and oversensing, and loss of capture. They unfortunately require repeat operation to rectify.

Pocket Hematoma and CIED Infections

Device infections include pocket infections and/or systemic presentations (including bacteremia, lead-associated endocarditis, and valvular endocarditis). Presentations of pocket infection vary considerably, including acute pain with pocket swelling due to inflammation and contained pus, subacute pain and inflammatory signs, chronic pain and induration, and generator (or lead) erosion. Infections may present from days to years after implant. Coagulase positive or negative staphylococci are the most common pathogens. Immediate preoperative antibiotics are considered mandatory as they have been shown to reduce infections. Pocket hematomas and repeat operation (such as for hematoma or other complication) markedly increase the risk of infection. Avoiding perioperative heparin, for example, by using uninterrupted warfarin or uninterrupted (or minimally interrupted) direct oral anticoagulant (DOAC) as opposed to heparin bridging reduces the risk of hematoma.[45,46] The management of either pocket infection or systemic infection requires full system removal, including lead extraction.[41,40] Although bacteremia can occur without incurring lead-associated endocarditis, the latter is more common with staphylococci[47] or if vegetations are identified. Recently, an antibiotic-impregnated, dissolvable envelope was found to reduce the risk of device infection, whereas a trial evaluating pocket instilled and additional antibiotics was not superior to a single preoperative antibiotic dose.[48,49]

Subcutaneous ICD Complications

Vascular access complications (pneumothorax, cardiac perforation, etc.) do not pertain to subcutaneous ICDs.[25] Pocket infection occurred in 1.1% of implants in a large series,[26] but systemic infections have not been reported. A trend toward lower total infections was seen in the Praetorian trial compared with transvenous ICDs.[27] Inappropriate shocks have been reduced with new sensing algorithms but still run higher than for transvenous ICDs.[26,27]

Leadless Pacemaker Complications

Leadless pacemaker implantation is not associated with pocket complications or pneumothorax, but can result in femoral access-related complications or cardiac perforation.[50] Initial studies found a higher rate of pericardial complications with leadless (1.0% to 1.5%) than transvenous pacemakers, but one study has shown a decline in such events possibly due to increased operator experience.[50,51] Tricuspid valve injury or regurgitation can occur especially for more basal insertions or from device removal.[52] Device dislodgement and embolization has occurred in 0% to 1.1% of implants. Pocket infection is of course eliminated, and intravascular infection appears to be much less likely even in cases of documented bacteremia, but one case has been reported.[50]

FOLLOW-UP AND MANAGEMENT

Remote Monitoring

The convergence of internet technology, improved telemetry, and enhanced CIED diagnostics permits remote monitoring of multiple device functions and improves patient management[53]. Currently, most ICDs and many pacemakers use "wireless telemetry" to transmit data automatically to a home monitor, which then relays the data to a server via an Internet connection. Smartphone-based applications are also coming into use for implanted devices. By convention, *remote interrogation* refers to scheduled, routine device interrogation at a distance, corresponding to in-clinic interrogation; *remote monitoring* refers to automatic data transmission based on device-generated alerts.[53] Colloquially, "remote monitoring" includes both. Routine, scheduled transmissions include battery status, pacing and sensing thresholds, lead impedances, and detected arrhythmias. Patients can also initiate transmissions in response to symptoms. Health care providers log into a Web server to review alerts and transmitted data. ICDs and some pacemakers provide programmable alerts for system malfunction (e.g., suspected lead failure), potential programming errors (e.g., VF detection or therapy "off"), or high-risk arrhythmias. Alerts may be transmitted daily or even immediately. Alerts may also notify the patient through audible tones or generator vibration. A "lead integrity alert" reduces inappropriate shocks caused by lead failure.[37]

CIED Diagnostics for Atrial Fibrillation

Remote monitoring can be used to monitor comorbidities if relevant data are stored in the device or input into the local hub from another source. AF is an important comorbidity that can be monitored reliably by CIEDs with an atrial lead. ICD patients with rapidly conducted AF have an increased risk of inappropriate shocks, and early diagnosis may permit treatment or reprogramming to prevent inappropriate therapy. Early treatment of new-onset, persistent AF may reduce exacerbations of HF. Alerts for AF facilitate early anticoagulation and adjustment of rate and rhythm control medications.[53] In CIED patients, asymptomatic AF episodes as short as 5 minutes are associated with an increased rate of stroke, although it is not clear if AF is causal. Present data are insufficient to determine if continuous device monitoring of patients with infrequent paroxysmal AF might permit safe withdrawal of anticoagulation or intermittent use of short-acting anticoagulants.

Device Clinic Follow-Up

Despite the ability to track device and patient status using remote monitoring, in-person follow-up remains helpful, particularly if troubleshooting, reprogramming, or optimization of device therapy is needed. Adjustments in pacing output may help to extend device longevity or maintain a capture safety margin. Inspection of rate histograms and atrial and ventricular pacing trends may indicate a need for sensor or AV delay programming optimization that can enhance exertional tolerance or reduce unnecessary ventricular pacing, respectively. Programming changes can be evaluated and, if needed, changed iteratively using in clinic walk testing. Typical in-person follow-up intervals for patients on remote monitoring are yearly for pacemakers and ICDs. More frequent in-person follow-up is advisable for patients not on remote monitoring (e.g., every 3 to 6 months) or those who are pacemaker-dependent (e.g., every 6 months). In-person follow-up remains necessary for reprogramming or evaluation of suspected malfunction.

Electromagnetic Interference

Ubiquitous electromagnetic waves sometimes interfere with CIEDs, potentially causing temporary or permanent inactivation, inappropriate

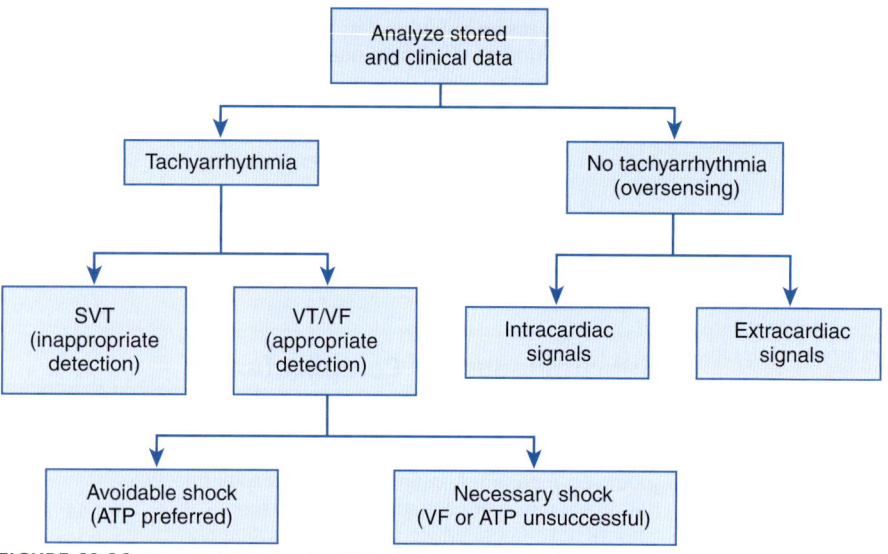

FIGURE 69.26 Differential diagnosis of ICD shocks. See text for details.

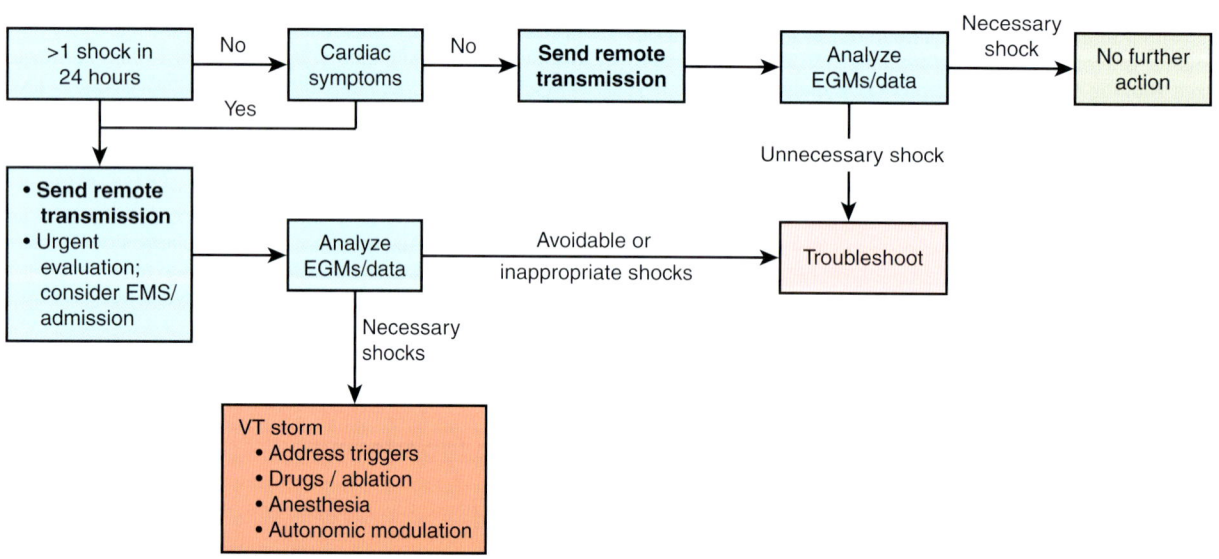

FIGURE 69.27 Approach to the patient with ICD shocks at home. Remote monitoring facilitates care of patients who receive shocks. In the absence of ongoing cardiac symptoms, a single appropriate shock (reviewed remotely) does not require further intervention. Multiple shocks or ongoing symptoms require urgent action to treat VT storm, treat SVT, or troubleshoot to prevent oversensing. (From Swerdlow CD, Friedman P. Implantable cardioverter-defibrillator: clinical aspects. In Zipes D, Jalife J, editors. Cardiac Electrophysiology: From Cell to Bedside. 7th ed. Philadelphia: Elsevier; 2018.)

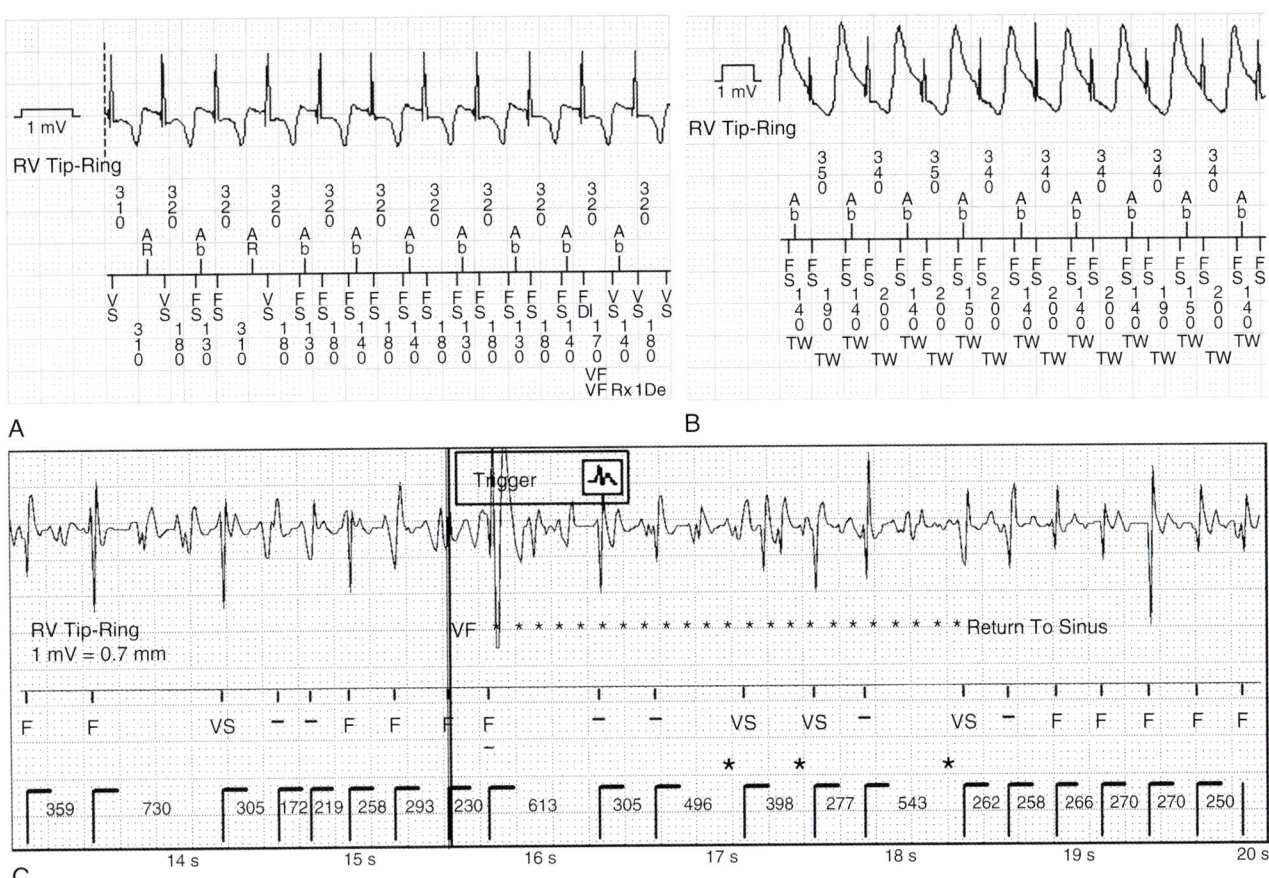

FIGURE 69.28 Abnormal sensing. Wide-band dedicated bipolar RV EGMs during sinus tachycardia with dual-chamber markers. Each EGM shows the characteristic pattern of alternating high-frequency and low-frequency sensed events, with two ventricular events for each atrial event. One millivolt (mV) calibration markers are shown at *left*. **A,** Oversensing of T waves causes inappropriate detection of ventricular fibrillation (VF). High-amplitude T waves cause intermittent oversensing despite adequate (10 mV base to peak) R waves. "VF Rx [Therapy] 1 De" at *lower right* denotes inappropriate detection of VF. **B,** Enhanced sensing algorithm identifies the pattern of T wave oversensing therapy (TW markers) and prevents inappropriate detection of VF despite consistent T wave oversensing. Low-amplitude (1.5 to 4.0 mV) R waves are the root cause of this T wave oversensing. **C,** Undersensing. Dedicated bipolar, filtered EGM is shown during ongoing VF. Between 15 and 18 seconds (s), there are fewer markers than true EGMs indicating undersensing. The single-zone VF detection interval is 360 msec and programmed minimum sensitivity 0.3 mV. Undersensing occurs primarily from amplitude of EGMs changing faster than dynamic sensitivity can adjust despite EGM amplitudes that exceed the minimum sensitivity. Shortly after detection of VF at vertical line (Trigger, VF), three consecutive classified intervals (separated by one unclassified interval) are classified in the sinus zone (VS, *asterisks*). This results in clinically incorrect termination of the device-defined VF episode (Return to Sinus) despite ongoing VF. The ICD subsequently performed a second initial detection of VF and delivered a successful shock. (From Swerdlow CD, Friedman P. Implantable cardioverter-defibrillator: clinical aspects. In Zipes D, Jalife J, editors. Cardiac Electrophysiology: From Cell to Bedside. 7th ed. Philadelphia: Elsevier; 2018.)

TABLE 69.6 Causes of Unsuccessful ICD Shocks

Successful Termination of VT/VF Misclassified by the ICD

VT/VF recurs before the device determines the VT/VF episode has terminated.
Failure to terminate SVT (e.g., sinus tachycardia)
Postshock rhythm is SVT in the VT rate zone.

Patient-Related Factors

Metabolic (hyperkalemia)
Ischemia
Progression of heart failure
Some antiarrhythmic drugs (e.g., amiodarone, type IC)
Pleural or pericardial effusions

Device System–Related Reasons

Insufficient programmed shock strength
Battery depletion
Failure of generator component or lead
Device-lead connection problem
Lead dislodgement
Delayed detection resulting in a prolonged VT/VF that increases required shock strength

ICD, Implantable cardioverter-defibrillator; *SVT,* supraventricular tachycardia; *VF,* ventricular fibrillation; *VT,* ventricular tachycardia.

pacing or inhibition of pacing or shocks, and inappropriate detection of VT/VF.[2]

Nonmedical Sources. Clinically significant EMI is extremely rare for household appliances. Although the risk is very low, patients should hold activated digital cellular phones to the contralateral ear and should avoid carrying phones in the ipsilateral breast pocket. CIED patients may walk through airport metal detectors and electronic article surveillance devices at a normal pace. Prolonged exposure can inhibit pacing and detection of VT/VF, cause inappropriate detection of VT/VF, or (rarely) program VT/VF detection "off."

Medical Sources. Medical sources of EMI are most frequently associated with electrosurgery (electrocautery) or MRI.

Perioperative Management of CIED Patients. A consensus statement requires preoperative determination of pacemaker dependency, device model, type of lead, and plans to use electrocautery to inform management[54]. The arterial pulse must be monitored intraoperatively. Intraoperative management strategies may include magnet application or perioperative reprogramming. When a magnet is placed over a pacemaker, it paces asynchronously. In contrast, a magnet placed over an ICD disables detection of VT/VF but does not alter pacing mode.

The risk of oversensing is greatest for monopolar electrocautery delivered between a pen and a remote dispersive ground electrode, especially when the surgical site is in proximity to the device or sensing electrodes.[54] If the surgical incision and dispersive ground pad are both

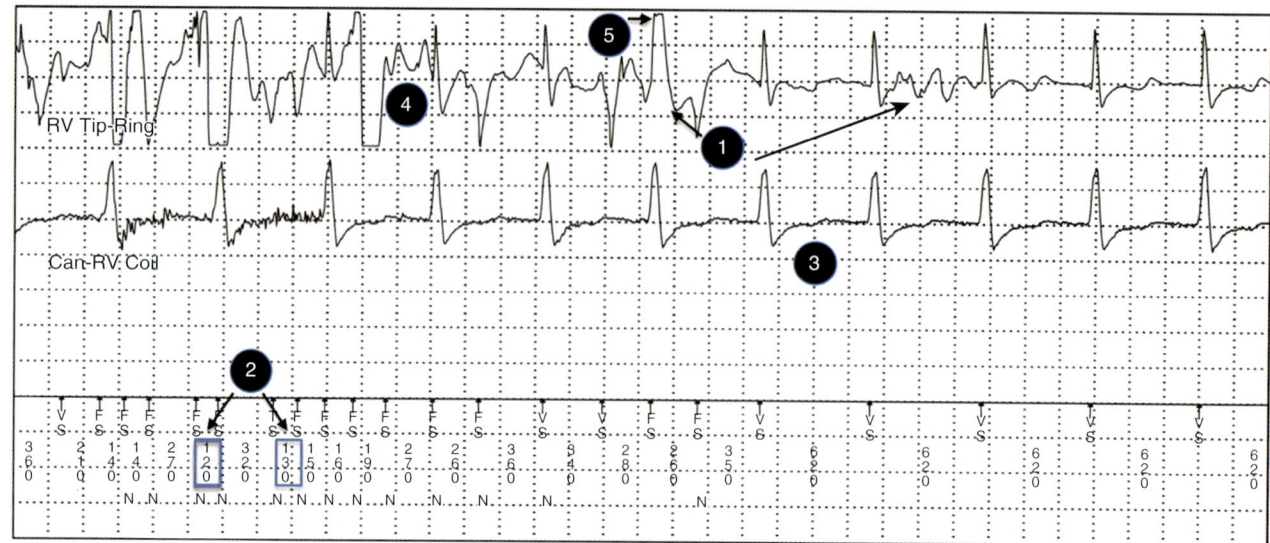

FIGURE 69.29 EGM conductor fracture or connection problem between DF1 lead and header. Characteristic features include (1) intermittent nonphysiologic signals, (2) "nonphysiologic" intervals too short to correspond to successive ventricular depolarizations, (3) no abnormal signals on shock channel of dedicated sensing bipole, (4) variable amplitude, morphology, and frequency, and (5) may saturate sensing amplifier. Enhanced sensing feature (lead noise algorithm) prevents inappropriate detection of VF, classifying intervals as "N" (noise) on marker channel. High-frequency signal superimposed on shock channel probably is caused by pectoral myopotentials, which are a normal finding on EGMs, including the can. (From Swerdlow CD, Friedman P. Implantable cardioverter-defibrillator: clinical aspects. In Zipes D, Jalife J, editors. Cardiac Electrophysiology: From Cell to Bedside. 7th ed. Philadelphia: Elsevier; 2018.)

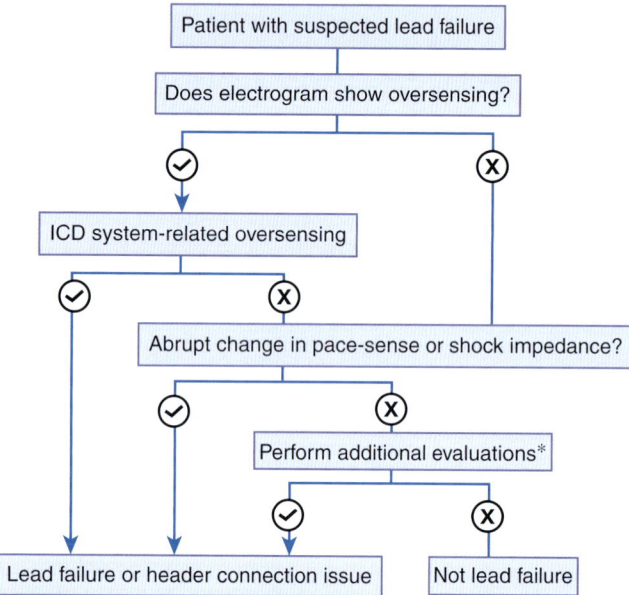

FIGURE 69.30 Deductive approach to suspected ICD lead failure. See text for details. *Additional evaluations include real-time, pace-sense electrograms with muscle exercise and pocket manipulation; shock EGMs; differential EGMs; and pacing and sensing thresholds. (From Swerdlow CD, et al. Implantable cardiac defibrillator lead failure and management. J Am Coll Cardiol 2016;67(11):1358-1368.)

below the umbilicus, the risk of EMI is low. Rate-adaptive sensors should be disabled.

Magnetic Resonance Imaging. MRI exposes CIED patients to risks resulting from mechanical forces generated by the static magnetic field, heat and current flow in the leads induced by the radiofrequency fields, and current induced by gradient magnetic fields. MRI-conditional pacemaker and ICD systems employ PGs and leads designed to permit safe imaging under specific MRI conditions when programmed to fixed rate (VOO, DOO) or nonpacing (ODO) modes.[55] MRI of patients with standard CIEDs may be performed safely by implementing rigorous risk mitigation strategies.[2]

Other Medical Procedures and Devices. When external cardioversion is required, defibrillation pads should be placed at least 8 inches (20 cm) from the PG. In ICD patients, cardioversion of AF can be attempted through the device. Ionizing radiation therapy can damage CIED circuitry, and CIEDs should be shielded or if necessary moved to the contralateral side when necessary (e.g., when exposure to the CIED device will exceed 5 Gy). Left ventricular assist devices (LVADs) cause specific forms of EMI.[2,56] Dialysis procedures pose potential infection risks, particularly if performed ipsilateral to an implanted CIED. If feasible, at implant, contralateral transvenous placement or subcutaneous ICD devices may be considered.

DEVICE LONGEVITY AND REPLACEMENT CONSIDERATIONS

Improvements in battery longevity have led to devices that can last 10 years or longer, depending on pacing use, shocks, and threshold requirements. Device indicators of battery depletion include measures of battery voltage. Devices can be programmed to issue a tone or vibration when elective replacement indicators are reached. Remote monitoring facilitates detection of these indicators. Generally several months of function remain when elective replacement indicators are reached, allowing a margin of time from detection to replacement.

Before device replacement, evaluation should include assessment of lead function to anticipate need for lead extraction, revision or replacement, and ventricular dysfunction that may indicate need for upgrade to an ICD or CRT device. In the event that addition of a lead is planned, venography may be needed. Another consideration is improvement in ventricular function in patients who had implanted ICDs for primary prevention of SCD due to ventricular dysfunction but who have had improvement in ventricular function. However, studies report that although arrhythmic events are reduced when ventricular function improves, risk for arrhythmic events is not entirely mitigated by improvements in ventricular function.[57] Thus, unless there is patient preference otherwise, ICDs are usually replaced with another ICD at time of battery depletion.

Common Clinical Issues in CIED Patients
Psychosocial Issues

ICD patients may experience anxiety about shocks, but they may also feel protected from the risk of sudden death. ICD recipients may benefit from interventions such as counseling, education, and support groups.[58] It is important to provide patients with a plan for what to do when a shock occurs. ICD patients benefit from counseling after shocks occur.[2] This includes reviewing what triggered the shock and what intervention has been taken to mitigate the trigger, estimating the likelihood of future shocks after this intervention, explaining that shocks are one of multiple challenges of living with heart disease, and usually emphasizing the value of returning to normal activity.

A consensus statement addresses legal and ethical issues related to withdrawal of CIED therapy to reduce suffering at the end of a patient's life.[2,59] This is important because 20% of ICD patients receive painful shocks in their last weeks of life. A patient (or legally defined surrogate decision maker) has the right to request withdrawal of any medical therapy, including CIED therapy, even if such withdrawal allows the patient to die naturally from an underlying disease.

Lifestyle Issues
Driving
Pacemaker patients are not restricted from driving after the perioperative period. Guidelines for ICD patients recommend that patients refrain from driving for 6 months after each shock for VT/VF and for 6 months after ICD implant for secondary prevention.[2] Primary prevention patients are not restricted from driving personal cars (versus commercial vehicles).

Participation in Sports
Exercise improves health and quality of life but may induce VT/VF in patients with specific diseases.[60] Decisions regarding sports participation should be based on the patient's underlying disease, indication for ICD therapy (e.g., primary versus secondary prevention, risk of exerciseinduced VT/VF), and risks of specific sports (e.g., ICD system damage in contact sports, risk of trauma with transient loss of consciousness).[60] Athletes with ICDs experience shocks for both VT/VF and SVT more frequently during sports than at rest, but the risk of injury or failure to terminate VT/VF is low.[2] Swimming presents the risk of drowning even if VT/VF is treated promptly.

Drug Interactions
Antiarrhythmic drugs are used in pacemaker patients to prevent AF and in ICD patients to prevent both AF and VT/VF. RCTs report reduction in VT/VF using either sotalol or the combination of amiodarone and beta blockers. However, antiarrhythmic and other drugs have important interactions with devices. Certain antiarrhythmic drugs (e.g., amiodarone, 1C agents) may increase pacing or DFTs. Beta blockers and other drugs that prolong AV conduction may increase RV pacing burden and thereby exacerbate HF. Antiarrhythmic drugs prescribed for VT/VF or AF (e.g., amiodarone) may slow the rate of VT and thus require decreasing the rate threshold to ensure that VT is detected.

REFERENCES
General Considerations
1. Kusumoto FM, Schoenfeld MH, Barrett C, et al. 2018 ACC/AHA/HRS guideline on the evaluation and management of patients with bradycardia and cardiac conduction delay. *J Am College Cardiol*. 2018.
2. Swerdlow CD, Wang PJ, Zipes DP. *Pacemakers and Implantable Cardioverter-Defibrillators. Braunwald's Heart Disease: A Textbook of Cardiovascular Medicine*. Mosby; 2018.
3. Roca-Luque I, Francisco-Pasqual J, Oristrell G, et al. Flecainide versus procainamide in electrophysiological study in patients with syncope and wide QRS duration. *JACC Clin Electrophysiol*. 2019;5:212–219.
4. Bradshaw PJ, Stobie P, Knuiman MW, et al. Trends in the incidence and prevalence of cardiac pacemaker insertions in an ageing population. *Open Heart*. 2014;1:e000177.
5. Galappaththige SK, Gray RA, Roth BJ. Cardiac strength-interval curves calculated using a bidomain tissue with a parsimonious ionic current. *PloS One*. 2017;12:e0171144.

Types of Pacemakers
6. Gaeta S, Bahnson TD, Henriquez C. Mechanism and magnitude of bipolar electrogram directional sensitivity: characterizing underlying determinants of bipolar amplitude. *Heart Rhythm*. 2020;17:777–785.
7. Josephson ME, Anter E. Substrate mapping for ventricular tachycardia: assumptions and misconceptions. *JACC Clin Electrophysiol*. 2015;1:341–352.
8. Worsnick SA, Sharma PS, Vijayaraman P. Right ventricular septal pacing: a paradigm shift. *J Innov Card Rhythm Manag*. 2018;9:3137–3146.
9. Vijayaraman P, Chung MK, Dandamudi G, et al. His bundle pacing. *J Am Coll Cardiol*. 2018;72:927–947.
10. Merchant FM, Mittal S. Pacing-induced cardiomyopathy. *Card Electrophysiol Clin*. 2018;10:437–445.
11. Vijayaraman P, Herweg B, Dandamudi G, et al. Outcomes of His-bundle pacing upgrade after long-term right ventricular pacing and/or pacing-induced cardiomyopathy: insights into disease progression. *Heart Rhythm*. 2019;16:1554–1561.
12. Sharma PS, Dandamudi G, Naperkowski A, et al. Permanent His-bundle pacing is feasible, safe, and superior to right ventricular pacing in routine clinical practice. *Heart Rhythm*. 2015;12:305–312.
13. Vijayaraman P, Naperkowski A, Subzposh FA, et al. Permanent His-bundle pacing: long-term lead performance and clinical outcomes. *Heart Rhythm*. 2018;15:696–702.
14. Burri H, Jastrzebski M, Vijayaraman P. Electrocardiographic analysis for His bundle pacing at implantation and follow-up. *JACC Clin Electrophysiol*. 2020;6:883–900.

Pacing Mode and Timing Cycles
15. Upadhyay GA, Cherian T, Shatz DY, et al. Intracardiac delineation of septal conduction in left bundle-branch block patterns. *Circulation*. 2019;139:1876–1888.
16. Vijayaraman P, Subzposh FA, Naperkowski A, et al. Prospective evaluation of feasibility and electrophysiologic and echocardiographic characteristics of left bundle branch area pacing. *Heart Rhythm*. 2019;16:1774–1782.
17. Auricchio A, Ellenbogen KA. Reducing ventricular pacing frequency in patients with atrioventricular block: is it time to change the current pacing paradigm? *Circ Arrhythm Electrophysiol*. 2016;9:e004404.
18. Tjong FV, Reddy VY. Permanent leadless cardiac pacemaker therapy: a comprehensive review. *Circulation*. 2017;135:1458–1470.
19. Wass SY, Kanj M, Mayuga K, et al. Proarrhythmic effects from competitive atrial pacing and potential programming solutions. *Pacing Clin Electrophysiol*. 2020;43:720–729.
20. Hussein AA, Wilkoff BL. Cardiac implantable electronic device therapy in heart failure. *Circ Res*. 2019;124:1584–1597.
21. Al-Khatib SM, Stevenson WG, Ackerman MJ, et al. AHA/ACC/HRS guideline for management of patients with ventricular arrhythmias and the prevention of sudden cardiac death: executive summary: a report of the American College of Cardiology/American Heart Association Task Force on Clinical Practice Guidelines and the Heart Rhythm Society. *J Am Coll Cardiol*. 2017.

Implantable Cardioverter-Defibrillators
22. Goldenberg I, Gillespie J, Moss AJ, et al. Long-term benefit of primary prevention with an implantable cardioverter-defibrillator: an extended 8-year follow-up study of the multicenter automatic defibrillator implantation trial II. *Circulation*. 2010;122:1265–1271.
23. Kusumoto FM, Calkins H, Boehmer J, et al. HRS/ACC/AHA expert consensus statement on the use of implantable cardioverter-defibrillator therapy in patients who are not included or not well represented in clinical trials. *J Am Coll Cardiol*. 2014.
24. Russo AM, Stainback RF, Bailey SR, et al. ACCF/HRS/AHA/ASE/HFSA/SCAI/SCCT/SCMR 2013 appropriate use criteria for implantable cardioverter-defibrillators and cardiac resynchronization therapy: a report of the American College of Cardiology Foundation Appropriate Use Criteria Task Force, Heart Rhythm Society, American Heart Association, American Society of Echocardiography, Heart Failure Society of America, Society for Cardiovascular Angiography and Interventions, Society of Cardiovascular Computed Tomography, and Society for Cardiovascular Magnetic Resonance. *J Am Coll Cardiol*. 2013.
25. Lewis GF, Gold MR. Safety and efficacy of the subcutaneous implantable defibrillator. *J Am Coll Cardiol*. 2016;67:445–454.
26. Gold MR, Lambiase PD, El-Chami MF, et al. Primary results from the understanding outcomes with the S-ICD in primary prevention patients with low ejection fraction (UNTOUCHED) trial. *Circulation*. 2021;143:7–17.
27. Knops RE, Olde Nordkamp LRA, Delnoy PHM, et al. Subcutaneous or transvenous defibrillator therapy. *N Engl J Med*. 2020;383:526–536.
28. Baccillieri MS, Gasparini G, Benacchio L, et al. Multicentre comparison of shock efficacy using single- vs. dual-coil lead systems and anodal vs. cathodaL polarITY defibrillation in patients undergoing transvenous cardioverter-defibrillator implantation. The MODALITY study. *J Interv Card Electrophysiol*. 2015;43:45–54.
29. Swerdlow CD, Asirvatham SJ, Ellenbogen KA, Friedman PA. Troubleshooting implanted cardioverter defibrillator sensing problems I. *Circ Arrhythm Electrophysiol*. 2014;7:1237–1261.
30. Wilkoff BL, Fauchier L, Stiles MK, et al. 2015 HRS/EHRA/APHRS/SOLAECE expert consensus statement on optimal implantable cardioverter-defibrillator programming and testing. *Heart Rhythm*. 2016;13:e50–86.
31. Schuger C, Daubert JP, Zareba W, et al. Reassessing the role of antitachycardia pacing in fast ventricular arrhythmias in primary prevention implantable cardioverter-defibrillator recipients: results from MADIT-RIT. *Heart Rhythm*. 2020.
32. Cakulev I, Efimov IR, Waldo AL. Cardioversion: past, present, and future. *Circulation*. 2009;120:1623–1632.
33. Chen PS, Shibata N, Dixon EG, et al. Comparison of the defibrillation threshold and the upper limit of ventricular vulnerability. *Circulation*. 1986;73:1022–1028.
34. Dixon EG, Tang AS, Wolf PD, et al. Improved defibrillation thresholds with large contoured epicardial electrodes and biphasic waveforms. *Circulation*. 1987;76:1176–1184.
35. Healey JS, Hohnloser SH, Glikson M, et al. Cardioverter defibrillator implantation without induction of ventricular fibrillation: a single-blind, non-inferiority, randomised controlled trial (SIMPLE). *Lancet*. 2015;385:785–791.
36. Tung R, Shivkumar K. Neuraxial modulation for treatment of VT storm. *J Biomed Res*. 2015;29:56–60.

Complications
37. Swerdlow CD, Kalahasty G, Ellenbogen KA. Implantable cardiac defibrillator lead failure and management. *J Am Coll Cardiol*. 2016;67:1358–1368.
38. Resnic FS, Majithia A, Dhruva SS, et al. Active surveillance of the implantable cardioverter-defibrillator registry for defibrillator lead failures. *Circ Cardiovasc Qual Outcomes*. 2020;13:e006105.
39. Pokorney SD, Mi X, Lewis RK, et al. Outcomes associated with extraction versus capping and abandoning pacing and defibrillator leads. *Circulation*. 2017.
40. Lewis RK, Pokorney SD, Hegland DD, Piccini JP. Hands on: how to approach patients undergoing lead extraction. *J Cardiovasc Electrophysiol*. 2020;31:1801–1808.
41. Kusumoto FM, Schoenfeld MH, Wilkoff BL, et al. 2017 HRS expert consensus statement on cardiovascular implantable electronic device lead management and extraction. *Heart Rhythm*. 2017.
42. Blomström-Lundqvist C, Traykov V, Erba PA, et al. European Heart Rhythm Association (EHRA) international consensus document on how to prevent, diagnose, and treat cardiac implantable electronic device infections-endorsed by the Heart Rhythm Society (HRS), the Asia Pacific Heart Rhythm Society (APHRS), the Latin American Heart Rhythm Society (LAHRS), International Society for Cardiovascular Infectious Diseases (ISCVID), and the European Society of Clinical Microbiology and Infectious Diseases (ESCMID) in collaboration with the European Association for Cardio-Thoracic Surgery (EACTS). *Eur Heart J*. 2020.
43. Carrillo R, Healy C. Clinical cardiac pacing, defibrillation and resynchronization therapy E-book. In: Ellenbogen KA, et al., eds. Elsevier; 2016: 1200.
44. Timmers L, Van Heuverswyn F, De Wilde H, Jordaens L. Evaluating current implantable cardioverter defibrillator implantation procedures: can common complications be minimised. *Expert Rev Cardiovasc Ther*. 2016;14:579–589.
45. Essebag V, Verma A, Healey JS, et al. Clinically significant pocket hematoma increases long-term risk of device infection: BRUISE CONTROL INFECTION study. *J Am Coll Cardiol*. 2016;67:1300–1308.
46. Birnie DH, Healey JS, Wells GA et al. Continued vs. interrupted direct oral anticoagulants at the time of device surgery, in patients with moderate to high risk of arterial thrombo-embolic events (BRUISE CONTROL-2). *Euro Heart J*. 2018ehy413-ehy413.
47. Maskarinec SA, Thaden JT, Cyr DD, et al. The risk of cardiac device-related infection in bacteremic patients is species specific: results of a 12-year prospective cohort. *Open Forum Infect Dis*. 2017;4:ofx132.
48. Tarakji KG, Mittal S, Kennergren C, et al. Antibacterial envelope to prevent cardiac implantable device infection. *N Engl J Med*. 2019;380:1895–1905.
49. Krahn AD, Longtin Y, Philippon F, et al. Prevention of arrhythmia device infection trial: the PADIT trial. *J Am Coll Cardiol*. 2018;72:3098–3109.
50. Lee JZ, Mulpuru SK, Shen WK. Leadless pacemaker: performance and complications. *Trends Cardiovasc Med*. 2018;28:130–141.

51. Roberts PR, Clementy N, Al Samadi F, et al. A leadless pacemaker in the real-world setting: the micra transcatheter pacing system post-approval registry. *Heart Rhythm.* 2017;14:1375–1379.
52. Beurskens NEG, Tjong FVY, de Bruin-Bon RHA, et al. Impact of leadless pacemaker therapy on cardiac and atrioventricular valve function through 12 Months of follow-up. *Circ Arrhythm Electrophysiol.* 2019;12:e007124.

Follow-up and Management

53. Slotwiner D, Varma N, Akar JG, et al. HRS Expert Consensus Statement on remote interrogation and monitoring for cardiovascular implantable electronic devices. *Heart Rhythm.* 2015;12:e69–e100.
54. Crossley GH, Poole JE, Rozner MA, et al. The Heart Rhythm Society (HRS)/American Society of Anesthesiologists (ASA) Expert Consensus Statement on the perioperative management of patients with implantable defibrillators, pacemakers and arrhythmia monitors: facilities and patient management this document was developed as a joint project with the American Society of Anesthesiologists (ASA), and in collaboration with the American Heart Association (AHA), and the Society of Thoracic Surgeons (STS). *Heart Rhythm.* 2011;8:1114–1154.
55. Indik JH, Gimbel JR, Abe H, et al. 2017 HRS expert consensus statement on magnetic resonance imaging and radiation exposure in patients with cardiovascular implantable electronic devices. *Heart Rhythm.* 2017.
56. Yalcin YC, Kooij C, Theuns DAMJ, et al. Emerging electromagnetic interferences between implantable cardioverter-defibrillators and left ventricular assist devices. *Europace.* 2020;22:584–587.
57. Yuyun M, Erqou S, Peralta A, et al. Ongoing risk of ventricular arrhythmias and all-cause mortality at implantable cardioverter defibrillator generator change: a systematic review and meta-analysis. *Circep.* 2021 (in press).
58. Lampert R. Managing with pacemakers and implantable cardioverter defibrillators. *Circulation.* 2013;128:1576–1585.
59. Lampert R, Hayes DL, Annas GJ, et al. HRS expert consensus statement on the management of Cardiovascular Implantable Electronic Devices (CIEDs) in patients nearing end of life or requesting withdrawal of therapy. This document was developed in collaboration and endorsed by the American College of Cardiology (ACC), the American Geriatrics Society (AGS), the American Academy of Hospice and Palliative Medicine (AAHPM); the American Heart Association (AHA), the European Heart Rhythm Association (EHRA), and the Hospice and Palliative Nurses Association (HPNA). *Heart Rhythm.* 2010;7:1008–1026.
60. Zipes DP, Link MS, Ackerman MJ, et al. Eligibility and disqualification recommendations for competitive athletes with cardiovascular abnormalities: Task force 9: arrhythmias and conduction defects: a scientific statement from the American Heart Association and American College of Cardiology. *Circulation.* 2015;132:e315–e325.

70 Cardiac Arrest and Sudden Cardiac Death

JEFFREY J. GOLDBERGER, CHRISTINE M. ALBERT, AND ROBERT J. MYERBURG

PERSPECTIVE, 1349

DEFINITIONS, 1349

EPIDEMIOLOGY, 1350
Epidemiologic Overview, 1350
Population Pools, Risk Gradients, and Time Dependence of Risk, 1351
Risk Factors for Sudden Cardiac Death, 1354

CAUSES OF SUDDEN CARDIAC DEATH, 1357
Coronary Artery Abnormalities, 1357
Ventricular Hypertrophy and Hypertrophic Cardiomyopathy, 1359
Cardiomyopathy and Systolic and Diastolic Heart Failure, 1359
Acute Heart Failure, 1360
Electrophysiologic Abnormalities, 1361
Sudden Infant Death Syndrome and Sudden Cardiac Death in Children, 1363

Sudden Cardiac Death in Competitive and Recreational Athletes and During Intense Exercise, 1363
Mechanisms and Pathophysiology, 1365
Pathophysiologic Mechanisms of Lethal Tachyarrhythmias, 1365
Bradyarrhythmias and Asystolic Arrest, 1366
Pulseless Electrical Activity, 1366

CLINICAL FEATURES OF PATIENTS WITH CARDIAC ARREST, 1367
Prodromal Symptoms, 1367
Onset of the Terminal Event, 1367
Cardiac Arrest, 1367
Progression to Biologic Death, 1368
Survivors of Cardiac Arrest, 1368

MANAGEMENT OF CARDIAC ARREST, 1369
In-Hospital Interventions, 1369
Community-Based Interventions, 1369

Initial Assessment and Basic Life Support, 1371
Advanced Life Support, 1373
Postcardiac Arrest Care and Postcardiac Arrest Syndrome, 1375
Long-Term Management of Survivors of Out-of-Hospital Cardiac Arrest, 1376

PREVENTION OF CARDIAC ARREST AND SUDDEN CARDIAC DEATH, 1377
Methods to Estimate Risk for Sudden Cardiac Death, 1377
Strategies to Reduce Risk for Sudden Cardiac Death, 1379
Application of Therapeutic Strategies to Specific Groups of Patients, 1380

SUDDEN DEATH AND PUBLIC SAFETY, 1383

REFERENCES, 1384

PERSPECTIVE

Sudden cardiac arrest (SCA), and its common consequence sudden cardiac death (SCD), is the common cardiac pathway for death. There are a diverse array of cardiac and noncardiac causes and mechanisms underlying the development of SCA and SCD. While SCA and SCD are most likely deterministic processes rather than true stochastic processes, the inability to delineate these processes presents a challenge in addressing this major public health problem. Current estimates for out-of-hospital SCDs are still in the range of 380,000/year in the United States alone,[1,2] with an additional 200,000 in-hospital cardiac arrests.[3] Generally, its impact is defined by the "rule of 50s": SCD accounts for 50% of all cardiovascular deaths, approximately 50% of all SCDs are unexpected first expressions of a cardiac disorder, and it often strikes during the victim's productive years, accounting for up to 50% of years of potential life lost due to heart disease.[4] Despite recognition of an association between forewarning symptoms of syncope and SCD dating to Hippocrates around 400 BC, advances in prediction, prevention, and management of unexpected SCA and SCD did not begin to emerge until approximately 50 years ago. It is anticipated that the major insights into causes, pathophysiology, and preventive and management strategies developed during the past few decades will continue to evolve.

DEFINITIONS

SCD is not a uniform entity resulting from a single precipitating diagnosis. SCD is natural death from cardiac causes heralded by abrupt loss of consciousness within 1 hour of the onset of an acute change in cardiovascular status. As such detailed information is often lacking, various definitions of SCD include up to a 24 hour period and death during sleep. Moreover, at least half of SCDs are unwitnessed, providing substantial uncertainty to the terminal events. Preexisting heart disease may or may not have been known to be present, but the time and mode of death are unexpected. This definition incorporates the key elements of natural, rapid, and most importantly unexpected death by a cardiac cause or mechanism. It consolidates previous definitions that

have conflicted, mainly because the most useful operational definition of SCD in the past differed for clinicians, cardiovascular epidemiologists, pathologists, and scientists attempting to define pathophysiologic mechanisms. As the epidemiology, clinical expression, causes, and mechanisms began to be understood, these differences merged.

To satisfy clinical, scientific, legal, and social considerations, four temporal elements must be considered: (1) prodromes, (2) onset, (3) cardiac arrest, and (4) biologic death (Fig. 70.1). Because the proximate cause of SCA is an abrupt disturbance in cardiovascular function resulting in loss of consciousness due to cessation of cerebral blood flow, any definition must recognize the brief time interval between onset of the mechanism *directly* responsible for cardiac arrest and the consequent loss of blood flow. The 1-hour definition primarily refers to the duration of the "terminal event," which defines the interval between the onset of symptoms signaling the pathophysiologic disturbance leading to cardiac arrest and the onset of the cardiac arrest itself. Based on human centrifuge studies carried out during the early years of the space program, the time between abrupt cessation of cerebral blood flow and loss of consciousness can be 10 seconds or less.

Prodromes, occurring weeks or months before an event, are generally predictors of an impending cardiac event, but not specific for SCA itself. The same premonitory signs and symptoms may be more specific for imminent cardiac arrest when they begin abruptly. Sudden onset of chest pain, dyspnea, or palpitations and other symptoms of arrhythmias often precede the onset of cardiac arrest and define the onset of the 1-hour terminal event period that brackets the cardiac arrest. The fourth element, biologic death, is an immediate consequence of cardiac arrest, unless there is a successful intervention, and usually occurs within minutes. The generally accepted clinical-pathophysiologic definition of up to 1 hour between onset of the terminal event and biologic death requires qualifications for specific circumstances. For example, since the development of community-based interventions and life support systems, patients may now remain biologically alive for a long period after the onset of a pathophysiologic process that has caused irreversible damage and will ultimately lead to death. In this circumstance, the causative pathophysiologic and clinical event is the cardiac arrest itself rather than the factors responsible for the delayed biologic death. Thus death remains defined biologically, legally, and literally as an absolute and irreversible event timed to cessation of all biologic functions, but most studies link the definition of SCD to the cardiac arrest rather than to a biologic death that occurs during hospitalization after cardiac arrest or within 30 days. Finally, forensic pathologists studying unwitnessed deaths continue to use the definition of sudden death for a person known to be alive and functioning normally 24 hours before, and this remains appropriate within obvious limits. Among the precautions is the recognition that not all sudden deaths are cardiac in origin.[5]

EPIDEMIOLOGY

Epidemiologic Overview

Epidemiologic studies of SCD are difficult to interpret for both theoretical and practical reasons. There are persisting inconsistencies about the definition and challenges in accessing data and adjudicating individual cases in data sets, in determining pathophysiologic mechanisms, and in making distinctions between population risk and individual risk.[6] In addition, the fact that SCA leading to SCD has short-term dynamics superimposed on a long-term static or dynamic substrate introduces unusual epidemiologic complexities, including long-term risk prediction based on the evolution of atherogenesis, myocardial hypertrophy, and ventricular muscle dysfunction over time and modulation by transient (short-term) variables such as ischemia, hemodynamic shifts, atherosclerotic plaque disruption and thrombosis, and autonomic variations. The differences between chronic disease evolution and transient events call for different forms of epidemiologic modeling (Table 70.1A). Furthermore, the emerging field of genetic epidemiology adds another dimension for consideration, and there is a need to focus on *interventional epidemiology*, a term coined to define the population dynamics of therapeutic outcomes.

In reference to risk for SCD from coronary heart disease, clinical categories ranging from general population risk to personalized risk profiling are paralleled by the partition of risk predictors into the pathophysiologic categories of substrate-based risk and expression-based risk (Table 70.1B). Substrate-based risk refers to prediction of the evolution or identification of vascular or myocardial substrates that establish risk for SCD (i.e., atherogenesis, scar patterns, remodeling) and to quantification of these risks. It should not be perceived as limited to anatomic features because risk substrates may exist at a molecular level, such as those characterized by the ion channelopathies that are associated with SCD. In contrast, expression-based risk refers to the identification of mechanisms and pathways that contribute to the clinical manifestation of the risk established by the substrate. This category includes plaque transition and acute coronary syndromes

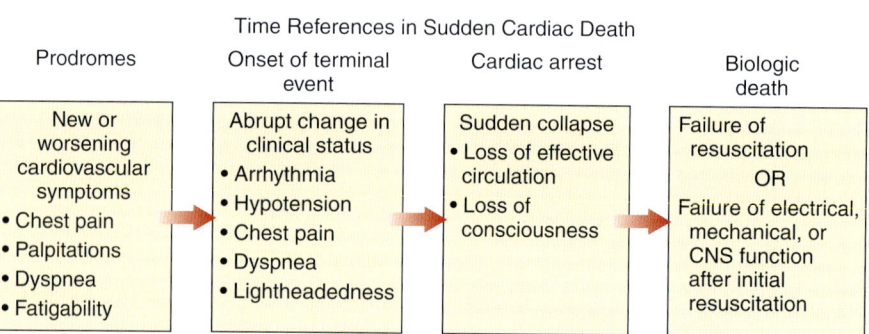

FIGURE 70.1 Sudden cardiac death viewed from four temporal perspectives: (1) prodromes, (2) onset of the terminal event, (3) cardiac arrest, and (4) progression to biologic death. Individual variability of the components influences clinical expression. Some victims experience no prodromes, with onset leading almost instantaneously to cardiac arrest; others may have an onset that lasts up to 1 hour before clinical arrest. Other patients may live days to weeks after the cardiac arrest before biologic death, often because of irreversible brain damage and dependence on life support. These factors influence interpretation of the 1-hour definition. The two most relevant clinical factors are onset of the terminal event and the clinical cardiac arrest itself; legal and social considerations focus on the time of biologic death. *CNS,* central nervous system.

TABLE 70.1 Pathophysiologic Epidemiology and Utility for Indicators of Risk for Sudden Cardiac Arrest

	A. UTILITY FOR RISK PREDICTION		
STRATEGY	**EXAMPLES**	**MEASURES**	**UTILITY**
Conventional risk factors	Framingham risk index	Prediction of evolution of disease	High for the population
			Low for the individual
Anatomic disease screening	Coronary calcium score and CT angiography	Identification of abnormal coronary arteries	High for anatomic identification
			Low for individual event prediction
Clinical risk profiling	Ejection fraction, stress testing, imaging techniques	Extent of disease	High for small, high-risk subgroups
			Low for large, low-risk subgroups
Transient risk predictors	Inflammatory markers; thrombotic cascade	Prediction of unstable plaques; acute changes in vascular status	Uncertain feasibility
Personalized risk predictors	Familial/genetic profiles	Individual SCD expression	Improved clinical precision
	B. PATHOPHYSIOLOGIC EPIDEMIOLOGY		
Substrate-based risk	Coronary heart disease		
	State of epicardial and intramyocardial vessels		
	Myocardial infarction		
	Myopathy, infiltration, inflammation, valvulopathy		
	Hypertrophy; myocardial fibrosis		
Expression-based risk	Left ventricular dysfunction and heart failure		
	Metabolic abnormalities		
	Autonomic dysfunction		
Mechanism-based causes	VF/pulseless VT		
	PEA		
	Asystole		

(plaque disruption and thrombogenesis) and their potential for specific expression as an arrhythmic event in susceptible individuals.

Incidence and the Population Burden of Sudden Cardiac Death

The worldwide incidence of out of hospital cardiac arrest (OHCA) leading to SCD is variable[7] and difficult to estimate because numbers vary as a function of reporting practices and the prevalence of coronary heart disease in different countries (see Chapter 2). The annual number of out-of-hospital SCDs in the United States is derived from multiple sources, such as retrospective death certificate data, American Heart Association (AHA) statistical updates based on data from the National Center for Health Statistics,[2] and extrapolations from population-based surveillance. Data from large surveillance studies, such as the Resuscitation Outcomes Consortium (ROC), have contributed additional insight into the subtleties of data collection and interpretation.

Statistical analyses from the same death certificate data sources have ranged from fewer than 250,000 SCDs annually when the etiologic definition is limited to coronary heart disease (International Classification of Diseases, ninth edition [ICD-9], classifications 410-414) to more than 460,000 SCDs/year when all causes are included.[8] Extrapolations from community-based sources set nationwide figures at fewer than 200,000,000 SCDs annually. Because these broad ranges and the reported regional differences in incidence and outcomes of cardiac arrest suggest that an accurate number can be found only by performing carefully designed prospective epidemiologic surveillance studies, the most widely cited estimates remain in the range of 380,000 SCDs annually, as suggested in the 2020 AHA statistical update.[9] These figures suggest an overall incidence of between one and two deaths/1000 persons in the general population. The annual number of emergency rescue (EMS) assessed OHCAs in people of any age in the United States in 2015 was 356,000.[2]

The temporal definition of sudden death strongly influences epidemiologic data. Retrospective death certificate studies have demonstrated that a temporal definition of sudden death of less than 2 hours after the onset of symptoms results in 12% to 15% of all natural deaths being defined as "sudden" and almost 90% of all natural sudden deaths having cardiac causes. In contrast, application of a 24-hour definition of sudden death increases the fraction of all natural deaths falling into the sudden category to more than 30% but reduces the proportion of all sudden natural deaths resulting from cardiac causes to 75%.

Prospective studies have demonstrated that approximately 50% of all deaths caused by coronary heart disease are sudden and unexpected and occur shortly (instantaneous to 1 hour) after the onset of symptoms. Because coronary heart disease is the dominant cause of both sudden and non-SCDs in the United States, the fraction of total cardiac deaths that are sudden is similar to the fraction of deaths from coronary heart disease that are sudden, although there does appear to be geographic variation in the fraction of coronary deaths that are sudden.[3,4] It is also of interest that the age-adjusted decline in mortality from coronary heart disease in the United States during the past half-century has not changed the fraction of coronary deaths that are sudden and unexpected.[4,10] Furthermore, the decreasing age-adjusted mortality does not imply a decrease in absolute numbers of cardiac or sudden deaths because of the growth and aging of the U.S. population and the increasing prevalence of chronic heart disease,[4] including heart failure. Yet a substantial 44% decline in the SCD rate in patients with heart failure and reduced ejection fraction enrolled in clinical trials from 1995 to 2014 has been observed.[11] It does not appear that the cumulative SCD burden in absolute numbers is tracking the age-adjusted decrease in cardiac deaths that has been evolving during the past 40 to 50 years.[12] In a prospective study of SCD victims in Finland undergoing autopsy between 1998 and 2012, while the proportion of SCDs resulting from coronary heart disease decreased, the concomitant increase in SCDs attributable to nonischemic causes maintained a relatively stable rate of SCD.[13] The landscape of SCD over time is further complicated by the suggested shift of mechanisms of out-of-hospital SCA from ventricular tachyarrhythmias to pulseless electrical activity/asystole, in part as a consequence of ICD efficacy.[4]

Population Pools, Risk Gradients, and Time Dependence of Risk

Three factors are of primary importance for identification of populations at risk and consideration of strategies for prevention of SCD: (1) the absolute numbers and event rates (incidence) among population subgroups (Fig. 70.2A), (2) the clinical subgroups in which SCDs occur (Fig. 70.2B), (3) competing risks, and (4) the time dependence of risk.

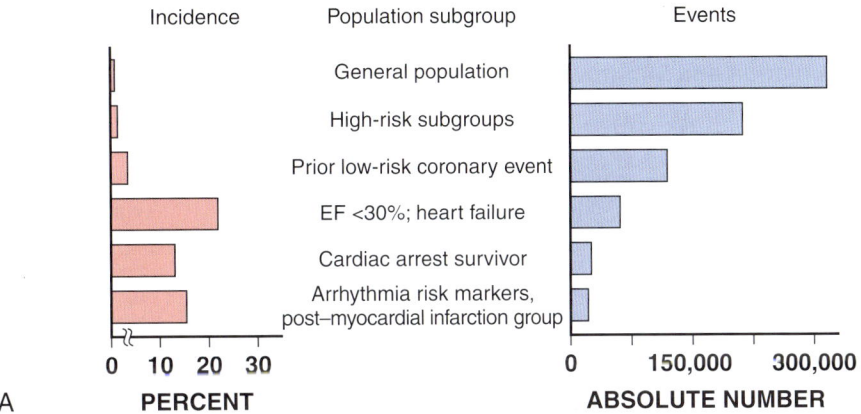

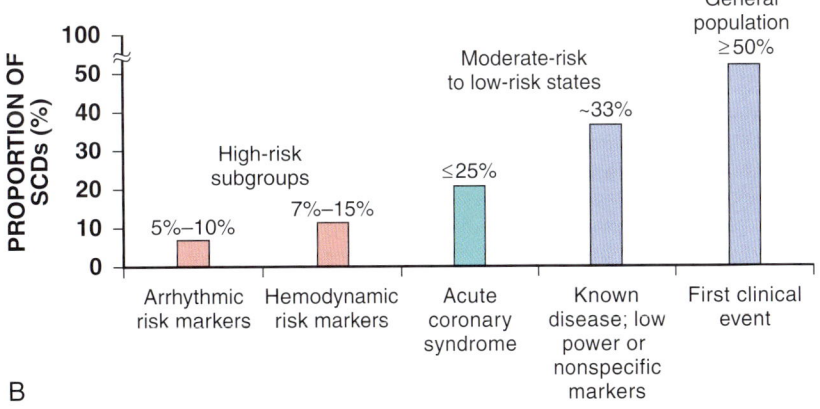

FIGURE 70.2 Impact of population subgroups and time from events on the clinical epidemiology of sudden cardiac death. **A,** Estimates of incidence (percent per year) and the total number of events per year for the general adult population in the United States and for increasingly high-risk subgroups. The overall adult population has an estimated incidence of sudden death of 0.1% to 0.2%/year, which accounts for a total of more than 300,000 events per year. With the identification of increasingly powerful risk factors, the incidence increases progressively, but this is accompanied by a progressive decrease in the total number of events represented by each group. The inverse relationship between incidence and the total number of events is due to the progressively smaller denominator pool in the highest subgroup categories. Successful interventions in larger population subgroups require identification of specific markers to increase the ability to identify specific patients who are at particularly high risk for a future event. (Note: The horizontal axis for the incidence figures is not linear and should be interpreted accordingly.) **B,** Distribution of the clinical status of victims at the time of SCD. Approximately 50% of all cardiac arrests caused by coronary heart disease occur as the first clinical event, and up to an additional 30% occur in the clinical setting of known disease in the absence of strong risk predictors. Less than 25% of victims have high-risk markers based on arrhythmic or hemodynamic parameters. *EF,* Ejection fraction. (**A** modified from Myerburg RJ, et al. Sudden cardiac death: structure, function, and time-dependence of risk. Circulation 1992;85(Suppl I):I2; **B** modified from Myerburg RJ: Sudden cardiac death: exploring the limits of our knowledge. J Cardiovasc Electrophysiol 2001;12:369.)

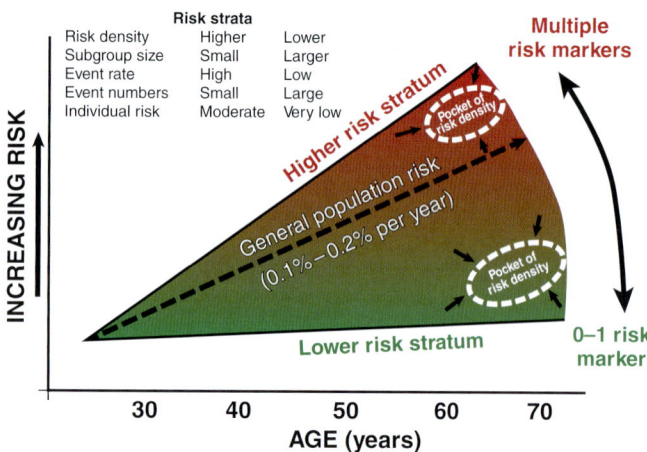

FIGURE 70.3 Stratification of risk as a continuum across the population as a function of age. The mean risk in the general population is demonstrated as a continuum across four decades. The mean risk of approximately 0.1% to 0.2%/year is bracketed by extremes of higher and lower risk strata, with the larger absolute numbers accumulated in the lower-risk strata. The ability to identify high–risk density subgroups within the general population would contribute to better individual risk prediction. (Modified from Myerburg RJ, Junttila MJ. Sudden cardiac death caused by coronary heart disease. Circulation 2012;125:1043.)

Population and Subgroup Risk Versus Individual Risk Assessment

When the estimated 380,000 SCDs that occur annually in the United States are viewed as a global figure for an unselected adult population 35 years and older, the overall incidence is calculated to be in the range of 0.1% to 0.2%/year (1 to 2/1000 population; Fig. 70.2A). This general population includes the large proportion of SCDs that occur as a first clinical manifestation of previously unrecognized heart disease, as well as SCDs that can be predicted with somewhat greater accuracy in higher risk subgroups (Fig. 70.2B), as it is impractical to plan an intervention designed for the general population that would be applied to the 999/1000 who do not have an event to reach and possibly influence the 1/1000 who will experience an event. Figure 70.2A highlights this problem by expressing the incidence (percent per year) of SCD among various subgroups and comparing the incidence figures with the total number of events that occur annually in each subgroup. Thus, despite the large absolute number at risk in the general population and the impact of preventive interventions on population risk for coronary artery disease, the precise ability to identify these individuals for targeted therapy for SCD prevention is an unmet challenge. The cost and risk-to-benefit uncertainties limit the nature of such broad-based interventions and demand a higher resolution of risk identification.[14] Two fundamental approaches for attacking this challenge can be followed: a general population strategy targeting prevention of acquired risk factors such as obesity (primordial prevention) and primary prevention by control of manifest risk factors and a more focused individual risk strategy based on identification and intervention in small subsets of the general population with a high density of risk (Fig. 70.3). Several population-based risk scores have been reported that provide an initial attempt to identify subsets within the general population who have heightened risk of SCD.[15,16] Based on data from the Atherosclerosis Risk in Communities (ARIC) Study, a race-adjusted risk score incorporating readily available variables from the medical record—age, sex, total cholesterol, lipid-lowering and hypertension medication use, blood pressure, smoking status, diabetes, and body mass index—provided good internal discrimination, which held up with external validation in the Framingham study.[17]

On moving from the total adult population to a subgroup at higher risk because of the presence of selected coronary risk factors, there may be a 10-fold or greater increase in the annual incidence of events, with the magnitude being dependent on the number and types of risk factors operating in specific subgroups. Higher resolution is desirable and can be achieved by identification of more specific subgroups. However, the corresponding absolute number of deaths may become progressively smaller as the subgroups become more focused (Fig. 70.2A),

unless the gradients of risk are steep. Applying the ARIC-based risk score[17] to the U.S. National Health and Nutrition Examination Survey, it was noted that there is an exponential rise in calculated risk by decile with a 10-fold gradient in risk between the highest and lowest decile.[18] Up to half of all SCDs attributable to coronary heart disease are first clinical events, and another 20% to 30% occur in subgroups of patients with known coronary heart disease who are profiled to be at relatively low risk for SCD on the basis of current clinically available markers (Fig. 70.2B). It is notable that when the ARIC-based risk score[17] was applied to a general population,[18] those in the highest risk deciles had a very high burden of risk factors. Moreover, these patients may have occult heart disease, providing an opportunity for early detection and treatment.[19] The principle of a high proportion of SCDs occurring as first events or in previously asymptomatic individuals with a high burden of risk factors also applies to SCD in the young (under age 35 years).[20]

Biologic and Clinical Time-Dependent Risk

Temporal elements in risk for SCD have been analyzed in the context of both biologic and clinical chronology. In the former, epidemiologic analyses of risk for SCD in populations have identified three patterns: diurnal, day of the week, and seasonal. General patterns of heightened risk during the morning hours, on Mondays, and during the winter months have been described.[12,21] An exception to the diurnal risk pattern is SCD in sleep apnea, in which the risk tends to be nocturnal.

Ambient temperature is an environmental factor associated with risk for SCD.[22,23] Both excessive cold and excessive heat have been linked to risk for cardiac arrest, although the studies did not determine whether temperature extremes are associated with ventricular tachyarrhythmias versus other mechanisms of cardiac arrest. However, significant cooling of the core temperature can lengthen the time course of repolarization of ventricular myocardium and prolong the QT interval, while sweating associated with increases in core temperature can alter electrolyte balance. Elevated temperature is a risk for SCA in patients with Brugada syndrome[24] (see Chapters 63 and 67). Another environmental variable, short-term ambient air pollution conditions, has been associated with increased risk of OHCA, but not consistently.[12,25,26] In patients with an implantable defibrillator, exposure to fine particulate material correlated significantly to episodes of ventricular tachycardia and fibrillation.[27] A sympathetically mediated mechanism has been postulated.

In the longer term, risk for SCD is not linear as a function of time after changes in cardiovascular status. Survival curves after major cardiovascular events, which identify risk for both SCD and total cardiac death, usually demonstrate that the most rapid rate of attrition occurs during the first 6 to 18 months after an index event. Thus, there is a time dependence of risk that focuses the potential opportunity for maximum efficacy of an intervention during the early period after a cardiovascular event. Even though the rate of attrition decreases after the early spike in mortality, a secondary delayed increase in risk occurs in post–myocardial infarction (MI) patients 2 to 5 years after an index event, probably related to ventricular remodeling and heart failure.

Age, Race, Sex, and Heredity
Age

The incidence of sudden death has two peak ages: within the first year of life (including sudden infant death syndrome [SIDS]; see Chapter 82) and between 45 and 75 years of age. Among the general populations of infants younger than 1 year and middle-aged or older adults, the incidence is surprisingly similar.[28] In adults older than 35 years, the incidence of SCD is in the range of 1/1000 persons/year (Fig. 70.4A), with an age-related increase in risk over time as the prevalence of coronary heart disease increases in parallel with advancing age.

The incidence in infants is 73/100,000 person-years and is most commonly associated with complex congenital heart disease, and the incidence in children and adolescents is approximately 4 to 6/100,000 person-years versus 125/100,000 person-years in adults (Fig. 70.4A).[28] One study demonstrated that approximately 40% of SCDs in this age category were unexplained, based on the absence of an autopsy or premortem clinical diagnosis, but postmortem genetic studies identified a likely cause in 27% of such cases that underwent studies.[29]

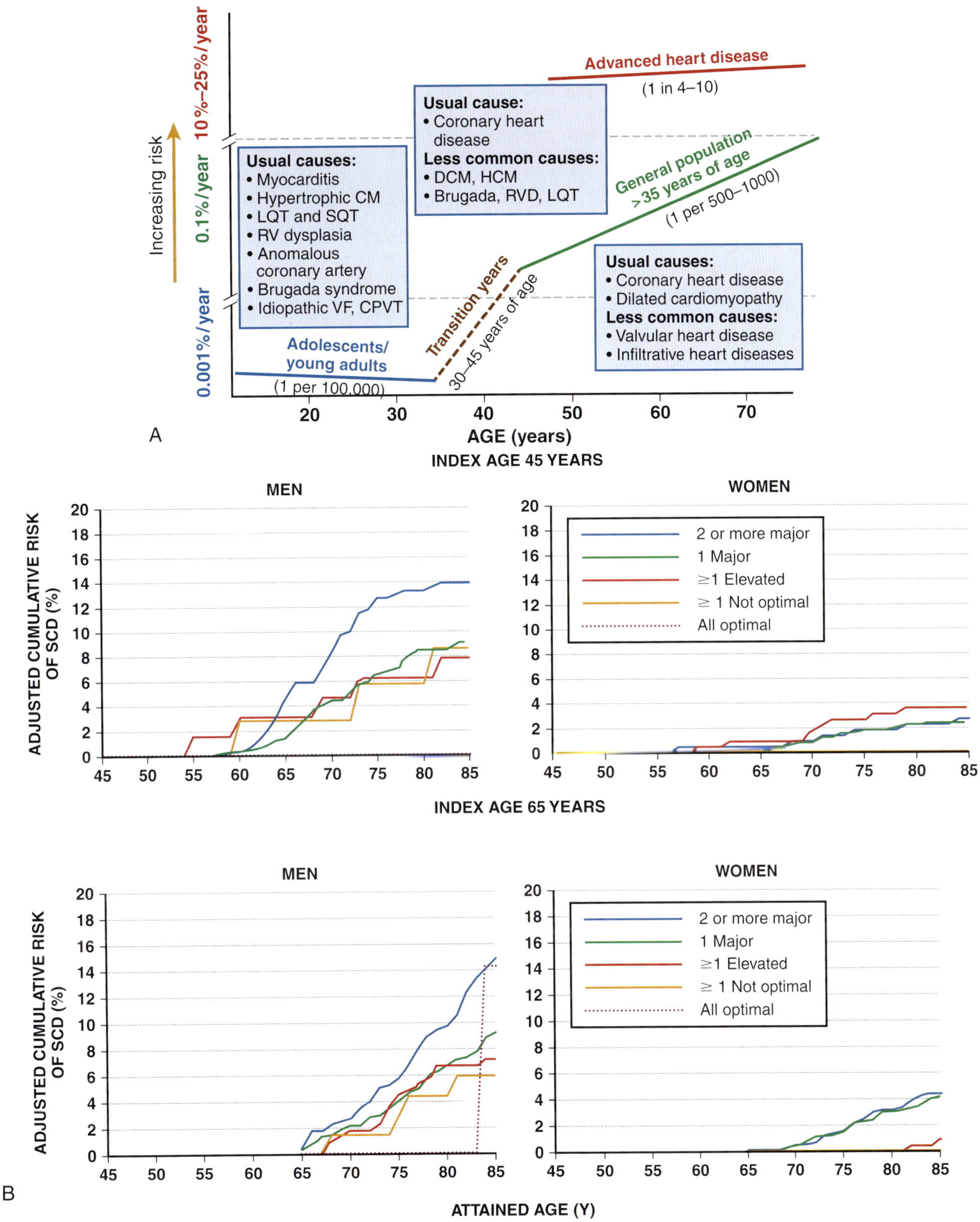

FIGURE 70.4 Age- and sex-specific risks for SCD. A, Age-related and disease-specific risk for SCD. For the general population 35 years and older, the risk for SCD is 0.1% to 0.2%/year (1/500 to 1000 population), with a wide spread in subgroup risk based on the number and power of individual risk factors. Causes are dominated by coronary heart disease and, to a lesser extent, nonischemic cardiomyopathy in this age range. The risk for SCD increases dramatically beyond the age of 35 years and continues to increase past the age of 70 years. In patients older than 30 years with advanced structural heart disease and markers of high risk for cardiac arrest, the event rate may exceed 25%/year, and the age-related risk is attenuated. In adolescents and adults younger than 30 years, the overall risk for SCD is 1/100,000 population or 0.001%/year, with a variety of causes such as inherited structural and electrical disorders, developmental defects, and myocarditis dominating. In adolescents and young adults at risk for SCD from specific identified causes, it is difficult to ascertain the risk in individual patients because of variable expression of the disease state (see text for details). In the transition range from 30 to 45 years of age, the relative frequency of the uncommon disease yields to the dominance of coronary heart disease and nonischemic cardiomyopathy, but both groups of potential causes must be entertained because many of the rare disorders are expressed in that age range. **B,** Lifetime risk for SCD risk as a function of index age (shown for age 45 and 65 years), sex, and risk factor burden derived from the Framingham Heart Study. Boxes show risk factors burden strata coded by colors. *CA,* cardiac arrest; *CM,* cardiomyopathy; *CPVT,* catecholaminergic polymorphic VT; *DCM,* dilated CM; *HCM,* hypertrophic CM; *LQT,* long-QT; *RV,* right ventricular; *RVD,* RV dysplasia; *SQT,* short QT; *VF,* ventricular fibrillation. (**B** from Bogle BM, et al. Lifetime risk for sudden cardiac death in the community. J Am Heart Assoc 2016;5(7):e002398.)

In contrast to incidence, however, the proportion of deaths caused by coronary heart diseases that are sudden and unexpected decreases with advancing age. In the 20- to 39-year age group, approximately 75% of the deaths attributable to coronary heart disease in men are sudden and unexpected, with the proportion falling to approximately 60% in the 45- to 54-year age group and hovering close to 50% thereafter. Age also influences the proportion of any cardiovascular cause among all causes of natural sudden death in that the proportion of coronary deaths and of all cardiac causes of death that are sudden is highest in the younger age groups whereas the fraction of total sudden natural deaths that result from any cardiovascular cause is higher in the older age groups. At the other end of the age range, only 19% of sudden natural deaths in children between 1 and 13 years of age have cardiac causes; the proportion increases to 30% in the 14- to 21-year age group.

In the transition age range between adolescence and young adulthood (to the age of 25 years) and in the middle and older ages (beginning at 35 years of age), coronary heart disease emerges to its position as the dominant cause of SCD. However, rare disorders, such as hypertrophic cardiomyopathy (HCM), Brugada syndrome, long-QT syndrome, right ventricular dysplasia, and idiopathic myocardial fibrosis, are significant contributors to the distribution of causes of SCD in this age group.

Race

A number of studies comparing racial differences in the relative risk for SCD in white and Black with coronary heart disease in the United States had yielded conflicting and inconclusive data. More recent studies demonstrate a higher risk for cardiac arrest and SCD in Blacks than in whites. Data from the ARIC and REGARD studies show that Blacks had an adjusted hazard ratio for SCD of 1.38 to 1.97 compared with whites.[30,31] SCD rates in Hispanic populations have been less well studied but do not appear to show increased risk (see Chapter 93).

Sex

SCD syndrome has a large preponderance in men relative to women during the young adult and early middle-age years because of the protection that women enjoy from coronary atherosclerosis before menopause (Fig. 70.4B). There is at least a threefold increase lifetime risk for SCD among men aged 45 to 65 years compared with women, with only mild attenuation of this accentuated risk at age 75 years.[32] Even though the overall risk for SCD is much lower in younger women, coronary artery disease is the most common cause of SCD in women older than 40 years, and the classic coronary risk factors, including cigarette smoking, diabetes, use of oral contraceptives, and hyperlipidemia, all influence risk in women (see Chapter 91).[4] In an autopsy study, the profile of women experiencing SCD differed significantly from men; women were older (70 versus 64 years), more commonly had nonischemic causes (28% versus 24%) and primary myocardial fibrosis (5.2% versus 2.6%), and more commonly had ECG evidence of left ventricular (LV) hypertrophy with or without repolarization abnormalities.[33]

Heredity

Familial patterns of risk for SCD, which result from known or suspected genetic variations, are emerging as important factors for risk profiling. This concept is generally applicable to both disease development and SCD expression in the common acquired disorders and in a specific sense to inherited arrhythmogenic conditions associated with SCD.[34] The various genetic associations can be separated into four categories (Table 70.2): uncommon inherited primary arrhythmic syndromes (e.g., long-QT syndromes, Brugada syndrome, catecholaminergic polymorphic ventricular tachycardia or fibrillation; see Chapter 63), uncommon inherited structural diseases associated with risk for SCD (e.g., HCM, right ventricular dysplasia; see Chapters 52 and 54), "acquired" or induced risk for arrhythmias (e.g., drug-induced long-QT interval or proarrhythmia, electrolyte disturbances), and common acquired diseases associated with risk for SCD (e.g., coronary heart disease, nonischemic cardiomyopathies; see Chapters 38, 39, and 50). Genetic variants mapped to loci on many chromosomes are being defined as the molecular bases for these entities and associations.

TABLE 70.2 Genetic Contributors to Risk for Sudden Cardiac Death

Genetically Based Primary Arrhythmia Disorders
Congenital long-QT syndrome, short-QT syndrome
Brugada syndrome
Catecholaminergic polymorphic VT/VF
J wave syndromes
Nonsyndromic VT/VF
Inherited Structural Disorders with Risk for Arrhythmic SCD
Hypertrophic cardiomyopathy
Right ventricular dysplasia/cardiomyopathy
Genetic Predisposition to Induced Arrhythmias and SCD
Drug-induced "acquired" long-QT syndrome (drugs, electrolytes)
Electrolyte and metabolic arrhythmogenic effects
Genetic Modulation of Complex Acquired Diseases
Coronary artery disease, acute coronary syndromes
Congestive heart failure, dilated cardiomyopathies

The multiple specific mutations at gene loci-encoding ion channel proteins associated with the various inherited arrhythmia syndromes (see Chapter 63) represent a major advance in the understanding of a genetic and pathophysiologic basis for these causes of sudden death. In addition, the role of modifier genes and mutation specificity in the severity of clinical phenotypes in long–QT interval syndromes (LQTS)[35] and structural diseases such as HCM is of increasing interest. These observations may provide screening tools for individuals at risk, as well as the potential to devise specific therapeutic strategies. In a study of screening ECGs for long-QT in children entering first grade and those in the seventh grade, and subsequent genetic testing in those children who were positive, there was a suggestion that the incidence of inherited LQT was considerably higher (~1/1000) at the age of 12 years (seventh graders) than earlier estimates from studies based on diagnoses from general clinical expressions.[36] Moreover, the cumulative risk of SCA among those with unrecognized or untreated LQTS was reported to be 13% before the age of 40 years.[37] In addition, gene loci identified by genome-wide association studies may also serve as candidates for investigation of the role of low-penetrance mutations or polymorphisms in SCD caused by more common conditions, such as coronary heart disease.[38]

To the extent that SCD is an expression of underlying coronary heart disease, hereditary factors that contribute to risk for coronary heart disease operate nonspecifically for the SCD syndrome. Various studies have identified mutations and relevant polymorphisms along multiple steps of the cascade, from atherogenesis to plaque destabilization, thrombosis, and arrhythmogenesis, each of which is associated with increased risk for a coronary event (Fig. 70.5). Several studies have suggested that SCD as the initial expression of coronary heart disease demonstrates familial clustering, including general population surveillance studies, family histories of cardiac arrest survivors in the community, studies of ventricular fibrillation (VF) during acute MI, and postmortem evaluation of SCD cases.

Risk Factors for Sudden Cardiac Death
General Profile of Risk for Sudden Cardiac Death

Risk prediction for SCD is far more challenging than simply profiling risk for coronary artery disease by means of the conventional risk factors for coronary atherogenesis (see Chapters 33 and 34). While the latter is useful for identifying levels of population risk and some aspects of individual risk, it is not sufficient for distinguishing individual patients at risk for SCD from those at risk for other manifestations of coronary heart disease (see Chapters 35 to 40).[6]

Multivariate analyses of selected risk factors (e.g., age, sex, diabetes mellitus, blood pressure/hypertension, current smoking, body mass index, lipid lowering medication use) have demonstrated that the majority of all SCDs occur in the upper deciles of risk (Fig. 70.6). It is likely that the interactions of multiple risk factors potentiates the sum of the individual risks. Comparison of risk factors in victims of SCD with those in people with any manifestation of coronary artery disease does not provide useful patterns to distinguish victims of SCD from the overall pool. However, a history of diabetes mellitus and a tendency to longer QTc intervals on random ECGs are suggested as potential markers of interest for prediction of SCD. ECG analyses by artificial intelligence merits investigation for SCD risk stratification (see Chapter 11). Familial clustering of SCD as a specific manifestation of the disease may lead to the identification of specific genetic abnormalities that predispose to SCD.[4]

Hypertension is a clearly established risk factor for coronary heart disease and also emerges as a highly significant risk factor in the incidence of SCD (see Chapter 26). However, there is no influence of increasing systolic blood pressure levels on the ratio of sudden deaths to total coronary heart disease deaths. No relationship has been observed between cholesterol concentration and the proportion of coronary deaths that were sudden. Neither the electrocardiographic pattern of LV hypertrophy nor nonspecific ST-T wave abnormalities influence the proportion of total coronary deaths that are sudden and unexpected; only intraventricular conduction abnormalities are suggestive of a disproportionate number of SCDs, an old observation reinforced by data from some device trials that suggest the importance of QRS duration as a risk marker, but one with low individual predictive ability.

The conventional risk factors used in early studies of SCD are risk factors for the evolution of coronary artery disease. The rationale is based on two facts: (1) Coronary disease has been considered the structural basis for 80% of SCDs in the United States, and (2) coronary risk factors are easy to identify because they tend to be present continuously over time (see Fig. 70.5). However, there is evolving evidence that the anatomic consequences of coronary artery disease may not account for as large a proportion of SCDs in adults as previously estimated, with hypertension, LV hypertrophy, and myocardial fibrosis being identified as dominant anatomic/pathophysiologic factors. In a Finnish autopsy study of SCD victims, there was a decline in coronary artery disease with an increase in hypertensive heart disease with LV hypertrophy (and no coronary artery disease).[13] A 10-year longitudinal study of clinical associations identified in hospitalized OHCA victims demonstrated a trend toward decreasing structural heart disease associations, paralleled by an increasing dominance of dynamic, transient pathophysiologic events.[4] Transient

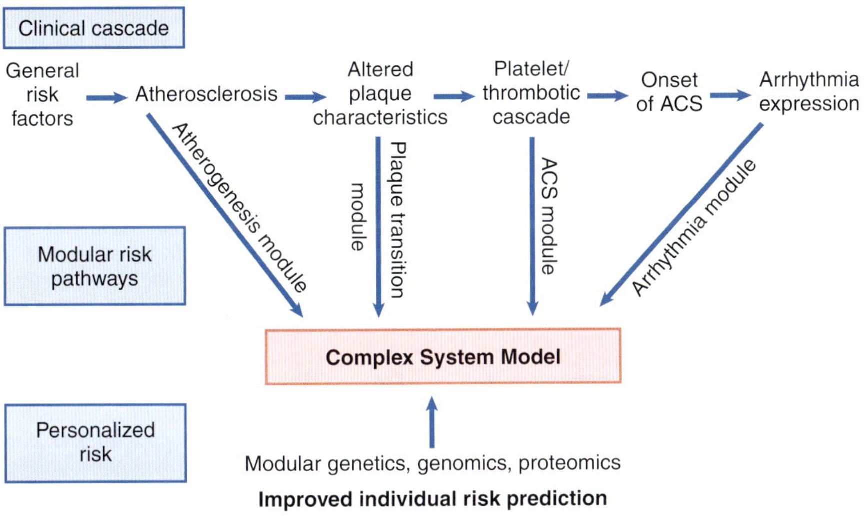

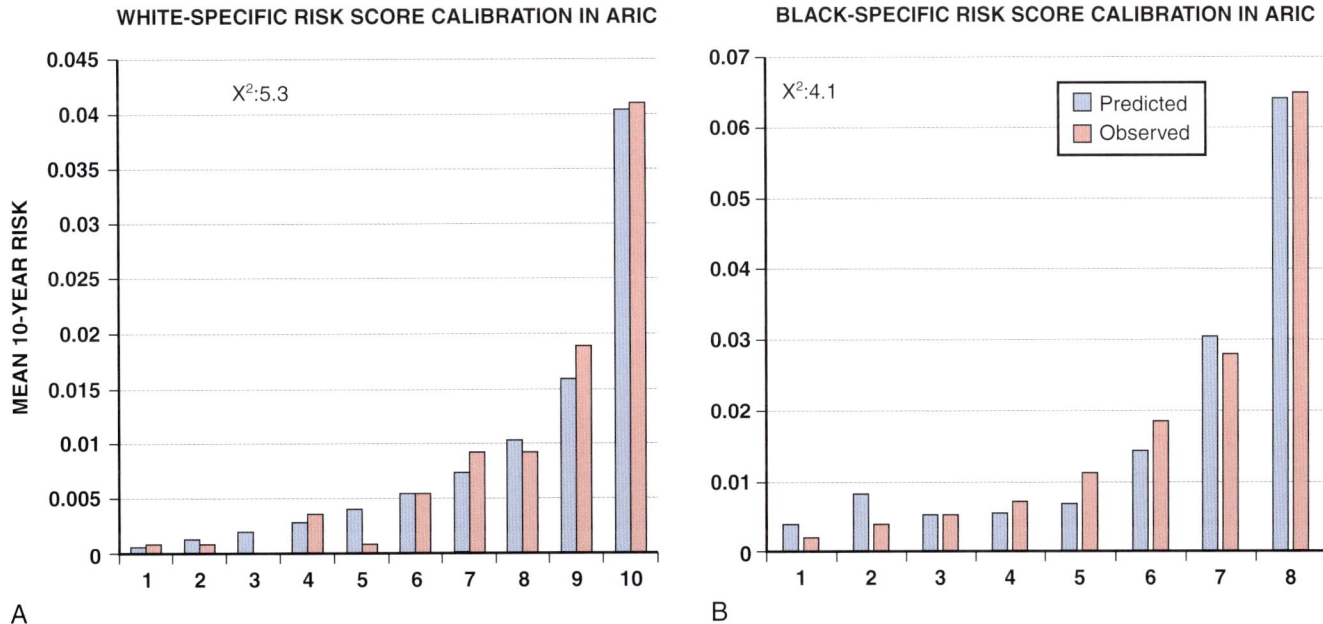

FIGURE 70.5 Coronary atherosclerosis cascade and genetic imprints on the progression to SCD. The cascade from conventional risk factors for coronary atherosclerosis to arrhythmogenesis in SCD related to coronary heart disease includes initiation and development, progression to an active state, initiation of acute coronary syndromes (ACSs), and finally, progression to the specific expression of life-threatening arrhythmias. Multiple factors enter at each level, including specific risk based on the genetic profiles of individual patients. Individual risk based on genetic profiles has been identified for atherogenesis, plaque evolution, the thrombotic cascade, and arrhythmia expression. Stepwise integration of these characteristics may lead to higher single-patient probabilities for individual SCD risk prediction. See text for details. (Modified from Myerburg RJ, Junttila MJ: Sudden cardiac death caused by coronary heart disease. Circulation 2012;125:1043.)

FIGURE 70.6 Risk for sudden death by decile of a multivariate risk score derived in the Framingham Heart Study and calibrated for white (**A**) and Black (**B**) Atherosclerosis Risk in Communities (ARIC) participants. Observed (*red*) and predicted (*blue*) mean 10-year risk of SCD are shown. (From Bogle BM, et al. A simple community-based risk-prediction score for sudden cardiac death. Am J Med 2018;131:532-539.)

pathophysiologic events are being modeled epidemiologically in an attempt to express and use them as clinical risk factors for both profiling and intervention. Nonetheless, data suggest that longitudinal and transient risk predictors may have their power blunted by clinical interventions, such as percutaneous coronary intervention during acute coronary syndromes and post-MI beta blocker therapy.

Identification of specific clinical markers of risk for SCD as a specific expression of both coronary heart disease and other cardiovascular disorders has been a goal for many years. LV ejection fraction has been the most popular of such markers for clinical trials but with limited sensitivity, encouraging investigators to seek additional markers. These additional markers are quite variable, depend on the underlying structural heart disease, and likely reflect the multifactorial basis for SCD.[39-42] Functional metrics such as LV size, strain, and functional status all have demonstrated prognostic significance. Electrical abnormalities in depolarization (QRS duration, fragmented QRS, late potentials) and repolarization, including QT interval, dispersion, and dynamicity, also have prognostic significance. Noninvasive measures of autonomic abnormalities have also demonstrated prognostic significance. Finally, imaging evidence of fibrosis/scarring and autonomic denervation have also demonstrated prognostic significance. Emerging data on the role of biomarkers and genetics may also provide important prognostication. It is notable that no single parameter has adequate predictive power to impact clinical decisions on an individual level.

The general framework for considering SCD risk is to consider the underlying substrate, potential triggers, and other modulating factors. The substrate may represent an anatomical or molecular (e.g., ion channel) abnormality. Common triggers include ventricular ectopic activity and exercise or other conditions of sympathoexcitation. While ventricular ectopic activity was once thought to represent a treatment target for prevention of SCD, the Cardiac Arrhythmia Suppression Trial (CAST) dispelled this notion. Exercise is a well known trigger for SCD, but it must be emphasized that habitual exercise dramatically lowers the risk. Nevertheless, many markers related to exercise have been found to be related to risk of SCD including the acceleration and deceleration of heart rate with and after exercise and exercise repolarization dynamics.[1]

Functional Capacity and Sudden Death

The Framingham Study demonstrated a striking relationship between functional classification and death during a 2-year follow-up period. However, the proportion of deaths that were sudden did not vary with the functional classification, including those free of clinical heart disease and those in functional class IV. Generally, it has been shown that mortality increases with functional class. Competing risk of death from heart failure and other causes does diminish the proportional risk of SCD.[43]

Lifestyle and Psychosocial Factors

A strong association has been found between cigarette smoking and all manifestations of coronary heart disease (see Chapter 28). The Framingham Study demonstrated that cigarette smokers have a two- to threefold increase in risk for sudden death in each decade of life at entry between 30 and 59 years and that this is one of the few risk factors in which the proportion of deaths attributable to coronary heart disease that are sudden increases in association with the risk factor. Importantly, smoking cessation can reverse the excess risk associated with smoking. In support of a direct effect of smoking on arrhythmogenesis, survivors of out-of-hospital cardiac arrest who continued to smoke had a higher recurrence of cardiac arrest than those who stopped.[4]

Alcohol has complex effects on the heart. Light to moderate alcohol consumption was associated with a reduced risk for SCD in the Physicians' Health Study, but there was no reduction in those consuming two or more drinks per day. Alcohol abuse is associated with increased risk of atrial fibrillation, MI, and congestive heart failure,[44] conditions associated with SCD. It is likely that there is a U-shaped relationship between alcohol consumption and SCD (see Chapter 84).

Obesity also influences the proportion of coronary deaths that occur suddenly. With increasing relative weight, the percentage of coronary heart disease deaths that were sudden and total coronary heart disease mortality in the Framingham Study increased linearly. In the ARIC study, obesity was associated with increased risk of SCD but only in nonsmokers (see Chapter 30).[45]

Associations between levels of physical activity and SCD have been studied with variable results. Epidemiologic observations have suggested a relationship between low levels of physical activity and increased risk for death from coronary heart disease. The Framingham Study, however, showed an insignificant relationship between low levels of physical activity and the incidence of sudden death but a high proportion of sudden to total cardiac deaths with higher levels of physical activity. An association between acute physical exertion and the onset of MI and SCD has been suggested, particularly in individuals who are habitually physically inactive. Analysis from the Physicians' Health Study demonstrated a 17-fold relative increase in SCD associated with vigorous exertion and the 30 minute postexertion period compared with periods of lower level activity or inactive states. However, the absolute risk for events was very low (one event/1.5 million exercise sessions). Habitual vigorous exercise markedly attenuated risk. A clue that intensity of exercise may play a role in SCA risk comes from an observation in college athletes, suggesting that division 1 basketball players are at higher risk than division 2 and division 3 athletes.[46] Information about physical activity relationships in various clinical settings, such as overt and silent disease states, is still lacking (see Chapter 32).

The role of social determinants of health on cardiac risk factors and mortality are well recognized, but no data specifically links this to SCD. There is an association with significant elevations in life change scores during the 6 months before a coronary event, and the association is particularly striking in victims of SCD. In women, it has been reported that those who die suddenly were less often married, had fewer children, and had greater educational discrepancies with their spouses than did age-related control subjects living in the same neighborhood. A history of psychiatric treatment, including phobic anxieties, cigarette smoking, and greater quantities of alcohol consumption than in control subjects also characterized the sudden death group. Behavioral changes (e.g., inactivity) secondary to depression appeared to relate more closely to event rates than did depression itself. Acute psychosocial stressors have been associated with a higher risk for cardiovascular events, including SCD. The risk appears to cluster around the time of the stress in victims with preexisting risk, with the stressor simply advancing the time of an impending event. Natural disasters, such as earthquakes and tsunamis, may be associated with a transient increase in SCD, though specific aggravation of ventricular tachyarrhythmias in patients with implantable defibrillators may not be noted.[47] The possibility of physical stress–induced coronary plaque disruption has been suggested.

Left Ventricular Ejection Fraction in Chronic Ischemic Heart Disease

A marked reduction in the LV ejection fraction is the most powerful of the known predictors of total mortality and SCD in patients with chronic ischemic heart disease, as well as in those at risk for SCD from other causes (see later). Increased mortality, independent of other risk factors, is measurable with ejection fractions higher than 40%, but the greatest rate of change in mortality occurs at levels between 30% and 40%. An ejection fraction of 30% or lower is the single most powerful independent predictor of SCD but has low sensitivity and specificity. Notably, relying on a low ejection fraction as the sole risk-stratifier misses a large number of SCDs that occur at lower incidence rates among the very large subset of patients with normal or moderately reduced ejection fractions and unrecognized disease.[48] Generally, ejection fraction measurements are highly variable, among imaging techniques and even in a given patient depending on loading conditions. Contractility is a major factor determining the ejection fraction and its role in SCD risk may be related to quantifying the extent of scar or myopathy. There are emerging data that LV fibrosis may be a better predictor of cardiac events than ejection fraction alone.[49-51]

Ventricular Arrhythmias in Chronic Ischemic Heart Disease

Most forms of ambient ventricular ectopic activity (premature ventricular complexes [PVCs] and short runs of nonsustained ventricular tachycardia [VT]) have a benign prognosis in the absence of structural heart disease (see Chapters 67 and 40). An exception is the polymorphic forms of nonsustained VT that occur in patients without structural heart disease but can have a molecular, functional, drug-related, or electrolyte-related basis for high-risk arrhythmias. When present in coronary disease-prone age groups, PVCs select a subgroup with a higher probability of coronary artery disease and SCD. Exercise-induced PVCs and short runs of nonsustained VT indicate some level of risk for SCD, even in the absence of recognizable structural heart disease. However, the data available to support this hypothesis are conflicting, with the possible exception of polymorphic runs of nonsustained VT. Additional data suggest that PVCs and nonsustained VT during both the exercise and recovery phases of a stress test predict increased risk. Arrhythmias in the recovery phase, previously thought to be benign, appear to predict higher risk than do arrhythmias in the exercise phase, and there is a gradient of risk with increasing severity of arrhythmias.

The occurrence of PVCs in survivors of MI, particularly if frequent and having complex forms such as repetitive PVCs, predicts an increased risk for SCD and total mortality during long-term follow-up. Data are conflicting on the role of measures of frequency and forms of ventricular ectopic activity as discriminators of risk, but most studies have cited a frequency cutoff of 10 PVCs/hour as a threshold level for increased risk. Several investigators have emphasized that the most powerful predictors among the various forms of PVCs are runs of nonsustained VT, although this relationship is now questioned. It is important to note that much of the foundational data that demonstrated the important prognostic role of ejection fraction after MI also demonstrated the similarly important role of PVC frequency.

While both ejection fraction and PVC frequency were shown to be important prognostic markers after MI, only PVCs were considered to be modifiable with antiarrhythmic drugs. The results of CAST (Cardiac Arrhythmia Suppression Trial; see Chapter 64), which was designed to test the hypothesis that suppression of PVCs by antiarrhythmic drugs alters the risk for SCD after MI, were surprising for two reasons. First, the death rate in the randomized placebo group was lower than expected, and second, the death rate among patients in the encainide and flecainide arms exceeded control rates by more than threefold. The excess death rates may be accounted for by drug-induced proarrhythmia during ischemic events. The SWORD (Survival with Oral *d*-Sotalol) study, a comparison of *d*-sotalol with placebo in a post-MI population with a low mortality rate, also demonstrated excess risk in the drug treated group. Whether the conclusions from CAST, CAST II, and SWORD extend beyond the drug studies or to other diseases remains to be learned. What is clear is that markers of risk for SCD do not necessarily represent appropriate treatment targets.

LV dysfunction is the major modulator of risk associated with chronic PVCs after MI. The risk for death predicted by post-MI PVCs is enhanced by the presence of LV dysfunction, which appears to exert its influence most strongly in the first 6 months after infarction. Delayed deterioration of LV function, probably because of remodeling after MI, may increase the risk further.

Emerging Markers of Risk for Sudden Cardiac Death
Decades of evaluations of ECG-based testing for abnormalities in depolarization, repolarization, and cardiac autonomic function provide consistent data linking these markers to mortality and/or SCD risk in populations but with little utility for individual risk prediction and clinical decision making. Emerging tests such as contrast-enhanced magnetic resonance imaging of the infarction, as well as noninfarct patterns of fibrosis seen on MRI delayed hyperenhancement, and sympathetic imaging with 11C-hydroxyephedrine or I-*m*-iodobenzylguanidine (MIBG) require further evaluation to assess utility for individual risk prediction (see Chapter 18). The potential of genetic risk profiling based on studies of familial clustering of SCD also requires further evaluation.[6]

CAUSES OF SUDDEN CARDIAC DEATH
Coronary Artery Abnormalities
Diseases of the coronary arteries and their consequences have been estimated to account for at least 80% of SCDs in Western countries, but recent observations suggest that the magnitude of this excess burden may be decreasing.[13] Coronary artery disease is also the most common cause in many areas of the world in which the prevalence of atherosclerosis is lower. As developing nations improve access to health care for communicable disease in the earlier years of life, coronary atherosclerosis and its consequences may emerge as a larger problem.[52] Continued focus on control of underlying risk factors will be key to prevention of SCD.

Despite the established dominant relationship between coronary atherosclerosis and SCD, complete understanding of SCD requires recognition that less common and often rare coronary vascular disorders (Table 70.3) may be identifiable before death and have therapeutic implications. Many of these entities are relatively more common causes of SCD in adolescents and young adults, in whom the prevalence of coronary heart disease-related SCDs is much lower before the age of 30 years[29] (see Fig. 70.4A).

Atherosclerotic Coronary Artery Disease
The structural and functional abnormalities of the coronary vasculature as a result of coronary atherosclerosis interact with the electrophysiologic alterations that result from the myocardial impact of an ischemic burden (see Chapters 37 to 40). The relationship between the vascular and myocardial components of this pathophysiologic model, as well as its modulation by hemodynamic, autonomic, genetic, and other influences, establishes multiple patterns of risk derived from the fundamental disease state (Fig. 70.7). Risk is modulated by multiple factors that can be either transient or persistent, and transient modulations may interact with persistent changes. The myocardial component of this pathophysiologic model is not static over time, and the term *persistent* must be viewed with caution because of the gradual effects of remodeling after an initial ischemic event and the effects of recurrent ischemic episodes. SCA and SCD resulting from transient ischemia or acute MI differ in physiology and prognosis from the risk for SCA implied by a previous MI with or without subsequent ischemic cardiomyopathy. In general, the short-term risk for life-threatening events is associated more closely with acute ischemia or the acute phase of MI, and longer-term risk is associated more with transient ischemia, myocardial scarring, remodeling, ischemic cardiomyopathy, alterations in autonomic modulation, and heart failure.

Nonatherosclerotic Coronary Artery Abnormalities
Nonatherosclerotic coronary artery abnormalities include congenital lesions, coronary artery embolism, coronary arteritis, and mechanical abnormalities of the coronary arteries. Among the congenital lesions, anomalous origin of a left coronary artery from the pulmonary artery (see Chapters 21 and 82) is relatively common and associated with an increased death rate in infancy and early childhood without surgical treatment. The early risk for SCD is not excessively high, but patients who survive to adolescence and young adulthood without surgical intervention are at risk for SCD. Other forms of coronary arteriovenous fistulas are much less frequent and associated with a low incidence of SCD.

Anomalous Origin of Coronary Arteries from the Wrong Sinus of Valsalva
These anatomic variants are associated with an increased risk for SCD, particularly during exercise. When the anomalous artery passes between the aortic and the pulmonary artery root, the takeoff angle of the anomalous ostium creates a slitlike opening of the vessel that reduces the effective cross-sectional area for blood flow. The less common origin of the left coronary artery from the right sinus of Valsalva is a higher risk variant, but the origin of the right coronary artery from the left sinus of Valsalva, while lower risk, accounts for a proportion of SCDs that should not be ignored, based on the incidence of this anomaly.[53] Congenitally hypoplastic, stenotic, or atretic left coronary arteries are uncommon abnormalities associated with a risk for MI in the young, but not for SCD.

TABLE 70.3 Causes of and Contributing Factors in Sudden Cardiac Death

I. **Coronary artery abnormalities**
   A. Coronary atherosclerosis
      1. Chronic coronary atherosclerosis with acute or transient myocardial ischemia—thrombosis, spasm, physical stress
      2. Acute myocardial infarction, onset and early phase
      3. Chronic atherosclerosis with a change in myocardial substrate, including previous myocardial infarction
   B. Congenital abnormalities of coronary arteries
      1. Anomalous origin from the pulmonary artery
      2. Other coronary arteriovenous fistula
      3. Origin of a left coronary artery from the right or noncoronary sinus of Valsalva (lower incidence; higher risk)
      4. Origin of the right coronary artery from the left sinus of Valsalva (higher incidence; lower risk)
      5. Hypoplastic or aplastic coronary arteries
      6. Coronary-intracardiac shunt
   C. Coronary artery embolism
      1. Aortic or mitral endocarditis
      2. Prosthetic aortic or mitral valves
      3. Abnormal native valves or left ventricular mural thrombus
      4. Platelet embolism
   D. Coronary arteritis
      1. Polyarteritis nodosa, progressive systemic sclerosis, giant cell arteritis
      2. Mucocutaneous lymph node syndrome (Kawasaki disease)
      3. Syphilitic coronary ostial stenosis
   E. Miscellaneous mechanical obstruction of the coronary arteries
      1. Coronary artery dissection in Marfan syndrome
      2. Coronary artery dissection in pregnancy (primarily labor/delivery)
      3. Prolapse of aortic valve myxomatous polyps into the coronary ostia
      4. Dissection or rupture of the sinus of Valsalva
   F. Functional obstruction of the coronary arteries
      1. Coronary artery spasm with or without atherosclerosis
      2. Myocardial bridges

II. **Hypertrophy of the ventricular myocardium**
   A. Left ventricular hypertrophy associated with coronary heart disease
   B. Hypertensive heart disease without significant coronary atherosclerosis
   C. Hypertrophic myocardium secondary to valvular heart disease
   D. Hypertrophic cardiomyopathy
      1. Obstructive
      2. Nonobstructive
   E. Primary or secondary pulmonary hypertension
      1. Advanced chronic right ventricular overload
      2. Pulmonary hypertension in pregnancy (highest risk peripartum)

III. **Myocardial diseases and dysfunction, with or without heart failure**
   A. Chronic congestive heart failure
      1. Ischemic cardiomyopathy
      2. Idiopathic dilated cardiomyopathy, acquired
      3. Hereditary dilated cardiomyopathy
      4. Alcoholic cardiomyopathy
      5. Hypertensive cardiomyopathy
      6. Postmyocarditis cardiomyopathy
      7. Peripartum cardiomyopathy
      8. Idiopathic fibrosis
   B. Acute and subacute cardiac failure
      1. Large acute myocardial infarction
      2. Myocarditis, acute or fulminant
      3. Acute alcoholic cardiac dysfunction
      4. Takotsubo syndrome (uncertain risk for sudden death)
      5. Ball valve embolism in aortic stenosis or prosthesis
      6. Mechanical disruptions of cardiac structures
         a. Rupture of the ventricular free wall
         b. Disruption of the mitral apparatus
            (1). Papillary muscle
            (2). Chordae tendineae
            (3). Leaflet
         c. Rupture of the interventricular septum
            (1). Acute pulmonary edema in noncompliant ventricles

IV. **Inflammatory, infiltrative, neoplastic, and degenerative processes**
   A. Viral myocarditis, with or without ventricular dysfunction
      1. Acute phase
      2. Postmyocarditis interstitial fibrosis
   B. Myocarditis associated with the vasculitides
   C. Sarcoidosis
   D. Progressive systemic sclerosis
   E. Amyloidosis
   F. Hemochromatosis
   G. Idiopathic giant cell myocarditis
   H. Chagas disease
   I. Cardiac ganglionitis
   J. Arrhythmogenic right ventricular dysplasia, right ventricular cardiomyopathy
   K. Neuromuscular diseases (e.g., muscular dystrophy, Friedreich ataxia, myotonic dystrophy)
   L. Intramural tumors
      1. Primary
      2. Metastatic
   M. Obstructive intracavitary tumors
      1. Neoplastic
      2. Thrombotic

V. **Diseases of the cardiac valves**
   A. Valvular aortic stenosis/insufficiency
   B. Mitral valve disruption
   C. Mitral valve prolapse
   D. Endocarditis
   E. Prosthetic valve dysfunction

VI. **Congenital heart disease**
   A. Congenital aortic (potentially high risk) or pulmonic (low risk) valve stenosis
   B. Congenital septal defects with Eisenmenger physiology
      1. Advanced disease
      2. During labor and delivery
   C. Late after surgical repair of congenital lesions (e.g., tetralogy of Fallot)

VII. **Electrophysiologic abnormalities**
   A. Abnormalities of the conducting system
      1. Fibrosis of the His-Purkinje system
         a. Primary degeneration (Lenègre disease)
         b. Secondary to fibrosis and calcification of the cardiac skeleton (Lev disease)
         c. Postviral conducting system fibrosis
         d. Hereditary conducting system disease
      2. Anomalous pathways of conduction (Wolff-Parkinson-White syndrome, short refractory period bypass tract)
   B. Abnormalities of repolarization
      1. Congenital abnormalities in duration of the QT interval
         a. Congenital abnormalities in duration of the QT interval
            (1). Romano-Ward syndrome (without deafness)
            (2). Jervell and Lange-Nielsen syndrome (with deafness)
      2. Congenital short QT interval syndrome
      3. Acquired (or provoked) long-QT interval syndromes
         a. Drug effect (enhanced by predisposition)
            (1). Cardiac, antiarrhythmic
            (2). Noncardiac
            (3). Drug interactions
         b. Electrolyte abnormality (response modified by genetic predisposition)
         c. Toxic substances
         d. Hypothermia
         e. Central nervous system injury, subarachnoid hemorrhage
      4. Brugada syndrome—right bundle branch block pattern and ST segment elevation in the absence of ischemia
      5. Early repolarization syndrome
   C. Ventricular fibrillation of unknown or uncertain cause
      1. Absence of identifiable structural or functional causes
         a. Idiopathic ventricular fibrillation
         b. Short-coupled torsades de pointes, polymorphic ventricular tachycardia
         c. Nonspecific fibrofatty infiltration in a previously healthy victim (variation of right ventricular dysplasia?)
      2. Sleep-death in Southeast Asians (Brugada syndrome)
         a. Bangungut
         b. Pokkuri
         c. Lai-tai

VIII. **Electrical instability related to neurohumoral and central nervous system influences**
   A. Catecholaminergic polymorphic ventricular tachycardia
   B. Other catecholamine-dependent arrhythmias
   C. Central nervous system related
      1. Psychic stress, emotional extremes (Takotsubo syndrome)
      2. Auditory related
      3. "Voodoo death" in primitive cultures
      4. Diseases of the cardiac nerves
      5. Arrhythmia expression in congenital long-QT syndrome

IX. **Sudden cardiac death in the young**
   A. Sudden cardiac death in newborns
      1. Complex congenital heart disease
      2. Neonatal myocarditis
   B. Sudden infant death syndrome
      1. Immature respiratory control function
      2. Long-QT syndrome
      3. Congenital heart disease
      4. Myocarditis
   C. Sudden death in children
      1. Eisenmenger syndrome, aortic stenosis, hypertrophic cardiomyopathy, pulmonary atresia
      2. After corrective surgery for congenital heart disease
      3. Myocarditis
      4. Genetic disorders of electrical function (e.g., long-QT syndrome)
      5. No identified structural or functional cause

X. **Miscellaneous**
   A. Sudden death during extreme physical activity (seek predisposing causes)
   B. Commotio cordis—blunt chest trauma
   C. Mechanical interference with venous return
      1. Acute cardiac tamponade
      2. Massive pulmonary embolism
      3. Acute intracardiac thrombosis
   D. Cardiorespiratory arrest secondary to mechanical asphyxia
   E. Dissecting aneurysm of the aorta
   F. Toxic and metabolic disturbances (other than the QT interval effects listed above)
      1. Electrolyte disturbances
      2. Metabolic disturbances
      3. Proarrhythmic effects of antiarrhythmic drugs
      4. Proarrhythmic effects of noncardiac drugs
   G. Mimics sudden cardiac death
      1. "Café coronary"
      2. Acute alcoholic states ("holiday heart")
      3. Acute asthmatic attacks
      4. Air or amniotic fluid embolism

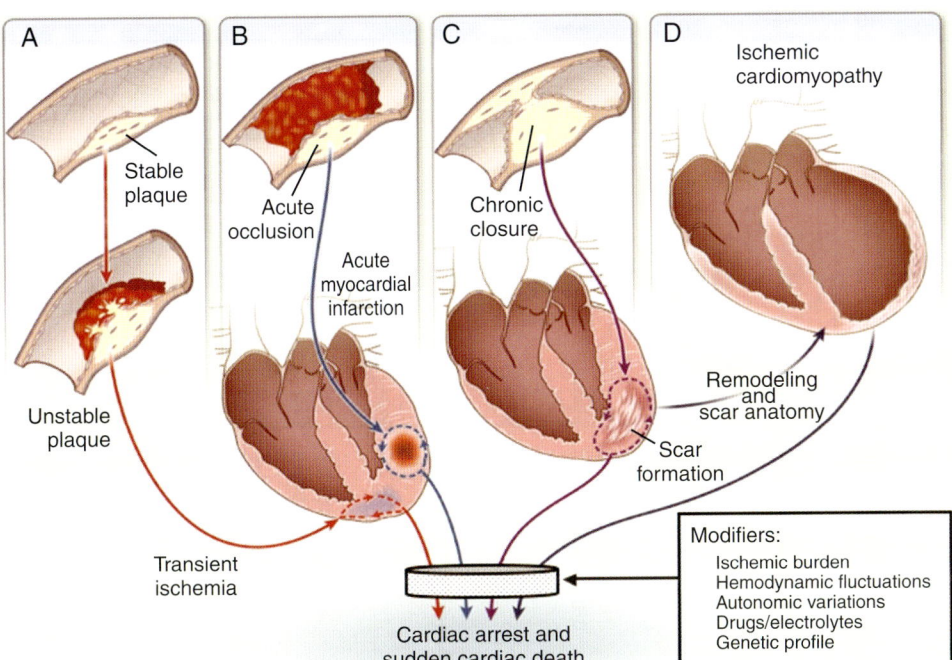

FIGURE 70.7 Pathophysiology of ventricular tachyarrhythmias in coronary heart disease. The short- and long-term risks for the development of VT or VF and recurrent events are related to the presence of transient or persistent physiologic factors. VT/VF caused by transient ischemia **(A)** and the acute phase (24 to 48 hours) of myocardial infarction **(B)** are not predictive of recurrent events if the recurrent ischemia is preventable. In contrast, VT/VF associated with healed myocardial infarction, with or without acute transient ischemia **(C)**, is associated with risk for recurrence. Longstanding ischemic cardiomyopathy **(D)**, especially when accompanied by heart failure, establishes a substrate associated with risk for VT/VF and recurrences over time. A series of modifying influences contribute to individual expression. (Modified from Myerburg RJ: Implantable cardioverter-defibrillators after myocardial infarction. N Engl J Med 2008;359:2245.)

to the Black population that are missed because of underrepresentation in control populations.[58]

Specific clinical markers have not been especially predictive of SCD in individual patients, although young age at onset, a strong family history of SCD in a first-degree relative, magnitude of the LV mass, wall thickness >3 cm, unexplained syncope, nonsustained VT, LV apical aneurysm, and LV systolic dysfunction appear to indicate higher risk. Both a substantial provocable gradient, regardless of the resting gradient, and a high resting gradient alone identify high risk for SCD.[59] The mechanism of SCD in patients with HCM was initially thought to involve outflow tract obstruction, possibly as a consequence of catecholamine stimulation, but later data have focused on lethal arrhythmias as the common mechanism of sudden death in this disease.

The pathogenesis of the arrhythmias in HCM is discussed in Chapter 54. The observation that patients with nonobstructive HCM, such as the diffuse, midcavitary, and to a lesser extent the apical variety, are also at risk for SCD suggests that an electrophysiologic mechanism secondary to the hypertrophied muscle itself plays a major role. In athletes younger than 35 years, HCM is the most common cause of SCD, in contrast to athletes older than 35 years, in whom coronary heart disease is the most common cause.

Ventricular Hypertrophy and Hypertrophic Cardiomyopathy

LV hypertrophy, an independent risk factor for SCD, is associated with many causes of SCD and may be a physiologic contributor to mechanisms of potentially lethal arrhythmias.[54] Underlying states resulting in LV hypertrophy include hypertensive heart disease with or without atherosclerosis, valvular heart disease, obstructive and nonobstructive HCM (see Chapter 54), primary pulmonary hypertension with right ventricular hypertrophy, and advanced right ventricular overload secondary to congenital heart disease. Each of these conditions is associated with risk for SCD, and it has been suggested that patients with severely hypertrophic ventricles are particularly susceptible to arrhythmic death.

Risk for SCD in patients with obstructive and nonobstructive HCM was identified in the early clinical and hemodynamic descriptions of this entity.[42,55] In patients who have the obstructive form, a majority of all deaths are sudden. However, survivors of cardiac arrest in this group may have a better long-term outcome than might survivors with other causes, and reports have suggested that the risk for primary cardiac arrest and SCD in those with HCM is lower than previously thought. It is suggested that it is now less than 1%/year, perhaps related to risk stratification based therapies such as the implantable cardioverter defibrillator.[42] Yet this is a significant cause for SCD in the young.[56,57]

A substantial proportion of patients with obstructive and nonobstructive HCM have a family history of affected relatives with premature SCDs of unknown cause. Genetic studies have confirmed autosomal dominant inheritance patterns, but with significant allelic and phenotypic heterogeneity. Most of the mutations are at loci that encode elements in the contractile protein complex, the most common being myosin binding protein C and beta-myosin heavy chain, which together account for more than half of identified abnormalities. The genetics of HCM is characterized by a large number of private mutations with variable expression. Possible interaction with modifier genes may account for variable expression among carriers of a specific variant, but there is also a possibility that a number of HCM variants thought to be disease-causing in the Black population are actually benign variants unique

Cardiomyopathy and Systolic and Diastolic Heart Failure

The advent of therapeutic interventions that provide better control of congestive heart failure has improved the long-term survival of these patients (see Chapters 50 to 52). However, the proportion of patients with heart failure who die suddenly is substantial, especially among those who appear clinically stable (i.e., functional class I or II). The mechanism of SCD may be tachyarrhythmic (VT or VF) or nonshockable bradyarrhythmias or asystole. The absolute risk for SCD increases with deteriorating LV function, but the ratio of sudden to nonsudden deaths is inversely related to the extent of functional impairment. In patients with cardiomyopathy who have good functional capacity (classes I and II), total mortality risk is considerably lower than in those with functional classes III and IV, but the probability that a death will be sudden is higher (Fig. 70.8). Unexplained syncope has been observed to be a powerful predictor of SCD in patients who have functional class III or IV symptoms, regardless of the cause of cardiomyopathy.

Heart failure with preserved ejection fraction (HFpEF) has a risk for mortality over time similar to that of heart failure with reduced ejection fraction (see Chapter 51). In a summary[60] of the cause specific mortality in HFpEF from the I-Preserve, CHARM-Preserved, and TOPCAT trials, 68% were cardiovascular. SCD accounted for approximately 40% of the cardiovascular deaths (27% of all deaths). The precise etiology remains unknown with both VT and bradyarrhythmias recorded in these patients.[61] To date, there have been no targeted interventions that have successfully reduced the risk of SCD in this population.

Ischemic cardiomyopathy provides the strongest association between chronic heart failure and SCD. The prevalence of ischemic cardiomyopathy had been increasing because of better acute MI survival statistics coupled with late remodeling. Other causes include "idiopathic" fibrosis, alcoholic and postmyocarditis cardiomyopathies, peripartum cardiomyopathy (see Chapter 92), and the familial pattern of dilated cardiomyopathy, many of the latter being associated with lamin A/C mutations.[62] Other gene loci have also been implicated. A residual group of undefined causes have been classified as idiopathic cardiomyopathy.

Acute Heart Failure

All causes of acute cardiac failure (see Chapters 47-49), in the absence of prompt interventions, can result in SCD as a result of the circulatory failure itself or secondary arrhythmias. The electrophysiologic mechanisms involved have been proposed to be caused by acute stretching of ventricular myocardial fibers or the His-Purkinje system on the basis of its experimentally demonstrated arrhythmogenic effects. However, the roles of neurohumoral mechanisms and acute electrolyte shifts have not been fully evaluated. Among the causes of acute cardiac failure associated with SCD are massive acute MI, acute myocarditis, acute alcoholic cardiac dysfunction, acute pulmonary edema in any form of advanced heart disease, and a number of mechanical causes of heart failure, such as massive pulmonary embolism, mechanical disruption of intracardiac structures secondary to infarction or infection, and ball valve embolism in aortic or mitral stenosis (see Table 70.3).

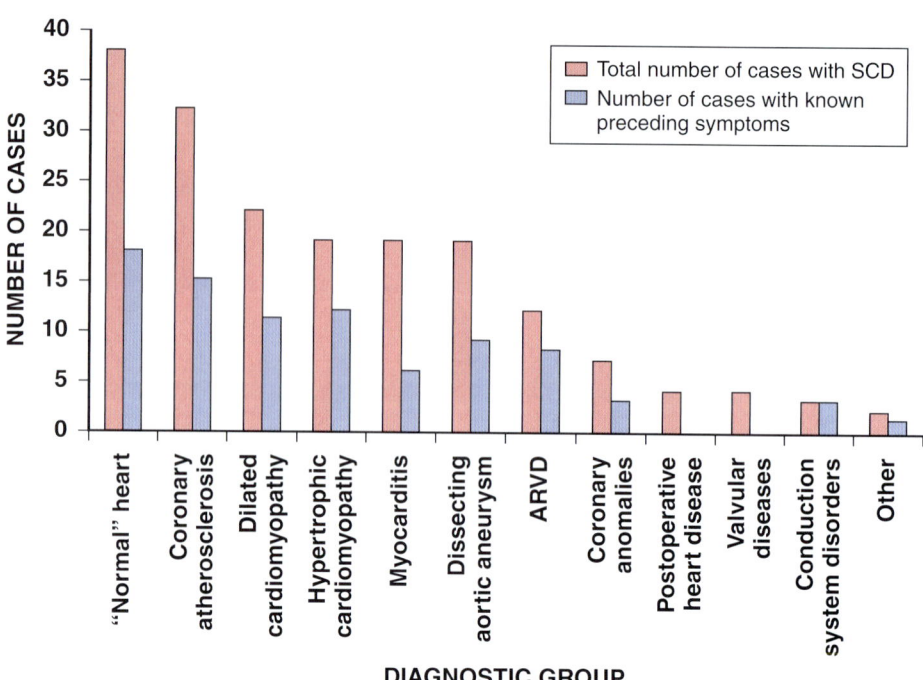

FIGURE 70.8 SCD in adolescents and young adults in Sweden. The frequency of preceding symptoms in 181 cases of SCD in persons 15 to 35 years old is shown by diagnostic group. *ARVD,* Arrhythmogenic right ventricular dysplasia. (Modified from Wisten A, et al. Sudden cardiac death in 15-35-year-olds in Sweden during 1992-99. J Intern Med 2002;252:529.)

Inflammatory, Infiltrative, Neoplastic, and Degenerative Diseases of the Heart.

Almost all diseases in this category have been associated with SCD, with or without concomitant cardiac failure. Acute viral myocarditis with LV dysfunction (see Chapters 52 and 55) is commonly associated with cardiac arrhythmias, including potentially lethal arrhythmias. Serious ventricular arrhythmias or SCD can occur in patients with myocarditis, even in the absence of clinical evidence of LV dysfunction. This has most recently been reported following SARS-CoV-2 infection during the COVID-19 pandemic.[63-67] In autopsy series of young people presenting with SCD, myocarditis may be found in up to 10%.[68] As noted during the COVID-19 pandemic, many individuals with myocarditis have no to minimal symptoms (Fig. 70.8). Most data available suggest a bias toward victims younger than 35 years. Focal myocarditis can be associated with SCD and may be missed on autopsy depending on the extent of the cardiac evaluation. Giant cell myocarditis and acute necrotizing eosinophilic myocarditis are particularly virulent for both myocardial damage and arrhythmias. Viral myocarditis can also cause damage isolated to the specialized conducting system and result in a propensity to arrhythmias; the rare association of this process with SCD has been reported. Varicella in adults is a rare cause of striking conduction system disorders, largely involving the intraventricular specialized conducting tissue with very prolonged QRS complexes. LV function is usually preserved, and its relationship to SCD is unclear.

Myocardial involvement in collagen-vascular disorders, tumors, chronic granulomatous diseases, infiltrative disorders, and protozoan infestations varies widely, but SCD can be the initial or terminal manifestation of the disease process in all cases. Among the granulomatous diseases, cardiac sarcoidosis stands out because of the frequency of associated SCD.[69] Clinical cardiac involvement in patients with sarcoidosis is approximately 5% with another 20% to 25% having asymptomatic involvement.[70] The risk for SCD has been related to the extent of cardiac involvement, but ambient arrhythmias, such as nonsustained VT, may indicate risk in such patients with lesser degrees of cardiac involvement. In a report of the pathologic findings in nine patients who died of progressive systemic sclerosis, eight who died suddenly had evidence of transient ischemia and reperfusion histologically, thus suggesting that this might represent spasm of the coronary vessels. Amyloidosis of the heart (see Chapter 53) can also cause sudden death. An incidence of 30% has been reported, and diffuse involvement of ventricular muscle or the specialized conducting system may be associated with SCD. Cardiac involvement can occur in both light chain (AL) and transthyretin (ATTR) amyloid. TTR-associated cardiac amyloid tends to express later in life, almost always after the age of 50 years, and observed in up to 4% of the Black population, with or without the disease. Despite a high incidence of treatment for VT/fibrillation, the role of the implantable defibrillator in improving survival has not been established.[71]

Arrhythmogenic Right Ventricular Dysplasia or Right Ventricular Cardiomyopathy.

This condition with a prevalence ranging between 1/1000 and 1/5000[72] is associated with a high incidence of ventricular arrhythmias, including polymorphic nonsustained VT and VF and recurrent sustained monomorphic VT (see Chapters 63 and 67). Importantly, this is a significant underlying etiology for SCD in young people, likely accounting for 10% to 20% of cases.[73] Importantly, in a high proportion of victims, perhaps as many as 80%, the first manifestation of arrhythmogenic right ventricular dysplasia or right ventricular cardiomyopathy (ARVD/C) is "unexplained" syncope or SCD. With more widespread screening and evaluation for ARVD/C, this is being identified among family members of probands who also have substantial risk for VT, but the clinical characteristics suggest a more aggressive course in the subset who present with SCD—occurring at a younger age, in a higher percent of males, and during high levels of exertion.[74]

SCD is often exercise related, and in some areas of the world where screening for HCM has excluded affected athletes from competition, ARVD/C has emerged as the most common cause of sports-related SCD. High-level competitive sports participation is not recommended for those with a confirmed diagnosis.[75] Although it is generally considered a right ventricular abnormality, with possible late involvement of the left ventricle in advanced cases, a left ventricle-dominant pattern has also been described.

ARVD/C is predominantly an inherited disorder in which the variants cause or predispose to the disease, interacting with high right ventricular strain during exercise. In addition, there is some basis for considering that RV arrhythmogenic responses may be caused by very high-intensity athletic activity as a result of repeated RV strain exposures.[76] The inheritance pattern is autosomal dominant, except in one geographically isolated cluster in which it is autosomal recessive (Naxos disease, plakoglobin locus on chromosome 17). Four loci-encoding components of the desmosome (plakoglobin, desmoplakin, plakophilin 2, and desmoglein 2) are collectively the most common known mutations associated with right ventricular dysplasia.[77] Autosomal dominant mutations have also been identified in the ryanodine receptor locus on chromosome 1 (1q42) (see Chapter 63).

Valvular Heart Disease

Before the advent of surgery for valvular heart disease, severe aortic stenosis was associated with high risk for mortality (see Chapter 72). Approximately 70% of deaths were sudden and accounted for an absolute SCD mortality rate of 15% to 20% among all affected patients. In the Contemporary Outcomes After Surgery and Medical Treatment in Patients With Severe Aortic Stenosis (CURRENT AS) registry,[78] the annual rate of SCD was 1.6%/year and 1.1%/year with and without censoring for surgical or transcatheter valve replacement. Even asymptomatic patients experienced a 1.4%/year rate of SCD. In patients with mild to moderate AS, a 0.39%/year rate of SCD has been reported.[79]

The advent of aortic valve replacement has reduced the incidence of SCD, but patients with prosthetic or heterograft aortic valve replacements remain at some risk for SCD caused by arrhythmias, prosthetic valve dysfunction, or coexistent coronary heart disease. The incidence peaks 3 weeks after surgery and then levels off after 8 months. A high incidence of ventricular arrhythmia has been observed during the follow-up of patients with valve replacement, especially those who had aortic stenosis, multiple valve surgery, or cardiomegaly. Among 3726 patients who underwent transcatheter aortic valve replacement, 5.6% were reported to have SCD at average 22 month follow-up.[80] New-onset left bundle branch block was a significant predictor of SCD, but not in those who received a pacemaker, suggesting that AV block may be a significant etiology for SCD in these patients. Similar observations have been made following surgical aortic valve replacement. An association between stenotic lesions of other valves and SCD has not been demonstrated.

Mitral valve prolapse has been associated with SCD. While mitral valve prolapse is common, the risk for SCD is extremely low. There may be a subset of patients with mitral valve prolapse that are particularly susceptible to ventricular arrhythmias and SCD. The estimated incidence of SCD is 0.2% to 0.4% per year.[81] Fibrosis of the papillary muscles and inferobasal left ventricle is noted in these patients. Mapping studies show a papillary muscle origin for ventricular ectopy in patients with mitral valve prolapse and evidence of late gadolinium enhancement in the papillary muscle,[82] though other LV origins for ventricular ectopy have also been noted. SCD is associated with marked redundancy of mitral leaflets, in conjunction with nonspecific ST-T wave changes in inferior leads.

Regurgitant lesions, particularly chronic aortic regurgitation and acute mitral regurgitation, may cause SCD, but the risk is lower than with aortic stenosis. Limited data suggest that inducibility of VT with programmed ventricular stimulation is a significant predictor of arrhythmic events.

> **Endocarditis of the Aortic and Mitral Valves.** This condition may be associated with rapid death resulting from acute disruption of the valvular apparatus (see Chapter 80), coronary embolism, or abscesses of valvular rings or the septum; however, such deaths are rarely true sudden deaths because conventionally defined tachyarrhythmic mechanisms are uncommon. Coronary embolism from valvular vegetations can trigger fatal ischemic arrhythmia on rare occasion.
>
> **Congenital Heart Disease.** The congenital lesions most commonly associated with SCD are aortic stenosis (see Chapter 82) and communications between the left and right sides of the heart with Eisenmenger physiology. In the latter, the risk for SCD is a function of the severity of pulmonary vascular disease; also, pregnant patients with Eisenmenger syndrome have an extraordinarily high risk for maternal mortality during labor and delivery (see Chapter 92). Potentially lethal arrhythmias and SCD have been described as late complications after surgical repair of complex congenital lesions, particularly tetralogy of Fallot, transposition of the great arteries, and atrioventricular (AV) canal defects. These patients should be observed closely and treated aggressively when cardiac arrhythmias are identified, although the late risk for SCD may not be as high as previously thought.

Electrophysiologic Abnormalities

Acquired disease of the AV node and His-Purkinje system and the presence of accessory AV pathways (see Chapter 68) may be associated with SCD. Clinical surveillance and follow-up studies have suggested that intraventricular conduction disturbances in coronary heart disease is one of the few factors that can increase the proportion of SCD in patients with coronary heart disease. Early studies demonstrated a very high risk for total mortality and SCD during the late in-hospital course and the first few months after hospital discharge in patients with anterior MIs and right bundle branch or bifascicular block. In a later study evaluating the impact of thrombolytic therapy versus the pre–thrombolytic era experience, the incidence of pure right bundle branch block was higher but that of bifascicular block was lower, as were late complications and mortality.

Primary fibrosis (Lenègre disease) or injury secondary to other disorders (Lev disease) of the His-Purkinje system is commonly associated with intraventricular conduction abnormalities and symptomatic AV block and less commonly with SCD. Identification of those at risk and the efficacy of pacemakers for prevention of SCD, rather than only amelioration of symptoms, have been subjects of debate. However, survival appears to depend more on the nature and extent of the underlying disease than on the conduction disturbance itself.

Patients with congenital AV block (see Chapter 68) or nonprogressive congenital intraventricular block, in the absence of structural cardiac abnormalities and with a stable heart rate and rhythm, have been characterized as being at low risk for SCD in the past. Later data have suggested that patients with the patterns of congenital AV block previously thought to be benign are at risk for dilated cardiomyopathy, and routine pacemaker implantation in patients older than 15 years, if not indicated sooner based on symptoms, has been suggested by at least one group. Confirmation from clinical trial data is not available. Hereditary forms of AV block have also been reported in association with a familial propensity to SCD. Sodium channel gene mutations have been associated with progressive conduction system disturbances and variants of Brugada syndrome (see Chapter 63). External ophthalmoplegia and retinal pigmentation with progressive conduction system disease (Kearns-Sayre syndrome), which is associated with mitochondrial DNA variants, may lead to high-grade heart block and pacemaker dependence.

The anomalous pathways of conduction in Wolff-Parkinson-White syndrome are commonly associated with nonlethal arrhythmias. However, when the anomalous pathways of conduction have short anterograde refractory periods, the occurrence of atrial fibrillation may allow the initiation of VF during very rapid conduction across the accessory pathway (see Chapter 65). Patients who have multiple pathways appear to be at higher risk for SCD, as do patients with a familial pattern of anomalous pathways and premature SCD.

Long-QT Syndromes

Congenital long-QT syndrome is a functional abnormality usually caused by mutations affecting ion channel proteins and is associated with environmental or neurogenic triggers that can initiate symptomatic or lethal arrhythmias (see Chapters 63 and 67).[83] Such mutations may occur de novo or more commonly may be transmitted from an apparently normal parent. Syncope is the most common manifestation in symptomatic patients. SCD is less common, although data are limited by the absence of information on undiagnosed carriers in whom fatal cardiac arrest is the first clinical event. For example, the prevalence of long-QT variants in the population is generally cited to be in the range of 1/2000 to 1/2500, but a study from Japan reporting on routine ECG screening among first- and seventh-grade school children provides an estimated prevalence of 1/988, more than double the generally accepted figure from referral populations.[36] Some patients have prolonged QT intervals throughout life without any manifest arrhythmias, whereas others are highly susceptible to symptomatic and potentially fatal ventricular arrhythmias. The concept of modifier genes interacting with the primary defect or physiologic contributors to expression is an area of active investigation.[84]

Higher levels of risk are associated with female sex, greater degrees of QT prolongation or QT alternans, unexplained syncope, family history of premature SCD, and documented torsades de pointes or previous VF. Patients with the syndrome require avoidance of drugs that are associated with QT lengthening and careful medical management, which may include implantable defibrillators. Moreover, it is important to identify and to manage relatives medically who carry the mutation and may be at risk (see Chapters 63, 64, and 67). While abnormalities in genes coding for ion channels are the most frequent causes of long-QT syndrome, there are now multiple LQT types coding for other proteins that are responsible for this syndrome (see Chapter 63).

Even in the absence of manifest long-QT syndrome, from an epidemiologic perspective, there is interest in whether QT interval abnormalities or the propensity thereto, interacting with acquired diseases, predisposes to SCD as a specific clinical expression. In many studies, QT prolongation has been associated with increased SCD, but it is interesting to note that individual components of the QT interval may bear more predictive utility.[85] The hypothesis that common genetic variants may modulate QTc in unselected populations has stimulated interest in the relationship to selective risk for SCD in individuals with acquired diseases. However, a number of rare variants may be even more important.

The acquired form of prolonged–QT interval syndrome refers to excessive lengthening of the QT interval and the potential for the development of torsades de pointes (TdP) in response to environmental influences. As with congenital LQTS, it is more common in women. The syndrome may be caused by drug effects or an individual patient's idiosyncrasies (particularly related to class IA or III antiarrhythmic drugs and psychotropic drugs; see Chapters 9 and 99), electrolyte abnormalities, hypothermia, toxic substances, bradyarrhythmia-induced QT adjustments, and central nervous system injury (most commonly subarachnoid hemorrhage). It had also been reported in intensive weight reduction programs that involved the use of certain liquid protein diets and in patients with anorexia nervosa. Lithium carbonate can prolong the QT interval and unmask Brugada syndrome and has been reported to be associated with an increased incidence of SCD in cancer patients with preexisting heart disease. Drug interactions have been recognized as a mechanism of prolongation of the QT interval and TDP. Inherited polymorphisms or mutations with low penetrance involving the same gene loci associated with phenotypically expressed long-QT syndrome may underlie the acquired form, in many cases. In acquired prolonged-QT syndrome, as in the congenital form, torsades de pointes is commonly the specific arrhythmia that triggers or degenerates into VF.

Short-QT Syndrome. A familial pattern of risk for SCD has been associated with abnormally short QT intervals, defined as a QTc shorter than 300 milliseconds (QT <280 milliseconds). Short-QT syndrome is much less common than long-QT syndrome, and there is little to guide risk profiling other than documented life-threatening arrhythmias and familial clustering of SCD. Several ion channel gene loci variants have been identified, but they account for a minority of cases (see Chapter 63).

Brugada Syndrome

This disorder, now considered part of the J wave syndromes, is characterized by an atypical right bundle branch block pattern and unusual forms of nonischemic ST-T wave elevations in the anterior precordial leads (Fig. 70.9). It is a familial disorder associated with risk for SCD and occurs most commonly in young and middle-aged men (see Chapters 63 and 67). Mutations involving the cardiac Na+ channel gene (SCN5A) are the most commonly observed variants but are identified in only a minority of cases, and a number of other ion channel defects have been associated with the syndrome. A variant in SCN10A has been observed in more than 16% of affected individuals. The right bundle branch block and ST-T wave changes may be intermittent and evoked or exaggerated by Na+ channel blockers (e.g., ajmaline, flecainide, procainamide). Individual risk for SCD is difficult to predict. Persistent type I electrocardiographic patterns, syncope, sex, and life-threatening arrhythmias, in various combinations, are thought to be the best predictors.[86] Though the role of programmed ventricular stimulation to identify patients at high risk for SCD is debated, a pooled analysis of eight studies incorporating 1312 patients found a hazard ratio of 2.66 (95% confidence interval [CI], 1.44 to 4.92) for inducible sustained or hemodynamically significant polymorphic VT or fibrillation.[4]

Early Repolarization and Sudden Cardiac Death

An association between the electrocardiographic pattern of early repolarization (ER) and risk for idiopathic VF has been described (J wave syndrome; see Chapter 67). ER was limited to the inferior and lateral leads, in contrast to the anterior leads, which associated with the conventional definition of benign ER. The magnitude of J point elevation was significantly greater in cardiac arrest survivors than in controls with ER. It has been estimated that ER accounts for an increase of 139.6 cardiac arrests per 100,000 subjects per year.[87]

The observation that excess risk is expressed later in life suggests a possible interaction between the physiology of ER and structural heart disease, such as coronary heart disease. An association between ER and a higher mortality during acute MI has been reported.[88]

Catecholaminergic Polymorphic Ventricular Tachycardia. Catecholaminergic polymorphic ventricular tachycardia (CPVT) is an inherited syndrome associated with catecholamine-dependent lethal arrhythmias in the absence of forewarning electrocardiographic abnormalities and with at least partial control by beta adrenoceptor-blocking agents (see Chapters 63 and 67). An autosomal dominant pattern involving the ryanodine receptor locus (RyR2) was initially described predominantly in younger patients, with bidirectional or polymorphic VT associated with risk for SCD. Another variant involving autosomal recessive inheritance of calsequestrin loci (CASQ2) is observed in approximately

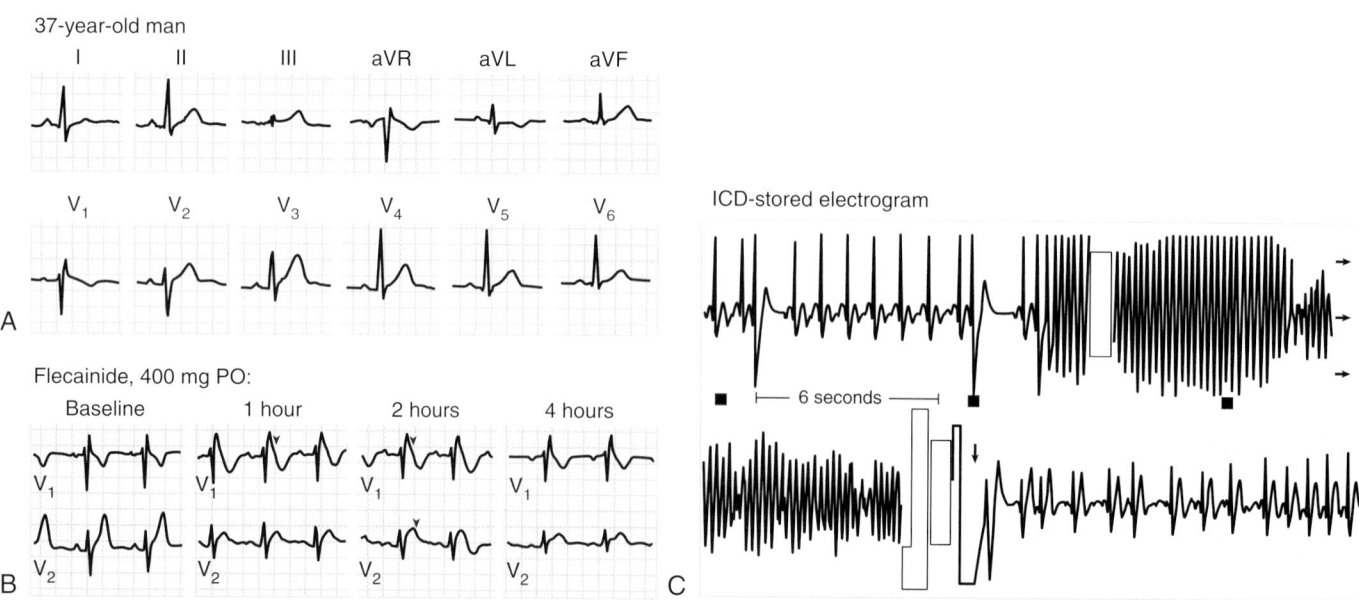

FIGURE 70.9 Electrocardiographic and clinical findings in a 37-year-old man with Brugada syndrome. The patient was resuscitated after out-of-hospital VF. No structural disease was identified. **A,** The 12-lead ECG shows an incomplete right bundle branch block pattern, which is not typical of Brugada syndrome. **B,** The typical repolarization changes associated with Brugada syndrome (*red arrowheads*) were elicited by a single oral dose of flecainide, 400 mg. The patient received an ICD and 6 months later had an appropriate shock (*arrow,* **C**), as shown on the accompanying electrogram stored in the device.

10% of genotyped cases and relatives. Overall incidence has been estimated at 1 in 10,000 with a high mortality in untreated patients.[83]

Electrical Instability Resulting from Neurohumoral and Central Nervous System Influences. The central nervous system can adversely effect cardiac electrophysiology to produce SCD (see Chapters 62 and 102). Epidemiologic data have also suggested an association between behavioral abnormalities and risk for SCD. Psychological stress and emotional extremes have been suggested for many years to be triggering mechanisms for advanced arrhythmias and SCD, but only limited, largely observational data support such associations (see Chapter 99). Takotsubo cardiomyopathy is a catecholamine-mediated condition with a generally good long-term prognosis, but the short-term risk for SCD during the acute phase remains uncertain and can be associated with QT prolongation. The possibility that it contributed to unexplained SCD in the young and middle aged population should be explored.

Stress-induced arrhythmias are better supported than stress-induced risk for mortality, which requires further study. Data from the 1994 Los Angeles earthquake identified an increased rate of fatal cardiac events on that day, but the event rate was reduced during the ensuing 2 weeks, thus suggesting triggering of events about to happen rather than independent causation. Other natural disasters have been associated with a transient increase in SCD.[4,47] Associations between auditory stimulation and auditory auras and SCD have been reported. Auditory abnormalities in some forms of congenital QT prolongation have also been observed.

A variant of TDP characterized by short coupling intervals between a normal impulse and the initiating impulse has been described. It appears to have familial trends and to be related to alterations in autonomic nervous system activity. The 12-lead ECG demonstrates normal QT intervals, but VF and sudden death are common (see Chapters 63 and 67).

The phenomenon of so-called voodoo death has been studied in pockets of isolation in underdeveloped countries. There appears to be an association between isolation from the tribe, a sense of hopelessness, severe bradyarrhythmias, and sudden death. Limited clinical observations and experimental data modeling voodoo death have suggested a mechanism related to parasympathetic overactivity, as opposed to the evidence of an adrenergic basis for syndromes related to acute emotional stress.

Sudden Infant Death Syndrome and Sudden Cardiac Death in Children

SIDS occurs between birth and 6 months of age, is more common in male infants, and had an incidence of 1.2 deaths per 1000 live births before widespread publication of appropriate sleep positions in at-risk infants. In 1992, the American Academy of Pediatrics recommended that infants be placed to sleep in a nonprone position to reduce the risk of SIDS. The SIDS rate dropped from 120 per 100,000 live births in 1992 to 56 per 100,000 live births in 2001.[89] This supports a major role for obstructive sleep apnea as a mechanism. Vulnerability as a result of various mechanisms of dysfunctional central respiratory control, both inherent and related to prematurity, is likely to interact with sleep position as a multicomponent mechanism.

Because of its abrupt nature, a primary cardiac mechanism had been suspected in some cases, and a large study of ECGs of infants suggested prolonged QT intervals associated with risk for SIDS. A near-miss survivor with a de novo mutation of the cardiac Na$^+$ channel gene (*SCN5A*) provided proof of concept that a long-QT may be a mechanism of SIDS. Subsequent data have supported the notion that as many as 15% of cases of SIDS may occur by this mechanism. Other very rare potential cardiac associations, such as accessory pathways and dispersed or immature AV nodal or bundle branch cells in the annulus, have also been described.

Sudden death in children beyond the SIDS age group and in adolescents and young adults is associated with structural heart disease in most cases. Approximately 25% of cases of SCDs in children occur in those who have undergone previous surgery for congenital cardiac disease. Of the remaining 75%, more than half occur in children who have one of four lesions: congenital aortic stenosis, Eisenmenger syndrome, pulmonary stenosis or atresia, or obstructive HCM (see Chapter 82). Other common causes included myocarditis, hypertrophic and dilated cardiomyopathy, congenital heart disease, and aortic dissection.

Sudden Cardiac Death in Competitive and Recreational Athletes and During Intense Exercise

SCD can occur during or after extreme physical activity in competing athletes or under special circumstances in the general population (see Chapter 32). Examples of the latter include intense conditioning exercise and basic military training. Among adolescent and young adult competitive athletes, the incidence was estimated to be in the range of 1/75,000 annually in Italy, as opposed to less than 1/125,000 for the general nonathlete population in the same age group. A more recent report from Italy revealed a rate of 1/100,000 among competitive athletes and 0.32/100,000 among those involved only in recreational or leisure activity.[90] In the National Collegiate Athletic Association (NCAA) database, there was 1 SCD per 53,703 athlete-years, with increased rates for males and Black athletes.[46] Differences by sport and NCAA division have been reported. The US National Registry similarly reports male predominance and higher prevalence in Blacks.[91]

While regular physical activity is associated with improved survival, there is an incremental risk related to the time period bounded by the exertion and its recovery period compared with other times—the "exercise paradox" for SCD. Overall, the risk is low, <20 per million per year,[46,92] with lower rates in women than men. Most athletes and nonathletes have a previously known or unrecognized cardiac abnormality. In middle-aged and older adults, in whom coronary disease dominates as the cause of SCD, exercise-related deaths appear to be associated with acute plaque disruption. Whether exercise contributed to the initiation of plaque disruption or preexisting disruption simply set the stage for the fatal response during exercise remains unclear. Among adolescent and young adult athletes, HCM with or without obstruction and occult congenital or acquired coronary artery disease are the most common causes identified after death,[59,91] with myocarditis contributing a significant minority. Other causes, such as ARVD/C, mitral valve prolapse, and dilated cardiomyopathy, were less common. In a report of a cohort of U.S. Air Force recruits, a surprisingly large fraction of those who died suddenly during exertion had unsuspected myocarditis. There is therefore general consensus that athletes with myocarditis should be restricted from exercise for 3 to 6 months.[93] With the advent of the COVID-19 pandemic, screening athletes for myocarditis to prevent exercise-induced SCD was widely undertaken. A study of SCA risk in marathon and half-marathon runners suggested that the overall incidence did not appear to be higher than that for the general population in the age group of participants (see Chapter 32).

Diseases attributed to molecular abnormalities, such as long-QT syndrome and right ventricular dysplasia, are increasingly being recognized as causes of SCD in athletes and exercising nonathletes. Blunt chest wall trauma by sports objects, such as baseballs and hockey pucks, can initiate lethal arrhythmias, a syndrome known as commotio cordis.[94]

Sudden death from true cardiac causes in athletes should not be confused with precipitous death related to noncardiac causes, such as acute stroke,[95] heat stroke, or malignant hyperthermia. In the latter, the victim has usually exercised excessively in hot weather, often with athletic gear that impairs heat dissipation and sometimes in association with the use of substances such as ephedrine that may cause vasoconstriction impairing heat exchange. This leads to collapse with markedly elevated core body temperatures and, ultimately, irreversible organ system damage. As a result, the U.S. Food and Drug Administration (FDA) has banned marketing of these substances for enhancement of athletic performance or weight loss.

Other Causes and Circumstances Associated with Sudden Death

A small group of victims has neither previously determined functional abnormality nor identifiable structural abnormalities at postmortem examination. Such events or deaths, when they are associated with documented VF, are classified as idiopathic. Although long-term survival after an idiopathic, potentially fatal event is still unclear, some degree of risk appears to remain. The idiopathic category is decreasing as the molecular causes become better defined, including recognition by postmortem genetic studies. Limited data suggest that higher risk persists primarily in patients with subtle cardiac structural abnormalities, in contrast to patients who are truly normal.

A number of noncardiac-related conditions can also cause or mimic SCD. Sleep apnea is associated with increased risk of SCD,[96] particularly nocturnal death, including deaths attributable to cardiac causes (see Chapter 89). The risk for death peaks during the night rather than in the early morning hours. Another respiratory system–based cause of sudden death is the so-called café coronary, in which food lodges in the oropharynx and causes an abrupt obstruction at the glottis. The holiday heart syndrome is characterized by cardiac arrhythmias, most commonly atrial fibrillation, as well as other cardiac abnormalities associated with alcohol consumption. It has not been determined whether potentially lethal arrhythmias occurring in such settings account for the reported sudden deaths associated with acute alcoholic states. Massive pulmonary embolism (see Chapter 87) can cause acute cardiovascular collapse and sudden death; sudden death in severe acute asthmatic attacks, without prolonged deterioration of the patient's condition, is well recognized. Air or amniotic fluid embolism at the time of labor and delivery may cause sudden death on rare occasion, with the clinical picture mimicking that of SCD.

Finally, a number of abnormalities that do not directly involve the heart may cause sudden deaths that mimic SCD. Such abnormalities include aortic dissection (see Chapter 42), acute cardiac tamponade (see Chapter 86), and rapid exsanguination. The electrical mechanism associated with these deaths is most commonly severe bradyarrhythmias, pulseless electrical activity (PEA), or asystole rather than VT or fibrillation.

Pathology and Pathophysiology. Protocols and observations from postmortem studies of SCD victims have changed in recent years. It is now recommended that cases of SCD that do not have obvious causes identified on routine postmortem studies or available clinical information, have post mortem examinations performed by specialized cardiac pathology centers. This is particularly important for younger populations with unexplained SCA. In a series of autopsy cases referred by a pathologist to an expert cardiac pathologist, there was divergence in final diagnoses. Notably, there was a tendency for the routine autopsy to overdiagnose cardiomyopathy as a cause of death, and CAD was less common than in other studies. However, the study was limited to some extent by being skewed to a younger population, limiting extrapolation of this observation to the overall population.[4] In addition, a number of studies now support the notion that postmortem genetic studies are useful for increasing the probability of identifying a cause that is unexplained based on anatomical findings.[29,97,98]

Earlier pathologic studies in SCD victims across a broad age range reflected the epidemiologic and clinical observations that coronary atherosclerosis is the major predisposing cause. All other causes of SCD (see Table 70.3) collectively account for no more than 20% of cases. In the Postmortem Systematic Investigation of SCD (POST SCD) study,[5] 55.8% of cases with World Health Organization defined SCD were determined to have sudden arrhythmic death. Coronary artery disease accounted for only 32% of all cases, with evidence of acute coronary syndrome in one-third. Noncardiac causes included occult overdose and neurologic causes. Cardiomyopathy and hypertrophy were other significant cardiac causes. The decline in the proportion of SCDs attributed to coronary artery disease, with a concomitant increase in hypertensive cardiomyopathy and idiopathic myocardial fibrosis has been demonstrated in a longitudinal autopsy series from Finland.[13] Continued attention to the postmortem evaluation of cases labelled as SCD is clearly needed to help guide further attempts at prevention.

Pathology of Sudden Death Caused by Coronary Artery Abnormalities

Coronary Arteries. Extensive atherosclerosis has long been recognized as the most common pathologic finding in the coronary arteries of victims of SCD. The combined results of a number of studies have suggested a general pattern of at least two coronary arteries with 75% or greater narrowing in more than 75% of the victims. Several studies have demonstrated no specific pattern of distribution of coronary artery lesions that preselect for SCD, but the extent of coronary artery narrowing at postmortem examination was greater in SCD victims than in control subjects.

The role of active coronary artery lesions, characterized by plaque fissuring, plaque erosion or rupture, platelet aggregation, and thrombosis, as a major pathophysiologic mechanism of the onset of cardiac arrest has emerged (see Chapters 24 and 37). Disruption, platelet aggregation, and thrombosis are associated with markers of inflammation and various conventional risk factors for coronary atherosclerosis, such as cigarette smoking and hyperlipidemia.

Some of the less common, nonatherosclerotic coronary artery abnormalities have specific pathologic features as well. Coronary artery spasm, an established cause of acute ischemia and SCD, is commonly associated with nonobstructive plaque (Fig. 70.10), and the consequences of spasm/reperfusion has been recognized at postmortem examination. When deep myocardial bridges are identified in association with SCD, patchy fibrosis in areas subserved by the affected vessel

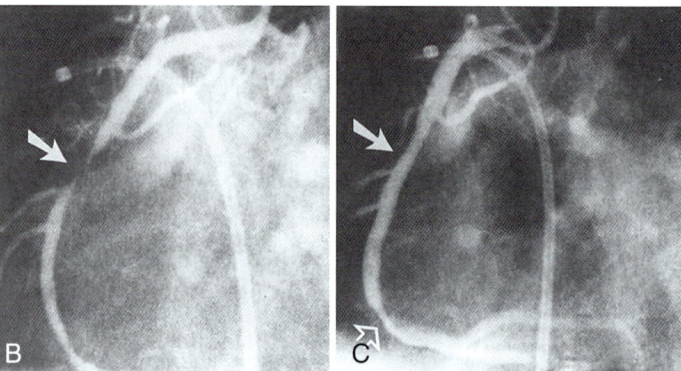

FIGURE 70.10 Life-threatening ventricular arrhythmias associated with acute myocardial ischemia related to coronary artery spasm and with reperfusion. **A,** Continuous lead II electrocardiographic monitor recording during ischemia (time, 0 to 55 seconds) caused by spasm of the right coronary artery **(B).** Following the administration of nitroglycerin at approximately 55 seconds, an abrupt transition from repetitive ventricular ectopy to a rapid polymorphic, prefibrillatory tachyarrhythmia occurs (time, 80 to 130 seconds) in association with reversal of the spasm **(C).** *Closed arrow* indicates the site of spasm before and after nitroglycerin; the *open arrow* indicates a lower grade distal lesion. (Modified from Myerburg RJ, et al: Life-threatening ventricular arrhythmias in patients with silent myocardial ischemia due to coronary artery spasm. N Engl J Med 1992;326:1451.)

is commonly seen at postmortem examination. Coronary vasculitis in association with various autoimmune disorders may cause diffuse myocardial abnormalities, but asymptomatic cardiac involvement or global myocardial dysfunction is more common than SCD.

Myocardium. Myocardial injury in SCD caused by coronary heart disease reflects the extensive atherosclerosis usually present. Studies of victims of out-of-hospital SCD have indicated that healed MI is a common finding in SCD victims, with most investigators reporting frequencies ranging from 40% to more than 70%. The incidence of acute MI is considerably lower, with cytopathologic evidence of recent MI found in approximately 20% of individuals. This estimate corresponds well with the frequency of new MI in of out-of-hospital cardiac arrest survivors. The POST SCD study noted that only one third of the cases attributed to coronary artery disease had evidence of acute coronary syndrome.[5] These pathologic observations do not provide insight into the likely possibility that many SCDs occur as a result of acute coronary syndrome mechanisms and progress from ischemia to fatal arrhythmias without time for structural markers to become visible. Since elevations in troponin levels occur during chest pain syndromes and also in a substantial proportion of cardiac arrest survivors, the determination whether myocardial injury preceded or resulted from the cardiac arrest is difficult to resolve in individual cases.

Ventricular Hypertrophy. Myocardial hypertrophy can coexist and interact with acute or chronic ischemia but appears to confer an independent risk for mortality. No close correlation has been found between increased heart weight and the severity of coronary heart disease in SCD victims; however, heart weight is higher in SCD victims than in those whose death is not sudden despite a similar prevalence of a history of hypertension before death. Risk for hypertrophy-associated mortality is also independent of LV function and the extent of coronary artery disease, and LV hypertrophy itself may predispose to SCD. Experimental data have also suggested increased susceptibility to potentially lethal ventricular arrhythmias in patients with LV hypertrophy and ischemia and reperfusion.

Specialized Conducting System in Sudden Cardiac Death. Fibrosis of the specialized conducting system may be observed in SCD victims. Although this process is associated with AV block or intraventricular conduction abnormalities, its role in SCD is uncertain. Lev disease, Lenègre disease, ischemic injury caused by small-vessel disease, and numerous infiltrative or inflammatory processes can result in such changes. In addition, active inflammatory processes such as myocarditis and infiltrative processes such as amyloidosis, scleroderma, hemochromatosis, and morbid obesity may damage or destroy the AV node, bundle of His, or both and result in AV block.[4]

Focal diseases such as sarcoidosis, rheumatoid arthritis, fibrotic or fatty infiltration of the AV node or His-Purkinje system with apparent discontinuities, Lyme disease, and very rarely Whipple disease (infection with *Tropheryma whipplei*), can also involve the conducting system (see Chapter 68). These various categories of conducting system disease have been considered possible pathologic substrates for SCD that might be overlooked because of the difficulty of performing careful postmortem examinations of the conducting system routinely; careful studies of the conducting system are necessary to identify up to 22% of otherwise unexplained SCDs under the age of 40 years.[99] Focal involvement of conducting tissue by tumors (especially mesothelioma of the AV node but also lymphoma, carcinoma, rhabdomyoma, and fibroma) has also been reported, and rare cases of SCD have been associated with these lesions. It has been suggested that abnormal postnatal morphogenesis of the specialized conducting system may be a significant factor in some cases of SCD in infants and children.

Cardiac Nerves and Sudden Cardiac Death. Intrinsic and extrinsic autonomic dysfunction mediated by altered cardiac innervation and/or neuro-cardiac interactions have a role in SCD (see Chapter 102).[100] Neural involvement can be the result of damage to neural elements within the myocardium (i.e., concomitant with MI leading to a secondary cardioneuropathy) or may be primary, as in diabetic cardiac autonomic neuropathy, which is associated with a 3.5-fold increased risk of SCD, or rarely a selective autonomic neuropathy. Alterations in autonomic function as a compensatory mechanism for cardiac disease, such as heart failure, is well described. Generally, sympathoexcitation, which can be noted with multiple techniques ranging from heart rate variability analysis, catecholamine levels, and direct neural recordings, is associated with poor prognosis and increased risk for ventricular tachyarrhythmias leading to SCD. The role of anatomic changes in neural innervation is also significant. Myocardial infarction has been shown to lead to areas of sympathetic denervation. These may contribute to arrhythmogenesis by a mechanism of denervation supersensitivity to catecholamines causing increased dispersion of refractoriness. Nerve sprouting due to released nerve growth factors after MI may be important[101,102] in determining changes in cardiac innervation in response to injury. Clinical techniques for sympathetic imaging suggest a changing pattern over time after MI.[103]

Mechanisms and Pathophysiology

Electrical mechanisms of cardiac arrest are divided into tachyarrhythmic and bradyarrhythmic-asystolic events, or conversely shockable versus nonshockable. The tachyarrhythmias include VF and pulseless sustained VT, in which a perceptible pulse may not be present (<60 mm Hg), and adequate blood flow is not maintained. Bradyarrhythmic-asystolic events include severe bradyarrhythmias, PEA (formerly called *electromechanical dissociation* [EMD]), and inability to generate a mechanical event because of complete absence of electrical activity (asystole). To qualify as a mechanism of cardiac arrest, severe bradyarrhythmias must be slow enough to result in an inability to adequately perfuse and maintain consciousness, which usually requires a heart rate of less than 20 beats/min. In PEA, the electrical rate can be considerably faster, but in general much slower than true pulseless VT, with either a narrow or wide QRS complex. The important distinction between PEA and pulseless VT is that pulseless VT is a shockable rhythm. Included in the classification of PEA are the slow agonal rhythms heralding death (random irregular depolarizations that do not generate a pulse), narrow and wide QRS rhythms at rates from 40 to >100 without a pulse. In PEA, there is no perfusion because of absent mechanical activity or mechanical obstruction to blood flow, as in massive pulmonary embolism. However, echocardiographic imaging during PEA has suggested that residual LV wall motion may persist but not be adequate for generating a pulse, as in pulseless VT. This phenomenon has implications for exploring new therapeutic approaches for PEA. Data from the Resuscitation Outcomes Consortium show that PEA accounts for approximately 20% of initial rhythms.[104] Asystole is the most common initial rhythm, though it is likely that many victims found to be asystolic at contact were initially in VF or VT. After a variable time, fibrillation may cease and asystole or less commonly PEA emerges. In contrast to earlier data, the most common initial recording documented in recent years is asystole or PEA.

The occurrence of potentially lethal tachyarrhythmias or severe bradyarrhythmia or asystole is the end of a cascade of pathophysiologic abnormalities that result from complex interactions between coronary vascular events, myocardial injury, variations in autonomic tone, and the metabolic and electrolyte state of the myocardium (see Fig. 70.5). There is no uniform hypothesis of mechanisms by which these elements interact to lead to the final pathway of lethal arrhythmias. However, Figure 70.7 shows models of the pathophysiologic process of SCD that include vascular, myocardial, and functional components. The risk for cardiac arrest is conditioned by the presence of structural abnormalities and modulated by functional variations.

Pathophysiologic Mechanisms of Lethal Tachyarrhythmias

Coronary Artery Structure and Function

Among the large fraction of SCDs associated with coronary atherosclerosis, an extensive distribution of chronic arterial narrowing has been well defined by pathologic studies. However, the specific mechanisms by which these lesions lead to potentially lethal disturbances in electrical stability are not simply the consequence of steady-state reductions in regional myocardial blood flow in association with variable demands (see Chapter 36). A simple increase in myocardial oxygen demand, in the presence of a fixed supply, may be a mechanism of exercise-induced arrhythmias and sudden death during intense physical activity. It is notable that asymptomatic ST depression during exercise testing in men without prevalent coronary artery disease is associated with a doubling of risk of SCD. Yet, the overall risk of SCD during exercise and/or exercise testing even with induced ischemia is extremely low, supporting recommendations for continued exercise in most patients with angina and/or provokable ischemia on stress testing.[105] However, the dynamic nature of the pathophysiologic mechanism of acute coronary events creates a setting in which alterations in the metabolic or electrolyte state of the myocardium may lead to disturbed electrical stability. Active vascular events resulting in an acute or transient reduction in regional myocardial blood flow in the presence of a normal or previously compromised circulation constitute a common mechanism of ischemia, angina pectoris, arrhythmias, and SCD. Coronary artery spasm or modulation of coronary collateral flow, predisposed to by local endothelial dysfunction, further exposes the myocardium to the double hazard of transient ischemia and reperfusion[106] (see Fig. 70.10). Neurogenic influences may also be contributory. Vessel susceptibility and humoral factors, particularly those related to platelet activation and aggregation, also appear to be important mechanisms.

Transition of stable atherosclerotic plaque to an "active" state because of plaque fissuring leading to platelet activation and aggregation followed by thrombosis, is a mechanism that appears to be present in many SCDs related to coronary heart disease (see Chapters 24 and 37). Inflammatory responses in atherosclerotic plaque are now viewed as the condition leading to lesion progression, including erosion, disruption, platelet activation, and thrombosis. In addition to causing a subacute or acute critical reduction in regional blood flow, these mechanisms produce a series of biochemical alterations that may enhance or retard susceptibility to VF by means of vasomotor modulation.

The step in the cascade of coronary artery pathophysiology leading to ischemia-induced arrhythmias that follows conversion to an active plaque involves the thrombotic module of platelet aggregation and thrombosis (see Figs. 70.5 and 70.7; see Chapter 24). However, there is a discrepancy between the relatively high incidence of platelet aggregation or acute thrombi in postmortem studies and the low incidence of evolution of new MI in survivors of out-of-hospital VF. The rapid initiation of lethal arrhythmias, the spontaneous thrombolysis, a dominant role of spasm induced by platelet products, or a combination of these factors may explain this observation.

Acute Ischemia and Initiation of Lethal Arrhythmias

The onset of acute ischemia produces immediate electrical, mechanical, and biochemical dysfunction of cardiac muscle. The specialized conducting tissue is more resistant to acute ischemia than working myocardium, and therefore the electrophysiologic consequences are less intense and delayed in onset in specialized conduction tissue. In addition to the direct effect of ischemia on normal or previously abnormal tissue, reperfusion after transient ischemia can cause lethal arrhythmias (see Fig. 70.10). Reperfusion of ischemic areas can occur by three mechanisms: (1) spontaneous thrombolysis, (2) recruitment of collateral vessels from other vascular beds in response to local ischemia, and (3) reversal of vasospasm. Some mechanisms of reperfusion-induced arrhythmogenesis appear to be related to the duration of ischemia before reperfusion. An array of pathophysiologic changes resulting in intracellular calcium overload is likely the underlying mechanism.[106]

Electrophysiologic Effects of Acute Ischemia. Within the first minutes after experimental coronary ligation, there is a propensity to ventricular arrhythmias that abates after 30 minutes and reappears after several hours (Chapter 62). The initial 30 minutes of arrhythmias is divided into two periods, the first of which lasts for approximately 10 minutes and is presumably directly related to the initial ischemic injury. The second period (20 to 30 minutes) may be related either to reperfusion of ischemic areas or to the evolution of different injury patterns in epicardial and endocardial muscle. Multiple mechanisms of reperfusion arrhythmias have been observed experimentally, including slow conduction and reentry and afterdepolarizations and triggered activity.

At the level of the myocyte, the immediate consequences of ischemia of particular interest are the possible continued influx of Ca^{2+}, which may produce electrical instability; responses to alpha or beta adrenoceptor stimulation, or both; and afterdepolarizations as triggering responses for Ca^{2+}-dependent arrhythmias. Other possible mechanisms studied experimentally include the formation of superoxide radicals in reperfusion arrhythmias and differential responses of endocardial and epicardial muscle activation times and refractory periods during ischemia or reperfusion. The adenosine triphosphate–dependent K^+ current ($I_{K,ATP}$), which is inactive during normal conditions, is activated during ischemia. Its activation results in a strong efflux of K^+ ions from myocytes and markedly shortening of the time course of repolarization, which leads to slow conduction and ultimately to inexcitability. The fact that this response is more marked in epicardium than in endocardium leads to a prominent dispersion of repolarization across the myocardium during transmural ischemia. At an intercellular level, ischemia alters the distribution of connexin-43, the primary gap junction protein between myocytes. This alteration results in uncoupling of myocytes, a factor that is arrhythmogenic because of altered patterns of excitation and regional changes in conduction velocity.

The state of the myocardium at the time of onset of ischemia is important. Tissue healed after previous injury appears to be more susceptible to the electrical destabilizing effects of acute ischemia, as is chronically hypertrophied muscle. Remodeling-induced local stretch, regional hypertrophy, or intrinsic cellular alteration may contribute to this vulnerability. Of more direct clinical relevance is the suggestion that potassium depletion by diuretics and clinical hypokalemia may make ventricular myocardium more susceptible to potentially lethal arrhythmias, in part by its effect on repolarization (QT) duration.

The association of metabolic and electrolyte abnormalities and neurophysiologic and neurohumoral changes with lethal arrhythmias emphasizes the importance of integrating changes in the myocardial substrate with systemic influences. Most direct among myocardial metabolic changes in response to ischemia are local acute increase in interstitial K^+ levels to values exceeding 15 mM, decrease in tissue pH to below 6.0, changes in adrenoceptor activity, and alterations in autonomic nerve traffic, all of which tend to create and maintain electrical instability, especially if it is regional in distribution. Other metabolic changes, such as elevation of cyclic adenosine monophosphate levels, accumulation of free fatty acids and their metabolites, formation of lysophosphoglycerides, and impaired myocardial glycolysis, have also been suggested as myocardial-destabilizing influences. These local myocardial changes integrate with systemic patterns of autonomic fluctuation that can be observed as patterns of altered heart rate variability and fractal dynamics, thus potentially identifying subsets of patients at higher risk for SCD during an acute ischemic event.[4]

Transition from Myocardial Instability to Lethal Arrhythmias

The combination of a triggering event and a susceptible myocardium is a fundamental electrophysiologic concept for the mechanism of initiation of potentially lethal arrhythmias (see Figs. 70.5 and 70.7). The triggering event for VT or VF can be electrophysiologic, ischemic, metabolic, or hemodynamic. For VF, the endpoint of their interaction is disorganization of patterns of myocardial activation into multiple uncoordinated reentrant pathways. Clinical, experimental, and pharmacologic data have suggested that triggering events in the absence of myocardial instability are unlikely to initiate lethal arrhythmias.

Bradyarrhythmias and Asystolic Arrest

The basic electrophysiologic mechanism in this form of arrest is failure of normal subordinate automatic activity to assume the pacing function of the heart in the absence of normal function of the sinus node, AV junction, or both. Asystolic arrest is more common in severely diseased hearts and in patients with a number of end-stage disorders, cardiac and noncardiac. These mechanisms may result, in part, from diffuse involvement of subendocardial Purkinje fibers in advanced heart disease.

Pulseless Electrical Activity

PEA is separated into primary and secondary forms. No one unifying definition for PEA, mechanistically or clinically, is recognized. The common denominator in both is the presence of organized cardiac electrical activity in the absence of effective mechanical function. The absence of rapid return of spontaneous circulation (ROSC) is important in that it excludes transient losses of cerebral blood flow, such as the various patterns of vasovagal reflex syncope, which have different clinical implications. The secondary form of PEA results from an abrupt cessation of cardiac venous return, such as massive pulmonary embolism, acute malfunction of prosthetic valves, exsanguination, and cardiac tamponade from hemopericardium. The primary form is the more familiar; in this form none of these obvious mechanical factors is present, but ventricular muscle fails to produce an effective contraction despite continued electrical activity. It usually occurs as an end-stage event in advanced heart disease, but it can occur in patients with acute ischemic events or, more commonly, after electrical resuscitation from prolonged cardiac arrest. Although it is not thoroughly understood, it appears that diffuse disease, metabolic abnormalities, or global ischemia provides the pathophysiologic substrate. The proximate mechanism for failure of electromechanical coupling may be abnormal intracellular Ca^{2+} metabolism, intracellular acidosis, or perhaps depletion of ATP.

CLINICAL FEATURES OF PATIENTS WITH CARDIAC ARREST

Although the pathologic anatomy associated with SCD caused by coronary artery disease often reflects the changes associated with acute myocardial injury, <20% of survivors of OHCA have clinical evidence of a new transmural MI. Nonetheless, many have elevations in enzyme levels along with nonspecific electrocardiographic changes suggesting myocardial damage, which may be caused by transient ischemia as a triggering event or a consequence of the loss of myocardial perfusion during the cardiac arrest. The recurrence rate is low in survivors of OHCA caused by transmural MI. In contrast, early studies demonstrated a 30% recurrence rate at 1 year and 45% at 2 years in the survivors who did not have a new transmural MI. Recurrence rates decreased subsequently, probably in part due to the result of long-term interventions.

Prodromal Symptoms

Patients at risk for SCD can have prodromes such as chest pain, dyspnea, weakness or fatigue, palpitations, syncope, and a number of nonspecific complaints. Several epidemiologic and clinical studies have demonstrated that such symptoms can presage coronary events, particularly MI and SCD, and result in contact with the medical system weeks to months before SCD.

Attempts to identify early prodromal symptoms specific for SCD risk have not been successful. Although several studies have reported that 12% to 46% of fatalities occur in patients who had seen a physician 1 to 6 months before death, such visits are more likely to presage MI or nonsudden death, and most complaints responsible for these visits are not heart related. However, patients who have chest pain as a prodrome to SCD appear to have a higher probability of intraluminal coronary thrombosis at postmortem examination. Fatigue has been a particularly common symptom in the days or weeks before SCD in a number of studies, but this symptom is nonspecific. The symptoms that occur within the last hours or minutes before cardiac arrest are more specific for heart disease and may include symptoms of arrhythmias, ischemia, and heart failure.

Onset of the Terminal Event

Ambulatory recordings fortuitously obtained during the onset of an unexpected cardiac arrest have indicated dynamic changes in cardiac electrical activity during the minutes or hours before the event. Increasing heart rate and advancing grades of ventricular ectopy are common antecedents of VF. Alterations in autonomic nervous system activity may also contribute to onset of the event. Studies of short-term variations in heart rate variability or related measures have identified changes that correlate with the occurrence of ventricular arrhythmias. Although these physiologic properties may be associated with transient electrophysiologic destabilization of the myocardium, the extent to which they are paralleled by clinical symptoms or events has been less well documented.

Cardiac Arrest

Cardiac arrest is characterized by abrupt loss of consciousness caused by lack of adequate cerebral blood flow as a result of failure of cardiac pump function. In contrast to previous data, the most common electrical mechanism of OHCA currently identified by Emergency Rescue Systems is asystole (50%), with VF/pulseless VT and PEA each estimated in the range of 20% to 25%.[104] The extent to which these proportions of first recorded rhythms reflect the rhythms that trigger the onset of SCA remains unknown because of the lag between onset and EMS arrival. Mechanical causes include rupture of the ventricle, cardiac tamponade, acute obstruction to flow, and acute disruption of a major blood vessel, each of which is more likely to present with PEA or asystole.

Among elderly persons, outcomes after community-based responses to OHCA are not as good as for younger victims. In one study comparing persons younger than 80 years (mean age, 64 years) with those in their 80s and 90s, the survival rate to hospital discharge in the younger group was 19.4% as opposed to 9.4% for octogenarians and 4.4% for nonagenarians. However, when the groups were analyzed according to markers favoring survival (e.g., VF, pulseless VT), the incremental benefit was even better for the elderly than for the younger patients (36%, 24%, and 17%, respectively), but the frequency of ventricular tachyarrhythmias versus nonshockable rhythms was lower in elderly persons. Overall, advanced age is only a weak predictor of an adverse outcome and should not be used in isolation as a reason to not resuscitate.[107] Long-term neurologic status and length of hospitalization were similar in older and younger surviving patients.

The potential for successful resuscitation is a function of the setting in which the cardiac arrest occurs, the mechanism of the arrest, and the underlying clinical status of the victim. The decision whether to attempt to resuscitate is closely related to the potential for success.[108]

At present, there are fewer low-risk patients with otherwise uncomplicated MIs accounting for in-hospital cardiac arrest (IHCA) than previously reported. Patients with IHCA associated with acute MI (AMI), typically had a history of congestive heart failure, and commonly had experienced previous cardiac arrests. Noncardiac-related clinical diagnoses were dominated by renal failure, pneumonia, sepsis, diabetes, and a history of cancer. The strong male preponderance consistently reported in out-of-hospital cardiac arrest studies is not present in in-hospital patients, but the better prognosis of VT or VF mechanisms than PEA or asystolic mechanisms persists (27% versus 8% survival rate). However, the proportion of arrests caused by in-hospital VT or VF is considerably less (33%), with the combination of respiratory arrest, asystole, and PEA dominating the statistics (61%). Similar findings were reported from China.[109] One year survival after IHCA is also influenced by age, sex, race, and presenting rhythm. Strategic factors affecting survival after IHCA include the location in the hospital, the type of hospital, daytime and evening events versus night and weekend events, and a rapid time to performance of defibrillation.[4,110]

A multihospital study of outcomes after IHCA in pediatric patients demonstrated a major improvement in survival to hospital discharge between 2000 and 2009, with a risk-adjusted improvement from 14.3% in 2000 to 43.4% in 2009. There was neither improvement nor worsening of the proportion with residual neurologic deficits. The proportion with VF or pulseless VT decreased from 22% in 2000 to 2003 to 9.7% in 2007 to 2009, and those with asystole decreased from 51.4% to 20%. In contrast, PEA increased from 26.6% to 70.3%. The reason for the dramatic increase in the proportion of PEA events is not clear because respiratory insufficiency as an initial condition increased only modestly, but may be related to the increased proportion of patients maintained on mechanical ventilators at the time of arrest.[4]

Survival after IHCA is lower for events that occur during weeknights and weekends than during the daytime and evening hours during the week and more rapid times to defibrillation are advantageous. Such data suggest the need for additional strategies for uniformly rapid in-hospital responses, as well as for the limitations reported for in-hospital early warning systems.

Progression to Biologic Death

The time course for progression from cardiac arrest to biologic death is related to the mechanism of the cardiac arrest, the nature of the underlying disease process, and the delay between onset and resuscitative efforts. The onset of irreversible brain damage usually begins within 4 to 6 minutes after loss of cerebral circulation, and biologic death follows quickly in unattended cardiac arrest. In large series, however, it has been demonstrated that a limited number of victims can remain biologically alive for longer periods and may be resuscitated after delays in excess of 8 minutes before beginning basic life support and in excess of 16 minutes before advanced life support. Despite these exceptions, it is clear that the probability of a favorable outcome—survival neurologically intact—deteriorates *rapidly* as a function of time after cardiac arrest. Younger patients with less severe cardiac disease and the absence of coexistent multisystem disease have a higher probability of a favorable outcome after such delays.

Irreversible injury to the central nervous system usually occurs before biologic death, and the interval may extend days to weeks and occasionally result in very prolonged persistent vegetative states in patients who are resuscitated during the temporal gap between brain damage and biologic death. IHCA caused by VF is less likely to have a protracted course between the arrest and biologic death, with patients surviving after a prompt intervention or succumbing rapidly because of inability to stabilize their cardiac and/or medical conditions. Overall, patients who have ROSC with persistent severe cerebral performance disability or who remain comatose (CPC-3 or -4) have a very low survival rate, both in-hospital and at 6 months postarrest.

Patients whose cardiac arrest is caused by sustained VT with cardiac output inadequate to maintain consciousness can remain in VT for considerably longer periods with blood flow that is marginally sufficient to maintain viability. Thus there is a longer interval between the onset of cardiac arrest and the end of the period that allows successful resuscitation. The lives of such patients usually end in VF or an asystolic event (PEA or asystole) if the VT is not reverted.

The progression in patients with asystole or PEA as the initiating event is more rapid. Such patients, whether in-hospital or out-of-hospital, have a poor prognosis because of advanced heart disease or coexistent multisystem disease. They tend to respond poorly to interventions, even if the heart is successfully paced. Although there has been an increase in survival from PEA in recent years, it is generally limited to the small subgroup of patients with reversible conditions (e.g., respiratory, electrolyte imbalances) that respond well to interventions, and most progress rapidly to biologic death. Cardiac arrests caused by mechanical factors such as tamponade, structural disruption, and impedance to flow by major thromboembolic obstructions to right or LV outflow are reversible only in patients in whom the mechanism is recognized and an intervention is feasible.

Survivors of Cardiac Arrest
Hospital Course

Cardiac arrests during the acute phase of MI may be primarily related to an electrical event, or secondarily to LV dysfunction or cardiogenic shock. Patients who are resuscitated immediately from primary VF associated with ST elevation MI usually stabilize promptly, and no long-term arrhythmia management is recommended based on the early arrhythmia (see Chapters 28 and 37). However, there are data linking early primary VF to heightened short- and long-term mortality.[111,112] The mechanism for excess mortality is not well delineated. Management after secondary cardiac arrest in patients with MI is dominated by the hemodynamic status of the patient.

Survivors of out-of-hospital cardiac arrest may have repetitive ventricular arrhythmias during the initial 24 to 48 hours of hospitalization. These arrhythmias have variable responses to antiarrhythmic therapy, depending on hemodynamic status. The overall rate of recurrent cardiac arrest is low, 10% to 20%, but the mortality rate in patients who have recurrent cardiac arrests is approximately 50%. Only 5% to 10% of in-hospital deaths after out-of-hospital resuscitation are caused by recurrent cardiac arrhythmias. Patients with recurrent cardiac arrest have a high incidence of new or preexisting AV or intraventricular conduction abnormalities.

The most common causes of death in hospitalized survivors of out-of-hospital cardiac arrest are noncardiac events related to central nervous system injury, including anoxic encephalopathy and sepsis related to prolonged intubation and hemodynamic monitoring lines. Approximately 40% of those who arrive at the hospital in coma never awaken after admission to the hospital and die after a median survival of 3.5 days. Two-thirds of those who regain consciousness have no gross deficits, and an additional 20% have persisting cognitive deficits only. Of the patients who do awaken, 25% do so by admission, 71% by the first hospital day, and 92% by the third day. A small number of patients have awakened after prolonged hospitalization. Among those who die in the hospital, 80% do not awaken before death. Therapeutic hypothermia in patients with postcardiac arrest coma is beneficial,[113] even for those with nonshockable rhythms[114] (see next section).

Cardiac causes of delayed death during hospitalization after out-of-hospital cardiac arrest are most commonly related to hemodynamic deterioration, which accounts for about a third of deaths in hospitals. Among all deaths, those that occurred within the first 48 hours of hospitalization were usually caused by hemodynamic deterioration or arrhythmias regardless of neurologic status; later deaths were dominated by neurologic complications. Admission characteristics most predictive of subsequent awakening included motor response, pupillary light response, spontaneous eye movement, and blood glucose level below 300 mg/dL.

Clinical Profile of Survivors of Out-of-Hospital Cardiac Arrest

The clinical features of survivors of out-of-hospital cardiac arrest are heavily influenced by the type and extent of the underlying disease associated with the event. Causation is dominated by coronary heart disease and cardiomyopathies. All other structural heart diseases plus functional abnormalities and toxic or environmental causes are responsible for the remainder.

In a study of 375 survivors of cardiac arrest with normal ejection fractions and no obvious heart disease, genetic testing was performed in 174 patients.[115] Pathogenic variants were identified in 17% of cases for long-QT syndrome, catecholaminergic polymorphic VT, right ventricular dysplasia, idiopathic VF, Brugada syndrome (9%), and HCM. A substantial number of variants of uncertain significance were identified. This highlights the role of genetic testing in the evaluation of the etiology of OHCA in those without structural heart disease.

Postresuscitation Electrocardiographic Changes

Among survivors of OHCA, the 12-lead ECG has proved to be of value only for discriminating risk for recurrence in those whose cardiac arrest was associated with new transmural MI. Patients in whom documented new Q waves develop in association with a clinical picture that supports acute ST-segment elevation MI as the mechanism of cardiac arrest itself are at lower risk for recurrence, unless they develop criteria for postinfarct primary prevention of SCD, such as EF <30% to 40%. In contrast, nonspecific electrocardiographic markers of ischemia, associated with elevation of troponin or creatine kinase MB levels, indicate higher risk for recurrence. Nonspecific repolarization abnormalities (e.g., ST-segment depression, flat T waves) are commonly present, often transiently, after a cardiac arrest. Transient prolongation of the QT interval, often associated with postresuscitation hypokalemia, can follow CPR, and associate with risk of recurrent arrhythmias. A prolonged QRS duration in association with a markedly reduced ejection fraction portends increased risk for mortality.

Left Ventricular Function

LV function is abnormal in most survivors of out-of-hospital cardiac arrest, often severely abnormal, but there is wide variation ranging from severe dysfunction to normal or almost normal function. The severity of myocardial dysfunction estimated shortly after cardiac arrest is due to a combination of myocardial stunning consequent to the cardiac arrest itself and the extent of preexisting dysfunction. Stunning commonly improves within the first 24 to 48 hours,[116] and the residual is assumed to be due to preexisting disease or to the acute injury leading to the cardiac arrest. Reliance on postarrest troponin elevations alone to determine whether MI caused a cardiac arrest can be treacherous because cardiac arrest and even nonlife-threatening sustained arrhythmias, as well as ICD shocks, can be associated with transient elevations. Moreover, troponin levels do not improve risk prediction beyond standard clinical variables. If the ejection fraction is severely reduced initially, failure to begin improvement within the first 48 hours is an adverse short-term prognostic sign. In the CREST model, ejection fraction <30% at the time of admission was a multivariate predictor of a circulatory etiology death.[117] Among survivors to hospital discharge, a reduced ejection fraction is an adverse long-term prognostic sign.

Coronary Angiography
Coronary angiography is performed with increasing frequency during initial hospitalization after OHCA. In a recent report based on data from the National Inpatient Sample, patients, 143,607 of 407,974 survivors (35.2%), underwent coronary angiography, increasing from 27.2% in 2000 to 43.9% 2012, and percutaneous coronary intervention increased from 9.5% in 2000 to 24.1% in 2012.[118] Survivors of OHCA tend to have extensive coronary disease but no specific pattern of abnormalities. Acute coronary lesions, often multifocal, are present in many survivors. Significant lesions in two or more vessels are present in at least 70% of patients who have any coronary lesion. In patients who have recurrent cardiac arrests, the incidence of triple-vessel disease is higher than in those who do not. However, the frequency of moderate to severe stenosis of the left main coronary artery does not differ between cardiac arrest survivors and the overall population of patients with symptomatic coronary heart disease.

Blood Chemistry
Lower serum potassium levels are observed in survivors of cardiac arrest than in patients with AMI or stable coronary heart disease. This finding is often a consequence of resuscitation interventions rather than a preexisting hypokalemic state because of chronic diuretic use or other causes. However, severe preexisting hypokalemia may aggravate the risk for VF and recurrent VF.[119] Among survivors who are hypokalemic during the first 12 to 24 hours after SCA, serum K^+ levels following stabilization should be checked to exclude a chronic potassium-wasting state. Low ionized calcium levels with normal total calcium levels were also observed during resuscitation from out-of-hospital cardiac arrest. Higher resting lactate levels have been reported in out-of-hospital cardiac arrest survivors than in normal subjects. Lactate levels correlated inversely with ejection fractions and directly with PVC frequency and complexity.

Long-Term Prognosis
Studies from Miami and Seattle in the early 1970s had indicated that the risk for recurrent cardiac arrest in the first year after survival of an initial VT/VF event was approximately 30% and at 2 years was 45%. Total mortality at 2 years was approximately 60% in both studies. More recent mortality data, including those from the control groups of secondary prevention ICD trials, have demonstrated improved survival.[120] The Israel ICD registry demonstrated one- and two-year mortality rates of 8% and 11%, respectively,[121] and a European cohort of patients with secondary prevention ICDs for ischemic or dilated cardiomyopathy had 5- and 10-year mortalities of 24% and 51%, respectively.[122] The apparent improved outcomes, independent of the benefit provided by ICD therapy, are probably attributable to the current interventions used in survivors, such as beta adrenoceptor blockers, statins and angiotensin converting enzyme inhibitor (ACEI)/angiotensin receptor blocker (ARBs), anti-ischemic procedures, and heart failure therapies that were not available or in general use at the earlier time. The risk for recurrent cardiac arrest and all-cause mortality is higher during the first 12 to 24 months after the index event and relates best to the ejection fraction during the first 6 months.

MANAGEMENT OF CARDIAC ARREST

The response to cardiac arrest is driven by two principles: (1) maintenance of continuous cardiopulmonary support until ROSC has been achieved and (2) achieve ROSC as quickly as possible. To achieve these goals, the management strategy is divided into five elements: (1) initial assessment by a witness/bystander and summoning of an emergency response team, (2) basic life support BLS, (3) early defibrillation by a first responder (if available), (4) advanced life support, and (5) post-cardiac arrest care. If successful, the algorithm is followed by a sixth element, long-term management. The initial elements can be applied by physicians and nurses, EMTs or paramedics, lay people trained in bystander interventions, and untrained bystanders prompted in CPR by 911 telecommunicators who are trained to prompt callers in BLS technique. Emerging data suggest that telephone prompts by 911 operators can improve survival with preserved neurologic status.[123] Further enhancements may include drones for deployment of automated external defibrillators (AEDs), mobile technology/social media to alert nearby potential responders, and specialized applications.[124-126] Requirements for specialized knowledge and skills increase progressively as the patient is moved through postcardiac arrest management into long-term follow-up care. These emergency response principles are intended for both in-hospital and community-based responses.

In-Hospital Interventions
Development of the coronary care unit resulted in an immediate reduction of in-hospital mortality risk during AMI from 30% to 15% based almost entirely on the reduction of cardiac arrests. Other specialized monitoring and intensive care units demonstrated various levels of benefit as well, but the impact has been less in general care hospital units and for cardiac arrests associated with complex comorbid states or occurring during off-hours.[127] A registry study in the decade from 2000 to 2009 provided trends for risk-adjusted rates of survival to discharge after cardiac arrest in monitored units and general hospital units. Among 84,625 subjects, 20.7% had VF or pulseless VT as the initial rhythm and 79.3% had asystole or PEA, with the proportion of cardiac arrests attributable to asystole/PEA increasing over time ($P < 0.001$). The overall survival rate to discharge increased from 13.7% in 2000 to 22.3% in 2009 ($P < 0.001$), with improvement in both the VT/VF and the PEA/asystole subsets (Fig. 70.11A). Absolute rates of survival to discharge remained higher for the VT/VF group, whereas improvement in survival occurred in the two rhythm groups. The improvement in survival appeared to be due to both improved acute resuscitation actions and postresuscitation care. A small decrease in rates of clinically significant neurologic disability in survivors occurred over time.

Community-Based Interventions
The initial out-of-hospital intervention experience in Miami and Seattle yielded only 14% and 11% rates of survival to discharge, respectively. Subsequent improvements correlated with the addition of emergency medical technicians as another tier of responders to provide CPR and earlier defibrillation. In general, rural areas have lower success rates, and the U.S. national success rate remains approximately 10%.[9] Regional variability is highlighted by a county level analysis from the CARES Surveillance Group and the HeartRescue Project demonstrating survival to discharge rates from 3.4% to 20.1%.[128] A large portion of this variability is explained by rates of bystander CPR, median age, and median household income. Rates of bystander CPR have been shown to increase with a mobile phone technology to alert nearby lay volunteers trained in CPR that there is a nearby OHCA.[124,126]

Reports from different areas in the United States show marked variations in outcomes.[129] Older data from Chicago and New York City provided disturbing outcome data. A study from Chicago reported that only 9% of out-of-hospital cardiac arrest victims survive to be hospitalized and only 2% are discharged alive. Moreover, outcomes in Blacks are worse than those in whites (0.8% versus 2.6%). The fact that a large majority had bradyarrhythmias, asystole, or PEA on initial contact with emergency medical services suggests prolonged times between collapse and arrival of the emergency medical service, absent or ineffective bystander interventions, or both. The New York City report indicated a survival to hospital discharge rate of only 1.4%. Among those who undergo bystander CPR, the rate increases to 2.9%, and bystander

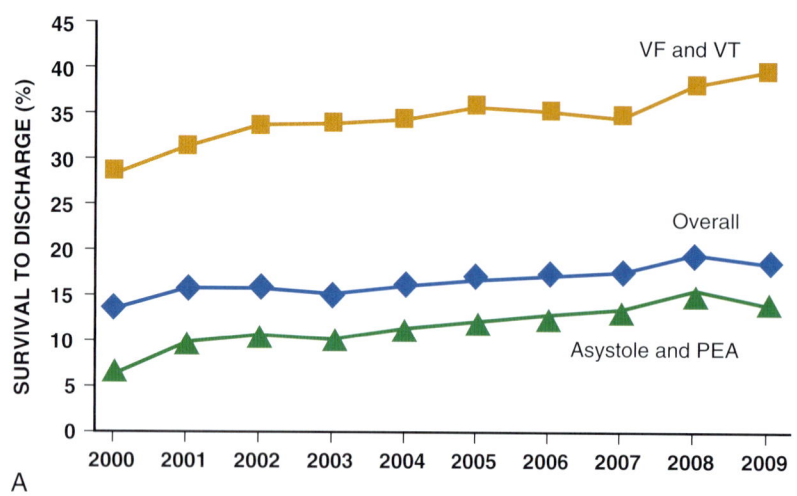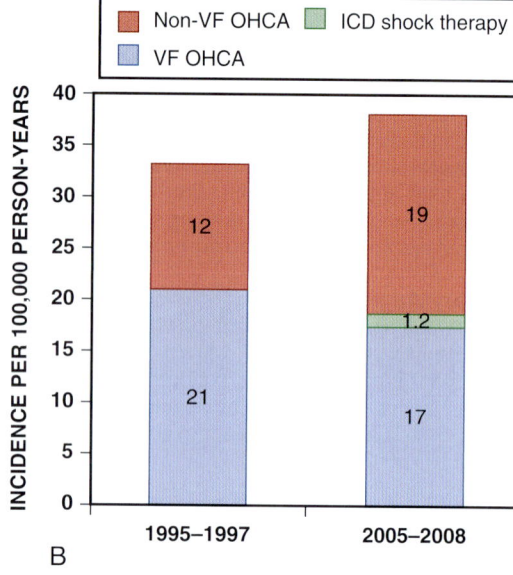

FIGURE 70.11 Changing incidence of shockable and nonshockable rhythms. **A,** Survival to discharge for VF and pulseless VT versus asystole and PEA between 2000 and 2009 ($P < 0.001$ for trend in each survival curve). **B,** In Holland, there was a decrease in the VF event rate with a concomitant increase in non-VF rhythms. Thus, the proportion of events with VF at initial contact is decreasing, as observed in several other studies. (**A** from Girotra S, et al. Trends in survival after in-hospital cardiac arrest. N Engl J Med 2012;367:1912-1920. **B** from Hulleman M, et al. Implantable cardioverter defibrillators have reduced the incidence of resuscitation for out of hospital cardiac arrest caused by lethal arrhythmias. Circulation 2012;126:815-821.)

CPR plus VF as the initial rhythm yields a further increase to 5.3%. Finally, for those whose arrests occurred after the arrival of emergency medical services, the success rate increases further to 8.5%. These trends support the concept that delays and breaks in the in the "chain of survival" have a major negative impact on the results of emergency medical services in densely populated areas. Cardiac arrest data from the COVID-19 pandemic support this observation. The rate of OHCA was substantially increased during comparable time periods before and during the pandemic, with increased mortality perhaps linked to increased time to EMS arrival and reduced frequency of bystander CPR, among other factors.[130] Even communities with low rates of infection demonstrated this pattern.[131] Both bystander CPR and EMS arrival time have been shown to influence survival,[132] providing support for the importance of these community interventions.

There are circumstances in which resuscitative effort in the out-of-hospital setting is deemed futile. A victim found unconscious after an unwitnessed collapse, reasonably assumed to be found after a prolonged interval (e.g., cool skin, rigor mortis), obviously fulfills this classification. However, studies have provided markers of futility under less stark circumstances. In a study involving trained responders with AEDs, only 0.5% of victims survived if (1) the arrest was not witnessed by emergency medical service personnel, (2) there was no ROSC, and (3) no shocks were delivered per protocol. Adding a response time longer than 8 minutes reduced the survival rate to 0.3%, and events unwitnessed by a bystander yielded no survivors.

Impact of Tiered Response Systems

Improvements in both out-of-hospital care and in-hospital technology and practices can contribute to better outcomes, as described in the chain-of-survival concept.[1] Of these two general factors, the influence of out-of-hospital care has been studied in more detail. The importance of early defibrillation for improving outcome has been supported by many studies. These observations have motivated a search for strategies that shorten response times, largely by the development of two-tiered systems in which nonconventional first responders, such as police, firefighters, security guards, and lay bystanders, deploy AEDs that are now commonly available in public places. Available data suggest that this strategy may improve outcome, primarily in public locations.[133]

In rural communities, earlier defibrillation by ambulance technicians yielded a 19% survival rate versus only 3% for standard CPR. In another report, an analysis of the relationship between response delay and survival to hospital discharge revealed a 48% survival rate for response times of 2 minutes or less and less than a 10% survival rate when responses were longer than 10 minutes. Another study showed survival decline by 5.2%/min for EMS arrival between 5 and 10 minutes and a further decline of 1.9%/min for arrival between 11 and 15 minutes after collapse.

A second element in out-of-hospital care that contributes to outcome is the role of bystander CPR by laypeople awaiting the arrival of EMS personnel.[134] It has been reported that although there was no significant difference in the percentage of patients successfully resuscitated and admitted to the hospital alive with (67%) or without (61%) bystander intervention, almost twice as many OHCA victims were ultimately discharged alive when they had undergone bystander CPR (43%) than when such support was not provided (22%). Central nervous system protection, expressed as early regaining of consciousness, is the major protective element of bystander CPR. It has been reported that more than 40% of victims whose defibrillation and other advanced life support activities were instituted more than 8 minutes after collapse survived if basic CPR had been initiated less than 2 minutes after onset of the arrest. While it has been suggested that a period of CPR before defibrillation may also be helpful, particularly if the time to defibrillation exceeds 4 minutes from the onset of arrest, the data are unclear.

Importance of Electrical Mechanisms. Several sources have identified a changing distribution of initial rhythms recorded by EMS personnel. When compared with data from the 1970s and 1980s, there has been a decrease in the number of events in which ventricular tachyarrhythmias are the initial rhythm recorded, with a consequent reduction in the proportion of victims who have rhythms amenable to cardioversion-defibrillation (see Fig. 70.11B). Similar observations have been reported in in-hospital settings. Some studies have now suggested that less than 50% of victims have shockable rhythms at initial contact. This could contribute to a reduction in cumulative survival probability with community-based interventions.[129] It is likely that pre-911 delays in recognition of and reaction to an event may be playing a role, in conjunction with longer response times based on geographic considerations. This suggests a need for more extensive public education programs. Thus response times may not accurately reflect true downtimes, and consequently the potential for success is impaired. The 4- to 6-minute time for a desirable response is not optimal. By 4 minutes, significant circulatory and ischemic changes have taken place, and conditions worsen rapidly beyond that time.

The electrical mechanism of out-of-hospital cardiac arrest, as defined by the initial rhythm recorded by EMS personnel, has a powerful impact

TABLE 70.4 Tachyarrhythmic and Nontachyarrhythmic Cardiac Arrest

PRIMARY ARRHYTHMIAS	ELECTRICAL MECHANISMS	MECHANICAL MECHANISMS
Tachyarrhythmic Cardiac Arrest		
Ventricular fibrillation	Absence of organized ventricular depolarization	Absence of LVWM
Pulseless ventricular tachycardia	Organized ventricular pattern; rapid rate	Absent LVWM or LVWM insufficient for organ perfusion
Secondary Arrhythmias		
Sinus tachycardia; other	Sinus or other supraventricular rhythm; narrow QRS	Obstruction to cardiac blood flow; hypovolemia
Nontachyarrhythmic Cardiac Arrest		
PEA, Primary (Initial Rhythm)		
With residual LV contraction	Organized QRS complexes, usually wide	LVWM insufficient for organ perfusion
Without LV contraction	Organized QRS complexes, usually wide	Absence of LVWM
PEA, Secondary		
Postshock	Regular or irregular QRS complexes, usually wide	Absent LVWM or LVWM insufficient for organ perfusion
Primary noncardiac	Regular or irregular QRS complexes, usually wide	Usually LVWM insufficient for organ perfusion; LVWM may be absent
Agonal PEA	Slow, usually irregular, wide QRS	Absence of LVWM
Ventricular asystole	Absent ventricular electrical activity; exclude fine ventricular fibrillation	Absence of LVWM

LV, Left ventricular; *LVWM*, left ventricular wall motion; *PEA*, pulseless electrical activity.
Modified from Myerburg RJ, et al. Pulseless electrical activity: definition, causes, mechanisms, management, and research priorities for the next decade. Report from a National Heart, Lung, and Blood Institute Workshop. Circulation 2013;128:2532.

on outcome. They are generally categorized as shockable (VF, and pulseless VT [pVT]) and nonshockable (PEA, asystole) rhythms (Table 70.4). The distinction between pVT and PEA is sometimes confused and has relevance because it impacts response strategies. The subgroup of patients who are in pVT at the time of first contact, although small, has the best outcome. Eighty-eight percent of patients in cardiac arrest related to VT were successfully resuscitated and admitted to the hospital alive, and 67% were ultimately discharged alive. However, this relatively low-risk group represents less than 10% of all cardiac arrests. Because of the inherent time lag between collapse and initial recordings, it is likely that many more cardiac arrests begin as rapid sustained VT and degenerate into VF before the arrival of rescue personnel.

Patients with a bradyarrhythmia or with asystole or PEA at initial contact have the worst prognosis; only 9% of such patients in the Miami study were admitted to the hospital alive, and none were discharged. In a later experience, some improvement in outcome was noted, although the improvement was limited to patients in whom the initial bradyarrhythmia recorded was an idioventricular rhythm that responded promptly to chronotropic agents in the field. In a large prospective observational in-hospital study of cardiac arrests in children and adults, children had a higher probability of asystole or PEA as the initial documented rhythm but had a better overall survival rate because they had better outcomes of interventions for these rhythms than adults did. Overall survival after PEA appears to be better in recent years, and may be somewhat better than for asystole.[135] Moreover, for patients with an initial nonshockable rhythm that converts to a shockable rhythm, there may also be improved outcomes, but this may depend on how early this conversion occurs and whether the initial rhythm was asystole or PEA.[136]

Bradyarrhythmias also have adverse prognostic implications after defibrillation from VF in the field. Patients with a heart rate lower than 60 beats/min after defibrillation, regardless of the specific bradyarrhythmic mechanism, had a poor prognosis, with 95% of such patients dying before hospitalization or in the hospital. The outcome in the group of patients in whom VF is the initial rhythm recorded is intermediate between the outcomes associated with sustained VT and with bradyarrhythmia and asystole. The proportion of each of the electrophysiologic mechanisms responsible for cardiac arrest varied among the earlier reports, with VF ranging from 65% to more than 90% of the study populations and bradyarrhythmia and asystole ranging from 10% to 30%. However, in reports from densely populated metropolitan areas, the ratios of tachyarrhythmic to bradyarrhythmic or pulseless activity events were reversed, and outcomes were far worse.

Initial Assessment and Basic Life Support

Activities at initial contact with the unconscious victim include diagnostic maneuvers and basic cardiopulmonary support interventions. The first action must be confirmation that collapse is the result of a cardiac arrest. A few seconds of evaluation for response to voice, observation for respiratory movements and skin color, and simultaneous palpation of major arteries for the presence or absence of a pulse yields sufficient information to determine whether a life-threatening incident is in progress. Once a life-threatening incident has been suspected or confirmed, contact with an available emergency medical rescue system (911) for out-of-hospital settings or a "code" team in the hospital should be an immediate priority.

The absence of a carotid or femoral pulse detected by a medical professional, particularly if it is confirmed by the absence of an audible heartbeat, is a primary diagnostic criterion. For lay responders, the pulse check is no longer recommended.[108] Skin color may be pale or intensely cyanotic. Absence of respiratory effort or the presence of only agonal respiratory effort in conjunction with an absent pulse is diagnostic of cardiac arrest; however, respiratory effort can persist for 1 minute or longer after onset of the arrest. In contrast, absence of respiratory effort or the presence of severe stridor with persistence of a pulse suggests a primary respiratory arrest that will lead to cardiac arrest in a short time. In the latter circumstance, initial efforts should include exploration of the oropharynx in search for a foreign body and performance of the Heimlich maneuver, particularly if the incident occurs in a setting in which aspiration is likely (e.g., restaurant death or café coronary).

Chest Thump

A blow to the chest (precordial thump, "thumpversion") may be attempted by a properly trained rescuer. It has been recommended that it be reserved as an advanced life support activity. Precordial thumps will rarely revert apparent VF, VT, and asystole. The use of the precordial thump does not impact ROSC or overall survival. The technique is considered optional for responding to a pulseless cardiac arrest in the absence of monitoring when a defibrillator is not immediately available. It should not be used unmonitored in a patient with a rapid tachycardia without complete loss of consciousness. The thumpversion technique involves one or two blows delivered firmly to the junction of the middle and lower thirds of the sternum from a height of 8 to 10 inches. The effort should be abandoned if a spontaneous pulse does not develop immediately. Another mechanical method, which requires that the patient still be conscious, is so-called cough-induced cardiac compression. It is a conscious act of forceful coughing by the patient that may support forward flow by cyclical increases in intrathoracic pressure during VF or may cause conversion of sustained VT. Available data supporting its successful use are limited; it is not an alternative to conventional techniques.

Basic Life Support—The Initial Steps in Cardiopulmonary Resuscitation

The goal of BLS is to maintain viability of the central nervous system, heart, and other vital organs until definitive ROSC can be achieved. BLS encompasses both the initial responses outlined earlier and their natural flow into establishing perfusion and ventilation. This range of activities can be carried out not only by professional and paraprofessional personnel but also by trained emergency technicians and laypeople. There should be minimal delay between diagnosis and preparatory effort in the initial response and institution of BLS. The first steps are to verify the environmental safety of the site and confirm that the victim is unresponsive. The responder should call for nearby help, activate an emergency response system (via mobile device, if appropriate), and send for an AED.

These principles have measurable impact for both OHCA and IHCA. The survival rate to discharge for IHCA, considering all causes and mechanisms, was reported to be 33% when CPR was initiated within the first minute versus 14% when the time was longer than 1 minute. When VF was the initial rhythm, the corresponding figures were 50% and 32%, respectively. In the out-of-hospital setting, if only one witness is present, notification of emergency personnel (calling 911) is the only activity that should precede BLS. The previous sequence of the "ABC" of BLS—airway, breathing, compression—has been changed to "CAB"—compression, airway, breathing—based on the recognition that compression alone is the better strategy because it minimizes interruptions in perfusion and avoids excessive ventilation.

Circulation

This element of BLS is intended to maintain blood flow (i.e., circulation) until definitive steps can be taken. The rationale is based on the hypothesis that chest compression allows the heart to maintain an externally driven pump function by sequential emptying and filling of its chambers, with competent valves favoring forward direction of flow. In fact, application of this technique has proved successful when it is used as recommended. The palm of one hand is placed over the lower half of the sternum and the heel of the other rests on the dorsum of the lower part of the hand. The sternum is then depressed, with the resuscitator's arms straight at the elbows to provide a less tiring and more forceful fulcrum at the junction of the shoulders and back. By use of this technique, sufficient force is applied to depress the sternum at least 2 inches (>5 cm). Compression is followed by abrupt relaxation, and the cycle is carried out at a rate of about 100 compressions/min.

Techniques of CPR based on the hypothesis that increased intrathoracic pressure is the prime mover of blood, rather than cardiac compression itself, have been evaluated, and the guidelines for conventional CPR ventilatory techniques were modified in 2005. For single responders to victims from infancy (excluding newborns) through adulthood, and for adults responded to by two rescuers, a compression-ventilation ratio of 30:2 is now recommended. For two-rescuer CPR in infants and children, the former compression-ventilation ratio of 15:2 is retained. A more recent modification intended to encourage more bystander participation in CPR and to allay concerns about mouth-to-mouth ventilation of unknown victims is the "hands-only" (compression-only) technique. This technique is particularly important for untrained or remotely trained bystanders who are not confident in their ability to perform compression-ventilation sequences. The 2005 changes in CPR recommendations, in which the number of successive shocks and pulse checks during initial responses is reduced (Electrotherapy for Cardiac Arrhythmias, Chapter 67), are retained in the current recommendations.[4] This is intended in part to increase the cumulative time of circulatory support during CPR before restoration of a spontaneous pulse.

Concept of Cardiocerebral Resuscitation

This concept, also referred to as minimally interrupted cardiac resuscitation, is based on the hypothesis that the primary benefit of CPR is its pumping action rather than the combination of compression and ventilation. It challenges the general guidelines, which assume a benefit of interrupting compression to provide ventilation and that an initial phase of ventilation before initial defibrillation improves outcomes when response times are longer than 4 or 5 minutes. Cardiocerebral resuscitation[137] emphasizes continuous chest compressions, interrupted primarily for single shocks and evaluation of responses to shocks and deferring and limiting ventilatory and certain pharmacologic actions. Despite interesting preliminary data, it is generally agreed that a randomized trial is needed before the minimal interruption concept can replace the current guidelines.

Even though conventional techniques produce measurable carotid artery flow with a record of successful resuscitations, the absence of a pressure gradient across the heart in the presence of an extrathoracic arteriovenous pressure gradient has led to the concept that it is not cardiac compression per se but rather a pumping action produced by changes in pressure in the entire thoracic cavity that optimizes systemic blood flow during resuscitation. Experimental work in which the chest is compressed during ventilations rather than between them (simultaneous compression-ventilation) has demonstrated better extra-thoracic arterial flow. However, increased carotid artery flow does not necessarily equate with improved cerebral perfusion, and the reduction in coronary blood flow caused by elevated intrathoracic pressure with the use of certain techniques may be too high a price for the improved peripheral flow. In addition, a high thoracoabdominal gradient has been demonstrated during experimental simultaneous compression-ventilation, which could divert flow from the brain in the absence of concomitant abdominal binding. On the basis of these observations, new mechanically assisted techniques, including an active decompression phase (i.e., active compression-decompression), have been evaluated for improved circulation during CPR.[138] An impedance threshold device for ventilation has also been developed that in combination with active compression-decompression enhances venous return to the heart. The combination of these two technologies has demonstrated improved survival. Further addition of a "head-up/torso-up" position improves cerebral perfusion and has been reported to almost double resuscitation rates in a community-based study.[139]

Airway

Clearing of the airway is a critical step in preparing for successful resuscitation. This process includes tilting the head backward and lifting the chin, in addition to exploring the airway for foreign bodies, including dentures, and removing them. The Heimlich maneuver should be performed if there is reason to suspect that a foreign body is lodged in the oropharynx. This maneuver entails wrapping the arms around the victim from the back and delivering a sharp thrust to the upper part of the abdomen with a closed fist. If it is not possible for the person in attendance to carry out the maneuver because of insufficient physical strength, mechanical dislodgment of the foreign body can sometimes be achieved by abdominal thrusts with the unconscious patient in a supine position. The Heimlich maneuver is not entirely benign; ruptured abdominal viscera in the victim have been reported, as has a case in which the rescuer disrupted his own aortic root and died. If there is strong suspicion that respiratory arrest precipitated cardiac arrest, particularly in the presence of a mechanical airway obstruction, a second precordial thump should be delivered after the airway has been cleared.

Breathing

With the head placed properly and the oropharynx clear, mouth-to-mouth resuscitation can be initiated if no specific rescue equipment is available. To a large extent the procedure used to establish ventilation depends on the site at which the cardiac arrest occurs. Various devices are available, including plastic oropharyngeal airways, esophageal obturators, masked Ambu bags, and endotracheal tubes. Intubation is the preferred procedure, but time should not be sacrificed, even in the in-hospital setting, while awaiting an endotracheal tube or a person trained to insert it quickly and properly. Thus, in the in-hospital setting, temporary support with Ambu bag ventilation is the usual method until endotracheal intubation can be carried out, and in the out-of-hospital setting, mouth-to-mouth resuscitation is used while awaiting EMS personnel. The effect of various infectious diseases, such as acquired immunodeficiency syndrome, hepatitis B, and SARS-CoV-2, on attitudes about mouth-to-mouth resuscitation by bystanders and even professional personnel in hospitals is an area of concern, likely impacting its use.

Early Defibrillation by First Responders

The time from the onset of cardiac arrest to advanced life support (ACLS) influences outcome. Both early neurologic status and survival are better in patients defibrillated by first responders than if one awaits the assistance of more highly trained paramedics. The term *first responder* refers to the person on scene providing initial CPR and has emerged from minimally trained emergency technicians allowed to carry out defibrillation in conjunction with BLS to nonconventional responders, such as trained security guards and police, and subsequently to lay bystanders knowledgeable in CPR with access to AEDs. Because the time to defibrillation plays a central role in determining outcome in cardiac arrest caused by VF, the development and deployment of AEDs (see Chapter 67) in public locations has had impact on outcomes. This technology is potentially applicable to a number of different strategic models, each with its own benefits and limitations.

Overall, AED use is associated with improved outcomes but the quality of the cumulative evidence had been low to very low.[140] Data from the Resuscitation Outcomes Consortium showed that patients shocked by an AED by a bystander were more likely to survive to discharge (66.5% versus 43.0%) than patients initially shocked by EMS with better functional outcome.[141] Among the strategies that have yielded various levels of identifiable survival benefit to date are deployment in police vehicles, airliners and airports, casinos, and more general community-based sites. Police AED deployment data have been inconsistent in various studies, possibly because of appropriateness for various types of communities and the specific deployment strategies used, but data suggest that it is beneficial in large metropolitan areas. Initial airline data were similarly uncertain, but a more recent report on data from a large airline with a well-organized system has suggested benefit. Similar encouraging results have been reported with the deployment of AEDs in the Chicago airport system. Finally, the special circumstance of casinos, in which continuous television monitoring alerts security officers to medical problems immediately, has yielded impressive survival rates (Fig. 70.12). However, there appears to be a great deal of variability in efficiency on the basis of expected event rates at different types of community sites, and deployment strategies have been suggested on the basis of projected event rates at various locations. Deployment in schools, accompanied by comprehensive response planning, is associated with good outcomes, even with relatively low event rates. A study of the deployment of AEDs in the homes of patients who recently had MIs and were not candidates for implantable defibrillators did not demonstrate benefit. Because the home is the most common site of cardiac arrest and survival rates are lower than those in public sites, additional strategies for both AEDs and other technologies should be tested. Further research on effective strategies is needed because most community-based cardiac arrests occur in the home. Novel approaches such as the use of drones to deploy AEDs where needed and mobile applications that can locate the nearest AED may alleviate some of these issues.[142]

As is the case with any medical device, malfunctions of AEDs may occur infrequently because of design or manufacturing defects or failure to adhere to manufacturers' recommendations for replacement of batteries and leads. It is an obligation of those responsible for maintaining AEDs to remain cognizant of FDA safety alerts and recalls and the shelf-lives of batteries and leads.

Advanced Life Support

This next step in the resuscitative sequence is designed to achieve stable ROSC and hemodynamic stabilization.[108] Implementation of advanced life support (ACLS) is not intended to suggest an abrupt cessation of BLS activities, but rather a transition from one level of activity to the next. In the past, ACLS required judgments and technical skills that removed it from the realm of activity of lay bystanders and even emergency medical technicians, instead limiting these activities to specifically trained paramedical personnel, nurses, and physicians. With further education of emergency technicians, most community-based CPR programs now permit them to carry out ACLS activities. However, some studies suggest that the addition of ACLS to an otherwise optimized out-of-hospital response system (i.e., bystander CPR and early defibrillation) does not improve survival. In this regard, the development and testing of AEDs that have the ability to sense and analyze cardiac electrical activity and to prompt the user to deliver definitive electrical intervention provide a role for rapid defibrillation by less highly trained rescue personnel (i.e., police, ambulance drivers) and even minimally trained lay bystanders.

The general goals of ACLS are to restore cardiac rhythm to one that is hemodynamically effective, to optimize ventilation, and to maintain and support the restored circulation. Thus, during advanced life support, the patient's cardiac rhythm is promptly cardioverted or defibrillated as the first priority, if appropriate equipment is immediately available. Although a short period of closed-chest cardiac compression immediately before defibrillation has been reported to enhance the probability of survival, especially if circulation has been absent for 4 to 5 or more minutes, the data are unclear. After the initial attempt to restore a hemodynamically effective rhythm, the patient is intubated and oxygenated, if needed, and the heart is paced if bradyarrhythmia or asystole occurs. An intravenous line is established to deliver medications. After intubation, the goal of ventilation is to reverse the hypoxemia and not merely to achieve high alveolar oxygen pressure (p_{O_2}). Thus oxygen rather than room air should be used to ventilate the patient; if possible, arterial P_{O_2} should be monitored. Respiratory support in the hospital by means of an endotracheal tube and Ambu bag—or facemasks in the out-of-hospital setting—is generally used.

Successful ROSC after IHCA is associated with a shorter median duration of resuscitation than is the case in nonsurvivors (12 minutes, interquartile range [IQR] of 6 to 21, versus 20 minutes, IQR of 14 to 30). Nonetheless, hospitals that habitually ran the longest maximum code runs (the median value in the longest quartile was 25 versus 16) generated a higher likelihood of ROSC and survival to discharge. This observation supports longer attempts at resuscitation in patients without do-not-resuscitate orders or futile medical status.

Defibrillation-Cardioversion

Rapid conversion to an effective cardiac electrical mechanism is a key step in successful resuscitation. Delay should be minimal, even when conditions for CPR are optimal. When VF or VT that is pulseless and/or accompanied by loss of consciousness is recognized on a monitor or by telemetry, defibrillation should be carried out immediately. An initial shock of 120 to 200 J by biphasic devices, with the energy level depending on the recommendations for the individual biphasic devices, should be delivered. Energies delivered through AEDs are generally preprogrammed and vary among the devices available. Failure

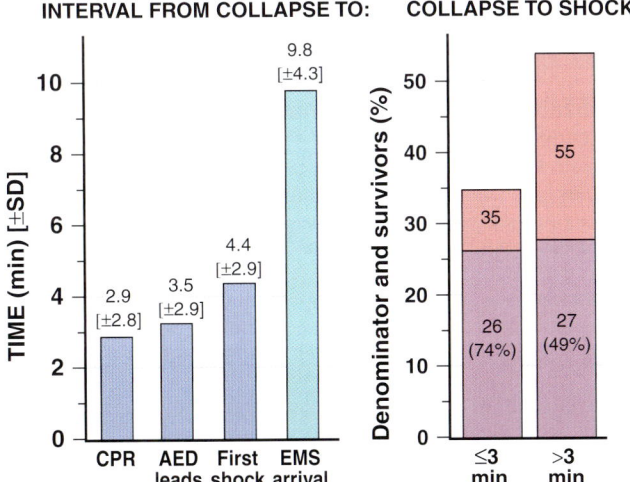

FIGURE 70.12 Results of AED deployment in the controlled environment of casinos. Because the onset of cardiac arrest can frequently be witnessed, short intervals from the onset of collapse to CPR and AED shocks were achieved. Response times were reduced by more than 50% in comparison to the standard emergency medical system (EMS). For those found in VT/VF, the survival rate approached 60% for VT/VF with a witnessed onset. When response time was less than 3 minutes, the survival rate after VT/VF was greater than 70%. (Modified from Valenzuela TD, et al: Outcomes of rapid defibrillation by security officers after cardiac arrest in casinos. N Engl J Med 2000;343:1206.)

of the initial shock to provide an effective rhythm is a poor prognostic sign. Failure of a single adequate shock to restore a pulse should be followed by continued CPR and a second shock delivered after five cycles of CPR. This supersedes the previous strategy of three successive shocks before resuming CPR. The intent is to maximize circulatory time by chest compressions until a pulse has been restored.

If cardiac arrest still persists, the patient is intubated and intravenous access achieved. Epinephrine is administered and followed by repeated defibrillation attempts at maximal output. Although its efficacy is not established, double sequential defibrillation—delivering shocks from two different defibrillators almost simultaneously—may be considered for patients who are refractory to defibrillation.[108] Epinephrine may be repeated at 3- to 5-minute intervals with a defibrillator shock in between. Vasopressin is an effective alternative to epinephrine. However, studies of the value of high-dose versus standard-dose epinephrine and epinephrine versus vasopressin have not demonstrated superiority of one strategy for survival to discharge or neurologic outcome, though some differences in ROSC were noted. In a placebo controlled trial from the United Kingdom, there was improved 30-day survival with epinephrine (3.2% versus 2.4%) but no difference in neurologic outcome as more patients in the epinephrine group had neurologic impairment.[143]

Simultaneously, the rescuer should focus on ventilation to improve oxygenation, reversal of acidosis, and improvement of the underlying electrophysiologic condition to make the heart more likely to reestablish a stable rhythm. Although adequate oxygenation of the blood is crucial in immediate management of the metabolic acidosis of cardiac arrest, additional correction by intravenous administration of sodium bicarbonate has been used. In a small study patients randomized to intravenous sodium bicarbonate or saline for patients undergoing CPR with pH <7.1 or bicarbonate <10 mEq/L, there was no improvement in ROSC or good neurologic survival at one month.[144] Sodium bicarbonate is generally not recommended except in certain conditions such as hyperkalemia and drug overdose.[145]

Pharmacotherapy

For patients who have persistent or recurrent VT or VF despite direct-current cardioversion after epinephrine, intravenous administration of antiarrhythmic agents has been recommended (Chapter 64) during continued resuscitative efforts. Based on a single controlled trial with a survival to hospital admission endpoint, intravenous amiodarone emerged as the initial treatment of choice. Bolus therapy (150 mg), followed by a maintenance dose during the next 18 hours and for several days if necessary, was recommended, depending on response. A bolus of lidocaine (60 to 100 mg) may be given intravenously and the dose repeated in 2 minutes for patients in whom amiodarone is unsuccessful and possibly for those who have an acute transmural MI as the triggering mechanism for the cardiac arrest. In a randomized, placebo controlled, double blind trial, the Resuscitation Outcomes Consortium compared intravenous amiodarone (150 mg, followed by a second bolus if necessary) or lidocaine (60 mg) against placebo. There was no difference between either drug or placebo for survival to discharge outcomes or survival with favorable neurologic status.[146] However, survival to hospital admission was significantly better with both active drugs compared with placebo. In addition, survival to discharge was improved with both drugs among the subgroup with bystander-witnessed arrest, but neither active drug was superior to the other. In another placebo controlled trial, the Resuscitation Outcomes Consortium compared intravenous and intraosseous administration of amiodarone and lidocaine and found that only intravenous administration improved outcomes.[147] Intravenous procainamide is rarely used in this setting any longer, but it may be tried for persisting, hemodynamically stable arrhythmias.

For patients in whom acute hyperkalemia is associated with resistant VF or for those who have hypocalcemia or are toxic from Ca^{2+} entry–blocking drugs, 10% calcium gluconate may be helpful. Calcium should not be used routinely during resuscitation, even though ionized calcium levels may be low during resuscitation from cardiac arrest. Some resistant forms of polymorphic VT or torsades de pointes, rapid monomorphic VT or ventricular flutter (rate ≥260/min), or resistant VF may respond to intravenous beta blocker therapy or intravenous magnesium sulfate. For patients with acute ventricular arrhythmias or VT storm associated with long-QT syndrome, intravenous magnesium sulfate is often an effective antiarrhythmic, even if it has no effect on QT duration.[145]

Bradyarrhythmic and Asystolic Arrest; Pulseless Electrical Activity

The approach to patients with bradyarrhythmic or asystolic arrest or with PEA differs from the approach to those with a tachyarrhythmic event. When this form of cardiac arrest is recognized, effort should focus first on establishing control of cardiorespiratory status (i.e., continue CPR, intubate, and establish intravenous access), reconfirming the rhythm (in two leads if possible), and finally taking action that favors the emergence of a stable spontaneous rhythm or attempt to pace the heart. Possible reversible causes, particularly for bradyarrhythmia and asystole, should be considered and excluded (or treated) promptly. Such causes include hypovolemia, hypoxia, cardiac tamponade, tension pneumothorax, preexisting acidosis, drug overdose, hypothermia, and hyperkalemia. Epinephrine is commonly used in an attempt to elicit spontaneous electrical activity or to increase the rate of a bradycardia. It has had only limited success, as has intravenous isoproterenol infusions in doses of up to 15 to 20 µg/min. In the absence of an intravenous line, epinephrine 1 mg (10 mL of a 1:10,000 solution) may be given by the intracardiac or intraosseous route, but there is danger of coronary or myocardial laceration with the former. Endotracheal delivery can be used if neither IV or IO can be achieved. The added value of high-dose epinephrine is unclear, as in the case of resistant VF. Atropine is no longer considered of value for PEA or asystole, although it may be of benefit for other bradyarrhythmic mechanisms.

Pacing of a bradyarrhythmic or asystolic heart has been limited in the past by the unavailability of personnel capable of carrying out such procedures at the scene of cardiac arrest. With the development of more effective external pacing systems, the role of pacing and its influence on outcome must now be reevaluated. Unfortunately, to date, no clear benefit to transcutaneous pacing has been established.[145]

The published standards for CPR and emergency cardiac care include a series of teaching algorithms to be used as guides to appropriate care. These general guides are not to be interpreted as inclusive of all possible approaches or contingencies. CPR in pregnant women requires attention to the influence of the gravid uterus on the mechanics of CPR. The pregnant patient should be placed in a left lateral decubitus position with left uterine displacement during CPR to relieve aorto-caval compression,[148] and standard defibrillation has no risk for the fetus. Acute antiarrhythmic drug therapy during ACLS is generally safe, although long-term amiodarone therapy raises concern for potential fetal organ toxicity.

Stabilization of Cardiac Rhythm after Initial Return of Spontaneous Circulation

If frequent PVCs and runs of nonsustained VT persist after restoration of a sinus mechanism, continuous infusion of an effective antiarrhythmic drug may be used, but this is based on the clinical situation and clinical judgement of the provider. Intravenous amiodarone is the preferred agent, but lidocaine is an option for arrhythmias caused by acute ischemic events. On occasion, continuous infusion of propranolol or esmolol is used, sometimes in conjunction with magnesium sulfate, especially for recurrent episodes of polymorphic VT or VT storm unresponsive to amiodarone.

Catecholamines are used for cardiac arrest not only in an attempt to achieve better electrical stability (e.g., conversion from fine to coarse VF or increasing the rate of spontaneous contraction during bradyarrhythmias) but also for their inotropic and peripheral vascular effects. Epinephrine is the first choice among the catecholamines for use in cardiac arrest because it increases myocardial contractility, elevates perfusion pressure, may convert electromechanical dissociation to electromechanical coupling, and improves the chances for successful defibrillation. Because of its adverse effects on renal and mesenteric flow, norepinephrine is a less desirable agent despite its inotropic effects. When the chronotropic effect of epinephrine is undesirable, dopamine or dobutamine is preferable to norepinephrine for inotropic effect. Isoproterenol may be used for the treatment of primary or postdefibrillation bradycardia when heart rate control is the primary goal of therapy intended to improve cardiac output. Calcium chloride is sometimes used in patients with PEA that persists after the administration of catecholamines. The efficacy of this intervention is uncertain. Stimulation of alpha adrenoceptors may be important during definitive resuscitative efforts. For example, the alpha adrenoceptor–stimulating effects of epinephrine and higher dosages of dopamine, which elevate aortic diastolic pressure by peripheral vasoconstriction with increased cerebral and myocardial flow, have been reemphasized.

Postcardiac Arrest Care and Postcardiac Arrest Syndrome

After return of spontaneous or stable assisted circulation, focus shifts to the diagnostic and therapeutic elements of postcardiac arrest syndrome, a field of pathophysiology and clinical intervention that emerged from the recognition that the various elements of injury following cardiac arrest should be organized into a multidisciplinary continuum. The four elements of postcardiac arrest syndrome include brain injury, myocardial dysfunction, systemic ischemia/reperfusion responses, and control of persistent precipitating factors. The therapeutic goal is to achieve and maintain stable electrical, hemodynamic, and central nervous system (CNS) status, based on complex algorithms. The specialized and multidisciplinary nature of postcardiac arrest care have led to the proposal and preliminary data supporting the concept of specialized cardiac centers for postcardiac arrest patients, analogous to trauma or stroke centers. When transporting the hemodynamically unstable or comatose patient, EMS responders would selectively bypass the nearest hospital, in favor of the closest facility having facilities and staff sufficient to manage postcardiac arrest complexities, assuming an added transport time of no more than 15 minutes. The profile of the patient ready for transport is matched to the capabilities of the institution to which the victim is transported, as outlined in Figure 70.13.

For successfully resuscitated cardiac arrest victims, whether the event occurred in or out of the hospital, postcardiac arrest care includes admission to an intensive care unit and continuous monitoring for a minimum of 48 to 72 hours. Some elements of postcardiac arrest syndrome are common to all resuscitated patients, but the prognosis and certain details of management are specific for the clinical setting in which the cardiac arrest occurred. The major management categories include (1) primary cardiac arrest in patients with AMI; (2) secondary cardiac arrest in patients with AMI; (3) cardiac arrest associated with noncardiac-related diseases, drug effects, or electrolyte disorders; and (4) survival after out-of-hospital cardiac arrest.

Cardiac Arrest in Patients with Hemodynamically Stable Acute Myocardial Infarction

VF in patients with AMI free of concomitant hemodynamic complications (i.e., primary VF; see Chapter 38) is now less common in hospitalized patients compared with the 15% to 20% incidence noted before the availability of cardiac care units. The events that do occur are almost always reverted successfully by prompt interventions in properly equipped emergency departments or cardiac care units. If ventricular arrhythmias persist after successful resuscitation, a lidocaine or amiodarone infusion is used. Antiarrhythmic drugs are generally discontinued after 24 hours if sustained arrhythmias do not recur. The occurrence of VF during the early phase of AMI (i.e., first 24 to 48 hours) does not identify long-term arrhythmic risk and is not an indication for long-term antiarrhythmic or device therapy. Polymorphic VT has similar implications.

Monomorphic VT, which may lead to cardiac arrest in AMI, has different implications as it may be due to the presence of a substrate that has long-term implications or transient electrophysiologic changes due to the acute ischemia and infarction. VF within 48 hours of MI was shown to be associated with a better prognosis than VT. Of those with VT who received an ICD, there was a high rate of appropriate ICD therapy in follow-up. Though monomorphic VT is uncommon in the setting of acute coronary syndromes, it has been shown to be an independent predictor of long-term survival, whereas nonmonomorphic VT was not.[149]

Cardiac arrest caused by bradyarrhythmias or asystole in acute *inferior* wall MI, in the absence of primary hemodynamic deterioration, is uncommon and may respond to atropine or pacing. The prognosis is good, with no special long-term care required in most cases. Persistent

Level	Patient Status	Hospital Resource Minimums
Level 1 🔴	Failure to restore circulation; ROSC without regaining consciousness ± hemodynamic instability ± acute coronary syndrome; ± recurrent arrhythmias	Local or regional facility capable of providing highest level of neurological, cardiovascular, and intensive care support 24/7 (ICU/CCU/NICU)
Level 2 🟠	ROSC with restoration of consciousness; Persistent hemodynamic instability ± acute coronary syndrome; ± recurrent arrhythmias	Nearest facility capable of providing high level cardiovascular and intensive care support 24/7; cardiac catheterization laboratory capable of providing PCI within 90 minutes
Level 3 🟢	ROSC with restoration of consciousness; hemodynamically stable Evidence of acute coronary syndrome; ± recurrent arrhythmias	Nearest facility with cardiac catheterization laboratory capable of providing PCI within 90 minutes - 24/7
Level 4 🔵	ROSC with restoration of consciousness; hemodynamically stable; no evidence of acute coronary syndrome ± recurrent arrhythmias	Nearest facility capable of providing standard ED, ICU/CCU; cardiac catheterization desirable with PCI capability within 24 hours

FIGURE 70.13 A four-tiered EMS bypass model aligning immediate postcardiac arrest status and level of required care is illustrated to reflect a priority-based hospital bypass system. The Copenhagen model provides a foundation for this additional level of coordination. Patients can be transported to the closest facility appropriate to the optimal or minimal care requirements. *CCU,* coronary care unit; *ED,* emergency department; *ICU,* intensive care unit; *NICU,* neurologic intensive care unit; *PCI,* percutaneous coronary intervention; *ROSC,* return of spontaneous circulation. (Modified from Myerburg RJ: Initiatives for improving out-of-hospital cardiac arrest outcomes. Circulation 2014;30:1840-1843.)

symptomatic bradyarrhythmias requiring permanent pacemakers rarely occur in such patients. In contrast, bradyarrhythmic cardiac arrest associated with large *anterior* wall infarctions (and AV or intraventricular block) has a poor prognosis.

Cardiac Arrest in Patients with Hemodynamically Unstable Acute Myocardial Infarction

Cardiac arrest occurring in association with, or as a result of, hemodynamic or mechanical dysfunction during the acute phase of MI has an immediate mortality rate ranging from 59% to 89%, depending on the severity of the hemodynamic abnormalities and size of the MI. Resuscitative efforts commonly fail in such patients, and when they are successful, postcardiac arrest management is often difficult. When secondary cardiac arrest occurs by the mechanisms of VT or VF in this setting, aggressive postresuscitation hemodynamic or anti-ischemic measures may help achieve rhythm stability. Intravenous amiodarone has emerged as the antiarrhythmic therapy of choice. Lidocaine may also be tried if the mechanism appears to be ischemic but is less likely to be successful in this setting than in primary VF. The success of interventions and prevention of recurrent cardiac arrest are closely related to the success in managing the patient's hemodynamic status. The proportion of cardiac arrests caused by bradyarrhythmias or asystole or by PEA is higher in hemodynamically unstable patients with AMI. Such patients usually have large MIs and major hemodynamic abnormalities and may be acidotic and hypoxemic. Even with aggressive therapy, the prognosis after asystolic arrest in such patients is poor, and they are resuscitated only rarely from PEA.

Cardiac Arrest Among In-Hospital Patients With Noncardiac Abnormalities. These patients fall into two major categories: (1) those with life-limiting diseases, such as malignant neoplasms, sepsis, organ failure, end-stage pulmonary disease, and advanced CNS disease, and (2) those with acute toxic or proarrhythmic states that are potentially reversible. In the former category, the ratio of tachyarrhythmic to bradyarrhythmic cardiac arrest is low, and the prognosis for survival of cardiac arrest is poor. Although the data may be somewhat skewed by the practice of assigning "do-not-resuscitate" orders to patients with end-stage disease, the data available for attempted resuscitations show poor outcomes. For the few successfully resuscitated patients in these categories, postarrest management is dictated by the underlying precipitating factors.

Risk Identification by QT Interval Prolongation after Cardiac Arrest

The initial management of survivors of OHCA centers on stabilizing cardiac electrical status, supporting hemodynamics, and providing supportive care for reversal of any organ damage that has occurred as a consequence of the cardiac arrest. The in-hospital risk for recurrent cardiac arrest is relatively low, and arrhythmias account for only 10% of in-hospital deaths after successful out-of-hospital resuscitation. However, the mortality rate during the index hospitalization is 50%, thus indicating that nonarrhythmic mortality dominates the mechanisms of early postresuscitation deaths (30% hemodynamic, 60% CNS related). Antiarrhythmic therapy, usually intravenous amiodarone, is used in an attempt to prevent recurrent cardiac arrest in patients who demonstrate recurrent arrhythmia during the first 48 hours of postarrest hospitalization. Patients who have preexisting or new AV or intraventricular conduction disturbances are at particularly high risk for recurrent cardiac arrest. The routine use of temporary pacemakers has been evaluated in such patients but has not been found to be helpful for prevention of early recurrent cardiac arrest. Invasive techniques for hemodynamic monitoring are used in patients whose condition is unstable but are not used routinely in those whose condition is stable on admission.

Anoxic encephalopathy is a strong predictor of in-hospital death or death within 6 months postdischarge. The induction of therapeutic hypothermia to reduce metabolic demands and cerebral edema should be applied promptly to a postarrest survivor who remains unconscious on hospital admission. A randomized study of prehospital intravenous hypothermia demonstrated a small reduction in ROSC and no benefit for survival to hospital discharge.[150] The initial temperature target was 32 to 34°C, but subsequent data suggest that a target of 36°C is equally effective and easier to achieve.

During the later convalescent period, continued attention to CNS status, including physical rehabilitation, is of primary importance for an optimal outcome. Respiratory support by conventional methods is used as necessary. Management of other organ system injury (e.g., renal, hepatic), as well as early recognition and treatment of infectious complications, also contributes to ultimate survival.

Long-Term Management of Survivors of Out-of-Hospital Cardiac Arrest

When a survivor of out-of-hospital cardiac arrest has awakened and achieved electrical and hemodynamic stability, usually within a few days if it is to occur at all, decisions must be made about the nature and extent of the workup required to establish a long-term management strategy. The goals of the workup are to identify the specific causative and triggering factors of the cardiac arrest, to clarify the functional status of the patient's cardiovascular system, and to establish long-term therapeutic strategies. Patients who have limited return of CNS function usually do not undergo extensive workups, and patients whose cardiac arrests were triggered by an acute transmural AMI have workups similar to those for other patients with AMI (see Chapter 38).

Survivors of OHCA not associated with AMI who have good return of neurologic function appear to have a long-term survival probability commensurate with their age, sex, and extent of disease when they are treated according to existing guidelines.[151] These patients should undergo diagnostic workups to define the cause of the cardiac arrest and to tailor long-term therapy, the latter targeted to the underlying disease and strategies for prevention of recurrent cardiac arrest or SCD. The workup includes cardiac catheterization with coronary angiography if coronary atherosclerosis is known or considered to be the possible cause of the event, evaluation of the functional significance of coronary lesions by stress imaging techniques if indicated, determination of functional and hemodynamic status, and assessment of whether the life-threatening arrhythmic event was caused by a transient risk associated with AMI or there is persisting risk based on clinical characteristics.

General Care

The general management of survivors of cardiac arrest is determined by the specific cause and the underlying pathophysiologic process. For patients with ischemic heart disease, interventions to prevent myocardial ischemia, optimization of therapy for LV function, and attention to general medical status are all addressed. Although limited data suggest that revascularization procedures may improve the recurrence rate and total mortality rates after survival from OHCA, no properly controlled prospective studies have validated this impression for bypass surgery or percutaneous interventions. The indications for revascularization after cardiac arrest are limited to those who have a generally accepted indication for angioplasty or surgery, including a documented ischemic mechanism of the cardiac arrest.

Although no data from placebo-controlled trials are available to define a benefit of various anti-ischemic strategies (including beta blockers or other medical anti-ischemic therapy) for long-term management after OHCA, medical, catheter interventional, or surgical anti-ischemic therapy, rather than antiarrhythmic drug therapy, is generally considered the primary approach to long-term management of the subgroup of prehospital cardiac arrest survivors in whom transient myocardial ischemia was the inciting event. Moreover, in an uncontrolled observation comparing cardiac arrest survivors who had ever received beta blockers after the index event with those who had not, a significant improvement in long-term outcome with beta blocker therapy was noted. Further evaluation of the specific role of revascularization procedures and anti-ischemic medical therapy after OHCA is needed.

Whether the various pharmacologic strategies (e.g., angiotensin-converting enzyme inhibitors, carvedilol and other beta-adrenergic blocking agents, and spironolactone) that have been shown to provide a clinical and mortality benefit in patients with LV dysfunction provide a specific SCD benefit separate from a total mortality benefit remains uncertain.

PREVENTION OF CARDIAC ARREST AND SUDDEN CARDIAC DEATH

Prevention of SCA can be classified into five clinical subgroup categories: (1) prevention of recurrent events in survivors of cardiac arrest (secondary prevention) (see Table 69.3); (2) prevention of an initial event in patients at high risk because of advanced heart disease, such as those with low ejection fractions and other markers of risk (primary prevention) (see Table 69.4); (3) primary prevention in patients with less advanced common or uncommon structural heart diseases; (4) primary prevention in patients with structurally normal hearts, subtle or minor structural abnormalities, or genetically based molecular disorders (Table 70.5); and (5) primary prevention in the general population. The last category includes the substantial proportion of SCDs that occur as a first cardiac event in victims previously free of known disease. While all-encompassing preventive strategies have been difficult to establish, the potential public health impact of prevention in the context of limited postcardiac arrest survival suggests that this needs to be incorporated into the global strategy for prevention of SCD (Fig. 70.14).

Four general antiarrhythmic strategies, which are not mutually exclusive, can be contemplated for patients at high risk for cardiac arrest: implantable defibrillators, antiarrhythmic drugs, catheter ablation, and antiarrhythmic surgery. While the mainstay of therapy for the highest risk patients is the implantable defibrillator, there are a variety of nontraditional antiarrhythmic medications that have shown survival benefit. These include beta blockers, angiotensin-converting enzyme (ACE) inhibitors, angiotensin receptor blockers, aldosterone receptor antagonists, combined angiotensin-neprilysin inhibitors, statins, polyunsaturated fatty acids, and SGLT2 inhibitors, among others.[152] The role of antiarrhythmic drug therapy (class I and class III) for secondary prevention of subsequent SCD, as opposed to adjunctive therapy, has not been established, though there is some supportive evidence for the use of amiodarone.[153]

The choice of a therapy, or combinations of therapies, is based on estimation of risk determined by evaluation of the individual patient by various risk-profiling techniques, coupled with available efficacy and safety data.

Methods to Estimate Risk for Sudden Cardiac Death

General Medical and Cardiovascular Risk Markers

The presence and severity of acquired medical disorders (such as coronary atherosclerosis and associated myocardial ischemia or magnetic resonance imaging–defined scar patterns, LV dysfunction and ventricular volume, and heart failure) and general medical conditions (such as hypertension, diabetes, dyslipidemias, chronic renal failure, and cigarette smoking) are integral to estimation of risk for SCD. Although lacking the specificity of individual SCD risk prediction, they provide general indicators of risk and data supporting the benefit of therapies, such as beta blockers, ACE inhibitors and receptor blockers, and statins, in appropriate subgroups of patients. In several recent reports, a series of easily identified markers was used to generate a risk score for SCD among subjects in two long-term population studies

TABLE 70.5 Selected Indications for Implantable Cardioverter-Defibrillators in Genetic Disorders Associated with Risk for Sudden Cardiac Death (Refer to Most Recent Guidelines)

DIAGNOSIS	ICD INDICATION	PRIMARY SOURCE OF DATA	RISK INDICATORS	GUIDELINES CLASSIFICATION	EVIDENCE
HCM	Secondary SCA protection	Registries, cohorts	Previous SCA, sustained VT	Class I	Level B
	Primary SCA protection	Registries, cohorts	For adults ≥1 major risk factor: family history of SCD, Left ventricular thickness ≥30 mm, syncope suspected to be arrhythmic, apical aneurysm, ejection fraction <50%	Class IIa	Level B
ARVD/RVCM	Secondary SCA protection	Registry, case series	Previous SCA, hemodynamically unstable sustained VT	Class I	Level B
			Hemodynamically stable sustained VT	Class IIa	Level B
			Unexplained syncope	Class IIa	Level B
	Primary SCA protection	Registry, case series	Three major, two major and two minor, or one major and four minor risk factors for ventricular arrhythmia*	Class IIa	Level B
				Class IIb	Level B
			Two major, one major and two minor, or four minor risk factors for ventricular arrhythmia*		
Congenital LQT	Secondary SCA protection	Registry, cohorts	Previous SCA	Class I	Level B
	Primary SCA protection	Registry, cohorts	Beta blocker ineffective/not tolerated (intensification is recommended—ICD is an option)	Class 1	Level B
			QTc >500 msec on beta blocker (intensification may be considered—ICD is an option)	Class IIb	Level B
Brugada syndrome	Secondary SCA protection	Case cohorts	SCA, sustained VT, recent syncope suspected to be arrhythmic	Class I	Level B
	Primary SCA protection	Case cohorts	Positive electrophysiology study (1-2 extra stimuli)	Class IIb	Level B
CPVT/F	Secondary SCA protection	Small case series	Previous SCA	Class I	Level B
	Primary SCA protection	Small case series	Syncope or VT while taking beta blockers, family history of premature SCA (?)	Class I	Level B

ARVD/RVCM, Arrhythmogenic right ventricular dysplasia/cardiomyopathy; *CPVT/F*, catecholaminergic polymorphic ventricular tachycardia/"idiopathic" ventricular fibrillation; *HCM*, hypertrophic cardiomyopathy; *LQT*, long-QT syndrome; *N-S*, nonsustained; *PVT*, polymorphic ventricular tachycardia; *SQT*, short-QT syndrome; *VA*, ventricular arrhythmia; *(?)*, uncertain.

*Major criteria: nonsustained ventricular tachycardia (NSVT), inducible VT, LVEF ≤49%. Minor criteria: male sex, >1000 premature ventricular complexes (PVCs)/24 hours, RV dysfunction, proband status, two or more desmosomal variants. If both NSVT and PVC criteria are present, then only NSVT can be used.

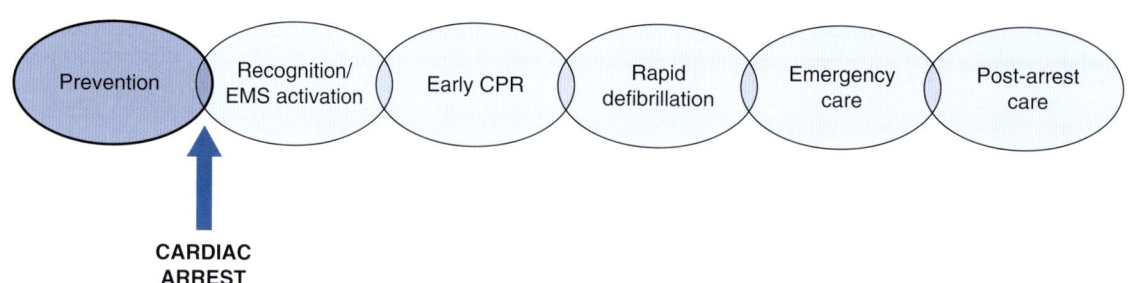

FIGURE 70.14 Prevention of cardiac arrest is an important element of addressing the public health burden of sudden cardiac death. On a case-by-case basis, prevention may be even more effective to improve survival than the well described import and impact of the postcardiac arrest chain of survival. *CPR*, Cardiopulmonary resuscitation; *EMS*, emergency medical services. (From Mitrani RD, Goldberger JJ. Cardiac arrests during the COVID-19 pandemic: the perfect storm. JACC: Clinical Electrophysiology 2021;7:12-15.)

without a history of cardiovascular disease.[16,17] Bogle et al. used only clinical information that is widely available in the electronic health record including age, sex, cholesterol, blood pressure, lipid and blood pressure medication use, diabetes, current smoking, and body mass index. The model demonstrated large, nonlinear, gradients of risk, with the major impact in the highest 1 to 2 deciles. The score yielded very good internal discrimination and very good external discrimination among Framingham participants. This type of model moves in the right direction for individual risk prediction, but it is limited by its effect sizes—approximately a 4% SCD risk over 10 years in the highest decile. This magnitude of risk is not sufficient to justify certain interventions and further risk stratification will be needed to identify even higher risk subgroups at sufficient risk to merit advanced therapies.

In patients with known or suspected coronary heart disease or nonischemic cardiomyopathy, other noninvasive markers of risk are being employed and/or explored, including ejection fraction and measures reflecting autonomic function, depolarization and repolarization abnormalities, and genetic influences on risk for SCD (see Risk Factors for Sudden Cardiac Death). While ejection fraction is the most widely studied and most widely used clinical measure to assess risk for SCD, it is now well appreciated that it lacks sensitivity and specificity. Electrocardiographic based tests for abnormal depolarization and repolarization have enjoyed tremendous enthusiasm and have been evaluated extensively. Abnormal depolarization provides information about conduction; areas of slow or delayed conduction are critical for reentrant tachyarrhythmias. While evaluations of QRS duration, late potentials on signal averaged electrocardiography, and fragmented QRS all show prognostic value, the individual predictive value is not high enough to be used clinically and these are not incorporated in the guidelines. Similarly, abnormal repolarization indices may indicate heterogeneities in repolarization and/or refractoriness that may also be a key requirement for the pathogenesis of reentrant tachyarrhythmias. While evaluations of QT interval duration, QT dispersion, QT alternans, and QT variability, among others, all show prognostic value, the individual predictive value is not high enough to be used clinically and these are not incorporated in the guidelines. Recent data suggest that scores composed of combinations of novel and/or standard ECG markers might add to SCD risk prediction in the general population and in patients with established coronary heart disease.

The role of the autonomic nervous system in the pathogenesis of ventricular tachyarrhythmias and SCD is well appreciated. ECG-based analyses of heart rate variability—time domain, frequency domain, and nonlinear techniques—and heart rate changes with exercise provide prognostic information, but the individual predictive value is not high enough to be used clinically. The only testing/findings currently included in the guidelines[151] are low ejection fraction, nonsustained VT, inducible ventricular tachycardia, and MRI findings of scar (discussed below). It should be noted that although several clinical trials incorporating the ECG-based markers have been negative, dampening enthusiasm for the clinical use of these techniques, these trials also typically incorporated a low ejection fraction which remains a clinically used technique. It may be that risk stratification strategies can be applied that utilize these methods in a strategic fashion.[154]

The potential importance of proper timing for evaluation of risk markers has been explored. There is a well-known time-dependence to risk of SCD following MI.[155] Overlaid on this is a changing proportion of presumed arrhythmic and mechanical causes for SCD, as noted in the VALIANT study.[4] It is therefore not surprising that there is time-dependence to risk stratification. The REFINE study suggested greater risk predictive power for post-MI adverse events when markers were evaluated after 8 weeks versus closer to the index event. Another study of a cohort of 231 patients with acute MI and an initial EF ≤35% reported that the distribution of EFs on echocardiograms at 90 days of follow-up remained at 35% or less in 43%, increased to 36% to 49% in 31%, and increased to 50% or more in 26%.[156] How this impacts future SCD risk remains to be determined.

Ambulatory Monitoring. Although ambulatory monitoring is not routinely recommended as a screening tool, it is used for profiling the risk for development of life-threatening sustained arrhythmias in individuals with certain forms of structural or electrophysiologic disease who are considered to be at high risk (Chapter 61). Notably, nonsustained VT is an actionable finding in certain conditions such as HCM[42,151] and ischemic cardiomyopathy with LV ejection fraction ≤40%.[151] Technologic advances making very long-term monitoring easier allows identification of episodic arrhythmias as causes of relevant symptoms, such as near-syncope and syncope. In addition to the common disorders associated with SCA, loop recorders may be useful for selected individuals with disorders such as HCM, long-QT syndrome, and right ventricular dysplasia and in patients with dilated cardiomyopathy or heart failure.

Programmed Electrical Stimulation for Risk Profiling. Despite a large, albeit somewhat conflicting data base on the role of electrophysiologic testing for risk profiling,[157] particularly in patients with advanced heart disease, its use is currently more limited than in the past. In primary prevention trials such as MADIT and MUSTT, programmed electrical stimulation studies were used to profile risk and suggested large benefits. MADIT II, subsequently enrolled patients with lower ejection fractions than did MADIT or MUSTT and did not use programmed stimulation or other arrhythmia markers; this study demonstrated a survival benefit of ICD therapy without the need for incorporating results of electrophysiologic testing in the treatment decision. This led to a dramatic decline in its use. Nevertheless, based on the criteria in MUSTT, it is currently included in the guidelines.[151] It is the most direct test to evaluate for the presence of substrate for monomorphic VT, but its utility to predict VF is more limited. The question of whether electrophysiologic testing is generally useful has yet to be fully resolved, although it appears to have a role in selected patients and clinical circumstances. Of interest, a follow-up study of patients in MADIT II suggested inducibility was associated with a higher incidence of VT and noninducibility was associated with a higher incidence of VF. The utility of programmed ventricular stimulation to assess for inducible VT was shown in the PRE-SERVE EF study.[154] In post-MI patients with LV ejection fraction ≥40%, programmed ventricular stimulation was performed if one noninvasive risk factor derived from the signal-averaged ECG and ambulatory 24-hour monitoring was positive. Patients with a positive noninvasive risk factor and inducible VT comprised approximately 7% of the population and experienced approximately an 8% annual rate of major arrhythmic events. The Programmed Ventricular Stimulation to Risk Stratify for Early Cardioverter-Defibrillator Implantation to Prevent Tachyarrhythmias following Acute Myocardial Infarction (PROTECT-ICD) is testing whether programmed ventricular stimulation in patients with LV ejection fraction ≤40% 2 to 40 days after AMI can identify patients who benefit from an ICD.[158] Finally, in patients with nonischemic dilated cardiomyopathy, the accumulated evidence is that programmed ventricular stimulation does provide moderate risk stratification with an approximate doubling of relative risk for those with inducible ventricular tachyarrhythmias.

The secondary prevention trials of cardiac arrest survivors did not seek to determine whether routine electrophysiologic testing offered predictive value. It is not a necessary component of the evaluation unless there is no structural heart disease or a suspicion for a supraventricular tachycardia as the initiating rhythm for cardiac arrest. In the latter patients, treatment targeting the supraventricular tachycardia should be pursued rather than ICD therapy. For the evaluation of precipitating ventricular arrhythmias, most previous studies had demonstrated limitations because of the relatively small fraction of cardiac arrest survivors (an average of less than 50% on the basis of multiple studies) who had inducible ventricular arrhythmias. Under conditions in which a potentially reversible trigger for cardiac arrest can be identified and perhaps in some cardiac arrest survivors in whom transient ischemia was the initiating mechanism and the ejection fraction is normal or near-normal, there might be a persistent limited role for electrophysiologic testing as a guide to therapy.

Cardiac MRI. Cardiac MRI has the ability to define reactive/interstitial fibrosis and replacement fibrosis with T1 mapping/extracellular volume fraction and delayed enhancement.[40] Many studies have related the findings of dense scar and "border zone" to arrhythmic outcomes in patients with ischemic heart disease. The rationale is that the infarct topology and/or size provides the anatomic platform or substrate for reentrant ventricular tachyarrhythmias. While infarct size is correlated with LV ejection fraction, the strength of the correlation is not high. The accumulated evidence over many studies is that late gadolinium enhancement is a strong predictor of arrhythmic events. In a meta-analysis,[50] the hazard ratio for ventricular arrhythmias and SCD associated with late gadolinium enhancement in ischemic cardiomyopathy was 3.87 and in nonischemic cardiomyopathy was 4.32. Importantly, LV ejection fraction above or below 35% did not significantly modulate this risk (hazard ratio 3.72 and 3.53, respectively). The CMR-Guide study is currently under way to assess whether late gadolinium enhancement in patients with ischemic or nonischemic cardiomyopathies with LV ejection fractions between 36% and 50% can be used to stratify arrhythmic risk and demonstrate utility of an ICD.[159]

The utility of substrate delineation in nonischemic and HCM has also been demonstrated. In a study of 339 patients with nonischemic dilated cardiomyopathy and ejection fraction ≥40% followed for a median of 4.6 years, 18% of those with late gadolinium enhancement experienced SCD or aborted SCD compared with 2% without late gadolinium enhancement.[51] After adjusting for age, New York Heart Association class, and ejection fraction, the hazard ratio was 9.2. The cumulative data from many studies is strongly supportive of the role of late gadolinium enhancement in nonischemic, dilated cardiomyopathy, even among those with better ejection fractions (e.g., between 35%-43%).[160] Annual rates for arrhythmic events for those with late gadolinium enhancement was over 6% regardless of ejection fraction and below 2% for those without late gadolinium enhancement. Newer methods for analysis of the substrate—for example the area of interface between scar and surviving myocardium—may also provide more direct pathophysiologic correlation to ventricular tachyarrhythmias.[161] Observational studies also support the value of late gadolinium enhancement in patients with HCM.[162] In a meta-analysis including almost 3000 patients, late gadolinium enhancement was associated with an odds ratio (OR) of 3.41 for SCD.[163] The extent of late gadolinium enhancement was also an important predictor. The guidelines currently do include the use of MRI in patients with nonischemic dilated cardiomyopathy and HCM for assessment of SCD risk but do not provide a recommendation on how to specifically use this information.

Novel Proteomic and Genomic Markers of Risk for Sudden Cardiac Death. Biomarkers released in the setting of inflammation, myocardial stretch, ischemia, hyperglycemia, and renal dysfunction have been associated with SCD in the general population as well as in selected subsets of high-risk patients with heart failure or coronary heart disease.[164] Several of these biologic markers have also been documented to be associated with ICD therapies for ventricular arrhythmias. Individual associations tend to be modest; and thus, biomarkers have yet to be used clinically for SCD risk prediction. However, elevations in these biomarkers may be useful for identifying individuals with undiagnosed coronary or structural heart disease and prompting further diagnostic evaluation and initiation of standard preventive therapies, which would be expected to impact SCD risk. Recent data suggest that individuals with high levels of several of these markers (TC:HDL, hsTnI, NT-proBNP, and hsCRP) in combination are at marked increased risk (HR = 6.9); however, the number of individuals at such high risk is quite small.[165] In addition to standard cardiac and renal biomarkers, levels of very long chain n-3 fatty acid, eicosapentaenoic acid (EPA) and docosahexaenoic acid (DHA), have also been associated with elevated risks of SCD. In four studies within the general population, levels of EPA and DHA have been associated with markedly lower risks of SCD (risk reduction [RR] = 0.20 to 0.50 for those in the highest versus lowest quartile/tertile).[166] Relationships with SCD appear to be stronger than those observed for other forms of cardiac death, and thus these fatty acids may be able to discriminate risk for SCD from that for other cardiovascular causes.

The genetic basis of SCD in the general population is poorly understood. Several studies have demonstrated a familial predisposition to SCD.[8,167] Three case-control studies demonstrate that a history of SCD among a first-degree relative is an independent risk factor for VF or SCD (e.g., reference[168]) in the setting of acute MI. Two large-scale genome-wide association studies[33,34] and several single candidate gene studies have identified several potential genetic variants associated with SCD risk,[35-42] but these results have not been replicated in larger studies.[169] Data are beginning to accumulate in support of utilizing combinations of genetic variants in the form of genetic risk scores (GRS) to advance SCD risk prediction in the general population[170] and in patients with coronary heart disease (CHD).[171] A GRS composed of 153 genetic variants associated with CHD at genome-wide significance was found to associate with SCD in the setting of CHD in three separate cohorts (OR 1.045 per SD of CHD risk score, $P = 1.7 \times 10^{-7}$) and to predict the occurrence of SCD in patients undergoing stress test, with an improvement in the net reclassification index (NRI) over standard risk factors.[171] In the largest genome-wide association study of SCD published to date, GRS for CHD, BMI, and QT interval were all associated with SCD, suggesting that these risk factors are causally associated with SCD.[169] Despite these promising data, the current role for genetic testing for SCD risk stratification is confined to select patients and families with suspected inherited arrhythmias such as LQTS, Brugada, and CPVT, and cardiomyopathies, such as ARVC, HCM, and DCM.

Strategies to Reduce Risk for Sudden Cardiac Death

Antiarrhythmic Drugs

Historically, the earliest approach to management of risk for out-of-hospital cardiac arrest and VT with hemodynamic compromise was the use of membrane-active antiarrhythmic agents. This approach was based initially on the assumption that a high frequency of ambient ventricular arrhythmias constituted a triggering mechanism for potentially lethal arrhythmias and that their suppression by antiarrhythmic drugs was protective. It was also assumed that electrophysiologic instability of the myocardium, likely associated with regional disease associated changes in refractory periods and conduction velocities, predisposed to potentially lethal arrhythmias and could be positively modified by these drugs. Suppression of inducibility of VT or VF during programmed electrical stimulation studies likely reflected this effect as well and had been a widespread strategy, particularly before the advent of the ICD. Suppression of ambient arrhythmias was demonstrated by the empiric use of amiodarone, beta-adrenergic–blocking agents, or membrane-active antiarrhythmic drugs, but scientifically valid demonstration of a survival benefit was lacking. The discrepancy between ambient arrhythmia suppression and survival benefit was clarified by the results of CAST, which showed that certain class I antiarrhythmic drugs increased mortality despite suppression of ambient ventricular ectopy. In contrast, beta blocker therapy might have some benefit in such patients, and amiodarone might also be effective for some patients, although it did not perform better than the control group in the heart failure patients studied in SCD-HeFT (Sudden Cardiac Death–Heart Failure Trial). A subgroup analysis of patients in AVID suggested that cardiac arrest survivors with EF >35% had identical outcomes with ICDs and amiodarone, but there was no untreated control group to determine both were beneficial versus ineffective. In summary, ambient arrhythmia suppression and empiric antiarrhythmic drug therapy enjoyed a short period of popularity as a strategy for reduction of risk in VT/VF survivors and in high-risk primary prevention candidates, but in time were shown to be ineffective for this purpose.

Surgical Intervention Strategies

Coronary artery bypass surgery can be an effective approach for prevention of SCD in patients with clear acute ischemia induced SCD due to critical coronary artery disease, but for most patients this is not effective as an isolated strategy. The previously popular antiarrhythmic surgical techniques now have limited applications. Intraoperative map-guided cryoablation may be used for patients who have inducible, hemodynamically stable, sustained monomorphic VT during electrophysiologic testing and ventricular and coronary artery anatomy amenable to catheter ablation. However, it has little applicability to survivors of OHCA because the type of arrhythmia favoring this surgical approach is infrequently observed in cardiac arrest survivors. It can be used as adjunctive therapy for ICD recipients whose arrhythmia burden requires frequent shocks.

Catheter Ablation Therapy
The use of catheter ablation techniques to prevent ventricular tachyarrhythmias has been most successful for benign focal tachycardias that may originate from preferential locations in the right or left ventricle (see Chapter 67) and for some reentrant VTs. With rare exceptions, catheter ablation techniques are not used for the treatment of higher risk ventricular tachyarrhythmias or for definitive therapy in patients at risk for progression of the arrhythmic substrate. For VT caused by bundle branch reentrant mechanisms, which occur in cardiomyopathies, as well as in other structural cardiac disorders, ablation of the right bundle branch to interrupt the reentrant cycle has been successful. However, this has limited applicability to the large number of patients with structural heart disease who are at risk for SCD or those who have survived a cardiac arrest. Nonetheless, catheter ablation is an appropriate adjunctive treatment strategy for patients with ICDs who are having multiple tachyarrhythmic events. Catheter-based substrate modification/ablation has been demonstrated to be useful in ICD recipients receiving multiple therapies and performed somewhat better than escalation of antiarrhythmic therapy.[172] Presently, this benefit is limited to reducing the number of patients receiving ICD therapies; further studies are needed to determine whether it has an expanded role for survival. Catheter ablation may have a role in prevention of cardiac arrest in patients with consistent premature ventricular beats that trigger VF, such as may be seen in a wide variety of conditions including idiopathic VF, acute ischemia, and Brugada syndrome. The Purkinje system is frequently a triggering source.[173-175]

Implantable Cardioverter Defibrillators
Development of the implantable cardioverter defibrillator (ICD) added a new dimension to the management of patients at high risk for cardiac arrest (see Chapter 69). After the initial reports of small case series of very high-risk patients in the early 1980s, a number of observational studies confirmed that ICDs can achieve rates of sudden death consistently less than 5% at 1 year and total death rates in the 10% to 20% range in populations at high risk for mortality, as predicted by mortality surrogates such as historical controls or time to the first delivered appropriate therapy. However, determination of the survival benefit of ICDs remained uncertain and was debated. More than 16 years elapsed between the first clinical use of an implanted defibrillator and publication of the first major randomized clinical trial comparing implantable defibrillator therapy with antiarrhythmic drug therapy. During that period, reports had documented the ability of ICDs to revert potentially fatal arrhythmias but could not identify a valid relative or absolute mortality benefit because of confounding factors, such as competing risks for sudden and non-sudden death and determination of whether appropriate shocks represented the interruption of an event that would have been fatal.

MADIT provided the first randomized trial data on the relative benefit of defibrillators over antiarrhythmic drug therapy (largely amiodarone) for primary prevention of SCD in a high-risk population. The outcome demonstrated a 59% reduction in the relative risk for total mortality at 2 years of follow-up (54% cumulative) and a 19% reduction in the absolute risk of dying at 2 years of follow-up. It was followed over a period of less than 10 years by a series of randomized trial reports evaluating ICD therapy for primary and secondary prevention of SCD in patients with previous MI, previous cardiac arrests, and heart failure.

Although these studies documented the ability of ICDs to revert potentially fatal arrhythmias and showed a relative benefit over amiodarone in some groups of patients, the absence of placebo-controlled trials still prevents quantitation of the true magnitude of any mortality benefit because of the inability of positive-controlled trials to identify the absolute benefit of an intervention. Despite these limitations, an ICD is now the preferred therapy for survivors of cardiac arrest at risk for recurrences and for primary prevention in patients in a number of high-risk categories.

Application of Therapeutic Strategies to Specific Groups of Patients

Secondary Prevention of Sudden Cardiac Death after Survival from Cardiac Arrest
As populations of OHCA survivors began to accumulate from community-based EMS activities, the development of therapeutic strategies intended to improve long-term survival emerged as a mandate for clinical investigators. This mandate is complicated by the inability to do randomized controlled trials and the confounding influence of specific cardiovascular therapies that may also improve survival. Early approaches to long-term therapy centered on the use of antiarrhythmic drugs, largely guided by the results of electrophysiologic testing or the empiric use of antiarrhythmic drugs, particularly amiodarone. Various observational and positive-controlled studies had suggested that suppression of inducible ventricular arrhythmias yielded a better outcome than did failure of suppression and that amiodarone was better than class I antiarrhythmic drugs. This approach is no longer widely used. The first adequately powered secondary prevention trial of ICDs versus antiarrhythmic drugs was published in 1997.[176] This study, the AVID Trial, demonstrated a 27% reduction in the relative risk for total mortality at 2 years of follow-up, with an absolute risk reduction of 7% (Fig. 70.15). It was followed shortly thereafter by reports of two other studies, CIDS (Canadian Implantable Defibrillator Study) and CASH (Cardiac Arrest Study Hamburg), both limited by their enrollment numbers but suggesting trends toward similar benefits (see Table 69.3). A meta-analysis of these data confirmed the benefit of ICDs for secondary prevention,

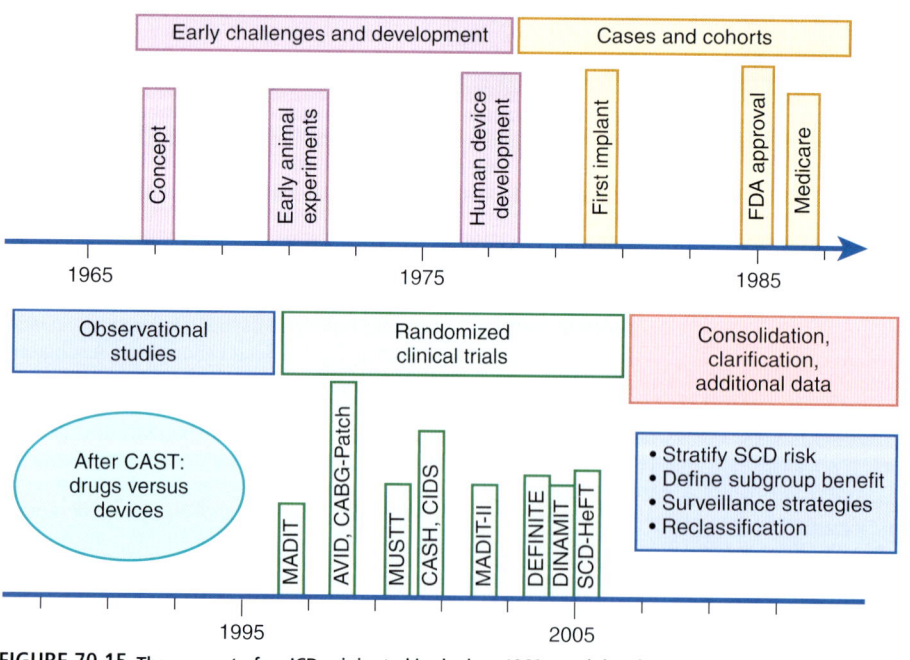

FIGURE 70.15 The concept of an ICD originated in the late 1960s, and development of the technology and proof of concept leading to the first clinical implant extended to 1980. From 1980 until late 1996, data supporting the benefit of ICDs were largely observational or based on small high-risk cohorts or case-control studies. All the major trials for both primary and secondary indications were published during an interval of 10 years between late 1996 and early 2005. Additional studies since then have aided in interpretation of the outcomes from the clinical trials, but there remains a need for consolidation and clarification and for additional data to better define the efficiency of therapy and targeted selection of individual candidates who have a high likelihood of benefit. (Modified from Myerburg RJ, et al. Indications for implantable cardioverter-defibrillators based on evidence and judgment. J Am Clin Cardiol 2009;54:747.)

although only AVID demonstrated a statistically significant survival benefit of an ICD over antiarrhythmic therapy, usually amiodarone. A retrospective subgroup analysis of AVID has also suggested that ICDs had no advantage over antiarrhythmic drugs for VT/VF survivors with ejection fractions >35%. Currently, despite these limitations, ICDs have emerged as the preferred therapy for survivors of OHCA or hemodynamically significant VT, regardless of the ejection fraction, in the absence of identifiable and correctable transient causes of cardiac arrest. The National Cardiovascular Data Registry (NCDR) ICD Registry provides a contemporary report on the outcomes of patients treated with ICD for secondary prevention of SCD.[177] Among 36,434 patients (mean age 65 years, ejection fraction 36%) who received a secondary prevention ICD, 65% for cardiac arrest, the 1- and 2-year mortalities were 10.9% and 16.5%, reflecting better overall survival than the antiarrhythmic drug therapy group in AVID, though this observation should be tempered by many factors including the dramatic change in medical and interventional therapies that have ensued between these reports.

Primary Prevention of Sudden Cardiac Death in Patients with Advanced Heart Disease

After the disturbing outcome of CAST and suggestions of a lack of efficacy or adverse effects of the class I antiarrhythmic drugs in general when used for primary or secondary prevention of SCD, interest shifted to the use of amiodarone and the ICD. Two major trials of amiodarone in post-MI patients, EMIAT and CAMIAT, one of which required ejection fractions lower than 40%, demonstrated no total mortality benefit, even though both trials demonstrated antiarrhythmic benefit, expressed as a reduction in arrhythmic deaths or resuscitated VF. Subgroup analyses have suggested that the concomitant use of beta blockers does confer a mortality benefit.

In parallel with the amiodarone trials, the first randomized controlled trial comparing antiarrhythmic therapy (primarily amiodarone) with ICD therapy (MADIT) was carried out (see Table 69.4). The randomly assigned patients had ejection fractions lower than 35%, nonsustained VT during ambulatory recording, and inducible VT that was not suppressible by procainamide. This very high-risk group demonstrated a 54% reduction in total mortality with ICD therapy versus drug therapy. At the same time, a trial comparing ICD implantation with no specific therapies for arrhythmias in patients with ejection fractions lower than 36% who were undergoing coronary bypass surgery (CABG Patch trial) demonstrated no benefit of defibrillators on total mortality. The only markers for arrhythmic risk required for entry into the study were a low EF and a positive signal-averaged ECG. A third trial, MUSTT, was a complex study designed to determine whether electrophysiologically guided therapy would lead to an improved outcome in patients with ambient nonsustained VT, inducible VT, history of previous MI, and ejection fraction lower than 40%. The results demonstrated that although a statistically significant beneficial effect on total mortality was achieved by guiding therapy according to the results of electrophysiologic testing, when compared with patients with inducible tachycardia who did not receive therapy, the subgroup of patients who received ICDs because they failed to respond to drug therapy accounted for all the benefit. MADIT II was next among the post-MI primary prevention trials, and demonstrated that ICD therapy provided a mortality benefit over conventional therapy in patients with previous MI and ejection fractions lower than 30%, with a relative risk reduction of 28% and an absolute risk reduction of 6% (22% versus 16%) at 2 years (see Fig. 70.15). During long-term follow-up, a constant annualized risk of approximately 8.5% was estimated in survivors, with the most powerful risk predictors being age greater than 65 years, class III or IV heart failure, diabetes, non–sinus rhythm, and elevated blood urea nitrogen levels.

MADIT and MADIT II had set entry requirements of >3 weeks and >1 month after the qualifying infarction, but the actual enrollment in these studies and MUSTT was considerably longer on average. Because both old and recent data suggested higher risk for SCD early after MIs, DINAMIT (Defibrillator in Acute Myocardial Infarction Trial) was designed to evaluate any possible benefit of ICD implantation early after MI in patients with ejection fractions of 35% or lower and other markers of risk. DINAMIT demonstrated no survival benefit attributable to early implantation of ICDs in patients randomly assigned at 6 to 40 days after MI (mean, 18 days) despite reduced arrhythmic mortality (see Table 69.4). There was also an unexplained increase in nonarrhythmic mortality over conventional therapy that needs to be explored in future studies. The IRIS (Immediate Risk Stratification Improves Survival) trial also evaluated ICD implantation early after a MI (entry criteria for days from infarct to randomization = 5 to 31; mean to randomization = 13 ± 7 days) in patients with either ejection fractions of 40% or lower and other markers of risk or nonsustained VT. No survival benefit was noted with ICD therapy. These data suggest that either some SCDs in the early post-MI period are due to a nonarrhythmic mechanism or that different risk predictors are required in this setting. Indeed, there are limited data supporting both of these possibilities. The VALIANT investigators evaluated autopsy findings in patients considered to be SCD and identified that approximately half of the SCDs in the early post-MI period were due to mechanical complications, with a large proportion of these being recurrent MI and ruptured ventricular aneurysms. Observational data from Australia support the potential for this approach to identifying risk for SCD in the early postinfarction period, and support the rationale for the ongoing PROTECT-ICD trial.[158] Further efforts to properly address SCD risk prediction in this critical time period are necessary.

The promise of early ICD benefit from the intervention studies cited above were all reported between 1996 and 2005 and had been designed and executed beginning in the early 1990s and extending to 2004. Modern day optimized therapy during and after MI, with "optimized" being defined as revascularization and the use of beta blockers, acetylsalicylic acid, statins, and ACE inhibitors, may beneficially influence risk for SCD during long-term follow-up after the event. Moreover, thrombolytic therapy and percutaneous coronary intervention during AMI and other changes in therapy that have occurred between 1995 and 2010 have improved 30-day mortality.

A 2009 to 2011 randomized trial, MADIT-RIT was designed to evaluate ICD therapy programming strategies on delivered shocks and mortality. Higher detection rates and longer detection times were associated with fewer shocks and improved survival compared with conventional programming. Interestingly, cumulative mortality at 24 months in the conventional programming group was 10% versus 16% in the original MADIT II cohort (1997 to 2001), thus suggesting beneficial influences other than ICDs on outcomes. More recent data also demonstrate dramatically lower rates of appropriate ICD therapy than were noted in the primary prevention randomized clinical trials. In the MADIT-RIT study of patients with reduced ejection fraction (mean 26%) who were all treated with an ICD, the incidence of appropriate ICD therapy in the optimally programmed group was 6% at a mean follow-up of 1.4 years. In the PROSE-ICD registry, there were 143 ICD shocks for adjudicated ventricular arrhythmias among 1177 patients (mean ejection fraction 23%) over a 59-month follow-up period (annualized 2.5%/year). The low rate of appropriate ICD shocks supports reconsideration of deployment strategies for ICDs. While the initial randomized clinical trials were critical in establishing the efficacy of the ICD for primary prevention of SCD, they were certainly not designed to ensure that the utilized strategy was optimal. Indeed, it has been demonstrated that within the currently indicated population for primary prevention ICD, there is likely a low-risk subgroup whose risk is low enough that there is no ICD benefit. Similarly, there is a high risk subgroup in whom the competing risks of death are high enough that there is also no clinical benefit to the ICD.[43,178-180] There is substantial opportunity to optimize data and clinical approaches to primary prevention of SCD.

In patients with nonischemic cardiomyopathy, the data for primary prevention are more variable. The DEFINITE study enrolled patients with a history of heart failure, ejection fractions of 35% or lower, and PVCs or nonsustained VT. The statistical significance for the outcome of survival benefit was not established ($P = 0.08$), but the study may have been underpowered. However, the reported results demonstrated a strong trend toward benefit, with a 35% reduction in relative risk and a 6% reduction in absolute risk during 2 years of follow-up. Subgroups with prolonged QRS durations, ejection fractions higher than 20%, and class III heart failure performed better than did the overall cohort data. SCD-HeFT was designed to test the potential benefit of

ICDs versus amiodarone and placebo in patients with functional class II or III congestive heart failure and ejection fractions lower than 35%. Nonischemic cardiomyopathy and ischemic cardiomyopathy were almost equally represented, with 85% of the patients with ischemic cardiomyopathy having a history of MI. The results of this study demonstrated a 23% reduction in relative risk and a 7% reduction in absolute risk during 5 years (Fig. 70.16). Amiodarone provided no added benefit over conventional therapy. In contrast to DEFINITE, the class II patients in SCD-HeFT had better outcomes than did the class III patients. In the Danish Study to Assess the Efficacy of ICDs in Patients with Non-ischaemic Heart Failure on Mortality (DANISH) trial, patients were randomized to receive an ICD or not.[181] Notably 58% of patients in both groups were treated with cardiac resynchronization therapy. No survival benefit was noted with an ICD. The cumulative data do support the efficacy of the ICD in this patient population.[182] However, demonstration of efficacy is not the same as demonstration that a strategy is optimal or efficient.

Primary Prevention in Patients With Less Advanced Common Heart Diseases or Uncommon Diseases. Primary prevention trials have been designed to enroll populations of patients with advanced heart disease who were estimated to be at very high risk for SCD and total mortality as a consequence of the severity of the underlying disease. Most clinical trials testing the question of the relative efficacy of antiarrhythmic versus ICD therapy have used the ejection fraction as the marker for advanced disease, with the upper limits of qualifying ejection fractions being between 30% and 40% and the majority set at 35%. The mean or median values of those actually enrolled ranged from 21% to 30%, and subgroups with ejection fractions higher than 30%, particularly those in the range of 35% to 40%, had lower if any benefit.

Although the risk for SCD and total mortality is highest in patients with advanced structural heart disease, characterized by low ejection fractions, impaired functional capacity, or both, a substantial proportion of the total SCD burden occurs in patients with coronary heart disease or the various nonischemic cardiomyopathies with ejection fractions between 35% and 40% and higher.[48] In the Pre-DETERMINE cohort of patients with established coronary artery disease without an indication for ICD, adjudicated sudden or arrhythmic death accounted for 56% of all cardiac deaths, with a 4-year cumulative incidence of 2.1%. Moderately reduced ejection fraction, heart failure severity, and age distinguished sudden arrhythmic death from nonsudden arrhythmic death. Clinical subgroups could be identified with differing profiles of total and proportional risk for sudden arrhythmic death which could be used as a guide for future risk profiling and intervention. In addition, in patients with heart failure related to various forms of cardiomyopathy, even though the total mortality risk is considerably lower in patients with functional class I or early class II than in those with late class III or class IV status, the probability of a death being sudden is higher in the former group. Despite this observation, no data are available to guide therapy for primary prevention of cardiac arrest in such patients. This limitation is confounded by the fact that patients in these categories generally have low event rates but cumulatively account for large numbers of SCD (see Fig. 70.2A and B). In addition, certain other structural entities associated with some elevation in risk for SCD in the absence of a severely reduced ejection fraction, such as some patterns of viral myocarditis, HCM, right ventricular dysplasia, and sarcoidosis, are managed without the benefit of clinical trials to guide therapeutic decisions (see Table 69.4). Patients with symptomatic ventricular arrhythmias related to structural disorders such as right ventricular dysplasia, in which most of the mortality risk is arrhythmic, are often advised to have an ICD, even in the absence of a previous cardiac arrest or hemodynamically significant VT. Whether antiarrhythmic therapy would be just as effective remains unknown, but the judgement of using defibrillators in patients with a disorder whose fatal expression is primarily arrhythmic carries the strength of logic, often supported by risk profiling based on observational data of clinical markers. Among the entities in which the family history is helpful in defining risk, clinical judgment is made easier in patients with a strong family history of SCD. Specific support for this approach is derived from genetic studies of individuals with HCM. In addition, clinical observational data have supported the use of ICDs in high-risk subsets of patients with HCM.

Primary Prevention in Patients with Structurally Normal Hearts or Molecular Disorders of Cardiac Electrical Activity

Clinically subtle or unapparent structural disorders and entities with pure electrophysiologic expression, such as the congenital long-QT syndromes, Brugada syndrome, and idiopathic VF, are receiving increasing attention with regard to preventive activities (see Chapter 63).[83] No randomized clinical trials evaluating the utility of ICDs in these patients have been performed, but there is some evidence of efficacy.[183]

The decision-making process for cardiac arrest or symptomatic VT survivors with long-QT syndrome is similar to that for other entities in that those who have survived a potentially fatal arrhythmia are generally treated with ICDs (see Table 70.5). In contrast, individuals who express the electrocardiographic phenotype of long-QT syndrome in the absence of symptomatic arrhythmias are generally

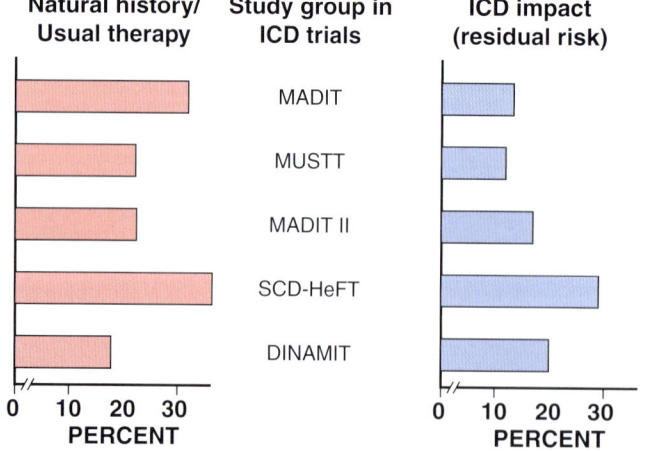

FIGURE 70.16 A, Relative and absolute benefits of ICDs in three ICD trials: a secondary prevention study (AVID) trial, a primary prevention trial (MADIT II), and a heart failure sudden death trial (SCD-HeFT); see text for definitions and trial descriptions. Relative risk reductions indicate proportional differences in outcomes between test and control populations, absolute reductions indicate proportional benefits for individuals, and residual risks indicate mortality remaining after accounting for ICD benefits. **B,** Residual risk after accounting for ICD-associated survival benefit in five major primary prevention ICD clinical trials. (**A** modified from Myerburg RJ, et al. Interpretation of outcomes of antiarrhythmic clinical trials: design features and population impact. Circulation 1998;97:1514.)

treated with beta blocker therapy. Beta blockers are also considered useful for affected family members who have not had an event and for subgroups of long-QT patients with syncope of undocumented mechanism. Between these extremes are asymptomatic affected family members of patients with symptomatic long-QT syndrome. The threshold for consideration of ICD therapy is decreasing, primarily among carriers who breakthrough with symptoms while on beta blocker therapy. Currently, many such clinical therapeutic decisions remain based on judgment rather than driven by data (see Chapter 63). QTc intervals ≥550 msec and syncope while on beta blocker therapy have been shown to be predictors of appropriate ICD shocks.[184]

Among the other molecular arrhythmia syndromes, Brugada syndrome is one for which management strategies remain problematic and debated.[83,86] An ICD is accepted as the secondary prevention strategy in SCA survivors and primary prevention therapy in symptomatic patients with type I Brugada patterns, even though it is based largely on observational data. Studies have suggested that syncope associated with electrocardiographic changes suggestive of the disorder at baseline is a marker of risk sufficient to warrant ICD therapy and that baseline electrocardiographic changes associated with inducibility of ventricular tachyarrhythmias during electrophysiologic testing may also be a marker of risk in some subgroups, although this remains debated. However, a family history of SCD is often considered in judgment-based decisions. Similar arguments, but supported by even fewer data, apply to affected family members of patients with right ventricular dysplasia.

Prediction and Primary Prevention in the General Population

Because SCD is frequently the first clinical expression of underlying structural heart disease or occurs in identified patients profiled to be at low risk (see Fig. 70.2B), there has been longstanding interest in risk profiling and therapeutic strategies targeted to primary prevention. To have a major impact on the problem of SCD in the general population, including adolescents and young adults, we need to move beyond the identification of high-risk patients who have specific clinical entities, advanced or subtle, that predict high risk for SCD. Rather, it is necessary to find small subgroups of patients in the general population at specific risk for SCD as a manifestation of underlying heart disease, if and when that disease becomes manifested. As an example, studies that have demonstrated familial clustering of SCD as the first expression of underlying coronary artery disease and thus suggesting a genetic or behavioral predisposition may provide some help for the future. If highly specific markers related to electrophysiologic properties or along multiple points in the cascade of coronary events (see Fig. 70.5) can be found, preventive therapy before the first expression of an underlying disease may have a major effect on the population burden of SCD. Short of that, successes will be limited to community-based intervention and to subgroups that are easier to identify and in whom it is more justifiable to use prophylactic interventional therapy on the basis of population size and magnitude of risk.

The clinical risk score developed in ARIC and validated in the Framingham study[17] has been implemented in the electronic health record to evaluate risk of SCD among 36,885 primary care patients. Those in the low SCD risk category (deciles 1 to 4) had a mean age of 55.3 ± 11.3 years, 65% were female, 35% were Hispanic, 60% had hypertension, and 65% had diabetes. Those in deciles 9 to 10 (highest risk) were 71.0 ± 9.8 years of age, 91% male, 32% Hispanic, 88% had hypertension, and 91% had diabetes. Among the 7256 patients who were classified in the highest SCD risk category (deciles 9 to 10), these patients were seen frequently by a primary care physician (82%), but only 35% were seen by a cardiologist, 36% had an echocardiogram, and 18% had a stress test. It is interesting to note that patients at the highest risk of SCD without known heart disease actually have a significant burden of occult heart disease, including late gadolinium enhancement, abnormal heart rate recovery after exercise, and pathogenic SNPs related to cardiomyopathy and/or arrhythmias.[19] This presents a potential pathway to identify high risk subgroups that may benefit from some intervention.

Adolescents and young adults, including athletes (see Chapter 32), constitute a group for special consideration. Risk for SCD in these groups is approximately 1% of the risk in the general adult population older than 35 years (see Fig. 70.3).[57] However, most causes of SCD in these populations are not characterized by advanced life-limiting structural heart disease, and therefore surviving cardiac arrest victims can, with appropriate long-term therapy, be expected to have significant extensions of life. Because most deaths are arrhythmic, the ability to identify individuals at risk in advance of a life-threatening arrhythmic event offers more long-term impact than in older populations. For both the general young population and athletes, identification of individuals at risk may lead to prevention of events triggered by physical activity. One study has demonstrated a reduction in SCDs in athletes with the use of widespread electrocardiographic screening. In the United States, strategies for screening of adolescents, young adults, and athletes to identify entities that create risk have largely been limited to medical and family histories and physical examination, although a consensus statement spearheaded by the NCAA has taken a more permissive position on ECG screening.[185] The European and the International Olympic Committee recommendations add electrocardiographic screening for athletes, which continues to be debated in the United States despite data indicating both feasibility and suggestions of cost-effectiveness. Electrocardiographic screening of the general adolescent population, including athletes, can identify many of those at potential risk because of congenital long-QT syndrome, HCM, right ventricular dysplasia, and Brugada syndrome. In Japan, where ECG screening of first and seventh grade school children is routine, the apparent incidence of LQT is considerably higher than recognized in the United States and Europe—1/3298 first graders and 1/988 by the seventh grade versus 1/2000 to 2500 in the general population elsewhere.[36] Although electrocardiographic screening in the adolescent and athletic subgroups is imperfect and usually accompanied by depolarization and repolarization patterns that may be difficult to interpret, this strategy can lead to further testing in appropriate individuals. Echocardiography has also been suggested as a screening method, but it is more expensive and less cost-efficient and does not recognize conditions such as long-QT syndrome and Brugada syndrome.

Risk for SCD must be evaluated in competitive athletes with previously known cardiovascular disorders or those discovered during preparticipation screening, as well as in those with known disorders who wish to participate in recreational sports. Recommendations for competitive athletes, based on the intensity of exercise,[186] the nature of the diseases,[75,187] response strategies,[188] and legal considerations,[189] are available; issues for recreational athletes are more complex because of absence of organizational infrastructures in most instances.

SUDDEN DEATH AND PUBLIC SAFETY

The unexpectedness of SCD has raised questions concerning secondary risk to the public created by people in the throes of cardiac arrest. No data from controlled studies are available to guide public policy regarding people at high risk for potentially lethal arrhythmias and for abrupt incapacitation. In a report of observations on 1348 sudden deaths caused by coronary heart disease in people 65 years or younger during a 7-year period in Dade County, FL, 101 (7.5%) of the deaths occurred in people who were engaged in activities at the time of death that were potentially hazardous to the public (e.g., driving a motor vehicle, working at altitude, piloting aircraft), and 122 (9.1%) of the victims had occupations that could create potential hazards to others if an abrupt loss of consciousness had occurred while they were at work. No catastrophic events occurred as a result of these cardiac arrests.

In specific reference to private automobiles, a study from Seattle identified 33 SCDs per year while driving the estimated 1.32 million vehicles in the community. An analysis of recurrent events in cardiac arrest survivors has suggested limitation of driving privileges for the first 8 months after the index event on the basis of the clustering of recurrent event rates early after the index event. Therefore, although there are likely to be isolated cases in which cardiac arrest causes public hazards, the risk appears to be small, and because it is difficult to identify specific individuals at risk, sweeping restrictions to avoid such risks appear to be unwarranted. The exceptions are people with multisystem disease, particularly senility, and individual circumstances that require specific consideration, such as patients with documented or substantial risk for loss of consciousness associated with the onset of arrhythmias and high-risk patients who have special responsibilities—school bus drivers, aircraft pilots, train operators, and truck drivers.

Among patients with primary prevention ICD implants, it was originally suggested that driving be avoided for 6 months postimplant, but a revision of the recommendations had reduced that to 1 week or more, depending on individual circumstances. Once a therapy has been delivered, the posttherapy guideline of up to 6 months still prevails, again with modification based on individual circumstances and preshock symptoms. Studies of temporal patterns of recurrent ICD shock therapies identified an acceleration of time to recurrent events after a first event has occurred, but with an overall low rate, an observation that may have implications for driving depending on associated symptoms in individual patients.[190,191]

REFERENCES

Perspectives/Definition

1. Berg KM, Cheng A, Panchal AR, et al. Part 7: systems of care: 2020 American Heart Association guidelines for cardiopulmonary resuscitation and emergency cardiovascular care. *Circulation*. 2020;142:S580–S604.
2. Virani SS, Alonso A, Benjamin EJ, et al. Heart disease and stroke statistics-2020 update: a report from the American Heart Association. *Circulation*. 2020;141:e139–e596.
3. Kolte D, Khera S, Aronow WS, et al. Regional variation in the incidence and outcomes of in-hospital cardiac arrest in the United States. *Circulation*. 2015;131:1415–1425.
4. Myerburg RJ, Goldberg JJ. Cardiac arrest and sudden cardiac death. In: Zipes DP, et al., ed. *Braunwald's Heart Disease*. 11 ed. Philadelphia: Elsevier; 2019.
5. Tseng ZH, Olgin JE, Vittinghoff E, et al. Prospective countywide surveillance and autopsy characterization of sudden cardiac death: post scd study. *Circulation*. 2018;137:2689–2700.

Epidemiology

6. Myerburg RJ, Goldberger JJ. Sudden cardiac arrest risk assessment: population science and the individual risk mandate. *JAMA Cardiol*. 2017;2:689–694.
7. Wong CX, Brown A, Lau DH, et al. Epidemiology of sudden cardiac death: global and regional perspectives. *Heart Lung Circ*. 2019;28:6–14.
8. Myerburg RJ, GJJ. Sudden cardiac arrest/death in adults. In: Zipes DP, Jalife J, Stevenson WG, eds. *Cardiac Electrophysiology: from Cell to Bedside*. 7th ed. Philadelphia, PA: Elsevier; 2018:937–948.
9. Virani SS, Alonso A, Aparicio HJ, et al. Heart disease and stroke statistics-2021 update: a report from the American Heart Association. *Circulation*. 2021;143:e254–e743.
10. Huikuri HV, Castellanos A, Myerburg RJ. Sudden death due to cardiac arrhythmias. *N Engl J Med*. 2001;345:1473–1482.
11. Shen L, Jhund PS, Petrie MC, et al. Declining risk of sudden death in heart failure. *N Engl J Med*. 2017;377:41–51.
12. Hayashi M, Shimizu W, Albert CM. The spectrum of epidemiology underlying sudden cardiac death. *Circ Res*. 2015;116:1887–1906.
13. Junttila MJ, Hookana E, Kaikkonen KS, et al. Temporal trends in the clinical and pathological characteristics of victims of sudden cardiac death in the absence of previously identified heart disease. *Circ Arrhythm Electrophysiol*. 2016;9.
14. Myerburg RJ, Ullmann SG. Alternative research funding to improve clinical outcomes: model of prediction and prevention of sudden cardiac death. *Circ Arrhythm Electrophysiol*. 2015;8:492–498.
15. Aro AL, Reinier K, Rusinaru C, et al. Electrical risk score beyond the left ventricular ejection fraction: prediction of sudden cardiac death in the Oregon sudden unexpected death study and the atherosclerosis risk in communities study. *Eur Heart J*. 2017;38:3017–3025.
16. Deo R, Norby FL, Katz R, et al. Development and validation of a sudden cardiac death prediction model for the general population. *Circulation*. 2016;134:806–816.
17. Bogle BM, Ning H, Goldberger JJ, et al. A simple community-based risk-prediction score for sudden cardiac death. *Am J Med*. 2018;131:532-539.e535.
18. Olson KA, Patel RB, Ahmad FS, et al. Sudden cardiac death risk distribution in the United States population (from nhanes, 2005 to 2012). *Am J Cardiol*. 2019;123:1249–1254.
19. Tamariz L, Palacio A, Myerburg R, et al. Asymptomatic patients without known heart disease have markers of occult heart disease. *Am J Cardiol*. 2020;125:1449–1450.
20. Jayaraman R, Reinier K, Nair S, et al. Risk factors of sudden cardiac death in the young: multiple-year community-wide assessment. *Circulation*. 2018;137:1561–1570.
21. Farioli A, Christophi CA, Quarta CC, et al. Incidence of sudden cardiac death in a young active population. *J Am Heart Assoc*. 2015;4:e001818.
22. Kang SH, Oh IY, Heo J, et al. Heat, heat waves, and out-of-hospital cardiac arrest. *Int J Cardiol*. 2016;221:232–237.
23. Onozuka D, Hagihara A. Extreme temperature and out-of-hospital cardiac arrest in Japan: a nationwide, retrospective, observational study. *Sci Total Environ*. 2017;575:258–264.
24. Abdelsayed M, Peters CH, Ruben PC. Differential thermosensitivity in mixed syndrome cardiac sodium channel mutants. *J Physiol*. 2015;593:4201–4223.
25. Dai J, Chen R, Meng X, et al. Ambient air pollution, temperature and out-of-hospital coronary deaths in Shanghai, China. *Environ Pollut*. 2015;203:116–121.
26. Zhao R, Chen S, Wang W, et al. The impact of short-term exposure to air pollutants on the onset of out-of-hospital cardiac arrest: a systematic review and meta-analysis. *Int J Cardiol*. 2017;226:110–117.
27. Folino F, Buja G, Zanotto G, et al. Association between air pollution and ventricular arrhythmias in high-risk patients (aria study): a multicentre longitudinal study. *Lancet Planet Health*. 2017;1:e58–e64.
28. Holmberg MJ, Ross CE, Fitzmaurice GM, et al. Annual incidence of adult and pediatric in-hospital cardiac arrest in the United States. *Circ Cardiovasc Qual Outcomes*. 2019;12:e005580.
29. Bagnall RD, Weintraub RG, Ingles J, et al. A prospective study of sudden cardiac death among children and young adults. *N Engl J Med*. 2016;374:2441–2452.
30. Deo R, Safford MM, Khodneva YA, et al. Differences in risk of sudden cardiac death between blacks and whites. *J Am Coll Cardiol*. 2018;72:2431–2439.
31. Zhao D, Post WS, Blasco-Colmenares E, et al. Racial differences in sudden cardiac death. *Circulation*. 2019;139:1688–1697.
32. Bogle BM, Ning H, Mehrotra S, et al. Lifetime risk for sudden cardiac death in the community. *J Am Heart Assoc*. 2016;5.
33. Haukilahti MAE, Holmstrom L, Vahatalo J, et al. Sudden cardiac death in women. *Circulation*. 2019;139:1012–1021.
34. Bezzina CR, Lahrouchi N, Priori SG. Genetics of sudden cardiac death. *Circ Res*. 2015;116:1919–1936.
35. Schwartz PJ, Crotti L, George Jr AL. Modifier genes for sudden cardiac death. *Eur Heart J*. 2018;39:3925–3931.
36. Yoshinaga M, Kucho Y, Nishibatake M, et al. Probability of diagnosing long QT syndrome in children and adolescents according to the criteria of the HRS/EHRA/APHRS expert consensus statement. *Eur Heart J*. 2016;37:2490–2497.
37. Myerburg RJ. Electrocardiographic screening of children and adolescents: the search for hidden risk. *Eur Heart J*. 2016;37:2498–2501.
38. Tamariz L, Balda J, Pareja D, et al. Usefulness of single nucleotide polymorphisms as predictors of sudden cardiac death. *Am J Cardiol*. 2019;123:1900–1905.
39. Deyell MW, Krahn AD, Goldberger JJ. Sudden cardiac death risk stratification. *Circ Res*. 2015;116:1907–1918.
40. Grani C, Benz DC, Gupta S, et al. Sudden cardiac death in ischemic heart disease: from imaging arrhythmogenic substrate to guiding therapies. *JACC Cardiovasc Imaging*. 2020;13:2223–2238.
41. Halliday BP, Cleland JGF, Goldberger JJ, et al. Personalizing risk stratification for sudden death in dilated cardiomyopathy: the past, present, and future. *Circulation*. 2017;136:215–231.
42. Ommen SR, Mital S, Burke MA, et al. 2020 AHA/ACC guideline for the diagnosis and treatment of patients with hypertrophic cardiomyopathy: a report of the American College of Cardiology/American Heart Association joint committee on clinical practice guidelines. *J Am Coll Cardiol*. 2020;76:e159–e240.
43. Bilchick KC, Wang Y, Cheng A, et al. Seattle heart failure and proportional risk models predict benefit from implantable cardioverter-defibrillators. *J Am Coll Cardiol*. 2017;69:2606–2618.
44. Whitman IR, Agarwal V, Nah G, et al. Alcohol abuse and cardiac disease. *J Am Coll Cardiol*. 2017;69:13–24.
45. Adabag S, Huxley RR, Lopez FL, et al. Obesity related risk of sudden cardiac death in the atherosclerosis risk in communities study. *Heart*. 2015;101:215–221.
46. Harmon KG, Asif IM, Maleszewski JJ, et al. Incidence, cause, and comparative frequency of sudden cardiac death in national collegiate athletic association athletes: a decade in review. *Circulation*. 2015;132:10–19.
47. Chan C, Daly M, Melton I, et al. Two major earthquakes in Christchurch were not associated with increased ventricular arrhythmias: analysis of implanted defibrillator diagnostics. *PloS One*. 2019;14:e0216521.
48. Chatterjee NA, Moorthy MV, Pester J, et al. Sudden death in patients with coronary heart disease without severe systolic dysfunction. *JAMA Cardiol*. 2018;3:591–600.
49. Disertori M, Rigoni M, Pace N, et al. Myocardial fibrosis assessment by lge is a powerful predictor of ventricular tachyarrhythmias in ischemic and nonischemic LV dysfunction: a meta-analysis. *JACC Cardiovasc Imaging*. 2016;9:1046–1055.
50. Ganesan AN, Gunton J, Nucifora G, et al. Impact of late gadolinium enhancement on mortality, sudden death and major adverse cardiovascular events in ischemic and nonischemic cardiomyopathy: a systematic review and meta-analysis. *Int J Cardiol*. 2018;254:230–237.
51. Halliday BP, Gulati A, Ali A, et al. Association between midwall late gadolinium enhancement and sudden cardiac death in patients with dilated cardiomyopathy and mild and moderate left ventricular systolic dysfunction. *Circulation*. 2017;135:2106–2115.

Causes of Sudden Death

52. Herrington W, Lacey B, Sherliker P, et al. Epidemiology of atherosclerosis and the potential to reduce the global burden of atherothrombotic disease. *Circ Res*. 2016;118:535–546.
53. Brothers JA, Frommelt MA, Jaquiss RDB, et al. Expert consensus guidelines: anomalous aortic origin of a coronary artery. *J Thorac Cardiovasc Surg*. 2017;153:1440–1457.
54. Shenasa M, Shenasa H. Hypertension, left ventricular hypertrophy, and sudden cardiac death. *Int J Cardiol*. 2017;237:60–63.
55. Adamczak DM, Oko-Sarnowska Z. Sudden cardiac death in hypertrophic cardiomyopathy. *Cardiol Rev*. 2018;26:145–151.
56. Ha FJ, Han HC, Sanders P, et al. Sudden cardiac death in the young: incidence, trends, and risk factors in a nationwide study. *Circ Cardiovasc Qual Outcomes*. 2020;13:e006470.
57. Ackerman M, Atkins DL, Triedman JK. Sudden cardiac death in the young. *Circulation*. 2016;133:1006–1026.
58. Manrai AK, Funke BH, Rehm HL, et al. Genetic misdiagnoses and the potential for health disparities. *N Engl J Med*. 2016;375:655–665.
59. Maron BJ, Maron MS. Contemporary strategies for risk stratification and prevention of sudden death with the implantable defibrillator in hypertrophic cardiomyopathy. *Heart Rhythm*. 2016;13:1155–1165.
60. Vaduganathan M, Patel RB, Michel A, et al. Mode of death in heart failure with preserved ejection fraction. *J Am Coll Cardiol*. 2017;69:556–569.
61. van Veldhuisen DJ, van Woerden G, Gorter TM, et al. Ventricular tachyarrhythmia detection by implantable loop recording in patients with heart failure and preserved ejection fraction: the VIP-HF study. *Eur J Heart Fail*. 2020;22:1923–1929.
62. Wahbi K, Ben Yaou R, Gandjbakhch E, et al. Development and validation of a new risk prediction score for life-threatening ventricular tachyarrhythmias in laminopathies. *Circulation*. 2019;140:293–302.
63. Clark DE, Parikh A, Dendy JM, et al. COVID-19 myocardial pathology evaluation in athletes with cardiac magnetic resonance (compete cmr). *Circulation*. 2021;143:609–612.
64. Martinez MW, Tucker AM, Bloom OJ, et al. Prevalence of inflammatory heart disease among professional athletes with prior COVID-19 infection who received systematic return-to-play cardiac screening. *JAMA Cardiol*. 2021.
65. Puntmann VO, Carerj ML, Wieters I, et al. Outcomes of cardiovascular magnetic resonance imaging in patients recently recovered from coronavirus disease 2019 (covid-19). *JAMA Cardiol*. 2020;5:1265–1273.
66. Rajpal S, Tong MS, Borchers J, et al. Cardiovascular magnetic resonance findings in competitive athletes recovering from COVID-19 infection. *JAMA Cardiol*. 2021;6:116–118.
67. Starekova J, Bluemke DA, Bradham WS, et al. Evaluation for myocarditis in competitive student athletes recovering from coronavirus disease 2019 with cardiac magnetic resonance imaging. *JAMA Cardiol*. 2021.
68. Ammirati E, Frigerio M, Adler ED, et al. Management of acute myocarditis and chronic inflammatory cardiomyopathy: an expert consensus document. *Circ Heart Fail*. 2020;13:e007405.
69. Ekstrom K, Lehtonen J, Nordenswan HK, et al. Sudden death in cardiac sarcoidosis: an analysis of nationwide clinical and cause-of-death registries. *Eur Heart J*. 2019;40:3121–3128.
70. Birnie D, Ha A, Kron J. Which patients with cardiac sarcoidosis should receive implantable cardioverter-defibrillators: some answers but many questions remain. *Circ Arrhythm Electrophysiol*. 2018;11:e006685.
71. Kim EJ, Holmes BB, Huang S, et al. Outcomes in patients with cardiac amyloidosis and implantable cardioverter-defibrillator. *Europace*. 2020;22:1216–1223.
72. Calkins H, Corrado D, Marcus F. Risk stratification in arrhythmogenic right ventricular cardiomyopathy. *Circulation*. 2017;136:2068–2082.
73. Finocchiaro G, Papadakis M, Robertus JL, et al. Etiology of sudden death in sports: insights from a United Kingdom regional registry. *J Am Coll Cardiol*. 2016;67:2108–2115.

74. Gupta R, Tichnell C, Murray B, et al. Comparison of features of fatal versus nonfatal cardiac arrest in patients with arrhythmogenic right ventricular dysplasia/cardiomyopathy. *Am J Cardiol*. 2017;120:111–117.
75. Zipes DP, Link MS, Ackerman MJ, et al. Eligibility and disqualification recommendations for competitive athletes with cardiovascular abnormalities: task force 9: arrhythmias and conduction defects: a scientific statement from the American Heart Association and American College of Cardiology. *Circulation*. 2015;132. e315-325.
76. La Gerche A, Claessen G, Dymarkowski S, et al. Exercise-induced right ventricular dysfunction is associated with ventricular arrhythmias in endurance athletes. *Eur Heart J*. 2015;36:1998–2010.
77. Bhonsale A, Groeneweg JA, James CA, et al. Impact of genotype on clinical course in arrhythmogenic right ventricular dysplasia/cardiomyopathy-associated mutation carriers. *Eur Heart J*. 2015;36:847–855.
78. Taniguchi T, Morimoto T, Shiomi H, et al. Sudden death in patients with severe aortic stenosis: observations from the current as registry. *J Am Heart Assoc*. 2018;7:e008397.
79. Minners J, Rossebo A, Chambers JB, et al. Sudden cardiac death in asymptomatic patients with aortic stenosis. *Heart*. 2020;106:1646–1650.
80. Urena M, Webb JG, Eltchaninoff H, et al. Late cardiac death in patients undergoing transcatheter aortic valve replacement: incidence and predictors of advanced heart failure and sudden cardiac death. *J Am Coll Cardiol*. 2015;65:437–448.
81. Basso C, Iliceto S, Thiene G, et al. Mitral valve prolapse, ventricular arrhythmias, and sudden death. *Circulation*. 2019;140:952–964.
82. Fulton BL, Liang JJ, Enriquez A, et al. Imaging characteristics of papillary muscle site of origin of ventricular arrhythmias in patients with mitral valve prolapse. *J Cardiovasc Electrophysiol*. 2018;29:146–153.
83. Singh M, Morin DP, Link MS. Sudden cardiac death in long QT syndrome (LQTS), Brugada syndrome, and catecholaminergic polymorphic ventricular tachycardia (CPVT). *Prog Cardiovasc Dis*. 2019;62:227–234.
84. Myerburg RJ. Physiological variations, environmental factors, and genetic modifications in inherited LQT syndromes. *J Am Coll Cardiol*. 2015;65:375–377.
85. O'Neal WT, Singleton MJ, Roberts JD, et al. Association between QT-interval components and sudden cardiac death: the aric study (atherosclerosis risk in communities). *Circ Arrhythm Electrophysiol*. 2017;10.
86. Adler A, Rosso R, Chorin E, et al. Risk stratification in Brugada syndrome: clinical characteristics, electrocardiographic parameters, and auxiliary testing. *Heart Rhythm*. 2016;13:299–310.
87. Cheng YJ, Lin XX, Ji CC, et al. Role of early repolarization pattern in increasing risk of death. *J Am Heart Assoc*. 2016;5.
88. Fan J, Yao FJ, Cheng YJ, et al. Early repolarization pattern associated with coronary artery disease and increased the risk of cardiac death in acute myocardium infarction. *Ann Noninvasive Electrocardiol*. 2020;25:e12768.
89. Moon RY, Task Force On Sudden Infant Death S. SIDS and other sleep-related infant deaths: evidence base for 2016 updated recommendations for a safe infant sleeping environment. *Pediatrics*. 2016;138.
90. Sollazzo F, Palmieri V, Gervasi SF, et al. Sudden cardiac death in athletes in Italy during 2019: Internet-based epidemiological research. *Medicina (Kaunas)*. 2021;57.
91. Maron BJ, Haas TS, Ahluwalia A, et al. Demographics and epidemiology of sudden deaths in young competitive athletes: from the United States National Registry. *Am J Med*. 2016;129:1170–1177.
92. Marijon E, Uy-Evanado A, Reinier K, et al. Sudden cardiac arrest during sports activity in middle age. *Circulation*. 2015;131:1384–1391.
93. Pelliccia A, Solberg EE, Papadakis M, et al. Recommendations for participation in competitive and leisure time sport in athletes with cardiomyopathies, myocarditis, and pericarditis: position statement of the sport cardiology section of the European Association of Preventive Cardiology (EAPC). *Eur Heart J*. 2019;40:19–33.
94. Link MS, Estes 3rd NAM, Maron BJ. Eligibility and disqualification recommendations for competitive athletes with cardiovascular abnormalities: task force 13: commotio cordis: a scientific statement from the American Heart Association and American College of Cardiology. *J Am Coll Cardiol*. 2015;66:2439–2443.
95. Kim AS, Moffatt E, Ursell PC, et al. Sudden neurologic death masquerading as out-of-hospital sudden cardiac death. *Neurology*. 2016;87:1669–1673.
96. Heilbrunn E, Ssentongo P, Chinchilli VM, et al. Sudden death in individuals with obstructive sleep apnoea: protocol for a systematic review and meta-analysis. *BMJ Open*. 2020;10:e039774.

Pathology and Pathophysiology

97. Anderson JH, Tester DJ, Will ML, et al. Whole-exome molecular autopsy after exertion-related sudden unexplained death in the young. *Circ Cardiovasc Genet*. 2016;9:259–265.
98. Quenin P, Kyndt F, Mabo P, et al. Clinical yield of familial screening after sudden death in young subjects: the French experience. *Circ Arrhythm Electrophysiol*. 2017;10.
99. Vassalini M, Verzeletti A, Restori M, et al. An autopsy study of sudden cardiac death in persons aged 1-40 years in Brescia (Italy). *J Cardiovasc Med*. 2016;17:446–453.
100. Goldberger JJ, Arora R, Buckley U, et al. Autonomic nervous system dysfunction: JACC focus seminar. *J Am Coll Cardiol*. 2019;73:1189–1206.
101. Huang WA, Boyle NG, Vaseghi M. Cardiac innervation and the autonomic nervous system in sudden cardiac death. *Card Electrophysiol Clin*. 2017;9:665–679.
102. Li CY, Li YG. Cardiac sympathetic nerve sprouting and susceptibility to ventricular arrhythmias after myocardial infarction. *Cardiol Res Pract*. 2015;2015:698368.
103. Gardner RT, Ripplinger CM, Myles RC, et al. Molecular mechanisms of sympathetic remodeling and arrhythmias. *Circ Arrhythm Electrophysiol*. 2016;9:e001359.
104. Kurz MC, Schmicker RH, Leroux B, et al. Advanced vs. Basic life support in the treatment of out-of-hospital cardiopulmonary arrest in the resuscitation outcomes consortium. *Resuscitation*. 2018;128:132–137.
105. Pelliccia A, Sharma S, Gati S, et al. 2020 ESC guidelines on sports cardiology and exercise in patients with cardiovascular disease. *Eur Heart J*. 2021;42:17–96.
106. van der Weg K, Prinzen FW, Gorgels AP. Editor's choice- reperfusion cardiac arrhythmias and their relation to reperfusion-induced cell death. *Eur Heart J Acute Cardiovasc Care*. 2019;8:142–152.

Clinical Features of Patients With Cardiac Arrest

107. Chan PS, McNally B, Nallamothu BK, et al. Long-term outcomes among elderly survivors of out-of-hospital cardiac arrest. *J Am Heart Assoc*. 2016;5:e002924.
108. Merchant RM, Topjian AA, Panchal AR, et al. Part 1: executive summary: 2020 American Heart Association guidelines for cardiopulmonary resuscitation and emergency cardiovascular care. *Circulation*. 2020;142:S337–S357.
109. Shao F, Li CS, Liang LR, et al. Incidence and outcome of adult in-hospital cardiac arrest in Beijing, China. *Resuscitation*. 2016;102:51–56.
110. Hirlekar G, Karlsson T, Aune S, et al. Survival and neurological outcome in the elderly after in-hospital cardiac arrest. *Resuscitation*. 2017;118:101–106.
111. Kosmidou I, Embacher M, McAndrew T, et al. Early ventricular tachycardia or fibrillation in patients with ST elevation myocardial infarction undergoing primary percutaneous coronary intervention and impact on mortality and stent thrombosis (from the harmonizing outcomes with revascularization and stents in acute myocardial infarction trial). *Am J Cardiol*. 2017;120:1755–1760.
112. Takada T, Shishido K, Hayashi T, et al. Impact of late ventricular arrhythmias on cardiac mortality in patients with acute myocardial infarction. *J Interv Cardiol*. 2019;2019:5345178.
113. Nolan JP, Soar J, Cariou A, et al. European resuscitation council and European society of intensive care medicine guidelines for post-resuscitation care 2015: section 5 of the European resuscitation council guidelines for resuscitation 2015. *Resuscitation*. 2015;95:202–222.
114. Lascarrou JB, Merdji H, Le Gouge A, et al. Targeted temperature management for cardiac arrest with nonshockable rhythm. *N Engl J Med*. 2019;381:2327–2337.
115. Mellor G, Laksman ZWM, Tadros R, et al. Genetic testing in the evaluation of unexplained cardiac arrest: from the CASPER (cardiac arrest survivors with preserved ejection fraction registry). *Circ Cardiovasc Genet*. 2017;10.
116. Jozwiak M, Bougouin W, Geri G, et al. Post-resuscitation shock: recent advances in pathophysiology and treatment. *Ann Intensive Care*. 2020;10:170.
117. Bascom KE, Dziodzio J, Vasaiwala S, et al. Derivation and validation of the crest model for very early prediction of circulatory etiology death in patients without ST-segment-elevation myocardial infarction after cardiac arrest. *Circulation*. 2018;137:273–282.
118. Patel N, Patel NJ, Macon CJ, et al. Trends and outcomes of coronary angiography and percutaneous coronary intervention after out-of-hospital cardiac arrest associated with ventricular fibrillation or pulseless ventricular tachycardia. *JAMA Cardiol*. 2016;1:890–899.
119. Rodriguez AP, Badiye A, Lambrakos LK, et al. Refractory ventricular tachycardia storm associated with severe hypokalemia in fanconi syndrome. *Heart Rhythm Case Rep*. 2019;5:374–378.
120. Sawyer KN, Camp-Rogers TR, Kotini-Shah P, et al. Sudden cardiac arrest survivorship: a scientific statement from the American Heart Association. *Circulation*. 2020;141:e654–e685.
121. Sabbag A, Suleiman M, Laish-Farkash A, et al. Contemporary rates of appropriate shock therapy in patients who receive implantable device therapy in a real-world setting: from the Israeli ICD registry. *Heart Rhythm*. 2015;12:2426–2433.
122. Schaer B, Kuhne M, Reichlin T, et al. Incidence of and predictors for appropriate implantable cardioverter-defibrillator therapy in patients with a secondary preventive implantable cardioverter-defibrillator indication. *Europace*. 2016;18:227–231.

Management of Cardiac Arrest

123. Bobrow BJ, Spaite DW, Vadeboncoeur TF, et al. Implementation of a regional telephone cardiopulmonary resuscitation program and outcomes after out-of-hospital cardiac arrest. *JAMA Cardiol*. 2016;1:294–302.
124. Andelius L, Malta Hansen C, Lippert FK, et al. Smartphone activation of citizen responders to facilitate defibrillation in out-of-hospital cardiac arrest. *J Am Coll Cardiol*. 2020;76:43–53.
125. Cheng A, Nadkarni VM, Mancini MB, et al. Resuscitation education science: educational strategies to improve outcomes from cardiac arrest: a scientific statement from the American Heart Association. *Circulation*. 2018;138:e82–e122.
126. Ringh M, Rosenqvist M, Hollenberg J, et al. Mobile-phone dispatch of laypersons for CPR in out-of-hospital cardiac arrest. *N Engl J Med*. 2015;372:2316–2325.
127. Ofoma UR, Basnet S, Berger A, et al. Trends in survival after in-hospital cardiac arrest during nights and weekends. *J Am Coll Cardiol*. 2018;71:402–411.
128. Girotra S, van Diepen S, Nallamothu BK, et al. Regional variation in out-of-hospital cardiac arrest survival in the United States. *Circulation*. 2016;133:2159–2168.
129. van Diepen S, Girotra S, Abella BS, et al. Multistate 5-year initiative to improve care for out-of-hospital cardiac arrest: primary results from the Heart Rescue Project. *J Am Heart Assoc*. 2017;6.
130. Lim ZJ, Ponnapa Reddy M, Afroz A, et al. Incidence and outcome of out-of-hospital cardiac arrests in the COVID-19 era: a systematic review and meta-analysis. *Resuscitation*. 2020;157:248–258.
131. Uy-Evanado A, Chugh HS, Sargsyan A, et al. Out-of-hospital cardiac arrest response and outcomes during the COVID-19 pandemic. *JACC Clin Electrophysiol*. 2021;7:6–11.
132. Mitrani RD, Goldberger JJ. Cardiac arrests during the COVID-19 pandemic: the perfect storm. *JACC Clin Electrophysiol*. 2021;7:12–15.
133. Malta Hansen C, Kragholm K, Pearson DA, et al. Association of bystander and first-responder intervention with survival after out-of-hospital cardiac arrest in North Carolina, 2010-2013. *J Am Med Assoc*. 2015;314:255–264.
134. Nakahara S, Tomio J, Ichikawa M, et al. Association of bystander interventions with neurologically intact survival among patients with bystander-witnessed out-of-hospital cardiac arrest in Japan. *J Am Med Assoc*. 2015;314:247–254.
135. Fukuda T, Ohashi-Fukuda N, Matsubara T, et al. Association of initial rhythm with neurologically favorable survival in non-shockable out-of-hospital cardiac arrest without a bystander witness or bystander cardiopulmonary resuscitation. *Eur J Intern Med*. 2016;30:61–67.
136. Luo S, Zhang Y, Zhang W, et al. Prognostic significance of spontaneous shockable rhythm conversion in adult out-of-hospital cardiac arrest patients with initial non-shockable heart rhythms: a systematic review and meta-analysis. *Resuscitation*. 2017;121:1–8.
137. Ewy GA. Cardiocerebral and cardiopulmonary resuscitation - 2017 update. *Acute Med Surg*. 2017;4:227–234.
138. Riess ML. New developments in cardiac arrest management. *Adv Anesth*. 2016;34:29–46.
139. Pepe PE, Scheppke KA, Antevy PM, et al. Confirming the clinical safety and feasibility of a bundled methodology to improve cardiopulmonary resuscitation involving a head-up/torso-up chest compression technique. *Crit Care Med*. 2019;47:449–455.
140. Holmberg MJ, Vognsen M, Andersen MS, et al. Bystander automated external defibrillator use and clinical outcomes after out-of-hospital cardiac arrest: a systematic review and meta-analysis. *Resuscitation*. 2017;120:77–87.
141. Pollack RA, Brown SP, Rea T, et al. Impact of bystander automated external defibrillator use on survival and functional outcomes in shockable observed public cardiac arrests. *Circulation*. 2018;137:2104–2113.
142. Delhomme C, Njeim M, Varlet E, et al. Automated external defibrillator use in out-of-hospital cardiac arrest: current limitations and solutions. *Arch Cardiovasc Dis*. 2019;112:217–222.
143. Perkins GD, Ji C, Deakin CD, et al. A randomized trial of epinephrine in out-of-hospital cardiac arrest. *N Engl J Med*. 2018;379:711–721.
144. Ahn S, Kim YJ, Sohn CH, et al. Sodium bicarbonate on severe metabolic acidosis during prolonged cardiopulmonary resuscitation: a double-blind, randomized, placebo-controlled pilot study. *J Thorac Dis*. 2018;10:2295–2302.
145. Panchal AR, Bartos JA, Cabanas JG, et al. Part 3: adult basic and advanced life support: 2020 American Heart Association guidelines for cardiopulmonary resuscitation and emergency cardiovascular care. *Circulation*. 2020;142:S366-S468.
146. Kudenchuk PJ, Brown SP, Daya M, et al. Amiodarone, lidocaine, or placebo in out-of-hospital cardiac arrest. *N Engl J Med*. 2016;374:1711–1722.
147. Daya MR, Leroux BG, Dorian P, et al. Survival after intravenous versus intraosseous amiodarone, lidocaine, or placebo in out-of-hospital shock-refractory cardiac arrest. *Circulation*. 2020;141:188–198.
148. Jeejeebhoy FM, Zelop CM, Lipman S, et al. Cardiac arrest in pregnancy: a scientific statement from the American Heart Association. *Circulation*. 2015;132:1747–1773.
149. Hai JJ, Un KC, Wong CK, et al. Prognostic implications of early monomorphic and non-monomorphic tachyarrhythmias in patients discharged with acute coronary syndrome. *Heart Rhythm*. 2018;15:822–829.
150. Bernard SA, Smith K, Finn J, et al. Induction of therapeutic hypothermia during out-of-hospital cardiac arrest using a rapid infusion of cold saline: the rinse trial (rapid infusion of cold normal saline). *Circulation*. 2016;134:797–805.

151. Al-Khatib SM, Stevenson WG, Ackerman MJ, et al. 2017 AHA/ACC/HRS guideline for management of patients with ventricular arrhythmias and the prevention of sudden cardiac death: executive summary: a report of the American College of Cardiology/American Heart Association task force on clinical practice guidelines and the heart rhythm society. *Circulation.* 2018;138:e210–e271.

Prevention of Cardiac Arrest and Sudden Cardiac Death

152. Fernandes GC, Fernandes A, Cardoso R, et al. Association of SGLT2 inhibitors with arrhythmias and sudden cardiac death in patients with type 2 diabetes or heart failure: a meta-analysis of 34 randomized controlled trials. *Heart Rhythm.* 2021.
153. Claro JC, Candia R, Rada G, et al. Amiodarone versus other pharmacological interventions for prevention of sudden cardiac death. *Cochrane Database Syst Rev.* 2015:CD008093.
154. Gatzoulis KA, Tsiachris D, Arsenos P, et al. Arrhythmic risk stratification in post-myocardial infarction patients with preserved ejection fraction: the preserve ef study. *Eur Heart J.* 2019;40:2940–2949.
155. Bui AH, Waks JW. Risk stratification of sudden cardiac death after acute myocardial infarction. *J Innov Card Rhythm Manag.* 2018;9:3035–3049.
156. Brooks GC, Lee BK, Rao R, et al. Predicting persistent left ventricular dysfunction following myocardial infarction: the predicts study. *J Am Coll Cardiol.* 2016;67:1186–1196.
157. Katritsis DG, Zografos T, Hindricks G. Electrophysiology testing for risk stratification of patients with ischaemic cardiomyopathy: a call for action. *Europace.* 2018;20:f148–f152.
158. Zaman S, Taylor AJ, Stiles M, et al. Programmed ventricular stimulation to risk stratify for early cardioverter-defibrillator implantation to prevent tachyarrhythmias following acute myocardial infarction (protect-icd): trial protocol, background and significance. *Heart Lung Circ.* 2016;25:1055–1062.
159. Selvanayagam JB, Hartshorne T, Billot L, et al. Cardiovascular magnetic resonance-guided management of mild to moderate left ventricular systolic dysfunction (CMR guide): study protocol for a randomized controlled trial. *Ann Noninvasive Electrocardiol.* 2017;22.
160. Di Marco A, Anguera I, Schmitt M, et al. Late gadolinium enhancement and the risk for ventricular arrhythmias or sudden death in dilated cardiomyopathy: systematic review and meta-analysis. *JACC Heart Fail.* 2017;5:28–38.
161. Balaban G, Halliday BP, Porter B, et al. Late-gadolinium enhancement interface area and electrophysiological simulations predict arrhythmic events in patients with nonischemic dilated cardiomyopathy. *JACC Clin Electrophysiol.* 2021;7:238–249.
162. Freitas P, Ferreira AM, Arteaga-Fernandez E, et al. The amount of late gadolinium enhancement outperforms current guideline-recommended criteria in the identification of patients with hypertrophic cardiomyopathy at risk of sudden cardiac death. *J Cardiovasc Magn Reson.* 2019;21:50.
163. Weng Z, Yao J, Chan RH, et al. Prognostic value of LGE-CMR in HCM: a meta-analysis. *JACC Cardiovasc Imaging.* 2016;9:1392–1402.
164. Dhindsa DS, Khambhati J, Sandesara PB, et al. Biomarkers to predict cardiovascular death. *Card Electrophysiol Clin.* 2017;9:651–664.
165. Everett BM, Moorthy MV, Tikkanen JT, et al. Markers of myocardial stress, myocardial injury, and subclinical inflammation and the risk of sudden death. *Circulation.* 2020;142:1148–1158.
166. Elagizi A, Lavie CJ, Marshall K, et al. Omega-3 polyunsaturated fatty acids and cardiovascular health: a comprehensive review. *Prog Cardiovasc Dis.* 2018;61:76–85.
167. Kaab S. Genetics of sudden cardiac death - an epidemiologic perspective. *Int J Cardiol.* 2017;237:42–44.
168. Jabbari R, Engstrom T, Glinge C, et al. Incidence and risk factors of ventricular fibrillation before primary angioplasty in patients with first ST-elevation myocardial infarction: a nationwide study in Denmark. *J Am Heart Assoc.* 2015;4:e001399.
169. Ashar FN, Mitchell RN, Albert CM, et al. A comprehensive evaluation of the genetic architecture of sudden cardiac arrest. *Eur Heart J.* 2018;39:3961–3969.
170. Huertas-Vazquez A, Nelson CP, Sinsheimer JS, et al. Cumulative effects of common genetic variants on risk of sudden cardiac death. *Int J Cardiol Heart Vasc.* 2015;7:88–91.
171. Hernesniemi JA, Lyytikainen LP, Oksala N, et al. Predicting sudden cardiac death using common genetic risk variants for coronary artery disease. *Eur Heart J.* 2015;36:1669–1675.
172. Sapp JL, Wells GA, Parkash R, et al. Ventricular tachycardia ablation versus escalation of antiarrhythmic drugs. *N Engl J Med.* 2016;375:111–121.
173. Gianni C, Burkhardt JD, Trivedi C, et al. The role of the purkinje network in premature ventricular complex-triggered ventricular fibrillation. *J Interv Card Electrophysiol.* 2018;52:375–383.
174. Haissaguerre M, Duchateau J, Dubois R, et al. Idiopathic ventricular fibrillation: role of purkinje system and microstructural myocardial abnormalities. *JACC Clin Electrophysiol.* 2020;6:591–608.
175. Nogami A. Mapping and ablating ventricular premature contractions that trigger ventricular fibrillation: trigger elimination and substrate modification. *J Cardiovasc Electrophysiol.* 2015;26:110–115.
176. Borne RT, Katz D, Betz J, et al. Implantable cardioverter-defibrillators for secondary prevention of sudden cardiac death: a review. *J Am Heart Assoc.* 2017;6.
177. Katz DF, Peterson P, Borne RT, et al. Survival after secondary prevention implantable cardioverter-defibrillator placement: an analysis from the NCDR ICD registry. *JACC Clin Electrophysiol.* 2017;3:20–28.
178. Lee DS, Hardy J, Yee R, et al. Clinical risk stratification for primary prevention implantable cardioverter defibrillators. *Circ Heart Fail.* 2015;8:927–937.
179. Merchant FM, Levy WC, Kramer DB. Time to shock the system: moving beyond the current paradigm for primary prevention implantable cardioverter-defibrillator use. *J Am Heart Assoc.* 2020;9:e015139.
180. Younis A, Goldberger JJ, Kutyifa V, et al. Predicted benefit of an implantable cardioverter-defibrillator: the MADIT-ICD benefit score. *Eur Heart J.* 2021;42:1676–1684.
181. Kober L, Thune JJ, Nielsen JC, et al. Defibrillator implantation in patients with nonischemic systolic heart failure. *N Engl J Med.* 2016;375:1221–1230.
182. Pathak RK, Sanders P, Deo R. Primary prevention implantable cardioverter-defibrillator and opportunities for sudden cardiac death risk assessment in non-ischaemic cardiomyopathy. *Eur Heart J.* 2018;39:2859–2866.
183. McNamara DA, Goldberger JJ, Berendsen MA, et al. Implantable defibrillators versus medical therapy for cardiac channelopathies. *Cochrane Database Syst Rev.* 2015:CD011168.
184. Biton Y, Rosero S, Moss AJ, et al. Primary prevention with the implantable cardioverter-defibrillator in high-risk long-QT syndrome patients. *Europace.* 2019;21:339–346.
185. Hainline B, Drezner JA, Baggish A, et al. Interassociation consensus statement on cardiovascular care of college student-athletes. *J Am Coll Cardiol.* 2016;67:2981–2995.
186. Levine BD, Baggish AL, Kovacs RJ, et al. Eligibility and disqualification recommendations for competitive athletes with cardiovascular abnormalities: task force 1: classification of sports: dynamic, static, and impact: a scientific statement from the American Heart Association and American College of Cardiology. *Circulation.* 2015;132:e262-266.
187. Maron BJ, Zipes DP, Kovacs RJ, et al. Eligibility and disqualification recommendations for competitive athletes with cardiovascular abnormalities: preamble, principles, and general considerations: a scientific statement from the American Heart Association and American College of Cardiology. *Circulation.* 2015;132:e256–261.
188. Link MS, Myerburg RJ, Estes 3rd NA, et al. Eligibility and disqualification recommendations for competitive athletes with cardiovascular abnormalities: task force 12: emergency action plans, resuscitation, cardiopulmonary resuscitation, and automated external defibrillators: a scientific statement from the American Heart Association and American College of Cardiology. *Circulation.* 2015;132:e334–338.
189. Mitten MJ, Zipes DP, Maron BJ, et al. Eligibility and disqualification recommendations for competitive athletes with cardiovascular abnormalities: task force 15: legal aspects of medical eligibility and disqualification recommendations: a scientific statement from the American Heart Association and American College of Cardiology. *Circulation.* 2015;132:e346–349.

Sudden Death and Public Safety

190. Kim MH, Zhang Y, Sakaguchi S, et al. Time course of appropriate implantable cardioverter-defibrillator therapy and implications for guideline-based driving restrictions. *Heart Rhythm.* 2015;12:1728–1736.
191. Merchant FM, Hoskins MH, Benser ME, et al. Time course of subsequent shocks after initial implantable cardioverter-defibrillator discharge and implications for driving restrictions. *JAMA Cardiol.* 2016;1:181–188.

71 Hypotension and Syncope

HUGH CALKINS, THOMAS H. EVERETT IV, AND PENG-SHENG CHEN

DEFINITION, 1387

CLASSIFICATION, 1387

VASCULAR CAUSES OF SYNCOPE, 1387
Orthostatic Hypotension, 1387
Reflex-Mediated Syncope, 1388
Neurally Mediated Hypotension or Syncope (Vasovagal Syncope), 1389
Carotid Sinus Hypersensitivity, 1389

CARDIAC CAUSES OF SYNCOPE, 1390

NEUROLOGIC CAUSES OF TRANSIENT LOSS OF CONSCIOUSNESS, 1390

METABOLIC CAUSES OF TRANSIENT LOSS OF CONSCIOUSNESS, 1390

DIAGNOSTIC TESTS, 1390
History, Physical Examination, and Carotid Sinus Massage, 1390
Laboratory Testing: Blood Tests, 1391
Tilt-Table Test, 1391
Cardiac Imaging, 1392
Stress Tests and Cardiac Catheterization, 1392
Electrocardiography, 1392
Electrophysiologic Testing, 1393

APPROACH TO THE EVALUATION OF PATIENTS WITH SYNCOPE, 1394

MANAGEMENT OF PATIENTS WITH SYNCOPE, 1394
Neurally Mediated Syncope, 1395

CARDIONEUROABLATION FOR TREATMENT OF NEURALLY MEDIATED SYNCOPE, 1396

FUTURE PERSPECTIVES, 1397

REFERENCES, 1397

DEFINITION

Syncope is a symptom that presents with abrupt, transient, complete loss of consciousness (LOC) associated with the inability to maintain postural tone, with rapid and spontaneous recovery. The presumed mechanism of syncope is cerebral hypoperfusion.[1,2] The metabolism of the brain, in contrast to that of many other organs, is exquisitely dependent on perfusion. Consequently, cessation of cerebral blood flow leads to LOC within approximately 10 seconds. Restoration of appropriate behavior and orientation after a syncopal episode is usually immediate. Retrograde amnesia, although uncommon, can be present in older adults. It is important to recognize that syncope, as previously defined, represents a subset of a much wider spectrum of conditions that can result in transient LOC, including conditions such as cerebrovascular accident (stroke) and epileptic seizures. Nonsyncopal causes of transient LOC differ in their mechanism and duration.[1,2]

Syncope is an important clinical problem because it is common, costly, and often disabling; can cause injury; and can be the only warning sign before sudden cardiac death (SCD) (see Chapter 70).[1-3] Patients with syncope account for 1% of hospital admissions and 3% of emergency department (ED) visits. Up to 50% of young adults report a previous episode of LOC, mostly isolated events that never come to medical attention. The prevalence of a first episode of syncope is particularly high between the ages 10 and 20, with additional peaks at approximately 60 and 80 years.[4] Patients who experience syncope also report greatly reduced quality of life; syncope can result in traumatic injury.

The prognosis of patients with syncope varies greatly with the diagnosis. Patients with syncope in the setting of structural heart disease or primary electrical disease have an increased incidence of SCD and overall mortality. Syncope caused by orthostatic hypotension is associated with a twofold increase in mortality, which reflects the presence of multiple comorbid conditions in this patient group. In contrast, young patients with neurally mediated syncope (NMS) have an excellent prognosis.

CLASSIFICATION

Tables 71.1 and 71.2 present the diagnostic considerations in patients with real or apparent transient LOC and in those with syncope, respectively. Syncope can be distinguished from most other causes of transient LOC by asking whether the LOC was transient, of rapid onset, of short duration, and followed by spontaneous recovery. If the answer to each of these questions is yes and the transient LOC did not result from head trauma, the diagnostic considerations include true syncope in which the mechanism of transient LOC is global cerebral hypoperfusion, epileptic seizures, psychogenic syncope, and other rare causes. It is important to consider nonsyncopal conditions when evaluating a patient with transient LOC, such as metabolic disorders, epilepsy, or alcohol, as well as conditions in which consciousness is only apparently lost (i.e., conversion reaction). These psychogenic causes of syncope, being recognized with increased frequency, are typically diagnosed in patients 40 years or younger and especially in those with a history of psychiatric disease.[1,5]

The differential diagnosis of syncope (see Table 71.2) most often involves vascular causes, followed by cardiac causes, most frequently arrhythmias. Although knowledge of the common conditions that can cause syncope is essential and allows the clinician to arrive at a probable cause of the syncope in most patients, it is equally important to be aware of several less common but potentially lethal causes of syncope, such as long-QT syndrome, arrhythmogenic right ventricular dysplasia, Brugada syndrome, hypertrophic cardiomyopathy, idiopathic ventricular fibrillation (VF), catecholaminergic polymorphic ventricular tachycardia (VT), short-QT syndrome, and pulmonary emboli (see Chapters 63 and 67).[1,6-11]

It is important to recognize that the distribution of causes of syncope varies both with patient age and with the clinical setting in which the patient is evaluated. NMS and other causes of reflex-mediated syncope are the most frequent causes of syncope at any age and in any setting. Cardiac causes of syncope, especially cardiac tachyarrhythmias and bradyarrhythmias, are the second most common causes of syncope. The incidence of cardiac causes of syncope is higher in older adults and in patients evaluated in the ED. Orthostatic hypotension is extremely uncommon in patients younger than 40 years but is common in much older adults (see Chapter 90).

VASCULAR CAUSES OF SYNCOPE

Vascular causes of syncope, particularly reflex-mediated syncope and orthostatic hypotension, are by far the most common causes and account for at least one third of all syncopal episodes.[12,13] In contrast, vascular steal syndromes are exceedingly uncommon causes of syncope.

Orthostatic Hypotension

Standing upright displaces 500 to 800 mL of blood to the abdomen and lower extremities, thereby resulting in an abrupt drop in venous return

TABLE 71.1 Causes of Real or Apparent Transient Loss of Consciousness

Syncope (see Table 71.2)
Neurologic or cerebrovascular disease
 Epilepsy
 Vertebrobasilar transient ischemic attack
Metabolic syndromes and coma
 Hyperventilation with hypocapnia
 Hypoglycemia
 Hypoxemia
 Intoxication with drugs or alcohol
 Coma
Psychogenic syncope
 Anxiety, panic disorder
 Somatization disorders

TABLE 71.2 Causes of Syncope

Vascular Causes

Anatomic
Vascular steal syndromes (subclavian steal syndrome)

Orthostatic
Autonomic insufficiency
Idiopathic
Volume depletion
Drug and alcohol induced

Reflex Mediated
Carotid sinus hypersensitivity
Neurally mediated syncope (common faint, vasodepressor, neurocardiogenic, vasovagal)
Glossopharyngeal syncope
Situational (acute hemorrhage, cough, defecation, laugh, micturition, sneeze, swallow, postprandial)

Cardiac Causes

Anatomic
Obstructive cardiac valve disease
Aortic dissection
Atrial myxoma
Pericardial disease, tamponade
Hypertrophic obstructive cardiomyopathy
Myocardial ischemia, infarction
Pulmonary embolism
Pulmonary hypertension

Arrhythmias
Bradyarrhythmias
 Atrioventricular block
 Sinus node dysfunction, bradycardia
Tachyarrhythmias
 Supraventricular tachycardia
  Atrial fibrillation
  Paroxysmal supraventricular tachycardia (AVNRT, WPW)
  Other
 Ventricular tachycardia
  Structural heart disease
  Inherited syndromes (ARVD, HCM, Brugada syndrome, long-QT syndrome)
 Drug-induced proarrhythmia
 Implanted pacemaker or ICD malfunction

Syncope of Unknown Origin

ARVD, Arrhythmogenic right ventricular dysplasia; *AVNRT*, atrioventricular nodal reentrant tachycardia; *HCM*, hypertrophic cardiomyopathy; *ICD*, implantable cardioverter-defibrillator; *WPW*, Wolff-Parkinson-White syndrome.

---

to the heart. This drop leads to a decrease in cardiac output and stimulation of aortic, carotid, and cardiopulmonary baroreceptors, which triggers a reflex increase in sympathetic outflow. As a result, heart rate, cardiac contractility, and vascular resistance increase to maintain stable systemic blood pressure (BP) on standing. *Orthostatic intolerance* is a term used to refer to the signs and symptoms of an abnormality in any portion of this BP control system. Orthostatic hypotension is defined as a 20-mm Hg drop in systolic BP or a 10-mm Hg drop in diastolic BP within 3 minutes of standing. Orthostatic hypotension can be asymptomatic or associated with syncope, lightheadedness/presyncope, tremulousness, weakness, fatigue, palpitations, diaphoresis, and blurred or tunnel vision. Many patients with orthostatic hypotension are asymptomatic despite substantial falls in systolic BP and low upright BPs.[14] These symptoms are often worse immediately on arising in the morning or after meals or exercise. Initial orthostatic hypotension is defined as less than a 40-mm Hg decrease in BP immediately on standing with rapid (<30 seconds) return to normal.[1,2,12] In contrast, *delayed progressive* orthostatic hypotension is characterized by a slow progressive decrease in systolic BP on standing. Syncope that occurs after meals, particularly in older adults, can result from a redistribution of blood to the gut. A decline in systolic BP of approximately 20 mm Hg approximately 1 hour after eating has been reported in up to one third of older adult nursing home residents. Although usually asymptomatic, it can result in lightheadedness or syncope.

Drugs that either cause volume depletion or result in vasodilation are the most common causes of orthostatic hypotension (Table 71.3). Older adult patients are particularly susceptible to the hypotensive effects of drugs because of reduced baroreceptor sensitivity, decreased cerebral blood flow, renal sodium wasting, and an impaired thirst mechanism that develops with aging (see Chapter 90). Orthostatic hypotension can also result from neurogenic causes, which can be subclassified into primary and secondary *autonomic failure* (see Chapter 102). Primary causes are generally idiopathic, whereas secondary causes are associated with a known biochemical or structural anomaly or are seen as part of a particular disease or syndrome.

There are three types of primary autonomic failure. *Pure autonomic failure* (Bradbury-Eggleston syndrome) is an idiopathic sporadic disorder characterized by orthostatic hypotension, usually in conjunction with evidence of more widespread autonomic failure, such as disturbances in bowel, bladder, thermoregulatory, and sexual function. Patients with pure autonomic failure have reduced supine plasma norepinephrine levels. *Multisystem atrophy* (Shy-Drager syndrome) is a sporadic, progressive, adult-onset disorder characterized by autonomic dysfunction, parkinsonism, and ataxia in any combination. The third type of primary autonomic failure is *Parkinson disease* with autonomic failure. A small subset of patients with Parkinson disease may also experience autonomic failure, including orthostatic hypotension. In addition to these forms of chronic autonomic failure is a rare, acute *panautonomic neuropathy*. This neuropathy generally occurs in young people and results in severe, widespread sympathetic and parasympathetic failure with orthostatic hypotension, loss of sweating, disruption of bladder and bowel function, fixed heart rate, and fixed dilated pupils.

Postural orthostatic tachycardia syndrome (POTS) is a clinical syndrome characterized by frequent symptoms that occur with standing (e.g., lightheadedness, palpitations, tremulousness, generalized weakness, blurred vision, exercise intolerance, fatigue), an increase in heart rate of 30 beats/min or more on standing (or ≥40 beats/min in those 12 to 19 years of age), and absence of a more than 20-mm Hg reduction in systolic BP.[1,2,13] The precise pathophysiologic basis for POTS has not been well defined. Some patients have both POTS and NMS.

Reflex-Mediated Syncope

Reflex-mediated, or *situational*, causes of syncope are listed in Table 71.2. In this group of conditions, the cardiovascular reflexes that control the circulation become inappropriate in response to a trigger, which results in vasodilation with or without bradycardia and a drop in BP and global cerebral hypoperfusion. In each case the reflex is composed of a trigger (the afferent limb) and a response (the efferent limb). This group of reflex-mediated

TABLE 71.3 Causes of Orthostatic Hypotension

Drugs

Diuretics

Alpha-adrenergic blocking drugs
 Terazosin (Hytrin), labetalol

Adrenergic neuron-blocking drugs
 Guanethidine

Angiotensin-converting enzyme inhibitors

Antidepressants
 Monoamine oxidase inhibitors

Alcohol

Ganglion-blocking drugs
 Hexamethonium, mecamylamine

Tranquilizers
 Phenothiazines, barbiturates

Vasodilators
 Prazosin, hydralazine, calcium channel blockers

Centrally acting hypotensive drugs
 Methyldopa, clonidine

Primary Disorders of Autonomic Failure

Pure autonomic failure (Bradbury-Eggleston syndrome)

Multisystem atrophy (Shy-Drager syndrome)

Parkinson disease with autonomic failure

Secondary Neurogenic Causes

Aging

Autoimmune disease
 Guillain-Barré syndrome, mixed connective tissue disease, rheumatoid arthritis
 Eaton-Lambert syndrome, systemic lupus erythematosus

Carcinomatosis autonomic neuropathy

Central brain lesions
 Multiple sclerosis, Wernicke encephalopathy
 Vascular lesions or tumors involving hypothalamus and midbrain

Dopamine beta-hydroxylase deficiency

Familial hyperbradykininism

General medical disorders
 Diabetes, amyloid, alcoholism, renal failure

Hereditary sensory neuropathies, dominant or recessive

Infections of the nervous system
 Human immunodeficiency virus infection, Chagas disease, botulism, syphilis

Metabolic disease
 Vitamin B_{12} deficiency, porphyria, Fabry disease, Tangier disease

Spinal cord lesions

Modified from Bannister SR, ed. *Autonomic Failure*. 2nd ed. Oxford: Oxford University Press; 1988:8.

syncopal syndromes has in common the response limb of the reflex, which consists of increased vagal tone and withdrawal of peripheral sympathetic tone and leads to bradycardia, vasodilation, and ultimately, hypotension, presyncope, or syncope. If hypotension secondary to peripheral vasodilation predominates, it is classified as a *vasodepressor-type* reflex response; if bradycardia or asystole predominates, it is classified as a *cardioinhibitory* response; and when both vasodilation and bradycardia play a role, it is classified as a *mixed* response. Specific triggers distinguish these causes of syncope. For example, micturition-induced syncope results from activation of mechanoreceptors in the bladder, defecation-induced syncope results from neural input from gut wall tension receptors, and swallowing-induced syncope results from afferent neural impulses arising from the upper gastrointestinal tract. The two most common types of reflex-mediated syncope, carotid sinus hypersensitivity and neurally mediated hypotension, are discussed later. Identification of the trigger is of importance because of its therapeutic implications, with avoidance of the trigger, where possible, preventing further syncopal episodes.

Neurally Mediated Hypotension or Syncope (Vasovagal Syncope)

The term *neurally mediated hypotension* or *syncope* (also known as neurocardiogenic, vasodepressor, and vasovagal syncope and "fainting") has been used to describe a common abnormality in regulation of BP characterized by an abrupt onset of hypotension with or without bradycardia. Triggers associated with the development of NMS include orthostatic stress, such as can occur with prolonged standing or a hot shower, and emotional stress, such as can result from the sight of blood.[1,2,13] Neurally mediated hypotension has shown to run in families and three genes have been associated.[15] While our understanding of the genetic basis for neurally mediated hypotension is in its early stages, this is an active area of research. A large proportion of patients with NMS may have minor psychiatric disorders. Patients with syncope caused by neurally mediated hypotension may also have psychogenic pseudosyncope.[5] It has been proposed that NMS results from a paradoxical reflex that is initiated when ventricular preload is reduced by venous pooling. This reduction leads to a decrease in cardiac output and BP, which is sensed by arterial baroreceptors. The resultant increased catecholamine levels, combined with reduced venous filling, leads to a vigorously contracting, volume-depleted ventricle. The heart itself is involved in this reflex by virtue of the presence of mechanoreceptors, or C fibers, consisting of nonmyelinated fibers found in the atria, ventricles, and pulmonary artery. It has been proposed that vigorous contraction of a volume-depleted ventricle leads to activation of these receptors in susceptible individuals. These afferent C fibers project centrally to the dorsal vagal nucleus of the medulla and can result in "paradoxical" withdrawal of peripheral sympathetic tone and an increase in vagal tone, which in turn causes vasodilation and bradycardia. The ultimate clinical consequence is syncope or presyncope. It has been speculated that the fall in BP seen during neurally mediated hypotension mimics a "fictitious hemorrhage." To protect against this fictitious hemorrhage, the brainstem triggers cardioinhibition as protection against the hypothetical loss of blood simulated by the reduction in venous return. The most effective solution to stopping blood loss is to stop the heart.[16] A recent study has shown that in patients who experienced a syncopal episode during a tilt-table test there was sympathetic activation before a syncopal event followed by sympathetic withdrawal and parasympathetic activation.[17] Not all NMS, however, results from activation of mechanoreceptors. In humans the sight of blood or extreme emotion can trigger syncope, thus suggesting that higher neural centers can also participate in the pathophysiology of vasovagal syncope. In addition, central mechanisms can contribute to the production of NMS.

Carotid Sinus Hypersensitivity

Syncope caused by carotid sinus hypersensitivity results from stimulation of carotid sinus baroreceptors located in the internal carotid artery above the bifurcation of the common carotid artery. It is diagnosed by the reproduction of clinical syncope during carotid sinus massage, with a cardioinhibitory response if asystole is longer than 3 seconds or AV block occurs; or a significant vasodepressor response if there is a more than 50-mm Hg drop in systolic BP; or a mixed cardioinhibitory and vasodepressor response.[1] Carotid sinus hypersensitivity is detected in approximately one third of older adult patients evaluated for syncope or falls.[2] It is important, however, to recognize that carotid sinus hypersensitivity is also frequently observed in asymptomatic older adult patients. Thus the diagnosis of carotid sinus hypersensitivity should be approached cautiously after excluding alternative causes of the syncope. Once diagnosed, dual-chamber pacemaker implantation is recommended for patients with recurrent syncope or falls resulting from carotid sinus hypersensitivity that is cardioinhibitory or mixed (class 2A/IIa, level of evidence [LOE] B-R).[1,2,18]

CARDIAC CAUSES OF SYNCOPE

Cardiac causes of syncope, particularly tachyarrhythmias and bradyarrhythmias, are the second most common cause of syncope and account for 10% to 20% of syncopal episodes (see Table 71.2 and Chapters 65 and 67). VT is the most common tachyarrhythmia that can cause syncope. Supraventricular tachycardia (SVT) can also cause syncope, although the great majority of patients with supraventricular arrhythmias have less severe symptoms, such as palpitations, dyspnea, and lightheadedness. Bradyarrhythmias that can result in syncope include sick sinus syndrome and atrioventricular (AV) block. Anatomic causes of syncope include obstruction to blood flow, such as massive pulmonary embolism (see Chapter 87), atrial myxoma (Chapter 98), or aortic stenosis (Chapter 72).

NEUROLOGIC CAUSES OF TRANSIENT LOSS OF CONSCIOUSNESS

Neurologic causes of transient LOC, including migraines, seizures, Arnold-Chiari malformations, and transient ischemic attacks, are surprisingly uncommon and account for less than 10% of all cases of syncope (see Chapters 45 and 100). Most patients in whom a "neurologic" cause of transient LOC is established are in fact found to have had a seizure rather than true syncope.

METABOLIC CAUSES OF TRANSIENT LOSS OF CONSCIOUSNESS

Metabolic causes of transient LOC are rare and account for less than 5% of syncopal episodes. The most common metabolic causes of syncope are hypoglycemia (see Chapter 31), hypoxia, and hyperventilation. Establishing hypoglycemia as the cause of apparent LOC requires demonstration of hypoglycemia during the syncopal episode. Although hyperventilation-induced syncope has generally been considered to result from a reduction in cerebral blood flow, one study demonstrated that hyperventilation alone was not sufficient to cause syncope. This observation suggests that hyperventilation-induced syncope may also have a psychological component. Psychiatric disorders can also cause syncope. Up to one fourth of patients with syncope of unknown origin may have psychiatric disorders for which apparent syncope is one of the initial symptoms (see Chapter 99).[1]

DIAGNOSTIC TESTS

Identification of the precise cause of the syncope is often challenging. Because syncope usually occurs sporadically and infrequently, it is extremely difficult to examine a patient or obtain an electrocardiogram (ECG) during an episode of syncope. For this reason, the primary goal in the evaluation of a patient with syncope is to arrive at a presumptive determination of the cause of the syncope.

History, Physical Examination, and Carotid Sinus Massage

The history and physical examination are by far the most important components of the evaluation of a patient with transient LOC and syncope and can be used to identify the cause in more than 25% of patients.[1,2,13,19–21] The 2017 ACC/AHA/HRS syncope guidelines provide a class I (LOE B-NR) recommendation for performing a detailed history and physical examination in patients with syncope.[1] Maximal information can be obtained from the clinical history when it is approached in a systematic and detailed manner. Initial evaluation should begin by determining whether the patient did in fact experience a syncopal episode by asking the following: (1) Did the patient experience complete LOC? (2) Was the LOC transient with a rapid onset and short duration? (3) Did the patient recover spontaneously, completely, and without sequelae? and (4) Did the patient lose postural tone? If the answer to one or more of these questions is negative, other nonsyncopal causes of transient LOC should be suspected. Although falls can be differentiated from syncope by the absence of LOC, an overlap between symptoms of falls and syncope has been reported,[2,22] because older adults may experience amnesia for the LOC episode. When evaluating a patient with syncope, particular attention should then be focused on (1) determining whether the patient has a history of cardiac disease or metabolic disease (i.e., diabetes) or a family history of cardiac disease, syncope, or sudden death; (2) identifying medications that may have played a role in syncope, especially those that may cause hypotension, bradycardia/heart block, or a proarrhythmic response (antiarrhythmics); (3) quantifying the number and chronicity of previous syncopal and presyncopal episodes; (4) identifying precipitating factors, including body position and activity immediately before syncope; and (5) quantifying the type and duration of prodromal and recovery symptoms. It is also useful to obtain careful accounts from witnesses to provide a detailed description of the episode, including how the patient collapsed and the patient's skin color and breathing pattern, duration of unconsciousness, and movements during the episode of unconsciousness. Table 71.4 summarizes features of the clinical history most helpful in differentiating neurally mediated hypotension, arrhythmia, seizures, and psychogenic syncope.

The clinical histories obtained from patients with syncope related to AV block and VT are similar. In each case, syncope typically occurs with less than 5 seconds of warning and few if any prodromal and recovery symptoms. Demographic features suggesting that the syncope results from an arrhythmia such as VT or AV block include male sex, fewer than three previous episodes of syncope, and increased age. Features of the clinical history that point toward a diagnosis of NMS include palpitations, blurred vision, nausea, warmth, diaphoresis, or lightheadedness before syncope and the presence of nausea, warmth, diaphoresis, or fatigue after syncope.

Features of the clinical history useful in distinguishing seizures from syncope include orientation following an event, a blue face or not becoming pale during the event, frothing at the mouth, aching muscles, feeling sleepy after the event, time of seizure relative to onset of syncope—early points to neurologic whereas late suggests arrhythmic cause—and a duration of unconsciousness of longer than 5 minutes.[20] Tongue biting strongly points toward a seizure rather than syncope as the cause of LOC. One recent study reported that a history of tongue biting during an episode of LOC had 33% sensitivity and 96% specificity in predicting a seizure as the cause of the LOC.[21] Other findings suggestive of a seizure as a cause of the syncopal episode include (1) an aura before the episode, (2) horizontal eye deviation during the episode, (3) elevated BP and pulse during the episode, and (4) a headache following the event. Urinary or fecal incontinence can be observed with either a seizure or a syncopal episode but occurs more often with a seizure. Grand mal seizures are usually associated with tonic-clonic movements. It is important to note that syncope caused by cerebral ischemia can result in decorticate rigidity with clonic movements of the arms. Akinetic or petit mal seizures can be recognized by the patient's lack of responsiveness in the absence of loss of postural tone. Temporal lobe seizures last several minutes and are characterized by confusion, changes in level of consciousness, and autonomic signs such as flushing. Vertebral basilar insufficiency should be considered as the cause of the syncope if it occurs in association with other symptoms of brainstem ischemia (i.e., diplopia, tinnitus, focal weakness or sensory loss, vertigo, or dysarthria). Migraine-mediated syncope is often associated with a throbbing unilateral headache, scintillating scotomata, and nausea.

Physical Examination

In addition to a complete cardiac examination, particular attention should be focused on whether structural heart disease is present, defining the patient's level of hydration, and detecting the presence of significant neurologic abnormalities suggestive of dysautonomia or a cerebrovascular accident. Orthostatic vital signs are a critical component of the evaluation. The patient's BP and heart rate should be determined while supine and then repeated each minute for approximately

TABLE 71.4 Differentiation of Syncope Caused by Neurally Mediated Hypotension, Arrhythmias, Seizures, and Psychogenic Causes

	NEURALLY MEDIATED HYPOTENSION	ARRHYTHMIAS	SEIZURES	PSYCHOGENIC
Demographics and clinical setting	Female > male sex Younger age (<55 years) More episodes (>2) Standing, warm room, emotional upset	Male > female sex Older age (>54 years) Fewer episodes (<3) During exertion or supine Family history of sudden death	Younger age (<45 years) Any setting	Female > male sex Occurs in presence of others Younger age (<40 years) Many episodes (often many episodes in a day) No identifiable trigger
Premonitory symptoms	Longer duration (>5 sec) Palpitations Blurred vision Nausea Warmth Diaphoresis Lightheadedness	Shorter duration (<6 sec) Palpitations less common	Sudden onset or brief aura (déjà vu, olfactory, gustatory, visual)	Usually absent
Observations during the event	Pallor Diaphoresis Dilated pupils Slow pulse, low BP Incontinence may occur Brief clonic movements may occur	Blue, not pale Incontinence may occur Brief clonic movements may occur	Blue face, no pallor Frothing at the mouth Prolonged syncope (duration > 5 min) Tongue biting Horizontal eye deviation Elevated pulse and BP Incontinence more likely* Tonic-clonic movements if grand mal	Normal color Not diaphoretic Eyes closed Normal pulse and BP No incontinence Prolonged duration (minutes) common
Residual symptoms	Residual symptoms common Prolonged fatigue common (>90%) Oriented	Residual symptoms uncommon (unless prolonged unconsciousness) Oriented	Residual symptoms common Aching muscles Disoriented Fatigue Headache Slow recovery	Residual symptoms uncommon Oriented

*May be observed with any of these causes of syncope but more common with seizures.
BP, Blood pressure.

3 minutes while standing. The two abnormalities that should be sought are (1) early orthostatic hypotension, defined as a 20-mm Hg drop in systolic BP or a 10-mm Hg drop in diastolic BP within 3 minutes of standing, and (2) POTS, an increase in heart rate of 30 beats/min or more on standing (or ≥40 beats/min in those 12 to 19 years of age), and absence of a more than 20-mm Hg reduction in systolic BP.[1,2,13] The significance of POTS lies in its close overlap with NMS.

Carotid Sinus Massage

Carotid sinus massage should be performed after checking for bruits by applying *gentle* pressure over the carotid pulsation, first one side and then the other, just below the angle of the jaw where the carotid bifurcation is located. Pressure should be applied for 5 to 10 seconds in both the supine and the upright position because an abnormal response to carotid sinus massage is present only in the upright position in up to one third of patients. Since the main complications associated with performing carotid sinus massage are neurologic, it should be avoided in patients with previous transient ischemic attacks, strokes within the past 3 months, and carotid bruits, except if significant stenosis has been excluded by carotid Doppler studies. A normal response to carotid sinus massage is a transient decrease in the sinus rate, prolongation of AV conduction, or both. Carotid sinus hypersensitivity is diagnosed by the reproduction of clinical syncope during carotid sinus massage and the responses previously noted.[1] Diagnosis of carotid sinus hypersensitivity as the cause of the syncope requires reproduction of the patient's symptoms during carotid sinus massage.

Laboratory Testing: Blood Tests

Routine use of blood tests, such as serum electrolytes, cardiac enzymes, glucose, and hematocrit levels, is of low diagnostic value in syncopal patients and therefore not recommended routinely. The 2017 ACC/AHA/HRS syncope guidelines state that targeted blood tests are reasonable in the evaluation of selected patients with syncope identified based on clinical assessment from history, physical examination, and ECG (class IIa, LOE B-NR).[1]

Tilt-Table Test

The tilt-table test is a valuable diagnostic test for evaluating patients with syncope,[1,2,13] with a positive response indicating susceptibility to NMS. The 2017 ACC/AHA/HRS syncope guidelines state that tilt-table testing can be useful for patients with suspected vasovagal syncope if the diagnosis is unclear after initial evaluation (class IIa, LOE B-NR).[1] Upright tilt testing is generally performed for 30 to 45 minutes following a 20-minute horizontal pretilt stabilization phase at an angle between 60 and 80 degrees (with 70 degrees being most common). The sensitivity of the test can be increased, along with an associated fall in specificity, by the use of longer tilt durations, steeper tilt angles, and provocative agents such as isoproterenol or nitroglycerin. When isoproterenol is used, it is recommended that the infusion rate be increased incrementally from 1 to 3 μg/min to increase the heart rate 25% greater than baseline. When nitroglycerin is used, a fixed dose of 300 to 400 μg of nitroglycerin spray should be administered sublingually after a 20-minute unmedicated phase with the patient in the upright position. These two provocative approaches are equivalent in diagnostic accuracy. In the absence of pharmacologic provocation, the specificity of the test has been estimated to be 90%; when provocative agents are used, specificity decreases significantly.

The main indication for upright tilt testing is to confirm a diagnosis of NMS when the initial evaluation was insufficient to establish this diagnosis. Tilt-table testing is also of value in diagnosing psychogenic pseudosyncope.[5] Upright tilt testing is not generally recommended in patients in whom the diagnosis can be established from the initial history and physical examination. However, for some patients, confirmation of the diagnosis with a positive response to upright tilt testing is very reassuring. Induction of reflex hypotension/bradycardia without reproduction of the syncope points toward a diagnosis of NMS but is a less specific response. If a patient has structural heart disease, other cardiovascular causes of syncope should be excluded before considering a positive response to upright tilt testing to be diagnostic of NMS. Upright tilt testing is also indicated in the evaluation of patients for whom the cause of the syncope has been determined (i.e., asystole), but the presence of NMS on upright tilt would influence treatment. Upright tilt testing has also been shown to be of value in patients with psychogenic causes of syncope in that it may trigger LOC in association with a normal BP and heart rate. Induction of LOC with no change in vital signs points strongly toward a diagnosis of psychogenic pseudosyncope. Upright tilt testing has no value in assessing the efficacy of treatment of NMS.

Cardiac Imaging

Echocardiograms are frequently used to evaluate patients with syncope (see Chapter 16), but current guidelines suggest that an echocardiogram should be performed only in patients suspected of having structural heart disease.[1,2] The 2017 ACC/AHA/HRS syncope guidelines state that echocardiography can be useful in selected patients presenting with syncope if structural heart disease is suspected (class IIa, LOE B-NR).[1] The guidelines also state that routine cardiac imaging is not useful in the evaluation of patients with syncope unless cardiac etiology is suspected on the basis of an initial evaluation including history, physical examination, or ECG (class 3/III, LOE B-NR).[1] These guidelines also recommend that computed tomography (CT) or magnetic resonance imaging (MRI) may be useful in selected patients presenting with syncope of suspected cardiac etiology (class IIb, LOE B-NR).[1] Studies have shown that the diagnostic yield of an echocardiogram in a syncope patient with a normal ECG and physical examination is extremely low. Therefore, routine echocardiograms are not advised in this setting. For example, an echocardiogram should be obtained in patients who have clinical features suggestive of a cardiac cause of the syncope, such as syncope with exertion or while supine, a family history of sudden death, or syncope of abrupt onset. Echocardiographic findings considered diagnostic of the cause of syncope include severe aortic stenosis, pericardial tamponade, aortic dissection, congenital abnormalities of the coronary arteries, and obstructive atrial myxomas or thrombi. Findings of impaired right or left ventricular function, evidence of right ventricular overload or pulmonary hypertension (pulmonary emboli), or the presence of hypertrophic cardiomyopathy (see Chapter 54) are of prognostic importance and justify additional diagnostic testing.

Stress Tests and Cardiac Catheterization

Myocardial ischemia is an unlikely cause of syncope and, when present, is usually accompanied by angina (see Chapters 35 and 40). The use of stress tests (see Chapter 15) is best reserved for patients in whom syncope or presyncope occurred during or immediately after exertion in association with chest pain or in a patient at high risk for coronary artery disease.[1,2] The 2017 ACC/AHA/HRS syncope guidelines state exercise stress testing can be useful to establish the cause of syncope in selected patients who experience syncope or presyncope during exertion (class IIa, LOE C-LD).[1] Syncope occurring during exercise is suggestive of a cardiac cause. In contrast, syncope following exercise is usually caused by NMS. Even in patients with syncope during exertion, exercise stress testing is highly unlikely to trigger another event. Coronary angiography is recommended in patients with syncope suspected to result, directly or indirectly, from myocardial ischemia.

Electrocardiography

The 12-lead ECG is another important component in the workup of a patient with syncope (see Chapter 14). The 2017 ACC/AHA/HRS syncope guidelines provide a class I (LOE B-NR) recommendation for performing an ECG in patients with syncope.[1] The initial ECG results in establishment of a diagnosis in approximately 5% of patients and suggests a diagnosis in another 5% of patients. Specific findings that can identify the probable cause of the syncope include QT prolongation (long-QT syndrome), the presence of a short PR interval and a delta wave (Wolff-Parkinson-White syndrome), the presence of a right bundle branch block pattern with ST-segment elevation (Brugada syndrome), or evidence of acute myocardial infarction, high-grade AV block, or T wave inversion in the right precordial leads (arrhythmogenic right ventricular dysplasia) (see Chapters 63, 65 and 67). Any abnormal finding on the baseline ECG is an independent predictor of cardiac syncope or increased mortality and suggests the need to pursue evaluation of cardiac causes of syncope.[1] Most patients with syncope have normal findings on ECGs, which is useful because it suggests a low likelihood of a cardiac cause of the syncope and is associated with an excellent prognosis, particularly when observed in a young patient with syncope. Despite the low diagnostic yield of electrocardiography, the test is inexpensive and risk free and is considered a standard part of the evaluation of virtually all patients with syncope.[1]

Cardiac Monitoring

Continuous ECG monitoring via telemetry or Holter monitoring is frequently performed in patients with syncope but is unlikely to identify the cause of the syncope (see Chapter 61). Over the past 5 years, patch monitoring and mobile cardiac telemetry have been developed to allow long-term continuous recording of heart rhythm. The mobile cardiac telemetry transmits real-time ECG recordings to a service center. The prescribing physicians are alerted when serious arrhythmias occur. The patch monitoring stores heart rhythm over a 1- to 2-week period for later off-line analyses but does not transmit data real time. Both types of devices may result in higher diagnostic yield in patients with syncope or presyncope than do the conventional event monitors just described. The information provided by ECG monitoring at the time of syncope is extremely valuable in that it allows an arrhythmic cause of syncope to be established or excluded. Another clinically useful finding is detection of symptoms in the absence of an arrhythmia, which is observed in up to 15% of patients undergoing continuous ECG monitoring. It is important to emphasize that the absence of an arrhythmia and symptoms during continuous ECG monitoring may not exclude an arrhythmia as the cause of the syncope. In patients suspected of having an arrhythmia as the cause of the syncope, additional evaluation, such as electrophysiologic (EP) testing or event monitoring, should be considered. Inpatient telemetry monitoring or continuous ECG monitoring is recommended for patients who have clinical or ECG features suggesting an arrhythmic syncope or a history of recurrent syncope with injury. Continuous ECG monitoring and inpatient telemetry monitoring are most likely to be diagnostic when used for the occasional patient with frequent (i.e., daily) episodes of syncope or presyncope.

In patients with extremely infrequent episodes of syncope (e.g., once or twice a year), a traditional non-invasive monitoring device is unlikely to record an event. Implantable event recorders address this problem by triggering automatically on the basis of programmed detection criteria, as well as with a handheld activator, and storing the ECG signal in a circular buffer (see Chapter 61). These devices, with battery lives up to 3 years, store data that can be also be downloaded with remote telemetry. They can be implanted with a minimally procedure in the outpatient clinic or in a procedure room. The main disadvantage of these devices is their cost. Implantable loop recorders have also been shown to improve the diagnostic yield in patients with syncope.[23] However, a Cochrane meta-analysis showed no impact of implantable loop recorders on mortality.[23]

TABLE 71.5 Indications for and Diagnostic Findings of Electrophysiologic Testing in Evaluation of Patients with Syncope

INDICATIONS/DIAGNOSTIC CRITERIA	CLASS	LEVEL OF EVIDENCE
Indications		
In patients with ischemic heart disease when the initial evaluation suggests an arrhythmic cause and there is no established indication for an ICD.	I	B
In patients with BBB, EPS should be considered when noninvasive tests do not establish a diagnosis.	IIa	B
In patients with syncope preceded by sudden and brief palpitations when noninvasive tests do not establish a diagnosis.	IIb	B
In patients with syncope and Brugada syndrome, ARVD, or hypertrophic cardiomyopathy, EPS is appropriate in selected cases.	IIb	C
In patients with high-risk occupations, in whom every effort to exclude a cardiovascular cause of syncope is warranted	IIb	C
EPS is not recommended in syncopal patients with normal findings on an ECG, no structural heart disease, and no palpitations.	III	B
Diagnostic Criteria		
EPS is diagnostic and no additional tests are required in the following situations:		
Sinus bradycardia and a prolonged CSNRT (>525 msec)	I	B
BBB and either a baseline H-V interval ≥100 msec or second- or third-degree His-Purkinje block during incremental atrial pacing or with pharmacologic challenge	I	B
Induction of sustained monomorphic VT in patients with a previous myocardial infarction	I	B
Induction of SVT with reproduction of the hypotensive or spontaneous symptoms	I	B
H-V interval between 70 and 100 msec should be considered diagnostic.	IIa	B
Induction of polymorphic VT or VF in patients with Brugada syndrome, patients with ARVD, or patients resuscitated from cardiac arrest	IIb	B
Induction of polymorphic VT or VF in patients with ischemic disease or DCM should not be considered a diagnostic finding.	III	B

ARVD, Arrhythmogenic right ventricular dysplasia; *BBB*, bundle branch block; *CSNRT*, corrected sinus node recovery time; *DCM*, dilated cardiomyopathy; *ECG*, electrocardiogram; *EPS*, electrophysiologic study; *H-V*, His-ventricular; *ICD*, implantable cardioverter-defibrillator; *SVT*, supraventricular tachycardia; *VF*, ventricular fibrillation; *VT*, ventricular tachycardia.
Modified from Moya A, Sutton R, Ammirati R, et al. Guidelines for the diagnosis and management of syncope 2009. *Eur Heart J.* 2009;30:2631.

The 2017 ACC/AHA/HRS syncope guidelines state that the choice of a specific cardiac monitor should be determined on the basis of the frequency and nature of the syncope events (class I, LOE C-EO). The guidelines also state that each of the monitors previously discussed can be useful to evaluate selected ambulatory patients with syncope of suspected arrhythmic etiology (class IIa, LOE B-NR).[1]

Electrophysiologic Testing

EP testing can provide important diagnostic information in patients with syncope by establishing a diagnosis of sick sinus syndrome, carotid sinus hypersensitivity, heart block, SVT, and VT (see Chapter 61). Table 71.5 presents indications for EP testing and diagnostic findings in the evaluation of patients with syncope.[2] The 2017 ACC/AHA/HRS syncope guidelines state that an electrophysiologic study (EPS) can be useful for evaluation of select patients with syncope of suspected arrhythmic etiology (class IIa, LOE B-NR). These guidelines further note that EPS is not recommended for syncope evaluation in patients with a normal ECG and normal cardiac structure and function, unless an arrhythmic etiology is suspected (class III, LOE B-NR).[1] It is generally agreed that EP testing should be performed in patients when the initial evaluation suggests an arrhythmic cause of the syncope,[2] such as those with abnormal findings on an ECG or structural heart disease, those whose clinical history suggests an arrhythmic cause of the syncope, and those with a family history of sudden death. EP testing should not be performed in patients with normal findings on an ECG and no heart disease and in whom the clinical history does not suggest an arrhythmic cause of the syncope. The class II indications for performing EPS are shown in Table 71.5, which indicates that EP testing is appropriate when the results may have an impact on treatment and also in patients with "high-risk" occupations, in whom every effort should be expended to determine the probable cause of the syncope. EP testing is no longer indicated for patients with a severely depressed ejection fraction, because in this setting an implantable cardioverter-defibrillator (ICD) is indicated regardless of the presence or mechanism of the syncope.[1,2]

Electrophysiologic Testing Protocol

A comprehensive EP evaluation should be performed in patients with syncope, including evaluation of sinus node function by measuring the sinus node recovery time (SNRT) and evaluation of AV conduction by measuring the His-ventricular (H-V) interval at baseline, with atrial pacing, and following pharmacologic challenge with intravenous procainamide. In addition, programmed electrical stimulation using standard techniques should be performed to evaluate the inducibility of ventricular and supraventricular arrhythmias. Although the minimal suggested EP protocol includes only double extra stimuli and two basic drive train cycle lengths, it is common practice in the United States to include triple extra stimuli and three basic drive train cycle lengths. It is also common practice to limit the shortest coupling interval to 200 milliseconds. In select patients in whom suspicion for ventricular arrhythmia is high, EP testing with atrial and ventricular programmed stimulation may be repeated following an infusion of isoproterenol, which is of particular importance for patients suspected of having a supraventricular arrhythmia, such as AV nodal reentrant tachycardia or orthodromic AV reciprocating tachycardia, as the cause of the syncope.

Sinus node function is evaluated during EP testing primarily by determining the SNRT. Identification of sinus node dysfunction as the cause of syncope is uncommon during EP tests (<5%). The sensitivity of an abnormal SNRT or corrected SNRT (CSNRT) is approximately 50% to 80%. The specificity of an abnormal SNRT or CSNRT is less than 95%. It is important to note that the absence of evidence of sinus node dysfunction during EP testing does not exclude a bradyarrhythmia as the cause of the syncope (see Chapter 68).

During EP testing, AV conduction is assessed by measuring the AV nodal–to–His bundle conduction time (A-H interval) and the His bundle–to–ventricular conduction time (H-V interval) and also by determining the response of AV conduction to incremental atrial pacing and atrial premature stimuli. If the results of an initial assessment of AV conduction in the baseline state are inconclusive, procainamide (10 mg/kg) can be administered intravenously and atrial pacing and programmed stimulation repeated. Findings on EPS that allow heart block to be established as the probable cause of the syncope are bundle branch block and a baseline H-V interval of 100 milliseconds or longer, or demonstration of second- or third-degree His-Purkinje block during incremental atrial pacing or provoked by an infusion of procainamide (see Table 71.5). An H-V interval of 70 to 100 milliseconds is of less certain diagnostic value. In studies of EP testing to evaluate patients with syncope, AV block was identified as the probable cause of syncope in approximately 10% to 15% of patients.

Although it is uncommon for SVT to result in syncope, this is an important diagnosis to establish because most types of supraventricular arrhythmias can be cured with catheter ablation (see Chapters 64 and 65). The usual setting in which SVT causes syncope is in a patient with underlying heart disease and/or limited cardiovascular reserve, a patient with SVT of abrupt onset and with an extremely rapid rate, or a patient who has a propensity for the development of NMS. The typical pattern is the development of syncope or near-syncope at the onset of the SVT because of an initial drop in BP. The patient often regains consciousness despite continuation of the arrhythmia as a result of activation of a compensatory mechanism. Completion of a standard EP test allows accurate identification of most types of supraventricular arrhythmias that may have caused the syncope, and it should be repeated during an isoproterenol infusion to increase the sensitivity of the study, particularly for detecting AV nodal reentrant tachycardia in a patient with dual–AV node physiology or catecholamine-sensitive atrial fibrillation. An EPS is considered diagnostic of SVT as the cause of syncope when induction of a rapid supraventricular arrhythmia reproduces the hypotensive or spontaneous symptoms (see Table 71.5). A supraventricular arrhythmia is diagnosed as the probable cause of syncope in fewer than 5% of patients who undergo EP testing for evaluation of syncope of unknown origin, but the probability is increased in patients who report a history of palpitations ("heart racing") before syncope.

VT is the most common abnormality uncovered during EP testing in patients with syncope and was identified as the probable cause in approximately 20% of patients (see Chapter 67). In general, an EP test is interpreted as positive for VT when sustained monomorphic VT is induced. Induction of polymorphic VT and VF may represent a nonspecific response to EP testing. The diagnostic and prognostic importance of induction of polymorphic VT or VF remains uncertain. An EPS is considered diagnostic of VT as the cause of the syncope when sustained monomorphic VT is induced (see Table 71.5),[2] with less certain diagnostic value with induction of polymorphic VT or VF in patients with Brugada syndrome or arrhythmogenic right ventricular dysplasia and in patients resuscitated from cardiac arrest. The role of EP testing and pharmacologic challenge with procainamide in syncope patients with suspected Brugada syndrome is controversial.[24]

Overall, approximately one third of patients with syncope referred for diagnostic EP testing have a presumptive diagnosis established.

Test to Screen for Neurologic Causes of Syncope

Syncope as an isolated symptom rarely has a neurologic cause. As a result, widespread use of tests to screen for neurologic conditions is rarely diagnostic.[1,2] In many institutions, CT scans, electroencephalograms (EEGs), and carotid duplex scans are overused; these are obtained in more than 50% of patients with syncope. A diagnosis is almost never uncovered that was not first suspected on the basis of a careful history and neurologic examination. A recent systematic review of CT imaging in patients who present with syncope found that more than half of syncope patients had a head CT performed and the diagnostic yield was 1.1% to 3.8%.[25] Transient ischemic attacks that result from carotid disease are not accompanied by LOC. No studies have suggested that carotid Doppler ultrasonography is beneficial in patients with syncope. EEGs should be obtained only in patients with a relatively high likelihood of epilepsy. CT and MRI should be avoided in patients with uncomplicated syncope (see Chapters 19 and 20). Although the low diagnostic yield of screening "neurologic tests" has been recognized for more than a decade, they continue to be overused and result in a dramatic increase in costs.

The 2017 ACC/AHA/HRS syncope guidelines state that MRI and CT of the head are not recommended in the routine evaluation of patients with syncope in the absence of focal neurologic findings or head injury that support further evaluation (class III, LOE B-NR). The guidelines also provide a class III recommendation for the routine use of carotid artery imaging and EEG in the evaluation of patients with syncope.[1]

APPROACH TO THE EVALUATION OF PATIENTS WITH SYNCOPE

Figure 71.1 outlines the approach to the diagnostic evaluation of a patient with syncope proposed by the 2017 ACC/AHA/HRS Syncope Guidelines.[1] This is consistent with the approach also recommended in the 2018 ESC guidelines.[2] The first step is to take a careful history, perform a physical examination, and obtain an ECG. In some patients the diagnosis can be established based on this limited evaluation. For most patients, the diagnosis is unclear and additional evaluation will be needed as outlined in the Figure 71.1.

The initial evaluation begins with a careful history, physical examination, supine and upright BP, and a 12-lead ECG, followed by additional testing in select patient subgroups, including carotid sinus massage, echocardiography, cardiac ECG monitoring, and tilt-table testing, as discussed earlier. The various types of neurologic testing are generally of little or no value except in the case of head trauma and when nonsyncopal causes of transient LOC such as epilepsy are suspected.

The European and ACC/AHA/HRS guidelines on management of syncope have called attention to the importance of a structured care pathway in the evaluation of patients with syncope.[1,2,26,27] Other studies have reported favorable outcomes when a syncope evaluation unit or standardized approach to the evaluation of syncope is used.[27,28]

MANAGEMENT OF PATIENTS WITH SYNCOPE

Treatment of a patient with syncope has three goals: (1) prolong survival, (2) prevent traumatic injuries, and (3) prevent recurrences of syncope. The approach to treatment of a patient with syncope depends largely on the cause and mechanism of the syncope. For example, the appropriate treatment of a patient with syncope related to AV block would be a pacemaker in most situations. However, a patient with syncope secondary to heart block in the setting of an inferior wall myocardial infarction will not usually require a permanent pacemaker because the heart block usually resolves spontaneously. Similarly, heart block resulting from NMS does not generally require pacemaker implantation. Treatment of a patient with syncope related to Wolff-Parkinson-White syndrome typically involves catheter ablation, and treatment of a patient with syncope related to VT or in the setting of ischemic or nonischemic cardiomyopathy would probably involve placement of an implantable defibrillator (see Chapter 69). However, ICD implantation may not be required for patients with VT/VF occurring within 48 hours of an acute myocardial infarction. For other types of syncope, optimal management may involve discontinuation of an offending pharmacologic agent, an increase in salt intake, or education of the patient.[29]

Other issues that need to be considered include the indication for hospitalization of a patient with syncope and the duration of driving restrictions. Current guidelines recommend that patients with syncope be hospitalized when there is known or suspected heart disease, ECG abnormalities suggestive of arrhythmic syncope, syncope with severe injury or during exercise, and syncope in patients with a family history of sudden death (Table 71.6).[1]

Physicians who care for patients with syncope are often asked to address the issue of driving risk. Patients who experience syncope while driving pose a risk both to themselves and to others. One study has reported that a prior hospitalization for syncope was associated with a small increase in the risk of a motor vehicle accident during follow-up.[30] Although some would argue that all patients with syncope should never drive again because of the theoretical possibility of recurrence, this is an impractical solution that would be ignored by many patients. Factors that should be considered when making a recommendation for a particular patient include: (1) the potential for

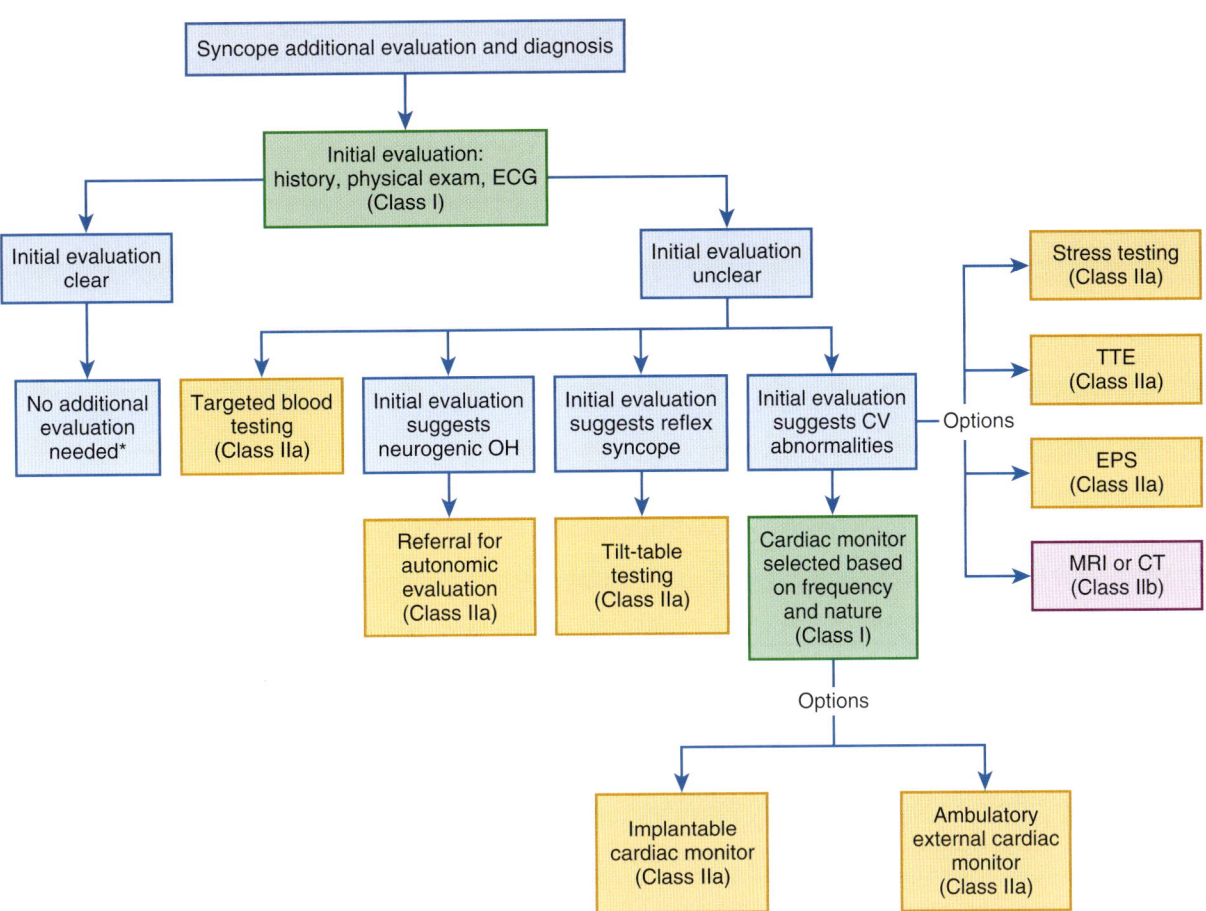

FIGURE 71.1 Diagnostic approach to the evaluation of patients with syncope. *Applies to patients with a normal evaluation, no significant cardiovascular morbidity, or significant injuries with syncope. The recommendation in the yellow boxes are for selected patients; see text for details (Adapted from Writing Committee Members; Shen WK, Sheldon RS, Benditt DG, et al. 2017 ACC/AHA/HRS guideline for the evaluation and management of patients with syncope: A report of the American College of Cardiology/American Heart Association Task Force on Clinical Practice Guidelines and the Heart Rhythm Society. J Am Coll Cardiol 70(5):e39-110.)

TABLE 71.6 Clinical Variables for Identification of High-Risk Syncope Patients Who May Benefit from Hospitalization or an Accelerated Outpatient Evaluation

Severe structural heart disease (low ejection fraction, previous myocardial infarction, heart failure)

Clinical or ECG features suggesting arrhythmic syncope
 Syncope during exertion or while supine
 Palpitations at the time of syncope
 Family history of sudden death
 Nonsustained ventricular tachycardia
 Bifascicular block or QRS >120 msec
 Severe sinus bradycardia (<50 beats/min) in the absence of medications or physical training
 Preexcitation
 Prolonged or very short QT interval
 Brugada ECG pattern (right bundle branch block with ST elevation in leads V_1–V_3)
 Arrhythmogenic right ventricular dysplasia ECG pattern (T wave inversion in leads V_1–V_3 with or without epsilon waves)
 ECG suggestive of hypertrophic dilated cardiomyopathy
 Clinical evidence or suspicion of a pulmonary embolus (clinical setting, sinus tachycardia, shortness of breath)
 Severe anemia

Important comorbid conditions
 Significant electrolyte abnormalities
 Severe anemia

ECG, Electrocardiogram.

recurrent syncope, (2) the presence and duration of warning symptoms, (3) whether syncope occurs while seated or only when standing, (4) how often and in what capacity the patient drives, and (5) whether any state laws may be applicable.

When considering these issues, physicians should note that acute illnesses, including syncope, are unlikely to cause a motor vehicle accident. The American Heart Association and the Canadian Cardiovascular Society have published guidelines concerning this issue. For noncommercial drivers, it is generally recommended that driving be restricted for several months. If the patient remains asymptomatic for several months, driving can then be resumed.

Neurally Mediated Syncope

Because NMS and reflex syncope are so common, treatment options are reviewed (Table 71.7).[1,2,13] Treatment of syncope resulting from neurally mediated hypotension begins with a careful history with particular attention on identifying precipitating factors, quantifying the degree of salt intake and current medication use, and determining whether the patient has a previous history of peripheral edema, hypertension, asthma, or other conditions that may alter the approach used for treatment. For most patients with NMS, particularly those with infrequent episodes associated with an identifiable precipitant, education plus reassurance is sufficient. Patients should be educated about common precipitating factors, such as dehydration, prolonged standing, alcohol, and medications (e.g., diuretics, vasodilators). Patients should also be taught to sit or lie down at the onset of symptoms and to initiate physical counterpressure

TABLE 71.7 Treatment of Neurally Mediated and Reflex-Mediated Syncope

TREATMENT	CLASS	LEVEL OF EVIDENCE
Patient education on diagnosis and prognosis	I	C-EO
Physical counterpressure maneuvers can be useful in patients with vasovagal syncope (VVS) who have a sufficiently long prodromal period.	IIa	B-R
Midodrine is reasonable in patients with recurrent VVS with no history of hypertension, heart failure, or urinary retention. Cardiac pacing should be considered with frequent recurrent reflex syncope, age >40 years, and documented spontaneous cardioinhibitory response during monitoring of recurrent syncope.	IIa	B-R
The use of orthostatic training is uncertain in patients with frequent VVS. Midodrine may be indicated in patients with neurally mediated syncope refractory to conservative treatment approaches.	IIb	B-R
Dual-chamber pacing might be reasonable in a select population of patients age 40 or older with recurrent VVS and prolonged spontaneous pauses.	IIb	B-R
Fludrocortisone might be reasonable for patients with recurrent VVS and inadequate response to salt and fluid intake, unless contraindicated.	IIb	B-R
Beta blockers might be reasonable in patients age 42 or older with recurrent VVS.	IIb	B-NR
Encouraging increased salt and fluid intake may be reasonable in select patients with VVS, unless contraindicated.	IIb	C-LD
In select patients with VVS, it may be reasonable to reduce or withdraw medications that can cause hypotension when appropriate.	IIb	C-LD
In select patients with VVS, a selective serotonin reuptake inhibitor might be considered.	IIb	C-LD
Beta blockers are not indicated in pediatric patients with VVS.	IIb	C-LD

Modified from Shen WK, Sheldon RS, Benditt DG, et al. 2017 ACC/AHA/HRS Guideline for the Evaluation and Management of Patients With Syncope: A Report of the American College of Cardiology/American Heart Association Task Force on Clinical Practice Guidelines and the Heart Rhythm Society. *J Am Coll Cardiol.* 2017;70:e39–e110.

maneuvers. One recent study reported that a standardized education protocol significantly reduced traumatic injuries and recurrence of syncope.[29] In this trial the syncope burden was reduced from 0.35 ± 0.3 at initial evaluation to 0.08 ± 0.02 during follow-up. Volume expansion by salt supplementation is also frequently recommended. Ingestion of approximately 500 mL of water acutely improves orthostatic tolerance to tilt in healthy persons and may be of value as prophylaxis for syncope in blood donors. The effectiveness of water ingestion alone in the management of patients with recurrent NMS has not been well studied.

A recent important shift in the approach used for the treatment of NMS has resulted from the effectiveness of "physical" measures and maneuvers in the treatment of patients with this condition.[1] Isometric physical counterpressure maneuvers such as leg crossing or handgrip with arm tensing can prevent syncope in many patients with neurally mediated hypotension. The 2017 ACC/AHA/HRS guidelines on management of syncope identify the following physical measures as class IIA treatments of NMS.[1] It has been reported that 2 minutes of an isometric handgrip maneuver initiated at the onset of symptoms during tilt testing rendered two thirds of patients asymptomatic. Other studies have demonstrated that tilt (standing) training is effective in the treatment of NMS. Standing training involves leaning against a wall with the heel 10 inches (25 cm) from the wall for progressively longer periods for 2 to 3 months. Standing time should initially be 5 minutes two times per day with a progressive increase to 40 minutes twice daily. Although the results of nonrandomized studies of standing training have been positive, the results of randomized trials suggest that standing training may have only limited effectiveness.

In contrast to these effective physical maneuvers, the value of pharmacologic agents is less certain. Medications that are generally relied on to treat NMS include beta blockers, fludrocortisone, serotonin reuptake inhibitors, and midodrine. Despite the widespread use of these agents, the quality and quantity supporting these medications in the treatment of NMS are limited. Table 71.7 shows the recommendation class for each of these medications based on the 2017 ACC/AHA/HRS syncope guidelines.[1] Even though beta blockers were previously considered by many to be first-line therapy, recent studies have reported that the beta blockers metoprolol, propranolol, and nadolol are no more effective than placebo.[13] A recent subanalysis of data from a randomized prospective study evaluating the effectiveness of fludrocortisone (Florinef) reported weak evidence that fludrocortisone may be of therapeutic value despite missing its primary endpoint.[31]

Even though pacemakers have also been found to be valuable in the treatment of some patients with NMS in nonrandomized and nonblinded clinical trials, blinded randomized clinical trials have shown that pacemakers have no benefit.[32–34] In contrast, one recent randomized trial demonstrated the benefit of implanted pacemakers in a select population of patients with NMS.[35] This double-blind placebo-controlled clinical trial randomly assigned 77 patients 40 years or older with recurrent NMS, documented by implantable loop monitor as associated with 3 seconds or longer of asystole or a 6-second or greater pause without syncope, to dual-chamber pacing with rate-drop hysteresis or to sensing only. The 2-year estimated syncope recurrence rate was 57% with pacing off and 25% with pacing on. Overall, the risk for recurrent syncope was reduced by 57% with pacing. The most recent study to examine PPM in neurally mediated syncope was the SPAIN study.[36] Forty-six patients older than 40 years of age with recurrent syncope due to neurally mediated hypotension and a tilt test demonstrating bradycardia less than 40 beats/min for 10 seconds or more than 3 seconds of asystole underwent placement of a dual-chamber pacemaker with closed-loop stimulation. Patients were randomized to DDD pacing with closed loop stimulation or DDI pacing at 30 beats/min for 12 months at a time. The study was positive and revealed that DDD pacing with closed-loop stimulation reduced the syncope burden and prolonged the time to first recurrence of syncope sevenfold. Critics of the study argue that it was not perfectly blinded as patients could sense the activation of the pacing algorithm. Based on the available literature and clinical experience the 2017 ACC/AHA/HRS syncope guidelines provide a class IIb indication for pacing in a specific subgroup of patients with neurally mediated syncope over 40 years of age (see Table 71.7).[1] When considering pacemaker implantation for patients with NMS, pacemakers that provide specialized pacing algorithms are often selected. These include rate-drop hysteresis or closed-loop stimulation[33,34] and closed-loop stimulation which is a form of rate-adaptive pacing that responds to myocardial contraction dynamics by measuring variations in right ventricular intracardiac impedance. When an incipient, neurally mediated syncopal episode is detected, the pacing rate is increased. The SPAIN trial provides important data to demonstrate the potential value of close loop stimulation.[36]

CARDIONEUROABLATION FOR TREATMENT OF NEURALLY MEDIATED SYNCOPE

In 2005 a paper was published describing a new treatment for NMS, referred to as "cardioneuroablation."[37] This report included six patients with NMS. RF ablation was used to ablate the three main cardiac ganglia. All patients responded to this treatment with a mean follow-up duration of 9 months.[37] Several years later this group published an expanded report, also with encouraging results.[38] A slightly different approach based on ablation of the typical autonomic ganglia that have been identified in patients with AF was published by a Chinese team.[39] Among 10 patients with NMS, all were free of recurrent syncope. This group has subsequently published an expanded series, also with excellent results.[40,41] The most recent report describes using the cryoballoon system to accomplish neuromodulation by targeting the four PVs, using a protocol identical to what would be used to ablate AF.[42] Among 26 patients, some of whom also had AF, 84% were free of recurrent NMS during follow-up.[42] A recent editorial has drawn attention to this new treatment strategy.[16] A major limitation of all available data is that no prospective randomized clinical trials have been performed. Clearly this is the next step before "cardioneuroablation" becomes a reality.

FUTURE PERSPECTIVES

As the US population ages and the prevalence of cardiac disease increases, it is inevitable that syncope will become an increasingly common and important problem that physicians of all types will need to address. The 2017 ACC/AHA/HRS syncope guidelines provide a timely, comprehensive update on syncope and also emphasize that further research is needed. A new generation of experts in syncope must help develop further knowledge regarding the diagnosis and management of patients with syncope. A particularly challenging problem is the management of patients with various types of orthostatic hypotension. One of the most exciting developments in this field is the potential that "cardioneuroablation" will emerge as a safe and effective treatment strategy.

REFERENCES

1. Shen WK, Sheldon RS, Benditt DG, et al. 2017 ACC/AHA/HRS guideline for the evaluation and management of patients with syncope. *Circulation*. 2017;136(5):e60–e122.
2. Brignole M, Moya A, de Lange FJ, et al. Guidelines for the diagnosis and management of syncope 2009. *Eur Heart J*. 2018;30.2631.
3. Sutton R, Benditt DG. Epidemiology and economic impact of cardiac syncope in western countries. *Future Cardiol*. 2012;8:467.
4. Ruwald MH, Hansen ML, Lamberts M, et al. The relation between age, sex, comorbidity, and pharmacotherapy and the risk of syncope: a Danish nationwide study. *Europace*. 2012;14:1506.
5. Blad H, Lamberts RJ, van Dijk GJ, Thijs RD. Tilt-induced vasovagal syncope and psychogenic pseudosyncope: overlapping clinical entities. *Neurology*. 2015;85(23):2006–2010.
6. Lieve KV, van der Werf C, Wilde AA. Catecholaminergic polymorphic ventricular tachycardia. *Arrhythm Electrophysiol Rev*. 2016;5(1):45–49.
7. Maron BJ, Rowin EJ, Casey SA, Maron MS. How hypertrophic cardiomyopathy became a contemporary treatable genetic disease with low mortality: shaped by 50 years of clinical research and practice. *JAMA Cardiol*. 2016;1(1):98–105.
8. Calkins H. Arrhythmogenic right ventricular dysplasia/cardiomyopathy: three decades of progress. *Circ J*. 2015;79(5):901–913.
9. Mizusawa Y, Wilde AA. Brugada syndrome. *Circ Arrhythm Electrophysiol*. 2012;5:606.
10. Napolitano C, Bloise R, Monteforte N, Priori SG. Sudden cardiac death and genetic ion channelopathies: long QT, Brugada, short QT, catecholaminergic polymorphic ventricular tachycardia, and idiopathic ventricular fibrillation. *Circulation*. 2012;125:2027.
11. Keller K, Beule J, Balzer JO, Dippold W. Syncope and collapse in acute pulmonary embolism. *Am J Emerg Med*. 2016;34(7):1251–1257.
12. Chisholm P, Anpalahan M. Orthostatic hypotension: pathophysiology, assessment, treatment, and the paradox of supine hypertension—a review. *Intern Med J*. 2017;47(4):370–379.
13. Sheldon RS, Grubb 2nd BP, Olshansky B. 2015 Heart Rhythm Society expert consensus statement on the diagnosis and treatment of postural tachycardia syndrome, inappropriate sinus tachycardia, and vasovagal syncope. *Heart Rhythm*. 2015;12(6):e41–e63.
14. Freeman R, Illigens BMW, Lapusca R, et al. Symptom recognition is impaired in patients with orthostatic hypotension. *Hypertension*. 2020;75(5):1325–1332.
15. Sheldon R, Sandhu R. The search for the genes of vasovagal syncope. *Front Cardiovasc Med*. 2019;6:175.
16. Pachon-M JC. Neurocardiogenic syncope: pacemaker or cardioneuroablation? *Heart Rhythm*. 2020:S1547–5271(20)30177-6.
17. Kumar A, Wright K, Uceda DE, et al. Skin sympathetic nerve activity as a biomarker for syncopal episodes during a tilt table test. *Heart Rhythm*. 2020 (in press).
18. Lopes R, Gonçalves A, Campos J, et al. The role of pacemaker in hypersensitive carotid sinus syndrome. *Europace*. 2011;13:572.
19. Sheldon R, Hersi A, Ritchie D, et al. Syncope and structural heart disease: historical criteria for vasovagal syncope and ventricular tachycardia. *J Cardiovasc Electrophysiol*. 2010;21:1358.
20. Sheldon R. How to differentiate syncope from seizure. *Cardiol Clin*. 2015;33(3):377–385.
21. Brigo F, Nardone R, Bongiovanni LG. Value of tongue biting in the differential diagnosis between epileptic seizures and syncope. *Seizure*. 2012;21:568.
22. Ungar A, Mussi C, Ceccofiglio A, et al. Etiology of syncope and unexplained falls in elderly adults with dementia: Syncope and Dementia (SYD) Study. *J Am Geriatr Soc*. 2016;64(8):1567–1573.
23. Solbiati M, Costantino G, Casazza G, et al. Implantable loop recorder versus conventional diagnostic workup for unexplained recurrent syncope. *Cochrane Database Syst Rev*. 2016;4:CD011637.
24. Myerburg RJ, Marchlinski FE, Scheinman MM. Controversy on electrophysiology testing in patients with Brugada syndrome. *Heart Rhythm*. 2011;8:1972.
25. Viau JA, Chaudry H, Hannigan A, et al. The yield of computed tomography of the head among patients presenting with syncope: a systematic review. *Acad Emerg Med*. 2019;26(5):479–490.
26. Costantino G, Sun BC, Barbic F, et al. Syncope clinical management in the emergency department: a consensus from the first international workshop on syncope risk stratification in the emergency department. *Eur Heart J*. 2016;37(19):1493–1498.
27. Brignole M, Ungar A, Casagranda I, et al. Syncope Unit Project (SUP) investigators. Prospective multicentre systematic guideline-based management of patients referred to the syncope units of general hospitals. *Europace*. 2010;12(1):109–118.
28. Sanders NA, Jetter TL, Brignole M, Hamdan MH. Standardized care pathway versus conventional approach in the management of patients presenting with faint at the University of Utah. *Pacing Clin Electrophysiol*. 2013;36:152.
29. Aydin MA, Mortensen K, Salukhe TV, et al. A standardized education protocol significantly reduces traumatic injuries and syncope recurrence: an observational study in 316 patients with vasovagal syncope. *Europace*. 2012;14:410.
30. Numé AK, Gislason G, Christiansen CB, et al. Syncope and motor vehicle crash risk: a Danish nationwide study. *JAMA Intern Med*. 2016;176(4):503–510.
31. Sheldon R, Raj SR, Rose MS, et al. Fludrocortisone for the prevention of vasovagal syncope: a randomized, placebo-controlled trial. *J Am Coll Cardiol*. 2016;68(1):1–9.
32. Connolly SJ, Sheldon R, Thorpe KE, et al. Pacemaker therapy for prevention of syncope in patients with recurrent severe vasovagal syncope: Second Vasovagal Pacemaker Study (VPS II): a randomized trial. *J Am Med Assoc*. 2003;289(17):2224–2229.
33. Sutton R, de Jong JSY, Stewart JM, et al. Pacing in vasovagal syncope: physiology, pacemaker sensors, and recent clinical trials-precise patient selection and measurable benefit. *Heart Rhythm*. 2020:S1547–5271(20)30084–9.
34. de Jong JSY, Jardine DL, Lenders JWM, Wieling W. Pacing in vasovagal syncope: a physiological paradox?. *Heart Rhythm*. 2019 Sep 24:S1547–5271(19)30855-0.
35. Brignole M, Menozzi C, Moya A, et al. Pacemaker therapy in patients with neurally mediated syncope and documented asystole. Third International Study on Syncope of Uncertain Etiology (ISSUE-3): a randomized trial. *Circulation*. 2012;125(21):2566–2571.
36. Baron-Esquivias G, Morillo CA, Moya-Mitjans A, et al. Dual-chamber pacing with closed loop stimulation in recurrent reflex vasovagal syncope: the Spain study. *J Am Coll Cardiol*. 2017;70(14):1720–1728.
37. Pachon JC, Pachon EI, Pachon JC, et al. Cardioneuroablation"—new treatment for neurocardiogenic syncope, functional AV block and sinus dysfunction using catheter RF-ablation. *Europace*. 2005;7(1):1–13.
38. Pachon JC, Pachon EI, Cunha Pachon MZ, et al. Catheter ablation of severe neurally mediated reflex (neurocardiogenic or vasovagal) syncope: cardioneuroablation long-term results. *Europace*. 2011;13(9):1231–1242.
39. Yao Y, Shi R, Wong T, et al. Endocardial autonomic denervation of the left atrium to treat vasovagal syncope: an early experience in humans. *Circ Arrhythm Electrophysiol*. 2012;5(2):279–286.
40. Sun W, Zheng L, Qiao Y, et al. Catheter ablation as a treatment for vasovagal syncope: long-term outcome of endocardial autonomic modification of the left atrium. *J Am Heart Assoc*. 2016;5(7):e003471.
41. Hu F, Zheng L, Liang E, et al. Right anterior ganglionated plexus: the primary target of cardioneuroablation? *Heart Rhythm*. 2019;16(10):1545–1551.
42. Maj R, Borio G, Osório TG, et al. Conversion of atrial fibrillation to sinus rhythm during cryoballoon ablation: a favorable and not unusual phenomenon during second-generation cryoballoon pulmonary vein isolation. *J Arrhythm*. 2020;36(2):319–327.

第八部分　心脏瓣膜疾病

王墨扬　吴永健　导读

心脏瓣膜疾病是心脏病领域常见的重要病种，其发病机制复杂，病理生理改变对心脏功能以及心肌重塑等具有深远影响。同时其临床症状表现多样，不同病变治疗干预时机及方式也不尽相同，而我国罹患心脏瓣膜疾病患者人群庞大，对于社会及健康负担严重，所以心脏瓣膜疾病是我们需要面对和解决的重要疾患。随着时代的发展，全球人口老龄化趋势明显，心脏瓣膜疾病谱发生改变，同时医疗技术及检查手段不断完善，其诊断及治疗方式在近年取得重大进步，尤其以微创介入治疗为主的新兴方式的发展使得很多心脏瓣膜疾病患者有了新的治疗机会和选择。本部分在系统性梳理经典心脏瓣膜疾病的流行病学、病理生理机制、临床诊断标准之外着重展示了在新时期瓣膜疾病治疗学的进展和未来方向，对主动脉瓣疾病、二尖瓣疾病到三尖瓣疾病及多瓣膜疾病均进行了深度的探讨，同时对于瓣膜感染性疾病以及风湿性疾病等特殊病种也进行了介绍。相信阅读本部分的内容会使读者像坐上了心脏瓣膜疾病领域发展长河中的一艘小船，在饱揽经典历史之后一起驶向未来的新技术海洋。

本部分共分为 10 个章节（72～81 章），第 72～73 章主要介绍了主动脉瓣狭窄与反流两种疾病的相关内容，条理清晰地介绍了其病因、流行病学特征、病理生理机制、临床表现、临床分期及治疗方法，尤其是针对复合影像学及功能学检查判定疾病程度及分期等进行了详细讲解。第 74 章介绍了目前心脏瓣膜疾病介入治疗最为成熟与具有代表性的经导管主动脉瓣置换术（TAVR）技术的发展历程，本章针对患者筛选、解剖评估、器械研发、植入策略等方面均进行了介绍，同时对于尚缺乏证据的二叶式主动脉瓣 TAVR、单纯主动脉瓣反流 TAVR 等难点热点进行了展望和分析。第 75～76 章重点介绍了二尖瓣狭窄和反流两种疾病，虽然目前以风湿性改变为主的二尖瓣狭窄在发达国家较为少见，但在我国仍然是临床常见的瓣膜疾病，其球囊扩张及外科干预的指征和治疗方法需要我们仔细研读。而二尖瓣反流是目前最具有发展前景的微创治疗瓣膜病种，第 76 章系统分析了不同二尖瓣反流机制的差异以及其治疗指征及方法的异同，对于理解二尖瓣介入治疗器械和手术方式具有重要的基石作用。第 77 章对于三尖瓣和多瓣膜受累疾病进行了介绍，作为最容易被遗忘的瓣膜，三尖瓣疾病近年越来越被学术界重视，本章对于右心系统血流动力学的特殊性及三尖瓣解剖进行了细致讲解，同时对于多瓣膜疾病的治疗方式进行了探讨。第 78 章针对二、三尖瓣介入治疗进行介绍，展现了目前瓣膜疾病治疗方式的最前沿内容，文章中列举了诸多最新的器械以及治疗方式，对不同解剖和适应证的原理进行了分析，是了解瓣膜疾病最新技术的最佳窗口。第 79 章主要内容为目前人工瓣膜的发展进程，器械进步是目前技术革新的重要组成部分，本章重点介绍了包括外科瓣膜及介入瓣膜的种类、特点以及研发方向。第 80～81 章则就心脏瓣膜疾病中特殊病种——感染性疾病及风湿性疾病进行了系统梳理，对于尚处于发展中的我国具有特殊意义，值得临床医生参考。

　　本部分对于心脏瓣膜疾病的介绍系统经典、内容翔实，同时结合了最前沿的治疗方式和器械研发，相信会给读者带来丰富的知识与思考启迪。

PART VIII DISEASES OF THE HEART VALVES

72 Aortic Valve Stenosis

BRIAN R. LINDMAN, ROBERT O. BONOW, AND CATHERINE M. OTTO

扫描二维码阅读
第72章中文导读

EPIDEMIOLOGY, 1399

CAUSES AND ETIOLOGY, 1399
Calcific Aortic Valve Disease, 1399
Bicuspid Aortic Valve Disease, 1399
Rheumatic Aortic Stenosis, 1400

PATHOPHYSIOLOGY, 1400
Valve Calcification and Obstruction, 1400
Left Ventricular Response: Structure and Function, 1401

Pulmonary and Systemic Vasculature Response, 1403

CLINICAL PRESENTATION, 1403
Symptoms, 1403
Physical Examination, 1406
Diagnostic Testing, 1406

DISEASE COURSE AND STAGING, 1408
Progressive Aortic Stenosis, 1409
Classification of Severe Aortic Stenosis, 1409

TREATMENT, 1412
Medical Management, 1412
Balloon Aortic Valvuloplasty, 1413
Aortic Valve Replacement, 1413

CLASSIC REFERENCES, 1417

REFERENCES, 1417

EPIDEMIOLOGY

In population-based echocardiographic studies, 1% to 2% of persons aged 65 or older and 12% of persons 75 or older had calcific aortic stenosis (AS)[1-3] (see Chapter 90). Among those older than 75, 3.4% (95% confidence interval [CI] 1.1% to 5.7%) have severe AS.[2] The prevalence of aortic valve sclerosis without stenosis, defined as irregular thickening or calcification of the aortic valve leaflets, increases with age and ranges from 9% in populations with a mean age of 54 years to 42% in populations with a mean age of 81 years.[4] The rate of progression from aortic sclerosis to stenosis is 1.8% to 1.9% per year. With the aging of the population, the number of individuals with AS is expected to increase twofold to threefold in developed countries in the coming decades.[3]

CAUSES AND ETIOLOGY

Valvular AS has three principal causes: a congenital bicuspid valve with superimposed calcification, calcification of a normal trileaflet valve, and rheumatic disease (Fig. 72.1). In a U.S. series of 933 patients undergoing aortic valve replacement (AVR) for AS, a bicuspid valve was present in more than 50%, including two thirds of those younger than 70 years and 40% of those older than 70 (see Classic References, Roberts and Ko).

In addition, AS may result from a congenital valve stenosis manifesting in infancy or childhood. Rarely, AS is caused by severe atherosclerosis of the aorta and aortic valve; this form of AS occurs most frequently in patients with severe hypercholesterolemia and is observed in children with homozygous type II hyperlipoproteinemia. Rheumatoid involvement of the valve is a rare cause of AS and results in nodular thickening of the valve leaflets and involvement of the proximal portion of the aorta. Ochronosis with alkaptonuria is another rare cause of AS.

Fixed obstruction to left ventricular (LV) outflow also may occur above the valve (supravalvular stenosis) or below the valve (discrete subvalvular stenosis) (see Fig. 16.41). Dynamic subaortic obstruction may be caused by hypertrophic cardiomyopathy (see Chapter 54).

Calcific Aortic Valve Disease

Calcific (formerly "senile" or "degenerative") aortic valve disease affecting a congenital bicuspid or normal trileaflet valve is now the most common cause of AS in adults. Aortic sclerosis, identified by either echocardiography or computed tomography (CT), is the initial stage of calcific valve disease and, even in the absence of valve obstruction or known cardiovascular disease, is associated with an increased risk of myocardial infarction (MI) and cardiovascular and all-cause mortality.[4] Epidemiologic associations have been documented between cardiovascular risk factors and calcific aortic valve disease, suggesting that treating or preventing these risk factors may lessen the risk of developing AS (Table 72.1).[1,5] Whether better control of modifiable risk factors may slow progression of AS is unknown.[6]

Bicuspid Aortic Valve Disease

Congenital malformations of the aortic valve may be unicuspid, bicuspid, or quadricuspid, or the anomaly may manifest as a dome-shaped diaphragm (see Chapter 82). Unicuspid valves typically produce severe obstruction in infancy and are the most common malformations found in fatal valvular AS in children younger than 1 year but also may be seen in young adults with an anatomy that mimics bicuspid valve disease. A congenital bicuspid aortic valve (BAV) is present in approximately 1% to 2% of the population, with a male predominance of approximately 3:1. Reflecting an underlying but complex genetic basis, a 9% prevalence of BAV has been reported in first-degree relatives of individuals with a BAV.

A BAV may be an isolated abnormality (approximately 50% of the time) or occur in the context of a genetic syndrome (e.g., Turner syndrome), alongside other congenital heart defects (e.g., hypoplastic left heart, coarctation of the aorta), or with a thoracic aortic aneurysm (most common nonvalvular manifestation).[7] The genetic etiologies of BAV are complicated and incompletely understood; several genes appear to play a role with different patterns of inheritance. Familial inheritance is complex and increased when nonvalvular abnormalities accompany a BAV.

The most prevalent anatomy for a bicuspid valve is two cusps with a right-left systolic opening, consistent with congenital fusion of the right and left coronary cusps, seen in 70% to 80% of patients (Fig. 72.2). An anterior-posterior orientation, with fusion of the right and noncoronary cusps, is less common, seen in approximately 20% to 30% of patients. Fusion of the left and noncoronary cusps is rarely seen. A prominent ridge of tissue or raphe may be present in the larger of the two cusps so that the closed valve in diastole may mimic a trileaflet valve. Echocardiographic diagnosis relies on imaging the systolic leaflet opening with only two aortic commissures, but CT is now commonly used to identify or confirm the bicuspid morphology of the valve (Fig. 72.3).

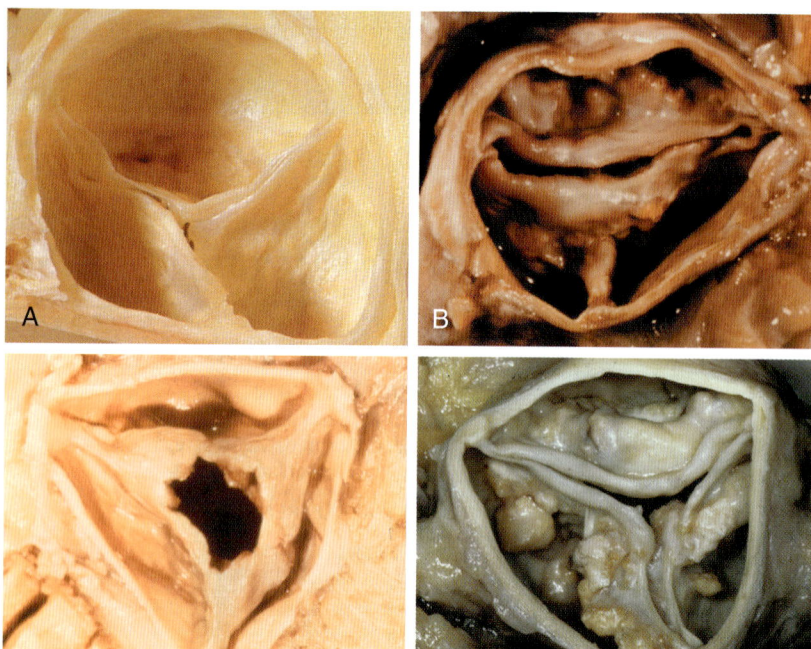

FIGURE 72.1 Major types of aortic valve stenosis. **A,** Normal aortic valve. **B,** Congenital bicuspid aortic stenosis. A false raphe is present at 6 o'clock. **C,** Rheumatic aortic stenosis. The commissures are fused with a fixed central orifice. **D,** Calcific aortic stenosis. (**A** from Manabe H, Yutani C, editors. *Atlas of Valvular Heart Disease*. Singapore: Churchill Livingstone; 1998:6, 131; **B-D** courtesy Dr. William C. Roberts, Baylor University Medical Center, Dallas, Tex.)

TABLE 72.1 Strength of Associations in Observational and Epidemiologic Studies of Clinical Risk Factors and Calcific Aortic Valve Disease (CAVD)

RISK FACTOR	CAVD ANALYSIS		
	CROSS-SECTIONAL	INCIDENT	PROGRESSION
Age	+++	+++	+++
Male sex	++/−	++	0
Height	++	++	0
Body mass index	++	++	0
Hypertension	++	++	0
Diabetes	+++	+++	0
Metabolic syndrome	++	++	+
Dyslipidemia	++	++	0
Smoking	++	++	+
Renal dysfunction	+	0	0
Inflammatory markers	+	0	0
Phosphorus levels	++	0	N/A
Calcium levels	0	0	N/A
Baseline calcium score	N/A	N/A	+++

+, Weak positive association; ++, modest positive association; +++, strong positive association; −, weak negative association; 0, no association seen; N/A, no/insufficient data available.
From Thanassoulis G. Clinical and genetic risk factors for calcific valve disease. In Otto CM, Bonow RO, editors. *Valvular Heart Disease: A Companion to Braunwald's Heart Disease*. 5th ed. Philadelphia: Saunders; 2021;66-78.

Unicuspid valves are distinguished from a bicuspid valve by having only one aortic commissure.

The clinical manifestations of a BAV tend to relate to the function of the aortic valve (stenosis or regurgitation), infection of the aortic valve (endocarditis), or damage to a dilated aorta related to an underlying aortopathy (dissection).[8] Often, the diagnosis is unknown until the physical examination reveals manifestations of valve dysfunction or the patient develops symptoms. The risk of aortic dissection in patients with BAV is five to nine times higher than in the general population, but the absolute risk is still quite low (see Chapter 42).[9,10]

Most bicuspid valves function normally until late in life, although a subset of patients present in childhood or adolescence with valve dysfunction. Overall, survival is no different from population estimates.[9,11] Patients with BAV also are at increased risk for endocarditis (0.4 per 100,000), accounting for approximately 1200 deaths per year in the United States. However, the most common cardiac event is need for AVR,[9] and most patients with BAV develop calcific valve stenosis later in life, typically presenting with severe AS after the age of 50 years. Although the histopathologic features of calcific stenosis of a BAV are no different from those of a trileaflet valve, the turbulent flow and increased leaflet stress caused by the abnormal architecture are postulated to result in accelerated valve changes, explaining the earlier average age at presentation in patients with a bicuspid, compared with trileaflet, stenotic valve. BAV disease accounts for greater than 50% of AVRs in the United States and is a common cause of calcific AS, even in older persons. The aortopathy associated with BAV disease often results in aortic dilation and carries an increased risk of aortic dissection. The magnitude of risk appears to vary depending on valve and aortic morphology and on a family history of aortic involvement.[12,13]

Rheumatic Aortic Stenosis

Rheumatic AS results from adhesions and fusions of the commissures and cusps and vascularization of the leaflets of the valve ring, leading to retraction and stiffening of the free borders of the cusps. Calcific nodules develop on both surfaces, and the orifice is reduced to a small, round or triangular opening (see Fig. 72.1C). As a consequence, the rheumatic valve often is regurgitant as well as stenotic. Patients with rheumatic AS invariably have rheumatic involvement of the mitral valve (see Chapter 81). With the decline in rheumatic fever in developed nations, rheumatic AS is decreasing in frequency, although it continues to be a major problem on a worldwide basis.

PATHOPHYSIOLOGY
Valve Calcification and Obstruction

Although calcific AS once was considered to represent the result of years of normal mechanical stress on an otherwise normal valve ("wear and tear"), it is now clear that active biological processes underlies the initiation and progression of calcific aortic valve disease (Fig. 72.4).[1,14-16] Differences in the biology driving the early versus later stages of calcific aortic valve disease could have important implications for medical therapies aimed at preventing, slowing, or reversing the path from aortic sclerosis to severe stenosis, both in terms of which pathways are relevant to target and when along the disease spectrum drugs targeting them are most likely to be effective.[15-17]

Normal valve leaflets comprise the fibrosa (facing the aorta), ventricularis (facing the ventricle), and spongiosa (located between the fibrosa and ventricularis). *Valve interstitial cells* (VICs) are the most predominant cell type; endothelial and smooth muscle cells are also present. Through a complex interplay of molecular events, the pliable, flexible valve becomes stiff and immobile, characterized grossly by fibrosis and calcification. The process is initiated by lipid infiltration and oxidative stress, which attract and activate inflammatory cells and promote the elaboration of cytokines (Fig. 72.5).[1] VICs undergo osteogenic reprogramming that promotes the mineralization of the extracellular matrix and the progression of fibrocalcific remodeling of the valve.

In addition to the genetic underpinnings of BAV, there is evidence indicating a genetic predisposition to valve calcification.[18] Genetic polymorphisms have been linked to the presence of calcific AS, including

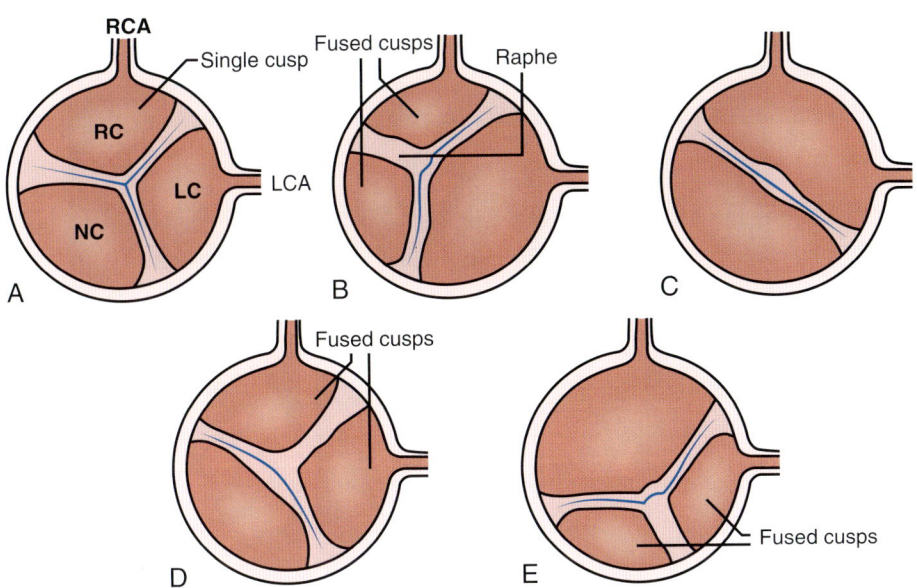

FIGURE 72.2 Comparison of tricuspid and bicuspid aortic valve structures. **A,** Schematic representation of a normal tricuspid aortic valve with the three cusps. *LC,* Left coronary; *LCA,* left coronary artery; *NC,* noncoronary; *RC,* right coronary; *RCA,* right coronary artery. **B,** Bicuspid valve with right noncoronary cusp fusion and one raphe (the line of union between the fused cusps). **C,** Bicuspid valve with fusion of the right and left coronary cusps and no raphe. **D,** Bicuspid valve with right-left coronary cusp fusion and one raphe. **E,** Bicuspid valve with fusion of the left and noncoronary cusps and one raphe. (From Lindman BR, et al. Calcific aortic stenosis. *Nat Rev Dis Primers.* 2016;2:16006.)

Hypertrophic Myocardial Remodeling. Maintenance of cardiac output in the face of an obstructed aortic valve imposes a chronic increase in LV pressure. In response, the ventricle typically undergoes hypertrophic remodeling characterized by myocyte hypertrophy and increased wall thickness (Fig. 72.6). LV remodeling may manifest as concentric remodeling, concentric hypertrophy, or eccentric hypertrophy. Based on the LaPlace law, LV remodeling reduces wall stress (afterload) and is considered one of the important compensatory mechanisms to maintain LV ejection performance, which is directly affected by afterload (see Classic References, Grossman).

Cardiac hypertrophy in response to pressure overload involves both adaptive and maladaptive processes.[36] Hypertrophic remodeling is not simply related to increased valvular afterload; several factors other than the severity of valve obstruction influence it, including sex, genetics, vascular load, and metabolic abnormalities.[37,38] Additionally, the degree to which LV hypertrophic remodeling is maladaptive versus adaptive and the resulting functional and clinical effects are not simply an issue of total LV mass and geometry; composition and energetics of the myocardium also are important.[36] Preclinical studies have demonstrated that blocking the hypertrophic response to pressure overload did not have deleterious effects on LV performance despite increased wall stress (see Classic References, Hill).

In patients with AS, several studies have now documented that increased LV hypertrophic remodeling is associated with more severe ventricular dysfunction and heart failure (HF) symptoms, as well as higher mortality.[39] In a recent study combining the largest patient numbers with the longest clinical follow-up to date, increased LV mass index before transcatheter aortic valve replacement (TAVR), particularly severe LV hypertrophy (LVH) was associated with increased mortality and rehospitalization over 5 years after the procedure.[40] Related to this, among patients with moderate or severe LVH treated with TAVR, greater LV mass index regression at 1 year is independently associated with lower death and rehospitalization rates out to 5 years.[41] Among those with moderate or severe LVH before TAVR, 39% still had severe LVH at 1 year and this degree of residual LVH was associated with a marked increase in subsequent mortality and rehospitalization rates.[41] Thus, although it may reduce wall stress, LV hypertrophic remodeling also may have longer-term deleterious effects that translate into impaired ventricular performance and worse clinical outcomes.

Myocardial Fibrosis. Although not routinely assessed in clinical practice, myocardial fibrosis is now well established as a risk factor for adverse clinical outcomes in patients with AS.[34,42-44] As a part of the hypertrophic remodeling process, diffuse and replacement myocardial fibrosis (not fibrosis from prior MI) may develop (see Chapter 19), although the incidence and extent of fibrosis are variable and unpredictable and the underlying biologic mechanisms not yet clarified (Fig. 72.7; see also Fig 72.6).[42,43,45] Diffuse fibrosis tends to regress after AVR, whereas replacement fibrosis does not.[34,45-47] Both the amount of diffuse fibrosis and the presence of replacement fibrosis are associated with subsequent mortality (Fig. 72.8).[34,42-44] Importantly, patients with severe fibrosis, despite a normal LV ejection fraction (LVEF), are more likely to have worse preoperative HF symptoms and less likely to experience improvement in symptoms midterm after AVR, compared to those with no or minimal fibrosis before valve replacement.[48]

Myocardial Ischemia. In patients with AS, the hypertrophied left ventricle, increased systolic pressure, and prolongation of ejection all elevate myocardial oxygen (O_2) consumption.[49] At the same time, even in the absence of epicardial coronary artery disease (CAD), decreased myocardial capillary density in the hypertrophied ventricle, endothelial cell loss, increased LV end-diastolic pressure (LVEDP), and a shortened diastole all serve to decrease the coronary perfusion pressure gradient and myocardial blood flow (see Chapter 36). Together, these conditions create an imbalance between myocardial O_2 supply and demand, yielding ischemia. Impaired myocardial flow reserve underlies symptoms of angina in patients with AS that is often indistinguishable from that caused by epicardial coronary obstruction.[50] Exercise or other states of increased O_2 demand may exacerbate this ischemic imbalance and

those involving the vitamin D receptor, interleukin (IL)-10 alleles, estrogen receptor, transforming growth factor (TGF)-β receptor, and the apolipoprotein E4 allele.[18] The most consistently observed genetic association is for lipoprotein(a) (Lp(a)). In a genome-wide association study (GWAS) based on a meta-analysis of data on nearly 7000 patients from three population-based cohorts, a single-nucleotide polymorphism (SNP) in Lp(a) was associated with aortic valve calcification, serum Lp(a) levels, and incident AS (hazard ratio [HR], 1.68; CI 1.32 to 2.15).[19] This association has been confirmed in several other cohorts.[20-22] Recent evidence suggests a potential link between Lp(a) and AS through lipoprotein-associated phospholipase A_2 (Lp-PLA$_2$) and ectonucleotide pyrophosphatase/phosphodiesterase family member 2 (ENPP2), also known as *autotaxin*.[23-27] Lp(a) transports both Lp-PLA$_2$ and autotaxin, and each of these is found in increased abundance in stenotic aortic valves.[25,26] Lp-PLA$_2$ transforms oxidized phospholipids species into lysophosphatidylcholine (lysoPC); in turn, autotaxin transforms lysoPC into lysophosphatidic acid (lysoPA), which appears to play a role in the osteogenic reprogramming of VICs.[26,27]

Key regulators of osteogenesis, including *BMP2* and *RUNX2*, are under the control of *NOTCH1*. Expression of BMP2 and RUNX2 are increased in diseased aortic valves. Heritable forms of calcific aortic valve disease have been linked to *NOTCH1* mutations; more recently, a role for NOTCH1 in idiopathic forms of calcific aortic valve disease was discovered.[28,29] Hypomethylation of the promoter region of long noncoding RNA *H19* led to overexpression of *H19*, which was associated with mineralized aortic valves and upregulation of *BMP2* and *RUNX2*. This was shown to be mediated by repression of *NOTCH1* as a result of *H19* preventing recruitment of p53 to the *NOTCH1* promoter. Subsequent investigations showed that cadherin 11 (*CDH11*), which is enriched in diseased aortic valves and overexpressed in VICs from *Notch1*+/− mice, mediates *NOTCH1*-induced calcific aortic valve disease.[30] The roles of DNA methylation and noncoding RNAs in the pathophysiology of calcific aortic valve disease have been reviewed.[31] Despite progress in elucidating pathobiology, there is no medical therapy for calcific aortic valve disease, but several potentially promising therapeutic targets have been reviewed.[15,17,32]

Over time, progressive fibrocalcific remodeling of the aortic valve leaflets makes them less pliable and obstruction to flow out of the left ventricle develops and increases. This yields a chronic pressure overload state that leads to myocardial remodeling and dysfunction and accompanying changes in the pulmonary and systemic vasculature.

Left Ventricular Response: Structure and Function

Progressive valve obstruction imposes a chronic pressure overload state that leads to numerous changes in the structure and function of the left ventricle and accompanying changes in the pulmonary and systemic vasculature.[33-35]

Classification	Characteristics	Double oblique transverse MPR	Volume-rendered en face view systole	Volume-rendered en face view diastole
Sievers Type 0/ bicommissural non–raphe type	• Two fairly symmetric cusps and two commissures • Each cusp has one most basal insertion point; thus there is a total of two most basal insertion points			
Sievers Type 1/ bicommissural raphe type	• Two of three cusps are conjoined by a raphe • Asymmetric cusp sizes with the cusp opposing the raphe (i.e., cusp not participating in raphe formation) being larger than in a tricuspid aortic valve • Raphe does not extend to the level of the STJ, which is the distinguishing characteristic compared to a non-opening commissure • Size of raphe and degree of calcification can vary *Upper row*: non-calcified raphe *Middle row*: Moderately calcified raphe *Lower row*: Severely calcified raphe			
Acquired/ functional bicuspid valve (underlying tricuspid anatomy)	• Underlying tricuspid anatomy with symmetric sinus of Valsalva • Non-opening commissure due to degenerative changes (here RL commissure) • Non-opening commissure reaches STJ, which is the distinguishing factor compared to a raphe			

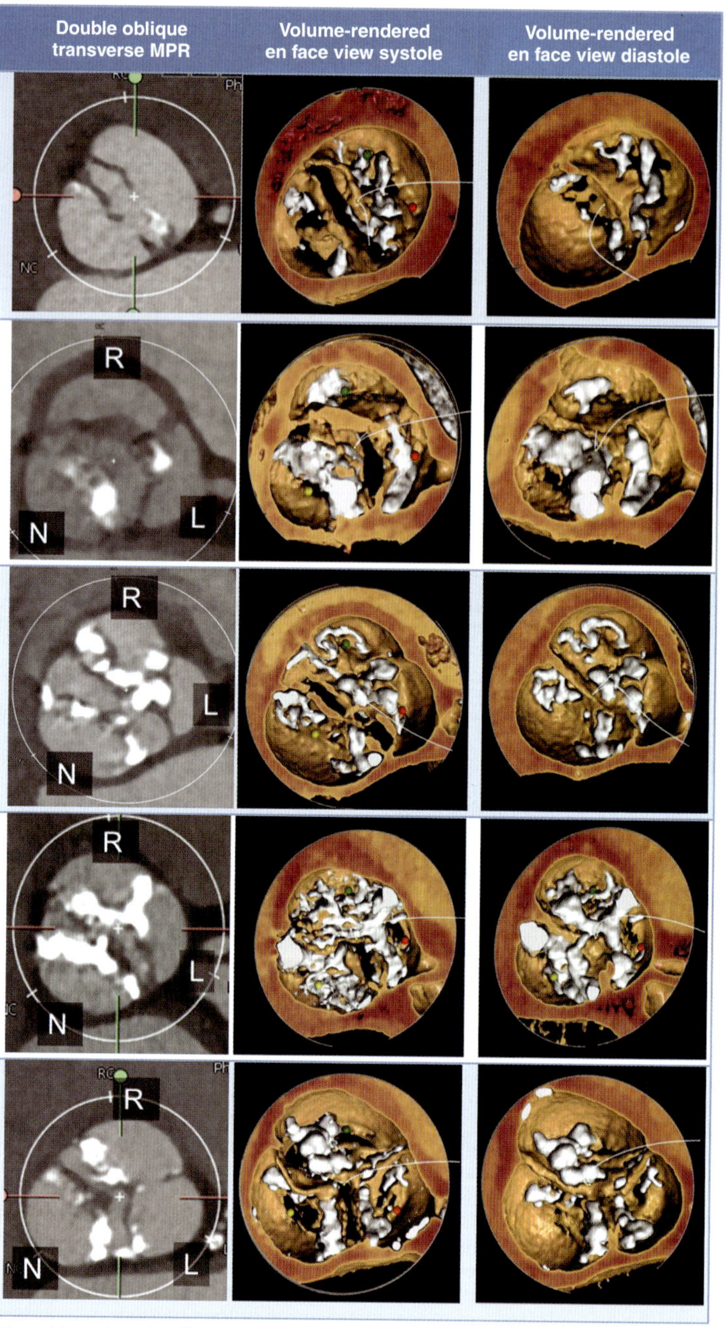

FIGURE 72.3 Differing morphologies and calcification patterns of bicuspid aortic valves by cardiac CT. *STJ*, Sinotubular junction. (From Blanke P, et al. Computed tomography imaging in the context of transcatheter aortic valve implantation (TAVI)/transcatheter aortic valve replacement (TAVR). *JACC Cardiovasc Imaging*. 2019;12:1-24.)

provoke angina that may not be experienced at rest. Myocardial flow reserve is independently associated with aerobic exercise capacity and HF functional class in severe AS and appears to be influenced by the extent of LV hypertrophic remodeling and fibrosis, endothelial cell loss, and severity of valve obstruction.[51,52]

Left Ventricular Diastolic Function. Hypertrophic remodeling also impairs diastolic myocardial relaxation and increases stiffness, as modulated by cardiovascular and metabolic comorbidities.[53] Higher cardiomyocyte stiffness, increased myocardial fibrosis, advanced-glycation end products, and metabolic abnormalities each contribute to increased chamber stiffness and higher end-diastolic pressures.[43] Atrial contraction plays a particularly important role in filling of the left ventricle in AS because it increases LVEDP without causing a concomitant elevation of mean left atrial pressure. This "booster pump" function of the left atrium prevents the pulmonary venous and capillary pressures from rising to levels that would produce pulmonary congestion, while maintaining LVEDP at the elevated level necessary for effective contraction of the hypertrophied left ventricle. Loss of appropriately timed, vigorous atrial contraction, as occurs in atrial fibrillation (AF) or atrioventricular (AV) dissociation, may result in rapid clinical deterioration in patients with severe AS. After relief of the pressure overload with AVR, diastolic dysfunction may revert toward normal with regression of hypertrophy, but some degree of long-term diastolic dysfunction typically persists.[53,54] Worse diastolic function before AVR and worse residual diastolic dysfunction after AVR have been associated with worse long-term outcomes.[53,54] The severity of diastolic dysfunction may also influence the clinical consequences of aortic regurgitation (AR) after TAVR.[55]

Left Ventricular Systolic Function. LV systolic function, as measured by the LVEF, generally remains preserved until late in the disease process in most patients with AS, but emerging data indicate that ejection fraction (EF) may begin to decline in patients before AS is considered severe.[1,56] What characterizes a "normal" or "preserved" EF in the setting of AS is not clear. Traditionally, it has been characterized as an EF 50% or greater, but accumulating evidence indicates that an EF <60% is associated with poor post-AVR outcomes, suggesting that the threshold indicative of impaired/

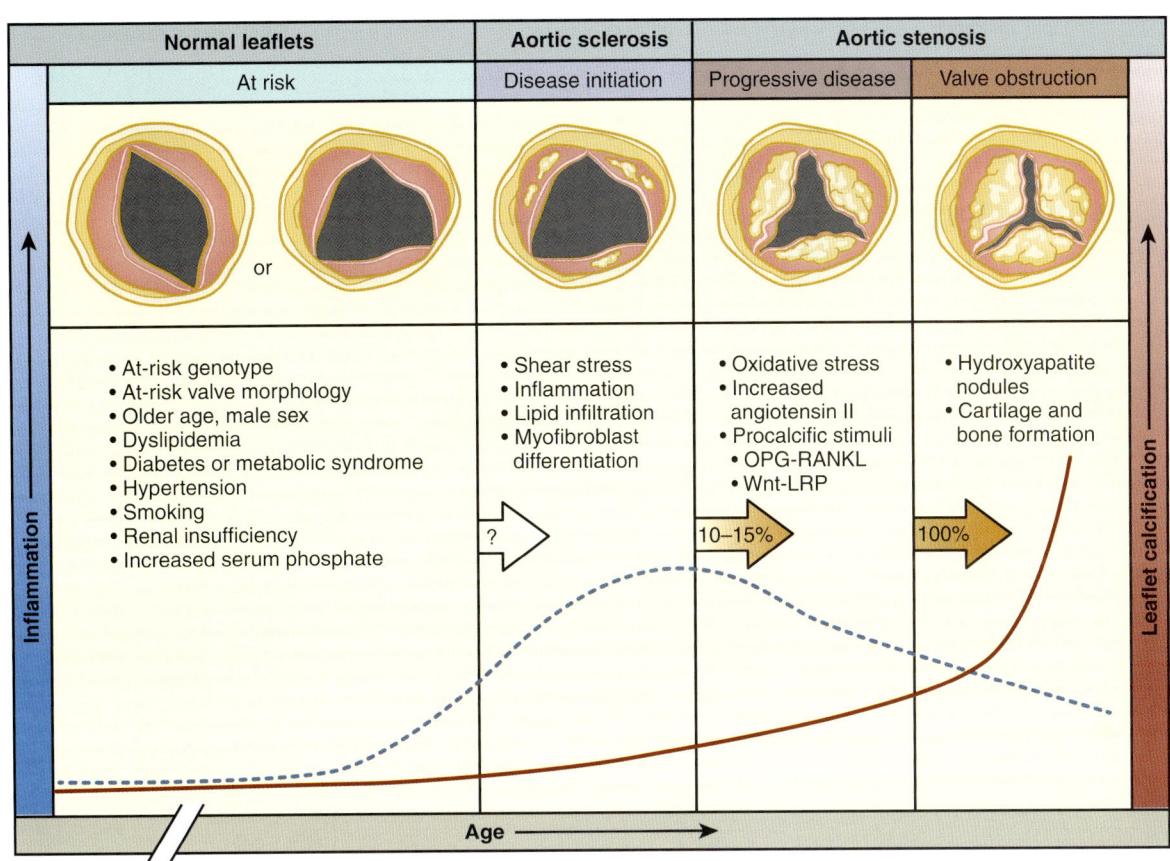

FIGURE 72.4 Disease mechanisms and time course of calcific aortic stenosis (AS): relationship among disease stage, valve anatomy, clinical risk factors, mechanisms of disease, and patient's age. Endothelial disruption with inflammation (*dashed line*) and lipid infiltration are key elements in the initiation of disease. There are few data on the prevalence of disease initiation in at-risk patients, and progressive disease develops in only a subgroup of these patients. Progressive leaflet disease, which is associated with several disease pathways, develops in approximately 10% to 15% of patients with AS. Once these disease mechanisms are activated, leaflet calcification results in severe AS in almost all patients. With end-stage disease, tissue calcification (*red line*) is the predominant tissue change, resulting in valve obstruction. Current imaging approaches are reliable only when substantial leaflet changes are present (in patients with progressive disease or valve obstruction), which limits clinical studies of interventions to prevent or slow the progression of early disease. *LRP*, Lipoprotein receptor–related protein complex; *OPG*, osteoprotegerin; *RANKL*, receptor activator of nuclear factor-κB ligand. (From Otto CM, Prendergast B. Aortic-valve stenosis: from patients at risk to severe valve obstruction. *N Engl J Med.* 2014;371:744-756.)

reduced EF in the setting of AS may need to be changed.[57-61] Before a reduction in EF occurs, more subtle systolic dysfunction can be detected as reduced longitudinal systolic strain, which is associated with worse outcomes in patients with severe AS[59,62] (see Chapter 16). The development and severity of systolic dysfunction results from a complex interplay of factors, including the severity of valve obstruction, metabolic abnormalities, vascular load, maladaptive hypertrophy (resulting in impaired contractility), ischemia, and fibrosis.[1,38,45] Eventually, a subset of patients develops overt systolic dysfunction manifested by a reduced LVEF. In these patients, systolic function usually improves after the ventricle is unloaded by AVR; the amount of recovery depends on many factors, including the degree to which systolic dysfunction was affected by afterload mismatch versus myocardial fibrosis and altered contractility.[63-65]

Pulmonary and Systemic Vasculature Response

The hypertrophied and pressure-overloaded left ventricle transmits increased pressure to the pulmonary vasculature, which leads to pulmonary hypertension in many patients with AS, becoming severe in 15% to 20%. Although patients may initially manifest pulmonary venous hypertension alone, some will go on to develop increased pulmonary vascular resistance, perhaps influenced by specific comorbidities and chronicity of pulmonary venous hypertension.[66-68] Among asymptomatic patients, exercise-induced pulmonary hypertension is associated with decreased event-free survival, and among patients undergoing TAVR or surgical AVR (SAVR), the presence and severity of pulmonary hypertension is associated with increased postoperative mortality.[67,68] Elevated pulmonary artery pressures decrease in some patients after AVR, but not all; residual pulmonary hypertension is associated with worse clinical outcomes.[69,70]

The systemic vasculature also makes an important contribution to total LV afterload.[33,66,71-73] Hemodynamic studies with agents that dilate the systemic vasculature show an acute increase in LV stroke volume, underscoring that changes in vascular properties can unload the left ventricle despite no change in the valvular obstruction[66,74] (see also Classic References, Khot). Measures of increased vascular load, including arterial stiffness, global load (integrating both valvular and vascular load), and systolic blood pressure, have been associated with adverse LV remodeling, impaired LV function, and worse clinical outcomes.[72,75] In patients with AS, characterization of systemic vascular properties is conditioned by upstream obstruction; valve replacement unmasks and induces stiffer vascular behavior (Fig. 72.9).[71] Accordingly, in patients with AS, the load on the LV is a combined load at the valvular and vascular level; increased vascular load may identify patients who benefit less from AVR and may be a target for adjunctive medical therapy to optimize outcomes.

CLINICAL PRESENTATION

The diagnosis of AS is most often made on auscultation of a murmur suggestive of AS, followed by confirmation with echocardiography. When AS is not severe and symptoms are absent, patients are reevaluated clinically and with echocardiography based on the AS severity. Generally, repeat imaging is performed every 6 to 12 months for severe AS, every 1 to 2 years for moderate AS, and every 3 to 5 years for mild AS, unless a change in signs or symptoms prompts repeat imaging sooner.[57]

Symptoms

The cardinal manifestations of acquired AS are exertional dyspnea, angina, syncope, and ultimately HF.[1,14] Many patients are diagnosed

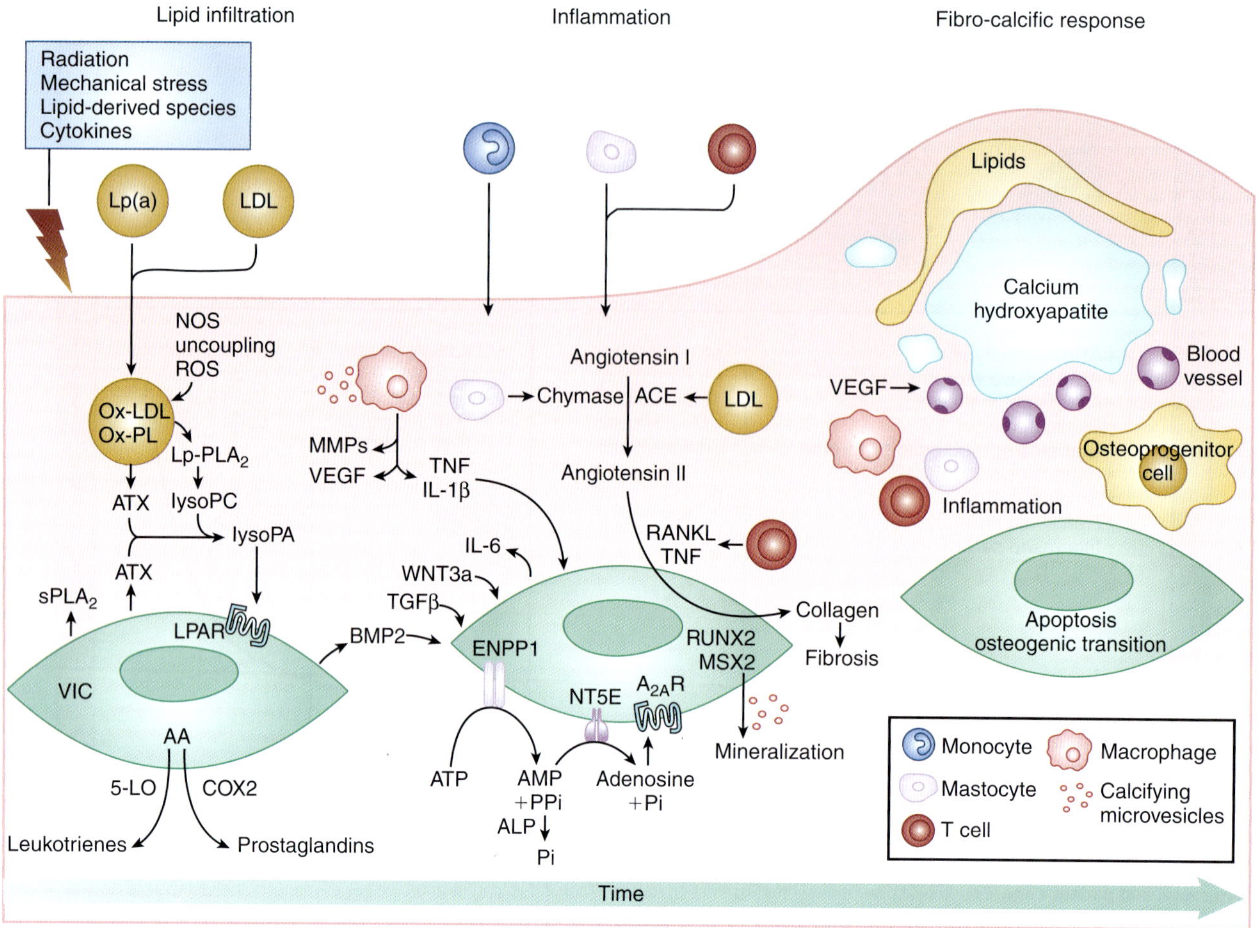

FIGURE 72.5 Pathogenesis of calcific aortic stenosis. Endothelial damage allows infiltration of lipids, specifically low-density lipoprotein (*LDL*) and lipoprotein(a) [*Lp(a)*], into the fibrosa and triggers the recruitment of inflammatory cells into the aortic valve. Endothelial injury can be triggered by several factors, including lipid-derived species, cytokines, mechanical stress, and radiation injury. The production of reactive oxygen species (*ROS*) is promoted by the uncoupling of nitric oxide synthase (*NOS*), which increases the oxidation of lipids and further intensifies the secretion of cytokines. Enzymes transported in the aortic valve by lipoproteins (i.e., LDL, Lp[a]) such as lipoprotein-associated phospholipase A_2 (*Lp-PLA_2*) and ectonucleotide pyrophosphatase/phosphodiesterase 2 (ENPP2), also known as autotoxin (*ATX*), produce lysophospholipid derivatives. ATX, which is also secreted by valve interstitial cells (*VICs*), transforms lysophosphatidylcholine (*lysoPC*) into lysophosphatidic acid (*lysoPA*). Several factors, including lysoPA, the receptor activator of nuclear factor-κB ligand (*RANKL*; also known as TNFSF11), and WNT3a, promote the osteogenic transition of VIC. Arachidonic acid (*AA*) generated by cytosolic PLA_2 promotes the production of eicosanoids such as prostaglandins and leukotrienes through prostaglandin G/H synthase 2 (PTGS2; also known as cyclooxygenase 2 [*COX2*]) and 5-lipoxygenase (*5-LO*) pathways, respectively. In turn, eicosanoids promote inflammation and mineralization. Chymase and angiotensin-converting enzyme (*ACE*) promote production of angiotensin II, which increases synthesis and secretion of collagen by VIC. Because of increased production of matrix metalloproteinases (*MMPs*) and decreased synthesis of tissue inhibitors of metalloproteinases (TIMPs), disorganized fibrous tissue accumulates within the aortic valve. Microcalcification begins early in the disease, driven by microvesicles secreted by VIC and macrophages. In addition, overexpression of ectonucleotidases—ENPP1, 5′-nucleotidase ecto (*NT5E*), and alkaline phosphatase (*ALP*)—promotes both apoptosis and osteogenic-mediated mineralization. Bone morphogenetic protein 2 (*BMP2*) leads to osteogenic transdifferentiation, which is associated with the expression of bone-related transcription factors (e.g., runt-related transcription factor 2 [*RUNX2*] and homeobox protein MSX2). Osteoblast-like cells subsequently coordinate calcification of the aortic valve as part of a highly regulated process analogous to skeletal bone formation. Deposition of mineralized matrix is accompanied by fibrosis and neovascularization, which is abetted by vascular endothelial growth factor (*VEGF*). In turn, neovascularization increases the recruitment of inflammatory cells and bone marrow-derived osteoprogenitor cells. $A_{2A}R$, Adenosine A_{2A} receptor; *sPLA_2*, secreted phospholipase A_2; *LPAR*, lysophosphatidic acid receptor; *Ox-PL*, oxidized phospholipid; *Ox-LDL*, oxidized LDL; *TGFβ*, transforming growth factor beta; *TNF*, tumor necrosis factor. (From Lindman BR, et al. Calcific aortic stenosis. Nat Rev Dis Primers. 2016;2:16006.)

before symptom onset on the basis of the finding of a systolic murmur on physical examination, with confirmation of the diagnosis by echocardiography. Symptoms can develop at any age but typically begin at age 50 to 70 years with BAV stenosis and in those older than 70 with calcific stenosis of a trileaflet valve, although even in this age group approximately 40% of patients with AS have a congenital BAV (see Classic References, Roberts and Ko).

The most common clinical presentation in patients with a known diagnosis of AS who are followed prospectively is a gradual decrease in exercise tolerance, fatigue, or dyspnea on exertion. However, in some cases, symptom onset can be more abrupt and severe.[76] The mechanism of exertional dyspnea may be LV diastolic dysfunction, with an excessive rise in end-diastolic pressure leading to pulmonary congestion. Alternatively, exertional symptoms may be a result of the limited ability to increase cardiac output with exercise. More severe exertional dyspnea, with orthopnea, paroxysmal nocturnal dyspnea, and pulmonary edema are relatively late symptoms in patients with AS; in current practice, intervention typically is undertaken before this disease stage.

Angina is a frequent symptom of patients with severe AS, indicates myocardial ischemia, and usually resembles the angina observed in patients with CAD in that it is usually precipitated by exertion and relieved by rest (see Chapters 35 and 40). In patients without CAD, angina results from the combination of the increased O_2 needs of hypertrophied myocardium and reduction of O_2 delivery due to decreased myocardial capillary density, endothelial cell loss, and increased LVEDP, which reduce the coronary perfusion pressure gradient and impair myocardial flow reserve. In patients with CAD, angina is caused by a combination of epicardial coronary artery obstruction and the O_2 imbalance characteristic of AS. Very rarely, angina results from calcific emboli to the coronary vascular bed.

Syncope most often is caused by the reduced cerebral perfusion that occurs during exertion when arterial pressure declines because of systemic vasodilation and an inadequate increase in cardiac output related to valvular stenosis. Syncope also has been attributed to malfunction of the baroreceptor mechanism in severe AS (see Chapter 102), as well as to a vasodepressor response to a greatly elevated LV systolic pressure during exercise. Premonitory symptoms of syncope are common. Exertional hypotension also may be manifested as "graying-out spells" or dizziness on effort. Syncope at rest may be caused by transient AF with loss of the atrial contribution to LV filling,

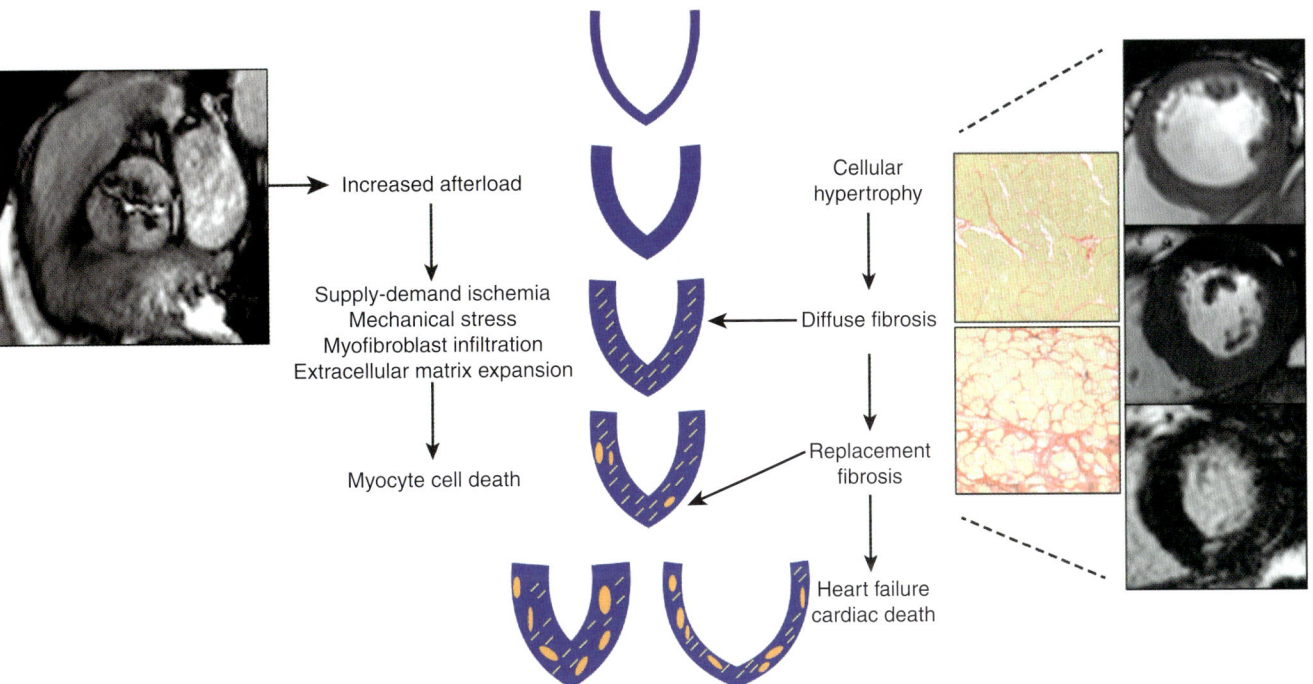

FIGURE 72.6 Hypertrophic remodeling in response to pressure overload from aortic stenosis. (From Bing R, et al. Imaging and impact of myocardial fibrosis in aortic stenosis. *JACC Cardiovasc Imaging.* 2019;12:283-296.)

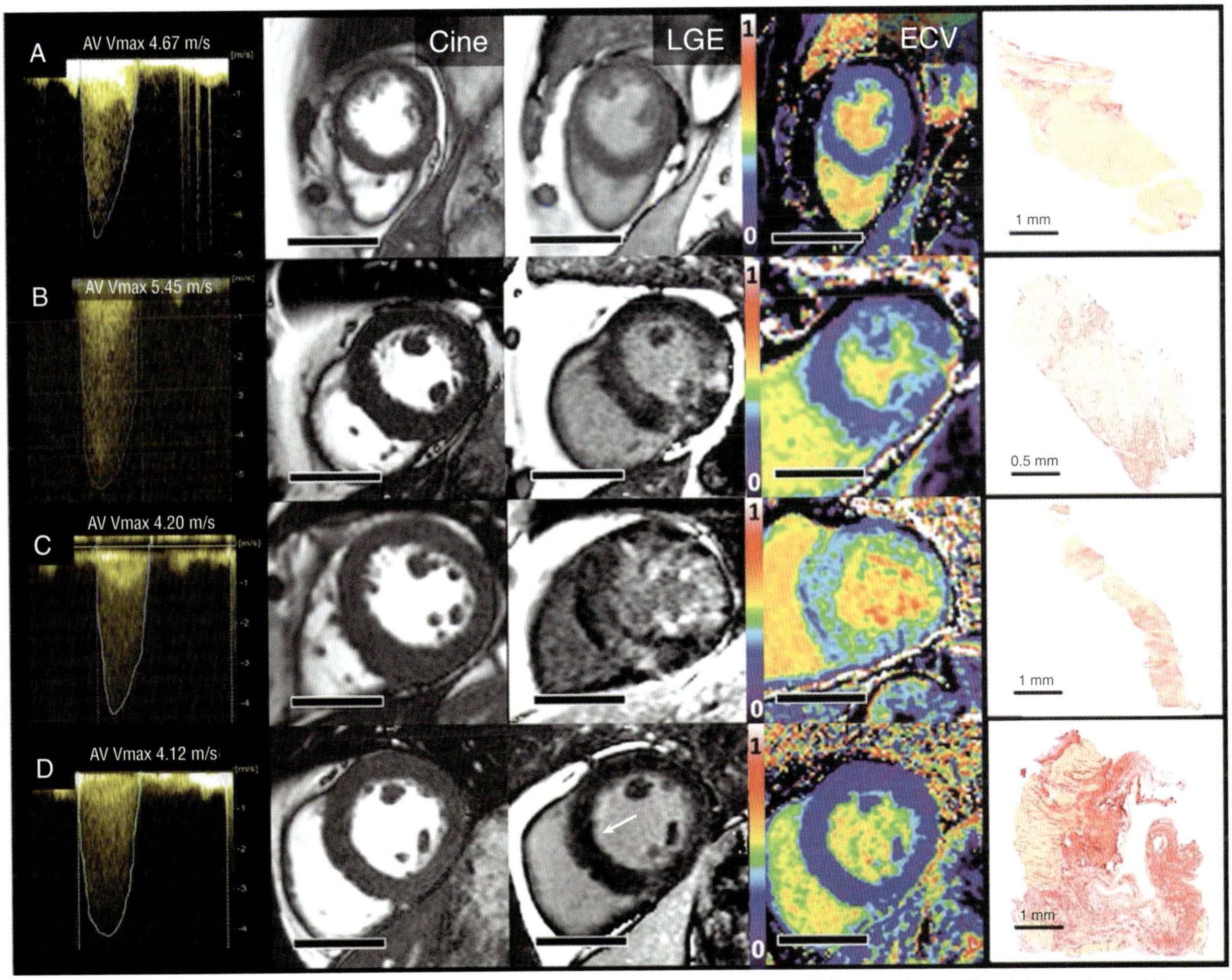

FIGURE 72.7 **Diffuse and replacement myocardial fibrosis in aortic stenosis.** Aortic stenosis, myocardial hypertrophy, and fibrosis by imaging and biopsy. *Column 1*, Four exemplar patients showing continuous-wave Doppler (maximum velocities >4 m/sec). *Column 2 (Cine)*, Short-axis cine stills demonstrating degrees of left ventricular hypertrophy. *Column 3 (LGE)*, Matching late gadolinium enhancement images. *Column 4 (ECV)*, Matching extracellular volume fraction. *Column 5*, Myocardial biopsy sample stained with picrosirius red (collagen volume fraction [CVF]). Patient **A** has minimal left ventricular hypertrophy [LVH], no LGE, an ECV of 28.4% and minimal biopsy subendocardial fibrosis (CVF 4.6%). Patient **B** has concentric LVH, patchy noninfarct LGE, an ECV of 29.9%, and moderate biopsy fibrosis (CVF 19.3%). Patient **C** has concentric LVH, widespread noninfarct LGE, an ECV of 36.5%, and severe biopsy fibrosis (CVF 24.5%). Patient **D** has mild concentric LVH, subtle subendocardial LGE (*arrow*), an ECV of 24.5%, thickened endocardium, and subendocardial scarring. Scale bars (columns 2–4) equal 5 cm. (From Treibel TA, et al. Reappraising myocardial fibrosis in severe aortic stenosis: an invasive and non-invasive study in 133 patients. *Eur Heart J.* 2018;39:699-709.)

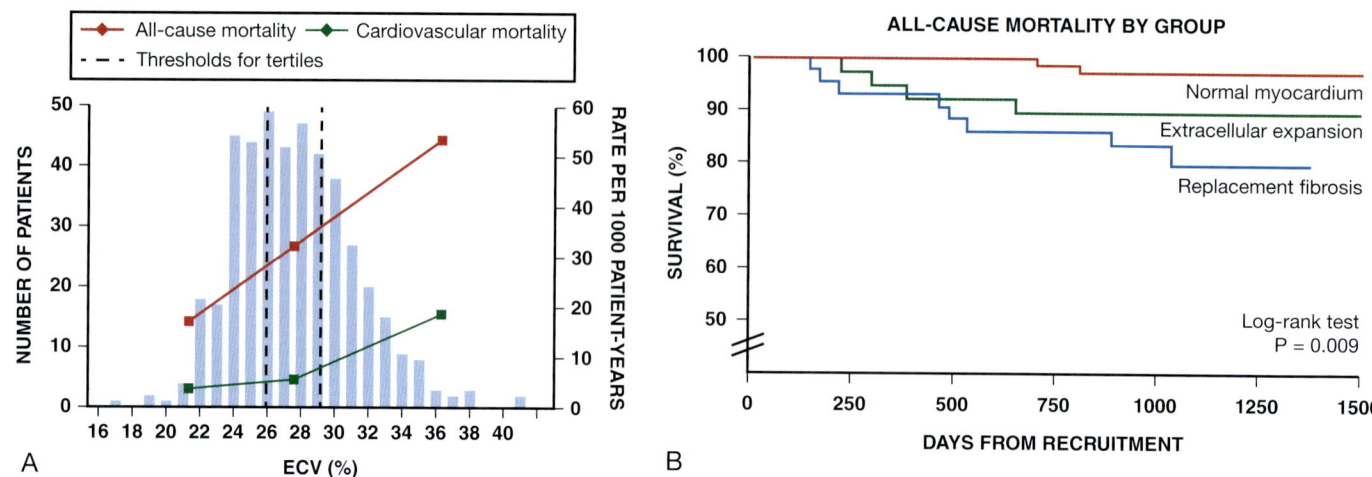

FIGURE 72.8 Myocardial fibrosis and mortality in aortic stenosis. **A,** Frequency distribution of magnitude of extracellular volume fraction (ECV, expressed as percent of left ventricular myocardium) in patients with aortic stenosis, and association of ECV with all-cause and cardiovascular mortality. **B,** Survival in subgroups of patients with AS defined by normal myocardium, extracellular expansion, and replacement fibrosis. (**A** from Everett RJ, et al. Extracellular myocardial volume in patients with aortic stenosis. *J Am Coll Cardiol.* 2020;75:304-316. **B** from Chin CWL, et al. Myocardial fibrosis and cardiac decompensation in aortic stenosis. *JACC Cardiovasc Imaging.* 2017;10:1320-1333.)

which causes a precipitous decline in cardiac output, or to transient AV block caused by extension of the calcification of the valve into the conduction system.

Gastrointestinal bleeding may develop in patients with severe AS, often associated with angiodysplasia (most frequently of the right colon) or other vascular malformations. This complication arises from shear stress–induced platelet aggregation with a reduction in high-molecular-weight multimers of von Willebrand factor and increases in proteolytic subunit fragments.[77] These abnormalities correlate with the severity of AS and are correctable by AVR.

An increased risk of infective endocarditis has been documented in patients with aortic valve disease, particularly in younger patients with a BAV (see Chapter 80). Cerebral emboli resulting in stroke or transient ischemic attacks may be caused by microthrombi on thickened BAVs. Calcific AS rarely may cause embolization of calcium to various organs, including the heart, kidneys, and brain.

Physical Examination

The key features of the physical examination in patients with AS are palpation of the carotid upstroke, evaluation of the systolic murmur, assessment of splitting of the second heart sound (S_2), and examination for signs of HF (see Chapters 13 and 49).

The carotid upstroke directly reflects the arterial pressure waveform. The expected finding with severe AS is a slow-rising, late-peaking, low-amplitude carotid pulse, the *parvus and tardus* carotid impulse. When present, this finding is specific for severe AS. However, many adults with AS have concurrent conditions, such as AR or systemic hypertension, that affect the arterial pressure curve and the carotid impulse. Thus, an apparently normal carotid impulse is not reliable for excluding the diagnosis of severe AS. In addition, with severe AS, radiation of the murmur to the carotid arteries may result in a palpable thrill or carotid shudder.

Auscultation

Overall, auscultation has relatively poor sensitivity and specificity for detecting AS, even among cardiologists.[78] The ejection systolic murmur of AS typically is late-peaking and heard best at the base of the heart, with radiation to the carotids. Cessation of the murmur before A_2 is helpful in differentiation from a pansystolic mitral murmur. In patients with calcified aortic valves, the systolic murmur is loudest at the base of the heart, but high-frequency components may radiate to the apex—the so-called *Gallavardin phenomenon*, in which the murmur may be so prominent that it is mistaken for the murmur of mitral regurgitation (MR). In general, a louder and later-peaking murmur indicates more severe stenosis. However, although a systolic murmur of grade 3 intensity or greater is relatively specific for severe AS, this finding is insensitive, and many patients with severe AS have only a grade 2 murmur. When the left ventricle fails and stroke volume falls, the systolic murmur of AS becomes softer; rarely, it disappears altogether.

Splitting of S_2 is helpful in excluding the diagnosis of severe AS, because normal splitting implies the aortic valve leaflets are flexible enough to create an audible closing sound (A_2). With severe AS, S_2 may be single because (1) calcification and immobility of the aortic valve make A_2 inaudible, (2) closure of the pulmonic valve (P_2) is buried in the prolonged aortic ejection murmur, or (3) prolongation of LV systole makes A_2 coincide with P_2. The intensity of the systolic murmur varies from beat to beat when the duration of diastolic filling varies, as in AF or after a premature contraction. This characteristic is helpful in differentiating AS from MR, in which the murmur usually is unaffected. The murmur of valvular AS is augmented by squatting, which increases stroke volume. It is reduced in intensity during the strain of the Valsalva maneuver and on standing, both of which reduce transvalvular flow.

Diagnostic Testing

Echocardiography

Echocardiography is the standard approach for evaluating and following patients with AS and selecting them for valve replacement (see Chapter 16). Echocardiographic imaging allows for characterization of valve anatomy, including the cause of AS (see Fig. 16.40), a qualitative impression of valve calcification (see Fig. 16.42), and sometimes allows direct imaging of the orifice area using three-dimensional imaging.[78] Echocardiographic imaging is also invaluable for the evaluation of LVH and systolic function, with calculation of EF, measurement of aortic sinus dimensions, and detection of associated AR and mitral valve disease. Longitudinal systolic strain imaging has emerged as a more sensitive measure of LV function and predicts adverse clinical events, including mortality.[59,62]

Doppler echocardiography allows measurement of indices to determine the severity of AS, including peak transvalvular jet velocity (which is used to calculate the peak transvalvular pressure gradient with the modified Bernoulli equation), mean transvalvular pressure gradient, and aortic valve area (AVA) (calculated using the continuity equation) (Fig 72.10).[79,80] Both AVA and pressure gradient calculations from Doppler data have been well validated compared with invasive

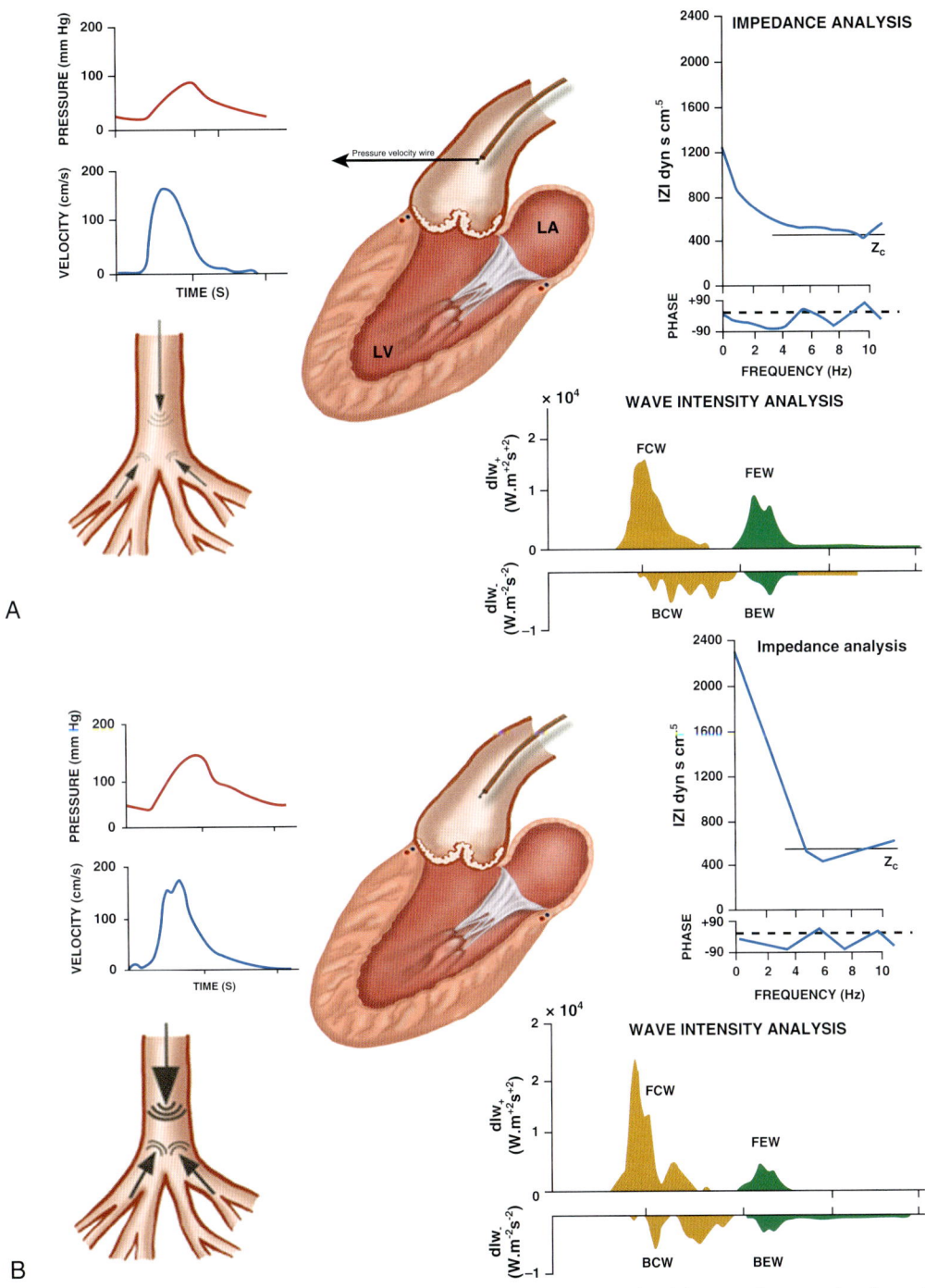

FIGURE 72.9 Aortic impedance and wave intensity analysis are shown in a patient before (A) and after (B) transcatheter aortic valve replacement (TAVR). Aortic systolic and pulse pressures increased after TAVR. Fourier decomposition of the simultaneous aortic pressure and velocity signals shows that SVR and the first three harmonic frequencies of the impedance spectrum (Z) increase after TAVR. Wave intensity analysis was used to separate total wave intensity into contributions from the forward (dIw+) and backward (dIw−) traveling waves. Compression waves (*gold*) increase pressure, and expansion waves (*green*) decrease aortic pressure. The forward compression wave (FCW) increases immediately after TAVR. *BCW,* Backward compression wave; *BEW,* backward expansion wave; *dIw,* wave intensity; *FEW,* forward expansion wave; *LA,* left atrium; *LV,* left ventricle; *SVR,* systemic vascular resistance. (From Yotti R, et al. Systemic vascular load in calcific degenerative aortic valve stenosis: insight from percutaneous valve replacement. *J Am Coll Cardiol.* 2015;65:423-433.)

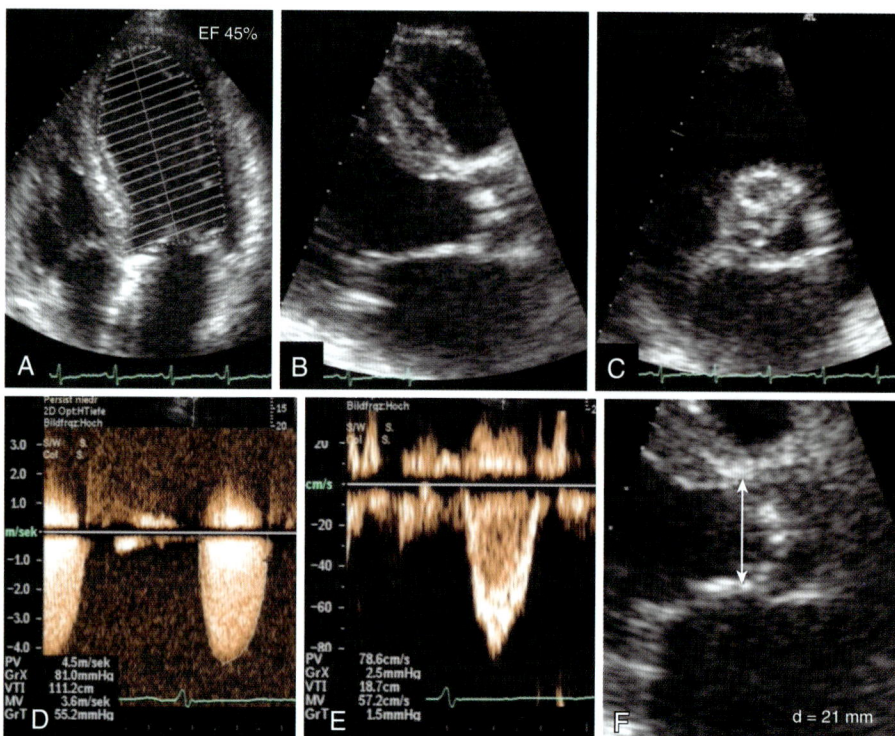

FIGURE 72.10 Assessment of aortic stenosis severity. **A,** The Simpson method is used to assess LV function by ejection fraction (EF). **B,** The long-axis view is used to assess the morphology, degree of calcification, and opening movement. **C,** The short axis further assesses morphology and the number of cusps. **D,** CW Doppler measures peak velocity, mean gradient, and the aortic velocity-time integral (VTI). **E,** Pulsed-wave Doppler is used to measure prestenotic velocity and the VTI in the LV outflow tract (LVOT). **F,** LVOT diameter (*d, double-headed arrow*) in zoom mode is used to calculate LVOT area. Images show a severely stenosed calcified tricuspid aortic valve with a mean gradient of 55 mm Hg, a calculated aortic valve area of 0.6 cm², and a reduced EF of 45%. (From Otto CM, ed. *The Practice of Clinical Echocardiography.* 6th ed. Philadelphia: Elsevier; 2022.)

hemodynamics and in terms of their ability to predict clinical outcome. However, the accuracy of these measures requires an experienced laboratory with meticulous attention to technical details. Evaluation of AS severity is affected by the presence of systemic hypertension, and reevaluation after blood pressure control may be necessary.[81] In patients with LV dysfunction and low cardiac output, assessing the severity of AS can be enhanced by assessing hemodynamic changes during dobutamine infusion (see later). In some patients, additional measures of AS severity may be necessary, such as correction for poststenotic pressure recovery or three-dimensional transesophageal echocardiography (TEE) of valve anatomy. The combination of pulsed, continuous-wave, and color flow Doppler echocardiography is helpful in detecting and determining the severity of AR (which coexists in approximately 75% of patients with predominant AS) and in estimating pulmonary artery pressure.

Exercise Stress Testing. Because patients may tailor their lifestyle to minimize symptoms or may ascribe fatigue and dyspnea to deconditioning or aging, they may not recognize early symptoms as important warning signals, although these symptoms often can be elicited by a careful history. Exercise testing may be helpful in apparently asymptomatic patients or when symptoms are vague (e.g., fatigue) to unmask symptoms or demonstrate limited exercise capacity or an abnormal blood pressure response.[57,82] Exercise stress testing should be attended by a physician and should be absolutely avoided in clearly symptomatic patients.

Cardiac Computed Tomography. The use and value of CT is rapidly expanding in patients with calcific aortic valve disease (see Chapter 20). CT is useful for evaluating aortic dilation in patients with evidence or suspicion of aortic root disease on echocardiography or chest radiography, particularly those with a bicuspid valve. Measurement of aortic dimensions at several levels, including the sinuses of Valsalva, sinotubular junction, and ascending aorta, is necessary for clinical decision making and surgical planning. CT is increasingly used to assess valve calcification to predict the rate of disease progression or, more often, when the severity of the stenosis is in doubt, particularly in those with low-flow, low-gradient AS (Fig. 72.11).[83-85] It is complementary to echocardiography in assessing valve morphology (see Fig. 20.20B) and provides valuable information on the location and extent of calcification; this can guide treatment decisions regarding transcatheter versus surgical valve replacement and, if a transcatheter approach is selected, valve choice (see Fig. 72.3).[86-89] CT is also a routine part of the preprocedural evaluation of patients undergoing SAVR or TAVR (see Chapter 74), principally to look for a porcelain aorta, as well as determine appropriate valve sizing and assess aortic and peripheral arterial anatomy for a potential transcatheter approach (see Fig. 20.23).[86] Finally, as the quality and resolution of CT have rapidly improved, a gated CT coronary angiogram (with assessment of fractional flow reserve as warranted) may be used to evaluate for CAD instead of routine invasive angiography before AVR.[90,91]

Cardiac Catheterization. In almost all patients, the echocardiographic examination provides the important hemodynamic information required for patient management. Cardiac catheterization is now recommended only when noninvasive tests are inconclusive, when clinical and echocardiographic findings are discrepant, and for coronary angiography before AVR[57] (see Chapters 21 and 22).

Other Imaging Modalities

Cardiac Magnetic Resonance Imaging. Cardiac magnetic resonance (CMR) is useful for assessing LV volume, function, and mass, especially in settings in which this information cannot be obtained readily from echocardiography (see Chapter 19).[92] CMR is also excellent for assessing aortic dimensions in patients with a bicuspid valve, particularly to avoid radiation when serial imaging is needed over many years. Given the adverse prognosis associated with the presence and severity of myocardial fibrosis, CMR with T1 mapping and late gadolinium enhancement (LGE) may be used to risk-stratify patients with AS (see Figs. 72.6 through 72.8).[34,42-47] CMR is also sometimes used instead of CT to assess valve morphology, vascular anatomy, and annular dimensions in preparation for TAVR, although CMR is not recommended for assessment of stenosis severity because of underestimation of transvalvular velocities.[92]

Positron Emission Tomography. Active uptake of ¹⁸F-fluoride in the aortic valve on positron emission tomography (PET) identifies active tissue calcification and ¹⁸F-fluorodeoxyglucose uptake is a marker of valvular inflammation (see Chapter 18). These tracers are associated with disease progression and predict changes in severity of aortic valve calcification on serial CT studies (Fig. 72.12).[93-95] This may become a useful surrogate end point for trials testing therapies to slow the progression of calcific aortic valve disease, but further studies are needed.

Multimodality Imaging for Cardiac Amyloidosis. Transthyretin cardiac amyloidosis (ATTR-CA) is increasingly recognized as a coexistent disease process in individuals with AS, particularly those with low-flow or low-gradient AS.[96-98] Up to 16% of patients undergoing TAVR have been identified as having ATTR-CA, which is associated with more advanced cardiac structural and functional abnormalities. Multiple imaging modalities (see Chapters 16, 18, and 19) may be helpful in assessing for ATTR-CM, including echocardiographic strain, cardiac MRI, and technetium pyrophosphate (Fig. 72.13; see also Figs. 18.34, 18.35, and 19.13).[34] Even emerging methods to assess extracellular volume with CT may be useful.[99] Although ATTR-CA in a patient with severe AS may not make TAVR futile, it may be associated with worse outcomes, and emerging therapies for ATTR-CA should be considered.[98,100] This is an evolving area that requires additional research to determine the best method(s) for screening and treatment.

DISEASE COURSE AND STAGING

The disease course for a patient with AS is characterized by (1) progressive narrowing/obstruction of the valve with its attendant consequences for myocardial and vascular remodeling/dysfunction and (2)

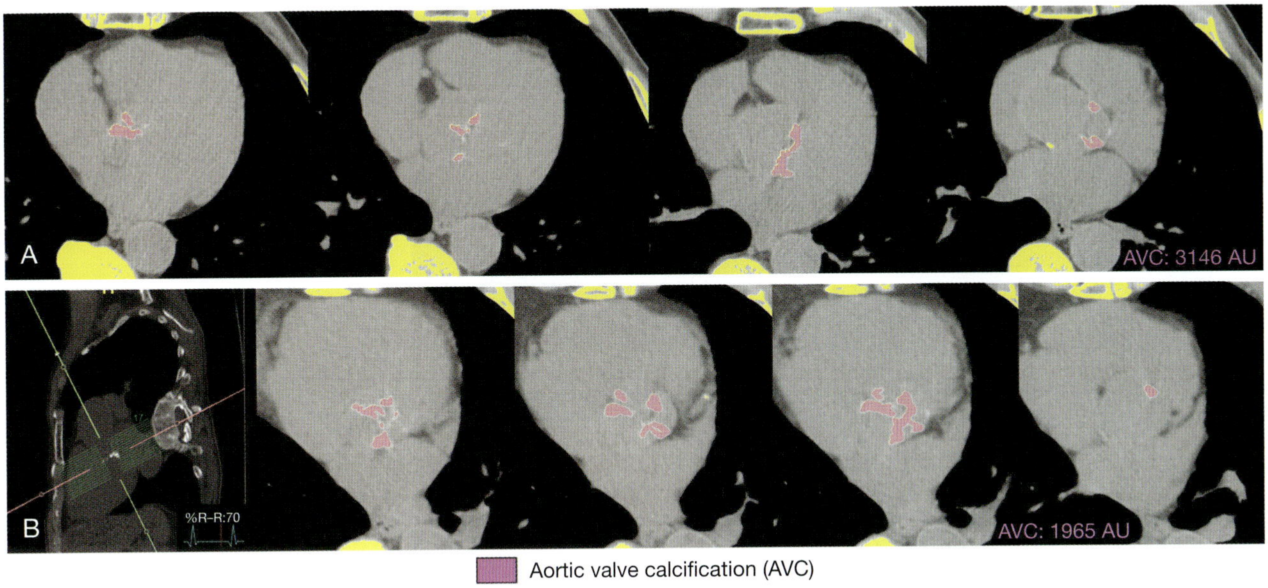

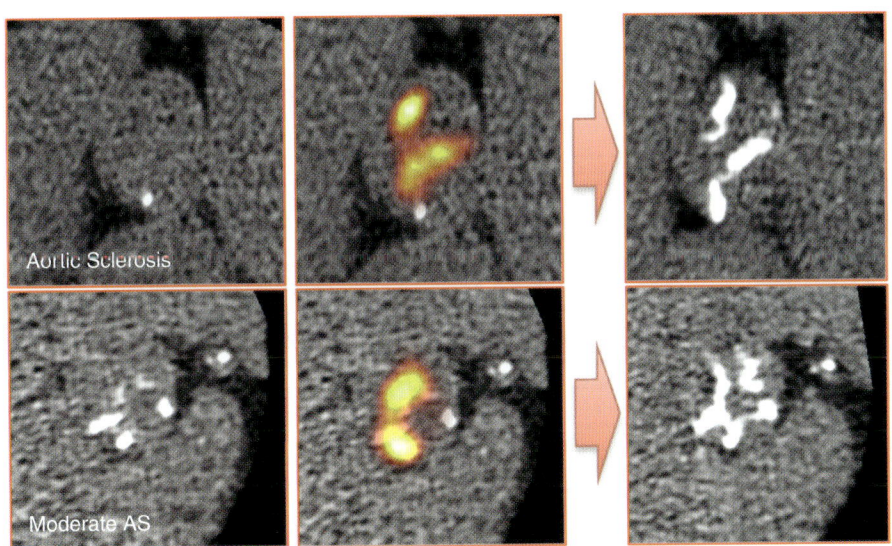

FIGURE 72.11 Aortic valve calcification quantified by cardiac CT. Multiplanar reformat images in "native" axial **(A)** and "en face" **(B)** views showing aortic valve calcification (AVC) (*pink*). Note that, with the use of the "en face" reconstructed view, the calcification score is decreased by 37% and that aortic stenosis severity would be classified as nonsevere. Thus, "en face" view measurement of aortic valve calcification must not be used to assess AVC severity. (From Pawade T, et al. Why and how to measure aortic valve calcification in patients with aortic stenosis. *JACC Cardiovasc Imaging.* 2019;12:1835-1848.)

FIGURE 72.12 Valvular 18F-fluoride uptake predicts the progression of calcification in aortic stenosis. Two patients with calcific aortic valve disease. *Left,* Baseline CT images. *Middle,* Fused positron emission tomography (PET)/CT images showing increased 18F-fluoride valvular uptake (*red/yellow areas*). *Right,* Repeat CT scans after 2 years with new areas of macroscopic calcium (*white areas*) in a similar distribution to that of baseline PET uptake. (From Jenkins WS, et al. Valvular (18)F-fluoride and (18)F-fluorodeoxyglucose uptake predict disease progression and clinical outcome in patients with aortic stenosis. *J Am Coll Cardiol* 2015;66:1200-1201.)

ultimately the development of symptoms. These are reflected in the staging nomenclature of the American College of Cardiology/American Heart Association (ACC/AHA) Valvular Heart Disease Guidelines (Table 72.2).[57] Stage A includes those at risk for AS; stage B includes progressive AS (mild to moderate valve obstruction); stage C includes individuals with severe AS but no symptoms with LVEF ≥50% (C1) or with overt LV dysfunction (LVEF <50%) (C2); and stage D includes individuals with severe AS and symptoms broken down into three different subgroups (D1, D2, and D3) based on differing hemodynamics.[57]

The degree of stenosis associated with symptom onset varies among patients. Although stenosis is on average more severe in symptomatic than in asymptomatic patients, marked overlap is evident in all measures of severity between these two groups. Once AS is severe, only about 50% of patients report symptoms.[101] Markers of more rapid symptom onset include greater valve calcification, higher transvalvular gradient, more rapid increase in transvalvular gradient, and higher B-type natriuretic peptide, among others.[57]

Progressive Aortic Stenosis (Stage B; Mild to Moderate Valve Obstruction)

In adults with calcific AS, a significant burden of leaflet disease is present before obstruction to outflow develops. However, once even mild obstruction is present, hemodynamic progression occurs in almost all patients, with the interval from mild to severe obstruction ranging from less than 5 to more than 10 years. There is substantial patient-to-patient variability in the rate of progression; factors associated with more rapid hemodynamic progression include older age, more severe leaflet calcification, renal insufficiency, hypertension, obesity, metabolic syndrome, smoking, hyperlipidemia, and elevated circulating levels of Lp(a) and increased activity of Lp-PLA$_2$.[1,23,24,57] A greater initial increase in transvalvular gradient portends faster progression.[102] *Moderate* AS is characterized by an aortic jet velocity of 3.0 to 3.9 m/sec or mean transvalvular pressure gradient of 20 to 39 mm Hg, usually with an AVA of 1.0 to 1.5 cm^2. *Mild* AS is characterized by an aortic jet velocity of 2.0 to 2.9 m/sec or mean transvalvular pressure gradient less than 20 mm Hg, usually with aortic orifice of 1.5 to 2.0 cm^2 (see Table 72.2).[57,79]

Classification of Severe Aortic Stenosis

Criteria have been developed for characterizing severe AS; they are useful for categorizing patients, but it is important to recognize their limitations and imprecision. They should not be rigidly adhered to in isolation when determining clinical management. Clinical decisions are based on consideration of symptom status, severity of AS as determined by echocardiography, and LV systolic function. In some cases, additional measures of valve calcification by CT and hemodynamic stress with B-type natriuretic peptide (BNP) or N-terminal (NT)-pro hormone BNP (NT-proBNP) can provide important data regarding AS severity and its effect on the left ventricle. Additional factors, such as energy loss index, valvular impedance, or evaluation with changing

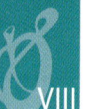

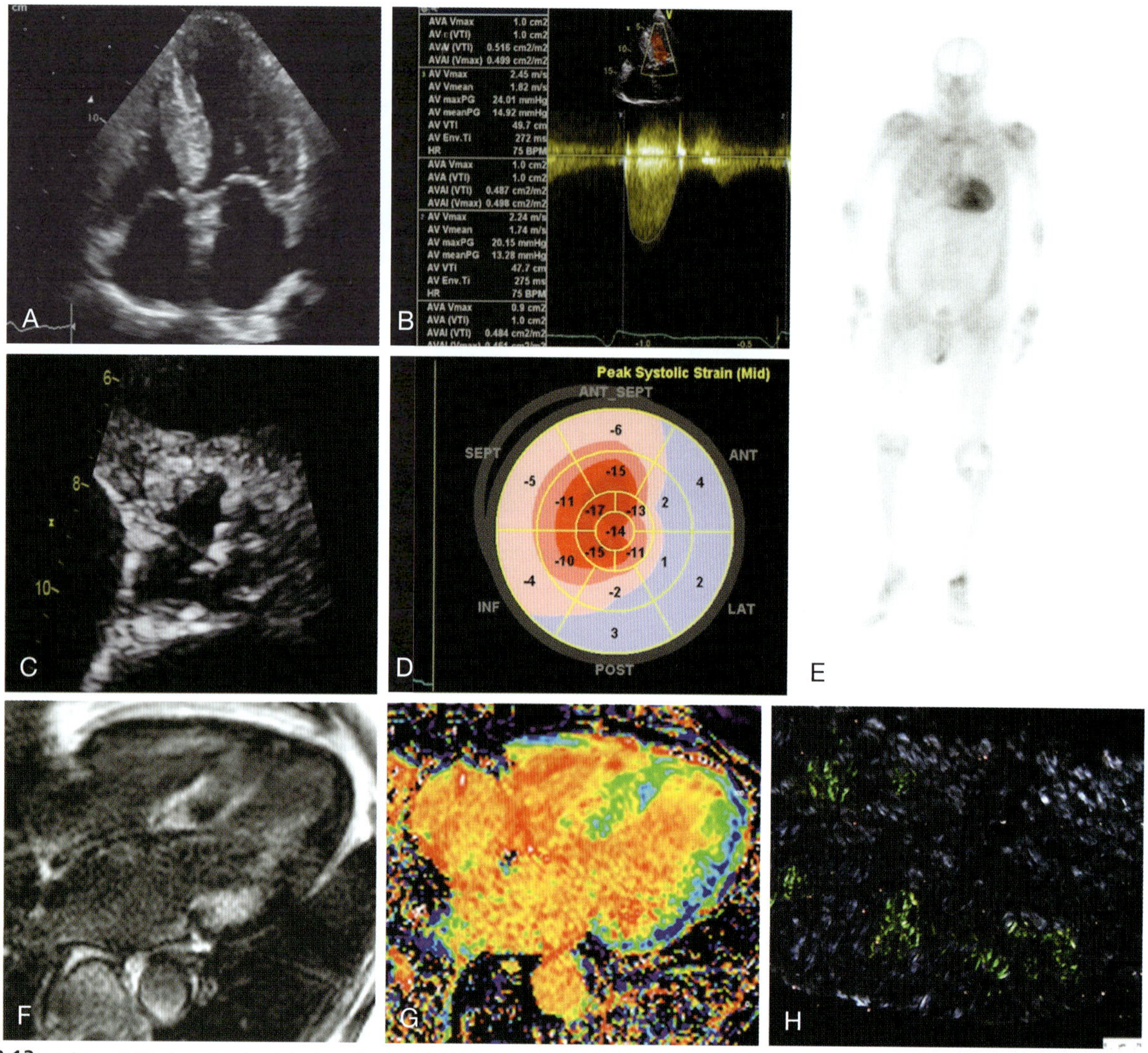

FIGURE 72.13 Multimodality imaging to detect cardiac amyloid in a patient with aortic stenosis. **A,** Although the echocardiogram showed left ventricular hypertrophy, this was attributed to the myocardial response to severe valve gradients **(B)** due to a heavily calcified tricuspid aortic valve **(C)**. **D,** Strain imaging showed a characteristic apical sparing. **E,** Bone scintigraphy showed Perugini grade 2 cardiac uptake. Cardiac magnetic resonance showed transmural late gadolinium enhancement with higher signal from the myocardium than from the blood pool **(F)**, and elevated native myocardial ECV **(G)**. **H,** Diagnosis was confirmed as transthyretin amyloidosis on cardiac biopsy. (From Treibel TA, et al. Multimodality imaging markers of adverse myocardial remodeling in aortic stenosis. *JACC Cardiovasc Imaging.* 2019;12:1532-1548.)

loading conditions (e.g., dobutamine stress) or with exercise, are under investigation for evaluation of disease severity.[74,103]

The most specific definition for severe AS is a peak jet velocity of 4.0 m/sec or greater or mean gradient of 40 mm Hg or greater, usually accompanied by an AVA of 1.0 cm^2 or less (see Table 72.2 and Fig. 72.10).[57] When aortic velocity or gradient meets these criteria, severe AS is present and classified as stage C in asymptomatic patients and stage D1 in symptomatic patients. Classification of stenosis severity is more complex when AVA is 1.0 cm^2 or less, but mean pressure gradient is less than 40 mm Hg and peak jet velocity is less than 4.0 m/sec. This apparent discordance in indices of AS severity occurs because at a normal flow rate, an AVA of 1.0 corresponds to a mean gradient of 30.[104,105] This is a common clinical conundrum because over one third of patients with severe AS with an AVA of 1.0 cm^2 or less have a peak jet velocity less than 4.0 m/sec or mean gradient less than 40 mm Hg (stages D2 and D3 in Table 72.2).[104-106] Clinical judgment and expert imaging are the keys to differentiating patients with severe low-flow, low-gradient AS from those with moderate AS.

Asymptomatic Severe Aortic Stenosis (Stage C)

Stage C1 is defined as high-gradient severe AS with no symptoms and preserved systolic function (see Table 72.2). The strongest predictor of progression to symptoms is the Doppler aortic jet velocity[106] (see also Classic References, Otto). Survival free of symptoms is 84% at 2 years when aortic velocity is less than 3 m/sec, compared with only 21% when velocity is greater than 4 m/sec (Fig. 72.14A). In adults with severe AS (Doppler velocity >4 m/sec), outcome can be further predicted by the magnitude of the Doppler velocity (Fig. 72.14B), as well as by the severity of aortic valve calcification.[84] In such studies, most events consisted of the development of symptoms prompting AVR and not sudden death in otherwise asymptomatic patients. However, retrospective studies have reported cases of sudden death in apparently asymptomatic adults with severe AS.[60]

Stage C2 is defined as high-gradient severe AS with no symptoms but overt LV systolic dysfunction with an LVEF <50%. However, several recent studies indicate that an LVEF of 50% to 60% is linked to a worse prognosis among patients with severe AS.[57-61] Accordingly, an LVEF of 60% is probably a better cutoff for indicating an LVEF below which abnormal function has developed in response to pressure overload from AS; expeditious AVR even in the absence of symptoms may be warranted below this higher LVEF threshold.

Symptomatic Severe Aortic Stenosis (Stage D)

Once even mild symptoms are present, survival is poor unless outflow obstruction is relieved. Expected survival for patients with severe symptomatic AS will differ somewhat based on the age, number of comorbidities,

TABLE 72.2 Stages of Valvular Aortic Stenosis (AS)

STAGE	DEFINITION	VALVE ANATOMY	VALVE HEMODYNAMICS	HEMODYNAMIC CONSEQUENCES	SYMPTOMS
A	At risk of AS	Bicuspid aortic valve (or other congenital valve anomaly) Aortic valve sclerosis	Aortic Vmax <2 m/sec with normal leaflet motion	None	None
B	Progressive AS	Mild to moderate leaflet calcification/fibrosis of a bicuspid or trileaflet valve with some reduction in systolic motion *or* Rheumatic valve changes with commissural fusion	**Mild AS:** Aortic Vmax 2.0-2.9 m/sec or mean ΔP <20 mm Hg **Moderate AS:** Aortic Vmax 3.0-3.9 m/sec or mean ΔP 20-39 mm Hg	Early LV diastolic dysfunction may be present Normal LVEF	None
C	Asymptomatic severe AS				
C1	Asymptomatic severe AS	Severe leaflet calcification/fibrosis or congenital stenosis with severely reduced leaflet opening	**Severe AS:** Aortic Vmax ≥4 m/sec or mean ΔP ≥40 mm Hg AVA typically is ≤1 cm² (or AVAi ≤0.6 cm²/m²) Very severe AS is an aortic Vmax ≥5 m/sec, or mean ΔP ≥ 60 mm Hg	LV diastolic dysfunction Mild LV hypertrophy Normal LVEF	None Exercise testing is reasonable to confirm symptom status
C2	Asymptomatic severe AS with LV systolic dysfunction	Severe leaflet calcification/fibrosis or congenital stenosis with severely reduced leaflet opening	Aortic Vmax ≥4 m/sec or mean ΔP ≥40 mm Hg AVA typically is ≤1 cm² (or AVAi ≤0.6 cm²/m²) but not required to define severe AS	LVEF <50%	None
D	Symptomatic severe AS				
D1	Symptomatic severe high-gradient AS	Severe leaflet calcification/fibrosis or congenital stenosis with severely reduced leaflet opening	**Severe AS:** Aortic Vmax ≥4 m/sec, or mean ΔP ≥40 mm Hg AVA typically is ≤1 cm² (or AVAi ≤0.6 cm²/m²), but may be larger with mixed AS/AR	LV diastolic dysfunction LV hypertrophy Pulmonary hypertension may be present	Exertional dyspnea or decreased exercise tolerance Exertional angina Exertional syncope or presyncope
D2	Symptomatic severe low-flow, low-gradient AS with reduced LVEF	Severe leaflet calcification/fibrosis with severely reduced leaflet motion	AVA ≤1 cm² with resting aortic Vmax <4 m/sec, or mean ΔP <40 mm Hg Dobutamine stress echo shows AVA ≤1 cm² with Vmax ≥4 m/sec at any flow rate	LV diastolic dysfunction LV hypertrophy LVEF <50%	HF Angina Syncope or presyncope
D3	Symptomatic severe low-gradient AS with normal LVEF or paradoxical low-flow severe AS	Severe leaflet calcification/fibrosis with severely reduced leaflet motion	AVA <1.0 cm² (AVAi <0.6 cm²/m²) with aortic Vmax <4 m/sec, or mean ΔP <40 mm Hg *and* stroke volume index <35 mL/m² Measured when patient is normotensive (systolic BP <140 mm Hg)	Increased LV relative wall thickness Small LV chamber with low stroke volume Restrictive diastolic filling LVEF ≥50%	HF Angina Syncope or presyncope

AVA, Aortic valve area; *AVAi*, AVA indexed to body surface area; *BP*, blood pressure; *HF*, heart failure; *LVEF*, left ventricular ejection fraction; ΔP, pressure gradient; *Vmax*, maximum aortic jet velocity.
From Otto CM, et al. 2020 AHA/ACC guideline for the management of patients with valvular heart disease: a report of the American College of Cardiology/American Heart Association Task Force on Practice Guidelines. *J Am Coll Cardiol.* 2021;77:e25-e197.

and severity of HF of the cohort examined, but average survival without AVR is only 1 to 3 years after symptom onset. Among symptomatic patients with severe AS, the outlook is poorest when the left ventricle has failed and the cardiac output and transvalvular gradient are both low. The risk of sudden death is high with symptomatic severe AS, so these patients should be promptly referred for AVR. In patients who do not undergo AVR, recurrent hospitalizations for angina and decompensated HF are common, associated with significant consumption of health care resources.[107]

Symptomatic Severe High-Gradient Aortic Stenosis (Stage D1)

Severe high-gradient AS is defined as peak jet velocity of 4.0 m/sec or greater or mean gradient of 40 mm Hg or greater, usually accompanied by an AVA of 1.0 cm² or less (or indexed AVA of 0.6 cm²/m² or less) (see Table 72.2). Occasionally, AVA may be larger with mixed AS and AR. With alignment of all hemodynamic indices of AS severity, these patients have the clearest evidence of severe AS and warrant prompt referral for AVR.

Symptomatic Severe Low-Flow, Low-Gradient Aortic Stenosis with Reduced LVEF (Stage D2)

Classic low-flow, low-gradient AS (stage D2) is defined as AVA of 1.0 cm² or less with an aortic velocity less than 4.0 m/sec or mean gradient less than 40 mm Hg and LVEF less than 50% (see Table 72.2). Patients with HF symptoms and stage D2 AS often create a diagnostic dilemma for the clinician because their clinical presentation

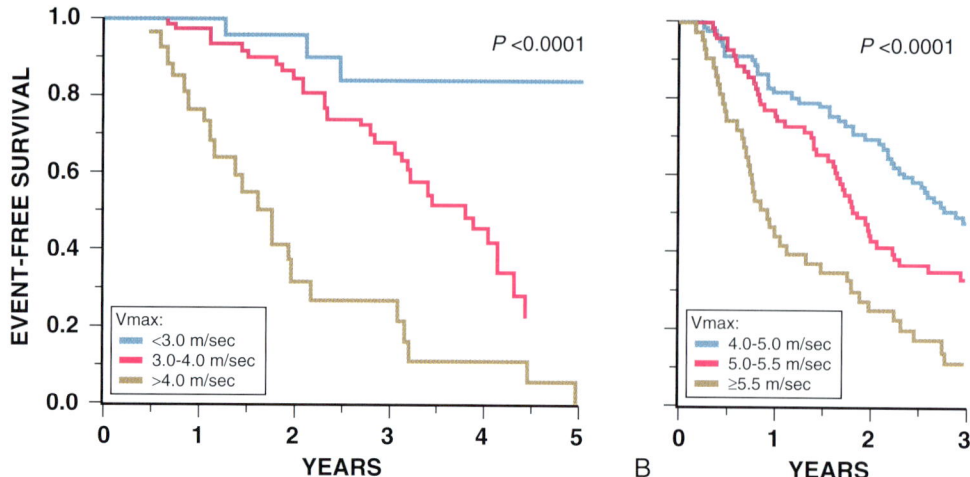

FIGURE 72.14 Event-free survival based on initial peak aortic jet velocity. **A,** Natural history as reflected by event-free survival in asymptomatic patients with aortic stenosis. Initial peak aortic jet velocity (Vmax) stratifies patients according to the likelihood that symptoms requiring valve replacement will develop over time. **B,** Outcomes with very severe aortic stenosis. Kaplan-Meier event-free survival rate for patients with Vmax of 4.0 m/sec or greater. In both **A** and **B,** most "events" consisted of the onset of symptoms warranting aortic valve replacement. (**A** from Otto CM, et al. A prospective study of asymptomatic valvular aortic stenosis: clinical, echocardiographic, and exercise predictors of outcome. *Circulation.* 1997;95:2262; **B** from Rosenhek R, et al. Natural history of very severe aortic stenosis. *Circulation.* 2010;121:151.)

and hemodynamic data may be indistinguishable from those of patients with dilated cardiomyopathy and a calcified valve that is not severely stenotic.[57,83] Severe AS can be distinguished from moderate AS with primary LV dysfunction based on the changes in valve hemodynamics during transient increases in flow, usually by increasing cardiac output with dobutamine[79,83] (see Chapter 16). Severe AS is present if there is an increase in aortic velocity to at least 4 m/sec at any flow rate, with AVA that remains less than 1.0 cm². Dobutamine echocardiography also provides evidence of myocardial contractile reserve (increase in stroke volume >20% from baseline), which historically has been an important predictor of operative risk and survival after SAVR in these patients.[83] However, even in patients who lack contractile reserve, SAVR is associated with better survival (approximately 50% at 5 years) than medical therapy, and more recent studies in patients undergoing TAVR have shown equivalent improvement in LVEF and survival in patients with and without contractile reserve.[65,108]

Symptomatic Severe Low-Flow, Low-Gradient Aortic Stenosis with Preserved LVEF (Stage D3)

Low-flow, low-gradient AS also can occur with a normal LVEF (≥50%) (see Table 72.2), typically in elderly patients with a small, hypertrophied left ventricle or those with concurrent hypertension. This is often referred to as "paradoxical" low-flow, low-gradient AS because despite a normal EF, transaortic flow is low (stroke volume index <35 mL/m²).[57,79,83] Distinguishing truly severe AS from moderate AS can be challenging. Measurement errors should be ruled out and small body size accounted for (an indexed AVA ≤0.6 cm²/m² is consistent with severe AS).[79] Dobutamine has been used to augment flow to distinguish truly severe AS from pseudosevere AS, but is less preferred in these patients with a small, hypertrophied ventricle and marked diastolic dysfunction.[109] Evaluation of valve hemodynamics after treatment of hypertension and, increasingly, CT assessment of valve calcification can be helpful in establishing the diagnosis of severe AS and is being used to identify patients with a severely calcified valve.[57,79,83]

TREATMENT

Medical Management

Medical therapy has thus far been shown to have no effect on disease progression in patients with AS.[1,14,32] Furthermore, both observational studies and randomized clinical trials (RCTs) convincingly demonstrate that AVR is superior to medical therapy in patients with severe symptomatic AS. The risk of sudden death increases dramatically once symptoms are present, and patients should be advised to report promptly the development of any symptoms possibly related to AS. In asymptomatic patients with AS of any degree, evaluation and treatment for conventional cardiovascular risk factors is recommended in accordance with established guidelines (see Chapter 25).

Hypertension accompanies AS in many patients.[110] Because of traditional teaching that AS is a disease with fixed afterload, there often has been reluctance to treat hypertension because of concerns that vasodilation would not be offset by an increase in stroke volume. However, several studies have demonstrated that vasodilation is accompanied by increases in stroke volume, even in patients with severe AS[66] (see also Classic References, Khot). Hypertension imposes an additional load on the left ventricle and is associated with more adverse hypertrophic LV remodeling. Although treatment of hypertension may not reduce AS-related events, it should be treated because of the well-known adverse association between hypertension and vascular events and mortality.[111] Whether blood pressure targets should be the same (versus slightly higher) for patients with AS as the general population is unclear.[111] There is no one class of medicines established as the preferred treatment of hypertension in patients with AS, but because the renin-angiotensin system is upregulated in the valve and ventricle of patients with AS, angiotensin-converting-enzyme (ACE) inhibitors or angiotensin receptor blockers (ARBs) may be preferentially considered. Small studies have demonstrated their safety, and some suggest a clinical benefit, but larger-scale randomized studies are needed.

Concomitant CAD is common in middle-aged and elderly patients with AS. Primary and secondary prevention guidelines should be followed, and the decision of whether to prescribe a statin medication should not be influenced by the presence of AS. RCTs testing the use of statins in patients with mild AS to more advanced disease were adequately powered and showed no improvement in mortality, time to AVR, or rate of AS progression in the treatment versus placebo groups.[15]

AF or atrial flutter develop in up to one third of older patients with AS, perhaps exacerbated by left atrial enlargement related to diastolic dysfunction. When such an arrhythmia is observed in a patient with AS, the possibility of associated mitral valvular disease should be considered. When AF occurs, the rapid ventricular rate may precipitate symptoms, and the loss of atrial contribution to LV filling and a sudden fall in cardiac output may cause serious hypotension. If this occurs, AF should be treated promptly, usually with cardioversion. New-onset AF in a previously asymptomatic patient with severe AS may be a marker of impending symptom onset. For those with AF and native valve AS, as well as those treated with a bioprosthetic valve more than 3 months ago, anticoagulation with a non–vitamin K oral anticoagulant is an effective alternative to warfarin.[57]

In patients with HF and volume overload, AVR is indicated, but diuretics may reduce congestion and provide some symptomatic relief before intervention. Patients with decompensated HF may benefit from medical therapy as a bridge to definitive therapy with AVR. Nitroprusside has been used during hemodynamic monitoring in the intensive care unit to unload the left heart, reduce congestion, and improve forward flow (see Classic References, Khot). Similarly, phosphodiesterase type 5 inhibition has been shown to provide acute improvements in pulmonary and systemic hemodynamics resulting in biventricular unloading.[66] These medications may improve the patient's hemodynamic status, allowing the AVR procedure to be performed more safely.

TABLE 72.3 Indications for Aortic Valve Replacement in Patients with Aortic Stenosis

COR	LOE	RECOMMENDATIONS
1	A	1. In adults with severe high-gradient AS (stage D1) and symptoms of exertional dyspnea, HF, angina, syncope, or presyncope by history or on exercise testing, AVR is indicated.
1	B-NR	2. In asymptomatic patients with severe AS and an LVEF <50% (stage C2). AVR is indicated.
1	B-NR	3. In asymptomatic patients with severe AS (stage C1) who are undergoing cardiac surgery for other indications, AVR is indicated.
1	B-NR	4. In symptomatic patients with low-flow, low-gradient severe AS with reduced LVEF (stage D2). AVR is recommended.
1	B-NR	5. In symptomatic patients with low-flow, low-gradient severe AS with normal LVEF (stage D3), AVR is recommended if AS is the most likely cause of symptoms.
2a	B-NR	6. In apparently asymptomatic patients with severe AS (stage C1) and low surgical risk, AVR is reasonable when an exercise test demonstrates decreased exercise tolerance (normalized for age and sex) or a fall in systolic blood pressure of ≥10 mm Hg from baseline to peak exercise.
2a	B-R	7. In asymptomatic patients with very severe AS (defined as an aortic velocity of ≥5 m/s) and low surgical risk, AVR is reasonable.
2a	B-NR	8. In apparently asymptomatic patients with severe AS (stage C1) and low surgical risk, AVR is reasonable when the serum B-type natriuretic peptide (BNP) level is greater than three times normal.
2a	B-NR	9. In asymptomatic patients with high-gradient severe AS (stage C1) and low surgical risk. AVR is reasonable when serial testing shows an increase in aortic velocity ≥0.3 m/s per year.
2b	B-NR	10. In asymptomatic patients with severe high-gradient AS (stage C1) and a progressive decrease in LVEF on at least three serial imaging studies to <60%, AVR may be considered.
2b	C-EO	11. In patients with moderate AS (stage B) who are undergoing cardiac surgery for other indications. AVR may be considered.

AS, Aortic stenosis; *AVR*, aortic valve replacement; *HF*, heart failure *LVEF*, left ventricular ejection fraction.
From Otto CM, et al. 2020 AHA/ACC guideline for the management of patients with valvular heart disease: a report of the American College of Cardiology/American Heart Association Task Force on Practice Guidelines. *J Am Coll Cardiol.* 2021;77:e25-e197.

Balloon Aortic Valvuloplasty

AVR is the procedure of choice for relief of outflow obstruction in adults with valvular AS. Balloon aortic valvuloplasty has only a modest hemodynamic effect in patients with calcific AS. It can provide short-term improvement in survival and quality of life, but these benefits are not sustained.[112] Accordingly, balloon aortic valvuloplasty is not recommended as an alternative to valve replacement for calcific AS. In selected cases, it might be reasonable as a bridge to definitive treatment with AVR in unstable patients or as a palliative procedure in patients who are not candidates for AVR.[57]

Aortic Valve Replacement

Recommendations regarding indications for and timing of AVR, type of valve used, and procedural approach require discussions within a multidisciplinary heart team and shared decision making with the patient and family.[57] Current recommendations for AVR in the 2020 revised ACC/AHA guidelines for management of valvular heart disease are shown in Table 72.3. AVR is recommended (Class I) for adults with symptomatic severe AS (stages D1, D2, and D3), even if symptoms are mild (Fig. 72.15).[57,113] AVR also is recommended (Class I) for severe AS with a LVEF less than 50% and for patients with severe asymptomatic AS who are undergoing coronary artery bypass grafting (CABG) or other forms of heart surgery. In addition, AVR is reasonable (Class IIa) for apparently asymptomatic patients with severe high-gradient AS when exercise testing provokes symptoms or a fall in blood pressure. AVR is also reasonable (Class IIa) in asymptomatic patients at low surgical risk when (1) AS is very severe (Vmax ≥5 m/sec), (2) there is rapid disease progression, or (3) BNP is greater than three times the upper limit of normal. AVR may be considered (Class IIb) when there is a progressive decrease in LVEF on at least three serial imaging studies to less than 60%.[57] Further studies are needed to determine whether other indexes of risk warrant earlier intervention in asymptomatic patients with severe AS. These include evidence of myocardial fibrosis, impaired longitudinal strain, pulmonary hypertension, and moderate or severe LVH, among others.[40,42,59,62]

The management of asymptomatic patients is the subject of ongoing study and debate.[114] A prospective observational study of initially asymptomatic Japanese patients with severe AS compared outcome in those who underwent early surgery versus a "watchful waiting" strategy.[115] With propensity matching to adjust for baseline differences between the two groups, the survival rate was significantly higher in the 291 patients with early surgery compared to the 291 initially followed conservatively. However, it is noteworthy that 31% of patients in the conservative group who developed symptoms did not undergo AVR, and this accounted for 17% of the deaths during "watchful waiting." Although this and other retrospective studies comparing prompt AVR versus medical therapy[116] are suggestive, propensity matching has its limitations. The nonperformance of AVR in many patients in the medical therapy group either initially or when criteria for AVR develop limit the value of these comparisons for informing optimal timing of AVR. Thus, the role of early AVR in asymptomatic patients can be determined only with appropriately designed RCTs.

Recently, a small trial randomized 145 asymptomatic patients with very severe AS (AVA ≤0.75 cm^2 and peak jet velocity ≥4.5 m/sec or higher or mean gradient ≥50 mm Hg or higher) to early SAVR (within 2 months of randomization) or conservative therapy with referral to SAVR when symptoms or overt LV dysfunction developed.[117] The primary end point of operative mortality or cardiovascular mortality occurred in 1% in the early surgery group and 15% in the conservative care group (HR 0.09, 95% CI 0.01 to 0.67); death from any cause occurred in 7% in the early surgery group and 21% in the conservative care group (HR 0.33, 95% CI 0.12 to 0.90). These randomized data are helpful in clarifying optimal timing of AVR in asymptomatic patients, but a couple of limitations should be considered: only younger, lower risk patients with very severe AS were included, and the small sample size with few events yielded wide confidence intervals. Several larger RCTs are under way testing the optimal timing of TAVR in asymptomatic patients; these include older, higher-risk patients and modestly less severe AS, albeit generally still high-gradient severe AS.[114] Additional RCTs are needed to

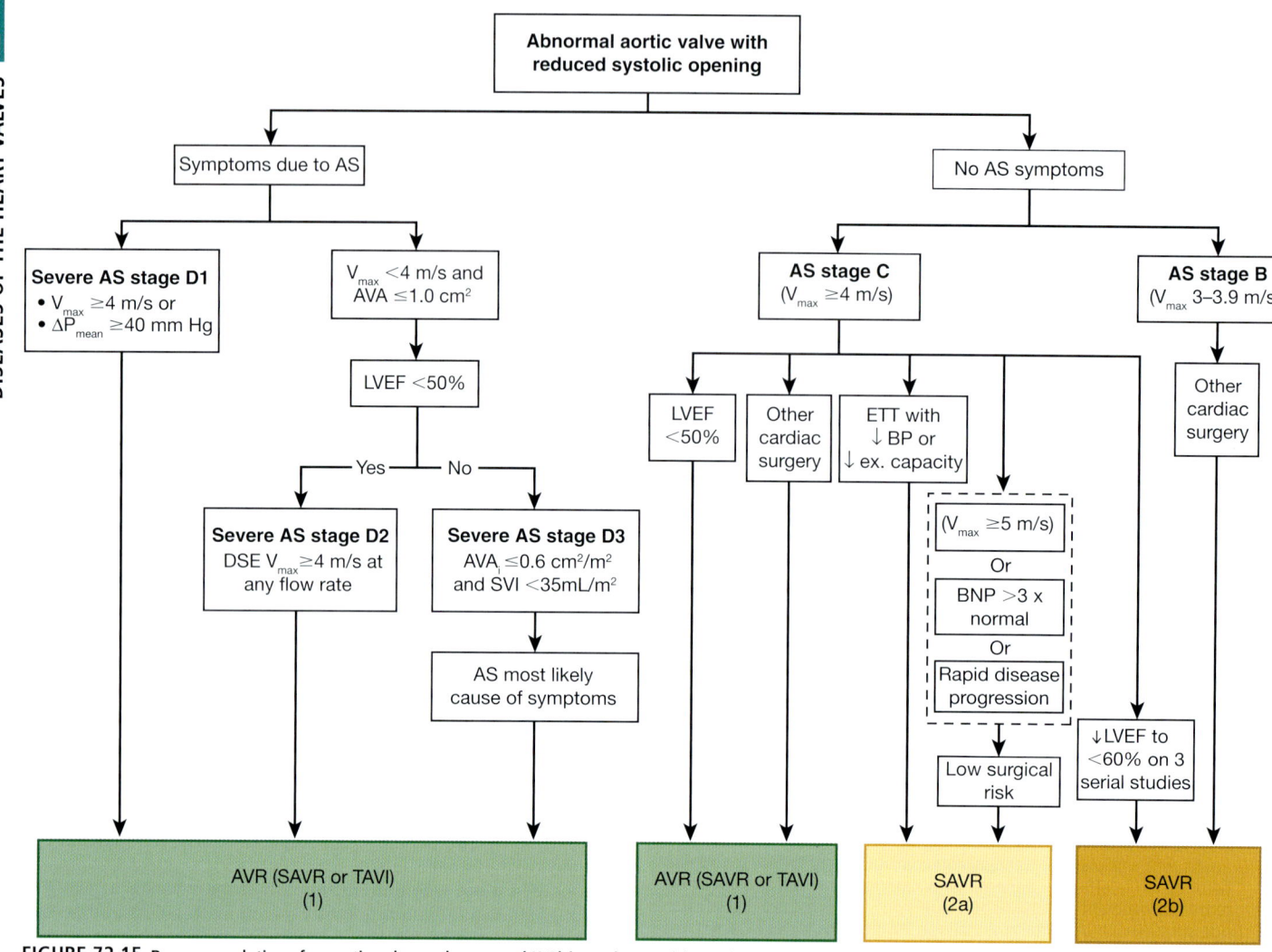

FIGURE 72.15 Recommendations for aortic valve replacement (*AVR*) in patients with aortic stenosis (*AS*). Colors correspond to Table 72.3. *Arrows* show the decision pathways that result in a recommendation for AVR. Periodic monitoring is indicated for all patients in whom AVR is not yet indicated, including those with asymptomatic (stage C) and symptomatic (stage D) AS and those with low-gradient AS (stage D2 or D3) who do not meet the criteria for intervention. See Fig 72.16 for choice of valve type (mechanical versus bioprosthetic [TAVI or SAVR]) when AVR is indicated. *AVA*, Aortic valve area; *AVA$_i$*, aortic valve area index; *BNP*, B-type natriuretic peptide; *BP*, blood pressure; *DSE*, dobutamine stress echocardiography; *ETT*, exercise treadmill test; *ex*, exercise; *LVEF*, left ventricular ejection fraction; ΔP_{mean}, mean systolic pressure gradient between LV and aorta; *SAVR*, surgical aortic valve replacement; *SVI*, stroke volume index; *TAVI*, transcatheter aortic valve implantation; *TAVR*, transcatheter aortic valve replacement; V_{max}, maximum velocity. (From Otto CM, et al. 2020 AHA/ACC guideline for the management of patients with valvular heart disease: a report of the American College of Cardiology/American Heart Association Task Force on Practice Guidelines. *J Am Coll Cardiol.* 2021;77:e25-197.)

clarify optimal timing of SAVR and TAVR in numerous subgroups of patients with moderate and severe AS.

In patients fulfilling current criteria for AVR, the next series of decisions revolves around a surgical or transcatheter approach. Current recommendations for SAVR or TAVR are shown in Table 72.4 and Fig. 72.16 (see also Fig. 72.15). For patients with life expectancy less than 1 year or anticipated poor quality of life not related to their AS, AVR is likely futile and palliative care is recommended.[57,118,119]

In general, AVR leads to an improvement in symptoms, quality of life, and functional capacity and lower rates of hospitalization and death. These clinical improvements are accompanied by reverse remodeling in the heart and improvements in LV function; however, cardiac recovery is variable and often incomplete with untoward consequences.[34,41,43,46,48,120]

Surgical Aortic Valve Replacement

The Society of Thoracic Surgeons (STS) 2020 update on outcomes (reporting data for the year 2018) cited an overall 30-day mortality rate of 1.9% in 25,274 patients undergoing isolated SAVR and 3.6% in 15,855 patients undergoing SAVR and CABG.[121] In patients younger than 70 with minimal comorbidities, the operative risk of mortality is less than 1% in many centers. Medicare data from the past decade indicate that the 30-day mortality after SAVR in patients aged 65 and older in the United States has decreased from 7.6% in 1999 to 4.2% in 2011, with the most marked decrease in patients aged 85 and older, in whom the 30-day mortality has decreased from 12.3% to 5.8%.[122] Therefore, advanced age should not be considered a contraindication to operation, although the majority of such patients are now treated with TAVR. Overall surgical volumes are declining as the volume of TAVR procedures steadily increases (63,361 in 2018).[121] This has the effect of also reducing SAVR mortality rates. The 30-day SAVR mortality rate also is significantly related to the number of AVR procedures performed at each hospital. Risk factors associated with a higher mortality rate include a high New York Heart Association functional class, impaired LV function, advanced age, the presence of associated CAD, and other comorbidities.

Transcatheter Aortic Valve Replacement

Over the last decade, TAVR has transformed the treatment of patients with calcific AS (see Chapter 74). Initial RCTs showed TAVR to be

TABLE 72.4 Recommendations for Choice of SAVR Versus TAVR for Patients for Whom a Bioprosthetic AVR Is Appropriate

COR	LOE	RECOMMENDATIONS
1	A	1. For symptomatic and asymptomatic patients with severe AS and any indication for AVR who are younger than 65 years of age or have a life expectancy >20 years, SAVR is recommended.
1	A	2. For symptomatic patients with severe AS who are 65 to 80 years of age and have no anatomic contraindication to transfemoral TAVI, either SAVR or transfemoral TAVI is recommended after shared decision making about the balance between expected patient longevity and valve durability.
1	A	3. For symptomatic patients with severe AS who are older than 80 years of age or for younger patients with a life expectancy <10 years and no anatomic contraindication to transfemoral TAVI, transfemoral TAVI is recommended in preference to SAVR.
1	B-NR	4. In asymptomatic patients with severe AS and an LVEF <50% who are 80 years of age or younger and have no anatomic contraindication to transfemoral TAVI, the decision between TAVI and SAVR should follow the same recommendations as for symptomatic patients in Recommendations 1, 2, and 3 above.
1	B-NR	5. For asymptomatic patients with severe AS and an abnormal exercise test, very severe AS, rapid progression, or an elevated BNP (COR 2a indications for AVR), SAVR is recommended in preference to TAVI.
1	A	6. For patients with an indication for AVR for whom a bioprosthetic valve is preferred but valve, vascular anatomy, or other factors are not suitable for transfemoral TAVI, SAVR is recommended.
1	A	7. For symptomatic patients of any age with severe AS and a high or prohibitive surgical risk, TAVI is recommended if predicted post-TAVI survival is >12 months with an acceptable quality of life.
1	C-EO	8. For symptomatic patients with severe AS for whom predicted post-TAVI or post-SAVR survival is <12 months or for whom minimal improvement in quality of life is expected, palliative care is recommended after shared decision making, including discussion of patient preferences and values.
2b	C-EO	9. In critically ill patients with severe AS, percutaneous aortic balloon dilation may be considered as a bridge to SAVR or TAVI.

AS, Aortic stenosis; *LVEF*, left ventricular ejection fraction; *SAVR*, surgical aortic valve replacement; *TAVI*, transcatheter aortic valve implantation.
From Otto CM, et al. 2020 AHA/ACC guideline for the management of patients with valvular heart disease: a report of the American College of Cardiology/American Heart Association Task Force on Practice Guidelines. *J Am Coll Cardiol.* 2021;77:e25-e197.

---

superior to medical therapy (usually accompanied by balloon aortic valvuloplasty) in patients who were at prohibitive risk for surgery. Subsequently, in patients deemed high, intermediate, and low risk for surgery, TAVR was shown to be noninferior and, in some trials/subgroups, superior to SAVR.[123-127] Accordingly, TAVR is approved for the treatment of severe AS at all level of levels of risk. The most common approach to valve implantation is *transfemoral* (~95% of cases), particularly as sheath size progressively decreases. Although 5-year data on transcatheter valve durability are encouraging, longer-term data are needed particularly as we move toward treating younger, lower-risk patients.[128]

Patient Selection for TAVR or SAVR

The choice of SAVR versus TAVR should come after a decision that AVR is indicated (see Fig. 72.15). Recommendations for type of valve (mechanical versus bioprosthetic) and type of procedure (surgical versus transcatheter) are outlined in detail in Fig. 72.16. Given the complexity of issues to consider, it is recommended that these decisions occur in the environment of a multidisciplinary heart valve team of cardiac surgeons, interventional cardiologists, clinical and imaging experts in valve disease, and nurses, anesthetists, and geriatricians as needed.[57] Shared decision making with the patient and family is also essential, so that their values and preferences can be incorporated into any treatment decision.[57,129,130] As the field, experience, and technology have evolved, the choice between TAVR and SAVR has become less about patient/surgical risk (because of comorbidities) and more about age, anatomy, and accompanying coronary, valve, or aortic pathology (Table 72.5). TAVR is favored for individuals 80 years and older and those at high or extreme surgical risk, whereas SAVR is favored in those younger than 65 years of age (see Fig. 72.16). Beyond that, multiple factors should be considered to match a specific patient with the right therapy; in many cases, either TAVR or SAVR will be reasonable options. A significant area of uncertainty relates to younger patient age due to uncertainty regarding transcatheter valve durability, higher need for pacemakers after TAVR, and the anticipated need for multiple lifetime procedures if a bioprosthetic valve is implanted. Related to that is uncertainty regarding how to treat patients with BAV anatomy because of uncertainties regarding TAVR efficacy in BAVs, which are encountered more frequently in young patients, and those with a BAV were routinely excluded from the randomized trials comparing TAVR to SAVR. However, TAVR has been performed in patients with a bicuspid valve with excellent results,[1,131-133] but patient age, valve anatomy, extent and location of calcification, and associated aortopathy all influence anticipated success with TAVR and degree of clinical equipoise between the two treatment options. Randomized trials are being considered to clarify optimal management of patients with bicuspid AS.

Postprocedural Issues

Even after treatment of AS with AVR, several issues remain important for clinical management to optimize patient outcomes. As is true after other cardiovascular events, participation in *cardiac rehabilitation* after heart valve surgery is associated with lower rates of death and rehospitalization over the first postprocedure year; however, only a minority participate.[134] In the case of *structural valve degeneration and valve thrombosis*, bioprosthetic valves, both surgical and transcatheter, are prone to develop valve thrombosis and/or degenerate (e.g., calcify, pannus, leaflet tearing) over time (see Chapter 79). The incidence, consequences, and treatment implications of valve thrombosis are still being examined.[135] In some cases, there will be a marked early increase in transvalvular gradient as a result of valve thrombosis that is often responsive to treatment with anticoagulation. Ongoing surveillance with echocardiography and, as indicated, four-dimensional CT is important to detect these issues early. Although AVR improves HF symptoms and quality of life on the whole, a sizeable minority has *residual HF* after AVR, resulting in rehospitalization and less or no improvement in quality of life.[119,136,137] Accordingly, rather than simply viewing AVR as the curative "fix" for AS, treatment of HF with a reduced or preserved EF with appropriate medical therapy is critical to optimize outcomes. Some studies suggest that blood pressure targets for patients treated with AVR for AS may need to be slightly higher than for the general population, although further studies are needed to clarify this issue.[72,138]

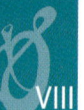

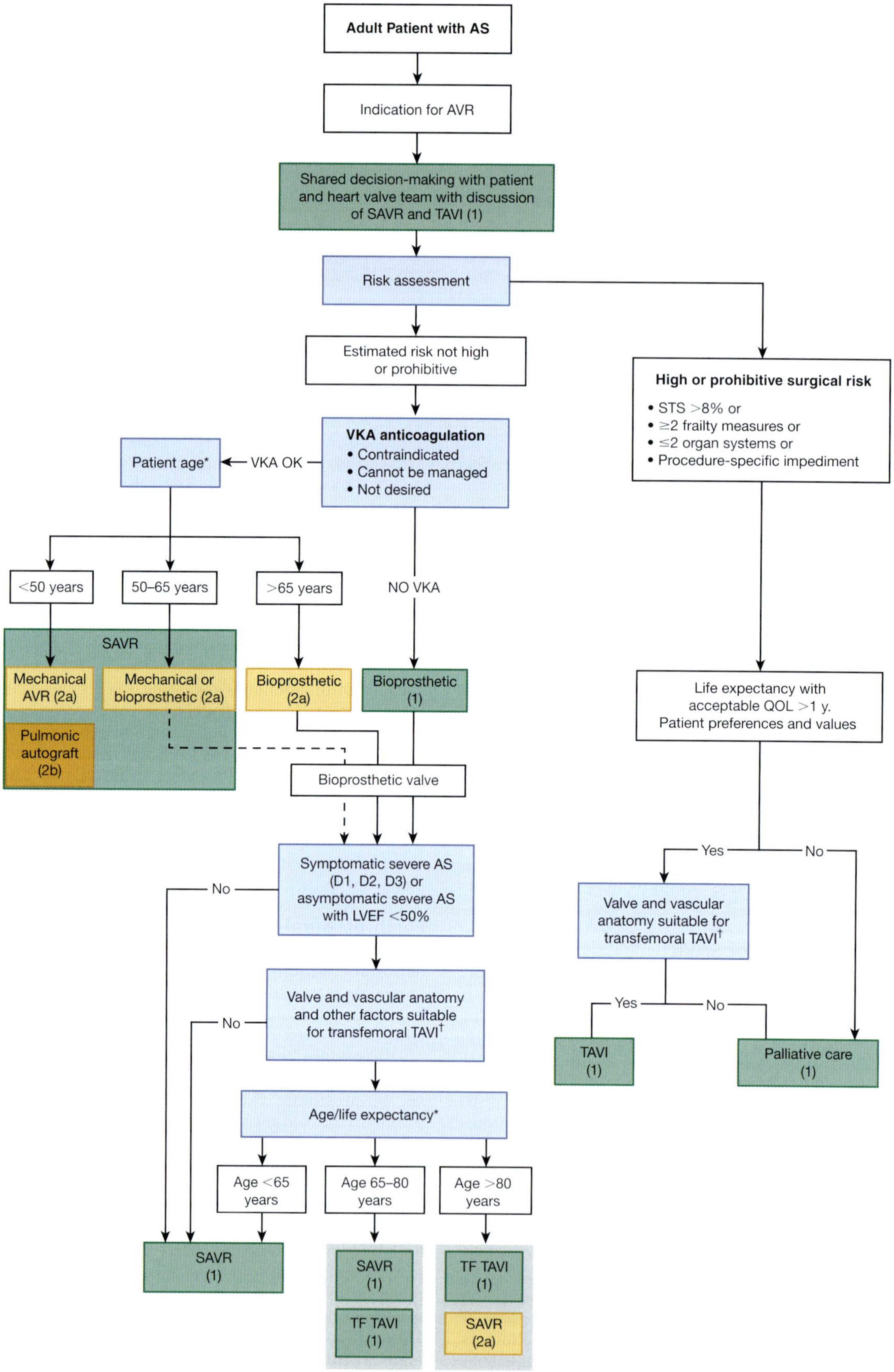

FIGURE 72.16 Selection of surgical versus transcatheter aortic valve replacement. Colors correspond to Table 72.3. *Approximate ages, based on U.S. Actuarial Life Expectancy tables, are provided for guidance. The balance between expected patient longevity and valve durability varies continuously across the age range, with more durable valves preferred for patients with a longer life expectancy. Bioprosthetic valve durability is finite (with shorter durability for younger patients), whereas mechanical valves are very durable but require lifelong anticoagulation. Long-term (20 years) data on outcomes with surgical bioprosthetic valves are available; robust data on transcatheter bioprosthetic valves extend to only 5 years, leading to uncertainty about longer-term outcomes. The decision about valve type should be individualized on the basis of patient-specific factors that might affect expected longevity. †Placement of a transcatheter valve requires vascular anatomy that allows transfemoral delivery and the absence of aortic root dilation that would require surgical replacement. Valvular anatomy must be suitable for placement of the specific prosthetic valve, including annulus size and shape, leaflet number and calcification, and coronary ostial height. *AS,* Aortic stenosis; *AVR,* aortic valve replacement; *LVEF,* left ventricular ejection fraction; *QOL,* quality of life; *SAVR,* surgical aortic valve replacement; *STS,* Society of Thoracic Surgeons; *TAVI,* transcatheter aortic valve implantation; *TF,* transfemoral; and *VKA,* vitamin K antagonist. (From Otto CM, et al. 2020 AHA/ACC guideline for the management of patients with valvular heart disease: a report of the American College of Cardiology/ American Heart Association Task Force on Practice Guidelines. *J Am Coll Cardiol.* 2021;77:e25-197.)

TABLE 72.5 Factors to Consider for Patient Selection for Transcatheter Versus Surgical Aortic Valve Replacement

Age

Bicuspid versus tricuspid valve

Valve calcification (amount, location)

Aortic size

Annulus size

Concomitant severe mitral or tricuspid valve disease

Extent, location, and complexity of coronary disease

Severity of left ventricular dysfunction

Transfemoral vascular access

CLASSIC REFERENCES

Grossman W, Jones D, McLaurin LP. Wall stress and patterns of hypertrophy in the human left ventricle. *J Clin Invest*. 1975;56:56–64.

Hill JA, Karimi M, Kutschke W, et al. Cardiac hypertrophy is not a required compensatory response to short-term pressure overload. *Circulation*. 2000;101:2863–2869.

Khot UN, Novaro GM, Popovic ZB, et al. Nitroprusside in critically ill patients with left ventricular dysfunction and aortic stenosis. *N Engl J Med*. 2003;348:1756–1763.

Otto CM, Burwash IG, Legget ME, et al. Prospective study of asymptomatic valvular aortic stenosis. Clinical, echocardiographic, and exercise predictors of outcome. *Circulation*. 1997;95:2262–2270.

Roberts WC, Ko JM. Frequency by decades of unicuspid, bicuspid, and tricuspid aortic valves in adults having isolated aortic valve replacement for aortic stenosis, with or without associated aortic regurgitation. *Circulation*. 2005;111:920–925.

REFERENCES

Epidemiology

1. Lindman BR, Clavel MA, Mathieu P, et al. Calcific aortic stenosis. *Nat Rev Dis Primers*. 2016;2:16006.
2. Osnabrugge RL, Mylotte D, Head SJ, et al. Aortic stenosis in the elderly: disease prevalence and number of candidates for transcatheter aortic valve replacement: a meta-analysis and modeling study. *J Am Coll Cardiol*. 2013;62:1002–1012.
3. d'Arcy JL, Coffey S, Loudon MA, et al. Large-scale community echocardiographic screening reveals a major burden of undiagnosed valvular heart disease in older people: the OxVALVE Population Cohort Study. *Eur Heart J*. 2016;37:3515–3522.
4. Coffey S, Cox B, Williams MJ. The prevalence, incidence, progression, and risks of aortic valve sclerosis: a systematic review and meta-analysis. *J Am Coll Cardiol*. 2014;63:2852–2861.
5. Yan AT, Koh M, Chan KK, et al. Association between cardiovascular risk factors and aortic stenosis: the CANHEART aortic stenosis study. *J Am Coll Cardiol*. 2017;69:1523–1532.
6. Lindman BR. Aortic stenosis: moving from treatment to prevention. *J Am Coll Cardiol*. 2017;69:1533–1535.
7. Prakash SK, Bosse Y, Muehlschlegel JD, et al. A roadmap to investigate the genetic basis of bicuspid aortic valve and its complications: insights from the International BAVCon (Bicuspid Aortic Valve Consortium). *J Am Coll Cardiol*. 2014;64:832–839.
8. Verma S, Siu SC. Aortic dilatation in patients with bicuspid aortic valve. *N Engl J Med*. 2014;370:1920–1929.
9. Michelena HI, Prakash SK, Della Corte A, et al. Bicuspid aortic valve: identifying knowledge gaps and rising to the challenge from the international Bicuspid Aortic Valve Consortium (BAVCon). *Circulation*. 2014;129:2691–2704.
10. Sherrah AG, Andvik S, van der Linde D, et al. Nonsyndromic thoracic aortic aneurysm and dissection outcomes with marfan syndrome versus bicuspid aortic valve aneurysm. *J Am Coll Cardiol*. 2016;67:618–626.
11. Masri A, Svensson LG, Griffin BP, et al. Contemporary natural history of bicuspid aortic valve disease: a systematic review. *Heart*. 2017;103:1323–1330.
12. Detaint D, Michelena HI, Nkomo VT, et al. Aortic dilatation patterns and rates in adults with bicuspid aortic valves: a comparative study with Marfan syndrome and degenerative aortopathy. *Heart*. 2014;100:126–134.
13. Braverman AC, Cheng A. The bicuspid aortic valve and associated aortic disease. In: Otto CM, Bonow RO, eds. *Valvular Heart Disease: A Companion to Braunwald's Heart Disease*. 5th ed. Philadelphia: Saunders; 2021:197–222.

Pathophysiology: Calcification and Obstruction

14. Otto C, Prendergast B. Aortic-valve stenosis–from patients at risk to severe valve obstruction. *N Engl J Med*. 2014;371:744–576.
15. Hutcheson JD, Aikawa E, Merryman WD. Potential drug targets for calcific aortic valve disease. *Nat Rev Cardiol*. 2014;11:218–231.
16. Zheng KH, Tzolos E, Dweck MR. Pathophysiology of aortic stenosis and future perspectives for medical therapy. *Cardiol Clin*. 2020;38:1–12.
17. Marquis-Gravel G, Redfors B, Leon MB, et al. Medical treatment of aortic stenosis. *Circulation*. 2016;134:1766–1784.
18. Thanassoulis G. Clinical and genetic risk factors for calcific valve disease. In: Otto CM, Bonow RO, eds. *Valvular Heart Disease: A Companion to Braunwald's Heart Disease*. 5th ed. Philadelphia: Saunders; 2021:66–78.
19. Thanassoulis G, Campbell CY, Owens DS, et al. Genetic associations with valvular calcification and aortic stenosis. *N Engl J Med*. 2013;368:503–512.
20. Kamstrup PR, Tybjærg-Hansen A, Nordestgaard BG. Elevated lipoprotein(a) and risk of aortic valve stenosis in the general population. *J Am Coll Cardiol*. 2014;63:470–477.
21. Cairns BJ, Coffey S, Travis RC, et al. A replicated, genome-wide significant association of aortic stenosis with a genetic variant for lipoprotein(a): meta-analysis of published and novel data. *Circulation*. 2017;135:1181–1183.
22. Perrot N, Theriault S, Dina C, et al. Genetic Variation in LPA, calcific aortic valve stenosis in patients undergoing cardiac surgery, and familial risk of aortic valve microcalcification. *JAMA Cardiol*. 2019;4:620–627.
23. Capoulade R, Chan KL, Yeang C, et al. Oxidized phospholipids, lipoprotein(a), and progression of calcific aortic valve stenosis. *J Am Coll Cardiol*. 2015;66:1236–4126.
24. Capoulade R, Mahmut A, Tastet L, et al. Impact of plasma Lp-PLA2 activity on the progression of aortic stenosis: the PROGRESSA study. *JACC Cardiovasc Imaging*. 2015;8:26–33.
25. Mahmut A, Boulanger MC, El Husseini D, et al. Elevated expression of lipoprotein-associated phospholipase A2 in calcific aortic valve disease: implications for valve mineralization. *J Am Coll Cardiol*. 2014;63:460–469.
26. Bouchareb R, Mahmut A, Nsaibia MJ, et al. Autotaxin derived from lipoprotein(a) and valve interstitial cells promotes inflammation and mineralization of the aortic valve. *Circulation*. 2015;132:677–690.
27. Rogers MA, Aikawa E. A Not-So-Little role for lipoprotein(a) in the development of calcific aortic valve disease. *Circulation*. 2015;132:621–362.
28. Hadji F, Boulanger MC, Guay SP, et al. Altered DNA methylation of long noncoding RNA H19 in calcific aortic valve disease promotes mineralization by silencing NOTCH1. *Circulation*. 2016;134:1848–1862.
29. Merryman WD, Clark CR. Lnc-ing NOTCH1 to idiopathic calcific aortic valve disease. *Circulation*. 2016;134:1863–1865.
30. Clark CR, Bowler MA, Snider JC, et al. Targeting cadherin-11 prevents notch1-mediated calcific aortic valve disease. *Circulation*. 2017;135:2448–2450.
31. Menon V, Lincoln J. The genetic regulation of aortic valve development and calcific disease. *Front Cardiovasc Med*. 2018;5:162.
32. Lindman BR, Merryman WD. Unloading the stenotic path to identifying medical therapy for calcific aortic valve disease: barriers and opportunities. *Circulation*. 2021;143:1455–1457.

Pathophysiology: Left Ventricular Response

33. Lindman BR. Left ventricular and vascular changes in valvular heart disease. In: Otto CM, Bonow RO, eds. *Valvular Heart Disease: A Companion to Braunwald's Heart Disease*. 5th ed. Philadelphia: Saunders; 2021:79–93.
34. Treibel TA, Badiani S, Lloyd G, et al. Multimodality imaging markers of adverse myocardial remodeling in aortic stenosis. *JACC Cardiovasc Imaging*. 2019;12:1532–1548.
35. Dweck MR, Boon NA, Newby DE. Calcific aortic stenosis: a disease of the valve and the myocardium. *J Am Coll Cardiol*. 2012;60:1854–1863.
36. Carabello BA. Is cardiac hypertrophy good or bad? The answer, of course, is yes. *JACC Cardiovasc Imaging*. 2014;7:1081–1083.
37. Petrov G, Dworatzek E, Schulze TM, et al. Maladaptive remodeling is associated with impaired survival in women but not in men after aortic valve replacement. *JACC Cardiovasc Imaging*. 2014;7:1073–1080.
38. Lindman BR, Arnold SV, Madrazo JA, et al. The adverse impact of diabetes mellitus on left ventricular remodeling and function in patients with severe aortic stenosis. *Circ Heart Fail*. 2011;4:286–292.
39. Beach JM, Mihaljevic T, Rajeswaran J, et al. Ventricular hypertrophy and left atrial dilatation persist and are associated with reduced survival after valve replacement for aortic stenosis. *J Thorac Cardiovasc Surg*. 2014;147:362–369.e8.
40. Gonzales H, Douglas PS, Pibarot P, et al. Left ventricular hypertrophy and clinical outcomes over 5 Years after TAVR: an analysis of the PARTNER trials and registries. *JACC Cardiovasc Interv*. 2020;13:1329–1339.
41. Chau KH, Douglas PS, Pibarot P, et al. Regression of left ventricular mass after transcatheter aortic valve replacement: the PARTNER trials and registries. *J Am Coll Cardiol*. 2020;75:2446–2458.
42. Everett RJ, Treibel TA, Fukui M, et al. Extracellular myocardial volume in patients with aortic stenosis. *J Am Coll Cardiol*. 2020;75:304–316.
43. Chin CWL, Everett RJ, Kwiecinski J, et al. Myocardial fibrosis and cardiac decompensation in aortic stenosis. *JACC Cardiovasc Imaging*. 2017;10:1320–1333.
44. Papanastasiou CA, Kokkinidis DG, Kampaktsis PN, et al. The prognostic role of late gadolinium enhancement in aortic stenosis: a systematic review and meta-analysis. *JACC Cardiovasc Imaging*. 2020;13:385–392.
45. Treibel TA, Lopez B, Gonzalez A, et al. Reappraising myocardial fibrosis in severe aortic stenosis: an invasive and non-invasive study in 133 patients. *Eur Heart J*. 2018;39:699–709.
46. Treibel TA, Kozor R, Schofield R, et al. Reverse myocardial remodeling following valve replacement in patients with aortic stenosis. *J Am Coll Cardiol*. 2018;71:860–871.
47. Bing R, Cavalcante JL, Everett RJ, et al. Imaging and impact of myocardial fibrosis in aortic stenosis. *JACC Cardiovasc Imaging*. 2019;12:283–296.
48. Weidemann F, Herrmann S, Stork S, et al. Impact of myocardial fibrosis in patients with symptomatic severe aortic stenosis. *Circulation*. 2009;120:577–584.
49. Naya M, Chiba S, Iwano H, et al. Myocardial oxidative metabolism is increased due to haemodynamic overload in patients with aortic valve stenosis: assessment using 11C-acetate positron emission tomography. *Eur J Nucl Med Mol Imaging*. 2010;37:2242–2248.
50. Ahn JH, Kim SM, Park SJ, et al. Coronary Microvascular dysfunction as a mechanism of angina in severe AS: prospective adenosine-stress CMR study. *J Am Coll Cardiol*. 2016;67:1412–1422.
51. Singh A, Jerosch-Herold M, Bekele S, et al. Determinants of exercise capacity and myocardial perfusion reserve in asymptomatic patients with aortic stenosis. *JACC Cardiovasc Imaging*. 2020;13:178–180.
52. Mahmod M, Chan K, Raman B, et al. Histological evidence for impaired myocardial perfusion reserve in severe aortic stenosis. *JACC Cardiovasc Imaging*. 2019;12:2276–2278.
53. Kampaktsis PN, Kokkinidis DG, Wong SC, et al. The role and clinical implications of diastolic dysfunction in aortic stenosis. *Heart*. 2017;103:1481–1487.
54. Ong G, Pibarot P, Redfors B, et al. Diastolic function and clinical outcomes after transcatheter aortic valve replacement: PARTNER 2 SAPIEN 3 registry. *J Am Coll Cardiol*. 2020;76:2940–2951.
55. Kampaktsis PN, Bang CN, Chiu Wong S, et al. Prognostic importance of diastolic dysfunction in relation to post procedural aortic insufficiency in patients undergoing transcatheter aortic valve replacement. *Catheter Cardiovasc Interv*. 2017;89:445–451.
56. Ito S, Miranda WR, Nkomo VT, et al. Reduced left ventricular ejection fraction in patients with aortic stenosis. *J Am Coll Cardiol*. 2018;71:1313–1321.
57. Otto CM, Nishimura RA, Bonow RO, et al. 2020 ACC/AHA guideline for the management of patients with valvular heart disease: a report of the American College of Cardiology/American Heart Association Joint Committee on Clinical Practice Guidelines. *J Am Coll Cardiol*. 2021;77:e25–e197.
58. Dahl JS, Eleid MF, Michelena HI, et al. Effect of left ventricular ejection fraction on postoperative outcome in patients with severe aortic stenosis undergoing aortic valve replacement. *Circ Cardiovasc Imaging*. 2015;8:e002917.
59. Dahl JS, Magne J, Pellikka PA, et al. Assessment of Subclinical left ventricular dysfunction in aortic stenosis. *JACC Cardiovasc Imaging*. 2019;12:163–171.
60. Lancellotti P, Magne J, Dulgheru R, et al. Outcomes of patients with asymptomatic aortic stenosis followed up in heart valve clinics. *JAMA Cardiol*. 2018;3:1060–1068.
61. Taniguchi T, Morimoto T, Shiomi H, et al. Prognostic impact of left ventricular ejection fraction in patients with severe aortic stenosis. *JACC Cardiovasc Interv*. 2018;11:145–157.
62. Magne J, Cosyns B, Popescu BA, et al. Distribution and Prognostic significance of left ventricular global longitudinal strain in asymptomatic significant aortic stenosis: an individual participant data meta-analysis. *JACC Cardiovasc Imaging*. 2019;12:84–92.
63. Elmariah S, Palacios IF, McAndrew T, et al. Outcomes of transcatheter and surgical aortic valve replacement in high-risk patients with aortic stenosis and left ventricular dysfunction: results from the Placement of Aortic Transcatheter Valves (PARTNER) trial (cohort A). *Circ Cardiovasc Interv*. 2013;6:604–614.
64. Dauerman HL, Reardon MJ, Popma JJ, et al. Early recovery of left ventricular systolic function after CoreValve transcatheter aortic valve replacement. *Circ Cardiovasc Interv*. 2016;9:e003425.

65. Maes F, Lerakis S, Barbosa Ribeiro H, et al. Outcomes from transcatheter aortic valve replacement in patients with low-flow, low-gradient aortic stenosis and left ventricular ejection fraction less than 30%: a Substudy from the TOPAS-TAVI registry. *JAMA Cardiol*. 2019;4:64–70.

Pathophysiology: Pulmonary and Systemic Vasculature Response

66. Lindman BR, Zajarias A, Madrazo JA, et al. Effects of phosphodiesterase type 5 inhibition on systemic and pulmonary hemodynamics and ventricular function in patients with severe symptomatic aortic stenosis. *Circulation*. 2012;125:2353–2362.
67. Lindman BR, Zajarias A, Maniar HS, et al. Risk stratification in patients with pulmonary hypertension undergoing transcatheter aortic valve replacement. *Heart*. 2015;101:1656–1664.
68. O'Sullivan CJ, Wenaweser P, Ceylan O, et al. Effect of pulmonary hypertension hemodynamic presentation on clinical outcomes in patients with severe symptomatic aortic valve stenosis undergoing transcatheter aortic valve implantation: insights from the new proposed pulmonary hypertension classification. *Circ Cardiovasc Interv*. 2015;8:e002358.
69. Testa L, Latib A, De Marco F, et al. Persistence of severe pulmonary hypertension after transcatheter aortic valve replacement: incidence and prognostic impact. *Circ Cardiovasc Interv*. 2016;9:e003563.
70. Masri A, Abdelkarim I, Sharbaugh MS, et al. Outcomes of persistent pulmonary hypertension following transcatheter aortic valve replacement. *Heart*. 2018;104:821–827.
71. Yotti R, Bermejo J, Gutierrez-Ibanes E, et al. Systemic vascular load in calcific degenerative aortic valve stenosis: insight from percutaneous valve replacement. *J Am Coll Cardiol*. 2015;65:423–433.
72. Lindman BR, Otto CM, Douglas PS, et al. Blood pressure and arterial load after transcatheter aortic valve replacement for aortic stenosis. *Circ Cardiovasc Imaging*. 2017;10:e006308.
73. Ben-Assa E, Brown J, Keshavarz-Motamed Z, et al. Ventricular stroke work and vascular impedance refine the characterization of patients with aortic stenosis. *Sci Transl Med*. 2019;11:eaaw0181.
74. Lloyd JW, Nishimura RA, Borlaug BA, et al. Hemodynamic response to nitroprusside in patients with low-gradient severe aortic stenosis and preserved ejection fraction. *J Am Coll Cardiol*. 2017;70:1339–1348.
75. Chirinos JA, Akers SR, Schelbert E, et al. Arterial properties as determinants of left ventricular mass and fibrosis in severe aortic stenosis: findings from ACRIN PA 4008. *J Am Heart Assoc*. 2019;8:e03742.

Clinical Presentation and Diagnostic Testing

76. Zilberszac R, Gabriel H, Schemper M, et al. Asymptomatic severe aortic stenosis in the elderly. *JACC Cardiovasc Imaging*. 2017;10:43–50.
77. Loscalzo J. From clinical observation to mechanism–Heyde's syndrome. *N Engl J Med*. 2012;367:1954–1956.
78. Thoenes M, Bramlage P, Zamorano P, et al. Patient screening for early detection of aortic stenosis (AS): review of current practice and future perspectives. *J Thorac Dis*. 2018;10:5584–5594.
79. Baumgartner H, Hung J, Bermejo J, et al. Recommendations on the echocardiographic assessment of aortic valve stenosis: a focused update from the European Association of Cardiovascular Imaging and the American Society of Echocardiography. *J Am Soc Echocardiogr*. 2017;30:372–392.
80. Hahn RT, Cavalcante JL. Imaging the aortic valve. In: Otto CM, Bonow RO, eds. *Valvular Heart Disease: A Companion to Braunwald's Heart Disease*. 5th ed. Philadelphia Saunders; 2013:124–155.
81. Eleid MF, Nishimura RA, Sorajja P, et al. Systemic hypertension in low-gradient severe aortic stenosis with preserved ejection fraction. *Circulation*. 2013;128:1349–1353.
82. Redfors B, Pibarot P, Gillam LD, et al. Stress testing in asymptomatic aortic stenosis. *Circulation*. 2017;135:1956–1976.
83. Clavel MA, Magne J, Pibarot P. Low-gradient aortic stenosis. *Eur Heart J*. 2016;37:2645–2657.
84. Pawade T, Clavel MA, Tribouilloy C, et al. Computed tomography aortic valve calcium scoring in patients with aortic stenosis. *Circ Cardiovasc Imaging*. 2018;11:e007146.
85. Pawade T, Sheth T, Guzzetti E, et al. Why and how to measure aortic valve calcification in patients with aortic stenosis. *JACC Cardiovasc Imaging*. 2019;12:1835–1848.
86. Blanke P, Weir-McCall JR, Achenbach S, et al. Computed tomography imaging in the context of Transcatheter Aortic Valve Implantation (TAVI)/Transcatheter Aortic Valve Replacement (TAVR): an expert consensus document of the society of cardiovascular computed tomography. *JACC Cardiovasc Imaging*. 2019;12:1–24.
87. Yoon SH, Lefevre T, Ahn JM, et al. Transcatheter aortic valve replacement with early- and New-Generation Devices in bicuspid aortic valve stenosis. *J Am Coll Cardiol*. 2016;68:1195–1205.
88. Yoon SH, Kim WK, Dhoble A, et al. Bicuspid aortic valve morphology and outcomes after transcatheter aortic valve replacement. *J Am Coll Cardiol*. 2020;76:1018–1030.
89. Okuno T, Asami M, Heg D, et al. Impact of left ventricular outflow tract calcification on procedural outcomes after transcatheter aortic valve replacement. *JACC Cardiovasc Interv*. 2020;13:1789–1799.
90. Michail M, Ihdayhid AR, Comella A, et al. Feasibility and Validity of computed tomography-derived fractional flow reserve in patients with severe aortic stenosis: the CAST-FFR study. *Circ Cardiovasc Interv*. 2021;14:e009586.
91. Strong C, Ferreira A, Teles RC, et al. Diagnostic accuracy of computed tomography angiography for the exclusion of coronary artery disease in candidates for transcatheter aortic valve implantation. *Sci Rep*. 2019;9:19942.
92. Cavalcante JL, Lalude OO, Schoenhagen P, et al. Cardiovascular magnetic resonance imaging for structural and valvular heart disease interventions. *JACC Cardiovasc Interv*. 2016;9:399–425.
93. Dweck MR, Jones C, Joshi NV, et al. Assessment of valvular calcification and inflammation by positron emission tomography in patients with aortic stenosis. *Circulation*. 2012;125:76–86.
94. Dweck MR, Jenkins WS, Vesey AT, et al. 18F-sodium fluoride uptake is a marker of active calcification and disease progression in patients with aortic stenosis. *Circ Cardiovasc Imaging*. 2014;7:371–378.
95. Jenkins WS, Vesey AT, Shah AS, et al. Valvular (18)F-fluoride and (18)F-fluorodeoxyglucose uptake predict disease progression and clinical outcome in patients with aortic stenosis. *J Am Coll Cardiol*. 2015;66:1200–1201.
96. Castano A, Narotsky DL, Hamid N, et al. Unveiling transthyretin cardiac amyloidosis and its predictors among elderly patients with severe aortic stenosis undergoing transcatheter aortic valve replacement. *Eur Heart J*. 2017;38:2879–2887.
97. Scully PR, Treibel TA, Fontana M, et al. Prevalence of cardiac amyloidosis in patients referred for transcatheter aortic valve replacement. *J Am Coll Cardiol*. 2018;71:463–464.
98. Cavalcante JL, Rijal S, Abdelkarim I, et al. Cardiac amyloidosis is prevalent in older patients with aortic stenosis and carries worse prognosis. *J Cardiovasc Magn Reson*. 2017;19:98.
99. Scully PR, Patel KP, Saberwal B, et al. Identifying cardiac amyloid in aortic stenosis: ECV quantification by CT in TAVR patients. *JACC Cardiovasc Imaging*. 2020;13:2177–2189.
100. Maurer MS, Schwartz JH, Gundapaneni B, et al. Tafamidis treatment for patients with transthyretin amyloid cardiomyopathy. *N Engl J Med*. 2018;379:1007–1016.

Disease Course and Staging

101. Genereux P, Stone GW, O'Gara PT, et al. Natural history, diagnostic approaches, and therapeutic strategies for patients with asymptomatic severe aortic stenosis. *J Am Coll Cardiol*. 2016;67:2263–2288.
102. Nayeri A, Xu M, Farber-Eger E, et al. Initial changes in peak aortic jet velocity and mean gradient predict progression to severe aortic stenosis. *Int J Cardiol Heart Vasc*. 2020;30:100592.
103. Bahlmann E, Gerdts E, Cramariuc D, et al. Prognostic value of energy loss index in asymptomatic aortic stenosis. *Circulation*. 2013;127:1149–1156.
104. Minners J, Allgeier M, Gohlke-Baerwolf C, et al. Inconsistent grading of aortic valve stenosis by current guidelines: haemodynamic studies in patients with apparently normal left ventricular function. *Heart*. 2010;96:1463–1468.
105. Berthelot-Richer M, Pibarot P, Capoulade R, et al. Discordant grading of aortic stenosis severity: echocardiographic predictors of survival benefit associated with aortic valve replacement. *JACC Cardiovasc Imaging*. 2016;9:797–805.
106. Linefsky JP, Otto CM. Aortic stenosis: clinical presentation, disease stages, and timing of intervention. In: Otto CM, Bonow RO, eds. *Valvular Heart Disease: A Companion to Braunwald's Heart Disease*. 5th ed. Philadelphia Saunders; 2013:124–155.
107. Clark MA, Arnold SV, Duhay FG, et al. Five-year clinical and economic outcomes among patients with medically managed severe aortic stenosis: results from a Medicare claims analysis. *Circ Cardiovasc Qual Outcomes*. 2012;5:697–704.
108. Ribeiro HB, Lerakis S, Gilard M, et al. Transcatheter aortic valve replacement in patients with low-flow, low-gradient aortic stenosis: the TOPAS-TAVI Registry. *J Am Coll Cardiol*. 2018;71:1297–1308.
109. Clavel MA, Ennezat PV, Marechaux S, et al. Stress echocardiography to assess stenosis severity and predict outcome in patients with paradoxical low-flow, low-gradient aortic stenosis and preserved LVEF. *JACC Cardiovasc Imaging*. 2013;6:175–183.

Treatment

110. Lindman BR, Otto CM. Time to treat hypertension in patients with aortic stenosis. *Circulation*. 2013;128:1281–1283.
111. Nielsen OW, Sajadieh A, Sabbah M, et al. Assessing optimal blood pressure in patients with asymptomatic aortic valve stenosis: the SEAS study. *Circulation*. 2016;134:455–468.
112. Kapadia S, Stewart WJ, Anderson WN, et al. Outcomes of inoperable symptomatic aortic stenosis patients not undergoing aortic valve replacement: insight into the impact of balloon aortic valvuloplasty from the PARTNER trial (Placement of AoRtic TraNscathetER Valve trial). *JACC Cardiovasc Interv*. 2015;8:324–333.
113. Baumgartner H, Falk V, Bax JJ, et al. 2017 ESC/EACTS Guidelines for the management of valvular heart disease. *Eur Heart J*. 2017;38:2739–2791.
114. Lindman BR, Dweck MR, Lancellotti P, et al. Management of asymptomatic severe aortic stenosis: evolving concepts in timing of valve replacement. *JACC Cardiovasc Imaging*. 2020;13:481–493.
115. Taniguchi T, Morimoto T, Shiomi H, et al. Initial surgical versus conservative strategies in patients with asymptomatic severe aortic stenosis. *J Am Coll Cardiol*. 2015;66:2827–2838.
116. Campo J, Tsoris A, Kruse J, et al. Prognosis of severe asymptomatic aortic stenosis with and without surgery. *Ann Thorac Surg*. 2019;108:74–80.
117. Kang DH, Park SJ, Lee SA, et al. Early surgery or conservative care for asymptomatic aortic stenosis. *N Engl J Med*. 2020;382:111–119.
118. Lindman BR, Alexander KP, O'Gara PT, et al. Futility, benefit, and transcatheter aortic valve replacement. *JACC Cardiovasc Interv*. 2014;7:707–716.
119. Arnold SV, Afilalo J, Spertus JA, et al. Prediction of poor outcome after transcatheter aortic valve replacement. *J Am Coll Cardiol*. 2016;68:1868–1877.
120. Kafa R, Kusunose K, Goodman AL, et al. Association of abnormal postoperative left ventricular global longitudinal strain with outcomes in severe aortic stenosis following aortic valve replacement. *JAMA Cardiol*. 2016;1:494–496.
121. Bowdish ME, D'Agostino RS, Thourani VH, et al. The society of thoracic surgeons adult cardiac surgery database: 2020 update on outcomes and research. *Ann Thorac Surg*. 2020;109:1646–1655.
122. Barreto-Filho JA, Wang Y, Dodson JA, et al. Trends in aortic valve replacement for elderly patients in the United States, 1999-2011. *J Am Med Assoc*. 2013;310:2078–2085.
123. Adams DH, Popma JJ, Reardon MJ, et al. Transcatheter aortic-valve replacement with a self-expanding prosthesis. *N Engl J Med*. 2014;370:1790–1798.
124. Leon MB, Smith CR, Mack MJ, et al. Transcatheter or surgical aortic-valve replacement in intermediate-risk patients. *N Engl J Med*. 2016;374:1609–1620.
125. Mack MJ, Leon MB, Thourani VH, et al. Transcatheter aortic-valve replacement with a balloon-expandable valve in low-risk patients. *N Engl J Med*. 2019;380:1695–1705.
126. Reardon MJ, Van Mieghem NM, Popma JJ, et al. Surgical or transcatheter aortic-valve replacement in intermediate-risk patients. *N Engl J Med*. 2017;376:1321–1331.
127. Popma JJ, Deeb GM, Yakubov SJ, et al. Transcatheter aortic-valve replacement with a self-expanding valve in low-risk patients. *N Engl J Med*. 2019;380:1706–1715.
128. Pibarot P, Ternacle J, Jaber WA, et al. Structural deterioration of transcatheter versus surgical aortic valve bioprostheses in the PARTNER-2 trial. *J Am Coll Cardiol*. 2020;76:1830–1843.
129. Coylewright M, O'Neill E, Sherman A, et al. The learning curve for shared decision-making in symptomatic aortic stenosis. *JAMA Cardiol*. 2020;5:442–448.
130. Lindman BR, Perpetua E. Incorporating the patient voice into shared decision-making for the treatment of aortic stenosis. *JAMA Cardiol*. 2020;5:380–381.
131. Makkar RR, Yoon SH, Leon MB, et al. Association between transcatheter aortic valve replacement for bicuspid vs tricuspid aortic stenosis and mortality or stroke. *J Am Med Assoc*. 2019;321:2193–2202.
132. Forrest JK, Kaple RK, Ramlawi B, et al. Transcatheter aortic valve replacement in bicuspid versus tricuspid aortic valves from the STS/ACC TVT Registry. *JACC Cardiovasc Interv*. 2020;13:1749–1759.
133. Halim SA, Edwards FH, Dai D, et al. Outcomes of transcatheter aortic valve replacement in patients with bicuspid aortic valve disease: a report from the Society of Thoracic Surgeons/American College of Cardiology transcatheter valve therapy Registry. *Circulation*. 2020;141:1071–1079.
134. Patel DK, Duncan MS, Shah AS, et al. Association of Cardiac Rehabilitation with decreased hospitalization and mortality risk after cardiac valve surgery. *JAMA Cardiol*. 2019;4:1250–1259.
135. Goel K, Lindman BR. Hypoattenuated leaflet thickening after transcatheter aortic valve replacement: expanding the evidence base but questions remain. *Circ Cardiovasc Imaging*. 2019;12:e010151.
136. Vemulapalli S, Dai D, Hammill BG, et al. Hospital resource utilization before and after transcatheter aortic valve replacement: the STS/ACC TVT Registry. *J Am Coll Cardiol*. 2019;73:1135–1146.
137. O'Leary JM, Clavel MA, Chen S, et al. Association of natriuretic peptide levels after transcatheter aortic valve replacement with subsequent clinical outcomes. *JAMA Cardiol*. 2020;5:1113–1123.
138. Lindman BR, Goel K, Bermejo J, et al. Lower blood pressure after transcatheter or surgical aortic valve replacement is associated with increased mortality. *J Am Heart Assoc*. 2019;8:e014020.

73 Aortic Regurgitation

ROBERT O. BONOW AND RICK A. NISHIMURA

CAUSES AND PATHOLOGY, 1419
Valvular Disease, 1419
Disease of the Aortic Root and Ascending Aorta, 1419

CHRONIC AORTIC REGURGITATION, 1419
Pathophysiology, 1419
Clinical Presentation, 1420
Diagnostic Testing, 1421
Disease Course, 1423

ACUTE AORTIC REGURGITATION, 1428
Pathophysiology and Clinical Presentation, 1428

CLASSIC REFERENCES, 1429

REFERENCES, 1429

CAUSES AND PATHOLOGY

Aortic regurgitation (AR) can result from primary disease of the aortic valve leaflets and/or dilation of the aortic root and ascending aorta (Table 73.1).[1] Among patients with isolated AR who undergo aortic valve replacement (AVR), the percentage with primary disease of the aorta has been increasing steadily during the past few decades; it now represents the most common cause, accounting for more than 50% of all such patients in some series.

Valvular Disease

There are two predominant groups of patients who present with AR caused by a primary valve abnormality that is at least moderately severe. One group is comprised of young adults with noncalcified bicuspid aortic valves (BAVs) age 20 through 40 with AR caused by incomplete closure and/or prolapse of a valve leaflet. The other group consists of patients age 60 or older with calcific aortic valve disease. Although these latter patients usually have aortic stenosis (AS) as the primary valve disorder (see Chapter 72), among patients with significant calcific AS some degree (usually mild) of AR is often present. Other common causes of valve disorders leading to AR include infective endocarditis (see Chapter 80), in which the infection may destroy or cause perforation of a leaflet, or the vegetations may interfere with proper coaptation of the cusps; chest trauma resulting in valve disruption or a tear of the ascending aorta leading to valve prolapse; and rheumatic heart disease, particularly in low and middle income countries in which rheumatic fever is endemic (see Chapter 81). In rheumatic aortic valve disease, fusion of the commissures and fibrotic retraction of leaflet tissue lead to a fixed orifice with a central defect often producing combined AS and AR (see Fig. 72.1C). Associated mitral valve involvement is usually present (see Chapter 75). Progressive AR may also occur in patients with congenital heart disease (see Chapter 82), including those with a large ventricular septal defect, as well as in patients with membranous subaortic stenosis and as a complication of percutaneous balloon aortic valvuloplasty. Progressive AR also may occur in patients with myxomatous proliferation of the aortic valve. Increasingly common causes of valvular AR are structural deterioration of a bioprosthetic valve (see Chapter 79) and both central and paravalvular AR in patients who have undergone transcatheter aortic valve replacement (TAVR) (see Chapter 74).

Less common valvular causes of AR include various forms of congenital AR, such as unicommissural and quadricuspid valves,[2,3] or rupture of a congenitally fenestrated valve, particularly in the presence of hypertension. AR may also occur in association with systemic lupus erythematosus, rheumatoid arthritis, ankylosing spondylitis, Jaccoud arthropathy, Takayasu disease, Whipple disease, Crohn disease, and, in the past, the use of certain anorectic drugs.

Disease of the Aortic Root and Ascending Aorta

AR secondary to marked dilation of the ascending aorta (see Chapter 42) is now more common than primary valve disease in patients undergoing AVR for isolated AR. The conditions responsible for aortic root disease include age-related (degenerative) aortic dilation, systemic hypertension, aortic dilation related to BAVs,[4,5] cystic medial necrosis of the aorta (either isolated or associated with classic Marfan syndrome), aortic dissection, osteogenesis imperfecta, syphilitic aortitis, ankylosing spondylitis, Behçet syndrome, psoriatic arthritis (see Chapter 97), arthritis associated with ulcerative colitis, relapsing polychondritis, reactive arthritis, and giant cell arteritis, as well as exposure to some appetite-suppressant drugs.

When the aortic annulus becomes greatly dilated, the aortic leaflets separate and AR may ensue. Dissection of the diseased aortic wall may cause or aggravate the AR. Dilation of the aortic root also may have secondary effects on the aortic valve because dilation causes tension and bowing of the individual cusps, which may thicken and retract. This defect leads to intensification of the AR, further dilating the ascending aorta and leading to a vicious cycle in which, as is the case for mitral regurgitation (MR) (see Chapter 76), more regurgitation leads to more regurgitation.

CHRONIC AORTIC REGURGITATION

Pathophysiology

Left Ventricular Remodeling and Function. In contrast with MR, in which a fraction of the left ventricular (LV) stroke volume is ejected into the low-pressure left atrium, in AR the entire LV stroke volume is ejected into a high-pressure chamber (i.e., the aorta), although the low aortic diastolic pressure does facilitate ventricular emptying during early systole (Fig. 73.1). In MR, especially acute MR, the reduction of wall tension (i.e., reduced afterload) allows more complete systolic emptying; in AR, the increase in LV end-diastolic volume (i.e., increased preload) provides hemodynamic compensation.

Severe AR may occur with a normal effective forward stroke volume and a normal LV ejection fraction (EF) ([forward plus regurgitant stroke volume]/[end-diastolic volume]), together with an elevated LV end-diastolic volume, pressure, and stress[6] (Fig. 73.2). In accord with Laplace's law, which indicates that wall tension is related to the product of the intraventricular pressure and radius divided by wall thickness (see Chapter 46), LV dilation also increases the LV systolic tension required to develop any level of systolic pressure. Thus in AR, there is an increase in both preload and afterload. LV systolic function is maintained through the combination of chamber dilation and hypertrophy. This leads to eccentric hypertrophy, with replication of sarcomeres in series and elongation of myocytes and myocardial fibers (see Classic References, Grossman et al.). In compensated AR, sufficient wall thickening results in a normal ratio of LV wall thickness to cavity radius. Under these conditions, end-diastolic wall stress is maintained at or returns to normal levels. In AS, in contrast, changes include pressure overload (concentric) hypertrophy with replication of sarcomeres, largely in parallel, and an increased ratio of wall thickness to radius, but in both AR and AS, an increase in interstitial connective tissue develops (see Chapter 72). In AR, LV mass usually is greatly increased, often to levels even higher than in isolated AS. As AR persists and increases in severity over time, however, wall thickening fails to keep pace with the hemodynamic load, and end-systolic wall stress rises. At this point, the afterload mismatch results in a decline in systolic function, and the LVEF falls (see Fig. 73.2).

TABLE 73.1 Causes of Aortic Regurgitation

Leaflet Abnormalities

Rheumatic disease

Aortic valve sclerosis and calcification

Congenital abnormalities (bicuspid, unicuspid, and quadricuspid valves; aortic regurgitation associated with discrete subaortic stenosis and ventricular septal defect)

Infective endocarditis

Myxomatous valve disease

Complicating balloon valvuloplasty and transcatheter aortic valve implantation

Rare causes (drugs, leaflet fenestration, irradiation, nonbacterial endocarditis, trauma)

Aortic Root Abnormalities

Chronic hypertension

Marfan syndrome

Annulo-aortic ectasia

Aortic dissection

Ehlers-Danlos syndrome

Osteogenesis imperfecta

Atherosclerotic aneurysm

Syphilitic aortitis

Other systemic inflammatory disorders (giant cell aortitis, Takayasu disease, Reiter syndrome)

Combined Valve and Aortic Root Abnormalities

Bicuspid aortic valve

Ankylosing spondylitis

From Evangelista A, et al. Aortic regurgitation: clinical presentation, disease stages, and management. In Otto CM, Bonow RO, editors. Valvular Heart Disese. A Companion to Braunwald's Heart Disease. 5th ed. Philadelphia: Elsevier; 2021, pp. 179-196.

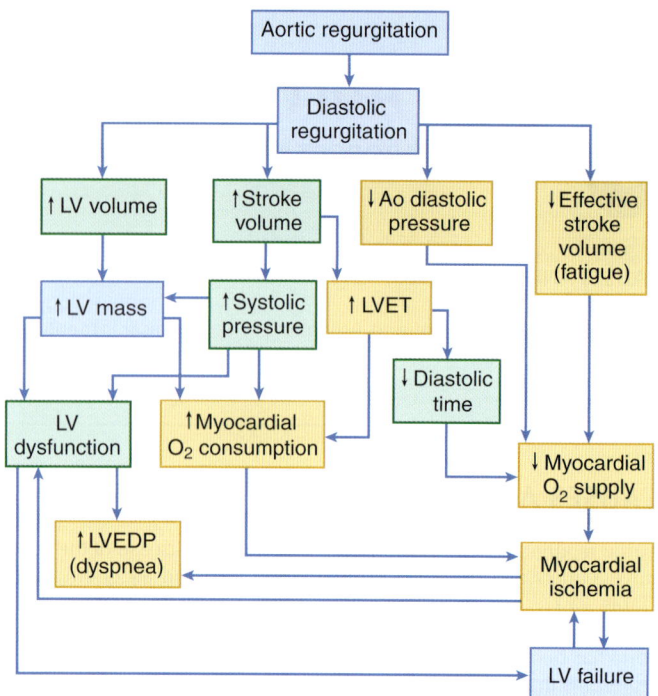

FIGURE 73.1 **Pathophysiology of aortic regurgitation.** Regurgitation results in an increased left ventricular (LV) volume, increased stroke volume, increased aortic (Ao) systolic pressure, and decreased effective stroke volume. Increased LV volume results in an increased LV mass, which may lead to LV dysfunction and failure. Increased LV stroke volume increases systolic pressure and prolongation of LV ejection time (LVET). Increased LV systolic pressure results in a decrease in diastolic time. Decreased diastolic time (myocardial perfusion time), diastolic aortic pressure, and effective stroke volume lead to reduced myocardial O_2 supply. Increased myocardial O_2 consumption and decreased myocardial O_2 supply produce myocardial ischemia, which further impairs LV function. *LVEDP*, Left ventricular end-diastolic pressure. (From Boudoulas H, Gravanis MB. Valvular heart disease. In Gravanis MB, editor. Cardiovascular Disorders: Pathogenesis and Pathophysiology. St Louis: Mosby; 1993, p. 64.)

Patients with severe chronic AR, left unchecked, can develop the largest LV end-diastolic volumes of any form of heart disease, resulting in so-called cor bovinum. However, end-diastolic pressure is not uniformly elevated (i.e., LV compliance often is increased; see Fig. 73.2). The adaptive response to gradually increasing, chronic AR permits the ventricle to function as an effective high-compliance pump, handling a large stroke volume, often with little increase in filling pressure. During exercise, peripheral vascular resistance declines and, with an increase in heart rate, diastole shortens and the regurgitation per beat decreases, facilitating an increment in effective (forward) cardiac output without substantial increases in end-diastolic volume and pressure. The EF and related ejection phase indices are often within normal limits, both at rest and during exercise, even though myocardial function, as reflected in the slope of the end-systolic pressure-volume relationship, is depressed.

As the left ventricle decompensates, interstitial fibrosis increases, compliance declines, and LV end-diastolic pressure and volume rise (see Fig. 73.2). In advanced stages of decompensation, left atrial, pulmonary artery wedge, pulmonary arterial, right ventricular (RV), and right atrial pressures rise and the effective (forward) cardiac output falls, at first during exercise and then at rest. The normal decline in LV end-systolic volume (ESV) or the rise in LVEF fails to occur during exercise. Symptoms of heart failure develop, particularly those secondary to pulmonary congestion.

Myocardial Ischemia

When acute AR is induced experimentally, myocardial oxygen requirements rise substantially, secondary to an increase in wall tension. In patients with chronic severe AR, total myocardial oxygen requirements also are augmented by the increase in LV mass (see Fig 73.1). Because the major portion of coronary blood flow occurs during diastole, when aortic pressure is lower than normal in AR, coronary perfusion pressure is reduced. Studies in experimentally induced AR have shown a reduction in coronary flow reserve, with a change in forward coronary flow from diastole to systole. The result, a combination of increased oxygen demands and reduced supply, sets the stage for the development of myocardial ischemia, especially during exercise. Thus patients with severe AR exhibit a reduction of coronary reserve, which may be responsible for myocardial ischemia and which may in turn play a role in the deterioration of LV function.

Clinical Presentation

The clinical stages of chronic AR are indicated in Table 73.2, demonstrating the progressive nature of the disease.[7]

Symptoms

In chronic severe AR, the left ventricle gradually enlarges while the patient remains asymptomatic.[1,7,8] Symptoms of reduced cardiac reserve or myocardial ischemia develop, most often in the fourth or fifth decade of life, and usually only after considerable cardiomegaly and myocardial dysfunction have occurred. The principal manifestations, including exertional dyspnea, orthopnea, and paroxysmal nocturnal dyspnea, usually develop gradually. Angina pectoris is prominent late in the course; nocturnal angina may be troublesome and often is accompanied by diaphoresis, which occurs when the heart rate slows and arterial diastolic pressure falls to extremely low levels. Patients with severe AR often complain of an uncomfortable awareness of the heartbeat, especially in supine position lying on left side, and thoracic discomfort caused by pounding of the heart against the chest wall. Tachycardia, occurring with emotional stress or exertion, may cause palpitations and head pounding. Premature ventricular contractions are particularly distressing because of the great heave of the volume-loaded left ventricle during the postextrasystolic beat. These complaints may be present for many years before symptoms of overt LV dysfunction develop.

Physical Examination

In patients with chronic, severe AR, the head may bob with each heartbeat (de Musset sign), and water hammer pulses, with abrupt distention and quick collapse (Corrigan pulse), are evident. The arterial pulse often is prominent and can be best appreciated by palpation of the radial artery with the patient's arm elevated (see Chapter 13). A bisferiens pulse may be present and is more readily recognized in the brachial and femoral arteries than in the carotid arteries. A variety of auscultatory

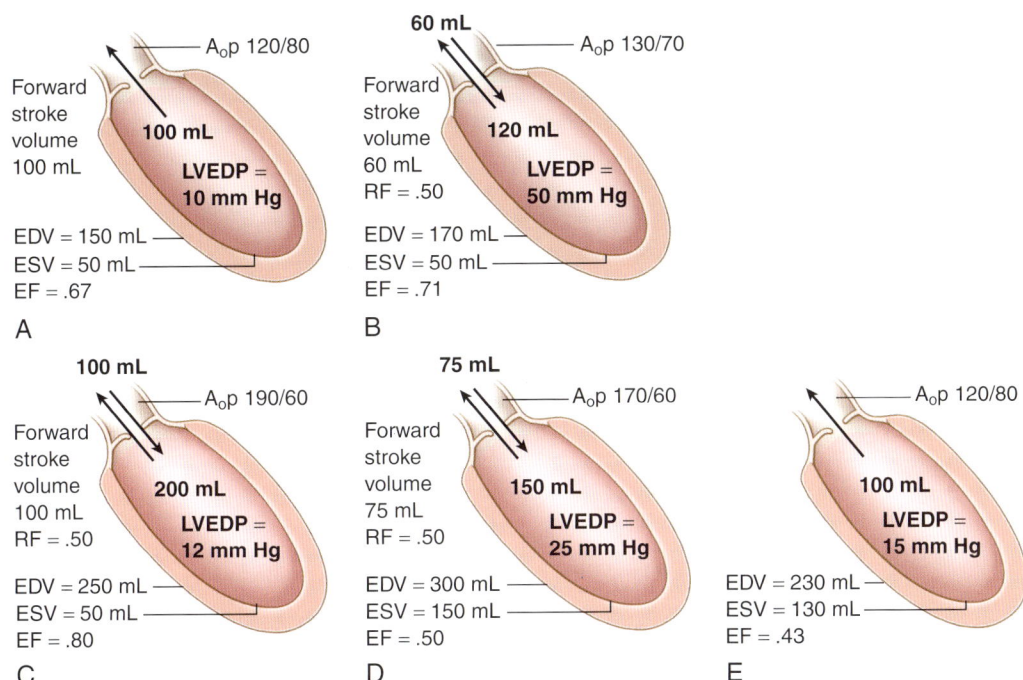

FIGURE 73.2 Hemodynamics of aortic regurgitation (AR). **A,** Normal conditions. **B,** The hemodynamic changes that occur in severe acute AR. Although total stroke volume is increased, forward stroke volume is reduced. Left ventricular end-diastolic pressure (LVEDP) rises dramatically. **C,** Hemodynamic changes occurring in chronic compensated AR. Eccentric hypertrophy produces increased end-diastolic volume (EDV), which permits an increase in total, as well as forward, stroke volume. The volume overload is accommodated, and LV filling pressure is normalized. Ventricular emptying and end-systolic volume (ESV) remain normal. **D,** In chronic decompensated AR, impaired LV emptying produces an increase in ESV and a fall in ejection fraction (EF), total stroke volume, and forward stroke volume. Further cardiac dilation and re-elevation of LV filling pressure occur. **E,** Immediately after valve replacement, preload estimated by EDV decreases, as does filling pressure. ESV also is decreased, but to a lesser extent. The result is an initial fall in EF. Despite these changes, elimination of AR leads to an increase in forward stroke volume, and with time, EF increases. A_op, Aortic pressure; *RF*, regurgitant fraction. (From Carabello BA. Aortic regurgitation: hemodynamic determinants of prognosis. In Cohn LH, DiSesa VJ, editors. Aortic Regurgitation: Medical and Surgical Management. New York: Marcel Dekker; 1986, pp. 99-101.)

early diastole and typically is high pitched and blowing. In severe AR, the murmur is holodiastolic and may have a rough quality. When the murmur is musical (cooing dove murmur), it usually signifies eversion or perforation of an aortic cusp. In patients with severe AR and LV decompensation, equilibration of aortic and LV pressures in late diastole abolishes the late diastolic component of the regurgitant murmur. When AR is caused by primary valvular disease, the diastolic murmur is heard best along the left sternal border in the third and fourth intercostal spaces. However, when it is caused mainly by dilation of the ascending aorta, the murmur often is more readily audible along the right sternal border.

Many patients with chronic AR have a harsh systolic outflow murmur caused by the increased total LV stroke volume and ejection rate, which often radiates to the carotid vessels. The systolic murmur often is more readily audible than the diastolic murmur. It may be higher pitched and less rasping than the murmur of AS but often is accompanied by a systolic thrill. Palpation of the carotid pulses will elucidate the cause of the systolic murmur and differentiate it from the murmur of AS.

A third heart sound (S_3) correlates with an increased LV end-diastolic volume. Its development may be a sign of impaired LV function, which is useful in identifying patients with severe AR who are candidates for surgical treatment. A mid-diastolic and late diastolic apical rumble, the *Austin Flint murmur*, is common in severe AR and may occur in the presence of a normal mitral valve. This murmur appears to be created by severe AR impinging on the anterior leaflet of the mitral valve or the free LV wall; convincing evidence for obstruction to mitral inflow in these patients is lacking.

findings provide confirmation of a wide pulse pressure. The Traube sign (also known as pistol shot sounds) refers to booming systolic and diastolic sounds heard over the femoral artery, the Müller sign consists of systolic pulsations of the uvula, and the Duroziez sign consists of a systolic murmur heard over the femoral artery when it is compressed proximally and a diastolic murmur when it is compressed distally. Capillary pulsations (the Quincke sign) can be detected by transmitting a light through the patient's fingertips or exerting gentle pressure on the tip of a fingernail.

Systolic arterial pressure is elevated, and diastolic pressure is abnormally low. The reduction in diastolic pressure reflects severity of AR and has prognostic implications.[9,10] Korotkoff sounds often persist to zero even though the intra-arterial pressure rarely falls below 30 mm Hg. The point of change in Korotkoff sounds (i.e., the muffling of these sounds in phase IV) correlates with the diastolic pressure. As heart failure develops, peripheral vasoconstriction may occur and arterial diastolic pressure may rise, even though severe AR is present.[9]

The apical impulse is diffuse and hyperdynamic and is displaced laterally and inferiorly. A rapid ventricular filling wave often is palpable at the apex. The augmented stroke volume may create a systolic thrill at the base of the heart or suprasternal notch, and over the carotid arteries. In many patients, a carotid shudder is palpable.

Auscultation
The diastolic murmur, the principal physical finding in AR, is of high frequency and begins immediately after A_2. It may be distinguished from the murmur of pulmonic regurgitation by its earlier onset (i.e., immediately after A_2 rather than after P_2) and usually by the presence of a widened pulse pressure. The murmur is heard best with the diaphragm of the stethoscope while the patient is sitting up and leaning forward, with the breath held in deep exhalation. In severe AR, the murmur reaches an early peak and then shows a dominant decrescendo pattern throughout diastole.

The severity of AR correlates better with the duration than with the intensity of the murmur. In mild AR, the murmur may be limited to

Diagnostic Testing
Echocardiography
Echocardiography (see Chapter 16) is essential in evaluating cause (Fig. 73.3) and severity of AR as it impacts LV volume and function.[1,11] Anatomic findings such a BAV, thickening of the valve cusps, other congenital abnormalities, prolapse of the valve, a flail leaflet, or vegetation (see Fig. 80.4) are usually well delineated. In addition to leaflet anatomy and motion, the size and shape of the aortic root can be evaluated, although visualization of the ascending aorta is not always adequate, necessitating additional imaging tests in some cases. Transthoracic imaging usually is satisfactory, but transesophageal echocardiography (TEE) often provides more detail, particularly of the aortic root.

TEE is useful for the measurement of LV end-diastolic and end-systolic dimensions and volumes, EF, and mass.[11,12] Current recommendations for assessment of LV dilation emphasize measurement of LV volumes as well as linear dimensions, and criteria for normal dimensions and volumes as well as mild, moderate, and severe LV dilation have been published by the American Society of Echocardiography (ASE).[13] Three-dimensional (3D) and contrast echocardiography will enhance the accuracy of the volume measurements.[14] Recent studies have suggested that LVESV, indexed to body surface area, is a strong predictor of adverse clinical outcomes.[15,16] These measurements, when made serially, are of great value in selecting the optimal time for surgical intervention. When LV volumes are measured, meticulous attention

TABLE 73.2 Clinical Stages of Chronic Aortic Regurgitation (AR)

STAGE	DEFINITION	VALVE ANATOMY	VALVE HEMODYNAMICS	HEMODYNAMIC CONSEQUENCES	SYMPTOMS
A	At risk of AR	Bicuspid aortic valve (or other congenital valve anomaly) Aortic valve sclerosis Diseases of the aortic sinuses or ascending aorta History of rheumatic fever or known rheumatic heart disease IE	AR severity none or trace	None	None
B	Progressive AR	Mild to moderate calcification of a trileaflet valve or bicuspid aortic valve (or other congenital valve anomaly) Dilated aortic sinuses Rheumatic valve changes Previous IE	**Mild AR:** Jet width <25% of LVOT Vena contracta <0.3 cm RVol <30 mL/beat RF <30% ERO <0.10 cm² Angiography grade 1+ **Moderate AR:** Jet width 25%-64% of LVOT Vena contracta 0.3-0.6 cm RVol 30-59 mL/beat RF 30%-49% ERO 0.10-0.29 cm² Angiography grade 2+	Normal LV systolic function Normal LV volume or mild LV dilation	None
C	Asymptomatic severe AR	Calcific aortic valve disease Bicuspid valve (or other congenital abnormality) Dilated aortic sinuses or ascending aorta Rheumatic valve changes IE with abnormal leaflet closure or perforation	**Severe AR:** Jet width ≥65% of LVOT Vena contracta >0.6 cm Holodiastolic flow reversal in proximal abdominal aorta RVol ≥60 mL/beat RF ≥50% ERO ≥0.3 cm² Angiography grade 3+ to 4+ In addition, diagnosis of chronic severe AR requires evidence of LV dilation	C1: Normal LVEF (>55%) and mild to moderate LV dilation (LVESD ≤50 mm) C2: Abnormal LV systolic function with depressed LVEF (≤55%) or severe LV dilation (LVESD >50 mm or indexed LVESD >25 mm/m²)	None; exercise testing is reasonable to confirm symptom status
D	Symptomatic severe AR	Calcific valve disease Bicuspid valve (or other congenital abnormality) Dilated aortic sinuses or ascending aorta Rheumatic valve changes Previous IE with abnormal leaflet closure or perforation	**Severe AR:** Doppler jet width ≥65% of LVOT Vena contracta >0.6 cm Holodiastolic flow reversal in the proximal abdominal aorta RVol ≥60 mL/beat RF ≥50% ERO ≥0.3 cm² Angiography grade 3+ to 4+ In addition, diagnosis of chronic severe AR requires evidence of LV dilation	Symptomatic severe AR may occur with normal systolic function (LVEF >55%), mild to moderate LV dysfunction (LVEF 40% to 55%), or severe LV dysfunction (LVEF <40%). Moderate to severe LV dilation is present	Exertional dyspnea or angina, or more severe HF symptoms

AR, Aortic regurgitation; *ERO*, effective regurgitant orifice; *HF*, heart failure; *IE*, infective endocarditis; *LVEF*, left ventricular ejection fraction; *LVESD*, left ventricular end-systolic dimension; *LVOT*, left ventricular outflow tract; *RF*, regurgitant fraction; *RVol*, regurgitant volume.
From Otto CM, et al. 2020 AHA/ACC guideline for the management of patients with valvular heart disease: a report of the American College of Cardiology/American Heart Association Task Force on Practice Guidelines. J Am Coll Cardiol. 2021;77:e25-197.

to detail is needed, ensuring that the endocardium is well seen and the apex is not foreshortened, according to the ASE guidelines.

Doppler echocardiography and color flow Doppler imaging are the most sensitive and accurate noninvasive techniques for the diagnosis and evaluation of AR. They readily detect mild degrees of AR that may be inaudible on physical examination. As the severity of AR increases, there will be a larger area of turbulence in the LV outflow tract on color flow imaging, but this is only a semi-qualitative measure. There are indirect Doppler findings in severe AR including a high LV outflow velocity, reversal of flow in the descending aorta, and a short

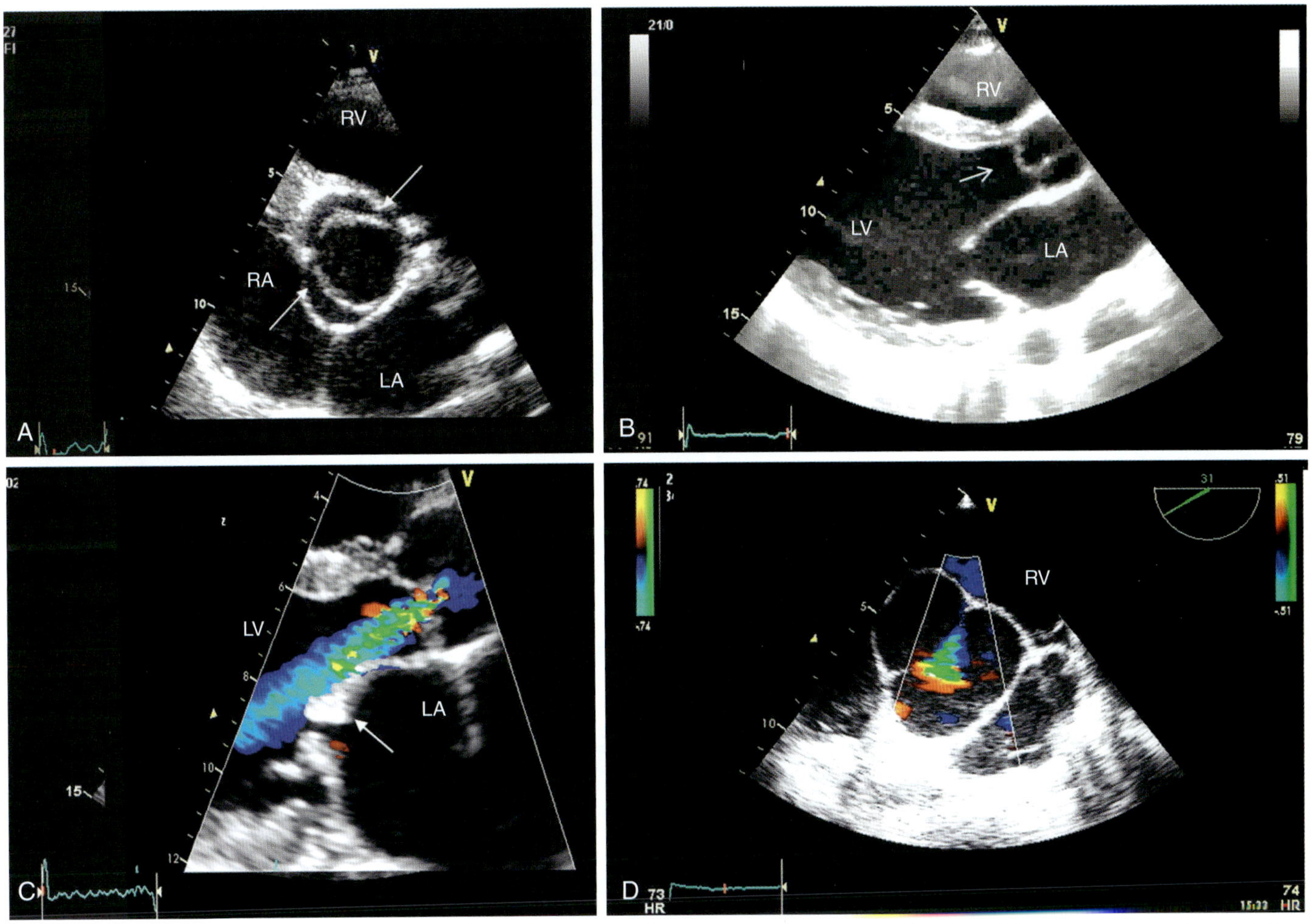

FIGURE 73.3 **A,** Transthoracic parasternal short-axis view shows a bicuspid aortic valve. **B,** Myxomatous aortic valve with prolapse of the right coronary cusp (*arrow*). **C,** Rheumatic valvular disease with mitral (*arrow*) and aortic involvement. **D,** Transesophageal echocardiography shows a central regurgitant orifice due to an annulo-aortic ectasia. *Ao,* Aorta; *LA,* left atrium; *LV,* left ventricle; *RV,* right ventricle. (From Evangelista A, et al. Aortic regurgitation: clinical presentation, disease stages, and management. In Otto CM, Bonow RO, editors. Valvular Heart Disease. A Companion to Braunwald's Heart Disease. 5th ed. Philadelphia: Elsevier; 2021, pp. 179-196.)

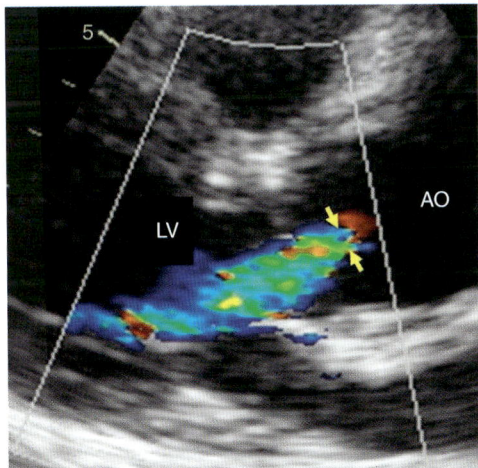

FIGURE 73.4 Parasternal long-axis view shows the vena contracta (*arrows*) of the regurgitant flow by Doppler in a patient with severe aortic regurgitation. *AO,* Aorta; *LV,* left ventricle. (From Evangelista A, et al. Aortic regurgitation: clinical presentation, disease stages, and management. In Otto CM, Bonow RO, editors. Valvular Heart Disease. A Companion to Braunwald's Heart Disease. 5th ed. Philadelphia: Elsevier; 2021, pp. 179-196.)

diastolic half-time of the AR continuous wave signal. Both the AR orifice size and AR flow can be estimated quantitatively[11] (Figs. 73.4 and 73.5; see also Fig 16.46), and such determinations are strongly recommended.[7,12] These quantitative data provide the basis for the definitions of mild, moderate, and severe AR in current guidelines (see Table 73.2). Serial studies permit determination of the progression of AR and its effect on the left ventricle.

Cardiac Magnetic Resonance

Cardiac magnetic resonance (CMR) (see Chapter 19) is useful for assessing the degree of aortic dilation in patients with BAV and other diseases affecting the aortic root and ascending aorta, and it provides accurate measurements of regurgitant volumes and the regurgitant orifice to assess severity of AR on the basis of the antegrade and retrograde flow volumes in the ascending aorta (Fig. 73.6; see also Fig. 19.16). CMR is the most accurate noninvasive technique for assessing LVESV, end-diastolic volume, and mass,[11,14,17-19] and is recommended when echocardiographic evaluation of LV size and function or severity of regurgitation is suboptimal.[7,12]

Angiography

For angiographic assessment of AR, contrast material should be injected rapidly (i.e., at 55 to 60 mL at 20 mL/sec/sec) into the aortic root, and filming should be carried out in the right and left anterior oblique projections (see Chapter 22). Opacification may be improved by filming during a Valsalva maneuver.

Disease Course

Asymptomatic Patients

Patients with mild or moderate AR who are asymptomatic with normal or only minimally increased cardiac size require no therapy but should be followed clinically and by echocardiography every 12 or 24 months. Asymptomatic patients with chronic severe AR and normal LV systolic function should be examined at intervals of approximately 6 months. In

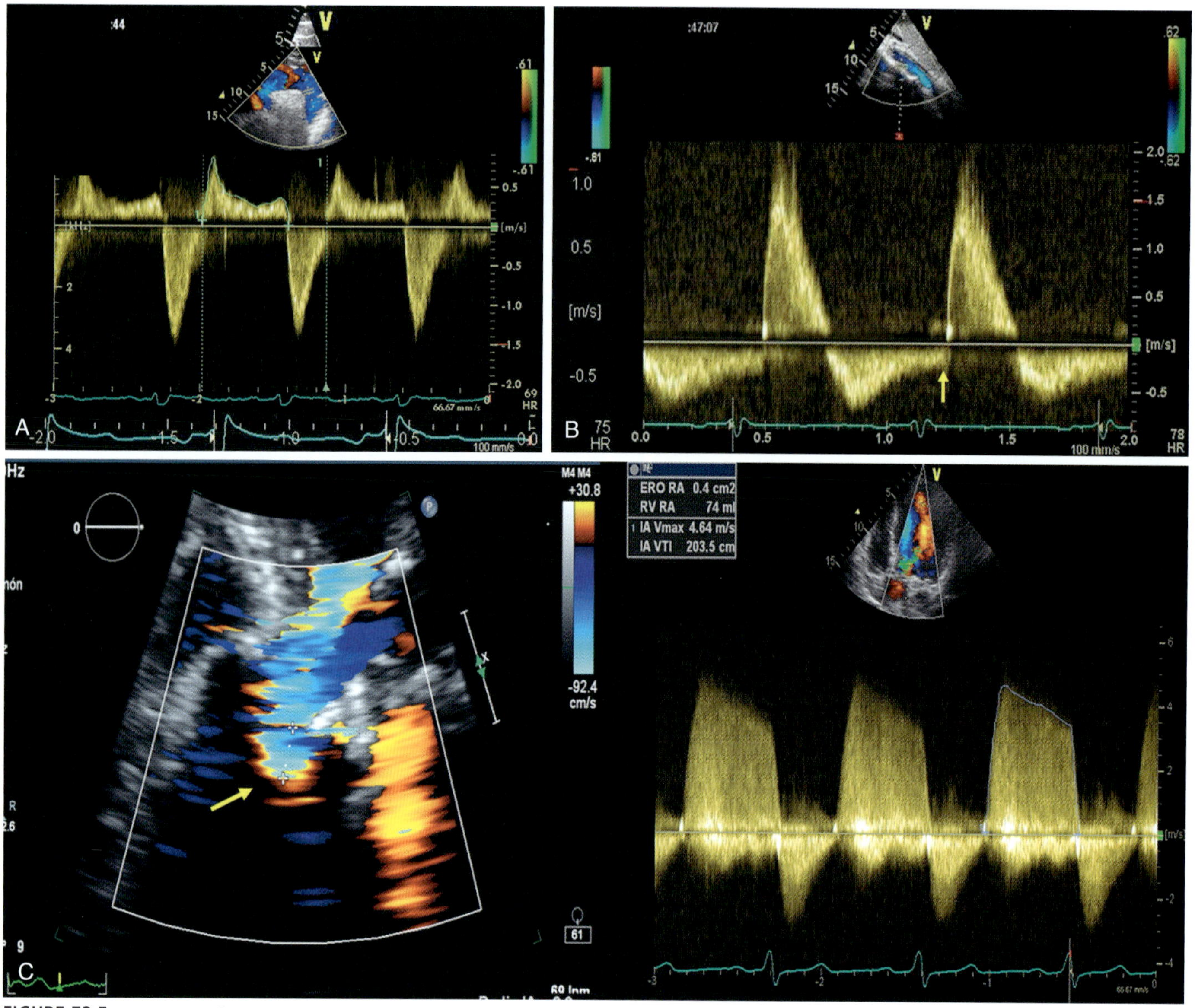

FIGURE 73.5 Assessment of severity of aortic regurgitation (AR). **A,** Diastolic flow reversal in the descending thoracic aorta by pulse-wave Doppler. The velocity-time integral is 22 cm, and end-diastolic velocity is greater than 20 cm/s. **B,** Holodiastolic flow reversal in the abdominal aorta (*arrow*) in a patient with severe AR. **C,** Quantitative assessment of AR severity using the proximal isovelocity surface area (PISA) method shows severe AR with effective regurgitant orifice area (EROA) of 0.40 cm^2 and regurgitant volume 74 mL/beat. (From Evangelista A, et al. Aortic regurgitation: clinical presentation, disease stages, and management. In Otto CM, Bonow RO, editors. Valvular Heart Disease. A Companion to Braunwald's Heart Disease. 5th ed. Philadelphia: Elsevier; 2021, pp. 179-196.)

addition to clinical examination, serial echocardiographic assessments of LV size and EF should be made. CMR usually is not necessary but may be useful in patients whose noninvasive test results are inconclusive or discordant with clinical findings or when further evaluation of aortic size is needed (see Fig. 73.6). Patients with mild to moderate AR and those with severe AR with a normal LVEF and only mild ventricular dilation may engage in aerobic forms of exercise. However, patients with AR who have limitations of cardiac reserve and/or evidence of declining LV function should not engage in competitive sports or strenuous activities.[20]

Moderately severe or even severe chronic AR often is associated with a generally favorable prognosis for many years. Quantitative measures of AR severity predict clinical outcome, and LV size and systolic function also are strong predictors of clinical outcome.[1,7,15,21-26] In a study of 251 asymptomatic patients (mean age, 61 years), the 10-year survival was 94% ± 4% in those with mild AR, compared with 69% ± 9% in those with severe AR (see Classic References, Detaint et al.) (Fig. 73.7). In contrast, in series involving younger asymptomatic patients (mean age, 39 years) with severe AR and a normal LVEF, the mortality rate was less than 1% per year,[7,8] and more than 45% of the patients remained asymptomatic with normal LV function at 10 years. The average rate of developing symptoms or LV systolic dysfunction in these latter series was less than 6% per year (see Classic References, Bonow et al.).

Gradual deterioration of LV function may occur even during the asymptomatic period, and some patients may incur significant impairment of systolic function before the onset of symptoms (see Table 73.2). Numerous surgical series over the past two decades have indicated that depressed LVEF is among the most important determinants of mortality after AVR, particularly as LV dysfunction may become irreversible and not improve after AVR.[7,8,22,23,25-27] LV dysfunction is more likely to be reversible if detected early, before EF becomes severely depressed, before the left ventricle becomes markedly dilated, and before significant symptoms develop. It is, therefore, important to intervene surgically before these changes have become irreversible.[1,7,8,23,27-29] Measures of LV systolic volume and systolic function are the most important predictors of clinical course in asymptomatic patients.[7,8,15] Biomarkers such as brain natriuretic peptide (BNP)[30] and assessment of myocardial strain[30-33] also may play a role in the future in identifying high-risk patients, based on small series published to date, but more work is necessary before these additional measures are recommended for routine management.

Symptomatic Patients

As is the case for AS (see Chapter 72) once the patient becomes symptomatic, the downhill course becomes rapidly progressive. Congestive heart failure, punctuated by episodes of acute pulmonary edema, and sudden

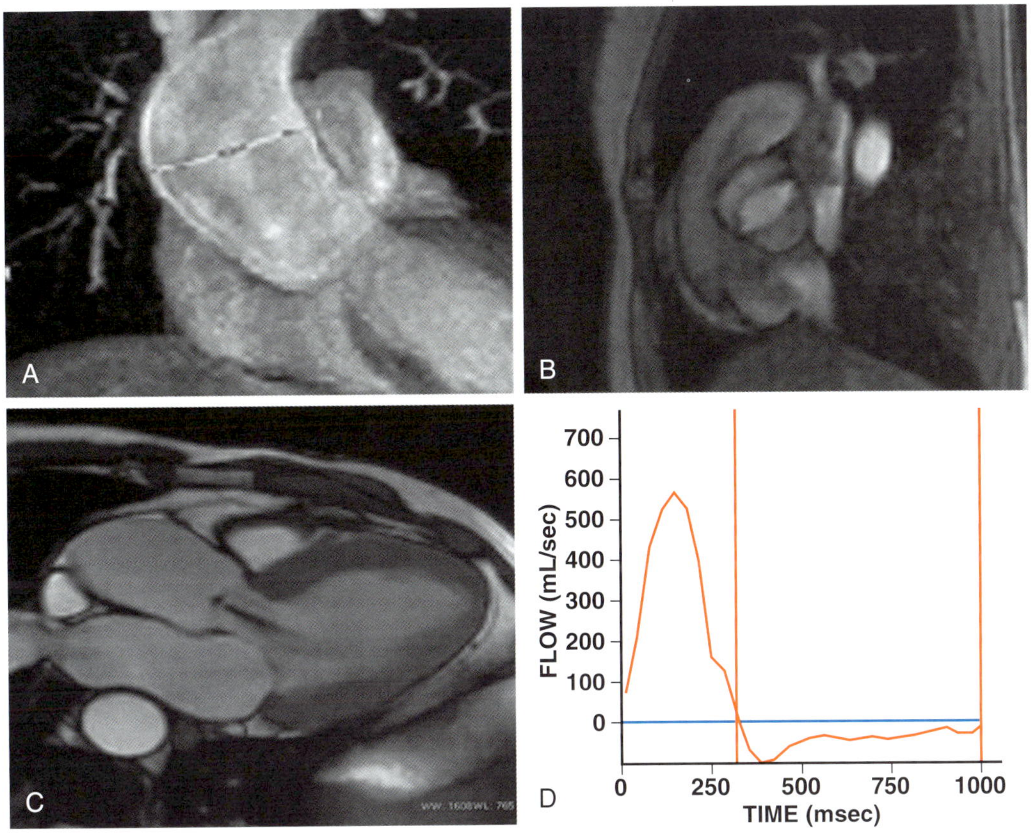

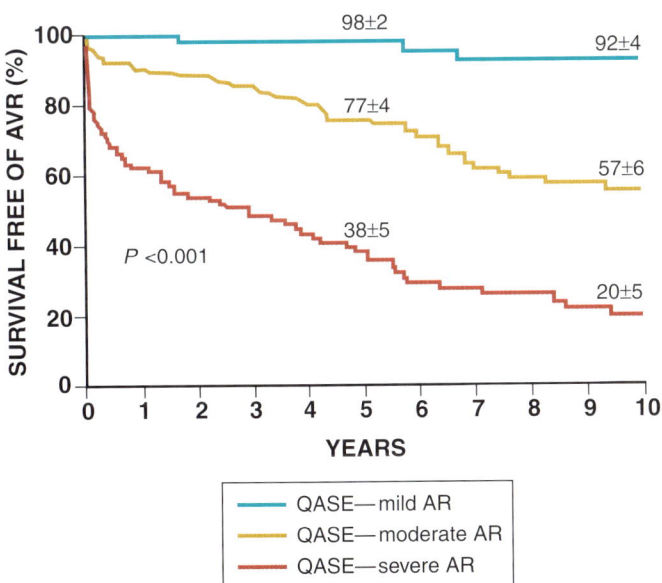

FIGURE 73.6 Cardiac magnetic resonance images showing a bicuspid aortic valve with aortic regurgitation and ascending aorta dilation. **A,** Fast single-shot steady-state free precession (SSFP) image in a coronal view. **B,** Retrospectively reconstructed magnitude image from a phase-contrast sequence showing a bicuspid aortic valve. **C,** Balanced SSFP image. Oblique axial left ventricle inflow-outflow view, showing grade 2 AR. **D,** Flow-versus-time plot for the ascending aorta. Antegrade flow was calculated at 140 mL/beat, retrograde flow at 40 mL/beat, and aortic regurgitant fraction of 33%. (From Tornos P, et al. Aortic regurgitation. In Otto CM, Bonow RO, editors. Valvular Heart Disease: A Companion to Braunwald's Heart Disease. 4th ed. Philadelphia: Saunders; 2013, pp. 163-178.)

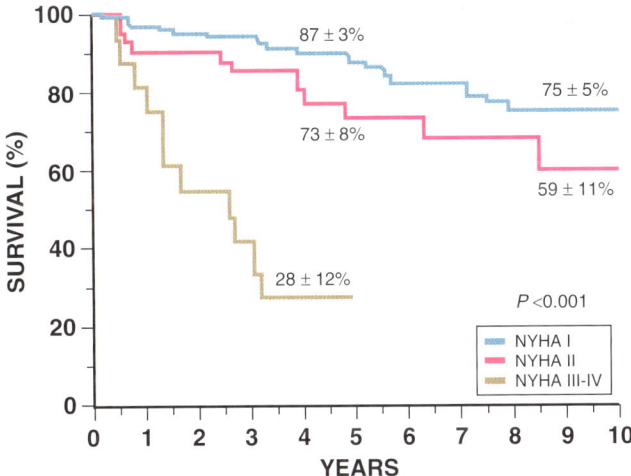

FIGURE 73.7 Composite endpoint of survival free of surgery for aortic regurgitation after diagnosis in asymptomatic patients. Patients are stratified according to quantitative criteria of the American Society of Echocardiography (QASE) for AR grading. The QASE–severe AR is defined as regurgitant volume (RV) greater than 60 mL/beat or effective regurgitant orifice (ERO) greater than 30 mm^2, the QASE–mild AR is defined as RV less than 30 mL/beat and ERO less than 10 mm^2, and the QASE–moderate AR is defined as greater than mild but not reaching QASE–severe criteria. The 5- and 10-year rates of the endpoint (± standard error) are indicated. Note the wide difference in outcomes according to QASE grading at baseline. *AVR,* Aortic valve replacement. (From Detaint D, et al. Quantitative echocardiographic determinants of clinical outcome in asymptomatic patients with aortic regurgitation: a prospective study. JACC Cardiovasc Imaging 2008;1:1-11.)

FIGURE 73.8 Survival without surgery in 242 patients with chronic aortic regurgitation, demonstrating the importance of symptoms in determining outcome. Patients with New York Heart Association (NYHA) class III or IV symptoms had a survival of only 28% at 4 years. In contrast, the 10-year survival in patients in NYHA class I was 75%, which was identical to that for an age-matched normal population. (From Dujardin KS, et al. Mortality and morbidity of aortic regurgitation in clinical practice: a long-term follow-up study. Circulation 1999;99:1851-1857.)

death may occur, usually in previously symptomatic patients who have considerable LV dilation. Data compiled in the presurgical era indicate that without surgical treatment, death usually occurred within 4 years after the development of angina pectoris and within 2 years after the onset of heart failure. Even in the current era, 4-year survival without surgery in patients with New York Heart Association (NYHA) class III or IV symptoms is only approximately 30% (see Classic References, Dujardin et al.) (Fig. 73.8).

TABLE 73.3 Indications for Aortic Valve Surgery in Patients with Aortic Regurgitation

COR	LOE	RECOMMENDATIONS
1	B-NR	1. In symptomatic patients with severe AR (stage D), aortic valve surgery is indicated regardless of LV systolic function
1	B-NR	2. In asymptomatic patients with chronic severe AR and LV systolic dysfunction (LVEF ≤55%) (stage C2), aortic valve surgery is indicated if no other cause for systolic dysfunction is identified
1	C-EO	3. In patients with severe AR (stage C or D) who are undergoing cardiac surgery for other indications, aortic valve surgery is indicated
2a	B-NR	4. In asymptomatic patients with severe AR and normal LV systolic function (LVEF >55%), aortic valve surgery is reasonable when the LV is severely enlarged (LVESD >50 mm or indexed LVESD >25 mm/m²) (stage C2)
2a	C-EO	5. In patients with moderate AR (stage B) who are undergoing cardiac or aortic surgery for other indications, aortic valve surgery is reasonable
2b	B-NR	6. In asymptomatic patients with severe AR and normal LV systolic function at rest (LVEF >55%; stage CI) and low surgical risk, aortic valve surgery may be considered when there is a progressive decline in LVEF on at least three serial studies to the low-normal range (LVEF 55% to 60%) or a progressive increase in LV dilation into the severe range (LVEDD >65 mm)
3: Harm	B-NR	7. In patients with isolated severe AR who have indications for SAVR and are candidates for surgery, TAVI should not be performed.

AR, Aortic regurgitation; *COR*, class of recommendation; *EO*, expert opinion; *LOE*, level of evidence; *LVEDD*, left ventricular end-diastolic dimension; *LVEF*, left ventricular ejection fraction; *LVESD*, left ventricular end-systolic dimension; *NR*, nonrandomized data; *SAVR*, surgical aortic valve replacement; *TAVI*, transcatheter aortic valve implantation.
From Otto CM, et al. 2020 AHA/ACC guideline for the management of patients with valvular heart disease: a report of the American College of Cardiology/American Heart Association Task Force on Practice Guidelines. J Am Coll Cardiol 2021;77:e25-197.

Treatment of Chronic Aortic Regurgitation
Medical Therapy

No specific therapy to prevent disease progression in chronic AR is currently available. Randomized clinical trials of dihydropyridine calcium channel antagonists and angiotensin-converting enzyme (ACE) inhibitors have not shown consistent clinical benefit in terms of blunting progression of LV dilation or delaying in need for AVR, and definitive recommendations regarding the indications for these drugs are not possible.[1,7]

Although there is no specific therapy to improve clinical outcomes in patients with chronic AR, it is recommended to treat hypertension (systolic blood pressure [SBP] >140 mm Hg), coronary artery disease (CAD), atrial arrhythmias, and any other cardiovascular comorbidities according to established guidelines.[7,23] For symptomatic patients, chronic medical therapy may be necessary for some patients who refuse surgery or are considered to have a prohibitive risk of surgery because of comorbid conditions. These patients should receive an aggressive evidence-based heart failure regimen (see Chapter 50) with ACE inhibitors (and perhaps other vasodilators), diuretics, and salt restriction; beta blockers may also be beneficial. Even though nitroglycerin and other nitrates are not as helpful in relieving anginal pain in patients with AR as they are in patients with CAD or AS, they are reasonable to try. In patients who are candidates for surgery but who have severely decompensated LV dysfunction, vasodilator therapy may be particularly helpful to stabilize patients prior to AVR.

Surgical Treatment

INDICATIONS FOR VALVE REPLACEMENT. Patients with chronic severe AR may be stable for years. However, long-standing volume overload will eventually result in irreversible LV dysfunction. In addition, the risk of isolated AVR has significantly decreased over the years, with an operative risk less than 3% when performed at experienced centers. Thus is it important to balance the immediate risks of AVR and continuing risks of an implanted prosthetic valve against the hazards of allowing a severe volume overload to irreversibly damage the left ventricle.

The current recommendations for AVR for patients with chronic severe AR in the 2020 American College of Cardiology (ACC)/American Heart Association (AHA) guidelines for the management of patients with valvular heart disease[7] are shown in Table 73.3, and the proposed management pathway is depicted in Fig. 73.9. Previous thresholds for depressed LVEF as an indication for surgery were set at 50%, but recent data indicate higher long-term postoperative risk in patients undergoing surgery with LVEF below 55% (in some series, 60%).[15,26,27] The 2020 revised guidelines have set the threshold for surgery at an LVEF of 55% or less.

SYMPTOMATIC PATIENTS. Because severe symptoms (NYHA class III or IV) are independent risk factors for poor postoperative survival, which has been confirmed in recent series,[22,25,26,27] surgery should be carried out in patients with even mild symptoms (NYHA class II) before severe LV dysfunction has developed.[1,7,8,23,34] Even after successful correction of AR, patients with severe LV dysfunction may have persistent cardiomegaly and depressed LV function. Such patients often exhibit persistent histologic changes in the left ventricle, including massive fiber hypertrophy and increased interstitial fibrous tissue. Therefore it is highly desirable to operate on patients before irreversible LV changes have occurred, and surgery is indicated for patients with severe chronic AR and any symptoms.

On the other hand, surgery should not be withheld in symptomatic patients with even moderate to severe LV systolic dysfunction, as outcomes are better with surgery than with medical therapy, and there is always the possibility of improvement in LV function following surgery with the addition of guideline-directed medical therapy.[35-37] Management with a multidisciplinary heart team and shared decision making with the patient and caregivers are essential in selecting high-risk patients for surgical intervention.[7,38]

ASYMPTOMATIC PATIENTS. In the absence of obvious contraindications or serious comorbidity, surgical treatment is advisable for asymptomatic patients with chronic severe AR with either an LVEF of 55% or less or a severe increase in LVESD (defined as end-systolic diameter [ESD] greater than 50 mm or indexed LVESD greater than 25 mm/m²),[7] as shown in Fig. 73.9. Because of their excellent prognosis in the short and medium term, operative correction should be deferred in patients with chronic severe AR without these indications for surgery. This includes those who are asymptomatic, exhibit good exercise tolerance, and have an LVEF greater than 55% without severe LV dilation as defined previously or progressive LV dilation on serial echocardiograms. Between these two ends of the clinical-hemodynamic spectrum are many patients in whom it may be difficult to balance the immediate risks of AVR and the continuing risks of an implanted prosthetic valve against the hazards of allowing a severe volume overload to damage the left ventricle. Once again, a multidisciplinary heart team should be consulted when difficult decisions must be made.[38]

Because AR has complex effects on preload and afterload, the selection of appropriate indices of ventricular contractility to identify patients for operation is challenging. Serial changes in LV end-diastolic and ESVs or dimensions can be used to detect the relative deterioration of LV function. Although LV end-diastolic and ESVs and ejection phase indices (e.g., LVEF) are strongly influenced by loading conditions, they are nonetheless useful empirical predictors of postoperative function. Global longitudinal strain has the advantage of being a less

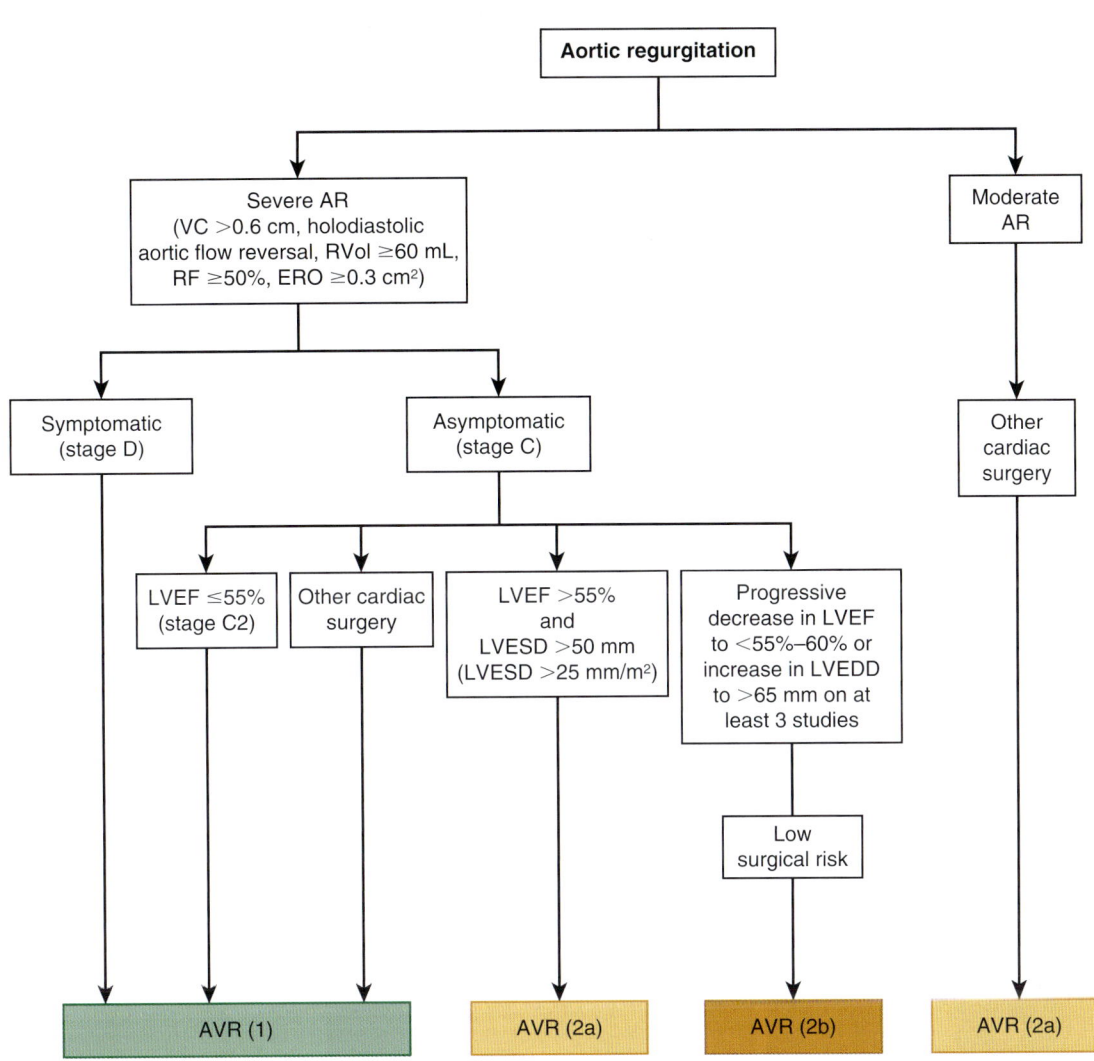

FIGURE 73.9 Management of patients with chronic aortic regurgitation. Colors correspond to Table 73.3. *AR*, Aortic regurgitation; *AVR*, aortic valve replacement; *EDD*, end-diastolic dimension; *EF*, ejection fraction; *ERO*, effective regurgitant orifice; *ESD*, end-systolic dimension; *LV*, left ventricular; *RF*, regurgitant fraction; *RVol*, regurgitant volume; *VC*, vena contracta. (From Otto CM, Nishimura, RA, Bonow RO, et al. 2020 AHA/ACC guideline for the management of patients with valvular heart disease: a report of the American College of Cardiology/American Heart Association Task Force on Practice Guidelines. J Am Coll Cardiol 2021;77:e25-197.)

load-dependent index of LV function,[30-33] but more data are needed before definitive recommendations can be made.

Serial echocardiographic measurements should be made with side-by-side comparison of previous serial studies. A consistent change in dimensions or volumes, greater than measurement variability, must be ensured before recommending AVR for asymptomatic patients on the basis of these numbers alone. This usually involves progressive changes over at least three sequential studies.

Although asymptomatic patients with chronic severe AR but normal LV function have an excellent prognosis over the short term, they need to be evaluated with frequent clinical evaluations and serial echocardiograms. LVESD is valuable in predicting outcome in asymptomatic patients. Patients with chronic severe AR and an ESD less than 40 mm almost invariably remain stable and can be followed without need for surgery in the near term (see Classic References, Bonow et al.). However, patients with an ESD of more than 50 mm have a 19% likelihood per year of developing symptoms of LV dysfunction, and those with an ESD more than 55 mm are at increased risk for development of irreversible LV dysfunction if they do not undergo AVR. Indexed LVESD or LVESV, which adjust for body size, may be more robust indicators for timing of surgical intervention than absolute dimensions and volumes.[7] Patients with an LVESD index of 2.5 cm/m^2 or LVESV index of 45 mL/m^2 or greater are at higher risk for adverse outcomes[15,16] (see also Classic References, Detaint et al.), and the LVESV index value of 45 mL/m^2 matches the ASE criteria for severe LV dilation.[13] Although the current guideline recommendations for surgical intervention are based on an LVESD index threshold of 25 mm/m^2 (see Table 73.3 and Fig. 73.9),[7] recent studies have consistently suggested that lower thresholds of LVESD index should be considered to optimize long-term survival after AVR (Fig. 73.10).[22,25,26] In addition, observational studies in asymptomatic patients with chronic severe AR and normal LV systolic function have reported greater long-term postoperative survival rates in those undergoing early AVR compared with those followed conservatively with AVR based on guidelines recommendations.[27,28] These data have fueled discussions regarding earlier intervention to enhance long-term prognosis of patients with chronic severe AR,[29,39] a topic that warrants future clinical trials.

The indications for AVR for patients with chronic severe AR secondary to aortic sinus or ascending aortic disease are similar to those for patients with primary valvular disease. In addition, in patients undergoing AVR for severe AR, concomitant surgery to repair the aortic sinuses or replace the ascending aorta is indicated if the amount of aortic dilation is greater than 45 mm.[7,23,40] As is the case for patients with other valvular lesions, adult surgical candidates who may have underlying CAD, based on symptoms, age, sex, and risk factors, should undergo preoperative coronary angiography. Those with significant proximal coronary artery stenoses should undergo revascularization at the time of AVR.

OPERATIVE PROCEDURES. The standard surgical approach for chronic AR is AVR. Concurrent aortic root replacement is performed when aortic dilation is the cause of or accompanies valve dysfunction. However, experience is accumulating with surgical aortic valve repair, which is a viable option for selected younger patients in experienced

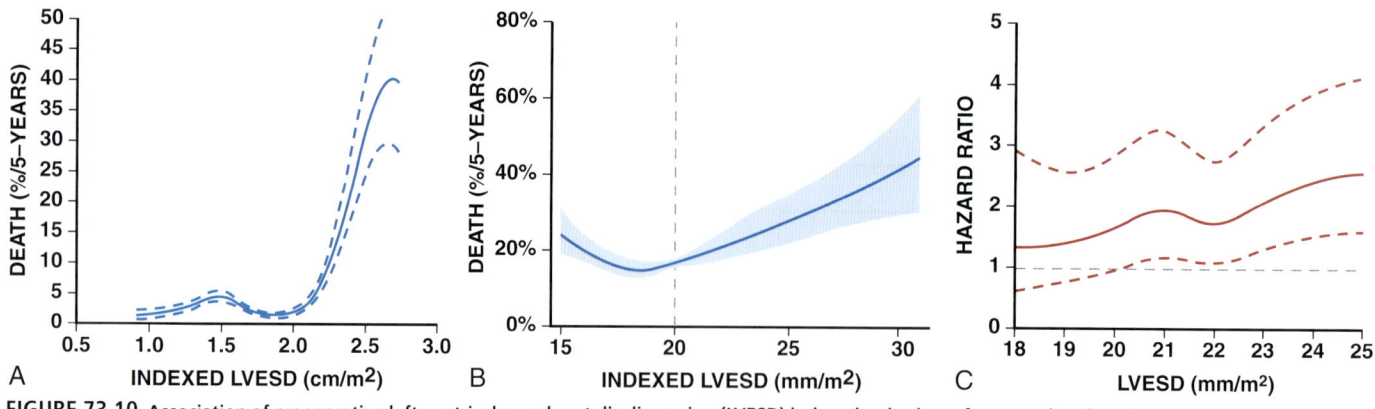

FIGURE 73.10 Association of preoperative left ventricular end-systolic dimension (LVESD) indexed to body surface area (BSA) and postoperative survival after aortic valve replacement. In all three series, postoperative risk rises as a continuous function above 20 mm/m² and thus lower than current recommendation for intervention of 25 mm/m². *Dashed lines* indicate confidence intervals. (**A** from Mentias A, et al. Long-term outcomes in patients with aortic regurgitation and preserved left ventricular ejection fraction. J Am Coll Cardiol 2016;68:2144-2153; **B** from Yang LT, et al. Outcomes in chronic hemodynamically significant aortic regurgitation and limitations of current guidelines. J Am Coll Cardiol 2019;73:1741-1752; and **C** from de Meester C, et al. Do guideline-based indications result in an outcome penalty for patients with severe aortic regurgitation? JACC Cardiovasc Imaging 2019;12:2126-2138.)

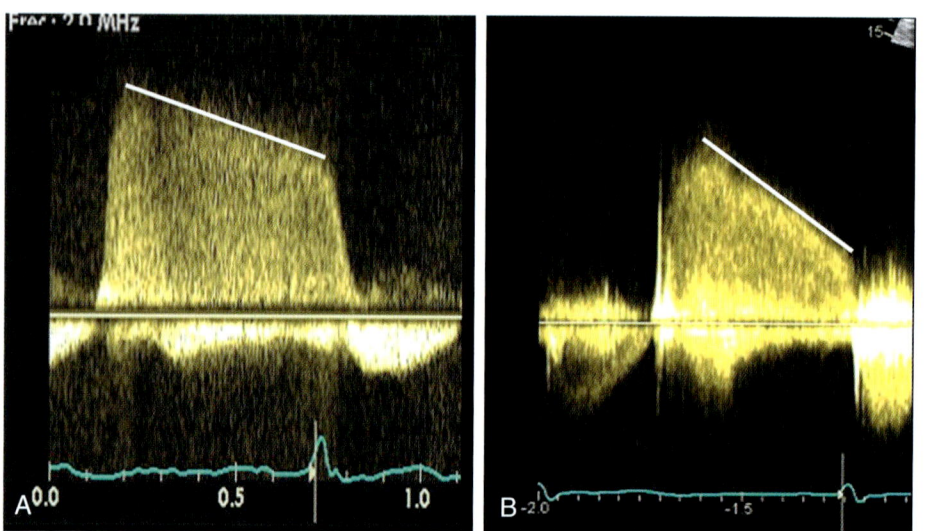

FIGURE 73.11 Diastolic Doppler signals. **A,** Chronic severe aortic regurgitation (AR). **B,** Acute severe AR. Notice the steeper deceleration slope in the acute phase, which is due to the equalization of LV and aortic diastolic pressures. (From Evangelista A, et al. Aortic regurgitation: clinical presentation, disease stages, and management. In Otto CM, Bonow RO, editors. Valvular Heart Disease. A Companion to Braunwald's Heart Disease. 5th ed. Philadelphia: Elsevier; 2021, pp. 179-196.)

centers, particularly those who are candidates for valve-sparing aortic root reconstruction.[41-44] However, unlike patients with chronic MR (see Chapter 76), the large majority of patients with pure AR will require AVR rather than repair. A Ross procedure is an option for selected young adults in centers of excellence skilled in this operation,[45-48] but the long-term results of the Ross procedure for AR are poorer than if performed for AS. TAVR for AR is under investigation but is not an established approach,[49,50] and it is not recommended in current guidelines (see Table 73.3).[7]

ACUTE AORTIC REGURGITATION

Pathophysiology and Clinical Presentation

Acute AR is caused most commonly by infective endocarditis, aortic dissection, or trauma (see Chapters 42 and 80). The characteristic features of acute AR are tachycardia and an increase in LV diastolic pressure. In contrast with the pathophysiologic events in chronic AR just described, in which the left ventricle can adapt over time to the increased hemodynamic load, in acute AR the regurgitant volume fills a ventricle of normal size that cannot accommodate the combined large regurgitant volume and inflow from the left atrium. Because the ability of total stroke volume to rise acutely is limited, forward stroke volume declines. The sudden increase in LV filling causes the LV diastolic pressure to rise rapidly above left atrial pressure during early diastole (see Fig. 73.2), causing the mitral valve to close prematurely in diastole. The tachycardia may compensate for the reduced forward stroke volume, and the LV and aortic systolic pressures may exhibit little change. However, acute severe AR may cause profound hypotension and cardiogenic shock. In light of the limited ability of the left ventricle to tolerate acute severe AR, patients with this valvular lesion often develop clinical manifestations of sudden cardiovascular collapse, including weakness, severe dyspnea, and profound hypotension secondary to the reduced stroke volume and elevated left atrial pressure. In some patients, the aortic diastolic pressure equilibrates with the elevated LV diastolic pressure.

Physical Examination. Patients with acute severe AR characteristically appear gravely ill, with tachycardia, severe peripheral vasoconstriction, cyanosis, and sometimes pulmonary congestion and edema. Depending on the etiology of the acute AR, signs suggestive of endocarditis or aortic dissection may be present. The peripheral signs of AR are often not impressive and certainly not as dramatic as in patients with chronic AR. The normal or only slightly widened pulse pressure may lead to significant underestimation of the severity of the valvular lesion. The LV impulse is normal or almost normal, and the rocking motion of the chest characteristic of chronic AR is not apparent. S_1 may be soft or absent because of premature closure of the mitral valve, and the sound of mitral valve closure in mid- or late diastole occasionally is audible. Closure of the mitral valve may be incomplete, however, and diastolic MR may occur.

The early diastolic murmur of acute AR is lower pitched and of shorter duration compared with that of chronic AR, because as LV diastolic pressure rises, the (reverse) pressure gradient between the aorta and left ventricle is rapidly reduced. A systolic murmur is common, resulting in to-and-fro sounds. The Austin Flint murmur often is present but is of brief duration and ceases when LV pressure exceeds left atrial pressure in diastole. With premature diastolic closure of the mitral valve, the presystolic portion of the Austin Flint murmur is eliminated.

Echocardiography. In acute AR, the echocardiogram reveals a dense, diastolic Doppler signal (Fig. 73.11) with a short diastolic half time and an end-diastolic velocity approaching zero. There may also be premature closure of the mitral valve with diastolic MR on the Doppler traces due to the LV diastolic pressure exceeding the left atrial pressure at late diastole. LV size and EF are usually normal, although contractility may be enhanced and EF increased due to the compensatory adrenergic surge. These findings contrast with those in chronic AR, in which end-diastolic dimensions and wall motion are increased. TEE is often useful to clarify the underlying reason for the acute regurgitation, particularly to identify an ascending aortic dissection or endocarditis.

Electrocardiography. In acute AR, the electrocardiogram (ECG) will usually show sinus tachycardia. If endocarditis is a possible etiology, progressive severity of heart block on serial ECGs may indicate the presence and expansion of an accompanying aortic root abscess.

Radiography. In acute AR, radiographic examination often reveals evidence of marked pulmonary edema. The cardiac silhouette usually is remarkably normal, although left atrial enlargement may be present, and depending on the cause of the AR, enlargement of the ascending aorta may be seen.

Management of Acute Aortic Regurgitation

Because early death caused by LV failure is frequent in patients with acute severe AR, prompt surgical intervention is indicated. Even a normal ventricle cannot sustain the burden of acute, severe volume overload. Therefore the risk of acute AR is much greater than that of chronic AR. While the patient is being prepared for surgery, treatment with an intravenous positive inotropic agent (dopamine or dobutamine) and/or a vasodilator (nitroprusside) often is necessary. The agent and dosage should be selected on the basis of arterial pressure (see Chapter 49). Beta blockers and intra-aortic balloon counterpulsation are contraindicated, because either lowering the heart rate or augmenting peripheral resistance during diastole can lead to rapid hemodynamic decompensation. In hemodynamically stable patients with acute AR secondary to active infective endocarditis, operation may be deferred to allow 5 to 7 days of intensive antibiotic therapy (see Chapter 80). However, AVR should be undertaken at the earliest sign of hemodynamic instability or if there is any evidence of abscess formation. If an acute aortic dissection is the cause for the AR, the aorta will also need to be fixed during surgery.

CLASSIC REFERENCES

Bonow R, Lakatos E, Maron B, Epstein S. Serial long-term assessment of the natural history of asymptomatic patients with chronic aortic regurgitation and normal left ventricular systolic function. *Circulation*. 1991;84:1625–1635.

Detaint D, Messika-Zeitoun D, Maalouf J, et al. Quantitative echocardiographic determinants of clinical outcome in asymptomatic patients with aortic regurgitation: a prospective study. *JACC Cardiovasc Imaging*. 2008;1:1–11.

Dujardin KS, Enriquez-Sarano M, Schaff HV, et al. Mortality and morbidity of aortic regurgitation in clinical practice: a long-term follow-up study. *Circulation*. 1999;99:1851–1857.

Grossman W, Jones D, McLaurin LP. Wall stress and patterns of hypertrophy in the human left ventricle. *J Clin Invest*. 1975;56:56–64.

REFERENCES

Causes and Pathology

1. Evangelista A, Tornos P, Bonow RO. Aortic regurgitation: clinical presentation, disease stages, and management. In: Otto CM, Bonow RO, eds. *Valvular Heart Disease. A Companion to Braunwald's Heart Disease*. 5th ed. Philadelphia: Elsevier; 2021:179–196.
2. Slostad BD, Witt CM, O'Leary PW, et al. Unicuspid aortic valve: demographics, comorbidities, echocardiographic features, and long-term outcomes. *Circulation*. 2019;140:1853–1855.
3. Tsang MYC, Abudiab MM, Ammash NM, et al. Quadricuspid aortic valve: characteristics, associated structural cardiovascular abnormalities, and clinical outcomes. *Circulation*. 2016;133:312–319.
4. Braverman AC, Cheng A. The bicuspid aortic valve and associated aortic disease. In: Otto CM, Bonow RO, eds. *Valvular Heart Disease: A Companion to Braunwald's Heart Disease*. 5th ed. Philadelphia Saunders; 2013:197–222.
5. Verma S, Siu SC. Aortic dilatation in patients with bicuspid aortic valve. *N Engl J Med*. 2014;370:1920–1929.

Chronic AR – Pathophysiology and Clinical Presentation

6. Zilberszac R, Gabriel H, Schemper M, et al. Outcome of combined stenotic and regurgitant aortic valve disease. *J Am Coll Cardiol*. 2013;61:1489–1495.
7. Otto CM, Nishimura RA, Bonow RO, et al. 2020 ACC/AHA guideline for the management of patients with valvular heart disease: a report of the American College of Cardiology/American Heart Association joint committee on clinical practice guidelines. *J Am Coll Cardiol*. 2021;77:e25–e197.
8. Bonow RO. Chronic mitral regurgitation and aortic regurgitation: have indications for surgery changed? *J Am Coll Cardiol*. 2013;61:693–701.
9. Yang LT, Pellikka PA, Enriquez-Sarano M, et al. Diastolic blood pressure and heart rate are independently associated with mortality in chronic aortic regurgitation. *J Am Coll Cardiol*. 2020;75:29–39.
10. Chambers J. Aortic regurgitation: the value of clinical signs. *J Am Coll Cardiol*. 2020;75:40–41.

Chronic AR – Diagnostic Testing

11. Hahn RT, Cavalcante JL. Imaging the aortic valve. In: Otto CM, Bonow RO, eds. *Valvular Heart Disease: A Companion to Braunwald's Heart Disease*. 5th ed. Philadelphia Saunders; 2013:124–155.
12. Zoghbi WA, Adams D, Bonow RO, et al. Recommendations for non-invasive evaluation of native valvular regurgitation. A report from the American Society of Echocardiography developed in collaboration with the Society for Cardiovascular Magnetic Resonance. *J Am Soc Echocardiogr*. 2017;30:303–371.
13. Lang RM, Badano LP, Mor-Avi V, et al. Recommendations for cardiac chamber quantification by echocardiography in adults: an update from the American Society of Echocardiography and the European Association of Cardiovascular Imaging. *J Am Soc Echocardiogr*. 2015;28:1–39.
14. Ewe SH, Delgado V, van der Geest R, et al. Accuracy of three-dimensional versus two-dimensional echocardiography for quantification of aortic regurgitation and validation by three-dimensional three-directional velocity-encoded magnetic resonance imaging. *Am J Cardiol*. 2013;112:560–566.
15. Yang LT, Anand V, Zambito E, et al. Association of echocardiographic left ventricular end-systolic volume and volume-derived ejection fraction with outcome in asymptomatic chronic aortic regurgitation. *JAMA Cardiol*. 2021;6:189–198.
16. Bonow RO, O'Gara PT. Left ventricular end-systolic volume in chronic aortic regurgitation – finally, a step forward. *JAMA Cardiol*. 2021;6:189–199.
17. Cavalcante JL, Lalude OO, Schoenhagen P, Lerakis S. Cardiovascular magnetic resonance imaging for structural and valvular heart disease interventions. *JACC Cardiovasc Interv*. 2016;9:399–425.
18. Harris AW, Krieger EV, Kim M, et al. Cardiac magnetic resonance imaging versus transthoracic echocardiography for prediction of outcomes in chronic aortic or mitral regurgitation. *Am J Cardiol*. 2017;119:1074–1081.
19. Kammerlander AA, Wiesinger M, Duca F, et al. Diagnostic and prognostic utility of cardiac magnetic resonance imaging in aortic regurgitation. *JACC Cardiovasc Imaging*. 2019;12:1474–1483.

Chronic AR – Disease Course and Treatment

20. Bonow RO, Nishimura R, Thompson PD, Udelson JE. Eligibility and disqualification recommendations for competitive athletes with cardiovascular abnormalities. Task Force 5: valvular heart disease. A scientific statement from the American Heart Association and American College of Cardiology. *J Am Coll Cardiol*. 2015;66:2385–2392.
21. Kusunose K, Cremer PC, Tsutsui RS, et al. Regurgitant volume informs rate of progressive cardiac dysfunction in asymptomatic patients with chronic aortic or mitral regurgitation. *JACC Cardiovasc Imaging*. 2015;8:14–23.
22. Mentias A, Feng K, Alashi A, et al. Long-term outcomes in patients with aortic regurgitation and preserved left ventricular ejection fraction. *J Am Coll Cardiol*. 2016;68:2144–2153.
23. Baumgartner H, Falk V, Bax JJ, et al. 2017 ESC/ EACTS guidelines for the management of valvular heart disease. *Eur Heart J*. 2017;38:2739–2791.
24. Yang LT, Enriquez-Sarano M, Michelena HI, et al. Predictors of progression in patients with stage B aortic regurgitation. *J Am Coll Cardiol*. 2019;74:2480–2492.
25. Yang LT, Michelena HI, Scott CG, et al. Outcomes in chronic hemodynamically significant aortic regurgitation and limitations of current guidelines. *J Am Coll Cardiol*. 2019;73:1741–1752.
26. de Meester C, Gerber BL, Vancraeynest D, et al. Do guideline-based indications result in an outcome penalty for patients with severe aortic regurgitation? *J Am Coll Cardiol Imaging*. 2019;12:2126–2138.
27. Murashita T, Schaff HV, Suri RM, et al. Impact of left ventricular systolic function on outcome of correction of chronic severe aortic valve regurgitation: implications for timing of surgical intervention. *Ann Thorac Surg*. 2017;103:1222–1228.
28. Wang Y, Jiang W, Liu J, et al. Early surgery versus conventional treatment for asymptomatic severe aortic regurgitation with normal ejection fraction and left ventricular dilatation. *Eur J Cardio Thorac Surg*. 2017;52:118–124.
29. Desai MY, Svensson L. Chronic severe aortic regurgitation: should we lower operating thresholds? *Circulation*. 2019;140:1045–1047.
30. Lee JKT, Franzone A, Lanz J, et al. Early detection of subclinical myocardial damage in chronic aortic regurgitation and strategies for timely treatment of asymptomatic patients. *Circulation*. 2018;137:184–196.
31. Kusunose K, Agarwal S, Marwick TH, et al. Decision making in asymptomatic aortic regurgitation in the era of guidelines incremental values of resting and exercise cardiac dysfunction. *Circ Cardiovasc Imaging*. 2014;7:352–362.
32. Ewe SH, Haeck MLA, Ng ACT, et al. Detection of subtle left ventricular systolic dysfunction in patients with significant aortic regurgitation and preserved left ventricular ejection fraction: speckle tracking echocardiographic analysis. *Eur Heart J Cardiovasc Imaging*. 2015;16:992–999.
33. Alashi AA, Khullar T, Mentias A, et al. Long-term outcomes after aortic valve surgery in patients with asymptomatic chronic aortic regurgitation and preserved LVEF: impact of baseline and follow-up global longitudinal strain. *JACC Cardiovasc Imaging*. 2020;13:12–21.
34. Bonow RO, Leon MB, Doshi D, Moat N. Management strategies and future challenges for aortic valve disease. *Lancet*. 2016;387:1312–1323.
35. Kaneko T, Ejiofor JI, Neely RC, et al. Aortic regurgitation with markedly reduced left ventricular function is not a contraindication for aortic valve replacement. *Ann Thorac Surg*. 2016;102:41–47.
36. Fiedler AG, Bhambhani V, Laikhter E, et al. Aortic valve replacement associated with survival in severe regurgitation and low ejection fraction. *Heart*. 2018;104:835–840.
37. McConkey HZR, Rajani R, Prendergast BD. Improving outcomes in chronic aortic regurgitation: timely diagnosis, access to specialist assessment and earlier surgery. *Heart*. 2018;104:794–795.
38. Nishimura RA, O'Gara PT, Bavaria JE, et al. 2019 AATS/ACC/ASE/SCAI/STS expert consensus systems of care document: a proposal to optimize care for patients with valvular heart disease: a joint report of the American Association for Thoracic Surgery, American College of Cardiology, American Society of Echocardiography, Society for Cardiovascular Angiography and Interventions, and Society of Thoracic Surgeons. *J Am Coll Cardiol*. 2019;73:2609–2635.
39. O'Gara PT, Sun YP. Timing of valve interventions in patients with chronic aortic regurgitation: are we waiting too long? *J Am Coll Cardiol*. 2019;73:1753–1755.
40. Hiratzka LF, Creager MA, Isselbacher EM, et al. Surgery for aortic dilatation in patients with bicuspid aortic valves: a statement of clarification from the American College of Cardiology/American Heart Association Task Force on clinical practice guidelines. *J Am Coll Cardiol*. 2016;67:724–731.

Chronic AR – Aortic Valve Repair, Ross Procedure, TAVR

41. El Khoury G, de Kerchove L. Principles of aortic valve repair. *J Thorac Cardiovasc Surg*. 2013;145:S26–S29.
42. Ugur M, Schaff HV, Suri R, et al. Late outcome of noncoronary sinus replacement in patients with bicuspid aortic valves and aortopathy. *Ann Thorac Surg*. 2014;97:1242–1246.
43. Ouzounian M, Rao V, Manlhiot C, et al. Valve-sparing root replacement compared with composite valve graft procedures in patients with aortic root dilation. *J Am Coll Cardiol*. 2016;68:1838–1847.
44. Schneider U, Hofmann C, Schöpe J, et al. Long-term results of differentiated anatomic reconstruction of bicuspid aortic valves. *JAMA Cardiol*. 2020;5:1366–1373.
45. Mazine A, El-Hamamsy I, Verma S, et al. Primer on the Ross procedure in adults for cardiologists and cardiac surgeons. *J Am Coll Cardiol*. 2018;72: 2761–2177.
46. Martin E, Mohammadi S, Jacques F, et al. Clinical outcomes following the Ross procedure in adults: a 25-year longitudinal study. *J Am Coll Cardiol*. 2017;70:1890–1899.
47. Romeo JLR Papageorgiou G, da Costa FFD, et al. Long-term clinical and echocardiographic outcomes in young and middle-aged adults undergoing the Ross procedure. *JAMA Cardiol*. 2021;6(5):539–548. https://doi.org/10.1001/jamacardio.2020.7434.
48. Aboud A, Charitos EI, Fujita B, et al. Long-term outcomes of patients undergoing the Ross procedure. *J Am Coll Cardiol*. 2021;77:1412–1422.
49. Sawaya FJ, Deutsch MA, Seiffert M, et al. Safety and efficacy of transcatheter aortic valve replacement in the treatment of pure aortic regurgitation in native valves and failing surgical bioprostheses: results from an International registry study. *JACC Cardiovasc Interv*. 2017;10:1048–1056.
50. Jiang J, Liu X, He Y, et al. Transcatheter aortic valve replacement for pure native aortic valve regurgitation: a systematic review. *Cardiology*. 2018;141:132–140.

74 Transcatheter Aortic Valve Replacement

MARTIN B. LEON AND MICHAEL J. MACK

EPIDEMIOLOGY, NATURAL HISTORY, AND TREATMENT ALTERNATIVES FOR VALVULAR AORTIC STENOSIS, 1430

HISTORY AND BACKGROUND OF TRANSCATHETER AORTIC VALVE REPLACEMENT (TAVR), 1430

THE EARLY YEARS OF TAVR, 1430

TAVR EVIDENCE-BASED CLINICAL RESEARCH, 1431

TAVR TECHNOLOGY EVOLUTION, 1433

TAVR PROCEDURAL MATURATION, 1435

TAVR-ASSOCIATED COMPLICATIONS, 1436

TAVR IN SURGICAL BIOPROSTHETIC AORTIC VALVE FAILURE, 1437

GAPS IN TAVR KNOWLEDGE AND ONGOING CONTROVERSIES, 1437

REFERENCES, 1439

EPIDEMIOLOGY, NATURAL HISTORY, AND TREATMENT ALTERNATIVES FOR VALVULAR AORTIC STENOSIS

Eepidemiology, natural history, and treatment alternatives for valvular aortic stenosis (AS) see Chapter 72.

HISTORY AND BACKGROUND OF TRANSCATHETER AORTIC VALVE REPLACEMENT (TAVR)

The combination of an aging population and accrued comorbidities rendered an enlarging segment of severe AS patients as poor candidates (real or perceived) for open surgical aortic valve replacement (AVR). Thus, a search for meaningful less-invasive catheter-based treatment options became a compelling clinical need.

Predicate Technologies Including Balloon Aortic Valvuloplasty

The first transcatheter approach embraced by interventional valve therapists for AS was balloon aortic valvuloplasty, introduced in 1986.[11] Early results from a U.S. registry of 492 patients demonstrated acute hemodynamic improvement, but mortality was 7.5% within 7 days and 34% within 1 year, and periprocedural complications were frequent.[12,13] The failure of balloon aortic valvuloplasty as a definitive therapy for AS was well documented in 165 patients with median follow-up of 3.9 years; freedom from either death, surgical AVR, or repeat balloon valvuloplasty at 1, 2, and 3 years was 40%, 19%, and 6%, respectively.[14] More recently, in the first PARTNER trial,[1] among the cohort of 102 patients randomized to standard therapy and receiving balloon aortic valvuloplasty within 30 days, despite acute hemodynamic improvement and few periprocedural complications, by 6 months and 1 year, mortality was 25.5% and 47.3% respectively.[15] Based upon these findings, balloon aortic valvuloplasty should not be considered as an alternative to surgical AVR for calcific AS and can only be recommended as a bridge to definitive AVR (surgical or transcatheter) in unstable patients or as short-term symptom palliation for patients who are not candidates for AVR.

The initial concept of an implantable bioprosthetic aortic valve mounted to a stent and delivered on a catheter was characterized in a closed-chested acute porcine model in 1992.[16] Excised porcine aortic valves, sewn to a homemade wire frame and crimped onto balloon catheters were delivered retrograde across the aortic valve and deployed at a transannular location after balloon inflation.[16] Several years later, a dedicated commercial program developed refined versions of this concept for durability testing, animal implants, human cadaver feasibility studies, and first-in-human cases. The early prototypes used three bovine pericardial leaflets, which were sewn to a tubular-slotted, balloon-expandable stainless-steel stent and crimped onto commercial noncompliant balloon valvuloplasty catheters. After accelerated pulse duplicator testing and 2 years of animal studies, the prototype devices were ready for compassionate-use human cases.

THE EARLY YEARS OF TAVR

Outcomes in Patients Not Suitable for Surgery Using Early TAVR Technologies

The acronyms TAVI (transcatheter aortic valve implantation) and TAVR (transcatheter aortic valve replacement) have been used interchangeably; TAVI used more frequently in Europe and TAVR used more frequently in the United States and Asia. After the first-human use experiences, TAVR with first-generation balloon-expandable valves was applied sparingly in compassionate-use patients who were rejected for surgery.

These early TAVR clinical experiences were negatively impacted by first-generation technology, evolving procedural methods with inexperienced operators, and patient selection favoring the poorest candidates for surgery, which amplified the frequency and severity of post-treatment complications and adverse clinical events.

Patient Surgical Risk Profiles and Comorbidity Assessments

Initially, the expectations for TAVR were to provide an acceptable alter-native for severe symptomatic AS patients who were not suitable for surgery. Implicit in the early case selection for TAVR was a stratification process for surgical risk. Multiple predictive risk scores have been developed and validated to help stratify a patient's risk for mortality or morbidity after aortic valve surgery, either alone or combined with coronary revascularization. The most frequently used model in the United States is the STS predictive risk of operative mortality (PROM).[22] Common comorbidities contributing to increased surgical risk include chronic kidney disease, chronic lung disease (especially oxygen dependent), prior stroke, and vascular disease (coronary and peripheral). Risk stratification of AS patients, according to the most recent STS database, indicated a predicted mortality of 1.4% in low-risk (STS-PROM <4%, 80% of all patients), 5.1% in intermediate-risk (STS-PROM 4% to 8%), and 11.8% in high-risk (STS-PROM >8%) patients.[10]

Introduction to the Heart Team

The use of multidisciplinary health care provider teams to manage complex medical problems has become a common theme in organ transplantation and oncology tumor boards. Likewise, the optimal management of severe AS in elderly patients with comorbid conditions has required a multidisciplinary "heart team" comprising the collective expertise of valve cardiologists, cardiac surgeons, interventional cardiologists trained in structural heart disease, imaging experts, gerontologists, other medical subspecialists, and advanced nursing practitioners. The roles of the heart team extend from the initial patient contact to valve clinic assessments, diagnostic decision making, inpatient procedural management, and subsequent follow-up care. The importance of the heart team was emphasized in the 2014 American College of Cardiology (ACC)/American Heart Association (AHA) guidelines for the management of valvular heart disease,[26] wherein the heart team was designated a class I recommendation for centers involved in TAVR care.

TAVR EVIDENCE-BASED CLINICAL RESEARCH

Randomized Clinical Trials According to Surgical Risk Strata

Having created an ecosystem for aortic valve research, a series of landmark randomized clinical trials with both balloon-expandable and selfexpanding TAVR systems were performed largely in the United States, which served to establish the evidence base for appropriate clinical indications. Based upon surgical risk stratification into de-escalating categories of prohibitive (or extreme), high, intermediate, and low risk for surgical valve replacement, available TAVR systems were randomized against standard therapies.

Primary Clinical Endpoints

The first randomized TAVR trial in AS was the PARTNER trial in elderly patients who were considered unsuitable candidates for surgery due to coexisting conditions with a 50% or more predicted probability of either death by 30 days after surgery or a serious irreversible complication[1]. In 358 patients with severe symptomatic AS, the rate of death from any cause at 1 year (the primary endpoint) was 30.7% with balloon-expandable TAVR compared with 50.7% with nonsurgical standard therapies, consisting of medical treatment and balloon aortic valvuloplasty (hazard ratio 0.55 with TAVR; 95% confidence interval [CI], 0.40 to 0.74; $P < 0.001$) (Fig. 74.1A). After 5 years' follow-up,[30] the absolute 20% difference in all-cause mortality favoring TAVR was maintained, resulting in an increase in median survival from 11.7 months with standard therapy to 31.0 months after TAVR ($P < 0.0001$). Similar outcomes were observed in extreme-risk AS patients after TAVR using a self-expanding bioprosthesis.[31]

Concurrent with the extreme-risk trials and balloon-expandable and self-expanding TAVR was randomized versus surgery in high-risk AS patients[32,33]. The primary endpoint, death from any cause at 1 year, was noninferior for the comparison of TAVR versus surgery (Fig. 74.1B and C), and the results were maintained after 5 years' follow-up.[34,35] Next, larger trials in intermediate-risk patients were performed with an expanded primary endpoint including all-cause death or disabling stroke after 2 years.[36,37] In the balloon-expandable TAVR intermediate-risk trial, 2032 patients were randomized to either TAVR or surgery and the rate of death or stroke at 2 years was similar in the TAVR (19.3%) and surgery (21.1%) groups ($P = 0.001$ for noninferiority)[36]. After 5 years' follow-up,[38] the overall primary endpoint results were still similar between the groups. However, in those TAVR patients requiring transapical access (23.7% of the study cohort) due to unfavorable anatomic factors precluding the transfemoral approach, surgical AVR was superior to TAVR. In the self-expanding TAVR intermediate-risk trial, 1746 were randomized and the estimated rate of death or stroke at 2 years (Bayesian analysis) was 12.6% in the TAVR group and 14.0% in the surgery group (posterior probability of noninferiority >0.999)[37]. Importantly, the high- and intermediate-risk AS patients treated in these trials were elderly ($\geq$ 80 years), with multiple comorbidities (STS scores ranged from 4% to 12%) and frequent frailty.

Given the favorable TAVR results in previous higher surgical risk trials, using current generation balloon-expandable and self-expanding TAVR systems and evolved procedural methods, trials were recently undertaken in younger, low-risk patients, which represents a high proportion of the patients currently being treated with severe AVR. Enrollment was confined to patients with tricuspid valve disease with transfemoral access and favorable anatomy for TAVR and surgery. The balloon-expandable low-risk PARTNER trial randomized 1000 patients with a mean age 73 years and mean STS score 1.9% to either transfemoral TAVR or surgery[39]. The primary composite endpoint of death, stroke, or cardiovascular rehospitalization within 1 year was significantly lower in the TAVR group than in the surgery group (8.5% versus 15.1%; $P = 0.001$ for superiority)[39] (Fig. 74.2A). The self-expanding TAVR low-risk trial randomized 1468 patients with a mean age 74 years and mean STS score 1.9%[40]. The primary endpoint of all-cause death or disabling stroke at 2 years was an estimated rate of 5.3% in the TAVR group and 6.7% in the surgery group (Bayesian methods, posterior probability of noninferiority > 0.999)[40] (Fig.74.2B).

Based on these early-term results in selected patients who are similar to those randomized in the clinical trials, TAVR should be considered as an alternative therapy to surgery for severe symptomatic AS (see guideline recommendations).

Key Secondary Outcomes

In addition to the clinical outcomes comprising the primary endpoint of randomized TAVR trials, other important secondary endpoints that impact patient morbidity, hospital stay, or late mortality must be considered when comparing the safety and efficacy of new versus standard therapies.[1,32,33,36,37,39,40]

Echocardiographic Findings

Using echocardiography-derived measurements, reduction in aortic valve gradients and improvement in aortic valve areas have been similar with both transcatheter and surgical bioprosthetic valves, as determined by core laboratory assessments from the randomized trials.[32,33,36,37,39,40] In fact, many studies suggest greater hemodynamic improvements with transcatheter compared to surgical valves[40]. Moreover, sustained improvement in antegrade hemodynamics for both transcatheter and surgical valves has been observed in studies with 5-year echocardiography follow-up[34,35,38] Other echo findings after relief of AS with both surgical and transcatheter replacement valves have been progressive regression of LV hypertrophy over time, reduction in functional mitral regurgitation, and improvement in LV ejection fraction, especially in patients with reduced baseline LV systolic function.

Paravalvular aortic regurgitation (PVR) after TAVR was commonly seen during the early registries and was increased compared with surgically implanted bioprostheses in the randomized trials[32,33,36,37,39,40]

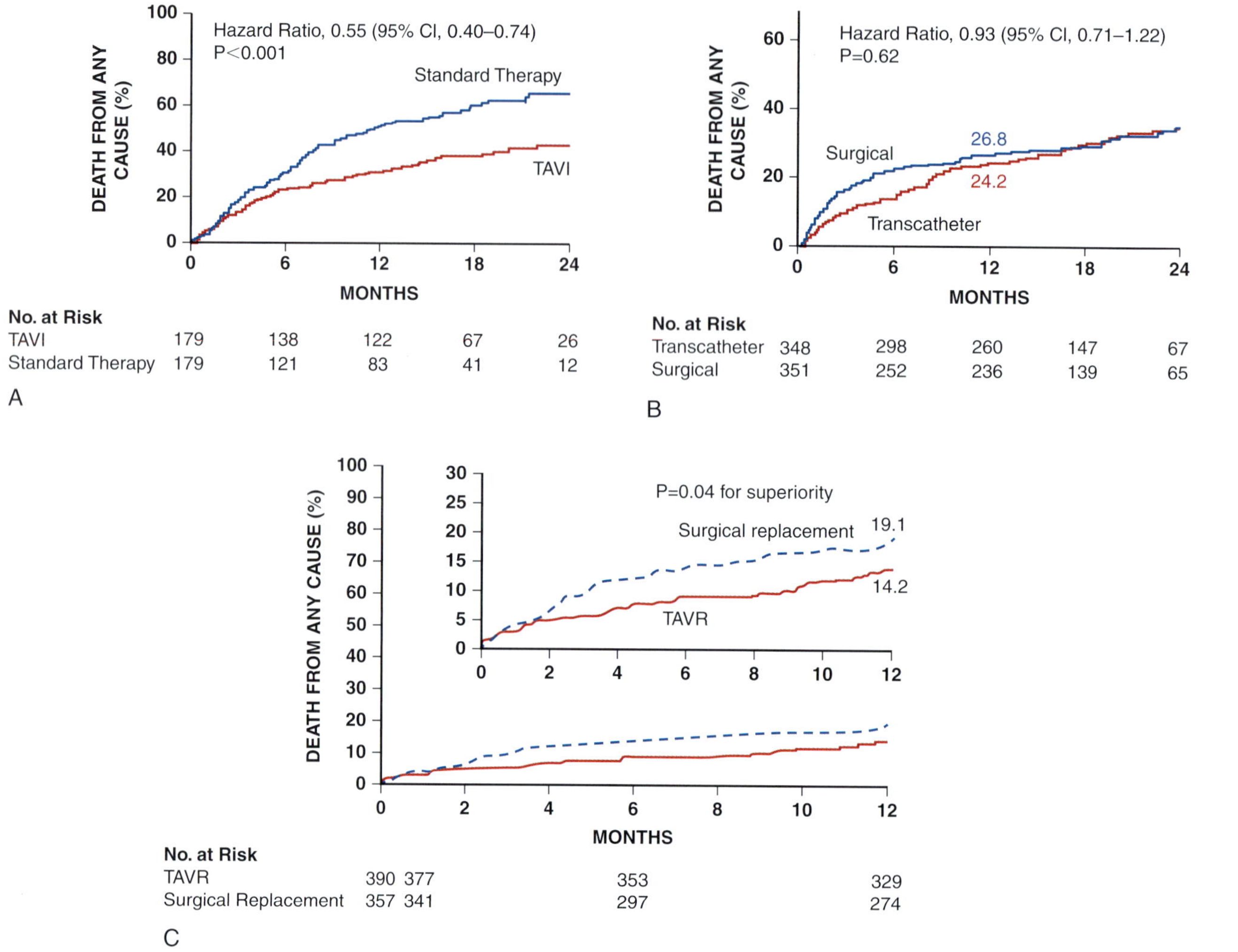

FIGURE 74.1 TAVR versus surgery randomized trials in extreme and high-risk patients; primary endpoint, all-cause death at 1 year. **A,** Extreme-risk patients with balloon-expandable TAVR. **B,** High-risk patients with balloon-expandable TAVR. **C,** High-risk patients with self-expanding TAVR. (From Leon MB, et al. Transcatheter aortic-valve implantation for aortic stenosis in patients who cannot undergo surgery. N Engl J Med 2010;363:1597-1607; Smith CR, et al. Transcatheter versus surgical aortic-valve replacement in high-risk patients. N Engl J Med 2011;364:2187-2198; Adams DH, et al. Transcatheter aortic-valve replacement with a self-expanding prosthesis. N Engl J Med 2014;370:1790-1798.)

In most studies, moderate or severe (but not mild) PVR was associated with increased late mortality after TAVR[36]. Due to technology and procedural enhancements, recent TAVR systems have shown a reduction in moderate or severe PVR, which is now comparable to surgical valves, but there remains a significant difference favoring surgery in mild PVR[39].

Quality-of-Life Assessments

Beginning with the highest surgical risk patients, TAVR resulted in a dramatic improvement in cardiac symptoms and functional capacity, as determined by a significant decrease in the New York Heart Association (NYHA) functional class. At baseline, 75% to 95% of patients had functional class III or IV symptoms, which was reduced to 15% to 25% within one month after treatment.

In the low-risk balloon-expandable TAVR randomized trial, when expressed as ordinal categorical improvement variables, TAVR was associated with greater symptom benefit compared to surgery, both early and late[44].

National TAVR Registries

After regulatory approval in Europe of early TAVR systems in 2007, many countries (most notably France, Germany, Italy, and the United Kingdom) established national registries to capture representative data from the emerging TAVR treatment experiences.

Perhaps the most comprehensive and useful of the national registries has been the United States joint initiative of the Society of Thoracic Surgeons (STS) and the ACC with multiple other stakeholders (e.g., industry sponsors) to form the Transcatheter Valve Therapy (TVT) registry soon after the initial U.S. Food and Drug Administration (FDA) approval of the first balloon-expandable TAVR system in the United States in 2011.[45]

The relationship of procedural volume and patient outcomes was described from the TVT registry.[47] An inverse volume–mortality association was observed for transfemoral TAVR procedures; mortality at 30 days was higher and more variable at hospitals with a low procedural volume than at hospitals with a high procedural volume.

The 2020 TVT registry comprehensive report included 276,316 TAVR patients representing 715 U.S. sites from 2011 through 2019, all three FDA-approved TAVR manufacturers, and all FDA-approved clinical indications.[48] During the TVT registry experience, TAVR volume has increased yearly from 14,000 to 73,000 cases per year, and the annual number of TAVR procedures exceeded the total number of surgical AVRs in 2018[48]. Changes over time in patient demographics included a reduction in patient median age from 84 to 80 years, an increase in transfemoral access cases from 47% to 95%, and lower median STS scores from 6.9% to 4.4%, indicating a lower proportion of high-risk patients. Concurrently, clinical outcomes improved significantly over time; 30-day mortality decreased from 7.5% to 2.5%, 30-day

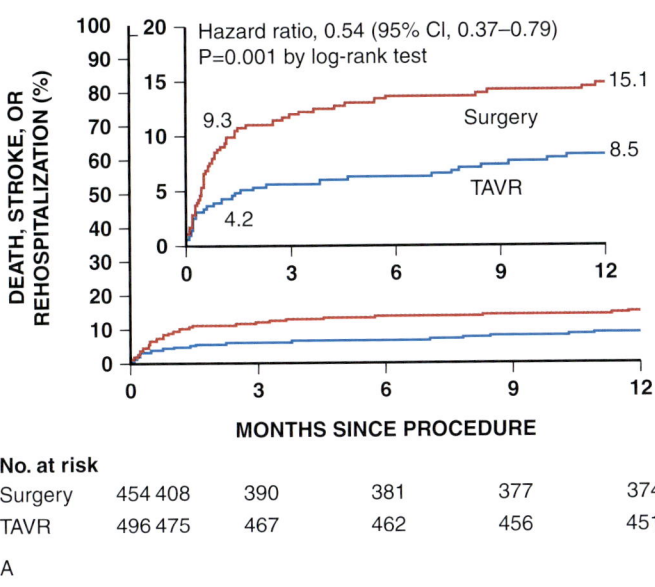

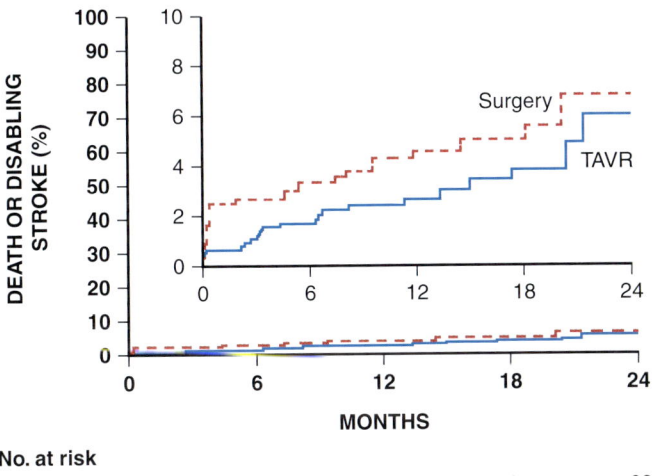

FIGURE 74.2 TAVR versus surgery randomized trials in low-risk patients. **A,** Primary endpoint, all-cause death or all stroke, or CV rehospitalization at 1 year; low-risk patients with balloon-expandable TAVR. **B,** Primary endpoint, all-cause death or disabling stroke at 2 years; low-risk patients with self-expanding TAVR. (From Mack MJ, et al. Transcatheter aortic-valve replacement with a balloon-expandable valve in low-risk patients. N Engl J Med 2019;380:1695-1705; Popma JJ, et al. Transcatheter aortic-valve replacement with a self-expanding valve in low-risk patients. N Engl J Med 2019;380:1706-1715.)

TABLE 74.1 Class 1 Recommendations for TAVR (ACC/AHA 2020 Guidelines)

COR	LOE	RECOMMENDATION
1	A	For symptomatic patients of any age with severe AS and a high or prohibitive surgical risk, TAVR is recommended if predicted post-TAVR survival is >12 months with an acceptable quality of life
1	A	For symptomatic patients with severe AS who are >80 years of age or for younger patients with a life expectancy <10 years and no anatomic contraindication to transfemoral access, TAVR is recommended
1	A	For symptomatic patients with severe AS who are 65 to 80 years of age and no anatomic contraindication to transfemoral access, after shared decision making, TAVR is an alternative to SAVR
1	B-NR	In asymptomatic patients with severe AS and an LVEF <50% who are ≤80 years of age and no anatomic contraindication to transfemoral access, TAVR is an alternative to SAVR (preference according to age)

COR, Class of recommendation; *LOE,* level of evidence; *LVEF,* left ventricular ejection fraction; *NR,* nonrandomized.
From Otto CM, et al. 2020 ACC/AHA Guideline for the management of patients with valvular heart disease: a report of the American College of Cardiology/American Heart Association Joint Committee on Clinical Practice Guidelines. J Am Coll Cardiol 2020.

strokes from 2.8% to 2.3%, the need for new pacemakers diminished from 15.1% to 10.8%, length of hospital stay diminished from a median of 7 to 2 days, and patients discharged post-TAVR to home increased from 62% to 90%. Undoubtedly, a portion of the improved outcomes has been due to expanding treatment cohorts with reduced risk profiles, but the combination of procedural simplification, technology advances, and increased operator and site experience are likely also playing significant roles.

Society-Based Guidelines and Appropriate Use Criteria

In patients with severe AS and indications for AVR using a bioprosthetic valve, the choice of either surgery or TAVR has evolved with increasing clinical trial evidence. The ACC/AHA 2020 valvular heart disease guidelines[8] have expanded the recommended use of TAVR (either preferred or as an alternative to surgery) to four class 1 categories (Table 74.1). TAVR is the preferred recommendation for symptomatic patients (1) with high or prohibitive surgical risk (regardless of age) if predicted post-TAVR survival is >12 months with an acceptable quality of life and (2) >80 years of age (or younger with a life expectancy <10 years) without contraindications to transfemoral TAVR. After shared decision making, TAVR is an alternative to surgery for (1) symptomatic patients from 65 to 80 years of age without contraindications to transfemoral TAVR and (2) asymptomatic patients with an LV ejection fraction <50% (preference according to age). Clearly, the choice of surgery or TAVR is determined by four factors: (1) age and life expectancy, favoring TAVR in older patients with reduced life expectancy and surgery in younger patients with longer life expectancy, due to less well-understood bioprosthetic valve durability with TAVR; (2) clinical comorbidities, which favor the less-invasive TAVR procedure; (3) anatomic constraints challenging the safety of surgery (e.g., hostile chest wall deformities) or TAVR (e.g., suitability for transfemoral access); and (4) shared decision making in which a careful discussion with patients includes lifestyle preferences and explanations of known and unknown factors accounting for risks and benefits of each procedure. A flow diagram, which incorporates the current ACC/AHA guideline recommendations depicting the nodal points for choosing surgery versus TAVR in AVR-indicated patients, is provided (Fig. 74.3).

Not infrequently, the complexity of individual case scenarios cannot be captured easily within the confines of formal recommendation categories. Case-based decisions often require greater flexibility and should incorporate clinical experience and judgment. An additional guidance tool for TAVR practitioners is the development of appropriate use criteria for numerous AS case situations,[49] which details expert opinions on reasonable clinical management decisions.

TAVR TECHNOLOGY EVOLUTION

Anatomy (Components) of a TAVR System

Development of a transcatheter system for bioprosthetic AVR requires the integration of three basic foundational components: a bioprosthetic trileaflet valve, mounted on an expandable metallic frame or scaffold, which is attached to and incorporated with a catheter delivery system. Bioprosthetic valve materials generally consist of predetermined thickness bovine or porcine pericardium of prespecified geometry treated with glutaraldehyde fixation and anticalcification processes.

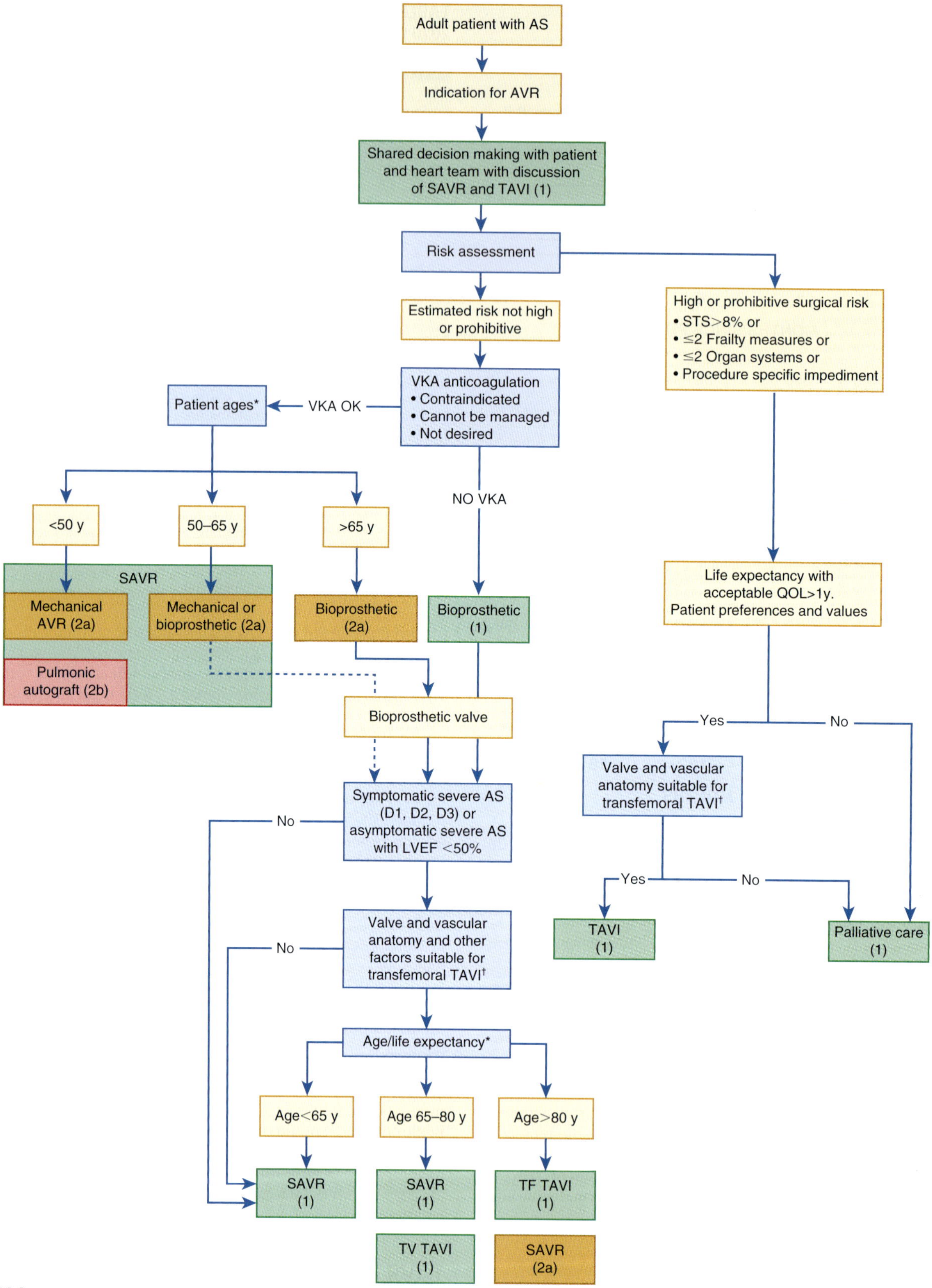

FIGURE 74.3 Choice of SAVR versus TAVI when AVR is indicated for valvular AS, based on the 2020 ACC/AHA valve guidelines recommendations. Green boxes denote class I recommendations. D1, Symptomatic severe high-gradient AS; D2, Symptomatic severe low-flow, low-gradient AS with reduced LVEF; D3, Symptomatic severe low-gradient AS with normal LVEF or paradoxical low-flow severe AS. *Approximate ages, based on US Actuarial Life Expectancy tables, are provided for guidance. The balance between expected patient longevity and valve durability varies continuously across the age range, with more durable valves preferred for patients with a longer life expectancy. †Placement of a transcatheter valve requires vascular anatomy that allows transfemoral delivery and the absence of aortic root dilation that would require surgical replacement. Valvular anatomy must be suitable for placement of the specific prosthetic valve, including annulus size and shape, leaflet number and calcification, and coronary ostial height. (From Otto CM, et al. 2020 ACC/AHA Guideline for the management of patients with valvular heart disease: a report of the American College of Cardiology/American Heart Association Joint Committee on Clinical Practice Guidelines. J Am Coll Cardiol 2020;77(4):e25-e197.)

The leaflets are sewn or attached to short, balloon-expandable metallic frames or to long, super-elastic nitinol self-expanding platforms. The valve-frame composite is compressed or crimped onto catheter delivery systems that facilitate frame expansion via either underlying noncompliant balloon inflation or overlying sheath retraction. After appropriate valve sizing (using CT-imaging formulas and accounting for 10% to 20% oversizing) and correct axial positioning within the aortic annulus, the valve-frame is deployed to the desired location with retention mediated by radial expansion of the frame against highfriction elements of the calcified native aortic valve complex. Various catheter-based delivery systems have been developed, some with directional steerability features, and all attempting to reduce overall system profiles to optimize use of the common femoral artery as the primary vascular access site. Other important features of TAVR systems include the implant location of the bioprosthetic valve, either intra-annular or supra-annular, the available valve sizes to match the range of annulus dimensions (from 18- through 30-mm mean diameter), and the frame length and geometry affecting catheter access to the coronary arteries.

Rapid Progression of TAVR Technologies to the Modern Era

Since the initial experiences with balloon-expandable and self-expanding TAVR systems,[11,20] there have been dramatic improvements in all TAVR components (Figs. 74.4 and 74.5).

Clearly, rapid technology evolution of both balloon-expandable and self-expanding TAVR systems have resulted in current generation devices that can treat almost all aortic annulus dimensions with userfriendly, low-profile delivery catheters for transfemoral access, repositionable features with predictable valve deployment, and reduced PVR.

Other TAVR Systems and Comparative Device versus Device Studies

Given the success of TAVR as a new therapy alternative for AS, there has been an explosion of novel technologies that have been developed and examined in clinical studies.

Accessory Devices for TAVR

The use of off-the-shelf or purpose-driven accessory devices to either facilitate or reduce complications associated with TAVR has rapidly matured over the past decade. Presently, the routine TAVR procedure may be performed with dedicated preshaped 0.035" guidewires of different shapes, special large-diameter balloon catheters for pre- and especially post-dilation to optimize valve implantation, new temporary pacing catheters for valve deployment, expandable and in-line vascular sheaths to assist with low-profile transfemoral access, large-hole vascular closure devices to assist with arterial closure after sheath removal, and catheter-based cerebral embolic protection devices to reduce periprocedural neurologic events.

From the earliest TAVR studies, among the most concerning complications were vascular events due to high-profile sheaths and/or catheters straining the limits of iliofemoral anatomy[52] and embolic strokes due to device interactions with the ascending aorta and/or aortic valve.[53]

The risk of brain injury associated with embolic particulate debris liberated during TAVR procedures depends on the specific definitions applied and the intensity of diagnostic neuroimaging studies.[55] Temporary catheter-based intravascular filters and deflectors have been used in clinical trials to protect the brain from embolic neurologic events during TAVR.

Importantly, significant clinical stroke reduction after TAVR has not been confirmed, so the systematic use of cerebral protection devices is left up to the physician's judgment until ongoing large, randomized strokestudiesarecompleted.

TAVR PROCEDURAL MATURATION

Computed Tomography Imaging for Procedural Planning

Computed tomography (CT) contrast imaging has become a funda-mental diagnostic and procedure planning tool for all TAVR procedures. Most critically, CT is routinely used to optimally select the transcatheter valve size[57] and to assess anatomic features of the iliofemoral arteries to determine the suitability of transfemoral access for a given TAVR system.

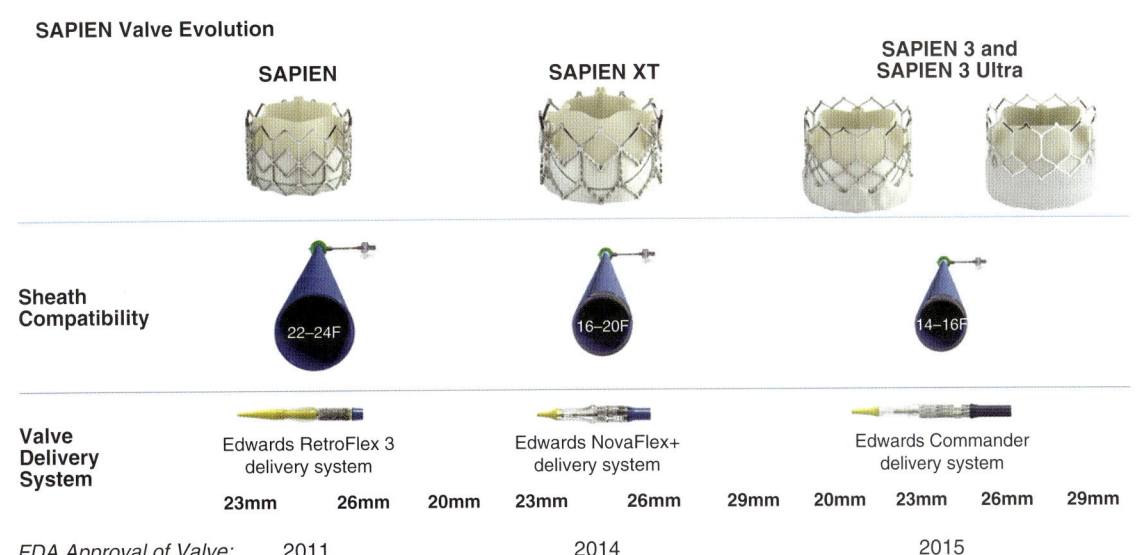

FIGURE 74.4 Evolution of balloon-expandable SAPIEN valves (Edwards Lifesciences), sheath compatibility, and valve delivery systems from initial FDA approval to the current generation.

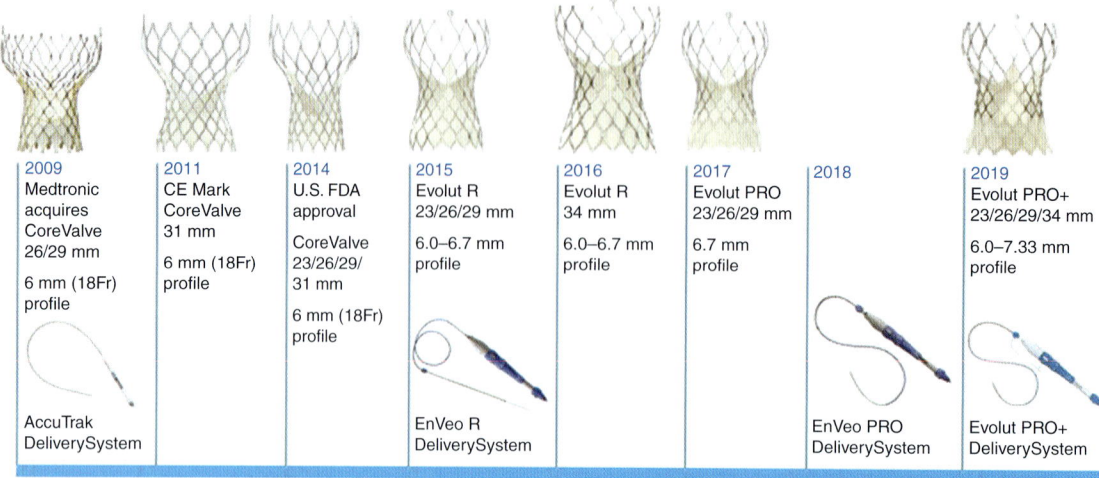

FIGURE 74.5 Evolution of self-expanding CoreValve-Evolut valves (Medtronic) and valve delivery systems from prior to initial FDA approval to the current generation.

Echocardiography for Diagnosis, Procedure-Planning and Follow-Up

The most useful and widely utilized imaging modality for evaluating aortic valve disease is transthoracic echocardiography (two- and three-dimensional). In the management of TAVR patients, echocardiography is used (1) pretreatment for diagnosis of stenosis severity and for procedure planning; (2) intra-procedure to determine the etiology of complications and to assess PVR; and (3) during follow-up as a clinical and research tool to assess long-term bioprosthetic valve function, especially in the setting of recurrent symptoms.[59] In addition, echocardiography provides critical quantitative and qualitative information to correctly stratify low-flow AS syndromes and to monitor LV mass regression, LV function (both systolic and diastolic), RV function, and concomitant mitral and tricuspid valve disease.[60] In post-TAVR patients, routine transthoracic echocardiograms are usually incorporated into follow-up clinical assessments, at 1- or 2-year intervals, or in response to symptom changes.

Minimalist Approach (Including Conscious Sedation Anesthesia)

Undoubtedly, among the most impactful advances in TAVR therapy has been the progressive evolution to a simplified or "minimalist" clinical care management strategy. The minimalist approach is meant to preserve patient safety while leveraging the less-invasive features of a transcatheter procedure to improve efficiencies, reduce costs, and create a more patient-friendly experience. An initially controversial but key aspect of the minimalist strategy was the elimination of routine general anesthesia with associated transesophageal echocardiography during the TAVR procedure, which was replaced by conscious sedation and transthoracic echocardiography.

Importantly, although many components of the minimalist TAVR strategy can be used in most patients, thoughtful screening and triage is necessary. A minority of AS patients have high-risk clinical or anatomic factors, wherein the use of general anesthesia with transesophageal echocardiography guidance or other precautionary measures are advisable to optimize patient safety.

Alternative Vascular Access Strategies

Currently, transfemoral access for TAVR procedures is performed in >95% of all patients treated in the United States,[48] largely related to markedly smaller arterial sheath size requirements. There has been a corresponding decline in transthoracic access TAVR procedures (either transapical or direct aorta entry sites) due to evidence for increased complications with inferior early and late clinical outcomes.[36] For those remaining TAVR patients in whom transfemoral access is not possible, depending on operator experience and training, the most frequently used alternatives are transaxillary, transcarotid, and transcaval approaches.

TAVR-ASSOCIATED COMPLICATIONS

Intraprocedural Complications

Intraprocedural major complications during TAVR have declined over time and are currently uncommon. In the 2020 TVT registry report of >275,000 TAVR procedures overall and 73,000 in 2019, the incidence of acute structural complications (annulus rupture, chamber perforation, and valve embolization), need for cardiopulmonary bypass support, and conversion to open heart surgery were all <0.5%.[48] The very low incidence of intraprocedural complications has allowed more procedures to be safely performed in catherization laboratory settings with less formal surgical backup requirements in many centers.

Coronary Obstruction

Acute coronary obstruction during TAVR is rare due to careful preoperative CT-imaging for risk assessment. Important CT-measurements are the coronary orifice height above the aortic annulus and size of the sinuses of Valsalva relative to the annulus and the ascending aorta relative to the type and size of the planned valve. In patients deemed to be at high risk for coronary obstruction, coronary protection with preemptive wiring of the at-risk coronary ostia and eventual stent implantation in cases of coronary flow impairment is a potential strategy to prevent coronary obstruction. In a recent international registry, preemptive wiring was employed in 2.2% of TAVR cases deemed high risk for coronary obstruction followed by coronary stent deployment in 61% of these cases.[64]

Vascular Complications

The most frequent intraprocedural complication is related to transfemoral access with major vascular complications reported in 1.5% of patients.[48] The combination of preprocedure planning with CT-imaging, utilization of suture-based vascular closure devices for percutaneous common femoral artery repair, and the expanding use of ultrasound guidance to perform controlled common femoral artery access has reduced the frequency of minor and major vascular complications during TAVR. If vascular complications do occur, most can be successfully managed by an experienced operator using an endovascular approach, with the seldom need for surgical cutdown and open repair.

Postprocedural Complications
Neurologic Events

The 2% incidence of periprocedural stroke after TAVR has remained constant over the past 5 years.[48] A recent propensity-matched study compared strokes after transfemoral TAVR and surgical AVR in randomized trials.[65]

Although cerebral embolic protection during TAVR is approved by the FDA,[56] the lack of definitive stroke prevention evidence has resulted in variable adoption with use in approximately 20% of cases in 2019.[48]

Conduction Disturbances

New atrioventricular conduction disturbances after TAVR remain an ongoing concern without complete resolution. The incidence of new permanent pacemaker (PPM) implantation due to high-degree atrioventricular block ranges from 6% to 7% with balloon-expandable valves to 17% to 18% with self-expanding valves, with an overall national rate of 11% for TAVR.[39,40,48] There has been a focus on procedural techniques to avoid oversizing the valve relative to the annulus and to minimize the depth of valve implantation to reduce trauma to the membranous septum, which have been shown to reduce the need for new PPM. Clinical management algorithms have been developed to guide optimal patient screening for advanced atrioventricular block after TAVR and the indications for PPM implantation.[66]

As younger patients with a longer life expectancy undergo TAVR, the importance of avoiding the need for permanent pacing increases. Another concern is an increase in the incidence of new left bundle branch block after TAVR, which has been demonstrated to be associated with decreased long-term survival.[67]

Paravalvular Regurgitation

The early TAVR randomized trials clearly indicated that PVR was more common after TAVR compared with surgery and was associated with increased late mortality.[68] The incidence of moderate-severe PVR post-TAVR has diminished significantly to approximately 1.5%, based on site reports in the most recent TVT registry.[48] There are a number of factors responsible for reduced PVR: (1) the routine use of CT-imaging to accurately assess annular dimensions for selection of the optimal valve size; (2) new generation transcatheter valve designs, which incorporate external wraps (polymers or biologic materials) to fill gaps and promote flush contact with the annulus; and (3) intraprocedure recognition of PVR and the use of post-dilation strategies which commonly resolves or greatly diminishes the severity of PVR. Placement of a second valve inside the initial valve (TAVR in TAVR) can help to resolve the PVR if initial placement location was imprecise. Finally, if moderate or severe PVR persists after the procedure, transcatheter device closure, most commonly using a vascular plug, can be performed and is usually successful.[69]

Prosthesis–Patient Mismatch

Prosthesis–patient mismatch is a condition where the effective orifice area (EOA) of a normally functioning prosthesis is too small in relation to the patient's body size and has been associated with worse outcomes after surgical AVR. Although TAVR prostheses generally have larger valve orifices, a recent analysis of the TVT registry demonstrated that severe and moderate prosthesis-patient mismatches were present following TAVR in 12% and 25% of patients, respectively.[70] Predictors of severe prosthesis-patient mismatch included small (≤ 23-mm diameter) valve prosthesis, valve-in-valve procedures, larger body surface area, female sex, younger age, non-white/Hispanic race, lower ejection fraction, atrial fibrillation (AF), and severe mitral or tricuspid regurgitation. Severe prosthesis-patient mismatch was associated with higher mortality and heart failure rehospitalization at 1 year. Recent studies have noted that Doppler echocardiography may overestimate the severity of prosthesis-patient mismatch post-TAVR due to pressure recovery considerations and assumptions made in calculating transvalvular gradients in a nonstenotic prosthetic valve. This has been demonstrated by a hemodynamic discordance, with systematically higher echocardiographic measurements of postprocedure transvalvular gradients compared with simultaneously measured invasive gradients.[71]

Other Complications

The incidence of other important complications after TAVR is low,[48] including major or life-threatening bleeding 4% to 5%, acute kidney injury ~ 1%, and endocarditis <1%. The frequency of endocarditis after TAVR is approximately the same as after surgical AVR.

TAVR IN SURGICAL BIOPROSTHETIC AORTIC VALVE FAILURE

The use of TAVR for the management of surgical bioprosthetic valve failure as an alternative to reoperative surgical AVR has become broadly adopted in clinical practice. The previously implanted surgical bioprosthesis serves as an ideal "landing zone" for TAVR implantation, and the risks of PVR and new PPMs are greatly reduced. The initial experience in the United States was reported in the TVT registry beginning in 2013 with 455 cases, and by 2019, there were almost 5000 valve-in-valve (ViV) cases performed.[48,85] The results of the PARTNER trial with ViV treatment in 365 high- and intermediate-risk patients using early generation balloon-expandable TAVR indicated a 1-year all-cause mortality of 12.4%, improved hemodynamics, and a dramatic improvement in quality-of-life measures.[86]

Current issues regarding aortic ViV procedures include the potential for coronary obstruction at the time of implant, prosthesis–patient mismatch, and unknown long-term valve durability. Patients who are at higher risk for coronary obstruction include those with surgical valves with externally mounted leaflets, low coronary artery orifices, and reduced space in the aortic sinuses around the surgical valve. The likelihood of coronary obstruction due to deflection of the surgical valve leaflet over the coronary ostia can be mitigated by splitting the leaflet of the surgical valve using a guidewire electrocautery technique, the so-called BASILICA procedure.[87] An ongoing clinical trial has demonstrated successful BASILICA pretreatment followed by uneventful ViV in patients at high risk for coronary obstruction. The presence or creation of prosthesis–patient mismatch especially with small surgical valves remains a limitation of the ViV procedure.[88] The use of supra-annular self-expanding TAVR systems is recommended in these challenging circumstances to achieve the lowest possible transvalvular gradients. Another approach is to fracture the surgical bioprosthesis with high-pressure noncompliant balloon inflations during ViV procedures, which further expands the surgical frame and results in improved hemodynamics after subsequent TAVR.[89] This technique has been used predominantly in patients with small surgical bioprostheses to enlarge the patient cohort for ViV therapy. Whether valve frame fracturing should be limited to smaller size surgical valves (19 and 21 mm) and in patients at risk for severe prosthesis-patient mismatch or should be performed routinely in all surgical valves to optimize the reduction in transvalvular gradients has been a point of controversy. A new surgical valve has also been developed, which is ideally suited to subsequent ViV, as the frame is designed to expand during subsequent ViV. The use of oral anticoagulants after ViV procedures due to possibly higher rates of valve thrombosis remains unknown. There is also increasing experience with placing TAVR valves within degenerated TAVR valves (TAV in TAV), a procedure likely to be more widely utilized in the coming years.[90]

GAPS IN TAVR KNOWLEDGE AND ONGOING CONTROVERSIES

Durability of TAVR Systems

Valve durability is now a critical issue as TAVR evolves to include younger, low-risk patients who are likely to survive for several decades after the procedure. The tissue from both surgical and transcatheter bioprostheses is prone to structural valve deterioration (SVD), which could lead to hemodynamic valve dysfunction. Durability is determined by numerous factors including tissue origin and thickness, anti-calcification treatments, leaflet and valve design, and clinical factors such as patient age and metabolic abnormalities. In studies of surgical valves, SVD commonly begins 8 years after implantation, with marked acceleration after 10 years.[91] Follow-up surgical series indicate that the overall freedom from reintervention or death in patients with surgical aortic valves is approximately 95% at 5 years, 70% to 90% at 10 years, and 50% to 80% at 15 years.[92]

Long-term durability and freedom from SVD are largely unknown for TAVR, especially since the bulk of the early TAVR experiences were in elderly patients with limited life expectancy. Recent reports from Denmark (NOTION trial) and the United Kingdom (UK-TAVI registry) using early TAVR systems have provided some durability information for TAVR between 5 and 10 years.[93,94] In the randomized NOTION trial through 6 years, SVD was significantly greater for surgical aortic valve replacement (SAVR) than TAVR, and bioprosthetic valve failure was extremely low and similar for both groups. The UK-TAVI observational registry reported 91% of surviving patients remaining free of SVD between 5 and 10 years post-implantation, and the incidence of moderate or severe SVD was approximately 9% at a mean of 6 years. Although these data are reassuring, caution is still warranted in extending the indications for TAVR to young, low-risk patients.

Treatment of Bicuspid Aortic Valve Disease

Patients with known bicuspid aortic valve disease (BAVD) were excluded from the pivotal randomized trials of TAVR due to the uncertainty of TAVR prosthesis performance in complex bicuspid anatomies. Concerns regarding TAVR in BAVD relate to the more oval shape of the aortic annulus and the bulky eccentric calcification of the leaflets, raphe, and LV outflow tract. Indeed, these concerns were borne out in the early experience with TAVR using first-generation devices that led to a higher incidence of annular rupture, moderate-severe PVR, and the need for new PPMs.[95] However, with greater experience, especially in properly selected patients with less hostile anatomy using newer generation devices, the outcomes have been similar to TAVR in patients with tricuspid AS.[96] The role of TAVR in BAVD will be of greater importance as TAVR is used to treat younger patients who have a higher incidence of BAVD. Based on CT-imaging and clinical experience, it appears that TAVR may be suitable for some BAVD patients with a non- or minimally calcified raphe and those without bulky eccentric calcification of the valve leaflets and LV outflow tract. Likewise, there is consensus that younger patients with bulky, eccentric calcification at risk for annular rupture, marked annular ovality, and ascending aortic aneurysmal disease are best treated with surgery. Whether a randomized trial to clearly define the best management strategies in BAVD patients between these two extremes has been an ongoing controversy.

TAVR for Aortic Regurgitation

TAVR devices have been used mainly for the treatment of calcific AS due to the reliance on calcified native valve tissue for secure prosthesis anchoring. There has been early experience with currently approved devices in patients with pure aortic regurgitation (AR). A registry report of 331 patients with severe AR showed improvement in clinical outcomes with later generation balloon-expandable and self-expanding TAVR systems, emphasizing the need for device over-expansion and careful case selection.[97] Novel TAVR designs for the treatment of AR with features to secure the prosthetic valve to the underlying native leaflets are promising and are in various stages of clinical evaluation in the United States and elsewhere.

Managing the Young, Low-Risk Patient with AS

The management of young, low-risk patients with AS is in a state of rapid evolution and will be based on further evidence development. Clearly, valve durability is of greater importance in younger patients and there are scant TAVR durability data beyond 5 years, although there is no signal of premature SVD in transcatheter bioprostheses. Also, younger patients have a higher incidence of BAVD, and the additional burdens of increased anatomic complexity must be considered. Based on current best available evidence, clinical management should apply an algorithm where the first decision is whether a tissue or mechanical valve is preferred. In general, patients <50 years are best treated with a mechanical valve if anticoagulation is acceptable, and in patients >60 to 65 years, a bioprosthetic valve is preferable. Shared decision making with patients in their 50s regarding the advantages and disadvantages of valve choice (anticoagulation versus durability) is appropriate. Once the decision for a tissue valve is made, the next decision is TAVR versus surgery, which also requires a careful shared decision-making process. Fewer than 10% of patients in the low-risk TAVR trials were <65 years, so long-term durability is unknown. The use of ViV TAVR after the first valve, be it a TAVR or surgery, may potentially lengthen the time to the next surgical intervention. Ongoing discussions are active among thought leaders regarding the lifetime management of young patients with AS, with a goal to generate evidence that can help to decide the most appropriate sequence for procedures (e.g., surgery or TAVR first).

Subclinical Leaflet Thrombosis

With the expanded use of CT-imaging, the detection of subclinical leaflet thrombosis on bioprosthetic valves has become readily available.[98] The sentinel imaging findings—hypoattenuated leaflet thickening (HALT) and reduced leaflet motion—were observed in approximately 20% of patients during the first year after TVR. To determine the frequency, natural history, and clinical relevance of these imaging findings, CT-surveillance substudies were imbedded in both low-risk randomized TAVR trials.[99,100] The PARTNER 3 CT-substudy[99] found that subclinical leaflet thrombosis was more frequent in transcatheter compared with surgical valves at 30 days but not at 1 year, a significant minority of patients had either resolution of 1-month HALT by 1 year or newly appearing HALT at 1 year, and the impact of HALT on thromboembolic complications and SVD was indeterminate and required long-term follow-up. Based on these studies, there is reasonable consensus that routine CT-evaluations or systematic anticoagulation therapy is not warranted after TAVR and should only be considered if thromboembolic complications are present (e.g., stroke or retinal artery embolus) or if there is an unexplained early increase in transvalvular aortic valve gradients.

Optimal Antithrombotic Therapies

Based on experience with coronary stents, dual antiplatelet therapy for 6 months became the early default antithrombotic management of patients after TAVR. However, multiple studies have demonstrated an increased incidence of bleeding complications with dual antiplatelet therapy compared with aspirin monotherapy without added benefit in reducing thromboembolic complications.[101] In a recent randomized trial, the direct factor Xa inhibitor rivaroxaban was associated with a higher incidence of death, thromboembolic complications, and bleeding compared with antiplatelet therapy. However, antithrombotic therapy was associated with a lower incidence of HALT in a substudy.[102,103] At the current time, aspirin monotherapy (or another single antiplatelet agent) is the preferred post-TAVR pharmacotherapy strategy in patients without recent coronary stents and without other indications for antithrombotic agents.

REFERENCES

Background

1. Leon MB, Smith CR, Mack M, et al. Transcatheter aortic-valve implantation for aortic stenosis in patients who cannot undergo surgery. *N Engl J Med*. 2010;363:1597–1607.
2. Genereux P, Pibarot P, Redfors B, et al. Staging classification of aortic stenosis based on the extent of cardiac damage. *Eur Heart J*. 2017;38:3351–3358.
3. Roberts WC, Ko JM. Frequency by decades of unicuspid, bicuspid, and tricuspid aortic valves in adults having isolated aortic valve replacement for aortic stenosis, with or without associated aortic regurgitation. *Circulation*. 2005;111:920–925.
4. d'Arcy JL, Coffey S, Loudon MA, et al. Large-scale community echocardiographic screening reveals a major burden of undiagnosed valvular heart disease in older people: the OxVALVE Population Cohort Study. *Eur Heart J*. 2016;37:3515–3522.
5. Osnabrugge RL, Mylotte D, Head SJ, et al. Aortic stenosis in the elderly: disease prevalence and number of candidates for transcatheter aortic valve replacement: a meta-analysis and modeling study. *J Am Coll Cardiol*. 2013;62:1002–1012.
6. Baumgartner H, Falk V, Bax JJ, et al. 2017 ESC/EACTS Guidelines for the management of valvular heart disease. *Eur Heart J*. 2017;38:2739–2791.
7. Nishimura RA, Otto CM, Bonow RO, et al. 2017 AHA/ACC focused update of the 2014 AHA/ACC guideline for the management of patients with valvular heart disease: a report of the American College of Cardiology/American Heart Association Task Force on Clinical Practice Guidelines. *Circulation*. 2017;135:e1159–e1195.
8. Otto CM, Nishimura RA, Bonow RO, et al. 2020 ACC/AHA guideline for the management of patients with valvular heart disease: a report of the American College of Cardiology/American Heart Association Joint Committee on Clinical Practice Guidelines. *J Am Coll Cardiol*. 2020;77(4):e25–e197.
9. Bonow RO. Improving outlook for elderly patients with aortic stenosis. *J Am Med Assoc*. 2013;310:2045–2047.
10. Thourani VH, Suri RM, Gunter RL, et al. Contemporary real-world outcomes of surgical aortic valve replacement in 141,905 low-risk, intermediate-risk, and high-risk patients. *Ann Thorac Surg*. 2015;99:55–61.
11. Cribier A, Savin T, Saoudi N, et al. Percutaneous transluminal valvuloplasty of acquired aortic stenosis in elderly patients: an alternative to valve replacement? *Lancet*. 1986;1:63–67.
12. McKay RG. The Mansfield scientific aortic valvuloplasty registry: overview of acute hemodynamic results and procedural complications. *J Am Coll Cardiol*. 1991;17:485–491.
13. O'Neill W W. Predictors of long-term survival after percutaneous aortic valvuloplasty: report of the Mansfield scientific balloon aortic valvuloplasty registry. *J Am Coll Cardiol*. 1991;17:193–198.
14. Lieberman EB, Bashore TM, Hermiller JB, et al. Balloon aortic valvuloplasty in adults: failure of procedure to improve long-term survival. *J Am Coll Cardiol*. 1995;26:1522–1528.
15. Kapadia S, Stewart WJ, Anderson WN, et al. Outcomes of inoperable symptomatic aortic stenosis patients not undergoing aortic valve replacement: insight into the impact of balloon aortic valvuloplasty from the PARTNER trial (Placement of AoRtic TraNscathetER Valve trial). *JACC Cardiovasc Interv*. 2015;8:324–333.
16. Andersen HR, Knudsen LL, Hasenkam JM. Transluminal implantation of artificial heart valves. Description of a new expandable aortic valve and initial results with implantation by catheter technique in closed chest pigs. *Eur Heart J*. 1992;13:704–708.
17. Cribier A, Eltchaninoff H, Bash A, et al. Percutaneous transcatheter implantation of an aortic valve prosthesis for calcific aortic stenosis: first human case description. *Circulation*. 2002;106:3006–3008.
18. Cribier A, Eltchaninoff H, Tron C, et al. Treatment of calcific aortic stenosis with the percutaneous heart valve: mid-term follow-up from the initial feasibility studies: the French experience. *J Am Coll Cardiol*. 2006;47:1214–1223.
19. Kodali SK, O'Neill WW, Moses JW, et al. Early and late (one year) outcomes following transcatheter aortic valve implantation in patients with severe aortic stenosis (from the United States REVIVAL trial). *Am J Cardiol*. 2011;107:1058–1064.
20. Grube E, Laborde JC, Zickmann B, et al. First report on a human percutaneous transluminal implantation of a self-expanding valve prosthesis for interventional treatment of aortic valve stenosis. *Catheter Cardiovasc Interv*. 2005;66:465–469.

Evolution of TAVR

21. Grube E, Schuler G, Buellesfeld L, et al. Percutaneous aortic valve replacement for severe aortic stenosis in high-risk patients using the second- and current third-generation self-expanding CoreValve prosthesis: device success and 30-day clinical outcome. *J Am Coll Cardiol*. 2007;50:69–76.
22. Shahian DM, Jacobs JP, Badhwar V, et al. The society of thoracic surgeons 2018 adult cardiac surgery risk models: part 1-background, design considerations, and model development. *Ann Thorac Surg*. 2018;105:1411–1418.
23. Fried LP, Tangen CM, Walston J, et al. Frailty in older adults: evidence for a phenotype. *J Gerontol A Biol Sci Med Sci*. 2001;56:M146–M156.
24. Green P, Woglom AE, Genereux P, et al. The impact of frailty status on survival after transcatheter aortic valve replacement in older adults with severe aortic stenosis: a single-center experience. *JACC Cardiovasc Interv*. 2012;5:974–981.
25. Afilalo J, Lauck S, Kim DH, et al. Frailty in older adults undergoing aortic valve replacement: the FRAILTY-AVR study. *J Am Coll Cardiol*. 2017;70:689–700.
26. Nishimura RA, Otto CM, Bonow RO, et al. 2014 AHA/ACC guideline for the management of patients with valvular heart disease: a report of the American College of Cardiology/American Heart Association Task Force on Practice Guidelines. *J Am Coll Cardiol*. 2014;63:e57–e185.
27. Leon MB, Piazza N, Nikolsky E, et al. Standardized endpoint definitions for transcatheter aortic valve implantation clinical trials: a consensus report from the valve academic research consortium. *J Am Coll Cardiol*. 2011;57:253–269.
28. Kappetein AP, Head SJ, Genereux P, et al. Updated standardized endpoint definitions for transcatheter aortic valve implantation: the Valve Academic Research Consortium-2 consensus document. *J Am Coll Cardiol*. 2012;60:1438–1454.
29. Genereux P, Piazza N, Alu MC, et al. Valve Academic Research Consortium 3: updated endpoint definitions for aortic valve clinical research. *Eur Heart J*. 2020.
30. Kapadia SR, Leon MB, Makkar RR, et al. 5-year outcomes of transcatheter aortic valve replacement compared with standard treatment for patients with inoperable aortic stenosis (PARTNER 1): a randomised controlled trial. *Lancet*. 2015;385:2485–2491.
31. Popma JJ, Adams DH, Reardon MJ, et al. Transcatheter aortic valve replacement using a self-expanding bioprosthesis in patients with severe aortic stenosis at extreme risk for surgery. *J Am Coll Cardiol*. 2014;63:1972–1981.
32. Smith CR, Leon MB, Mack MJ, et al. Transcatheter versus surgical aortic-valve replacement in high-risk patients. *N Engl J Med*. 2011;364:2187–2198.
33. Adams DH, Popma JJ, Reardon MJ, et al. Transcatheter aortic-valve replacement with a self-expanding prosthesis. *N Engl J Med*. 2014;370:1790–1798.
34. Mack MJ, Leon MB, Smith CR, et al. 5-year outcomes of transcatheter aortic valve replacement or surgical aortic valve replacement for high surgical risk patients with aortic stenosis (PARTNER 1): a randomised controlled trial. *Lancet*. 2015;385:2477–2484.
35. Gleason TG, Reardon MJ, Popma JJ, et al. 5-Year outcomes of self-expanding transcatheter versus surgical aortic valve replacement in high-risk patients. *J Am Coll Cardiol*. 2018;72:2687–2696.
36. Leon MB, Smith CR, Mack MJ, et al. Transcatheter or surgical aortic-valve replacement in intermediate-risk patients. *N Engl J Med*. 2016;374:1609–1620.
37. Reardon MJ, Van Mieghem NM, Popma JJ, et al. Surgical or transcatheter aortic-valve replacement in intermediate-risk patients. *N Engl J Med*. 2017;376:1321–1331.
38. Makkar RR, Thourani VH, Mack MJ, et al. Five-year outcomes of transcatheter or surgical aortic-valve replacement. *N Engl J Med*. 2020;382:799–809.
39. Mack MJ, Leon MB, Thourani VH, et al. Transcatheter aortic-valve replacement with a balloon-expandable valve in low-risk patients. *N Engl J Med*. 2019;380:1695–1705.
40. Popma JJ, Deeb GM, Yakubov SJ, et al. Transcatheter aortic-valve replacement with a self-expanding valve in low-risk patients. *N Engl J Med*. 2019;380:1706–1715.
41. Reynolds MR, Magnuson EA, Wang K, et al. Health-related quality of life after transcatheter or surgical aortic valve replacement in high-risk patients with severe aortic stenosis: results from the PARTNER (Placement of AoRTic TraNscathetER Valve) Trial (Cohort A). *J Am Coll Cardiol*. 2012;60:548–5558.
42. Arnold SV, Reynolds MR, Wang K, et al. Health status after transcatheter or surgical aortic valve replacement in patients with severe aortic stenosis at increased surgical risk: results from the CoreValve US pivotal trial. *JACC Cardiovasc Interv*. 2015;8:1207–1217.
43. Baron SJ, Arnold SV, Wang K, et al. Health status benefits of transcatheter vs surgical aortic valve replacement in patients with severe aortic stenosis at intermediate surgical risk: results from the PARTNER 2 randomized clinical trial. *JAMA Cardiol*. 2017;2:837–845.
44. Baron SJ, Magnuson EA, Lu M, et al. Health status after transcatheter versus surgical aortic valve replacement in low-risk patients with aortic stenosis. *J Am Coll Cardiol*. 2019;74:2833–2842.
45. Carroll JD, Edwards FH, Marinac-Dabic D, et al. The STS-ACC transcatheter valve therapy national registry: a new partnership and infrastructure for the introduction and surveillance of medical devices and therapies. *J Am Coll Cardiol*. 2013;62:1026–1034.
46. Holmes Jr DR, Nishimura RA, Grover FL, et al. Annual outcomes with transcatheter valve therapy: from the STS/ACC TVT registry. *J Am Coll Cardiol*. 2015;66:2813–2823.
47. Vemulapalli S, Carroll JD, Mack MJ, et al. Procedural volume and outcomes for transcatheter aortic-valve replacement. *N Engl J Med*. 2019;380:2541–2550.
48. Carroll JD, Mack MJ, Vemulapalli S, et al. STS-ACC TVT registry of transcatheter aortic valve replacement. *J Am Coll Cardiol*. 2020;76:2492–2516.
49. Bonow RO, Brown AS, Gillam LD, et al. ACC/AATS/AHA/ASE/EACTS/HVS/SCA/SCAI/SCCT/SCMR/STS 2017 appropriate use criteria for the treatment of patients with severe aortic stenosis: a report of the American College of Cardiology Appropriate Use Criteria Task Force, American Association for Thoracic Surgery, American Heart Association, American Society of Echocardiography, European Association for Cardio-Thoracic Surgery, Heart Valve Society, Society of Cardiovascular Anesthesiologists, Society for Cardiovascular Angiography and Interventions, Society of Cardiovascular Computed Tomography, Society for Cardiovascular Magnetic Resonance, and Society of Thoracic Surgeons. *J Am Coll Cardiol*. 2017;70:2566–2598.
50. Feldman TE, Reardon MJ, Rajagopal V, et al. Effect of mechanically expanded vs self-expanding transcatheter aortic valve replacement on mortality and major adverse clinical events in high-risk patients with aortic stenosis: the REPRISE III randomized clinical trial. *J Am Med Assoc*. 2018;319:27–37.
51. Makkar RR, Cheng W, Waksman R, et al. Self-expanding intra-annular versus commercially available transcatheter heart valves in high and extreme risk patients with severe aortic stenosis (PORTICO IDE): a randomised, controlled, non-inferiority trial. *Lancet*. 2020;396:669–683.

Complications of TAVR

52. Genereux P, Webb JG, Svensson LG, et al. Vascular complications after transcatheter aortic valve replacement: insights from the PARTNER (Placement of AoRTic TraNscathetER Valve) trial. *J Am Coll Cardiol*. 2012;60:1043–1052.
53. Schaff HV. Transcatheter aortic-valve implantation–at what price? *N Engl J Med*. 2011;364:2256–2258.
54. Wood DA, Krajcer Z, Sathananthan J, et al. Pivotal clinical study to evaluate the safety and effectiveness of the MANTA percutaneous vascular closure device. *Circ Cardiovasc Interv*. 2019;12:e007258.
55. Lansky AJ, Messe SR, Brickman AM, et al. Proposed standardized neurological endpoints for cardiovascular clinical trials: an academic research consortium initiative. *J Am Coll Cardiol*. 2017;69:679–691.
56. Kapadia SR, Kodali S, Makkar R, et al. Protection against cerebral embolism during transcatheter aortic valve replacement. *J Am Coll Cardiol*. 2017;69:367–377.
57. Blanke P, Pibarot P, Hahn R, et al. Computed tomography-based oversizing degrees and incidence of paravalvular regurgitation of a new generation transcatheter heart valve. *JACC Cardiovasc Interv*. 2017;10:810–820.
58. Blanke P, Weir-McCall JR, Achenbach S, et al. Computed tomography imaging in the context of Transcatheter Aortic Valve Implantation (TAVI)/Transcatheter Aortic Valve Replacement (TAVR): an expert consensus document of the society of cardiovascular computed tomography. *JACC Cardiovasc Imaging*. 2019;12:1–24.
59. Douglas PS, Leon MB, Mack MJ, et al. Longitudinal hemodynamics of transcatheter and surgical aortic valves in the PARTNER trial. *JAMA Cardiol*. 2017;2:1197–1206.
60. Pibarot P, Salaun E, Dahou A, et al. Echocardiographic results of transcatheter versus surgical aortic valve replacement in low-risk patients: the PARTNER 3 trial. *Circulation*. 2020;141:1527–1537.
61. Babaliaros V, Devireddy C, Lerakis S, et al. Comparison of transfemoral transcatheter aortic valve replacement performed in the catheterization laboratory (minimalist approach) versus hybrid operating room (standard approach): outcomes and cost analysis. *JACC Cardiovasc Interv*. 2014;7:898–904.
62. Wood DA, Lauck SB, Cairns JA, et al. The Vancouver 3M (multidisciplinary, multimodality, but minimalist) clinical pathway facilitates safe next-day discharge home at low-, medium-, and high-volume transfemoral transcatheter aortic valve replacement centers: the 3M TAVR study. *JACC Cardiovasc Interv*. 2019;12:459–469.
63. Lederman RJ, Greenbaum AB, Rogers T, et al. Anatomic suitability for transcaval access based on computed tomography. *JACC Cardiovasc Interv*. 2017;10:1–10.
64. Palmerini T, Chakravarty T, Saia F, et al. Coronary protection to prevent coronary obstruction during TAVR: a multicenter international registry. *JACC Cardiovasc Interv*. 2020;13:739–747.
65. Kapadia SR, Huded CP, Kodali SK, et al. Stroke after surgical versus transfemoral transcatheter aortic valve replacement in the PARTNER trial. *J Am Coll Cardiol*. 2018;72:2415–2426.
66. Rodes-Cabau J, Ellenbogen KA, Krahn AD, et al. Management of conduction disturbances associated with transcatheter aortic valve replacement: JACC scientific expert panel. *J Am Coll Cardiol*. 2019;74:1086–1106.
67. Nazif TM, Chen S, George I, et al. New-onset left bundle branch block after transcatheter aortic valve replacement is associated with adverse long-term clinical outcomes in intermediate-risk patients: an analysis from the PARTNER II trial. *Eur Heart J*. 2019;40:2218–2227.
68. Kodali S, Pibarot P, Douglas PS, et al. Paravalvular regurgitation after transcatheter aortic valve replacement with the Edwards sapien valve in the PARTNER trial: characterizing patients and impact on outcomes. *Eur Heart J*. 2015;36:449–456.
69. Calvert PA, Northridge DB, Malik IS, et al. Percutaneous device closure of paravalvular leak: combined experience from the United Kingdom and Ireland. *Circulation*. 2016;134:934–944.
70. Herrmann HC, Daneshvar SA, Fonarow GC, et al. Prosthesis-patient mismatch in patients undergoing transcatheter aortic valve replacement: from the STS/ACC TVT registry. *J Am Coll Cardiol*. 2018;72:2701–2711.

71. Abbas AE, Mando R, Hanzel G, et al. Invasive versus echocardiographic evaluation of transvalvular gradients immediately post-transcatheter aortic valve replacement. *Circ Cardiovasc Interv*. 2019;12:e007973.
72. Alperi A, Voisine P, Kalavrouziotis D, et al. Aortic valve replacement in low-risk patients with severe aortic stenosis outside randomized trials. *J Am Coll Cardiol*. 2021;77:111–123.
73. Chiche O, Rodes-Cabau J, Campelo-Parada F, et al. Significant mitral regurgitation in patients undergoing TAVR: mechanisms and imaging variables associated with improvement. *Echocardiography*. 2019;36:722–731.
74. Freitas-Ferraz AB, Lerakis S, Barbosa Ribeiro H, et al. Mitral regurgitation in low-flow, low-gradient aortic stenosis patients undergoing TAVR: insights from the TOPAS-TAVI registry. *JACC Cardiovasc Interv*. 2020;13:567–579.
75. Lindman BR, Maniar HS, Jaber WA, et al. Effect of tricuspid regurgitation and the right heart on survival after transcatheter aortic valve replacement: insights from the Placement of Aortic Transcatheter Valves II inoperable cohort. *Circ Cardiovasc Interv*. 2015;8(4). https://doi.org/10.1161/CIRCINTERVENTIONS.114.002073 e002073.
76. Okuno T, Hagemeyer D, Brugger N, et al. Valvular and nonvalvular atrial fibrillation in patients undergoing transcatheter aortic valve replacement. *JACC Cardiovasc Interv*. 2020;13:2124–2133.
77. Faroux L, Guimaraes L, Wintzer-Wehekind J, et al. Coronary artery disease and transcatheter aortic valve replacement: JACC state-of-the-art review. *J Am Coll Cardiol*. 2019;74:362–372.
78. Witberg G, Zusman O, Codner P, et al. Impact of coronary artery revascularization completeness on outcomes of patients with coronary artery disease undergoing transcatheter aortic valve replacement: a meta-analysis of studies using the residual syntax score (synergy between PCI with taxus and cardiac surgery). *Circ Cardiovasc Interv*. 2018;11:e006000.
79. Vilalta V, Asmarats L, Ferreira-Neto AN, et al. Incidence, clinical characteristics, and impact of acute coronary syndrome following transcatheter aortic valve replacement. *JACC Cardiovasc Interv*. 2018;11:2523–2533.
80. Magne J, Mohty D. Paradoxical low-flow, low-gradient severe aortic stenosis: a distinct disease entity. *Heart*. 2015;101:993–995.
81. Clavel MA, Burwash IG, Pibarot P. Cardiac imaging for assessing low-gradient severe aortic stenosis. *JACC Cardiovasc Imaging*. 2017;10:185–202.
82. Fischer-Rasokat U, Renker M, Liebetrau C, et al. 1-Year survival after TAVR of patients with low-flow, low-gradient and high-gradient aortic valve stenosis in matched study populations. *JACC Cardiovasc Interv*. 2019;12:752–763.
83. Kataoka A, Watanabe Y, Kozuma K, et al. Prognostic impact of low-flow severe aortic stenosis in small-body patients undergoing TAVR: the OCEAN-TAVI registry. *JACC Cardiovasc Imaging*. 2018;11:659–669.
84. Ribeiro HB, Lerakis S, Gilard M, et al. Transcatheter aortic valve replacement in patients with low-flow, low-gradient aortic stenosis: the TOPAS-TAVI registry. *J Am Coll Cardiol*. 2018;71:1297–1308.
85. Tuzcu EM, Kapadia SR, Vemulapalli S, et al. Transcatheter aortic valve replacement of failed surgically implanted bioprostheses: the STS/ACC registry. *J Am Coll Cardiol*. 2018;72:370–382.
86. Webb JG, Mack MJ, White JM, et al. Transcatheter aortic valve implantation within degenerated aortic surgical bioprostheses: PARTNER 2 valve-in-valve registry. *J Am Coll Cardiol*. 2017;69:2253–2262.
87. Khan JM, Bruce CG, Babaliaros VC, et al. TAVR roulette: caution regarding BASILICA laceration for TAVR-in-TAVR. *JACC Cardiovasc Interv*. 2020;13:787–789.
88. Pibarot P, Simonato M, Barbanti M, et al. Impact of pre-existing prosthesis-patient mismatch on survival following aortic valve-in-valve procedures. *JACC Cardiovasc Interv*. 2018;11:133–141.
89. Chhatriwalla AK, Allen KB, Saxon JT, et al. Bioprosthetic aortic valve fracture improves the hemodynamic results of valve-in-valve transcatheter aortic valve replacement. *Circ Cardiovasc Interv*. 2017;10.
90. Landes U, Webb JG, De Backer O, et al. Repeat transcatheter aortic valve replacement for transcatheter prosthesis dysfunction. *J Am Coll Cardiol*. 2020;75:1882–1893.
91. Foroutan F, Guyatt GH, O'Brien K, et al. Prognosis after surgical replacement with a bioprosthetic aortic valve in patients with severe symptomatic aortic stenosis: systematic review of observational studies. *BMJ*. 2016;354:i5065.
92. Pibarot P, Dumesnil JG. Prosthetic heart valves: selection of the optimal prosthesis and long-term management. *Circulation*. 2009;119:1034–1048.
93. Blackman DJ, Saraf S, MacCarthy PA, et al. Long-term durability of transcatheter aortic valve prostheses. *J Am Coll Cardiol*. 2019;73:537–545.
94. Sondergaard L, Ihlemann N, Capodanno D, et al. Durability of transcatheter and surgical bioprosthetic aortic valves in patients at lower surgical risk. *J Am Coll Cardiol*. 2019;73:546–553.
95. Yoon SH, Lefevre T, Ahn JM, et al. Transcatheter aortic valve replacement with early- and new-generation devices in bicuspid aortic valve stenosis. *J Am Coll Cardiol*. 2016;68:1195–1205.
96. Makkar RR, Yoon SH, Leon MB, et al. Association between transcatheter aortic valve replacement for bicuspid vs tricuspid aortic stenosis and mortality or stroke. *J Am Med Assoc*. 2019;321:2193–2202.
97. Yoon SH, Schmidt T, Bleiziffer S, et al. Transcatheter aortic valve replacement in pure native aortic valve regurgitation. *J Am Coll Cardiol*. 2017;70:2752–2763.
98. Makkar RR, Fontana G, Jilaihawi H, et al. Possible subclinical leaflet thrombosis in bioprosthetic aortic valves. *N Engl J Med*. 2015;373:2015–2024.
99. Makkar RR, Blanke P, Leipsic J, et al. Subclinical leaflet thrombosis in transcatheter and surgical bioprosthetic valves: PARTNER 3 cardiac computed tomography substudy. *J Am Coll Cardiol*. 2020;75:3003–3015.
100. Blanke P, Leipsic JA, Popma JJ, et al. Bioprosthetic aortic valve leaflet thickening in the Evolut low risk sub-study. *J Am Coll Cardiol*. 2020;75:2430–2442.

Future Direction

101. Rodes-Cabau J, Masson JB, Welsh RC, et al. Aspirin versus aspirin plus clopidogrel as antithrombotic treatment following transcatheter aortic valve replacement with a balloon-expandable valve: the ARTE (aspirin versus aspirin + clopidogrel following transcatheter aortic valve implantation) randomized clinical trial. *JACC Cardiovasc Interv*. 2017;10:1357–1365.
102. Dangas GD, Tijssen JGP, Wohrle J, et al. A controlled trial of rivaroxaban after transcatheter aortic-valve replacement. *N Engl J Med*. 2020;382:120–129.
103. De Backer O, Dangas GD, Jilaihawi H, et al. Reduced leaflet motion after transcatheter aortic-valve replacement. *N Engl J Med*. 2020;382:130–139.

Anticoagulant and Antiplatelet Management post-TAVR

104. Resor CD, Bhatt DL. Polymeric heart valves: back to the future? *Matter*. 2019;1:30–32.
105. Scherman J, Bezuidenhout D, Ofoegbu C, et al. TAVI for low to middle income countries. *Eur Heart J*. 2017;38:1182–1184.
106. Everett RJ, Clavel MA, Pibarot P, et al. Timing of intervention in aortic stenosis: a review of current and future strategies. *Heart*. 2018;104:2067–2076.
107. Lancellotti P, Magne J, Dulgheru R, et al. Outcomes of patients with asymptomatic aortic stenosis followed up in heart valve clinics. *JAMA Cardiol*. 2018;3:1060–1068.
108. Kang DH, Park SJ, Lee SA, et al. Early surgery or conservative care for asymptomatic aortic stenosis. *N Engl J Med*. 2020;382:111–119.
109. Strange G, Stewart S, Celermajer D, et al. Poor long-term survival in patients with moderate aortic stenosis. *J Am Coll Cardiol*. 2019;74:1851–1863.
110. Vannan MA, Pibarot P, Lancellotti P. Aortic stenosis: the emperor's new clothes. *J Am Coll Cardiol*. 2019;74:1864–1867.
111. van Gils L, Clavel MA, Vollema EM, et al. Prognostic implications of moderate aortic stenosis in patients with left ventricular systolic dysfunction. *J Am Coll Cardiol*. 2017;69:2383–2392.
112. Vollema EM, Amanullah MR, Ng ACT, et al. Staging cardiac damage in patients with symptomatic aortic valve stenosis. *J Am Coll Cardiol*. 2019;74:538–549.
113. Tastet L, Tribouilloy C, Marechaux S, et al. Staging cardiac damage in patients with asymptomatic aortic valve stenosis. *J Am Coll Cardiol*. 2019;74:550–563.

75 Mitral Stenosis

Y.S. CHANDRASHEKHAR

EPIDEMIOLOGY AND SECULAR TRENDS, 1441
Rheumatic Mitral Stenosis, 1441
Nonrheumatic Mitral Stenosis, 1441

DEFINITION OF DISEASE AND SEVERITY, 1441

RHEUMATIC MITRAL STENOSIS, 1442
Pathology, 1442
Clinical Pathophysiology, 1442
Natural History, 1443
Diagnosis, 1444
Associated Conditions, 1446
Treatment, 1448

NONRHEUMATIC MITRAL STENOSIS, 1450
Degenerative MS Related to Mitral Annular Calcification, 1450
Radiotherapy-Induced MS, 1452
MS Following Interventional and Surgical Therapies, 1453

CLASSIC REFERENCES, 1453

REFERENCES, 1453

Mitral stenosis (MS), known in the literature since at least the 1669 description by John Mayow and a major manifestation of rheumatic heart disease (RHD), remains an important problem worldwide. While the developed world has all but eliminated RHD, it continues to be a major cause of heart disease, morbidity, and mortality in the low and middle income countries (LMICs; 5.6 billion people or 80% of humanity) (see Chapter 81), especially affecting children and young adults in their most productive age.[1] It has, however, not disappeared entirely from the West—rheumatic MS (RMS) is occasionally seen in some under-resourced communities and among immigrants from areas with high prevalence of rheumatic fever; more importantly, nonrheumatic forms of MS are being increasingly seen—the degenerative MS (DMS) associated with mitral annular calcification (MAC), MS after radiation to the chest, and MS after surgical or percutaneous mitral valve interventions. Classic RMS can be prevented with good secondary prophylaxis for acute rheumatic fever (ARF) and can also be diagnosed as well as treated with relative ease. Nonrheumatic MS is more difficult to diagnose and may need specialized treatment options. It is, therefore, very important to recognize and understand multiple etiologic subsets of MS since they have very different natural history and strategies of prevention and treatment.

EPIDEMIOLOGY AND SECULAR TRENDS

Rheumatic Mitral Stenosis

There is, unfortunately, scarcity of good data on the prevalence of RHD and MS. A 2015 Global Burden of Disease modeling estimate puts the total prevalence of RHD at approximately 33.4 million cases (see Chapter 81),[1] and the mitral valve is involved most commonly in RHD. Subclinical disease, detectable by echocardiographic screening, is seven to eight times more common than clinically detectable disease[2] and would reveal an even larger prevalence of MS.

RMS is now largely concentrated among the LMICs that are endemic for group A Streptococcus (GAS) pharyngitis and ARF.[3] ARF-related carditis often occurs among children in the second decade and MS follows a couple of decades later. Classic RMS is more common in women, even though ARF is equally common in both sexes. Repeated episodes of untreated GAS pharyngeal infection accelerate its progression. The mechanism for valve damage is not clear but is thought to be autoimmune response to GAS moieties that mimic valve antigens and involves both humoral and cellular immune mechanisms.[4] There are some differences in how RMS behaves in endemic (South and East Asia, sub-Saharan Africa, and indigenous populations of Oceania) and nonendemic regions.[5] The former seesa more aggressive course: Patients are symptomatic at a younger age, often presenting in the second to fourth decade, approximately 75% of the patients don't recall an ARF episode, and the disease progresses more rapidly with higher mitral valve gradients that need earlier intervention.[3] Patients in the nonendemic regions seem to present with a more indolent course: They have slower progression and present much later (fifth to seventh decades), with suboptimal morphology for intervention, generally lower gradients and multiple other comorbidities (see Classic References, Shaw et al.).

Nonrheumatic Mitral Stenosis

DMS is most common in the Western world and is mainly MAC related,[6] although MS after mitral valve interventions[7] is increasingly seen in tertiary care centers. MAC-associated DMS has not been studied as extensively as RMS and its prevalence is not known, but it is thought to occur in about 1% to 2% of patients with MAC.[8] In a recent series, DMS due to MAC constituted 41% of patients with severe MS on echocardiography.[6] DMS is also being recognized increasingly (11% to 18%) in patients with aortic stenosis (AS) referred for transcatheter aortic valve replacement (TAVR). Other causes of MS are extremely rare and do not have good epidemiologic data.

DEFINITION OF DISEASE AND SEVERITY

Increased resistance at any level in the atrioventricular circuit (net AV resistance) can generate the MS physiology: obstruction to left atrial (LA) outflow and pressure gradient across the mitral valve, with consequent remodeling in the LA and pulmonary bed. Understanding this complexity is important since it may call for therapeutic approaches to DMS that differ from those applicable to patients with RMS.[9-11] The normal mitral valve area (MVA) is ≥4.0 cm^2. A gradient across the mitral valve starts to form with reduction in MVA to 2.0 cm^2, considered mild MS, and symptoms begin to appear, initially with exercise. Symptoms, more consistently develop at ≤1.5 cm^2 and are associated with a 5 to 10 mm Hg gradient. Significant hemodynamic changes (gradients in excess of 10 mm Hg) and resting symptoms are common at MVA ≤1.0 cm^2.[9] Guidelines consider "severe" MS based on when symptoms occur and where intervention can improve them, and ≤1.5 cm^2 is the recommended threshold for this.[9,10] However, some patients can develop significant symptoms with just moderate MS (MVA between 1.5 and 2.0 cm^2) and can be selectively considered for intervention if other causes for their symptoms are excluded. Gradients depend on many hemodynamic variables including heart rate or flow and are not generally used to define severity. MAC-associated DMS currently uses the same definition as RMS, but the relation between MVA, gradients, and symptoms is much different than in RMS and might need an updated definition. MS due to a prosthetic valve is generally defined as resting mean valve gradient ≥ 5 mm Hg, peak mitral inflow velocity ≥ 1.9 msec, or effective orifice area ≤ 2 cm^2.

RHEUMATIC MITRAL STENOSIS

Pathology

Cardiac valve involvement in ARF starts with inflammation at the valve edges. It progresses to leaflet thickening and retraction along with variable degrees of calcification, all of which can lead to loss of flexibility. The main abnormality is fusion of the mitral leaflets in critical areas at their medial and lateral edges (commissural fusion), and the valve opening, narrowest at the valve tips, becomes a rigid structure that is oval or fish mouth shaped (Fig. 75.1; see also Fig. 16.32). The proximal and mid parts of the leaflets preserve some flexibility which results in the hockey stick appearance of the anterior leaflet in diastole. More severe disease extends into the subvalvular apparatus creating a dense mat of fused and shortened chordae that adds an additional level of resistance. Understanding pathology is crucial for clinical management.

Clinical Pathophysiology

The clinical consequences of MS depend on the degree of stenosis and consequent elevation in LA pressure (Fig. 75.2).[11] RMS is characterized by commissural fusion rather than just stiff valve leaflets and hence a relatively fixed orifice, and unlike AS, changes very little with varying hemodynamic conditions. An increased LA pressure is then needed to maintain left ventricular (LV) filling and preserve cardiac output.

Left Atrial Pressure

While MVA defines anatomic severity, it is the LA pressure that determines clinical symptoms[11] and improvement after definitive therapies like percutaneous balloon mitral valvuloplasty (BMV; see Fig. 78.1) or surgery.[11,12] LA pressure (measured indirectly as the gradient across the mitral valve), however, is highly variable (Fig. 75.3) depending on the time allowed for diastolic filling (heart rate) and flow (cardiac output). Tachycardia is one of the most important factors in increasing LA pressures since it significantly reduces diastolic filling time and compromises forward flow, which is immediately seen as high mitral valve gradients and worsening symptoms. Atrial contraction helps overcome the resistance at the mitral valve level and preserve forward flow in MS—not surprisingly, the loss of atrial contraction and tachycardia during atrial fibrillation (AF) can precipitate clinical worsening even in patients previously asymptomatic. Since the gradient across the mitral valve increases as a square of the flow, small increases in the latter can have large effects on the gradient and its resulting symptoms, as seen in pregnancy, severe anemia, thyrotoxicosis, systemic infection, and other hyperdynamic states.

Chamber compliance (LA and to some extent, LV) also plays a role in development of symptoms, abnormal exercise hemodynamics, pulmonary hypertension (PAH), and degree of relief after relief of stenosis. A newly recognized subset termed low gradient MS (MVA <1.5 cm^2, mean gradient <10 mm Hg, and significant symptoms) is now being recognized in the developed world and may account for a significant proportion of patients coming to BMV in some centers. Some patients with these hemodynamic findings—constituting 11% of BMV patients in one series[12]—appear to have a physiology akin to heart failure with preserved ejection fraction superimposed on MS (see Chapter 51) and is characterized by older individuals with normal intrinsic LV contractility, decreased LV compliance, and high arterial afterload. They respond suboptimally to BMV, highlighting that reduced LV compliance may explain symptoms that do not respond to treatment of MS alone.[12]

Backward transmission of high LA pressures results in pulmonary venous hypertension and increased lung water; lung congestion explains exercise intolerance and dyspnea (and pulmonary edema in the most severe cases), and its relief, with diuretics or definitive MS treatment, is associated with immediate clinical benefit through reversing these changes. Signs of low cardiac output (due to severe flow restriction at the mitral valve and PAH) appear only at a much later stage.

Some compensatory mechanisms alter the relationship between LA pressure increase and symptoms. Chronically elevated LA pressure results in alveolar/interstitial thickening that limits alveolar edema, and increased lymphatic drainage helps redistribute alveolar fluid. This can improve symptoms for a short period before progressive MS overcomes these mechanisms. The development of PAH also ameliorates these symptoms but at the expense of right heart overload and possibly low cardiac output. Long-standing adverse changes in the lung and pulmonary vasculature can persist after relief of MS, explaining the lack of a direct relationship between hemodynamic improvement and changes in pulmonary function or exercise capacity. Prolonged elevation of LA pressure and LA remodeling can result in LA fibrosis that affects LA compliance. This may not be reversible after BMV, and low net AV compliance, which reflects the LA-LV as a unit, predicts both need for intervention and worse prognosis after BMV.

Left Atrial Function

The LA cannot empty readily in MS and remodels as a consequence of both increased pressure and volume. LA function is variably affected depending on severity of MS and degree of fibrosis and can be a form of atrial myopathy. LA volume is increased and LA emptying fraction is reduced. LA strain abnormalities are an early marker for LA dysfunction, can be seen in asymptomatic subjects with moderate MS, and are common in both RMS and DMS. Conduit strain is affected particularly in RMS and both reservoir strain (reflecting LA filling) and conduit strain (a marker for early diastolic emptying) are reduced, especially in patients with MAC. Abnormal peak atrial longitudinal strain (PALS) is associated with reduced

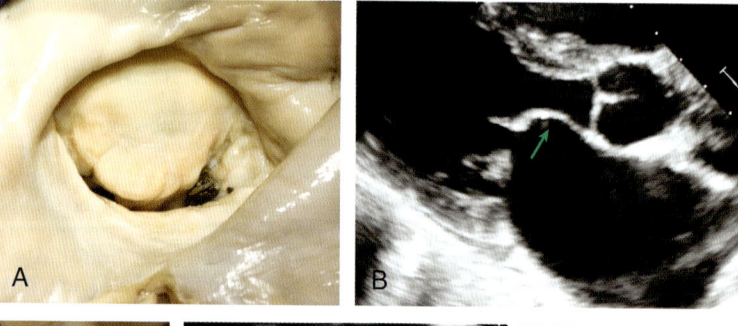
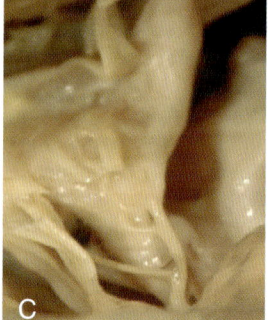
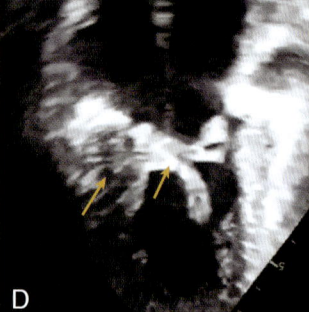
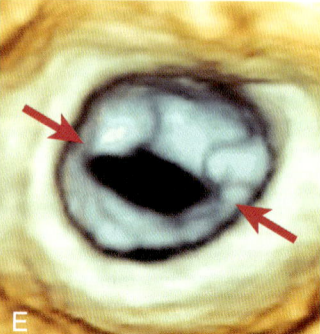

FIGURE 75.1 Pathology of mitral stenosis and imaging correlations. **A,** Fused commissures are the hallmark of rheumatic MS. Fusion starts along the valve tips and progresses to limit the opening from both ends. **B,** Some pliability of the rest of the leaflet causes a hockey stick appearance of the anterior leaflet on 2D echocardiography (*arrow*). **C,** Fibrosis and fusion extend to the sub-valvular apparatus resulting in matted and retracted chordae, which (**D**) can be seen on echocardiography (*arrows*). **E,** Fusion of the commissures (*arrows*) creates a fish-mouth appearance as demonstrated on 3D echocardiography

functional capacity, predicts future AF, and identifies adverse prognosis in asymptomatic subjects with moderate MS.

Left Ventricular Function

LV function is abnormal in some studies and is hypothesized to be due to multiple mechanisms (inflammatory process, tethering due to the rigid valve apparatus, altered LV compliance). However, it is not prominent in most patients with RMS but may be more prevalent in DMS due to coexisting comorbidities. LV deformation, a more sensitive parameter for LV function, however, is commonly abnormal in RMS and improves rapidly after BMV. Deformation parameters are normal when indexed to LV end-diastolic volume, suggesting this to be an effect of loading conditions rather than intrinsic myocardial dysfunction. Preliminary evidence suggests that impaired LV global longitudinal strain (GLS) might predict progression in milder forms of MS and outcomes after BMV over and above traditional measures. Post-BMV improvement in GLS is smaller in patients with suboptimal outcomes and often associated with an increase in LV end-diastolic pressure (LVEDP) after BMV, suggesting some degree of intrinsic diastolic dysfunction. Nevertheless, there is no immediately actionable clinical correlate for this subtle degree of LV dysfunction. LV diastolic dysfunction is difficult to diagnose in patients with MS and most indices including those with speckle tracking cannot accurately detect elevated LVEDP, an important marker of poor outcomes after BMV.

Right Ventricular Function

Overt RV dysfunction occurs late in the course of MS and is often a consequence of PAH. RV enlargement and elevated PA pressures track the severity of MS. These findings convey adverse prognosis even in patients treated with BMV or surgery. RV strain is emerging as a useful marker for subtle RV dysfunction even before onset of other signs, and it improves rapidly after BMV. Whether deformation imaging can be used to fine tune timing of intervention is not known at present.

Natural History

The stages of RMS as defined in the 2020 ACC/AHA guidelines for the management of patients with valvular heart disease[9] are shown in Table 75.1. Unlike rheumatic mitral regurgitation (MR) that starts proximate to the ARF episode, MS is a late presentation, is unlikely to regress, and progresses in severity in the majority of patients. Data on the natural history of untreated MS are very old[11] and have little relevance for patients seen today. In addition, the natural history of MS has diverged between LMICs (RMS) and the developed world (very little RMS and increasing DMS). A few things to take away from these studies include the following:

1. Valve area in RMS decreases approximately 0.09 cm^2 per year. Age, hemodynamic severity at diagnosis, and degree of valve deformity seem to predict progression. About a third show higher rate of progression, but this is not easily predictable from traditional clinical variables. Recurrent episodes of ARF mediate faster progression in LMICs but this evolution can occur even without repeated episodes suggesting some role for other factors like hemodynamic damage and scarring.

2. Symptoms are an important trigger for definitive therapy and have strong prognostic value. It takes approximately one to two decades to develop significant MS. About half of the

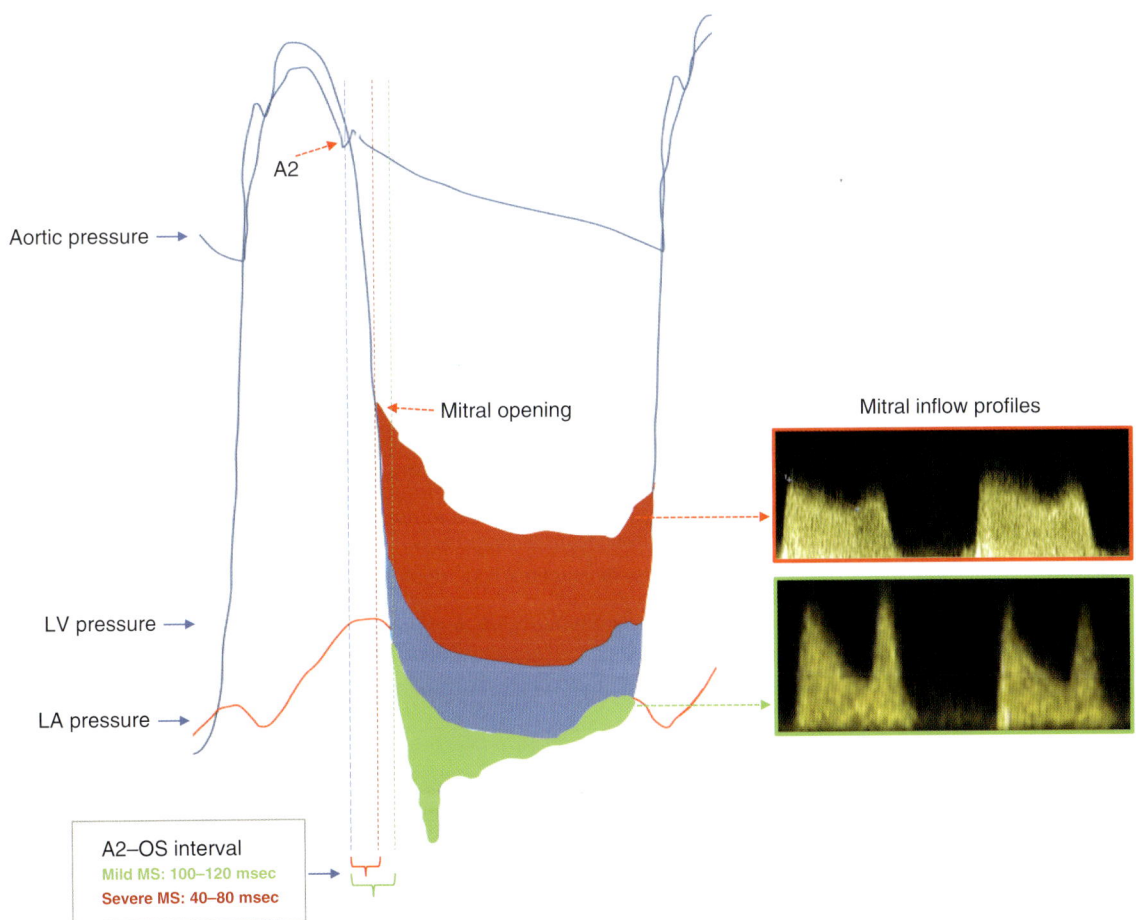

FIGURE 75.2 Hemodynamics of mitral stenosis. Severity of MS determines the magnitude of the diastolic pressure gradient between left atrium (LA) and left ventricle (LV). As MS progress from mild (*green*) to moderate (*blue*) to severe (*red*), the increasing pressure gradient causes the opening snap (OS) to occur earlier, thus shortening the time interval between aortic valve closure (A2) and OS. The corresponding Doppler inflow profiles show longer deceleration time and reduction in atrial augmentation as LA pressure increases.

asymptomatic patients with MS then develop symptoms over the next decade and most are symptomatic in two decades after onset of MS.
3. Symptomatic patients with severe MS do poorly without intervention, with a mortality that varies from 8% to 13% per year in the first 5 years. Severe symptoms denote worse prognosis—untreated, only 15% of patients in New York Heart Association (NYHA) functional Class IV and 60% in NYHA Class III survived for 5 years. Treating severe symptomatic MS with surgery in the pre-BMV era improved this otherwise dismal natural history.
4. Patients can first present with AF; almost 20% presented with an embolic episode in the past but early detection of AF in MS and aggressive use of oral anticoagulants (OACs) has markedly reduced this complication.
5. Latent RHD, diagnosed through screening echocardiography, identifies patients at risk for progression, especially without prophylaxis (see Chapter 81). Approximately 15% to 20% will progress especially if they have clear structural heart disease.

Diagnosis
Clinical Presentation
Clinical features of RMS, to some extent, depend on where patients live. There is no better description of signs and symptoms of classic MS than in the famous writings of Paul Wood (see Classic References, Wood) but that now apply mainly to subjects in locations with high endemic burden of ARF and suboptimal care. These patients are younger, have higher gradients, have lower MVA, and have low prevalence of AF and thus present with more typical signs and symptoms of MS. Patients from higher income countries[11-14] are often likely to be older, hypertensive, overweight and in AF; they can have comorbidities that can obscure the classic signs and symptoms of MS and present with lower gradients.

Dyspnea, initially on exertion and then at rest, is the usual presentation in MS. Paroxysmal nocturnal dyspnea and orthopnea are seen in severe symptomatic MS but may become less common with longer duration of untreated illness, as compensatory mechanisms in the lung and pulmonary circulation attenuate alveolar edema. Transition to the symptomatic phase is often precipitated by tachycardia or conditions generating increased flow across the valve—AF and pregnancy commonly bring asymptomatic patients to attention in LMICs. Clinical presentation is influenced by age, other comorbidities (like diastolic dysfunction), and presence of PAH. Onset of significant PAH, or aggressive use of diuretics and beta blockers, may reduce dyspnea but increase fatigue and symptoms of low cardiac output. Traditionally, a rise in LA pressure during exercise was thought to mediate exercise intolerance, but the correlation between MVA, gradient, and exercise capacity is imperfect. Newer data[15] suggest that exercise intolerance is mainly due to a combination of abnormalities comparable to those in patients with

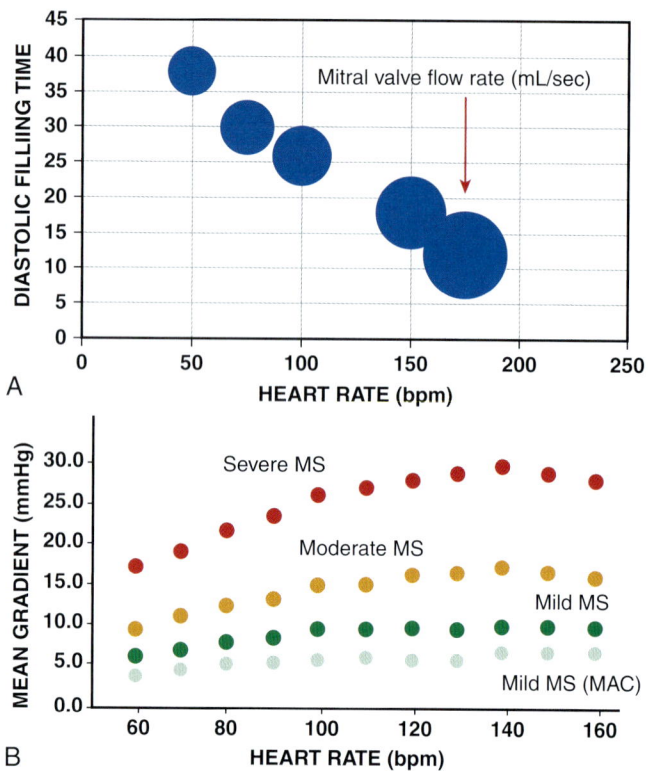

FIGURE 75.3 Relation between heart rate, diastolic filling time, and pressure gradient in mitral stenosis. **A,** Increasing heart rate causes sequential reduction in diastolic filling period. **B,** The reduced diastolic filling time at increasing heart rates is associated with exacerbation of the mitral pressure gradient, which is most marked with severe MS. Thus, higher heart rates are likely to precipitate symptoms.

TABLE 75.1 Stages of Mitral Stenosis (MS)

STAGE	DEFINITION	VALVE ANATOMY	VALVE HEMODYNAMICS*	HEMODYNAMIC CONSEQUENCES	SYMPTOMS
A	At risk for MS	Mild valve doming during diastole	Normal transmitral flow velocity	None	None
B	Progressive MS	Rheumatic valve changes with commissural fusion and diastolic doming of mitral valve leaflets Planimetered MVA >1.5 cm²	Increased transmitral flow velocities MVA >1.5 cm² Diastolic pressure half-time <150 msec	Mild to moderate LA enlargement Normal pulmonary pressure at rest	None
C	Asymptomatic severe MS	Rheumatic valve changes with commissural fusion and diastolic doming of mitral valve leaflets Planimetered MVA ≤1.5 cm²	MVA ≤1.5 cm² Diastolic pressure half-time ≥150 msec	Severe LA enlargement Elevated PASP >50 mm Hg	None
D	Symptomatic severe MS	Rheumatic valve changes with commissural fusion and diastolic doming of mitral valve leaflets Planimetered MVA ≤1.5 cm²	MVA ≤1.5 cm² Diastolic pressure half-time ≥150 msec	Severe LA enlargement Elevated PASP >50 mm Hg	Decreased exercise tolerance Exertional dyspnea

*The transmitral mean pressure gradient should be obtained to determine the full hemodynamic effect of the MS and usually is greater than 5 to 10 mm Hg in severe MS; however, because of the variability of the mean pressure gradient with heart rate and forward flow, it has not been included in the criteria for severity.
LA, Left atrial; *MVA,* mitral valve area; *PASP,* pulmonary artery systolic pressure.
From Otto CM, et al. 2020 AHA/ACC guideline for the management of patients with valvular heart disease: a report of the American College of Cardiology/American Heart Association Task Force on Practice Guidelines. J Am Coll Cardiol 2021;77:e25-197.

heart failure (chronotropic incompetence, abnormal stroke volume reserve, impaired ventilation, and low peak A–VO$_2$ difference). Palpitations, often a consequence of AF, are seen in the later stages of the disease and increase with age. Pulmonary edema is now seen rarely, except in LMICs, especially in pregnant patients with previously undetected disease. Severe PAH can result in angina or symptoms of right heart failure. The dilated LA (Ortner syndrome—hoarseness due to compression of the recurrent laryngeal nerve) or pulmonary artery can cause pressure effects. Stroke (especially in undetected AF) and hemoptysis (from pulmonary venous hypertension or ruptured bronchial veins) were not uncommon symptoms in the past but are now seen infrequently.

Physical Examination

Bedside physical signs of RMS can be divided into those arising from the pathologic mitral valve itself and those that are consequences of severe MS. The former includes a loud S_1 (and a tapping apex), the opening snap (OS), and mid-diastolic murmur with presystolic accentuation. The latter include the usual signs of AF, pulmonary venous and arterial hypertension, tricuspid regurgitation (TR), right heart failure, and, in late stages, systemic hypoperfusion.

The S_1 is often loud with a pliable mitral valve, but significant leaflet restriction (with fibrosis, calcification or subvalvular pathology) can decrease its intensity. The OS is a classic feature of RMS and arises at the peak of a rapid and forced opening of the restricted mitral leaflet by high LA pressure. It denotes two important things: (1) its presence along with a loud S_1 implies a pliable mitral valve that is likely to be a good candidate for BMV; (2) its timing helps in assessing severity of MS (see Fig. 75.2)—a higher LA pressure opens the mitral valve earlier, and, therefore, time between aortic closure sound and mitral OS (A2-OS interval) is inversely proportional to the severity of MS. As with a loud S_1, increasing calcification and rigidity of the body of the leaflets diminishes OS and might indicate unfavorable anatomy for percutaneous intervention.

The murmur in MS is difficult to hear and needs practice and a quiet room for best detection; tachycardia with mild exercise can bring out the findings. It is a low pitched diastolic rumble, best heard at the apex with the bell of the stethoscope while the patient is in the left lateral position. Its onset follows the OS, but may be heard just during presystolic accentuation in mild MS and gradually increases in length with increasing severity of stenosis. A presystolic accentuation (coinciding with atrial contraction) is prominent unless the patient is in AF. The RMS murmur is less discernable in patients with obesity, chronic obstructive pulmonary disease (COPD), or AF with a rapid ventricular response. The length of the murmur correlates with severity of MS but the intensity does not. Severe MS can occasionally have a thrill. S_3 (which occurs later in diastole, is softer and not generally confused with OS) and S_4 are not usually audible and their presence excludes severe MS. MR murmurs are not common in severe MS although a TR murmur (in the left lower sternal area that increases in inspiration) might be prominent in patients with significant PAH and RV enlargement. Some murmurs may mimic MS—those from high flow across the mitral valve (severe MR, some shunts like ventricular septal defect, or patent ductus arteriosus with high Qp/Qs or other high flow conditions) can be differentiated from MS by their clinical context, short murmurs, lack of an OS, and often the presence of an S_3. The Austin Flint murmur of aortic regurgitation (AR) usually does not have a loud S_1, OS, or presystolic accentuation and there are clear signs of significant AR (see Chapter 73). Tricuspid stenosis can accompany MS and has a diastolic murmur that increases with inspiration. Physical examination also helps to address two pertinent clinical questions at the bedside: how severe is the MS and how suitable is the valve for BMV. A short A2-OS interval followed by a long murmur starting earlier in diastole with prominent presystolic accentuation and signs of PAH or RV overload in a patient with limiting symptoms suggests severe MS. Loud S_1 and prominent OS indicates a pliable valve that could be suitable for BMV.

Echocardiography

Echocardiography is the mainstay of diagnosis in all forms of MS[11] (see Chapter 16)—it is the best modality to detect the presence and severity of LA outflow obstruction and evaluate its severity as well as hemodynamic consequences (Fig. 75.4; see also Fig. 16.34). It identifies the etiology of MS and is crucial for determining suitability of various interventions. Finally, it allows evaluation of other valve and myocardial disease that might affect the course of MS.

Each etiology has characteristic echo signatures but questions about severity of obstruction (MVA and gradients) are common to all conditions. MVA is best assessed with planimetry in all patients with RMS since it is the most accurate method if done correctly (tracing the inner edge at valve tips in mid-diastole of a completely seen, enface orifice of good image quality) and less subject to effect of changing loading conditions. However, two-dimensional (2D) echo may underestimate severity and is less optimal for understanding anatomy (e.g., commissural morphology pre and postintervention); 3D overcomes many of these limitations, is more reproducible, and should be used where possible (see Fig. 16.33).[16] Planimetry is not a good option for MVA in DMS and the continuity equation may work better. Pressure half time is useful to assess valve area in RMS but is not accurate in valves with prior intervention or in DMS since it is influenced by chamber compliance and multiple other factors. The proximal isovelocity surface area (PISA) method and continuity equation (see Fig. 16.35) can provide good measurements but are more complex and the latter is not useful if there is either AR or MR. MS following previous intervention like BMV poses special issues, and planimetry, especially with 3D, is the best option.

Gradients measured from Doppler tracings are reasonably accurate in reflecting the hemodynamic conditions at that given moment and are suitable for all kinds of MS, including DMS. It is important to recognize that gradients are heart rate and flow dependent and thus

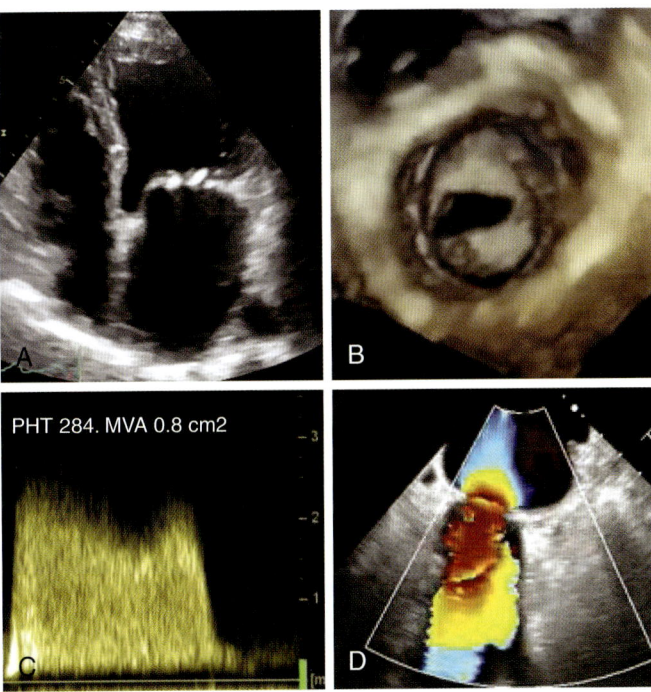

FIGURE 75.4 Echocardiography for diagnosing MS. 2D and 3D echocardiography is the best method to define morphology, assess severity (valve area and gradients), complications like left atrial thrombus and other valve pathology. **A,** Thickened mitral valve leaflets and large left atrium identified on four-chamber 2D echo view. **B,** Commissural fusion and fish mouth deformity seen on 3D echo. **C,** High inflow velocities, longer pressure half time, persisting gradient during diastasis and reduction in atrial contribution are characteristics of severe MS. **D,** Transesophageal echo showing clear flow convergence (PISA shell) with higher velocities.

could change appreciably between studies. All echo measurements should be interpreted in the correct clinical context, and discrepancies between MVA, gradients, and symptoms should be adjudicated thoughtfully by appropriately synthesizing multiple parameters. Transesophageal echocardiography (TEE), both 2D and 3D (see Chapter 16), provides greater details of valve anatomy and is very useful for excluding LA clot, although computed tomography (CT) can substitute for this. TEE is often used during BMV to guide the procedure as well as assess immediate results and complications.

An important role of echocardiography is to assess suitability for intervention, and at least four scoring systems for RMS are in use. Scoring systems have limitations including semiquantitative assessment and suboptimal reproducibility, and they do not reflect the contribution of each individual component of adverse outcome with equal accuracy. No single scoring method is preferable over another,[16] and ultimately, most centers use scores with which they are comfortable. The most often used score is the Wilkins score that combines leaflet mobility and calcification along with leaflet and subvalvular thickening into a numerical score (see Table 16.9 and Classic References, Wilkins et al.). It has good predictive accuracy for both short- and long-term outcome (see Fig. 78.2) but misses the effect of commissural calcification and the degree of preexisting MR and is not very effective in prognosticating the midrange of scores. Patients with suboptimal scores are not automatically destined for bad outcomes, and many centers successfully perform BMV in moderately suboptimal scores. Leaflet and commissural calcification and subvalvular pathology might have a disproportionate effect on outcomes and permit better triage of patients even with optimal Wilkins scores. A newer score, incorporating leaflet displacement and asymmetry in commissural remodeling,[17] was found to be better at predicting procedural outcome than Wilkins scores, and another one using 3D might be capable of identifying structural abnormalities better.

Additional Diagnostic Investigations
EKG and Chest X-Ray
Both EKG and chest x-ray can show consequences of MS in the form of LA enlargement (P mitrale) and RV pressure overload. In the later stages, the EKG can show AF and x-ray can show the presence and degree of pulmonary congestion.

Exercise Testing in MS
Exercise testing can be performed safely in most patients with MS and plays an important role in evaluating patients with severe MS who are asymptomatic or have equivocal symptoms and those who are symptomatic with moderate MS.[9,10] Stress echo can document exercise limitation and resolve discordance between symptoms and clinical or echocardiographic severity, and finding exercise-induced PAH can indicate need for BMV (see Chapter 16). In asymptomatic patients, exercise testing can also predict prognosis in multiple forms of MS including RMS, DMS, and prosthetic valve MS.[7] Dobutamine stress has been used in the past but is not currently a good option in most patients.

Other Diagnostic Tests
CT or cardiac magnetic resonance can provide information about valve anatomy and function but are rarely needed and are used when there is some other indication for them. Cardiac catheterization is rarely needed unless there are other specific clinical questions that it can best answer (e.g., coronary artery disease).

Associated Conditions
Atrial Fibrillation
AF is a dreaded complication of MS—it is common, increases with age and severity of MS, worsens hemodynamic as well as clinical status, is an important determinant of the high risk of stroke, and can limit survival in patients with RMS.[5,11,18] AF seems to be driven by both LA stretch and possibly inflammation, which together can cause structural and electrical remodeling (see Chapter 66). LA size

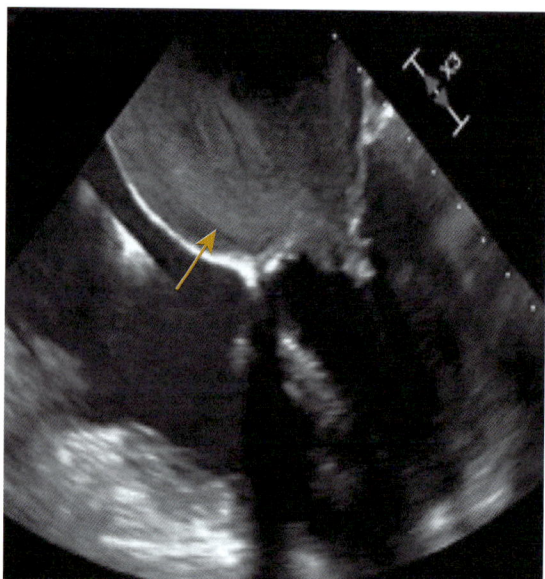

FIGURE 75.5 Severe MS promotes left atrial stasis. Blood stasis (*arrow*) promotes left atrial thrombosis and predisposes to embolic stroke.

and hemodynamic abnormalities relate to its occurrence and persistence. LA fibrosis is common, and subtle changes in LA function in the form of reduced PALS might precede onset of AF. AF worsens symptoms through a loss of atrial contribution to LV filling and cardiac output as well as the effect of fast heart rates. It facilitates stroke risk by further promoting stasis (Fig. 75.5). Age has a strong influence on its occurrence. AF is uncommon (<5%) in young patients with RMS coming for BMV in the LMICs but is very prevalent (>60%) in the aging MS population in the West. The incidence of new AF in RMS is unclear but almost 20% developed AF over a median of 6-year follow-up in a recent study[19]; the average annual event rate was 3.5 % per year and increased to 6.0 % per year with even mildly increased LA size and pressure, with a correspondingly high event rate (embolism and death). Larger LA dimension and MVA of 1.5 cm^2 or less were good predictors for new-onset AF. The combination of MS and AF poses considerable risk for embolic events; patients with MS and AF are many times more likely to have embolic complications than MS without AF or AF without MS, and risk may be as high as patients with prosthetic valves—consequently, OACs (warfarin and not direct acting OACs) are strongly recommended in such patients irrespective of lesion severity or $CHADS_2$ VASc scores.[9,10] Threshold to use OACs is lower than in other forms of valvular heart disease since AF can be intermittent, and even transient episodes (<30 sec) detected on ambulatory monitoring significantly increase risk of thromboembolic events. Moreover, patients with MS have been occasionally shown to have evidence of LA thrombus or may experience embolic events even when in sinus rhythm. The European guidelines even recommend considering OACs in patients with RMS in sinus rhythm if they have dense spontaneous LA echocardiographic contrast (see Fig. 75.5) and/or LA dilation.[10] Rate control is difficult to achieve in RMS but strategies are similar to those in the other patients with AF. Ivabradine has been used with some success. Restoring sinus rhythm is more likely in the presence of a small LA, short duration of AF, and less severe MS. Rhythm control improves quality of life and exercise tolerance, especially in those with small LA and durable results. Unless needed urgently, electrical cardioversion is best done after BMV. AF with MS has a high recurrence after cardioversion and antiarrhythmic drugs, especially amiodarone, are often needed for maintaining sinus rhythm. Pulmonary vein isolation is not as well studied in patients with RMS as in those with AF without MS, but there is some evidence of efficacy in these patients. Restoring sinus rhythm with a surgical maze procedure increases chances of remaining in sinus rhythm and reduces risk of embolism. AF does not appreciably affect success of BMV but adversely influences long-term event-free survival. AF is not consistently prevented with BMV, supporting efforts to reduce its occurrence in the first place; however, BMV in patients with AF is associated with less systemic embolism. Nonetheless, patients continue to have significant residual risk (approximately 20% embolic event rate in the next 5 years) and need adequate anticoagulation.

Pulmonary Hypertension

PAH is quite common in patients with symptomatic RMS, but prevalence depends on age, as well as duration and severity of MS. Some degree of PAH is seen in almost 80% of patients coming to BMV in various series and one-third have systolic PA pressure (PAP) greater than 50 mm Hg. The prevalence may be even higher for PAH during exercise or if the newest PAH definition is used (see Chapter 88). While primarily dependent on the severity of MS, mitral gradients correlate imperfectly with PAP, and net AV compliance might better reflect its genesis. PAH often is post capillary (mean PAP ≥25 mm Hg, mean pulmonary artery wedge pressure (PAWP) >15 mm Hg, low transpulmonary gradient, pulmonary vascular resistance (PVR) ≤3 WU) and is a consequence of pulmonary venous hypertension. However, chronically elevated PAP, especially in some hyperresponders, can mediate structural remodeling in the pulmonary arterial system, resulting in a combination of pre and postcapillary hypertension (mean PAP ≥25 mm Hg, mean PAWP >15 mm Hg, PVR >3 WU). Remodeling in PAH is mediated by mechanical stretch as well as inflammatory cytokine and growth factors and affects both arterioles and venules. PAH mediates RV dysfunction and TR, but the correlation with RV failure is not linear. PAH adversely affects long-term prognosis, even in patients treated with BMV or surgical mitral valve repair or replacement. However, patients with severe PAH have good immediate results with BMV in that PAH resolves in most patients quite rapidly and continues to improve further in the next few months unless there is suboptimal relief of MS, worsening MR, or valve restenosis. PAH may persist in a small proportion of patients despite optimal BMV results, and this might depend on whether the remodeling was reversible (mainly involving venules with vessel edema, or loose fibrosis) or irreversible (severe arteriolar hyperplasia and plexiform lesions), but these factors are difficult to identify a priori. Given its adverse influence, PAH is a class IIa trigger for therapeutic intervention in asymptomatic patients with PA systolic pressure >50 mm Hg in the both the U.S. and European guidelines.[9,10] While some drugs can influence PAH temporarily, relief of MS is the only proven treatment.

Pregnancy

Worldwide, MS is one of the most common valve conditions in pregnant women with structural heart disease.[20,21] In the European Registry of Pregnancy and Cardiac Disease (ROPAC), 10% of cases were MS, and MS was first detected during pregnancy in 25%.[20] This problem is magnified in those living in the world's poorest countries such as sub-Saharan Africa and the indigenous people of Oceania. Pregnancy poses a special burden in patients with MS given the unfavorable confluence of tachycardia and increased cardiac output. Cardiac output peaks in the second trimester (see Chapter 92), and patients with MS are often first detected at this time or present with worsening symptoms around 24 to 30 weeks of gestation. Delivery is the other dangerous time period; a third of pregnant patients developing heart failure due to MS become symptomatic around the time of delivery and in the first week postpartum, often in the first 72 hours, due to high LA pressures caused by increased venous return following relief of inferior vena cava (IVC) compression and autotransfusion of blood from the utero-placental circuit after delivery. Pregnant patients with mild MS usually tolerate the stress of pregnancy but need careful attention since 16% to 24% of patients can develop symptomatic heart failure.[20] Complications occur mainly in patients with symptomatic (NYHA II or greater) moderate to severe MS, of whom almost 40% to 50% require hospitalization, mainly for heart failure, compared to a quarter in those with asymptomatic moderate MS. Moderate or severe MS should, therefore, be detected and corrected if possible before pregnancy, as patients have four times fewer adverse events if intervention is undertaken prior to conception.[20] The modified WHO risk stratification algorithm appropriately classifies untreated severe MS as a Class IV risk (pregnancy is contraindicated)

Diagnosis and Treatment

Diagnosis of MS remains largely the same as in the nonpregnant patient but with some nuances. Physiologic changes of pregnancy (peripheral vasodilation, hyperdynamic circulation, increased blood volume, tachycardia, anemia, elevated diaphragm, compression of IVC) can cause dyspnea, leg edema, loud S_1, and mitral murmurs (see Chapter 92)—these can mimic RMS but normal pregnancy is not accompanied by prominent diastolic murmurs or an OS; echocardiography remains diagnostic even though the gradient might be affected by hemodynamic conditions. Pressure half time is not as validated in this population and planimetry remains the reference standard as in the nonpregnant patient. There are few good prospective data but systematic reviews suggest that severe MS during pregnancy is adverse for both the mother and the child. Age, significant PAH, heart failure, and reduced ejection fraction are factors associated with poor maternal and fetal outcome. Maternal mortality is increased (3% range with severe MS and 0% to 2% with moderate MS), and is especially worse with PAH and in resource poor countries. There is an excess of stillbirth and neonatal death (2% to 4%) as well as preterm birth (up to 20%), related to compromised uteroplacental flow. Much of the morbidity can be minimized with adequate prepregnancy evaluation/counseling and early access to better care. Activity is allowed as tolerated but those with severe PAH might need some restriction.[21] Management of tachycardia and diuresis for dyspnea are the foundation of conservative treatment. AF is not uncommon in pregnant patients with severe MS (16%) and can precipitate symptoms, pulmonary edema, and rarely a cerebral vascular accident.[20] Drugs used to control rate, rhythm, and thrombotic risk have unique effects on the fetus. Beta blockers can cause fetal bradycardia, hypoglycemia, and a mild increase in premature births, but no major congenital abnormalities have been conclusively identified. Intrauterine growth restriction has been described especially for atenolol used in the second trimester. Calcium channel blockers can be used for rate control (FDA Category D) but amiodarone is contraindicated. Diuretics can affect uteroplacental perfusion and amniotic volume but have been used with few major adverse effects. Direct current cardioversion can be performed, if needed urgently. Anticoagulation needs thoughtful planning and use per guidelines.[9,22]

A significant portion of the excess mortality associated with severe MS occurs during delivery. Careful planning and proper medical supervision, however, results in good outcomes in the majority of patients. Vaginal delivery is the best option for patients with mild MS and mild symptoms (NYHA I-II) and asymptomatic moderate MS. Caesarean delivery is indicated in those with severe symptoms (NYHA III-IV) or moderate symptoms with significant PAH, and when BMV could not be undertaken previously.[10]

Percutaneous Balloon Mitral Valvuloplasty

BMV is safe and very effective for treating severe MS during pregnancy. Success rates are very high with minimal mortality (except in patients with florid heart failure), fluoroscopy times are under 10 minutes, and gradients fall immediately with excellent symptomatic improvement. Fetal development and growth and development of the child are unaffected. These results are far superior to those obtained with surgical intervention in pregnant patients. Not surprisingly, BMV is the treatment of choice for managing such patients but the success depends on the time of intervention. BMV before 20 weeks of gestation has poorer fetal outcomes and should be delayed as much as reasonable, optimally to after 24 weeks. Standard criteria for intrapregnancy BMV for MS include severe MS, NYHA Class III or IV symptoms while on optimal medical treatment, and suitable valve anatomy. Contraindications remain the same as in nonpregnant patients. Mitral valve surgery is used in refractory NYHA Class IV heart failure if BMV is not possible but has a high risk (9% of mothers and almost one-third of babies do not survive the procedure) and needs careful thought before proceeding.

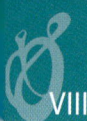

Treatment

Patients with RMS should, whenever possible, be treated according to the current ACC/AHA and European guidelines.[9,10]

Medical Therapy

Severe symptomatic RMS is clearly a mechanical obstruction that needs structural intervention (either BMV or surgery). Medical therapy does not change the progression of the disease but can be a reasonable temporary measure before definitive therapy and is also useful in some mildly symptomatic patients who are not yet candidates for definitive therapy or as a palliative measure in those not suitable for any intervention. It mainly involves rate control, management of secondary conditions that could worsen MS (including AF, anemia, thyrotoxicosis, or infection), and judicious diuresis in patients who still continue to have exercise intolerance. At the same time, secondary prophylaxis for ARF and OACs to prevent embolic events should be meticulously offered per guideline recommendations. Patients with RMS with any incidence of AF and those in sinus rhythm with history of prior thromboembolism or LA thrombus should receive OACs. It is reasonable to consider OACs in patients with severely dilated LA or those with severe spontaneous contrast in the LA per European guidelines (no U.S. recommendation). Direct-acting OACs are not recommended. Rate control with any suitable drug is indicated in patients with AF and a rapid ventricular response and may help in patients in sinus rhythm who develop significant symptoms during exercise. Beta blockers decrease heart rates, thus creating longer diastolic filling time and reduced gradients but have not been consistently shown to improve exercise capacity.[15] Ivabradine might better control tachycardia during exercise than beta blockers. Digoxin is helpful only in patients with AF.

Transcatheter Interventional Therapy

Indications for intervention in RMS in the 2020 ACC/AHA guidelines are shown in Table 75.2 and Fig. 75.6. BMV and surgery (mostly open valve repair and rarely valve replacement) are effective but have particular indications. BMV is a very efficacious as well as cost effective treatment and is the preferred modality in most patients with valve area <1.5 cm^2 and suitable anatomy (see Chapter 78). It might be considered in those with valve area >1.5 cm^2 if symptoms can be clearly attributed to MS, especially if they develop high PAP. BMV might also be considered rather than offering surgery in patients with somewhat unfavorable anatomy, particularly those at high surgical risk, if performed at a comprehensive valve center.[9] Asymptomatic patients are not currently recommended intervention unless they have severe PAH (>50 mm Hg) or new-onset AF and have favorable anatomy. Additional factors that might be considered in asymptomatic patients include those with very high thromboembolic risk, are considering pregnancy, or scheduled to undergo major noncardiac surgery. Some preliminary observational studies support earlier performance of BMV in asymptomatic subjects with moderate stenosis and good valve morphology but there are no randomized trials to support this. Surgery is offered only in patients when BMV cannot be done safely due to adverse valve morphology or major contraindication, when the patient is having cardiac surgery for other reasons, or when the patient needs treatment for MS but there are other concomitant conditions that require surgical therapy like moderate to severe MR or TR, AS, or coronary artery disease (CAD).

The ideal patient is one with good valve morphology scores, MR <grade II, and few comorbidities. An LA thrombus is a contraindication for the procedure even though some experienced centers have safely performed BMV after 2 to 3 months of OAC. BMV has high success rates in patients with favorable morphology (>90%). Predictors of procedural success include extent of valve thickening, mobility and subvalvular involvement, uneven leaflet thickening, commissural asymmetry, and calcification (Fig. 75.7). Although none of the scores based on echocardiography are very good at predicting outcomes, a Wilkins score <8 in general predicts good outcomes (see Fig. 78.2), while those with a score >11 are best treated with surgery.[9] Patients with intermediate scores (between 9 and 11) can still have reasonable results and should be considered for BMV in experienced centers. The more recently designed scores[17,23,24] seemed to reclassify risk and predict long-term outcomes more robustly. The use of 3D echo is likely to improve triage to BMV.[16]

An MVA ≥ 1.5 cm^2 and MR ≤ 2/4 (without in-hospital major adverse cardiac and cerebrovascular events) are considered to be a good result after BMV.[23] Increase in MVA and reduction in gradient and PAP are durable over the long term in the majority of patients. The results are more durable in patients with favorable anatomy before BMV.[23] A post-procedure area of >1.8 cm^2 seems to predict good long-term outcomes. There has been a trend toward offering BMV in a larger pool of patients, especially in higher income countries.[13] Over the years, patients coming to BMV are older, have more AF and PAH, have a higher NYHA functional class, and have more suboptimal valve morphology (valvular and subvalvular calcification, MR and previous intervention).[14] As a result, while almost 90% of the patients in Western series had a good outcome after BMV in the past, more recent data show a success rate

TABLE 75.2 Recommendations for Intervention for Rheumatic Mitral Stenosis

COR	LOE	RECOMMENDATIONS
1	A	1. In symptomatic patients (NYHA Class II, III, or IV) with severe rheumatic MS (mitral valve area ≤1.5 cm^2, Stage D) and favorable valve morphology with less than moderate (2+) MR* in the absence of LA thrombus. PMBC is recommended if it can be performed at a comprehensive valve center.
1	B-NR	2. In severely symptomatic patients (NYHA Class III or IV) with severe rheumatic MS (mitral valve area ≤1.5 cm^2, Stage D) who (1) are not candidates for PMBC, (2) have failed a previous PMBC, (3) require other cardiac procedures, or (4) do not have access to PMBC, mitral valve surgery (repair, commissurotomy, or valve replacement) is indicated.
2a	B-NR	3. In asymptomatic patients with severe rheumatic MS (mitral valve area ≤1.5 cm^2, Stage C) and favorable valve morphology with less than 2 + MR in the absence of LA thrombus who have elevated pulmonary pressures (pulmonary artery systolic pressure >50 mm Hg), PMBC is reasonable if it can be performed at a comprehensive valve center.
2b	C-LD	4. In asymptomatic patients with severe rheumatic MS (mitral valve area ≤1.5 cm^2, Stage C) and favorable valve morphology with less than 2f/ MR* in the absence of LA thrombus who have new onset of AF, PMBC may be considered if it can be performed at a comprehensive valve center.
2b	C-LD	5. In symptomatic patients (NYHA Class II, III, or IV) with rheumatic MS and a mitral valve area >1.5 cm^2, if there is evidence of hemodynamically significant rheumatic MS on the basis of a pulmonary artery wedge pressure >25 mm Hg or a mean mitral valve gradient >15 mm Hg during exercise, PMBC may be considered if it can be performed at a comprehensive valve center.
2b	B-NR	6. In severely symptomatic patients (NYHA Class III or IV) with severe rheumatic MS (mitral valve area ≤1.5 cm^2, Stage D) who have a suboptimal valve anatomy and who are not candidates for surgery or are at high risk for surgery, PMBC may be considered if it can be performed at a comprehensive valve center.

*2+ on a 0 to 4+ scale according to Sellar's criteria or less than moderate by Doppler echocardiography.
PMBC, Percutaneous mitral balloon commissurotomy.
(From Otto CM, et al. 2020 AHA/ACC guideline for the management of patients with valvular heart disease: a report of the American College of Cardiology/American Heart Association Task Force on Practice Guidelines. J Am Coll Cardiol 2021;77:e25-197.)

of about 75%.[14] Cardiac complications (5%) including strokes (3%) are also slightly higher than in previous decades, as is the need for surgery (6%).[13] Success rates in LMICs continue to remain much higher (over 90%) and juvenile patients seem to have a particularly effective treatment with BMV.

Complications
Some degree of mild MR or worsening MR has been reported in 20% of patients in recent series.[24] It generally is tolerated well and remains stable or improves. MR arising from commissural splitting actually predicts a good outcome. Acute severe MR is one of the most feared complication of BMV but is rare (<1% to 2%). Severe MR due to tear of the anterior leaflet central scallop or damage to the subvalvular apparatus usually requires early surgery. Most other patients tolerate severe MR initially with only a minority needing emergency intervention. Significant MR, however, affects long-term outcomes adversely. A small interatrial shunt develops within 48 hours of BMV in 60% to 70% of patients, but this persists in less than 10% over the long term, especially if the MS is relieved.

Long-Term Results
Age and procedural success determine long-term outcomes.[14,17] Nearly 80% of patients undergoing BMV remain free of death, need for mitral surgery, or repeat BMV over the next 15 years[25] and about two-thirds remain so after 20 years. However, results also depend on the age of the patient and the era when BMV was performed. A study from France (patient age 49 ± 14) reported that the 20-year rate of good functional results (survival without cardiovascular death, severe symptoms [NYHA Class III-IV], mitral surgery, or repeat BMV) was only 30.2 ± 2.0%.[23] Greater age, higher NYHA class, and suboptimal relief of MS during the initial procedure were factors associated with outcome. Post-BMV restenosis, which is strongly related to suboptimal immediate results, affects long-term outcomes.[26] It develops over many years and can be treated with repeat BMV with reasonable success if the mechanism is once again fusion of commissures. In patients with restenosis, results of repeat BMV are comparable to surgery but may be less successful if MS is due to valve leaflet rigidity and degeneration.

Surgical Intervention
Surgery is indicated in patients with contraindication for BMV, in those in whom BMV was unsuccessful, and in those with other conditions that would warrant surgery (TR, AS, or CAD).[9] A maze procedure and LA ligation can be performed concomitantly to reduce AF burden and related morbidity. Three types of surgery are offered for MS: closed mitral valvotomy (CMV), open mitral valvotomy (OMV), and mitral valve replacement (MVR). There is good long-term experience with all the three methods, and the results are durable with low rates of MR and reoperation. CMV is not practiced widely except in LMICs where it is economical and has reasonably good results in experienced centers; however, increases in MVA are less and outcomes suboptimal compared to OMV or BMV. Hence, BMV should be chosen over CMV, when both are available. OMV is the surgical procedure of choice, especially in the young. It has excellent results that are comparable to MVR but avoids many of the long-term issues with prosthetic valves. OMV is associated with mortality rates under 2%, excellent relief of symptoms, excellent long-term survival (96% at 10 years), and freedom from reoperation (98% at 9 years). Unless there are distinct indications for its use, MVR is the least preferred option due to higher risk, need for anticoagulation with mechanical valves, and high bioprosthesis failure rate in young patients. MVR has higher operative mortality (3% to 10%) and lower 10-year survival than OMV, but these statistics might reflect a more suboptimal patient substrate.

Comparison with BMV
Randomized clinical trials with limited-term follow-up show that results of BMV are as good or perhaps better than surgery. Robust long-term

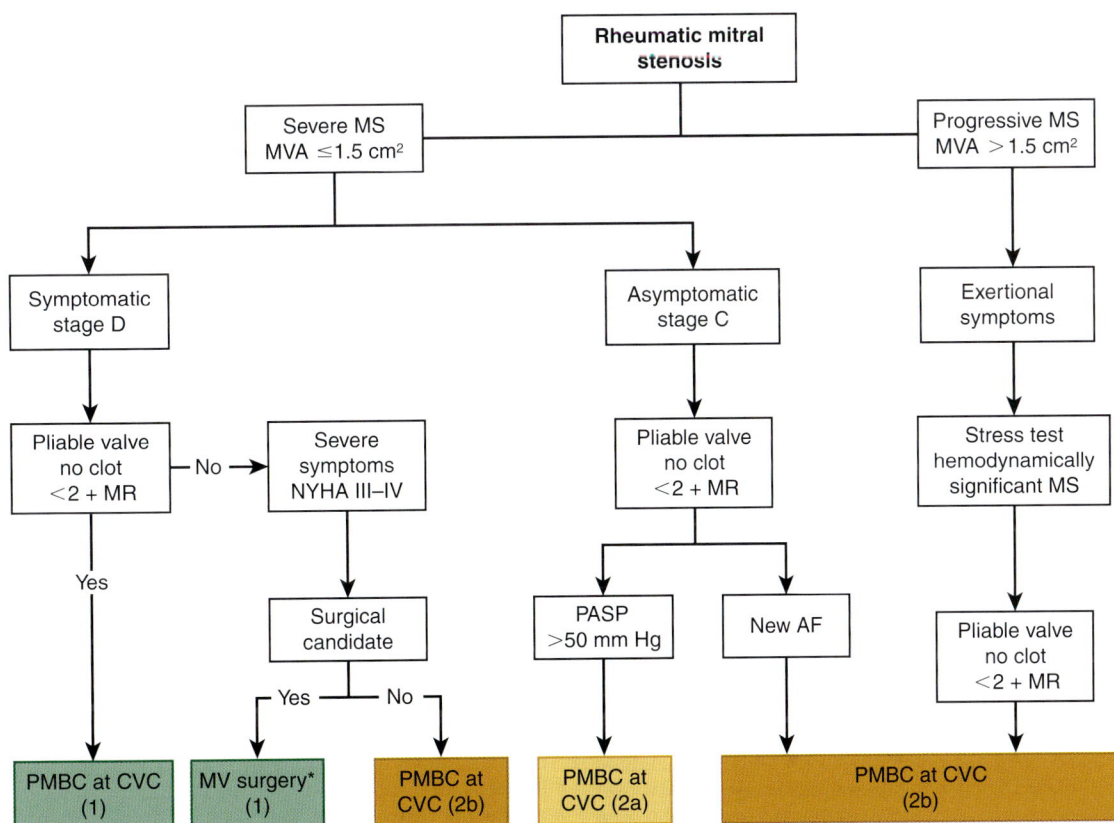

FIGURE 75.6 Management strategy for rheumatic mitral stenosis. Colors correspond to Table 75.2. *MV surgery could be repair, commissurotomy, or valve replacement. *AF*, Atrial fibrillation; *CVC*, comprehensive valve center; *MR*, mitral regurgitation; *MS*, mitral stenosis; *MV*, mitral valve; *MVA*, mitral valve area; *NYHA*, New York Heart Association; *PASP*, pulmonary artery systolic pressure; *PMBC*, percutaneous mitral balloon commissurotomy. (From Otto CM, et al. 2020 AHA/ACC guideline for the management of patients with valvular heart disease: a report of the American College of Cardiology/American Heart Association Task Force on Practice Guidelines. J Am Coll Cardiol 2021;77:e25-197.)

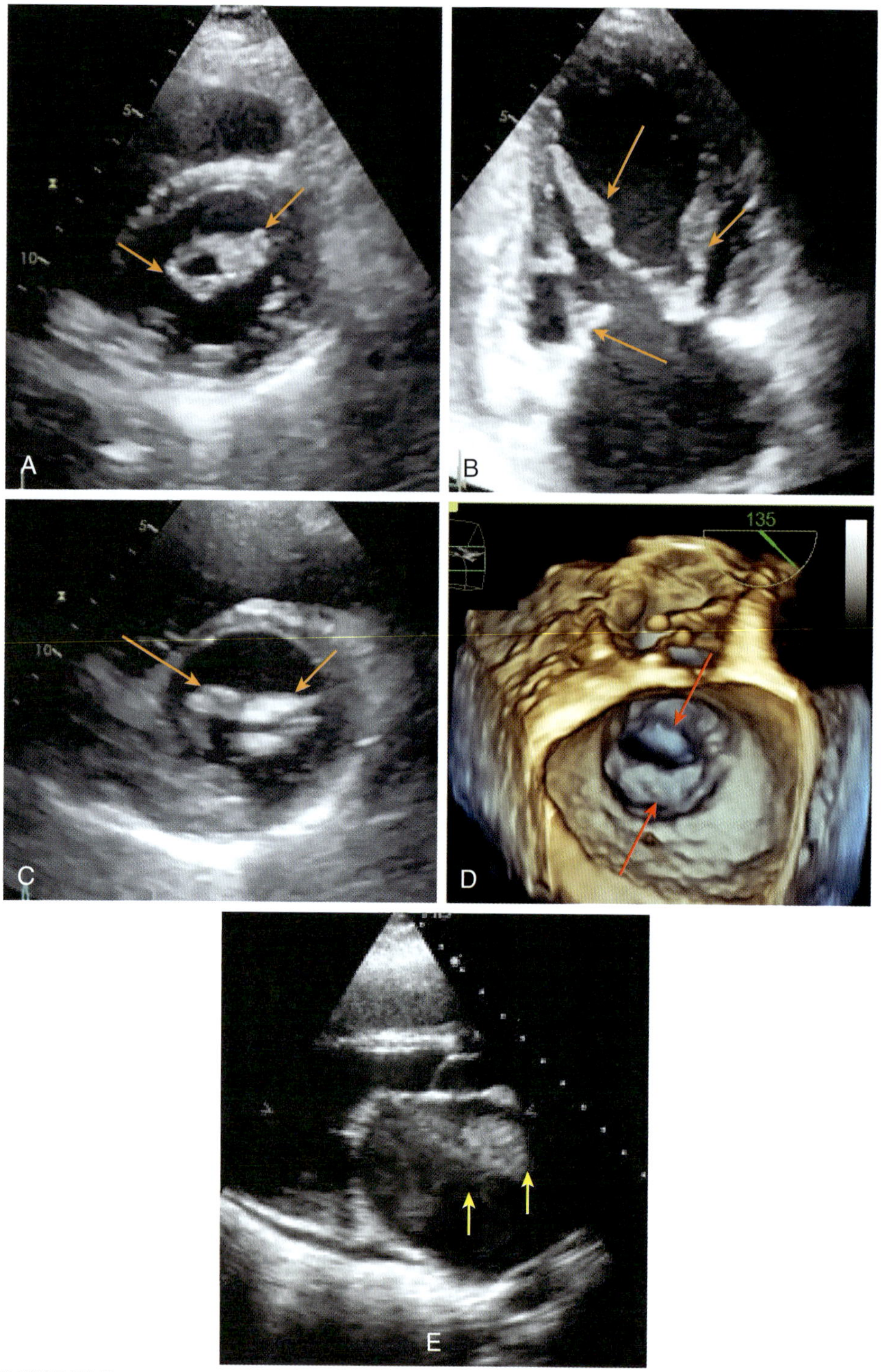

NONRHEUMATIC MITRAL STENOSIS

A number of conditions can cause nonrheumatic MS, and they each have many nuances of their own.

Degenerative MS Related to Mitral Annular Calcification

MAC is a chronic process that causes extensive calcification of the mitral valve annulus with extension into the base of both leaflets (see Fig. 17.6). It is now becoming an important cause of MS in the developed world. MAC increases as the population ages and, not surprisingly, MAC related MS is increasingly observed in aging societies. It has many atypical features, has pathophysiology that is somewhat different from RMS, is difficult to diagnose, and has limited treatment options.

The exact mechanism for MS is not clear but a number of factors including reduced diastolic annular expansion and stiff leaflets have been postulated. Both severity and pattern of distribution of MAC influence the degree of LA outflow obstruction. MAC in the anterior annulus, involvement of the anterior leaflet and in particular the A2 scallop, and extension into more than half of the leaflet length seem to predict development and severity of MS. Unlike RMS, there is no commissural fusion or subvalvular involvement (Fig. 75.8). The posterior leaflet is often very restricted due to significant calcification but the tips of both leaflets remain mobile. The mitral gradient due to MAC increases variably, roughly 0.8 ± 2.4 mm Hg/year and MVA decreases 0.05 cm^2/year, which is slower than in RMS.[11] PAH can be severe (>50 mm Hg), but only a small proportion (roughly 20%) of patients progress to systolic PAP >50 mm Hg.[6]

Diagnosis of hemodynamically significant DMS is difficult. The classic patients are older adults, often women, with multiple comorbidities including hypertension, heart failure with preserved ejection fraction (see Chapter 51), AF, COPD, and significant LV hypertrophy that make diagnosis difficult.[11] There may occasionally be a short diastolic rumble, but not the classical signs of RMS such as a loud S$_1$ or OS. Symptomatic patients with severe DMS have modest gradients and higher MVA (e.g., 8.0 ± 3.8 mm Hg and 1.26 ± 0.19 cm^2, respectively in the Mayo series[6]) than RMS. Defining severity of MS and proving it is the proximate cause for the patient's symptoms are quite challenging.[28] The main abnormality in DMS involves the base of the valve leaflets rather than the tips as in RMS and is unevenly distributed around the valve inflow. Early mitral filling is often preserved and late diastolic gradients can become minimal in beats with long RR intervals, unlike in RMS (Fig. 75.9). In addition, comorbidities reduce LA compliance and increase LV stiffness, both of which can lead to elevated LA pressure despite smaller Doppler gradients across the

FIGURE 75.7 Echocardiographic features identifying poor suitability for percutaneous balloon mitral valvuloplasty (BMV). 2D and 3D echo is the best method to define less favorable morphology, risk of complications, and contraindications. **A,** Severe asymmetric commissural fusion could indicate that BMV may distribute force nonuniformly, thus increasing risk of suboptimal results and noncommissural tears. **B,** Severe fusion and matting of the subvalvular apparatus is a marker for increased risk of persistent gradient and complications after BMV. **C,** Asymmetric calcification of leaflets and commissures is a marker of risk of MR after BMV. **D,** Fibrotic leaflets with uneven leaflet thickening can influence results of BMV. **E,** Left atrial thrombus (*arrows*) is an absolute contraindication for BMV.

head-to-head comparisons with BMV are lacking, but intermediate outcomes of BMV and surgery are largely similar with higher procedural morbidity after surgery.[27] Long-term survival advantage of BMV over surgery has not been conclusively shown in the past and will be even more difficult to show in future, given that patients referred for surgery are usually those who are not favorable candidates for BMV. Surgery for restenosis carries a higher risk due to older age and other comorbidities, and BMV should be the first option whenever feasible.[26]

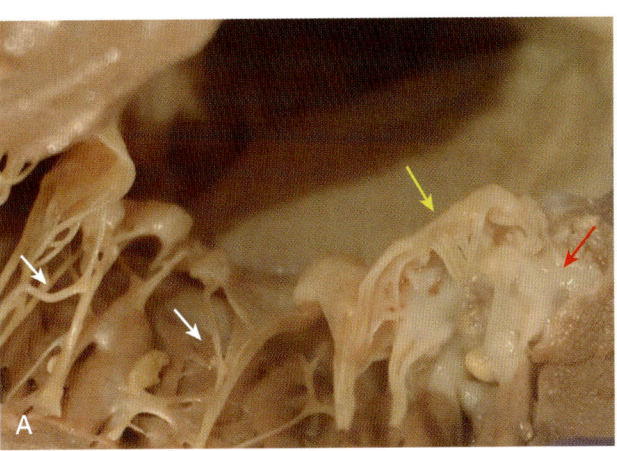
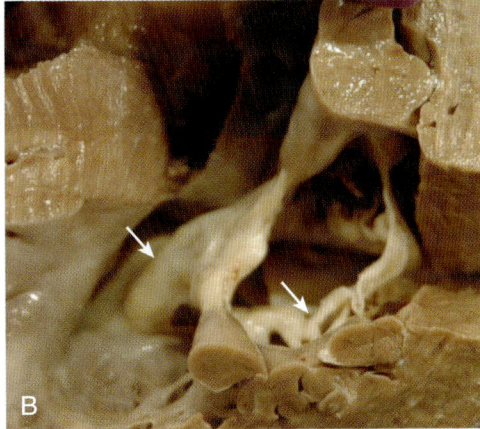

FIGURE 75.8 Pathologic distinction between degenerative and rheumatic MS. **A,** In this example of degenerative MS, the posterior annulus has severe mitral annular calcification (MAC; *red arrow*) that extends into the posterior mitral leaflet (PML; *yellow arrow*). The PML is thick and rigid, adding resistance to left atrial outflow. In severe cases, MAC extends into the anterior mitral leaflet, making MS more likely. The rest of the valve, including its tips, are spared and opens normally. The subvalvular apparatus is also unaffected (*white arrows*) and commissures are not fused. The narrowed valve orifice thus is at the base of the valve rather than at the leaflet tips, and BMV is not an option. **B,** In rheumatic MS, the annulus is unaffected and the pathology is in the valve edges, commissures and the subvalvular apparatus (*arrows*). The narrowed valve orifice is thus at the tips of the leaflets, and valve areas tend to be smaller than those of degenerative MS caused by MAC.

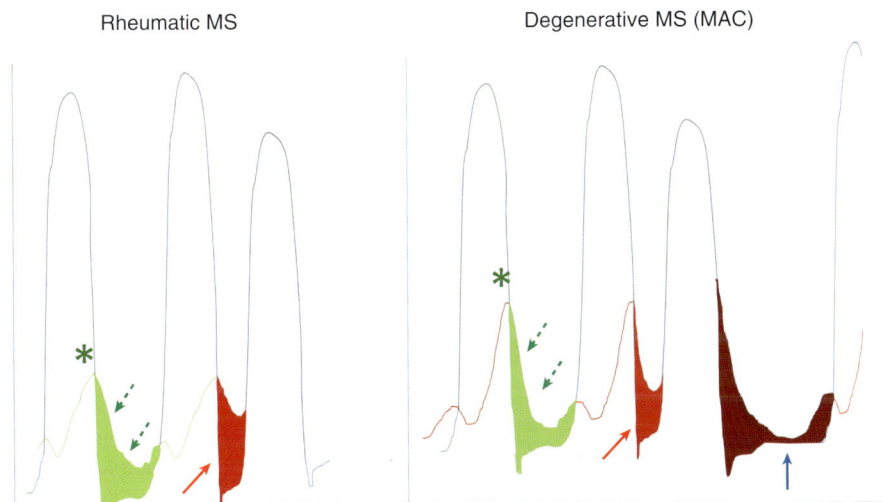

FIGURE 75.9 Pathophysiology of rheumatic MS versus degenerative MS caused but mitral annular calcification (MAC). **Left,** In rheumatic MS, the mitral valve area (MVA) is fixed and the early rapid filling phase is slow (*green arrows*) with significant gradient continuing during diastasis and atrial contraction. A premature beat (or tachycardia) will shorten diastole and increase the transmitral gradient (*red*). **Right,** In degenerative MS caused by MAC, the orifice is not as fixed and is comparatively larger than that in rheumatic MS. The left atrial (LA) and left ventricular end-diastolic pressure (LVEDP) are greater, but early rapid filling is better preserved (*green arrows*). The elevated LVEDP increases LA pressure above that due to mitral valve resistance alone. A premature beat has less of an impact on LA pressures. Long RR intervals allow more complete LA emptying, and significantly lower LA pressure, and the gradient is appreciably reduced during diastasis (*blue arrow*), something that is not usually seen in severe rheumatic MS. *Mitral valve opening.

discrepancy between echocardiographic MVA, gradients, and symptoms. The 3D planimetry lacks robust validation in DMS. Finally, mitral valve diastolic PISA is useful in calculating MVA in RMS, but this has not been well validated in DMS. In patients without significant MR or AR, a careful analysis using the continuity equation is probably the best way to diagnose severe DMS. Exercise testing might help clarify the hemo-dynamic effects of DMS in patients with symptoms but unclear severity of DMS.[7] CT is being used increasingly in studying MAC since it provides exquisite details about location, severity, circumferential extent and distribution of calcification into the mitral leaflets (see Fig. 75.10) that are far better than obtained from echocardiography. It may allow planimetry and calcium quantitation[30] that has clinical implications. Furthermore, it is a prerequisite for planning MAC related interventions.

Associated Aortic Stenosis

MAC is commonly seen in patients with AS (50% have MAC and 11% to 18% have MS, majority due to DMS) (see Chapter 72), and associated DMS, even if mild, affects short- and long-term outcomes, including stroke, with or without intervention for AS.[31,32] Recognizing MS is thus vital in patients with AS being considered for intervention, but the presence of both can make evaluation of MS difficult. AS can result in low flow-low gradient MS. Planimetry may not be accurate due to significant calcification, and pressure half time is unreliable. MS severity even with use of the continuity equation is commonly overestimated in patients with AS. Half of patients with concomitant AS and MS show increased MVAs after treatment of AS, suggesting low stroke volume before aortic intervention created a pseudo-MS. True DMS in the other half (predicted by preintervention MVA <1.5 cm², and a rigid annulus with calcification that extended into both leaflets) adversely influences outcome after AS intervention.[31]

Natural History

The natural history of MAC-related DMS is incompletely understood. DMS is associated with poor survival, mainly a consequence of the extensive comorbidities, with 1-year mortality in the 32% range. The majority of patients (60%) with severe DMS in a contemporary series[6] had symptoms, with dyspnea being the most common, while asymptomatic patients developed symptoms at the rate of 7% to 8% per year. Adverse events are fairly common (47% at 1 year, almost 75% over longer follow-up), and almost 50% of the patients died during the short follow-up of 2.8 ± 3.0 years.

mitral valve; it is sometimes difficult to be certain that MAC related mitral inflow obstruction rather than comorbidities is the dominant cause of symptoms. Not surprisingly, elevated LA and LV end-diastolic pressures often continue to be seen in some patients even after successful interventions.

Multiple techniques are often used to image and understand the etiology of symptoms (Fig. 75.10) in patients with MAC.[29] Planimetry, the reference standard for RMS, may not work well since MS is not a fixed obstruction at one level (e.g., at the leaflet tip in RMS) but is a result of increased resistance at the level of the leaflet base and annulus level as well as reduced opening angle of the calcified leaflet base. The difference in shape of the stenosed valve (dome shape in RMS and tubular funnel shape in DMS) can have differential effects on pressure loss and result in different effective MVAs or gradients. Extensive calcium can obscure the valve orifice outlines so planimetry is difficult. Pressure half time is affected by LV and LA compliance, which leads to an overestimate of the MVA, creating a

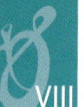

associated with adverse outcomes including AV groove disruption. In addition, surgical risk is heightened by patient age and comorbidities. Complication rates, not surprisingly, tend to be high and rarely, procedures like mitral valve bypass (LA to LV conduit) might be needed. Many patients do report reduced symptoms if they survive surgery, but long-term survival studies are lacking. Transcatheter techniques are under development, and transcatheter mitral valve replacement (TMVR) and (ViMAC) with balloon-expandable transcatheter aortic valves have shown some promise. These are currently reserved for highly symptomatic patients with significant surgical risk. Early results from the TMVR in MAC Global Registry[33] in 116 severely symptomatic patients at extreme surgical risk indicate procedural success in 76.7% of patients but 15% needed a second valve due to suboptimal results (migration or severe MR). One year all-cause mortality was 54%, and the majority of the survivors (72%) were in NYHA functional Class I or II. The mean mitral gradient was reduced from 11.5 mm Hg to 5.8 mm Hg, the mean MVA increased from 1.3 cm^2 to 1.9 cm^2, and 75% of patients had no or trace MR. TMVR is feasible in patients with severe MAC but is associated with high 30-day and 1-year mortality, with LV outflow tract (LVOT) obstruction being the most dreaded complication (11.2%). Another multicenter study also confirmed suboptimal results in ViMAC compared to excellent outcomes for patients with transcatheter valve-in-valve for degenerated bioprostheses despite similar high surgical risk.[34] Early and midterm mortality after transcatheter ViMAC were high (35% and 63%, respectively). These early disappointing results may improve in the future with more optimal use of multimodality imaging for predicting LVOT obstruction and optimal valve sizing, dedicated MAC-related valve designs and more precise anticoagulation protocols.

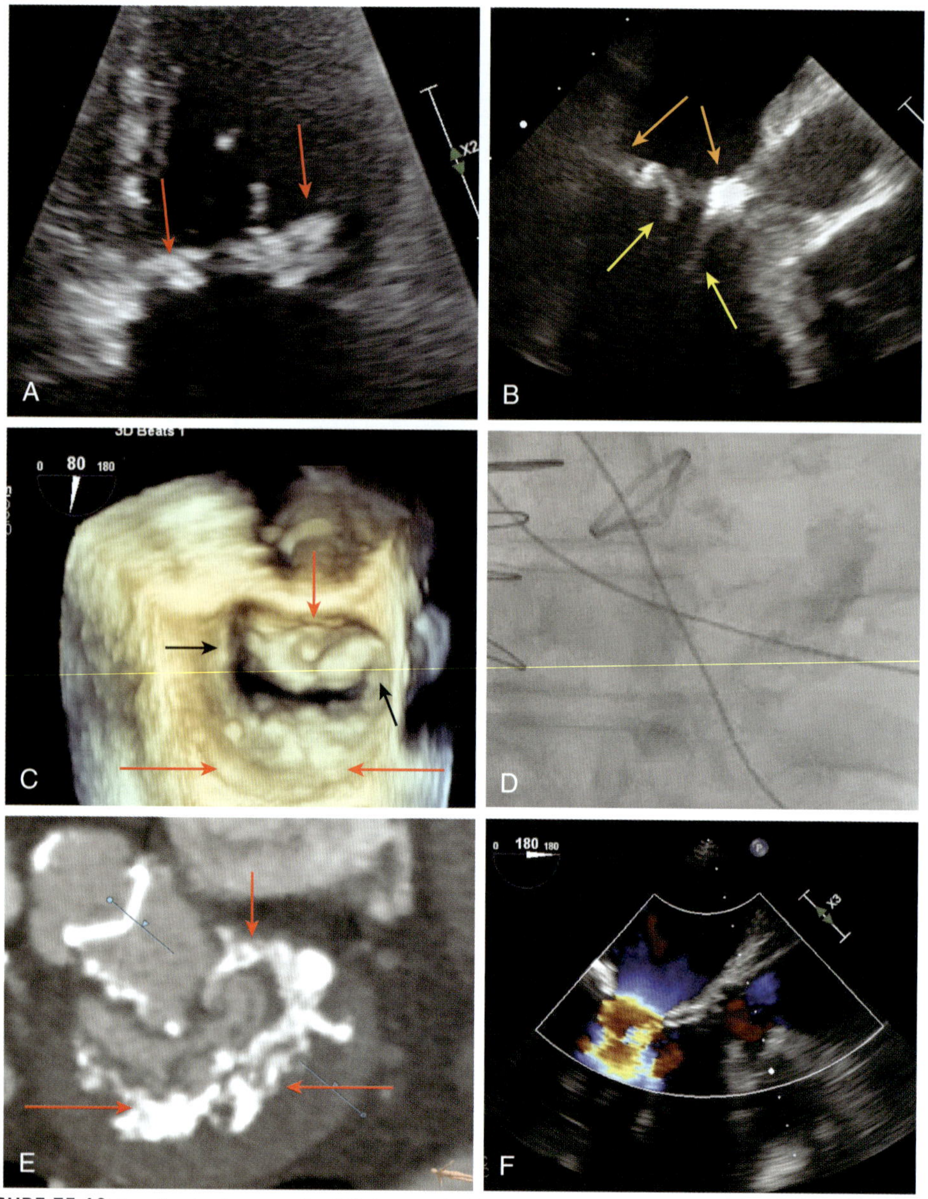

FIGURE 75.10 Imaging in degenerative MS due to mitral annular calcification (MAC). **A,** Extensive MAC (*arrows*) in a patient with MAC associated MS. **B,** The MAC starts from the annulus and extends for some length into the base of the leaflets (*orange arrows*), making them stiff. The rest of the leaflet is spared (*yellow arrows*). **C,** 3D echo shows extensive MAC (*red arrows*). Unlike rheumatic MS there is no commissural fusion (*black arrows*). **D,** MAC is well visualized on x-ray. **E,** CT is the best modality for quantitation. **F,** Flow convergence shell is not impressive, suggesting lower gradient and relatively larger valve area despite severe symptoms.

Treatment

Therapeutic options in DMS are limited but evolving. A lack of good quality data prevents clear recommendations for treating DMS, unlike in RMS.[9-11] Medical therapy, in the form of diuretics and beta blockers to slow the heart rate, is commonly used in symptomatic DMS. However, mortality remains high with medical therapy.[6] Despite this dismal prognosis, MAC-related interventional procedures are performed only in a minority of patients, even in major medical centers. As an example, only 16% of such symptomatic patients underwent nonmedical therapies, of which 85% were surgical MVR.[6] BMV is not an option in DMS given that the abnormality does not involve commissural fusion. There are no effective methods to decalcify MAC and replacing the valve, either surgically or with transcatheter valve in MAC (ViMAC) using a transcatheter aortic valve device (see Chapter 78) are the only choices at this time. Surgical options have suboptimal results due to difficulty in suturing the new valve into heavily calcified segments, and extensive debriding of the annulus to adequately seat a valve is often

Radiotherapy-Induced MS

Valvular heart disease, including MS, is a time- and dose-dependent complication of chest radiation, particularly when using protocols that did not adequately shield nontarget structures. It takes decades to rise to clinical attention and can be a combination of MR and MS, the latter happening about two decades after exposure. Severe calcification of the cardiac fibrous skeleton, especially in the aortomitral curtain, the anterior annulus and anterior leaflet, is common but is not accompanied by subvalvular involvement or commissural fusion (Fig. 75.11). Radiation-associated MS is often accompanied by involvement of the aortic valve as well as restrictive myocardial disease. Treatment of radiation-associated MS is suboptimal but general principles remain the same as with other forms of MS.

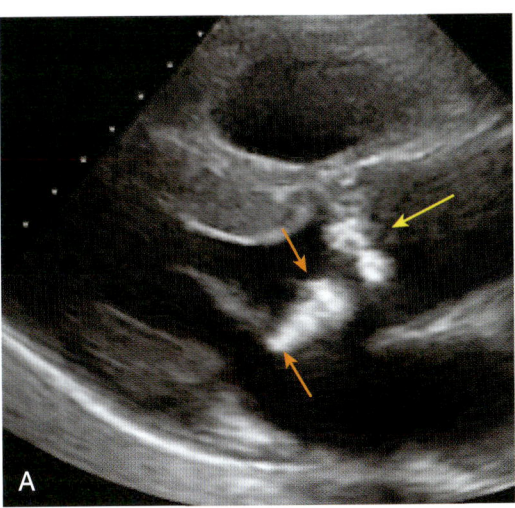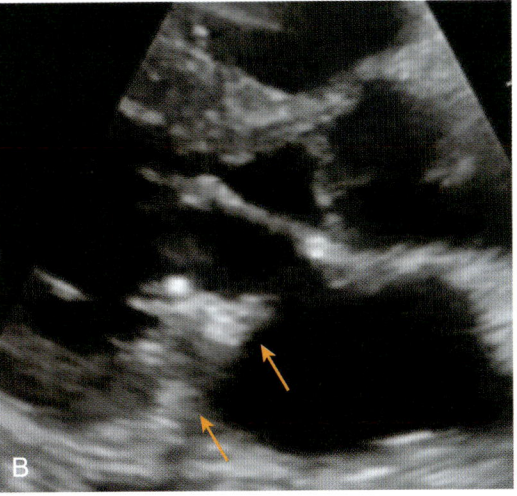

FIGURE 75.11 Nonrheumatic MS due to prior radiation therapy. **A,** Extensive calcification in a patient with radiation associated MS is predominantly in the "aortic-mitral curtain" (*orange arrows*), which is a classic sign of radiation induced valvular damage. In addition, the patient has calcific aortic stenosis (*yellow arrow*), which occurs before the onset of MS. Commissural fusion does not occur and hence balloon dilation is not an option. **B,** In contrast, degenerative MS related to mitral annular calcification most commonly involves the posterior annulus and then extends around the annulus and into the base of the leaflets. Aorto-mitral curtain calcification is not prominent.

MS Following Interventional and Surgical Therapies

A number of mitral valve interventions both surgical (prosthetic valves, Alfieri stitch, or mitral repair with annuloplasty) and percutaneous mitral valve clips (see Chapters 76 and 78) are becoming an important cause for MS in the Western world; indeed, MS related to prosthetic valve dysfunction was more common than even calcific DMS in the most recent experience at a major tertiary center.[7] Surgical series report MVA <1.5 cm^2 in approximately 20% of patients after surgical mitral valve repair for primary MR. These patients require a very nuanced evaluation since identifying prosthesis-related dysfunction as the main cause of LA outflow obstruction is difficult. However, it needs to be diagnosed correctly since it has specific therapeutic options, and intervention seems to improve mortality. Prosthetic valves can cause an MS-like syndrome either with disease affecting the operating valve orifice (thrombus, pannus, leaflet thickening and degeneration, or calcification and very rarely commissural fusion) or prosthesis-patient mismatch (PPM) (see Chapter 79). Both repeat surgical MVR and transcatheter mitral valve-in-valve replacement are options for treating MS due to degenerated mitral bioprostheses. These options seem to have largely similar outcomes in preliminary studies despite a 2 mm Hg higher gradient in the valve-in-valve group.[35] Data in 1529 high-risk patients (50% with MS) from the Society of Thoracic Surgeons/American College of Cardiology Transcatheter Valve Therapy Registry showed very high procedural success of transcatheter valve-in-valve (96.8%), good valve function that was maintained at 1 year, and low risks of valve thrombosis, LVOT obstruction (0.9%), and all-cause mortality (16.7% at 1 year).[36] The choice of therapy depends on the risk-benefit profile of the patient, expertise of the heart team, and need for other surgery (such as treatment of TR, which is seen in up to 50% of patients with prosthetic mitral valve stenosis). Smaller bioprosthetic valves (<23 mm) may perhaps be best treated with surgery to avoid higher gradients after transcatheter valve-in-valve. This transcatheter option was initially offered only to patients at high risk for repeat cardiac surgery but is now being used increasingly in patients who are somewhat lower risk (see Chapter 78). However, durability of the procedure and whether small residual valve gradients have future consequences need to be resolved.

PPM after MVR is fairly common, ranging between 30% and 85% by effective orifice area criteria (see Chapter 79). Unlike aortic valve PPM, there is conflicting data whether PPM after MVR significantly influences long-term prognosis. Clinically significant PPM is treated surgically but newer valve designs may provide other options in future.

Annuloplasty procedures during surgical repair of MR, especially when using a smaller-sized ring, can cause functional MS, which mediates PAH, new-onset AF, lower exercise capacity, and poorer quality of life even after abolishing the MR.[37] Treatment is often repeat surgery, but there is growing experience with transcatheter valve-in-ring procedures, which might be a reasonable option in some selected patients. About one-quarter to one-third of patients develop mitral valve gradients greater than 5 mm Hg (most in the 5 to 10 mm Hg range) after transcatheter edge-to-edge mitral clip procedures (see Chapter 78).[38] Preprocedure MVA <4 cm^2, preexisting gradients, significant leaflet calcification, and implanting >2 clips predict development of gradients of this magnitude. Clip-related MS, especially in patients with primary MR,[39] has poorer long-term outcomes including risk of death, AF, and reintervention. Residual MR has adverse outcomes but MS (>5 mm Hg) may be worse,[38] and both together are even more detrimental; there is thus a delicate balance between how aggressive one can be with clips to abolish MR and the risk of an unfavorable gradient. Diagnosing MS in the presence of a clip and two orifices is difficult. Measuring the hemodynamics of the larger orifice or averaging both has been suggested, but no single method has been well validated. Surgery provides definitive therapy; the valve can be repaired in 50% to 60% of cases but this becomes more difficult with an increasing number of clips. There is a 9% risk of early mortality, depending on urgency of surgery and the extent of patient comorbidities, and a 60% to 70% survival at 1 to 2 years.

CLASSIC REFERENCES

Shaw TR, Sutaria N, Prendergast B. Clinical and haemodynamic profiles of young, middle aged, and elderly patients with mitral stenosis undergoing mitral balloon valvotomy. *Heart.* 2003;89: 1430–1436.

Wilkins GT, Weyman AE, Abascal VM, et al. Percutaneous balloon dilatation of the mitral valve: an analysis of echocardiographic variables related to outcome and the mechanism of dilatation. *Br Heart J.* 1988;60:299–308.

Wood P. An appreciation of mitral stenosis. I. Clinical features. *Br Med J.* 1954;1(4870):1051–1063.

REFERENCES

Epidemiology and Secular Trends

1. Watkins DA, Johnson CO, Colquhoun SM, et al. Global, regional, and national burden of rheumatic heart. Disease, 1990–2015. *New Engl J Med.* 2017;377:713–722.
2. Rothenbuhler M, O'Sullivan CJ, Stortecky S, et al. Active surveillance for rheumatic heart disease in endemic regions: a systematic review and meta-analysis of prevalence among children and adolescents. *Lancet Glob Health.* 2014;2:e717–e726.
3. Zuhlke L, Engel ME, Karthikeyan G, et al. Characteristics, complications, and gaps in evidence-based interventions in rheumatic heart disease: the Global Rheumatic Heart Disease Registry (the REMEDY study). *Eur Heart J.* 2015;36:1115–1122.
4. Tandon R, Sharma M, Chandrashekhar Y, et al. Revisiting the pathogenesis of rheumatic fever and carditis. *Nat Rev Cardiol.* 2013;10:171–177.
5. Zuhlke L, Karthikeyan G, Engel ME, et al. Clinical outcomes in 3343 children and adults with rheumatic heart disease from 14 low- and middle-income countries: two-year follow-up of the global Rheumatic Heart Disease Registry (the REMEDY study). *Circulation.* 2016;134:1456–1466.
6. Kato N, Padang R, Scott CG, et al. The natural history of severe calcific mitral stenosis. *J Am Coll Cardiol.* 2020;75:3048–3057.
7. Gentry JL, Parikh PK, Alashi A, et al. Characteristics and outcomes in a contemporary group of patients with susepcted significant mitral stenosis undergoing treadmill stress echocardiography. *Circ Cardiovasc Imaging.* 2019;12:e009062.
8. Nishimura RA, Vahanian A, Eleid MF, Mack MJ. Mitral valve disease—current management and future challenges. *Lancet.* 2016;387:1324–1334.
9. Otto CM, Nishimura RA, Bonow RO, et al. 2020 ACC/AHA guideline for the management of patients with valvular heart disease: executive summary: a report of the American College of Cardiology/American Heart Association joint committee on clinical practice guidelines. *J Am Coll Cardiol.* 2021;77:e25–197.
10. Baumgartner H, Falk V, Bax JJ, et al. 2017 ESC/EACTS Guidelines for the management of valvular heart disease. *Eur Heart J.* 2017;38:2739–2791.

Rheumatic Mitral Stenosis: Pathophysiology, Natural History, Diagnosis
11. Chandrashekhar Y, Westaby S, Narula J. Mitral stenosis. *Lancet.* 2009;374:1271–1283.
12. El Sabbagh A, Reddy YN, Barros-Gomes S, et al. Low-gradient severe mitral stenosis: hemodynamic profiles, clinical characteristics, and outcomes. *J Am Heart Assoc.* 2019;8:e010736.
13. Badheka AO, Shah N, Ghatak A, et al. Balloon mitral valvuloplasty in the United States: a 13-year perspective. *Am J Med.* 2014;127(1126).e1–12.
14. Desnos C, Iung B, Himbert D, et al. Temporal trends on percutaneous mitral commissurotomy: 30 years of experience. *J Am Heart Assoc.* 2019;8:e012031.
15. Laufer-Perl M, Gura Y, Shimiaie J, et al. Mechanisms of effort intolerance in patients with rheumatic mitral stenosis. *JACC Cardiovasc Imaging.* 2017;10:622–633.
16. Wunderlich NC, Beigel R, Siegel RJ. Management of mitral stenosis using 2D and 3D echo-Doppler imaging. *JACC Cardiovasc Imaging.* 2013;6:1191–1205.
17. Nunes MC, Tan TC, Elmariah S, et al. The echo score revisited: impact of incorporating commissural morphology and leaflet displacement to the prediction of outcome for patients undergoing percutaneous mitral valvuloplasty. *Circulation.* 2014;129:886–895.

Rheumatic Mitral Stenosis: Atrial Fibrillation, Pregnancy
18. Iung B, Leenhardt A, Extramiana F. Management of atrial fibrillation in patients with rheumatic mitral stenosis. *Heart.* 2018;104:1062–1068.
19. Kim H, Cho G, Kim Y, et al. Development of atrial fibrillation in patients with rheumatic mitral valve disease in sinus rhythm. *Int J Cardiovasc Imaging.* 2015;31:735–742.
20. van Hagen IM, Thorne SA, Taha N, et al. Pregnancy outcomes in women with rheumatic mitral valve disease: results from the registry of pregnancy and cardiac disease. *Circulation.* 2018;137:806–816.
21. Elkayam U, Goland S, Pieper PG, Silverside CK. High-risk cardiac disease in pregnancy: Part 1. *J Am Coll Cardiol.* 2016;68:396–410.
22. Regit-Azgrosek V, Roos-Hesselink JW, Bauersachs J, ESC Scientific Document Group, et al. 2018 ESC guidelines for the management of cardiovascular diseases during pregnancy. *Eur Heart J.* 2018;39:3165–3241.

Rheumatic Mitral Stenosis: Treatment
23. Bouleti C, Iung B, Laouenan C, et al. Late results of percutaneous mitral commissurotomy up to 20 years: development and validation of a risk score predicting late functional results from a series of 912 patients. *Circulation.* 2012;125:2119–2127.
24. Nunes MCP, Levine RA, Braulio R, et al. Mitral regurgitation after percutaneous mitral valvuloplasty: insights into mechanisms and impact on clinical outcomes. *JACC Cardiovasc Imaging.* 2020;13:2513–2526.
25. Meneguz-Moreno RA, Costa JR, Gomes NL, et al. Very long term follow-up after percutaneous balloon mitral valvuloplasty. *JACC Cardiovasc Interv.* 2018;11:1945–1952.
26. Bouleti C, Iung B, Himbert D, et al. Reinterventions after percutaneous mitral commissurotomy during long-term follow-up, up to 20 years: the role of repeat percutaneous mitral commissurotomy. *Eur Heart J.* 2013;34:1923–1930.
27. Singh AD, Mian A, Devasenapathy N, et al. Percutaneous mitral commissurotomy versus surgical commissurotomy for rheumatic mitral stenosis: a systematic review and meta-analysis of randomised controlled trials. *Heart.* 2020;106:1094–1101.

Degenerative Mitral Stenosis Due to Mitral Annular Calcification
28. Reddy YVN, Murgo JP, Nishimura RA. Complexity of defining severe "stenosis" from mitral annular calcification. *Circulation.* 2019;140:523–525.
29. Eleid MF, Foley TA, Said SM, et al. Severe mitral annular calcification: multimodality imaging for therapeutic strategies and interventions. *JACC Cardiovasc Imaging.* 2016;9:1318–1337.
30. Guerrero M, Wang DD, Pursnani A, et al. A cardiac computed tomography-based score to categorize mitral annular calcification severity and predict valve embolization. *JACC Cardiovasc Imaging.* 2020;13:1945–1957.
31. Kato N, Padang R, Pislaru C, et al. Hemodynamics and prognostic impact of concomitant mitral stenosis in patients undergoing surgical or transcatheter aortic valve replacement for aortic stenosis. *Circulation.* 2019;140:1251–1260.
32. Asami M, Windecker S, Praz F, et al. Transcatheter aortic valve replacement in patients with concomitant mitral stenosis. *Eur Heart J.* 2019;40:1342–1351.
33. Guerrero M, Urena M, Himbert D, et al. 1-Year outcomes of transcatheter mitral valve replacement in patients with severe mitral annular calcification. *J Am Coll Cardiol.* 2018;71:1841–1853.

Mitral Stenosis Following Surgical or Transcatheter Mitral Valve Procedures
34. Yoon SH, Whisenant BK, Bleiziffer S, et al. Outcomes of transcatheter mitral valve replacement for degenerated bioprostheses, failed annuloplasty rings, and mitral annular calcification. *Eur Heart J.* 2019;40:441–451.
35. Kamioka N, Babaliaros V, Morse MA, et al. Comparison of clinical and echocardiographic outcomes after surgical redo mitral valve replacement and transcatheter mitral valve-in-valve therapy. *JACC Cardiovasc Interv.* 2018;11:1131–1138.
36. Whisenant B, Kapadia SR, Eleid MF, et al. One-year outcomes of mitral valve-in-valve using the SAPIEN 3 transcatheter heart valve. *JAMA Cardiol.* 2020;5:1245–1252.
37. Kawamoto N, Fujita T, Fukushima S, et al. Functional mitral stenosis after mitral valve repair for type II dysfunction: determinants and impacts on long-term outcome. *Eur J Cardio Thorac Surg.* 2018;54:453–459.
38. Neuss M, Schau T, Isotani A, et al. Elevated mitral valve pressure gradient after MitraClip implantation deteriorates longterm outcome in patients with severe mitral regurgitation and severe heart failure. *JACC Cardiovasc Interv.* 2017;10:931–939.
39. Patzelt J, Zhang W, Sauter R, et al. Elevated mitral valve pressure gradient is predictive of long-term outcome after percutaneous edge-to-edge mitral valve repair in patients with degenerative Mitral Regurgitation (MR), but not in functional MR. *J Am Heart Assoc.* 2019;8:e011366.

76 Mitral Regurgitation

REBECCA TUNG HAHN AND ROBERT O. BONOW

MITRAL VALVE ANATOMY, 1455
Mitral Annulus, 1455
Mitral Leaflets, 1455
Mitral Valve Chordae and Papillary Muscles, 1455

MECHANISMS OF MITRAL REGURGITATION, 1456
Normal Mitral Valve Physiology, 1456

Mitral Regurgitation Morphologic Classifications, 1456

PRIMARY MITRAL REGURGITATION, 1458
Clinical Presentation, 1458
Natural History, 1462
Management of Primary Mitral Regurgitation, 1463

SECONDARY MITRAL REGURGITATION, 1465

Pathophysiology, 1465
Clinical Presentation, 1466
Management of Secondary Mitral Regurgitation, 1467

ACUTE MITRAL REGURGITATION, 1470
Clinical Presentation, 1470

CLASSIC REFERENCES, 1471

REFERENCES, 1471

The prevalence of valvular heart disease increases with age, and population studies have shown mitral regurgitation (MR) of either primary or secondary cause is the most prevalent valvular disorder, occurring in 9% to 10% of elderly patients in United States (see Nkomo et al., Classic References). Prognosis and treatment, however, are distinctly different based on the cause of the MR,[1] and thus accurate diagnosis of valve morphology is an important first step in determining the appropriate treatment options.[2] The following chapter will review mitral valve (MV) anatomy, characterize morphologic and etiologic features and outcomes associated with primary and secondary disease, and then discuss current and investigational treatment options.

MITRAL VALVE ANATOMY

The MV is a complex three-dimensional structure involving multiple, anatomically distinct components (see Perloff and Roberts, Classic References). Coordinated interaction of the annulus, commissures, leaflets, chordae tendineae, papillary muscles, and left ventricle is crucial for MV functional integrity (Fig. 76.1). Abnormalities of any of these structures may cause MR.

Mitral Annulus

The mitral annulus is not a single, well-defined ring of connective tissue but is instead a multifaceted structure made up of the convergence of several components: the atrial and ventricular muscular walls, the hinge line of the mitral leaflets, the epicardial adipose tissue, a discontinuous semi-circle of fibrous tissue on its posterior aspect, and a band of connective tissue at its anterior aspect.[3] The annulus is often described as saddle-shaped on three-dimensional studies with anterior and posterior peaks and nadirs near the medial and lateral fibrous trigones (see Levine et al., Classic References). The anterior "horn" of the saddle is composed of the curved band of connective tissue that adjoins the annulus of the aorta at the level of the left and noncoronary cusps, referred to as the "aorto-mitral curtain" by surgeons and the 'intervalvular fibrosa' by imagers.[4] This band of tissue is continuous with the anterior MV leaflet, which hinges where the left atrial (LA) wall joins the leaflet. This hinge-point is more apical, usually below the fibrous trigones; thus, measurement of the annulus by multimodality imaging often demarcates the anterior annulus by cutting off the aorto-mitral curtain superior to the trigone-to-trigone line, making the annulus D-shaped: the straight component is conventionally named the anterior mitral annulus, and the curved component is the posterior mitral annulus.[5] The posterior annulus is less fibrotic and moves with myocardial contraction, allowing for systolic bending and apical displacement of the medial and lateral horns, increasing saddle height but reducing circumferential area. The mitral annulus is innervated and supplies blood vessels to the leaflets.[6] Because it forms the convergence of the atrial and ventricular myocardium, the posterior annulus may dilate in the setting of either left ventricular (LV) or LA dilation and is also prone to age-related degenerative calcification.

Mitral Leaflets

Due to the oblique orientation of the mitral apparatus relative to the anatomic axes of the body, the anterior and posterior MV leaflets are oriented in a more anterosuperior and posteroinferior position.[7] The anterior leaflet is longer radially and thicker than the posterior leaflet, because it must withstand significantly higher tensile load. The posterior leaflet is longer circumferentially and more flexible. Two leaflet segmentation schemes have been proposed. The most commonly used classification scheme was proposed by Carpentier (Fig. 76.2A; see also Fig. 16.31) (see Carpentier, Classic References). Because the posterior leaflet typically has two well-defined indentations, there are three separate sections or "scallops" referred to as P1 (anterolateral), P2 (middle), and P3 (posteromedial). The anterior leaflet typically is devoid of indentations, so the anterior leaflet opposing P1 is designated as A1 (anterior segment), the segment opposite to P2 is A2 (middle segment), and the segment opposite to P3 is A3 (posterior segment). A modification of the Carpentier scheme (see Fig. 76.2B) divides the large middle segment into lateral (A2L and P2L) and medial (A2M and P2M) halves, which respects the separate chordal origins of the leaflets. The anterior and posterior leaflets come into direct continuity at the anterolateral and posteromedial commissures; commissural tissue may range from a few millimeters to distinct leaflets or scallops.

Mitral Valve Chordae and Papillary Muscles

The chordae tendineae are responsible for determining the position and tension on the leaflets at LV end-systole. The chordae are composed of collagen and elastin, are surrounded by a layer of endothelium, and originate from the heads of the papillary muscles or infrequently from the inferolateral ventricular wall. There are multiple chordal classification systems based on the origin (i.e., apical or basal portion of the papillary muscles), attachment site within the mitral complex (i.e., leaflet, interpapillary, myocardial wall), and insertion site on the mitral leaflets, to name a few.[8] The classification by leaflet insertion is the most often used with marginal or primary chordae inserting on the free margin of the mitral leaflets and secondary chordae inserting on the ventricular (rough zone) surface of the leaflets preventing billowing while reducing tension on the leaflet tissues. "Strut" chordae are thicker, secondary chordae and attach to the anterior MV leaflet with a broad, muscular base. These chordae have greater viscoelasticity than marginal chordae[9] and may play a role in determining dynamic ventricular shape and function due to their contribution to

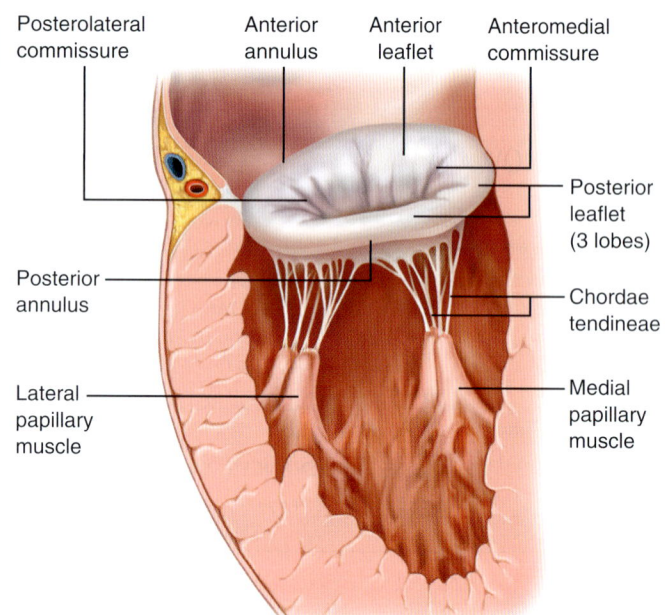

FIGURE 76.1 Continuity of the mitral apparatus and the left ventricular (LV) myocardium. Mitral regurgitation (MR) may be caused by any condition that affects the leaflets or the structure and function of the left ventricle. Similarly, a surgical procedure that disrupts the mitral apparatus in an attempt to correct MR will have adverse effects on LV geometry, volume, and function. (From Otto CM. Evaluation and management of chronic mitral regurgitation. *N Engl J Med.* 2001;345:740-746.)

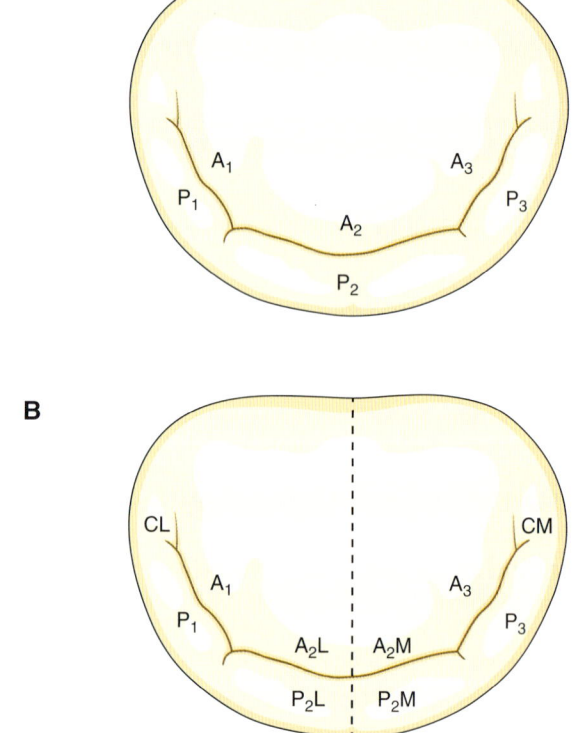

FIGURE 76.2 Classification of mitral valve segmentation, viewed from the atrial aspect of the valve. **A,** Segmentation model of Carpentier. **B,** Proposed adaptation by Shah. *CL,* lateral commissure; *CM,* medial commissure. (**A** modified from Carpentier A. Cardiac valve surgery: the "French correction." *J Thorac Cardiovasc Surg.* 1983;86:323-337; **B** modified from Shah PM. Current concepts in mitral valve prolapse: diagnosis and management. *J Cardiol.* 2010;56:125-133.)

ventricular-valve continuity. *Tertiary or basal chordae* insert on the posterior leaflet base and mitral annulus.

There are two papillary muscles; the anterolateral arises from the apicolateral third of the LV, and the posteromedial arises from the middle of the LV inferior wall. The anterolateral papillary muscle is composed of an anterior and posterior head, and the posteromedial papillary muscle is usually composed of anterior, intermediate, and posterior heads. Because the papillary muscles connect directly to the LV, any geometric change in LV shape can change the axial relationship of the chordae and leaflets, resulting in poor leaflet coaptation. The posteromedial papillary muscle gives chordae to the medial half of both leaflets (i.e., posteromedial commissure, A3, P3, A2M, and P2M). Similarly, the anterolateral papillary muscle chordae attach to the lateral half of the MV leaflets (i.e., anterolateral commissure, A1, P1, A2L, and P2L). The midline of the valve is a relatively chordal-free zone.

MECHANISMS OF MITRAL REGURGITATION

Normal Mitral Valve Physiology

The MV complex described earlier must work in concert to close the annular orifice in systole without permitting regurgitation while maximizing forward flow during diastole under low pressure conditions. An appreciation of the dynamic nature of the MV is integral to the understanding of the morphologic abnormalities resulting in MR. In addition, the MV apparatus is thought to have the capacity to modify its structure in response to both genetic and biomechanical stresses.[10]

Three-dimensional imaging studies have shown that during the isovolumic contraction period in early systole, anteroposterior contraction occurs with accentuated folding across the fixed intercommissural diameter such that the annular saddle shape (with anteroposterior high points and mediolateral low points) is accentuated with resulting approximation of anterior and posterior leaflets. With LV contraction and longitudinal LV shortening, the annulus moves toward the apex while the papillary muscles contract to maintain the distance between the mitral annulus and papillary muscle tips. The papillary muscles that attach to the posterior half of the LV maintain leaflet closure in the posterior LV cavity away from the LV outflow tract (LVOT). At the same time, the mitral annulus and aortic annulus angle becomes more acute during systole to facilitate blood flow out the LVOT.

Mitral Regurgitation Morphologic Classifications

The 2020 American College of Cardiology/American Heart Association (ACC/AHA) guideline for the management of patients with valvular heart disease[1] and the 2020 focused update of the 2017 ACC expert consensus decision pathway on the management of MR[2] emphasize the importance of an initial assessment of its cause, mechanism, and severity. The major causes of MR include myxomatous degeneration (mitral valve prolapse [MVP] and ruptured mitral chordae), rheumatic heart disease, infective endocarditis, hypertrophic cardiomyopathy, annular calcification, dilated cardiomyopathy, and ischemic heart disease (Table 76.1). Less common causes of MR include collagen vascular diseases, trauma, the hypereosinophilic syndrome, carcinoid, and exposure to certain drugs. The morphologic classification for MR described by Carpentier (see Carpentier, Classic References) are based on the mobility of the MV leaflets (Fig. 76.3). A variety of causes are associated with each type of leaflet motion.

Type I MR involves normal mobility of leaflets with poor coaptation due to annular dilation or perforation or cleft/indentations of a leaflet. Etiologies associated with leaflet disruption are considered primary MR and include endocarditis and iatrogenic trauma. Congenital isolated cleft MV leaflets or deep indentations also may be associated with significant MR.[11] Atrial and annular dilation causing MR or atriogenic MR (Fig. 76.4, upper left), is a morphologic subtype of secondary MR and is usually associated with chronic atrial fibrillation (AF) or heart failure (HF) with preserved ejection fraction (EF), both resulting in progressive remodeling of the LA.[12-14] The LV dimensions, papillary muscles, chordae, and leaflets are typically intrinsically normal; however, in the setting of chronic AF or increased LA pressures, a number of anatomic derangements result in MR: LA dilation results in annular dilation and flattening, insufficient leaflet remodeling or leaflet thickening exceeds the increase in mitral annular area, and abnormal atrial-annular dynamics reduce normal leaflet coaptation mechanics.[14,15] Studies have suggested that maintenance of sinus rhythm may result in reduction of MR.[16] A possible subtype of atriogenic MR is atriogenic leaflet tethering.[17] This entity is still associated with LA and annular dilation, but because the posterior leaflet is attached to the junction of the LA and LV myocardium, progressive annular dilation may result in deviation of the leaflet attachment toward the outer wall of

TABLE 76.1 Causes of Acute and Chronic Mitral Regurgitation

Acute	Chronic
Mitral Annulus Disorders	**Inflammatory**
• Infective endocarditis (abscess formation)	• Rheumatic heart disease
• Trauma (valvular heart surgery)	• Systemic lupus erythematosus
• Paravalvular leak caused by suture interruption (surgical technical problems or infective endocarditis)	• Scleroderma
	Degenerative
Mitral Leaflet Disorders	• Myxomatous degeneration of mitral valve leaflets (Barlow click-murmur syndrome, prolapsing leaflet, mitral valve prolapse)
• Infective endocarditis (perforation or interfering with valve closure by vegetation)	• Marfan syndrome
• Trauma (tear during percutaneous balloon mitral valvotomy or penetrating chest injury)	• Ehlers-Danlos syndrome
• Tumors (atrial myxoma)	• Pseudoxanthoma elasticum
• Myxomatous degeneration	• Calcification of mitral valve annulus
• Systemic lupus erythematosus (Libman-Sacks lesion)	**Infective**
Rupture of Chordae Tendineae	• Infective endocarditis affecting normal, abnormal, or prosthetic mitral valves
• Idiopathic (e.g., spontaneous)	**Structural**
• Myxomatous degeneration (mitral valve prolapse, Marfan syndrome, Ehlers-Danlos syndrome)	• Ruptured chordae tendineae (spontaneous or secondary to myocardial infarction, trauma, mitral valve prolapse, endocarditis)
• Infective endocarditis	• Rupture or dysfunction of papillary muscle (ischemia or myocardial infarction)
• Acute rheumatic fever	• Dilation of mitral valve annulus and left ventricular cavity (congestive cardiomyopathies, aneurysmal dilation of left ventricle)
• Trauma (percutaneous balloon valvotomy, blunt chest trauma)	• Hypertrophic cardiomyopathy
Papillary Muscle Disorders	• Paravalvular prosthetic leak
• Coronary artery disease (causing dysfunction and rarely rupture)	**Congenital**
• Acute global left ventricular dysfunction	• Mitral valve clefts or fenestrations
• Infiltrative diseases (amyloidosis, sarcoidosis)	• Parachute mitral valve abnormality in association with:
• Trauma	• Endocardial cushion defects
Primary Mitral Valve Prosthetic Disorders	• Endocardial fibroelastosis
• Porcine cusp perforation (endocarditis)	• Transposition of great arteries
• Porcine cusp degeneration	• Anomalous origin of left coronary artery
• Mechanical failure (strut fracture)	
• Immobilized disc or ball of the mechanical prosthesis	

Data from Jutzy KR, Al-Zaibag M. Acute mitral and aortic valve regurgitation. In: Al-Zaibag M, Duran CMG, eds. *Valvular Heart Disease*. New York: Marcel Dekker; 1994:345-362; and Haffajee CI. Chronic mitral regurgitation. In: Dalen JE, Alpert JS, eds. *Valvular Heart Disease*. 2nd ed. Boston: Little, Brown; 1987;112

the LV myocardium and result in restriction of posterior leaflet motion in both systole and diastole with malcoaptation of the anterior leaflet and a posteriorly directed MR jet.

Type II MR involves excessive motion of the margin of a leaflet segment above the annular plane. This has been referred to as degenerative MR, also a morphologic subtype of primary MR. The two classic subtypes are MVP and leaflet flail with ruptured chordae. The two phenotypes related to these morphologic subtypes are fibroelastic deficiency and myxomatous degeneration. Fibroelastic deficiency is seen as a degenerative disease, and thus patients are older and the disease is typically localized to one or two segments and can involve ruptured chordae with leaflet redundancy and thickening primarily on the flail segment (typically posterior, especially P2). Although considered a "specific" sign of significant MR according to American Society of Echocardiography (ASE) guidelines,[18] a flail mitral leaflet is not synonymous with severe MR and can be associated with only mild or moderate MR.[19] In fibroelastic deficiency, leaflet area remains constant throughout the cardiac cycle with relatively normal annular dynamics and often holosystolic MR. Conversely, myxomatous disease is seen in younger patients with familial clustering and a variety of genetic abnormalities have been identified.[20] Myxomatous valves usually show generalized redundancy, cellular proliferation, and increased matrix production, resulting in thickening of both leaflets (Fig. 76.5), involving multiple segments and prolapse volume and height increases in late systole (see Fig. 76.4, upper right). In myxomatous disease, the mitral annulus is typically dilated and annular dynamics may be altered with the largest annular area in late systole, contributing to the presence of late-systolic MR.[21] In addition, there is loss of early-systolic area contraction and saddle-shape deepening that may also contribute to leaflet malcoaptation. It is uncertain whether these diseases are variants along a single pathophysiologic spectrum; however, recent data showing distinct physiologic differences suggest that they are related but separate entities. A ruptured chordae and flail segment may occur with either phenotype.

Type III disease is associated with restricted mobility of leaflets, resulting in coaptation of leaflets in the ventricular level. This attenuated mobility can be diastolic and systolic (type IIIa) or just systolic (type IIIb). The first type (type IIIa) is the result of thickening and shortening of leaflets, chordae, or annulus secondary to inflammatory or congenital disease and is considered a form of primary MR. Classic etiologies associated with this mechanism are rheumatic heart disease (see Fig. 76.4, lower left), carcinoid, radiation induced, and mitral annular calcification–related MR. These entities share the same pathomorphologic changes: thickening, retraction, and rigidity of leaflets and attached chordae, which restricts both systolic and diastolic leaflet motion. In type IIIb the attenuated mobility is entirely systolic and is associated with LV enlargement, displacement of papillary muscles away from the mitral annulus, and systolic tethering of mitral leaflets transferred through the tensed chordae tendineae. This is the second morphologic subtype, considered secondary MR. A loss of annular folding across the intercommissural axis and the loss of saddle shape accentuation in early systole, play a role in early-systolic type IIIb MR just as it does in myxomatous MV disease.[22]

In general, types II and IIIa usually are caused by primary disorders of the MV leaflets, whereas types I and IIIb have relatively normal leaflets, which are distorted by LV and annular remodeling, resulting in secondary MR.

Dysfunction	Ventricular View	Atrial View	Etiologic Disorder
Type I Normal leaflet motion	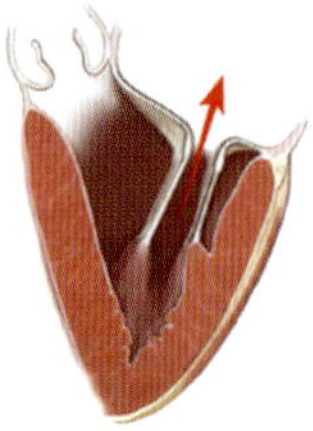	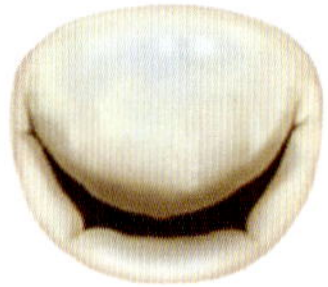	Ischemic cardiomyopathy Dilated cardiomyopathy Endocarditis Congenital
Type II Increased leaflet motion (leaflet prolapse)	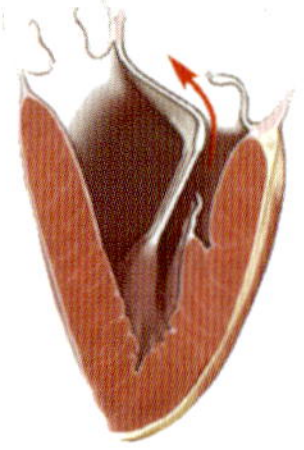	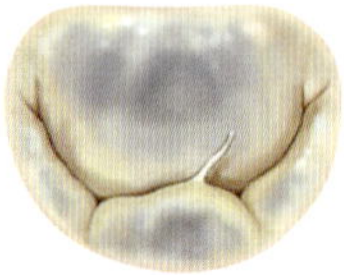	Degenerative disease Fibroelastic deficiency Marfan syndrome Forme fruste Barlow Barlow disease Endocarditis Rheumatic disease Trauma Ischemic cardiomyopathy Ehlers-Danlos syndrome
Type IIIA Restricted leaflet motion (restricted opening)	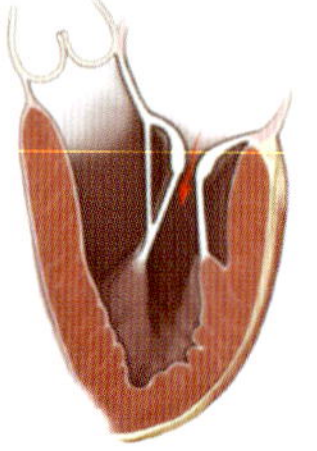	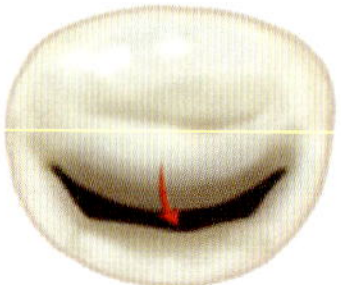	Rheumatic disease Carcinoid disease Radiation Lupus erythematosus Ergotamine use Hypereosinophilic syndrome Mucopolysaccharidosis
Type IIIB Restricted leaflet motion (restricted closure)	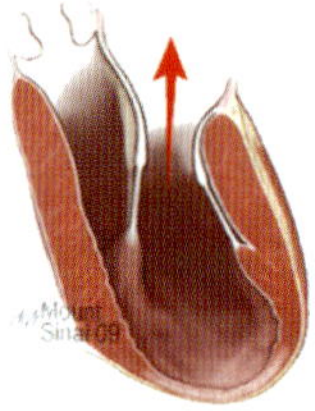	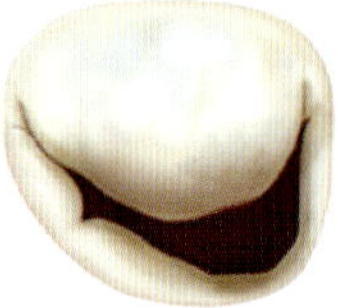	Ischemic cardiomyopathy Dilated cardiomyopathy

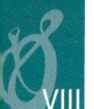

FIGURE 76.3 Pathophysiologic triad approach to mitral regurgitation (MR) and its multifactorial etiology. The mechanism of leaflet dysfunction defines the three types of MR. (From Castillo JG, Adams DH. Mitral valve repair and replacement. In: Otto CM, Bonow RO, eds. *Valvular Heart Disease: A Companion to Braunwald's Heart Disease*. Philadelphia: Saunders; 2013:327-340.)

PRIMARY MITRAL REGURGITATION

Clinical Presentation

The clinical stages of primary chronic degenerative MR are indicated in Table 76.2, demonstrating the progressive nature of the disease.

Symptoms

The nature and severity of symptoms in patients with chronic MR are functions of a combination of interrelated factors, including the severity of MR, rate of its progression, level of LA, pulmonary venous, and pulmonary arterial (PA) pressure, presence of episodic or chronic atrial tachyarrhythmias, and presence of associated valvular, myocardial, or coronary artery disease. In addition, there may be symptoms related to the underlying pathogenic cause of the MR (e.g., endocarditis, lupus, or Marfan syndrome). Many patients with severe MR remain completely asymptomatic, though close questioning of the patient or family may reveal subtle reductions in functional capacity (i.e., chronic weakness or fatigue). Symptoms may occur with preserved LV contractile function in patients with chronic MR who have severely elevated pulmonary venous pressures or AF. In other patients, symptoms herald LV decompensation.

Physical Examination (see Chapter 13)

Palpation of the arterial pulse is helpful in differentiating aortic stenosis (AS) from MR, both of which may produce a prominent systolic murmur at the base of the heart and apex (see Chapter 13). The carotid arterial upstroke is sharp in severe MR and delayed in AS; the volume of the pulse may be normal or reduced in the presence of HF. The cardiac impulse, like the arterial pulse, is brisk and hyperdynamic. It is displaced to the left, and a prominent LV filling wave is frequently palpable in thin patients.

Auscultation. S_1, produced by MV closure, is often diminished in patients with primary MR and defective valve leaflets. Wide splitting of S_2 is common and results from shortening of LV ejection and an earlier A_2 as a consequence of reduced resistance to LV ejection. In patients with severe pulmonary hypertension, P_2 is louder than A_2. The abnormal increase in the flow rate across the mitral orifice during the rapid filling phase is often associated with an S_3, which should not be interpreted as a feature of HF in these patients, and this may be accompanied by a brief diastolic rumble.

The systolic murmur is the most prominent physical finding; it must be differentiated from the systolic murmur of AS, tricuspid regurgitation, and ventricular septal defect. In most patients with severe MR, the systolic murmur commences immediately after the soft S_1 and continues beyond and may obscure A_2 because of the persisting pressure difference between the LV and LA after aortic valve closure. The holosystolic murmur of chronic MR is usually constant in intensity, blowing, high-pitched, and loudest at the apex, with frequent radiation to the left axilla and left infrascapular area, particularly with posteriorly directed jets. Radiation toward the sternum or aortic area, however, may occur with abnormalities of the posterior leaflet associated with an anteriorly directed regurgitant jet and is particularly common in patients with MVP and flail involving this leaflet (see Fig. 16.26). The murmur shows little change, even in the presence of large beat-to-beat variations of LV stroke volume, as in AF. This finding contrasts with that in most midsystolic (ejection) murmurs, such as in AS, which vary greatly in intensity with stroke volume and therefore with the duration of diastole. Little correlation has been found between the intensity of the systolic murmur and severity of MR.

The murmur of MR may be holosystolic, late systolic, or early systolic. When the murmur is confined to late systole, the regurgitation usually is secondary to MVP and may follow one or more mid-systolic clicks and typically is not severe. Such late systolic MR is often associated with a normal S_1 because initial closure of the MV cusps may be unimpaired. A midsystolic click preceding a mid- to late-systolic murmur, and the response of that murmur to a number of maneuvers helps establish the diagnosis of MVP (discussed subsequently). Early systolic murmurs are typical of acute MR. When the LA v wave is markedly elevated in acute MR, the murmur may diminish or disappear in late systole as the reverse pressure gradient declines. As noted, a short, low-pitched diastolic murmur following S_3 may be audible in patients with severe MR, even without accompanying MS, due to increased early diastolic flow.

Dynamic Auscultation. Auscultation during positional changes or the Valsalva maneuver can be quite helpful in characterizing the MR murmur. When MR is holosystolic, it typically varies little during respiration. However, sudden standing usually diminishes the murmur, whereas squatting augments it. The late systolic murmur of MVP behaves in the opposite direction, decreasing in duration with squatting and increasing in duration with standing. Similarly, with the Valsalva maneuver, MVP clicks may occur earlier in systole with lengthening of the murmur. Holosystolic MR murmur is often softer during the strain of the Valsalva maneuver and shows a left-sided response (i.e., a transient overshoot that occurs six to eight beats after release of the strain). The murmur of MR usually is intensified by isometric exercise, differentiating it from the systolic murmurs of valvular AS and obstructive hypertrophic cardiomyopathy, both of which are reduced by this intervention.

Echocardiography (see Chapter 16)

Echocardiography plays an integral role in the diagnosis of primary MR, in determining its cause and potential for repair, and in quantifying its severity (see Chapter 16). Assessment of MR severity by echocardiography can be divided into four general categories: structural, qualitative, semi-quantitative, and quantitative.[18] Structural assessment of patients with severe MR, includes not only the determination of valve morphology and mechanisms of MR (see Figs, 16.36, 16.37, and 80.5), but should also provide measures of LV systolic function, severity of dilation of the LV and LA, and right heart size and function. Quantification of mitral leaflet lengths, severity of tethering, and the severity of leaflet displacement into the atrium may be important for determining the success of surgical or transcatheter interventions.

All other assessments of MR severity rely on a number of Doppler echocardiographic modalities. Doppler echocardiography in MR characteristically reveals a highvelocity systolic jet in the LA during systole.[23] Qualitative assessment of MR severity uses color Doppler to assess the color jet area and flow convergence (vena contracta), and continuous wave Doppler to evaluate the density and shape of the regurgitant jet spectral profile.

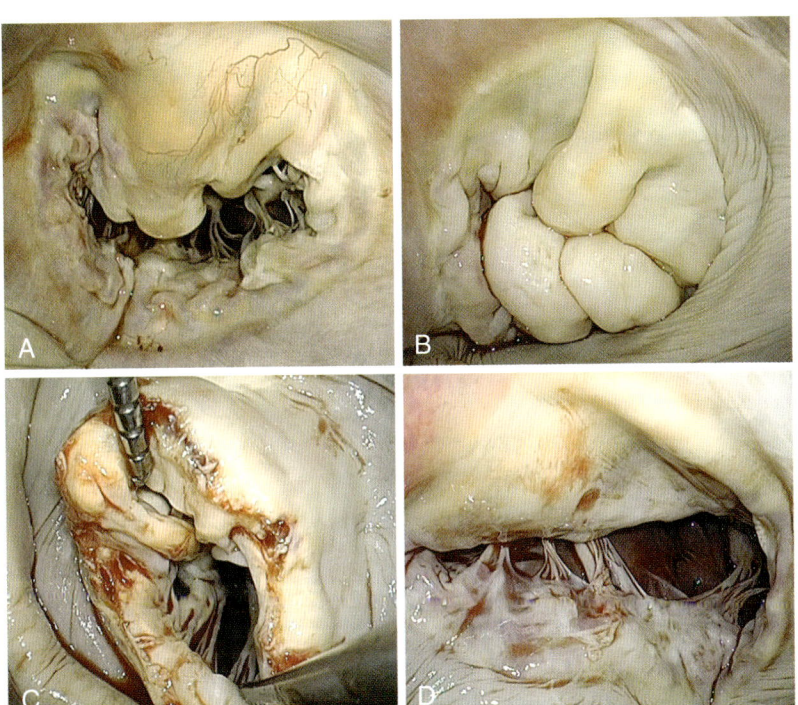

FIGURE 76.4 Valve lesions in mitral regurgitation. **A,** Severe annular dilation leading to type I dysfunction. **B,** Severe myxomatous changes with redundant, thick, and bulky segments in a patient with Barlow disease and type II dysfunction. **C,** Rheumatic mitral valve disease with classic "fish mouth" appearance and type IIIA dysfunction. **D,** Ischemic mitral valve disease caused by severe tethering of the P_3 scallop leading to type IIIB dysfunction. (From Castillo JG, Adams DH. Mitral valve repair and replacement. In: Otto CM, Bonow RO, eds. *Valvular Heart Disease: A Companion to Braunwald's Heart Disease.* 5th ed. Philadelphia: Saunders; 2021:370-379.)

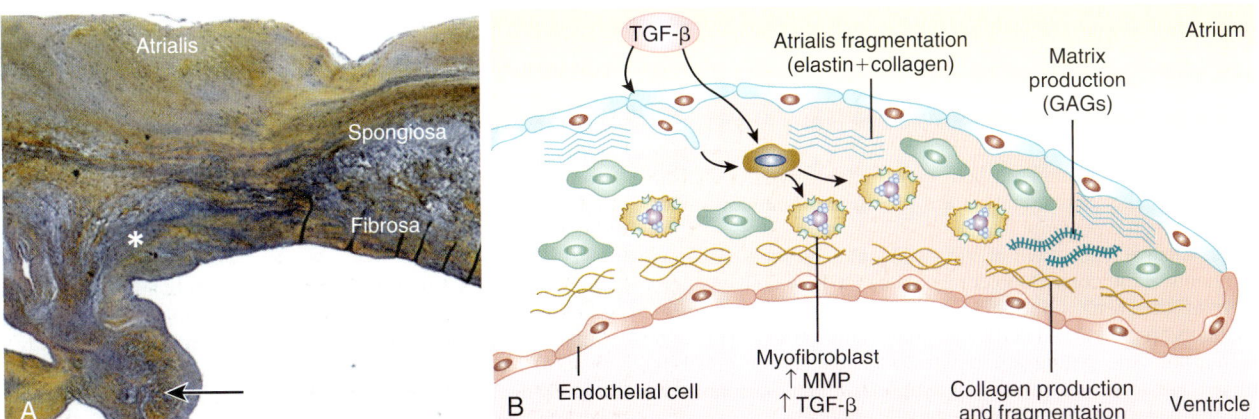

FIGURE 76.5 Mechanisms of mitral valve prolapse (MVP). **A,** Mitral valve stained with hematoxylin and eosin to define the lesion of MVP as disruption of the fibrosa by myxoid extracellular matrix (*), which also infiltrates the collagen core of the chordae tendineae, one of which was ruptured (*arrow*). The elastin lamina beneath the atrialis is also disrupted **B,** Schematic showing the mechanism of myxomatous degeneration, with activation of valve interstitial cells to myofibroblasts that increase matrix production and turnover, secrete MMPs that drive collagen and elastin fragmentation, and release transforming growth factor (TGF)-β, which in turn promotes further cell proliferation and myofibroblast differentiation. *GAGs,* Glycosaminoglycans; *MMP,* matrix metalloproteinase. (From Levine RA, et al. Mitral valve disease: morphology and mechanisms. *Nat Rev Cardiol.* 2015;12:689-710.)

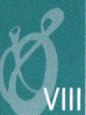

TABLE 76.2 Stages of Chronic Primary Mitral Regurgitation

STAGE	DEFINITION	VALVE ANATOMY	VALVE HEMODYNAMICS*	HEMODYNAMIC CONSEQUENCES	SYMPTOMS
A	At risk for MR	Mild MVP with normal coaptation Mild valve thickening and leaflet restriction	No MR jet or small central jet area <20% LA on Doppler Small vena contracta <0.3 cm	None	None
B	Progressive MR	Moderate to severe MVP with normal coaptation Rheumatic valve changes with leaflet restriction and loss of central coaptation Previous IE	Central jet MR 20%-40% LA or late systolic eccentric jet MR Vena contracta <0.7 cm Rvol <60 mL RF <50% ERO <0.40 cm^2 Angiographic grade 1-2+	Mild LA enlargement No LV enlargement Normal pulmonary pressure	None
C	Asymptomatic severe MR	Severe MVP with loss of coaptation or flail leaflet Rheumatic valve changes with leaflet restriction and loss of central coaptation Previous IE Thickening of leaflets with radiation heart disease	Central jet MR >40% LA or holosystolic eccentric jet MR Vena contracta ≥0.7 cm Rvol ≥60 mL RF ≥50% ERO ≥0.40 cm^2 Angiographic grade 3-4+	Moderate or severe LA enlargement LV enlargement Pulmonary hypertension may be present at rest or with exercise. C1: LVEF >60% and LVESD <40 mm C2: LVEF ≤60% and LVESD ≥40 mm	None
D	Symptomatic severe MR	Severe MVP with loss of coaptation or flail leaflet Rheumatic valve changes with leaflet restriction and loss of central coaptation Previous IE Thickening of leaflets with radiation heart disease	Central jet MR >40% LA or holosystolic eccentric jet MR Vena contracta ≥0.7 cm Rvol ≥60 mL RF ≥50% ERO ≥0.40 cm^2 Angiographic grade 3-4+	Moderate or severe LA enlargement LV enlargement Pulmonary hypertension present	Decreased exercise tolerance Exertional dyspnea

ERO, Effective regurgitant orifice; *IE,* infective endocarditis; *LA,* left atrium; *LV,* left ventricle; *LVEF,* left ventricular ejection fraction; *LVESD,* left ventricular end-systolic dimension; *MR,* mitral regurgitation; *MVP,* mitral valve prolapse; *RF,* regurgitant fraction; *Rvol,* regurgitant volume.
*Several valve hemodynamic criteria are provided for assessment of MR severity, but not all criteria for each category will be present in each patient. Classification of MR severity as mild, moderate, or severe depends on data quality and integration of these parameters in conjunction with other clinical evidence.
From Otto CM, et al. 2020 AHA/ACC guideline for the management of patients with valvular heart disease: a report of the American College of Cardiology/American Heart Association Task Force on Practice Guidelines. *J Am Coll Cardiol.* 2021;77:e25-197.

Because color flow jet areas are significantly influenced by the driving pressure (LV-LA gradient) and momentum within the LA, hemodynamic factors (i.e., blood pressure, LA and LV compliance), jet eccentricity, as well as instrument factors (i.e., transmit power and frequency, receiver gain, Nyquist limit, and wall filter) limit the accuracy of this approach.[23] Importantly, though, the color Doppler jet duration and direction can give important clues as to the mechanism of the MR. In primary MR, the jet may be late systolic with a direction typically away from the most significant anatomic lesion, so posterior prolapse or flail typically produces an anterior jet and vice versa. With secondary MR, regurgitation is frequently bimodal, peaking in both early and late systole, with or without directionality depending on the presence of anterior leaflet override of a tethered posterior leaflet.

Semi-quantitative assessment of MR severity include measurements of components of the color Doppler regurgitant jet: flow convergence, jet width at the vena contracta, and jet area. Because these measurements are performed at a single point in the cardiac cycle and assume a symmetric regurgitant orifice, semi-quantitative methods become less accurate in the setting of temporal variability, nonplanar leaflet conformation and noncircular regurgitant orifices.

Quantification of MR Severity

Quantitative methods to measure regurgitant fraction, regurgitant volume (Rvol), and regurgitant orifice area have greater accuracy when done carefully (Fig. 76.6), and these methods are strongly recommended (see Table 76.2).[1,2,18] There are three methods for quantifying MR severity: proximal isovelocity surface area (PISA), volumetric Doppler, and three-dimensional direct planimetry of the vena contracta area.

The PISA method is perhaps the most practical quantitative method for daily use (see Chapter 16).[18,23] It exploits the predictable flow acceleration leading into the MV, which forms roughly hemispheric isovelocity shells that can be highlighted by shifting the aliasing velocity of the color display and identified where the color changes from blue to red (see Fig. 16.38). If the radial distance is r from the vena contracta to the contour with velocity v, then the flow rate Q will be given by

$$Q = 2\pi r^2 v$$

from which the effective regurgitant orifice area (EROA) can be obtained by dividing Q by the maximal velocity through the orifice obtained by continuous-wave (CW) Doppler (Vmax). A handy simplification that works in the majority of cases assumes approximately 100 mm Hg driving pressure across the regurgitant orifice (leading, via the Bernoulli equation, to a 5 m/sec maximal jet velocity). If the aliasing velocity is set to (approximately) 40 cm/sec, the math simplifies to EROA = $r^2/2$. An approximation to Rvol can be obtained by multiplying EROA by the velocity time integral of the regurgitant CW signal.

There are some important caveats to use of the PISA equation, the most critical of which involves nonholosystolic jets, such as those occurring with MVP in which the MR does not begin until the latter half of systole. In this case, the MR is much less severe than a single frame showing either the largest jet, vena contracta, or convergence zone would imply. Additional pitfalls include situations in which there are two or more regurgitant jets. Finally, the PISA method quantifies EROA with calculation of the Rvol. Regurgitant fraction requires a measure of total LV stroke volume and thus cannot be directly measured by this technique.

The volumetric Doppler method (see Fig 16.39) quantifies Rvol as the difference between the diastolic stroke volume across the MV and the forward stroke volume (typically using the LV outflow stroke volume). The expertise required to accurately measure these stroke volumes make this method less practical for general use. However, this method is not limited by MR temporal variability, multiple jets, or elliptical orifice. In addition, this method allows the quantitation of all three measures of MR severity important for making decisions about intervention: regurgitant fraction, Rvol, and EROA. This is the preferred method in many comprehensive valve centers.

Finally, improvements in three-dimensional imaging permit acquisition of color Doppler volumes for direct planimetry of the vena contracta area. This method is more difficult for transthoracic compared with transesophageal echocardiography.

Supportive evidence for MR severity can be found in pulmonary venous flow. The normal pattern of systolic (S) wave greater than diastolic (D) wave generally indicates mild MR, frank systolic reversal indicates severe MR, but the common "blunted" pattern (S < D) may be seen in all degrees of MR. A transmitral E-wave >1.2 m/sec is supportive of severe MR, whereas a pattern with E < A virtually excludes severe MR. Doppler echocardiography also is an important tool to estimate the PA systolic pressure and to determine the presence and severity of associated aortic or tricuspid regurgitation.

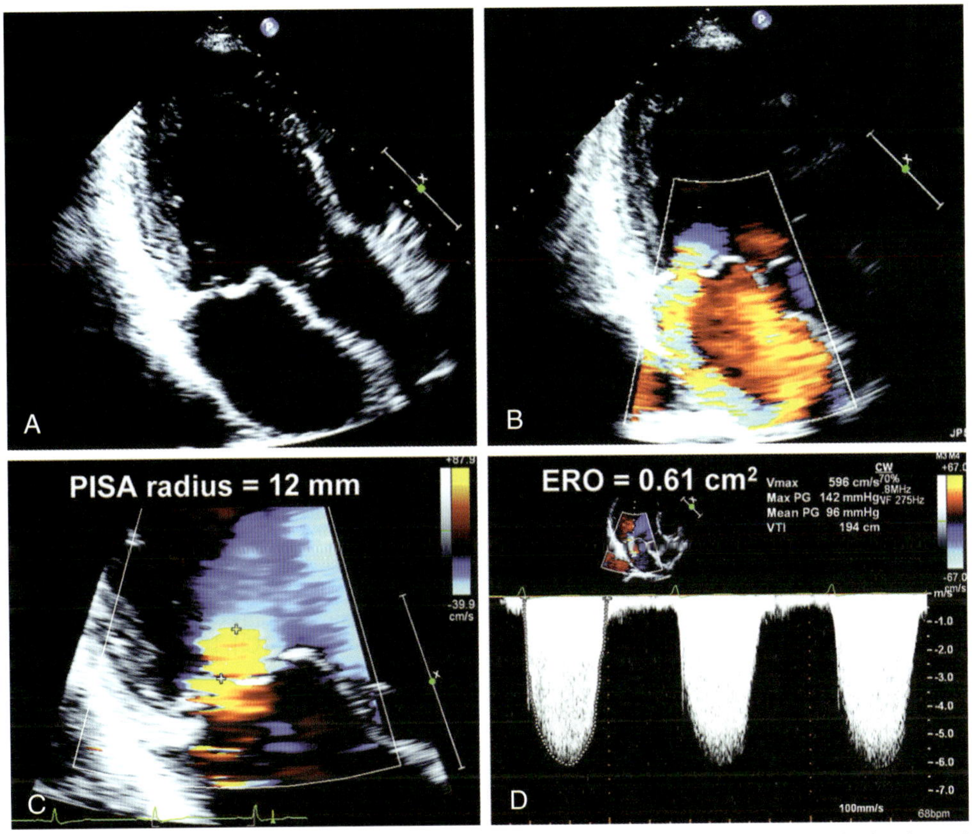

FIGURE 76.6 Severe mitral regurgitation (MR) caused by prolapse of the mitral valve with quantitative determination of effective regurgitant orifice area (ERO) on echocardiography. **A** and **B**, Severe prolapse of the mitral valve with severe MR. **C** and **D**, ERO was calculated with the proximal isovelocity surface area (PISA) radius and peak velocity of the MR jet. (From Kang DH, et al. Comparison of early surgery versus conventional treatment in asymptomatic severe mitral regurgitation. *Circulation*. 2009;119:797-804.)

Transesophageal Echocardiography

Transesophageal echocardiography (TEE) may be needed in addition to transthoracic imaging for assessment of the detailed anatomy of the regurgitant MV, the mechanisms of MR, and the severity of MR in some patients (see Chapter 16). Because the MV is in the far-field of all transthoracic imaging planes, TEE has significant advantages for imaging the morphology of the valve and severity of MR, particularly when transthoracic imaging is limited or discordant with clinical presentation. TEE imaging is also recommended for patients in whom surgical or transcatheter intervention is contemplated to assess anatomic suitability.[1] Three-dimensional imaging and three-dimensional color Doppler[24] help elucidate the mechanism and severity of MR (Fig. 76.7; see also Fig. 16.36) but also becomes an essential tool to guide interventions.

Exercise Echocardiography

Assessment of LV function, MR severity, and PA systolic pressure can be extremely helpful in determining severity of MR and hemodynamic abnormalities (e.g., pulmonary hypertension) during exercise.[25] This is a useful objective means to evaluate symptomatic patients who appear to

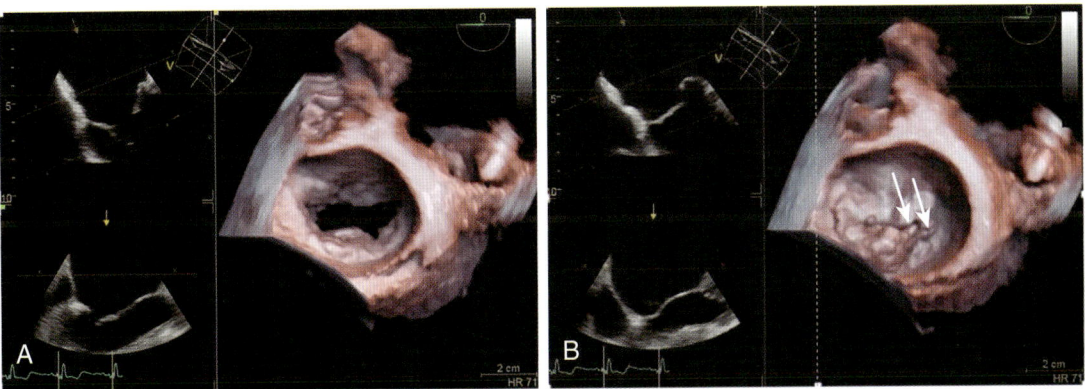

FIGURE 76.7 Three-dimensional echocardiography now allows direct visualization of the pathology, here demonstrating ruptured chordae to P_2 and P_3 (*arrows*). **A**, Ventricular diastole. **B**, Systole.

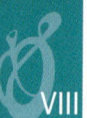

have less than severe MR at rest and, alternatively, to determine functional status and dynamic changes in hemodynamics in patients who otherwise appear stable and asymptomatic with severe MR (see section on Symptoms). Late-systolic MR may become more holosystolic with exercise, particularly if PA pressure rises significantly. Treadmill or bicycle exercise is appropriate in patients with MR. When ordering a treadmill exercise echo, one should provide guidance to the sonographer as to the priority for the various datasets to be obtained after exercise, because it is often impossible to obtain diagnostic mitral and tricuspid imaging and wall motion assessment while heart rate is still optimally high. If the focus is on the MV, rapid acquisition of mitral color and CW Doppler and tricuspid CW Doppler will usually be the priority. Semi-supine exercise testing on an appropriate tilted table allows continuous echocardiographic monitoring for quantifying changes in valvular regurgitation severity, LV function, and pulmonary pressure, offering significant advantages for the assessment of MR patients. Dobutamine echocardiography has little role in assessing organic MR but may be useful for ischemia or viability assessment in secondary MR (see section on Secondary Mitral Regurgitation).

OTHER DIAGNOSTIC EVALUATION MODALITIES (SEE PART III)
Electrocardiography
The principal electrocardiogram (ECG) findings are LA enlargement and AF. ECG evidence of LV enlargement occurs in approximately one third of patients with severe MR. Approximately 15% of patients exhibit ECG evidence of right ventricular (RV) hypertrophy, a change that reflects the presence of pulmonary hypertension of sufficient severity to counterbalance the hypertrophied LV in patients with MR.

Radiography
Cardiomegaly with LV enlargement, and particularly with LA enlargement, is a common finding in patients with chronic severe MR. Although the LA may be severely enlarged, little correlation has been found between LA size and pressure. Interstitial edema with Kerley B lines frequently is seen in patients with acute MR or with progressive LV failure.

Calcification of the mitral annulus, an important cause of MR in older adults, is most prominent in the posterior third of the cardiac silhouette. The lesion is best visualized on chest films exposed in the lateral or right anterior oblique projections (see Chapter 17), in which it appears as a dense, coarse, C-shaped opacity.

Cardiac Magnetic Resonance
Cardiac magnetic resonance (CMR) (see Chapter 19) provides accurate measurements of regurgitant flow that correlates well with quantitative Doppler imaging. It also is the most accurate noninvasive technique for measuring LV end-diastolic volume (EDV), end-systolic volume (ESV), and mass,[26] and is included in guidelines for imaging in valvular regurgitation.[18] Although detailed visualization of MV structure and function is obtained more reliably with echocardiography, particularly TEE, CMR offers a promising approach for accurate assessment of regurgitant severity and its impact on chamber size.[27]

CMR also has an evolving role for identifying the presence and severity of myocardial fibrosis for risk stratification of patients with MVP who have ventricular tachyarrhythmias and/or mitral annular disjunction (see section on Mitral Annular Disjunction).

Cardiac Computed Tomography
Cardiac CT imaging can provide useful structural information about the regurgitant MV (see Chapter 20),[28-30] with particular value in sizing the mitral annulus and quantifying the degree of annular calcification.[31] It appears to be particularly useful in planning for percutaneous MV replacement[32] and has been used in conjunction with three-dimensional printing to ensure an adequate fit of the proposed valve within the mitral apparatus.[33,34] Some have proposed CT imaging for quantification of the chamber volumes and regurgitant severity, specifically the planimetered size of the anatomic regurgitant orifice area, but this will likely remain adjunctive given the availability of echocardiography and CMR.

Left Ventricular Angiography
Given the availability of echocardiography and CMR, there is little reason to perform left ventriculography for the purpose of characterizing MR. The prompt appearance of contrast material in the LA after its injection into the LV indicates the presence of MR. The injection should be rapid enough to permit LV opacification but slow enough to avoid the development of premature ventricular contractions, which can induce spurious regurgitation (see Chapter 22). The Rvol can be estimated from the difference between the total LV stroke volume, estimated by angiocardiography, and the simultaneous measurement of the effective forward stroke volume by the Fick method.

Natural History
Although primary MR may be caused by Carpentier type I (perforation or cleft) and type IIIA (leaflet/chordal thickening) diseases, MVP is the most common cause of chronic primary MR in developed countries and is defined by an overriding of the annulus by a leaflet edge with displacement of the coaptation point into the atrium. Leaflet "flail" implies coaptation failure with eversion of the free edge of a leaflet into the LA, usually consequent to chordal rupture (see Fig. 76.7; see also Fig. 16.36). Echocardiography has been central to the diagnosis of MVP and flail (see Chapter 16). Because of the normal saddle shape of the annulus, diagnostic criteria for MVP were refined to include single-leaflet or bileaflet displacement >2 mm beyond the long-axis annular plane, with >5 mm leaflet thickening.[35,36] Using this more specific criteria, the prevalence of echocardiographically diagnosed MVP is ~2% to 3%. Multimodality imaging is useful to confirm the severity of regurgitation and assess myocardial fibrosis, which can accompany variants of this disease.[18,36,37]

Although screening of the general population indicates that many individuals with MVP have few clinical symptoms in large clinical populations, the disease is strongly associated with HF, need for valve surgery, development of AF, and increased mortality.[38] In a community-based study of 833 asymptomatic patients with MVP, 10-year all-cause mortality was 19% ± 2% and cardiovascular mortality was 9% ± 2% (see Avierinos et al., Classic References). In a retrospective analysis of patients presenting with moderate or severe MR, a primary etiology was identified in approximately one-third of patients, of whom >70% had MVP.[39] Compared with patients with secondary MR, patients with moderate or severe primary MR had larger Rvol, moderate cardiac remodeling, normal stroke volume index, and mildly elevated pulmonary pressure, yet had a 40% 5-year HF rate and increased risk of mortality (risk ratio, 1.83 [1.50 to 2.22]; $P < 0.0001$).[39] An increase in mortality with MVP is related to the quantitative severity of MR (adjusted hazard ratio [HR], 1.15; 95% confidence interval [CI], 1.10 to 1.20; $P < 0.0001$ per 10 mm^2).[40]

Left Ventricular Volumes and Systolic Function
In addition to severity of MR, outcomes are associated with LV size, with mortality risk increasing linearly with LV end-systolic dimension (ESD) >40 mm (HR, 1.15; 95% CI 1.04 to 1.27 per 1-mm increment) or LVESD index ≥22 mm/m^2 (adjusted HR 1.12; 95% CI, 1.01 to 1.23 per 1-mm/m^2 LVESD increment; $p = 0.01$).[41] Although surgery was associated with reduced mortality (adjusted HR, 0.62; 95% CI, 0.45 to 0.86; $p = 0.0035$), LVESD ≥40 mm was an independent predictor of reduced postsurgical survival.

In the setting of chronic severe MR, the LV end-diastolic volume (LVEDV) increases, which, by means of the Laplace principle, results in increased systolic LV wall stress, a stimulus for eccentric hypertrophy. Initially the reduced afterload is associated with increased ejection phase indices of myocardial contractility (i.e., LV ejection fraction [LVEF], fractional fiber shortening, and velocity of circumferential fiber shortening). However, prolonged hemodynamic overload ultimately leads to myocardial decompensation, an increase in LV end-diastolic pressure, and eventually a decrease in LV contractility despite only modest decreases in LVEF, which often remains in the normal or near-normal range. Long-term follow-up of 1875 patients with significant MR secondary to flail MV in the Mitral Regurgitation International Database (MIDA) registry,[42] patients with LVEF of 45% to 60% represented a large proportion of patients (23%), who rarely exhibited overt symptoms, and had higher mortality compared with EF >60%. An LVEF <60% was associated with an adjusted HR of 1.51 (1.22 to 1.87) and an EF <45% with an adjusted HR of 2.46 (1.67 to 3.61). The benefit of surgery was significant in the groups with EF <45% (adjusted HR, 0.28 [0.17 to

0.56]) and with EF of 45% to 60% (adjusted HR, 0.34 [0.21 to 0.64]).[42,43] A measure of longitudinal LV mechanics, global longitudinal strain (GLS) may be a more sensitive and accurate measurement of LV function than LVEF (see Chapter 16). In a study of 593 patients with severe primary MR (Barlow disease, fibroelastic deficiency, or forme fruste) who underwent MV surgery, LV-GLS ≥−20.6% (more impaired) showed significantly worse survival than did patients with LV-GLS ≤−20.6% ($p < 0.001$) and GLS LV-GLS had incremental prognostic value over clinical risk factors for long-term survival.[44] The role of GLS in determining the timing of surgery remains unexplored.

Mitral Annular Disjunction

Mitral annular disjunction (MAD) has received growing awareness as a marker for risk of ventricular arrhythmias and sudden death in patients with MVP. This term describes abnormal spatial displacement of the point of insertion of the posterior MV leaflet, which results in a wide separation between the LA wall and MV junction and the LV attachment.[37,45] MAD has gained attention in recent years because of its association with frequent premature ventricular beats and nonsustained ventricular tachycardia, suggesting that it may be a marker of a "malignant" form of MVP. Although the incidence of sudden cardiac death is low among patients with MVP (estimated to be 0.2% to 0.4% per year),[46] this incidence is 3 times higher than that in the general population; thus, the prevalence of MVP of 2% to 3% suggests that the absolute number at risk is considerable. CMR imaging has shown late gadolinium enhancement indicative of myocardial fibrosis in patients with arrhythmias and MAD.[27,47,48] Additional risk findings include inverted or biphasic T waves, QT dispersion, QT prolongation, and premature ventricular contractions originating from the LVOT and papillary muscles, paradoxal systolic increase of the mitral annulus diameter, and increased tissue Doppler velocity of the mitral annulus.[37,46] In early studies, MAD was reported as a specific finding in patients with MVP, but more recent studies suggest that MAD associated with arrhythmias can occur in those without MVP and may be a separate morphologic entity.[47] Although arrhythmogenic MVP has been associated with increased MR severity,[47] recent data have shown no association with either MR severity or LV systolic dysfunction.[49]

Symptoms

The onset of symptoms in patients with severe chronic primary MR, regardless of LV function, is also associated with poor outcomes. Although "watchful waiting" often has been the treatment strategy for asymptomatic patients with severe organic MR, there is growing evidence that patients with severe primary MR who have no or minimal symptoms not only have lower operative mortality but would have improved long-term outcomes if surgery was performed before the onset of symptoms,[43,50] with societal recommendations to consider early surgery in patients who are candidates for MV repair.[1,2,51] Propensity score matching of early surgery and initial medical management groups in the MIDA registry confirmed higher survival after early surgery (HR, 0.52; 95% CI, 0.35 to 0.79; $P = 0.002$).[43] In the absence of symptoms, 10-year survival was also better with early surgery (84%; 95% CI, 78% to 90%) compared with initial medical management (78%; 95% CI, 72% to 85%; $P = 0.04$). There was also an independent protective effect associated with early surgery upon late HF risk. Notably in this study, 93% of patients had MV repair performed. Similarly, in a study of 1234 patients with primary MR who underwent MV repair, long-term (median 13 years) survival was significantly associated with severity of symptoms, with highest survival rates among those who were asymptomatic before surgery (Fig. 76.8).[50] There is growing use of exercise testing to either elicit symptoms in asymptomatic patients with severe MR or confirm the cause of symptoms in patients with less than severe MR.[1,25]

A MIDA score has been proposed in which clinical parameters are used to assess mortality risk, which would be applicable to both medical and surgical treatment.[52] The several clinical parameters of the MIDA score and their point assignments (determined by Cox proportional hazard, competing risk, and competing risk with imputation models) are age ≥65 years (3 points), symptoms (3 points), RV systolic pressure >50 mm Hg (2 points), AF (1 point), LA diameter ≥55 mm (1 point), LV end-systolic diameter ≥40 mm (1 point), and LVEF ≤60% (1 point). MIDA score was associated with long-term risk of death under

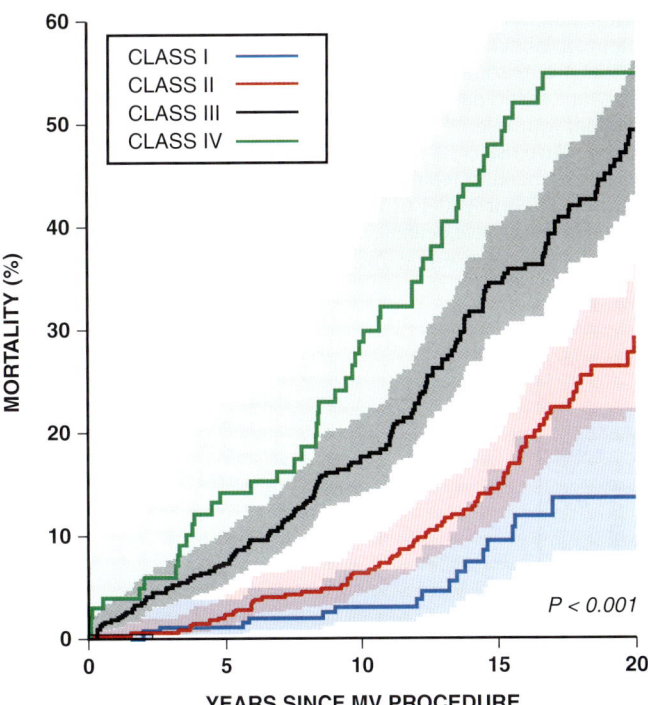

FIGURE 76.8 Survival over the course of 2 decades after mitral valve (MV) repair among 1234 patients with severe primary mitral regurgitation. Long-term postoperative survival was significantly associated with presence and severity of preoperative symptoms. (From David TE, et al. Long-term results of mitral valve repair for regurgitation due to leaflet prolapse. *J Am Coll Cardiol*. 2019;74:1044-1053.)

medical management (adjusted HR [95% CI] per unit 1.13 [1.01 to 1.22]; $P < 0.001$) (c = 0.81; standard deviation [SD] 0.03) and postsurgical outcome (adjusted HR [95% CI] per unit 1.35 [1.19 to 1.54]; $P < 0.001$). Although a simple risk score for both medical and surgical treatment (and that outperforms the standard surgical risk scores) will be of use to the clinician, the importance of integrating these and other comorbidities and weighing them against the expected benefit of surgical repair cannot be overemphasized. Both U.S. and European guidelines strongly support the involvement of the multidisciplinary heart team, for consensus decision making and with shared decision making with patient and family.[1,51]

Management of Primary Mitral Regurgitation

Medical Therapy for Primary Mitral Regurgitation

In the setting of a primary valvular disorder, medical management is limited and there are no specific recommendations for medical therapy of chronic primary MR. Treatment of hypertension is warranted according to standard guidelines for management of high blood pressure, and notably in doing so severity of MR will be reduced. However, vasodilator therapy is not indicated in normotensive patients with chronic primary MR and normal LVEF. Reduced preload and/or afterload may actually worsen MR in MVP. A meta-analysis of 19 studies evaluating the use of angiotensin-converting enzyme inhibitors and angiotensin receptor blockers (ARBs) showed only a modest change in regurgitant fraction (~8%)[53] and there is no strong evidence of benefit on clinical outcomes.[54] In the setting of reduced LVEF (<60%), however, standard guideline-directed medical therapy is indicated.

With acute, hemodynamically significant primary MR (i.e., flail), vasodilator therapy can increase forward flow but is often limited by systemic hypotension. In these instances, intra-aortic balloon counterpulsation can be helpful to treat acute severe MR.

Surgical Therapy for Primary Mitral Regurgitation

As noted previously, surgical intervention is warranted in patients with severe primary MR who are symptomatic or who have LV systolic dysfunction, defined as LVEF <60% or LVESD >40 mm.[1,51] Both U.S. and European guidelines recommendations are also concordant in stating that it is reasonable (Class IIa) to proceed with surgical MV repair in asymptomatic patients with severe primary MR and preserved LV function, with referral to centers that can provide durable repair at low operative risk (<1% mortality). Patients should be referred to centers experienced in repair, and patients with more complex forms of MR (e.g., anterior leaflet or bileaflet prolapse) should be referred to comprehensive valve centers.[1,2] Repair success increases with surgical volume and expertise (Fig. 76.9), which should be considered when referring a patient for surgery.[55-57] In addition, MV repair has superior outcomes to biological or mechanical MV replacement.[58] Unfortunately, national data persist in showing that many patients who are candidates for repair are treated with MV replacement, particularly at lower volume institutions.[59]

Indications for surgical intervention for chronic primary MR according to the revised ACC/AHA guidelines on management of patients with valvular heart disease[1] are listed in Table 76.3, along with a schema for patient management based on these guidelines recommendations (Fig. 76.10).

Transcatheter Therapy for Primary Mitral Regurgitation
Edge-to-Edge Repair

Transcatheter MV repair using an edge-to-edge clip between the anterior and posterior leaflets (see Fig. 78.3) is safe and effective in reducing severity of primary MR (see Chapter 78). Surgical MV repair is more effective at reducing or eliminating MR compared with the clip, but in randomized trials the clinical outcomes with the transcatheter repair were not inferior to outcomes with surgery.[60] In addition, anticipated progressive worsening after clip therapy has not been observed.

Studies of the MV clip have demonstrated improved symptoms and a reduction in MR by 2 to 3 grades leading to reverse remodeling of the LV. The revised 2020 ACC/AHA guidelines indicate that it is reasonable to perform transcatheter MV edge-to-edge repair (Class IIa) in severely symptomatic patients with primary MR who are considered at high or prohibitive surgical risk, if MV anatomy is favorable for the repair procedure and patient life expectancy is at least 1 year (see Table 76.3 and Fig. 76.10).

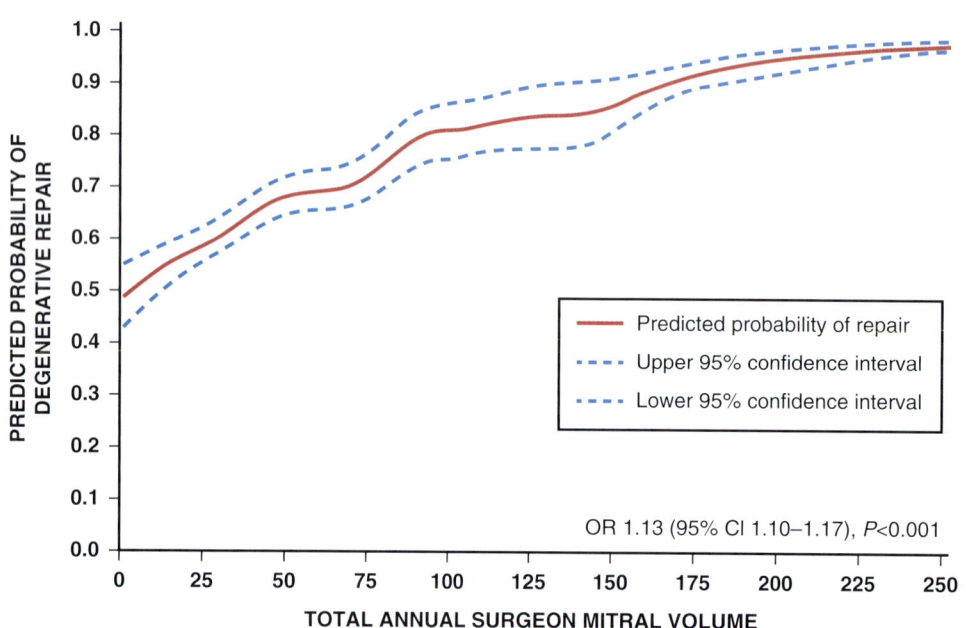

FIGURE 76.9 Predicted probability of mitral repair for primary mitral regurgitation (MR) according to total annual surgeon mitral valve volume. After adjustment for preoperative risk factors, degenerative repair probability is significantly associated with total annual mitral valve surgeon volume. Data based on 5475 patients undergoing surgery by 313 surgeons in 41 hospitals in New York State. *CI,* Confidence interval; *OR,* odds ratio. (From Chikwe J, et al. Relation of mitral valve surgery volume to repair rate, durability, and survival. *J Am Coll Cardiol.* 2017;69:2397-2406.)

TABLE 76.3 Recommendations for Intervention for Chronic Primary Mitral Regurgitation.

COR	LOE	RECOMMENDATIONS
1	B-NR	1. In symptomatic patients with severe primary MR (stage D), mitral valve intervention is recommended irrespective of LV systolic function.
1	B-NR	2. In asymptomatic patients with severe primary MR and LV systolic dysfunction (LVEF ≤60%, LVESD ≥40 mm) (stage C2), mitral valve surgery is recommended.
1	B-NR	3. In patients with severe primary MR for whom surgery is indicated, mitral valve repair is recommended in preference to mitral valve replacement when the anatomic cause of MR is degenerative disease, if a successful and durable repair is possible.
2a	B-NR	4. In asymptomatic patients with severe primary MR and normal LV systolic function (LVEF ≥60% and LVESD ≤40 mm) (stage C1), mitral valve repair is reasonable when the likelihood of a successful and durable repair without residual MR is >95% with an expected mortality rate of <1%, when it can be performed at a primary or comprehensive valve center.
2b	C-LD	5. In asymptomatic patients with severe primary MR and normal LV systolic function (LVEF >60% and LVESD <40 mm) (stage C1) but with a progressive increase in LV size or decrease in EF on ≥3 serial imaging studies, mitral valve surgery may be considered irrespective of the probability of a successful and durable repair.
2a	B-NR	6. In severely symptomatic patients (NYHA Class III or IV) with primary severe MR and high or prohibitive surgical risk, transcatheter edge-to-edge repair (TEER) is reasonable if mitral valve anatomy is favorable for the repair procedure and patient life expectancy is at least 1 year.
2b	B-NR	7. In symptomatic patients with severe primary MR attributable to rheumatic valve disease, mitral valve repair may be considered at a comprehensive valve center by an experienced team when surgical treatment is indicated, if a durable and successful repair is likely.
3: Harm	B-NR	8. In patients with severe primary MR in which leaflet pathology is limited to less than half the posterior leaflet, mitral valve replacement should not be performed unless mitral valve repair has been attempted at a primary or comprehensive valve center and was unsuccessful.

EF, Ejection fraction; *LV,* left ventricle; *LVEF,* LV ejection fraction; *LVESD,* LV end-systolic dimension; *MR,* mitral regurgitation; *NYHA,* New York Heart Association.
From Otto CM, et al. 2020 AHA/ACC guideline for the management of patients with valvular heart disease: a report of the American College of Cardiology/American Heart Association Task Force on Practice Guidelines. *J Am Coll Cardiol.* 2021;77:e25-197.

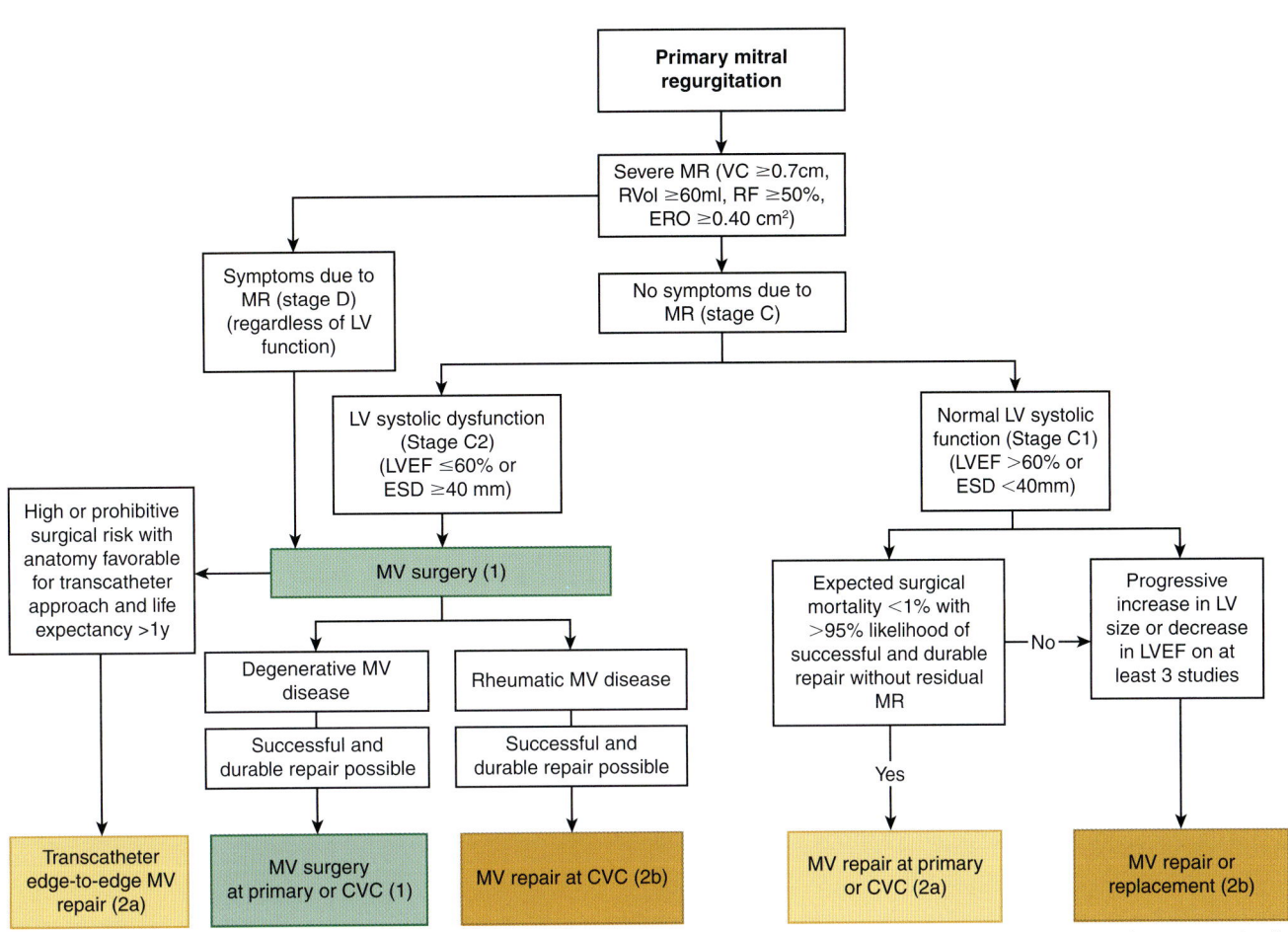

FIGURE 76.10 Management strategy for intervention for primary mitral regurgitation. Colors correspond to Table 76.3. *CVC,* Comprehensive valve center; *ERO,* effective regurgitant orifice; *ESD,* end-systolic dimension; *LVEF,* ejection fraction; *MR,* mitral regurgitation; *MV,* mitral valve; *MVR,* mitral valve replacement; *RF,* regurgitant fraction; *RVol,* regurgitant volume; *VC,* vena contracta. (From Otto CM, et al. 2020 AHA/ACC guideline for the management of patients with valvular heart disease: a report of the American College of Cardiology/American Heart Association Task Force on Practice Guidelines. *J Am Coll Cardiol.* 2021;77:e25-e197.)

A retrospective study of 100 low- to intermediate-risk elderly patients with primary MR treated with edge-to-edge repair compared with 206 patients with isolated surgical repair, showed that transcatheter repair resulted in lower acute postoperative complications and improved 1-year survival compared with surgery. However, the transcatheter approach was associated with greater MR recurrence and reduced survival beyond 1 year.[61] Another study that assigned patients to surgical versus transcatheter repair based on recommendations of a heart team[62] showed that such an individualized treatment strategy was effective. Low-risk patients with favorable anatomy were assigned to surgical repair, whereas high-risk patients with favorable anatomy for edge-to-edge repair underwent transcatheter therapy, and those with unfavorable anatomy were assigned to surgical replacement. Overall, surgical repair patients had higher 4-year survival (HR, 0.40; 95% CI, 0.26 to 0.63); $p < 0.001$) and fewer combined endpoints (HR, 0.51; 95% CI, 0.32 to 0.80; $p < 0.001$) compared with the other interventions, but the 4-year mortality for edge-to-edge repair for primary MR was low (~10%). Results of a meta-analysis of nine studies investigating the 1-year outcome of transcatheter edge-to-edge repair in patients with secondary versus primary MR ($n = 2615$) showed no significant differences in mortality rate (RR 1.26; 95% CI: 0.90 to 1.77; $p = 0.18$).[63]

The ideal anatomy for edge-to-edge repair for nonrheumatic primary MR come from the EVEREST trial and include involvement limited to the A2/P2 scallop, absence of calcium in the grasping zone, baseline MV area ≥ 4 cm^2, flail width <15 mm and flail gap <10 mm.[64] Several authors, however, have shown the feasibility of expanding these criteria.[65-67]

Investigational Devices

A number of other devices are under investigation for transcatheter repair of both primary and secondary MR. These include edge-to-edge devices, chordal repair therapies, and annuloplasty devices (see Fig. 78.6). In addition, trials of transcatheter approaches to MV replacement (TMVR) are in progress. These devices are discussed in detail in Chapter 78.

SECONDARY MITRAL REGURGITATION

Pathophysiology

The two main etiologies of secondary MR are annular dilation or atriogenic MR (Carpentier type I) and leaflet tethering from a ventricular disease (Carpentier IIIA) (see Fig 76.2). Atriogenic MR has gained increasing recognition as the etiology of MR in the setting of normal LV mechanics. Recent studies suggest the underlying mechanism is related to insufficient leaflet growth, LA dilation and annular dilation with altered annular dynamics.[15,17,68] In patients with HF and preserved EF (HFpEF), the Acute Decompensated Heart Failure Syndromes (ATTEND) registry found a significantly higher risk of reaching the clinical endpoint in patients with mild or moderate/severe secondary MR compared with patients without MR. Abe et al.[69] showed a prevalence of MR of ~8% in a HFpEF population, a significantly higher prevalence of adverse events (cardiac death, hospitalization from worsening HF, or mitral/tricuspid valve surgery) with a HR of 4.0; 95% CI, 2.3 to 7.0 per 1-grade increase. Although specific treatment of atriogenic MR in the setting of HFpEF has not been systematically studied, rhythm control may play a role. Atriogenic MR decreases in response to restoration of sinus rhythm after AF cardioversion and ablation.[16,70]

Secondary MR stemming from LV dilation and systolic dysfunction, often with concomitant mitral annular dilation, is a common consequence of ischemic and nonischemic cardiomyopathies (see Chapters 40 and 52).[71,72] The clinical stages of secondary MR are indicated in Table 76.4. In the setting of LV dysfunction and dilation, secondary MR results from displacement of the papillary muscles, tethering of the MV leaflets, and alteration of annular mechanics.[10,38] The etiology of LV dysfunction can be either ischemic or nonischemic (see Fig. 16.27B). A number of mechanisms may contribute to malcoaptation of the MV leaflets in secondary MR (Fig. 76.11; see also Fig. 16.37): (1) global and/or regional LV dilation/dysfunction that decreases the closing forces of the leaflets, (2) displacement of the papillary muscles with tethering of the leaflets into the ventricular cavity, which outweighs the closing forces, (3) dilation and dysfunction of the annulus, and (4) inadequate leaflet adaptation to ventricular or atrial enlargement.[10,73,74] The anatomic features associated with these mechanisms thus predict the severity of MR and recurrence after surgical repair: mitral leaflet tethering and restricted closure, asymmetric displacement and abnormal contraction of the LV wall underlying the papillary muscles, decreased shortening of the distance between the papillary muscles, and increased LV sphericity.[10]

Clinical Presentation

Symptoms

Patients with secondary MR related to LV dysfunction often present with HF symptoms, but many are asymptomatic (at least with regard to the MR), with MR detected incidentally on physical examination or echocardiography. AF is common.

Physical Examination. An apical S_3 is a common finding. Unlike primary MR, the systolic murmur of secondary MR related to LV dilation

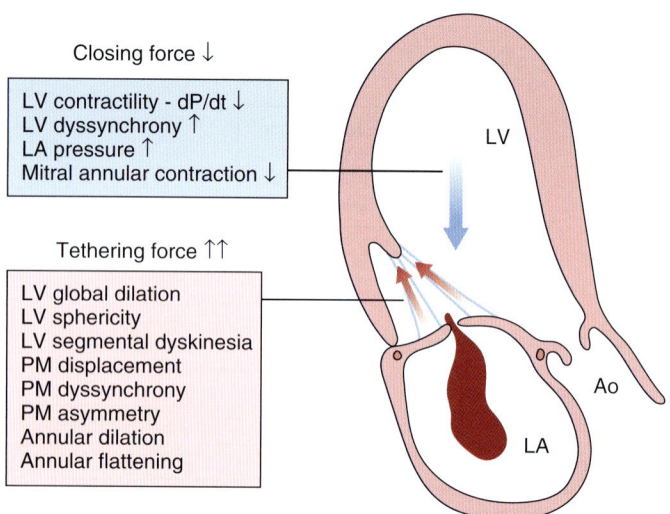

FIGURE 76.11 Tethering and closing forces. The imbalance between tethering and closing forces result in secondary mitral regurgitation. (From Bertrand PB, et al. Exercise dynamics in secondary mitral regurgitation: pathophysiology and therapeutic implications. *Circulation.* 2017;135:297-314.)

TABLE 76.4 Stages of Chronic Secondary Mitral Regurgitation

STAGE	DEFINITION	VALVE ANATOMY	VALVE HEMODYNAMICS*	ASSOCIATED CLINICAL FINDINGS	SYMPTOMS
A	At risk of MR	Normal valve leaflets, chords, and annulus in a patient with coronary disease or cardiomyopathy	No MR jet or small central jet area <20% LA on Doppler Small vena contracta <0.30 cm	Normal or mildly dilated LV size with fixed (infarction) or inducible (ischemia) regional wall motion abnormalities Primary myocardial disease with LV dilation and systolic dysfunction	Symptoms attributable to coronary ischemia or HF may be present that respond to revascularization and appropriate medical therapy
B	Progressive MR	Regional wall motion abnormalities with mild tethering of mitral leaflet Annular dilation with mild loss of central coaptation of the mitral leaflets	ERO† <0.40 cm² Rvol <60 mL RF <50%	Regional wall motion abnormalities with reduced LV systolic function LV dilation and systolic dysfunction attributable to primary myocardial disease	Symptoms attributable to coronary ischemia or HF may be present that respond to revascularization and appropriate medical therapy
C	Asymptomatic severe MR	Regional wall motion abnormalities and/or LV dilation with severe tethering of mitral leaflet Annular dilation with severe loss of central coaptation of the mitral leaflets	ERO† ≥0.40 cm² Rvol ≥60 mL RF ≥50%	Regional wall motion abnormalities with reduced LV systolic function LV dilation and systolic dysfunction attributable to primary myocardial disease	Symptoms attributable to coronary ischemia or HF may be present that respond to revascularization and appropriate medical therapy
D	Symptomatic severe MR	Regional wall motion abnormalities and/or LV dilation with severe tethering of mitral leaflet Annular dilation with severe loss of central coaptation of mitral leaflets	ERO† ≥0.40 cm² Rvol ≥60 mL RF ≥50%	Regional wall motion abnormalities with reduced LV systolic function LV dilation and systolic dysfunction attributable to primary myocardial disease	HF symptoms attributable to MR persist even after revascularization and optimization of medical therapy Decreased exercise tolerance Exertional dyspnea

ERO, Effective regurgitant orifice; *HF,* heart failure; *LA,* left atrium; *LV,* left ventricular; *MR,* mitral regurgitation; *RF,* regurgitant fraction; *Rvol,* regurgitant volume.
*Several valve hemodynamic criteria are provided for assessment of MR severity, but not all criteria for each category will be present in each patient. Categorization of MR severity as mild, moderate, or severe depends on data quality and integration of these parameters in conjunction with other clinical evidence.
†The measurement of the proximal isovelocity surface area (PISA) by two-dimensional transthoracic echocardiography (TTE) in patients with secondary MR underestimates the true ERO because of the crescentic shape of the proximal convergence.
From Otto CM, et al. 2020 AHA/ACC guideline for the management of patients with valvular heart disease: a report of the American College of Cardiology/American Heart Association Task Force on Practice Guidelines. *J Am Coll Cardiol.* 2021;77:e25-197.

may be soft and barely audible, particularly in those patients with non-holosystolic MR that becomes minimal in midsystole. Thus, the physical examination can be misleading regarding the presence and severity of secondary MR. The murmur of papillary muscle dysfunction may occur in late systole and is highly variable, often accentuated or holosystolic during acute myocardial ischemia and absent when ischemia is relieved.

Echocardiography
Quantifying the severity of secondary MR by echocardiography has a number of limitations that resulted in the past in conflicting criteria in the American and European guidelines. Using the standard PISA method to assess MR severity, an EROA of 0.2 cm² has been associated with worse prognosis in secondary MR (Fig. 76.12) (see Grigioni et al., Classic References). Thus, European guidelines have used this cutoff to define "severe" disease.[51] However, underestimation of MR severity by this method may arise given the dynamic nature and crescent shape of the orifice in secondary MR.[75] Recognizing this issue, as well as needing to differentiate between prognostically severe and quantitatively severe secondary MR, both ASE and ACC/AHA guidelines grade severe secondary MR and primary MR the same using the cutoffs of EROA ≥0.4 cm², Rvol ≥60 mL and regurgitant fraction ≥50%.[1,2,18]

The various quantitative echocardiographic criteria may be discordant in secondary MR, making an assessment of severity more difficult (see Chapter 16). Rvol is dependent on loading conditions and chamber function and compliance. For instance, for the same regurgitant orifice, a higher LV systolic pressure may result in a larger Rvol and in the setting of LV dysfunction with reduced stroke volume, a low Rvol may be associated with a high regurgitant fraction. In a recent study of 423 patients with HF, Bartko et al. used the PISA method to measure EROA and Rvol, and the biplane Simpson LV volume to calculate regurgitant fraction.[76] Importantly, there was increased 5-year mortality associated with each of the measures of severity with HRs ranging from 1.37 to 1.50 (P < 0.001). Spline-curve analyses showed a linearly increasing risk enabling the ability to stratify patients into low-risk (EROA <20 mm² and Rvol <30 mL), intermediate-risk (EROA 20 to 29 mm² and Rvol 30 to 44 mL), and high-risk (EROA ≥30 mm² and Rvol ≥45 mL) groups. In the intermediate-risk group, a regurgitant fraction ≥50% was an indicator of hemodynamic severe secondary MR associated with poor outcome (p = 0.017). These cutoffs should be evaluated in larger patient populations and prospective trials.

Kamperidis et al.,[77] demonstrated that LV GLS is an early and more sensitive marker of LV systolic dysfunction than LVEF in patients with nonischemic dilated cardiomyopathy and significant secondary MR. In addition, Namazi and associates showed the incremental prognostic value of LV GLS (in addition to LVEF) in secondary MR.[78] Patients with a more impaired LV GLS (> −7.0%) experienced higher mortality rates than those with a more preserved LV GLS (≤ −7.0%).

Cardiac Magnetic Resonance
CMR is useful in assessing severity of LV remodeling and contractile dysfunction as well as the pattern of myocardial fibrosis as it relates to regional dysfunction and papillary muscle dysfunction[18,79] (see Chapter 19, particularly Fig. 19.17).

Management of Secondary Mitral Regurgitation

Medical Therapy for Secondary Mitral Regurgitation
Patients with secondary MR stemming from LV dilation and dysfunction should undergo aggressive evidence-based medical management for LV systolic dysfunction[80] (see Chapter 50). In contrast to primary MR, a beneficial effect of medical therapy in patients with secondary MR, with respect to both valve function and clinical outcomes, is well established. However, this benefit is mainly attributed to a favorable impact of medical therapy on the underlying disease. Medical therapies have been shown to reduce MR in up to 40% of patients and are associated with improved outcomes.[81] Guideline-directed medical therapy (GDMT) including inhibitors of the renin-angiotensin-aldosterone system (RAAS) and beta-adrenergic blockers can significantly reduce secondary MR in 30% to 40% of patients with HF. In addition, HF guidelines have been updated to include the use of angiotensin receptor neprilysin inhibition (ARNI) in the treatment of symptomatic LV systolic dysfunction,[80] and treatment with sacubitril/valsartan has been associated with reduction in EROA related to reduction in LVEDV index (p= 0.044).[82] Significant reductions in secondary MR also occur with cardiac resynchronization therapy (CRT)[83] (see Chapters 50 and 58). Bartko et al.[84] showed that restoration of longitudinal papillary muscle synchronicity correlated with regression of secondary MR, which was associated with a better prognosis during the 8-year follow-up period compared with patients with no improvement in MR (adjusted HR, 0.41; 95% CI, 0.18 to 0.91; p = 0.028). Finally, guideline-directed management of significant coronary artery disease in the setting of ischemic MR should be instituted.[85,86]

Surgical Therapy for Secondary Mitral Regurgitation
In atriogenic secondary MR, small single-site case series[87] report good short-term outcomes after annuloplasty. However, the need for surgical intervention to treat atriogenic MR beyond rhythm control has been questioned.[16]

MV surgery is recommended at the time of coronary artery bypass surgery (CABG) in patients with LV dysfunction and severe ischemic MR. Whether concomitant MV repair should be performed during CABG in patients with moderate ischemic MR was addressed in the randomized trial conducted by the Cardiothoracic Surgical Trials Network (CTSN).[88] This trial randomized 301 patients with moderate MR (defined for this study as EROA between 0.2 and 0.4 cm²) all requiring CABG to MV repair (with annuloplasty) versus CABG alone. Although there were significantly more patients with moderate or greater MR at 12 months in the no-repair group (31.0% versus 11.2%; p< 0.001), there was no difference between groups in the prespecified primary endpoint of postoperative LV end-systolic volume (ESV), nor was there any difference in mortality or major adverse cardiac events (Fig. 76.13).[88]

These results illustrate that in patients with secondary MR, the primary problem is disease of the LV myocardium, and prognosis is strongly influenced by the degree of LV dysfunction and residual ischemia. MV repair or replacement in these latter patients has a less beneficial effect on long-term outcome, particularly in those with ischemic MR, than in patients with primary MR. Thus, the indications for MV surgery are less clear for secondary MR than for primary MR, exemplified by there being no Class I or IIa indications for isolated surgery in secondary MR in the current ACC/AHA guidelines.[1] Moreover, unlike repair of primary MR caused by myxomatous disease or fibroelastic deficiency, in which an experienced surgeon can

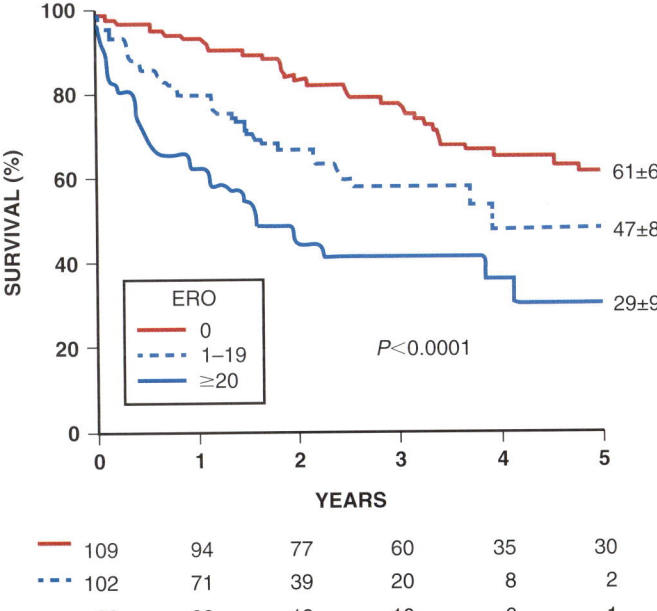

FIGURE 76.12 Survival in 303 patients with previous myocardial infarction and mean ejection fraction 34%, subgrouped by effective regurgitant orifice (ERO) according to presence and severity of ischemic mitral regurgitation (MR). Any degree of ischemic MR was associated with worse outcome than no MR. (From Grigioni F, et al. Ischemic mitral regurgitation: long-term outcome and prognostic implications with quantitative Doppler assessment. *Circulation*. 2001;103:1759-1764.)

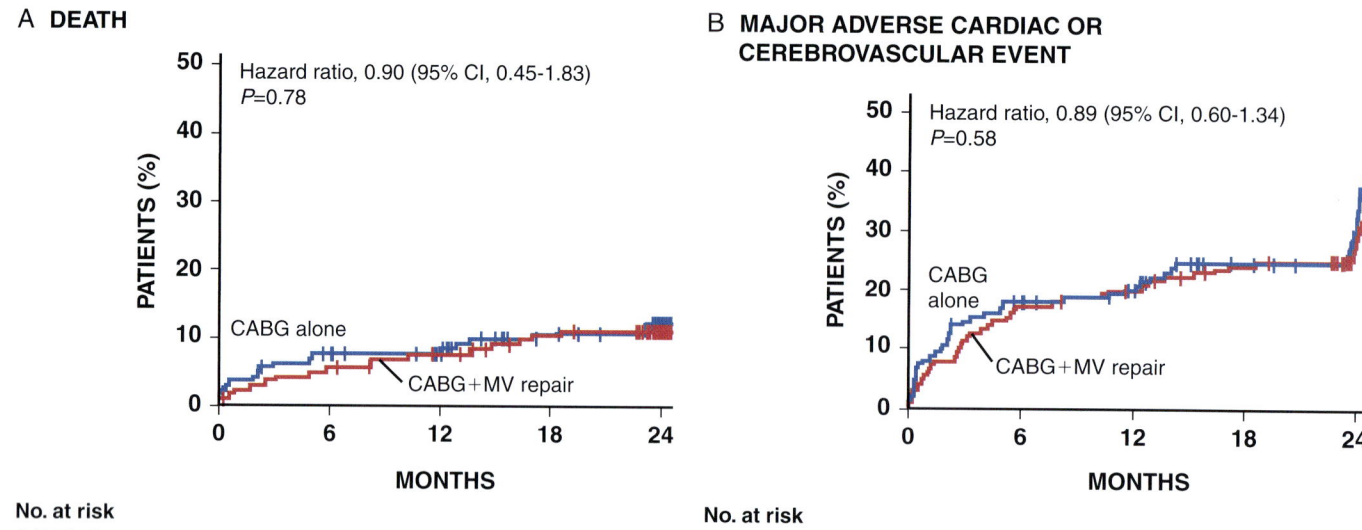

FIGURE 76.13 Two-year outcomes of patients with moderate mitral regurgitation undergoing coronary artery bypass graft (CABG) who were randomized to CABG alone versus CABG plus mitral valve (MV) repair. **A,** Death. **B,** Composite endpoint of major adverse cardiac or cerebrovascular events. (From Michler RE, et al. Two-year outcomes of surgical treatment of moderate ischemic mitral regurgitation. *N Engl J Med.* 2016;374:1932-1941.)

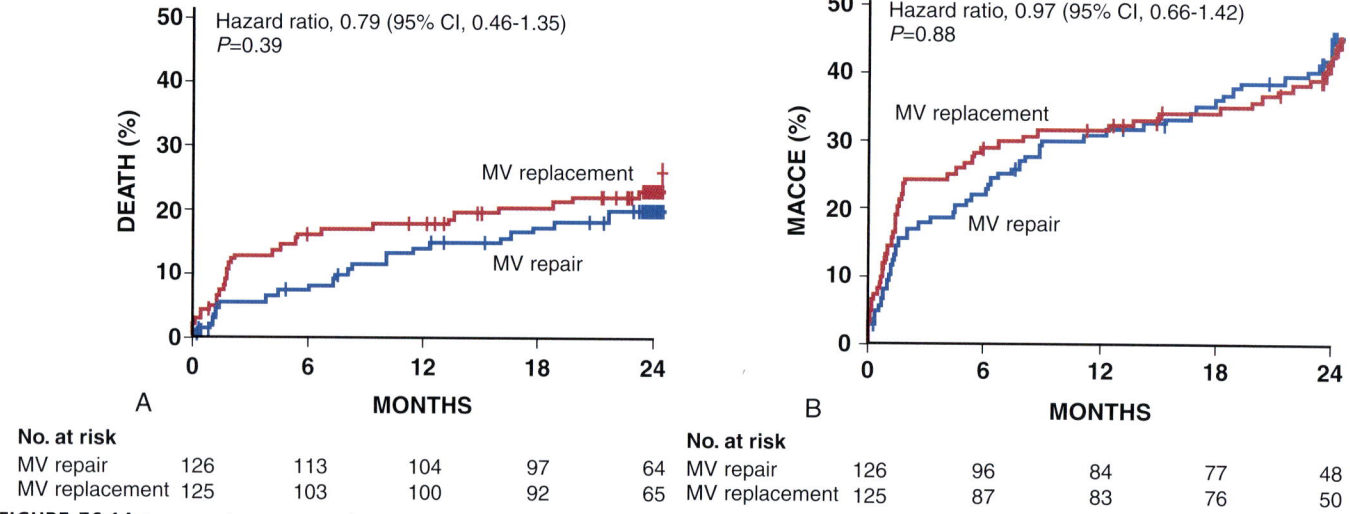

FIGURE 76.14 Postoperative outcomes of patients with ischemic mitral regurgitation randomly assigned to mitral valve (MV) repair versus replacement. **A,** Mortality. **B,** Composite endpoint of death, stroke, repeat MV surgery, hospitalization for heart failure, and increase in NYHA functional class by 1 or more. *MACCE,* major adverse cardiac or cerebrovascular events. (From Goldstein D, et al. Two-year outcomes of surgical treatment of severe ischemic mitral regurgitation. *N Engl J Med.* 2016;374:344–353.)

produce results that are durable for decades, MV repair of secondary MR is often not durable because of progression of the underlying LV myocardial disease. This has fueled suggestions that MV replacement might provide a more durable surgical solution to secondary MR with reduced recurrence rates. This hypothesis was addressed in a CTSN prospective randomized clinical trial of MV repair versus replacement in 251 patients with severe ischemic MR,[89] which demonstrated that MV replacement achieved equivalent degrees of reduction in LV volume compared with repair, with less recurrent MR during the follow-up period out to 2 years (Fig. 76.14). This result was driven by the 32.6% of repair patients who developed recurrent moderate or greater MR at 1 year, rising to 58.8% at 2 years. Among the patients with recurrent MR, LVESV index was significantly larger than in those without recurrence (62.6 ± 26.9 and 42.7 ± 26.4 mL, respectively; $p< 0.001$). These data have informed predictive models to identify patients most likely to fail a MV repair,[90] including those with larger EROA, outward tethering of the valve, and inferobasal aneurysms. In multivariate analysis, the ratio of LVESD to annuloplasty ring diameter was most predictive of recurrent MR.[91] Such patients appear to be better served by a chordal-sparing MV replacement.

Transcatheter Therapy for Secondary Mitral Regurgitation

One of the major new recommendations in the 2020 ACC/AHA guidelines is the indication for transcatheter edge-to-edge MV repair in patients with secondary MR.[1] The Cardiovascular Outcomes Assessment of the MitraClip Percutaneous Therapy for Heart Failure Patients with Functional Mitral Regurgitation (COAPT) trial,[92] which randomized patients with LV dysfunction and secondary MR to GDMT alone versus GDMT plus transcatheter edge-to-edge repair showed a significant reduction in the primary endpoint, rehospitalization for HF, and secondary endpoints of reduction in mortality, and combined endpoints of mortality and rehospitalization for HF (see Fig. 78.5). This seminal trial led the U.S. Food and Drug Administration to approve the edge-to-edge repair device for severe secondary MR as well as a Class IIa recommendation in the revised guidelines (Table 76.5 and Fig. 76.15). However, the Multicentre Study of Percutaneous Mitral Valve Repair MitraClip Device in Patients With Severe Secondary Mitral Regurgitation (MITRA-FR) trial,[93] which also randomized patients with LV dysfunction and secondary MR to GDMT alone versus GDMT plus transcatheter edge-to-edge repair, reported no significant benefit to edge-to-edge repair in the primary combined endpoint of survival or rehospitalization for HF (Fig. 76.16).

TABLE 76.5 Recommendations for Intervention for Chronic Secondary Mitral Regurgitation

COR	LOE	RECOMMENDATIONS
2a	B-R	1. In patients with chronic severe secondary MR related to LV systolic dysfunction (LVEF <50%) who have persistent symptoms (NYHA Class II, III, or IV) while on optimal GDMT for HF (stage D), TEER is reasonable in patients with appropriate anatomy as defined on TEE and with LVEF between 20% and 50%, LVESD ≤70 mm, and pulmonary artery systolic pressure ≤70 mm Hg.
2a	B-NR	2. In patients with severe secondary MR (stages C and D), mitral valve surgery is reasonable when CABG is undertaken for the treatment of myocardial ischemia.
2b	B-NR	3. In patients with chronic severe secondary MR from atrial annular dilation with preserved LV systolic function (LVEF ≥50%) who have severe persistent symptoms (NYHA Class III or IV) despite therapy for HF and therapy for associated AF or other comorbidities (stage D), mitral valve surgery may be considered.
2b	B-NR	4. In patients with chronic severe secondary MR related to LV systolic dysfunction (LVEF <50%) who have persistent severe symptoms (NYHA class III or IV) while on optimal GDMT for HF (stage D), mitral valve surgery may be considered.
2b	B-R	5. In patients with CAD and chronic severe secondary MR related to LV systolic dysfunction (LVEF <50%) (stage D) who are undergoing mitral valve surgery because of severe symptoms (NYHA class III or IV) that persist despite GDMT for HF, chordal-sparing mitral valve replacement may be reasonable to choose over downsized annuloplasty repair.

CABG, Coronary artery bypass graft; *CAD*, coronary artery disease; *GDMT*, guideline-directed medical therapy; *HF*, heart failure; *LVEF*, left ventricular ejection fraction; *LVESD*, left ventricular end-systolic dimension; *MR*, mitral regurgitation; *NYHA*, New York Heart Association; *TEE*, transesophageal echocardiography; *TEER*, transcatheter edge-to-edge repair.
From Otto CM, et al. 2020 AHA/ACC guideline for the management of patients with valvular heart disease: a report of the American College of Cardiology/American Heart Association Task Force on Practice Guidelines. *J Am Coll Cardiol.* 2021;77:e25-197.

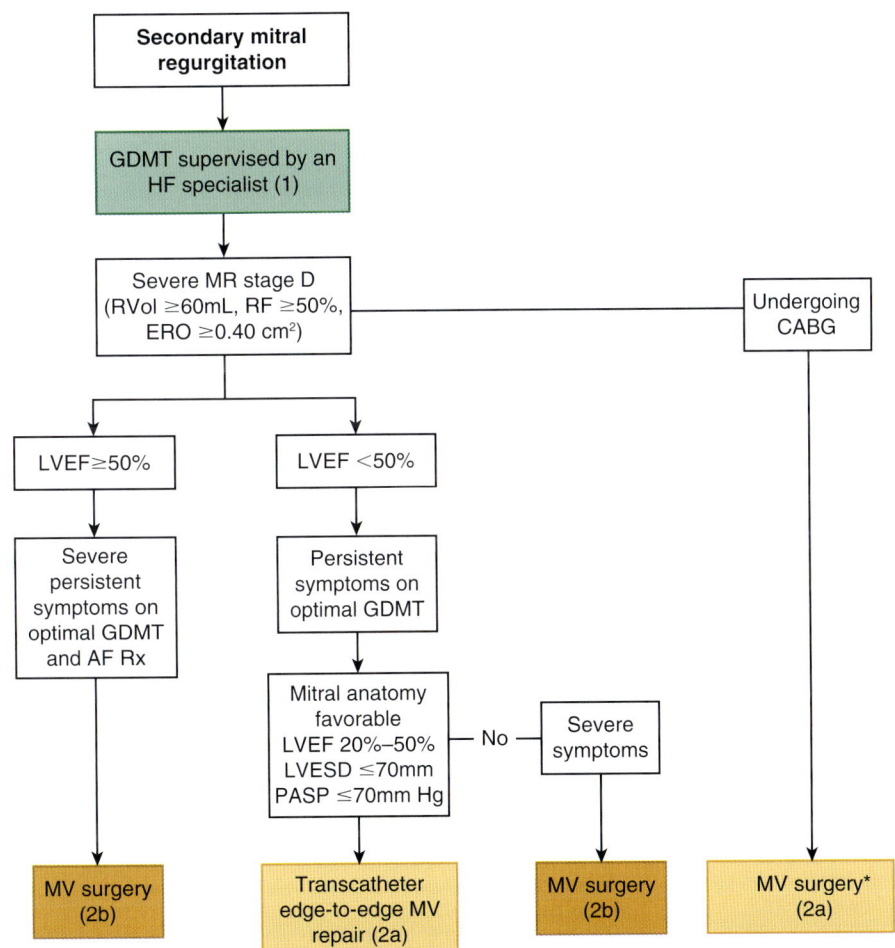

FIGURE 76.15 Management strategy for intervention for secondary mitral regurgitation. Colors correspond to Table 76.5. *AF*, Atrial fibrillation; *CABG*, coronary artery bypass graft; *ERO*, effective regurgitant orifice; *GDMT*, guideline-directed management and therapy; *HF*, heart failure; *LVEF*, left ventricular ejection fraction; *LVESD*, left ventricular end-systolic dimension; *MR*, mitral regurgitation; *MV*, mitral valve; *PASP*, pulmonary artery systolic pressure; *RF*, regurgitant fraction; *Rvol*, regurgitant volume; *Rx*, medication. (From Otto CM, et al. 2020 AHA/ACC guideline for the management of patients with valvular heart disease: a report of the American College of Cardiology/American Heart Association Task Force on Practice Guidelines. *J Am Coll Cardiol.* 2021;77:e25-197.)

These discordant results have led to extensive discussion and reevaluation of trial design, inclusion criteria, and patient populations that could explain the differences in results, as well as determine the appropriate patient populations for this therapy.

Differences in the COAPT and MITR-FR trial design and inclusion criteria may help explain the apparent discordance between the trials.[94] Randomization for COAPT occurred only after aggressive GDMT was achieved, including CRT as indicated, and stable for 3 months, and the primary efficacy outcome was rehospitalization for heart failure within 24 months; a relatively low percent of patients received ARB or ARNI therapy. Randomization for the MITRA-FR trial, however, occurred after identification of appropriate LVEF and MR criteria, and GDMT could continue to be fine-tuned during the course of the trial for both randomized cohorts; and a higher percentage of patients in both arms were treated with RAAS blockers. All-cause mortality rates at 1 year were similar for both treatment groups between the two trials. However, by 2 years the mortality rate for the GDMT arm in COAPT was worse (46% in COAPT versus 34% in MITRA-FR).[92,95]

Inclusion criteria for the trials was also different given the different thresholds for MR severity in the guidelines at the time of trial design. Because the EROA of the COAPT population was larger than that in MITRA-FR (~40 mm^2 compared with ~30 mm^2) and the LVEDV index was smaller (~101 mL/m^2 versus ~135 mL/m^2), the concept of proportionate and disproportionate secondary MR was proposed as a possible physiologic construct to understand the differences in the trials. To support this theory, Grayburn et al.[96] showed a linear relationship between MR severity (EROA) to LVEDV based on the Gorlin equation, using constant LVEF of 30% and regurgitant fraction of 50%. Using an EROA/EDV ratio of 0.14, the COAPT trial population had a disproportionately greater degree of MR relative to EDV, whereas the MITRA-FR patients had a proportionate degree of MR.[97] Thus, the argument was made that the COAPT patients were more likely to benefit from treatments to reduce MR severity than the MITRA-FR patients. In an opposing analysis, Gaasch et al.[98] used the Rvol/EDV ratio to argue that both trial populations had proportionate MR. Understandably, the physiologic relationship of MR severity to LV size depends not only on the etiology of the MR (ischemic versus

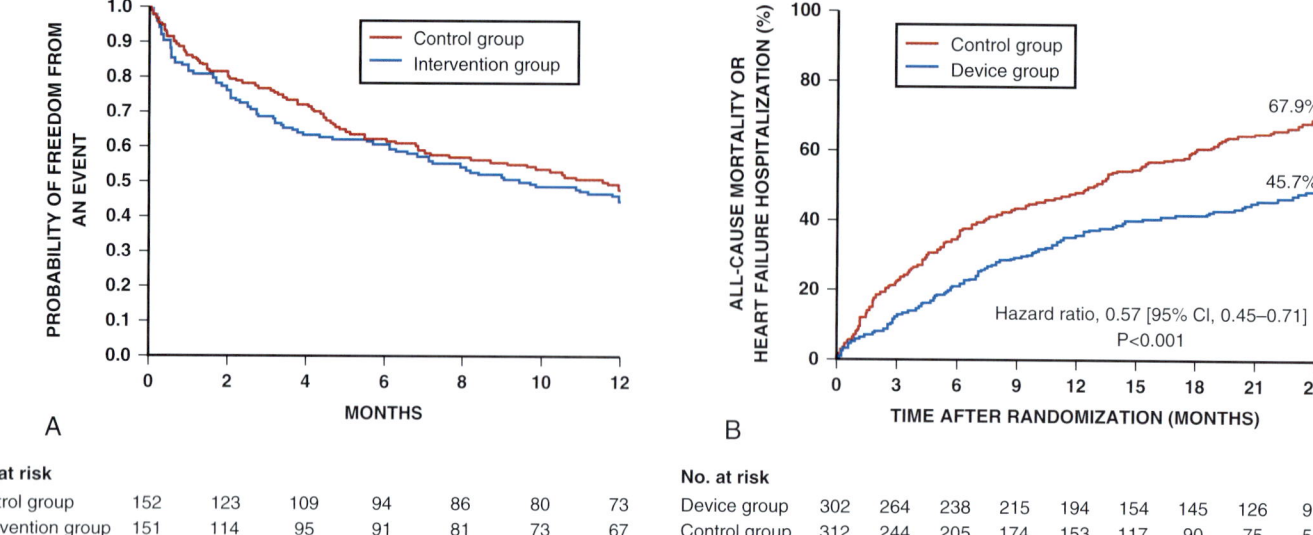

FIGURE 76.16 Outcomes of the MITRA-FR and COAPT trials. **A,** Freedom from death or hospitalization for heart failure in the MITRA-FR trial, the primary endpoint. **B,** Incidence of death or hospitalization for heart failure in the COAPT trial, a secondary endpoint. The primary endpoint in COAPT was hospitalization for heart failure. The secondary endpoint is shown here to compare outcomes to those with MITRA-FR using similar endpoints. (**A** from Obadia J-F, et al. Percutaneous repair or medical treatment for secondary mitral regurgitation. *N Engl J Med.* 2018;379:2297-2306; **B** from Stone GW, et al. Transcatheter mitral-valve repair in patients with heart failure. *N Engl J Med.* 2018;379:2307-2318.)

nonischemic) but also on hemodynamic load (preload and afterload), LV volume and function, and ventricular/atrial compliance, which may also be affected by disease duration, presence of AF, and underlying LV pathology.[99] More recent analyses of both trials,[100,101] including longer follow-up of the COAPT trial[102] and single site experience[103] suggest that severity of MR, LV remodeling, or their combination may not readily predict response to edge-to-edge repair in secondary MR.

Investigational Devices
A number of devices are under investigation for treatment of secondary MR (see Chapter 78), with focus on both transcatheter MV repair and TMVR.[104] As with surgery for secondary MR, TMVR has theoretical advantages compared with MV repair, because TMVR is applicable to a number of different anatomies and will virtually eliminate MR (see Fig. 78.7).

ACUTE MITRAL REGURGITATION
The causes of acute MR (see Table 76.1) are diverse and represent acute manifestations of disease processes that may, under other circumstances, cause chronic MR. Especially important causes of acute MR are spontaneous rupture of chordae tendineae (see Fig. 76.7), infective endocarditis with disruption of valve leaflets or chordal rupture (see Fig. 16.74A), ischemic dysfunction or rupture of a papillary muscle (see Fig. 16.21A), and malfunction of a prosthetic valve (see Fig. 79.5G).

Clinical Presentation
Acute severe MR causes a marked reduction in forward stroke volume, slight reduction in ESV, and increase in EDV. One major hemodynamic difference between acute and chronic MR derives from the differences in LA compliance. Patients who develop acute severe MR usually have a normal-size LA, with normal or reduced LA compliance. The LA pressure rises abruptly, which often leads to pulmonary edema, marked elevation of pulmonary vascular resistance, and right-sided heart failure.

Because the *v* wave is markedly elevated in patients with acute severe MR, the reverse pressure gradient between the LV and LA declines at the end of systole, and the murmur may be decrescendo rather than holosystolic, ending well before A_2. It usually is lower pitched and softer than the murmur of chronic MR. A left-sided S_4 frequently is found. Pulmonary hypertension, which is common in patients with acute MR, may increase the intensity of P_2, and the murmurs of pulmonary regurgitation and tricuspid regurgitation also may develop, along with a right-sided S_4. In patients with severe, acute MR, a *v* wave (late systolic pressure rise) in the pulmonary artery pressure pulse may rarely cause premature closure of the pulmonary valve, an early P_2, and paradoxical splitting of S_2. Acute MR, even if severe, often does not increase overall cardiac size, as seen on the chest radiograph, and may produce only mild LA enlargement despite marked elevation of LA pressure.

In addition, the echocardiogram may show little initial increase in the internal diameter of the LA or LV, but increased systolic motion of the LV is prominent. Characteristic features on Doppler echocardiography are the severe jet of MR and elevation of the pulmonary artery systolic pressure. Similar to the physical examination, the high atrial *v* wave can lead to early cessation of MR and a triangular CW Doppler profile instead of the usual parabolic shape. Careful interrogation of the valve by both transthoracic and transesophageal echo is essential to identify the mechanism and underlying etiology of the acute valve dysfunction (see Chapter 16).

In severe MR secondary to acute myocardial infarction, pulmonary edema, hypotension, and frank cardiogenic shock may develop. It is essential to determine the cause of the MR, which may be a ruptured papillary muscle, annular dilation from severe LV dilation, or papillary muscle displacement with leaflet tethering.[105]

Medical Management of Acute Mitral Regurgitation
Afterload reduction is particularly important in treating patients with acute MR. Intravenous nitroprusside may be lifesaving in patients with acute MR caused by rupture of the head of a papillary muscle complicating an acute myocardial infarction. It may permit stabilization of clinical status, thereby allowing coronary arteriography and surgery to be performed with the patient in optimal condition. In patients with acute MR who are hypotensive, an inotropic agent such as dobutamine should be administered with the nitroprusside. Intra-aortic balloon counterpulsation may be necessary to stabilize the patient while preparations for surgery are made.

Surgical Treatment of Acute Mitral Regurgitation
Emergency surgical treatment may be required for patients with acute LV failure caused by acute severe MR. Emergency surgery is associated with higher mortality rates than those for elective surgery for chronic MR.[106] However, unless patients with acute severe MR and heart failure are treated aggressively, a fatal outcome is almost certain.

Acute papillary muscle rupture requires emergency surgery with MV repair or replacement. In patients with papillary muscle dysfunction, initial treatment should consist of hemodynamic stabilization, usually with the aid of an intra-aortic balloon pump, and surgery should be considered for those patients who do not experience improvement with aggressive medical therapy. If patients with MR can be stabilized by medical treatment, it is preferable to defer operation until 4 to 6 weeks after the infarction if possible. Vasodilator treatment may be useful during this period. However, medical management should not be prolonged if multisystem (renal and/or pulmonary) failure develops.

Surgical mortality rates also are higher in patients with acute MR and refractory HF (NYHA Class IV), those with prosthetic valve dysfunction, and those with active infective endocarditis (of a native or prosthetic valve). Despite the higher surgical risks, the efficacy of early operation has been established in patients with infective endocarditis complicated by medically uncontrollable congestive heart failure and/or recurrent emboli.

Transcatheter Treatment of Acute Mitral Regurgitation

Experience is limited with percutaneous approaches to acute MR, although early reports support the selective use of the MitraClip in postinfarct MR[107] and even endocarditis, once the infection has been cleared.[108]

CLASSIC REFERENCES

Avierinos J-F, Gersh BJ, Melton LJ, et al. Natural history of asymptomatic mitral valve prolapse in the community. *Circulation*. 2002;106:1355–1361.

Carpentier A. Cardiac valve surgery–the "French correction". *J Thorac Cardiovasc Surg*. 1983;86:323–337.

Grigioni F, Enriquez-Sarano M, Zehr KJ, et al. Ischemic mitral regurgitation: long-term outcome and prognostic implications with quantitative doppler assessment. *Circulation*. 2001;103:1759–1764.

Levine RA, Handschumacher MD, Sanfilippo AJ, et al. Three-dimensional echocardiographic reconstruction of the mitral valve, with implications for the diagnosis of mitral valve prolapse. *Circulation*. 1989;80:589–598.

Nkomo VT, Gardin JM, Skelton TN, et al. Burden of valvular heart diseases: a population-based study. *Lancet*. 2006;368:1005–1011.

Perloff JK, Roberts WC. The mitral apparatus. Functional anatomy of mitral regurgitation. *Circulation*. 1972;46(2):227–239.

REFERENCES

1. Otto CM, Nishimura RA, Bonow RO, et al. 2020 AHA/ACC guideline for the management of patients with valvular heart disease: a report of the American College of Cardiology/American Heart Association task force on practice guidelines. *J Am Coll Cardiol*. 2021;77:e25–e197.
2. Bonow RO, O'Gara PT, Adams DH, et al. 2020 Focused update of the 2017 ACC expert consensus decision pathway on the management of mitral regurgitation. A report of the American College of Cardiology solution set oversight committee. *J Am Coll Cardiol*. 2020;75:2236–2270.

Mitral Valve Anatomy and Mechanisms of Regurgitation

3. Faletra FF, Leo LA, Paiocchi VL, et al. Anatomy of mitral annulus insights from non-invasive imaging techniques. *Eur Heart J Cardiovasc Imaging*. 2019;20:843–587.
4. Maréchaux S, Illman JE, Huynh J, et al. Functional anatomy and pathophysiologic principles in mitral regurgitation: non-invasive assessment. *Prog Cardiovasc Dis*. 2017;60:289–304.
5. Blanke P, Naoum C, Webb J, et al. Multimodality imaging in the context of transcatheter mitral valve replacement: establishing consensus among modalities and disciplines. *JACC Cardiovasc Imaging*. 2015;8:1191–1208.
6. Dal-Bianco JP, Levine RA. Anatomy of the mitral valve apparatus: role of 2D and 3D echocardiography. *Cardiol Clin*. 2013;31:151–164.
7. Theriault-Lauzier P, Andalib A, Martucci G, et al. Fluoroscopic anatomy of left-sided heart structures for transcatheter interventions: insight from multislice computed tomography. *JACC Cardiovasc Interv*. 2014;7:947–957.
8. Gunnal SA, Wabale RN, Farooqui MS. Morphological study of chordae tendinae in human cadaveric hearts. *Heart Views*. 2015;16:1–12.
9. Wilcox AG, Buchan KG, Espino DM. Frequency and diameter dependent viscoelastic properties of mitral valve chordae tendineae. *J Mech Behav Biomed Mater*. 2014;30:186–195.
10. Levine RA, Hagége AA, Judge DP, et al. Mitral valve disease—morphology and mechanisms. *Nat Rev Cardiol*. 2015;12:689–710.
11. Narang A, Addetia K, Weinert L, et al. Diagnosis of isolated cleft mitral valve using three-dimensional echocardiography. *J Am Soc Echocardiogr*. 2018;31:1161–1167.
12. Tang Z, Fan YT, Wang Y, et al. Mitral annular and left ventricular dynamics in atrial functional mitral regurgitation: a three-dimensional and speckle-tracking echocardiographic study. *J Am Soc Echocardiogr*. 2019;32:503–513.
13. Muraru D, Guta AC, Ochoa-Jimenez RC, et al. Functional regurgitation of atrioventricular valves and atrial fibrillation: an elusive pathophysiological link deserving further attention. *J Am Soc Echocardiogr*. 2020;33:42–53.
14. Kagiyama N, Mondillo S, Yoshida K, et al. Subtypes of atrial functional mitral regurgitation: imaging insights into their mechanisms and therapeutic implications. *JACC Cardiovasc Imaging*. 2020;13:820–835.
15. Deferm S, Bertrand PB, Verbrugge FH, et al. Atrial functional mitral regurgitation: JACC review topic of the week. *J Am Coll Cardiol*. 2019;73:2465–2476.
16. Gertz ZM, Raina A, Saghy L, et al. Evidence of atrial functional mitral regurgitation due to atrial fibrillation: reversal with arrhythmia control. *J Am Coll Cardiol*. 2011;58:1474–1481.
17. Silbiger JJ. Mechanistic insights into atrial functional mitral regurgitation: far more complicated than just left atrial remodeling. *Echocardiography*. 2019;36:164–169.
18. Zoghbi WA, Adams D, Bonow RO, et al. Recommendations for noninvasive evaluation of native valvular regurgitation: a report from the American Society of Echocardiography Developed in Collaboration with the Society for Cardiovascular Magnetic Resonance. *J Am Soc Echocardiogr*. 2017;30:303–371.
19. Kehl DW, Rader F, Siegel RJ. Echocardiographic features and clinical outcomes of flail mitral leaflet without severe mitral regurgitation. *J Am Soc Echocardiogr*. 2017;30:1162–1168.
20. Le Tourneau T, Mérot J, Rimbert A, et al. Genetics of syndromic and non-syndromic mitral valve prolapse. *Heart*. 2018;104:978–984.
21. Lee AP, Hsiung MC, Salgo IS, et al. Quantitative analysis of mitral valve morphology in mitral valve prolapse with real-time 3-dimensional echocardiography: importance of annular saddle shape in the pathogenesis of mitral regurgitation. *Circulation*. 2013;127:832–841.
22. Topilsky Y, Vaturi O, Watanabe N, et al. Real-time 3-dimensional dynamics of functional mitral regurgitation: a prospective quantitative and mechanistic study. *J Am Heart Assoc*. 2013;2:e000039.

Primary Mitral Regurgitation: Echocardiography and Other Diagnostic Modalities

23. Narang A, Puthumana J, Thomas JD. Diagnostic evaluation of mitral regurgitation. In: Otto CM, Bonow RO, eds. *Valvular Heart Disease: A Companion to Braunwald's Heart Disease*. 5th ed. Philadelphia: Saunders; 2021:289–310.
24. Tsang W, Freed BH, Lang RM. Three-dimensional anatomy of the aortic and mitral valves. In: Otto CM, Bonow RO, eds. *Valvular Heart Disease. A Companion to Braunwald's Heart Disease*. 5th ed. Philadelphia: Saunders; 2013:22–42.
25. Lancellotti P, Pellikka PA, Budts W, et al. The clinical use of stress echocardiography in non-ischaemic heart disease: recommendations from the European Association of Cardiovascular Imaging and the American Society of Echocardiography. *Eur Heart J Cardiovasc Imaging*. 2016;17:1191–1229.
26. Kawel-Boehm N, Maceira A, Valsangiacomo-Buechel ER, et al. Normal values for cardiovascular magnetic resonance in adults and children. *J Cardiovasc Magn Reson*. 2015;17:29.
27. Uretsky S, Gillam L, Lang R, et al. Discordance between echocardiography and MRI in the assessment of mitral regurgitation severity: a prospective multicenter trial. *J Am Coll Cardiol*. 2015;65:1078–1088.
28. Naoum C, Blanke P, Cavalcante JL, et al. Cardiac computed tomography and magnetic resonance imaging in the evaluation of mitral and tricuspid valve disease: implications for transcatheter interventions. *Circ Cardiovasc Imaging*. 2017:10;pii: e005331. https://doi.org/10.1161/CIRCIMAGING.116.005331.
29. Koo HJ, Yang DH, Oh SY, et al. Demonstration of mitral valve prolapse with CT for planning of mitral valve repair. *Radiographics*. 2014;34:1537–1552.
30. van Rosendael PJ, Katsanos S, Kamperidis V, et al. New insights on Carpentier I mitral regurgitation from multidetector row computed tomography. *Am J Cardiol*. 2014;114:763–768.
31. Mak GJ, Blanke P, Ong K, et al. Three-dimensional echocardiography compared with computed tomography to determine mitral annulus size before transcatheter mitral valve Implantation. *Circ Cardiovasc Imaging*. 2016:9:pii: e004176. https://doi.org/10.1161/CIRCIMAGING.115.004176.
32. Blanke P, Dvir D, Cheung A, et al. Mitral annular evaluation with CT in the context of transcatheter mitral valve replacement. *JACC Cardiovasc Imaging*. 2015;8:612–615.
33. Vukicevic M, Mosadegh B, Min JK, et al. Cardiac 3D printing and its future directions. *JACC Cardiovasc Imaging*. 2017;10:171–184.
34. Vukicevic M, Puperi DS, Grande-Allen KJ, et al. 3D Printed modeling of the mitral valve for catheter-based structural interventions. *Ann Biomed Eng*. 2017;45:508–519.

Primary Mitral Regurgitation: Natural History

35. Delling FN, Vasan RS. Epidemiology and pathophysiology of mitral valve prolapse. *Circulation*. 2014;129:2158–2170.
36. Parwani P, Avierinos JF, Levine RA, et al. Mitral valve prolapse: multimodality imaging and genetic insights. *Prog Cardiovasc Dis*. 2017;60:361–369.
37. Basso C, Iliceto S, Thiene G, et al. Mitral valve prolapse, ventricular arrhythmias, and sudden death. *Circulation*. 2019;140:952–964.
38. El Sabbagh A, Reddy YNV, Nishimura RA. Mitral valve regurgitation in the contemporary era: insights into diagnosis, management, and future directions. *JACC Cardiovascular Imaging*. 2018;11:628–643.
39. Dziadzko V, Dziadzko M, Medina-Inojosa JR, et al. Causes and mechanisms of isolated mitral regurgitation in the community: clinical context and outcome. *Eur Heart J*. 2019;40:2194–2202.
40. Antoine C, Benfari G, Michelena HI, et al. Clinical outcome of degenerative mitral regurgitation: critical importance of echocardiographic quantitative assessment in routine practice. *Circulation*. 2018;138:1317–1326.
41. Tribouilloy C, Grigioni F, Avierinos JF, et al. Survival implication of left ventricular end-systolic diameter in mitral regurgitation due to flail leaflets. A Long-Term Follow-Up Multicenter Study. *J Am Coll Cardiol*. 2009;54:1961–1968.
42. Tribouilloy C, Rusinaru D, Grigioni F, et al. Long-term mortality associated with left ventricular dysfunction in mitral regurgitation due to flail leaflets: a multicenter analysis. *Circ Cardiovasc Imaging*. 2014;7:363–370.
43. Suri RM, Vanoverschelde JL, Grigioni F, et al. Association between early surgical intervention vs watchful waiting and outcomes for mitral regurgitation due to flail mitral valve leaflets. *J Am Med Assoc*. 2013;310:609–616.
44. Hiemstra YL, Tomsic A, van Wijngaarden SE, et al. Prognostic value of global longitudinal strain and etiology after surgery for primary mitral regurgitation. *JACC: Cardiovasc Imaging*. 2020;13:577–585.
45. Enriquez-Sarano M. Mitral annular disjunction: the forgotten component of myxomatous mitral valve disease. *JACC Cardiovasc Imaging*. 2017;10:1434–1436.
46. Muthukumar L, Jahangir A, Jan MF, et al. Association between malignant mitral valve prolapse and sudden cardiac death: a review. *JAMA Cardiol*. 2020;5:1053–1061.
47. Dejgaard LA, Skjølsvik ET, Lie ØH, et al. The mitral annulus disjunction arrhythmic syndrome. *J Am Coll Cardiol*. 2018;72:1600–1609.
48. Perazzolo Marra M, Basso C, De Lazzari M, et al. Morphofunctional abnormalities of mitral annulus and arrhythmic mitral valve prolapse. *Circ Cardiovasc Imaging*. 2016;9:e005030.
49. Essayagh B, Sabbag A, Antoine C, et al. Presentation and outcome of arrhythmic mitral valve prolapse. *J Am Coll Cardiol*. 2020;76:637–649.
50. David TE, David CM, Tsang W, et al. Long-Term results of mitral valve repair for regurgitation due to leaflet prolapse. *J Am Coll Cardiol*. 2019;74:1044–1053.

Primary Mitral Regurgitation: Management

51. Baumgartner H, Falk V, Bax JJ, et al. 2017 ESC/EACTS guidelines for the management of valvular heart disease: the Task Force for the management of valvular heart disease of the European Society of Cardiology (ESC) and the European Association for Cardio-Thoracic Surgery (EACTS). *Eur Heart J*. 2017;38:2739–2791.
52. Grigioni F, Clavel MA, Vanoverschelde JL, et al. The MIDA Mortality Risk Score: development and external validation of a prognostic model for early and late death in degenerative mitral regurgitation. *Eur Heart J*. 2018;39:1281–1291.
53. Strauss CE, Duval S, Pastorius D, Harris KM. Pharmacotherapy in the treatment of mitral regurgitation: a systematic review. *J Heart Valve Dis*. 2012;21:275–285.
54. Katsi V, Georgiopoulos G, Magkas N, et al. The role of arterial hypertension in mitral valve regurgitation. *Curr Hypertens Rep*. 2019;21:20.
55. LaPar DJ, Ailawadi G, Isbell JM, et al. Mitral valve repair rates correlate with surgeon and institutional experience. *J Thorac Cardiovasc Surg*. 2014;148:995–1003.
56. Chikwe J, Toyoda N, Anyanwu AC, et al. Relation of mitral valve surgery volume to repair rate, durability, and survival. *J Am Coll Cardiol*. 2017;69:2397–2406.
57. Badhwar V, Vemulapalli S, Mack MA, et al. Volume-Outcome association of mitral valve surgery in the United States. *JAMA Cardiol*. 2020;5:1092–1101.
58. Lazam S, Vanoverschelde JL, Tribouilloy C, et al. Twenty-year outcome after mitral repair versus replacement for severe degenerative mitral regurgitation. *Circulation*. 2017;135:410–422.
59. Gammie JS, Chikwe J, Badhwar V, et al. Isolated mitral valve surgery: the society of thoracic surgeons adult cardiac surgery database analysis. *Ann Thorac Surg*. 2018;106:716–727.
60. Feldman T, Kar S, Elmariah S, et al. Randomized comparison of percutaneous repair and surgery for mitral regurgitation: 5-year results of EVEREST II. *J Am Coll Cardiol*. 2015;66:2844–2854.
61. Buzzatti N, Maisano F, Latib A, et al. Comparison of outcomes of percutaneous MitraClip versus surgical repair or replacement for degenerative mitral regurgitation in octogenarians. *Am J Cardiol*. 2015;115:487–492.
62. Külling M, Corti R, Noll G, et al. Heart team approach in treatment of mitral regurgitation: patient selection and outcome. *Open Heart*. 2020;7:e001280. https://doi.org/10.1136/openhrt-2020-001280.
63. Chiarito M, Pagnesi M, Martino EA, et al. Outcome after percutaneous edge-to-edge mitral repair for functional and degenerative mitral regurgitation: a systematic review and meta-analysis. *Heart*. 2018;104:306–312.
64. Feldman T, Foster E, Glower DD, et al. Percutaneous repair or surgery for mitral regurgitation. *N Engl J Med*. 2011;364:1395–1406.

65. Attizzani GF, Ohno Y, Capodanno D, et al. Extended use of percutaneous edge-to-edge mitral valve repair beyond EVEREST (Endovascular Valve Edge-To-Edge Repair) criteria: 30-day and 12-month clinical and echocardiographic outcomes from the GRASP (Getting Reduction of Mitral Insufficiency by Percutaneous Clip Implantation) registry. *JACC Cardiovasc Interv*. 2015;8:74–82.
66. Bottari VE, Tamborini G, Bartorelli AL, Alamanni F, Pepi M. MitraClip implantation in a previous surgical mitral valve edge-to-edge repair. *JACC Cardiovasc Interv*. 2015;8:111–113.
67. Hahn RT. Transcathether valve replacement and valve repair: review of procedures and intraprocedural echocardiographic imaging. *Circ Res*. 2016;119:341–356.

Secondary Mitral Regurgitation: Pathophysiology

68. Machino-Ohtsuka T, Seo Y, Ishizu T, et al. Novel mechanistic insights into atrial functional mitral regurgitation: 3-dimensional echocardiographic study. *Circ J*. 2016;80:2240–2248.
69. Abe Y, Akamatsu K, Ito K, et al. Prevalence and prognostic significance of functional mitral and tricuspid regurgitation despite preserved left ventricular ejection fraction in atrial fibrillation patients. *Circ J*. 2018;82:1451–1458.
70. Reddy ST, Belden W, Doyle M, et al. Mitral regurgitation recovery and atrial reverse remodeling following pulmonary vein isolation procedure in patients with atrial fibrillation: a clinical observation proof-of-concept cardiac MRI study. *J Interv Card Electrophysiol*. 2013;37:307–315.
71. Grayburn PA. Secondary (functional) mitral regurgitation in ischemic and dilated cardiomyopathy. In: Otto CM, Bonow RO, eds. *Valvular Heart Disease: A Companion to Braunwald's Heart Disease*. 5th ed. Philadelphia: Saunders; 2013:354–369.
72. O'Gara PT, Mack MJ. Secondary mitral regurgitation. *N Engl J Med*. 2020;383:1458–1467.
73. Bertrand PB, Schwammenthal E, Levine RA, et al. Exercise dynamics in secondary mitral regurgitation: pathophysiology and therapeutic implications. *Circulation*. 2017;135:297–314.
74. Kimura T, Roger VL, Watanabe N, et al. The unique mechanism of functional mitral regurgitation in acute myocardial infarction: a prospective dynamic 4D quantitative echocardiographic study. *Eur Heart J Cardiovasc Imaging*. 2019;20:396–406.

Secondary Mitral Regurgitation: Echocardiography and Other Diagnostic Modalities

75. Grayburn PA, Carabello B, Hung J, et al. Defining "severe" secondary mitral regurgitation: emphasizing an integrated approach. *J Am Coll Cardiol*. 2014;64:2792–2801.
76. Bartko PE, Arfsten H, Heitzinger G, et al. A unifying concept for the quantitative assessment of secondary mitral regurgitation. *J Am Coll Cardiol*. 2019;73:2506–2517.
77. Kamperidis V, Marsan NA, Delgado V, et al. Left ventricular systolic function assessment in secondary mitral regurgitation: left ventricular ejection fraction vs. speckle tracking global longitudinal strain. *Eur Heart J*. 2016;37.811–681.
78. Namazi F, van der Bijl P, Hirasawa K, et al. Prognostic value of left ventricular global longitudinal strain in patients with secondary mitral regurgitation. *J Am Coll Cardiol*. 2020;75:750–758.
79. Chinitz JS, Chen D, Goyal P, et al. Mitral apparatus assessment by delayed enhancement CMR: relative impact of infarct distribution on mitral regurgitation. *JACC Cardiovasc Imaging*. 2013;6:220–234.

Secondary Mitral Regurgitation: Management

80. Yancy CW, Jessup M, Bozkurt B, et al. 2017 ACC/AHA/HFSA focused update of the 2013 ACCF/AHA guideline for the management of heart failure: a report of the American College of Cardiology/American Heart Association Task Force on Clinical Practice Guidelines and the Heart Failure Society of America. *Circulation*. 2017;136:e137–e161.
81. Nasser R, Van Assche L, Vorlat A, et al. Evolution of functional mitral regurgitation and prognosis in medically managed heart failure patients with reduced ejection fraction. *JACC Heart Fail*. 2017;5:652–659.
82. Kang DH, Park S-J, Shin SH, et al. Angiotensin receptor neprilysin inhibitor for functional mitral regurgitation. *Circulation*. 2019;139:1354–1365.
83. Levine RA, Nagata Y, Dal-Bianco JP. Left ventricular dyssynchrony and the mitral valve apparatus: an orchestra that needs to play in sync. *JACC Cardiovasc Imaging*. 2019;12:1738–1740.
84. Bartko PE, Arfsten H, Heitzinger G, et al. Papillary muscle dyssynchrony-mediated functional mitral regurgitation: mechanistic insights and modulation by cardiac resynchronization. *JACC Cardiovasc Imaging*. 2019;12:1728–1737.
85. Fihn SD, Blankenship JC, Alexander KP, et al. 2014 ACC/AHA/AATS/PCNA/SCAI/STS focused update of the guideline for the diagnosis and management of patients with stable ischemic heart disease: a report of the American College of Cardiology/American Heart Association Task Force on Practice Guidelines, and the American Association for Thoracic Surgery, Preventive Cardiovascular Nurses Association, Society for Cardiovascular Angiography and Interventions, and Society of Thoracic Surgeons. *J Am Coll Cardiol*. 2014;64:1929–4199.
86. Knuuti J, Wijns W, Saraste A, et al. 2019 ESC Guidelines for the diagnosis and management of chronic coronary syndromes: the task force for the diagnosis and management of chronic coronary syndromes of the European Society of Cardiology (ESC). *Eur Heart J*. 2019;41:407–747.
87. Takahashi Y, Abe Y, Sasaki Y, et al. Mitral valve repair for atrial functional mitral regurgitation in patients with chronic atrial fibrillation. *Interact Cardiovasc Thorac Surg*. 2015;21:163–168.
88. Michler RE, Smith PK, Parides MK, et al. Two-year outcomes of surgical treatment of moderate ischemic mitral regurgitation. *N Engl J Med*. 2016;374:1932–1941.
89. Goldstein D, Moskowitz AJ, Gelijns AC, et al. Two-year outcomes of surgical treatment of severe ischemic mitral regurgitation. *N Engl J Med*. 2016;374:344–353.
90. Kron IL, Hung J, Overbey JR, et al. Predicting recurrent mitral regurgitation after mitral valve repair for severe ischemic mitral regurgitation. *J Thorac Cardiovasc Surg*. 2015;149:752–761e1.
91. Capoulade R, Zeng X, Overbey JR, et al. Impact of left ventricular to mitral valve ring mismatch on recurrent ischemic mitral regurgitation after ring annuloplasty. *Circulation*. 2016;134:1247–1256.
92. Stone GW, Lindenfeld J, Abraham WT, et al. Transcatheter mitral-valve repair in patients with heart failure. *N Engl J Med*. 2018;379:2307–2318.
93. Obadia JF, Messika-Zeitoun D, Leurent G, et al. Percutaneous repair or medical treatment for secondary mitral regurgitation. *N Engl J Med*. 2018;379:2297–2306.
94. Nishimura RA, Bonow RO. Percutaneous repair of secondary mitral regurgitation: a tale of two trials. *N Engl J Med*. 2018;379:2374–2376.
95. Iung B, Armoiry X, Vahanian A, et al. Percutaneous repair or medical treatment for secondary mitral regurgitation: outcomes at 2 years. *Eur J Heart Fail*. 2019;21:1619–1627.
96. Grayburn PA, Carabello B, Hung J, et al. Defining "severe" secondary mitral regurgitation: emphasizing an integrated approach. *J Am Coll Cardiol*. 2014;64:2792–2801.
97. Packer M, Grayburn PA. New evidence supporting a novel conceptual framework for distinguishing proportionate and disproportionate functional mitral regurgitation. *JAMA Cardiol*. 2020;5:469–475.
98. Gaasch WG, Aurigemma GP, Meyer TE. An appraisal of the association of clinical outcomes with the severity of regurgitant volume relative to end-diastolic volume in patients with secondary mitral regurgitation. *JAMA Cardiol*. 2020;5:469–475.
99. Hahn RT. Disproportionate emphasis on proportionate mitral regurgitation: are there better measures of regurgitant severity? *JAMA Cardiol*. 2020;5:377–379.
100. Grayburn PA, Sannino A, Cohen DJ, et al. Predictors of clinical response to transcatheter reduction of secondary mitral regurgitation: the COAPT trial. *J Am Coll Cardiol*. 2020;76:1007–1014.
101. Messika-Zeitoun D, Iung B, Armoiry X, et al. Impact of mitral regurgitation severity and left ventricular remodeling on outcome after MitraClip implantation: results from the mitra-FR trial. *JACC Cardiovasc Imaging*. 2021;14:742–752.
102. Lindenfeld J, Abraham WT, Grayburn PA, et al. Association of effective regurgitation orifice area to left ventricular end-diastolic volume ratio with transcatheter mitral valve repair outcomes: a secondary analysis of the COAPT trial. *JAMA Cardiol*. 2021;6:427–436.
103. Adamo M, Cani DS, Gavazzoni M, et al. Impact of disproportionate secondary mitral regurgitation in patients undergoing edge-to-edge percutaneous mitral valve repair. *EuroIntervention*. 2020;16:413–420.
104. Mangieri A, Laricchia A, Giannini F, et al. Emerging technologies for percutaneous mitral valve repair. *Front Cardiovasc Med*. 2019;6:161.

Acute Mitral Regurgitation

105. Bajaj A, Sethi A, Rathor P, et al. Acute complications of myocardial infarction in the current era: diagnosis and management. *J Investig Med*. 2015;63:844–855.
106. Chatterjee S, Rankin JS, Gammie JS, et al. Isolated mitral valve surgery risk in 77,836 patients from the society of thoracic surgeons database. *Ann Thorac Surg*. 2013;96:1587–1595.
107. Adamo M, Curello S, Chiari E, et al. Percutaneous edge-to-edge mitral valve repair for the treatment of acute mitral regurgitation complicating myocardial infarction: a single centre experience. *Int J Cardiol*. 2017;234:53–57.
108. Chandrashekar P, Fender EA, Al-Hijji MA, et al. Novel use of MitraClip for severe mitral regurgitation due to infective endocarditis. *J Invasive Cardiol*. 2017;29:E21–E22.

77 Tricuspid, Pulmonic, and Multivalvular Disease

PATRICIA A. PELLIKKA AND VUYISILE T. NKOMO

TRICUSPID STENOSIS, 1473
Causes and Pathology, 1473
Pathophysiology, 1473
Clinical Presentation, 1473
Management, 1475

TRICUSPID REGURGITATION, 1475
Causes and Pathology, 1475

Clinical Presentation, 1476
Management, 1478

PULMONIC STENOSIS, 1479
Causes and Pathology, 1479
Clinical Presentation, 1479

PULMONIC REGURGITATION, 1479
Causes and Pathology, 1479

Clinical Presentation, 1479
Management, 1481

MULTIVALVULAR DISEASE, 1481

REFERENCES, 1483

TRICUSPID STENOSIS
Causes and Pathology
Tricuspid stenosis (TS) is almost always rheumatic in origin, although rheumatic valve disease more commonly affects left-sided valves.[1] Other causes of obstruction to right atrial emptying are unusual and include congenital tricuspid atresia (see Chapter 82); right atrial tumors, which may produce a clinical picture suggesting rapidly progressive TS; and device leads, which more often are associated with tricuspid regurgitation (TR) but can become looped and fused to the tricuspid valve apparatus, and if multiple could cause obstruction. The carcinoid syndrome (see Chapter 52) and use of ergot-related drugs more frequently produce TR, which if severe, contributes to a gradient across the tricuspid valve.[2] Dysfunction, including thrombosis, of a tricuspid mechanical or bioprosthetic valve can result in stenosis. Rarely, endomyocardial fibrosis, tricuspid valve vegetations, or extracardiac tumors cause obstruction to right ventricular (RV) inflow. Localized compression of the right atrium by a pericardial effusion may also lead to RV inflow obstruction and may be unrecognized if the effusion is mistaken for the right atrium (Fig. 77.1).

Most patients with rheumatic tricuspid valve disease have TR or a combination of TS and TR. Isolated rheumatic tricuspid valve disease is uncommon, and this lesion generally accompanies mitral valve disease, which dominates the presentation (see Chapters 75 and 76). In many patients with TS, the aortic valve also is involved (i.e., trivalvular stenosis is present). TS is found at autopsy in approximately 15% of patients with rheumatic heart disease but is of clinical significance in only approximately 5%. Organic tricuspid valve disease is more common in India, Pakistan, and other developing nations near the equator than in North America or Western Europe. The anatomic changes of rheumatic TS resemble those of mitral stenosis (MS), with fusion and shortening of the chordae tendineae and fusion of the leaflets at their edges, producing a diaphragm with a fixed central aperture, typically without calcification. Like MS, TS is more common in women. The right atrium often is greatly dilated in TS, and its walls are thickened. There may be evidence of severe passive congestion, with enlargement of the liver and spleen, and right atrial thrombus formation which may extend into the vena cava or cause pulmonary embolism.

Pathophysiology
A diastolic pressure gradient between the right atrium and ventricle—the hemodynamic expression of TS—is augmented when the transvalvular blood flow increases during inspiration or exercise and is reduced when the blood flow declines during expiration. A relatively modest diastolic pressure gradient (i.e., a mean gradient of only 5 mmHg) usually is sufficient to elevate the mean right atrial pressure to levels that result in systemic venous congestion and, unless sodium intake has been restricted or diuretics have been given, is associated ultimately with jugular venous distention, ascites, and edema.

In patients with sinus rhythm, the right atrial *a* wave may be very tall. Resting cardiac output usually is markedly reduced and fails to rise during exercise. This accounts for the normal or only slightly elevated left atrial, pulmonary arterial, and RV systolic pressures, despite the frequent presence of accompanying mitral valvular disease.

A mean diastolic pressure gradient across the tricuspid valve as low as 2 mmHg and the typical echocardiographic appearance of leaflet restriction or doming is sufficient to establish the diagnosis of TS. Exercise, deep inspiration, and the rapid infusion of fluids or the administration of atropine may greatly enhance a borderline pressure gradient in a patient with TS. The diagnosis is generally made with transthoracic echocardiography; occasionally, transesophageal echocardiography (TEE) or other imaging such as cardiac magnetic resonance imaging (CMR) or computed tomography (CT) is necessary. Invasive assessment is rarely necessary.

Clinical Presentation
Symptoms. The low cardiac output in TS causes fatigue, and patients often experience discomfort from hepatomegaly, ascites, and anasarca (see Table 77.1). The severity of these symptoms, which are secondary to an elevated systemic venous pressure, is out of proportion to the degree of dyspnea. Some patients complain of a fluttering discomfort in the neck, caused by giant *a* waves in the jugular venous pulse. Occasionally, the symptoms of MS (severe dyspnea, orthopnea, and paroxysmal nocturnal dyspnea) may be masked by severe TS because the latter prevents surges of blood into the pulmonary circulation behind the stenotic mitral valve. The absence of symptoms of pulmonary congestion in a patient with obvious MS should suggest the possibility of TS.

Physical Examination (see Chapter 13). Because of the high frequency with which MS occurs in patients with TS, the similarity in the physical findings between the two valvular lesions, and the subtlety of physical findings in TS, echocardiography is essential to diagnose TS. The physical findings of TS may be attributed to MS, which is more common and associated with a louder murmur. Therefore a high index of clinical suspicion is required to detect TS. In the presence of sinus rhythm, the *a* wave in the jugular venous pulse is tall, and a presystolic hepatic pulsation often is palpable. The *y* descent is slow and barely appreciable. The lung fields are clear and, despite engorged neck veins

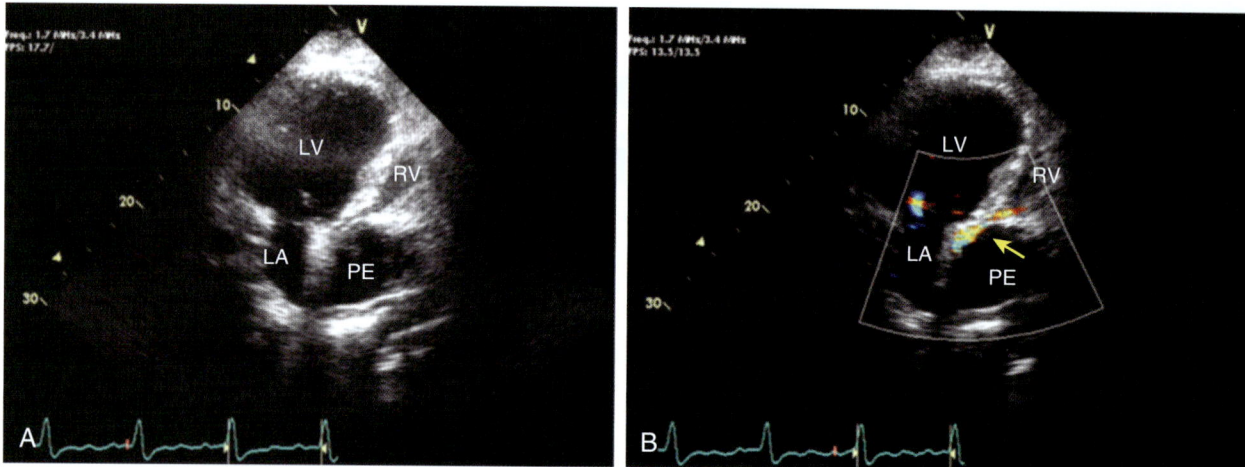

FIGURE 77.1 A, Apical four-chamber view showing localized pericardial effusion (PE) compressing the right atrium and assuming the shape of the right atrium. **B,** There is compression and significant narrowing of right ventricular inflow with a slit-like opening confirmed by color Doppler (*arrow*). Clinically the patient was in shock and underwent redo sternotomy and removal of a large hematoma around the diaphragmatic surface which was causing extrinsic compression of the right atrium. *LA,* Left atrium; *LV,* left ventricle; *RV,* right ventricle; *PE,* pericardial effusion.

TABLE 77.1 Clinical and Laboratory Features of Rheumatic Tricuspid Stenosis

History
- Progressive fatigue, edema, anorexia
- Minimal orthopnea, paroxysmal nocturnal dyspnea
- Rheumatic fever in two thirds of patients
- Female preponderance
- Pulmonary edema and hemoptysis rare

Physical Findings
- Signs of multivalvular involvement
- Diastolic rumble at lower left sternal border, increasing in intensity with inspiration
- Often confused with mitral stenosis
- Peripheral cyanosis
- Neck vein distention, with prominent *a* waves and slow *y* descent
- Absent right ventricular lift
- Associated murmurs of mitral and aortic valve disease
- Hepatic pulsation
- Ascites, peripheral edema

Imaging Findings
- ECG—tall right atrial P waves and no right ventricular hypertrophy
- Chest radiograph—dilated right atrium without enlarged pulmonary artery segment
- Echocardiogram—diastolic doming of tricuspid valve leaflets, thickening of valve, diastolic pressure gradient across tricuspid valve, right atrial enlargement

Modified from Ockene IS. Tricuspid valve disease. In Dalen JE, Alpert JS, eds. *Valvular Heart Disease.* 2nd ed. Boston: Little, Brown; 1987:356, 390.

and the presence of ascites and anasarca, the patient may be comfortable while lying flat. Thus, the diagnosis of TS may be suspected from inspection of the jugular venous pulse in a patient with MS but without clinical evidence of pulmonary hypertension. This suspicion is strengthened when a diastolic thrill is palpable at the lower left sternal border, particularly if the thrill appears or becomes more prominent during inspiration.

The auscultatory findings of the accompanying MS usually are prominent and often overshadow the more subtle signs of TS. A tricuspid opening snap (OS) may be audible but often is difficult to distinguish from a mitral OS. However, the tricuspid OS usually follows the mitral OS and is localized to the lower left sternal border, whereas the mitral OS usually is most prominent at the apex and radiates more widely. The diastolic murmur of TS is also commonly heard best along the lower left parasternal border in the fourth intercostal space and usually is softer, higher-pitched, and shorter in duration than the murmur of MS. The presystolic component of the TS murmur has a scratchy quality and a crescendo-decrescendo configuration that diminishes before S_1. The diastolic murmur and OS of TS both are augmented by maneuvers that increase trans-tricuspid valve flow, including inspiration, the Mueller maneuver (forced inspiration against a closed glottis), assumption of the right lateral decubitus position, leg raising, inhalation of amyl nitrite, squatting, and isotonic exercise. They are reduced during expiration or the strain of the Valsalva maneuver and return to control levels immediately (i.e., within two or three beats) after the Valsalva release.

Echocardiography. The tricuspid valve should be carefully inspected at the time of echocardiography in any patient with known or suspected rheumatic heart disease or other valve disease known to affect multiple valves. The echocardiographic changes (see Chapter 16) of the tricuspid valve in rheumatic TS resemble those observed in the mitral valve in rheumatic MS (see Fig. 16.47). Two-dimensional echocardiography characteristically shows diastolic doming of the leaflets, thickening and restricted motion of the other leaflets, reduced separation of the tips of the leaflets, and a reduction in diameter of the tricuspid orifice. The presence of commissural fusion and the anatomy of the valve and subvalvular apparatus should also be assessed, as these features may impact therapy. TEE allows added delineation of the details of valve structure. Doppler echocardiography can be helpful in assessment of the tricuspid valve even when 2-dimensional images are suboptimal. In TS, Doppler shows a prolonged slope of antegrade flow and compares well with cardiac catheterization in the quantification of TS and assessment of associated TR. Doppler evaluation of TS has largely replaced the need for catheterization to assess severity. Severe TS is characterized by a valve area of $\leq 1 cm^2$ as assessed by the continuity equation. The pressure half-time is generally greater than 190 msec, and the right atrium and inferior vena cava are dilated. The mean pressure gradient across the tricuspid valve varies with heart rate, but a mean gradient ≥ 5 mm Hg is consistent with significant TS.[3] Additional assessment of valve morphology may be provided by three-dimensional echocardiography, which allows en face views of the tricuspid valve from the atrial and ventricular aspects with simultaneous views of all three leaflets.

Other Diagnostic Evaluation Modalities

Electrocardiography. In the absence of atrial fibrillation (AF) in a patient with valvular heart disease, TS is suggested by the presence of electrocardiographic evidence of right atrial enlargement (see Chapter 14). The P wave amplitude in leads II and V_1 exceeds 0.25 mV. Because most patients with TS have mitral valve disease, the electrocardiographic signs of biatrial enlargement commonly are seen. The amplitude of the QRS complex in lead V_1 may be reduced by the dilated right atrium.

Radiography. The key radiologic finding is marked cardiomegaly with conspicuous enlargement of the right atrium (i.e., prominence of the right heart border), which extends into a dilated superior vena cava and azygos vein, but without conspicuous dilation of the pulmonary artery. The vascular changes in the lungs characteristic of mitral valvular disease may be masked, with little or no interstitial edema or vascular redistribution, but left atrial enlargement may be present.

The stenotic tricuspid valve can also be visualized with CMR or computed tomographic imaging and right atrial and ventricular volumes quantified.

Cardiac Catheterization. Invasive hemodynamic assessment of TS is rarely needed but is appropriate in the symptomatic patient in whom the physical findings and noninvasive data are discordant. It may occasionally be undertaken in patients undergoing invasive hemodynamic assessment for another indication. Right atrial and RV pressures can be recorded simultaneously, using two catheters or a single catheter with a double lumen, with one lumen opening on either side of the tricuspid valve.

Management

Although the fundamental approach to the management of severe TS is surgical treatment, intensive sodium restriction and diuretic therapy may diminish those symptoms secondary to the accumulation of excess salt and water. If AF is present, ventricular rate control is needed to improve diastolic filling. A preparatory period of diuresis may diminish hepatic congestion, thereby improving hepatic function sufficiently to diminish the risks of subsequent operation.

Most patients with TS have coexisting valvular disease that requires surgery. Surgical treatment of TS should be carried out at the time of mitral valve repair or replacement in patients with TS in whom the mean diastolic pressure gradient exceeds 5 mm Hg and the tricuspid orifice is less than approximately 2.0 cm^2. The final decision concerning surgical treatment is sometimes made at the operating table.

Because TS almost always is accompanied by some TR, simple finger fracture valvotomy may not result in significant hemodynamic improvement but may merely substitute severe TR for TS. However, open valvotomy or commissurotomy in which the stenotic tricuspid valve is converted into a functionally bicuspid valve may result in improvement, but annuloplasty may also be necessary if annular dilatation is present.[4] The commissures between the anterior and septal leaflets and between the posterior and septal leaflets are opened. It is not advisable to open the commissure between the anterior and posterior leaflets for fear of producing severe TR. If open valvotomy does not restore reasonably normal valve function, the tricuspid valve may have to be replaced. A large bioprosthesis is preferred to a mechanical prosthesis in the tricuspid position because of the high risk of thrombosis of the latter and the longer durability of bioprostheses in the tricuspid than in the mitral or aortic positions. Tricuspid balloon valvuloplasty is feasible, but has limited efficacy as it may result in significant TR. It may be considered in the rare patient without TR, but because of lack of long-term outcome data, surgical therapy is preferred.

TRICUSPID REGURGITATION

Causes and Pathology

A trivial to mild degree of TR is commonly seen with echocardiography in patients with a normal right heart and structurally normal tricuspid valve. This is of no consequence and under normal conditions, does not increase in severity. However, various conditions can lead to greater degrees of TR. The most common cause of TR is not intrinsic involvement of the valve itself (i.e., primary TR) but rather dilation of the right ventricle and of the tricuspid annulus causing secondary (functional) TR (see Table 77.2).[5] Right heart dilatation may result from volume overload as seen with left-to-right shunts in atrial septal defects or anomalous pulmonary venous connections. Dilatation may be a complication of RV failure of any cause (see Fig. 16.48). It is observed in patients with RV hypertension secondary to any form of cardiac or pulmonary vascular disease. Thus, secondary TR may be seen in left-sided valve disease, acute or chronic pulmonary thromboembolic disease, or chronic obstructive lung disease.[6,7] In general, a RV systolic pressure greater than 55 mm Hg will cause functional TR. TR can also occur secondary to RV infarction, congenital heart disease (e.g., pulmonic stenosis [PS] and pulmonary hypertension secondary to Eisenmenger syndrome; see Chapter 82), primary pulmonary hypertension (see Chapter 88) and cor pulmonale. In infants, TR may complicate RV failure secondary to neonatal pulmonary diseases and pulmonary hypertension with persistence of the fetal pulmonary circulation. In all these cases, TR reflects the presence of, and in turn aggravates, severe RV failure. Functional TR may diminish or disappear as the right ventricle decreases in size with the treatment of heart failure. TR can also occur as a consequence of dilation of the annulus in the Marfan syndrome, in which RV dilation secondary to pulmonary hypertension is not present. Acute or chronic AF can also lead to functional TR from tricuspid annulus dilatation, and AF is an important cause of isolated TR.[6,8]

A variety of disease processes can affect the tricuspid valve apparatus directly and lead to regurgitation (primary TR).[1,5] Organic TR may occur on a congenital basis (see Chapter 82), as part of Ebstein anomaly, defects involving the atrioventricular canal, when the tricuspid valve is involved in the formation of an aneurysm of the ventricular septum, or in corrected transposition of the great arteries, or it may occur as an isolated congenital lesion. Rheumatic fever may involve the tricuspid valve directly. When this occurs, it usually causes scarring of the valve leaflets and/or chordae tendineae, leading to limited leaflet mobility and either isolated TR or a combination of TR and TS. Rheumatic involvement of the mitral, and often aortic, valves coexist.

TR may result from prolapse of the tricuspid valve caused by myxomatous changes in the valve and chordae tendineae; prolapse of the

TABLE 77.2 Causes and Mechanisms of Pure Tricuspid Regurgitation

Causes

Anatomically Abnormal Valve

- Rheumatic
- Nonrheumatic
  Infective endocarditis
  Ebstein anomaly
  Floppy (prolapse)
  Congenital (non-Ebstein anomaly)
  Carcinoid
  Papillary muscle dysfunction
  Trauma
  Connective tissue disorders (Marfan syndrome)
  Rheumatoid arthritis
  Radiation injury

Anatomically Normal Valve (Functional, dilated annulus)

- Elevated right ventricular systolic pressure
- Chronic atrial fibrillation
- Restrictive cardiomyopathy

Mechanisms

CONDITION	LEAFLET AREA	ANNULAR CIRCUMFERENCE	LEAFLET INSERTION
Floppy	↑	↑	Normal
Ebstein anomaly	↑	↑	Abnormal
Pulmonary/right ventricular systolic hypertension	Normal	↑	Normal
Papillary muscle dysfunction	Normal	Normal	Normal
Carcinoid	↓/Normal	Normal	Normal
Rheumatic	↓/Normal	Normal	Normal
Infective endocarditis	↓/Normal	Normal	Normal

Modified from Waller BF. Rheumatic and nonrheumatic conditions producing valvular heart disease. In Frankl WS, Brest AN, eds. *Cardiovascular Clinics: Valvular Heart Disease: Comprehensive Evaluation and Management*. Philadelphia, FA: Davis; 1989:35, 95.

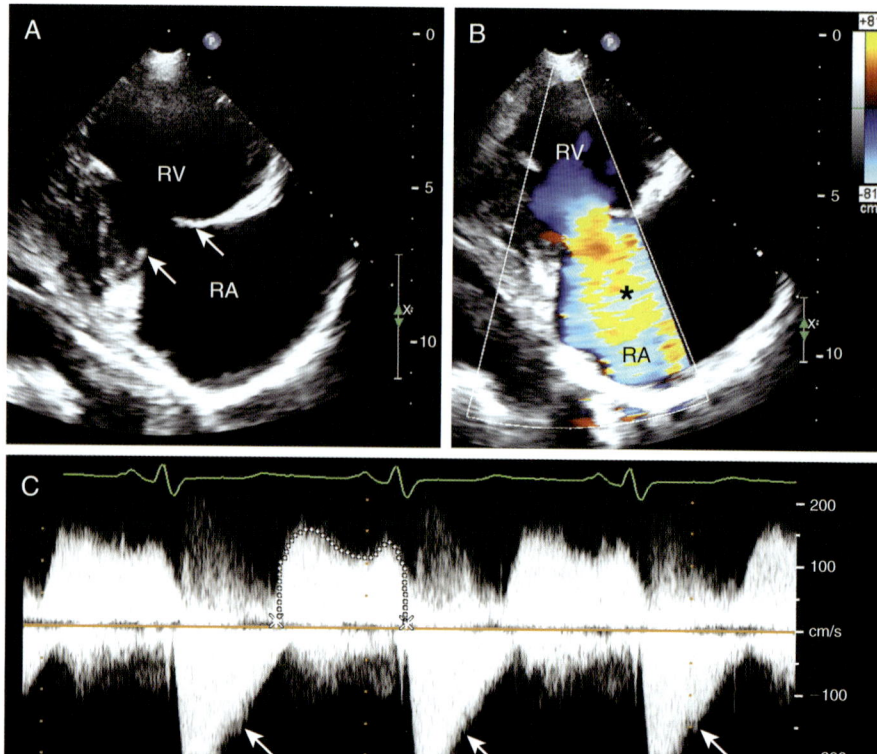

FIGURE 77.2 Transthoracic echocardiographic images of the tricuspid valve in a patient with carcinoid valvular heart disease. **A,** Two-dimensional parasternal long axis image of the tricuspid valve inflow view in mid-systole demonstrating a marked thickening and restriction of the tricuspid valve leaflets (*arrow*) resulting in failure of leaflet closure. **B,** Color Doppler imaging of the tricuspid valve in the parasternal long axis tricuspid valve inflow view in mid-systole demonstrating a broad regurgitant jet which occupies the entire right atrium consistent with severe tricuspid valve regurgitation (*asterisk*). **C,** Continuous wave Doppler imaging across the tricuspid valve demonstrating a dense, systolic, "dagger-shaped" tricuspid regurgitant jet consistent with severe tricuspid valve regurgitation (*arrows*). Less severe forms of tricuspid regurgitation are typically associated with parabolic shaped regurgitant jets. *RA,* Right atrium; *RV,* right ventricle. (From Luis SA, Pellikka PA. Carcinoid heart disease: diagnosis and management. *Best Pract Res Clin Endocrinol Metab.* 2016;30:149–158. https://doi.org/10.1016/j.beem.2015.09.005\.)

mitral valve is usually present in these patients as well. Prolapse of the tricuspid valve has been estimated to occur in 20% of all patients with mitral valve prolapse (MVP), but compared to MVP, diagnostic criteria are less well-defined. Tricuspid valve prolapse also may be associated with atrial septal defect.

Distortion of the tricuspid leaflets by transvenous pacemaker and defibrillator leads is an increasingly common cause of clinically significant TR.[9,10] Injury to the tricuspid valve or subvalvular apparatus may complicate endomyocardial biopsy.

TR or the combination of TR and TS is an important feature of the carcinoid syndrome (Fig. 77.2; see also Fig. 16.49), which leads to focal or diffuse deposits of fibrous tissue on the endocardium of the valvular cusps and cardiac chambers and on the intima of the great veins and coronary sinus (see Chapter 52). The white, fibrous carcinoid plaques are most extensive on the right side of the heart, where they usually are deposited on the ventricular surfaces of the tricuspid valve and cause the cusps to adhere to the underlying RV wall, thereby producing TR. A similar process may affect the tricuspid valve in patients who have used drugs that increase serotonin levels or simulate its effect on serotonin receptors. These include the anorectic drugs, fenfluramine and phentermine; ergot derivatives used for treating migraine headaches (ergotamine and methylsergide) or Parkinson disease (pergolide or cabergoline); or the synthetic stimulant and hallucinogen, 3,4-methylenedioxymethamphetamine (Ecstasy).

Other causes of TR include penetrating and nonpenetrating trauma,[11] dilated cardiomyopathy, and infective endocarditis (particularly staphylococcal endocarditis in intravenous drug users). Endomyocardial fibrosis with shortening of the tricuspid leaflets and chordae tendineae is an important cause of TR in tropical Africa, Asia, and South America. Less common causes of TR include cardiac tumors (particularly right atrial myxoma), endomyocardial fibrosis, methysergide-induced valvular disease, and systemic lupus erythematosus involving the tricuspid valve.

Clinical Presentation

The clinical stages of TR are depicted in Table 77.3.[3]

Symptoms. In the absence of pulmonary hypertension or RV failure, TR generally is well tolerated. When pulmonary hypertension and TR coexist, cardiac output declines and the manifestations of right-sided heart failure become intensified. Thus, the symptoms of TR result from a reduced cardiac output and from ascites, painful congestive hepatomegaly, and massive edema. Occasionally, patients exhibit throbbing pulsations in the neck, which intensify on effort and are caused by jugular venous distention, and systolic pulsations of the eyeballs also have been described. In the many patients with TR who have mitral valve disease, the symptoms of the latter usually predominate. Symptoms of pulmonary congestion may abate as TR develops but are replaced by weakness, fatigue, and other manifestations of a depressed cardiac output.

Physical Examination (see Chapter 13). In patients with severe TR, evidence of weight loss and cachexia, cyanosis, and jaundice are often present on inspection. AF is common. Jugular venous distention also is evident, the normal x and x' descents disappear, and a prominent systolic wave—a c-v wave (or s wave)—is apparent. The descent of this wave, y descent, is sharp and becomes the most prominent feature of the venous pulse except with coexisting TS, in which case it is slowed. A venous systolic thrill and murmur in the neck may be present in patients with severe TR. The RV impulse is hyperdynamic and thrusting in quality. Initially, systolic pulsations of an enlarged tender liver are frequent. However, in patients with chronic TR and congestive cirrhosis, the liver may become firm and nontender. Ascites and edema are frequent.

On auscultation, the murmur of mild TR may be absent or very subtle and of short duration. When TR occurs in the absence of pulmonary hypertension (e.g., infective endocarditis or after trauma), the murmur usually is of low intensity and limited to the first half of systole. With greater degrees of TR, auscultation usually reveals an S_3 originating from the right ventricle, which is accentuated by inspiration. When TR is associated with and secondary to pulmonary hypertension, P_2 is accentuated as well. When TR occurs in the presence of pulmonary hypertension, the systolic murmur usually is high-pitched, pansystolic, and loudest in the fourth intercostal space in the parasternal region but occasionally is loudest in the subxiphoid area. When the right ventricle is greatly dilated and occupies the anterior surface of the heart, the murmur may be prominent at the apex and difficult to distinguish from that produced by mitral regurgitation (MR).

TABLE 77.3 Stages of Tricuspid Regurgitation

STAGE	DEFINITION	VALVE HEMODYNAMICS	HEMODYNAMIC CONSEQUENCES	CLINICAL SYMPTOMS AND PRESENTATION
B	Progressive TR	Central jet ≤50% RA Vena contracta width ≤0.7 cm ERO ≤0.4 cm^2 R Vol ≤45 mL	None	None
C	Asymptomatic severe TR	Central jet >50% RA Vena contracta width >0.7 cm ERO >0.4 cm^2 R Vol >45 mL Dense CW signal with dagger shape Hepatic vein systolic flow reversal	Dilated RV and RA Elevated RA with cV wave	Elevated venous pressure No symptoms
D1	Symptomatic severe TR	Central jet >50% RA Vena contracta width >0.7 cm ERO >0.4 cm^2 R Vol >45 mL Dense CW signal with dagger shape Hepatic vein systolic flow reversal	Dilated RV and RA Elevated RA with cV wave	Elevated venous pressure Dyspnea on exertion, fatigue, ascites, edema

CW, Continuous wave Doppler signal; *ERO*, effective regurgitant orifice; *RA*, right atrium; *RV*, right ventricle; *R Vol*, regurgitant volume; *TR*, tricuspid regurgitation.
From Otto, Nishimura, RA, Bonow RO, CM, et al. 2020 AHA/ACC guideline for the management of patients with valvular heart disease: a report of the American College of Cardiology/American Heart Association Task Force on Practice Guidelines. *J Am Coll Cardiol*. 2021. doi.org/10.1016/j.jacc.2020.11.018.

The response of the systolic murmur to respiration and other maneuvers is of considerable aid in establishing the diagnosis of TR. The murmur characteristically is augmented during inspiration (Carvallo sign) with inspiration being associated with an increase in RV size and tricuspid valve annulus dimension, as well as an increase in regurgitant orifice area.[12] However, when the failing ventricle can no longer increase its stroke volume with the patient in the recumbent or sitting position, the inspiratory augmentation may be elicited by standing. The murmur also increases during the Mueller maneuver (see earlier), exercise, leg raising, and hepatic compression. It demonstrates an immediate overshoot after release of the Valsalva strain but is reduced in intensity and duration in the standing position and during the strain of the Valsalva maneuver. Increased atrioventricular flow across the tricuspid orifice in diastole may cause a short early diastolic flow rumble in the left parasternal region following S_3. Tricuspid valve prolapse, like MVP, causes nonejection systolic clicks and late systolic murmurs. In tricuspid valve prolapse, however, these findings are more prominent at the lower left sternal border. With inspiration, the clicks occur later and the murmurs intensify and become shorter in duration.

Echocardiography. The goal of echocardiography is to estimate the severity of TR and assess pulmonary arterial pressure and RV function.[13,14] In patients with TR secondary to dilation of the tricuspid annulus, the right atrium, right ventricle, and tricuspid annulus all usually are greatly dilated on echocardiography.[15] Doppler of the hepatic vein in severe TR shows systolic flow reversals (Fig. 77.3). There is evidence of RV diastolic overload with paradoxical motion of the ventricular septum similar to that observed in atrial septal defect. Severity of TR can be assessed by measuring vena contracta (Fig. 77.4) and regurgitant volume and effective regurgitant area quantified by quantitative Doppler or proximal isovelocity surface area method. Exaggerated motion and delayed closure of the tricuspid valve are evident in patients with Ebstein anomaly. Prolapse of the tricuspid valve caused by myxomatous degeneration may be evident on echocardiography. Echocardiographic indications of tricuspid valve abnormalities, especially TR by Doppler examination, can be detected in the vast majority of patients with carcinoid heart disease (see Fig. 77.2). A similar appearance of the tricuspid valve may be seen in patients who have used drugs that increase serotonin levels or simulate its effect on serotonin receptors. In patients with TR caused by endocarditis, echocardiography may reveal vegetations on the valve or a flail valve. TEE enhances detection of TR, but the degree of TR may be reduced compared to transthoracic echocardiography because of sedation given during TEE. Doppler echocardiography is a sensitive technique for visualizing the TR jet. The magnitude of TR can be quantified using techniques similar to those used to evaluate MR.[13,15]

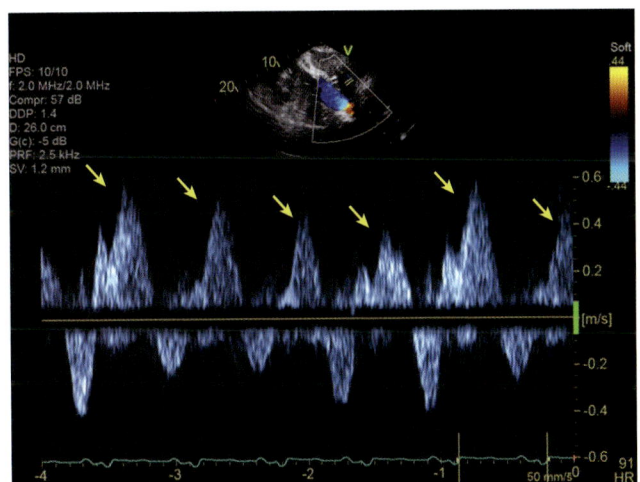

FIGURE 77.3 Pulsed-wave Doppler of the hepatic vein in a patient with severe tricuspid valve regurgitation showing significant hepatic vein systolic flow reversals (*arrows*).

Other Diagnostic Evaluation Modalities

Electrocardiography. ECG changes usually are nonspecific and characteristic of the lesion causing TR. Incomplete right bundle branch block, Q waves in lead V_1, and AF commonly are found.

Radiography. Marked cardiomegaly and a prominent right atrium are usually evident in patients with functional TR. Evidence of elevated right atrial pressure may include distention of the azygos vein and the presence of a pleural effusion. Ascites with upward displacement of the diaphragm may be present. Systolic pulsations of the right atrium may be present on fluoroscopy.

Cardiac Magnetic Resonance and Computed Tomography. CMR and CT are both useful for determining the three-dimensional geometric relationships between the right ventricle and the tricuspid annulus and leaflets in patients with functional TR.[16]

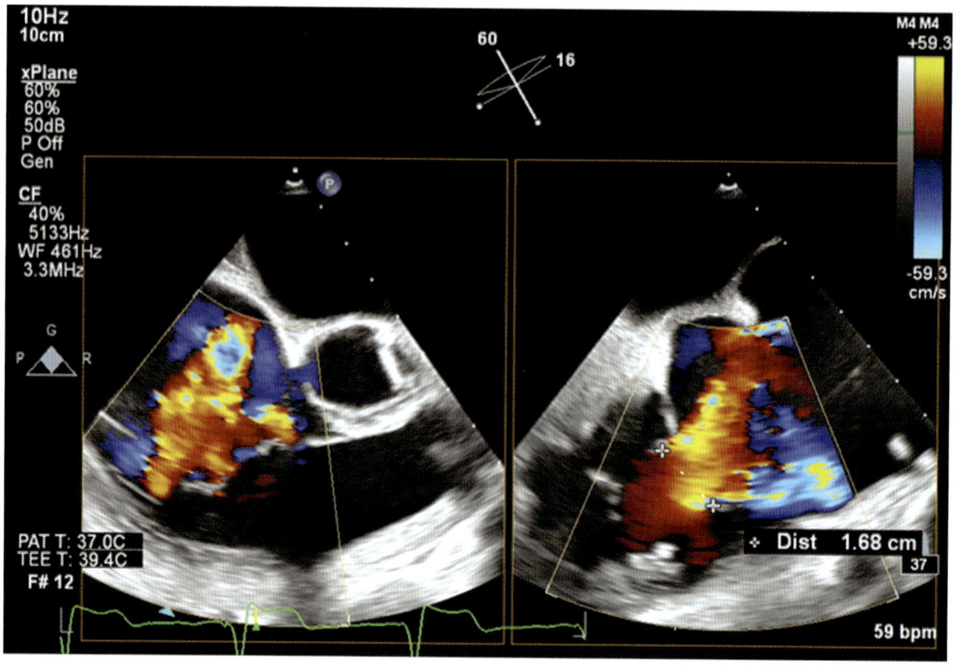

FIGURE 77.4 Transesophageal orthogonal views of the tricuspid valve showing severe tricuspid valve regurgitation with a large vena contracta of 1.68 cm in a patient with long-standing atrial fibrillation and functional tricuspid valve regurgitation from severe right atrial enlargement and tricuspid annulus dilation.

TABLE 77.4 ACC/AHA Guidelines for Intervention for Tricuspid Regurgitation

COR	LOE	INDICATION
1	B-NR	In patients with severe TR (Stages C and D) undergoing left-sided valve surgery, tricuspid valve surgery is recommended
2a	B-NR	In patients with progressive TR (Stage B) undergoing left-sided valve surgery, tricuspid valve surgery can be beneficial in the context of either (1) tricuspid annular dilation (tricuspid annulus end diastolic diameter >4.0 cm) or (2) prior signs and symptoms of right-sided HF
2a	B-NR	In patients with signs and symptoms of right-sided HF and severe primary TR (Stage D), isolated tricuspid valve surgery can be beneficial to reduce symptoms and recurrent hospitalizations
2a	B-NR	In patients with signs and symptoms of right-sided HF and severe isolated secondary TR attributable to annular dilation (in the absence of pulmonary hypertension or left-sided disease) who are poorly responsive to medical therapy (Stage D), isolated tricuspid valve surgery can be beneficial to reduce symptoms and recurrent hospitalizations.
2b	C-LD	In asymptomatic patients with severe primary TR (Stage C) and progressive RV dilation or systolic dysfunction, isolated tricuspid valve surgery may be considered
2b	B-NR	In patients with signs and symptoms of right-sided HF and severe TR (Stage D) who have undergone previous left-sided valve surgery, reoperation with isolated tricuspid valve surgery may be considered in the absence of severe pulmonary hypertension or severe RV systolic dysfunction

HF, heart failure; *LD,* limited data; *LOE,* level of evidence; *NR,* based on non-randomized studies; *RV,* right ventricular; *TR,* tricuspid regurgitation; *TS,* tricuspid stenosis.
From Otto CM, Nishimura, RA, Bonow RO, et al. 2020 AHA/ACC guideline for the management of patients with valvular heart disease: a report of the American College of Cardiology/American Heart Association Task Force on Practice Guidelines. *J Am Coll Cardiol.* 2021. doi.org/10.1016/j.jacc.2020.11.018.

Hemodynamic Findings. The right atrial and RV end-diastolic pressures often are elevated in TR, whether the condition is caused by organic disease of the tricuspid valve or is secondary to RV systolic overload. The right atrial pressure tracing usually reveals absence of the x descent and a prominent v or c-v wave (ventricularization of the atrial pressure). Absence of these findings essentially excludes moderate or severe TR. As the severity of TR increases, the contour of the right atrial pressure pulse increasingly resembles that of the RV pressure pulse. A rise or no change in right atrial pressure on deep inspiration, rather than the usual fall, is a characteristic finding.[17] Determination of the pulmonary arterial (or RV) systolic pressure may be helpful in deciding whether the TR is primary (caused by disease of the valve or its supporting structures) or functional (secondary to RV dilation). A pulmonary arterial or RV systolic pressure less than 40 mm Hg favors a primary cause, whereas a pressure greater than 55 mm Hg suggests that TR is secondary.

Management

TR in the absence of pulmonary hypertension is initially well tolerated. However, if TR is severe and sustained, eventually right heart failure will endure, which is associated with increased hospitalizations and excess mortality[18,19]; thus, appropriate consideration of and timing for surgery are indicated (see Table 77.4). Functional TR in the setting of pulmonary hypertension is associated with heart failure and poor survival.[20]

With the development of annuloplasty techniques, with or without an annuloplasty ring, surgical treatment of acquired TR secondary to annular dilation has greatly improved.[21,22] Repair rates have continued to increase significantly in the context of concomitant cardiac surgery; isolated tricuspid valve repair or replacement remains substantially underutilized.[23] At the time of mitral valve surgery in patients with TR secondary to pulmonary hypertension, the severity of the regurgitation should be assessed. It should be determined whether the TR is secondary to pulmonary hypertension, in which case the valve is normal, or whether it is secondary to other disease processes. Patients with mild TR without annular dilation usually do not require surgical treatment; pulmonary vascular pressures decline after successful mitral valve surgery, and the mild TR tends to disappear. However, even mild TR should be repaired if there is dilation of the tricuspid annulus, because the TR is likely to progress in severity if left untreated.[3,22] Excellent results have been reported in patients with mild to moderate TR using suture annuloplasty of the posterior (unsupported) portion of the annulus.[24] Patients with severe TR require ring annuloplasty.[25] Surgical mortality rates have continued to decrease over time. Contemporary data shows positive long-term outcomes associated with concomitant tricuspid valve repair at the time of left-heart valve surgery or coronary artery bypass surgery, irrespective of degree of TR,[26] although a doubling of risk of permanent pacemaker implantation was noted with use of tricuspid ring annuloplasty during mitral valve surgery.[26] Residual TR after tricuspid annuloplasty is determined principally by the degree of preoperative tricuspid leaflet tethering.[27] If these procedures do not provide a good functional result at the operating table, as assessed by TEE, valve replacement using a large bioprosthesis may be required. Transcatheter approaches to tricuspid valve repair and replacement using various methods and devices (see Chapter 78) are feasible and currently being studied in clinical trials.[28-30]

When organic disease of the tricuspid valve (Ebstein anomaly or carcinoid heart disease) causes TR severe enough to require surgery, valve replacement usually is needed. The risk of thrombosis of mechanical prostheses is greater in the tricuspid than in the mitral or aortic positions, presumably because pressure and flow rates are lower in the right side of the heart. For this reason, the artificial valve of choice for the tricuspid position in adults is a bioprosthesis. Graft durability of more than 10 years has been established. Postoperative vitamin K antagonist therapy is recommended after bioprosthetic tricuspid valve replacement in patients with carcinoid heart disease, because of a potential for thrombosis.[31]

In treating the difficult problem of tricuspid endocarditis in intravenous drug users (see Chapter 80), total excision of the tricuspid valve without immediate replacement generally can be tolerated by these patients, who usually do not have associated pulmonary hypertension. However, management decisions should be made by a heart valve team, including cardiology, cardiac surgery, and infectious disease specialists. Diseased valvular tissue should be excised to eradicate the endocarditis, and antibiotic treatment can then be continued. RV dysfunction will eventually occur if the resultant severe TR is untreated. A bioprosthetic valve may therefore be inserted several months after valve excision and control of the infection.

PULMONIC STENOSIS

Causes and Pathology

Congenital PS is the most common etiology of PS with an estimated worldwide birth prevalence of 0.5 per 1000 live births, and a higher prevalence in Asia.[32] Noonan syndrome is associated with PS, and PS may be seen with tetralogy of Fallot, Williams syndrome, and with other congenital heart defects. The pulmonary valve may be bicuspid, unicommissural, acommissural, or dysplastic. Manifestations in children and adults are discussed in Chapter 82. Rheumatic inflammation of the pulmonic valve is very uncommon, is usually associated with involvement of other valves, and rarely leads to serious deformity. Carcinoid heart disease often involves the pulmonary valve, and plaques, similar to those involving the tricuspid valve, are often present in the outflow tract of the right ventricle of patients with malignant carcinoid. The plaques result in constriction of the pulmonic valve annulus, retraction, thickening and fusion of the valve cusps, and a combination of PS and pulmonic regurgitation (PR) (see Fig. 77.3).[2] Another cause of PS is extrinsic compression by cardiac tumors or by aneurysm of the sinus of Valsalva.

Clinical Presentation

It is not until PS is severe that symptoms develop. These symptoms include fatigue, dyspnea, exertional pre-syncope or syncope, and eventually, right heart failure.

Physical Examination

The systolic ejection murmur of PS is heard at the left base and increases with inspiration. With increasing severity of PS, the ejection click moves closer to the first heart sound; the click disappears in severe PS. With severe PS, the jugular venous pulse shows a prominent a wave. A RV lift becomes palpable.

Management

Management of congenital PS focuses on balloon dilation when PS is severe or the patient is symptomatic (see Chapter 82). For the mixed stenosis and regurgitation of carcinoid involvement of the pulmonic valve, patch annuloplasty at the time of pulmonic valve replacement is frequently advisable.[31] Transcatheter pulmonary valve replacement is increasingly being used for pulmonary stenosis, atresia, or regurgitation.[33] Long-term outcome after surgical treatment of PS is excellent.[34]

PULMONIC REGURGITATION

Causes and Pathology

PR can result from dilation of the valve ring secondary to pulmonary hypertension (of any cause) or from dilation of the pulmonary artery. Infective endocarditis can involve the pulmonic valve, resulting in valve regurgitation. As more patients with congenital heart disease survive to adulthood, there is an increasing population of young adults with residual PR after surgical treatment of tetralogy of Fallot (Fig. 77.5) or surgical or transcatheter treatment of congenital PS. PR also may result from various lesions that directly affect the pulmonic valve. These include congenital malformations, such as absent, malformed, fenestrated, or supernumerary leaflets. These anomalies may occur as isolated lesions but more often are associated with other congenital anomalies, particularly tetralogy of Fallot, ventricular septal defect, and pulmonary valvular stenosis. Less common causes include trauma, carcinoid syndrome, in which leaflet thickening and retraction results in mixed stenosis and regurgitation (Fig. 77.6; see also Fig. 16.49), rheumatic involvement, injury produced by a pulmonary artery flow-directed catheter, syphilis, and chest trauma.

Clinical Presentation

Like TR, isolated PR causes RV volume overload and may be tolerated for many years without difficulty unless it complicates, or is complicated by, pulmonary hypertension. In this case, PR usually is accompanied by and aggravates RV failure. Patients with PR caused by infective endocarditis who develop septic pulmonary emboli and pulmonary hypertension often exhibit severe RV failure. In most patients, the clinical manifestations of the primary disease are severe and usually overshadow the PR.

Physical Examination.
The right ventricle is hyperdynamic and produces palpable systolic pulsations in the left parasternal area, and an enlarged pulmonary artery often produces systolic pulsations in the second left intercostal space. Sometimes systolic and diastolic thrills are felt in the same area. A tap reflecting pulmonic valve closure is usually palpable in the second intercostal space in patients with pulmonary hypertension and secondary PR.

Auscultation.
P_2 is not audible in patients with congenital absence of the pulmonic valve; however, this sound is accentuated in patients with PR secondary to pulmonary hypertension. Wide splitting of S_2 caused by prolongation of RV ejection accompanying the augmented RV stroke volume may be noted. A nonvalvular systolic ejection click generated by the sudden expansion of the pulmonary artery by the augmented RV stroke volume frequently initiates a midsystolic ejection murmur, most prominent in the second left intercostal space. An S_3 and S_4 originating from the right ventricle are often audible in the fourth intercostal space at the left parasternal area, and are augmented by inspiration.

In the absence of pulmonary hypertension, the diastolic murmur of PR is low-pitched and usually is heard best at the third and fourth left intercostal spaces adjacent to the sternum. The regurgitant murmur reflects the diastolic pressure gradient between the pulmonary artery and the right ventricle; as these pressures are usually lower than left-sided pressures, the murmur of PR is less likely to be heard than that of a similar grade of aortic regurgitation (AR). The PR murmur commences when pressures in the pulmonary artery and right ventricle diverge, approximately 0.04 second after P_2. The murmur becomes louder during inspiration.

When systolic pulmonary arterial pressure exceeds approximately 55 mm Hg, dilation of the pulmonic annulus produces a high-velocity regurgitant jet resulting in the audible murmur of PR, or Graham Steell

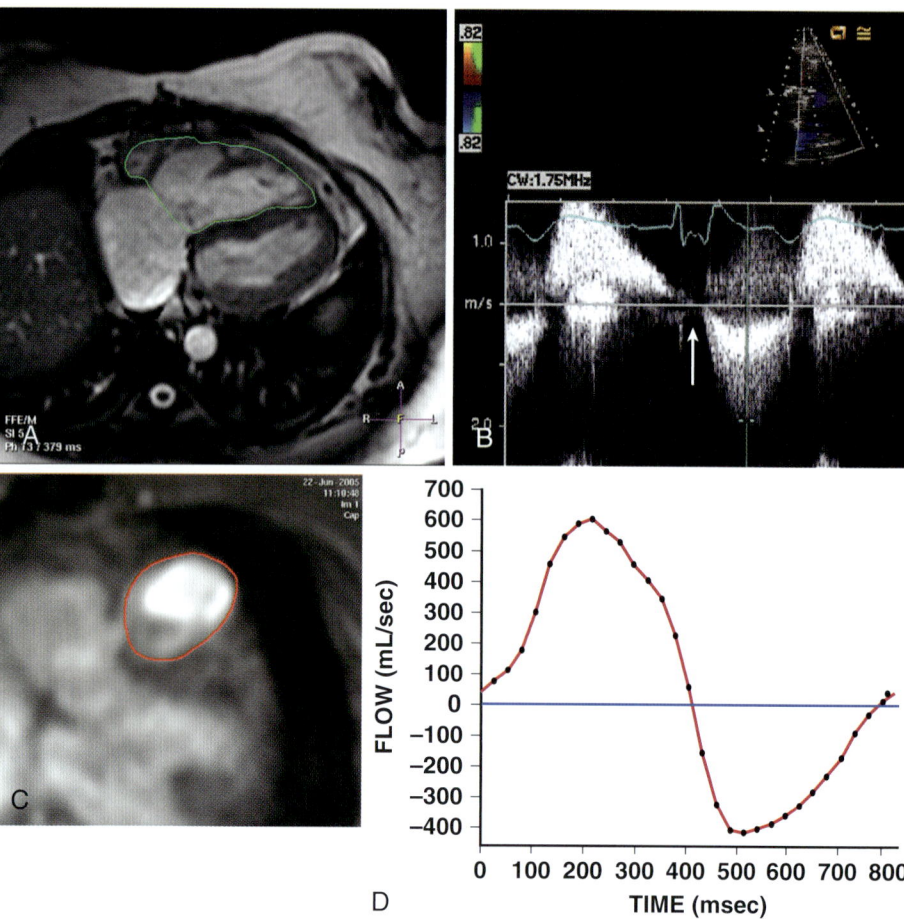

FIGURE 77.5 Cardiac magnetic resonance imaging (CMR) and Doppler echocardiographic evaluation in a 40-year-old woman who underwent repair of tetralogy of Fallot as a child. She was asymptomatic, but significant right ventricular (RV) enlargement was seen on echocardiography. **A,** RV dilation (*green circled area*) was confirmed in the CMR images, with a calculated RV end-diastolic volume of 444 mL. **B,** The Doppler tracing shows a dense signal in diastole with a steep deceleration slope that reaches the baseline before the end of diastole (*arrow*). **C,** Interrogation of pulmonary artery flow in the CMR phase-velocity images was performed by drawing a region of interest (*red circle*) around the pulmonary artery. **D,** Graph of the pulmonary artery flow within the region of interest indicated in **C** demonstrates both antegrade and retrograde flow. The total RV stroke volume was 245 mL, with antegrade flow of 98 mL, yielding a regurgitant fraction of 67%.

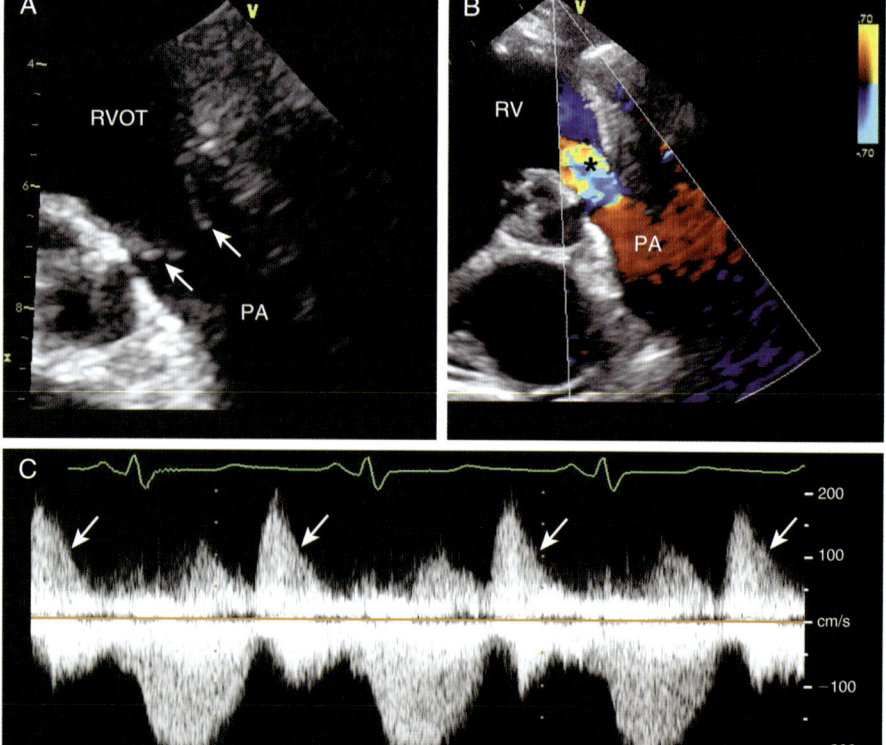

FIGURE 77.6 Transthoracic echocardiographic images of the pulmonary valve in a patient with carcinoid heart disease. **A,** Zoomed two-dimensional parasternal short axis image of the pulmonary in mid-diastole demonstrating a marked thickening with restriction of the pulmonary valve leaflets (*arrows*) resulting in failure of leaflet closure. **B,** Color Doppler imaging of the pulmonary valve in a modified parasternal short axis view demonstrating a broad regurgitant jet occupying the entire width of the right ventricular outflow tract consistent with severe pulmonary valve regurgitation (*asterisk*). **C,** Continuous wave Doppler imaging across the pulmonary valve demonstrating a dense, diastolic, pulmonary regurgitant jet which returns to baseline prior to the end of diastole consistent with severe pulmonary valve regurgitation (*arrows*). *RV,* Right ventricle; *RVOT,* right ventricular outflow tract; *PA,* pulmonary artery. (From Luis SA, Pellikka PA. Carcinoid heart disease: diagnosis and management. *Best Pract Res Clin Endocrinol Metab.* 2016;30:149–158. https://doi.org/10.1016/j.beem.2015.09.005.)

murmur. This murmur is high-pitched, blowing, and decrescendo, beginning immediately after P_2, and is most prominent in the left parasternal region in the second to fourth intercostal spaces. Thus, although it resembles the murmur of AR, it usually is accompanied by severe pulmonary hypertension—that is, an accentuated P_2 or fused S_2, an ejection sound, and a systolic murmur of TR, and not by a widened arterial pulse pressure. Sometimes, a low-frequency presystolic murmur is present, originating from increased diastolic flow across the tricuspid valve.

The murmur of PR secondary to pulmonary hypertension usually increases in intensity with inspiration, is diminished during the Valsalva strain, and returns to baseline intensity almost immediately after release of the Valsalva strain. This PR murmur resembles and may be confused with the diastolic blowing murmur of AR. However, a diastolic blowing murmur along the left sternal border in patients with rheumatic heart disease and pulmonary hypertension (even in the absence of peripheral signs of AR) usually is caused by AR rather than PR.

Echocardiography. A trivial or mild degree of PR can be detected by Doppler echocardiography in most normal patients. With more severe degrees, two-dimensional echocardiography shows RV dilation, and RV hypertrophy, in patients with pulmonary hypertension. RV function can be evaluated. Abnormal motion of the septum characteristic of volume overload of the right ventricle in diastole and/or septal flutter may be evident. The motion of the pulmonic valve may point to the cause of the PR. Absence of a waves and systolic notching of the posterior leaflet suggest pulmonary hypertension; large a waves indicate PS. Doppler echocardiography is extremely accurate in detecting PR and in helping estimate its severity (see Fig. 77.6; see also Fig. 16.50). Severe PR is associated with a reduced pressure half-time, indicating rapid equalization of pressure in the right ventricle and pulmonary artery. Additionally, the density of the Doppler profile of the jet is increased, and reversal of flow in the pulmonary artery by color flow imaging can be detected a distance from the valve. Abnormal Doppler signals in the RV outflow tract with velocity sustained throughout diastole are generally observed in patients in whom PR is caused by dilation of the valve ring secondary to pulmonary hypertension. When the velocity falls during diastole, the pulmonary artery pressure is usually normal, and the regurgitation is caused by an abnormality of the valve itself.

Other Diagnostic Evaluation Modalities

Electrocardiography. In the absence of pulmonary hypertension, PR is seen on an ECG as RV diastolic overload—an rSr (or rsR) configuration in the right precordial leads. PR secondary to pulmonary hypertension is usually associated with ECG evidence of RV hypertrophy.

Radiography. The pulmonary artery and right ventricle are usually enlarged, but these signs are nonspecific. Fluoroscopy may demonstrate pronounced pulsation of the main pulmonary artery.

CMR may be used to assess pulmonic valve anatomy, recognize any obstruction above or below the valve, measure pulmonary artery dilation, and quantify PR severity (see Fig. 77.5). CMR also is useful in evaluating RV dilation and systolic function.[35] Alternatively, cardiac CT may be used.[35]

Management

Except in patients with previous surgery for tetralogy of Fallot or similar RV outflow obstruction, or carcinoid heart disease, PR alone is seldom severe enough to require specific treatment. Treatment of the primary condition, such as infective endocarditis, or the lesion responsible for the pulmonary hypertension, such as surgery for mitral valvular disease, often ameliorates the PR. The timing of surgery for severe PR is based on the degree of RV dilation and evidence of systolic dysfunction.[3,36] In these patients, valve replacement may be carried out, preferably with a pulmonary allograft. There is growing experience with catheter-based approaches to pulmonic valve replacement in native pulmonic valve disease and in PR after surgical correction of congenital heart defects (see Chapter 82).[33]

MULTIVALVULAR DISEASE

Various clinical and hemodynamic syndromes can be produced by different combinations of valvular abnormalities. Multivalvular involvement has diverse causes (Table 77.5). It is frequently caused by rheumatic fever but is also seen in congenital heart disease, carcinoid heart disease, radiation heart disease, and connective tissue disorders. Degenerative calcific valve disease of the elderly is increasingly recognized to impact multiple valves. Myxomatous MR and prolapse may be associated with tricuspid valve prolapse and TR, or with pulmonary hypertension, tricuspid annulus dilation and TR. Marfan syndrome and other connective tissue disorders may cause multivalve prolapse and dilation, resulting in multivalvular regurgitation. Degenerative calcification of the aortic valve may be associated with degenerative mitral annular calcification, resulting in concomitant aortic stenosis (AS) and MR. Different pathologic conditions may affect two valves in the same patient (e.g., infective endocarditis on the aortic valve causing AR and ischemia causing MR).

In patients with multivalvular disease, the clinical manifestations depend on the relative severity of each lesion. When the valvular abnormalities are of approximately equal severity, clinical manifestations produced by the more proximal (upstream) of the two valvular lesions (i.e., the mitral valve in patients with combined mitral and aortic valvular disease and the tricuspid valve in patients with combined tricuspid and mitral valvular disease) are generally more prominent than those produced by the distal lesion. Thus, the proximal lesion tends to mask the distal lesion.

It is important to recognize multivalvular involvement preoperatively because failure to correct all significant valvular disease at the time of surgery increases mortality. Specific recommendations exist for concomitant valve surgery in patients undergoing surgery on another valve.[3,37] In patients with multivalvular disease, the relative severity of each lesion may be difficult to estimate by clinical examination because one lesion may mask the manifestations of the other. Therefore, patients suspected of having multivalvular involvement and who are being considered for surgical treatment should undergo careful clinical evaluation and full Doppler echocardiographic evaluation. Stress echocardiography is well suited to assess multivalvular disease and may be especially useful when the patient's symptoms are disproportionate to the resting hemodynamics. Mixed stenotic and regurgitant lesions can be assessed with a combination of two- or three-dimensional imaging, including planimetry of stenotic orifices, color flow imaging and Doppler. Multiple valves can be systematically assessed during exercise[38]; this is

TABLE 77.5 Causes of Multivalvular Heart Disease

Acquired

Systemic diseases
- Infective endocarditis
- Carcinoid heart disease
- Systemic lupus erythematosus

Cardiac diseases
- Infective endocarditis
- Rheumatic heart disease

Degenerative
- Calcific diseases, increased with age, prior radiation, chronic kidney disease

Iatrogenic
- Adverse drug effects—ergot-related antagonists
- Radiation therapy

Functional (annulus dilatation)
- Due to ischemic heart disease, hypertensive heart disease, chronic arrhythmia, pulmonary hypertension, cardiomyopathy

Congenital

Connective tissue disorders
- Marfan syndrome, Ehlers-Danlos syndrome

Other
- Trisomy 18, 13, and 15
- Shone syndrome
- Ochronosis

Mixed

Multiple conditions may contribute to valve dysfunction
- Degenerative diseases may lead to associated functional disease
- Congenital heart disease may predispose to infective endocarditis or degenerative disease

particularly helpful in assessing patients with exertional symptoms, especially when these seem disproportionate to findings on imaging at rest. Right and left cardiac catheterization may occasionally be necessary. If there is any question concerning the presence of significant AS in patients undergoing mitral valve surgery, the aortic valve should be inspected because overlooking this condition can lead to a high perioperative mortality. Similarly, it is useful to palpate the tricuspid valve at the time of mitral valve surgery. Intraoperative TEE is also important to assess the impact of repair of one valve lesion on another.

Mitral Stenosis and Aortic Valve Disease
Aortic valve involvement is present in approximately one third of patients with rheumatic MS. Rheumatic aortic valve disease may result in primary regurgitation, stenosis, or mixed stenosis and regurgitation. AR is evident on physical examination in approximately two thirds of patients with severe MS, but only approximately 10% of patients with MS have severe rheumatic AR. On physical examination, a proximal lesion may mask signs of a distal lesion. For example, significant AR may be missed in patients with severe MS because the widened pulse pressure may be absent. An accentuated S_1 and an OS in a patient with AR should suggest the possibility of mitral valvular disease. AS is evident on physical examination based on the typical murmur, even when MS is present; however, the cardiac output tends to be reduced more than that in patients with isolated AS. On physical examination, a S_4 (which is common in patients with pure AS) usually is not present. The midsystolic murmur characteristic of AS may be reduced in intensity and duration because the stroke volume is reduced by the MS.

Echocardiography is of decisive value in evaluating patients with rheumatic disease and allows accurate diagnosis of the presence and severity of multivalve involvement, taking into consideration the altered flow conditions with serial lesions. In the setting of severe AS, MS severity may be overestimated, especially when indexed stroke volume is reduced. True MS in patients with severe AS can be recognized by Doppler-derived mitral valve area ≤1.5 cm^2 and the extension of calcification to both anterior and posterior mitral leaflets and is associated with excess mortality.[39]

Because double-valve replacement is associated with increased short- and long-term risks, balloon mitral valvuloplasty (BMV) can be the first procedure if MS is the predominant lesion, with subsequent aortic valve replacement (AVR) when needed. If percutaneous BMV is not an option or concurrent AVR is needed, surgical valvotomy may be considered.

It is vital to recognize the presence of hemodynamically significant aortic valvular disease (i.e., AS and/or AR) preoperatively in patients who are to undergo BMV. This procedure may be hazardous because it can impose a sudden hemodynamic load on the left ventricle that had previously been protected by the MS and may lead to acute pulmonary edema.

Aortic Stenosis and Mitral Regurgitation
AS is often accompanied by MR caused by MVP, annular calcification, rheumatic disease, or functional MR. The increased left ventricular (LV) pressure secondary to LV outflow obstruction may augment the volume of MR flow, whereas the presence of MR may diminish the ventricular preload necessary to maintain the LV stroke volume in patients with AS. The result is a reduced forward cardiac output and marked left atrial and pulmonary venous hypertension. Significant MR is one explanation for low output AS (see Chapter 72).[40] The development of AF (caused by left atrial enlargement) has an adverse hemodynamic effect in the presence of AS. Physical findings may be confusing because it may be difficult to recognize two distinct systolic murmurs. However, on echocardiography, the cause and severity of AS and MR can be accurately diagnosed. In most cases, MR is mild to moderate and it is appropriate to treat AS alone. When MR is severe or there is significant structural mitral valve disease, concurrent mitral repair (whenever possible) or valve replacement at the time of AVR should be considered.

Aortic Regurgitation and Mitral Regurgitation
The relatively infrequent combination of AR and MR may be caused by rheumatic heart disease, prolapse of the aortic and mitral valves secondary to myxomatous degeneration, or dilation of both annuli in patients with connective tissue disorders, or IE. The clinical features of AR usually predominate, and it is sometimes difficult to determine whether the MR is caused by organic involvement of this valve or by dilation of the mitral valve ring secondary to LV enlargement. When both valvular leaks are severe, this combination of lesions is poorly tolerated. The normal mitral valve ordinarily serves as a backup to the aortic valve, and premature (diastolic) closure of the mitral valve limits the volume of reflux that occurs in patients with acute AR. With severe combined regurgitant lesions, regardless of the cause of the mitral lesion, blood may reflux from the aorta through both chambers of the left side of the heart into the pulmonary veins. Physical and laboratory examinations usually show evidence of both lesions. An S_3 and a brisk arterial pulse frequently are present. The relative severity of each lesion can be assessed best by Doppler echocardiography, especially using proximal isovelocity surface area or vena contracta methods, three-dimensional imaging, or contrast angiography. This combination of lesions leads to severe LV dilation. MR that occurs in patients with AR secondary to LV dilation often regresses after AVR alone. If severe, the MR may be corrected by annuloplasty at the time of AVR. An intrinsically normal mitral valve that is regurgitant because of a dilated annulus should not be replaced.

Surgical Treatment of Multivalvular Disease
Timing and indication for surgery is typically driven by the more severe predominant valve lesion.[3,37,41] The long-term survival following multivalvular surgery depends strongly on the preoperative functional status. Patients operated on for combined AR and MR have poorer outcomes than patients undergoing double-valve replacement for any of the other combinations of lesions, presumably because both AR and MR may produce irreversible LV damage. Surgical or transcatheter mitral valve repair for MR or balloon mitral valvotomy for MS performed in combination with AVR may be preferable to double-valve replacement and should be considered. Moreover, most patients will experience some decrease in functional MR severity after AVR. In the setting of planned AVR, management of coexistent MR should take into consideration the severity of MR, its mechanism, operative risks and co-morbidities. Risk factors that reduce long-term survival after double-valve replacement include advanced age, less favorable functional status, decreased LV ejection fraction, greater LV enlargement, and accompanying ischemic heart disease requiring coronary artery bypass grafting.

In view of the higher risks, a higher threshold is required for multivalvular versus single-valve surgery. Thus, patients generally are advised not to undergo multivalvular surgery until they reach late New York Heart Association (NYHA) functional class II or class III, unless they exhibit evidence of declining LV function. Despite a detailed noninvasive and invasive workup, the decision to treat more than one valve often is made on the basis of findings on palpation or direct inspection at the operating table, or the findings on intraoperative TEE.

Triple- and Quadruple-Valve Disease
Hemodynamically significant disease involving the mitral, aortic, and tricuspid valves is uncommon and typically is caused by rheumatic heart disease. Carcinoid heart disease can sometimes involve three or four valves.[31] Patients with multivalvular disease may present in advanced heart failure with marked cardiomegaly, and surgical correction of all significant valvular lesions is imperative. However, triple- or quadruple-valve replacement is a long and complex operation. Early in the experience with this procedure, the mortality rate was 20% for patients in NYHA class III and 40% for patients in class IV. More recently, the mortality rate has declined but is still substantial and should be reserved for high-volume cardiac surgical centers.[42] In many patients with triple-valvular disease, it is possible to replace the aortic valve, repair the mitral valve, and perform a tricuspid annuloplasty or valvuloplasty.

Patients who survive triple- or quadruple-valve replacement surgery usually experience substantial clinical improvement during the early postoperative period, and postoperative catheterization studies show marked reductions in pulmonary arterial and capillary pressures. However, some patients die of arrhythmias or congestive heart failure in the late postoperative period despite normally functioning prostheses. The cause of cardiac failure in this situation is unknown, but may be related to intraoperative myocardial ischemia, microemboli from the multiple prostheses, or continued subclinical episodes of rheumatic myocarditis.

When multiple prosthetic valves must be inserted, it is logical to select two bioprostheses or two mechanical prostheses for the left side of the heart. If the patient is to be exposed to the hazards of anticoagulants for one mechanical prosthesis, it seems unreasonable to add the potential risks of early failure of a bioprosthesis. However, if two mechanical prostheses are selected for the left side of the heart, the use of a bioprosthesis in the tricuspid position is suggested. Repair instead of replacement of the mitral and tricuspid valves during triple valve surgery is associated with improved short-term outcomes.[43] Percutaneous therapies are a growing alternative to surgical intervention when valve lesions are amenable to percutaneous intervention and surgical risk is increased (see Chapters 74 and 78).[41]

REFERENCES

Tricuspid Stenosis

1. Rodes-Cabau J, Taramasso M, O'Gara PT. Diagnosis and treatment of tricuspid valve disease: current and future perspectives. *Lancet*. 2016;388:2431–2442.
2. Luis SA, Pellikka PA. Carcinoid heart disease: diagnosis and management. *Best Pract Res Clin Endocrinol Metab*. 2016;30:149–158.
3. Otto CM, Nishimura RA, Bonow RO, et al. 2020 AHA/ACC guideline for the management of patients with valvular heart disease: a report of the American College of Cardiology/American Heart Association Task Force on Practice guidelines. *J Am Coll Cardiol*. 2021. https://doi.org/10.1016/j.jacc.2020.11.018.
4. Cevasco M, Shekar PS. Surgical management of tricuspid stenosis. *Ann Cardiothorac Surg*. 2017;6:275–282.

Tricuspid Regurgitation—Pathophysiology and Clinical Presentation

5. Asmarats L, Taramasso M, Rodes-Cabau J. Tricuspid valve disease: diagnosis, prognosis and management of a rapidly evolving field. *Nat Rev Cardiol*. 2019;16:538–554.
6. Benfari G, Antoine C, Miller WL, et al. Excess mortality associated with functional tricuspid regurgitation complicating heart failure with reduced ejection fraction. *Circulation*. 2019;140:196–206.
7. Essayagh B, Antoine C, Benfari G, et al. Functional tricuspid regurgitation of degenerative mitral valve disease: a crucial determinant of survival. *Eur Heart J*. 2020;41:1918–1929.
8. Topilsky Y, Nkomo VT, Vatury O, et al. Clinical outcome of isolated tricuspid regurgitation. *JACC Cardiovasc Imaging*. 2014;7:1185–1194.
9. Hoke U, Auger D, Thijssen J, et al. Significant lead-induced tricuspid regurgitation is associated with poor prognosis at long-term follow-up. *Heart*. 2014;100:960–968.
10. Ebrille E, Chang JD, Zimetbaum PJ. Tricuspid valve dysfunction caused by right ventricular leads. *Card Electrophysiol Clin*. 2018;10:447–452.
11. Zhang Z, Yin K, Dong L, et al. Surgical management of traumatic tricuspid insufficiency. *J Card Surg*. 2017;32:342–346.
12. Topilsky Y, Tribouilloy C, Michelena HI, et al. Pathophysiology of tricuspid regurgitation: quantitative Doppler echocardiographic assessment of respiratory dependence. *Circulation*. 2010;122:1505–1513.
13. Topilsky Y, Michelena HI, Messika-Zeitoun D, Enriquez Sarano M. Doppler-echocardiographic assessment of tricuspid regurgitation. *Prog Cardiovasc Dis*. 2018;61:397–403.
14. Badano LP, Hahn R, Rodriguez-Zanella H, et al. Morphological assessment of the tricuspid apparatus and grading regurgitation severity in patients with functional tricuspid regurgitation: thinking outside the box. *JACC Cardiovasc Imaging*. 2019;12:652–664.
15. Hahn RT, Thomas JD, Khalique OK, et al. Imaging assessment of tricuspid regurgitation severity. *JACC Cardiovasc Imaging*. 2019;12:469–490.
16. Naoum C, Blanke P, Cavalcante JL, Leipsic J. Cardiac computed tomography and magnetic resonance imaging in the evaluation of mitral and tricuspid valve disease: implications for transcatheter interventions. *Circ Cardiovasc Imaging*. 2017;10. https://doi.org/10.1161/CIRCIMAGING.116.005331.
17. Syed FF, Schaff HV, Oh JK. Constrictive pericarditis–a curable diastolic heart failure. *Nat Rev Cardiol*. 2014;11:530–544.

Tricuspid Regurgitation—Management

18. Topilsky Y, Maltais S, Medina Inojosa J, et al. Burden of tricuspid regurgitation in patients diagnosed in the community setting. *JACC Cardiovasc Imaging*. 2019;12:433–442.
19. Fender EA, Petrescu I, Ionescu F, et al. Prognostic importance and predictors of survival in isolated tricuspid regurgitation: a growing problem. *Mayo Clin Proc*. 2019;94:2032–2039.
20. Chen L, Larsen CM, Le RJ, et al. The prognostic significance of tricuspid valve regurgitation in pulmonary arterial hypertension. *Clin Respir J*. 2018;12:1572–1580.
21. Hamandi M, Smith RL, Ryan WH, et al. Outcomes of isolated tricuspid valve surgery have improved in the modern era. *Ann Thorac Surg*. 2019;108:11–15.
22. Antunes MJ, Rodriguez-Palomares J, Prendergast B, et al. Management of tricuspid valve regurgitation: position statement of the European Society of Cardiology working groups of cardiovascular surgery and valvular heart disease. *Eur J Cardio Thorac Surg*. 2017;52:1022–1030.
23. Alqahtani F, Berzingi CO, Aljohani S, et al. Contemporary trends in the use and outcomes of surgical treatment of tricuspid regurgitation. *J Am Heart Assoc*. 2017;6. https://doi.org/10.1161/JAHA.117.007597.
24. Pagnesi M, Montalto C, Mangieri A, et al. Tricuspid annuloplasty versus a conservative approach in patients with functional tricuspid regurgitation undergoing left-sided heart valve surgery: a study-level meta-analysis. *Int J Cardiol*. 2017;240:138–144.
25. Parolari A, Barili F, Pilozzi A, Pacini D. Ring or suture annuloplasty for tricuspid regurgitation? A meta-analysis review. *Ann Thorac Surg*. 2014;98:2255–2263.
26. Badhwar V, Rankin JS, He M, et al. Performing concomitant tricuspid valve repair at the time of mitral valve operations is not associated with increased operative mortality. *Ann Thorac Surg*. 2017;103:587–593.
27. Yiu KH, Wong A, Pu L, et al. Prognostic value of preoperative right ventricular geometry and tricuspid valve tethering area in patients undergoing tricuspid annuloplasty. *Circulation*. 2014;129:87–92.
28. Taramasso M, Pozzoli A, Guidotti A, et al. Percutaneous tricuspid valve therapies: the new frontier. *Eur Heart J*. 2017;38:639–647.
29. Nickenig G, Weber M, Lurz P, et al. Transcatheter edge-to-edge repair for reduction of tricuspid regurgitation: 6-month outcomes of the TRILUMINATE single-arm study. *Lancet*. 2019;394:2002–2011.
30. Nickenig G, Weber M, Schueler R, et al. 6-Month outcomes of tricuspid valve reconstruction for patients with severe tricuspid regurgitation. *J Am Coll Cardiol*. 2019;73:1905–1915.
31. Connolly HM, Schaff HV, Abel MD, et al. Early and late outcomes of surgical treatment in carcinoid heart disease. *J Am Coll Cardiol*. 2015;66:2189–2196.

Pulmonic Stenosis and Pulmonic Regurgitation

32. van der Linde D, Konings EE, Slager MA, et al. Birth prevalence of congenital heart disease worldwide: a systematic review and meta-analysis. *J Am Coll Cardiol*. 2011;58:2241–2247.
33. Alkashkari W, Alsubei A, Hijazi ZM. Transcatheter pulmonary valve replacement: current state of art. *Curr Cardiol Rep*. 2018;20:27.
34. Cuypers JA, Menting ME, Opic P, et al. The unnatural history of pulmonary stenosis up to 40 years after surgical repair. *Heart*. 2017;103:273–279.
35. Chambers JB, Myerson SG, Rajani R, et al. Multimodality imaging in heart valve disease. *Open Heart*. 2016;3:e000330.
36. Cramer JW, Ginde S, Hill GD, et al. Tricuspid repair at pulmonary valve replacement does not alter outcomes in tetralogy of Fallot. *Ann Thorac Surg*. 2015;99:899–904.

Multivalvular Disease

37. Baumgartner H, Falk V, Bax JJ, et al. 2017 ESC/EACTS Guidelines for the management of valvular heart disease. *Eur Heart J*. 2017;38:2739–2791.
38. Lancellotti P, Pellikka PA, Budts W, et al. The clinical use of stress echocardiography in non-ischaemic heart disease: recommendations from the European Association of Cardiovascular Imaging and the American Society of Echocardiography. *Eur Heart J Cardiovasc Imaging*. 2016;17:1191–1229.
39. Kato N, Padang R, Pislaru C, et al. Hemodynamics and prognostic impact of concomitant mitral stenosis in patients undergoing surgical or transcatheter aortic valve replacement for aortic stenosis. *Circulation*. 2019;140:1251–1260.
40. Pislaru SV, Pellikka PA. The spectrum of low-output low-gradient aortic stenosis with normal ejection fraction. *Heart*. 2016;102:665–671.
41. Unger P, Pibarot P, Tribouilloy C, et al. Multiple and mixed valvular heart diseases. *Circ Cardiovasc Imaging*. 2018;11:e007862.
42. Pagni S, Ganzel BL, Singh R, et al. Clinical outcome after triple-valve operations in the modern era: are elderly patients at increased surgical risk? *Ann Thorac Surg*. 2014;97:569–576.
43. Suri RM, Thourani VH, Englum BR, et al. The expanding role of mitral valve repair in triple valve operations: contemporary North American outcomes in 8,021 patients. *Ann Thorac Surg*. 2014;97:1513–1519; discussion 1519.

78 Transcatheter Therapies for Mitral and Tricuspid Valvular Heart Disease

HOWARD C. HERRMANN AND MICHAEL J. REARDON

MITRAL STENOSIS, 1484
Mitral Balloon Valvuloplasty, 1484

MITRAL REGURGITATION, 1485
Rationale for Transcatheter Therapy, 1485
Leaflet Repair with MitraClip Device, 1485

Transcatheter Mitral Valve Replacement, 1488

TRICUSPID REGURGITATION, 1489
Pathophysiology, 1490
Treatment, 1490

SUMMARY, 1492
CONCLUSION, 1493
CLASSIC REFERENCES, 1493
REFERENCES, 1493

The impetus for the development of transcatheter therapies for valvular heart disease (VHD) arises from two major factors. First, a transcatheter therapy can avoid the risks associated with more invasive surgical approaches, particularly those associated with cardiopulmonary bypass and median sternotomy, while preserving or enhancing outcomes. Second, the patient wants to avoid the invasiveness and prolonged recovery associated with major surgery. However, these factors must always be balanced with the efficacy of the transcatheter approach. In this regard, the patient will always prefer a transcatheter approach that is less invasive, provides a faster patient recovery, and has similar efficacy to a more invasive surgical approach. However, a less efficacious approach, even if safer and associated with faster recovery, will require more complex decision making that takes into account the patient's age, comorbidities, and goals of care.

Historically, the first and quite successful transcatheter therapy for VHD was balloon valvuloplasty for congenital pulmonic stenosis, developed by Dr. Jean Kan in 1982. That led to a decade of extension of balloon therapies to the treatment of mitral stenosis (MS) and aortic stenosis (AS), transcatheter aortic valve replacement (TAVR) for severe aortic stenosis, and opened the door to other transcatheter therapies for regurgitation lesions, such as MitraClip (Abbott Vascular, Santa Clara, California) repair for mitral regurgitation (MR) and new innovative approaches under development for tricuspid regurgitation (TR). The success of TAVR with both balloon-expandable and self-expanding prostheses for severe, symptomatic AS and MitraClip for MR has ushered in an entire medical specialty focused on transcatheter therapy of VHD. This chapter addresses the indications, techniques, and clinical and investigational therapies available for MS, MR, and TR.

MITRAL STENOSIS (SEE CHAPTER 75)

In the patient with severe and symptomatic MS, transthoracic echocardiography (TTE) is key to diagnose and confirm the functional severity of the stenosis (see Chapter 14).

Mitral Balloon Valvuloplasty

Determining the morphology of the mitral valve and subvalvular apparatus is important in preprocedural planning for mitral balloon valvuloplasty (MBV). The suitability of a valve for MBV can be determined using a morphologic score; the most widely used is the system of Wilkins (see Classic References), which assigns a score of 1 to 4 for leaflet mobility, valve thickening, calcification, and subvalvular thickening (see Table 14.9). Recently, the incorporation of additional echocardiographic measures including commissural calcification and asymmetry and leaflet displacement have allowed refinement and improved accuracy for predicting outcome.[1] The severity of concomitant MR is also a key determining factor for MBV, both as it relates to the final result, which may increase up to one grade, and to confirm that the patient's symptoms are indeed caused by valvular obstruction and not concomitant regurgitation. In the latter case, surgical mitral valve replacement may be a better option for symptomatic relief. Transesophageal echocardiography (TEE) is a final step to assess further the severity of MR and valve morphology and to ensure the absence of left atrial (LA) thrombus before MBV. Some patients with severe calcification of the mitral annulus and leaflets, who are not candidates for balloon valvuloplasty, may be candidates for placement of a balloon-expandable transcatheter mitral valve replacement with a device initially approved for TAVR for AS. However, in a report of more than 100 such patients, the 30-day and 1-year mortality was high at 25% and 54%, respectively.[2] For other patients with less calcification and a suboptimal balloon morphology or mixed stenosis and regurgitation, a dedicated transcatheter mitral valve replacement may be another alternative.[3]

Indications

MBV is indicated in symptomatic MS patients who have at least moderate to severe MS, favorable valve morphology, absence of LA thrombus, and less than moderate to severe MR. In patients with rheumatic MS and calcified nonpliable valves who are at high risk or unsuitable for open surgery, MBV may be a reasonable alternative to provide palliative symptomatic relief. MBV may also be considered in asymptomatic patients with moderate to severe MS and new-onset atrial fibrillation after excluding LA thrombus (class IIb). In patients with symptoms and mild MS (mitral valve area [MVA] >1.5 cm^2), MBV can be considered if there is evidence of significant MS with exercise testing (class IIb).[4] The mechanism of benefit is separation of the fused commissures, which relieves the physical obstruction, thereby reducing the gradient and increasing MVA.

Procedure. The transvenous antegrade transseptal route is typically used to gain access to the left atrium to perform MBV. Inoue first used a self-positioning latex balloon wrapped with a nylon mesh to allow phased balloon expansion in 1982 and described the technique in 1984 (see Classic References). The double-balloon technique involves two peripheral arterial balloons tracked over separate guidewires placed in the left ventricle and simultaneously inflated.

The double-balloon technique was the first one used in the United States. Following transseptal catheterization and therapeutic anticoagulation, a balloon-tipped end-hole catheter is used to traverse the mitral valve via the transseptal puncture site. This catheter is navigated to the apex of the left ventricle, and once positioned, a 260-cm guidewire is

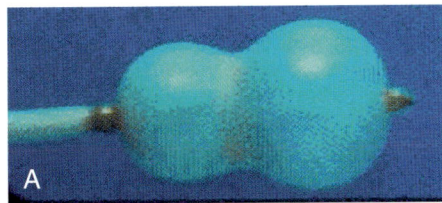
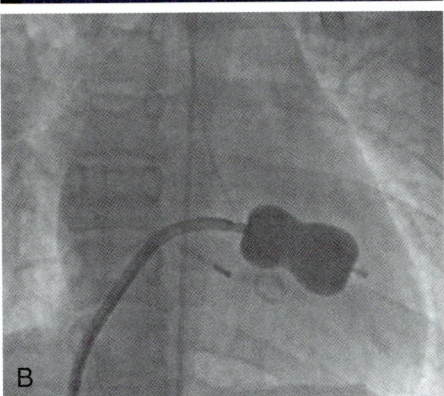

FIGURE 78.1 **A,** Inoue mitral balloon valvuloplasty catheter and three-stage balloon. **B,** Partially inflated Inoue balloon positioned across the mitral valve. Note an intracardiac echocardiographic catheter in the right ventricle and a pigtail catheter in the left ventricle.

then placed in the LV apex or looped across the aortic valve into the descending aorta. A second guidewire is placed using a similar technique or by using a dual-lumen catheter. Two 18- or 20-mm dilation balloons are tracked and positioned on the wires and inflated simultaneously to dilate the valve.

The Inoue technique has mostly replaced the double-balloon technique, in part because there is no risk of left ventricular (LV) perforation with the Inoue balloon (Fig. 78.1). The initial size of the Inoue balloon is based on patient's height. Once inserted over a guidewire into the left atrium, it can be steered across the mitral valve orifice with an internal stylet and then sequentially inflated multiple times over a 4-mm diameter range, with both hemodynamic and echocardiographic results assessed, to achieve the maximal dilation with the least increase in grade of MR. As such, it is important to evaluate carefully for severe commissural calcium preprocedurally. Calcium does not split with balloon inflation but does increase the potential for tearing the leaflets creating MR.

A reduction in mean mitral valve gradient by 50% or an increase in MVA greater than 1.5 cm^2 is considered a successful result and can be achieved in more than 80% of appropriately selected patients. An increase in MR by more than one grade after balloon inflation should signal an end to the procedure despite a residual gradient. Event-free survival after MBV is influenced by valve morphology. In a large study of 879 North American patients with a mean follow-up of 4.2 ± 3.7 years, there was a greater immediate increase in MVA after MBV and improved long-term survival (82% versus 57%; P < 0.0001) in patients with a Wilkins score of 8 or less (Fig. 78.2). Patients with higher echocardiographic scores have more events in the long term, including need for repeat MBV, need for mitral valve surgery, and death (Fig. 78.2B). In multivariate analysis, age, post-MBV MR grade of 3+ or higher, prior surgical commissurotomy, New York Heart Association (NYHA) Class IV symptoms, and elevated post-MBV pulmonary artery systolic pressure were all independently associated with worse outcome at follow-up.

The most common complication from MBV, severe MR, occurs in 2% to 10% of patients, with no significant difference between the Inoue and double-balloon techniques. Overall procedural mortality is approximately 1%. Other, less common procedural complications include pericardial tamponade, embolic events, vascular complications, arrhythmias, bleeding, stroke, myocardial infarction, residual atrial septal defect, and LV perforation.

Echocardiography is essential for many aspects of MBV, including the transseptal puncture and assessment of postprocedural results and complications (see Chapter 14). TEE is considered the gold standard, and 3D TEE has been shown to be superior to TTE in reducing fluoroscopy time and the interval from first transseptal puncture to first balloon inflation.[5] Intracardiac echocardiography can also be used, with the advantage of avoiding the endotracheal intubation and general anesthesia usually required for TEE.

MITRAL REGURGITATION

Unlike MS, which is caused primarily by rheumatic fever, MR is a more diverse disease that results from dysfunction of any of the portions of the complex mitral valve apparatus, including the leaflets, chords, annulus, and left ventricle. As discussed in Chapter 76, MR is often further classified into *primary* (organic or degenerative) disease, which affects the leaflets (e.g., fibromuscular dysplasia, mitral valve prolapse, and rheumatic disease), and *secondary* (ischemic or functional) disease, which spares the leaflets (e.g., diseases of atrium and ventricle, including ischemic dysfunction and dilated cardiomyopathy). Patients with severe MR have decreased survival, whether symptomatic or not, and surgery is often recommended.[6] In asymptomatic patients with primary MR and preserved LV function, a "watchful waiting" or "active surveillance" approach can be considered until the development of symptoms, LV dysfunction, pulmonary hypertension, or atrial fibrillation,[7] and current guidelines recommend surgery in patients who have reached these endpoints.[4] Surgery may also be considered for asymptomatic patients with normal LV function in whom there is a high likelihood of successful mitral valve repair.[4]

Rationale for Transcatheter Therapy

Surgery improves survival in observational studies but is associated with mortality rates of 1% to 5% and additional morbidity rates of 10% to 20%, including stroke, reoperation, renal failure, and prolonged ventilation.[8] The risks of surgery are particularly high in patients who are elderly or have LV dysfunction and secondary MR. In one study of more than 30,000 patients undergoing mitral valve replacement, mortality increased from 4.1% in those younger than 50 years to 17.0% in octogenarians,[9] although these outcomes improved in a more recent report.[10] The risks and morbidity of surgery coupled with patient preference have stimulated attempts to develop less invasive solutions.

When considering percutaneous or transcatheter approaches for mitral repair, it is useful to classify them according to the major structural abnormality that they address.[11] Unlike the extensive toolbox available to the mitral surgeon, transcatheter approaches are much more limited and often able to address only a single major element of the dysfunctional valve that contributes to MR.[12]

Table 78.1 lists some of the devices, their manufacturers, and current state of development.

Leaflet Repair with MitraClip Device

MitraClip (Abbott Vascular) was the first transcatheter mitral valve repair technology to receive CE (Conformité Européenne) Mark approval (European Union) and has now also received FDA approval for patients with primary (degenerative) MR and prohibitive surgical risk as well as for heart failure patients with left ventricular dysfunction (secondary MR) despite optimal medical therapy (Fig. 78.3). This system replicates the Alfieri stitch operation, in which the middle scallops of the posterior and anterior leaflets (P2 and A2, respectively) are sutured together to create a double-orifice mitral valve. The operation, although usually performed with adjunctive ring annuloplasty, has proved effective and durable in a wide variety of pathologies as well as in select patients without annuloplasty.[13]

Trials with MitraClip have confirmed its feasibility (e.g., Endovascular Valve Edge-to-Edge Repair Study [EVEREST] I), and its safety and efficacy were compared with those of surgical repair in a randomized trial (EVEREST II).[14] The procedure is performed with standard catheterization techniques using a transseptal approach from the right femoral vein.[15] The clip delivery system is introduced through a 24F sheath into the left atrium, where it can be guided by TEE using a series of turning knobs through the mitral valve into the left ventricle. A properly aligned and oriented clip can grasp the P2 and A2 segments of the leaflets from

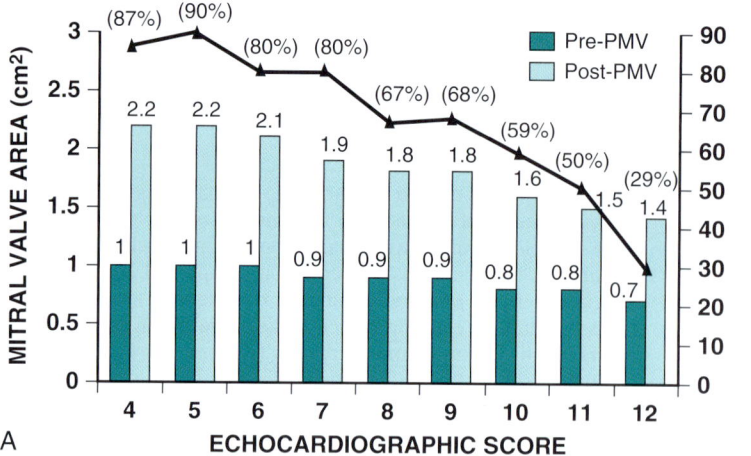

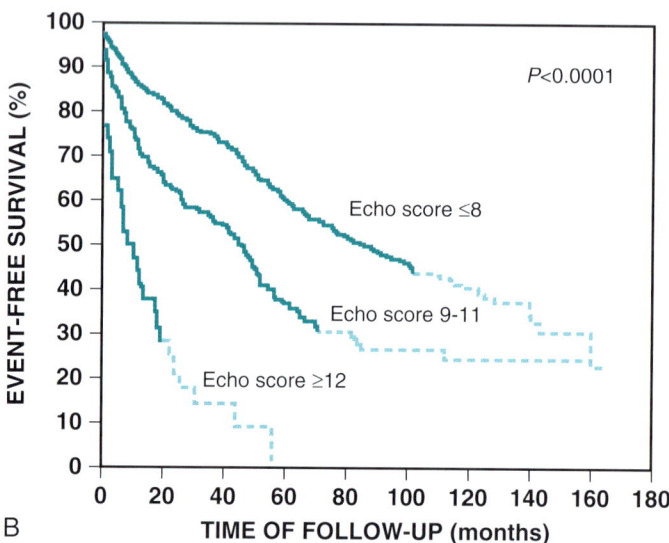

FIGURE 78.2 Results of mitral balloon valvuloplasty relative to preprocedural Wilkins score derived from echocardiography. **A,** Bars indicate mitral valve area before and after percutaneous mitral valvuloplasty (PMV) as a function of the echocardiographic score, and the connected *triangles* indicate procedural success rate. **B,** Association between echocardiographic score and postprocedural event-free survival. (From Palacios IF, et al. Which patients benefit from percutaneous mitral valvuloplasty? Prevalvuloplasty and postvalvuloplasty variables that predict long-term outcome. Circulation 2002;105:1465-1471. Copyright 2002 American Heart Association Inc.)

the ventricular side to create leaflet apposition. Once leaflet insertion is confirmed by echocardiography, the clip can be released. If a suboptimal grasp occurs, the leaflet can be released, allowing repositioning before a second grasp attempt. Additionally, a second or more clips can be placed as needed for optimal MR reduction.

In the randomized EVEREST II trial, 184 patients received MitraClip therapy and 95 underwent surgical repair or replacement.[16] These patients were almost a decade older (mean age, 67 years) than in usual surgical series and had more comorbidities. Major adverse events at 30 days were significantly less frequent with MitraClip therapy (9.6% versus 57% with surgery; $P < 0.0001$), although much of the difference could be attributed to the greater need for blood transfusions with surgery. The freedom from the combined outcome of death, mitral valve surgery, and MR severity greater than 2+ at 12 months was higher with surgery (73%) than with MitraClip therapy (55%; $P = 0.0007$). In patients with acute MitraClip therapy success, the result appears durable, with a very low rate of later mitral valve surgery.[17]

Subsequent analyses of this study and additional registries have demonstrated persistent reductions in MR grade, improvement in NYHA functional class, and reduction in LV dimensions with MitraClip therapy.[17] Other studies have shown a lack of MS, no effect of initial rhythm on results, and importantly, greater benefit than with surgery for higher-risk patients (Fig. 78.4). Although the EVEREST II trial failed to demonstrate efficacy equivalent to that of surgery for a diverse group of patients with varied risk and etiology, the EVEREST High-Risk Registry and prohibitive-risk patient subset, combined with the experience outside the United States, indicate a more appropriate role in high-risk patients.

A new indication has recently emerged for MitraClip therapy in heart failure patients with secondary MR based on the results of the COAPT (Clinical Outcomes Assessment of the MitraClip Percutaneous Therapy for High Surgical Risk Patients) trial. This landmark trial compared the MitraClip device with medical therapy in patients with secondary MR in 614 patients after initial optimal medical therapy.[18] After 24 months of follow-up, there was a close to 50% reduction in the annualized rate of all hospitalizations for heart failure and an approximately 40% reduction in all-cause mortality with a very low rate of device-related complications (4%) (Fig. 78.5). In contrast, a similar French study failed to demonstrate a difference between heart failure patients treated with MitraClip and optimal medical management at 12 months of follow-up.[19] There are a number of reasons why these two similar trials had conflicting results, including different inclusion and exclusions, primary endpoints, operator experience, and procedural results.[20] An additional trial in this space (RESHAPE HF2) has not yet been reported and may add further clarity to who are the best candidates for MitraClip repair. Several other devices, designed to provide leaflet repair, including NeoChord, Mitra-Spacer, and MitraFlex, are in preclinical or phase I evaluation (see Table 78.1). The PASCAL edge-to-edge repair device has some similarities to MitraClip in that it is used to create a double orifice mitral valve, but has wider grasping elements and a central spacer.[21] In an initial report of 62 patients treated with this device, 98% and 86% had MR grade ≤2+ and ≤1+, respectively at 30 days.[21] A comparison of this device and MitraClip (The CLASP Study of Edwards PASCAL Transcatheter Mitral Valve Repair System Study; NCT03170349) is underway.

Indirect Annuloplasty

The venous anatomy of the heart is of particular interest for treating MR because of the ease of access (from the right internal jugular vein) and the location of the great cardiac vein in proximity to the posterior mitral annulus. Some of the first attempts to treat MR without surgery consisted of mimicking surgical ring annuloplasty through placement of devices in the coronary sinus, so-called indirect or percutaneous coronary sinus annuloplasty. The goal of this approach is to remodel the posterior annulus, cinching the great cardiac vein or pushing on the posterior annulus from the vein to improve leaflet coaptation.

The CARILLON XE2 Mitral Contour System (Cardiac Dimensions) has CE Mark and uses anchors placed in the coronary sinus that are pulled toward each other with a cinching device to reduce the mitral annular dimension by traction (Fig. 78.6). Early evaluation in the Amadeus study demonstrated feasibility, with implantation in 30 of 48 patients and modest improvement in quantitative measures of MR with a small risk of coronary compromise (15%) and death (one patient). More recently, a redesigned device was tested in the TITAN (Transcatheter Implantation of Carillon Mitral Annuloplasty Device) trial.[22] Among 65 patients with secondary MR (62% ischemic), the device was implanted successfully in 36 patients, with a mean age of 62 years, mean ejection fraction (EF) of 29%, predominantly NYHA Functional Class III symptoms, and 2+ (30%), 3+ (55%), or 4+ (15%) grade MR. Quantitative measures of MR were better at 6 and 12 months than in 17 patients who did not receive implants. In the most recent randomized, blinded, and sham-controlled evaluation of this device (REDUCE FMR, NCT02325830), a statistically significant modest difference in MR volume was observed at 1 year despite many missing echocardiograms.[23]

In general, indirect annuloplasty devices may be able to provide modest MR reduction in select patients, but likely less than that achievable surgically with a complete ring placed directly on the annulus. The limited efficacy is related to the location of the coronary sinus relative to the annulus (up to

TABLE 78.1 Devices for Transcatheter Mitral Valve Repair and Replacement

TYPE/INDICATION	BRAND NAME	MANUFACTURER	STATUS
Leaflet/chordal	MitraClip	Abbott Vascular, Abbott Park, Ill	CE Mark
			FDA approved
	NeoChord DS1000 System	NeoChord, Eden Prairie, Minn	CE Mark
			U.S. IDE trial
	Harpoon NeoChord	Edwards Lifesciences, Irvine, Calif	Phase 1 (OUS)
	Mitra-Spacer	Cardiosolutions, West Bridgewater, Mass	Phase 1 (OUS)
	MitraFlex	TransCardiac Therapeutics, Atlanta, Ga	Preclinical
	Middle Peak Medical	Middle Peak Medical, Palo Alto, Calif	Phase 1 (OUS)
Indirect annuloplasty	CARILLON XE2 Mitral Contour System	Cardiac Dimensions, Kirkland, Wis	CE Mark
	Kardium MR	Kardium, Richmond, British Columbia, Canada	Preclinical
	Cerclage annuloplasty	National Heart, Lung and Blood Institute, Bethesda, Md	Phase 1 (OUS)
Direct or left ventricular annuloplasty	Mitralign Percutaneous Annuloplasty System	Mitralign, Tewksbury, Mass	CE Mark
	GDS Accucinch System	Guided Delivery Systems, Santa Clara, Calif	Phase 1 (OUS)
	Boa RF Catheter	QuantumCor, Laguna Niguel, Calif	Preclinical
	Cardioband	Valtech Cardio, Or Yehuda, Israel	CE Mark
	Millipede System	Millipede, Santa Rosa, Calif	Phase 1 (OUS)
	Arto System	MVRx, Belmont, Calif	Phase 1 (OUS)
Hybrid surgical	Adjustable Annuloplasty Ring	Mitral Solutions, Fort Lauderdale, Fla	Phase 1 (OUS)
	enCor ring	MiCardia Corporation, Irvine, Calif	CE Mark
			Phase 1
Left ventricular remodeling	The Basal Annuloplasty of the Cardia Externally (BACE)	Mardil Medical, Minneapolis, Minnesota	Phase 1 (OUS)
	Tendyne Repair	Tendyne Holdings, Baltimore, Md	Preclinical
	MitraSpacer	Cardiosolutions, Stoughton, Mass	Phase 1 (OUS)
Replacement	CardiAQ-Edwards	Edwards Lifesciences, Irvine, Calif	Phase 1 (OUS)
			U.S. EFS
	Tendyne	Abbott Vascular, Chicago	Phase 1 (OUS)
			U.S. EFS
	Tiara	Neovasc, Richmond, British Columbia, Canada	Phase 1 (OUS)
			U.S. EFS
	Intrepid (Twelve)	Medtronic, Minneapolis, Minn	Phase 1 (OUS)
			U.S. EFS
	Caisson	Caisson Interventional, Maple Grove, Minn	U.S. EFS

CE, Conformité Européenne (European Union); *EFS*, early feasibility study; *FDA*, U.S. Food and Drug Administration; *IDE*, investigational device exemption; *OUS*, outside United States.

10 mm more cranial), great individual anatomic variability, and limited benefit of partial annular remodeling. Whether this level of efficacy will result in sufficient symptomatic improvement and LV remodeling to justify the procedure requires further study. Some "super-responders" may be identified on the basis of anatomic considerations before the procedure. The risks of this approach must also be considered. In addition to the risk for damage to the cardiac venous system, devices in this location can compress the left circumflex or diagonal coronary arteries, which traverse between the coronary sinus and the mitral annulus in most patients.[22,23]

In this regard, one novel indirect approach to reduce the septal-lateral dimension that deserves further consideration is the *cerclage annuloplasty* technique, which recently entered clinical evaluation. This approach attempts to create a more complete circumferential annuloplasty by placing a suture from the coronary sinus through a septal perforator vein into the right atrium or ventricle, where it is snared and tensioned with the proximal end from the right atrium to create a closed pursestring suture.[24] The procedure is guided by cardiac MRI and also uses a novel rigid protection device to avoid coronary compression.

Direct Annuloplasty and Left Ventricular Remodeling Techniques

Several devices have been developed to remodel more directly the mitral annulus, in part because of the limitations of indirect coronary sinus annuloplasty described earlier (see Table 78.1). The Mitralign Percutaneous Annuloplasty System (Mitralign) was originally based on the surgical techniques of Paneth's posterior suture plication. In this procedure a transaortic catheter is advanced to the left ventricle and used to deliver pledgeted anchors through the posterior annulus that can be pulled together to shorten (plicate) the annulus up to 17 mm (with two implants) (Fig. 78.6B). In 50 of 71 patients successfully treated in a phase I trial, septal-lateral dimension was reduced about 2 mm, MR grade at 6 months was reduced by a mean of 1.3 grades in 50% of patients, and modest symptomatic improvement was observed.[25] The Accucinch (Guided Delivery Systems) device utilizes a catheter approach to place up to 12 anchors along the ventricular myocardium just below the valve plane (percutaneous ventriculoplasty). This approach may be able to reduce MR as well as improve LV function in patients with heart failure. In a preliminary report of 21 patients, reductions in LV end-systolic volume (28%), effective regurgitant orifice area (37%), and an increase in LV ejection fraction (33%) were observed at 6 months.[26]

More recently, the Cardioband annuloplasty system (Valtech Cardio, Or Yehuda, Israel) received CE Mark. This is an adjustable, catheter-delivered, sutureless device that is inserted transseptally and directly anchored on the atrial side of the annulus with subsequent adjustment (Fig. 78.6C). In a phase I European study, 31 high-risk patients with severe secondary MR received treatment.[27] Mean septal-lateral

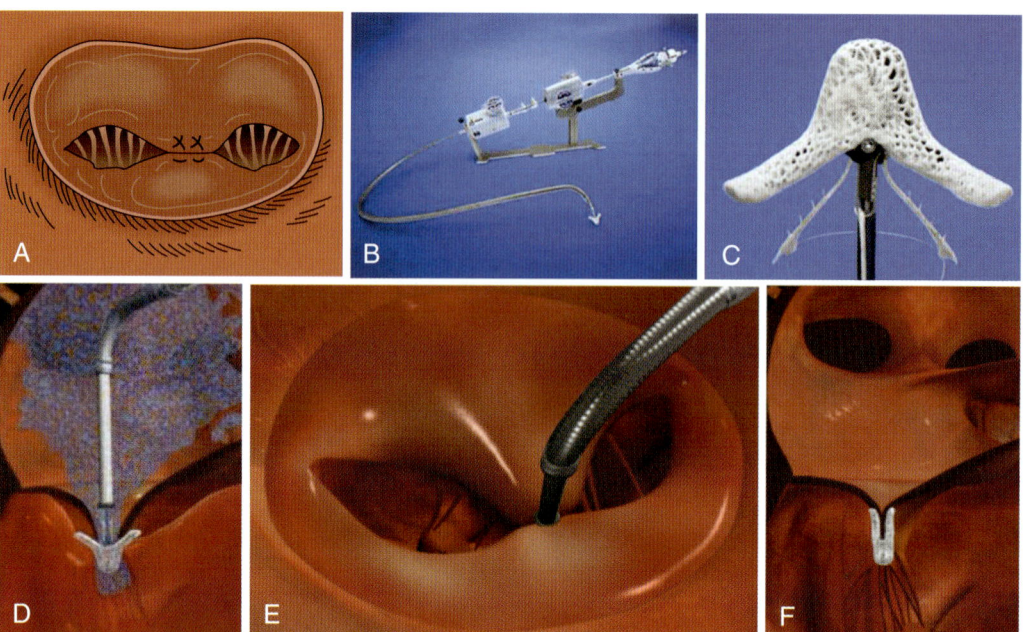

FIGURE 78.3 MitraClip leaflet coaptation system (Abbott Vascular) creates a bridge between the P2 and A2 segments of the mitral valve similar to the Alfieri stitch operation (**A**) utilizing a clip delivery system (**B**) and the MitraClip NT (**C**). Drawings of side (**D**) and left atrial (**E**) views of the clip delivery system as it is advanced through the mitral valve in the open position prior to grasping of the leaflets. **F**, The final result is illustrated after the clip has been released and the delivery system removed. (Courtesy Abbott Vascular, Inc.)

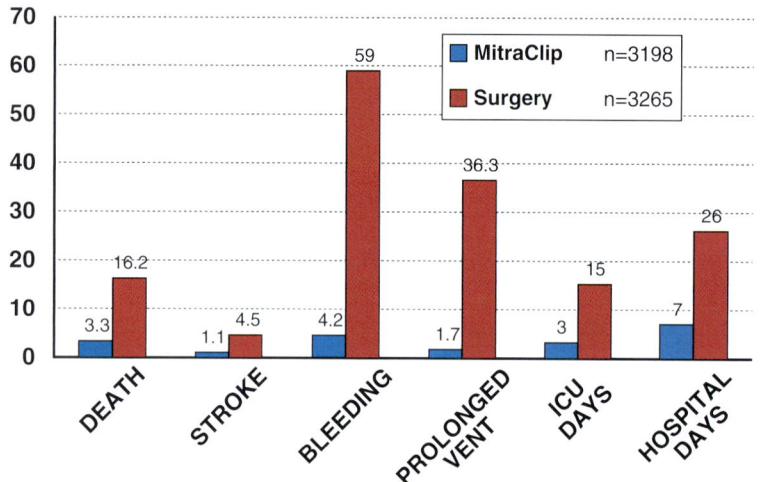

FIGURE 78.4 Meta-analysis of outcomes of the MitraClip compared with mitral valve surgery in high-risk patients. *ICU*, Intensive care unit; *Vent*, ventilation. (From Philip F, et al. MitraClip for severe symptomatic mitral regurgitation in patients at high surgical risk. Catheter Cardiovasc Interv 2014;84:581-590.)

dimension was reduced from 37 to 29 mm, with initial reduction in MR grade to "trace" or "mild" in 93% of patients and to moderate MR or less at 30 days in 88%.[27] In a subsequent report of 60 patients with a procedural success rate of 68%, moderate or less MR at 1 year was observed in 61% of patients and was associated with improvements in functional status and quality of life.[28] The basis for devices to treat MR by affecting the shape of the left ventricle arises from the pathophysiology of secondary ischemic or functional MR (see Chapter 76). Changes in the inferior and lateral left ventricle from infarction can lead to tethering or tenting of the posterior leaflet, allowing anterior leaflet override as the mechanism of MR. Similarly, failure of leaflet coaptation from global LV enlargement causing annular distention is the major mechanism for MR in dilated cardiomyopathy.[18] Although ring annuloplasty can often ameliorate MR caused by LV distortion, procedures that also address the underlying LV pathology may be more beneficial. The Basal Annuloplasty of the Cardia Externally (BACE) device (Mardil) is a surgically implanted external tension band placed around the heart externally to treat ischemic MR at the time of coronary artery bypass graft (CABG) surgery. In a preliminary report of 11 patients treated in India, MR grade was reduced acutely from grade 3.3 to 0.6. Preclinical work with a transcatheter approach to approximate the papillary muscles is also in development (Tendyne Repair).

Transcatheter Mitral Valve Replacement

The rationale for transcatheter mitral valve replacement (TMVR) is based on several lessons learned from surgical valve replacement[29,30] and results thus far with transcatheter mitral valve repair. With the current state of technologic development and clinical experience, transcatheter repairs do not appear to reduce MR to the same extent as surgical repairs. Moreover, in patients with secondary ischemic MR, mitral valve replacement (MVR) appears to provide more complete and durable elimination of MR than valve repair. In a surgical trial of 251 patients with severe ischemic MR randomized to mitral repair versus chordal-sparing MVR,[31] recurrent moderate or severe MR was higher at 12 months in the repair group (32.6%) than the replacement group (2.3%).

Early experience with valve-in-valve treatment using TAVR devices in previously implanted degenerating surgical mitral bioprostheses and annuloplasty rings has confirmed the feasibility of this approach. Balloon-expandable TAVR prostheses were initially implanted in degenerating bioprostheses and surgical annuloplasty rings via a transapical approach.[32] Subsequently, the feasibility of transseptal delivery and transatrial delivery has been demonstrated. Complications, including valve embolization, bleeding, and death, have been reported, but the early results have generally been favorable, with excellent reduction in MR grade and low residual transmitral gradients, resulting in the Sapien 3 device receiving FDA approval for this indication.[33]

Despite these initial demonstrations of the feasibility of transcatheter mitral valve-in-valve implantation, de novo placement of such devices in native valves, even those with mitral annular calcification, has proved more challenging.[34] Compared with TAVR, mitral devices need to be larger, and fixation to the diseased mitral apparatus is hampered by the greater valve complexity, lack of calcium, potential need for orientation, and noncircular annular shape.

Most current designs use a stent-based bioprosthesis that is self-expanding, anchors to attach to the annulus and/or leaflets, and a sealing skirt. Because the size of the mitral annulus requires a large prosthesis, initial experience has been with transapical delivery systems, although early experience with several transseptal and transatrial delivery approaches is underway. Novel devices that use a two-stage deployment with separate anchoring and valve portions are also being tested.[30]

At least five TMVR devices have entered early feasibility investigation clinically in the United States (Fig. 78.7; see also Table 78.1), and more than 30 are in early development. The initial experience with TMVR has been challenging, in part from inclusion of compassionately treated patients with multiple comorbidities and predominantly

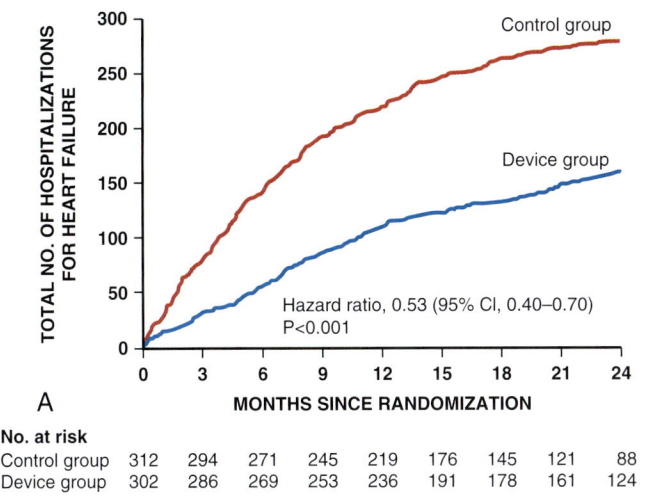
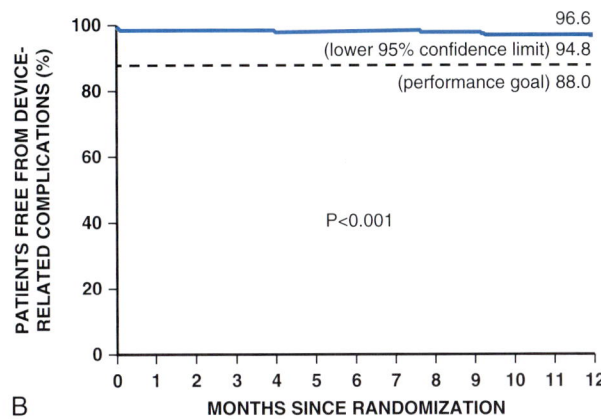
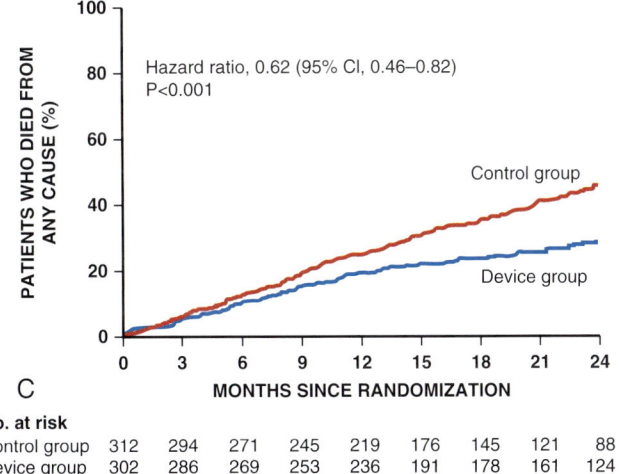

FIGURE 78.5 Primary effectiveness and safety end points and death in patients with secondary mitral regurgitation and heart failure from the COAPT trial. **A,** The cumulative incidence of the primary effectiveness end point of all hospitalizations for heart failure within 24 months of follow-up among patients who underwent transcatheter mitral-valve repair and received guideline-directed medical therapy (device group) and among those who received guideline-directed medical therapy alone (control group). The data shown here do not account for the competing risk of death, which was considered in the joint frailty model. A total of 160 hospitalizations for heart failure occurred in 92 patients in the device group, and a total of 283 hospitalizations for heart failure occurred in 151 patients in the control group. **B,** The rate of the primary safety endpoint of freedom from device-related complications at 12 months among the 293 patients in whom device implantation was attempted, as compared with an objective performance goal. **C,** Time-to-event curves for all-cause mortality in the device group and the control group. (From Stone GW, et al. Transcatheter mitral-valve repair in patients with heart failure. N Engl J Med 2018;379:2307-2318.)

treated with a relatively invasive transapical approach. Current trials are therefore targeting high-risk, but not inoperable, patients with both primary and secondary MR. Phase II study investigators will address that most patients with secondary MR do not have high short-term mortality and therefore are frequently medically managed. Overcoming procedural complications of TMVR will be essential to realize the symptomatic benefits compared with medical care. Patient comorbidities, cardiac and noncardiac, could hamper and confound comparative evaluations.

In the largest study of such a device to date, Sorajja and colleagues[35] treated 30 patients at high risk for surgery with a transcatheter transapical self-expanding nitinol prosthesis supporting a trileaflet porcine pericardial valve (Tendyne Mitral Valve System, Abbott Vascular, Roseville, Minnesota). The device was successfully implanted in 97 of 100 patients (97%) with no procedural deaths. The 30-day rates of mortality and stroke were 6% and 2%, respectively. At 1 year, MR was absent in 98% of patients and associated with significant improvements in symptoms and quality of life. Based on these results, this became the first TMVR device to attain CE Mark approval, and it is currently being evaluated in a pivotal US trial comparing it to MitraClip (SUMMIT trial, NCT03433274).

It is hoped that improvements in devices, operator and procedural experience, and patient selection will lead to better outcomes. The potential advantages of this approach include the avoidance of both the surgical incision and the effects of cardiopulmonary bypass. Such devices could be fully sparing of the subvalvular apparatus and provide MR reduction that is equivalent to that achieved with surgical valve replacement. However, the early high mortality, although in very-high-risk patients receiving the device as a compassionate approach, has tempered some of the early enthusiasm for TMVR.[36]

In this regard, it is useful to emphasize that TMVR is not a "mitral TAVR."[36,37] The mitral valve is more complex than the aortic valve, and MR has a vast array of etiologies. Unlike AS, MR is not as often a disease of elderly persons, and repair (not replacement) is the preferred surgical therapy, especially for patients with primary MR. Replacement may have less favorable effects on normal vortex flow and LV remodeling than successful repair.[38] Transcatheter prostheses in the mitral position will likely have lower durability, more risks associated with paravalvular leak,[39] and a greater risk of embolization, LV outflow tract obstruction, and thrombosis. Finally, the more frequent association with TR, which may need to be addressed, and the lower short-term mortality will be impediments to the design of rigorous clinical trials.[33,36]

TRICUSPID REGURGITATION

Tricuspid regurgitation (TR) is a common valve lesion that increases with age and affects about 1.6 million people in the United States and more than 70 million worldwide.[40,41] Focused analysis of the population of Olmsted County showed a prevalence of 0.55% for moderate or greater TR,[42] which would give an estimate of 160,000 to 240,000 cases of moderate or greater TR in the United States.[43] The majority of TR cases are functional and are associated with increased mortality.[42-45] Despite this high prevalence and association with increased mortality, <10,000 surgeries a year are performed in the United States for tricuspid valve disease, and in Olmsted County, only 2.6% of the patients with moderate or greater TR had surgery during the follow-up period.[42] Much of the apparent reticence to operate on isolated TR comes from the reported mortality in the surgical literature, which has ranged from 8% to 16%,[46-49] although mortality as low as 3.3% has been reported in a contemporary surgical series.[50] This reluctance to operate on patients with TR has led to the tricuspid valve being referred to as the "forgotten valve." In addition, the poor surgical outcomes in many series have fostered late referral for treatment. Many patients, by the time they are referred for potential intervention, have developed comorbidities, including liver failure, renal failure, coagulopathy, and end-stage heart failure, further increasing the risk of any intervention. The remodeling associated with TR results in increased annular and right ventricular size further increasing leaflet restriction and TR. Tricuspid regurgitation begets worsening tricuspid regurgitation. Understanding this has

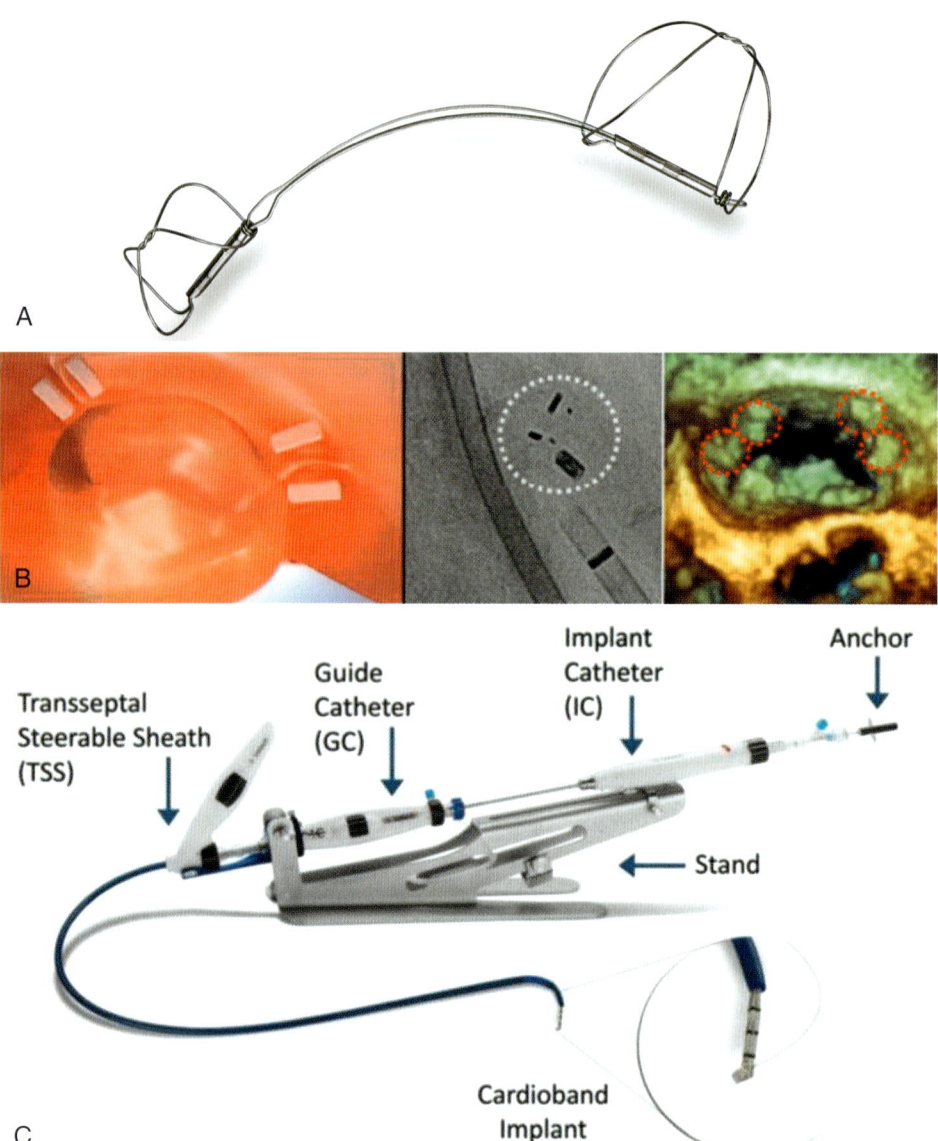

FIGURE 78.6 Evolving devices for mitral valve repair. **A,** Carillon XE2 Mitral Contour System (Cardiac Dimensions) **B,** Mitralign Percutaneous Annuloplasty System (Mitralign, Tewksbury, Mass). **C,** Cardioband annuloplasty system (Valtech Cardio, Or Yehuda, Israel). (From Nickenig G, et al. Treatment of functional mitral valve regurgitation with a percutaneous annuloplasty system. J Am Coll Cardiol 2016;67:2927-2936.)

helped reignite interest in tricuspid valve intervention for TR, particularly with a less invasive transcatheter approach.[51]

Pathophysiology

The tricuspid valve is the largest and most caudal of the cardiac valves. Tricuspid regurgitation is primary in about 10% of cases, but less common in developed countries.[52] Primary TR can occur in congenital anomalies such as Ebstein anomaly, trauma, or carcinoid syndrome. Increasing causes of primary TR in developed countries are pacemaker and defibrillator leads across the valve and endocarditis, especially IV drug–related cases. Secondary or functional TR accounts for 90% of the cases. Secondary TR is the result of a negative remodeling of the right ventricle with normal valve leaflets. This leads to increased annular size and leaflet tethering producing TR.[53] Left-sided heart disease and pulmonary hypertension are common causes of negative remodeling and TR. Chronic atrial fibrillation can cause annular enlargement rather than right ventricular remodeling as a cause of TR.[54]

Treatment

In very early experience, TR was largely managed medically with the belief that it would improve with treatment of the underlying cause.[55] Current evidence suggests that this is not correct and that TR that is moderate or greater is an independent risk for mortality (Fig. 78.8).[42,43,52,56] Even with this mortality risk, current guidelines only have a class I recommendation for TR surgery if left-sided valve surgery is being done.[57] When tricuspid valve repair is added to surgery for mitral valve repair in patients with moderate or greater TR, there is no increase in mortality but there is a significantly lower late rate of TR and better right ventricular recovery.[58] There is a clear undertreatment of significant TR, suggesting a large unmet need. Recognizing this unmet need has led clinicians to refocus on what has been often referred to as the forgotten valve. Transcatheter tricuspid valve intervention (TTVI) is emerging as a potential less invasive option to treat TR. It is hoped that this less invasive transcatheter approach, especially if it can prove safer, will lead to earlier intervention for TR to slow the progression of the associated heart failure. Most TTVI procedures mimic surgical procedures already in use. Isolated surgical tricuspid valve repair has a lower mortality than isolated surgical tricuspid valve replacement.[47,59] It is unknown if this difference will extend to transcatheter approaches as well, but this would seem likely as long as the repair is successful in decreasing the TR and durable. Transcatheter TR correction devices fall into several broad categories of annular remodeling, leaflet remodeling, spacers, and novel approaches such as caval valves or tricuspid valve replacement (Fig. 78.9). It is early in the development of TTVI procedures, and data are currently limited and the specific devices are likely to change with time, but the categories remain consistent. The tricuspid valve presents several physiologic and anatomic challenges for the interventionist. Anatomically, the tricuspid valve borders the right coronary artery and the atrioventricular node, placing both at risk for injury. Most TR is functional in nature and more related to right ventricular and TV annular enlargement than actual valve pathology. Surgical repair of functional atrioventricular valve pathology has not proven as consistent or durable as repair of primary lesions. At this time, it is also unknown if this applies to TTVI. Physiologically, TR is often associated with right heart failure and congestive liver failure and its consequences. An increased Model of End-Stage Liver Disease (MELD) score from liver congestion is associated with an increase in mortality for tricuspid valve interventions.[60] Choosing patients with right heart function that is likely to recover and allow the patient to survive and benefit from the procedure is crucial.

Annuloplasty Devices

Surgeons have used annuloplasty bands and rings for mitral valve repair in both primary and secondary mitral regurgitation. Transcatheter annuloplasty devices attempt to replicate the annular remodeling achieved by surgical devices. Although transcatheter approaches, particularly with partial annuloplasty and bicuspidization techniques, may not be as efficacious as rigid surgical rings, the freedom from at least moderate TR at long-term follow-up was still achievable in the majority of patients[61] (Fig. 78.10).

The Cardioband transcatheter annuloplasty device fixes a partial annuloplasty band to the valve annulus with anchors using a transseptal approach that can then be tightened or cinched. The results with Cardioband were presented in the TRI-REPAIR (Tricuspid Regurgitation Repair With Cardioband Transcatheter System) study (NCT02981953).[62] This was a 30-patient prospective feasibility study with a primary performance endpoint of successful access, deployment, and positioning of the device with reduction of the septolateral annular diameter. The cases were carefully selected for anatomic and physiologic suitability and patients with pacemaker leads crossing the valve were excluded. Technical success was 100% with a 6.8% mortality at 30 days and 10% at 6 months. TR improved, but at 6 months, four patients still had torrential TR. Of note, three patients had a right coronary artery injury that was corrected with angioplasty in two of these patients and one was left untreated and led to the death of the patient. Other annuloplasty devices include the IRIS annuloplasty ring is a complete rigid ring anchored on the supravalvular annulus and then can be differentially cinched down to an appropriate annulus size and shape,[63,64] and the TriCinch device, which attempts to replicate the surgical Kay procedure, eliminating the posterior TV leaflet and converting the valve into a bileaflet valve.[63,64] This is a two-component device. The first part is a stainless-steel corkscrew implant, to be placed in the anterior annulus of the TV, in proximity to the anteroposterior commissure, which is connected to a self-expanding nitinol stent that is deployed below the hepatic region of the inferior vena cava. Once the corkscrew is deployed, the nitinol stent is pulled down into the inferior vena cava until the appropriate tension on the tricuspid valve annulus reduces the posterior leaflet to approximate a Kay repair. The stent is then deployed locking the system into place. The Percutaneous 4TECH TriCinch Coil Tricuspid Valve Repair System early feasibility study is ongoing (NCT03632967). The TriAlign system also attempts to replicate the Kay repair. The device is a transjugular suture-based tricuspid valve annuloplasty system that reduces tricuspid annular diameter by plication of the posterior leaflet.[65] The early results with this device were reported in the SCOUT

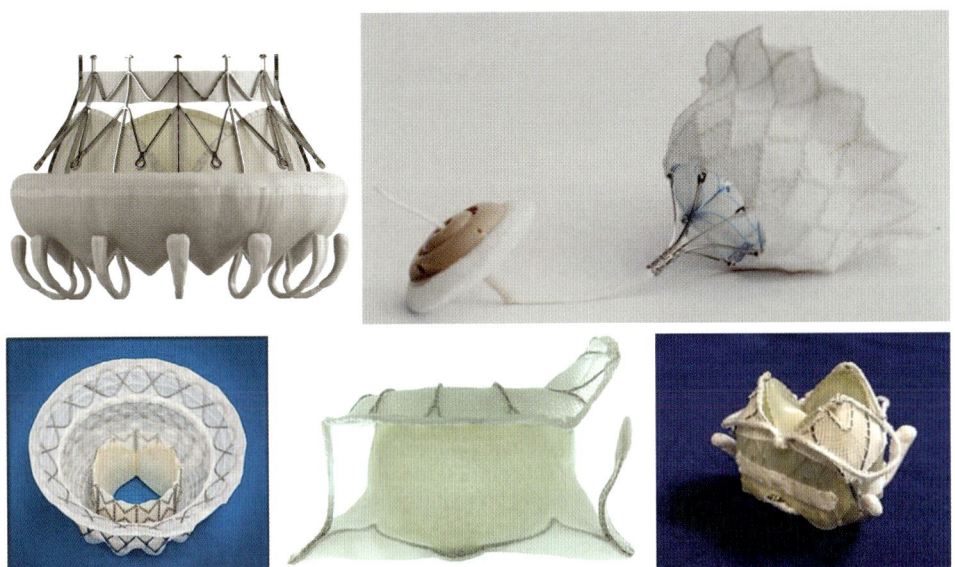

FIGURE 78.7 Transcatheter mitral valve replacement devices in early U.S. feasibility evaluation. *Top row,* CardiAQ-Edwards Transcatheter Mitral Valve (Edwards Lifesciences, Irvine, Calif) and Tendyne (Courtesy Abbott). *Bottom row,* Intrepid (Medtronic, Minneapolis, Minn), Tiara (Neovasc, Richmond, BC, Canada), and Caisson (Caisson Interventional, Maple Grove, Minn).

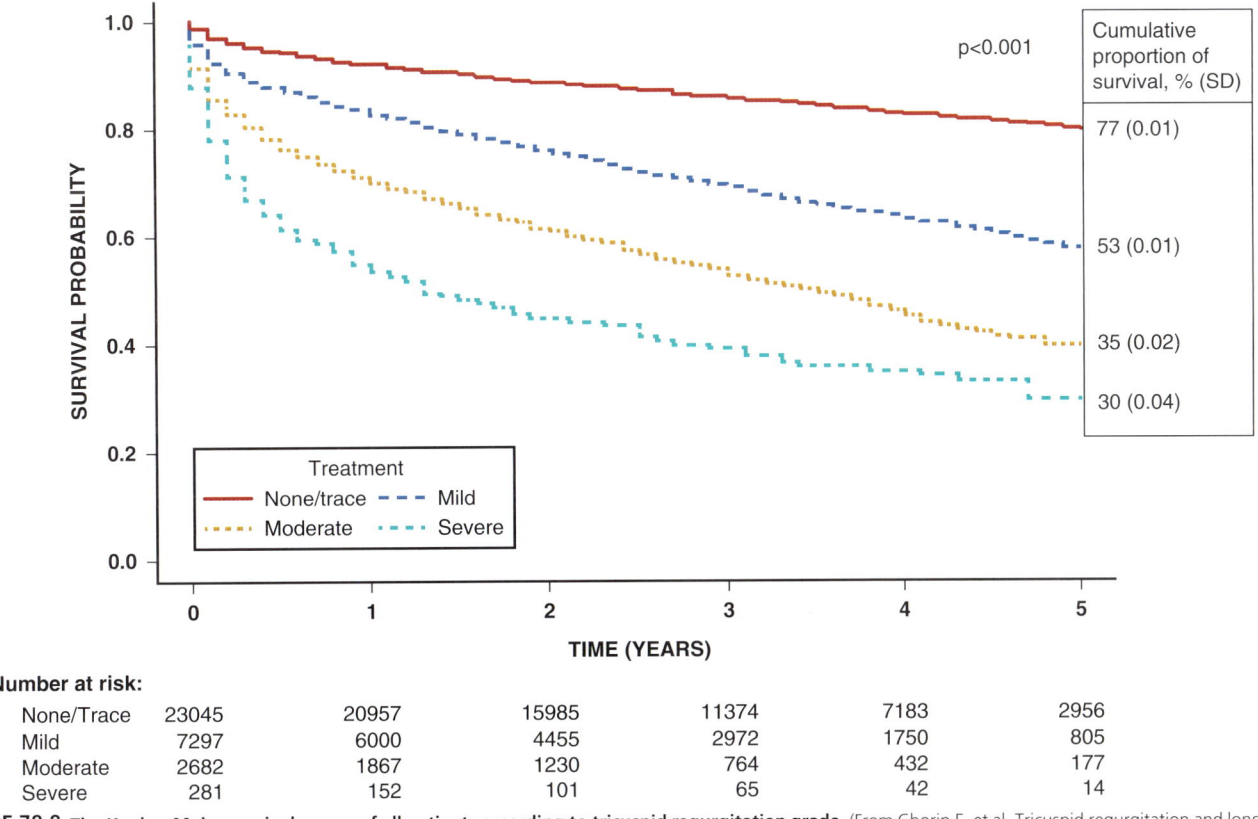

FIGURE 78.8 The Kaplan-Meier survival curves of all patients according to tricuspid regurgitation grade. (From Chorin E, et al. Tricuspid regurgitation and long-term clinical outcomes. Eur Heart J Cardiovasc Imaging 2020;21:157-165.)

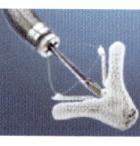
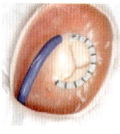
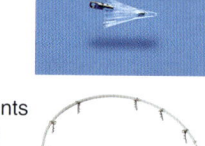
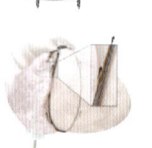
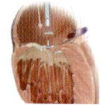

FIGURE 78.9 Current devices for transcatheter tricuspid valve repair. MitraClip, Abbott, Abbott Park, IL; PASCAL, Cardioband, Edwards Lifesciences, Irvine, CA; IRIS, Millipede, Santa Rosa, CA; MIA-T Percutaneous Tricuspid Annuloplasty System, Micro Interventional Devices, Newtown, PA; Cardiac Implants Tricuspid Annuloplasty System, Tarrytown, NY; TRAIPTA, from *JACC Cardiovasc Interv.* 2015;8(3):483-491; PASTA, from *Catheter Cardiovasc Interv.* 2018;92(3):E175-E184.)

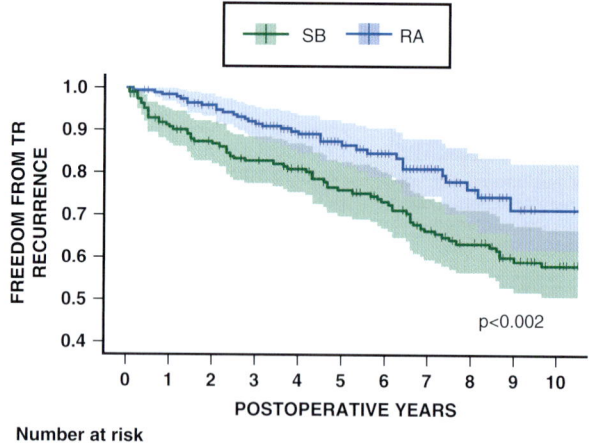

FIGURE 78.10 Freedom from TR recurrence (≥ moderate) with surgical ring annuloplasty (RA) versus suture bicuspidization (SB). (From Hirji S, et al. Outcomes after tricuspid valve repair with ring versus suture bicuspidization annuloplasty. *Ann Thorac Surg* 2020;110(3):821-828.)

(Percutaneous Tricuspid Valve Annuloplasty System for Symptomatic Chronic Functional Tricuspid Regurgitation) trial (NCT03225612).[66] Fifteen patients were treated with this device, with a technical success of 80% at 30 days.

Finally, a minimally invasive annuloplasty (MIA) device that utilizes proprietary anchors with a suture cinching approach is being studied in a OUS trial (STTAR, Study of Transcatheter Tricuspid Annuloplasty, Microinterventional Devices, Inc., Newtown, Penn). More than 30 patients have been treated with this device with reportedly good safety and efficacy, and a U.S. trial is planned.

Leaflet Clip Devices

Both the MitraClip and Pascal clip devices are being tested in the tricuspid position, usually clipping the anterior and septal leaflets.[63] The results for MitraClip from the TRIVALVE registry included 249 patients with a technical success rate of 96%.[67] The rate of TR of 3+ or more was decreased from 97% preprocedure to 23% at discharge. Preexisting pacemaker was present in 30% of these patients. This trial also excluded preexisting pacemakers. The hospital mortality was 2.8%. Mortality at 1 year was 20.3% and the 1-year combined endpoint of mortality or rehospitalization occurred in 31% of patients. The TRILUMINATE trial (NCT03227757) is a prospective, single-arm, multicenter study at 21 sites in Europe and the United States using MitraClip in severe TR and is currently ongoing.

Valve Spacer Devices

The FORMA system consists of a spacer and a rail, which is anchored within the right ventricular apex under echocardiography guidance. The spacer will passively expand using holes within the shaft. The spacer gives the valve leaflets something to coapt against to reduce TR.[63,68,69] The device is being tested in the SPACER trial (NCVT02787408).

Caval Devices

Heterotopic implantation of valve(s) into the inferior vena cava alone or with the superior vena cava also has been done to protect the hepatic and renal venous circulation from the high pressures related to TR without actually eliminating the TR.[70,71] Two early trials, HOVER (NCT2339974) and TRICAVAL (NC02387696), are assessing this approach.

Tricuspid Valve Replacement Devices

Finally, valves for complete TV replacement are being developed and are early in their use. The NaviGate valve is an early stented, trileaflet valve fabricated from equine pericardium and a self-expanding tapered nitinol stent.[72] The valve is placed thru a small right anterior thoracotomy and early compassionate use in five patients has been reported with all patients having a successful implant.[73] The LUV_VALVE (Jenscare Biotechnology) and Trisol valve (Mor Research Applications) are two addition valve replacement platforms beginning early feasibility testing.[74] Finally, the Edwards EVOQUE mitral transcatheter valve and Medtronic's Intrepid device are also undergoing U.S. early feasibility evaluation for the treatment of TR.

SUMMARY

All of the transcatheter tricuspid valve device systems are early in their development and use. Preliminary results suggest safety and that TR does not need to be completely corrected to improve the patient's clinical status. Comparing transcatheter tricuspid intervention to medical therapy suggests that intervention provides better survival as well as less heart failure hospitalization (Fig. 78.11).[75] This will prompt continued work in this area.

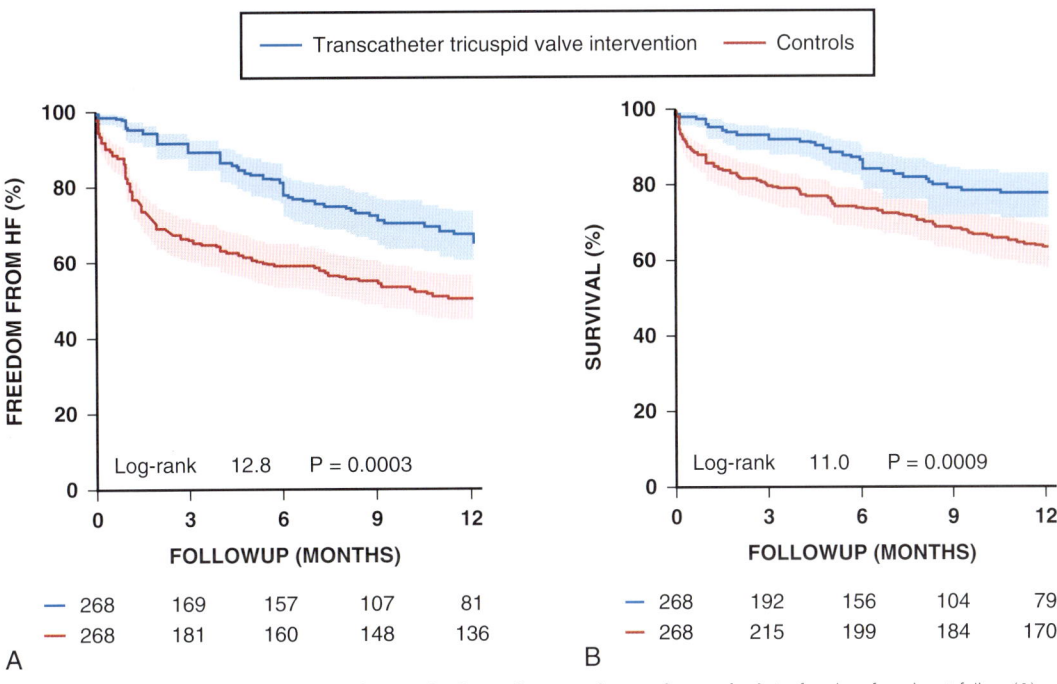

FIGURE 78.11 Transcatheter treatment of severe tricuspid regurgitation, primary and secondary endpoints: freedom from heart failure (**A**) and survival (**B**). (From Taramasso M, et al. Transcatheter versus medical treatment of patients with symptomatic severe tricuspid regurgitation. J Am Coll Cardiol 2019;74:2998-3000.)

CONCLUSION

Transcatheter therapy of VHD is an exciting, evolving, and growing area of cardiovascular medicine and surgery. The initial success of balloon valvuloplasty for stenotic lesions leading to the more recent growth of TAVR revolutionized the modern approach to AS. The complexity of the mitral valve apparatus and the myriad causes of mitral regurgitation led to slower growth and success of transcatheter mitral valve repair and replacement. However, fueled by the ever-growing prevalence of heart failure in the aging U.S. population[76]—most of these older patients with heart failure have significant MR—and aided by the ingenuity of physicians and engineers, we can anticipate that transcatheter mitral and tricuspid valve therapies will become an available option for many patients in the near future.

CLASSIC REFERENCES

Andersen HR, Knudsen LL, Hasemkam JM. Transluminal implantation of artificial heart valves: description of a new expandable aortic valve and initial results with implantation by catheter technique in closed chest pigs. *Eur Heart J.* 1992;13:704–708.

Cribier A, Eltchaninoff H, Bash A, et al. Percutaneous transcatheter implantation of an aortic valve prosthesis for calcific aortic stenosis: first human case description. *Circulation.* 2002;106:3006–3008.

Cribier A, Savin TSN, Rocha PBJ, Letac B. Percutaneous transluminal valvuloplasty of acquired aortic stenosis in elderly patients: an alternative to valve replacement? *Lancet.* 1986;1:63–67.

Harken DE, Scroff MS, Taylor MC. Partial and complete prostheses in aortic insufficiency. *J Thorac Cardiovasc Surg.* 1960;40:744–762.

Inoue K, Owaki T, Nakamura T, et al. Clinical application of transvenous mitral commissurotomy by a new balloon catheter. *J Thorac Cardiovasc Surg.* 1984;87:394–402.

National Heart, Lung and Blood Institute (NHLBI). Percutaneous balloon aortic valvuloplasty: acute and 30 day follow up results in 674 patients from the NHLBI Balloon Valvuplasty Registry. *Circulation.* 1991;84:2383–2397.

Wilkins GT, Weyman AE, Abascal VM, et al. Percutaneous balloon dilatation of the mitral valve: an analysis of echocardiographic variables related to outcome and the mechanism of dilatation. *Br Heart J.* 1988;60:299–308.

REFERENCES

Mitral Stenosis

1. Nunes MCP, Tan TC, Elmariah S, et al. The Echo score revisited. *Circulation.* 2014;129:886–895.
2. Guerrero M, Urena M, Himbert D, et al. 1-Year outcomes of transcatheter mitral valve replacement in patients with severe mitral annular calcification. *J Am Coll Cardiol.* 2018;71:1841–1853.
3. Fiorilli PN, Herrmann HC. Transcatheter mitral valve replacement: rationale and current status. *Annu Rev Med.* 2020;71:249–261.
4. Nishimura RA, Otto CM, Bonow RO, et al. 2014 AHA/ACC guideline for the management of patients with valvular heart disease: a report of the American College of Cardiology/American Heart Association task force on practice guidelines. *J Am Coll Cardiol.* 2014;63:e57–e185.
5. Eng MH, Salcedo EE, Kim M, et al. Implementation of real-time three-dimensional transesophageal echocardiography for mitral balloon valvuloplasty. *Catheter Cardiovasc Interv.* 2013;82:994–998.

Mitral Regurgitation

6. Glower DD. Surgical approaches to mitral regurgitation. *J Am Coll Cardiol.* 2012;60:1315–1322.
7. Rosenhek R, Rader F, Klaar U, et al. Outcome of watchful waiting in asymptomatic severe mitral regurgitation. *Circulation.* 2006;113:2238–2244.
8. Gammie JS, O'Brien SM, Griffith BP, et al. Influence of hospital procedural volume on care process and mortality for patients undergoing elective surgery for mitral regurgitation. *Circulation.* 2007;115:881–887.
9. Mehta RH, Eagle KA, Coombs LP, et al. Influence of age on outcomes in patients undergoing mitral valve replacement. *Ann Thorac Surg.* 2002;74:1459–1467.
10. Chatterjee S, Rankin JS, Gammie JS, et al. Isolated mitral valve surgery risk in 77,836 patients from the Society of Thoracic Surgeons database. *Ann Thorac Surg.* 2013;96:1587–1594.
11. Chaim PTL, Ruiz CE. Percutaneous mitral valve repair: a classification of the technology. *JACC Cardiovasc Interv.* 2011;4:1–13.
12. Herrmann HC, Maisano F. Transcatheter therapy of mitral regurgitation. *Circulation.* 2014;130:1712–1722.
13. Maisano F, Caldarola A, Blasio A, et al. Midterm results of edge-to-edge mitral valve repair without annuloplasty. *J Thorac Cardiovasc Surg.* 2003;126:1987–1997.
14. Feldman T, Foster E, Glower D, et al. Percutaneous repair or surgery for mitral regurgitation. *N Engl J Med.* 2011;364:1395–1406.
15. Silvestry FE, Rodriguez LL, Herrmann HC, et al. Echocardiographic guidance and assessment of percutaneous repair for mitral regurgitation with the Evalve MitraClip: lessons learned from EVEREST 1. *J Am Soc Echocardiogr.* 2007;20:1131–1140.
16. Feldman T, Kar S, Elmariah S, et al. Randomized comparison of percutaneous repair and surgery for mitral regurgitation. *J Am Coll Cardiol.* 2015;66:2844–2854.
17. Philip F, Athappan G, Tuzcu EM, et al. MitraClip for severe symptomatic mitral regurgitation in patients at high surgical risk. *Catheter Cardiovasc Interv.* 2014;84:581–590.
18. Stone GW, Lindenfeld JA, Abraham WT, et al. Transcatheter mitral-valve repair in patients with heart failure. *N Engl J Med.* 2018;379:2307–2318.
19. Obadia JF, Messika-Zeitoun D, Iung LB, et al. Percutaneous repair or medical treatment for secondary mitral regurgitation. *N Engl J Med.* 2018;379:2297–2306.
20. Pibarot P, Delgado V, Bax JJ. MITRA-FR vs. COAPT: lessons from two trials with diametrically opposed results. *Eur Heart J Cardiovasc Imaging.* 2019;20:620–624.
21. Lim DS, Kar S, Spargias K, et al. Transcatheter valve repair for patients with mitral regurgitation. *JACC Cardiovasc Interv.* 2019;12:1369–1378.
22. Siminiak T, Wu JC, Haude M, et al. Treatment of functional mitral regurgitation by percutaneous annuloplasty: results of the TITAN Trial. *Eur J Heart Fail.* 2012;14:931–938.
23. Witte KK, Lipiecki J, Siminiak T, et al. The REDUCE FMR trial. *JACC Heart Fail.* 2019;7:945–955.
24. Kim JH, Kocaturk O, Ozturk C, et al. Mitral cerclage annuloplasty, a novel transcatheter treatment for secondary mitral valve regurgitation: initial results in swine. *J Am Coll Cardiol.* 2009;54:638–651.
25. Nickenig G, Schueler R, Dager A, et al. Treatment of functional mitral regurgitation with a percutaneous annuloplasty system. *J Am Coll Cardiol.* 2016;67:2927–2936.
26. Reisman M, Wudel J, Martin S, et al. TCT-88 6-month outcomes of an early feasibility study of the AccuCinch left ventricular repair system in patients with heart failure and functional mitral regurgitation. *J Am Coll Cardiol.* 2019;74(suppl 13):B88 (abstract).
27. Maisano F, Taramasso M, Nickenig G, et al. Cardioband, a transcatheter surgical-like direct mitral valve annuloplasty system: early results of the feasibility trial. *Eur Heart J.* 2016;37:817–825.
28. Messika-Zeitoun D, Nickenig G, Latib A, et al. Transcatheter mitral valve repair for functional mitral regurgitation using the Cardioband system: 1 year outcomes. *Eur Heart J.* 2019;40:466–472.
29. Herrmann HC. Transcatheter mitral valve implantation. *Cardiac Interv Today.* 2009:82–85.
30. Fiorilli PN, Herrmann HC. Transcatheter mitral valve replacement: rationale and current status. *Annu Rev Med.* 2020;71:249–261.
31. Acker MA, Parides MK, Perrault LP, et al. Mitral valve repair versus replacement for severe ischemic mitral regurgitation. *N Engl J Med.* 2014;370:23–32.
32. Cheung A, Webb JG, Barbanti M, et al. 5-Year experience with transcatheter transapical mitral valve-in-valve implantation for bioprosthetic valve dysfunction. *J Am Coll Cardiol.* 2013;61:1759–1766.
33. Grover FL, Vemulapalli S, Carroll JD, et al. 2016 annual report of the Society of Thoracic Surgeons/American College of Cardiology transcatheter valve therapy registry. *J Am Coll Cardiol.* 2017;69:1215–1230.
34. Guerrero M, Dvir D, Himbert D, et al. Transcatheter mitral valve replacement in native mitral valve disease with severe mitral annular calcification. *JACC Cardiovasc Interv.* 2016;9:1361–1371.
35. Sorajja P, Moat N, Badhwar V, et al. Initial feasibility study of a new transcatheter mitral prosthesis. *J Am Coll Cardiol.* 2019;73:1250–1260.
36. Herrmann HC, Chitwood WR. Transcatheter mitral valve replacement clears the first hurdle. *J Am Coll Cardiol.* 2017;69:392–394.

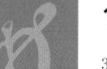

37. Anyanwu AC, Adams DH. Transcatheter mitral valve replacement. *J Am Coll Cardiol.* 2014;64:1820–1824.
38. Pedrizzetti G, La Canna G, Alfieri O, et al. The vortex: an early predictor of cardiovascular outcome? *Nat Rev Cardiol.* 2014;11:545–553.
39. Taramasso M, Maisano F, Denti P, et al. Surgical treatment of paravalvular leak: long-term results in a single center experience (up to 14 years). *J Thorac Cardiovasc Surg.* 2015;149:1270–1275.

Tricuspid Regurgitation

40. Singh JP, Evans JC, Levy D, et al. Prevalence and clinical determinants of mitral, tricuspid, and aortic regurgitation (the Framingham Heart Study). *Am J Cardiol.* 1999;83:897–902.
41. Demir OM, Razzoli D, Mangieri A, et al. Transcatheter tricuspid valve replacement: principles and design. *Front Cardiovasc Med.* 2018;5:129.
42. Topilsky Y, Maltais S, Medina Inojosa J, et al. Burden of tricuspid regurgitation in patients diagnosed in the community setting. *JACC Cardiovasc Imaging.* 2019;12:433–442.
43. Enriquez-Sarano M, Messika-Zeitoun D, Topilsky Y, et al. Tricuspid regurgitation is a public health crisis. *Prog Cardiovasc Dis.* 2019;62:447–451.
44. Kazum SS, Sagie A, Shochat T, et al. Prevalence, echocardiographic correlations, and clinical outcome of tricuspid regurgitation in patients with significant left ventricular dysfunction. *Am J Med.* 2019;132:81–87.
45. Benfari G, Antoine C, Miller WL, et al. Excess mortality associated with functional tricuspid regurgitation complicating heart failure with reduced ejection fraction. *Circulation.* 2019;140:196–206.
46. Zack CJ, Fender EA, Chandrashekar P, et al. National trends and outcomes in isolated tricuspid valve surgery. *J Am Coll Cardiol.* 2017;70:2953–2960.
47. Alqahtani F, Berzingi CO, Aljohani S, et al. Contemporary trends in the use and outcomes of surgical treatment of tricuspid regurgitation. *J Am Heart Assoc.* 2017;6(12):e007597.
48. Axtell AL, Bhambhani V, Moonsamy P, et al. Surgery does not improve survival in patients with isolated severe tricuspid regurgitation. *J Am Coll Cardiol.* 2019;74:715–725.
49. Ejiofor JI, Neely RC, Yammine M, et al. Surgical outcomes of isolated tricuspid valve procedures: repair versus replacement. *Ann Cardiothorac Surg.* 2017;6:214–222.
50. Hamandi M, Smith RL, Ryan WH, et al. Outcomes of isolated tricuspid valve surgery have improved in the modern era. *Ann Thorac Surg.* 2019;108:11–15.
51. Taramasso M, Pozzoli A, Guidotti A, et al. Percutaneous tricuspid valve therapies: the new frontier. *Eur Heart J.* 2017;38:639–647.
52. Arsalan M, Walther T, Smith 2nd RL, Grayburn PA. Tricuspid regurgitation diagnosis and treatment. *Eur Heart J.* 2017;38:634–638.
53. Dreyfus GD, Martin RP, Chan KM, et al. Functional tricuspid regurgitation: a need to revise our understanding. *J Am Coll Cardiol.* 2015;65:2331–2336.
54. Topilsky Y, Khanna A, Le Tourneau T, et al. Clinical context and mechanism of functional tricuspid regurgitation in patients with and without pulmonary hypertension. *Circ Cardiovasc Imaging.* 2012;5:314–323.
55. Braunwald NS, Ross Jr J, Morrow AG. Conservative management of tricuspid regurgitation in patients undergoing mitral valve replacement. *Circulation.* 1967;35:163–169.
56. Chorin E, Rozenbaum Z, Topilsky Y, et al. Tricuspid regurgitation and long-term clinical outcomes. *Eur Heart J Cardiovasc Imaging.* 2020;21:157–165.
57. Nishimura RA, Otto CM, Bonow RO, et al. 2014 AHA/ACC guideline for the management of patients with valvular heart disease: executive summary: a report of the American College of Cardiology/American Heart Association task force on practice guidelines. *J Am Coll Cardiol.* 2014;63:2438–2488.
58. Chikwe J, Itagaki S, Anyanwu A, Adams DH. Impact of concomitant tricuspid annuloplasty on tricuspid regurgitation, right ventricular function, and pulmonary artery hypertension after repair of mitral valve prolapse. *J Am Coll Cardiol.* 2015;65:1931–1938.
59. Wong WK, Chen SW, Chou AH, et al. Late outcomes of valve repair versus replacement in isolated and concomitant tricuspid valve surgery: a Nationwide Cohort Study. *J Am Heart Assoc.* 2020:e015637.
60. Ailawadi G, Lapar DJ, Swenson BR, et al. Model for end-stage liver disease predicts mortality for tricuspid valve surgery. *Ann Thorac Surg.* 2009;87:1460–1467. discussion 1467-8.
61. Hirji S, Yazdchi F, Kiehm S, et al. Outcomes after tricuspid valve repair with ring versus suture bicuspidization annuloplasty. *Ann Thorac Surg.* 2020;110(3):821–828.
62. Nickenig G, Weber M, Schueler R, et al. 6-Month outcomes of tricuspid valve reconstruction for patients with severe tricuspid regurgitation. *J Am Coll Cardiol.* 2019;73:1905–1915.
63. Kolte D, Elmariah S. Current state of transcatheter tricuspid valve repair. *Cardiovasc Diagn Ther.* 2020;10:89–97.
64. Rogers JH, Boyd WD, Bolling SF. Tricuspid annuloplasty with the Millipede ring. *Prog Cardiovasc Dis.* 2019;62(6):486–487.
65. Besler C, Meduri CU, Lurz P. Transcatheter treatment of functional tricuspid regurgitation using the Trialign device. *Interv Cardiol.* 2018;13:8–13.
66. Hahn RT, Meduri CU, Davidson CJ, et al. Early feasibility study of a transcatheter tricuspid valve annuloplasty: SCOUT trial 30-day results. *J Am Coll Cardiol.* 2017;69:1795–1806.
67. Mehr M, Taramasso M, Besler C, et al. 1-Year outcomes after edge-to-edge valve repair for symptomatic tricuspid regurgitation: results from the TriValve Registry. *JACC Cardiovasc Interv.* 2019;12:1451–1461.
68. Puri R, Rodes-Cabau J. The FORMA repair system. *Interv Cardiol Clin.* 2018;7:47–55.
69. Asmarats L, Perlman G, Praz F, et al. Long-term outcomes of the FORMA transcatheter tricuspid valve repair system for the treatment of severe tricuspid regurgitation: insights from the first-in-human experience. *JACC Cardiovasc Interv.* 2019;12:1438–1447.
70. Lauten A, Dreger H, Schofer J, et al. Caval valve implantation for treatment of severe tricuspid regurgitation. *J Am Coll Cardiol.* 2018;71:1183–1184.
71. O'Neill BP. Caval valve implantation: are 2 valves better than 1? *Circ Cardiovasc Interv.* 2018;11:e006334.
72. Elgharably H, Harb SC, Kapadia S, et al. Transcatheter innovations in tricuspid regurgitation: navigate. *Prog Cardiovasc Dis.* 2019;62:493–495.
73. Hahn RT, George I, Kodali SK, et al. Early single-site experience with transcatheter tricuspid valve replacement. *JACC Cardiovasc Imaging.* 2019;12:416–429.
74. Asmarats L, Taramasso M, Rodes-Cabau J. Tricuspid valve disease: diagnosis, prognosis and management of a rapidly evolving field. *Nat Rev Cardiol.* 2019;16:538–554.
75. Taramasso M, Benfari G, van der Bijl P, et al. Transcatheter versus medical treatment of patients with symptomatic severe tricuspid regurgitation. *J Am Coll Cardiol.* 2019;74:2998–3008.

Conclusion

76. Benjamin EJ, Blaha MJ, Chiuve SE, et al. Heart disease and stroke statistics—2017 update. A report from the American Heart Association. *Circulation.* 2017;135:e146–e603.

79 Prosthetic Heart Valves

PHILIPPE PIBAROT AND PATRICK T. O'GARA

TYPES OF PROSTHETIC HEART VALVES, 1495
Mechanical Valves, 1495
Tissue Valves, 1495
Comparison of Mechanical and Tissue Valves, 1497

CHOICE OF VALVE REPLACEMENT PROCEDURE AND PROSTHESIS, 1498
Choice of Procedure, 1498
Choice of Prosthetic Valve, 1498

MEDICAL MANAGEMENT AND SURVEILLANCE AFTER VALVE REPLACEMENT, 1498
Antithrombotic Therapy, 1498
Pregnancy, 1499
Infective Endocarditis Prophylaxis, 1499
Clinical Assessment, 1499
Echocardiography, 1500

EVALUATION AND TREATMENT OF PROSTHETIC VALVE DYSFUNCTION AND COMPLICATIONS, 1500

Prosthesis-Patient Mismatch, 1500
Structural Valve Deterioration, 1501
Paravalvular Leak, 1501
Infective Endocarditis, 1503
Hemolytic Anemia, 1503

CLASSIC REFERENCES, 1503

REFERENCES, 1503

The past six decades have witnessed extraordinary advancements in patient survival and functional outcomes following heart valve replacement surgery. Continued refinements in prosthetic valve design and performance, surgical and percutaneous techniques, myocardial preservation, systemic perfusion, cerebral protection, and anesthetic management have enabled the application of surgical and transcatheter valve therapy to an increasingly wider spectrum of patients. Minimally invasive surgical approaches and the use of primary valve repair for mitral or aortic valve pathology when anatomically appropriate are now the routine in the vast majority of comprehensive valve centers.[1] Heart valve teams provide multidisciplinary assessment and treatment of complex patients, including with the use of transcatheter interventions when appropriate. Over 57,000 aortic valve replacement (AVR) and over 19,000 mitral valve replacement (MVR) operations (with or without coronary artery bypass) were reported to the Society of Thoracic Surgeons (STS) National Adult Cardiac Database in calendar year 2019, whereas 72,991 transcatheter aortic valve replacements (TAVRs) and 1164 transcatheter mitral valve replacements (TMVRs, all within the confines of clinical trials) were reported to the STS/American College of Cardiology (ACC) Transcatheter Valve Therapy Registry in calendar year 2019.[2,3] The COVID-19 pandemic was associated with a significant decrease in the volume of valve replacement procedures reported to both registries in the calendar year 2020. Familiarity with the specific hemodynamic attributes, durability, thrombogenicity, and inherent limitations of currently available heart valve substitutes, as well as their potential for long-term complications, is critical for appropriate clinical decision making in patients in whom repair is not appropriate or feasible. The choice of valve prosthesis is inherently a trade-off between durability and risk of thromboembolism, with the associated hazards and lifestyle limitations of anticoagulation. The ideal heart valve substitute remains an elusive goal.

TYPES OF PROSTHETIC HEART VALVES

Mechanical Valves
There are three basic types of mechanical prosthetic valves: bileaflet, tilting disc, and ball-cage (Fig. 79.1). The St. Jude bileaflet valve is the most frequently implanted mechanical prosthesis worldwide. It consists of two pyrolytic semi-circular "leaflets" or discs with a slit-like central orifice between the two leaflets and two larger semi-circular orifices laterally. The opening angle of the leaflets relative to the annulus plane ranges from 75 to 90 degrees. The Carbomedics valve is a variation of the St. Jude prosthesis that can be rotated to prevent limitation of leaflet excursion by subvalvular tissue. For a given valve annulus size, the effective orifice areas (EOAs) are generally larger and transprosthetic pressure gradients are lower for the bileaflet mechanical valves compared with the tilting disc valves. Because the central orifice is smaller than the lateral orifices in bileaflet valves, the blood flow velocity may be locally higher within the inflow aspect of the central orifice; this phenomenon may yield to overestimation of gradient and underestimation of EOA by transthoracic echocardiography (TTE) (see Chapter 16).[4,5] Bileaflet valves typically have a small amount of normal regurgitation ("washing jet") designed in part to decrease the risk of thrombus formation. A small central jet and two converging jets emanating from the hinge points of the disc can be visualized on color Doppler flow imaging.

Tilting disc or monoleaflet valves use a single circular disc that rotates within a rigid annulus to occlude or open the valve orifice. The disc is secured by lateral or central metal struts. The opening angle of the disc relative to the valve annulus ranges from 60 to 80 degrees, resulting in two orifices of different size. The nonperpendicular opening angle of the valve occluder tends to slightly increase the resistance to blood flow, particularly in the major orifices. Tilting disc valves also have a small amount of regurgitation, arising from small gaps at the perimeter of the valve.

The bulky Starr-Edwards ball-cage valve, the oldest commercially available prosthetic heart valve first used in 1965, is no longer implanted. The ball-cage valve is more thrombogenic and has less favorable hemodynamic performance characteristics than either bileaflet or tilting disc valves.

Currently available mechanical valves have excellent long-term durability, with up to 45 years for the Starr-Edwards valve and more than 35 years for the St. Jude valve. Structural deterioration, exemplified by some older generation Bjork-Shiley (strut fracture with disc embolization) and Starr-Edwards (ball variance) prostheses, is now extremely rare. Ten-year freedom from valve-related death exceeds 90% for both St. Jude and Carbomedics bileaflet valves. All patients with mechanical valves require lifelong anticoagulation with a vitamin K antagonist (VKA).[6] Long-term issues associated with mechanical valves include infective endocarditis, paravalvular leaks, hemolytic anemia, valve thrombosis/thromboembolism, pannus ingrowth, and hemorrhagic complications related to anticoagulation (Fig. 79.2).

Tissue Valves
Tissue or biological valves include stented and stentless bioprostheses (porcine, bovine), homografts (or allografts) from human cadaveric sources, and autografts of pericardial or pulmonic valve origin (see Fig. 79.1). They provide an alternative, less thrombogenic heart valve substitute for which long-term anticoagulation in the absence of additional risk factors for thromboembolism is not required.

Stented Bioprosthetic Valves
The traditional design of a heterograft valve consists of three biologic leaflets made from the porcine aortic valve or bovine pericardium treated with glutaraldehyde to reduce its antigenicity. The leaflets are

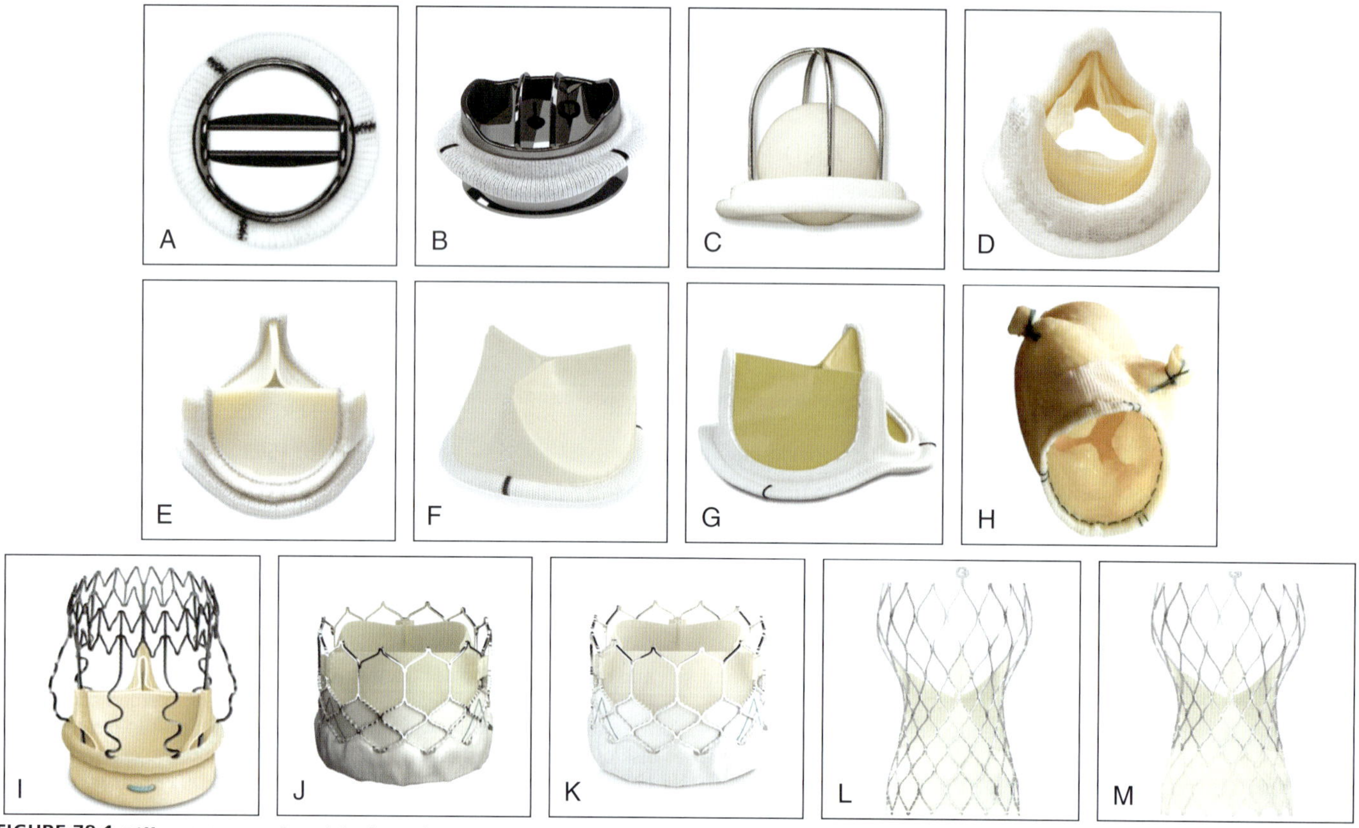

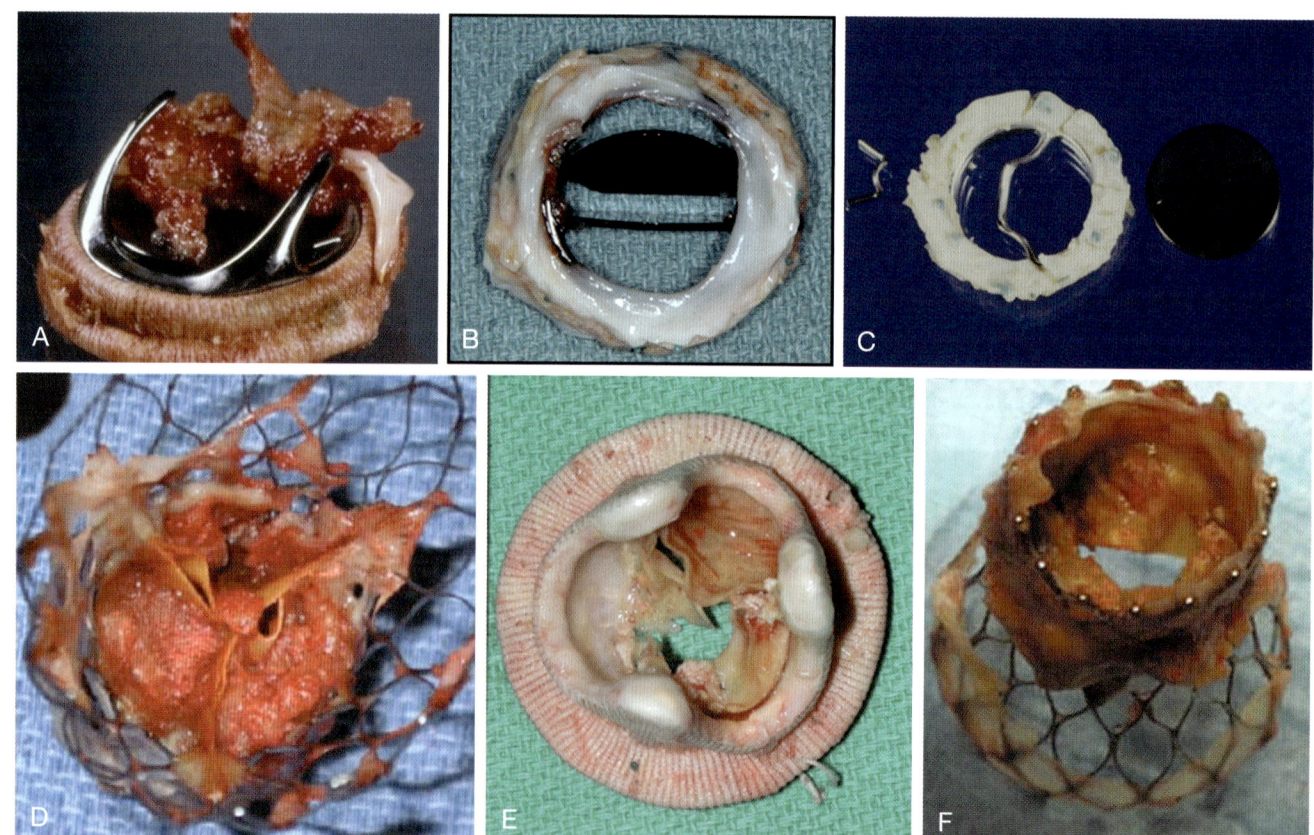

FIGURE 79.1 Different types and models of prosthetic valves. **A,** Bileaflet St. Jude mechanical valve. **B,** On-X heart valve (with permission of CryoLife). **C,** Caged ball Starr-Edwards mechanical valve. **D,** Stented porcine Medtronic Mosaic bioprosthetic valve. **E,** Stented bovine pericardial Edwards Magna bioprosthetic valve. **F,** Stented bovine pericardial Abbott Trifecta bioprosthetic valve. **G,** Stented bovine pericardial Edwards Inspiris bioprosthetic valve. **H,** Stentless porcine Medtronic Freestyle bioprosthetic valve. **I,** Sutureless Sorin Perceval bioprosthetic valve. **J,** Transcatheter balloon-expandable Edwards SAPIEN 3 bioprosthetic valve. **K,** Transcatheter balloon-expandable Edwards SAPIEN 3 Ultra bioprosthetic valve. **L,** Transcatheter self-expanding Medtronic CoreValve Evolut R bioprosthetic valve. **M,** Transcatheter self-expanding Medtronic CoreValve Evolut PRO bioprosthetic valve.

FIGURE 79.2 Prosthetic valve complications. **A,** Obstructive thrombosis of a Lillehei-Kaster tilting disc mechanical valve. **B,** Pannus ingrowth interacting with leaflet opening in a St. Jude Medical bileaflet mechanical valve. **C,** Rupture of the outlet strut and leaflet escape in a Björk-Shiley mechanical valve. **D,** Thrombosis in a self-expanding transcatheter aortic valve. **E,** Leaflet calcific degeneration and tear in a porcine bioprosthesis. **F,** Leaflet calcific degeneration and stenosis in a self-expanding transcatheter aortic valve. (Courtesy Dr. Siamak Mohammadi, Québec Heart & Lung Institute, Québec (**A** and **C**); Dr. Christian Couture, Québec Heart & Lung Institute, Québec (**B**); Dr. Gosta Petterson, Cleveland Clinic, Cleveland (**E**); **D** from Latib A, et al. Treatment and clinical outcomes of transcatheter heart valve thrombosis. Circ Cardiovasc Interv 2015;8:1-8; **F** from Seeburger J, et al. Structural valve deterioration of a CoreValve prosthesis 9 months after implantation. Eur Heart J 2013;34:1607.)

mounted on a metal or polymeric stented ring; they open to a circular orifice in systole, resembling the anatomy of the native aortic valve (see Fig. 79.1). The vast majority of bioprosthetic valves are treated with anti-calcifying agents or processes. The Inspiris Resilia Aortic Valve (Edwards LifeSciences, Irvine, CA) incorporates newer anti-calcification technology and an expandable sewing ring to accommodate future valve-in-valve implantation for symptomatic, severe structural valve deterioration (SVD).[7,8] The Perceval valve (LivaNova, London, UK) is a sutureless bioprosthetic valve designed to reduce intraoperative times.[8a,8b] The current generation of bovine pericardial valves offers improved hemodynamic performance compared with earlier generations.[9-14] A small degree of regurgitation can be detected by color Doppler flow imaging in 10% of normally functioning bioprostheses. One limitation of earlier generations of bioprosthetic valves was their limited durability due to SVD, typically beginning within 5 to 7 years after implantation but varying by position and age at implant, with tissue changes characterized by calcification, fibrosis, tears, and perforations. SVD occurs earlier for mitral than for aortic bioprosthetic valves, perhaps due to exposure of the mitral prosthesis to relatively higher left ventricular (LV) closing pressures. The process of SVD is accelerated in younger patients, in those with disordered calcium metabolism (end-stage renal disease), and, possibly, in pregnant women independent of younger age. With current generation bioprosthetic pericardial valves, durability is excellent, with SVD rates of 2% to 10% at 10 years, 10% to 20% at 15 years, and 40% at 20 years.[9,10] Premature SVD, however, was an issue with the certain models of the Sorin Mitroflow valve.[15]

Stentless Bioprosthetic Valves

The rigid sewing ring and stent-based construction of certain bioprostheses allow for easier implantation and maintenance of the three-dimensional relationships of the leaflets. However, these features also contribute to impaired hemodynamic performance. Stentless porcine valves (see Fig. 79.1) were developed in part to address these issues. Their use has been restricted to the aortic position. Implantation is technically more challenging, whether deployed in a subcoronary position or as part of a mini-root, and hence they are preferred by only a minority of surgeons. Early postoperative mean gradients can be <15 mm Hg with further improvement in valve performance over time due to aortic root remodeling, resulting in lower peak exercise transvalvular gradients and more rapid reduction in LV mass.[16]

Homografts

Aortic valve homografts are harvested from human cadavers within 24 hours of death and are treated with antibiotics and cryopreserved at −196°C. They are most commonly implanted in the form of a total root replacement with reimplantation of the coronary arteries. Homograft valves appear resistant to infection and are preferred by some surgeons for management of aortic valve and root endocarditis in the active phase (see Chapter 80). Neither immune suppression nor routine anticoagulation is required. Despite earlier expectations, long-term durability beyond 10 years is not superior to that for current generation pericardial valves[17] and reoperation may be technically more challenging due to calcification of the cylinder.

Autografts

In the Ross procedure, the patient's own pulmonic valve (or autograft) is harvested as a small tissue block containing the pulmonic valve, annulus, and proximal pulmonary artery and inserted in the aortic position usually as a complete root replacement with reimplantation of the coronary arteries.[17] The pulmonic valve and right ventricular outflow tract are then replaced with either an aortic or a pulmonic homograft. Thus, the procedure requires two separate valve operations, a longer time on cardiopulmonary bypass, and a steep learning curve. With appropriate selection of young patients by expert surgeons at experienced centers of excellence, operative mortality rates are <1% and 20-year survival rates as high as 95% and similar or slightly lower to the general population.[18,19] Advantages of the autograft include the ability to increase in size during childhood growth, excellent hemodynamic performance characteristics, lack of thrombogenicity, and resistance to infection. The hemodynamic performance characteristics of the pulmonary autograft are similar to those of a normal, native aortic valve. The procedure is usually reserved for children and young adults but should be avoided in patients with dilated aortic roots given the unacceptably high incidence of accelerated degeneration, pulmonary autograft dilation, and significant regurgitation.[20] The critical requirements of surgical skill and institutional experience cannot be overstated.[6]

Transcatheter Bioprosthetic Valves

TAVR is a valuable alternative to surgical AVR in patients across the surgical risk spectrum (see Chapters 72 and 74). Two main types of transcatheter aortic valves are currently used: balloon-expandable valves (BEV) and self-expanding valves (SEV) (see Fig. 79.1).

The Edwards LifeSciences (Irvine, CA) SAPIEN 3 and SAPIEN 3 Ultra BEVs consist of a three-leaflet pericardial bovine valve mounted in a cobalt chromium frame. These valves are available in several sizes. The Medtronic (Minneapolis, MN) EVOLUT-R and EVOLUT-Pro+ SEVs consist of three leaflets of porcine pericardium seated relatively higher in a nitinol frame to provide supra-annular placement and are also available in several sizes.

The vast majority of TAVR procedures are performed via a transfemoral approach, which is associated with lower mortality, fewer complications, and quicker recovery compared with alternative access site approaches (e.g., subclavian, carotid, transcaval, transaortic, apical). The choice of SEV versus BEV is highly operator dependent, though there are anatomic and echocardiographic considerations to be taken into account. Intermediate term durability appears similar, though the risk of permanent pacemaker implantation is higher with SEVs. Other risk factors for the development of high-grade AV block after TAVR have been identified.[21] Leaflet thrombosis can be recognized by the appearance of hypoattenuated leaflet thickening (HALT) on ECG-gated computed tomography (CT) and occurs in 10% to 20% of patients 30 days after TAVR, compared with approximately 5% to 15% after surgical AVR (SAVR).[22-24] Subclinical leaflet thrombosis, that is HALT in the absence of thromboembolic complications or a progressive increase in the transvalvular gradient, appears to be a dynamic phenomenon for which indications for treatment are uncertain.

For a given aortic annulus size, TAVR valves often have larger EOAs, lower gradients, and lower incidence of severe prosthesis-patient mismatch compared with SAVR valves.[25-28] Paravalvular leak (PVL) is, however, more frequent following TAVR and may result in adverse long-term consequences depending on its severity.[29] The risk of PVL has decreased over time with iterative improvements in valve design, preprocedural imaging, patient selection and intraprocedural techniques.[28,30] Some studies have suggested that SEVs have slightly larger EOAs and lower gradients but somewhat higher rates of PVL than BEVs.[31] The rate of SVD over short- to intermediate-term follow-up for the SAPIEN 3 valve is comparable to that of bioprosthetic SAVR valves.[32]

COMPARISON OF MECHANICAL AND TISSUE VALVES

Obvious differences between valve types relate to durability (i.e., theoretically indefinite for mechanical versus limited for tissue valves) and need for anticoagulation (i.e., obligatory use for mechanical versus none for tissue valves absent other risk factors for thromboembolism). Short- to intermediate-term hemodynamic performance characteristics with low-profile mechanical prostheses (e.g., St. Jude) are comparable to those with stented tissue valves of similar size. There are no important differences in rates of prosthetic valve endocarditis (PVE), though some series have suggested a higher incidence of early (<1 year) infection with mechanical valves versus bioprostheses.[33] In the Veterans Affairs randomized trial conducted between 1977 and 1982, patients undergoing AVR had a better 15-year survival with a mechanical valve than with a bioprosthetic valve, whereas there was no difference in survival with mechanical versus biological MVR (see Classic Reference, Hammermeister et al.). With AVR, the increased mortality among patients treated with a bioprosthesis was driven largely by the higher rate of SVD. There was an increased risk of bleeding with mechanical valve replacement, but no significant differences were observed for other valve-related complications such as thromboembolism or PVE. A smaller randomized trial of patients 55 to 70 years of age with aortic valve disease also showed no difference in late survival between newer generation mechanical and bioprosthetic valves, with higher rates of SVD and reoperation in patients with bioprostheses but no other differences in secondary endpoints.[34] In an analysis of over 39,000 AVR patients aged 65 to 80 years reported to the STS Adult Cardiac Surgery Database and linked to Medicare, patients receiving a bioprosthesis had a similar adjusted risk for death, higher risks for reoperation and endocarditis, and lower risks for stroke and bleeding, compared with patients receiving a mechanical valve.[35] Two propensity-matched analyses from New York's Statewide Planning and Research Cooperative System (SPARCS) reported no survival differences for patients 50 to 69 years of age undergoing mechanical versus bioprosthetic, AVR, or MVR.[36,37] Rates of stroke and bleeding were higher, whereas rates of reoperation were lower, among mechanical valve recipients. A survival advantage among patients in this age group who underwent mechanical rather than bioprosthetic valve replacement was, however, reported from the Swedish system for the Enhancement and Development of Evidence-based care in Heart disease Evaluated According to Recommended Therapies (SWEDEHEART) register.[38] Stroke risk was similar between the groups, though bleeding rates were higher and need for reoperation lower after mechanical valve replacement. Overall survival and rates of reoperation, stroke, and bleeding after bioprosthetic versus mechanical valve replacement were examined in a 2017 report from the California Office of Statewide Health Planning and Development.[39] Among patients 45 to 54 years of age who underwent SAVR, receipt of a biological prosthesis was associated with a significantly higher 15-year mortality rate than receipt of a mechanical prosthesis. Among patients undergoing surgical MVR, use of a mechanical valve was associated with lower mortality up to age 69. There was significant decrease in the use of mechanical valves over the 17-year period examined (1996 to 2013). Rates of reoperation were lower but rates of bleeding and stroke were higher for those who received a mechanical valve.[39]

CHOICE OF VALVE REPLACEMENT PROCEDURE AND PROSTHESIS

Once the indication for valve intervention is established, the next step is to select the type of procedure (repair versus replacement) and the type of prosthetic valve to be used should replacement be necessary. The 2020 AHA/ACC guidelines for the management of patients with valvular heart disease advocate shared decision making regarding the choice of intervention (repair or replacement, transcatheter or surgical) as well as the type of prosthetic valve (mechanical valve or bioprosthesis).[6] This choice is based on consideration of several factors including patient age, expected longevity and comorbidities, valve durability, expected hemodynamics for a specific valve type and size, surgical or interventional risk, the potential need for and safety of long-term anticoagulation, and patient preferences.

CHOICE OF PROCEDURE

For patients meeting an indication for AVR, the choice of TAVR versus SAVR begins with assessment of surgical risk considering patient age and life expectancy (see Chapters 72 and 74). The ultimate choice also hinges on technical factors related to access (transfemoral versus alternative route), aortic valve and root anatomy, the extent and severity of calcification, the height of the coronary arteries, and the need for additional cardiac surgery (e.g., root or ascending aortic replacement, coronary artery bypass grafting). TAVR is preferred for prohibitive or high surgical risk patients provided life expectancy with reasonable quality exceeds 1 year. SAVR is preferred for low or intermediate surgical risk patients younger than 65 due to the paucity of data regarding TAVR valve durability beyond 5 years. For patients 65 to 80 years of age, the choice between TAVR and SAVR is largely driven by patient preference and the need for concomitant surgery. TAVR is generally preferred for patients over age 80.[6] Recommendations regarding TAVR apply primarily to patients with trileaflet aortic stenosis, although the use of TAVR for selected patients with bicuspid aortic valve stenosis has increased rapidly.

In patients with chronic severe primary mitral regurgitation (MR) who meet an indication for mitral valve surgery, mitral valve repair is recommended in preference to MVR when a successful and durable repair can be accomplished (see Chapter 76).[6] Transcatheter mitral valve repair using an edge-to-edge clip device is reserved for prohibitive surgical risk patients with primary MR. In patients with severe chronic secondary MR in the setting of ischemic cardiomyopathy referred for coronary artery bypass graft, concomitant MVR may be superior to mitral valve repair because it is associated with lower rates of recurrent moderate to severe regurgitation.[40] Transcatheter edge-to-edge repair (TEER) is reasonable for selected patients with heart failure, reduced ejection fraction and moderately severe to severe MR (see Chapter 78).[6,41]

Tricuspid valve annuloplasty repair is frequently performed at the time of left-sided valve surgery when secondary tricuspid regurgitation (TR) is severe or when there is significant tricuspid annular dilation (>40 mm) despite only mild or moderate degrees of TR or a history of right-sided heart failure) (see Chapter 77).[42] Tricuspid valve replacement is undertaken for severe primary tricuspid valve disease that cannot be repaired, such as with advanced rheumatic disease, carcinoid, or destructive endocarditis.[6] Surgical or transcatheter pulmonic valve replacement in the adult is rare.

CHOICE OF PROSTHETIC VALVE

A bioprosthesis is recommended in patients of any age for whom anticoagulant therapy is contraindicated, cannot be managed appropriately, or is not desired. A mechanical prosthesis is reasonable for SAVR in patients <50 years old who do not have a contraindication to anticoagulation, whereas a bioprosthesis is reasonable in SAVR patients >65 years old.[6] Either a bioprosthetic or mechanical valve is reasonable in SAVR patients between 50 and 65 years old. When MVR is necessary, a mechanical prosthesis is reasonable for patients <65 years old and a bioprosthesis is reasonable for patients ≥65 years old. For women contemplating pregnancy, a bioprosthesis is preferred to avoid the hazards of anticoagulation. The choice of prosthesis in patients with end-stage renal disease is challenging and should take into account life expectancy.

MEDICAL MANAGEMENT AND SURVEILLANCE AFTER VALVE REPLACEMENT

Antithrombotic Therapy

General Principles

Table 79.1 presents the antithrombotic regimens included in the 2020 AHA/ACC guideline for different types of procedures and prosthetic valves.[6] All patients with mechanical heart valves require lifelong anticoagulation with a VKA, the intensity of which varies as a function of valve type or thrombogenicity, valve position and number, and the presence of additional risk factors for thromboembolism, such as atrial fibrillation, LV systolic dysfunction, a history of thromboembolism, and hypercoagulable state (see Table 79.1). Anticoagulant therapy with non-vitamin K oral anticoagulants (NOACs) should not be used in patients with mechanical prostheses, although they can be used in patients with bioprosthetic valves or annuloplasty rings at a distance from surgery.[6] The addition of low-dose aspirin to VKA therapy can be considered in patients with mechanical valves when dictated by another indication. Although there is no clear consensus, a VKA may be used even in the absence of risk factors for thromboembolism for the first 3 to 6 months after bioprosthetic AVR or MVR.[6] Longer-term treatment of low thromboembolic risk bioprosthetic AVR and MVR patients consists of low-dose aspirin, although there are no randomized data to support this practice. In the absence of an indication for anticoagulation, single-agent antiplatelet therapy with low-dose aspirin is reasonable after TAVR.[6,43,44] For patients with an indication for anticoagulation, monotherapy with either a VKA or NOAC is reasonable after TAVR.[6] Treatment following TAVR with low-dose rivaroxaban (10 mg daily) plus aspirin (75 to 100 mg daily for the first 3 months) is contraindicated.[45]

Interruption of Antithrombotic Therapy

In the planned interruption of VKA therapy for noncardiac surgery, the following must be taken into account: the nature of the procedure; the magnitude of risk of thromboembolism based on valve type, position, and number; underlying patient risk factors; the length of time over which therapy is to be interrupted; and the competing risk of periprocedural hemorrhage.[6] Low-risk patients with low-profile bileaflet or tilting disc valves in the aortic position can usually stop VKA therapy 3 to 5 days before noncardiac surgery and then resume it postoperatively as soon as it is considered safe, without the need for a heparin "bridge." In all other patients, either low-molecular-weight heparin (LMWH) or intravenous unfractionated heparin

TABLE 79.1 Antithrombotic Therapy in Patients with Prosthetic Valves

COR**	LOE		VKA (TARGET INR)	ASPIRIN (75-100 MG)	CLOPIDOGREL (75 MG)
		Mechanical Valves			
I	B-NR	AVR–Bileaflet or current generation single tilting disc valves and no risk factors for thromboembolism*	Yes (INR: 2.5)	If indicated‡	
I	B-NR	AVR–Older-generation valves† and/or any risk factor for thromboembolism*	Yes (INR: 3.0)	If indicated‡	
I	B-NR	MVR–Mechanical valves	Yes (INR: 3.0)	If indicated‡	
IIb	B-NR	AVR–On-X valve and no risk factors for thromboembolism	Yes (INR: 1.5-2.0) §	Yes	
		Surgical Bioprosthetic Valves			
IIa	B-NR	AVR or MVR–Initial 3-6 months	Yes (2.5)		
IIa	B-NR	AVR or MVR–Lifelong		Yes	
		Transcatheter Aortic Valves			
IIb	B-NR	TAVR–Initial 3-6 months¶		Yes	Yes
IIb	B-NR	TAVR–Initial 3-6 months¶	Yes		
IIa	B-NR	TAVR–Lifelong		Yes	

AVR, Aortic valve replacement; *MVR*, mitral valve replacement; *INR*, international normalized ratio; *VKA*, vitamin K antagonist; *TAVR*, transcatheter aortic valve implantation.
*Risk factors for thromboembolism: Atrial fibrillation, LV dysfunction (LVEF ≤35%), LA dilation (LA diameter ≥50 mm), previous thromboembolism, and hypercoagulable condition.
†Ball-in-cage valves, older generation of single tilting-disc valves.
‡Addition of low-dose aspirin in low bleeding risk patients may be predicated on development of independent indication during follow-up, such as intra-coronary stent implantation.
§INR goal 2.5 for the first 3 months after On-X SAVR; INR goal 1.5-2.0 thereafter with lifelong continuation of low-dose aspirin.
¶If low risk of bleeding, one of the two antithrombotic therapies (aspirin + clopidogrel or VKA) but not both may be considered.
**COR refers to the AHA/ACC 2020 Valvular Heart Disease Class of Recommendation for each scenario. Class I indicates that the recommendation should be followed and the treatment given. Class IIa indicates that the recommendation is reasonable, and Class IIb indicates that the recommendation may be considered.
From Otto CM, et al. 2020 AHA/ACC guideline for the management of patients with valvular heart disease: a report of the American College of Cardiology/American Heart Association Task Force on Practice Guidelines. J Am Coll Cardiol 2021;77:e25-197.

(UFH) should be given on an individualized basis both before and after surgery, as directed by the surgeon. The use of LMWH avoids the need for preoperative hospitalization. For patients with a bioprosthetic valve or annuloplasty ring receiving an anticoagulant, it is reasonable to consider the need for bridging on the basis of the CHA_2DS_2-VASc score and the risk of bleeding. There is a paucity of randomized trial data and significant institutional and operator variability in the use of bridging strategies for noncardiac surgery in patients with prosthetic valves.

Pregnancy (see Chapter 92)

Pregnant patients with prosthetic valves should be followed carefully because of the increased hemodynamic burden that can cause or worsen heart failure if there is prosthetic valve dysfunction and also because of the hypercoagulable state related to pregnancy that increases the risk of valve thrombosis. All antithrombotic regimens carry an increased risk to the fetus, an increased risk of miscarriage, and an increased risk of hemorrhagic complications for the mother. Hence, patients require appropriate counseling, close monitoring, and adjustment of anticoagulation therapy. In pregnant patients with mechanical valves, warfarin is reasonable in the first trimester if the dose is ≤5 mg/day and is recommended to achieve a therapeutic international normalized ratio (INR) target in the second and third trimesters.[6] Discontinuation of warfarin with initiation of intravenous UFH is recommended before planned vaginal delivery in pregnant patients with a mechanical valve.

Infective Endocarditis Prophylaxis (see Chapter 80)

Patients with prosthetic valves are at increased risk for infective endocarditis because of the foreign valve surface and sewing ring (see Chapter 80). Antibiotic prophylaxis is indicated for patients with prosthetic valves who undergo dental procedures that involve manipulation of gingival tissue, the periapical region of teeth, or perforation of the oral mucosa, and it is not recommended for non-dental procedures such as transesophageal echocardiography, esophagogastroduodenoscopy, colonoscopy, or cystoscopy (unless there is active infection in these areas).[6,33]

Clinical Assessment

Postoperative visits should begin approximately 3 to 4 weeks after valve implantation. The first visit is focused on ensuring a smooth transition from hospital/rehabilitation facility to home, reconciling medications, and assessing neurocognitive function, wound healing, volume status, heart rhythm, and the auscultatory characteristics of prosthetic valve function. The history at subsequent visits is tailored to detect symptoms suggestive of heart failure or reduced functional capacity, arrhythmia, thromboembolism, or infection. Adherence to the recommended schedule of INR determinations and the relative time spent in the therapeutic range should be assessed in all VKA anticoagulated patients. Problems with bleeding should be identified. A focused cardiovascular examination is repeated at each visit. Instructions regarding antibiotic prophylaxis are repeated. After the 6-month mark, follow-up visits can be conducted annually unless interim problems arise.

A chest radiograph is obtained by the surgeon at the first visit to assess for residual pleural fluid, pneumothorax, lung aeration, and heart size. An electrocardiogram is routinely performed and should be reviewed for rhythm, conduction, and dynamic repolarization changes. Postoperative baseline values for hemoglobin, hematocrit, lactate dehydrogenase (LDH), and bilirubin should be established for patients with mechanical heart valves, allowing future comparisons should hemolysis be suspected. It is less useful to follow the serum haptoglobin. Other laboratory studies are performed as clinically relevant.

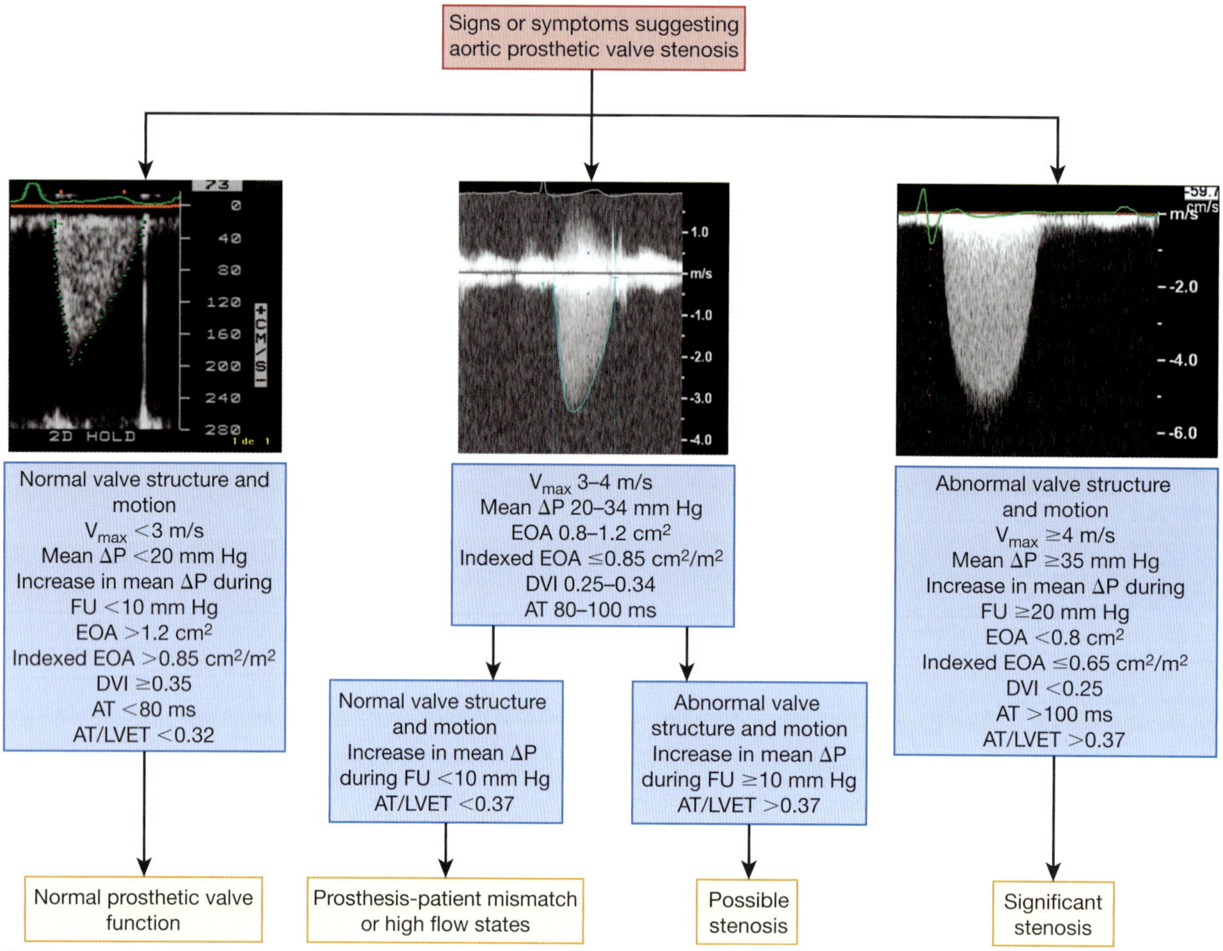

FIGURE 79.3 Evaluation of aortic prosthetic valve stenosis. A practical approach to evaluation of possible prosthetic aortic stenosis is to begin with standard measures of stenosis severity, including maximal velocity (V_{max}), mean pressure gradient (ΔP), effective orifice area (EOA), and Doppler velocity index (DVI: ratio of left ventricular outflow tract to aortic velocity). Normal values for each valve type and size should be referenced, but simple thresholds of 3 and 4 m/s for V_{max} and 20 and 35 mm Hg for mean ΔP are a quick first step. For patients with intermediate measures of stenosis severity, the assessment of valve structure and motion and of the changes in ΔP, EOA, and DVI during follow-up (FU) can be helpful to differentiate normal prosthetic valve function with concomitant prosthesis-patient mismatch or high flow states versus prosthetic valve stenosis. The shape of the transprosthetic flow velocity curve may also be helpful with a triangular shape (short acceleration time [AT], i.e., time to peak velocity relative to LV ejection time [LVET]) suggesting normal valve function and a rounded waveform (increased AT/LVET ratio) suggesting significant stenosis. Additional imaging including transesophageal echocardiography, cinefluoroscopy, or cardiac CT may be needed to assess valve leaflet structure and motion.

Echocardiography (see Chapter 16)

An initial TTE examination performed 6 weeks to 3 months after prosthetic valve implantation is recommended to assess the results of surgery and serve as a baseline for comparison should complications or deterioration occur later (see Figs. 16.51, 16.52, and 16.53).[6] Repeat TTE (as well as transesophageal echocardiography (TEE), fluoroscopy, or gated cardiac CT) is recommended if there is a change in clinical symptoms or signs suggesting valve dysfunction. In patients with a bioprosthetic surgical valve, routine TTE follow-up is recommended at 5 and 10 years and then annually thereafter. Presently, annual TTE studies are recommended for TAVR patients.[6] Studies estimate that 25% to 30% of patients with a bioprosthesis implanted for less than 10 years in the aortic position have some degree of valve degeneration/dysfunction.[10] In patients with mechanical valves, routine annual echocardiography is not indicated in the absence of a change in clinical status.

A complete echocardiogram includes two-dimensional imaging of the prosthetic valve; evaluation of the valve leaflet/occluder morphology and mobility; measurement of the transprosthetic velocity and gradients, valve EOA, and Doppler velocity index; estimation of the degree of regurgitation; evaluation of LV size and systolic function; and calculation of systolic pulmonary arterial pressure (see Chapter 16).[4,5,46,47] Paravalvular regurgitation is more common following TAVR than SAVR and the measurement of valve EOA is more challenging in transcatheter valves than in surgical valves due to the presence of the valve stent in the LV outflow tract.[6,48]

EVALUATION AND TREATMENT OF PROSTHETIC VALVE DYSFUNCTION AND COMPLICATIONS

The suspicion of prosthetic valve dysfunction may be heightened by the appreciation of a new murmur or symptom in a patient with a prosthetic valve or the incidental finding of abnormally high flow velocities and gradients detected during routine echocardiography. Doppler-echocardiography is the method of choice to evaluate prosthetic valve function, identify and quantitate prosthetic valve stenosis or regurgitation, and identify prosthesis-patient mismatch (PPM) (Figs. 79.3 and 79.4).[4,5,46] Cinefluoroscopy and ECG-gated cardiac CT may also be helpful to evaluate leaflet mobility in mechanical and bioprosthetic valves, respectively.[5] Prosthetic valve stenosis may be caused by thrombus formation, pannus ingrowth (or a combination of both) (see Figs. 16.55 and 20.21), leaflet calcification in the case of bioprosthetic valves, and vegetations. Prosthetic valve regurgitation may be related to thrombus formation (mechanical valves), leaflet tear (bioprostheses), vegetations, or PVL.

Prosthesis-Patient Mismatch

PPM occurs when the size of a normally functioning prosthetic valve is too small in relation to the patient's body size and thus to the patient's cardiac output requirements, resulting in abnormally high postoperative gradients. PPM is defined as an indexed EOA <0.85 cm² (severe:

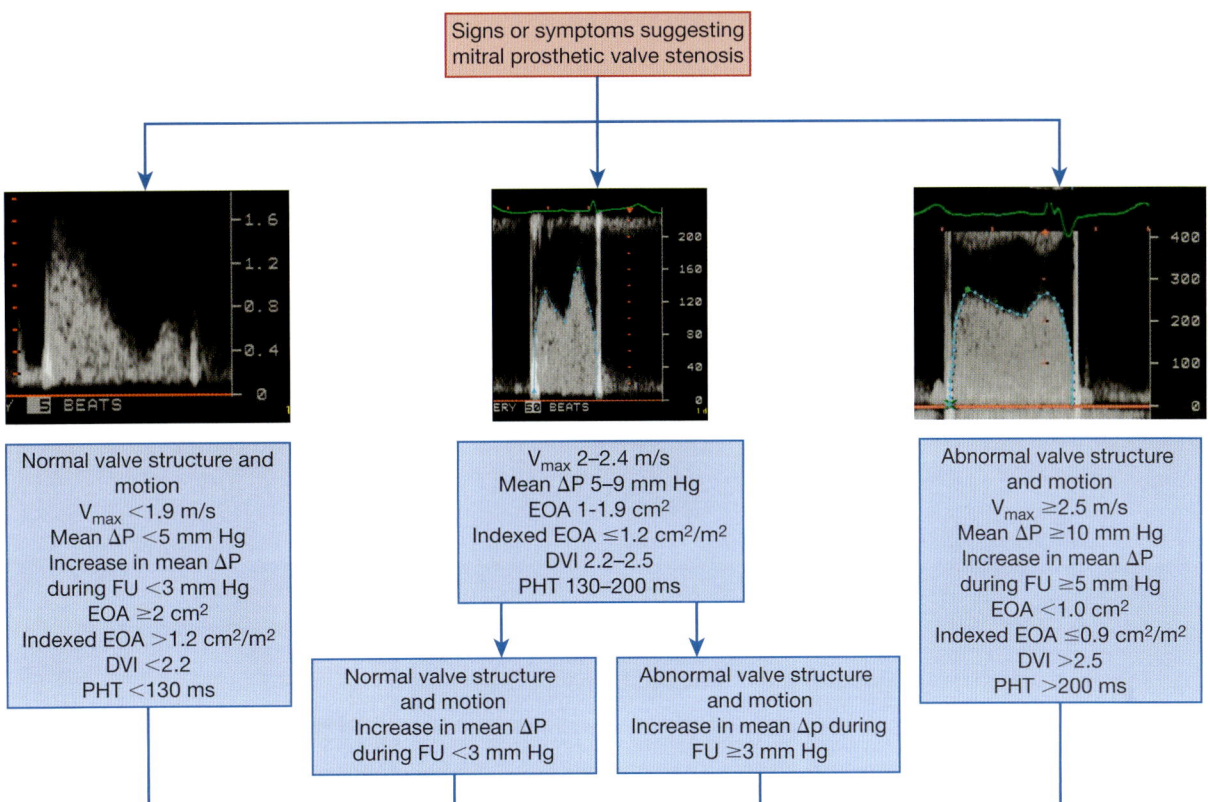

FIGURE 79.4 Evaluation of mitral prosthetic valve stenosis. The evaluation starts with standard measures of stenosis severity including maximal velocity (V_{max}), mean pressure gradient (mean ΔP), effective orifice area (EOA), and pressure half-time (PHT). Doppler velocity index (DVI) is the ratio of mitral to left ventricular outflow tract velocity, and therefore an elevated value is abnormal. Normal values for each valve type and size should be referenced, but the thresholds shown are a quick first step. In patients with intermediate measures of stenosis severity, the differential diagnosis includes significant stenosis, prosthesis-patient mismatch (PPM), and a high flow state. Additional imaging including transesophageal echocardiography, cinefluoroscopy, or cardiac CT may be needed to assess valve leaflet structure and motion. *FU*, Follow-up.

<0.65 cm^2) for aortic prosthetic valves and EOA <1.2 cm^2 (severe: <0.9 cm^2) for mitral prosthetic valves. The prevalence of moderate PPM ranges from 20% to 70% and that of severe PPM from 2% to 10% following AVR or MVR, respectively.[49] Patients with aortic PPM have higher functional class and worse exercise capacity, reduced regression of LV hypertrophy, more adverse cardiac events, and increased risk of both perioperative and late mortality after SAVR when compared with patients who do not have PPM.[49] Patients with mitral PPM have persisting pulmonary hypertension and increased incidence of congestive heart failure and death. A greater clinical impact of aortic PPM is also observed in specific groups of patients such as those with preexisting LV dysfunction or severe LV hypertrophy, and/or concomitant MR, as well as in those <65 to 70 years old. PPM is less frequent with TAVR compared with SAVR, particularly in the subset of patients with a small aortic annulus.[25,50] To reduce the incidence of postoperative PPM, aortic root enlargement is often performed to allow for implantation of a larger prosthesis. Figures 79.3 and 79.4 provide algorithms for differentiating between normal prosthetic valve function, PPM, and intrinsic valve dysfunction due to SVD, thrombus, or pannus.

Structural Valve Deterioration

Mechanical prostheses have an excellent durability, and SVD is extremely rare with contemporary valves. On the other hand, SVD due to leaflet calcification and/or collagen fiber disruption is the major cause of bioprosthetic valve failure. SVD may lead to leaflet stiffening and progressive stenosis or leaflet tear with transvalvular regurgitation[13,51] (Fig. 79.5; see also Fig. 16.56). Although SVD of bioprostheses has long been considered a purely passive degenerative process, more recent studies suggest that active and potentially modifiable processes may be involved including lipid infiltration, inflammation, immune rejection, and active mineralization. Transcatheter valve-in-valve implantation offers a valuable alternative to surgery for patients with failed bioprosthetic valves who are at higher risk for reoperation (see Chapters 74 and 78). Nearly 4500 valve-in-valve implants were reported to the STS/ACC TVT Registry in 2019.[2]

Paravalvular Leak

PVL occurs external to the prosthetic valve at the interface between the valve ring and the native valve annulus (see Fig. 79.5). It can occur as a result of inadequate technique, suture dehiscence, compromised native tissue integrity (dense calcification, extensive myxomatous degeneration), infection, or chronic abrasion of the sewing ring against a calcified or rigid annulus. The magnitude of the regurgitant volume will depend on the size of the orifice. A small and hemodynamically inconsequential PVL is usually discovered incidentally during routine TTE with color Doppler flow imaging. No change in management would be indicated. Small PVLs may, however, be associated with significant intravascular hemolysis and anemia as red blood cells are forced through a narrow orifice at high velocities. Despite a high clinical index of suspicion in this circumstance, a new, regurgitant murmur may not be audible. TEE may be necessary to differentiate paravalvular versus transvalvular regurgitation and to visualize the defect appropriately, especially with mitral prostheses. Larger PVLs may result in significant volume overload and heart failure, to an extent that reoperation or catheter closure with an occluder device might be indicated. Significant PVL may develop during the late postoperative period and if such is the case, this is often the result of endocarditis. Management can prove quite challenging and a conservative approach with medical therapy may be chosen.

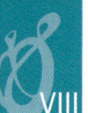

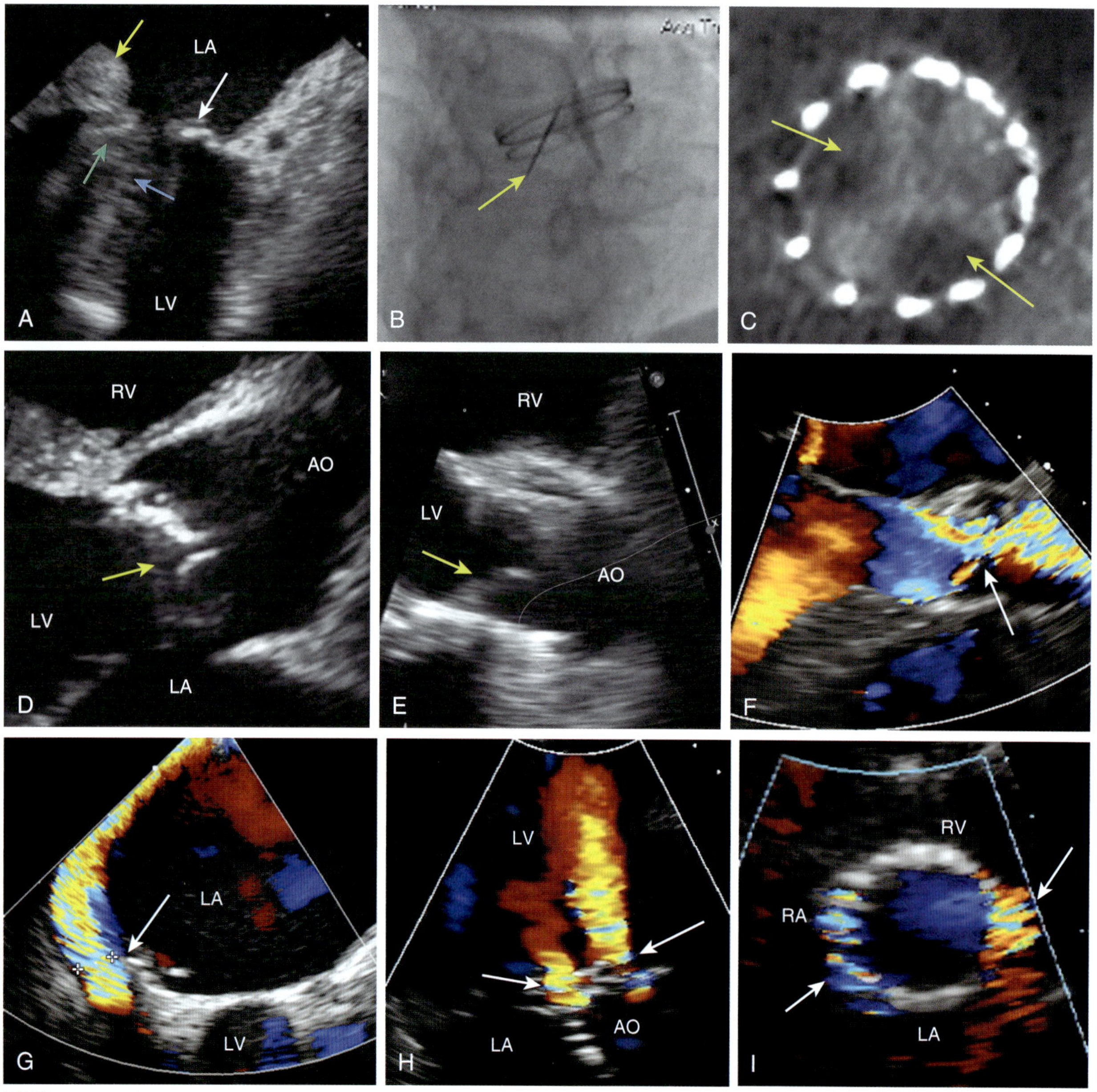

FIGURE 79.5 Imaging of prosthetic valve dysfunction. **A,** Transesophageal echocardiographic view of an obstructed mitral bileaflet mechanical valve. *Yellow arrow,* large-size thrombus; *white arrow,* pannus; *blue arrow,* mobile leaflet; *green arrow,* immobile leaflet. **B,** Cinefluoroscopy of bileaflet mechanical valve showing an immobile leaflet (*yellow arrow*). **C,** Multi-detector computed tomography with contrast injection showing an area of hypoattenuation (*yellow arrows*) indicating thrombi on two of the leaflets of a balloon expandable transcatheter valve. **D,** Transthoracic echocardiographic view of a stented bioprosthetic valve with calcific degeneration, thickening, and reduced mobility of the leaflets (*yellow arrow*). **E** and **F,** Transthoracic echocardiographic views of an obstructive valve leaflet thrombus in a balloon-expandable transcatheter aortic valve. The leaflets are thickened (**E,** *yellow arrow*) and the width of the transprosthetic flow jet on color-Doppler is narrowed (**F,** *white arrow*); **G,** Transesophageal color Doppler echocardiographic view of a severe paravalvular leak (*white arrow*) in a mitral mechanical valve; **H** and **I,** Transthoracic color Doppler echocardiographic views (**H,** apical three-chamber; **I,** parasternal short-axis) of two paravalvular regurgitant jets (*white arrows*) in a transcatheter aortic valve. (Courtesy Dr. Steven A. Goldstein, Washington Hospital Center **(A)**; Dr. John Chambers, Guy's and St. Thomas Hospitals, London, UK **(D)**; and Dr Arsène Basmadjian, Montreal Heart Institute, Montreal, Canada **(G)**.)

PVL is more frequent following TAVR compared with SAVR (see Chapter 74); its incidence is significantly lower with newer generation TAVR bioprostheses.[26,52,53] Because PVL jets after TAVR are often multiple, irregular, and eccentric, the imaging and grading of PVL can be challenging (see Fig. 79.5; see also Fig. 16.57). A multi-window, multi-parametric, integrative approach is essential to assess the severity of PVL by Doppler-echocardiography (see Chapter 16).[46-48] Other imaging modalities, such as cineangiography, cardiac CT, and cardiac magnetic resonance, as well as serum biomarkers, may also be useful to complement or corroborate the findings on TTE and TEE. The use of corrective procedures such as repeat balloon dilation, valve-in-valve implantation, and/or transcatheter leak closure may be considered depending on the severity of PVL and the risk of procedural complications.

Thromboembolism and Bleeding

Thromboembolisms are a major source of morbidity in patients with prosthetic heart valves. The incidence of clinically recognizable events ranges from 0.6% to 2.3% per patient-year,[6] an estimate that does not account for any subclinical episodes, which might be detected with sensitive imaging techniques.[54] Thromboembolic incidence rates are similar for nonanticoagulated patients with bioprostheses and appropriately anticoagulated patients with mechanical valves. Risk factors for thromboembolism include the inherent thrombogenicity of the prosthesis, valve position (mitral > aortic), valve number, time spent out of the therapeutic range of VKA anticoagulation, a history of thromboembolism, hypercoagulable state, atrial fibrillation, left atrial enlargement, and LV systolic dysfunction. The risk of bleeding, estimated at 1% per patient-year, increases with age and the intensity of anticoagulation. In patients with uncontrollable bleeding who require reversal of anticoagulation, administration of prothrombin complex concentrate is reasonable.[6] Antidotes to oral anti-Xa and antithrombin agents are also available.

Management of a thromboembolic event in patients with mechanical valves generally proceeds along one or more of the following lines: (1) For patients whose INR is subtherapeutic, the dose of the VKA is advanced to achieve the intended INR range; (2) for patients whose INR is in the therapeutic range, the dose of the VKA is advanced to achieve a higher INR range and/or low-dose aspirin is added if not already used; (3) the patient and family are informed about the increased risks of bleeding; (4) the potential for drug interactions is reviewed. Reoperation to implant a less thrombogenic valve is rarely undertaken for patients with recurrent thromboemboli despite aggressive antithrombotic therapy.

Prosthetic Valve Thrombosis (see Chapter 20)

The incidence of mechanical valve thrombosis is estimated at 0.3% to 1.3% per patient-year in high-income countries, but as high as 6% per patient-year in low- to middle-income countries.[6] Thrombosis of a mechanical heart valve can have devastating consequences (see Figs. 79.2 and 79.5; see also Fig. 16.54). Bioprosthetic (surgical or transcatheter) valve thrombosis is less common but does occur (see Figs. 20.21 and 20.24). A CT substudy of the PARTNER 3 trial observed a 30-day incidence of 13% among TAVR patients versus 5% for SAVR patients (see Chapter 74).[22] However, 56% of patients with HALT at 30 days showed resolution by 1 year, whereas 21% of patients without HALT at 30 days had evidence of leaflet thrombosis at 1 year. The 1-year prevalence of HALT was 28% for TAVR patients and 20% for SAVR patients.[22] The CT substudy of the EVOLUT Low Risk trial reported similar incidence of HALT in TAVR versus SAVR at 30 days (17.3% versus 16.5%) and 1 year (31% versus 27%).[24] Oral anticoagulation is reasonable for patients with bioprosthetic valve thrombosis and clinical symptoms (thromboembolism) or progressive prosthetic valve gradients with evidence of leaflet dysfunction; a VKA may be preferred.[6] The clinical significance and benefit of treatment for subclinical leaflet thrombosis is less clear (see Figs. 79.2 and 79.5).[22,23,55]

Clinical suspicion of mechanical prosthetic valve thrombosis should be raised by symptoms of heart failure, thromboembolism, and/or low cardiac output, coupled with a decrease in the intensity of the valve closure sounds new and pathologic murmurs and/or documentation of inadequate anticoagulation. Thrombosis is more common in the mitral and tricuspid positions than in the aortic position. Although differentiation from pannus formation can be difficult, the clinical context usually allows accurate diagnosis. Evaluation with TTE/TEE can help guide management decisions.[4,5] Confirmation of abnormal leaflet or disc excursion in the presence of an occluding thrombus can also be obtained with cinefluoroscopy or ECG-gated cardiac CT (see Fig. 79.5; see also Fig 20.20D).[5,22,24,56]

Emergency surgery is reasonable for patients with left-sided mechanical valve thrombosis and shock or New York Heart Association (NYHA) functional class III to IV symptoms and for patients with a large thrombus burden (≥0.8 cm² on TEE).[6] Slow infusion, low-dose fibrinolytic therapy is reasonable for patients with recent onset (<2 weeks) NYHA class I to II symptoms and small thrombus burden (<0.8 cm²) or for sicker patients with larger thrombi when surgery is either not available or inadvisable. Fibrinolytic therapy is generally recommended for patients with right-sided prosthetic valve thrombosis.[6] Some patients with no or minimal symptoms and small thrombi can often be managed with intravenous UFH alone and then converted to fibrinolytic therapy if unsuccessful. Any course of fibrinolytic therapy is followed at the appropriate interval by a continuous infusion of UFH during the transition to VKA therapy targeted to a higher INR with or without low-dose aspirin. Serial TTE studies are useful to assess the response to treatment.

Infective Endocarditis (see Chapter 80)

PVE is the most severe form of infective endocarditis and occurs in 1% to 6% of patients with valve prostheses accounting for 10% to 30% of all cases of infective endocarditis (see Chapter 80).[33,57] PVE is an extremely serious condition with high in-hospital mortality rates (20% to 50%). The diagnosis based on the Modified Duke Criteria relies predominantly on the combination of positive blood cultures and echocardiographic evidence of prosthetic valve infection, including vegetations, paravalvular abscess, or a new paravalvular regurgitation.[33] TEE is essential in patients with prosthetic valves because of its greater sensitivity in detecting these abnormalities (see Figs. 80.6 and 80.7). Increased uptake of ¹⁸Fluorodeoxyglucose measured by positron emission tomography CT (PET-CT) may improve the early diagnosis of PVE (see Figs. 18.40 and 18.41).[58-60] Despite prompt and appropriate antibiotic treatment, many patients with PVE will eventually require surgery. Medical treatment alone is more likely to succeed in late PVE (occurring >6 months after surgery) and in nonstaphylococcal infections. Surgery should be considered in the following situations: heart failure; failure of antibiotic treatment; hemodynamically significant prosthetic valve regurgitation, especially if associated with deterioration of LV function; large vegetations (>10 mm in size); persistently positive blood cultures on therapy; recurrent emboli with persistent vegetations; and intracardiac fistula formation.[6] PVE after TAVR occurs predominantly within the first year after the procedure. Its incidence is low (0.5% to 1% per patient-year) but in-hospital (~35%) and 2-year (~67%) mortality rates are high,[61] likely reflective of patient age and comorbidities.

Hemolytic Anemia

The development of a non-immune hemolytic anemia after valve replacement or repair is usually attributable to PVL with intravascular red blood cell destruction. Diagnosis is based on a high index of suspicion, coupled with laboratory evidence of hemolysis, including the characteristic changes in red blood cells morphology (schistocytes), elevated indirect bilirubin and LDH, a high reticulocyte count, and depressed serum haptoglobin. Reoperative surgery or catheter closure of the defect is indicated when heart failure, a persistent transfusion requirement, or poor quality of life intervenes. Empiric medical measures include iron and folic acid replacement therapy and beta-adrenoreceptor blockers. It is important to exclude PVE as a cause.

CLASSIC REFERENCES

Hammermeister K, Sethi GK, Henderson WG, et al. Outcomes 15 years after valve replacement with a mechanical versus a bioprosthetic valve: final report of the veterans affairs randomized trial. *J Am Coll Cardiol.* 2000;36:1152–1158.

REFERENCES

1. Nishimura RA, O'Gara PT, Bavaria JE, et al. 2019 AATS/ACC/ASE/SCAI/STS expert consensus systems of care document: a proposal to optimize care for patients with valvular heart disease: a joint report of the American Association for Thoracic Surgery, American College of Cardiology, American Society of Echocardiography, Society for Cardiovascular Angiography and Interventions and Society of Thoracic Surgeons. *J Am Coll Cardiol.* 2019;73:2609–2635.
2. Carroll JD, Mack MJ, Vemulapalli S, et al. STS-ACC TVT registry of transcatheter aortic valve replacement. *J Am Coll Cardiol.* 2020;76:2492–2516.
3. Vemulapalli S, Dai D, Hammill BG, et al. Hospital resource utilization before and after transcatheter aortic valve replacement: the STS/ACC TVT registry. *J Am Coll Cardiol.* 2019;73:1135–1146.

Types of Prosthetic Heart Valves

4. Zoghbi WA, Chambers JB, Dumesnil JG, et al. Recommendations for evaluation of prosthetic valves with echocardiography and Doppler ultrasound: a report from the American Society of Echocardiography's guidelines and standards committee and the task force on prosthetic valves, developed in conjunction with the American College of Cardiology Cardiovascular Imaging Committee, Cardiac Imaging Committee of the American Heart Association, the European Association of Echocardiography, a registered branch of the European Society of Cardiology, the Japanese Society of Echocardiography and the Canadian Society of Echocardiography, endorsed by the American College of Cardiology Foundation, American Heart Association, European Association of Echocardiography, a registered branch of the European Society of Cardiology, the Japanese Society of Echocardiography, and Canadian Society of Echocardiography. *J Am Soc Echocardiogr.* 2009;22:975–1014.
5. Lancellotti P, Pibarot P, Chambers J, et al. Recommendations for the imaging assessment of prosthetic heart valves: a report from the European Association of Cardiovascular imaging endorsed by the Chinese Society of Echocardiography, the Interamerican Society of Echocardiography and the Brazilian Department of Cardiovascular Imaging. *Eur Heart J Cardiovasc Imaging.* 2016;17:589–590.
6. Otto CM, Nishimura RA, Bonow RO, et al. 2020 ACC/AHA guideline for the management of patients with valvular heart disease: executive summary: a report of the American College of Cardiology/American Heart Association joint committee on clinical practice guidelines. *J Am Coll Cardiol.* 2021;77:e25–e197.
7. Puskas JD, Bavaria JE, Svensson LG, et al. The COMMENCE trial: 2-year outcomes with an aortic bioprosthesis with RESILIA tissue. *Eur J Cardio Thorac Surg.* 2017;52:432–439.
8. Meuris B, Borger MA, Bourguignon T, et al. Durability of bioprosthetic aortic valves in patients under the age of 60 years - rationale and design of the international INDURE registry. *J Cardiothorac Surg.* 2020;15:119.
8a. Lorusso R, Folliguet T, Shrestha M, et al. Sutureless versus stented bioprostheses for aortic valve replacement: the randomized PERSIST-AVR study design. *Thorac Cardiovasc Surg.* 2020;68:114–123.
8b. Szecel D, Eurlings R, Rega F, et al. Perceval sutureless aortic valve implantation: mid-term outcomes. *Ann Thorac Surg.* 2021;111:1331–1337.
9. Johnston DR, Soltesz EG, Vakil N, et al. Long-term durability of bioprosthetic aortic valves: implications from 12,569 implants. *Ann Thorac Surg.* 2015;99:1239–1247.
10. Bourguignon T, Bouquiaux-Stablo AL, Candolfi P, et al. Very long-term outcomes of the Carpentier-Edwards Perimount valve in aortic position. *Ann Thorac Surg.* 2015;99:831–837.
11. Rodriguez-Gabella T, Voisine P, Dagenais F, et al. Long-term outcomes following surgical aortic bioprosthesis implantation. *J Am Coll Cardiol.* 2018;71:1401–1412.
12. Salaun E, Mahjoub H, Dahou A, et al. Hemodynamic deterioration of surgically implanted bioprosthetic aortic valves. *J Am Coll Cardiol.* 2018;72:241–251.
13. Salaun E, Clavel MA, Rodés-Cabau J, Pibarot P. Bioprosthetic aortic valve durability in the era of transcatheter aortic valve implantation. *Heart.* 2018;104:1323–1332.

14. Sondergaard L, Costa G. Transcatheter aortic valve replacement in patients with aortic stenosis and low surgical risk. *J Am Coll Cardiol.* 2019;74:1541–1542.
15. Sénage T, Le Tourneau T, Foucher Y, et al. Early structural valve deterioration of Mitroflow aortic bioprosthesis: mode, incidence, and impact on outcome in a large cohort of patients. *Circulation.* 2014;130:2012–2020.
16. Kunadian B, Vijayalakshmi K, Thornley AR, et al. Meta-analysis of valve hemodynamics and left ventricular mass regression for stentless versus stented aortic valves. *Ann Thorac Surg.* 2007;84:73–78.
17. El-Hamamsy I, Eryigit Z, Stevens LM, et al. Long-term outcomes after autograft versus homograft aortic root replacement in adults with aortic valve disease: a randomised controlled trial. *Lancet.* 2010;376:524–531.
18. David TE, David C, Woo A, Manlhiot C. The Ross procedure: outcomes at 20 years. *J Thorac Cardiovasc Surg.* 2014;147:85–93.
19. Martin E, Mohammadi S, Jacques F, et al. Clinical outcomes following the Ross procedure in adults: a 25-year longitudinal study. *J Am Coll Cardiol.* 2017;70:1890–1899.

Transcatheter Bioprosthetic Valves

20. Mazine A, El-Hamamsy I, Verma S, et al. Ross procedure in adults for cardiologists and cardiac surgeons: JACC state-of-the-art review. *J Am Coll Cardiol.* 2018;72:2761–2777.
21. Lilly SM, Deshmukh AJ, Epstein AE, et al. 2020 ACC expert consensus decision pathway on management of conduction disturbances in patients undergoing transcatheter aortic valve replacement: a report of the American College of Cardiology Solution Set Oversight committee. *J Am Coll Cardiol.* 2020;76:2391–2411.
22. Makkar RR, Blanke P, Leipsic J, et al. Subclinical leaflet thrombosis in transcatheter and surgical bioprosthetic valves: PARTNER 3 cardiac computed tomography substudy. *J Am Coll Cardiol.* 2020;75:3003–3015.
23. De Backer O, Dangas GD, Jilaihawi H, et al. Reduced leaflet motion after transcatheter aortic-valve replacement. *N Engl J Med.* 2020;382:130–139.
24. Blanke P, Leipsic JA, Popma JJ, et al. Bioprosthetic aortic valve leaflet thickening in the Evolut low risk sub-study. *J Am Coll Cardiol.* 2020;75:2430–2442.
25. Pibarot P, Weissman N, Stewart W, et al. Reduced incidence of prosthesis-patient mismatch and its sequelae in transcatheter versus surgical valve replacement in high-risk patients with severe aortic stenosis: a PARTNER trial Cohort A analysis. *Circulation.* 2013;61:E1865.
26. Mack MJ, Leon MB, Thourani VH, et al. Transcatheter aortic-valve replacement with a balloon-expandable valve in low-risk patients. *N Engl J Med.* 2019;380:1695–1705.
27. Popma JJ, Deeb GM, Yakubov SJ, et al. Transcatheter aortic-valve replacement with a self-expanding valve in low-risk patients. *N Engl J Med.* 2019;380:1706–1715.
28. Pibarot P, Salaun E, Dahou A, et al. Echocardiographic results of transcatheter versus surgical aortic valve replacement in low-risk patients: the PARTNER 3 trial. *Circulation.* 2020;141:1527–1537.
29. Kodali SK, Williams MR, Smith CR, et al. Two-Year outcomes after transcatheter or surgical aortic-valve replacement. *N Engl J Med.* 2012;366:1686–1695.
30. Thourani VH, Kodali S, Makkar RR, et al. Transcatheter aortic valve replacement versus surgical valve replacement in intermediate-risk patients: a propensity score analysis. *Lancet.* 2016;387:2218–2225.
31. Abdel-Wahab M, Mehilli J, Frerker C, et al. Comparison of balloon-expandable vs self-expandable valves in patients undergoing transcatheter aortic valve replacement: the CHOICE randomized clinical trial. *J Am Med Assoc.* 2014;311:1503–1514.
32. Pibarot P, Ternacle J, Jaber WA, et al. Structural deterioration of transcatheter versus surgical aortic valve bioprostheses in the PARTNER-2 trial. *J Am Coll Cardiol.* 2020;76:1830–1843.

Comparison of Mechanical and Tissue Valves and Choice of Procedure and Prosthesis

33. Habib G, Lancellotti P, Antunes MJ, et al. 2015 ESC Guidelines for the management of infective endocarditis: the task force for the management of infective endocarditis of the European Society of Cardiology (ESC) endorsed by: European Association for Cardio-Thoracic Surgery (EACTS), the European Association of Nuclear Medicine (EANM). *Eur Heart J.* 2015;36:3075–3128.
34. Stassano P, Tommaso LD, Monaco M, et al. Aortic valve replacement: a prospective randomized evaluation of mechanical versus biological valves in patients ages 55 to 70 years. *J Am Coll Cardiol.* 2009;54:1868.
35. Brennan JM, Edwards FH, Zhao Y, et al. Long-term safety and effectiveness of mechanical versus biologic aortic valve prostheses in older patients: results from the Society of Thoracic Surgeons Adult Cardiac Surgery National Database. *Circulation.* 2013;127:1647–1655.
36. Chiang YP, Chikwe J, Moskowitz AJ, et al. Survival and long-term outcomes following bioprosthetic vs mechanical aortic valve replacement in patients aged 50 to 69 years. *J Am Med Assoc.* 2014;312:1323–1329.
37. Chikwe J, Chiang YP, Egorova NN, et al. Survival and outcomes following bioprosthetic vs mechanical mitral valve replacement in patients aged 50 to 69 years. *J Am Med Assoc.* 2015;313:1435–1442.
38. Glaser N, Jackson V, Holzmann MJ, et al. Aortic valve replacement with mechanical vs. biological prostheses in patients aged 50-69 years. *Eur Heart J.* 2016;37:2658–2667.
39. Goldstone AB, Chiu P, Baiocchi M, et al. Mechanical or biologic prostheses for aortic-valve and mitral-valve replacement. *N Engl J Med.* 2017;377:1847–1857.
40. Acker MA, Parides MK, Perrault LP, et al. Mitral-valve repair versus replacement for severe ischemic mitral regurgitation. *N Engl J Med.* 2014;370:23–32.
41. Stone GW, Lindenfeld J, Abraham WT, et al. Transcatheter mitral-valve repair in patients with heart failure. *N Engl J Med.* 2018;379:2307–2318.
42. Agricola E, Asmarats L, Maisano F, et al. Imaging for tricuspid valve repair and replacement. *JACC Cardiovasc Imaging.* 2021;14:61–111.

Medical Management and Surveillance After Valve Replacement

43. Brouwer J, Nijenhuis VJ, Delewi R, et al. Aspirin with or without clopidogrel after transcathetera Aortic-valve implantation. *N Engl J Med.* 2020;383:1447–1457.
44. Nijenhuis VJ, Brouwer J, Delewi R, et al. Anticoagulation with or without clopidogrel after transcatheter aortic-valve implantation. *N Engl J Med.* 2020;382:1696–1707.
45. Dangas GD, Tijssen JGP, Wöhrle J, et al. A controlled trial of rivaroxaban after transcatheter aortic-valve replacement. *N Engl J Med.* 2020;382:120–129.
46. Zoghbi WA, Asch FM, Bruce C, et al. Guidelines for the evaluation of valvular regurgitation after percutaneous valve repair or replacement: a report from the American Society of Echocardiography developed in collaboration with the Society for Cardiovascular Angiography and interventions, Japanese Society of Echocardiography, and Society for Cardiovascular Magnetic Resonance. *J Am Soc Echocardiogr.* 2019;32:431–475.
47. Pibarot P, Hahn RT, Weissman NJ, Monaghan MJ. Assessment of paravalvular regurgitation following TAVR: a proposal of unifying grading scheme. *JACC Cardiovasc Imaging.* 2015;8:340–360.
48. Kappetein AP, Head SJ, Généreux P, et al. Updated standardized endpoint definitions for transcatheter aortic valve implantation: the Valve Academic Research Consortium-2 consensus document. *Eur J Cardio Thorac Surg.* 2012;42:S45–S60.

Prosthetic Valve Dysfunction and Complications

49. Pibarot P, Dumesnil JG. Valve prosthesis-patient mismatch, 1978 to 2011: from original concept to compelling evidence. *J Am Coll Cardiol.* 2012;60:1136–1139.
50. Zorn 3rd GL, Little SH, Tadros P, et al. Prosthesis-patient mismatch in high-risk patients with severe aortic stenosis: a randomized trial of a self-expanding prosthesis. *J Thorac Cardiovasc Surg.* 2016;151:1014–1023.e3.
51. Rodriguez-Gabella T, Voisine P, Puri R, et al. Aortic bioprosthetic valve durability incidence, mechanisms, predictors, and management of surgical and transcatheter valve degeneration. *J Am Coll Cardiol.* 2017;70:1013–1028.
52. Thiele H, Kurz T, Feistritzer HJ, et al. Comparison of newer generation self-expandable vs. balloon-expandable valves in transcatheter aortic valve implantation: the randomized SOLVE-TAVI trial. *Eur Heart J.* 2020;41:1890–1899.
53. Kolte D, Vlahakes GJ, Palacios IF, et al. Transcatheter versus surgical aortic valve replacement in low-risk patients. *J Am Coll Cardiol.* 2019;74:1532–1540.
54. Al-Atassi T, Lam K, Forgie M, et al. Cerebral microembolization after bioprosthetic aortic valve replacement: comparison of warfarin plus aspirin versus aspirin only. *Circulation.* 2012;126:S239–S244.
55. Latib A, Naganuma T, Abdel-Wahab M, et al. Treatment and clinical outcomes of transcatheter heart valve thrombosis. *Circ Cardiovasc Interv.* 2015;8:1–8.
56. Makkar RR, Fontana G, Jilaihawi H, et al. Possible subclinical leaflet thrombosis in bioprosthetic aortic valves. *N Engl J Med.* 2015;373:2015–2024.
57. Habib G, Erba PA, Iung B, et al. Clinical presentation, aetiology and outcome of infective endocarditis. Results of the ESC-EORP EURO-ENDO (European Infective Endocarditis) registry: a prospective cohort study. *Eur Heart J.* 2019;40:3222–3232.
58. Saby L, Laas O, Habib G, et al. Positron emission tomography/computed tomography for diagnosis of prosthetic valve endocarditis: increased valvular 18F-fluorodeoxyglucose uptake as a novel major criterion. *J Am Coll Cardiol.* 2013;61:2374–2382.
59. San S, Ravis E, Tessonier L, et al. Prognostic value of (18)F-fluorodeoxyglucose positron emission tomography/computed tomography in infective endocarditis. *J Am Coll Cardiol.* 2019;74:1031–1040.
60. Regueiro A, Linke A, Latib A, et al. Association between transcatheter aortic valve replacement and subsequent infective endocarditis and in-hospital death. *J Am Med Assoc.* 2016;316:1083–1092.
61. Summers MR, Leon MB, Smith CR, et al. Prosthetic valve endocarditis after TAVR and SAVR: insights from the PARTNER trials. *Circulation.* 2019;140:1984–1994.

80 Infectious Endocarditis and Infections of Indwelling Devices

LARRY M. BADDOUR, NANDAN S. ANAVEKAR, JUAN A. CRESTANELLO, AND WALTER R. WILSON

INFECTIVE ENDOCARDITIS, 1505
Epidemiology, 1505
Pathogenesis, 1507
Clinical Presentation, 1507
Symptoms, 1508
Physical Examination, 1508
Diagnosis, 1510
Indications for and Timing of Surgery, 1523
Outpatient Management and Follow-Up Evaluation, 1525

CARDIOVASCULAR IMPLANTABLE ELECTRONIC DEVICE INFECTIONS, 1526
Epidemiology, 1526
Clinical Syndromes, 1526
Microbiology, 1526
Pathogenesis, 1526
Diagnosis, 1526
Management, 1526
Prophylaxis, 1528

LEFT VENTRICULAR ASSIST DEVICE INFECTIONS, 1528
Microbiology, 1528
Management, 1528
Prevention, 1528

REFERENCES, 1529

Infections involving the heart valves (infectious endocarditis [IE]) and those that involve cardiovascular devices, including permanent pacemakers, implantable cardioverter-defibrillators (ICDs), coronary stents, and ventricular assist devices, are associated with substantial morbidity and mortality. As indications for devices continue to expand, infectious complications, including those that may require device removal, are becoming more commonplace. Because IE and other types of cardiovascular infections are often caused by multidrug-resistant (MDR) organisms acquired in the health care setting, there are fewer drugs are available for treating these infections and increased likelihood of drug-related toxicities. In addition, longer durations of therapy may be needed, which can increase the rate of drug-induced adverse events. These factors call for a multidisciplinary approach to cardiac infections.

INFECTIVE ENDOCARDITIS

IE has the proclivity to cause complications both at the cardiac valve site and at extracardiac locations that can predispose affected patients to serious morbidity and mortality. Management of IE therefore requires a team approach, which generally includes, at a minimum, specialists in infectious diseases, cardiovascular medicine, and cardiovascular surgery with particular expertise in IE. Thus every patient with IE should be managed in the inpatient setting of a medical center with experienced medical and surgical specialists to provide care, which often includes emergent diagnostic and surgical interventions. This "team" approach in IE management is warranted in medical centers that care for IE patients, and this approach of diagnosis and management has resulted in improved outcomes.

Epidemiology

The global burden of disease from IE is largely unknown. Much of the world's population lives in developing countries, where many people do not have routine access to advanced medical care, and usually no local or national infrastructure exists for disease reporting (see Chapter 2). Thus the clinical characterization of IE is biased, shaped by the collective experiences at large teaching facilities in countries where patient access is available and disease reporting is done. However, even in many developed countries, including the United States, IE is not included among the diagnoses requiring mandatory reporting to public health agencies that would define a statewide or national disease incidence or burden.

IE is a heterogeneous syndrome that is heavily influenced by the epidemiology of the infection. For example, in developing countries where rheumatic fever is still endemic, younger adults with longstanding rheumatic heart disease frequently present with a subacute clinical course spanning several weeks that involves left-sided native valve infection caused by viridans group streptococci (VGS). In contrast, in large, teaching, tertiary care centers in developed countries, patients with previous health care exposure frequently present with an acute illness that can be measured in days and is caused primarily by *Staphylococcus aureus*, with numerous anatomic sites of metastatic foci of infection and worse outcomes. Injection drug use (IDU) as a complication of the opioid epidemic currently active in the United States is another factor contributing to the escalating rate of IE due to *S. aureus* and has been prominent in rural settings. All types of care centers have provided care for these patients who are often seen in primary care settings initially with subsequent transfer to larger institutions with IE expertise.

The incidence of IE is influenced by multiple host factors that modify the risk of infection. Such factors include the underlying anatomic (usually valvular) cardiac conditions that result in turbulent blood flow and endothelial cell disruption (see later, Pathogenesis). In addition, aging of the population in developed countries has resulted in more patients with myxomatous degeneration of the mitral valve, with subsequent prolapse and insufficiency (see Chapter 76). At the same time, a dramatic fall in the incidence of rheumatic fever in developed countries has reduced the overall risk of IE in younger persons. Advances in medicine also alter the incidence of IE. For example, reduced use of tunneled catheters and increasing use of arteriovenous fistulas for chronic hemodialysis will reduce the risk of bloodstream infection and complicating IE. Improvement in oral health in developed countries also may affect the incidence of IE, but this notion remains to be proven.

Population-based studies[1,2] have been used to estimate both the incidence of IE and its clinical characterization, but complete case ascertainment is difficult to secure. For example, in the United States, patients may receive medical care in locations that are not in their place of residence. Thus large medical centers that have unique team expertise in IE management may be unable to obtain complete case ascertainment in a population because of changing referral patterns or second-party coverage. Data generated from a population-based investigation will have limited applicability (generalizability) if the cohort under study is not representative of other populations in demographic or clinical features.

Incidence studies of IE are limited in number and in geographic coverage of populations. Adjusted annual incidence rates reported among more recent surveys from Western Europe and Olmsted County, Minnesota, have varied and have ranged from approximately 3 to 14 cases per 100,000 persons annually.[3] Incidence trends have slowly increased in some countries with an expected increase due to increased IDU in the United States (see later). Historically, a sex predilection has been noted, with males more often affected by IE, and has been, in part, due to IDU, which more frequently is reported among men. This male predominance may be fading; an increasing prevalence of female IDU with IE has been noted in many rural areas in the United States in the current opioid epidemic.[4] In addition, the female incidence had increased with a high level of health care exposure cited as a predisposing condition for the development of IE in a recent analysis.[2] Health care exposure, including both nosocomial and non-nosocomial exposure, has been recognized only recently[2,5,6] as a major contributor to the development of IE. Not only do indwelling central venous catheters and hemodialysis predispose to bloodstream infection, but infection with antimicrobial resistant pathogens is more likely to occur as a consequence of health care–related exposure. The virulence of some of these pathogens, in particular methicillin-resistant S. aureus (MRSA), is notable and is associated with increased mortality in patients with IE.

As alluded to previously in this section, people who inject drugs (PWID) are a unique group at increased risk for IE and the current opioid epidemic has magnified the effect of IDU on IE in the United States. Surgery for drug use–associated IE increased 2.7-fold from 2011 to 2018, with higher rates observed in the East South Central and South Atlantic regions.[7] These patients tend to be young, male, and otherwise healthy, except for having hepatitis C virus infection, which is highly prevalent. The prevalence of human immunodeficiency virus (HIV) infection has been considerably less to date. The contact of these patients with the health care system often is limited to short stays in an emergency department (ED).

MICROBIOLOGY

A vast array of bacteria and fungi can cause IE,[8] as is evident in novel case reports and literature reviews of IE caused by unusual organisms. Although changes in the prevalence of pathogens causing IE have emerged in recent years because of critical changes in the epidemiology of IE in developed countries,[2,9] the overall distribution of infecting organisms has remained the same, with gram-positive cocci being predominant. These include streptococcal, staphylococcal, and enterococcal species. Important virulence factors unique to each genus group appear to be operative in infection pathogenesis (see later). It is therefore not surprising that the modified Duke criteria[10] listed only these three groups of pathogens as "typical microorganisms" in the designation of the major criterion of "blood culture positive" for IE (see later).

Streptococcal Species

Among streptococci, the VGS are the predominant organisms that cause IE. A "subacute" presentation is typical, with symptoms of infection present for weeks to a few months, with low-grade fever, night sweats, and fatigue being common. These organisms normally are found in the mouth of humans and tend to cause indolent infections. Sustained bacteremia due to this group of bacteria should prompt a consideration of the diagnosis of IE, as few other infection syndromes cause sustained bloodstream infection. The viridans group includes several evolving species of streptococci and currently includes *sanguis, oralis (mitis), salivarius, mutans, intermedius, anginosus,* and *constellatus.* The latter three species have been referred to the "*Streptococcus anginosus* or *S. milleri* group" and are unique in that they have a proclivity to produce abscess formation and metastatic infection foci, both within the heart and in extracardiac locations in IE patients.

The genera of *Gemella, Abiotrophia,* and *Granulicatella* have generally been included in discussions of VGS. For *Gemella,* one species designated as *morbillorum* was previously listed in the *Streptococcus* genus. These organisms can cause IE and exhibit metabolic characteristics similar to those previously referred to "nutritionally variant streptococci," and have been reassigned to *Abiotrophia* and *Granulicatella* genera. The recommended medical therapy for infections caused by these unique organisms is discussed later (see Antimicrobial Therapy).

The VGS constitute a predominant cause of native valve infection acquired in the community setting, in both developing and developed nations. A common substrate for infection from these organisms has been rheumatic valvular disease, but as mentioned, the incidence of acute rheumatic fever has fallen dramatically in developed countries.

Similar to other bacteria, VGS have developed resistance to some antibiotics. Fortunately, resistance to penicillin is seen in a small minority of IE isolates. Resistance is not based on beta-lactamase production, and the definitions used[8] to characterize strains as being "penicillin resistant" are not the same as the break points recommended by the Clinical and Laboratory Standards Institute (CLSI). This distinction can be confusing because selection of antibiotic therapy is based on in vitro susceptibility results.

In contrast to VGS, beta-hemolytic streptococci typically cause an acute presentation of IE. PWID and elderly persons are two at-risk groups. Complications are common and often involve valve destruction and extracardiac sites, frequently musculoskeletal, of infection. The prevalence of beta-hemolytic streptococci among cases of IE is less than 10%. Beta-hemolytic streptococci have remained uniquely susceptible to penicillin, with extremely rare exceptions. Nevertheless, it is prudent to obtain susceptibility testing on all IE-related isolates. Surgery is often required for management of severe valvular and perivalvular involvement (see later).

Streptococcus gallolyticus (formerly known as *S. bovis*) deserves particular attention. The organism usually is found in the gastrointestinal (GI) tract, and when recovered from blood culture, whether related to IE or not, an examination for an underlying GI lesion, including colon cancer, should be performed. Although it currently is the cause of less than 10% of cases of IE, the expectation is that it will become more prominent in aging populations and those with increasing restrictions on cancer prevention screening.

Historically, IE from *Streptococcus pneumoniae* has received considerable attention. Although it continues to be a common cause of community-acquired bloodstream infection that often is related to pneumonia, it is a rare cause of IE today. When *S. pneumoniae* does cause IE, the clinical presentation is usually acute and associated with valve destruction. It can be associated with meningitis as well as other intracranial complications. Invasive isolates of pneumococci tend to be penicillin susceptible, but susceptibility testing is required to confirm this notion. As with IE from beta-hemolytic streptococci, surgery often is required to address valve-related complications.

Staphylococcal Species

Staphylococci are gram-positive cocci that are well recognized as causes of IE. *S. aureus* is a common cause of both native and prosthetic valve endocarditis (PVE).[8,9] The presentation in cases caused by *S. aureus* is acute in onset and often associated with considerable systemic toxicity. In cases of left-sided heart infection, morbidity and mortality rates are high, despite appropriate therapy, including surgical intervention. Right-sided heart infection, predominantly of the tricuspid valve in PWID, has a much higher cure rate than that for left-sided heart infection, and mortality rates are low, unless bilateral infection is present. Unfortunately, the rate of IE from *S. aureus* is increasing, in part because of an increased exposure to health care and IDU. *S. aureus* predominates in both PWID and non–drug users with IE and accounted for 42.1% of IE related to drug use versus 24.3% of non–drug use IE cases who underwent valve surgery in one large series.[7] In addition, resistance to oxacillin and other antibiotics also has increased, which has made treatment more difficult.

Although coagulase-negative staphylococci are recognized as frequent pathogens of prosthetic valve infection, they also can infrequently cause native valve infection. Although these infections usually are subacute in presentation, the morbidity and mortality associated with IE caused by coagulase-negative staphylococci are considerable. Of the more than 30 species of coagulase-negative staphylococci, two deserve special attention. *Staphylococcus epidermidis* is the most commonly identified species to cause bacteremia and IE. *Staphylococcus lugdunensis* is another species that causes both native and PVE and tends to be more virulent than the other species of coagulase-negative staphylococci. Because this group of organisms is the most common cause of contaminated blood cultures, a delay in diagnosis can be due to misinterpretation of blood culture results. Multiple sets of blood culture specimens should therefore be collected to better distinguish contamination from bloodstream infection. Except for *S. lugdunensis*, which usually is penicillin susceptible, other species of coagulase-negative staphylococci are more drug resistant, and, accordingly, fewer treatment options exist.

Enterococcal Species

Age is strongly associated with the development of IE caused by enterococcal species, with the prevalence of these organisms in IE cases doubling among elderly persons compared with young adults.

The large majority of IE cases is by *Enterococcus faecalis* and is associated with genitourinary (GU) tract abnormalities. In the past, enterococcal IE was community acquired, and enterococci were well recognized as part of the normal gut flora in humans. More recently, enterococcal species associated with health care exposure and central venous catheter use have caused IE, and typically presents subacutely. MDR enterococcal species, in particular *Enterococcus faecium*, can cause IE that is difficult to cure; this includes infection caused by vancomycin-resistant strains collectively termed *vancomycin-resistant enterococci* (VRE).

HACEK Organisms
HACEK organisms are fastidious gram-negative bacilli comprising *Haemophilus* species (other than *H. influenzae*); *Aggregatibacter actinomycetemcomitans* (formerly *Actinobacillus actinomycetemcomitans*) and *Aggregatibacter aphrophilus* (formerly *Haemophilus aphrophilus*); *Cardiobacterium hominis*; *Eikenella corrodens*; and *Kingella kingae* and *Kingella denitrificans*. They colonize the oropharynx and upper respiratory tract, causing subacute IE presentation that is community acquired. Most of the organisms in blood cultures may require several days of incubation. Because of the indolent clinical course, diagnosis often is delayed, with the formation of large vegetations observed at echocardiography. As a result, embolism to the brain or other systemic sites occurs frequently.

Aerobic Gram-Negative Bacilli
In view of their universal causation of bloodstream infection, it is noteworthy that IE caused by aerobic gram-negative bacilli is rare. This observation attests to the particular virulence factors that characterize gram-positive cocci in IE pathogenesis and are not found in gram-negative bacilli. This group includes *Escherichia coli*, *Klebsiella* spp., *Enterobacter* spp., *Pseudomonas* spp., and others. In cases of IE caused by these organisms, presentations generally have been acute and sometimes associated with systemic toxicity, including sepsis and its complications. IE can be either community or health care associated. Outcomes of IE caused by aerobic gram-negative bacilli are characterized by increased morbidity and mortality rates.

Fungi
Fungi are extremely rare causes of IE. Identification of these organisms often is difficult because some do not grow in routine blood culture media. Even when selected culture media are used, fungal isolation may not be achieved. Thus fungi can cause either blood culture–positive or culture-negative IE.

The bulk of these infections are caused by *Candida* spp., although a broad array of fungi may cause IE. These infections usually are health care associated and involve prosthetic valves, often arising as a result of a central venous catheter infection. An indwelling right-heart catheter, such as a flotation catheter, can denude a valve and nonvalvular endothelial surface, predisposing the patient to fungal (or bacterial) right-sided IE. In addition, IDU is a well-recognized risk factor for fungal IE; in one multicenter investigation, fungal IE was twice as common in drug users (3.13%) as compared with that (1.5%) in non–drug users.[7]

Clinical presentations range in severity from acute to subacute. Complications are frequent, and surgical intervention is recommended as a routine intervention, particularly with infections caused by molds such as *Aspergillus* spp. Because relapsing IE is a concern and can be delayed in onset, many clinicians advocate the use of lifelong oral antifungal suppressive therapy, usually with an azole, after initial parenteral therapy is completed.

Culture-Negative Endocarditis
In most cases designated as blood culture–negative endocarditis, the pathogen is not recovered from blood cultures due to a patient's recent exposure to an antimicrobial that had suppressive or killing activity against the pathogen. In addition, with some uncommon causes of culture-negative endocarditis, the pathogen either will not grow in routine blood culture media or grows slowly in the media and is not detected in the time used for blood cultures. In the former scenario, nothing can be done. In the latter, blood cultures can be held for an extended period, at least 14 days, to determine if an isolate is recovered. Other techniques, such as special culture methods or serologic studies, also are used to isolate or identify infection. Organisms that should be included in this category include fungi, *Coxiella burnetii*, *Bartonella* spp., *Brucella* spp., *Tropheryma whippelii*, *Cutibacterium* (previously known as *Propionibacterium*) spp., and *Legionella* spp.

Pathogenesis
Two overarching aspects of endocarditis pathogenesis have been identified.[8] Already noted is a primary predilection for development of IE from an underlying valvular or nonvalvular cardiac structural abnormality that results in blood flow turbulence, endothelial disruption, and platelet and fibrin deposition. This lesion, termed *nonbacterial thrombotic endocarditis* (NBTE), serves as a nidus for subsequent adhesion by bacteria or fungi in the bloodstream. This pathway is thought to account for a majority of cases of IE, most often related to left-sided valvular stenosis or regurgitation. This picture of pathogenesis is mirrored, in many ways, in the animal model of endocarditis that has been used for decades to examine the pathogenesis, treatment, and prevention of IE. The microbiologic and histopathologic findings in infected animals reflect those seen in humans. A second factor is that infection may involve normal valves. Some reservations regarding this pathway of infection seem appropriate, because it is impossible to know if a valve is completely normal, including its endothelial surface, before onset of valve infection. In addition, animals do not develop experimental endocarditis after an intravascular challenge with a relatively large inoculum of virulent organisms, in particular *S. aureus*, in the absence of a previous disruption of the cardiac endothelial surface. Nevertheless, in vitro endothelial cell cultures studies have demonstrated uptake of organisms by endothelial cells.

The predominance of gram-positive cocci as causing IE deserves additional comment. Advances in molecular biologic techniques have resulted in the ability to define virulence factors that are unique to these organisms.[11] Infectivity studies that have compared "wild-type" parent strains to molecularly "engineered" strains using an experimental IE model have been of critical importance in defining virulence factors among strains of staphylococci, streptococci, and enterococci. Some of these factors serve as "adhesins" and are largely responsible for initial bacterial attachment to an NBTE nidus or to endothelial cells. They also are responsible for the attachment to medical devices, including prosthetic valves and cardiovascular implantable electronic device (CIED) leads. In this regard, biofilm formation occurs with some of these organisms and is important in both native tissue and prosthetic valve infections, in the context of factors responsible for the propagation of IE after initial bacterial attachment.

The findings from these investigations are expected to affect future treatment and prevention of IE. Novel vaccines containing bacterial proteins that function as adhesins and are good immunogens are being examined, for example, and already have proven to be efficacious in the prevention of experimental IE. In this case, the protein (FimA) is expressed by several VGS species in the pathogenesis of IE. In addition, it is conceivable that work focusing on treatment and prevention of dental caries by VGS could have some role in the management and prevention of IE.

Clinical Presentation
Predisposing Cardiac Conditions
Our understanding of predisposing conditions to IE has evolved over the decades since early clinical series were reported. More recently, the International Collaboration on Endocarditis–Prospective Cohort Study (ICE-PCS)[9] has detailed the clinical presentation in 2781 patients with definite IE. Native valve IE was predominant (72%), followed by PVE (21%) and permanent pacemaker or ICD IE (7%). Consistent with numerous earlier series, this international cohort study found that IE manifests with definite vegetations most frequently in the mitral valve position (41%), followed by the aortic valve position (38%), whereas the tricuspid (12%) and pulmonary (1%) valves were much less frequently involved.[9]

Preexisting valvular regurgitant lesions are much more prone to infection than stenotic lesions. It has been suggested that the incidence of IE is directly related to the impact of pressure on the closed valve, with shear stress disruption of the valvular endothelium in the vicinity of the egressing regurgitant jet. In the presence of the Venturi effect, circulating organisms are deposited within the high-velocity, lowered-pressure eddy zones of the regurgitant orifice of the receiving chamber, leading to the typical localization of vegetations on the upstream aspect of the infected valve.

Mitral regurgitation associated with degenerative mitral valve prolapse (MVP), particularly with advanced myxomatous leaflet thickening, is the most common predisposing condition for IE and is far more common than rheumatic mitral valve disease.[9] A recent population-based study demonstrated that an increased incidence of IE in patients with MVP was associated with either preexisting mitral regurgitation of at least moderate severity, or flail mitral leaflet.[12] Functional mitral regurgitation, associated with left ventricular (LV) remodeling causing malcoaptation of intrinsically normal mitral leaflets in a low-pressure, low-cardiac-output state (see Chapter 76), is quite uncommonly complicated by IE. The second most common native valve lesion predisposing to IE is aortic regurgitation. The risk of IE in patients with bicuspid aortic valve (BAV) is low (see Chapter 72), with an incidence of approximately 2% during follow-up periods ranging from 9 to 20 years.[13,14] BAV, however, is relatively common (16% to 43%) in case series of confirmed aortic valve IE,[15,16] is associated with a high incidence of periannular complications of IE (50% to 64%), and is a strong independent predictor of perivalvular extension of infection, where the infection extends beyond the valve annulus to involve adjacent cardiac structures.[15] In patients older than 65 years of age, nonrheumatic aortic stenosis is seen as the aortic valve lesion in IE at a rate almost three times that of younger patients (28% and 10%, respectively).[17] Structurally normal valves may also be affected in IE, with risk associations of advanced age, renal failure requiring hemodialysis, and infection caused by *S. aureus* or enterococci.[18]

Congenital heart disease (CHD) (see Chapter 82), other than BAV disease, is a predisposing condition to IE in approximately 5% to 12% of cases.[1,9,19] Unrepaired ventricular septal defects are the most frequent CHD lesions associated with IE, followed by ventricular outflow tract obstructive lesions, such as with tetralogy of Fallot.[20] Any highly turbulent shunt lesion can predispose affected patients to IE, as can the presence of prosthetic material used for palliative shunts, conduits, or shunt closures, particularly if a residual shunt is present after intervention. Low-velocity, low-turbulence shunt lesions, such as secundum atrial septal defect, are much less prone to endocardial disruption and are associated with a very low incidence of IE.[20]

Additional conditions contribute to the anatomic cardiac lesions in the predisposition to risk of IE. These include a history of previous IE, the presence of chronic intravenous (IV) access, IV drug abuse, and indwelling endocavitary devices. Predisposing general medical conditions include diabetes mellitus, underlying malignancy, renal failure requiring hemodialysis, and chronic immunosuppressive therapy.[9,19] A history of an invasive or dental procedure can be identified in approximately 25% of patients within 60 days of clinical presentation with IE.[9] A history of cardiac disease may be present in approximately 50% to 65% of patients.[21] Superimposed and of mounting concern is the increasing frequency of health care–associated IE. In a report from the ICE-PCS investigators,[22] 19% of the cases in a study cohort of 1622 patients with IE were considered to be nosocomial (defined as related to hospitalization for more than 2 days before presentation with IE). An additional 16% of cases were related to non-nosocomial health care (e.g., outpatient hemodialysis, IV chemotherapy, wound care, or residence in a long-term care facility) received within 30 days of onset of symptoms of IE.

A recent study demonstrated that a portal of pathogen entry responsible for IE could be identified in almost 75% of patients if a systematic search was pursued.[23] In this study, the most common entry site was cutaneous (40%), associated with health care delivery, such as vascular access or a surgical site, or sites used for IV drug abuse. The second most common (29%) portal of entry was oral/dental, with an active infection implicated much more frequently than a prior dental procedure. Thirdly, a GI source was detected in 23% of patients, in the majority with colonic neoplasm, or less commonly, ulcerative or inflammatory disease. Far less (<5%) frequently, a GU, otorhinolaryngologic, or respiratory portal of entry was detected.[23]

Symptoms

The presentation of IE encompasses a broad spectrum of symptoms and is influenced by multiple contributing factors (Figs. 80.1 and 80.2).

These factors would include (1) the virulence of the infecting organism and persistence of bacteremia, (2) extent of local tissue destruction of the involved valve(s) and hemodynamic sequelae, (3) perivalvular extension of infection, (4) septic embolization to any organ in the systemic arterial circulation or to the lungs, as in the case of right-sided IE, and (5) the consequences of circulating immune complexes and systemic immunopathologic factors.

The diverse potential symptoms associated with IE are listed in Table 80.1. The frequency of symptoms has been approximated from numerous clinical series in both the older and more contemporary literature. Fever (>38°C) is the most common presenting symptom, in up to 95% of patients, but may be absent in up to 20% of cases, particularly in elderly persons,[17] the immunocompromised, patients treated with previous empiric antibiotic therapy, or patients with CIED infections.[24,25] Fever defervescence usually occurs within 5 to 7 days of appropriate antibiotic therapy. Persistence of fever may indicate progressive infection with perivalvular extension such as abscess, septic embolization, an extracardiac site of infection (native or prosthetic), infected indwelling catheters or devices, inadequate antibiotic treatment of a resistant organism, or even an adverse reaction to the antibiotic therapy itself.

Other nonspecific constitutional symptoms of infection, such as chills, sweats, cough, headache, malaise, nausea, myalgias, and arthralgias, are less common accompanying symptoms and may be noted in approximately 20% to 40% of patients. In more protracted subacute cases of IE, symptoms and signs such as anorexia, weight loss, weakness, arthralgias, and abdominal pain may also occur in 5% to 30% of patients, misleading the clinician to pursue incorrect diagnoses such as malignancy, connective tissue disease, or other chronic infection or systemic inflammatory disorders.

Dyspnea is important to recognize because they may indicate a severe hemodynamic lesion, usually left-sided valvular regurgitation. Associated symptoms of orthopnea and paroxysmal nocturnal dyspnea herald the onset of heart failure (HF). Early recognition of HF symptoms is imperative because it is the most common complication of IE, has the greatest impact on prognosis, is the most frequent indication for surgical intervention, and is the most important predictor of poor outcome with surgical therapy for IE.[26] HF complicates the course of approximately 30% to 50% of patients with IE,[9,19,27,28] and even with early surgical intervention, still doubles in-hospital mortality to almost 25%.[28]

A variety of chest pain syndromes can accompany IE. Pleuritic chest pain may result from septic pulmonary embolization and infarction complicating tricuspid IE. Much less common is angina pectoris related to embolization of vegetation fragments into the coronary circulation, which complicates IE in approximately 1% of the cases. Musculoskeletal chest symptoms related to systemic infection or superimposed infectious pneumonitis also would be in the differential diagnosis.

Physical Examination (see Chapter 13)

Potential findings on physical examination are delineated in Table 80.2. These data are approximated from both older and more recently reported clinical series.[9,19,22,26-28] A definite murmur is audible in at least 80% of patients on presentation, particularly with left-sided IE. In the large ICE-PCS collaboration, the murmur was new in almost 50% of the patients.[9] The same cohort study found that worsening of a preexisting murmur occurred in 20% of cases. The presence of a new heart murmur also is noted more frequently in patients with IE complicated by HF[26] and an S_3 gallop and pulmonary rales would further substantiate this diagnosis. Murmurs are detected in less than half of patients with IE complicating an implanted cardiac device[24] and are infrequently heard in patients with right-sided IE. Heart murmurs associated with acute IE complicated by extensive left-sided valvular destruction with acute, severe regurgitation may also be deceptively unimpressive because of rapid equalization of pressures between the chambers that diminishes the substrate for turbulent flow. Precipitous HF, pulmonary edema, and cardiogenic shock are most often associated with severe acute aortic regurgitation associated with IE, less so by severe acute mitral regurgitation. Severe tricuspid regurgitation, even as an acute complication of IE, is much better tolerated.

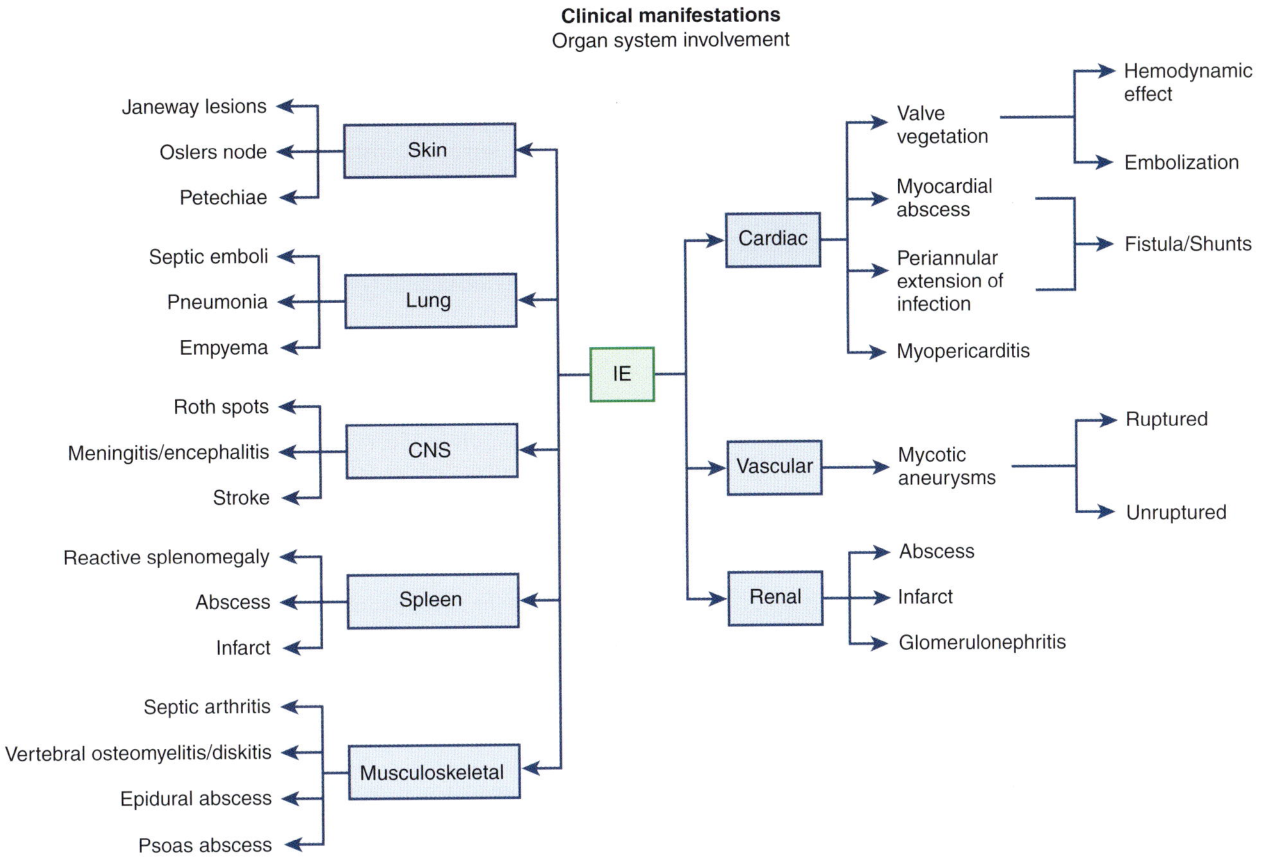

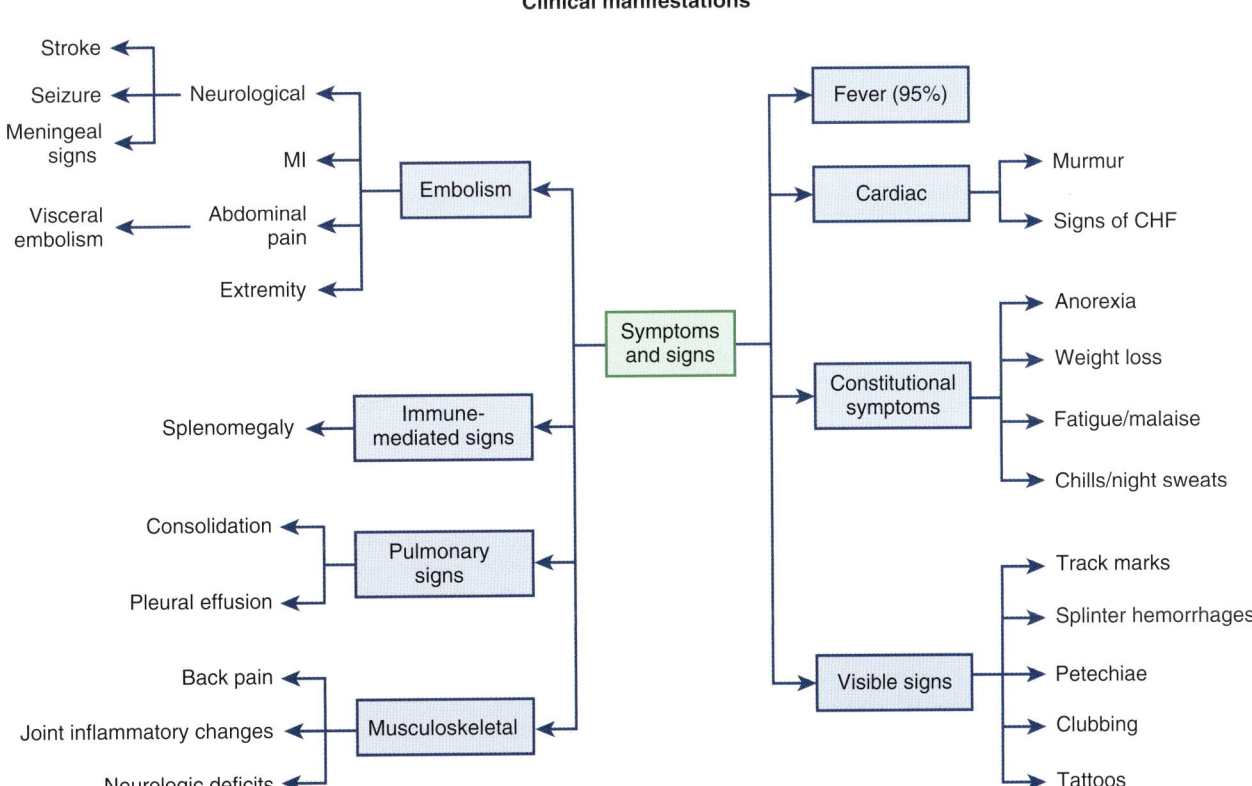

FIGURE 80.1 Clinical manifestations of organ system involvement due to infective endocarditis.

FIGURE 80.2 Signs and symptoms of infective endocarditis and its complications.

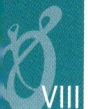

TABLE 80.1 **Symptoms in Infective Endocarditis**

SYMPTOM	PATIENTS AFFECTED (%)
Fever	80–95
Chills	40–70
Weakness	40–50
Malaise	20–40
Sweats	20–40
Anorexia	20–40
Headache	20–40
Dyspnea	20–40
Cough	20–30
Weight loss	20–30
Myalgia/arthralgia	10–30
Stroke	10–20
Confusion/delirium	10–20
Nausea/vomiting	10–20
Edema	5–15
Chest pain	5–15
Abdominal pain	5–15
Hemoptysis	5–10
Back pain	5–10

TABLE 80.2 **Physical Findings in Infective Endocarditis**

FINDING	PATIENTS AFFECTED (%)
Fever	80–90
Heart murmur	75–85
New murmur	10–50
Changing murmur	5–20
Central neurologic abnormality	20–40
Splenomegaly	10–40
Petechiae/conjunctival hemorrhage	10–40
Splinter hemorrhages	5–15
Janeway lesions	5–10
Osler nodes	3–10
Retinal lesion or Roth spot	2–10

A central neurologic abnormality can often be identified, and focal deficits consistent with stroke may be detected in 10% to 20% of patients (see Chapter 45).[9,26] In subacute, indolent IE, an acute stroke typically is the event that prompts the patient to seek medical attention. Most frequently, the stroke is cardioembolic in nature but may infrequently result from complications of intracranial cerebrovascular mycotic aneurysm, such as hemorrhagic rupture. Seizures, visual deficits, cranial nerve deficits, subarachnoid hemorrhage, and toxic encephalopathy are other potential neurologic complications of IE. The development of neurologic deterioration during the course of IE is associated with significantly increased mortality.

Abdominal examination may elicit nonspecific findings of tenderness and discomfort, particularly in the left upper quadrant, suggestive of splenic embolization and infarction, particularly if complicated by splenic abscess. The spleen is a common site of septic embolization. This most often is not identified by localized symptoms or findings but is discovered incidentally on computed tomography (CT) or using other imaging techniques. Splenomegaly usually is seen in subacute IE and is reported in approximately 10% of patients in more recent clinical series in which the diagnosis is established earlier in the course of the disease.[9,19,22]

As a result of advances leading to earlier diagnosis and therapy, the classic peripheral manifestations of IE are now infrequently observed. Petechiae are the most common, occurring on the conjunctivae, oral mucosa, or extremities. Janeway lesions are painless hemorrhagic macules with a predilection for the soles or palms and are sequelae of peripheral septic embolization, most often associated with staphylococcal IE. Splinter subungual hemorrhages also are painless, dark-red linear lesions in the proximal nailbed and may coalesce. Brown distal splinter lesions at the tips of the nails are quite common in patients who perform manual labor and are caused by trauma, not infection. *Osler nodes* are painful, erythematous, nodular lesions usually located in the pads of the fingers and toes and are the result of immune complex deposition and focal vasculitis. *Roth spots* are retinal hemorrhages with a pale center of coagulated fibrin and also are related to immune complex–mediated vasculitis secondary to IE. An immune complex–mediated diffuse glomerulonephritis rarely may be associated with these findings. Both Osler nodes and Roth spots can be observed with other disorders, such as systemic lupus erythematosus (SLE), leukemia, and nonbacterial endocarditis. Aside from petechiae and conjunctival hemorrhage, these peripheral findings were detected in less than 10% of patients in the recent ICE-PCS cohort.[9] A recent multicenter prospective cohort study of 1804 patients with IE confirmed similar results as pertains to the spectrum of clinical presentations and physical examination findings.[29]

Diagnosis

The protean clinical presentations and manifestations of IE encompass a broad differential diagnosis in the patient presenting with fever without a readily apparent cause. Other primary cardiac diagnoses that may potentially mimic IE include acute rheumatic fever, left atrial (LA) myxoma, antiphospholipid antibody syndrome, and nonbacterial thrombotic or marantic endocarditis. A number of connective tissue disorders, including SLE, reactive arthritis, polymyalgia rheumatica, and vasculitides, may be additional diagnostic considerations in select patients, as well as many other serious syndromes of infectious disease. The index of suspicion for IE incrementally increases in the presence of predisposing cardiac conditions, new or changing murmurs, bloodstream infection, clinical evidence of embolic phenomena, and evolving HF or certain other hemodynamic abnormalities.

In 1994, Durack and associates proposed diagnostic criteria, subsequently known as the Duke criteria, to establish the diagnosis of definite or possible IE, and also to reject the diagnosis of IE. These criteria incorporated direct histopathologic evidence of IE or major clinical criteria, namely, blood culture positivity and evidence of endocardial involvement, supplemented by minor clinical criteria, for the definite diagnosis of IE. Thereafter, multiple clinical series using the Duke criteria in the diagnosis of IE reported the sensitivity to be in the range of 80%, with both specificity and negative predictive value (NPV) exceeding 90%.[8,26] Recognizing the increasing impact of *S. aureus* IE, the potential for IE associated with *C. burnetii* infection, and the evolving role of transesophageal echocardiography (TEE) in the diagnosis of IE, Li and colleagues[10] proposed the modified Duke criteria (Table 80.3). *Major clinical criteria* include (1) blood culture positivity for bacteria typically associated with IE, or persistently positive cultures for organisms uncommonly associated with IE, or a blood culture or serology clearly positive for *C. burnetii* and (2) evidence of endocardial involvement by echocardiography demonstrating vegetation, significantly new valvular regurgitation, dehiscence of a prosthetic valve, or findings consistent with perivalvular extension of infection, such as abscess. *Minor clinical criteria* include (1) predisposing cardiac conditions or IV drug use; (2) persistent fever with temperatures greater than 38°C without an alternative explanation; (3) vascular phenomena such as systemic or pulmonary embolism, mycotic aneurysm, or intracranial or cutaneous hemorrhagic lesions; (4) immunologic phenomena such as Osler nodes, Roth spots, or glomerulonephritis; and (5) positive blood culture status not meeting major criteria or serologic evidence of active infection with an organism that could be associated with IE. By this diagnostic classification, a *definite* clinical diagnosis of IE is established in the presence of (a) two major criteria or (b) one

TABLE 80.3 Definition of Infective Endocarditis: Modified Duke Criteria

Definite Infective Endocarditis

Pathologic Criteria

- Microorganisms demonstrated by results of cultures or histologic examination of a vegetation, a vegetation that has embolized, or an intracardiac abscess specimen; or
- Pathologic lesions; vegetation, or intracardiac abscess confirmed by results of histologic examination showing active endocarditis

Clinical Criteria

- 2 major criteria, or
- 1 major criterion and 3 minor criteria, or
- 5 minor criteria

Possible Infective Endocarditis

- 1 major criterion and 1 minor criterion, or
- 3 minor criteria

Rejected Diagnosis of Infective Endocarditis

- Firm alternate diagnosis explaining evidence of suspected IE, or
- Resolution of IE syndrome with antibiotic therapy for ≤4 days, or
- No evidence of IE at surgery or autopsy, on antibiotic therapy for ≤4 days, or
- Does not meet criteria for possible IE

Definition of Terms Used in the Modified Duke Criteria for Diagnosis of Infective Endocarditis

Major Criteria

Blood culture findings positive for IE
  Typical microorganisms consistent with IE from two separate blood cultures:
  - Viridans streptococci, *Streptococcus gallolyticus* (formerly known as *S. bovis*), *Staphylococcus aureus*, HACEK group, or
  - Community-acquired enterococci, in the absence of a primary focus, or
  Microorganisms consistent with IE from persistently positive blood culture findings, defined as:
  - ≥2 positive culture findings of blood samples drawn >12 hr apart, or
  - 3 or most of ≥4 separate culture findings of blood (with first and last sample drawn ≥1 hr apart)
  - Single positive blood culture for *Coxiella burnetii* or anti–phase I IgG titer ≥1:800

Evidence of endocardial involvement
  Echocardiographic findings positive for IE (TEE recommended in patients with prosthetic valves, rated at least possible IE by clinical criteria or complicated IE [paravalvular abscess]; TTE as first test in other patients), defined as follows:
  - Oscillating intracardiac mass on valve or supporting structures, in the path of regurgitant jets, or on implanted material in the absence of an alternative anatomic explanation, or
  - Abscess, or
  - New partial dehiscence of prosthetic valve
  New valvular regurgitation; worsening or changing of preexisting murmur not sufficient

Minor Criteria

- Predisposition, predisposing heart condition, or intravenous drug use
- Fever—temperature >38°C
- Vascular phenomena, major arterial emboli, septic pulmonary infarcts, mycotic aneurysm, intracranial hemorrhage, conjunctival hemorrhages, and Janeway lesions
- Immunologic phenomena: glomerulonephritis, Osler nodes, Roth spots, and rheumatoid factor
- Microbiologic evidence: positive blood culture finding but does not meet a major criterion as noted above (excludes single positive culture findings for coagulase-negative staphylococci and organisms that do not cause endocarditis) or serologic evidence of active infection with organism consistent with IE

HACEK, Haemophilus spp., other than H. influenzae; Aggregatibacter actinomycetemcomitans [formerly Actinobacillus actinomycetemcomitans], Aggregatibacter aphrophilus [formerly Haemophilus aphrophilus]; Cardiobacterium hominis; Eikenella corrodens; Kingella kingae and Kingella denitrificans; IE, infective endocarditis; TEE, transesophageal echocardiography; TTE, transthoracic echocardiography.
Modified from Li JS, Sexton DJ, Mick N, et al. Proposed modifications to the Duke criteria for the diagnosis of infective endocarditis. *Clin Infect Dis.* 2000;30:633.

---

major and three minor criteria, or (c) five minor criteria. A *possible* clinical diagnosis of IE is appropriate in the presence of (a) one major and one minor criterion or (b) three minor criteria. The diagnosis of IE is *rejected* if clinical evaluation (a) does not meet criteria for possible IE or (b) reveals complete resolution of a suspected IE syndrome or absence of anatomic evidence for IE on a course of antibiotic therapy for 4 days or less, or if (c) an alternative diagnosis explaining the initial presentation is confirmed.

Since their publication in 2000, the modified Duke criteria have been validated in subsequent investigations of diagnostic accuracy (confirmed to be high) and also clinical and epidemiologic utility and have been endorsed by guideline documents pertinent to the evaluation and management of the patient with IE.[8,26] In view of the vast heterogeneity of clinical presentations of IE, the modified Duke criteria must always be used in combination with circumspect clinical judgment.

Diagnostic Testing

MICROBIOLOGY

The microbiology and epidemiology of pathogens that cause IE are detailed earlier in this chapter. As determined from data summarized from contemporary cohort series,[9,22,30-33] organisms identified in patients with IE in a variety of clinical settings are listed in Table 80.4. In community-acquired IE, VGS remain the most frequently isolated organism, followed closely by *S. aureus*, which is the predominant organism implicated in health care–associated IE, accounting for more than 40% of cases both in and out of the hospital environment. A defined portal of entry, such as an intravascular catheter or tissue disruption from a recent surgical or dental procedure, can be implicated in 25% to 67% of such cases.[19,22,30] MRSA IE is much more common in health care–associated than in community-acquired IE (47% versus 12%, respectively).[22] In IE associated with IV drug abuse, S. aureus accounts for almost 70% of cases.[9]

In patients with prosthetic valves (see Chapter 79), early PVE has been defined as occurring as early as 60 days or less[31] up to 1 year[26,32,33] after surgery. S. aureus also is the leading pathogen in early PVE, accounting for approximately 35% of cases, of which approximately one-fourth are MRSA,[31] followed closely by coagulase-negative staphylococci. Streptococcal early PVE is unusual. Late PVE is caused less often by staphylococci, which nevertheless are still the most common infecting organism, and a higher occurrence of infections with both VGS and *S. gallolyticus* (formerly *S. bovis*) has been documented. As with community-acquired native valve IE, enterococcal infections account for approximately 10% of cases of both early and late PVE.

Negative blood culture results are observed in approximately 5% to 15% of the cases for both native and prosthetic valve IE. In the large ICE-PCS, 62% of patients with culture-negative IE had received antibiotic therapy within 7 days of obtaining the initial blood culture.[9] Other reasons for blood culture negativity would include IE caused by fastidious organisms or unusual pathogens such as *Bartonella* or *Legionella* spp., *C. burnetii*, or fungi, as stated earlier Rapid detection of pathogens associated with IE by polymerase chain reaction (PCR) techniques may become a reliable alternative to standard blood culture techniques in such cases.[34]

OTHER BLOOD TESTING

The complete blood count often is abnormal in IE. In patients with subacute IE, a normochromic normocytic anemia of variable severity is detected in a majority of patients, often with low serum iron and total iron-binding capacity. Even with the systemic infection of IE, a leukocytosis with a left differential shift may be detected in only 50% to 60% of patients[32] and is more common with acute than with subacute IE. Leukopenia also may infrequently occur with subacute IE and usually is associated with splenomegaly. Thrombocytopenia may occur in approximately 10% of patients and has been found to be a predictor of early adverse outcome in IE. Sy and colleagues[35] reported a hazard ratio (HR) of approximately 1.13 for each 20×10^9/L decrement in the platelet count as a multivariate predictor of mortality from days 1 to 15 after presentation with IE.[35]

The erythrocyte sedimentation rate (ESR) usually is elevated in patients with IE, and in ICE-PCS, was elevated in 61% of patients. This large cohort study found that an elevated ESR was independently associated with a decreased risk of in-hospital death, presumably because of an association with subacute IE with a more indolent course.[9] The same study found that the C-reactive protein (CRP) also was elevated in approximately 60% of patients, whereas the rheumatoid factor concentration was abnormal in 5%[9]—the latter usually a feature of protracted subacute IE, not acute IE. Inclusion of ESR and CRP in the minor modified Duke criteria for the diagnosis of IE has been proposed but is not endorsed by current guideline recommendations.[8]

Procalcitonin (PCT) is another protein that rises in response to a proinflammatory stimulus, particularly with severe bacterial infection. A meta-analysis of six studies, including 1006 patients with suspected IE, found PCT to be only 64% sensitive and 73% specific for the diagnosis of IE, and was less accurate than CRP.[36] PCT and other bacteremia-activated markers, such as cellular and vascular adhesion molecules, are currently not recommended as routine biomarkers for the diagnosis of IE.[37]

A new elevation in serum creatinine occurs in 10% to 30% of patients with IE[26] and may be related to multifactorial reasons including renal hypoperfusion from severe sepsis or HF, embolic renal infarction, immune complex–mediated glomerulonephritis, and toxicity from either antibiotic therapy or contrast agents used for imaging. Renal dysfunction developing within the first 8 days of presentation is independently predictive of early IE mortality, with HR of 1.13 per incremental increase in serum creatinine of 0.23 mg/dL,[35] and persistent serum creatinine elevation to greater than 2 mg/dL is predictive of 2-year mortality.[29] Urinalysis usually demonstrates hematuria and proteinuria. In cases of immune complex glomerulonephritis, red blood cell casts are evident, associated with depressed serum complement levels.

Limited studies conducted with small numbers of patients have assessed the prognostic value of cardiac biomarkers in IE. The cardiac troponins may be elevated from ventricular wall stress in HF, myocardial injury with myocardial abscess or embolic infarction, or septicemia alone. An increase in troponin I level to greater than 0.4 ng/mL significantly increases the risk of in-hospital mortality and need for early valve replacement.[38] A subset analysis of ICE-PCS demonstrated that in patients with IE, a troponin T level of 0.08 ng/mL or higher was associated with increased risk of cardiac abscess, central nervous system (CNS) events, and death IE.[39] An elevation of the B-type natriuretic peptide (BNP) level to 400 pg/mL or higher also has been associated with a fourfold risk of the same three complications of IE, even with exclusion of patients with LV dysfunction or severe left-sided valve regurgitation.[40] In another study, elevation of the NT-proBNP level to 1500 pg/mL or higher at hospital admission was an independent predictor of need for surgical intervention or death within 30 days.[41]

Electrocardiogram

The 12-lead electrocardiogram (ECG) usually demonstrates nonspecific findings in patients with uncomplicated IE (Fig. 80.3). Because of the close proximity of the atrioventricular node and proximal intraventricular conduction system to the aortic valve and root, perivalvular extension of infection from this location is the most common cause of new atrioventricular block (AVB) of any degree or bundle branch block (BBB). With perivalvular extension of infection, the incidence of AVB ranges from 10% to 20%, whereas new BBB occurs in approximately 3%.[22,32] The occurrence of a new conduction abnormality also is a multivariate risk predictor for death associated with IE.[22] In a

TABLE 80.4 Microbiology of Infective Endocarditis

| | NATIVE VALVE | | | | PROSTHETIC VALVE | |
| | | HEALTH CARE–ASSOCIATED IE (%) | | | | |
ORGANISM	COMMUNITY-ACQUIRED IE (%) (n = 1201)[23,30]	NOSOCOMIAL (n = 370)[22,53]	NON-NOSOCOMIAL (n = 254)[22]	INTRAVENOUS DRUG USERS WITH IE (%) (n = 237)[9]	EARLY IE (%) (n = 140)[31,33]	LATE IE (%) (n = 390)[31,33]
Staphylococcus aureus	21	45	42	68	34	19
Coagulase-negative staphylococci	6	12	15	3	28	20
Enterococcus species	10	14	16	5	10	13
Viridans group streptococci	26	10	6	10	1	11
Streptococcus gallolyticus*	10	3	3	1	1	7
HACEK	3	0	0	0	0	2
Fungi	0	2	2	1	6	3
Other	13	7	10	7	6	15
Negative blood culture	11	7	6	5	14	10

*Formerly *Streptococcus bovis*.
HACEK, *Haemophilus* spp., other than *H. influenzae*; *Aggregatibacter actinomycetemcomitans* [formerly *Actinobacillus actinomycetemcomitans*], *Aggregatibacter aphrophilus* [formerly *Haemophilus aphrophilus*]; *Cardiobacterium hominis*; *Eikenella corrodens*; *Kingella kingae* and *Kingella denitrificans*; IE, infective endocarditis.

minority of patients, perivalvular extension complicating aortic valve IE may compromise proximal coronary artery patency, or emboli from aortic valve vegetations may cause damage, resulting in ischemic ECG changes or even ST-segment elevation acute coronary syndromes.[26] Ischemic ECG changes may also manifest secondary to hemodynamic sequelae resulting in coronary arterial demand supply mismatch. Other atrial and ventricular arrhythmias may potentially complicate structural or hemodynamic complications of IE, especially in the context of underlying LV dysfunction. In a recent investigation that included 507 patients with left-sided native valve IE, new-onset atrial fibrillation was independently associated with HF and in-hospital mortality.[42]

Imaging
Imaging for Diagnosis of Infective Endocarditis

A major clinical criterion for the diagnosis of IE based on the modified Duke criteria is the demonstration of endocardial involvement with vegetations, perivalvular extension of infection, or evidence of disruption of the integrity of either native or prosthetic valves (see Table 80.3). Echocardiography has been and remains the cornerstone of diagnostic imaging in the context of infective endocarditis (see Chapter 16) (see Fig. 80.3). Using early-generation imaging systems, initial studies reported a sensitivity of transthoracic echocardiography (TTE) as 40% to 60% for the detection of native valvular vegetations, and substantially less for prosthetic valve vegetations.[43] With evolving advances in harmonic imaging and numerous other techniques to improve spatial image resolution, sensitivity of current TTE imaging techniques for detection of native valve IE recently has been 82% and as high as 89% if high-quality TTE images are available (Fig. 80.4; see also Fig. 16.74A).[44] The specificity for TTE in the diagnosis of IE has been reported as 70% to 90%.[28,43-45] The absence of regurgitant lesions of the mitral or aortic valves makes endocarditic involvement of these valves less likely.

TEE circumvents multiple potential impediments to TTE imaging, such as body habitus, pulmonary disease, and other sources of acoustic interference between the chest wall and heart. Owing to much closer proximity of the transducer to the heart, TEE is performed with higher-frequency imaging, greatly enhancing spatial resolution (Fig. 80.5; see also Fig. 16.74B). With numerous imaging projections available, multiplane two-dimensional and three-dimensional TEE can characterize vegetations with a resolution size of approaching 2 to 3 mm, with a sensitivity in the range of 90% to 100% and specificity exceeding 90%.[43-46] PVE, characterized by a lower incidence of valvular vegetations (60% to 70%) and higher incidence of periannular infection and associated complications (30% to 50%), is difficult to detect with TTE, generally with a sensitivity of less than 50%.[26] Valvular vegetations have been more frequently identified with IE involving transcatheter-implanted aortic bioprostheses (see Chapter 74), with perivalvular complications less common than for surgically implanted prostheses.[47,48] With sensitivity reported in the range of 80% to 95% and specificity greater than 90%,[28,49] TEE clearly is the imaging procedure of choice for the evaluation of suspected PVE (Figs. 80.6 and 80.7).

In general, TTE is more readily available, entirely noninvasive, and provides a complete cardiovascular hemodynamic profile. Furthermore, TTE may perform similarly to TEE in evaluating anterior structures of the heart, including the tricuspid valve and right ventricular

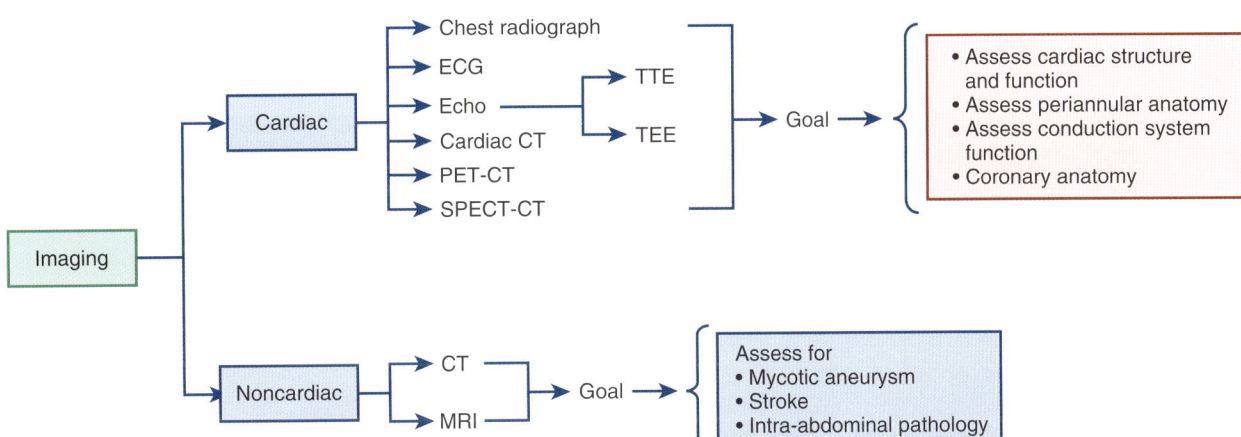

FIGURE 80.3 Imaging techniques in the diagnosis and management of infective endocarditis and its complications.

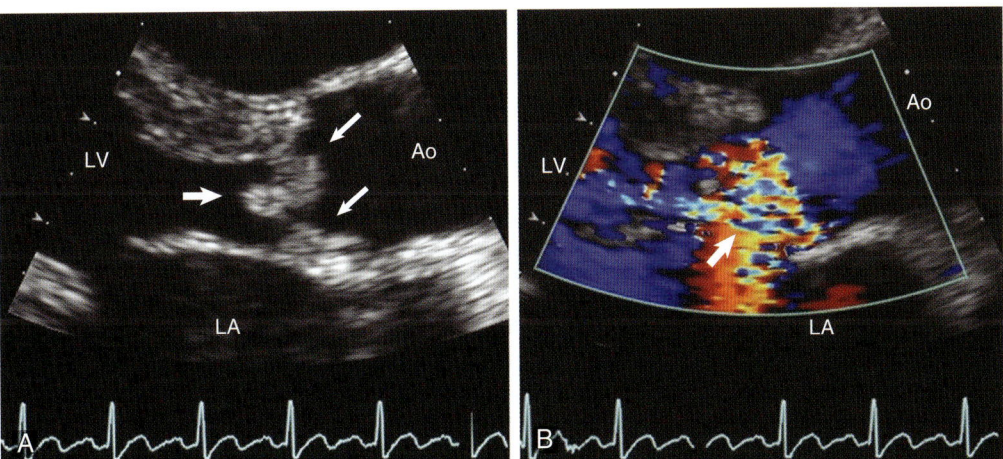

FIGURE 80.4 Infective endocarditis of the native aortic valve. **A,** Transthoracic echocardiography shows vegetations (*small arrows*) attached to the left ventricular aspects of the valve cusps and prolapsing into the left ventricular outflow tract (*large arrow*) during diastole. **B,** Severe aortic regurgitation (*arrow*) is shown by color Doppler. *Ao,* Ascending aorta; *LA,* left atrium; *LV,* left ventricle.

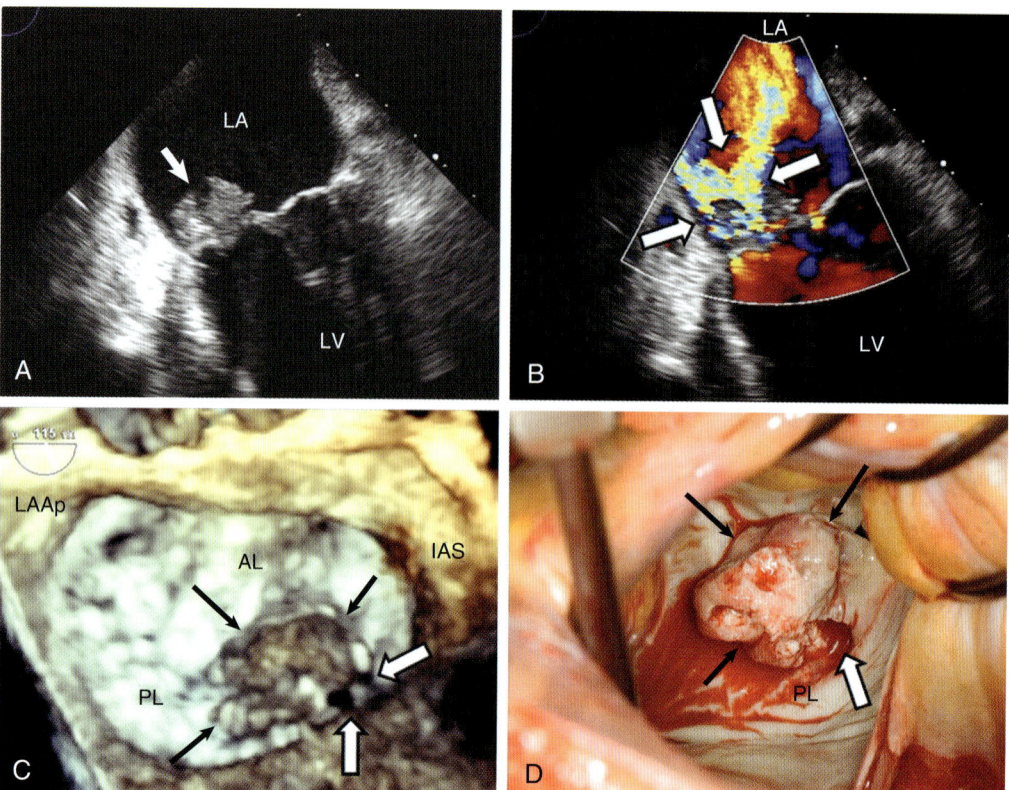

FIGURE 80.5 Infective endocarditis involving the mitral valve. **A,** Transesophageal echocardiography (TEE) image shows a large vegetation (*arrow*) attached to the atrial aspect of the posterior leaflet. **B,** Color Doppler image demonstrates a complex jet of mitral regurgitation (*arrows*) coursing through the body of the posterior mitral leaflet and vegetative mass, consistent with leaflet perforation. **C,** Three-dimensional TEE image of the mitral valve, as viewed from the left atrium (*LA*). Large vegetations (*black arrows*) are attached to the medial aspect of the posterior leaflet (*PL*), with perforation (*white arrows*) at the margin of the posteromedial commissure. **D,** Intraoperative visualization of the mitral valve as viewed from the left atriotomy. The large vegetative mass (*black arrows*) is attached to the posterior leaflet, and the posteromedial perforation (*white arrow*) is confirmed. *AL,* Anterior leaflet; *IAS,* interatrial septum; *LAAp,* left atrial appendage; *LV,* left ventricle.

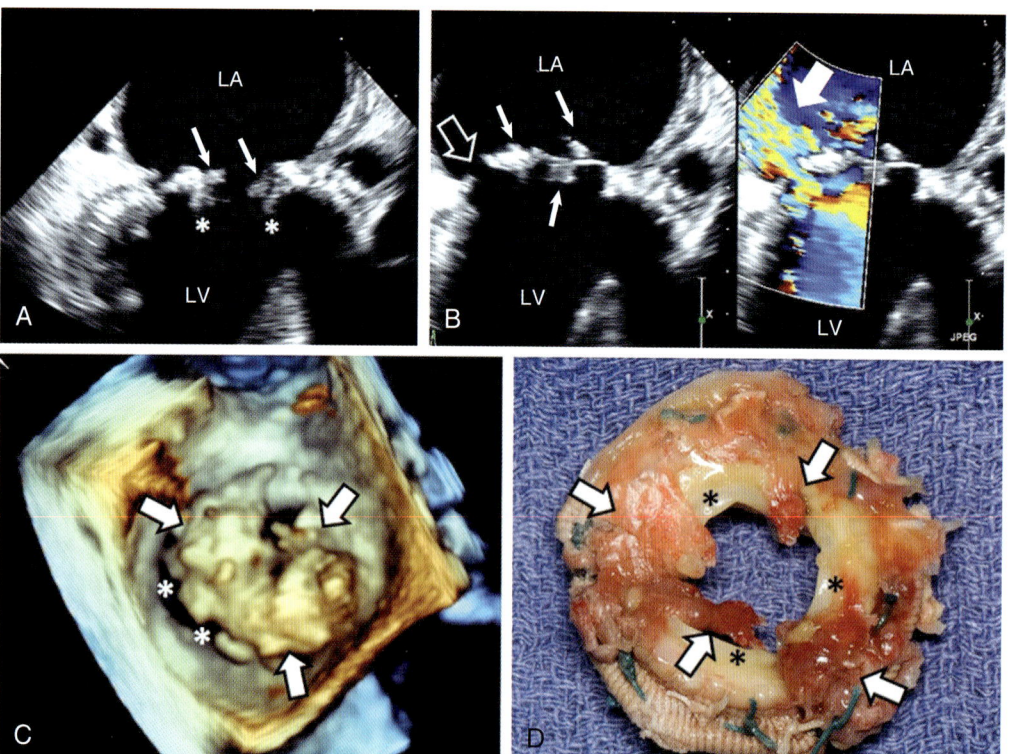

FIGURE 80.6 Infective endocarditis of a mitral bioprosthesis. **A,** On transesophageal echocardiography (TEE), multiple vegetations (*arrows*) can be seen within the inflow orifice of the bioprosthesis (*) during diastole. **B, Left,** During systole, a zone of inferolateral periannular prosthetic dehiscence (*large open arrow*) is evident with rocking motion of the prosthesis. Vegetations are present on the closed bioprosthetic leaflets and prosthetic annulus (*small arrows*). **Right,** Color Doppler image shows severe, eccentric periprosthetic mitral regurgitation (*large white arrow*) emanating from the zone of periannular dehiscence. *LA,* Left atrium; *LV,* left ventricle. **C,** Three-dimensional TEE view from the left atrium shows an extensive mass of vegetations encompassing the periannular margins (*arrows*), which was not fully appreciated by two-dimensional imaging. A large crescentic zone of periannular dehiscence (*) is well visualized. **D,** The surgically excised mitral bioprosthesis shows extensive vegetations (*arrows*) attached to the atrial aspects of the prosthesis. Pannus ingrowth (*) into the prosthetic orifice also is present.

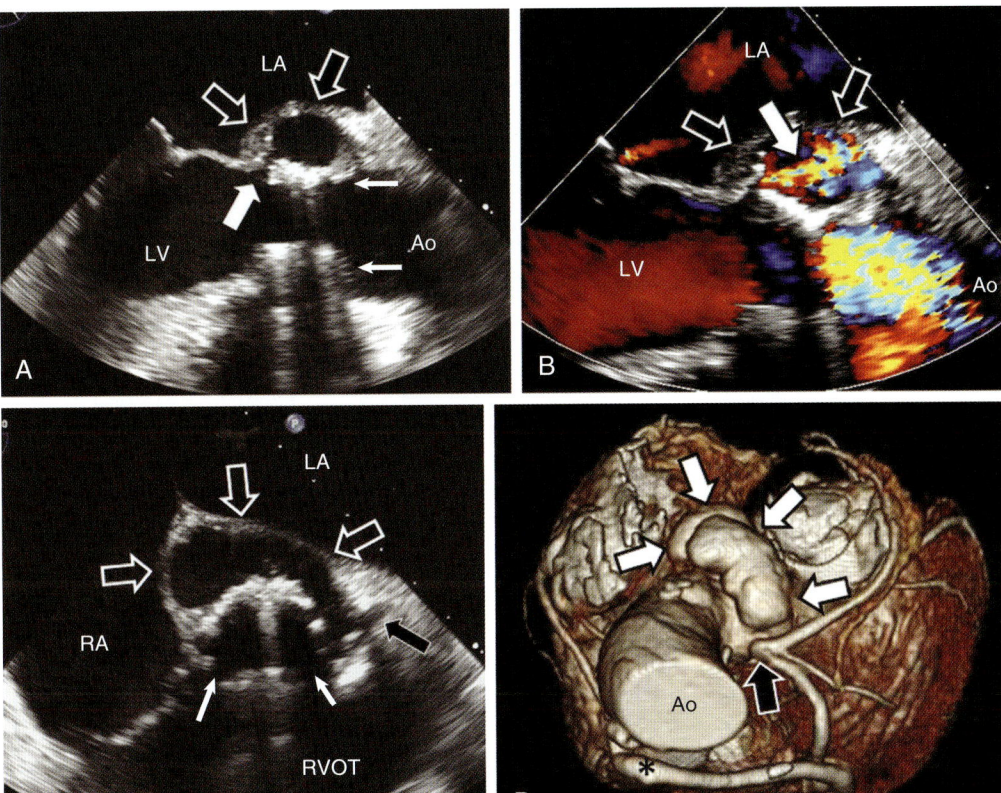

FIGURE 80.7 Periannular extension of infection complicating mechanical aortic prosthetic valve endocarditis. **A,** Transesophageal echocardiography (TEE) image shows a large, mycotic false aneurysm (*open arrows*) within the mitral-aortic intervalvular fibrosa adjacent to the prosthesis (*small arrows*). Communication with the left ventricular outflow tract is evident (*large white arrow*). **B,** Color Doppler image demonstrates flow communication (*arrow*) into the mycotic false aneurysm (*open arrows*) during systole, at which time the larger, color flow signal exits the aortic prosthesis into the ascending aorta (*Ao*). **C,** Short-axis TEE imaging of the mechanical aortic prosthesis (*small arrows*) indicates that the large mycotic false aneurysm (*large open arrows*) extends posteriorly adjacent to the left atrium (*LA*), bulges toward the right atrium (*RA*), and extends to the left main coronary artery (*black arrow*). **D,** Computed tomography with three-dimensional reconstruction, viewed from above and tilted anteriorly to show the posterior aortic root, shows the large posterolateral mycotic false aneurysm (*white arrows*) extending from the aortic root and encroaching upon the left main coronary artery (*black arrow*). A saphenous vein bypass graft (*) to the left anterior descending coronary artery also is seen. *LV,* Left ventricle; *RVOT,* right ventricular outflow tract.

outflow tract. In a study of IV drug users with suspected right-sided endocarditis, TTE performed as well as TEE in the detection of vegetations.[50] Because TTE and TEE provide complementary information, the most recent American Heart Association (AHA) guidelines[8] recommend both TTE and TEE be obtained in cases of suspected IE (Fig. 80.8). Variably mobile echodensities may be observed with echocardiography, particularly TEE. A differential diagnosis would include degenerative changes in a native valve, such as Lambl excrescences, endocardial fenestrations, ruptured or retracted chordae, and even acoustic artifacts reflected by calcified tissue. Valvular thickening, myxomatous changes, and sclerotic lesions move in concert with leaflet or cusp motion, without independent mobility of a vegetation, but may be difficult to discern from sessile vegetations. Filamentous valvular strands may be seen on both native and prosthetic valves. Thrombus associated with prosthetic valves may or may not be infected. Valvular neoplasms, such as papillary fibroelastoma or rarely myxomas, also are included in the differential. Vegetations of IE typically are located on the upstream, lower-pressure side of the regurgitant valve, have soft tissue echocardiographic density (particularly early in the course of infection) and often are multiple and lobulated, with motion independent of the valve structure. Hyperrefractile, discretely nodular, or filamentous echodensities located on the downstream side of the valve are much less likely to represent vegetations associated with IE.

In addition to confirming the diagnosis of IE, echocardiography provides important information regarding complications of IE that indicate the potential need for surgery (Table 80.5). In patients with suspect IE of a mechanical prosthetic valve, particularly in the mitral position, TEE is the diagnostic test of choice because of shadowing that could obscure standard TTE imaging. Cardiac CT can also be used to assess vegetations (see later) (see Fig. 80.3).

Imaging for Delineation of Complications of Endocarditis
LOCAL VALVULAR DESTRUCTION. Caused most frequently by left-sided valvular regurgitant lesions, HF may complicate the course of approximately 30% to 40% of patients with IE, is three times more common in native than in prosthetic valve IE, and is the primary indication for early surgery in at least 50% to 60% of these patients.[26,28,50] New York Heart Association (NYHA) Functional Class III or IV HF complicating IE has the greatest impact on both medical and surgical prognosis, with reported in-hospital mortality rates in the range of 55% and 25%, respectively, in ICE-PCS.[50] HF most frequently is associated with aortic valve IE (30%), followed by mitral valve (20%) and tricuspid valve (<10%).[8]

New, moderate to severe valvular regurgitation may be detected by TEE in up to 70% of patients presenting with IE.[19] On imaging with TTE, and particularly with TEE, mechanisms contributing to valvular regurgitation include perforation, prolapse, and flail of the involved cusp or leaflet. Native valve perforations develop in 10% to 30% of patients with IE.[15,19,27,51] Even with TEE, which is much more sensitive than TTE (90% vs. 45%), perforations can be difficult to visualize using two-dimensional imaging alone. Three-dimensional TEE imaging can significantly enhance detection of valvular perforations complicating IE (see Fig. 80.5).[46] Color Doppler imaging can readily identify a perforation, with color flow convergence entraining into the perforation from the exiting chamber and a regurgitant jet traversing through the body of a cusp or leaflet. Saccular mycotic aneurysms, most often present on the atrial aspect of the mitral valve, may rupture, leaving a large defect in the leaflet. Extensive vegetations may also impede valvular coaptation, leading to regurgitation, or rarely may cause stenosis.

Infectious destruction of left-sided native valvular cusp or leaflet integrity and disruption of the valvular support apparatus can lead to acute severe valvular regurgitation complicated by precipitous HF, pulmonary edema, and hemodynamic instability (see Chapters 73 and 76). In addition to identifying the mechanism(s) of regurgitation, echocardiographic imaging typically demonstrates normal LV size and ejection fraction (EF). In acute severe aortic regurgitation, Doppler assessment will demonstrate evidence of rapid elevation of LV diastolic filling pressures with very short aortic regurgitant pressure half-times and a restrictive pattern of mitral inflow. Such hemodynamics are associated with premature closure of the mitral valve before the onset of systole. In acute severe mitral regurgitation, truncation of the usual parabolic continuous-wave Doppler regurgitant signal indicates

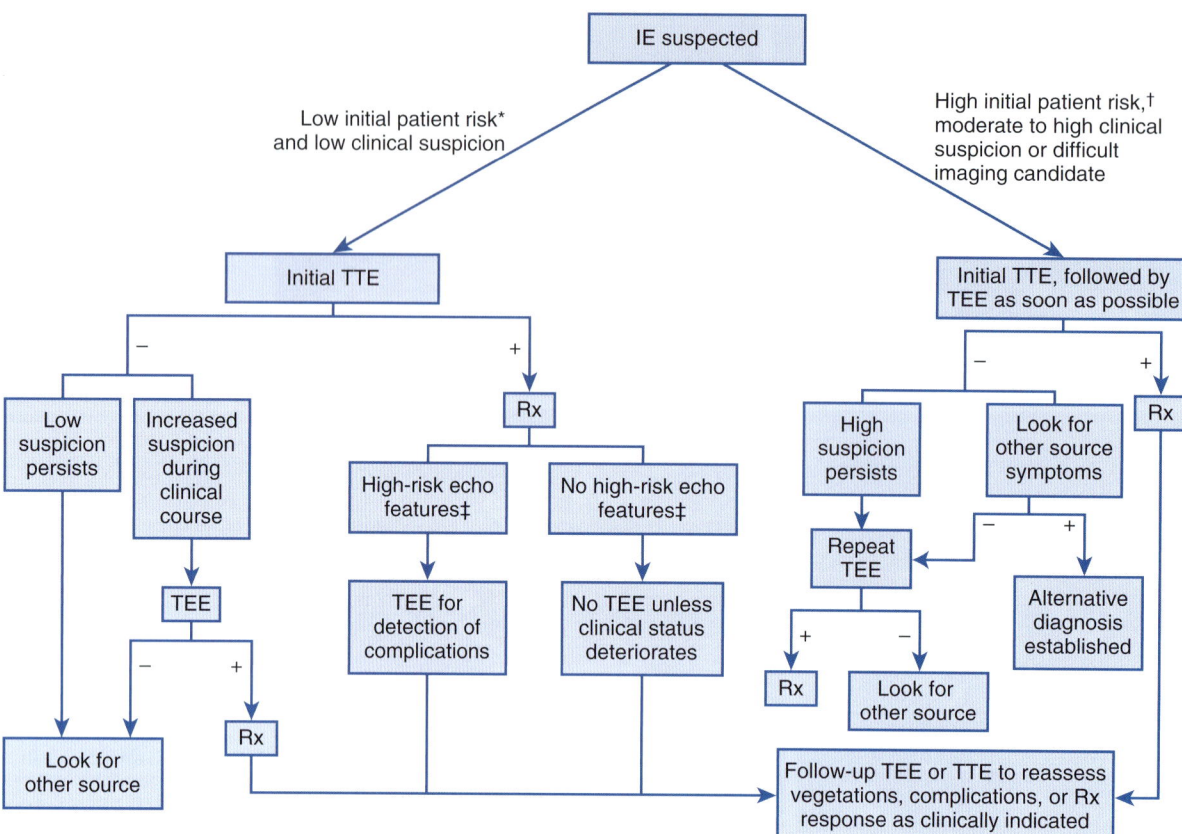

FIGURE 80.8 An approach to the diagnostic use of echocardiography (echo). *Rx,* Prescription; *TEE,* transesophageal echocardiography; *TTE,* transthoracic echocardiography. *For example, a patient with fever and a previously known heart murmur and no other stigmata of infective endocarditis (IE). [†]High initial patient risks include prosthetic heart valves, many congenital heart diseases, previous endocarditis, new murmur, heart failure, or other stigmata of endocarditis. [‡]High-risk echocardiographic features include large or mobile vegetations, valvular insufficiency, suggestion of perivalvular extension, or secondary ventricular dysfunction (see text). (Modified from Baddour LM, Wilson WR, Bayer AS, et al. Infective endocarditis in adults: diagnosis, antimicrobial therapy, and management of complications. A scientific statement for healthcare professionals from the American Heart Association. *Circulation.* 2015;132:1435; and Habib G, et al. 2015 ESC guidelines for the management of infective endocarditis. The Task Force for the Management of Infective Endocarditis of the European Society of Cardiology. *Eur Heart J.* 2015;36:3075.)

TABLE 80.5 Echocardiographic Features That Suggest Potential Need for Surgical Intervention

Vegetation
Persistent vegetation after systemic embolization
Anterior mitral valve leaflet vegetation, particularly if it is highly mobile with size >10 mm*
One or more embolic events during the first 2 weeks of antimicrobial therapy*
Increase in vegetation size despite appropriate antimicrobial therapy*,[†]
Valvular Dysfunction
Acute aortic or mitral insufficiency with signs of ventricular failure[†]
Heart failure unresponsive to medical therapy[†]
Valve perforation or rupture[†]
Perivalvular Extension
Valvular dehiscence, rupture, or fistula[†]
New heart block[†,‡]
Large abscess or extension of abscess despite appropriate antimicrobial therapy[†]

*Surgery may be required because of risk of embolization.
[†]Surgery may be required because of heart failure or failure of medical therapy.
[‡]Echocardiography should not be the primary modality used to detect or monitor heart block.
See text for more complete discussion of indications for surgery based on vegetation characterizations.

PERIVALVULAR EXTENSION OF INFECTION.
Perivalvular extension in IE includes the complications of periannular or intramyocardial abscess, mycotic false aneurysm, and fistula. The incidence of perivalvular extension ranges from 10% to almost 30% in native valve IE and at least 30% to 55% in PVE (see Figs. 80.6 and 80.7).[27,31] IE involving a transcatheter-implanted aortic bioprosthesis has been reported to have a lower incidence of complications from perivalvular extension of infection, such as abscess (15%), aortic mycotic pseudoaneurysm (4%), or aortoatrial fistula (4%).[47] Earlier series have reported the incidence of perivalvular extension of infection to approach 100% for aortic PVE.[8,26] Independent predictors of perivalvular extension are PVE, aortic valve involvement, and staphylococcal infection (from both coagulase-negative strains and *S. aureus*).[8,26] Periannular abscess has been reported in up to 50% of patients with native BAV IE (see Fig. 16.74C), versus 20% in those with a tricuspid aortic valve.[15] Persistent fever, ongoing bacteremia despite appropriate antibiotic therapy, chest pain, a new heart murmur, recurrent embolism, or HF all should alert the clinician to the possible presence of perivalvular extension. After HF, perivalvular extension of infection is the second most common indication for early surgical intervention for IE, and although surgery clearly confers an early survival benefit,[51] perivalvular extension remains an independent predictor of increased in-hospital and 1-year mortality.[9,26,27,50] In left-sided native valve *S. aureus* IE, the echocardiographic findings of perivalvular extension of infection, such as intracardiac abscess, and LVEF less than 40% have been strong independent predictors of in-hospital early mortality.[52]

It is recognized that the sensitivity of TTE for the diagnosis of perivalvular extension is at best 50%, and even less in PVE. TEE has a reported sensitivity of 80% to 90%, specificities of greater than 90%, with positive predictive value (PPV) and NPV of 85% to 90% for diagnosis of perivalvular extension.[8,45] Although TEE is quite sensitive for the diagnosis of aortic perivalvular extension, mitral annular calcification may obscure

late-systolic LV and LA pressure equilibration, consistent with a giant *v* wave noted on LA catheterization. Quantitative Doppler methods are quite useful to confirm the presence of acute severe regurgitation, because qualitative color flow jets may be complex, eccentric, or rapidly dissipating because of the loss of transvalvular pressure gradients.

small regions of mitral perivalvular extension, particularly in the posterior aspects of the annulus.[53] On echocardiographic imaging, early perivalvular abscess usually appears as a nonhomogeneous, soft tissue, echodense thickening that distorts the margins of normal periannular anatomy.

With IE in the aortic valve position, a high predilection for perivalvular extension of infection to involve the *mitral-aortic intervalvular fibrosa* (MAIF) has been recognized. The MAIF is the fibrous zone of continuity between the noncoronary cusp of the aortic valve and insertion of the anterior mitral valve leaflet. Being one of the least vascular structures of the heart, the MAIF is more susceptible to infection and mycotic false aneurysm formation. On echocardiographic imaging of these false aneurysms, systolic expansion of an echolucent cavity can be appreciated within the infected MAIF (see Fig. 80.7), with color Doppler flow communication usually evident from the subvalvular LV outflow tract. Potential complications of MAIF mycotic false aneurysms include fistulous communications into the left atrium or aorta, extension around the aortic root, compression of the proximal left coronary arteries with resultant myocardial ischemia, systemic embolization, and rupture into the pericardial space.[53] Fistulas from aortic perivalvular extension of infection may track into any cardiac chamber and are best identified with TEE color flow Doppler techniques. Mitral valve IE complicated by perivalvular extension is less common, with much lower frequency of structural and conduction system sequelae. Prosthetic valve dehiscence is another manifestation of perivalvular extension of infection and usually is seen without impressive vegetations on the prosthesis itself (see Fig. 80.7). Imaging by TEE demonstrates crescentic defect adjacent to the sewing ring, variable rocking of the prosthesis, and periprosthetic regurgitation.

APPROACH TO ECHOCARDIOGRAPHIC IMAGING. Clinical risk assessment of the patient with suspected IE is the first step in deciding which echocardiographic imaging modality to use for evaluation (see Fig. 80.8 and Table 80.6). Patients with undifferentiated febrile syndromes, a chronic unchanged murmur, no physical examination findings suggestive of IE, and no high-risk cardiac anatomy (e.g., prosthetic valves or complex CHD) are characterized as being at initially low patient risk with a lower pretest likelihood of IE. High initial patient risk characteristics that present a high pretest probability of IE and likelihood of adverse outcome include clinical findings of a significant new heart murmur, peripheral stigmata of IE, new HF, *S. aureus* bacteremia, and high-risk cardiac anatomy, including the presence of a prosthetic valve or complex CHD.[2,8] Independent risk factors for IE (established in 10% to 15% of cases) in the presence of *S. aureus* bacteremia include community-acquired status, IV drug abuse, significant preexisting native valve disease, intracardiac prosthesis or CIED, prolonged (>72 hours) bacteremia, secondary foci of infection, and embolic event.[54-56]

As shown in Figure 80.8, patients at low initial risk should undergo TTE. In the absence of significant preexisting native valve disease or any prosthetic or implanted devices, adequate- or better-quality images detecting no vegetations exclude the diagnosis of IE, with NPV of 97% and sensitivity exceeding 90%.[54] With preexisting valve disease, the sensitivity approaches 60% but with a similar NPV if TTE image quality is adequate.[57] Even with *S. aureus* bacteremia, initial TTE imaging is reasonable in the absence of the previous risk factors.[8,56,58,59] If TTE images are limited or inadequate, TEE should be pursued. If TTE detects high-risk findings such as large (>10 mm in diameter) or highly mobile vegetations, suggests the presence of perivalvular extension of infection, or identifies new grade III to IV valvular regurgitation or new LV dysfunction, TEE should be promptly performed for further evaluation with the aim to definitively characterize the anatomic extent of infection and complications thereof. Patients at high risk (e.g., new-onset HF, significant new murmur, clinical stigmata of IE, prior IE, prosthetic heart valves/devices, complex CHD, *S. aureus* bacteremia) should undergo initial imaging with TEE (see Fig. 80.8), with supplemental TTE for complete semiquantitation of valvular regurgitation and delineation of left- and right-sided hemodynamics and ventricular function. If TEE is not immediately possible or available, TTE should be pursued first to avoid delay in imaging evaluation and diagnosis.

Provided that initial TTE images are of diagnostic quality and are negative for IE, if a low clinical suspicion for IE persists, other diagnoses should be pursued (see Fig. 80.8). With increased clinical suspicion for IE throughout the patient's clinical course, an initially negative TTE should be followed up with TEE. If the initial TTE is positive for IE but high-risk findings as noted previously are lacking, TEE should not be mandatory, unless the patient is clinically unresponsive to antibiotic therapy or deteriorates during the clinical course. Any high-risk finding on TTE would warrant further evaluation with TEE.

As outlined in Figure 80.8, if the initial TEE is negative for IE and there is diminishing clinical suspicion of IE, other diagnoses should be evaluated. If IE remains high in the differential diagnosis, repeat TEE should be performed in 3 to 5 days, recognizing that NPV of two sequential TEE studies is 98%.[8] After an initial TEE is positive for IE, it should be repeated throughout the patient's course as clinically indicated, to assess response to antibiotic therapy or evaluate clinical or hemodynamic deterioration.

At the completion of antibiotic therapy, repeat echocardiography is indicated to establish a new post-treatment fingerprint of valvular morphology, residual vegetations, valvular regurgitation, and other hemodynamic factors and to assess ventricular function (see Table 80.6). Provided that images are of diagnostic quality, TTE should be adequate for this purpose. With complex anatomy, or if prosthetic valve function remains in question, TEE usually is indicated.

OTHER ADVANCED IMAGING. CT may be helpful in the evaluation of complications of endocarditis, including abscesses and pseudoaneurysms, and may be beneficial in surgical planning (see Fig. 80.3).[20] CT with angiography (multidetector computed tomographic angiography, or MDCTA) is a sensitive alternative imaging procedure for the evaluation of IE and perivalvular extension of infection (see Chapter 20). In a small group of patients with suspected IE, cardiac MDCTA was 96% sensitive for the detection of valvular vegetations, identical to that of multiplanar TEE, compared with intraoperative findings.[60] Both imaging techniques had specificity and PPV/NPV exceeding 95%. Excellent correlation was found between MDCTA and TEE in the determination of vegetation size and mobility; however, TEE was

TABLE 80.6 Use of Echocardiography During Diagnosis and Treatment of Infective Endocarditis

Early
Echocardiography as soon as possible (<12 hr after initial evaluation)
TEE preferred; obtain TTE views of any abnormal findings for later comparison
TTE if TEE is not immediately available
TTE may be sufficient in small children
Repeat Echocardiography
TEE after positive TTE as soon as possible in patients at high risk for complications
TEE 7–10 days after initial TEE if suspicion exists without diagnosis of IE or with worrisome clinical course during early treatment of IE
Intraoperative
Prepump
Identification of vegetations, mechanism of regurgitation, abscesses, fistulas, and pseudoaneurysms
Postpump
Confirmation of successful repair of abnormal findings
Assessment of Residual Valve Dysfunction
Elevated afterload if necessary to avoid underestimating valve insufficiency or presence of residual abnormal flow
Completion of Therapy
Establish new baseline for valve function and morphology and ventricular size and function
TTE usually adequate; TEE or review of intraoperative TEE may be needed for complex anatomy to establish new baseline

IE, Infective endocarditis; *TEE*, transesophageal echocardiography; *TTE*, transthoracic echocardiography.

superior for the detection of small vegetations (≤4 mm) and valvular perforations. The sensitivity of MDCTA for the detection of perivalvular extension of infection confirmed at surgery was 100%, versus 89% for TEE, and it provided additional information regarding the extent of perivalvular extension that was not detected by TEE.[60] Similar findings have been reported in a series of patients with aortic PVE, with good accuracy of MDCTA in the detection of early perivalvular extension of infection (see Fig. 80.7), periannular abscess, false aneurysm, and prosthetic valve dehiscence compared with TEE and surgery.[61] The greatest advantage of cardiac CT in the setting of IE is its ability to couple the detection of complex cardiac anatomic abnormalities with coronary artery delineation, serving two important components of the diagnostic evaluation, particularly among patients who will require surgical intervention due to IE complications. In a study of 255 adults who underwent surgery for IE, TEE had statistically higher detection of vegetations (95.6% versus 70.0%, p < 0.0001) and leaflet perforations (81.3% versus 42.9%, p = 0.02) as compared with cardiac CTA; however, for detection of abscess/pseudoaneurysm, TEE had a similar sensitivity to cardiac CTA (90.5% versus 78.4%, p = 0.21).[52] There was no significant difference in perioperative outcomes whether coronary arteries were evaluated by CTA or ICA. Therefore there is a strong argument to consider cardiac CT as an alternate coronary artery imaging modality in IE patients with low to intermediate risk of disease but meet guideline recommendations for coronary artery imaging.

Recently, positron emission tomography (CT imaging with fluorine 18–fluorodeoxyglucose (^{18}F-FDG) has incrementally improved the diagnostic accuracy in evaluation of suspected PVE, particularly CIED IE, increasing the sensitivity from approximately 60% to 70% with the modified Duke criteria and TEE imaging alone to 87% to 97% with the addition of ^{18}F-FDG PET/CT (see Figs. 18.40 and 18.41).[62,63] This resulted primarily from enhanced identification of infection in the tissue spaces adjacent to the prosthetic valve or implanted device, and less from the identification of sites of secondary infection. This imaging technique has been proposed as an additional major Duke criterion for the diagnosis of prosthetic device IE,[62] but because of the current lack of large studies, routine use of ^{18}F-FDG PET/CT has not been endorsed by guideline-writing committees to date.[8,26] Moreover, ^{18}F-FDG PET/CT has not been of incremental value in the diagnosis of native valve IE.[64]

EMBOLISM. Embolic events are common early in the course of IE, particularly before the institution of appropriate antibiotic therapy. Over the past two decades, numerous studies have reported an overall incidence of embolic events that has ranged from 20% to 50%.[8,26] In more recent clinical series, the reported incidence of acute stroke complicating IE ranged from 10% to 23%,[9,17,19,22,27] with rates of 15% to 25% reported for other embolic events not causing stroke.[9,15,17] Both stroke and other embolic events complicating IE occur more frequently in patients younger than 65 years[17] and are adverse predictors of outcome and survival in IE.[8,26] In a multicenter study using admission-screening CT imaging in 384 patients presenting with IE, 26% had one site of embolism, and another 9% had multiple sites of embolism in the following distribution: CNS (38%), spleen (30%), renal (13%), lung (10%), peripheral artery (6%), mesenteric (2%), and coronary (1%). The embolic event was clinically silent in 15% of all patients. The incidence of cerebral embolic events probably is significantly underestimated by clinical assessment. In a study of 130 patients with definite or possible IE based on the modified Duke criteria, cerebral magnetic resonance imaging (MRI) detected acute ischemic lesions in 52% of patients and only 12% had acute neurologic symptoms.[65] In this study, MRI also demonstrated cerebral microhemorrhages in 57%, other hemorrhagic lesions in 8%, asymptomatic mycotic aneurysms in 8%, and abscesses in 6%. Screening cerebral MRI led to significant modification of the diagnosis or treatment plan in 28% of the entire study group.[65]

Peripheral embolization with or without metastatic infection also may be detected with PET/CT, and clinically unsuspected lesions of this nature were observed in 28% of patients in one small series.[66] Imaging with PET/CT also is useful in the detection of perivalvular extension of infection, particularly of the aortic root, and for identification of CIED infections.

Numerous studies have examined the ability of echocardiographic characterization of vegetations to predict risk of embolic events in IE. More recent analyses have consistently shown that vegetations more than 10 mm in greatest dimension are independent predictors of embolism, with considerably higher risk with dimensions above 15 mm.[8,26,67–69] Before initiation of appropriate antibiotic therapy, large vegetations are associated with a greater than 40% risk of a clinically evident or silent embolic event. Pedunculated and highly mobile vegetations also are independently associated with embolic risk.[45] Both vegetation length of more than 10 mm and severe vegetation mobility are multivariate predictors of embolism, even after initiation of antibiotic therapy. Mitral valve vegetations, particularly on the anterior leaflet in native valve IE, are more likely to embolize than those in the aortic position; the embolic risk generally is equivalent in native and in prosthetic valve IE.[8,45,70]

The infecting organism also has an impact on embolic risk. *S. aureus* IE has been consistently implicated as an independent risk predictor for embolism; IE from *S. gallolyticus* and VGS is less implicated.[70] The presence of intracardiac perivalvular abscess is another independent risk factor for stroke associated with IE.[61]

Prediction of symptomatic embolism in IE has been proposed with the derivation and validation of a risk calculator using the variables of age, diabetes mellitus, atrial fibrillation, embolism before initiation of antibiotic therapy, vegetation length, and the presence of *S. aureus* infection. This calculator, known as the Embolic Risk French Calculator, is available online. Using this calculator, a 70-year-old patient with *S. aureus* IE, having all clinical risk variables present and vegetation size greater than 10 mm in length, would have an estimated 7-day embolic risk of 23%. The same-age patient with *S. aureus* IE but no clinical risk variables and vegetation size less than 10 mm would have an estimated 2% 7-day embolic risk.[71]

Over the past several decades, multiple clinical series have shown that the risk of embolism decreases dramatically, generally to less than 10% to 15%, within 1 week after initiation of appropriate antibiotic therapy.[8,26] The occurrence of stroke has been shown to fall to 3% after the first week of antibiotic therapy, with the overall incidence decreasing from 4.82 to 1.71 per 1000 patient-days during the second week of therapy.[70] With this documented response to antibiotic therapy, preemptive surgical intervention for potentially high-embolic-risk vegetations has not been previously advised unless there are recurrent embolic events despite ongoing appropriate antibiotic therapy.[8,26] This position has been challenged by a small study of patients with left-sided vegetations greater than 10 mm in diameter randomized to conventional management versus early surgery (within 48 hours).[72] On admission, almost 30% of each group had evidence of cerebral emboli and had no other indications for urgent surgical intervention. In patients randomized to conventional therapy, recurrent cerebral embolic events occurred in 13%, with an overall embolic event rate of 21% at 6 weeks, compared with a 0% over the same period for the early surgical patients; the in-hospital mortality was 3% for both groups.[72]

Recurrent embolic events or progressive increase in vegetation size despite appropriate antibiotic therapy, especially in the presence of significant perivalvular extension of infection or HF, would constitute clear indications for early surgical intervention.[8,26]

Thus far, no randomized controlled trials (RCTs) support the initiation of either antiplatelet or anticoagulant therapy to decrease embolic risk in IE. A retrospective analysis has suggested a lower occurrence of embolic events in patients who continue to receive antiplatelet therapy taken before the onset of IE.[73] In a larger prospective cohort analysis, established antiplatelet therapy did not reduce the incidence of cerebrovascular complications associated with IE but also did not increase the occurrence of hemorrhagic complications.[69] Therefore the initiation of aspirin or other antiplatelet agents as adjunctive therapy in IE is not currently recommended; however, the continuation of long-term antiplatelet therapy at the time of development of IE with no bleeding complications may be considered. Snygg-Martin et al.[59] reported that previously prescribed warfarin therapy, continued through the clinical course of left-sided native valve IE, was associated with a lower incidence of stroke, transient ischemic attack (TIA), and cerebral infections compared with those not receiving warfarin therapy (6% versus 26%, respectively), with the incidence of hemorrhagic complications being 2% in both groups.

ANTIMICROBIAL THERAPY

Not only is it important to diagnose IE, but it also is critical that an etiologic diagnosis be obtained to ensure that optimal antimicrobial therapy is provided for attempted cure.[8,75] Because of the rarity of presentation, diagnosis of IE often eludes nonspecialists, which results in the administration of empiric therapy for a variety of more common febrile illnesses. This empiricism can greatly reduce the sensitivity of subsequent blood cultures when the IE diagnosis is eventually considered. Thus initial empiricism results in a blood culture–negative presentation, which prompts administration of empiric antimicrobial therapy for IE. This scenario is a bane of infectious diseases specialists, who have traditionally cared for patients with IE. The antimicrobial regimen selected for therapy on the basis of the culture-negative state may not be curative. Moreover, the empiric regimen may include drugs, in particular aminoglycosides, that pose toxicity risks that might have been avoided had a pathogen been identified. Ultimately, this could result in a worst-case scenario in which a microbiologic cure is not achieved and irreversible toxicity occurs.

Some of the regimens employed in the treatment of IE are based on clinical trials with small numbers (dozens) of patients. Many of the regimens, however, are based on consensus opinion that is outlined in guidelines promulgated by societies or associations worldwide. Not surprisingly, these guidelines differ in their recommendations, which can be confusing for the practicing clinician.

Several tenets of medical management are important in defining an optimal antimicrobial regimen in each case of IE. First, consultation with a physician who is experienced in the care of patients with IE is mandatory; this usually involves a specialist trained in infectious diseases. Second, selection and dosing of antimicrobial therapy are based on both pharmacokinetic and pharmacodynamic characteristics of specific drugs and in vitro susceptibility testing results of an isolated pathogen in blood or tissue specimen culture-positive cases. Third, antimicrobial treatment should be prolonged (over weeks), high dose, parenteral, and "cidal" in its activity against a patient's isolate. Although important data were recently published regarding treatment regimens that include partial oral antibiotic dosing, more study is needed before regimens that include orally dosed antibiotics can be advocated for left-sided IE.[76] These aspects of medical therapy are necessary primarily because organisms in infected vegetations downregulate their metabolism once a relatively high concentration of organisms accumulate in vegetation tissue, which is an avascular structure.

Streptococci

Viridans Group Streptococci and *Streptococcus gallolyticus* (formerly *S. bovis*). Treatment regimens vary, depending on type of valve (native or prosthetic) and whether the streptococcal isolate is penicillin susceptible or not.[8] Regarding the latter issue, the definition of susceptibility to penicillin, as addressed previously, is based on minimum inhibitory concentrations (MICs) that are specific to treatment of the syndrome of IE; *highly penicillin-susceptible* status is defined as that of an isolate with an MIC of 0.12 µg/mL or less to penicillin. Therapy with either aqueous crystalline penicillin G sodium or ceftriaxone sodium should be microbiologically curative in 98% or more of patients with native valve IE who complete 4 weeks of treatment (Table 80.7). Because of the ease of administration of one dose per day of ceftriaxone parenterally, the bulk of therapy is with this agent rather than with intravenously administered aqueous crystalline penicillin G, which requires four to six doses per day. The once-a-day dosing of ceftriaxone sodium has been pivotal in some cases in allowing patients to avoid nursing home placement for multiple doses of antibiotic administration on a daily basis. The administration of one dose of ceftriaxone sodium each day is done in a variety of outpatient venues that routinely administer parenteral medications.

Vancomycin is recommended in patients who cannot tolerate penicillin or cephalosporin therapy because of a history of immunoglobulin E (IgE)-mediated allergic reactions (see Table 80.7). Before the preferred therapies of aqueous crystalline penicillin G or ceftriaxone are abandoned, consultation with an allergy specialist should be obtained, which may include oral amoxicillin challenge and/or skin testing to confirm that beta-lactam regimens are not a treatment option. Vancomycin should be administered intravenously for 4 weeks with serial, usually weekly, monitoring of serum trough levels, if the dose is stable and the renal status is not changing. The desired serum trough level is 10 to 15 µg/mL; serum peak vancomycin levels are not required for treatment.

TABLE 80.7 Therapy of Native Valve Endocarditis Caused by Highly Penicillin-Susceptible Viridans Group Streptococci and *Streptococcus gallolyticus*

REGIMEN	DOSE* AND ROUTE	DURATION (WEEKS)	STRENGTH OF RECOMMENDATION	COMMENTS
Aqueous crystalline penicillin G sodium	12–18 million U/24 hr IV either continuously or in 4 or 6 equally divided doses	4	Class IIa, LOE: B	Preferred in most patients >65 years or patients with impairment of eighth cranial nerve function or renal function
				Ampicillin, 2 g IV every 4 hr, is reasonable alternative to penicillin if a penicillin shortage exists.
Or				
Ceftriaxone sodium	2 g/24 hr IV/IM in 1 dose	4	Class IIa, LOE: B	
Aqueous crystalline penicillin G sodium	12–18 million U/24 hr IV either continuously or in 6 equally divided doses	2	Class IIa, LOE: B	Two-week regimen not intended for patients with known cardiac or extracardiac abscess or for those with creatinine clearance of <20 mL/min, impaired eighth cranial nerve function, or *Abiotrophia, Granulicatella,* or *Gemella* spp. infection; gentamicin dose should be adjusted to achieve peak serum concentration of 3–4 µg/mL and trough serum concentration of <1 µg/mL when 3 divided doses are used; there are no optimal drug concentrations for single daily dosing.[†]
or				
Ceftriaxone sodium	2 g/24 hr IV or IM in 1 dose	2	Class IIa, LOE: B	
Plus				
Gentamicin sulfate[‡]	3 mg/kg/24 hr IV or IM in 1 dose	2		
Vancomycin hydrochloride[§]	30 mg/kg/24 hr IV in 2 equally divided doses	4	Class IIa, LOE: B	Vancomycin therapy is reasonable only for patients unable to tolerate penicillin or ceftriaxone; vancomycin dose should be adjusted to a trough concentration range of 10–15 µg/mL.

*Doses recommended are for patients with normal renal function.
[†]Data for once-daily dosing of aminoglycosides for children exist, but no data for treatment of infective endocarditis (IE) exist.
[‡]Other potentially nephrotoxic drugs (e.g., nonsteroidal antiinflammatory drugs) should be used with caution in patients receiving gentamicin therapy. Although it is preferred that gentamicin (3 mg/kg) be given as a single daily dose to adult patients with endocarditis caused by viridans group streptococci, as a second option, gentamicin can be administered daily in three equally divided doses.
[§]Vancomycin dosages should be infused during the course of at least 1 hour to reduce the risk of histamine-release "red man" syndrome.
Minimum inhibitory concentration (MIC) is ≤0.12 µg/mL. The subdivisions differ from Clinical and Laboratory Standards Institute–recommended break points that are used to define penicillin susceptibility.
IM, Intramuscularly; *IV*, intravenously; *LOE*, level of evidence.
From Baddour LM, Wilson WR, Bayer AS, et al. Infective endocarditis in adults: diagnosis, antimicrobial therapy, and management of complications. A scientific statement for healthcare professionals from the American Heart Association. *Circulation.* 2015;132:1435–1486.

For selected patients, a 2-week treatment regimen can be used, but this should be based on input from an infectious disease specialist. The combination regimen includes either aqueous crystalline penicillin G sodium or ceftriaxone sodium plus gentamicin sulfate (see Table 80.7). The 2-week regimen should be limited to cases of uncomplicated native valve IE caused by VGS or *S. gallolyticus* strains that are highly susceptible to penicillin. The regimen would not be appropriate in patients with underlying renal or eighth cranial nerve dysfunction. If the ceftriaxone-containing regimen is used, then the single daily dose of the drug should be administered immediately before or after gentamicin dosing. No recommended guidelines for monitoring serum gentamicin concentrations are currently available.

Penicillin resistance is divided into two categories for VGS and *S. gallolyticus* infection in patients with native valve IE. In one category, relative resistance to penicillin is defined as a penicillin MIC greater than 0.12 μg/mL to less than 0.5 μg/mL. In this group, 4 weeks of therapy is recommended with either aqueous crystalline penicillin G or ceftriaxone plus gentamicin once daily for the first 2 weeks of treatment (Table 80.8). Vancomycin can be used in patients who are not candidates for beta-lactam therapy. In the other category, penicillin resistance is defined as a penicillin MIC greater than 0.5 μg/mL. Fortunately, native valve IE due to these penicillin-resistant strains is rarely seen. In patients with these infections, a more aggressive course of therapy is recommended and is the same regimen as that used in the treatment of native valve IE caused by penicillin- and aminoglycoside-susceptible enterococci (see Table 80.7). Monotherapy with vancomycin should be administered in patients who are not candidates for the combination regimen.

Patients who have IE involving a prosthetic valve or prosthetic material (e.g., annuloplasty ring) due to VGS or *S. gallolyticus* should receive 6 weeks of antibiotic therapy (Table 80.9). In those infected with strains that are highly susceptible to penicillin (MIC <0.12 μg/mL), the addition of gentamicin for the first 2 weeks of either penicillin or ceftriaxone therapy is optional. In patients infected with streptococci that harbor any level of resistance to penicillin (MIC >0.12 μg/mL), combination therapy for 6 weeks is recommended. In patients who do not tolerate beta-lactam therapy, vancomycin as monotherapy should be administered for 6 weeks.

Bacteria Formerly Known as "Nutritionally Variant Streptococci." Because of their previous designation as "nutritionally variant streptococci," a discussion of organisms now included in nonstreptococcal categories is warranted, although the frequency of these organisms causing IE is low. *Abiotrophia defectiva* and *Granulicatella* spp. and *Gemella* spp. have unusual metabolic characteristics that can result in diminished activity of cell wall–active antibiotics to kill these organisms and thus decreased cure rates. Moreover, because of this characteristic, the ability to perform in vitro susceptibility testing is adversely affected, with potentially unreliable results.

Thus a regimen recommended for treatment of native valve IE is advocated (see Table 80.7).

Beta-Hemolytic Streptococci. Unlike IE caused by VGS and *S. gallolyticus*, IE caused by beta-hemolytic streptococci typically is characterized by an acute onset with rapid valve destruction and other complications that often require cardiovascular surgical intervention. Consultation with a specialist in infectious diseases and cardiology is recommended. Because IE is infrequently caused by these organisms, prospective clinical trial data for therapeutic decisions are lacking. Nevertheless, recommended therapy for IE caused by *Streptococcus pyogenes* (group A) includes either aqueous crystalline penicillin G or ceftriaxone or cefazolin, and treatment is for at least 4 weeks. For the other types (groups B, C, F, and G) of beta-hemolytic streptococcal infections, gentamicin is advocated by some clinicians for the first 2 weeks of treatment.

Staphylococci. As noted previously, staphylococci have become more prominent as causes of IE in developed countries. In addition, antibiotic resistance has dramatically increased over the years, and for many patients, therapeutic choices are limited, although use of these agents has been largely unexamined in prospective clinical trials.

Infections caused by oxacillin-susceptible staphylococci can be treated with either nafcillin or oxacillin that is administered intravenously over 6 weeks for left-sided native valve IE or complicated right-sided IE (Table 80.10). Although previously included as an optional agent to be given over the first 3 to 5 days of therapy,[8] gentamicin is no longer advocated because of nephrotoxicity risk.[76] Cefazolin is an option for patients with left-sided infection who are intolerant of penicillins but have not had an IgE-mediated allergic reaction to penicillins. Some experts advocate for the use of cefazolin over the antistaphylococcal penicillins.

For uncomplicated right-sided native valve IE caused by oxacillin-susceptible staphylococci, 2 weeks of antibiotic therapy with nafcillin or oxacillin is an option. For patients who are intolerant of beta-lactam therapy, vancomycin can be used, but many favor a longer treatment. Daptomycin, 6 mg/kg/day intravenously, is another treatment option in patients intolerant of beta-lactam therapy.

Defining an optimal treatment regimen for native valve IE, including left- and right-sided infection, caused by oxacillin-resistant staphylococci is a more difficult task. Currently, IV vancomycin is recommended, but cure rates are less than desired. Daptomycin and ceftaroline are treatment options in patients intolerant of or nonresponsive to vancomycin, but prospective trial data including large cohorts are lacking. In addition, combination therapy with daptomycin plus a variety of beta-lactams is undergoing evaluation.

Therapy for PVE caused by staphylococci involves more complex regimens because of the difficulty in curing infections involving prosthetic valve material. For oxacillin-susceptible strains, nafcillin or oxacillin is given for at least 6 weeks in combination with rifampin, which can be administered either intravenously or orally (Table 80.11). Cefazolin

TABLE 80.8 Therapy of Native Valve Endocarditis Caused by Strains of Viridans Group Streptococci and *Streptococcus gallolyticus* Relatively Resistant to Penicillin

REGIMEN	DOSE* AND ROUTE	DURATION (WEEKS)	STRENGTH OF RECOMMENDATION	COMMENTS
Aqueous crystalline penicillin G sodium	24 million U/24 hr IV either continuously or in 4–6 equally divided doses	4	Class IIa, LOE: B	It is reasonable to treat patients with IE caused penicillin-resistant (MIC ≥0.5 μg/mL) VGS strains with a combination of ampicillin or penicillin plus gentamicin as done for enterococcal IE with infectious diseases consultation. (Class IIa, LOE: C)
				Ampicillin, 2 g IV every 4 hr, is a reasonable alternative to penicillin if a penicillin shortage exists.
Plus				
Gentamicin sulfate†	3 mg/kg/24 hr IV or IM in 1 dose	2		Ceftriaxone may be a reasonable alternative treatment option for VGS isolates that are susceptible to ceftriaxone. (Class IIb, LOE: C)
Vancomycin hydrochloride‡	30 mg/kg/24 hr IV in 2 equally divided doses	4	Class IIa, LOE: C	Vancomycin therapy is reasonable only for patients unable to tolerate penicillin or ceftriaxone therapy.

*Doses recommended are for patients with normal renal function.
†See Table 80.7 for appropriate dose of gentamicin. Although it is preferred that gentamicin (3 mg/kg) be given as a single daily dose to adult patients with endocarditis caused by VGS, as a second option, gentamicin can be administered daily in three equally divided doses.
‡See Table 80.7 for appropriate dosage of vancomycin.
Minimum inhibitory concentration (MIC) is greater than 0.12 to less than 0.5 μg/mL for penicillin. The subdivisions differ from Clinical and Laboratory Standards Institute–recommended break points that are used to define penicillin susceptibility.
IE, Infective endocarditis; *IM*, intramuscularly; *IV*, intravenously *LOE*, level of evidence; *VGS*, Viridans Group Streptococci.
From Baddour LM, Wilson WR, Bayer AS, et al. Infective endocarditis in adults: diagnosis, antimicrobial therapy, and management of complications. A scientific statement for healthcare professionals from the American Heart Association. *Circulation*. 2015;132:1435–1486.

can be used if the patient is intolerant of penicillins and has not had an IgE-mediated allergic reaction. Gentamicin is recommended for the initial 2 weeks of treatment as well. In patients intolerant of gentamicin, or if the infecting isolate is resistant to gentamicin and other aminoglycosides, levofloxacin can be given, provided that the isolate is susceptible to this agent. For PVE caused by oxacillin-resistant strains, IV vancomycin should be given in combination with rifampin for at least 2 weeks and gentamicin for 2 weeks.

Enterococci. Enterococci are common causative organisms in IE, particularly in the elderly population and those with health care–associated infections, and treatment requires both penicillin or ampicillin and an aminoglycoside (usually gentamicin) for attempted cure of infection.

TABLE 80.9 Therapy for Endocarditis of Prosthetic Valves or Other Prosthetic Material Caused by Viridans Group Streptococci and *Streptococcus gallolyticus*

REGIMEN	DOSE* AND ROUTE	DURATION (WEEKS)	STRENGTH OF RECOMMENDATION	COMMENTS
Penicillin-Susceptible Strain (≤0.12 µg/mL)				
Aqueous crystalline penicillin G sodium	24 million U/24 hr IV either continuously or in 4–6 equally divided doses	6	Class IIa, LOE: B	Penicillin or ceftriaxone together with gentamicin has not demonstrated superior cure rates compared with monotherapy with penicillin or ceftriaxone for patients with highly susceptible strain.
Or				
Ceftriaxone	2 g/24 hr IV or IM in 1 dose	6	Class IIa, LOE: B	Ampicillin, 2 g IV every 4 hr, is reasonable alternative to penicillin if a penicillin shortage exists.
with or without				
Gentamicin sulfate†	3 mg/kg/24 hr IV or IM in 1 dose	2		Gentamicin therapy should not be administered to patients with creatinine clearance <30 mL/min.
Vancomycin hydrochloride‡	30 mg/kg/24 hr IV in 2 equally divided doses	6	Class IIa, LOE: B	Vancomycin is reasonable only for patients unable to tolerate penicillin or ceftriaxone.
Penicillin Relatively or Fully Resistant Strain (MIC >0.12 µg/mL)				
Aqueous crystalline penicillin sodium	24 million U/24 hr IV either continuously or in 4–6 equally divided doses	6	Class IIa, LOE: B	Ampicillin, 2 g IV every 4 hr, is a reasonable alternative to penicillin if a penicillin shortage exists.
Or				
Ceftriaxone	2 g/24 hr IV/IM in 1 dose	6	Class IIa, LOE: B	
Plus				
Gentamicin sulfate	3 mg/kg per 24 hr IV/IM in 1 dose	6		
Vancomycin hydrochloride	30 mg/kg/24 hr IV in 2 equally divided doses	6	Class IIa, LOE: B	Vancomycin is reasonable only for patients unable to tolerate penicillin or ceftriaxone.

*Doses recommended are for patients with normal renal function.
†See Table 80.7 for appropriate dose of gentamicin. Although it is preferred that gentamicin (3 mg/kg) be given as a single daily dose to adult patients with endocarditis resulting from VGS, as a second option, gentamicin can be administered daily in 3 equally divided doses.
‡See text and Table 80.7 for appropriate dose of vancomycin.
IM, Intramuscularly; *IV,* intravenously; *LOE,* level of evidence; *MIC,* minimum inhibitory concentration; *VGS,* Viridans Group Streptococci.
From Baddour LM, Wilson WR, Bayer AS, et al. Infective endocarditis in adults: diagnosis, antimicrobial therapy, and management of complications. A scientific statement for healthcare professionals from the American Heart Association. *Circulation.* 2015;132:1435–1486.

TABLE 80.10 Therapy for Endocarditis Caused by Staphylococci in the Absence of Prosthetic Materials

REGIMEN	DOSE* AND ROUTE	DURATION (WEEKS)	STRENGTH OF RECOMMENDATION	COMMENTS
Oxacillin-Susceptible Strains				
Nafcillin or oxacillin	12 g/24 hr IV in 4–6 equally divided doses	6	Class I, LOE: C	For complicated right-sided IE and for left-sided IE. For uncomplicated right-sided IE, 2 weeks (see text).
For penicillin-allergic (nonanaphylactoid-type) patients:				Consider skin testing for oxacillin-susceptible staphylococci and questionable history of immediate-type hypersensitivity to penicillin.
Cefazolin	6 g/24 hr IV in 3 equally divided doses	6	Class I, LOE: B	Cephalosporins should be avoided in patients with anaphylactoid-type hypersensitivity to beta-lactams; vancomycin should be used in these cases.
Oxacillin-Resistant Strains				
Vancomycin†	30 mg/kg/24 hr IV in 2 equally divided doses	6	Class I, LOE: C	Adjust vancomycin dose to achieve trough concentration of 10–20 µg/mL (see text for vancomycin alternatives).
Daptomycin	≥8 mg/kg/dose	6	Class IIb, LOE: B	Await additional study data to define optimal dosing.

*Doses recommended are for patients with normal renal function.
†For specific dosing adjustment and issues concerning vancomycin, see Table 80.7 footnotes.
IE, Infective endocarditis; *IV,* intravenously; *LOE,* level of evidence.
From Baddour LM, Wilson WR, Bayer AS, et al. Infective endocarditis in adults: diagnosis, antimicrobial therapy, and management of complications. A scientific statement for healthcare professionals from the American Heart Association. *Circulation.* 2015;132:1435–1486.

TABLE 80.11 Therapy for Endocarditis of Prosthetic Valves or Other Prosthetic Material Caused by Staphylococci

REGIMEN	DOSE* AND ROUTE	DURATION (WEEKS)	STRENGTH OF RECOMMENDATION	COMMENTS
Oxacillin-Susceptible Strains				
Nafcillin or oxacillin	12 g/24 hr IV in 6 equally divided doses	≥6	Class I, LOE: B	Vancomycin should be used in patients with immediate-type hypersensitivity reactions to beta-lactam antibiotics (see Table 80.7 for dosing guidelines).
plus				
Rifampin	900 mg/24 hr IV or orally in 3 equally divided doses	≥6		Cefazolin may be substituted for nafcillin or oxacillin in patients with non–immediate-type hypersensitivity reactions to penicillins.
plus				
Gentamicin[†]	3 mg/kg/24 hr IV or IM in 2 or 3 equally divided doses	2		
Oxacillin-Resistant Strains				
Vancomycin	30 mg/kg/24 hr in 2 equally divided doses	≥6	Class I, LOE: B	Adjust vancomycin to a trough concentration of 10–20 µg/mL.
Plus				
Rifampin	900 mg/24 hr IV/PO in 3 equally divided doses	≥6		
Plus				
Gentamicin	3 mg/kg/24 hr IV/IM in 2 or 3 equally divided doses	2		See text for gentamicin alternatives.

*Doses recommended are for patients with normal renal function.
[†]Gentamicin should be administered in close proximity to vancomycin, nafcillin, or oxacillin dosing. See Table 80.7 for appropriate dose of gentamicin.
IM, Intramuscularly; *IV*, intravenously; *LOE*, level of evidence; *PO*, orally.
From Baddour LM, Wilson WR, Bayer AS, et al. Infective endocarditis in adults: diagnosis, antimicrobial therapy, and management of complications. A scientific statement for healthcare professionals from the American Heart Association. *Circulation.* 2015;132:1435–1486.

E. faecalis accounts for the bulk (approximately 97%) of IE cases and are typically penicillin susceptible, while *E. faecium* and other enterococcal species are uncommon and may be resistant to penicillin and other agents. Because of the recommended 4 to 6 weeks of therapy, it often is difficult to complete the aminoglycoside-containing regimen in these older patients without the development of nephrotoxicity and/or ototoxicity. These adverse events are a greater concern in patients who are not candidates for penicillin therapy, usually because of previous allergic reaction, in whom vancomycin is combined with an aminoglycoside.

For native valve IE caused by strains that are susceptible to both penicillin and gentamicin, 4 weeks of antibiotic treatment is recommended in patients with symptoms for 3 months or less; 6 weeks is recommended for symptoms of IE longer than 3 months or for PVE. If an isolate is gentamicin resistant and streptomycin susceptible, streptomycin should be given with either ampicillin or penicillin.

When the isolate is *faecalis* species and resistant to all aminoglycosides or the patient is unable or unlikely to tolerate an aminoglycoside-containing regimen, a combination of "high-dose" ceftriaxone (4 g daily in two divided doses) with ampicillin has been successfully used,[77,78] but no head-to-head trials have been conducted to determine if the double–beta-lactam regimen is comparable in efficacy to the aminoglycoside-containing regimen. Nevertheless, historical data suggest comparable outcomes with the two regimens; thus double–beta-lactam therapy for IE caused by *E. faecalis* is a treatment option and has been included as a recommended regimen in the current AHA guidelines.[8,26] The beta-lactam combination should be administered for 6 weeks.

Some enterococcal isolates are penicillin resistant; most do not produce beta-lactamase as the mechanism of penicillin resistance and should be treated with a combination of vancomycin plus gentamicin. For the extremely rare isolate that produces beta-lactamase, ampicillin-sulbactam can be used with gentamicin. For enterococcal strains resistant to vancomycin (VRE) and penicillin, optimal treatment regimens are undefined, and therapy should be defined by a consulting infectious diseases expert. Often, daptomycin or linezolid is selected for use with other agents, depending on additional susceptibility results, which may require sending an isolate to a reference laboratory.

HACEK Organisms. The primary choice of therapy for IE caused by the HACEK group of organisms is ceftriaxone, given for 4 weeks for native valve infection and 6 weeks for PVE. Cefotaxime and ampicillin-sulbactam are acceptable alternative therapeutic agents, but their use has been limited because of the ease of dosing (once daily) with ceftriaxone, which is not shared by these other two treatment options. Fluoroquinolones should be efficacious as second-line agents, but clinical experience in IE treatment is limited.

Aerobic Gram-Negative Bacilli and Fungi. Although they rarely cause IE, coverage of both aerobic gram-negative bacilli and fungi is included here because many experts recommend a combined medical and surgical approach to management of IE caused by these pathogens.[26] Infectious diseases, cardiology, and cardiovascular surgery consultations should be sought in these cases. A lack of clinical trial data, reflecting in part the rarity of these syndromes, makes defining an optimal treatment regimen difficult.

Nevertheless, for IE caused by aerobic gram-negative bacilli, a combination of beta-lactam with an aminoglycoside is recommended, and the selection of these agents should be based on in vitro susceptibility testing results. A fluoroquinolone that is active against the isolated pathogen can be used instead of an aminoglycoside if the infecting isolate is aminoglycoside resistant or if the patient is intolerant of aminoglycosides.

Fungal IE primarily involves prosthetic valves and is characterized by poor outcomes. In some cases the infecting organism does not grow in routine blood cultures, and the infection can manifest as culture-negative endocarditis (discussed next). As noted previously, a majority of cases are caused by *Candida* spp., and many of the infections are health care associated. Because clinical trial data do not exist, defining an optimal treatment regimen is difficult, and drug therapy, which usually includes an amphotericin B–containing product, is associated with both infusion-related (rigors, fever, back pain, hypotension, bronchospasm, tachyarrhythmias) and delayed (nephrotoxicity, anemia, cation-wasting) adverse events that can be severe and limit use of these agents.[26] Moreover, relapse rates are high, even if valve surgery is done. The echinocandins (caspofungin, micafungin, and anidulafungin) have been useful in some patients who cannot tolerate an amphotericin B–containing regimen. Thus many experts advocate the use of long-term oral suppressive therapy once initial "induction" therapy is completed and an active oral agent is identified. Azole agents, including fluconazole and voriconazole, have been used most often. Unfortunately, none of the echinocandins is available for oral use. The complexity of antifungal selection warrants consultation with an expert in infectious diseases.

Culture-Negative Endocarditis. Empiricism begets empiricism. In most cases, when no pathogen is isolated in blood cultures or in other specimens (embolism, valve tissue), empiric antimicrobial therapy is started before specimen collection. Therefore selecting an optimal treatment regimen for these patients is difficult. Certainly, epidemiologic features of each case should be evaluated to assist in defining a treatment regimen (Table 80.12). In addition, the course of illness associated with the endocarditis presentation may offer clues to the cause of the infection and to the specific antibiotics already administered that might have

TABLE 80.12 Epidemiologic Clues in Etiologic Diagnosis of Culture-Negative Endocarditis

EPIDEMIOLOGIC FEATURE	COMMON MICROORGANISM
Injection drug use (IDU)	*Staphylococcus aureus*, including community-acquired oxacillin-resistant strains
	Coagulase-negative staphylococci
	Beta-hemolytic streptococci
	Fungi
	Aerobic gram-negative bacilli, including *Pseudomonas aeruginosa*
	Polymicrobial
Indwelling cardiovascular medical devices	*S. aureus*
	Coagulase-negative staphylococci
	Fungi
	Aerobic gram-negative bacilli
	Corynebacterium spp.
Genitourinary disorders, infection, and manipulation, including pregnancy, delivery, and abortion	*Enterococcus* spp.
	Group B streptococci (*S. agalactiae*)
	Listeria monocytogenes
	Aerobic gram-negative bacilli
	Neisseria gonorrhoeae
Chronic skin disorders, including recurrent infections	*S. aureus*
	Beta-hemolytic streptococci
Poor dental health, dental procedures	Viridans group streptococci (VGS)
	Nutritionally variant streptococci
	Abiotrophia defective
	Granulicatella spp.
	Gemella spp.
	HACEK organisms
Alcoholism, cirrhosis	*Bartonella* spp.
	Aeromonas spp.
	Listeria spp.
	Streptococcus pneumonia
	Beta-hemolytic streptococci
Burns	*S. aureus*
	Aerobic gram-negative bacilli, including *P. aeruginosa*
	Fungi
Diabetes mellitus	*S. aureus*
	Beta-hemolytic streptococci
	S. pneumoniae
Early (≤1 year) prosthetic valve placement	Coagulase-negative staphylococci
	S. aureus
	Aerobic gram-negative bacilli
	Fungi
	Corynebacterium spp.
	Legionella spp.
Late (>1 year) prosthetic valve placement	Coagulase-negative staphylococci
	S. aureus
	Viridans group streptococci
	Enterococcus spp.
	Fungi
	Corynebacterium spp.
Dog or cat exposure	*Bartonella* spp.
	Pasteurella spp.
	Capnocytophaga spp.
Contact with contaminated milk or infected farm animals	*Brucella* spp.
	Coxiella burnetii
	Erysipelothrix spp.
Homeless, body lice	*Bartonella* spp.
HIV/AIDS	*Salmonella* spp.
	S. pneumonia
	S. aureus
Pneumonia, meningitis	*S. pneumoniae*
Solid-organ transplantation	*S. aureus*
	Aspergillus fumigatus
	Enterococcus spp.
	Candida spp.
Gastrointestinal lesions	*Streptococcus gallolyticus* (bovis)
	Enterococcus spp.
	Clostridium septicum

HACEK, Haemophilus spp., *Aggregatibacter* spp., *Cardiobacterium hominis, Eikenella corrodens,* and *Kingella* spp.; *HIV/AIDS,* human immunodeficiency virus infection and acquired immunodeficiency syndrome.
From Baddour LM, Wilson WR, Bayer AS, et al. Infective endocarditis in adults: diagnosis, antimicrobial therapy, and management of complications. A scientific statement for healthcare professionals from the American Heart Association. *Circulation.* 2015;132:1435–1486.

accounted for negative specimen (usually blood) cultures. In addition, an evaluation of blood and tissue should be done to determine if rare causes of endocarditis could account for a culture-negative presentation, particularly in patients who did not receive recent antimicrobial therapy. An evaluation of these rare causes of culture-negative endocarditis is outlined earlier.

Based on epidemiologic features and the most likely cadre of pathogens, a strategy for selection of antimicrobial therapy can be devised with input from an infectious diseases physician who has expertise in IE management. Considerations include the type of valve—native or prosthetic—and, with prosthetic valves, time since implantation of the valve. These regimens are necessarily broad to cover the most likely pathogens, which include the streptococci, staphylococci, enterococci, and HACEK organisms. Certain epidemiologic features may dictate broader coverage. The most troubling aspects of this approach are that the selected empiric therapy may not be adequate for a specific pathogen, and antimicrobials that would not be administered if the pathogen were identified will be given, with the potential for development of toxicity that may not be fully reversible.

Indications for and Timing of Surgery

The frequency with which surgery is used in the treatment of IE increased on average by 7% per decade between 1969 and 2000, with an attendant decrease in early mortality. In a recent study surgery for IE increased by 1.7-fold from 2011 to 2018 driven by drug use IE that increased 2.7-fold while non–drug use IE increased 1.4-fold (Geirsson et al).[7] In the current era, surgery is the mainstay of therapy for complicated IE. Current practice guidelines (largely based on observational series and expert opinion) advise that surgery should be considered in the presence of (1) HF, (2) features suggestive of a high risk of embolism, and (3) uncontrolled infection.[26,79] A review by Bannay and colleagues[80] demonstrated that early surgery led to significant improvements in survival after treatment for left-sided IE (adjusted HR for mortality, 0.55; 95% confidence interval [CI] 0.35 to 0.87;

$P = 0.01$). This benefit was further confirmed by a large, prospective, multinational study of the effect of early surgery on in-hospital mortality, accounting for treatment selection, survivorship, and hidden biases.[81] The investigators found that early surgery plus antimicrobial therapy (compared with medical management alone) was associated with a significant reduction in mortality in the overall cohort (12.1% versus 20.7%), as well as after propensity-based matching and adjustment for survivor bias (absolute risk reduction [ARR], −5.9%; $P < 0.001$). The results of these and other studies have led to management algorithms recommending the early consideration of surgical intervention after recognition of native valve IE.

Acute decompensated HF is the most frequently encountered reason for consideration of urgent surgical treatment. HF may be caused by severe regurgitation (aortic or mitral), intracardiac fistulas, or less often, vegetation-related valve obstruction. Emergent surgery for HF unresponsive to medical management is crucial, and swift intervention also is recommended, even if temporary stabilization of the patient can be achieved. Delayed surgery may be considered in the absence of HF after healing of acute endocarditic lesions, which in some circumstances may increase the likelihood of native valve repair.

Uncontrolled infection, the next most likely reason for surgical intervention, can be characterized broadly by increasing vegetation size, abscess formation, false aneurysms, or the creation of fistulas. Persistent fever frequently is associated with these anatomic findings. Early surgery is indicated in the setting of uncontrolled infection associated with persistent fever and positive blood cultures despite an appropriate antibiotic regimen, but surgery ideally should be delayed until after exclusion of extracardiac sources of infection. Perivalvular extension of infection is more common in aortic valve IE (10% to 40% in native valve IE and 56% to 100% in PVE). Some clinicians have noted that perivalvular abscesses most frequently occur in the posterior or lateral portions of the mitral annulus, whereas in aortic IE, extension can occur through the intervalvular fibrosa. The predictors of intervalvular fibrosa invasion include presence of a prosthetic valve (see Fig. 80.7), aortic location, and infection with coagulase-negative staphylococci. Pseudoaneurysms and fistula formation occur on average in 1.6% of cases and are more frequently related to *S. aureus* infection (46%). Other, less frequent manifestations of extension include ventricular septal defect, third-degree AVB, and acute coronary syndrome. Urgent surgery generally is recommended to treat perivalvular extension of infection (except in rare circumstances) and in cases of IE due to fungi, MDR organisms, and gram-negative bacteria. In general, perivalvular extension or infection with aggressive microorganisms warrants early surgery in the absence of severe comorbid disease that would otherwise be prognosis-limiting.

IE-related embolism is common (20% to 50% of cases) and can be fatal. Occult embolism may occur in approximately 20% of patients. A 2007 report indicated that the risk of embolism was highest in the first week after initiation of antibiotic therapy (4.8/1000 patient-days) and decreases thereafter (1.7/1000 patient-days).[82] Some experts therefore suggest that the greatest benefit to patient survival is the prevention of systemic embolization, which can best be realized during the first week of antibiotic therapy.

The exact timing of surgical intervention for embolism prevention should be based on the presence or absence of previous embolic events, other complications of IE, size and mobility of the vegetation, likelihood of conservative surgery (valve repair), and duration of antibiotic therapy.[80] Ultimately, extrapolation of surgical benefits also must consider factors of patient viability, comorbid conditions, potential consequences of conservative management, and patient preferences.

Surgery generally is recommended in the presence of large, mobile vegetations (>10 mm),[69] particularly after an embolic event occurring during treatment with appropriate antibiotics. Even if embolization has not occurred, the presence of HF, severe valvular dysfunction, persistent infection despite appropriate antibiotic therapy, or perivalvular abscess plus a large vegetation (>10 mm) constitutes an indication for earlier surgery. Only one small, randomized trial has evaluated the role of valve surgery in IE management.[69] Patients underwent valve surgery within 48 hours of randomization. There were several exclusion criteria for enrollment, and patients had left-sided IE, severe valvular regurgitation without HF, and vegetations larger than 10 mm to be included in the study. Valve surgery patients had fewer embolic events in follow-up, but other outcome measures, including mortality and infection relapse rates, did not differ between the two groups (each with <40 patients).

When an indication for early surgical intervention is met, the next issue becomes the risk of surgery in the context of the illness and manifest complications, most importantly, neurologic complications. When an indication for surgical management is present, the timing of surgery is an important consideration. The European and U.S. guidelines on management of infective endocarditis differ on their definitions regarding surgical timing. In the European Society of Cardiology (ESC) guidelines, surgical timing is defined as either emergent (within 24 hours), urgent (within a few days) or elective (after 1 to 2 weeks of antibiotic therapy).[8,24] Despite these differences, both guidelines recommend avoiding a delay in surgical management of IE in the setting of progressive HF, uncontrolled infection, and prevention of embolism. Evidence for timing of surgical management of IE came from a randomized clinical trial from South Korea in which patients with left-sided, native valve endocarditis and severe valve disease with large vegetations were assigned to either early surgery (defined as within 48 hours of randomization) or conventional treatment.[69] The primary outcome was a composite of in-hospital death or embolic events within 6 weeks of randomization. Among the patients in the conventional treatment arm, 77% underwent surgery either at some point during the hospitalization or in follow up. Those who underwent early surgery had a significant reduction in the composite endpoint (HR 0.10; 95% CI, 0.01 to 0.82; $P = 0.03$). The benefit of early surgery was confirmed by other observational studies, one of which used propensity score matching to show that patients with native valve endocarditis who had surgery during index hospitalization had lower in-hospital mortality than those treated medically.[51]

A unique challenge is surgical timing in patients with prior stroke, especially hemorrhagic stroke, as postsurgical mortality in these patients is high in the first 4 weeks. In a retrospective analysis of a cohort of patients with left-sided endocarditis, patients with brain hemorrhage had a higher mortality when surgery was performed within 4 weeks as compared with delayed surgery.[83] The recommendation from the AHA guidelines states that it is reasonable to delay surgical intervention for at least 4 weeks in patients with major stroke or intracranial hemorrhage (ICH).[8]

Despite a progressive emphasis on earlier surgical intervention in distinct subgroups of patients with IE, a significant proportion still do not receive surgery even in the absence of stroke. In a prospective cohort of 863 patients with left-sided endocarditis and an indication for cardiac surgery, 24% did not undergo surgery with stroke being cited as the reason in nearly a quarter of cases.[84] Several risk score models are available to assist with the decision regarding surgical management.[85,86] and worse outcomes were present in older patients with multiple comorbidities including diabetes and renal disease.

Considerable debate surrounds the performance of surgical intervention with a history of recent neurologic embolization. Iung and coauthors[87] systematically performed cerebral and abdominal MRI in early IE and found neurologic lesions in 82% of cases (ischemic lesions in 25, microbleeds in 32, and silent aneurysms in 6), and abdominal lesions in 20 patients (34%). Of importance, these findings led to modifications of classification and/or therapy in 28% of patients. Rossi and colleagues[88] detailed a best-evidence summary of whether there is an ideal time for surgery in IE with cerebrovascular complications, including ICH, ruptured mycotic aneurysm, TIA, meningitis, encephalopathy, and brain abscess. The investigators recommended 1 to 2 weeks of antibiotic treatment before cardiac surgery is indicated. However, earlier surgery is indicated in HF (class I, level of evidence [LOE]: B) and uncontrolled infection (class I, LOE: B) and for prevention of embolic events (class I, LOE: B/C). After stroke, surgery should not be delayed in the absence of coma and once cerebral hemorrhage has been excluded by cranial CT (class IIa LOE: B). After a TIA or a silent cerebral embolism, surgery is recommended without delay (class I, LOE: B). After diagnosis of ICH, surgery should ideally be postponed for at least

1 month (class I, LOE: C). In the case of surgery for PVE, the general principles outlined for native valve IE should be followed. Every patient should have a repeated head CT scan immediately before the operation to rule out preoperative hemorrhagic transformation of a brain infarction. Presence of a hematoma warrants neurosurgical consultation and consideration of cerebral angiography to rule out a mycotic aneurysm.

Medical therapy in the setting of right-sided native valve IE is the mainstay of treatment, and surgical intervention most often can be deferred in the absence of (1) diuretic-resistant right-sided HF associated with severe tricuspid regurgitation, (2) fastidious organisms resistant to antimicrobial treatment (i.e., fungemia or persistent bacteremia for >7 days), or (3) vegetations larger than 20 mm in diameter associated with multiple pulmonary emboli and possible right-sided HF.

Surgical Intervention

Before surgical intervention, several considerations in addition to the confirmation of appropriate antibiotic therapy are important. First, coronary artery assessment using either cardiac catheterization or CT angiography is recommended, to ascertain whether concomitant coronary revascularization is necessary. Before the performance of cardiac surgery, identification of primary or secondary extracardiac sites of infection should be undertaken, and extirpation should be performed if practically possible.

The primary principles guiding surgical management of IE are (1) excision of infected material along with sterilization of remaining tissue and instruments, followed by (2) reconstruction of cardiac or valve structures to permit normal heart function. Valve repair almost always is a favored option in the treatment of valvular IE.[85] If the extent of débridement necessary to eradicate infection precludes valve reconstruction, prosthetic valve replacement may be necessary.

The specific techniques used are tailored to the anatomy encountered at operation. Perforations in a valve cusp or leaflet are reconstructed using pericardial patch or other matrix substances. In general, the use of prosthetic material should be minimized; however, in settings where valve replacement is required, consensus documents do not routinely recommend one particular valve substitute over another (i.e., mechanical vs. biologic).[89]

Reports have varied regarding frequency of mitral valve repair procedures. Data from one investigation suggest that mitral valve IE can be repaired in up to 80% of patients, particularly by experienced teams at referral centers.[90] Mitral valve repair in the United States was performed in only 25.8% of patients requiring valve surgery in one large, multicenter experience that included both IDU and non-IDU with IE.[7] A combination of traditional valvuloplasty techniques is utilized,[91] and results are assessed by intraoperative TEE (Table 80.13). Although theoretically appealing, mitral valve homografts and pulmonary autografts have failed to gain widespread acceptance.

In the setting of acute IE, mechanical or biologic (xenograft) aortic valve replacement may be required, with few early demonstrated differences between device types.[92,93] Homografts or stentless root xenograft conduits are selectively used to reconstruct severely affected aortic sinuses, repair abscess-related destruction, or correct aortoventricular discontinuity.[94]

Postsurgical outcomes depend on the etiologic microorganism, the extent of tissue destruction, the presence of systolic or diastolic HF, and comorbid conditions. Early operative mortality ranges between 5% and 15%.[95] A 2008 report suggested that surgery within the first week of antibiotic therapy is associated with in-hospital mortality rate of 15%, and the main predictor was periannular extension of disease; risk of recurrent IE was 12%.[96] With isolated infection of leaflets or cusps (particularly in the subacute/chronic phase), early mortality is lower and approaches that seen in normal valve repair and replacement surgery.

Postoperative complications in this high-risk patient population typically include profound intraoperative coagulopathy necessitating mediastinal reexploration, acute renal failure, stroke, low cardiac output, pneumonia, and AVB necessitating pacemaker implantation.[86,95,97]

Outpatient Management and Follow-Up Evaluation

Antimicrobial treatment of IE is done in the outpatient setting once microbiologic control of infection is obtained, and after surgical or other interventions, if required, are completed and clinical recovery is observed.[8] Parenteral therapy is delivered in a variety of settings, related in part to the individual patient's health care coverage; often, therapy is done in a patient's home by a family member who has received instruction regarding (usually) IV infusions. Serial laboratory monitoring for evidence of drug-related toxicity and serum concentrations of drugs, when applicable, is mandatory and can be accomplished in a variety of settings, including home health agencies, primary care offices, and infectious diseases clinics. Monitoring also includes serial visits with an experienced clinician to assess clinical status and evidence of drug tolerance and complications related to an indwelling venous catheter. As outlined earlier, beta-lactam antibiotics frequently are used in the treatment of IE caused by a variety of bacterial infections. These agents are well recognized to have various adverse effects, including diarrhea, which may or may not be caused by *Clostridioides difficile* infection, as well as rash, fever, neutropenia, and less often, hepatobiliary or renal toxicities.

Once parenteral antimicrobial therapy is completed (Table 80.14), the indwelling venous catheter should be removed because it can be a nidus of subsequent infection or of other, noninfectious complications, unless there is another need for the device. At completion of therapy, an echocardiogram should be obtained to serve as a baseline (see Table 80.6), because patients who have had an initial bout of IE, regardless of whether or not the valve was replaced, are at high risk for subsequent IE relapse or recurrence. Consultation with a cardiologist should determine whether TTE versus TEE is preferred. Daily dental hygiene and dental visits should be done to promote dental health.

Patients and their family members should be educated about aspects of IE,[8] in particular the importance of obtaining three sets of blood culture specimens if the patient develops fever any time in the future before taking any antibiotic. The critical aspect of securing multiple sets of blood cultures before initiating antibiotic therapy cannot be overemphasized. If a bloodstream infection is confirmed as the cause of the fever, an evaluation for relapsing or recurrent IE is necessary, which generally will include TEE in the evaluation for a source of the infection, in addition to initiating treatment for infection.

For PWID with IE, it is critical that addiction medicine consultation be obtained, preferably before hospital discharge, because these patients are at increased risk of recurrent IE with poorer outcomes, including mortality.[98]

TABLE 80.13 Frequency and Types of Operative Procedures in Patients with and Without Drug Use

VARIABLE	OVERALL (N = 34,905)	DRUG USE (N = 11,756)	NO DRUG USE (N = 23,149)	P-VALUE
First cardiovascular surgery	25,782 (73.9%)	9,654 (82.1%)	16,128 (69.7%)	<0.001
Aortic valve procedure	19,854 (56.9%)	5,253 (44.7%)	14,601 (63.1%)	<0.001
Mitral valve procedure	16,808 (48.2%)	4,636 (39.4%)	12,172 (52.6%)	<0.001
Tricuspid valve procedure	6,982 (20.0%)	4,624 (39.3%)	2,358 (10.2%)	<0.001
Pulmonary valve procedure	281 (0.8%)	138 (1.2%)	143 (0.6%)	<0.001
Multiple valve procedures	8,195 (23.5%)	2,621 (22.3%)	5,574 (24.1%)	

TABLE 80.14 Patient Care During and After Completion of Antimicrobial Treatment

Initiation Before or at Completion of Therapy

Echocardiography to establish new baseline

Drug rehabilitation referral for patients who use illicit injection drugs

Education on the signs of endocarditis and need for antibiotic prophylaxis for certain dental/surgical/invasive procedures

Thorough dental evaluation and treatment if not performed earlier in evaluation

Prompt removal of intravenous catheter at completion of antimicrobial therapy

Short-Term Follow-Up

At least three sets of blood cultures from separate sites for any febrile illness and before initiation of antibiotic therapy

Physical examination for evidence of heart failure

Evaluation for toxicity resulting from current/previous antimicrobial therapy

Long-Term Follow-Up

At least three sets of blood cultures from separate sites for any febrile illness and before initiation of antibiotic therapy

Evaluation of valvular and ventricular function (echocardiography)

Scrupulous oral hygiene and frequent dental professional office visits

From Baddour LM, Wilson WR, Bayer AS, et al. Infective endocarditis in adults: diagnosis, antimicrobial therapy, and management of complications. A scientific statement for healthcare professionals from the American Heart Association. *Circulation.* 2015;132:1435–1486.

CARDIOVASCULAR IMPLANTABLE ELECTRONIC DEVICE INFECTIONS

The number of patients with CIEDs has dramatically increased over the past two decades, and this trend will continue as the indications for their use expand (see Chapters 58 and 69) and the population continues to age. With this expansion of CIED placement, a concomitant increase in infections of these devices has been documented.[99-101] The accompanying morbidity, mortality, and financial burden from CIED infection have been substantial.

Epidemiology

Several database surveys suggest that the rate of CIED infection has increased more than the rate of device implantation.[101-103] Factors associated with increased CIED infection risk include device placement in older patients and those with more comorbidities (particularly renal failure), more leads placed per patient, increased need for device revision or replacement, and complications at the pocket site after device placement or revision, particularly hematoma formation and delayed or poor wound healing. Factors that reduce the likelihood of device infection include the administration of surgical site prophylaxis at the time of device placement or revision and a higher volume of devices implanted by the physician performing the procedure.

Clinical Syndromes

The most common presentation of CIED infections is that of erosion and/or inflammatory changes at the shoulder generator pocket site, with or without systemic manifestations of infection.[102] For others, systemic manifestations of infection prompt clinical evaluation with or without local findings of infection at the pocket site. Pulmonary manifestations, including pleuritic pain, lung infiltrates, and lung abscess, can develop. In addition, cardiac and peripheral stigmata of IE occur in patients with CIED infection, and there may be associated valve infection.

Microbiology

Staphylococcal species predominate as causes of CIED infection, accounting for 60% to 80% of infections in most series.[99-103] Both *S. aureus* and coagulase-negative staphylococci are common pathogens and often are oxacillin resistant. Other gram-positive cocci, including streptococcal and enterococcal species, can cause CIED infection. Aerobic gram-negative bacilli and fungi are identified as pathogens in only a small minority of cases. Rarely, nontuberculous mycobacteria have been identified as causes of CIED infection.

Pathogenesis

Device infection pathogenesis involves the interactions of device, pathogen, and host.[103] Regarding the host, risk factors associated with infection have been outlined previously. For both the device and the pathogen, certain characteristics may not be unique to CIED infection but are considered operative in all types of device infections. Important among the pathogen-related mechanisms is biofilm formation. Bacteria and yeasts can attach and accumulate on the surface of a device, with eventual formation of a layer of organisms and amorphous material that harbors living organisms, able in this setting to evade normal host immune response and antimicrobial therapy. In addition to the mechanical barrier of the biofilm, organisms that accumulate in biofilms in this setting may alter their metabolic activities, protecting them from the static and cidal effects of certain antimicrobials.

On the basis of the proven efficacy of surgical site prophylaxis at CIED implantation, most CIED infections are believed to result from bacterial or fungal contamination of the device at placement. A less frequent mode of device contamination is lead infection occurring as a complication of bloodstream infection from an ectopic nidus such as an infected intravascular catheter.

Ongoing investigations are examining the surface components and physical and chemical aspects of a device and how those features interact with a pathogen's cell surface structures to either enhance or inhibit initial organism adherence to the device. Elucidation of mechanisms of initial pathogen adherence could lead to the development of devices that are more resistant to infection. Moreover, adjunctive therapies that could be administered at device placement or as vaccines before device placement may become available in the future to further reduce infection risks.

Diagnosis

The diagnosis of CIED infection is straightforward in cases where percutaneous device erosion has occurred or purulent drainage is present at a pocket site. Erythema, swelling, and pain at the pocket site also indicate infection. Distinguishing local findings due to early postoperative healing versus those due to infection can sometimes be challenging and may require serial patient examinations to determine the etiology of the local manifestations.

Blood cultures should be obtained in all cases of CIED infection, including those with clinical manifestations limited to the pocket site. The possibility of CIED infection should be considered in all patients with bloodstream infection. In patients with positive blood cultures, TEE should be performed. The sensitivity of TEE in detecting lead- and valve-related infection is superior to that of TTE.[99,100] A documented limitation of TEE, however, is that lead infection can occur with no abnormalities detected on the TEE image. Moreover, TEE identifies clots on leads in 5% to 10% of patients who have no infection. In select cases of CIED-IE, PET/CT may be helpful where pocket infection is not apparent and no alternative source of bloodstream infection is identified.

Ultimately, intraoperative findings and Gram staining and culture of deep pocket tissue and device samples obtained at complete device removal are useful in confirming CIED infection.

Management

A primary tenet of management of CIED infection includes complete device removal, if infection cure is the goal.[100,104] Despite the well-recognized risks of lead extraction,[104,105] it is essential to reduce the likelihood of relapsing infection. A management algorithm has been developed to assist in the care of patients with CIED infections (Figs. 80.9 and 80.10). Duration of antimicrobial therapy is based on the clinical syndrome of CIED infection and the identified pathogen. The recommended duration of antimicrobial therapy for the different infection syndromes is

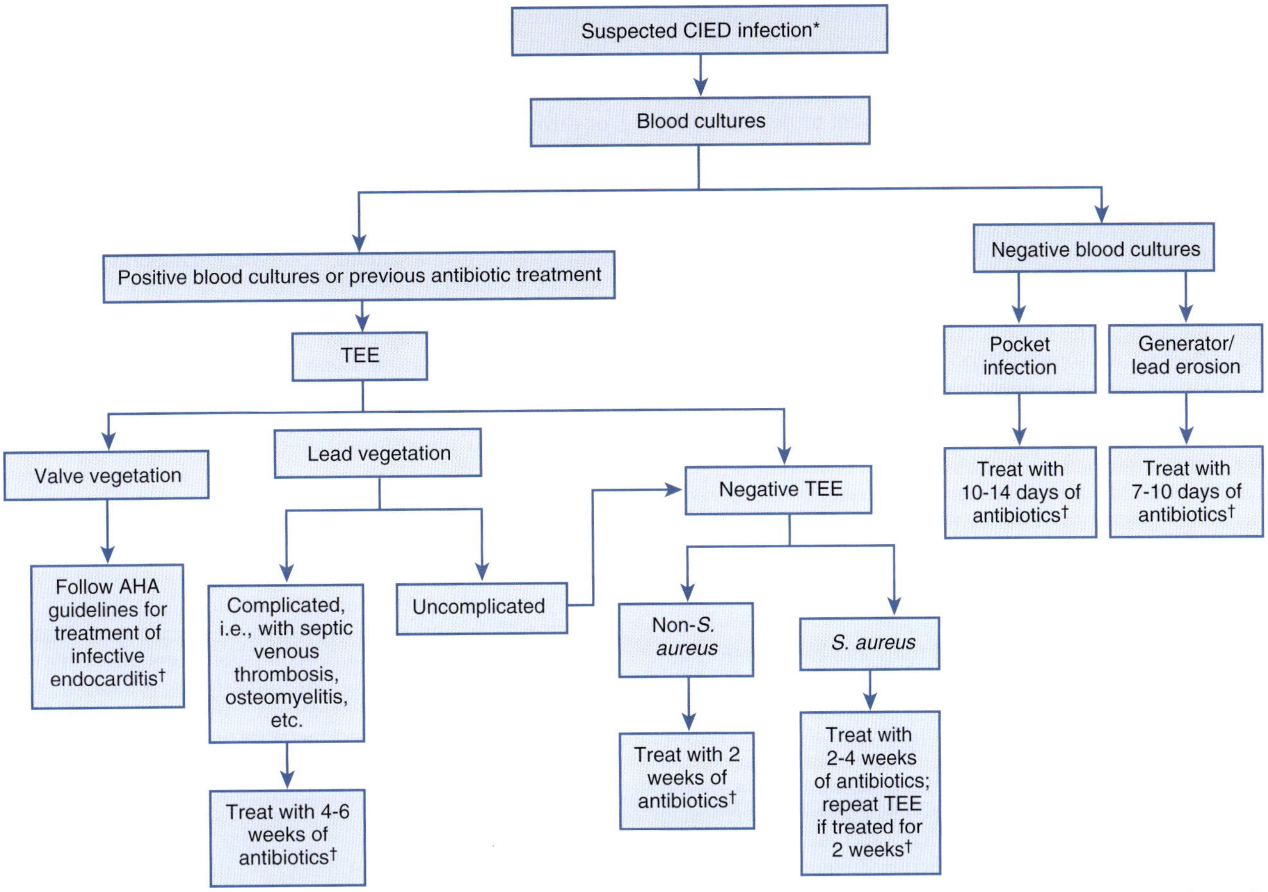

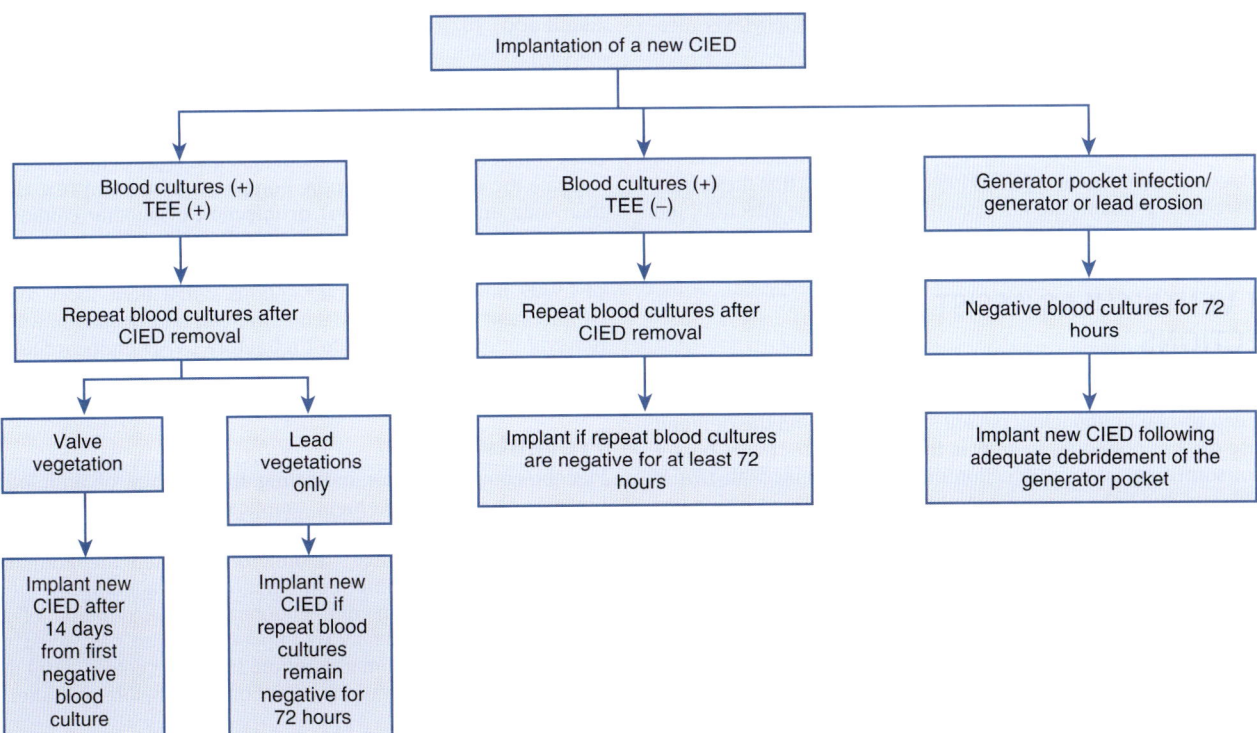

FIGURE 80.9 Approach to management of adults with cardiovascular implantable electronic device (CIED) infection. *A history, physical examination, chest radiograph, electrocardiogram, and echocardiographic device interrogation are standard baseline procedures before CIED removal. †Duration of antibiotics should be counted from the day of device explantation. Treatment can be extended to 4 or more weeks in the setting of metastatic septic complications (i.e., osteomyelitis, organ or deep abscess) or sustained bloodstream infection despite CIED removal. *AHA*, American Heart Association; *TEE*, transesophageal echocardiography. (Modified from Sohail MR, Uslan DZ, Khan AH, et al. Management and outcome of permanent pacemaker and implantable cardioverter-defibrillator infections. *J Am Coll Cardiol.* 2007;49:1851.)

FIGURE 80.10 Approach to implantation of a new device in patients after removal of an infected cardiovascular implantable electronic device (CIED). *TEE*, Transesophageal echocardiography. (Modified from Sohail MR, Uslan DZ, Khan AH, et al. Management and outcome of permanent pacemaker and implantable cardioverter-defibrillator infections. *J Am Coll Cardiol.* 2007;49:1851.)

not evidence based. Moreover, no evidence-based data are available to indicate the preferred route of therapy. In cases with complications such as valvular IE, duration of therapy can extend for 6 weeks or longer.

The optimal timing of new device placement is undefined. Each patient should undergo individualized assessment to determine the need for a new device. Some experts have advocated that a new device can be implanted 72 hours after removal of the infected device, provided that blood cultures are negative, no valvular IE is present, and control of infection at the pocket site is secured.[100,102]

Management of patients with bloodstream infection as the *sole* manifestation of an infection is more difficult.[100] In such patients a thorough evaluation, including TEE, identifies no nidus responsible for bloodstream infection. The obvious concern is that either the CIED is infected and serves as a source of bloodstream infection, or the bloodstream infection could secondarily infect the CIED. Decisions regarding device removal are complex. If the device is not removed, relapsing bloodstream infection is inevitable once antimicrobial therapy is completed, if the device is the source of bloodstream infection. Conversely, if the CIED is removed but was not infected, the patient was exposed to the risk and complications of device removal without benefit, as well as incurring considerable expense for the procedure.

Prophylaxis

Prospective, placebo-controlled, clinical trials and case-control and meta-analysis studies[106] consistently indicate that the preoperative administration of an antistaphylococcal antibiotic, usually cefazolin, given intravenously 30 to 60 minutes before device placement or revision, is effective in reducing the risk of CIED infection. If vancomycin is deemed a more appropriate choice, the IV administration should begin 2 hours before the procedure. Subsequent postoperative dosing is not recommended with either cefazolin or vancomycin.

Two "prevention" trials deserve particular comment. The PADIT examined a regimen that included preprocedural cefazolin *plus* vancomycin, intraoperative bacitracin pocket wash, and a 2-day postprocedural oral cephalexin course and demonstrated no benefit of this incremental treatment strategy in reducing CIED infections as compared with that of conventional single-dose, preprocedural cefazolin.[107] The WRAP-IT evaluated an antibacterial envelope that was placed at the time of generator implantation of CIED.[108] Major device infections were reduced as compared with that of standard prophylaxis measures and the envelope, which was absorbable, was well tolerated.

Antimicrobial prophylaxis is not recommended for patients with CIEDs who undergo invasive procedures, such as dental, GI, or GU procedures, because evidence-based data indicating that such procedures carry a risk of CIED infection are lacking. The predominance of staphylococci as the agents of CIED infection suggests that these invasive procedures probably are not responsible for device infection, and "secondary" prophylaxis is not warranted.

LEFT VENTRICULAR ASSIST DEVICE INFECTIONS

Major advances in the technologic aspects of LV assist devices (LVADs) have been pivotal in impacting patient survival,[109,110] and the demand for these devices continues to grow in the United States (see Chapter 59). Not surprisingly, device infection occurs in patients with LVADs and will continue to be a major complication of LVAD use as long as it remains a percutaneous device. The most dramatic change in infection risk among cardiac devices may be that associated with LVADs. Infection risks have fallen, largely because of improvements in device design, including reduction in size.

Characterizing the incidence, epidemiology, and risk factors associated with LVAD infections is difficult because of the striking design changes in these devices since their inception.[109,110] The first-generation, pulsatile-flow, volume-displacement devices, including Novacor, Heartmate XVE, and other Thoratec devices, have been associated with higher rates of infection than the more recently reported rates with the second-generation, continuous-flow devices, including Heartmate II, VentrAssist, and MicroMed DeBakey.

Three categories of LVAD infections have been identified based on the portion of the device that is infected. These designations are somewhat arbitrary, however, because infection can involve more than one portion of an LVAD. The most common presentation is that of driveline infection. Erythema and drainage at the driveline site, with or without systemic manifestations of infection, usually are present.

Pump pocket infection is a second infection presentation and can be a complication of driveline infection. Local pain or discomfort with systemic manifestations is present, and abnormal fluid collection is demonstrated on ultrasound examination or CT. Fluid aspiration or surgical drainage procedures yield purulent material.

LVAD-associated IE is the least often diagnosed of the three presentations, but some cases may go undiagnosed (or may be diagnosed only at autopsy) because diagnostic tools such as TEE lack sensitivity. This diagnosis should be considered in all patients with sustained bloodstream infection and no other cardiovascular device that could serve as a nidus for sustained bacteremia or fungemia.

Microbiology

Staphylococcal species are the predominant causes of LVAD infection,[109,110] and oxacillin resistance is common. Less often, a panoply of other bacteria, encompassing enterococci (including VRE) and *Pseudomonas* spp., and fungi (*Candida* spp.) are identified as pathogens. Treatment options, particularly as oral therapy, usually are limited because of the MDR profiles of these pathogens.

Management

The medical management of LVAD infections is difficult. Ideally, the device would be completely removed, but this approach requires surgical intervention and is associated with considerable morbidity and mortality. Therefore antimicrobial therapy is the mainstay of management and often is used for prolonged periods on a recurrent basis. In addition, antimicrobial selection is difficult because of the characteristic multidrug resistance of infecting pathogens and the underlying comorbidities that increase the likelihood of drug toxicity (e.g., chronic renal failure and colistin or aminoglycoside use for MDR *Pseudomonas aeruginosa* infection).

Regardless of site of device infection, blood culture specimens should be obtained in every case of LVAD infection. Positive blood cultures can occur in patients without systemic signs of infection and can indicate the presence of a more complicated infection (e.g., IE rather than only driveline infection) or infection of another cardiovascular device, such as a prosthetic valve or CIED.

A variety of surgical interventions are used in the management of LVAD infection. Such interventions range from local soft tissue débridement for driveline infection to heart transplantation with LVAD removal in an effort to control refractory LVAD endocarditis and its associated complications.

Prevention

Placebo-controlled trials indicating the efficacy of antibiotic prophylaxis at LVAD placement (surgical site prophylaxis) are lacking. Nevertheless, the adoption of this practice is universal,[109,110] and multiple (up to five) antimicrobials often are administered, typically including some combination of vancomycin, rifampin, cefepime, ciprofloxacin, and fluconazole. The duration of antimicrobial prophylaxis after LVAD implantation also has varied widely, with 24 hours as a minimal duration. In some centers, nasal mupirocin also is used for a variable duration both before and after LVAD implantation.

Meticulous daily care at the driveline exit site is advocated. Patient and family education and serial visits with specialized caregivers are critical in infection prevention and in securing an early diagnosis.

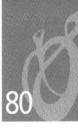

REFERENCES

Epidemiology

1. Tleyjeh IM, Abdel-Latif A, Rahbi H, et al. A systematic review of population-based studies of infective endocarditis. *Chest*. 2007;132:1025–1035.
2. de Sa DDC, Tleyjeh IM, Anavekar NS, et al. Epidemiological trends of infective endocarditis: a population-based study in Olmsted County, Minnesota. *Mayo Clin Proc*. 2010;85:422–426.
3. Keller K, Hobohm L, Munzel T, Ostad MA. Incidence of infective endocarditis before and after the guideline modification regarding a more restrictive use of prophylactic antibiotics therapy in the USA and Europe. *Minerva Cardioangiol*. 2019;67:200–206.
4. Schranz AJ, Fleischauer A, Chu VH, et al. Trends in drug use-associated infective endocarditis and heart valve surgery, 2007 to 2017: a study of statewide discharge data. *Ann Intern Med*. 2019;170:31–40.
5. Siegman-Igra Y, Koifman B, Porat R, et al. Healthcare associated infective endocarditis: a distinct entity. *Scand J Infect Dis*. 2008;40:474–480.
6. Fedeli U, Schievano E, Buonfrate D, et al. Increasing incidence and mortality of infective endocarditis: a population-based study through a record-linkage system. *BMC Infect Dis*. 2011;11:48.
7. Geirsson A, Schranz A, Jawitz O, et al. The evolving burden of drug use associated infective endocarditis in the United States. *Ann Thorac Surg*. 2020;110(4):1185–1192.

Pathophysiology, Presentation, and Diagnosis

8. Baddour LM, Wilson WR, Bayer AS, et al. Infective endocarditis in adults: diagnosis, antimicrobial therapy, and management of complications: a scientific statement for healthcare professionals from the American Heart Association. *Circulation*. 2015;132:1435–1486.
9. Murdoch DR, Corey GR, Hoen B, et al. Clinical presentation, etiology, and outcome of infective endocarditis in the 21st century: the international collaboration on endocarditis–prospective cohort study. *Arch Int Med*. 2009;169:463–473.
10. Li JS, Sexton DJ, Mick N, et al. Proposed modifications to the Duke criteria for the diagnosis of infective endocarditis. *Clin Infect Dis*. 2000;30:633–638.
11. Holland TL, Baddour LM, Bayer AS, et al. Infective endocarditis. *Nat Rev Dis Primers*. 2016;2:16059.
12. Katan O, Michelena HI, Avierinos J-F, et al. Incidence and predictors of infective endocarditis in mitral valve prolapse: a population-based study. *Mayo Clin Proc*. 2016;91:336–342.
13. Tzemos N, Therrien J, Yip J, et al. Outcomes in adults with bicuspid aortic valves. *J Am Med Assoc*. 2008;300:1317–1325.
14. Michelena HI, Desjardins VA, Avierinos JF, et al. Natural history of asymptomatic patients with normally functioning or minimally dysfunctional bicuspid aortic valve in the community. *Circulation*. 2008;117:2776–2784.
15. Tribouilloy C, Rusinaru D, Sorel C, et al. Clinical characteristics and outcome of infective endocarditis in adults with bicuspid aortic valves: a multicentre observational study. *Heart*. 2010;96:1723–1729.
16. Kahveci G, Bayrak F, Pala S, et al. Impact of bicuspid aortic valve on complications and death in infective endocarditis of native aortic valves. *Tex Heart Inst J*. 2009;36:111–116.
17. Durante-Mangoni E, Bradley S, Selton-Suty C, et al. Current features of infective endocarditis in elderly patients: results of the international collaboration on endocarditis prospective cohort study. *Arch Intern Med*. 2008;168:2095–2103.
18. Sun BJ, Choi S-W, Park K-H, et al. Infective endocarditis involving apparently structurally normal valves in patients without previously recognized predisposing heart disease. *J Am Coll Cardiol*. 2015;65:307–309.
19. Lopez J, Revilla A, Vilacosta I, et al. Age-dependent profile of left-sided infective endocarditis: a 3-center experience. *Circulation*. 2010;121:892–897.
20. Knirsch W, Nadal D. Infective endocarditis in congenital heart disease. *Eur J Pediatr*. 2011;170:1111.
21. Duval X, Delahaye F, Alla F, et al. Temporal trends in infective endocarditis in the context of prophylaxis guideline modifications: three successive population-based surveys. *J Am Coll Cardiol*. 2012;59:1968–1976.
22. Benito N, Miró JM, de Lazzari E, et al. Health care–associated native valve endocarditis: importance of non-nosocomial acquisition. *Ann Intern Med*. 2009;150:586–594.
23. Delahaye F, M'Hammedi A, Guerpillon B, et al. Systematic search for present and potential portals of entry for infective endocarditis. *J Am Coll Cardiol*. 2016;67:151–158.
24. Sohail MR, Uslan DZ, Khan AH, et al. Infective endocarditis complicating permanent pacemaker and implantable cardioverter-defibrillator infection. *Mayo Clin Proc*. 2008;83:46–53.
25. Athan E, Chu VH, Tattevin P, et al. Clinical characteristics and outcome of infective endocarditis involving implantable cardiac devices. *J Am Med Assoc*. 2012;307:1727–1735.
26. Habib G, Lancellotti P, Antunes MJ, et al. 2015 ESC guidelines for the management of infective endocarditis: the task Force for the management of infective endocarditis of the European Society of Cardiology (ESC)endorsed by: European Association for Cardio-Thoracic Surgery (EACTS), The European Association of Nuclear Medicine (EANM). *Eur Heart J*. 2015;36:3075–3128.
27. López J, Fernández-Hidalgo N, Revilla A, et al. Internal and external validation of a model to predict adverse outcomes in patients with left-sided infective endocarditis. *Heart (British Cardiac Society)*. 2011;97:1138–1142.
28. Nadji G, Rusinaru D, Rémadi J-P, et al. Heart failure in left-sided native valve infective endocarditis: characteristics, prognosis, and results of surgical treatment. *Eur J Heart Fail*. 2009;11:668–675.
29. Muñoz P, Kestler M, De Alarcon A, et al. Current epidemiology and outcome of infective endocarditis: a multicenter, prospective, cohort study. *Medicine*. 2015;94:e1816.
30. Hill EE, Herijgers P, Claus P, et al. Infective endocarditis: changing epidemiology and predictors of 6-month mortality: a prospective cohort study. *Eur Heart J*. 2007;28:196–203.
31. Wang A, Athan E, Pappas PA, et al. Contemporary clinical profile and outcome of prosthetic valve endocarditis. *J Am Med Assoc*. 2007;297:1354–1361.
32. López J, Revilla A, Vilacosta I, et al. Definition, clinical profile, microbiological spectrum, and prognostic factors of early-onset prosthetic valve endocarditis. *Eur Heart J*. 2007;28:760–765.
33. Hill EE, Herregods M-C, Vanderschueren S, et al. Management of prosthetic valve infective endocarditis. *Am J Cardiol*. 2008;101:1174–1178.
34. Que Y-A, Moreillon P. Infective endocarditis. *Nat Rev Cardiol*. 2011;8:322–336.
35. Sy RW, Chawantanpipat C, Richmond DR, Kritharides L. Development and validation of a time-dependent risk model for predicting mortality in infective endocarditis. *Eur Heart J*. 2009;32:2016–2026.
36. Yu C-W, Juan L-I, Hsu S-C, et al. Role of procalcitonin in the diagnosis of infective endocarditis: a meta-analysis. *Am J Emerg Med*. 2013;31:935–941.
37. Snipsøyr MG, Ludvigsen M, Petersen E, et al. A systematic review of biomarkers in the diagnosis of infective endocarditis. *Int J Cardiol*. 2016;202:564–570.
38. Tsenovoy P, Aronow WS, Joseph J, Kopacz MS. Patients with infective endocarditis and increased cardiac troponin I levels have a higher incidence of in-hospital mortality and valve replacement than those with normal cardiac troponin I levels. *Cardiology*. 2009;112:202–204.
39. Stancoven AB, Shiue AB, Khera A, et al. Association of troponin T, detected with highly sensitive assay, and outcomes in infective endocarditis. *Am J Cardiol*. 2011;108:416–420.
40. Shiue AB, Stancoven AB, Purcell JB, et al. Relation of level of B-type natriuretic peptide with outcomes in patients with infective endocarditis. *Am J Cardiol*. 2010;106:1011–1015.
41. Kahveci G, Bayrak F, Mutlu B, et al. Prognostic value of N-terminal pro-B-type natriuretic peptide in patients with active infective endocarditis. *Am J Cardiol*. 2007;99:1429–1433.
42. Ferrera C, Vilacosta I, Fernández C, et al. Usefulness of new-onset atrial fibrillation, as a strong predictor of heart failure and death in patients with native left-sided infective endocarditis. *Am J Cardiol*. 2016;117:427–433.
43. Tornos P, Gonzalez-Alujas T, Thuny F, Habib G. Infective endocarditis: the European viewpoint. *Curr Prob Cardiol*. 2011;36:175–222.

Echocardiography

44. Casella F, Rana B, Casazza G, et al. The potential impact of contemporary transthoracic echocardiography on the management of patients with native valve endocarditis: a comparison with transesophageal echocardiography. *Echocardiography*. 2009;26:900–906.
45. Habib G, Badano L, Tribouilloy C, et al. Recommendations for the practice of echocardiography in infective endocarditis. *Eur J Echo*. 2010;11:202–219.
46. Hansalia S, Biswas M, Dutta R, et al. The value of live/real time three-dimensional transesophageal echocardiography in the assessment of valvular vegetations. *Echocardiography*. 2009;26:1264–1273.
47. Amat-Santos IJ, Messika-Zeitoun D, Eltchaninoff H, et al. Infective endocarditis after transcatheter aortic valve implantation. *Circulation*. 2015;131:1566–1574.
48. Latib A, Naim C, De Bonis M, et al. TAVR-associated prosthetic valve infective endocarditis: results of a large, multicenter registry. *J Am Coll Cardiol*. 2014;64:2176–2178.
49. Banchs J, Yusuf SW. Echocardiographic evaluation of cardiac infections. *Expert Rev Cardiovasc Ther*. 2012;10:1–4.
50. Román JS, Vilacosta I, Zamorano J, et al. Transesophageal echocardiography in right-sided endocarditis. *J Am Coll Cardiol*. 1993;21:1226–1230.
51. Kiefer T, Park L, Tribouilloy C, et al. Association between valvular surgery and mortality among patients with infective endocarditis complicated by heart failure. *J Am Med Assoc*. 2011;306:2239–2247.
52. Lauridsen TK, Park L, Tong SYC, et al. Echocardiographic findings predict in-hospital and 1-year mortality in left-sided native valve *Staphylococcus aureus* endocarditis. *Circ Cardiovasc Imag*. 2015;8:e003397.
53. Hill EE, Herijgers P, Claus P, et al. Abscess in infective endocarditis: the value of transesophageal echocardiography and outcome: a 5-year study. *Am Heart J*. 2007;154:923–928.
54. Showler A, Burry L, Bai AD, et al. Use of transthoracic echocardiography in the management of low-risk staphylococcus aureus bacteremia: results from a retrospective multicenter cohort study. *JACC Cardiovasc Imaging*. 2015;8:924–931.
55. Palraj BR, Baddour LM, Hess EP, et al. Predicting Risk of Endocarditis Using a Clinical Tool (PREDICT): scoring system to guide use of echocardiography in the management of Staphylococcus aureus bacteremia. *Clin Infect Dis*. 2015;61:18–28.
56. Tubiana S, Duval X, Alla F, et al. The VIRSTA score, a prediction score to estimate risk of infective endocarditis and determine priority for echocardiography in patients with Staphylococcus aureus bacteremia. *J Infect*. 2016;72:544–553.
57. Barton TL, Mottram PM, Stuart RL, et al. Transthoracic echocardiography is still useful in the initial evaluation of patients with suspected infective endocarditis: evaluation of a large cohort at a tertiary referral center. *Mayo Clin Proc*. 2014;89:799–805.

Complications

58. Snygg-Martin U, Rasmussen RV, Hassager C, et al. The relationship between cerebrovascular complications and previously established use of antiplatelet therapy in left-sided infective endocarditis. *Scand J Infect Dis*. 2011;43:899–904.
59. Snygg-Martin U, Rasmussen RV, Hassager C, et al. Warfarin therapy and incidence of cerebrovascular complications in left-sided native valve endocarditis. *Eur J Clin Microbiol Infect Dis*. 2011;30:151–157.
60. Sudhakar S, Sewani A, Agrawal M, Uretsky BF. Pseudoaneurysm of the Mitral-Aortic Intervalvular Fibrosa (MAIVF): a comprehensive review. *J Am Soc Echocardiogr*. 2010;23:1009–1018.
61. Feuchtner GM, Stolzmann P, Dichtl W, et al. Multislice computed tomography in infective endocarditis: comparison with transesophageal echocardiography and intraoperative findings. *J Am Coll Cardiol*. 2009;53:436–444.
62. Sims JR, Anavekar NS, Chandrasekaran K, et al. Utility of cardiac computed tomography scanning in the diagnosis and pre-operative evaluation of patients with infective endocarditis. *Int J Cardiovasc Imaging*. 2018;34:1155–1163.
63. Fagman E, Perrotta S, Bech-Hanssen O, et al. ECG-gated computed tomography: a new role for patients with suspected aortic prosthetic valve endocarditis. *Eur Radiol*. 2012;22:2407–2414.
64. Saby L, Laas O, Habib G, et al. Positron emission tomography/computed tomography for diagnosis of prosthetic valve endocarditis: increased valvular 18F-fluorodeoxyglucose uptake as a novel major criterion. *J Am Coll Cardiol*. 2013;61:2374–2382.
65. Pizzi MN, Roque A, Fernandez-Hidalgo N, et al. Improving the diagnosis of infective endocarditis in prosthetic valves and intracardiac devices with 18F-fluordeoxyglucose positron emission tomography/computed tomography angiography: initial results at an infective endocarditis referral center. *Circulation*. 2015;132:1113–1126.
66. Millar BC, Habib G, Moore JE. New diagnostic approaches in infective endocarditis. *Heart*. 2016;102:796–807.
67. Duval X, Iung B, Klein I, et al. Effect of early cerebral magnetic resonance imaging on clinical decisions in infective endocarditis: a prospective study. *Ann Intern Med*. 2010;152:497–504.

Management

68. Van Riet J, Hill EE, Gheysens O, et al. 18F-FDG PET/CT for early detection of embolism and metastatic infection in patients with infective endocarditis. *Eur J Nucl Med Molec Imaging*. 2010;37:1189–1197.
69. Kang D-H, Kim Y-J, Kim S-H, et al. Early surgery versus conventional treatment for infective endocarditis. *N Engl J Mede*. 2012;366:2466–2473.
70. Berdejo J, Shibayama K, Harada K, et al. Evaluation of vegetation size and its relationship with embolism in infective endocarditis. *Circ Cardiovasc Imaging*. 2014;7:149–154.
71. Pfister R, Betton Y, Freyhaus FT, et al. Three-dimensional compared to two-dimensional transesophageal echocardiography for diagnosis of infective endocarditis. *Infection*. 2016;44:725–731.
72. Dickerman SA, Abrutyn E, Barsic B, et al. The relationship between the initiation of antimicrobial therapy and the incidence of stroke in infective endocarditis: an analysis from the ICE Prospective Cohort Study (ICE-PCS). *Am Heart J*. 2007;154:1086–1094.
73. Hubert S, Thuny F, Resseguier N, et al. Prediction of symptomatic embolism in infective endocarditis: construction and validation of a risk calculator in a multicenter cohort. *J Am Coll Cardiol*. 2013;62:1384–1392.
74. Anavekar NS, Tleyjeh IM, Anavekar NS, et al. Impact of prior antiplatelet therapy on risk of embolism in infective endocarditis. *Clin Infect Dis*. 2007;44:1180–1186.
75. Thuny F, Grisoli D, Collart F, et al. Management of infective endocarditis: challenges and perspectives. *Lancet*. 2012;379:965–975.
76. Iversen K, Ihlemann N, Gill SU, et al. Partial oral versus intravenous antibiotic treatment of endocarditis. *New Engl J Med*. 2018;380:415–424.
77. Cosgrove SE, Vigliani GA, Fowler Jr VG, et al. Initial low-dose gentamicin for staphylococcus aureus bacteremia and endocarditis is nephrotoxic. *Clin Inf Dis*. 2009;48:713–721.
78. Gavaldà J, Len O, Miró JM, et al. Brief communication: treatment of enterococcus faecalis endocarditis with ampicillin plus ceftriaxone. *Ann Intern Med*. 2007;146:574–579.

79. Nishimura RA, Otto CM, Bonow RO, et al. 2014 AHA/ACC guideline for the management of patients with valvular heart disease: executive summary. *Circulation*. 2014;129:2440–2492.
80. Bannay A, Hoen B, Duval X, et al. The impact of valve surgery on short- and long-term mortality in left-sided infective endocarditis: do differences in methodological approaches explain previous conflicting results? *Eur Heart J*. 2009;32:2003–2015.
81. Lalani T, Cabell CH, Benjamin DK, et al. Analysis of the impact of early surgery on in-hospital mortality of native valve endocarditis. *Circulation*. 2010;121:1005–1013.
82. Thuny F, Beurtheret S, Mancini J, et al. The timing of surgery influences mortality and morbidity in adults with severe complicated infective endocarditis: a propensity analysis. *Eur Heart J*. 2009;32:2027–2033.
83. García-Cabrera E, Fernández-Hidalgo N, Almirante B, et al. Neurological complications of infective endocarditis. *Circulation*. 2013;127:2272–2284.
84. Chu VH, Park LP, Athan E, et al. Association between surgical indications, operative risk, and clinical outcome in infective endocarditis. *Circulation*. 2015;131:131–140.
85. Martínez-Sellés M, Muñoz P, Arnáiz A, et al. Valve surgery in active infective endocarditis: a simple score to predict in-hospital prognosis. *Int J Cardiol*. 2014;175:133–137.
86. Gaca JG, Sheng S, Daneshmand MA, et al. Outcomes for endocarditis surgery in North America: a simplified risk scoring system. *J Thorac Cardiovasc Surg*. 2011;141:98–106.e2.
87. Iung B, Klein I, Mourvillier B, et al. Respective effects of early cerebral and abdominal magnetic resonance imaging on clinical decisions in infective endocarditis. *Eur Heart J Cardiovasc Imaging*. 2012;13:703–710.
88. Rossi M, Gallo A, De Silva RJ, Sayeed R. What is the optimal timing for surgery in infective endocarditis with cerebrovascular complications? *Interact Cardiovasc Thorac Surg*. 2011;14:72–80.
89. Fernández-Hidalgo N, Almirante B, Gavaldà J, et al. Ampicillin plus ceftriaxone is as effective as ampicillin plus gentamicin for treating enterococcus faecalis infective endocarditis. *Clin Infect Dis*. 2013;56:1261–1268.
90. Prendergast BD, Tornos P. Surgery for infective endocarditis. *Circulation*. 2010;121:1141–1152.
91. Suri RM, Burkhart HM, Daly RC, et al. Robotic mitral valve repair for all prolapse subsets using techniques identical to open valvuloplasty: establishing the benchmark against which percutaneous interventions should be judged. *J Thorac Cardiovasc Surg*. 2011;142:970–979.
92. Minakata K, Schaff HV, Zehr KJ, et al. Is repair of aortic valve regurgitation a safe alternative to valve replacement? *J Thorac Cardiovasc Surg*. 2004;127:645–653.
93. Avierinos J-F, Thuny F, Chalvignac V, et al. Surgical treatment of active aortic endocarditis: homografts are not the cornerstone of outcome. *Ann Thorac Surg*. 2007;84:1935–1942.
94. Lopes S, Calvinho P, de Oliveira F, Antunes M. Allograft aortic root replacement in complex prosthetic endocarditis. *Eur J Cardio Thorac Surg*. 2007;32:126–132.
95. David TE, Gavra G, Feindel CM, et al. Surgical treatment of active infective endocarditis: a continued challenge. *J Thorac Cardiovasc Surg*. 2007;133:144–149.
96. Thuny F, Beurtheret S, Gariboldi V, et al. Outcome after surgical treatment performed within the first week of antimicrobial therapy during infective endocarditis: a prospective study. *Arch Cardiovasc Dis*. 2008;101:687–695.
97. de Kerchove L, Vanoverschelde J-L, Poncelet A, et al. Reconstructive surgery in active mitral valve endocarditis: feasibility, safety and durability. *Eur J Cardio Thorac Surg*. 2007;31:592–599.
98. Nguemeni Tiako MJ, Mori M, Bin Mahmood SU, et al. Recidivism is the leading cause of death among intravenous drug users who underwent cardiac surgery for infective endocarditis. *Semin Thorac Cardiovasc Surg*. 2019;31:40–45.

Implantable Device Infections

99. Baddour LM, Cha Y-M, Wilson WR. Infections of cardiovascular implantable electronic devices. *N Engl J Med*. 2012;367:842–849.
100. Baddour LM, Epstein AE, Erickson CC, et al. Update on cardiovascular implantable electronic device infections and their management. *Circulation*. 2010;121:458–477.
101. Greenspon AJ, Patel JD, Lau E, et al. 16-Year trends in the infection burden for pacemakers and implantable cardioverter-defibrillators in the United States: 1993 to 2008. *J Am Coll Cardiol*. 2011;58:1001–1006.
102. Sohail MR, Uslan DZ, Khan AH, et al. Management and outcome of permanent pacemaker and implantable cardioverter-defibrillator infections. *J Am Coll Cardiol*. 2007;49:1851–1859.
103. Nagpal A, Baddour LM, Sohail MR. Microbiology and pathogenesis of cardiovascular implantable electronic device infections. *Circ Arrhythm Electrophysiol*. 2012;5:433–441.
104. Wilkoff BL, Love CJ, Byrd CL, et al. Transvenous lead extraction: Heart Rhythm Society Expert consensus on facilities, training, indications, and patient management: this document was endorsed by the American Heart Association (AHA). *Heart Rhythm*. 2009;6:1085–1104.
105. Bracke F. Complications and lead extraction in cardiac pacing and defibrillation. *Neth Heart J*. 2008;16:S28–S31.
106. de Oliveira JC, Martinelli M, Nishioka SA, et al. Efficacy of antibiotic prophylaxis before the implantation of pacemakers and cardioverter-defibrillators: results of a large, prospective, randomized, double-blinded, placebo-controlled trial. *Circ Arrhythm Electrophysiol*. 2009;2:29–34.
107. Krahn AD, Longtin Y, Philippon F, et al. Prevention of arrhythmia device infection trial: the PADIT trial. *J Am Coll Cardiol*. 2018;72:3098–3109.
108. Tarakji KG, Mittal S, Kennergren C, et al. Antibacterial envelope to prevent cardiac implantable device infection. *N Engl J Med*. 2019;380:1895–1905.
109. Nienaber JJC, Kusne S, Riaz T, et al. Clinical manifestations and management of left ventricular assist device–associated infections. *Clin Infect Dis*. 2013;57:1438–1448.
110. O'Horo JC, Abu Saleh OM, Stulak JM, et al. Left ventricular assist device infections: a systematic review. *ASAIO J*. 2018;64:287–294.

Guidelines

111. Wilson WR, Gewitz M, Lockhart PB, et al; American Heart Association Young Hearts Rheumatic Fever, Endocarditis and Kawasaki Disease Committee of the Council on Lifelong Congenital Heart Disease and Heart Health in the Young; Council on Cardiovascular and Stroke Nursing; and the Council on Quality of Care and Outcomes Research. Prevention of Viridans Group Streptococcal Infective Endocarditis: A Scientific Statement From the American Heart Association. *Circulation*. 2021;143(20):e963-e978.
112. Otto CM, Nishimura RA, Bonow RO, et al. 2020 ACC/AHA Guideline for the Management of Patients With Valvular Heart Disease: Executive Summary: A Report of the American College of Cardiology/American Heart Association Joint Committee on Clinical Practice Guidelines. *J Am Coll Cardiol*. 2021;77(4) 450–500.

81 Rheumatic Fever

ANA OLGA MOCUMBI

扫描二维码阅读
第81章中文导读

EPIDEMIOLOGY, 1531

PATHOGENESIS, 1531
The Agent, 1532
The Host, 1532
The Environment, 1532
Pathogenesis of Acute Rheumatic Fever, 1532
Pathologic Features, 1532

CLINICAL FEATURES, 1533
Arthritis, 1533
Carditis, 1534
Sydenham Chorea, 1534
Cutaneous and Subcutaneous Features, 1534

Other Manifestations, 1535

DIAGNOSIS, 1535
Evidence of Preceding GAS Infection, 1535
Revised Jones Criteria, 1535
Other Tests, 1535
Differential Diagnosis, 1536
Recurrences, 1536

NATURAL HISTORY, 1536

MANAGEMENT, 1536
General Management, 1536
Antibiotic Treatment, 1536

Aspirin and Other Anti-Inflammatory Drugs, 1537
Antibiotic Prophylaxis, 1537

PREVENTION, 1537
Primordial Prevention, 1537
Primary Prevention, 1537
Secondary Prevention, 1538

FUTURE PERSPECTIVES, 1538

CLASSIC REFERENCES, 1538

REFERENCES, 1539

Rheumatic fever (RF) is a leading cause of acquired heart disease in children and young adults worldwide. It is an illness preceded by a pharyngeal infection with group A beta-hemolytic streptococci (GAS), occurring most often between 5 and 15 years. The inflammatory process causes damage to collagen fibrils and connective tissue ground substance, resulting typically in combinations of arthritis, carditis, erythema marginatum, subcutaneous nodules, and chorea. The diagnosis is based on applying the modified Jones criteria to information gleaned from the history, examination, laboratory testing, individual risk, and, more recently, echocardiographic data (see "Diagnosis"). The treatment includes aspirin or other nonsteroid anti-inflammatory drugs, corticosteroids during severe carditis, and antimicrobials to eradicate residual streptococcal infection and prevent reinfection.

In allusion to the fleeting arthritis and damaging carditis that is characteristic of RF, the French physician Ernst-Charles Lasegue famously said, in 1884, that *"rheumatic fever licks the joints but bites the heart."* Indeed, it is the destructive effect on the heart that leads to the chronic sequelae of the RF—rheumatic heart disease (RHD)—a preventable cause of health failure, stroke, endocarditis, and premature deaths in highly endemic areas.

EPIDEMIOLOGY

The burden of RF remains uncertain due to the complexity of its diagnosis, which includes epidemiologic considerations, a high level of awareness, trained health professionals who can recognize subtle signs, and complementary tests that are not always readily available.

The burden of RF and RHD is most salient within marginalized communities in developed nations as well as in low- and middle-income regions.[1] Worldwide, incidence is 19/100,000 (range, 5 to 51/100,000), with lowest rates (<10/100,000) in North America and Western Europe and highest rates (>10/100,000) in Eastern Europe, the Middle East, Asia, Africa, Australia, and New Zealand.[2] The condition is more prevalent among young people, particularly between the ages of 5 to 30, and although its occurrence is similar between women and men, the inherent biological factors, the risk of illness during pregnancy, exposure to GAS through child rearing, and poor accessibility to resources make women approximately 1.8 times more susceptible to developing RHD.[3]

Four changing patterns for the burden of RF have been recognized over the past 150 years (Fig. 81.1). Curve A is typical of industrialized countries and represents the preantibiotic fall in RF incidence. This decrease preceding the introduction of antibiotics in the 1940s is almost certainly the result of improved socioeconomic standards, less overcrowded housing, and improved access to medical care; for example, in the United States, the incidence per 100,000 population was 100 at the start of the 20th century, was 45 to 65 between 1935 and 1960, and is currently estimated at less than 10 cases per 100,000.[4] Curve B shows persistently high incidence of RF in developing regions and among indigenous populations of some developed countries, such as Australia and New Zealand. The incidence of RF per 100,000/year among 5- to 14-year-old indigenous Australian children is as high as 162 in men and 228 in women.[5] This hyperendemic pattern is found in the majority of the population living in Africa, the Middle East, Asia, Eastern Europe, South America, and indigenous communities of Australasia. However, in Curve C, some developing countries—Cuba, Costa Rica, Martinique, Guadeloupe, and Tunisia—have experienced a fall in the incidence of RF after implementation of comprehensive public health programs of primary and secondary prevention of RF.[6] Finally, outbreaks of RF have been reported in affluent communities in the United States and Italy[7] (see also Veasy et al., Classic References). In Curve D, there is a sustained resurgence of RF and RHD in central Asia,[8] where the incidence of RF had fallen to the same levels as Japan in the 1970s but rose sharply in the post-Soviet period to levels associated with developing countries. This may reflect weakening of the primary care system and the economic crisis of the post-Soviet period (see Tulchinsky and Varavikova, Classic References).

The attack rate, defined as the percentage of patients with untreated GAS pharyngitis who develop acute RF (ARF), varies from <1.0% to 3.0%. Higher attack rates occur with certain streptococcal M protein serotypes and a stronger host immune response, likely resulting from undefined genetic predisposition[2] and factors such as the carrier state.[1,9]

Rheumatic arthritis was found in around 10% of family members of RHD cases undergoing cardiac surgery in Egypt,[10] and cardiac sequelae were detected in asymptomatic children during active community-based screening.[11] The strict application of the updated Jones criteria[12] still leads to underdiagnosis of RF in highly endemic regions[13]; the most effective predictors—arthritis, carditis, chorea, aortic regurgitation, significant mitral regurgitation, thick anterior mitral valve leaflets, elevated acute phase reactants, positive family history, and prolonged PR interval—show an overall prediction accuracy of 81.4%, with high sensitivity of 93% and specificity of 62%.[13]

PATHOGENESIS

RF is a multifactorial disease that follows GAS *(the agent)* pharyngitis in a susceptible individual *(the host)* who lives under deprived social conditions *(the environment)*. The theory of molecular mimicry holds

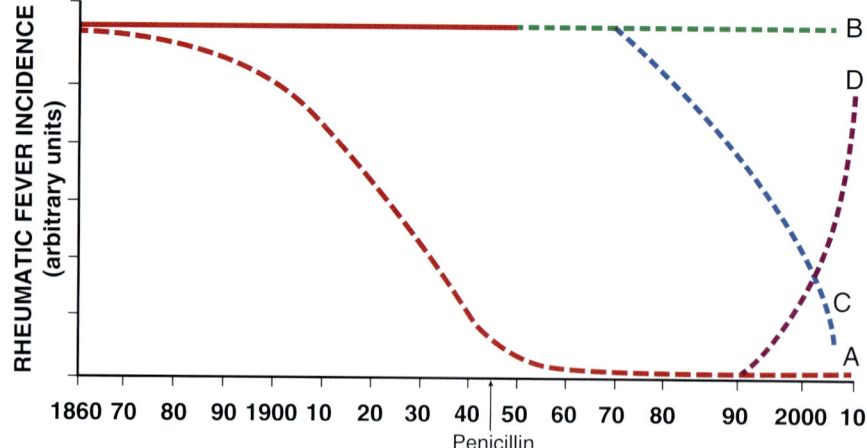

FIGURE 81.1 Incidence of rheumatic fever (RF): four patterns over the past 150 years. Curve A represents the preantibiotic fall in incidence of RF that is typical of industrialized countries. Curve B is typical of the persistent high incidence in regions of the world with no comprehensive program for prevention such as Africa and South Asia. Curve C shows the postantibiotic fall in the incidence of RF in countries that instituted comprehensive programs for primary and secondary prevention of RF, such as Cuba, Costa Rica, Martinique, and Guadeloupe. Curve D shows the fall and rise in the incidence of RF in the formerly Soviet republics of Central Asia. (Modified from Parry E, et al., editors. Principles of Medicine in Africa. 3rd ed. Cambridge: Cambridge University Press; 2004, p 861.)

that GAS pharyngitis triggers an autoimmune response in susceptible individuals by cross-reacting with similar epitopes in the heart, brain, joints, and skin, and that repeated episodes of RF lead to RHD.[1,14] In situations of untreated epidemic GAS pharyngitis, up to 3% of patients develop the disease.[15] The risk of RF is substantially reduced by effective antibiotic therapy.

The Agent
Epidemiologic data, immunologic observations, and the preventive effect of antibiotic treatment for pharyngitis demonstrated in clinical trials strongly support the causative role of untreated GAS pharyngitis in RF (see Dajani, Classic References). There is also growing evidence regarding the potential role of GAS skin infections in causing ARF, either alone or in combination with GAS pharyngitis.[16] Initial suggestions came from a report of RF following streptococcal wound infection (see Popat and Riding, Classic References). This may be particularly important in Africa, where excoriation of highly endemic scabies lesions can lead to secondary pyoderma infection, most commonly by Staphylococcus aureus and GAS.[17]

The hypothesis of molecular mimicry in the pathogenesis of RF[1] state that patients with RHD have cross-reactive autoantibodies that target the dominant GAS epitope of the group A carbohydrate, N-acetyl-beta-d-glucosamine (GlcNAc), and laminin and laminar basement membrane in heart valve endothelium. T cells in peripheral blood and heart valves of RHD patients cross-react with streptococcal M protein and cardiac myosin. Furthermore, autoantibodies against the GAS carbohydrate epitope GlcNAc and cardiac myosin appear during progression of RHD. In addition, autoantibodies against collagen that are cross-reactive may form because of the release of collagen from damaged valves.

The *two-hit hypothesis* for the initiation of disease proposes that antibody attack of valve endothelium facilitates the extravasation of T cells through activated epithelium into valve tissue, leading to the formation of granulomatous nodules called Aschoff bodies, characteristic of rheumatic myocarditis (Fig. 81.2). The area of central necrosis is surrounded by a ring of plump histiocytes, called Anitschkow cells. These nodules were discovered by Ludwig Aschoff and Paul Rudolf Geipel and thus are occasionally called Aschoff-Geipel bodies.

Human monoclonal antibodies (mAbs) derived from patients with disease target GlcNAc, gangliosides, and dopamine receptors on the surface of neuronal cells in the brain. Human mAbs and autoantibodies in Sydenham chorea activate calcium/calmodulin-dependent protein kinase II (CaMKii) in neuronal cells and recognize the intracellular protein biomarker tubulin.

The Host
Genetic predisposition to RF and RHD has been hypothesized by findings from familial studies, as well as observed associations between genes located in the human leukocyte antigens (HLA) on chromosome 6p21.3 and elsewhere in the genome. Currently, several lines of epidemiologic evidence support the role of hereditary factors in susceptibility to RF. First, the lifetime cumulative incidence of RF in populations exposed to rheumatogenic GAS infection is constant at 3% to 6% regardless of geography or ethnicity,[18] suggesting that the proportion of susceptible individuals is the same in all continental populations worldwide.[12] Second, the chance of an individual with a family history of RF acquiring the disease is nearly five times greater than that of an individual who has no such hereditary predisposition.[12] This familial aggregation of RHD has been supported by a study of children raised separately from parents with RHD, who had a relative risk of 2.93 for the development of RF compared with children whose parents did not have RHD.[12] The heritability of RF, at 60%, highlights the importance of heredity as a major susceptibility factor of the disease.

Studies conducted to search for specific genetic susceptibility factors in RF have targeted genes controlling the adaptive immune response (e.g., HLA class II alleles, cytotoxic T-cell lymphocyte antigen 4), the innate immune response (e.g., ficolin 2, mannose-binding lectin 2, receptor for Fc fragments of IgG, Toll-like receptor 2), cytokine genes (e.g., tumor necrosis factor-α, transforming growth factor-β, interleukin-1 receptor A, interleukin-10), and B-cell alloantigens. Significant associations have been found between genetic factors and RF, but studies either conflict or are not replicated.[12] Therefore, it is not possible at the present to predict the individuals who are at risk of developing RF following an episode of untreated GAS pharyngitis.

The Environment
RF is generally associated with low socioeconomic status. The incidence of RF has been falling consistently in industrialized countries since the mid-19th century, independently of the advent of penicillin, possible related to less crowding, improved housing and nutritional status, higher levels of parental employment, and better access to health care (see Fig. 81.1, Curve A). In endemic regions, the risk of RF is linked to high levels of deprivation based on household income, access to telephone and car, education level, and housing, as well as overcrowding and unemployment.

Pathogenesis of Acute Rheumatic Fever
The reason for the difference in complications resulting from GAS infections of the pharynx and of other areas of the body is not well understood. Pharyngeal infection with GAS leads to activation of the innate immune system. Neutrophils, macrophages, and dendritic cells phagocytose the bacteria and then present antigens to T cells; this leads to activation of humoral (antibodies) and cellular immune responses (CD4+ T-cell activation). The driving mechanism of ARF is the immune response becoming cross-reactive with human tissues: Carditis is caused by both cross-reactive antibodies and T cells, arthritis by immune complex deposition, chorea by antibody binding to neuronal cells and the skin, and subcutaneous manifestations by a delayed hypersensitivity reaction.[19]

Pathologic Features
The pathology of ARF varies by site with the joints, heart, skin, and central nervous system (CNS) being most often affected. Cardiac involvement manifests as carditis, typically affecting valves and endocardium, then myocardium, and finally pericardium. In ARF, Aschoff bodies (Fig. 81.2) often develop in the myocardium and other parts of the heart; the incidental finding of Aschoff nodules diagnoses acute rheumatic myocarditis.[20] Fibrinous nonspecific pericarditis, sometimes with effusion, occurs only in patients with endocardial inflammation and usually subsides without permanent damage.

Joint involvement manifests as nonspecific synovial inflammation; if biopsied, it sometimes shows small foci resembling Aschoff bodies (granulomatous collections of leukocytes, myocytes, and interstitial collagen). Unlike the cardiac findings, however, the abnormalities of the joints are not chronic and do not leave scarring or residual abnormalities.

Subcutaneous nodules appear indistinguishable from those of juvenile idiopathic arthritis (JIA), but biopsy shows features resembling Aschoff bodies. Erythema marginatum differs histologically from other skin lesions with similar macroscopic appearance (e.g., the rash of systemic JIA, Henoch-Schönlein purpura, erythema chronicum migrans, and erythema multiforme). Perivascular neutrophilic and mononuclear infiltrates of the dermis is usually found.

Sydenham chorea manifests as hyperperfusion and increased metabolism in the basal ganglia. Increased levels of antineuronal antibodies have also been shown.[21]

CLINICAL FEATURES

The typical attack of RF follows an episode of GAS infection—usually symptoms of GAS pharyngitis—after a latent period of 2 to 3 weeks, during which there are no clinical or laboratory evidence of active inflammation. However, as many as one-third of patients who develop RF do so after asymptomatic GAS, and in outbreaks up to 58% of patients have no symptoms of pharyngitis. Preceding symptomatic pharyngitis is recognized in only about two-thirds of patients with ARF in high-income countries, and even less in endemic regions.

A first episode of ARF can occur at any age but occurs most often between 4 and 15 years, ages that are also the peak years for streptococcal pharyngitis. However, in developing countries there are reports of RHD occurring at age 3 to 5 years. ARF typically involves some combination of the joints, heart, skin, and CNS. The most common major sign is polyarthritis, which occurs in two-thirds to three-quarters of patients, followed by carditis and chorea. The illness usually begins with high fever, but in some patients the fever may be low-grade or absent.

Arthritis

Joint involvement is more common and more severe in young adults (100%) than in teenagers (82%) and children (66%). At the onset of the illness the joint involvement is asymmetric and usually affects the lower limbs initially before spreading to the upper limbs. *Migratory polyarthritis* is the most common manifestation of ARF, occurring in about 35% to 66% of children, often accompanied by fever. In some cases the joint involvement may be additive rather than migratory, with several joints affected simultaneously; thus in untreated patients the number of joints affected varies between 6 and 16. The affected joint may be inflamed for only a few days to 1 week before inflammation subsides. The polyarthritis is severe for approximately 1 week in two-thirds of the patients and may last for another 1 or 2 weeks in the remainder, before it resolves completely. If the joint swelling persists after 4 weeks, it becomes necessary to consider other conditions, such as JIA or systemic lupus erythematosus (SLE).

Monarthritis occurs in high-risk indigenous populations (e.g., in Australia, India, Fiji), as has been reported in 17% to 25% of patients. Joints become extremely painful and tender; these symptoms are often out of proportion to the modest warmth and swelling present on examination (this is in contrast to the arthritis of Lyme disease, in which the examination findings tend to be more severe than the symptoms). The large joints such as ankles, knees, elbows, and wrists are usually involved. Shoulders, hips, and small joints of the hands and feet may also be involved, but almost never alone. If vertebral joints are affected, another disorder should be suspected. Joint pain and fever usually subside within 2 weeks and seldom last more than 1 month.

The synovial fluid has characteristics of sterile inflammation. There may be reduction in complement components C1q, C3, and C4, suggesting their consumption by immune complexes. Radiographs may show features of a join effusion, but no other abnormality is noted.

Jaccoud arthritis or arthropathy (or chronic post-RF arthropathy) is a rare manifestation of RF characterized by deformities of the fingers and toes (Fig. 81.3). The condition may occur after repeated attacks of RF and results from recurrent inflammation of the fibrous articular capsule. There is ulnar deviation of the fingers, especially the fourth and fifth fingers, flexion of the metacarpophalangeal joints, and hyperextension of the proximal interphalangeal joints (i.e., swan neck deformity). The hand is usually painless, and there are no signs of inflammation. The deformities usually correctible but may become fixed in the later stages. There are no true erosions on radiography, and the rheumatoid factor is usually negative. A similar form of arthropathy is seen in patients with SLE.

Because the arthritis of RF responds promptly to nonsteroidal anti-inflammatory drugs (NSAIDs), the classic presentation of a migratory polyarthritis may be infrequent in regions where NSAID self-medication or prescription is common; this may explain the apparent fall in incidence of RF in some developing countries.[22]

Poststreptococcal reactive arthritis (PSRA) is diagnosed in patients who have arthritis that is not typical of RF but who have evidence of recent streptococcal infection. This condition occurs after a shorter latent period than RF, is less responsive to NSAIDs, may be associated with renal manifestations, and evidence of carditis is infrequent. The distinction between PSRA and RF is unclear, and many would recommend that a diagnosis of PSRA not be made in populations where RF is common. Even if the diagnosis is considered, it is appropriate to offer a period of secondary prophylaxis with penicillin, as for episodes of acute RF, in such populations.

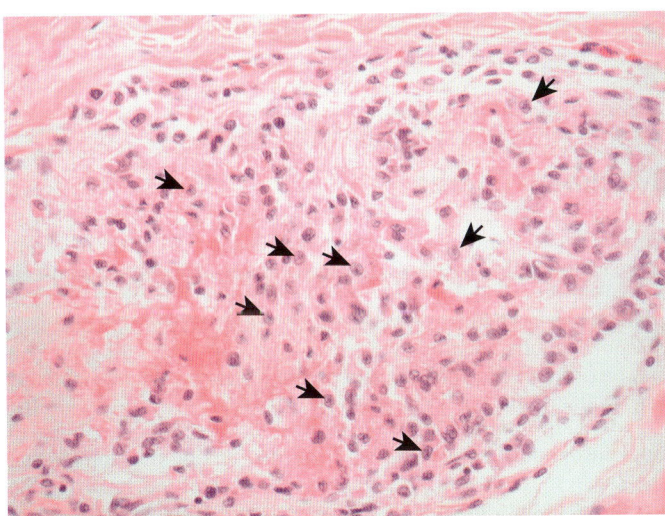

FIGURE 81.2 The Aschoff body of rheumatic fever. Photomicrography of an Aschoff nodule from the heart in a case of acute rheumatic fever. The nodule is composed of Anitschkow cells; these have clear nuclei with a central bar of chromatin, said to resemble a caterpillar. There is a central area of fibrin. This central necrosis is further surrounded by a mononuclear cell infiltrate. Myocardial fibers adjacent to the Aschoff body are undergoing destruction. (From Sebire NJ, et al., editors. Diagnostic Pediatric Surgical Pathology. London: Churchill Livingstone; 2010.)

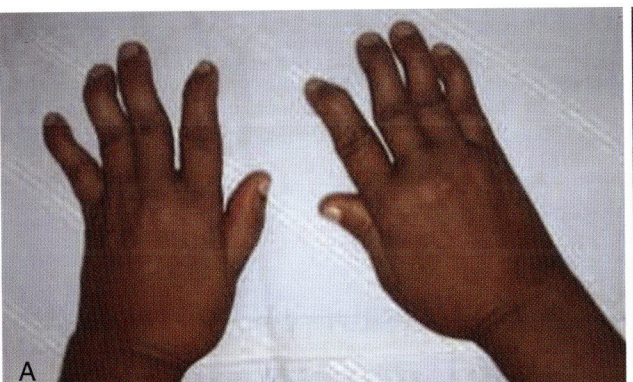
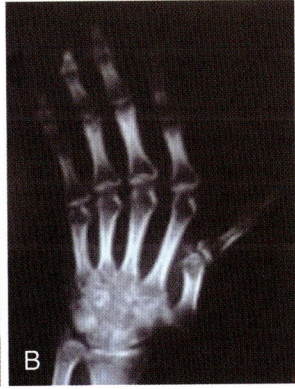

FIGURE 81.3 Post-rheumatic fever Jaccoud arthropathy. **A,** Swan neck deformity in Jaccoud arthropathy, with ulnar deviation and metacarpophalangeal subluxation. **B,** Plain radiograph of the left hand showing deformities but not erosions. (From Santiago MB. Jaccoud's arthropathy. Best Prac Res Rheumatol 2011;25:715.)

TABLE 81.1 World Heart Federation Minimum Criteria for the Diagnosis of Pathologic Valvular Regurgitation Caused by Rheumatic Carditis

ECHOCARDIOGRAPHIC FEATURES IN RHEUMATIC VALVULITIS			
DOPPLER FINDINGS		**MORPHOLOGIC FINDINGS**	
Pathologic mitral regurgitation*	Pathologic aortic regurgitation*	Acute mitral valve changes	Aortic valve changes in carditis or chronic RHD
Seen in at least two views	Seen in the least two views	Annular dilatation	Irregular or focal leaflet thickening
		Chordal elongation	
Jet length ≥2 cm in at least one view†	Jet length ≥1 cm in at least one view†	Chordal rupture resulting in flail leaflet with severe mitral regurgitation	Coaptation defect
Peak velocity > 3 m/sec	Peak velocity >3 m/sec	Anterior (or less commonly posterior leaflet tip prolapse)	Restricted leaflet motion
Pansystolic jet in the least one envelope	Pandiastolic jet in at least one envelope	Beading/nodularity of leaflet tips	Leaflet prolapse

*All four criteria must be met.
†A regurgitant jet length should be measured from the vena contracta to the last pixel of regurgitant color (blue or red) on the nonmagnified (nonzoomed) images. The listed criteria provide a set of objective measures to distinguish physiologic valvular regurgitation from pathologic regurgitation but are not specific for rheumatic carditis. Morphologic abnormalities presented may or may not be present.
RHD, Rheumatic heart disease.
Adapted from Remenyi B, et al. World Heart Federation criteria for echocardiographic diagnosis of rheumatic heart disease: an evidence-based guideline. Nat Rev Cardiol 2012;9:297-309; Dougherty S, et al. Acute Rheumatic Fever and Rheumatic Heart Disease. 1st ed. Philadelphia: Elsevier; 2020.

Carditis

The incidence of carditis during the initial attack of RF varies from 40% to 91% depending on the selection of patients, the age of patient, and whether the diagnosis is made on clinical assessment alone or combined with echocardiography.[11] Carditis is the most serious manifestation of RF because it may lead to chronic RHD. It may be asymptomatic and detected during clinical examination of patients with arthritis or chorea. Heart failure results from a combination of carditis and valvular dysfunction and occurs in 5% to 10% of the initial episodes, more frequently during recurrences of RF. Patients may have high fever, chest pain, or both; tachycardia is common, especially during sleep. In about 50% of cases, cardiac damage (i.e., persistent valve dysfunction) occurs much later. The symptoms and signs depend on whether there is involvement of the pericardium, myocardium, or heart valves. Although considered to be a pancarditis, valvulitis is the most consistent feature of ARF, and if it is not present, the diagnosis should be reconsidered.

Valvulitis

The clinical diagnosis of valvulitis has classically been made by auscultation of murmurs, but subclinical cases detected by echocardiography may occur in up to 18% of cases of ARF. When heart murmurs are not heard at initial examination, repeated clinical examinations and echocardiography are recommended. The most common valvular lesion is mitral regurgitation; aortic regurgitation is less common. Stenotic lesions are uncommon in the early stages of RF, but a transient apical mid-diastolic murmur (Carey-Coombs) may occur in association with the murmur of mitral regurgitation. Murmurs often persist indefinitely; if no worsening occurs during the next 2 to 3 weeks, new manifestations of carditis seldom follow. In the presence of history of previous RHD, a change in the character of the murmurs or the appearance of a new murmur is indicative of acute rheumatic carditis.

Myocarditis

Inflammation of the myocardium is unlikely to be rheumatic in origin in the absence of valvulitis. Patients with myocarditis develop cardiomegaly or congestive heart failure, which may be severe and life threatening. Electrocardiographic abnormalities include varying degrees of heart block.

Pericarditis

Pericarditis occurs in approximately 10% of patients and may be manifested by anterior chest pain and a pericardial friction rub. The pericardial effusion may sometimes be large, but cardiac tamponade is rare and constrictive pericarditis does not occur.

Echocardiography is recommended for all patients with suspected or definite ARF, as it is more sensitive and specific than cardiac auscultation for detection of acute rheumatic carditis. (See Vasan et al., Classic References.) Table 81.1 outlines the World Heart Federation minimum echocardiographic criteria for pathologic regurgitation caused by rheumatic carditis.

Sydenham Chorea

The CNS is affected in up to 40% of children with RF,[23] predominating in females after puberty. The latent period between GAS pharyngitis and chorea is longer (6 to 8 weeks) than for arthritis and carditis; its onset is typically insidious and may be preceded by inappropriate laughing or crying. It can last for up to 2 years (usually 8 to 15 weeks); if it occurs in isolation, all inflammatory markers may be normal and the diagnosis may be overlooked as an indicator of ARF. It does not occur simultaneously with arthritis but may coexist with carditis.

Sydenham chorea, also referred to as St. Vitus dance, consists of rapid, involuntary, purposeless, and irregular jerking movements that may begin in the hands but often become generalized, involving the feet and face and interfering with voluntary activity; they disappear during sleep. The purposeless movements are associated with hypotonia, weakness (sometimes mistaken for paralysis), and loss of fine motor control.

Characteristic findings include fluctuating grip strength (milkmaid's grip), tongue fasciculations or tongue darting (patients intermittently involuntarily withdraw the tongue when attempting to protrude it for 30 seconds, the so-called jack-in-the-box tongue), facial grimacing, and explosive speech with or without tongue clucking. Emotional lability manifests in personality changes, with inappropriate behavior, restlessness, outburst of anger and crying, and learning difficulties; previously undiagnosed obsessive-compulsive behavior may be unmasked in many patients. The term pediatric autoimmune neuropsychiatric disorders associated with streptococcal infections (PANDAS) is used for children with tic or obsessive-compulsive disorders triggered by GAS infection, without cardiac valve damage. In populations at high risk of RF the suspicion of PANDAS should be considered as a manifestation of ARF and managed with secondary prophylaxis.

Cutaneous and Subcutaneous Features

Rarely, subcutaneous nodules and erythema marginatum develop in patients already having carditis, arthritis, or chorea; they almost never occur alone. The subcutaneous nodules of RF occur most frequently on the extensor surfaces of large joints. They may be detected over the occiput, elbows, knees, ankles, and Achilles tendons. Ordinarily, the

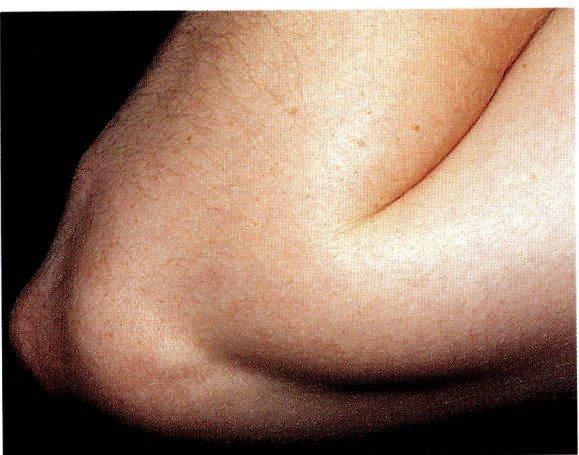

FIGURE 81.4 Subcutaneous nodules of rheumatic fever over the bony prominences of the elbow. (From Beeman LB, et al. Cardiology. In Zetelli BJ, et al., editors. Atlas of Pediatric Physical Diagnosis. 6th ed. Philadelphia: Saunders; 2012.)

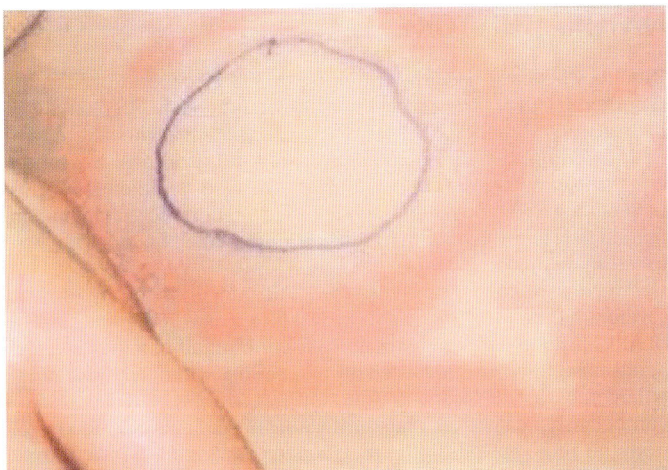

FIGURE 81.5 Erythema marginatum in acute rheumatic fever. The pen mark shows the location of the rash approximately 60 minutes previously. (From Cohen J, Powderly WG. Infectious Diseases. 2nd ed. St Louis: Mosby; 2004.)

nodules are firm, painless, and freely movable over the subcutaneous tissue; they vary in size from 0.5 to 2 cm and tend to occur in crops that may be related to the severity of the carditis (Fig. 81.4). They are transitory (seldom more than 1 month) and respond to treatment of joint or heart inflammation. Fewer than 10% of children with ARF have nodules.

Erythema Marginatum

Erythema marginatum occurs as a serpiginous, flat or slightly raised, nonscarring, and painless rash in fewer than 6% of children. The rash usually appears on the trunk and proximal extremities but not the face (Fig. 81.5), and is evanescent, pink, and nonpruritic. It extends centrifugally while the skin at the center returns to normal, always with an irregular serpiginous border. It sometimes lasts less than 1 day and may become more prominent after a shower. Its appearance is often delayed after the inciting streptococcal infection, with or after the other manifestations of rheumatic inflammation.

Other Manifestations

Fever (≥38.5°C), tachycardia during sleep, tachycardia out of proportion to fever, anorexia, and malaise can be prominent but are not specific. The temperature usually decreases within 1 week, rarely lasting more than 4 weeks. Abdominal pain and anorexia can occur because of the hepatic involvement in heart failure or because of concomitant mesenteric adenitis; rarely, the situation may resemble acute appendicitis.

DIAGNOSIS

No specific test exists to confirm conclusively a diagnosis of RF, which is based on the Jones criteria modified several times since T. Duckett Jones in 1944 first formulated them (see Bland and Jones, Classic References). The American Heart Association published the most recent revision in 2015[14] (Table 81.2). Diagnosis of a first episode of ARF is based on two major criteria, or one major and two minor criteria, each along with evidence of preceding GAS infection. Sydenham chorea alone (i.e., without minor criteria) fulfills diagnostic criteria if other causes of movement disorder are ruled out. Recent scarlet fever is highly suggestive.

Evidence of Preceding GAS Infection

Recent GAS infection is suggested by a recent history of pharyngitis and confirmed by one or more of the following: throat swab culture (positive in about 11% of patients with diagnosis of RF), an increased—or preferably rising—antistreptolysin O (ASO) titer, or a positive rapid antigen detection test (RADT) in a child with clinical manifestations suggestive of streptococcal pharyngitis. However, it is extremely difficult to distinguish patients with true GAS pharyngitis from carriers who have viral pharyngitis when throat swab culturing alone is used to diagnose GAS pharyngitis. Most studies assessing the incidence of GAS pharyngitis use throat swabbing and culture; while a RADT may be used, laboratory culture is still considered the most specific means of GAS confirmation.

Clinical symptoms are combined with RADT or culturing when diagnosing GAS pharyngitis. At present, serologic testing of antistreptolysin and anti-DNase B antibody titers in two blood samples taken 2 to 4 weeks apart with seroconversion is thought to distinguish true GAS pharyngitis from pharyngeal GAS carriers.[16] Throat cultures and RADT tests are often negative by the time ARF manifests, whereas ASO titers and anti-DNase B typically peak 3 to 6 weeks after GAS pharyngitis; about 80% of children with ARF have a significantly elevated ASO titer. As throat swab cultures have limited accuracy for ARF diagnosis (10% to 20%), polymerase chain reaction (PCR) based tests have been used with more than 90% specificity.

Revised Jones Criteria

The 2015 revised Jones criteria incorporate three main changes. First, subclinical valvulitis detected by echocardiography is accepted as a major criterion for the diagnosis of ARF in all patient populations. Second, there is recognition that the clinical utility of the Jones criteria is determined by the pretest probability and background disease prevalence in the population. To avoid over diagnosis in low-incidence populations (ARF incidence <2/100,000 school-aged children, usually 5 to 14 years old, per year, or all-age prevalence of RHD of >1/1000 population per year) and underdiagnosis in high-risk populations, variability in applying diagnostic criteria in low-risk versus high-risk populations has been introduced in line with the Australian guidelines.[12] Finally, in moderate- to high-risk communities, monoarthritis and polyarthralgia have been added to polyarthritis as major criteria, and a temperature of 38°C and monoarthralgia are the revised minor criteria (Table 81.2). The clinical entity "possible" RF is appropriate for clinical judgment in parts of the world where RF remains common and where it is not possible to fulfill the criteria due to lack of laboratory facilities to conduct all investigations to exclude RF.[12,19] Suspected RF in high-incidence setting warrants secondary prophylaxis for 12 months and reevaluation based on history, physical examination, and echocardiogram.

Other Tests

Electrocardiogram (ECG) reveals a prolonged PR interval in only 35% of children with ARF; higher-degree heart block may occur but is uncommon. Other ECG abnormalities may be due to pericarditis, enlargement of ventricles or atria, or arrhythmias.

Echocardiography can detect evidence of carditis even in patients without apparent murmurs. It is recommended for all patients with confirmed or suspected ARF to detect subclinical carditis in patients with apparently isolated Sydenham chorea and to monitor the status of patients with recurrences of carditis or chronic RHD. Not all echocardiographic abnormalities represent rheumatic carditis; isolated trivial

TABLE 81.2 2015 American Heart Association Revised Jones Criteria for Diagnosis of Acute Rheumatic Fever

A. FOR ALL PATIENT POPULATIONS WITH EVIDENCE OF PRECEDING GAS INFECTION	
Diagnosis: Initial ARF	Two major manifestations or one major plus two minor manifestations
Diagnosis: Recurrent ARF	Two major, or one major and two minor, or three minor manifestations

B. MAJOR CRITERIA	
Low-Risk Populations*	**Moderate and High-Risk Populations**
Carditis[†]	Carditis[†]
• Clinical and/or subclinical	• Clinical and/or subclinical
Arthritis	Arthritis
• Polyarthritis only	• Monoarthritis or polyarthritis
	• Polyarthralgia[‡]
Chorea	Chorea
Erythema marginatum	Erythema marginatum
Subcutaneous nodules	Subcutaneous nodules

C. MINOR CRITERIA	
Low-Risk Populations*	**Moderate and High-Risk Populations**
Polyarthralgia	Monoarthralgia
Fever ≥ 38.5°C	Fever ≥ 38°C
ESR ≥60 mm in the first hour and/or CRP ≥ mg/dL[§]	ESR ≥30 mm/hr and/or CRP ≥3.0 mg/dL[§]
Prolonged PR interval after accounting for age variability (unless carditis is a major criterion)	Prolonged PR interval after accounting for age variability (unless carditis is a major criterion)

From Dougherty S, et al. Acute Rheumatic Fever and Rheumatic Heart Disease. 1st ed. Elsevier; 2020.
*Annual acute rheumatic fever (ARF) incidence of <2/100,000 school-aged children or all-age rheumatic heart disease (RHD) prevalence of <1/1000 people per year.
[†]Defined as echocardiographic valvulitis (Table 81.1).
[‡]Polyarthralgia should only be considered as a major manifestation in moderate- and high-risk populations after exclusion of other causes.
[§]C-reactive protein (CRP) value must be greater than the normal laboratory upper limit. In addition, because the erythrocyte sedimentation rate (ESR) might evolve during the course of ARF, peak ESR values should be used.
Joint manifestations are only considered in either the major or the minor category, but not in both categories in the same patient.

valvar regurgitation or trivial pericardial effusion may be nonspecific. To maintain specificity, echocardiographic and Doppler results should meet the criteria for acute rheumatic carditis (Table 81.1).

Chest X-rays can detect cardiomegaly, a common manifestation of carditis in ARF.

Erythrocyte sedimentation rate (ESR) and serum C-reactive protein (CRP) are sensitive but not specific. The ESR is typically >60 mm/hr, while CRP is >30 mg/L and often >70 mg/L. Because it rises and falls faster than ESR, a normal CRP may confirm that inflammation is resolving in a patient with prolonged ESR elevation after acute symptoms have subsided. In the absence of carditis, ESR usually returns to normal within 3 months. Evidence of acute inflammation, including ESR, usually subsides within 5 months in uncomplicated carditis.

The *white blood cell (WBC)* count reaches 12,000 to 20,000/μL and may go higher with corticosteroid therapy. *Serum cardiac marker* levels may be obtained; normal cardiac troponin I levels exclude prominent myocardial damage.

Joint aspiration may be needed to exclude other causes of arthritis (e.g., infection). The joint fluid is usually cloudy and yellow, with an elevated WBC count composed primarily of neutrophils; culture is negative. Complement levels are usually normal or slightly decreased, compared with decreased levels in other inflammatory arthritis.

Biopsy of a subcutaneous nodule can aid in early diagnosis, especially when other major clinical manifestations are absent.

Differential Diagnosis

The differential diagnosis of ARF includes JIA (especially systemic and, less so, polyarticular), Lyme disease, reactive arthritis, arthropathy of sickle cell disease, leukemia or other cancer, SLE, embolic bacterial endocarditis, serum sickness, Kawasaki disease, drug reactions, and gonococcal arthritis. These are usually distinguished by history or specific laboratory tests. Absence of previous GAS infection, diurnal variation of the fever, evanescent rash, and prolonged symptomatic joint inflammation usually distinguish systemic JIA from ARF.

Recurrences

Recurrent episodes of ARF often mimic the initial attack; carditis tends to recur in patients who have had moderate to severe carditis in the past, and chorea without carditis recurs in patients who had chorea without carditis initially. The diagnosis of recurrent ARF requires two major, one major and two minor, or three minor criteria. While the Jones criteria were designed for the evaluation of ARF (rather than for a possible recurrence), if patients have a reliable history of ARF or RHD and GAS infection is documented, they may be used to establish the presence of a recurrence. Finally, in established RHD, a recurrence of ARF can be diagnosed by the presence of two minor criteria plus evidence of a preceding GAS infection.

NATURAL HISTORY

Patients who have had RF have about a 50% likelihood of having a recurrence if they have another episode of untreated GAS pharyngitis. In endemic areas for RHD it is usual to see patients with severe RHD and superimposed ARF, particularly carditis. Episodes of Sydenham chorea usually last several months and resolve completely in most patients, but about one-third of patients have recurrences. Joint inflammation may take one month to subside if not treated but does not lead to residual damage.

Prognosis following an episode of ARF depends mostly on how severely the heart is affected, and whether it is a recurrent episode of ARF. Murmurs eventually disappear in about half of patients whose acute episodes were manifested by mild carditis without major cardiac enlargement or decompensation; however, chronic valvular disease can occur, typically over years or decades, in patients who recovered from the acute episode with no evidence of valvular disease. Chronic RHD is the cause of 25% to 45% of all cardiovascular disease and a major cause of heart failure in developing countries.

MANAGEMENT

The primary goals of the treatment of a proven attack of ARF are to suppress the inflammatory response and minimize its effects on the heart and joints, to eradicate GAS from the pharynx, to provide relief of acute symptoms, and to initiate prophylaxis to prevent recurrent heart disease. The management of ARF is summarized in Table 81.3.

General Management

Patients should limit their activities if they have symptoms of arthritis, chorea, or heart failure. Strenuous exertion should be avoided, especially in patients with carditis. In asymptomatic carditis, strict bed rest has no proven value, despite its traditional usage. Bed rest appears to be appropriate to lessen joint pain, and its duration should be individually determined. Ambulation can usually be started once fever has subsided and acute-phase reactants are returning to normal.

Antibiotic Treatment

Although poststreptococcal inflammation is well developed by the time ARF is detected, and throat swabs are rarely positive for GAS, a 10-day course of oral penicillin or amoxicillin, or a single injection of intramuscular benzathine penicillin (or erythromycin if allergic to penicillin) is used to eradicate any lingering organisms; however, this conventional strategy is untested. Thereafter, secondary prophylaxis should be commenced as described later.

TABLE 81.3 Management Protocol for Acute Rheumatic Fever

Diagnosis
- Admission to hospital
- Investigation to confirm ARF and to exclude other pathologies
- Blood tests including acute-phase reactants and serology for the streptococcal organism
- Electrocardiogram
- Echocardiographic evaluation

Eradication of GAS
- Oral penicillin V* for 10 days OR single dose of intramuscular benzathine penicillin G
- Treatment of coexisting streptococcal impetigo

Arthritis/Arthralgia and Symptomatic Treatment
- Paracetamol until the diagnosis has been confirmed
- NSAIDs (naproxen is preferably used)
- Corticosteroids in cases where NSAIDs cannot be used

Carditis/Heart Failure
- Bed rest, fluid restriction, heart failure medications (furosemide, spironolactone, ACEI)
- Corticosteroids for severe heart failure if surgery is not indicated or unavailable
- Surgery for intractable heart failure associated with severe mitral or aortic regurgitation; preferable to defer surgery until acute rheumatic activity has resolved

Chorea
- Penicillin V* orally or intramuscular benzathine penicillin G
- Haloperidol or carbamazepine can be considered if the abnormal movements interfere with daily activities
- Valproic acid reserved for refractory cases
- Multidisciplinary input as required for significant motor or neuropsychiatric manifestations

Discharge Procedure
- Discharge once there is clinical improvement and reduction in ESR or CRP
- Notification to health authorities
- Patient and family education
- Secondary prophylaxis
- Outpatient follow-up

*Also known as phenoxymethylpenicillin or penicillin V potassium (PVK).
ACEI, Angiotensin-converting enzyme inhibitor; CRP, C-reactive protein; ESR, erythrocyte sedimentation rate; GAS, group A streptococcal; NSAIDs, nonsteroidal anti-inflammatory drugs.
From Dougherty S, et al. Acute Rheumatic Fever and Rheumatic Heart Disease. 1st ed. Elsevier; 2020:31-54.

Aspirin and Other Anti-Inflammatory Drugs

Anti-inflammatory agents used include salicylates, NSAIDs, and corticosteroids. Eight randomized clinical trials (RCTs), involving 996 people and conducted between 1950 and 2001, compared antiinflammatory agents (e.g., aspirin, corticosteroids, immunoglobulins, pentoxifylline) with placebo or controls and anti-inflammatory agents with one another, in both adults and children with ARF (according to Jones or modified Jones criteria)[24]; several steroidal agents were compared to aspirin, placebo, or no treatment. Overall, there was no significant difference in the risk of cardiac disease at 1 year between the corticosteroid-treated and aspirin-treated groups. Thus, there is little evidence of benefit of using corticosteroids or IV immunoglobulins to reduce the risk of heart valve lesions in patients with ARF.[24] However, these trials assessed cardiac involvement on clinical grounds only, and thus observer error and interobserver variability of clinical methodology could invalidate the results. Moreover, the short duration of the follow-up does not guarantee that important cardiac sequelae did not develop in the ensuing decades.

Aspirin controls fever and pain and should be given to all patients with arthritis and/or mild carditis. Although aspirin has been used for many decades, there are surprisingly few data from RCTs to define the optimal dosing schedule. Symptomatic ARF responds dramatically to aspirin and if no improvement is seen after 24 to 48 hours of high-dose aspirin therapy, the diagnosis of ARF should be reconsidered. Salicylate toxicity is the limiting factor to aspirin therapy and is manifested by tinnitus, headache, or hyperpnea; it may not appear until after 1 week of therapy. Salicylate levels are measured only to manage toxicity. Enteric-coated, buffered, or complex salicylate molecules provide no advantage.

Other NSAIDs have been reported to be effective in small trials; naproxen (7.5 to 10 mg/kg po bid) is the most studied. However, other NSAIDs have few advantages over aspirin, especially in the first week of therapy when salicylism is uncommon.

Prednisone is recommended instead of aspirin for patients with moderate to severe carditis, as judged by a combination of clinical findings, presence of cardiac enlargement, and possibly by severely abnormal echocardiography results. The appropriate dosage is 1 to 2 mg/kg/day oral (up to 60 mg/day) divided in two or three doses. If inflammation is not suppressed after 2 days or for cases of severe heart failure, an IV corticosteroid pulse of methylprednisolone succinate (30 mg/kg IV once/day, maximum 1 g/day for 3 successive days) may be given. Oral corticosteroids are typically given for 2 to 4 weeks and then tapered over another 2 to 3 weeks. Aspirin should be started during the corticosteroid taper and continued for 2 to 4 weeks after the corticosteroid has been stopped.

The duration of therapy depends on the severity of the attack, presence of carditis, and rate of response to treatment. Milder attacks with little or no carditis may be treated with salicylates for approximately 1 month or until inflammation (clinical and laboratory evidence) has subsided. More severe cases may require 2 to 3 months of corticosteroid therapy before this can be gradually weaned. Up to 5% of patients may still have rheumatic activity despite 6 months of therapy. Occasionally a "rebound" of inflammatory activity can occur when anti-inflammatory agents are reduced and may require salicylate treatment. Inflammatory markers such as ESR and CRP may be used to monitor disease activity and response to treatment. Recurrences of mild cardiac inflammation (indicated by fever or chest pain) may subside spontaneously; anti-inflammatory drugs should be resumed if recurrent symptoms last longer than a few days or if heart failure is uncontrolled by standard management.

Antibiotic Prophylaxis

Antistreptococcal prophylaxis (with penicillin) should be maintained continuously after the initial episode of ARF to prevent recurrences. See section titled Secondary Prevention.

PREVENTION

Primordial Prevention

Improvement of social conditions and increasing access to primary health care have been associated with dramatic fall in the incidence of RF even before the advent of antibiotics (see Fig. 81.1, Curve A). Therefore, primordial prevention requires improving the broad determinants of health in people at high risk, including environmental, economic, social, behavioral, and cultural.

Primary Prevention

Antibiotic treatment of proven or presumed GAS pharyngitis with intramuscular (IM) penicillin appears to reduce the attack rate by as much as 80%.[15] Eradication of GAS from the upper respiratory tract can usually be achieved with a single IM injection of benzathine penicillin or by a 10-day course of oral penicillin.[15] Although the use of IM penicillin is supported by clinical trials, few trials have tested the efficacy of oral

TABLE 81.4 Drug Regimens for Primary and Secondary Prevention of Rheumatic Fever

AGENT	ANTIBIOTICS FOR GROUP A STREPTOCOCCAL PHARYNGITIS				
	DOSE		ROUTE	DURATION	RATING
Penicillins					
Penicillin V (phenoxymethyl penicillin)	**Children** (≤27 kg [≤60 lb]) 250 mg 2-3 times daily **Children** (>27 kg [>60 lb]) **Adolescents and adults:** 500 mg 2-3 times daily		Oral	10 days	IB
Amoxicillin	50 mg/kg once daily (maximum 1 g)		Oral	10 days	IB
Benzathine penicillin G	600,000 U for patients ≤27 kg (≤60 lb), 1,200,000 U for patients >27 kg (>60 lb)		Intramuscular	Once	IB
For Individuals Allergic to Penicillin					
Narrow-spectrum cephalosporin* (cephalexin, cefadroxil)	Variable		Oral	10 days	IB
Clindamycin	20 mg/kg per day divided in three doses (maximum 1.8 g/day)		Oral	10 days	IIaB
Azithromycin	12 mg/kg once daily (maximum 500 mg)		Oral	5 days	IIaB
Clarithromycin	15 mg/kg per day divided bid (maximum 250 mg bid)		Oral	10 days	IIaB

Recommendations for Secondary Prevention of Acute Rheumatic Fever

- Secondary prophylaxis of acute rheumatic fever (ARF) and rheumatic heart disease (RHD) comprises long-term antibiotic therapy for an individual's diagnosis with ARF or RHD to prevent ARF recurrences triggered by recurrent group A streptococcal (GAS) infection and therefore prevent the development of RHD or worsening of existing RHD.
- International guidelines differ slightly on recommendations of antibiotic choice, duration, and patient groups in whom it is indicated.
- Key standard recommendations usually include use of parental (intramuscular) benzathine penicillin G (BPG) every 4 weeks in individuals diagnosed with ARF and/or RHD for minimum 5- to 10-year period after diagnosis of the most recent ARF episode, or to the age of 21, whichever comes later. In some countries, duration for severe cases is lifelong.

*To be avoided in those with immediate (type I) hypersensitivity to penicillin.
Rating indicates classification of recommendation and level of evidence (LOE) (e.g., IB indicates class I, LOE B); bid bis in die (twice per day).
Adapted from Dougherty S, et al. Acute Rheumatic Fever and Rheumatic Heart Disease. 1st ed. Elsevier; 2020:31–54.

penicillin for the primary prevention of RF. Table 81.4 presents drug regimens of choice for primary prevention.

A cluster-randomized RCT in Nepal tested the utility of echocardiographic screening and primary prevention as a public health strategy to prevent ARF,[11] and there has been successful application of primary prevention within a comprehensive public health program in Cuba, Costa Rica, and the French islands of Martinique and Guadeloupe (see Fig. 81.1, Curve C).[6] Finally, a study conducted in South Africa showed that a strategy of using a clinical decision rule to diagnose GAS pharyngitis without culturing, associated with provision of treatment with a single IM benzathine penicillin (BPG) injection, was cost-effective in a high-risk community,[25] where culturing for RF is prohibitively expensive. Evidence from the clinical trial on primary prevention[15] and this cost-effectiveness study[25] support the treatment of symptomatic cases of GAS pharyngitis diagnosed on clinical grounds as a cost-effective public health strategy for primary prevention of RF in the context of a comprehensive national prevention program. Potential barriers to the effectiveness of primary prevention of RF solely with antibiotic therapy of GAS pharyngitis include the fact that as many as one-third of patients who develop RF do not recall any symptoms of pharyngitis, and that in outbreaks, symptoms of pharyngitis are absent in up to 58% of those infected.

Secondary Prevention

RCTs strongly support the superiority of IM compared with oral penicillin for prevention of RF recurrences (see Manyemba and Mayosi, Classic References). Shorter intervals between injections are more effective. Evidence strongly supports injections every 2 weeks (with an almost 50% reduction in the risk of RF recurrence compared with injections every 4 weeks), while it is less strong for injections taken every 3 weeks.

Recommendations for the optimal duration of secondary prophylaxis are largely empiric and based on observational studies. The duration should be individualized, taking into account the socioeconomic conditions, the risk of exposure to GAS, and the previous history of carditis with or without valve involvement. Children without carditis should receive prophylaxis for 5 years or until age 21, whichever is longer; those with carditis with mild mitral regurgitation or healed carditis should receive prophylaxis for 10 years or until age 25 (whichever is longer). Children with carditis and evidence of residual heart damage, or those who had valve surgery, should receive prophylaxis indefinitely or, alternatively, until age 40. Finally, prophylaxis should be lifelong in all patients with severe valvular disease who have close contact with young children because these have a high rate of GAS carriage.

FUTURE PERSPECTIVES

Comprehensive programs that include primary and secondary prevention interventions are effective in reducing the incidence of ARF and RHD in endemic countries[7] and thus are recommended by the World Health Organization.

However, the diagnosis of ARF is complex, and despite involving clinical, laboratory, and echocardiographic measurements, the Jones criteria are not very sensitive or specific in countries with a high incidence. An understanding of the molecular genetic mechanisms underlying host susceptibility to enhance the Jones criteria has been hampered by the relatively small number of candidate genes in RF/RHD. There is thus the need for large-scale multicenter studies with different populations to obtain reliable and reproducible findings.[26]

There is a clear case for development of vaccines against streptococci given the large disease burden, and there are multiple vaccine candidates in clinical and preclinical development.[27-29] Demonstration of vaccine efficacy against pharyngitis and skin infections constitutes a key near-term strategic goal, which will need investments and collaborative partnerships to diversify and advance vaccine candidates.

CLASSIC REFERENCES

Bland EF, Duckett Jones T. Rheumatic fever and rheumatic heart disease; a twenty year report on 1000 patients followed since childhood. *Circulation*. 1951;4:836–843.
Dajani AS. Current status of nonsuppurative complications of group A Streptococci. *Pediatr Infect Dis J*. 1991;10:S25–S27.

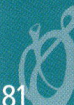

Manyemba J, Mayosi BM. Intramuscular penicillin is more effective than oral penicillin in secondary prevention of rheumatic fever: a systematic review. *S Afr Med J.* 2003;93:212–218.

Popat K, Riding W. Acute rheumatic fever following streptococcal wound infection. *Postgrad Med J.* 1976;52:165–170.

Tulchinsky TH, Varavikova EA. Addressing the epidemiologic transition in the former Soviet Union: strategies for health system and public health reform in Russia. *Am J Public Health.* 1996;86:313–320.

Vasan RS, Shrivastava S, Vijayakumar M, et al. Echocardiographic evaluation of patients with acute rheumatic fever and rheumatic carditis. *Circulation.* 1996;94:73–82.

Veasy LG, Wiedmeirer SE, Orsmond GS, et al. Resurgence of acute rheumatic fever in the intermountain area of the United States. *N Engl J Med.* 1987;316:421–427.

REFERENCES

Pathogenesis

1. Carapetis JR, McDonald M, Wilson NJ. Acute rheumatic fever. *Lancet.* 2005;366:155–168.
2. Watkins DA, Johnson CO, Colquhoun SM, et al. Global, regional, and national burden of rheumatic heart disease, 1990–2015. *N Engl J Med.* 2017;377:713–722.
3. Zühlke LJ, Beaton A, Engel ME, et al. Group A Streptococcus, acute rheumatic fever and rheumatic heart disease: epidemiology and clinical considerations. *Curr Treat Options Cardiovasc Med.* 2017;19:15.
4. Carapetis JR, Beaton A, Cunningham MW, et al. Acute rheumatic fever and rheumatic heart disease. *Nat Rev Dis Primers.* 2016;2:15084.
5. Lawrence JG, Carapetis JR, Griffiths K, et al. Acute rheumatic fever and rheumatic heart disease: incidence and progression in the Northern Territory of Australia, 1997 to 2010. *Circulation.* 2013;128:492–501.
6. Mayosi BM. Screening for rheumatic heart disease in eastern Nepal. *JAMA Cardiol.* 2016;1:96–97.
7. Pastore S, De Cunto A, Benettoni A, et al. The resurgence of rheumatic fever in develop country area: the role of echocardiography. *Rheumatology.* 2011;50:396–400.
8. Nulu S, Bukhman G, Kwan GF. Rheumatic heart disease: the unfinished global agenda. *Cardiol Clin.* 2017;35:165–180.
9. Yokchoo N, Patanarapeelert N, Patanarapeelert K. The effect of group A streptococcal carrier on the epidemic model of acute rheumatic fever. *Theor Biol Med Model.* 2019;16:14.
10. Ghamrawy A, Ibrahim NN, Abd El-Wahab EW. How accurate is the diagnosis of rheumatic fever in Egypt? Data from the national rheumatic heart disease prevention and control program (2006-2018). *PLoS Negl Trop Dis.* 2020;14(8):e0008558. https://doi.org/10.1371/journal.pntd.0008558.
11. Karki P, Uranw S, Bastola S, et al. Effectiveness of systematic echocardiographic screening for rheumatic heart disease in Nepalese school children: a cluster randomized comparison. *JAMA Cardiol.* 2021. https://doi.org/10.1001/jamacardio.2020.7050.
12. Gewitz MH, Baltimore RS, Tani LY, et al. Revision of the Jones Criteria for the diagnosis of acute rheumatic fever in the era of doppler echocardiography: a scientific statement from the American Heart Association. *Circulation.* 2015;131:1806–1818.
13. Aty-Marzouk PA, Hamza H, Mosaad N, et al. New guidelines for diagnosis of rheumatic fever: do they apply to all populations? *Turk J Pediatr.* 2020;62:411–423.

Pathogenesis

14. Bright PD, Mayosi BM, Martin WJ. An immunological perspective on rheumatic heart disease pathogenesis: more questions than answer. *Heart.* 2016;102:1527–1532.
15. Lennon D, Stewart J, Aderson P. Primary prevention of rheumatic fever. *Pediatr Infect Dis J.* 2016;35:820.
16. Bennett J, Moreland NJ, Oliver J, et al. Understanding group A streptococcal pharyngitis and skin infections as causes of rheumatic fever: protocol for a prospective disease incidence study. *BMC Infect Dis.* 2019;19:633.
17. Armitage EP, Senghore E, Darboe S, et al. High burden and seasonal variation of paediatric scabies and pyoderma prevalence in the Gambia: a cross-sectional study. *PLoS Negl Trop Dis.* 2019;13:e0007801. https://doi.org/10.1371/journal.pntd.0007801.
18. Woldu B, Bloomfield GS. Rheumatic heart disease in the twenty-first century. *Curr Cardiol Rep.* 2016;18:96.
19. Dougherty S, Nascmento B, Carapetis J. Clinical evaluation and diagnosis of acute rheumatic fever. In: Dougherty S, et al., ed. *Acute Rheumatic Fever and Rheumatic Heart Disease.* 1st ed. Elsevier; 2020:31–54.
20. Spina GS, Sampaio RO, Branco CE, et al. Incidental histological diagnosis of acute rheumatic myocarditis: case report and review of the literature. *Front Pediatr.* 2014;2:126.
21. Chain JL, Alvarez K, Mascaro-Blanco A, et al. Autoantibody biomarkers for basal Ganglia Encephalitis in Sydenham chorea and pediatric autoimmune neuropsychiatric disorder associated with streptococcal infections. *Front Psychiatry.* 2020;11:564.

Clinical Features, Diagnosis, Treatment, Prevention

22. Branco CE, Sampaio RO, Branco MM, et al. Rheumatic fever: neglected and underdiagnosed disease- new perspective on diagnosis and prevention. *Arq Bras Cardiol.* 2016;107:482–484.
23. Beier K, Pratt DP. Sydenham Chorea. 2020 Jul 21. In: *StatPearls [Internet].* Treasure Island (FL): StatPearls Publishing; 2020 Jan–. PMID: 28613588.
24. Cilliers A, Manyemba J, Adler AJ, Saloojee H. Autoinflammatory treatment for carditis in acute rheumatic fever. *Cochrane Database Syst Rev.* 2012;(6):CD003176.
25. Irlam J, Mayosi BM, Engel M, Gaziano T. Primary prevention of acute rheumatic fever and rheumatic heart disease with penicillin in South Africa children with pharyngitis: a cost-effectiveness analysis. *Circ Cardiovasc Qual Outcomes.* 2013;6:343–351.

Future Perspectives

26. Muhamed B, Shaboodien G, Engel ME. Genetic variants in rheumatic fever and rheumatic heart disease. *Am J Med Genet C Semin Med Genet.* 2020;184:159–177.
27. Steer AC, Carapetis JR, Dale JB, et al. Status of research and development of vaccines for streptococcus pyogenes. *Vaccine.* 2016;34:2953–2958.
28. Rivera-Hernandez T, Carnathan DG, Jones S, et al. An Experimental group A Streptococcus vaccine that reduces pharyngitis and Tonsillitis in a Nonhuman primate model. *mBio.* 2019;10(2):e00693-19. https://doi.org/10.1128/mBio.00693-19.
29. Vekemans J, Gouvea-Reis F, Kim JH, et al. The Path to group A Streptococcus vaccines: world health Organization research and development Technology Roadmap and Preferred Product characteristics. *Clin Infect Dis.* 2019;69:877–883.

第九部分　心肌、心包和肺血管系统疾病

赵青　柳志红　导读

本部分主要围绕先天性心脏病（先心病）、心肌病、心包疾病和各种肺血管系统疾病进行逐一阐述，具体包括以下八章内容：第82章　青少年和成人先天性心脏病、第83章　基于导管的成人先天性心脏病治疗、第84章　药物或毒素引起的心肌病、第85章　HIV感染者的心血管异常、第86章　心包疾病、第87章　肺栓塞和深静脉血栓形成、第88章　肺动脉高压、第89章　睡眠呼吸障碍与心血管疾病。

青少年和成人先天性心脏病（ACHD）患者日益增长，第82章强调此类患者应转至专业的先心病中心管理。从ACHD患者病变的解剖学分类和病理生理出发，归纳了先天性心脏病的命名法和其疾病的发生发展机制，详细讲解了各种简单及复杂ACHD患者临床症状和诊断方法、治疗策略选择，以及疾病的长期预后和并发症管理。

成人先天性心脏病的介入治疗已然成为大型医疗中心的常规疗法，极大地改善了患者的长期预后与生存质量。第83章详尽阐述了各种成人先天性心脏病的介入治疗，包括肺动脉瓣成形术、肺动脉瓣置换术、肺血管成形术、主动脉狭窄支架植入术、房间隔缺损封堵术、室间隔缺损封堵术、动脉导管未闭封堵术等。导管技术飞速发展，相信会给该领域的各位医者带来全面的认识与崭新的收获。

药物或毒素性心肌病是由天然和人工合成的物质以及环境暴露对心血管系统造成的不良后果。主要的毒物和药物包括酒精、电子烟、可卡因和大麻、咖啡因等。第84章重点围绕以上药物和毒物的药理学、病理生理机制、心血管系统损害和心血管疾病的发生风险进行讲解。深入讲解药物或毒物导致心血管系统疾病的具体病理生理机制，有助于我们更好地控制应用这些物质所带来的问题和经济负担。

第85章介绍HIV感染者的心血管危险因素以及HIV相关的心血管疾病。随着HIV治疗手段的不断进步，HIV患者的心血管疾病谱也将持续变化。HIV患者心血管危险因素的发生率明显高于普通人群，多种因素共同促进HIV患者中动脉粥样硬化的发生发展，另外HIV感染还可能会引起肺动脉高压、心律失常、心脏性猝死以及卒中等心脑血管疾病。

心包疾病则是心包发生生理或病理改变而引起临床症状的一系列疾病。第86章详细探讨了心包的解剖和生理学、急性和复发性心包炎、心包积液和心脏压塞、缩窄性和渗出-缩窄性心包炎等内容，相信读者在仔细阅读后会对心包疾病有更深刻的认识和体会。

静脉血栓栓塞症包括肺栓塞和深静脉血栓形成，由于其高发病率、致残率和致死率引起了临床上的广泛关注。第87章从流行病学、发病机制、危险因素、病理生理、临床分型、临床表现、危险分层、诊断治疗以及预防等方面全面地介绍了肺栓塞和深静脉血栓形成的相关内容。

肺动脉高压是一类以肺动脉压力升高为特征的异质性疾病。第88章对肺动脉高压的定义、分类、病理生理和分子生物学机制进行了详细阐述。肺动脉高压的临床症状缺乏特异性，需要通过多项化验检查手段，对患者进行确诊、分类分型和风险分层，肺动脉高压的治疗策略因不同的临床分型而存在差异，需要多学

科综合管理。如今，肺动脉高压虽然风险极高，但是可防可控。

睡眠呼吸障碍（SDB）主要包括阻塞性睡眠呼吸暂停（OSA）和中枢性睡眠呼吸暂停（CSA）。OSA可以引起一系列病理生理紊乱，对心脏结构和功能产生不利影响，与高血压、冠心病、心力衰竭、心律失常等心血管疾病及心脑血管事件的发生有关。对SDB病理生理机制进行表型和分级的优化，针对性地提出个体化诊治方案，或将有利于进一步改善心血管疾病合并SDB患者的疾病严重程度及预后。

PART IX DISEASES OF THE MYOCARDIUM, PERICARDIUM, AND PULMONARY VASCULATURE BED

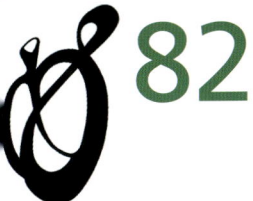

82 Congenital Heart Disease in the Adolescent and Adult

ANNE MARIE VALENTE, ADAM L. DORFMAN, SONYA V. BABU-NARAYAN, AND ERIC V. KRIEGER

扫描二维码阅读
第82章中文导读

GENERAL CONSIDERATIONS, 1541
Access and Delivery of ACHD Care, 1541
Transition to ACHD Care, 1541
Clinical Evaluation, 1542
Noncardiac Complications in the ACHD Patient, 1543

CONGENITAL ANATOMY, 1544
Congenital Nomenclature, 1544
Cardiac Development, 1545
Genetic Considerations, 1545

LONG-TERM CONSIDERATIONS, 1545
Arrhythmias in Adult Congenital Heart Disease, 1545
Heart Failure, Transplantation, and Mechanical Circulatory Support, 1549
Medical Therapy, 1550
Mechanical Circulatory Support, 1551
Palliative Care, 1551

Aortopathies in Congenital Heart Disease, 1551
Pregnancy in Women With Congenital Heart Disease, 1552
Exercise and Sports Participation, 1553

SPECIFIC DEFECTS, 1554
Left-to-Right Shunt Lesions, 1554
Atrial Septal Defects and Partial Anomalous Pulmonary Veins, 1554
Atrioventricular Septal Defects, 1557
Ventricular Septal Defects, 1558
Patent Ductus Arteriosus, 1559
Ebstein Anomaly of the Tricuspid Valve, 1560
Pulmonary Stenosis, 1562
Tetralogy of Fallot, 1563
Transposition of the Great Arteries, 1566
Congenitally Corrected Transposition of the Great Arteries, 1569
Double Outlet Right Ventricle, 1570

Truncus Arteriosus, 1572
Cor Triatriatum, 1572
Subvalvular Left Ventricular Outflow Tract Obstruction, 1573
Supravalvar Aortic Stenosis, 1573
Coarctation of the Aorta, 1575
Interrupted Aortic Arch, 1576
Vascular Rings, 1577
Anomalous Coronary Artery From the Pulmonary Artery, 1578
Single Ventricle, 1578

PULMONARY HYPERTENSION AND EISENMENGER SYNDROME, 1582
Demographics and Prognosis, 1582
Classification, 1582

REFERENCES, 1585

GENERAL CONSIDERATIONS

The number of adults living with congenital heart disease (CHD) is growing faster than the number of children with CHD, and now is estimated to be at least 1.4 million adults in the United States alone.[1,2] At least 20% of these adult congenital heart disease (ACHD) patients have complex cardiovascular anatomy and suffer from multi-system organ involvement. Lifelong follow-up in coordination with, or directly by, clinicians with expertise in ACHD is recommended. This chapter describes the long-term complications of living with CHD and highlights many of the potential comorbidities, discusses CHD nomenclature and cardiac development, and summarizes the more common CHD lesions that may be encountered in adulthood.

Access and Delivery of ACHD Care

In 2001, the 32nd Bethesda Conference addressed the changing profile of adults living with CHD by developing guidelines for delivery of care. In this document, congenital heart defects are grouped according to anatomic complexity. As the field has grown, there has been a recognition of the limitations of this system, which does not incorporate comorbidities or physiology into the levels of anatomic complexity. Therefore, in 2018, the American College of Cardiology (ACC) and the American Heart Association (AHA) released an updated set of ACHD guidelines which incorporates not only the anatomical classification (Table 82.1A) but also the physiological stage (Table 82.1B) of each patient.[3] This classification scheme is used throughout the guidelines to provide lesion-specific frequency of follow-up, testing, and general management.

Inherent in these guidelines is the expectation that any adult with CHD who has anything other than simple, unrepaired, isolated lesions or fully repaired shunt lesions should be managed in conjunction with an ACHD cardiologist. There is also emphasis that the most complex ACHD patients should receive the majority of their care at a center with dedicated ACHD expertise, as data confirms that ACHD patients cared for in specialized centers have lower mortality than those receiving care in centers lacking specific ACHD programs.[4] In 2020, revised guidelines for management of ACHD patients were released by the European Society of Cardiology.[5] This document includes sections on staffing requirements for ACHD expert centers, consideration of palliative care planning, expanded recommendations on arrhythmia and pulmonary hypertension (PH) management, and the emerging role of biomarkers and catheter-based interventions in ACHD patients.

Transition to ACHD Care

Due to advances in the management of CHD, a once life-threatening childhood illness is now often transformed into a chronic adult condition. With early surgical intervention, the majority of patients are repaired but not cured and require lifelong surveillance. Therefore, there is a critical need for successful transition and transfer of CHD patients from pediatric to adult CHD care. However, multiple barriers prevent effective transition. These barriers range from lack of a structured transition program to provider-patient/parent attachment, or unavailability of ACHD providers.[6] Pediatric cardiology programs should partner with an ACHD program to allow for successful transition and transfer of care. Transition discussions should begin at the age of 12 years, with the expectation of complete transfer to ACHD care

TABLE 82.1A Anatomic Classification of Congenital Heart Conditions

CHD ANATOMY*		
I: Simple	**II: Moderate Complexity**	**III: Great Complexity (or Complex)**
Native disease <ul><li>Isolated small ASD</li><li>Isolated small VSD</li><li>Mild isolated pulmonic stenosis</li></ul> **Repaired conditions** <ul><li>Previously ligated or occluded ductus arteriosus</li><li>Repaired secundum ASD or sinus venosus defect without significant residual shunt or chamber enlargement</li><li>Repaired VSD without significant residual shunt or chamber enlargement</li></ul>	**Repaired or unrepaired conditions** <ul><li>Aorto-left ventricular fistula</li><li>Anomalous pulmonary venous connection, partial or total</li><li>Anomalous coronary artery arising from the pulmonary artery</li><li>Anomalous aortic origin of a coronary artery from the opposite sinus</li><li>AVSD (partial or complete, including primum ASD)</li><li>Congenital aortic valve disease</li><li>Congenital mitral valve disease</li><li>Coarctation of the aorta</li><li>Ebstein anomaly (disease spectrum includes mild, moderate, and severe variations)</li><li>Infundibular right ventricular outflow obstruction</li><li>Ostium primum ASD</li><li>Moderate and large unrepaired secundum ASD</li><li>Moderate and large persistently patent ductus arteriosus</li><li>Pulmonary valve regurgitation (moderate or greater)</li><li>Pulmonary valve stenosis (moderate or greater)</li><li>Peripheral pulmonary stenosis</li><li>Sinus of Valsalva fistula/aneurysm</li><li>Sinus venosus defect</li><li>Subvalvar aortic stenosis (excluding HCM; HCM not addressed in these guidelines)</li><li>Supravalvar aortic stenosis</li><li>Straddling atrioventricular valve</li><li>Repaired tetralogy of Fallot</li><li>VSD with associated abnormality and/or moderate or greater shunt</li></ul>	<ul><li>Cyanotic congenital heart defect (unrepaired or palliated, all forms)</li><li>Double-outlet ventricle</li><li>Fontan procedure</li><li>Interrupted aortic arch</li><li>Mitral atresia</li><li>Single ventricle (including double inlet left ventricle, tricuspid atresia, hypoplastic left heart, any other anatomic abnormality with a functionally single ventricle)</li><li>Pulmonary atresia (all forms)</li><li>TGA (classic or d-TGA; CCTGA or l-TGA)</li><li>Truncus arteriosus</li><li>Other abnormalities of atrioventricular and ventriculoarterial connection (i.e., crisscross heart, isomerism, heterotaxy syndromes, ventricular inversion)</li></ul>

*This list is not meant to be comprehensive; other conditions may be important in individual patients.
ACHD, Adult congenital heart disease; *AP*, anatomic and physiological; *ASD*, atrial septal defect; *AVSD*, atrioventricular septal defect; *CCTGA*, congenitally corrected transposition of the great arteries; *CHD*, congenital heart disease; *d- TGA*, dextro-transposition of the great arteries; *FC*, functional class; *HCM*, hypertrophic cardiomyopathy; *l-TGA*, levo-transposition of the great arteries; *NYHA*, New York Heart Association; *TGA*, transposition of the great arteries; *VSD*, ventricular septal defect.
Modified from Stout KK, Daniels CJ, Aboulhosn J, et al. 2018 AHA/ACC Guideline for the Management of Adults With Congenital Heart Disease: A report of the American College of Cardiology/American Heart Association Task Force on Clinical Practice Guidelines. J Am Coll Cardiol. 2019;73(12):1494–1563.

TABLE 82.1B Physiologic Stages of Adult Congenital Heart Disease Patient Classification

	A	B	C	D
Symptoms	NYHA FC I symptoms	NYHA FC II symptoms	NYHA FC III symptoms	NYHA IV symptoms
Valvular Disease		Mild	Significant	
Arrhythmias		Not requiring treatment	Controlled with treatment	Refractory to treatment
Hemodynamic Sequelae		Mild (mild aortic enlargement, mild ventricular enlargement, mild ventricular dysfunction)	Moderate or greater ventricular dysfunction (systemic, pulmonic, or both)	Severe aortic enlargement
			Moderate aortic enlargement	
Exercise Capacity	Normal	Abnormal objective cardiac limitation to exercise		
Other	Normal renal, hepatic, and pulmonary function	Trivial or small shunt (not hemodynamically significant)	Venous or arterial stenosis	Severe hypoxemia (almost always associated with cyanosis)
			Mild or moderate hypoxemia/cyanosis	Severe pulmonary hypertension
			Hemodynamically significant shunt	Eisenmenger syndrome
			Pulmonary hypertension	Refractory end-organ dysfunction
			End-organ dysfunction responsive to therapy	

Modified from Stout KK, Daniels CJ, Aboulhosn JA, et al. 2018 AHA/ACC Guideline for the Management of Adults With Congenital Heart Disease: A report of the American College of Cardiology/American Heart Association Task Force on Clinical Practice Guidelines. J Am Coll Cardiol. 2019;73(12):1494–1563.

by 21 years of age. The probability of a successful transfer is directly related to documentation of the need for such in the medical record and formal educational interventions geared at understanding self-management skills.[7]

Clinical Evaluation

In caring for adults with CHD, it is helpful to understand some of the common terminology regarding congenital anatomy and prior procedures (Table 82.2). Many ACHD patients have had surgical interventions as children, and it is essential to understand the specific procedures and potential sequelae from these interventions. The physical examination of ACHD patients may also provide unique clues to prior procedures when the recorded history is unclear. Location of surgical scars will indicate whether a patient has had a lateral thoracotomy, such as with a patent ductus arteriosus (PDA) ligation or aortic coarctation repair. Additionally, absence of a radial pulse on the ipsilateral arm as a thoracotomy scar may suggest that the subclavian artery was sacrificed in the repair (such as a subclavian flap repair for coarctation of the aorta or a prior classic Blalock-Taussig-Thomas [BTT] shunt).

TABLE 82.2 Common Congenital Heart Disease Eponyms

ANATOMY EPONYMS	ANATOMIC DESCRIPTION
Bland-White-Garland syndrome	Anomalous left coronary artery from the pulmonary artery (ALCAPA)
Eisenmenger syndrome	Pulmonary hypertension with cyanosis due to right to left shunting
Gerbode defect	Septal defect resulting in direct left ventricle to right atrium shunt
Holmes Heart	Double inlet left ventricle with D-looped ventricles and normally related great vessels
Raghib defect	Coronary sinus septal defect in the presence of a left superior vena cava
Scimitar syndrome	Partial anomalous pulmonary venous connections of the right lower pulmonary vein to the IVC-RA junction, often accompanied by pulmonary artery hypoplasia and aortopulmonary collateral formation.
Shone syndrome	Series of left-sided obstructive lesions
Taussig-Bing Malformation	Form of double outlet right ventricle with D-malposed, side-by-side great vessels, sub-pulmonary VSD, hypoplastic aortic arch

SURGICAL EPONYMS	PROCEDURE DESCRIPTION
Baffes procedure	Early palliative procedure for transposition of the great arteries, with the inferior vena cava directed to the left atrium via homograft
Blalock-Taussig(-Thomas) shunt	"Classic"—direct end to end anastomosis of subclavian artery to pulmonary artery
	"Modified"—tube graft from subclavian artery to pulmonary artery
Brock Procedure	Closed infundibular resection for relief of pulmonary stenosis
Fontan or Fontan-Kreutzer	Atriopulmonary anastomosis for single ventricle heart disease
Fontan-Björk Modification	Includes the right ventricle into the pulmonary circulation, was the unique modification for tricuspid atresia
Glenn	"Classic"—end to end anastomosis of superior vena cava to right pulmonary artery
	"bidirectional"—end to side anastomosis of superior vena cava to right pulmonary artery
Kawashima	Bidirectional Glenn in context of interrupted inferior vena cava with azygos continuation to the superior vena cava
Lecompte Maneuver	Anterior translocation of the pulmonary arteries, so that both branch pulmonary arteries run anterior to the aorta. Most commonly used as part of the arterial switch operation
Mustard/Senning	Atrial switch operations for transposition of the great arteries, with atrial baffling using native atrial (Senning) or pericardial (Mustard) tissue to redirect systemic and pulmonary venous flow
Nikaidoh	In double outlet right ventricle, posterior translocation of the aortic root towards the left ventricle, with baffling of the left ventricle to the aorta in its new position
Norwood	Neonatal palliative procedure for hypoplastic left heart syndrome including aortic arch reconstruction with anastomosis of the native aorta to the pulmonary artery, which becomes the "neo-aorta," as well as atrial septectomy and a modified BT shunt
Potts shunt	Direct anastomosis of the left pulmonary artery to the descending aorta
Rastelli	Intra-cardiac routing of the left ventricle to the aorta, which arose from the right ventricle. Usually accompanied by a right ventricle to pulmonary artery conduit.
Takeuchi repair	Intrapulmonary baffle of the left coronary artery performed for anomalous left coronary artery from the pulmonary artery
Waterston shunt	Direct anastomosis of the right pulmonary artery to the ascending aorta

IVC, Inferior vena cava; *RA*, right atrium; *VSD*, ventricular septal defect.

The physical examination is also revealing in adult patients with newly discovered CHD, such as fixed splitting of the second heart sound in a patient with an unrepaired atrial septal defect (ASD), or diminished lower extremity pulses in a patient with an aortic coarctation. A classic physical examination finding in a patient with pulmonary stenosis is a systolic ejection click which decreases in intensity with inspiration.

The electrocardiogram (ECG) is an important tool in the assessment of CHD. The heart rhythm and rate, as well as the atrioventricular (AV) conduction, can be evaluated (see Chapter 14). Table 82.3 lists some of the common arrhythmias and ECG findings in various CHD conditions. The chest radiograph is an additional valuable tool in the assessment of the patient with CHD. Cardiac imaging plays an essential role in the management of ACHD patients. In 2020, Appropriate Use Criteria for multimodality imaging for follow-up care of CHD was released. This document presents 1035 unique scenarios to consider and rates various noninvasive imaging modalities into three categories: appropriate, may be appropriate, or rarely appropriate.[8]

The choice of when to obtain an echocardiogram, cardiac magnetic resonance (CMR), computed tomography (CT), nuclear scintigraphy, cardiac catheterization with x-ray angiography, or a combination of these modalities is dictated by the pertinent clinical question(s) and by a host of patient- and modality-related factors. Echocardiography remains the cornerstone of cardiac imaging in the CHD patient (see also Chapter 16). However, as patients age, acoustic windows may be suboptimal, and the other imaging modalities such as CMR (see also Chapter 19) or cardiac CT (CCT, see also Chapter 20) are advantageous. Due to the need for serial imaging, cumulative exposure to ionizing radiation should be taken into account as ACHD patients have increased risk for malignancy, perhaps related to these procedures. Cardiopulmonary exercise testing and measurement of biomarkers play an important role in the serial follow-up and the timing of intervention and re-intervention. Cardiac catheterization (see also Chapter 21) is recommended in any ACHD patient with signs of elevated pulmonary artery (PA) pressure to determine pulmonary vascular resistance (PVR). There should be a low threshold for cardiac catheterization in any ACHD patient with new symptoms not explained with noninvasive testing, particularly in complex CHD patients.

Noncardiac Complications in the ACHD Patient

As ACHD patients age, extracardiac complications become increasingly prevalent and affect patients' long-term outcomes.[9] These

TABLE 82.3 Common Arrhythmias and Typical ECG Abnormalities Seen in Adults with Congenital Heart Disease

ACHD CONDITION	COMMON ARRHYTHMIAS	TYPICAL ECG ABNORMALITIES
D-loop TGA, status post atrial switch (Mustard or Senning)	• Sinus node dysfunction • IART • Sudden death	• Right axis deviation • Right ventricular hypertrophy with strain
L-loop TGA	• Complete heart block	• Q-waves in right precordial leads and absent septal Q waves in the left precordial leads • PR prolongation or AV block
Fontan circulation	• Sinus node dysfunction • IART • Atrial fibrillation	• Depends on intracardiac anatomy
Atrioventricular septal defects	• Complete heart block • IART	• Left axis deviation • Right bundle branch block
Ebstein anomaly	• Accessory pathways and pre-excitation • IART • Atrial fibrillation	• Right atrial enlargement • Right bundle branch block with QRS fragmentation • Low-amplitude QRS • First-degree AV block but PR interval can be short if accessory pathways present
Tetralogy of Fallot	• Ventricular tachycardia • IART • Sudden death	• Right atrial enlargement • Right axis deviation • Right bundle branch block with QRS fragmentation
Eisenmenger syndrome	• IART • Sudden death	• Right atrial enlargement • Right axis deviation • Right ventricular hypertrophy

ACHD, Adult congenital heart disease; *AV,* atrioventricular; *IART,* interatrial re-entrant tachycardia; *TGA,* transposition of the great arteries.

noncardiac complications may be present in ACHD patients, regardless of their level of complexity and may involve any organ system (Table 82.4). Many ACHD patients live with subclinical levels of organ dysfunction and small perturbations in their hemodynamics may result in dramatic decline in function. Abnormal lung function is common in ACHD patients, and up to 40% of ACHD patients have abnormal pulmonary function tests. There are multiple mechanisms for abnormal pulmonary mechanics in ACHD patients, such as restrictive lung disease in postoperative patients. Other patients may have diaphragmatic paralysis due to phrenic nerve injury, asymmetric pulmonary blood flow due to branch PA abnormalities or acquired conditions, such as sleep apnea. ACHD patients are more prone to develop pulmonary thrombosis and embolism, pulmonary hemorrhage, and pneumonia. Pneumonia is one of the leading causes of noncardiac death in ACHD patients.[10] There are specific pulmonary complications that may be seen in certain ACHD conditions, such as plastic bronchitis in patients living with Fontan physiology. Hemoptysis may occur in up to one-third of ACHD patients with Eisenmenger syndrome. PH is found in up to 10% of ACHD patients and is strongly associated with increased morbidity and mortality (see section on Pulmonary Hypertension and Eisenmenger Syndrome).

Renal dysfunction is common in ACHD patients and has been shown to be a primary driver of high-resource utilization for ACHD hospitalizations, accounting for up to one-third of hospital charges.[11] While cyanotic ACHD patients have the highest prevalence of impaired renal function, non-cyanotic ACHD patients also develop renal insufficiency with age, and renal impairment is directly associated with mortality in these patients. Therefore, it is prudent to assess renal function at regular intervals in aging ACHD patients. Cystatin C-based estimated glomerular filtration rate (eGFR) more accurately predicts clinical effects in ACHD patients than creatinine-based eGFR.[12]

The prevalence of liver disease among ACHD patients is poorly characterized and most likely underestimated. The majority of the evidence of hepatic dysfunction in ACHD patients has been focused on Fontan-associated liver disease (FALD).[13] The pathologic findings can range from congestive hepatopathy to frank cirrhosis. Patients may have varying degrees of fibrosis with nodular regeneration. The etiology of hepatic dysfunction is most likely multifactorial, with systemic venous congestion and/or ischemia coupled with non-hemodynamic factors such as drug or viral-induced injury (see section on Fontan-Associated Liver Disease). Hepatitis C remains an important cause of liver disease in older ACHD patients, particularly those who received blood transfusions prior to 1992. Hematologic abnormalities in ACHD patients are common and include anemia, which is associated with increased mortality. Abnormalities of the coagulation system are observed in patients with Fontan physiology and are associated with bleeding and thrombotic complications. Cyanotic patients with erythrocytosis are at risk for hyperviscosity symptoms (see Eisenmenger section). Endocrinopathies and metabolic disorders are common in ACHD patients and may include thyroid disorders, obesity, diabetes, dyslipidemia, and disorders of calcium metabolism. Cancer is the second leading cause of non-cardiovascular death in ACHD patients,[10] with certain malignancies having an increased prevalence in specific CHD conditions, that is, hepatocellular carcinoma in adults with Fontan physiology. There is an increased risk of infectious and immunological complications in the ACHD population. The incidence of stroke is higher in ACHD patients than the general population.[14] Lastly, there is a growing body of evidence on the association of neurocognitive defects and CHD. At least one-third of ACHD patients report a mood or anxiety related disorder and many patients have deficits in executive function. These cognitive defects and psychosocial challenges have an impact on health status, education, employment, and quality of life.

CONGENITAL ANATOMY

Congenital Nomenclature

One of the challenges in caring for adults with CHD is the inconsistent terminology used to describe the anatomy and several classification systems have been proposed. Drs. Stella and Richard Van Praagh

TABLE 82.4 Noncardiac Complications in Adult Congenital Heart Disease

Neurologic	Increased incidence of occult or clinically evident strokes
	Decreased level of executive functioning skills
	Anxiety, post-traumatic stress disorder, depression
	Psychosocial disorders
	Neurodevelopmental deficits
Lungs	Restrictive lung disease
	Pulmonary vascular disease
	Pulmonary hypertension
	Pulmonary hemorrhage
	Plastic bronchitis
Immunology/infectious disease	Protein-losing enteropathy
	Infective endocarditis
	Pneumonia
	Brain abscess
Renal	Decreased perfusion
	Chronic kidney disease
	Cardiorenal syndrome
Hepatic	Liver fibrosis
	Congestive hepatopathy
	Cardiac cirrhosis
	Fontan associated liver disease
Endocrine	Thyroid
	Calcium hemostasis/Bone health
	Obesity/Metabolic syndrome
	Diabetes
	Dyslipidemia
Vascular	Chronic venous insufficiency
	Cerebrovascular disease
	Aortopathy
	Endothelial dysfunction
	Hypertension
	Peripheral venous/arterial disease
Orthopedic	Scoliosis
	Kyphosis
Hematologic	Anemia
	Coagulopathies
	Secondary erythrocytosis/iron deficiency/hyperuricemia (cyanotic CHD)
	Thromboembolism
Oncology	Low-dose ionizing radiation and malignancy
	Hepatocellular carcinoma
	Age-appropriate cancer screening

championed the segmental approach for description of congenital anatomy. In this approach, the heart is composed of several segments that are analyzed separately before formulating a comprehensive diagnosis. The principal segments are the atria, the ventricles, and the great arteries, which are joined together by the AV canal and the conus (infundibulum). In the normal heart, the right ventricle (RV) is right-sided and organized inflow-to-outflow from right to left, while the left ventricle (LV) is left-sided and organized inflow-to-outflow from left to right. It is important to determine the segmental alignments: that is, what drains into what. For example, in the normal heart the right atrium (RA) is aligned with the RV and the RV is aligned with the PA. Similarly, in a normal heart the left atrium (LA) is aligned with the LV and the LV is aligned with the aorta. Finally, the segmental connections, the way in which adjacent segments are physically linked to each other, are described. For example, in the normal heart the RV is connected to the PA by a complete muscular conus (infundibulum), while the LV is connected to the aorta by aortic-mitral fibrous continuity (without a complete conus). Alignment and connection are distinct concepts and both are important, especially in complex defects.

Cardiac Development (Fig. 82.1)

The heart starts to form in the third week of gestation and is nearly fully formed by 8 weeks gestation. Mesodermal precardiac cells migrate to form the cardiac crescents (primary heart fields) in anterior lateral plate mesoderm, which are then brought together to form a primary linear heart tube by ventral closure of the embryo. Cells of the second heart field continue to proliferate outside the heart and are added to the heart tube over the course of embryogenesis, contributing to the atria, the RV, and outflow tract. Additionally, cardiac neural crest cells migrate into the developing heart in the 5th to 6th weeks and are essential for septation of the outflow, formation of the semilunar valves, and patterning of the aortic arches. Once formed, the heart tube grows and elongates by addition of cells from the second heart field. The ends of the heart tube are relatively fixed by the pericardial sac so that as it elongates it must loop (bend), and in the vast majority of hearts the loop falls to the right (D-loop). Further elongation pushes the mid-portion of the tube (future ventricles) inferior or caudal to the inflow, resulting in the normal relationship between the atria and ventricles. Further growth pushes the outflow medially and is associated with outflow rotation, both processes essential for normal alignment of the outflow. Finally, the proximal part of the outflow is incorporated in the RV, shortening the outflow in association with further rotation. While this remodeling is occurring, the outflow is undergoing septation under the influence of cardiac neural crest cells. Septation proceeds from distal to proximal, culminating in formation and muscularization of the infundibular, or muscular, outflow septum, which inserts onto the superior endocardial cushion at the rightward rim of the outflow foramen, walling the aorta into the LV via the outflow foramen and the PA directly into the RV.

Genetic Considerations

CHD is the most commonly occurring birth defect and genetic etiologies are increasingly being recognized. Several hundred genes have been identified to either cause or contribute to CHD.[15] Epidemiological studies have suggested that a genetic or environmental cause can be identified in up to 30% of CHD cases. Single-gene disorders are found in 3% to 5%, gross chromosomal anomalies/aneuploidy in 8% to 10%, and pathogenic copy number variants in up to 25% of CHD cases. Environmental causes are identifiable in 2% of CHD cases. The remainder of CHD is presumed to be multifactorial.[16]

Sequence variants in CHD genes can cause both sporadic and inherited forms of CHD. Sequence variants in the same genes may be associated with different cardiac phenotypes, not only between families but also within families. Additionally, there is evolving evidence that some of the outcomes in patients with CHD may be influenced by the underlying genetic cause.[17]

Down syndrome is the most common aneuploidy and is usually caused by trisomy 21. It is also the most common chromosome abnormality associated with CHD. Fifty percent of children born with Down syndrome have CHD, most commonly defects in the AV canal. Table 82.5 lists certain genetic syndromes and associated congenital cardiac conditions.

LONG-TERM CONSIDERATIONS

Arrhythmias in Adult Congenital Heart Disease
Demographics and Prognosis

Arrhythmias are prevalent in ACHD patients. The frequency of arrhythmias increases with age and disease complexity. Arrhythmia causes

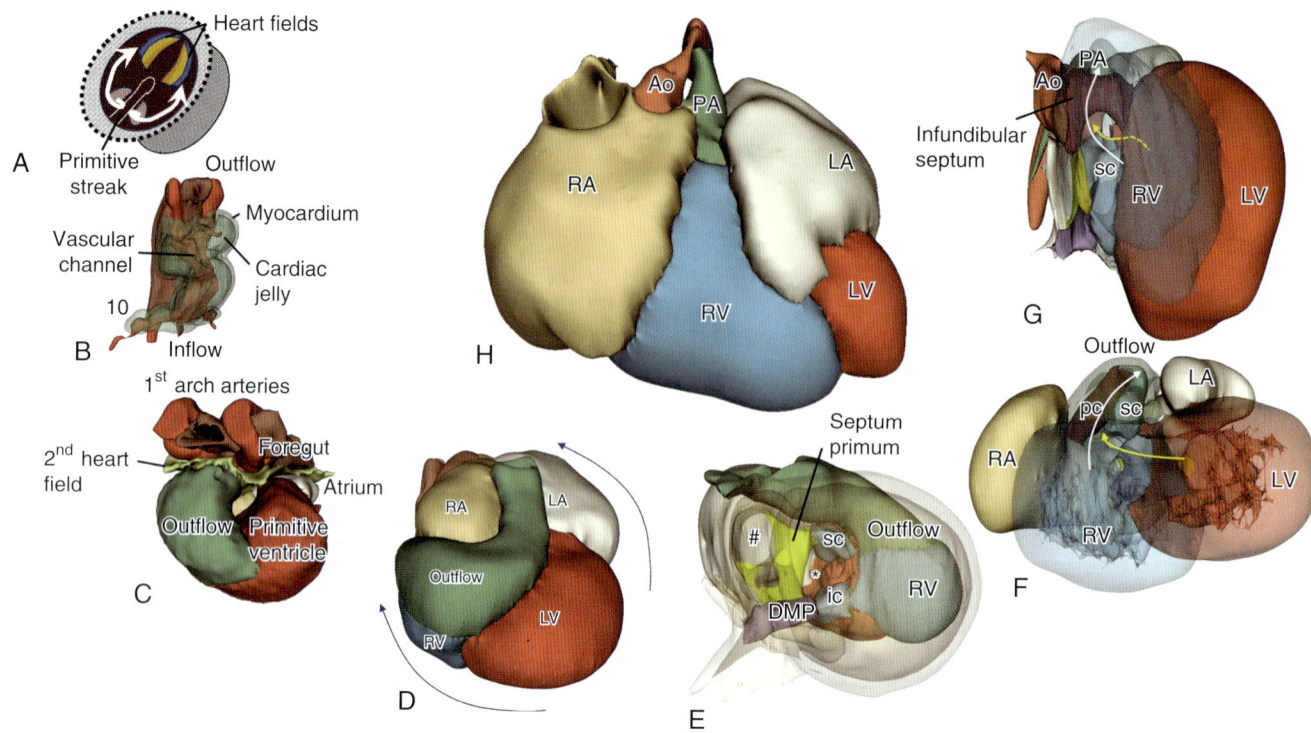

FIGURE 82.1 Developmental highlights. **A,** Carnegie stage (CS) 7-disc embryo during mid 3rd week illustrating gastrulation through the primitive streak to form the mesoderm and rostral migration of pre-cardiac mesoderm to form the 1st *(blue)* and 2nd *(yellow)* heart fields. **B,** CS 10 heart in the early 4th week showing the newly formed tubular heart. The vascular channel is seen through the semitransparent myocardium and cardiac jelly. **C,** CS 11 heart at mid 4th week. The heart tube is enlarged and lengthened by addition of cells from the proliferating 2nd heart field at both the outflow and inflow ends. As it lengthens in the confined pericardial space the heart tube bends or loops, usually to the right (**D** or dextral looping), leading to the final shape of the heart with ventricles caudal and atria rostral. **D,** CS 13 heart at the beginning of the 5th week showing chamber development by ballooning outgrowth of proliferating myocytes at specified points around the outer or greater curvature of the looped heart tube. Lengthening of the outflow pushes it centrally between the developing atria (*LA*, left atrium; *LV*, left ventricle; *RA*, right atrium; *RV*, right ventricular). **E,** CS 15 heart at the beginning of the 6th week. Looking through the semitransparent right posterior wall of the right atrium shows the septum primum (primary atrial septum) in yellow and the dorsal mesenchymal protrusion (DMP) in purple, the main components of the atrial septation complex. The DMP, a prong of cells originating from 2nd heart field, will continue to invade, filling the space between the superior *(sc)* and inferior *(ic)* endocardial cushions and closing ostium primum *(*)*, completing atrial septation and contributing to division of the atrioventricular (AV) canal into left (mitral) and right (tricuspid) orifices. By this stage ostium secundum *(#)* or the foramen ovale has formed by breakdown of the septum primum at its origin from the posterior-superior atrial wall. The AV canal has begun to expand rightward so that it drains both atria into only the left ventricle (LV). **F,** CS 17 heart at the beginning of the 7th week viewed from the apex with the ventricles and outflow semitransparent showing the shortened and partially rotated outflow, resulting in spiraling of the parietal (pc) and septal (sc) outflow cushions or ridges about each other. The cushions have begun to fuse together distally under the influence of neural crest cells dividing the outflow into an anterior pulmonary *(white arrow)* and a posterior aortic *(yellow arrow)* pathway. Further anticlockwise rotation will bring the aortic pathway closer to the interventricular foramen, the eventual LV outflow. **G,** CS 19 heart at the end of the 7th week viewed from right and anterior with the RV semitransparent and the RA removed. Complete septation of the outflows is accomplished by formation and muscularization of the infundibular septum as the proximal parts of the outflow cushions fuse. The membranous septum forms where the developing infundibular septum joins the superior endocardial cushion *(sc)*. The LV pathway to the aorta *(yellow arrow)* through the interventricular foramen is on the far side of the infundibular septum and the pathway from RV to pulmonary artery *(white arrow)* is on the near side. **H,** CS 23 heart at the end of embryogenesis (end of 8th week) showing the completed but still immature fetal heart.

morbidity and mortality in adults with CHD and is the most frequent cause for hospital admission in adults with CHD. Patients with CHD with arrhythmia have a worse prognosis than those without.

New arrhythmias in a patient with CHD should prompt a careful evaluation to determine whether there is a hemodynamic cause for the arrhythmia. In many cases worsening ventricular dysfunction, valve dysfunction, or filling pressures can precipitate new rhythm disturbances. Echocardiography may yield information but in some catheterization is required.

The demographics and mechanisms of arrhythmia are very different in ACHD patients compared to adults with acquired heart disease: ACHD patients develop arrhythmia at a much younger age, frequently in their late teens or early 20s for patients with complex forms of CHD. Patients with ACHD are likely to have re-entrant arrhythmia related to surgical scars or around patches although diffuse fibrosis may predispose to arrhythmias as well. Patients with CHD are often intolerant of arrhythmia and in most instances restoration of sinus rhythm is preferred over rate control. In 2014 the Pediatric and Congenital Electrophysiology Society and the Heart Rhythm Society published a comprehensive consensus statement on the management of arrhythmias in adults with CHD.[18] Arrhythmias are discussed further in the sections on individual lesions.

Diagnostic Testing

Resting ECG is indicated in most patients with CHD. Common ECG abnormalities are shown in Table 82.3. Because rhythm disturbances become more prevalent with increasing age, serial ECG monitoring is needed for patients at high risk for arrhythmia such as those with tetralogy of Fallot (TOF), Ebstein anomaly, Fontan circulation, transposition of the great arteries (TGA), and others.

Ambulatory ECG monitoring is useful to investigate palpitations and to screen for occult arrhythmia in asymptomatic patients. In patients with TOF asymptomatic nonsustained ventricular tachycardia (VT) recorded on Holter monitoring predicts clinical VT. In other CHD lesions, however, the clinical significance of asymptomatic arrhythmias seen on ambulatory ECG remains unknown. Exercise ECG monitoring is useful for patients with exercise-induced symptoms. Implantable loop recorders can be used for patients with infrequent but worrisome symptoms of arrhythmia.

The need for invasive electrophysiology (EP) study with programmed stimulation and electroanatomic mapping should be determined on a case-by-case basis. Inducible sustained VT is a risk factor for clinical VT and sudden death in patients with repaired TOF and is discussed in more detail in the section on Tetralogy of Fallot. The prognostic value of programmed electrical stimulation has not been determined in other forms of CHD and, in some conditions such as TGA, is not of prognostic value.[18]

Types of Arrhythmia

The type of arrhythmia encountered depends both on the native CHD lesion as well as the type of surgical repair (see Table 82.3).

TABLE 82.5 Genetic Syndromes and Congenital Heart Disease

SYNDROME	GENE(S)	CARDIAC DISEASE	% CONGENITAL HD	ASSOCIATED FINDINGS
Alagille	JAG1, Notch2	Pps, tof, pa	>90	Bile duct paucity, butterfly vertebrae, renal defects
CHARGE	CHD7	TOF, PDA, DORV, AVSD, VSD	75–85	Coloboma, choanal atresia, genital hypoplasia, ear anomalies, hearing loss, developmental delay, growth retardation, intellectual disability
22q11.2DS	TBX1	Conotruncal defects, VSD, IAA, ASD, VR	74–85	Cleft palate, bifid uvula, velopharyngeal insufficiency, microcephaly, hypocalcemia, immune deficit, psychiatric disorder, learning disability
Ellis-van Creveld	EVC, EVC2	Common atrium	60	Skeletal dysplasia, short limbs, polydactyly, short ribs, dysplastic nails, respiratory insufficiency
Holt-Oram	TBX5	VSD, ASD, AVSD, conduction defects	50	Absent, hypoplastic, or triphalangeal thumbs; phocomelia; defects of radius; limb defects more prominent on left
Kabuki	KMT2D, KDM6A	CoA, BAV, VSD, TOF, TGA, HLHS	50	Growth deficiency, wide palpebral fissures, large protuberant ears, fetal finger pads, intellectual disability, clinodactyly
Noonan	PTPN11, SOS1, RAF1, KRAS, NRAS, RIT1, SHOC2, SOS2, BRAF	Dysplastic PVS, ASD, TOF, AVSD, HCM, VSD, PDA	75	Short stature, hypertelorism, down-slanting palpebral fissures, ptosis, low posterior hairline, pectus deformity, bleeding disorder, chylothorax, cryptorchidism
VACTERAL association	Unknown	VSD, ASD, HLHS, PDA, TGA, TOF, TA	53–80	Vertebral anomalies, anal atresia, tracheoesophageal fistula, renal anomalies, radial dysplasia, thumb hypoplasia, single umbilical artery
Williams-Beuren	7q11/23 deletion (ELN)	SVAS, PAS, VSD, ASD	80	Unusual facies, thick lips, strabismus, stellate iris pattern, intellectual disability

ASD, Atrial septal defect; AVSD, atrioventricular septal defect; BAV, bicuspid aortic valve; CoA, coarctation of the aorta; DORV, double outlet right ventricle; HCM, hypertrophic cardiomyopathy; HLHS, hypoplastic left heart syndrome; IAA, interrupted aortic arch; PA, pulmonary atresia; PAS, pulmonary artery stenosis; PDA, patent ductus arteriosus; PPS, peripheral pulmonary stenosis; PVS, pulmonary valve stenosis; TOF, tetralogy of Fallot; VR, vascular ring; VSD, ventricular septal defect; TGA, transposition of the great arteries; TA, truncus arteriosus; SVAS, supravalvular aortic stenosis.
Modified from Pierpont ME, Brueckner M, Chung WK, et al. Genetic basis for congenital heart disease: revisited: a scientific statement from the American Heart Association. Circulation. 2018;138(21):e653–e711.

Bradyarrhythmia
Sinus Node Dysfunction
Sinus node dysfunction is most commonly related to surgical injury. Sinus node dysfunction is commonly encountered in patients with D-loop TGA who have undergone a Mustard or Senning operation and is also common following repair for ASD or sinus venosus defects. Patients with Glenn shunt or Fontan circulation may have sinus node dysfunction.

Atrial pacing is required for symptomatic sinus node dysfunction. Transvenous pacing is usually preferred but may be technically difficult in patients who have had surgical manipulation of the superior vena cava (SVC) (who are the same patients who are predisposed to sinus node dysfunction). Patients who have had a Fontan operation with an extracardiac conduit and those with open atrial shunts typically require epicardial pacing. Transvenous atrial pacing may be possible in patients with a lateral tunnel or atriopulmonary Fontan. Transvenous pacing is typically possible following the Mustard or Senning procedure or after repair of a superior sinus venosus defect but endocardial leads increase the risk of SVC stenosis or obstruction.

Heart Block
Heart block is common in patients with L-loop TGA as the AV node is superiorly and anteriorly displaced. The incidence of complete heart block in L-loop TGA is 2% per year. Patients with double-inlet LV also have a high incidence of heart block. Heart block is common in adults who had surgical repair of an atrioventricular septal defect (AVSD) as the AV node and His bundles are displaced posteriorly and can be injured by ventricular septal defect (VSD) closure, although modern surgical techniques have decreased the likelihood of heart block in this population. Finally, complete heart block is a common post-surgical complication from patients who have had resection of a subaortic membrane or multiple operations on the left ventricular outflow tract (LVOT).

Pacemakers are used to treat heart block. Transvenous pacemakers are preferred when technically feasible. Biventricular pacing with cardiac resynchronization may be desirable for patients with underlying ventricular dysfunction or a systemic RV who require chronic ventricular pacing.

Tachyarrhythmias
Interatrial Re-Entrant Tachycardia
Interatrial re-entrant tachycardia (IART) is the most common tachyarrhythmia in CHD, accounting for 62% of atrial arrhythmias.[19] The cumulative incidence of IART approaches 50% by age 65 and occurs in a wide variety of CHD lesions.[20] IART can conduct around an anatomic obstacle such as an ASD patch or an atriotomy scar. While it may occur in children, frequency increases by young adulthood as progressive atrial fibrosis contributes to arrhythmogenesis. IART is exceedingly common in patients who have had a Mustard or Senning operation and for those with an atriopulmonary Fontan. In patients who have undergone the atrial switch operation, IART is a dangerous arrhythmia which may convert to polymorphic VT or pulseless electrical activity as the noncompliant interatrial baffles and systemic RV perform poorly at high heart rates. Patients with Fontan circulation also tolerate chronic

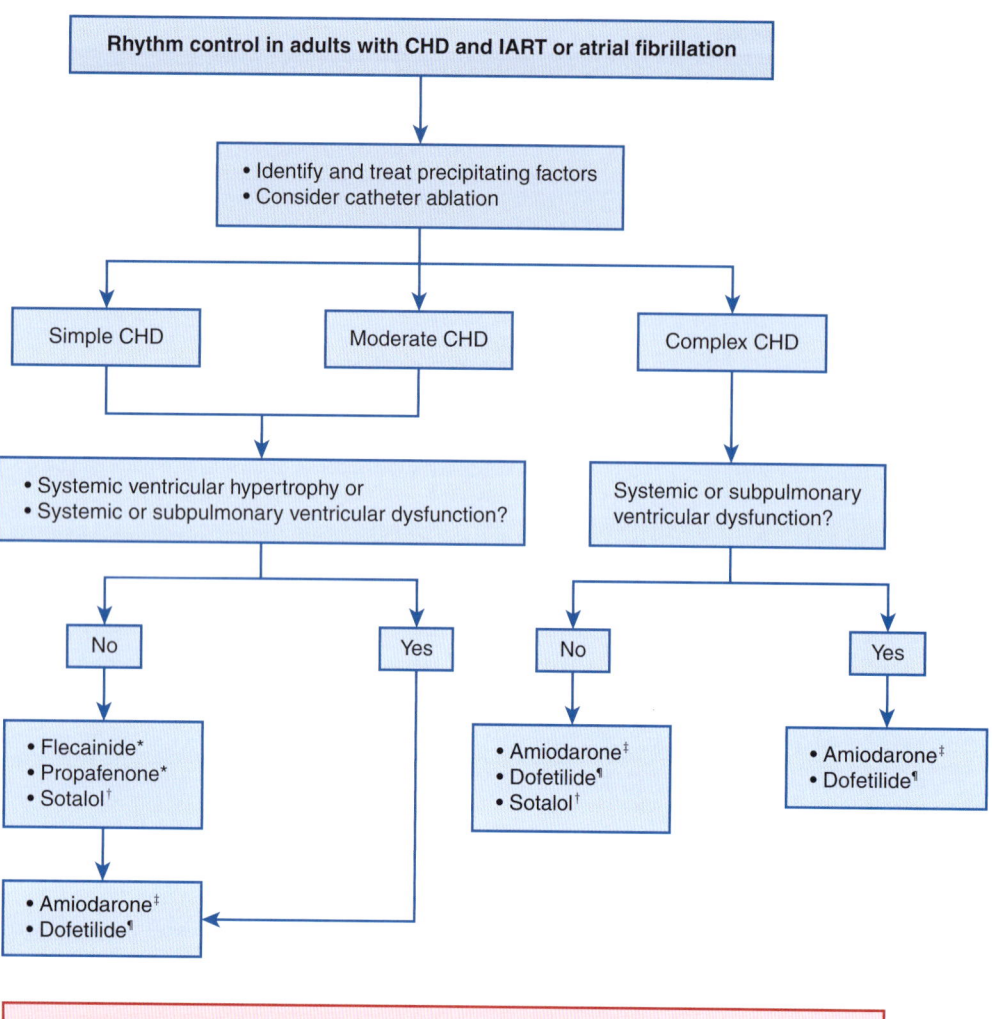

FIGURE 82.2 Rhythm control in adults with congenital heart disease (CHD) and intra-atrial reentrant tachycardia (IART) or atrial fibrillation. (From Khairy P, Van Hare GF, Balaji S, et al. PACES/HRS expert consensus statement on the recognition and management of arrhythmias in adult congenital heart disease. *Heart Rhythm.* 2014;11:e102–e665.)

patient's underlying congenital anatomy and consider risk factors for pro-arrhythmia such as ventricular dysfunction or QTc prolongation (Fig. 82.2). Sotalol and dofetilide are often preferred in patients with complex CHD. Amiodarone has considerable cumulative toxicity so is usually not a preferred first-line antiarrhythmic in younger patients but is sometimes required for patients with ventricular dysfunction.

Which patients with atrial arrhythmia and CHD require long-term anticoagulation remains an area of active investigation. Risk models such as CHA_2DS_2-VASc are not validated in CHD and should not be relied upon because CHD patients have a much higher rate of thromboembolism than similarly aged patients with acquired heart disease, even in the absence of conventional risk factors.[22] Patients with Fontan circulation and IART should receive long-term anticoagulation. Patients with atrial arrhythmia and complex CHD should be considered for long-term anticoagulation as well. Both vitamin K antagonists and direct oral anticoagulants have been used successfully in adult patients with CHD.[23]

Atrial Fibrillation (see Chapter 66)

As patients with CHD age, atrial fibrillation becomes more common and is the most common atrial arrhythmia in adults with CHD older than age 50. Adults with CHD have a greater than 20-fold increased risk of developing atrial fibrillation compared to age matched controls; by age 42 greater than 8% of CHD patients have a diagnosis of atrial fibrillation.[19] Atrial fibrillation is most common in those with traditional risk factors such as obesity, tobacco use, and hypertension. Atrial fibrillation is common in patients with AV valve regurgitation, LVOT obstruction, Ebstein anomaly, Fontan circulation, ASDs, and AVSDs.

Compared with IART, atrial fibrillation is less reliably treated with catheter ablation. However, other principles related to rhythm control and anticoagulation, as discussed above, are broadly similar.

Ventricular Tachycardia and Sudden Death (see Chapters 67 and 70)

Sudden death is the second most common cause of cardiac death in adults with CHD following heart failure, and accounts for approximately 20% of death in patients with CHD, occurring at a rate of ~0.1% per patient year. Patients with TOF, TGA with a systemic RV, Fontan circulation, Eisenmenger syndrome, and complex forms of CHD are at the highest risk for ventricular arrhythmias and sudden cardiac death. Fortunately, the frequency of sudden death may be declining due to improved risk stratification, implantable cardioverter defibrillators (ICDs), and improvements in surgical technique (such as earlier definitive surgical repair and avoidance of ventriculotomies).[10,20] Ventricular arrhythmias are often macroreentrant scar-based arrhythmias. Discrete or diffuse replacement fibrosis also contributes to ventricular arrhythmia.

IART poorly and restoration of sinus rhythm is desirable. Patients with atrial arrhythmias have a 50% increased risk of mortality and double the morbidity compared to patients without atrial arrhythmia.[21] Acute termination of arrhythmia is usually performed with electrical cardioversion after atrial thrombus has been excluded with transesophageal echocardiography (TEE) or gated CCT. Pace termination or pharmacologic cardioversion can be performed in selected patients. Anticoagulation is required for at least 4 weeks following cardioversion.

Rhythm control is usually preferred over rate control for adults with CHD and IART. Catheter ablation is often effective and used as first-line therapy when IART is recurrent. Ablation should be performed by an electrophysiologist with experience in CHD as the mechanisms of re-entry are due to surgical patches and unconventional anatomy not typically seen in acquired heart disease. Trans-baffle punctures are often required in patients with Mustard/Senning operations or Fontan circulation where the majority of patients have multiple IART circuits.

Medical therapy is a useful adjunct to catheter ablation or can be used when ablation is unsuccessful. AV nodal blockade with beta-blockers or calcium blockers is reasonable to prevent rapid ventricular response. Anti-arrhythmic drug choice must be tailored to the

Risk stratification to predict which patients are at risk for sudden death is challenging. Patients with a systemic LV and severe systolic dysfunction are thought to be high risk. A combination of clinical, ECG, and imaging parameters identify high-risk patients with repaired TOF and is discussed in detail in the section on Tetralogy of Fallot. Invasive EP studies further identify patients with repaired TOF but have not been shown to be predictive in other forms of CHD.

Secondary prevention ICDs are appropriate for patients with clinical sustained VT or aborted sudden cardiac death. Antiarrhythmic drugs may be adjunctive and catheter ablation can reduce the risk of ICD shocks. Results of catheter ablation for VT in repaired TOF are discussed separately.

Pacemakers and Implantable Defibrillators (see Chapter 69)

Pacemakers and ICDs are required in many patients with CHD. Indications for pacemakers are sinus node dysfunction and heart block. Indications for primary and secondary prevention ICDs are shown in Table 82.6.

Unfortunately, patients with CHD are at high risk for device complications such as lead fractures or device infections, which occur in up to 26% of adults with CHD. Both appropriate and inappropriate shocks are common in ACHD patients with ICDs. In a meta-analysis, appropriate shock rate was 22% at 3.3 years and inappropriate shock rate was 35% at 4.3 years follow-up, each higher than is seen in acquired heart disease.[24] Improvements in device algorithms and programming may reduce the risk of inappropriate shocks in contemporary cohorts.

Device implantation can be difficult in patients with surgically manipulated or variant venous anatomy (such as following Mustard/Senning procedures). Pacemakers should be epicardial in patients with intracardiac shunts, single ventricle, or ventricular leads in Fontan circulation. Cardiac resynchronization leads may be technically difficult due to variation in the location of the coronary sinus (CS) os. A proposed algorithm for cardiac resynchronization therapy (CRT) in CHD is shown in Fig. 82.3.

Because of the higher risk of device complications, both appropriate and inappropriate shocks, and the challenges with device implantation, the risk-benefit ratio of devices needs to be weighed carefully and in conjunction with ACHD providers and electrophysiologists experienced in CHD.

Heart Failure, Transplantation, and Mechanical Circulatory Support (see Part VI)

Epidemiology

Despite continued improvements in outcomes for those born with CHD, most adults with CHD, particularly for those with moderate or complex CHD, die from cardiac causes. Heart failure remains a major source of morbidity and the dominant cause of death for adults with CHD in the modern era, accounting for up to 40% of the ACHD mortality.[10]

The rate of heart failure hospitalizations among adults with CHD is increasing at a rapid rate. Hospitalizations for adults with CHD is associated with longer length of stay, high resource utilization, and poor in-hospital and long-term outcomes.[25] Heart failure is most common in patients with high anatomic or physiologic complexity including single ventricle anatomy, systemic RV, PH, and cyanosis. However, even patients with simple forms of CHD are at increased long-term risk of heart failure.[26]

Clinical Features

The clinical presentation of heart failure in patients with CHD is diverse. Typical symptoms such as pulmonary congestion, edema, and dyspnea on exertion may not be present. Often arrhythmia, hypoxemia, or exertional fatigue may be the presenting symptoms of heart failure in patients with CHD. Many patients with CHD have adapted to their lifelong cardiac condition and may under-report functional limitations. Cardiopulmonary exercise testing is useful to elicit sub-clinical deterioration, even in patients who report that they feel well. Patients with CHD and heart failure often have elevated biomarkers. Elevations in brain natriuretic peptide (BNP), troponin, and other biomarkers are associated with heart failure and poor outcomes in adults with CHD.[27]

TABLE 82.6 Indications for Implantable Defibrillators in Adults With Congenital Heart Disease

COR	LOE	RECOMMENDATION
SECONDARY PREVENTION		
I	B	ICD therapy is indicated in adults with CHD who are survivors of cardiac arrest due to ventricular fibrillation or hemodynamically unstable VT after evaluation to define the cause of the event and exclude any completely reversible etiology
I	B	ICD therapy is indicated in adults with CHD and spontaneous sustained VT who have undergone hemodynamic and electrophysiologic evaluation.
	C	Catheter ablation or surgery may offer a reasonable alternative or adjunct to ICD therapy in carefully selected patients
PRIMARY PREVENTION		
I	B	ICD therapy is indicated in adults with CHD and a systemic left ventricular ejection fraction ≤ 35%, biventricular physiology, and NYHA Class II or III symptoms
IIa	B	ICD therapy is reasonable in selected adults with tetralogy of Fallot and multiple risk factors for sudden cardiac death such as left ventricular systolic or diastolic dysfunction, nonsustained VT, QRS duration ≥180 ms, extensive right ventricular scarring, or inducible sustained VT at electrophysiologic study
IIb	C	ICD therapy may be reasonable in adults with a single or systemic right ventricular ejection fraction <35%, particularly in the presence of additional risk factors such as complex ventricular arrhythmias, unexplained syncope, NYHA functional Class II or III symptoms, QRS duration ≥140 msec, or severe systemic atrioventricular valve
		Regurgitation
IIb	B	ICD therapy may be considered in adults with CHD and syncope of unknown origin with hemodynamically significant sustained ventricular tachycardia or fibrillation inducible at electrophysiologic study
IIb	C	ICD therapy may be considered for adults with syncope and moderate or complex CHD in whom there is a high clinical suspicion of ventricular arrhythmia and in whom thorough invasive and noninvasive investigations have failed to define a cause
IIb	C	ICD therapy may be considered in adults with CHD and a systemic ventricular ejection fraction <35% in the absence of overt symptoms (NYHA class I) or other known risk factors

CHD, congenital heart disease; COR, class of recommendation; ICD, implantable cardioverter-defibrillator; LOE, level of evidence; NYHA, New York Heart Association; VT, ventricular tachycardia.
Adapted from Khairy P, Van Hare GF, Balaji S, et al. PACES/HRS expert consensus statement on the recognition and management of arrhythmias in adult congenital heart disease. *Heart Rhythm.* 2014;11(10):e102–e165.

Pathophysiology

The etiology and pathophysiology of heart failure in adults with CHD is often quite different from that of adults with acquired cardiovascular disease. The majority of heart failure in adults with acquired cardiovascular disease is secondary to left ventricular systolic or diastolic dysfunction; this is not true in adults with CHD. Adults with CHD are more likely to have a single ventricle, systemic RV, associated pulmonary vascular disease, residual shunt, or residual outflow obstruction as an underlying etiology of heart failure.

The pathophysiologic basis of heart failure differs depending on the underlying lesions. Volume loading from shunts and valvular regurgitation cause ventricular dilation and, if untreated, ventricular dysfunction. Residual outflow obstruction can result from sub-valvular or valvular stenosis as well as peripheral arterial narrowing, such as aortic

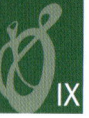

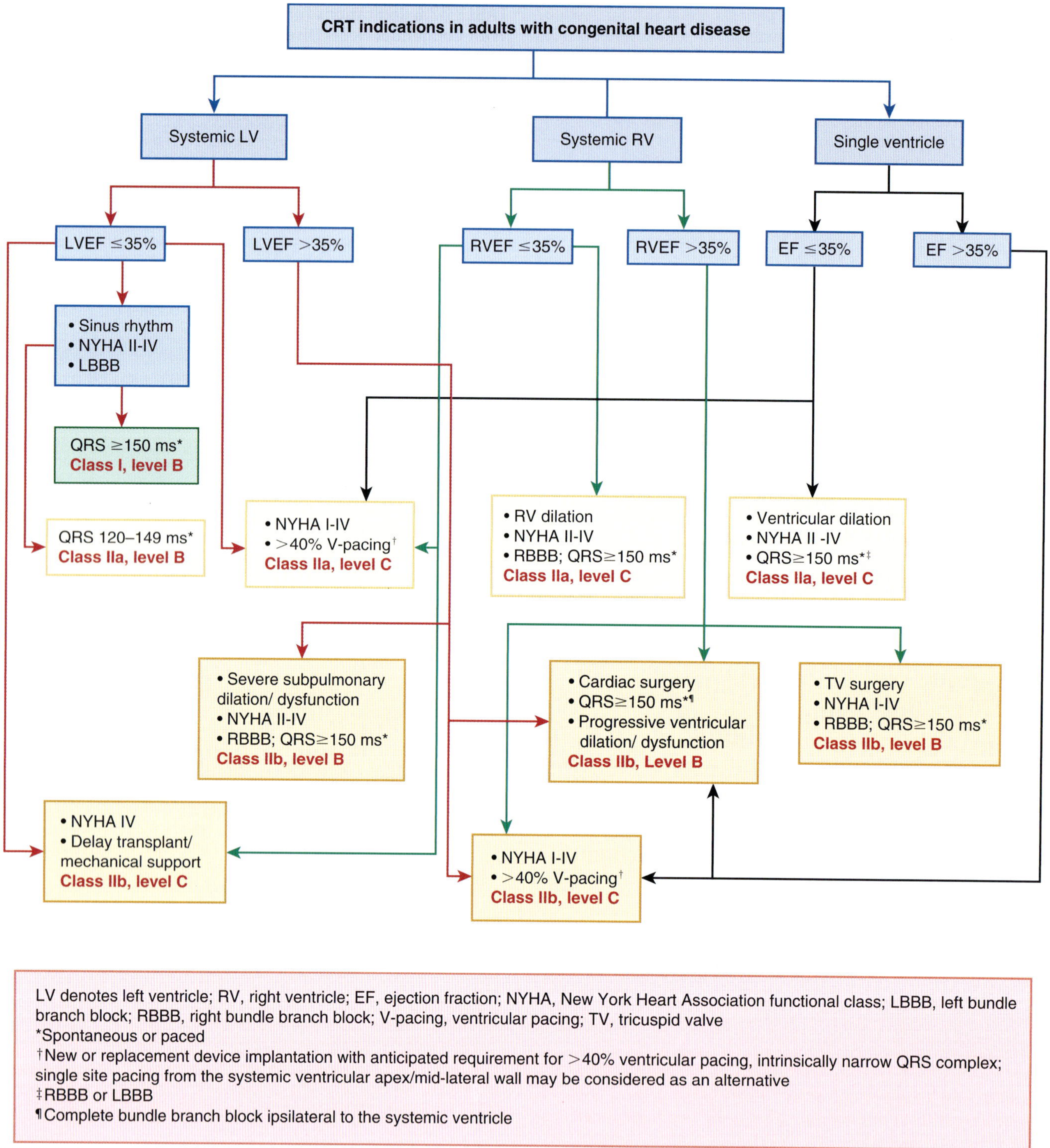

FIGURE 82.3 Recommendations for cardiac resynchronization therapy (CRT) in adults with congenital heart disease. (From Khairy P, Van Hare GF, Balaji S, et al. PACES/HRS expert consensus statement on the recognition and management of arrhythmias in adult congenital heart disease. *Heart Rhythm.* 2014;11:e102–e665.)

coarctation. Obstructive lesions can induce ventricular hypertrophy and dysfunction.

Patients with a systemic RV (such as those with D-loop TGA treated with an atrial switch procedure or those with L-loop TGA) are at high risk for ventricular dysfunction. The systemic RV is predisposed to systolic dysfunction due to unfavorable myocardial fiber orientation, nonconical shape, coronary supply-demand mismatch, and volume loading from tricuspid regurgitation.

Heart failure is exceedingly common in adults who have undergone the Fontan operation; transplant-free survival is less than 70% 25 years after the Fontan operation and most patients develop heart failure by age 40.[28] The mechanisms for heart failure after the Fontan operation are multifactorial and incompletely understood. Not all patients have overt ventricular or valvular dysfunction. Fontan failure is characterized by chronically elevated central venous pressure, low cardiac output, cyanosis due to collaterals, ascites, and cirrhosis.

Medical Therapy

Patients with CHD and heart failure should be managed at a specialty CHD center. The pathophysiologic basis of heart failure in CHD differs from that of acquired heart failure, therefore, it is often difficult to know which treatments are effective in CHD. Patients with CHD have been excluded from most heart failure trials and few studies have examined CHD patients specifically. Nonetheless, clinicians must make decisions about how to use medical therapy in patients with CHD, even in the absence of definitive data.

Prior to turning to medical therapy for heart failure, residual hemodynamic lesions such as shunts, valve dysfunction, and outflow obstruction should be sought out and treated. In many cases, transthoracic echocardiography (TTE) is insufficient and cross-sectional imaging or invasive hemodynamics are needed to define the cause of symptoms.

Standard guideline-directed medical therapy (GDMT) is likely effective when taken by CHD patients with a systemic LV who have heart failure due to left ventricular systolic dysfunction after residual hemodynamic lesions have been addressed. The efficacy of GDMT in other populations is less well established. Angiotensin blockade is commonly used in patients with a systemic RV and systolic dysfunction. However, the largest trial of Renin-Angiotensin-Aldosterone System (RAAS) blockade in patients with a systemic RV did not improve right ventricular ejection fraction. There is very little data to suggest that beta-blockers are beneficial for patients with a systemic RV. Pulmonary vasodilators, including PDE5-inhibitors and endothelin receptor antagonists, have been shown to improve functional class and exercise capacity in patients with Fontan circulation.[29] Newer heart failure medications such as sacubitril/valsartan, ivabradine, and dapagliflozin have not been prospectively studied in patients with CHD. Finally, modifiable risk factors such as hypertension, diabetes, obesity, and sleep apnea should be aggressively treated in CHD patients with heart failure.

Cardiac Resynchronization

CRT via multi-site pacing is appropriate for patients with a systemic LV, spontaneous or pacing-induced left bundle-branch block, and heart failure. The role of CRT in other forms of CHD is not as well established.[30]

Patients with a systemic RV (particularly those with L-loop TGA) have a high incidence of heart block as well as frequent need for ventricular pacing. Multiple observational studies suggest benefit of CRT in patients with a systemic RV, although the data are generally retrospective and uncontrolled. Placing CRT leads is technically more difficult in patients with a systemic RV due to variability in the location of the CS os, variant coronary vein anatomy, and the presence of surgical interatrial baffles. It is reasonable to consider placement of epicardial multi-site pacing leads in selected patients if they are going for cardiac surgery for other indications.

The benefit of CRT in patients with single ventricle anatomy following the Fontan operation is not well established. Additionally, multi-site pacing requires epicardial lead placement.

Transplantation

Patients with CHD and heart failure refractory to medical therapy should be considered for heart transplantation. Since 2000, the number of ACHD patients listed for transplantation and ultimately transplanted has doubled. Adult CHD patients account for more than 4% of adult heart transplantations done in the United States.

Compared to patients with acquired heart failure, CHD patients listed for heart transplantation are younger, more likely to have a prior sternotomy, less likely to have coronary artery disease, and less likely to have a left ventricular assist device. Alloimmunization secondary to prior transfusions or homograft implantation can prolong waitlist times, require desensitization, or make some patients ineligible for transplantation. Many patients with CHD have important comorbidities such as cirrhosis, chronic kidney disease, restrictive lung disease (as a consequence of prior chest surgery), or pulmonary vascular disease which may make them high-risk, or even ineligible for cardiac transplantation. For all these reasons, many patients with CHD and advanced heart failure are never listed for heart transplantation. Even those patients who are ultimately listed for transplantation are more likely to be delisted or die without transplantation than patients with acquired cardiovascular disease.[31]

Due to the high complexity and prevalence of comorbidities in CHD patients with advanced heart failure, a multidisciplinary team consisting of ACHD specialists, advanced heart failure specialists, and cardiac surgeons with experience in both congenital and transplant surgery should evaluate all ACHD patients considered for transplantation. Necessarily, this process should take place at an ACHD specialty center.

Patients with CHD are listed at UNOS Status 4 in the allocation system adopted in 2018. They share status urgency with ambulatory patients with a left ventricular assist device, patients with cardiac amyloidosis, and those awaiting re-transplantation. Many of the criteria used to justify higher-urgency status, such as poor hemodynamics, inotropic support, or mechanical circulatory support may not be applicable to patients with ACHD. Therefore, patients with ACHD may require an exception to be listed at higher urgency in order to reflect their acuity and higher waitlist mortality.[32]

Patients with CHD have high operative risk which is reflected by increased in-hospital and 1-year mortality following transplantation. This early risk is mitigated by low late graft failure and mortality compared to those with acquired heart disease so that long-term survival is not lower for ACHD patients undergoing transplantation (Fig. 82.4).[33,34] For this reason, organ allocation to ACHD patients results in acceptable utility of donor hearts. Because of the high surgical risk and complexity of transplant in CHD, transplant should be performed at specialty ACHD centers.[35] When performed at high-volume ACHD transplant centers, outcomes are improved.

Mechanical Circulatory Support

ACHD patients with advanced heart failure have higher anatomic and physiologic complexity than those with acquired heart failure, therefore, mechanical circulatory support may not provide the same benefit. Left ventricular assist devices are appropriate for patients with advanced heart failure due to left ventricular systolic dysfunction who meet conventional indications for mechanical support. In carefully selected patients, ventricular assist devices can be used in patients with Fontan circulation, systemic RVs, or complex anatomy but this requires careful surgical planning and a multidisciplinary approach. ACHD patients have higher mortality after ventricular assist device placement than those with acquired heart disease.[36]

Palliative Care

It is important to acknowledge each patient's desires for care, as in ACHD patients nearing end-of-life the frequency of hospitalizations, intensive care admission, and increased length of hospital stay appear greater (despite younger age) than for adults with cancer. In a retrospective study of ACHD patients who died during a hospitalization, only a minority had engaged in end-of-life discussions with their providers. Data suggests that both adults with CHD, as well as their providers, would like to participate in advanced care planning and discussion of palliative care.[37]

Aortopathies in Congenital Heart Disease

Aortic dilation is common in adults with CHD, particularly in patients with bicuspid aortic valve (BAV) and conotruncal defects.[38] BAV is prevalent in 2% of the general population. The most common complications in BAV are stenosis or regurgitation of the valve, however, ascending aortic dilation occurs in at least 50% of patients (see Chapter 42). Aortopathy is a common finding in patients with conotruncal anomalies because the arterial walls are derived from cardiac neural crest and second heart field cells, either or both of which can be abnormal in these defects. For example, marked histologic abnormalities have been documented in the aortic root and ascending aorta present from infancy in patients with TOF. Aortic dilation is common in adults with repaired TOF, with up to 25% of adults with repaired TOF having an aortic

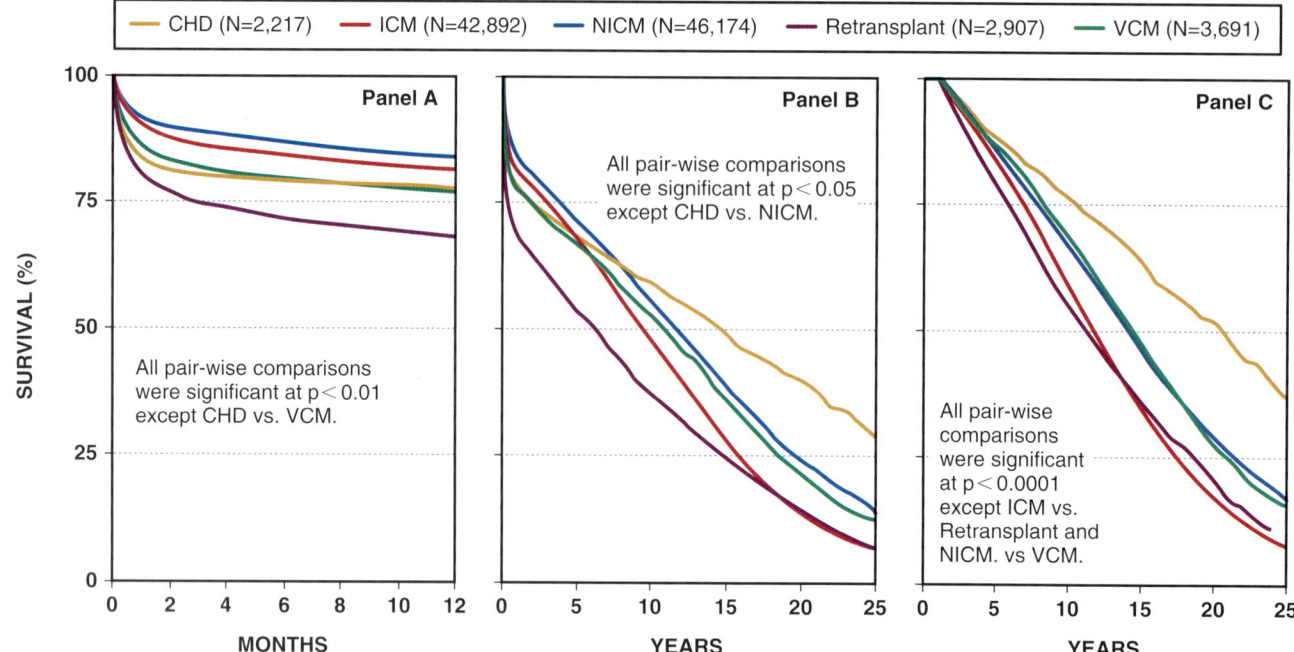

FIGURE 82.4 Kaplan-Meier curve demonstrating 1-year survival (**A**), long-term survival (**B**), and long-term survival conditional on survival to 1 year by diagnosis (**C**). January 1982–June 2014. *CHD*, Congenital heart disease; *ICM*, ischemic cardiomyopathy; *NICM*, non-ischemic cardiomyopathy; *VCM*, valvular cardiomyopathy. (From Lund LH. The Registry of the International Society for Heart and Lung Transplantation. Thirty-Third Adult Heart Transplantation Report—2016; Focus Theme: Primary Diagnostic Indications for Transplant. *J Heart Lung Transplant*. 2016;35[10]:1158–1169.)

root diameter larger than 4 cm; however, only 6.6% have *indexed* aortic values above the expected limits. Similarly, 50% of children with D-loop TGA have aortic root dilation 10 years after arterial switch operation; however, this dilation does not appear to be progressive. Despite the high prevalence of dilated ascending aorta in patients with conotruncal anomalies aortic dissection is exceedingly rare.

In following CHD patients serially over time, one must recognize that aortic measurements will vary depending on the specific imaging modality and measurement technique. Echocardiography labs may have various imaging protocols for aortic measurements that must be considered when comparing serial studies. The current multimodality imaging guidelines for the thoracic aorta in adults advocate obtaining aortic root measurements at end-diastole with a leading edge–to–leading edge technique, whereas imaging guidelines for pediatric echocardiograms, which are often used in echocardiography labs specializing in CHD, suggest obtaining aortic root measurements in mid-systole with an inner edge–to–inner edge technique.[39]

Subacute Bacterial Endocarditis

Patients with ACHD have an increased risk of developing subacute bacterial endocarditis (SBE), and this is associated with significant morbidity and mortality (see Chapter 80).[40] The most common pathogens responsible for SBE include *Streptococcus viridans*, *Staphylococcus* species, and *Enterococcus* species. Antibiotic prophylaxis is recommended prior to dental procedures for ACHD patients with high-risk characteristics, which include: (1) prior episodes of SBE, (2) prosthetic valves (including transcatheter), (3) valve repair using a prosthetic ring, (4) residual intracardiac shunts adjacent to prosthetic material, (5) cyanotic CHD, (6) any CHD repaired with prosthetic material up to 6 months after the procedure or lifelong if residual shunt or valvular regurgitation remains, and (7) for cardiac transplant recipients who develop cardiac valvulopathy. In a registry of over 14,000 ACHD patients, the incidence of SBE was 1.33 cases per 1000-person years. Valve-containing prosthetics were found to be an important independent risk factor for SBE, both short and long term after implantation, whereas non-valve-containing prosthetics (including valve repair) are associated with greater risk only in the short term (<6 months) after implantation (Fig. 82.5).[41] ACHD patients should be educated about symptoms of SBE and the importance of good oral hygiene and of obtaining blood cultures before starting antibiotic treatment in situations with concerning features for infection.

Pregnancy in Women With Congenital Heart Disease (see Chapter 92)

Profound hemodynamic changes occur during pregnancy, which are usually well tolerated by women with structurally normal hearts; however, these changes may not be tolerated as well in women with underlying CHD. Despite the fact that most women do not have cardiac complications during pregnancy, cardiovascular disease is the leading cause of indirect maternal mortality. All women with CHD should receive preconception counseling to determine maternal cardiac, obstetrical, and fetal risks, and potential long-term risks to the mother. Additionally, an individualized plan of care that addresses expectations and contingencies should be developed for and with women with CHD who are pregnant or who may become pregnant and shared with the patient and all caregivers (AHA/ACC Class I recommendation, level of evidence C-LD).

Men and women of childbearing age with CHD should be counseled on the risk of CHD recurrence in offspring and fetal echocardiography offered if either parent has CHD.

Several risk stratification scores have been developed for maternal cardiac conditions. The CARPREG 2 investigators reported the maternal outcomes of 1938 pregnancies in women with cardiac disease (63% CHD), and 16% of women experienced an adverse cardiac outcome, primarily heart failure and arrhythmias. The highest-weighted risk factors (weight of three points) include a prior history of cardiac events or arrhythmias, decreased functional status (New York Heart Association, NYHA, Class ≥III), and presence of a mechanical heart valve. Risk factors that account for two points include: ventricular dysfunction, high-risk left-sided valve disease/LVOT obstruction, PH, coronary artery disease, and high-risk aortopathy. One point was assigned for late pregnancy assessment or no prior cardiac intervention. The predicted risks for cardiac events stratified according to point score were ≤1 point (5%), 2 points (10%), 3 points (15%), 4 points (22%), and >4 points (41%).[42]

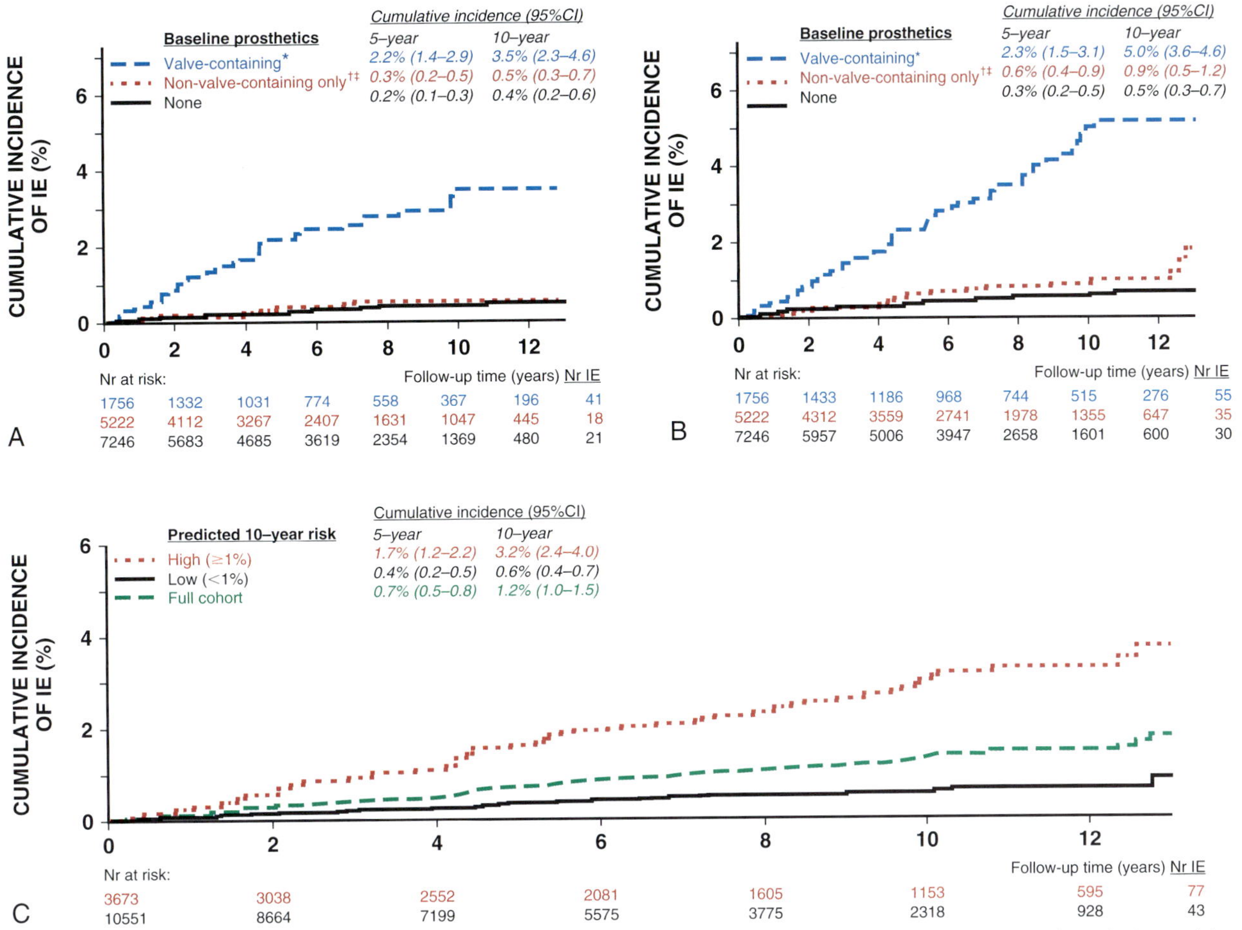

FIGURE 82.5 Cumulative incidence of infectious endocarditis (IE) in adults with congenital heart disease during follow-up by presence of prosthetic material at baseline (**A** and **B**) and predicted risk category (**C**). (From Kuijpers JM, Koolbergen DR, Groenink M, et al. Incidence, risk factors, and predictors of infective endocarditis in adult congenital heart disease: focus on the use of prosthetic material. *Eur Heart J.* 2017;38:2048–2056.)

The European Society of Cardiology published an extensive set of guidelines for management of cardiovascular diseases during pregnancy which includes the modified WHO risk classification, listed in Table 82.7. The recommended follow-up for women with WHO risk category II is every trimester; women with WHO risk category ≥III should be seen monthly or bimonthly.[43] Women with a high risk of maternal morbidity or mortality, including women with pulmonary arterial hypertension (PAH), Eisenmenger syndrome, severe systemic ventricular dysfunction, severe left-sided obstructive lesions, or in physiological stage D should be counselled against pregnancy and consider termination if they become pregnant.[44]

Exercise and Sports Participation (see Chapter 32)
Benefits of Physical Exercise
Virtually all patients with CHD should be encouraged to be physically active, exercise, and maintain physical fitness. Physical activity promotes cardiovascular and mental health; people who exercise regularly have an improved quality of life, better exercise capacity, and are less likely to suffer from obesity or type 2 diabetes. Even patients with complex CHD, such as Fontan circulation, derive benefits from regular physical exercise.[45]

Despite the benefits of exercise, physicians, parents, or patients may have concerns about the risk of sudden death with exercise and restrict physical activity or competitive sports. The risk of sudden death during exercise is very low for adults with CHD and observational studies do not suggest that exercise restriction reduces the risk of sudden death, perhaps because the majority of sudden death in patients with CHD occurs at rest, not with exercise.[46] At least in part due to these exercise restrictions, patients with CHD have lower levels of physical activity than patients without CHD and only 30% of patients with CHD achieve the recommended levels of physical activity.[47]

Individualized Exercise Programs
Patients with CHD require individualized counseling regarding exercise recommendations or restrictions.[48] In general, patients with CHD have lower exercise capacity than patients without CHD and there is considerable heterogeneity across different diagnoses (Fig. 82.6).[49] Patients with moderate or complex anatomy or physiology may benefit from formal exercise testing to establish baseline exercise capacity and demonstrate safety of exercise. Patients with high-risk anatomy or physiology should be discouraged from participating in high-intensity sports and counseled toward lower-intensity physical activity (Table 82.8).

Low-risk patients can begin a training program at approximately 70% maximal predicted heart rate at least three times per week (totaling 150 minutes/week) and increase intensity or duration over time.

Competitive Sports
There are important differences between competitive sports and recreational exercise. In competitive sports, participants cannot reliably self-regulate effort and require high-intensity burst efforts imposed by coaches or playing conditions. For these reasons, competitive sports are thought to pose greater risk.

The AHA and ACC published a consensus statement on eligibility for participation in competitive sports in 2015.[50] Sports are graded in terms of their static and dynamic components and appropriateness for competition depends on the native anatomy and the presence of residual sequelae following repair. In many patients, pre-participation stress testing can provide useful information about the patient's exercise capacity, hemodynamics with exercise, and the presence of exercise-induced arrhythmias that can help guide decision making. Particularly

TABLE 82.7 Modified WHO Classification for Maternal Cardiac Risk

	mWHO I	mWHO II	mWHO II–III	mWHO III	mWHO IV
Diagnosis (if otherwise well and uncomplicated)	Small or mild • Pulmonary stenosis • Patent ductus arteriosus • Mitral valve prolapse • Successfully repaired simple lesions (atrial or ventricular septal defect, patent ductus arteriosus, anomalous pulmonary venous drainage) • Atrial or ventricular ectopic beats, isolated	Unoperated atrial or ventricular septal defect Repaired tetralogy of Fallot Most arrythmias (supraventricular arrhythmias) Turner syndrome without aortic dilatation	Mild left ventricular impairment (EF > 45%) Hypertrophic cardiomyopathy Native or tissue valve disease not considered WHO I or IV (mild mitral stenosis, moderate aortic stenosis) Marfan or other HTAD syndrome without aortic dilatation Aorta < 45 mm in bicuspid aortic valve pathology Repaired coarctation Atrioventricular septal defect	Moderate left ventricular impairment (EF 30%–45%) Previous peripartum cardiomyopathy without any residual left ventricular impairment Mechanical valve Systemic right ventricle with good or mildly decreased ventricular function Fontan circulation If otherwise the patient is well and the cardiac condition uncomplicated Unrepaired cyanotic heart disease Other complex heart disease Moderate mitral stenosis Severe asymptomatic aortic stenosis Moderate aortic dilatation (40–45 mm in Marfan syndrome or other HTAD; 45–50 mm in bicuspid aortic valve, Turner syndrome ASI 20–25 mm/m², tetralogy of Fallot <50 mm) Ventricular tachycardia	Pulmonary arterial hypertension Severe systemic ventricular dysfunction (EF < 30% or NYHA Class III–IV) Previous peripartum cardiomyopathy with any residual left ventricular impairment Severe mitral stenosis Severe symptomatic aortic stenosis Systemic right ventricle with moderate or severely decreased ventricular function Severe aortic dilatation (>45 mm in Marfan syndrome or other HTAD, > 50 mm in bicuspid aortic valve, Turner syndrome ASI > 25/mm/m², tetralogy of Fallot > 50 mm) Vascular Ehlers-Danlos Severe (re)coarctation Fontan with any complication
Risk	No detectable increased risk of maternal mortality and no/mild increased risk in morbidity	Small increased risk of maternal mortality or moderate increase in morbidity	Intermediate increased risk of maternal mortality or moderate to severe increase in morbidity	Significantly increased risk of maternal mortality or severe morbidity	Extremely high risk of maternal mortality or severe morbidity

Modified from Regitz-Zagrosek V, Roos-Hesselink JW, Bauersachs J, et al. 2018 ESC guidelines for the management of cardiovascular diseases during pregnancy. *Eur Heart J*. 2018;39:3165–3241.

for teenagers and adults shared decision making is often required following a detailed conversation about risks.

SPECIFIC DEFECTS

Left-to-Right Shunt Lesions

The physiology of a left-to-right shunt involves flow of pulmonary venous, or oxygenated, blood toward systemic venous, or deoxygenated, chambers or vessels. The degree of left-to-right shunting determines the amount of chamber dilation and is dictated by the size of the defect as well as the diastolic properties of the heart and the resistance in the great arteries. In general, shunt lesions proximal to the tricuspid valve (such as ASDs and anomalous pulmonary venous return) cause right heart dilation, those below the tricuspid valve (such as VSDs and PDAs) cause left heart dilation (Table 82.9). Small shunts may close spontaneously during childhood or remain small and hemodynamically insignificant. However, larger shunts that are not corrected early in life have the potential to cause elevations in PVR with reversal of the direction of flow from right-to-left leading to cyanosis and Eisenmenger syndrome (see section on Eisenmenger Syndrome).

The invasive evaluation of cardiac shunts should include the calculation of pulmonary and systemic vascular resistance (SVR). The ratio of pulmonary blood flow (Qp) to systemic blood flow (Qs) may be determined either noninvasively or by cardiac catheterization. Fig. 82.7 displays invasive hemodynamics in such a patient, with calculations of Qp/Qs and vascular resistance.

Atrial Septal Defects and Partial Anomalous Pulmonary Veins

Anatomic Description and Prevalence

There are multiple locations for interatrial communications, and a detailed understanding of the atrial septal anatomy is needed. Fig. 82.8 illustrates various locations of ASDs. The prevalence of ASD is 0.88 per 1000 adults. The most common type of ASD is a secundum ASD (Fig. 82.9), which is a true deficiency in the atrial septum, in the region of the fossa ovalis. This should be differentiated from a patent foramen ovale (PFO), which is persistence of patency of the flap valve of the fossa ovalis (not associated with right-sided cardiac dilation) and persists in up to 25% of adults. Primum ASDs may be considered in the spectrum of AVSDs (Fig. 82.10) and involve a deficiency in the region of the AV valves and are associated with a cleft in the mitral valve. Sinus venosus defects occur in the sinus venosus septum posterior to the true atrial septum and usually involve anomalous right-sided pulmonary venous return (Fig. 82.11). CS defects (also called unroofed CSs) are rare and involve direct communication of the CS and the LA due to complete or partial unroofing of the CS and are often accompanied by a persistent left-sided SVC.

Patients may also have anomalous pulmonary venous connections not associated with an ASD, known as partial anomalous pulmonary venous connection (PAPVC). PAPVC may be associated with either right- or left-sided pulmonary veins which can have several possible anomalous connections, with the most common being a left upper pulmonary vein to an ascending vertical vein into the brachiocephalic

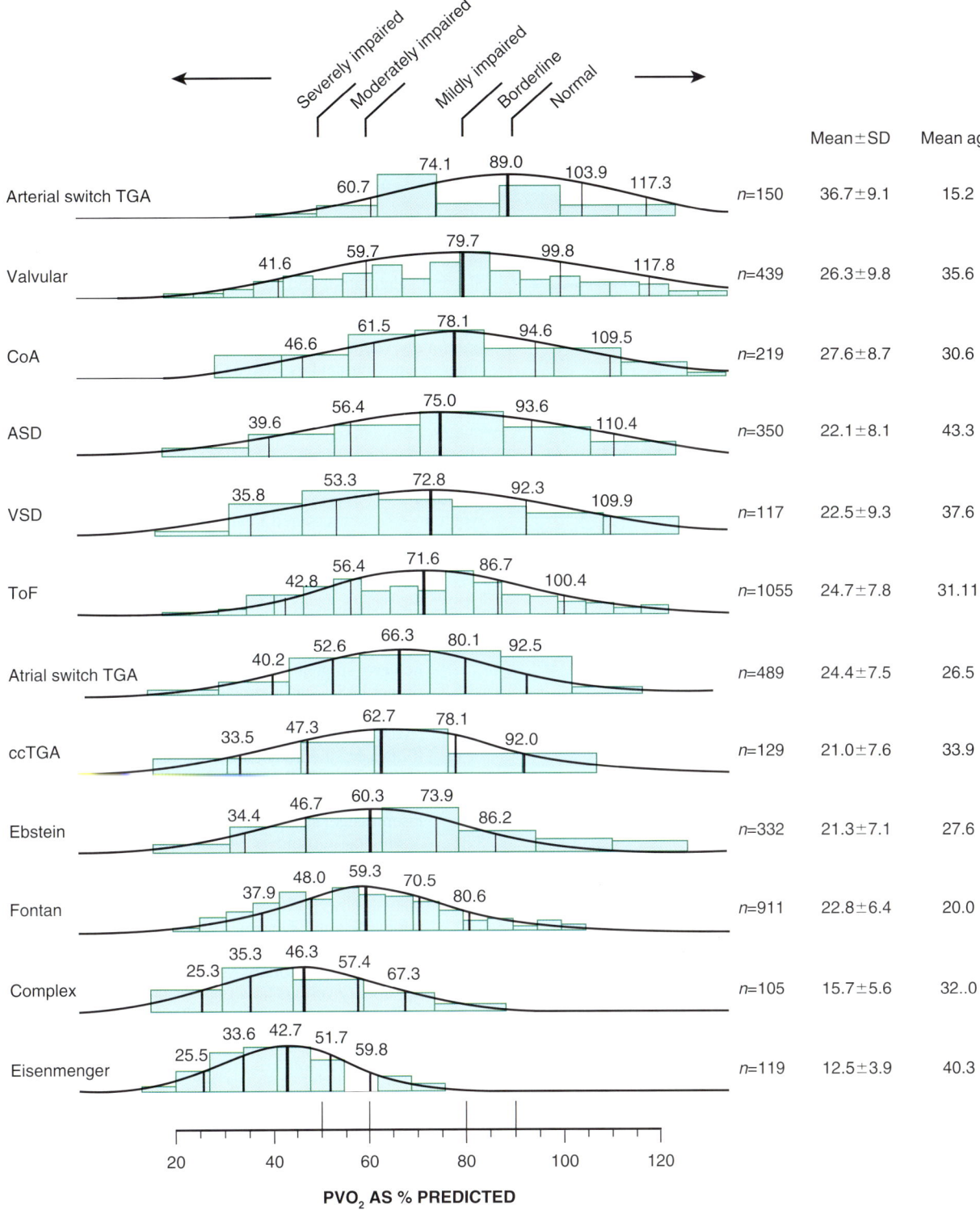

FIGURE 82.6 Range of peak oxygen consumption values in various types of adult congenital heart disease (ACHD) patients. *ASD*, Atrial septal defect; *ccTGA*, congenitally corrected transposition of the great arteries; *CoA*, coarctation of the aorta; *pVO₂*, peak oxygen consumption; *TGA*, transposition of the great arteries; *ToF*, tetralogy of Fallot; *VSD*, ventricular septal defect. (From Kempny A, Dimopoulos K, Uebing A, et al. Reference values for exercise limitations among adults with congenital heart disease. Relation to activities of daily life—single centre experience and review of published data. *Eur Heart J.* 2012;33:1386–396.)

vein or the right upper pulmonary vein draining to the SVC (Fig. 82.12). In the latter case, careful attention should be paid to ensure that there is not an associated sinus venosus defect. When the right-sided pulmonary veins connect to the inferior vena cava (IVC), this is called a scimitar vein. Isolated PAPVC involving a single pulmonary vein may cause mild degrees of right heart overload, but rarely require surgical correction.

Clinical Features

It is not uncommon for adults to have an ASD incidentally discovered at the time of imaging for unrelated issues. Symptoms, when they occur, most commonly include exercise intolerance, palpitations, or dyspnea with exertion. Supraventricular arrhythmias develop by 40 years of age in about 10% of patients and become increasingly prevalent with advancing age. The presence of cyanosis should alert one to the possibility of shunt reversal and Eisenmenger syndrome or, alternatively, to a prominent eustachian valve directing the inferior vena caval flow to the LA via a secundum ASD or sinus venosus defect of the inferior vena caval type. Pulse oximetry at rest and during exercise is recommended for evaluation of adults with unrepaired or repaired ASD with residual shunt to determine the direction and magnitude of the shunt.

The classic physical examination of an ASD is a wide, fixed splitting of the second heart sound, which is due to prolonged RV ejection and increased PA capacitance, which, in turn, delay pulmonary valve closure. Pulmonary flow murmurs are common. The ECG commonly displays a rightward QRS axis and an incomplete right bundle branch block (RBBB). The classic chest radiograph features are of cardiomegaly (from right atrial and right ventricular enlargement), and dilated central pulmonary arteries with pulmonary congestion. Cardiac imaging is essential in determining the anatomy of the atrial septum and pulmonary venous drainage. TTE is the initial imaging test, however, other imaging modalities, such as TEE, CMR, and CCT may be needed to confirm the anatomy. The 2020 Appropriate Use Criteria guidelines rate these modalities as always appropriate for the evaluation prior to planned surgical repair for sinus venous defects or for patients with a change in clinical status or new symptoms.

TABLE 82.8 Congenital Conditions* in Which High-Intensity Exercise Should be Avoided

Cyanosis
High risk coronary anomalies
Hypoxemia
Severe aortic dilation
Severe outflow tract obstruction
Severe pulmonary hypertension
Severe ventricular dysfunction
Ventricular arrhythmias

*This list does not include non–adult congenital heart disease (ACHD) high-risk lesions such as hypertrophic cardiomyopathy, channelopathies, or arrhythmogenic cardiomyopathy. See Chapters 52, 54 and 63.

TABLE 82.9 Expected Chamber Enlargement With Cardiac Shunts

SHUNT	RA	RV	PA	LA	LV	AORTA
ASD	+	+	+			
VSD		±	+	+	+	
PDA			+	+	+	+

Repairs

When an ASD is discovered in an adult, if there is any degree of right heart dilation associated with symptoms, closure should be considered.[51] It is important to verify the direction of the shunt as left-to-right.

The next step is to verify that the PVR is less than ⅓ the SVR, the PA systolic pressure is less than 50% systemic, there is right heart enlargement, and the Qp/Qs is at least 1.5:1. The majority of secundum ASDs may be closed percutaneously (Fig. 82.13), however, surgical closure is required for sinus venosus defects, primum ASDs, or CS septal defects. It is reasonable to close an ASD in an asymptomatic patient with right heart enlargement (AHA/ACC Class IIa recommendation, level of evidence C-LD). If invasive hemodynamic assessment confirms significant elevations in PVR and/or pulmonary pressure, collaboration between ACHD and PH providers is important (see section on Eisenmenger syndrome).

Surgical closure is typically performed using a patch of autologous pericardium or synthetic material with an open sternotomy and cardiopulmonary bypass. The operative mortality is low, however, postoperative complications of postpericardiotomy syndrome or atrial arrhythmias may occur. Special attention must be paid to those defects with partial anomalous pulmonary venous drainage, as redirecting the pulmonary venous flow may result in pulmonary vein stenosis. In patients with primum ASDs, care must be taken in closing the mitral valve cleft to avoid mitral stenosis or residual regurgitation.

Transcatheter closure is now widely accepted as an alternative to surgical repair for the majority of secundum ASDs. Several devices are available and range in size and configuration. Adequate rims of the defect must be demonstrated to ensure safe transcatheter closure. Post-procedural complications include atrial arrhythmias, heart block, thrombus formation on the device, and rarely device mobilization or erosion.

Long-Term Outcomes and Complications

Patients who undergo ASD repair prior to the age of 25 years have favorable outcomes. However, surgical repair does not provide proven benefit in reducing arrhythmia burden in older adults. Following closure, patients with significant residual shunt, valvular or ventricular dysfunction, arrhythmias, and/or PH should be followed at regular intervals with TTE. The imaging recommendations for patients following transcatheter ASD closure are dictated by the specific manufacturer, but in general, TTE is performed at 1 week, 1 month, and then annually for at least 5 years following closure. Any patient who has had a transcatheter ASD device placed who presents with chest pain

A. Cardiac Output

Systemic blood flow (L/min)

$$Qs = \frac{VO_2}{\frac{(13.6)(Hb)(Ao\ O^2\ sat - SVC\ O_2\ sat)}{100}}$$

Pulmonary blood flow (L/min)

$$Qp^* = \frac{VO_2}{\frac{(13.6)(Hb)(Ao\ O^2\ sat - SVC\ O_2\ sat)}{100}}$$

*Last, Qp can be inaccurate when there are multiple sources of pulmonary blood flow with differing oxygen contents and their relative contribution to flow is unknown.

B. Shunt Fraction

$$\frac{Qp}{Qs} = \frac{(Ao\ O_2\ sat - MVS\ O_2\ sat)}{(PV\ O_2\ sat - PA\ O_2\ sat)}$$

C. Vascular Resistance (mmHg/L/min)

Systemic Vascular Resistance (SVR) = $\frac{\text{Mean Aop} - \text{Mean RAp}}{Qs}$

Pulmonary Vascular Resistance (PVR) = $\frac{\text{Mean PAp} - \text{Mean LAp}}{Qp}$

FIGURE 82.7 Calculations of flow and resistance. **A,** Calculations of blood flow based on the Fick principle, oxygen consumption (VO_2) equals the delivered oxygen (cardiac output × arterial O_2 content) minus the returned oxygen (cardiac output × venous O_2 content). Rearranging this equation, the cardiac output (Qs) can be calculated. In room air, the contribution of dissolved oxygen is minimal, and left out of the equation. **B,** The shunt fraction (Qp/Qs) accounts for effective blood flow and provides the contribution of intracardiac shunts. The net shunt Qp:Qs summarizes the excess/deficit of flow across the pulmonary vascular bed relative to systemic, reflecting the totality of all unique sources of left-to-right, and right-to-left, intra- and extracardiac shunts. **C,** The vascular resistance across the systemic and pulmonary vascular beds and is calculated by the change in mean pressure divided by the flow through the circulatory bed. It is measured in Wood units (mm Hg/L/min), and is often indexed to body surface area (m²). *Ao,* Aorta; *Aop,* aortic pressure; *Hb,* hemoglobin; *LAp,* left atrial pressure; *MVS,* mixed venous saturation; O_2 sat, oxygen saturation; *PA,* pulmonary artery; *PAp,* pulmonary artery pressure; *PV,* pulmonary venous; *PVR,* pulmonary vascular resistance; *Qp,* pulmonary blood flow; *Qs,* systemic blood flow; *RAp,* right atrial pressure; *SVC,* superior vena cava; *SVR,* systemic vascular resistance; VO_2, oxygen consumption.

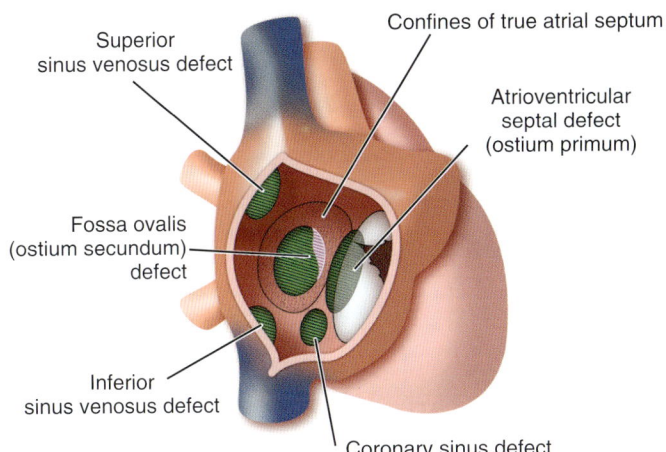

FIGURE 82.8 Various atrial level shunts. (From Webb GA, et al. Congenital heart disease in the adult and pediatric patient. In: Zipes P, et al., eds. *Braunwald's Heart Disease*. 11th ed. Philadelphia: Elsevier; 2019.)

Atrioventricular Septal Defects

Anatomic Description and Prevalence

AVSDs are a spectrum of lesions that involve deficiencies of the AV septum, often accompanied by anomalies of the AV valves. AVSDs are the result of failed fusion of the endocardial cushions, and comprise up to 5% of CHD. These include primum ASDs, partial or complete AV canal defects (Fig. 82.14). Complete AVSDs are characterized by both an atrial and ventricular level defect with a common AV valve, usually comprised of five leaflets. A partial AVSD does not have a VSD component, and almost always has a cleft in the anterior mitral valve leaflet. A unique anatomic feature in patients with AVSD is elongation of the LVOT, due to the aortic valve being displaced anteriorly. This results in a scooped-out appearance of the ventricular septum and a shortened LV inlet, creating a "goose neck" appearance (Fig. 82.15). The severity of the defect is dictated by several factors including size of the shunt, extent of AV valve abnormalities, size discrepancy of the ventricle, and presence of additional anomalies, including LVOT obstruction.

Clinical Features

The great majority of patients with AVSD undergo repair in childhood. Older patients with large AVSDs which have not been repaired early in life usually develop irreversible pulmonary vascular disease and Eisenmenger syndrome, precluding complete repair. More commonly, adults with a history of AVSD repair in childhood present with symptoms from residual left AV valve regurgitation and stenosis, LVOT obstruction, or atrial arrhythmias.

should have an urgent evaluation to rule out device erosion, which occurs in 1 in 1000 cases.

Patients with ASD and elevated PVR require closely monitored management as PAH can progress even after ASD closure.

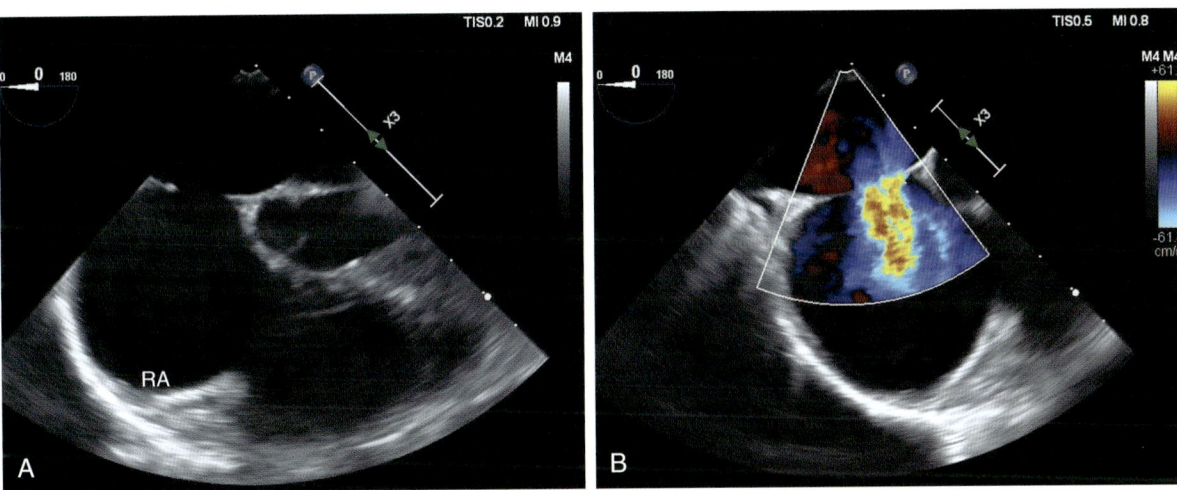

FIGURE 82.9 Transesophageal echocardiogram in the transverse plane. **A,** 2-D image of a secundum atrial septal defect (ASD). **B** Color Doppler showing flow through the ASD from the left atrium to the right atrium. *LA,* Left atrium; *RA,* right atrium.

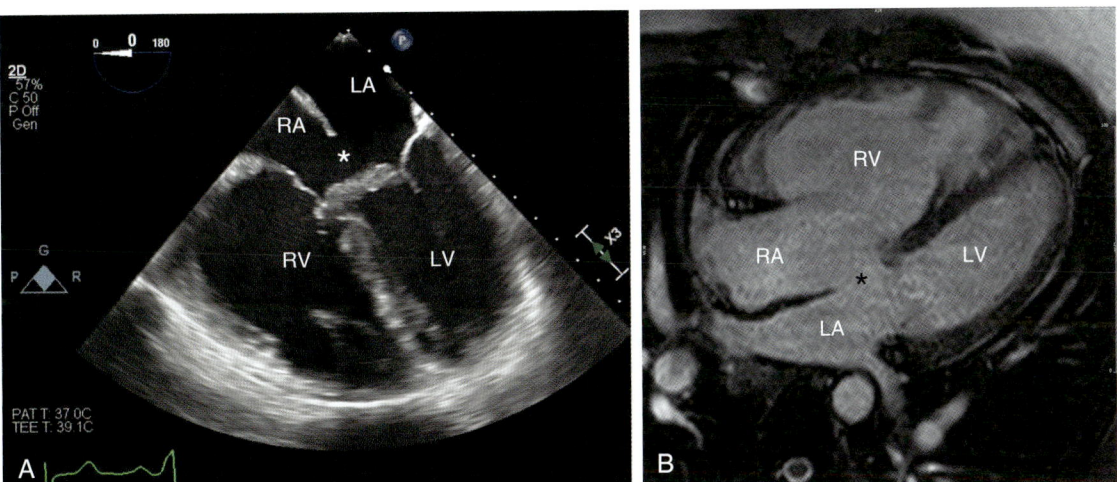

FIGURE 82.10 Ostium primum atrial septal defect shown by transesophageal echocardiogram (**A**) and cardiac magnetic resonance imaging (**B**). *LA,* Left atrium; *LV,* left ventricular; *RA,* right atrium; *RV,* right ventricle; *asterisk,* atrial septal defect.

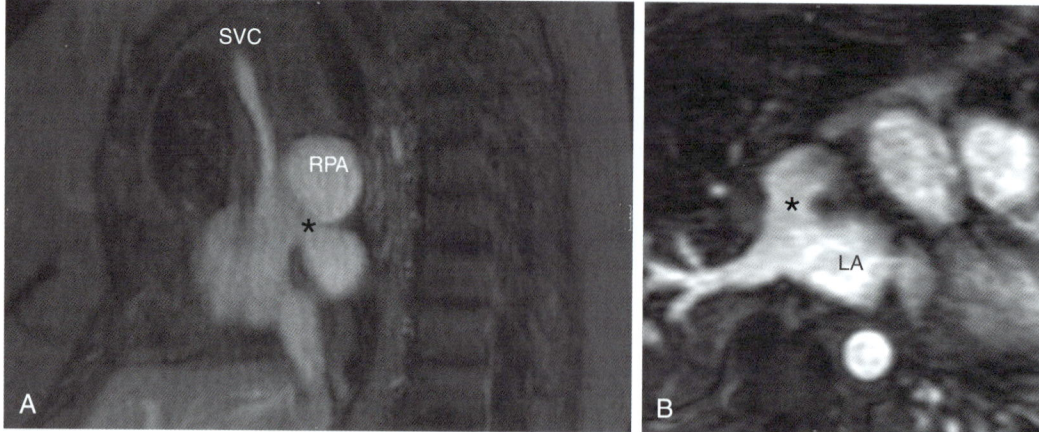

FIGURE 82.11 Gadolinium-enhanced 3-D MR angiogram of a superior-type sinus venosus defect **(A)**, sagittal oblique projection showing the superior vena cava (SVC) in its length and the defect superior to the true atrial septum *(asterisk)*. Note the dilated right pulmonary artery (RPA) in this patient with pulmonary hypertension and longstanding pulmonary overcirculation. **B**, Axial oblique image demonstrating the distal SVC with the defect at its posterior margin *(asterisk)* and communication with the left atrium (LA).

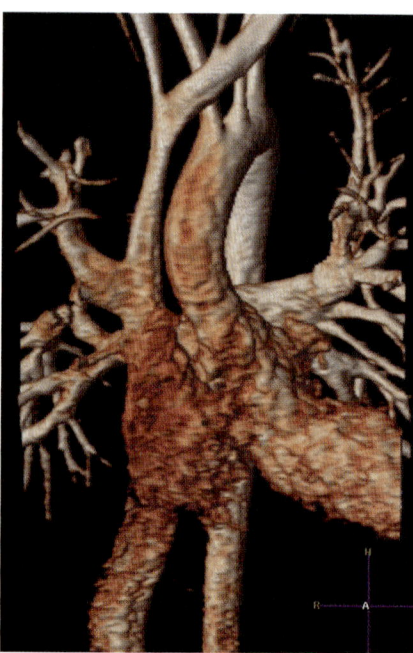

FIGURE 82.12 3-D reconstruction of gadolinium-enhanced MR angiogram in coronal view showing partial anomalous pulmonary venous connection of the right upper pulmonary vein to the superior vena cava.

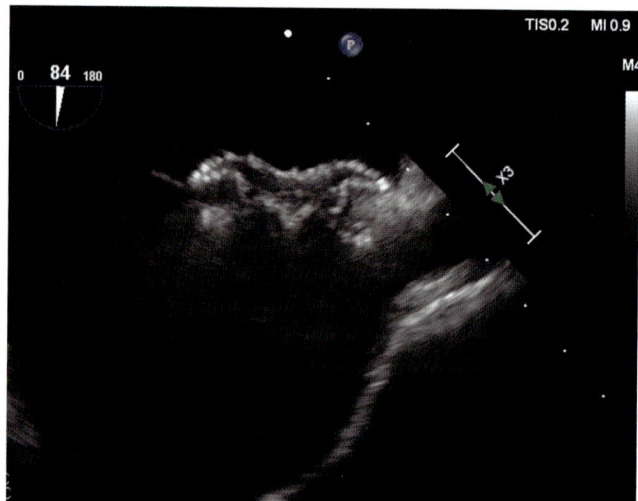

FIGURE 82.13 Transesophageal echo image in the near-vertical plane showing an Amplatzer septal occluder device positioned in a secundum ASD. The SVC is to the right of the image. *SVC*, Superior vena cava.

Surgical Repairs
Indications for surgical intervention of AVSD in adults are similar to those for ASD closure. These include a net left-to-right shunt (Qp:Qs ≥1.5:1), PA systolic pressure less than 50% systemic, and PVR less than one third systemic. Pre-operative cardiac catheterization may be required to assess for PH. For adults with prior repair, left AV valve regurgitation is the most common reason for later surgical reintervention.

Long-Term Outcomes and Complications
Survival after AVSD defects repair is good, yet reoperation for left AV valve disease and LVOT obstruction remains significant.[52] Other late complications include patch dehiscence or residual septal defects and development of complete heart block. Those adults with repaired AVSD and any degree of PH must be followed closely.

Ventricular Septal Defects
Anatomic Description and Prevalence
VSDs are the most common form of CHD, and the reported incidence of isolated VSDs varies widely, from 1.5 to 53 per 1000 live births. There are several classification schemes used to describe VSDs (Table 82.10). Fig. 82.16 demonstrates the locations of VSDs.

Clinical Features
Many isolated muscular and perimembranous VSDs are small and close spontaneously in childhood. However, there are several clinical presentations of VSDs in adults (Fig. 82.17). Patients living with small, restrictive VSDs are usually asymptomatic with a harsh holosystolic murmur on exam. Continuous wave Doppler through these defects reveals a high velocity, often greater than 5 msec, which confirms the pressure-restrictive physiology. In this case, the left-to-right shunt is minimal, and there is usually not left ventricular dilation. Other adults may present with prior VSD surgical repair in childhood, some of whom have residual patch margin leaks. A small number of adults will present with moderate- or large-size VSDs which have not undergone closure. These patients must be assessed for elevated PVR and the presence of Eisenmenger syndrome.

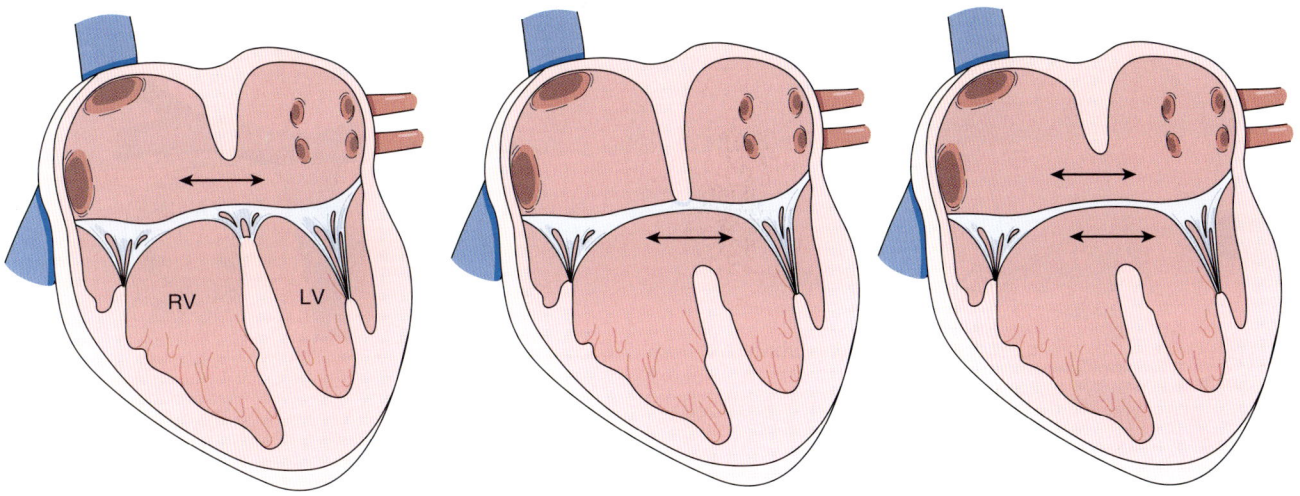

FIGURE 82.14 Various types of atrioventriucular canal (AVC) defects. The right diagram illustrates an exclusively atrial level communication, with the common atrioventricular (AV) valve densely attached to the ventricular septum. The type of AVC is termed a *primum atrial septal defect (ASD)*. The middle diagram has an exclusively ventricular communication. The common AV valve is fused with the inferior limbic band of septum secundum, and thus there is no primum ASD. The left diagram has both atrial and ventricular defects and is termed *complete common AVC defect*. *LV*, Left ventricle; *RV*, right ventricle. (Modified from Libby P. *Essential Atlas of Cardiovascular Disease*. New York: Springer; 2009.)

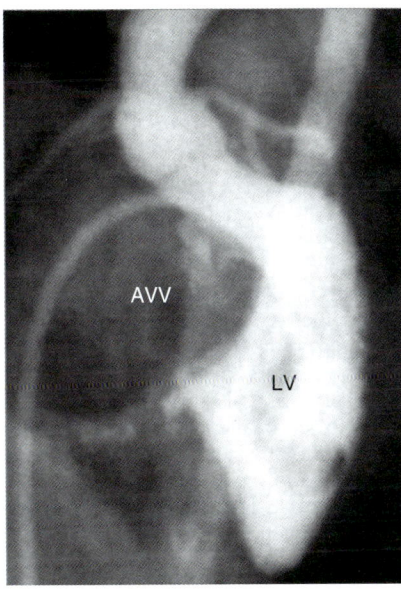

FIGURE 82.15 Angiogram of the left ventricular outflow tract demonstrating the classic "gooseneck" deformity in a patient with a primum atrial septal defect. This appearance is the result of the inlet dimension of the left ventricle being shorter than the outlet dimension. *AVV*, Atrioventricular valve; *LV*, left ventricle. (Modified from Libby P. *Essential Atlas of Cardiovascular Disease*. New York: Springer; 2009.)

TABLE 82.10 Ventricular Septal Defect Nomenclature

CHS	VAN PRAAGH	ANDERSON	OTHER
Perimembranous	Conoventricular*	Perimembranous outlet	Subaortic
Subarterial	Conal septal		Supracristal
Inlet	Atrioventricular canal	Juxta-arterial	Inlet
Muscular		Perimembranous	
	Muscular	Muscular	

*Not all conoventricular defects are in the perimembranous septum.

Patent Ductus Arteriosus

Anatomic Description and Prevalence
The ductus arteriosus, derived from the distal left sixth primitive arch, connects the PA to the descending aorta in fetal life and normally closes within the first day of life. It may remain patent, particularly in premature infants. A PDA is found in about 0.3% to 0.8% of term infants.

Clinical Features
A PDA can range from a small hemodynamically insignificant lesion that is not heard on auscultation to one that is large enough to cause congestive heart failure and PH and Eisenmenger syndrome. Measurement of oxygen saturation should be performed in feet and both hands in adults with a PDA to assess for the presence of right-to-left shunting, as cyanosis is caused by right-to-left shunting in PDA predominantly downstream from the ductal insertion into the aorta. Adults with a hemodynamically significant PDA typically have a wide pulse pressure. On auscultation, a classic murmur is heard best just below the left clavicle and typically extends from systole past the second heart sound into diastole and peripheral pulses may be bounding.

Repairs
PDA closure in adults is recommended if left atrial or LV enlargement is present and attributable to PDA with net left-to-right shunt, PA systolic pressure is less than 50% systemic, and PVR less than one third systemic. Closure is usually feasible by transcatheter techniques.

Long-Term Outcomes and Complications
Patients with device occlusion or after surgical closure should be examined periodically for possible recanalization. Those patients with post-procedural left pulmonary artery (LPA) or aortic obstruction should be imaged at regular intervals. Endocarditis prophylaxis is recommended for 6 months following PDA device closure for life if any residual defect persists following device closure. Patients with a silent or small PDA do not require endocarditis prophylaxis.

Repairs
Adults with a VSD and evidence of left ventricular volume overload and hemodynamically significant shunts (Qp:Qs ≥ 1.5:1) should undergo VSD closure if PA systolic pressure is less than 50% systemic and PVR is less than one third systemic (AHA/ACC Class I recommendation, level of evidence B-NR). It is reasonable to close conal septal VSDs in the presence of significant aortic regurgitation. The gold standard for VSD closure remains surgical direct suture closure or patch. However, transcatheter device occlusion of selected muscular and perimembranous defects is possible with favorable outcomes.[53]

Long-Term Outcomes and Complications
The prognosis for adults with surgically closed VSDs is generally favorable. However, studies have demonstrated these patients may have impaired ventricular contractility, compromised ventilatory response, reduced cardiac output during exercise, and lower functional capacity.[54]

Long-term surveillance is recommended for adults with prior VSD closure and any valvular dysfunction, ventricular dysfunction, arrhythmias, or PH.

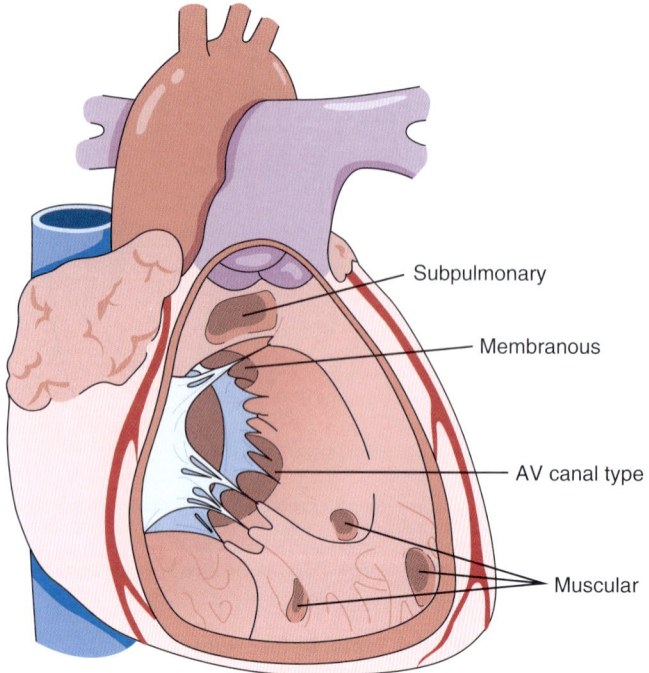

FIGURE 82.16 Diagram showing the interventricular septum from the right ventricular side. The locations of specific types of ventricular septal defects are labeled. (Modified from Libby P. *Essential Atlas of Cardiovascular Disease*. New York: Springer: 2009.)

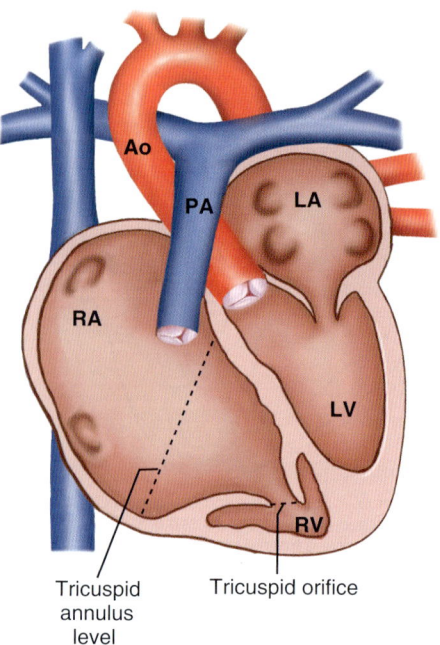

FIGURE 82.18 Diagram of Ebstein anomaly. *Ao*, Aorta; *LA*, left atrium; *LV*, left ventricle; *PA*, pulmonary artery; *RA*, right ventricle; *RV*, right ventricle. (From Mullins CE, Mayer DC. *Congenital Heart Disease: A Diagrammatic Atlas*. New York: Wiley-Liss; 1988.)

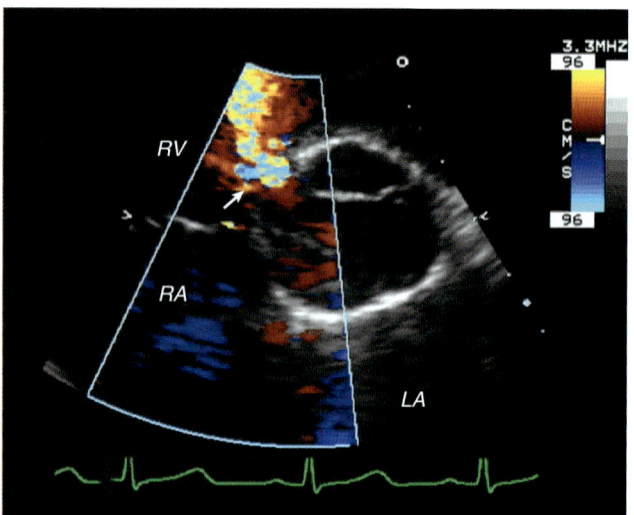

FIGURE 82.17 Parasternal short-axis echocardiogram view of a small membranous ventricular septal defect (VSD; *arrow*) with left-to-right flow by color Doppler. *LA*, Left atrium; *RA*, right atrium; *RV*, right ventricle. (Modified from Libby P. *Essential Atlas of Cardiovascular Disease*. New York: Springer; 2009.)

Ebstein Anomaly of the Tricuspid Valve
Anatomic Description and Prevalence
Ebstein anomaly is characterized by apical displacement of the septal tricuspid valve leaflets from the AV junction into the RV resulting from failure of delamination of the tricuspid valve leaflets from the underlying RV endocardium during cardiac development (Fig. 82.18). A distance between insertion sites of the two AV valves greater than 8 mm/m^2 is required for the diagnosis of Ebstein malformation of the tricuspid valve, or a maximum displacement of more than 20 mm in an adult. The inferior and occasionally the anterior leaflet may also be displaced and rotated. In severe cases the displacement is associated also with rotation toward the right ventricular outflow tract (RVOT) and pulmonary valve. The anterior leaflet is elongated, may be fenestrated, and is frequently partly redundant appearing "sail-like." The leaflets may be dysplastic or tethered altering surgical options. There is dilatation of the right AV junction. The RV is frequently referred to as having two parts, a basal "atrialized" RV component with its proximal limit the AV groove and the "functional RV." The RV is myopathic and beneath the atrialized portion may be very thin. Associated anomalies include PFO/ASD, accessory pathways including Mahaim-type pathways, pulmonary stenosis, VSD, PDA, mitral valve disease, BAV, subaortic stenosis, and coarctation of the aorta. Patients that present neonatally may have pulmonary atresia, pulmonary stenosis, or subpulmonary stenosis but this is seen in < 10% of those who present in adulthood. Ebstein-like anomaly of the tricuspid valve is a common association in L-loop TGA. Left ventricular noncompaction, in addition to RV myocardial disease, may be present.

Ebstein anomaly is rare. The incidence of Ebstein malformation of the tricuspid valve is 1 per 200,000 live births.

Clinical Features and Diagnostic Testing
Clinical manifestations of Ebstein anomaly are highly variable as may be expected given the high variation in the severity of the structural and functional abnormality of the tricuspid valve and the spectrum of associated abnormalities. Ebstein anomaly may be lethal in utero or present with cyanosis and cardiomegaly in children. But older adults may remain asymptomatic even with severe tricuspid regurgitation, may have been followed up medically without intervention or after previous tricuspid valve repair or replacement.

Patients are typically followed lifelong on a yearly basis or less frequently depending on their clinical status. Those with impaired RV function, cyanosis, cardiomegaly, recurrent atrial arrhythmia, and with severe tricuspid regurgitation after tricuspid valve repair, or with already dysfunctional tricuspid valve bioprosthetic or mechanical valves require closer follow-up.

Adult presentation may be with severe tricuspid regurgitation with RV dysfunction, arrhythmia, exercise intolerance, fatigue, or paradoxical embolism or cyanosis. A normal jugular venous pressure is usual at physical examination even with significant tricuspid regurgitation because of the large and compliant RA and atrialized RV.

The 12-lead ECG is frequently abnormal due to arrhythmias, conduction defects, or enlarged right heart chambers. Features to look for include low voltage QRS, peaked tall P waves (>2.5 mm) in leads II and VI due to right atrial enlargement or "Himalayan" p waves (>5 mm height), prolonged PR interval, or importantly a short PR interval and delta wave reflective of pre-excitation from an accessory pathway. Complete or incomplete RBBB is common in adults. An RSR pattern consistent with right ventricular conduction delay is typically seen in lead V1. Atrial flutter or fibrillation are common. The chest radiograph may show cardiomegaly, decreased pulmonary vascular markings, a small aorta and pulmonary trunk shadow, and may classically be described as showing a "boxed shaped" heart. Echocardiography (Fig. 82.19) must characterize the valve leaflets and subvalvar apparatus, the presence and flow direction in any PFO or ASD, and quantify tricuspid regurgitation. At TEE the tricuspid valve anterior leaflet and its distal tethering points are quite far from the probe and the combination of TTE and TEE or CMR may be necessary to fully evaluate valve morphology, function, and suitability for different surgical approaches. CMR is used to assess the degree of displacement and rotation of the tricuspid valve, quantify tricuspid regurgitation, RV volumes and RV systolic function, LV volumes which may be small, cardiac output which may be low, and Qp:Qs for measurement of cardiac shunt. CMR-derived RV and LV systolic dysfunction are associated with mortality and sustained VT.[35] Reduced or deteriorating exercise tolerance seen on cardiopulmonary exercise testing may prompt repair.

Long-term Outcomes and Complications
Unrepaired Ebstein Anomaly
Natural history outcomes for 72 adults with unoperated Ebstein anomaly demonstrated decreased survival due to biventricular failure or sudden death which were predicted by younger age at diagnosis, male gender, increased cardiothoracic ratio ≥0.65, and severity of valve displacement.[56] In a similar sized cohort major adverse cardiovascular events in adults with Ebstein anomaly were preceded by atrial tachycardia in the vast majority, which itself was often preceded by RV dilation and systolic dysfunction, and more anatomically severe Ebstein anomaly. LV or RV systolic dysfunction predicts adverse events. Atrial arrhythmia increases in prevalence with age. Atrioventricular reentrant tachycardia (AVRT) is the most common. In patients with symptomatic arrhythmias, or pre-excitation on the ECG, electrophysiologic testing followed by ablation is recommended. It is preferable to treat arrhythmia with ablation before surgery as following tricuspid valve surgery access to right-sided accessory pathways and the slow pathway in AV node re-entry tachycardia may be hindered.[5] Multiple accessory pathways in conjunction with atrial tachycardia and atrial fibrillation are associated with sudden death. Identification of Ebstein patients at high risk for late life-threatening arrhythmias requires improvement.

Tricuspid Valve Repair and Replacement Surgery
The goal of surgery is to increase pulmonary blood flow, minimize tricuspid regurgitation, eliminate interatrial shunting, and improve RV function. Surgery is recommended for symptoms, heart failure attributed to tricuspid valve disease, exercise intolerance demonstrated by exercise testing, or progressive systolic dysfunction. It may also be considered for progressive RV enlargement, desaturation from right to left shunt, paroxysmal embolism, or atrial tachyarrhythmia. Timing of surgery is challenging especially for patients who are minimally symptomatic.

Tricuspid valve repair is preferred when feasible. The RV is usually plicated, shunts are closed, and adjunctive ablation may be performed. A large mobile anterior leaflet with a free leading edge and sufficient septal leaflet tissue is favorable for repair. The degree to which the inferior posterior chordae are shortened and tethered, of leaflet adherence, and rotation of the leaflets into the RVOT are determinants of whether the valve can be repaired or whether it must be replaced. Repair should be performed by a congenital surgeon with specific experience in Ebstein surgery.

There are many different types of valve repair described for Ebstein anomaly.

Tricuspid valve repair with the cone reconstruction was first proposed in 2004 and involves delamination of the anterior tricuspid valve leaflet from the RV endocardium, detaching and rotating it to bring the redundant leaflets to the level of the true tricuspid annulus to form a cone-shaped valve and longitudinal plication of the atrialized RV to restore RV geometry and function. A bidirectional Glenn procedure may be added as part of a "one and a half ventricle repair" when the RV is judged incapable to support the pulmonary circulation due to small size or poor function. Bidirectional Glenn may improve the chances of successful tricuspid valve repair by decreasing RV preload and increasing LV preload. In adults the creation of a Glenn shunt reduces the volume returning to the right heart by about one third. Reintervention may be required for recurrent tricuspid regurgitation post repair or failure of prosthetic tricuspid valves.

Transcatheter Atrial Septal Defect/Patent Foramen Ovale Closure
Device closure of ASD/PFO should be considered for paradoxical embolism but requires careful evaluation before intervention to exclude induction of RA pressure increase or fall in cardiac output. Intervention for cyanosis is considered in highly selected cases as it

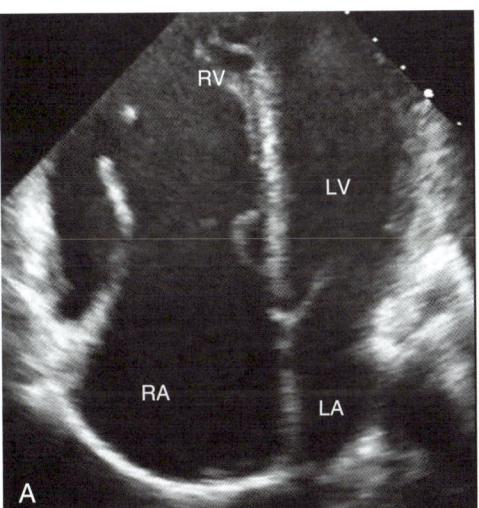
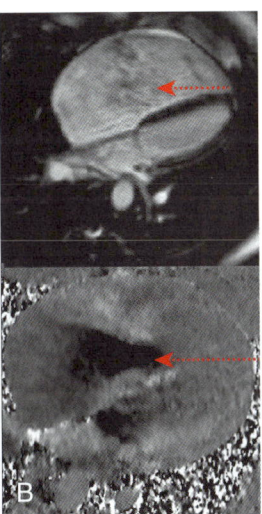
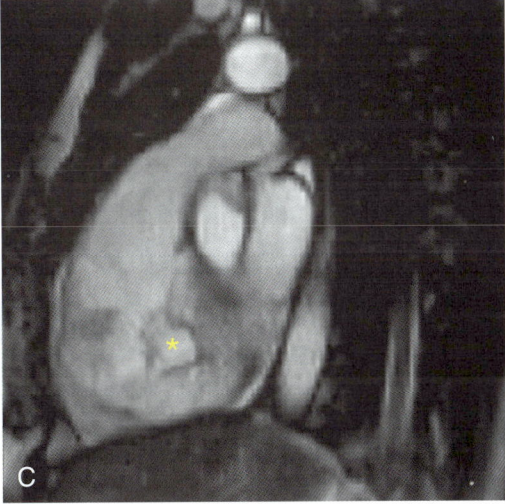

FIGURE 82.19 Ebstein malformation of the tricuspid valve. Four-chamber transthoracic echo showing mild apical displacement of the septal leaflet of the tricuspid valve compared to the origin of the mitral valve, with tricuspid annular dilatation and failure of coaptation of the tricuspid valve leaflets. The severe TR jet (*arrow*) is also seen on the four-chamber cardiac magnetic resonance cine (**B,** *top*) and by inplane velocity mapping (**B,** *bottom*). The valve leaflets are rotated toward the RV outflow tract (**C**) with an obvious coaptation gap (*asterisk*). *LA,* Left atrium; *LV,* left ventricle; *RA,* right atrium; *RV,* right ventricle.

can result in further increase in right heart pressures and decrease in systemic cardiac output.

Ventricular Dysfunction, Heart Failure, and Transplantation
It is easy to overestimate RV contractility in Ebstein anomaly as systolic ejection of stroke volume is also to the low-pressure RA. When the left ventricle is underfilled or compressed it may be unable to generate a normal cardiac output despite preserved contractility. Cardiac transplantation is considered for patients with severe LV or severe biventricular dysfunction.

Pulmonary Stenosis
Anatomic Description and Prevalence
Isolated valvular pulmonary stenosis is one of the more common forms of CHD. The valve is typically formed abnormally; it may be bicuspid or monocuspid and may include dysplastic leaflets, incomplete opening of the commissures and systolic doming, or some combination of these. The severity of the lesion is defined by the echocardiography estimated peak instantaneous gradient, with mild stenosis less than or equal to 36 mm Hg (3 msec), moderate as 36 to 64 mm Hg (3 to 4 msec), and severe as greater than 64 mm Hg (4 msec). Severe pulmonary stenosis will typically be intervened upon during childhood. Mild and sometimes moderate disease may present in adulthood without prior intervention. The adult presenting with congenital valvular pulmonary stenosis may have some combination of pulmonary stenosis, pulmonary regurgitation, or both, depending on their original lesion and whether they underwent intervention during childhood.

Pulmonary valve disease can be seen in association with several genetic and chromosomal lesions. These can include Noonan syndrome or Williams syndrome.[57] While this lesion can be seen in association with some chromosomal non-disjunction syndromes, it would be quite rare for a patient with trisomy 13 or 18 to survive to adulthood.

Clinical Features and Diagnostic Testing
Patients are often asymptomatic. However, longstanding pulmonary stenosis will often lead to a hypertrophied and stiff RV, which may present with progressive exercise intolerance or signs and symptoms of heart failure. If there is an associated PFO or ASD, the noncompliant RV can lead to right-to-left shunting at the atrial level and cyanosis, particularly with exercise. Physical findings reflect pulmonary valve and RV disease. Cardiovascular exam will include a crescendo-decrescendo systolic ejection murmur of variable intensity and often a systolic ejection click. This click becomes softer with inspiration. The non-compliant RV will lead to a lift on palpation and a prominent jugular a wave. Hepatomegaly is uncommon except with advanced disease. Patients with significant pulmonary regurgitation will have a low-pitched diastolic decrescendo murmur, which can become higher pitched in the presence of PH. Mixed disease leads to a "to-and-fro" murmur of pulmonary stenosis and regurgitation.

Echocardiography is the mainstay of diagnosis for pulmonary stenosis (Fig. 82.20). In patients with moderate stenosis or greater, TTE is appropriate to perform yearly.[3] Echo can assess for severity of stenosis and regurgitation, as well as for qualitative change in RV size and function. Signs of increased RV filling pressure include RA dilation, IVC dilation, and increased A wave reversal in the hepatic veins. End diastolic forward flow in the PA suggests impaired RV compliance.

CMR can quantify RV size and function. CMR is particularly useful for patients who have had intervention and developed pulmonary regurgitation as RV function and pulmonary regurgitation can both be assessed. Compared to patients with repaired TOF and severe pulmonary regurgitation, this patient population may have equal RV dilation but typically have more preserved RV systolic function.[58]

Cardiopulmonary exercise testing is recommended every 2 years for moderate valve disease. Serial decline in exercise capacity may prompt intervention.

Surgical Repairs
Repair of valvular pulmonary stenosis can be performed by transcatheter balloon valvuloplasty or with open surgical techniques. Balloon pulmonary valvuloplasty is usually preferred in the contemporary era, but many adults had surgical valvotomy in childhood. Less frequent is the Brock procedure, a blind surgical valvotomy performed through the infundibulum, which has fallen out of use. The result of any of these procedures is often pulmonary regurgitation; complete relief of stenosis is often accompanied by moderate or greater regurgitation, and some patients have no residual valve function whatsoever.

Long-Term Outcomes and Complications
Overall outcomes of valvar pulmonary stenosis as well as pulmonary regurgitation as a result of valve intervention are quite good. Patients with mild pulmonary stenosis rarely progress or require intervention. More significant valve dysfunction can lead to impairment of RV systolic and diastolic function, with complications related to the RV disease.

Indications for Intervention or Re-Intervention
The indications for primary intervention on pulmonary stenosis are straightforward. The 2018 ACC/AHA guidelines for the management of the adult with congenital heart disease recommend intervention as a class I indication for moderate or severe valvar pulmonary stenosis in the presence of symptoms including heart failure, exercise intolerance, or cyanosis. Primary intervention by balloon valvuloplasty is recommended, with surgical repair recommended for patients who have a contraindication to or have failed the transcatheter intervention. For asymptomatic patients with severe valvar pulmonary stenosis, intervention is considered reasonable, as a class IIa indication.

The indications for pulmonary valve replacement in the patient with mixed pulmonary stenosis and regurgitation are less clear. Pulmonary

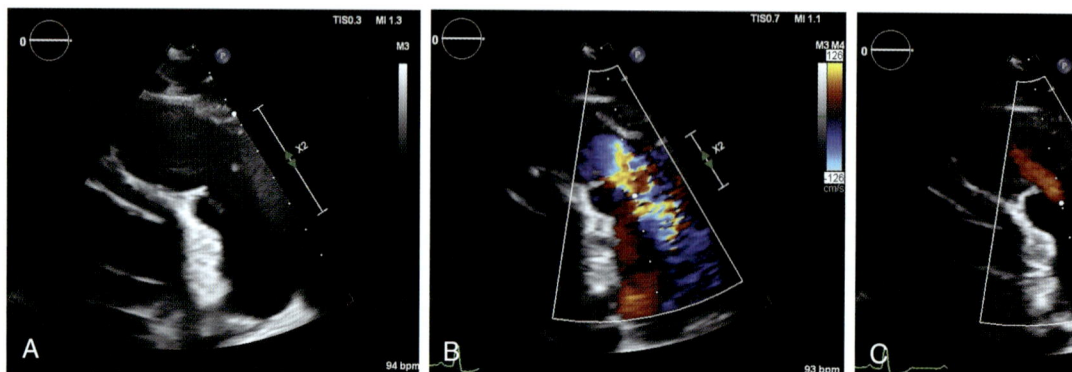

FIGURE 82.20 Transthoracic echocardiogram in the parasternal long axis view. **A**, 2-D image of the right ventricular outflow tract with the pulmonary valve open in systole. Note the thickened and mildly doming valve leaflet and dilated main pulmonary artery. **B**, Color Doppler image of antegrade flow through the stenotic pulmonary valve with turbulent and aliased flow. **C**, Color Doppler image in diastole of a narrow regurgitant jet through the pulmonary valve.

valve replacement is indicated for the patient with at least moderate regurgitation, RV dilation, and the presence of symptoms that can be attributed to the heart disease. In the absence of symptoms, there are not clear indications for valve replacement. Intervention may be reasonable in the patient with progressive changes in RV dilation or dysfunction, or with decreasing exercise capacity. Thresholds for intervention in TOF should not necessarily be extrapolated to patients with pulmonary stenosis.

Tetralogy of Fallot
Anatomic Description and Prevalence
TOF is the most common cyanotic congenital heart defect, comprising a "tetrad" of overriding aorta, VSD, pulmonary stenosis, and right ventricular hypertrophy (Fig. 82.21). Anterocephalad deviation of the outlet septum together with hypertrophy of the septoparietal trabeculations causes subpulmonary stenosis. The pulmonary valve, main and branch pulmonary arteries may also be narrow. Hypoplasia of the pulmonary arteries has been reported to be as frequent as 50%. Associated anomalies include right aortic arch, present in about 25% of patients, and anomalous course of the coronary arteries, the most common with a left anterior descending artery that originates from the right coronary artery and crosses the RVOT. This may be of surgical importance, sometimes necessitating the use of a RV-to-PA conduit. An ASD, a second muscular inlet VSD, or an AVSD—usually in the setting of Down syndrome—can coexist with TOF.

There are important anatomic variations of TOF. TOF with pulmonary atresia with major aortopulmonary collateral arteries (MAPCAs) is an extreme form of TOF present in approximately 15% of all cases. There is absence of any direct connection between the heart and the pulmonary arterial tree, a large VSD and two ventricles. Prior to repair blood reaches the pulmonary bed through the PDA and or MAPCAs. Repair is via unifocalization of MAPCAs, closure of the VSD, and RVOT reconstruction with a conduit.

Another anatomic variant is TOF with absent pulmonary valve, in which there is marked stenosis of the pulmonary valve annulus with poorly formed or absent valve leaflets and severely dilated or aneurysmal pulmonary arteries which may produce airway compression at birth.

Patients with repaired TOF constitute one of the largest groups of ACHD patients surviving into adulthood. Life expectancy depends on the precise underlying anatomy and nature and timing of previous interventions and is excellent for those with uncomplicated anatomy, early primary repair, and good biventricular function.

Clinical Features and Diagnostic Testing
Patients are followed lifelong at varying intervals depending on their clinical status. Symptoms include shortness of breath on exertion, palpitations, or syncope. The clinical examination will typically include normal oxygen saturations. A diastolic to-and-fro murmur in the pulmonary area signifies pulmonary regurgitation. An RV heave and a single second heart sound are present if pulmonary regurgitation is severe. Overt signs of right heart failure such as hepatomegaly, increased jugular venous pressure, and edema are uncommon. ECG will commonly show complete right bundle branch in older adults dependent on the reparative surgical technique. BNP is predictive of mortality.[59] Other diagnostic testing may include chest radiograph, echocardiography, CMR, and cardiopulmonary exercise testing. Ambulatory ECG monitoring, CCT, cardiac catheterization, and diagnostic electrophysiological studies are performed by clinical indication.

Knowledge of the patient's surgical history and most recent physiological status is critical for influencing appropriate frequency of diagnostic imaging and vital for decision-making related to indications for intervention for pulmonary regurgitation, RVOT obstruction, residual VSD, ascending aortic dilatation with aortic regurgitation, RV and LV dysfunction, arrhythmia, or endocarditis.

Echocardiography is routinely used for all patients including screening for significant pulmonary regurgitation and right heart dilatation and for assessing ventricular function. Severity of RVOT obstruction, tricuspid regurgitation, and diastolic dysfunction and presence of residual VSD are optimally assessed with echocardiography. Quantification of right atrial size is helpful as large right atrial area has been associated with sustained tachyarrhythmias in these patients.[60] Furthermore, Doppler can identify the presence of a restrictive RV with the presence

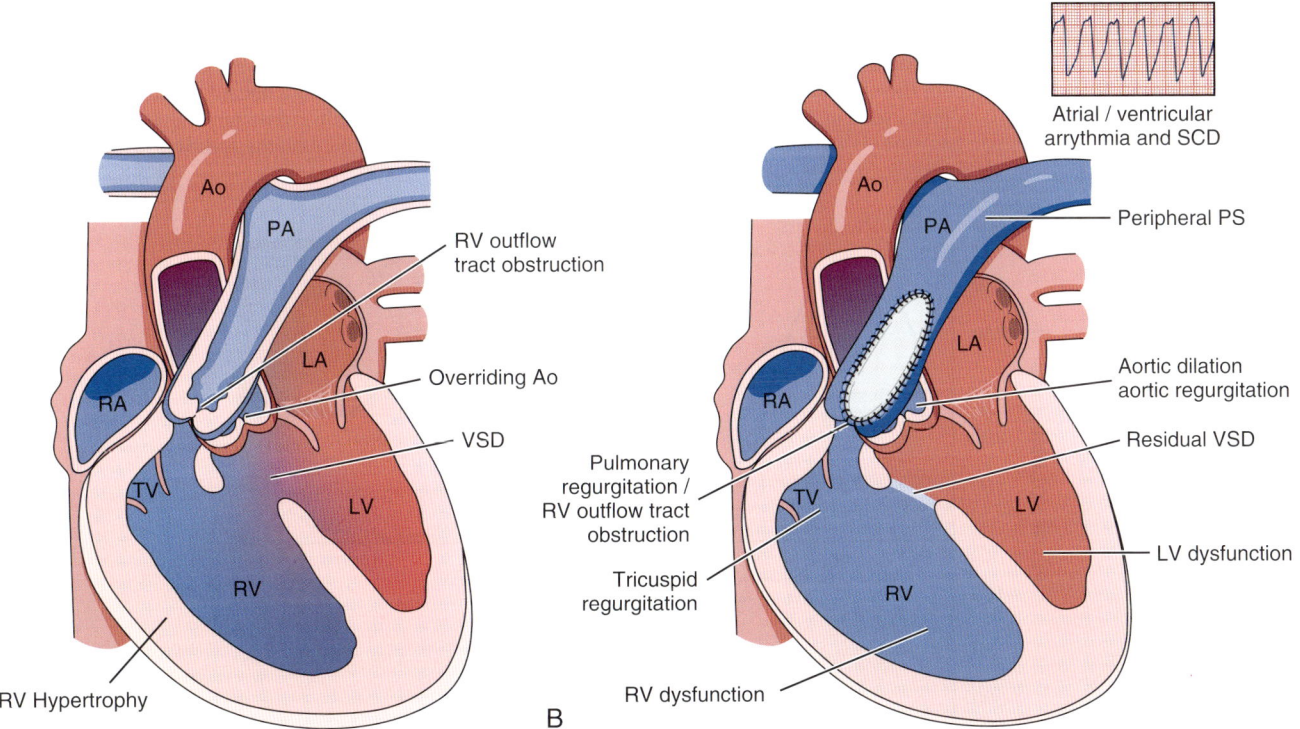

FIGURE 82.21 A, Native anatomy of tetralogy of Fallot. **B,** Anatomy of tetralogy of Fallot repair, with ventricular septal defect (VSD) patch and right ventricular outflow tract patch. Note the indication of various possible complications following surgery. *Ao,* Aorta; *LA,* left atrium; *LV,* left ventricle; *PA,* pulmonary artery; *PS,* pulmonary stenosis; *RA,* right atrium; *RV,* right ventricle; *SCD,* sudden cardiac death; *TV,* tricuspid valve. (From Baumgartner H, De Backer J. 2020 ESC guidelines for the management of adult congenital heart disease. *Eur Heart J.* 2020;42[6]:563–645.)

of an antegrade "a" wave (end-diastolic forward flow) in the RVOT on pulse wave Doppler throughout the respiratory cycle demonstrating a filled, non-compliant RV which is unable to distend further (Fig. 82.22).

CMR imaging is used for accurate assessment of right ventricular volume and function, severity of pulmonary regurgitation (Fig. 82.23), the entire RVOT including branch pulmonary arteries and the course of the proximal coronary arteries, size of both the aortic root and ascending aorta, quantification of tricuspid and aortic regurgitation, and if redo surgery is being planned shows the proximity of these structures to the sternum. RVOT regional wall motion abnormalities and aneurysms (Fig. 82.24) are common; the RVOT akinetic area length predicts the onset of sustained ventricular arrhythmia. RV volumes quantified by CMR in the context of moderate or severe pulmonary regurgitation are followed serially for progressive dilatation and to inform optimal timing for pulmonary valve replacement. Late gadolinium enhancement imaging correlates with adverse prognosis in adults with repaired TOF, hence may be useful in selected cases for decision-making. Cardiopulmonary exercise testing is crucial for objective measure of exercise capacity which is related to prognosis and facilitates decision-making regarding valve replacement. CCT is used primarily for coronary artery relationships to the RVOT, extent of calcification and RVOT and PA dimensions in the planning of transcatheter pulmonary valve implantation, and for coronary artery assessment preoperatively in older patients or delineation of MAPCAs in selected patients. Ambulatory ECG monitoring, event recorders, and diagnostic EP study are used in patients with arrhythmia symptoms or who are considered high risk or suspected high risk for arrhythmia. Inducible VT during EP study has prognostic value for future clinical VT and sudden cardiac death.

Cardiac catheterization for diagnostic purposes alone is rarely indicated for asymptomatic TOF patients. Preoperative assessment of TOF with pulmonary atresia with MAPCAs usually includes delineation of the arterial supply to both lungs by selective catheterization and angiography to show the course and segmental supply from the collateral arteries and central pulmonary arteries.

Surgical Repair

Those born in developed countries have usually undergone surgical repair with closure of the VSD and relief of pulmonary stenosis with resection of RV muscle bundles in the RVOT with or without more extensive right ventricular outflow reconstruction. Since surgical repair of TOF was introduced in the 1950s[61] survival rates of greater than 90% are expected beyond 40 years from repair. Therefore, repaired TOF constitutes one of the most common conditions seen in ACHD outpatient care.[62] The surgical strategy for repair has evolved with time: Previously many infants received a BTT shunt prior to repair but now early primary repair is common. Due to recognition of the deleterious effects of pulmonary regurgitation, transannular patch is avoided where possible to preserve the integrity of the pulmonary valve. Patients with TOF with pulmonary atresia and those with anomalous left coronary artery from the right sinus may undergo a RV-to-PA artery conduit repair.

Long-Term Outcomes and Complications
Anatomic Sequalae

Table 82.11 lists the common sequelae of repaired TOF. Pulmonary regurgitation is a common sequela in repaired TOF patients particularly in patients who received a transannular patch repair. Patients with repaired TOF and pulmonary regurgitation are often asymptomatic for several decades; however, if untreated, severe pulmonary regurgitation results in RV dilatation and dysfunction, arrhythmia, heart failure, and even death.

In the past several decades, advancements have been made to determine the optimal timing of pulmonary valve replacement prior to symptoms and irreversible RV dysfunction. Symptomatic patients with significant pulmonary regurgitation should undergo valve replacement. The optimal threshold for elective pulmonary valve replacement for asymptomatic patients with significant pulmonary regurgitation is a subject of ongoing research. Pulmonary valve replacement is considered when RV end-systolic volume indexed to body surface area

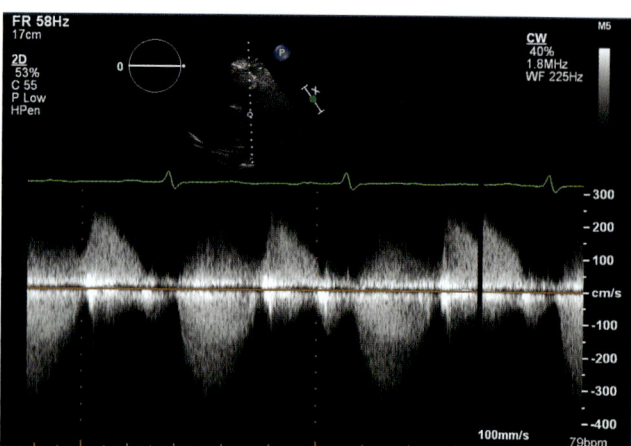

FIGURE 82.22 Spectral Doppler tracing of the main pulmonary artery in repaired tetralogy of Fallot; forward flow is seen in systole and retrograde flow of pulmonary regurgitation in diastole. Note the end diastolic forward flow in the main pulmonary artery corresponding to atrial systole, just before the QRS complex.

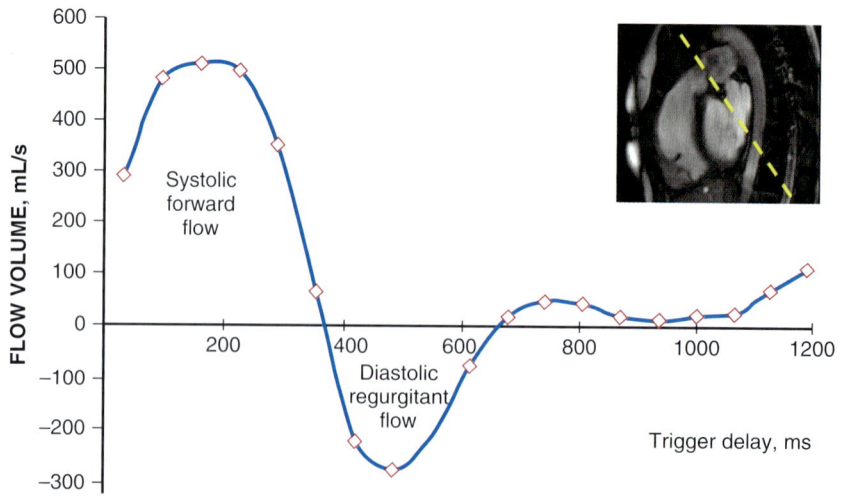

FIGURE 82.23 Cardiac magnetic resonance (CMR) quantification of pulmonary regurgitation after repair of tetralogy of Fallot. Pulmonary regurgitation is quantified by CMR in a cross section transecting the main pulmonary artery in the plane shown inset. The resultant through-plane phase contrast velocity mapping acquisition is used to plot forward flow to the lungs and to derive a pulmonary regurgitant fraction from integration of areas contained by forward and reversed flow curves. Typically, significant pulmonary regurgitation has a pulmonary regurgitant fraction ≥40%; this is greater with distal pulmonary obstruction or increased pulmonary artery compliance and less with subpulmonary stenosis or restrictive RV physiology. *ms*, milliseconds.

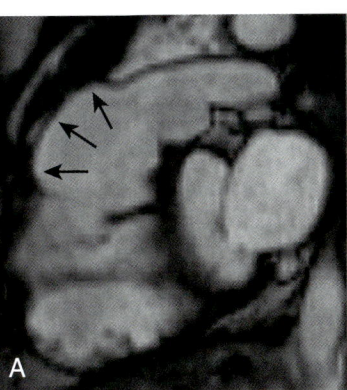 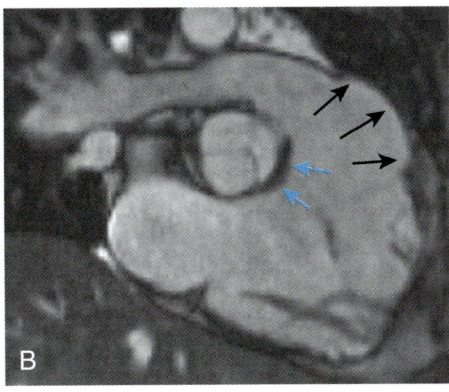 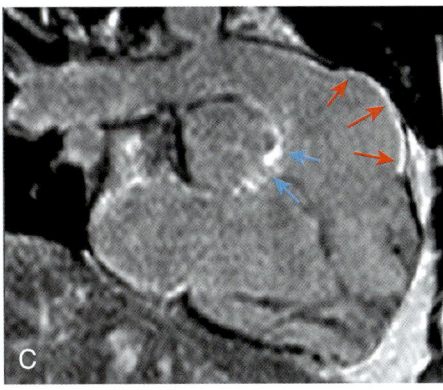

FIGURE 82.24 Right ventricular (RV) outflow tract aneurysmal or akinetic regions following tetralogy of Fallot repair. In older adults, RV outflow tract akinetic and or aneurysmal regions are common, are due to previous more generous resection of RV muscle bands with or without RV outflow tract or transannular patch augmentation, and contribute to worse RV ejection fraction. In the same patient this large akinetic RV outflow tract region is indicated by arrows in RV outflow tract **(A)** and RV in out **(B)** cine planes and its length was nearly 50 mm. **C,** Late gadolinium enhancement cardiac magnetic resonance (CMR) demonstrates fibrosis corresponding to the regional wall motion abnormality *(red arrows)* and there is fibrosis at the ventricular septal defect closure site *(blue arrows)*.

TABLE 82.11 Common Long-Term Issues in Repaired Tetralogy of Fallot

RV volume overload
Pulmonary regurgitation
Tricuspid regurgitation
Left-to-right shunt
- VSD
- Atrial septal defect
- Systemic-to-pulmonary collaterals

RV pressure overload
RVOT obstruction or pulmonary artery stenosis
Pulmonary vascular disease
Pulmonary venous hypertension secondary to LV diastolic dysfunction

RV systolic or diastolic dysfunction

LV systolic or diastolic dysfunction

Aortic regurgitation

Ventricular conduction delay and dyssynchrony

Arrhythmias
Atrial flutter
Atrial fibrillation
Ventricular tachycardia

LV, Left ventricle; *RV*, right ventricle; *RVOT*, right ventricular outflow tract; *VSD*, ventricular septal defect.

reaches 80 mL/m^2 (or end-diastolic volume index reaches 160 mL/m^2) as these RV volume thresholds predict normalization of RV volume following intervention. Right ventricular dysfunction is an indication for valve replacement.[3,63–65]

Transcatheter pulmonary valve implantation is an option when the anatomy of the RVOT and coronary arteries is favorable for available valves. Patients after previous surgical pulmonary valve replacement with a homograft or xenograft are usually suitable for transcatheter pulmonary valve implantation.

Symptomatic patients with severe RVOT obstruction require intervention. In those without symptoms intervention is indicated depending on objective exercise capacity, decreased or decreasing RV function, increasing tricuspid regurgitation, and presence of right-to-left shunting. Patients with discrete branch pulmonary stenosis, increased RV pressure, and reduced lung perfusion at CMR may benefit from branch PA dilatation and stenting.

Residual VSD may occur in up to 10% of repaired TOF patients and is often due to incomplete repair or VSD patch dehiscence.

Aortic dilatation not only at sinus level but of the ascending aorta is common after repaired TOF particularly after later repair, palliative shunt, with right aortic arch, and in men. Reassuringly progression is slow and acute aortic dissection in the setting of repaired TOF is extremely rare.[66] Aortic dilatation may be associated with aortic regurgitation.

Ventricular Dilation and Dysfunction and Heart Failure

Heart failure is the most common cause of death in patients with repaired TOF.[10] Patients may have systolic or diastolic dysfunction of the LV or the RV. Pulmonary regurgitation can lead to RV dilatation and dysfunction. Tricuspid regurgitation may be a complication of previous surgical VSD closure or secondary to RV dilatation. LV dysfunction is present in greater than 20% of patients with repaired TOF and may result from ventricular-ventricular interaction, electromechanical dyssynchrony, or ischemia. LV dysfunction is more common in patients with previous palliative shunt, late repair, or aortic regurgitation and is associated with increased mortality.

Randomized controlled trials of medical therapies targeted at right ventricular dysfunction have been small, underpowered, and have not shown benefit.

Arrhythmia and Risk Stratification for Sudden Cardiac Death

Both atrial and ventricular arrhythmia increase in prevalence after around 35 years of age. The most common is IART related to the cavotricuspid isthmus, right atriotomy, and dilatation of the RA which is amenable to ablation. Atrial fibrillation from the LA can be difficult to treat. Monomorphic or polymorphic sustained VT may be fatal, the former typically associated with ventricular dysfunction.[67]

Ventricular arrhythmia is an important cause of sudden death, putative risk factors for which include prior LV systolic and diastolic dysfunction, sustained ventricular and atrial tachyarrhythmia, systolic RV dysfunction, excessive RV hypertrophy, QRS duration ≥180 milliseconds, QRS fragmentation, LV systolic or diastolic dysfunction, extensive fibrosis at CMR, and inducible VT at EP testing.[3,63,68] The latter invasive testing is performed in selected patients with multiple non-invasively derived risk factors. The INDICATOR study of 873 repaired TOF patients showed that CMR derived impaired RV and LV ejection fraction and increased RV mass/volume ratio together with history of sustained atrial arrhythmia predicted mortality and sustained VT during follow-up.[69]

Targeting anatomical isthmuses prophylactically by VT catheter ablation may be an effective way to obliterate the usual VT substrates but any role in patient-specific risk stratification requires further investigation. VT ablation may be a treatment of choice in patients with good RV and LV function in centers with appropriate expertise.[70] For patients surviving sustained VT or cardiac arrest an ICD is usually indicated for secondary prevention. Preoperative RV dysfunction and RV hypertrophy may confer ongoing risk of mortality and sustained VT even after pulmonary valve replacement.[71]

Robust algorithms to appropriately weight risk factors for individuals for indications for primary prevention ICD remain lacking. As in all cardiology these are likely to benefit selected patients with at least 3.5%/year mortality risk. Clinical practice is to consider automatic implantable cardioverter defibrillators (AICDs) in selected repaired TOF patients with multiple VT risk factors among LV dysfunction, non-sustained and symptomatic VT, QRS duration ≥180 milliseconds, extensive RV scarring on CMR, or inducible VT at programmed electrical stimulation and remains controversial.

Transposition of the Great Arteries
Anatomic Description and Prevalence
In D-loop TGA the aorta arises from the RV and the PA arises from the LV; that is ventriculo-arterial discordance. With this anatomy the pulmonary and systemic circulations are in parallel rather than in series; de-oxygenated blood recirculates through the systemic circulation while oxygenated blood recirculates through the pulmonary circulation (Fig. 82.25). Therefore, without mixing or correction, TGA is not survivable. TGA occurs in approximately 30/100,000 live births, accounting for approximately 6% of congenital heart defects making it the second most common cyanotic congenital heart defect, following TOF.

In the vast majority of patients with TGA, the atria are normally positioned and the AV connections are normal. Venous return is typically normal. The great arteries are transposed with the aortic valve anterior and rightward to the pulmonic valve (D-loop transposition). In some, the aortic valve is directly anterior to the pulmonic valve or the valves can be side-by-side.

TGA is frequently associated with other congenital malformations. Approximately 35% of patients have a concomitant VSD. The VSD is most typically malalignment, peri-membranous, or muscular. LVOT obstruction (native pulmonic or sub-pulmonic obstruction) is common. Mechanisms for LVOT obstruction include a discrete fibrous membrane in the LVOT, systolic anterior motion of the mitral valve, and valvular pulmonic stenosis.

Coronary artery anomalies are very common in TGA, and of clinical importance in those repaired with an arterial switch operation, discussed below. Approximately ⅔ of patients have a "typical" coronary artery pattern in which the left coronary arises from the left posterior sinus and the right coronary arises from the right posterior sinus. A single coronary artery is present in 10% and intra-arterial course is present in approximately 5%.

Unless repaired, TGA is lethal within the first year of life. Therefore, virtually all adults with TGA will have undergone a prior surgical repair.

Clinical Features
Unrepaired TGA in the adult is exceedingly rare. The physical exam will be dominated by profound cyanosis and erythrocytosis. The physical findings of the repaired patient depend entirely on the type of repair.

Surgical Repairs
Atrial Switch Operation
The atrial switch operation was the surgical repair for TGA from 1957 until the 1980s at which point it was replaced by the arterial switch operation (discussed below). The atrial switch procedure is often referred to by the eponyms Mustard procedure or Senning procedure. In the atrial switch, venous return is re-directed to create a circulation in series and resolve cyanosis. The SVC and IVC are re-routed leftward toward the mitral valve and the LV via inter-atrial baffles. The pulmonary veins are re-routed anteriorly and rightward, toward the tricuspid valve and the RV. Following the atrial switch operation, de-oxygenated blood flows from the SVC/IVC through the mitral valve, to the sub-pulmonic LV, where it is pumped to the PA and the lungs. Oxygenated blood returns via pulmonary veins, flows to the tricuspid valve and the systemic RV, and is pumped to the aorta. Therefore, following the atrial switch operation, the RV is the systemic ventricle, the tricuspid valve is the systemic AV valve, and the LV and mitral valve support the pulmonary circulation (Fig. 82.25B).

Arterial Switch Operation
In the contemporary era the arterial switch operation is the preferred treatment for TGA because it results in a systemic LV. In the arterial switch operation, the surgeon transects the great arteries above the sinuses and anastomoses them to the contralateral root. The coronary arteries must be removed from the native aortic root and re-anastomosed to the neo-aortic root, the most technically challenging portion of the operation and a source of operative morbidity in the early years of the arterial switch. Often draping the pulmonary arteries over the ascending aorta is required. Following the arterial switch operation, the LV supports the systemic circulation and the RV supports the pulmonary circulation (Fig. 82.25C).

Rastelli Operation
The Rastelli operation is a surgical option for infants with TGA, large VSD, and pulmonic stenosis. The surgeon over-sews the native pulmonic valve and places an angled VSD patch to direct oxygenated blood from the LV, across the VSD, and to the aortic valve. A RV-to-PA conduit provides for pulmonary blood flow (Fig. 82.25D).

Long-Term Outcomes and Complications Following the Atrial Switch Operation
While the atrial switch operation (Mustard or Senning) was revolutionary in that it allowed infants born with TGA to survive childhood, late complications are common in adults who have been treated with these operations (Table 82.12).

Ventricular Dysfunction
Following the atrial switch operation, the RV is the systemic ventricle. While systemic right ventricular systolic dysfunction is relatively uncommon in childhood, progressive deterioration is typical. By age 30 years, only a minority of patients are NYHA Functional Class I and up to a quarter have clinical heart failure.[72,73] There are multiple reasons why the RV is predisposed to systolic dysfunction when exposed to high afterload including unfavorable myocardial fiber orientation, non-conical ventricular geometry, and tricuspid (systemic AV valve) regurgitation imposing additional volume loading. Right ventricular dilation and dysfunction lead to annular enlargement and secondary tricuspid (systemic AV valve) regurgitation. The superimposed volume load on the systemic RV accelerates ventricular dysfunction and makes patients more likely to develop heart failure with reduced ejection fraction.

Systolic function of the systemic RV can be evaluated qualitatively by TTE. Quantitative assessment of systemic right ventricular systolic function is difficult by echocardiography: Parameters such as TAPSE, fractional area change, and tissue Doppler are not well validated in patients with a systemic RV. Cardiac MR remains the gold standard for quantification of RV systolic function.

Medical management of systemic right ventricular systolic dysfunction is discussed in more detail in the section on heart failure in CHD. There is no conclusive evidence that standard GDMT impacts ejection fraction, functional class, or clinical outcomes; however, ACE inhibitors and angiotensin receptor antagonists are commonly used in patients with a systemic RV and clinical heart failure with systolic dysfunction.

Baffle Complications
The interatrial baffles which divert pulmonary and systemic venous blood to the contralateral ventricle are predisposed to malfunction as well. The pathways can become narrowed, most commonly in the SVC limb (Fig. 82.26). Some patients may present with symptoms of SVC syndrome such as facial swelling or headache, although most are asymptomatic due to decompression down the azygous vein. Percutaneous stents usually effectively relieve symptomatic pathway obstruction so surgical baffle reconstruction is rarely required. Transvenous pacemaker or defibrillator leads are risk factors for SVC pathway obstruction and, when possible, are extracted prior to stent implantation to avoid jailing the lead between the SVC and the stent. Obstruction within the pulmonary venous pathway is less common and would present with symptoms of pulmonary edema. Pathway obstruction within the IVC limb is

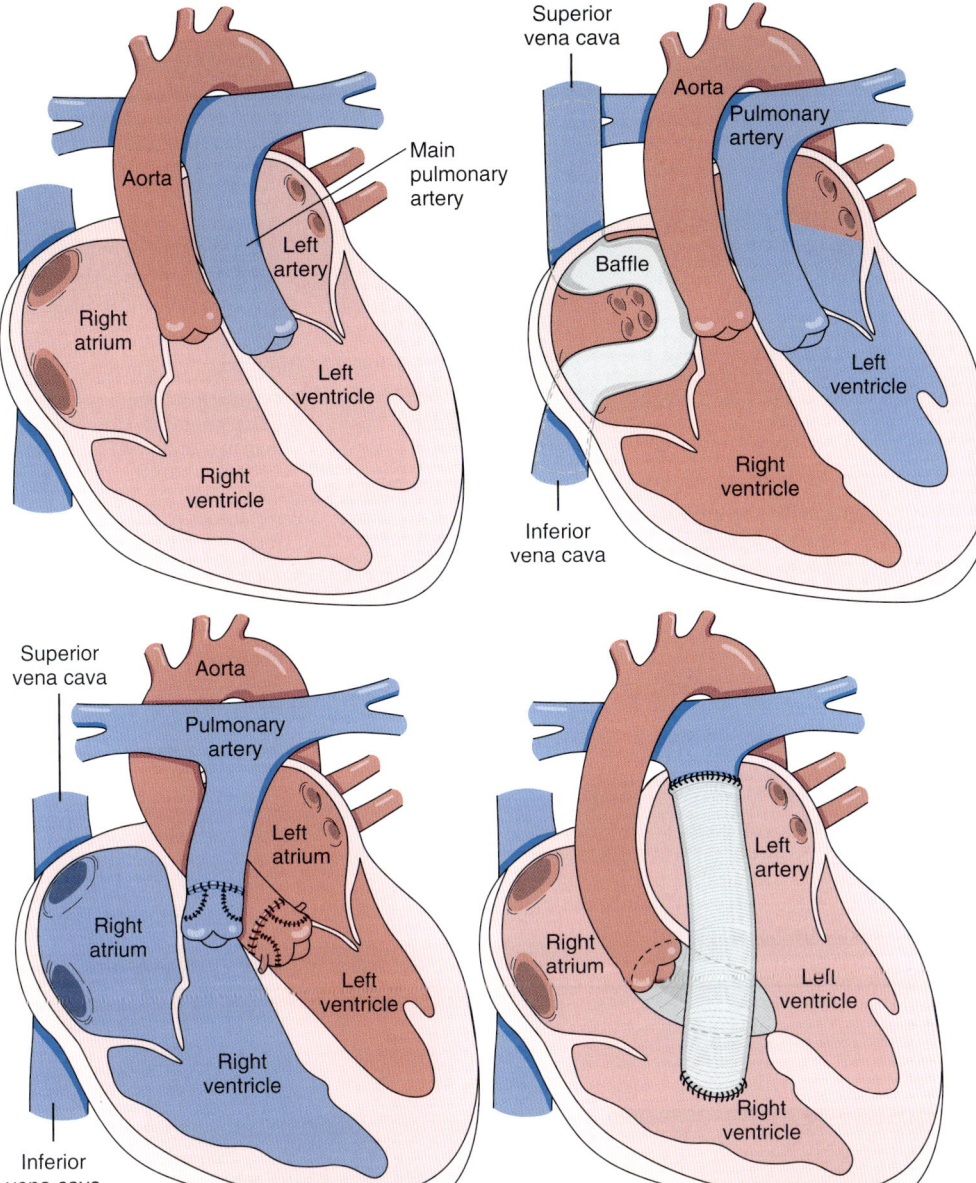

FIGURE 82.25 A, D-loop transposition of the great arteries, unrepaired with intact ventricular septum. The aorta is anterior and rightward of the pulmonary artery, and arising from the right ventricle. **B,** Following the atrial switch operation, the aorta continues to arise from the right ventricle; the systemic venous return has been baffled to the mitral valve and left ventricle, and the pulmonary venous return runs posterior to the systemic venous baffle to the tricuspid valve and right ventricle. **C,** Following the arterial switch operation, there is now ventriculo-arterial concordance, with the neo-aorta arising from the left ventricle. Note the suture lines above the coronary arteries on the neo-aorta and on the neo-pulmonary artery. **D,** Following Rastelli operation, a patch has been placed to direct the left ventricle through a ventricular septal defect to the native aorta, which sits above the right ventricle. A conduit has been placed from the right ventricle to the pulmonary arteries.

relatively rare but presents with lower extremity edema, ascites, or hepatic congestion.

A communication between the systemic venous pathway and the pulmonary venous pathway is called a baffle leak. Baffle leaks can lead to resting or exertional desaturation and can present with exercise intolerance, chamber dilation, or paradoxical embolism. Shunts are often bidirectional. Agitated saline injection on TTE show opacification of the systemic RV. Baffle leak is a risk for paradoxical embolism. Baffle leaks can be closed percutaneously, either with an ASD occluder device or a covered stent.

Atrial Arrhythmia

The extensive atrial suture lines used to create interatrial baffles predispose patients to developing atrial arrhythmias. Interatrial re-entry tachycardia is common in adults who have undergone atrial switch procedure. Atrial tachyarrhythmias are associated with sudden cardiac death so should be treated aggressively, either with ablation or antiarrhythmic drugs.[74] Over 1/3 of patients with an atrial switch procedure have sinus node dysfunction or other bradyarrhythmia requiring a pacemaker. Transvenous pacemaker leads are a risk factor for SVC pathway obstruction.

Long-Term Complications Following the Arterial Switch Operation

Late outcomes after the arterial switch are favorable compared to the atrial switch (see Table 82.12). Following the arterial switch the LV is the systemic ventricle and there are no interatrial baffles. Consequently, the risk of heart failure and arrhythmia is low after the arterial switch operation.

Coronary Artery Stenosis

The most technically difficult aspect of the arterial switch operation is the coronary transfer from the native aortic root to the neo-aortic root. The surgery is more challenging in patients with variant coronary artery patterns, single coronary arteries, or intramural coronary arteries, approximately 1/3 of patients with TGA. Coronary artery ostial stenosis typically presents within the first year after the arterial switch operation but can present in adolescence or adulthood with ventricular dysfunction, angina, ventricular arrhythmia, or sudden cardiac death. Patients with any of these symptoms should undergo coronary evaluation with invasive angiography, CT angiography, or stress testing. Percutaneous and surgical revascularization are both reasonable treatment options.

Aortic Dilation and Regurgitation

Following the arterial switch operation, the neo-aortic valve and root (native pulmonic valve and root) are predisposed to dilation and secondary neo-aortic valve regurgitation. The rate of dissection is not known following the arterial switch operation, but there are very few reports of aortic dissection or rupture following the arterial switch operation. Indications for surgery on neo-aortic valve regurgitation mirror that for intervention for native aortic regurgitation and are based on symptoms, ventricular dilation, or the presence of ventricular dysfunction.

Supravalvar Pulmonic Stenosis

Supravalvar pulmonic stenosis can occur just above the pulmonic valve or in the branch pulmonary arteries. Proximal supravalvar pulmonic stenosis is well demonstrated by TTE but branch PA stenosis may be difficult to visualize by echocardiography; a high parasternal or suprasternal notch imaging can show the branch pulmonary arteries splayed over the mid-ascending aorta. MR angiography visualizes the degree of stenosis and using phase contrast MR in the branch pulmonary arteries provides quantitative flow data to each lung. When branch PA stenosis causes symptoms or right ventricular hypertension, percutaneous angioplasty with stenting is typically effective treatment.

TABLE 82.12 Common Complications Following Repair of Transposition of the Great Arteries

SURGICAL CORRECTION	COMPLICATION	TYPICAL SIGNS AND SYMPTOMS	DIAGNOSTIC EVALUATION	TYPICAL TREATMENT
Atrial switch operation (Mustard or Senning)	Baffle leak	Exercise intolerance, cyanosis, erythrocytosis, paradoxical embolism	TTE with agitated saline, TEE, gated cardiac CT, cardiac MR	Transcatheter closure with covered stent or ASD occlude device
	Pathway obstruction	Facial swelling, headaches, often asymptomatic	CT or MR angiography. Invasive angiography	If symptomatic, angioplasty with stenting; may require pacemaker lead extraction
	Interatrial re-entrant tachycardia	Palpitations, syncope	ECG, ambulatory monitoring, invasive EP study	Ablation, antiarrhythmic drugs
	Sinus node dysfunction	Exercise intolerance, syncope	ECG, ambulatory monitoring	Pacemaker
	Ventricular dysfunction	Exercise intolerance, congestive heart failure	TTE, cardiac MR	RAAS inhibition (although efficacy not well documented), diuretics, advanced HF pathway
Arterial switch operation	Ostial coronary artery stenosis	Angina, ventricular arrhythmias	Stress testing, CT, or invasive coronary angiography	Percutaneous or surgical revascularization
	Branch pulmonary artery stenosis	Exercise intolerance, chest discomfort; systolic murmur	TTE, CT, or MR angiography; quantitative nuclear lung perfusion scan	Balloon angioplasty with stenting; surgical pulmonary artery reconstruction
	Neo-aortic root dilation	None	TTE, CT, or MR angiography	Surgical neo-aortic root replacement for severe enlargement
	Neo-aortic valve regurgitation	Exercise intolerance; diastolic murmur	TTE, cardiac MR	Surgical neo-aortic valve replacement
Rastelli operation	Right ventricle to pulmonary artery conduit stenosis	Exercise intolerance, systolic murmur (often ≥ grade 3), right ventricular dysfunction	TTE	Transcatheter pulmonary valve implantation or surgical conduit replacement
	Right ventricle to pulmonary artery conduit regurgitation	Exercise intolerance, diastolic murmur, right ventricular dysfunction	TTE, cardiac MR	Transcatheter pulmonary valve implantation; occasionally surgical conduit revision

CT, Computed tomography; *EP*, electrophysiology; *HF*, heart failure; *MR*: Magnetic resonance; *RAAS*: Renin-angiotensin-aldosterone; *TEE*, Transesophageal echocardiography; *TTE*, transthoracic echocardiography.

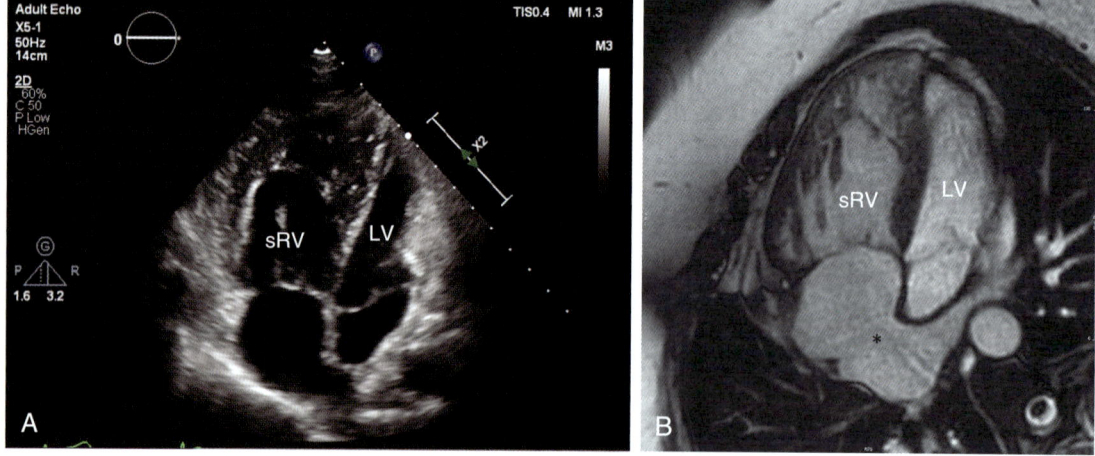

FIGURE 82.26 D-loop transposition of the great arteries s/p atrial switch operation. **A,** Transthoracic echocardiogram from apical view showing a hypertrophied and dilated systemic right ventricle and a thin-walled and pancaked left ventricle (LV). **B,** Steady state free precession cardiac MRI image in a similar plane showing the pulmonary venous pathway *(asterisk)* to the systemic, hypertrophied right ventricle.

Long-Term Complications Following the Rastelli Operation

Following the Rastelli operation, the LV is the systemic ventricle and the RV supplies the lungs via a RV-to-PA conduit. Children often require multiple conduit revisions during childhood as the conduit does not grow with the child. Late morbidity in adulthood is typically due to conduit stenosis, regurgitation, or mixed dysfunction (see Table 82.12).

Symptoms of conduit dysfunction include exercise intolerance and patients may show signs of right-sided heart failure. Conduit stenosis generates a systolic murmur (often grade III or higher) and conduit regurgitation generates a diastolic decrescendo murmur. Usually, echocardiography is useful to visualize the conduit and is particularly useful for quantifying obstruction. In some patients the conduit is obscured by the sternum. CMR with phase contrast and contrast enhanced angiography provide information on conduit anatomy and can be used to quantify regurgitation. In many patients with conduit dysfunction, transcatheter pulmonary valve implantation is effective for both stenosis and regurgitation. In some patients the conduit may be too small for percutaneous therapy. In others, conduit expansion results in coronary artery compression. In these patients surgical conduit replacement is required. Occasionally, following the Rastelli operation, patients may have residual VSD.

Congenitally Corrected Transposition of the Great Arteries

Anatomic Description and Prevalence

L-loop TGA, also called congenitally corrected TGA (ccTGA), is an uncommon congenital heart defect, accounting for less than 1% of CHD. L-loop TGA is characterized by AV discordance and ventriculo-arterial discordance; deoxygenated blood goes from the vena cavae to the RA, through the mitral valve to the LV, and then to the PA. Oxygenated blood returns via the pulmonary veins to the LA, through the tricuspid valve to the RV, and then is ejected to the aorta (Fig. 82.27). Therefore, L-loop TGA is a non-cyanotic congenital heart defect. Unoperated patients with L-loop TGA have a systemic RV. In the most common form of L-loop TGA the atria are normally situated, and there is ventricular inversion with the RV lying leftward and posterior. The great arteries are L-transposed with the aortic valve anterior and leftward of the pulmonic valve. Approximately 10% of patients with L-loop TGA have atrial situs inversus and mirror image dextrocardia; the physiology is unaltered by this variation.

The majority of patients with L-loop TGA have associated cardiovascular defects. More than half have a VSD. Subpulmonic or valvular pulmonic stenosis are common. The majority have a congenitally abnormal tricuspid (systemic AV) valve which shares features of Ebstein anomaly.

Clinical Features

Patients with L-loop TGA and no associated cardiac defects may remain asymptomatic and even go undiagnosed for decades. Those with ventricular dysfunction may have exercise intolerance or signs of heart failure. Because the AV node is displaced, patients with L-loop TGA have an abnormal conduction system which predisposes to complete heart block at a rate of 2% per year. The physical examination in L-loop TGA without associated lesions may be nearly normal with the exception of a single second heart sound (as the pulmonic closure sound is obscured by its posterior location). ECG shows absent septal Q-waves in the left precordial leads. AV block may be present. Chest radiograph typically shows a narrow and straight mediastinal silhouette. Patients with concomitant valve dysfunction will have associated murmurs. Fig. 82.28 illustrates imaging examples of L-loop TGA.

Surgical Repairs

Patients with L-loop TGA and no associated cardiac anomalies do not necessarily require surgery, although this will leave them with a systemic RV.

The double switch operation (Fig. 82.29) is a technically complex surgery which results in the LV in the sub-aortic position. In patients without a VSD, this consists of an atrial switch procedure (Mustard or Senning) and an arterial switch procedure. In patients with a VSD, the double switch can be achieved via an atrial switch and Rastelli operation.

Some patients with L-loop TGA and a pulmonic stenosis undergo a LV-to-PA conduit (and VSD closure, if indicated). This is a simpler surgery than the double-switch operation, but leaves the patient with a systemic RV and tricuspid valve.

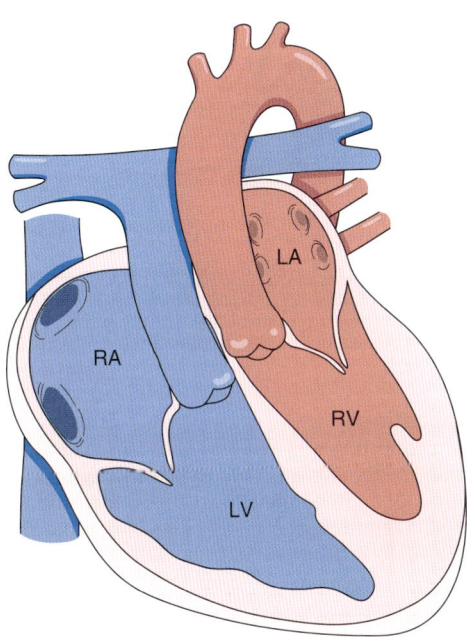

FIGURE 82.27 Diagram of L-loop transposition of the great arteries, demonstrating atrioventricular and ventriculoarterial discordance. Note the shading showing deoxygenated blood in the left ventricle and oxygenated blood in the right ventricle. *LA*, Left atrium; *LV*, Left ventricle, *RA*, right atrium; *RV*, right ventricle. (Modified from Libby P. *Essential Atlas of Cardiovascular Disease*. New York: Springer; 2009.)

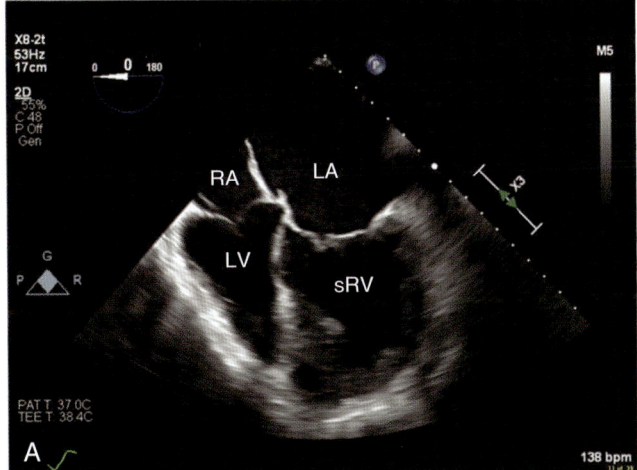 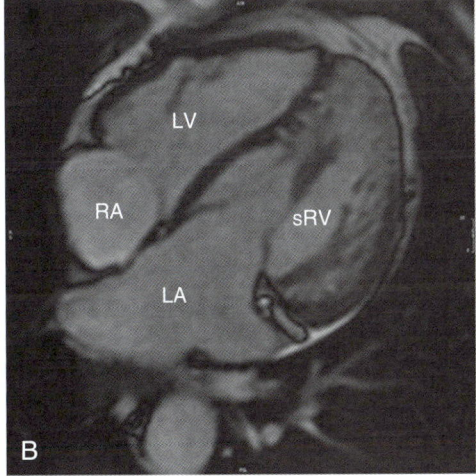

FIGURE 82.28 L-loop transposition of the great arteries. **A,** Transesophageal echocardiogram in transverse view showing atrioventricular discordance. **B,** Cardiac MRI steady state free precession cine imaging in a similar horizontal long axis plane. *LA*, Left atrium, *LV*, left ventricle, *RA*, right atrium, *sRV*, systemic right ventricle.

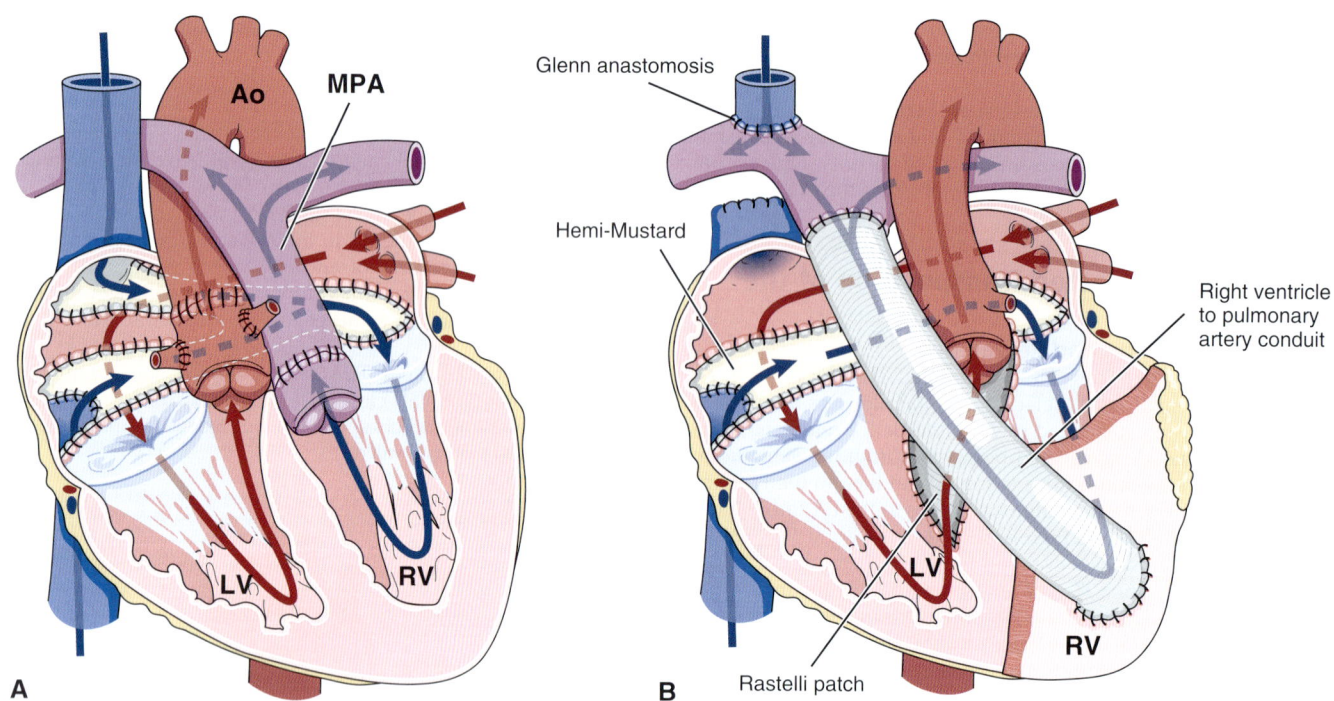

FIGURE 82.29 Diagram of two surgical options for L-loop transposition of the great arteries. **A**, Double switch operation, consisting of an atrial level switch and arterial switch. Note the superior vena cava (SVC) and inferior vena cava (IVC) blood baffled to the left-sided tricuspid valve and right ventricle (with *blue arrows*) and pulmonary venous blood flowing to the right-sided mitral valve and left ventricle (with *red arrows*). Suture lines are seen on the neo-aorta and neo-pulmonary artery following arterial switch. **B**, Hemi-Mustard and Rastelli operations. In this panel, the IVC blood is baffled to the left-sided tricuspid valve and right ventricle (*blue arrows*) and the SVC is directly anastomosed to the right pulmonary artery in end-to-side fashion (bidirectional Glenn). The right-sided left ventricle has been baffled through the native ventricular septal defect to the L-transposed aorta, forming a pathway for oxygenated blood. There is a conduit placed from the right ventricle to the pulmonary artery. *Ao*, Aorta; *LV*, left ventricle; *MPA*, main pulmonary artery; *RV*, right ventricle. (From Otto CM, ed. *The Practice of Clinical Echocardiography*. 5th ed. Philadelphia: Elsevier; 2017.)

Late Complications

Patients with L-loop TGA and no prior surgical repair are susceptible to regurgitation of the systemic tricuspid valve, systolic dysfunction of the systemic RV, and complete heart block. Tricuspid regurgitation is usually organic and results from a congenitally abnormal tricuspid valve with Ebstein-like features. Patients with symptomatic tricuspid regurgitation should be considered for valve replacement surgery as valve repair has poor long-term outcomes.[75,76] Because tricuspid regurgitation drives right ventricular systolic dysfunction, valve replacement should also be considered in the asymptomatic patient. Outcomes are better when valve replacement is performed in patients with preserved right ventricular systolic function, particularly with a right ventricular ejection fraction greater than 40%.

Medical management of systemic right ventricular systolic dysfunction is discussed in more detail in the section on heart failure in CHD.

Because of the abnormal location of the AV node and the conduction system in L-loop TGA, patients are predisposed to complete heart block. Serial monitoring with ECG and ambulatory monitors is warranted, as the incidence of complete heart block is as high as 2%/year and permanent pacemaker implantation may be required.

Patients who have undergone the double-switch procedure have a systemic LV, so they are less susceptible to ventricular dysfunction and less impacted by tricuspid regurgitation. However, they may develop any of the problems associated with the double switch such as baffle complications, coronary ostial stenosis, or conduit dysfunction. These complications, appropriate testing, and management are discussed in the section on D-loop TGA.

Double Outlet Right Ventricle

Anatomic Description and Prevalence

Double outlet RV (DORV) is a conotruncal anomaly in which both great arteries are completely or nearly completely aligned with the RV. DORV varies in complexity from a simple form that is physiologically like a VSD to extremely complex defects associated with heterotaxy syndrome. The key anatomic features of DORV are the VSD, the infundibular septum, and the position of the arterial roots. The location of the VSD is almost always the same—between the limbs of the septal band. The commitment of the VSD to an arterial root is dependent on the orientation and size of the infundibular septum and the position of the arterial roots. Fig. 82.30 illustrates the relationship between the VSD and arterial roots in some common forms of DORV. Most often the VSD is aligned with the rightward aorta because the infundibular septum attaches to the muscular septum leftward and superior to the VSD, shielding the PA from the VSD. In 30% of cases the VSD is aligned with the PA because the infundibular septum extends anterior and rightward away from the muscular septum and under the aorta, shielding it from the VSD. If the infundibular septum is hypoplastic or absent, there is nothing to shield either arterial root from the VSD and it is doubly committed. In rare cases, the VSD is distant from the arterial roots and uncommitted to either. These are usually muscular or inlet defects.

The position of the great arteries is also important in determining the relationship between the VSD and the arterial roots. The aorta is usually posterior to or side by side with the PA if there is a subaortic VSD. However, in cases with a subpulmonic VSD, the aorta is usually side by side or anterior to the PA. In rare cases the aorta is to the left of the PA, so what would usually be a subpulmonary VSD becomes subaortic and vice versa.

There are four common physiologic variations of DORV that dictate the clinical presentation and approach to surgical repair:

1. VSD physiology: DORV with large subaortic VSD and no pulmonic stenosis
2. TOF physiology: DORV with subaortic VSD and pulmonic stenosis
3. TGA physiology: DORV with subpulmonary VSD with or without aortic obstruction
4. Single ventricle physiology: DORV with mitral atresia, severely unbalanced AV canal defect, or other cause of significant ventricular hypoplasia

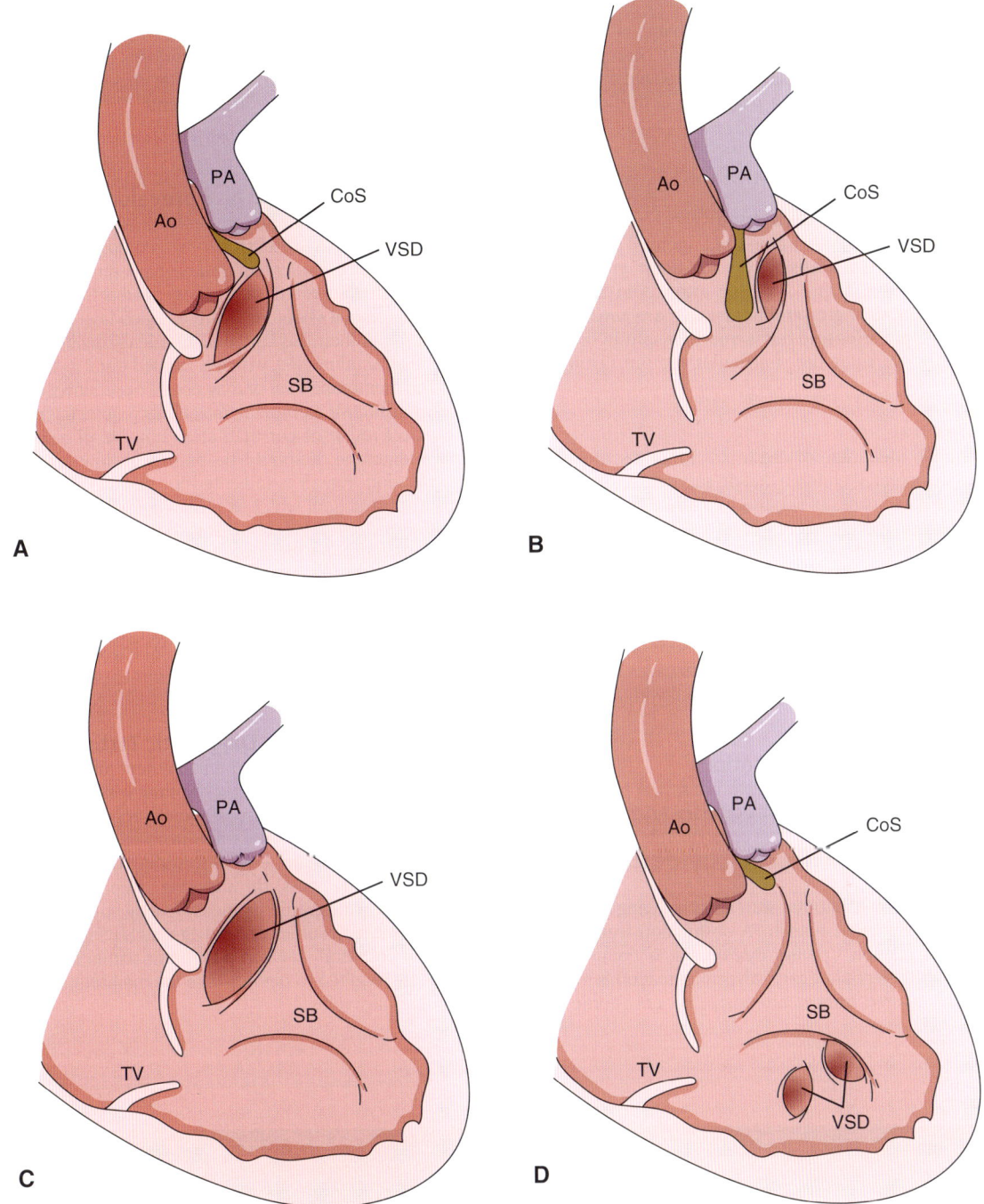

FIGURE 82.30 The relationship between the ventricular septal defect *(VSD)* and arterial roots in some common forms of double-outlet right ventricle (RV). **A,** Subaortic VSD. **B,** Subpulmonary VSD. **C,** Doubly committed VSD. **D,** Remote VSD. *Ao,* Aorta; *CoS,* conal septum; *PA,* pulmonary artery; *SB,* septal band; *TV,* tricuspid valve. (Modified from Lopez L. Double outlet ventricles. In: Lai WW, Mertens MM, Cohen MS, Geva T, eds. *Echocardiography in Pediatric and Congenital Heart Disease: From Fetus to Adult.* Wiley-Blackwell; 2009.)

A specific subset of DORV patients with subpulmonary VSD, bilateral conus, and side-by-side semilunar valves is known as "Taussig-Bing" anomaly. These patients often require frequent interventions in adult life to address residual obstruction in both outflow tracts.

Clinical Features
The clinical presentation of a child with DORV is dependent on the lesion with the most similar anatomy and physiology (TOF or TGA physiology).

Repairs
The surgical approach to DORV depends on the intracardiac anatomy. The position of the VSD and relationship to the great arteries is critical to the surgical approach. In the most common form (subaortic VSD), the surgical goals include establishing LV to aortic continuity by patching the VSD to tunnel the LV to the aorta. This pathway is often long and tortuous and, in some cases, the VSD must be enlarged to create this tunnel. Care must be taken to avoid creation of LVOT obstruction, which may result in the need for reoperation. If there is pulmonary stenosis (PS), relief of obstruction must be accomplished by either patch enlargement of the RVOT, valvotomy, or insertion of a conduit to establish RV-to-PA continuity.

For patients with DORV and a subpulmonary VSD, the surgical repair is similar to those with D-loop TGA with a baffle from the LV to the pulmonary valve and arterial switch operation. For patients with unfavorable anatomy for a biventricular repair, patients are staged to a Fontan palliation.

Long-Term Outcomes and Complications

There is limited data on long-term outcomes of patients with DORV. Reinterventions are most commonly done for LVOT obstruction. The mechanism of LVOT obstruction is believed to be related to subaortic membrane and muscle hypertrophy or restriction at the level of the VSD.[77]

Truncus Arteriosus
Anatomic Description and Prevalence

Truncus arteriosus is an uncommon type of congenital heart defect in which a single arterial trunk arises from the heart, giving origin to the coronary arteries, PAs, and systemic arteries, in that order. In most cases, a VSD and single semilunar valve are present. This semilunar valve is usually tricuspid but is quadricuspid in one-third of cases and usually overrides the ventricular septum through an outlet VSD.

Clinical Features

Without treatment, the mean age of death is 2.5 months, most often from heart failure. Unoperated children that do survive usually develop PH. Although rare, isolated cases of survival into adulthood with unrepaired truncus arteriosus have been reported, and these patients usually have Eisenmenger syndrome.

Repairs

Earlier surgical intervention is preferred. The surgical repair involves removing the PAs from the truncal root, patch closure of the VSD, and placement of a conduit between the RV and PAs. In cases in which the truncal valve is dysfunctional, repair or replacement with a homograft is performed.

Long-Term Outcomes and Complications

Important risk factors for perioperative death are severe truncal valve regurgitation, an interrupted aortic arch, coronary artery anomalies, and age at initial operation older than 100 days. Patients with only one PA are especially prone to early development of severe pulmonary vascular disease.

Postoperatively, patients are followed with serial imaging to monitor for RV-to-PA conduit dysfunction, branch PA obstruction, truncal valve dysfunction, and root dilation. Conduit dysfunction is common and replacement, or transcatheter pulmonary valve implantation, is required in most adults with repaired truncus arteriosus. Truncal (aortic) root dilation is common and can cause truncal valve regurgitation. Dissection is rare.

In adults with prior truncus arteriosus repair, decreased right ventricular ejection fraction and smaller ascending aorta on CMR were associated with adverse clinical events.[78]

Cor Triatriatum
Anatomic description and prevalence

Cor triatriatum is a rare lesion in which a membrane separates the LA *(sinister)* or the RA *(dexter)* into two compartments. The remainder of this section will consider the left atrial type. Anatomically, the membrane is proximal to the left atrial appendage, so that the pulmonary veins drain into the proximal chamber and the appendage and mitral valve are in the distal chamber. This landmark classically divides cor triatriatum from a supravalvar mitral ring, which is located distal to the left atrial appendage. The membrane may or may not be obstructive; a nonobstructive or mildly obstructive membrane may never require intervention.

Surgical repair of cor triatriatum consists of resection of the intraatrial membrane. It should be done with low levels of morbidity or complication. Repair is indicated for patients showing signs or symptoms of obstruction, which is physiologically analogous to pulmonary vein stenosis, leading to congestive heart failure, respiratory symptoms, lung pathology, and PH. Atrial flutter or fibrillation is not uncommon.[79] The membrane should also be resected in a patient presenting to the operating room for associated cardiac disease, such as ASD or VSD. Repair may also be considered for the asymptomatic patient with a high gradient across the membrane, which would commonly be considered in the 8 to 10 mm Hg range, although this is not based on strong published outcomes data.

Clinical Features and Diagnostic Testing

The ECG may show left atrial enlargement and depending on severity of disease could have findings consistent with PH. Echo is the mainstay of diagnosis (Fig. 82.31). Transthoracic echo can clearly demonstrate the obstructive membrane, often from parasternal long axis or short axis and apical 4-chamber views. Adding color Doppler shows where blood flow can pass through the membrane and assesses for obstruction, with gradients measured by spectral Doppler. If acoustic windows are insufficient for diagnosis, TEE is an excellent choice to show the posteriorly located membrane within the LA. Rarely, CMR or CT can be required to demonstrate the membrane and the anatomy of the pulmonary veins.

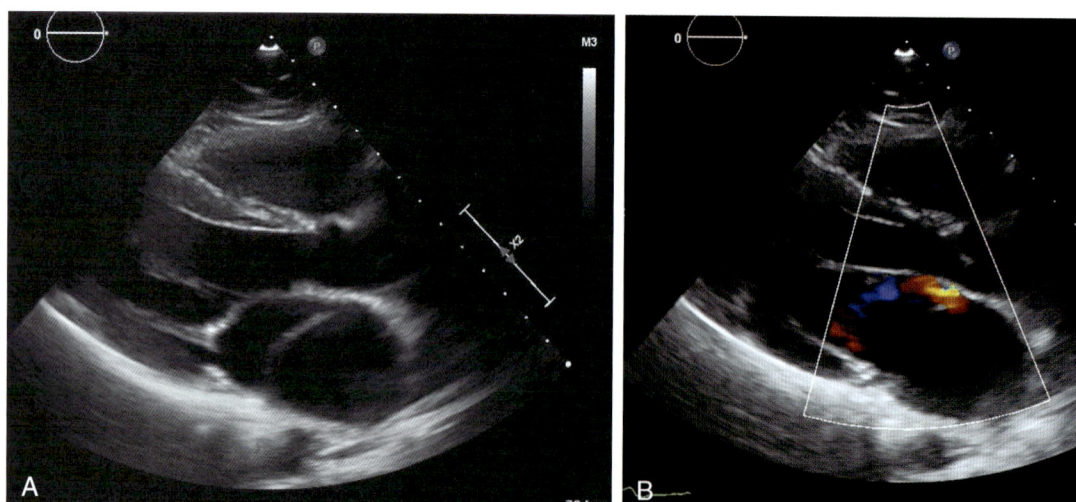

FIGURE 82.31 A, Transthoracic echocardiogram in the parasternal long axis view demonstrating cor triatriatum membrane within the left atrium. **B,** Color Doppler from the same window demonstrating a small flow jet around the obstructive membrane.

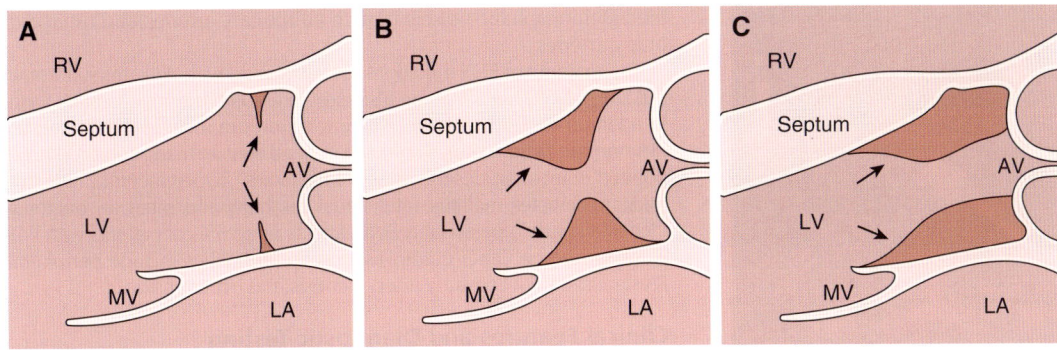

FIGURE 82.32 Types of subaortic stenosis. **A,** Discrete subaortic membrane *(arrows)*. **B,** Thick fibromuscular ridge *(arrows)*. **C,** Tunnel or tubular *(arrows)*. *AV,* Aortic valve; *LA,* left atrium; *LV,* left ventricle; *MV,* mitral valve; *RV,* right ventricle. (From Devabhaktuni SR, Chakfeh E, Malik AO, et al. Subvalvular aortic stenosis: a review of current literature. *Clin Cardiol*. 2018;41[1]:131–136.)

Long-term Outcomes and Complications
Outcomes following repair of cor triatriatum are generally excellent. There is an incidence of pulmonary vein stenosis following repair, which should be investigated in any patient with recurrent symptoms.

Subvalvular Left Ventricular Outflow Tract Obstruction
Anatomic Description and Prevalence
LVOT obstruction proximal to the aortic valve can occur from a variety of different mechanisms including a discrete subaortic membrane, a fibromuscular ridge, or tunnel-like LVOT obstruction due to outflow tract hypoplasia (Fig. 82.32). LVOT obstruction due to hypertrophic cardiomyopathy is discussed separately (see Chapter 54.)

Subaortic obstruction due to a discrete subaortic membrane is a frequent cause of LVOT obstruction in children and is more common in males. It rarely occurs in infancy but may become manifest in early childhood or in adult years. It usually consists of a ridge of fibrous or fibromuscular tissue in the LVOT. The membrane is often circumferential extending both onto the septal surface anteriorly and the base of the anterior leaflet of the mitral valve posteriorly. The fibrous tissue may extend onto the aortic valve leaflets contributing to concomitant aortic regurgitation. Subaortic membranes or fibromuscular tunnels may exist with other left-sided obstructive lesions such as cor triatriatum sinister, supra-annular mitral ring, BAV, and aortic coarctation as part of Shone syndrome.

Subaortic obstruction can occur as a component of other forms of CHD as well. Patients with an AVSD may have LVOT obstruction due to elongation of the LVOT and chordal attachments of the left AV valve to the septum. Patients with a VSD may have prolapse of the tricuspid valve through the VSD or bowing of the membranous portion of the septum into the LVOT.

Clinical Features and Diagnostic Testing
Patients with isolated subaortic stenosis may present with dyspnea on exertion or with an asymptomatic harsh systolic ejection murmur. ECG may show left ventricular hypertrophy if the obstruction is severe. Untreated LVOT obstruction causes LV hypertrophy and, if severe, LV systolic and diastolic dysfunction.

The high-velocity jet from a subaortic membrane causes barotrauma to the aortic valve leaflets which induces leaflet thickening and fibrosis and predisposing to aortic regurgitation. Aortic regurgitation is present in the majority of patients with significant LVOT obstruction from a subaortic membrane and is usually mild. Aortic regurgitation is most common in patients with high outflow gradients. At the time of surgery in one large series, only 27% were free from aortic regurgitation.[80]

Echocardiography is the most useful test to determine the anatomy and severity of LVOT obstruction. A subaortic membrane typically appears as a linear membrane below the level of the aortic valve. It is seen from the parasternal long-axis view or the apical 3-chamber view on TTE. Color Doppler and pulsed-wave Doppler determines the level of obstruction. Continuous-wave Doppler echocardiography determines the severity of obstruction. Concomitant aortic regurgitation is common and color and spectral Doppler should be used to determine the aortic regurgitation severity. The aortic valve is typically tricommissural. However, eccentric flow from the LVOT obstruction can cause asymmetric opening, giving the impression of a BAV.

TEE is often helpful in distinguishing subaortic stenosis from valvular aortic stenosis, and determining whether the membrane encroaches onto the aortic valve leaflets (Fig. 82.33). CCT, cardiac MRI, and cardiac catheterization are rarely required for the evaluation of subaortic stenosis and are reserved for patients with inadequate echocardiographic windows. Cardiac MRI to evaluate LVOT obstruction due to hypertrophic cardiomyopathy is discussed elsewhere. Exercise testing can help determine the functional impact of LVOT obstruction in patients without overt symptoms.

Repairs
Symptomatic patients with severe LVOT obstruction (maximum gradient > 50 mm Hg, mean gradient > 30 mm Hg) should be referred for repair. Repair is also appropriate for patients with severe obstruction and reduced exertional capacity on exercise testing. Patients with subaortic stenosis and heart failure should also undergo repair,[3] even with moderate gradients (maximum gradient 30 to 50 mm Hg) because the low cardiac output from heart failure may lead to reduced gradients, even if obstruction is severe. Because high gradients are associated with progressive aortic regurgitation, asymptomatic patients with high gradients and aortic regurgitation can consider subaortic membrane resection in order to prevent progressive aortic regurgitation.

The treatment for LVOT obstruction is surgical. Surgery involves membrane resection with enucleation to the base of the membrane; some surgeons advocate for a concomitant limited myectomy. Occasionally LVOT enlargement with a Konno or Manougian procedure is needed. Patients with severe aortic regurgitation require valve replacement. Surgical mortality is low and immediate postoperative results are usually excellent.

Long-Term Outcomes and Complications
Late recurrence of LVOT obstruction and re-growth of a subaortic membrane is common. Following resection, the average rate of gradient increase is ~ 1.4 mm Hg/year and is more likely to recur in older patients and in females. Some (but not all) studies have suggested that combining myectomy with membrane resection results in less likelihood of recurrence and avoids the need for reoperation.[81] However, myectomy increases the risk of heart block (up to 4%) and iatrogenic VSD. Many patients require repeat surgery for recurrence of subaortic membrane years or decades after their initial intervention. It remains uncertain whether resection of the subaortic membrane prevents progression of aortic regurgitation.[82] For these reasons, long-term follow-up with serial echocardiography is needed for all patients who have undergone prior intervention for subaortic stenosis.

Supravalvar Aortic Stenosis
Anatomic Description and Prevalence
Supravalvar aortic stenosis (SVAS) refers to a narrowing in the ascending aorta. Morphologically it is most commonly an hourglass-shaped narrowing but can also occur from a fibrous ridge, or tubular hypoplasia of the proximal ascending aorta.

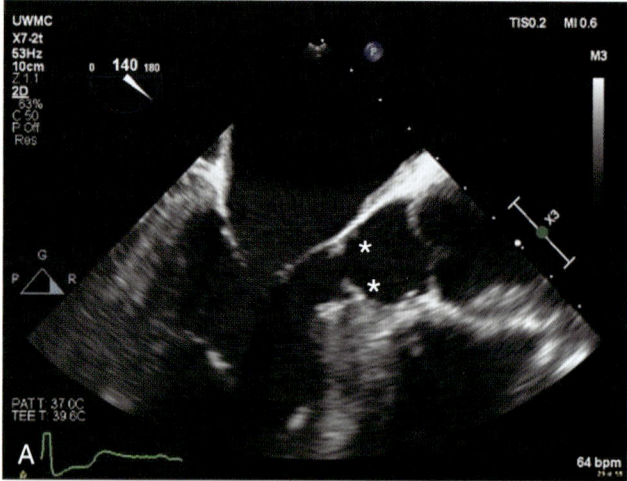
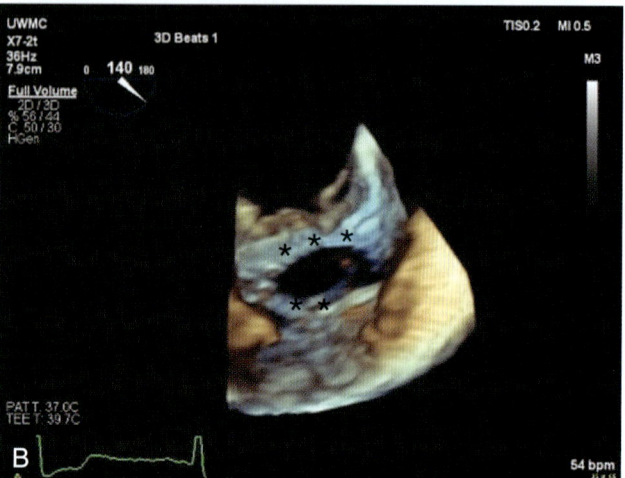
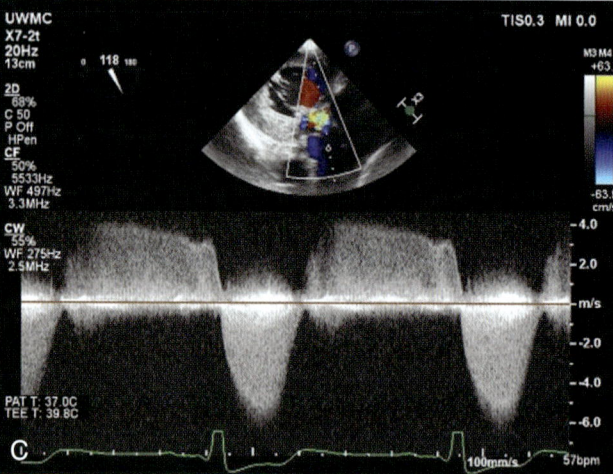

FIGURE 82.33 Transesophageal echocardiogram of a patient with a discrete subaortic membrane. **A**, Mid-esophageal window at 140 degrees showing the circumferential membrane on the septum and the base of the anterior leaflet of the mitral valve (asterisk). **B**, Three-dimensional view from the left ventricle looking out toward the aortic valve. **C**, Deep transgastric window with continuous wave Doppler across the left ventricular outflow tract showing severe left ventricular outflow tract obstruction (peak velocity 5.8 msec) and mild aortic regurgitation.

the brachiocephalic vessels, branch pulmonary arteries, and ostial coronary arteries.

The majority of ELN mutations are associated with Williams syndrome (OMIM 194050) but SVAS can also exist in a non-syndromic familial form. In addition to SVAS stenosis, Williams syndrome includes characteristic dysmorphic facial features (broad forehead, stellate irises, upturned nose, pointed chin; often described as "elfin" facies), hypercalcemia, hypothyroidism, diabetes mellitus, intellectual disability, and often an outgoing ("cocktail party") personality. SVAS affects up to 65% of patients with Williams syndrome. Other cardiovascular abnormalities include peripheral PA stenosis, ostial coronary artery stenosis, and hypertension.

Clinical Features and Diagnostic Testing

Physical examination findings may reveal hypertension. Four extremity blood pressures should be performed with the patient supine; if pressure is lower in the legs than the arms, hypoplasia of the descending aorta should be suspected. Patients with hypoplasia of the descending aorta may have an abdominal bruit and peripheral pulses may be diminished. SVAS results in a systolic ejection murmur. Patients with peripheral PA stenosis will have a murmur which radiates to the intrascapular regions. Facial and physical features of Williams syndrome may be present. There is a high incidence of sudden cardiac death in patients with Williams syndrome. Sudden death often occurs during noncardiac procedures and with induction of anesthesia. Careful periprocedural preparation is required. Patients who are at highest risk include young children, those with severe outflow tract obstruction, those with documented coronary artery involvement, or patients with prior history of arrhythmia or cardiovascular event.[84,85]

ECG reflects left ventricular pressure overload and may demonstrate LV hypertrophy. QTc prolongation is common in Williams syndrome.

Echocardiography is the primary imaging modality used to evaluate the morphology and severity of outflow tract obstruction in patients with SVAS. 2D imaging from the parasternal long axis view can usually define the anatomy and spectral Doppler is used to measure the degree of obstruction. Echocardiography is also appropriate to evaluate for LV hypertrophy in patients with SVAS or hypertension. Continuous wave Doppler from the high right parasternal window often yields the highest gradients. Right ventricular systolic pressures should also be calculated during echocardiography due to the high frequency of supravalvar PS and peripheral PA stenosis. CT or MR angiography is superior to echocardiography at imaging the branch pulmonary arteries and the head-and-neck vessels, particularly in adults.

Patients with ventricular dysfunction or symptoms of angina should be evaluated for coronary artery stenosis. Stenosis is often ostial but can also include diffuse stenosis or segments of ectasia and stenosis. Aortic valve leaflets may have unusual attachments to the ascending aorta which can also contribute to coronary artery obstruction. Coronary angiography remains the gold standard for the diagnosis of ostial coronary artery stenosis, but gated CCT scan can be diagnostic in many cases.

Repair

Surgery remains the mainstay of treatment. Patch arterioplasty is effective to treat most instances of SVAS and peripheral PA stenosis. Surgery usually provides more durable results than catheter intervention, which can be predisposed to in-stent restenosis.

Long-term Outcomes and Complications

Hypertension should be managed aggressively. Anatomic contributors, such as renal artery stenosis or diffuse hypoplasia of the descending thoracic aorta should be excluded. Medical therapy with calcium channel blockers or beta-blockers is appropriate. ACE inhibitors or angiotensin receptor blockers are appropriate for patients after renal artery stenosis has been excluded.

Due to the risk of sudden cardiac death with induction of anesthesia careful preparation is required. A cardiologist and anesthesia team familiar with Williams syndrome should evaluate the patient prior to procedures. Patients should maintain euvolemia whenever possible and agents which abruptly drop preload or afterload should be avoided whenever possible.

SVAS results as a consequence of mutations of ELN, the gene which encodes for the elastin protein, on chromosome 7q11.23. Most cases of SVAS result from new mutations but can also be transmitted in an autosomal dominant fashion. SVAS results from a combination of smooth muscle hyperplasia and deficient circumferential growth in the affected arteries.[83] In addition to causing supravalvar stenosis, ELN mutation frequently causes stenosis in other proximal arteries such as

Coarctation of the Aorta

Anatomic Description and Prevalence

Coarctation of the aorta, first described by Morgagni in 1760, involves a localized or tubular narrowing in the aorta or aortic interruption. It is characterized by a generalized arteriopathy with decreased aortic compliance. Thus, systemic hypertension is common in adults even after excellent results from repair.[86]

Typically, coarctation is juxtaductal, located at the junction of the distal aortic arch and the descending aorta beyond the origin of the left subclavian artery. Rarely it occurs elsewhere in the aorta. Coarctation is formed by a localized shelf in the posterior and lateral aortic wall opposite or close to the ductus arteriosus. It can be tubular extending toward the origin of the subclavian artery and can involve the transverse aortic arch. Hypoplastic aortic arch is common and this or a "Gothic-shaped arch" is particularly associated with hypertension without residual obstruction at the coarctation site. Associated anomalies are common and include BAV (50% to 85%), VSD, mitral valve abnormalities, subaortic obstruction, anomalous origin of the right subclavian artery, and intracranial aneurysm (particularly Berry aneurysms in the Circle of Willis). Coarctation is common in certain syndromes, including Shone, Turners, Williams-Beuren, Noonan, hypoplastic left heart syndrome (HLHS), and other complex CHD. Shone syndrome is the association with coarctation of the aorta with mitral valve disease (parachute or supramitral ring) and multilevel left-sided outflow tract obstruction (subaortic or aortic valve stenosis).

Clinical Features and Diagnostic Testing

Coarctation of the aorta presents with a bimodal distribution. Severe coarctation may present as a neonate with shock and/or heart failure and a ductal-dependent circulation. Less severe forms of coarctation can present in adulthood discovered incidentally while screening for causes of systemic hypertension. Adults living with coarctation have impaired long-term survival and in particular there is morbidity related to hypertension, aortic valve disease, and post-repair complications at the site of the coarctation including aneurysmal dilatation, rupture, or dissection. Left heart failure, endocarditis, premature coronary artery and cerebral artery disease also occur as well as complications related to associated lesions.[86]

Symptoms in adults with coarctation when present include systemic hypertension, headache, and leg claudication. On physical examination, blood pressure measurements should be taken in the right arm as left arm blood pressure may be misleadingly low if the left subclavian artery was sacrificed in the repair. Lower extremity blood pressure measurement should also be made as a systolic blood pressure gradient between the right arm and lower limb ≥ 20 mm Hg indicates significant coarctation. Femoral pulses may be reduced and there may be brachial-femoral delay. If present, a murmur associated with discrete coarctation is systolic and best heard from the back. Continuous interscapular murmurs are suggestive of collateral arterial flow. Fundoscopy may show hypertensive retinopathy.

The 12-lead ECG should be assessed for features of left ventricular hypertrophy, left atrial enlargement, and ischemia. Chest radiograph may show erosion of the undersurface of the outer third of a posterior 2nd to 9th rib due to collaterals called rib notching. This may be present unilaterally if either the left or right subclavian artery arises distal to the coarctation. The "figure 3" sign of coarctation refers to the silhouette of aortic dilatation both before (pre-stenotic) and after (post-stenotic) the coarctation site (Fig. 82.34). Ambulatory 24-hour right arm blood pressure measurement is useful for screening for hypertension during follow-up which is important even in those without important residual coarctation. Echocardiography is used to assess the aortic valve, aortic root, coarctation site, LV function, and mass. Evidence of increased velocity at the coarctation site can be sought with the use of continuous wave Doppler from suprasternal views (Fig. 82.35). Doppler evidence of a diastolic tail in the descending thoracic aorta and continuous-flow pattern in the abdominal aorta suggests significant stenosis at the level of coarctation. CMR is routine in coarctation diagnosis, assessing suitability for transcatheter stenting or hybrid repair and follow-up, and is cost effective. CMR is used for quantification of LV mass, evaluating the entire aorta including for arch hypoplasia or Gothic angulation, severity of coarctation, and quantification of collateral flow. It also identifies complications post repair (e.g., aneurysms, false aneurysms, recoarctation, or residual stenosis), presence of aberrant subclavian arteries, and for the morphology and function of the aortic valve. All adults with coarctation should undergo cross-sectional imaging (usually CMR) at least once. Cardiac CT is more suited for assessing stent lumen and fracture, and coronary arteries. Exercise testing may reveal exercise-induced hypertension which is prognostically important in patients with repaired coarctation, as it has been linked to adverse ventricular remodeling (left ventricular hypertrophy). At cardiac catheterization, a peak-to-peak gradient across the coarctation site ≥ 20 mm Hg in the absence of well-developed collateral circulation is considered significant.

When an extensive collateral circulation is present increased systolic and diastolic gradient assessed by echocardiography or peak velocity at CMR are not reliable to detect severe coarctation nor is pressure gradient at cardiac catheterization.

Long-Term Outcomes and Complications

Lifelong expert surveillance for late complications is essential with cross-sectional imaging at intervals of at least 3 to 5 years.[87] Hypertension is a major determinant of late mortality after coarctation repair.[88] Hypertension prior to treatment of coarctation may resolve at first but recur or persist in over 50% of adults especially if intervention was at an older age. When there is new hypertension the coarctation should be reassessed to determine if there is a hemodynamic target for intervention. Hypertension is common without any residual coarctation as the aorta proximal to the coarctation site is abnormal with decreased compliance. Medical treatment choices for hypertension are

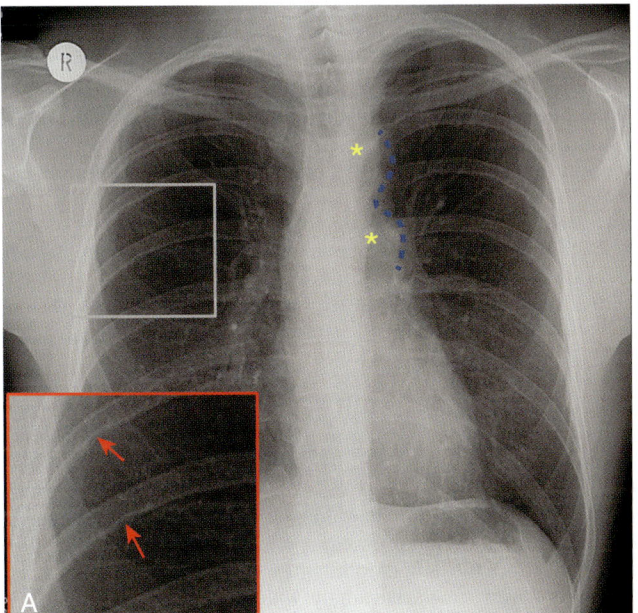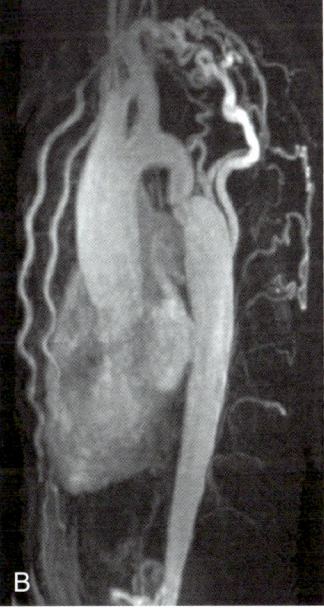

FIGURE 82.34 A, Chest radiograph reveals rib notching *(arrows)* in the 3rd to 5th ribs bilaterally as shown. The "figure 3" mediastinal silhouette *(blue)* is associated with coarctation and made by the distal aortic arch/dilated left subclavian artery and the post-stenotic dilatation of the descending aorta *(asterisks)*. **B,** CMR contrast enhanced angiography confirmed coarctation of the aorta with collaterals.

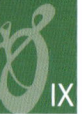

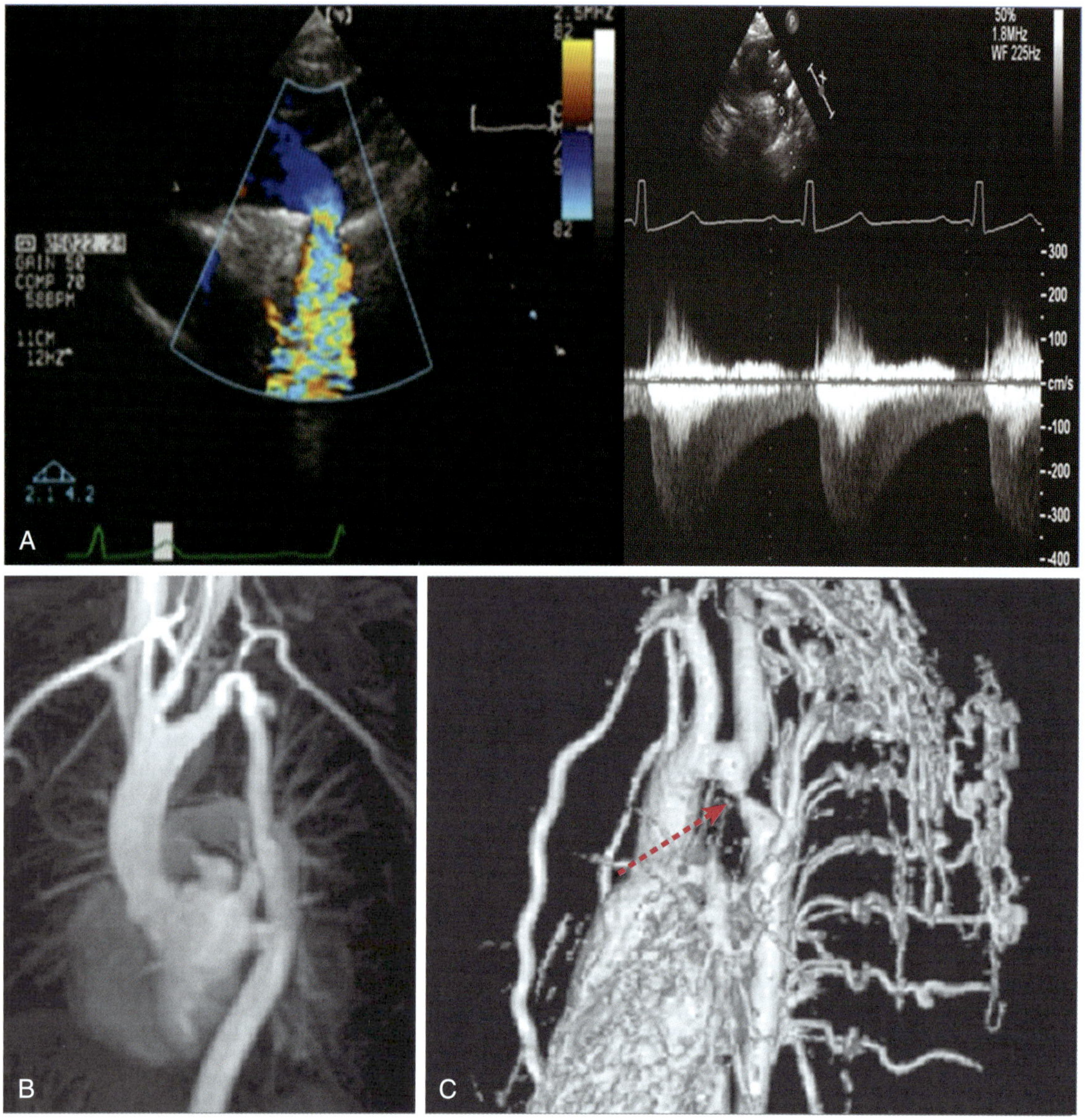

FIGURE 82.35 **A,** Turbulent color flow in the descending aorta with peak velocity above 3.5 msec. In the suprasternal continuous wave Doppler there is a double envelope reflecting both flow proximal to the aorta and high velocity flow across the coarctation site and there is a diastolic tail. **B,** Complex coarctation with hypoplastic arch, acute angulation, and tortuosity between the proximal arch and the descending aorta and a long (~8 cm) length segment of tubular hypoplasia. **C,** Severe coarctation with multiple large collaterals *(arrow)*.

as per standard guidelines. Proactive and aggressive control of blood pressure, and hyperlipidemia if present, is important given the need to prevent atherosclerotic heart disease and cerebral vascular disease.

The decision to intervene for coarctation or recoarctation of the aorta depends on blood pressure, gradient, and stenosis morphology. In adults, surgery is rarely needed and stenting is the treatment of choice when technically feasible. Repair (endovascular or surgical) of coarctation or recoarctation is indicated in hypertensive patients with an invasive peak-to-peak gradient ≥20 mm Hg. Coarctation stenting is also considered when feasible for hypertensive patients with a coarctation diameter ≤50% of the aortic diameter at the diaphragm regardless of peak-to-peak gradient and in normotensive coarctation with peak-to-peak gradient ≥20 mm Hg. Covered stents have been developed to prevent and treat acute wall injury associated with aortic coarctation.[89] Surgery to repair coarctation in adults may be indicated to treat more complex anatomy including interrupted aortic arch and long segment coarctation with options including an interposition graft and bypass grafts including ascending to descending aorta conduits.

Patients who have undergone balloon dilatation without stenting of coarctation at a younger age commonly need reintervention. Balloon dilatation can result in aneurysm formation at the site of coarctation or dissection. These complications are reduced by primary stenting which is the usual first-line treatment for adults. Aneurysms at the site of the surgical coarctation repair also occur and this is particularly concerning for adults with a history of Dacron patch aortoplasty (Fig. 82.36). The aortic wall opposite to the patch becomes aneurysmal and the false aneurysm at the suture line can also occur. Interposition grafts are at particular risk of false aneurysm. Associated ascending aortopathy with aneurysmal dilatation often related to a BAV and aortic valve disease itself may progress and require intervention.

Interrupted Aortic Arch

Interrupted aortic arch is a rare (<1.5% of all congenital heart defects) and severe CHD also associated with DiGeorge syndrome. Interrupted aortic arch occurs distal to the left subclavian artery (type A), between the left carotid artery and the left subclavian artery (type B) and uncommonly (<1%) between the brachiocephalic trunk and the left carotid artery (type C). It is associated with aberrant right subclavian artery which often arises distal to the interruption.

Adult survivors will usually have had previous childhood surgery with an interposition graft and possibly closure of VSD and subaortic stenosis resection. Associated intracardiac lesions typically include

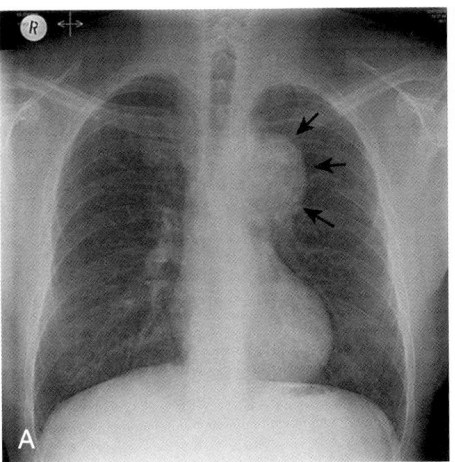 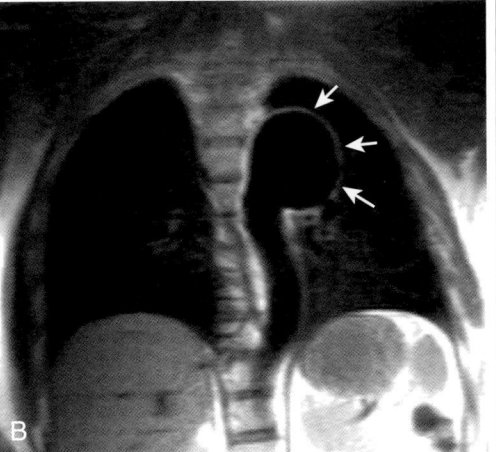 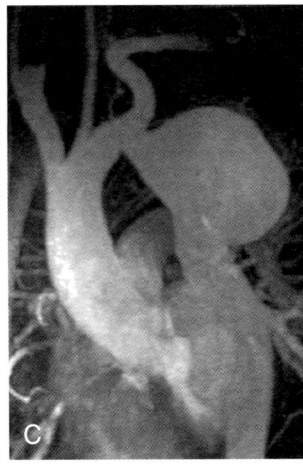

FIGURE 82.36 Dacron patch coarctation site aneurysm. **A,** Chest radiography done as routine surveillance after Dacron patch repair of coarctation shows alarming dilatation of the aorta *(arrows)* also revealed with the corresponding coronal plane MR image (**B,** *arrows*). **C,** The large, rounded aneurysm is just below the left subclavian artery branch, measures 53 × 55 × 64 mm, and is likely a contained false aneurysm. There is no residual coarctation.

VSD (80% to 90%), PDA, BAV, and complex congenital heart conditions, namely aortopulmonary window, double outlet RV, TGA, truncus arteriosus, single ventricle, or AVSD. Posterior deviation of the outlet septum in those with a VSD can result in LV outflow tract obstruction. During follow-up, reintervention for either LV outflow tract obstruction or recurrent aortic arch obstruction may be needed.

Vascular Rings
Anatomic Description and Prevalence
A vascular ring is an abnormality of aortic arch development which is defined as complete surrounding of the esophagus and trachea by vascular structures. This is distinct from an LPA sling, in which the LPA passes posterior to the trachea but anterior to the esophagus. The vessels comprising a vascular ring may all be patent or may include fibrous ligamenta, such as a ductal ligament or atretic arch.

A detailed discussion of the embryology of vascular ring formation is beyond the scope of this chapter. Briefly, there are six paired arches that form early in embryology; several of these arches fully or partially regress, while others form the aortic arch, its primary brachiocephalic branches, the proximal PAs, and ductus arteriosus. Errors in the pattern of regression can result in various forms of vascular ring.

The most common forms of vascular ring include double aortic arch and right aortic arch with aberrant left subclavian artery (Fig. 82.37). In the former, the right aortic arch is nearly always the dominant vessel, with a hypoplastic or atretic left aortic arch completing the ring. In the latter, there is a diverticulum of Kommerell at the origin of the aberrant subclavian vessel from the proximal descending aorta, which is a dilated proximal portion of the vessel due to the origin of the ductus arteriosus from that area and the high amount of ductal flow during fetal life. The presence of this diverticulum signifies that if the ductus is not patent, there is a ductal ligament arising from this region. There are several other rarer forms of vascular ring, but concepts for management are the same.

Vascular rings are rare lesions overall, although the true prevalence is probably not known due to a percentage of these lesions that never present clinically. Additionally, as repair is indicated for those lesions that present with symptoms, the vast majority of symptomatic rings are repaired in childhood. However, there is rare incidence of new symptoms first presenting in adulthood, as well as scattered cases that may have been symptomatic but eluded medical attention during childhood. There are also rare cases who may present with recurrent symptoms of respiratory changes or dysphagia in adulthood following correction in childhood.

Clinical Features and Diagnostic Testing
The most common symptomatic presentation for an adult with a vascular ring is dysphagia. Respiratory symptoms more commonly present in childhood, but adults can present with wheezing or stridor, particularly with exertion, as well as dyspnea on exertion. Vascular rings can also present incidentally, such as with the discovery of a right aortic arch by chest x-ray leading to additional testing. Physical exam may include the aforementioned respiratory signs, but is otherwise typically not revealing.

The presence of a vascular ring is classically demonstrated by a barium swallow, with the finding of a posterior indentation of the esophagus. Most patients now receive further testing prior to considering surgery.

Echocardiography is often suggestive, but overall limited for this diagnosis, particularly in the presence of poor acoustic windows. Imaging at the suprasternal notch should demonstrate arch sidedness or a double aortic arch. An aberrant subclavian artery can be very difficult to visualize directly, but absence of normal bifurcation of the innominate artery is suggestive. In addition, the presence of a right aortic arch in an otherwise anatomically normal heart is highly suspicious for a vascular ring. Cross-sectional imaging by CT or MRI is diagnostic for a vascular ring and best characterizes the individual components of the anatomy; the presence of a ductal or arch ligament cannot be directly visualized except in the unusual case of extensive calcification, but can be inferred by the remainder of the anatomy. CT is superior for imaging the airway directly but MRI can also diagnose related airway compression.

Surgical Repairs
The classic surgical management of a vascular ring consists of releasing the ring by ligation and division of a patent vascular structure, or division of a ductal or aortic arch ligamentum. Opening the ring allows the vessels to release and affords greater space for the trachea and esophagus and is usually curative. This is performed via thoracotomy on whichever side the structure is found for division, usually the left.

There are some who advocate for more extensive surgery for vascular rings that include a diverticulum of Kommerell, such as a right aortic arch with aberrant left subclavian artery.[90] This typically includes translocation of the aberrant subclavian artery to the ipsilateral carotid artery, along with resection of the diverticulum of Kommerell. Note that this procedure has to include division of the ductal ligamentum, or the vascular ring has not been released and symptoms will not be relieved. It has been described via thoracotomy as a single procedure, or in two stages with a lower neck incision followed by thoracotomy.[90,91] This has also been described as hybrid repair, in which the subclavian artery is surgically translocated to the carotid artery, followed by endovascular exclusion of the diverticulum with embolization material and/or stent grafting of the descending aorta across the diverticulum. The argument in favor of the more extensive operation is that the diverticulum of Kommerell can compress the airway even after release of the vascular

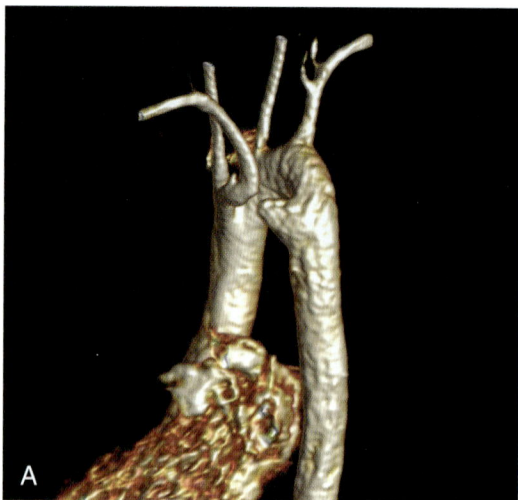 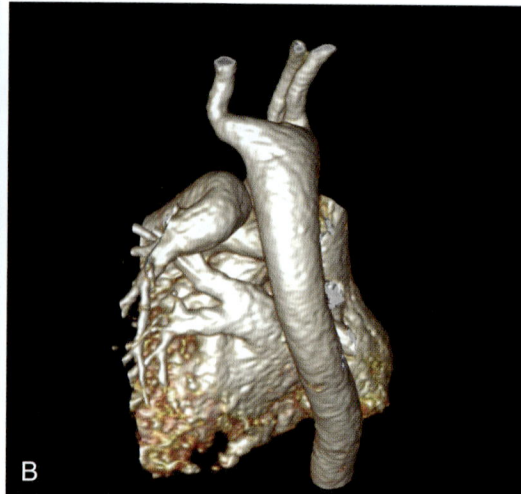

FIGURE 82.37 3-D reconstructions of gadolinium-enhanced MR angiograms. **A**, View from posterior and to the left of a double aortic arch with atresia of the distal left arch distal to the left subclavian artery. **B**, Posterior view of a right aortic arch with diverticulum of Kommerell and aberrant left subclavian artery; note the dilated diverticulum of Kommerell arising from the distal aortic arch.

ring, leading to recurrent symptoms, or can become aneurysmal and even rupture, causing a catastrophic event. The true incidence of diverticulum of Kommerell aneurysm and/or rupture is not known given the unclear incidence of vascular rings.

Diverticulum of Kommerell in the context of a left aortic arch with aberrant right subclavian artery almost always does not comprise a vascular ring but can cause dysphagia and can also become aneurysmal or rupture. There is a wealth of literature on the management of this condition, with serial imaging and sometimes surgical or endovascular repair, which remains somewhat controversial with a wide spectrum of approaches.[92] Surgical series in the literature are selected for more severe disease and the true incidence and therefore rate of complication remains unknown. However, it is crucial when assessing a patient with a diverticulum of Kommerell to discern whether there is the concomitant presence of a vascular ring (usually with a right aortic arch). If so, endovascular repair without surgical release of the ring will not relieve symptoms.

Long-Term Outcomes and Complications

Outcomes of vascular ring repair are excellent overall. However, as the vast majority of childhood repairs will have no further symptoms, those presenting to adult cardiology are selected for late or recurrent symptoms. After repair in adulthood, recurrent dysphagia has been reported in 14% of patients.[90] While this can have an anatomic basis, there may also be a functional component of esophageal dysmotility related to long-standing compression. As discussed, the rate of complications for a diverticulum of Kommerell is not known.

Anomalous Coronary Artery From the Pulmonary Artery

A coronary artery arising from the PA is an uncommon coronary anomaly. Anomalous left coronary artery from the pulmonary artery (ALCAPA) is more common than anomalous right coronary artery from the pulmonary artery (ARCAPA).

In patients with ALCAPA or ARCAPA, myocardial perfusion is via the coronary artery which arises normally from the aorta and is typically quite dilated. The anomalous coronary artery is supplied retrograde via collaterals and then drains into the PA. Because coronary artery pressure is higher than PA pressure, the anomalous coronary does not receive anterograde flow from the PA.

The degree of myocardial ischemia present in patients with ALCAPA or ARCAPA depends on the degree of collateralization and the coronary perfusion pressure. Most patients with ALCAPA present in infancy or early childhood with left ventricular systolic dysfunction, arrhythmias, or ischemic mitral regurgitation. Patients with ARCAPA typically have a more favorable clinical course and may escape detection until adulthood.

Diagnosis should be suspected in infants or young children with ventricular dysfunction or secondary mitral regurgitation. Adults may show a dilated coronary artery or robust collaterals on echocardiography (Fig. 82.38). Coronary angiography demonstrates a dilated coronary artery arising from the aorta which fills the anomalous artery via collaterals and drains into the PA (Fig. 82.39). CT angiography is useful to delineate the coronary anatomy and facilitate surgical planning (Fig. 82.40).

Surgery is indicated for patients with ALCAPA and patients with ARCAPA who have ventricular dysfunction, angina, or demonstrable ischemia. Options for surgical repair depend on the anatomy and the proximity of the anomalous coronary to the aorta. Direct reimplantation of the anomalous coronary artery into the aorta is preferred when technically feasible. Otherwise, the coronary artery can be supplied via an intrapulmonary tunnel to baffle the coronary to the aorta (Takeuchi repair). In some patients ligation and coronary artery bypass surgery is required. Operations in ALCAPA and ARCAPA should be performed by a congenital heart surgeon.

Single Ventricle

Anatomic Description and Prevalence

Single ventricle heart disease comprises several distinct anatomic lesions, which may represent a true anatomic single ventricle lesion, or a functional single ventricle lesion, in which a 2nd ventricle is present but is not adequate to supply the systemic or pulmonary circulation. Except in the rare case of congenital balance between the systemic and pulmonary circulations, these lesions require early palliative surgery for survival.

Tricuspid atresia is a functional single ventricle lesion, in which the tricuspid valve does not form. It is uncommon, with an incidence of approximately 1.2 per 10,000 live births.[93] This lesion is categorized by the relationship of the great vessels and the degree of pulmonary stenosis present at birth. There is typically a hypoplastic RV, and the great vessels can be in normal (S) position, D-transposed, or L-transposed. Decision making for neonatal surgery is dependent on the degree of obstruction to systemic or pulmonary outflow.

HLHS consists of a spectrum of left-sided obstructive lesions from mitral and aortic stenosis with a small LV to mitral and aortic atresia with a nearly absent left ventricular cavity. The incidence of this lesion is approximately 1.6 per 10,000 live births. HLHS typically includes severe hypoplasia of the aorta, requiring surgical reconstruction. Neonatal surgery includes aortic reconstruction with anastomosis to the

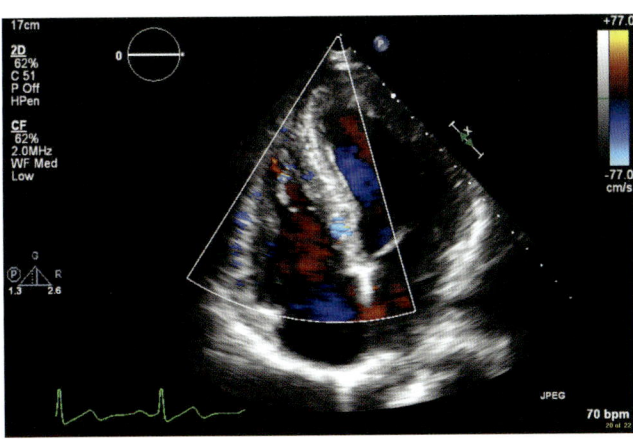

FIGURE 82.38 Transthoracic echocardiogram in apical 4-chamber view with color Doppler in a patient with anomalous right coronary artery from the pulmonary artery (ARCAPA). Note the extensive coronary collaterals seen by color Doppler.

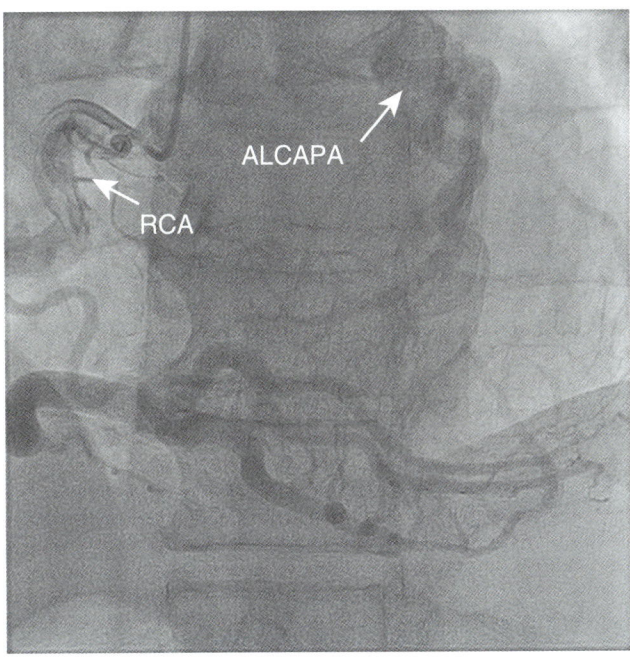

FIGURE 82.39 Coronary angiography in the right coronary artery (RCA) in a patient with anomalous left coronary artery from the pulmonary artery (ALCAPA). Note the dilated right coronary artery and left coronary artery which fills retrograde via collaterals and drains to the pulmonary artery.

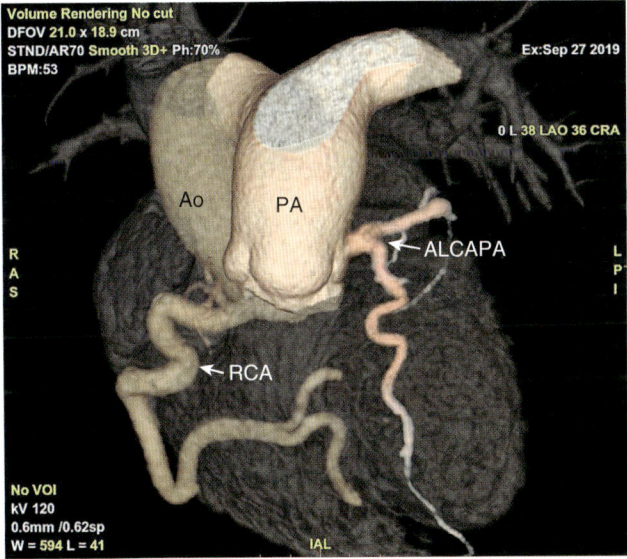

FIGURE 82.40 Volume rendered image from a gated CT angiogram from a patient with anomalous left coronary artery from the pulmonary artery (ALCAPA). Note the dilated right coronary artery (RCA) arising from the aorta (Ao) and the ALCAPA draining into the pulmonary artery (PA).

native PA to create a systemic outflow from the RV, opening of the atrial septum, and providing pulmonary blood flow from one of several surgical shunt options.

Double inlet LV is an anatomic single ventricle lesion in which both AV valves are in continuity with the LV. The sinus of the RV does not form, though there remains an infundibular outflow tract connected by a bulboventricular foramen to the LV. The ventricles can be D- or L-looped, and the great vessels can be in normal (S), D-transposed, or L-transposed position, so that either the aorta or the PA can be related to the hypoplastic infundibular outflow. These relationships help determine decision making for initial palliative surgery. Double inlet/double outlet RV is a very rare example of true anatomic single ventricle disease, in which there is an embryonic RV associated with both AV valves and both systemic and pulmonary outlets, with no vestigial LV.

There are several other congenital defects that include two ventricles, but sometimes require single ventricle palliation, depending on details of the anatomy. Complete AV canal defect can be unbalanced; that is, the common valve can sit nearly entirely over one or the other ventricle, leaving a hypoplastic second ventricle and no option for a two-ventricle type of repair. Transposition of the great vessels can be complicated by other lesions such as VSDs and pulmonary outflow obstruction. A two-ventricle repair may not be achievable if the pulmonary valve is not usable as a "neo-aortic" valve and if a surgical pathway cannot be constructed from the LV through the VSD to the native aortic valve. Straddling of AV valves can also complicate a two-ventricle repair in this lesion. In these cases, an eventual Fontan palliation may be pursued.

Surgical Palliation

This section will not discuss patients who had single ventricle heart disease but have since received a heart transplant. Nearly all adult congenital patients with single ventricle heart disease will have received what is widely known as a Fontan palliation (Fig. 82.41), after the original surgical description by Drs. Fontan and Baudet in 1971.[94] This is generally reached in staged palliation, with the ultimate result of all systemic venous return bypassing the heart to flow passively directly to the pulmonary circulation, while the single functional ventricle acts as the systemic pump. There are several versions of the Fontan circulation, which will be discussed below.

The current surgical approach often includes neonatal surgery to achieve a stable systemic outflow and balance between systemic and pulmonary circulation to provide adequate oxygenation but protect the pulmonary circulation from pressure or volume overload, followed by a superior cavopulmonary anastomosis later in the first year of life, after which pulmonary circulation is provided by direct, passive flow of the superior systemic venous return to the lungs. This is ultimately followed by the Fontan procedure, which depending on version of procedure and individual center preference, is typically performed sometime between 18 months and 4 years of age. It is important to have some understanding of the stages of palliation, as some patients are unable to proceed down this pathway due to problems such as increased PVR, and rarely may present in adulthood with physiology of an aortopulmonary shunt or superior cavopulmonary anastomosis, typically with severe cyanosis.

The details of the Fontan palliation have gone through multiple iterations. The type of operation seen in an individual patient may have implications related to the likelihood of various complications in adulthood. The three most commonly seen versions of the Fontan circulation in adults include the extracardiac Fontan, the lateral tunnel Fontan, and direct right atrial to PA anastomosis, which is closer to the original described operation and has fallen out of favor. There

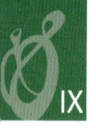

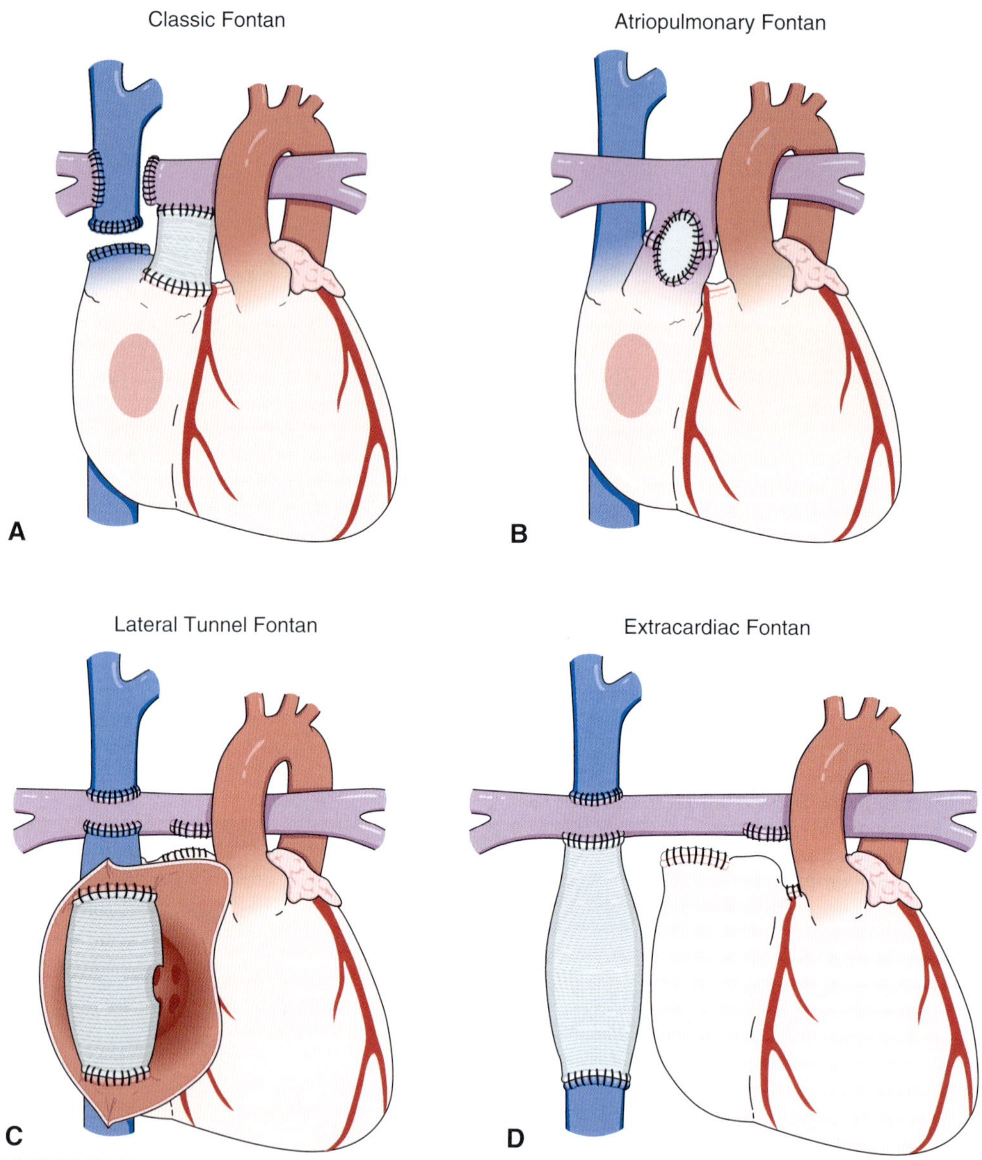

FIGURE 82.41 Diagrammatic representation of the various types of Fontan surgeries. **A**, The classic style Fontan, which consists of a conduit from the inferior vena cava to the left pulmonary artery and a classic right Glenn procedure (superior vena cava to the right pulmonary artery). **B**, The atriopulmonary connection has been largely abandoned due to dilation of the right atrium predisposing to thrombosis and atrial arrhythmias. **C**, Lateral tunnel is widely used in part due to the ease of creating a fenestration in this type. **D**, Extracardiac conduits are often used as it does not create extensive atrial sutures and may be performed off bypass. (Modified from Libby P. *Essential Atlas of Cardiovascular Disease.* New York: Springer; 2009.)

to the right atrial appendage. This often led to marked dilation of the RA due to exposure to chronic high pressure.

Clinical Features and Diagnostic Testing

The adult with a Fontan circulation may frequently present with dyspnea with activity, from exercise to basic activities of daily living. There is inherently less ability to augment stroke volume with demand in this circulation, and many patients may have chronotropic incompetence by adulthood as well. Palpitations are also a frequent complaint. Other symptoms may be related to end-organ damage from long-term impaired cardiac output.

There can be many findings on exam that are important to assess. Signs of chronic cyanosis such as clubbing of the digits may be present in patients with a Fontan, and are near-ubiquitous in adults with single ventricle disease who do not have a Fontan operation. Cardiac exam will show a single S1 and S2 on auscultation. Rhythm may reveal a rapid intra-atrial reentrant tachycardia or premature atrial or ventricular contractions. Any murmurs heard are typically pathologic, potentially related to AV or semilunar valve regurgitation or another inefficiency of the intracardiac circulation. A patient with an aortopulmonary shunt will have a continuous murmur. A small percentage of patients will have dextrocardia detected on exam. Hepatomegaly is frequently observed, and may be accompanied by ascites. Lower extremity edema is less common.

The routine care of the patient with a Fontan circulation includes considered use of cardiac-specific testing as well as monitoring for complications related to other organs. Routine history and physical exam should be performed at least yearly, more frequently for active problems.

Electrocardiography is routine with yearly clinic follow-up, as well as in the assessment for patients presenting with palpitations or other signs of arrhythmia.

Imaging assessment with either echocardiography or CMR is considered a Class I indication annually for this patient population, with CMR performed in lieu of echo typically every 2 to 3 years.[3] Echocardiography is useful for assessment of ventricular size and function, valve stenosis, and regurgitation, and the Fontan pathway and presence of a fenestration. Acoustic windows can limit the usefulness of echocardiography in this patient population. CMR also visualizes ventricular function and is a superior option for quantification of right ventricular size and function in particular (Fig. 82.42). Valve regurgitation can be quantified. CMR also provides superior visualization of the complete Fontan pathway and branch pulmonary arteries, including flow assessment for differential pulmonary blood flow and aorto-pulmonary or veno-venous collateralization. Placement of stainless-steel embolization coils in the past can severely limit CMR visualization due to magnetic susceptibility artifact. CT scanning overcomes artifacts related to coils and other implants and can also be used to provide excellent visualization of

are some other rarely seen versions of this circulation with variations in how the systemic venous blood is routed to the pulmonary circulation.

The extracardiac Fontan is currently in wide use. Surgically, this consists of a conduit placed outside of the heart, routing the IVC and hepatic veins directly to the pulmonary arteries. This is most typically preceded by a superior cavopulmonary anastomosis commonly known as a bidirectional Glenn operation, which is an end-to-side anastomosis of the SVC to the right pulmonary artery (RPA) (this can also be done on the left in the presence of a left SVC).

The lateral tunnel Fontan has become less prevalent but was the most common version of the Fontan operation and as such, is seen in many adults with single ventricle heart disease. In this operation the IVC and hepatic flow is tunneled through the RA, usually using the atrial wall as part of the tunnel, and anastomosed directly to the pulmonary arteries. This operation was often performed with a fenestration in the wall of the tunnel, enabling a small right-to-left shunt and mild systemic desaturation.

Direct right atrial to PA anastomosis was usually used specifically for patients with tricuspid atresia. In this version of the Fontan operation, the atrial septum was closed and the pulmonary arteries anastomosed

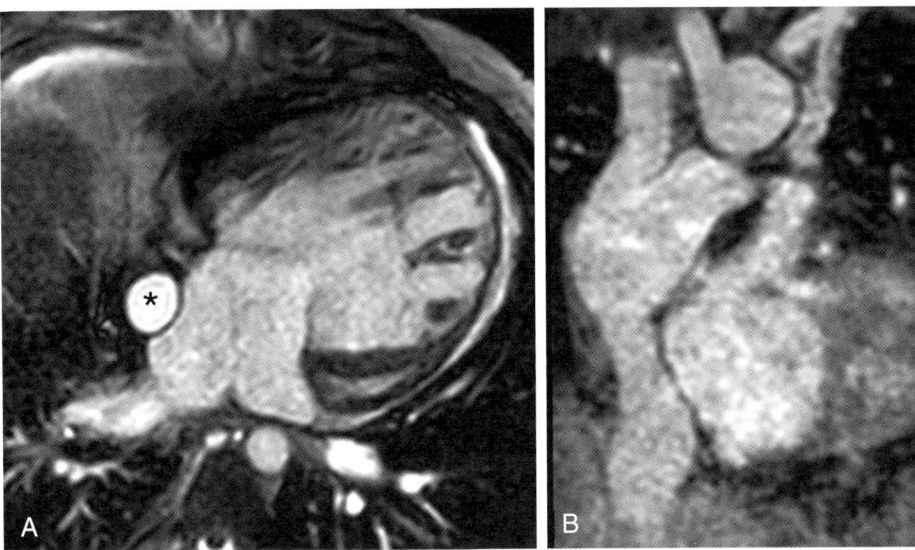

FIGURE 82.42 A, Still image from a cine steady state free precession MRI sequence in the horizontal long axis view; hypoplastic left heart syndrome s/p lateral tunnel Fontan. The right ventricle (RV) is dilated; the tricuspid valve is open at the beginning of diastole. There is a severely hypoplastic left ventricle seen. The Fontan pathway *(asterisk)* is at the rightward aspect of the right atrium; no fenestration is seen in this plane. **B,** 3-D steady state free precession image in the coronal oblique projection showing the Fontan pathway with inferior vena cava (IVC) and superior vena cava (SVC) draining into the lateral tunnel; the pulmonary arteries in this patient arise from the pathway to the left of the SVC after a previous hemi-Fontan procedure.

the Fontan pathway and pulmonary arteries, with less physiologic information compared to CMR.

Exercise testing is recommended every 1 to 3 years depending on severity of an individual patient's disease state.[3] This can comprise full cardiopulmonary exercise testing or a 6-minute walk test. Trends in exercise ability over time can be useful for medical management.

Cardiac catheterization provides the best assessment of intracardiac and Fontan pathway pressures and PVR. Patients undergoing Fontan revision surgery should have a pre-operative catheterization. For symptomatic patients, cardiac catheterization is considered a Class IIa indication if imaging does not provide adequate information.[3]

Basic metabolic profile testing, bNPPT/INR, total cholesterol, and complete blood count can be performed every 1 to 2 years and are considered a class IIa indication for Fontan patients. Testing provides greater information regarding liver and kidney function, as well as changes in hematocrit that can be related to chronic cyanosis or iron deficiency.

Liver ultrasound or MRI is indicated to assess the status of FALD. Expert consensus recommends hepatic imaging every 1 to 2 years.[95]

Long-Term Outcomes and Complications

Overall 20-year survival following the Fontan operation in two large series was 61% and 74%.[96,97] Survival has improved over time, and it is estimated that current 30-year survival for a child newly receiving a Fontan operation is approximately 85%. Complications are common and varied.

Ventricular Dilation, Dysfunction, and Heart Failure

The development of ventricular dilation in the Fontan patient is a marker for bad outcomes.[98] Dilation can result directly from pump failure and adaptation to decreased ejection fraction, but more commonly from lesions that volume-load the single ventricle. The single morphologic RV has been associated with decreased long-term survival, often with AV valve regurgitation as the precipitating and progressive lesion leading to single RV dilation and dysfunction.[28] Other volume loading lesions that can lead to progressive ventricular dilation, dysfunction, and failure include aortic or neo-aortic regurgitation and extensive aortopulmonary collateral vessels. CMR is an excellent imaging modality for the quantification of ventricular size and function, as well as for identifying potential etiologies for ventricular dilation.

Failure of the Fontan circulation can result from numerous hemodynamic insults. Primary pump failure may be a common final pathway resulting from valve regurgitation, volume overload from collateral flow, or chronic myocardial damage which could be related to multiple operations on cardiopulmonary bypass during childhood, chronic hypoxia in some patients, or coronary artery insufficiency. In addition, the nature of the Fontan physiology is such that increasing pressure in the Fontan pathway can result from increased ventricular diastolic pressure, increased atrial pressure related to AV valve regurgitation, or increased PVR. Chronically high (>20 mm Hg) pressure in the Fontan pathway will eventually lead to other complications. There is interest in the use of pulmonary vasodilators in patients with a Fontan; there are some data suggesting this can improve exercise performance but no data suggesting changes in mortality or serious complications.[99]

Cardiac transplantation is ultimately indicated for failure of the Fontan circulation that is not amenable to medical or other interventional therapy. This can be related to pump failure, to high pressures in the Fontan circuit, or to other complications discussed below, such as FALD or protein-losing enteropathy (PLE). Importantly, transplantation of a Fontan patient is complex. The anatomy of systemic and pulmonary veins and arteries can vary widely, leading to challenging surgical situations for anastomosis of the donor heart to the recipient blood vessels. This requires a surgeon experienced in transplant of CHD patients. Physiology can also lead to complications, as Fontan patients for whom transplantation is indicated often have numerous comorbidities. These challenges lead to worse outcomes compared to standard transplantation. A recent analysis of national discharge data showed far higher in-hospital mortality for adult Fontan transplant patients compared to other adult transplants, 26.3% versus 5.3%.[100]

Arrhythmia

The development of atrial tachyarrhythmias in the Fontan patient is frequent. Notably, this has changed with time as newer surgical approaches to the Fontan have significantly altered the substrate for generating intra-atrial re-entrant tachycardia. The progression from atriopulmonary to lateral tunnel to extra-cardiac Fontan has brought benefit in a reduction in incidence of atrial arrhythmia, which was one of the driving factors in the development of these newer techniques. Still, periodic home Holter monitoring is routine for these patients. For patients with an atriopulmonary Fontan, the development of arrhythmia is nearly ubiquitous by the third decade of life.[101] IART is most common, but atrial fibrillation is also seen. The lateral tunnel Fontan improved substantially on this incidence, with a 15-year freedom from atrial tachyarrhythmia of 83%, and the extracardiac Fontan more so, with a 15-year freedom of 92%.[102] Need for pacemaker, usually for sinoatrial node dysfunction, is not infrequent. However, this too is more common in the atriopulmonary Fontan, with incidence of 21.5% at late follow-up, compared to 11% for lateral tunnel and 3.5% for extracardiac, meaning that the overall incidence will likely decrease as the newer forms of the operation progressively account for greater percentages of the adult Fontan population.[103]

Cyanosis

The Fontan circulation ideally includes complete separation of the pulmonary and systemic circulations. Therefore, cyanosis in the Fontan patient is a concerning finding. There are several anatomic factors that can lead to cyanosis. The lateral tunnel Fontan often includes a surgical fenestration to allow pulmonary to systemic shunting to relieve pressure on the pulmonary circulation. These fenestrations often close spontaneously, or may be closed with trans-catheter device placement. The adult with a patent fenestration, or other leak in a lateral tunnel Fontan baffle, will have a degree of cyanosis, depending on the size of the shunt. Increasing cyanosis with a stable fenestration or baffle leak could suggest an increase in PVR. This diagnosis can often be made by TTE. If acoustic windows are limiting, TEE can often be diagnostic.

Patients may present with cyanosis due to the development of systemic vein to pulmonary vein collateral vessels. These also form in part as a response to abnormal pressure within the systemic veins. These collateral vessels can become markedly dilated and tortuous. They can sometimes be diagnosed by echocardiography, but this can be difficult. MRI or CT can noninvasively diagnose veno-venous collaterals, and MRI has the added benefit of flow analysis to measure degree of shunting. If indicated, veno-venous collaterals can often be closed with embolization coils or other devices by catheterization.

Cyanosis in the Fontan patient can also be due to formation of pulmonary arteriovenous malformations (AVMs). These are most likely to occur when there is an imbalance of systemic venous blood to the lungs such that hepatic venous effluent goes only to one lung. The existence of a "hepatic factor" that inhibits AVM formation has been widely postulated, although not identified; the lung that does not receive flow of hepatic venous blood is at risk of AVM formation. Pulmonary AVMs can be diagnosed by echocardiography with agitated saline contrast. There is typically rapid return of contrast via the pulmonary veins to the LA, within 2 to 3 beats of the contrast arriving in the Fontan pathway. Localization of AVMs to the left or right lung can be accomplished in the catheterization lab, with direct injection of agitated saline into the LPA and RPA with simultaneous echo visualization of the heart. Treatment is challenging. A surgical revision of the Fontan pathway can help reroute hepatic venous blood to the affected lung.

Protein-Losing Enteropathy and Plastic Bronchitis

PLE is a severe complication of the Fontan, carrying high levels of morbidity and significant mortality, although the latter has improved over time. It is difficult to cure and is typically managed as a chronic disease with acute-on-chronic exacerbations. In PLE, protein is lost into the intestinal lumen, probably via abnormal lymphatic channels. This results in reduced serum oncotic pressure and systemic edema, as well as complications from the specific proteins lost, such as immune deficiency from loss of immunoglobulin. The etiology is not precisely known, but likely includes components of high systemic venous pressure, chronic inflammation, and chronic low cardiac output. There are no clear methods to predict which Fontan patients will develop this complication. This can be diagnosed clinically, with confirmation by stool alpha-1 antitrypsin levels. Treatment of exacerbations is largely symptomatic, consisting largely of albumin infusions combined with diuresis to repair fluid imbalance.[95] Other medications used include enteral corticosteroids for direct enteral anti-inflammatory properties, spironolactone, perhaps as another anti-inflammatory agent or as a diuretic. Unfractionated heparin is sometimes effective but not consistently so. More definitive treatment is invasive, with some effect of fenestration creation, although this leads to increased cyanosis, various direct interventions on the lymphatic system, or ultimately, heart transplantation.

Plastic bronchitis has a lower prevalence than PLE. This condition is similarly related to lymphatic abnormalities, leading to protein drainage into the airways and the formation of bronchial casts. These are often coughed up by the patient but can lead to acute airway decompensation. Treatment focuses on pulmonary toilet, including inhaled tissue plasminogen activator and percussive vests. Like PLE, the Fontan circulation is also assessed and invasive treatment to improve hemodynamics may be helpful, also including heart transplantation.

Abnormalities of the Aorta and Pulmonary Arteries

Many patients with a Fontan circulation had one or more interventions during childhood on their pulmonary arteries and/or their aorta. There may be residual or progressive lesions in those vessels as a result. Many single ventricle patients, particularly single RV, require aortic reconstruction as neonates. They may present as adults with aortic coarctation or aneurysm. Diagnosis is typically first made with echocardiography, but CT or MRI can be more definitive at times and is particularly important for surgical planning. Treatment of recurrent coarctation is usually by balloon angioplasty and possible stenting in the catheterization laboratory. Aneurysm of the ascending aorta or transverse arch typically requires surgical repair, which can carry considerable morbidity and mortality. PA pathology often comprises discrete narrowings or diffuse hypoplasia. Patients who required aortic arch reconstruction are at higher risk for diffuse hypoplasia of the LPA. Echo imaging of the pulmonary arteries can be technically challenging due to limited acoustic windows. Most often, screening CT or MRI is used to make these diagnoses. MRI has the added benefit of calculating differential antegrade pulmonary blood flow. Discrete lesions can be addressed in the catheterization laboratory, usually with stenting. Diffusely hypoplastic vessels may not have a clear interventional option.

Fontan-Associated Liver Disease

Hepatic disease is eventually ubiquitous in Fontan patients. This is primarily related to a lifetime of elevated central venous pressure to the mid-teens and higher, leading to passive congestion and eventually cardiac cirrhosis. In adults who had surgery in the 1970s and 1980s, this may be compounded by chronic hepatitis C infection. Additionally, the Fontan patient often has impaired cardiac output and is in a chronic inflammatory state, all of which may lead to hepatic disease. Serum biomarkers are often not specifically diagnostic. Synthetic function is typically preserved until late stage of disease, and transaminases and gamma-glutamyl transferases (GGT) may often be mildly elevated. Regular imaging with ultrasound or MRI is indicated every 1 to 2 years. Hepatocellular carcinoma is a rare complication of FALD and can be suspected based on serum screening for alpha-fetoprotein and diagnosed with imaging. There is increasing experience with combined heart-liver transplantation, with small single center studies showing good survival.[104,105]

PULMONARY HYPERTENSION AND EISENMENGER SYNDROME

Demographics and Prognosis

More than 5% of ACHD patients have concurrent PH, as defined by a mean pulmonary arterial pressure of greater than 20 mm Hg.[106] ACHD patients with PH have more symptoms, worse exercise capacity, and are more likely to be hospitalized than ACHD patients without PH. Mortality is increased in ACHD patients who have PH. While PH can complicate almost any form of ACHD, it is most common in patients with shunt lesions, late repair, Down syndrome, and female gender.

Classification

Several distinct mechanisms contribute to PH in patients with CHD. It is critical to define the pathophysiology of PH in order to appropriately evaluate and treat the patient. The 6th World Symposium on Pulmonary Hypertension updated the classification of PH in patients with CHD (Table 82.13). In most cases, PH can be separated into pre-capillary and post-capillary etiologies, although mixed and complex forms exist. Pre-capillary PH (or PAH) is characterized by mPAP greater than 20 mm Hg, pulmonary capillary wedge pressure (PCWP) ≤ 15 mm Hg, and an elevated transpulmonary gradient (TPG) and PVR ≥ 3 Wood units (WU). PAH is most commonly seen in patients with shunt lesions and results from adverse pulmonary vascular remodeling characterized by vasoconstriction, smooth muscle hypertrophy, and intimal proliferation which is histopathologically indistinguishable from other forms of WHO Group 1 PAH (see Chapter 88). In its most severe form, pre-capillary PAH results in markedly elevated PVR, shunt reversal, and Eisenmenger syndrome (see below). Post-capillary PH is characterized by mPAP greater than 20 mm Hg with an elevated PCWP (>15 mm Hg) and a normal TPG and normal PVR less than 3 WU. Post-capillary PH is caused by left heart disease such as ventricular dysfunction, inflow or outflow obstruction, or severe regurgitant lesions. Often patients have overlapping etiologies of PH with combined pre- and post-capillary PH with elevations in PCWP, TPG, and PVR.

TABLE 82.13 Classification of Pulmonary Hypertension in Patients With Congenital Heart Disease

GROUPING ACCORDING TO SIXTH WORLD SYMPOSIUM ON PULMONARY HYPERTENSION	SUBGROUP
Group 1	(A) Eisenmenger syndrome
	(B) PAH associated with systemic-to-pulmonary shunt
	(C) PAH and coincidental/small defect
	(D) PAH following corrective surgery/defect closure
Group 2	Left heart disease (e.g., systemic ventricular dysfunction, valve disease)
	Pulmonary vein stenosis
	Isolated
	Associated (BPD, prematurity)
	Cor triatriatum
	Obstructed total anomalous pulmonary venous return
	Mitral/aortic stenosis (including supra-/subvalvular)
	Coarctation of the aorta
Group 3	BPD
	Lung disease (e.g., restrictive lung defect)
	OSA/nocturnal hypoventilation
Group 4	PH due to pulmonary artery obstructions
	Congenital
	Related to previous surgery
	Related to other conditions (e.g., sarcoidosis)
Group 5 (complex CHD)	Segmental PH
	Isolated pulmonary artery of ductal origin
	Absent pulmonary artery
	Pulmonary atresia with VSD and MAPCAs
	Hemitruncus
	Other
	Single ventricle
	Unoperated
	Operated
	Scimitar syndrome

BPD, Bronchopulmonary dysplasia; *CHD*, congenital heart disease; *MAPCA*, major aortopulmonary collateral artery; *PAH*, pulmonary arterial hypertension; *PH*, pulmonary hypertension; *VSD*, ventricular septal defect.
Based on the updated clinical classification of pulmonary hypertension from the *Proceedings of the 6th World Symposium on Pulmonary Hypertension*. Modified from Constantine A, Dimopoulos K, Opotowsky AR. Congenital heart disease and pulmonary hypertension. *Cardiol Clin.* 2020:38(3):445–456.

Patients with ACHD and suspected PH require invasive cardiac catheterization to define the severity and mechanism of the patient's PH. In patients with open shunt lesions, a "shunt run" is required and the systemic and pulmonary blood flow must be calculated separately in order to accurately calculate resistances. Using standard sampling techniques will lead to spurious results for PVR calculations. Patients with CHD and pre-capillary PH should be managed in conjunction with a PH specialist.

Eisenmenger Syndrome

Eisenmenger syndrome occurs when patients with a left-to-right shunt develop irreversible pulmonary vascular injury and severe PAH in response to pulmonary over-circulation. When PVR surpasses SVR shunt direction reverses leading to cyanosis. Eisenmenger syndrome is most common in patients with large unrepaired post-tricuspid shunts such as AVSDs, VSD, or PDA in which cases Eisenmenger syndrome develops during the first few years of life. Eisenmenger syndrome can also exist in patients with complex intracardiac anatomy and is commonly seen in patients with truncus arteriosus, if unrepaired. A minority of patients (<10%) with unrepaired pre-tricuspid shunts, such as an ASD, also develop Eisenmenger syndrome. In these cases, Eisenmenger syndrome typically develops in adulthood. It is unknown why some patients with pre-tricuspid shunts develop Eisenmenger syndrome, but it is more common in women and other genetic or environmental factors may contribute. Due to improved diagnosis and treatment of CHD, Eisenmenger syndrome is rare in high-income nations but remains prevalent in regions where access to congenital heart surgery is limited.

Eisenmenger syndrome is a multi-organ systemic disease (Table 82.14). Chronic cyanosis induces a secondary erythrocytosis which leads to iron deficiency and hyperviscosity.[107] Hematologic dysregulation results in predisposition to both hemorrhage and thrombosis. Patients are therefore at risk for hemoptysis but also at risk for paradoxical embolism and cerebrovascular accidents.

Clinical Features

Patients with Eisenmenger syndrome demonstrate central cyanosis and digital clubbing (Fig. 82.43). Physical examination findings and laboratory abnormalities common in Eisenmenger syndrome can be found in Table 82.15.

TABLE 82.14 Noncardiac Complications of Eisenmenger Syndrome

Hematologic	Erythrocytosis
	Iron deficiency
	Leukopenia
	Thrombocytopenia
	Hyperviscosity
Rheumatologic	Hyperuricemia
	Gout
	Arthritis
	Myalgias
Infectious	Endocarditis
	Pneumonia
	Intracranial abscesses
Pulmonary	Hemoptysis

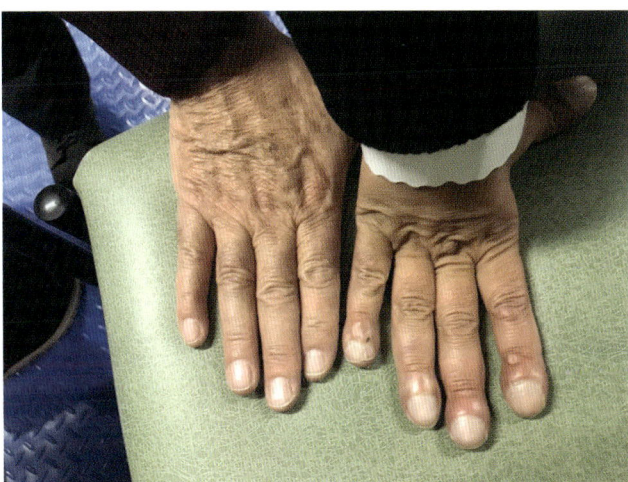

FIGURE 82.43 Cyanosis and digital clubbing in a patient with Eisenmenger syndrome *(right side of image)* compared to a healthy family member *(left side of image)*.

TABLE 82.15 Physical and laboratory findings typical for Eisenmenger syndrome

Vital Signs	Hypoxemia
Physical Exam	Central cyanosis
	Hypertrophic osteoarthropathy (digital clubbing)
	Prominent jugular venous a-wave
	Right parasternal heave or lift
	Loud P2
	S3 or S4
	High-pitched diastolic murmur of pulmonary regurgitation
	Systolic murmurs may be faint or absent
Laboratory	Erythrocytosis
	Iron deficiency
	Thrombocytopenia
	Leukopenia
	Elevated BNP
	Hyperuricemia
Chest radiograph	Dilation of pulmonary arteries
	Peripheral pulmonary artery pruning
	Right atrial and right ventricular enlargement
ECG	Right atrial enlargement
	Right axis deviation
	Biventricular hypertrophy
	ST-T wave abnormalities
Transthoracic echocardiography	Right ventricular enlargement
	Right ventricular hypertrophy
	Pulmonary artery enlargement
	Pulmonary hypertension
	Large shunt defect with low-velocity flow; PDA can be difficult to visualize

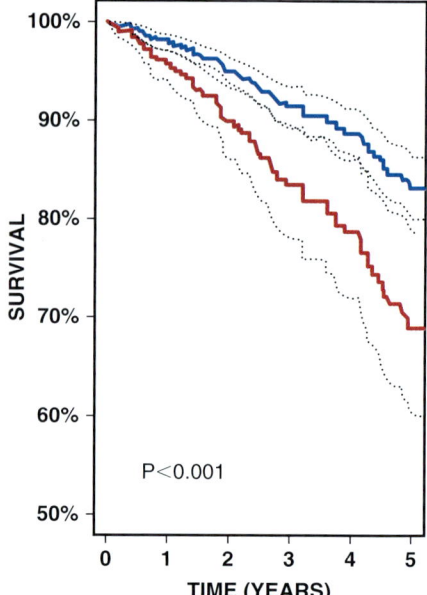

FIGURE 82.44 Survival by underlying shunt type in patients with Eisenmenger syndrome. Adjusted survival curves for patients with pre-tricuspid lesions *(red)* and post-tricuspid or complex shunts *(blue)* with 95% confidence intervals. (From Kempny A. Predictors of death in contemporary adult patients with Eisenmenger syndrome: a multicenter study. *Circulation.* 2017;135[15]:1432–1440.)

TABLE 82.16 Conditions to Avoid in Eisenmenger Syndrome

CONDITION TO AVOID	RATIONALE
Volume depletion	May worsen hyperviscosity
Excessive heat	May worsen hyperviscosity
Nonessential noncardiac surgery	High risk of operative morbidity or mortality. Anesthesia should be provided by cardiac anesthesiologist familiar with Eisenmenger syndrome.
Iron deficiency	May worsen hyperviscosity. Worsens symptoms. Patients should be tested for iron deficiency and iron should be replaced judiciously, with frequent monitoring.
Routine phlebotomy	Increases risk of stroke. Worsens iron deficiency. Phlebotomy should be reserved for symptomatic patients with adequate iron stores when symptoms are refractory to hydration.
Endocardial pacing	Increases risk of stroke
Pregnancy	High risk of maternal mortality (>30%). High risk of spontaneous abortion or miscarriage
Estrogen containing contraception	Increases risk of thrombotic complication.

Exercise capacity is markedly reduced in patients with Eisenmenger syndrome, worse than all other forms of ACHD. Symptoms may be nonspecific and include fatigue, dyspnea, arthralgias, chest pain, syncope, headache, hemoptysis, or stroke.

The prognosis of patients with Eisenmenger is variable, but better than other forms of severe PAH. Death during childhood is rare but becomes much more common during the 4th decade of life or later.[108] In a large multi-center study of patients with Eisenmenger syndrome including 1098 patients, on multivariable analysis, mortality was higher in patients with pre-tricuspid shunts, older age, lower resting oxygen saturations, non-sinus rhythm, and pericardial effusions (Fig. 82.44).[108] As with other forms of PAH, poor functional status and reduced 6-minute walk distance are also predictors of mortality. The most common causes of death include sudden death, congestive heart failure, and pulmonary hemorrhage. Patients are at risk from death during noncardiac surgery or infections, particularly brain abscesses. Antibiotic prophylaxis is required in all patients with Eisenmenger syndrome.

Management of Eisenmenger Syndrome

Patients with Eisenmenger syndrome should be managed at a comprehensive ACHD center with expertise in both CHD and PH. Patients should be seen at least annually with imaging and laboratory assessment. Much of the management of Eisenmenger syndrome is supportive. Patients should be counseled to avoid scenarios which are known to worsen outcomes in patients with Eisenmenger syndrome (Table 82.16). Specifically, patients should be counseled against volume depletion, extreme exercise, and extreme heat, as these can worsen hyperviscosity.

Pregnancy is absolutely contraindicated in Eisenmenger syndrome as it is associated with very high levels of maternal mortality (>30%) and fetal loss.[109] Effective non-estrogen containing contraception is required for women with Eisenmenger; options include intrauterine devices (IUDs), Depo-Provera injections, and progesterone eluting subcutaneous implantations (e.g., Nexplanon). Surgical sterilization is less commonly performed with the advent of less invasive contraception options. If pregnancy occurs, early termination should be encouraged.

Most patients with Eisenmenger syndrome develop a secondary erythrocytosis as an adaptive response to chronic cyanosis. The degree of erythrocytosis is proportional to the degree of cyanosis. Hematocrit greater than 60% is common, but in the compensated state rarely leads to hyperviscosity. Routine phlebotomy in asymptomatic patients is contraindicated as it increases the risk of stroke.

For patients who are experiencing symptoms suggestive of hyperviscosity (headache, lethargy, visual disturbances, paresthesia, myalgias) iron deficiency should first be excluded. Iron deficiency is common in patients with Eisenmenger syndrome and symptoms overlap with those of hyperviscosity. Volume depletion should also be excluded and corrected; this is usually effective at relieving the symptoms of hyperviscosity. In patients who are iron replete and volume replete but still have moderate or severe symptoms of hyperviscosity there is a limited role for therapeutic phlebotomy. Phlebotomy should be accompanied by simultaneous volume expansion with saline and frequent hemodynamic monitoring.

Pulmonary vasodilators should be considered in patients with Eisenmenger syndrome. The BREATH-5 randomized double-blind placebo-controlled trial demonstrated that bosentan improved exercise capacity and hemodynamics compared to placebo in patients with Eisenmenger syndrome to ASD, VSD, or PDA. However, the more recent MAESTRO trial did not show similar benefit with the use of macitentan[110] in a more heterogenous group of Eisenmenger patients. Epidemiologic data and smaller trials suggest benefit from sildenafil in Eisenmenger syndrome. Calcium channel blockers should not be used due to their negative inotropic effects.

Patients with Eisenmenger syndrome and advanced symptoms refractory to medical therapy can be considered for combined heart-lung transplantation or lung transplantation with repair of the cardiac defect. Outcomes in Eisenmenger syndrome are comparable to combined heart-lung transplantation in other conditions. A recent multinational study identified 63 patients who underwent heart-lung or lung transplantation for Eisenmenger syndrome. Early mortality was 11% and 15-year survival following transplantation was 41%.[111]

REFERENCES
General Considerations
1. Marelli AJ, Ionescu-Ittu R, Mackie AS, et al. Lifetime prevalence of congenital heart disease in the general population from 2000 to 2010. *Circulation*. 2014;130:749–756.
2. Gilboa SM, Devine OJ, Kucik JE, et al. Congenital heart defects in the United States: estimating the magnitude of the affected population in 2010. *Circulation*. 2016;134:101–109.
3. Stout KK, Daniels CJ, Aboulhosn JA, et al. 2018 AHA/ACC guideline for the management of adults with congenital heart disease: executive summary: a report of the American College of cardiology/American heart association Task Force on clinical practice guidelines. *J Am Coll Cardiol*. 2018.
4. Mylotte D, Pilote L, Ionescu-Ittu R, et al. Specialized adult congenital heart disease care: the impact of policy on mortality. *Circulation*. 2014;129:1804–1812.
5. Baumgartner H, Bonhoeffer P, De Groot NM, et al. ESC Guidelines for the management of grown-up congenital heart disease (new version 2010). *Eur Heart J*. 2010;31:2915–2957.
6. Fernandes SM, Marelli A, Hile DM, Daniels CJ. Access and delivery of adult congenital heart disease care in the United States: quality-driven team-based care. *Cardiol Clin*. 2020;38:295–304.
7. Mackie AS, Rempel GR, Kovacs AH, et al. Transition intervention for adolescents with congenital heart disease. *J Am Coll Cardiol*. 2018;71:1768–1777.
8. Sachdeva R, Valente AM, Armstrong AK, et al. ACC/AHA/ASE/HRS/ISACHD/SCAI/SCCT/SCMR/SOPE 2020 appropriate use criteria for multimodality imaging during the follow-up care of patients with congenital heart disease: a report of the American College of Cardiology Solution Set Oversight Committee and Appropriate Use Criteria Task Force, American Heart Association, American Society of Echocardiography, Heart Rhythm Society, International Society for Adult Congenital Heart Disease, Society for Cardiovascular Angiography and Interventions, Society of Cardiovascular Computed Tomography, Society for Cardiovascular Magnetic Resonance, and Society of Pediatric Echocardiography. *J Am Coll Cardiol*. 2020;75:657–703.

Long-Term Considerations
9. Lui GK, Saidi A, Bhatt AB, et al. Diagnosis and management of noncardiac complications in adults with congenital heart disease: a scientific statement from the American heart association. *Circulation*. 2017;136:e348–e392.
10. Diller GP, Kempny A, Alonso-Gonzalez R, et al. Survival prospects and circumstances of death in contemporary adult congenital heart disease patients under follow-up at a large tertiary centre. *Circulation*. 2015;132:2118–2125.
11. Bhatt AB, Rajabali A, He W, Benavidez OJ. High resource use among adult congenital heart surgery admissions in adult hospitals: risk factors and association with death and comorbidities. *Congenit Heart Dis*. 2015;10:13–20.
12. Opotowsky AR, Carazo M, Singh MN, et al. Creatinine versus cystatin C to estimate glomerular filtration rate in adults with congenital heart disease: results of the Boston Adult Congenital Heart Disease Biobank. *Am Heart J*. 2019;214:142–155.
13. Wu FM, Kogon B, Earing MG, et al. Liver health in adults with Fontan circulation: a multicenter cross-sectional study. *J Thorac Cardiovasc Surg*. 2017;153:656–664.
14. Lanz J, Brophy JM, Therrien J, et al. Stroke in adults with congenital heart disease: incidence, cumulative risk, and predictors. *Circulation*. 2015;132:2385–2394.
15. Zaidi S, Brueckner M. Genetics and genomics of congenital heart disease. *Circ Res*. 2017;120:923–940.
16. Pierpont ME, Brueckner M, Chung WK, et al. Genetic basis for congenital heart disease: revisited: a scientific statement from the American heart association. *Circulation*. 2018;138:e653–e711.
17. Gelb BD. History of our understanding of the causes of congenital heart disease. *Circ Cardiovasc Genet*. 2015;8:529–536.
18. Khairy P, Van Hare GF, Balaji S, et al. PACES/HRS expert consensus statement on the recognition and management of arrhythmias in adult congenital heart disease: developed in partnership between the Pediatric and Congenital Electrophysiology Society (PACES) and the Heart Rhythm Society (HRS). Endorsed by the governing bodies of PACES, HRS, the American College of Cardiology (ACC), the American Heart Association (AHA), the European Heart Rhythm Association (EHRA), the Canadian Heart Rhythm Society (CHRS), and the International Society for Adult Congenital Heart Disease (ISACHD). *Heart Rhythm*. 2014;11:e102–e165.
19. Labombarda F, Hamilton R, Shohoudi A, et al. Increasing prevalence of atrial fibrillation and permanent atrial arrhythmias in congenital heart disease. *J Am Coll Cardiol*. 2017;70:857–865.
20. Moore JP, Khairy P. Adults with congenital heart disease and arrhythmia management. *Cardiol Clin*. 2020;38:417–434.
21. Bouchardy J, Therrien J, Pilote L, et al. Atrial arrhythmias in adults with congenital heart disease. *Circulation*. 2009;120:1679–1686.
22. Masuda K, Ishizu T, Niwa K, et al. Increased risk of thromboembolic events in adult congenital heart disease patients with atrial tachyarrhythmias. *Int J Cardiol*. 2017;234:69–75.
23. Yang H, Bouma BJ, Dimopoulos K, et al. Non-vitamin K antagonist oral anticoagulants (NOACs) for thromboembolic prevention, are they safe in congenital heart disease? Results of a worldwide study. *Int J Cardiol*. 2020;299:123–130.
24. Vehmeijer JT, Brouwer TF, Limpens J, et al. Implantable cardioverter-defibrillators in adults with congenital heart disease: a systematic review and meta-analysis. *Eur Heart J*. 2016;37:1439–1448.
25. Burchill LJ, Gao L, Kovacs AH, et al. Hospitalization trends and health resource use for adult congenital heart disease-related heart failure. *J Am Heart Assoc*. 2018;7:e008775.
26. Videbaek J, Laursen HB, Olsen M, et al. Long-term nationwide follow-up study of simple congenital heart disease diagnosed in otherwise healthy children. *Circulation*. 2016;133:474–483.
27. Baggen VJ, van den Bosch AE, Eindhoven JA, et al. Prognostic value of N-terminal pro-B-type natriuretic peptide, troponin-T, and growth-differentiation factor 15 in adult congenital heart disease. *Circulation*. 2017;135:264–279.
28. Moon J, Shen L, Likosky DS, Sood V, et al. Relationship of ventricular morphology and atrioventricular valve function to long-term outcomes following fontan procedures. *J Am Coll Cardiol*. 2020;76:419–431.
29. Hebert A, Mikkelsen UR, Thilen U, et al. Bosentan improves exercise capacity in adolescents and adults after fontan operation: the TEMPO (Treatment with Endothelin Receptor Antagonist in Fontan Patients, a Randomized, Placebo-Controlled, Double-Blind Study Measuring Peak Oxygen Consumption) study. *Circulation*. 2014;130:2021–2030.
30. Moore JP, Cho D, Lin JP, et al. Implantation techniques and outcomes after cardiac resynchronization therapy for congenitally corrected transposition of the great arteries. *Heart Rhythm*. 2018;15(12):1808–1815.
31. Alshawabkeh LI, Hu N, Carter KD, et al. Wait-list outcomes for adults with congenital heart disease listed for heart transplantation in the U.S. *J Am Coll Cardiol*. 2016;68:908–917.
32. OPTN/UNOS Thoracic Organ Transplantation Committee. *Review Board (RB) Guidance for Adult Congenital Heart Disease (CHD) Exception Requests*; 2017.
33. Menachem JN, Lindenfeld J, Schlendorf K, et al. Center volume and post-transplant survival among adults with congenital heart disease. *J Heart Lung Transplant*. 2018;37:1351–1360.
34. Lund LH, Edwards LB, Dipchand AI, et al. The registry of the International Society for heart and lung transplantation: thirty-third adult heart transplantation report-2016; focus Theme: primary diagnostic indications for transplant. *J Heart Lung Transplant*. 2016;35:1158–1169.
35. Nguyen VP, Dolgner SJ, Dardas TF, et al. Improved outcomes of heart transplantation in adults with congenital heart disease receiving regionalized care. *J Am Coll Cardiol*. 2019;74:2908–2918.
36. VanderPluym CJ, Cedars A, Eghtesady P, et al. Outcomes following implantation of mechanical circulatory support in adults with congenital heart disease: an analysis of the Interagency Registry for Mechanically Assisted Circulatory Support (INTERMACS). *J Heart Lung Transplant*. 2018;37:89–99.
37. Schwerzmann M, Goossens E, Gallego P, et al. Recommendations for advance care planning in adults with congenital heart disease: a position paper from the ESC Working group of adult congenital heart disease, the Association of Cardiovascular Nursing and Allied Professions (ACNAP), the European Association for Palliative Care (EAPC), and the International Society for Adult Congenital Heart Disease (ISACHD). *Eur Heart J*. 2020.
38. Kuijpers JM, Mulder BJ. Aortopathies in adult congenital heart disease and genetic aortopathy syndromes: management strategies and indications for surgery. *Heart*. 2017;103:952–966.
39. Lopez L, Colan SD, Frommelt PC, et al. Recommendations for quantification methods during the performance of a pediatric echocardiogram: a report from the pediatric measurements writing group of the American Society of echocardiography pediatric and congenital heart disease council. *J Am Soc Echocardiogr*. 2010;23:465–495; quiz 576-7.
40. Tutarel O, Alonso-Gonzalez R, Montanaro C, et al. Infective endocarditis in adults with congenital heart disease remains a lethal disease. *Heart*. 2018;104:161–165.
41. Kuijpers JM, Koolbergen DR, Groenink M, et al. Incidence, risk factors, and predictors of infective endocarditis in adult congenital heart disease: focus on the use of prosthetic material. *Eur Heart J*. 2017;38:2048–2056.
42. Silversides CK, Grewal J, Mason J, et al. Pregnancy outcomes in women with heart disease: the CARPREG II study. *J Am Coll Cardiol*. 2018;71:2419–2430.
43. Regitz-Zagrosek V, Roos-Hesselink JW, Bauersachs J, et al. 2018 ESC Guidelines for the management of cardiovascular diseases during pregnancy. *Eur Heart J*. 2018;39:3165–3241.
44. Stout KK, Daniels CJ, Aboulhosn JA, et al. 2018 AHA/ACC guideline for the management of adults with congenital heart disease: a report of the American College of cardiology/American heart association Task Force on clinical practice guidelines. *J Am Coll Cardiol*. 2019;73(12):1494–1563.
45. Holbein CE, Veldtman GR, Moons P, et al. Perceived health mediates effects of physical activity on quality of life in patients with a fontan circulation. *Am J Cardiol*. 2019;124:144–150.
46. Jortveit J, Eskedal L, Hirth A, et al. Sudden unexpected death in children with congenital heart defects. *Eur Heart J*. 2016;37:621–626.
47. Ko JM, White KS, Kovacs AH, et al. Physical activity-related drivers of perceived health status in adults with congenital heart disease. *Am J Cardiol*. 2018;122:1437–1442.
48. Buber J, Shafer K. Cardiopulmonary exercise testing and sports participation in adults with congenital heart disease. *Heart*. 2019;105:1670–1679.
49. Kempny A, Dimopoulos K, Uebing A, et al. Reference values for exercise limitations among adults with congenital heart disease. Relation to activities of daily life–single centre experience and review of published data. *Eur Heart J*. 2012;33:1386–1396.
50. Van Hare GF, Ackerman MJ, Evangelista JA, et al. Eligibility and disqualification recommendations for competitive athletes with cardiovascular abnormalities: task Force 4: congenital heart disease: a scientific statement from the American heart association and American College of cardiology. *Circulation*. 2015;132:e281–e291.

Specific Defects
51. Oster M, Bhatt AB, Zaragoza-Macias E, et al. Interventional therapy versus medical therapy for secundum atrial septal defect: a systematic review (Part 2) for the 2018 AHA/ACC guideline for the management of adults with congenital heart disease: a report of the American College of cardiology/American heart association Task Force on clinical practice guidelines. *Circulation*. 2019;139:e814–e830.
52. Mery CM, Zea-Vera R, Chacon-Portillo MA, et al. Contemporary results after repair of partial and transitional atrioventricular septal defects. *J Thorac Cardiovasc Surg*. 2019;157:1117–1127.e4.
53. Bergmann M, Germann CP, Nordmeyer J, et al. Short- and long-term outcome after interventional VSD closure: a single-center experience in pediatric and adult patients. *Pediatr Cardiol*. 2020.
54. Maagaard M, Eckerstrom F, Boutrup N, Hjortdal VE. Functional capacity past age 40 in patients with congenital ventricular septal defects. *J Am Heart Assoc*. 2020;9:e015956.
55. Rydman R, Shiina Y, Diller GP, et al. Major adverse events and atrial tachycardia in Ebstein's anomaly predicted by cardiovascular magnetic resonance. *Heart*. 2018;104:37–44.

56. Attie F, Rosas M, Rijlaarsdam M, et al. The adult patient with ebstein anomaly - outcome in 72 unoperated patients. *Medicine*. 2000;79:27–36.
57. De Backer J, Bondue A, Budts W, et al. Genetic counselling and testing in adults with congenital heart disease: a consensus document of the ESC Working group of grown-up congenital heart disease, the ESC working group on aorta and peripheral vascular disease and the European Society of Human genetics. *Eur J Prev Cardiol*. 2020;27:1423–1435.
58. Joynt MR, Yu S, Dorfman AL, et al. Differential impact of pulmonary regurgitation on patients with surgically repaired pulmonary stenosis versus tetralogy of Fallot. *Am J Cardiol*. 2016;117:289–294.
59. Heng EL, Bolger AP, Kempny A, et al. Neurohormonal activation and its relation to outcomes late after repair of tetralogy of Fallot. *Heart*. 2015;101:447–454.
60. Bonello B, Kempny A, Uebing A, et al. Right atrial area and right ventricular outflow tract akinetic length predict sustained tachyarrhythmia in repaired tetralogy of Fallot. *Int J Cardiol*. 2013;168:3280–3286.
61. Lillehei CW, Cohen M, Warden HE, Varco RL. The direct-vision intracardiac correction of congenital anomalies by controlled cross circulation; results in thirty-two patients with ventricular septal defects, tetralogy of Fallot, and atrioventricularis communis defects. *Surgery*. 1955;38:11–29.
62. Cuypers JA, Menting ME, Konings EE, et al. Unnatural history of tetralogy of Fallot: prospective follow-up of 40 years after surgical correction. *Circulation*. 2014;130:1944–1953.
63. Baumgartner H, De Backer J. 2020 ESC Guidelines for the management of adult congenital heart disease. *Eur Heart J*. 2020;42(6):563–645.
64. Bokma JP, Geva T, Sleeper LA, et al. A propensity score-adjusted analysis of clinical outcomes after pulmonary valve replacement in tetralogy of Fallot. *Heart*. 2018;104:738–744.
65. Heng EL, Gatzoulis MA, Uebing A, et al. Immediate and midterm cardiac remodeling after surgical pulmonary valve replacement in adults with repaired tetralogy of Fallot: a prospective cardiovascular magnetic resonance and clinical study. *Circulation*. 2017;136:1703–1713.
66. Bonello B, Shore DF, Uebing A, et al. Aortic dilatation in repaired tetralogy of Fallot. *JACC Cardiovasc Imaging*. 2018;11:150–152.
67. Gatzoulis MA, Balaji S, Webber SA, et al. Risk factors for arrhythmia and sudden cardiac death late after repair of tetralogy of Fallot: a multicentre study. *Lancet*. 2000;356:975–981.
68. Khairy P, Van Hare GF, Balaji S, et al. PACES/HRS expert consensus statement on the recognition and management of arrhythmias in adult congenital heart disease: developed in partnership between the Pediatric and Congenital Electrophysiology Society (PACES) and the Heart Rhythm Society (HRS). Endorsed by the governing bodies of PACES, HRS, the American College of Cardiology (ACC), the American Heart Association (AHA), the European Heart Rhythm Association (EHRA), the Canadian Heart Rhythm Society (CHRS), and the International Society for Adult Congenital Heart Disease (ISACHD). *Can J Cardiol*. 2014;30:e1–e63.
69. Valente AM, Gauvreau K, Assenza GE, et al. Contemporary predictors of death and sustained ventricular tachycardia in patients with repaired tetralogy of Fallot enrolled in the INDICATOR cohort. *Heart*. 2014;100:247–253.
70. Kapel GF, Reichlin T, Wijnmaalen AP, et al. Re-entry using anatomically determined isthmuses: a curable ventricular tachycardia in repaired congenital heart disease. *Circ Arrhythm Electrophysiol*. 2015;8:102–109.
71. Geva T, Mulder B, Gauvreau K, et al. Preoperative predictors of death and sustained ventricular tachycardia after pulmonary valve replacement in patients with repaired tetralogy of Fallot enrolled in the INDICATOR cohort. *Circulation*. 2018.
72. Couperus LE, Vliegen HW, Zandstra TE, et al. Long-term outcome after atrial correction for transposition of the great arteries. *Heart*. 2019;105:790–796.
73. Cuypers JA, Eindhoven JA, Slager MA, et al. The natural and unnatural history of the Mustard procedure: long-term outcome up to 40 years. *Eur Heart J*. 2014;35:1666–1674.
74. Khairy P, Harris L, Landzberg MJ, et al. Sudden death and defibrillators in transposition of the great arteries with intra-atrial baffles: a multicenter study. *Circ Arrhythm Electrophysiol*. 2008;1:250–257.
75. Koolbergen DR, Ahmed Y, Bouma BJ, et al. Follow-up after tricuspid valve surgery in adult patients with systemic right ventricles. *Eur J Cardio Thorac Surg*. 2016;50:456–463.
76. Deng L, Xu J, Tang Y, et al. Long-term outcomes of tricuspid valve surgery in patients with congenitally corrected transposition of the great arteries. *J Am Heart Assoc*. 2018;7.
77. Oladunjoye O, Piekarski B, Baird C, et al. Repair of double outlet right ventricle: midterm outcomes. *J Thorac Cardiovasc Surg*. 2019.
78. Robinson Vimala L, Hanneman K, et al. Characteristics of cardiovascular magnetic resonance imaging and outcomes in adults with repaired truncus arteriosus. *Am J Cardiol*. 2019;124:1636–1642.
79. Rudiene V, Hjortshoj CMS, Glaveckaite S, et al. Cor triatriatum sinistrum diagnosed in the adulthood: a systematic review. *Heart*. 2019;105:1197–1202.
80. van der Linde D, Roos-Hesselink JW, Rizopoulos D, et al. Surgical outcome of discrete subaortic stenosis in adults: a multicenter study. *Circulation*. 2013;127:1184–1191.e1-4.
81. Tefera E, Gedlu E, Bezabih A, et al. Outcome in children operated for membranous subaortic stenosis: membrane resection plus aggressive septal myectomy versus membrane resection alone. *World J Pediatr Congenit Heart Surg*. 2015;6:424–428.
82. Tal N, Golender J, Rechtman Y, et al. Long-term aortic valve function in patients with or without surgical treatment for discrete subaortic stenosis. *Pediatr Cardiol*. 2021;42(2):324–330.
83. Jiao Y, Li G, Korneva A, et al. Deficient circumferential growth is the primary determinant of aortic obstruction attributable to partial elastin deficiency. *Arterioscler Thromb Vasc Biol*. 2017;37:930–941.
84. Collins 2nd RT. Cardiovascular disease in Williams syndrome. *Curr Opin Pediatr*. 2018;30:609–615.
85. Latham GJ, Ross FJ, Eisses MJ, et al. Perioperative morbidity in children with elastin arteriopathy. *Paediatr Anaesth*. 2016;26:926–935.
86. Lee MGY, Babu-Narayan SV, Kempny A, et al. Long-term mortality and cardiovascular burden for adult survivors of coarctation of the aorta. *Heart*. 2019;105:1190–1196.
87. Choudhary P, Canniffe C, Jackson DJ, et al. Late outcomes in adults with coarctation of the aorta. *Heart*. 2015;101:1190–1195.
88. Rinnstrom D, Dellborg M, Thilen U, et al. Hypertension in adults with repaired coarctation of the aorta. *Am Heart J*. 2016;181:10–15.
89. Taggart NW, Minahan M, Cabalka AK, et al. Immediate outcomes of covered stent placement for treatment or prevention of aortic wall injury associated with coarctation of the aorta (COAST II). *JACC Cardiovasc Interv*. 2016;9:484–493.
90. Saran N, Dearani J, Said S, et al. Vascular rings in adults: outcome of surgical management. *Ann Thorac Surg*. 2019;108:1217–1227.
91. Luciano D, Mitchell J, Fraisse A, et al. Kommerell diverticulum should Be removed in children with vascular ring and aberrant left subclavian artery. *Ann Thorac Surg*. 2015;100:2293–2297.
92. Vinnakota A, Idrees JJ, Rosinski BF, et al. Outcomes of repair of Kommerell diverticulum. *Ann Thorac Surg*. 2019;108:1745–1750.
93. Hoffman JI, Kaplan S. The incidence of congenital heart disease. *J Am Coll Cardiol*. 2002;39:1890–1900.
94. Fontan F, Baudet E. Surgical repair of tricuspid atresia. *Thorax*. 1971;26:240–248.
95. Rychik J, Atz AM, Celermajer DS, et al. Evaluation and management of the child and adult with fontan circulation: a scientific statement from the American heart association. *Circulation*. 2019; CIR0000000000000696.
96. Pundi KN, Johnson JN, Dearani JA, et al. 40-Year follow-up after the fontan operation: long-term outcomes of 1,052 patients. *J Am Coll Cardiol*. 2015;66:1700–1710.
97. Downing TE, Allen KY, Glatz AC, et al. Long-term survival after the Fontan operation: twenty years of experience at a single center. *J Thorac Cardiovasc Surg*. 2017;154:243–253 e2.
98. Rathod RH, Prakash A, Kim YY, et al. Cardiac magnetic resonance parameters predict transplantation-free survival in patients with fontan circulation. *Circ Cardiovasc Imaging*. 2014;7:502–509.
99. Goldberg DJ, Zak V, Goldstein BH, et al. Results of the FUEL trial. *Circulation*. 2020;141:641–651.
100. Hernandez GA, Lemor A, Clark D, et al. Heart transplantation and in-hospital outcomes in adult congenital heart disease patients with Fontan: a decade nationwide analysis from 2004 to 2014. *J Card Surg*. 2020;35:603–608.
101. Quinton E, Nightingale P, Hudsmith L, et al. Prevalence of atrial tachyarrhythmia in adults after Fontan operation. *Heart*. 2015;101:1672–1677.
102. Ben Ali W, Bouhout I, Khairy P, et al. Extracardiac versus lateral tunnel fontan: a meta-analysis of long-term results. *Ann Thorac Surg*. 2019;107:837–843.
103. Dennis M, Zannino D, du Plessis K, et al. Clinical outcomes in adolescents and adults after the fontan procedure. *J Am Coll Cardiol*. 2018;71:1009–1017.
104. Vaikunth SS, Concepcion W, Daugherty T, et al. Short-term outcomes of en bloc combined heart and liver transplantation in the failing Fontan. *Clin Transplant*. 2019;33:e13540.
105. Reardon LC, DePasquale EC, Tarabay J, et al. Heart and heart-liver transplantation in adults with failing Fontan physiology. *Clin Transplant*. 2018;32:e13329.
106. Simonneau G, Montani D, Celermajer DS, et al. Haemodynamic definitions and updated clinical classification of pulmonary hypertension. *Eur Respir J*. 2019;53.

Eisenmenger Syndrome

107. Arvanitaki A, Giannakoulas G, Baumgartner H, Lammers AE. Eisenmenger syndrome: diagnosis, prognosis and clinical management. *Heart*. 2020;106:1638–1645.
108. Kempny A, Hjortshoj CS, Gu H, et al. Predictors of death in contemporary adult patients with eisenmenger syndrome: a multicenter study. *Circulation*. 2017;135:1432–1440.
109. Duan R, Xu X, Wang X, et al. Pregnancy outcome in women with Eisenmenger's syndrome: a case series from west China. *BMC Pregnancy Childbirth*. 2016;16:356.
110. Gatzoulis MA, Landzberg M, Beghetti M, et al. Evaluation of macitentan in patients with eisenmenger syndrome. *Circulation*. 2019;139:51–63.
111. Hjortshoj CS, Gilljam T, Dellgren G, et al. Outcome after heart-lung or lung transplantation in patients with Eisenmenger syndrome. *Heart*. 2020;106:127–132.

83 Catheter-Based Treatment of Congenital Heart Disease in Adults

SHABANA SHAHANAVAZ, JOHN M. LASALA, AND DAVID T. BALZER

VALVULAR INTERVENTIONS, 1587
Pulmonary Valvuloplasty, 1587
Pulmonary Valve Replacement, 1587
Pulmonary Valve Systems, 1588

ARTERIAL INTERVENTIONS, 1588
Pulmonary Angioplasty, 1588
Stenting for Coarctation of the Aorta, 1589

SEPTAL INTERVENTIONS, 1589
Techniques for Closure of Atrial Septal Defects, 1589
Techniques for Closure of Superior Sinus Venosus Atrial Septal Defects, 1590
Techniques for Closure of Ventricular Septal Defects, 1590
Treatment of Patent Ductus Arteriosus, 1591

FUTURE PERSPECTIVES, 1591
REFERENCES, 1592

Advances in surgical and medical care have led to rapid growth in the number and state of adults living with congenital heart disease (see Chapter 82). Consequently there has been an increase in the volume and variety of transcatheter interventional procedures applicable to adult congenital heart disease (ACHD) patients. ACHDs span a wide spectrum with heterogeneous anomalies involving all aspects of cardiovascular physiology such that specialized training has become a necessity for anyone caring for such patients. Multiple professional societies including ACC, AHA, and SCAI have published recommendations regarding the delivery of ACHD interventional care. Current consensus explicitly states that interventional procedures should be performed at regional ACHD centers by qualified and experienced ACHD specialists, and in laboratories with appropriate staffing and experience to fulfill this task.[1,2] In addition, because of the complexity of disorders in these patients, any site undertaking the care of adults with congenital heart disease must have a well-established multidisciplinary team that includes congenital cardiothoracic surgeons, cardiac anesthesiologists, cardiac intensivists, and congenital cardiologists.[1,2] Pediatric interventional cardiologists are also key persons on the team, and partnerships between adult congenital interventionalists and pediatric interventional cardiologists are mandatory. As the capabilities of the congenital catheterization laboratory continue to evolve, the line between surgical and catheter-based interventions will become more and more blurred. Many interventions already take place in highly specialized hybrid operating suites whereby interventional cardiologists work alongside their cardiothoracic surgery colleagues. This combined model of intervention will continue to be adapted for adult congenital interventions, and it is this ongoing evolution that makes the field so exciting. Furthermore, as interventional approaches change, the indications for intervention become a "moving target." As a result, national guidelines outdate sooner than later; therefore, interventional cardiologists who treat adults must remain current about the ever-changing medical literature on this topic. In this chapter, we review major areas in which catheter-based interventions have become well established for adults with congenital heart disease. The topic of congenital heart disease in adults is reviewed in Chapter 82.

VALVULAR INTERVENTIONS

The first static pulmonary balloon valvuloplasty was performed in 1982; successful catheter-based interventions have since been performed on all types of cardiac valves.[3–5] Although valvuloplasty defined the early era of congenital interventional catheterization, valve replacement is defining the current era.

Pulmonary Valvuloplasty

Congenital valvular pulmonary stenosis accounts for 5% to 10% of all congenital heart disease.[6] In most cases, the stenosis is due to fusion of commissures with normal valve leaflets leading to "doming" of the valve leaflets, but rarely due to dysplastic leaflets. Static pulmonary valvuloplasty (aimed at separating the fused leaflets) was first performed in the early 1980s and has replaced surgical valvotomy as the initial intervention in cases of typical isolated valvar pulmonary stenosis.[5] Valvuloplasty for thick and/or dysplastic valves is less successful; moreover, balloon dilation will be unsuccessful in relieving any muscular subvalvar stenosis. Indications for pulmonary valvuloplasty in adults with congenital heart disease have been outlined elsewhere (see Chapter 82).[1] Before pulmonary valvuloplasty is performed, a complete right heart catheterization should be performed, followed by right ventricular (RV) angiography to profile the right ventricular outflow tract (RVOT). Angiographic measurements of the pulmonary annulus allows for the selection of the appropriately sized balloon, which is approximately 120% of the measured pulmonary annulus. Successful balloon valvuloplasty can usually be achieved with low pressure inflation of a compliant balloon. In patients with large annulus, double balloons can be used to achieve adequate dilation.[7] After dilation of the pulmonary valve, repeat angiography should be performed to rule out vascular injury. Pulmonary regurgitation is best assessed on post procedure echocardiography.

OUTCOMES AND COMPLICATIONS

Case selection is critical for optimizing outcomes. Patients with typical pulmonary valve stenosis will have relatively thin leaflets with partial fusion and will respond well to balloon valvuloplasty.[5] The most common complication of pulmonary valvuloplasty is pulmonary regurgitation (<10% with 2+ or greater pulmonary regurgitation), which is usually well tolerated. Major adverse events or unplanned surgeries were not reported for patients with typical valvar stenosis in the most recent report from the National Cardiovascular Data Registry (NCDR).[8]

Pulmonary Valve Replacement

Patients presenting for pulmonary valve replacement typically have a history of congenital heart disease and may have undergone multiple cardiac surgeries. The most common initial pathologies present in these patients are tetralogy of Fallot with associated pulmonary atresia, stenosis, or absence of the pulmonary valve, pulmonary valve dysfunction following a Ross procedure and truncus arteriosus.[9] The unifying component of the surgical repair in these patients is the frequent presence of a RV to pulmonary artery conduit, which is a prosthetic or tissue graft that is placed to bypass or reconstruct the

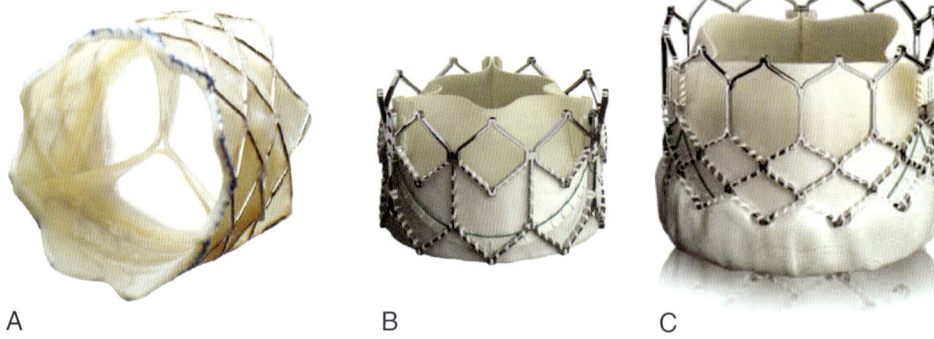

FIGURE 83.1 Transcatheter valves. **A,** Melody valve (Medtronic, Minneapolis, MN). **B,** Edwards SAPIEN XT valve (Edwards Lifesciences LLC, Irvine, CA). **C,** Edwards SAPIEN S3 valve (Edwards Lifesciences LLC, Irvine, CA).

RVOT. Over time, these conduits often develop progressive stenosis, regurgitation or a combination of these. Patients can present with symptoms of exercise intolerance, congestive heart failure and dysrhythmias heralding significant RV dysfunction. In an effort to avoid such dysfunction, relief of stenosis and placement of a competent valve are warranted. Determining the optimal timing for pulmonary valve replacement remains an issue; there are currently several indications in symptomatic[1] and asymptomatic[10] patients with pulmonary valve disease (see Chapter 82).

Pulmonary Valve Systems

There are currently two available valve systems approved by the Food and Drug Administration (FDA) for transcatheter pulmonary valve replacement (TPVR): Melody Transcatheter Pulmonary Valve (Medtronic, Inc., Minneapolis), and SAPIEN XT Pulmonic Valve (Edwards Lifesciences, Irvine, CA). Each has its own unique strengths and weaknesses.

Melody Valve

In 2000, Bonhoeffer and colleagues published the first successful percutaneous placement of his prototype stent-mounted valve in the pulmonary valve.[11] The rights to Bonhoeffer's valve design were acquired by Medtronic, Inc. (Minneapolis, MN) to develop the Melody valve (Fig. 83.1A). The Melody valve is composed of a valved segment of bovine internal jugular vein that is fixed with glutaraldehyde and then sutured to a platinum-iridium stent frame.[12] A percutaneous introducer, Ensemble Delivery sheath (Medtronic, Inc., Minneapolis, MN) covers the valve and is used to deliver the valve. Once in proper position, the sheath on the Ensemble system is pulled back to expose the valve, and via two sequential balloon dilations, the valve is deployed. RVOT stenting is routinely performed prior to valve deployment to prevent stent fractures of the Melody valve frame. There are currently two sizes of Melody valves available: 20 and 22 mm, with the delivery system available in three sizes: 18, 20, and 22 mm.

SAPIEN Valve

The Edwards SAPIEN transcatheter heart valve (Irvine, CA) was originally designed for placement in the aortic position, but was found to have high success rates when placed in the pulmonary valve position, with the first successful pulmonary implantation in 2006.[13,14] This device is composed of bovine pericardium of three equal-sized leaflets that are hand-sewn to a cobalt chromium balloon-expandable stent with a polyethylene terephthalate fabric cuff (Fig. 83.1B). Additionally, the S3 has a new outer polyethylene terephthalate skirt which decreases the incidence of paravalvular leak. The Sapien XT and S3 system is crimped onto the Novaflex and Commander delivery system (Edwards Lifesciences, Irvine, CA), respectively (Fig. 83.1C). The delivery systems minimize profile by allowing the valve to be crimped onto the shaft of the balloon and then pushed onto the balloon *in vivo* once advanced through the introducer sheath. The Sapien delivery system does not cover the valve as it is advanced through the right heart. The SAPIEN valve comes in larger diameters of 23, 26, and 29 mm. These larger valve sizes allow for percutaneous intervention in patients with large native RVOTs, transannular patches, and large RV to PA conduits. The Sapien XT valve has received FDA approval for percutaneous placement in pulmonary conduits since 2012. The Sapien S3 valve has completed primary endpoint data collection under the COMPASSION S3 trial (NCT02744677) for placement in stenotic conduits. There is ongoing enrollment for Sapien S3 placement in bioprosthetic valves.

OUTCOMES AND COMPLICATIONS

The Melody valve received US Food and Drug Administration approval under a Humanitarian Device Exemption (HDE) in 2010 and Pre–Market Approval in 2015 for the treatment of conduit dysfunction. In 2016, it received approval for valve-in-valve placement to combat bioprosthetic valve dysfunction. Early and intermediate[15] outcome data have demonstrated excellent procedural success and freedom from RVOT reintervention at rates of 98% at 3 years and 91% at 5 years from intervention. SAPIEN valves have had similarly good early outcomes[16] and favorable comparisons with the Melody valve.[17] Valve selection is influenced by patient cohort (conduit versus transannular patch), ease of use of the delivery system (stiffness and lack of flexibility of the delivery system for the Sapien), and operator experience/preference. Important procedural complications include vascular injury, conduit disruption, pulmonary artery perforation, stent or valve embolization, coronary artery compression, ventricular arrhythmias, and tricuspid valve injury. Long-term complications include stent frame fracture (Melody valve), valve dysfunction, and endocarditis.[16–18]

ARTERIAL INTERVENTIONS

The pathologic "arterial" conditions encountered most frequently by congenital interventionalists are related to anatomic lesions in the pulmonary arterial tree, followed by coarctations of the aorta. As in other interventional areas, technologic advances have increased the breadth of catheter-based treatments for congenital heart disease, as well as the quality and durability of the outcomes. In adult patients, stenting has become a well-established companion to angioplasty and has improved acute and long-term outcomes.

Pulmonary Angioplasty

Pulmonary artery abnormalities can be isolated or in association with other cardiac defects, and occur in 2% to 3% of all patients with congenital heart disease. Depending on the obstruction site, these lesions can result in elevated RV pressure or significant flow discrepancies between lung segments, thereby causing isolated lung hypertension. Indications for pulmonary arterial intervention have been described elsewhere (see Chapter 82).[1] There are currently no stents approved by the FDA for use in pulmonary arteries; however, Palmaz Genesis stents (Cordis, Milpitas, CA) and the EV3 family of stents (Covidien/Medtronic, Minneapolis, MN) have been used and have shown good radial strength, low profiles, and achievable diameters. In children or in small or distal pulmonary arteries in adults, it is reasonable to use premounted stents.

OUTCOMES AND COMPLICATIONS

The heterogeneous nature of pulmonary arterial disease has resulted in a wide spectrum of clinical outcomes following catheter-based interventions.[19,20] Both the anatomic location of the stenosis and its

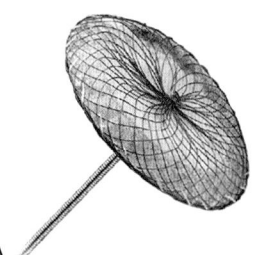 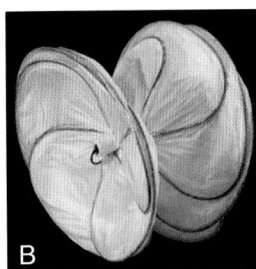 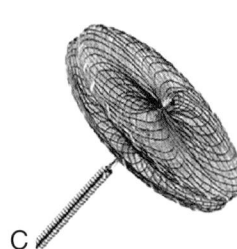 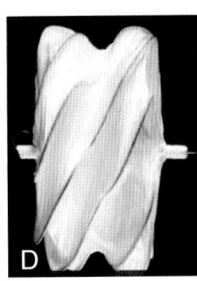

FIGURE 83.2 Various closure devices for atrial septal defects. **A,** Amplatzer Cribriform device (Abbott Inc., St. Paul, MN). **B,** GORE Cardioform Septal Occluder (W.L. GORE and Associates, Inc., Flagstaff, AZ). **C,** Amplatzer Septal Occluder (Abbott Inc., St. Paul, MN). **D,** Gore Cardioform ASD occlude (W.L. GORE and Associates, Inc., Flagstaff, AZ).

less than 10 mm Hg.[8] Complications include access injuries, vascular tears or dissections, stent embolization or malpositioning, restenosis, and aneurysm; and even death. For adults in the NCDR, 8.6% experienced an adverse event, but only one major adverse event occurred in 92 patients.[8] Long-term follow-up will continue to reveal the true risk of late aneurysm and restenosis in these patients. For children who are not fully grown, future dilations should be anticipated to keep pace with somatic growth.

circumstances of formation as a congenital or postoperative greatly contribute to the differences in clinical outcomes. Complications include vascular tears, stent embolization or malpositioning, pulmonary edema, and the need for unanticipated procedures or surgeries; some patients may not survive. A report from the NCDR revealed reasonable safety; in 245 procedures across all age-groups, adverse events were reported in 13.2% of cases and major adverse events in 1.2% of cases, and 2 patients died.[8]

Stenting for Coarctation of the Aorta

Coarctation is characterized by discrete narrowing of the thoracic aorta adjacent to where the ductus arteriosus was once inserted (see Chapter 82). Although it can present as an isolated lesion, it is also commonly found in genetic syndromes (Turner and Williams syndrome).[21] Hence, detailed investigation for the presence of coarctation should be made in these patients. The most common cardiovascular malformation associated with CoA is bicuspid aortic valve (BAV). Current guidelines recommend that patients with CoA undergo evaluation for intracranial aneurysms.[22] The increase in afterload imposed by the coarctation can result in left ventricular (LV) dysfunction and cardiogenic shock, which often develop in early infancy. More frequently, the body develops extensive collaterals through the chest wall, which minimize the increase in afterload and preserve systolic function. Over time, patients with coarctation will develop hypertension in varying degrees and, eventually, coronary artery disease and LV diastolic dysfunction. Transcatheter approach with stenting of the aorta is now considered a mainstay in the management of adults with native CoA and recoarctation. Coarctation stenting is typically performed by a retrograde approach via the femoral artery. After measuring the baseline gradient, angiography is performed and measurements of the distal aortic arch and thoracic aorta (at the level of the diaphragm) are recorded. The covered Cheatham pulmonary (CP) stent (NuMED, Inc., Hopkinton, NY) is approved by the FDA for use in coarctation, but other stents are often used off-label. The diameter of the implanted balloon should not be larger than that of the surrounding aorta or 3.5 times the narrowest dimension.[23] Stents are most frequently placed by balloon-in-balloon catheters because of their improved control. Once a stiff guidewire is positioned across the coarctation, a long sheath is positioned above the narrowed area and a mounted stent is advanced into position at the site of coarctation. The stent is uncovered and deployed with inflation of the balloon catheter. After successful placement of the stent, additional serial dilations of any residual waist may be considered. Follow-up angiography should be performed to rule out dissection or aneurysm before measuring the final pressure gradient. Indications for coarctation intervention are discussed elsewhere (see Chapter 82).[1] Comparisons between balloon angioplasty, aortic stenting, and surgical resection have been done, and catheter-based stenting has emerged as the preferred treatment modality for older children and adults.

OUTCOMES AND COMPLICATIONS

Coarctation stenting is safe and compares favorably with surgery in regard to its ability to eliminate the pressure gradient.[8,23] The NCDR report noted more frequent stenting in older children and adults, with nearly 84% of stented patients achieving a postprocedural gradient of

SEPTAL INTERVENTIONS

Techniques for Closure of Atrial Septal Defects

Atrial septal defects (ASDs) are the third most common form of congenital heart disease. They occur in 56 to 100 live births per 100,000 infants.[6,24] Isolated ASDs will result in left-to-right shunting, with the magnitude of the shunt determined by ventricular compliance and atrioventricular valve stenosis. Significant left-to-right shunts result in RV dilation; if they are left unrepaired, they may ultimately result in pulmonary arterial muscularization and elevations in the pulmonary vascular resistance by the sixth decade of life. In an effort to avoid irreversible changes in pulmonary vascular resistance, early closure of significant ASDs has become standard practice. Transcatheter devices and techniques have evolved substantially since the first case was reported in 1976 by King and colleagues.[24] The currently available devices each have unique strengths and weaknesses (Fig. 83.2).[25] Indications for intervention have been previously outlined.[1]

Amplatzer Devices

Originally introduced in the mid-1990s, the Amplatzer Septal Occluder (ASO) (Abbott Inc., St. Paul, MN) has been used in thousands of cases worldwide. The ASO is made of woven nitinol wire that forms a self-centering device, with left and right atrial discs, and a central waist. The device is filled with interwoven Dacron polyester fibers to facilitate platelet aggregation and endothelialization. The device is secured to a delivery cable and introduced into the left atrium via the appropriately sized, proprietary TorqVue sheath. ASOs can treat ASDs of variable sizes as long as the atrial septal rim is substantial enough to allow for a secured placement of the. If the septal rim is deficient (<5 mm in contiguous zones), stable positioning will be more difficult to achieve and at times may not be possible. Numerous deployment techniques can be used if the septal rim is deficient, but are out of the scope of this chapter.[26–28] Shortly after the introduction of the ASO, Amplatzer developed the Cribriform device. In contrast to the ASO, the Cribriform device does not have a waist and is therefore not self-centering. Its primary benefit is that it can be placed in a small central defect and also covers numerous satellite defects. Its deployment is identical to that of the ASO, using the same TorqVue sheaths and delivery cables. The Amplatzer PFO occluder has been approved by the FDA for PFO closure in the context of cryptogenic stroke. It is made of two nitinol woven discs with integral Dacron patches and a fixed short waist (see Fig. 83.2). The Dacron patches are designed to stimulate endothelialization. The device comes in multiple sizes with the right atrial disc being larger than the left atrial disc. The Amplatzer Trevisio intravascular delivery system is a second generation delivery cable that has three sections with varying flexibility to decrease device distortion once positioned across the defect. The proximal portion is a stainless steel cable with moderate pushability. The middle part of the wire has a stainless steel cable with loosely wound stainless steel coil, and the distal part of the wire has a nitinol core with loosely wound stainless steel coil. The more flexible distal cable enables better assessment of final device position and is especially helpful in larger defects. Device sizing for the ASO should be based on the stop flow method of balloon sizing. In order to decrease the risk of device erosion, over inflation of the balloon should be avoided (not >1.5 × the static echocardiographic dimension). Device selection should be the same size (or at most 1 size larger) than the stop flow dimension. Defects with a deficient retroaortic rim (<5 mm) are considered higher risk for an erosion.

OUTCOMES AND COMPLICATIONS

The ASO demonstrated superior safety and similar closure rates when compared to surgery in the US Pivotal Trial. The postmarket approval study and multicenter community use trial have further solidified the ASO's position as a safe and effective device for transcatheter closure of an ASD or a patent foramen ovale (PFO).[29,30] Major adverse events reported include arrhythmias, device embolization, device erosion, device fracture, stroke, and left arterial thrombus. One of the most significant adverse events is device erosion. After the first reported case in 2002, AGA/St. Jude revised the ASO guidelines, but erosions continued to be reported to the Manufacturer and User Facility Device Experience (MAUDE) database. In response to ongoing erosion reports (<0.05% of worldwide sales, estimated to be approximately 0.1% of implants), the FDA and AGA/St. Jude made additional changes to the guidelines in an effort to minimize the erosion risk, and recommended closer follow-up with more frequent echocardiograms. In addition to erosion, several case reports in children and adults have demonstrated delayed endothelialization in the setting of endocarditis, and concerns have been raised regarding the optimal length of time for subacute bacterial endocarditis prophylaxis following device placement.[31] The RESPECT clinical trial (evaluating PFO closure with the Amplatzer PFO Occluder) showed that among adults with a history of a cryptogenic ischemic stroke, closure of a PFO was associated with a lower rate of recurrent ischemic strokes than medical therapy alone during extended follow-up.[32]

GORE Devices

The GORE Helex device (no longer commercially available) was approved in 2006. It was not self-centering and therefore was relatively limited with regard to the sizes of defects it could effectively treat. GORE redesigned its septal occluder system which is now marketed as the GORE Cardioform Septal Occluder (GSO) (W.L. Gore and Associates, Flagstaff, AZ). The new device consists of a five-wire nitinol frame, which adds radial strength and improves structural integrity, and it is covered with the same expanded polytetrafluoroethylene (ePTFE) membrane as the original Helex device (see Fig. 83.2B). The redesigned delivery system is much more intuitive, and it maintains its novel retention cord mechanism. Owing to its non–self-centering design, the GSO can only close defects up to 18 mm in diameter. Similar to the GSO, the GORE Cardioform ASD occluder (GCA) is composed of a platinum–filled nitinol wire frame covered with ePTFE. The principal modification from the original GSO is its anatomically adaptable "intra–disc occluder" which expands to conform to the ASD size and shape, allowing different devices to treat a range of ASD diameters. The current device is locked by a nitinol pin running through the central eyelets, and has a retrieval cord attached to the right atrial eyelet. The available sizes are 27, 32, 37, 44, and 48 mm and are designed to treat defects ranging from 8 to 35 mm. These devices are not contraindicated in defects with deficient retroaortic rim since there is no erosion risk.

OUTCOMES AND COMPLICATIONS

The GSO was approved by the FDA in 2012 and has demonstrated comparable safety and efficacy to the ASO in closure of PFO and ASD.[33] In contrast to the ASO, there is no report of device erosion following implantation of a GORE device. Overall, percutaneous device placement has emerged as the preferred intervention for ASDs because of its excellent outcomes and safety records. The Gore ASSURED clinical study was a prospective single arm registry that evaluated the safety and efficacy of the GCA device. The study showed excellent technical success with 100% closure rate and low adverse event rates.[34] The REDUCE study determined safety and efficacy of PFO closure with the GORE CARDIOFORM Septal Occluder or GORE HELEX Septal Occluder plus antiplatelet medical management compared to antiplatelet medical management alone in patients with a PFO and history of cryptogenic stroke.[35] The risk of subsequent ischemic stroke was lower among those assigned to PFO closure combined with antiplatelet therapy than those assigned to antiplatelet therapy alone. Current recommendations from the American Academy of Neurology states that clinicians can recommend closure following a discussion of potential benefits (absolute recurrent stroke risk reduction of 3.4% at 5 years) and risks (periprocedural complication rate of 3.9% and increased absolute rate of non-periprocedural atrial fibrillation of 0.33% per year) in patients <60 years of age with a PFO and embolic infarct and no other mechanism of stroke identified (level C).[36]

Techniques for Closure of Superior Sinus Venosus Atrial Septal Defects

The superior sinus venosus ASD is a congenital abnormality that is caused by a deficiency of the common wall between the superior vena cava (SVC) and the right sided pulmonary veins (see Chapter 82). This defect is frequently associated with an anomalous drainage of the right-sided pulmonary veins to the SVC. Traditionally, this defect is treated by surgical correction. However, advances in current covered stent technology has led to a transcatheter approach. This novel technique uses a covered stent deployed in the SVC-RA, closing the interatrial communication and redirecting pulmonary venous flow to the left atrium. In the presence of anomalous drainage of the right sided pulmonary veins higher in the SVC, surgical repair with reimplantation of the veins and patch closure of the sinus venosus ASD is recommended.[37]

Techniques for Closure of Ventricular Septal Defects

Ventricular septal defects (VSDs) are the most common congenital heart defects and can range in size from tiny pinholes to near absence of the septum (see also Chapter 82). VSDs can be an isolated finding or associated with other complex congenital heart diseases, primarily conotruncal defects (e.g., tetralogy of Fallot, double-outlet right ventricle, transposition of the great arteries). The ventricular septum has four primary regions: inlet, outlet, perimembranous area, and muscular area. Defects can occur in any location and extend to adjacent regions. The shunt through a VSD is predicated on ventricular outflow obstruction and downstream vascular resistance. The management of VSD is a complex topic beyond the scope of this chapter, and indications for intervention have been previously described (see Chapter 82).[1] Catheter-based device closure of muscular, traumatic, postoperative residual, and postinfarct VSDs has become a reasonable alternative to surgery. Perimembranous VSD remains controversial because of the associated risk of heart block. Inlet VSDs are not amenable to transcatheter techniques because there is no circumferential tissue for secured placement of device.[38] Percutaneous closure of VSDs that are secondary to myocardial infarction has been attempted with a variety of devices (Amplatzer Septal Occluder and Amplater muscular VSD device). The Amplatzer Post Infarct muscular VSD device (Abbott Inc., St. Paul, MN) has larger disks and a longer waist (10 mm) than the Amplatzer muscular VSD device, in order to accommodate the thicker adult interventricular septum. This indication has received FDA approval. Details regarding timing of post infarct VSD intervention are outside the scope of this chapter.

OUTCOMES AND COMPLICATIONS

Complications specific to transcatheter device closure of VSDs include aortic regurgitation, tricuspid regurgitation, rhythm disturbances, and atrioventricular (AV block); death occurs rarely. In a review of the European registry of transcatheter VSD devices, Carminati and associates[39] found that VSDs in the perimembranous location were at increased risk for developing complete AV block. When similar devices were used, others found similar rates of AV block, ranging from 2% to 6%.[40–42] Interestingly, a lower risk of AV block has been seen in some cases

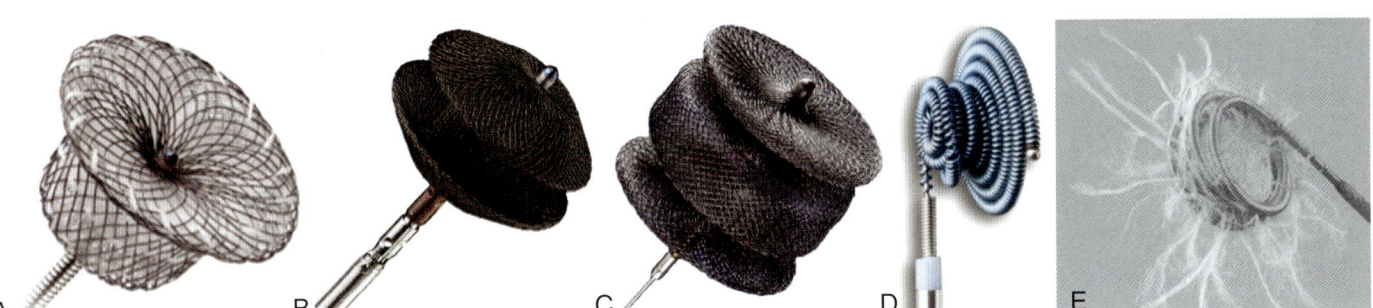

FIGURE 83.3 Various closure devices for patent ductus arteriosus. **A,** Amplatzer Ductal Occluder (St. Jude Medical, St. Paul, MN). **B,** Amplatzer Ductal Occluder II (St. Jude Medical, St. Paul, MN). **C,** Amplatzer Vascular Plug II (St. Jude Medical, St. Paul, MN). **D,** Nit-Occlud PDA Occluder (PFM Medical AG, Köln, Germany).

when the first-generation Amplatzer ductal occluders were used.[43] Review of outcomes for device closure of VSD's post myocardial infarction show that the mortality among overall surgical repair and percutaneous closure was significantly lower than medical management alone (P< 0.001 for all comparisons). The overall mortality with percutaneous closure was lower compared with late surgical closure (P < 0.0001).[44]

Treatment of Patent Ductus Arteriosus

Patent ductus arteriosus (PDA) is a frequent congenital heart defect that is most commonly detected in infancy through the associated murmur (see also Chapter 82). After birth, several important physiologic changes lead to early functional closure of the ductus followed by an anatomic closure in subsequent weeks to months. For patients in whom the ductus persists, the elevation in systemic vascular resistance and drop in pulmonary vascular resistance promotes a left-to-right shunt with resultant pulmonary overcirculation and left heart dilation. Left untreated, a large PDA can lead to significant heart failure, atrial arrhythmias (secondary to atrial hypertension), and pulmonary hypertension. PDA can be a site for infective endarteritis in rare cases.[45] Prior to catheter-based interventions, significant PDAs were ligated surgically via posterolateral thoracotomy. Indications for intervention have been outlined elsewhere.[1] From coils to vascular plugs to dedicated occlusion devices, the interventionalist has multiple options for PDA occlusion (Fig. 83.3). There is consensus regarding the indication for closure in large PDAs with associated left heart dilation despite a current controversy with respect to the need for closing "silent" PDAs.[46]

Amplatzer Duct Occluders (First- and Second-Generation)

The ADO-I device is made of a nitinol wire mesh packed with Dacron polyester fabric to facilitate platelet aggregation and endothelialization. The second-generation ADO-II has symmetric retention skirts, which allow it to be placed in an antegrade or a retrograde fashion. The ADO-II is not packed with polyester fibers because the nitinol wire weave is tighter than in ADO-I.

Amplatzer Vascular Plugs (Second- and Fourth-Generation)

In patients with long, tubular ducts, a vascular plug may be the optimal occlusion device. Vascular plugs have a conveniently low profile and work well in ducts with sufficient length to ensure that the left pulmonary artery and aorta are not obstructed. The AVP-II has a wide assortment of sizes (3 to 22 mm). The AVP-IV has fewer available sizes (4 to 8 mm) and is slightly longer than AVP-II, but it offers an even lower profile, to easily navigate tortuous anatomy.

Nit-Occlud Device

The Nit-Occlud device (PFM Medical, Carlsbad, CA) has a single nitinol wire coil, which can be wound in a funnel shape when it is advanced from the catheter. The Nit-Occlud device can be delivered via a 4 Fr guide catheter with a controlled-release mechanism. The Nit-Occlud comes in multiple sizes with variable levels of wire stiffness.

Standard Coiling

After small ducts have been crossed, they can be reliably occluded with simple coils or detachable coils.

OUTCOMES AND COMPLICATIONS

Transcatheter closure of PDA has become a reliable procedure with excellent technical success and good efficacy.[6] Numerous articles have reviewed the outcomes of detachable coils and the Amplatzer devices, and found the overall closure rate to be approximately 94%.[8,47] Serious adverse events are extremely rare.[6] Minor complications (vascular injuries, device embolization, residual shunts, blood loss requiring transfusion, hemolysis, and aortic or pulmonary artery narrowing not requiring intervention) occur in the young, but rarely in adults.[6]

FUTURE PERSPECTIVES

The transcatheter management of structural congenital heart disease in adults has undergone rapid advances over the past decade. Pulmonary valve implants have become standard therapy for patients with pulmonic valve stenosis and/or regurgitation in circumferential conduits and within bioprosthetic valves. Currently approved therapies to manage circumferential RVOTs include surgically placed conduits, and TPVR with bioprosthetic valves. In addition to standard valve-in-valve therapy, intentional fracture of the surgical bioprosthetic valve frame using ultra-high-pressure balloons can be a means of facilitating further expansion of the valve in the aortic, pulmonary, and tricuspid positions.[48]

Unfortunately, most patients with dysfunctional RVOTs have large, compliant, non-circumferential outflow tracts previously modified by either surgical placement of a transannular patch or catheter-based balloon valvuloplasty. In recent years, several self-expanding, percutaneous valve devices have been designed and are in various stages of clinical testing for patients with these types of RVOT. The Harmony TPV is a porcine pericardial tissue valve mounted on a self-expanding nitinol frame (Fig. 83.4). The Harmony valve recently was studied as a part of an early feasibility trial where 20 patients underwent device implantation.[49] In contrast, the Alterra Adaptive Prestent (Edwards Lifesciences) is a valveless stent designed to be used as a docking adaptor for the 29 mm SAPIEN 3 THV within the RVOT. It is comprised of a covered self-expanding nitinol frame assembly that has 40-mm symmetrical inflow and outflow diameters and a 27-mm central section that serves as a landing zone for a 29 mm SAPIEN 3 valve.[50] Both of these devices are promising catheter-based treatment plans of congenital heart disease in adults.

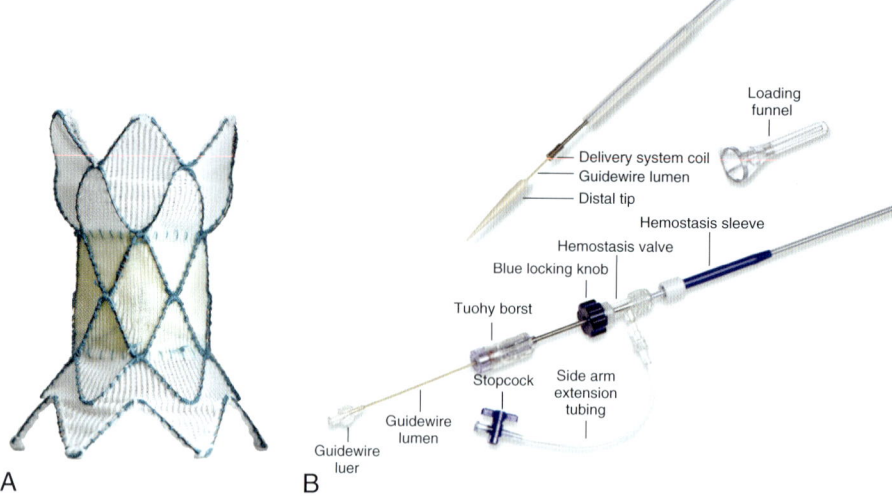

FIGURE 83.4 A, Harmony TPV porcine pericardial tissue valve mounted on a self expanding nitinol stent. **B,** The delivery system is a 25 Fr coil loading catheter with an integrated sheath.

REFERENCES
Valvular Interventions
1. Warnes CA, Williams GR, Bashore TM, et al. ACC/AHA 2008 guidelines for the management of adults with congenital heart disease: a report of the American College of Cardiology/American Heart Association task Force on Practice guidelines (Writing Committee to develop guidelines on the management of adults with congenital heart disease). Developed in Collaboration with the American Society of Echocardiography, heart rhythm society, International society for adult congenital heart disease, society for cardiovascular angiography and interventions, and society of thoracic surgeons. *J Am Coll Cardiol.* 2008;52(23):e143–e263.
2. Aboulhosn JA, Hijazi ZM, Kavinsky CJ, et al. SCAI position statement on adult congenital cardiac interventional training, competencies and organizational recommendations. *Catheter Cardiovasc Interv.* 2020;96(3):643–650.
3. Nishimura RA, Otto CM, Bonow RO, et al. 2014 AHA/ACC guideline for the management of patients with valvular heart disease: a report of the American College of Cardiology/American Heart Association task Force on Practice guidelines. *J Am Coll Cardiol.* 2014;63(22):e57–e185.
4. Kan JS, White RI, Mitchell SE, Gardner TJ. Percutaneous balloon valvuloplasty: a new method for treating congenital pulmonary valve stenosis. *N Engl J Med.* 1982;307:540–542.
5. Rao PS. Percutaneous balloon pulmonary valvuloplasty: state of the art. *Catheter Cardiovasc Interv.* 2007;69(5):747–763.
6. Hoffman JI, Kaplan S. The incidence of congenital heart disease. *J Am Coll Cardiol.* 2002;39(12):1890–1900. https://doi.org/10.1016.
7. Mullins CE, Nihill MR, Vick GW III, et al. Double balloon technique for dilation of valvular or vessel stenosis in congenital and acquired heart disease. *J Am Coll Cardiol.* 1987;10:107–114.
8. Moore JW, Vincent RN, Beekman RH, et al. Procedural results and safety of common interventional procedures in congenital heart disease: initial report from the National Cardiovascular Data Registry. *J Am Coll Cardiol.* 2014;64(23):2439–2451.
9. Marelli AJ, Ionescu-Ittu R, Mackie AS, et al. Lifetime prevalence of congenital heart disease in the general population from 2000 to 2010. *Circulation.* 2014;130(9):749–756.
10. Geva T. Indications for pulmonary valve replacement in repaired tetralogy of Fallot: the quest continues. *Circulation.* 2013;128(17):1855–1857.
11. Bonhoeffer P, Boudjemline Y, Saliba Z, et al. Percutaneous replacement of pulmonary valve in a right-ventricle to pulmonary-artery prosthetic conduit with valve dysfunction. *Lancet.* 2000;356:1403–1405.
12. McElhinney DB, Hennesen JT. The Melody(R) valve and Ensemble(R) delivery system for transcatheter pulmonary valve replacement. *Ann N Y Acad Sci.* 2013;1291:77–85.
13. Leon MB, Smith CR, Mack M, et al. Transcatheter aortic-valve implantation for aortic stenosis in patients who cannot undergo surgery. *N Engl J Med.* 2010;363(17):1597–1607.
14. Garay F, Webb J, Hijazi ZM. Percutaneous replacement of pulmonary valve using the Edwards-Cribier percutaneous heart valve: first report in a human patient. *Catheter Cardiovasc Interv.* 2006;67:659–662.
15. Cheatham JP, Hellenbrand WE, Zahn EM, et al. Clinical and hemodynamic outcomes up to 7 years after transcatheter pulmonary valve replacement in the US Melody valve investigational device exemption trial. *Circulation.* 2015;131(22):1960–1970.
16. Holzer RJ, Hijazi ZM. Transcatheter pulmonary valve replacement: state of the art. *Catheter Cardiovasc Interv.* 2016;87(1):117–128.
17. McElhinney DB, Hellenbrand WE, Zahn M, et al. Short- and medium-term outcomes after transcatheter pulmonary valve placement in the expanded multicenter US Melody valve trial. *Circulation.* 2010;122(5):507–516.
18. McElhinney DB, Benson LN, Eicken A, et al. Infective endocarditis after transcatheter pulmonary valve replacement using the Melody valve: combined results of 3 prospective North American and European studies. *Circ Cardiovasc Interv.* 2013;6(3):292–300.
19. Bergersen L, Gauvreau K, Lock JE, Jenkins KJ, et al. Recent results of pulmonary arterial angioplasty: the differences between proximal and distal lesions. *Cardiol Young.* 2005;15(6):597–604.
20. Bergersen L, Gauvreau K, Justino H, et al. Randomized trial of cutting balloon compared with high-pressure angioplasty for the treatment of resistant pulmonary artery stenosis. *Circulation.* 2011;124(22):2388–2396.

Arterial Interventions
21. Lin AE, Craig TB, Elizabeth G, et al. Adults with genetic syndromes and cardiovascular abnormalities: clinical history and management. *Genet Med.* 2008;10(7):469–494.
22. Thompson BG, Brown Jr RD, Amin-Hanjani S, et al. Guidelines for the management of patients with unruptured intracranial aneurysms: a guideline for healthcare professionals from the American Heart Association/American Stroke Association. *Stroke.* 2015;46:2368–2400.
23. Salcher M, et al. Balloon dilatation and stenting for aortic coarctation: a systematic review and meta-analysis. *Circ Cardiovasc Interv.* 2016;9(6):e003153.

Septal Interventions
24. King TD, Thompson SL, Steiner C, et al. Secundum atrial septal defect. Nonoperative closure during cardiac catheterization. *J Am Med Assoc.* 1976;235:2506–2509.
25. Geva T, Martins JD, Wald RM. Atrial septal defects. *Lancet.* 2014;383(9932):1921–1932.
26. Dalvi B. Balloon assisted technique for closure of large atrial septal defects. *Images Paediatr Cardiol.* 2008;10(4):5–9.
27. Pinto R, Jain S, Dalvi B. Transcatheter closure of large atrial septal defects in children using the left atrial disc engagement-disengagement technique (LADEDT): technical considerations and short term results. *Catheter Cardiovasc Interv.* 2013;82(6):935–943.
28. Varma C, et al. Outcomes and alternative techniques for device closure of the large secundum atrial septal defect. *Catheter Cardiovasc Interv.* 2004;61(1):131–139.
29. Turner DR, et al. Closure of secundum atrial septal defects with the Amplatzer Septal Occluder: a prospective, multicenter, post-approval study. *Circ Cardiovasc Interv.* 2017;10:e004212.
30. Everett AD, et al. Community use of the Amplatzer atrial septal defect occluder: results of the multicenter MAGIC atrial septal defect study. *Pediatr Cardiol.* 2009;30(3):240–247.
31. Nguyen AK, et al. Endocarditis and incomplete endothelialization 12 years after Amplatzer septal occluder deployment. *Tex Heart Inst J.* 2016;43(3):227–231.
32. Saver JL, Carroll JD, Thaler DE, et al. Long-term outcomes of patent foramen ovale closure or medical therapy after stroke. *N Engl J Med.* 2017;377:1022–1032.
33. Grohmann J, et al. Transcatheter closure of atrial septal defects in children and adolescents: single-center experience with the GORE septal occluder. *Catheter Cardiovasc Interv.* 2014;84(6):E51–E57.
34. Sommer RJ, Love BA, Paolillo JA, et al. ASSURED clinical study: new GORE® CARDIOFORM ASD occluder for transcatheter closure of atrial septal defect [published online ahead of print, 2020 Jan 14]. *Catheter Cardiovasc Interv.* 2020;95(7):1285–1295.
35. Søndergaard L, Kasner SE, Rhodes JF, et al. Patent foramen ovale closure or antiplatelet therapy for cryptogenic stroke [published correction appears in N. *Engl J Med.* 2020;382(10):978.
36. Steven RM, Gary SG, David MK, et al, and Kasner. Practice advisory update summary: patent foramen ovale and secondary stroke prevention. *Rep Guideline Subcommittee of the American Academy of Neurology* First published April 29. 2020. https://doi.org/10.1212.
37. Hansen JH, Duong P, Jivanji SGM, et al. Transcatheter correction of superior sinus venosus atrial septal defects as an alternative to surgical treatment. *J Am Coll Cardiol.* 2020;75(11):1266–1278.
38. Yang L, Tai BC, Khin LA, et al. A systematic review on the efficacy and safety of transcatheter device closure of ventricular septal defects (VSD). *J Interv Cardiol.* 2014;27(3):260–272.
39. Carminati M, Butera G, Chessa M, et al. Transcatheter closure of congenital ventricular septal defects: results of the European Registry. *Eur Heart J.* 2007;28(19):2361–2368.
40. Fu Y-C, Bass J, Amin Z, et al. Transcatheter closure of perimembranous ventricular septal defects using the new Amplatzer membranous VSD occluder: results of the U.S. phase I trial. *J Am Coll Cardiol.* 2006;47(2):319–325.
41. Butera G, Carminati M, Chessa M, et al. Transcatheter closure of perimembranous ventricular septal defects: early and long-term results. *J Am Coll Cardiol.* 2007;50(12):1189–1195.
42. Butera G, Gaio G, Carminati M. Is steroid therapy enough to reverse complete atrioventricular block after percutaneous perimembranous ventricular septal defect closure? *J Cardiovasc Med (Hagerstown).* 2009;10(5):412–414.
43. Mahimarangaiah J, Subramanian A, Hemannasetty S, et al. Transcatheter closure of perimembranous ventricular septal defects with ductal occluders. *Cardiol Young.* 2015;25(5):918–926.
44. Omar S, Morgan GL, Panchal HB, et al. Management of post-myocardial infarction ventricular septal defects: a critical assessment. *J Interv Cardiol.* 2018;31(6):939–948. https://doi.org/10.1111.
45. Sabzi F, Faraji R. Adult patent ductus arteriosus complicated by endocarditis and hemolytic anemia. *Colomb Méd.* 2015;46(2):80–83.
46. Fortescue EB, Lock JE, Galvin T, et al. To close or not to close: the very small patent ductus arteriosus. *Congenit Heart Dis.* 2010;5(4):354–365.
47. Jin M, Liang Y-M, Wang X-F, et al. A retrospective study of 1,526 cases of transcatheter occlusion of patent ductus arteriosus. *Chin Med J.* 2015;128(17):2284–2289.

Future Perspectives
48. Shahanavaz S, Asnes JD, Grohmann J, et al. Intentional fracture of bioprosthetic valve frames in patients undergoing valve-in-valve transcatheter pulmonary valve replacement. *Circ Cardiovasc Interv.* 2018;11(8):e006453. https://doi.org/10.1161.
49. Bergersen L, Benson LN, Gillespie MJ, et al. Harmony feasibility trial: acute and short-term outcomes with a self-expanding transcatheter pulmonary valve. *JACC Cardiovasc Interv.* 2017;10(17):1763–1773.
50. Zahn EM, Chang JC, Armer D, Garg R. First human implant of the Alterra Adaptive PrestentTM: a new self-expanding device designed to remodel the right ventricular outflow tract. *Catheter Cardiovasc Interv.* 2018;91(6):1125–1129.

84 Cardiomyopathies Induced by Drugs or Toxins

ROBERT A. KLONER AND SHEREIF REZKALLA

ALCOHOL, 1593
History, 1593
Epidemiology, 1593
Pharmacology and Pathophysiology, 1593
Alcoholic Cardiomyopathy, 1593
Cardiac Arrhythmias, 1594
Alcohol and Lipid Metabolism, 1594
Alcohol and Coronary Artery Disease, 1594
Alcohol and Hypertension, 1595

ELECTRONIC CIGARETTES, 1595
The Effect of Electronic Cigarettes/Vaping on the Cardiovascular System, 1595
E-Cigarette or Vaping Product Use Associated Lung Injury, 1596

COCAINE, 1596
History and Epidemiology, 1596
Pathophysiology, 1596
Clinical Presentation, 1597
Aortic Dissection, 1598
Myocardial Dysfunction, 1598
Cardiac Arrhythmias, 1598

OTHER CARDIAC STIMULANTS, 1599
Amphetamines and Methamphetamines, 1599
Khat and Cathinones, 1599

MARIJUANA, 1599
Atrial Arrhythmias, 1599
Ventricular Arrhythmias, 1599

Acute Coronary Syndromes, 1600
Neurologic Events, 1600
Cannabidiol Oil, 1600

ENERGY DRINKS AND CAFFEINE, 1600

OPIATES, 1601

HEAVY METALS, 1601

FUTURE DIRECTIONS, 1601

ACKNOWLEDGMENT, 1601

REFERENCES, 1601

Many natural and synthetic substances and environmental exposures may affect the heart adversely. Accordingly, it is important to understand the myriad ways in which these substances may influence the cardiovascular system. Many of these substances are used and abused by people throughout the world. With better understanding of the full extent of the pathophysiology of these toxins, we may be able to curb the problems associated with the use of these substances, as well as their associated economic burden. Chapter 56 discusses the toxicities of various chemotherapeutic agents.

ALCOHOL

History
Ancient Egyptians were one of the first civilizations to manufacture beer for both pleasure and religious rituals. In ancient China, rice wine was a tradition and consumed in moderation.[1] In the 16th century, distilled liquor was prepared and termed *alcohol*. The potential beneficial effects that alcohol could have on the heart were first described in medieval times. In the United States, the 21st amendment was added to the Constitution, which ended prohibition; since then, alcohol has become a widely available product.

For several decades, the deleterious effects of excessive alcohol intake on organ systems, including the cardiovascular system, have become widely recognized, and alcohol abuse is now considered a major cause of morbidity, mortality, and burden to the economics of society. The following section discusses the types of damage that excess alcohol causes to the heart and blood vessels.

Epidemiology
Alcohol is the most commonly used and abused substance across the globe. Approximately 40% of adults use alcohol worldwide. In the United States, approximately 70% of adults use alcohol. Eastern Europe and the former Soviet Union report the highest rates of alcohol consumption, at 10 L of pure alcohol per person per year, while the lowest areas of consumption are southeast Asia and the Middle East, at less than 2.5 L per person per year of pure alcohol.[2] Because of the heavy economic burden of alcohol abuse, the World Health Organization had a goal of decreasing alcohol consumption by 10%. Unfortunately, that goal was not achieved, and in fact, alcohol consumption is on the rise.

Although men consume significantly more alcohol compared with women, the latter are more sensitive to the drug, and the prevalence of alcoholic cardiomyopathy is equal between men and women. Moderate drinking is considered up to one drink per day in women and up to two drinks per day in men. Binge drinking (four drinks for women and five drinks for men in approximately 2 hours, resulting in blood alcohol concentration to 0.08 g/dL or greater) is becoming an increasing problem. Binge drinking in the elderly is on the rise, and it is estimated to occur in approximately 10% of adults older than 65 years of age.[3] Definitions of heavy drinking (Centers for Disease Control and Prevention [CDC]) include 15 drinks or more per week for men and 8 drinks or more per week for women. Both binge drinking and heavy drinking are associated with alcohol use disorder or alcoholism, the inability to control drinking related to both physical and emotional dependence upon alcohol consumption. There have been recent concerns that isolation during the COVID-19 pandemic crisis of 2020 may be associated with an increase in alcohol abuse.

Pharmacology and Pathophysiology
When ingested, ethanol is oxidized by the enzyme alcohol dehydrogenase into acetaldehyde. Acetaldehyde is then oxidized into acetic acid and acetate by the enzyme aldehyde dehydrogenase. These metabolites have an impact on cardiac myocytes, impairing mitochondrial function, enhancing oxidative stress, and increasing myocyte apoptosis,[4] ultimately leading to both systolic and diastolic cardiac dysfunction. The deleterious effects of alcohol drinking depend on the amount consumed and the duration of consumption. The degree of alcohol-induced cardiac effects varies by individual based on many genotypic and phenotypic variants. Although various manifestations of alcoholic heart disease are mainly associated with chronic heavy alcohol abuse, acute binge drinking may also cause myocardial injury, enhance inflammation, and result in cardiac arrhythmias. Other factors that contribute to the cardiac effects of alcohol include associated nutritional deficiencies as well as many additives that may be found in different alcoholic drinks.

Alcoholic Cardiomyopathy
Heavy alcohol drinking for prolonged periods of time affects systolic and diastolic heart function and may lead to overt heart failure (see Chapter 52).[5] The amount of alcohol drinking to be considered an

alcoholic is generally more than 90 g/day of alcohol for 5 years or more. William MacKenzie first described the cardiac effects of alcohol in 1902, calling it alcoholic heart disease. As many as 30% of chronic alcoholics have evidence of left ventricular (LV) dysfunction by two-dimensional echocardiography. Alcoholic cardiomyopathy represents approximately 20% to 30% of cases of nonischemic dilated cardiomyopathy. The incidence is affected by both phenotypic and genotypic factors. Increased amounts of alcohol consumed per day and a long duration of alcohol use are associated with higher incidence of cardiomyopathy. Women are more susceptible to the development of the disease. The clinical picture of this disease ranges from asymptomatic cardiac abnormalities to clinically advanced congestive heart failure with symptoms of dyspnea, fatigue, and exercise intolerance; the clinical findings on physical examination include jugular venous congestion, rales in the lungs, and peripheral edema (see also Chapter 48). In history taking, the term *social drinking* does not capture the extent of alcohol use. The type, number of drinks per day, and the duration of drinking is essential in evaluating such patients. A 12-lead electrocardiogram (ECG) may show sinus tachycardia (particularly during acute intoxication), nonspecific ST and T wave abnormality, right and left bundle branch block, and various atrial and ventricular arrhythmias. Chest radiography shows cardiomegaly and pulmonary congestion when patients are in decompensated heart failure.[6] Echocardiography is an important noninvasive diagnostic modality. The earliest echocardiographic abnormality in heavy alcohol drinkers is diastolic dysfunction, present in at least one-third of asymptomatic patients. With progression of the disease, global systolic dysfunction ensues, and the echocardiogram may be indistinguishable from advanced idiopathic nonischemic cardiomyopathy. Atrial and ventricular thrombi may be detected in advanced cases, resulting in systemic embolization. Longitudinal, circumferential, and radial strain echocardiography can detect very early cases of alcoholic cardiomyopathy, which will aid in early detection and management of the disease.[7]

The histopathology of alcoholic cardiomyopathy is similar to dilated cardiomyopathy, except there is lower myocyte count in histologic sections in the former compared to the latter.[8] Guzzo-Merello et al.[9] followed 94 consecutive patients with alcoholic cardiomyopathy for a median follow-up of approximately 5 years. In that study, 5% of patients died from heart failure, 8.5% had sudden death, and 15% ended up with cardiac transplant. The remaining patients either remained clinically stable or improved after reducing alcohol intake. Atrial fibrillation, absence of beta blocker therapy, and QRS duration longer than 120 milliseconds were associated with poor prognosis.

Management of alcoholic cardiomyopathy parallels the treatment for heart failure with a reduced ejection fraction (see Chapter 50). Abstinence of alcohol drinking should be the first major component of treatment. Patients who stopped drinking or even decreased drinking to mild or moderate levels demonstrated improvement in LV ejection fraction upon follow-up. Patients who completely stop drinking alcohol may normalize their ejection fraction in 1 year. Factors that were associated with the best recovery of ejection fraction included narrow QRS, beta blocker therapy, and lack of use or need for diuretic therapy.[10]

Cardiac Arrhythmias

Frequent atrial and ventricular arrhythmias reported with alcohol drinking are secondary to the effect of alcohol on atrial muscle and ventricular myocytes as well as electrolyte abnormalities. The most common abnormality, and the one that needs more attention in the clinical setting, is atrial fibrillation.[11] Low levels of alcohol intake, with only one standard drink per day, is not associated with increased incidence of atrial fibrillation. Moderate drinking increases the incidence of atrial fibrillation in males only, whereas heavy drinking is associated with atrial arrhythmias in both sexes. The Framingham study showed an increase in the incidence of atrial fibrillation in 34% of patients who consumed more than three standard drinks per day. In a randomized study, 140 patients who consumed at least 10 drinks per week and had atrial fibrillation were randomized to either continuing drinking or no drinking. Those who stopped drinking had significantly lower incidence of atrial fibrillation.[12]

Several decades ago, "holiday heart" syndrome was described as cardiac arrhythmias that were mainly atrial flutter and atrial fibrillation.[13] This syndrome describes patients who consume excessive alcohol on weekends and holidays, who then develop these arrhythmias a day or two later. It is more common in men than in women, occurs in patients with an apparently normal heart, and has a relatively benign prognosis.

Ventricular arrhythmias occur with heavy alcohol drinking and may be fatal. A V-shaped or J-shaped curve that characterizes the relationship between alcohol drinking and mortality has been described. Mild to moderate drinking is associated with lower cardiovascular mortality, whereas heavy drinking leads to increased mortality.[14] Alcohol drinking was followed in 33,593 healthy volunteers who drank alcohol for 26 years. Significant alcohol drinking was associated with higher mortality (Fig. 84.1).[15] Alcohol drinking in the presence of left bundle branch block and decreased ventricular function are determinants of malignant ventricular arrhythmias.[16]

Alcohol and Lipid Metabolism

Alcohol increases high-density lipoprotein (HDL) and may reduce low-density lipoprotein (LDL). It may even have some favorable effect on lipoprotein(a) (Fig. 84.2).[17] In addition, moderate intake of beer enhances the antioxidative properties of HDL; thus it prevents lipid deposition in blood vessel walls. Severe alcohol consumption may increase triglyceride levels, blunting the beneficial effect of moderate alcohol drinking.[18,19]

Alcohol and Coronary Artery Disease

In addition to a potential benefit on HDL levels, alcohol may have other protective effects that limit coronary atherosclerosis. Systemic inflammation is shown to promote atherosclerosis. Alcohol has antioxidant and antiinflammatory effects.[20] It is associated with a decrease in C-reactive protein as well as interleukin-6.[21] The beneficial effect is limited to low to moderate drinking,[22] and it appears to be more pronounced in men compared with women. In heavy drinkers, the opposite occurs. Heavy drinking and binge drinking are associated with an increase in inflammatory markers.[23] After mild to moderate alcohol drinking, there is a decrease in platelet aggregation. However, binge drinking may have the opposite effect, which may account for the increase in cardiac events following binge drinking. Some alcoholic beverages, specifically wine, contain resveratrol, which has an antioxidant effect that stimulates mitochondria biogenesis.[24] It is quite clear that low to moderate alcohol consumption is associated with a decreased risk of atherosclerotic burden.[25] Mild alcohol drinking, particularly wine, is associated with a decrease in cardiovascular risk. There is a favorable effect on mortality when mild alcohol

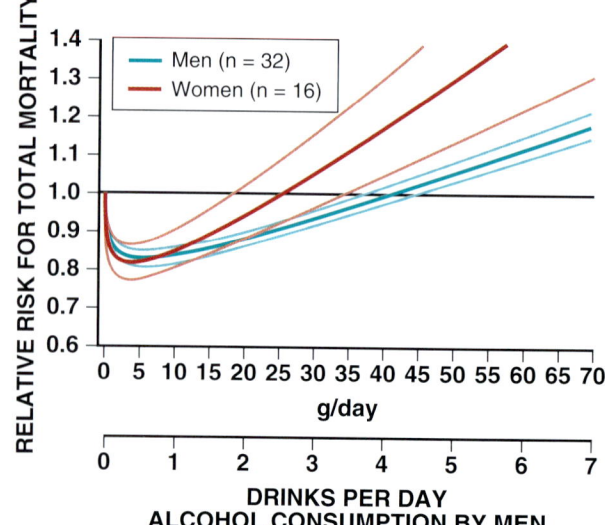

FIGURE 84.1 Risk of total mortality and its relationship to alcoholic drinks per day in both men and women. (From Di Castelnuovo A, Costanzo S, Bagnardi V, et al. Alcohol dosing and total mortality in men and women: an updated meta-analysis of 34 prospective studies. *Arch Intern Med.* 2006;166[22]:2437–2445.)

drinking is combined with other healthy lifestyle factors such as no smoking, a healthy diet, and moderate physical activity.[26] The American Heart Association (AHA) suggests that if a person already drinks, their intake be limited, with one or two drinks per day for men and only one drink for women. A "drink" is considered to be 12 ounces of beer, 5 ounces of wine, or a mixed drink containing 1.5 ounces of hard liquor. However, the AHA does not recommend that people start drinking to lower their cardiovascular risk.

Alcohol and Hypertension

Mild alcohol drinking does not affect blood pressure. However, heavy alcohol drinking, which initially may cause vasodilation, may later result in an increase in blood pressure. It is expected that controlling excessive alcohol drinking in people 40 to 60 years of age will result in a decrease in hypertension, and that is expected in both men and women.[27] In a randomized study, 25 normotensive volunteers received either 375 mL of red wine or a nonalcoholic beverage. Blood pressure fell 4 hours after drinking alcohol but was significantly higher 24 hours later as compared with the control subjects. When drinking is combined with weight gain and smoking, the effect on blood pressure is accentuated. The deleterious and protective effects of alcohol on the cardiovascular system are summarized in Figure 84.3.

ELECTRONIC CIGARETTES

The Effect of Electronic Cigarettes/Vaping on the Cardiovascular System

It is well known that smoking tobacco cigarettes leads to a number of health problems including ischemic heart disease, lung cancer, other forms of cancer, chronic obstructive lung disease, and peripheral vascular disease. Tobacco smoking accelerates atherosclerosis and leads to myocardial infarction (MI), stroke, and peripheral arterial disease. Carbon monoxide in tobacco smoke reduces oxygen availability. The nicotine in tobacco smoke is known to stimulate the sympathetic nervous system, which results in an increase in heart rate, blood pressure, heart contractility, and coronary vasoconstriction. Nicotine lowers HDL cholesterol, increases triglyceride levels, and induces endothelial dysfunction. Tobacco smoke results in oxidant chemicals, particulates, and combustion products that cause inflammation, endothelial dysfunction, and activates clotting mechanisms.

There is a common perception that electronic (e-)cigarettes may be safer than tobacco cigarettes because they lack the tars that cause cancer and do not contain as many of the over 4000 chemical compounds that are created by a burning tobacco cigarette. It is also thought that they might help smokers quit tobacco smoking. E-cigarettes consist of a liquid cartridge that typically contains propylene glycol and vegetable glycerin and may contain nicotine at various doses (including very high doses). The e-liquid may also contain flavorings, some of which are fruit flavored and sweet and appeal to young people. The e-cigarette devices also include a sensor, a microprocessor, and a battery. The electronic cigarette is activated with inhalation by the sensor or by pushing a button; this triggers the heating of coils, which then vaporizes

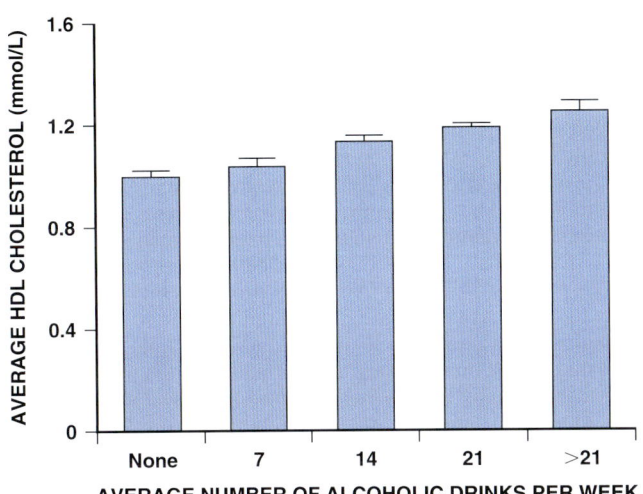

FIGURE 84.2 Relationship between average high-density lipoprotein (HDL) levels and average number of alcoholic drinks per week. (Modified from Suh I, Shaten BJ, Cutler JA, et al. Alcohol use and mortality from coronary heart disease: the role of high-density lipoprotein cholesterol. *Ann Intern Med.* 1992;116:881–887.)

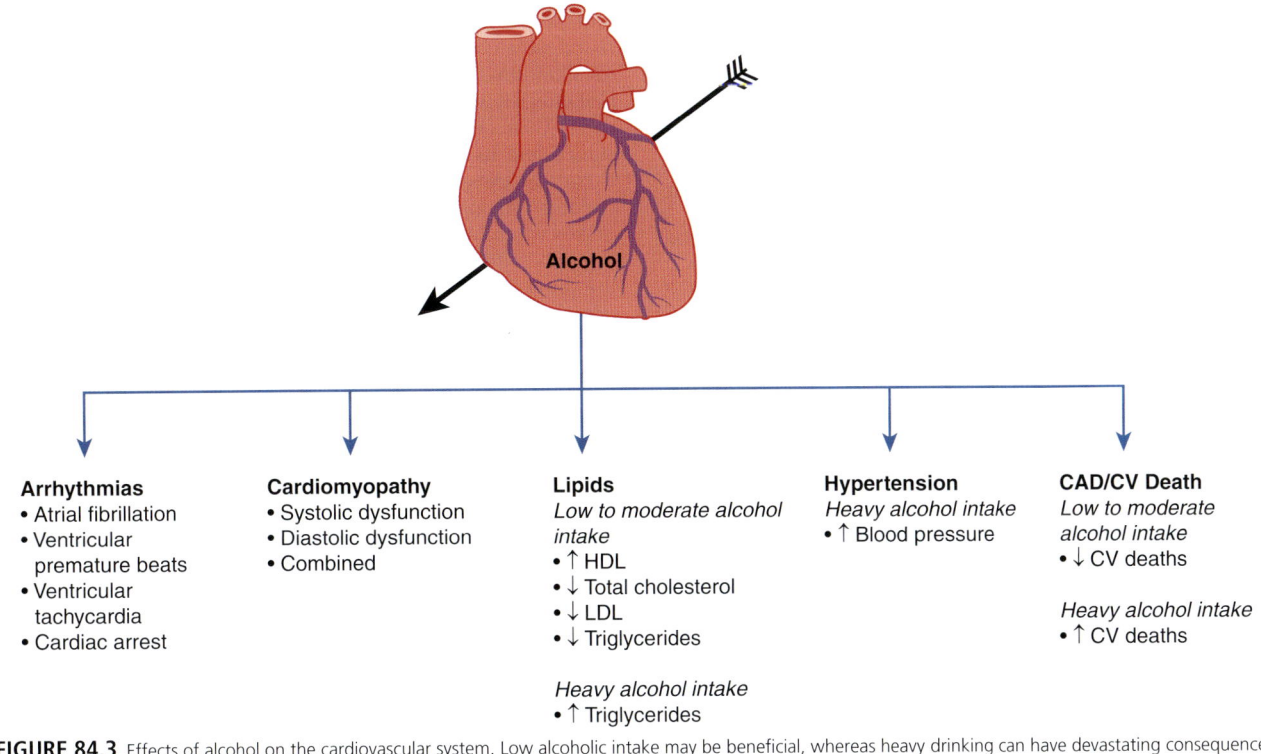

FIGURE 84.3 Effects of alcohol on the cardiovascular system. Low alcoholic intake may be beneficial, whereas heavy drinking can have devastating consequences.

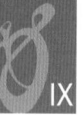

the e-liquid within the cartridge. E-cigarette vapors reach the mouth or the air and condense into particles that form an aerosol. Some of the devices have a light that simulates the glow of a lit cigarette, which is turned on by the microprocessor. Although e-cigarettes do not contain tar or generate carbon monoxide as do tobacco cigarettes,[28] when the e-liquid is heated the results may include formation of formaldehyde, acetaldehyde, and acrolein, which result in reactive oxygen species and inflammation that can contribute to an acceleration of atherosclerosis and clotting. Electronic cigarettes are commonly used as a nicotine delivery device. Nicotine can result in the cardiovascular effects described earlier and is addictive. In addition, the high temperatures of e-cigarettes can result in the generation of very small particulate matter that can enter the lungs and possibly the vasculature to a greater extent than tobacco cigarettes and contribute to vascular damage. Metals and flavoring contained in e-cigarette vapor can contribute to adverse cardiovascular effects including inflammation.[29]

Electronic cigarettes have been around since approximately 2003, and they have become increasingly popular, even as overall tobacco smoking has declined. It is estimated that approximately 9 million adults in the United States vape on a regular basis. In 2019, approximately 28% of high school students reported using e-cigarettes, while only 5.8% reported smoking tobacco cigarettes. Approximately 10.5% of middle school students reported using e-cigarettes. E-cigarette use increased from 12% to 21% among high school students from 2017 to 2018.

Preclinical and clinical studies have examined the effects of e-cigarettes on the cardiovascular system. Variable effects on hemodynamics such as blood pressure and heart rate have been reported. One study showed that in people who smoked an e-cigarette with nicotine or standard cigarettes, both demonstrated an increase in blood pressure.[30] Blood pressure was elevated for a longer time (45 minutes) after using an e-cigarette with nicotine than with a standard cigarette (15 minutes). Those who smoked e-cigarettes without nicotine did not have an increase in blood pressure. Studies of heart rate variability have shown the use of e-cigarettes with nicotine was associated with a marked shift in cardiac sympathovagal balance towards sympathetic predominance, whereas this shift did not occur with e-cigarettes without nicotine. Some studies have suggested that e-cigarette vapor causes endothelial dysfunction with reduced flow-mediated vasodilation, increased vascular resistance, vascular stiffness, and reduced distal blood flow velocity. Although some studies suggested that nicotine was the cause, others suggested that the e-cigarette vapor itself was causing vascular abnormalities including abnormalities in endothelial cells. Other studies suggested that e-cigarettes increased low density lipoprotein oxidation and increased platelet activation. Flavoring, especially cinnamon flavoring, has been associated with abnormalities induced by e-cigarettes in an experimental model.[31] In these studies, e-cigarette flavoring caused decreased endothelial cell viability, increased reactive oxygen species levels, and increased inflammatory cytokine expression in human-induced pluripotent stem cell–derived endothelial cells. The long-term effects of e-cigarettes on the cardiovascular system are largely unknown.

One study suggested that e-cigarettes were more effective than standard, already approved nicotine replacement therapies for smoking cessation.[32] However, the AHA recommended using e-cigarettes for smoking cessation only as a last resort. They recommended behavioral support, nicotine patches, bupropion, or varenicline. In an observational study of over 69,000 participants from the National Health Interview Surveys, daily use of e-cigarettes was an independent factor associated with increased odds of suffering from a myocardial infarction (nearly double that of conventional tobacco smoking). There was a fivefold risk of having a myocardial infarction in individuals who used both standard cigarettes plus e-cigarettes compared with those who did not use either.[33] In a cross-sectional study of 400,000 participants from a 2016 behavioral risk factor surveillance study, the odds of having a stroke were 71% higher in e-cigarette users versus nonusers. In addition, the incidence of myocardial infarction was 59% greater in e-cigarette users than nonusers, and the incidence of angina pectoris was 40% higher in e-cigarette users than nonusers.[34] Thus, although e-cigarettes might help with smoking cessation, there may be consequences, including increased rates of myocardial infarction, stroke, endothelial dysfunction, increased platelet aggregation, and possible other cardiovascular effects.

E-Cigarette or Vaping Product Use Associated Lung Injury (see Chapter 28)

Beginning in July 2019, a new form of lung injury was described in people who vape and has now exploded into a true epidemic.[35] The condition is now known as E-cigarette or vaping product use associated lung injury (EVALI). As of January 14, 2020, there have now been over 2660 clinical cases of EVALI reported, with 60 deaths in the United States. Over 90% of victims have been hospitalized, and over 30% required respirators. Cases have been reported in nearly all states in the United States. The typical victim is a young male who has been using e-cigarettes (vaping) within days to weeks of the illness. The patients present with respiratory distress including shortness of breath, cough, chest pain, fever, fatigue, and gastrointestinal symptoms including nausea, vomiting, and diarrhea. The patients are often hypoxic. Chest radiography typically shows ground glass–appearing bilateral pulmonary infiltrates. Histology has shown pneumonitis, bronchiolitis, and diffuse alveolar damage. Some reports have described lipid-laden macrophages. The phenomenon has been observed in people using a wide variety of e-cigarette liquid brands, substances, and devices. The exact cause of EVALI remains to be determined. Of note, over 80% of cases included use of tetrahydrocannabinol (THC). One leading theory suggested by the CDC is that contaminants such as vitamin E acetate oil, which is often used to dilute THC, may be responsible for EVALI. However, although studies have shown that there is an association between the presence of vitamin E acetate in the lungs of victims and the presence of EVALI, these studies have not clearly demonstrated that vitamin E is responsible for the pulmonary problems that develop. Over 60% of the victims of EVALI also used e-liquid that contained nicotine. Although vitamin E acetate and nicotine may contribute to EVALI, additional studies will be necessary to determine the role of these agents. Other than stopping vaping, there is no specific treatment, as yet, for EVALI other than supportive measures and hospitalization if needed. Influenza testing should be considered, and other causes of pneumonia and respiratory distress (including COVID-19) should be ruled out and treated. Some patients have responded to corticosteroids.

COCAINE

History and Epidemiology

Cocaine is an active chemical found in the plant *Erythroxylon coca* and has been used since the Inca empire 5000 years ago. Alfred Neimann isolated cocaine in 1860, and the drug was initially used as a local anesthetic. Because of its special properties, including its stimulant effect, it was mixed with wine (Vin Mariani, 1865) and soft drinks (Coca-Cola, 1888). In 1914, it was legally classified as a narcotic substance, and its use was largely limited to addicts. In the early 1980s, a cheap, potent form of crystallized cocaine, referred to as crack cocaine (so named because of the crackling or popping sound it makes when heated) was introduced, which has led to an increase in cardiac events related to cocaine use.[36] Although cocaine use in the general population is trending downward, it is still one of the most commonly used illicit drugs in subjects seeking care in hospital emergency departments, and it is one of the most frequent causes of drug-related deaths reported by medical examiners in the United States. Importantly, cocaine use is rising among high school students, with a prevalence of approximately 5%.[37]

Pathophysiology

The onset and duration of cocaine's effects depend on its route of use, which consequently leads to varying cardiovascular and hemodynamic effects.[38] In general, the intravenous and inhaled (i.e., smoked) routes have a very rapid onset of action (seconds) and short-lived (30 minutes) duration when compared with the mucosally absorbed (e.g., oral, nasal [i.e., snorted], rectal, vaginal) routes. When applied locally, cocaine acts as an anesthetic by virtue of its inhibition of membrane permeability to sodium during depolarization, thereby blocking the initiation and transmission of electrical signals. When given systemically, it blocks the presynaptic reuptake of norepinephrine and dopamine, thereby producing an excess of these neurotransmitters at the site of the postsynaptic receptor (Fig. 84.4A). Experimental studies in dogs showed cocaine injection led to diffuse coronary artery spasm, reduced regional coronary blood flow, and a marked decrease in both systolic and diastolic cardiac function within minutes.[36] Cocaine induces vasoconstriction in normal coronary arteries but exerts a particularly marked vasoconstrictive effect in diseased segments (Fig. 84.4B). As a result, cocaine users with atherosclerotic coronary artery disease probably have an especially high risk for an ischemic event after cocaine use. Cocaine-induced coronary arterial vasoconstriction results primarily from the stimulation of coronary arterial alpha-adrenergic receptors because it is reversed by phentolamine (an alpha-adrenergic antagonist) and exacerbated by propranolol (a beta-adrenergic antagonist). Although it was suspected initially that the decrease in coronary blood flow was solely responsible for the myocardial dysfunction, rigorous time analysis studies suggested that cocaine has a direct negative effect on cardiac myocytes that can lead to cardiac dysfunction. Cocaine acts as a powerful sympathomimetic agent, with increases in circulating catecholamine levels leading to increases in blood pressure and heart rate, both of which increase oxygen demand.[36] The increase in oxygen demand combined with a decrease in blood supply due to coronary artery vasoconstriction explains various ischemic events temporally related to cocaine use. The effect of intranasal cocaine use in 42 smokers was studied in the catheterization laboratory. Cocaine resulted in an increase in the rate-pressure product, as well as a decrease in the diameter of the diseased segments of the coronary arteries. This combination of increased oxygen demand and decreased myocardial oxygen supply may explain the deleterious effects of cocaine on the human heart.[39] Additional studies suggested that cocaine enhances platelet aggregation, a mechanism that may contribute to the development of MI (Fig. 84.4B).

Clinical Presentation

Considering the deleterious effects that cocaine can have on disrupting the oxygen supply/demand balance in the heart, it is not surprising that chest pain is the chief complaint in cocaine abusers presenting to emergency departments. The risk of MI increases up to 24-fold in the first hour after cocaine abuse.[39] Chest pain may be related to cardiac involvement including acute MI, or alternatively, be noncardiac in nature. Two large-scale registries revealed that the incidence of MI among cocaine abusers who presented with chest pain was only 6%, suggesting that there are likely extracardiac cocaine-related causes of chest pain (e.g., pleuritic, musculoskeletal).

Based on the earlier observations, a stepped approach is recommended for the evaluation of patients presenting with cocaine-related chest pain, to reduce unnecessary hospitalizations and interventions. As shown in Figure 84.5, these patients should be first evaluated by history, physical examination, and vital signs, followed by an ECG and measurement of cardiac troponins. A recent review of 363,143 hospitalized patients with cocaine-induced chest pain revealed that only 0.69% suffered an acute MI. Moreover, the mortality rate in these patients was low (0.09%), suggesting that patients without ST-segment elevation can be safely observed in the emergency department.[40] The current American College of Cardiology (ACC)/AHA guidelines recommend that stable patients with cocaine-related chest pain should be observed for at least 12 hours (see Chapter 39).

Patients with ECG evidence of persistent ST-segment elevation that is nonresponsive to nitrates should be directly referred for coronary angiography, for consideration for possible angioplasty and stent implantation. Management of cocaine-induced MI is similar to non–drug-related MI (see Chapters 37, 38, and 39), with some exceptions. Immediate use of aspirin and clopidogrel is recommended because of the increased platelet aggregation and increased coronary thrombosis (see Fig. 84.4B). Although drug-eluting stents are occasionally used

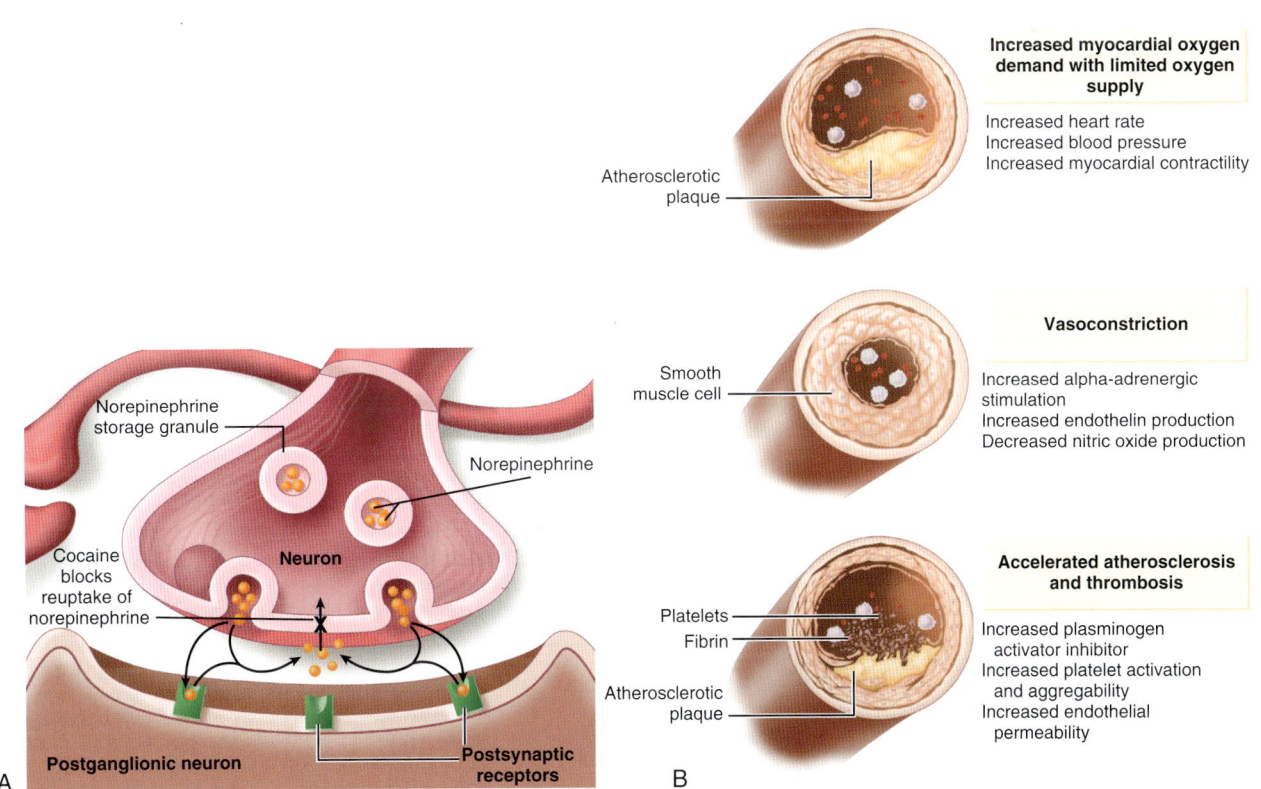

FIGURE 84.4 Mechanisms of cocaine toxicity. **A,** Mechanism by which cocaine alters sympathetic tone. Cocaine blocks the reuptake of norepinephrine by the preganglionic neuron (X), thereby resulting in excess amounts of this neurotransmitter at postganglionic receptor sites. **B,** Mechanisms by which cocaine may induce myocardial ischemia or infarction. Cocaine may induce myocardial ischemia or infarction by increasing the determinants of myocardial oxygen demand in the setting of limited oxygen supply *(top)*, causing intense coronary arterial vasoconstriction *(middle)* or inducing accelerated atherosclerosis and thrombosis *(bottom)*.

in the management of cocaine abusers, the majority of these patients usually receive bare-metal stents, and both the 2008 and 2012 ACC/AHA scientific statements recommend the use of bare-metal stents in cocaine users.[39] If immediate percutaneous intervention is not available, thrombolytic therapy should be initiated, unless otherwise contraindicated. If the patient's history suggests a low risk for cardiac events, the 12-lead ECG is normal, and the troponin level is within normal limits, then outpatient follow-up is adequate (see Fig. 84.5).

Nitrates, phentolamine (an alpha-receptor blocker), and verapamil (a calcium channel blocker) have been shown to reverse cocaine-induced coronary vasoconstriction in the controlled setting of the cardiac catheterization laboratory and are used to manage cocaine-induced chest pain. Although beta blockers represent an essential therapy in the mitigation of hyperadrenergic states and are known to reduce myocardial oxygen demand, the use of beta blockers in the setting of cocaine-induced vasoconstriction is still debated because of the concern that β_1/β_2-blockade might lead to unopposed alpha-stimulation, resulting in coronary artery vasoconstriction. ACC/AHA guidelines recommend against using beta-blockers in the setting of acute coronary syndromes with signs of acute cocaine intoxication (class III, Level of Evidence: C) unless patients are receiving a vasodilator. More recent studies examining beta blocker use in cocaine-exposed patients with acute coronary syndromes have shown that beta blockers are safe and potentially efficacious.[41] The 2012 AHA/ACC guidelines endorse the use of nonselective beta blockers in patients with persistent hypertensive or tachycardia after cocaine use, provided the patients are treated with a vasodilator (Class IIb, Level of Evidence: C). Although combined beta blocker and alpha blockers (e.g., labetalol and carvedilol) should theoretically be safer than nonselective beta blockers because they avoid unopposed alpha-stimulation, head-to-head comparisons of combined beta blocker and alpha blockers versus nonselective beta blockers have not been performed in patients with cocaine-induced chest pain.

Aortic Dissection

Because aortic dissection or rupture has been temporally related to cocaine use, it should be considered a possible cause of chest pain in cocaine users (see also Chapter 42). Cocaine has been implicated as a causative factor in 0.5% to 37% of cases of aortic dissection, with an average interval from cocaine use to the onset of symptoms of 12 hours (range, 0 to 24). Dissection probably results from a cocaine-induced increase in systemic arterial pressure. In addition to aortic rupture, cocaine-related rupture of mycotic and intracerebral aneurysms has been reported. Also, in patients with suspected MI, the possibility of aortic dissection should be considered before the use of thrombolytic therapy.

Myocardial Dysfunction

Long-term cocaine abuse has been associated with LV hypertrophy, as well as with LV diastolic and/or systolic dysfunction. The presence of LV dysfunction may be related to the occurrence of MI or repetitive episodes of myocardial ischemia. In addition, cocaine exerts a depressant effect on cardiac myocytes in animal studies, as well as in human myocytes. Cases of Takotsubo cardiomyopathy have been described following cocaine use (see Chapter 52).[42] Treatment of symptomatic heart failure arising after cocaine use follows the same guidelines for treating non-cocaine users with heart failure (see Chapter 50).[43] Stopping the use of cocaine may result in a significant improvement of LV function.

Cardiac Arrhythmias

Cardiac arrhythmias are a frequent finding in cocaine users presenting to the emergency department, including various atrial arrhythmias and ventricular arrhythmias such as ventricular extrasystoles, ventricular tachycardia, and ventricular fibrillation. Arrhythmias may be secondary to myocardial ischemia and MI as well as LV dysfunction. Cocaine may affect the generation and conduction of cardiac impulses by several mechanisms. First, its sympathomimetic properties may increase ventricular irritability and lower the threshold for fibrillation. Second, it inhibits action potential generation and conduction (i.e., it prolongs the QRS and QT intervals) as a result of its sodium channel–blocking effects. In so doing, it acts in a manner similar to that of a class I antiarrhythmic agent. Accordingly, Brugada-type electrocardiographic features and torsades de pointes have been observed following cocaine use. Third, cocaine increases the intracellular calcium concentration, which may result in afterdepolarizations and triggered ventricular arrhythmias. Fourth, it reduces vagal activity, thereby potentiating its sympathomimetic effects.

Acute cocaine use may result in ischemic strokes in young adults.[44] The enhanced sympathetic activity, prothrombotic effects, and cerebral vasoconstriction may be contributing factors. Another clinical manifestation of cocaine use is pulmonary hypertension. Similar to systemic hypertension, a retrospective study showed a fivefold increase in pulmonary hypertension in cocaine users compared with an age-sex-race–matched control group.[45]

COCAETHYLENE

In individuals who use cocaine in temporal proximity to the ingestion of ethanol, hepatic transesterification leads to the production of cocaethylene, a unique metabolic by-product of cocaine. Cocaethylene has a similar mechanism of action to cocaine, but it is more potent. Similar to cocaine, cocaethylene blocks reuptake of dopamine at the synaptic cleft, thereby possibly potentiating the systemic toxic

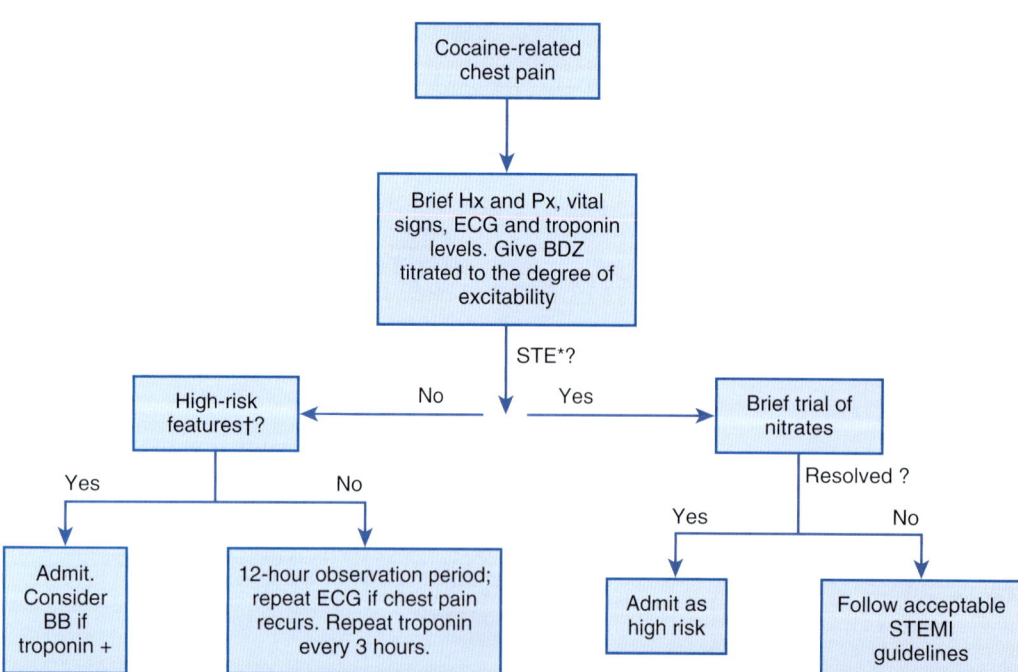

FIGURE 84.5 Algorithm for management of cocaine-induced chest pain in the emergency department. *STE is defined as ST-segment elevation of ≥2 mm. †High-risk features: hemodynamic instability, positive cardiac troponin, recurrent chest pain. *BB*, Beta blocker; *BDZ*, benzodiazepine; *ECG*, electrocardiogram; *STEMI*: ST elevation myocardial infarction. (From Havakuk O, Rezkalla SH, Kloner RA. The cardiovascular effects of cocaine. *J Am Coll Cardiol.* 2017;70:101–113.)

effects of cocaine. People who use cocaine and drink alcohol present with an exaggerated clinical presentation of cocaine use and have a higher mortality rate when compared with either drug alone.[46]

OTHER CARDIAC STIMULANTS

In addition to cocaine, there are a host of other stimulant drugs that can affect the heart.[47] Prescription drugs such as amphetamines and illicitly produced drugs such as methamphetamines and methylenedioxymethamphetamine (MDMA, ecstasy) are examples of some of these agents. These drugs are psychoactive stimulants that can result in sensations of euphoria, empathogenic-entactogenic (feelings of oneness, emotional communion, relatedness, empathy, sympathy), and hallucinations.

Amphetamines and Methamphetamines

The first amphetamines were marketed for nasal congestion, followed by the use amphetamines for narcolepsy and attention-deficit hyperactivity disorders. Some forms of amphetamines are sold illegally, for example, crystal methamphetamine or ice. These agents are central nervous system stimulants that release catecholamines, including norepinephrine, dopamine, and serotonin from presynaptic nerve terminals and prevent their reuptake, resulting in a hyperadrenergic state. These agents can increase heart rate and blood pressure and have been associated with a number of cardiac problems such as chest pain and acute coronary artery syndromes, including acute MI, vasospasm, cardiomyopathy, and acute pulmonary edema.

In a study of 230 patients with a history of acute amphetamine and methamphetamine abuse and positive urine tests (mainly young males), the most common electrocardiographic findings were sinus tachycardia, prolonged QT interval, and arrhythmia (supraventricular and ventricular). Additionally, there were elevations in creatine kinase-MB and troponin I levels. Most patients had normal echocardiograms, while a small number (7%) had LV systolic and/or diastolic dysfunction.[48]

In a retrospective study from New Zealand, 30 patients with a history of amphetamine abuse admitted with heart failure and echocardiographic features of cardiomyopathy (LV ejection fraction 22 ± 8%) were identified. At presentation, four were in cardiogenic shock and five required ICU admission for inotropic support and mechanical ventilation. Most did not recover LV function despite optimal treatment, and five died from end stage heart failure.[49] In another study, investigators used the SphygmoCor system to assess the degree of arterial stiffening in users of recreational amphetamines such as "speed," "ecstasy," and "ice." Amphetamine users, both men and women, demonstrated evidence of accelerated cardiovascular aging, even when adjusting for other cardiovascular risk factors.[50]

An analysis of 894 cases of methamphetamine-related deaths in Australia revealed a mean age of 38 years, with 79% being male. Of the deaths, 76% were associated with enlarged hearts, and LV hypertrophy was present in 19% of cases. Of all cases, 19% had severe coronary artery disease, and 20% had replacement fibrosis within the cardiac walls. Evidence of hypertension based on histologic findings was present in 33% of cases. The conclusion of this autopsy analysis was that cardiovascular disease was highly prevalent in these patients who used methamphetamine, despite their young age. In another study, young male methamphetamine users were found to have higher blood pressure, greater LV mass, and impaired diastolic ventricular function by echocardiographic measures, compared with age-matched male controls. Additionally, the methamphetamine abusers had evidence of reduced myocardial perfusion by myocardial contrast echocardiography.[51]

Methamphetamine use has also now been associated with a dissection of multiple coronary arteries, heart failure, and severe ischemic cardiomyopathy. Experimental studies showed that methamphetamine induces cardiac damage by increasing apoptosis (programmed cell death) in cardiomyocytes and reducing protein expression of melusin (a protein that is a mechanotransducer and is important in maintaining normal cardiac function).[52]

Pulmonary hypertension has also been associated with methamphetamine use (see Chapter 88).[53] In contrast to patients with idiopathic pulmonary hypertension, patients with methamphetamine-associated pulmonary hypertension were more likely to be males, have more severe symptoms of heart failure, have higher right atrial pressure, and demonstrate lower stroke volume index. The patients with methamphetamine-related pulmonary hypertension had more than double the risk of deteriorating clinically and dying compared with patients with idiopathic pulmonary hypertension. The authors concluded that methamphetamine-associated pulmonary artery hypertension is an especially severe form of pulmonary hypertension that is progressive and has a poor outcome.

Khat and Cathinones

Khat is a flowering plant used for its neurostimulant effect. It has two active ingredients: cathine and cathinone. The plant is native to East Africa and the Arabian peninsula and is used in cultural and social situations. Khat is chewed like tobacco, can be made into tea or chewable paste, or can be smoked or added to food. Like other stimulants, it has sympathomimetic properties and is associated with increased heart rate and blood pressure. Khat has been linked to MIs, dilated cardiomyopathy, hypertension, and stroke. Synthetic cathinones, often marketed as "bath salts," have also been associated with cardiac disease, including sudden death and myocarditis.[54]

MARIJUANA

Marijuana is a psychoactive substance produced by drying the leaves and flowering tops of several species of the cannabis plant. It contains several endogenous cannabinoids, the most studied of which is trans-Δ^9-tetrahydrocannabinol (Δ–9–THC). THC is the active component of marijuana that is responsible for its psychoactive properties; it also has sympathomimetic effects that have been linked to cardiovascular side effects.[55] The cannabinoids in marijuana exert their effects by binding two cannabinoid receptors: cannabinoid receptor 1 (CB_1) and cannabinoid receptor 2 (CB_2). CB_1 and CB_2 both belong to a superfamily of metabotropic G protein–coupled receptors. CB_1 receptors are found predominantly in neurons of the brain, whereas CB_2 receptors are present in immune cells, vascular smooth muscle cells, and cardiac myocytes.

The effect of smoking marijuana on the cardiovascular system has been studied in healthy volunteers. Marijuana use resulted in an increase in pulse rate (thereby increasing myocardial oxygen demand) and various electrocardiographic changes, such as P wave abnormalities, as well as nonspecific ST and T wave abnormalities shortly after use. These effects were blocked by beta blockers.[55] The cardiovascular and many other side effects led the Surgeon General of the United States to issue a warning about the cardiac toxicity of marijuana use more than four decades ago. Despite that, and despite federal government laws declaring marijuana use illegal, many states in the United States have legalized marijuana use for recreational purposes. By early 2021, 16 states and the District of Columbia legalized the drug for such recreational purposes, and 36 states plus the District of Columbia legalized the use of medical marijuana. This section of the chapter focuses on various reported cardiovascular effects of marijuana use. It should be noted that the current medical literature is based on temporal associations between marijuana use and increased cardiovascular events, and the safety of marijuana has not been evaluated in controlled studies.

Atrial Arrhythmias

Various atrial arrhythmias have been reported following marijuana use.[56] Both tachycardias and sinus bradycardia have been reported after smoking the drug. The patients often were relatively young, without known risk factors, and the atrial arrhythmias were temporally related to the drug use. The most commonly reported atrial arrhythmia is atrial fibrillation, which was reported in 26% of published cases.[57]

Ventricular Arrhythmias

Ventricular arrhythmias, such as premature ventricular beats and ventricular tachycardia, have been reported to occur in people following marijuana use. The authors reported a case of syncope after marijuana use, associated with inducible ventricular tachycardia during electrophysiology study and no-reflow during coronary angiography. After the patient stopped using marijuana, no-reflow resolved and the ventricular tachycardia was no longer inducible.[58] There are no controlled studies determining the incidence of ventricular tachycardias in marijuana users.

Abouk et al.[59] studied the rate of death attributed to the cardiovascular system in the states that legalized marijuana. They compared death rates before and then after legalizing marijuana. There was a significant increase in death rate after legalizing marijuana, which was more pronounced in men. Whether this observation was secondary to ventricular arrhythmias, coronary artery disease, or other causes is not known. Other reports described unexpected sudden cardiac death following marijuana use, as well as synthetic cannabinoid use.[60]

Acute Coronary Syndromes

Marijuana inhalation results in increased myocardial oxygen demand in addition to creation of reactive oxygen radicals, endothelial dysfunction, and effects on human platelets. Most reports strongly suggest an increase in the incidence of acute coronary syndromes following marijuana use. Patients tend to be younger, with no other significant risk factors for the development of MI. Angiography during presentation of ST-segment elevation MI showed coronary thrombosis in normal coronary arteries or at sites in mildly atherosclerotic arteries. Some cases had normal appearing epicardial coronary arteries with coronary artery no-reflow.

Colorado was one of the earlier states to legalize marijuana use. Review of emergency department records in Colorado showed an increase in cardiovascular events following legalization of recreational use of marijuana.[61] In a report from France, there was an increase in patients who presented to the emergency department following marijuana use. When compared with nonusers who presented with similar cardiovascular complications, there was a 25% increase in mortality in those who were marijuana users. The increase in marijuana use in the United States, and indeed in many other countries across the world, and the emergence of more potent marijuana plants and synthetic cannabinoids clearly compound the problem. A study using hospital records from the national inpatient sample in the United States showed an increase in the number of marijuana users who were admitted with acute cardiovascular events. Figure 84.6 illustrates the cardiovascular complications of marijuana. Not all reports suggest a relation between marijuana use and cardiovascular events, however. A long-term follow-up of the CARDIA study followed young marijuana users for 25 years. Neither recent use nor cumulative lifetime marijuana use was associated with increased incidence of cardiovascular events.[62] However, this study may represent older preparations of marijuana and lower THC concentrations than are now present in contemporary marijuana preparations.

Neurologic Events

Marijuana use may result in cognitive dysfunction, behavioral problems, and memory attention disorders. Additionally, reports of ischemic strokes, and rarely hemorrhagic strokes, were reported. Transient ischemic attacks were reported as well. The mechanisms of such events are not well elucidated but are likely similar to that of cardiac ischemic events. Data from the Behavioral Risk Factor Surveillance System show that marijuana use for therapeutic and recreational purposes results in increased stroke incidence in young adults with recent use.[63] The odds of stroke occurrence increased in subjects who used the drug frequently compared with those who only occasionally used the drug.

Cannabidiol Oil

Cannabidiol (CBD) oil is a product derived from the plant cannabis sativa. CBD is another component of marijuana, but it lacks the psychoactive effect of THC. It has a favorable effect as a pain reliever, anti-inflammatory, and anxiety-relieving agent. No cardiac side effects were noticed during the use of CBD oils, and there are reports that it may reduce both resting and stress-induced hypertension.[64]

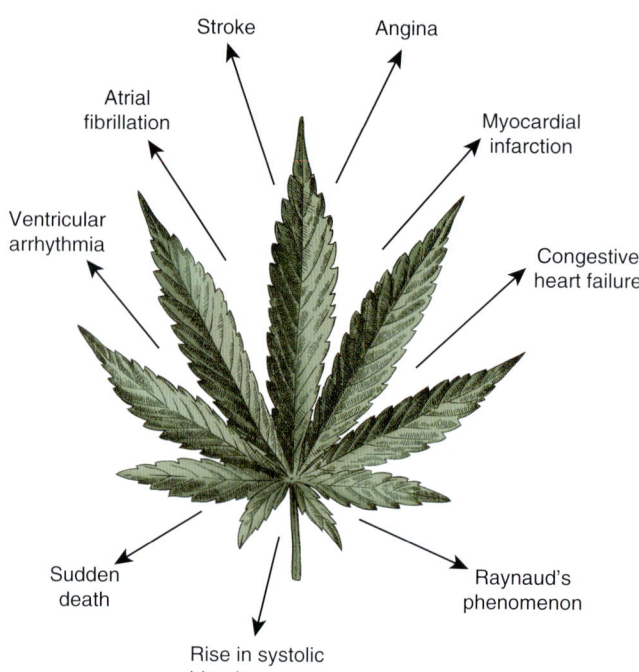

FIGURE 84.6 Cardiovascular complications of marijuana. (Modified from Rezkalla S, Kloner RA. Cardiovascular effects of marijuana. *Trends Cardiovasc Med.* 2019;29:403–407.)

ENERGY DRINKS AND CAFFEINE

Energy drinks have become increasingly popular as a dietary supplement among young people in the United States. They are often used to enhance physical performance, mental acuity, and concentration, to induce weight loss, to improve energy level, and to counteract the effects of alcohol. They contain a number of stimulants, primarily caffeine, which is usually present in much higher concentrations than in coffee or other beverages. For example, energy drinks may contain between 154 and 505 mg of caffeine in a 16- to 24-ounce can, whereas a 6.5-ounce cup of coffee contains 80 to 120 mg of caffeine, tea has 50 mg, and a 12-ounce can of cola has no more than 65 mg of caffeine.[65] Other stimulants found in energy drinks may include guarana, a plant from South America (also known as Brazilian cocoa) that is also high in caffeine content but is typically not included in the total estimate of caffeine in energy drinks. These beverages also contain taurine, sugars, ginseng (which can increase blood pressure), B vitamins, and other additives. Caffeine has sympathomimetic effects and increases cytosolic calcium concentration by inhibiting calcium reuptake in the sarcoplasmic reticulum. It can increase sinus rate, but in doses associated with moderate coffee drinking it does not stimulate atrial fibrillation, nor is it associated with ventricular arrhythmias at moderate doses. However, caffeine overdose is associated with tachycardia, arrhythmias, and hypertension. Energy drinks, especially when taken in excess, can be associated with cardiac arrhythmias, prolonged QT interval, MI, cardiac death, and aortic dissection.[66] Increases in heart rate, blood pressure, and stroke volume and contractility can occur with energy drink excess. Svatikova et al.[67] studied 25 healthy volunteers randomized to receive either placebo or a commercially available energy drink. In this study, the energy drink increased systolic, diastolic, and mean blood pressure and increased norepinephrine levels, but did not increase heart rate. Some reports of acute MI associated with energy drinks revealed patent coronary arteries at the time of catheterization, while one was associated with an intracoronary thrombus. Coronary vasospasm and/or increased platelet aggregation due to energy drinks have been considered possible mechanisms by which MI occurred. In one systematic study of platelet aggregation, volunteers were given water or energy drinks, and platelet function was measured before and 60 minutes after consumption. Energy drinks caused a significant increase in platelet aggregability to arachidonic acid–induced activation, but not with several other activating factors.[68] Practitioners and consumers should be made aware of the potential cardiac dangers of energy drinks.

OPIATES

Opioids are drugs used for pain relief, but their use is often abused, and in recent years this has resulted in increased use with deleterious consequences and the "opioid crisis" in the United States. Examples of opioids include opium, morphine, heroin, hydrocodone, oxycodone, and fentanyl. One of the leading side effects of opioids is respiratory depression that can lead to respiratory arrest. However, opioids have important adverse cardiovascular effects as well. Some of these drugs prolong the QT interval, a phenomenon that can result in the life-threatening ventricular arrhythmia, torsades de pointes, which can cause sudden cardiac death. Methadone is high risk for causing QT prolongation and ventricular arrhythmias, even at low doses. Tramadol, fentanyl, and oxycodone are intermediate in risk and may be more of a problem at higher doses. Morphine and buprenorphine are lower risk and do not usually cause QT prolongation or torsades de pointes at routine dosing levels. Other arrhythmias have been reported in opium consumers including supra-ventricular arrhythmias, atrial fibrillation, sinus bradycardia, and heart block, especially in those with underlying heart disease.[69] Opioids can also cause hypotension, bradycardia, and can reduce cardiac contractility. One study showed that opioids and sedatives represent independent risk factors for in-hospital cardiopulmonary arrest and resuscitation.[70] High doses of opioids should be used with caution, and periodic monitoring of the ECG and QT interval should be considered in high-risk users and patients participating in opioid maintenance treatment programs, where they are exposed to these drugs on a chronic basis. There has been concern that opioids might be associated with an increase in atherosclerotic diseases. In a large prospective cohort study of over 29,000 participants over 5 years, female prescription opioid users—but not male users—had a higher risk of coronary heart disease and cardiovascular death. There was no increase in stroke among opioid users.[71]

HEAVY METALS

Heavy metals have been implicated in heart disease, but many of the studies are older and may include exposures that are now outdated (e.g., cobalt in beer). A recent meta-analysis showed exposure to the heavy metals arsenic, lead, cadmium, and copper was associated with increased cardiovascular disease including coronary artery disease and stroke. However, mercury was not associated with an increase in cardiovascular disease.[72] Heavy metal exposure (including exposure to cadmium, lead, and mercury) has been implicated as contributing to metabolic syndrome. A recent analysis concluded that, although heavy metals may contribute to this syndrome, data were inconclusive and sometimes conflicting; the authors recommended a need for better prospective, standardized studies to determine the importance of heavy metals in the mechanism of metabolic syndrome.[73] People can be exposed to cadmium through food, cigarette smoke, air pollution, or occupational exposure. Cadmium increases reactive oxygen species and depletes natural antioxidants. Exposure to this heavy metal has been associated with endothelial and smooth muscle dysfunction, hypertension, atherosclerosis, and diabetes. Although chelation therapy is one approach to removing cadmium, recent studies suggest that the antioxidants curcumin and tetrahydrocurcumin may play a protective role in dealing with cadmium exposure.[74] A recent analysis showed that prenatal exposure to lead was a risk factor for congenital heart disease in the child (see Chapter 82).[75] Iron overload or hemochromatosis of the cardiovascular system is discussed in other sections of this book (see Chapter 52).

FUTURE DIRECTIONS

In this chapter, we discussed a variety of natural and synthetic drugs and toxins linked to significant deleterious cardiac events. Unfortunately, the precise mechanism of their effects is often unknown, and as a result, effective treatment is not established. This information is essential to avoid agents that interfere with specific molecular pathways that regulate cardiac function and to develop therapy that limits cardiotoxicity. Health care providers and the patients or subjects who use these drugs would benefit from a true understanding of their potential risks to the cardiovascular system. Finally, when new medications are approved for use, postmarketing studies should be required to identify any cardiotoxic effects that may occur infrequently and hence are not evident when the drug is studied in limited numbers of subjects, or only in the presence of concomitant conditions.

ACKNOWLEDGMENT

The authors gratefully acknowledge the editing and technical support of Marie Fleisner in the preparation of this chapter.

REFERENCES

Alcohol

1. Maisch B. Alcoholic cardiomyopathy. The result of dosage and individual predisposition. *Herz*. 2016;41:484–493.
2. Axley PD, Richardson CT, Singal AK. Epidemiology of alcohol consumption and societal burden of alcoholism and alcoholic liver disease. *Clin Liver Dis*. 2019;23:39–50.
3. Han BH, Moore AA, Ferris R, Palamar JJ. Binge drinking among older adults in the United States, 2015-2017. *J Am Geriatr Soc*. 2019;67:2139–2144.
4. Steiner JL, Lang CH. Etiology of alcoholic cardiomyopathy: mitochondria, oxidative stress and apoptosis. *Int J Biochem Cell Biol*. 2017;89:125–135.
5. Piano MR. Alcohol's effects on the cardiovascular system. *Alcohol Res*. 2017;38:219–241.
6. Mirijello A, Tarli C, Vassallo GA, et al. Alcoholic cardiomyopathy: What is known and what is not known. *Eur J Intern Med*. 2017;43:1–5.
7. Wang Y, Li G, Sun Y, et al. Left ventricular strain and rotation by 2-D speckle tracking echocardiography identify early alcoholic cardiomyopathy. *Ultrasound Med Biol*. 2016;42:1741–1749.
8. Li X, Nie Y, Lian H, Hu S. Histopathologic features of alcoholic cardiomyopathy compared with idiopathic dilated cardiomyopathy. *Medicine (Baltim)*. 2018;97:e12259.
9. Guzzo-Merello G, Segovia J, Dominguez F, et al. Natural history and prognostic factors in alcoholic cardiomyopathy. *JACC Heart Fail*. 2015;3:78–86.
10. Amor-Salamanca A, Guzzo-Merello G, Gonzalez-Lopez E, et al. Prognostic impact and predictors of ejection fraction recovery in patients with alcoholic cardiomyopathy. *Rev Esp Cardiol*. 2018;71:612–619.
11. Gallagher C, Hendriks JM, Elliott AD, et al. Alcohol and incident atrial fibrillation—a systemic review and meta-analysis. *Int J Cardiol*. 2017;246:46–52.
12. Voskoboinik A, Kalman JM, De Silva A, et al. Alcohol abstinence in drinkers with atrial fibrillation. *N Engl J Med*. 2020;382:20–28.
13. Brown KN, Yelamanchili VS, Goel A. Holiday heart syndrome. In: *StatPearls*. Treasure Island (FL): StatPearls Publishing; 2020.
14. Haseeb S, Alexander B, Baranchuk A. Wine and cardiovascular health: a comprehensive review. *Circulation*. 2017;136:1434–1448.
15. Whitfield JB, Heath AC, Madden PAF, et al. Effects of high alcohol intake, alcohol-related symptoms and smoking on mortality. *Addiction*. 2018;113:158–166.
16. Guzzo-Merello G, Dominguez F, Gonzalez-Lopez E, et al. Malignant ventricular arrhythmias in alcoholic cardiomyopathy. *Int J Cardiol*. 2015;199:99–105.
17. Vu KN, Ballantyne CM, Hoogeveen RC, et al. Causal role of alcohol consumption in an improved lipid profile: the Atherosclerosis Risk in Communities (ARIC) Study. *PLoS One*. 2016;11:e0148765.
18. Padro T, Muñoz-García N, Vilahur G, et al. Moderate beer intake and cardiovascular health in overweight individuals. *Nutrients*. 2018;10:1237.
19. You M, Arteel GE. Effect of ethanol on lipid metabolism. *J Hepatol*. 2019;70:237–248.
20. Migliori M, Panichi V, de la Torre R, et al. Anti-inflammatory effect of white wine in CKD patients and healthy volunteers. *Blood Purif*. 2015;39:218–223.
21. Relja B, Menke J, Wagner N, et al. Effects of positive blood alcohol concentration on outcome and systemic interleukin-6 in major trauma patients. *Injury*. 2016;47:640–645.
22. Giacosa A, Barale R, Bavaresco L, et al. Mediterranean way of drinking and longevity. *Crit Rev Food Sci Nutr*. 2016;56:635–640.
23. Orio L, Anton M, Rodriguez-Rojo IC, et al. Young alcohol binge drinkers have elevated blood endotoxin, peripheral inflammation and low cortisol levels: neuropsychological correlations in women. *Addict Biol*. 2018;23:1130–1144.
24. Xia N, Daiber A, Forstermann U, Li H. Antioxidant effects of resveratrol in the cardiovascular system. *Br J Pharmacol*. 2017;174:1633–1646.
25. Golan R, Shai I, Gepner Y, et al. Effect of wine on carotid atherosclerosis in type 2 diabetes: a 2-year randomized controlled trial. *Eur J Clin Nutr*. 2018;72:871–878.
26. Li Y, Pan A, Wang DD, et al. Impact of healthy lifestyle factors on life expectancies in the US population. *Circulation*. 2018;138:345–355.
27. Rehm J, Gmel G, Sierra C, Gual A. Reduction of mortality following better detection of hypertension and alcohol problems in primary health care in Spain. *Adicciones*. 2018;30:9–18.

E-Cigarettes

28. MacDonald A, Middlekauff HR. Electronic cigarettes and cardiovascular health: what do we know so far? *Vasc Health Risk Manag*. 2019;15:159–174.
29. Buchanan ND, Grimmer JA, Tanwar V, et al. Cardiovascular risk of electronic cigarettes: a review of preclinical and clinical studies. *Cardiovasc Res*. 2020;116:40–50.
30. Franzen KF, Willig J, Cayo Talavera S, et al. E-Cigarettes and cigarettes worsen peripheral and central hemodynamics as well as arterial stiffness: a randomized, double-blinded pilot study. *Vasc Med*. 2018;23:419–425.

31. Lee WH, Ong S-G, Zhou Y, et al. Modeling cardiovascular risks of e-cigarettes with human-induced pluripotent stem cell-derived endothelial cells. *J Am Coll Cardiol*. 2019;73:2722–2737.
32. Hajek P, Phillips-Waller A, Przulj D, et al. A randomized trial of E-cigarettes versus nicotine-replacement therapy. *N Engl J Med*. 2019;380:626–637.
33. Alzahrani T, Pena I, Temesgen N, Glantz SA. Association between electronic cigarette use and myocardial infarction. *Am J Prev Med*. 2018;55:455–461.
34. Ndunda PM. Electronic cigarette use is associated with a higher risk of stroke. *Stroke*. 2019; 50:A9.
35. Layden JE, Ghinai I, Pray I, et al. Pulmonary illness related to E-cigarette use in Illinois and Wisconsin—Final Report. *N Engl J Med*. 2020;382:903–916.

Cocaine

36. Stankowski RV, Kloner RA, Rezkalla SH. Cardiovascular consequences of cocaine use. *Trends Cardiovasc Med*. 2015;25:517–526.
37. Schneider KE, Krawczyk N, Xuan Z, Johnson RM. Past 15-year trends in lifetime cocaine use among US high school students. *Drug Alcohol Depend*. 2018;183:69–72.
38. Anderson JL, Adams CD, Antman EM, et al. 2012 ACCF/AHA focused update incorporated into the ACCF/AHA 2007 guidelines for the management of patients with unstable angina/non-ST-elevation myocardial infarction: a report of the American College of Cardiology Foundation/American Heart Association Task Force on Practice Guidelines. *J Am Coll Cardiol*. 2013;61:e179–e347.
39. Havakuk O, Rezkalla SH, Kloner RA. The cardiovascular effects of cocaine. *J Am Coll Cardiol*. 2017;70:101–113.
40. Singh V, Rodriguez AP, Thakkar B, et al. Hospital admissions for chest pain associated with cocaine use in the United States. *Am J Med*. 2017;130:688–698.
41. Pham D, Addison D, Kayani W, et al. Outcomes of beta blocker use in cocaine-associated chest pain: a meta-analysis. *Emerg Med J*. 2018;35:559–563.
42. Gill D, Sheikh N, Ruiz VG, Liu K. Case report: cocaine-induced takotsubo cardiomyopathy. *Hellenic J Cardiol*. 2018;59:129–132.
43. Nguyen P, Kamran H, Nasir S, et al. Comparison of frequency of cardiovascular events and mortality in patients with heart failure using versus not using cocaine. *Am J Cardiol*. 2017;119:2030–2034.
44. Cheng YC, Ryan KA, Qadwai SA, et al. Cocaine use and risk of ischemic stroke in young adults. *Stroke*. 2016;47:918–922.
45. Alzghoul BN, Abualsuod A, Alqam B, et al. Cocaine use and pulmonary hypertension. *Am J Cardiol*. 2020;125:282–288.
46. Jones AW. Forensic drug profile: cocaethylene. *J Anal Toxicol*. 2019;43:155–160.

Other Stimulants

47. Duflou J. Psychostimulant use disorder and the heart. *Addiction*. 2020;115:175–183.
48. Bazmi E, Mousavi F, Giahchin L, et al. Cardiovascular complications of acute amphetamine abuse. Cross-sectional study. *Sultan Qaboos Univ Med J*. 2017;17:e31–e37.
49. Kueh S-HA, Gabriel RS, Lund M, et al. Clinical characteristics and outcomes of patients with amphetamine-associated cardiomyopathy in South Aukland, New Zealand. *Heart Lung Circ*. 2016;25:1087–1093.
50. Reece AS, Norman A, Hulse GK. Acceleration of cardiovascular-biological age by amphetamine exposure is a power function of chronological age. *Heart Asia*. 2017;9:30–38.
51. Darke S, Duflou J, Kaye S. Prevalence and nature of cardiovascular disease in methamphetamine-related death: a national study. *Drug Alcohol Depend*. 2017;179:174–179.
52. Sun X, Wang Y, Xia B, et al. Methamphetamine produces cardiac damage and apoptosis by decreasing melusin. *Toxicol Appl Pharmacol*. 2019;378:114543.
53. Zamanian RT, Hedlin H, Greuenwald P, et al. Features and outcomes of methamphetamine-associated pulmonary arterial hypertension. *Am J Respir Crit Care Med*. 2018;197:788–800.
54. Zaami S, Giorgetti R, Pichini S, et al. Synthetic cathinones related fatalities: an update. *Eur Rev Med Pharmacol Sci*. 2018;22:268–274.

Marijuana

55. Rezkalla S, Kloner RA. Cardiovascular effects of marijuana. *Trends Cardiovasc Med*. 2019;29:403–407.
56. Kariyanna PT, Wengrofsky P, Jayarangaiah A, et al. Marijuana and cardiac arrhythmias: a scoping study. *Int J Clin Res Trials*. 2019;4:132.
57. Adegbala O, Adejumo AC, Olakanmi O, et al. Relation of cannabis use and atrial fibrillation among patients hospitalized for heart failure. *Am J Cardiol*. 2018;122:129–134.
58. Rezkalla S, Stankowski R, Kloner RA. Cardiovascular effects of marijuana. *J Cardiovasc Pharmacol Ther*. 2016;21:452–455.
59. Abouk R, Adams S. Examining the relationship between medical marijuana laws and cardiovascular deaths in the US. *Int J Drug Policy*. 2018;53:1–7.
60. Drummer OH, Gerostamoulos D, Woodford NW. Cannabis as a cause of death: a review. *Forensic Sci Int*. 2019;298:298–306.
61. Roberts BA. Legalized cannabis in Colorado emergency departments: a cautionary review of negative health and safety effects. *West J Emerg Med*. 2019;20:557–572.
62. Reis JP, Auer R, Bancks MP, et al. Cumulative lifetime marijuana use and incident cardiovascular disease in middle age: the Coronary Artery Risk Development in Young Adults (CARDIA) study. *Am J Public Health*. 2017;107:601–606.
63. Parekh T, Pemmasani S, Desai R. Marijuana use among young adults (18–44 Years of age) and risk of stroke: a behavioral risk factor surveillance system survey analysis. *Stroke*. 2020;51:308–310.
64. Sultan SR, O'Sullivan SE, England TJ. The effects of acute and sustained cannabidiol dosing for seven days on the haemodynamics in healthy men: a randomised controlled trial. *Br J Clin Pharmacol*. 2020;86:1125–1138.

Energy Drinks and Caffeine

65. Sifferlin A. What's in your energy drink? *Time Magazine*. Feb 04, 2013. https://healthland.toime.com/2013/02/04whats-in-your-energy-drink/.
66. Mangi MA, Rehman H, Rafique M, Illovsky M. Energy drinks and the risk of cardiovascular disease: a review of current literature. *Cureus*. 2017;9:e1322.
67. Svatikova A, Covassin N, Somers KR, et al. A randomized trial of cardiovascular responses to energy drink consumption in healthy adults. *J Am Med Assoc*. 2015;314:2079–2082.
68. Pommerening MJ, Cardenas JC, Radwan ZA, et al. Hypercoagulability after energy drink consumption. *J Surg Res*. 2015;199:635–640.

Opiates and Heavy Metals

69. Behzadi M, Joukar S, Beik A. Opioids and cardiac arrhythmia: a literature review. *Med Princ Pract*. 2018;27:401–414.
70. Overdyk FJ, Dowling O, Marino J, et al. Association of opioids and sedatives with increased risk of in-hospital cardiopulmonary arrest from an Administrative Database. *PloS One*. 2016;11:e0150214.
71. Khodneva Y, Muntner P, Kertesz S, et al. Prescription opioid use and risk of coronary heart disease, stroke, and cardiovascular death among adults from a prospective cohort (REGARDS study). *Pain Med*. 2016;17:444–455.
72. Chowdhury R, Ramond A, O'Keeffe LM, et al. Environmental toxic metal contaminants and risk of cardiovascular disease: systemic review and meta-analysis. *BMJ*. 2018;362:k3310.
73. Planchart A, Green A, Hoyo C, Mattingly CJ. Heavy metal exposure and metabolic syndrome: evidence from human and model system studies. *Curr Environ Health Rep*. 2018;5:110–124.
74. Kukongviriyapan U, Apakjit K, Kukongviriyapan V. Oxidative stress and cardiovascular dysfunction associated with cadmium exposure: beneficial effects of curcumin and tetrahydrocurcumin. *Tohuku J Exp Med*. 2016;239:25–38.
75. Ou Y, Bloom MS, Nie Z, et al. Associations between toxic and essential trace elements in maternal blood and fetal congenital heart defects. *Environ Int*. 2017;106:127–134.

85 Cardiovascular Abnormalities in HIV-Infected Individuals

PRISCILLA Y. HSUE AND DAVID D. WATERS

CARDIOVASCULAR RISK FACTORS IN PEOPLE LIVING WITH HIV, 1603
Dyslipidemia, 1603
Lipodystrophy, the Metabolic Syndrome, and Obesity, 1604
Diabetes, 1605
Hypertension and Chronic Kidney Disease, 1605
Smoking, 1605

MECHANISMS OF HIV-RELATED ATHEROGENESIS, 1605
Features of Atherosclerosis in People with HIV, 1607

CORONARY DISEASE IN HIV SUBJECTS, 1607
Epidemiology, 1607
Clinical Presentation, 1608
Treatment, 1608
Antiretroviral Therapy and Cardiovascular Disease, 1608
Treatment of Lipids in the Setting of HIV, 1609

RISK ASSESSMENT AND SCREENING FOR CORONARY DISEASE, 1610

OTHER CARDIOVASCULAR CONDITIONS ASSOCIATED WITH HIV, 1610
Pulmonary Hypertension, 1610
Heart Failure, 1612
Arrhythmias and Sudden Cardiac Death, 1612
Cerebrovascular Disease, 1613

REFERENCES, 1613

Approximately 37,900,000 people were living with human immunodeficiency virus (HIV) infection at the end of 2018, and 1,700,000 had become newly infected that year.[1] An estimated 23,300,000 people living with HIV were accessing antiretroviral therapy (ART), up from 7,700,000 in 2010.[1] The introduction of ART in 1996 and its increasingly widespread availability since then have dramatically reduced HIV-related mortality rates and has transformed HIV into a chronic disease for those receiving treatment. As a consequence, between 2010 and 2030 the proportion of people with HIV infection aged 50 years or older will increase from 28% to 73%, and the proportion with cardiovascular disease (CVD) from 19% to 78%.[2] Over the same period the proportion taking a cardiovascular (CV) drug is projected to increase from 9% to 50%.

The types of CVD associated with HIV have changed from the pre-ART to the ART eras, (Fig. 85.1) and will likely evolve further.[3] In the pre-ART era, people with acquired immunodeficiency syndrome (AIDS) often had pericardial effusions and dilated cardiomyopathy; these complications still occur in persons without access to ART. Following the introduction of protease inhibitors (PIs) in the late 1990s, manifestations of atherosclerosis, specifically myocardial infarction (MI) and stroke, became prominent, and heart failure (HF), atrial fibrillation (AF), and sudden cardiac death have emerged.

CARDIOVASCULAR RISK FACTORS IN PEOPLE LIVING WITH HIV

People living with HIV have elevated traditional coronary risk factors, particularly those receiving ART, compared with noninfected persons. Dyslipidemia, metabolic syndrome, hypertension, and cigarette smoking are all more prevalent among subjects with HIV, leading to higher calculated Framingham risk scores in this group than in noninfected individuals. In the North American AIDS Cohort Collaboration on Research and Design, smoking, hypercholesterolemia, and hypertension were calculated to account for 37%, 44%, and 42% of MIs, respectively.[4] These risk factors also contributed to cancers and end-stage renal disease. Thus CV risk factors should merit aggressive treatment in people with HIV.

Dyslipidemia

The onset of HIV infection associates with a decrease in total cholesterol, low-density lipoprotein cholesterol (LDL-C), and high-density lipoprotein cholesterol (HDL-C), and an increase in triglyceride levels.[5] The effect of ART on lipid levels varies among the classes of ART drugs and even varies among drugs within the same class. Two or three ART drugs are usually used in combination to block replication of the virus by more than one mechanism. As a consequence, the effect of single drugs can be difficult to ascertain. As a general rule, PIs, non-nucleoside reverse transcriptase inhibitors (NNRTIs), and nucleoside reverse transcriptase inhibitors (NRTIs) increase triglyceride levels and may increase LDL-C levels.[5] The probability that each ART drug will adversely affect lipid levels is classified as low, intermediate, or high (Table 85.1).

PIs increase triglyceride levels; in particular, ritonavir can cause extreme hypertriglyceridemia exceeding 1000 mg/dL. Ritonavir-saquinavir, ritonavir-lopinavir, and ritonavir-tipranavir combinations can also increase triglycerides. Atazanavir, either alone or in combination with ritonavir, associates less with an increase in triglycerides compared with these other PIs. Older PIs such as ritonavir also increase LDL-C, probably by increasing intestinal cholesterol absorption and not by increased synthesis. PIs have variable effects on HDL-C levels, which are often already low in persons with HIV due to smoking.

NNRTIs also increase LDL-C levels but do not depress HDL-C levels.[5] Among NNRTIs, efavirenz associates with slightly more subjects developing hypercholesterolemia and hypertriglyceridemia in one study compared with nevirapine. Efavirenz can associate with greater increases in LDL-C but not total to HDL-C ratio compared with atazanavir-ritonavir. The newer NNRTI rilpivirine generally associates with lower total, HDL-C, LDL-C, and triglyceride levels than efavirenz. The NRTI tenofovir alafenamide, a newer formulation of tenofovir disoproxil fumarate (TDF), is associated with higher levels of LDL-C and HDL-C but similar total cholesterol to HDLC ratios compared with TDF.[5]

The integrase strand transfer inhibitors (INSTIs), raltegravir, elvitegravir, and dolutegravir, and the C-C chemokine receptor type 5 coreceptor antagonist maraviroc have favorable effects on lipids, particularly compared with older forms of ART. Switching from a ritonavir-boosted PI regimen to darunavir/cobicistat can reduce triglyceride levels.[6]

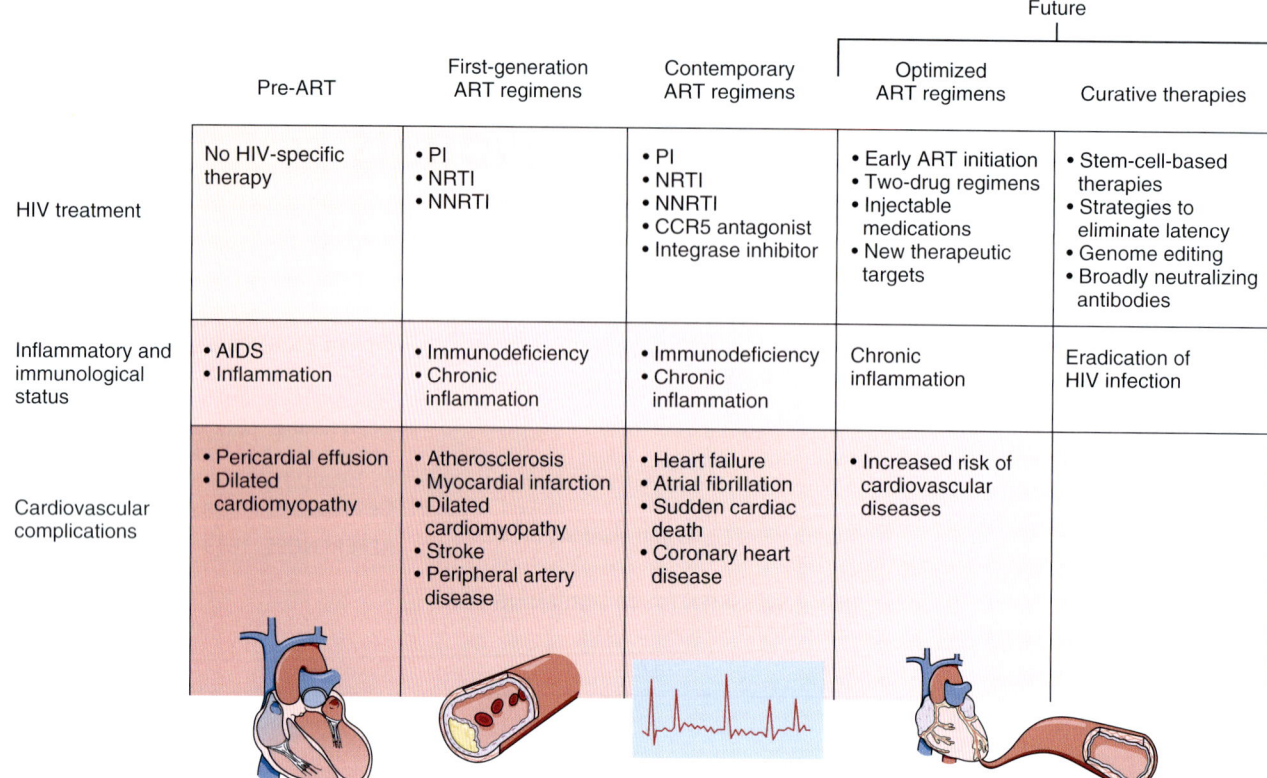

FIGURE 85.1 Overview of changes in HIV treatment and HIV-associated cardiovascular diseases. The types of cardiovascular complications associated with HIV infection have changed in the pre-antiretroviral therapy (ART) and ART eras and are likely to continue evolving in the future as new medications and treatment approaches emerge. In the pre-ART era, dilated cardiomyopathy and pericardial effusions were the most commonly reported cardiovascular issues in patients living with HIV. After the introduction of protease inhibitors in the late 1990s, atherosclerotic complications including myocardial infarction were described. More recently, reports of heart failure and rhythm abnormalities are now emerging in the setting of HIV infection. In the future, among individuals with access to ART, HIV infection will be a chronic disease state with increased risk of coronary artery disease. *CCR5,* CC-chemokine receptor 5; *NNRTI,* non-nucleoside reverse-transcriptase inhibitor; *NRTI,* nucleoside reverse-transcriptase inhibitor.

TABLE 85.1 Probability of Adverse Effects on Lipid Levels with HIV Drugs

LIPID EFFECTS	PI	NRTI	NNRTI	INSTI	OTHER CLASSES
Low	Atazanavir	Tenofovir	Nevirapine	Raltegravir	Maraviroc
	Atazanavir/Ritonavir	Abacavir	Etravirine	Elvitegravir	Enfuvirtide
		Lamivudine	Rilpivirine	Dolutegravir	Ibalizumab
		Emtricitabine	Doravirine	Bictegravir	
Intermediate	Saquinavir/Ritonavir	Zidovudine	Efavirenz		Cobicistat
	Darunavir/Ritonavir	Didanosine			
	Fosamprenavir/Ritonavir				
High	Lopinavir/Ritonavir	Stavudine			
	Tipranavir/Ritonavir				
	indinavir/ritonavir				

HIV, Human immunodeficiency virus; *INSTI,* integrase strand transfer inhibitors; *NNRTI,* non-nucleoside reverse transcriptase inhibitor; *NRTI,* nucleoside reverse transcriptase inhibitor; *PI,* protease inhibitor.

Most of the studies examining the effects of ART on lipid levels were of relatively short duration and were usually carried out in North American or European populations. However, ART is now initiated most often in people living in sub-Saharan Africa, where less data are available on the metabolic effects of treatment. In a recent meta-analysis of 14 trials of 21,023 individuals assessed between 2003 and 2014 from this region, ART associated with an increased risk of hypertriglyceridemia (RR 2.05, 95% CI, 1.51 to 2.77).[7] No consistent associations were seen between ART and raised blood pressure, glucose, hemoglobin A_{1c}, and other lipids across these studies.

The use of newer ART with fewer adverse lipid consequences might lead to a reduction in CV risk among patients living with HIV. However, although not affecting lipids, integrase inhibitors cause weight gain,[8] which may increase CV risk particularly after long-term use.

Lipodystrophy, the Metabolic Syndrome, and Obesity

Lipodystrophy is a syndrome characterized by fat accumulation in the dorsocervical region and an increase in or preservation of visceral fat, with subcutaneous and peripheral fat loss, resulting in relative central adiposity. Early PIs and the NRTIs stavudine and didanosine associated with lipodystrophy in at least 20% to 35% of persons taking these drugs long term, but newer PIs such as atazanavir do not appear to induce lipodystrophy.

Lipodystrophy in people with HIV commonly associates with features of the metabolic syndrome: insulin resistance, impaired glucose tolerance, hypertriglyceridemia, low HDL-C levels, and hypertension. The prevalence of the metabolic syndrome in subjects with HIV varies from 8.5% to 52% in published reports, with rates at the higher end of this range reported in Latin American countries and rates at the lower end in multicenter studies where patients had less exposure to ART.[9] Development of the metabolic syndrome was common in the first 3 years after initiation of an ART regimen that included stavudine or lopinavir/ritonavir, but is less common with newer drugs. Most studies indicate that the metabolic syndrome predicts for CVD and death in persons with HIV.[9]

A growing body of recent evidence suggests that INSTIs cause weight gain and an increased prevalence of obesity.[10] In some circumstances, weight gain might not be viewed as harmful; for example, someone with advanced HIV beginning treatment, where weight gain would be part of a return-to-health phenomenon, or weight gain after switching from a regimen that caused anorexia or nausea and vomiting. In a pooled analysis of weight gain in eight randomized, controlled trials of 5680 treatment-naïve subjects with HIV, INSTI use associated with more weight gain than were PIs or NNRTIs, with dolutegravir and bictegravir associated with more weight gain than elvitegravir/cobicistat.[11] Among NNRTIs, rilpivirine was linked to more weight gain than efavirenz. Among NRTIs, tenofovir alafenamide associated with more weight gain than TDF, abacavir, or zidovudine. Weight gain was more common in women, African Americans, and those with lower CD4 cell counts. The long-term implications of weight gain in the setting of integrase inhibitors and HIV on CVD have not been well studied at this time.

Diabetes

Whether HIV infection itself associates with an increased risk of diabetes or whether the increased risk relates only to specific ART drugs has been controversial. The PIs indinavir and lopinavir/ritonavir and the thymidine analogue stavudine can cause insulin resistance[9]; however, these drugs are no longer recommended for initial treatment of HIV owing to their toxicity. In a large cohort study from Denmark, the risk of diabetes among patients with HIV infection was nearly triple that of the general population in 1996–1999, but this excess was absent in 1999–2010. The difference in risk in the two periods is likely due to a decreased use of drugs with adverse metabolic consequences.

In a meta-analysis of 39 studies of CV risk factors in 13,698 people with HIV, the prevalence of diabetes was 7.24% but ranged from 0.5% to 39.1%.[12] Diabetes is more prevalent in persons with HIV compared with controls in some studies; for example, in an HIV cohort in Malawi where subjects had received ART for more than 10 years, the prevalence of diabetes was higher than in controls at all ages studied, and at age 60 or older was 13.2% in persons with HIV compared with 1.7% in controls.[13]

Among people with HIV, physical inactivity associates strongly with CV risk factors, including diabetes. In a study of 11,719 individuals with HIV, only 13% reported high levels of physical activity.[14] Compared with this group, those reporting very low levels of physical activity were more likely to have elevated triglycerides, obesity, hypertension, and diabetes. Other factors may play a role in the development of diabetes, including chronic inflammation, poor control of HIV disease, hepatitis C co-infection, along with demographic factors such as older age and male gender.

Hypertension and Chronic Kidney Disease

The prevalence of hypertension among persons with HIV averaged 19.8%, ranging from 4.8% to 63.3%, in the recent, large meta-analysis, mentioned earlier, where the prevalence of diabetes was 7.24%.[12] In studies comparing subjects living with HIV to uninfected controls, hypertension is not consistently higher in the HIV groups; however, both hypertension and prehypertension increase the risk of MI in the presence of HIV, just as in uninfected persons.[15]

In a meta-analysis comprising 61 studies and more than 200,000 subjects with HIV, with balanced geographic distribution, the prevalence of chronic kidney disease (CKD) varied from 6.4% with the MDRD equation, 4.8% with CKD-EPI, and 12.3% with Cockcroft-Gault.[16] CKD was more prevalent in Africa and less prevalent in Europe compared with other regions. CKD associated with hypertension and diabetes but not sex, hepatitis B or C co-infection, CD4 count, or ART status.

When CKD is defined as either albuminuria or a decreased glomerular filtration rate, it associates with an increased risk of CV events in people with HIV. Among 35,357 subjects with HIV in the D:A:D cohort, lower glomerular filtration rate associated strongly with a higher risk of CVD.[17] The development of CKD in persons with previously normal renal function has been reported with some forms of ART; specifically, TDF and the PIs atazanavir/ritonavir and lopinavir/ritonavir.[18]

Smoking

Smoking rates are two to three times higher in HIV cohorts compared with the general population, in the range of 40% to 70% in most studies, and with a high average number of pack-years.[19] Vaping is also prevalent among people with HIV but has as yet received little attention in the literature. Among 3251 subjects from the Danish HIV Cohort Study and 13,004 controls from the Copenhagen General Population Study, the population-attributable fraction of current or past smoking for MI was 72% (95% CI 55% to 82%) for HIV-infected individuals and 24% (95% CI, 3% to 40%) for controls.[19] If all current smokers stopped smoking, 42% (95% CI 21% to 57%) and 21% (95% CI 12% to 28%) of all MIs could potentially be avoided in the HIV and control populations.

In a previous study these investigators calculated that more life-years were lost from smoking than with HIV: 12.3 life-years (95% CI 8.1 to 16.4) compared with 5.1 life-years (95% CI 1.6 to 8.5). A 35-year-old living with HIV had a median life expectancy of 62.6 years if a smoker and 78.4 years if a non-smoker. These numbers illustrate the importance of stopping smoking in the context of HIV. Smoking cessation programs have the same modest success rates in people with HIV infection as in individuals without HIV. In a meta-analysis of eight trials including 1822 patients with HIV who were smokers, behavioral interventions increased abstinence rates by half.[20] Intensive group therapy can double the rate of quitting, to 13% compared with 6.6% in controls in one study of subjects with HIV, but the difference had dissipated by 6 months.[21] In another recent study of HIV subjects, the doubling of the quit rate persisted to 3 years, albeit at low levels, 10.3% versus 4.2% of controls.[22]

Potential drug-drug interactions between ART and smoking cessation drugs have not been well studied. Reports of varenicline, bupropion, and nicotine-replacement therapy in people with HIV infection have generally been small, short, and uncontrolled but have shown similar safety and success rates to reports in individuals without HIV infection.

Smoking may contribute to worsening of HIV-related damage in the heart, kidney, and brain. Neurocognitive defects are common among older people living with HIV and are more prevalent and severe in smokers than in non-smokers.[23] A quarter to half of persons living with HIV have deficits in multiple cognitive domains, including memory, verbal fluency, processing speed, and executive function, impairing their ability to accomplish many common tasks of daily living. Nicotine has antiinflammatory properties, and nicotine withdrawal may worsen neurocognitive defects.[23] The presence of neurocognitive defects predicts failure of smoking cessation. Smoking thus impairs quality of life, as well as markedly shortening the duration of life in subjects with HIV. Smoking cessation reduces CV events in subjects living with HIV.[3] The incidence of MI decreases within the first year and at 2 to 3 years was much reduced, although still double the rate of non-smokers with HIV. Thus, smoking cessation is a very desirable goal.

MECHANISMS OF HIV-RELATED ATHEROGENESIS

The pathogenesis of atherosclerosis in the setting of HIV infection is complicated and incompletely understood. Contributing mechanisms include the effects of the HIV proteins on immune and vascular cells, the immunodeficiency caused by the HIV infection, co-infection with cytomegalovirus (CMV), translocation of microbial products from the gut, chronic inflammation, and immune activation (Fig. 85.2).

In individuals receiving ART with undetectable levels of the virus, the HIV infection is not cured and low-level transcription of HIV genes persists. HIV-encoded proteins such as transactivator of transcription

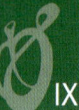

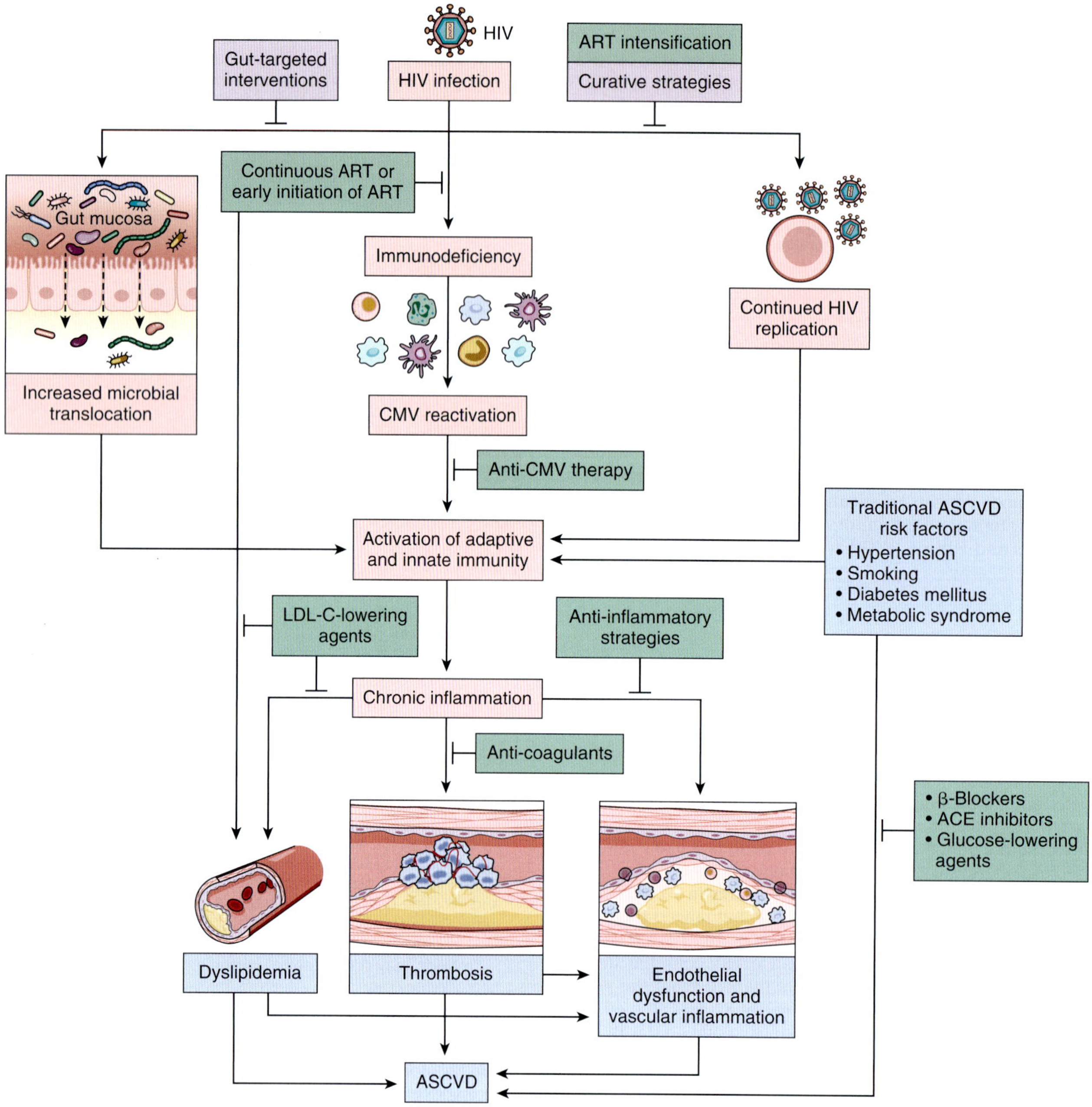

FIGURE 85.2 Pathophysiology and management of HIV-associated atherosclerotic cardiovascular disease. Schematic representation of the effects of HIV infection (*pink*) and the available strategies (*green*), as well as approaches under investigation (*purple*), for reducing the risk of atherosclerotic cardiovascular disease (ASCVD) and chronic inflammation in this patient population. In the setting of HIV infection, the increased microbial translocation from the gut, the continued HIV viral replication, and the HIV-induced immunodeficiency, along with traditional ASCVD risk factors, contribute to immune cell activation and chronic inflammation. HIV-specific interventions to reduce the risk of ASCVD include strategies targeted at co-infections (such as cytomegalovirus infection), use of newer antiretroviral therapies (ARTs) and intensification of ART. Strategies aimed at eradicating the HIV infection are under investigation. Treatments targeting traditional ASCVD risk factors, such as hypertension, diabetes mellitus, smoking and metabolic syndrome, are also critical for reducing the risk of ASCVD in patients living with HIV. Use of anticoagulants, beta blockers, angiotensin-converting enzyme (ACE) inhibitors and LDL cholesterol (LDL-C)-lowering agents (such as statins and PCSK9 inhibitors) reduce the risk of ASCVD in patients with cardiovascular disease without HIV infection and might, therefore, be useful in reducing the risk of HIV-associated ASCVD. Finally, strategies to lower inflammation, such as canakinumab, which has been reported to reduce cardiovascular events significantly in a non–HIV patient population, might also reduce the risk of HIV-associated ASCVD.

(Tat) and negative factor (Nef) induce inflammation and endothelial dysfunction.[24] In addition, the HIV envelope protein gp120 can stimulate endothelin-1 production.

CD4+ T cell depletion is the hallmark of HIV infection, and nadir CD4+ T cell count is a rough marker of the severity of immunodeficiency. Nadir CD4+ T cell count has been linked to increased carotid intima-media thickness (IMT), increased arterial stiffness, and incident MI.[3] The CD4:CD8 ratio, a marker of immunosenescence, predicts CV events in some but not in other studies. Thus, markers of immune system damage and viral detectability relate to CV events in HIV. Immune abnormalities persist in individuals with HIV infection even after successful treatment with ART. The mechanisms linking immune system damage to atherosclerosis have not been elucidated. Although non–AIDS-related events, such as MI and stroke, are less common with complete viral suppression, such events still occur at rates higher than in an uninfected population.

Co-infection with CMV might play a part in HIV-associated atherosclerosis. Compared with uninfected individuals, subjects with HIV consistently have a higher proportion of CMV-specific CD8+ T cells, with the highest levels seen in those receiving long-term ART with HIV suppression. CMV co-infection links strongly to HIV viral persistence and may also have a role in chronic immune activation and inflammation by expansion of the HIV reservoir. These CMV-specific T cell responses also correlate with markers of atherosclerosis, such as coronary artery calcification (CAC) and carotid IMT.[25] In the setting of HIV infection, high antibody titers to CMV, and to herpes simplex and varicella-zoster virus, associate with higher levels of biomarkers that accelerate inflammation and atherosclerosis.

Impairment of the gut barrier is an early feature of HIV infection, leading to microbial translocation, a process whereby microbial products leak through the intestinal barrier and cause immune activation.[3,26] Plasma levels of markers of microbial translocation such as soluble CD14 and lipopolysaccharide independently predict HIV disease progression and mortality in individuals not receiving ART. Whether these markers predict adverse outcomes in ART-treated individuals is unsettled; however, gut damage and microbial translocation persist even when HIV infection is suppressed by ART.[26] Plasma levels of the inflammatory markers interleukin-6 (IL-6) and tumor necrosis factor may be higher in individuals with higher levels of markers of microbial translocation. Although microbial translocation is thus another mechanism that might contribute to HIV-associated atherogenesis, interventions targeting this mechanism, specifically sevelamer, rifaximin, probiotics, and mesalamine, have not consistently lowered inflammatory markers or T cell activation.[3]

The three mechanisms discussed earlier, latent HIV infection, coinfection with other viruses, and microbial translocation, all stimulate atherogenesis by increasing inflammation. HIV infection associates with high plasma levels of inflammatory and coagulation markers, specifically C-reactive protein (CRP), IL-6, and D-dimer, and these biomarkers strongly predict CV events and all-cause mortality in individuals with HIV infection.[27] Subjects with HIV infection have higher arterial and lymph node inflammation as assessed by FDG-PET and CT imaging than uninfected individuals, and this marker of increased inflammation correlates with higher circulating levels of CRP, IL-6, and activated monocytes.[28]

Inflammation is a therapeutic target to reduce CV events in individuals with or without HIV infection (see Fig. 85.2). Statin therapy reduces inflammation, but the effects of statins on inflammatory markers seem to be attenuated in the presence of HIV infection.[29] Neither intensification of ART nor changing PI-based regimens to integrase inhibitors consistently reduces inflammatory markers. Short studies of aspirin treatment also had no effect on inflammatory markers in HIV infection.[30] Taken together, these findings suggest that strategies beyond ART and treatment of traditional CV risk factors are needed to reduce inflammation with the aim of lowering the risk of atherosclerosis in the setting of HIV infection.

Canakinumab, a monoclonal antibody targeting IL-1β, reduces CV events in patients with previous MI and a high-sensitivity CRP level of ≥2 mg/L.[31] In an on-treatment analysis, canakinumab-treated subjects who had a CRP reduction to <2 mg/L had significant reductions in CV endpoints, whereas no significant reduction in these outcomes was observed in patients who did not achieve a CRP reduction to this level.[32] Similar success was reported for individuals who achieved on-treatment IL-6 levels less than the study median value but not for those who did not.[33]

Would canakinumab reduce CV events in the setting of HIV? In a small study of subjects with HIV infection, canakinumab significantly reduced plasma IL-6 and CRP levels, with no effect on CD4, CD8, or RNA viral levels.[34] Inflammation in the bone marrow and arterial inflammation fell after canakinumab administration. By contrast, in the general population with stable atherosclerosis, methotrexate did not reduce inflammatory markers or improve clinical outcomes.[35] In a clinical trial in treated HIV, methotrexate lowered CD8 T cells and did not impact inflammation or endothelial function.[36] These small preliminary studies with inflammatory biomarkers as surrogate endpoints will hopefully lead to larger clinical trials of antiinflammatory therapies with CV endpoints in the population living with HIV.

Markers of inflammation and coagulation predict CV and other adverse events in individuals with HIV infection (Table 85.2).[37,38] The strong relationship between these markers and outcomes appears consistently across diverse HIV-infected populations including men, women, and different age groups. In combined data from three large cohorts of individuals with HIV infection, a 25% decrease in IL-6 or D-dimer levels in plasma associated independently with a 37% reduction in non-AIDS events or mortality.[39]

Biomarkers in HIV infection tend to group into clusters, with each cluster related to a cardiac phenotype.[40] The inflammatory phenotype is characterized by higher levels of CRP, IL-6, and D-dimer, whereas the cardiac cluster comprises higher levels of protein ST2 (also known as IL-1 receptor-like 1), N-terminal pro-B-type natriuretic peptide and growth/differentiation factor 15. Diastolic dysfunction is common with the inflammatory cluster of biomarkers, and pulmonary hypertension (PH) is more common in the cardiac cluster. Both groups associate with a threefold increase in mortality over a 6.9-year follow-up after adjustment for other prognostic variables.[40] These biomarker clusters in patients with HIV might be helpful for selecting patients for appropriate therapy to prevent CV events.

The most obvious mechanism by which ART increases atherosclerosis is by worsening blood lipid levels. Interestingly, even after adjustment for blood lipid levels in the large D:A:D study, cumulative exposure to the NRTIs abacavir or didanosine or to the PIs lopinavir-ritonavir or indinavir associated with an increased risk of MI.

ART might also increase the risk of CV events through other mechanisms. Insulin resistance, lipodystrophy, and other patterns of fat distribution can contribute to atherogenesis. The NRTI abacavir has been linked to an increased risk of MI in some but not all studies. This increased risk has been attributed to increased platelet reactivity and to endothelial dysfunction. In the D:A:D study, a difference in the risk of MI was noted between two widely used PIs, with atazanavir being associated with a lower risk than darunavir. This reduced risk of MI may result from a protective effect of atazanavir because it increases bilirubin levels and elevated bilirubin levels independently predict lower incident CVD in HIV.[41] Overall, although current ART regimens appear to confer a much lower risk of CV events than older ART, longer-term data on newer regimens will be needed to ascertain this benefit.

Features of Atherosclerosis in People with HIV

Cardiac computed tomography (CCT) provides insight into the features of coronary disease in HIV patients.[42] The prevalence of CAC by CCT was not higher in HIV-infected individuals compared with controls across seven studies. However, CT angiographic studies reveal that noncalcified plaques are much more common in persons living with HIV than in uninfected controls.[43] In a meta-analysis of nine studies including 1229 HIV patients and 1029 controls, the prevalence of coronary stenosis greater than 30% or greater than 50%, or calcified plaques did not differ between HIV patients and controls.[44] However, noncalcified plaques were more than three times more likely to be present in HIV patients, 58% compared with 17%. Noncalcified plaques are more likely to be lipid-laden and inflammatory and exhibit imaging features associated with plaque rupture. HIV subjects with higher levels of arterial inflammation as assessed by FDG-PET imaging were more likely than those with lower levels of inflammation to have plaques with high-risk features.[45]

In non-HIV cohorts, carotid IMT associates with prevalent CVD and risk factors as well as increased risk of future stroke and MI. Many observational studies have compared carotid IMT in individuals with HIV and in controls.[42] Across these studies, carotid IMT averaged 0.04 mm thicker (95% CI 0.02 to 0.06 mm, p < 0.001) in subjects with HIV than in uninfected controls.[42] This conclusion should be viewed with caution due to differences among the studies in population characteristics, study designs, sample sizes, and ultrasound techniques. In some studies with serial measurements, carotid IMT progressed more rapidly in the HIV group than in controls. Carotid plaque also occurs more commonly in HIV patients compared with uninfected controls across six studies.[42] Carotid IMT independently predicts mortality in HIV.[46]

CORONARY DISEASE IN HIV SUBJECTS

Epidemiology

A recent systematic review that included 80 longitudinal studies with 793,635 individuals with HIV found a relative risk of CVD in persons living with HIV of 2.16 (95% CI 1.68 to 2.77) compared with uninfected individuals.[47] This risk resembles that of hypertension, diabetes, lipids, and smoking.[48] Over the past 26 years, the global population-attributable fraction of CVD due to HIV has tripled and now approaches 1%, with the greatest impact in sub-Saharan African and the Asia Pacific regions.[47] Thus the contribution of HIV to CVD is still small overall, but in an HIV-infected individual, HIV is as potent as any classical risk factor.

TABLE 85.2 Biomarkers of Inflammation and Coagulation Are Associated with Adverse Events in HIV Infection

STUDY (YEAR)	STUDY POPULATION	NUMBER OF PATIENTS	FOLLOW-UP	FINDINGS
SMART (2008)	Subjects with well-controlled HIV from 33 countries	5472	3700 person-years	IL-6 and D-dimer levels in plasma were strongly associated with all-cause mortality
				IL-6, CRP, and D-dimer levels in plasma were associated with increased risk of CVD
FRAM (2010)	Subjects with HIV	922	5 years	Fibrinogen and CRP levels were strong and independent predictors of mortality
ALLRT (2014)	Subjects with HIV and virologic suppression <1 yr after ART initiation	143	48–64 weeks after ART initiation	High IL-6, sTNFRI, sTNFRII, and D-dimer plasma levels and KT ratio at 1 year were associated with increased risk of non-AIDS events
VACS (2016)	Subjects with HIV and uninfected controls	2350	6.9 years	HIV infection was associated with elevated IL-6, sCD14, and D-dimer levels in plasma, which are associated with mortality
MACS (2016)	Subjects with well-controlled HIV	670	Up to 18 years	IL-6 and sCD14 levels in plasma were predictive of mortality
START (2017)	Subjects with HIV from 35 countries	4299	3.2 years	Baseline IL-6 and D-dimer levels in plasma were associated with the risk of AIDS, serious non-AIDS events or death

ART, Antiretroviral therapy; *CRP,* C-reactive protein; *CVD,* cardiovascular disease; *HIV,* human immunodeficiency virus; *IL-6,* interleukin-6; *KT,* kynurenine:tryptophan; *sCD14,* soluble CD14; *sTNFRI,* soluble tumor necrosis factor receptor type I; *sTNFRII,* soluble tumor necrosis factor receptor type II.

In addition to the elevated risk of an acute coronary syndrome (ACS), subjects with HIV have involvement of other vascular beds. The incidence of ischemia stroke increased by 25% in HIV-infected men compared with uninfected subjects in the Veterans Aging Cohort Study.[49] Peripheral arterial disease as assessed by ankle-brachial index was higher in subjects living with HIV compared with controls in a study from Copenhagen, and the difference persisted after adjustment for classic CV risk factors.[50]

Clinical Presentation

The clinical presentation of ACS differs in HIV-infected compared with uninfected individuals. HIV-infected individuals with ACS are on average more than a decade younger and are more likely to be men, to be current smokers, and to have low HDL-cholesterol levels. Their risk scores tend to be lower, and they are more likely to have single- rather than multiple-vessel coronary artery disease. In general, subjects with HIV hospitalized with ACS have excellent immediate outcomes.

In earlier studies, people with HIV had substantially higher rates of restenosis after percutaneous coronary interventions with bare metal stents, compared with uninfected individuals. More recent studies in which most patients received drug-eluting stents show similar medium-term outcomes between HIV subjects and matched controls.[51] A report from the Nationwide Inpatient Sample detected no increase in in-hospital mortality among 9771 HIV-infected individuals undergoing cardiac surgery, including coronary bypass, compared with matched, uninfected controls.[52] Long-term outcome studies after coronary bypass surgery have not been reported in large cohorts of persons living with HIV.

Some data indicate that HIV status of ACS patients influences the likelihood of receiving guideline-directed investigations and treatments. For example, in a U.S. Nationwide Impatient Sample from 2002 to 2011, comparing nearly 4000 HIV MI patients with more than 1.3 million uninfected MI patients, subjects with HIV were less likely to undergo invasive management (adjusted odds ratio [OR] 0.59, 95% CI 0.55 to 0.65), to undergo coronary bypass surgery (OR 0.66, 95% CI 0.57 to 0.76) or to receive drug-eluting stents (OR 0.83, 95% CI 0.76 to 0.92).[53] In a cohort of HIV subjects, 388 of 812 (48%) adjudicated MI were classified as type 2 MI (related to demand ischemia), a much higher rate than those reported in non-HIV populations.[54]

Treatment

The treatment of CHD in HIV-infected individuals should largely be guided by existing recommendations for uninfected patients in the absence of clinical trial data specific to HIV. However, two aspects specific to HIV deserve mention: (1) the potential contribution of ART to CVD, and (2) the treatment of lipid levels in HIV disease, for which separate guidelines have been devised.

Antiretroviral Therapy and Cardiovascular Disease

Since ART first became available in the 1990s, the indications for treatment and specific drug regimens have evolved rapidly. In earlier years, when the benefits of ART were more limited and treatment-related adverse effects were more common, the initiation of treatment was often delayed until subjects were at increased risk of immunosuppression. More recent studies suggest that the chronic immune stimulation and inflammation that accompanies early asymptomatic HIV infection can result in long-term morbidity. Thus, whereas treatment was initially restricted to those with low CD4 counts, it is now widely accepted that treatment should be started in all individuals with HIV infection with detectable viremia irrespective of CD4 cell count.[55] Initiation of ART is recommended as soon as possible in the setting of acute HIV infection because initiation prior to the development of HIV antibody positivity reduces the size of the latent HIV reservoir, reduces immune activation, and may protect against infection of central memory T cells. Early compared with deferred initiation of ART reduced AIDS-related and non–AIDS-related events in the START trial; this benefit did not reach statistical significance for CV outcomes, however.[56] Furthermore, early initiation of ART associated with increases in total and LDL-C but also decreased use of blood pressure medication.[57] The impact of early ART on CVD and CV risk in HIV remains unknown.

Planned discontinuation of early ART after a specific treatment duration is not recommended because the benefits do not persist and the subsequent viral rebound associates with increased clinical events and the potential for transmission.[55] Initiation of ART in elite controllers, defined as subjects with confirmed HIV infection and persistent undetectable HIV RNA without ART, remains controversial.[58] Of note, elite controllers are more likely to be hospitalized than individuals with controlled HIV, with CV hospitalizations being the most common.[59]

What combinations of drugs are recommended for initial therapy? The INSTIs have moved into a key role as first-line therapy because they are highly effective, with higher and more rapid rates of virologic suppression compared with PIs and NNRTIs, the previous mainstays of ART. INSTIs have the additional advantage of being extremely well tolerated. As discussed previously, weight gain is being increasingly recognized as a disquieting feature of modern ART combinations, with INSTIs being the main culprit.

TABLE 85.3 Metabolic Pathways of Statins and Interactions with ART

DRUG	METABOLISM	LIPOPHILIC	ART INTERACTIONS	COMMENT
Lovastatin	CYP3A4	Yes	PI, NNRTI	Limited potency
Simvastatin	CYP3A4	Yes	PI, NNRTI	Contraindicated
Pravastatin	Partial hepatic	No	PI	Limited potency
Fluvastatin	CYP2CY, CYP3A4	Yes		Limited potency
Atorvastatin	CYP3A4	Yes	PI	More potent
Rosuvastatin	CYP2C9 (<10%)	No	PI	More potent
Pitavastatin	Glucuronidation	Yes		Least D-D interaction; limited potency

ART, Antiretroviral therapy; *D-D*, drug-drug; *NNRTI*, non-nucleoside reverse transcriptase inhibitor; *PI*, protease inhibitor.

Guidelines recommend initial ART combinations.[55] Up to 96% of individuals who remain in care and receive ART have undetectable plasma HIV RNA levels. Several non–INSTI-containing regimens suppress HIV RNA in most subjects who adhere to therapy. These may be chosen based on individual clinical features, preferences, financial considerations, or unavailability of INSTIs.[55]

Pregnant women, those with hepatitis B or C co-infection, or those with opportunistic infections require modifications to ART.[55] Osteoporosis and fractures increase with HIV infection. During the first year or two after initiation of ART, patients may lose 2% to 6% of their bone mineral density. TDF-containing regimens associate with a greater initial decline in bone mineral density than TAF- or abacavir-containing regimens; thus, TDF is not recommended for patients with osteopenia or osteoporosis.[55]

Monitoring of kidney function with eGFR, urinalysis, and testing for glycosuria and albuminuria or proteinuria is recommended when ART is initiated or changed and every 6 months (along with HIV RNA) once HIV RNA is stable. TDF, especially with a boosted PI, increased the risk of CKD in cohort studies and thus is not recommended for subjects with an eGFR of less than 60 mL/min. Long-term data on TAF in subjects with preexisting renal disease are limited. TDF or TAF should be discontinued if renal function worsens, particularly if there is evidence of proximal tubular dysfunction.[55] Switching from TDF to TAF associates with an increase in lipids, mainly LDL-C and triglycerides.[60]

Improvements in ART have reduced the frequency of needing to switch drugs because of virologic failure and drug resistance. However, these improvements provide a rationale for switching therapy in some individuals who have virologic suppression with older regimens that are less convenient or that have more adverse effects. Reasons for considering switching therapy in such individuals include the development of adverse effects, the desire to reduce dosages or the number of pills taken, the occurrence of drug-drug interactions, or pregnancy. Some individuals may benefit from switching even if they are doing well on their current treatment. For instance, switching is reasonable for those taking regimens containing stavudine, didanosine, or zidovudine, because of long-term toxic effects, or older PIs that have higher pill burdens and greater metabolic toxicities than darunavir or atazanavir. Some drugs that are no longer recommended for initial use may be safely continued if well tolerated. For example, although nevirapine and efavirenz have substantial early toxic effects, they are safe and tolerable in the long term.[55]

Recommendations for laboratory monitoring include as close to the time of HIV diagnosis as possible and before beginning ART, measurement of: CD4 cell count; plasma HIV RNA level; serologic studies for hepatitis A, B, and C; serum chemistries, estimated creatinine clearance; complete blood cell count, and urine glucose and protein and genotyping for resistance to reverse transcriptase and PIs. Routine pretreatment screening for integrase resistance is not currently recommended. Screening for syphilis and mucosal nucleic acid amplification testing for chlamydia infection and gonorrhea should also be done at the time of HIV diagnosis, and a lipid profile should be obtained. Other laboratory assessments should be individualized, in keeping with current guidelines. If ART is initiated on the first visit, all laboratory specimens should be drawn before the first dose.

Treatment of Lipids in the Setting of HIV

Diet and lifestyle optimization should form the foundation for treatment of lipids in persons living with HIV.[5] As with all overweight individuals, caloric restriction and exercise should be used to attain ideal body weight. Reducing carbohydrate intake can improve triglyceride levels. In one report, fasting triglyceride levels and adipose tissue mass decreased, and muscle mass increased in HIV-infected men with hypertriglyceridemia after 16 weeks of resistance training. Nevertheless, diet and exercise by themselves rarely suffice to achieve adequate control.

A large number of controlled clinical trials have documented that LDL-C lowering, usually with statins, reduces the risk of CV events across a broad spectrum of patients without HIV infection. Similar data are not yet available for people living with HIV; however, the Randomized Trial to Prevent Vascular Events in HIV (REPRIEVE; clinicaltrials.gov NCT02344290) will address this issue. This trial has enrolled 7700 HIV-infected subjects without known CVD and randomized them to pitavastatin 4 mg/d or to placebo. The primary endpoint of REPRIEVE is a composite of CV events, and the trial is scheduled to be completed in early 2023.

Until recently, guidelines for cholesterol management have not specifically addressed individuals living with HIV. The 2016 European Society of Cardiology (ESC)/European Atherosclerosis Society (EAS) guidelines devote a short section to individuals with HIV infection and recommend dietary changes and exercise, as well as switching, when feasible, to a more lipid-friendly ART.[61] These guidelines also state that statin therapy should be considered to achieve the target LDL-C level of less than 2.6 mmol/L (100 mg/dL), the same target that is recommended for other patients at high risk of CVD.

The U.S. National Lipid Association recommended considering HIV infection as an independent risk factor for selecting drug therapy to lower LDL-C levels[62] but do not set specific LDL-C targets for subjects with HIV. Unfortunately, the 2013 American College of Cardiology/American Heart Association (ACC/AHA) guidelines based treatment recommendations on risk assessment tools that appear to be inaccurate in the setting of HIV. For example, in one recent study, high-risk coronary plaque morphology was seen on coronary CT angiography in 36% of 108 HIV patients, but the guidelines would recommend treatment for only 19% of them.[63] Similarly, in another study the guidelines failed to recommend therapy for two-thirds of individuals with HIV who had carotid plaque on ultrasound imaging.[64] The 2018 updated ACC/AHA guidelines state that HIV infection can be considered a CVD risk enhancer, which would favor starting moderate-intensity or high-intensity statin therapy.[65] These guidelines also recommend that a risk assessment, including fasting lipid profile, be done before and 4 to 12 weeks after starting ART.

Drug-drug interactions must be considered when using lipid-lowering drugs in persons living with HIV (Table 85.3). A systemic review of 18 clinical trials in HIV-infected subjects receiving ART confirmed that statin administration is safe when drug-drug interactions are taken into account.[66] Lovastatin and simvastatin are contraindicated with PIs because of the risk of rhabdomyolysis from high statin blood levels.[5] For the same reason, no more than 40 mg/day of atorvastatin should be used for individuals taking ritonavir-boosted PIs. Rosuvastatin blood levels increase when used with atazanavir/ritonavir and lopinavir/ritonavir, so limiting the rosuvastatin dose to 10 mg is advisable with these drugs. Pravastatin and fluvastatin are safe but do not lower LDL-C as much as atorvastatin or rosuvastatin. These weaker statins were widely used after the introduction of ART but are less popular now because of the growing realization, reflected in contemporary guidelines, that greater degrees of LDL-C lowering produce greater CV event reduction.[5] The proportion of subjects with HIV who had contraindicated statin use from PI has decreased from 2007 to 2015 but has increased in the setting of cobicistat-containing ART regimens,[54] which has similar interactions with statins to ritonavir.

Despite a lack of clinical trial outcomes data, pitavastatin is a good choice for individuals living with HIV because at higher doses its LDL-C–lowering effect is moderate, and because its metabolism is via glucuronidation, drug-drug interactions are avoided.[5] In a randomized, double-blind comparison study in 252 subjects with HIV, pitavastatin 4 mg/day reduced LDL-C by 31% and pravastatin 40 mg/day reduced LDL-C by 21%, with similar low rates of adverse events in the two treatment groups.[67]

As with other patients, statins should be the mainstay of lipid-lowering drug therapy for persons living with HIV. Several studies indicate that statins are underused in the setting of HIV even among eligible individuals.[68] In individuals with HIV who do not tolerate statins, ezetimibe is a safe option, albeit with limited LDL-C–lowering potency. Ezetimibe should be considered as add-on therapy for very-high-risk individuals with HIV who do not achieve sufficient LDL-C lowering with statins. Bile acid sequestrants are not recommended in the context of HIV because they increase triglyceride levels and their effects on the absorption of ART drugs have not been studied.[5] Add-on therapy can be problematic for individuals with HIV because they often already suffer from a high pill burden from ART and other medications.

Proprotein convertase subtilisin/kexin type 9 (PCSK9) inhibitors have not been widely studied in the setting of HIV but have several inherent advantages in this condition, including profound LDL-C lowering, a reduction in pill burden, avoidance of the drug-drug interactions of statins, and ease of use in patients with chronic liver disease, a common problem in this population. PCSK9 levels may be higher in persons with HIV compared with uninfected controls.[5] Switching ART to drugs that do not adversely affect lipid levels is a worthwhile strategy as long as viral suppression is maintained. Switching from older PIs to INSTIs can improve lipid levels but at the cost of an increased risk of virologic failure and thus is not recommended for individuals with a history of virologic failure.[5] Adding a statin might be preferable to switching for those not already taking a statin; in one study the addition of rosuvastatin 10 mg per day yielded better lipid results and was better tolerated compared with switching.[69]

Hypertriglyceridemia is a common finding in individuals with HIV and probably increases the risk of a CV event. Reducing alcohol and carbohydrate intake has a favorable effect in people with or without HIV infection. Consideration should be given to a change in ART to drugs that induce less hypertriglyceridemia. Fibrates reduce triglycerides, often at low doses, but have a drug-drug interaction with statins and some types of ART; for example, the lopinavir-ritonavir PI combination greatly reduces gemfibrozil absorption.[5] Monitoring of hepatic enzymes and creatine phosphokinase levels is advised for patients taking ART, a statin, and a fibrate. When triglycerides are greater than 1000 mg/dL, pancreatitis is a serious risk and urgent treatment is required.

Omega-3 fatty acids found in fish oil reduce triglyceride levels in persons with HIV and hypertriglyceridemia and has the advantage of no important drug-drug interactions; however, some fish oil preparations increase LDL-C levels modestly.[5] The Reduction of Cardiovascular Events with Icosapent Ethyl–Intervention Trial (REDUCE-IT) tested the effect of icosapent ethyl, a purified and quality-controlled pharmaceutical-grade eicosapentaenoic acid preparation, 2 g twice daily as add-on therapy with statins in 8179 patients with CVD or diabetes and other CV risk factors, and a fasting triglyceride level of 150 to 499 mg/dL.[70] After a median follow-up of 4.9 years, the primary endpoint, a composite of CV events, occurred in 17.2% of the icosapent ethyl patients compared with 22.0% of the placebo patients (HR 0.75, 95% CI 0.68 to 0.83). Although outcome data such as this are not available in the context of HIV, icosapent ethyl should now be considered as treatment for such persons with triglyceride levels in this range.

RISK ASSESSMENT AND SCREENING FOR CORONARY DISEASE

The tools used to calculate CV risk in the general population, (Framingham Risk Score, Systematic Coronary Risk Evaluation [SCORE] and the ACC/AHA pooled cohort equation), function poorly in HIV-infected cohorts.[71] A prediction model specific to HIV includes clinical variables, lipid levels, CD4 lymphocyte count, and ART history; a reduced model omits ART.[72] In the hands of its developers, the model performed better than the Framingham Risk Score, even after the Framingham score had been recalibrated to the HIV population. Studies comparing different models have reported that they yield quite different results with less overlap than would be expected. A recent AHA statement concluded that a clear best risk estimation model for HIV has not been identified.[73] Whatever risk assessment tool is use may underestimate true risk in the HIV population.

A 2019 AHA statement proposed a pragmatic approach to CV risk assessment in individuals with HIV (Fig. 85.3). The presence and extent of CAC as assessed by a CT scan strongly predict CV events in the general population and may be a useful risk assessment tool in subjects with HIV and intermediate risk.[73]

The 2019 AHA statement recommends consideration of selected CV risk enhancers identified in the 2018 ACC/AHA cholesterol clinical practice guidelines as likely atherosclerotic cardiovascular disease (ASCVD) risk enhancers in HIV (see Fig. 85.3).[73] These include early family history of MI or stroke (men, age <55 years; women, age <65 years), persistently elevated LDL-C ≥160 mg/dL, CKD, preeclampsia or premature menopause, subclinical atherosclerosis on imaging (including CAC), and high levels of selected biomarkers associated with elevated CV risk independently of traditional risk factors, specifically lipoprotein(a), CRP, and apolipoprotein B.

Cardiac screening for coronary disease may be cost-effective in intermediate risk subjects with HIV.[74] Of note, the ACC/AHA guidelines failed to recommend statin in more than two-thirds of HIV-infected individuals with evidence of carotid plaque >1.5 mm.[75] Depending on the clinical features of a patient, either screening for CAC, IMT, or a stress test would be an appropriate first step. An electrocardiogram should be done in all HIV-infected adults, and an echocardiogram is reasonable because of the high prevalence of left ventricular (LV) hypertrophy and LV dysfunction in this population (discussed later).

OTHER CARDIOVASCULAR CONDITIONS ASSOCIATED WITH HIV

Pulmonary Hypertension (see also Chapter 88)

The prevalence of idiopathic PH in the general population is estimated to be 1 to 2 persons per million, but in the setting of HIV the prevalence is several thousand times higher (0.5%). Studies where subjects with HIV were screened with Doppler echocardiography suggest that many more have asymptomatic mild PH and that the true prevalence considerably exceeds 0.5%. A revised definition of PH proposed in 2018 included a mean PA pressure greater than 20 mm Hg, a PA wedge pressure of 15 mm Hg or less, and a pulmonary vascular resistance of 3 Wood units or higher.[76] Implementation of this definition would increase the proportion of people with HIV who also have PH.

The pathology of PH associated with HIV infection is similar to that seen in PH patients without HIV. It includes intimal thickening of small pulmonary arteries with plexogenic lesions in the media, leading ultimately to obstruction of small pulmonary arteries. As with idiopathic PH, no single cause of HIV-associated PH has been identified, but many factors may contribute. Levels of inflammatory markers such as vascular endothelial growth factor-A, platelet-derived growth factor, and IL-1 and IL-6 increase in HIV-associated PH. Certain HIV proteins can activate endothelial cells indirectly, such as the envelope glycoprotein-120, which associate with higher levels of endothelin-1. Levels of endothelin-1 correlate with pulmonary artery systolic pressure among HIV-infected subjects with PH,[77] suggesting that this potent vasoconstrictor plays a central role in the pathogenesis of PH-HIV. Another potential mechanism is asymmetric dimethylarginine (ADMA)-induced endothelial

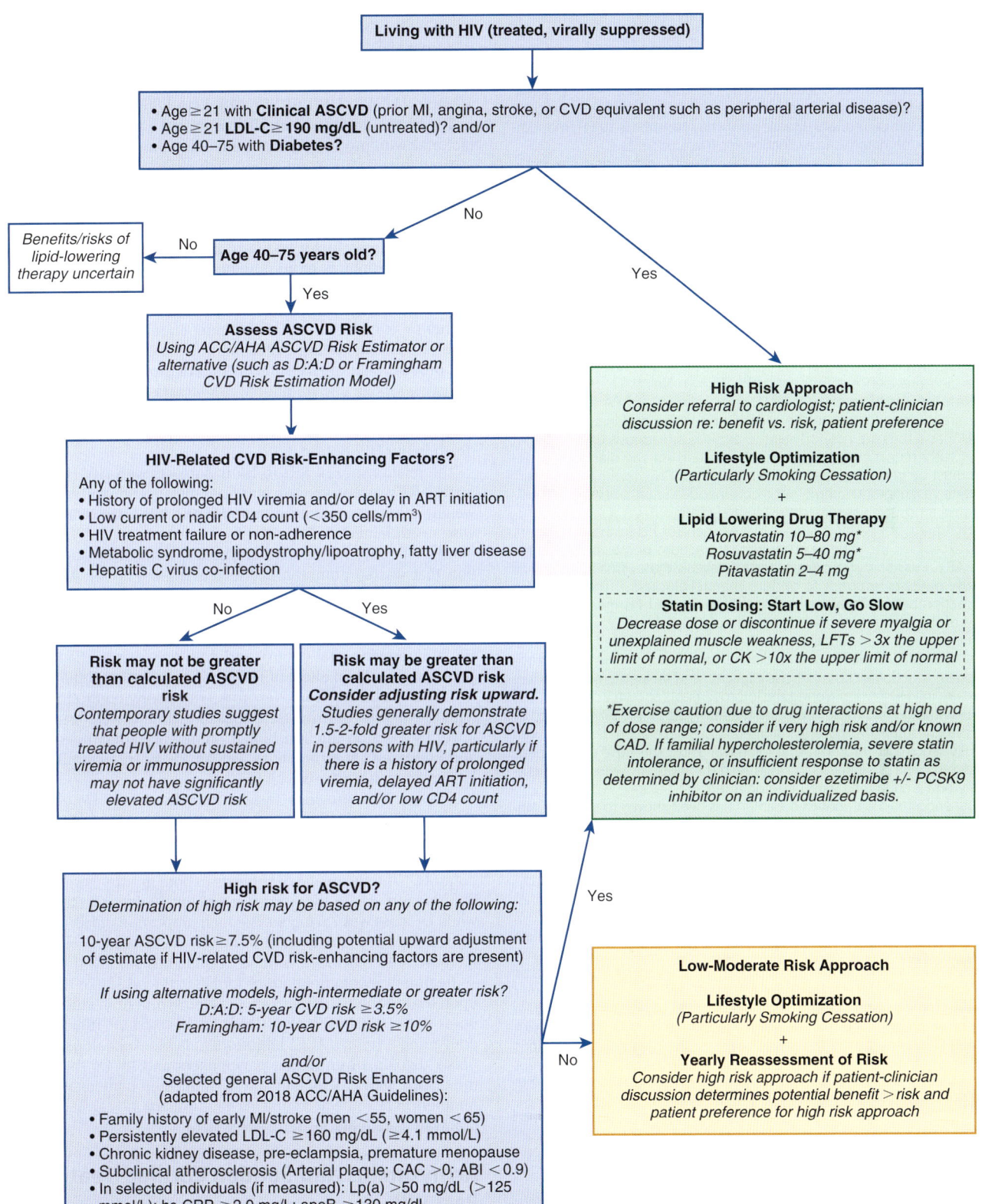

FIGURE 85.3 Pragmatic approach to atherosclerotic cardiovascular disease (ASCVD) risk assessment and prevention in treated HIV infection. This figure applies to people with treated HIV. For people with uncontrolled HIV, the first priority is appropriate HIV therapy to achieve viral suppression. Thresholds are based on findings of elevated CVD risk at current or nadir CD4 count less than 200, less than 350, and less than 500 cells/mm³. Hazard ratios and incidence rate ratios of 1.4–2.1 for myocardial infarction (MI) for people living with HIV (PLWH) versus uninfected people has been demonstrated in several studies. The hazard ratio of stroke for PLWH versus uninfected people was 1.40 in one study. *ABI*, Ankle-brachial index; *ACC/AHA*, American College of Cardiology/American Heart Association; *apoB*, apolipoprotein B; *ART*, antiretroviral therapy; *CAC*, coronary artery calcium; *CAD*, coronary artery disease; *CK*, creatine kinase; *CVD*, cardiovascular disease; *D:A:D*, Data Collection on Adverse Events of Anti-HIV Drugs; *hs-CRP*, high sensitivity C-reactive protein; *LFT*, liver function test; *LDL-C*, low-density lipoprotein cholesterol; *Lp(a)*, lipoprotein A; *PCSK9*, proprotein convertase subtilisin-kexin type 9. (From Feinstein MJ, et al. Characteristics, prevention, and management of cardiovascular disease in people living with HIV: a scientific statement from the American Heart Association. *Circulation.* 2019;140:e98-e124, Fig 4.)

dysfunction, because elevated ADMA levels have been reported in HIV-associated PH.[78] Finally, a genetic predisposition to HIV-associated PH has been suggested, and some evidence indicates that autoimmunity may contribute.

Severe PH leads to worsening dyspnea, curtailed exercise capacity, right HF, and sudden cardiac death. PH may occur at any stage of HIV infection and does not appear to relate to CD4 count, ART, or other HIV-related factors. As the population with HIV ages, other conditions such as chronic pulmonary disease or HF may contribute to PH, mandating a thorough diagnostic evaluation for these patients.[79]

PH worsens outcomes in individuals with HIV, although asymptomatic subjects have a much better prognosis than do those with advanced dyspnea and reduced exercise tolerance. Death in PH-HIV is usually sudden or due to right HF and is rarely due to other HIV complications.[79] In one series of 77 PH-HIV subjects treated from 2000 to 2008, survival at 1, 3, and 5 years was 88%, 72%, and 63%, respectively. Predictors of survival were a cardiac index greater than 2.8 L/min/m^2 and a CD4 count of greater than 200 cells/μL. ART has not been shown to improve survival.[79]

Echocardiographic screening for PH is now recommended independent of symptoms for individuals with HIV and one of the following risk factors: female sex, intravenous drug or cocaine use, hepatitis C infection, high-prevalence country of origin, known Nef or Tat HIV proteins, and African-American patients.[80] Doppler estimates of PA systolic pressure are inaccurate both in the general population and in subjects with PH-HIV and thus are not sufficient to exclude a diagnosis of PH.[79] Right heart catheterization is the reference standard for the diagnosis of PH and must be performed before the initiation of PH-specific treatment.[79] Routine vasodilator testing is not recommended in patients with PH-HIV because a positive vasodilator test is rarely found.[79]

Treatment of PH-HIV is similar to treatment of PH in the absence of HIV, except for the issue of drug-drug interactions between PH therapy and ART. Pulmonary vasodilator testing reveals that a small minority of PH-HIV patients responds to calcium channel blockers.[81] The drug-drug interaction between calcium channel blockers and PIs means that the dose of the calcium channel blocker should be limited.

In case reports and small series, the phosphodiesterase type-5 inhibitors sildenafil, tadalafil, and vardenafil have been shown to improve dyspnea, functional class, exercise capacity, and mean pulmonary artery pressure in PH-HIV,[81] mirroring the improvements shown in clinical trials in PH without HIV. These drugs are metabolized by the 3A4 isoform of the cytochrome P450 system and interactions have been described with the PIs saquinavir, ritonavir, and indinavir. Thus, the dose of phosphodiesterase type-5 inhibitors in HIV-infected individuals who are concurrently on PIs should be carefully monitored.

The endothelin antagonist bosentan has been shown to improve pulmonary vascular resistance and exercise tolerance over 1 year of treatment, similar to the response expected in uninfected PH patients. The recommended dose of bosentan for individuals taking PIs is 62.5 mg/day or every other day instead of the usual dose of 125 mg twice daily. Studies of the selective endothelin receptor antagonists ambrisentan and sitaxsentan are limited to case reports in PH-HIV.

Several small series demonstrate that prostacyclin analogues induce hemodynamic benefit in PH-HIV.[82] Subcutaneous treprostinil and inhaled iloprost have improved functional capacity in the very small numbers of HIV-infected PH subjects that have been reported. Selexipag is a newer prostacyclin receptor agonist that was studied in 1156 patients in a randomized controlled trial; however, it included only 10 patients with PH-HIV.[83] In general, the treatment of PH in HIV-infected subjects does not appear to differ much from treatment in uninfected patients, except that specific clinical trial data are lacking in PH-HIV, and concomitant PI therapy introduces the problem of drug-drug interactions.

Heart Failure (see Part VI)

HF is a common accompaniment of HIV infection and portends a poor prognosis.[83] In the pre-ART era, HF generally resulted from HIV-associated cardiomyopathy and manifested as symptomatic systolic dysfunction with LV dilatation and a poor short-term outcome. This type of HF is still common with advanced HIV disease and AIDS in geographic areas where ART is not readily available.

In contrast, in the current era the diagnosis of HF includes many asymptomatic people living with HIV and often refers only to systolic or diastolic dysfunction detected by echocardiography. In a large cohort study of uninfected and HIV-infected U.S. veterans, where 2636 HF events occurred over 7.1 years of follow-up, HF with preserved ejection fraction (HFpEF) accounted for 34.6% of these, borderline HFpEF accounted for 15.5%, HF with reduced ejection fraction (HFrEF) for 37.1%, and HF of unknown type for 12.8%.[84] Compared with uninfected veterans, HIV-infected veterans had an increased risk of HFpEF (HR 1.21, 95% CI 1.03 to 1.41), borderline HFpEF (HR 1.37, 95% CI 1.09 to 1.72), and HFrEF (HR 1.61; 95% CI 1.40 to 1.86).

The pathophysiology of HIV-associated cardiomyopathy is multifactorial, with proposed causes including direct HIV infection with or without myocarditis, co-infection with other viruses such as Coxsackie virus B3 and CMV, opportunistic infections, and nutritional disorders.[83] HIV infection of the heart impairs systolic function. HIV gene products, such as tat, probably also contribute. Proinflammatory cytokines such as tumor necrosis factor and IL-1β also depress LV systolic function.

LV hypertrophy is more common in HIV-infected subjects than in controls. In a study from our group, HIV-infected participants had a mean 8 g/m^2 larger LV mass index compared with controls (p < 0.001). Higher LV mass index associated independently with lower nadir CD4 T cell count, suggesting that immunodeficiency might play a role in this process. Half of HIV subjects had diastolic dysfunction, and after adjusting for age and traditional risk factors, they were 2.4 times more likely to have diastolic dysfunction than controls. Both diastolic dysfunction and reduced ejection fraction predicted sudden cardiac death in our HIV cohort.[85]

The relationship of ART to HF in subjects with HIV is multifaceted. Some ART worsens glucose and lipid metabolism and associates with weight gain, factors that promote HF. ART has been blamed for otherwise unexplained LV hypertrophy in persons with HIV. On the other hand, ART prevents the cardiomyopathy and severe systolic dysfunction that was so common in the pre-ART era.[83] One ART, TDF, might reduce the risk of developing HF: in a large cohort of US veterans with HIV, HF risk was markedly lower in current TDF users (HR 0.68, 95% CI 0.53 to 0.86) compared with never users.[86] TDF might reduce the risk of HF by improving viral control and thus decreasing inflammation. The potential beneficial effect of TDF in HF requires confirmation.

In a cohort study from New York, with poorly controlled HIV and a high prevalence of drug use, PI-based regimens were associated with lower LV ejection fraction, higher pulmonary artery systolic pressure, and increased CV mortality as well as 30-day HF readmission among HIV-infected individuals with HF.[87]

Cardiac MRI provides insight into the subtle LV abnormalities that contribute to HF in the context of HIV. In one study, late gadolinium enhancement on cardiac MRI, a marker of cardiac fibrosis, was detected in 83% of 103 HIV subjects compared with only 16% of 92 controls.[88] The mean age of subjects in both groups was 45 years; ejection fraction was in the normal range but 6% lower in the HIV group, while LV mass was 7% higher. The high proportion of HIV subjects with myocardial fibrosis may not only contribute to incident HF but also the increased risk of sudden cardiac death in this group.

Treatment recommendations for HF in the setting of HIV are based upon trials done in uninfected HF patients and from guidelines based upon these trials (see also Chapters 48 to 51).[83] Thus, angiotensin-converting enzyme (ACE) inhibitors, beta blockers, aldosterone antagonists, digoxin, biventricular pacemakers, and AICDs should be used in persons with HIV as they are in uninfected patients with HF. Small numbers of HIV-infected subjects have undergone cardiac transplantation with excellent long-term survival.[89]

Arrhythmias and Sudden Cardiac Death (see Part VII)

HIV accentuates the risk of cardiac arrhythmias. The incidence of AF is rising as people with HIV age in the era of ART. In a large registry of U.S. veterans followed for a mean of 6.8 years from 1996 to 2011, 2.6% patients developed AF. Markers of HIV disease severity, specifically low CD4 count and high viral load, independently associate with the development of AF, along with expected clinical factors such concomitant coronary disease, HF, alcoholism, renal dysfunction, and hypothyroidism. HIV infection associates with an increased risk for AF with an HR of 1.46, a magnitude of risk that is similar to established AF risk factors.[90]

As in the general population, management of AF aims to control the ventricular rate and to prevent embolic events. Scores to assess embolic risk do not appear to perform well in persons with AF and HIV.[91] Drugs used for rate control (diltiazem, verapamil) and newer anticoagulants (apixaban, rivaroxaban, ticagrelor) are metabolized by the CYP3A4 hepatic metabolism and thus interact with ART.[92] Although there are limited data available in HIV, dabigatran may have the least drug-drug interactions with ART.[93] Caution is therefore warranted in dose selection, and a dose adjustment may be indicated.

Subjects with HIV appear to be more susceptible to sudden cardiac death than uninfected persons. In a consecutive series of 2860 HIV patients followed for a mean of 3.7 years, the mean sudden cardiac death rate was 2.6 per 1000 person-years (95% CI 1.8 to 3.8), 4.5-fold higher than expected.[80] Sudden cardiac death patients had a higher prevalence of previous MI, cardiomyopathy, HF, and arrhythmias. LV systolic dysfunction and diastolic dysfunction, especially in the presence of detectable HIV RNA levels, predicted sudden cardiac death.[80] AICD implantation may be beneficial in subjects with HIV who meet criteria for a device. In one study comparing 59 HIV AICD subjects with 267 uninfected AICD controls, discharge rate over a mean follow-up of 19 months was higher in the HIV group (39% versus 20%, $P = 0.001$).[94]

Cerebrovascular Disease (see also Chapter 45)

As with ACS, the clinical features of ischemic stroke differ in HIV subjects compared with uninfected individuals. HIV stroke patients tend to be younger and male. Risk factors for ischemic stroke in the general population (i.e., hypertension, diabetes, smoking and dyslipidemia) are also risk factors for stroke in the setting of HIV. In the Veterans Aging Cohort Study the risk of ischemia stroke increased by 25% in HIV-infected men compared with uninfected subjects.[49] After adjustment, the risk of ischemic stroke was attenuated but still higher among HIV-infected men (HR 1.17, 95% CI 1.01 to 1.36, $P = 0.04$). HIV appears to increase the risk of ischemic stroke more in women than in men, with a risk that was almost doubled (HR 1.93, 95% CI 1.31 to 2.85) in one of the few studies of stroke incidence in HIV-infected women.[95] In a large series from the U.S. National Inpatient Sample, in-hospital mortality was higher in HIV-infected stroke than in uninfected stroke patients (7.6% versus 5.2%).[96]

The incidence of intracerebral hemorrhage is also higher in the setting of HIV, with an unadjusted incidence rate ratio of 1.85 (95% CI 1.37 to 2.47, $p < 0.001$).[97] In a multivariable model, HIV infection associated independently with a higher hazard of ICH, although its effect diminished with increasing age. A low CD4 count may associate with intracerebral hemorrhage.

More than one-third of strokes in persons with HIV are intracranial, as opposed to extracranial origin.[66] HIV crosses the blood-brain barrier early in the course of the infection and promotes inflammation of small vessels. During the first 6 months of ART in immunosuppressed individuals, the risk of stroke increases, perhaps due to small vessel thinning and erosion due to remodeling and neuroinflammation.[66] The relative contributions of atherosclerosis and inflammation to intracranial stroke in the context of HIV require further investigation.

The data linking ART to an increased risk of stroke are less compelling than the data for MI, possibly due to the lower incidence of stroke. A high viral load and a low CD4 count increase the risk of stroke. Yet even treated individuals with well-controlled infection show evidence of inflammation and immune activation and likely have increased risk for stroke.

The acute and long-term treatment of stroke in persons with HIV resembles that in uninfected individuals.[98] Primary and secondary prevention of stroke in subjects with HIV has great importance because of the increased risk in these individuals and because of their high prevalence of modifiable risk factors, notably smoking, dyslipidemia, and hypertension.

REFERENCES

General

1. Global HIV & AIDS Statistics—2019 Fact Sheet. https://www.unaids.org/en/resources/fact-sheet.
2. Smit M, Brinkman K, Geerlings S, et al. Future challenges for clinical care of an ageing population infected with HIV: a modelling study. *Lancet Infect Dis.* 2015;15:810–818.
3. Hsue PY, Waters DD. HIV infection and coronary heart disease: mechanisms and management. *Nat Rev Cardiol.* 2019;16:745–759.

Cardiovascular Risk Factors in People Living with HIV

4. Althoff KN, Gebo KA, Moore RD, et al. North American AIDS Cohort Collaboration on Research and Design. Contributions of traditional and HIV-related risk factors on non-AIDS-defining cancer, myocardial infarction, and end-stage liver and renal diseases in adults with HIV in the USA and Canada: a collaboration of cohort studies. *Lancet HIV.* 2019;6:e93–e104.
5. Waters DD, Hsue PY. Lipid abnormalities in persons living with HIV infection. *Can J Cardiol.* 2019;35:249–259.
6. Gori A, Antinori A, Vergori A, et al. Effectiveness of switching to darunavir/cobicistat in virologically-suppressed HIV-positive patients receiving ritonavir-boosted protease inhibitor-based regimen: the "STORE" study. *J Acquir Immune Defic Syndr.* 2020. (online ahead of print).
7. Ekoru K, Young EH, Dillon DG, et al. HIV treatment is associated with a two-fold higher probability of raised triglycerides: pooled analyses in 21023 individuals in sub-Saharan Africa. *Glob Health Epidemiol Genom.* 2018;3:e7.
8. Eckard AR, McComsey GA. Weight gain and integrase inhibitors. *Curr Opin Infect Dis.* 2020;33(1):10–19.
9. Nix LM, Tien PC. Metabolic syndrome, diabetes, and cardiovascular risk in HIV. *Curr HIV AIDS Rep.* 2014;11(3):271–278.
10. Hill A, Waters L, Pozniak A. Are new antiretroviral treatments increasing the risks of clinical obesity? *J Virus Erad.* 2019;5:41–43.
11. Sax PE, Erlandson KM, Lake JE, et al. Weight gain following initiation of antiretroviral therapy: risk factors in randomized comparative clinical trials. *CID.* 2019. (in press).
12. Grand M, Bia D, Diaz A. Cardiovascular risk assessment in people living with HIV: a systematic review and meta-analysis of real-life data. *Curr HIV Res.* 2020;18:5–18.
13. Mathabire Ru¨cker SC, Tayea A, Bitiliny J, et al. High rates of hypertension, diabetes, elevated low-density lipoprotein cholesterol, and cardiovascular disease risk factors in HIV- infected patients in Malawi. *AIDS.* 2018;32:253–260.
14. Willig AL, Webel AR, Westfall AO, et al. Physical activity trends and metabolic health outcomes in people living with HIV in the US, 2008-2015. *Prog Cardiovasc Dis.* 2020. https://doi.org/10.1016/j.pcad.2020.02.005. (on line ahead of print).
15. Armah KA, Chang CC, Baker JV, et al. Prehypertension, hypertension, and the risk of acute myocardial infarction in HIV-infected and -uninfected veterans. *Clin Infect Dis.* 2014;58(1):121–129.
16. Ekrikpo UE, Kengne AP, Bello AK, et al. Chronic kidney disease in the global adult HIV-infected population: a systematic review and meta-analysis. *PloS One.* 2018;13(4):e0195443.
17. Ryom L, Lundgren JD, Ross M, et al. Renal impairment and cardiovascular disease in HIV- positive individuals: the D:A:D study. *J Infect Dis.* 2016;214:1212–1220.
18. Mocroft A, Lundgren JD, Ross M, et al. Current and cumulative exposure to potentially nephrotoxic antiretrovirals and development of chronic kidney disease in HIV-positive individuals with a normal baseline estimated glomerular filtration rate: a prospective international cohort study. *Lancet HIV.* 2016;3(1):e23–e32.
19. Rasmussen LD, Helleberg M, May MT, et al. Myocardial infarction among Danish HIV-infected individuals: population-attributable fractions associated with smoking. *Clin Infect Dis.* 2015;60(9):1415–1423.
20. Keith A, Dong Y, Shuter J, et al. Behavioral interventions for tobacco use in HIV-infected smokers: a meta-analysis. *J Acquir Immune Defic Syndr.* 2016;72:527–533.
21. Stanton CA, Kumar PN, Moadel AB, et al. A multicenter randomized controlled trial of intensive group therapy for tobacco treatment in HIV-infected cigarette smokers. *J Acquir Immune Defic Syndr.* 2020;83(4):405–414.
22. Shuter J, Kim RS, Durant S, Stanton CA. Long-term follow-up of smokers living with HIV after an intensive behavioral tobacco treatment intervention. *J Acquir Immune Defic Syndr.* 2020. (on line ahead of print).
23. Ghura S, Gross R, Jordan-Sciutto K, et al. Bidirectional associations among nicotine and tobacco smoke, neuroHIV, and anti-viral therapy. *J Neuroimmune Pharmacol.* 2019. https://doi.org/10.1007/s11481-019-09897-4. (on line ahead of print).

Mechanisms of HIV-Related Atherogenesis

24. Faust TB, Binning JM, Gross JD, Frankel AD. Making sense of multifunctional proteins: human immunodeficiency virus type 1 accessory and regulatory proteins and connections to transcription. *Annu Rev Virol.* 2017;4(1):241–260.
25. Knudsen A, Kristoffersen US, Panum I, et al. Coronary artery calcium and intima-media thickness are associated with level of cytomegalovirus immunoglobulin G in HIV-infected patients. *HIV Med.* 2018;20:60–62.
26. Tincati C, Douek DC, Marchetti G. Gut barrier structure, mucosal immunity and intestinal microbiota in the pathogenesis and treatment of HIV infection. *AIDS Res Ther.* 2016;13:19.
27. Borges AH, O'Connor JL, Phillips AN, et al. Interleukin 6 is a stronger predictor of clinical events than high-sensitivity C-reactive protein or D-dimer during HIV infection. *J Infect Dis.* 2016;214(3):408–416.
28. Tawakol A, Ishai A, Li D, et al. Association of arterial and lymph node inflammation with distinct inflammatory pathways in human immunodeficiency virus infection. *JAMA Cardiol.* 2017;2:163–171.
29. Toribio M, Fitch KV, Sanchez L, et al. Effects of pitavastatin and pravastatin on markers of immune activation and arterial inflammation in HIV. *AIDS.* 2017;31(6):797–806.
30. O'Brien MP, Hunt PW, Kitch PW, et al. A randomized placebo controlled trial of aspirin effects on immune activation in chronically human immunodeficiency virus-infected adults on virologically suppressive antiretroviral therapy. *Open Forum Infect Dis.* 2017;4(1):ofw278.
31. Ridker PM, Everett BM, Thuren T, et al. Antiinflammatory therapy with canakinumab for atherosclerotic disease. *N Engl J Med.* 2017;377:1119–1131.
32. Ridker PM, MacFadyen JG, Everett BM, et al. Relationship of C-reactive protein reduction to cardiovascular event reduction following treatment with canakinumab: a secondary analysis from the CANTOS randomised controlled trial. *Lancet.* 2018;391:319–328.
33. Ridker PM, Libby P, MacFadyen JG, et al. Modulation of the interleukin-6 signalling pathway and incidence rates of atherosclerotic events and all- cause mortality: analyses from the Canakinumab Anti- Inflammatory Thrombosis Outcomes Study (CANTOS). *Eur Heart J.* 2018;39:3499–3507.
34. Hsue PY, Li D, Ma Y, et al. IL-1beta inhibition reduces atherosclerotic inflammation in HIV infection. *J Am Coll Cardiol.* 2018;72:2809–2811.
35. Ridker PM, Everett BM, Pradhan A, et al. Low-dose methotrexate for the prevention of atherosclerotic events. *N Engl J Med.* 2019;380(8):752–762.
36. Hsue PY, Ribaudo HJ, Deeks SG, et al. Safety and impact of low-dose methotrexate on endothelial function and inflammation in individuals with treated human immunodeficiency virus: AIDS Clinical Trials Group Study A5314. *Clin Infect Dis.* 2019;68(11):1877–1886.
37. Borges AH, O'Connor JL, Phillips AN, et al. Interleukin 6 is a stronger predictor of clinical events than high-sensitivity C-reactive protein or D-dimer during HIV infection. *J Infect Dis.* 2016;214:408–416.
38. Nordell AD, McKenna M, Borges ÁH, et al. Severity of cardiovascular disease outcomes among patients with HIV is related to markers of inflammation and coagulation. *J Am Heart Assoc.* 2014;3:e000844.
39. Grund B, Baker JV, Deeks SG, et al. Relevance of interleukin-6 and D-dimer for serious non-AIDS morbidity and death among HIV-positive adults on suppressive antiretroviral therapy. *PloS One.* 2016;11:e0155100.
40. Scherzer R, Shah SJ, Secemsky E, et al. Association of biomarker clusters with cardiac phenotypes and mortality in patients with HIV infection. *Circ Heart Fail.* 2018;11:e004312.

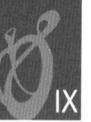

41. Marconi VC, Duncan MS, So-Armah K, et al. Bilirubin is inversely associated with cardiovascular disease among HIV-positive and HIV-negative individuals in VACS (Veterans Aging Cohort Study). *J Am Heart Assoc*. 2018;7(10):e007792.

Atherosclerosis in People with HIV/AIDS

42. Stein JH, Currier JS, Hsue PY. Arterial disease in patients with human immunodeficiency virus infection: what has imaging taught us? *JACC Cardiovasc Imaging*. 2014;7:515–525.
43. Post WS, Budoff M, Kingsley L, et al. Associations between HIV infection and subclinical coronary atherosclerosis: the Multicenter AIDS Cohort Study (MACS). *Ann Intern Med*. 2014;160:458–467.
44. D'Ascenzo F, Cerrato E, Calcagno A, et al. High prevalence at computed coronary tomography of non-calcified plaques in asymptomatic HIV patients treated with HAART: a meta-analysis. *Atherosclerosis*. 2015;240:197–204.
45. Tawakol A, Lo J, Zanni MV, et al. Increased arterial inflammation relates to high-risk coronary plaque morphology in HIV-infected patients. *J Acquir Immune Defic Syndr*. 2014;66(2):164–171.
46. Hsu DC, Ma YF, Narwan A, et al. Plasma tissue factor and immune activation are associated with carotid intima-media thickness progression in treated HIV infection. *AIDS*. 2020;34(4):519–528.
47. Shah ASV, Stelzle D, Lee KK, et al. Global burden of atherosclerotic cardiovascular disease in people living with HIV: systematic review and meta-analysis. *Circulation*. 2018;138:1100–1112.
48. Hsue PY, Waters DD. Time to recognize HIV infection as a major cardiovascular risk factor. *Circulation*. 2018;138:1113–1115.
49. Sico JJ, Chang CC, So-Armah K, et al. HIV status and the risk of ischemic stroke among men. *Neurology*. 2015;84:1933–1940.
50. Knudsen AD, Gelpi M, Afzal S, et al. Brief report: prevalence of peripheral artery disease is higher in persons living with HIV compared with uninfected controls. *J Acquir Immune Defic Syndr*. 2018;79(3):381–385.
51. Badr S, Minha S, Kitabata H, et al. Safety and long-term outcomes after percutaneous coronary intervention in patients with human immunodeficiency virus. *Catheter Cardiovasc Interv*. 2015;85:192–198.
52. Robich MP, Schiltz N, Johnston DR, et al. Outcomes of patients with human immunodeficiency virus infection undergoing cardiovascular surgery in the United States. *J Thorac Cardiovasc Surg*. 2014;148:3066–3073.
53. Smilowitz NR, Gupta N, Guo Y, et al. Influence of human immunodeficiency virus seropositive status on the in-hospital management and outcomes of patients presenting with acute myocardial infarction. *J Invasive Cardiol*. 2016;28(10):403–409.
54. Rosenson RS, Colantonio LD, Burkholder GA, Chen L, Muntner P. Trends in utilization of statin therapy and contraindicated statin use in HIV-infected adults treated with antiretroviral therapy from 2007 through 2015. *J Am Heart Assoc*. 2018;7(24):e010345.
55. Günthard HF, Saag MS, Benson CA, et al. Antiretroviral drugs for treatment and prevention of HIV infection in adults. 2016 recommendations of the International Antiviral Society–USA Panel. *JAMA Med Assoc*. 2016;316:191–210.
56. Lundgren JD, Babiker AG, Gordin F, et al. Initiation of antiretroviral therapy in early asymptomatic HIV infection. *N Engl J Med*. 2015;373(9):795–807.
57. Baker JV, Sharma S, Achhra AC, et al. Changes in cardiovascular disease risk factors with immediate versus deferred antiretroviral therapy initiation among HIV-positive participants in the START (Strategic Timing of Antiretroviral Treatment) Trial. *J Am Heart Assoc*. 2017;6(5):e004987.
58. Promer K, Karris MY. Current treatment options for HIV elite controllers: a review. *Curr Treat Options Infect Dis*. 2018;10(2):302–309.
59. Crowell TA, Gebo KA, Blankson JN, et al. Hospitalization rates and reasons among HIV elite controllers and persons with medically controlled HIV infection. *J Infect Dis*. 2015;211(11):1692–1702.
60. Milinkovic A, Berger F, Arenas-Pinto A, Mauss S. Reversible effect on lipids by switching from tenofovir disoproxil fumarate to tenofovir alafenamide and back. *AIDS*. 2019;33(15):2387–2391.
61. Landmesser U, Chapman MJ, Stock JK, et al. Update of ESC/EAS Task Force on practical clinical guidance for proprotein convertase subtilisin/kexin type 9 inhibition in patients with atherosclerotic cardiovascular disease or in familial hypercholesterolaemia. *Eur Heart J*. 2017;39:1131–1143. 2017.
62. Jacobson TA, Maki KC, Orringer CE, et al. National Lipid Association recommendations for patient-centered management of dyslipidemia: Part 2. *J Clin Lipidol*. 2015;9(suppl 6):S1–S122.
63. Zanni MV, Fitch KV, Feldpausch M, et al. 2013 American College of Cardiology/American Heart Association and 2004 Adult Treatment Panel III cholesterol guidelines applied to HIV-infected patients with/without subclinical high-risk coronary plaque. *AIDS*. 2014;28:2061–2070.
64. Phan BA, Weigel B, Ma Y, et al. Utility of 2013 American College of Cardiology/American Heart Association cholesterol guidelines in HIV-infected adults with carotid atherosclerosis. *Circ Cardiovasc Imaging*. 2017;10:e005995.
65. Grundy SM, Stone NJ, Bailey AL, et al. 2018 AHA/ACC/AACVPR/AAPA/ABC/ACPM/ADA/AGS/APhA/ASPC/NLA/PCNA guideline on the management of blood cholesterol: a report of the American College of Cardiology/American Heart Association task force on clinical practice guidelines. *Circulation*. 2019;139:e1082–e1143.
66. Feinstein MJ, Achenbach CJ, Stone NJ, et al. A systematic review of the usefulness of statin therapy in HIV-infected patients. *Am J Cardiol*. 2015;115:1760–1766.
67. Aberg JA, Sponseller CA, Ward DJ, et al. Pitavastatin versus pravastatin in adults with HIV-1 infection and dyslipidaemia (INTREPID): 12 week and 52 week results of a phase 4, multicentre, randomised, double-blind, superiority trial. *Lancet HIV*. 2017;4:e284–e294.
68. Clement ME, Park LP, Navar AM, et al. Statin utilization and recommendations among HIV- and HCV-infected veterans: a cohort study. *Clin Infect Dis*. 2016;63(3):407–413.
69. Lee FJ, Monteiro P, Baker D, et al. Rosuvastatin vs. protease inhibitor switching for hypercholesterolaemia: a randomized trial. *HIV Med*. 2016;17:605–614.
70. Bhatt DL, Steg G, Miller M, et al. Cardiovascular risk reduction with icosapent ethyl for hypertriglyceridemia. *N Engl J Med*. 2019;380:11–22.
71. Triant VA, Perez J, Regan S, et al. Cardiovascular risk prediction functions underestimate risk in HIV infection. *Circulation*. 2018;137:2203–2214.
72. Friis-Møller N, Ryom L, Smith C, et al. An updated prediction model of the global risk of cardiovascular disease in HIV-positive persons: the Data-collection on Adverse Effects of Anti-HIV Drugs (D:A:D) study. *Eur J Prev Cardiol*. 2016;23:214–223.
73. Feinstein MJ, Hsue PY, Benjamin LA, et al. Characteristics, prevention, and management of cardiovascular disease in people living with HIV: a scientific statement from the American Heart Association. *Circulation*. 2019;140:e98–e124.
74. Nolte JE, Neumann T, Manne JM, et al. Cost-effectiveness analysis of coronary artery disease screening in HIV-infected men. *Eur J Prev Cardiol*. 2014;21:972–729.
75. Phan BAP, Weigal B, Ma Y, et al. Utility of 2013 American College of Cardiology/American Heart Association cholesterol guidelines in HIV-infected adults with carotid atherosclerosis. *Circ Cardiovasc Imaging*. 2017;10(7):e005995.

Other Cardiovascular Conditions Associated with HIV

76. Simonneau G, Montani D, Celermajer DS, et al. Haemodynamic definitions and updated clinical classification of pulmonary hypertension. *Eur Respir J*. 2019;53(1).
77. Parikh RV, Ma Y, Scherzer R, et al. Endothelin-1 predicts hemodynamically assessed pulmonary artery hypertension in HIV infection. *PloS One*. 2016;11:e0146355.
78. Parikh RV, Scherzer R, Nitta EM, et al. Increased levels of asymmetric dimethylarginine are associated with pulmonary arterial hypertension in HIV infection. *AIDS*. 2014;28:511–519.
79. Basyal B, Jarrett H, Barnett CF. Pulmonary hypertension in HIV. *Can J Cardiol*. 2019;35:288–298.
80. Moyers BS, Secemsky EA, Vittinghoff E, et al. Effect of left ventricular dysfunction and viral load on risk of sudden cardiac death in patients with human immunodeficiency virus. *Am J Cardiol*. 2014;113(7):1260–1265.
81. Chinello P, Petrosillo N. Pharmacological treatment of HIV-associated pulmonary hypertension. *Expert Rev Clin Pharmacol*. 2016;9:715–725.
82. Sitbon O, Channick R, Chin KM, et al. Selexipag for the treatment of pulmonary arterial hypertension. *N Engl J Med*. 2015;373:2522–2533.
83. Hsue PY, Waters DD. Heart failure in persons living with HIV infection. *Curr Opin HIV AIDS*. 2017;12:534–539.
84. Freiberg MS, Chang CH, Skanderson M, et al. Association between HIV infection and the risk of heart failure with reduced ejection fraction and preserved ejection fraction in the antiretroviral therapy era: results from the veterans aging cohort study. *JAMA Cardiol*. 2017;2:536–546.
85. Moyers BS, Secemsky EA, Vittinghoff E, et al. Effect of left ventricular dysfunction and viral load on risk of sudden cardiac death in patients with human immunodeficiency virus. *Am J Cardiol*. 2014;113:1260–1265.
86. Chen R, Scherzer R, Hsue PY, et al. Association of tenofovir use with risk of incident heart failure in HIV-infected patients. *J Am Heart Assoc*. 2017;6:e005387.
87. Alvi RM, Neilan AM, Tariq N, et al. Protease inhibitors and cardiovascular outcomes in patients with HIV and heart failure. *J Am Coll Cardiol*. 2018;72(5):518–530.
88. Ntusi N, O'Dwyer E, Dorrell L, et al. HIV-1-related cardiovascular disease is associated with chronic inflammation, frequent pericardial effusions, and probable myocardial edema. *Circ Cardiovasc Imaging*. 2016;9:e004430.
89. Agüero F, Castel MA, Cocchi S, et al. An update on heart transplantation in human immunodeficiency virus-infected patients. *Am J Transplant*. 2016;16(1):21–28.
90. Sardana M, Hsue PY, Tseng ZH, et al. Human immunodeficiency virus infection and incident atrial fibrillation. *J Am Coll Cardiol*. 2019;74(11):1512–1514.
91. Chau KH, Scherzer R, Grunfeld C, et al. CHA2DS2-VASc score, warfarin use, and risk for thromboembolic events among HIV-infected persons with atrial fibrillation. *J Acquir Immune Defic Syndr*. 2017;76(1):90–97.
92. West TA, Perram J, Holloway CJ. Use of direct oral anticoagulants for treatment of atrial fibrillation in patients with HIV: a review. *Curr Opin HIV AIDS*. 2017;12(6):554–560.
93. Perram J, O'Dwyer E, Holloway C. Use of dabigatran with antiretrovirals. *HIV Med*. 2019;20(5):344–346.
94. Alvi RM, Neilan AM, Tariq N, et al. Incidence, predictors, and outcomes of implantable cardioverter-defibrillator discharge among people living with HIV. *J Am Heart Assoc*. 2018;7(18):e009857.
95. Chow FC, Regan S, Zanni MV, et al. Elevated ischemic stroke risk among women living with HIV infection. *AIDS*. 2018;32(1):59–67.
96. Sweeney EM, Thakur KT, Lyons JL, et al. Outcomes of intravenous tissue plasminogen activator for acute ischaemic stroke in HIV-infected adults. *Eur J Neurol*. 2014;21:1394–1399.
97. Chow FC, He W, Bachetti P, et al. Elevated rates of intracerebral hemorrhage in individuals from a US clinical care HIV cohort. *Neurology*. 2014;83(19):1705–1711.
98. Nguyen I, Kim AS, Chow FC. Prevention of stroke in people living with HIV. *Prog Cardiovasc Dis*. 2020; Jan 31;S0033-0620(20)30028_1.

86 Pericardial Diseases

MARTIN M. LEWINTER, PAUL C. CREMER, AND ALLAN L. KLEIN

ACUTE PERICARDITIS, 1616
Definition, Causes, Epidemiology, and Pathophysiology, 1616
History and Differential Diagnosis, 1616
Physical Examination, 1616
Laboratory Testing, 1616
Diagnosis, Natural History, and Management, 1618
Recurrent Pericarditis, 1619

PERICARDIAL EFFUSION AND CARDIAC TAMPONADE, 1620
Etiology, 1620
Pathophysiology and Hemodynamics, 1620
Clinical Presentation, 1621
Laboratory Testing, 1622
Management of Pericardial Effusion and Tamponade, 1623
Pericardial Fluid Analysis, 1624
Pericardioscopy and Percutaneous Biopsy, 1625

CONSTRICTIVE PERICARDITIS, 1625
Physical Examination, 1626
Laboratory Testing, 1627
Echocardiography-Doppler Examination, 1627
Cardiac Catheterization and Angiography, 1627
Computed Tomography and Cardiac Magnetic Resonance, 1627
Differentiating Constrictive Pericarditis from Restrictive Cardiomyopathy, 1628
Management, 1628

EFFUSIVE-CONSTRICTIVE PERICARDITIS, 1630

REFERENCES, 1633

The pericardium is involved in a wide variety of diseases which result in some of the classic physical, imaging, and hemodynamic findings in cardiology. In this chapter we discuss the anatomy and physiology of the pericardium, acute and recurrent pericarditis, pericardial effusion and tamponade, constrictive and effusive-constrictive pericarditis (ECP), and selected specific etiologies.[1,2]

ANATOMY AND PHYSIOLOGY OF THE PERICARDIUM

The pericardium is composed of two layers,[3] the *visceral* pericardium, a monolayer of mesothelial cells and collagen and elastin fibers adherent to the epicardial surface of the heart, and the fibrous *parietal* pericardium, which is normally about 2 mm thick and surrounds most of the heart (Fig. 86.1). The parietal pericardium is largely acellular and contains collagen and elastin fibers. The visceral pericardium reflects back near the origins of the great vessels and is continuous with and forms the inner layer of the parietal pericardium. The pericardial space or sac is contained within these two layers, and normally contains up to 50 mL of serous fluid. The visceral-parietal reflection is a few centimeters proximal to the junctions of the cavae with the right atrium (RA); thus, portions of the caval vessels lie within the pericardial sac. Posterior to the left atrium (LA), the reflection occurs at the oblique sinus of the pericardium. The LA is largely extra-pericardial. The parietal pericardium has ligamentous attachments to the diaphragm, sternum, and other structures.

While its removal has no obvious negative consequences, the pericardium does function to maintain a relatively constant position of the heart in the thorax and provides a barrier to infection.[3] The pericardium is well-innervated with mechano- and chemoreceptors and phrenic afferent receptors which participate in reflexes arising from pericardium and/or epicardium (e.g., the Bezold-Jarisch reflex) and transmission of pericardial pain. The pericardium also secretes prostaglandins and related substances that may modulate neural traffic and coronary tone.

The best-characterized mechanical function of the pericardium is its *restraining* effect on cardiac volume.[3] This reflects the mechanical properties of the parietal pericardium. At low stresses the tissue is very elastic. With further stretch, it abruptly becomes stiff and resistant to further stretch. The point on the stress-strain relation where this transition occurs is near the upper range of physiologic cardiac volumes. The *pressure-volume relation* of the pericardial sac reflects the properties of the tissue[3], that is, a flat, compliant segment transitioning relatively abruptly to a noncompliant segment around the upper limit of normal total cardiac volume. Thus, the sac has a relatively small reserve volume. When exceeded, the pressure within the sac operating on the surface of the heart increases rapidly and is transmitted into the cardiac chambers. The shape of the pericardial pressure-volume relation dictates that once a critical level of effusion is reached relatively small amounts of additional fluid will cause large increases in intra-pericardial pressure and markedly affect cardiac function. Conversely, removal of small amounts of fluid can result in striking benefit. The shape of the pericardial pressure-volume relation also suggests that it *normally* restrains cardiac volume, that is, the force it exerts on the surface of the heart limits filling, with a component of *intra-cavitary* pressure reflecting the surface pressure. Studies with specially designed balloons[3] demonstrate a substantial surface pressure, especially when the upper limit of normal cardiac volume is exceeded.

Pericardial contact pressure has also been estimated by quantifying the shift in the right and left heart diastolic *pressure-volume relation* before and after pericardiectomy.[3] A decrease in pressure at a given volume is the *effective* pericardial pressure at that volume. Studies in normal canine hearts indicate negligible pressure at low normal filling volumes, with pressures in the 2 to 4 mm Hg range at the upper end of normal. At filling volumes above normal the pressure rapidly increases. Thus, at left-sided filling pressure approximately 25 mm Hg, contact pressure is approximately 10 mm Hg. Patients undergoing pericardiotomy during heart surgery develop mild postoperative increases in cardiac volume, consistent with relief of underlying, normal pericardial restraint to filling.

The normal pericardium also contributes to diastolic interaction,[3] defined here as transmission of intra-cavitary filling pressure to adjoining chambers. Thus, for example, a portion of right ventricular (RV) diastolic pressure is transmitted to the left ventricle (LV) across the interventricular septum and contributes to LV diastolic pressure. The overall effect of the pericardium is to more tightly couple right- and left-sided filling pressures. As cardiac volume increases the pericardium contributes increasingly to intra-cavitary filling pressures due to both external contact pressure and increased diastolic interaction. When the cardiac chambers dilate rapidly, the restraining effect of the pericardium and its contribution to diastolic interaction are augmented, resulting in a hemodynamic picture with features of both cardiac tamponade and constrictive pericarditis (CP), an example being RV myocardial infarction (MI).[3] Here, the right heart dilates rapidly such that total heart volume exceeds pericardial reserve volume. As a result, left- and right-sided filling pressures equilibrate at elevated levels and a paradoxical pulse and inspiratory increase in systemic venous pressure (Kussmaul's sign) may occur. Other conditions with similar effects include acute pulmonary embolus and sub-acute mitral regurgitation.[3]

Chronic cardiac dilatation, for example, dilated cardiomyopathy or regurgitant valvular disease, can result in total cardiac volume well in excess of the pericardial reserve volume yet exaggerated restraining effects are not observed. Thus, the pericardium adapts to accommodate chronic increases in cardiac volume. In experimental chronic volume overload, the pericardial pressure-volume relation shifts to the right and its slope decreases, that is, it becomes more compliant, along with an increase in area and mass and a decreased effect on the diastolic pressure-volume relation.[3]

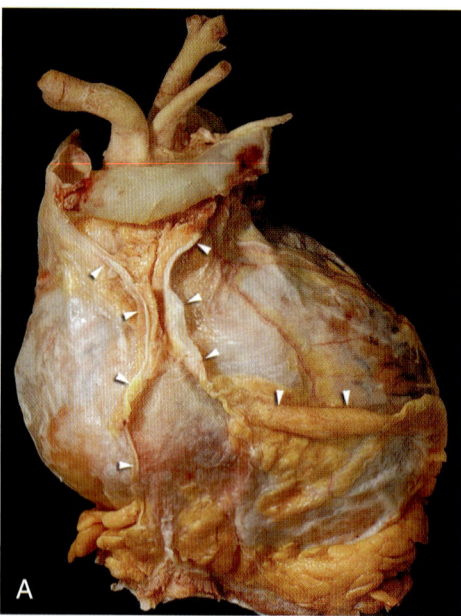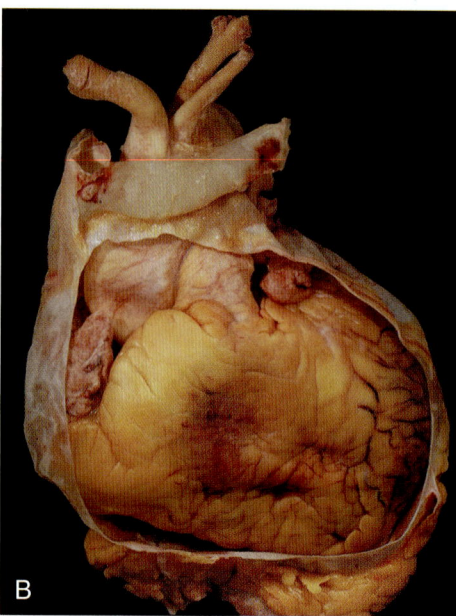

FIGURE 86.1 A, Anterior view of the intact parietal pericardial sac. The mediastinal pleura invest the lateral portion of the fibrous pericardium, with reflections indicated by the *arrowheads*. The space between the arrowheads corresponds to the attachment of the pericardium to the posterior surface of the sternum. Superiorly, the left innominate vein is seen merging with the superior vena cava. The branches of the aortic arch are just dorsal to the innominate vein. **B,** Anterior portion of the pericardial sac has been removed to show the heart and great vessels. The proximal segments of the great arteries are intrapericardial. (From Klein AL, Abbara S, Agler DA, et al. American Society of Echocardiography clinical recommendations for multimodality cardiovascular imaging of patients with pericardial disease: endorsed by the Society for Cardiovascular Magnetic Resonance and Society of Cardiovascular Computed Tomography. *J Am Soc Echocardiogr.* 2013;26(9):965–1012.e1015.)

ACUTE PERICARDITIS

Definition, Causes, Epidemiology, and Pathophysiology

Acute pericarditis is an inflammatory syndrome with or without pericardial effusion with a wide variety of causes (Table 86.1).[4-6] The prevalence of tuberculosis (TB) is a key element in the assessment of a suspected case of pericarditis. In developing regions where TB is endemic, it is the most common cause of pericarditis and effusion. TB is rare in developed countries and therefore a far less important consideration.[4-6]

There are limited epidemiological data documenting the incidence and prevalence of acute pericarditis. At autopsy, the frequency is approximately 1%.[4,5] Pericarditis is common in the emergency department, accounting for up to 5% of patients with nonischemic chest pain.[5] A review of etiologies in published series is presented in Table 86.2. In developed countries, presumed viral and idiopathic etiologies are most common. We use *idiopathic* to denote acute pericarditis for which no specific cause is identified with routine diagnostic testing, as outlined below. Idiopathic cases are presumed to be viral. Testing for specific viruses is costly and has low yield and impact on management.[7,8] Such a term, although an admission of ignorance, is clinically meaningful if nonviral causes of pericarditis have been excluded, because treatment with antiinflammatory therapy is similar for all cases and prognosis is good.[9,10]

In a contemporary series from Northern Italy, the incidence of acute pericarditis was 27.7 cases/100,000 population/year with concomitant myocarditis in about 15%.[11] In hospitalized patients with acute pericarditis from Finland, the incidence rate of hospitalization was 3.32/100,000 population/year.[12] Men aged 16 to 65 years were at higher risk than women (RR 2.02). Acute pericarditis was the cause of 0.20% of all cardiovascular admissions. The proportion of admissions declined in younger patients. In-hospital mortality rate was 1.1% and increased with age and severe infections such as pneumonia or septicemia.

Most of the various causes of pericardial inflammation result in a response characterized by edema, thickening of the parietal layer, production of exudative pericardial fluid, and increased friction between the layers.[9] Acute pericarditis and myocarditis share common viral etiologies and, as noted, as many as 15% of pericarditis cases are associated with myocarditis.[4,5,9,13] Coexistent myocarditis is usually manifested by modest release of cardiac biomarkers such as troponin (see Chapter 55). LV dysfunction is rare and the long-term prognosis of pericarditis complicated by myocarditis is excellent.[9,13] When ventricular function is normal the term "myopericarditis" is used. Cases with impaired function are labeled "perimyocarditis."

History and Differential Diagnosis

In greater than 90% of cases, the main symptom of acute pericarditis is chest pain, often quite severe.[4,5] It is usually retrosternal but may be localized to the left anterior chest and radiate to the neck, shoulders, and arms. Classically, the pain radiates to the trapezius ridge. Pericardial pain is pleuritic and worsened by lying down. Associated symptoms include dyspnea, cough, and occasionally hiccups. An antecedent history suggesting a viral illness is common. The history may provide clues to specific causative diagnoses. For example, a known malignancy or autoimmune disorder, high fevers with shaking chills, or weight loss suggest specific, nonidiopathic etiologies.

The differential diagnosis of chest pain is lengthy (see Chapters 35). Diagnoses most easily confused with pericarditis include myocardial ischemia/infarction, pneumonia with pleurisy, pulmonary embolism/infarction, costochondritis, and gastroesophageal reflux. Acute pericarditis is usually easily distinguished from myocardial ischemia, but further testing may be required. Other considerations include aortic dissection, intraabdominal processes, pneumothorax, and herpes zoster pain before skin lesions appear. Rarely, pericarditis can signal a preceding, silent MI.

Physical Examination

Patients with *uncomplicated* acute pericarditis often appear uncomfortable and anxious, with low-grade fever (<38°C) and sinus tachycardia. Arrhythmias are uncommon, although atrial fibrillation/flutter are reported in approximately 5% of cases.[14] The pathognomonic physical sign of acute pericarditis is the friction rub, reported in about one third of cases. Rubs are typically evanescent and may require repeated auscultation for detection.[5] The rub is ascribed to friction between pericardial layers. The classic rub consists of three components corresponding to ventricular systole, early diastole, and atrial contraction, and can be likened to the sound made when walking on crunchy snow. The rub is usually loudest at the lower left sternal border and best heard with the patient leaning forward. It is important to perform a thorough physical examination to look for clues to specific causative diagnoses as well as findings suggesting significant pericardial effusion.

Laboratory Testing

The electrocardiogram (ECG) is a key test for diagnosing acute pericarditis (see Chapter 14). The classic finding is "diffuse" ST-segment elevation (Fig. 86.2). The ST-segment vector points leftward, anterior, and inferior, with ST-segment elevation in all leads except aVR and often V_1. Usually, the ST segment is curved upward and resembles the current of injury of transmural ischemia. The distinction between acute pericarditis and transmural ischemia is usually not difficult because of more extensive lead involvement and lack of evolution to pathologic Q waves in pericarditis, and more prominent reciprocal ST depression in ischemia. However, ST elevation in pericarditis can at times involve a smaller number of leads and in some cases the ST segment more

TABLE 86.1 Categories of Diseases That Can Involve the Pericardium and Selected Specific Etiologies

Idiopathic*

Infectious

Viral* (echovirus, coxsackievirus, adenovirus, cytomegalovirus, hepatitis B, infectious mononucleosis, HIV/AIDS, SARS-CoV-2)

Bacterial* (*Mycobacterium tuberculosis, Mycobacterium avium-intracellulare,* pneumococcus, staphylococcus, streptococcus, mycoplasma, Lyme disease, *Haemophilus influenzae, Neisseria meningitides,* and many others)

HIV-associated*

Fungal (histoplasmosis, coccidioidomycosis, candida)

Protozoal

Inflammatory

Autoimmune diseases* (systemic lupus erythematosus, rheumatoid arthritis, scleroderma, dermatomyositis, Sjogren syndrome, inflammatory bowel disease, mixed)

Drug-induced autoimmune diseases* (procainamide, hydralazine, isoniazid, cyclosporine, etc.)

Arteritis (polyarteritis nodosa, temporal arteritis)

Post-cardiotomy/thoracotomy,* post-cardiac injury,* early and late post-myocardial infarction (Dressler syndrome*)

Autoinflammatory diseases* (tumor necrosis factor receptor-1 associated periodic syndrome, familial Mediterranean fever, others)

Miscellaneous: Sarcoidosis, Erdheim-Chester disease, Churg-Strauss disease, immunoglobulin G4 related diseases

Cancer

Primary: mesothelioma, fibrosarcoma, lipoma, etc.

Secondary*: breast and lung carcinoma, lymphomas, Kaposi sarcoma

Radiation-induced*

Early post-cardiac surgery and post-orthotopic heart transplantation

Hemopericardium

Trauma

Post-myocardial infarction free wall rupture

Endomyocardial biopsy

Dissecting aortic aneurysm

Device and procedure-related: percutaneous coronary procedures, implantable defibrillators and pacemakers, arrhythmia ablation, atrial septal defect closure, left atrial appendage isolation, percutaneous valve repair/replacement, laparoscopic hiatal hernia repair

Oral anticoagulants

Congenital

Cysts, diverticula, congenital absence

Miscellaneous

Stress cardiomyopathy

Cholesterol ("gold paint") pericarditis

Chronic renal failure, dialysis-associated*

Chylopericardium

Hypo- and hyperthyroidism

Amyloidosis

Pneumopericardium

Polycystic kidney disease

Pulmonary arterial hypertension

*Etiologies that can present as the syndrome of acute pericarditis.

TABLE 86.2 Etiology of Pericarditis in Major Series

ETIOLOGY	REPORTED FREQUENCY (%)
Idiopathic	15% (Africa) to 80%–90% (Europe)
Infectious pericarditis	
Viral	Largely unknown
Bacterial:	
Tuberculosis	1%–4% developed countries, up to 70% (Africa)
Purulent	<1% developed countries, 2%–3% Africa
Other infectious causes	Rare, largely unknown
Noninfectious pericarditis	
Neoplastic	5%–9% to 35% (in tertiary referral centers)
Autoimmune	2%–24%
Other noninfectious causes	Rare (largely unknown)

closely resembles early repolarization. As with the rub, ECG changes can be dynamic. Frequent recordings can yield a diagnosis in patients who initially have neither rub nor ST elevation. PR-segment depression is also common and considered the earliest ECG sign of acute pericarditis, reflecting pericardial involvement overlying the atria (see Fig. 86.2). PR-depression can occur without ST elevation and be the initial or sole ECG manifestation. Typical ECG evolution follows four stages: (1) PR depression and/or diffuse ST segment elevation, (2) normalization of ST segment, (3) T wave inversion with or without ST segment depression, and (4) normalization. The ECG often evolves without all four stages.

Although usually considered a hallmark of pericarditis, typical ECG changes reflect concomitant involvement of the myocardium, because the pericardium is electrically silent. For that reason, ECG changes are reported in no more than 60% of cases and are more common (>90%) with concomitant myocarditis.[13] Additional ECG changes that may constitute clues to the cause of pericarditis or associated findings include atrioventricular block in Lyme disease, pathologic Q waves signifying a previous, silent MI, and low-voltage or electrical alternans pointing toward significant effusion.

Many patients with acute pericarditis have a modestly elevated white blood cell count (WBC).[4,5] WBCs in excess of 13,000 to 14,000/mm^3 suggest a specific etiology. As noted earlier, as many as 15% of patients have coexistent myocarditis based on elevations in cardiac biomarkers such as troponin (see Chapter 55). Patients with myocarditis usually have ST-segment elevation.[13] Another concern in patients with elevated injury biomarkers is a prior silent MI followed by subsequent pericarditis. The latter usually occurs after large or late-presenting MIs with transmural ECG changes.[15]

Serum C-reactive protein (CRP) is elevated in approximately three-fourths of patients with acute pericarditis.[16] Normal values generally occur in patients seen very early or who have previously received anti-inflammatory drugs including corticosteroids. CRP usually normalizes within 1 week and in almost all cases by 4 weeks after initial evaluation. Failure to normalize CRP is independently associated with recurrent symptoms.[9] In addition to aiding in diagnosis, CRP can be used to monitor disease activity and individualize duration of therapy.[4,16] Although the utility of CRP for this purpose has not been prospectively validated, the association of elevated values with recurrences provides a rationale for measurement initially and when it is uncertain how long treatment should be maintained.

Chest radiograms are normal in uncomplicated acute pericarditis.[5] Occasionally, small pulmonary infiltrates or pleural effusions are present, presumably related to the underlying causative infection. Because small to moderate effusions may not cause an abnormal cardiac silhouette, even modest cardiac enlargement is of concern and generally associated with an effusion greater than 300 mL.

The echocardiographic-Doppler examination (see Chapter 16) is completely normal in approximately 40% of patients with acute pericarditis.[1,7] It is performed mainly to determine if an effusion is present and recommended in all patients with suspected pericarditis.[1,4] Pericardial effusion is reported in about 60% of cases of acute pericarditis and is usually small (<10 mm on semiquantitative echocardiographic assessment). Moderate (10 to 20 mm) or large effusions (>20 mm) are unusual and may signal a diagnosis other than *idiopathic* pericarditis. An effusion in a patient with a history consistent with acute pericarditis is confirmatory of the diagnosis.

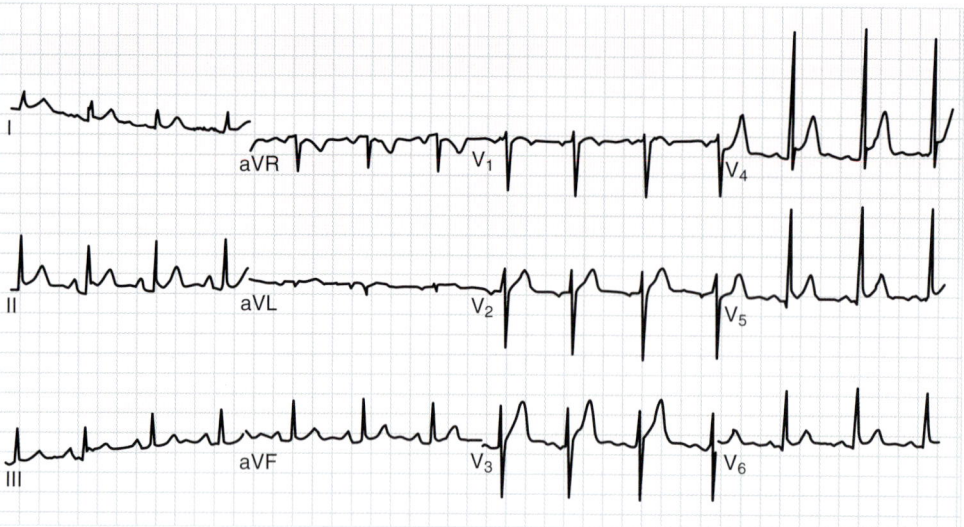

FIGURE 86.2 The electrocardiogram in acute pericarditis. Note both diffuse ST-segment elevation and PR-segment depression.

TABLE 86.3 Initial Approach to the Patient with Definite or Suspected Acute Pericarditis

1. If the diagnosis is suspected but not certain, listen often for pericardial rub and obtain ECGs frequently to check for diagnostic findings.

2. If the diagnosis is suspected or certain, obtain the following tests to help confirm the diagnosis (if necessary) and determine whether a specific causative diagnosis and/or significant associated conditions and/or complications are present:
   Hemogram
   hsCRP
   Troponin I
   Chest radiograph
   Echocardiogram
   Consider additional testing on the basis of clinical suspicion of a specific (non-idiopathic) etiology.

3. If the diagnosis is likely or certain, initiate therapy with an NSAID plus colchicine.

4. If diagnosis still uncertain consider CT scan or cardiac MRI to document pericardial inflammation.

CT, Computed tomography; *ECG,* electrocardiogram; *NSAID,* nonsteroidal antiinflammatory drugs.

Echocardiography is also useful in unusual cases where associated myocarditis is severe enough to alter ventricular function and to detect a previously silent MI. In uncomplicated acute pericarditis, it is rarely necessary to use imaging modalities other than echocardiography. However, in difficult cases computed tomography (CT) and/or cardiac magnetic resonance (CMR) imaging can help to detect pericardial thickening and/or active inflammation.[17,18]

Diagnosis, Natural History, and Management

ESC guidelines include the results of the first randomized clinical trials in pericarditis as well as more recent observational studies.[4] However, objective data to support recommendations for management of acute pericarditis and other pericardial diseases remain limited; most are based on expert opinion and consensus. According to the guidelines, the clinical diagnosis of acute pericarditis requires at least two of the following: (1) chest pain, (2) pericardial friction rub, (3) ECG changes consisting of typical ST elevation and/or PR depression, and (4) pericardial effusion.

In atypical presentations, additional imaging can be helpful in establishing the diagnosis. CT may show thickening or hyperattenuation of the pericardium. CMR may show pericardial edema based on fat-suppressed T2-weighted dark blood images, or delayed pericardial hyperenhancement indicative of ongoing inflammation.[17,18] Elevation of biomarkers of inflammation (e.g., CRP) is supportive of the diagnosis, but not definitive.

Initial management is focused on confirming the diagnosis, screening for specific causes that would alter management, detection of effusion and other echocardiographic abnormalities, alleviation of symptoms, and directed treatment if a specific cause is discovered (Table 86.3). Certain features are associated with an increased risk of complications (mainly tamponade) (*inset,* Fig. 86.3). On this basis, triage of patients is possible after initial evaluation. We recommend the following routine testing: ECG, CBC, serum creatinine, CRP (or hsCRP), cardiac troponin, chest radiograph, and echocardiogram. Additional testing is guided by suspicion of a specific cause or complication. For example, if there are signs or symptoms concerning for systemic lupus erythematosus (SLE), an anti-nuclear antibody (ANA) titer is appropriate. However, low ANA titers are common in patients with *recurrent* idiopathic pericarditis without SLE criteria.[19] Thus, the significance of low ANA titers can be uncertain. Figure 86.3 and Table 86.3 summarize our recommendations for triage and initial management of patients with definite or suspected acute pericarditis.

Acute idiopathic pericarditis is a self-limited disease without significant complications or recurrence in 70% to 90% of patients.[5,9] If laboratory data do not contradict the diagnosis of *idiopathic* pericarditis, symptomatic treatment with nonsteroidal antiinflammatory drugs (NSAIDs) is recommended.[4,5,9] Restriction of physical activity until resolution of symptoms and normalization of CRP occurs is recommended. For athletes, return to sports is recommended after an arbitrary term of 3 months and only after symptoms have fully resolved and CRP, ECG, and echocardiogram have normalized.[4]

The choice of an antiinflammatory regimen is based on concomitant therapies (e.g., favoring aspirin [ASA] if antiplatelet therapy is required), patient preferences, and medical history (allergies, intolerances, etc.). Two alternative regimens with an excellent safety profile are recommended (Table 86.4): ibuprofen 600 to 800 mg orally three times daily, or ASA 750 to 1000 mg orally three times daily. Gastric protection in the form of a proton pump inhibitor should be provided. Many patients have satisfactory responses to the first few doses of an NSAID. A majority respond fully after 10 to 14 days and need no additional treatment. As noted, using normalization of CRP to guide duration of therapy is a reasonable alternative to a predetermined time course.[4,16] Once the patient is asymptomatic and CRP normalized, tapering rather than abrupt cessation of antiinflammatory drugs should be considered in an attempt to reduce recurrences (see Table 86.4).

Colchicine is recommended for 3 months as an adjunct to NSAIDs. When added to standard antiinflammatory therapy, colchicine reduces recurrences by approximately half[20] and speeds resolution of symptoms. Colchicine is thought to exert an antiinflammatory effect by blocking microtubule assembly in WBCs and inhibiting the inflammasome.[9] Weight-adjusted doses (0.5 to 0.6 mg orally every 12 hours or 0.5 to 0.6 mg once daily for patients <70 kg) are recommended.[4,20]

Patients with no more than small effusion and no high-risk features do not need to be admitted to hospital (see Fig. 86.3). Patients who do not respond well to initial treatment, have larger effusions, high-risk features, or a concerning etiology should be hospitalized for observation, further diagnostic testing, and treatment (see Fig. 86.3). In those who respond slowly to an NSAID and colchicine, analgesics allow time for a more complete response. Initial use of the IV route of administration for NSAIDs can be considered to more quickly alleviate symptoms.[4,21]

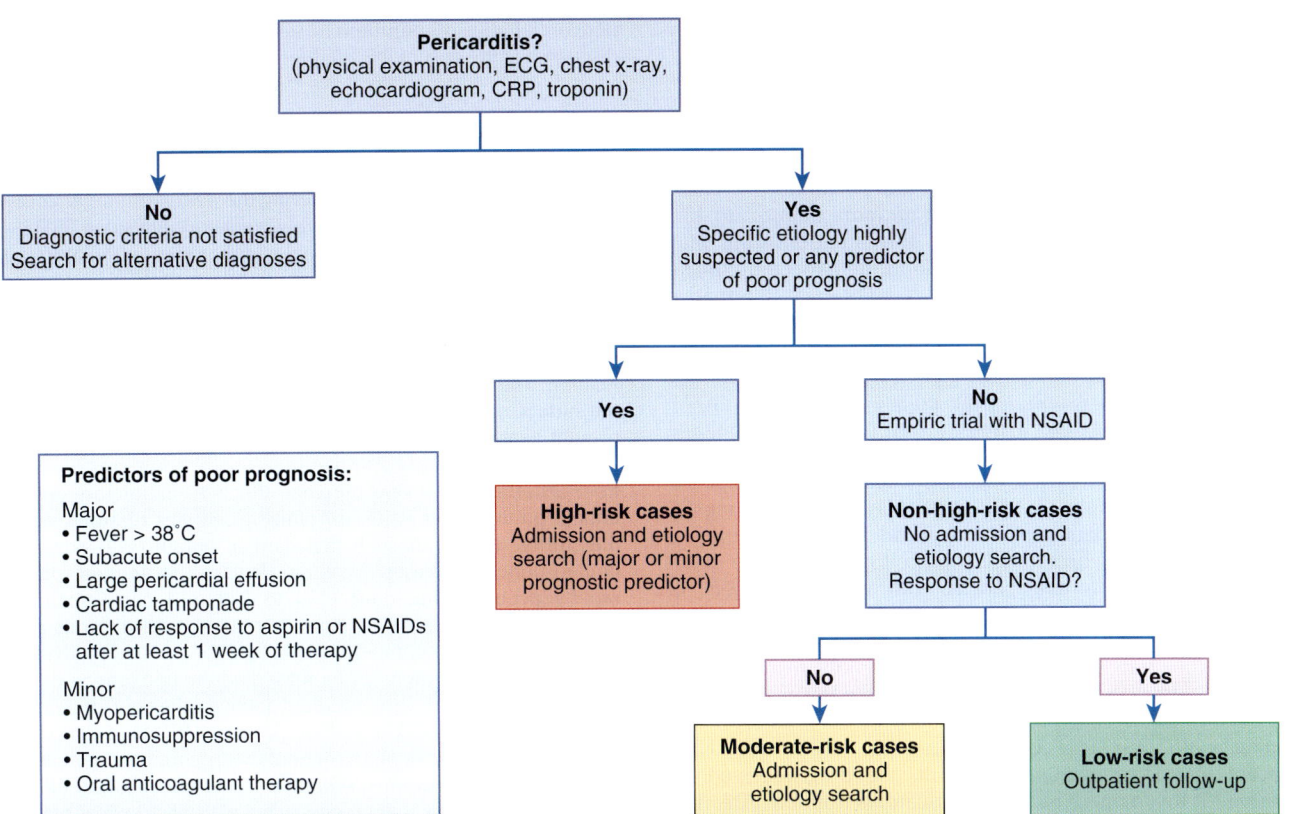

FIGURE 86.3 A proposed scheme for the triage and initial management of patients with suspected pericarditis, including markers of elevated risk (*box at left*). (From Adler Y, Charron P, Imazio M, et al. 2015 ESC Guidelines for the diagnosis and management of pericardial diseases: The Task Force for the Diagnosis and Management of Pericardial Diseases of the European Society of Cardiology (ESC)Endorsed by: The European Association for Cardio-Thoracic Surgery (EACTS). *Eur Heart J.* 2015;36[42]:2921–2964.)

TABLE 86.4 Empiric Antiinflammatory Therapy for Acute Idiopathic Pericarditis

DRUG	USUAL DOSING	INITIAL DURATION	TAPERING*
Aspirin	750–1000 mg every 8 hr	1–2 weeks	Decrease doses every week for 2–3 weeks, then discontinue
Ibuprofen	600–800 mg every 8 hr	1–2 weeks	Decrease doses every week for 2–3 weeks, then discontinue
Colchicine	0.5–0.6 mg once (<70 kg) or 0.5–0.6 mg twice daily (≥70 kg)	3 months	Optional, over 2–3 weeks

*Therapy duration is individualized and guided by symptoms and hsCRP. Maintain initial dose and taper only when asymptomatic and hsCRP is normalized.

Corticosteroid use should be minimized in patients with acute pericarditis because they may impair the clearance of infectious agents and short, high-dose courses may increase the risk of recurrence.[4,5,9] However, there are selected indications for their use: (1) contraindications to or failure of NSAID/colchicine, (2) underlying conditions (e.g., autoimmune diseases) whose primary treatment is corticosteroids, (3) concomitant diseases (e.g., renal failure), (4) pregnancy, and (5) concomitant therapies constituting relative contraindications to NSAIDs and/or colchicine (e.g., oral anticoagulants).[9,22] When used, relatively low doses of corticosteroids are recommended (e.g., prednisone 0.2 to 0.5 mg/kg daily) to minimize complications. Higher doses of corticosteroids are associated with major side effects in about one quarter of patients, leading to drug withdrawal, more hospitalizations, and more recurrences.[23] Tapering should be gradual, typically over 6 to 12 weeks, and guided by symptomatic response and CRP. Concurrent colchicine should be administrated during corticosteroid therapy.

Complications of acute pericarditis include effusion, tamponade, constriction, and recurrences. As noted earlier, small effusions are common. Relatively little is known about the incidence of more significant complications. In one study, over an average 31-month follow-up, tamponade developed in 3.1% and constriction in 1.5%.[24] Most complications occurred in patients with identified specific causes. In another study with longer follow-up, constriction developed in 1.8%. In the 83% of patients with idiopathic pericarditis, constriction developed in only 0.48%.[25] Thus, patients with idiopathic pericarditis can be reassured that development of constriction is exceedingly unlikely.

Recurrent Pericarditis

Recurrences occur in 15% to 30% of patients with idiopathic acute pericarditis.[5,9,26] Recurrences may seriously affect quality of life. They have not been associated with evolution to constriction.[25] A diagnosis of recurrent pericarditis requires new symptoms and signs of disease activity (friction rub, ECG changes, new or worsening pericardial effusion, elevation of CRP) after a symptom-free interval of at least 4 to 6 weeks.[4,5] It is not unusual for patients to have recurrent pain without objective evidence of disease activity. These patients may respond to repeated treatment but should not be classified as having a definite recurrence.

For recurrences, we recommend NSAID and colchicine in the same doses used for an initial episode. Therapy should be continued until complete resolution of symptoms and normalization of CRP, if elevated. At this point, the NSAID should be gradually tapered. If this therapy fails, corticosteroids may replace NSAID or may be added as "triple therapy." As for an initial episode, doses of 0.2 to 0.5 mg/kg/day of prednisone or equivalent are recommended for at least 2 to 4 weeks until resolution of symptoms and normalization of CRP, followed by gradual tapering every 2 to 4 weeks. Colchicine should be included for at least 6 months and up to 12 months for difficult cases.[9] For recurrence during corticosteroid tapering, we recommend maintaining the same dose if possible and controlling the recurrence by adding or increasing NSAID and/or starting colchicine if this has not been done. Some patients have recurrences which are mild and easily managed with re-institution of an NSAID for a brief period of time. These patients often do not have objective evidence of inflammation; an increase in corticosteroid dose or more intensive immunosuppressive therapy is not necessary.

For patients with colchicine-resistant and/or corticosteroid-dependent disease, additional therapies are available.[9,21] These patients are relatively rare, representing no more than 5% to 10% of recurrent pericarditis cases.[9,27] In this situation, CMR may help identify higher-risk patients and inform the expected clinical course and duration of treatment.[17,28–30] Potential alternative therapies include azathioprine (1 mg/kg/day with gradual dose increases and monitoring of WBC, transaminases, and amylase) and human intravenous immunoglobulin (400 to 500 mg/kg/day for 5 days with a possible repeat course after 1 month).[4,31] Interleukin-1 antagonists are a newer, very promising additional therapy for recurrent pericarditis.[21] Anakinra, a recombinant short-acting IL-1 α and IL-1 β cytokine receptor blocker, which is off-label, is one example (1 to 2 mg/kg/day up to 100 mg SC daily).[32] Optimal duration of therapy and whether tapering is required and if so how best to accomplish it have yet to be determined.[33] We generally treat patients with anakinra for 9 to 12 months followed by slow tapering. Recently, rilonacept (loading dose of 320 mg SC followed by 160 mg SC weekly), an IL-1 α and IL-1 β cytokine trap, has been shown to rapidly resolve acute episodes of recurrent pericarditis and markedly lower the risk of future recurrence by 96%.[33a,33b] Standard of care medications, including corticosteroids, were successfully discontinued as rilonacept was introduced. As a result, the drug received an indication for treatment of recurrent pericarditis from the FDA. The optimal duration of rilonacept is not known; however, the median duration in the RHAPSODY trial was 9 months (maximum 14 months), and tapering of rilonacept may not be required due to the gradual washout pharmacokinetics of the drug.[33c] For physicians who do not ordinarily prescribe these drugs, it is prudent to enlist the help of colleagues experienced in their use. In patients with pericarditis refractory to medical therapies, pericardiectomy may be considered.[34]

PERICARDIAL EFFUSION AND CARDIAC TAMPONADE

Etiology

Virtually any disease that involves the pericardium can cause an effusion (see Table 86.1).[3,4,7,35] In the developing world TB remains a major cause. In the developed world idiopathic pericarditis, malignancy, and percutaneous procedural complications are the most common causes of significant effusions.[4,35]

Effusions are common for several weeks to a few months following cardiac surgery and transplantation[4] but tamponade is unusual. Various miscellaneous, noninflammatory diseases can cause effusion (see Table 86.1), including transudates in patients with severe circulatory congestion. Bleeding into the pericardial sac occurs after blunt and penetrating trauma, following post-MI rupture of the LV free wall, and as a complication of various percutaneous cardiac procedures. Retrograde bleeding is a major cause of death due to aortic dissection (see Chapter 42). Effusions are also common in patients with pulmonary hypertension.[2] Asymptomatic pericardial effusions are sometimes discovered when a chest X-ray or echocardiogram is performed for unrelated indications, often in otherwise healthy individuals.[4]

Effusions with a high likelihood of progression to tamponade include bacterial, HIV-associated infections (see Chapter 80), bleeding, and neoplastic disease. Large effusions due to acute idiopathic pericarditis are infrequent, but account for significant numbers of tamponade cases because this diagnosis is so common. About 20% of large, symptomatic effusions without an obvious etiology following routine evaluation represent the initial presentation of a cancer.[4,36] Details of pericardial effusion pertinent to selected, specific disease entities are discussed at the end of this chapter.

Pathophysiology and Hemodynamics

Formation of an effusion is usually a response to inflammatory, infectious, or neoplastic diseases involving the pericardium. Other diseases that can occasionally cause *noninflammatory* effusions include lymphomas with enlarged mediastinal lymph nodes,[3] circulatory congestion, and metabolic diseases including hypothyroidism and protein malnutrition.[3,4,7]

When an effusion accumulates, the pressure in the pericardial sac depends on the amount of fluid and the pericardial pressure-volume relation. The mechanical consequences of a high pressure acting on the surface of the heart mainly result from compression and collapse of right heart. Left heart underfilling then ensues from reduced right heart output. Clinically, cardiac tamponade comprises a continuum from an effusion causing minimal effects to circulatory collapse. A critical point occurs when an effusion reduces diastolic volume of the cardiac chambers such that cardiac output (CO) declines. The limited pericardial reserve volume dictates that modest amounts of rapidly accumulating fluid (150 to 200 mL) can impair cardiac function. In contrast, large, slowly accumulating effusions are often well-tolerated. The compensatory response to a hemodynamically significant effusion includes increased adrenergic tone and parasympathetic withdrawal. The resultant tachycardia and increased contractility[3] maintain CO and blood pressure (BP) for a period of time, but eventually they decline. Patients who cannot mount an adrenergic response are more susceptible to the effects of an effusion. In terminal tamponade, a depressor reflex with paradoxical bradycardia may supervene.

As fluid accumulates, left- and right-sided atrial and ventricular diastolic pressures rise and in severe tamponade equalize at a pressure similar to that in the pericardial sac, typically 20 to 25 mm Hg (Fig. 86.4). Equalization is closest during inspiration. Thus, *transmural* filling pressures are markedly reduced. Correspondingly, cardiac volumes progressively decline. The small end-diastolic ventricular volume (decreased preload) mainly accounts for reduced stroke volume (SV). Because of compensatory increases in contractility, end-systolic volume also decreases, but not enough to maintain SV.

In addition to elevated and equal intra-cavitary filling pressures, low transmural filling pressures, and small cardiac volumes, two other hemodynamic abnormalities are characteristic of tamponade.[3] One is loss of the y descent of the RA or systemic venous pressure wave (see Fig.86.4). *x* and *y descents* correspond to periods when venous flow is increasing. Loss of the *y* descent has been explained based on the concept that total heart volume is fixed in severe tamponade.[3] Thus, blood can enter the heart only when blood is simultaneously leaving. The normal *y* descent begins when the tricuspid valve opens, that is, blood is not leaving. In tamponade inflow cannot increase and the descent is lost. The *x* descent occurs during ventricular ejection. Because blood is leaving the heart, inflow can increase and the *x* descent is retained. Loss of the *y* descent in systemic venous or RA pressure recordings is a useful clue to the presence of tamponade. An absent *y* descent and loss of diastolic venous inflow are considered classic.[3] However, in many cases in the modern era pulsed wave Doppler recordings reveal some degree of venous inflow into the right heart during ventricular diastole.[1,2] These patients may have ECP, with a mixed hemodynamic picture.

The second characteristic finding is the paradoxical pulse (Fig. 86.5), an abnormally large drop (>10 mm Hg) in systolic arterial pressure during inspiration. Other causes of *pulsus paradoxus* include CP, pulmonary embolus, and pulmonary disease with large variations in intra-thoracic pressure. The mechanism of the paradoxical pulse is multifactorial, but respiratory changes in systemic venous return are important.[3] In tamponade, in contrast to constriction, the normal inspiratory *increase* in systemic venous return is present and the normal inspiratory *decline* in systemic venous pressure is retained (Kussmaul's

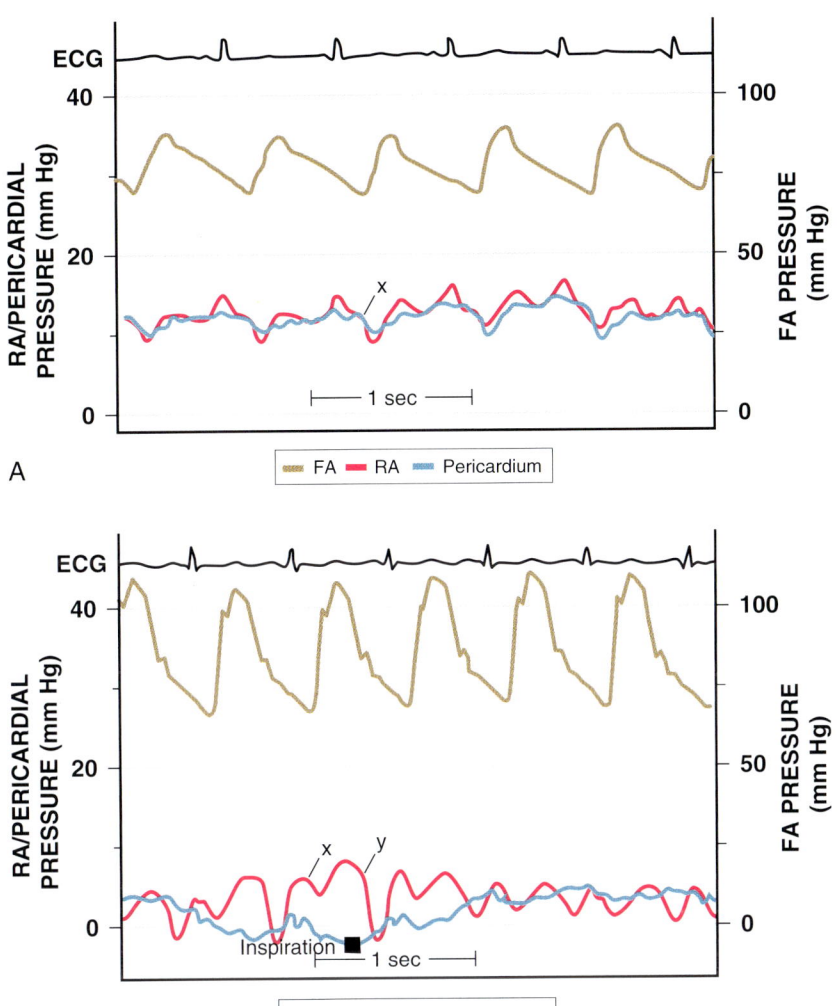

FIGURE 86.4 Femoral arterial (FA), right atrial (RA), and pericardial pressure before (**A**) and after (**B**) pericardiocentesis in a patient with cardiac tamponade. RA and pericardial pressure are about 15 mm Hg before pericardiocentesis. There is a minimal paradoxical pulse. RA x descent is present but y descent is absent before pericardiocentesis. Pericardiocentesis results in marked increase in FA pressure and decrease in RA pressure. During inspiration, pericardial pressure becomes negative, there is clear separation between RA and pericardial pressure, and y descent is now prominent, suggesting an effusive-constrictive picture. (From Baim DS, Grossman W, eds. *Grossman's Cardiac Catheterization, Angiography, and Intervention.* Philadelphia: Lippincott Williams & Wilkins, 2000:840.)

sign is *absent*). The increase in right heart filling pressure occurs, once again, under conditions where total heart volume is fixed and left heart volume markedly reduced. The interventricular septum shifts to the left in exaggerated fashion on inspiration, encroaching on the LV such that SV and pressure generation are further reduced (see Fig. 86.5). This is termed exaggerated ventricular interaction[1,7,35,36] (in distinction to the previous definition of ventricular interaction). Although the inspiratory increase in right heart volume (preload) increases RV SV, a few cardiac cycles are required to increase LV filling and SV and counteract the septal shift. Other factors that may contribute include increased afterload caused by transmission of negative intrathoracic pressure to the aorta and traction on the pericardium caused by descent of the diaphragm. Associated with these mechanisms, left and right heart pressure and SV variations are exaggerated and 180 degrees out of phase (see Figs. 86.4 and 86.5). Table 86.5 lists hemodynamic findings in tamponade compared with constriction. When there are preexisting elevations in diastolic pressures and/or volume, tamponade can occur without a paradoxical pulse.[3] Examples include chronic LV dysfunction, aortic regurgitation, and atrial septal defect. In patients with retrograde bleeding into the pericardial sac due to aortic dissection,[4] tamponade may occur without a paradoxical pulse because of aortic valve disruption and regurgitation.

Although mean left- and right-sided filling pressures are typically 20 to 25 mm Hg, tamponade can occur at lower filling pressures, that is, low-pressure tamponade.[3,4,35] Low-pressure tamponade often occurs when there is a decrease in blood volume in the setting of a preexisting effusion which would not otherwise be significant. A modestly elevated pericardial pressure can lower transmural filling pressure to levels where SV is compromised. Because venous pressure is only modestly elevated or normal, the diagnosis may be missed. Low-pressure tamponade may be observed during hemodialysis, in patients with blood loss and volume depletion, and when diuretics are administered to patients with effusions. As many as 10% of patients undergoing closed pericardiocentesis may meet criteria for low-pressure tamponade. Compared with conventional tamponade, these patients are less often critically ill and signs of tamponade are less prominent.

Pericardial effusions can be loculated or localized, resulting in regional tamponade, most commonly after cardiac surgery.[3,4] Although reports are scarce, regional tamponade may cause atypical hemodynamic findings, for example, reduced CO with unilateral filling pressure elevation. Regional tamponade should be considered whenever there is hypotension in a setting where a loculated effusion is present. Rarely, large pleural effusions and pneumopericardium can compress the heart and cause tamponade.[3,4]

Clinical Presentation

A history pertinent to a specific disease etiology may be elicited. As noted earlier, asymptomatic effusions may be discovered in otherwise healthy individuals.[4] Specific etiologies are rarely found in these cases. Effusions per se do not cause symptoms without tamponade, although patients may have pain due to pericarditis. Patients with tamponade often complain of dyspnea (the mechanism is uncertain because there is no pulmonary congestion) and are more comfortable sitting forward. Other symptoms reflect the severity of CO and BP reduction.

The physical examination in pericardial effusion may provide clues to its etiology. In pericardial effusion without tamponade, the cardiovascular examination is normal except if the effusion is large, the cardiac impulse is difficult to palpate and heart sounds are muffled. A friction rub may of course be present. Tubular breath sounds may be heard in the left axilla or base due to bronchial compression. *Beck's triad*, hypotension, muffled heart sounds, and elevated jugular venous pressure, suggests severe tamponade. Patients with tamponade appear uncomfortable and display signs of reduced CO and shock, including tachypnea, diaphoresis, cool extremities, peripheral cyanosis, and depressed sensorium.[3,4,35] Hypotension is usually present, although in early stages compensatory mechanisms maintain BP. Some patients with subacute tamponade are initially *hypertensive*.[37] A paradoxical pulse is the rule, but it is important to be alert to situations where it may be absent. The paradox is quantified by cuff sphygmomanometry as the difference between the pressure at which Korotkoff sounds first appear and that at which they are present with each contraction. Tachycardia is also the rule unless heart rate lowering drugs have been administered, conduction system disease coexists, or a pre-terminal bradycardic reflex has supervened. The jugular venous pressure is markedly elevated except in low-pressure tamponade, and the y descent is usually absent. The normal decrease in venous pressure on inspiration is retained. Examination of the heart is simply consistent with effusion. Tamponade can be confused with anything that causes hypotension, shock, and elevated venous pressure, including decompensated heart failure, pulmonary embolus and other causes of pulmonary hypertension, and RV MI.

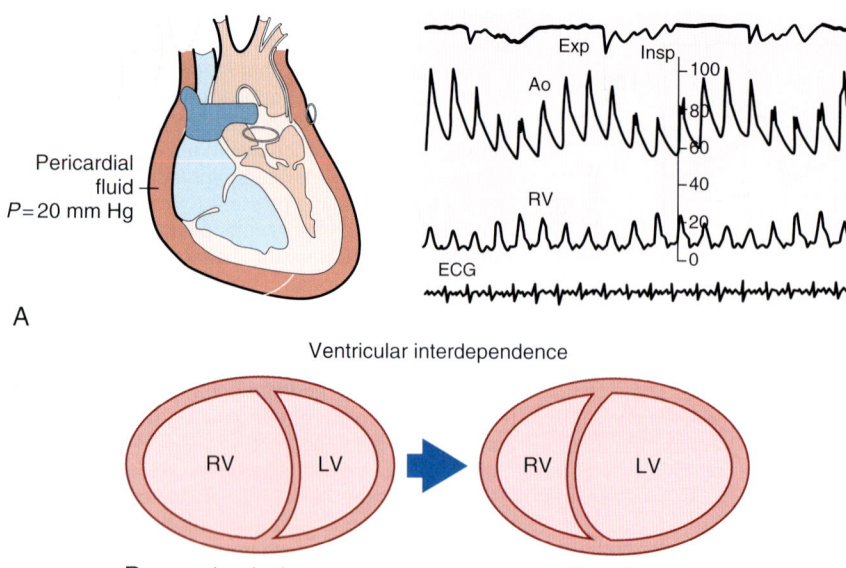

FIGURE 86.5 **A**, *Left*, illustration of leftward septal shift with encroachment of left ventricular (LV) volume during inspiration in cardiac tamponade. *Right*, respiration marker and aortic and right ventricular (RV) pressure tracings in cardiac tamponade. Note paradoxical pulse and 180 degrees out of phase respiratory variation in right and left-sided pressures. **B**, Exaggerated interventricular dependence in tamponade. On inspiration (*left*) there is a shift of the ventricular septum toward the LV, and on expiration (*right*) there is a shift of the ventricular septum toward the RV. (From Shabetai R. *The Pericardium*. New York: Grune & Stratton; 1981:266; and From Atherton JJ, Moore TD, Thomson HL, et al. *J Am Coll Cardiol.* 1998;31:413–418.)

TABLE 86.5 Hemodynamics in Cardiac Tamponade and Constrictive Pericarditis

	TAMPONADE	CONSTRICTION
Paradoxical pulse	Usually present	Present in approximately 1/3
Equal left/right filling	Present	Present pressures
Systemic venous wave morphology	Absent y descent	Prominent y descent (M or W shape)
Inspiratory change in systemic venous pressure	Decrease (normal)	Increase or no change (Kussmaul's sign)
"Square root" sign in ventricular pressure	Absent	Present

Laboratory Testing

ECG abnormalities include reduced voltage and electrical alternans.[3,4] Reduced voltage is nonspecific and can be caused by emphysema, infiltrative myocardial disease, and pneumothorax. Electrical alternans is specific but relatively insensitive and caused by anterior-posterior swinging of the heart with each contraction. When pericarditis coexists, usual ECG findings may be present.

The chest radiograph reveals a normal cardiac silhouette until effusions are at least moderate in size. With larger effusions the antero-posterior cardiac silhouette assumes a rounded, flask-like appearance. Lateral views may reveal the fat pad sign, a linear lucency at least 2 mm in width between chest wall and anterior surface of the heart caused by separation of epicardial from anterior mediastinal fat by the effusion. The lungs are oligemic.

M-mode and two-dimensional Doppler echocardiography are standard noninvasive methods for detection of effusion and tamponade (see also Chapter 16).[1,2,7,35,38] A significant effusion appears as a lucent separation between parietal and visceral pericardium for the entire cardiac cycle (Fig. 86.6 and Video 86.1). Small effusions are usually first evident over the posterobasal LV. With increasing effusions, the fluid spreads anteriorly, laterally, and behind the LA, where it is limited by the visceral pericardial reflection. Ultimately, the separation becomes circumferential. Effusions are graded as trivial (only seen in systole), small (echo free space in diastole <10 mm), moderate (10 to 20 mm), large (>20 mm), and very large (>25 mm) (see Fig. 86.6).[7,35] Because speed of accumulation is critical, the hemodynamic significance of an effusion may not be correlated with its size. However, it is very unusual for tamponade to occur without a circumferential effusion. Frond-like or shaggy appearing structures in the pericardial space on echocardiography suggest clots, chronic inflammation, or neoplastic processes. CT and CMR are more accurate than transthoracic echocardiography for estimating pericardial thickness, although *transesophageal* echocardiography (TEE) is comparable.[1,2,7,35]

Several echocardiographic findings indicate that an effusion is large enough to cause hemodynamic compromise.[1,2,6,7] These include early diastolic collapse of RV, late diastolic indentation or collapse of RA, and exaggerated respiratory variation in RV and LV size and interventricular septal shifting during inspiration (septal bulge or "bounce"). Early diastolic RV collapse (Fig. 86.7, *right*) and late diastolic RA collapse (see Fig. 86.7, *left*) usually appear relatively early during tamponade,[1,2,7,35] when pericardial pressure transiently exceeds intra-cavitary pressure. Rarely, a large *pleural* effusion can cause right-sided chamber collapse.[7,35] Isolated *LV* and *LA* chamber collapse can occur with pericardial hematomas after cardiac surgery.[1,7,35] Cardiac chambers are small in tamponade and, as noted, the heart may swing antero-posteriorly. Distention of the inferior vena cava that does not diminish with inspiration is an important confirmatory finding. Doppler recordings demonstrate exaggerated respiratory variation in right- and left-sided venous and valvular flow, with inspiratory increases on the right and decreases on the left.[1,2,7,35] Caval inflow occurs largely during ventricular systole. These flow patterns are at least as sensitive for tamponade as M-mode and two-dimensional echocardiographic features.

With most effusions, transthoracic echocardiography provides sufficient diagnostic information for management decisions. TEE provides better quality images but is usually impractical in sick patients unless they are intubated. Fluoroscopy is useful in the cardiac catheterization laboratory for detection of procedure-related effusions that cause damping or abolition of cardiac pulsation. CT (see Chapter 20) and CMR (see Chapter 19) are useful adjuncts to echocardiography in characterizing effusion and tamponade,[39,40] but neither is ordinarily required and/or advisable in sick patients. They have a role when hemodynamics are atypical, other conditions complicate interpretation, the severity of tamponade is uncertain, or echocardiography is technically inadequate.

CT and MRI provide more detailed quantitation and regional localization of effusions than echocardiography and are useful with loculated and coexistent pleural effusions.[1,2,39,40] Pericardial thickness can be measured with both methods, allowing indirect assessment of the severity and chronicity of inflammation; MRI with gadolinium directly identifies inflammation. Clues to the nature of pericardial fluid can be gained from CT attenuation coefficients.[41] Attenuation similar to water suggests transudative effusion; attenuation denser than water suggests malignant, bloody or purulent fluid; and attenuation less dense than water, a chylous effusion. Malignant effusions are associated with a thicker pericardium than benign effusions. Finally, cine CT or CMR provides information similar to echocardiography for assessment of tamponade, for example, septal shifting, chamber collapse.

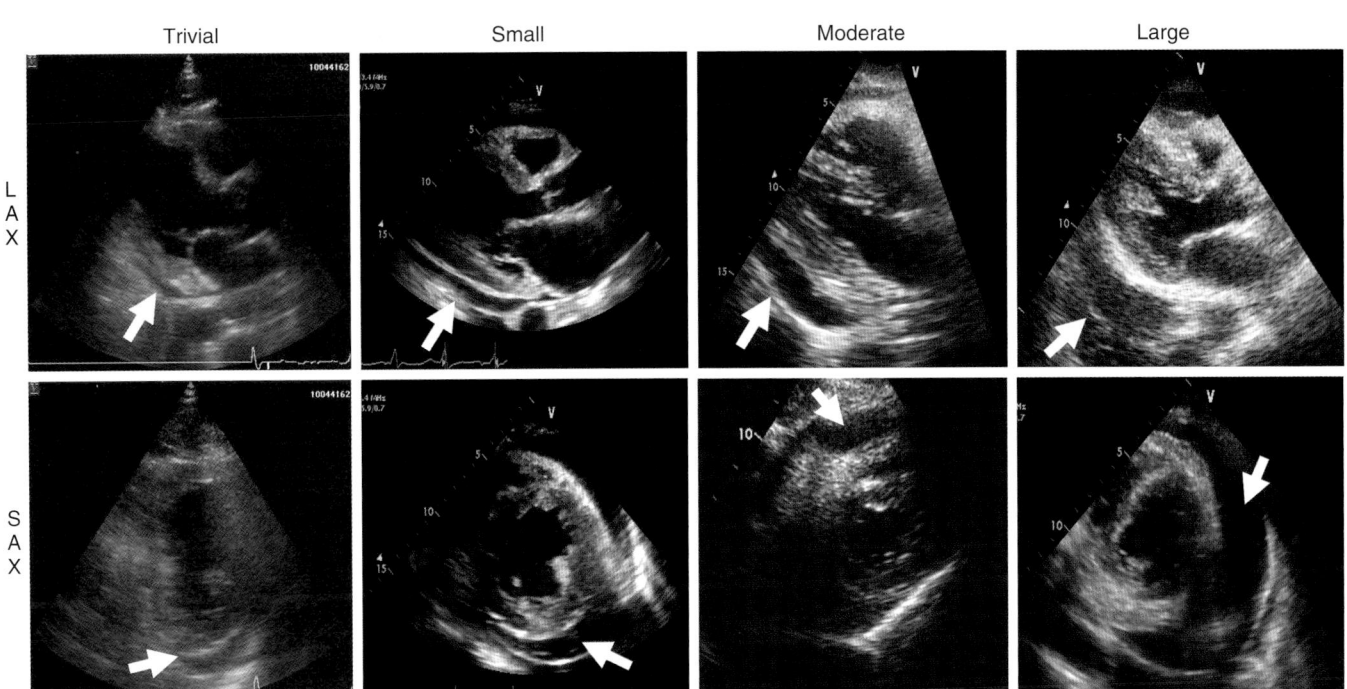

FIGURE 86.6 Trivial, small, moderate, and large pericardial effusions. Parasternal long axis (LAX) and short axis (SAX) views. (From Klein AL, Abbara S, Agler DA, et al. American Society of Echocardiography clinical recommendations for multimodality cardiovascular imaging of patients with pericardial disease: endorsed by the Society for Cardiovascular Magnetic Resonance and Society of Cardiovascular Computed Tomography. *J Am Soc Echocardiogr.* 2013;26:965–1012.e1015.)

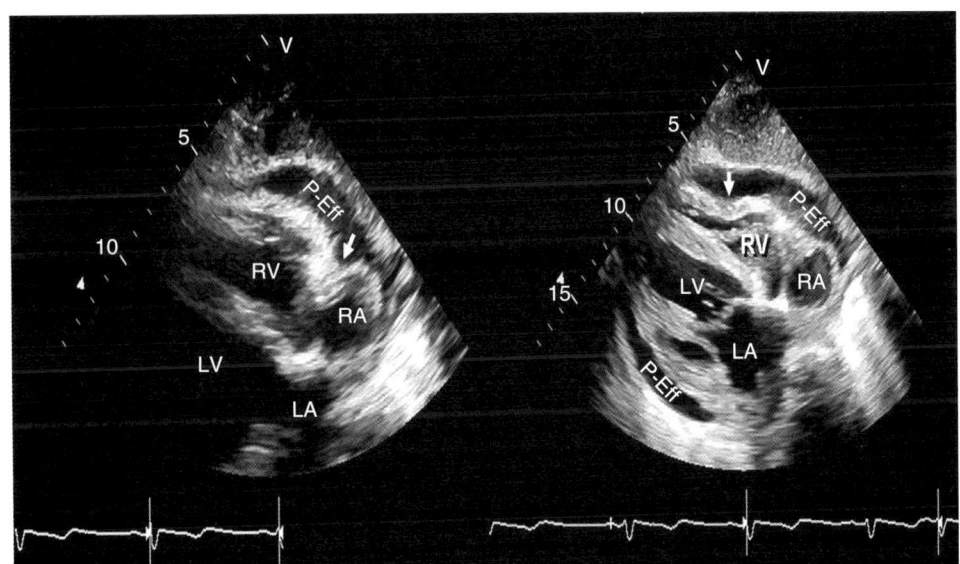

FIGURE 86.7 Two-dimensional echocardiographic subcostal view in a patient with cardiac tamponade showing right atrium (RA) *(left side)* and right ventricular (RV) *(right side)* indentation or "collapse" *(arrows)*. In RA and RV, indentation occurs during their respective relaxation when pressure is lowest, transiently falling below pericardial pressure. RA indentation occurs during early ventricular systole, whereas RV indentation occurs in early diastole. (From Klein AL, Abbara S, Agler DA, et al. American Society of Echocardiography clinical recommendations for multimodality cardiovascular imaging of patients with pericardial disease: endorsed by the Society for Cardiovascular Magnetic Resonance and Society of Cardiovascular Computed Tomography. *J Am Soc Echocardiogr.* 2013;26:965–1012.e1015.)

Management of Pericardial Effusion and Tamponade

Management is primarily dictated by whether tamponade is already present or has a high chance of developing (Table 86.6).[1,3,4,35] Situations where tamponade is a near-term threat include suspected bacterial pericarditis, hemopericardium, and any moderate to large effusion that is not thought to be chronic and/or is increasing in size. When tamponade is present or threatened, decision-making requires urgency and a low threshold for pericardiocentesis (see Table 86.6). *In the absence of actual or threatened tamponade,* management can be more leisurely. This includes several categories of patients. Some have acute pericarditis with a small to moderate effusion detected as part of routine evaluation. Others do not have symptoms or signs of pericarditis or effusion but undergo echocardiography because of the presence of diseases known to involve the pericardium. The rest are asymptomatic and have effusions detected when tests are performed for reasons other than suspected pericardial disease, for example, screening, evaluation of an enlarged cardiac silhouette. Klein and colleagues[1] propose a three-step scoring system for pericardial effusion that awards points based on etiology, clinical presentation, and imaging to arrive at a cumulative score whose value dictates whether *urgent* drainage is warranted.

In many cases of effusion where tamponade is neither present nor threatened, an etiology will be evident or suggested based on the history and/or previous diagnostic tests. When the diagnosis is unclear, an assessment of specific etiologies should be undertaken, including diagnostic tests recommended for acute pericarditis and anything else dictated by the clinical picture, for example, neoplastic and autoimmune diseases, infections, and hypothyroidism.

In patients without actual or imminent tamponade, closed pericardiocentesis or, occasionally, surgical drainage (possibly with biopsy and/or creation of a window) may be undertaken for diagnostic purposes but is often not required. As discussed above, in many cases a diagnosis will either be obvious or become evident during initial investigations. Moreover, in this setting routine analysis of pericardial fluid has a low diagnostic yield.[4,35] In situations where pericardiocentesis is felt to be necessary for diagnosis, consideration should be given to open drainage with biopsy.

TABLE 86.6 Initial Approach to the Patient with a Pericardial Effusion

1. Determine if tamponade is present or threatened based on history, physical examination, echocardiogram.
2. If tamponade is not present or threatened:
   - if etiology not apparent, consider diagnostic tests as for acute pericarditis
   - if effusion is large, consider course of an NSAID + colchicine or corticosteroid and, if no response, consider closed pericardiocentesis
3. If tamponade is present or threatened:
   - urgent or emergent closed pericardiocentesis or careful monitoring if trial of medical treatment to reduce effusion is considered appropriate

Otherwise healthy patients with large, asymptomatic effusions and no evidence of tamponade or a specific etiology are a special category.[4,41] The effusions are by definition chronic and in general stable, but a minority (perhaps 20% to 30%) develop tamponade unpredictably. After closed pericardiocentesis the effusions may not reaccumulate. Thus, there is a rationale for pericardiocentesis following routine evaluation for specific etiologies as outlined above. Before undertaking pericardiocentesis a brief course of an NSAID or corticosteroid combined with colchicine may be considered. However, absent evidence of inflammation (increased CRP, gadolinium uptake on CMR), antiinflammatory regimens are not likely to be efficacious. Recurrence of this type of effusion after closed pericardiocentesis is considered an indication for a pericardial window or pericardiectomy.[4,41]

Patients with actual or threatened tamponade constitute medical emergencies. With the exception of those who do not wish prolongation of life (e.g., metastatic cancer), hospital admission and careful hemodynamic and echocardiographic monitoring is mandatory. The great majority require pericardiocentesis to treat or prevent tamponade, but there are some exceptions. Patients with acute, apparently idiopathic pericarditis with no more than mild tamponade can be treated for a brief period of time under careful monitoring with an NSAID and/or a corticosteroid combined with colchicine in an attempt to rapidly shrink the effusion. Patients with known inflammatory/autoimmune diseases can be treated similarly (there is no evidence that corticosteroids increase recurrences in these patients). Patients with suspected bacterial infections or hemopericardium *with small effusions (<10 mm)* should be considered to have threatened tamponade because of the etiology. These patients are appropriate for initial conservative management and careful monitoring because of the elevated risk of closed pericardiocentesis with smaller effusions.

Hemodynamic monitoring with a central venous or pulmonary artery catheter is often useful, especially in patients with threatened or mild tamponade in whom pericardiocentesis is deferred. Monitoring is also helpful *after* pericardiocentesis to assess reaccumulation and detect underlying constriction (see Fig. 86.4). Insertion of a catheter in the central circulation should not delay definitive therapy in critically ill patients.

For most patients in this category urgent or emergent pericardiocentesis is indicated. Once actual or threatened tamponade is diagnosed, intravenous hydration with normal saline should be instituted.[4,41] However, hydration as well as positive inotropes are temporizing measures that should not delay pericardiocentesis. In the vast majority of cases, echocardiographically guided *closed* pericardiocentesis is the method of choice. Before proceeding it is important to ensure that there is indeed an effusion large enough to cause tamponade that is amenable to a closed approach. Loculated effusions or effusions containing clots or fibrinous material increase the risk and difficulty of closed pericardiocentesis.

Whether to perform closed versus open pericardiocentesis in patients with *hemopericardium* is a difficult decision.[4,41] The danger of a closed approach is that lowering intra-pericardial pressure will allow more bleeding without affording an opportunity to correct its source. In cases of trauma or post-MI LV rupture, closed pericardiocentesis should usually be avoided. If bleeding is slower, closed pericardiocentesis is generally indicated because bleeding may stop spontaneously and/or the procedure can provide temporary relief before definitive repair. Closed pericardiocentesis in patients with hemopericardium due to type A aortic dissection has been considered contraindicated. However, in one report closed pericardiocentesis using intermittent cycles of drainage dictated by systolic BP appeared safe and effective for stabilization.[42]

The usual approach to closed pericardiocentesis is para-apical needle insertion with echocardiographic guidance to minimize risks of myocardial puncture and assess completeness of fluid removal.[4] Occasionally, a sub-xyphoid site is preferred. Once the needle has entered the pericardial space, a modest amount of fluid is removed (perhaps 50 to 100 mL) in an effort to produce rapid improvement. A guidewire is then inserted and the needle replaced with a pigtail catheter, which is manipulated to maximize fluid removal. When possible, closed pericardiocentesis should be performed in an ICU procedure room or cardiac catheterization laboratory with experienced personnel available. Echocardiographically guided pericardiocentesis has a greater than 95% success rate and less than 2% serious complication rate.[43,44] Rarely, patients suffer "pericardial decompression syndrome" following closed or open drainage,[45] a poorly understood but life-threatening syndrome characterized by combinations of pulmonary edema and shock.

CT guidance is a valuable alternative to both echocardiographic guidance and open pericardiocentesis.[46] Its success rate and safety are comparable to echocardiographic guidance. It is particularly well suited for regional and/or loculated effusions and effusions where the usual needle insertion sites are felt to be unsafe.

If a pulmonary artery catheter has been inserted, RA and pulmonary capillary wedge pressure and CO should be monitored before, during, and after the procedure. Ideally, pericardial fluid pressure should also be measured. Hemodynamic monitoring is useful for several reasons. Initial measurements confirm and document severity of tamponade. Measurements after completion establish a baseline to assess reaccumulation. Some patients with tamponade have coexisting constriction (ECP), which is difficult to detect when an effusion dominates but becomes apparent after pericardiocentesis. Following pericardiocentesis, repeat echocardiography and in many cases continued hemodynamic monitoring should be used to assess reaccumulation. Intra-pericardial catheters should ideally be left in place for 2 to 3 days to allow continued drainage and minimize recurrence.[4,35,47]

Open pericardiocentesis is occasionally preferred for initial removal of fluid. Bleeding due to trauma and rupture of the LV free wall have been mentioned previously. Loculated effusions and/or effusions that are borderline in size are drained more safely in the operating room or using CT guidance. Recurring effusions, especially those causing tamponade, may initially be drained using a closed approach due to logistical considerations. However, open pericardiocentesis with possible biopsy and creation of a window are usually preferred for recurrences causing tamponade.[4,48]

Percutaneous balloon pericardiotomy and periocardioscopy have been used to drain fluid, create pericardial windows, and perform pericardial biopsy.[4,49] Balloon pericardiotomy is useful for malignant effusions and other situations where recurrence is common and a more definitive approach without surgery desirable. These methods appear safe and effective, but experience is confined to a few centers.

Pericardial Fluid Analysis

Normal pericardial fluid has the features of a plasma ultrafiltrate.[3] Lymphocytes are the predominant cell type. Although routine analysis does not have a very high yield for disease etiology, it is rewarding with bacterial infections and malignant effusions.[4,50] Measurements include WBC and differential, hematocrit glucose levels, and protein content. Although most effusions are exudates, detection of a transudate reduces diagnostic possibilities. Sanguineous appearing fluid is nonspecific and does not necessarily indicate active bleeding. Chylous effusions can occur after traumatic or surgical injury to the thoracic duct or obstruction by neoplasms. Cholesterol-rich ("gold paint") effusions occur in hypothyroidism. Pericardial fluid should be stained and cultured for bacteria and as much fluid as possible submitted for detection of malignant cells.

If TB pericarditis is suspected, several other tests are useful,[4,50,51] including unstimulated interferon-gamma (uIFN-γ), adenosine deaminase (ADA), lysozyme levels, and polymerase chain reaction (PCR). When TB is suspected at least one of these tests should be routine because of the time required for bacteriologic diagnosis.

Newer approaches for analysis of pericardial fluid have been investigated. There may be a role for measurement of tumor markers as a screen for malignant effusion.[4,52] Selected cytokine and related biomarkers measured in both pericardial fluid and serum[52] have shown promise in distinguishing various types of inflammatory effusions, but their roles are uncertain. In a small study, anti-myolemmal antibodies in pericardial fluid and serum were found to be predictive of recurrence in patients with chronic effusions.[53]

Pericardioscopy and Percutaneous Biopsy

Pericardioscopic-guided drainage of pericardial effusions was discussed earlier. When standard methods to evaluate the etiology of pericardial effusions are unsuccessful, extended pericardioscopically guided biopsies combined with immunological and molecular methods applied to both fluid and tissue (e.g., PCR)[49] have been advocated to improve diagnostic and management. This approach appears safe, but experience is limited.

CONSTRICTIVE PERICARDITIS

ETIOLOGY

CP is the end stage of an inflammatory process involving the pericardium. Many diseases listed in Table 86.1 can cause constriction. In the developed world common etiologies are idiopathic, post-surgical, and radiation injury.[3,4] TB was very common before the advent of effective therapy and remains important in developing countries.[54] Constriction can follow an initial insult by as little as several months and occasionally less, but typically takes years to develop. The end result is fibrosis, often calcification, and adhesions of parietal and visceral pericardium. Figure 86.8 (top) illustrates the reciprocal relationship between the intense inflammation seen in acute and often in ECP (see below) and end-stage CP as inflammation diminishes and scarring and fibrosis gradually supervene. CMR images (see Fig. 86.8, bottom), discussed subsequently, demonstrate corresponding degrees of inflammation during this progression. Scarring is usually more or less symmetric and impedes filling of all heart chambers. Most patients have a thickened pericardium, but 18% are reported to have normal thickness on direct histopathologic examination and 28% on CT.[1,4,55] In a subset of patients with subacute inflammation constriction is transient and/or reversible by antiinflammatory drugs. This is observed early after cardiac surgery and in other patients with severe pericardial inflammation (discussed below).[3,9,17,28,56,57]

PATHOPHYSIOLOGY

The consequence of pericardial scarring and/or severe thickening is markedly restricted filling of the heart.[3,4] This results in elevated and equal filling pressures in all chambers and systemic and pulmonary veins. In early diastole the ventricles fill rapidly due to markedly elevated atrial pressures and accentuated ventricular suction related to small end-systolic volumes. During early to mid-diastole, filling abruptly ceases when cardiac volume reaches the limit set by the pericardium. Thus, almost all filling occurs early in diastole. Systemic venous congestion results in hepatic congestion, peripheral edema, ascites, anasarca, and cardiac cirrhosis. Reduced CO results from impaired filling and causes fatigue, muscle wasting, and weight loss. In "pure" constriction, ventricular contractile function is preserved, although ejection fraction (EF) can be reduced due to a small end-diastolic volume. In occasional patients, the myocardium is involved in inflammation and fibrosis, leading to contractile dysfunction that predicts a poor result after pericardiectomy.[4,58,59]

Failure of transmission of intrathoracic respiratory pressure changes to the cardiac chambers through the thickened pericardium is an important contributor to the pathophysiology of CP (Fig. 86.9, top panel). On inspiration the drop in intrathoracic pressure is transmitted to the pulmonary veins but not the left heart. Consequently, the small pulmonary venous to LA pressure gradient that normally drives left heart filling is reduced, resulting in decreased transmitral inflow. The inspiratory decrease in LV filling allows an increase in RV filling and a leftward

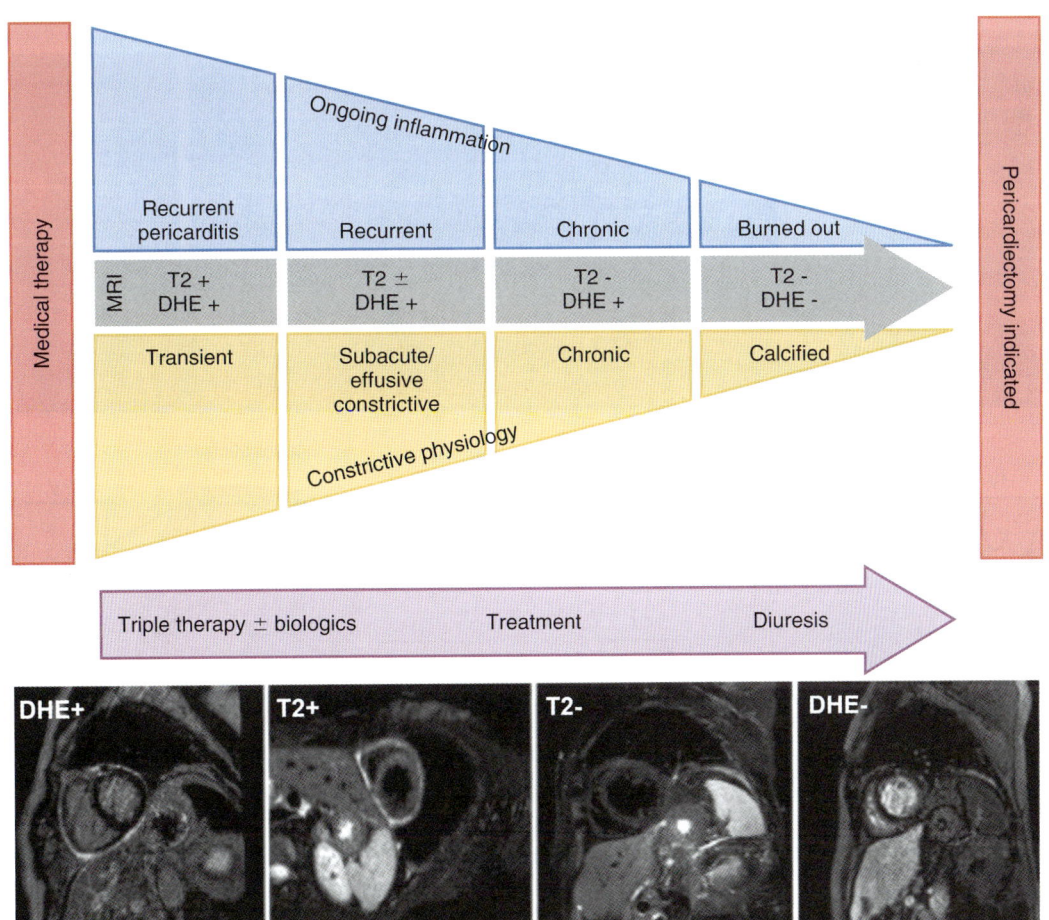

FIGURE 86.8 The spectrum of pericardial disease and its relation to inflammation (**top**, see text). Cardiac MRI (**bottom**) demonstrates the continuum of inflammatory disease starting with an acute phase and ending in burnt-out and/or calcific constrictive pericarditis. *DHE*, Delayed hyperenhancement. (From Chetrit M, et al. *J Am Coll Cardiol Imag*. 2020;13:1422–1437.)

interventricular septal shift. The opposite occurs with expiration (see Fig. 86.9, *middle and bottom panels*).[60-62] Similar to tamponade, these changes result in exaggerated respiratory variation in mitral and tricuspid inflow and LV and RV systolic and diastolic pressure and volumes (see Fig. 86.9, *bottom*). High systemic venous pressure and reduced CO induce renal retention of sodium and water. Inhibition of natriuretic peptides may exacerbate increased filling pressures.[63]

CLINICAL PRESENTATION

The usual presentation consists of signs and symptoms of right heart failure, lower extremity edema, vague abdominal complaints, and passive hepatic congestion, which can progress to ascites, anasarca, and jaundice due to cardiac cirrhosis. Signs and symptoms of left heart failure, dyspnea, cough, and orthopnea may also appear. Atrial fibrillation and tricuspid regurgitation, which further exacerbate venous pressure elevation, are common at this stage. At the end stage, effects of a chronically low CO are prominent, including fatigue, muscle wasting, and cachexia. Other findings include recurrent pleural effusions and syncope. CP can be mistaken for any cause of right heart failure, for example, RV systolic dysfunction, and end-stage liver disease.[60,61]

Physical Examination (see Chapter 13)

Physical findings include elevated jugular venous pressure with a prominent, rapidly collapsing *y*-descent. This, combined with a normal *x* descent, results in an M or W-shaped venous pressure contour. In patients with atrial fibrillation the *x* descent is lost, leaving only the prominent *y* descent. The latter is difficult to distinguish from tricuspid regurgitation which, as noted above, may also be present. *Kussmaul's sign*, an inspiratory increase in mean venous pressure, is usually present,[3] or pressure may simply fail to decrease on inspiration. Kussmaul's sign reflects loss of the normal increase in right heart venous return on inspiration, even though tricuspid flow increases. A paradoxical pulse occurs in perhaps one-third of patients, especially with an

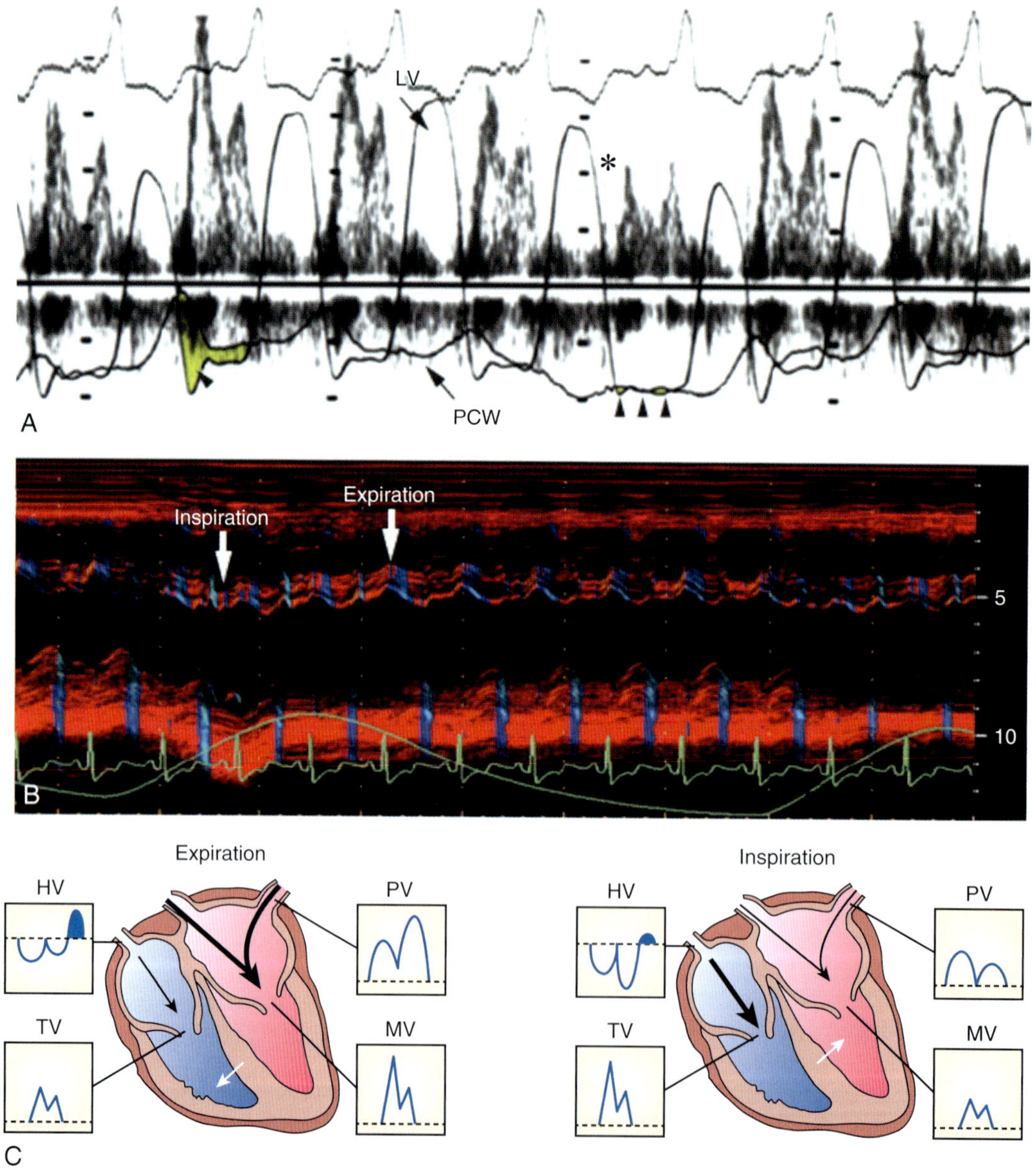

FIGURE 86.9 Ventricular interdependence and dissociation of intrathoracic and intracardiac pressure in patients with CP. **A,** LV and PCW pressures with simultaneous Doppler echocardiography of mitral inflow in a patient with constriction. Inspiration is associated with reduced left-sided filling gradient (*three arrowheads*) compared with the increased gradient with expiration (*yellow*) as the fall in intrathoracic pressure is transmitted to the pulmonary veins, but poorly to the LV. This is reflected by a fall in early mitral inflow velocity (*). **B,** Color M-mode echocardiogram with respirometer tracing showing septal bounce and ventricular interdependence in CP. Posterior displacement of the interventricular septum in early diastole is seen (*blue*). A posterior shift of the interventricular septum toward the LV during inspiration and toward the RV during expiration demonstrates ventricular interdependence. **C,** Typical changes of interventricular septal motion during respiration (*white arrows*) and blood velocities (*black arrows*). Insets show typical Doppler velocity versus time tracings across mitral (MV) and tricuspid (TV) valves and pulmonary (PV) and hepatic (HV) veins. (From Syed FF, et al. *Nat Rev Cardiol.* 2014;11:530–544.)

effusive-constrictive picture. It is probably best explained by the aforementioned lack of transmission of decreased intra-thoracic pressure to the left heart.[64] Table 86.5 reviews hemodynamic findings in tamponade versus constriction.

The most notable cardiac physical finding is the pericardial knock, an early diastolic sound best heard at the left sternal border and/or cardiac apex. It occurs slightly earlier and has a higher frequency content than a third heart sound and corresponds to early, abrupt cessation of ventricular filling. Widening of second sound splitting may also be present, as well as a tricuspid regurgitant murmur. Abdominal examination reveals hepatomegaly, often with palpable venous pulsations, and often ascites. Other signs of hepatic congestion/cirrhosis include jaundice, spider angiomata, and palmar erythema. Lower extremity edema is the rule. Muscle wasting, cachexia, and massive ascites and anasarca occur with end-stage constriction.

Laboratory Testing

There are no specific ECG findings. Nonspecific T wave abnormalities, reduced voltage, and left atrial enlargement may be present. Atrial fibrillation is common. On chest radiography, the cardiac silhouette can be enlarged due to a coexisting effusion. Pericardial calcification[65,66] is seen in a minority of patients and suggests TB but is not diagnostic of constrictive physiology. Pleural effusions are common and can be a presenting sign. If left heart filling pressures are markedly elevated pulmonary vascular congestion and redistribution may be present.

Echocardiography-Doppler Examination

M-mode and two-dimensional transthoracic and Doppler echocardiography and strain imaging are primary modalities for evaluating CP (see Chapter 16). Major findings include pericardial thickening and calcification (best appreciated with TEE), abrupt displacement of the interventricular septum during early diastole (septal "bounce") (see Fig. 86.9, middle), and systemic venous congestion (dilated hepatic veins, inferior vena caval distention with blunted respiratory variation).[1,2,67] Premature pulmonic valve opening resulting from elevated RV early diastolic pressure and exaggerated septal shifting during respiration are common. As discussed above, LV EF is usually normal unless there is a marked decrease in end-diastolic volume or myocardial involvement. Mild to moderate biatrial enlargement is common.

Lack of transmission of intra-thoracic pressure to the cardiac chambers and resulting mitral/tricuspid inflow patterns have been discussed earlier. In accordance with these patterns, Doppler measurements usually reveal exaggerated respiratory variation in both mitral and tricuspid inflow velocity and tricuspid-mitral inflow velocity differences, with the latter 180 degrees out of phase (Fig. 86.9, bottom). Although there is some overlap with tamponade, these patterns have good sensitivity and specificity for diagnosing constriction and differentiating restrictive cardiomyopathy.[1,55,67,68] Typically, patients with CP demonstrate ≥ a 25% increase in mitral E velocity during expiration versus inspiration and increased diastolic flow reversal with expiration in the hepatic veins. Mitral E wave deceleration time is usually less than 160 milliseconds. Up to 20% of patients with CP do not exhibit typical respiratory changes, most likely because of markedly increased left atrial pressure and/or a mixed constrictive-restrictive pattern due to myocardial involvement. In patients without typical respiratory mitral-tricuspid flow findings, examination after maneuvers that decrease preload (head-up tilt, sitting) can unmask characteristic respiratory variations.

Respiratory mitral inflow variations similar to those in CP can be observed in chronic obstructive pulmonary disease (COPD), RV MI, pulmonary embolism, and pleural effusion.[1] These conditions have clinical and echocardiographic features that differentiate them from constriction. Superior vena caval flow velocities are helpful in distinguishing constriction from COPD. COPD patients display an increase in inspiratory superior vena caval systolic forward flow velocity not seen in constriction. As discussed earlier, TEE is superior to transthoracic echocardiography for estimating pericardial thickness and correlates well with CT.[1,2,67]

Tissue Doppler and strain (deformation) imaging are useful adjuncts for diagnosing CP and distinguishing it from restrictive cardiomyopathy (see below).[1,2,67] Tissue Doppler reveals increased e′ velocity of the medial mitral annulus and septal abnormalities corresponding to the "bounce." Lateral mitral annular e′ is lower than medial annular e′, termed "annulus reversus". In restrictive cardiomyopathy, the characteristic tall and narrow transmitral E is present, but e′ is reduced. Regional variations in deformation and strain include reduced LV circumferential strain, torsion, and early diastolic untwisting, with preserved longitudinal strain. In contrast, in restriction circumferential strain and untwisting are preserved but reduced in the longitudinal direction. Regional longitudinal strain ratios of lateral LV wall/septum and RV free wall/septum indicative of pericardial-myocardial tethering are useful in differentiating constriction from constriction and improve after pericardiectomy (strain reversus).[69]

Cardiac Catheterization and Angiography (see Chapter 21)

Cardiac catheterization in patients with suspected CP provides documentation of hemodynamics and assists in distinguishing constriction from restrictive cardiomyopathy and in assessing myocardial involvement.[4,60] Coronary angiography is ordinarily performed in patients being considered for pericardiectomy. Rarely, external pinching or compression of a coronary artery by the pericardium is detected.

RA, RV diastolic, pulmonary capillary wedge, and pre-a wave LV diastolic pressures are elevated and equal, or nearly so, at around 20 to 25 mm Hg (Fig. 86.10). Differences of more than 3 to 5 mm Hg between left and right heart filling pressures are rare. The RA pressure tracing shows a preserved x descent, a prominent y descent, and roughly equal a and v wave heights, with resultant M or W configuration. RV and LV pressures reveal an early, marked diastolic dip and plateau ("square root" sign) (see Fig. 86.10).[60] Respiratory variation in LV and RV systolic and diastolic pressure is exaggerated. This has been quantified using the "systolic area index," the ratio of RV to LV systolic pressure × time[70] on inspiration versus expiration (see Fig. 86.10). A ratio greater than 1.1 strongly suggests constriction. Pulmonary artery and RV systolic pressures are often modestly elevated to 35 to 45 mm Hg. Greater elevation is not a feature of constriction. A ratio of RA pressure/ PCWP greater than 0.77 is an indicator of pericardial constraint that may distinguish pure constriction from constriction with myocardial involvement.[59,71] Hypovolemia, for example, due to diuretic therapy, can mask hemodynamic findings. Rapid infusion of 1 L of normal saline over 6 to 8 minutes may reveal typical features. SV is reduced but CO can be preserved because of tachycardia.

Computed Tomography and Cardiac Magnetic Resonance

ECG synchronized CT and EMR are important adjuncts to echocardiography-Doppler examinations in evaluating CP. CT (see Chapter 20) is helpful in detecting even minute amounts of pericardial calcification[1,17,55,66,67] and is the most accurate method for measuring thickness (normal <2 mm).[9] These features make CT well-suited for preoperative planning. CT may also obviate the need for invasive coronary angiography if vessels appear normal. Its major disadvantage is the frequent need for contrast medium to best display pericardial pathology. CMR (see Chapter 19) provides a detailed examination of the pericardium without the need for contrast or ionizing radiation. It is less sensitive for detecting calcification than CT and less accurate for measuring thickness. The "normal" pericardium visualized by CMR is up to 3 to 4 mm in thickness. This most likely reflects the entire pericardial "complex," with physiologic fluid representing a component of measured thickness. Cine acquisition MRI or CT are useful for detecting common findings of constriction (septal "bounce," ventricular interaction) when echocardiography is technically inadequate. Additional CT/CMR findings include distorted

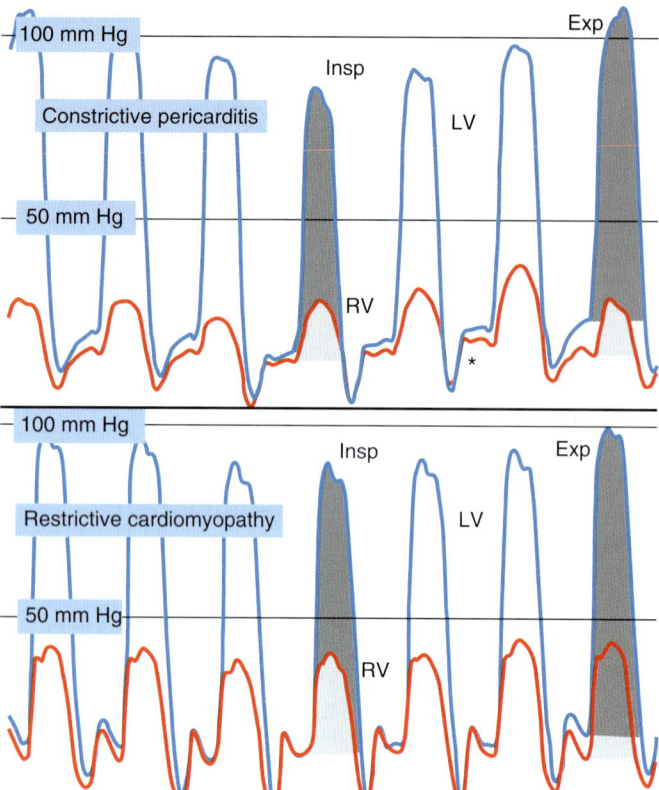

FIGURE 86.10 Top: LV (*blue*) and RV (*red*) pressure tracings in constrictive pericarditis. End-diastolic pressures are elevated and a "square root" sign (*) is present in both chambers. Enhanced ventricular interdependence is illustrated by visualization of the RV (*light gray*) and LV (*dark gray*) systolic areas under the curve for inspiration (*Insp*) and expiration (*Exp*). During inspiration the RV pressure curve area increases, whereas the LV pressure curve area decreases. **Bottom:** LV and RV pressures in restrictive cardiomyopathy. Although end-diastolic pressures are elevated and a "square root" sign (*) is present there is no evidence of enhanced ventricular interdependence; that is, changes in LV and RV pressure curve areas are parallel. (From Geske JB, Anavekar NS, Nishimura RA, et al. Differentiation of constriction and restriction: complex cardiovascular hemodynamics. *J Am Coll Cardiol.* 2016;68(21):2329–2347.)

ventricular contours, hepatic venous congestion, ascites, and pleural effusions.[17]

A thickened pericardium indicates acute and/or chronic pericarditis. Pericardial edema on T2 STIR and late gadolinium enhancement on CMR is more specific for active inflammation and may be useful in identifying patients who are candidates for management with antiinflammatory drugs (Fig. 86.11; see below).[3,9,17,28,56,57] Evidence of impaired diastolic filling and pericardial thickening, especially with calcification, is virtually diagnostic of constriction. Normal thickness argues against constriction but does not exclude it. Most patients with CP and normal thickness have calcification and distorted ventricular contours. The pericardium can be globally or focally thickened. Localized constriction caused by focal thickening is reported. In patients being considered for pericardiectomy, delineation of the location and severity of thickening and calcification by CT or CMR aids in risk stratification and surgical planning.

Differentiating Constrictive Pericarditis from Restrictive Cardiomyopathy

Because treatment differs, distinguishing CP from restrictive cardiomyopathy is important (Table 86.7).[60,72] Restrictive cardiomyopathy is increasingly recognized, in part due to the subgroup of patients with heart failure with preserved EF in whom transthyretin amyloidosis is diagnosed using technetium PYP scanning. The presentation and course of constriction and restriction overlap in many respects. A pericardial knock points to constriction. ECG and chest radiographic findings are mostly nonspecific. However, a calcified pericardium indicates constriction, whereas low QRS voltage suggests amyloidosis. Echocardiographic distinctions are very helpful. Patients with restriction usually have thick-walled ventricles due to infiltrative processes or hypertrophy. Marked biatrial enlargement is typical of restriction but not constriction. In constriction, the most distinctive finding is the septal "bounce" and respirophasic shift.[68] As discussed above, the pericardium is usually but not invariably thickened in constriction.

Doppler flow measurements are also useful.[1,55,67] Enhanced respiratory variation in mitral inflow velocity (>25%) is seen in constriction but varies by less than 10% in restriction. In restriction, pulmonary venous systolic flow is blunted and diastolic flow is increased; this is not observed in constriction. Hepatic veins demonstrate enhanced expiratory flow reversal with constriction, in contrast to increased inspiratory flow reversal in restriction. Tissue Doppler and strain imaging can aid in differentiation.[1,55,67] Recently proposed criteria (respirophasic ventricular shift, preserved or increased medial mitral annulus e′ velocity [>9 cm/sec], increased hepatic vein expiratory diastolic flow ratio [≥0.79]) distinguish constriction from restriction with sensitivity of 87% and specificity of 91%.[62,68]

Invasive hemodynamic differentiation between constriction and restrictive cardiomyopathy can be difficult. However, careful attention to the hemodynamic profile usually allows their distinction (see Table 86.6). In both, RV and LV diastolic pressures are markedly elevated. In restriction, LV diastolic pressure is usually higher than RV by at least 3 to 5 mm Hg, whereas in constriction LV and RV diastolic pressures track closely and rarely differ by more than 3 to 5 mm Hg. Severe pulmonary hypertension is sometimes observed in restriction but not in constriction. The absolute level of atrial or ventricular diastolic pressure is also useful, with extremely high pressures (>25 mm Hg) more common in restriction.[55,67,71] Finally, the systolic area index[70] is greater in constriction than restriction and reported to have high sensitivity and specificity for distinguishing between them.

CT or CMR, because of their ability to provide detailed assessment of pericardial thickness and calcification, are very useful in differentiating constriction from restriction,[2,67,71,73] although once again patients with constriction occasionally have normal thickness. PYP scanning has emerged as the primary means to diagnose cardiac. Brain natriuretic peptide (BNP) levels are elevated in restrictive cardiomyopathy but usually normal in constriction.[60]

Management

CP has a progressive but variable course. Radical surgical pericardiectomy is the definitive treatment in most patients. Pericardiectomy has been considered to have a relatively high perioperative mortality, ranging from 2 to nearly 20% in modern series.[74–76] However, this depends on the etiology of the constriction with a low mortality in idiopathic patients.

Risk factors for poor results include radiation-induced disease, comorbidities, especially COPD and renal insufficiency, coronary artery disease and prior cardiac surgery, reduced LV EF, cardiopulmonary bypass, and NYHA stage IV symptoms. Severely debilitated patients with stage IV symptoms in general have a prohibitively high risk. Relatively healthy older patients with mild constriction may be managed nonsurgically, with pericardiectomy held in reserve until the disease progresses. Otherwise, surgery should not be delayed once the diagnosis is made. Diuretics and salt restriction relieve volume overload, but patients ultimately become refractory. Because sinus tachycardia is compensatory, drugs that slow the heart rate should be avoided. In patients with atrial fibrillation and a rapid ventricular response, digoxin is recommended for rate control.

Pericardiectomy is performed through a median sternotomy, clamshell incision, or bilateral thoracotomy with or without cardiopulmonary bypass.[4,76] The visceral pericardium can be resected if involved. A more aggressive approach with complete removal of the pericardium has been advocated to facilitate access to the lateral, diaphragmatic, and posterior surfaces of the heart.[76] Ultrasonic or laser débridement[4] is an adjunct to conventional débridement or as the sole technique in patients with extensive, calcified adhesions. The "waffle" procedure,[77] in which multiple transverse and longitudinal incisions are made in

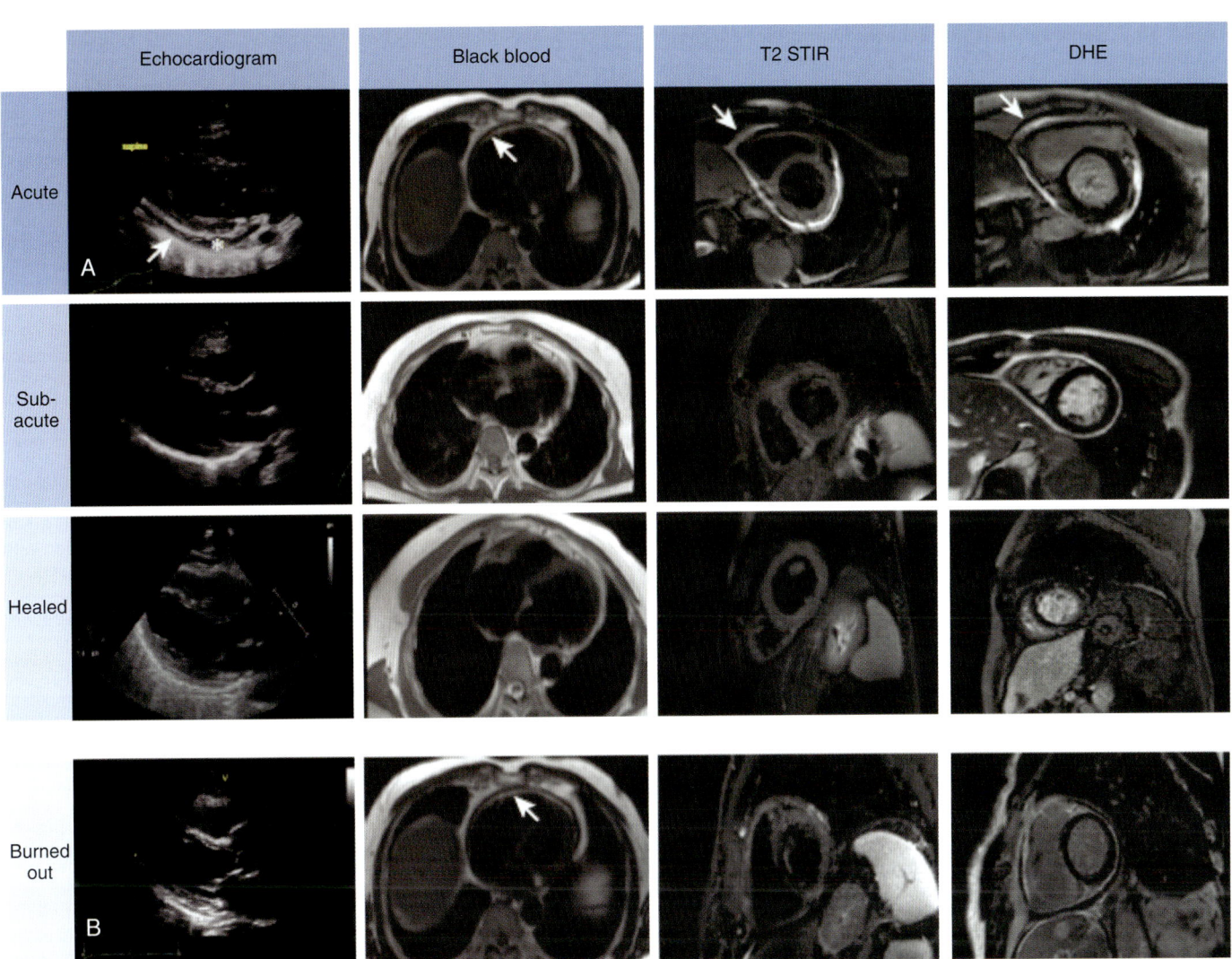

FIGURE 86.11 Changes in inflammation during the course of pericardial disease in a 27-year-old woman first seen after a recurrence of acute pericarditis. **A,** Initial (***acute***) stage echocardiogram shows a thickened pericardium (*) and a small effusion (*arrow*). Cardiac magnetic resonance shows acute inflammation with a thickened pericardium on black blood images (*arrow*), pericardial enhancement on T2 STIR and delayed images (DHE) (*arrow*). Triple therapy was intensified and anakinra introduced. Subsequent imaging showed a normal pericardial thickness, black blood sequences with interval resolution of T2 STIR enhancement but persistence of DHE signal suggesting a ***subacute*** stage of inflammation. After 8 months of treatment there was resolution of DHE with a normal-appearing pericardium on echocardiogram and black-blood sequences and normal T2 STIR suggesting a ***healed*** pericardium. **B,** Images from a 44-year-old man with idiopathic constrictive pericarditis. The echocardiogram appears normal, but black-blood sequences show a thickened pericardium (*arrow*). Furthermore, there is no signal on T2 STIR and DHE, which suggests "burned-out" disease. (From Chetrit M, et al. *J Am Coll Cardiol Imag.* 2020;13:1422–1437.)

the epicardial layer, is an alternative in patients with extensive epicardial involvement and can be done without cardiopulmonary bypass.

Hemodynamic and symptomatic improvement following pericardiectomy is achieved in some patients very soon after surgery. In others improvement may be delayed for weeks to months. There have been several recent reports of longterm results of pericardiectomy for CP.[75,76] One-year survival ranges from 81% to 91%, five-year 64% to 85%, and 10-year 49% to 81%. Most survivors are free of adverse cardiovascular outcomes. Long-term results are worst in patients with radiation-induced disease, impaired renal function, reduced LV EF, moderate or severe tricuspid regurgitation, low serum sodium, and advanced age. LV diastolic function returns to normal in about 40% of patients early and 60% late after surgery. Poor responses to pericardiectomy have been attributed to myocardial atrophy or fibrosis, incomplete resection, and development of recurrent cardiac compression by mediastinal inflammation and fibrosis. Tricuspid regurgitation usually does not improve.

There have been several reports of transient or reversible CP.[3,9,17,28,56,57] Etiologies are diverse, but patients presenting early post-cardiac surgery appear to be common. Although features of constriction dominate, many patients have coexistent effusions and can be classified as ECP (see below). Because reported patients have been treated with various antiinflammatory regimens, it is possible the syndrome might disappear spontaneously. Reversible constriction typically resolves in 3 to 6 months or longer.[17] CMR gadolinium enhancement has been correlated with severity of inflammation in operative specimens.[17] Intensity of enhancement as well as pericardial thickness ≥3 mm on late enhancement images is predictive of a response to antiinflammatory drugs with resolution of constriction (see Figs. 86.8 and 86.11).[17] Responders also have higher hsCRP. It is not clear if patients with reversible constriction are as common as suggested in reported series,[17] which have been small and highly selected. Nonetheless, patients with intense late gadolinium enhancement on MRI, especially those with pericardial thickness greater than 3 mm, should be considered for a trial of antiinflammatory therapy, especially if they have had recent cardiac surgery, symptoms have appeared relatively rapidly, hsCRP is elevated, and there is not extensive calcification. NSAIDs, colchicine, and corticosteroids have been used separately and in various combinations with no clearly preferred regimen. As a practical matter, any antiinflammatory regimen should be administered for up to 6 months or longer if necessary to allow time for success but not so long that surgery is excessively delayed and/or significant side effects occur. Although there is no specific evidence to support it, we

TABLE 86.7 Hemodynamic and Echocardiographic Features of Constrictive Pericarditis Compared with Restrictive Cardiomyopathy

	CONSTRICTION	RESTRICTION
Prominent *y* descent in venous pressure	Present	Variable
Paradoxical pulse	Approximately 1/3 cases	Absent
Pericardial knock	Present	Absent
Equal right-left side filling pressures > right	Present	Left at least 3–5 mm Hg
Filling pressures >25 mm Hg	Rare	Common
Pulmonary artery systolic pressure >60 mm Hg	No	Common
"Square root" sign	Present	Variable
Respiratory variation in left-right pressures/flows	Exaggerated	Normal
Ventricular wall thickness	Normal	Usually increased
Pericardial thickness	Increased	Normal
Atrial size	Possible left atrium enlargement	Biatrial enlargement
Septal "bounce"	Present	Absent
Tissue Doppler E' velocity	Increased	Reduced
Speckle tracking	Normal longitudinal, decreased circumferential restoration	Decreased longitudinal, normal circumferential restoration

suggest "triple" therapy (NSAIDs, colchicine, and prednisone) in doses similar to those recommended for recurrent pericarditis. In the authors' experience, approximately 60% of these patients will not require surgery.

EFFUSIVE-CONSTRICTIVE PERICARDITIS

ECP combines elements of effusion/tamponade and constriction. Constrictive features usually are detected after pericardiocentesis.[4,78,79] Many cases of "transient" and/or medically treatable CP represent ECP. The course is quite variable, but usually subacute, from a few weeks to several months. An inflammatory effusion typically dominates early with constriction more prominent later, but there are many variations. The visceral pericardium is usually prominently involved. Figure 86.11 shows CMR images demonstrating varying effusion, pericardial thickening, and inflammation in a patient with a prolonged course of acute pericarditis leading to ECP (top three panels). For contrast, a patient with "burnt-out" CP is shown in the bottom of Figure 86.11. A proposed definition of underlying constriction is failure of RA pressure to decline by at least 50% to a level below 10 mm Hg when pericardial pressure is reduced to almost 0 mm Hg by pericardiocentesis and/or all detectable fluid is removed. A recent report revealed that echocardiographic-Doppler findings of constriction (respiratory variation in mitral inflow, hepatic vein expiratory diastolic flow reversal, respiratory septal shift) were most commonly seen before pericardiocentesis for effusion in those who *subsequently* developed effusion-constriction.[78,80,81] The reported incidence of ECP in patients with pericardial effusion varies from 1% to 15% in different series and may be especially high in TB.[78,79]

The most common causes of ECP are idiopathic, malignancy, radiation, post-pericardiotomy, and connective tissue diseases. TB is the leading cause in sub-Saharan Africa.[4,78,79] Physical, hemodynamic, and echocardiographic findings are mixtures of those associated with effusion and constriction and may vary with time as the syndrome progresses. Etiologic diagnosis occasionally requires acquisition of pericardial fluid and biopsy if the cause is not obvious and tamponade does not mandate pericardiocentesis. Management is tailored to the specific cause, if known. In idiopathic and post-pericardiotomy cases, antiinflammatory treatment as described for noneffusive CP may provide a gratifying result with avoidance of pericardiectomy, but no guidance is available in regard to a specific approach. CMR with gadolinium uptake and measurement of hsCRP can be useful to identify patients with active inflammation who are more likely to respond to an antiinflammatory regimen. Pericardiectomy is ultimately required in many patients.

SPECIFIC ETIOLOGIES OF PERICARDIAL DISEASE

The pericardium is involved in numerous diseases (see Table 86.1), with selected etiologies discussed in the following sections.

Infectious Diseases

Viral Pericarditis. Viral pericarditis is presumed to be the most common infection in countries with low TB prevalence.[4] Numerous viruses have been implicated (see Table 86.1). Definitive diagnosis requires identification of viral particles or genomic material in pericardial fluid or tissue or antibody rises. This is impractical and/or unnecessary in almost all cases of acute pericarditis because management of immunocompetent patients is not affected by a specific viral diagnosis.

As of this writing, knowledge of pericardial involvement in COVID-19 is emerging. CT scans reveal pericardial effusions in a significant minority of patients; most are critically ill.[82,83] There is one published case report of pericardial effusion and tamponade, in association with myocarditis.[84] Others have been posted online. Reluctance to perform formal echocardiography (as opposed to point of care) has probably limited knowledge of natural history and clinical features of pericardial involvement. The mechanism of pericardial involvement is unclear.

Bacterial Pericarditis. In sub-Saharan Africa the most common bacterial cause of pericardial disease is TB. In the developed world TB and other forms of bacterial pericarditis are unusual in immunocompetent patients.

TB Pericarditis. TB pericarditis represents a secondary localization of a primary infection (usually pleural-pulmonary).[85] Specifics of the cytokine-mediated inflammatory response have been elucidated in recent years, with γ-interferon (IFN-γ) and IL-10 implicated.[85] Clinical presentations include acute pericarditis with effusion, isolated effusion, ECP, and CP. Acute pericarditis without effusion is very uncommon. Making the correct diagnosis is critical because mortality is 20% to 40% within 6 months of diagnosis absent effective treatment.

Diagnosis: A *definitive* diagnosis is based on detection of tubercle bacilli in pericardial fluid or tissue.[4,85] A *probable* diagnosis is based on evidence of disease elsewhere and/or a lymphocytic pericardial exudate with elevated IFN-γ, ADA or lysozyme levels. A presumptive diagnosis without evidence as outlined above is appropriate only in countries with high TB prevalence, followed by a positive response to therapy.[4,85]

Therapy: Rifampicin, isoniazid, pyrazinamide, and ethambutol for at least 2 months, followed by isoniazid and rifampicin for a total of 6 months is recommended. Treatment longer than 9 months gives no better results, increases costs, and risks poor compliance.[4,85,86]

Prognosis: In addition to its high untreated mortality, TB pericarditis has a 20% to 40% risk of evolving to constriction, often within 6 months.[4,85] Prompt antibiotic therapy is essential to prevent this. Additional treatments that may prevent constriction include intrapericardial urokinase[4] and adjunctive prednisolone for 6 weeks.[85,86] Corticosteroids should be avoided in HIV patients because they may increase HIV-associated malignancies. The role of colchicine is uncertain.[86] Even with optimal therapy the mortality of TB pericarditis remains high. Pericardiectomy is recommended if the patient's condition is not improving or is deteriorating after 4 to 8 weeks of therapy,[4] and in appropriately selected patients with more long-standing constriction.

Non-Tuberculous Bacterial Pericarditis. In developed countries, non-tuberculous bacterial pericarditis is rare, amounting to less than 1% cases. It is generally seen in the course of a critical febrile illness.[4] If bacterial pericarditis is suspected, urgent pericardiocentesis is mandatory for diagnosis, providing effusions are of sufficient size. Blood cultures should be obtained in any patient with pericarditis and fever greater than 38°C.[4]

Diagnosis: Pericardial fluid is usually purulent, with low glucose concentration and high WBC and neutrophil count. The diagnosis is made by microscopic detection of bacteria and/or positive cultures.[4]

Medical Therapy: IV antimicrobial therapy should be started empirically until bacteriological results are available. Prolonged drainage is crucial. Purulent effusions are often heavily loculated and likely to re-accumulate. Intrapericardial thrombolysis may help achieve adequate drainage before resorting to surgery. Subxiphoid pericardiostomy and rinsing of the pericardial sac should be considered.[4]

Prognosis: Bacterial pericarditis has a high mortality if untreated, and a high risk of evolving to constriction.[4]

Fungal Pericarditis. There has been a handful of case reports of fungal pericarditis. It is difficult to generalize about clinical features. Reported patients have presented with effusions and have had major comorbidities. Aspergillus and candida are among the organisms implicated.

Pericardial Disease and Human Immunodeficiency Virus

Various pericardial diseases have been reported in HIV patients (see Chapter 85). In the developed world, the epidemiology has been altered by highly active antiretroviral therapy (HAART). HAART has reduced all forms of cardiac involvement except for hypertensive heart disease and coronary artery disease, which are now the most common cardiac diseases in these patients.[87,88] Pericardial effusion, formerly the most common cardiovascular manifestation of HIV, is now rare. Patients receiving HAART have similar pericardial disease etiologies and prognosis as patients without HIV. In contrast, pericardial diseases are more complex and have a much poorer prognosis in untreated HIV and AIDS patients.[4,89] Small, asymptomatic effusions of uncertain etiology are common in untreated patients. TB remains the most common cause of larger effusions in African HIV-infected patients.[89] Less common forms of pericardial disease include various neoplasms, typical acute pericarditis, and myopericarditis. Constriction is rare.

Pericarditis in Patients with Renal Disease

Pericardial disease in patients with end-stage renal disease (ESRD) is less common in the era of widespread dialysis, but remains a significant problem and should be considered in patients with appropriate signs and symptoms.[4,90] Its pathophysiology is complex and probably multifactorial.[90] There are three main presentations[4,90]: (1) uremic pericarditis, often with moderate to large effusions, occurs before dialysis is initiated or within 8 weeks of initiation and is thought to be related to toxic metabolites; (2) "dialysis" pericarditis, occurring more than 8 weeks after dialysis initiation; and, rarely (3) CP. It is unclear if uremic and "dialysis" pericarditis truly differ from a pathophysiologic standpoint.

Some features of pericardial disease in patients with ESRD are distinctive. Chest pain is infrequent and one-third of patients are asymptomatic, and ECG changes are usually absent. Pericardial effusions are often bloody because of uremic coagulopathy. Tamponade is uncommon because effusions tend to develop gradually.

Intensive dialysis is effective in uremic pericarditis; in patients already receiving dialysis, intensification is less effective but remains a mainstay of treatment. Pericardiocentesis should be considered in patients unresponsive to dialysis and of course in those with tamponade. There are few data to guide use of antiinflammatory agents in ESRD.[4,90] Current guidelines[4] recommend NSAIDs, specifically 1 to 2 weeks of aspirin (750 to 1000 mg every 8 hours) or indomethacin (600 mg every 8 hours) as first-line therapy. NSAID bleeding complications are heightened in ESRD. Colchicine is relatively contraindicated but can be used on a short-term basis. Prednisone (0.2 to 0.5 mg/kg daily) may be prescribed to patients unresponsive or with contraindication/adverse effects to NSAIDs.

Pericardial Involvement in Autoimmune and Autoinflammatory Diseases

Autoimmune diseases SLE, rheumatoid arthritis, scleroderma, sarcoidosis, inflammatory bowel disease) not infrequently cause pericarditis and/or effusion.[4,91,92] As many as 10% of patients with acute pericarditis may have an autoimmune disease. SLE accounts for the largest number; rarely, pericardial disease is its first manifestation. Pericardial involvement is usually related to activity of the underlying disease. Concomitant myocarditis may be present. CP is rare, but most common in rheumatoid arthritis.[4] Treatment of pericardial involvement is directed toward optimally treating the underlying disease and is best accomplished with close coordination between cardiologists, rheumatologists, and clinical immunologists.

Another group of patients, especially children, are affected by rare, auto-inflammatory periodic fevers (PFs).[4,93,94] PFs cause recurrent polyserositis, frequently including pericarditis. Most are caused by mutations resulting in dysregulation of inflammatory responses mediated by inflammasome IL-1β production, which is also implicated in recurrent idiopathic pericarditis. The most common PFs are familial Mediterranean fever (FMF) and tumor necrosis factor receptor-associated periodic syndrome. A positive family history for pericarditis or PFs, especially in a pediatric patient, a poor response to colchicine (in some PFs), and the need for corticosteroids or immunosuppressive agents such as anakinra are clues to these diseases. Genetic testing is required for diagnosis.

Various antiinflammatory regimens have been used for PFs.[93,94] Inflammasome-directed therapy, for example, anti-I-L1 α/β blockers (anakinra, rilonacept, canakinumab) or anti-TNF agents are highly effective for selected PFs.

Post-Cardiac Injury Syndromes. Post-cardiac injury syndromes (PCISs) include post-MI pericarditis, post-pericardiotomy syndrome (PPS), and posttraumatic pericarditis.[4,95-97] With the exception of early post-MI pericarditis, all are presumed to have an immune pathogenesis triggered by damage to pericardial tissue and/or blood in the pericardial sac associated with myocardial necrosis (late post-MI pericarditis), surgical trauma (PPS), or iatrogenic trauma (pericarditis after percutaneous procedures including coronary intervention [PCI], valve repair, arrhythmia ablation, device implantations, and left atrial isolation).

An immune-mediated pathogenesis is supported by a latent period, typically a few weeks, response to antiinflammatory drugs, and potential for recurrences. PCIS is an emerging cause of pericarditis because of an aging population and expansion of cardiac procedures.

Definition and Diagnostic Criteria: According to proposed criteria diagnosis of PCIS after cardiac injury requires at least two of the following[4,95]: (1) fever without an alternative cause, (2) pleuritic chest pain, (3) pericardial/pleural rubs, (4) pericardial effusion, (5) elevated CRP.

Specific considerations apply to post-MI pericarditis (see also Chapter 38). Two forms are recognized.[4] Early post-MI pericarditis occurs 1 to 3 days after MI. It is rare in the primary PCI era and is now seen after large, transmural MIs due to absent or late/failed reperfusion. Late post-MI pericarditis (Dressler syndrome) is also rare (<1% of MIs in the modern era) and also most common after large MIs.

Early post-MI pericarditis is usually asymptomatic and diagnosed by auscultation of a rub 1 to 3 days after the index event. Cardiac tamponade is rare. However, tamponade does occur with LV free wall rupture. Because of its association with large MIs, early post-MI pericarditis should alert the clinician to possible rupture, especially if an effusion is present. In the occasional symptomatic patient, pleuritic chest pain appears within the above time frame. It is important to distinguish pericardial from recurrent ischemic discomfort. Ordinarily, this is not difficult on clinical grounds. Typical ECG changes of acute pericarditis are uncommon. ECG changes usually involve subtle ST segment re-elevation in originally involved leads. Atypical T wave evolution (persistent upright T waves or early normalization of inverted T waves) appears to be sensitive for early post-MI pericarditis.[4] Late post-MI pericarditis occurs from 1 week to a few months after MI. Symptoms include fever and pleuritic chest pain. Physical examination may reveal pleural and/or pericardial rubs. The chest radiograph reveals pleural effusion and/or enlargement of the cardiac silhouette. The ECG often demonstrates typical acute pericarditis. Effusions are common but tamponade unusual.

Medical Therapy: Treatment guidelines recommend empiric antiinflammatory regimens as outlined for viral/idiopathic pericarditis.[4] Asymptomatic early post-MI pericarditis does not require treatment. Acetaminophen or aspirin are preferred for symptomatic patients.

Prognosis: The prognosis of PCIS is generally good. Long-term follow-up is warranted because CP has been reported in about 3% of cases.[25]

Pericardial Disease in Patients with Cancer

Most pericardial involvement in cancer occurs in the setting of metastatic disease, and may present as acute pericarditis, isolated effusion, ECP, or CP.[4,36,98] Malignant effusions are often moderate to large and frequently cause tamponade. They are usually caused by direct pericardial implants resulting from hematogenous spread and less commonly by lymphatic involvement. Virtually any metastatic cancers can involve the pericardium. Lung and breast carcinomas are most common. Lymphomas, leukemias, melanomas, and cancers of contiguous organs (e.g., esophagus) make up most of the rest. Cancer patients can also develop chemotherapy-related and radiation pericardial disease and are at risk for bacterial pericarditis.

The diagnosis of metastatic pericardial disease is based on confirmation of malignant infiltration of the pericardium by pericardial fluid cytology or biopsy.[4,36,98] A probable diagnosis is achieved by detection of tumor markers in pericardial fluid (CEA, GATA3, VEGF, and others).[4,52] None are accurate enough to definitively distinguish malignant from benign effusions. Evidence of malignant disease elsewhere with concomitant pericarditis and/or effusion is very suggestive. In almost two-thirds of patients with documented malignancy, pericardial effusion is due to nonmalignant causes, for example, radiation and other therapies or infections.[36,98]

Medical Therapy: Management of these patients requires a multidisciplinary approach including cardiologists, oncologists, and radiotherapists.[4,36,98,99]

General principles include the following:
1. Appropriate antineoplastic therapy.
2. Therapeutic and diagnostic pericardiocentesis for tamponade and as a diagnostic tool for moderate to large, suspicious effusions. Prolonged drainage is recommended to reduce the high recurrence rate (>40% to 50%). Additional interventions for recurrent effusions include surgical pericardial window and percutaneous balloon pericardiotomy.
3. Intrapericardial instillation of cytostatic/sclerosing agents is sometimes effective in preventing recurrences. The agent should be tailored to the type of cancer.
4. Radiation for controlling effusions in patients with radiosensitive cancers such as lymphomas and leukemias. Management is often palliative in patients with advanced disease and aimed at symptom relief rather than aggressive treatment of the underlying cancer.

Adverse pericardial effects of conventional cancer chemotherapeutic agents are rare and confined to case reports of acute pericarditis and/or effusion.[99] Several agents have been implicated including bleomycin and anthracyclines. Various adverse cardiovascular effects have been ascribed to kinase targeted drugs.[99] The main offender is dasatinib, used to treat leukemias. Dasatinib has been associated with pleural/pericardial effusions, including some cases of tamponade. Other kinase inhibitors appear to have less cardiovascular effects.

Pericardial disease has also been observed with several types of immunotherapy. IL-2, a T lymphocyte growth factor, is used to treat cancers such as renal cell carcinoma and melanoma. Myocarditis and pericarditis have been reported. More recently, immune checkpoint inhibitors (ICIs) have been used to treat various cancers. ICIs are antibodies directed against checkpoint or "brake" receptors on T-lymphocytes, important regulators of tumor growth. Resultant activation of the immune system has beneficial effects. About 1% of patients receiving ICIs have adverse cardiovascular effects, most commonly myocarditis and pericarditis with effusion and occasional tamponade.[99] Although the percentage of patients receiving ICIs who develop cardiovascular effects is small, this is an emerging problem because of the numbers of patients receiving these drugs and the seriousness of the effects. Pericardial tissue examination has revealed infiltration of lymphocytes and macrophages.

Pericarditis occurring as an adverse response to cancer treatment is treated with discontinuation of the offending agent and otherwise similarly to idiopathic pericarditis, that is, NSAIDs and colchicine, with corticosteroids used in poorly responsive patients. Patients with ICI-mediated pericarditis and severe myocarditis may require high-dose corticosteroids. Effusion and tamponade are treated as in other patients with malignant pericardial involvement.

Radiation-Induced Pericarditis

Chest radiation remains a significant cause of pericardial disease.[4,100,101] Radiation may also affect myocardium, valves, coronary arteries, and other mediastinal structures, promoting fibrosis.[100,101] Most cases occur in Hodgkin lymphoma, breast, or lung cancer patients. Modern treatment, including lower doses, better shielding, and dose calculation has reduced cardiovascular complications to about 2.5%.[4,100,101]

Radiation can induce early, transient, often sub-clinical acute or sub-acute pericarditis with or without effusion. CP is rare and may appear 2 to 20 years after treatment. Late constriction is dose-dependent and associated with an effusion late in the acute phase. Therapy for symptomatic pericarditis during the acute phase is similar to that for idiopathic pericarditis.[4] Concomitant myocardial damage contributes to poor outcomes after pericardiectomy for constriction.[4]

Thyroid-Associated Pericardial Disease

Pericardial effusions develop in 25% to 35% of patients with severe hypothyroidism (see Chapter 96).[4,102] These can be large but rarely cause tamponade. Hypothyroid effusions often have high concentrations of cholesterol. They gradually resolve with thyroid replacement. Rarely, effusion can occur in hyperthyroidism.

Pericardial Diseases in Pregnancy and Lactation

Insignificant pericardial effusions are observed in approximately 40% of healthy pregnant women (see Chapter 92).[102] Pregnancy does not influence the incidence, cause, or course of pericardial disease but it does impact management.[4,102] Acute pericarditis has a good prognosis with outcomes similar to the general population. NSAIDs may be prescribed during the first and early second trimester. After gestational week 20, all NSAIDs (except aspirin ≤100 mg/day) can cause constriction of the ductus arteriosus and should either not be started or withdrawn. Relatively low-dose corticosteroids (e.g., prednisone 0.2 to 0.5 mg/kg/day) are an option that can be adopted for the entire duration of pregnancy. Absent a specific indication (e.g., FMF), colchicine is contraindicated during pregnancy.[4,102] Acetaminophen is allowed throughout pregnancy and breastfeeding as are proton pump inhibitors. During lactation, ibuprofen, indomethacin, naproxen, and prednisone are allowable. Colchicine is considered contraindicated, although in FMF patients no adverse effects on fertility, pregnancy, or fetal development have been reported.[4,102]

Pericardial Diseases in Children

Pericarditis is a significant cause of chest pain in children, accounting for about 5% of such patients in emergency departments.[4,103] The etiologic distribution differs from adults, with specific causes more common, including bacterial, auto-inflammatory diseases, and PCIS following surgical repair of congenital defects.[4,103] Children often have a more marked systemic inflammatory response, with a higher incidence of fever, pleuro-pulmonary involvement, and elevation of inflammatory markers.

There have been no randomized clinical trials in pediatric settings. Management follows the general scheme for adults, with appropriate dose adjustments.[4,103] Aspirin should generally be avoided because of the risk of Reye syndrome. Colchicine can be used, but corticosteroids should be restricted even more than in adults given particularly deleterious side effects (e.g., striae rubra, growth impairment). Biological agents such as anakinra and intravenous immunoglobulin have been advocated as alternatives.[104,105] Exercise restriction is difficult for children, especially in recurrent cases. Long-term prognosis is generally good, albeit related to the etiology of the underlying pericardial syndrome.

Stress Cardiomyopathy

Stress cardiomyopathy (Takotsubo syndrome) has been recognized for over two decades. Reversible ballooning of the apical LV was originally described, but variants are common. There are a number of case reports of pericarditis, effusion, and even cardiac tamponade.[106] The overall incidence of pericardial involvement is uncertain, but probably quite low. The mechanism is likely epicardial inflammation.

Hemopericardium

Any form of chest trauma can cause hemopericardium (see Chapter 71).[4] Post-MI free wall rupture occurs within several days of transmural MI (see Chapter 37). Hemopericardium due to retrograde bleeding into the pericardial sac is an important complication of type I aortic dissections (see Chapter 42). These patients may also have combined aortic regurgitation due to disruption of the aortic valve and tamponade without a paradoxical pulse. The role of pericardiocentesis has been discussed above.

Percutaneous cardiology procedures can be complicated by hemopericardium due to perforation of a cardiac chamber (with the exception of PCI).[4] Because these same procedures can cause PCIS, it is possible that blood in the pericardial sac can itself cause or worsen PCIS. Because of the proliferation of these procedures, they are now an important cause of hemopericardium. With experience the incidence of hemopericardium declines. Puncture of atrial or ventricular walls can occur during mitral valvuloplasty and during insertion of devices to correct mitral regurgitation.[4,107] Small pericardial effusions are observed rarely after device closure of atrial septal defects, most of which are asymptomatic.[108] Earlier reports of insertion of the Watchman left atrial appendage device and other left atrial isolation procedures indicated a relatively high incidence of perforation and effusions.[109] The Watchman has become the most commonly used device. Recent registry data indicate that rates of effusion have decreased, 0.2% for patients in atrial fibrillation and 1.5% for patients in sinus rhythm. Transcutaneous aortic valve implantation is complicated by about a 1% to 2% incidence of pericardial effusion/tamponade.[110]

Pericardial effusion and tamponade due to coronary perforation during PCI is now rare (see Chapter 41), with an incidence of 0.1% to 0.6%.[4,111] The clinical presentation is typically rapidly progressive cardiac decompensation, although occasionally it is delayed. The diagnosis is usually made by extravasation of dye from a coronary vessel. Loss of cardiac pulsation on fluoroscopy indicates a significant effusion. Management requires sealing the perforation, pericardiocentesis, and reversal of anticoagulation.[4,111] If a perforation cannot be managed percutaneously emergency surgery is indicated. Endomyocardial biopsy is occasionally complicated by perforation, but tamponade is unusual.[4]

Pericardial effusion and tamponade can occur as a complication of catheter-based arrhythmia procedures.[4,112,113] The incidence of effusion following atrial fibrillation ablation is on the order of 2% to 3%. Many patients can be managed conservatively and closed drainage is usually sufficient. Atrial flutter ablations have a 1% to 2% incidence of effusion; for supraventricular tachycardia ablations the incidence is 0.1% to 1.3%. Endocardial ventricular tachycardia ablations have a 1% to 3% risk of pericardial effusion. Epicardial ablations have a similar risk of effusion but a relatively high risk of tamponade.[113] RV perforation occasionally complicates pacemaker and implantable defibrillator lead insertion, but rarely causes tamponade.[114] Finally, tamponade is a rare complication of laparoscopic gastroesophageal surgery.[115] The incidence of *recurrent* pericarditis after percutaneous cardiac procedures is unknown. The authors believe this is an emerging problem.

Congenital Anomalies of the Pericardium

Pericardial cysts are rare, benign congenital malformations,[4,116] typically located at the right or left cardiophrenic angle. Cysts are typically round or elliptical and range from a few to greater than 20 cm. They are usually discovered as an incidental finding on imaging studies. They occasionally become symptomatic due to hemorrhage or infection, increasing in size and compressing adjacent structures.[116] On CT imaging, cysts appear as round or elliptical masses with the same density as water. Absent complications, cysts do not demonstrate contrast enhancement or delayed gadolinium uptake.

Surgery is not ordinarily recommended for pericardial cysts unless they become symptomatic. However, approximately 10% of apparent cysts actually represent pericardial diverticula with a persistent connection to the pericardial sac.[117] This may not be apparent on imaging studies and only identified at surgery. These lesions may cause atypical symptoms that are only relieved after surgery. Minimally invasive thoracoscopic resection or percutaneous aspiration are nonsurgical alternatives.

Congenital absence of the pericardium is very rare (see Chapter 82).[4,118] Usually part or all of the left parietal pericardium is absent, but partial absence of the right side is also reported. Partial absence of left pericardium is associated with atrial septal defect, bicuspid aortic valve, and pulmonary malformations. While usually asymptomatic, herniation of portions of the heart through the defect and/or torsion of great vessels can occur, with life-threatening consequences. Patients can have chest pain, syncope, or even sudden death. The ECG typically reveals incomplete right bundle branch block. Absence of all or most of the left pericardium results in a chest radiograph with a leftward shift of the cardiac silhouette and an elongated left heart border. Echocardiography reveals paradoxical septal motion and RV enlargement. CT or MRI establishes the diagnosis. Pericardiectomy ameliorates symptoms and prevents herniation.

Primary Pericardial Tumors

Various rare primary pericardial neoplasms have been reported, including mesotheliomas, fibrosarcomas, lymphangiomas, hemangiomas, teratomas, neurofibromas, and lipomas.[4] Many are locally invasive and/or compress cardiac structures or are detected because of an abnormal cardiac silhouette on chest radiograph. Mesotheliomas and fibrosarcomas are lethal, whereas others are benign. CT and CMR are helpful in delineating the anatomy of these tumors, but surgery is usually required for diagnosis and treatment.

REFERENCES

1. Klein AL, Abbara S, Agler DA, et al. American society of echocardiography clinical recommendations for multimodality cardiovascular imaging of patients with pericardial disease: endorsed by the society for cardiovascular magnetic resonance and society of cardiovascular computed tomography. *J Am Soc Echocardiogr*. 2013;26(9):965-1012.e1015.
2. Cosyns B, Plein S, Nihoyanopoulos P, et al. European Association of Cardiovascular Imaging (EACVI) position paper: multimodality imaging in pericardial disease. *Eur Heart J Cardiovasc Imaging*. 2015;16(1):12-31.
3. Shabetai R. *The Pericardium*. Norwell, MA: Kluwer Academic Publishers; 2003.
4. Adler Y, Charron P, Imazio M, et al. 2015 ESC guidelines for the diagnosis and management of pericardial diseases: the Task force for the diagnosis and management of pericardial diseases of the European Society of Cardiology (ESC) Endorsed by: The European Association for Cardio-Thoracic Surgery (EACTS). *Eur Heart J*. 2015;36(42):2921-2964.
5. Imazio M, Gaita F, LeWinter M. Evaluation and treatment of pericarditis: a systematic review. *J Am Med Assoc*. 2015;314(14):1498-1506.
6. Imazio M, Gaita F. Diagnosis and treatment of pericarditis. *Heart*. 2015;101(14):1159-1168.
7. Vakamudi S, Ho N, Cremer PC. Pericardial effusions: causes, diagnosis, and management. *Prog Cardiovasc Dis*. 2017;59(4):380-388.
8. Gouriet F, Levy PY, Casalta JP, et al. Etiology of pericarditis in a prospective cohort of 1162 cases. *Am J Med*. 2015;128(7).784.e781-788.
9. Cremer PC, Kumar A, Kontzias A, et al. Complicated pericarditis: understanding risk factors and pathophysiology to inform imaging and treatment. *J Am Coll Cardiol*. 2016;68(21):2311-2328.
10. Brucato A, Imazio M, Cremer PC, et al. Recurrent pericarditis: still idiopathic? The pros and cons of a well-honoured term. *Intern Emerg Med*. 2018;13(6):839-844.
11. Imazio M, Cecchi E, Demichelis B, et al. Myopericarditis versus viral or idiopathic acute pericarditis. *Heart*. 2008;94(4):498-501.
12. Kytö V, Sipilä J, Rautava P. Clinical profile and influences on outcomes in patients hospitalized for acute pericarditis. *Circulation*. 2014;130(18):1601-1606.
13. Imazio M, Brucato A, Barbieri A, et al. Good prognosis for pericarditis with and without myocardial involvement: results from a multicenter, prospective cohort study. *Circulation*. 2013;128(1):42-49.
14. Imazio M, Lazaros G, Picardi E, et al. Incidence and prognostic significance of new onset atrial fibrillation/flutter in acute pericarditis. *Heart*. 2015;101(18):1463-1467.
15. Imazio M, Hoit BD. Post-cardiac injury syndromes. An emerging cause of pericardial diseases. *Int J Cardiol*. 2013;168(2):648-652.
16. Imazio M, Brucato A, Maestroni S, et al. Prevalence of C-reactive protein elevation and time course of normalization in acute pericarditis: implications for the diagnosis, therapy, and prognosis of pericarditis. *Circulation*. 2011;123(10):1092-1097.
17. Chetrit M, Xu B, Kwon DH, et al. Imaging-guided therapies for pericardial diseases. *JACC Cardiovasc Imaging*. 2019.
18. Chetrit M, Xu B, Verma BR, Klein AL. Multimodality imaging for the assessment of pericardial diseases. *Curr Cardiol Rep*. 2019;21(5):41.
19. Imazio M, Brucato A, Doria A, et al. Antinuclear antibodies in recurrent idiopathic pericarditis: prevalence and clinical significance. *Int J Cardiol*. 2009;136(3):289-293.
20. Imazio M, Brucato A, Cemin R, et al. A randomized trial of colchicine for acute pericarditis. *New Engl J Med*. 2013;369(16):1522-1528.
21. Xu B, Harb SC, Cremer PC. New insights into pericarditis: mechanisms of injury and therapeutic targets. *Curr Cardiol Rep*. 2017;19(7):60.
22. Rehman KA, Betancor J, Xu B, et al. Uremic pericarditis, pericardial effusion, and constrictive pericarditis in end-stage renal disease: insights and pathophysiology. *Clin Cardiol*. 2017;40(10):839-846.
23. Imazio M, Brucato A, Cumetti D, et al. Corticosteroids for recurrent pericarditis: high versus low doses: a nonrandomized observation. *Circulation*. 2008;118(6):667-671.
24. Imazio M, Cecchi E, Demichelis B, et al. Indicators of poor prognosis of acute pericarditis. *Circulation*. 2007;115(21):2739-2744.
25. Imazio M, Brucato A, Maestroni S, et al. Risk of constrictive pericarditis after acute pericarditis. *Circulation*. 2011;124(11):1270-1275.
26. Imazio M, Belli R, Brucato A, et al. Efficacy and safety of colchicine for treatment of multiple recurrences of pericarditis (CORP-2): a multicentre, double-blind, placebo-controlled, randomised trial. *Lancet*. 2014;383(9936):2232-2237.
27. Imazio M, Lazaros G, Brucato A, Gaita F. Recurrent pericarditis: new and emerging therapeutic options. *Nat Rev Cardiol*. 2016;13(2):99-105.
28. Cremer PC, Tariq MU, Karwa A, et al. Quantitative assessment of pericardial delayed hyperenhancement predicts clinical improvement in patients with constrictive pericarditis treated with anti-inflammatory therapy. *Circ Cardiovasc Imaging*. 2015;8(5):e003125.
29. Kumar A, Sato K, Yzeiraj E, et al. Quantitative pericardial delayed hyperenhancement informs clinical course in recurrent pericarditis. *JACC Cardiovasc Imaging*. 2017;10(11):1337-1346.
30. Kumar A, Sato K, Verma BR, et al. Quantitative assessment of pericardial delayed hyperenhancement helps identify patients with ongoing recurrences of pericarditis. *Open Heart*. 2018;5(2):e000944.
31. Imazio M, Lazaros G, Picardi E, et al. Intravenous human immunoglobulins for refractory recurrent pericarditis: a systematic review of all published cases. *J Cardiovasc Med*. 2016;17(4):263-269.
32. Brucato A, Imazio M, Gattorno M, et al. Effect of anakinra on recurrent pericarditis among patients with colchicine resistance and corticosteroid dependence: the AIRTRIP randomized clinical trial. *J Am Med Assoc*. 2016;316(18):1906-1912.
33. Imazio M, Andreis A, De Ferrari GM, et al. Anakinra for corticosteroid-dependent and colchicine-resistant pericarditis: the IRAP (International Registry of Anakinra for Pericarditis) study. *Eur J Prev Cardiol*. 2019.2047487319879534.
33a. Klein AL, Lin D, Cremer PC, et al. Efficacy and safety of rilonacept for recurrent pericarditis: results from a phase II clinical trial. *Heart*. 2021;107:488-496.
33b. Klein AL, Imazio M, Cremer P, et al. Phase 3 trial of tnterleukin-1 trap rilonacept in recurrent pericarditis. *N Engl J Med*. 2021;384:31-41.
33c. Klein AL, Imazio M, Paolini JF. Correspondence: Phase 3 trial of tnterleukin-1 trap rilonacept in recurrent pericarditis. *N Engl J Med*. 2021;384:1474-1476.
34. Khandaker MH, Schaff HV, Greason KL, et al. Pericardiectomy vs medical management in patients with relapsing pericarditis. *Mayo Clin Proc*. 2012;87(11):1062-1070.
35. Hoit BD. Pericardial effusion and cardiac tamponade in the new millennium. *Curr Cardiol Rep*. 2017;19(7):57.
36. Imazio M, Colopi M, De Ferrari GM. Pericardial diseases in patients with cancer: contemporary prevalence, management and outcomes. *Heart*. 2020;106(8):569-574.
37. Argulian E, Herzog E, Halpern DG, Messerli FH. Paradoxical hypertension with cardiac tamponade. *Am J Cardiol*. 2012;110(7):1066-1069.
38. Shabetai R, Oh JK. Pericardial effusion and compressive disorders of the heart: influence of new technology on unraveling its pathophysiology and hemodynamics. *New Braunwald_Cardiol Clin*. 2017;35(4):467-479.
39. O'Leary SM, Williams PL, Williams MP, et al. Imaging the pericardium: appearances on ECG-gated 64-detector row cardiac computed tomography. *Br J Radiol*. 2010;83(987):194-205.
40. Aldweib N, Farah V, Biederman RWW. Clinical utility of cardiac magnetic resonance imaging in pericardial diseases. *Curr Cardiol Rev*. 2018;14(3):200-212.
41. Imazio M, Adler Y. Management of pericardial effusion. *Eur Heart J*. 2013;34(16):1186-1197.
42. Hayashi T, Tsukube T, Yamashita T, et al. Impact of controlled pericardial drainage on critical cardiac tamponade with acute type A aortic dissection. *Circulation*. 2012;126(11 suppl 1):S97-S101.
43. Akyuz S, Zengin A, Arugaslan E, et al. Echo-guided pericardiocentesis in patients with clinically significant pericardial effusion. Outcomes over a 10-year period. *Braunwald_ Herz*. 2015;40(suppl 2):153-159.
44. Maggiolini S, Gentile G, Farina A, et al. Safety, efficacy, and complications of pericardiocentesis by real-time echo-monitored procedure. *Am J Cardiol*. 2016;117(8):1369-1374.
45. Pradhan R, Okabe T, Yoshida K, et al. Patient characteristics and predictors of mortality associated with pericardial decompression syndrome: a comprehensive analysis of published cases. *Eur Heart J Acute Cardiovasc Care*. 2015;4(2):113-120.
46. Vilela EM, Ruivo C, Guerreiro CE, et al. Computed tomography-guided pericardiocentesis: a systematic review concerning contemporary evidence and future perspectives. *Ther Adv Cardiovasc Dis*. 2018;12(11):299-307.
47. El Haddad D, Iliescu C, Yusuf SW, et al. Outcomes of cancer patients undergoing percutaneous pericardiocentesis for pericardial effusion. *J Am Coll Cardiol*. 2015;66(10):1119-1128.
48. Horr SE, Mentias A, Houghtaling PL, et al. Comparison of outcomes of pericardiocentesis versus surgical pericardial window in patients requiring drainage of pericardial effusions. *Am J Cardiol*. 2017;120(5):883-890.
49. Maisch B, Rupp H, Ristic A, Pankuweit S. Pericardioscopy and epi- and pericardial biopsy—a new window to the heart improving etiological diagnoses and permitting targeted intrapericardial therapy. *Heart Fail Rev*. 2013;18(3):317-328.
50. Azarbal A, LeWinter MM. Pericardial effusion. *Cardiol Clin*. 2017;35(4):515-524.
51. Abu Fanne R, Banai S, Chorin U, et al. Diagnostic yield of extensive infectious panel testing in acute pericarditis. *Cardiology*. 2011;119(3):134-139.

52. Karatolios K, Pankuweit S, Maisch B. Diagnostic value of biochemical biomarkers in malignant and non-malignant pericardial effusion. *Heart Fail Rev.* 2013;18(3):337–344.
53. Karatolios K, Pankuweit S, Richter A, et al. Anticardiac antibodies in patients with chronic pericardial effusion. *Dis Markers.* 2016;2016:9262741.
54. Uchi T, Hakuno D, Fukae T, et al. Armored heart because of tuberculous constrictive pericarditis. *Circ Cardiovasc Imaging.* 2019;12(3):e008726.
55. Cosyns B, Plein S, Nihoyanopoulos P, et al. European Association of Cardiovascular Imaging (EACVI) position paper: multimodality imaging in pericardial disease. *Eur Heart J Cardiovasc Imaging.* 2015;16(1):12–31.
56. Feng D, Glockner J, Kim K, et al. Cardiac magnetic resonance imaging pericardial late gadolinium enhancement and elevated inflammatory markers can predict the reversibility of constrictive pericarditis after antiinflammatory medical therapy: a pilot study. *Circulation.* 2011;124(17):1830–1837.
57. Gentry J, Klein AL, Jellis CL. Transient constrictive pericarditis: current diagnostic and therapeutic strategies. *Curr Cardiol Rep.* 2016;18(5):41.
58. Busch C, Penov K, Amorim PA, et al. Risk factors for mortality after pericardiectomy for chronic constrictive pericarditis in a large single-centre cohort. *Eur J Cardio Thorac Surg.* 2015;48(6):e110–e116.
59. Yang JH, Miranda WR, Borlaug BA, et al. Right atrial/pulmonary arterial wedge pressure ratio in primary and mixed constrictive pericarditis. *J Am Coll Cardiol.* 2019;73(25):3312–3321.
60. Geske JB, Anavekar NS, Nishimura RA, et al. Differentiation of constriction and restriction: complex cardiovascular hemodynamics. *J Am Coll Cardiol.* 2016;68(21):2329–2347.
61. Welch TD. Constrictive pericarditis: diagnosis, management and clinical outcomes. *Heart.* 2018;104(9):725–731.
62. Qamruddin S, Alkharabsheh SK, Sato K, et al. Differentiating constriction from restriction (from the mayo clinic echocardiographic criteria). *Am J Cardiol.* 2019;124(6):932–938.
63. Karaahmet T, Yilmaz F, Tigen K, et al. Diagnostic utility of plasma N-terminal pro-B-type natriuretic peptide and C-reactive protein levels in differential diagnosis of pericardial constriction and restrictive cardiomyopathy. *Congest Heart Fail.* 2009;15(6):265–270.
64. Miranda WR, Oh JK. Constrictive pericarditis: a practical clinical approach. *Prog Cardiovasc Dis.* 2017;59(4):369–379.
65. Bogaert J, Meyns B, Dymarkowski S, et al. Calcified constrictive pericarditis: prevalence, distribution patterns, and relationship to the myocardium. *JACC Cardiovasc Imaging.* 2016;9(8):1013–1014.
66. Senapati A, Isma'eel HA, Kumar A, et al. Disparity in spatial distribution of pericardial calcifications in constrictive pericarditis. *Open Heart.* 2018;5(2):e000835.
67. Alajaji W, Xu B, Sripariwuth A, et al. Noninvasive multimodality imaging for the diagnosis of constrictive pericarditis. *Circ Cardiovasc Imaging.* 2018;11(11):e007878.
68. Welch TD, Ling LH, Espinosa RE, et al. Echocardiographic diagnosis of constrictive pericarditis: mayo Clinic criteria. *Circ Cardiovasc Imaging.* 2014;7(3):526–534.
69. Kusunose K, Dahiya A, Popovic ZB, et al. Biventricular mechanics in constrictive pericarditis comparison with restrictive cardiomyopathy and impact of pericardiectomy. *Circ Cardiovasc Imaging.* 2013;6(3):399–406.
70. Talreja DR, Nishimura RA, Oh JK, Holmes DR. Constrictive pericarditis in the modern era: novel criteria for diagnosis in the cardiac catheterization laboratory. *J Am Coll Cardiol.* 2008;51(3):315–319.
71. Klein AL, Xu B. Constrictive pericarditis: differentiating the "purebred" from the "mixed bag". *J Am Coll Cardiol.* 2019;73(25):3322–3325.
72. Garcia MJ. Constrictive pericarditis versus restrictive cardiomyopathy? *J Am Coll Cardiol.* 2016;67(17):2061–2076.
73. Chetrit M, Natalie Szpakowski N, Desai MY. Multimodality imaging for the diagnosis and treatment of constrictive pericarditis. *Expert Rev Cardiovasc Ther.* 2019:1–10.
74. Vistarini N, Chen C, Mazine A, et al. Pericardiectomy for constrictive pericarditis: 20 Years of experience at the montreal heart institute. *Ann Thorac Surg.* 2015;100(1):107–113.
75. Biçer M, Özdemir B, Kan İ., et al. Long-term outcomes of pericardiectomy for constrictive pericarditis. *J Cardiothorac Surg.* 2015;10. 177-177.
76. Gillaspie EA, Stulak JM, Daly RC, et al. A 20-year experience with isolated pericardiectomy: analysis of indications and outcomes. *J Thorac Cardiovasc Surg.* 2016;152(2):448–458.
77. Matsuura K, Mogi K, Takahara Y. Off-pump waffle procedure using an ultrasonic scalpel for constrictive pericarditis. *Eur J Cardio Thorac Surg.* 2015;47(5):e220–e222.
78. Kim KH, Miranda WR, Sinak LJ, et al. Effusive-constrictive pericarditis after pericardiocentesis: incidence, associated findings, and natural history. *JACC Cardiovasc Imaging.* 2018;11(4):534–541.
79. Klein AL, Cremer PC. Ephemeral effusive constrictive pathophysiology. *JACC Cardiovasc Imaging.* 2018;11(4):542–545.
80. Miranda WR, Newman DB, Oh JK. Effusive-constrictive pericarditis: doppler findings. *Curr Cardiol Rep.* 2019;21(11):144.
81. Miranda WR, Newman DB, Sinak LJ, et al. Pre- and post-pericardiocentesis echo-Doppler features of effusive-constrictive pericarditis compared with cardiac tamponade and constrictive pericarditis. *Eur Heart J Cardiovasc Imaging.* 2018.
82. Salehi S, Abedi A, Balakrishnan S, Gholamrezanezhad A. Coronavirus disease 2019 (COVID-19): a systematic review of imaging findings in 919 patients. *AJR Am J Roentgenol.* 2020:1–7.
83. Li K, Wu J, Wu F, et al. The clinical and chest CT features associated with severe and critical COVID-19 pneumonia. *Invest Radiol.* 2020;55(6):327–331.
84. Hua A, O'Gallagher K, Sado D, Byrne J. Life-threatening cardiac tamponade complicating myopericarditis in COVID-19. *New Braunwald_Eur Heart J.* 2020;41(22):2130.
85. Wiysonge CS, Ntsekhe M, Thabane L, et al. Interventions for treating tuberculous pericarditis. *Cochrane Database Syst Rev.* 2017;9(9):Cd000526.
86. Isiguzo G, Du Bruyn E, Howlett P, Ntsekhe M. Diagnosis and management of tuberculous pericarditis: what is new? *Curr Cardiol Rep.* 2020;22(1):2.
87. Manga P, McCutcheon K, Tsabedze N, et al. HIV and nonischemic heart disease. *J Am Coll Cardiol.* 2017;69(1):83–91.
88. Hsue PY. Mechanisms of cardiovascular disease in the setting of HIV infection. *Can J Cardiol.* 2019;35(3):238–248.
89. Noubiap JJ, Agbor VN, Ndoadoumgue AL, et al. Epidemiology of pericardial diseases in Africa: a systematic scoping review. *Heart.* 2019;105(3):180–188.
90. Rehman KA, Betancor J, Xu B, et al. Uremic pericarditis, pericardial effusion, and constrictive pericarditis in end-stage renal disease: insights and pathophysiology. *Clin Cardiol.* 2017;40(10):839–846.
91. Prasad M, Hermann J, Gabriel SE, et al. Cardiorheumatology: cardiac involvement in systemic rheumatic disease. *Nat Rev Cardiol.* 2015;12(3):168–176.
92. Lee KS, Kronbichler A, Eisenhut M, et al. Cardiovascular involvement in systemic rheumatic diseases: an integrated view for the treating physicians. *Autoimmun Rev.* 2018;17(3):201–214.
93. Rigante D, Cantarini L, Imazio M, et al. Autoinflammatory diseases and cardiovascular manifestations. *Ann Med.* 2011;43(5):341–346.
94. Krainer J, Siebenhandl S, Weinhausel A. Systemic autoinflammatory diseases. *J Autoimmun.* 2020;109:102421.
95. Tamarappoo BK, Klein AL. Post-pericardiotomy syndrome. *Curr Cardiol Rep.* 2016;18(11):116.
96. Verma BR, Banerjee K, Noll A, et al. Pericardial complications and postcardiac injury syndrome after cardiovascular implantable electronic device placement : a meta-analysis and systematic review. *Herz.* 2019.
97. Verma BR, Chetrit M, Gentry Iii JL, et al. Multimodality imaging in patients with post-cardiac injury syndrome. *Heart.* 2020;106(9):639–646.
98. Lestuzzi C, Berretta M, Tomkowski W. 2015 update on the diagnosis and management of neoplastic pericardial disease. *Expert Rev Cardiovasc Ther.* 2015;13(4):377–389.
99. Ala CK, Klein AL, Moslehi JJ. Cancer treatment-associated pericardial disease: epidemiology, clinical presentation, diagnosis, and management. *Curr Cardiol Rep.* 2019;21(12):156.
100. Szpakowski N, Desai MY. Radiation-associated pericardial disease. *Curr Cardiol Rep.* 2019;21(9):97.
101. Donnellan E, Jellis CL, Griffin BP. Radiation-associated cardiac disease: from molecular mechanisms to clinical management. *Curr Treat Options Cardiovasc Med.* 2019;21(5):22.
102. Chahine J, Ala CK, Gentry JL, et al. Pericardial diseases in patients with hypothyroidism. *Heart.* 2019;105(13):1027–1033.
103. Bergmann KR, Kharbanda A, Haveman L. Myocarditis and pericarditis in the pediatric patient: validated management strategies. *Pediatr Emerg Med Pract.* 2015;12(7):1–22. quiz 23.
104. Brucato A, Emmi G, Cantarini L, et al. Management of idiopathic recurrent pericarditis in adults and in children: a role for IL-1 receptor antagonism. *Intern Emerg Med.* 2018;13(4):475–489.
105. del Fresno MR, Peralta JE, Granados MA, et al. Intravenous immunoglobulin therapy for refractory recurrent pericarditis. *Pediatrics.* 2014;134(5):e1441–e1446.
106. Nagamori Y, Hamaoka T, Murai H, et al. Takotsubo cardiomyopathy complicated by cardiac tamponade due to non-hemorrhagic pericardial effusion: a case report. *BMC Cardiovasc Disord.* 2020;20(1):67.
107. Gheorghe L, Ielasi A, Rensing B, et al. Complications following percutaneous mitral valve repair. *Front Cardiovasc Med.* 2019;6:146.
108. Wang J, Patel M, Xiao M, et al. Incidence and predictors of asymptomatic pericardial effusion after transcatheter closure of atrial septal defect. *EuroIntervention.* 2016;12(2):e250–256.
109. Schmidt B, Betts TR, Sievert H, et al. Incidence of pericardial effusion after left atrial appendage closure: the impact of underlying heart rhythm-Data from the EWOLUTION study. *J Cardiovasc Electrophysiol.* 2018;29(7):973–978.
110. Hodson RW, Jin R, Ring ME, et al. Intrathoracic complications associated with trans-femoral transcatheter aortic valve replacement: implications for emergency surgical preparedness. *Catheter Cardiovasc Interv.* 2019.
111. Bauer T, Boeder N, Nef HM, et al. Fate of patients with coronary perforation complicating percutaneous coronary intervention (from the Euro heart survey percutaneous coronary intervention registry). *Am J Cardiol.* 2015;116(9):1363–1367.
112. Bhaskaran A, Chik W, Thomas S, et al. A review of the safety aspects of radio frequency ablation. *Int J Cardiol Heart Vasc.* 2015;8:147–153.
113. Liu XH, Chen CF, Gao XF, Xu YZ. Safety and efficacy of different catheter ablations for atrial fibrillation: a systematic review and meta-analysis. *Pacing Clin Electrophysiol.* 2016;39(8):883–899.
114. Ohlow MA, Lauer B, Brunelli M, Geller JC. Incidence and predictors of pericardial effusion after permanent heart rhythm device implantation: prospective evaluation of 968 consecutive patients. *Circ J.* 2013;77(4):975–981.
115. Sugumar H, Kearney LG, Srivastava PM. Pericardial tamponade: a life threatening complication of laparoscopic gastro-oesophageal surgery. *Heart Lung Circ.* 2012;21(4):237–239.
116. Khayata M, Alkharabsheh S, Shah NP, Klein AL. Pericardial cysts: a contemporary comprehensive review. *Curr Cardiol Rep.* 2019;21(7):64.
117. Money ME, Park C. Pericardial diverticula misdiagnosed as pericardial cysts. *J Thorac Cardiovasc Surg.* 2015;149(6):e103–e107.
118. Khayata M, Alkharabsheh S, Shah NP, et al. Case series, contemporary review and imaging guided diagnostic and management approach of congenital pericardial defects. *Open Heart.* 2020;7(1):e001103.

87 Pulmonary Embolism and Deep Vein Thrombosis

SAMUEL Z. GOLDHABER AND GREGORY PIAZZA

EPIDEMIOLOGY, 1635
General Considerations, 1635
Clinical Risk Factors, 1636
Cancer and Venous Thromboembolic, 1636
Venous Thromboembolic in the Pediatric Population, 1636
Hypercoagulable States, 1637
Other Conditions Associated with Venous Thromboembolic, 1637
Long-term Complications of Venous Thromboembolic and Risk of Subsequent Adverse Events, 1637
Pulmonary Embolism in COVID-19 Infection, 1637

PATHOPHYSIOLOGY, 1637

CLASSIFICATION OF PULMONARY EMBOLISM, 1639
High-Risk Pulmonary Embolism, 1639
Intermediate-Risk Pulmonary Embolism, 1639
Low-Risk Pulmonary Embolism, 1639
Pulmonary Infarction, 1639
Paradoxical Embolism, 1639
Nonthrombotic Pulmonary Embolism, 1639
Post-Pulmonary Embolism Syndrome, 1639
Chronic Thromboembolic Pulmonary Hypertension, 1640

DIAGNOSIS, 1641

Clinical Presentation, 1642
Differential Diagnosis, 1642
Nonimaging Diagnostic Methods, 1642
Imaging Methods, 1643
Overall Strategy: An Integrated Diagnostic Approach, 1644

THERAPY, 1644
Risk Stratification, 1644
Parenteral Anticoagulation, 1645
Unfractionated Heparin, 1646
Low-Molecular-Weight Heparin, 1646
Warfarin Anticoagulation, 1646
Warfarin Overlap with Heparin, 1647
Dosing and Monitoring of Warfarin, 1647
Novel Oral Anticoagulants, 1647
Managing Bleeding Complications from Anticoagulants, 1647

OPTIMAL DURATION OF ANTICOAGULATION AND SELECTION OF OPTIMAL ANTICOAGULANT, 1648
Risk of Recurrent Venous Thromboembolism after Discontinuation of Anticoagulation, 1648
How to Determine the Optimal Duration of Anticoagulation, 1648
Selection of an Optimal Oral Anticoagulant for Extended-Duration Anticoagulation, 1648

ADVANCED THERAPY FOR ACUTE PULMONARY EMBOLISM, 1648
High-Risk Pulmonary Embolism, 1648
Advances in Catheter-Based Therapy, 1649
Surgical Embolectomy, 1650
Deep Vein Thrombosis Interventions, 1650
Emotional Support, 1651

PREVENTION, 1651
Rationale for In-Hospital Venous Thromboembolism Prophylaxis, 1651
Rationale for Venous Thromboembolism Prophylaxis at Hospital Discharge, 1651
In-Hospital Risk Factors for Venous Thromboembolism and Bleeding, 1652
Primary Prevention of Venous Thromboembolism in High-Risk Patients with Active Cancer, 1652
Mechanical Prophylaxis in Medically Ill Patients, 1652
Advances in Venous Thromboembolism Prophylaxis in Major Orthopedic Surgery, 1652

FUTURE PERSPECTIVES, 1652

REFERENCES, 1653

Venous thromboembolic disease (VTE), comprising both pulmonary embolism (PE) and deep vein thrombosis (DVT), contributes to substantial cardiovascular morbidity and mortality. PE causes more than 100,000 deaths annually in the United States, and the death rate is increasing (Fig. 87.1). Recently, there have been several advances in our understanding of these diseases and increasing recognition of the elevated VTE risk in certain groups, including patients with cancer and those in chronic care facilities, as well as greater understanding of risks and potential therapies in the pediatric population. There has also been increasing recognition of the role of inflammation in the pathogenesis of VTE, which shares pathophysiologic similarities with atherothrombosis.[1] This line of reasoning has uncovered a wide range of unconventional inflammation-related risk factors for PE, including sepsis, which is associated with a particularly high rate of VTE despite the use of thromboprophylaxis. Our knowledge of VTE genetics is also expanding rapidly, and recent large genetic studies have identified novel loci and led to development of polygenic risk scores for VTE.

Advances in diagnostic, therapeutic, and preventive strategies, coupled with novel perspectives on VTE pathophysiology, are emerging at an unprecedented pace. Clinical and electronic decision tools facilitate early VTE detection and improve prevention strategies. Novel oral anticoagulants (NOACs) such as dabigatran, rivaroxaban, apixaban, and edoxaban allow PE and DVT to be managed with fewer bleeding complications than with warfarin. Moreover, distinct advantages of NOAC therapy, including fixed dosing, the absence of drug-food interactions, the minimal number of drug-drug interactions, and the lack of need for testing blood coagulation levels simplify and enhance the safety of anticoagulation.

Finally, VTE and PE are being increasingly recognized as part of the syndrome associated with COVID-19, the disease caused by the SARS-CoV-2 virus and appear to be driven by the unique and thus far poorly understood inflammatory and thrombotic complications associated with the disease. Therapy for these patients has been particularly challenging and rapidly evolving.

EPIDEMIOLOGY

General Considerations

The incidence of VTE in North America and Europe is approximately 1.5 cases per 1000 person-years. About two-thirds of cases are DVT, and the rest are PE with or without DVT. Incidence increases with age and is similar in men and women. Approximately half of VTE occurs without antecedent trauma, surgery, immobilization, or cancer.

Death due to PE is increasing in the United States, particularly among young and middle-aged adults and has plateaued among those 65 years of age and older. In contrast, between 2000 and 2015 in Europe, age-standardized annual PE-related mortality rates decreased linearly from 12.8 to 6.5 deaths per 100,000.[2] These differences may reflect differences in patient demographics and comorbidities. In the United States, socioeconomically disadvantaged older adults hospitalized with PE have higher long-term mortality rates than their non-disadvantaged counterparts and are more likely to be readmitted within 30 and 90 days of discharge.[3] Most deaths in hospitalized patients with PE are sudden, characterized by pulseless electrical activity or resulting from multisystem organ failure caused by right heart dysfunction. Among

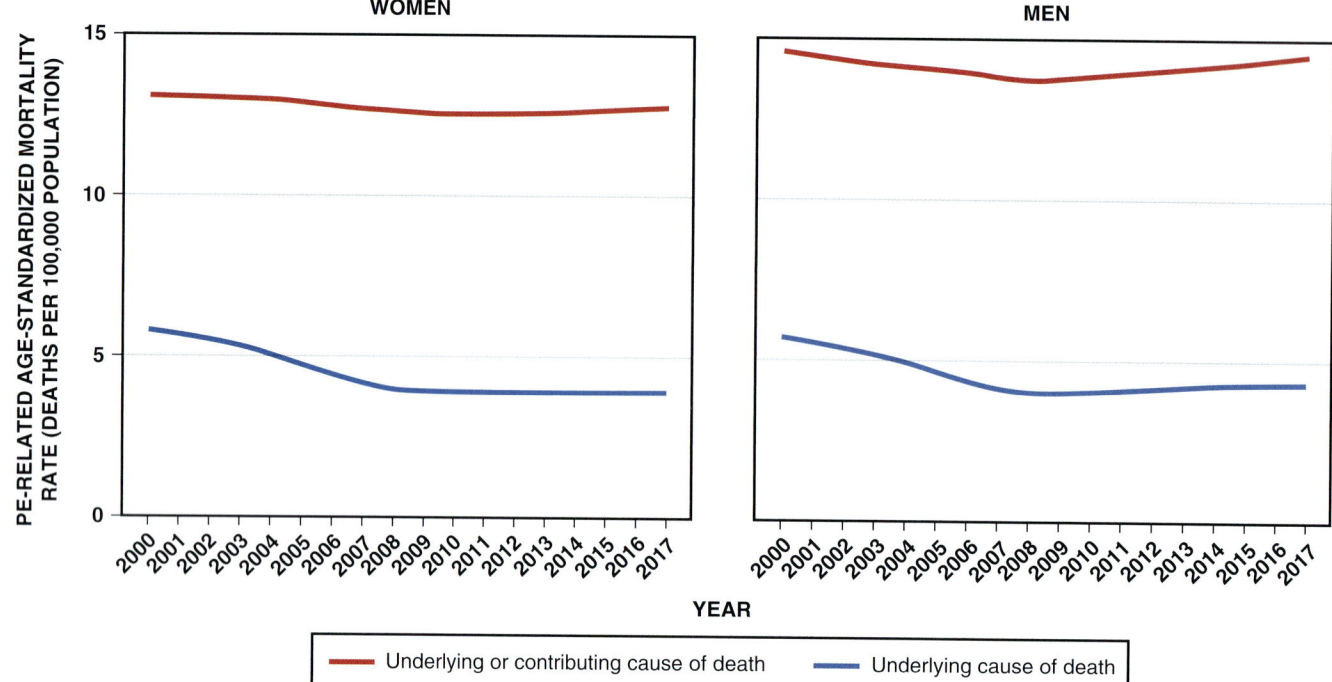

FIGURE 87.1 PE-related mortality in the United States, stratified by age and gender.

adults aged ≥65 years in the United States, the in-hospital case-fatality rate is approximately 4%, the 30-day readmission rate is 15%, and the 6-month mortality rate jumps to 20%.[4]

Clinical Risk Factors

Risk factors for VTE include advancing age, cancer, previous VTE, venous insufficiency, pregnancy, trauma, frailty, and immobility. Of those suffering VTE in the Worcester Venous Thromboembolism Study, 23% had undergone surgery, and 36% had been hospitalized within the preceding 3 months. Among those patients, less than 50% had received anticoagulant prophylaxis.[5]

Cardiovascular risk factors are associated with VTE. A meta-analysis of 63,552 patients with VTE and control subjects found that the relative risk for VTE was 2.3 for obesity, 1.5 for hypertension, 1.4 for diabetes mellitus, 1.2 for cigarette smoking, and 1.2 for hypercholesterolemia.[6] Heart failure (both reduced ejection fraction and preserved ejection fraction) triples the long-term risk of VTE.[7] Given the overlap between venous and arterial thrombosis risk factors, clinicians can counsel patients on steps to reduce VTE and coronary heart disease risk simultaneously.

Population-based cohort studies have shown that older age, smoking, and adiposity have been consistently linked to higher VTE risk.[8] In a study of more than 1 million women with a mean age of 56 years in the United Kingdom, VTE risk increased with increasing body mass index (BMI). Women with a BMI of 35 kg/m^2 or greater, for example, were three to four times more likely to develop VTE than women with a BMI between 22 and 25 kg/m^2.[9] A Spanish VTE registry called RIETE (Registro Informatizado de Enfermedad TromboEmbólica) included 18,023 patients with PE. Immobilized patients had a more than twofold increased risk of fatal PE. Of RIETE patients dying from PE, 43% had a history of recent immobilization for 4 days or longer.[10]

VTE is also a women's health issue. In the United States, PE accounts for 9% of all pregnancy-related deaths or approximately 1.5 deaths per 100,000 live births. Maternal deaths and maternal morbidity due to PE are more common among women who deliver by cesarean section.[11] Pregnancy, hormonal contraception, and postmenopausal hormonal therapy each contribute to increased risk. Use of progesterone-only birth control pills is not associated with increased VTE risk.

Long-haul air travel is a frequently discussed acquired risk factor, although the associated risk of fatal PE is less than 1/1 million air travelers. When death occurs, however, it is dramatic and especially tragic because the victim is often an otherwise healthy young person.

It has also been recognized that certain populations are at higher risk for VTE. Nursing home residency has been identified as an independent risk factor for VTE. Within Olmsted County, Minnesota, a Mayo Clinic study found that VTE incidence appears to be highest during the first week after admission to a nursing facility. The rate of VTE was 2.3%—nearly 30-fold higher than the incidence of VTE among all residents of Olmsted County. Nursing home residents with VTE had a twofold higher mortality rate compared with those who did not have VTE.[12] Unfortunately, appropriate guidelines for VTE prevention in nursing homes are lacking.

Cancer and Venous Thromboembolic

Some risk factors for VTE are not readily modifiable (Table 87.1). Cancer patients have a fourfold increased risk of VTE compared with the general population.[13] When unprovoked VTE occurs, there is about a 5% chance that occult cancer will be detected within the ensuing year.[14] For treatment of acute VTE in patients with established cancer, the National Comprehensive Cancer Network (NCCN) guidelines now recommend consideration of an NOAC rather than low molecular weight heparin (LMWH) monotherapy.[15]

As VTE patients with cancer survive longer due to advances in oncologic therapy, the frequency of VTE is increasing because cancer patients have a markedly increased incidence of VTE (see Chapter 57). Cancer-chemotherapy-associated VTE is common. Increased VTE risk is associated with solid tumors, especially adenocarcinomas of the pancreas, stomach, lung, esophagus, prostate, and colon. Less well known is that VTE risk also increases with "liquid tumors" such as myeloproliferative disorders, lymphoma, and leukemia.

Venous Thromboembolic in the Pediatric Population

Although the frequency of PE and DVT increases with age, VTE also afflicts infants, children, and teenagers.[16] VTE is increasingly diagnosed in pediatric patients, and anticoagulant use in this population has become common, despite the absence of US Food and Drug Administration (FDA) approval for this indication (see below). The increase in VTE diagnosis in children and adolescents

TABLE 87.1 Major Risk Factors for Venous Thromboembolism That Are Not Readily Modifiable

- Advanced age
- Arterial disease, including carotid and coronary disease
- Personal or family history of venous thromboembolism
- Recent surgery, trauma, or immobility, including stroke
- Congestive heart failure
- Chronic obstructive pulmonary disease
- Acute infection
- Blood transfusion
- Erythropoietin-stimulating factor
- Chronic inflammation (e.g., inflammatory bowel disease)
- Chronic kidney disease
- Air pollution
- Long-haul air travel
- Pregnancy, oral contraceptive pills, or postmenopausal hormone replacement therapy
- Pacemaker, implantable cardioverter-defibrillator leads, or indwelling central venous catheter
- Hypercoagulable states
- Factor V Leiden resulting in activated protein C resistance
- Prothrombin gene mutation 20210
- Antithrombin deficiency
- Protein C deficiency
- Protein S deficiency
- Antiphospholipid antibody syndrome (acquired, not inherited)

is probably due, in part, to increased awareness, improved imaging, and more frequent use of indwelling central venous catheters for chemotherapy and nutrition.

Hypercoagulable States

The two most common identified genetic causes of thrombophilia are factor V Leiden and the prothrombin gene mutation (see Chapter 95). Normally, a specified amount of activated protein C (aPC) can be added to plasma to prolong the activated partial thromboplastin time (aPTT). Patients with "aPC resistance" exhibit blunted aPTT prolongation and are predisposed to the development of PE and DVT. The phenotype of aPC resistance is associated with a single-point mutation, designated factor V Leiden, in the factor V gene. Factor V Leiden triples the risk of VTE and is associated with recurrent pregnancy loss, probably because of placental vein thrombosis. Use of oral estrogen-containing contraceptives by patients with factor V Leiden increases the VTE risk by at least 10-fold. A single-point mutation in the 3′untranslated region of the prothrombin gene (G-to-A transition at nucleotide position 20210) is associated with increased levels of prothrombin. The prothrombin gene mutation doubles the risk of VTE.

Antiphospholipid syndrome, the most common acquired thrombophilia, is a prothrombotic disorder that can cause venous or arterial thrombosis, thrombocytopenia, recurrent fetal loss, or acute ischemic encephalopathy. One of the following antiphospholipid antibodies must be present for at least 12 weeks to make the diagnosis: IgG or IgM anticardiolipin antibodies, anti-beta2-glycoprotein I, antiprothrombin, or lupus anticoagulant. The antiphospholipid syndrome heightens susceptibility to recurrent venous or arterial thrombosis if anticoagulation is discontinued. The antiphospholipid syndrome is often associated with other systemic autoimmune diseases such as systemic lupus erythematosus. However, primary antiphospholipid syndrome commonly occurs without other autoimmune manifestations.[17]

Obtaining a family history remains the fastest and most cost-effective method to identify a predisposition to venous thrombosis. Investigation with blood tests to detect known causes of hypercoagulability can be misleading. Consumption coagulopathy caused by venous thrombosis, for example, may be misdiagnosed as deficiency of antithrombin, protein C, or protein S. Heparin administration can depress antithrombin levels. Use of warfarin ordinarily causes a mild deficiency of protein C or protein S. Oral contraceptives and pregnancy also depress protein S levels.

Other Conditions Associated with Venous Thromboembolic

Chronic kidney disease is also associated with VTE,[18] probably because impaired kidney function heightens oxidative stress and inflammation. Other inflammation-based risk factors for VTE include Crohn disease, ulcerative colitis, rheumatoid arthritis, psoriasis, pneumonia, urinary tract infections, influenza, diabetes mellitus type 2, and inflammatory mediators such as transfused blood or erythropoietin stimulating factor.

Long-term Complications of Venous Thromboembolic and Risk of Subsequent Adverse Events

Major long-term complications of VTE include recurrent VTE, post-PE syndrome,[19] chronic thromboembolic pulmonary hypertension (CTEPH),[20] and postthrombotic syndrome (PTS, also called chronic venous insufficiency) of the legs.[21] PTS patients compared with controls report worse long-term physical health, mental health, and quality of life.[22] The most likely pathophysiological trigger for the development of CTEPH and PTS is thrombus persistence.[23]

The risk of subsequent arterial cardiovascular events doubles in VTE patients compared with controls.[24] Among 1023 Australian patients initially hospitalized with PE, the cumulative mortality rate was 32% over 5 years, with 40% of the deaths attributed to cardiovascular causes. Postdischarge mortality was 2.5 times higher than in an age- and gender-matched population.[25] In a Norwegian observational study of 29,506 participants with a median follow-up of 16 years, 1853 participants suffered myocardial infarction (MI), and 699 were diagnosed with VTE. MI was associated with a 72% increased risk of PE.[26] Heart failure[7] and chronic obstructive pulmonary disease (COPD) are also potent risk factors for in-hospital death among patients with VTE.

Pulmonary Embolism in COVID-19 Infection

VTE and PE are being increasingly recognized among patients diagnosed with COVID-19, the disease caused by the novel coronavirus SARS-CoV-2 (see Chapter 94). Patients triaged to the intensive care unit (ICU) have a high prevalence of PE as well as in situ pulmonary arterial thrombosis. In a multicenter prospective study of COVID-19 patients, the rate of VTE was 37% and was associated with an increased length of stay and a trend toward higher death rates due to PE.[27] Among 107 patients admitted to the Lille (France) University Hospital ICU with COVID-19 pneumonia, 21% suffered PE. The median time from ICU admission until a PE diagnosis was 6 days.[28] PE has also been reported in outpatients with COVID-19.[29] Proposed mechanisms for the development of macrovascular (Fig. 87.2A) and microvascular in situ thrombosis in the pulmonary vessels (Fig. 87.2B) include conventional risk factors such as immobility, pneumonia, fever, and obesity, as well as the inflammatory response (Fig. 87.2C), causing endothelial dys-function and cytokine storm, which are known to occur in COVID-19.[30]

PATHOPHYSIOLOGY

ROLE OF COAGULATION AND PLATELETS IN VENOUS THROMBOEMBOLIC

VTE and atherothrombosis have intertwining risk factors and pathophysiology. The historical characterization of PE as a "red clot" disease, compared to atherothrombosis as a "white clot" disease, is no longer

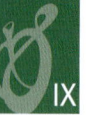

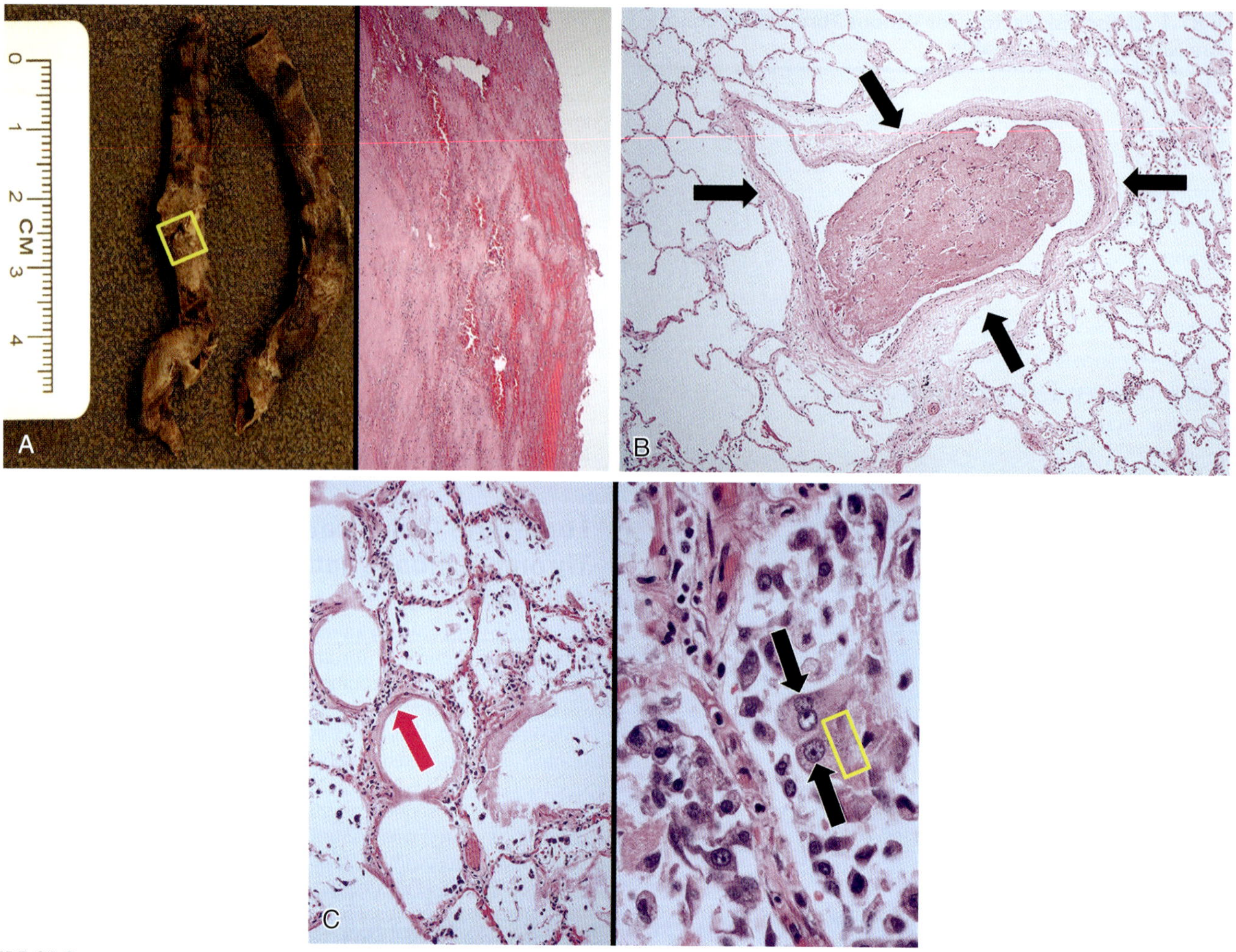

FIGURE 87.2 A, COVID-19 thrombosis: macroscopic thrombosis. *Left panel:* Right ventricular macroscopic thrombus originating in deep leg veins; yellow boxed area delineates a "chevron" with the imprint of venous valve markings. *Right panel:* Laminated microscopic thrombus. **B,** COVID-19 thrombosis: microscopic thrombosis. Microthrombus within a venule (*arrows*). **C,** COVID-19 thrombosis: acute respiratory distress syndrome triggers an inflammatory response that leads to arterial and venous thrombosis. *Left panel: Arrow* points to the hyaline membrane of an alveolus filled with transudative fluid. *Right panel: Arrows* point to two activated macrophages. Within the *yellow rectangle* there are multiple viral inclusion bodies. (Images kindly provided by Richard N. Mitchell, MD, PhD, and Robert F. Padera, MD, PhD.)

tenable. VTE is part of a pan-cardiovascular syndrome that includes coronary artery disease and cerebrovascular disease (Fig. 87.3). Virchow's triad of stasis, hypercoagulability, and endothelial injury often activates the pathophysiologic cascade leading to VTE. Inflammation is not included in Virchow's triad but is also a key precipitant. Infection and associated inflammation lead to the recruitment of platelets—one of the first steps necessary for thrombus initiation. Activated platelets release polyphosphates, procoagulant microparticles, and proinflammatory mediators. These activated platelets bind neutrophils and stimulate them to release nuclear material and form web-like extracellular networks containing DNA, histones, and neutrophil granule constituents. These networks are called *neutrophil extracellular traps* (NETs) and consist of DNA extruded from leukocytes to contain infections. These extracellular webs of chromatin, microbicidal proteins, and oxidant enzymes are prothrombotic and procoagulant. Histones stimulate platelet aggregation and promote platelet-dependent thrombin generation. As venous thrombi start to organize, neutrophils infiltrate the NETs. As thrombi mature, NETs provide the scaffold that binds red blood cells and promotes further platelet aggregation.[31] When not properly regulated, NETs have the potential to propagate inflammation and microvascular thrombosis, particularly in the lungs of patients with acute respiratory distress syndrome.[32]

Venous thrombi contain fibrin, red blood cells, platelets, and neutrophils. These thrombi flourish in an environment of stasis, low oxygen tension, oxidative stress, increased expression of proinflammatory gene products, and impaired endothelial cell regulatory capacity. Inflammation resulting from infection, transfusion, or erythropoietin-stimulating factor[33] activates a cascade of biochemical reactions in the vein endothelium that promotes thrombosis.[34]

The high recurrence rate of VTE in the absence of anticoagulation supports the hypothesis that venous thrombosis can persist as a subclinical and perhaps chronic inflammatory state that becomes clinically apparent intermittently, when activated platelets degranulate and release preformed proinflammatory mediators. In the JUPITER trial, an initially healthy cohort of 17,802 asymptomatic subjects with elevated baseline high-sensitivity C-reactive protein (hsCRP) levels was treated with rosuvastatin 20 mg daily and had a 43% reduction in symptomatic VTE.[35] The principal postulated mechanism of action was rosuvastatin's antiinflammatory effect, evidenced by its reduction of hsCRP levels.

MOLECULAR GENETICS AND VTE

The Million Veteran Program and the UK Biobank collaborated to perform a genome-wide association study on 26,066 cases and 624,053 controls. They identified 22 previously unknown loci and then developed a genome-wide polygenic risk score for VTE that identifies 5% of the population as at-risk carriers.[36] Common polymorphisms such as factor V Leiden and the prothrombin gene mutation account for an additional 5% of VTE heritability. Another research consortium identified 16 novel susceptibility loci for VTE, some of which were outside known coagulation pathways.[37] A polygenic risk score has been developed that identifies patients at greater than twofold increased risk for VTE.[38]

CARDIOPULMONARY DYNAMICS

PE can elicit a complex cardiopulmonary response that includes: (1) increased pulmonary vascular resistance due to vascular obstruction, hypoxemia, neurohumoral agents, and pulmonary artery baroreceptors; (2) impaired gas exchange caused by increased alveolar dead space

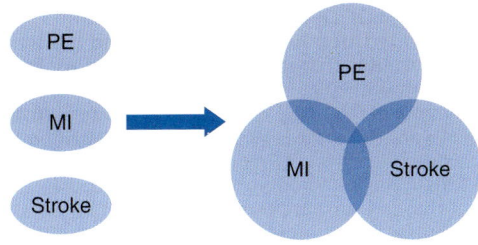

FIGURE 87.3 Pulmonary embolism (PE) is part of a pan-cardiovascular syndrome that includes myocardial infarction (MI) and stroke. Inflammation is a common underlying process.

from vascular obstruction and hypoxemia from alveolar hypoventilation and right-to-left shunting, as well as impaired carbon monoxide transfer caused by loss of gas exchange surface area; (3) alveolar hyperventilation caused by reflex stimulation of irritant receptors; (4) increased airway resistance due to bronchoconstriction; and (5) decreased pulmonary compliance due to edema, alveolar hemorrhage, and loss of surfactant.

The extent of pulmonary vascular obstruction, the presence of underlying cardiopulmonary disease, and the neurohumoral response determine whether and to what extent right ventricular dysfunction ensues. As pulmonary vascular resistance increases, pulmonary artery pressure rises. In response to pressure overload, the right ventricle (RV) releases cardiac biomarkers such as N-terminal prohormone-brain type natriuretic peptide (NT-proBNP), brain-type natriuretic peptide (BNP), and troponin, all of which portend an increased likelihood of adverse clinical outcomes.

The sudden rise in pulmonary artery pressure abruptly increases right ventricular afterload, with consequent elevation of right ventricular wall tension followed by right ventricular dilation and dysfunction (Fig. 87.4). As pressure in the RV increases further, the interventricular septum shifts toward the left, leading to underfilling and decreased left ventricular diastolic distensibility. With impaired filling of the left ventricle (LV), systemic cardiac output and systolic arterial pressure both decline, decreasing coronary perfusion and causing myocardial ischemia. Elevated right ventricular wall tension can reduce right coronary artery perfusion and increase right ventricular myocardial oxygen demand, causing ischemia. Perpetuation of this cycle can lead to right ventricular infarction, circulatory collapse, and death.

CLASSIFICATION OF PULMONARY EMBOLISM

Classification of acute PE (Table 87.2) can assist with prognostication and clinical management.[39] High-risk, also known as massive, PE accounts for 5% to 10% of cases. Catastrophic, or "super-massive," PE patients have refractory cardiogenic shock or require ongoing cardiopulmonary resuscitation. They may need mechanical circulatory support such as extracorporeal membrane oxygenation (ECMO) followed by surgical pulmonary embolectomy. Intermediate-risk or submassive PE is more common, occurring in approximately 20% to 25% of patients. Low-risk PE constitutes most PE cases—approximately 65% to 70%.

High-Risk Pulmonary Embolism

Patients with high-risk PE are susceptible to cardiogenic shock and multisystem organ failure. Renal insufficiency, hepatic dysfunction, and altered mentation are common findings. Their mortality rate approaches one-third.[40] PE is typically present bilaterally, sometimes as a "saddle" PE in the main pulmonary artery. Dyspnea is usually the most prominent symptom; chest pain and transient cyanosis occur less often; and systemic arterial hypotension requiring pressor support occurs frequently. Excessive fluid boluses may worsen right-sided heart failure, rendering therapy more difficult. These patients may require heroic efforts to enable survival, such as venoarterial ECMO.[41]

Intermediate-Risk Pulmonary Embolism

Intermediate-risk PE patients present with normal systemic arterial pressure. The European Society of Cardiology (ESC) PE Guidelines subdivide intermediate-risk PE into intermediate-high- and intermediate-low-risk.[39] Patients with intermediate-high-risk PE present with both right ventricular hypokinesis and elevated cardiac biomarkers such as troponin, NT-proBNP, or BNP. Those with intermediate-low-risk PE present with right ventricular dysfunction, elevated cardiac biomarkers, or neither, but not both. Usually, one-third or more of the pulmonary artery vasculature is obstructed in intermediate-risk PE patients. Sudden onset of moderate pulmonary arterial hypertension and right ventricular enlargement is common. If patients have no previous history of cardiopulmonary disease, they may appear clinically well, but this initial impression may be misleading. They are at risk for recurrent PE, even with adequate anticoagulation. Most survive, but some will deteriorate clinically and require escalation of therapy with pressor support or advanced therapy.[42]

Low-Risk Pulmonary Embolism

Patients with low-risk PE do not exhibit markers of an adverse prognosis. They present with normal systemic arterial pressure and normal right ventricular function and do not have elevated cardiac biomarkers. They often have anatomically small PEs and appear clinically stable. Adequate anticoagulation usually results in an excellent clinical outcome. A subset with a reliable social network and clinical follow-up may be appropriate for home therapy.[43]

Pulmonary Infarction

Pulmonary infarction is characterized by pleuritic chest pain that may be unremitting or may wax and wane. The pleurisy is occasionally accompanied by hemoptysis. The embolus typically lodges in the peripheral pulmonary arterial tree, near the pleura (Fig. 87.5). Tissue infarction usually occurs 3 to 7 days after embolism. Signs and symptoms often include fever, leukocytosis, elevated erythrocyte sedimentation rate, and radiologic evidence of a wedge-shaped or pleural-based infiltrate.

Paradoxical Embolism

Paradoxical embolism may manifest with a sudden stroke, which may be misdiagnosed as "cryptogenic." The cause is a DVT that embolizes to the arterial system, usually through a patent foramen ovale or atrial septal defect. The DVT can be small and break away completely from a tiny leg vein, leaving no residual evidence of thrombosis that can be imaged on venous ultrasound examination.[44]

Nonthrombotic Pulmonary Embolism

Sources of embolism other than thrombus are uncommon. They include fat, tumor, air, and amniotic fluid. Fat embolism most often occurs after blunt trauma complicated by long bone fractures.[45] Air embolus can occur during placement or removal of a central venous catheter. Amniotic fluid embolism may be catastrophic and is characterized by respiratory failure, cardiogenic shock, and disseminated intravascular coagulation. Intravenous drug abusers sometimes self-inject contaminants such as hair, talc, and cotton; they are susceptible to septic PE.

Post-Pulmonary Embolism Syndrome

The post-PE syndrome is characterized by persistent symptoms, including chest pain and dyspnea, functional limitation, and exercise intolerance in the absence of pulmonary hypertension.[46] The impact of advanced therapies (i.e., systemic fibrinolysis or catheter-based intervention) on the frequency of post-PE syndrome remains unclear. However, in long-term follow-up from the PEITHO trial, systemic fibrinolysis did not decrease symptom burden or functional limitation in patients with intermediate-risk PE.[47]

Chronic Thromboembolic Pulmonary Hypertension (see Chapter 88)

CTEPH is characterized by persistent pulmonary arterial obstruction, pulmonary vasoconstriction, and a secondary small-vessel arteriopathy that results in chronic dyspnea, functional limitation, and progressive right ventricular failure.[48] CTEPH occurs in 2% to 4% of patients after PE. There are evolving therapeutic approaches for operable and inoperable disease.[49] Pulmonary thromboendarterectomy is the most effective and durable therapy. Pulmonary vasodilators, such as riociguat, can potentially improve symptoms and functional capacity in patients with inoperable disease or post-thromboendarterectomy pulmonary hypertension.[50] Balloon pulmonary angioplasty offers an additional option for patients who are not surgical candidates.[51] Because the evaluation and treatment are complex and evolving, patients with CTEPH should be referred to specialized centers of excellence.

CLASSIFICATION OF DEEP VEIN THROMBOSIS

Lower-Extremity Deep Vein Thrombosis and the Relationship Between Deep Vein Thrombosis and Pulmonary Embolism

Patients present with DVT symptoms about twice as frequently as with PE symptoms. Leg DVT occurs approximately 10 times more often than upper-extremity DVT. The more proximal the thrombus is within the deep leg veins, the more likely it is to embolize and cause acute PE. When venous thrombi detach from their sites of formation, they travel through the venous system toward the vena cava. They pass through the right atrium and RV and then enter the pulmonary arterial circulation. An extremely large embolus may lodge at the bifurcation of the pulmonary artery, forming a saddle embolus (Fig. 87.6). In many patients with large PEs, ultrasonographic evidence of DVT is lacking, likely because the clot has already embolized to the lungs.

Isolated Calf Deep Vein Thrombosis

The clinical significance and treatment of isolated calf DVT have been the focus of ongoing investigation and debate. A randomized trial of injectable anticoagulation for 6 weeks in low-risk patients with isolated calf DVT did not reduce adverse outcomes, including extension of calf DVT, contralateral proximal DVT, and symptomatic PE at day 42 versus no treatment (3% vs. 5%; p=0.54), but did result in bleeding (4% vs. 0%; p=0.025).[52] In contrast, a meta-analysis found anticoagulation to be associated with a 50% reduction in recurrent VTE risk (6.5% vs. 12.0%; RR, 0.50; 95% CI, 0.31 to 0.79), without increasing the risk of major bleeding (0.4% vs. 0.7%; RR, 0.64; 95% CI, 0.15 to 2.73).[53] Anticoagulant therapy is typically prescribed in patients with symptomatic calf DVT.

Upper-Extremity Deep Vein Thrombosis

Upper-extremity DVT is an increasingly important clinical entity owing to more frequent placement of pacemakers and implantable cardioverter-defibrillators, as well as growing use of chronic indwelling catheters for chemotherapy and nutrition. The likelihood of upper-extremity DVT increases as the size and number of lumens of a peripherally inserted central catheter increase.[54] Catheter-based thrombosis is a major source of COVID-19-associated DVT.

A hospital initiative to use smaller-diameter catheters and to minimize the number of lumens can reduce the frequency of catheter-associated DVT.[55] Patients with upper-extremity DVT are at risk for PE, superior vena cava syndrome, loss of vascular access, and central venous stenosis of the subclavian or

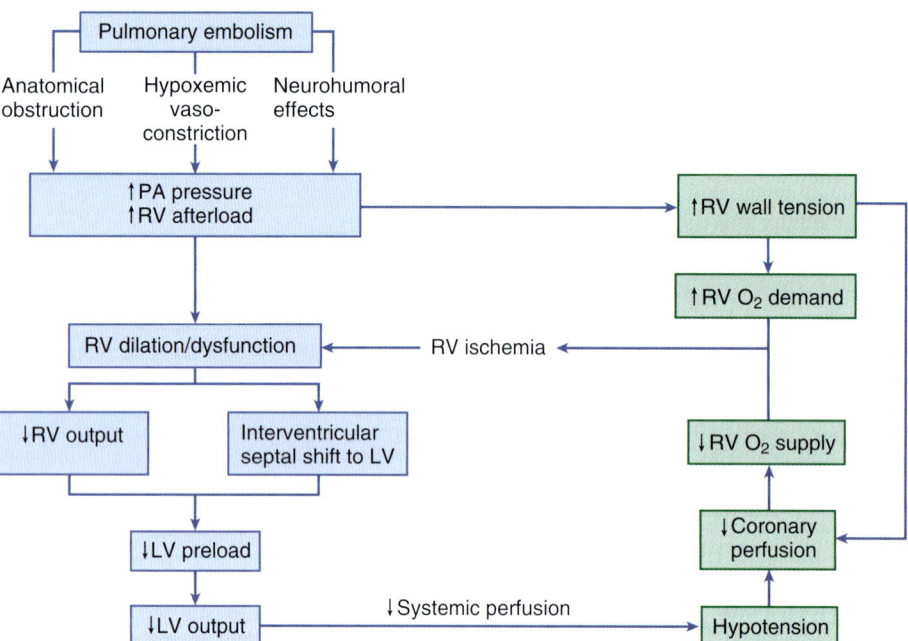

FIGURE 87.4 Pathophysiology of right ventricular dysfunction and its deleterious effects of causing decreased systemic arterial pressure, decreased coronary perfusion, and deteriorating ventricular function. *LV*, left ventricle/ventricular; *PA*, pulmonary artery; *RV*, right ventricle/ventricular.

TABLE 87.2 Classification of Acute Pulmonary Embolism

EUROPEAN SOCIETY OF CARDIOLOGY (ESC, 2019)	AMERICAN HEART ASSOCIATION (AHA, 2011)	HEMODYNAMIC STATUS	PE SEVERITY INDEX (PESI) (OR SIMPLIFIED PESI)	EVIDENCE OF DYSFUNCTION	TREATMENT
High risk	Massive	Unstable	High	Typically abnormal RV on imaging, elevated troponin, OR both	Anticoagulation and advanced therapy
Intermediate-high risk	Submassive	Stable	High	Abnormal RV on imaging, AND elevated troponin	Anticoagulation with advanced therapy if clinical deterioration
Intermediate-low risk			High	May have abnormal RV on imaging OR elevated troponin BUT not both	Anticoagulation
Low risk	Low risk	Stable	Low	None	Anticoagulation with home therapy in subset with reliable follow-up

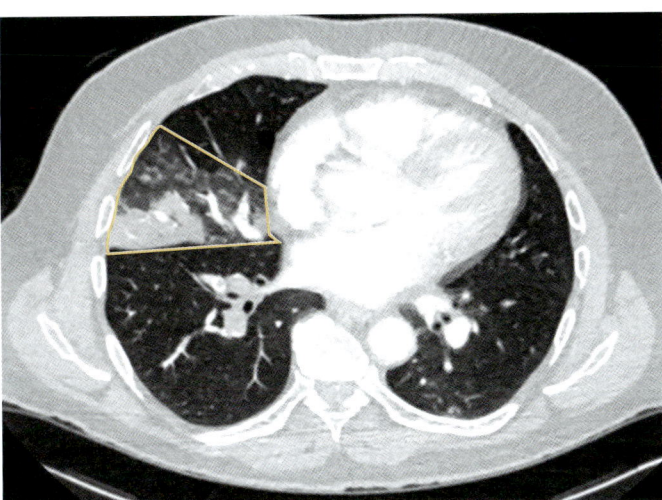

FIGURE 87.5 Chest computed tomography (CT) image showing a large, wedge-shaped (*outline*), right-sided pulmonary infarction.

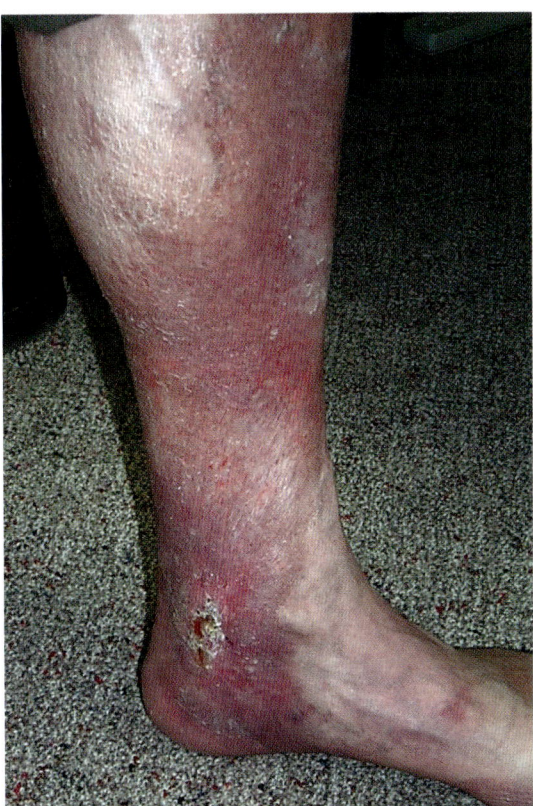

FIGURE 87.7 Left medial malleolus venous ulcer due to postthrombotic syndrome in a 57-year-old man with a history of left iliofemoral deep vein thrombosis (DVT) and extensive tobacco use. Note the extensive erythema of the skin of the left lower leg. (Courtesy Suresh Vedantham, MD.)

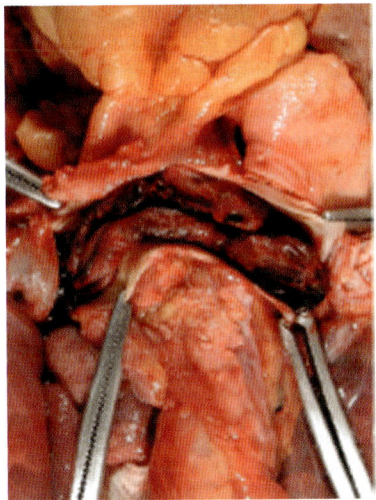

FIGURE 87.6 A 41-year-old woman with poorly controlled hypertension suffered an intracerebral hemorrhage, complicated 6 days later by acute pulmonary embolism. Emergency catheter embolectomy was unsuccessful, and she suffered cardiac arrest. At autopsy, a large saddle embolus extended from the root of the pulmonary artery into the left and right lungs.

brachiocephalic veins. In a study of 3790 patients receiving peripherally inserted central catheters during hospitalization, central catheter use tripled the likelihood of upper-extremity DVT and increased the likelihood of leg DVT by about 50%.[56]

Postthrombotic Syndrome and Chronic Venous Insufficiency
Valve dysfunction in the deep venous system often results from damage due to DVT. Obstruction of the deep veins may further limit the outflow of blood, causing venous hypertension with leg muscle contraction. Abnormal hemodynamics in the large veins of the leg are transmitted into the microcirculation, causing venous microangiopathy. Patients with DVT who develop PTS have higher measured levels of inflammatory markers compared with those who do not.[57] Risk factors for PTS include iliofemoral DVT, recurrent ipsilateral DVT, persistent symptoms after 1 month of anticoagulation, increased BMI, advanced age, and suboptimal anticoagulation during the first 3 months after DVT diagnosis.[58] Physical findings may include varicose veins, abnormal pigmentation of the medial malleolus, and venous ulceration (Fig. 87.7). The economic impact of PTS is high[59] because of time lost from work and the expense of medical diagnosis and treatment. Chronic venous disease is associated with a reduced quality of life because of pain, decreased physical function, and decreased mobility. Vascular compression stockings (below-knee, 20 to 30 mm Hg or 30 to 40 mm Hg) do not prevent the development of PTS after an acute proximal DVT.[60] However, for patients with venous insufficiency, vascular compression stockings are a mainstay of therapy, improving venous hemodynamics, reducing edema, alleviating calf discomfort, and minimizing skin discoloration. Supervised exercise training may have a role in treatment of PTS.[61]

Differentiating Lymphedema from Venous Insufficiency
Lymphedema may be misdiagnosed as chronic venous insufficiency. Leg discomfort due to lymphedema is usually caused by leg swelling or increased limb weight. In contrast, pain from venous insufficiency typically occurs during standing and is alleviated by leg elevation. Swelling from venous insufficiency tends to be symmetric in both legs and is often most marked in the calves. In contrast, lymphedema swelling affects the entire leg and foot but is rarely symmetric. Unlike venous insufficiency, swelling due to lymphedema does not decrease during the night. Some patients with lymphedema have a positive Kaposi-Stemmer sign—the skin on the dorsum of the base of the second toe cannot be pinched as a fold between the fingers.

Superficial Venous Thrombosis
Superficial venous thrombosis (thrombophlebitis) is associated with a small but finite risk of DVT and PE. In a large Danish population-based case-control study, the risk of VTE was 3.4% in the 3 months following diagnosis of superficial venous thrombosis. The risk of VTE remained at a fivefold increase for more than 5 years after the initial superficial venous thrombosis.[62] Treatment of superficial venous thrombosis has been studied in recent randomized trials (see below).

DIAGNOSIS

PE is notorious for masquerading as other illnesses, such as asthma, pneumonia, pleurisy, acute coronary syndrome, and congestive heart failure. PE often occurs concomitantly with other illnesses, especially pneumonia, asthma, and heart failure, thereby confounding the diagnostic workup. The most useful approach is a clinical assessment of likelihood, based on presenting symptoms and signs, in conjunction with judicious use of laboratory testing and diagnostic imaging.

Clinical Presentation

Symptoms and signs of PE are nonspecific. Hence, awareness of VTE risk factors and a clinical suspicion for PE are of paramount importance in guiding diagnostic testing. Dyspnea is the most frequent symptom, and tachypnea is the most frequent sign (Table 87.3). Severe dyspnea, syncope, or cyanosis portends a life-threatening PE. Severe pleuritic pain often signifies a PE located in the distal pulmonary arterial system, near the pleural lining.

Clues to a possible hemodynamically significant PE include: (1) acute cor pulmonale (acute right ventricular failure), with features such as distended neck veins, right-sided S_3 gallop, right ventricular heave, tachycardia, or tachypnea, especially if (2) there are echocardiographic findings of right ventricular dilation and hypokinesis or electrocardiographic evidence of acute cor pulmonale manifested by a new $S_1Q_3T_3$ pattern (Fig. 87.8), new right bundle branch block, or right ventricular ischemia with inferior T wave inversion or with T wave inversion in leads V_1 through V_4. Clinical decision rules can stratify patients into groups with high clinical likelihood or non-high clinical likelihood of PE, using a set of seven bedside assessment questions known as the Wells criteria (Table 87.4).

Differential Diagnosis

The differential diagnosis of PE covers a wide spectrum, from life-threatening conditions—such as MI—to anxiety states (Table 87.5). Concomitant illnesses should be considered. For example, if pneumonia or heart failure does not respond to appropriate therapy, the possibility of coexisting PE should be considered. Idiopathic pulmonary arterial hypertension may manifest with sudden exacerbations that mimic acute PE.

Nonimaging Diagnostic Methods
Plasma D-Dimer Assay

The plasma D-dimer assay is a blood-screening test that relies on the following principle: most patients with PE have ongoing endogenous fibrinolysis that is not effective enough to prevent PE but that nevertheless breaks down some of the fibrin clot to D-dimers, cross-linked fragments of the fibrin protein that are present following fibrinolysis. Although elevated plasma concentrations of D-dimers are sensitive for the diagnosis of PE, they are not specific. Even in the absence of PE, levels are elevated for at least 1 week postoperatively and are abnormally high in patients with MI, sepsis, cancer, or almost any other systemic illness. This test is generally not useful for screening acutely ill hospitalized inpatients, because their D-dimer levels are usually elevated. However, the plasma D-dimer assay is ideally suited for screening outpatients or emergency department patients who have suspected PE but no coexisting acute systemic illness.

A normal plasma D-dimer enzyme-linked immunosorbent assay (ELISA) usually rules out PE in the absence of high clinical suspicion. These patients rarely warrant diagnostic imaging. However, when PE is strongly suspected or the patient has been hospitalized, a D-dimer ELISA should not be obtained, and one should proceed directly to chest computed tomography (CT) imaging.[63] Although the traditional upper limit of normal (ULN) for a D-dimer screening test is 500 ng/mL, the ULN should be increased for patients older than 50 years to 10 times the patient's age.[64] In addition to being a screening test for PE, an elevated D-dimer is an independent correlate of increased mortality and subsequent VTE across a broad variety of disease states.[65]

TABLE 87.3 Most Common Symptoms and Signs of Pulmonary Embolism

Symptoms
Dyspnea
Chest pain, especially pleuritic or "positional"
Anxiety
Cough
Hemoptysis
Leg swelling and pain

Signs
Tachypnea
Tachycardia
Low-grade fever
Jugular venous distension
Tricuspid regurgitant murmur
Accentuated P_2
Leg edema, erythema, tenderness

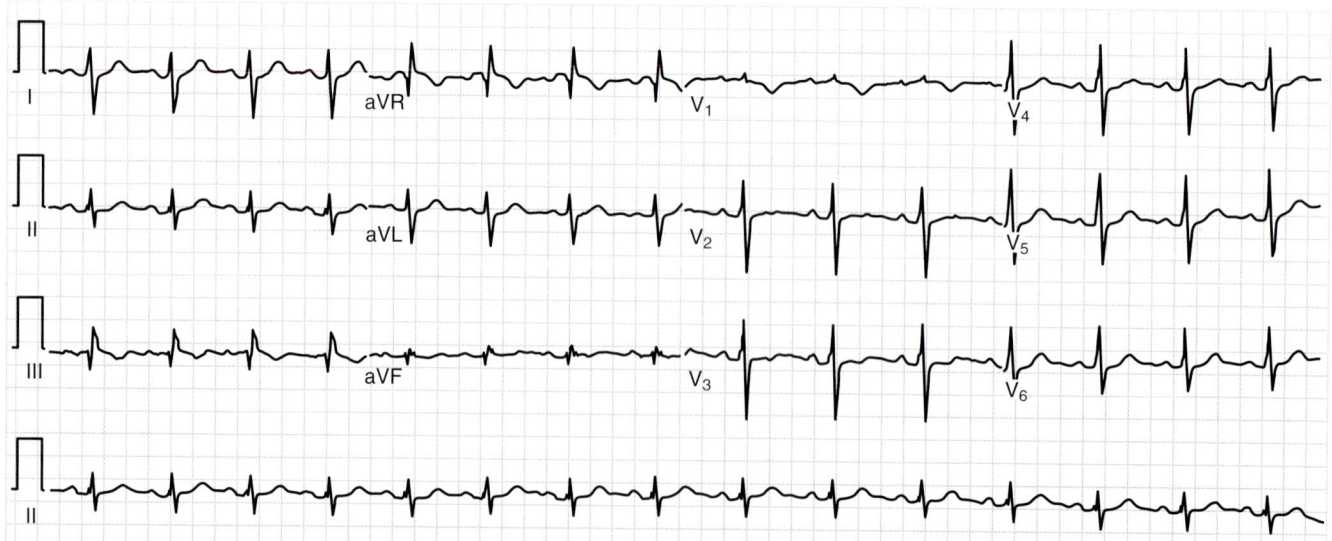

FIGURE 87.8 Electrocardiogram (ECG) from a 33-year-old man who presented with a left main pulmonary artery embolism on chest CT scan. He was hemodynamically stable, with normal right ventricular function on echocardiography. His troponin and brain-type natriuretic peptide (BNP) levels were normal. He was managed with anticoagulation alone. The initial ECG tracing shows an $S_1Q_3T_3$ (leads I and III) with an S wave in lead I, Q wave in lead III, and inverted T wave in lead III, and incomplete right bundle branch block, with inverted or flattened T waves in leads V_1 through V_4.

TABLE 87.4 Classic Wells Criteria to Assess Clinical Likelihood of Pulmonary Embolism

CRITERION	SCORING*
DVT symptoms or signs	3
An alternative diagnosis is less likely than PE	3
Heart rate >100 beats/min	1.5
Immobilization or surgery within 4 weeks	1.5
Previous DVT or PE	1.5
Hemoptysis	1
Cancer treated within 6 months or metastatic	1

DVT, Deep vein thrombosis; *PE*, pulmonary embolism.
*>4 score points = high probability; ≤4 score points = non–high probability.

TABLE 87.5 Differential Diagnosis of Pulmonary Embolism

Acute coronary syndromes
Chronic obstructive pulmonary disease exacerbation
Aortic dissection
Pneumonia
Acute bronchitis
Decompensated heart failure
Pulmonary hypertension
Pericardial disease
Intrathoracic malignancy
Musculoskeletal pain
Pneumothorax
Anxiety
Hepatobiliary or splenic pathology

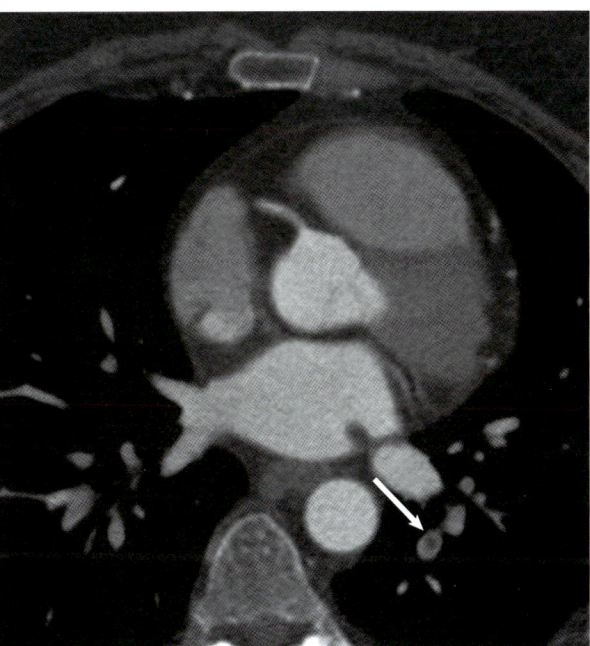

FIGURE 87.9 Small peripheral pulmonary embolism in the left lower lobe (*arrow*). (Courtesy U. Joseph Schoepf, MD.)

Electrocardiogram

The electrocardiogram (ECG) helps exclude other conditions that may present similarly to acute PE, including acute MI and acute pericarditis. This test may lead the clinician toward a PE diagnosis in patients with electrocardiographic manifestations of right-sided heart strain. The most famous sign of right heart strain is the S1Q3T3 pattern, which consists of a deep S wave in lead I, a Q wave in lead III, and an inverted T wave in lead III, but the most common signs are sinus tachycardia and T wave inversion in leads V_1 to V_4 (see Fig. 87.8). Right-sided heart strain is not specific for PE and may be observed in patients with asthma, COPD, or idiopathic pulmonary hypertension. In patients with PE, the ECG may not be especially remarkable and may exhibit only sinus tachycardia, slight ST-segment and T wave abnormalities, or even an entirely normal appearance.

Imaging Methods
Chest Radiography
A near-normal radiographic appearance in the setting of severe respiratory compromise is highly suggestive of PE. Major chest radiographic abnormalities are uncommon. Focal oligemia (Westermark sign) indicates large central embolic occlusion. A peripheral wedge-shaped density above the diaphragm (Hampton hump) usually indicates pulmonary infarction (see Fig. 87.5). A subtle abnormality suggestive of PE is enlargement of the descending right pulmonary artery. The chest radiograph also can help identify patients with diseases that mimic PE, such as lobar pneumonia and pneumothorax, but patients with these illnesses also can have concomitant PE.

Lung Ultrasound
Point-of-care lung ultrasound has gained popularity in the evaluation of patients with dyspnea or chest pain in the emergency department and critical care settings.[66] PE may be suggested by subpleural parenchymal consolidations visible on lung ultrasound when a pulmonary artery occlusion occurs.[67] Peripheral pulmonary consolidations identified on lung ultrasound can be observed in greater than 75% of patients having a PE.[67] While chest CT is still the best modality for PE diagnosis, point-of-care lung ultrasound may be a valuable alternative when clinical suspicion is high and the patient is not stable enough to travel safely to the CT scanner or CT is unavailable.[68] Lung ultrasound can also help distinguish PE from conditions such as heart failure, where B-lines will be present (see Chapter 16, echocardiography).

Chest Computed Tomography (see Chapter 20)
Chest CT has supplanted pulmonary radionuclide perfusion scintigraphy (see below) as the initial imaging test in most patients with suspected PE. Multidetector-row CT scanners can rapidly image the entire chest with submillimeter resolution. Three-dimensional images can be reconstructed, and color can be added electronically to enhance details of thrombus localization. The CT scan helps determine surgical or catheter accessibility to the thrombus in addition to alternative diagnoses that may require different therapy.[69] One cautionary note is that the CT scan may lead to overdiagnosis of PE due to breathing motion artifact or beam-hardening artifact.[70]

The latest generation of scanners can image thrombus in sixth-order vessels. These thrombi are so tiny that their clinical significance is uncertain (Fig. 87.9). The chest CT scan can also detect other pulmonary diseases that manifest in conjunction with PE or explain a clinical presentation that mimics PE. These diseases include pneumonia, atelectasis, pneumothorax, and pleural effusion, which may not be well-visualized on the chest radiograph.

For patients with suspected PE, the CT scan serves as a prognostic and diagnostic test. It shows a 4-chamber view of the heart and images the pulmonary arteries. Careful evaluation of the CT scan can detect signs of right ventricular dysfunction by analyzing (1) right ventricular-to-left ventricular end-diastolic diameter ratio (Fig. 87.10), (2) RV-to-LV volume ratio, (3) interventricular septal bowing toward the LV, and (4) reflux of contrast medium into the inferior vena cava (IVC).[71]

Right ventricular enlargement on CT correlates with right ventricular dysfunction and portends a complicated hospital course often marked by clinical deterioration. A RV-to-LV dimensional ratio of 0.9 or greater on a chest CT scan is abnormal and indicates right ventricular enlargement, correlating with right ventricular dysfunction on echocardiography.

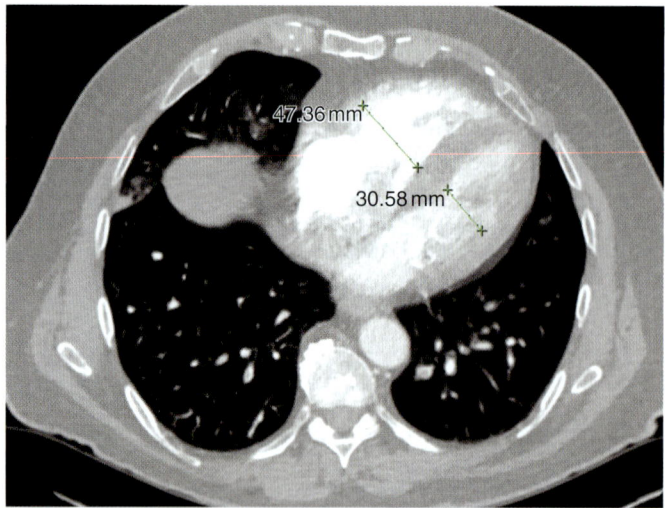

FIGURE 87.10 Enlarged right ventricle on chest CT in a patient with pulmonary embolism (PE). Normally, the ratio of the diameters of the right ventricle and the left ventricle is less than 0.9. This patient has an end-diastolic RV diameter of 47 mm and an end-diastolic LV diameter of 31 mm. The RV-to-LV diameter ratio of 1.5 is abnormally high and correlates with a poor prognosis. *LV*, Left ventricular; *RV*, right ventricular.

Echocardiography (see also Chapter 16)
Echocardiographic findings are normal in approximately half of unselected patients with acute PE, so echocardiography is not recommended as a routine diagnostic test for PE. Echocardiography is, however, a rapid, practical, and sensitive technique for detection of right ventricular overload among patients with established PE and helps identify patients who are at high risk for adverse events following PE. Moderate or severe right ventricular hypokinesis, persistent pulmonary hypertension, patent foramen ovale, and free-floating thrombus in the right atrium (Fig. 87.11A–E) or RV[72] are factors associated with high risk of death or recurrent thromboembolism. The presence of a specific pattern of regional right ventricular dysfunction, known as the "McConnell sign" and characterized by akinesis or dyskinesis of the mid right ventricular free wall with relative sparing of the base and apex, is highly specific for PE and often immediately recognizable by echocardiography (see also Chapter 16, Echocardiography). Echocardiography also can help identify illnesses that may mimic PE, such as MI and pericardial disease.

Venous Ultrasonography
The primary diagnostic criterion for DVT on ultrasound imaging is loss of vein compressibility (Fig. 87.12). Normally, the vein collapses completely when gentle pressure is applied to the overlying skin. Upper-extremity DVT can be more difficult to diagnose than leg DVT because the clavicle can hinder attempts to compress the subclavian vein. At least half of PE patients have no imaging evidence of DVT, probably because the entire DVT embolized to the pulmonary arteries. Therefore, if the level of clinical suspicion of PE is moderate or high, patients without evidence of DVT should undergo further investigation for PE.

Lung Scanning
Pulmonary radionuclide perfusion scintigraphy (lung scanning) uses radiolabeled aggregates of albumin or microspheres that lodge in the pulmonary microvasculature. Patients with large PE often have multiple perfusion defects. If ventilation scanning is performed on a patient with PE but no intrinsic lung disease, a normal ventilation study result is expected, yielding ventilation-perfusion mismatch that is interpreted as a high probability of PE. However, many patients with low-probability scans but with clinical findings strongly suggestive of PE do, in fact, have PE proven by invasive pulmonary angiography. Thus, clinical probability assessment helps to correctly interpret the scan results.

Most lung scans are nondiagnostic. An unequivocal normal or high-probability scan is the exception, not the rule. Interobserver variability is common, even among experts. Two principal indications for obtaining a lung scan are renal insufficiency and an anaphylactic reaction to an intravenous contrast agent that cannot be suppressed with high-dose corticosteroids.

Magnetic Resonance Imaging
Gadolinium-enhanced magnetic resonance angiography (MRA) is far less sensitive than CT for the detection of PE, but unlike chest CT or catheter-based pulmonary angiography, MRA does not require ionizing radiation or injection of an iodinated contrast agent. Pulmonary MRA also can assess right ventricular size and function. Three-dimensional MRA can be performed during a single breath-hold and may provide high resolution from the main pulmonary artery through the segmental pulmonary artery branches. MRA has limited sensitivity for detection of distal PE and cannot be used as a stand-alone test to exclude PE.[73]

Pulmonary Angiography
Invasive pulmonary angiography formerly was the reference standard for the diagnosis of PE but is now rarely performed as a diagnostic test. However, use of this modality is routine when advanced interventions such as pharmacomechanical catheter-assisted therapy are planned. New thrombus usually has a concave edge. Chronic thrombus leads to bandlike defects called webs, in addition to intimal irregularities and abrupt narrowing or occlusion of lobar vessels.

Contrast Venography
Although contrast phlebography was once the reference standard for DVT diagnosis, venograms are rarely obtained now for diagnostic purposes. Venography is the first step, however, for evaluating patients with large femoral or iliofemoral DVT who will undergo invasive pharmacomechanical catheter-directed therapy.

Overall Strategy: An Integrated Diagnostic Approach
Suspected PE can be investigated with a wide array of diagnostic tests. The first step in an integrated diagnostic strategy (Fig. 87.13) is a directed history and physical examination to assess the clinical likelihood of acute PE. The finding of non-high clinical probability is followed by D-dimer testing; a normal D-dimer assay usually rules out PE. If the D-dimer is elevated, chest CT usually provides the definitive diagnosis or exclusion of PE. Electronic decision support at the time of ordering chest CT scans can reduce unwarranted imaging and increase the proportion of test results that are positive for PE.[74]

THERAPY

Risk Stratification (see Chapter 95)
PE manifests with a wide spectrum of acuity ranging from mild to severe. Therefore, rapid and accurate risk stratification is of paramount importance. Summoning the hospital's multidisciplinary PE response team (PERT) may be helpful in this regard.[75] Low-risk patients have an excellent prognosis with anticoagulation alone. High-risk patients may require intensive hemodynamic and respiratory support with pressors, mechanical ventilation, or ECMO.[76,77] In addition to anticoagulation, advanced management[78,79] options include systemic thrombolysis, pharmacomechanical catheter-assisted therapy, vena cava filter placement, or surgical embolectomy (Fig. 87.14).[80,81] The three key components for risk stratification are: (1) clinical evaluation, (2) assessment of right ventricular size and function, and (3) analysis of cardiac biomarkers to determine whether there is right ventricular microinfarction.

Clinical evaluation is straightforward if the PE patient looks and feels well and has no evidence of right ventricular dysfunction. The Pulmonary Embolism Severity Index (PESI) identifies 11 features from demographics, history, and clinical findings that can be weighted and scored to identify low-risk and high-risk patients (Table 87.6).[82] Clinicians should try to detect right ventricular dysfunction on physical examination by looking for distended jugular veins, a palpable

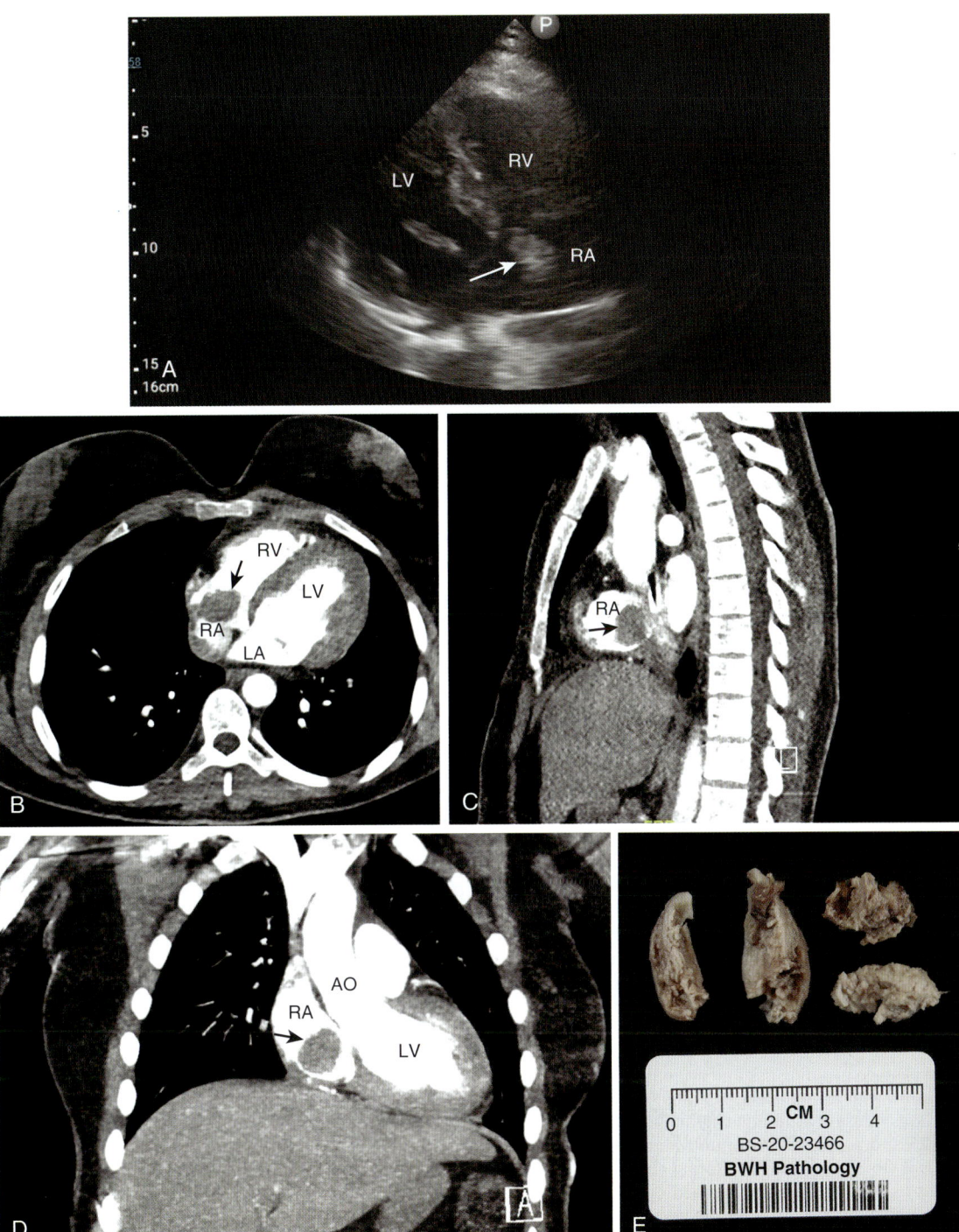

FIGURE 87.11 A, Right atrial thrombus on ECHO in a 60-year-old man with AML, myopericarditis, and cytokine storm due to chemotherapy, with an irregularly shaped 21 × 11 mm mobile mass in the right atrium. The mass intermittently prolapses partially through the tricuspid valve. There is no clear stalk or visible connection to the right atrial wall, interatrial septum, or tricuspid valve. **B** to **D,** Right atrial thrombus on chest CT of a 27-year-old woman with sickle cell disease who suffered three episodes of syncope heralded by lightheadedness and dizziness. Contrast-enhanced chest computed tomogram demonstrates clot-in-transit (black arrow) in a 27-year-old woman with sickle cell anemia. A large 26 × 18 mm filling defect in the right atrium is visualized in the axial (**B**), sagittal (**C**), and coronal views (**D**). *AO,* Aorta; *LA,* left atrium; *LV,* left ventricle; *RA,* right atrium; *RV,* right ventricle. The attending surgeon who excised the mass said, "I think her syncope was due to right ventricular inflow obstruction. The mass at surgery was bobbing in and out in front of the tricuspid valve, shutting down substantial flow into the right ventricle when in certain positions." **E,** Surgically excised right atrial thrombus seen on chest CT in **B** to **D**. It was *pink-red* and friable and measured 4.6 × 3.7 × 2.1 cm. The pathologist stated, "It does look mostly chronic with only a little bit of fresher thrombus." (Kindly provided by Robert F. Padera, MD, PhD, and Richard N. Mitchell, MD, PhD.)

left parasternal lift, a systolic murmur of tricuspid regurgitation, or an accentuated P_2. Clinical evaluation should integrate the results of electrocardiography that might show a right ventricular strain pattern (right bundle branch block, $S_1Q_3T_3$, negative T waves in leads V_1 through V_4), chest CT, echocardiography, and cardiac biomarkers of right ventricular microinfarction.

Parenteral Anticoagulation

Anticoagulation is the cornerstone of treatment for acute PE. Heparin, the most commonly used parenteral anticoagulant, acts primarily by binding to antithrombin, a protein that inhibits the coagulation factors thrombin (factor IIa) and factors Xa, IXa, XIa, and XIIa. Heparin subsequently promotes a conformational change

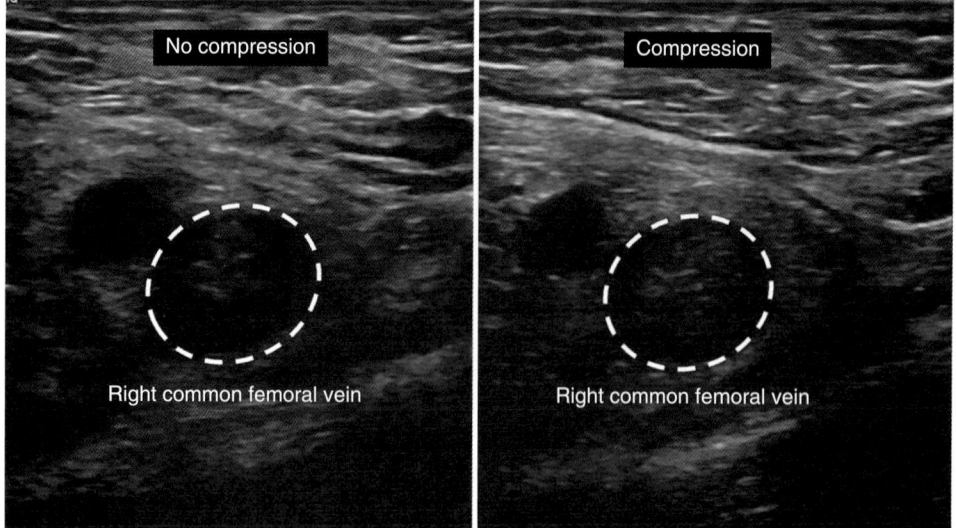

FIGURE 87.12 Acute right common femoral deep vein thrombosis (DVT) diagnosed by venous ultrasound examination of the leg. *Left:* Without compression. A cross-section of the right common femoral vein. The right common femoral vein is dilated. Thrombotic material can be visualized within the vein. The right common femoral artery is a smaller vessel, pulsating in real time, and is located at about 10 o'clock relative to the right common femoral vein. *Right:* With compression. Thrombotic material can be visualized within the vein. The dilated right common femoral vein fails to compress despite the technologist's firm pressure over the vein. Failure to compress the vein with manual pressure is the primary criterion for the diagnosis of DVT with venous ultrasound imaging. (Courtesy Gregory Piazza, MD, MS.)

in antithrombin that accelerates its activity approximately 100- to 1000-fold, thus preventing additional thrombus formation. Heparin does *not* directly dissolve thrombus. However, endogenous fibrinolytic mechanisms may lyse some of the previously formed thrombus. Beyond its anticoagulant activity, heparin also exerts pleiotropic effects, including antiinflammatory[83] and vasodilatory properties.[84]

Unfractionated Heparin

Unfractionated heparin (UFH) is a highly sulfated glycosaminoglycan that is partially purified, most often from pig intestinal mucosa. The intensity of continuous infusion intravenous UFH anticoagulation can be titrated by adjusting the infusion rate to reach a goal aPTT. The short half-life of UFH is advantageous for patients who may require subsequent insertion of an IVC filter, systemic thrombolysis, catheter-directed pharmacomechanical therapy, or surgical embolectomy.

For patients with average bleeding risk and normal hepatic function, UFH should be started with an intravenous bolus of 80 units/kg, followed by a continuous infusion at 18 units/kg/hr. The aPTT should be targeted between 1.5 and 2.5 times the control value. The therapeutic range commonly is 60 to 80 seconds. Monitoring continuous intravenous UFH infusions using anti-Xa assays (instead of aPTT) has some advantages, particularly in ill patients with multisystem organ failure, because this approach measures heparin's effect directly. It is especially useful for patients with a baseline elevated aPTT, such as those with lupus anticoagulant. The target level for therapeutic dosing is 0.3 to 0.7 units/mL.

Low-Molecular-Weight Heparin

LMWH consists of fragments of UFH that exhibit less binding to plasma proteins and endothelial cells. It therefore has greater bioavailability, with a more predictable dose response and a longer half-life compared with UFH. These features permit weight-based LMWH dosing without laboratory tests because no dose adjustment is needed in most cases. LMWH is gaining popularity for initial anticoagulation of intermediate-risk and high-risk PE because of the concern that administration of UFH does not rapidly and consistently achieve full therapeutic efficacy. The kidneys metabolize LMWH, and patients with renal impairment require downward adjustment of LMWH dosing. If a quantitative assay is desired, an anti-Xa level can be obtained. Whether use of anti-Xa levels improves efficacy and safety remains controversial.

Fondaparinux

Fondaparinux is an anticoagulant pentasaccharide that specifically inhibits activated factor X. It can be thought of as an ultra-low-molecular-weight heparin. Fondaparinux's predictable and sustained pharmacokinetic properties allow a fixed-dose, once-daily subcutaneous injection, without the need for coagulation laboratory monitoring or dose adjustment. Fondaparinux has a 17-hour half-life, and its elimination is prolonged in patients with renal impairment. Fondaparinux is indicated for the initial treatment of acute PE and acute DVT. It is often used off-label for the management of suspected or proven heparin-induced thrombocytopenia (HIT) because it does not cross-react with heparin-induced antibodies.[85]

Heparin-Induced Thrombocytopenia

HIT is an immune-mediated complication of heparin.[86] It occurs more often with UFH than with LMWH. Immunoglobulin G antibodies bind to a heparin-platelet factor 4 complex to activate platelets, causing the release of prothrombotic microparticles. The microparticles promote excessive thrombin generation, which can result in paradoxical thrombosis despite thrombocytopenia. The thrombosis usually manifests as extensive and often bilateral DVT (sometimes affecting one upper extremity and one lower extremity) or PE, but presentations of MI, stroke, and unusual arterial thrombosis (such as mesenteric arterial thrombosis) also have been described.

The "4T Point Score" is a semiquantitative clinical screening test for HIT.[87] The four components are (1) **T**hrombocytopenia, (2) **T**iming of decrease in platelet count, (3) **T**hrombosis or other sequelae such as skin necrosis, and (4) absence of o**T**her explanation. HIT should be suspected when the platelet count decreases to less than 100,000 or to less than 50% of baseline. The thrombocytopenia is usually mild, in the range of 40,000 to 70,000. Typically, HIT occurs after 5 to 10 days of heparin exposure, most often in cardiac surgical ICUs. ELISA testing quantifies antiplatelet factor 4 (PF4)/heparin antibody levels, which are measured in optical density (OD) units. The higher the OD value, the more likely the diagnosis of HIT with thrombosis.[88] The serotonin release assay is the gold standard laboratory test for HIT.

When HIT is diagnosed, UFH or LMWH should be discontinued immediately, and patients should not receive platelet transfusions. Heparin "flushes" of intravenous lines should also be discontinued. For HIT with thrombosis, a parenteral direct thrombin inhibitor such as argatroban or bivalirudin should be used.

Warfarin Anticoagulation

Warfarin is a vitamin K antagonist, first approved for clinical use in 1954. It prevents gamma-carboxylation activation of coagulation factors II, VII, IX, and X. The full anticoagulant effect of warfarin becomes evident after 5 to 7 days, even if the prothrombin time, used to monitor warfarin's effect, becomes elevated more rapidly. For patients with VTE, the usual target INR range is between 2.0 and 3.0. Self-monitoring of INRs improves patient satisfaction and quality of life and may reduce the rate of bleeding and thromboembolic events.

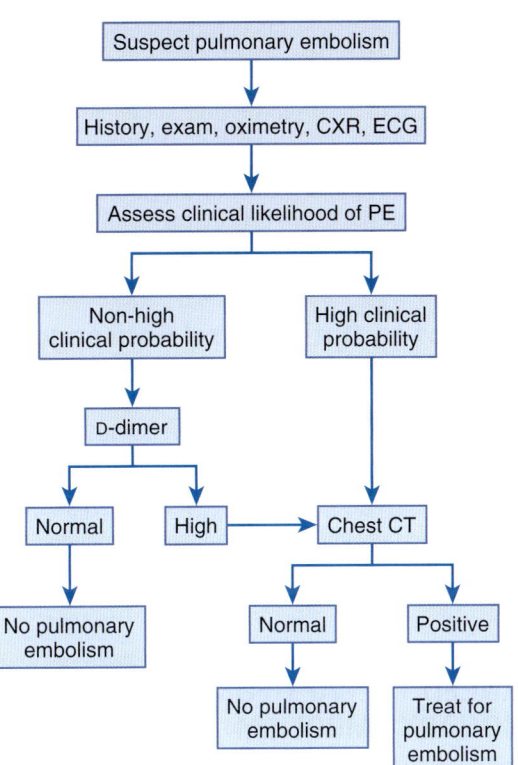

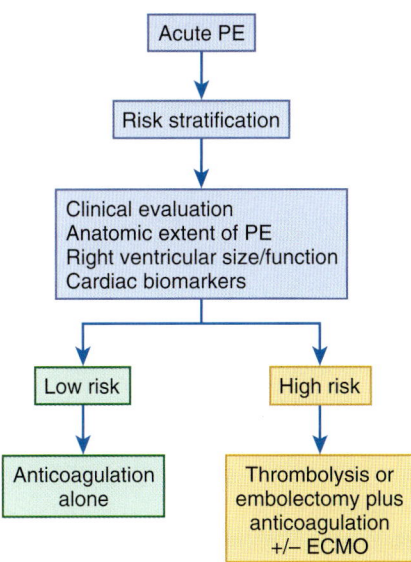

FIGURE 87.14 Management strategy for acute pulmonary embolism (PE), based on risk stratification. *ECMO*, Extracorporeal membrane oxygenation.

FIGURE 87.13 Integrated diagnostic approach for acute PE. *CXR*, Chest x-ray.

Warfarin Overlap with Heparin

Initiation of warfarin as monotherapy to treat acute VTE without UFH, LMWH, or fondaparinux may paradoxically exacerbate hypercoagulability, increasing the likelihood of recurrent thrombosis, by decreasing the levels of two endogenous anticoagulants, proteins C and S. Overlapping warfarin for at least 5 days with an immediately effective parenteral anticoagulant counteracts the procoagulant effect of unopposed warfarin.

Dosing and Monitoring of Warfarin

Dosing warfarin is both an art and a science. Warfarin traditionally is dosed using an "educated guess" coupled with trial and error. Many physicians begin with 5 mg daily. Debilitated or older adult patients require a reduced dose. High INRs from excessive warfarin predispose to bleeding complications. Warfarin-related major bleeding is the most common reason for adverse drug events and subsequent emergency hospitalization in older Americans. In contrast, subtherapeutic dosing makes patients vulnerable to recurrent VTE. All patients taking warfarin should wear a medical alert bracelet or necklace in case they require rapid reversal of warfarin. Warfarin also can have nonhemorrhagic side effects, such as alopecia and increased levels of arterial calcification.[89] In addition, warfarin may induce osteoporotic fractures.[90] Some patients complain of fatigue and "feeling cold".

Warfarin therapy is further plagued by multiple drug-drug and drug-food interactions. Centralized anticoagulation clinics, staffed by nurses or pharmacists, have eased the administrative burden of prescribing warfarin and have facilitated safer and more effective anticoagulation.

Warfarin "Bridging"

When patients undergo elective surgery or procedures such as colonoscopy, warfarin is temporarily discontinued. To ensure continued perioperative anticoagulation, "bridging" with LMWH used to be prescribed preoperatively while the warfarin activity washed out. However, the BRIDGE trial of atrial fibrillation patients showed that forgoing bridging was associated with a 59% reduction in major bleeding complications.[91] Subsequently, the practice of routine bridging has fallen out of favor.[92] Now, we forgo bridging with only a few exceptions, such as extreme thrombophilia or mechanical heart valves. For almost all patients, we instruct them to hold warfarin preoperatively (usually for 4 days) and on the day of surgery.

Novel Oral Anticoagulants

NOACs (see also Chapter 95) have a rapid onset of action and provide full anticoagulation within several hours of ingestion. They are prescribed in fixed doses without laboratory coagulation monitoring and have minimal drug-drug or drug-food interactions. These agents have a short half-life, so when they are stopped for an invasive diagnostic or surgical procedure, no bridging is needed. We usually instruct patients to hold NOACs for two days preoperatively and on the day of surgery. For VTE treatment, NOACs are noninferior to warfarin for efficacy and are superior to warfarin for safety.[93] In a meta-analysis of 24,455 patients with acute VTE, NOACs compared with warfarin had a 40% reduction in major bleeding, 61% reduction in nonfatal intracranial bleeding, and 64% reduction in fatal bleeding.[94]

Evolution of Oral Anticoagulants for Pulmonary Embolism and Deep Vein Thrombosis Treatment

Four NOACs are licensed for VTE treatment: dabigatran (an oral thrombin inhibitor),[95,96] and three factor Xa inhibitors[97]: rivaroxaban,[98,99] apixaban,[100] and edoxaban (Table 87.7).[101] For extended therapy after an initial 6-month course of anticoagulation, dabigatran was compared with warfarin and with placebo.[102] Rivaroxaban[98] and apixaban[103] were also compared against placebo in extended-therapy trials. These randomized trials showed that NOACs—in the doses tested—are safe and effective for extended-duration anticoagulation.

In children, the first major study of NOACs versus warfarin was undertaken with rivaroxaban. This global study included children from 107 pediatric hospitals in 28 countries. They all had documented acute VTE and had started heparin in the hospital. They were randomized to rivaroxaban versus warfarin in this 3-month, open-label trial. Rivaroxaban resulted in a similar low VTE recurrence risk and similar bleeding rate compared with standard warfarin anticoagulation.[104]

Managing Bleeding Complications from Anticoagulants

Protamine sulfate can be given for life-threatening bleeding caused by UFH or LMWH. Life-threatening bleeding caused by warfarin can be

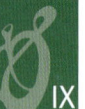

TABLE 87.6 Pulmonary Embolism Severity Index and Simplified Pulmonary Embolism Severity Index: Predictors of Prognostic Risk

PESI Criteria*	
Age >80 years	Age in years
Male gender	+10
History of cancer	+30
History of heart failure	+10
History of chronic lung disease	+10
Heart rate ≥110 beats/min	+20
Systolic blood pressure <100 mm Hg	+30
Respiratory rate ≥30 breaths/min	+20
Temperature <36°C	+20
Altered mental status	+60
Arterial oxygen saturation <90%	+20
Simplified PESI† Criteria	
Age >80 years	+1
History of cancer	+1
History of heart failure or chronic lung disease	+1
Heart rate ≥110 beats/min	+1
Systolic blood pressure <100 mm Hg	+1
Arterial oxygen saturation <90%	+1

PE, Pulmonary embolism; *PESI*, Pulmonary Embolism Severity Index.
*Class 1 = ≤65; class 2 = 66 to 85; class 3 = 86 to 105; class 4 = 106 to 125; class 5 ≥126. In the PESI score, classes 1 and 2 are considered low risk, and classes 3 to 5 are considered high risk.
†Patients with a score of 0 are considered to be at low risk for PE; those with scores ≥1 are considered at high risk.

managed with prothrombin complex concentrates (PCC) to achieve immediate hemostasis.[105] For major bleeding, use idarucizumab to reverse dabigatran[106,107] and andexanet alfa to reverse rivaroxaban, apixaban, or edoxaban[108,109]

OPTIMAL DURATION OF ANTICOAGULATION AND SELECTION OF OPTIMAL ANTICOAGULANT

Risk of Recurrent Venous Thromboembolism after Discontinuation of Anticoagulation

VTE is associated with a high risk of recurrence after discontinuation of anticoagulation. Cardiovascular inflammation may explain the recurrent nature of VTE.[110] Accordingly, VTE is a chronic illness for many individuals, recurring in about 30% to 40% of patients who stop anticoagulation within 10 years after an initial event.[111–113] After discontinuing anticoagulation, men suffer recurrent VTE more often than women. In a meta-analysis of 7515 patients from 18 studies, men had a 41% recurrent VTE rate versus 29% for women at 10 years following the initial VTE.[114]

Persistent thrombus imaged on chest CT does not predict recurrent PE. Approximately half of patients with PE will have persistent thrombus on chest CT 6 months after the initial event. Abnormally elevated D-dimer levels after withdrawal of anticoagulation may signify ongoing hypercoagulability. However, the risk for recurrence in patients with a first unprovoked VTE who have a subsequent negative D-dimer result is not low enough to justify stopping anticoagulant therapy. In 319 patients with a negative D-dimer after completing 3 to 7 months of anticoagulation, the rate of recurrent VTE was 6.7% per patient-year.[115]

How to Determine the Optimal Duration of Anticoagulation

Until recently, most evidence-based clinical practice guidelines have dichotomized VTE into "provoked" and "unprovoked" silos. Such guidelines recommended extended treatment in patients with "unprovoked," or idiopathic, VTE. However, the definition of "provoked" VTE is challenging because triggers may be subtle, and recurrence risk can be high in those with clear provocation but enduring predisposing factors.[113,116] Accordingly, the 2019 ESC guidelines no longer endorse the terminology "provoked" and "unprovoked."[39] Instead, an individualized risk assessment is proposed in which only patients with an estimated recurrence risk of less than 3% per year should receive time-limited anticoagulant therapy. Attempts to refine prediction, including gender-specific models, have been proposed.[117,118]

Selection of an Optimal Oral Anticoagulant for Extended-Duration Anticoagulation

Apixaban, rivaroxaban, dabigatran, and warfarin have all been shown to safely and effectively reduce VTE recurrence in randomized trials of extended treatment (see Table 87.7). Low-intensity DOAC regimens offer enhanced safety while maintaining efficacy for long-term secondary prevention.[119,120] Low-dose aspirin has been investigated as an alternative for extended treatment but is only recommended for patients who refuse or are unable to tolerate anticoagulation.[39] Meta-analyses have confirmed the net clinical benefit of DOACs over warfarin, aspirin, or placebo.[121,122]

ADVANCED THERAPY FOR ACUTE PULMONARY EMBOLISM

Patients with high-risk PE or intermediate-high-risk PE that decompensates or fails to improve on anticoagulation generally warrant advanced therapy. Options include full-dose systemic fibrinolysis, half-dose systemic fibrinolysis, catheter-based therapy with or without fibrinolysis, surgical embolectomy, and IVC filter placement.

High-Risk Pulmonary Embolism

Multidisciplinary PERTs are being set up throughout the United States to immediately evaluate patients who present with high- or intermediate-high-risk PE. Team members have subspecialized cognitive and technical skills in PE, and the team approach promotes consensus and a unified, reasoned plan for the individual patient.[123,124]

Systemic Fibrinolysis Administered Through a Peripheral Vein. Fibrinolysis reverses right-sided heart failure by physical dissolution of anatomically obstructing pulmonary arterial thrombus. The hallmarks of successful therapy are reduction of right ventricular pressure overload and prevention of continued release of serotonin and other neurohumoral factors that exacerbate pulmonary hypertension.

When prescribing fibrinolysis, there are three dosing intensities: (1) full-dose systemic (licensed), (2) half-dose systemic (prescribed "off-label"), or (3) low-dose catheter-directed therapy.[78] The FDA has approved alteplase for high-risk PE, in a dose of 100 mg delivered through a peripheral vein as a continuous infusion over 2 hours, without concomitant heparin. Patients who receive fibrinolysis up to 14 days after onset of new symptoms or signs can derive benefit. Intracranial hemorrhage is the most feared and severe complication.

A meta-analysis examined patients randomized to fibrinolytic therapy versus anticoagulation alone, with most patients classified as intermediate-risk PE (1775 out of a total of 2115) because they had hemodynamic stability despite right ventricular dysfunction. Fibrinolysis resulted in a 47% reduction in all-cause mortality, a 60% decrease in recurrent PE, a 2.7-fold increased risk of major bleeding, and a 4.6-fold increased risk of intracranial hemorrhage.[125]

An alternative strategy has focused on half-dose systemic fibrinolysis. However, propensity-score-matched studies comparing outcomes in 3768 patients receiving 50 mg versus full-dose 100 mg of alteplase for PE demonstrated that half-dose fibrinolysis was associated with an increased requirement for treatment escalation (53.8% vs. 41.4%; p < 0.01), driven largely by rescue fibrinolysis (25.9% vs. 7.3%; p < 0.01) and catheter-directed therapy (14.2% vs. 3.8%; p< 0.01).[126] Furthermore, rates of hospital mortality (13% vs. 15%; p = 0.3), intracranial bleeding

TABLE 87.7 Novel Oral Anticoagulants for Venous Thromboembolism

DRUG/STUDY NAME	NOAC	WARFARIN
Dabigatran/ RE-COVER	(N = 1274)	(N = 1265)
	2.4% recurrence	2.1% recurrence
Dabigatran/ RE-MEDY	(N = 1430)	(N = 1426)
	1.8% recurrence	1.3% recurrence
Dabigatran/ RE-COVER II	(N = 1279)	(N = 1289)
	2.3% recurrence	2.2% recurrence
Rivaroxaban/ EINSTEIN Acute DVT	(N = 1731)	(N = 1718)
	2.1% recurrence	3.0% recurrence
Rivaroxaban/ EINSTEIN-PE	(N = 2420)	(N = 2413)
	2.1% recurrence;	1.8% recurrence;
	1.1% major bleeding	2.2% major bleeding
Apixaban AMPLIFY	(N = 2691)	(N = 2704)
	2.3% recurrence	2.7% recurrence
	0.6% major bleeding	1.8% major bleeding
Edoxaban/Hokusai—VTE	(N = 4143)	(N = 4149)
	3.2% recurrence	3.5% recurrence
	8.5% clinically relevant bleeding	10.3% clinically relevant bleeding
DRUG/STUDY NAME	**NOAC**	**PLACEBO**
Dabigatran/RE-SONATE	(N = 681)	(N = 662)
	0.4% recurrence	5.6% recurrence
Rivaroxaban/EINSTEIN DVT Continued Treatment	(N = 602)	(N = 594)
	1.3% recurrence	7.1% recurrence
Apixaban Extension VTE	(N = 829)	(N = 840)
	1.7% recurrence	8.8% recurrence
Einstein Choice	Rivaroxaban 20 mg (N = 1107)	Aspirin 100 mg (N = 1131)
	1.5%	4.4%
	Rivaroxaban 10 mg (N = 1127)	
	1.2%	

(0.5% vs. 0.4%; p = 0.67), gastrointestinal hemorrhage (1.6% vs. 1.6%; p = 0.99), and anemia (6.9% vs. 4.6%; p = 0.11) were similar.

Advances in Catheter-Based Therapy

The 1% to 3% rate of intracranial hemorrhage in patients with PE receiving systemic fibrinolysis has dampened enthusiasm for this potential life-saving therapy. Catheter-based reperfusion, however, holds the promise of efficacy, with lower rates of major bleeding owing to lower doses of a fibrinolytic agent or no need for fibrinolysis at all. Catheter-based therapy for acute PE includes pharmacomechanical therapy, catheter-directed fibrinolysis, and mechanical embolectomy. Catheter-based therapy that combines local fibrinolysis with mechanical thrombus "conditioning" may increase the efficacy of thrombus dissolution via higher local fibrinolytic drug concentrations and a greater exposed thrombus surface area. Because higher local drug concentration is achieved with a lower overall dose of fibrinolytic agent, catheter-based fibrinolysis may offer the advantage of decreased hemorrhagic complications.

Ultrasound-facilitated, catheter-directed fibrinolysis has been the most rigorously studied of these catheter-based techniques. In a European-based randomized controlled trial of 59 patients with intermediate-risk PE, ultrasound-facilitated, catheter-directed fibrinolysis with 20 mg of t-PA plus anticoagulation reduced a surrogate endpoint, RV-diameter-to-LV-diameter (RV-to-LV) ratio, from baseline to 24 hours to a greater extent than anticoagulation.[127] In the US-based, single-arm, multicenter SEATTLE II trial, the safety and efficacy of ultrasound-facilitated, catheter-directed fibrinolysis (24 mg t-PA) was assessed in 150 patients with high- (N = 31) or intermediate-risk (N = 119) PE.[128] Mean RV-to-LV ratio decreased by 25%, mean pulmonary artery systolic pressure decreased by 30%, and mean modified Miller angiographic obstruction index diminished by 30% from pre-procedure to 48 hours post-procedure. Major bleeding occurred in 10% of patients with no intracranial hemorrhage. In 2014, the FDA cleared ultrasound-facilitated, catheter-directed fibrinolysis for PE treatment. In a subsequent dose-ranging trial, four accelerated-dosing regimens (8 mg/2 hours, 8 mg/4 hours, 12 mg/6 hours, and 24 mg/6 hours) for ultrasound-facilitated, catheter-directed fibrinolysis were evaluated in 101 patients with intermediate-risk PE.[129] All four regimens improved RV function comparable to 24 mg of t-PA administered over 12 to 24 hours, based on the CT-measured RV-to-LV ratio from baseline to 48 hours. A study utilizing a novel technique for three-dimensional reconstruction of the pulmonary vasculature from chest CT data obtained in the SEATTLE II trial showed that reduction in RV volume correlated with increased blood volume through the small peripheral, rather than large proximal, pulmonary arteries.[130] These data suggest that ultrasound-facilitated, catheter-directed fibrinolysis may relieve RV pressure overload via distal pulmonary artery reperfusion.

Purely mechanical catheter embolectomy techniques may have a niche in PE patients with contraindications to fibrinolytic therapy. The FlowTriever system (Inari Medical, Irvine, CA) is a large-bore device that mechanically engages thrombus via three self-expanding nitinol disks and then aspirates the thrombus. In a US-based, single-arm, multicenter study of 106 patients with intermediate-risk PE, embolectomy with the FlowTriever system resulted in a 25% reduction

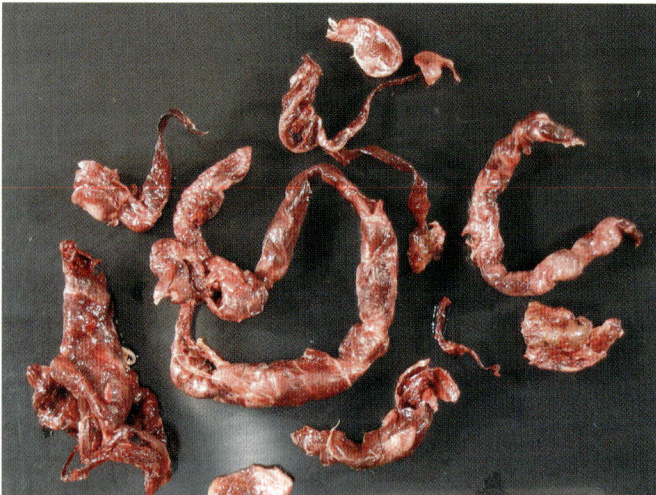

FIGURE 87.15 Surgical pulmonary embolectomy specimen in a 72-year-old woman who presented with presyncope, hypotension, and hypoxia. She was diagnosed with massive pulmonary embolism (PE) by chest CT scan and underwent successful emergency pulmonary embolectomy.

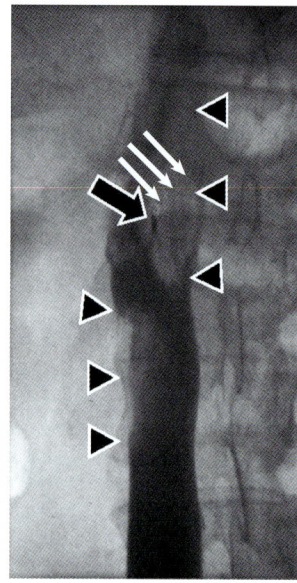

FIGURE 87.16 Large pulmonary embolism (PE)-in-transit, with thrombus (*arrowheads*) trapped below and visualized above the Bard Eclipse inferior vena cava filter. The force of the embolizing deep vein thrombosis (DVT) displaced one of the filter struts (*white arrows*). The "hook" to retrieve the filter is marked with the *black arrow*.

in CT-measured RV-to-LV ratio and 10% decrease in mean modified Miller index.[131] In the study, six major adverse events occurred within 48 hours of the procedure, including one major hemorrhage. The FlowTriever device received FDA clearance for treatment of PE in 2018. The Indigo Thrombectomy System (Penumbra, Inc, Alameda, CA) is a smaller-bore aspiration catheter that does not require fibrinolytic administration and was evaluated in a single-arm study of 119 patients with intermediate-risk PE (ClinicalTrials.gov identifier: NCT03218566). The Indigo System is intended for the removal of fresh, soft emboli and thrombi from vessels of the peripheral and venous systems using continuous aspiration. Treatment with the Indigo device resulted in a 27% reduction in the mean CT-measured RV-to-LV diameter ratio and was associated with three major adverse events.[132] It received FDA clearance in 2019.

Catheter-directed fibrinolysis without mechanical thrombus disruption has undergone limited prospective evaluation and may be a consideration for patients with high-risk or intermediate-high-risk PE,[133] although the data remain limited.[134] The 2019 ESC Guidelines offer catheter-based therapy as an alternative to surgical embolectomy for patients with high-risk PE in whom systemic fibrinolysis has failed or is contraindicated (Class IIa; Level of Evidence C) and as an alternative to systemic fibrinolysis in other PE patients who have experienced hemodynamic deterioration despite anticoagulation (Class IIa; Level of Evidence C).[39]

Surgical Embolectomy

Surgical embolectomy has reemerged for the management of patients with high-risk PE or intermediate-high-risk PE with severe right ventricular dysfunction and clinical deterioration despite anticoagulation, in whom contraindications preclude thrombolysis (Fig. 87.15). This procedure is also suitable for patients with acute PE who require surgical excision of a right atrial thrombus, closure of a patent foramen ovale, or excision of a clot-in-transit (Fig. 87.16). Surgical embolectomy can also be used as rescue therapy for patients whose PE is refractory to thrombolysis. Results are best when patients undergo surgery before they become pressor-dependent and before the onset of cardiogenic shock and multisystem organ failure.[135] Avoiding blind instrumentation of the fragile pulmonary arteries is imperative. Extraction is limited to directly visible clots. In experienced centers, surgical pulmonary embolectomy has been shown to be safe and effective.[136]

Inferior Vena Cava Filters

IVC filter insertion is considered in acute VTE patients (regardless of the size or clinical severity of the VTE) with contraindications to anticoagulation or with recurrent PE despite therapeutic anticoagulation.

Until recently, IVC filter insertion had also been considered on an individual basis for patients with intermediate- or high-risk PE who were tolerating therapeutic anticoagulation but in whom there was concern that a subsequent PE would likely be fatal. Such an indication was the focus of the PREPIC2 trial which randomly assigned 399 normotensive patients with acute PE, concomitant lower-extremity DVT, and at least 1 risk factor for adverse outcomes to retrievable IVC filter implantation plus anticoagulation versus anticoagulation alone.[137] Adjunctive insertion of a retrievable IVC filter, compared with anticoagulation alone, failed to reduce the risk of symptomatic recurrent PE or mortality at 3 or 6 months. In a meta-analysis of randomized controlled trials and prospective observational studies, IVC filters appear to reduce the short-term risk of subsequent PE, increase the long-term risk for DVT, and have no impact on overall mortality.[138]

Data demonstrate that retrievable IVC filters can be removed safely and easily, yet up to 50% remain permanently indwelling.[139] Device-related complications include strut fracture, filter migration, strut embolization, device tilt, IVC penetration, perforation of surrounding structures, PE, DVT, and IVC thrombosis. To avoid these complications, IVC filters should be retrieved as soon as no longer necessary and after anticoagulation has been safely started.

Deep Vein Thrombosis Interventions

Indications for catheter-directed DVT thrombolysis remain uncertain but usually include extensive iliofemoral and upper-extremity venous thrombosis. In Norway, the CaVenT study randomly assigned 209 patients with iliofemoral DVT to receive catheter-directed thrombolysis versus conventional therapy with LMWH bridging to warfarin. At 24 months, the frequency of PTS was 56% in the conventionally treated group, compared with 41% in the intervention group (p= 0.047). Iliofemoral patency was present in 66% of the intervention group, compared with 47% of the group receiving conventional anticoagulation.[140] The US-based ATTRACT trial randomly assigned 692 patients with acute iliofemoral or femoral DVT to receive either anticoagulation alone (LMWH or UFH) or anticoagulation and pharmacomechanical therapy.[141] Pharmacochemical therapy did not reduce the risk of PTS (47% in the intervention group vs. 48% in the anticoagulation alone group; RR, 0.96; 95% CI, 0.82 to 1.11), and resulted in a higher risk of major hemorrhage (1.7% vs. 0.3%; RR, 6.18; 95% CI, 0.78 to 49.2). Patients treated with catheter-directed thrombolysis had decreased rates of moderate-to-severe PTS, but quality of life did not differ. Based on these findings, pharmacomechanical therapy for acute lower-extremity DVT should be performed in experienced centers and reserved for highly selected patients with iliofemoral disease, severe symptoms or limb-threatening disease, and a low risk of bleeding.

Therapy in Patients with Cancer

LMWH has been traditionally prescribed as monotherapy without oral anticoagulation for cancer patients with VTE. In one randomized trial, dalteparin monotherapy reduced the recurrent VTE rate by about half compared with warfarin.[142] In a subsequent trial of tinzaparin monotherapy versus warfarin in cancer patients, tinzaparin-treated patients had an approximate 40% lower bleeding rate than those treated with warfarin.[143]

For cancer patients with acute VTE, NOACs are supplanting LMWH monotherapy, especially in patients who do not have gastrointestinal cancers. In the HOKUSAI-VTE Cancer trial of edoxaban versus dalteparin, edoxaban had less recurrent VTE than dalteparin but also had more major bleeding, primarily gastrointestinal.[144] Similarly, in the SELECT-D trial of rivaroxaban versus dalteparin, rivaroxaban had a lower rate of recurrent VTE but a higher rate of clinically relevant non-major bleeding than dalteparin.[145] The NCCN gave a top-tier recommendation to consider edoxaban or rivaroxaban when treating cancer patients with acute VTE and gave a limited recommendation to consider dabigatran or apixaban in situations where LMWH monotherapy was contraindicated or when patients declined LMWH injections.[20] Subsequently, the Caravaggio trial of apixaban versus dalteparin in 1155 cancer patients with acute VTE found that apixaban was noninferior to dalteparin both in preventing recurrent VTE and with respect to major bleeding.[146] There was a 5.6% recurrence rate with apixaban compared with a 7.9% recurrence rate with dalteparin (HR, 0.63; 95% CI, 0.37 to 1.07; p < 0.001 for noninferiority).

Treatment of Superficial Thrombophlebitis

Short-term use of fondaparinux (2.5 mg once daily for 45 days) is the best validated anticoagulation strategy.[147] In a randomized, open-label, noninferiority study of fondaparinux 2.5 mg daily versus rivaroxaban 10 mg daily for patients with superficial thrombophlebitis, rivaroxaban was found to be noninferior to fondaparinux and was not associated with more major bleeding.[140]

Therapy in Patients with Antiphospholipid Syndrome and Factor V Leiden

Antiphospholipid syndrome patients have an acquired, not a genetic, thrombophilia. They are susceptible to MI and stroke as well as to VTE. These patients are traditionally anticoagulated with warfarin rather than with NOACs. If anticoagulation is discontinued after a PE or DVT has occurred, these patients are at very high risk of suffering a recurrent event, with an incidence of at least 8% per year. In a randomized trial of rivaroxaban versus warfarin in patients with *severe* antiphospholipid syndrome, the trial was stopped early because rivaroxaban patients suffered more frequent thromboembolism than warfarin patients (12% vs. zero) and more major bleeding complications (7% vs. 3%).[149] However, with *mild* or *moderately severe* antiphospholipid syndrome, clinicians are prescribing NOACs rather than warfarin with increasing frequency.

Factor V Leiden is the most frequently diagnosed thrombophilia. It is genetic (autosomal dominant), not acquired. These patients are at higher-than-average risk of suffering a first-time acute PE or DVT. VTE is especially common if these individuals are taking estrogen-containing contraceptives. During pregnancy, they are susceptible to first-trimester miscarriage, presumed due to placental vein thrombosis, as well as to VTE. Two poorly understood observations about factor V Leiden are: (1) DVTs have a low embolization rate and if they do embolize, the PEs are typically smaller and less life-threatening than average; (2) the rate of recurrent VTE is not higher among Leiden patients compared with non-Leiden patients.

Therapy in Pediatric Populations

Guidelines for the use of anticoagulants in pediatrics are largely extrapolated from large randomized controlled trials in adults, smaller dose-finding and observational studies in children, and expert opinion. Randomized clinical trials of NOACs in pediatric VTE are ongoing.[150] More than 200 children participated in an open-label, single-arm, prospective cohort trial of dabigatran. Pharmacokinetics and pharmacodynamics of dabigatran were similar to those in adult VTE patients. Dabigatran showed a favorable safety profile for treating VTE in children aged ≥3 months to < 18 years.[151]

Emotional Support

PE impairs quality of life. In young adults diagnosed with VTE, the prescription of psychotropic drugs doubled compared with age- and gender-matched controls. Antidepressants were most frequently prescribed (53%), followed by sedatives (22%), anxiolytics (20%), and antipsychotics (5%).[152] VTE exacts a psychological toll on patients; many wonder if they will suffer a recurrent event and worry about the potential burden on their families, a diminished quality of life, and a shortened life span.[153]

Patients find PE to be emotionally draining, and they, along with their families, want to be reassured that they can expect good outcomes once the diagnosis has been established. Those affected by PE must confront issues such as genetic predisposition, potential long-term disability, changes in lifestyle related to anticoagulation, and the possibility of suffering a recurrent event. Clinicians can help allay this emotional burden by discussing the implications of PE with patients and their families, and PE support groups can help allay patient and family anxiety.

PREVENTION

Rationale for In-Hospital Venous Thromboembolism Prophylaxis

PE is the most preventable cause of in-hospital death. It may be difficult to detect, expensive and burdensome to treat, and potentially fatal. Fortunately, low fixed-dose anticoagulant prophylaxis is effective and safe during hospitalization (Table 87.8). Commonly used regimens include minidose UFH 5000 units three times daily, enoxaparin 40 mg daily, and dalteparin 5000 units daily. A multifaceted approach including electronic alerts, sharing comparative physician metrics, and continuing medical education can increase the frequency of appropriate VTE prophylaxis and reduce the incidence of 90-day symptomatic VTE.[154]

Rationale for Venous Thromboembolism Prophylaxis at Hospital Discharge

In the United States, about 7 million acutely ill medical patients at increased risk for VTE are hospitalized annually with conditions such as pneumonia, heart failure, and COPD. They account for more than 20% of the attributable risk for VTE. Thromboprophylaxis can halve their rate of VTE while hospitalized. However, venous stasis and immobilization tend to increase after hospital discharge because patients remain too weak and debilitated to walk at home. Prophylactic anticoagulation is discontinued at discharge, yet the peak incidence of acute VTE occurs within the first month after hospital stay.

To determine whether extended-duration administration of anticoagulation is superior to a standard course of prophylaxis with enoxaparin, the APEX trial compared the anti-Xa NOAC betrixaban, administered for 35 to 42 days, versus 6 to 14 days of enoxaparin, in 7513 hospitalized medically ill patients at risk for VTE. There was a 24% reduction in VTE among the extended-duration betrixaban patients compared with those assigned to enoxaparin. There was no difference in major bleeding between the two groups.[155] Ancillary APEX studies showed that betrixaban halved the rate of stroke compared with enoxaparin,[156] reduced the rate of cardiovascular mortality, MI, and stroke by 31%,[157] and halved the rate of rehospitalization.[158] Another ancillary APEX study showed that asymptomatic DVT is associated with an

TABLE 87.8 Regimens for Venous Thromboembolism Prevention

CONDITION	PROPHYLAXIS
Hospitalization with medical illness	Unfractionated heparin 5000 units SC bid or tid or Enoxaparin 40 mg SC qd or Dalteparin 2500 units or 5000 units SC qd or Fondaparinux 2.5 mg SC qd with normal renal function (in patients with a heparin allergy such as heparin-induced thrombocytopenia) or Rivaroxaban 10 mg qd started at hospital discharge and continued for 5 weeks
General surgery	Unfractionated heparin 5000 units SC bid or tid or Enoxaparin 40 mg SC qd or Dalteparin 2500 or 5000 units SC qd
Major orthopedic surgery	Warfarin (target INR 2.5) or Enoxaparin 30 mg SC bid or Enoxaparin 40 mg SC qd or Dalteparin 2500 or 5000 units SC qd or Fondaparinux 2.5 mg SC qd or Rivaroxaban 10 mg qd or Aspirin 81 mg BID or Rivaroxaban 10 mg qd for 5 days and then aspirin 81 mg daily thereafter Dabigatran 220 mg qd or Apixaban 2.5 mg twice daily

SC, Subcutaneous.

TABLE 87.9 Padua Prediction Score for Identification of Hospitalized Patients at Risk for Venous Thromboembolism

RISK FACTOR	SCORING
Cancer	3
Previous VTE	3
Immobility	3
Thrombophilia	3
Trauma/surgery	2
Age ≥70 years	1
Heart/respiratory failure	1
Acute MI or stroke	1
Infection/rheumatologic disorder	1
Obesity	1
Hormonal treatment	1

High risk for developing pulmonary embolism is defined as 4 score points or greater. *VTE*, Venous thromboembolic.

increased risk of death.[159] Betrixaban received FDA approval in 2017 for extended-duration VTE prophylaxis. However, the manufacturer withdrew it from the market for commercial reasons.

The MAGELLAN study of extended-duration VTE prophylaxis—rivaroxaban for 35 days versus enoxaparin for 10 days in medically ill patients being discharged from the hospital—showed that extended-duration rivaroxaban reduced the risk of VTE 23% more than enoxaparin. However, major bleeding complications were twice as frequent with rivaroxaban. Fatal bleeding occurred in 5 rivaroxaban patients compared with 1 enoxaparin patient.[160] Nevertheless, the benefit-risk profile of rivaroxaban became favorable when five groups at high bleeding risk were excluded: those with (1) active cancer, (2) dual antiplatelet therapy, (3) bronchiectasis/ pulmonary cavitation, (4) gastroduodenal ulcer, and (5) bleeding within 3 months of randomization.[161] In addition, rivaroxaban was compared against placebo in the MARINER trial of 12,024 medical patients being discharged from the hospital. The rivaroxaban group developed symptomatic VTE at half the rate of the placebo group. Major bleeding occurred more frequently in the rivaroxaban group but the difference with placebo was not statistically significant.[162] In 2019, the FDA approved rivaroxaban for extended-duration VTE prophylaxis at hospital discharge. In an ancillary MARINER study, rivaroxaban, like betrixaban, also reduced major adverse cardiovascular events by 28% compared with placebo.[163]

Whether extended-duration VTE prophylaxis is used in the United States remains to be seen. So far the uptake has been minimal. The absolute reduction in VTE is low, and cost-benefit analyses have not convinced clinicians or hospital administrators that the effort and expense to implement an extended-duration VTE prophylaxis program is worth the time and the money.[164]

In-Hospital Risk Factors for Venous Thromboembolism and Bleeding

The Padua Prediction Score is the most widely used risk assessment tool to aid clinicians in deciding whether to administer VTE prophylaxis to hospitalized medical patients. It has a point scoring system based on 11 variables (Table 87.9). A score of 4 or more points denotes a high risk for developing VTE. A simpler validated risk assessment model, developed at Intermountain Medical Center in Utah, predicts high risk if a patient has at least one of the following four risk factors: (1) previous VTE, (2) a medical indication for bed rest, (3) a peripherally inserted central venous catheter, or (4) cancer.[165] Pharmacologic thromboprophylaxis is generally withheld if the bleeding risk is excessively high due to threatened, active, or recent major bleeding or thrombocytopenia.

Primary Prevention of Venous Thromboembolism in High-Risk Patients with Active Cancer

The double-blind, randomized AVERT trial with apixaban[166] and the CASSINI trial with rivaroxaban[167] compared NOACs with placebo to prevent VTE in high-risk patients with cancer. Both trials showed a substantial reduction in VTE, and both had low rates of major bleeding. It remains uncertain whether these trials will change clinical practice.[168]

Mechanical Prophylaxis in Medically Ill Patients

Unless there is an absolute contraindication to low-dose UFH or LMWH, hospitalized patients at high risk for developing VTE should receive pharmacological prophylaxis rather than mechanical prophylaxis. In a critical care unit trial of 2003 patients, all of whom were receiving thromboprophylaxis, the addition of adjunctive intermittent pneumatic compression did not lower the incidence of proximal leg DVT.[169]

Advances in Venous Thromboembolism Prophylaxis in Major Orthopedic Surgery

Extended prophylaxis after hospital discharge decreases the risk of PE and DVT among patients undergoing major orthopedic surgery, particularly total hip or knee replacement. There is evidence to support the use of almost any prophylactic measure in these patients.[170] Approved approaches include LMWH, warfarin, NOACs, and aspirin. The PEPPER Trial [NCT02810704] is randomizing about 20,000 patients undergoing total knee or hip replacement to warfarin (target INR 2.0) versus rivaroxaban 10 mg daily versus aspirin 81 mg twice daily for 30 days to determine whether any one of these three modalities has superior efficacy and safety.[171]

FUTURE PERSPECTIVES

PE is an illness we thought we understood well. However, new concepts are rapidly evolving regarding VTE pathophysiology in COVID-19, anticoagulation management, advanced therapy with thrombolysis, surgical embolectomy, and ECMO. Novel approaches to VTE prophylaxis are also being tested and challenged.

We used to celebrate the 50% decline of in-hospital PE mortality from 8% to 4%. Unfortunately, the overall US mortality rate, including the death rate from PE, is now increasing. The median age of death from PE has decreased from 73 years in 2000 to 68 years in 2017. Socioeconomically disadvantaged older adults hospitalized with PE have higher long-term mortality rates than their non-disadvantaged counterparts and are more likely to be readmitted within 30 days of hospital discharge.

Our understanding of VTE in patients with COVID-19 will continue to evolve. Moreover, as we begin to better understand the mechanisms underlying this disease, our treatment of thrombotic complications, including PE and VTE, will change.

With respect to the optimal duration of anticoagulation, the ESC PE Guidelines recommend that we no longer use the terms "provoked" and "unprovoked" when describing VTE and predicting the risk of recurrence. The guidelines also support a bold and novel directive: we should no longer provide a definitive "stop date" for anticoagulation, except for major trauma or major surgery. This is a major paradigm shift.

New anticoagulants are being developed that are expected to have a more favorable safety profile than currently available drugs. Two promising targets are inhibitors of factor XIa and factor XIIa. For those with congenital factor XIa deficiency, spontaneous bleeding is rare. Factor XIIa helps achieve thrombosis but has no role in hemostasis.[172] Major strides are being made in advanced therapies for high-risk PE as well. These include dose reduction of fibrinolytic agents and the deployment of novel catheters that either deliver drugs directly to the thrombus or remove large clots without the use of any fibrinolytic agent.

In prevention, implementation of in-hospital VTE prophylaxis is far-reaching. But now we must confront COVID-19, which causes PE despite thromboprophylaxis. The last frontier of VTE prevention is during the risky first 4 to 6 weeks after hospital discharge. While orthopedic and cancer surgeons have used postoperative extended-duration VTE prophylaxis for decades, this strategy is not endorsed by many healthcare providers who care for acute medically ill patients after hospital discharge.

We are privileged to witness such positive and rapid change in the field of PE and DVT. Clinicians, laboratory scientists, government agencies, business representatives, philanthropists, patients, and the public are working together to improve VTE awareness and to implement newly developed cutting-edge technologies, drugs, and best practices.

REFERENCES

1. Riva N, Donadini MP, Ageno W. Epidemiology and pathophysiology of venous thromboembolism: similarities with atherothrombosis and the role of inflammation. *Thromb Haemost.* 2015;113:1176–1183.

Epidemiology

2. Barco S, Mahmoudpour SH, Valerio L, et al. Trends in mortality related to pulmonary embolism in the European Region, 2000-15: analysis of vital registration data from the WHO Mortality Database. *Lancet Respir Med.* 2020;8:277–287.
3. Wadhera RK, Secemsky EA, Wang Y, et al. Association of socioeconomic disadvantage with mortality and readmissions among older adults hospitalized for pulmonary embolism in the United States. *J Am Heart Assoc.* 2021;10(13):e021117. https://doi.org/10.1161/JAHA.121.021117. Epub 2021 Jul 2.
4. Minges KE, Bikdeli B, Wang Y, et al. National trends in pulmonary embolism hospitalization rates and outcomes for adults aged >/=65 Years in the United States (1999 to 2010). *Am J Cardiol.* 2015;116:1436–1442.
5. Spencer FA, Lessard D, Emery C, et al. Venous thromboembolism in the outpatient setting. *Arch Intern Med.* 2007;167:1471–1475.
6. Ageno W, Becattini C, Brighton T, et al. Cardiovascular risk factors and venous thromboembolism: a meta-analysis. *Circulation.* 2008;117:93–102.
7. Fanola CL, Norby FL, Shah AM, et al. Incident heart failure and long-term risk for venous thromboembolism. *J Am Coll Cardiol.* 2020;75:148–158.
8. Gregson J, Kaptoge S, Bolton T, et al. Cardiovascular risk factors associated with venous thromboembolism. *JAMA Cardiol.* 2019;4:163–173.
9. Parkin L, Sweetland S, Balkwill A, et al. Body mass index, surgery, and risk of venous thromboembolism in middle-aged women: a cohort study. *Circulation.* 2012;125:1897–1904.
10. Nauffal D, Ballester M, Reyes RL, et al. Influence of recent immobilization and recent surgery on mortality in patients with pulmonary embolism. *J Thromb Haemost.* 2012;10:1752–1760.
11. Abe K, Kuklina EV, Hooper WC, Callaghan WM. Venous Thromboembolism as a cause of severe maternal morbidity and mortality in the United States. *Semin Perinatol.* 2019;43:200–204.
12. Petterson TM, Smith CY, Emerson JA, et al. Venous Thromboembolism (VTE) incidence and VTE-associated survival among olmsted county residents of local nursing homes. *Thromb Haemost.* 2018;118:1316–1328.
13. Hisada Y, Geddings JE, Ay C, Mackman N. Venous thrombosis and cancer: from mouse models to clinical trials. *J Thromb Haemost.* 2015;13:1372–1382.
14. van Es N, Le Gal G, Otten HM, et al. Screening for occult cancer in patients with unprovoked venous thromboembolism: a systematic review and meta-analysis of individual patient data. *Ann Intern Med.* 2017;167:410–417.
15. Streiff MB, Holmstrom B, Angelini D, et al. NCCN guidelines insights: cancer-associated venous thromboembolic disease, version 2.2018. *J Natl Compr Canc Netw.* 2018;16:1289–1303.
16. Sabapathy CA, Djouonang TN, Kahn SR, et al. Incidence trends and mortality from childhood venous thromboembolism: a population-based cohort study. *J Pediatr.* 2016;172:175–180.e171.
17. Garcia D, Erkan D. Diagnosis and management of the antiphospholipid syndrome. *N Engl J Med.* 2018;378:2010–2021.
18. Mahmoodi BK, Gansevoort RT, Naess IA, et al. Association of mild to moderate chronic kidney disease with venous thromboembolism: pooled analysis of five prospective general population cohorts. *Circulation.* 2012;126:1964–1971.
19. Dzikowska-Diduch O, Kostrubiec M, Kurnicka K, et al. The post-pulmonary syndrome—results of echocardiographic driven follow up after acute pulmonary embolism. *Thromb Res.* 2020;186:30–35.
20. Klok FA, Dzikowska-Diduch O, Kostrubiec M, et al. Derivation of a clinical prediction score for chronic thromboembolic pulmonary hypertension after acute pulmonary embolism. *J Thromb Haemost.* 2016;14:121–128.
21. Kahn SR, Comerota AJ, Cushman M, et al. The postthrombotic syndrome: evidence-based prevention, diagnosis, and treatment strategies: a scientific statement from the American Heart Association. *Circulation.* 2014;130:1636–1661.
22. Lubberts B, Paulino Pereira NR, et al. What is the effect of venous thromboembolism and related complications on patient reported health-related quality of life? A meta-analysis. *Thromb Haemost.* 2016;116.
23. Winter MP, Schernthaner GH, Lang IM. Chronic complications of venous thromboembolism. *J Thromb Haemost.* 2017;15:1531–1540.
24. Becattini C, Vedovati MC, Ageno W, et al. Incidence of arterial cardiovascular events after venous thromboembolism: a systematic review and a meta-analysis. *J Thromb Haemost.* 2010;8:891–897.
25. Ng AC, Chung T, Yong AS, et al. Long-term cardiovascular and noncardiovascular mortality of 1023 patients with confirmed acute pulmonary embolism. *Circ Cardiovasc Qual Outcomes.* 2011;4:122–128.
26. Rinde LB, Lind C, Smabrekke B, et al. Impact of incident myocardial infarction on the risk of venous thromboembolism: the Tromso Study. *J Thromb Haemost.* 2016;14:1183–1191.
27. Kaplan D, Casper TC, Elliott CG, et al. VTE incidence and risk factors in patients with severe sepsis and septic shock. *Chest.* 2015;148:1224–1230.
28. Poissy J, Goutay J, Caplan M, et al. Pulmonary embolism in COVID-19 patients: awareness of an increased prevalence. *Circulation.* 2020 Apr 24. https://doi.org/10.1161/CIRCULATIONAHA.120.047430.
29. Bompard F, Monnier H, Saab I, et al. Pulmonary embolism in patients with Covid-19 pneumonia. *Eur Respir J.* 2020:2001365. https://doi.org/10.1183/13993003.01365-2020.
30. Bikdeli B, Madhavan MV, Jimenez D, et al. COVID-19 and thrombotic or thromboembolic disease: implications for prevention, antithrombotic therapy, and follow-up. *J Am Coll Cardiol.* 2020.
31. Savchenko AS, Martinod K, Seidman MA, et al. Neutrophil extracellular traps form predominantly during the organizing stage of human venous thromboembolism development. *J Thromb Haemost.* 2014;12:860–870.
32. Zuo Y, Yalavarthi S, Shi H, et al. Neutrophil extracellular traps in COVID-19. *JCI Insight.* 2020;5(11):138999. https://doi.org/10.1172/jci.insight.138999.
33. Rogers MA, Levine DA, Blumberg N, et al. Triggers of hospitalization for venous thromboembolism. *Circulation.* 2012;125:2092–2099.
34. Tichelaar YI, Kluin-Nelemans HJ, Meijer K. Infections and inflammatory diseases as risk factors for venous thrombosis. A systematic review. *Thromb Haemost.* 2012;107:827–837.
35. Glynn RJ, Danielson E, Fonseca FA, et al. A randomized trial of rosuvastatin in the prevention of venous thromboembolism. *N Engl J Med.* 2009;360:1851–1861.
36. Klarin D, Busenkell E, Judy R, et al. Genome-wide association analysis of venous thromboembolism identifies new risk loci and genetic overlap with arterial vascular disease. *Nat Genet.* 2019;51:1574–1579.
37. Lindstrom S, Wang L, Smith EN, et al. Genomic and transcriptomic association studies identify 16 novel susceptibility loci for venous thromboembolism. *Blood.* 2019;134:1645–1657.
38. Marston NA, Gurmu Y, Melloni GEM, et al. The effect of PCSK9 (Proprotein Convertase Subtilisin/Kexin Type 9) inhibition on the risk of venous thromboembolism. *Circulation.* 2020;141:1600–1607.

Classification of Pulmonary Embolism

39. Konstantinides SV, Meyer G, Becattini C, et al. 2019 ESC Guidelines for the diagnosis and management of acute pulmonary embolism developed in collaboration with the European Respiratory Society (ERS). *Eur Heart J.* 2019.
40. Casazza F, Becattini C, Bongarzoni A, et al. Clinical features and short term outcomes of patients with acute pulmonary embolism. The Italian Pulmonary Embolism Registry (IPER). *Thromb Res.* 2012;130:847–852.
41. Yusuff HO, Zochios V, Vuylsteke A. Extracorporeal membrane oxygenation in acute massive pulmonary embolism: a systematic review. *Perfusion.* 2015;30:611–616.
42. Sista AK, Horowitz JM, Goldhaber SZ. Four key questions surrounding thrombolytic therapy for submassive pulmonary embolism. *Vasc Med.* 2016;21:47–52.
43. Hendriks SV, Klok FA, den Exter PL, et al. RV/LV ratio measurement seems to have no role in low risk patients with pulmonary embolism treated at home triaged by hestia criteria. *Am J Respir Crit Care Med.* 2020 Mar 23. https://doi.org/10.1164/rccm.202002-0267LE.
44. Windecker S, Stortecky S, Meier B. Paradoxical embolism. *J Am Coll Cardiol.* 2014;64:403–415.
45. Kosova E, Bergmark B, Piazza G. Fat embolism syndrome. *Circulation.* 2015;131:317–320.
46. Kahn SR, Akaberi A, Granton JT, et al. Quality of life, dyspnea, and functional exercise capacity following a first episode of pulmonary embolism: results of the ELOPE cohort study. *Am J Med.* 2017;130:990 e999-990 e921.
47. Konstantinides SV, Vicaut E, Danays T, et al. Impact of thrombolytic therapy on the long-term outcome of intermediate-risk pulmonary embolism. *J Am Coll Cardiol.* 2017;69:1536–1544.
48. Piazza G, Goldhaber SZ. Chronic thromboembolic pulmonary hypertension. *N Engl J Med.* 2011;364:351–360.
49. Mahmud E, Madani MM, Kim NH, et al. Chronic thromboembolic pulmonary hypertension: evolving therapeutic approaches for operable and inoperable disease. *J Am Coll Cardiol.* 2018;71:2468–2486.
50. Ghofrani HA, D'Armini AM, Grimminger F, et al. Riociguat for the treatment of chronic thromboembolic pulmonary hypertension. *N Engl J Med.* 2013;369:319–329.
51. Kataoka M, Inami T, Kawakami T, et al. Balloon pulmonary angioplasty (Percutaneous Transluminal Pulmonary Angioplasty) for chronic thromboembolic pulmonary hypertension: a Japanese perspective. *JACC Cardiovasc Interv.* 2019;12:1382–1388.
52. Righini M, Galanaud JP, Guenneguez H, et al. Anticoagulant therapy for symptomatic calf deep vein thrombosis (CACTUS): a randomised, double-blind, placebo-controlled trial. *Lancet Haematol.* 2016;3:e556–e562.
53. Franco L, Giustozzi M, Agnelli G, Becattini C. Anticoagulation in patients with isolated distal deep vein thrombosis: a meta-analysis. *J Thromb Haemost.* 2017;15:1142–1154.
54. Evans RS, Sharp JH, Linford LH, et al. Risk of symptomatic DVT associated with peripherally inserted central catheters. *Chest.* 2010;138:803–810.
55. Evans RS, Sharp JH, Linford LH, et al. Reduction of peripherally inserted central catheter-associated DVT. *Chest.* 2013;143:627–633.
56. Greene MT, Flanders SA, Woller SC, et al. The association between PICC use and venous thromboembolism in upper and lower extremities. *Am J Med.* 2015;128:986–993.e981.
57. Rabinovich A, Cohen JM, Cushman M, et al. Inflammation markers and their trajectories after deep vein thrombosis in relation to risk of post-thrombotic syndrome. *J Thromb Haemost.* 2015;13:398–408.
58. Galanaud JP, Righini M, Le Collen L, et al. Long-term risk of postthrombotic syndrome after symptomatic distal deep vein thrombosis: the CACTUS-PTS study. *J Thromb Haemost.* 2020;18:857–864.

59. Kachroo S, Boyd D, Bookhart BK, et al. Quality of life and economic costs associated with post-thrombotic syndrome. *Am J Health Syst Pharm*. 2012;69:567–572.
60. Kahn SR, Shapiro S, Wells PS, et al. Compression stockings to prevent post-thrombotic syndrome: a randomised placebo-controlled trial. *Lancet*. 2014;383:880–888.
61. Kahn SR, Shrier I, Shapiro S, et al. Six-month exercise training program to treat post-thrombotic syndrome: a randomized controlled two-centre trial. *CMAJ (Can Med Assoc J)*. 2011;183:37–44.
62. Cannegieter SC, Horvath-Puho E, Schmidt M, et al. Risk of venous and arterial thrombotic events in patients diagnosed with superficial vein thrombosis: a nationwide cohort study. *Blood*. 2015;125:229–235.

Diagnosis

63. Le Gal G, Righini M, Wells PS. D-dimer for pulmonary embolism. *J Am Med Assoc*. 2015;313:1668–1669.
64. Parpia S, Takach Lapner S, et al. Clinical pre-test probability adjusted versus age-adjusted D-dimer interpretation strategy for DVT diagnosis: a diagnostic individual patient data meta-analysis. *J Thromb Haemost*. 2020;18:669–675.
65. Halaby R, Popma CJ, Cohen A, et al. D-Dimer elevation and adverse outcomes. *J Thromb Thrombolysis*. 2015;39:55–59.
66. Picano E, Scali MC, Ciampi Q, Lichtenstein D. Lung ultrasound for the cardiologist. *JACC Cardiovasc Imaging*. 2018;11:1692–1705.
67. Squizzato A, Galli L, Gerdes VE. Point-of-care ultrasound in the diagnosis of pulmonary embolism. *Crit Ultrasound J*. 2015;7:7.
68. Bekgoz B, Kilicaslan I, Bildik F, et al. BLUE protocol ultrasonography in emergency department patients presenting with acute dyspnea. *Am J Emerg Med*. 2019;37:2020–2027.
69. Moore AJE, Wachsmann J, Chamarthy MR, et al. Imaging of acute pulmonary embolism: an update. *Cardiovasc Diagn Ther*. 2018;8:225–243.
70. Hutchinson BD, Navin P, Marom EM, et al. Overdiagnosis of pulmonary embolism by pulmonary CT angiography. *AJR Am J Roentgenol*. 2015;205:271–277.
71. Kang DK, Ramos-Duran L, Schoepf UJ, et al. Reproducibility of CT signs of right ventricular dysfunction in acute pulmonary embolism. *AJR Am J Roentgenol*. 2010;194:1500–1506.
72. Koc M, Kostrubiec M, Elikowski W, et al. Outcome of patients with right heart thrombi: the Right Heart Thrombi European Registry. *Eur Respir J*. 2016;47:869–875.
73. Li J, Feng L, Li J, Tang J. Diagnostic accuracy of magnetic resonance angiography for acute pulmonary embolism - a systematic review and meta-analysis. *Vasa*. 2016;45:149–154.
74. Raja AS, Ip IK, Prevedello LM, et al. Effect of computerized clinical decision support on the use and yield of CT pulmonary angiography in the emergency department. *Radiology*. 2012;262:468–474.

Anticoagulation Therapy

75. Carroll BJ, Beyer SE, Mehegan T, et al. Changes in care for acute pulmonary embolism with a multidisciplinary pulmonary embolism response team: PE response team. *Am J Med*. 2020; S0002-9343(20)30374-0. https://doi.org/10.1016/j.amjmed.2020.03.058.
76. Aso S, Matsui H, Fushimi K, Yasunaga H. In-hospital mortality and successful weaning from venoarterial extracorporeal membrane oxygenation: analysis of 5,263 patients using a National inpatient database in Japan. *Crit Care*. 2016;20:80. https://doi.org/10.1186/s13054-016-1261-1.
77. Meneveau N, Guillon B, Planquette B, et al. Outcomes after extracorporeal membrane oxygenation for the treatment of high-risk pulmonary embolism: a multicentre series of 52 cases. *Eur Heart J*. 2018;39:4196–4204.
78. Konstantinides SV, Warntges S. Acute phase treatment of venous thromboembolism: advanced therapy. Systemic fibrinolysis and pharmacomechanical therapy. *Thromb Haemost*. 2015;113:1202–1209.
79. Zhang R, Kobayashi T, Pugliese S, et al. Interventional therapies in acute pulmonary embolism. *Interv Cardiol Clin*. 2020;9:229–241.
80. Keeling WB, Bundt T, Leacche M, et al. Outcomes after surgical pulmonary embolectomy for acute pulmonary embolus: a multi-institutional study. *Ann Thorac Surg*. 2016;102(5):1498–1502.
81. Percy ED, Shah R, Hirji S, et al. National outcomes of surgical embolectomy for acute pulmonary embolism. *Ann Thorac Surg*. 2020;110(2):441–447.
82. Chan CM, Woods C, Shorr AF. The validation and reproducibility of the pulmonary embolism severity index. *J Thromb Haemost*. 2010;8:1509–1514.
83. Poterucha TJ, Libby P, Goldhaber SZ. More than an anticoagulant: do heparins have direct anti-inflammatory effects? *Thromb Haemost*. 2017;117(3):437–444.
84. Black SA, Cohen AT. Anticoagulation strategies for venous thromboembolism: moving towards a personalised approach. *Thromb Haemost*. 2015;114:660–669.
85. Kang M, Alahmadi M, Sawh S, et al. Fondaparinux for the treatment of suspected heparin-induced thrombocytopenia: a propensity score-matched study. *Blood*. 2015;125:924–929.
86. Salter BS, Weiner MM, Trinh MA, et al. Heparin-induced thrombocytopenia: a comprehensive clinical review. *J Am Coll Cardiol*. 2016;67:2519–2532.
87. Greinacher A. Clinical practice. heparin-induced thrombocytopenia. *N Engl J Med*. 2015;373:252–261.
88. Baroletti S, Hurwitz S, Conti NA, et al. Thrombosis in suspected heparin-induced thrombocytopenia occurs more often with high antibody levels. *Am J Med*. 2012;125:44–49.
89. Poterucha TJ, Goldhaber SZ. Warfarin and vascular calcification. *Am J Med*. 2016;129:635.e631–e634.
90. Binding C, Bjerring Olesen J, Abrahamsen B, et al. Osteoporotic fractures in patients with atrial fibrillation treated with conventional versus direct anticoagulants. *J Am Coll Cardiol*. 2019;74:2150–2158.
91. Douketis JD, Spyropoulos AC, Kaatz S, et al. Perioperative bridging anticoagulation in patients with atrial fibrillation. *N Engl J Med*. 2015;373:823–833.
92. Baumgartner C, de Kouchkovsky I, Whitaker E, Fang MC. Periprocedural bridging in patients with venous thromboembolism: a systematic review. *Am J Med*. 2019;132:722–732.e727.
93. Beyer-Westendorf J, Ageno W. Benefit-risk profile of non-vitamin K antagonist oral anticoagulants in the management of venous thromboembolism. *Thromb Haemost*. 2015;113:231–246.
94. van der Hulle T, Kooiman J, den Exter PL, et al. Effectiveness and safety of novel oral anticoagulants as compared with vitamin K antagonists in the treatment of acute symptomatic venous thromboembolism: a systematic review and meta-analysis. *J Thromb Haemost*. 2014;12:320–328.
95. Schulman S, Kearon C, Kakkar AK, et al. Dabigatran versus warfarin in the treatment of acute venous thromboembolism. *N Engl J Med*. 2009;361:2342–2352.
96. Schulman S, Kakkar AK, Goldhaber SZ, et al. Treatment of acute venous thromboembolism with dabigatran or warfarin and pooled analysis. *Circulation*. 2014;129:764–772.
97. Yeh CH, Gross PL, Weitz JI. Evolving use of new oral anticoagulants for treatment of venous thromboembolism. *Blood*. 2014;124:1020–1028.
98. Investigators E, Bauersachs R, Berkowitz SD, et al. Oral rivaroxaban for symptomatic venous thromboembolism. *N Engl J Med*. 2010;363:2499–2510.
99. Einstein-EP Investigators, Buller HR, Prins MH, et al. Oral rivaroxaban for the treatment of symptomatic pulmonary embolism. *N Engl J Med*. 2012;366:1287–1297.
100. Agnelli G, Buller HR, Cohen A, et al. Oral apixaban for the treatment of acute venous thromboembolism. *N Engl J Med*. 2013;369:799–808.
101. Hokusai VTEI, Buller HR, Decousus H, et al. Edoxaban versus warfarin for the treatment of symptomatic venous thromboembolism. *N Engl J Med*. 2013;369:1406–1415.
102. Schulman S, Kearon C, Kakkar AK, et al. Extended use of dabigatran, warfarin, or placebo in venous thromboembolism. *N Engl J Med*. 2013;368:709–718.
103. Agnelli G, Buller HR, Cohen A, et al. Apixaban for extended treatment of venous thromboembolism. *N Engl J Med*. 2013;368:699–708.
104. Male C, Lensing AWA, Palumbo JS, et al. Rivaroxaban compared with standard anticoagulants for the treatment of acute venous thromboembolism in children: a randomised, controlled, phase 3 trial. *Lancet Haematol*. 2020;7:e18–e27.
105. Hickey M, Gatien M, Taljaard M, et al. Outcomes of urgent warfarin reversal with frozen plasma versus prothrombin complex concentrate in the emergency department. *Circulation*. 2013;128:360–364.
106. Pollack Jr CV, Reilly PA, Eikelboom J, et al. Idarucizumab for dabigatran reversal. *N Engl J Med*. 2015;373:511–520.
107. Pollack Jr CV, Reilly PA, Weitz JI. Dabigatran reversal with idarucizumab. *N Engl J Med*. 2017;377:1691–1692.
108. Siegal DM, Curnutte JT, Connolly SJ, et al. Andexanet alfa for the reversal of factor Xa inhibitor activity. *N Engl J Med*. 2015;373:2413–2424.
109. Connolly SJ, Crowther M, Eikelboom JW, et al. Full study report of andexanet alfa for bleeding associated with factor Xa inhibitors. *N Engl J Med*. 2019;380:1326–1335.
110. Libby P, Hansson GK. From focal lipid storage to systemic inflammation: JACC review topic of the week. *J Am Coll Cardiol*. 2019;74:1594–1607.
111. Huang W, Goldberg RJ, Anderson FA, et al. Secular trends in occurrence of acute venous thromboembolism: the Worcester VTE study (1985-2009). *Am J Med*. 2014;127:829–839.e825.
112. Sogaard KK, Schmidt M, Pedersen L, et al. 30-year mortality after venous thromboembolism: a population-based cohort study. *Circulation*. 2014;130:829–836.
113. Albertsen IE, Nielsen PB, Sogaard M, et al. Risk of recurrent venous thromboembolism: a Danish Nationwide Cohort Study. *Am J Med*. 2018;131:1067–1074.e1064.
114. Khan F, Rahman A, Carrier M, et al. Long term risk of symptomatic recurrent venous thromboembolism after discontinuation of anticoagulant treatment for first unprovoked venous thromboembolism event: systematic review and meta-analysis. *BMJ*. 2019;366:l4363.
115. Kearon C, Spencer FA, O'Keeffe D, et al. D-dimer testing to select patients with a first unprovoked venous thromboembolism who can stop anticoagulant therapy: a cohort study. *Ann Intern Med*. 2015;162:27–34.
116. Kearon C, Ageno W, Cannegieter SC, et al. Categorization of patients as having provoked or unprovoked venous thromboembolism: guidance from the SSC of ISTH. *J Thromb Haemost*. 2016;14:1480–1483.
117. Rodger MA, Le Gal G, Anderson DR, et al. Validating the HERDOO2 rule to guide treatment duration for women with unprovoked venous thrombosis: multinational prospective cohort management study. *BMJ*. 2017;356:j1065.
118. Albertsen IE, Sogaard M, Goldhaber SZ, et al. Development of sex-stratified prediction models for recurrent venous thromboembolism: a Danish Nationwide Cohort Study. *Thromb Haemost*. 2020;120:805–814.
119. Agnelli G, Buller HR, Cohen A, et al. Apixaban for extended treatment of venous thromboembolism. *N Engl J Med*. 2013;368:699–708.
120. Weitz JI, Lensing AWA, Prins MH, et al. Rivaroxaban or aspirin for extended treatment of venous thromboembolism. *N Engl J Med*. 2017;376:1211–1222.
121. Vasanthamohan L, Boonyawat K, Chai-Adisaksopha C, Crowther M. Reduced-dose direct oral anticoagulants in the extended treatment of venous thromboembolism: a systematic review and meta-analysis. *J Thromb Haemost*. 2018;16:1288–1295.
122. Mai V, Guay CA, Perreault L, et al. Extended anticoagulation for VTE: a systematic review and meta-analysis. *Chest*. 2019;155:1199–1216.

Advanced Therapy

123. Dudzinski DM, Piazza G. Multidisciplinary pulmonary embolism response teams. *Circulation*. 2016;133:98–103.
124. Kolte D, Parikh SA, Piazza G, et al. Vascular teams in peripheral vascular disease. *J Am Coll Cardiol*. 2019;73:2477–2486.
125. Chatterjee S, Chakraborty A, Weinberg I, et al. Thrombolysis for pulmonary embolism and risk of all-cause mortality, major bleeding, and intracranial hemorrhage: a meta-analysis. *J Am Med Assoc*. 2014;311:2414–2421.
126. Kiser TH, Burnham EL, Clark B, et al. Half-dose versus full-dose alteplase for treatment of pulmonary embolism. *Crit Care Med*. 2018;46:1617–1625.
127. Kucher N, Boekstegers P, Muller OJ, et al. Randomized, controlled trial of ultrasound-assisted catheter-directed thrombolysis for acute intermediate-risk pulmonary embolism. *Circulation*. 2014;129:479–486.
128. Piazza G, Hohlfelder B, Jaff MR, et al. A prospective, single-arm, multicenter trial of ultrasound-facilitated, catheter-directed, low-dose fibrinolysis for acute massive and submassive pulmonary embolism: the SEATTLE II study. *JACC Cardiovasc Interv*. 2015;8:1382–1392.
129. Tapson VF, Sterling K, Jones N, et al. A randomized trial of the optimum duration of acoustic pulse thrombolysis procedure in acute intermediate-risk pulmonary embolism: the OPTALYSE PE trial. *JACC Cardiovasc Interv*. 2018;11:1401–1410.
130. Rahaghi FN, Estepar RSJ, Goldhaber SZ, et al. Quantification and significance of pulmonary vascular volume in predicting response to ultrasound-facilitated, catheter-directed fibrinolysis in acute pulmonary embolism (SEATTLE-3D). *Clin Cardiovasc Imaging*. 2019;12(12):e009903. https://doi.org/10.1161/CIRCIMAGING.119.009903. Epub 2019 Dec 17.
131. Tu T, Toma C, Tapson VF, et al. A prospective, single-arm, multicenter trial of catheter-directed mechanical thrombectomy for intermediate-risk acute pulmonary embolism: the FLARE study. *JACC Cardiovasc Interv*. 2019;12:859–869.
132. VIVA 2019: Penumbra Indigo Aspiration system IDE trial for acute PE meets primary safety and efficacy endpoints. [Electronic article]. *Vascular News*. 2019. *https://vascularnews.com/viva19-penumbra-indigo-aspiration-system-ide-trial-for-acute-pe-meets-primary-safety-and-efficacy-endpoints/*. Published 6 November 2019. Accessed 21 April 2020.
133. Kuo WT, Banerjee A, Kim PS, et al. Pulmonary Embolism Response to Fragmentation, Embolectomy, and Catheter Thrombolysis (PERFECT): initial results from a prospective multicenter registry. *Chest*. 2015;148:667–673.
134. Giri J, Sista AK, Weinberg I, et al. Interventional therapies for acute pulmonary embolism: current status and principles for the development of novel evidence: a scientific statement from the American Heart Association. *Circulation*. 2019;140:e774–e801.
135. Poterucha TJ, Bergmark B, Aranki S, et al. Surgical pulmonary embolectomy. *Circulation*. 2015;132:1146–1151.
136. Kolkailah AA, Hirji S, Piazza G, et al. Surgical pulmonary embolectomy and catheter-directed thrombolysis for treatment of submassive pulmonary embolism. *J Card Surg*. 2018;33:252–259.
137. Mismetti P, Laporte S, Pellerin O, et al. Effect of a retrievable inferior vena cava filter plus anticoagulation vs anticoagulation alone on risk of recurrent pulmonary embolism: a randomized clinical trial. *J Am Med Assoc*. 2015;313:1627–1635.
138. Bikdeli B, Chatterjee S, Desai NR, et al. Inferior vena cava filters to prevent pulmonary embolism: systematic review and meta-analysis. *J Am Coll Cardiol*. 2017;70:1587–1597.
139. Sutphin PD, Reis SP, McKune A, et al. Improving inferior vena cava filter retrieval rates with the define, measure, analyze, improve, control methodology. *J Vasc Interv Radiol*. 2015;26:491–498.e491.
140. Enden T, Haig Y, Klow NE, et al. Long-term outcome after additional catheter-directed thrombolysis versus standard treatment for acute iliofemoral deep vein thrombosis (the CaVenT study): a randomised controlled trial. *Lancet*. 2012;379:31–38.

141. Vedantham S, Goldhaber SZ, Julian JA, et al. Pharmacomechanical catheter-directed thrombolysis for deep-vein thrombosis. *N Engl J Med*. 2017;377:2240–2252.
142. Lee AY, Levine MN, Baker RI, et al. Low-molecular-weight heparin versus a coumarin for the prevention of recurrent venous thromboembolism in patients with cancer. *N Engl J Med*. 2003;349:146–153.
143. Lee AY, Kamphuisen PW, Meyer G, et al. Tinzaparin vs warfarin for treatment of acute venous thromboembolism in patients with active cancer: a randomized clinical trial. *J Am Med Assoc*. 2015;314:677–686.
144. Raskob GE, van Es N, Verhamme P, et al. Edoxaban for the treatment of cancer-associated venous thromboembolism. *N Engl J Med*. 2018;378:615–624.
145. Young AM, Marshall A, Thirlwall J, et al. Comparison of an oral factor Xa inhibitor with low molecular weight heparin in patients with cancer with venous thromboembolism: results of a randomized trial (SELECT-D). *J Clin Oncol*. 2018;36:2017–2023.
146. Agnelli G, Becattini C, Meyer G, et al. Apixaban for the treatment of venous thromboembolism associated with cancer. *N Engl J Med*. 2020;382:1599–1607.
147. Cosmi B. Management of superficial vein thrombosis. *J Thromb Haemost*. 2015;13:1175–1183.
148. Beyer-Westendorf J, Schellong SM, Gerlach H, et al. Prevention of thromboembolic complications in patients with superficial-vein thrombosis given rivaroxaban or fondaparinux: the open-label, randomised, non-inferiority SURPRISE phase 3b trial. *Lancet Haematol*. 2017;4:e105–e113.
149. Pengo V, Denas G, Zoppellaro G, et al. Rivaroxaban vs warfarin in high-risk patients with antiphospholipid syndrome. *Blood*. 2018;132:1365–1371.
150. Witmer C, Raffini L. Treatment of venous thromboembolism in pediatric patients. *Blood*. 2020;135:335–343.
151. Brandao LR, Albisetti M, Halton J, et al. Safety of dabigatran etexilate for the secondary prevention of venous thromboembolism in children. *Blood*. 2020;135:491–504.
152. Hojen AA, Gorst-Rasmussen A, Lip GY, et al. Use of psychotropic drugs following venous thromboembolism in youth. A nationwide cohort study. *Thromb Res*. 2015;135:643–647.
153. Hojen AA, Sorensen EE, Dreyer PS, et al. Long-term mental wellbeing of adolescents and young adults diagnosed with venous thromboembolism: results from a multistage mixed methods study. *J Thromb Haemost*. 2017;15:2333–2343.

Prevention

154. Woller SC, Stevens SM, Evans RS, et al. Electronic alerts, comparative practitioner metrics, and education improves thromboprophylaxis and reduces thrombosis. *Am J Med*. 2016;129:1124. e1117–e1126.
155. Cohen AT, Harrington RA, Goldhaber SZ, et al. Extended thromboprophylaxis with betrixaban in acutely ill medical patients. *N Engl J Med*. 2016;375:534–544.
156. Gibson CM, Chi G, Halaby R, et al. Extended-duration betrixaban reduces the risk of stroke versus standard-dose enoxaparin among hospitalized medically ill patients: an APEX trial substudy (Acute Medically Ill Venous Thromboembolism Prevention With Extended Duration Betrixaban). *Circulation*. 2017;135:648–655.
157. Nafee T, Gibson CM, Yee MK, et al. Reduction of cardiovascular mortality and ischemic events in acute medically ill patients. *Circulation*. 2019;139:1234–1236.
158. Chi G, Yee MK, Amin AN, et al. Extended-duration betrixaban reduces the risk of rehospitalization associated with venous thromboembolism among acutely ill hospitalized medical patients: findings from the APEX trial (Acute Medically Ill Venous Thromboembolism Prevention With Extended Duration Betrixaban Trial). *Circulation*. 2018;137:91–94.
159. Kalayci A, Gibson CM, Chi G, et al. Asymptomatic deep vein thrombosis is associated with an increased risk of death: insights from the APEX trial. *Thromb Haemost*. 2018;118:2046–2052.
160. Cohen AT, Spiro TE, Buller HR, et al. Rivaroxaban for thromboprophylaxis in acutely ill medical patients. *N Engl J Med*. 2013;368:513–523.
161. Spyropoulos AC, Lipardi C, Xu J, et al. Improved benefit risk profile of rivaroxaban in a subpopulation of the MAGELLAN study. *Clin Appl Thromb Hemost*. 2019;25:1076029619886022.
162. Spyropoulos AC, Ageno W, Albers GW, et al. Rivaroxaban for thromboprophylaxis after hospitalization for medical illness. *N Engl J Med*. 2018;379:1118–1127.
163. Spyropoulos AC. Post-discharge prophylaxis with rivaroxaban reduces fatal and major thromboembolic events in medically ill patients. *J Am Coll Cardiol*. 2020;75(25):3140–3147. https://doi.org/10.1016/j.jacc.2020.04.071. PMID: 32586587.
164. Goldhaber SZ. Thromboembolism prophylaxis for patients discharged from the hospital: easier said than done. *J Am Coll Cardiol*. 2020;75(25):3148–3150. https://doi.org/10.1016/j.jacc.2020.05.023. PMID: 32586588.
165. Woller SC, Stevens SM, Jones JP, et al. Derivation and validation of a simple model to identify venous thromboembolism risk in medical patients. *Am J Med*. 2011;124:947–954.e942.
166. Carrier M, Abou-Nassar K, Mallick R, et al. Apixaban to prevent venous thromboembolism in patients with cancer. *N Engl J Med*. 2019;380:711–719.
167. Khorana AA, Soff GA, Kakkar AK, et al. Rivaroxaban for thromboprophylaxis in high-risk ambulatory patients with cancer. *N Engl J Med*. 2019;380:720–728.
168. Agnelli G. Direct oral anticoagulants for thromboprophylaxis in ambulatory patients with cancer. *N Engl J Med*. 2019;380:781–783.
169. Arabi YM, Al-Hameed F, Burns KEA, et al. Adjunctive intermittent pneumatic compression for venous thromboprophylaxis. *N Engl J Med*. 2019;380:1305–1315.
170. Xu K, Chan NC, Ibrahim Q, et al. Reduction in mortality following elective major hip and knee surgery: a systematic review and meta-analysis. *Thromb Haemost*. 2019;119:668–674.
171. Pellegrini Jr VD, Eikelboom J, McCollister Evarts C, et al. Selection bias, orthopaedic style: knowing what we don't know about aspirin. *J Bone Joint Surg Am*. 2020;102:631–633.
172. Weitz JI, Chan NC. Novel antithrombotic strategies for treatment of venous thromboembolism. *Blood*. 2020;135:351–359.

88 Pulmonary Hypertension

BRADLEY A. MARON

NORMAL PULMONARY CIRCULATION, 1656
Pulmonary Circulatory Physiology, 1656
Pulmonary Venous System, 1657
Pulmonary Circulatory Physiology During Exercise, 1657

CLASSIFICATION OF PULMONARY HYPERTENSION, 1657
Hemodynamic Classifications, 1658
Isolated Post-Capillary Pulmonary Hypertension Clinical Classifications, 1659
Pre-Capillary Pulmonary Hypertension Clinical Classifications, 1660
Combined Pre- and Post-Capillary Pulmonary Hypertension, 1662

PATHOLOGY, 1662

PATHOBIOLOGY, 1662

PATHOPHYSIOLOGY, 1665
Right Ventricular Dysfunction, 1665
Systemic Manifestations of Pulmonary Hypertension, 1665

PATIENT PRESENTATION AND CLINICAL ASSESSMENT, 1665
Patient Medical History, 1665
Physical Examination Findings, 1665
Approach to Diagnosis, 1667
Risk Stratification, 1670

INTEGRATED APPROACH TO DIAGNOSING PULMONARY HYPERTENSION, 1671
Pulmonary Venoocclusive Disease, 1671
Chronic Thromboembolic Pulmonary Hypertension, 1672

TREATMENT, 1672

Pulmonary Arterial Hypertension, 1672
Chronic Thromboembolic Pulmonary Hypertension, 1674
Pulmonary Hypertension from Left Heart Disease, 1674

SPECIAL CLINICAL CIRCUMSTANCES, 1674
High-Altitude Pulmonary Edema, 1674
Sarcoidosis, 1676
Sickle Cell Disease, 1676
Pregnancy, 1676
Perioperative Management, 1676

FUTURE PERSPECTIVES, 1676

ACKNOWLEDGMENTS, 1676

REFERENCES, 1676

Pulmonary hypertension (PH) is a specific although heterogeneous clinical disorder defined foremost by elevated pulmonary artery pressure. Pathogenic remodeling of medium and small pulmonary arterials increases pulmonary vascular resistance (PVR), which accompanies the hemodynamic pattern encountered in most PH patients clinically. Predominately, PH is caused by left heart disease or parenchymal lung disease. Pulmonary arterial hypertension (PAH), which was formerly termed *primary pulmonary hypertension*, is a distinct albeit uncommon subgroup of PH.[1] In PAH, interplay between genetic and molecular factors results in a classic plexogenic pulmonary arteriopathy occurring in the absence of other diseases that affect pulmonary artery pressure.

The pathophysiology of PH extends beyond the pulmonary circulation, and often includes right ventricular (RV) dysfunction, chronic kidney disease, overactivation of neurohumoral signaling pathways, and many other processes that impair global cardiovascular function and fitness.[2] This constellation of features forebodes disease burden, and informs treatment timing and escalation. Several recent advances have contemporized aspects central to PH epidemiology, diagnosis, prognosis, and patient management. For example, fresh insight on PH risk factors, the contribution of right ventricular-pulmonary arterial (RV-PA) uncoupling to right heart failure, and a widened cardiopulmonary hemodynamic risk spectrum have modernized the clinical profile of PH and caused a strategic shift emphasizing early diagnosis. Additionally, newly available medical and procedural therapies for PAH highlight continued progress toward improving quality of life and lifespan in patients affected by a disease once considered uniformly fatal. This chapter will begin by discussing the normal pulmonary circulation to provide an anatomic and physiological bases for understanding: (1) the classification of PH, (2) the pathology and pathobiology of PH, (3) the pathophysiology of PH, (4) and the clinical presentation, assessment, and treatment of patients with PH and PAH.

NORMAL PULMONARY CIRCULATION

The pulmonary vascular circuit originates from the main pulmonary artery, which measures approximately 2.7 to 2.9 cm in diameter, and divides into the right and left main pulmonary arteries. Iterative branching occurs proximal to distal along a course that tracks with each successive generation of bronchus. The main pulmonary arteries give rise to lobar arteries that branch into segmental, subsegmental, and intralobar arteries. Collectively, these aspects of the pulmonary circulatory tree comprise elastic arterials that are distensible at low transmural pressures, greater than 500 μm in diameter, and largely spared from adverse remodeling that underlies most pulmonary circulatory diseases.

By contrast, muscular pulmonary arteries and arterioles measure 100 to 500 μm and less than 100 μm in diameter, respectively, and are the principal structures affected in pulmonary circulatory diseases.[3] The wall of muscular arteries includes the single cell endothelial layer and muscular media, which is separated by the internal and external elastic laminae and densely populated with pulmonary artery smooth muscle cells. The adventitia is the outer most layer of muscular arteries and is comprised of fibroblasts, macrophage, progenitor cells, and vaso-vasorum. Pulmonary arterioles are pre-capillary structures that consist of a thin intima and single elastic lamina only. Alveolar capillaries measure 5 to 10 μm in diameter and are lined with a continuous layer of endothelium enveloped by pericytes at focal connections, but do not include pulmonary artery smooth cells and, thus, are noncontractile.

Pulmonary Circulatory Physiology

The anatomy of the pulmonary vasculature is oriented in a parallel circuit, which permits high blood flow, low pressure, and low resistance (Fig. 88.1A). This is in contradistinction to the systemic vasculature that is organized as a circuit in series and designed to distribute cardiac output (CO) to regional beds. In the pulmonary circulation, multiplicative branching with successive smaller caliber vessels maximizes surface area to optimize gas exchange at the alveolar-capillary interface. Indeed, there are 280 billion capillaries, which outnumbers individual alveoli by a factor of 900-fold to cover 85% of all available alveolar surface area. The PVR reflects the ratio of change in pulmonary artery pressure (ΔP) to mean pulmonary blood flow (Q) (L/min); when this value is multiplied by 80, the result is expressed as mm Hg/L/min and referred to as a Wood unit (alternatively, resistance expressed as dyne*sec*cm^{-5} divided by 80 yields a Wood unit).[4] The calculated PVR may also be determined in clinical practice as: (mean pulmonary artery pressure [mPAP]-left atrial pressure)/CO). Because routine left atrial sampling is not practical, the pulmonary artery wedge pressure (PAWP) is used as a surrogate of this measurement.

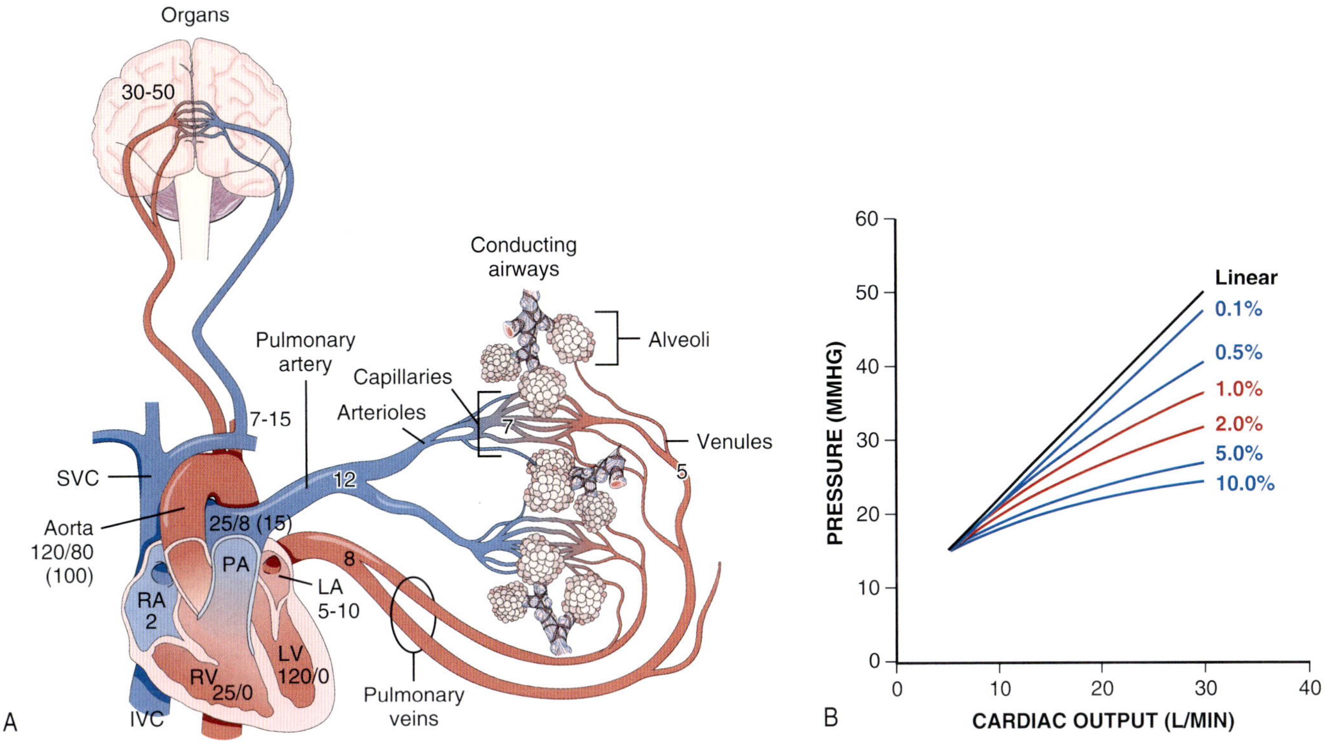

FIGURE 88.1 Pulmonary vascular anatomy and distensibility. **A,** Low pressure and low resistance characteristics of the pulmonary circulation permit optimal surface for gas exchange at the alveolar-capillary interface. Normal systolic and diastolic blood pressure values are presented in various compartments. *IVC,* Inferior vena cava; *LA,* left atrium; *LV,* left ventricle; *PA,* pulmonary artery; *RA,* right atrium; *RV,* right ventricle; *SVC,* superior vena cava. **B,** Modeled mean pulmonary arterial pressure–cardiac output relationships during dynamic exercise with progressively increased distensibility coefficients (α). The normal range of α values is 1% to 2%. (**A** adapted from Chamarthy MR et al. *Cardiovasc Diagn Ther* 2018 Jun;8(3):208–213; **B** from Lewis GD et al. *Circulation* 2013;128:1470–1479.)

Effect of Aging on the Pulmonary Circulation

Beyond the age of 35 years, there is a gradual decline in extensibility of the conduit pulmonary arteries, and an increase in muscularization of medium and small vessels. This is characterized by collagen deposition and deterioration of elastin, which, collectively causes mild fibrotic remodeling of the intima and vascular stiffening. The main pulmonary artery dilates slightly with age,[5] and the consequences of these age-related anatomical and histologic changes include a subtle rise in average mean mPAP and PVR, most evident in the seventh decade of life or greater.[6]

Pulmonary Venous System

A pulmonary venous network emerges from the alveolar-capillary interface with vessel diameter and branching ratios comparable to the arterial tree, totaling 15 enumerations.[7] Ultimately, three or four bronchial veins converge to a main pulmonary vein, in a pair per lung hilum. Overall, a total of four pulmonary veins articulate into the posterior left atrium. Small intra-pulmonary veins include a smooth muscle media, adventitia with vaso-vasorum, and elastin casing. Large pulmonary veins generally lack an elastic lamina and are muscular but are 60% less thick than pulmonary arteries with relatively more extracellular matrix. Sclerosis, fibrosis, and muscularization of pulmonary veins is recognized increasingly in the pathogenesis of left heart failure and other PH syndromes once considered to be exclusively due to arterial remodeling.[8]

Pulmonary Circulatory Physiology During Exercise

The average pulmonary blood flow at rest is 3.5 L/min/m², and at any moment 300 mL/m² of blood is in the pulmonary circulation of which approximately 25% occupies capillaries.[7] However, during exercise the cardiopulmonary apparatus must accommodate a fivefold or greater increase in CO. This dramatic shift affects mPAP via the direct effect of increased CO on intravascular blood volume and left atrial pressure.[9] It is important that the relationship between mPAP and CO is curvilinear in vivo (Fig. 88.1B). This allows the pulmonary circulatory unit to accommodate increased blood volume without a proportional increase in pulmonary artery pressure, which would have a detrimental effect on RV afterload. The CO-mPAP relationship hinges on preserved distensibility, however, and pathological processes that impair normal pulmonary vascular compliance (even subtly) stand to disrupt cardiopulmonary physiology leading to a pathological state manifest by impaired exercise tolerance.[10]

CLASSIFICATION OF PULMONARY HYPERTENSION

In the 1950s, the British cardiologist Dr. Paul Wood assembled the first comprehensive data on PH patients. This classic work included observations from his own cohort at the National Heart and Brompton Hospitals, seminal descriptive publications on "primary pulmonary hypertension" by Castleman and Bland (1946), and pulmonary vascular pathology reports by Edwards (1950). Wood concluded upon six PH types: passive, hyperkinetic, obstructive, obliterative, vasoconstrictive, and polygenic (i.e., multifactorial). Given the rudimentary technology of that time compared to today, the sustained usefulness of this initial PH framework is quite remarkable. Indeed, the current PH classification overlaps with this scheme by Wood,[11] but now the cardiopulmonary hemodynamic profile is integrated directly with information on clinical disorders that predispose to pulmonary vascular disease. This collective, in turn, informs the pathophysiology (and presumed pathobiology) of an individual patient at point of care.

There are two broad, inter-related strategies by which to classify patients with PH.[12] First, the cardiopulmonary hemodynamic profile is used to assign patients into one of three categories: pre-capillary, isolated post-capillary, and combined pre- and post-capillary PH (Table 88.1). These designations aim to distinguish PH originating due to a pulmonary arterial lesion (pre-capillary) from disorders originating in the pulmonary venous bed or structures distal (post-capillary). Combined pre- and post-capillary PH refers to a post-capillary process that causes pulmonary arterial remodeling (indicated by increased PVR). Second, the comorbidity and demographic profile is used to assign individual patients into an

TABLE 88.1 Overlap Between Hemodynamic and Clinical Classification of Pulmonary Hypertension

DEFINITIONS	CHARACTERISTICS	PH CLINICAL GROUPS
Pre-capillary PH	mPAP >20 mm Hg	PAH
	PAWP ≤15 mm Hg	Lung disease
	PVR ≥3 WU	Sleep-disordered breathing
		Miscellaneous causes
Isolated post-capillary PH (IpcPH)	mPAP >20 mm Hg	Left heart disease
	PAWP >15 mm Hg	Miscellaneous causes
	PVR <3 WU	
Combined pre- and post-capillary PH (CpcPH)	mPAP >20 mm Hg	Left heart disease
	PAWP >15 mm Hg	Miscellaneous causes
	PVR ≥3 WU	

mPAP, Mean pulmonary artery pressure; *PAH*, pulmonary arterial hypertension; *PAWP*, pulmonary artery wedge pressure; *PH*, pulmonary hypertension; *PVR*, pulmonary vascular resistance.
Adapted from Simonneau G, et al. *Eur Respir J.* 2019;53(1):180191.

TABLE 88.2 Revised Clinical Classification of Pulmonary Hypertension

1 PAH
 1.1 Idiopathic PAH
 1.2 Heritable PAH
 1.3 Drug- and toxin-induced PAH
 1.4 PAH associated with:
  1.4.1 Connective tissue disease
  1.4.2 HIV infection
  1.4.3 Portal hypertension
  1.4.4 Congenital heart disease
  1.4.5 Schistosomiasis
 1.5 PAH long-term responders to calcium channel blockers
 1.6 PAH with overt features of venous/capillaries (PVOD/PCH) involvement
 1.7 Persistent PH of the newborn syndrome

2 PH due to left heart disease
 2.1 PH due to heart failure with preserved LVEF
 2.2 PH due to heart failure with reduced LVEF
 2.3 Valvular heart disease
 2.4 Congenital/acquired cardiovascular conditions leading to post-capillary PH

3 PH due to lung diseases and/or hypoxia
 3.1 Obstructive lung disease
 3.2 Restrictive lung disease
 3.3 Other lung disease with mixed restrictive/obstructive pattern
 3.4 Hypoxia without lung disease
 3.5 Developmental lung disorders

4 PH due to pulmonary artery obstructions
 4.1 Chronic thromboembolic PH
 4.2 Other pulmonary artery obstructions

5 PH with unclear and/or multifactorial mechanisms
 5.1 Hematological disorders
 5.2 Systemic and metabolic disorders
 5.3 Others
 5.4 Complex congenital heart disease

HIV, Human immunodeficiency virus; *LVEF*, left ventricular ejection fraction; *PAH*, pulmonary arterial hypertension; *PCH*, pulmonary capillary hemangiomatosis; *PH*, pulmonary hypertension; *PVOD*, pulmonary venoocclusive disease.
Adapted from Simonneau G, et al. *Eur Respir J.* 2019;53(1):801913.

appropriate clinical PH group (Table 88.2). It is important to note that certain clinical-hemodynamic combinations are not compatible; for example, PAH is exclusive of post-capillary PH.[1]

Hemodynamic Classifications

Elevated mPAP greater than 20 mm Hg diagnosed by invasive right heart catheterization (RHC) measured supine at rest is the sine qua non of PH. This is based on early-era normative data in 1,187 healthy research subjects showing that the median mPAP at rest was 14.0 ± 3.1 mm Hg. Using two times the SD, the upper limit of normal mPAP is 19 to 20 mm Hg.[13] These findings converge with results from large RHC databases suggesting that clinical risk emerges at mPAP approximately 19 mm Hg.[14] The relationship between mPAP and mortality is continuous, and patients referred for RHC with mPAP approximately 20 to 24 mm Hg and greater than 25 mm Hg have an all-cause adjusted mortality risk that is 1.23-fold and 2.16-fold greater, respectively, compared to mPAP less than 19 mm Hg. However, the association between mPAP and outcome is not homogenous throughout the mPAP continuum, as an increase by 1 mm Hg influences outcome risk to a greater extent between 20 and 25 mm Hg compared to levels indicative of severe disease (e.g., mPAP >40 mm Hg) (Fig. 88.2). It is also important to note that the normal mPAP increases slightly with age and may be as high as 22 mm Hg among those greater than 50 years. This should be considered when interpreting cardiopulmonary hemodynamics in symptomatic patients within this age range.[6,13]

A major branch point in the hemodynamic classification of PH patients is delineating pre-capillary PH from post-capillary PH. This is generally accomplished by turning to the PAWP, which transmits left ventricular end-diastolic pressure (LVEDP) in the absence of mitral valve disease or other mechanical obstruction between the pulmonary capillary network and LV. A PAWP greater than 15 mm Hg (or more conservatively >12 mm Hg) suggests pulmonary venous hypertension and post-capillary PH, whereas PAWP ≤ 15 mm Hg (or ≤ 12 mm Hg) indicates pre-capillary PH.[12] If a direct LVEDP measurement is performed, greater than 15 mm Hg is generally used to diagnose post-capillary PH (see section below on performing cardiac catheterization).

The most common form of PH that cardiologists will encounter in contemporary medical practice is in the setting of left heart disease. This includes patients with left ventricular systolic or diastolic dysfunction, mitral valvular disease of any type, stiff left atrial syndrome, and LV outflow tract or aortic valvular lesions, including obstructive hypertrophic cardiomyopathy. Virtually any left heart structural or functional abnormality from the ascending aorta to pulmonary venous bed may predispose patients to post-capillary PH. Thus, traditional risk factors for coronary artery disease, cardiomyopathy, left-sided structural heart disease, and mitral/aortic valvular heart disease are implicated directly or indirectly as PH risk factors as well. Notable examples include obstructive sleep apnea (OSA), tobacco use, connective tissue disease, and prior or active cardiotoxic chemotherapy. Processes that promote pathological remodeling of pulmonary arterials proximal to the lung capillary interface predispose patients to pre-capillary PH. Broadly, this encompasses patients with PAH, hypoxic lung or sleep disordered breathing conditions, and chronic thromboembolic pulmonary hypertension (CTEPH).

The prognostic implications of elevated mPAP have been affirmed in numerous studies involving patients with PH from almost all etiologies, particularly heart failure with reduced LV ejection fraction (HFrEF), mitral stenosis, idiopathic pulmonary fibrosis, chronic obstructive pulmonary disease (COPD), and sickle cell disease.[15,16] Nonetheless, physiological or easily reversible causes of mPAP greater than 20 mm Hg have been reported, such as anemia, pregnancy, and increased pulmonary blood flow states (e.g., highly conditioned athletes). To address this dilemma, PVR is used as a hemodynamic surrogate of pulmonary vascular disease, and the addition of PVR to mPAP increases the specificity of diagnosing PH compared to mPAP alone. A cut-off PVR equal to or greater than 3.0 Wood units (WU) distinguishes pulmonary vascular disease in PH patients; however, this demarcation is largely historical or based on observational studies in selected subgroups, such as those with idiopathic PAH, congenital heart defects with intracardiac shunt, and pulmonary fibrosis. Emergent data on the spectrum of PVR associated with adverse outcome suggests that greater than 2.2 WU may be sufficient to identify a pathogenic rise in mPAP, which differs in magnitude between pre- and post-capillary PH patients.[17] Combined pre- and post-capillary PH is an overlapping pathophenotype that is characterized by pulmonary arterial remodeling due to chronic pulmonary venous hypertension, and in these patients mPAP

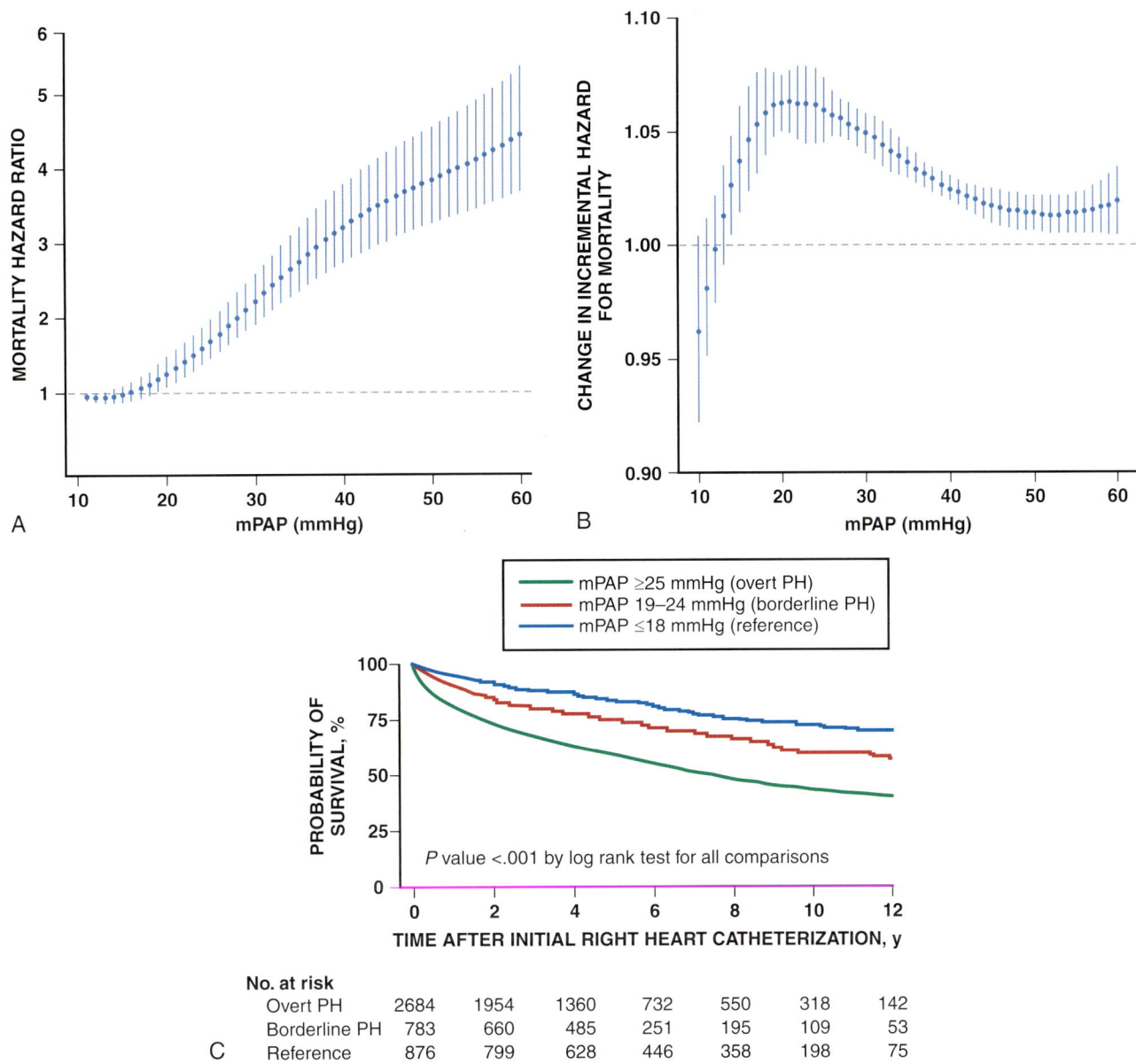

FIGURE 88.2 The association between pulmonary artery pressure and mortality. **A**, Data from a U.S. national cohort of patients referred for right heart catheterization were collected and the mean pulmonary artery pressure (mPAP) was modeled as a continuous variable. The association between all-cause mortality and mPAP emerges approximately 19 mm Hg and increases through approximately 60 mm Hg. **B**, Compared to mPAP levels at the high end of the continuum, an incremental increase by 1 mm Hg between approximately 20 and 25 mm Hg is associated with a greater change in clinical risk. **C**, The relationship between mildly elevated mPAP (>19 mm Hg) and adverse clinical outcome has been validated in several populations, demonstrated here by a Kaplan Meier analysis from patients referred for right heart catheterization (RHC) at Vanderbilt University. *PH*, Pulmonary hypertension. (**A** and **B** from Maron BA et al. *Circulation* 2016;133:1240–1248; **C** from Assad TR et al. *JAMA Cardiol* 2017;2:1361–1368.)

greater than 20 mm Hg, PAWP greater than 15 mm Hg, and PVR equal to or greater than 3.0 WU is used for diagnosis (see Table 88.1).[12]

Isolated Post-Capillary Pulmonary Hypertension Clinical Classifications
Heart Failure and Cardiomyopathy
The prevalence of PH in HFrEF populations is 30% to 50% when considering a pulmonary artery systolic pressure (PASP) cut-off greater than 45 mm Hg estimated echocardiographically.[18] This corresponds to a mPAP approximately 30 mm Hg, using the conversion method of Syyed: mPAP = 0.65 × PASP + 0.55 mm Hg. A stepwise increase in mortality risk of 6% to 8% is generally observed per 5 mm Hg rise in PASP. Catheter-based studies, which may be subject to referral bias, indicate that PH is present in 62% to 77% of HFrEF patients. Compared to idiopathic cardiomyopathy, patients with ischemic, infiltrative, hypertensive, or substance abuse cardiomyopathy tend to have higher mPAP at diagnosis. The adjusted mortality risk per 5 mm Hg increase in mPAP is 85% in myocarditis compared to non-myocarditis patients.

In heart failure with preserved LV ejection fraction (HFpEF), the prevalence of PH is substantial and of greater clinical risk.[19] By some estimates, approximately 80% of HFpEF patients have PH (defined by an estimated PASP >35 mm Hg), which correlates with PAWP, and associates with a 30% mortality risk increase per 10 mm Hg PASP. Population studies in which RHC was used to directly measure cardiopulmonary hemodynamics suggest that more than half of patients have mPAP greater than 25 mm Hg, and compared to non-PH counterparts this group is at 33% higher risk for heart failure hospitalization rates. In obstructive hypertrophic cardiomyopathy, PH is observed in over half of patients referred for anterior septal myectomy.[20]

Valvular Heart Disease
The spectrum of PH severity reported in valvular heart disease is wide, which akin to data in cardiomyopathy patients is likely due to

variable patient selection, method of assessment, and study enrollment criteria.[21,22] Across echocardiographic and RHC population studies, between 30% and 36% of asymptomatic aortic stenosis patients have at least mild PH, with severe PH observed in 20% of affected patients. In mitral stenosis, PH affects greater than 50% of patients, tracks strongly with symptoms, is a key determinant of management, and prognosticates outcome. Mitral stenosis patients with PASP greater than 60 mm Hg, for example, have a higher long-term rate of restenosis following mitral balloon valvuloplasty, and decreased 3-year survival following valvotomy compared to similar patients without severe PH. There is a positive association between mitral regurgitation grade and regurgitant orifice area with PASP. Moderate or severe PH is observed in greater than 50% of patients with severe primary mitral regurgitation, and is higher in subgroups with increased symptom burden. The average 5-year survival rate among primary mitral regurgitation patients is 25% less with PH compared to similar patients without PH. In secondary mitral valvular regurgitation, PH prevalence aligns with findings from HFrEF, in which approximately 40% of patients are affected. Stiff left atrial syndrome is probably underrecognized clinically, and certainly overlooked as a cause of PH even though impaired atrial compliance is a direct determinant of pulmonary venous congestion.[23]

Pre-Capillary Pulmonary Hypertension Clinical Classifications

Pulmonary Arterial Hypertension

Most PAH is idiopathic (iPAH) and prevalence depends somewhat on the methods for collecting population data. In studies from France, United Kingdom, Spain, Scotland, United States, and Ireland, the PAH prevalence is approximately 15 to 52 in 1 million population with an incidence of 2.4 to 7.1 cases per million per year.[24] The clinical profile of prevalent patients has evolved substantially since the initial NIH registry of PAH between 1981 and 1986. In that study, the mean age was 36 ± 15 years and the female to male ratio was 1.7.[1] Then, descriptions of PAH focused on women of childbearing age with connective tissue disease. However, modern registries suggest PAH affects patients across a broader age range: the Registry to Evaluate Early And Long-term PAH disease management (REVEAL),[25] inclusive of 54 U.S. centers, reported age at enrollment of 53 ± 15 years. Although the case distribution by gender remains stable compared with earlier reports, men tend to present with more severe disease burden compared with women, especially when diagnosis is made before age 45.[26,27] The female-predominant prevalence of PAH appears to be greater in black patients, although it remains unclear if this reflects a true racial trend or bias in access to care, or other factors.

Longitudinal outcome data from the NIH registry was in the era prior to pulmonary vasodilator therapies, and treatment was limited mainly to digoxin and diuretics. Accordingly, prognosis was dismal: the 1-, 3-, and 5-year survival rates were 68%, 48%, and 34%, respectively. Today, the 3-year survival approaches 84% in cross-sectional studies among patients treated with multiple drugs, although lifespan and quality of life remain greatly limited in most PAH patients.[28]

Hereditary Pulmonary Artery Hypertension

In 2001, Drs. John Newman and Jim Loyd and colleagues reported that a T354G variant in the *BMPR2* gene was common to 6 of 10 PAH patients across 5 subfamilies with affected members (reviewed in ref. 29). This large kindred genotype analysis gave rise to the field of hereditary PAH, which is a term that includes familial PAH (e.g., two or more affected family members) and simplex PAH (e.g., single occurrence in a family) when a pathogenic variant has been identified. Today, a BMRP2 variant is recognized as the most common genetic risk factor for PAH, identifiable in 70% of families with PAH and 10% of sporadic iPAH cases. However, a

TABLE 88.3 Key Genes Implicated in the Pathogenesis of Pulmonary Arterial Hypertension

GENES	NAME	BIOFUNCTIONALITY/PATHOGENICITY	CLINICAL PHENOTYPE
BMPR2	Bone Morphogenetic Protein Receptor Type 2	Pulmonary artery smooth muscle cell proliferation	Hereditary/familial PAH (germline)
		Endothelial dysfunction	PAH (de novo)
		Apoptosis-resistance	
		Dysregulated cellular metabolism	
ACVRL1	Activin A Receptor Like Type 1	Cell-surface receptor for the TGF-β superfamily of ligands	PAH associated with Hemorrhagic telangiectasia type 2
ENG	Endoglin	Regulates endothelial binding of TGF-β-1 and β-1 peptides	PAH associated with Hemorrhagic telangiectasia type 2
EIF2AK4	Eukaryotic Translation Initiation Factor 2 Alpha Kinase 4	Intimal fibrosis	Pulmonary venoocclusive disease
		Endothelial proliferation	Pulmonary capillary hemangiomatosis
GDF2	Growth differentiation factor 2	Regulates vascular quiescence	Hereditary/familial PAH
		Anti-apoptotic	
		Anti-proliferative	
		Inhibits vascular permeability	
TBX4	T-Box Transcription Factor 4	Developmental processes	Pediatric PAH
			Associated with small patella syndrome
ATP13A3	ATPase Family Homolog Up-Regulated In Senescence Cells 1	Cellular senescence	iPAH
SOX17	SRY-box 17	Erk an Wnt signaling	iPAH
		Immune response	
AQP1	Aquaporin 1	Pulmonary arterial smooth muscle cell migration and proliferation	Hereditary/familial PAH
		β-catenin signaling	
CAV1	Caveolin-1	Regulates physical colocalization of BMP receptors	Hereditary/familial PAH
		TGF-β signaling	
KCNK3	Potassium channel subfamily K member 3	Regulates membrane potential	Hereditary/familial PAH iPAH
		Vascular tone	

iPAH, Idiopathic pulmonary arterial hypertension; *TGF-β*, transforming growth factor-beta.

variant in any of 12 genes is considered pathogenic in PAH (Table 88.3), and evidence exists to implicate the involvement of 5 other potential genes.[29] Notable examples include variants in *ENG* and *ACVRL1* that code for endoglin and activin receptor-like kinase 1 (ALK-1), respectively, which are linked mechanistically to dysfunctional BMPR-2 and implicated in hereditary hemorrhagic telangiectasia-PAH. Most variants, including those affecting the BMPR-2 gene, are inherited in an autosomal dominant pattern, but exhibit reduced penetrance. Overall, fewer than 30% of PAH patients have single variants in causative genes.

Toxin-Induced Pulmonary Artery Hypertension

There is an established association between PAH and the anorexigens fenfluramine and dexfenfluramine, resulting in the discontinuation of these drugs for public use in 1997. Illicit methamphetamine use (in many cases leading to addiction), is a newly recognized worldwide epidemic affecting greater than 1% of the population aged 15 to 64 years in the United States, Australia, South Africa, and the United Kingdom among other countries (Fig. 88.3). Methamphetamines may account for up to 18% of non-idiopathic PAH, but data on the true prevalence of this population are lacking.[30] Pulmonary vascular remodeling from a mechanical injury induced by the drug packing material or as a result of molecular interactions with drug metabolites are proposed to cause PAH. Based on available data, the prognosis for methamphetamine PAH is concerning with a twofold risk of clinical worsening compared to iPAH and event-free survival at 5 years of 47%. The tyrosine kinase inhibitor dasatinib is associated with PAH, although this is unlikely a drug class effect.

Systemic Sclerosis with Pulmonary Artery Hypertension

Connective tissue disease-associated PAH accounts for approximately one in four cases of PAH overall, with systemic sclerosis (SSc) as the most common subtype. The overall prevalence of SSc-PAH is likely underestimated, but is at least 24 cases per million, which again is far greater than iPAH. Among SSc patients, the prevalence of PAH is 12% and up to 20% in patients with evidence of impaired lung diffusion capacity. However, PAH is the leading cause of death in SSc, and the mortality rate is fourfold greater than for iPAH.[31] The overall SSc syndrome includes immune dysfunction, inflammation, increased extracellular matrix remodeling, and fibrosis resulting in multiorgan injury, which provides a pathobiological basis for pulmonary vascular involvement. Although PAH may be observed in either the diffuse or limited cutaneous SSc subtypes, interstitial lung disease (pulmonary fibrosis) is particularly common in diffuse SSc. Therefore, it is important to determine if abnormal cardiopulmonary hemodynamics are in the setting of SSc-PAH or, conversely, due to PH from interstitial lung disease.

Infectious Pulmonary Artery Hypertension Subtypes

Schistosomiasis is a flatworm fluke parasite endemic to 52 countries, particularly Brazil and African nations, infecting between 200 and 300 million worldwide.[32] *Schistosomiasis mansoni* has a mandatory two-host life cycle that includes avian and snail. The cercariae are released by snail into fresh water, and gain access to humans via transdermal penetration. The result is an immune complex hypersensitivity reaction (i.e., Katayama fever) which self-resolves over 4 to 6 weeks. However, the worms mate in the portal circulation and the eggs themselves are transported to the pulmonary vasculature where granulomatous remodeling ensues resulting in a PAH clinical syndrome. The actual prevalence of Schistosomiasis-PAH is not known, but this is undoubtedly the most common cause of precapillary PH in developing countries. Pre-existing hepatosplenic disease increases PAH risk of infected hosts exponentially.

Pulmonary vascular dysfunction is a well-documented complication of human immunodeficiency virus (HIV), although uncertainty persists to the extent to which PAH, rather than elevated pulmonary artery pressure due to comorbid or iatrogenic causes, explain dyspnea or PH. From 7648 consecutive HIV-positive adults in France, 0.46% had PAH confirmed by RHC. Within HIV populations, the odds ratio of increased pulmonary artery pressure is 1.27 and 1.28 in patients with viral load greater than 500 copies/mL and CD4 cell count less than 200 cells/μL, respectively, which is associated with a risk-adjusted mortality increase of 78%.[33] Convincing evidence to suggest the virus directly infects pulmonary vascular cells is lacking, although vascular injury induced by viral proteins is plausible. Reports early in the COVID-19 pandemic suggest pulmonary vascular involvement in some patients, including key features consistent with end-stage disease such as frank right heart failure.[34] Understanding the longitudinal implications of COVID-19 on the development of PH, however, remain forthcoming.

Congenital Heart Disease

Pathogenic pulmonary vascular remodeling may develop in any patient with a large volume left-to-right intra- or extra-cardiac shunt, or an anatomic catastrophe that affects inflow or outflow (see Chapter 82). From a Dutch nationwide epidemiological study over a 15-year period, PH was reported in 63.7 per million children, which included 34% that had shunts amenable to immediate surgical correction. Among those patients with long-term PAH, 72% had a form of congenital heart disease.[35] As congenital heart disease patients

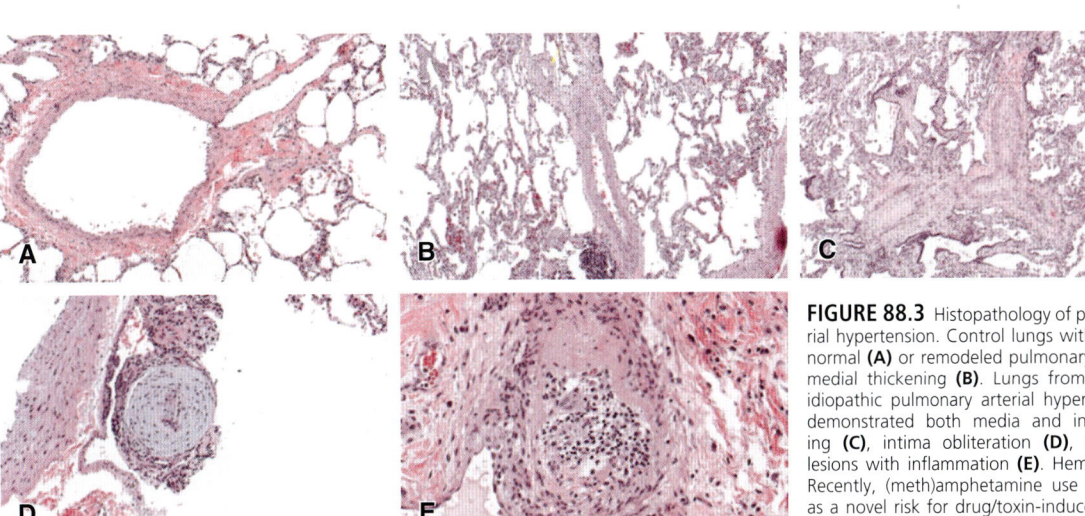

FIGURE 88.3 Histopathology of pulmonary arterial hypertension. Control lungs with histologically normal **(A)** or remodeled pulmonary arterials with medial thickening **(B)**. Lungs from patients with idiopathic pulmonary arterial hypertension (iPAH) demonstrated both media and intimal thickening **(C)**, intima obliteration **(D)**, and plexiform lesions with inflammation **(E)**. Hematoxylin-eosin. Recently, (meth)amphetamine use was identified as a novel risk for drug/toxin-induced PAH. (From Tuder RM et al. *Clin Chest Med* 2013;34:650.)

continue to live longer into adulthood, PAH will remain an important consideration for clinicians managing these patients. Indeed, cases discovered in the greater than or equal to seventh decade of life are well documented.

Lung Disease and Sleep Disordered Breathing
Approximately 90% of COPD patients have mPAP greater than 20 mm Hg, but only 5% have mPAP greater than 40 mm Hg.[36] Thus, severe PH in COPD is uncommon but when present is a risk factor for *cor pulmonale*. Similarly, PH is reported in 8% to 15% of mild idiopathic pulmonary fibrosis but may affect two-thirds of end-stage patients. Chronic PH is an uncommon manifestation of OSA, is almost always mild, and may be reversible with noninvasive ventilation (see Chapter 89). Nonetheless, given the expanding rate of obesity in the United States and other industrialized countries, OSA is an important and often overlooked PH risk factor.

Chronic Thromboembolic Pulmonary Hypertension
Thrombotic in situ pulmonary vascular remodeling resulting in PH occurs in approximately 3% of patients following luminal pulmonary embolism (see Chapter 87). Risk factors for developing CTEPH are not known, although elevated levels of factor VIII have been demonstrated in about 40% of patients. The clinical burden of CTEPH is mitigated fully in patients who are eligible and undergo successful surgical pulmonary thromboendarterectomy, which represents approximately two-thirds of patients. Surgical, medical, and percutaneous therapies for CTEPH are discussed below.

Pulmonary Venoocclusive Disease
Muscularization and sclerotic changes of pulmonary venules are the cornerstone findings of pulmonary venoocclusive disease (PVOD), which has an estimated annual incidence of 0.1 to 0.2 per million people.[37] Risk factors include auto-immune disorders, organic solvent exposure, medical therapy with alkylating agents (particularly mitomycin and cyclophosphamide), and certain genetic predispositions. No gender predominance has been established for the prevalence of PVOD.

Portopulmonary Hypertension
Portal hypertension with pre-capillary PH and PVR equal to or greater than 3.0 WU defines portopulmonary hypertension. Approximately 5% of cirrhotic patients have PH, although the prevalence is 16% in liver transplant referral populations. The detrimental effects of high CO and endotoxin release from liver dysfunction are proposed to underlie portopulmonary hypertension.[38] This is distinct from hepatopulmonary syndrome, for which hypoxemia from intrapulmonary vasodilation and impaired hypoxic vasoconstriction (without PH) is the hallmark feature.

Combined Pre- and Post-Capillary Pulmonary Hypertension
Left Heart Structural and Functional Disorders
Elevated PVR in patients with post-capillary PH is observed in many of the same circumstances associated with isolated post-capillary PH. Thus, there is overlap in the risk factors between these phenotypes, including diabetes mellitus; causes of LV dysfunction such as ischemic heart disease; valvular disease; and HFpEF. Although the genetic profile between these groups differs, it is not clear how genetic risk may protect or predispose to either clinical phenotype.[39] The combined pre-/post-capillary PH phenotype accounts for approximately 15% of all PH patients, although outcome is similar between this group and isolated post-capillary PH patients.[12,39]

PATHOLOGY

All forms of persistent PH are associated with pathogenic vascular remodeling, and most subtypes involve hypertrophic concentric muscularization, as well as fibrotic and (micro)thrombotic effacement of distal pulmonary arterials. The main-, lobar-, and intra-lobar pulmonary arteries are usually phenotypically normal. Exceptions to this include congenital pulmonary stenosis, and proximal pulmonary arterial involvement in patients with CTEPH. In iPAH, certain forms of congenital heart disease, HIV-PAH, and Schistosomiasis-PAH there is a unique plexogenic vasculopathy (see Fig. 88.3). These focal but dense lesions are characterized by endothelial proliferation, the formation of microchannel networks, and irregular smooth muscle cell orientation in a glomeruloid pattern. The functional significance of these malformations is contested, but, nonetheless, their appearance is pathognomonic for PAH on autopsy.

Pulmonary venous remodeling is a classic feature of PVOD, which is a rare form of PH that overlaps histopathologically with pulmonary capillary hemangiomatosis (PCH). In both PVOD and PCH, arterial medial hypertrophy and/or intimal fibrosis, hemosiderosis, venulitis, and mild lymphocytic infiltrate are observed. In PVOD, obliteration of small pulmonary veins occurs due to sclerotic and fibrous thickening. A biallelic mutation in the *EIF2AK4* gene is associated with PVOD, and although chest radiation or other toxic exposures are related weakly to prevalence, definitive risk factors are lacking.[29] Autopsy specimens from patients with left heart failure show increased arterialization of pulmonary veins, including medial and intimal thickening that is largely concentric, and variable within the lung. These remodeling patterns correlate strongly with pulmonary artery pressure, providing a histopathological basis for the combined pre- and post-capillary PH hemodynamic pattern observed in some HFpEF and HFrEF patients.[8]

Unique pathology of CTEPH. Organized clot, defined by heavily fibrotic and obstructive lesions involving the intima and medial layers of distal pulmonary arterials, is a cornerstone feature of CTEPH. Strictures, webbing, dearborization, and collateralization with bronchial arterials is often also observed. It is important to note that vascular segments distal to the site of initial embolic injury are involved commonly, raising speculation that a propagative vasculopathy ultimately underlies the complete CTEPH pathophenotype.

PATHOBIOLOGY

The molecular basis of PAH is complex, and in blood vessels driven by interplay between signaling pathways that involve pulmonary artery endothelial cells, smooth muscle cells, pericytes, and adventitial fibroblasts (Fig. 88.4). Dysregulated cellular metabolism, specifically the preferential synthesis of lactic acid even under oxygen-rich circumstances (Warburg effect), apoptosis-resistance, post-transcriptional regulation of pro-fibrotic proteins, and epigenetic events underlie pathogenic changes to the ultrastructure of pulmonary arterioles.[40] A unifying, inciting trigger that perturbs vasoactive signaling pathways across patients is unlikely. Instead, susceptibility, in part genetic, to maladaptive responses following a stressor is more likely. Abnormalities in T cell (Treg cell)-dependent self-tolerance in PAH following an inflammatory insult leads to vascular infiltration of macrophages, mast cells, and B cells. This pathway may explain some forms of PAH, such as in HIV and SSc.

Activation of hypoxia signaling pathways (even in the absence of frank hypoxemia), nutritional (vitamin C) deficiencies, toxins, and other acquired risk factors stimulate pathogenetic events through alternative pathways. The accumulation of vascular reactive oxygen species is implicated in numerous maladaptive events that drive the PAH pathophenotype. For example, mitochondrial dysfunction perturbs the redox balance of pulmonary artery smooth muscle cells following hypoxia inducible factor (HIF)-1α stimulation, and increases cell survival through dynamin related protein-1/cyclin B1 signaling. Oxidative post-translational modification of a functionally essential cysteine in the SMAD3 docking region of NEDD9 results in pulmonary endothelial fibrillar collagen deposition and is identified recently as a potentially modifiable molecular mediator of PAH.[41] A predilection to metabolic dysfunction and overactivation of neurohumoral systems underlies the pathobiology of PAH (Fig. 88.5).

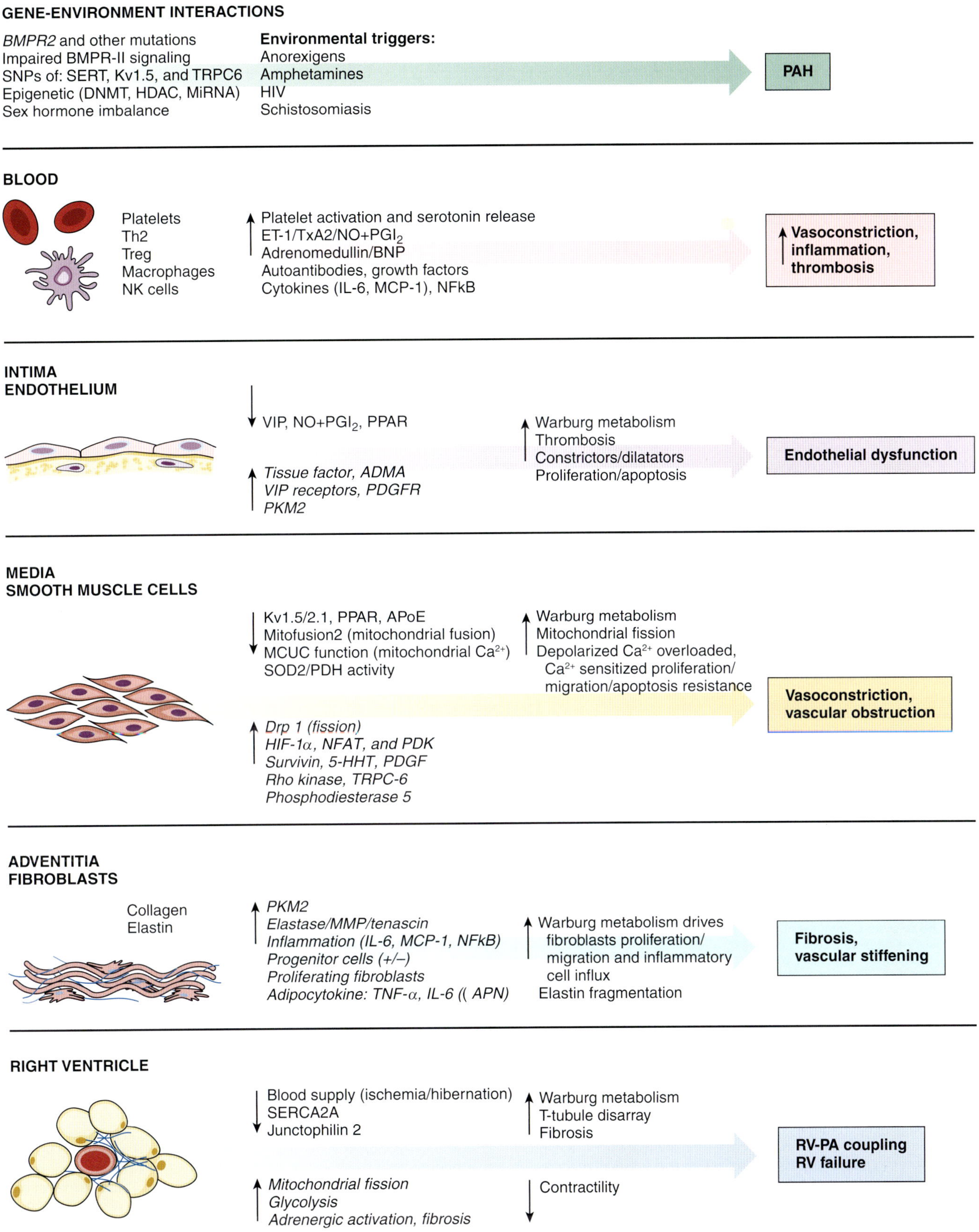

GENE-ENVIRONMENT INTERACTIONS

BMPR2 and other mutations
Impaired BMPR-II signaling
SNPs of: SERT, Kv1.5, and TRPC6
Epigenetic (DNMT, HDAC, MiRNA)
Sex hormone imbalance

Environmental triggers:
Anorexigens
Amphetamines
HIV
Schistosomiasis

→ **PAH**

BLOOD

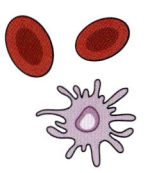

Platelets
Th2
Treg
Macrophages
NK cells

↑ Platelet activation and serotonin release
ET-1/TxA2/NO+PGI$_2$
Adrenomedullin/BNP
Autoantibodies, growth factors
Cytokines (IL-6, MCP-1), NFkB

→ ↑ **Vasoconstriction, inflammation, thrombosis**

INTIMA
ENDOTHELIUM

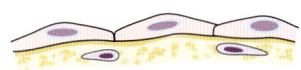

↓ VIP, NO+PGI$_2$, PPAR

↑ Tissue factor, ADMA
VIP receptors, PDGFR
PKM2

↑ Warburg metabolism
Thrombosis
Constrictors/dilatators
Proliferation/apoptosis

→ **Endothelial dysfunction**

MEDIA
SMOOTH MUSCLE CELLS

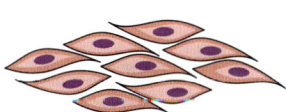

↓ Kv1.5/2.1, PPAR, APoE
Mitofusion2 (mitochondrial fusion)
MCUC function (mitochondrial Ca^{2+})
SOD2/PDH activity

↑ Warburg metabolism
Mitochondrial fission
Depolarized Ca^{2+} overloaded,
Ca^{2+} sensitized proliferation/
migration/apoptosis resistance

↑ Drp 1 (fission)
HIF-1α, NFAT, and PDK
Survivin, 5-HHT, PDGF
Rho kinase, TRPC-6
Phosphodiesterase 5

→ **Vasoconstriction, vascular obstruction**

ADVENTITIA
FIBROBLASTS

Collagen
Elastin
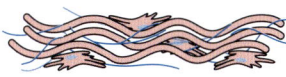

↑ PKM2
Elastase/MMP/tenascin
Inflammation (IL-6, MCP-1, NFkB)
Progenitor cells (+/−)
Proliferating fibroblasts
Adipocytokine: TNF-α, IL-6 (↓ APN)

↑ Warburg metabolism drives
fibroblasts proliferation/
migration and inflammatory
cell influx
Elastin fragmentation

→ **Fibrosis, vascular stiffening**

RIGHT VENTRICLE

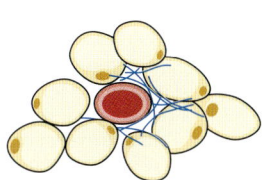

↓ Blood supply (ischemia/hibernation)
↓ SERCA2A
↓ Junctophilin 2

↑ Warburg metabolism
T-tubule disarray
Fibrosis

↑ Mitochondrial fission
Glycolysis
Adrenergic activation, fibrosis

↓ Contractility

→ **RV-PA coupling
RV failure**

FIGURE 88.4 FOR LEGEND SEE PAGE 1664.

FIGURE 88.4 Mechanisms implicated in pathogenesis of pulmonary arterial hypertension (PAH). PAH is a panvasculopathy, meaning that all layers of the vascular wall are involved. PAH is also reflective of gene environment interactions and has important genetic and epigenetic mechanisms. This figure shows abnormalities in the gene environment, blood, and each layer of the pulmonary artery, from intima (endothelial cells) to media (pulmonary arterial smooth muscle cells—PASMCs) to adventitia (fibroblasts). Because of the many reports that inform this composite figure, individual sources for the information are not referenced. The normal state is shown on the left side, the abnormalities that occur in PAH are highlighted in the middle section, and the consequences of these abnormalities are shown on the right. The net effect of these abnormalities is a state of vasoconstriction, inflammation, thrombosis with a hyperproliferative, apoptosis-resistant PASMC population, which promotes vasoconstriction and vascular obstruction, and excessive fibrosis, which reduces vascular compliance. These vascular changes ultimately increase RV afterload and impair RV-pulmonary artery coupling, leading to RV failure. *5-HHT*, 5 hydroxytryptamine; *ADMA*, asymmetric dimethylarginine; *APN*, adiponectin; *BMPR2*, bone morphogenetic protein receptor 2; *BNP*, brain natriuretic peptide; Ca^{2+}, calcium; *DNAMT*, DNA methyltransferase; *Drp-1*, dynamin related protein 1; *ET-1*, endothelin-1; *HDAC*, histone deacetylases; *HIF*, hypoxia inducible factor; *IL*, interleukin; *MCP-1*, monocyte chemoattractant protein-1; *MCUC*, mitochondrial calcium uniporter complex; *miRNA*, micro RNA; *MMP*, matrix metalloproteinase; *NFAT*, nuclear factor of activated T cells; *NF-κB*, nuclear factor kappa light chain enhancer of activated B cells; *NK*, natural killer cells; *NO*, nitric oxide; *PDGFR*, platelet derived growth factor receptor; *PDGR*, platelet derived growth factor; *PDH*, pyruvate dehydrogenase; *PDK*, pyruvate dehydrogenase kinase; PGI_2, prostacyclin-I_2; *PKM-2*, pyruvate kinase M2; *PPAR*, peroxisome proliferator activated receptor; *SERCA*, sarco-endoplasmic reticulum Ca^{2+} ATPase; *SERT*, serotonin transporter; *SNP*, single nucleotide polymorphism; *SOD*, superoxide dismutase; *Th2*, T helper cells; *TNF*, tumor necrosis factor; *T-reg*, regulatory T cells; *TRPC*, transient receptor potential cation channel; *TxA2*, thromboxane A2; *VIP*, vasoactive intestinal peptide. (From Thenappan T et al. *BMJ* 2018;360:5492.)

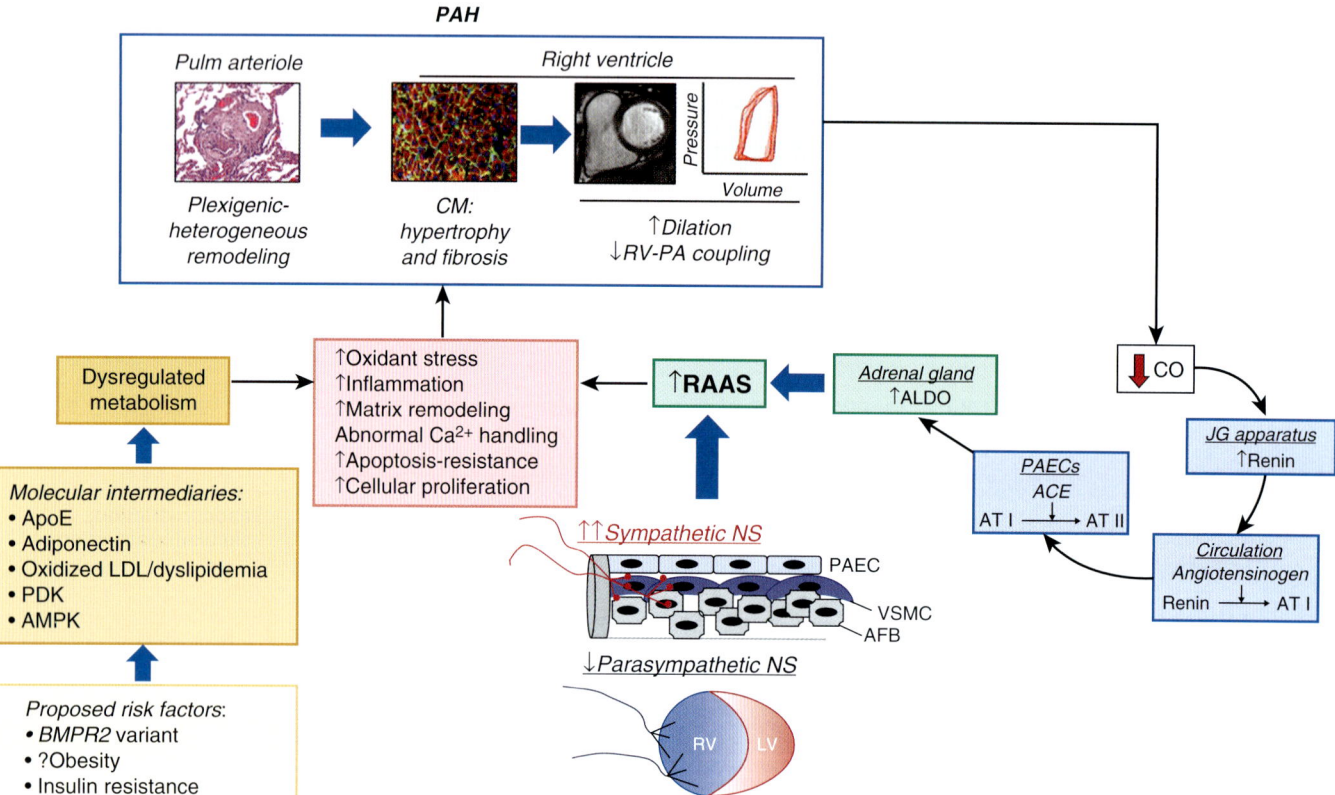

FIGURE 88.5 Dysregulated neurohumoral and metabolic signaling promote pulmonary arterial hypertension (PAH). Acquired and genetic risk factors predispose to dysregulated cellular metabolism involving pulmonary artery endothelial cells, pulmonary artery smooth muscle cells, and right ventricular (RV) cardiomyocytes. This induces various intermediate pathophenotypes involved in the progression of PAH (*red box*). Similarly, chronic elevation in RV afterload in PAH results in cavitary dilation and impaired efficiency, including decreased right ventricular–pulmonary arterial (RV–PA) coupling. A decrease in cardiac output up-regulates the renin–angiotensin–aldosterone system (RAAS), which is independently associated with cardiovascular remodeling and PAH progression. Abnormal sympathetic and parasympathetic nervous system (NS) increase pulmonary arterial tone and impair RV diastolic function, respectively, although the precise cellular targets modulating these effects remain incompletely characterized. *AFB*, Adventitial fibroblast; *ApoE*, apolipoprotein E; *Ang*, angiotensin; *BPMR2*, bone morphogenetic protein receptor–2; *CM*, cardiomyocyte; *CO*, cardiac output; *JG*, juxtaglomerular; *LV*, left ventricle; *PAEC*, pulmonary artery endothelial cell; *PDK*, pyruvate dehydrogenase kinase; *VSMC*, vascular smooth muscle cell. (From Maron BA et al. *Br J Pharmacol* 2020;177:1457–1471.)

ENDOTHELIN-1

Endothelin-1 (ET-1) is a 21-amino acid vasoactive peptide secreted from the endothelium and targets two G-protein coupled receptor isoforms. In pulmonary artery smooth muscle cells, simulation of the ET_A receptors by ET-1 leads to phospholipase C-β activation and subsequent increases in intracellular calcium (Ca^{2+}) bioavailability or, alternatively, influx of Ca^{2+} through plasma membrane channels. This mechanism induces an extremely potent vasoconstrictor as well as pro-mitogenic response. In pulmonary artery endothelial cells, stimulation of the ET_B-receptor activates endothelial nitric oxide synthase and subsequent nitric oxide (NO·) synthesis. Overall, these vasoconstrictor/pro-proliferative effects of ET_A-dependent signaling dominate ET-1 biofunctionality in pulmonary arterials. It is notable that increased ET-1 is not exclusive to PAH; in left heart failure there is a parabolic, positive association between ET-1 concentration and pulmonary artery pressure thereby implicating vascular congestion in the pulmonary release of ET-1.

PROSTAGLANDIN-I_2

Prostaglandin-I_2 (PGI_2) is a potential vasodilator, anti-platelet, and anti-inflammatory biochemical derivative of arachidonic acid, which under normal conditions is released from the endothelial membrane following phospholipid hydrolysis by phospholipase A2 in a reaction that requires cyclooxygenase. In PAH, endothelial dysfunction causes a depletion of bioactive PGI_2, which is associated with increased vascular tone and microthrombus. Additionally, 5-lipooxygenase, 5-hydroperoxyeicosatetraenoic acid, and leukotriene A_4 are lipoxygenase-dependent arachidonic acid metabolites that increase pulmonary vascular tone, induce pulmonary artery smooth muscle cells chemotaxis, and recruit mast cells.

NITRIC OXIDE

Activation of the heterodimeric protein soluble guanylyl cyclase in pulmonary artery smooth muscle cells by NO· results in the conversion of guanosine-5'-triphosphate (GTP) to the second messenger molecule cyclic guanosine monophosphate (cGMP). In turn, cGMP is either hydrolyzed to inactive 5′-GMP by the phosphodiesterase type-V (PDE-V) enzyme isoform, or stimulates protein kinase G-dependent blood vessel relaxation, platelet inhibition, and transcriptional changes that regulate ion channel conductance and cell survival favorably. In PAH and most other forms of PH, bioavailable NO· is decreased due to impaired endothelial nitric oxide synthase activity or via a scavenger effect by reactive oxygen species that converts NO· to peroxynitrite (ONOO⁻) and other higher oxidative species.

SEROTONIN
This neurotransmitter is synthesized primarily by enterochromaffin cells of the gut from L-tryptophan, and is metabolized primarily by the liver (first pass) and lung.[42] However, expression of pulmonary endothelial tryptophan hydroxylase, which catalyzes the first step in serotonin synthesis, is increased in PAH and endothelial serotonin targets pulmonary artery smooth muscle cells via paracrine signaling to promote vasoconstriction, proliferation, mitogenesis, and inhibition of bone morphogenetic protein (BMP) signaling. Patients with PAH also have increased serotonin, and anorexigenic-PAH was described originally in the context of serotonergic weight-loss drugs (e.g., fenfluramine).

PATHOPHYSIOLOGY

The pulmonary vascular bed is a parallel circuit densely packed with blood vessels, evolved to maximize surface area for gas exchange at the alveolar interface, and is, therefore, a high-flow, low-resistance system. Pathogenic changes in the architecture of pulmonary arterials causes an early decline in pulmonary arterial compliance (RV stroke volume/pulmonary artery pulse pressure) prior to elevation in PVR, ultimately leading to increased pulmonary artery blood pressure.[43] It is important to recognize that pressure in the pulmonary circuit is determined, in part, by RV contractility. If RV failure is present, pulmonary artery pressure may be only mildly elevated despite severe pulmonary vascular remodeling (Fig. 88.6A). Alternatively, mildly elevated mPAP is observed in some physiological or immediately reversible states. Thus, staging PAH (and many forms of PH) is accomplished by considering PVR, which is related inversely to CO and may be viewed as an indirect hemodynamic surrogate of arterial remodeling severity.

Right Ventricular Dysfunction
The importance of RV performance in PH pathophysiology cannot be overemphasized, because diminished systolic function, decreased ejection fraction, cavitary dilation, and in some cases hypertrophy are prognostic for adverse outcome. In contrast to the LV, the RV is triangular, contracts in a predominately longitudinal plane, and is not governed by classical Frank-Starling mechanics. Furthermore, physiologic parameters familiar to anticipating load-dependent changes in LV contractility do not depict intrinsic RV function. Instead, understanding and predicting RV function hinges on the concept of efficient energy utilization. Specifically, the extent to which RV cardiac function and pulmonary vascular blood flow are matched is of central importance. Broadly, this is determined by the contribution of RV contractility that is dedicated to perfusing the lungs relative to RV work needed to maintain intravascular pulmonary arterial pressure. This relationship is referred to as RV-PA coupling (Fig. 88.6B).

Constructing the RV-PA coupling relationship requires direct measurement of the RV pressure-volume relationship, from which the end-systolic elastance (Ees) is determined by the slope of the end-systolic pressure versus the end-systolic volume.[44] Ventricular afterload is estimated from the pressure-volume relationship as arterial elastance (Ea), which is a measure of intrinsic (i.e., ventricular-independent) PVR. The Ees/Ea ratio quantifies RV-PA coupling. With increasing PVR, hypertrophic RV remodeling permits a matched increase in contractility. Ultimately, further hypertrophy is not possible or contra-productive. Cavitary dilation then ensues as a maladaptive response to defend stroke volume. In advanced-stage PH, the Ees/Ea ratio declines. Overall, the adult RV lacks pre-programmed molecular pathways that respond to pressure loading conditions in the same adaptive way that is observed for the LV. It is important to recognize that RV dysfunction is observed as a consequence of pre-capillary, isolated post-capillary, and combined pre-/post-capillary PH.

Systemic Manifestations of Pulmonary Hypertension
The clinical phenotypic spectrum of PH, and, more specifically, PAH, has widened substantially in comparison to early reports focusing exclusively on pulmonary vascular remodeling. Regardless of the underlying cause, chronic RV dysfunction due to pulmonary vascular disease impacts nearly all organ systems.[2] In most cases, symptoms are secondary to end-organ damage from impaired CO that decreases perfusion in resistance (systemic) vascular beds. Examples include acute or exacerbation of chronic renal failure, leaky bowel syndrome, volitional muscle atrophy including diaphragmatic weakness, and cognitive impairment, or passive hepatic congestion due to elevated right atrial pressure. In PAH, neurohumoral overactivation, including increased circulating catecholamine levels and secondary hyperaldosteronism, associate with central cardiopulmonary hemodynamics and heart failure burden severity.[45] In turn, new onset depression, diabetes mellitus, and metabolic syndrome are common tertiary consequences of pulmonary vascular disease through impaired exercise tolerance or other life-limiting symptoms.

Beyond the secondary and tertiary manifestations of PH, it appears that some PAH subtypes involve primary but extra-pulmonary vascular mechanisms. Compared to iPAH, for example, patients with SSc-PAH demonstrate impaired RV-PA coupling at much lower RV afterload levels. This finding is linked to increased interstitial RV cardiac fibrosis and decreased maximal calcium-activated force, implying an intrinsic pathogenic feature of SSc-PAH that involves RV cardiomyocytes.[46] Other potential organs proposed in the primary PAH syndrome include (i) blood, by virtue of thrombocytopenia affecting 20% of PAH patients and microthrombosis observed at autopsy, and (ii) thyroid dysfunction, which is observed in up to approximately 25% of iPAH without a different explanation.[2]

PATIENT PRESENTATION AND CLINICAL ASSESSMENT

Patient Medical History
The presenting symptoms for PAH most often are shortness of breath, fatigue, abdominal distension, lower extremity edema, weakness, exercise limitation, or dyspnea with bending (bendopnea). Cardiac angina (due to either RV ischemia or left main coronary artery compression) and syncope (due to severely decreased CO) are high-risk presenting symptoms that are equivalent to a PAH emergency. Nevertheless, most PAH symptoms are nonspecific, which is a major barrier to timely diagnosis. In one-fifth of patients, the lag between initial presentation and diagnosis is greater than 2 years, particularly among those encountered before the age of 36 years. Pursuit of an explanation by which to account for symptoms in older patients may end after excluding more common cardiovascular diseases such as coronary artery disease, and PAH in often overlooked or misdiagnosed.

Physical Examination Findings
Although a "classic" physical examination for pulmonary hypertension (or PAH) does not exist, physicians should monitor for findings suggesting the presence or consequences of right-sided pressure and volume overload (see also Chapter 13). A loud or paradoxical P2 component of the second heart sound indicates accentuation of pulmonic closure. In severe PH, right-sided S3, RV lift, increased jugular venous pressure, and pulsatile liver may be observed. In *cor pulmonale*, decompensated right heart failure is the end-stage result of severe RV-PA uncoupling and should be considered in patients with systemic hypotension and cool lower extremities associated with severe functional limitation, heart failure symptoms at rest or with minimal activity, and/or mental status changes.

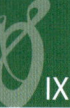

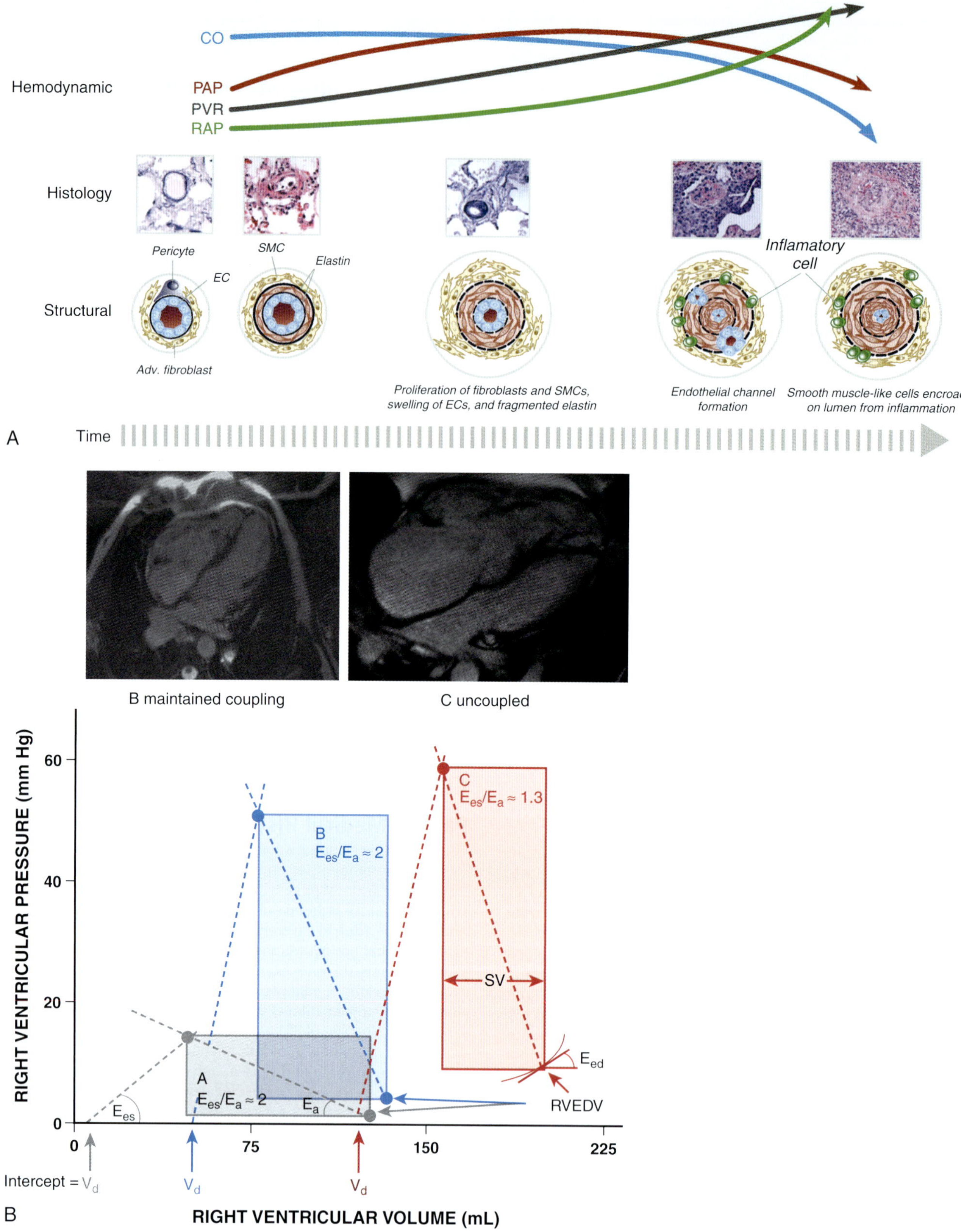

FIGURE 88.6 Hemodynamic and right ventricular pressure-volume relationship trajectory in pulmonary arterial hypertension. **A,** The trajectory of cardiopulmonary hemodynamics over time in patients with pulmonary arterial hypertension, overlaid with changes in the histology and structure of pulmonary arterials. (Adapted from Maron BA, et al. *Am J Respir Crit Care Med*. 2017;195:292–301.) **B** (*Top*), Right ventricular (RV) volumes at coupled stage and uncoupled stage in pulmonary hypertension (PH); (*Bottom*), Representative pressure-volume loops of control, PH with maintained coupling (early stage), and PH with increased RV volume. In regions A and B, E_{es}/E_a is within normal range, ventriculoarterial coupling is maintained, and wall stress is similar. In region C, volume is increased, E_{es}/E_a is decreased (uncoupling), and wall stress is increased. E_a, Measure of arterial load; E_{ed}, ventricular elastance at end-diastole; E_{es}, slope of the end-systolic pressure volume relation as a measure of RV contractility; *PVR*, pulmonary vascular resistance; *RVEDV*, right ventricular end-diastolic volume; *SV*, stroke volume; *Vd*, intercept with the volume axis. (From Vonk Noordegraaf A et al. *J Am Coll Cardiol* 2017;69:236–243.)

Approach to Diagnosis

The initial assessment of patients with suspected PH includes an electrocardiogram (ECG), chest roentgenogram, and echocardiogram (Fig. 88.7A–C).[38] In "real-world" practice, however, the possibility of PH is often deduced from results of these and other tests ordered for a different reason. Therefore, it is important to maintain a high clinical index of suspicion for PH when reviewing primary data and test results.

ECG. The pattern on ECG may indicate geometric changes in right heart structures such as right atrial enlargement or RV hypertrophy, which is suggested by an R/S ratio greater than 1 in lead V1 without other causes, or if the R wave amplitude in lead V1 is greater than 7 mm (see Chapter 14). An RV strain pattern (defined by RV hypertrophy with ST segment depression in V1 to V3) may be evident in advanced disease stages. In turn, LV hypertrophy and left atrial enlargement may point toward left heart disease PH rather than PAH.

Chest roentgenogram. The chest x-ray is abnormal in 90% of PAH patients, and findings include central pulmonary artery dilation, peripheral dearborization, right atrial and RV enlargement (see Chapter 17).[38] The presence of lung hyperinflation, pneumonia, or other features of primary lung disease, as well as features suggesting PE (e.g., Westermark sign, Hampton hump) may guide diagnosis.

Two-dimensional transthoracic echocardiography. Transthoracic echocardiography provides quantitative data noninvasively that is used to screen patients for PH, including PAH (see Chapter 16). However, this method *estimates* PASP by Doppler interrogation of a tricuspid regurgitant jet and does not determine right atrial pressure, PVR, or PAWP accurately, all of which are important for assessing PH clinically (Fig. 88.7D–G). In population studies, the Pearson correlation coefficient (r) for PASP estimated by echocardiography versus direct measurement using RHC (the gold standard diagnostic test, see below) ranges between 0.60 and 0.77 even when the two studies are performed in close temporal proximity. Wide chest anterior-posterior dimension, obstructive lung disease, and other factors that limit the acoustic windows may explain this finding. Furthermore, in one-third of patients with proven PH, a sufficient tricuspid jet is lacking and PASP is unmeasurable.[47] Thus, echocardiography alone is insufficient for diagnosing, classifying, and fully prognosticating patients.

Despite limitations associated with ultrasonographic assessment of hemodynamics, much key data on cardiac structure and function is acquired from echocardiography and useful in staging PH. For example, RV cavitary dilation, RV hypertrophy, hepatic vein dilation or blunted respirophasic dilation, and pericardial effusion inform right heart pathophysiology. Decreased pulmonary vascular distensibility results in the formation of a "notch" in the RV outflow tract Doppler envelope as well as decreased pulmonary artery acceleration time. When these are observed in the setting of a normal left atrial dimension, increased PVR greater than 3.0 WU may be present.

Because RV contraction occurs along a longitudinal rather than circumferential plane, calculating ejection fraction accurately from two-dimensional imaging is not possible. Instead, quantifying RV function can be accomplished by measuring "lunge" of the RV free wall at the level of the tricuspid valve. The tricuspid annular plane of systolic excursion (TAPSE) is generally measured in the apical 4-chamber view by aligning an M-mode cursor parallel to the RV free wall at the tricuspid annulus. The distance measured between end-diastole and end-systole is the TAPSE, and when ≤1.7 cm prognosticates adverse clinical outcome in PAH (Fig. 88.8H and I).[38] Other RV functional measures reported in PH assessment include longitudinal myocardial velocity (S'), fractional area change (FAC), Tei index speckle tracking, and ejection fraction by three-dimensional echocardiography (Table 88.4).

Left atrial diameter greater than 4.4 cm measured in the parasternal long axis view is often associated with left atrial hypertension, and this can be useful for calibrating the likelihood of PH from left heart disease. Agitated saline-enhanced echocardiography is warranted in patients with PH and structural cardiac abnormalities that predispose to intracardiac shunt or in whom unexplained hypoxemia is observed at rest or during exercise.

Pulmonary function tests and sleep study. Comorbid obstructive and restrictive lung disease is reported in up to 75% of cross-sectional populations enriched for prevalent cardiovascular diseases including heart failure, myocardial infarction, cardiac angina, and stroke. PH in patients with overlapping left heart and parenchymal lung disease is also common, and, therefore, it is important to consider diagnostic testing that characterizes lung structure and function in at-risk patients. Generally, pulmonary function test with spirometry and lung diffusion capacity of carbon monoxide (DLCO) is recommended in all patients suspected of PH. Patients with PAH may demonstrate modestly reduced lung volumes in the absence of marked obstructive, restrictive, or combined ventilatory defects that are more characteristic of parenchymal lung disease. Decreased DLCO is associated with pathogenic remodeling of the alveolar-capillary interface, and is therefore observed in PAH as well as many parenchymal lung diseases that do not include PH. Nonetheless, decreased DLCO is prognostic in PAH. OSA, which through hypoventilation predisposes to nocturnal

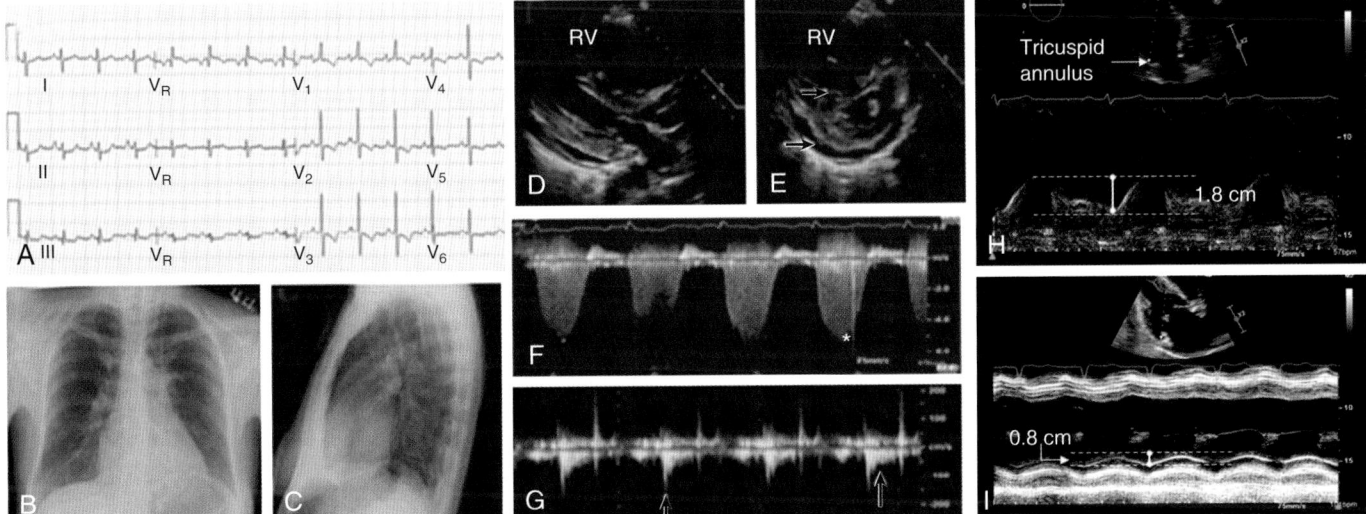

FIGURE 88.7 Representative findings from initial diagnostic tests in pulmonary arterial hypertension (PAH). Images obtained in a 43-year-old woman with idiopathic PAH. **A,** S1Q3T3 pattern noted consistent with right ventricle strain. T-wave inversion on anterior leads and ST depression is also suggestive of right ventricular hypertrophy (RVH) with strain (note early R wave predominance in V_1 to V_2 consistent with RVH). **B,** Chest roentgenography showing enlarged pulmonary artery and pruning of the distal pulmonary vasculature. **C,** Lateral chest roentgenography showing filling of the retrosternal space by an enlarged RV. **D,** Parasternal long axis echocardiography view showing dilated RV. **E,** Parasternal short axis echocardiography view showing flatted interventricular septum (*upper arrow*), severely dilated RV and pericardial effusion (*lower arrow*). **F,** Tricuspid regurgitation velocity (*asterisk*) is proportional to right ventricular systolic pressure and estimated by Bernoulli's equation. **G,** Measurement of pulmonary artery acceleration time (PAAT) (time from onset of flow to peak velocity) (*left arrow*) acquired from the RV outflow tract. Note the notching of the PA Doppler envelope, suggestive of pulmonary vascular hypertension (*right arrow*). **H,** The tricuspid plane of systolic excursion (TAPSE) that is normal (>1.7 cm). **I,** Abnormal in a patient with severe pulmonary hypertension. (**A-G** from Ryan JJ et al. *Pulm Circ* 2012;2:107–121; **H** and **I** courtesy Dr. Jayashri Aragam.)

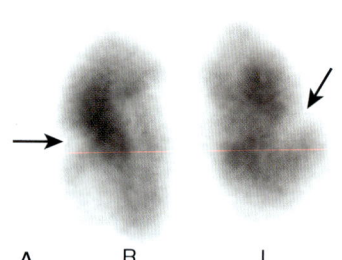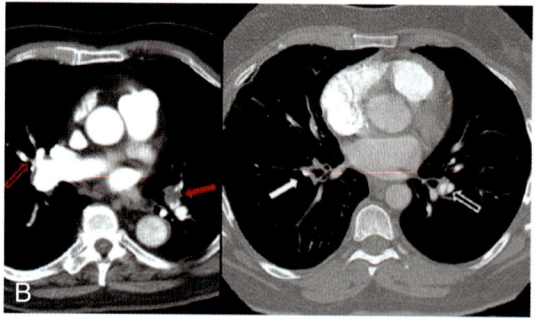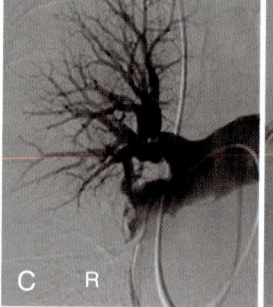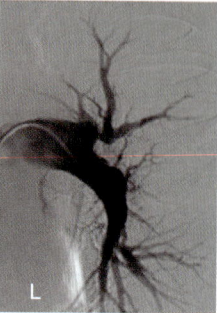

FIGURE 88.8 Imaging in chronic thromboembolic pulmonary hypertension (CTEPH). **A,** Nuclear ventilation/perfusion (V/Q) scintigraphy shows numerous mismatched perfusion defects (*arrows*). **B,** Computed tomographic pulmonary angiographic features of chronic thromboembolic disease. Left panel shows right middle lobe vessel narrowing (*open red arrow*) with lining thrombus versus intimal thickening involving the right descending pulmonary artery. Recanalized thrombus is seen in the left descending pulmonary artery (*solid red arrow*). Right panel shows marked vessel narrowing from organized clot in the right descending pulmonary artery (*solid white arrow*) and web in a proximal left lower lobe segmental vessel (*open white arrow*) **C,** Invasive pulmonary angiography demonstrates web and stricture filling defects, an occlusive arteriopathy in the central vasculature, as well as significant dearborization of distal pulmonary arterials bilaterally. (**B** and **C** from Mahmud E et al. *J Am Coll Cardiol* 2018;71:2468–2486.)

TABLE 88.4 Parameters Assessing Right Heart Structure and Function by Echocardiography Useful in Assessing Pulmonary Hypertension

ECHOCARDIOGRAPHIC RV PARAMETER	DESCRIPTION	DEFINITION	USE IN PH/PAH
Tricuspid annular plane systolic excursion (TAPSE)	Longitudinal movement of the RV free wall at the level of the tricuspid valve	Δ end-diastolic- end-systolic measurements acquired usually by M-mode in the apical 4-chamber view	<1.8 cm is prognostic for mortality in PAH
Longitudinal myocardial velocity	Peak velocity of RV longitudinal movement, indicating regional RV contractility	Doppler tissue imaging measures peak velocity (S') of longitudinal movement of the tricuspid lateral annulus at systolic phase and representative of regional RV systolic function	<10 cm/sec is a marker of RV dysfunction
Right atrial area index	Right atrial size expressed as area, indexed to patient	Apical 4-chamber view at end-systole, corrected for height.	Prognosticates mortality and lung transplantation in PAH per ↑ 5 cm^2
Myocardial performance (Tei) index	Measure of global RV performance	Sum of the isovolumic contraction and relaxation times divided by the ejection time.	>0.36 associates with PAH diagnosis; overall correlates with invasive hemodynamic measures, including mPAP and selected exercise parameters
RV fractional area change	Two-dimensional measure of global RV systolic function	(RV end-diastolic area − RV end-systolic area)/RV end-systolic area × 100	<35% suggests RV systolic dysfunction
RV strain and strain rate	Geometric changes to RV cavitary dimensions due to increased afterload	Angle-independent assessment of global and regional RV contractility	For < −12%: ↑ Clinical worsening ↑ 1- and 4-year mortality

mPAP, Mean pulmonary artery pressure; *PAH,* pulmonary arterial hypertension; *RV,* Right ventricle.

hypoxemia, and, thus, pulmonary vasoconstriction, should also be assessed by overnight oximetry or polysomnography in PAH patients or in those with otherwise unexplained PH.

Computed tomographic chest imaging and nuclear ventilation/perfusion (V/Q) scintigraphy. Noncontrast enhanced computed tomographic imaging of the lung is useful to delineate vascular from lung structural and parenchymal causes of PH, such as idiopathic pulmonary fibrosis. Mismatched perfusion defects on ventilation-perfusion (V/Q) scintigraphy is highly suggestive of CTEPH. When these imaging features are present, combining intermediate- and high-probability scan data results in a sensitivity and specificity of V/Q scan for CTPEH of approximately 100% and 86% to 90%, respectively (Fig. 88.8A).[48] In one study of 340 patients with severe PH, a proper V/Q scintigraphy was part of the diagnostic evaluation in only 16% of patients, emphasizing the need for clinicians to consider CTEPH in patients without a definitive cause of PH.[49] Staging CTEPH may require contrast-enhanced computed tomographic or digital subtraction pulmonary angiography, because operative candidacy hinges on anatomic distribution of *in situ* thrombosis that may not be fully evident by nuclear perfusion scanning alone (Fig. 88.8B,C).

Cardiac magnetic resonance (CMR) imaging. Quantitative assessment of RV ejection by CMR is useful for staging PH. This is a particularly important modality in patients for whom poor acoustic windows limit visualizing right heart structures by echocardiography. In PAH, the RV ejection fraction at baseline and in response to treatment prognosticates mortality, particularly when less than 35%. Similarly, there is an inverse association between RV ejection fraction and clinical outcome in patients with PH from left heart disease. Additionally, CMR integrates images across three dimensions, thereby providing optimal resolution for quantifying right atrial and RV chamber volume. Increased RV end-systolic and end-diastolic volumes are phenotypic patterns that correspond to uncoupled RV-PA pathophysiology but require CMR (or three-dimensional echocardiography) for assessing. Late gadolinium enhancement of the RV insertion points on T1 mapping, 4-dimensional quantitative pulmonary artery flow, and 3-dimensional magnetic resonance flow are next-generation imaging packages that show promise for optimizing right pathophenotype assessment in PH.

Positron emission tomography. Lung parenchymal uptake of fluorodeoxyglucose bound to 18-fluorine detected by positron emission tomography (^{18}FDG-PET) is increased in iPAH patients compared to healthy controls. This supports mechanistic data on dysregulated cellular metabolism in pulmonary endothelial, pulmonary artery smooth muscle, and adventitial fibroblast cells from PAH patients (see Fig 88.4), suggesting that PET may ultimately offer an imaging correlate to stage the pathobiology of individual patients. Detection of the mannose receptor expressed on lung macrophages by PET has also been shown in pre-clinical models to detect early PAH,[50] but overall PET remains an investigational tool without defined clinical usefulness at present.

Exercise testing. Functional assessment using a 6-minute walk distance (6-MWD) or standard (noninvasive) cardiopulmonary exercise test (CPET) is critical to the management of patients with PH. In PAH particularly, symptom-limited functional capacity prognosticates key clinical events including need for therapy escalation, hospitalization, lung transplantation, and mortality. The 6-MWD should be performed according to American Thoracic Society guidelines (https://www.thoracic.org/statements/resources/pfet/sixminute.pdf) because performance is heavily influenceable under nonstandardized conditions. Performance on 6-MWD correlates with workload, heart rate, oxygen saturation, and dyspnea response (i.e., symptom burden), but is dependent on gait speed, age, weight, and muscle mass among other anthropometric variables.[51] In the Naughton-Balke treadmill protocol, incremental increases in workload by 1 metabolic equivalent at successive 2-minute stages is used to assess functional capacity.[51] In contrast to 6-MWD, performance on this test is less modifiable by external cues such as coaching or internal factors such as motivation.

Exercise is a highly integrated process that beyond mechanical propulsion depends on O_2 uptake across the alveolar-capillary interface, normal O_2 delivery to target organs via CO, and preserved O_2 flux via diffusion across the skeletal muscle cell membrane. Peak volume of oxygen consumption (pVO_2) is a global determinant of cardiopulmonary and skeletal muscle fitness, and when measured using CPET correlates inversely with mortality in PAH and left heart failure patients.[52] In addition, CPET allows for assessment of the (assumed) anaerobic threshold, determined based on depletion of circulating bicarbonate that buffers excess protons (H^+) generated as a byproduct of lactic acid synthesis. This is identifiable by a succinct shift in the ratio of expired carbon dioxide to pVO_2, and when abnormal may suggest a pulmonary vascular limit to exercise. Additional CPET parameters that provide insight into pulmonary circulatory pathophysiology include an increase in the ratio of the peak minute ventilation to maximal voluntary ventilation (VE/MVV), widening of the difference between end-tidal partial pressure of oxygen (PETO_2), and end-tidal partial pressure of carbon dioxide (PETCO_2), and an increase in the ratio of minute ventilation to expired carbon dioxide ratio (VE/VCO_2), which suggest a pulmonary mechanical limit to exercise, intracardiac (or pulmonary) shunt, and poor aerobic fitness, respectively.

Cardiac catheterization. As time and financial pressures tilt emphasis to interventional opportunities, RHC seems to have been deemphasized in the current era (see Chapter 22). Nonetheless, perhaps no other widely available study in medicine provides as much integrated, real-time physiological data for use clinically, and a meticulous study is required to classify PH appropriately (see Table 88.1). Additional RHC indications include shock, guidance for pericardial disease, assessing constrictive versus restrictive cardiomyopathy, and quantifying shunt. A complete study includes the following three parts: oxyhemoglobin saturation (SaO_2) analysis in different vascular compartments, intravascular and intracardiac pressure measurement, CO assessment, and PAWP measurement (eTable 88.1). It is important to position the patient appropriately and "zero" the air-fluid interface in line with the phlebostatic axis (Fig. 88.9A–D).

Profiling the SaO_2 at different points within the superior vena cava (SVC), inferior vena cava (IVC), right atrium (RA), RV, and pulmonary artery (the latter referred to as the mixed venous SaO_2) is necessary to exclude intra- or extra-cardiac shunt. In turn, a "step-up" in SaO_2

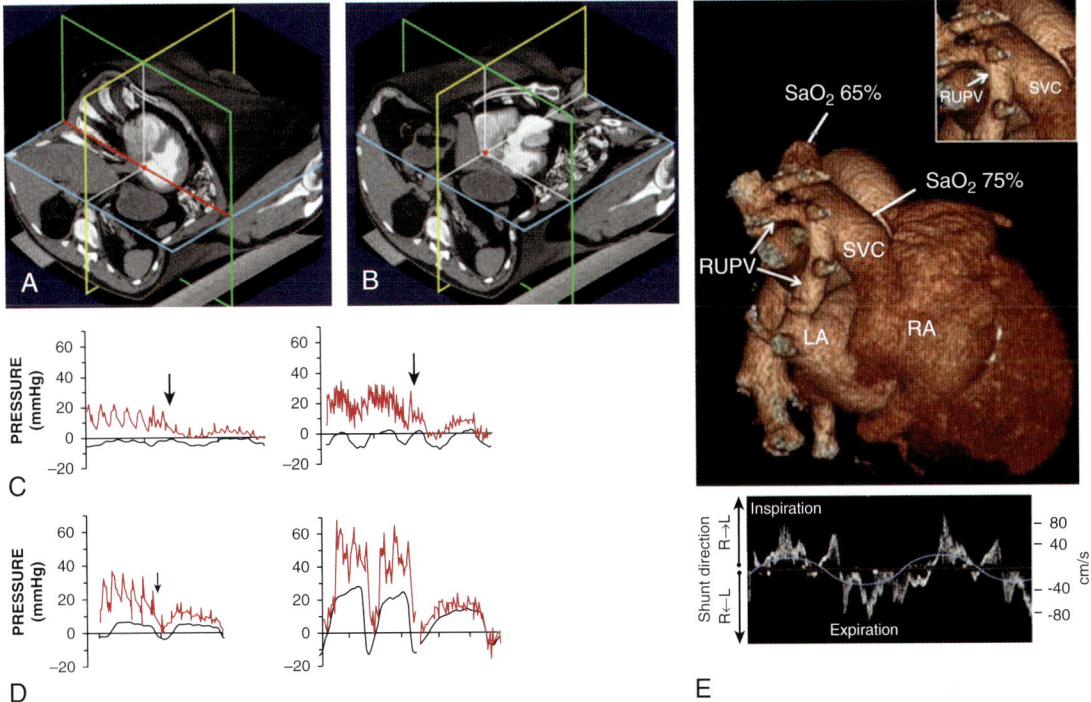

FIGURE 88.9 Anatomical and physiological considerations during right heart catheterization. **A,** Phlebostatic axis (*red line*): an axis running through the thorax at the junction of a transverse plane (*green*) passing through the fourth anterior intercostal space with a frontal plane (*blue*) passing midway between the posterior surface of the body and the base of the xiphoid process of the sternum. Suggested reference point (*red point*) defined by the intersection of the frontal plane (*blue*) at the midthoracic level, the transverse plane (*green*) at the level of fourth anterior intercostal space, and the midsagittal plane (*yellow*). In this patient, the reference point would be within the left atrium. **B,** Phlebostatic reference point (*red point*) defined by the intersection of the following planes: (1) midsagittal plane (*yellow*); (2) frontal plane (*blue*) anterior to the back 0.61 times the thickness of the chest; (3) transverse plane (*green*) caudal to the sternal notch 0.77 times the distance from the sternal notch to the tip of the xiphoid process. The reference point is within the right ventricle. **C,** Pulmonary artery pressure (*red line*) followed by pulmonary artery wedge pressure (*arrow*) in a normal subject at rest (*left*) and during exercise (*right*). Pleural pressure (*black line*) is on average negative with respiratory swings, which are amplified during exercise. **D,** Pulmonary artery pressure (*red line*) followed by pulmonary artery wedge pressure (*arrow*) in a patient with chronic obstructive pulmonary disease at rest (*left*) and during exercise (*right*). Pleural pressure (*black line*) shows respiratory swings, which appear transmitted to pulmonary vascular pressures. **E,** Multislice 3-dimensional reconstructive computed tomographic angiography performed in a 67-year-old man with newly diagnosed pulmonary hypertension due to a congenital anomalous pulmonary vein reveals an abnormal communication between the right upper pulmonary vein (RUPV) and superior vena cava (SVC) (provided at increased magnification in the *inset*) with normal insertion of the RUPV into the left atrium (LA). There is an oxyhemoglobin saturation "step-up" across the abnormal articulation point of the RUPV at the SVC. The Doppler signal demonstrates respirophasic bidirectional blood flow (i.e., shunt) through the RUPV. (**A,B** adapted from Kovacs G et al. *Am J Respir Crit Care Med* 2014;190:252–257; **C,D** from Naeije R, Boerrigter BG. *Eur Respir J* 2013;41:1002–1004; **E** adapted from Clarke JC et al. *Circ Cardiovasc Imaging* 2013;6(2):349–351.)

averaged across greater than 1 measurements between SVC-RA, RA-RV, or RV-PA of ≥7%, ≥5%, ≥5%, respectively, suggests the introduction of oxygenated blood to the right heart circulation through an anatomical shunt (Fig. 88.9E).[53] Characterizing shunt provides invaluable insight to PAH from Eisenmenger physiology (and subsequent right-to-left shunting), which in addition to specific congenital anatomic lesions is discussed in greater detail in Chapter 82.

In the absence of congenital pulmonic stenosis, a meaningful transpulmonary valvular gradient is not expected at rest. However, the compliance of the RV and pulmonary artery differs greatly, and, therefore, the diastolic measurements in these compartments are quite different normally. A RV end-diastolic pressure less than 10 mm Hg generally implies preserved RV function.

The CO is measured by direct pVO_2 analysis using a Douglas bag or metabolic cart; however this equipment is specialized and may be unavailable. More commonly, CO is measured indirectly using the estimated Fick (eFick) equation or thermodilutional (Td) method. The cardiac index corrects CO for body surface area and is often more useful clinically than CO alone for profiling the (dys)functional effects of cardiac performance. Accurate CO is critical, as these data bear on risk stratifying all forms of PH and guide the therapeutic approach to PAH in specific. Furthermore, the CO is used to calculate PVR, which itself is central to patient classification (see Table 88.1). Despite the importance of CO clinically there is only modest agreement between eFick and Td, and controversy exists regarding which is preferred in PH. One recent study using the national Veterans Affair catheterization database showed that Td or the average of eFick + Td was superior to eFick alone for predicting future mortality.[54]

The PAWP is a measure of LVEDP in the absence of mitral valve disease or pulmonary venous remodeling. Confirming optimal catheter placement in the wedge position may be challenging using the hemodynamic tracing alone but can be verified by measuring the wedge SaO_2 to confirm a venous sample.[55] Alternatively, a direct LVEDP measurement is recommended in cases where concordance between multiple PAWP measurements is lacking or the PAWP SaO_2 is less than 90%. It is essential to record the PAWP at end-expiration because wide undulation of the thorax (particularly in COPD) is associated with a transient decrease in PAWP levels. This, in turn, biases results toward over-diagnosing pre-capillary PH. Taken together, a diastolic transpulmonary gradient (calculated as the diastolic PAP − PAWP) ≥ 7 mm Hg and/or PVR ≥3 WU with PAWP or LVEDP ≥15 mm Hg suggests a contribution of left heart disease to PH.[55]

CARDIAC CATHETERIZATION DIAGNOSTIC MANEUVERS
Vasoreactivity Testing
Patients with idiopathic, hereditary, and drug/toxic-associated PAH should undergo vasoreactivity testing with inhaled NO•, intravenous prostacyclin, or intravenous adenosine. A positive test is defined by a decrease in mPAP ≥10 mm Hg to reach an mPAP ≤40 mm Hg with a decrease (or no change) in CO, and observed in approximately 5% of PAH patients.[1] However, identifying this patient subgroup has important implications on pharmacotherapeutic selection and outcome (see Approach to Treatment section below).

Confrontational Fluid Challenge
Differentiating PAH from PH-left heart disease may be challenging, especially in patients with borderline abnormal PAWP (13 to 15 mm Hg), risk factors for HFpEF, and/or on diuretic therapy. In these circumstances, monitoring a change in PAWP following the administration of 500 mL normal saline over 5 min may be useful for eliciting occult LV lusitropic impairment to uncover PH.[55] A rise in PAWP to greater than 18 mm Hg is suggestive of pulmonary PH-left heart disease, although universally accepted diagnostic criteria remain lacking.

Invasive Cardiopulmonary Exercise Testing
Supine or upright cycle ergometry with a pulmonary artery catheter, pneumotachograph, and radial artery catheter are the fundamental components of invasive cardiopulmonary exercise testing (iCPET), which is useful for interrogating the pathophysiological basis of unexplained dyspnea. In iCPET, continuous gas exchange data are integrated with serial invasive hemodynamic readings (including PAWP) as well as peripheral blood lactate, pH, and arterial content of oxygen among other variables. This approach aims to identify patients with the following potential disorders provoked by physical activity: pulmonary vascular disease with or without a component of left heart disease, peripheral oxygen extraction disorders (most often due to mitochondrial dysfunction), or neurovascular syndromes that may affect venous return to the RV (Table 88.5).[56] In 20% of patients referred for iCPET, a diagnosis of HFpEF is made demonstrating limitations to static cardiopulmonary hemodynamic assessment using only conventional RHC.

Risk Stratification
Standardized point-of-care risk assessment tools in PAH are available to guide clinical decision-making, including treatment escalation, and include the French Pulmonary Hypertension Network risk equation, REVEAL risk equation (v2.0), and the 2015 ESC/ERS Pulmonary Hypertension Guideline risk table.[38,57] These scales generally integrate clinical, functional, echocardiographic, and biochemical data to generate a composite profile that corresponds to prognosis, but also provides a strategy to inform goal-directed therapy. The overarching goal of therapy is to achieve the lowest risk level possible, which generally means: 6-MWD greater than 440 m or pVO_2 greater than 15 mL/min/kg, right atrial area less than 18 cm^2, cardiac index greater than 2.5 L/min/m^2, and absent or low symptom burden with routine physical activity.[38]

TABLE 88.5 Hemodynamic Framework to Inform Exercise Intolerance Phenotypes

	AGE (Year)	PEAK MPAP (mm Hg)	PEAK PAWP (mm Hg)	PEAK PVR (WU)
PVD	≤50	>30	≤19	>1.34
	>50	>33	≤17	>2.10
LHD+PVD	≤50	—	>19	>1.34
	>50	—	>17	>2.10
LHD-noPVD	≤50	—	>19	≤1.34
	>50	—	>17	≤2.10

	pVO_2	PEAK CO	Ca-Vo_2/Hb	PEAK RAP (mm Hg)	PEAK PAWP (mm Hg)	PEAK MPAP (mm Hg)
Peripheral O_2 extraction disorder	<80% Predicted	≤80% Predicted	<0.80	—	—	—
Low ventricular filling	<80% Predicted	<80% Predicted	—	<9	<14	<30
Presumed normal	≥80% Predicted	≥80% Predicted	≥0.8	Per age-specific cutoffs in above table		

Exercise hemodynamic, peripheral blood metabolic, and peak VO_2 data criteria that are useful toward diagnosing exercise intolerance from otherwise unexplained dyspnea, although universally accepted diagnostic criteria for these patient subgroups remain lacking.
Ca-vO_2, Content of oxygen in arterial minus venous blood; CO, cardiac output; Hb, hemoglobin; LHD, left heart disease; mPAP, mean pulmonary artery pressure; PAWP, pulmonary artery wedge pressure; Peak, peak exercise; PVD, pulmonary vascular disease; pVO_2, peak volume of O_2 extraction; PVR, pulmonary vascular resistance; RAP, right atrial pressure.
From Oldham WM, et al. Circ Res. 2018;122(6):864–876.

INTEGRATED APPROACH TO DIAGNOSING PULMONARY HYPERTENSION

Patients with suspected PH based on symptoms should be evaluated further with ECG, chest roentgenography, and echocardiography (Fig. 88.10). Clinicians should focus on assessing comorbid lung and cardiovascular disease to explain findings suggesting PH; to this end, pursuing computed chest CT, pulmonary function testing with DLCO, and arterial blood gas analysis should be considered on an individualized basis. Exercise testing with 6-MWD or CPET is important to characterize symptom burden objectively, and doing so may also expand the profile of an individual patient by discovering helpful findings that are absent at rest, such as exertional hypoxemia or a pulmonary mechanical limit to exercise. Ultimately, diagnosing, classifying, and risk stratifying PH requires a complete RHC. Patients with otherwise unexplained dyspnea that do not meet a hemodynamic classification of PH may benefit from exercise RHC or iCPET to unmask HFpEF or other etiologies as a cause of symptoms. In such patients, increased left atrial size greater than 4.4 cm, obesity, atrial fibrillation, age greater than 60 years, treatment with ≥2 anti-hypertensive drugs, echocardiographic E/e' ratio, or estimated PASP greater than 35 mm Hg may be sufficient to avoid invasive testing, as the presence of these features point toward HFpEF.[58]

It is incumbent on clinicians to integrate the totality of data from diagnostic testing, including RHC, for determining the most appropriate PH clinical classification. In the case of PAH, this is often informed by the absence of other cardiopulmonary diseases or known PH risk factors, and is suggested by a family history, drug/toxin exposure, or associated diseases such as SSc, HIV, or cirrhotic liver disease. Differentiating PAH from other PH phenotypes may be challenging in specific cases, including patients with left heart disease risk factors who present with severe PH, elevated PVR, and normal PAWP. Determining the contribution of standing diuretic therapy or other volume loading conditions on left heart disease can be determined by confrontational fluid challenge or exercise testing, as described above. In patients suspected of idiopathic, hereditary, or drug/toxin PAH, a positive hemodynamic response to testing with iNO is diagnostic for vasoreactive PAH (although a negative response does not *exclude* PAH). Compared to non-vasoreactive PAH patients, this subgroup is associated with a favorable prognosis including disease resolution in some patients when managed appropriately (Fig. 88.11).

Pulmonary Venoocclusive Disease

Diagnosing PVOD is a major challenge in clinical practice because the symptoms and hemodynamic pattern are often indistinguishable

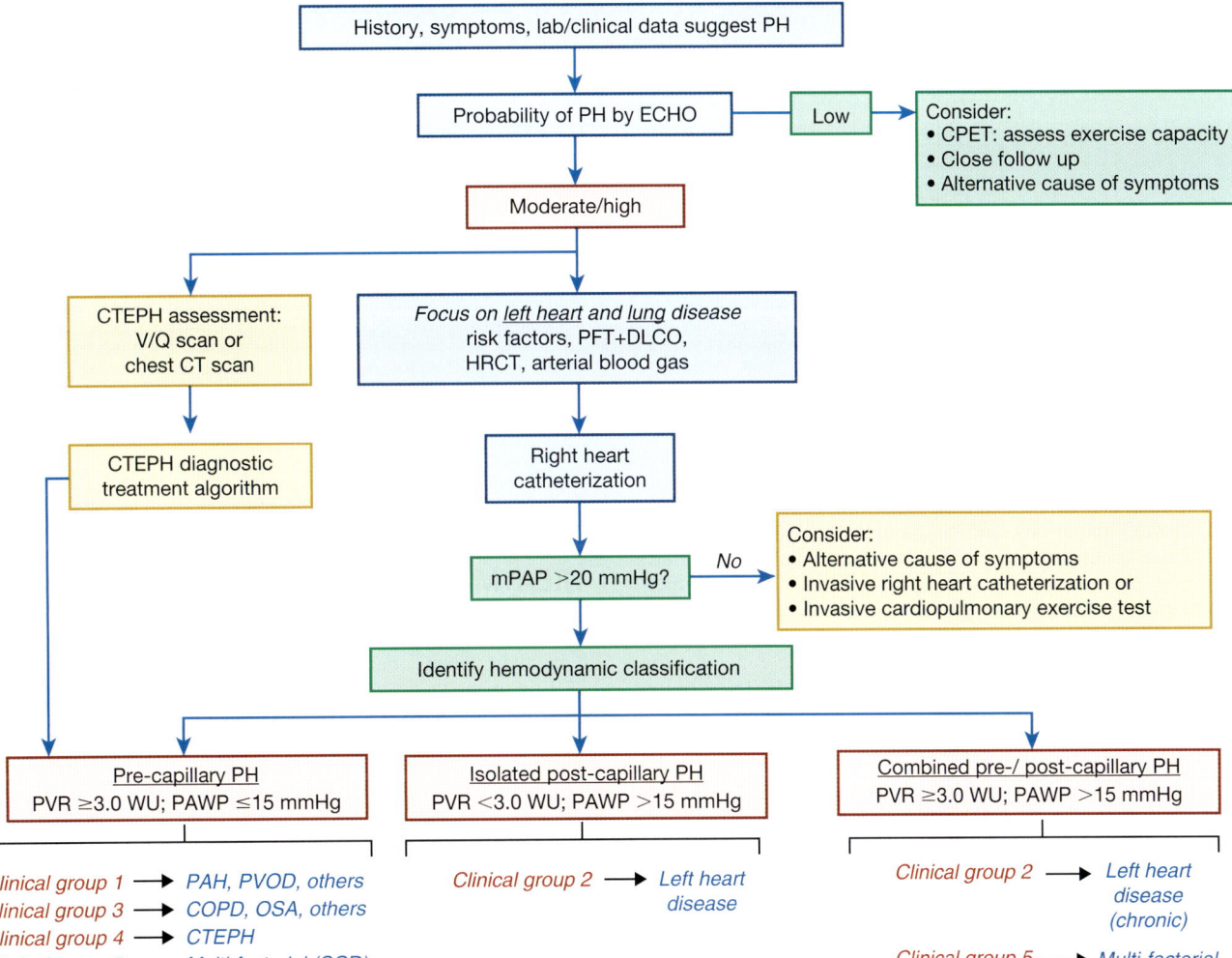

FIGURE 88.10 Integrated pathway for diagnosing pulmonary hypertension. In patients suspected of having pulmonary hypertension (PH) based on history, physical examination, and initial diagnostic testing (e.g., electrocardiogram, chest x-ray), a transthoracic echocardiogram (ECHO) is often used as the first quantitative test. In patients with moderate or high probability of PH based on echocardiography, assessment of left heart disease and pulmonary disease is warranted through various diagnostic tests, including pulmonary function testing with diffusion capacity for carbon monoxide (PFT+DLCO) and high-resolution computed tomography (HRCT). Patients should also be assessed for chronic thromboembolic pulmonary hypertension (CTEPH), initially by nuclear ventilation/perfusion (V/Q) scanning or contrast enhanced chest CT. The diagnosis of PH is made by right heart catheterization and requires a mean pulmonary artery pressure (mPAP) greater than 20 mm Hg. Patients are then classified by hemodynamic category (see Table 88.1 for details), which together with the clinical profile and other supporting data (e.g., serology, genetic testing) is used to determine the PH clinical group (see Table 88.2 for details). *COPD*, Chronic obstructive pulmonary disease; *CPET*, cardiopulmonary exercise test; *OSA*, obstructive sleep apnea; *PAH*, pulmonary arterial hypertension; *PAWP*, pulmonary artery wedge pressure; *PVOD*, pulmonary venoocclusive disease; *PVR*, pulmonary vascular resistance; *SCD*, sickle cell disease.

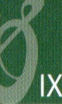

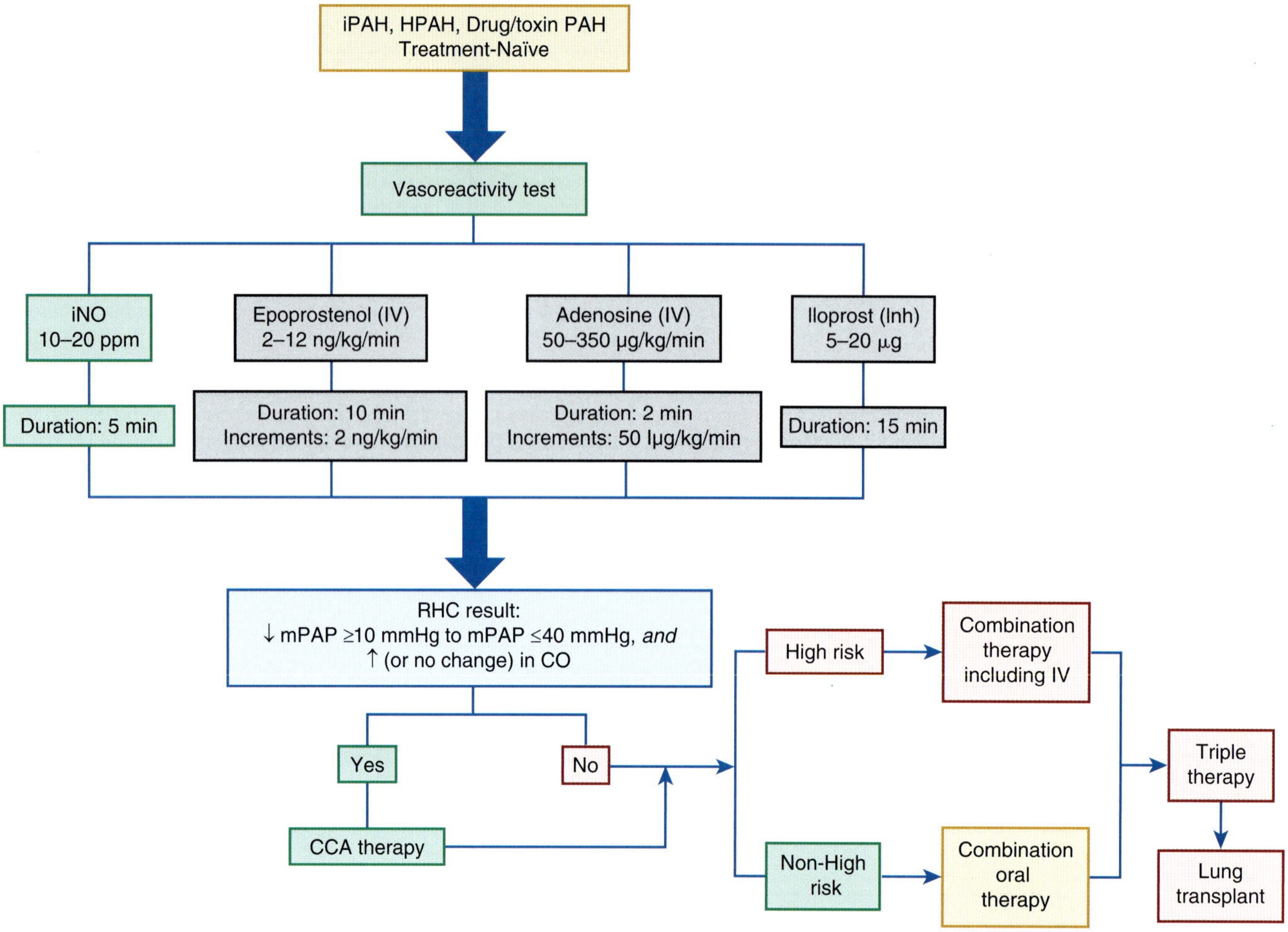

FIGURE 88.11 Vasoreactivity testing and overview of treatment in pulmonary arterial hypertension. Vasoreactivity is indicated in patients with idiopathic pulmonary arterial hypertension (iPAH), hereditary PAH (HPAH), and drug/toxin PAH. Inhaled nitric oxide (iNO) is the preferred agent for testing, although adenosine and prostacyclin analogues are suitable. In patients with a positive vasoreactivity test, high-dose calcium channel antagonist (CCA) therapy is first-line treatment in the absence of high-risk features. In patients without a positive vasoreactivity test, therapy selection is based on risk. Regardless of vasoreactivity results, chest pain, syncope, low cardiac index, and severe symptom burden are indications for intravenous (IV) prostacyclin therapy. Patients without both a positive vasoreactivity result and high-risk clinical features may be candidates for combination oral therapy. Suboptimal clinical response or clinical deterioration warrants consideration to triple therapy, and, if necessary lung transplantation. *CO*, cardiac output; *mPAP*, mean pulmonary artery pressure; *RHC*, right heart catheterization.

from PAH. Ultimately, the probability of PVOD hinges on a combination of factors, including clinical suspicion, genetic risk (e.g., biallelic *EIF2AK4* mutation), and subpleural thickened septal lines, centrilobular ground-glass opacities, and mediastinal lymphadenopathy on chest computed tomographic imaging (Table 88.6). Simultaneous measurement of LVEDP with multiple PAWP recordings from different pulmonary artery branches showing elevated PAWP:LVEDP ratio in some segments and normal ratio in other segments is suggestive, but not diagnostic of PVOD.[51] Lung biopsy remains the gold standard diagnostic test, but is generally avoided owing to the risk of major complication.[38] Unfortunately, PVOD may emerge as the operative diagnosis in patients that develop pulmonary edema following administration of pulmonary vasodilator therapy due to increased hydrostatic pressure proximal to fixed venous stenosis.

Chronic Thromboembolic Pulmonary Hypertension

A diagnosis of CTEPH must be suspected in any patient with prior PE and otherwise unexplained dyspnea or PH. The diagnostic approach to CTEPH is outlined in Figure 88.12, and integrates clinical data with imaging from V/Q, contrast enhanced chest CT, and pulmonary angiography. A subset of patients with symptoms (e.g., dyspnea and functional limitation) and evidence of pulmonary thromboembolic remodeling will present without PH. In this subgroup, chronic thromboembolic disease (CTED), ventilatory defects such as increased dead space ventilation and (near) normal cardiopulmonary hemodynamics are reported.

TREATMENT

Pulmonary Arterial Hypertension

A multi-disciplinary care strategy is needed to optimize outcome in PAH, and patients should be evaluated prior to treatment at an expert referral center whenever possible. Supportive care with loop diuretics and supplemental oxygen attenuates pulmonary vascular congestion and hypoxic pulmonary vasoconstriction, which otherwise aggravate symptoms and worsen RV function. Approximately one-third of PAH patients in clinical trials are reported to use potassium-sparing diuretics (e.g., spironolactone, eplerenone), which may resolve hypokalemia and exert salutary clinical benefit by inhibiting aldosterone-mediated pulmonary vascular injury.[45] Digoxin may increase CO by as much as 10% in patients with RV failure due to PH, and attenuates the adverse effect of increased circulating norepinephrine on pulmonary vascular function. Vaccination against influenza and pneumococcal pneumonia is not evidenced-based, but is recommended owing to untoward complications from pneumonia in PAH patients. Routine anticoagulation is not recommended currently as part of the standard therapeutic approach.

Prescription exercise is a proven, albeit underused strategy for treating PAH. This may be due to delayed diagnosis, which is common and linked to advanced symptom burden at the time of presentation, or

TABLE 88.6 Comparison of Distinguishing Features Between Pulmonary Arterial Hypertension and Pulmonary Venoocclusive Disease

	PAH	PVOD
Genetics	Autosomal dominant (see Table 3)	Autosomal recessive (EIF2AK4)
Epidemiology	Approximately 15 cases/million Female predominance (~2:1)	1–2 cases/million No gender predominance
Acquired risk factors	Anorexigens, Dasatinib Interferon Methamphetamines	Chemotherapy (alkylating agents)
Associated conditions	Connective tissue disease, HIV infection, portal hypertension	Systemic sclerosis
Clinical Examination		
Hemoptysis	±	±
Pleural effusion	±	±
Right Heart Catheterization		
mPAP	↑	↑
PAWP	Normal	Normal
PVR	↑	↑
Pulmonary vasoreactivity	~5% in iPAH (predicts long-term CCA response)	~5% (not a predictor of CCA response)
Pulmonary Function Testing		
FEV_1, FVC, TLC	Normal	Normal
DLCO	Normal or mild ↓	↓↓↓
Resting PaO_2	Normal or mild ↓	↓↓↓
Exercise-desaturation	Often present	↓↓↓
Imaging		
Chest HRCT	Usually normal	Centrilobular ground-glass opacities, septal lines, mediastinal lymph node enlargement
V/Q scan	Usually normal	Usually normal
Treatment	Targeted PAH therapy is supported by RCTs	Risk of pulmonary edema; conflicting data on targeted PAH therapy, limited to small case series

DLCO, Diffusion capacity of carbon monoxide; FEV_1, forced expiratory volume in 1 second; FVC, forced vital capacity; HIV, human immunodeficiency virus; HRCT, high resolution computed tomography; iPAH, idiopathic pulmonary arterial hypertension; mPAP, mean pulmonary artery pressure; PAH, pulmonary arterial hypertension; PaO_2, partial pressure of oxygen; PAWP, pulmonary artery wedge pressure; PVOD, pulmonary venoocclusive disease; PVR, pulmonary vascular resistance; RCTs, randomized controlled trials; TLC, total lung capacity; V/Q, ventilation-perfusion.
Adapted from Montani D, et al. Eur Respir J. 2016;47:1334–1335.

perhaps the misconception that moderated physical activity is dangerous. In one meta-analysis of 469 PAH patients, exercise improved 6-MWD by +53.3 m, pVO_2 by +1.8 mL/kg, and PASP by −3.7 mm Hg at week 15.[59] Inspiratory muscle training, too, is associated with an improvement in PAH endpoints.

At present, there are 14 U.S. Food and Drug Administration-approved PAH therapies that target NO· signaling, the endothelin receptor axis, or prostacyclin deficiency spanning oral, inhaled, subcutaneous (injectable and implantable), and intravenous delivery methods (Fig. 88.13A).[1] In patients without a positive vasoreactivity test, therapy selection is guided by clinical status: New York Heart Association Functional Class (NYHA FC) IV, cardiogenic shock by clinical or hemodynamic criteria (e.g., signs of impaired distal perfusion, cardiac index <2.1 l/min/m²), syncope, or chest pain (indicative of either RV ischemia or LMCA compression) are indications for continuous parenteral prostacyclin therapy.[38] For patients with a positive vasoreactivity test, high-dose calcium channel antagonist therapy is the initial treatment in the absence of high-risk findings.

Initial Management of Treatment-Naïve Pulmonary Arterial Hypertension Patients

An evidenced-based strategic shift in the approach to patients with newly diagnosed PAH (without an indication for immediate parenteral therapy) has emerged over the previous 5 years favoring the initiation of two oral PAH therapies. The Ambrisentan and Tadalafil in Patients with Pulmonary Arterial Hypertension (AMBITION) trial demonstrated a clear benefit in hard-clinical events among incident, treatment-naïve PAH patients administered combination ambrisentan (selective endothelin receptor-type A antagonist) plus tadalafil (PDE-V inhibitor) compared with monotherapy with either agent.[60] At a median of 517 days, an endpoint of death, hospitalization for PAH, disease progression, or unsatisfactory clinical response occurred in 18%, 34%, and 28% of patients randomized to combination therapy, ambrisentan monotherapy, and tadalafil monotherapy, respectively. The benefit of combination therapy corresponding to a 50% reduction in the hazard for achieving the composite endpoint (Fig. 88.13B–D). Data from observational cohort studies implies that the salutary benefit of combination therapy may not be exclusive to these drugs per se, and the evidence base is expanding in support of up-front treatment to triple therapy in highly selected patients. Conversely, monotherapy may be reasonable for patients that were initially administered one PAH drug and remain clinically stable or in whom prognosis is particularly favorable. Overall, personalizing a treatment plan for PAH should be done in collaboration with an expert referral center.

Therapeutic Escalation and End-Stage Disease

Generally, a low threshold to escalate therapy (e.g., dose uptitration or sequential addition of a new drug class) is warranted in PAH patients who demonstrate disease progression or, in turn, fail to demonstrate evidence of improvement. Hospitalization for heart failure and end-organ damage, particularly renal failure, are especially worrisome events that portend further decline and warrant adjustment to care. Indeed, referral for bilateral lung transplant evaluation should be considered in patients with suboptimal clinical response to the initial therapeutic approach. Although the 5-year post-transplant survival rate has improved in some series to 75% for PAH patients, availability of suitable donor lungs remains limited.[38] Temporizing (bridging) measures to transplantation in PAH include RV assist device or veno-arterial extracorporeal membrane oxygenation (V-A ECMO), although the precise indications and clinical profile that is best suited for these extreme measures is not clear. Balloon atrial septostomy, other interventional approaches that create a right-to-left shunt such as percutaneous Potts shunt, and salvage medical therapies may be considered to palliate symptoms in patients who are not candidates for lung transplant.

Genetic Counseling

Patients with idiopathic, familial, or anorexigen-associated PAH as well as PVOD/PCH should be considered for genetic counseling and testing. Generally, testing is focused first on the patient. Results are helpful if a pathogenetic variant is discovered in the patient, but not in unaffected family members. In this scenario, the risk of developing PAH in the unaffected family member is akin to the general population. Detecting the pathogenic variant harbored by a patient in a phenotype-negative family member is associated with an increased lifetime risk of developing PAH, although quantifying this risk with certainty is challenging due to the incomplete penetrant pattern of inheritance for most PAH variants. In the case of PVOD, identifying a biallelic EIF2AK4 mutation has direct implication on clinical management, as these patients tend to present at an earlier age and can be diagnosed and risk stratified for lung transplantation earlier by virtue of genetic testing results.

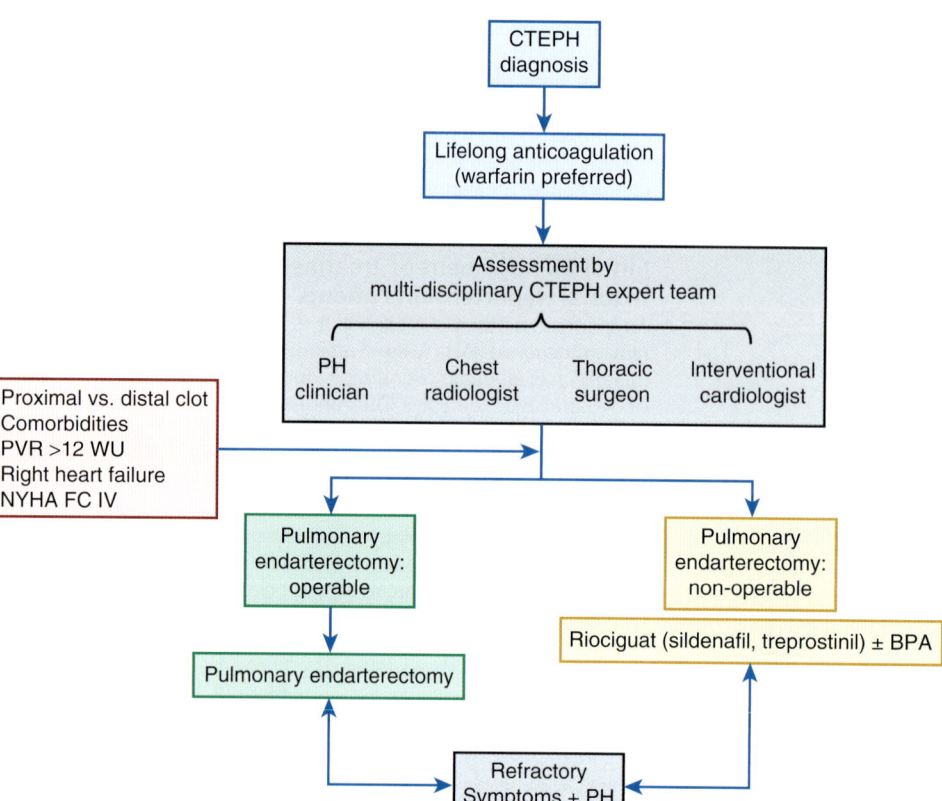

FIGURE 88.12 Chronic thromboembolic pulmonary hypertension (CTEPH) treatment algorithm. In patients diagnosed with CTEPH, lifelong anticoagulation with warfarin is generally indicated. Clinical decision-making requires a multi-disciplinary expert team including a PH specialist, chest radiologist, (high pulmonary endarterectomy volume) thoracic surgeon, and interventional cardiologists (or interventional radiologist). Surgical pulmonary endarterectomy is the preferred treatment option, although operative candidacy may be mitigated by various high-risk features. In nonoperative patients, medical therapy and/or balloon pulmonary angioplasty (BPA) should be considered. *NHYA*, New York Heart Association; *PVR*, pulmonary vascular resistance.

Chronic Thromboembolic Pulmonary Hypertension (see Chapter 87)

Upon diagnosing CTEPH, all patients should be considered for surgical pulmonary thromboendarterectomy.[61] This is based on several lines of data indicating that surgery provides a distinct survival advantage and opportunity for complete or near complete resolution of symptoms. In one prospective study of 679 newly diagnosed CTEPH patients, the 3-year survival rate was 89% in operated patients compared to 70% in nonoperated patients.[62] Pulmonary thromboendarterectomy is performed through a median sternotomy and requires cardiopulmonary bypass as well as periods of hypothermic circulatory arrest to allow optimal visualization of clot. Technical success hinges on surgical accessibility and, importantly, the experience of the operator and surgical team. The probability of an optimal therapeutic response to surgery aligns with the relationship between the PH severity by cardiopulmonary hemodynamics and burden of thrombotic disease on imaging. Thus, distal disease, particularly subsegmental arterial involvement, raises anatomic concerns to the potential for therapeutic benefit. Other factors that may influence peri-operative risk include cardiovascular comorbidity burden, right heart failure, NYHA FC IV, and patients with very elevated PVR (>12 WU).[61]

In patients that are poor surgical candidates, have inoperable disease, or decline surgery, percutaneous balloon pulmonary angioplasty (BPA) at an expert referral center is a modern-day treatment option (Fig. 88.14). Matching data from digital subtraction pulmonary angiography with lung perfusion findings is used to assist in identifying target lesions, which otherwise may be difficult to discern owing to the complex and multifocal vasculopathy of CTEPH. Although angiographic evidence showing improvement in post-stenotic blood flow following BPA is often evident immediately, achieving significant clinical benefits from BPA requires multiple procedural attempts, generally requiring separate hospitalizations.[63] Additionally, peri-procedural complications such as reperfusion injury, hemoptysis, or pulmonary artery perforation is reported in 15% of patients.[62] When these occur, pulmonary edema, hypoxemia, respiratory failure, and mortality are potential outcomes. In patients who are inoperable or in whom pulmonary thromboendarterectomy is associated with residual PH, therapy with the soluble guanylyl cyclase stimulator riociguat or the nonselective ERA macitentan can be useful for improving functional status and PVR.

Pulmonary Hypertension from Left Heart Disease

In PH from left heart disease (or any other specific cause), the principal goal of treatment is to optimize the underlying condition. This should include consideration to undiagnosed comorbid disease, such as COPD in patients with left heart disease, or vice-versa, including sleep apnea that is common to both. Conversely, PH drives decision-making in certain clinical scenarios, such as asymptomatic mitral valve regurgitation in which PASP greater than 50 mm Hg is a strong indication for valve repair or replacement. For management of PH due to conventional HFpEF or HFrEF, diuretic therapy remains the mainstay treatment (see Chapters 49 and 50). Implanting CardioMEMS heart failure system, which provides real-time pulmonary artery pressure monitoring, to guide diuretic dosing is an option for patients with a narrow therapeutic window (see Chapter 58). Efforts to repurpose pulmonary vasodilator therapy to either PH from cardiac or lung disease have been met mainly with negative or, at best, mixed data.[64] One exception is the minority of advanced heart failure patients post-left ventricular assist device implant with sustained PH. In this subgroup, PDE-V inhibitor therapy is effective for decreasing PVR as one strategy by which to delay, defer, or optimize candidacy for orthotropic heart transplantation.

There is a graded association between pre-operative PVR and peri-operative mortality following orthotopic heart transplantation that is particularly evident greater than 4 WU (and transpulmonary gradient greater than 15 mm Hg, calculated by the difference between mPAP and PAWP). In turn, PVR greater than 5 WU and transpulmonary gradient greater than 16 mm Hg is a relative contra-indication to heart transplantation. Acute vasodilator challenge should be performed if sPAP greater than 50 mm Hg, and either transpulmonary gradient ≥15 mm Hg (calculated by: mPAP − PAWP) or PVR greater than 3 WU and systemic systolic arterial pressure greater than 85 mm Hg.[55] However, consensus is lacking on the best vasodilator to use for testing in these circumstances, and data are variable on the relationship between PVR post-vasodilator challenge and outcome post-heart transplant. This scenario is complicated further by the fact that in many patients a reduction in PVR is accountable by increased PAWP.

SPECIAL CLINICAL CIRCUMSTANCES

High-Altitude Pulmonary Edema

At high altitude, particularly but not exclusively ≥2500 m, there are several environmental changes compared to sea level that bear directly on pulmonary vascular function, particularly hypobaric hypoxia. A fall in oxygen tension (measured as the partial pressure of O_2) detected at the

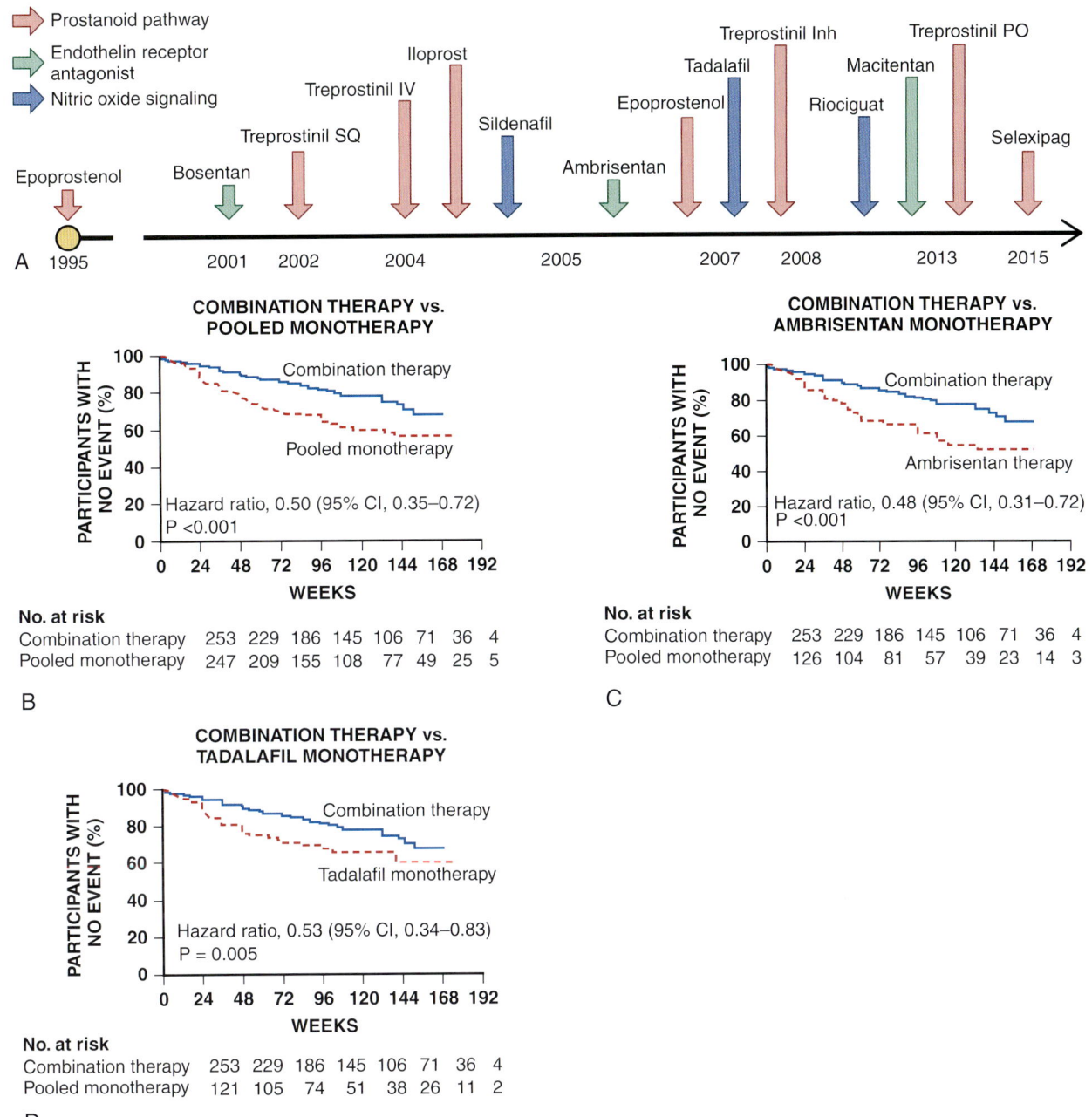

FIGURE 88.13 Pulmonary arterial hypertension therapies. **A,** Chronology of pulmonary arterial hypertension (PAH) therapies, organized by molecular pathway target. *IV,* Intravenous; *PO,* per oral; *SQ,* subcutaneous. Selexipag is a prostacyclin counterreceptor agonist, which differs from other same-class drugs that replace prostacyclin deficiency. **B-D,** Treatment-naïve PAH patients enrolled in the Ambrisentan and Tadalafil in Patients with Pulmonary Arterial Hypertension (AMBITION) trial were randomized to receive up-front monotherapy with the endothelin-type A receptor antagonist ambrisentan or the phosphodiesterase type-V inhibitor tadalafil, or the combination of both drugs. Kaplan-Meier curve for the primary endpoint, which was a time-to-event analysis of clinical failure, defined as death, hospitalization for worsening pulmonary arterial hypertension, disease progression, or unsatisfactory long-term clinical response. These data show comparisons in outcome for combination therapy vs. pooled monotherapy (**B**), ambrisentan monotherapy (**C**), and tadalafil monotherapy (**D**). (**B-D** from Galiè N et al. *N Engl J Med* 2015;373:834–844.)

level of the alveolar capillary is a major trigger of hypoxic pulmonary vasoconstriction. This occurs through membrane depolarization that propagates proximally, from capillary to arterials, leading to increased intrapulmonary artery smooth muscle cell Ca^{2+} levels. Teleologically, this appears necessary to shunt blood flow to lung regions that are "better" ventilated. There is a parabolic relationship between mPAP and altitude between 2000 and 4,500 m that ranges from 15 to 30 mm Hg, respectively.[65] Although this profile is compatible with normal living, the cardiopulmonary hemodynamic response to altitude varies substantially between individuals. Inhomogeneous hypoxic pulmonary vasoconstriction associated with rapid ascent causes high-altitude pulmonary edema (HAPE) arising from changes in capillary membrane permeability that lead to exudative effusion. The clinical syndrome includes shortness of breath and cough; treatment beyond prevention includes descent to a lower altitude, supplemental oxygen, and/or nifedipine.

The PH typical of high altitude is generally mild and tolerated clinically. In a population of Kyrgyz highlanders who dwell at approximately 3000 m above sea level, 14% have evidence of RV hypertrophy on ECG.[65] In patients with high-altitude PH, descent to lower altitude is important and may be lifesaving when the syndrome is complicated by heart failure. PDE-V inhibitor and acetazolamide therapies have also been reported effective at improving PH severity. The HAPE and high-altitude PH syndromes are distinct from acute or chronic mountain sickness, which are characterized by neurological symptoms in association with hypoventilation-induced overproduction of red blood cells and vasogenic cerebral edema.

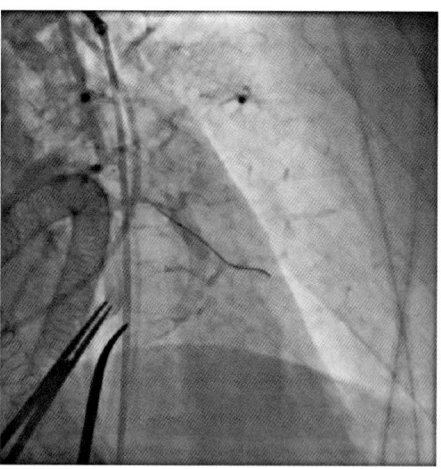 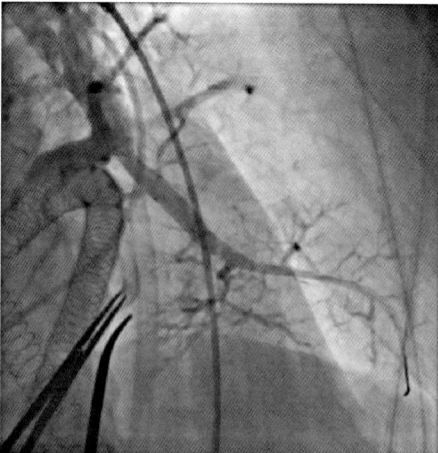

Pre-PBA　　　　　Post-PBA

FIGURE 88.14 Pulmonary balloon angioplasty (PBA) for chronic thromboembolic pulmonary hypertension (CTEPH). In inoperable CTEPH patients or in those with a suboptimal surgical result and residual symptoms, percutaneous pulmonary balloon angioplasty is a therapeutic option when performed at a PH center of excellence. Compared to pre-BPA, image of left pulmonary artery post-BPA demonstrates increased contrast flow to the lung periphery. (Adapted from Wiedenroth CB et al. *J Heart Lung Transpl* 2016;35:591–596.)

Sarcoidosis

Coalescing, non-necrotizing granulomas in clusters defines the pathology of sarcoidosis, which affects multiple organ systems including the lung parenchyma. The prevalence of PH in sarcoid patients varies widely and is biased by patient selection and method of assessment. Approximately 50% of sarcoid patients with exercise intolerance also have PH. Patients may present with either pre-capillary or post-capillary PH.[66] In the former, parenchymal fibrosis leading to arterial remodeling/destruction or direct granulomatous involvement of the vasculature underlies PH. In the latter, fibrosing mediastinitis, pulmonary venous involvement, or cardiac sarcoid including LV dysfunction should be considered. In one randomized clinical trial over 16 weeks, treatment with bosentan (nonselective endothelin receptor antagonist) did not improve 6-MWD or quality of life measures significantly.[66]

Sickle Cell Disease

Chronic hemolytic anemia is an important complication of sickle cell disease with direct ramifications on cardiopulmonary hemodynamics. The average basal CO for sickle cell disease patients approaches 11 liters/min, driven by low hemoglobin content (47 to 100 g/liter). It follows that PVR is low in sickle cell disease patients, which may be 50% of nonanemic healthy controls at baseline. Indeed, the upper limit of normal PVR in sickle cell disease is approximately 2.0 WU.[67] Red blood cell sickling itself is associated with increased release of intraerythrocytic hemoglobin that decreases NO· bioavailability and promotes the accumulation of vascular reactive oxygen species. This disruption in the redox balance of vascular cells underlies endothelial dysfunction, pulmonary artery smooth muscle cell proliferation, and in situ thrombosis. Indeed, pre-capillary PH is an established aspect of the sickle cell disease spectrum, affecting approximately 30% of patients. Longstanding high CO and plasma expansion from anemia also causes LV cavitary remodeling due to chronically elevated stroke volume. Over time, LV dysfunction may ensue, leading to pulmonary venous hypertension and post-capillary PH.

Overall, a stepwise increase in mPAP by 10 mm Hg is associated with a 1.7-fold increase in the mortality hazard. The pro-thrombotic potential in sickle cell disease elevates PVR (thus contributing to pre-capillary PH) and increases the risk of developing CTEPH. In fact, among sickle cell disease patients with PH, up to 25% are diagnosed with CTEPH. Therapy for sickle cell disease-PH should focus on correcting underlying anemia with hydroxyurea and blood transfusion. PDE-V inhibitor therapy may improve cardiopulmonary hemodynamics in this population but increases sickle cell vasoocclusive pain, and, therefore, should not be considered outside the advice and management of an expert referral center.[67]

Pregnancy (see Chapter 92)

Mortality or heart failure requiring lung transplantation is reported in 20% of pregnant women with PAH; therefore, it is recommended that patients avoid conception. Endothelin receptor antagonist therapy is teratogenic, and women of child-bearing age require counseling and a declaration of birth control prior to treatment. Pregnant PAH patients should be managed in a referral center with expertise in maternal-fetal medicine and pulmonary vascular disease.

Perioperative Management

Perioperative complication risk for noncardiac and nonobstetric surgeries is increased in PH; in one series of 114 PAH patients, major complications and mortality occurred in 6.1% and 3.5% of patients, respectively.[68] For PAH patients, general anesthesia should be avoided when possible. In patients requiring general anesthesia, an individualized care plan including cardiac anesthesia, intraoperative pulmonary artery catheter monitoring, and a plan to use inhaled therapies may prove useful.

FUTURE PERSPECTIVES

The PH field continues to evolve, including insight into the hemodynamic spectrum of clinical risk, a strategic shift in favor of aggressive early therapy in newly diagnosed PAH patients, and percutaneous interventions for selected patients affected by CTEPH. In particular, the mPAP threshold to diagnose PH is now greater than 20 mm Hg, placing emphasis on early diagnosis. Developing therapies specific to PH from left heart disease or lung disease remains a major goal. Overall, however, PH, including the PAH subtype, has emerged in the current era as a high-risk but manageable disease that should be considered in all patients with cardiopulmonary symptoms.

ACKNOWLEDGMENTS

Dr. Maron would like to acknowledge Dr. Stuart Rich, who authored an earlier version of this chapter which inspired many young physicians and students including Dr. Maron to pursue pulmonary hypertension in clinical and research endeavors.

Dr. Maron reports being a consultant for Actelion, and co-inventor on the following patents or patent application that are related to pulmonary hypertension (U.S. Patent #9,605,047; PCT/US2015/029672; Provisional ID: #62475955; Provisional ID: #24624; Provisional ID: #24622).

REFERENCES
Overview and Pulmonary Circulation
1. Maron BA, Galie N. Diagnosis, treatment, and clinical management of pulmonary arterial hypertension in the contemporary era: a review. *JAMA Cardiol.* 2016;1:1056–1065.
2. Rosenkranz S, Howard LS, Gomberg-Maitland M, Hoeper MM. Systemic consequences of pulmonary hypertension and right-sided heart failure. *Circulation.* 2020;141:678–693.
3. Tuder RM. Pulmonary vascular remodeling in pulmonary hypertension. *Cell Tissue Res.* 2017;367:643–649.
4. Rosenkranz S, Preston IR. Right heart catheterisation: best practice and pitfalls in pulmonary hypertension. *Eur Respir Rev.* 2015;24:642–652.
5. Raymond TE, Khabbaza JE, Yadav R, Tonelli AR. Significance of main pulmonary artery dilation on imaging studies. *Ann Am Thorac Soc.* 2014;11:1623–1632.
6. Kovacs G, Olschewski A, Berghold A, Olschewski H. Pulmonary vascular resistances during exercise in normal subjects: a systemic review. *Eur Respir J.* 2012;39:319–328.
7. Townsley MI. Structure and composition of pulmonary arteries, capillaries, and veins. *Compr Physiol.* 2012;2:675–709.
8. Fayyaz AU, Edwards WD, Maleszewski JJ, et al. Global pulmonary vascular remodeling in pulmonary hypertension associated with heart failure and preserved or reduced ejection fraction. *Circulation.* 2018;137:1796–1810.
9. Kovacs G, Herve P, Barbera JA, et al. An official European Respiratory Society statement: pulmonary haemodynamics during exercise. *Eur Respir J.* 2017;50:1700578.
10. Ho JE, Zern EK, Lau ES, et al. Exercise pulmonary hypertension predicts clinical outcomes in patients with dyspnea on effort. *J Am Coll Cardiol.* 2020;75:17–26.

Classification of Pulmonary Hypertension

11. Newman JH. Pulmonary hypertension by the method of Paul Wood. *Chest*. 2020;S0012-3692: 30428-1.
12. Simonneau G, Montani D, Celermajer DS, et al. Haemodynamic definitions and updated clinical classification of pulmonary hypertension. *Eur Respir J*. 2019;53:1801913.
13. Kovacs G, Douschan P, Maron BA, et al. Mildly increased pulmonary arterial pressure: a new disease entity or just a marker of poor prognosis? *Eur J Heart Fail*. 2019;21:1057–1061.
14. Maron BA, Hess E, Maddox TM, et al. Association of borderline pulmonary hypertension with mortality and hospitalization in a large patient cohort: insights from the Veterans Affairs Clinical Assessment, Reporting and Tracking program. *Circulation*. 2016;133:1240–1248.
15. Nishihara T, Yamamoto E, Tokitsu T, et al. New definition of pulmonary hypertension in patients with heart failure with preserved ejection fraction. *Am J Respir Crit Care Med*. 2019;200:386–388.
16. Nouraie M, Little JA, Hildesheim M, et al. Validation of a composite vascular high-risk profile for adult patients with sickle cell disease. *Am J Hematol*. 2019;94:E312–E314.
17. Maron BA, Brittain EL, Hess E, et al. The association between pulmonary vascular resistance and clinical outcomes in patients with pulmonary hypertension: a retrospective cohort study. *Lancet Respir Med*. 2020;S2213-2600(20)30317–9.
18. Guhaa A, Amione-Guerrab J, Park MH. Epidemiology of pulmonary hypertension in left heart disease. *Prog Cardiovasc Dis*. 2016;59:3–10.
19. Shah AM, Cikes M, Prasad N, et al. Echocardiographic features of patients with heart failure and preserved left ventricular ejection fraction. *J Am Coll Cardiol*. 2019;74:2858–2873.
20. Covella M, Rowin EJ, Hill NS, et al. Mechanism of progressive heart failure and significance of pulmonary hypertension in obstructive hypertrophic cardiomyopathy. *Circ Heart Fail*. 2017;10:e003689.
21. Magne J, Pibarot P, Sengupta PP, et al. Pulmonary hypertension in valvular disease: a comprehensive review on pathophysiology to therapy from the HAVEC Group. *JACC Cardiovasc Imaging*. 2015;8(1):83–99. https://doi.org/10.1016/j.jcmg.2014.12.003.
22. Nishimura RA, Otto CM, Bonow RO, et al. 2014 AHA/ACC guideline for the management of patients with valvular heart disease: executive summary: a report of the American College of Cardiology/American Heart Association Task Force on Practice Guidelines. *J Am Coll Cardiol*. 2014;63:2438–2488.
23. Caravita S, Mariani D, Blengino S, et al. Pulmonary hypertension due to a stiff left atrium: speckle tracking equivalents of large V-waves. *Echocardiography*. 2018;35:1464–1466.
24. Weatherald J, Reis A, Sitbon O, Humbert M, et al. Pulmonary arterial hypertension registries: past, present and into the future. *Eur Respir Rev*. 2019;28(154):190128.
25. Farber HW, Miller DP, Poms AD, et al. Five-Year outcomes of patients enrolled in the reveal registry. *Chest*. 2015;148:1043–1054.
26. Foderaro A, Ventetuolo CE. Pulmonary arterial hypertension and the sex hormone paradox. *Curr Hypertens Rep*. 2016;18:84.
27. Ventetuolo CE, Praestgaard A, Palevsky HI, et al. Sex and haemodynamics in pulmonary arterial hypertension. *Eur Respir J*. 2014;43:523–530.
28. Sitbon O, Sattlerr C, Bertoletti L, et al. Initial dual oral combination therapy in pulmonary arterial hypertension. *Eur Respir J*. 2016;47:1727–1736.
29. Morrell NW, Aldred MA, Chung WK, et al. Genetics and genomics of pulmonary arterial hypertension. *Eur Respir J*. 2019;53(1):1801899.
30. Zamanian RT, Hedlin H, Greuenwald P, et al. Features and outcomes of methamphetamine-associated pulmonary arterial hypertension. *Am J Respir Crit Care Med*. 2018;197:788–800.
31. Hassoun PM. The right ventricle in scleroderma (2013 Grover conference series). *Am J Respir Crit Care Med*. 2018;197:788–800.
32. Graham BB, Kumar R. Schistosomiasis and the pulmonary vasculature (2013 Grover Conference series). *Pulm Circ*. 2014;4:353–362.
33. Brittain EL, Duncan MS, Chang J, et al. Increased echocardiographic pulmonary pressure in HIV-infected and -uninfected individuals in the veterans aging cohort study. *Am J Respir Crit Care Med*. 2018;197:923–932.
34. Creel-Bulos C, Hockstein M, Amin N. Acute cor pulmonale in critically ill patients with Covid-19. *N Engl J Med*. 2020;382(21):e70.
35. van Loon RLE, Roofthooft MTR, Hillege HL, et al. Pediatric pulmonary hypertension in The Netherlands: epidemiology and characterization during the period 1991–2005. *Circulation*. 2011;124:1755–1764.
36. Nathan SD, Barbera JA, Gaine SP, et al. Pulmonary hypertension in chronic lung disease and hypoxia. *Eur Respir J*. 2019;53:1801914.
37. Montani D, Lau EEM, Dorfmuller P, et al. Pulmonary veno-occlusive disease. *Eur Respir J*. 2016;47:1518–1534.
38. Galiè N, Humbert M, Vachiery JL, et al. 2015 ESC/ERS Guidelines for the diagnosis and treatment of pulmonary hypertension. *Eur Respir J*. 2015;46:903–975.
39. Assad TR, Hemnes AR, Larkin EK, et al. Clinical and biological insights into combined post- and pre-capillary pulmonary hypertension. *J Am Coll Cardiol*. 2016;68(23):2525–2536.

Pathology, Pathobiology, and Pathophysiology

40. Archer SL. Acquired mitochondrial abnormalities, including epigenetic inhibition of superoxide dismutase 2, in pulmonary hypertension and cancer: therapeutic implications. *Adv Exp Med Biol*. 2016;903:29–53.
41. Samokhin AO, Stephens BA, Wertheim BM, et al. NEDD9 targets COL3A1 to promote endothelial fibrosis and pulmonary arterial hypertension. *Sci Transl Med*. 2018;10:445.
42. MacLean MR. The serotonin hypothesis in pulmonary hypertension revisited: targets for novel therapies (2017 Grover conference series). *Pulm Circ*. 2018;8: 2045894018759125.
43. Tedford RJ, Mudd JO, Girgis RE, et al. Right ventricular dysfunction in systemic sclerosis-associated pulmonary arterial hypertension. *Circ Heart Fail*. 2013;6:953–963.
44. Vonk Noordegraaf A, Westerhof BE, Westerhof N. The relationship between the right ventricle and its load in pulmonary hypertension. *J Am Coll Cardiol*. 2017;69:236–243.
45. Maron BA, Leopold JA. Emerging concepts in the molecular basis of pulmonary arterial hypertension: part ii: neurohormonal signaling contributes to the pulmonary vascular and right ventricular pathophenotype of pulmonary arterial hypertension. *Circulation*. 2015;131:2079–2091.
46. Hsu S, Kokkonen-Simon KM, Kirk JA, et al. Right ventricular myofilament functional differences in humans with systemic sclerosis-associated versus idiopathic pulmonary arterial hypertension. *Circulation*. 2018;137:2360–23670.

Integrated Approach to Diagnosis and Treatment

47. O'Leary JM, Assad TR, Xu M, et al. Lack of a tricuspid regurgitation Doppler signal and pulmonary hypertension by invasive measurement. *J Am Heart Assoc*. 2018;7:e009362.
48. Kim NH, Delcroix M, Jais X, et al. Chronic thromboembolic pulmonary hypertension. *Eur Respir J*. 2019;53:1801915.
49. Maron BA, Choudhary G, Khan UA, et al. Clinical profile and underdiagnosis of pulmonary hypertension in us veteran patients. *Circ Heart Fail*. 2013;6:906–912.
50. Park J-B, Suh M, Park J-Y, et al. Assessment of inflammation in pulmonary artery hypertension by 68 Ga-Mannosylated human serum albumin. *Am J Respir Crit Care Med*. 2020;201:95–106.
51. Rich JD, Rich S. Clinical diagnosis of pulmonary hypertension. *Circulation*. 2014;130:1820–1830.
52. Berry NC, Manyoo A, Oldham W, et al. Protocol for exercise hemodynamic assessment: performing an invasive cardiopulmonary exercise test in clinical practice. *Pulm Circ*. 2015;5:610–618.
53. Opotowsky AR. Clinical evaluation and management of pulmonary hypertension in the adult with congenital heart disease. *Circulation*. 2015;131:200–210.
54. Opotowsky AR, Hess E, Maron BA, et al. Thermodilution vs estimated fick cardiac output measurement in clinical practice: an analysis of mortality from the Veterans Affairs Clinical Assessment, Reporting, and Tracking (VA CART) program and Vanderbilt University. *JAMA Cardiol*. 2017;2:1090–1099.
55. Vachiéry JL, Tedford RJ, Rosenkranz S, et al. Pulmonary hypertension due to left heart disease. *Eur Respir J*. 2019;53:1801897.
56. Oldham WM, Oliveira RK, Wang RS, et al. Network analysis to risk stratify patients with exercise intolerance. *Circ Res*. 2018;122:864–876.
57. Benza RL, Gomberg-Maitland M, Elliott CG, et al. Predicting survival in patients with pulmonary arterial hypertension: the reveal risk score calculator 2.0 and comparison with ESC/ERS-based risk assessment strategies. *Chest*. 2019;156:323–337.
58. Reddy YNV, Carter RE, Obokata M, et al. A simple, evidence-based approach to help guide diagnosis of heart failure with preserved ejection fraction. *Circulation*. 2018;138:861–870.
59. Pandey A, Garg S, Khunger M, et al. Efficacy and safety of exercise training in chronic pulmonary hypertension. *Circ: Heart Fail*. 2015;8:1032–1043.
60. Galiè N, Barbera JA, Frost AE, et al. Initial use of ambrisentan plus tadalafil in pulmonary arterial hypertension. *N Engl J Med*. 2015;373:834–844.
61. Kim NH, Delcroix M, Jais X, et al. Chronic thromboembolic pulmonary hypertension. *Eur Respir J*. 2019;53:1801915.
62. Lang IM, Madani M. Update on chronic thromboembolic pulmonary hypertension. *Circulation*. 2014;130:508–518.
63. Auger WR. Surgical and percutaneous interventions for chronic thromboembolic pulmonary hypertension. *Cardiol Clin*. 2020;38:257–268.
64. Maron BA, Ryan JJ. A concerning trend for patients with pulmonary hypertension in the era of evidence-based medicine. *Circulation*. 2019;139(16):1861–1864.
65. Wilkins MR, Ghofrani H-A, Weissmann N, et al. Pathophysiology and treatment of high-altitude pulmonary vascular disease. *Circulation*. 2015;131:582–590.
66. Boucly A, Cottin V, Nunes H, et al. Management and long-term outcomes of sarcoidosis-associated pulmonary hypertension. *Eur Respir J*. 2017;50:1700465.
67. Gladwin MT. Cardiovascular complications and risk of death in sickle-cell disease. *Lancet*. 2016;387(10037):2565–2574.
68. Meyer S, McLaughlin VV, Seyfarth H-J, et al. Outcomes of noncardiac, nonobstetric surgery in patients with PAH: an international prospective survey. *Eur Respir J*. 2013;41:1302–1307.

89 Sleep-Disordered Breathing and Cardiac Disease

SUSAN REDLINE

DEFINITIONS, 1678

PATHOPHYSIOLOGY, 1678
Pathophysiology of Obstructive Sleep Apnea, 1678
Pathophysiology of Central Sleep Apnea, 1679
Risk Factors for and Recognition of Sleep-Disordered Breathing, 1679

Pathophysiologic Mechanisms That Link Sleep-Disordered Breathing to Cardiovascular Diseases, 1681

SLEEP-DISORDERED BREATHING AND HYPERTENSION, 1681

SLEEP-DISORDERED BREATHING AND CORONARY HEART DISEASE, 1682

SLEEP-DISORDERED BREATHING, CARDIAC FUNCTION, AND HEART FAILURE, 1683

SLEEP-DISORDERED BREATHING AND CARDIAC ARRHYTHMIAS, 1684

FUTURE PERSPECTIVES, 1685

REFERENCES, 1685

Sleep-disordered breathing (SDB) is prevalent in patients with cardiac diseases, contributing to a reduced quality of life, a reduced functional capacity, and poor health. SDB causes acute and chronic physiologic stressors that can exacerbate cardiac ischemia, reduce systolic and diastolic function, cause cardiac structural and electrical remodeling, and increase the risk of cardiac arrhythmias and sudden death. Despite strong evidence linking SDB to cardiovascular disease (CVD), and the vulnerability of the cardiac patient to SDB-related stressors, SDB often goes unrecognized in cardiology practice, so there is potential for improved recognition and initiation of interventions. This chapter reviews aspects of SDB recognition, pathophysiology, and health outcomes relevant to cardiac disease.

DEFINITIONS

SDB refers to a spectrum of sleep-related breathing disorders that includes obstructive sleep apnea (OSA), central sleep apnea (CSA), Cheyne-Stokes respiration, and sleep-related hypoventilation. The mechanisms and risk factors for these disorders have overlapping as well as unique characteristics. Each is associated with impaired ventilation during sleep and sleep disruption, but differ with regard to degree of abnormalities in neuromuscular respiratory drive and airway collapsibility. The constellation of symptoms, the diagnostic criteria, and their associations with CVD are summarized in Table 89.1.

Typical symptoms of OSA include loud or disruptive snoring, snorting or gasping during sleep, poor sleep quality, unrefreshed sleep, and excessive daytime sleepiness. Diagnosis requires objective sleep testing using an in-laboratory polysomnograph or a home sleep apnea test, with demonstration of recurrent episodes of apneas and/or hypopneas. An apnea indicates a near absence of airflow during the period of upper airway obstruction for at least 10 seconds, while a hypopnea signifies a reduction in airflow relative to baseline accompanied by drop in oxygen saturation or a cortical arousal (Fig. 89.1).[1] Apneas and hypopneas are further classified as "obstructive" based on the occurrence of concurrent respiratory effort during periods of reduced or absent airflow, and otherwise as "central". Diagnostic criteria for OSA are: (1) symptoms of breathing disturbances during sleep (snoring, snorting, gasping, or breathing pauses) *or* daytime sleepiness or fatigue, despite sufficient opportunities to sleep and unexplained by other medical problems; *and* (2) five or more apneas or hypopneas per hour of sleep (apnea-hypopnea index [AHI]). OSA may be diagnosed in the absence of symptoms if the AHI is greater than 15). OSA severity is judged based on the frequency of breathing disturbances (AHI level), degree of hypoxemia and sleep disruption, and associated symptoms.

Excessive daytime sleepiness, in particular, marks severe disease that is associated with an increased risk of adverse CVD outcomes, as well as better adherence with OSA treatment. CSA often overlaps with OSA and is identified when more than 50% of respiratory disturbances are unaccompanied by respiratory effort.

The AHI and other indices of sleep are measured with multichannel overnight recordings. Polysomnography performed in the sleep laboratory records airflow, breathing effort and oxygen saturation, as well as data from the electroencephalogram, electrocardiogram, and leg muscles; providing the ability to identify apneas and hypopneas as well as stage sleep, quantify sleep fragmentation, and identify other sleep-related phenomena such as arrhythmias and periodic leg movements. Home-based sleep apnea tests collect data on breathing parameters, but do not typically record additional information. Although home sleep apnea tests are increasingly used due to their lower cost, in-laboratory polysomnography still serves to evaluate patients with complex comorbidities, such as heart failure (HF). When interpreting the results of home sleep apnea tests, it is important to note that they can underestimate the AHI by approximately 12%,[2] and larger misclassifications are likely in patients with poor sleep quality, such as those with HF, and in women, who typically have shorter respiratory events with less desaturation than men.

PATHOPHYSIOLOGY

Pathophysiology of Obstructive Sleep Apnea

The pharyngeal airway has no bony or cartilaginous support, and its size and shape change dynamically with each expiration and inspiration (when negative intraluminal pressure causes the airway to be "sucked" inward). Its patency therefore depends on the activation of pharyngeal dilator muscles, which decreases with sleep onset. Whether an apnea occurs depends on whether the level of neuromuscular activation of the upper airway muscles is adequate to overcome forces that promote airway collapse during sleep. The presence of an anatomically small airway (e.g., micrognathia, fat deposition in the lateral pharyngeal walls) and lying in the supine position (when gravitational and positional factors alter the position of the tongue and other soft tissues) increase the level of neuromuscular drive needed to maintain airway patency. Therefore, patients with small oropharyngeal airways due to craniofacial factors or excessive airway soft tissue have an increased risk for OSA. When a person is in the recumbent position, there can be a rostral redistribution of peripheral fluid from the lower extremities to the neck area, contributing to airway narrowing during sleep, and this factor can predispose patients

TABLE 89.1 Key Features of Obstructive Sleep Apnea and Central Sleep Apnea

	OBSTRUCTIVE SLEEP APNEA	CENTRAL SLEEP APNEA
Common presenting symptoms	Snoring, observed apneas, gasping or snorting during sleep, daytime sleepiness	Observed apneas, gasping or snorting during sleep, frequent awakenings, unrefreshed sleep, fatigue
Diagnosis	Home sleep apnea test or polysomnography showing AHI >5 with a predominance of obstructive apneas or hypopneas (>50%)	Polysomnography showing a predominance of central apneas or hypopneas (>50%) with a central apnea hypopnea index >5 Cheyne-Stokes respiration: ≥3 consecutive central apneas/central hypopneas separated by crescendo and decrescendo change in breathing amplitude with a cycle length ≥40 sec associated with central AHI >5
Associated risk factors	Obesity, male, middle-older age	Male, older age
Associated cardiovascular disease*	Resistant hypertension, stroke, heart failure (preserved and reduced ejection fraction), atrial fibrillation, coronary artery disease	Atrial fibrillation, heart failure (reduced or preserved ejection fraction), stroke, pulmonary hypertension, coronary artery disease

*Order shown indicating approximate relative strength of association.

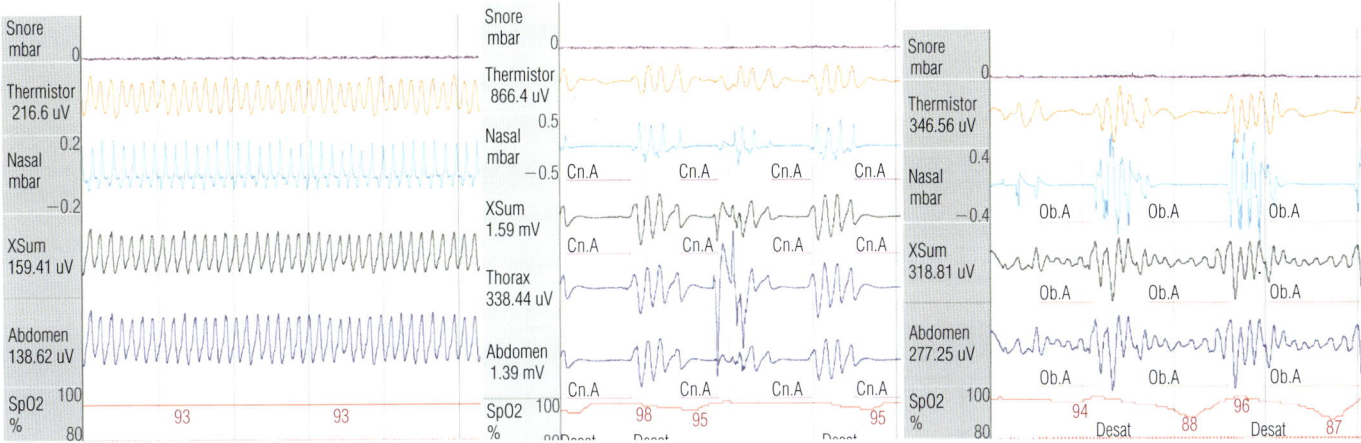

FIGURE 89.1 Examples from an overnight sleep study, displaying respiratory channels. The first panel shows normal breathing with stable oxygen saturation values. The second panel shows repetitive central apneas, characterized by 15- to 40-second periods of absent airflow (shown on the nasal and thermistor channels), with no associated respiratory effort of snoring, and oxyhemoglobin desaturation of 3% with each event. The third panel shows obstructive apneas, characterized by absent airflow with persistent effort on the thorax and abdominal channels, with deep desaturations (each panel is approximately 3 minutes long).

with HF and even mild peripheral edema or venous stasis to OSA.[3] Lung volume influences pharyngeal wall stiffness through tractional forces; therefore, reduced lung volumes, as may occur in obesity or with pulmonary congestion, can exacerbate propensity for OSA. Conversely, high lung volumes, as in chronic obstructive lung disease, may modestly protect against OSA. Increased nasal resistance (e.g., due to nasal septal deviation, polyps) promotes airway collapse by increasing the negative intraluminal suction pressure and is a risk factor for OSA in conditions such as pregnancy or allergy associated with nasal swelling.

Pharyngeal muscle activation depends both on the sensitivity of central and peripheral respiratory chemoreceptors and on neuromuscular responsiveness to CO_2 (Fig. 89.2).[4] During sleep, the blood CO_2 typically increases mildly, and this helps to activate respiratory muscles and stiffen airway dilators, protecting the upper airway (i.e., increasing critical closing pressure, P_{crit}). Depressed chemosensitivity and arousal response may prevent appropriate termination of apneas, prolonging the duration of the apnea and the severity of oxyhemoglobin desaturation. This ventilatory control problem can cause pathologic CO_2 retention and acidosis during sleep, a phenomenon common in obesity-hypoventilation and sleep-hypoventilation syndromes. Conversely, an overly sensitive response to CO_2 (i.e., reflecting high loop gain) can cause wide fluctuations in the ventilatory drive, resulting in central nervous system arousal and sleep fragmentation. Episodic hyperventilation can drive CO_2 levels to below the apneic threshold, precipitating cycles of apneas. This mechanism also occurs in CSA, and in its most extreme form is manifested as Cheyne-Stokes respiration.[5]

The severity of OSA can vary by sleep stage and position. During rapid eye movement (REM) sleep, the neuromuscular drive is low and fluctuating, sympathetic tone is high, and apneic events tend to be longest and associated with the most severe oxyhemoglobin desaturation. "REM-dependent" OSA, characterized by a predominance of respiratory events in REM as compared to non-REM sleep, better predicts incident hypertension and mortality compared to the overall AHI level.[6] OSA also can worsen following acute ingestion of alcohol, which reduces neuromuscular activation, and when a person is in the supine position.

Pathophysiology of Central Sleep Apnea

In adults, CSA often occurs in association with cardiac or cerebrovascular disease. Its pathogenesis relates to a heightened sensitivity to CO_2 and a prolonged circulation delay between the pulmonary capillaries and carotid chemoreceptors, causing instability in breathing. Periods of hyperventilation cause CO_2 levels to fall below the apneic threshold, precipitating apneas and hypopneas. The occurrence of cycles of crescendo-decrescendo breathing is recognized as Cheyne-Stokes respiration; cycle lengths of 60 seconds are characteristic of patients with HF.

Risk Factors for and Recognition of Sleep-Disordered Breathing

OSA affects 34% of males and 17% of females between the ages of 30 to 70 years.[7] OSA and CVD commonly co-occur, reflecting both shared risk factors (e.g., central obesity) and causal relationships; therefore, the prevalence of OSA is as high as 40% to 80% in patients with hypertension, HF, or coronary heart disease (CHD).[5] Male sex, older age, and obesity are well-recognized OSA risk factors. OSA is two- to fourfold more prevalent in men than in women.[8] Factors that predispose men

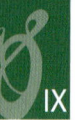

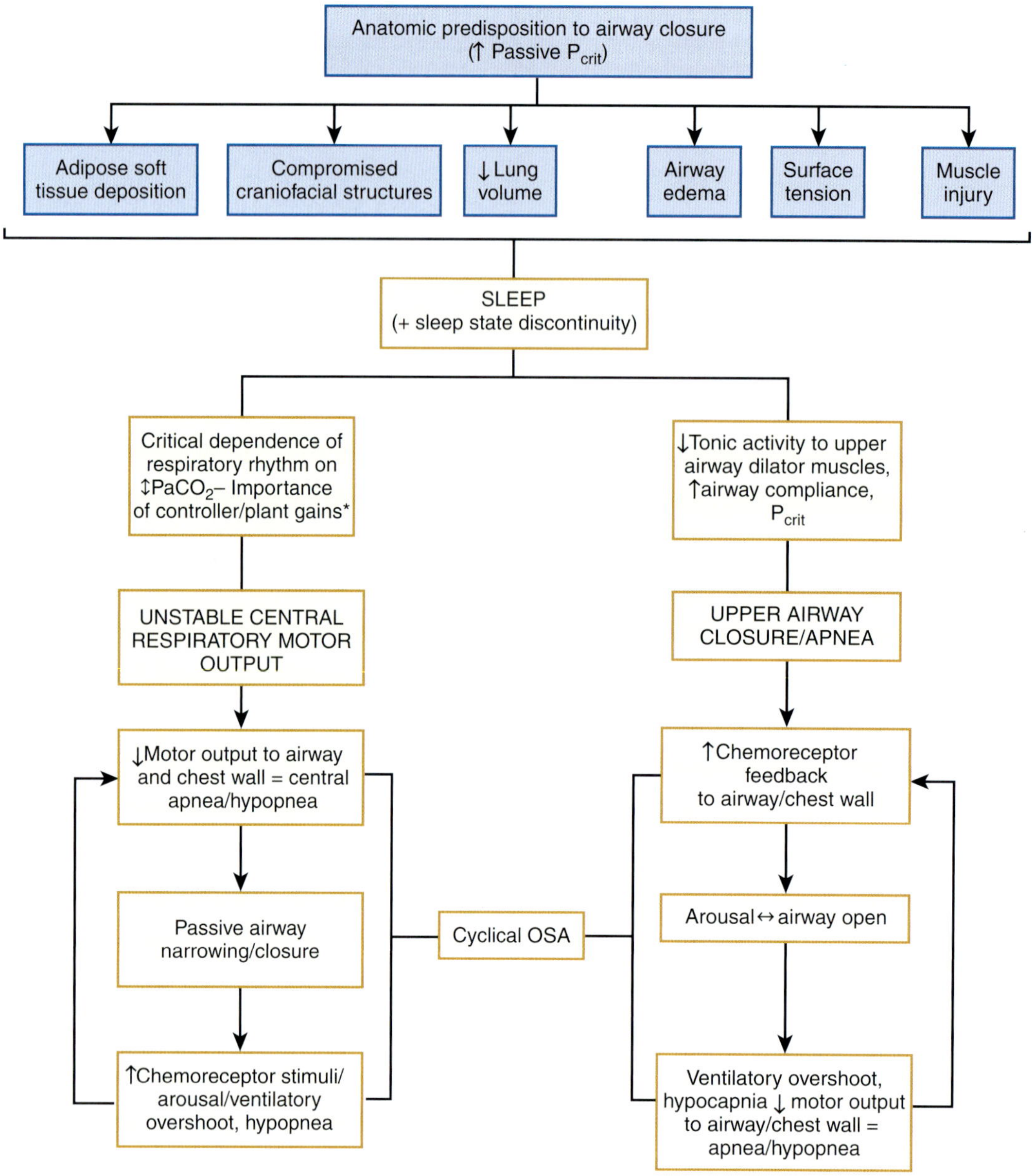

FIGURE 89.2 Pathogenetic mechanisms leading to obstructive apneas. *Controller/plant gains refer to the negative feedback loops that influence ventilation in response to a ventilatory disturbance (e.g., an apnea or change in pCO2). *Plant gain* refers to background drive to breathe; *controller gain* refers to the slope of changing ventilation in response to changes in pCO2 level. P_{crit}, critical closing pressure in the airway: the pressure at which the airway collapses. Passive P_{crit} is determined by the mechanical properties of the airway and surrounding tissues. A decrease in tonic activity to the airway dilator muscles refers to active P_{crit}. (From Dempsey JA, Veasey SC, Morgan BJ, O'Donnell CP. Pathophysiology of sleep apnea. *Physiol Rev.* 2010;90:47–112.)

to OSA include android patterns of adiposity (which predisposes to upper airway fat deposition) and relatively long pharyngeal length, which predisposes to collapsibility. OSA prevalence increases in women following menopause, and hormone replacement therapy is associated with reduced AHI levels, consistent with a role for sex hormones in modulating risk.[9] OSA severity increases not only in older women but also in older men, reflecting age-related comorbidities (e.g., cardiac diseases, neurologic diseases) and other age-related effects on airway stiffness and ventilation. OSA in elderly persons may differ from that in middle-aged individuals, with less prominent associations with snoring, obesity, autonomic system dysregulation, and CVD reported. It is not known whether differences in studies of middle-aged populations compared with older populations result from study biases or are true differences in OSA etiology and pathophysiology across the population.

Being overweight or obese accounts for approximately 40% to 60% of cases of OSA. Obese middle-aged individuals are fourfold or more likely to have OSA as compared with normal-weight individuals. Obesity contributes to OSA through effects on airway narrowing caused by fat deposition in the tongue and parapharyngeal tissues and by reducing chest wall compliance and lung volumes. Obesity-associated cytokine levels also may influence ventilatory control and promote daytime sleepiness. Even a modest weight loss or weight gain can have an impact on the severity of OSA. For example, a 1% increase in the body mass index (BMI, kg/m^2) is estimated to increase the AHI by 3%; this finding emphasizes the importance of weight management in OSA.[10] Approximately 20% of OSA patients are *not* obese, however, and the absence of obesity should not preclude an appropriate evaluation of patients with OSA symptoms. Other risk factors for OSA are craniofacial features that narrow the oropharyngeal airway, upper airway dilator muscle dysfunction, and abnormalities in ventilatory control.

A first-degree relative of a patient with OSA has an approximately twofold increased risk of OSA compared with someone without an affected relative.[11] Over 60% of the genetic variance explaining OSA is not associated with obesity, indicating the importance of multiple etiologic factors. Several genetic variants associated with OSA may also be associated with cardiac disease and abnormal lipid and glucose

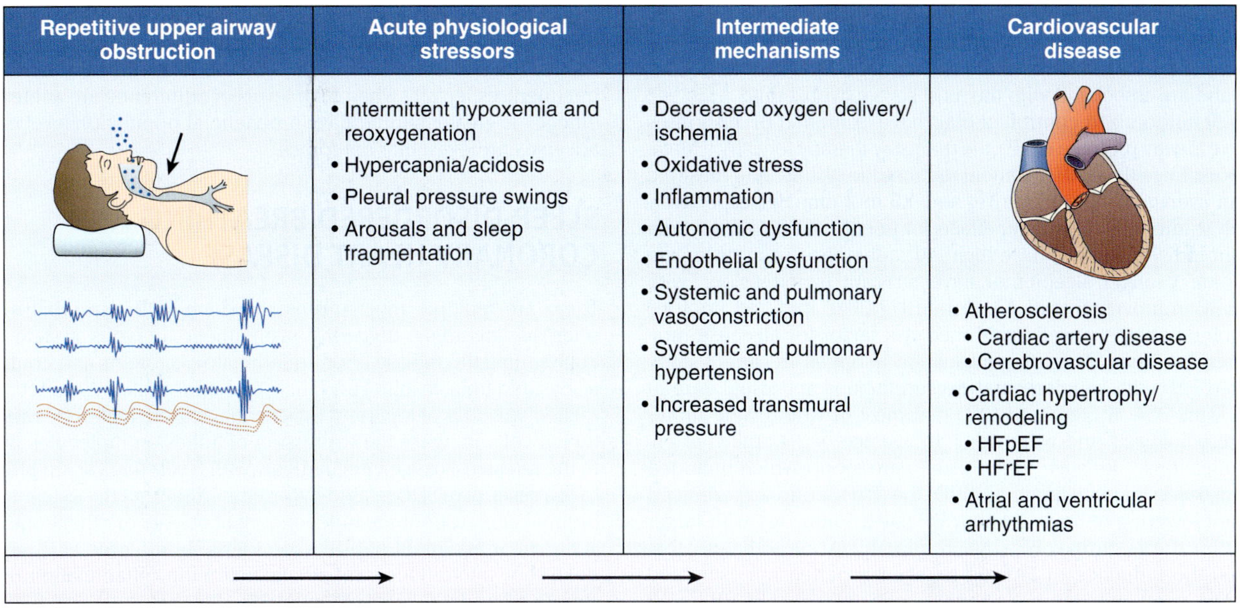

Repetitive upper airway obstruction	Acute physiological stressors	Intermediate mechanisms	Cardiovascular disease

	• Intermittent hypoxemia and reoxygenation
	• Hypercapnia/acidosis
	• Pleural pressure swings
	• Arousals and sleep fragmentation
		• Decreased oxygen delivery/ischemia
		• Oxidative stress
		• Inflammation
		• Autonomic dysfunction
		• Endothelial dysfunction
		• Systemic and pulmonary vasoconstriction
		• Systemic and pulmonary hypertension
		• Increased transmural pressure
			• Atherosclerosis
			  • Cardiac artery disease
			  • Cerebrovascular disease
			• Cardiac hypertrophy/remodeling
			  • HFpEF
			  • HFrEF
			• Atrial and ventricular arrhythmias

FIGURE 89.3 Mechanisms by which obstructive sleep apnea leads to physiological stressors, which then increase risk of atherosclerosis, cardiac remodeling, and arrhythmias.

levels, suggesting overlapping genetic mechanisms ("pleiotropy") for OSA and cardiac disease.[12] Sexual dimorphisms in genetic variants for OSA have been identified, similar to reports of sex-based differences in genetic variants for adiposity and cardiac disease.

Despite improved public awareness of OSA, it is estimated that more than 80% of individuals with moderate or severe OSA are undiagnosed.[13] Even among those diagnosed, more than 30% of patients report that the period between onset of symptoms and diagnosis exceeded 10 years.[14] Under-recognition is high among ethnic and minority groups and elderly individuals, particularly African Americans and older Asian Americans, groups also at risk for cardiometabolic diseases. Under-recognition in women may result from the preferential reporting of symptoms of fatigue rather than sleepiness, and the frequency of comorbid insomnia that can confound the diagnosis and reduce the sensitivity of screening questionnaires. Women often display REM-predominant OSA and may experience apneas that result in arousal without desaturation, findings that home sleep tests may miss.[15]

Risk factors for CSA are male sex, hypocapnia during wakefulness, and older age, as well as HF, CVD, and atrial fibrillation (AF).[16] Due to elevations in sympathetic drive, patients with CSA may not report sleepiness, and rather report symptoms of insomnia, such as difficulty falling asleep and frequent awakenings.

The role of routine screening for sleep apnea is not established. In 2017, The U.S. Preventive Services Task Force concluded that there was insufficient evidence to recommend routine screening for sleep apnea in primary care settings.[17] However, patients with diagnosed sleep apnea frequently report prolonged delays between the onset of symptoms and diagnosis and treatment, indicating a need to improve recognition. Screening questions or web-based algorithms that combine information on snoring frequency, age, BMI, and sex for calculating OSA risk[18] should be considered in cardiology practices, settings where sleep apnea prevalence is high, to improve identification and expedite treatment of this disorder.

Pathophysiologic Mechanisms That Link Sleep-Disordered Breathing to Cardiovascular Diseases

During healthy sleep, individuals experience a decrease in sympathetic nervous system activity and an increase in parasympathetic activity, with associated reductions in blood pressure (BP) and heart rate. Repetitive collapse of the upper airway that disrupts sleep continuity and causes arousal disturbs these patterns, resulting in surges in sympathetic activity and acute BP elevations.[19] Impaired gas exchange with intermittent hypoxia further affects the autonomic nervous system, as well as triggers the release of acute-phase proteins and reactive oxygen species. The release of these mediators may favor an augmented inflammatory and hypercoagulable state, exacerbating insulin resistance and lipolysis.[20] Hypoxia and autonomic nervous system alterations can contribute to electrical remodeling of the heart and myocyte injury. Oxyhemoglobin desaturation further compromises oxygenation of myocardial tissue. Inspiratory efforts against a closed glottis (with OSA) additionally cause wide swings in intrathoracic pressure, negatively affecting preload and afterload and left ventricular (LV) transmural pressure, increasing myocardial oxygen consumption, and impeding stroke volume. The pathophysiologic consequences of OSA are shown schematically in Figure 89.3, and summarized later in this chapter.

SLEEP-DISORDERED BREATHING AND HYPERTENSION

Approximately 30% of patients with essential hypertension (see also Chapter 26) and 80% of patients with resistant hypertension have OSA. Conversely, more than 50% of patients with OSA have hypertension.[21] Although the aggregation of hypertension and OSA partially reflects common risk factors, experimental animal and human data indicate that OSA is causally associated with hypertension.

OSA has both acute and chronic effects on BP. Acutely, BP and heart rate increase within 10 seconds of the termination of an apnea or hypopnea, corresponding to peak times of the arousal, ventilation, and oxygen saturation nadir. Frequent arousals trigger chemoreflexes and sympathetic output to the peripheral blood vessels, with consequent vasoconstriction, and altered renin-angiotensin-aldosterone system activity. Transient increases in BP can persist into the daytime. Chronic intermittent surges in BP also cause vascular remodeling.

OSA is associated with a non-dipping overnight BP pattern, increases in daytime BP to pre-hypertensive and hypertensive ranges, and an increased risk of poorly controlled and resistant hypertension. "Dose-response" associations are reported. Specifically, a 1-unit increase in the AHI is estimated to increase the odds of non-dipping systolic BP by 4%.[22] The Wisconsin Cohort Study, a prospective study of state employees, reported that the odds ratio, adjusted for obesity and other confounders, for the presence of hypertension after 4 years of follow-up was 2.9 for moderate or severe OSA.[23] The apneas and hypopneas occurring in REM sleep, rather than the AHI occurring across all sleep stages, appear to be most strongly associated with hypertension incidence.[6] During REM sleep, the sympathetic drive is highest, the muscular tone is lowest, and the respiratory events tend to last the longest and are associated with the most severe hypoxemia.

Over 30 randomized controlled trials have examined BP responses to positive airway pressure (PAP), the mainstay therapy for OSA.[24] Meta-analyses estimate that PAP treatment reduces the systolic and diastolic BP by an average of 2 to 3 mm Hg and 1.5 to 2 mm Hg, respectively. Generally, studies reported larger effects for nocturnal BP than daytime BP, and in individuals who have high PAP adherence or more severe OSA, or are younger, sleepier, or have resistant hypertension (with average BP improvements of 4 to 9 mm Hg). PAP also can improve non-dipping patterns, a well-established risk factor for all-cause mortality rates. The Heart Biomarker Evaluation in Apnea Treatment study compared PAP with supplemental oxygen therapy and usual care in patients with OSA at increased CVD risk, most of whom were under care of cardiologists and were using an average of 2.4 antihypertensive medications.[25] Relative to the usual care group, which included guideline-based management of CVD, the PAP group experienced significant lowering of mean 24-hour BP (by 2.4 mm Hg), with larger changes for the nocturnal BP (by 3.5 mm Hg). A meta-analysis that evaluated the influence of PAP on resistant hypertension estimated that PAP reduced ambulatory 24-hour systolic and diastolic BP by 7.2 and 5.0 mm Hg, respectively.[26] To address the role of PAP in reducing the incidence of hypertension, a multicenter trial conducted in Spain randomized 723 patients with moderate OSA but without significant sleepiness to PAP or usual care.[27] Over a median of 4 years of follow-up, an intention-to-treat analysis showed no reduction in the incidence of hypertension or CVD events with PAP. However, in an analysis of patients who used PAP for 4 hours or more per night, a 31% reduction in incident hypertension or CVD was observed and the magnitude of the 24-hour BP improvement was related directly to the hours of PAP use (each additional hour of PAP use resulted in a decrease in the average systolic BP of 1.3 mm Hg.)

The existing clinical trials highlight the importance of treatment adherence in achieving BP improvement. Other sources of variability in responses to OSA treatment include differences in residual apneic activity with treatment, severity of OSA, age, and cause of hypertension. The level of PAP adherence needed to obtain a significant BP reduction is unknown. Although a minimum threshold of 4 hours of CPAP use per night is commonly targeted, more than 6 hours of PAP use per night, including use during the late-night hours in REM sleep, is likely more effective. Suboptimal responses to PAP also may reflect delayed initiation of treatment; specifically, individuals with untreated OSA for years may undergo chronic remodeling of the vascular bed and changes in BP regulatory mechanisms that are not readily reversed with PAP. A variety of pathophysiologic processes contribute to hypertension, including insulin resistance, obesity, autonomic nervous system dysfunction, and variations in salt and fluid balance. OSA likely affects these mechanisms differently, and thus OSA treatment is expected to be more effective in certain subgroups. Biomarkers that reflect molecular mechanisms for CVD and/or sensitivity to hypoxemia may play a future role for risk stratification. Such an approach is supported by an initial report that three microribonucleic acids associated with CVD predicted BP responses in patients with OSA and resistant hypertension.[28]

Alternative strategies, such as combined therapies (PAP, medications, and lifestyle) or physiologically targeted interventions, may prove to be superior to single therapies for some patients with both OSA and hypertension. The addition of PAP, when used for 4 hours or more per night, enhances the effects of pharmacotherapy in improving the BP.[29] Among obese patients with moderate OSA and elevations of C-reactive protein (CRP), a combination of weight loss plus PAP proved more effective in lowering the BP than PAP alone, suggesting the importance of concomitant lifestyle interventions in high-risk groups.[30] Early studies suggest that spironolactone[24] or renal denervation[24] may reduce both the severity of OSA and lower BP in patients with resistant hypertension.

Based on the existing evidence, the Seventh Report of the Joint National Committee on Prevention, Detection, Evaluation, and Treatment of High Blood Pressure (JNC 7) identified OSA as a treatable cause of hypertension.[31] Although average treatment effects are modest, long-term improvements of systolic BP by 2 to 3 mm Hg may reduce the risk of stroke and CHD by as much as 10%. Therefore, OSA treatment, especially when high levels of adherence are achieved and efficacy is greater, should have a beneficial population-level effect on adverse cardiovascular outcomes.

SLEEP-DISORDERED BREATHING AND CORONARY HEART DISEASE

There are multiple mechanisms by which SDB exacerbates atherosclerosis, including triggering sympathetic nervous system activity, augmenting the release of proinflammatory proteins and contributing to dyslipidemia, insulin resistance, and endothelial dysfunction. SDB-related episodes of recurrent hypoxemia activate leukocytes and endothelial cells, increase the expression of adhesion molecules, and lead to the release of oxygen free radicals, with levels that vary in proportion to the severity of SDB-related hypoxemia. Although the extent to which biomarker elevations are independent of obesity or other confounders is not clear, treatment of SDB, even for as short a time as 2 weeks, has been shown to reduce sympathetic activation, inflammation, oxidative stress, and endothelial dysfunction.[32]

OSA also may contribute to acute ischemia because of both decreased oxygen delivery (secondary to obstructed breathing) and increased oxygen consumption (due to elevated diastolic and transmural pressures and cardiac hypertrophy). Ischemic stressors may be most notable during the rebreathing phase of obstructive apneas, when large hemodynamic changes occur. The fractional flow reserve, a quantitative measurement of coronary artery stenosis, can dynamically vary with obstructive apneas because of fluctuations in the intrathoracic pressure that affect the venous and aortic pressures and coronary perfusion.[33] Patients with intermediate coronary lesions may experience intermittent myocardial ischemia as a result of cyclical changes in the coronary blood flow. Endothelial damage and compromised coronary vascular conductance may ensue due to surges in the BP and heart rate associated with sympathetic activation and reduced endothelial production of nitric oxide. Subclinical ischemia can be manifested on overnight electrocardiograms of patients with OSA, showing ST segment depression, which indicates nocturnal myocardial ischemia, and changes in QT dispersion, as well as paroxysms of ventricular tachycardia or AF that are associated temporally with the occurrence of apneas. Women with OSA have elevated levels of high-sensitivity troponin, a marker of subclinical myocardial injury; the level of troponin is one factor in the risk for HF or death in untreated OSA.[34]

Evidence for SDB as a CHD risk factor is found in large cohort studies that demonstrate that SDB is associated with an increased incidence of CHD and cardiovascular death. In over 5000 participants in the Multi-Ethnic Study of Atherosclerosis (MESA) who were free of known CVD at baseline and followed for 7.5 years, a physician-diagnosis of sleep apnea was associated with a 1.9 increased adjusted hazard ratio for incident cardiovascular events and a 2.4-fold higher mortality rate.[35] Several studies from Spain followed patients referred to sleep laboratories for periods of 5 to 10 years. Among men, untreated severe OSA was associated with a 2.9-fold increased risk of fatal cardiovascular events and a 3.2-fold increased risk of nonfatal cardiovascular events when compared with a control group. Among women followed for a median time of 72 months, the mortality rate was 3.5-fold higher in women with severe OSA than in female controls.[36] In the Sleep Heart Health Study cohort, moderate to severe SDB defined by an AHI ≥15 was associated with a 35% increased incidence of CHD over 8 years; among men younger than age 70 years, this risk was 70%.[37] In a prospective analysis of more than 10,000 individuals, patients with significant nocturnal hypoxemia had a nearly twofold increase in the risk of sudden cardiac death after potential confounders had been considered.[38] Use of quantitative metrics of hypoxia burden show particular promise for predicting those at risk for developing CHD-related death: individuals with the most severe degree of sleep-apnea hypoxic burden (in the highest quintile) had an approximately twofold increased risk of cardiovascular death compared to individuals with less hypoxia, even after adjusting for the AHI level and multiple other confounders.[39] Temporal support for a causal link between OSA and CHD comes from a study showing that individuals with OSA compared with those without OSA were more likely to experience a morning-peak onset of myocardial infarction[40] and die suddenly between midnight and 6:00 AM, the hours when apneas and hypopneas occur.[41]

Subclinical markers of atherosclerosis are also elevated in individuals with OSA compared to controls. In analyses adjusted for multiple confounders, coronary artery calcium burden (CAC Agatston score >400) was 40% more common in individuals with sleep apnea than in controls.[42] Furthermore, over 8 years, the CAC was more likely to progress in individuals with OSA compared to those without OSA.[43]

SDB appears to contribute to adverse outcomes among patients with CHD; patients with CHD who have OSA experience higher rates of major acute cardiovascular events than patients without OSA.[44,45] OSA is implicated in both plaque instability[47] and plaque vulnerability. Untreated OSA is associated with an increased need for a revascularization procedure as compared with rates in patients without OSA.[46] Infarct sizes are reported to be higher 3 months after myocardial infarction salvage procedures in patients with OSA than in patients without OSA.[47] In contrast, some research findings suggest that patients with SDB may develop collateral coronary blood flow from periods of intermittent hypoxemia, with resultant angiogenesis,[48] which may reduce the extent of myocardial injury immediately following an ischemic event.

Large observational studies demonstrate that patients with severe OSA treated with PAP have significantly reduced rates of fatal and nonfatal CVD compared to untreated patients. Patients with CHD treated with PAP are reported to have lower rates of nocturnal ischemia, acute coronary syndrome, need for coronary revascularization, and death from CVD compared to untreated patients with OSA. However, the data from several randomized controlled trials do not provide support for PAP in secondary prevention of CVD in patients with moderate to severe OSA. Interventions were PAP (or auto-titrating PAP) or conservative therapy. All studies excluded patients with significant sleepiness, and one also excluded those with severe overnight hypoxemia, reducing the generalizability of the results. Modest PAP adherence limited all studies, and the studies were underpowered to detect moderate improvements. The first study, following 725 patients without CVD for a median of 4 years, did not find a benefit for the PAP group. However, patients who used PAP for 4 hours or more per night experienced a significant improvement in the composite study outcome (incidence density ratio, 0.72; 95% confidence interval [CI], 0.52 to 0.98) compared with controls and nonadherent patients.[49] The Randomized Intervention with Continuous Positive Airway Pressure in Coronary Artery Disease and OSA (RICCADSA), randomized 244 non-sleepy patients with established CHD and moderate or severe OSA to PAP or usual care in a single European center.[50] At a median follow-up time of 57 months, the PAP group compared with the usual-care group had a 20% non-statistically significant reduction in the primary composite endpoint. When restricted to patients using PAP for 4 hours or more per night, a significant 80% decrease in event rates was observed (HR, 0.29; 0.10 to 0.86). The multicenter international Sleep Apnea Cardiovascular Endpoints (SAVE) trial followed 2717 patients with a history of coronary artery or cerebrovascular disease for a mean of 3.7 years.[51] This study did not observe a difference in the primary composite CVD endpoint. A sub-analysis, however, showed that individuals adherent to PAP had a 40% significant reduction in cerebrovascular events compared with a propensity-matched subgroup from the usual-care group. The better effect for cerebrovascular disease than for the composite endpoint or CHD is in agreement with observational data showing stronger associations between OSA and cerebrovascular disease compared with CHD. Most recently, the Impact of Sleep Apnea Syndrome in the Evolution of Acute Coronary Syndrome (ISAACC) study randomized 1264 patients hospitalized with acute coronary syndrome with moderate to severe OSA to receive PAP therapy or usual care. Over a median follow-up of 3.4 years, the composite cardiovascular outcome did not significantly differ by intervention group (Hazard Ratio: 0.89 [95%CI, 0.68 to 1.17]).[52] The existing data suggest that PAP is unlikely to improve CVD outcomes unless it is used for at least 4 hours per night. However, the SAVE study demonstrated that even suboptimal PAP use can improve quality of life and mood and result in fewer days of missed work, as well as possible cerebrovascular benefits, indicating positive effects in patients with CVD. The results of these studies emphasize the need to provide adherence support for patients prescribed PAP. In patients with CVD, adjunctive behavioral therapies (e.g., motivational education and problem solving) have demonstrated improvements of PAP use by an average of 90 minutes per night.

SLEEP-DISORDERED BREATHING, CARDIAC FUNCTION, AND HEART FAILURE

Both CSA and OSA are common in HF, present in up to 60% of HF patients.[53] CSA is the most common SDB variant associated with HF with a reduced ejection fraction (HFrEF), but OSA is predominant in HF with a preserved ejection fraction (HFpEF). Both OSA and CSA can occur in the same individual, underscoring the complex etiology and treatment of these disorders.

There is a bidirectional relationship between HF and SDB (Fig. 89.4). In patients with HF, pulmonary vascular congestion, elevated peripheral and central chemosensitivities, and a prolonged circulation time can cause hyperventilation, with instability in ventilation leading to apneas. Conversely, SDB may adversely affect cardiac function by contributing to systemic and pulmonary hypertension, non-dipping BP, atherosclerosis and ischemic injury, hypoxemia- and catecholamine-related myocyte injury, and cardiac remodeling. Hypoxia can trigger pulmonary vasoconstriction, which may increase the right ventricular afterload, cause right ventricular distention and leftward shift of the ventricular septum during diastole, impair LV filling, and reduce the stroke volume and cardiac output. SDB is increasingly recognized as a common cause of diastolic dysfunction, with effects attributable to chronic pressure overload, impaired coronary flow reserve, and inflammation leading to cardiac interstitial fibrosis.[54] Population studies show that the LV mass and LV mass-volume ratio (concentric remodeling) increase in proportion to the severity of SDB, with associations stronger in adults younger than 65 years of age.[55] Indices of diastolic dysfunction, including an increased E/A ratio, reduced mitral deceleration, and isovolumic relaxation, are higher in patients with SDB compared with controls.

Prospective studies demonstrate that SDB independently predicts new-onset HF. Middle-aged men with severe SDB (predominantly OSA) are estimated to have a 60% increased 8-year incidence of HF compared with men without SDB.[37] A 14-year prospective analysis of data from the Atherosclerosis Risk in Communities Study (ARIC) demonstrated that women with SDB have an approximately 30% increased incidence of HF or death compared with women without SDB, and also have an increased risk for developing LV hypertrophy.[34] In older men, the Outcomes of Sleep Disorders in Older Men Study demonstrated that the presence of SDB predicted a nearly twofold increased incidence of HF.[56] However, in this study, the risk was related to the presence of CSA or Cheyne-Stokes respiration rather than OSA. In patients with HF, SDB predicts HF exacerbations and progression, including an impaired quality of life, increased fatigue, a reduced functional status, more frequent hospitalizations, arrhythmias, and death.[57]

Current treatment strategies for OSA or CSA in patients with HF include optimization of cardiac function, with a focus on minimizing the fluid overload, and weight loss as appropriate. Exercise and elastic stockings can help prevent rostral redistribution of fluid. PAP treatment, by improving oxygenation, sympathetic activation, 24-hour BP profiles, subendocardial ischemia, preload and afterload, and inflammatory and oxidative stress, could improve cardiac function. Short-term studies demonstrate that PAP can reduce HF symptoms and improve quality of life and functional status. Small randomized controlled studies in HF also demonstrated that PAP improved the vascular and myocardial sympathetic nerve function, myocardial energetics, and diastolic dysfunction.[5] A meta-analysis estimated that PAP treatment in OSA and HF was associated with a 5.2% improvement in the LV ejection fraction.[58]

PAP therapies, however, have not been demonstrated to reduce mortality or the occurrence of cardiac events in rigorous clinical trials.

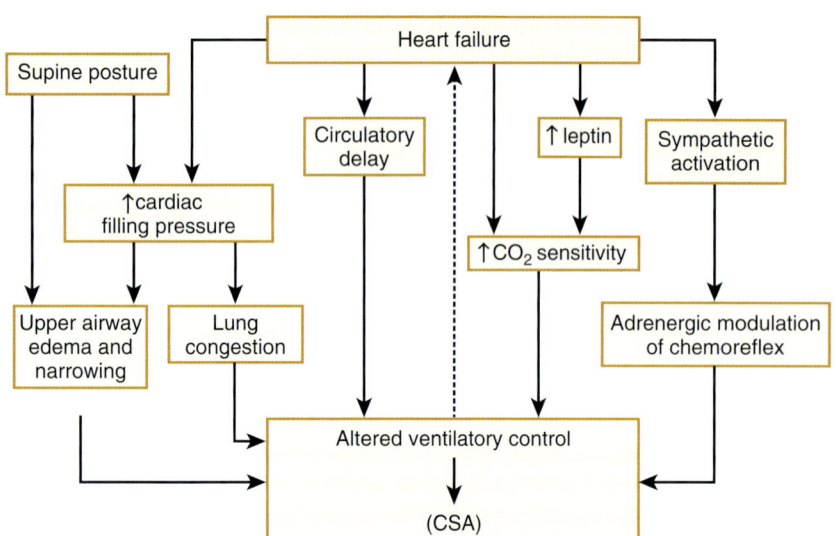

FIGURE 89.4 Possible mechanisms underlying development of CSA and the possible feedback from CSA resulting in exacerbation of heart failure. (From Somers VK, White DP, Amin R, et al. Sleep Apnea and Cardiovascular Disease: An American Heart Association/American College of Cardiology Foundation Scientific Statement From the American Heart Association Council for High Blood Pressure Research Professional Education Committee, Council on Clinical Cardiology, Stroke Council, and Council on Cardiovascular Nursing. *J Am Coll Cardiol*. 2008;52(8):686–717.)

Although a retrospective analysis of approximately 30,000 Medicare beneficiaries with newly diagnosed HF showed that treatment of SDB decreased rates of readmission, costs of health care, and mortality;[59] subsequent randomized controlled studies did not confirm these benefits. The first randomized controlled study—the Canadian Positive Airway Pressure (CANPAP) study—demonstrated that PAP improved several intermediate endpoints in patients with CSA and HFrEF (ejection fraction, catecholamines), but did not change mortality.[60] A potential explanation for this finding was that PAP did not adequately suppress central apneas, resulting in a suboptimal intervention. In support of this, a post hoc analysis suggested improved heart transplant–free survival in the subset of patients in whom CSA was suppressed.[61] Subsequently, two multinational studies were initiated to evaluate the role of a newer therapy—adaptive servoventilation (ASV)—a pressure device that delivers auto-adjusting pressure support on a breath-by-breath basis designed to suppress both obstructive and central apneas. The results of the first ASV trial, Treatment of Sleep-Disordered Breathing with Predominant Central Sleep Apnea by Adaptive Servo Ventilation in Patients with Heart Failure (SERVE-HF), conducted in 1345 patients with symptomatic HF and moderate to severe CSA, showed an unexpected 34% *increase* in CVD mortality rate with ASV as compared to usual care.[62] An advisory was subsequently issued against the use of ASV for treatment of patients with predominant CSA who have HFrEF with an ejection fraction of less than 45%. A second ongoing trial, Effect of ASV on Survival and Hospitalizations (ADVENT-HF), is testing an alternative ASV device in patients with OSA or CSA. Current consensus is that PAP can be used to treat symptoms of SDB such as sleepiness in patients with OSA or CSA who have HF, but that ASV should be avoided in patients with CSA with an ejection fraction less than 45%. This approach is reflected in the 2017 updated AHA/ACC Heart Failure Guidelines,[63] which highlighted (1) the importance of a formal sleep assessment to distinguish obstructive from CSA in patients with HF and symptoms of SDB or sleepiness; (2) use of PAP as a treatment strategy for improving sleep quality and daytime sleepiness; and (3) avoidance of ASV in patients with CSA and reduced ejection fraction.

The challenges of using pressure support therapies in patients with HF have stimulated investigations of alternative interventions. Nocturnal oxygen supplementation (NOS), which can stabilize breathing in patients with CSA and improve intermediate markers of cardiac function and quality of life, is under evaluation for use in patients with CSA and HFrEF in an ongoing multi-center trial (NCT03745898). Diaphragmatic stimulation, used to directly trigger or augment breathing efforts, is another approach potentially useful for treating CSA. An implantable unilateral transvenous phrenic nerve stimulator (PNS;

remedē, Respicardia) was tested in 151 patients with CSA, 64% of whom had HF. The initial study results showed that more than half of a treatment group experienced more than a 50% reduction in the AHI at 6-months as well as experienced improved sleep quality and sleepiness, with effects stable for as long as 36 months.[64] Although small improvements in ejection fraction were observed, data on long term effects on survival are not available. The FDA granted pre-market approval for commercial use of the device in 2017 for treatment of moderate to severe CSA, with use restricted to centers with specific clinical expertise. Longer-term follow-up and assessment of the role of PNS across the spectrum of HF phenotypes are needed.

SLEEP-DISORDERED BREATHING AND CARDIAC ARRHYTHMIAS

Patients with SDB are predisposed to ventricular and atrial arrhythmias because of underlying cardiac risk factors and cardiac disease, as well as to the specific SDB-related stressors of intermittent hypoxemia, acidosis, sympathetic nervous system surges, and swings in intrathoracic pressures. Bradycardia and atrioventricular block may occur secondary to vagal stimulation accompanying apneas and hypoxemia. Susceptibility to atrial arrhythmias also reflects the vulnerability of the atrial walls to swings in intrathoracic pressure and mechanoreceptor activation, as well as sensitivity of the pulmonary vein ganglia to autonomic stimulation.[65] The degree of hypoxemia appears to be a potent stimulus for ventricular arrhythmias, sudden cardiac death, and recurrence of AF following cardioversion. Although the molecular mechanisms underlying these associations are not well understood, connexin remodeling, dysregulation of myocardial excitation/coupling, and phosphorylation of sodium channels are implicated in SDB-related atrial fibrosis and conduction and sinus node abnormalities.[66–68]

Abnormalities of P wave morphology and QT dispersion, indicative of underlying electrical conduction problems, have been observed in the overnight recordings of patients with SDB.[69] Moreover, apneas and hypopneas appear to be direct triggers of paroxysms of ventricular tachycardia and AF. Analysis of the temporal patterns of overnight arrhythmias demonstrated a 17-fold increased rate of arrhythmias occurring after an episode of apnea compared with a period of normal breathing.[70] Based on this analysis, a patient with moderate OSA (AHI 25) is estimated to experience one episode of a significant arrhythmia every 6 months attributable to apneic activity. In community studies, moderate or severe OSA was associated with a two- to fourfold increased risk of nocturnal arrhythmias; this finding suggested a basis for the observed increase in nocturnal sudden cardiac death in SDB.[71]

Of the arrhythmias, the link between OSA and AF has received the most study (see Chapter 66). OSA occurs in 21% to 74% of patients with AF[72] and is associated with increased hospitalization rates and symptom burden,[73] and recurrent AF after cardioversion.[74] Meta-analyses estimate that untreated OSA is associated with a 31% increased AF recurrence after catheter ablation.[75,76] A meta-analysis of observational studies estimated that PAP use in patients with OSA reduces the AF risk by 44%.[77] Observational studies also estimate that PAP can reduce risk of recurrent AF after cardioversion or catheter ablation to levels comparable to those in individuals without OSA and reduces the likelihood of progression to more permanent forms of AF.[74–76] A lower recurrence rate following ablation therapy in OSA patients treated with CPAP was reported to parallel PAP-related reductions in BP, atrial size, and ventricular mass,[78] supporting a physiological benefit of PAP. A consensus panel has identified OSA as an AF risk factor.[79] The high rate of AF recurrence in untreated patients has discouraged the use of ablation procedures until OSA is treated with PAP. However, it is important to note that there are no RCTs to support benefit: only one small RCT was conducted that was designed to address this question, which was negative,[80] and the SAVE trial provided no evidence for a benefit of PAP on an AF secondary outcome.[51]

FUTURE PERSPECTIVES

SDB is highly prevalent in patients with hypertension, coronary artery disease, HF (with or without a reduced ejection fraction), and atrial and ventricular arrhythmias. The profound nightly disturbances that occur with SDB cause a range of physiologic disturbances that adversely affect cardiac structure and function, and likely exacerbate the incidence and progression of these diseases. Treatment of OSA can improve the BP, ejection fraction, ventricular ectopy, and recurrence rate of AF, and can also improve the quality of life and mood in patients with CVD. The existing data indicate that patients with OSA who successfully use PAP have reduced rates of resistant hypertension and experience improved outcomes, including fewer cardiac and cerebrovascular events and lower mortality rates. Although the impact of directly treating CSA on cardiovascular outcomes remains uncertain, the presence of CSA predicts increased mortality rates as well as incident AF, and patients with CSA and HF may benefit from intensive HF therapy. Cardiologists may be increasingly involved in recognizing SDB and can use information on its pathophysiologic effects to tailor interventions and inform chronic disease management strategies.

REFERENCES

Epidemiology

1. Berry RB, Budhiraja R, Gottlieb DJ, et al. Rules for scoring respiratory events in sleep: update of the 2007 AASM manual for the scoring of sleep and associated events. Deliberations of the sleep apnea definitions task force of the American Academy of Sleep Medicine. *J Clin Sleep Med*. 2012;8(5):597–619.
2. Chai-Coetzer CL, Antic NA, Rowland LS, et al. A simplified model of screening questionnaire and home monitoring for obstructive sleep apnoea in primary care. *Thorax*. 2011;66(3):213–219.
3. White LH, Bradley TD. Role of nocturnal rostral fluid shift in the pathogenesis of obstructive and central sleep apnoea. *J Physiol (Lond)*. 2013;591(5):1179–1193.
4. Dempsey JA, Veasey SC, Morgan BJ, O'Donnell CP. Pathophysiology of sleep apnea. *Physiol Rev*. 2010;90(1):47–112.
5. Javaheri S, Barbe F, Campos-Rodriguez F, et al. Sleep apnea: types, mechanisms, and clinical cardiovascular consequences. *J Am Coll Cardiol*. 2017;69(7):841–858.
6. Mokhlesi B, Finn LA, Hagen EW, et al. Obstructive sleep apnea during REM sleep and hypertension. Results of the Wisconsin Sleep Cohort. *Am J Respir Crit Care Med*. 2014;190(10):1158–1167.
7. Peppard PE, Young T, Barnet JH, et al. Increased prevalence of sleep-disordered breathing in adults. *Am J Epidemiol*. 2013;177(9):1006–1014.
8. Redline S, Strohl KP. Recognition and consequences of obstructive sleep apnea hypopnea syndrome. *Otolaryngol Clin North Am*. 1999;32(2):303–331.
9. Wimms A, Woehrle H, Ketheeswaran S, et al. Obstructive sleep apnea in women: specific issues and interventions. *BioMed Res Int*. 2016;2016:1764837.
10. Peppard PE, Young T, Palta M, et al. Longitudinal study of moderate weight change and sleep-disordered breathing. *J Am Med Assoc*. 2000;284(23):3015–3021.
11. Patel SR, Tishler PV. Familial and genetic factors. In: Kushida CA, ed. *Obstructive Sleep Apnea: Pathophysiology, Comorbidities, and Consequences*. New York: Informa Healthcare; 2007.
12. Chen H, Cade BE, Gleason KJ, et al. Multiethnic meta-analysis Identifies RAI1 as a possible obstructive sleep apnea-related quantitative trait locus in men. *Am J Respir Cell Mol Biol*. 2018;58(3):391–401.
13. Chen X, Wang R, Zee P, et al. Racial/ethnic differences in sleep disturbances: the Multi-Ethnic Study of Atherosclerosis (MESA). *Sleep*. 2015;38(6):877–888.
14. Redline S, Baker-Goodwin S, Bakker JP, et al. Patient partnerships transforming sleep medicine research and clinical care: perspectives from the sleep apnea patient-centered outcomes network. *J Clin Sleep Med*. 2016;12(7):1053–1058.
15. Won CHJ, Reid M, Sofer T, et al. Sex differences in obstructive sleep apnea phenotypes, the multi-ethnic study of atherosclerosis. *Sleep*. 2020;43(5).
16. Lyons OD, Bradley TD. Heart failure and sleep apnea. *Can J Cardiol*. 2015;31(7):898–908.
17. Jonas DE, Amick HR, Feltner C, et al. Screening for obstructive sleep apnea in adults: evidence report and systematic review for the US preventive services task force. *J Am Med Assoc*. 2017;317(4):415–433.
18. Shah N, Hanna DB, Teng Y, et al. Sex-specific prediction models for sleep apnea from the Hispanic community health study/study of Satinos. *Chest*. 2016;149(6):1409–1418.
19. Baltzis D, Bakker JP, Patel SR, Veves A. Obstructive sleep apnea and vascular diseases. *Compr Physiol*. 2016;6(3):1519–1528.
20. Orrù G, Storari M, Scano A, et al. Obstructive Sleep Apnea, oxidative stress, inflammation and endothelial dysfunction-An overview of predictive laboratory biomarkers. *Eur Rev Med Pharmacol Sci*. 2020;24(12):6939–6948.
21. Pedrosa RP, Drager LF, Gonzaga CC, et al. Obstructive sleep apnea: the most common secondary cause of hypertension associated with resistant hypertension. *Hypertension*. 2011;58(5):811–817.
22. Seif F, Patel SR, Walia HK, et al. Obstructive sleep apnea and diurnal nondipping hemodynamic indices in patients at increased cardiovascular risk. *J Hypertens*. 2014;32(2):267–275.
23. Peppard PE, Young T, Palta M, Skatrud J. Prospective study of the association between sleep-disordered breathing and hypertension. *N Engl J Med*. 2000;342(19):1378–1384.

Management

24. Liu L, Cao Q, Guo Z, Dai Q. Continuous positive airway pressure in patients with obstructive sleep apnea and resistant hypertension: a meta-analysis of randomized controlled trials. *J Clin Hypertens*. 2016;18(2):153–158.
25. Gottlieb DJ, Punjabi NM, Mehra R, et al. CPAP versus oxygen in obstructive sleep apnea. *N Engl J Med*. 2014;370(24):2276–2285.
26. Iftikhar IH, Valentine CW, Bittencourt LRA, et al. Effects of continuous positive airway pressure on blood pressure in patients with resistant hypertension and obstructive sleep apnea: a meta-analysis. *J Hypertens*. 2014;32(12):2341–2350; discussion 2350.

27. Martínez-García M-A, Capote F, Campos-Rodríguez F, et al. Effect of CPAP on blood pressure in patients with obstructive sleep apnea and resistant hypertension: the HIPARCO randomized clinical trial. *J Am Med Assoc*. 2013;310(22):2407–2415.
28. Sánchez-de-la-Torre M, Khalyfa A, Sánchez-de-la-Torre A, et al. Precision medicine in patients with resistant hypertension and obstructive sleep apnea: blood pressure response to continuous positive airway pressure treatment. *J Am Coll Cardiol*. 2015;66(9):1023–1032.
29. Thunström E, Manhem K, Rosengren A, Peker Y. Blood pressure response to losartan and continuous positive airway pressure in hypertension and obstructive sleep apnea. *Am J Respir Crit Care Med*. 2016;193(3):310–320.
30. Chirinos JA, Gurubhagavatula I, Teff K, et al. CPAP, weight loss, or both for obstructive sleep apnea. *N Engl J Med*. 2014;370(24):2265–2275.
31. National High Blood Pressure Education Program. *The Seventh Report of the Joint National Committee on Prevention, Detection, Evaluation, and Treatment of High Blood Pressure*. Bethesda (MD): National Heart, Lung, and Blood Institute (US); 2004.
32. Baessler A, Nadeem R, Harvey M, et al. Treatment for sleep apnea by continuous positive airway pressure improves levels of inflammatory markers - a meta-analysis. *J Inflamm*. 2013;10:13.
33. Mak GS, Kern MJ, Patel PM. Influence of obstructive sleep apnea and treatment with continuous positive airway pressure on fractional flow reserve measurements for coronary lesion assessment. *Catheter Cardiovasc Interv*. 2010;75(2):207–213.
34. Roca GQ, Redline S, Claggett B, et al. Sex-specific association of sleep apnea severity with subclinical myocardial injury, ventricular hypertrophy, and heart failure risk in a community-dwelling cohort: the atherosclerosis risk in communities-sleep heart health study. *Circulation*. 2015;132(14):1329–1337.
35. Yeboah J, Redline S, Johnson C, et al. Association between sleep apnea, snoring, incident cardiovascular events and all-cause mortality in an adult population: MESA. *Atherosclerosis*. 2011;219(2):963–968.
36. Campos-Rodriguez F, Martinez-Garcia MA, Reyes-Nuñez N, et al. Role of sleep apnea and continuous positive airway pressure therapy in the incidence of stroke or coronary heart disease in women. *Am J Respir Crit Care Med*. 2014;189(12):1544–1550.
37. Gottlieb DJ, Yenokyan G, Newman AB, et al. Prospective study of obstructive sleep apnea and incident coronary heart disease and heart failure: the sleep heart health study. *Circulation*. 2010;122(4):352–360.
38. Gami AS, Olson EJ, Shen WK, et al. Obstructive sleep apnea and the risk of sudden cardiac death: a longitudinal study of 10,701 adults. *J Am Coll Cardiol*. 2013;62(7):610–616.
39. Azarbarzin A, Sands SA, Stone KL, et al. The hypoxic burden of sleep apnoea predicts cardiovascular disease-related mortality: the Osteoporotic Fractures in Men Study and the Sleep Heart Health Study. *Eur Heart J*. 2019;40(14):1149–1157.
40. Nakashima H, Henmi T, Minami K, et al. Obstructive sleep apnoea increases the incidence of morning peak of onset in acute myocardial infarction. *Eur Heart J Acute Cardiovasc Care*. 2013;2(2):153–158.
41. Gami AS, Howard DE, Olson EJ, Somers VK. Day-night pattern of sudden death in obstructive sleep apnea. *N Engl J Med*. 2005;352(12):1206–1214.
42. Lutsey PL, McClelland RL, Duprez D, et al. Objectively measured sleep characteristics and prevalence of coronary artery calcification: the Multi-Ethnic Study of Atherosclerosis Sleep study. *Thorax*. 2015;70(9):880–887.
43. Kwon Y, Duprez DA, Jacobs DR, et al. Obstructive sleep apnea and progression of coronary artery calcium: the multi-ethnic study of atherosclerosis study. *J Am Heart Assoc*. 2014;3(5):e001241.
44. Mazaki T, Kasai T, Yokoi H, et al. Impact of sleep-disordered breathing on long-term outcomes in patients with acute coronary syndrome who have undergone primary percutaneous coronary intervention. *J Am Heart Assoc*. 2016;5(6).
45. Nakashima H, Kurobe M, Minami K, et al. Effects of moderate-to-severe obstructive sleep apnea on the clinical manifestations of plaque vulnerability and the progression of coronary atherosclerosis in patients with acute coronary syndrome. *Eur Heart J Acute Cardiovasc Care*. 2015;4(1):75–84.
46. Lee C-H, Sethi R, Li R, et al. Obstructive sleep apnea and cardiovascular events after percutaneous coronary intervention. *Circulation*. 2016;133(21):2008–2017.
47. Buchner S, Satzl A, Debl K, et al. Impact of sleep-disordered breathing on myocardial salvage and infarct size in patients with acute myocardial infarction. *Eur Heart J*. 2014;35(3):192–199.
48. Shah N, Redline S, Yaggi HK, et al. Obstructive sleep apnea and acute myocardial infarction severity: ischemic preconditioning? *Sleep Breath*. 2013;17(2):819–826.
49. Barbé F, Durán-Cantolla J, Sánchez-de-la-Torre M, et al. Effect of continuous positive airway pressure on the incidence of hypertension and cardiovascular events in nonsleepy patients with obstructive sleep apnea: a randomized controlled trial. *J Am Med Assoc*. 2012;307(20):2161–2168.
50. Peker Y, Glantz H, Eulenburg C, et al. Effect of positive airway pressure on cardiovascular outcomes in coronary artery disease patients with nonsleepy obstructive sleep apnea. The RICCADSA randomized controlled trial. *Am J Respir Crit Care Med*. 2016;194(5):613–620.
51. McEvoy RD, Antic NA, Heeley E, et al. CPAP for prevention of cardiovascular events in obstructive sleep apnea. *N Engl J Med*. 2016;375(10):919–931.
52. Sánchez-de-la-Torre M, Sánchez-de-la-Torre A, Bertran S, et al. Effect of obstructive sleep apnoea and its treatment with continuous positive airway pressure on the prevalence of cardiovascular events in patients with acute coronary syndrome (ISAACC study): a randomised controlled trial. *Lancet Respir Med*. 2020;8(4):359–367.

Heart Failure

53. Pearse SG, Cowie MR. Sleep-disordered breathing in heart failure. *Eur J Heart Fail*. 2016;18(4):353–361.
54. Bodez D, Damy T, Soulat-Dufour L, et al. Consequences of obstructive sleep apnoea syndrome on left ventricular geometry and diastolic function. *Arch Cardiovasc Dis*. 2016;109(8–9):494–503.
55. Javaheri S, Sharma RK, Wang R, et al. Association between obstructive sleep apnea and left ventricular structure by age and Gender: the multi-ethnic study of atherosclerosis. *Sleep*. 2016;39(3):523–529.
56. Javaheri S, Blackwell T, Ancoli-Israel S, et al. Sleep-disordered breathing and incident heart failure in older men. *Am J Respir Crit Care Med*. 2016;193(5):561–568.
57. Khayat R, Jarjoura D, Porter K, et al. Sleep disordered breathing and post-discharge mortality in patients with acute heart failure. *Eur Heart J*. 2015;36(23):1463–1469.
58. Sun H, Shi J, Li M, Chen X. Impact of continuous positive airway pressure treatment on left ventricular ejection fraction in patients with obstructive sleep apnea: a meta-analysis of randomized controlled trials. *PloS One*. 2013;8(5):e62298.
59. Javaheri S, Caref EB, Chen E, et al. Sleep apnea testing and outcomes in a large cohort of Medicare beneficiaries with newly diagnosed heart failure. *Am J Respir Crit Care Med*. 2011;183(4):539–546.
60. Bradley TD, Logan AG, Kimoff RJ, et al. Continuous positive airway pressure for central sleep apnea and heart failure. *N Engl J Med*. 2005;353(19):2025–2033.
61. Arzt M, Floras JS, Logan AG, et al. Suppression of central sleep apnea by continuous positive airway pressure and transplant-free survival in heart failure: a post hoc analysis of the Canadian Continuous Positive Airway Pressure for Patients with Central Sleep Apnea and Heart Failure Trial (CANPAP). *Circulation*. 2007;115(25):3173–3180.
62. Cowie MR, Woehrle H, Wegscheider K, et al. Adaptive servo-ventilation for central sleep apnea in systolic heart failure. *N Engl J Med*. 2015;373(12):1095–1105.

63. Yancy CW, Jessup M, Bozkurt B, et al. ACC/AHA/HFSA focused update of the 2013 ACCF/AHA guideline for the management of heart failure: a report of the American College of Cardiology/American Heart Association task force on clinical practice guidelines and the heart failure Society of America. *J Am Coll Cardiol.* 2017;70(6):776–803. 2017.
64. Fox H, Oldenburg O, Javaheri S, et al. Long-term efficacy and safety of phrenic nerve stimulation for the treatment of central sleep apnea. *Sleep.* 2019;42(11).
65. Linz D, Woehrle H, Bitter T, et al. The importance of sleep-disordered breathing in cardiovascular disease. *Clin Res Cardiol.* 2015;104(9):705–718.
66. Dimitri H, Ng M, Brooks AG, et al. Atrial remodeling in obstructive sleep apnea: implications for atrial fibrillation. *Heart Rhythm.* 2012;9(3):321–327.
67. Bare DJ, Yan J, Ai X. Evidence of CaMKII-regulated late INa in atrial fibrillation patients with sleep apnea: one-Step closer to finding Plausible Therapeutic Targets for atrial fibrillation? *Circ Res.* 2020;126(5):616–618.
68. Lebek S, Pichler K, Reuthner K, et al. Enhanced CaMKII-dependent late INa induces atrial proarrhythmic activity in patients with sleep-disordered breathing. *Circ Res.* 2020;126(5):603–615.
69. Maeno K, Kasagi S, Ueda A, et al. Effects of obstructive sleep apnea and its treatment on signal-averaged P-wave duration in men. *Circ Arrhythm Electrophysiol.* 2013;6(2):287–293.
70. Monahan K, Storfer-Isser A, Mehra R, et al. Triggering of nocturnal arrhythmias by sleep-disordered breathing events. *J Am Coll Cardiol.* 2009;54(19):1797–1804.
71. Mehra R, Stone KL, Varosy PD, et al. Nocturnal Arrhythmias across a spectrum of obstructive and central sleep-disordered breathing in older men: outcomes of sleep disorders in older men (MrOS sleep) study. *Arch Intern Med.* 2009;169(12):1147–1155.
72. Linz D, McEvoy RD, Cowie MR, et al. Associations of obstructive sleep apnea with atrial fibrillation and continuous positive airway pressure treatment: a review. *JAMA Cardiol.* 2018;3(6):532–540.
73. Holmqvist F, Guan N, Zhu Z, et al. Impact of obstructive sleep apnea and continuous positive airway pressure therapy on outcomes in patients with atrial fibrillation-Results from the Outcomes Registry for Better Informed Treatment of Atrial Fibrillation (ORBIT-AF). *Am Heart J.* 2015;169(5):647–654.e2.
74. Kanagala R, Murali NS, Friedman PA, et al. Obstructive sleep apnea and the recurrence of atrial fibrillation. *Circulation.* 2003;107(20):2589–2594.
75. Li L, Wang Z, Li J, et al. Efficacy of catheter ablation of atrial fibrillation in patients with obstructive sleep apnoea with and without continuous positive airway pressure treatment: a meta-analysis of observational studies. *Europace.* 2014;16(9):1309–1314.
76. Ng CY, Liu T, Shehata M, et al. Meta-analysis of obstructive sleep apnea as predictor of atrial fibrillation recurrence after catheter ablation. *Am J Cardiol.* 2011;108(1):47–51.
77. Qureshi WT, Nasir UB, Alqalyoobi S, et al. Meta-analysis of continuous positive airway pressure as a therapy of atrial fibrillation in obstructive sleep apnea. *Am J Cardiol.* 2015;116(11):1767–1773.
78. Neilan TG, Farhad H, Dodson JA, et al. Effect of sleep apnea and continuous positive airway pressure on cardiac structure and recurrence of atrial fibrillation. *J Am Heart Assoc.* 2013;2(6):e000421.
79. Estes NAM, Sacco RL, Al-Khatib SM, et al. American Heart Association atrial fibrillation research summit: a conference report from the American Heart Association. *Circulation.* 2011;124(3):363–372.
80. Caples SM, Mansukhani MP, Friedman PA, Somers VK. The impact of continuous positive airway pressure treatment on the recurrence of atrial fibrillation post cardioversion: a randomized controlled trial. *Int J Cardiol.* 2019;278:133–136.

第十部分 特定人群的心血管疾病

王汝涛 陶凌 导读

心血管疾病是人类健康的主要杀手，心血管医生不仅要关注普通人群的心血管健康，更需要关注特定人群的心血管疾病。心血管疾病在老年、女性、怀孕及不同种族和民族多样化人群中存在自身的特点，在临床诊疗过程中需要仔细评估，针对特定人群给予相应的个体化治疗。本部分详细阐述了老年、女性、怀孕及不同种族和民族多样化人群中心血管疾病的病理生理、疾病诊断、风险评估、患者管理以及预防等方面的知识，为临床医生在处理特定人群的心血管疾病方面提供了依据。

随着社会进步，世界范围内的人口老龄化逐渐加重，而衰老会增加年龄相关性心血管疾病的发生。老年患者增高的心血管疾病发病率造成了住院、手术、成本和医疗资源利用在年龄段方面的不成比例，加重了社会负担。了解和掌握老年人的心血管疾病的病理生理过程，对于该人群心血管疾病的防治意义重大。老年人心血管疾病的发生通常是处于多种合并症、虚弱、肌肉减少症、认知能力下降以及其他非心血管疾病的背景下，而这些合并疾病的存在也显著增加老年患者疾病管理的复杂性。本部分的老年人的心血管疾病章节（第90章）为我们提供了详细的阐述，从病理生理特点到疾病的复杂性，再到老年患者心血管疾病不同类型的流行病学、临床表现、疾病诊断以及处理原则，为临床上处理老年人的心血管疾病提供了指导性建议。

心血管疾病仍然是女性死亡的主要原因。女性和男性在心血管疾病和结局方面存在性别（生物学和社会文化层面）差异，这可能是由于多种因素造成的，包括传统心血管危险因素的差异、性别特异性心血管疾病危险因素的差异、心血管疾病的病理生理差异以及一级预防和二级预防方面的差异。充分了解女性心血管疾病的特点对于改善其预后尤为重要。本部分的女性心血管疾病章节（第91章）为我们详细介绍了女性心血管疾病的特点。文中详细阐述了女性心血管疾病的危险因素及其风险评估，介绍了女性缺血性心脏病的诊断和治疗，重点阐述了非阻塞性缺血性心脏病在女性患者中的发生发展、可能的病理生理机制以及诊断治疗。

在过去的几十年中，由于医疗条件的进步，越来越多的患有心血管疾病的年轻女性得到了及时救治。因此患有心血管疾病的女性的怀孕人数也在不断增加。妊娠会导致血流动力学和激素紊乱，从而增加患有心脏病的女性出现并发症的风险。因此，充分了解怀孕和心脏病，做好怀孕前和怀孕期间的评估尤为重要。本部分的妊娠和心脏病章节（第92章）对这一问题进行了详细介绍。对患有心脏病的女性在孕前孕中及时进行风险评估和分层可以降低风险、改善预后。同时对妊娠合并高血压、心肌病、缺血性心脏病、心脏瓣膜疾病、人工瓣膜和抗凝策略、心律失常、先天性心脏病、肺动脉高压、马方综合征和遗传性主动脉疾病等特殊情况也做了详细介绍。最后该章还对不同的避孕措施进行了介绍，强调了各种避孕措施的优缺点，应根据患者本身采取合适的避孕措施。

和性别差异一样，在不同种族和民族中，心血管疾病的负担也存在差异。黑人患致命性冠心病及死亡率均高于白人，西班牙裔/拉丁裔、黑人和亚洲人的糖尿病患病率要高于白种人。除了种族方面的差异，在患有心理疾病和性少数群体中由于其心血管风险更高也需要心血管医生的更多关注。研究发现心血管疾病还是无家可归者死亡的主要原因，在该群体中成年人的心血管死亡率是普通人群的 2～3 倍。对于种族和多样化人群的心血管疾病，需要根据现有的在此类人群中的循证医学证据和指南推荐进行管理和治疗。

PART X: CARDIOVASCULAR DISEASE IN SELECT POPULATIONS

90 Cardiovascular Disease in Older Adults

DANIEL E. FORMAN, JEROME L. FLEG, NANETTE KASS WENGER, AND MICHAEL W. RICH

WHAT IS AGING?, 1687

AGE-ASSOCIATED CHANGES IN CARDIOVASCULAR STRUCTURE AND FUNCTION, 1687

GERIATRIC DOMAINS PERTINENT TO CARDIOVASCULAR CARE, 1690

PRECEPTS OF PATIENT-CENTERED CARE IN OLDER ADULTS, 1693

CORONARY HEART DISEASE, 1695

ACUTE CORONARY SYNDROMES (ACS), 1696

HEART FAILURE, 1697

VALVULAR HEART DISEASE, 1699

CARDIAC RHYTHM ABNORMALITIES, 1701

VENOUS THROMBOEMBOLIC DISEASE, 1702

SYNCOPE, 1703

PREVENTION, 1703

NONCARDIAC SURGERY AND PERIOPERATIVE MANAGEMENT CONSIDERATIONS IN OLDER ADULTS, 1706

REFERENCES, 1707

The population of older adults is expanding throughout the world. In the United States the population age ≥65 years, barely 3 million total in 1900, has climbed to about 46 million and is expected to reach almost 84 million by 2050.[1] The population age ≥85, only about 0.2% of the total in 1900, is anticipated to reach 5% to 6% by 2050. Across the European Union, 20% of the population is over age 65, and more than 29% of Japan's population is in this age group.[2] Extended lifespan increases exposure to mounting cardiovascular disease (CVD) risk factors and leads to injurious effects that are cumulative over time[3]; in addition, intrinsic age-related cellular and subcellular physiologic changes increase susceptibility to CVD incidence and progression.[4] Prevalence of almost every type of CVD increases with age, including many conditions that develop predominantly in older adults (e.g., degenerative aortic stenosis [AS], heart failure [HF] with preserved ejection fraction [HFpEF], sick sinus syndrome). Furthermore, CVD in older adults tends to be more complex than in younger populations, both in underlying pathophysiology and because it is more likely to occur in combination with multiple comorbidities. Approximately 70% of adults age ≥65 years in the United States have CVD, including 85% of those age ≥80 years,[5] with disproportionate hospitalizations, procedures, costs, and health care resource utilization. Adults age ≥75 years old comprise only about 6% of the current U.S. population but account for >50% of CVD deaths.

The biologic processes that predispose to CVD in old age also foster higher susceptibility to concomitant diseases and geriatric syndromes.[6] CVDs in older individuals thus occur in a context of comorbidities, frailty, sarcopenia, cognitive decline, and other non-CVDs that add to management complexity. In addition to increased morbidity and mortality, CVD in older adults is associated with higher vulnerability to functional decline and progressive disability, which in turn increase risk for CVD.[7]

WHAT IS AGING?

Although aging is customarily measured in chronologic years, more fundamental determinants of aging entail biologic stress over time (e.g., oxidative stress) in juxtaposition to diminishing homeostatic capacities contingent on telomeres, epigenetics, proteostasis, autophagy, and other subcellular factors.[8] Cellular senescence and the related phenomenon of inflammaging, or chronic low-grade inflammation, also increase with age[9] and catalyze development of CVD, comorbidities, and geriatric syndromes. Yet progression of subcellular aging phenomena and clinical manifestations are moderated by each person's lifelong health habits (e.g., nutrition, physical activity, sleep, alcohol), CVD risk factors, comorbidities, social structure (e.g., spouse, children), and intrinsic functional capacities (e.g., physical, cognitive). Although chronologic years are immutable, other aspects of aging can often be modified. Habitual exercise and/or caloric restriction, for example, reduce the trajectory of aging and susceptibility to age-related CVD.

AGE-ASSOCIATED CHANGES IN CARDIOVASCULAR STRUCTURE AND FUNCTION

Normal aging is associated with alterations in cellular function, molecular signaling, proteostasis, and other mechanistic variations that lead to progressive changes in cardiovascular (CV) structure and function. These changes induce localized and systemic neurohormonal responses, such as release of proinflammatory cytokines and upregulation of the renin-angiotensin-aldosterone system, that set the stage for age-related CVDs (Fig. 90.1).[4]

Vasculature

Prominent structural and functional changes affect the arterial system in older adults, even among those with no apparent CVD. The arterial wall media thickens due to smooth muscle cell hypertrophy, extracellular matrix accumulation, and calcium deposition. Intimal-medial thickness (IMT) increases almost threefold between ages 20 and 90 years in normotensive individuals.[8] The range of IMT also increases with age, suggesting a variable response to aging, likely due to different genetic and lifestyle factors.

Along with increased IMT, advancing age leads to fraying of elastic fibers as well as increases in collagen content and enzymatic cross-linking of extracellular matrix molecules in the arterial media that reduce distensibility and increase stiffness.[10] Irreversible non-enzymatic glycation-based crosslinking of collagen forms advanced glycation end products (AGEs) that exacerbate the stiffening.

Changes in both vasodilating nitric oxide (NO) and vasoconstricting angiotensin II also contribute to vascular aging. Age-dependent reductions in endothelium-dependent vasodilation have been attributed to reduced NO production.[10] Animal studies show both lower NO levels

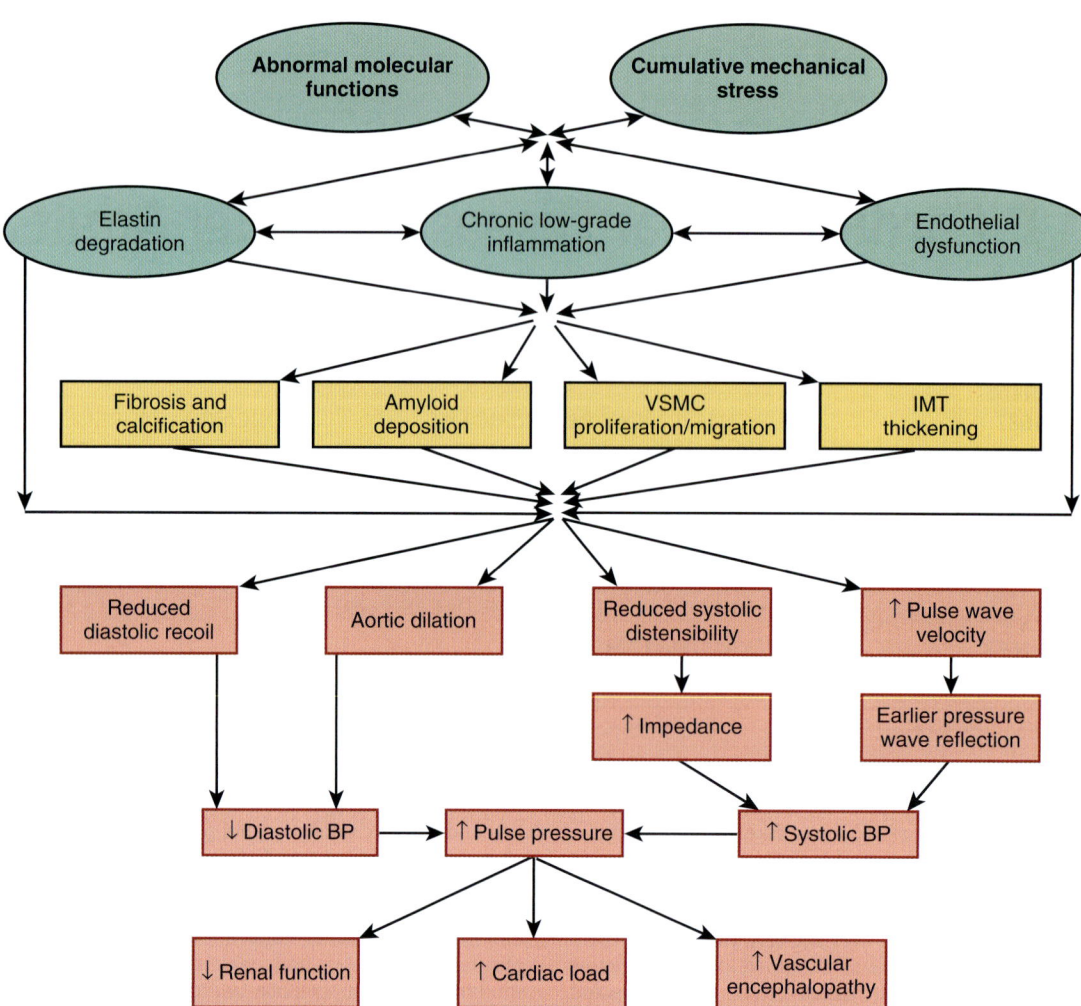

FIGURE 90.1 Conceptual model of arterial aging and its downstream effects. Age-associated molecular disorders and cumulative mechanical stress lead to a state of chronic inflammation, elastin degradation, and endothelial and vascular smooth muscle cell (VSMC) dysfunction. Downstream effects result in arterial wall calcification, fibrosis, amyloid deposition, VSMC proliferation, and intimal-medial thickening (IMT). These structural changes lead to functional alterations resulting in increased systolic blood pressure (BP) decreased diastolic BP, and widened pulse pressure. The increase in pulsatility leads to increased left ventricular load as well as elevated risks for chronic kidney disease and vascular dementia. (Adapted from Lakatta EG. So! What's aging? Is cardiovascular aging a disease? J Mol Cell Cardiol 2015;83:1-13.)

and reduced NO, consistent with reduced endothelial NO synthesis. Conversely, angiotensin II in the vessel wall increases 1000-fold with substantially increased angiotensin II signaling.

Both oxidative stress and chronic low-grade inflammation are key mediators of the structural and functional changes in the arterial wall with aging (see Chapter 24). Oxidative stress results from excessive generation of reactive oxygen species by enzymes such as NADPH oxidase, uncoupled NO synthase, and xanthine oxidase by the mitochondrial transport chain and from reduced antioxidant capacity. Increased reactive oxygen species and dysfunctional endothelial NO synthase contribute to age-associated decrements in endothelium-mediated vasodilation. Elevated oxidative stress also leads to enhanced protein oxidation, activation of inflammatory and endoplasmic reticulum stress responses, and apoptosis.

As a result of structural and functional changes in the arterial walls, stiffening of large- and medium-sized arteries occurs with aging, independent of disease. Systolic blood pressure (SBP) generally rises (see Chapter 26). In contrast, diastolic blood pressure (DBP) tends to rise until the sixth decade and declines thereafter due to reduced elastic recoil from the stiffer large arteries.[10] Pulse pressure, the difference between SBP and DBP, also increases with age, augmenting the pulsatile load on the heart and vasculature Pulse wave velocity (PWV), the speed with which an arterial pulse wave traverses the arterial tree, is another index of arterial stiffness. Aorto-femoral PWV increases two- to threefold across the adult lifespan in normotensive populations (see Chapter 43).

Left Ventricular (LV) Composition and Mass

With aging there is a decrease in the total number of cardiomyocytes, likely due to apoptosis, and an increase in their individual size (i.e., hypertrophy).[8] In both animal and human studies, apoptotic myocytes were more prevalent in the hearts of older men compared with women, paralleling an age-related decline of LV mass in men but not in women. Within the connective tissue, collagen content, fibrosis, and deposition of cardiac amyloid and lipofuscin all increase. The heart therefore becomes more fibrotic and stiffer with age.[11]

LV Wall Thickness, Cavity Size, and Shape

Despite the absence of an increase in cardiac mass with aging, there is a significant increase in myocardial thickness[11] due to increased cardiomyocyte size. Although concentric LV hypertrophy occurs, the interventricular septum increases in thickness more than the free wall, and there is a change in LV shape to a more spherical configuration. A more spherical ventricle is exposed to higher wall stress and is associated with higher incidence of LV dysfunction and HF (see Chapter 47). LV diastolic and systolic volumes decline with age and the LV mass/volume ratio increases in both sexes.[11]

Resting Cardiac Function

In healthy normotensive adults, resting LV shortening fraction and LV ejection fraction (LVEF), the two most commonly used measures of global LV systolic performance, are not affected by age.[11] Prolonged contractile activation of the thickened LV wall maintains a normal ejection time, and compensates for the late systolic augmentation of blood pressure (BP), preserving systolic LV pump function despite increased arterial stiffness. However, there is a modest decline in transmural global longitudinal strain and an increase in global circumferential strain with age. The increase in circumferential strain is likely a compensatory mechanism to maintain global LVEF.

TABLE 90.1 Relationship of Cardiovascular Aging in Healthy Humans to Cardiovascular Disease

AGE-ASSOCIATED CHANGES	PLAUSIBLE MECHANISMS	POSSIBLE RELATIONSHIP TO DISEASE
CV Structural Remodeling		
↑Vascular intimal thickness	↑ VSMC migration	Early stages of atherosclerosis matrix production
↑ Arterial stiffness	Elastin fragmentation and ↑ elastase activity	Systolic hypertension
	↑ Collagen production and cross-linking	
	Altered growth factor regulation and tissue repair	Atherosclerosis
↑ LV wall thickness	↑ LV myocyte size	↓ Early LV diastolic filling
	↓ Myocyte number and focal collagen deposition	↑ LV filling pressure/dyspnea
↑ Left atrial size	↑ Left atrial volume and pressure	↑ Risk of atrial fibrillation
Calcium deposits in valves and conduction system	Mechanical stress	Aortic stenosis
		Atrioventricular block
CV functional changes		
Altered vascular tone	↓ NO production/effects	Vascular stiffening and hypertension
	↓ βAR responses	
↓ CV reserve	↑Vascular load	Lower threshold for heart failure

βAR, Beta adrenergic receptor; *CV*, cardiovascular; *LV*, left ventricular, *VSMC*, vascular smooth muscle cell.

In contrast to systolic function, LV diastolic performance is prominently altered by aging. Whereas LV diastolic filling occurs primarily in early diastole in younger adults, transmitral early diastolic peak-filling rate declines by 30% to 50% between ages 20 and 80 years.[11] Conversely, there is an age-associated increase in peak A-wave velocity, which represents late LV filling facilitated by atrial contraction. The increase in late LV filling is mediated via a modest age-associated increase in left atrial size.[11] Tissue Doppler imaging in older adults shows lower E, e' and s', and greater E/e' compared with young individuals in both sedentary and trained persons.

Although age-related delays in early diastolic filling rate do not usually compromise end-diastolic volume and stroke volume at rest, stress-induced tachycardia (e.g., with exercise, fever, or other physiologic stress) is likely to exacerbate diastolic filling abnormalities. Tachycardia not only disproportionately shortens the time available for diastolic filling but also exacerbates impaired energy-dependent uptake of calcium into the sarcoplasmic reticulum. Therefore, fast heart rates are commonly associated with diastolic filling abnormalities, and the higher LV diastolic pressure is transmitted into the lungs despite normal resting LV systolic function. These findings are commonly manifested as HFpEF, especially when superimposed on other common age-associated comorbidities such as hypertension, diabetes, coronary heart disease (CHD), and atrial fibrillation (AF) (see Chapter 51).

The enlargement of the left atrium that occurs as a function of age and diastolic dysfunction occurs primarily after age 70 years[11] and increases susceptibility of older adults to AF. Whereas AF is often well tolerated in younger adults, it is more likely to provoke symptoms and clinical events among older individuals. Not only is AF commonly associated with poorly tolerated fast ventricular rates, but the AF-induced loss of the atrial boost to diastolic filling aggravates age-related diastolic filling impairment. Thus, older patients with AF are more likely than younger patients to incur reduced cardiac output and resultant dyspnea and fatigue (see Chapter 66).

Age-associated myocardial changes also predispose some older adults to myocardial ischemia and HF. A thicker LV predisposes to subendocardial ischemia by increasing the distance between the epicardial coronary arteries and the subendocardial myocytes. In addition, capillary growth and flow regulation in older hearts may not match the oxygen demands of the hypertrophied myocytes. These intramyocardial changes in capillarity and flow-dynamics are compounded by peripheral arterial stiffening and accelerated PWV (i.e., faster reflected pressure waves in systole), such that subendocardial perfusion is no longer bolstered by augmented pressures in diastole,[10] leading to a decline in coronary perfusion pressure.

Amidst the aforementioned age-associated changes in the vasculature and heart (Table 90.1), especially when compounded by prolonged exposure to other CVD risk factors, CVD increases markedly in older adults. Intrinsic vulnerability to atherosclerosis in the vasculature predisposes to myocardial ischemia, MI, stroke, and peripheral arterial disease (PAD). Heart failure with reduced ejection fraction (HFrEF) may develop as the result of ischemic coronary events or prolonged hypertension, either of which can impair LV systolic function. However, HFpEF is more likely to develop in the setting of ventricular stiffening, especially in association with hypertension, AF, and diabetes, all of which increase with age. Furthermore, CV aging occurs in a context of other age-related changes that compound the effects of CVD (Table 90.2) (see Chapter 51). Risks associated with myocardial ischemia, HF and other CVD become significantly worsened in the presence of concomitant renal, metabolic, hematologic, pulmonary, and other noncardiac physiologic changes.

TABLE 90.2 Common Age-Related Changes that Compound CVD Risks

Kidneys	↓ Glomerular filtration rate
	↓ Renal metabolism
Lungs	↓ Ventilatory capacity
	↑ Ventilation/perfusion mismatching
Musculoskeletal	↓ Skeletal muscle mass and function (sarcopenia)
	↓ Protein reserves
	↓ Bone mass
Immune function	↑ Susceptibility to infections
Hematopoietic	↑ Levels of coagulation factors
	↑ Platelet aggregability
	↑ Inhibitors of fibrinolysis
	↑ Anemia
Neurohormonal	↓ Cerebral autoregulatory
Liver	↓ Hepatic metabolism
Mood	↑ Depression
	↑ Anxiety
Sleep	↑ Obstructive sleep apnea

CV Response to Exercise

The ability to perform physical activity is highly relevant in clinical evaluation, especially in older adults. The CV response to aerobic exercise remains useful as a diagnostic and prognostic tool and is also strongly predictive of the ability of older individuals to withstand major procedures or aggressive therapies (see Chapter 32).

Aerobic Exercise Capacity. Cardiorespiratory fitness (defined by oxygen consumption [VO$_2$] max per kg weight at peak exercise) declines progressively with age. In cross-sectional studies, the decline is ~50% from the third to ninth decade. In longitudinal studies, a more

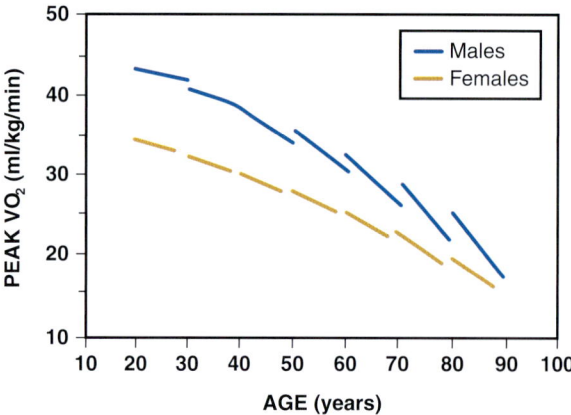

FIGURE 90.2 Longitudinal changes in peak oxygen (VO_2) consumption and maximal heart rate in healthy volunteers. Although the decrease in heart rate remained relatively constant over time at ~5% per decade, an accelerated age-associated decline occurs in peak VO_2 and oxygen pulse. (From Fleg JL, et al. Accelerated longitudinal decline of aerobic capacity in healthy older adults. Circulation. 2005 Aug 2;112(5):674-682.)

pronounced age-associated VO_2max decline is evident, regardless of habitual physical activity levels (Fig. 90.2).[11] The decline is only partially explained by changes in maximal heart rate and other CV parameters. Sarcopenia (i.e., atrophy and weakening of skeletal muscle) contributes significantly to age-associated decrease in VO_2 max. Age-related sarcopenia involves reduced number, size, and function of muscle fibers. By age 75 years, muscle mass typically represents ~15% of body weight compared with 30% in young adults. Fast twitch fibers atrophy to a greater extent than slow twitch fibers, which likely contributes to decrements in strength that are proportionally greater than the loss of muscle mass. Increased intramuscular fat and decreased mitochondrial bioenergetics contribute to reduced muscle function.[12] Furthermore, CVD has additional effect on skeletal muscle (most notably in HF) that compound impact of sarcopenia.[13]

The accelerated decline of aerobic capacity with age has important implications regarding functional independence and quality of life (QOL). Because many of the activities of daily living require fixed aerobic expenditures, they require a significantly larger percent of VO_2max in older than younger adults. When the energy required for an activity approaches or exceeds the aerobic capacity of an older individual, he or she will be less able and likely to perform it.[7]

Cardiac Function During Aerobic Exercise. In healthy adults, a ~50% decline in peak VO_2 between ages 20 and 80 years is accompanied by ~30% declines in cardiac output and ~20% declines in arteriovenous oxygen uptake. The decrease in cardiac index with age at maximal effort is due primarily to reduced heart rate.[11] Older individuals also have blunted capacity to reduce LV end-systolic volume (ESV) and to thereby augment LVEF with exercise to sustain higher capacity function (in part due to an age-related decline in adrenergic responsiveness). Some studies suggest this deficit may be offset by achieving a larger end-diastolic volume (EDV),[11] that is, the slower heart rate allows more time for LV filling, thereby providing a greater amount of blood in the heart at end-diastole. Nonetheless, maximum maximal LVEF often still diminishes with age due to insufficient diastolic expansion, reduced intrinsic myocardial contractility, increased arterial afterload, arterial-ventricular load mismatching, and blunted sympathetic modulation of LV contractility and arterial afterload.[10,11] The net effect of these changes is a marked reduction in CV reserve, such that even healthy older individuals free of CVD tend to become less able to maintain CV homeostasis in response to stress (e.g., major surgery or acute illness).

GERIATRIC DOMAINS PERTINENT TO CARDIOVASCULAR CARE

As described above, geriatric syndromes develop from the same biologic milieu as CVD in older adults. CVD in old age is likely to occur in combination with geriatric health care challenges that confound the standards of care that pertain primarily to younger and/or relatively more robust older populations (Table 90.3).

Multimorbidity

Multimorbidity or "multiple chronic conditions" denotes a situation in which two or more chronic conditions are active simultaneously. Multimorbidity shifts the therapeutic paradigm away from one that is oriented primarily to CVD-specific care to one that considers CVD in the context of competing conditions and priorities. For CVD therapies to achieve outcomes perceived as beneficial by a patient with multimorbidity, they must remain effective amidst conditions for which they were not intended or studied.[6]

Multimorbidity, prevalent in more than 70% of adults age ≥75 years[6] and in up to 90% of older HF patients, challenges the basic principles underlying conventional CV management. "Evidence-based" CVD guidelines typically rely on investigations that excluded study populations with significant comorbidities. Traditional therapy may be less applicable to patients with multiple diseases and concomitant medications. In a study of Medicare patients,[14] in those with HF, stroke, or AF, 50% had five or more comorbidities (Fig. 90.3). Moreover, the number of comorbidities correlates strongly with hospitalizations, cost of care, and mortality.

Management of CVD must be considered with added precautions as conventional therapies may provoke adverse effects; for example, antihypertensive medications are more likely to provoke falls in older patients with sarcopenia, Parkinson disease, or vision impairment. Furthermore, outcomes of older patients with CVD are often more likely to be affected by non-CVD comorbidities. For example, rehospitalization for HF may be caused by an infection or renal disease.

Frailty and Sarcopenia

Frailty denotes a state of vulnerability to stressors with limited reserves to stabilize declines across multiple physiologic systems.[15] Prevalence of frailty ranges from 10% to 70% in different CVD populations. Frail adults are prone to developing CVD and have worse outcomes and greater risks for harmful sequelae from standard therapies. With the advent of transcatheter aortic valve replacement (TAVR), interest in frailty accelerated among cardiology proceduralists as frailty often serves as a key selection criterion by which TAVR is considered (see Chapter 74). Subsequently, in the importance of frailty in informing personalized management has expanded to include care for acute coronary syndromes (ACS), CHD, and many other types of CVD.[15]

While the optimal assessment tool for frailty remains undefined, frailty is increasingly thought to be a biologic manifestation of inflammation[9]; circulating inflammatory biomarkers (high-sensitivity C-reactive protein and interleukin [IL]-6), as well as inflammatory cells (neutrophils and monocytes) are increased in frail individuals. Thus, CVD and frailty share inflammatory pathophysiology and tend to occur together. Older adults with CVD are more likely to be frail, and vice versa. Although geroscience insights implicate multiple subcellular mechanisms,[8] cellular senescence and associated inflammaging are significant components,[9,16] linking CVD, multimorbidity, frailty, and sarcopenia.

Sarcopenia is defined as a reduction in muscle strength and mass that is abnormally severe for an individual's age.[9] Whereas muscle atrophy is common with aging, sarcopenia entails muscle atrophy and weakening (dynapenia) that tends to be more common amid frailty and CVD. Inflammation is associated with reduced synthesis and activity of insulin-like growth factor 1 (IGF1), essential for muscle regeneration and maintenance of muscle integrity, and that also plays a role in mitigating plaque instability in atherosclerosis. In observational studies, high levels of IL-6 and low levels of IGF1 correlate with lower muscle strength and power, predicting frailty and associated risks of disability and death.

Two general approaches to identify frailty have evolved[17]: frailty conceptualized as an observable phenotype and frailty conceptualized as a numerical index. Fried advanced the premise of a "frailty phenotype" by identifying five specific physical characteristics that could be systematically assessed: weakness, low energy, slowed walking speed, decreased physical activity, and weight loss. Rockwood has championed an alternative approach in which frailty is conceptualized as an "index" of deficits of candidate variables, that is, a ratio of physical deficits as well as morbidities, disability, and other clinical variables that accumulate and progressively burden an individual. The magnitude and speed that deficits accumulate is applied as a gauge of vulnerability and risk. Variations on Fried's composite of physical phenotypic features include single-measure performance assessments including gait speed, handgrip strength, balance, or chair rise. Composite assessments such as the Timed Up and Go (TUG) and Sit to Stand tests[7] are also popular as they integrate multiple functional capabilities but usually entail more time and training to administer. A frailty tool app developed by Afilalo demonstrates their application (https://apps.apple.com/us/app/frailty-tool/id1330330931).

TABLE 90.3 Geriatric Syndromes and Clinical Implications

GERIATRIC SYNDROME	DIAGNOSIS/PREVALENCE	PROGNOSIS	DISEASE MANAGEMENT
Multimorbidity	Two or more chronic conditions (cardiac and noncardiac) that are active simultaneously Prevalence: 63% of those 65-74 years of age, 77% of those 75-84 years of age, and 83% of those ≥85 years of age	↑ Short and long-term prognostic risks due to CVD as well as non-CVD instability	Confounds customary CVD symptoms and signs Multiple diseases and providers often result in desynchronized or even contradictory aspects of care ↑ Likelihood that patients will experience high therapeutic burden
Frailty	State of vulnerability relating to diminished physiologic reserves across multiple physiologic systems Definition controversial: some define frailty as a phenotype, whereas others define frailty as an index of cumulative clinical deficits Prevalence: ranges from 10% to 60%, depending on the CVD burden, as well as the tool and cutoff chosen to define frailty.	↑ Risk from CVD as well as medical, device, percutaneous catheter, and surgical therapies used to treat CVD. ↑ Risks disability, falls, rehospitalization, poor quality of life, mortality	Guidelines-based therapy and procedures commonly overlook the impact of frailty on recommendations. Intensive care, bed rest, and functional decrements associated with many conventional therapies can exacerbate frailty and functional decline. Nutrition and exercise may help mitigate frailty and risks of frailty
Cognitive decline	Mild cognitive impairment (MCI)→ ↓ cognitive function without loss of function Prevalence estimates vary with the population and methods, but it rises with age, generally in the range of 2%-5% in those 60-55 to >20%-40% in those ≥90 years. Dementia → severe memory loss that interferes with daily life and loss of functional independence Prevalence increases with age, from ~5.0% of those aged 71-79 years to 35%-40% of those aged 90 and older.	↓ Independence ↓ Adherence ↓ Shared decision making ↓ QOL ↑ Hospitalization ↑ Mortality	Often confounds assessments of symptoms Often confounds accounts of present illness and PMHx Often confounds adherence Does not negate the potential value of therapeutic intervention, but it impacts the decision and implementation process
Delirium	Disturbance in cognition, attention, and consciousness or perception with fluctuating course Can manifest as agitated state or quiet and withdrawn High prevalence in older adults who are hospitalized, i.e., ~30%-60%.	↑ LOS ↑ Rehospitalization ↑ Functional decline ↑ Falls ↑ Long-term care ↑ Mortality	Predisposing risks include cognitive deficit, sensory limitations, and disorienting medications Treat by optimizing environment to increase orientation, avoid sedation, reduce meds, reduce pain
Polypharmacy	Multiple medications that have unintended interactive effects Polypharmacy usually considered four or more chronic medications 40% of older adults take ≥4 medications	↑ Adverse events (errors and drug interactions) ↑ Rehospitalizations ↑ Mortality	↑ Medication errors ↑ Drug–drug and drug–body interactions ↓ Adherence is common ↑ Under- and overtreatment both commonly occur Deprescribing is a relevant consideration
Disability	The inability to care for oneself or to manage one's own home	↑ Risk progressive functional and cognitive declines ↓ Self-reliance and self-efficacy ↑ Long-term care ↑ Mortality	Conventional care for CVD often contributes to a cycle of progressive disability, which highlights rationale for shared decision making for each aspect of therapy Suboptimal transitions are common contributors to disability, (e.g., hospital to home, and even hospital to postacute care)
Sensory loss	Vision and hearing deficits are common	↑ Risk progressive functional and cognitive declines ↓ Self-reliance and self-efficacy ↑ Long-term care ↑ Mortality	Conventional care for CVD often contributes to a cycle of progressive disability, which highlights rationale for shared decision making for each aspect of therapy Suboptimal transitions are common contributors to disability, (e.g., hospital to home, and even hospital to postacute care)
Incontinence	Urinary incontinence is common and often worsened by diuretics and other CVD meds		
Falls	Falls are common in older CVD patients as they can be provoked by environmental as well as syncopal etiologies and are often exacerbated by other geriatric syndromes such as polypharmacy, frailty, delirium, and visual deficits		

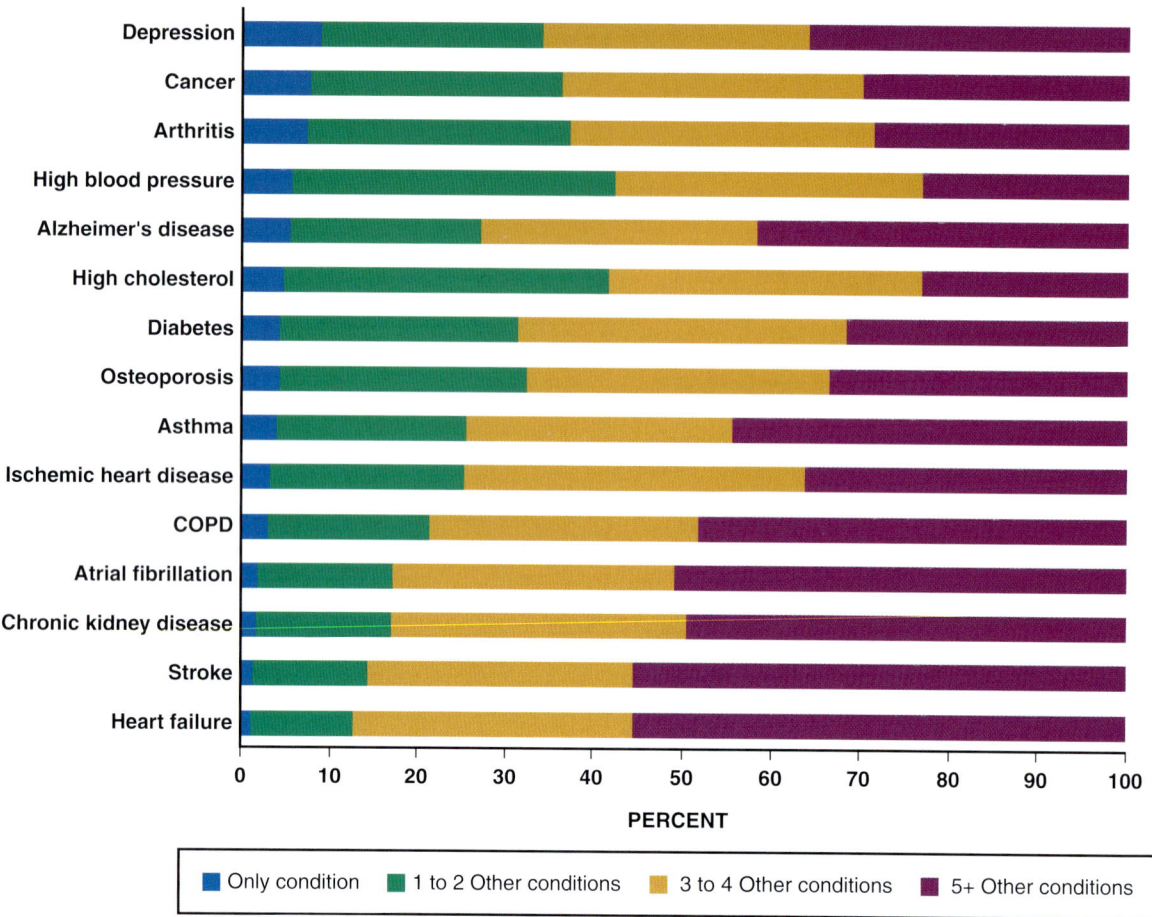

FIGURE 90.3 Number of coexisting chronic conditions among Medicare fee-for-service (FFS) beneficiaries with common cardiovascular diagnoses. *COPD*, Chronic obstructive pulmonary disease. (From Centers for Medicare and Medicaid Services. Chronic Conditions Among Medicare Beneficiaries. Chartbook, 2012 Edition. Baltimore, 2012.)

Cognitive Impairment

Whereas dementia affects fewer than 5% of the population at 65 years, it affects more than 40% of those living past 85.[18] Prevalence is even higher in those with CVD, with causal relationships attributable to vascular disease, HF, AF, hypertension, hypotension, and frailty; relevant pathophysiology includes perfusion abnormalities, thrombosis, inflammation, mitochondrial dysfunction, and other factors.[19] For many older adults, cognitive decline may be insidious and subtle, often masked by a protective family and/or by a gradual withdrawal from activities and engagements that were previously routine. For those with overt dementia as well as those with subtle progressions of dementia, managing CVD often becomes disproportionately challenging. Clinical challenges relate to eliciting symptoms and past medical histories, making informed decisions, navigating diagnostic testing and procedures, and achieving reliable adherence and follow-up. Formalized testing of cognition may provide value, especially when cognition changes are subtle. Screening with the Montreal Cognitive Assessment (MoCA), Mini-Mental State Exam (MMSE), and miniCog are feasible options that can be integrated as part of CV care, with referral to a geriatrician or neurocognitive expert for further evaluation if indicated.

Delirium

Delirium is a disorder of disturbed attention that can manifest as agitated disruptive behavior or as quiet and withdrawn behavior that is less likely to elicit attention and corrective response. Delirium occurs in one-third of hospitalized patients ≥70 years, including 50% of those undergoing cardiac surgery and over 75% of those who require mechanical ventilation in an intensive care unit (ICU)[20] (see "Special Considerations" under "Noncardiac Surgery and Perioperative Management Considerations in Older Adults"). Baseline cognitive impairment significantly increases risks that delirium may occur. Mortality, morbidity, length of stay, cost, and discharge to a facility are all increased in those who become delirious. Multiple factors of hospitalization are likely to trigger it, including the stress of a new environment, poor sleep, new medications, withdrawal from home medications, pain, dehydration, hypoxia, and metabolic shifts. Anticipatory screening by the Confusion Assessment Method (CAM) is a validated tool for screening in a hospital setting[21] and provides opportunity to mitigate precipitating factors.

Polypharmacy

Polypharmacy is common among older adults, with significant and sometimes dire consequences.[22] The Sloan survey showed that 44% of older men and 57% of older women received five or more prescription medications. In some cases polypharmacy relates to multimorbidity as multiple clinicians prescribe evidence-based medications oriented to different diseases. While disease guidelines are each supported by evidence, there is no guideline that addresses medications amidst multiple concurrent diseases and aggregate medical regimens.[23] Nonetheless, "quality indicators" used to assess the quality of care for individual diseases commonly reinforce tendencies for clinicians to prescribe guidelines-based medications irrespective of comorbidity and the total number of medications the patient is taking. Although most CVD guidelines acknowledge that clinical judgment is necessary to integrate evidence-based standards with each patient's circumstances, they do not provide a refined strategy to achieve such tailored care.

The safety risks associated with mounting numbers of medications in older adults are also affected by age-related changes in pharmacokinetics and pharmacodynamics[22] (see Chapter 9). The most significant age-related changes of pharmacokinetics pertain to renal metabolism. Glomerular filtration rate (GFR) decreases about 10% per decade in men and women. By age 80 years, GFR is typically one-half to two-thirds of that in younger adults. This reduction can be masked by overestimation of GFR using the Modified Diet in Renal Disease (MDRD) formula and the Chronic Kidney Disease Epidemiology Collaboration (CKD-EPI). The Cockroft-Gault is usually a preferred GFR equation; it accounts for age, sex, and weight, and characterizes a linear decrease of renal function. The dosage of many medications cleared by the kidney must be reduced in older patients with impaired renal function (e.g., digoxin, low-molecular-weight heparin [LMWH], glycoprotein IIb/IIIa inhibitors and, in some cases, direct-acting oral anticoagulants [DOACs]) (see Chapter 101).

Pharmacodynamic alterations are especially common amidst age-related changes in neuroautoregulation. Changes in thirst, temperature regulation, autonomic reflexes, sympathetic and cholinergic receptors, and cell signaling all impact the effects of medications, with greater susceptibility to orthostasis, syncope, falls, and other clinical sequelae.[24]

Drug–drug interactions are typical amidst polypharmacy, particularly when medications are metabolized by the same pathway.[25] Amiodarone, for example, inhibits CYP oxidative enzymes and increases drug levels of those medications that would normally be metabolized by this pathway (see Chapter 9). Adverse effects may also occur if clinical actions of medications are additive (e.g., administering aspirin, clopidogrel, and apixaban together will exacerbate bleeding risks) or competing (e.g., administering liraglutide and steroids together will decrease glucose control).

Drug–disease interactions occur as medications that benefit one chronic disease adversely affect another disease or syndrome. Beta blockers for cardiac ischemia may, for example, trigger bronchospasm in patients with concomitant chronic obstructive pulmonary disease (COPD). Calcium channel blockers can exacerbate chronic constipation, which is usually further compounded by sedentariness. Diuretics can aggravate incontinence and related social isolation and depression.

Disability

Disability refers to a physical or mental condition that limits a person's movements, senses, or activities. Whereas younger adults with CVD are usually able to rebound after a successful CVD hospitalization or therapy, an older adult has greater risks of new or worsening disability. Multimorbidity, frailty, sarcopenia, polypharmacy, and other geriatric syndromes predispose to disability in hospitalized older adults, especially in the context of deconditioning, cognitive impairment, malnutrition, and other burdens in older patients with CVD. The impact of hospital-related disability[26] is widespread and in some respects paradoxical, as older adults are especially vulnerable to morbid effects from the hospitalizations that are used to deliver care.

Notably, many CVD guideline-based therapies may inadvertently increase susceptibility to disability (e.g., increasing myalgias with statins and/or fatigue with beta blockers) especially among adults. Recent CV trials reflect the growing recognition that the therapeutic priorities of many older patients differ from those who are young. In the ASPirin in Reducing Events in the Elderly (ASPREE)[27] trial, instead of focusing principally on thromboembolic events, bleeding and other disease metrics, the main endpoint was a "disability-free life," including freedom from dementia, for which there was no benefit of aspirin therapy.

PRECEPTS OF PATIENT-CENTERED CARE IN OLDER ADULTS

Although there is a tendency to refer to older adults as a distinct population with uniform health challenges, the variability between patients increases with age. Over a lifetime each individual encounters a diverse array of experiences, engages in a wide range of behaviors affecting health for better or worse, accumulates a highly variable list of health conditions of differing severity and impact, develops individualized attitudes about health care and preferences for care, and does all of these things in the context of uniquely personal psychosocial and family dynamics. As a result, people become progressively more heterogeneous with age. A fundamental challenge in caring for older patients with CVD is to integrate all of these factors, including prevalent geriatric syndromes, into a management plan that provides greatest weight to what is most important to the patient while maintaining sensitivity to competing non-CV comorbidities and social milieu that may greatly influence the patient's health care goals.

Diagnosis and Risk Assessment

Older adults are at increased risk for CVD due to age-related changes in CV physiology and the high prevalence of traditional CV risk factors at older age, especially hypertension, dyslipidemia, diabetes, obesity, and sedentary lifestyle. However, older patients are also more likely to have ambiguous symptoms (i.e., symptoms with multiple often coexisting potential causes), atypical symptoms, or no symptoms despite advanced disease. Thus, a high index of suspicion for CVD is appropriate, and the clinician should be alert for subtle signs and symptoms that might suggest a new or worsening CV disorder. For example, a change in activity level or alterations in mood, cognition, or sleep and eating habits may reflect HF, severe CHD, or AF. Conversely, these same symptoms could be due to a host of other conditions, including depression, pulmonary or thyroid disease, or medication side effects. It is incumbent on the clinician to consider these possibilities before ordering a battery of diagnostic tests. Test selection, when indicated, should also include consideration of the clinical implications of test results. While this is true in patients of all ages, it is a consideration that becomes more germane in older adults. For example, an echocardiogram that is clearly warranted to assess LVEF to determine eligibility for an implantable cardioverter-defibrillator (ICD) in a middle-aged patient with HF becomes inappropriate for an 87-year-old woman who indicates that she does not want an ICD or in an older adult with limited life expectancy due to advanced comorbid illness.

Disease Management and Care Coordination

Given the likelihood of CVD occurring in a context of multimorbidity, most older patients have multiple providers, including physicians, advanced practice nurses, physician assistants, pharmacists, nutritionists, and therapists. While multiple providers offer complementary expertise, they predispose to fragmented care. The potential for mixed messaging, conflicting therapeutic plans, patient confusion, polypharmacy, and nonadherence is high. Although the primary care provider often assumes the role of medical "quarterback" to integrate care across multiple providers, decisions regarding medications, devices, procedures, and ongoing monitoring typically require CV expertise. Thus, CV clinicians must be skilled to work within such complex team relationships. Effective interpersonal skills and organization are increasingly requisite for effective CV care in older patients.

Application of Guidelines

Evidence-based practice CVD guidelines are based principally on randomized clinical trials in which older patients are underrepresented; those who are enrolled tend to be healthier with fewer comorbidities and geriatric syndromes than those encountered in clinical practice.[28] An additional limitation of guidelines is that recommendations are generally disease-specific and fail to adequately consider the impact of multimorbidity, cognitive impairment, or frailty. Other factors that may limit the relevance of guidelines to older patients include time-to-benefit versus time-to-harm, life expectancy, and patient burden. For many therapies, time-to-benefit is delayed, whereas adverse events may occur early during treatment. For example, ICD implantation is associated with an upfront procedural risk that is higher in patients ≥80 years, whereas the lifesaving benefit of an ICD may be delayed for years, if it occurs at all. Similarly, medication side effects often occur early after initiation, but benefit may not accrue for months to years. In the same way, patients with limited life expectancy due to very advanced age (i.e., ≥90 years) or competing illness may not survive long enough to derive benefit from some treatments. In addition, adherence to guideline recommendations often imposes burden on patients in the form of testing or additional medications that the patient, given the choice, would opt to forego. Importantly, in recent years many CV guidelines have acknowledged the above limitations and have advocated shared decision making in situations where applicability of recommendations is uncertain.

Shared Decision Making

Shared decision making (SDM) is a process by which an informed patient actively participates in decisions affecting the patient's health care.[29] The role of the clinician is to initially provide an unbiased

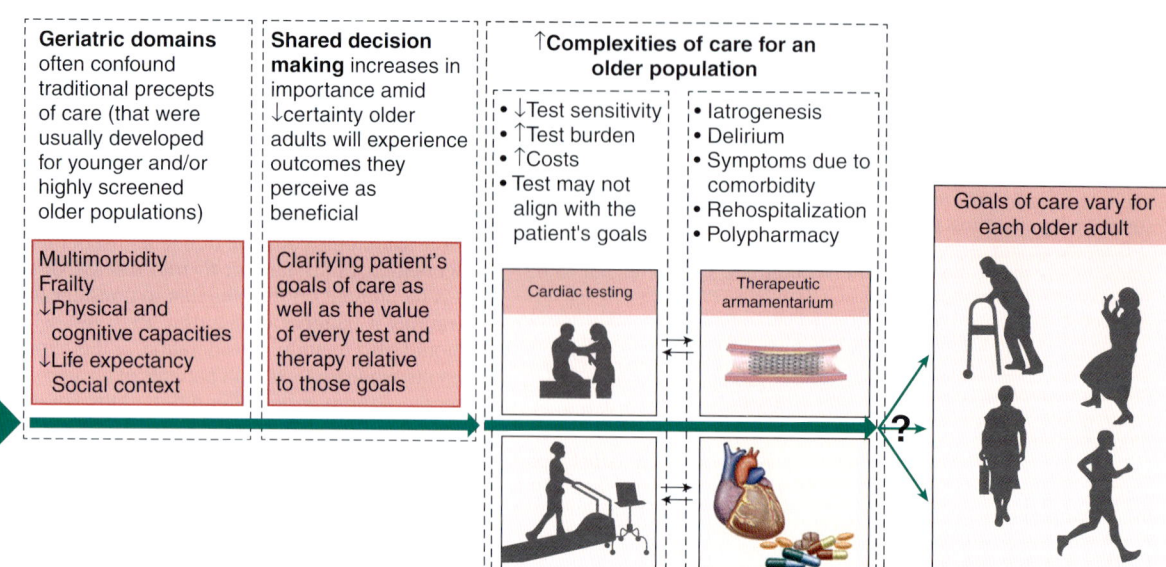

FIGURE 90.4 Among older adults with cardiovascular disease (CVD), clinical goals are more typically oriented to functional gains, independence, and quality of life (QOL), often with less priority ascribed to traditional CVD endpoints of major adverse cardiovascular events (MACE) that are emphasized in most major trials. Therapeutic risks are also relatively greater for older adults, particularly as geriatric syndromes compound the potential for harm. Given this ambiguous context, inclinations and oppositions for CVD therapy often vary from one patient to another, and shared decision-making becomes increasingly important. Nonetheless, shared decision-making is also challenged by common age-related limitations of health literacy and cognition.

summary of available options including advantages, disadvantages, and implications (in the case of testing). Following discussion with attention to patient concerns and questions, as well as incorporation of goals of care (e.g., QOL vs. length of life) and health care preferences (e.g., avoidance of risk and minimization of burden vs. willingness to accept risk and burden to achieve primary goal), a decision is made jointly by the patient (and family if appropriate) and the provider (Fig. 90.4). In most cases, decisions are not irrevocable and can be modified as circumstances, such as symptoms and comorbidities, evolve. In many cases, older patients, after being informed of the options and asking questions, will seek guidance from the clinician in reaching a decision. At this point, it is appropriate for the clinician to make a recommendation that is best aligned with the patient's goals and preferences.

Care Transitions, Skilled Nursing Facilities, and Long-Term Care

Care transition refers to any change in location of care delivery, for example, from hospital to postacute care or from skilled nursing facility to home. Older adults, especially those with multimorbidity, cognitive impairment, or frailty, are especially vulnerable to adverse outcomes during care transitions, including functional decline, medication errors, and delirium.[26] These perturbations often lead to rehospitalization and spiraling functional decline and progressive disability. To reduce the risk of adverse outcomes, effective care coordination is essential. In particular, meticulous medication reconciliation is required to ensure that the patient is taking all appropriately prescribed medications, but no medications that have been discontinued or which are no longer indicated. Minimizing polypharmacy and attention to potentially inappropriate medications in older adults, as defined by the Beers Criteria, is especially important.[30] A clinical pharmacist with experience in geriatric prescribing can play an invaluable role in ensuring safe and effective drug prescription and better medication adherence. Additional interventions that facilitate successful care transitions include frequent in-person or telephone follow-up and continuity of the care provider before, during, and after the transition.[31]

The role of postacute care for CVD patients is changing. In the past, older and sicker patients were routinely hospitalized for prolonged periods and were stable upon discharge to postacute care. As contemporary incentives encourage more rapid discharges from acute hospitalizations, increased numbers of older CVD patients are being discharged to skilled nursing facilities (SNFs). Of the more than 1 million hospital discharges for HF each year in the United States, approximately 20% are discharged to SNFs. These patients often have residual volume overload, fluctuating renal function, and evolving medication regimens. Yet SNF staff often lack adequate training and are uncomfortable caring for moderately ill and potentially unstable CVD patients. In addition, systematized access to CVD clinicians may be limited. CMS has imposed mandatory quality metrics for SNFs to improve and standardize care, but apart from medication review, these metrics are not directly applicable to CV conditions.

CVD is highly prevalent in patients in long-term care facilities. This is a particularly vulnerable population with high prevalence of cognitive dysfunction, physical disability, frailty, and multiple coexisting medical conditions. However, data on optimal management of CVD in long-term care residents is sparse, as these patients have routinely been excluded from CV trials and few observational studies have focused on this group.

Palliative Care and End-of-Life Care

Palliative care focuses on alleviating symptoms, reducing physical and emotional suffering, and improving QOL; these are integral components of almost all medical care.[32] In addition to managing symptoms, palliative care addresses psychosocial and spiritual needs. It provides an extra layer of support, often in association with standard care. Palliative care improves QOL and may increase survival.[33] It is distinct from hospice care, which is oriented to patients with a prognosis of <6 months of expected survival, and who have agreed to forgo more aggressive treatment.

In some respects, geriatric cardiology and palliative care overlap. Many patients referred for palliative care are older and have CVD in the context of frailty, disability, and other care complexities that require a tailored approach to CV management. Although palliative care does not preclude standard care, including procedures such as percutaneous coronary intervention (PCI) or TAVR that may markedly improve QOL, most patients who choose to pursue palliative care have prioritized QOL and comfort over length of life. In other situations, geriatric cardiologists are at the crossroads of management and must facilitate decisions about which older, complex, frail patients may still benefit from prevention and intervention strategies that may forestall or reverse decline.

Among people ≥75 years, CVD is the leading cause of death, exceeding all other causes of death combined. As a result, CV providers and their patients often face end-of-life decisions, including decisions about resuscitation, thresholds of futility, and strategies to help families/surrogate caregivers if patients lose capacity to make their own decisions. In most instances it is effective to encourage and support older adults to develop an advance directive, clarifying what medical care they would or would not want in the event of a life-threatening or terminal illness, as well as designating durable power of attorney for health care. It is also useful when patients discuss these issues with their families or health care proxies so that there is clear understanding of their preferences. It is helpful for clinicians of older patients with CVD to initiate these discussions as part of routine care delivery (i.e., "normalize" the conversation). Studies have shown that most patients, especially those with advanced symptoms (e.g., New York Heart Association [NYHA] Class III–IV), prefer having these conversations with their trusted clinicians.

Deprescribing

Deprescribing is the process of reducing the dose or discontinuing medications that have become burdensome to the patient (e.g., due to side effects), are no longer aligned with the patient's goals of care, or are no longer likely to provide benefit or to have a favorable benefit-to-risk ratio.[34] Deprescribing is an integral component of good prescribing practice with the goals of reducing medication burden, decreasing risk of drug–drug and drug–disease interactions, and eliminating medications no longer likely to be beneficial or consistent with patients' goals and preferences. Older adults with declining life expectancy, high self-perceived medication burden, advanced dementia, or multiple competing comorbidities are good candidates for deprescribing, but even more vigorous adults can potentially benefit. Care transitions with comprehensive medication reconciliation offer an excellent opportunity for deprescribing, but all contacts with providers should include a medication review with consideration of medications that might be discontinued.

CORONARY HEART DISEASE

Epidemiology

Age-related vascular changes in conjunction with increasing prevalence and duration of traditional cardiac risk factors predispose to the development of CHD at older age, and age is the strongest risk factor for incident CHD (see Chapter 25). Similarly, the prevalence and mortality rates of CHD increase progressively with age. The Global Burden of Disease Study indicates that in men, approximately 50% of deaths attributable to CHD occur in those over age 70, whereas in women, almost 50% of CHD deaths occur among those over age 80.[35]

Presentation

Compared with younger individuals, older adults with stable CHD, especially those over age 80, are less likely to experience exertional angina and more likely to report shortness of breath, fatigue, or lack of energy as manifestations of myocardial ischemia. Similarly, dyspnea is the most common presenting symptom of acute MI in patients over age 80, and the prevalence of atypical symptoms, including indigestion, dizziness, and altered mentation increases with age. In addition, many older patients with CHD are asymptomatic, in part due to sedentary lifestyle, and the incidence of silent or clinically unrecognized MI increases with age (see Chapter 35). Older patients also tend to minimize symptoms or attribute them to age or other causes, especially when comorbid diseases complicate the experience.

Risk Stratification and Diagnosis

Neither the Pooled Cohorts Equations nor the Framingham Risk Score permit estimation of risk for CVD events in patients ≥80 years, but even in the absence of other risk factors or symptoms, patients in this age group are at increased risk. Similarly, the majority of men over age 65 and women over age 70 in the United States are in the intermediate risk category, as defined by current guidelines.[36] Further risk stratification in older adults thus requires consideration of concomitant risk factors and symptoms.

The decision to pursue CHD evaluation in older adults is predicated on the pretest likelihood of disease, the probability that the test results will alter management, and patient preferences. In patients with relatively low pretest likelihood of severe CHD, mild to moderate symptoms that could potentially be controlled with medications, or clearly stated preference to avoid testing if possible, a conservative approach designed to control symptoms and risk factors is appropriate. For other patients, the decision-making process should start with a discussion of the advantages, disadvantages, and limitations of further testing in the context of the patient's goals of care. Results of two recent trials can be used to inform these discussions. In the PROMISE trial, 10,003 symptomatic patients with intermediate pretest likelihood of CHD were randomized to anatomical testing with coronary computed tomographic angiography (CCTA) or to functional testing (i.e., a stress test).[37] Over a median follow-up of 25 months, the primary outcome of death, MI, hospitalization for unstable angina, or major procedural complication occurred in 3.3% of the CCTA group and 3.0% of the stress test group, with no difference between groups and similar findings in patients younger or older than age 65. These findings indicate that the risk of a major adverse cardiac event during a 2-year follow-up period is quite low, and suggest that a conservative strategy, without testing, is reasonable for patients who prefer to avoid testing. The second study, the ISCHEMIA trial, randomized 5179 patients with moderate to severe ischemia on stress testing to an initial invasive strategy with coronary angiography and revascularization if indicated, or to an initial conservative strategy with intensive medical therapy.[38] Over a median follow-up of 3.2 years, there was no difference between groups in the primary outcome of CV death or MI, with similar findings across age groups. Patients randomized to the invasive strategy had better QOL, especially if they were more symptomatic at baseline. These results again provide rationale for conservative management, even in patients with moderate to severe symptoms, if the patient prefers to avoid testing and subsequent procedures.

In older patients who chose to proceed with further testing, the indications for stress testing, CCTA, and invasive angiography are similar to those in younger patients. If feasible, an exercise stress test is preferable to pharmacologic stress testing due to the important information derived on functional status, hemodynamic response to exercise, and occurrence of exercise-induced arrhythmias.[39] If appropriate, the exercise protocol should be modified to accommodate lower exercise capacity in older adults (i.e., starting at lower intensity and using smaller workload increments). Coronary CT angiography is less accurate in assessing lesion severity in older patients due to their high prevalence of coronary artery calcium (CAC).[39]

Management

Management of CHD (see Chapter 40) is similar in older and younger patients and includes control of risk factors, alleviation of symptoms, and prevention of complications (i.e., MI, death). Older patients are at increased risk for adverse effects from most medications, including bleeding with aspirin and other antithrombotic agents; bradycardia and hypotension with beta blockers; bradycardia, hypotension, pedal edema, constipation, and incontinence with calcium channel blockers (agent-specific); impaired renal function and hyperkalemia with ACE inhibitors (ACEI) and angiotensin receptor blockers (ARBs); and postural hypotension with nitrates. Statins in moderate- and high-intensities are recommended for adults >75 years, but risks of myalgias, fatigue, and reduced physical activity are increased.[40]

Invasive coronary angiography and revascularization are recommended for older adults with refractory symptoms, particularly those with significant ischemia on noninvasive diagnostic tests. In the Trial of Invasive versus Medical therapy in Elderly patients (TIME) study, symptom relief and exercise capacity during 4-year follow-up were better with revascularization than with optimized medical therapy alone in older patients with

CHD.[41] Similarly, the ISCHEMIA trial demonstrated improved QOL with revascularization in patients with high symptom burden.[39]

In older adults, PCI is associated with a modestly higher rate of procedural complications than in younger adults, including bleeding, stroke, and contrast-induced kidney injury. Dual antiplatelet therapy is associated with increased bleeding and transfusion risk in older patients. Bleeding risks can be minimized by using the radial artery approach and by weight- and renal dose-adjustments of anticoagulant and antiplatelet agents.

The choice of PCI versus coronary artery bypass grafting (CABG) involves consideration of the anatomy, comorbidities, functional capacity, frailty, and patient preferences. Although studies suggest that CABG is usually associated with less recurrence of symptoms and need for repeat revascularization, it also usually requires longer recovery and has a higher risk of stroke and procedure-related neurologic complications, including postoperative delirium.[41] Patients with diabetes or left main disease appear to have superior long-term outcomes with CABG. Although persistent cognitive decline following CABG has been reported, studies indicate this may primarily reflect unrecognized prior cognitive dysfunction.[42]

In assessing perioperative risk in older adults, physiologic status has greater import than chronologic age. The Euro SCORE and the Society of Thoracic Surgery (STS) risk score now include metrics of mobility and frailty (gait speed), respectively, in addition to surgical parameters and comorbidities, to help gauge short-term procedural risks and longer-term QOL outcomes. As discussed later (see "Cardiac Rehabilitation"), cardiac rehabilitation is also an integral component of CHD management.

Ischemia with Nonobstructive Coronary Arteries (INOCA)

INOCA is a multifactorial vascular syndrome in which an imbalance between oxygen supply and demand leads to ischemia in the absence of obstructive CHD.[43] Increasing age and age-related arterial stiffness are risk factors for INOCA, particularly in women, which in turn is associated with increased risk for CV events and impaired QOL. Many older adults have coronary microvascular dysfunction and diminished coronary flow reserve, as detected by positron emission tomography (PET), magnetic resonance imaging, or invasive coronary angiography. Treatment includes antiangina therapy and control of CV risk factors. A related syndrome, MI with nonobstructive coronary arteries (MINOCA), is more common in younger patients. However, in contrast to MINOCA, type 2 MI is more common in older adults. Type 2 MIs also result from supply–demand mismatch in the absence of obstructed coronary arteries when physiologic stresses (e.g., tachycardia, anemia, infections, hypertension) overwhelm limited CV flow reserves.

ACUTE CORONARY SYNDROMES (ACS) (SEE CHAPTERS 37 TO 39)

Epidemiology

In the United States, the average age at first acute MI is 65.6 years in men and 72.0 years in women.[44] In men, the incidence of MI peaks in the 65 to 74 year age group and declines at older ages, whereas the incidence in women increases progressively with age, surpassing that in men after age 85. The prevalence of MI in men increases from 2.8% at ages 40 to 59 to 11.5% at ages 60 to 79 and to 17.3% after age 80; comparable figures for women are 2.1%, 4.2%, and 12.7%. About 60% of hospitalizations for ACS are in patients ≥65 years, with approximately 85% of ACS mortality occurring in this age group; 32% to 43% of non-ST elevation (NSTE)-ACS admissions and 24% to 28% of ST-elevation MI (STEMI) admissions are in patients ≥75 years.[45] NSTE-ACS is far more prevalent than STEMI in the older population, as is type 2 MI.

Presentation

Older patients with ACS are less likely than younger patients to present with typical ischemic chest pain but more likely to experience dyspnea, diaphoresis, nausea and vomiting, presyncope or syncope, weakness, altered mental status, or confusion, even when chest discomfort is present. Chest pain is reported in only ~40% of those >85 years compared with almost 80% in those <65 years, often leading to delays in diagnosis and initiation of therapy. Heart failure, pulmonary edema, AF, bradyarrhythmias, hypotension, and shock all occur more frequently in older patients with ACS than in younger individuals, in part reflecting the marked reduction in CV reserve inherent to the aging process.

Diagnosis

Because older patients often present with atypical symptoms and NSTE-ACS, a heightened index of suspicion for ACS is required. The ECG may be nondiagnostic due to prior MI, conduction abnormalities, or paced rhythm, but ischemic ST-T changes carry the same implications as in younger patients. Older individuals tend to have higher baseline levels of troponin (cTn), such that 20% of community-dwelling adults >70 years have levels above the 99th percentile, and baseline levels tend to be higher in men than in women. These factors should be considered in evaluating the clinical significance of slight cTn elevations in older patients.[39] The emergence of high-sensitivity cTn (hs-cTn) could lead to over-diagnosis of ACS in older adults, with increased hospitalization and downstream testing, but additional data are needed.

Management

Older patients present complex challenges because of atypical symptomatology, high prevalence of cardiac and noncardiac comorbidities, age-related alterations in CV structure and physiology, and increased risk for adverse drug events and interactions due to polypharmacy. Although treatment standards for ACS do not differ with age, medication side effects, especially bleeding from antiplatelet and antithrombotic therapy, are more common in older patients.

Revascularization-STEMI

Timely reperfusion is the cornerstone of care for older patients with STEMI, with absolute benefits equal or greater than in younger patients given their higher mortality risks. However, older patients have more contraindications to reperfusion, and even if eligible are less likely to receive it. Primary PCI with stent placement is preferred over thrombolysis in older adults as it results in greater survival benefit, reduced reinfarction and need for repeat revascularization, and less intracranial hemorrhage. Fibrinolytic therapy has also been associated with an increased risk of myocardial rupture after age 75. If primary PCI cannot be performed within 120 minutes of symptom onset, fibrinolytic therapy is a reasonable option in carefully selected older patients with STEMI. In patients over age 75, streptokinase is associated with less intracranial bleeding than more fibrin-specific agents.

Revascularization-NSTE-ACS

Whereas randomized trials have shown benefit of an early invasive approach in high-risk ACS, including very old patients, management is frequently complicated by issues of multimorbidity, frailty, and geriatric domains that are coupled to MI pathophysiology.

Several trials have compared an invasive strategy to conservative management in older adults with NSTE-ACS with mixed results. In the After Eighty study, 457 patients ≥80 years were randomized to early catheterization and revascularization if indicated or to optimal medical therapy. During a median follow-up of 1.5 years, the invasive strategy was superior to the conservative strategy for the composite outcome of MI, need for urgent revascularization, stroke, or death.[46] The magnitude of benefit declined with age, and the small number of nonagenarians had no apparent benefit. There was no difference in bleeding complications, likely related to the predominant use of radial PCI access.[46]

Post-ACS Care and Discharge Planning

Older patients have longer lengths of stay following ACS, and frail individuals have even longer hospital stays and increased rates of discharge to institutional care. Older patients also have a high risk of rehospitalization and death, with a 50% increased mortality risk per 10-year increase in age starting at age 65. Utilization of recommended therapies mitigates these risks. Beta blockers have greater absolute benefit at older age in preventing subsequent MI and death than in younger groups. ACEIs and ARBs are beneficial in older patients, particularly those with HF or reduced LV systolic function. Statins are beneficial for secondary prevention in patients up to their early 80s but have not been adequately studied after age 80.[40] Dual antiplatelet therapy after PCI/stenting presents a challenge in older adults who also require anticoagulation for AF, deep vein thrombosis, mechanical heart valve, or other reasons. Recent studies and meta-analyses suggest that therapy with a P2Y12 inhibitor plus an oral anticoagulant, omitting aspirin, may be as effective as triple therapy in preventing MI, CV death, and ischemic stroke, with decreased bleeding.[47,48]

Comprehensive discharge planning includes the patient and family, and must address comorbidity, polypharmacy, and frailty, often in the context of impaired communication and cognition. Failure to understand and comply with the plan of care contributes to unreliable adherence, high rates of readmissions, and poor outcomes. The proportion of patients with ACS discharged to a postacute care facility or to home with home health services increases with age and with prevalent comorbidities, especially frailty and cognitive impairment. Cardiac rehabilitation (CR) has a Class IA recommendation following MI, PCI, or CABG, as well as in patients with stable CHD.[49] The benefits of CR extend to older adults and include reduced mortality, decreased hospitalizations, increased exercise tolerance, and improved QOL.

HEART FAILURE

Heart failure (see Part IV) epitomizes a convergence of CVD and geriatrics. The incidence and prevalence of HF rise exponentially with age, and entail the predisposing aspects of physiologic CV aging, mounting CVD risk factors over a lifetime, and geriatric syndromes. In addition, HF pathophysiology affects multiple systems (i.e., the heart as well as the vasculature, lungs, kidneys, and skeletal muscle).

Epidemiology

In the United States, HF is projected to increase from about 6.2 million currently to almost 8 million by 2030.[44] Prevalence more than doubles from 6% in those age 60 to 79 years to approximately 14% in those age ≥80 years; the mean age of patients with HF exceeds 70 years.[50] Whereas HF prevalence is higher in men than women through septuagenarian years, women predominate by age 80 and beyond. Incidence of HFpEF increases particularly rapidly among the very old[51]; underlying diastolic LV filling changes as well as high prevalence of hypertension, diabetes, AF, and other predisposing comorbid risks are all pervasive in older adults, intensifying susceptibility to HFpEF.[52] Hospital discharges for HF approximate 900,000 per year in the United States, comprising the most common reason for hospitalization in Medicare recipients, and progressively escalate as age increases. National Center for Health Statistics data show HF hospitalizations were 85.7/10,000 in adults age 65 to 74 years, 214.6/10,000 at age 75 to 84 years, and 430.7/10,000 for those age 85 years and older.[5]

Mortality rates from HF also increase with age, from <10/100,000 in adults age 45 to 49 years to 150/100,000 in octogenarians. Median survival was only 20 months for 825 patients ≥85 years versus 50 months for those <85 years in a study of 8507 hospitalized HF patients.[53] Atrial fibrillation, lower LVEF, and renal insufficiency were associated with greater long-term mortality. Risks for HF related to cumulative comorbid diseases are similar in older and younger adults, but the higher prevalence of comorbidity in older adults results in a higher attributable risk (i.e., prevalence times the relative risk) for developing HF despite a lower relative risk. Among Medicare beneficiaries, 65% of those with HF have five or more comorbidities, 25% have three to four comorbidities, and only 10% have two or fewer comorbidities.[14] High comorbidity burden is also associated with higher readmission rates and health care expenditures. The relationship between multimorbidity and HF is explained in part by the stresses induced by conditions superimposed upon age-related reduction in CV reserve. Inflammation associated with mounting comorbidity also exacerbates HF risks, particularly HFpEF.[52] Lifestyle factors (e.g., smoking, obesity, and low physical activity) add to HF risk in both older and younger populations.

Pathophysiology

Numerous population-based observational studies have demonstrated important age-related differences in the clinical profile and pathophysiology of HF[54] (see Chapter 47). More than half of older HF patients have a normal or near normal LVEF (i.e., HFpEF); in contrast, HF with reduced LVEF (HFrEF) represents the dominant form of HF in younger patients.

Diagnosis

Because HF affects multiple organ systems, no single test or procedure can definitively diagnose HF or exclude it (see Chapter 48). The specificity of one of the major Framingham diagnostic criteria for HF, orthopnea, or paroxysmal nocturnal dyspnea is low in older adults because these classic manifestations of HF can also be found in non-HF disorders such as pulmonary disease, deconditioning, and depression. Many older adults may attribute their HF symptoms to aging, thus delaying presentation until symptoms are more severe. Cognitive or sensory impairments may delay the diagnosis of HF in older adults.

Objective laboratory criteria are helpful in establishing the diagnosis of HF in older patients. A chest x-ray showing pulmonary venous hypertension and/or interstitial pulmonary edema is diagnostic. B-type natriuretic peptide (BNP) and N-terminal pro-BNP (NT-proBNP) levels increase with age, and higher cut points to diagnose HF are needed in older patients.[39] BNP levels are generally lower in HFpEF than HFrEF, making them less reliable as a diagnostic index for older adults, in whom HFpEF predominates.

Lifestyle HF Management

While lifestyle factors such as diet, physical activity, and patient/caregiver education retain an important role in older adults, rigid sodium and fluid restriction in older patients may reduce an already low caloric intake and exacerbate malnutrition and sarcopenia, both common in older HF patients and associated with adverse outcomes. In one trial, a sodium intake of 2.7 g/day reduced the rate of death or hospitalization by 25% compared with intake of 1.8 g/day.[55] Current guidelines suggest limiting sodium intake to <3 g/day in patients with stage C or D HF.[56]

Numerous trials have shown that exercise training in older patients with HFrEF improves functional capacity to a similar relative degree as in younger patients without increased safety concerns. The 2331 patient HF: A Controlled Trial Investigating Outcomes of Exercise Training (HF-ACTION) trial reported a similar modest improvement in a combined endpoint of all-cause mortality and hospitalizations as well as in combined CV mortality and HF hospitalizations in the 435 patients age ≥70 years compared with younger patients in a program of 36 supervised exercise sessions followed by home training for up to 4 years.[57] Based on the HF-ACTION results, Medicare approved outpatient supervised CR for stable HFrEF patients. Incorporating resistance exercises as well as flexibility and balance training is especially useful to counter age- and disease-associated deficits in these domains. In the absence of a formal training program, regular walking or other moderate intensity exercise is encouraged. Although an event-driven trial for exercise training in HFpEF is not available, many smaller trials suggest benefits, which may relate principally to improvements in peripheral mechanisms of disease (e.g., skeletal muscle and peripheral perfusion).

Because of the high hospitalization rates and their associated costs in older HF patients, much attention has been directed toward developing disease management programs to optimize HF patient care and improve outcomes. A meta-analysis of 47 trials including 10,869 older patients recently hospitalized for HF found that case management and multidisciplinary interventions probably reduced all-cause mortality, but clinic-based interventions had little or no effect on all-cause mortality. Case-management interventions, typically involving home visits and/or telephone follow-up, reduced HF readmissions at both 6 and 12 months' follow-up.[58] Multiple trials have also confirmed improved QOL from such programs. In older patients with NYHA Class III HF, an implanted pulmonary artery pressure sensor resulted in more medication changes and a 58% decrease in 30-day all-cause readmissions and 49% decrease in HF hospitalizations over 515 days mean follow-up.[59]

Pharmacotherapy for Chronic HFrEF (see Chapter 50)

Although ACEIs, ARBs, and beta blockers reduce CV events and improve survival in patients with HFrEF, this evidence base derives from RCTs that enrolled only modest numbers of patients age >75 years, and very few patients age ≥80. Benefits of each medication must be weighed against the risks associated with implicit polypharmacy of complex regimens in an older population prone to frailty, cognitive impairments, and other geriatric vulnerabilities. Frequent follow-up for adverse effects and need for medication adjustment is essential.

Diuretics. Diuretics remain the cornerstone for treatment of congestive signs and symptoms in chronic HFrEF despite the absence of RCT data that they reduce CV mortality. Observational studies suggest that chronic use may be associated with adverse outcomes, likely mediated by activation of neurohormones and electrolyte imbalances. Any of the three commonly used loop diuretics, furosemide, bumetanide, and torsemide may be considered for older adults, although absorption of bumetanide and torsemide is superior to furosemide. Doses are best started low and slowly uptitrated to achieve euvolemia; after which dose reduction can be tried. Serum electrolytes and renal function require more careful monitoring in older patients to reduce the risk for hypokalemia, hyponatremia, and prerenal azotemia. Concerns regarding incontinence and/or frequent voiding are also pertinent and may diminish an older patient's treatment experience and willingness to adhere to the medication.

ACEI OR ARB. Based on strong clinical trial evidence, older HFrEF patients who have no history of allergy or intolerance to an ACEI or ARB should be prescribed one of these drugs, starting at low doses. ARBs generally have fewer side effects. Close monitoring is required to avoid hypotension, hyperkalemia, or azotemia, especially in the first few weeks after initiating or up-titrating therapy. In RCTs, the average daily dose of ACEI or ARB was lower in older than younger patients.

Sacubitril-Valsartan Combination. The 2014 PARADIGM-HF study showed that the combination of the neprilysin inhibitor sacubitril and the ARB valsartan reduced total mortality by 16%, CV death by 20%, and HF hospitalization risk by 21% compared with the ACEI enalapril in 8442 patients with NYHA Class II to IV HFrEF. These benefits were similar in the 1563 patients >75 years as in younger groups.[60] Although hypotension, renal impairment, and hyperkalemia increased with age in both treatment arms, findings of more hypotension but less renal impairment or hyperkalemia with sacubitril-candesartan were consistent across age groups.

Beta Blockers. Unlike ACEI and ARB, a class effect is not evident for beta blockers in HFrEF. Clinical trial data supports only carvedilol, metoprolol succinate extended release, bisoprolol, nebivolol, and bucindolol, but the latter two drugs are not approved for HF in the United States. Although major RCTs of beta blockers included few patients ≥80 years, benefits appear similar across age. In hypertensive older patients with HFrEF, carvedilol may be a better beta blocker choice than metoprolol succinate or bisoprolol because of its vasodilating properties and tendency to lower BP more effectively. Side effects of beta blockers such as fatigue and/or chronotropic insufficiency are common in older patients, limiting maximal tolerated doses.

Aldosterone Antagonists. Despite powerful RCT evidence for efficacy of aldosterone antagonists in HFrEF, these drugs should be used with caution in older adults, with careful monitoring of renal function and serum potassium. While a high proportion of older participants participated in the Randomized Aldactone Evaluation Study (RALES), those enrolled were relatively healthy, and only about 20% of real-world very old HFrEF patients would have been eligible to enroll.[54] Generally, older patients with class III to IV HF should be started and maintained on spironolactone 12.5 mg daily or eplerenone 25 mg daily (or every other day if renal insufficiency is evident). Although hyperkalemia is a major limiting factor in older adults, the availability of the oral potassium-binding drug patiromer may enable more older individuals to benefit from aldosterone antagonists, but the risk of a prescribing cascade remains a concern.[22]

Digoxin. Even after two centuries of use, digitalis in HF patients is controversial. Despite its narrow therapeutic window and lack of life-prolonging benefits, the large DIG trial showed that digoxin reduced HF hospitalizations in HFrEF patients in sinus rhythm, including those ≥80 years. Because this trial antedated the widespread use of beta blockers and aldosterone antagonists, the benefit of digoxin in the current era is unclear. Recommended digoxin doses in older HFrEF patients are 0.125 mg/day or lower, which are likely to provide maximum clinical benefit with low risk of toxicity. While routine checking of serum digoxin concentration is not recommended, levels are indicated when symptoms or signs of digoxin toxicity are suspected.

Sodium Glucose Cotransport (SGLT)-2 Inhibitors. These drugs, originally developed as hypoglycemic agents, inhibit the reabsorption of both glucose and sodium from the distal renal tubule. Several recent studies have shown benefit of these drugs in HF patients with or without diabetes. In the DAPA-HF trial, dapagliflozin reduced the primary composite outcome of HF hospitalization, urgent HF visit, or CV death to a similar extent in age groups <55 years, 55 to 64, 65 to 74, and ≥75 years with HFrEF over an 18-month median follow-up without any age-related reduction in tolerability and safety compared with placebo.[61] Similar findings have been reported with empagliflozin.[62]

Other Pharmacologic Therapies. Although a RCT demonstrated a reduction of CV events with the combination of hydralazine and isosorbide dinitrate in younger (mean age 57 years) African Americans with HFrEF, adequate data in older patients is lacking. Intravenous inotropic agents, including dobutamine, milrinone, and levosimendan, have not been shown to improve clinical outcomes in patients with HF but may be considered as a palliative strategy in older patients with severe symptoms.

Nonmedicinal Options for Chronic HFrEF

Cardiac transplantation has been used successfully in highly selected patients in their 60s and early 70s with slightly higher surgical complications and mortality but fewer rejection episodes than in younger patients. Patients in their eighth decade and beyond are not generally cardiac transplant candidates. However, long-term or permanent LV assist devices (LVADs) have been shown to improve survival and QOL in such patients with end-stage HF. Risks of bleeding, infection, and thrombosis have been reduced with advent of continuous flow LVADs. An analysis of 1149 continuous flow LVAD recipients showed similar 1-year mortality in the 163 patients ≥70 years compared with younger patients, although gastrointestinal bleeding risk was higher in the older group.[63] Health-related QOL improved to a similar extent in 493 LVAD recipients age ≥70 years as in 977 younger recipients. Appropriate patient selection in experienced centers is critical for favorable outcomes.

Functionally active older HFrEF patients may benefit from cardiac surgical procedures. In one study, CABG improved survival in persons with reduced LVEF due to CHD, although the benefit was greater in younger individuals.[64] CABG may be considered for older HFrEF patients with multivessel CHD and evidence of ongoing myocardial ischemia with symptoms despite optimal medical therapy. Similarly, surgical or TAVR in older patients with HF due to severe AS is accompanied by markedly improved survival and functional status compared with medical therapy, although with higher bleeding and stroke risks and greater need for pacemaker implantation than in younger patients. Device therapy is discussed under "Cardiac Rhythm Abnormalities,"

Heart Failure with Preserved Ejection Fraction

More than half of older HF patients have HFpEF (see Chapter 51), and the prevalence is substantially higher in women than in men. The majority of patients with HFpEF have antecedent hypertension (60% to 80%). Multimorbidity is ubiquitous and often includes other CV disorders, such as CHD, AF, and valvular heart disease, as well as a wide range of non-CV conditions. Indeed, although HFpEF was once viewed as primarily a disorder of abnormal LV diastolic function, it is now considered to be a multifactorial systemic illness with complex pathogenesis involving aging, inflammation, multimorbidity, lifestyle, and genetic predisposition.[51] The prognosis for HFpEF is somewhat better than for HFrEF, but symptoms, QOL, and hospitalization rates are similar between the two forms of HF. However, despite multiple clinical trials investigating numerous agents, to date no pharmacologic or device-based interventions have demonstrated unequivocal efficacy in HFpEF. In the TOPCAT trial involving 3445 patients with HFpEF, spironolactone failed to reduce the primary composite endpoint of CV death, aborted cardiac arrest, or HF hospitalization but reduced HF hospitalization by a significant 17%.[65] In a posthoc subgroup analysis, spironolactone reduced the primary outcome by a significant 18% among patients enrolled in the Americas (United States, Canada, Brazil, Argentina), but not in those enrolled in Eastern Europe (Russia, Georgia), with similar results across the age spectrum, including patients age ≥75 years.[66] In the PARAGON-HF trial, 4822 patients with HFpEF (mean age 73 years, 53% women) were randomized to sacubitril-valsartan or to valsartan alone.[67] Although there was a 13% reduction in the composite primary outcome of CV mortality and total HF hospitalizations, the difference was not significant ($P = 0.06$). Prespecified subgroup analyses suggested that women and individuals with EF less than the median value of 57% benefitted from combined therapy.

Currently the management of HFpEF focuses on optimizing BP control, treating ischemia in patients with concomitant CHD, controlling heart rate in patients with AF, and avoiding excess dietary salt and fluid intake. In addition, aerobic exercise improves exercise tolerance in older adults with HFpEF, and weight loss with caloric restriction provides additional benefit in obese patients.[68] Diuretics are indicated to maintain euvolemia and minimize symptoms of shortness of breath and edema but must be used judiciously to avoid overdiuresis, which may lead to reduced organ perfusion and prerenal azotemia.

Cardiac Amyloidosis (see Chapter 53)

Transthyretin amyloid cardiomyopathy (ATTR) due to deposition of misfolded transthyretin protein in the myocardial interstitium, is an increasingly recognized cause of HFpEF in older adults.[69] Wild-type ATTR (ATTRwt) is an age-related disorder (formerly senile cardiac amyloid) that may contribute to 10% to 15% of HFpEF cases in older adults with a strong male predominance (>80% of cases). Hereditary ATTR (ATTRh) is related to specific genetic mutations, with the most common variant being present in 3% to 4% of African Americans. The cardiac manifestations of amyloid heart disease are similar to other forms of HFpEF, but noncardiac manifestations often include peripheral neuropathy, autonomic neuropathy (with orthostatic hypotension), bilateral carpal tunnel syndrome, and lumbar spinal stenosis. Low QRS voltage on electrocardiography is a classic feature of cardiac amyloid but is present in <50% of cases. Elevated cTn and NT-proBNP are common and correlate with prognosis but are nonspecific. Characteristic findings on echocardiography include increased LV wall thickness with normal or small LV cavity, markers of diastolic dysfunction, and abnormal global longitudinal strain with an "apical sparing" pattern. Recently bone-avid nuclear imaging has emerged as the noninvasive test of choice with high sensitivity and moderate specificity.[70] In patients in whom a light chain monoclonal gammopathy has been ruled out, a strongly positive bone-avid nuclear scan is diagnostic for ATTR, and biopsy is not required. In other cases, myocardial biopsy is needed to confirm the diagnosis.

Until recently there was no effective therapy for cardiac amyloid and the prognosis was poor, with a median survival of 2 to 4 years depending on type. However, tafamidis, a transthyretin-binding agent, was recently approved for treatment of ATTR amyloid based on the results of the ATTR-ACT trial.[71] In this study of 441 patients with ATTR cardiomyopathy (median age 75 years, 90% male, 81% white) tafamidis was associated with a 30% reduction in all-cause mortality, 32% reduction in CV-related hospitalizations, and better exercise tolerance and HF-related QOL over 30 months compared with placebo; tafamidis was generally well tolerated. Several other promising therapies for amyloidosis are currently under investigation.

Pulmonary Hypertension

Pulmonary hypertension (PH) (see Chapter 88) is increasingly recognized among older adults and is usually secondary to LV dysfunction. Differentiation of PH from HF or pulmonary disease is a key challenge, and specialized centers have evolved that focus on this differential.[72] HFpEF accompanied by pulmonary venous hypertension is associated with increased mortality as well as worse symptoms and diminished QOL.[73]

Pulmonary arterial hypertension (PAH) was once considered a disease that primarily affected young women, but it is increasingly recognized in the geriatric population. Recent Registry data show an increase in the proportion of older patients with PAH, particularly men. Given that <20% of patients who were enrolled in the clinical trials of the newer oral and parenteral therapies were older, extrapolation of the conclusions to older adults is uncertain.[74]

VALVULAR HEART DISEASE (SEE PART VIII)

Parallel to other age-associated changes in CV structure that may predispose to developing overt CVD, the cardiac valves undergo myxomatous degeneration and collagen infiltration, especially in the left heart. In the aortic valve, these processes manifest as valvular sclerosis, detected on physical exam by a short ejection murmur, and confirmed on echocardiography by leaflet thickening without calcification or orifice narrowing. Aortic sclerosis was observed in about half of individuals ≥85 years in the CHS. In ~2% of older adults, progressive calcification of the aortic leaflets results in valvular narrowing and AS. Aortic valvular regurgitation (AR), found in over a quarter of octogenarians, is usually due to annular dilation caused by chronic hypertension or leaflet calcification. In the mitral valve, myxomatous degeneration usually manifests as mitral regurgitation (MR) and is the primary mechanism for primary MR in older persons. Calcific deposits may also occur in the mitral valve leaflets, but more often in the mitral annulus, particularly in older women. Functional (i.e., secondary) MR is also common in seniors, usually due to ischemia-related papillary muscle dysfunction or to mitral annular dilation resulting from LV enlargement. Less common causes of mitral or aortic valvular regurgitation are endocarditis, rheumatic heart disease, mitral chordal rupture, aortic dissection, or trauma.

Aortic Stenosis

AS (see Chapter 72) is the prototypical valvular lesion in older adults, present in ~15% of those ≥65 years and is severe, as defined by a valve area <1 cm^2 or 0.6 cm^2/m^2 body surface area, in ~2%. In the majority, AS is secondary to calcification of a trileaflet AV; patients with congenital bicuspid valves generally present one to two decades earlier. Patients are usually asymptomatic on initial presentation with a harsh late-peaking systolic ejection murmur. In older sedentary individuals, the cardinal symptoms of angina, exercise intolerance, or syncope may not be reported because exertion sufficient to precipitate them occurs less frequently. The second heart sound is usually diminished and may be absent if calcification is extensive. In contrast to younger adults, the carotid artery upstroke is often not delayed because of large artery stiffening. The diagnosis is confirmed by Doppler echocardiography, which demonstrates the stenotic, calcified AV with a high transvalvular Doppler flow velocity, and a calculated AV area <1.0 cm^2. LV hypertrophy is generally present as well as reduced early diastolic LV filling rate. However, these latter findings are nonspecific because they are often present in older adults due to aging changes and hypertension.

The classic findings of severe AS on Doppler echocardiography are a stenotic, heavily calcified valve with restricted leaflet motion. A mean gradient across the AV ≥40 mm Hg and a peak flow velocity >4 m/sec with a LV stroke volume index ≥35 mL/m^2 signifies the most common hemodynamic pattern (high flow, high gradient). However, >40% of older patients have lower mean transvalvular gradients and/or peak velocities, that is, low gradient AS. About half of this latter group also have LV stroke volume indices of <35 mL/m^2, so called low flow, low gradient AS. This hemodynamic pattern is more common in women with small LV cavities and in patients with AF.[75] All-cause mortality over long-term follow-up is similar in medically treated patients with low flow, low gradient AS to that in the more typical high flow, high gradient pattern; both groups experience significant mortality reduction from AVR. However, the subset with high flow and low gradient does not generally have a mortality benefit from AVR.[75]

More robust older adults can generally undergo surgical AVR with acceptable morbidity and mortality. The 2020 ACC/AHA Guideline for the Management of Patients with Valvular Heart Disease[75a] recommends surgical AVR or transcatheter AVR after shared decision making among symptomatic patients ages 65 to 80 years. A tissue valve is generally preferred over a mechanical valve in older individuals to avoid the need for anticoagulation. Deterioration of bioprosthetic valves generally occurs more slowly in older than younger patients, increasing the likelihood that the prosthetic valve will not need to be replaced during the patient's remaining lifespan.

Transcatheter AVR (TAVR) has been transformative as an alternative for the sizable proportion of older patients with severe AS in a context of high surgical risks. In the initial PARTNER trial, 1-year mortality in otherwise inoperable patients with severe AS (mean age, 83 years; 54% women) randomized to TAVR was 30% compared with 50% in the medically treated group. Subsequent trials in patients at high and intermediate surgical risk showed similar 30-day and 1-year survival in patients randomized to TAVR vs. surgical AVR. In low risk patients (mean age, 73 years), the composite risk of death, stroke, or hospitalization at 1 year was significantly lower (8.5% vs. 15.1%) in patients randomized to TAVR compared to surgical AVR, as was hospital stay and risk of new-onset AF at 30 days.[76] Risks of stroke, vascular complications, permanent pacemaker implantation, and paravalvular leak are generally higher with TAVR, although strokes and vascular complication rates have decreased in recent trials.

In the Transcatheter Valve Therapy Registry, 30-day mortality after TAVR declined from 4% to 3% between 2013 and 2015 and 1-year mortality declined from 26% to 22%.[77] After TAVR, substantial improvement is seen in functional capacity, NYHA class, and QOL similar to surgical AVR. Excellent durability of TAVR, as defined by stability of the AV gradient and valve area, has been demonstrated to 5 years.

In the 2020 Guideline for the Management of Patients with Valvular Heart Disease,[75a] TAVR is recommended among symptomatic patients of any age with high or prohibitive surgical risk if predicted survival after intervention is >12 months with an acceptable quality of life. TAVR is also recommended for patients >80 years or any patient with life expectancy <10 years. As with other bioprosthetic valves, daily aspirin 75 to 100 mg is recommended as antithrombotic therapy.

Aortic Regurgitation

The prevalence of AR increases with age. Common causes of AR in older adults are valvular disease (degenerative or infectious) or aortic root dilation due to hypertension, connective tissue disease, aortic dissection, or trauma. Severe AR may be asymptomatic for many years; however, life expectancy without surgery is about 2 years in older individuals once HF develops. Left ventricular dilation, reduced EF, and moderate or greater PH predict higher mortality.

The classic diastolic high-pitched blowing murmur of AR is generally heard best at the lower left sternal border if due to valvular disease and at the upper right sternal border if due to aortic root disease. Presence of a widened pulse pressure is not as helpful an ancillary sign of AR in older adults because they often have widened pulse pressure due to arterial stiffening. Definitive diagnosis of AR is made by quantifying the regurgitant jet on Doppler echocardiography. Chronic severe AR accompanied by a systolic LV dimension >4.5 cm or LVEF <50% is an indication for AVR even in the absence of symptoms.[78] Older patients are more likely to develop HF symptoms and LV dysfunction earlier in the disease course and have higher postoperative mortality than younger individuals. Operative mortality in older patients varies with LV function, increasing from <5% with normal function to 14% for LVEF <35%. Although moderate or severe AR has been a contraindication for TAVR to date, small series have shown successful treatment of AR by TAVR.[79] TAVR may become a reliable alternative to surgical AVR in high-risk older individuals with severe AR.

Mitral Stenosis

With the dramatic reduction in rheumatic heart disease in developed countries, mitral stenosis (MS) (see Chapter 75), the hallmark lesion of this disease, has become uncommon and is mostly confined to foreign-born older adults, typically women, often with a prior mitral commissurotomy. Congestive symptoms generally indicate significant transmitral obstruction and a valve area <1.0 cm². Associated AF is more common in older patients with MS due to superimposed age-related left atrial enlargement and electrophysiologic changes. The resultant stasis of blood in the left atrium, especially the appendage, significantly increases risk for systemic thromboembolism, including stroke.

The pathognomonic low-pitched diastolic murmur of MS may be absent or of low intensity in older adults due to increased anteroposterior chest diameter or low stroke volume. In addition, the first heart sound may not be loud and the opening snap may be absent due to a fibrotic calcified mitral valve. Echocardiography is essential to confirm the diagnosis of MS, determine its severity, and characterize the extent of leaflet calcification and presence of associated MR.

In symptomatic older adults with severe MS, an intervention to increase mitral valve area is usually indicated. A percutaneous balloon valvulotomy may be suitable if the valve leaflets are not heavily calcified and their motion not severely restricted. However, success rates are below 50% in older patients and procedural complications and mortality are increased; cardiac tamponade occurs in ~5% and thromboembolism and death each in ~3%. Risks from mitral valve replacement (MVR) are also increased in older adults, with perioperative mortality ≥10%.

Mitral Annular Calcification

Mitral annular calcification (MAC) is an age-associated degenerative process that is more common in older women than men. It has been reported in about ~10% of community-dwelling adults age 45 to 84 years and much higher in those ≥85. The process parallels that in the AV, including the association with common atherosclerotic risk factors. Older patients with severe CKD have a particularly high rate of MAC. When MAC is extensive, it compromises the sphincter function of the mitral annulus and may stretch the mitral leaflets during systole, causing MR. Although MS may result from severe MAC that protrudes into the valve orifice, the MS is rarely severe. Calcific deposits from MAC may extend into the membranous ventricular septum, causing conduction disturbances. MAC increases the risk for endocarditis, especially perivalvular abscesses due to the avascularity of the annular tissue. Several studies have shown an increased risk of stroke or silent brain infarction in older patients with MAC. Although the net benefit of anticoagulation in patients with MAC is unclear, individuals with associated AF, MS, or severe MR are usually considered for such therapy.

Mitral Regurgitation

MR is common in older adults, with >10% of individuals age ≥75 years having at least moderate MR (see Chapter 76). Myxomatous degeneration is the most frequent structural etiology, with endocarditis, rheumatic heart disease, and papillary muscle rupture after MI less frequent causes. Functional MR is most often due to chronic LV and annular dilation or to ischemic papillary muscle dysfunction. Whereas myxomatous degeneration in younger populations typically presents as chest pain and mitral valve prolapse and is most common in women, in later life MR and congestive symptoms comprise the most common presentation, with similar prevalence in men and women. Chronic MR is often asymptomatic in older adults until it becomes severe. Presenting symptoms are initially exercise intolerance and fatigue, progressing to congestive symptoms as systolic LV function declines. Secondary PH is common in severe MR, and may result in right-sided HF.

Physical findings with significant MR are not generally altered by age; Doppler echocardiography quantifies the size of the regurgitant jet and provides insights regarding the etiology of MR based on leaflet and annular morphology and LV size and function. The prognosis of older patients with MR depends on its severity and etiology. Patients with acute MR secondary to papillary muscle rupture after an acute MI are an especially high-risk group due to the underlying myocardial insult and hemodynamic instability. Emergent surgical MVR with resection of the damaged papillary muscle and infarct zone is the treatment of choice. Patients with severe chronic MR and LV systolic dysfunction and/or dilation are also at high risk of adverse outcomes. Medical therapy for such patients should include ACEI/ARB and beta blockers, diuretics to relieve congestive symptoms, and rate or rhythm control of AF.

The 2020 ACC/AHA Guideline for the Management of Patients With Valvular Heart Disease recommends surgical repair in preference to valve replacement, provided that a successful and durable repair is technically feasible. In asymptomatic patients, surgery is recommended if LV ejection fraction (LVEF) ≤60% and/or LV end-systolic diameter ≥40 mm.[75a] Mitral valve repair is usually preferred over MVR for patients in their 70s and 80s, as results are similar to or better than MVR, including mortality ~5% or less and 70% to 80% 5-year survival. Functional status and

QOL are improved to a similar degree after MV repair or replacement. However, MVR is indicated when MV leaflets are fused, are extensively fibrotic or calcified, and have chordal shortening or fusion.

In parallel to the development of TAVR for treatment of severe AS, transcather mitral valve repair, now referred to as *transcatheter edge-to-edge repair* (TEER), provides a less invasive approach for severe MR. A MitraClip device "clips" the leaflets together, thereby reducing orifice size without affecting the annulus. In the Endovascular Valve Edge-to-Edge Repair Study (EVEREST) II, 351 older patients (mean age 76 years) with calculated surgical mortality risk ≥12% underwent MitraClip insertion. At 30 days, cardiac death occurred in 5%, MI in 1%, and stroke in 2.6%. At 12 months postprocedure, NYHA class and QOL had improved substantially, LV volumes were reduced, and MR severity was <2+ in 84% of patients.[80] A subsequent study of 564 patients of mean age 83 years reported 30-day mortality of 6%, strokes in 2%, and bleeding in 3%, with reduction of MR to grade <2 in 93%.[81] In older patients (mean age 72 years) with HF and moderate-to-severe or severe secondary MR who remained symptomatic despite maximal doses of guideline-directed medical therapy, transcatheter mitral-valve repair resulted in a lower rate of HF hospitalization and all-cause mortality over mean follow-up of 24 months compared with medical therapy alone.[82] Thus, TEER is an attractive option for a large proportion of high-risk older patients with severe MR. In the 2020 ACC/AHA Guideline for Management of Patients with Valvular Heart Disease, TEER is considered reasonable in patients with appropriate anatomy as defined on TEE and with LVEF between 20% and 50%, left ventricular end systolic diameter <70 mmHg, and pulmonary artery systolic pressure <70 mm Hg.[75a]

Endocarditis

Endocarditis (see Chapter 80) in older adults typically occurs as a result of indwelling vascular catheters, genitourinary or gastrointestinal instrumentation, pacemaker or ICD leads, prosthetic implants, or MAC. Diabetes and genitourinary and gastrointestinal cancer are major predisposing conditions. The most common pathogens in older adults are *Staphylococcus aureus*, often methicillin-resistant, *Streptococcus bovis*, and *Enterococci*. Morbidity and mortality from endocarditis are higher in older persons, due in part to comorbidities. In one large series, endocarditis incidence after TAVR was similar to that after surgical AVR and incurred a 36% in-hospital mortality.[83] Indications for endocarditis prophylaxis are similar regardless of age and include prosthetic valve implants, prior endocarditis, and cardiac transplantation.

CARDIAC RHYTHM ABNORMALITIES

Cardiac rhythm disorders (see Part VII) increase with age and become increasingly important contributors to morbidity and mortality.[84] Age-related changes in the heart and cardiac conduction system and the high prevalence of CVD provide substrates for arrhythmias. Fibrous, fatty, and calcific infiltration of the conduction system; calcification of the cardiac fibrous skeleton; reduction in the number of functioning sinus node pacemaker cells; impaired intracellular calcium handling; and blunted adrenergic responsiveness all increase the susceptibility to arrhythmias.[84] Cardiac amyloidosis is also increasingly recognized as etiologic for advanced AV block in older adults. Right and left bundle branch block increase with age.

Though the resting heart rate does not change with age, maximal heart rate decreases as a result of reduced sinus node responsivity to beta-adrenergic sympathetic stimulation[85]; beat-to-beat variability also decreases with age. Atrial ectopy occurs in about 10% of older individuals in the absence of known cardiac disease, with ventricular ectopy in 6% to 11% on resting ECG.

Supraventricular Arrhythmias
Atrial Fibrillation

Atrial fibrillation (see Chapter 66) occurs in about 12% of patients age ≥75 years and 18% of patients ≥85 years.[86] The high prevalence of AF relates to age-related changes in the atrial tissues, including fibrosis and conduction abnormalities that provide the substrate for electrical disarray. Hypertension and structural heart disease add to maladaptive atrial changes, which further predispose to AF.

The 2019 AHA/ACC/HRS Guideline for the Management of Patients with AF estimates that approximately one-third of patients with AF are ≥80 years.[87] Compared with younger adults, AF is more likely to occur in older adults in the absence of underlying heart disease. Common chronic comorbid conditions associated with AF include hypertension, CHD, obesity, sleep apnea, hyperlipidemia, and HF.

Symptoms of AF may include palpitations, light-headedness, chest discomfort, shortness of breath, fatigue, or decreased activity tolerance. Nonetheless, palpitations are less common than in younger patients and symptoms are frequently minimal or atypical. Acute pulmonary edema may occur with an abrupt loss of the atrial contribution to ventricular filling in a stiff LV. Less commonly, AF may be initially manifest as syncope, fall, or stroke.

The U.S. Preventive Services Task Force considers evidence insufficient for ECG screening for AF in old age, suggesting pulse palpation and confirmatory ECG.[88] The ESC guideline recommends AF screening at age ≥65 by pulse taking or an ECG rhythm strip (Class I); systematic ECG screening at age ≥75 is a Class IIb recommendation.[89] Wearable devices in the Apple Heart Study[90] suggest its utility to improve screening in older as well as younger adults.

Nonvalvular AF is associated with a fivefold increase in stroke. Strokes are often severe, and adverse outcomes are likely even after controlling for age and comorbidities. Increasing age is a potent risk factor for stroke, as highlighted in the CHA$_2$DS$_2$-VASc score, which assigns 1 point for age 65 to 74 years and 2 points for age ≥75 years. Thus, all persons age ≥75 years have a CHA$_2$DS$_2$-VASc score of ≥2 and are candidates for anticoagulation irrespective of whether the AF is paroxysmal, persistent, or permanent. In addition to the increased risk of stroke and HF, AF in older adults is associated with decreased physical performance and cognition,[91] shorter disability-free survival, and increased mortality.

Utility of anticoagulation is counterbalanced by increased risk of bleeding, particularly in older age. The HAS-BLED score reflects age-related bleeding risk, with "old age" defined as >65 years. The decision to initiate anticoagulation must integrate risks for stroke versus bleeding, as both increase with age. The frequent concomitant CHD may contribute to increased bleeding risk when dual antiplatelet agents are combined with anticoagulation. Multiple recent studies suggest the utility of using only a P2Y12 inhibitor (i.e., avoiding aspirin) in combination with warfarin[92] or a DOAC[93] with reduced bleeding events as compared with dual antiplatelet therapy.

Warfarin has been the traditional anticoagulant, with target international normalized ratio (INR) between and 2 and 2.5 recommended at older age. The estimated maintenance dose of warfarin is lower in senior adults, typically 2 to 5 mg daily, often initiated without a loading dose or with a loading dose of 5 mg. The requirements for regular INR surveillance as well as dietary limitations constitute significant challenges for older patients. Multiple drug interactions with warfarin pose added problems. Risk of osteoporosis also increases.[94] DOACs, dabigatran, rivaroxaban, apixaban, and edoxaban constitute favorable alternatives to warfarin without the need for dietary restriction or INR monitoring. Among patients ≥75 years, DOACs demonstrated similar or better stroke prevention efficacy with similar or less bleeding compared with warfarin.[95] Dose adjustment may be required based on age, body weight, and/or renal function. For older patients who are not candidates for anticoagulation, an alternative may be percutaneous left atrial appendage closure with the WATCHMAN device.[96]

Symptoms of AF may be managed by rate or rhythm control. Since rate control strategy is safer and usually as effective as pharmacologic rhythm control, it is the recommended first-line treatment in asymptomatic or mildly symptomatic patients of all ages. Class I options for achieving rate control include beta blockers and nondihydropyridine calcium channel blockers. Digoxin can aid in rate control in relatively sedentary individuals. Dronedarone is also useful. However, both nondihydropyridine calcium channel blockers and dronedarone are contraindicated in systolic HF. Given the vulnerability of older adults to medication-induced heart block, particularly with amiodarone and digitalis, the Rate Control Efficacy in Permanent Atrial Fibrillation (RACE) II trial assessed a more lenient rate control strategy. Therapy targeting heart rate <110 beats/min in older adults (Class IIb) without significant symptoms, CHD, or HF was comparable to strict rate control (<80 beats/min),[97] which may help to reduce need for cardiac pacing secondary to bradycardia.

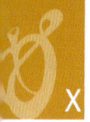

Antiarrhythmic drugs have a higher incidence of adverse events in older adults due to the potential for drug interactions, unpredictable pharmacokinetics and pharmacodynamics, and variable renal function. A rhythm control strategy was associated with increased mortality in older adults in the Atrial Fibrillation Follow-up Investigation of Rhythm Management (AFFIRM) trial.[87] Since a rhythm control strategy does not obviate the need for anticoagulation, a rate control strategy is preferable in older adults. Nonetheless, maintenance of sinus rhythm has been associated with a better QOL and many clinicians still try to restore sinus rhythm in older adults at least once.

Atrioventricular node ablation to create complete heart block with pacemaker implantation has a Class IIa recommendation to achieve a regular rhythm in symptomatic patients in whom pharmacologic therapy has failed. Catheter or surgical AF ablation are also compelling considerations. Older adults commonly have large atria and chamber fibrosis that may reduce the likelihood of restoring and maintaining sinus rhythm. Nonetheless, the Catheter Ablation vs Antiarrhythmic Drug Therapy for Atrial Fibrillation (CABANA) trial suggests the potential of catheter ablation to improve QOL in older subgroups.[98] Radiofrequency ablation in patients with atrial flutter showed the success rate (86%) was comparable in patients ≥80 years to younger patients.[99]

Supraventricular Tachycardia (SVT). Episodes of supraventricular tachycardia (SVT; see Chapter 65) (short atrial runs, atrial tachycardia, atrioventricular nodal reentrant tachycardia [AVNRT] and atrioventricular reciprocating tachycardia [AVRT]) occur in up to 50% of the older population in 24-hour monitoring studies.[85] Management is similar to younger adults. Multifocal atrial tachycardia (MAT) is especially common in the setting of decompensated pulmonary disease; patients are often quite ill and symptomatic. Management of MAT is often constrained by poor tolerance of beta blockers and amiodarone and limitation of use of nondihydropyridine calcium channel blockers when there is LV dysfunction. The best outcome is achieved by control of the underlying pulmonary disease.

Bradyarrhythmias. Bradyarrhythmias (see Chapter 68) increase with age, primarily due to sinus node dysfunction and atrioventricular (AV) block. The number of sinus node pacemaker cells decreases to <10% functional cells by age 75.[85] Medications (e.g., donepezil for dementia) compound vulnerability to bradyarrhythmias. Similarly, bradyarrhythmia may be provoked by treatment for a tachyarrhythmia (e.g., tachybrady variant of sick sinus syndrome). Hemodynamic effects may result from decreased cardiac output with dizziness, lightheadedness, falls, and syncope common sequelae, although symptoms may also include dyspnea, exercise intolerance, fatigue, or rarely chest pain. The ECG is the first diagnostic study, with a Holter monitor, event monitor, or implantable loop recorder also useful for detecting bradyarrhythmias. Assessment for chronotropic incompetence by exercise testing may be useful for patients with activity-related symptoms.

The initial management involves discontinuation of relevant medications (e.g., beta blockers, calcium channel blockers), if feasible. Presence of hypothyroidism and Lyme disease should also be considered. For persistent symptomatic bradycardia, permanent cardiac pacing is usually indicated (see Chapter 68). Greater than 75% of pacemaker implantations occur in patients age ≥65 years, with half >75 years. Pacemaker implantation has a Class I indication for sinus node dysfunction with documented symptomatic bradycardia or chronotropic incompetence, and Class II indication for symptoms at heart rate <40 beats/min.[100] Pacemaker implantation has a Class I indication for third-degree or advanced second-degree AV block with symptomatic bradycardia, an escape rhythm originating below the AV node or with a rate <40 beats/min, pauses ≥5 seconds, or after cardiac surgery without expectation for resolution.

Dual-chamber pacing improves QOL in older patents, likely because programmable pacing of both the atrial and ventricular rates improves diastolic flow and cardiac output, which are more dependent on the atrial contribution to ventricular filling in this population. Dual chamber pacing also reduces incidence of AF and decreases the rate of hospitalizations. Cardiac resynchronization therapy (CRT) has benefit for selected patients with symptomatic systolic HF (EF ≤35%) and a prolonged (≥150 msec) QRS as well as those with mild systolic dysfunction with an anticipated high pacing frequency (>40%). Class I indications for CRT are similar in older and younger patients.[100] Few patients age >75 years were enrolled in CRT trials; subgroup analyses from Cardiac Resynchronization-Heart Failure (CARE-HF), age <66 versus >66,[101] and Comparison of Medical Therapy, Pacing, and Defibrillation in Heart Failure (COMPANION), age ≤65 versus >65, suggest that older patients derive similar mortality benefit. In addition, CRT therapy improves gait speed, QOL, and frailty score in older HFrEF patients.

Ventricular Arrhythmias. Although the incidence of all ventricular arrhythmias (see Chapter 67) increases with age, sudden cardiac death (SCD) appears to decline after age 80 years, largely due to competing causes of death. No specific treatment is required for ventricular premature complexes (VPCs) in the absence of bothersome symptoms. Symptomatic VPCs often respond to low-dose beta blockade. Potentially life-threatening ventricular arrhythmias (i.e., sustained ventricular tachycardia and ventricular fibrillation) virtually always occur with structural heart disease such as ischemic or hypertensive cardiomyopathy.

Implantable Cardioverter Defibrillators and Cardiac Resynchronization Therapy: (See Chapter 69). The updated ACC/AHA/HRS 2008 Guidelines for device therapy of cardiac rhythm abnormalities do not have age-based indications and acknowledge that few clinical trials of device-based therapy have enrolled enough aged patients to reliably estimate the benefits. Relevance of comorbidities, limited life expectancy, and QOL issues are emphasized when considering ICDs for older adults.[100] In the Multicenter Automatic Defibrillator Implantation Trial (MADIT) II trial involving patients with a LVEF ≤30% and prior MI, ICD therapy improved survival in those age >70 years of age by more than 30% compared with conventional therapy. Nonetheless, the potential durability of ICD benefit is shorter and the risk of procedural complications higher in older patients. In a meta-analysis of the three major secondary prevention ICD trials (CASH, CIDS, AVID), patients ≥75 years old were more likely to die a nonarrhythmic death and there was no benefit from an ICD.[102]

The Guidelines address end-of-life issues and recommend that ICDs not be considered for patients with a life expectancy <1 year.[100] Implanting physicians are encouraged to discuss end-of-life issues before implantation and to encourage patients to complete advance directives and specifically address device management and deactivation if the patient becomes terminally ill.[103] Device deactivation in hospice care prevents multiple potentially painful shocks in terminally ill patients and may enable painless sudden death. While subcutaneous ICDs may have theoretical value for older patients, no trials of subcutaneous ICDs specifically address older adults.

VENOUS THROMBOEMBOLIC DISEASE

Epidemiology and Diagnosis

Deep vein thrombosis (DVT) and venous thromboembolism (VTE) (see Chapter 87), including pulmonary embolism (PE), increase exponentially with advancing age; increased blood thrombotic factors, limited mobility, and laxity of large venous valves contribute to risk. More than half of VTE follow surgery, injury, serious medical illness, or prolonged bed rest or occur with malignancy. A sharp increase in risk occurs after age 65, with a hazard ratio of 1.7 for every decade thereafter. Half of all patients with acute VTE are >70 years, and one-fourth are ≥80.[104] PE is more common than DVT in old age. There is increased hospital mortality with acute PE in older adults, with 1-year mortality of 39%, or 10% to 30% excess compared with younger individuals.[105]

In older adults, DVT has less typical symptoms such as lower extremity discomfort or difficulty with ambulation than at younger age, likely due to greater occurrence of proximal DVT without calf involvement. PE requires a high index of suspicion in any older patient admitted for shortness of breath. Pleuritic chest pain and hemoptysis are less common with PE than cough or syncope. Older adults with PE are more likely to have ECG abnormalities including tachycardia, $S_1Q_3T_3$, RBBB, AF, and anterior T wave abnormalities.[106]

Color flow imaging, in addition to duplex Doppler ultrasound, is highly accurate for diagnosis of DVT. D-dimer tests are highly sensitive for thrombus formation and can be used to exclude PE in patients with a low clinical probability. Application of age-adjusted cutoff values substantially increases the specificity without modifying the sensitivity.[107] In the age-adjusted D-dimer cutoff levels to rule out PE (ADJUST-PE) study, compared with a fixed D-dimer cutoff of 500 micrograms per liter, the combination of a pretest probability assessment with age-adjusted D-dimer cutoff, defined as age x 10, was associated with a larger number of patients in whom PE could be ruled out with a low likelihood of subsequent clinical VTE.[107]

Management

Aggressive VTE prophylaxis is the most important intervention, particularly early mobilization for hospitalized patients. Thromboprophylaxis with LMWH or low-dose unfractionated heparin is recommended, with extensive studies validating use in old age.[108] Fondaparinux is also effective. Intermittent pneumatic compression (IPC) and compression stockings are alternatives when anticoagulant bleeding risk is excessive, although IPC can cause skin injury, especially in frail older patients. Notably, routine use of compression stockings to prevent post-thrombotic syndrome in acute VTE is no longer recommended in the 2016 Guidelines.

The number of patients ≥75 years who require anticoagulation for DVT and VTE is rising. Management is challenging because both thrombosis and bleeding risks are high. Initial heparin therapy is requisite when starting warfarin. LMWH is preferable to unfractionated heparin because of simplicity of administration, less major bleeding risk, and lower mortality; LMWH also facilitates early hospital discharge and home management. Dose adjustment to body weight and renal function in older adults is essential. A meta-analysis of randomized trials confirmed that DOACs are associated with equal or greater efficacy than warfarin in older adults, with reduced bleeding and lower risk of VTE or VTE-related deaths.[109] Conventional anticoagulation for DVT lasts 3 months, but bleeding risks, particularly in patients >75 years and/or with concomitant cognitive impairments, falls, or other complexities often impact treatment duration. Unprovoked VTE is reasonably treated for longer duration when bleeding risk is acceptable.

Recently released American Society of Hematology guidelines recommend thromboprophylaxis in hospitalized medical patients with cancer, including LMWH or fondaparinux for surgical patients, LMWH or DOACs in ambulatory patients receiving systemic therapy at high risk of VTE, LMWH or DOAC for initial treatment of VTE, DOACs for the short-term treatment of VTE, and LMWH or DOACs for the long-term treatment of VTE.[109a]

Older adults are at high risk for PE and for adverse clinical outcomes and treatment-related complications. In an acutely ill PE patient with hypotension and hemodynamic instability, systemic thrombolysis, catheter-assisted thrombus removal or catheter-based thrombolysis are recommended.[110] For subsegmental PE and no proximal DVT, clinical surveillance is recommended rather than anticoagulation, with a low risk of recurrent VTE. However, anticoagulation is advised in patients with a high VTE risk.[108] Although the value of inferior vena cava filters (IVCFs) is controversial, an IVCF is recommended in patients with acute PE and contraindications to anticoagulation or active bleeding.

SYNCOPE

Background

Older adults are at increased risk for syncope (see Chapter 71) due to age-related changes in the CV system, including diminished baroreceptor responsiveness, impaired adrenergic responsiveness, and altered LV diastolic function, as well as increasing prevalence of CV and non-CV conditions and medications that predispose to syncope.[111] Prevalence of syncope exceeds 20% among adults aged ≥75 years; the annual incidence approaches 2% in those ≥80 years[112] and is substantially higher among nursing home residents. Prognosis of syncope worsens with age, with 2-year mortality rates of 25% to 30% in patients over 75 years. Syncope is also an important cause of injurious falls and associated disability in older adults.

Clinical Features and Etiology

The presentation of syncope is similar across the age spectrum, but older patients are less likely to recall preceding events. Amnesia for syncope is also common in older adults who fall, leading to misclassification of the etiology of falls and underdiagnosis of syncope.

Syncope in older adults is often multifactorial, reflecting the interplay between age-related CV changes, multimorbidity, and medications. Neurally-mediated syncope is the most frequent etiology in older adults, followed by orthostatic hypotension, dysautonomia, and CV etiologies. Neurally-mediated causes may be neurocardiogenic (vasovagal) or related to carotid sinus hypersensitivity (CSH), which is common in older adults although usually asymptomatic. Common causes of orthostatic hypotension and dysautonomia in older adults include diabetes, Parkinson disease, postprandial postural hypotension, dehydration, and prolonged bedrest (e.g., during hospitalization). Bradyarrhythmias due to sick sinus syndrome, conduction abnormalities, or medications are the most common cardiac causes of syncope in older adults. Supraventricular and ventricular tachyarrhythmias, as well as valvular heart disease (especially AS) and cardiomyopathies (hypertrophic cardiomyopathy, amyloid) are other important CV causes. The prognosis of cardiogenic syncope is worse than for other causes.

Evaluation

As in younger patients, a careful history is the cornerstone of the initial evaluation of syncope in older adults. However, the history in older patients may be less reliable due to impaired recall, cognitive impairment, anxiety, or medication side effects. A detailed assessment of medications is essential, including any recent changes in medications, adherence, and use of over-the-counter drugs and supplements. A complete physical examination should include measurement of heart rate and BP in the supine, sitting, and standing positions. Carotid sinus massage may be helpful if CSH is suspected.

Laboratory evaluation of syncope should be targeted to the most likely etiologies. If a cardiac cause is suspected, an echocardiogram and a period of ECG monitoring are usually appropriate. In patients with recurrent unexplained syncope, the implantable loop recorder has been associated with high diagnostic yield for an arrhythmic cause. Tilt-table testing may be helpful in evaluation of neurally-mediated syncope, but sensitivity and specificity are modest. Carotid duplex, head CT, EEG, brain MRI, and cardiac stress testing have very low diagnostic yield and should only be incorporated into the syncope evaluation in highly selected situations.[113]

Management

Management of syncope is oriented to the presumed etiology and is generally similar in younger and older patients. However, management of older patients is often complicated by age-related physiologic changes, comorbidities and geriatric syndromes, and polypharmacy. Optimal treatment of older adults requires consideration of each of these factors.

Syncope is a common cause of falls in older adults, and 35% of syncopal falls are associated with injury. Thus, a syncopal event should prompt a full evaluation of fall risk, including gait and balance testing, muscle strength, foot exam and assessment of footwear, review of predisposing medications (especially CV and psychoactive drugs) and neurologic exam to evaluate for neuropathy, Parkinson disease, and other neurologic deficits.

Numerous medications used to treat CV conditions may increase risk for syncope due to their effects on BP, heart rate, or heart rhythm. Medications that can prolong QTc, particularly when used in combination with other QTc-prolonging drugs, can induce syncope. Cholinesterase inhibitors used to treat Alzheimer disease (e.g., donepezil) may cause bradycardia, hypotension, and syncope, as can levodopa-carbidopa, a standard treatment for Parkinson disease. Alcohol, recreational drugs, and pain medications are additional potential causes of syncope. Deprescribing of potentially contributing medications, if clinically appropriate, should be considered.

Sarcopenia, frailty, malnutrition, cognitive impairment, and incontinence may contribute to syncope and should be treated as part of a holistic strategy to reduce risk of falls and syncope and improve function and QOL. Incontinence can contribute to syncope as a result of sudden standing in an attempt to get to the bathroom. Diuretics frequently exacerbate the problem, and dose adjustment is an important consideration. Referral to a geriatrician or urologist for further evaluation and management may be warranted.

PREVENTION

Efforts to prevent new or recurrent CV events in older adults center on control of modifiable factors known to facilitate development or progression of CV disease. Notably, most landmark clinical trials that established the treatment benefit included few if any individuals older than 70 to 75 years or only those without the comorbidities typically found in this age group. Competing risks for mortality from non-CV disorders may reduce the likelihood of demonstrating a survival benefit in older adults. However, benefits in respect to reducing CV events, preserving function, preserving cognition, reducing hospitalizations, and sustaining QOL are important rationales for prevention for many older adults.

Hypertension

Hypertension (see Chapter 26) is the most common CV risk factor among older men and women, with prevalence rates of ~70% in those aged 75 years and older.[10] Hypertension has the greatest population-attributable risk for CHD, cerebrovascular disease, and PAD among older adults. Over 70% of older adults with incident MI, stroke, acute aortic syndromes, and HF have preexisting hypertension. Hypertension is the most prevalent antecedent of HF, especially with preserved LVEF, and of chronic kidney disease.[5]

Before the 1980s, the age-associated elevation of SBP in older adults was generally considered a normal finding that did not warrant treatment. However, numerous observational studies have since documented that elevated SBP confers increased risk for CV morbidity and mortality.[114] After age 70 years, isolated systolic hypertension (ISH) accounts for >90% of all patients with hypertension.[10]

Multiple clinical trials in older cohorts have shown benefits of hypertension treatment.[115] Although only two trials showed significant reductions in total mortality, several showed substantial reductions in stroke and HF. The landmark HYpertension in the Very Elderly Trial (HYVET) demonstrated a 39% significant decrease in fatal stroke, 21% significant decrease in all-cause mortality, and 64% significant decrease in HF over 1.8 years mean follow-up in 3845 patients ≥80 years old with systolic BP ≥160 mm Hg treated with the thiazide-like diuretic indapamide to a target BP of 150/80 mm Hg versus placebo.[116] More recently, the Systolic Blood Pressure Intervention Trial (SPRINT) showed a 34% reduction in CV events and 33% reduction in mortality in 2636 patients aged ≥75 years with SBP >130 mm Hg randomized to a target of 120 mm Hg versus 140 mm Hg.[117] Based in part on these findings, the 2017 Update to the Hypertension Guidelines Committee recommended a target BP ≤130 mm Hg for persons in this age group.[114] In older patients with CHD, however, excessive lowering of DBP should be avoided to avert deleterious reductions in coronary blood flow. Some studies have found higher CHD rates when diastolic BP is reduced below 60 to 65 mm Hg.

Hypertension Management

Nonpharmacologic interventions are recommended as initial therapy to manage mild hypertension (see Chapter 26). Such an approach is especially useful in older adults to avoid or reduce the number and doses of antihypertensive drugs and their potential for adverse effects, biochemical changes, and high costs. For milder hypertension, lifestyle modifications may be the only treatment needed. These include aerobic exercise; reductions in excess body weight, mental stress, and intake of sodium and alcohol; smoking cessation; and adoption of the Dietary Approaches to Stop Hypertension (DASH) eating plan.[114]

Current guidelines recommend four major classes of antihypertensive drugs as first-line therapy: diuretics, ACEI, ARB, and calcium channel blockers. Two or more drugs will be required to achieve target BP levels in approximately two-thirds of seniors with hypertension. Combination therapy often allows lower individual drug dosages, minimizing dose-dependent side effects, and achieving longer duration of action and additive target organ protection,[114] although it also contributes to polypharmacy. The choice of specific agents is dictated by efficacy, tolerability, specific comorbidities, and cost. Given the age-related predisposition to orthostatic hypotension and changes in absorption, distribution, metabolism, and excretion of pharmacologic agents, therapy in older adults is best initiated at the lowest doses with gradual increments as tolerated. It is also important to assess resultant BP both seated and standing.

Dyslipidemia

Dyslipidemia (see Chapter 27) remains an important CV risk factor in older adults, although the relative risk imparted by lipid disorders may be attenuated compared with younger populations. Multiple cohort studies have shown that both total cholesterol and low density lipoprotein cholesterol (LDL-C) correlated significantly with fatal CHD in both sexes across a broad age range, including adults ≥65 years but with very few ≥80.[118] Despite the voluminous literature demonstrating reduction in CV events in both primary and secondary prevention populations receiving medications to lower LDL-C (primarily statins), the majority of patients in these trials were age <65 years old, with smaller enrollments in predominantly younger strata of older adults (Table 90.4).[40]

TABLE 90.4 Lipid Lowering Trials Supporting Secondary Prevention in Older Adults

TRIAL NAME	MEDICATION	N	AGE RANGE (YEAR)	% OLDER PATIENTS	FOLLOW-UP (YEARS)	OUTCOMES
4S	Simvastatin	4444	35-70	≥65 years (23%)	5.4	• 34% RRR in all-cause mortality
						• 34% RRR in MACE
HPS	Simvastatin	20,536	40-80	≥70 years (29%)	5	• 25% RRR in death or MI
CARE	Pravastatin	4159	21-75	≥65 years (31%)	5	• 24% RRR in death or MI
LIPID	Pravastatin	9014	31-75	≥65 years (36%)	6.1	• 24% RRR in all-cause mortality and cardiac mortality
						• 29% RRR in nonfatal MI
						• 20% RRR in coronary revascularization
PROSPER	Pravastatin	2565	70-82	≥70 years (100%)	3.2	• 20% RRR in CHD, nonfatal MI, and stroke*
TNT	Atorvastatin	10,001	35-75	≥65 years (38%)	4.9	• 19% RRR in composite endpoint of MACE, CHD-related death, nonfatal MI, or stroke
SAGE	Pravastatin vs. Atorvastatin	893	65-85	≥65 years (100%)	1	• 29% RRR in MACE and 67% RRR in death in atorvastatin group
ODYSSEY	Alirocumab	18,924	≥40	≥65 years (27%)	2.8	• 15% RRR in MACE with alirocumab
REDUCE-IT	Icosapent ethyl	8179	≥45	>65 years (46%)	4.9	• 25% RRR in MACE with icosapent ethyl

*Benefit was in the secondary prevention cohort with no benefit for the primary prevention cohort.
CHD, Coronary heart disease; MACE, major adverse cardiovascular events; MI, myocardial infarction; RRR, relative risk reduction.

Based on the available data, the 2018 ACC/AHA Prevention Guidelines continue to recommend statin therapy, designed to lower LDL-C by 30% to 49%, in patients older than 75 years with known CV disease and LDL-C of 70 to 189 mg/dL.[40] Recommendations are supported by data showing benefit in reducing major adverse CV events (MACE), including mortality, MI, strokes, and PAD for those expected to live sufficiently long to derive benefit. While recommendations differ from recommendations to initiate high-intensity statin therapy in adults 40 to 75 years old (with goals to lower LDL-C at least 50%), they do not recommend lowering doses when an older adult is already taking a high-dose statin and tolerating it well. High-intensity statin therapy is recommended for individuals with LDL-C ≥190 mg/dL regardless of age. In older individuals with CVD and LDL-C 70 to 189 mg/dL, the potential benefit of long-term statin therapy must be weighed against cost, inconvenience, and possible side effects. The Guidelines indicate that it may be reasonable to stop statin therapy when functional decline, multimorbidity, frailty, or reduced life expectancy limits the potential benefits of statin therapy.

The benefits of statins for primary prevention in older adults are less clear. In a meta-analysis of 28 statin trials involving over 186,000 patients, the proportional reduction in major vascular events was similar, irrespective of age, among patients with preexisting vascular disease, but appeared smaller among older than among younger individuals not known to have vascular disease (P trend = 0.05).[119] A recent propensity-adjusted analysis in a study of over 300,000 veterans age ≥75 years (mean 81.1 years, 97% men) without known atherosclerotic cardiovascular disease (ASCVD) stands out by showing that statin use was associated with significant reductions in all-cause mortality (25%), CV mortality (20%), and composite ASCVD events (8%).[120] Findings were consistent across subgroups by age, including patients age ≥90 years. While the 2018 Guidelines currently provide only a Class IIb recommendation for statin therapy as primary prevention in older adults,[40] the Pragmatic Evaluation of Events and Benefits of Lipid-Lowering in Older Adults (PREVENTABLE) trial is expected to provide better data to guide management (NCT04262206).

The most common side effect observed with statins is myalgia, which occurs in about 5% of patients. Myopathy documented by elevated muscle enzyme levels is much less common, occurring in 0.01% to 0.05%. The most severe adverse effect, rhabdomyolysis, has an incidence of 3.4/100,000 person-years. Age is not an independent risk factor for these complications.

In older patients intolerant of statins or who cannot achieve their LDL-C goal on maximally tolerated statin doses, ezetimibe may be a useful adjunct. Ezetimibe reduces cholesterol absorption from the gut, generally reducing LDL-C 15% to 20%. Ezetimibe is generally well tolerated in older adults, though it reduced CV events by a modest 6% in the Improved Reduction of Outcomes: Vytorin Efficacy International Trial (IMPROVE-IT).[121]

Proprotein convertase subtilisin–kexin type 9 (PCSK9) inhibition represents another option to substantially lower LDL-C levels in patients who do not achieve guideline-recommended goals. In the Evaluation of Cardiovascular Outcomes After an Acute Coronary Syndrome During Treatment with Alirocumab (ODYSSEY OUTCOMES) trial, the PCSK9 inhibitor alirocumab added to high-intensity or maximum-tolerated statin treatment, reduced the primary composite endpoint of death from CHD, nonfatal MI, ischemic stroke, or unstable angina requiring hospitalization compared with placebo in 18,924 patients with a recent ACS. The 15% reduction in CV events was similar across age groups, including individuals ≥75 years old,[122] and adverse effects were not increased relative to placebo. Similar findings have been reported with evolocumab.[123] This newer drug class therefore represents an important advance in reducing CV events in older adults with CHD, although the current high cost is an impediment. Although fibrates are sometimes used to raise low HDL-C or to reduce elevated triglycerides, evidence supporting their benefit in reducing CVD events is sparse. The combination of gemfibrozil and statins is associated with an increased risk of rhabdomyolysis (0.12%) and should usually be avoided, especially in older adults. Niacin (nicotinic acid), the most effective drug available to raise HDL-C, also reduces elevated triglycerides but showed no benefit in reducing CV events in clinical trials. In the REDUCE-IT trial, icosapent ethyl, a highly purified eicosapentaenoic acid ethyl ester, lowered elevated triglyceride levels an average of 18% and reduced major CV events by 25%. However, the benefit was blunted in patients ≥65 years (HR = 0.87) compared with those <65 years (HR = 0.65), interaction P = 0.004.[124]

Diabetes

Advancing age is accompanied by reduced insulin sensitivity and secretion, contributing to greater glucose intolerance and higher rates of type 2 diabetes mellitus (see Chapter 31) in older adults. Approximately 15% of adults ≥65 years have been diagnosed diabetes, and in another 7% diabetes is undiagnosed.[118] An estimated 30% of older adults with diabetes have clinical CHD, double the prevalence in age-matched nondiabetics. Older adults with diabetes and CVD are at high risk for adverse macrovascular and microvascular outcomes as well as functional disability and geriatric syndromes (e.g., frailty and falls).

The primary treatment goals for older adults with diabetes include managing hyperglycemia and reducing risk of adverse clinical outcomes. Lifestyle modification is paramount. Weight loss can reduce insulin resistance and improve glycemic control. Dietary interventions that optimize macronutrient content as well as calorie count help improve glycemic control, independent of weight change. Regular aerobic and resistance exercise lower HbA_{1c} by 0.5% to 1.0% in older adults, even without changes in body weight or fat mass.

Despite the benefits of lifestyle interventions, most older patients with diabetes require medications to achieve glycemic control. Because several large clinical trials have found either no effect or even increased mortality in older patients receiving intensive glycemic therapy, a less intensive target HbA_{1c} of 7% to 7.9% is recommended for most older adults, especially those with longstanding diabetes and chronic comorbidities including CVD. Even higher targets may be considered for older patients with frailty or short life expectancy.[125]

Metformin has been favored as a first-line therapy due to its low risk for hypoglycemia and other adverse effects. Additional options include the short-acting sulfonylurea, glipizide, and the short-acting insulin secretagogue, repaglinide.[118] Two new agents worthy of consideration are the sodium-glucose cotransporter 2 inhibitors and the glucagon-like peptide-1 analogues, which reduced CV events in large RCTs. The reduced CV risk with empagliflozin was especially prominent in patients ≥65 years old.[126] If insulin therapy is needed, ultra-long-acting basal and very-short-acting prandial insulins are strongly preferred over intermediate-acting insulin formulations. Although tighter glycemic control in diabetes may help to avoid microvascular complications, greater CV risk reduction may be achieved from control of concurrent risk factors such as hypertension and dyslipidemia.[118]

Tobacco

Although only 8.4% of Americans ≥65 years were current smokers in 2018, 49.4% of men and 30.6% of women ≥65 years were former smokers.[5] Numerous studies have demonstrated that continued smoking increases the rate for recurrent coronary and vascular events in both younger and older patients; reduced CV event rates are seen among those who quit smoking. Over 12 years of follow-up, older men in the Oslo II study who quit smoking between screenings had 31% lower mortality than those who smoked at both screening visits.[127] A meta-analysis of 17 general population studies in over 1.2 million persons age ≥60 years from seven countries showed dose-dependent increased all-cause mortality rates in current smokers, with a mean relative mortality of 1.83 compared with never-smokers. Among former smokers, the mortality risk was attenuated to 1.34. Risk reduction from smoking cessation was seen even in persons age ≥80 years.[128] In a registry of patients with CHD, mortality rate was markedly lower in recent quitters than in persistent smokers. Smoking cessation also reduces the risk of new or recurrent stroke and improves claudication symptoms.

Physical Inactivity

Physical inactivity (see Chapter 25) is a well-established risk factor for multiple chronic diseases, including hypertension, type 2 diabetes, CHD, stroke, PAD, depression, osteoporosis, and certain cancers. Physical inactivity is also associated with increased CV mortality.[118] Because the biologic and clinical repercussions of a sedentary lifestyle exacerbate age-related pathophysiologic changes, the health consequences and societal costs of physical inactivity are especially relevant to older adults. Physical inactivity results in decreased functional capacity, increased risk of falling, worsened psychological status, and reduced cognitive function. In older adults, decreased physical activity constitutes the most common modifiable CV risk factor after hypertension. Only 18% of persons ≥75 years old report regular moderate or vigorous physical activity, and only 14% of men and 8% of women ≥65 years old report aerobic and muscle strengthening activities that meet the 2008 Federal physical activity guidelines. Patel et al. reported increased total mortality, especially CV mortality, over 14-year follow-up in men and women 50 to 74 years old who sat >6 hours/day compared with those sitting only 3 hours/day[129]; similar findings have been reported in other studies.[118]

Numerous observational studies and RCTs demonstrate that older adults benefit from initiating an exercise program; benefits include greater functional capacity, cognitive and psychological functioning, less mobility disability, better QOL, reduced recurrent CV events, and an increase in active life expectancy.[118] Consistently, regular physical activity mitigates CHD risk factors (including body weight, BP, serum lipids, and insulin sensitivity), improves bone density, and improves muscular strength, all key elements of health and well-being in older adults.[118] Even modest physical activity in older adults has been associated with lower CV risk.[130]

Physical Activity Prescription

The most important considerations when counseling regarding physical activity is to help shape a program that is pleasurable and achievable and that avoids injury or exacerbation of comorbid problems. Aerobics, strength, balance, and flexibility are all vital components. For adults willing to enter a formal exercise program, specific exercises can help improve tolerance of the physical demands of daily living and recreational activities. Generally, work intensities start lower than in younger patients, with smaller increments over time, especially in those with significant comorbidities that limit mobility (e.g., arthritis, pulmonary disease, and PAD). Increasing frequency and duration of exercise sessions should supersede increases in intensity to reduce the potential for overuse injuries. For adults who are disinclined to exercise in a program, increasing activity as part of daily living is also beneficial. Regular leisure activities such as walking, yoga, and gardening are all healthful.

Accumulating evidence suggests that activity benefits may increase in proportion to intensity. Reports in patients with established heart disease, including one study of patients with a mean age of 75 years, suggest that high intensity aerobic interval training can elicit greater improvement in exercise capacity than continuous exercise at a lower intensity.[118] Despite these encouraging data, such training is more complex than traditional training, necessitating more supervision for implementation and safety. Larger studies are needed to establish the efficacy and safety of high intensity interval training in older patients.

Cardiac Rehabilitation

Cardiac rehabilitation (CR; see Chapter 33) consists of structured exercise training combined with secondary prevention reinforcement, including individualized exercise prescription as well as close supervision and support.[118] It can be particularly helpful in catalyzing physical activity and wellness in adults who are sedentary amidst illness, deconditioning, and entrenched behavior patterns. Older adults with CHD who participated in supervised CR experienced 21% to 34% lower mortality than nonusers over the subsequent 5 years, independent of other risk factors.[131] Patients also benefit in increased physical capacity, independence, and self-efficacy after a hospitalization and/or CVD exacerbation, mitigating risks of posthospitalization disability.[49] Unfortunately, the vast majority of older patients do not participate in CR due to multiple factors, including lack of referral, logistical barriers, or socioeconomic barriers. Failure to refer, particularly for women, is a major contributor to the low participation of older adults. Participation in CR by Medicare eligible recipients is only ~12%.[118] Growing utilization of home-based CR may increase participation for some older adults, but geriatric complexities (e.g., frailty, cognitive impairments) may make home-based options more difficult for others.

Obesity (see Chapter 30)

An estimated two-thirds of seniors are overweight (body mass index [BMI] 25 to 30 kg/m^2) or obese (BMI ≥30 kg/m^2), closely paralleling rates in the general population. Data from NHANES suggest that 35% of noninstitutionalized women and 40% of men 65 to 74 years old are obese, as well as 27% of women and 26% of men ≥75 years.[5] Between 1988 and 1994 and from 2007 to 2008, obesity rates increased 30% to 40% in older women and 67% to 100% in older men.

Although overweight and obesity are associated with mildly increased mortality,[5] the risk ratio decreases as age advances. In obese patients with established CVD, multiple studies have demonstrated an obesity paradox; overweight and obese patients show greater survival than those of normal weight. Similar findings have been observed in older populations with CVD, but most of these studies have not differentiated between fat and lean mass, which likely plays an important role in health effects in old age. Sarcopenic obesity in an older adult does not confer mortality benefit.[132]

Diet (see Chapter 29)

Undernutrition is more common in older than younger individuals due to a combination of medical and socioeconomic factors: 5% to 10% of community dwelling persons aged >70 years are undernourished and prevalence increases to 30% to 65% in institutionalized older adults. Vitamin and mineral deficiencies are common in seniors due to inadequate intake, decreased absorption, and the effects of disease and medications. Vitamin D deficiency is particularly common in older adults due to low sunlight exposure and reduced synthesis by the skin and has been associated with increased CV mortality.[118] However, of the value of vitamin D supplementation remains unsubstantiated.[133]

It is useful for cardiologists and primary care providers to assess dietary intake of older patients, provide general dietary advice, and refer to a nutritionist if major dietary deficiencies or malnutrition are suspected. The Mediterranean diet (i.e., fruits, vegetables, whole grains, and nuts plus low intake of saturated fat) has been associated with beneficial effects on CV risk factors and outcomes in both older and younger adults. Some of these benefits may derive from flavonoids, which are abundant in fruits, vegetables, nuts, tea, and wine, and have anti-inflammatory and antioxidant effects. Higher flavonoid intake was associated with a lower risk of CV death in a population of 98,000 adults of initial mean age 70 years.[134]

NONCARDIAC SURGERY AND PERIOPERATIVE MANAGEMENT CONSIDERATIONS IN OLDER ADULTS

Background

As the population ages, the number of older adults undergoing surgical interventions has increased markedly and continues to expand. Physiologic age-related changes in all organ systems in conjunction with increasing comorbidity contribute to higher risk for perioperative complications and increase complexity of perioperative management in older patients. These factors should be considered in relation to the potential benefits of a surgical procedure and in the context of the older patient's overall goals of care. Patients should be encouraged to develop an advance directive and identify a health care proxy. Suspending a do-not-resuscitate designation is common during procedures, but management plans should be clarified in case there is a serious adverse event. Practice guidelines for optimal preoperative assessment and perioperative care of older adults undergoing surgery have been developed by the American College of Surgeons (ACS) in collaboration with the American Geriatrics Society (AGS).[135]

Risk Assessment

Several tools to evaluate risk of perioperative CV complications have been developed and validated. However, most of these instruments fail to consider geriatric conditions, including sarcopenia, frailty, functional limitations, multimorbidity, and cognitive impairment that heighten risk for adverse CV and non-CV outcomes following major surgery. Thus, the ACS/AGS Guideline for preoperative evaluation recommends that, in addition to CV risk assessment, older adults should be screened for history of falls, functional impairment, cognitive impairment, nutritional status, depression, and alcohol or substance abuse.[135]

Gait speed, as assessed by a timed walk over a measured distance (e.g., 5 meters), is a marker of frailty that has been shown to predict adverse surgical outcomes beyond standard assessments. Slow gait speed (<0.8 m/sec) adds significantly to conventional risk scores, such as the STS score,[15] and patients unable to perform the gait speed test are at highest surgical risk.

Perioperative Management

Age-related changes alter drug pharmacodynamics and pharmacokinetics, rendering older patients more vulnerable to anesthetic and analgesic complications. Although regional (epidural) anesthesia does not decrease mortality or risk of postoperative delirium or cognitive dysfunction, it is associated with better peripheral vascular circulation, less blood loss, improved pain control, reduced ileus, attenuation of thromboembolic complications, fewer respiratory complications, reduced postoperative narcotic requirements, and reduced surgical stress response.

Specific Complications

In addition to increased risk for cardiopulmonary complications following surgery, older adults are at risk for delirium, falls, functional and cognitive decline, urinary tract infections, acute kidney injury, poor nutrition, bowel disorders, pressure ulcers, hypothermia, and venous thromboembolism.[136]

Delirium, an acute decline in orientation and attention, occurs in up to 50% of older adults undergoing major surgery, and in over 80% of those who require mechanical ventilation in an ICU. Postoperative delirium is associated with increased length of stay and costs, falls, functional and cognitive decline, and mortality. An estimated 30% to 40% of delirium is avoidable through nonpharmacologic measures, including maintaining a normal sleep/wake cycle, presence of family, early mobilization, provision of hearing and vision aids, avoidance of restraints, and adequate hydration and pain management. It is essential to avoid deliriogenic medications, especially benzodiazepines and related drugs, antihistamines, and anticholinergics. The primary treatment for delirium involves correction of avoidable factors predisposing to its development. Short-term use of low-dose antipsychotic medication may be used to treat agitated or distressed patients who pose a risk of harm to themselves or others.

Postoperative cognitive dysfunction (POCD) entails deterioration in memory and executive function in the days to weeks after surgery, but confusion is not usually present. Incidence following major surgery has been reported to be >50%, but several studies suggest that POCD may reflect unrecognized baseline cognitive deficiencies,[42] highlighting the need for thorough preoperative assessments. POCD is associated with increased hospital stay and diminished QOL.

Decubitus ulcers are also common in older surgical patients. Risks include loss of subcutaneous tissue and decreased elasticity of the aged skin that predispose to damaged superficial tissues when skin is compressed for prolonged periods. There may be secondary infection, delayed recovery, and prolonged hospitalization, often with discharge to a transitional care facility. Preventive measures include routine postoperative skin examination, frequent repositioning, use of pressure redistributing support surfaces, pressure-relieving overlays in the operating room, and use of foam alternatives and heel protectors.

Older adults are susceptible to hypothermia due to impaired central and peripheral thermoregulatory function and the effects of anesthesia. It is particularly common among underweight or frail older adults and may contribute to electrolyte abnormalities, platelet dysfunction, increased risk for wound infection, and impaired drug metabolism. Warming to a core temperature of about 36°C is recommended with correction of electrolyte abnormalities.

Over 30% of hospitalized older adults experience functional decline during admission, and fewer than 50% return to their prior level of function within 1 year after discharge. Early mobilization is vital to minimize deconditioning, frailty, and sarcopenia. Early mobilization has also been associated with improved cardiac output and hemodynamics and reduced bone loss, hypocalcemia, joint contractures, constipation, incontinence, DVT, pressure ulcers, sensory deprivation, atelectasis, hypoxemia, pneumonia, depression, delirium, anxiety, and insomnia.

Postoperative aspiration pneumonia is also common, with risks compounded by cognitive decline, delirium, and sedation. Urinary tract infections and acute kidney injury can be minimized by avoiding nephrotoxins and urinary catheters and maintaining hydration.

Discharge Planning

Risk assessment at discharge must include consideration of hospitalization-associated disability, frailty, deconditioning, malnutrition, and altered cognition; all may provoke loss of independence and a cycle of functional decline. Postdischarge rehabilitation is critical whether delivered by home health or physical therapy and in an SNF or a rehabilitation facility.

REFERENCES

General Considerations

1. Ortman JV, Velkoff VA, Hogan H. The Older Population in the United States. http://www.censu s.gov/library/publications/2014/demo/p25-1140.html.
2. https://www.cia.gov/library/publications/the-world-factbook/fields/341.html.
3. Domanski MJ, Tian X, Wu CO, et al. Time course of LDL cholesterol exposure and cardiovascular disease event risk. *J Am Coll Cardiol*. 2020;76(13):1507–1516.
4. Lakatta EG. So! What's aging? Is cardiovascular aging a disease? *J Mol Cell Cardiol*. 2015;83:1–13.
5. Mozaffarian D, Benjamin EJ, Go AS, et al. Heart disease and stroke Statistics 2016 update: a report from the American heart association. *Circulation*. 2016;133(4):e38–360.
6. Forman DE, Maurer MS, Boyd C, et al. Multimorbidity in older adults with cardiovascular disease. *J Am Coll Cardiol*. 2018;71(19):2149–2161.
7. Forman DE, Arena R, Boxer R, et al. Prioritizing functional capacity as a principal end point for therapies oriented to older adults with cardiovascular disease: a scientific statement for Healthcare Professionals from the American heart association. *Circulation*. 2017;135(16):e894–e918.
8. Paneni F, Diaz Cañestro C, et al. The aging cardiovascular system: understanding it at the cellular and clinical levels. *J Am Coll Cardiol*. 2017;69(15):1952–1967.
9. Ferrucci L, Fabbri E. Inflammageing: chronic inflammation in ageing, cardiovascular disease, and frailty. *Nat Rev Cardiol*. 2018;15(9):505–522.
10. Aronow WS, Fleg JL, Pepine CJ, et al. ACCF/AHA 2011 expert consensus document on hypertension in the elderly: a report of the American College of cardiology Foundation Task Force on clinical expert consensus documents. *Circulation*. 2011;123(21):2434–2506.
11. Fleg JL, Strait J. Age-associated changes in cardiovascular structure and function: a fertile milieu for future disease. *Heart Fail Rev*. 2012;17(4–5):545–554.
12. Addison O, Marcus RL, Lastayo PC, Ryan AS. Intermuscular fat: a review of the consequences and causes. *Int J Endocrinol*. 2014;2014:309570.
13. Kitzman DW, Nicklas B, Kraus WE, et al. Skeletal muscle abnormalities and exercise intolerance in older patients with heart failure and preserved ejection fraction. *Am J Physiol Heart Circ Physiol*. 2014;306(9):H1364–H1370.
14. Arnett DK, Goodman RA, Halperin JL, et al. AHA/ACC/HHS strategies to enhance application of clinical practice guidelines in patients with cardiovascular disease and comorbid conditions: from the American Heart Association, American College of Cardiology, and U.S. Department of Health and Human Services. *J Am Coll Cardiol*. 2014;64(17):1851–1856.
15. Afilalo J, Alexander KP, Mack MJ, et al. Frailty assessment in the cardiovascular care of older adults. *J Am Coll Cardiol*. 2014;63(8):747–762.
16. Boccardi V, Mecocci P. The importance of cellular senescence in frailty and cardiovascular diseases. *Adv Exp Med Biol*. 2020;1216:79–86.
17. Forman DE, Alexander KP. Frailty: a vital sign for older adults with cardiovascular disease. *Can J Cardiol*. 2016;32(9):1082–1087.
18. Harada CN, Natelson Love MC, Triebel KL. Normal cognitive aging. *Clin Geriatr Med*. 2013;29(4):737–752.
19. Justin BN, Turek M, Hakim AM. Heart disease as a risk factor for dementia. *Clin Epidemiol*. 2013;5:135–145.
20. Marcantonio ER. Delirium in hospitalized older adults. *N Engl J Med*. 2017;377(15):1456–1466.
21. Damluji AA, Forman DE, van Diepen S, et al. Older adults in the cardiac intensive care unit: factoring geriatric syndromes in the management, prognosis, and process of care: a scientific statement from the American Heart Association. *Circulation*. 2020;141(2):e6–e32.

Medication Consideration

22. Schwartz JB, Schmader KE, Hanlon JT, et al. Pharmacotherapy in older adults with cardiovascular disease: report from an American College of cardiology, American geriatrics society, and National Institute on aging Workshop. *J Am Geriatr Soc*. 2019;67(2):371–380.
23. Allen LA, Fonarow GC, Liang L, et al. Medication initiation burden required to comply with heart failure guideline recommendations and hospital quality measures. *Circulation*. 2015;132(14):1347–1353.
24. Budnitz DS, Lovegrove MC, Shehab N, Richards CL. Emergency hospitalizations for adverse drug events in older Americans. *N Engl J Med*. 2011;365(21):2002–2012.
25. Rossello X, Pocock SJ, Julian DG. Long-term Use of cardiovascular drugs: challenges for Research and for patient care. *J Am Coll Cardiol*. 2015;66(11):1273–1285.
26. Krumholz HM. Post-hospital syndrome–an acquired, transient condition of generalized risk. *N Engl J Med*. 2013;368(2):100–102.
27. McNeil JJ, Woods RL, Nelson MR, et al. Effect of aspirin on disability-free survival in the healthy elderly. *N Engl J Med*. 2018;379(16):1499–1508.

Management Precepts

28. Rich MW, Chyun DA, Skolnick AH, et al. Knowledge Gaps in cardiovascular care of the older adult population: a scientific statement from the American heart association, American College of cardiology, and American geriatrics society. *Circulation*. 2016;133(21):2103–2122.
29. Boyd C, Smith CD, Masoudi FA, et al. Decision making for older adults with multiple chronic conditions: executive summary for the American geriatrics society guiding principles on the care of older adults with multimorbidity. *J Am Geriatr Soc*. 2019;67(4):665–673.
30. American geriatrics society 2019 updated AGS Beers Criteria® for potentially inappropriate medication use in older adults. *J Am Geriatr Soc*. 2019;67(4):674–694.
31. Tomlinson J, Cheong VL, Fylan B, et al. Successful care transitions for older people: a systematic review and meta-analysis of the effects of interventions that support medication continuity. *Age Ageing*. 2020;49(4):558–569.
32. Sullivan MF, Kirkpatrick JN. Palliative cardiovascular care: the right patient at the right time. *Clin Cardiol*. 2020;43(2):205–212.
33. Meyers DE, Goodlin SJ. End-of-Life decisions and palliative care in advanced heart failure. *Can J Cardiol*. 2016;32(9):1148–1156.

Ischemic Heart Disease

34. Krishnaswami A, Steinman MA, Goyal P, et al. Deprescribing in older adults with cardiovascular disease. *J Am Coll Cardiol*. 2019;73(20):2584–2595.
35. Moran AE, Forouzanfar MH, Roth GA, et al. Temporal trends in ischemic heart disease mortality in 21 world regions, 1980 to 2010: the Global Burden of Disease 2010 study. *Circulation*. 2014;129(14):1483–1492.
36. Mortensen MB, Fuster V, Muntendam P, et al. A simple disease-guided approach to personalize ACC/AHA-Recommended statin allocation in elderly people: the BioImage study. *J Am Coll Cardiol*. 2016;68(9):881–891.
37. Douglas PS, Hoffmann U. Outcomes of anatomical versus functional testing for coronary artery disease. *N Engl J Med*. 2015;372(1):1291–1300.
38. Maron DJ, Hochman JS, Reynolds HR, et al. Initial invasive or conservative strategy for stable coronary disease. *N Engl J Med*. 2020;382(15):1395–1407.
39. Forman DE, de Lemos JA, Shaw LJ, et al. Cardiovascular biomarkers and imaging in older adults: JACC Council Perspectives. *J Am Coll Cardiol*. 2020;76(13):1577–1594.
40. Grundy SM, Stone NJ, Bailey AL, et al. 2018 AHA/ACC/AACVPR/AAPA/ABC/ACPM/ADA/AGS/APhA/ASPC/NLA/PCNA guideline on the management of blood cholesterol: a report of the American College of cardiology/American heart association Task Force on clinical practice guidelines. *Circulation*. 2019;139(25):e1082–e1143.
41. Madhavan MV, Gersh BJ, Alexander KP, et al. Coronary artery disease in patients ≥80 Years of age. *J Am Coll Cardiol*. 2018;71(18):2015–2040.
42. Selnes OA, Gottesman RF, Grega MA, et al. Cognitive and neurologic outcomes after coronary-artery bypass surgery. *N Engl J Med*. 2012;366(3):250–257.
43. Bairey Merz CN, Pepine CJ, Walsh MN, Fleg JL. Ischemia and No obstructive coronary artery disease (INOCA): developing evidence-based therapies and Research Agenda for the Next decade. *Circulation*. 2017;135(11):1075–1092.
44. Virani SS, Alonso A, Benjamin EJ, et al. Heart disease and stroke statistics-2020 update: a report from the American Heart Association. *Circulation*. 2020;141(9):e139–e596.
45. Dai X, Busby-Whitehead J, Alexander KP. Acute coronary syndrome in the older adults. *J Geriatr Cardiol*. 2016;13(2):101–108.
46. Tegn N, Abdelnoor M, Aaberge L, et al. Invasive versus conservative strategy in patients aged 80 years or older with non-ST-elevation myocardial infarction or unstable angina pectoris (After Eighty study): an open-label randomised controlled trial. *Lancet*. 2016;387(10023):1057–1065.
47. Ravi V, Pulipati P, Vij A, Kodumuri V. Meta-analysis comparing double versus triple antithrombotic therapy in patients with atrial fibrillation and coronary artery disease. *Am J Cardiol*. 2020;125(1):19–28.
48. Lopes RD, Heizer G, Aronson R, et al. Antithrombotic therapy after acute coronary syndrome or PCI in atrial fibrillation. *N Engl J Med*. 2019;380(16):1509–1524.
49. Schopfer DW, Forman DE. Cardiac rehabilitation in older adults. *Can J Cardiol*. 2016;32(9):1088–1096.

Heart Failure

50. Gorodeski EZ, Goyal P, Hummel SL, et al. Domain management approach to heart failure in the geriatric patient: present and future. *J Am Coll Cardiol*. 2018;71(17):1921–1936.
51. Upadhya B, Kitzman DW. Heart failure with preserved ejection fraction: new approaches to diagnosis and management. *Clin Cardiol*. 2020;43(2):145–155.
52. Paulus WJ, Tschope C. A novel paradigm for heart failure with preserved ejection fraction: comorbidities drive myocardial dysfunction and remodeling through coronary microvascular endothelial inflammation. *J Am Coll Cardiol*. 2013;62(4):263–271.
53. Mogensen UM, Ersboll M, Andersen M, et al. Clinical characteristics and major comorbidities in heart failure patients more than 85 years of age compared with younger age groups. *Eur J Heart Fail*. 2011;13(11):1216–1223.
54. Pirmohamed A, Kitzman DW, Maurer MS. Heart failure in older adults: embracing complexity. *J Geriatr Cardiol*. 2016;13(1):8–14.
55. Paterna S, Gaspare P, Fasullo S, et al. Normal-sodium diet compared with low-sodium diet in compensated congestive heart failure: is sodium an old enemy or a new friend? *Clin Sci (Lond)*. 2008;114(3):221–230.
56. Yancy CW, Jessup M, Bozkurt B, et al. 2013 ACCF/AHA guideline for the management of heart failure: a report of the American College of cardiology Foundation/American heart association Task Force on practice guidelines. *J Am Coll Cardiol*. 2013;62(16):e147–239.
57. Forman DE, Sanderson BK, Josephson RA, et al. Heart failure as a newly approved diagnosis for cardiac rehabilitation: challenges and opportunities. *J Am Coll Cardiol*. 2015;65(24):2652–2659.
58. Takeda A, Martin N, Taylor RS, Taylor SJ. Disease management interventions for heart failure. *Cochrane Database Syst Rev*. 2019;1(1):Cd002752.
59. Adamson PB, Abraham WT, Stevenson LW, et al. Pulmonary artery pressure-guided heart failure management reduces 30-day readmissions. *Circ Heart Fail*. 2016;9(6).
60. Jhund PS, Fu M, Bayram E, et al. Efficacy and safety of LCZ696 (sacubitril-valsartan) according to age: insights from PARADIGM-HF. *Eur Heart J*. 2015;36(38):2576–2584.
61. Martinez FA, Serenelli M, Nicolau JC, et al. Efficacy and safety of dapagliflozin in heart failure with reduced ejection fraction according to age: insights from DAPA-HF. *Circulation*. 2020;141(2):100–111.
62. Packer M, Anker SD, Butler J, et al. Cardiovascular and renal outcomes with empagliflozin in heart failure. *N Engl J Med*. 2020.
63. Kim JH, Singh R, Pagani FD, et al. Ventricular assist device therapy in older patients with heart failure: characteristics and outcomes. *J Card Fail*. 2016;22(12):981–987.
64. Petrie MC, Jhund PS, She L, et al. Ten-year outcomes after coronary artery bypass grafting according to age in patients with heart failure and left ventricular systolic dysfunction: an analysis of the extended follow-up of the STICH trial (surgical treatment for ischemic heart failure). *Circulation*. 2016;134(18):1314–1324.
65. Pitt B, Pfeffer MA, Assmann SF, et al. Spironolactone for heart failure with preserved ejection fraction. *N Engl J Med*. 2014;370(15):1383–1392.
66. Pfeffer MA, Claggett B, Assmann SF, et al. Regional variation in patients and outcomes in the treatment of preserved cardiac function heart failure with an aldosterone antagonist (TOP-CAT) trial. *Circulation*. 2015;131(1):34–42.
67. Solomon SD, McMurray JJV, Anand IS, et al. Angiotensin-neprilysin inhibition in heart failure with preserved ejection fraction. *N Engl J Med*. 2019;381(17):1609–1620.
68. Kitzman DW, Brubaker P, Morgan T, et al. Effect of caloric restriction or aerobic exercise training on peak oxygen consumption and quality of life in obese older patients with heart failure with preserved ejection fraction: a randomized clinical trial. *J Am Med Assoc*. 2016;315(1):36–46.
69. Ruberg FL, Grogan M, Hanna M, et al. Transthyretin amyloid cardiomyopathy: JACC state-of-the-art review. *J Am Coll Cardiol*. 2019;73(22):2872–2891.
70. Castano A, Haq M, Narotsky DL, et al. Multicenter study of planar Technetium 99m Pyrophosphate cardiac imaging: predicting survival for patients with ATTR cardiac amyloidosis. *JAMA Cardiol*. 2016;1(8):880–889.
71. Maurer MS, Schwartz JH, Gundapaneni B, et al. Tafamidis treatment for patients with transthyretin amyloid cardiomyopathy. *N Engl J Med*. 2018;379(11):1007–1016.
72. Berra G, Noble S, Soccal PM, et al. Pulmonary hypertension in the elderly: a different disease? *Breathe*. 2016;12(1):43–49.
73. Guazzi M, Gomberg-Maitland M, Arena R. Pulmonary hypertension in heart failure with preserved ejection fraction. *J Heart Lung Transplant*. 2015;34(3):273–281.
74. Campean IA, Lang IM. Treating pulmonary hypertension in the elderly. *Expert Opin Pharmacother*. 2020;21(10):1193–1200.
75. Bavishi C, Balasundaram K, Argulian E. Integration of flow-gradient patterns into clinical decision making for patients with suspected severe aortic stenosis and preserved LVEF: a systematic review of evidence and meta-analysis. *JACC Cardiovasc imaging*. 2016;9(11):1255–1263.

Valvular Heart Disease

75a. Otto CM, Nishimura RA, Bonow RO, et al. 2020 ACC/AHA Guideline for the Management of Patients With Valvular Heart Disease: Executive Summary: A Report of the American College of Cardiology/American Heart Association Joint Committee on Clinical Practice Guidelines. *J Am Coll Cardiol*. 2021;77(4):450–500.
76. Mack MJ, Leon MB, Thourani VH, et al. Transcatheter aortic-valve replacement with a balloon-Expandable valve in low-risk patients. *N Engl J Med*. 2019;380(18):1695–1705.
77. Grover FL, Vemulapalli S, Carroll JD, et al. 2016 annual report of the society of Thoracic Surgeons/American College of cardiology transcatheter valve therapy registry. *J Am Coll Cardiol*. 2016.
78. Nishimura RA, Otto CM, Bonow RO, et al. 2014 AHA/ACC guideline for the management of patients with valvular heart disease: executive summary: a report of the American College of Cardiology/American Heart Association Task Force on Practice Guidelines. *J Am Coll Cardiol*. 2014;63(22):2438–2488.
79. Franzone A, Piccolo R, Siontis GC, et al. Transcatheter aortic valve replacement for the treatment of pure native aortic valve regurgitation: a systematic review. *JACC Cardiovasc Interv*. 2016;9(22):2308–2317.
80. Glower DD, Kar S, Trento A, et al. Percutaneous mitral valve repair for mitral regurgitation in high-risk patients: results of the EVEREST II study. *J Am Coll Cardiol*. 2014;64(2):172–181.
81. Sorajja P, Mack M, Vemulapalli S, et al. Initial experience with commercial transcatheter mitral valve repair in the United States. *J Am Coll Cardiol*. 2016;67(10):1129–1140.
82. Stone GW, Lindenfeld J, Abraham WT, et al. Transcatheter mitral-valve repair in patients with heart failure. *N Engl J Med*. 2018;379(24):2307–2318.
83. Regueiro A, Linke A, Latib A, et al. Association between transcatheter aortic valve replacement and subsequent infective endocarditis and in-hospital death. *J Am Med Assoc*. 2016;316:1083–1092.

Arrhythmia

84. Curtis AB, Karki R, Hattoum A, Sharma UC. Arrhythmias in patients ≥80 Years of age: pathophysiology, management, and outcomes. *J Am Coll Cardiol*. 2018;71(18):2041–2057.
85. Chow GV, Marine JE, Fleg JL. Epidemiology of arrhythmias and conduction disorders in older adults. *Clin Geriatr Med*. 2012;28(4):539–553.
86. Hirsh DS, Wenger N. Atrial fibrillation in the elderly. *ESC CardioMed*. 2018:2221–2223.
87. January CT, Wann LS, Calkins H, et al. 2019 AHA/ACC/HRS focused update of the 2014 AHA/ACC/HRS guideline for the management of patients with atrial fibrillation: a report of the American College of cardiology/American heart association Task Force on clinical practice guidelines and the heart rhythm society in collaboration with the society of Thoracic Surgeons. *Circulation*. 2019;140(2):e125–e151.
88. Curry SJ, Krist AH, Owens DK, et al. Screening for atrial fibrillation with electrocardiography: US preventive services Task Force recommendation statement. *J Am Med Assoc*. 2018;320(5):478–484.
89. Kirchhof P, Benussi S, Kotecha D, et al. 2016 ESC Guidelines for the management of atrial fibrillation developed in collaboration with EACTS. *Eur Heart J*. 2016;37(38):2893–2962.
90. Perez MV, Mahaffey KW, Hedlin H, et al. Large-scale Assessment of a Smartwatch to identify atrial fibrillation. *N Engl J Med*. 2019;381(20):1909–1917.
91. Magnani JW, Wang N, Benjamin EJ, et al. Atrial fibrillation and declining physical performance in older adults: the health, aging, and body composition study. *Circ Arrhythm Electrophysiol*. 2016;9(5):e003525.
92. Khan SU, Osman M, Khan MU, et al. Dual versus triple therapy for atrial fibrillation after percutaneous coronary intervention: a systematic review and meta-analysis. *Ann Intern Med*. 2020;172(7):474–483.
93. Brunetti ND, Tricarico L, De Gennaro L, et al. Meta-analysis study on direct oral anticoagulants vs warfarin therapy in atrial fibrillation and PCI: dual or triple approach? *Int J Cardiol Heart Vasc*. 2020;29:100569.
94. Huang HK, Liu PP, Hsu JY, et al. Risk of osteoporosis in patients with atrial fibrillation using non-vitamin K antagonist oral anticoagulants or warfarin. *J Am Heart Assoc*. 2020;9(2):e013845.
95. Malik AH, Yandrapalli S, Aronow WS, et al. Meta-analysis of direct-acting oral anticoagulants compared with warfarin in patients >75 Years of age. *Am J Cardiol*. 2019;123(12):2051–2057.
96. Freeman JV, Varosy P, Price MJ, et al. The NCDR left atrial appendage occlusion registry. *J Am Coll Cardiol*. 2020;75(13):1503–1518.
97. Groenveld HF, Tijssen JG, Crijns HJ, et al. Rate control efficacy in permanent atrial fibrillation: successful and failed strict rate control against a background of lenient rate control: data from RACE II (Rate Control Efficacy in Permanent Atrial Fibrillation). *J Am Coll Cardiol*. 2013;61(7):741–748.
98. Packer DL, Mark DB, Robb RA, et al. Effect of catheter ablation vs antiarrhythmic drug therapy on mortality, stroke, bleeding, and cardiac arrest among patients with atrial fibrillation: the CABANA randomized clinical trial. *J Am Med Assoc*. 2019;321(13):1261–1274.
99. Brembilla-Perrot B, Olivier A, Sellal JM, et al. Influence of advancing age on clinical presentation, treatment efficacy and safety, and long-term outcome of pre-excitation syndromes: a retrospective cohort study of 961 patients included over a 25-year period. *BMJ Open*. 2016;6(5):e010520.
100. Epstein AE, DiMarco JP, Ellenbogen KA, et al. 2012 ACCF/AHA/HRS focused update incorporated into the ACCF/AHA/HRS 2008 guidelines for device-based therapy of cardiac rhythm abnormalities: a report of the American College of cardiology Foundation/American heart association Task Force on practice guidelines and the heart rhythm society. *Circulation*. 2013;127(3):e283–352.
101. Cleland JG, Freemantle N, Erdmann E, et al. Long-term mortality with cardiac resynchronization therapy in the Cardiac Resynchronization-Heart Failure (CARE-HF) trial. *Eur J Heart Fail*. 2012;14:628–634.
102. Vohra J. Implantable cardioverter defibrillators (ICDs) in octogenarians. *Heart Lung Circ*. 2014;23(3):213–216.

103. Hess PL, Matlock DD, Al-Khatib SM. Decision-making regarding primary prevention implantable cardioverter-defibrillators among older adults. *Clin Cardiol*. 2020;43(2):187–195.

Venous Thromboembolism

104. Boey JP, Gallus A. Drug treatment of venous thromboembolism in the elderly. *Drugs Aging*. 2016;33(7):475–490.
105. Lange N, Méan M, Stalder O, et al. Anticoagulation quality and clinical outcomes in multimorbid elderly patients with acute venous thromboembolism. *Thromb Res*. 2019;177:10–16.
106. Ali MS, Czarnecka-Kujawa K. Venous thromboembolism in the elderly. *Curr Geriatrics Rep*. 2016:132–139.
107. Righini M, Van Es J, Den Exter PL, et al. Age-adjusted D-dimer cutoff levels to rule out pulmonary embolism: the ADJUST-PE study. *J Am Med Assoc*. 2014;311(11):1117–1124.
108. Kearon C, Akl EA, Ornelas J, et al. Antithrombotic therapy for VTE disease: CHEST guideline and expert panel report. *Chest*. 2016;149(2):315–352.
109. Song ZK, Cao H, Wu H, et al. Current status of rivaroxaban in elderly patients with pulmonary embolism (Review). *Exp Ther Med*. 2020;19(4):2817–2825.
109a. Lyman GH, Carrier M, Ay C, et al. American Society of Hematology 2021 guidelines for management of venous thromboembolism: prevention and treatment in patients with cancer. *Blood Adv*. 2021;5(4):927–974.
110. Kim JS, Patel MHE, et al. Case series of elderly patients treated with catheter directed thrombolysis (CDT) for pulmonary embolism (PE) at large tertiary care center. *Am J Respir Crit Care Med*. 2020 (in press).
111. Goyal P, Maurer MS. Syncope in older adults. *J Geriatr Cardiol*. 2016;13(5):380–386.
112. O'Brien HAKR. Syncope in the elderly. *Eur Cardiol*. 2014;9(1):28–36.
113. Shen WK, Sheldon RS, Benditt DG, et al. 2017 ACC/AHA/HRS guideline for the evaluation and management of patients with syncope: a report of the American College of cardiology/American heart association Task Force on clinical practice guidelines and the heart rhythm society. *Circulation*. 2017;136(5):e60–e122.
114. Whelton PK, Carey RM, Aronow WS, et al. 2017 ACC/AHA/AAPA/ABC/ACPM/AGS/APhA/ASH/ASPC/NMA/PCNA guideline for the prevention, detection, evaluation, and management of high blood pressure in adults: executive summary: a report of the American College of cardiology/American heart association Task Force on clinical practice guidelines. *Circulation*. 2018;138(17):e426–e483.
115. Fleg JL, Aronow WS, Frishman WH. Cardiovascular drug therapy in the elderly: benefits and challenges. *Nat Rev Cardiol*. 2011;8(1):13–28.
116. Beckett NS, Peters R, Fletcher AE, et al. Treatment of hypertension in patients 80 years of age or older. *N Engl J Med*. 2008;358(18):1887–1898.
117. Williamson JD, Supiano MA, Applegate WB, et al. Intensive vs standard blood pressure control and cardiovascular disease outcomes in adults aged ≥75 Years: a randomized clinical trial. *J Am Med Assoc*. 2016;315(24):2673–2682.
118. Fleg JL, Forman DE, Berra K, et al. Secondary prevention of atherosclerotic cardiovascular disease in older adults: a scientific statement from the American Heart Association. *Circulation*. 2013;128(22):2422–2446.
119. Efficacy and safety of statin therapy in older people: a meta-analysis of individual participant data from 28 randomised controlled trials. *Lancet*. 2019;393(10170):407–415.
120. Orkaby AR, Driver JA, Ho YL, et al. Association of statin Use with all-cause and cardiovascular mortality in US Veterans 75 Years and older. *J Am Med Assoc*. 2020;324(1):68–78.
121. Cannon CP, Blazing MA, Giugliano RP, et al. Ezetimibe added to statin therapy after acute coronary syndromes. *N Engl J Med*. 2015;372(25):2387–2397.
122. Sinnaeve PR, Schwartz GG, Wojdyla DM, et al. Effect of alirocumab on cardiovascular outcomes after acute coronary syndromes according to age: an ODYSSEY OUTCOMES trial analysis. *Eur Heart J*. 2020;41(24):2248–2258.
123. Sever P, Gouni-Berthold I, Keech A, et al. LDL-cholesterol lowering with evolocumab, and outcomes according to age and sex in patients in the FOURIER Trial. *Eur J Prev Cardiol*. 2020. 2047487320902750.
124. Bhatt DL, Steg PG, Miller M, et al. Cardiovascular risk reduction with icosapent ethyl for hypertriglyceridemia. *N Engl J Med*. 2019;380(1):11–22.
125. Farrell B, Black C, Thompson W, et al. Deprescribing antihyperglycemic agents in older persons: evidence-based clinical practice guideline. *Can Fam Physician*. 2017;63(11):832–843.
126. Zinman B, Wanner C, Lachin JM, et al. Empagliflozin, cardiovascular outcomes, and mortality in type 2 diabetes. *N Engl J Med*. 2015;373(22):2117–2128.
127. Holme I, Anderssen SA. Increases in physical activity is as important as smoking cessation for reduction in total mortality in elderly men: 12 years of follow-up of the Oslo II study. *Br J Sports Med*. 2015;49(11):743–748.
128. Gellert C, Schottker B, Brenner H. Smoking and all-cause mortality in older people: systematic review and meta-analysis. *Arch Intern Med*. 2012;172(11):837–844.
129. Patel AV, Bernstein L, Deka A, et al. Leisure time spent sitting in relation to total mortality in a prospective cohort of US adults. *Am J Epidemiol*. 2010;172(4):419–429.
130. LaCroix AZ, Bellettiere J, Rillamas-Sun E, et al. Association of light physical activity measured by Accelerometry and incidence of coronary heart disease and cardiovascular disease in older women. *JAMA Netw Open*. 2019;2(3):e190419.
131. Suaya JA, Stason WB, Ades PA, et al. Cardiac rehabilitation and survival in older coronary patients. *J Am Coll Cardiol*. 2009;54(1):25–33.
132. Wannamethee SG, Atkins JL. Muscle loss and obesity: the health implications of sarcopenia and sarcopenic obesity. *Proc Nutr Soc*. 2015;74(4):405–412.
133. Manson JE, Cook NR, Lee IM, et al. Vitamin D supplements and prevention of cancer and cardiovascular disease. *N Engl J Med*. 2019;380(1):33–44.
134. McCullough ML, Peterson JJ, Patel R, et al. Flavonoid intake and cardiovascular disease mortality in a prospective cohort of US adults. *Am J Clin Nutr*. 2012;95(2):454–464.
135. Mohanty S, Rosenthal RA, Russell MM, et al. Optimal perioperative management of the geriatric patient: a best practices guideline from the American College of Surgeons NSQIP and the American geriatrics society. *J Am Coll Surg*. 2016;222(5):930–947.
136. Wolfe JD, Wolfe NK, Rich MW. Perioperative care of the geriatric patient for noncardiac surgery. *Clin Cardiol*. 2020;43(2):127–136.

91 Cardiovascular Disease in Women

MARTHA GULATI AND C. NOEL BAIREY MERZ

BACKGROUND, 1710

SEX, GENDER, AND GENETIC DIFFERENCES IN CARDIOVASCULAR DISEASE, 1710

CARDIOVASCULAR RISK FACTORS IN WOMEN, 1710

CARDIOVASCULAR DISEASE RISK ASSESSMENT, 1714

ISCHEMIC HEART DISEASE IN WOMEN, 1714
Symptoms of Ischemia, 1714
Delays in Care of Women, 1715
Diagnosis of Ischemia in Women, 1715
Interventions and Medical Therapy for Ischemic Heart Disease in Women, 1715

ISCHEMIC HEART DISEASE: BEYOND OBSTRUCTIVE CORONARY ARTERY DISEASE, 1716
Ischemia with No Obstructive Coronary Artery Disease, 1716
Myocardial Infarction with Nonobstructive Coronary Artery Disease, 1717
Takotsubo Cardiomyopathy, 1717

CARDIAC SURGERY, 1718
Coronary Artery Bypass Graft, 1718
Valvular Heart Surgery, 1718
Transcatheter Aortic Valve Intervention, 1718
Transcatheter Mitral Valve Repair, 1718

PERIPHERAL ARTERIAL DISEASE, 1718

HEART FAILURE, 1718
Peripartum Cardiomyopathy, 1719
Heart Failure Diagnosis, 1719
Heart Failure Treatment, 1719
Device Use in Heart Failure, 1719
Mechanical Circulatory Support, 1719
Cardiac Transplantation, 1719

ARRYTHMIA AND SUDDEN CARDIAC DEATH, 1719

CARDIOVASCULAR DISEASE PREVENTION, 1720

ACKNOWLEDGMENTS, 1721

REFERENCES, 1721

BACKGROUND

Cardiovascular disease (CVD) remains the leading cause of death among women, accounting for 420,184 deaths in women in 2018, and accounts for 1 in every 4 female deaths in the United States.[1] Approximately 60 million women are living with some form of CVD and the lifetime risk of developing CVD for a 40-year-old woman is estimated to be 1 in 2, with 1 in 3 at risk of developing coronary heart disease 1 in 5 developing heart failure (HF), and 1 in 5 having a stroke in their lifetime.[1] Since 2001, there had been a continuous decline in mortality from heart disease in women until 2010, where after mortality for CVD has risen in both sexes.[1] Nonetheless, the mortality rate from CVD in younger women (under the age of 55 years) has demonstrated no significant improvement in the last 2 decades, and these youngest women with CVD have the highest mortality rates.[2]

There are both sex (biological) and gender (sociocultural) differences in CVD and outcomes between women and men due to a number of variables including differences in the impact of traditional risk factors, sex-specific CVD risk factors, differences in treatment and management strategies for women for both primary and secondary prevention of CVD, and pathophysiological differences in CVD.

Prevention of CVD in women is influenced by awareness of the issue. Although more women have been dying from CVD than men in the United States, it was not until 1991 that the National Institutes of Health (NIH) established a policy that all NIH-funded trials must include both women and men in studies of conditions that affect both genders. In 2016 the NIH made it mandatory to include both sexes in cell and animal studies. While awareness of CVD as the leading cause of death in women has improved over time, it remains suboptimal, particularly in racial and ethnic minorities.[3] A nationally representative survey done by the Women's Health Alliance showed that even though 74% of women had one or more CVD risk factors, only 16% of women were informed that they were at risk for heart disease. Physician awareness, education, and assessment of women's CVD risk is also far from expected. This same survey showed that primary care physicians prioritized weight and breast health over concerns for CVD. Additionally, only 22% of primary care physicians and 42% of cardiologists felt well-equipped to assess CVD in women, and very few implemented the guidelines for CVD risk assessment in their practice in their women patients (16% of primary care physicians, 22% of cardiologists; p=NS).[3]

SEX, GENDER, AND GENETIC DIFFERENCES IN CARDIOVASCULAR DISEASE

The Institute of Medicine has defined *sex* as "the classification of living things, generally as male or female according to their reproductive organs and functions assigned by the chromosomal complement."[4] Sex differences result from true biological differences in the structure and function of the cardiovascular systems of men and women, in contrast with gender differences that stem from a person's self-representation resulting in psychosocial roles and behaviors imposed by society. Certainly, gender differences play a role in treatment of CVD and hence, impact outcomes but are very different from sex differences that arise from the genetic differences between men and women. Sex differences arise from the chromosomal differences between men (XY) and women (XX).

Genetic markers predictive of CVD remain undefined to date in women. The Multi-Ethnic Study of Atherosclerosis (MESA) is a study of subclinical CVD and risk factors that predict progression to clinically overt CVD and that predict progression of subclinical disease itself, in a diverse, population-based sample of 6814 men and women aged 45 to 84 unaffected with CVD. A genetic risk score (GRS) calculated using a literature-derived list of 46 SNPs predicted CHD in males but not women in MESA.[5] Currently there is no known genetic marker that can be used to improve risk assessment in women, beyond traditional methods.

CARDIOVASCULAR RISK FACTORS IN WOMEN (see Chapters 25 and 30)

TRADITIONAL CARDIOVASCULAR DISEASE RISK FACTORS AND THEIR IMPACT ON WOMEN

Age

Age powerfully predicts CVD, and specifically CHD. The prevalence of CVD increases with age in both men and women, but CHD events lag at least 10 years in women compared to men.[1] CHD increases in women after the age of 60, with 1 in 3 women having evidence of CHD after the age of 65 years, in contrast with 1 in 8 women aged 45 to 64. The atherosclerotic CVD (ASCVD) risk score increases with increasing age.[6] The highest sex difference in CHD mortality occurs in relatively young and middle-aged women, with relative stagnation in rates in contrast

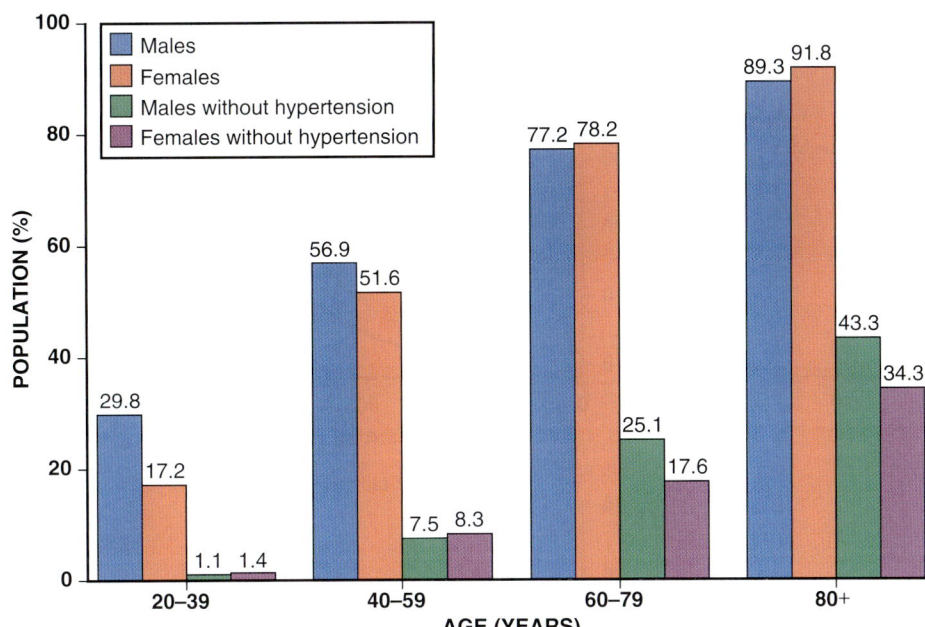

FIGURE 91.1 Prevalence of cardiovascular disease in US adults with and without hypertension (NHANES 2013–2016). (From Virani SS, et al. American Heart Association Council on Epidemiology and Prevention Statistics Committee and Stroke Statistics Subcommittee Heart Disease and Stroke Statistics-2020 Update: A Report from the American Heart Association. *Circulation.* 2020;141:e139–e596.)

with declines and no sex difference among older adult women and men.[7]

Family History
A history of CHD in a first-degree relative imparts risk on an individual. The 2018 American College of Cardiology/American Heart Association (ACC/AHA) guidelines on the treatment of blood cholesterol to reduce atherosclerotic cardiovascular risk in adults recommends consideration of a premature family history of CVD when assessing risk in asymptomatic adults.[8]

Hypertension (see also Chapter 26)
The definition of hypertension has changed, and as a result the prevalence of hypertension has increased with a lower threshold for the diagnosis of hypertension.[9] Based on the National Health and Nutrition Examination Survey (NHANES) 2017–2018, the overall prevalence of hypertension was similar among men (51.0%) and women (39.7%), which increases with age in both sexes. Women over the age of 60 have the same prevalence of hypertension compared with men (73.9% vs. 75.2%, respectively).[10] Women are more likely than men to have their hypertension controlled (53% vs. 46%), which does not change with age, in contrast with men where it worsens.[11] Hypertension rises two- to threefold in women taking second- and third-generation oral contraceptives, which raise blood pressure 7 to 8 mm Hg on average, however fourth-generation with drospirenone lower blood pressure.[12]

Hypertension has a greater adverse impact on CVD in women over the age of 60 when compared with men (Fig. 91.1).[1] Hypertension has an increased risk of the development of congestive HF, which is relatively greater in women. Women who present with strokes more likely have a history of hypertension than men. Indeed, the lifetime risk of stroke is greater in women compared with men, related to their greater life expectancy and the rise in stroke rates with age.

The effect of aging on blood pressure is not just a change due to menopause in women, as previously thought. Recent work has shown significant sex differences in blood pressure trajectories, where blood pressure actually increases more rapidly in women and begins early in life (Fig. 91.2).[13] The biological differences may explain the subsequent distinct pathophysiologic effects of hypertension, in addition to the variability in responsiveness to medications in women.

Diabetes (see also Chapter 31)
Diabetes increases the risk of CHD and confers greater risk for CHD in women than men, increasing a woman's risk of CHD by three-to sevenfold with only a two- to threefold increase in diabetic men. In addition, the risk of fatal CHD in a diabetic woman increases 3.5 times versus nondiabetic woman, and higher than in diabetic men (relative risk of fatal CHD is 2.0 that of a nondiabetic man).[14] Importantly, even women with type 1 diabetes have twice the risk of fatal and nonfatal cardiovascular events, and a 40% greater risk of all-cause mortality compared with men.[15]

The American Diabetes Association suggests consideration of diabetes screening for women and men over the age of 45 years, and then every 3 years if the results are normal.[16] For women with a history of gestational diabetes, screening for diabetes should occur 6 to 12 weeks postpartum, with lifelong testing every 3 years. Additionally, the 2020 guidelines recommend screening women with polycystic ovarian syndrome (PCOS) if they are overweight or obese.[16]

Dyslipidemia (see also Chapter 27)
Dyslipidemia is common in women but steadily decreasing over time, based on the NHANES 2015–2018 data.[17] Elevated total cholesterol (>240 mg/dL) is present in 12.1% of adult women, compared with 10.5% of men. The only age group of women that had a lower total cholesterol than men are those under the age of 40. Overall, this may reflect undertreatment of dyslipidemia in women. There is evidence that women who are eligible for statin therapy are less likely to be treated with any statin or the recommended intensity of statin.[18] The reasons are both due to less prescribing of appropriate therapy and women declining or discontinuing treatment more frequently compared with men.

High-density lipoprotein (HDL) levels are higher in women,[17] and on average HDL-C levels in women are approximately 10 mg/dL higher than men throughout their lives. HDL is inversely associated with ASCVD events. Nonetheless, HDL as a target of therapy has to date not improved outcomes, and is not the target of the ASCVD risk assessment.

The ASCVD risk assessment focuses on low-density lipoprotein cholesterol (LDL-C) as the primary target of lipid-lowering therapy to reduce risk of CVD.[8] The use of nuclear magnetic resonance (NMR) spectroscopy lipoprofiles, apolipoproteins, particle size, and density are not endorsed by the current cholesterol guidelines in either men or women for cardiovascular risk assessment.[8]

Notably in women, adverse changes in the lipid profile accompany menopause and include increased levels of total cholesterol, LDL-C, and triglycerides and decreased levels of HDL-C, although it remains unclear how much risk factor worsening is related to aging as opposed to menopause-related hormonal changes.[19]

Cigarette Smoking
Cigarette smoking is the leading cause of preventable cardiovascular deaths. The use of cigarettes continues to decline in the United States, due to effective public health measures. Based on 2018 data, 16% of men and 12% of women reported tobacco use.[20] Although women smoke less than men, smoking cigarettes may be more detrimental in women than men. Female smokers die 14.5 years earlier than female nonsmokers and male smokers die 13.2 years earlier than male nonsmokers.[21] The use of oral contraceptives and cigarette use imparts an even greater risk of myocardial infarction than smoking alone, likely related to pro-thrombotic effects.

Cessation of smoking substantially reduces CVD risk in women; mortality risk among former smokers decreases nearly to that of never smokers.[22] It is important to recognize that smoking cessation works differently in women compared with men. Men have more nicotine receptors in their brain and nicotine replacement is more effective in men compared with women. Varenicline, on the other hand, has been shown to be more effective as a smoking cessation aid in women.[23]

Physical Activity/Physical Fitness (see also Chapters 32 and 33)
Physical activity benefits cardiovascular health but physical inactivity is common, with women more likely to report not meeting the physical activity guidelines than men (47% vs. 38%), which worsens with age.[24] Nonetheless, gender bias exists in physical activity measurement

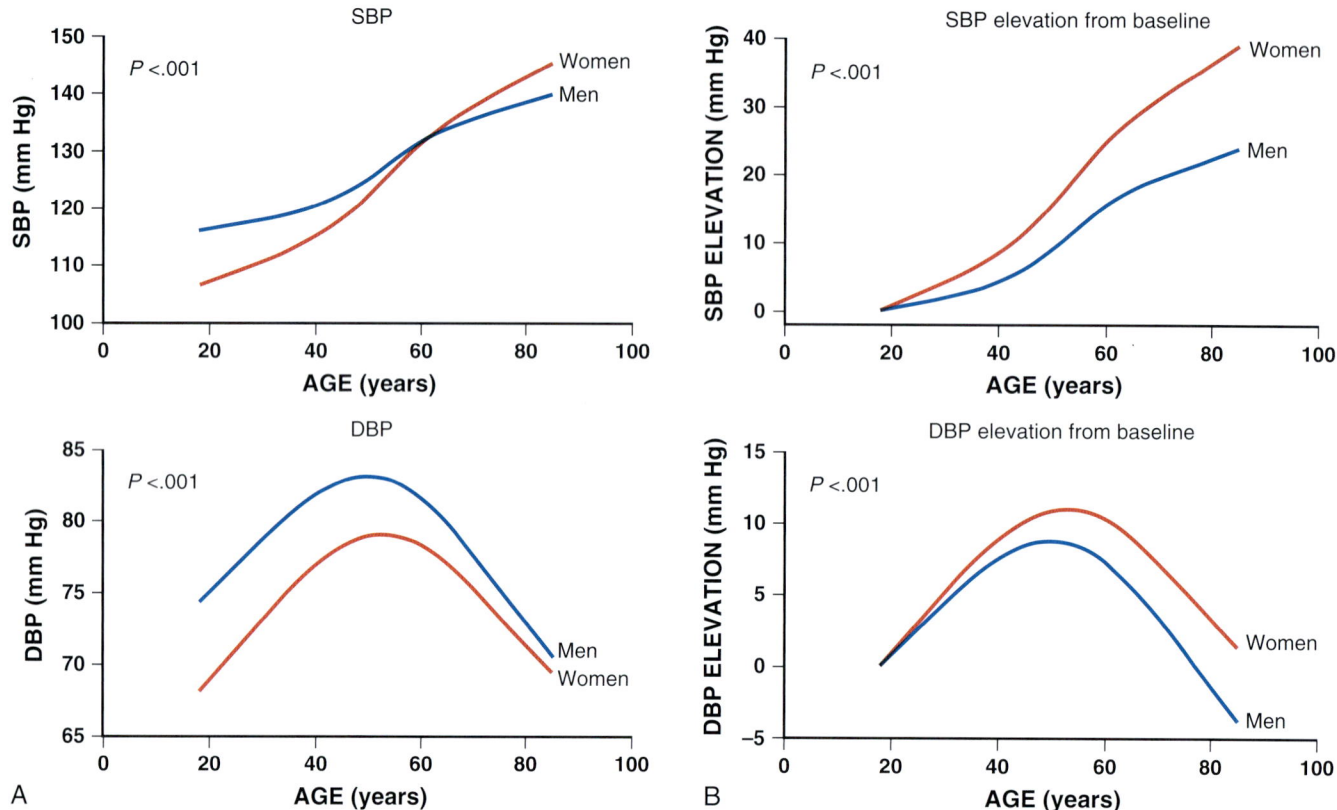

FIGURE 91.2 Sex-specific blood pressure changes over time in adults. (From Ji H, Kim A, Ebinger JE, et al. Sex differences in blood pressure trajectories over the life course. *JAMA Cardiol.* 2020;5[3]:19–26.)

instruments that do not collect domestic activities such as cooking, cleaning, and childcare, which may account for these observed differences. Using the 2008 U.S. federal physical activity guidelines, in every age group adult women reported performing less leisure-time physical activity than men in the 2017 National Health Interview Survey. Physical inactivity associates with higher blood pressure, worse cholesterol, poorer glucose metabolism, poorer mental health, and obesity. Physical inactivity, quantified by prolonged sitting time, has been shown to be an independent risk factor for CVD in women beyond leisure-time physical activity.[25]

Exercise capacity, also known as physical fitness, strongly and independently predicts all-cause mortality in asymptomatic women and can be quantified. In 4137 self-referred apparently healthy adults (2326 men, 1811 women; mean age: 42.8 ± 12.2 years) who underwent cardiopulmonary fitness testing, the low-fit women had a higher risk of dying from all-causes, CVD, and cancer during follow-up than those with moderate fitness and high fitness. At any point in time, low-fit women had a 28%, 34%, and 34% increased risk of dying from all-causes, CVD, and cancer compared with high-fit women (p < 0.01), respectively. In women, this relationship remained significant for all-cause and cancer mortality in the multivariable model (hazards ratio [HR] 1.63, p < 0.05 and HR 3.94, p < 0.01, respectively).[26]

Metabolic Syndrome (see also Chapters 30 and 31)
NHANES data from 2003 to 2014 indicate that 33.3% of women met the criteria for the metabolic syndrome, similar to that seen in men (35.3%, *P < 0.01*).[27] Those with the metabolic syndrome have an increased risk of developing CVD, and the association with the risk of MI has been demonstrated to be greater in women compared with men but no sex differences in the risk of stroke based on the presence of the metabolic syndrome.[28]

Obesity (see also Chapter 25)
Obesity, defined as a body mass index (BMI) of greater than 30 kg/m^2, is epidemic in the United States, with the 2017–2018 NHANES estimation of obesity in women at 41.8%, similar to that seen in men.[29] The rising incidence of diabetes associates closely with obesity. In the Nurses' Health Study, obesity was the most powerful predictor of diabetes, with women with a BMI ≥35 kg/m^2 having a relative risk for diabetes almost 40-fold greater than women with a BMI less than 23 kg/m^2. The pattern of obesity appears to be related to CVD, whereby elevated waist circumference above 35 inches, waist-to-hip ratio, and waist-to-height ratio, indicative of visceral obesity, is related to elevated CVD risk, whereas elevated BMI alone is not.[30]

Although obesity has also been associated with an increased mortality from CVD and shortened life expectancy from CVD, obesity is not an independent risk factor for CVD given that obesity is strongly associated with many of the traditional CHD risk factors. Notably, overweight, defined as a BMI of greater than 25 but less than 30 kg/m^2, is associated with lower mortality and CVD death compared to leaner counterparts. Obesity may simply be a marker for low physical activity and fitness levels. Prior work in women where both obesity and physical fitness were measured suggests that physically fit obese women are not at elevated risk, and conversely lean women who are not physically fit have elevated risk.[31]

High-Sensitivity C-Reactive Protein (see also Chapters 10 and 25)
Although high-sensitivity C-reactive protein (hsCRP) is not a causal risk factor for CVD, it may improve risk detection in women. Measuring hsCRP is not recommended in routine risk assessment of women, but rather as an option in those persons in the intermediate risk range based on the ASCVD risk score. An elevated hsCRP (>2.0 mg/L) is considered an ASCVD risk-enhancing factor.[6]

Sleep Apnea
Although sleep apnea is more prevalent in men compared with women, it is a very common issue in women and under-recognized in terms of its impact on CVD. In women, untreated obstructive sleep apnea is associated with an increased risk of hypertension, coronary artery disease (CAD), stroke, and atrial fibrillation.[32] Sleep apnea is believed to induce severe intermittent hypoxemia and CO_2 retention during sleep, with oxygen saturation sometimes dropping to ≤60%, disrupting the normal autonomic and hemodynamic responses to sleep.

Apnea often occurs repetitively through the night, and toward the end of an apneic episode, blood pressure rises and can reach levels as high as 240/130 mm Hg. This hemodynamic stress occurs simultaneously with severe hypoxemia, hypercapnia, and adrenergic activation, which in turn acts to promote CVD. Untreated sleep apnea in women is associated with 3.5 times greater risk of dying from CVD, yet this risk was reduced to the same as a woman without sleep apnea with appropriate treatment and continuous positive airway pressure.[32]

SEX-SPECIFIC RISK FACTORS
Age of Menarche
Age at onset of menarche is associated with ASCVD risk. Early menarche (occurring at or before the age of 12 years) and late onset menarche (>15 years) have both been shown to increase risk for adverse cardiovascular outcomes including myocardial infarction, stroke, and HF hospitalizations. In a 648-woman cohort from the WISE (Women's Ischemia Syndrome Evaluation) study, history of menarche at age ≤10 years and ≥15 years showed adverse cardiovascular events HR of 4.53 (95% CI 2.13 to 9.63) and 2.58 (95% CI 1.28 to 5.21), respectively, compared to women with menarche at age 12 years.[33]

Pregnancy-Associated Conditions:
Preterm Delivery. Preterm delivery, defined as births prior to 37 weeks gestation, complicates about 11% of deliveries worldwide. The underlying causes and mechanisms are not entirely clear but there is a strong association with preterm delivery and maternal risk of coronary heart disease and stroke, with the greatest risk associated with preterm deliveries before 32 weeks gestation.[34]

Eclampsia, Pre-eclampsia, and Pregnancy-Associated Hypertension (see also Chapter 92). Gestational hypertension of any sort associates with an increased risk of hypertension, chronic kidney disease, diabetes, stroke, and CVD (including HF, stroke, and myocardial infarction).[35] From the prospective UK Biobank cohort of over 220,000 women, those who reported hypertension during pregnancy were not just at greater risk of chronic hypertension, but also had a great risk of developing CAD, HF, aortic stenosis (AS), and mitral regurgitation over a median follow-up of 7 years (Fig. 91.3). From a causal standpoint, 64% of those with CAD and 49% of HF was driven by chronic hypertension, meaning treating hypertension in this group is of critical importance.[36]

Women with hypertensive disorders during pregnancy have a greater risk for stroke with the median age of a stroke in these women being ≤50 years, demonstrating an acceleration of CVD, despite premenopausal status and presumed low risk lessening emphasis on screening or treating of CVD risk factors.[37] Despite the association with elevated CVD events and labeling of pregnancy as a "stress test" for future CV events, some research suggests that the risk of CVD results from shared pre-pregnancy risk factors rather than any direct influence of the hypertensive disorder that occurred during pregnancy.[38] Hypertension during pregnancy is recognized as a risk-enhancing factor by the 2018 guidelines on the management of blood cholesterol.[8]

Gestational Diabetes (see also Chapter 92). Gestational diabetes increases the risk of future diabetes, but also increases the risk of CVD. A pooled analysis of nine studies that included over 5 million women demonstrated that women with gestational diabetes had a two-fold greater risk of cardiovascular events in the first 10 years postpartum, compared with women without gestational diabetes, even in those women who did not develop Type II diabetes.[39]

Small-for-Gestational-Age Infant. Small-for-gestational-age (SGA) delivery has been shown to be associated with an increased maternal risk of ASCVD. An SGA infant appears to be dose dependent, according to the severity of SGA as well as the number of SGA infants.[35]

Assisted Reproductive Therapies. Fertility hormonal therapies are estimated to be used in approximately 1% of births. The limited data available currently does not support an increased risk of ASCVD in women who undergo assisted reproductive therapy. In a systematic review of 41,910 women who received fertility therapy and 1,400,202 women who did not, there was no increased risk of a cardiac event (pooled HR: 0.91; 95% CI 0.67 to 1.25; I^2 = 36.6%) or diabetes mellitus (pooled HR 0.93, 95% CI 0.87 to 1.001; I^2 = 0%), however there was a trend toward higher risk of stroke (pooled HR 1.25, 95% CI 0.96 to 1.63; I^2 = 0%).[40] Although to date there has been no increase in subsequent ASCVD events in women who require reproductive therapies, there is a noted increase in hypertension while pregnant.

At this time, use of fertility therapy is not considered an independent risk factor for ASCVD. However, there is an early signal to suggest that women who have failed fertility therapy have an increased risk for future ASCVD events.[41] It is plausible that failed fertility therapy could be an indicator for future ASCVD risk as it poses a unique cardiometabolic stress test. This hypothesis warrants further investigation.

Polycystic Ovary Syndrome
Unique to women, PCOS associates with the development of many of the features of metabolic syndrome as well as insulin resistance, although first-degree male relatives also appear to have more insulin resistance. Women with PCOS have an increased prevalence of impaired glucose tolerance, the metabolic syndrome, and diabetes compared to women without PCOS.[42] Nonetheless, it remains unclear if PCOS is an independent risk factor for premature CVD in women. Based on the NHLBI-sponsored WISE (Women's Ischemia Syndrome Evaluation) study of postmenopausal women with PCOS and suspected myocardial ischemia, there was no greater risk of CVD or mortality over 10 years of follow-up.[42]

Functional Hypothalamic Amenorrhea (see also Chapter 96)
Up to 10% of premenopausal women have documented ovarian dysfunction with a larger proportion having subclinical hormonal dysfunction that may increase CVD risk. Functional hypothalamic amenorrhea (FHA) is a cause of a premenopausal ovarian dysfunction and occurs when gonadotropin-releasing hormone increases thereby increasing luteinizing hormone in a pulse frequency causing amenorrhea and hypoestrogenemia. Psychological stressors or metabolic insults such as caloric restriction or excessive exercise can induce FHA. Endothelial dysfunction, unfavorable lipid profiles, and premature CVD have been demonstrated in studies of young women with FHA.[43]

Premature Menopause and Premature Ovarian Insufficiency
The most common theory regarding the delayed onset of CAD in women compared with men is the role of circulating estrogen and its cardio-protective role. A meta-analysis concluded that women who had menopause at age younger than 45 years were more likely to have an incident coronary heart disease event (RR 1.50 [1.28 to 1.76]) compared to women undergoing menopause at ages ≥45 years.[44] The UK Biobank demonstrated that the earlier natural menopause occurs, the greater the risk of CHD and stroke.[45]

Premature ovarian insufficiency (POI) differs from premature menopause. It is defined as ovarian failure before the age of 40 years and results in a prolonged exposure of estrogen insufficiency. Reports have associated POI with an increased risk of CVD.[46] A meta-analysis from 10 observational studies with over 190,000 women demonstrated that POI was modestly associated with an increased incidence of coronary heart disease events (HR 1.69; p = 0.0001) but not with stroke.[47]

Premature menopause (before age 40 years) is a recognized risk-enhancing factor in the current ACC/AHA cholesterol guidelines.[8] Noting the presence of POI and the age of menopause should be part of any woman's ASCVD risk assessment.

Reproductive Hormones
Oral Contraceptive Therapy. For most women who are healthy and free of CVD and cardiovascular risk factors, the use of combination estrogen-progestin oral contraceptives associates with low relative and absolute risks of CVD. Women who are smokers over the age of 35, women with uncontrolled hypertension, a history of thromboembolic disease, or a history of ischemic heart disease (IHD) have an unacceptable level of CVD risk associated with oral contraceptives.[48]

Post-menopausal Hormone Therapy. A majority of CVD occurs after menopause in older women, in association with an increased burden of established CVD risk factors, hence the hypothesis that post-menopause hormone therapy reduces CVD risk, as supported by observational data. Nonetheless, randomized trials, such as Heart and Estrogen/Progestin Replacement Study (HERS) I, HERS II, Women's Health Initiative (WHI), and Raloxifene Use for The Heart (RUTH) did not find that hormone therapy or selective estrogen receptor modulators (SERMs) prevent either primary or secondary CVD events. Hormone replacement therapy and SERMS should not be used for the primary or secondary prevention of CVD.[49]

SEX-PREDOMINANT CARDIOVASCULAR DISEASE RISK FACTORS
Autoimmune Disease (see also Chapter 97)
Systemic inflammation in autoimmune disease, including rheumatoid arthritis (RA) and systemic erythematous lupus (SLE), may accelerate atherosclerosis and IHD and these diseases occur more frequently in women.[50] RA, SLE, and scleroderma associate with a significantly increased risk for CVD mortality.[50] Cardiovascular events often occur in younger women with SLE, with a risk for acute myocardial infarction 9- to 50-fold greater than the general population.[50] Traditional risk factors such as smoking, family history of premature CHD, hypertension, and elevated cholesterol do not completely account for the increased risk of CHD in patients with SLE. The 2018 ACC/AHA cholesterol guidelines include chronic inflammatory disorders as ASCVD risk enhancers which favor initiation of statin therapy for individuals with borderline ASCVD risk score.[8]

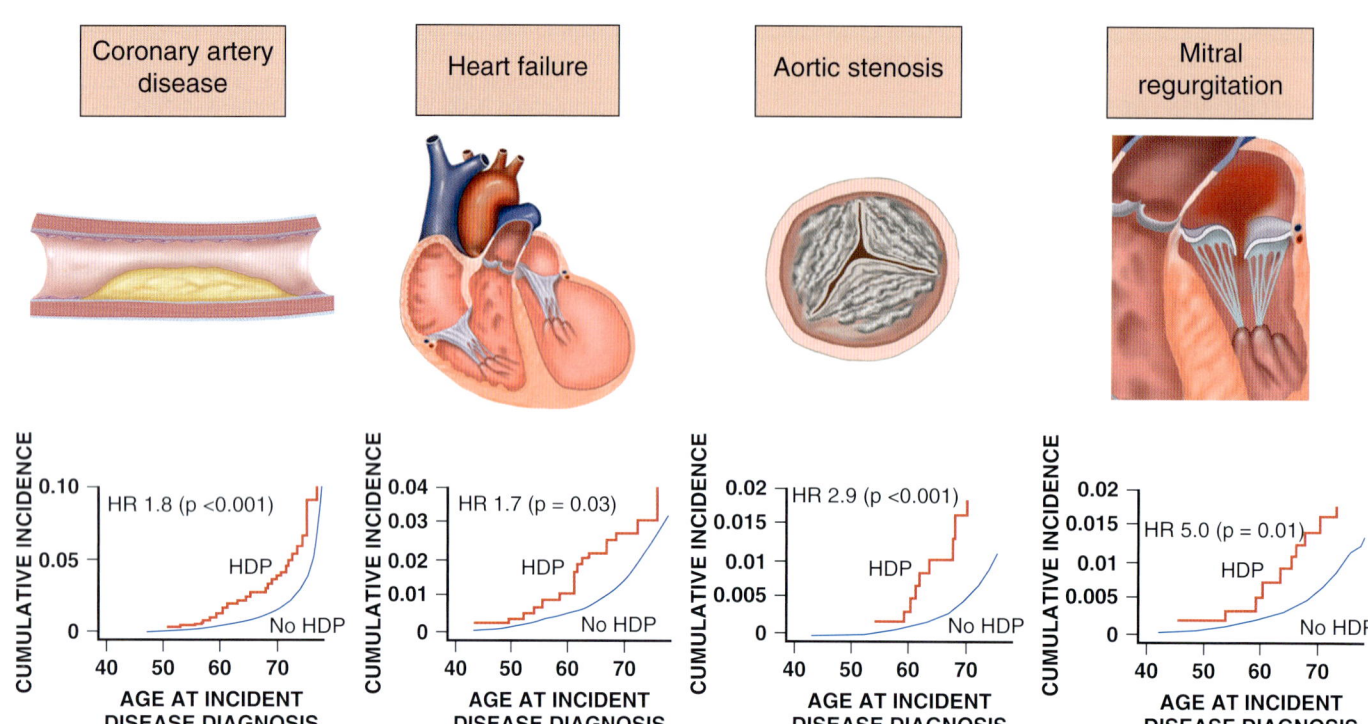

FIGURE 91.3 Hypertensive disorders in pregnancy and their relationship with cardiovascular disease. (From Honigberg MC, Zekavat SM, Aragam K, et al. Long-term cardiovascular risk in women with hypertension during pregnancy. *J Am Coll Cardiol.* 2019;74:2743–2754.)

Breast Cancer Therapy (see also Chapters 56 and 57)

Recent advancements in breast cancer treatment have led to improved survival but elevated risk of CVD.[51] The reasons for an increased risk of CVD appears to be the result of shared risk factors between breast cancer and CVD, in addition to the potential of direct cardiovascular injury that may accelerate atherosclerosis or HF.[52] Commonly used chemotherapeutic agents, such as anthracycline and trastuzumab, increase the risk of HF. In a large retrospective analysis of Medicare data of more than 45,000 older women who had early-stage breast cancer, the risk of developing HF was increased in women who received either trastuzumab (32.1/100 patients) or anthracycline plus trastuzumab (41.9/100 patients) compared with no adjuvant therapy (18.1/100 patients, p < 0.001). The addition of trastuzumab to anthracycline therapy added 12.1, 17.9, and 21.7 HF/cardiomyopathy events per 100 patients over 1, 2, and 3 years of follow-up, respectively. These rates are far higher than reported in early trials that established the use of trastuzumab.[52] Radiation therapy has an established association with the development of IHD. Exposure of the heart to ionizing radiation during radiotherapy for breast cancer increases the risk of IHD. The risk is directly proportional to the mean radiation dose to the heart, with an increase in CVD events of 7.4%/Gray (Gy) of radiation (95% CI, 2.9 to 14.5, p < 0.001). The risk of IHD begins within a few years after exposure and appears to continue for at least 20 years after the exposure. As expected, the risk for IHD is highest in women with pre-existing CVD risk factors.[52]

This period of breast cancer diagnosis and treatment is therefore an important window to provide ASCVD risk assessment, given that breast cancer is considered an ASCVD risk-enhancing factor.[8] Furthermore, a long-term post-treatment surveillance strategy needs to be implemented among these for monitoring late cardiotoxicity and/or non–therapy–related CVD event risk.

CARDIOVASCULAR DISEASE RISK ASSESSMENT (see also Chapter 25)

The role of ASCVD risk assessment is to identify those at highest risk of developing ASCVD, allowing guidance of appropriate intensity of screening and allocation of preventive therapy. Although there are a number of risk assessment tools available, the tool chosen should have been validated on the population on which it is being applied to. The risk estimator of choice in the United States remains the 2013 Pooled Cohort Equations (PCE), despite its acknowledged limitations in certain populations.[6] The 2018 ACC/AHA guidelines on the treatment of blood cholesterol to reduce ASCVD in adults relies on the PCE as the initial step in risk estimation, but incorporates nontraditional risk factors to refine the risk assessment.[8] The ASCVD risk estimator allows lifetime risk estimation for those aged 20 to 59 years, and 10-year risk estimation for those aged 40 to 75 years. Risk-enhancing factors allow individuals to be reclassified, and this includes the sex-specific and sex-predominant risk enhancers that impact women specifically.

ISCHEMIC HEART DISEASE IN WOMEN

Symptoms of Ischemia (see also Chapter 35)

Both sexes can experience the classic symptoms of myocardial ischemia. The perception that women may not experience chest pain or chest discomfort was based on retrospective data.[53,54] The National Registry of Myocardial Infarction demonstrated that women were more likely than men to present with a myocardial infarction without any chest pain at all (42 % vs. 31%, *P < 0.001*), particularly younger women who have the highest hospital mortality rates.[53] Nonetheless, more contemporary data has shown that symptoms of women and men are more alike than different. The Variation in Recovery: Role of Gender on Outcomes of Young AMI Patients (VIRGO) study reported presenting symptoms in women and men under the age of 55 years and found no differences in the report of chest pain by sex (87.2% women, 89.5% men) with AMI.[53] Young women were more likely to experience three or more associated symptoms, when compared with men. Similar findings were seen at all ages of AMI in the High-STEACS (High Sensitivity Troponin in the Evaluation of Patients with Acute Coronary Syndrome) trial. Those women diagnosed with AMI reported chest pain 92% of the time, comparable to the men at 91%.[55] Additionally, other "typical" symptoms were seen more in women compared with men (77% vs. 59%; *p = 0.007*) with AMI.

Certainly, for some women, the symptoms of ischemia may often be more nonspecific or less severe and can include shortness of breath; pain or discomfort in other body locations, such as that localized to the arm(s), shoulder, middle back, jaw, or epigastrium; indigestion; nausea or vomiting; diaphoresis; faintness or dizziness or syncope; fatigue; generalized weakness; or palpitations.[54] Nonetheless, most women do report chest pain or discomfort, along with additional symptoms. It is important to be aware of their risk and consider ischemia in the differential when women report such symptoms.

Delays in Care of Women

One barrier to the diagnosis of ischemia is delays in initiating care for women. This is a result of delays in women seeking care, in addition to delays in recognizing women being at risk by the healthcare team. The VIRGO study showed that young women also have delays in seeking care, and are more likely to present with AMI 6 or more hours after onset of symptoms, compared with men.[53] Additional delays occur upon presentation, with numerous studies documenting delays in care of women, particularly in initiating STEMI treatment and interventions, given public reporting of specific measures. Other work documents delays in reperfusion in women compared with men.[56] In-hospital and transfer times for percutaneous coronary intervention (PCI) were more likely to be exceeded in women compared with men (odds ratio [OR] 1.65, 95% CI 1.27 to 2.16), particularly when requiring transfer.

Diagnosis of Ischemia in Women

The classification of IHD risk in women refers to those females presenting for evaluation of suspected CAD who have chest discomfort or some ischemic equivalent including excessive dyspnea. Broadly characterized, pre-menopausal women with symptoms are typically low risk. Symptomatic women in their fifth decade of life should be considered at low-intermediate IHD risk, if they are capable of performing routine activities of daily living (ADL). If performance of routine ADL is compromised, a woman in her 50s should be elevated to the intermediate IHD risk category. Women in their 60s are also generally considered as intermediate IHD risk whereas women 70 and older are considered at high risk for CAD.[57] The low-intermediate or intermediate-risk woman is a candidate for an exercise ECG if they have a functional capacity estimate ≥5 METs (metabolic equivalent tests) using the Duke Activity Status Inventory (DASI). Intermediate-high IHD risk women with an abnormal 12 lead rest ECG should be referred for a CAD noninvasive imaging modality including pharmacologic stress myocardial perfusion imaging (MPI), Echo, or cardiovascular magnetic resonance (CMR) imaging or coronary computed tomography angiogram (CCTA). High-IHD–risk women with stable symptoms may be referred for a stress imaging modality for functional assessment of their ischemic burden and to guide post-test anti-ischemic therapies.[57]

These guidelines emphasize the usefulness of the traditional exercise stress test without imaging as the initial test of choice for women with a normal ECG and able to exercise. Although the ST segment depression with exercise may be less diagnostic of obstructive CAD in women, a negative exercise ECG stress test has significant diagnostic value. A markedly abnormal exercise ECG demonstrating 2 or more mm of ST segment changes, in particular when occurring at low workloads (<5 METs) or persisting for greater than 5 minutes into recovery, associates with a high likelihood of obstructive CAD for both women and men. It is important to note that the predictive value of stress testing is based on predicting obstructive CAD; an abnormal stress test in symptomatic women may still be consistent with IHD that is non-obstructive.

Although the IHD guidelines have not been recently updated, there are a number of trials that included women demonstrating the role of other imaging modalities. The Prospective Multicenter Imaging Study for Evaluation of Chest Pain (PROMISE) trial was a randomized trial that demonstrated that although coronary CTA (CCTA) was not superior to stress testing in low-to-intermediate–risk patients, it is an alternative test for evaluation of chest pain. In women, a positive CCTA (vs. negative CCTA) was more predictive of events (HR 5.9, 95% CI 3.3 to 10.4) than a positive stress test (vs. a negative stress test) (HR 2.3, 95% CI 1.2 to 4.3).[58] The role of CCTA is further enhanced by the randomized controlled SCOT-HEART (Scottish Computed Tomography of the Heart) trial, where CCTA imaging was associated with a significant reduction in nonfatal MI and deaths for coronary heart disease at 5 years, when compared with standard of care in those presenting with stable chest pain.[59]

With any imaging modality used in women, considerations must be made regarding the amount of radiation exposure. Many cardiac diagnostic procedures—including stress MPI, CCTA, and coronary angiography—expose women to varying doses of ionizing radiation. In those women for whom the benefit of IHD risk detection far exceeds the small projected cancer risk following exposure to ionizing radiation, radiation exposure should not be a consideration in physician decision-making.[60] For all other women, in particular low-risk pre-menopausal women, alternative tests without radiation exposure (i.e., exercise ECG) or a no-testing strategy should be applied. Applying appropriate use criteria can limit radiation exposure in women, lowering cancer risks due to imaging in the population. Emphasis on shared decision-making with patients on the impact of radiation exposure should be part of the process before testing is performed.

Interventions and Medical Therapy for Ischemic Heart Disease in Women

Optimal medical therapy for women with IHD does not differ from that for men. Nonetheless women often receive less intensive medical therapy and secondary preventive therapies, lifestyle counseling, or referral to cardiac rehabilitation, which ultimately influences outcomes.[61] SWEDEHEART (Swedish Web System for Enhancement and Development of Evidence–Based Care in Heart Disease Evaluated According to Recommended Therapies) included every hospital system in Sweden between 2003 and 2013 and demonstrated an excess mortality related to underuse of guideline-indicated therapies in those women with STEMI and NSTEMI, compared with men, after adjusting for age and comorbidities. Once adjusted for the sex disparities in medications, the excess mortality disappeared for NSTEMI at 1 year but persisted at 5 years (excess mortality risk ratio [EWMRR] 1.07, 95% CI 1.02 to 1.12) and for STEMI at 1 (EMRR 1.43, 95% CI 1.26 to 1.62) and 5 years (EMRR 1.31, 95% CI 1.19 to 1.43).[62] Gaps in outcomes could be reduced in women by using guideline-directed medical therapies in ACS.

In addition to the difference in medical therapy, there are sex differences in use of cardiac catheterization and revascularization use and timing (as discussed above), which associate with poorer outcomes in women with ACS. Based on the Acute Coronary Treatment and Intervention Outcomes Network Registry-Get with the Guidelines (ACTION Registry-GWTG) database for the treatment of STEMI and NSTEMI, there are sex and racial differences in not just medical therapy but also interventional therapies. In NSTEMI particularly, there were lower rates of invasive and interventional procedures, particularly pronounced in Black women.[63] In-hospital mortality after AMI remains higher in women compared with men in the ACTION-GWTG registry in those with obstructive CAD.[64] The Nationwide Inpatient Sample in a contemporary matched cohort found a significantly lower number of women underwent PTCA and other supportive procedures, which appears to be associated with significantly higher in-hospital mortality.[65] More recent analysis of the Nationwide Inpatient Sample looking at a more contemporary time from 2010 to 2016 demonstrated a persistence in disparities in reperfusion and revascularization therapies after STEMI in women, resulting in higher in-hospital mortality compared with men. Women had a higher overall in-hospital mortality than men (11% vs. 6.8%; OR 1.039, CI 1.003 to 1.007) which persisted with multi-variable adjustment. When stratified by age, this relationship persisted in the youngest (age 19 to 49 years) with a 25% elevated in-hospital mortality compared with men (adj OR 1.259, 95% CI 1.083 to 1.464).[66]

Furthermore, in randomized controlled PCI trials, women fare more poorly than men. In a pooled analysis of 10 randomized controlled PCI trials that included 2632 patients (22% women), women were older and had greater delays in reperfusion, but had better early post-MI left ventricular ejection fraction (LVEF) and similar infarct size to men.[67] Women still had higher adjusted 1-year rates of death or HF hospitalizations (HR 2.13, 95% CI 1.34 to 3.38), which were not explained by LVEF or infarct size.[67]

There is evidence that women do worse with incomplete revascularization compared with men after STEMI. A study of 589 consecutive STEMI patients followed for a median of 3.6 years demonstrated that women were equally likely to be incompletely revascularized (residual

SYNTAX score >8) compared with men, despite a lower burden of disease. These women who were incompletely revascularized were almost twice as likely as men to have repeat MI or die from cardiac causes, even after adjusting for risk (adjusted HR 1.77, 95% CI 1.13 to 2.77, p = 0.01).[68] This emphasizes the need for complete revascularization in women after STEMI.

Studies document increased bleeding risk in women undergoing PCI who receive glycoprotein IIb/IIIa inhibitors. The GLOBAL LEADERS randomized control trial that compared 1 month of dual antiplatelet therapy (DAPT) followed by 23 months of ticagrelor monotherapy with 12 months of DAPT following 21 months of aspirin found no difference in the efficacy or safety after 2 years with either antiplatelet regime.[69] Women experience an increased risk of bleeding and hemorrhagic stroke with either therapy, whereas men had lower risk of bleeding with ticagrelor monotherapy. Sex remains an independent predictor of bleeding post-PCI and has been demonstrated in the Nationwide Inpatient Sample of over 6.6 million patients with women having both an increased risk post PCI of in-hospital mortality (OR 1.20, 95% CI 1.16 to 1.23) and major bleeding (OR 1.81, 95% CI 1.77 to 1.86).[70]

A persistent pattern of higher mortality and poorer cardiovascular outcomes in women compared with men with IHD remains, mostly attributable to suboptimal use of guideline therapy in at-risk women, despite evidence that application of guideline therapy post-ACS reduces the mortality disparity in women, and that management of ACS and chronic angina with intensive medical therapy benefits both sexes equally.[71]

ISCHEMIC HEART DISEASE: BEYOND OBSTRUCTIVE CORONARY ARTERY DISEASE

Women have less anatomical obstructive CAD and relatively more preserved left ventricular function in the setting of both stable IHD and ACS.[72] Ischemia with no obstructive CAD is referred to as INOCA. Myocardial infarction with nonobstructive CAD is referred to as MINOCA. The traditional definition of obstructive CAD was any coronary stenosis greater than 70%,[73] but has been updated to include lesions of 50% to 70% where there is inducible ischemia or physiologic significant stenosis.

Ischemia with No Obstructive Coronary Artery Disease

INOCA is more frequently appreciated, with the recognition that obstructive lesions are not a prerequisite for ischemia. It can overlap with many features of MINOCA but exclusively refers to non-MI syndromes (Fig. 91.4).

Prevalence: In those who present with IHD and undergo angiography, approximately 50% have INOCA, with a higher prevalence in women compared with men (65% vs. 32%).[74] In a single-center study of all consecutive non-emergent cardiac angiograms, although women had a similar prevalence and extent of ischemia as men, women were more likely than men to have INOCA.[75] The odds of obstructive CAD in women undergoing coronary angiography is approximately half that compared with men, for an estimated prevalence of 2 to 3 million women with INOCA.

Pathophysiology: Studies have implicated adverse coronary reactivity, CMD, and plaque erosion/distal micro-embolization as contributory to INOCA pathophysiology. The prevalence may be increasing due to an increased recognition of these issues, in contrast with prior documentation of "false positive" ischemic imaging when no obstructive CAD was found. Additionally, more sensitive diagnostics, specifically advanced imaging techniques, are better able to detect IHD.

Prognosis: The lack of obstructive CAD does not imply a benign prognosis. Data from WISE has shown that symptomatic women with documented ischemia and nonobstructive CAD had a 10-year all-cause mortality and cardiac mortality of 17% and 11%, respectively.[76] In those women with normal coronary arteries but documented ischemia, the 10-year all-cause mortality and cardiac mortality was 10% and 6%, respectively.[76]

There are notable sex differences in outcomes in INOCA, with women having poorer outcomes when compared with men. Women with INOCA are four times more likely to be readmitted within 180 days for ACS when compared with men.[74] Coronary flow reserve (CFR) less than 2.5 is a significant incremental predictor of major adverse cardiac event (MACE) in both men and women, and by such stratification low CFR was a predictor of increased MACE rate (HR 1.06, 95% CI 1.01–1.12, p = 0.021), whereas low CBF was associated with increased risk of mortality (HR 1.12, 95% CI 1.01–1.24, p=0.038) and MACE in women undergoing invasive testing.[77]

Treatment: There is limited data regarding effectiveness of unique therapies for INOCA-related to outcomes. Nonetheless, treatment of stable IHD is necessary, but those with INOCA remain undertreated. When examining a number of studies, less than half of those with IHD are treated with guideline-recommended medical therapies for ischemia, including angiotensin-converting enzyme inhibitors

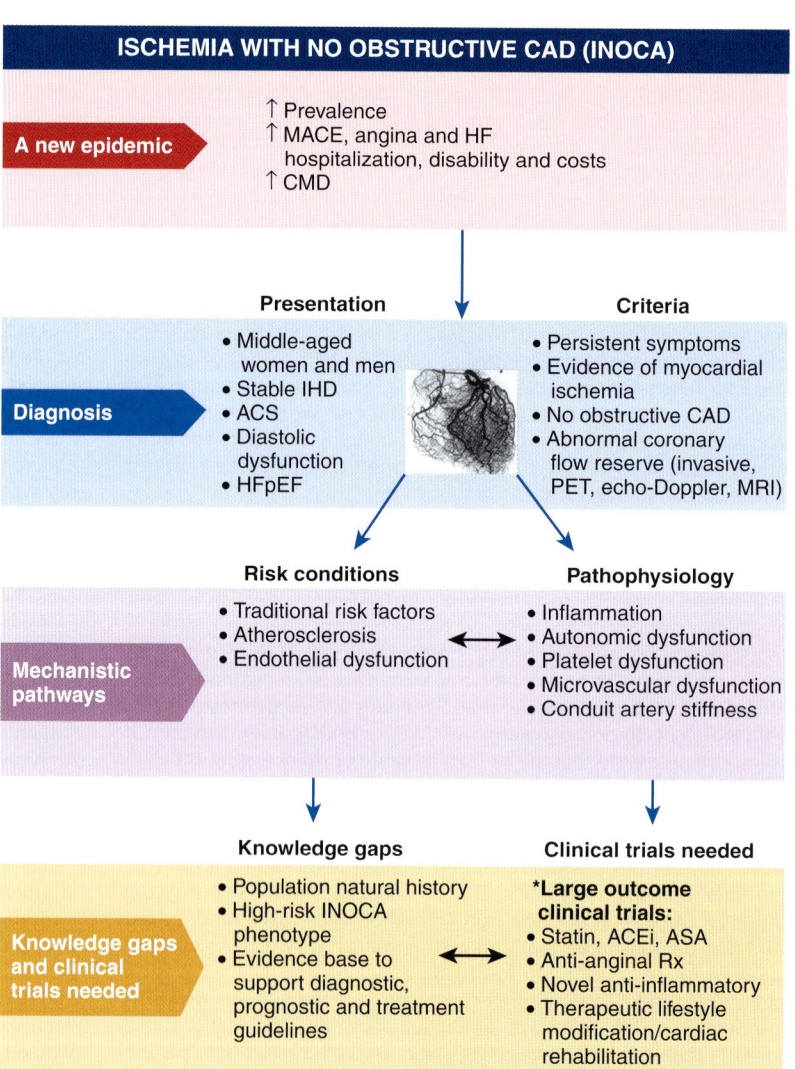

FIGURE 91.4 Ischemia with no obstructive coronary artery disease (INOCA). *ACEi*, Angiotensin-converting enzyme inhibitor; *ASA*, aspirin; *CAD*, coronary artery disease; *CMD*, coronary microvascular dysfunction; *HF*, heart failure; *HFpEF*, heart failure with preserved ejection fraction; *IHD*, ischemic heart disease; *MACE*, major adverse cardiac event; *MRI*, magnetic resonance imaging; *Rx*, prescription; *PET*, positron emission tomography. (From Bairey Merz CN, Pepine CJ, Walsh MN, Fleg JL. Ischemia and no obstructive coronary artery disease (INOCA): developing evidence-based therapies and research agenda for the next decade. *Circulation*. 2017;135(11):1075–1092.)

TABLE 91.1 Clinical Presentations with a Working Diagnosis of Myocardial Infarction with Nonobstructive Coronary Artery Disease

	UNDERLYING MECHANISM/ CLINICAL DISORDER	DIAGNOSTIC INVESTIGATIONS	TARGETED/EMPIRICAL THERAPIES
Noncoronary causes mimicking MINOCA	Supply-demand mismatch	History, identification of potential stressors	Treatment of underlying condition
	Takotsubo cardiomyopathy	Left ventricular angiogram, contrast MRI	GDMT for HF, ACE-I, beta blocker, mechanical circulatory support as needed
	Cardiomyopathies	Contrast cMRI	GDMT for HF, treatment of underlying cause
	Myocarditis	Contrast cMRI	GDMT for HF/myocarditis
Coronary causes of MINOCA	Plaque erosion/rupture	Angiogram review, consider IVUS/OCT	Aspirin, high-intensity statin, beta blocker, ACE-I, consider P2Y12 inhibitor
	Coronary vasospasm	Resolution with vasodilators, provocation testing, history of migraine medications or cocaine use	CCB, nitrates, cilostazol, consider statins
	Microvascular dysfunction	Invasive or noninvasive (PET) coronary blood flow and coronary flow reserve, cMRI	Lifestyle modification especially exercise, consider statin, ACE-I, beta blockers, L-arginine supplementation
	Coronary embolism/thrombus	Angiogram review, consider IVUS/OCT, thrombophilia screen/workup	Consider anticoagulation, treatment of underlying thrombotic condition
	SCAD	Angiogram review, consider IVUS/OCT	Aspirin, beta-blocker, consider P2Y12 inhibitor

ACE-I, Angiotensin-converting enzyme inhibitor; *ARB*, angiotensin receptor blocker; *CCB*, calcium channel blocker; *cMRI*, cardiac magnetic resonance imaging; *GDMT*, guideline-directed medical therapy; *IVUS*, intravascular ultrasound; *MINOCA*, myocardial infarction in the absence of obstructive coronary artery disease; *OCT*, optical coherence tomography; *PET*, positron emission tomography; *SCAD*, spontaneous coronary artery dissection.
Adapted from Tamis-Holland JE, Jneid H, Reynolds HR, et al. Contemporary Diagnosis and Management of Patients With Myocardial Infarction in the Absence of Obstructive Coronary Artery Disease: A Scientific Statement From the American Heart Association. *Circulation*. 2019;139:e891–e908.

or angiotensin receptor blockers, beta blockers, calcium channel blockers, or statin therapies.[74] The under-treatment may be a result of diagnostic and therapeutic uncertainty, resulting in fewer secondary preventive therapies.

Myocardial Infarction with Nonobstructive Coronary Artery Disease

The increasing recognition of MI in those without obstructive CAD is now commonly referred to as MINOCA. MINOCA is not a single disease process and requires further evaluation to make a diagnosis and also exclude noncoronary etiologies of AMI (Table 91.1).[64]

Prevalence: MI in the absence of obstructive CAD occurs in 5% to 6% of all AMI, seen in both contemporary registries and prior ACS trials.[64] Women with ACS are twice as likely to have "normal" angiograms or demonstrate no obstructive CAD when compared with men, while the average of MINOCA is 58 years, compared with 61 years in those with AMI with obstructive CAD.[78] Given there are 1.4 million ACS events per year, 600,000 of which are women, this translates to 60,000 to 150,000 women with ACS and nonobstructive CAD.

Pathophysiology: MINOCA can be caused by both atherosclerotic and nonatherosclerotic causes (see Table 91.1).[79] Because it does not reflect only one disease process, not all MINOCA cases will have electrocardiographic changes and troponin elevations may be smaller than seen in obstructive AMI. Additionally, myocardial injury that is nonischemic (i.e., myocarditis, Takotsubo cardiomyopathy) can mimic myocardial infarction, and this distinction needs to be clarified by additional diagnostic testing because both injury and infarction will have elevations in troponin.[79]

Based on the Scientific Statement from the American Heart Association on Contemporary Diagnosis and Management of Patients with MINOCA, the underlying pathophysiology can be due to coronary vasospasm, CMD, coronary embolism or thrombosis, spontaneous coronary artery dissection (SCAD), and supply-demand mismatch.[79]

Prognosis: In the setting of an ACS, "normal" coronary arteries do not have a benign prognosis.[79] All-cause mortality appears to be lower in MINOCA compared with MI with obstructive CAD but is substantial (in-hospital mortality: 1.1 vs. 3.2%, *P = 0.001*; 12-month mortality: 6.7% vs. 3.5%, *P = 0.003*).[78]

Treatment: The current guidelines that exist for STEMI and NSTEMI do not differ by sex and no studies to date support the value of specific therapies of MINOCA, hence efforts to improve the application of guidelines in practice could improve MI and IHD outcomes in women. The management of MINOCA has a limited evidence-based literature and as described above, has multiple different possible pathophysiologies. To date, there are no prospective randomized, controlled trials for management of any of these. It is important to try to define the likely cause of MINOCA and assess for potential myocardial injury causes. Acute management should involve emergency supportive care, cardioprotective therapies irrespective of the cause of MINOCA, in addition to cause-targeted therapies. Secondary ASCVD preventive therapies should also be initiated.

Takotsubo Cardiomyopathy (see also Chapters 37 and 38)

Takotsubo cardiomyopathy accounts for 4% of those presenting with presumed ACS,[80] although the prevalence is higher in women, particularly post-menopausal women (5.9% to 7.5%), and female sex is one of the seven parameters of the diagnostic score. Takotsubo cardiomyopathy should be considered in women as part of the differential diagnosis of acute coronary syndrome.[80] Other names for this syndrome include "transient ventricular ballooning syndrome," "left ventricular apical ballooning syndrome," "stress-induced cardiomyopathy," "ampulla cardiomyopathy," and "broken heart syndrome." Women account for 90% of all Takotsubo cardiomyopathy cases.[80] The Fourth Universal Definition of MI does not consider Takotsubo cardiomyopathy an AMI and recognizes it as a separate syndrome, therefore it is not classified as a form of MINOCA.[81]

There are no randomized controlled trials assessing therapeutic options for Takotsubo cardiomyopathy. Beta blockers appear to provide no benefit for the index event or prevention of subsequent episodes.[82] There is some observational benefit of ACE-I with improved 1-year survival, but no guidance to duration of treatment necessary.[83] Although it is often thought that Takotsubo cardiomyopathy was benign because it was often reversible, in-hospital and long-term mortality is 4.1% and 5.6%, respectively based on the International Takotsubo Registry (InterTAK).[83] The Mayo Clinic Takotsubo registry demonstrated a 1-year survival of 94% but the leading cause of death was cancer, and cardiac deaths only accounted for 5% of all deaths. Although for Takotsubo cardiomyopathy is often reversible, it may recur in up to 5% to 10%.[80]

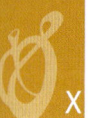

CARDIAC SURGERY

Coronary Artery Bypass Graft

Coronary artery bypass graft (CABG) surgery is a common procedure for the treatment of obstructive CAD for both men and women in the United States. Women undergo approximately 32% of CABG procedures annually.[1] For over 40 years, there has been a persistent sex disparity in outcomes with CABG, with women having higher perioperative morbidity and mortality after CABG than men.[84] When examining five US states from 2007 to 2014 which included 340,080 patients, women were 32% more likely to die compared with men, after adjusting for other factors including age, race, insurance, income, comorbidity index, surgical volumes, and year of procedure (adjusted OR 1.32, 95% CI 1.25 to 1.40). Women also had significantly greater risk of 30-day and 90-day readmissions. These sex differences noted have typically been explained by baseline differences in age, body size, coronary artery diameter, ASCVD risk factors, and other comorbidities. Nonetheless, risk assessment score includes sex as part of estimating risk of CABG, independent of other predictors. In an analysis of 72,824 patients women had significantly higher age–standardized mortality rate than men after CABG and combined CABG/mitral valve surgery. Men had lower rates of long-term mortality than women after isolated mitral valve repair, whereas women had lower rates of long-term mortality than men after isolated mitral valve replacement. There was a statistically significant association between female sex and long-term mortality after adjustment for key risk factors.[85] Data has been mixed in terms of outcomes based on sex, when off-pump CABG is performed. More contemporary cohorts have not shown a protective effect of off-pump CABG for women.

Valvular Heart Surgery

There are no sex-specific guidelines for valvular heart disease and valve surgery, although there are sex-specific outcome data after valve surgery. AS is the most common indication for valve replacement and women are older than men when presenting with symptomatic AS, have more exertional dyspnea, higher frailty scores, and more severe AS.[86] Smaller body size may also impact prosthetic valve size and affect outcomes, and as expected short-term survival is worse for women who undergo surgical replacement of the aortic valve.[86] Nonetheless, long-term outcomes suggest no gender differences in outcomes, and may even potentially favor women.

For mitral valve replacement surgery, regardless of type of valve replacement (mechanical or bioprosthetic), the evidence is inconsistent, with studies demonstrating women do worse than men, some with no difference in outcomes based on sex, and yet other studies demonstrating women have better long-term survival compared with men.[87] All risk calculators take sex into consideration and the risk scores are elevated for women compared with men.

Transcatheter Aortic Valve Intervention

Women referred for transcatheter aortic valve intervention (TAVI) have the same risk profile as women who are referred for surgical AVR. Female anatomy affects TAVI as well, including shorter distances from the coronary ostia to the annulus, increased calcification, and a more horizontal aorta, which can result in coronary obstruction necessitating conversion to open surgery.[88] On the other hand, small annuli in women results in less paravalvular regurgitation. Early TAVI trials limited transfemoral access in women due to lack of small sheath sizes but over time, the equipment has evolved.

In the early PARTNER trial of high-risk and inoperable patients with severe AS (1220 women and 1339 men), women had lower rates of renal disease, smoking, hyperlipidemia, and diabetes, yet higher STS mortality risk compared with men. Despite noting increased vascular and major bleeding complication in women, women had lower 1-year mortality rates with TAVI compared with men (19.0% vs. 25.6%, $P < 0.001$).[89] Women undergoing TAVI in a number of trials have demonstrated equal 30-day survival, but better long-term survival compared with men.[88-90]

Transcatheter Mitral Valve Repair

Recent data regarding transcatheter mitral valve repair (TMVR) with percutaneous edge-to-edge repair (MitraClip) has shown no difference by sex in terms of rehospitalization for HF but superior long-term survival in women compared with men.[91]

PERIPHERAL ARTERIAL DISEASE (see also Chapter 43)

Peripheral arterial disease (PAD) has a high prevalence in women in the United States, increasing with age and ranging from 2% at age 40 to as high as 25% in women 80 years or older, with more women with PAD over the age of 40 years compared with men. The incidence of PAD in women with chronic kidney disease has demonstrated significant sex differences, with women having a 1.53-fold greater adjusted PAD risk, compared to men in the Chronic Renal Insufficiency Cohort ($P < 0.001$).[92] Lower extremity PAD associates with equal morbidity and mortality and comparable health costs as IHD and ischemic stroke. PAD can be assessed using the ankle-brachial index (ABI), with the diagnosis of PAD when the ABI is less than 0.9.

There are sex differences in PAD symptoms. Women with PAD can lack the classical symptom of intermittent claudication and women are more likely to be asymptomatic than men. Like other CVD, there appears to be a long "latent phase" that can progress over time in women. In the K–VIS ELLA registry, a nationwide, multicenter, observational study that includes 3073 PAD patients undergoing endovascular therapy, women had higher rates of death, myocardial infarction, and major amputation than men and higher rates of complex lesions, procedural complications, and limb–specific adverse events.[93]

Women had lower amputation rates but still have persistent higher mortality than men.[94] Some studies have demonstrated that women with PAD that undergo endovascular therapy have poorer outcomes. Sex differences on survival after lower extremity PAD revascularization have been inconsistent but gender is often confounded by morbidity, age, and procedural factors that impact perioperative mortality. Women remain underrepresented in studies of PAD, contributing to the lack of sex-specific data or therapies.

Other forms of PAD also demonstrate sex differences. A single center in Canada has shown retrospectively that thoracic aortic aneurysms grow twice as fast in women, with aortic stiffness associated with the aneurysm growth in women but not in men.[95] Renal artery stenosis and abdominal aortic aneurysms are more common in men than women. Because abdominal aortic aneurysms are four times more likely in men, and less frequently associated with deaths in women, screening in asymptomatic women is not recommended, in contrast with men.[96]

HEART FAILURE (see also Chapters 47–52)

HF prevalence is increasing, and affects 3.2 million women in the United States, accounting for 54% of all people living with HF.[1] In 2016, there were 43,656 deaths in women due to HF, which accounted for more deaths in women compared with men (54.2% vs. 45.8%). Community surveillance data show that rates of hospitalization for HF are increasing over time, due to an increase in heart failure with preserved ejection fraction (HFpEF), which occurs more frequently in women.[97]

The risk factors associated with HF and its underlying pathophysiology differ by sex. Traditional risk factors, such as diabetes, obesity, hypertension, and tobacco use impact the risk of HF more in women than men. Additionally, psychological stress, a cause of Takotsubo cardiomyopathy, appears to have a greater impact on women than men. Women with HF have more hypertension, valvular heart disease, and thyroid disorders than men, but are less likely to have obstructive CAD. Even though obstructive CAD is less frequent in women, when it is present it is a stronger risk factor for the development of HF than hypertension. Risk factors selective for women include cardiac toxicity from chemotherapeutic drugs and radiation used for treatment of breast cancer and reproductive factors that can result in peripartum cardiomyopathy. Women who present with acute decompensated HF are twice as likely as men to have preserved left ventricular function or HFpEF,[98] with obesity being a significant risk factor for women with HFpEF, particularly in African American women.[98] Even those women with an impaired LVEF will have a higher LVEF when compared with men. Notably, women with HF have a lower quality of life, lower functional capacity, more hospitalizations for HF, and more frequent depression. Nonetheless, overall survival is better for women compared with men with HF. This is not just a result of women having more HFpEF because mortality rates from HF do not relate to preserved or impaired ejection fraction in either sex, although those with ischemic cardiomyopathy have a worse prognosis.[99]

Peripartum Cardiomyopathy (see also Chapter 92)

Peripartum cardiomyopathy causes impaired LVEF that occurs in the last month of pregnancy or in the months after delivery (although the exact timing remains ill-defined) with no pre-existing cardiac disease and no identifiable cause.[100] Its incidence is estimated to be 1 in 4000 pregnancies and is associated with risk factors including advanced maternal age, African descent, high parity, twin pregnancy, usage of tocolytics, and poverty. After the diagnosis, about half recover their LVEF within 6 months, however 20% deteriorate and either die or require heart transplantation. Recovery appears to be related to a less severe decline in LVEF.[101] The risk of recurrence during subsequent pregnancy is greater in those with persistent left ventricular dysfunction (48% with significant deterioration, 16% died), although even those who recover have a high risk of recurrence (27% showed deterioration, no deaths).[102]

Heart Failure Diagnosis

There appear to be sex differences in the biomarker brain natriuretic peptide (BNP) used to diagnose HF and markers of cardiac stretch (natriuretic peptides) and fibrosis (galectin-3) are higher in women, whereas markers of cardiac injury (cardiac troponins) and inflammation (sST2) are higher in men.[103] Such differences may reflect sex-specific pathogenic processes associated with HF risk, but may also arise as a result of differences in sex hormone profiles and fat distribution. From a clinical perspective, sex-related differences in biomarker levels may affect the objectivity of biomarkers in HF management because what is considered to be "normal" in one sex may not be so in the other. Further studies are needed to delineate and understand the sex differences in HF biomarkers.

Heart Failure Treatment

Treatment for HF may benefit both sexes equally, however the underrepresentation of women in HF trials and the more prevalent HFpEF in women contributes to our lack of evidence regarding treatment of HF in women. The CHARM trials, along with others, showed women were more likely to have preserved left ventricular function (50%) than men (35%).[98] More recently, the PARAGON-HF trial demonstrated that angiotensin neprilysin inhibitor sacubitril/valsartan appeared to benefit women with HFpEF more than men.[104] Although the study did not show a difference overall in its primary outcomes of total HF hospitalization and CV deaths, it did show a significant 28% reduction in this endpoint in women, when compared to valsartan alone (rate ratio 0.73, 95% CI 0.59 to 0.90). Women with HFpEF are more symptomatic and have worse quality of life, but had lower mortality and fewer HF hospitalizations (Fig. 91.5).[105]

Device Use in Heart Failure

Implantable cardioverter-defibrillator (ICD) devices are underused in both sexes with HF, but particularly in women. None of the randomized trials for ICDs enrolled sufficient numbers of women to permit conclusions regarding sex differences and hence, have not demonstrated a mortality benefit in women. The differences may result in part from sex differences in body size and delayed presentation in women. Women are less likely to receive a defibrillator or CRT than men.[105] Examining ICD implantation for primary prevention in 11 countries in Europe between 2002 and 2014 finds fewer women received an ICD (19% of all ICD implantations). Nonetheless, women had a significantly lower mortality but also received fewer appropriate ICD shocks than men.[106]

CRT also shows benefit in both women and men with HF and wide QRS complex, but observational data from the National Cardiovascular Data Registry demonstrated that the mortality benefit is more pronounced in women, confirming earlier randomized trials that compared CRT to medical therapy alone.[107] Nonetheless, these devices are underused in women, as demonstrated in the Nationwide Inpatient Sample and Medicare/Medicaid Data.[108]

Mechanical Circulatory Support

Mechanical circulatory support (MCS) can bridge an HF patient to transplant or extend life. The commonest form of MCS is a left ventricular assist device (LVAD), and most LVADs are implanted into men (79%).[109] Looking at the Nationwide Inpatient Sample from 2004 to 2016, although LVADs are used more and have gotten smaller and more durable, women received these devices even less frequently, representing 26% of LVADs in 2004 and 22% by 2016.[110]

Cardiac Transplantation

Women are less likely to be listed for transplant and are less likely to receive a transplant, despite shorter waiting times for women. As of 2016, only 26% of all heart transplants in the United States occurred in women.[111] This, despite that fact that there appears to be no significant survival difference based on sex.[112] The survival difference is when waiting for transplantation. Women on LVAD support are less likely to be transplanted (62% vs. 76%, $P < 0.001$) and more likely to die or be removed from the transplant list as a result of worsening clinical status.[109] Female sex was a significant predictor of waitlist mortality (HR 1.51, $P < 0.001$).

Women who undergo heart transplantation have lower-risk features than men, with less IHD, diabetes, hypertension, smoking history, or prior cardiac surgery than men.[112] Women who eventually get a heart transplant do equally as well as men, despite the fact that women often get higher-risk transplanted hearts than men.[112]

ARRYTHMIA AND SUDDEN CARDIAC DEATH

Important sex differences in cardiac electrophysiology can impact arrhythmias and sudden cardiac death. Starting at puberty, women have higher resting heart rates compared to men. Women also have longer QT intervals, and a greater risk for drug-induced torsades de pointes. There are sex differences in the supraventricular tachycardias (SVTs). Atrioventricular (AV) nodal reentrant tachycardia (AVNRT) is twice as common in women as compared to men, compared to AV reentrant tachycardia as seen in the Wolff-Parkinson-White syndrome which is more common in men. Atrial and ventricular fibrillation also occur more frequently in men with Wolff-Parkinson-White syndrome. Globally, there continues to be an increase in the incidence and prevalence of atrial fibrillation for both men and women, but age-adjusted mortality due to atrial fibrillation has been shown to be comparable in women and men.[113] Compared to men, women with atrial fibrillation tend to be more symptomatic, have a higher risk of stroke and mortality, are less likely to receive anticoagulation and ablation procedures than men, and yet fare worse when treated with antiarrhythmic medications.[114] Women who experience sudden cardiac death are

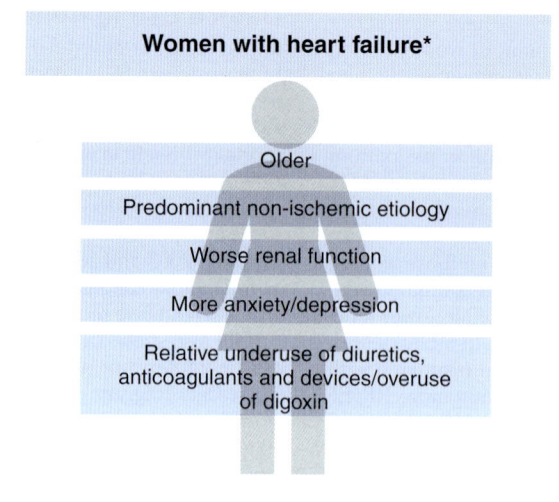
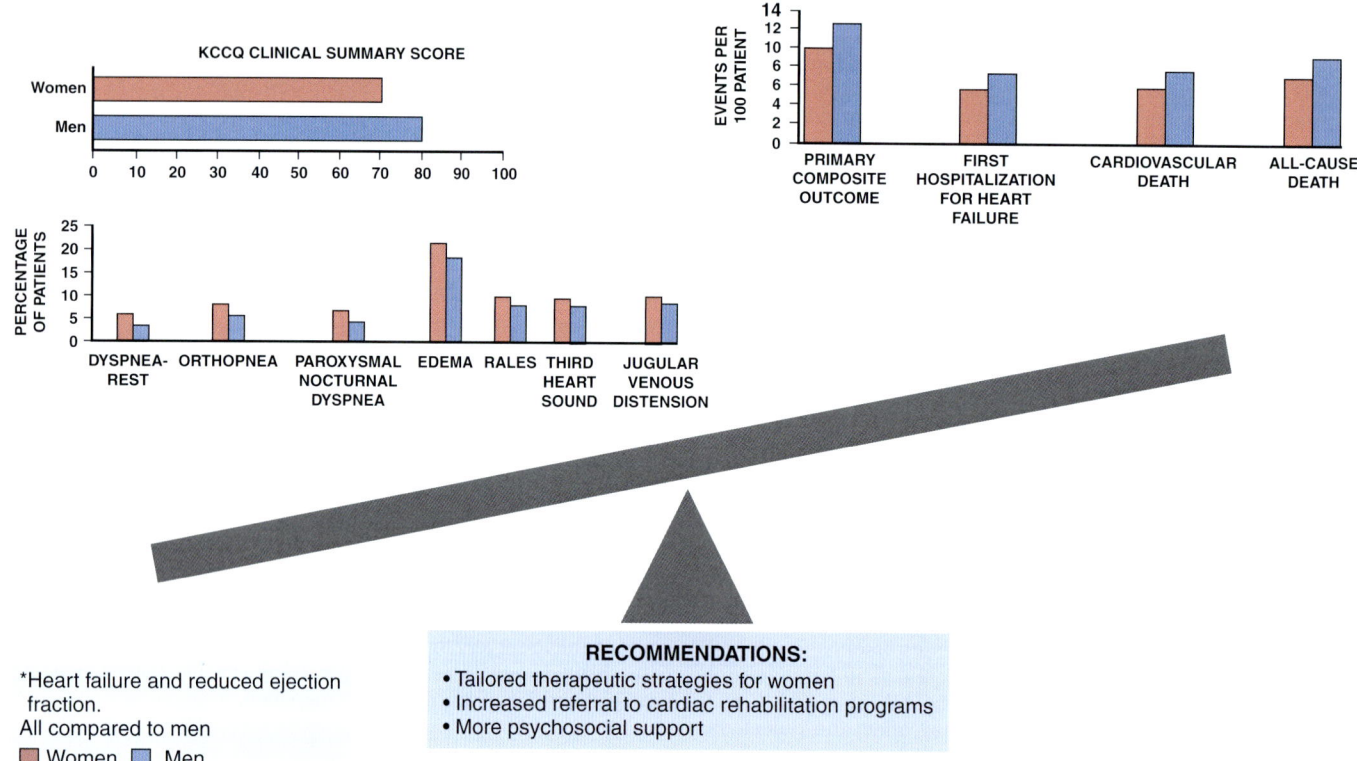

FIGURE 91.5 Women with heart failure with reduced ejection fraction. (From Dewan P, Rørth R, Jhund PS, et al. Differential impact of heart failure with reduced ejection fraction on men and women. *J Am Coll Cardiol.* 2019;73:29–40.)

older than men, and are less likely to have ischemic causes of sudden cardiac death.[115] Although women have an overall lower risk of sudden cardiac death, women with cardiac arrest who receive therapeutic hypothermia have significantly better outcomes than men, but are less likely than men to get recommended treatment after an out-of-hospital cardiac arrest.[116]

CARDIOVASCULAR DISEASE PREVENTION

Guidelines for CVD prevention in women were largely based on the "Effectiveness-Based Guidelines for the Prevention of Cardiovascular Disease in Women—2011 Update" but have been replaced by the 2018 ACC/AHA evidence-based guidelines on the treatment of blood cholesterol to reduce ASCVD in adults[8] and the 2019 ACC/AHA guidelines on the primary prevention of CVD.[7] These guidelines apply to both women and men, with the focus on primary prevention of CVD. Secondary CVD prevention must be implemented once a diagnosis of CVD has been made.

An important component of secondary CVD prevention includes cardiac rehabilitation (see also Chapter 33). Cardiac rehabilitation improves functional capacity, decreases anginal symptoms, facilitates CVD risk reduction, and improves psychosocial well-being in both sexes. It also improves quality of life and medication compliance and reduces morbidity and mortality. Both sexes should be referred to cardiac rehabilitation after experiencing angina, any type of MI, post-coronary revascularization (either CABG or PCI), after valvular heart surgery, and those with chronic HF.[117] Nonetheless, cardiac rehabilitation is remarkably underused in the United States, with an estimated participation rate of only 10% to 20% of eligible patients, with women particularly under-referred and less likely to complete cardiac rehabilitation even if they enroll.[61]

ACKNOWLEDGMENTS

This work was supported by contracts from the National Heart, Lung and Blood Institutes, nos. N01-HV-68161, N01-HV-68162, N01-HV-68163, N01-HV-68164, grants U0164829, U01 HL649141, U01 HL649241, T32HL69751, 1R03AG032631 from the National Institute on Aging, GCRC grant MO1-RR00425 from the National Center for Research Resources and grants from the Gustavus and Louis Pfeiffer Research Foundation, Danville, NJ, The Women's Guild of Cedars-Sinai Medical Center, Los Angeles, CA, the Ladies Hospital Aid Society of Western Pennsylvania, Pittsburgh, PA, and QMED, Inc., Laurence Harbor, NJ, the Edythe L. Broad Women's Heart Research Fellowship, Cedars-Sinai Medical Center, Los Angeles, California, the Barbra Streisand Women's Cardiovascular Research and Education Program, Cedars-Sinai Medical Center, Los Angeles, The Society for Women's Health Research (SWHR), Washington, D.C. and the Linda Joy Pollin Women's Heart Health Program, and the Erika Glazer Women's Heart Health Project, Cedars-Sinai Medical Center, Los Angeles, California (CNBM).

REFERENCES

Epidemiology

1. Virani SS, et al. Heart disease and stroke statistics-2021 update: a report from the American Heart Association. *Circulation*; 2021:143(8):e254–e743.
2. Arora S, Stouffer GA, Kucharska-Newton AM, et al. Twenty year trends and sex differences in young adults hospitalized with acute myocardial infarction. *Circulation*. 2019;139:1047–1056.
3. Bairey Merz CN, Andersen H, Sprague E, et al. Knowledge, attitudes, and beliefs regarding cardiovascular disease in women: the women's heart alliance. *J Am Coll Cardiol*. 2017;70:123–132.
4. *Exploring the Biological Contributions to Human Health: Does Sex Matter?* The National Academies Press; 2001.
5. Hajek C, Guo X, Yao J, et al. Coronary heart disease genetic risk score predicts cardiovascular disease risk in men, not women. *Circ Genom Precis Med*. 2018;11:e002324.

Risk Factors

6. Arnett DK, Blumenthal RS, Albert MA, et al. 2019 ACC/AHA guideline on the primary prevention of cardiovascular disease: executive summary: a report of the American College of Cardiology/American heart association task force on clinical practice guidelines. *J Am Coll Cardiol*. 2019;74:1376–1414.
7. Wilmot KA, O'Flaherty M, Capewell S, et al. Coronary heart disease mortality declines in the United States from 1979 through 2011: evidence for stagnation in young adults, especially women. *Circulation*. 2015;132:997–1002.
8. Grundy SM, Stone NJ, Bailey AL, et al. 2018 AHA/ACC/AACVPR/AAPA/ABC/ACPM/ADA/AGS/APhA/ASPC/NLA/PCNA guideline on the management of blood cholesterol: a report of the American College of Cardiology/American heart association task force on clinical practice guidelines. *J Am Coll Cardiol*. 2019;73:e285–e350.
9. Whelton PK, Carey RM, Aronow WS, et al. 2017 ACC/AHA/AAPA/ABC/ACPM/AGS/APhA/ASH/ASPC/NMA/PCNA guideline for the prevention, detection, evaluation, and management of high blood pressure in adults: executive summary: a report of the American College of Cardiology/American heart association task force on clinical practice guidelines. *J Am Coll Cardiol*. 2018;71:2199–2269.
10. Ostchega Y, Fryar CD, Nwankwo T, Nguyen DT. *Hypertension Prevalence Among Adults Aged 18 and over: United States, 2017–2018*; 2020.
11. Fryar CD, Ostchega Y, Hales CM, et al. *Hypertension Prevalence and Control Among Adults: United States, 2015–2016*. NCHS Data Brief; 2017:1–8.
12. Giribela CR, Consolim-Colombo FM, Nisenbaum MG, et al. Effects of a combined oral contraceptive containing 20 mcg of ethinylestradiol and 3 mg of drospirenone on the blood pressure, renin-angiotensin-aldosterone system, insulin resistance, and androgenic profile of healthy young women. *Gynecol Endocrinol*. 2015;31:912–915.
13. Ji H, Kim A, Ebinger JE, et al. Sex differences in blood pressure trajectories over the life course. *JAMA Cardiol*. 2020.
14. Regensteiner JG, Golden S, Huebschmann AG, et al. Sex differences in the cardiovascular consequences of diabetes mellitus: a scientific statement from the American heart association. *Circulation*. 2015;132:2424–2447.
15. Huxley RR, Peters SA, Mishra GD, Woodward M. Risk of all-cause mortality and vascular events in women versus men with type 1 diabetes: a systematic review and meta-analysis. *Lancet Diabetes Endocrinol*. 2015;3:198–206.
16. Professional Practice Committee. Standards of medical care in diabetes-2020. *Diabetes Care*. 2020;43:S3.
17. Carroll MD, Fryar CD. *Total and High-Density Lipoprotein Cholesterol in Adults: United States, 2015–2018*; 2020.
18. Nanna MG, Wang TY, Xiang Q, et al. Sex differences in the use of statins in community practice. *Circ Cardiovasc Qual Outcomes*. 2019;12:e005562.
19. Polotsky HN, Polotsky AJ. Metabolic implications of menopause. *Semin Reprod Med*. 2010;28:426–434.
20. Creamer MR, Wang TW, Babb S, et al. Tobacco product use and cessation indicators among adults—United States, 2018. *MMWR Morb Mortal Wkly Rep*. 2019;68:1013–1019.
21. Palmer J, Lloyd A, Steele L, et al. Differential risk of ST-segment elevation myocardial infarction in male and female smokers. *J Am Coll Cardiol*. 2019;73:3259–3266.
22. Pirie K, Peto R, Reeves GK, et al. The 21st century hazards of smoking and benefits of stopping: a prospective study of one million women in the UK. *Lancet*. 2013;381:133–141.
23. McKee SA, Smith PH, Kaufman M, et al. Sex differences in varenicline efficacy for smoking cessation: a meta-analysis. *Nicotine Tob Res*. 2016;18:1002–1011.
24. Centers for Disease Control and Prevention. *Participation in Leisure-Time Aerobic and Muscle-Strengthening Activities that Meet the Federal 2008 Physical Activity Guidelines for Americans Among Adults Aged 18 and over, by Selected Characteristics: United States, Selected Years 1998–2017*; 2017:2020.
25. Chomistek AK, Cook NR, Rimm EB, et al. Physical activity and incident cardiovascular disease in women: is the relation modified by level of global cardiovascular risk? *J Am Heart Assoc*. 2018;7.
26. Imboden MT, Harber MP, Whaley MH, et al. Cardiorespiratory fitness and mortality in healthy men and women. *J Am Coll Cardiol*. 2018;72:2283–2292.
27. Shin D, Kongpakpaisarn K, Bohra C. Trends in the prevalence of metabolic syndrome and its components in the United States 2007–2014. *Int J Cardiol*. 2018;259:216–219.
28. Kazlauskiene L, Butnoriene J, Norkus A. Metabolic syndrome related to cardiovascular events in a 10-year prospective study. *Diabetol Metab Syndr*. 2015;7:102.
29. Hales CM, Carroll MD, Fryar CD, Ogden CL. *Prevalence of Obesity and Severe Obesity Among Adults: United States, 2017–2018*. NCHS Data Brief; 2020.
30. Manrique-Acevedo C, Chinnakotla B, Padilla J, et al. Obesity and cardiovascular disease in women. *Int J Obes (Lond)*. 2020;44:1210–1226.
31. Farrell SW, Barlow CE, Willis BL, et al. Cardiorespiratory fitness, different measures of adiposity, and cardiovascular disease mortality risk in women. *J Womens Health (Larchmt)*. 2020;29:319–326.
32. da Silva Paulitsch F, Zhang L. Continuous positive airway pressure for adults with obstructive sleep apnea and cardiovascular disease: a meta-analysis of randomized trials. *Sleep Med*. 2019;54:28–34.

Pregnancy and Endocrine Considerations

33. Lee JJ, Cook-Wiens G, Johnson BD, et al. Age at menarche and risk of cardiovascular disease outcomes: findings from the national heart Lung and blood institute-sponsored women's ischemia syndrome evaluation. *J Am Heart Assoc*. 2019;8:e012406.
34. Wu P, Gulati M, Kwok CS, et al. Preterm delivery and future risk of maternal cardiovascular disease: a systematic review and meta-analysis. *J Am Heart Assoc*. 2018;7.
35. Haas DM, Ehrenthal DB, Koch MA, et al. Pregnancy as a window to future cardiovascular health: design and implementation of the nuMoM2b heart health study. *Am J Epidemiol*. 2016;183:519–530.
36. Honigberg MC, Zekavat SM, Aragam K, et al. Long-term cardiovascular risk in women with hypertension during pregnancy. *J Am Coll Cardiol*. 2019;74:2743–2754.
37. Lo CCW, Lo ACQ, Leow SH, et al. Future cardiovascular disease risk for women with gestational hypertension: a systematic review and meta-analysis. *J Am Heart Assoc*. 2020:e013991.
38. Benschop L, Duvekot JJ, Roeters van Lennep JE. Future risk of cardiovascular disease risk factors and events in women after a hypertensive disorder of pregnancy. *Heart*. 2019;105:1273–1278.
39. Kramer CK, Campbell S, Retnakaran R. Gestational diabetes and the risk of cardiovascular disease in women: a systematic review and meta-analysis. *Diabetologia*. 2019;62:905–914.
40. Dayan N, Filion KB, Okano M, et al. Cardiovascular risk following fertility therapy: systematic review and meta-analysis. *J Am Coll Cardiol*. 2017;70:1203–1213.
41. Udell JA, Lu H, Redelmeier DA. Failure of fertility therapy and subsequent adverse cardiovascular events. *CMAJ*. 2017;189:E391–E397.
42. Merz CN, Shaw LJ, Azziz R, et al. Cardiovascular disease and 10-year mortality in postmenopausal women with clinical features of polycystic ovary syndrome. *J Womens Health (Larchmt)*. 2016;25:875–881.
43. Shufelt CL, Torbati T, Dutra E. Hypothalamic amenorrhea and the long-term health consequences. *Semin Reprod Med*. 2017;35:256–262.
44. Muka T, Oliver-Williams C, Kunutsor S, et al. Association of age at onset of menopause and time since onset of menopause with cardiovascular outcomes, intermediate vascular traits, and all-cause mortality: a systematic review and meta-analysis. *JAMA Cardiol*. 2016;1:767–776.
45. Peters SA, Woodward M. Women's reproductive factors and incident cardiovascular disease in the UK Biobank. *Heart*. 2018;104:1069–1075.
46. Christ J, Gunning M, Palla G, et al. Prolonged estrogen deprivation is associated with increased cardiovascular disease risk among women with primary ovarian insufficiency. *Fertil Steril*. 2017;108:e392.
47. Roeters van Lennep JE, Heida KY, Bots ML, et al. Cardiovascular disease risk in women with premature ovarian insufficiency: a systematic review and meta-analysis. *Eur J Prev Cardiol*. 2016;23:178–186.
48. Curtis KM, Jatlaoui TC, Tepper NK, et al. U.S. Selected practice recommendations for contraceptive use, 2016. *MMWR Recomm Rep (Morb Mortal Wkly Rep)*. 2016;65:1–66.
49. The 2017 hormone therapy position statement of the North American Menopause Society. *Menopause*. 2018;25:1362–1387.
50. Faccini A, Kaski JC, Camici PG. Coronary microvascular dysfunction in chronic inflammatory rheumatoid diseases. *Eur Heart J*. 2016;37:1799–1806.
51. Bradshaw PT, Stevens J, Khankari N, et al. Cardiovascular disease mortality among breast cancer survivors. *Epidemiology*. 2016;27:6–13.
52. Gulati M, Mulvagh SL. The connection between the breast and heart in a woman: breast cancer and cardiovascular disease. *Clin Cardiol*. 2018;41:253–257.
53. Lichtman JH, Leifheit EC, Safdar B, et al. Sex differences in the presentation and perception of symptoms among young patients with myocardial infarction: evidence from the VIRGO study (variation in recovery: role of gender on outcomes of young AMI patients). *Circulation*. 2018;137:781–790.
54. McSweeney JC, Rosenfeld AG, Abel WM, et al. Preventing and experiencing ischemic heart disease as a woman: state of the science: a scientific statement from the American Heart Association. *Circulation*. 2016;133:1302–1331.
55. Ferry AV, Anand A, Strachan FE, et al. Presenting symptoms in men and women diagnosed with myocardial infarction using sex-specific criteria. *J Am Heart Assoc*. 2019;8:e012307.
56. Bugiardini R, Ricci B, Cenko E, et al. Delayed care and mortality among women and men with myocardial infarction. *J Am Heart Assoc*. 2017;6.
57. Hendel RC, Jabbar AY, Mahata I. Initial diagnostic evaluation of stable coronary artery disease: the need for a patient-centered strategy. *J Am Heart Assoc*. 2017;6.
58. Hemal K, Pagidipati NJ, Coles A, et al. Sex differences in demographics, risk factors, presentation, and noninvasive testing in stable outpatients with suspected coronary artery disease: insights from the PROMISE trial. *JACC Cardiovasc Imaging*. 2016;9:337–346.

Ischemic Heart Disease

59. SCOT-Heart Investigators, Newby DE, Adamson PD, et al. Coronary CT angiography and 5-year risk of myocardial infarction. *N Engl J Med*. 2018;379:924–933.
60. Douglas PS, Hoffmann U, Patel MR, et al. Outcomes of anatomical versus functional testing for coronary artery disease. *N Engl J Med*. 2015;372:1291–1300.
61. Li S, Fonarow GC, Mukamal K, et al. Sex and racial disparities in cardiac rehabilitation referral at hospital discharge and Gaps in long-term mortality. *J Am Heart Assoc*. 2018;7.
62. Alabas OA, Gale CP, Hall M, et al. Sex differences in treatments, relative survival, and excess mortality following acute myocardial infarction: national cohort study using the SWEDEHEART registry. *J Am Heart Assoc*. 2017;6.
63. Anstey DE, Li S, Thomas L, et al. Race and sex differences in management and outcomes of patients after ST-elevation and non-ST-elevation myocardial infarct: results from the NCDR. *Clin Cardiol*. 2016;39:585–595.
64. Smilowitz NR, Mahajan AM, Roe MT, et al. Mortality of myocardial infarction by sex, age, and obstructive coronary artery disease status in the ACTION registry-GWTG (acute coronary treatment and intervention outcomes network registry-get with the guidelines). *Circ Cardiovasc Qual Outcomes*. 2017;10:e003443.
65. Malik JS, Jenner C, Ward PA. Maximising application of the aerosol box in protecting healthcare workers during the COVID-19 pandemic. *Anaesthesia*. 2020;75:974–975.
66. Liu J, Elbadawi A, Elgendy IY, et al. Age-stratified sex disparities in care and outcomes in patients with ST-elevation myocardial infarction. *Am J Med*. 2020.
67. Kosmidou I, Redfors B, Selker HP, et al. Infarct size, left ventricular function, and prognosis in women compared to men after primary percutaneous coronary intervention in ST-segment

elevation myocardial infarction: results from an individual patient-level pooled analysis of 10 randomized trials. *Eur Heart J.* 2017;38:1656–1663.
68. Burgess SN, Juergens CP, Nguyen TL, et al. Comparison of late cardiac death and myocardial infarction rates in women Vs. Men with ST-elevation myocardial infarction. *Am J Cardiol.* 2020;128:120–126.
69. Chichareon P, Modolo R, Kerkmeijer L, et al. Association of sex with outcomes in patients undergoing percutaneous coronary intervention: a subgroup Analysis of the GLOBAL LEADERS randomized clinical trial. *JAMA Cardiol.* 2019;1–10.
70. Potts J, Sirker A, Martinez SC, et al. Persistent sex disparities in clinical outcomes with percutaneous coronary intervention: Insights from 6.6 million PCI procedures in the United States. *PloS One.* 2018;13:e0203325.
71. Zhao M, Vaartjes I, Graham I, et al. Sex differences in risk factor management of coronary heart disease across three regions. *Heart.* 2017;103:1587–1594.
72. Tamis-Holland JE, Jneid H, Reynolds HR, et al. Contemporary diagnosis and management of patients with myocardial infarction in the absence of obstructive coronary artery disease: a scientific statement from the American heart association. *Circulation.* 2019;139:e891–e908.
73. Knuuti J, Wijns W, Aet al S. 2019 ESC Guidelines for the diagnosis and management of chronic coronary syndromes: the task force for the diagnosis and management of chronic coronary syndromes of the European Society of Cardiology (ESC). *Eur Heart J.* 2019;41:407–477.
74. Bairey Merz CN, Pepine CJ, Walsh MN, Fleg JL. Ischemia And No Obstructive Coronary Artery Disease (INOCA): developing evidence-based therapies and research agenda for the next decade. *Circulation.* 2017;135:1075–1092.
75. Ouellette ML, Loffler AI, Beller GA, et al. Clinical characteristics, sex differences, and outcomes in patients with normal or Near-normal coronary arteries, non-obstructive or obstructive coronary artery disease. *J Am Heart Assoc.* 2018;7.
76. Kenkre TS, Malhotra P, Johnson BD, et al. Ten-year mortality in the WISE study (Women's Ischemia Syndrome Evaluation). *Circ Cardiovasc Qual Outcomes.* 2017;10.
77. AlBadri A, Bairey Merz CN, Johnson BD, et al. Impact of abnormal coronary reactivity on long-term clinical outcomes in women. *J Am Coll Cardiol.* 2019;73:684–693.
78. Pasupathy S, Air T, Dreyer RP, et al. Systematic review of patients presenting with suspected myocardial infarction and nonobstructive coronary arteries. *Circulation.* 2015;131:861–870.
79. Tamis-Holland JE, Jneid H, Reynolds HR, et al. Contemporary diagnosis and management of patients with myocardial infarction in the absence of obstructive coronary artery disease: a scientific statement from the American Heart Association. *Circulation.* 2019;139:e891–e908.
80. El-Battrawy I, Santoro F, Stiermaier T, et al. Incidence and clinical impact of recurrent takotsubo syndrome: results from the GEIST registry. *J Am Heart Assoc.* 2019;8:e010753.
81. Thygesen K, Alpert JS, Jaffe AS, et al. Fourth universal definition of myocardial infarction (2018). *Circulation.* 2018;138:e618–e651.
82. Manginas A, Rigopoulos AG, Bigalke B, et al. Takotsubo syndrome—adding pieces to a complex puzzle. *BMC Cardiovasc Disord.* 2017;17:296.
83. Tornvall P, Collste O, Ehrenborg E, Jarnbert-Petterson H. A case-control study of risk markers and mortality in takotsubo stress cardiomyopathy. *J Am Coll Cardiol.* 2016;67:1931–1936.
84. Gupta S, Lui B, Ma X, et al. Sex differences in outcomes after coronary artery bypass grafting. *J Cardiothorac Vasc Anesth.* 2020.
85. Johnston A, Mesana TG, Lee DS, et al. Sex differences In long-term survival after major cardiac surgery: a population-based cohort study. *J Am Heart Assoc.* 2019;8:e013260.

Vascular Disease

86. Chaker Z, Badhwar V, Alqahtani F, et al. Sex differences in the utilization and outcomes of surgical aortic valve replacement for severe aortic stenosis. *J Am Heart Assoc.* 2017;6.
87. Mantovani F, Clavel MA, Michelena HI, et al. Enriquez-Sarano M. Comprehensive imaging in women with organic mitral regurgitation: implications for clinical outcome. *JACC Cardiovasc Imaging.* 2016;9:388–396.
88. Chandrasekhar J, Dangas G, Yu J, et al. Sex-based differences in outcomes with transcatheter aortic valve therapy: TVT registry from 2011 to 2014. *J Am Coll Cardiol.* 2016;68:2733–2744.
89. Kodali S, Williams MR, Doshi D, et al. Sex-specific differences at presentation and outcomes among patients undergoing transcatheter aortic valve replacement: a cohort study. *Ann Intern Med.* 2016;164:377–384.
90. Vlastra W, Chandrasekhar J, Garcia Del Blanco B, et al. Sex differences in transfemoral transcatheter aortic valve replacement. *J Am Coll Cardiol.* 2019;74:2758–2767.
91. Tigges E, Kalbacher D, Thomas C, et al. Transcatheter mitral valve repair in surgical high-risk patients: gender-specific acute and long-term outcomes. *BioMed Res Int.* 2016;2016:3934842.

Peripheral Arterial Disease

92. Wang GJ, Shaw PA, Townsend RR, et al. Sex differences in the incidence of peripheral artery disease in the chronic renal insufficiency cohort. *Circ Cardiovasc Qual Outcomes.* 2016;9:S86–S93.
93. Jackson EA, Munir K, Schreiber T, et al. Impact of sex on morbidity and mortality rates after lower extremity interventions for peripheral arterial disease: observations from the Blue Cross Blue Shield of Michigan Cardiovascular Consortium. *J Am Coll Cardiol.* 2014;63:2525–2530.
94. Schramm K, Rochon PJ. Gender differences in peripheral vascular disease. *Semin Intervent Radiol.* 2018;35:9–16.
95. Boczar KE, Cheung K, Boodhwani M, et al. Sex differences in thoracic aortic aneurysm growth. *Hypertension.* 2019;73:190–196.
96. Ali MU, Fitzpatrick-Lewis D, Miller J, et al. Screening for abdominal aortic aneurysm in asymptomatic adults. *J Vasc Surg.* 2016;64:1855–1868.

Heart Failure

97. Chang PP, Wruck LM, Shahar E, et al. Trends in hospitalizations and survival of acute decompensated heart failure in four US Communities (2005–2014): ARIC study community surveillance. *Circulation.* 2018;138:12–24.
98. Lam CSP, Arnott C, Beale AL, et al. Sex differences in heart failure. *Eur Heart J.* 2019;40:3859–3868c.
99. Beale AL, Nanayakkara S, Segan L, et al. Sex differences in heart failure with preserved ejection fraction pathophysiology: a detailed invasive hemodynamic and echocardiographic analysis. *JACC Heart Fail.* 2019;7:239–249.
100. Arany Z, Elkayam U. Peripartum cardiomyopathy. *Circulation.* 2016;133:1397–1409.
101. Davis MB, Arany Z, McNamara DM, et al. JACC state-of-the-art review. *J Am Coll Cardiol.* 2020;75:207–221.
102. McNamara DM, Elkayam U, Alharethi R, et al. Clinical outcomes for peripartum cardiomyopathy in North America: results of the IPAC study (investigations of pregnancy-associated cardiomyopathy). *J Am Coll Cardiol.* 2015;66:905–914.
103. Suthahar N, Meems LMG, Ho JE, de Boer RA. Sex-related differences in contemporary biomarkers for heart failure: a review. *Eur J Heart Fail.* 2020;22:775–788.
104. Solomon SD, McMurray JJV, Anand IS, et al. Angiotensin-neprilysin inhibition in heart failure with preserved ejection fraction. *N Engl J Med.* 2019;381:1609–1620.
105. Dewan P, Rorth R, Jhund PS, et al. Differential impact of heart failure with reduced ejection fraction on men and women. *J Am Coll Cardiol.* 2019;73:29–40.
106. Sticherling C, Arendacka B, Svendsen JH, et al. Sex differences in outcomes of primary prevention implantable cardioverter-defibrillator therapy: combined registry data from eleven European countries. *Europace.* 2018;20:963–970.
107. Zusterzeel R, Spatz ES, Curtis JP, et al. Cardiac resynchronization therapy in women versus men: observational comparative effectiveness study from the National Cardiovascular Data Registry. *Circ Cardiovasc Qual Outcomes.* 2015;8:S4–S11.
108. Randolph TC, Hellkamp AS, Zeitler EP, et al. Utilization of cardiac resynchronization therapy in eligible patients hospitalized for heart failure and its association with patient outcomes. *Am Heart J.* 2017;189:48–58.
109. DeFilippis EM, Truby LK, Garan AR, et al. Sex-related differences in use and outcomes of left ventricular assist devices as bridge to transplantation. *JACC Heart Fail.* 2019;7:250–257.
110. Joshi AA, Lerman JB, Sajja AP, et al. Sex-based differences in left ventricular assist device utilization: insights from the nationwide inpatient sample 2004 to 2016. *Circ Heart Fail.* 2019;12:e006082.
111. Colvin M, Smith JM, Hadley N, et al. OPTN/SRTR 2016 Annual data report: heart. *Am J Transplant.* 2018;18(suppl 1):291–362.
112. Moayedi Y, Fan CPS, Cherikh WS, et al. Survival outcomes after heart transplantation: does recipient sex matter? *Circ Heart Fail.* 2019;12:e006218.
113. Magnussen C, Niiranen TJ, Ojeda FM, et al. Sex differences and similarities in atrial fibrillation epidemiology, risk factors, and mortality in community cohorts: results from the biomarcare consortium (biomarker for cardiovascular risk assessment in Europe). *Circulation.* 2017;136:1588–1597.
114. Westerman S, Wenger N. Gender differences in atrial fibrillation: a review of epidemiology, management, and outcomes. *Curr Cardiol Rev.* 2019;15:136–144.
115. Haukilahti MAE, Holmstrom L, Vahatalo J, et al. Sudden cardiac death in women. *Circulation.* 2019;139:1012–1021.
116. Mumma BE, Umarov T. Sex differences in the prehospital management of out-of-hospital cardiac arrest. *Resuscitation.* 2016;105:161–164.
117. Thomas RJ, Balady G, Banka G, et al. 2018 ACC/AHA clinical performance and quality measures for cardiac rehabilitation: a report of the American College of Cardiology/American Heart Association task force on performance measures. *J Am Coll Cardiol.* 2018;71:1814–1837.

92 Pregnancy and Heart Disease

SAMUEL C. SIU AND CANDICE K. SILVERSIDES

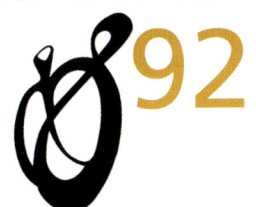

CARDIOVASCULAR CHANGES IN PREGNANCY, 1723
EVALUATION PRIOR TO PREGNANCY AND DURING PREGNANCY, 1724
  Cardiac Findings During Normal Pregnancy, 1724
  Role of Cardiac Testing During Pregnancy, 1725
  Evaluation and Counseling Prior to and During Pregnancy, 1725
GENERAL MANAGEMENT PRINCIPLES, 1729
SPECIFIC CARDIOVASCULAR CONDITIONS, 1731

Hypertension, 1731
CARDIOMYOPATHIES, 1732
MYOCARDIAL INFARCTION AND ISCHEMIC HEART DISEASE, 1733
NATIVE VALVULAR HEART DISEASE, 1734
PROSTHETIC VALVES AND MANAGEMENT OF ANTICOAGULATION, 1735
ARRHYTHMIAS, 1737
CONGENITAL HEART DISEASE, 1737
  Cardiac Shunts, 1737
  Left-Sided Obstruction, 1738

Complex Congenital Lesions, 1738
Unoperated Complex Congenital Lesions, 1738
Complex Congenital: Repaired, 1738
Cyanotic Congenital Heart Lesions, 1739
PULMONARY HYPERTENSION, 1740
MARFAN SYNDROME AND INHERITED AORTOPATHIES, 1740
CONTRACEPTION, 1740
REFERENCES, 1741

Pregnancy results in hemodynamic and hormonal stress, which increases the risk of complications in women with heart disease. Over the past few decades, the number of pregnancies in women with cardiovascular disease has grown due to increases in the population of young women surviving with pediatric heart disease, older maternal age, and a higher prevalence of chronic medical conditions such as hypertension. Although many women are aware of their cardiovascular diagnosis prior to pregnancy, pregnancy can also unmask heart disease, and women can present with cardiovascular complications for the first time during pregnancy. Less commonly, pregnancy leads to de novo cardiac conditions, such as peripartum cardiomyopathy (PPCM) or coronary artery dissection. Along with increases in the population of pregnant women with cardiovascular disease, the field of cardio-obstetrics has grown, the medical community has a better understanding of pregnancy risks and treatment options, and standards of care have been established.[1-5] There is also increasing recognition that some pregnancy complications, such as preeclampsia, are associated with long-term maternal cardiovascular risks.[6]

The etiology of cardiac disease in women of childbearing age differs when compared with other cardiac cohorts. In high-income countries, congenital heart disease is the most common preexisting cardiac condition in pregnant women.[7,8] In contrast, rheumatic heart disease is much more common in low- and middle-income countries.[7] Arrhythmic disorders and cardiomyopathies are other commonly encountered cardiac conditions in cardio-obstetric clinics. Women may also have cardiovascular risk factors such has hypertension or diabetes, and these conditions are associated with adverse pregnancy outcomes.

During pregnancy, maternal morbidity and mortality are increased in women with heart disease.[8-10] Although maternal mortality secondary to cardiac disease is rare in high-income countries, when it occurs, it is frequently due to cardiovascular conditions such as cardiomyopathy, aortic dissection, or myocardial infarction (MI).[11,12] Maternal mortality is higher in low- and middle-income countries, and,[7] even in high-income countries, there are important racial differences.[13] In comparison, maternal cardiac morbidity is common and, depending on the population studied, occurs in 5% to 20% of pregnancies in women with heart disease.[7,8,14,15] The most common cardiac complications in women with heart disease are arrhythmias and heart failure. Timing of complications varies; arrhythmias typically occur in the second and third trimester, whereas heart failure occurs at the time of peak cardiac output, beginning at the end of second trimester and as well in the postpartum period (Fig. 92.1).[15] Some conditions, such as coarctation of the aorta, are associated with high rates of hypertensive disorders of pregnancy and preeclampsia. A significant proportion of maternal cardiovascular complications that occur in women with heart disease are preventable.[16,17]

Pregnancy complications may have late effects on maternal cardiovascular health. Pregnancy can lead to deterioration in ventricular or valve function, and, although these often return to normal after delivery, on occasion, deterioration can be permanent. For instance, pregnant women with atrial switch operations for complete transposition of the great arteries are at risk for permanent deterioration in subaortic right ventricular systolic function and worsening atrioventricular valve regurgitation.[18] Women with congenital heart disease who develop cardiac complications during pregnancy are at a higher risk of cardiovascular events later in life.[19] Similarly, women who develop complications related to placental dysfunction, such as preeclampsia and preterm birth, are at higher risk of maternal cardiovascular disease years after pregnancy compared with pregnant women who did not have complications.[6]

In addition to cardiac risks, pregnant women with cardiovascular disease are also at higher risk of obstetric and perinatal complications when compared with women without heart disease. For instance, women with Fontan operations or cyanotic heart disease and those using anticoagulants are at increased risk of postpartum hemorrhage.[20] Women with heart disease have higher rates of miscarriage, stillbirth, and neonatal death compared with women without heart disease.[8] Premature births and low birth weight babies are more common in women with heart disease, especially in women with complex congenital heart disease or pulmonary hypertension. In mothers and fathers with inherited cardiac conditions, transmission of heart disease to offspring can occur. The increased risk of obstetric and perinatal complications highlights the need for multidisciplinary care teams including maternal fetal medicine specialists, obstetric anesthetists, and neonatologists.

CARDIOVASCULAR CHANGES IN PREGNANCY

Pregnancy is associated with hemodynamic changes that are usually well tolerated in women with normal hearts. However, the hemodynamic changes of pregnancy can lead to cardiovascular complications, especially in women with preexisting heart disease. The hemodynamic changes of pregnancy begin as early as the sixth week of gestation, with increases in plasma volume (Table 92.1).[21] Early in pregnancy, the peripheral vascular resistance decreases and there is a corresponding small drop in blood pressure (BP) by 5 to 10 mm Hg below baseline until the third trimester, when the BP increases back to baseline. The heart rate increases by approximately

10 beats/min above pre-pregnancy levels, and,[22] in combination with increases in stoke volume, there is a resultant increase in cardiac output by 30% to 50% (see Table 92.1). Twin pregnancies can increase the cardiac output by a further 10% to 15%. At the time of labor and delivery and immediately postpartum, cardiac output increases a further 60% to 80%. Catecholamines, release of inferior vena cava compression, autotransfusion from uterine contractions, and blood loss all contribute to further hemodynamic changes. Mobilization of fluid during the first week after delivery can result in heart failure in women with cardiomyopathy or severe outflow tract obstruction. Many of the hemodynamic changes resolve in the first 2 weeks after delivery, although complete resolution may take as long as 6 months. In addition to the hemodynamic changes, pregnancy results in increases in renal blood flow and glomerular filtration rate, cholesterol levels, insulin resistance, and clotting (see Table 92.1).

EVALUATION PRIOR TO PREGNANCY AND DURING PREGNANCY

Cardiac Findings During Normal Pregnancy

Fatigue, dyspnea, light-headedness, and palpitations are symptoms that can be associated with normal pregnancy.[23] Normal pregnancy results in cardiac examination findings including: (1) collapsing arterial pulses; (2) prominent jugular venous pulsations without elevation of jugular venous pressure; (3) laterally displaced apical impulse; (4) palpable right ventricle or pulmonary trunk; and (5) soft, short ejection systolic murmur best heard over the pulmonic area or left sternal border.[24] When it is difficult to differentiate between pregnancy-associated changes versus early cardiac decompensation, echocardiography, or B-type natriuretic peptide (BNP) level can be useful (a BNP value of 111 pg/mL has been proposed as having a positive likelihood ratio of 2.5 and a negative likelihood ratio of 0.1 for heart failure).[25] Pregnant women with heart disease have a higher BNP level than pregnant women without heart disease, and a BNP less than 100 pg/mL in the heart disease group had a 100% negative predictive value for cardiac complications.[26] Normal pregnancy is associated with electrocardiographic (sinus tachycardia, premature atrial or ventricular complexes, left QRS axis deviation, inferior Q waves, T wave flattening, ST depression, increased R/S ratio on right precordial leads) and chest radiographic (pleural effusion, straightening of left upper cardiac border, horizontal positioning of heart, increased lung vascular

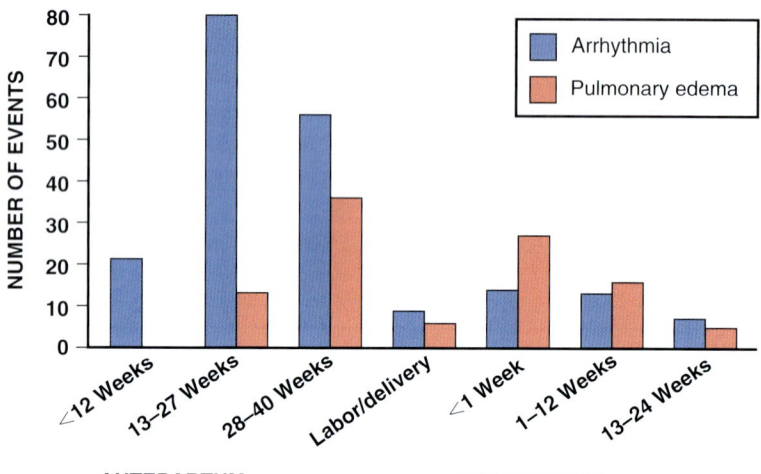

FIGURE 92.1 Timing of complications in women who develop arrhythmias or pulmonary edema during pregnancy. The *y* axis shows the total number of adverse events. The *x* axis shows the timing of presentation in women who develop pulmonary edema *(red bars)* or arrhythmias *(blue bars)*. (From Silversides CK, Grewal J, Mason J, et al. Pregnancy outcomes in women with heart disease: the CARPREG II study. *J Am Coll Cardiol*. 2018;71:2419–2430.)

TABLE 92.1 Normal Physiologic Changes in Pregnancy and Implications in Cardiovascular Conditions

ORGAN SYSTEM	NORMAL PHYSIOLOGIC CHANGES	IMPLICATIONS IN CARDIOVASCULAR CONDITIONS
Cardiovascular	During pregnancy: • ↑ Plasma flow (75%) ↑ cardiac output (CO) (30%–50%) ↓ systemic and pulmonary vascular resistance (SVR) and (PVR) During labor: • ↑ CO by 30% in active stage of labor • Increased circulating blood volume (300–500 mL) due to uterine contractions	• Cardiac complications in women with lesions that cannot tolerate volume loading (cardiomyopathy), decreases in SVR (Eisenmenger with intracardiac shunts) or with fixed obstruction (aortic or mitral stenosis) • Impaired hemodynamic adaptation • ↑ Mean arterial pressures (MAPs), SVR and ↓ CO in preeclampsia
Respiratory	• ↑ Metabolic rate and oxygen consumption • Mild compensated respiratory alkalosis	• Feeling of breathlessness during pregnancy • ↑ Minute ventilation in preeclampsia • Difficulty intubating in those who develop serious cardiac complications
Renal	• ↑ Plasma flow (75%) • ↑ Glomerular filtration rate (GFR) (40%–50%) • ↑ Proteinuria	• ↓ GFR ↓ uric acid clearance ↑ proteinuria in preeclampsia • Drug dosing may need to be adjusted based on GFR
Hematologic	• ↑ Plasma volume (50%) and red cell mass • ↑ Coagulation factors • ↓ Protein C • Compression of the inferior vena cava	• Physiologic anemia • ↑ Risk of thromboembolism in women with prosthetic heart valves, atrial fibrillation, Fontan circulation • ↓ Life span of platelets in and hemolysis in severe preeclampsia (HELLP syndrome)
Lipid metabolism	• ↑ Triglycerides, total cholesterol (50%) and in low-density lipoprotein cholesterol (LDL) (50%) and ↓ high-density lipoprotein cholesterol (HDL)	• ↑ Dyslipidemia with ↓ HDL ↑ free fatty acids in preeclampsia • Existing maternal dyslipidemia is associated with adverse pregnancy outcomes
Glucose metabolism	• ↑ Insulin resistance, mild diabetogenic state	• Gestational diabetes

From Sharma G, Ying Y, Silversides CK. The importance of cardiovascular risk assessment and pregnancy heart team in the management of cardiovascular disease in pregnancy. *Cardiol Clin*. 2020.

markings) findings that can mimic cardiac disease.[3,24] Similarly, one should be aware of the changes in echocardiographic data with normal pregnancy,[27] including: (1) increase in dimensions of all four cardiac chambers without changes in left ventricular ejection fraction; (2) increase in left ventricular wall thickness; (3) increasing degree of tricuspid regurgitation (TR) which usually does not exceed more than moderate in degree; and (4) changes in left ventricular mechanics (strain, twist, untwisting) and left atrial strain reflective of adaptive changes in LV volumes, mass, and loading conditions with advancing gestational age. Importantly the left ventricular diastolic dimension may exceed the normal limits reported in nonpregnant patients.[27]

Role of Cardiac Testing During Pregnancy

Transthoracic echocardiogram is the preferred imaging method in pregnancy, but imaging may be more technically challenging with cardiac displacement. When transesophageal echocardiography is performed in pregnancy to obtain data that cannot be obtained by transthoracic echocardiography, the imaging protocol should be abbreviated to minimize the potential risk of vomiting/aspiration due to delayed gastric emptying in pregnancy.[24] Exercise testing, with or without echocardiography, usually performed prior to pregnancy, should be limited to submaximal test if performed during pregnancy (peak heart rate not to exceed 70% to 80% of predicted maximum).[3,24] The use of dobutamine as a stress agent should be avoided.

The risk of fetal adverse outcome is highest with radiation exposure during the period of organogenesis during the first trimester.[28] A fetal exposure dose of less than 50 mGy is considered to be negligible risk. The fetal dose from chest radiography is less than 0.0001 mGy; however, maternal shielding should be used. Lung imaging with point of care ultrasound is an alternative when assessing for possible pulmonary edema or pulmonary pathology. Chest computed tomography (CT), if necessary for evaluation of pulmonary embolism or aortic pathology, should use low-radiation protocols (typically 0.01 to 0.66 mGy for CT pulmonary angiogram protocols). Cardiac magnetic resonance is an alternate to ionizing radiation imaging modalities, and gadolinium-based contrast should be avoided,[29] but may be less well tolerated due to greater time requirement for imaging. When cardiac catheterization is performed during pregnancy, radial approach is generally preferable (other than for suspected coronary artery dissection, see section on MI during pregnancy) and should be delayed until after period of organogenesis (>12 weeks gestational age)[3]; mean radiation exposure to the unshielded abdomen has been estimated to be 1.5 mGy with less than 20% reaching the fetus.[3] Electrophysiologic procedures for arrhythmias should best be deferred until after pregnancy or performed using a nonfluoroscopic system during pregnancy for refractory cases.[3,30]

Evaluation and Counseling Prior to and During Pregnancy

Pre-pregnancy counseling should be offered to females with heart disease who are of childbearing age, ideally during transition to adult cardiac care.[31] In those women who do not present until they are pregnant, counseling should be performed as early in pregnancy as possible.[16] Preconception counseling is universally recommended for all women with heart disease, preferably by a cardiac-obstetric or pregnancy heart team.[5] Physicians who provide this counseling should include, as a minimum, a cardiologist with expertise in management of pregnancy in women with heart disease, as well as an obstetrician with expertise in maternal fetal medicine.[8,31] The purposes of pre-pregnancy or pregnancy counseling are to provide risk assessment, risk reduction, and management planning to optimize risk or mitigate effects of complications.[2,16,31] Table 92.2 summarizes the general approach to evaluation and counseling. There is preliminary evidence that establishment of a cardio-obstetric clinic was associated with a reduction in the incidence of pulmonary edema.[15]

Risk Stratification

Heart failure and cardiac tachyarrhythmia comprised most of the non-fatal cardiac complications reported in large studies, with maternal mortality rate of 1% or less.[7,15,32,33] The rate of maternal cardiac complication is much higher in low- to middle-income countries or in populations with reduced access to health care.[8] Predictors of maternal cardiovascular complications (summarized in Table 92.3) can be obtained from cardiac history, maternal New York Heart Association (NYHA) functional class, oxygen saturation, and echocardiography. Comprehensive transthoracic echocardiography should be performed and interpreted by personnel experienced in the assessment of congenital and acquired heart disease. Of the various risk stratification approaches that incorporate individual predictors into an overall risk for maternal cardiac complications in women with spectrum of cardiac lesions, two are risk scores derived and validated from the prospective Canadian Cardiac Disease in Pregnancy Study (CARPREG).[8] The original CARPREG risk score incorporated four predictors, to classify pregnancies as being at low, intermediate, or high risk for maternal cardiovascular complications (Fig. 92.2, *left panel*). The CARPREG II risk score calculates the risk of maternal cardiovascular complications by functional, lesion specific, and process of care predictors (Fig. 92.2, *right panel*).[8] The third risk stratification tool, the modified

TABLE 92.2 Approach to Evaluation, Counseling, and Management: Before, During, and After Pregnancy

Preconception

Risk Assessment and Reduction
- Discuss maternal pregnancy risks (cardiac, obstetric, fetal)
- Discuss long-term maternal cardiac prognosis
- Discuss offspring risks including transmission of heart disease
- Referral to genetics when appropriate
- Modify medications as needed
- Smoking cessation and consideration of cardiac intervention prior to conception

Management Planning
- Referral to cardio-obstetric center
- Address assisted reproductive therapy safety in women with infertility
- Consider alternatives to pregnancy (surrogacy or adoption) in women with prohibitive pregnancy risks
- Discuss contraception options for women who want to avoid pregnancy
- Management during antepartum and peripartum period (see below)

Pregnancy and Delivery
- Referral to a cardio-obstetric center
- Consults with the pregnancy heart team including maternal fetal medicine and obstetric anesthesia
- Clinical surveillance throughout pregnancy with frequency of visits based on severity of disease
- Transthoracic echocardiographic surveillance during pregnancy
- Create and circulate a delivery plan including recommendations on the mode of delivery, induction, analgesia, safety of pushing, cardiac and postpartum monitoring
- Organize multidisciplinary conferences for complex or high-risk cases

Postpartum
- Ensure postpartum follow-up
- Medication modification for breastfeeding mothers
- Reestablish baseline in women with structural heart disease at 6 months postpartum
- Arrange postpartum cardiovascular risk assessment for women with pregnancy hypertension or maternal placental syndrome
- For women considering another pregnancy, reevaluate pregnancy risks
- Discuss contraception options

TABLE 92.3 Predictors of Pregnancy Associated Complications in Women with Heart Disease

HOW PREDICTOR IS IDENTIFIED	MATERNAL CARDIAC COMPLICATIONS	FETAL AND NEONATAL COMPLICATIONS	GESTATIONAL HYPERTENSION	POSTPARTUM HEMORRHAGE
Baseline Clinical Assessment				
Cardiac events before pregnancy	Yes			
Cardiovascular medications before pregnancy	Yes	Yes		
NYHA functional class III or IV	Yes	Yes		
Anticoagulation		Yes		Yes
Cyanosis	Yes	Yes		Yes
Smoking during pregnancy	Yes	Yes		
Nulliparity			Yes	
Multiple gestation		Yes		
Cardiac Imaging (Primarily by Transthoracic Echocardiography) and Other Assessments				
Left heart obstruction	Yes	Yes		
Reduced systemic ventricular systolic dysfunction	Yes			
Pulmonary atrioventricular valve regurgitation (moderate/severe)	Yes			
Systemic atrioventricular valve regurgitation (moderate/severe)	Yes			
Pulmonary regurgitation or depressed subpulmonary ventricular function	Yes			
B-type natriuretic peptide level	Yes			
Cardiopulmonary test prior to pregnancy	Yes			
Maternal Cardiac Lesion				
Uncorrected or corrected cyanotic heart disease	Yes	Yes		
High-risk aortopathy	Yes			
Coronary artery disease	Yes			
Pulmonary hypertension	Yes	Yes		
Aortic coarctation			Yes	
Maternal systemic lupus erythematosus			Yes	
Aortic valve disease			Yes	
Mechanical prosthesis	Yes	Yes		
Modified World Health Organization Class	Yes			
Process of Care				
No prior cardiac interventions	Yes			
Late presentation for care	Yes			
Serial Assessments During Pregnancy				
Abnormal Uteroplacental Doppler		Yes		
Reduction in cardiac output between 1st and 3rd trimester		Yes		

NYHA, New York Heart Association.
From Grewal J, Windram J, Bottega et al; Canadian Cardiovascular Society: Clinical practice update on cardiovascular management of the pregnant patient. *Can J Cardiol.* 2021 Jul 1:S0828-282X(21)00356-1. https://doi.org/10.1016/j.cjca.2021.06.021; Silversides CK, Siu SC. Heart disease in pregnancy. In: Otto CH, ed. *The Practice of Clinical Echocardiography.* 6th ed. Philadelphia: Elsevier; 2020.

World Health Organization (mWHO) classification system, used an expert consensus approach to classify maternal cardiac lesions into five risk classes corresponding to increasing maternal cardiovascular risks (Table 92.4).[3] In a Canadian study, the CARPREG II risk score had superior predictive accuracy compared with the mWHO classification system.[34]

Risk scores and risk classification approaches should always be combined with clinical judgment. One approach is to identify pregnancies in women with cardiac lesions associated with high mortality risk or with devastating implications even if there is prompt intervention (Fig. 92.3).[8] Pregnancy should be discouraged in women with high-risk cardiac lesions (as listed on Fig. 92.3), and termination should be considered if pregnancy occurs. Pregnant women with high-risk lesions should receive their care by a maternal heart team and deliver at a referral center.

For pregnancies in women without the aforementioned high-risk lesions, a CARPREG II risk score could be used, with subsequent modification after integrating patient (including exercise testing, compliance, comorbid conditions, socioeconomic status, anticoagulation) and lesion (i.e., type of cardiac lesions, type of operative repair, and late sequelae) specific information. For clinicians who prefer the mWHO risk-classification system, we recommend that general predictors of cardiovascular complications (e.g., prior history of heart failure and arrhythmias) be incorporated, which further stratify risk within each mWHO category (Fig. 92.4). Importantly, the cardiovascular complication rate can be as high as 5% in the low-risk group.[8] Assisted reproductive technologies (ARTs) confer additional risk to women with heart disease (see "Assisted Reproductive Technologies").[31]

Risk stratification should also include assessing the risk of noncardiac complications and long-term prognosis (see Table 92.3).[8] Maternal cardiovascular and fetal neonatal complications are related, likely reflecting the inability of the placenta to autoregulate blood flow. The likelihood of fetoneonatal complications

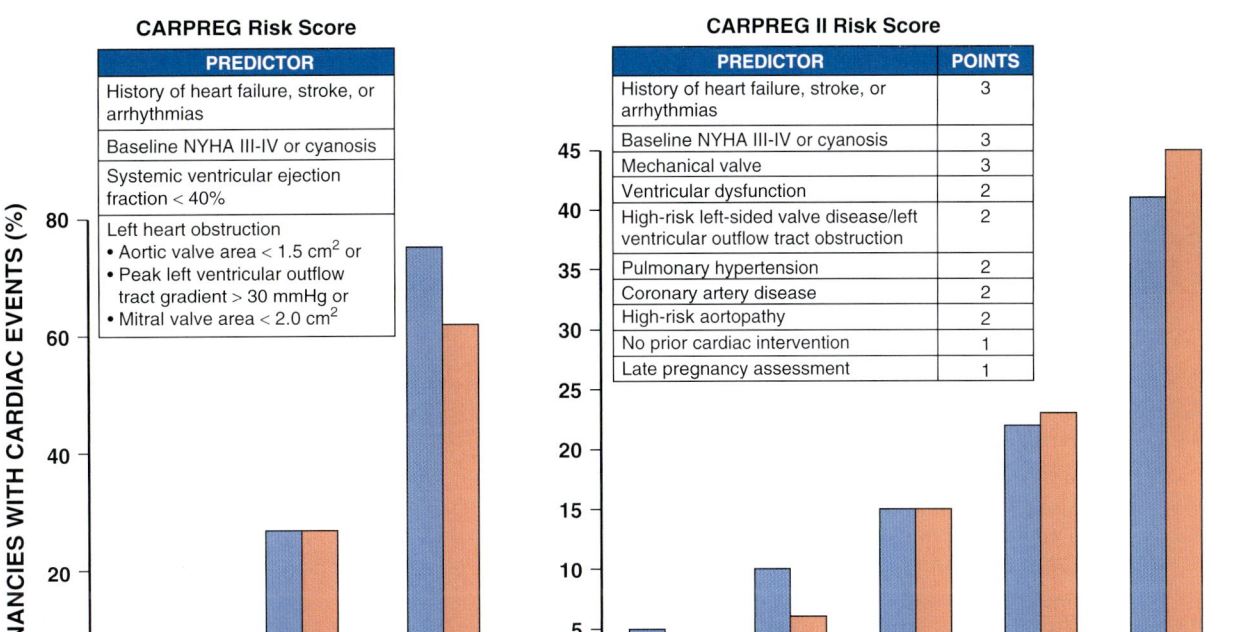

FIGURE 92.2 Predicted and observed frequency of maternal cardiovascular event rates in the two Canadian Cardiac Disease in Pregnancy Study (CARPREG) risk scores.[15,31] **Left**, The original CARPREG risk score is based on four predictors, shown in the Predictor box. The predicted frequency of maternal cardiac events (in *blue*) is 5%, 27%, and 75%, corresponding to 0, 1, and greater than 1 predictor. The observed frequency of events in the validation group is shown in *red*. **Right**, The CARPREG II risk score is based on 10 variables, shown in the box. Each variable is assigned a weighted score (points). The sum of the points for all 10 variables represents the risk score. Risk scores are categorized into the five groups shown on the x axis: risk score of 0–1 points, score of 2 points, score of 3 points, score of 4 points, and score greater than 4 points, corresponding to predicted frequency of cardiac events (in *blue*) of 5%, 10%, 15%, 22%, and 41%, respectively. The observed frequency of cardiac events in the validation groups is in *red*. (From Silversides CK, Grewal J, Mason J, et al. Pregnancy outcomes in women with heart disease: the CARPREG II study. *J Am Coll Cardiol*. 2018;71:2419–2430; and Haberer K, Silversides CK. Congenital heart disease and women's health across the life span: focus on reproductive issues. *Can J Cardiol*. 2019;35:1652–1663.)

is increased when there are concurrent obstetric risk factors.[8] The obstetric and fetoneonatal risks emphasize the vital role of the multidisciplinary team in comprehensive risk assessment and counseling.[31] Pregnancy may accelerate subsequent progression to symptoms or cardiac decompensation in women with certain cardiac lesions.[8]

Management Planning

Preconception counseling provides opportunities to optimize risk by: (1) better defining the nature of the cardiac lesion and or functional capacity by exercise or cardiopulmonary testing, imaging, or cardiac catheterization; (2) stopping medications that are contraindicated in pregnancy (e.g., afterload reducing agents in heart failure treatment) for a trial period prior to pregnancy to ascertain clinical stability; (3) interventions such as smoking cessation or intervention for severe aortic/mitral stenosis (MS); and (4) genetic consultation if the women, her first-degree relative, or her partner has congenital a heart defect.[31,35] Regardless of when the counseling occurs, the following areas need to be discussed and management recommendations provided:

(A) Cardiovascular medications: Cardiovascular medications that are safe versus contraindicated during pregnancy (see general management section).[5,35]
(B) Site of pregnancy care/delivery: There are three possible options: (1) Exclusive care and delivery at referral center by maternal heart team (recommended for high-risk pregnancies); (2) Joint care by local cardiology or obstetric practitioners with delivery at local center, after initial evaluation by pregnancy heart team (non–high-risk pregnancies); or (3) Initial review by pregnancy heart team and local obstetric care (for low-risk pregnancies).[5,36]
(C) Fetal echocardiogram for same indications as for genetic counseling (see earlier).
(D) Management during labor and delivery (see also section on general management):
   (i) Vaginal delivery versus cardiac indications for cesarean delivery.[2]
   (ii) Spontaneous onset of labor versus induction
   (iii) Indications for invasive hemodynamic monitoring
   (iv) Continuous telemetry for patients with uncontrolled arrhythmias
   (v) Postpartum monitoring of the mother in coronary or intensive care units for women in high cardiac risk group, including women who required hemodynamic monitoring during labor and delivery.

For patients with pregnancy who are at high risk, a multidisciplinary meeting should be convened in the antepartum period to develop and document management plan during the peripartum and early postpartum periods.

ASSISTED REPRODUCTIVE TECHNOLOGIES

As with the general population, ARTs are being increasingly used for treatment of infertility and subfertility. In the cardiac population, some women, such as those with Fontan operations, cyanotic heart disease, or Turner syndrome, have higher rates of infertility.[20] Although ARTs improve the chances of pregnancy, they are associated with complications that may be dangerous for women with heart disease.

ARTs such as in vitro fertilization or intrauterine insemination usually follow medical treatment to stimulate ovulation, and this can result in ovarian hyperstimulation syndrome. Ovarian hyperstimulation syndrome, directly related to superovulation protocols, can be particularly problematic for women with heart disease as it leads to fluid shifts

TABLE 92.4 2018 Version of Modified World Health Organization Classification of Maternal Cardiovascular Risk

mWHO CLASS	CARDIAC LESIONS	MATERNAL CARDIAC RISK ASSIGNED BY 2018 GUIDELINES AUTHORS*	CLINICAL APPLICATION
Class I	• Small or mild pulmonary stenosis, patent ductus arteriosus, mitral valve prolapse • Successfully repaired simple lesions (atrial or ventricular septal defect, patent ductus arteriosus, anomalous pulmonary venous connection) • Atrial or ventricular ectopic beats, isolated	2.5%–5%	No detectable increased risk of maternal mortality and no/mild increase in morbidity
Class II	• Unoperated atrial or ventricular septal defect • Repaired tetralogy of Fallot • Most arrhythmias (supraventricular arrhythmias) • Turner syndrome without aortic dilation	5.7%–10.5%	Small increase in maternal risk mortality or moderate increase in morbidity
Class II or III	• Mild left ventricular impairment (EF > 45%) • Hypertrophic cardiomyopathy • Native or tissue valvular heart disease not considered WHO I or IV (mild mitral stenosis, moderate aortic stenosis) • Marfan or other HTAD syndrome without aortic dilatation • Aorta <45 mm in association with bicuspid aortic valve pathology • Repaired coarctation • Atrioventricular septal defect	10%–19%	Intermediate increased risk of maternal mortality or moderate to severe increase in morbidity
Class III	• Moderate left ventricular impairment (EF 30%–45%) • Previous peripartum cardiomyopathy without residual left ventricular impairment • Mechanical valve • Systemic right ventricle with good or mildly decreased ventricular function • Fontan circulation if otherwise well and the cardiac condition uncomplicated • Unrepaired cyanotic heart disease • Other complex congenital heart disease • Moderate mitral stenosis • Severe asymptomatic aortic stenosis • Moderate aortic dilation (40–45 mm in Marfan syndrome or other HTAD, 45–50 mm in bicuspid aortic valve, Turner syndrome ASI 20–25 mm/m^2, tetralogy of Fallot <50 mm) • Ventricular tachycardia	19%–27%	Significantly increased risk of maternal mortality or severe morbidity.
Class IV	• Pulmonary arterial hypertension • Severe systemic ventricular dysfunction (EF <30% or NYHA class III–IV) • Previous peripartum cardiomyopathy with any residual left ventricular impairment • Severe mitral stenosis • Severe symptomatic aortic stenosis • Systemic right ventricle with moderate or severely decreased ventricular function • Severe aortic dilatation (>45 mm in Marfan syndrome or other HTAD, >50 mm in bicuspid aortic valve, Turner syndrome ASI >25 mm/m^2, tetralogy of Fallot >50 mm) • Vascular Ehlers-Danlos • Severe (re)coarctation • Fontan with any complication	40%–100%	Extremely high risk of maternal mortality or severe morbidity

*Basis of risk estimates not provided.
ASI, Aortic size index; *EF*, ejection fraction; *HTAD*, heritable thoracic aortic disease; *mWHO*, modified World Health Organization; *NYHA*, New York Heart Association functional class.
From Regitz-Zagrosek V, Roos-Hesselink JW, Bauersachs J, et al. 2018 ESC Guidelines for the management of cardiovascular diseases during pregnancy. *Eur Heart J.* 2018;39:3165–3241.

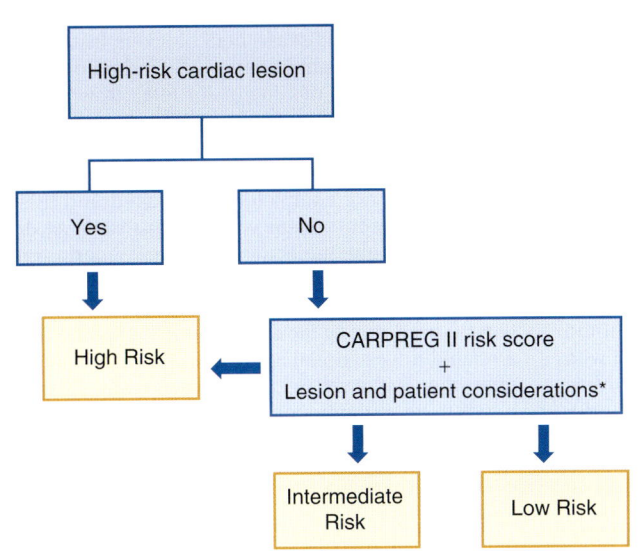

FIGURE 92.3 A proposed approach for assessing risk of maternal cardiovascular complications in pregnant women with heart disease. *Denotes exercise testing, cardiac imaging data, compliance, comorbid conditions, and socioeconomic status, medications including anticoagulants. (From D'Souza RD, Silversides CK, Tomlinson GA, Siu SC. Assessing cardiac risk in pregnant women with heart disease: how risk scores are created and their role in clinical practice. *Can J Cardiol.* 2020;36:1011–1021.)

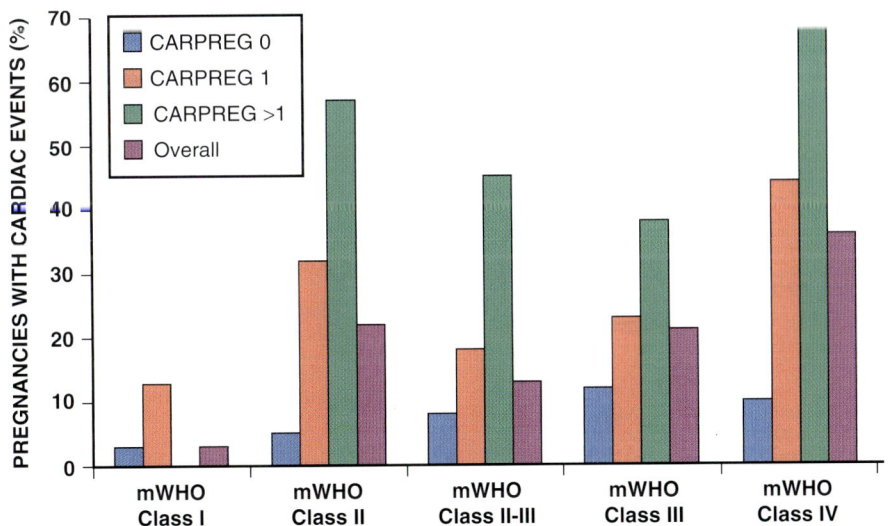

FIGURE 92.4 CARPREG Risk Score further stratifies risk within each mWHO Class. The x axis shows each modified World Health Organization (mWHO) class with the corresponding frequency of adverse primary maternal cardiovascular events (y axis). The overall maternal cardiac event rate during pregnancy for mWHO I, mWHO II, mWHO II to III, mWHO III, and mWHO IV was 3%, 22%, 13%, 21%, and 36%, respectively. There was a 12.5% event rate in pregnancies in which the mWHO class could not be determined. Each of the mWHO classes is further stratified according to CARPREG risk scores: 0, 1, and greater than 1. CARPREG denotes Cardiac Disease in Pregnancy Study. (From Silversides CK, Grewal J, Mason J, et al. Pregnancy outcomes in women with heart disease: the CARPREG II study. *J Am Coll Cardiol.* 2018;71:2419–2430.)

Multifetal gestations are more common in women receiving ARTs and are associated with increased hemodynamic stress when compared with singleton pregnancies. The additional hemodynamic stress may be poorly tolerated in women with severe forms of heart disease. In addition, twins and higher-order pregnancies are associated with higher rates of preeclampsia, preterm births, low birth weight babies, and neonatal mortality. One small study of fertility therapy in women with heart disease reported high rates of maternal and perinatal complications.[37] Although fertility therapy has not been shown to be associated with long-term cardiovascular risks, failed fertility therapy is associated with higher long-term cardiovascular events.[38]

Guidance is lacking on the optimal evaluation and treatment selection for women with heart disease. When making decisions about patient selection for ART, input from the cardiologist and the fertility specialist is crucial. Pregnancy is contraindicated in the presence of some serious cardiac conditions, and ARTs should be contraindicated in these same conditions.

into the extravascular space and thrombosis. Fluid shifts may be poorly tolerated in women with the Fontan operation and thrombosis poorly tolerated in women with mechanical valves. Therefore planning of superovulation protocols is important in women with heart disease and infertility. Women receiving in vitro fertilization are also at increased risk for pulmonary emboli, preeclampsia, and gestational hypertension.

GENERAL MANAGEMENT PRINCIPLES

Care of the pregnant women with heart disease requires a multidisciplinary team often referred to as the pregnancy heart team.[1,31] The pregnancy heart team includes cardiologists, maternal fetal medicine specialists, obstetric anesthetists, and nursing staff with expertise in pregnancy and heart disease. Other medical specialists (i.e., hematologists), geneticists, neonatologists, and social workers are required for specific cases. The goal of the pregnancy heart team is to provide preconception counseling, coordinate pregnancy surveillance, treat complications, develop and disseminate delivery plans, and ensure appropriate postpartum follow-up (see Table 92.2).

The frequency of surveillance during pregnancy is based on the severity of the cardiac lesion and the maternal and fetal risk.[3,5] Women at low risk for cardiac complications are often seen once or twice during pregnancy with plans to deliver at a local obstetric center. Women at moderate or high risk for cardiac complications are followed more closely. In addition to clinic visits, pregnancy surveillance includes electrocardiograms, transthoracic echocardiograms, fetal ultrasounds, and, in some cases, placental ultrasounds or serial biomarkers such as BNP. Women with congenital heart disease should be offered a fetal echocardiogram at 18 to 22 weeks' gestation to assess for congenital cardiac malformation.

When using medications during pregnancy, consideration of the maternal benefit needs to be weighed against the potential for fetal toxicity. Most cardiac drugs cross the placental barrier and expose the fetus to the drug, and therefore the lowest possible dose should be used. Benefits and side effects of drugs should be discussed with all women receiving drugs during pregnancy. Teratogenic cardiac drugs should be stopped and switched to safer alternative drugs prior to pregnancy (Fig. 92.5). Drug safety during breastfeeding is based on the concentration of drug in the breast milk and may differ when compared with drug safety during pregnancy. The effectiveness of medications can be altered by the pregnancy associated changes in the volume of distribution, drug absorption, metabolism, and binding.[3,35] The doses of some medications, such as beta blockers, may need to be increased during pregnancy to achieve heart rate or BP control.

The safety profile of cardiovascular medications during pregnancy/lactation are summarized in Figure 92.5.[5,35] Medications that are contraindicated during pregnancy because of fetal toxicity or teratogenicity are: (1) atenolol; (2) angiotensin-converting enzyme inhibitors (ACE-Is) and angiotensin II receptor blockers (ARBs); (3) aldosterone antagonists; (4) statins; (5) direct oral anticoagulants; and (6) bosentan (endothelin receptor antagonists).[35] ACE-Is and ARBs cause second-trimester fetal nephrotoxicity, and ACE-Is are teratogenic. The recommendation to avoid atenolol, particularly in the first trimester, is based on concerns regarding higher rates of fetal growth restriction compared with other beta blockers. However, for women with heart disease, beta blockers usually do not have major effects on birth weight (mean weight reduction 191 g) when adjusted for other maternal risk factor for fetal growth restriction.[39] Recommendations to avoid statins in pregnancy may evolve with additional safety data in the future.[35]

For many of the newer cardiovascular medications, the fetal risk profile is not completely established and their use represent a balance between benefit versus fetal risk. Most drugs, except high-molecular-weight molecules such as heparin, cross the placenta and equilibrate in the fetal circulation over time. Importantly, some medications (ACE-Is) that are contraindicated during pregnancy can be used during lactation. The risk of some medications may be a related to gestational age. Warfarin is associated with an embryopathy when exposure occurs between 6 and 12 weeks' gestation and needs to be discontinued prior to 6 weeks' gestation. In the treatment of acute pericarditis during pregnancy, both aspirin (ASA) and nonsteroidal antiinflammatory drugs (NSAIDs) cross the placenta. Classic NSAIDs (ibuprofen, indomethacin, naproxen) or high-dose ASA can be used early in the pregnancy. After the 20th gestational week, all NSAIDs (except enteric coated ASA [ECASA] ≤100 mg daily) have the potential of causing constriction of the ductus arteriosus and impact fetal renal function and should be withdrawn by the 32nd gestational week.[40] Lowest effective doses of prednisone may be used during pregnancy. Ibuprofen, indomethacin, naproxen, and prednisone may be considered for lactating women. Colchicine is considered to be contraindicated during pregnancy and lactation, but data are incomplete.[40]

Drugs that are considered safe:

Arrhythmia
Adenosine, bisoprolol, digoxin*, lidocaine, metoprolol, nadolol, propranolol

Hypertension
Labetalol, methyl-dopa, metoprolol, nifedipine

Heart failure
Bumetanide, carvedilol, furosemide, metoprolol, dobutamine, dopamine, norepinephrine

Anticoagulation/antiplatelets/thrombolytics
Aspirin, low molecular weight heparin, unfractionated heparin

Drugs that are considered contraindicated:

Arrhythmia
Amiodarone**, atenolol, ivabradine

Hypertension/heart failure
ACE-inhibitors, aldosterone antagonists, ARBs, SGLT-2 inhibitors

Anticoagulation/antiplatelets/thrombolytics
Direct oral anticoagulants

Pulmonary hypertension/others
Bosentan and other endothelin receptor antagonists (ERA), statins

Drugs with limited/conflicting data/use with caution:

Arrhythmia
Diltiazem, flecainide, procainamide, propafenone, sotalol, verapamil

Hypertension/heart failure
Amlodipine, hydralazine, nitrates, nitroprusside, hydrochlorothiazide, metolazone, milrinone, torsemide

Anticoagulation/antiplatelets/thrombolytics
Clopidogrel, ticagrelor, warfarin, argatroban, bivalirudin, fondaparinux, alteplase, streptokinase, tenecteplase

Pulmonary hypertension/others
Epoprostenol, iloprost, sildenafil, treprostinil

Drugs to avoid when breast feeding:
(again discuss the risks vs benefits of each agent)

Arrhythmia
Amiodarone, Ivabradine, sotalol

Hypertension/heart failure
ACE-inhibitors other than captopril, lisinopril or enalapril, aldosterone antagonists, ARBs, SGLT-2 inhibitors

Anticoagulation/antiplatelets/thrombolytics
Clopidogrel, direct oral anticoagulants

Pulmonary hypertension/others
Statins, bosentan & other ERAs

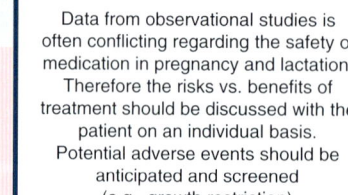

Data from observational studies is often conflicting regarding the safety of medication in pregnancy and lactation. Therefore the risks vs. benefits of treatment should be discussed with the patient on an individual basis. Potential adverse events should be anticipated and screened (e.g., growth restriction).

*Digoxin serum levels are unreliable during pregnancy. **May be used if other therapies have failed.

FIGURE 92.5 Safety profile of cardiovascular medications during pregnancy and lactation.[5,35] Summary of recent reviews of the use of cardiovascular medications during pregnancy and lactation.

When possible, a spontaneous vaginal delivery is preferred. Induction is usually reserved for logistical reasons (patient lives a long distance away from the hospital) or if a delivery is complex and a specific team is required to be present during delivery. Cesarean delivery is rarely required for cardiac indications except in women who do not have warfarin discontinued at least 2 weeks prior to delivery due to the risk of neonatal intracranial hemorrhage, those with severely dilated thoracic aortas, severe refractory heart failure, or hemodynamic instability. Vaginal deliveries can be conducted in the left lateral position to avoid compression of the inferior vena cava and optimize venous return. In women at high risk for complications, delivery planning should be made in conjunction with the pregnancy heart team and should take place at a cardiac and obstetric referral center. For some women, an assisted second stage of labor (i.e., with low forceps or vacuum extraction) may be helpful to prevent a long labor. Although routine endocarditis prophylaxis is no longer recommended for all pregnant women with heart disease, infective endocarditis prophylaxis is recommended at the time of labor and delivery in those at highest risk for endocarditis, such as women with prior endocarditis, mechanical valves, or cyanotic heart disease.

Most cardiac complications during pregnancy can be treated medically.[5] Heart failure should be treated with fluid and salt restriction and diuretics. It is important to identify and treat any precipitating factors such as tachyarrhythmias, infection, iatrogenic volume administration, and postpartum fluid shifts. Although ACE-Is and ARBs need to be stopped during pregnancy, afterload reduction with hydralazine and isosorbide dinitrate can be used.[36] Women who develop heart failure during pregnancy require close follow-up. Delivery needs to be planned carefully in women with antepartum complications, and treatment of heart failure prior to delivery is optimal. Hemodynamic monitoring with an arterial line should be considered for selected high-risk patients (severe left ventricular systolic dysfunction, severe aortic or MS, or pulmonary hypertension). Central venous and pulmonary artery catheters are rarely indicated and should be performed by an experienced operator after careful consideration of risk versus benefits.[3,24] Other than for obstetric and fetal indication, planned preterm delivery (<37 weeks' gestation) is seldom warranted for maternal cardiac reasons. Women with severe heart failure should be delivered at a center with availability of mechanical circulatory support as well as a transplant team.

Treatment of arrhythmias needs to be tailored to the individual and is based on the type of arrhythmia and the presence of underlying structural heart disease. Electrical cardioversion is safe during pregnancy, and women with tachyarrhythmias who are hemodynamically unstable require cardioversion. Bradycardias are less common during pregnancy. Pacemaker and implantable cardioverter defibrillators are safe during pregnancy and delivery. If cautery is used at the time of delivery, oversensing by the pacemaker is possible and therefore magnets should be available in the delivery room to use to eliminate oversensing.

Occasionally, women with refractory symptoms require a percutaneous or surgical intervention. Maternal abdominal lead shielding, radial approach, and procedural techniques can minimize radiation exposure to the fetus. Women with severe mitral, aortic, or pulmonary stenosis who have symptoms refractory to medical therapy may require a balloon valvuloplasty or, in very select cases, percutaneous valve insertion to relieve the outflow track obstruction. These procedures should be performed only at experienced centers because acute heart failure, arrhythmias, tamponade, and death have been reported. Obstetric back-up is required because precipitous labor can occur. Cardiac surgery during pregnancy should only be performed if no other options are available, because fetal mortality can occur in approximately 20% of cases. Urgent surgery, maternal comorbidities, and early gestational age are associated with the highest fetal risk.[3,41] Fetal risk can be mitigated by pulsatile perfusion, high pump flow, avoidance of hypothermic extracorporeal circulation, minimizing bypass times, and fetal monitoring.[3] Later in gestation, delivery followed by cardiac surgery is preferred if there is adequate fetal maturity. In comparison, maternal surgical risks are similar to the nonpregnant population. A multidisciplinary pregnancy heart team with cardiology, cardiac surgery, anesthesia, obstetrics, and neonatology is necessary to optimize mother and offspring outcomes.

Cardiac arrest during pregnancy is managed similarly to the nonpregnant arrest, with the following modifications: (1) lateral uterine displacement during an arrest is required after 20 weeks' gestation; (2) intubation may be more difficult due to changes in airway mucosa; and (3) emergency cesarean delivery should be initiated if there has been no return of spontaneous circulation within 4 minutes of the onset of arrest in a pregnant women with a fundus height at or above the umbilicus.[42]

SPECIFIC CARDIOVASCULAR CONDITIONS

Hypertension (see Chapter 26)

Hypertensive disorders of pregnancy are one of the leading causes of maternal and perinatal mortality worldwide and responsible for 16% of maternal deaths in high-income countries.[2,43,44] They can be classified into four categories: preeclampsia/eclampsia, gestational hypertension, chronic hypertension, and chronic hypertension with superimposed preeclampsia. Although obstetric providers usually manage hypertensive disorders in pregnant women, cardiovascular practitioners should be aware of the overall management approach. Hypertension in pregnancy is defined as systolic blood pressure (SBP) of 140 mm Hg or greater or diastolic blood pressure (DBP) of 90 mm Hg or greater on two measurements at least 4 hours apart, with the proviso that the second measurement can be obtained within 15 minutes if the BP is severely elevated (SBP ≥ 160 mm Hg or DBP ≥ 110 mm Hg). The BP should be remeasured from the arm with the higher BP after an interval of at least 15 minutes if there is nonsevere elevation of BP.[2,43,44] Tobacco or caffeine use within 30 minutes prior to measurement can temporarily increases BP. Many women with first BP reading of 140/90 or greater will subsequently be found to have normal BP on repeated measurement.[45] Ambulatory BP monitoring can separate white coat versus chronic hypertension for women with persistent BP elevation of 140/90 mm Hg or less at less than 20 weeks' gestation. Patients with preexisting hypertension may have a falsely normal BP due to the reduced systemic vascular resistance that manifests by the 12th gestational week. Pregnant women with severe hypertension (BP ≥ 160/110 persistent for 15 minutes) should be triaged expeditiously and pharmacotherapy initiated to reduce risk of heart failure, stroke, or renal disease (Fig. 92.6).[44,45]

Preeclampsia is defined as: (1) hypertension (defined earlier) after 20 weeks' gestation in persons who were previously normotensive and (2) new-onset proteinuria **or** new-onset end-organ damage. In the presence of new-onset end-organ manifestations, proteinuria is not needed to establish a diagnosis. One caveat is that gestational hypertension can manifest prior to 20 weeks, and previously undiagnosed chronic hypertension can present after 20 weeks, when the BP rises from its nadir in second trimester.[43,44] The current proposed mechanism for preeclampsia is uteroplacental ischemia resulting in imbalances in angiogenic and antiangiogenic factors.[44] Severe preeclampsia is an obstetrical emergency. The more severe form of preeclampsia, HELLP (hemolysis, elevated liver enzymes, and low platelet count) syndrome, usually presents in the third trimester and can present or progress in the postpartum period. Eclampsia, defined as new-onset seizures, the convulsive manifestation of preeclampsia, is a significant cause of maternal death, especially in low-resources settings. In a significant minority of cases, HELLP and eclampsia may not be preceded by hypertension or proteinuria.[44]

For those with less severe hypertension, pharmacotherapy can be initiated with any first-line agent (see Fig. 92.6). Current guidelines differ as to the threshold for initiation of pharmacotherapy in those women with less severe hypertension, as well as the optimal BP to be

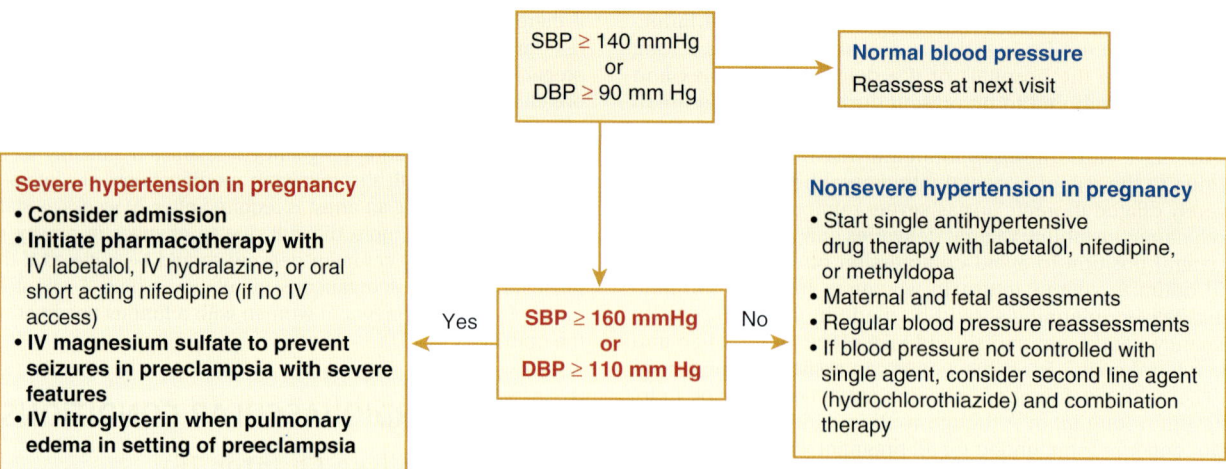

FIGURE 92.6 Management algorithm for hypertension in pregnancy.[2,45] Summary of North American recommendations for initial management of women with hypertensive disorders of pregnancy.

achieved with treatment.[44–47] Tight control of BP (DBP <85 mm Hg) did not confer an improved maternal or perinatal outcome compared with less tight control of BP but did reduce the risk of developing severe hypertension.[45] Currently, the optimal goal for BP therapy varies between United States (range of 140 to 150/90 to 100 mm Hg), European (<140/90 mm Hg), and Canadian (<85 mm Hg diastolic BP) recommendations.[2,45,47] An important consideration is that hemoconcentration, rather than hypervolemia, is a frequent finding in patients with preeclampsia.

For prevention of preeclampsia, low-dose ASA should be initiated between 12 and 16 weeks' gestation (and ideally, no later than 20 weeks) and continued until at least 36 weeks' gestation in women in women with any high risk factors (chronic hypertension, prior preeclampsia, multifetal gestation, diabetes mellitus, renal disease, autoimmune disease, or preterm birth <34 weeks' gestation) or in women with more than 1 moderate risk factor (nulliparity, body mass index >30, family history of preeclampsia, age ≥35 years, socioeconomic status, or personal history factors).[2,44,48,49] In women with gestational hypertension or preeclampsia, the decision to deliver versus expectant treatment needs to consider the absence/presence of severe features of preeclampsia and gestational age.[44] Ambulatory follow-up and/or home BP monitoring should be continued in the postpartum period and therapy should be continued in those with postpartum hypertension (≥ 150/100 mm Hg).[2] Women with hypertension during pregnancy require longitudinal follow-up and risk factor modification because they are at elevated risk of developing hypertension or cardiovascular disease later in life.

CARDIOMYOPATHIES (SEE PART VI)

Common preexisting cardiopathies in women of childbearing age are dilated cardiomyopathy (DCM), hypertrophic cardiomyopathy (HCM), and cardiomyopathies related to congenital heart disease or valvular heart disease. Less common causes include: ischemic cardiomyopathy, tachycardiac-induced cardiomyopathy, arrhythmogenic right ventricular cardiomyopathy, noncompaction cardiomyopathy, restrictive cardiomyopathy, and Chagas disease in endemic areas. PPCM develops de novo during pregnancy. Pregnant women with cardiomyopathies are at risk for maternal and fetal complications and require careful preconception risk stratification and counseling.

DCM in women of childbearing age may be idiopathic or secondary to genetic defects (i.e., lamin A/C [*LMNA*], beta-myosin heavy chain [*MYH7*], or cardiac troponin T [*TNNT2*] mutation), prior myocarditis, or drug exposure (i.e., Adriamycin exposure).[50] Genetic counseling should be offered to women with DCM who have a family history of cardiomyopathy. Women with DCM are at risk of worsening left ventricular systolic function, clinical heart failure, atrial or ventricular arrhythmia, thromboembolic complications, or, rarely, death.[3,51] Women with DCM who have good functional capacity and mild left ventricular systolic function often do well during pregnancy. Conversely, women with NYHA functional class III or IV and/or moderate or severe LV systolic dysfunction have high rates of cardiac complications including heart failure and arrhythmias.[51] Pregnancy is contraindicated in women with DCM and severe left ventricular systolic dysfunction.[3]

HCM is an inherited cardiomyopathy with autosomal dominant transmission, and transmission of HCM to offspring should be discussed at the time of the preconception visit because some women may wish to consider pre-implantation genetic screening. The HCM phenotype is variable and may have left ventricular outflow tract obstruction, diastolic or systolic dysfunction, or significant mitral regurgitation (MR). Atrial fibrillation (AF) and heart failure are the most common complications in pregnant women with HCM.[52] Maternal mortality, although rare, has been reported in women with high-risk features.[3] Most women with mild or moderate forms of HCM do not develop cardiac complications during pregnancy. Women with high-risk features such as severe left ventricular hypertrophy, syncope, prior ventricular tachycardia (VT), or severe left ventricular outflow tract obstruction can develop cardiac complications during pregnancy and require careful preconception assessment. In women with severe left ventricular outflow tract obstruction, epidural anesthesia should be used cautiously because it can result in hypotension and worsening of the outflow tract obstruction. Similarly, oxytocin may cause hypotension and tachycardia and should be given as a slow infusion. In women with obstructive HCM, avoidance of Valsalva and a facilitated second stage of labor is recommended at the time of labor and delivery.

PPCM is a cardiomyopathy that occurs de novo during pregnancy. Women typically present later in pregnancy or in the first few months postpartum with left ventricular systolic dysfunction (left ventricular ejection fraction [LVEF] <45%), heart failure, and embolic events. PPCM is a diagnosis of exclusion.[53] Older maternal age, Africa-American race, multigestation pregnancy, preeclampsia, and hypertension are risk factors for PPCM. The cause of PPCM is not known, but proposed mechanisms have included nutritional deficiencies, viral myocarditis, and autoimmune and vascular-hormonal processes. Treatment is similar to that for heart failure in general with diuresis, beta blockers, and afterload reduction. A mouse model for PPCM identified a 16-kDa prolactin fragment that resulted in vascular and myocardial dysfunction. Based on that finding and small human studies, bromocriptine, a suppressor of prolactin secretion, has been used as a therapy for PPCM.[53] Maternal recovery of left ventricular systolic function have been variable. In the North American Investigators of Pregnancy-Associated Cardiomyopathy (IPAC) study, approximately 70% of women had a left ventricular ejection fraction greater than

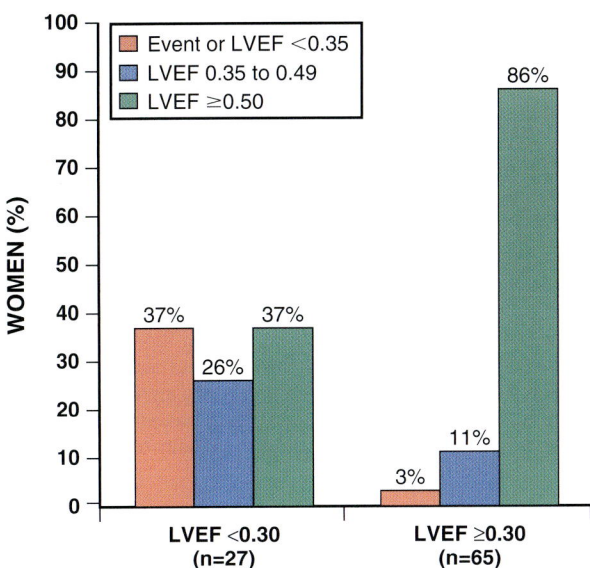

FIGURE 92.7 Recovery of left ventricular systolic function in women with peripartum cardiomyopathy. Comparison of left ventricular systolic function at 1 year post presentation based on the initial left ventricular ejection fraction. *Red column,* percentage of women with no recovery (event or final ejection fraction <0.35); *blue column,* percentage of women with partial recovery (final ejection fraction 0.35 to 0.49); *green column,* percentage of women with complete recovery (final ejection fraction ≥ 0.50). LVEF denotes left ventricular ejection fraction. (From McNamara DM, Elkayam U, Alharethi R, et al. Clinical outcomes for peripartum cardiomyopathy in North America: results of the IPAC study (investigations of pregnancy-associated cardiomyopathy). *J Am Coll Cardiol.* 2015;66:905–914.)

50% 1 year after their index presentation. Baseline left ventricular ejection fraction greater than 0.30 and left ventricular end diastolic dimensions less than 6.0 cm at presentation are prognostic markers associated with good recovery (Fig. 92.7).[54] One year after the index presentation in the IPAC study, 13% had experienced either a major cardiac event or had severe cardiomyopathy (LVEF <0.35). Higher mortality rates are reported in African Americans. Subsequent pregnancies carry risk, particularly in women in whom the left ventricular systolic function does not recover, and pregnancy is contraindicated in women with residual left ventricular systolic dysfunction because of the significant maternal mortality.[53]

Pregnancy after a heart transplant can be successful with careful planning. Pregnancy is not advised until at least 1 year after heart transplant and is contraindicated in women at high risk of rejection or with baseline graft dysfunction. All women should have preconception counseling so they can understand pregnancy risks and make medication modifications if necessary. A discussion about maternal life expectancy should be included as part of preconception counseling. Mycophenolate mofetil is teratogenic and should be stopped prior to conception. Alternatives to azathioprine should be used when possible. For those women who become pregnant, frequent surveillance of immunosuppressive medications is critical because changes in volume of distribution and metabolism may require dose adjustments during pregnancy and postpartum. Potential complications include rejection, graft dysfunction, and infection.[55] Hypertensive disorders of pregnancy occur in approximately 26% of pregnancies, and preeclampsia occurs in 18% of pregnancies.[55] Preterm deliveries occur in more than half of all pregnancies.[55] Immunosuppressive medications can impact the neonate, and therefore breastfeeding is not recommended.

MYOCARDIAL INFARCTION AND ISCHEMIC HEART DISEASE

Pregnancy is a risk factor for cardiac ischemic events,[2,56] relating to elevated pregnancy-associated increase in low-density lipoprotein (LDL) cholesterol levels, hypercoagulable state, inflammatory changes associated with preeclampsia/infection, hormonal weakening of the arterial wall, increased vascular reactivity, or use of prostaglandin analog in postpartum hemorrhage.[57] Although ischemic heart disease was rarely encountered in the past, it is expected to increase in frequency with rising maternal age and increasing prevalence of atherosclerotic risk factors. The incidence of MI is estimated to be approximately 3 per 100,000 pregnancies, with a case fatality rate of approximately 5%.[58] Coronary atherosclerotic disease accounts for up to 40% of cases, spontaneous coronary artery dissection (SCAD) has been responsible for up to 43% of cases, and the remainder have been attributed to intracoronary thrombus (up to 17%) or coronary spasm (approximately 2%).[2,57] Majority of acute MI presented in the third trimester or postpartum period.[59] The diagnosis of MI during pregnancy is similar to that of nonpregnant patient[60] and may be misdiagnosed as dyspepsia or reflux.[57] ST elevation MI is more common than non–ST elevation MI, and up to two-thirds of MIs are anterior.

SCAD results in formation of an intramural hematoma which encroaches on the true coronary artery lumen.[57,61,62] Of the three types of SCAD, type 1 (typical appearance, multiple lumens, arterial wall stain) was encountered in less than one-third of cases. Confirming the diagnosis of type 2 (diffuse smooth stenosis, most common) and type 3 (mimic atherosclerosis; least common) SCAD usually requires intravascular ultrasound or optical coherence tomography.[61] Urgent angiography should be performed for suspected SCAD and for those presenting with ST elevation MI.[61] Because SCAD is a common cause of ST elevation MI in pregnant women, thrombolysis for acute ST-segment elevation myocardial infarction [STEMI] is not recommended. Thrombolytic agents do not cross the placenta but can cause maternal and placental bleeding. The risk of iatrogenic catheter-induced coronary artery dissection is higher (approximately 3%) than for standard coronary angiography, attributed to underlying vascular frailty in patients with SCAD. The risk of iatrogenic coronary dissection was higher with radial approach; thus the femoral approach may be preferred in the pregnant patient.[61] Technical recommendations have been proposed to reduce the risk of causing a new dissection or propagating an existing dissection.[63] Cardiac catheterization and coronary interventions in pregnant women should be performed by experienced operators at a referral center. It is reasonable to perform coronary angiography for a pregnant patient with non–ST elevation MI or acute coronary syndrome, but this need not be done emergently. A negative coronary CT angiography does not exclude SCAD.[61]

Although at least 70% of patients with SCAD will have angiographic healing on repeat angiography, these data are not based on consecutive sample or pregnant patients.[61] Medical therapy is the preferred strategy for SCAD, with inpatient monitoring for an extended period because up to 10% of conservatively managed patients may have extension of dissection within the first 7 days. Percutaneous coronary intervention (PCI) in patients with SCAD has consistently been reported to increase risk of complications and poor outcomes, likely related to increased coronary frailty. PCI or coronary artery bypass grafting (CABG) should be considered for those women with active or ongoing ischemia, hemodynamic instability, left main, or severe proximal two vessel dissection.[61] Meticulous angiographic and specific PCI techniques, designed to restore coronary flow without further propagating the dissection, have been proposed.[61] Patients with PCI should be on dual platelet therapy, and clopidogrel is viewed as the only "safe" inhibitor. Coronary artery surgery was not protective against recurrent SCAD, with the risk of graft occlusion from competitive flow from healing of the native coronary arteries.

Patients with MI should be on beta blockers and low-dose ASA. The indications for clopidogrel in patient who have not undergone PCI is less certain due to potential increase in bleeding risk. Nitrates and calcium channel blockers can be used for angina therapy. ACE-Is/ARBs and statins are not recommended during pregnancy. Nitrates, beta blockers, or low-molecular-weight or unfractionated heparin can be used for acute MI during pregnancy.[2,35,61] Doses of nitrates will need to be carefully titrated to avoid excessive maternal hypotension because the placenta cannot autoregulate BP. Pregnancy and delivery should be at a referral center with involvement of the maternal heart team. Current recommendation is for vaginal delivery with epidural anesthesia, with minimization of maternal efforts during vaginal delivery. Given that pregnancy is a risk factor for developing SCAD and the 3-year risk of major cardiac events for patients with SCAD in general is up to 30%,[61] future pregnancies should be discouraged.

Women with preexisting coronary artery disease or prior MI currently constitute a small proportion of pregnant women with heart disease.[15] However, a systematic review reported ischemic events occurred in 9% of pregnancies and the mortality rate was 2%; only 21% of pregnancies were uncomplicated (no maternal or fetal/neonatal complications).[56] Prior to pregnancy, women with coronary artery disease should undergo treatment of any correctable lesions that are associated with ischemia. For those women with significant coronary stenosis but further intervention is not possible, avoidance of pregnancy should be considered. Similar to patients with SCAD or MI during pregnancy, this high-risk group of patients should receive care by a pregnancy heart team and deliver at a center that can perform coronary revascularization and provide advanced cardiac therapies.[2] Low-dose ASA, beta$_1$ selective blockers, nitrates, and clopidogrel can be continued during pregnancy.[35] ACE-I can be reinitiated in the postpartum period, and some are safe for lactation (see general management section). Statins can be restarted in the postpartum period for women who are not lactating.[35]

NATIVE VALVULAR HEART DISEASE (SEE PART VIII)

Rheumatic MS is the most common type of valvular heart disease encountered in pregnant women globally.[64] Pregnancy-associated increase in stroke volume and heart rate results in elevation of the transmitral gradient and left atrial pressure, thereby increasing the likelihood of functional class deterioration, pulmonary edema, and atrial arrhythmia. The hypercoagulable state associated with pregnancy increases the risk of left atrial thrombus. The fetus is at increased rate of preterm birth, intrauterine growth restriction, and death, attributed to inability to augment cardiac

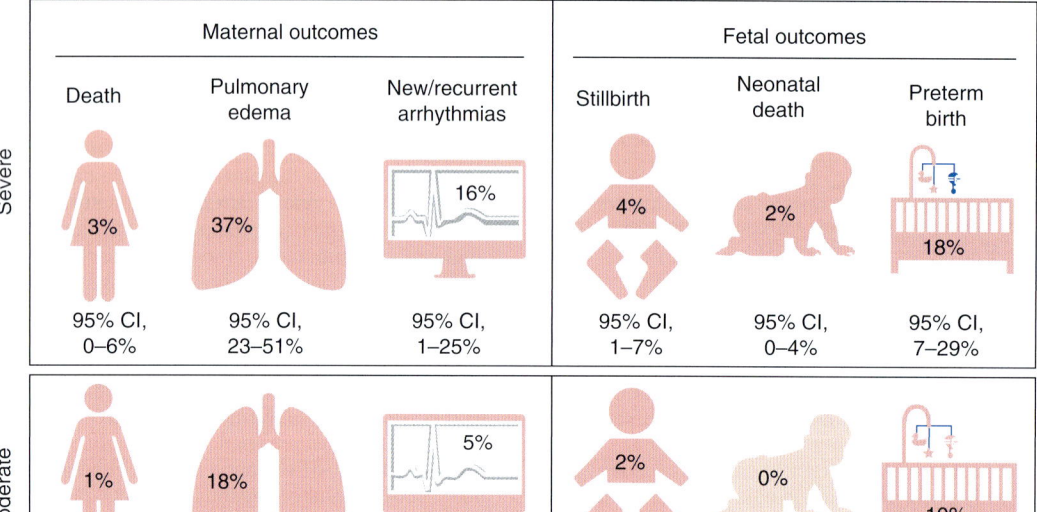

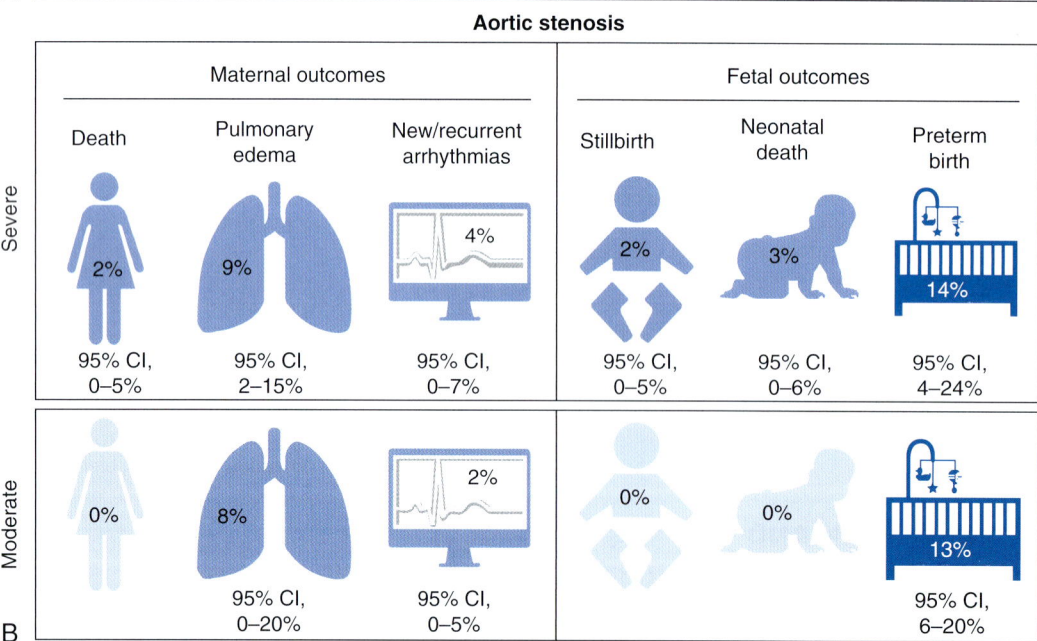

FIGURE 92.8 Maternal and fetal/neonatal outcomes by valve lesion and severity. Maternal and fetal complications in women with mitral (**A**) and aortic (**B**) stenosis as stratified by lesion severity. *CI,* Confidence interval. (From Ducas RA, Javier DA, D'Souza R, et al. Pregnancy outcomes in women with significant valve disease: a systematic review and meta-analysis. *Heart.* 2020;106:512–519.)

output and uteroplacental insufficiency. The frequency of complications generally corresponded to the severity of MS (Fig. 92.8A), and the risk within each class may be further elevated by symptoms, left ventricular systolic dysfunction, prior heart failure, or pulmonary artery hypertension.[65,66] Recent guidelines have reclassified mitral valve area of 1.5 cm^2 or less as severe or significant MS, which encompasses mitral valve area of 1.1 to 1.5 cm^2, which was formerly classified as moderate MS.[67] In countries with high prevalence of rheumatic heart disease and limited health care access, the mortality rate was 34%[68]; in contrast to the lower mortality reported in middle-high income countries (see Fig. 92.8A).[69]

Present guidelines have recommended percutaneous balloon valvuloplasty or mitral valve surgery prior to pregnancy for women with mitral valve area of 1.5 cm^2 or less,[3,67,70] to reduce the development of heart failure and AF. However, this strategy may not be applicable in women with access to specialty care and normal exercise tolerance, who are not at high thromboembolic risk and do not have pulmonary hypertension.[71] Pregnant women with MS should be followed serially during pregnancy, with a minimum frequency of at least once during the first trimester and again during the third trimester; those with severe MS will require more frequent follow-up. Mitral valve gradients will increase with increasing cardiac output during pregnancy, so assessment of MS severity should be by mitral valve area.[65] Beta$_1$ selective blockers are recommended,[67] especially in those with significant (moderate or severe) MS or symptoms. Deterioration in functional class may be an early warning sign of impending heart failure, and loop diuretics and increasing dose of beta blockers (or digoxin if intolerant to beta blockers) should be initiated along with restriction of activities. Exact heart rate goals with beta blockers have not been established. Atrial tachyarrhythmia is a frequent precipitant of maternal heart failure, especially in the third trimester.[5] Anticoagulation is recommended in those with AF, left atrial thrombus, or prior embolism. In those with significant MS and who are in sinus rhythm, anticoagulation is a consideration if there is spontaneous echocardiographic contrast in the left atrium, large left atrium ($\geq$ 60 mL/m^2), or congestive heart failure.[3] Mitral valvuloplasty can be performed during pregnancy but is usually reserved for refractory symptoms or heart failure despite maximal medical therapy and hospitalization.

The risk of maternal and fetal mortality is lower in pregnancies in women with isolated MR.[66,69] However, moderate to severe MR is associated with heart failure in 23% of pregnancies in women with rheumatic heart disease and is an independent predictor of maternal cardiac complications regardless of etiology.[15,66] Therefore patients with moderate or severe MR should have serial follow-up in the antepartum period similar to patients with MS. Clinicians should also be aware that the reduced systemic vascular resistance during the antepartum may reduce the magnitude of MR during second to third trimester, leading to underestimation of its severity. We recommend that a single dose of intravenous loop diuretics be administered during the first several hours after delivery in patient with moderate or severe MR or MS, to reduce the likelihood of redistribution edema from autotransfusion following birth. For patients with predominant mitral valve disease, vaginal delivery with epidural anesthesia is the preferred mode of delivery, with cesarean delivery considered for patients with NYHA functional class III to IV or pulmonary hypertension, despite medical therapy. Mitral valve prolapse is considered to be a low-risk condition unless there is moderate or severe MR.

Aortic stenosis (AS) most commonly occurs as a result of bicuspid aortic valve (BAV) and limits the ability of the heart to increase cardiac output or adjust to changes in loading conditions during pregnancy,[23] increasing propensity for heart failure, ischemia, or hypotension.[23] Asymptomatic women with mild AS typically will tolerate pregnancy well. Women with moderate or severe AS are at risk for heart failure, arrhythmias, and angina, although the mortality risk in those with severe AS is low in the current era (Fig. 92.8B).[69] For subvalvular AS, a resting gradient greater than 30 mm Hg is considered to be hemodynamically significant.[15]

Current guidelines recommend exercise testing to risk stratify asymptomatic women with severe AS.[3,67] Aortic valve replacement is recommended in women with symptomatic AS or asymptomatic women with left ventricular ejection fraction less than 50% or abnormalities during exercise testing.[3,67] Although pre-pregnancy aortic valve replacement has been recommended in asymptomatic women with severe AS, this decision should be individualize based on left ventricular function and results of exercise testing.[3] Anatomic feasibility for a Ross procedure, with avoidance of long-term anticoagulation and potential for long-term valve longevity, would be an additional consideration.

Patients with AS require follow-up similar to mitral lesion, with diuretics treatment for heart failure. How to deliver a woman with AS has not been established,[69] although cesarean is believed to reduce stress on the mother,[71] as well as facilitating logistics when there are plans for hemodynamic monitoring. Percutaneous valvuloplasty can be performed as a temporizing measure in those patients with refractory symptoms in the antepartum period. Valve replacement can be performed during pregnancy, or timed with a cesarean delivery, for life-threatening symptoms and where percutaneous approach is not possible.[4] Transcutaneous aortic valve replacement may be a potential option.

Aortic regurgitation is generally better tolerated than AS, and a small study reported that 29% of pregnancies in women with severe aortic regurgitation were complicated by pulmonary edema.[69] Functional deterioration will usually respond to loop diuretics.

Most women with significant valvular pulmonic stenosis would have been treated with percutaneous valvuloplasty in childhood. The small number of patients with severe pulmonic stenosis reported in studies have had generally good outcomes, with infrequent occurrence of right heart failure or deterioration in functional class.[71,18] Severe pulmonic regurgitation (PR) is also well tolerated, perhaps with the reduced pulmonary vascular resistance during pregnancy. Although there have been reports of right heart failure in patients with severe PR, many have been associated with right ventricular systolic dysfunction in patients with complex congenital lesions.[72] Isolated tricuspid stenosis is uncommonly encountered, and systematic outcome data are not available. With dilatation of tricuspid annulus with right ventricular enlargement during pregnancy, there can be an increase in TR,[27] and it is not unusual to see moderate TR during normal pregnancy. Women with isolated severe TR usually tolerate pregnancy well, when the right ventricle is not the systemic (subaortic) ventricle, although systematic data are absent. In patients with congenital cardiac lesions, moderate to severe TR was an independent predictor of cardiac complications,[72] but this finding has not been replicated by prospective studies.[15,73] Patients with right heart failure, or experiencing functional deterioration from right-sided valvular lesions, usually respond to loop diuretics; cardiac interventions can be deferred until after pregnancy.[71]

PROSTHETIC VALVES AND MANAGEMENT OF ANTICOAGULATION

Women with prosthetic valves are at risk for complications in pregnancy, and women should have preconception counseling for risk stratification and to discuss these risks. Compared with women with mechanical valves, those with bioprosthetic valves are at less risk for pregnancy-related complications as the valves are less thrombogenic and anticoagulation is not required.[74] Women with normal functioning bioprosthetic valves, good functional class, and normal left ventricular systolic function are at low risk for maternal cardiac complications. However, because valve degeneration occurs over time, some women with older valve implants may have abnormal valve function which increases pregnancy risk. Although pregnancy experience is limited, women with a Ross procedure (pulmonary valve autograft and bioprosthetic pulmonary valve) also have good pregnancy outcomes.[3]

Pregnancy in women with mechanical valves is associated with significant maternal and fetal risks. The most serious maternal complication is valve thrombosis, which can result in maternal mortality (Table 92.5).[75] The risk of valve thrombosis is related to a number of factors, including the type of anticoagulant used during pregnancy (warfarin less risk than heparin), the type of valve (newer generation valves less risk than older generation valves) and valve position (aortic position less risk than mitral position). There are three

TABLE 92.5 Maternal and Fetal Risk in Women with Mechanical Heart Valves

Anticoagulation Regimen	PRIMARY MATERNAL AND FETAL OUTCOMES			
	Maternal Mortality Estimate % (95% CI)	Thromboembolism Estimate % (95% CI)	Live Births Estimate % (95% CI)	Anticoagulant-Related Fetal and Neonatal Adverse Events Estimate % (95% CI)
Vitamin K antagonists (INR target 2.5–3.5)	0.9 (0.1, 1.6)	2.7 (1.4, 4.0)	64.5 (48.8, 80.2)*	2.0 (0.3, 3.7)*
Sequential treatment	2.0 (0.8, 3.1)	5.8 (3.8, 7.7)	79.9 (74.3, 85.6)	1.4 (0.3, 2.5)†
LMWH alone	2.9 (0.2, 5.7)	8.7 (3.9, 13.4)	92.0 (86.1, 98.0)	NA
UFH alone	3.4 (0, 7.7)	11.2 (2.8, 19.6)	69.5 (37.8, 100)	7.6 (0.1, 15.0)

*Of these, 7/407 (0.8% [0.0, 1.7]) represent embryopathy and 5/197 (2.1% [0.1, 4.1]) represent fetopathy.
†All cases represent fetopathy.
Estimates are presented as proportions per 100 affected pregnancies with 95% confidence intervals.
CI, Confidence intervals; INR, international normalized ratio; LMWH, low-molecular-weight heparin; NA, not applicable; UFH, unfractionated heparin.
From D'Souza R, Ostro J, Shah PS, Silversides CK, et al. Anticoagulation for pregnant women with mechanical heart valves: a systematic review and meta-analysis. Eur Heart J. 2017;38(19):1509-1516.

TABLE 92.6 International Recommendations for the Management of Anticoagulation in Pregnant Women with Mechanical Heart Valves[3,67,76]

	2018 EUROPEAN SOCIETY OF CARDIOLOGY GUIDELINES	2014 AMERICAN HEART ASSOCIATION/AMERICAN COLLEGE OF CARDIOLOGY GUIDELINES	2012 AMERICAN COLLEGE OF CHEST PHYSICIANS GUIDELINES
1st trimester	Warfarin dose <5 mg/day (or phenprocoumon <3 mg/day or acenocoumarol <2 mg/day) 1. VKA* 2. Adjusted-dose LMWH twice daily with monitoring of anti-Xa levels 4–6 hr post dose): Target anti-Xa level depends on valve site. Pre-dose target provided in recommendation footnotes 3. Adjusted-dose intravenous UFH (aPTT ≥2x control) Warfarin dose >5 mg/day 1. Adjusted-dose LMWH* twice daily with monitoring of anti-Xa levels 4–6 hr post dose: Target anti-Xa level depends on valve site. 2. Adjusted-dose intravenous UFH* (aPTT ≥ 2x control) 3. Continuation of VKA	Warfarin dose ≤5 mg/day 1. Warfarin* 2. Dose-adjusted LMWH ≥ two times daily (target anti-Xa level 0.8–1.2 U/mL 4–6 hr post dose) 3. Dose-adjusted continuous infusion UFH (aPTT at least 2 × control) Warfarin dose >5 mg/day 1. Dose-adjusted LMWH ≥ two times daily (target anti-Xa level 0.8-1.2 U/mL 4-6 hr post dose) * 2. Dose adjusted continuous infusion UFH (aPTT at least 2× control) *	Any of the following anticoagulant regimens are recommended: 1. Adjusted-dose bid LMWH throughout pregnancy, with doses adjusted to achieve the manufacturer's peak anti-Xa level 4 hr post dose 2. Adjusted-dose subcutaneous UFH throughout pregnancy administered every 12 hr in doses adjusted to keep the mid interval aPTT at least twice control or attain an anti-Xa heparin level of 0.35–0.70 units/mL 3. UFH or LMWH (as above) until the 13th week with substitution by VKA until close to delivery when UFH or LMWH is resumed. For women judged to be at very high risk of thromboembolism in whom concerns exist about the efficacy and safety of UFH or LMWH as dosed above (e.g., older-generation prosthesis in the mitral position or history of thromboembolism), VKA throughout pregnancy with replacement by UFH or LMWH (as above) close to delivery.
2nd and 3rd trimesters	1. VKA until 36 weeks' gestation†	1. Warfarin	
Addition of aspirin		Low-dose aspirin (75–100 mg daily) at the beginning of the 2nd trimester	Low-dose aspirin (75–100 mg daily)
Prior to delivery	1. Discontinue VKAs and start adjusted-dose intravenous UFH (aPTT ≥2× control) or adjusted-dose LMWH at 36 weeks' gestation 2. Replace LMWH with intravenous UFH (aPTT ≥ 2× control) at least 36 hr before planned delivery	1. Discontinue warfarin and dose-adjusted continuous infusion of UFH (aPTT at least 2× control)	1. UFH or LMWH is resumed close to delivery

*Option that received the highest grade of recommendation from among the competing options during that period of pregnancy.
†Option that received the highest grade of recommendation during the 2nd and 3rd trimesters, from among the competing options in the group with high dose of VKA.
aPTT, Activated partial thromboplastin time; INR, international normalized ratio; LMWH, low-molecular-weight heparin; UFH, unfractionated heparin; VKA, vitamin K antagonist (warfarin, phenprocoumon, or acenocoumarol).

anticoagulation options for pregnant women with mechanical valves: (a) warfarin or other vitamin K antagonists, (b) low-molecular-weight heparins, and (c) intravenous unfractionated heparin (Table 92.6). Direct oral anticoagulants are not safe for pregnant patients with mechanical valves. For pregnant women with mechanical valves, there is no perfect anticoagulant that is equally safe for both the mother and her child. Warfarin is associated with the lowest risk of valve thrombosis and maternal mortality for the mother but crosses the placenta and can cause warfarin embryopathy when used in the first trimester and fetopathy when used later in pregnancy. Warfarin embryopathy appears to be dose dependent, with lower rates of embryopathy reported in women taking daily warfarin doses less than 5 mg.[72] Heparin does not cross the placenta and is therefore a safer alternative for the fetus but is less effective at preventing valve thrombosis and is associated with higher rates of maternal mortality.[75] One treatment strategy is to replace warfarin with low-molecular-weight heparin during embryogenesis (6 to 12 weeks' gestation) to prevent embryopathy. Use of low-molecular-weight heparin throughout pregnancy is an option for women who wish to avoid warfarin altogether, but this requires close follow-up throughout pregnancy because many of the reported cases of valve thrombosis were related to inadequate dosing and monitoring of anti-Xa levels. Peak anti-Xa levels should be measured frequently, with experts suggesting weekly to monthly anti-Xa monitoring during pregnancy.[3,67,76] In addition, some experts advocate measurement of trough levels to ensure consistently therapeutic anti-Xa levels and have developed a detailed treatment algorithm that considers valve position and type.[72] Anticoagulation surveillance during pregnancy in women with mechanical valves is often best done in conjunction with a hematologist with expertise in pregnancy. Unfractionated heparin is associated with high rates of valve thrombosis when given subcutaneously. Its use is recommended only when administered as a continuous intravenous infusion, in a hospital setting. At the time of delivery, women on anticoagulants are at risk for postpartum hemorrhage and should be monitored closely. Both heparin and warfarin are safe in the breastfeeding mother. Recommendations for anticoagulation in pregnant women with mechanical valves have been published by the American Heart Association/American College of Cardiology,[67] the American College of Chest Physicians,[76] and the European Society of Cardiology[3] (see Table 92.6). In view of the competing maternal and fetal risks, shared decision-making with women is required when choosing an anticoagulation regimen. All women should be followed in a tertiary care center by an experienced pregnancy heart team.

Mechanical valve thrombosis can be fatal and should be excluded in any pregnant women with new cardiac symptoms, heart failure, or significant increases in valve gradients on their echocardiogram. Diagnosis of a thrombosed valve is usually confirmed using transesophageal echocardiography or fluoroscopy. The choice of treatment options (heparin, thrombolytics, or surgery) is determined by the clinical stability of the patient, the size of the thrombus, and the availability of surgery.[72] An algorithm for treatment of left-sided mechanical valve thrombosis is shown.[77] Right-sided valve thrombosis is often treated with heparin or thrombolytics.

ARRHYTHMIAS (SEE PART VII)

Increases in plasma volume, hormonal-mediated changes in action potential, and autonomic changes are potential mechanisms contributing to an increased propensity to arrhythmias during pregnancy. Women who present with arrhythmias during pregnancy should have an echocardiogram to exclude structural heart disease and a Holter monitor to determine the burden of arrhythmias. The most frequently detected arrhythmias in pregnancy are atrial and ventricular premature beats, and generally these do not require therapy. Treatment of tachyarrhythmias needs to be tailored to the individual with consideration of the type of arrhythmia, the underlying heart disease, ventricular function, and the severity of symptoms.

Supraventricular tachycardia (SVT) is the most common arrhythmia in pregnant women and usually occurs in women with structurally normal hearts.[5] Women may present for the first time during pregnancy, or they may have a history of SVT. Women with a history of SVT and structural heart disease have approximately 50% recurrence rates during pregnancy.[78] Most women with SVT can be treated medically.[5,79] In women with acute SVT who are hemodynamically stable, vagal maneuvers and adenosine can used to terminate the arrhythmias. For women with a contraindication to adenosine or in whom adenosine is ineffective, intravenous beta blockers such as metoprolol or propranolol can be used. Experience with other antiarrhythmic agents is more limited and is usually reserved for those women who are highly symptomatic despite beta blockers or calcium channel blockers.

AF and atrial flutter (AFL) often occur in the setting of structural heart disease such as MS or congenital heart disease.[78,80] In general, in women who develop AF or AFL, rate control is preferred over rhythm control. Pregnant women with acute unstable AF or AFL require cardioversion.[5] In pregnant women who are stable with rapid ventricular rates, beta blockers, or digoxin can be given to control the ventricular rate. As in the nonpregnant patient, pregnant women with AF/AFL for more than 48 hours or of unknown duration require a transesophageal echocardiogram or 3 weeks of therapeutic anticoagulation prior to cardioversion. Pharmacologic cardioversion should be individualized, and the choice of antiarrhythmic should be based on the presence of structural heart disease and the left ventricular systolic function. Management of AF in patients with Wolff-Parkinson-White (WPW) requires special consideration as the rhythm can degenerate into an unstable preexcited rhythm if drugs such as beta blockers, calcium channel blockers, or digoxin are given as these drugs increase conduction over the accessory pathway. Therefore antiarrhythmic drugs that slow or block conduction over the pathway, such as flecainide, should be used to treat AF. Consideration of thromboembolism prophylaxis should be given to women who develop AF/AFL, especially those with structural heart disease or elevated $CHADS_2$ scores. Warfarin is associated with warfarin embryopathy when used between 6 and 12 weeks' gestation, and therefore low-molecular-weight heparin is often used during pregnancy. Direct oral anticoagulants are not recommended in pregnancy.

VT and ventricular fibrillation (VF) are rare during pregnancy. VT may be idiopathic, or it may occur in the setting of structural heart disease such as cardiomyopathies, valve disease, and congenital heart disease.[7,15] VT may be secondary to primary electrical diseases such as long QT syndrome (LQTS). Rarely, VT occurs in the setting of hypomagnesemia or hypertensive crises. Acute unstable VT or VF in pregnant women should be treated similarly to the nonpregnant patient with cardioversion or defibrillation. Pharmacologic cardioversion with procainamide, amiodarone, or lidocaine may be appropriate in some cases of hemodynamically stable VT. Idiopathic VT is a monomorphic VT that typically originates from the right ventricular outflow tract. It is usually successfully treated with beta blockers or verapamil.[3] The risk of VT in women with LQTS, specifically LQT2 mutation, increases in the postpartum period.[81] Beta blockers are effective in preventing cardiac events in pregnant women with LQTS, and all women should be treated with beta blockers during pregnancy and postpartum.[81] VT in the setting of structural heart disease is more complex and requires and individualize approach to therapy. Amiodarone can affect fetal thyroid function and should be used only to treat recurrent VT and when other antiarrhythmic drugs are not suitable. In pregnant women with drug-refractory VT, catheter ablation may be considered and referral to a center that can offer radiofrequency catheter ablation without fluoroscopic guidance should be considered.

CONGENITAL HEART DISEASE (SEE CHAPTER 82)

The involvement of an adult congenital cardiologist, preferably as part of the pregnancy heart team, is recommended in the preconceptual counseling or care of pregnant women with congenital heart lesion. Review of prior clinical and procedural records will guide diagnostic tests and enable pregnancy management to be individualized.

Cardiac Shunts

Women with successful closure of isolated left-to-right shunts are at low risk for complications during pregnancy. In the absence of other risk factors such as cardiac arrhythmias, cardiac events after closure, systemic ventricular dysfunction, or pulmonary hypertension, women with repaired shunts can deliver at their local hospital. Women with unoperated atrial septal defect (ASD) usually tolerate pregnancy well. Overall frequency of arrhythmia, right heart failure, and thromboembolism is low.[3] In women of childbearing age, most unoperated ventricular septal defects (VSDs) or patent ductus arteriosus (PDA) are likely small (restrictive) as those with untreated significant shunts would have progressed to pulmonary hypertension in childhood. Women with small (restrictive) VSD or PDA, without other general risk factors, do not require additional cardiac precautions during the antepartum and peripartum period. For unrepaired ASD or VSD, repaired ASD or VSD with residual shunting, or patent foramen ovale, we recommend the use of air/particulate filters for indwelling IVs at time of labor and delivery, to reduce the chance of paradoxical right-to-left shunt.[23]

Cardiac shunts associated with pulmonary hypertension are discussed in the pulmonary hypertension section.

Left-Sided Obstruction

BAV is a common etiology of AS and aortic regurgitation (AR) in women in childbearing age. The management of AS and AR during pregnancy has been discussed earlier. An important association of BAV is ascending aorta dilatation and coarctation. Aortic dissection has been reported in women with BAV and aortopathy, although overall risk is lower than in women with aortopathy associated with Marfan syndrome.[23] The approach to the aortopathy associated with BAV is discussed in the aortopathy section.

Significant aortic coarctation impedes delivery of blood distally with adverse impact on the placental circulation, and increases the risk of intrauterine growth restriction and premature labor. Upper body hypertension and concomitant aortic valve disease pose additional risks. Maternal mortality has been reported, but this is rare in contemporary series.[23] Overtreatment of upper body hypertension during pregnancy could potentially result in hypotension distal to the coarctation site with adverse impact on fetal well-being. Even with successful coarctation repair, abnormal aortic compliance increases the risk of developing gestational hypertension.[23] An elevated descending aorta gradient may be a result of increase in flow, abnormal compliance, hypoplasia of the aorta, or true coarctation. Prolongation of the gradient into diastole (diastolic tail) as seen in the abdominal or descending aorta Doppler increases the certainty that true coarctation is present. Women with unrepaired coarctation or residual coarctation are at risk for aortic complication including dissection,[3] for which we offer empiric beta blockers therapy. Percutaneous intervention for residual or recurrent coarctation is best deferred until after pregnancy.[3]

Left-sided or systemic atrioventricular valvular regurgitation is treated similarly in those with acquired heart disease. Although isolated systemic atrioventricular valvular regurgitation may be well tolerated with heart failure/arrhythmia reported with low mortality, concomitant systemic ventricular systolic dysfunction will increase risk by impairing maternal adaptation to the regurgitant load during pregnancy. Those patients with moderate or severe regurgitation will need serial follow-up with consideration of postpartum intravenous loop diuretics to reduce the risk of redistribution pulmonary edema. Pulmonic and tricuspid valve disease has already been previously discussed in the section on native valvular disease.

Complex Congenital Lesions

The management considerations for selected complex congenital cardiac lesions are summarized on Table 92.7. Patients with complex congenital lesions represent a heterogeneous group, and their management during pregnancy has been extensively reviewed.[3,4,18,72] Women with complex congenital cardiac lesions should be followed by the pregnancy heart team, with the site of delivery determined by maternal risk, stability during pregnancy, and logistical considerations.

Unoperated Complex Congenital Lesions
Ebstein Anomaly

Acyanotic women with milder anatomic variations of Ebstein can expect to have an uncomplicated pregnancy, whereas women with severe Ebstein anomaly may be unable to tolerate the increased preload and cardiac output of pregnancy and are at risk for functional deterioration, right heart failure, and arrhythmia.[23] The overall frequency of cardiac complications during pregnancy is low (from 0% to ≤12%).[23,82] The associated lesions of preexcitation and interatrial shunting will increase cardiac risk during pregnancy. Those with the associated ASD or patent foramen ovale (PFO) may demonstrate reversal or increase in right-to-left shunting with pregnancy, leading to worsening cyanosis, with the risk of fetal loss, prematurity, or intrauterine growth restriction. Risk of preterm delivery and fetal mortality is increased.

Congenitally Corrected Transposition of Great Arteries

Systemic ventricular systolic dysfunction and significant systemic atrioventricular valvular regurgitation are common findings in adults with congenitally corrected transposition of the arteries. Importantly, significant systemic atrioventricular valvular regurgitation will mask systemic ventricular systolic dysfunction. Heart failure, endocarditis, stroke, or MI have been reported.[3,23] Pregnancy should be discouraged in patients with poor functional class, severe systemic ventricular systolic function, or severe systemic atrioventricular valvular regurgitation.[3]

Complex Congenital: Repaired
Repaired Tetralogy of Fallot

Pregnancy is usually well tolerated in women after repaired tetralogy, but risk is increased in the presence of left ventricular systolic dysfunction and/or severe PR with right ventricular dysfunction. Although right heart failure and arrhythmias have been reported in up to 12% of pregnancies, other series have reported lower complication rates.[3,23] Patients with VSD patch leak and residual right ventricular outflow tract obstruction usually tolerate pregnancy well as long as they are not cyanotic.[23,83]

Repaired Transposition of Great Arteries

Women born with repaired complete transposition of the great arteries would have undergone an atrial redirection operation (Mustard or Senning), an arterial switch operation (Jatene), or, less commonly, a Rastelli repair. Late complications after atrial redirection (baffle) operations include sinus node dysfunction, atrial arrhythmias, systemic ventricular dysfunction, and systemic atrioventricular valve regurgitation. Arrhythmias are the most common cardiac complication during pregnancy, and there is an increased risk of heart failure. Fetoneonatal complications are higher than in normal pregnancy. Pregnancy has been associated with progressive subaortic right ventricular dilation and deterioration in subaortic right ventricular function after pregnancy.[3,23] Baffle leak has been underrecognized (see Table 92.7). Pulmonary artery catheters should be discouraged due to potential problems with trapping of the catheter through the baffles. Reported experience during pregnancy in women treated with the arterial switch operation procedure remains limited,[3] but no maternal cardiovascular complications were observed in preliminary studies.[3,84] The main residua in those with Rastelli repair is right ventricular outflow tract conduit stenosis, which is usually well tolerated during pregnancy; those with severe conduit stenosis may experience functional deterioration, but right heart failure is uncommon.

Fontan

The ability of the heart to increase cardiac output during pregnancy is impaired following the Fontan operation, which directs systemic venous return to the pulmonary artery and bypasses the trabecular (or muscular) portion of the subpulmonary ventricle. Associated scarring and remodeling of the atria increase the risk of atrial arrhythmias while systemic venous stasis increases risk of atrial thrombi, particularly with atrial tachyarrhythmia. Importantly, adults with Fontan procedure may manifest reduced oxygen desaturation or cyanosis due to systemic to pulmonary collaterals or residual right to left shunt at the atrial level. Despite these concerns, low maternal mortality has been observed in pregnant women with Fontan procedure, likely reflecting patient selection as those with prior cardiac events, reduced systemic ventricular systolic function, or protein losing enteropathy were likely appropriately discouraged from pregnancy.[85] An overview reported SVT (9%) and heart failure (4%) with no maternal deaths.[20] Fetal and neonatal adverse outcomes remain common, with miscarriages complicating 45% of pregnancies and a high rate of antepartum bleeding (including abruptio placenta), prematurity, and cesarean delivery (11%, 59%, and 57%, respectively). Pregnant Fontan patients should deliver at a referral center and be cared for by a maternal heart team. Antiplatelet thromboprophylaxis should be considered (low-dose ECASA), with the use of low-molecular-weight heparin for those with prior history of embolism or atrial arrhythmias. Vaginal delivery is preferred.[3]

TABLE 92.7 Potential Complications and Management Recommendations for Pregnant Women with Complex Congenital Heart Lesions

CARDIAC LESION	CARDIAC COMPLICATIONS	MANAGEMENT RECOMMENDATIONS
Ebstein anomaly (unrepaired and repaired)	• Arrhythmias • Right heart failure • Paradoxical emboli • Oxygen desaturation from interatrial shunt	• Clinical and echocardiographic surveillance during pregnancy and postpartum including oxygen saturation • Echocardiographic monitoring of right ventricular systolic function • Air/particulate filters during labor and delivery for women with interatrial communications • Vaginal delivery preferred
Repaired tetralogy of Fallot	• Arrhythmias • Right heart failure	• Clinical and echocardiographic surveillance during pregnancy and postpartum • Echocardiographic monitoring of the right ventricular size, right ventricular systolic function, and pulmonary artery pressures • Autosomal dominant transmission of heart disease to offspring in women with 22q11.2 deletion syndrome • Vaginal delivery preferred
Arterial switch operation	• Arrhythmias • Aortic dilation or dissection • Heart failure in women with aortic regurgitation	• Clinical and echocardiographic surveillance during pregnancy and postpartum • Vaginal delivery preferred unless there is significant aortic dilation
Systemic right ventricle • Atrial switch operation (Mustard or Senning operation) • Congenitally corrected transposition of great arteries (unrepaired)	• Deterioration in ventricular function • Heart failure • Worsening systemic atrioventricular valve regurgitation • Arrhythmias • Heart failure	• Frequent clinical and echocardiographic surveillance during pregnancy and postpartum • Echocardiographic monitoring of the subaortic right ventricular size, systolic function, and atrioventricular valve regurgitation • Vaginal delivery with early epidural and a facilitated second stage of labor • Air/particulate filters during labor and delivery for women with atrial switch procedures • Avoid pulmonary catheters in women with atrial switch procedures • Postpartum monitoring for arrhythmias and heart failure
Fontan operation	• Arrhythmias • Heart failure • Thromboembolic complications • Bleeding complications	• Frequent clinical and echocardiographic surveillance during pregnancy and postpartum • Echocardiographic monitoring of subaortic ventricular function and atrioventricular valve regurgitation • Low-dose aspirin and consideration of anticoagulation for women at risk for thromboembolic complications • Prompt treatment of atrial arrhythmias • Prepare for preterm labor, which is common • Vaginal delivery with early epidural and a facilitated second stage of labor • Maintain adequate preload during delivery • Postpartum monitoring for arrhythmias and heart failure
Cyanotic congenital heart disease	• Mortality • Heart failure • Arrhythmias • Thromboembolism • Bleeding complications	• Frequent clinical and echocardiographic surveillance during pregnancy and postpartum including oxygen saturation • Supplemental oxygen and activity limitation • Air/particulate filters during labor and delivery • Consider thromboprophylaxis • Consider following brain natriuretic peptide • Preterm labor common • Vaginal delivery often possible • Postpartum monitoring for heart failure and arrhythmias

Cyanotic Congenital Heart Lesions

The cardiac causes of cyanosis in pregnant women without pulmonary artery hypertension are large shunts at atrial or ventricular levels, systemic venous to pulmonary venous collaterals, or reduced pulmonary blood flow. Maternal cardiovascular complications have been reported in approximately 30% of pregnancies and are related to maternal oxygen level. If the maternal oxygen saturation was 85% or less, the live birth rate was only 12%.[3] Supplemental oxygen and activity restriction are recommended. Thromboembolic prophylaxis has been proposed but must be balanced with the bleeding risk associated with cyanosis.[3]

Cyanosis is associated with abnormal thrombotic and bleeding tendency, and these patients are at risk for postpartum hemorrhage. Care by the pregnancy heart team and delivery at a referral center are recommended for pregnant women with cyanotic heart disease.

PULMONARY HYPERTENSION

Pulmonary arterial hypertension (PAH), from any cause, is associated with very high pregnancy risks. PAH is defined as a mean resting pulmonary arterial pressure greater than 25 mm Hg, and higher pulmonary arterial pressures are associated with higher risk. Maternal cardiac decompensation occurs because of the volume load on the right ventricle, the increased flow in the high-resistance pulmonary vascular bed, changes in intracardiac shunt flow with resulting desaturations, and thromboembolic events secondary to the prothrombotic effects of pregnancy. At delivery, adverse effects from anesthetic drugs and volume overload from intravenous fluids and volume shifts can further lead to cardiac decompensation. A review of pregnancy outcomes in women with PAH delivering between 1997 and 2007 reported a maternal mortality of 17%, 28%, and 33% in women with idiopathic PAH, congenital heart disease, and other causes, respectively.[86] Maternal mortality is the result of a number of causes, including right-sided heart failure, sudden death, pulmonary hypertensive crisis, and pulmonary embolism. Most maternal deaths occur within the first month after delivery. Although more favorable outcomes have been reported in women treated with pulmonary vasodilator therapy,[18,87-89] because of the high mortality risk, women with PAH should be advised against pregnancy and safe and reliable contraception should be provided. While women with idiopathic PAH or Eisenmenger syndrome are at the highest risk during pregnancy, pregnancy risks are high even when pulmonary hypertension is secondary to left heart disease.[90] Pregnant women with pulmonary hypertension are also at elevated risk of eclampsia, preterm delivery, and fetal death.[91]

For those women who become pregnant, termination often remains the safest option.[3] Those who choose to continue pregnancy require close antenatal follow-up with frequent clinic visits, transthoracic echocardiograms, and serum BNP levels.[18] Bosentan and other endothelin receptor antagonists are teratogenic and should be discontinued, ideally prior to pregnancy. Calcium channel blockers, phosphodiesterase-5 inhibitors, and prostacyclins have been used during pregnancy. During pregnancy and after delivery, fluid status should be followed closely to prevent right-sided heart failure. Joint care by the pregnancy heart and pulmonary hypertension team is important. All women should deliver at a tertiary care center with postpartum monitoring in the coronary/intensive care unit and careful diuresis. Women who are clinically stable can undergo vaginal delivery with early epidural anesthesia and an assisted second stage of delivery. Delivery is usually planned prior to 37 weeks' gestation.[18] Extended postpartum monitoring in hospital is recommended because many of the cardiac complications occur in the first postpartum week.

MARFAN SYNDROME AND INHERITED AORTOPATHIES

Increased cardiac output, hypervolemia, and the pregnancy-related changes in aorta media contribute to increased risk of aortic dilation and dissection.[18] Aortic dissection has been described in pregnant women with Marfan syndrome, Loeys-Dietz syndrome, vascular Ehlers-Danlos syndrome, Turner syndrome, and BAV.[92] The highest risk of dissection occurs in the third trimester or early postpartum.[18] The risk for complications varies according to the particular lesion.

In women with Marfan syndrome, the incidence of aortic dissection or rupture during pregnancy and postpartum period is eightfold higher than those who were not pregnant.[93] The overall risk of aortic dissection is approximately 3%, ranging from 1% in women with aortic diameters less than 40 mm, to approximately 10% in women with an aortic diameter greater than 40 mm, rapid dilatation, or previous ascending aortic dissection.[18] Aortic root replacement prior to pregnancy is not protective from distal aortic dissection.[94,95] Similarly, it is possible for dissection to occur in an aorta that appears "normal" by imaging.

Loeys-Dietz syndrome is a high-risk lesion during pregnancy. Vascular dissection or rupture can occur in the presence of normal aorta dimensions and can occur despite aortic root replacement and optimal medical therapy. Pooled data reported a vascular dissection or rupture in 11% of pregnancies.[96] Uterine rupture has been reported. Vascular Ehlers-Danlos syndrome is extremely high risk, and like Loeys-Dietz syndrome (LDS), vascular rupture can occur despite normal aorta dimensions. Pregnant women with Turner syndrome are at significant risk of aortic dissection, preeclampsia, premature birth, low birth weight, and need for cesarean delivery.[97] Concurrent cardiac lesions (e.g., BAV or coarctation) increase the dissection risk.[18] Aorta measurements must be indexed to body surface area to adjust for the smaller stature in some patients with Turner syndrome. Aortic dissection has been described in women with Turner syndrome with prior root replacement as well as during ART-associated pregnancies.[3,97] Aortic dissection is much less common in women with BAV and aortopathy.[18] Early data on SMAD 3 mutation have reported favorable outcomes, but the patient numbers were small.[98]

All women with aortopathies considering pregnancy or already pregnant should be evaluated by and receive care by a maternal heart team at a referral center with echocardiographic assessment of the aorta, preferably supplemented by cardiac MR or CT before pregnancy. Pregnancy is contraindicated in Marfan and Loeys-Dietz syndrome with an ascending aorta greater than 45 mm, all patients with vascular Ehlers-Danlos syndrome, bicuspid associated aorta greater than 50 mm, and Turner syndrome with high-risk features (aortic size index [ASI] >2.5 cm/m^2 or history of aortic dissection).[3,72,97] Women with Marfan, Ehlers-Danlos, and Loeys-Dietz syndrome have a 50% chance of transmitting the syndrome to offspring. In addition, they are at increased risk for obstetric and fetoneonatal complications. Obstetric and neonatal complications (including preterm delivery from premature rupture of membranes and neonatal death) occur in approximately 40% of pregnancy in women with Marfan syndrome.[18]

For all aortopathies, serial echocardiographic evaluation of the aorta is recommended at least once during each trimester and increasing up to every 4 to 6 weeks in patients with aortic diameter greater than 40 mm, history of aortic surgery, or with progressive dilatation. TEE or cardiac magnetic resonance imaging (CMR) without gadolinium can be used for assessment if transthoracic echocardiogram is suboptimal.[18] Optimal hypertension control is crucial. Cesarean delivery is recommended in those with Marfan syndrome with aorta diameter greater than 40 mm (or progressive dilatation during pregnancy or prior aortic dissection repair), bicuspid aortopathy with aortic diameter greater than 45 mm, and Turner syndrome with ASI greater than 20 mm/m^2.[18] Plans for regional anesthesia should consider the high prevalence of dural ectasia in patients with Marfan syndrome. Prophylactic beta blockers (reducing heart rate by at least 20 beats/min) is recommended for pregnant patients with Marfan syndrome[18] and should be considered for Loey-Dietz, Turner syndrome, and in other aortopathies.[96,97] Beta blockers should also be considered when these patients undergo ARTs. A management algorithm for suspected aortic dissection during pregnancy is summarized.[5]

CONTRACEPTION

There are multiple contraception formulations, including barrier method, estrogen-containing oral contraceptive pills, progestin-only contraceptives (oral and implantable), patches, subdermal implants, intrauterine devices, and sterilization procedures. Each of these contraceptive options has benefits, risks, and variable failure rates.[2] For women with heart disease, some forms of contraception can have important side effects and should be avoided. Barrier methods (male and female condoms, diaphragms, cervical caps) are safe for women with heart disease but have high failure rates and are therefore not suitable for women at high risk for complications who need reliable contraception. Estrogen-containing contraceptives, available as oral preparations, transdermal patches, and vaginal rings, have relatively low failure rates; however, the associated increased thromboembolic risks limit the use of these contraceptives in women with mechanical valves, Fontan circulation, severe left ventricular systolic dysfunction, coronary disease, or a history of thromboembolism. Progestin-only forms of contraception are not associated with thrombosis; however, progestin can lead to fluid retention, and progestin-only pills have higher failure rates than combined oral contraceptives and should not be used in women in whom pregnancy risks are prohibitive. Intrauterine devices have low failure rates and are effective for long periods of time, but implantation carries risk and can result in a profound vagal reaction which can be dangerous for women with pulmonary hypertension or Fontan circulation. For women with these high-risk conditions, intrauterine devices should be implanted in a monitored setting. In instances where pregnancy is contraindicated, permanent forms of contraception should be considered by the patient or her partner. Women with severe heart disease may have limited life expectancy, and it is important to consider that women may be outlived by their spouse, who may then want to father children in the future.

REFERENCES

Risk Assessment

1. Davis MB, Walsh MN. Cardio-obstetrics. *Circ Cardiovasc Qual Outcomes*. 2019;12:e005417.
2. Mehta LS, Warnes CA, Bradley E, et al. Cardiovascular considerations in caring for pregnant patients: a scientific statement from the American heart association. *Circulation*. 2020;141:e884–e903.
3. Regitz-Zagrosek V, Roos-Hesselink JW, Bauersachs J, et al. ESC Guidelines for the management of cardiovascular diseases during pregnancy. *Eur Heart J*. 2018;39:3165–3241. 2018.
4. Canobbio MM, Warnes CA, Aboulhosn J, et al. Management of pregnancy in patients with complex congenital heart disease: a scientific statement for healthcare professionals from the American heart association. *Circulation*. 2017;135:e50–e87.
5. Windram J, Grewal J, Bottega N, et al. Clinical practice update on cardiovascular management of the pregnant patient. *Can J Cardiol*. 2021 (in press).
6. Lane-Cordova AD, Khan SS, Grobman WA, et al. Long-term cardiovascular risks associated with adverse pregnancy outcomes: JACC review topic of the week. *J Am Coll Cardiol*. 2019;73:2106–2116.
7. Roos-Hesselink JW, Ruys TP, Stein JI, et al. Outcome of pregnancy in patients with structural or ischaemic heart disease: results of a registry of the European Society of Cardiology. *Eur Heart J*. 2013;34:657–665.
8. D'Souza RD, Silversides CK, Tomlinson GA, Siu SC. Assessing cardiac risk in pregnant women with heart disease: how risk scores are created and their role in clinical practice. *Can J Cardiol*. 2020;36:1011–1021.
9. Schlichting LE, Insaf TZ, Zaidi AN, et al. Maternal comorbidities and complications of delivery in pregnant women with congenital heart disease. *J Am Coll Cardiol*. 2019;73:2181–2191.
10. Ramage K, Grabowska K, Silversides C, et al. Association of adult congenital heart disease with pregnancy, maternal, and neonatal outcomes. *JAMA Netw Open*. 2019;2:e193667.
11. MBRRACE-UK. Saving lives, improving mothers' care: lessons learned to inform maternity care from the UK and Ireland confidential enquiries into maternal deaths and morbidity. 2015–17. 2019.
12. Main EK, McCain CL, Morton CH, et al. Pregnancy-related mortality in California: causes, characteristics, and improvement opportunities. *Obstet Gynecol*. 2015;125:938–947.
13. Petersen EE, Davis NL, Goodman D, et al. Racial/Ethnic disparities in pregnancy-related deaths—United States, 2007–2016. *MMWR Morb Mortal Wkly Rep*. 2019;68:762–765.
14. Drenthen W, Boersma E, Balci A, et al. Predictors of pregnancy complications in women with congenital heart disease. *Eur Heart J*. 2010;31:2124–2132.
15. Silversides CK, Grewal J, Mason J, et al. Pregnancy outcomes in women with heart disease: the CARPREG II study. *J Am Coll Cardiol*. 2018;71:2419–2430.
16. Pfaller B, Sathananthan G, Grewal J, et al. Preventing complications in pregnant women with cardiac disease. *J Am Coll Cardiol*. 2020;75:1443–1452.
17. Slomski A. Why do hundreds of us women die annually in childbirth? *J Am Med Assoc*. 2019;321:1239–1241.
18. Elkayam U, Goland S, Pieper PG, Silversides CK. High-risk cardiac disease in pregnancy: Part II. *J Am Coll Cardiol*. 2016;68:502–516.
19. Balint OH, Siu SC, Mason J, et al. Cardiac outcomes after pregnancy in women with congenital heart disease. *Heart*. 2010;96:1656–1661.
20. Garcia Ropero A, Baskar S, Roos Hesselink JW, et al. Pregnancy in women with a fontan circulation: a systematic review of the literature. *Circ Cardiovasc Qual Outcomes*. 2018;11:e004575.
21. Sharma G, Ying Y, Silversides CK. The importance of cardiovascular risk assessment and pregnancy heart team in the management of cardiovascular disease in pregnancy. *Cardiol Clin*. 2021;39:7–19.

Management

22. Green LJ, Mackillop LH, Salvi D, et al. Gestation-specific vital sign reference ranges in pregnancy. *Obstet Gynecol*. 2020;135:653–664.
23. Haberer K, Silversides CK, Colman JM, Siu SC. Pregnancy in young women with congenital heart disease. In: Allen HD, ed. *Moss & Adams' Heart Disease in Infants, Children, and Adolescents*. 10 ed. Baltimore: Lippincott Williams and Wildkins; 2021.
24. Elkayam U. Cardiovascular evaluation during pregnancy. In: Elkayam U, ed. *Cardiac Problems in Pregnancy*. 4th ed. Hoboken: Wiley Blackwell; 2018:19–31.
25. Malhame I, Hurlburt H, Larson L, et al. Sensitivity and specificity of B-type natriuretic peptide in diagnosing heart failure in pregnancy. *Obstet Gynecol*. 2019;134:440–449.
26. Tanous D, Siu SC, Mason J, et al. B-type natriuretic peptide in pregnant women with heart disease. *J Am Coll Cardiol*. 2010;56:1247–1253.
27. Silversides CK, Siu SC. Heart disease in pregnancy. In: Otto CM, ed. *The Practice of Clinical Echocardiography*. 6th ed. Phladelphia: Elsevier; 2020.
28. Colletti PM, Lee KH, Elkayam U. Cardiovascular imaging of the pregnant patient. *AJR Am J Roentgenol*. 2013;200:515–521.
29. Ray JG, Vermeulen MJ, Bharatha A, et al. Association between MRI exposure during pregnancy and fetal and childhood outcomes. *J Am Med Assoc*. 2016;316:952–961.
30. Brugada J, Katritsis DG, Arbelo E, et al. ESC Guidelines for the management of patients with supraventricular tachycardia the Task Force for the management of patients with supraventricular tachycardia of the European Society of Cardiology (ESC). *Eur Heart J*. 2020;41:655–720. 2019.
31. Haberer K, Silversides CK. Congenital heart disease and women's health across the life span: focus on reproductive issues. *Can J Cardiol*. 2019;35:1652–1663.
32. Lima FV, Yang J, Xu J, Stergiopoulos K. National trends and in-hospital outcomes in pregnant women with heart disease in the United States. *Am J Cardiol*. 2017;119:1694–1700.
33. van Hagen IM, Boersma E, Johnson MR, et al. Global cardiac risk assessment in the Registry of Pregnancy and Cardiac disease: results of a registry from the European Society of Cardiology. *Eur J Heart Fail*. 2016;18:523–533.
34. Siu SC, Evans KL, Foley MR. Risk assessment of the cardiac pregnant patient. *Clin Obstet Gynecol*. 2020;63:815–827.
35. Halpern DG, Weinberg CR, Pinnelas R, et al. Use of medication for cardiovascular disease during pregnancy: JACC state-of-the-art review. *J Am Coll Cardiol*. 2019;73:457–476.
36. Grewal J, Silversides CK, Colman JM. Pregnancy in women with heart disease: risk assessment and management of heart failure. *Heart Fail Clin*. 2014;10:117–129.
37. Dayan N, Laskin CA, Spitzer K, et al. Pregnancy complications in women with heart disease conceiving with fertility therapy. *J Am Coll Cardiol*. 2014;64:1862–1864.
38. Udell JA, Lu H, Redelmeier DA. Failure of fertility therapy and subsequent adverse cardiovascular events. *CMAJ (Can Med Assoc J)*. 2017;189:E391–E397.
39. Grewal J, Siu SC, Lee T, et al. Impact of beta-blockers on birth weight in a high-risk cohort of pregnant women with CVD. *J Am Coll Cardiol*. 2020;75:2751–2752.
40. Adler Y, Charron P, Imazio M, et al. ESC guidelines for the diagnosis and management of pericardial diseases: the Task Force for the diagnosis and management of pericardial diseases of the European Society of Cardiology (ESC)Endorsed by: The European Association for Cardio-Thoracic Surgery (EACTS). *Eur Heart J*. 2015;36:2921–2964. 2015.
41. John AS, Gurley F, Schaff HV, et al. Cardiopulmonary bypass during pregnancy. *Ann Thorac Surg*. 2011;91:1191–1196.
42. Lavonas EJ, Drennan IR, Gabrielli A, et al. Part 10: special circumstances of resuscitation: 2015 American Heart Association guidelines update for cardiopulmonary resuscitation and emergency cardiovascular care. *Circulation*. 2015;132:S501–S518.
43. ACOG Practice Bulletin No. Chronic hypertension in pregnancy. *Obstet Gynecol*. 2019;133:e26–e50. 203.
44. American College of Obstetricians and Gynecologists' Committee on Practice Bulletins-Obstetrics. Gestational hypertension and preeclampsia: ACOG practice Bulletin, number 222. *Obstet Gynecol*. 2020;135:e237–e260.
45. Butalia S, Audibert F, Cote AM, et al. Hypertension Canada's 2018 guidelines for the management of hypertension in pregnancy. *Can J Cardiol*. 2018;34:526–531.
46. Brown MA, Magee LA, Kenny LC, et al. The hypertensive disorders of pregnancy: ISSHP classification, diagnosis & management recommendations for international practice. *Pregnancy Hypertens*. 2018;13:291–310.
47. Williams B, Mancia G, Spiering W, et al. ESC/ESH Guidelines for the management of arterial hypertension. *Eur Heart J*. 2018;39:3021–3104. 2018.
48. D'Souza R, Kingdom J. Preeclampsia. *CMAJ*. 2016;188:1178.
49. Rolnik DL, Wright D, Poon LC, et al. Aspirin versus placebo in pregnancies at high risk for preterm preeclampsia. *N Engl J Med*. 2017;377:613–622.
50. Nolan M, Oikonomou EK, Silversides CK, et al. Impact of cancer therapy-related cardiac dysfunction on risk of heart failure in pregnancy. *JACC CardioOncol*. 2020;2:153–162.
51. Grewal J, Siu SC, Ross HJ, et al. Pregnancy outcomes in women with dilated cardiomyopathy. *J Am Coll Cardiol*. 2009;55:45–52.
52. Goland S, van Hagen IM, Elbaz-Greener G, et al. Pregnancy in women with hypertrophic cardiomyopathy: data from the European Society of Cardiology initiated Registry of Pregnancy and Cardiac disease (ROPAC). *Eur Heart J*. 2017;38:2683–2690.
53. Davis MB, Arany Z, McNamara DM, et al. Peripartum cardiomyopathy: JACC state-of-the-art review. *J Am Coll Cardiol*. 2020;75:207–221.
54. McNamara DM, Elkayam U, Alharethi R, et al. Clinical outcomes for peripartum cardiomyopathy in North America: results of the IPAC study (investigations of pregnancy-associated cardiomyopathy). *J Am Coll Cardiol*. 2015;66:905–914.
55. Acuna S, Zaffar N, Dong S, et al. Pregnancy outcomes in women with cardiothoracic transplants: a Systematic review and meta-analysis. *J Heart Lung Transplant*. 2020;39:93–102.
56. Lameijer H, Burchill LJ, Baris L, et al. Pregnancy in women with pre-existent ischaemic heart disease: a systematic review with individualised patient data. *Heart*. 2019;105:873–880.
57. Cauldwell M, Baris L, Roos-Hesselink JW, Johnson MR. Ischaemic heart disease and pregnancy. *Heart*. 2019;105:189–195.
58. Gibson P, Narous M, Firoz T, et al. Incidence of myocardial infarction in pregnancy: a systematic review and meta-analysis of population-based studies. *Eur Heart J Qual Care Clin Outcomes*. 2017;3:198–207.
59. Elkayam U, Jalnapurkar S, Barakkat MN, et al. Pregnancy-associated acute myocardial infarction: a review of contemporary experience in 150 cases between 2006 and 2011. *Circulation*. 2014;129:1695–1702.
60. Thygesen K, Alpert JS, Jaffe AS, et al. Fourth universal definition of myocardial infarction (2018). *Circulation*. 2018;138:e618–e651.
61. Hayes SN, Kim ESH, Saw J, et al. Spontaneous coronary artery dissection: current state of the science: a scientific statement from the American Heart Association. *Circulation*. 2018;137:e523–e557.
62. Tamis-Holland JE, Jneid H, Reynolds HR, et al. Contemporary diagnosis and management of patients with myocardial infarction in the absence of obstructive coronary artery disease: a scientific statement from the American Heart Association. *Circulation*. 2019;139:e891–e908.
63. Elkayam U, Havakuk O. Acute myocardial infarction and pregnancy. In: Elkayam U, ed. *Cardiac Problems in Pregnancy*. 4th ed. Hoboken: Wiley Blackwell; 2018:201–219.
64. French KA, Poppas A. Rheumatic heart disease in pregnancy: global challenges and clear opportunities. *Circulation*. 2018;137:817–819.
65. Silversides CK, Colman JM, Sermer M, Siu SC. Cardiac risk in pregnant women with rheumatic mitral stenosis. *Am J Cardiol*. 2003;91:1382–1385.
66. van Hagen IM, Thorne SA, Taha N, et al. Pregnancy outcomes in women with rheumatic mitral valve disease: results from the registry of pregnancy and cardiac disease. *Circulation*. 2018;137:806–816.
67. Nishimura RA, Otto CM, Bonow RO, et al. AHA/ACC guideline for the management of patients with valvular heart disease: a report of the American College of cardiology/American heart association Task Force on practice guidelines. *Circulation*. 2014;129:e521–e643. 2014.
68. Diao M, Kane A, Ndiaye MB, et al. Pregnancy in women with heart disease in sub-Saharan Africa. *Arch Cardiovasc Dis*. 2011;104:370–374.
69. Ducas RA, Javier DA, D'Souza R, et al. Pregnancy outcomes in women with significant valve disease: a systematic review and meta-analysis. *Heart*. 2020;106:512–519.
70. Baumgartner H, Falk V, Bax JJ, et al. ESC/EACTS Guidelines for the management of valvular heart disease. *Eur Heart J*. 2017;38:2739–2791. 2017.
71. Elkayam U. Native valvular heart disease and pregnancy. In: Elkayam U, ed. *Cardiac Problems in Pregnancy*. 4th ed. Hoboken: Wiley Blackwell; 2018:75–89.
72. Elkayam U, Goland S, Pieper PG, Silverside CK. High-risk cardiac disease in pregnancy: Part I. *J Am Coll Cardiol*. 2016;68:396–410.
73. Siu SC, Sermer M, Colman JM, et al. Prospective multicenter study of pregnancy outcomes in women with heart disease. *Circulation*. 2001;104:515–521.
74. North RA, Sadler L, Stewart AW, et al. Long-term survival and valve-related complications in young women with cardiac valve replacements. *Circulation*. 1999;99:2669–2676.
75. D'Souza R, Ostro J, Shah PS, et al. Anticoagulation for pregnant women with mechanical heart valves: a systematic review and meta-analysis. *Eur Heart J*. 2017;38(19):1509–1516.

76. Bates SM, Greer IA, Middeldorp S, et al. VTE, thrombophilia, antithrombotic therapy, and pregnancy: antithrombotic therapy and prevention of thrombosis, 9th ed: American college of chest physicians evidence-based clinical practice guidelines. *Chest*. 2012;141:e691S–e736S.
77. Bhagra CJ, D'Souza R, Silversides CK. Valvular heart disease and pregnancy part II: management of prosthetic valves. *Heart*. 2017;103:244–252.
78. Silversides CK, Harris L, Haberer K, et al. Recurrence rates of arrhythmias during pregnancy in women with previous tachyarrhythmia and impact on fetal and neonatal outcomes. *Am J Cardiol*. 2006;97:1206–1212.
79. Ghosh N, Luk A, Derzko C, et al. The acute treatment of maternal supraventricular tachycardias during pregnancy: a review of the literature. *J Obstet Gynaecol Can*. 2011;33:17–23.
80. Salam AM, Ertekin E, van Hagen IM, et al. Atrial fibrillation or flutter during pregnancy in patients with structural heart disease: data from the ROPAC (registry on pregnancy and cardiac disease). *JACC Clin Electrophysiol*. 2015;1:284–292.
81. Seth R, Moss AJ, McNitt S, et al. Long QT syndrome and pregnancy. *J Am Coll Cardiol*. 2007;49:1092–1098.
82. Lima FV, Koutrolou-Sotiropoulou P, Yen TY, Stergiopoulos K. Clinical characteristics and outcomes in pregnant women with Ebstein anomaly at the time of delivery in the USA: 2003–2012. *Arch Cardiovasc Dis*. 2016;109:390–398.
83. Egbe AC, El-Harasis M, Miranda WR, et al. Outcomes of pregnancy in patients with prior right ventricular outflow interventions. *J Am Heart Assoc*. 2019;8:e011730.
84. Stoll VM, Drury NE, Thorne S, et al. Pregnancy outcomes in women with transposition of the great arteries after an arterial switch operation. *JAMA Cardiol*. 2018;3:1119–1122.
85. Davis MB, Rogers IS. Pregnancy after fontan palliation: caution when details are lost in translation. *Circ Cardiovasc Qual Outcomes*. 2018;11:e004734.
86. Bedard E, Dimopoulos K, Gatzoulis MA. Has there been any progress made on pregnancy outcomes among women with pulmonary arterial hypertension? *Eur Heart J*. 2009;30:256–265.
87. Kiely DG, Condliffe R, Webster V, et al. Improved survival in pregnancy and pulmonary hypertension using a multiprofessional approach. *BJOG*. 2010;117:565–574.
88. Duarte AG, Thomas S, Safdar Z, et al. Management of pulmonary arterial hypertension during pregnancy: a retrospective, multicenter experience. *Chest*. 2013;143:1330–1336.
89. Jais X, Olsson KM, Barbera JA, et al. Pregnancy outcomes in pulmonary arterial hypertension in the modern management era. *Eur Respir J*. 2012;40:881–885.
90. Sliwa K, van Hagen IM, Budts W, et al. Pulmonary hypertension and pregnancy outcomes: data from the Registry of Pregnancy and Cardiac Disease (ROPAC) of the European Society of Cardiology. *Eur J Heart Fail*. 2016;18:1119–1128.
91. Thomas E, Yang J, Xu J, et al. Pulmonary hypertension and pregnancy outcomes: insights from the national inpatient sample. *J Am Heart Assoc*. 2017;6.
92. Kamel H, Roman MJ, Pitcher A, Devereux RB. Pregnancy and the risk of aortic dissection or rupture: a cohort-crossover analysis. *Circulation*. 2016;134:527–533.
93. Roman MJ, Pugh NL, Hendershot TP, et al. Aortic complications associated with pregnancy in Marfan syndrome: the NHLBI national registry of genetically triggered thoracic aortic aneurysms and cardiovascular conditions (GenTAC). *J Am Heart Assoc*. 2016;5.
94. Johnson MR, Roos Hesselink JW. Pregnancy, Marfan syndrome, and type-B aortic dissection. *BJOG*. 2018;125:494.
95. Sayama S, Takeda N, Iriyama T, et al. Peripartum type B aortic dissection in patients with Marfan syndrome who underwent aortic root replacement: a case series study. *BJOG*. 2018;125:487–493.
96. Frise CJ, Pitcher A, Mackillop L. Loeys-Dietz syndrome and pregnancy: the first ten years. *Int J Cardiol*. 2017;226:21–25.
97. Silberbach M, Roos-Hesselink JW, Andersen NH, et al. Cardiovascular health in turner syndrome: a scientific statement from the American Heart Association. *Circ Genom Precis Med*. 2018;11:e000048.
98. van Hagen IM, van der Linde D, van de Laar IM, et al. Pregnancy in women with SMAD3 mutation. *J Am Coll Cardiol*. 2017;69:1356–1358.

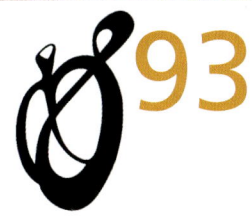

93

Heart Disease in Racially and Ethnically Diverse Populations

ALANNA A. MORRIS AND MICHELLE A. ALBERT

EPIDEMIOLOGY OF CARDIOVASCULAR DISEASE IN HETEROGENEOUS POPULATIONS, 1743
Cardiovascular Disease in Racial and Ethnic Groups, 1743
Cardiovascular Disease in Other Population Groups, 1743

CARDIOVASCULAR DISEASE MANAGEMENT, 1744
Hypertension, 1745
Coronary Heart Disease, 1747
Heart Failure, 1747

POTENTIAL FOR EMERGING SCIENTIFIC RESEARCH TO ADDRESS GROUP DISPARITIES IN CARDIOVASCULAR DISEASE, 1748

ACKNOWLEDGMENTS, 1748

REFERENCES, 1748

EPIDEMIOLOGY OF CARDIOVASCULAR DISEASE IN HETEROGENEOUS POPULATIONS

Cardiovascular Disease in Racial and Ethnic Groups

According to the 2017 National Center for Health Statistics (NHIS), the burden of coronary heart diseases (CHDs) varies by racial or ethnic group.[1] Although death rates from heart disease are declining for all race/ethnic groups, the rate of decline has been slower for race-ethnic minorities. In 2000, the age-adjusted death rate for heart disease was 326.5 per 100,000 people among non-Hispanic (NH) Blacks compared with 253.6 deaths per 100,000 among NH whites.[2] In 2017, the age-adjusted death rate had declined to 208.0 per 100,000 people among NH Blacks compared with 168.9 deaths per 100,000 among NH whites, thus preserving the higher rate of death for Blacks observed in 2000.[3] For Blacks and whites in the Atherosclerosis Risk In Communities (ARIC), Cardiovascular Health Study (CHS), and Reasons for Geographic And Racial Differences in Stroke (REGARDS) study, Black men were twice as likely to experience fatal CHD as white men (age-adjusted hazard ratio [HR], 2.09; 95% confidence interval [CI], 1.42 to 3.06), and Black women were more than twice as likely experience fatal CHD than white women (HR, 2.61; 95% CI, 1.57 to 4.34).[4] These differences in fatal CHD were largely attributable to social determinants of health and cardiovascular risk factors. Disparities in stroke prevalence and incidence are even greater.[1]

Hypertension (see also Chapter 26)

Blacks have higher rates of hypertension than other racial or ethnic groups.[5] Several proposed mechanisms may contribute to an increased incidence in Blacks (Fig. 93.1). Figure 93.2 presents the epidemiology of hypertension awareness, treatment, and control (see Fig. 93.3A-C) in the United States. Although rates of awareness in Blacks are higher (see Fig. 93.3A) than in other groups, and Blacks are more likely to be on treatment (see Fig. 93.3B) and use more medications to treat hypertension, Blacks have a lower rate of control than other racial or ethnic groups (see Fig. 93.3C).[6] American Indian/Alaska Natives (27.2%) also have higher rates of hypertension than Native Hawaiian or Other Pacific Islander (PI) (24.0%), Hispanic or LatinX (23.7%), white (24.8%), or Asian adults (21.9%).[1]

Among Hispanics/LatinXs, the hypertension prevalence varies considerably by subgroup. In the Hispanic Community Health Study/Study of LatinXs (HCHS/SOL), which measured blood pressure in 16,415 Hispanics/LatinXs (but does not include a comparison population of NHs), rates were highest among participants from Cuban, Puerto Rican, and Dominican ethnic backgrounds.[7] Hispanics/LatinXs are less likely to be aware of their hypertension and less likely to be treated than NH whites.[6,7]

National estimates of hypertension prevalence based on measured blood pressure in Asian Americans are lacking. Amongst the six largest Asian American populations (Asian Indian, Chinese, Filipino, Japanese, Korean, Vietnamese), Filipinos have particularly high rates of hypertension (53.2% to 59.9%), with poor awareness and control rates.[8] Filipino patients of older age, those with comorbid medical conditions, and those who did not smoke had improved hypertension treatment, and patients with health insurance had better blood pressure control. These findings suggest that better access to health care and an approach targeted toward multiple risk factors are needed to decrease the hypertension prevalence and risk among Filipinos.[9]

Type 2 Diabetes (see also Chapter 31)

The overall age-standardized prevalence of diabetes in the U.S. population is 14.6%, but Hispanics/LatinXs (16.6%), Blacks (18.3%), and Asians (16.4%) have a higher prevalence than NH whites (13.3%).[10]

The diabetes prevalence largely parallels the "epidemic" of obesity and physical inactivity, with evidence of disparities emerging even in childhood.[11,12] In the Hispanic/LatinX community, Dominicans, Puerto Ricans, and Mexicans (17% to 18%) seem to have a higher prevalence than South Americans and Cubans (10% to 13%).[13] Emerging research comparing the relative contributions of socioeconomic, environmental, and psychosocial factors, plus ancestry, to diabetes disparities has indicated that socioeconomic factors make up the largest group of mediating factors.[14]

Although the prevalence of diabetes generally parallels the obesity epidemic in most race/ethnic groups,[11] this has not been the case for Asian Americans. Asian Americans have on average a lower body mass index than other racial or ethnic groups but also display evidence of insulin resistance at lower values of body mass index which may be partly explained by differences in body fat distribution (see also Chapter 30).[11,15] PIs, South Asians, and Filipinos have prevalence of diabetes at least twofold to threefold higher than NH whites; prevalence of diabetes is also greater in Chinese, Japanese, Korean, and Southeast Asian adults compared with whites, although the magnitude of difference is less.[16] Filipinos and South/East Asians have higher rates of treatment than NH whites.

Cardiovascular Disease in Other Population Groups

Persons with psychological conditions and sexual minorities warrant increased attention because of their elevated risks of cardiovascular disease and its effects on health disparities. Psychological conditions including but not limited to anxiety, major depressive disorder, and bipolar disorder affected at least 46.6 million adults in 2017, with numerous others who are suffering but are undiagnosed and untreated.[17] This epidemic includes especially vulnerable populations, such as persons of lower socioeconomic status, the homeless, and military veterans.[18] An elevated cardiovascular risk is associated with adverse risk behaviors, isolation, limited contact with the health care system, and downward socioeconomic mobility; medications used to control some forms of mental illness can lead to weight gain and/or sedation, factors that contribute to decreases in motivation for physical activity (see also Chapter 99).[19]

Persons whose sexual orientation is lesbian, gay, bisexual, or transgender (LGBT) have not historically been considered "minorities," but they have emerged as sizeable social communities. Attention to the unique health needs in the LGBTQ population have traditionally focused on sexual health and less commonly on cardiovascular disease prevention and management. One exception that reflects the intersection between sexual and cardiovascular health relates to the shift of acquired immunodeficiency syndrome (AIDS) from an acute illness to a chronic illness, and its associated cardiovascular risks (see also Chapter 85). Although the burden of HIV/AIDS is not restricted to sexual minorities, the largest proportion of affected individuals are practicing male homosexuals and non-white minority women.[20] Medications used to manage HIV/AIDS have performed well in sparing associated wasting syndromes but as a result have yielded a higher burden of overweight and obesity and consequent metabolic disorders, including hypertension and diabetes.[21] HIV+ status (vs. HIV- status) associates with reduced systolic heart function and an increased prevalence of left ventricular hypertrophy, even after adjustments have been made for metabolic factors. These cardiac changes may predispose individuals with HIV/AIDS to heart failure.[22,23]

Cardiovascular disease is a major cause of death among homeless adults, with mortality rates twofold to threefold higher than the general population.[24] Various factors contribute to the worse outcomes, including substance use, high burden of traditional and nontraditional cardiovascular risk factors, and limited access to health care.[25] Importantly, men (60%) and Black persons (39%) are overrepresented among homeless populations,[26] and 19% of persons who are transgender or gender-nonconforming have experienced homelessness at some point in their lives.[27]

CARDIOVASCULAR DISEASE MANAGEMENT

Lifestyle modification through behavioral intervention that focuses on weight loss, reduced sodium intake, increased physical activity, and reduced alcohol consumption remains the cornerstone of cardiovascular disease prevention and management.[28] When examining Life Simple 7 scores (an American Heart Association lifestyle metric) in National Health and Nutrition Examination Survey (NHANES) participants,

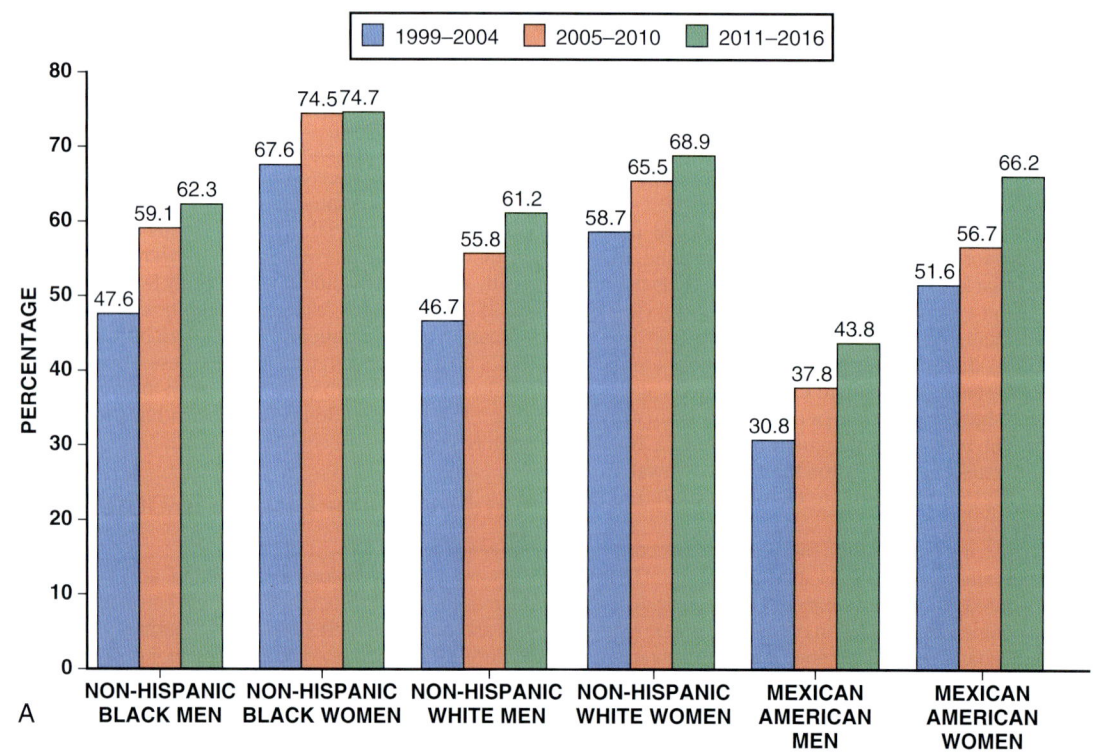

FIGURE 93.1 Proposed mechanisms for the increased incidence of hypertension in Blacks.

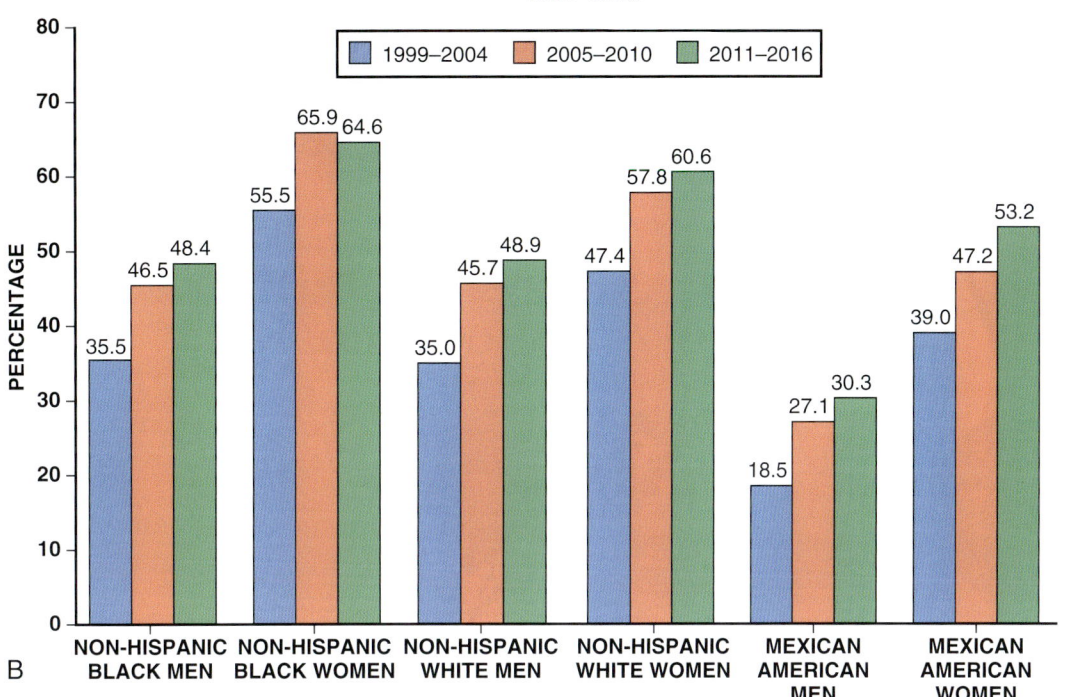

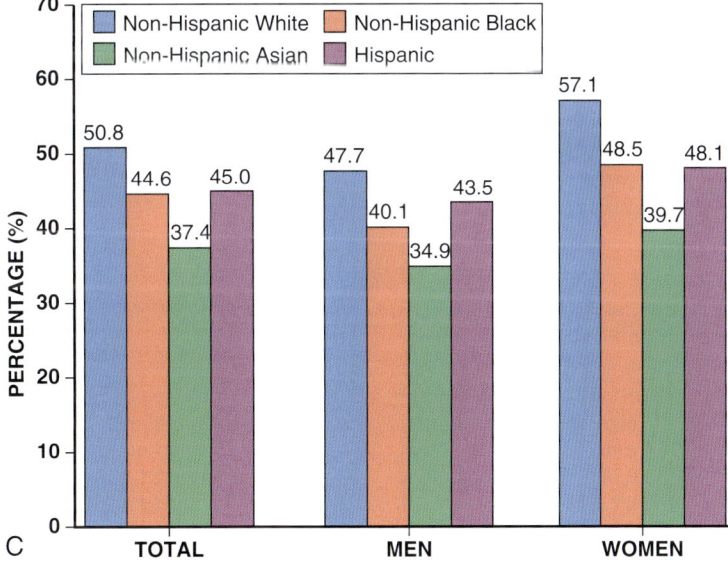

FIGURE 93.2 Epidemiology of adults with hypertension by race/ethnicity, United States. (**A** and **B** based on American Heart Association Heart Disease and Stroke Statistics—2020 Update. *Circulation.* 2020;141:e139–e596. DOI: 10.1161/CIR.0000000000000757; **C**, adapted from Fryar CD, et al. Hypertension prevalence and control among adults, United States, 2015-2016, NCHS Data Brief 2017, no 289.)

Black and Mexican-American women scored significantly lower compared with white women, while differences between Black and white men were smaller and mostly nonsignificant.[29] Moreover, despite higher body mass index and/or atherosclerotic cardiovascular disease risk, Black women (adjusted odds ratio [OR] 0.8, 95% CI, 0.7 to 0.9) were less likely to attempt weight loss, and Hispanic women (adjusted OR 0.8, 95% CI 0.6 to 0.9) were less likely to report physical activity than white women. Black women (adjusted OR 0.6, 95% CI 0.5 to 0.7) were less likely than white women, and Hispanics (women adjusted OR 0.6, 95% CI 0.5 to 0.7; men adjusted OR 0.7, 95% CI 0.6 to 0.9) were less likely than whites to report a healthy diet.[30]

Social determinants of health, including housing instability, food insecurity, and access to safe facilities to engage in leisure time physical activity, can impact the ability for socioeconomically disadvantaged to engage in healthy lifestyle behaviors, and impede the efficacy of proven prevention recommendations.

Hypertension (see also Chapter 26)

The Systolic Blood Pressure Intervention Trial (SPRINT) studied antihypertensive drug therapy that focused on lowering the systolic blood pressure (SBP) to less than 120 mm Hg rather than to less than

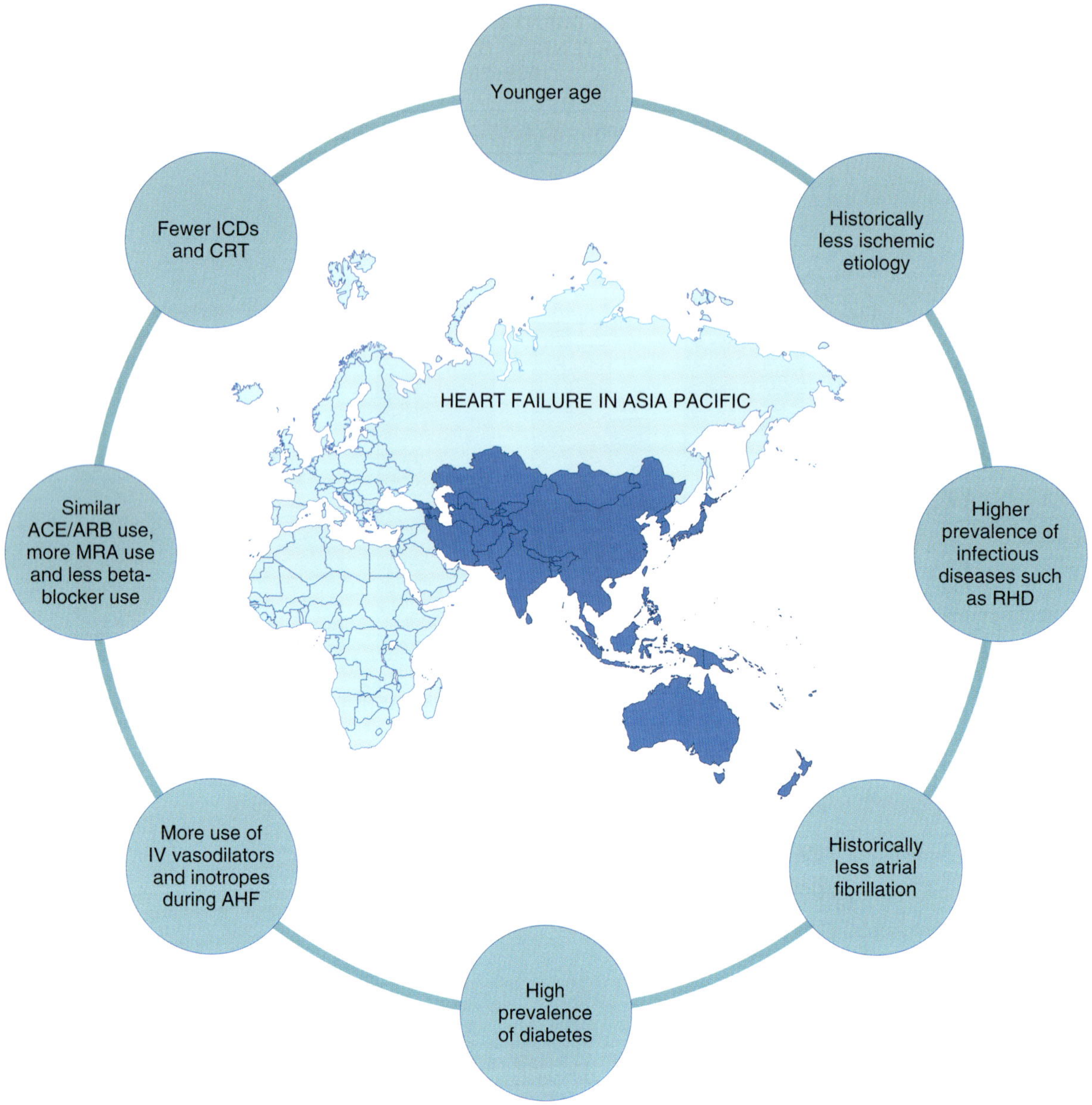

FIGURE 93.3 Heart failure phenotype in the Asian diaspora. (Adapted from Mentz RJ, Roessig L, Greenberg BH, et al. Heart failure clinical trials in East and Southeast Asia: understanding the importance and defining the next steps. *JACC Heart Fail*. 2016;4[6]:419–427.)

140 mm Hg in 9361 nondiabetic/stroke-free individuals whose SBP was 130 to 180 mm Hg and who had an increased cardiovascular disease risk (approximately 2%/year). The overall results showed that in the intensive therapy arm a 25% lower rate of combined outcomes for myocardial infarction (MI), acute coronary syndrome without MI, stroke, acute decompensated heart failure, or cardiovascular disease death, and a 27% reduced rate of all-cause mortality.[15] Stratified analyses revealed similar results in Blacks and non-Blacks, with a CI that included 1.0 among Blacks, and Blacks required an average of approximately 0.3 more antihypertensive medications.[31] Generalizability of the SPRINT population to the U.S. adult population 50 years old or older using NHANES data showed that 4% to 5% of Hispanics and Blacks compared with 9% of whites meet eligibility criteria for the study.[32] Nonetheless, only approximately 8.5% of Blacks and 14.2% of Hispanics with treated hypertension met the blood pressure targets identified in the SPRINT study, a finding that suggests there is substantial room for a hypertension-related cardiovascular disease risk reduction in these groups.

Pharmacotherapy informed by race or ethnicity for Black patients favors thiazide-type diuretics and calcium channel blocker drugs as first-line therapy in a majority of Blacks without contraindications (Table 93.1). A recent analysis of the NHANES suggests that Blacks were more likely to receive combination antihypertensive therapy (including diuretics and calcium channel blockers) compared with whites and Hispanics, and had the highest average number of antihypertensive medications (1.91, 95% CI, 1.84 to 1.97).[6] Despite this, only 31% of Blacks had their blood pressure controlled to recommended targets, as compared with 43% of whites. Hispanics were also less likely to have their blood pressure at recommended targets compared with whites but were less likely to be on antihypertensive therapy. Ongoing barriers to successful hypertension management in Black patients include lack of ambulatory self-monitoring of blood pressure, menthol cigarette smoking, lack of regular health care visits, and underinsurance.[33,34]

SPRINT included a substantial sample of race-ethnic minorities, and enrolled 984 (11%) Hispanics in the U.S. mainland and Puerto Rico.[35] Hispanics recruited into SPRINT were more likely to be uninsured and were on lower numbers of antihypertensive medications at baseline than NH subjects. Approximately 50% of Hispanic subjects in SPRINT had their blood pressure controlled to less than 140/90 mm Hg at baseline, similar to the NH subjects; better blood pressure control was more likely among those with a history of clinical cardiovascular disease. Many argue that because diabetes disproportionately affects the Hispanic population, use of a therapy targeted at the renin-angiotensin-aldosterone system may be more appropriate in Hispanics/LatinXs.[36]

TABLE 93.1 **Hypertension Guidelines and Recommendations: Initial Drug Selection**

GUIDELINE	EVIDENCE REVIEW METHODOLOGY	GENERAL ADULT POPULATION	GENERAL AFRICAN AMERICAN ADULT POPULATION	DIABETES MELLITUS	CHRONIC KIDNEY DISEASE
2017 Guideline for the Prevention, Detection, Evaluation, and Management of High Blood Pressure in Adults	Systematic review	ACE-I, ARB, CCB, thiazide	Thiazide, CCB	ACE-I, ARB, CCB, thiazide	ACE-I, ARB
International Society of Hypertension (2020)	Systematic review	ACE-I, ARB, CCB	ACE-I, ARB, CCB Thiazide-like diuretic	ACE-I, ARB, CCB, diuretics	ACE-I, ARB, CCB, diuretics
National Institute for Health and Care Excellence (2019)	Systematic review	≥55: CCB, ACE-I, ARB thiazide <55: ACE-I, ARB, CCB, thiazide	CCB, ACE-I, ARB, thiazide	ACE-I, ARB, CCB, thiazide	ACE-I, ARB
European Society of Hypertension and European Society of Cardiology (2018)	Consensus (graded)	ACE-I, ARB, CCB, diuretic, (consider BB if resistant)	Thiazide, CCB	ACE-I, ARB, CCB, diuretics	ACE-I, ARB, CCB, diuretics
Hypertension Canada Guidelines for Diagnosis, Risk Assessment, Prevention, and Treatment of Hypertension in Adults and Children (2018)	Consensus	ACE-I, ARB, CCB, thiazide	ACE-I are not recommended as first line	ACE-I, ARB, CCB, diuretic	ACE-I, ARB, diuretic
International Society on Hypertension in Blacks (2010)	Consensus	NA	Diuretic or CCB, RAS inhibitor plus CCB preferred over RAS inhibitor plus thiazide unless edema or high volume	ACE-I, ARB	ACE-I, ARB

ACE-I, Angiotensin-converting enzyme inhibitor; *ARB,* angiotensin-receptor blocker; *BB,* beta blocker; *CCB,* calcium channel blocker; *RAS,* renin-angiotensin system.
Adapted from Still CH, Ferdinand KC, Ogedegbe G, Wright JT Jr. Recognition and management of hypertension in older persons: focus on African Americans. *J Am Geriatr Soc.* 2015;63(10):2130–2138.

The general features of hypertension across the heterogeneous Asian diaspora appear similar. High salt intake, increased salt sensitivity, and more sustained 24-hour blood pressure elevations likely contribute to elevated risks of stroke compared with CHD among Asians.[37] The Japanese Society of Hypertension recommends the use of calcium channel blockers, angiotensin-converting enzyme inhibitors, and diuretics as first-line therapy for patients without other compelling indications.[13] Diuretics are recommended for salt-sensitive elderly Japanese patients. Like Blacks, South Asian patients develop hypertension at an earlier age and have accelerated end-organ damage compared with whites. Because morbidity and mortality data in South Asians are lacking, management principles resemble those of the general population, including early screening and use of combination therapy.[38]

Coronary Heart Disease

Almost 1 million percutaneous coronary interventions (PCIs) are performed annually in the United States for CHD. Blacks and Hispanics have longer wait times and are less likely to undergo PCI than whites, regardless of their insurance status.[39] Data from a large national improvement quality registry, ACTION Registry-GWTG of ST-segment elevation myocardial infarction (STEMI) and non-ST segment elevation myocardial infarction (NSTEMI) patients, showed that rates of catheterization were lower for NSTEMI and similar for STEMI in Blacks compared with whites.[40] Black patients were also less likely to have coronary artery bypass grafting (CABG). In general, Blacks and Hispanics have poorer revascularization outcomes, related to multidimensional influences, including individual, provider, hospital, and societal factors. For example, poorer CABG outcomes among Blacks and Hispanics relate in part to hospital quality and socioeconomic factors because poor and racial or ethnic minority patients receive care at lower-performing hospitals, according to standardized quality measures.[41,42] After enactment of the Massachusetts health care reform act in 2006, racial and ethnic disparities in those who received cardiovascular interventional care persisted.[43] However, counties in expansion states that participated in Medicaid expansion under the Affordable Care Act had fewer deaths per year from cardiovascular causes after Medicaid expansion compared with counties in nonexpansion states.[44]

Use of secondary prevention medications also varies by race and ethnicity. In the TReatment with ADP receptor iNhibitorS: Longitudinal Assessment of Treatment Patterns and Events after Acute Coronary Syndrome (TRANSLATE-ACS) study, race/ethnicity was not an independent predictor of medication nonadherence at 6 weeks post-MI. Financial hardship and depression associated with a higher risk of medication nonadherence, factors that may be more common in race/ethnic minorities. At 1 year post-MI, Black and Hispanic women seem to adhere least to medication regimens, suggesting that there is substantial room for improvement in post-MI care and understanding of treatment barriers in these patients.[45,46] Medication discontinuation is associated with side effects and physician discontinuation advice; higher rates of adherence are related to having private insurance, having assistance with paying for prescriptions, and having an outpatient follow-up appointment scheduled before hospital discharge.

In the context of dual antiplatelet therapy use after drug-eluting stent placement for acute coronary syndrome, there is limited specific data about racial and ethnic groups showing the effectiveness of the drugs and the adverse events that may occur, such as major bleeding. For example, the optimal duration of dual antiplatelet therapy after PCI may differ in East Asians compared with other groups, as there is some concern for higher bleeding risk in East Asians.[47] In addition, the efficacy of clopidogrel as an antiplatelet agent in Asians is of concern.[48]

Heart Failure

Blacks have a higher prevalence of heart failure, with an earlier onset and presentation than other racial and ethnic groups. Compared with whites, Blacks have almost a threefold increased risk for developing dilated cardiomyopathy, which is not fully explained by confounding variables such as hypertension or socioeconomic factors.[49] Emerging work suggests that there are complex relationships between heart failure with preserved ejection fraction (HFpEF) and race and ethnicity. Several key risk factors for HFpEF, including obesity, diabetes, and hypertension, are more common in Blacks. However, recent data suggest that amyloid deposition may be present in a substantial proportion of patients with clinical HFpEF, particularly with advanced age (see also Chapter 53).[50] The hereditary form of transthyretin (TTR)-related cardiac amyloidosis disproportionately affects Blacks, because the valine-to-isoleucine substitution at position 122 (V122I) mutation is carried by 3% to 5% of Black Americans.[51,52] Although the presence of the V122I variant associates strongly with the risk of heart failure, few Black patients are recognized as having a TTR-related cardiomyopathy or undergo genetic testing for TTR variants in routine clinical practice.[52,53]

Impaired vascular function caused by reduced endothelial nitric oxide synthesis and resultant endothelial dysfunction appears to contribute to the heart failure pathophysiology in Blacks.[54] The landmark African-American Heart Failure Trial (A-HeFT) study in 1052 Black patients with New York Heart Association Class III or IV heart failure showed a 43% reduction in deaths with fixed-dose isosorbide dinitrate and hydralazine treatment compared with placebo against a background of standard heart failure therapy.[55] In a subsequent Genetic Risk Assessment of Heart Failure (GRAHF) substudy of A-HeFT ($n = 350$ patients), a common GNB3 polymorphism, C825T associated with enhanced alpha$_2$-adrenergic receptor signaling, was associated with greater therapeutic effect of isosorbide dinitrate and hydralazine.[56]

Data regarding the prevalence of heart failure and effectiveness of therapeutic options in other race/ethnic groups are lacking despite their high prevalence of risk factors and structural heart disease. Among persons of Hispanic/LatinX background in the Echocardiographic Study of LatinXs (ECHO-SOL), left ventricular systolic and diastolic dysfunction were 3.6% and 50.3%, respectively, with more than 90% of the cardiac dysfunction categorized as subclinical or unrecognized.[57] Central Americans and Cuban Americans had a greater prevalence of diastolic dysfunction than Mexican Americans. Information about heart failure in Asians is sparse. Figure 93.3 illustrates the potential features of heart failure in Asia. In the United States, data from the GWTG-HF registry showed that Asians with heart failure were more likely to be younger males; to have hypertension, diabetes, and renal disease; and to be uninsured compared with whites.[58] Current Heart Failure Society of America/American Heart Association/American College of Cardiology (AHA/ACC) guidelines do not propose specific therapy for heart failure based on Hispanic ethnicity or Asian race.

Disparities in clinical heart failure outcomes exist based on race/ethnicity. Blacks have the highest risk of heart failure–related death.[59] The rate of heart failure hospitalization for Blacks is nearly 2.5-fold higher than the rate for whites, with costs that are significantly higher in the first year after an index hospitalization.[60,61] An analysis of the National Inpatient Sample showed the rate of heart failure hospitalization was 229% higher for Black males (P-for-trend = 0.141) and 240% higher for Black females (P-for-trend = 0.725) with reference to whites in 2013, with no significant change from 2002 to 2013.[60] Hispanic males had a 32% higher rate of heart failure hospitalization in 2002, and the difference narrowed to 4% (P-for-trend = 0.047) greater in 2013 relative to whites. For Hispanic females the rate was 55% greater in 2002 and narrowed to 8% greater (P-for-trend = 0.004) in 2013 relative to whites. Asian/PI males had a 27% lower rate in 2002 that improved to 43% (P-for-trend = 0.040) lower in 2013 relative to whites. For Asian/PI females the hospitalization rate was 24% lower in 2002 and improved to 43% (P-for-trend = 0.021) lower in 2013 relative to whites.

POTENTIAL FOR EMERGING SCIENTIFIC RESEARCH TO ADDRESS GROUP DISPARITIES IN CARDIOVASCULAR DISEASE

Despite what we have learned about the origin of disparities over the past few decades, disparities appear to be growing rather than shrinking. For areas with available clinical trial data for therapies that effectively treat cardiovascular disease in different racial and ethnic groups, comprehensive delivery and adherence present important challenges. Diversification of the workforce and increasing community outreach may also help, as prior research has shown that increasing the number of doctors who are race/ethnic minorities can improve adherence and the quality of communication experienced by patients.[62–64] Administering care in nontraditional settings in the community can also improve clinical outcomes. In a recent randomized controlled trial of Black male barbershop clients with uncontrolled hypertension, Black men randomized to a pharmacist-led intervention (in which barbers encouraged meetings in barbershops with specialty-trained pharmacists who prescribed drug therapy) achieved larger reductions in blood pressure than Black men randomized to an active control approach where barbers encouraged lifestyle modification and doctor appointments.[64] Moreover, efforts to realize the potential of "precision" and "personalized" medicine should also target populations that experience the greatest burden of health disparities, lest unmet needs become more pronounced. In addition, longitudinal information is needed on recent immigrant populations, including those from Asia, where the cardiovascular risk varies markedly by country of origin, and those from Africa, where there is a burgeoning epidemic of cardiovascular disease associated with urbanization (see also Chapter 2. Specific issues in the near future include scaling, dissemination, and implementation of known effective strategies for prevention and treatment of cardiovascular disease in high-risk heterogeneous populations. Finally, the COVID-19 pandemic has unearthed the effect of CVD disparities contributing to the overwhelming impact of this pandemic in racial/ethnic minority and socioeconomically disadvantaged groups. The prevalence of certain conditions such as cardiomyopathy and CVD-related mortality will likely increase over time due to the impact of COVID-19 and thus research and interventions targeting the most affected populations is required.

ACKNOWLEDGMENTS

The authors thank Mercedes Carnethon, coauthor of this chapter from the previous edition of *Heart Disease*, for her contributions.

REFERENCES

Epidemiology

1. National Center for Health Statistics. *Summary Health Statistics Tables for US Adults.* National Health Interview Survey; 2018. http://ftp.cdc.gov/pub/Health_Statistics/NCHS/NHIS/SHS/2018_SHS_Table_A-1.pdf.
2. Miniño A, Arias E, Kochanek K, et al. Final Data for 2000. National Vital Statistics Reports. Vol 50 No 15. Hyattsville, Maryland: National Center for Health Statistics; 2002. https://www.cdc.gov/Nchs/data/nvsr/nvsr50/nvsr50_15.pdf.
3. National Center for Health Statistics Health, United States. *2017: With Special Feature on Mortality.* Hyattsville, MD: National Center for Health Statistics; 2018. https://www.cdc.gov/nchs/data/hus/hus17.pdf.
4. Colantonio LD, Gamboa CM, Richman JS, et al. Black-white differences in incident fatal, nonfatal, and total coronary heart disease. *Circulation*. 2017;136:152–166.
5. Prevalence of self-reported hypertension and antihypertensive medication use among adults—United States, 2017. *MMWR Morb Mortal Wkly Rep*. 2020;69:393–398. https://doi.org/10.15585/mmwr.mm6914a1. (Accessed May 1, 2020, 2020).

Hypertension

6. Gu A, Yue Y, Desai Raj P, Argulian E. Racial and ethnic differences in antihypertensive medication use and blood pressure control among US adults with hypertension. *Circ Cardiovasc Qual Outcomes*. 2017;10:e003166.
7. Sorlie PD, Allison MA, Avilés-Santa ML, et al. Prevalence of hypertension, awareness, treatment, and control in the hispanic community health study/study of LatinXs. *Am J Hypertens*. 2014;27:793–800.
8. Zhao B, Jose PO, Pu J, et al. Racial/ethnic differences in hypertension prevalence, treatment, and control for outpatients in Northern California 2010–2012. *Am J Hypertens*. 2014;28:631–639.
9. Ursua R, Aguilar D, Wyatt L, et al. Awareness, treatment and control of hypertension among Filipino immigrants. *J Gen Intern Med*. 2014;29:455–462.

Diabetes

10. Cheng YJ, Kanaya AM, Araneta MRG, et al. Prevalence of diabetes by race and ethnicity in the United States, 2011–2016. *J Am Med Assoc*. 2019;322:2389–2398.
11. Ogden CL, Carroll MD, Kit BK, Flegal KM. Prevalence of childhood and adult obesity in the United States, 2011-2012. *J Am Med Assoc*. 2014;311:806–814.
12. Dabelea D, Mayer-Davis EJ, Saydah S, et al. Prevalence of type 1 and type 2 diabetes among children and adolescents from 2001 to 2009. *J Am Med Assoc*. 2014;311:1778–1786.
13. Schneiderman N, Llabre M, Cowie CC, et al. Prevalence of diabetes among Hispanics/LatinXs from diverse backgrounds: the Hispanic community health study/study of LatinXs (HCHS/SOL). *Diabetes Care*. 2014;37:2233–2239.

Vulnerable Populations

14. Piccolo RS, Subramanian SV, Pearce N, et al. Relative contributions of socioeconomic, local environmental, psychosocial, lifestyle/behavioral, biophysiological, and ancestral factors to racial/ethnic disparities in type 2 diabetes. *Diabetes Care*. 2016;39:1208–1217.
15. Hsu WC, Araneta MRG, Kanaya AM, et al. BMI cut points to identify at-risk Asian Americans for type 2 diabetes screening. *Diabetes Care*. 2015;38:150–158.
16. Gordon NP, Lin TY, Rau J, Lo JC. Aggregation of Asian-American subgroups masks meaningful differences in health and health risks among Asian ethnicities: an electronic health record based cohort study. *BMC Publ Health*. 2019;19:1551.
17. National Institute of Mental Health. Prevalence of Any Mental Illness. https://www.nimh.nih.gov/health/statistics/mental-illness.shtml#part_154785.
18. The 2019 Annual Homeless Assessment Report (AHAR) to Congress. https://files.hudexchange.info/resources/documents/2019-AHAR-Part-1.pdf.
19. Mental Health Medications. https://www.nimh.nih.gov/health/topics/mental-health-medications/index.shtml.
20. Centers for Disease Control and Prevention. *HIV Surveillance Report*; 2017:29. Published November 2018. http://www.cdc.gov/hiv/library/reports/hiv-surveillance.html.
21. Koethe JR, Jenkins CA, Lau B, et al. Rising obesity prevalence and weight gain among adults starting antiretroviral therapy in the United States and Canada. *AIDS Res Hum Retroviruses*. 2016;32:50–58.

22. Freiberg MS, Chang C-CH, Skanderson M, et al. Association between HIV infection and the risk of heart failure with reduced ejection fraction and preserved ejection fraction in the antiretroviral therapy era: results from the veterans aging cohort study. *JAMA Cardiol*. 2017;2:536–546.
23. Womack JA, Chang CCH, So-Armah KA, et al. HIV infection and cardiovascular disease in women. *J Am Heart Assoc*. 2014;3:e001035.
24. Slockers MT, Nusselder WJ, Rietjens J, van Beeck EF. Unnatural death: a major but largely preventable cause-of-death among homeless people? *Eur J Public Health*. 2018;28:248–252.
25. Baggett TP, Liauw SS, Hwang SW. Cardiovascular disease and homelessness. *J Am Coll Cardiol*. 2018;71:2585.
26. Henry M, Watt R, Rosenthal L, et al. *The 2016 Annual Homeless Assessment Report (AHAR) to Congress: Part 1: Point-in-Time Estimates of Homelessness*. Washington DC: US Department of Housing and Urban Development; 2016.
27. LGBTQ Homelessness. Published by the National Coalition for the Homeless; 2017. https://nationalhomeless.org/wp-content/uploads/2017/06/LGBTQ-Homelessness.pdf.

Management Considerations

28. Arnett DK, Blumenthal RS, Albert MA, et al. 2019 ACC/AHA guideline on the primary prevention of cardiovascular disease: a report of the American College of Cardiology/American heart association task force on clinical practice guidelines. *Circulation*. 2019;140:e596–e646.
29. Pool LR, Ning H, Lloyd–Jones DM, Allen NB. Trends in racial/ethnic disparities in cardiovascular health among US adults from 1999–2012. *J Am Heart Assoc*. 2017;6:e006027.
30. Morris AA, Ko YA, Hutcheson SH, Quyyumi A. Race/ethnic and sex differences in the association of atherosclerotic cardiovascular disease risk and healthy lifestyle behaviors. *J Am Heart Assoc*. 2018;7:e008250.
31. Still CH, Rodriguez CJ, Wright Jr JT, et al. Clinical outcomes by race and ethnicity in the Systolic Blood Pressure Intervention Trial (SPRINT): a randomized clinical trial. *Am J Hypertens*. 2017;31:97–107.
32. Bress AP, Tanner RM, Hess R, et al. Generalizability of SPRINT results to the U.S. Adult population. *J Am Coll Cardiol*. 2016;67:463–472.
33. Still CH, Ferdinand KC, Ogedegbe G, Wright Jr JT. Recognition and management of hypertension in older persons: focus on African Americans. *J Am Geriatr Soc*. 2015;63:2130–2138.
34. Egan BM, Bland VJ, Brown AL, et al. Hypertension in African Americans aged 60 to 79 Years: statement from the international society of hypertension in blacks. *J Clin Hypertens*. 2015;17:252–259.
35. Rodriguez CJ, Still CH, Garcia KR, et al. Baseline blood pressure control in Hispanics: characteristics of Hispanics in the systolic blood pressure intervention trial. *J Clin Hypertens (Greenwich)*. 2017;19:116–125.
36. Campbell PT, Krim SR, Lavie CJ, Ventura HO. Clinical characteristics, treatment patterns and outcomes of Hispanic hypertensive patients. *Prog Cardiovasc Dis*. 2014;57:244–252.
37. Kario K. Key points of the Japanese society of hypertension guidelines for the management of hypertension in 2014. *Pulse (Basel)*. 2015;3:35–47.
38. Brewster LM, van Montfrans GA, Oehlers GP, Seedat YK. Systematic review: antihypertensive drug therapy in patients of African and South Asian ethnicity. *Intern Emerg Med*. 2016;11:355–374.
39. Graham G, Xiao Y-YK, Rappoport D, Siddiqi S. Population-level differences in revascularization treatment and outcomes among various United States subpopulations. *World J Cardiol*. 2016;8:24–40.
40. Anstey DE, Li S, Thomas L, et al. Race and Sex differences in management and outcomes of patients after ST-Elevation and non-ST-Elevation myocardial infarct: results from the NCDR. *Clin Cardiol*. 2016;39:585–595.
41. Rangrass G, Ghaferi AA, Dimick JB. Explaining racial disparities in outcomes after cardiac surgery: the role of hospital quality. *JAMA Surgery*. 2014;149:223–227.
42. Khera R, Vaughan-Sarrazin M, Rosenthal GE, Girotra S. Racial disparities in outcomes after cardiac surgery: the role of hospital quality. *Curr Cardiol Rep*. 2015;17:29.
43. Albert MA, Ayanian JZ, Silbaugh TS, et al. Early results of Massachusetts healthcare reform on racial, ethnic, and socioeconomic disparities in cardiovascular care. *Circulation*. 2014;129:2528–2538.
44. Khatana SAM, Bhatla A, Nathan AS, et al. Association of Medicaid expansion with cardiovascular mortality. *JAMA Cardiol*. 2019;4:671–679.
45. Lauffenburger JC, Robinson JG, Oramasionwu C, Fang G. Racial/Ethnic and gender gaps in the use of and adherence to evidence-based preventive therapies among elderly Medicare Part D beneficiaries after acute myocardial infarction. *Circulation*. 2014;129:754–763.
46. Albert MA. Not there yet. Medicare Part D and elimination of cardiovascular medication usage sociodemographic disparities after myocardial infarction. *Circulation*. 2014;129:723–724.
47. Ki Y-J, Kang J, Park J, et al. Efficacy and safety of long-term and short-term dual antiplatelet therapy: a meta-analysis of comparison between Asians and non-Asians. *J Clin Med*. 2020;9:652.
48. Brown SA, Pereira N. Pharmacogenomic impact of CYP2C19 variation on clopidogrel therapy in precision cardiovascular medicine. *J Pers Med*. 2018;8(1):8.
49. Bozkurt B, Colvin M, Cook J, et al. Current diagnostic and treatment strategies for specific dilated cardiomyopathies: a scientific statement from the American Heart Association. *Circulation*. 2016;134:e579–e646.
50. Mohammed SF, Mirzoyev SA, Edwards WD, et al. Left ventricular amyloid deposition in patients with heart failure and preserved ejection fraction. *JACC Heart Fail*. 2014;2:113–122.
51. Quarta CC, Buxbaum JN, Shah AM, et al. The amyloidogenic V122I transthyretin variant in elderly Black Americans. *N Eng J Med*. 2014;372:21–29.
52. Shah KB, Mankad AK, Castano A, et al. Transthyretin cardiac amyloidosis in Black Americans. *Circ Heart Fail*. 2016;9(6):e002558.
53. Damrauer SM, Chaudhary K, Cho JH, et al. Association of the V122I hereditary transthyretin amyloidosis genetic variant with heart failure among individuals of African or Hispanic/LatinX ancestry. *J Am Med Assoc*. 2019;322:2191–2202.
54. Ozkor MA, Rahman AM, Murrow JR, et al. Differences in vascular nitric oxide and endothelium-derived hyperpolarizing factor bioavailability in blacks and whites. *Arterioscler Thromb Vasc Biol*. 2014;34:1320–1327.
55. Taylor AL, Ziesche S, Yancy C, et al. Combination of isosorbide dinitrate and hydralazine in blacks with heart failure. *N Eng J Med*. 2004;351:2049–2057.
56. McNamara DM, Taylor AL, Tam SW, et al. G-protein beta-3 subunit genotype predicts enhanced benefit of fixed-dose isosorbide dinitrate and hydralazine: results of A-HeFT. *JACC Heart Fail*. 2014;2:551–557.
57. Mehta H, Armstrong A, Swett K, et al. Burden of systolic and diastolic left ventricular dysfunction among Hispanics in the United States: insights from the echocardiographic study of LatinXs. *Circ Heart Fail*. 2016;9:e002733-e.
58. Qian F, Fonarow GC, Krim SR, et al. Characteristics, quality of care, and in-hospital outcomes of Asian-American heart failure patients: findings from the American Heart Association get with the guidelines-heart failure program. *Int J Cardiol*. 2015;189:141–147.
59. Glynn P, Lloyd-Jones DM, Feinstein MJ, et al. Disparities in cardiovascular mortality related to heart failure in the United States. *J Am Coll Cardiol*. 2019;73:2354–2355.
60. Ziaeian B, Kominski GF, Ong MK, et al. National differences in trends for heart failure hospitalizations by Sex and race/ethnicity. *Circ Cardiovasc Qual Outcomes*. 2017;10:e003552.
61. Ziaeian B, Heidenreich PA, Xu H, et al. Medicare expenditures by race/ethnicity after hospitalization for heart failure with preserved ejection fraction. *JACC Heart Fail*. 2018;6:388.
62. Alsan M, Garrick O, Graziani G. Does diversity matter for health? Experimental evidence from Oakland. *Am Econ Rev*. 2019;109:4071–4111.
63. Shen MJ, Peterson EB, Costas-Muñiz R, et al. The effects of race and racial concordance on patient-physician communication: a systematic review of the literature. *J Racial Ethn Health Disparities*. 2018;5:117–140.
64. Victor RG, Lynch K, Li N, et al. A Cluster-randomized trial of blood-pressure reduction in Black barbershops. *N Eng J Med*. 2018;378:1291–1301.

第十一部分　心血管疾病和其他器官疾病

王文尧　唐熠达　导读

非心血管系统疾病对心血管疾病的影响日益受到重视。在本书的该部分章节中，就病毒性疾病、凝血系统疾病、内分泌功能异常、风湿性疾病、心脏局部肿瘤、精神心理疾病、神经肌肉疾病、肾脏疾病以及自主神经功能紊乱对心血管系统的影响进行了详细阐述。这些内容对于心血管疾病患者的综合管理而言是至关重要的。在心血管疾病诊疗工作中，除了多学科合作以处理这些多系统疾病外，心血管医生如果作为患者的首诊者，应当对于其他系统疾病对心血管系统的影响有比较充分认识，方能在治疗过程中避免漏诊和延误治疗。该部分内容值得心脏专科医师认真学习，同时对于其他专科医师也是很好的参考资料。

在病毒性疾病章节中，重点介绍了常见的流行性感冒病毒与近些年爆发的COVID-19对心血管疾病的影响，其中有关COVID-19的循证内容更新至2021年9月15日。作为心脏病学领域的经典书籍，其与时俱进的编写理念令人眼前一亮。

凝血系统异常、内分泌功能异常以及肾脏疾病对心血管疾病的影响相对明确，在相关章节中，作者对致病机制及治疗选择进行了详细的阐述。凝血系统异常章节还简要概述了处于发展后期的新型抗血栓药物，对未来的药物选择提供借鉴。内分泌功能异常章节则讨论了与内分泌功能障碍相关的心血管发病率和死亡率的流行病学研究和荟萃分析，为读者呈现更为宏观的视角，以充分认识心血管代谢这一交叉领域。在肾脏疾病章节中，介绍了不同肾功能状态下心血管疾病的风险，同时强调了心血管疾病用药及介入治疗过程中的肾脏损伤风险和防范措施。

风湿性疾病对心血管系统的影响是广泛而复杂的。以炎症为基础，风湿性疾病可以参与到血管疾病、瓣膜疾病、心包疾病以及心肌损伤的病理生理过程中。本书系统性地介绍了多种风湿性疾病累及心血管的表现及治疗推荐。重点强调了严格评估预防策略，及早识别、诊断和治疗心血管并发症风险最高的风湿性疾病患者。

心脏及其周围的局部肿瘤相对少见，临床医生往往对其认识不足。本书介绍了提示心脏肿瘤的初始症状和体征、常见的心脏肿瘤组织学特点和预后，对指导临床早期发现心脏肿瘤和及时做出应对措施提供了很好的指导。

该部分内容尚包括精神和社会心理方面、神经肌肉疾病、自主神经功能紊乱对心血管系统的影响。概述了压力和精神疾病的心血管后果，并讨论了评估和管理心脏病患者精神病共病的方法。回顾了与重要心血管表现或后遗症相关的神经系统疾病。此外，还介绍了原发性和继发性心血管自主神经功能障碍。

在临床分科日益精细的今天，充分评估患者的综合病情是改善患者生活质量和治疗效果的重要一环。本书的该部分内容介绍了常见的影响心血管疾病的其他系统功能异常，提供了详实的机制阐述与治疗推荐。

PART XI CARDIOVASCULAR DISEASE AND DISORDERS OF OTHER ORGANS

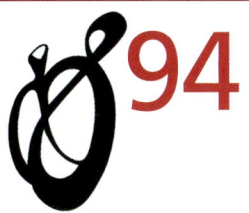

94 Endemic and Pandemic Viral Illnesses and Cardiovascular Disease: Influenza and COVID-19

ORLY VARDENY, MOHAMMAD MADJID, AND SCOTT D. SOLOMON

INTRODUCTION, 1751

INFLUENZA AND CARDIOVASCULAR RISK AND DISEASE, 1751
Epidemiology of Influenza and Cardiovascular Disease, 1752
Influenza Prevention and Therapy, 1754

SARS-CoV-2 AND COVID-19, 1754
Epidemiology of COVID-19 and Risk Factors, 1755
Clinical Cardiovascular Manifestations of COVID-19, 1757
Treatment of COVID-19 and COVID-19-Related Complications, 1762

Other Management Considerations, 1762
Prevention of COVID-19: Vaccines, 1763
Postacute Sequelae SARS-CoV-2 Infection, 1763

REFERENCES, 1763

INTRODUCTION

Over the past decade appreciation has grown that viral diseases can affect the cardiovascular system and contribute to cardiovascular disease (CVD). Influenza accounts for a substantial number of hospitalizations and deaths worldwide, and it has become increasingly evident that patients with CVD may have particular vulnerability to influenza-related complications and that influenza infection itself may contribute directly to CVD progression and events, including myocardial infarction (MI) and heart failure (HF). This association becomes even more evident when a large number of individuals in the population become infected, as has occurred several times in the past century in the setting of pandemics. In addition to influenza, other viruses, including respiratory syncytial virus (RSV), parainfluenza virus, adenovirus, human metapneumovirus, parvovirus, and enterovirus infections, have been implicated in CVD.

In late 2019, a novel coronavirus was found to be the cause of a cluster of cases of severe respiratory illness in Wuhan, China. This virus, SARS-CoV-2, and the disease it caused, COVID-19, quickly spread throughout the globe and was dubbed a global pandemic by the World Health Organization (WHO) on March 11, 2020. In addition to severe respiratory disease, often leading to a requirement for intensive care, mechanical ventilation, or death, this disease often affects the entire cardiovascular system, which may play a central role in the pathogenesis.

This chapter reviews the influence of endemic and pandemic viral infections, including influenza and COVID-19, on CVD. Several other viruses that directly affect the cardiovascular system, including parvovirus and coxsackie virus, are covered in other chapters (see Chapters 52 and 55). Due to the rapidly changing nature of our understanding of the pathophysiology and therapeutic options for COVID-19, this chapter focuses on established pathophysiology and treatment options at the time of writing (September 15, 2021) and will be updated online as more information becomes available.

INFLUENZA AND CARDIOVASCULAR RISK AND DISEASE

Influenza Virology
Influenza viruses are enveloped, negative-sense, single-stranded RNA viruses (~13.5-kb genome) that are characterized based on surface antigens and exist as A and B strains.[1] The hemagglutinin (HA) protein facilitates viral entry into the host cell and binds to the glycoprotein terminal sialic acid and glycolipid receptors. The neuraminidase protein (NA) facilitates viral release and affects viral evolution in concert with the HA protein. These two glycoproteins localize on the surface of the virus particle and are the main targets for protective antibodies generated from influenza virus infection or vaccination.

The segmental configuration of the influenza virus genome allows for reassortment, or interchange, of genetic RNA segments when two viruses of the same type infect the same cell. Thus influenza viruses undergo rapid antigenic *drifts* (defined as genetic variations in antigen structures stemming from point mutations in the HA and NA genes over time) and *shifts* (sudden genetic reassortment between two closely related influenza viral strains), which allow them to evade the host immune system. Although influenza B viruses primarily infect humans, the influenza A viruses (IAVs) are endemic in several species, including humans, birds, and pigs. Animal reservoirs offer a source of antigenically diverse HA and NA genes that can exchange between viral strains, creating virus variation, and occasionally forming novel influenza viruses that contain HA or NA segments from animals.[2] Reassortment of the influenza A pdm09 virus in which the HA H2 and polymerase PB1 genes of the avian H2N2 virus were replaced by two new avian H3 and PB1 genes led to a pandemic in 2009.[3] However, cases of swine- and avian-based zoonotic human transmission of influenza are rare, and are mainly confined to the avian H5N1 and H7N9 and the H3N2 variant viruses.

Pandemic influenza occurs every 20 to 50 years and stems from a viral strain that differs antigenically from previous strains. Because the human immune system is naive to the new virus, the overall lack of immunity in the population correlates with disease severity and excess mortality. Since 1918, the IAVs have caused four pandemics. The first and most severe pandemic in recent history, known as "Spanish influenza," occurred in 1918, was caused by an H1N1 IAV strain, and led to approximately 500 million infections and 50 to 100 million deaths worldwide. In 1957, the "Asian influenza" caused by an H2N2 IAV strain resulted in ~1.1 million deaths worldwide. In 1968, the "Hong Kong flu" caused by an A/H3N2 strain resulted in ~1 million deaths worldwide. The fourth pandemic in 2009, caused by the influenza A (H1N1) pdm09 virus, led to 151,700 to 575,400 deaths worldwide from 2009 to 2010. Since that time, this novel IAV has continued to spread as a seasonal influenza virus. Influenza B co-circulates with influenza A each year. Typically, outbreaks of influenza A and B in the northern and southern hemispheres can lead to as many as 5 million cases of severe influenza and up to 500,000 deaths worldwide in a single season.

The major societal burden from influenza is caused by influenza A and B through seasonal outbreaks, mostly during winter months when transmission conditions are more favorable due to low temperatures and humidity. Most infections occur in the pediatric population, although the most severe cases occur in younger children or in older adults. Children appear to be the main transmitters of influenza virus, evidenced by reduced incidence of severe influenza among older adults when children are vaccinated.[4]

Symptoms from influenza virus infection can vary from a mild upper respiratory disease limited to fever, sore throat, runny nose, cough, headache, muscle aches, and fatigue, to severe, in some cases leading to lethal influenza-induced pneumonia or due to a secondary bacterial infection. Influenza virus infection can also precipitate a wide range of nonrespiratory complications, including acute cardiovascular events.

Epidemiology of Influenza and Cardiovascular Disease

Several risk factors predispose patients to severe or lethal influenza infection. Due to lack of previous exposures, young children are more likely to develop worse symptoms and a higher fever and tend to shed larger amounts of virus for longer after being infected. Older adults are also at risk for more severe symptoms and infection-related complications, including hospitalizations, due to immunosenescence (reduced immune function with aging) and chronic conditions.[5] In addition to extremes of age, other groups at risk for severe disease, hospitalization, or death include those with concomitant pulmonary or cardiac conditions, neuromuscular disease, diabetes mellitus, and conditions that render patients immunocompromised. Obesity is associated with enhanced viral replication, and those with morbid obesity have increased risk for secondary bacterial infections and a reduced immune response to influenza vaccination. Pregnancy is also a risk factor for severe disease, possibly related to altered immune function coupled with increased cardiopulmonary demand; the risk appears to increase more with each trimester.[1]

Influenza and Acute Myocardial Infarction

Numerous observational studies utilizing case-control or case-only designs have reported associations between infection with influenza and other respiratory illnesses and acute MI, including a large self-controlled case series study including 115,112 individuals hospitalized for acute MI or stroke, which noted a fivefold increased risk for MI and a threefold increased risk for stroke within the first 3 days of an outpatient visit for various acute respiratory or urinary infections, including influenza.[6,7] Overall, influenza may account for between 3% and 6% of attributable risk for MI-related deaths. A patient-level study examining the relationship between laboratory-confirmed respiratory diagnosis and hospitalization for MI using insurance databases and public microbiology testing results found a 5-fold increased risk of acute MI within 7 days of influenza A and a 10-fold increased risk with influenza B. A significant time-dependent association was also detected with other respiratory viruses, including RSV, coronavirus, parainfluenza virus, adenovirus, human metapneumovirus, and enterovirus infections, adding to the evidence that various viral pathogens can precipitate atherothrombotic events.[8]

Influenza and Heart Failure

Influenza is also associated with increased risk for HF events. Increased overall hospitalization rates have been observed during influenza seasons compared with non-influenza seasons (adjusted hazard ratio [HR], 1.11; 95% confidence interval [CI], 1.03 to 1.20; P = 0.005).[9] In an analysis relating Centers for Disease Control and Prevention (CDC)-defined influenza-like illness (ILI) in four U.S. communities to rates of hospitalizations for HF or MI between 2010 and 2014, a 5% monthly absolute increase in influenza activity was associated with a 24% adjusted increase in hospitalizations for HF within the same month (incidence rate ratio (IRR), 1.24; 95% CI, 1.11 to 1.38; P < 0.001) (Fig. 94.1).[10] Patients with HF also have increased risk for other adverse outcomes when hospitalized with influenza. In over 8 million HF patients from a national inpatient sample, those with influenza (0.67%) had an increased risk for in-hospital mortality (odds ratio [OR], 1.15; 95% CI, 1.03 to 1.30), acute respiratory failure (OR, 1.95; 95% CI 1.83 to 2.07), and requirement for mechanical ventilation (OR, 1.75; 95% CI, 1.62 to 1.89).[11]

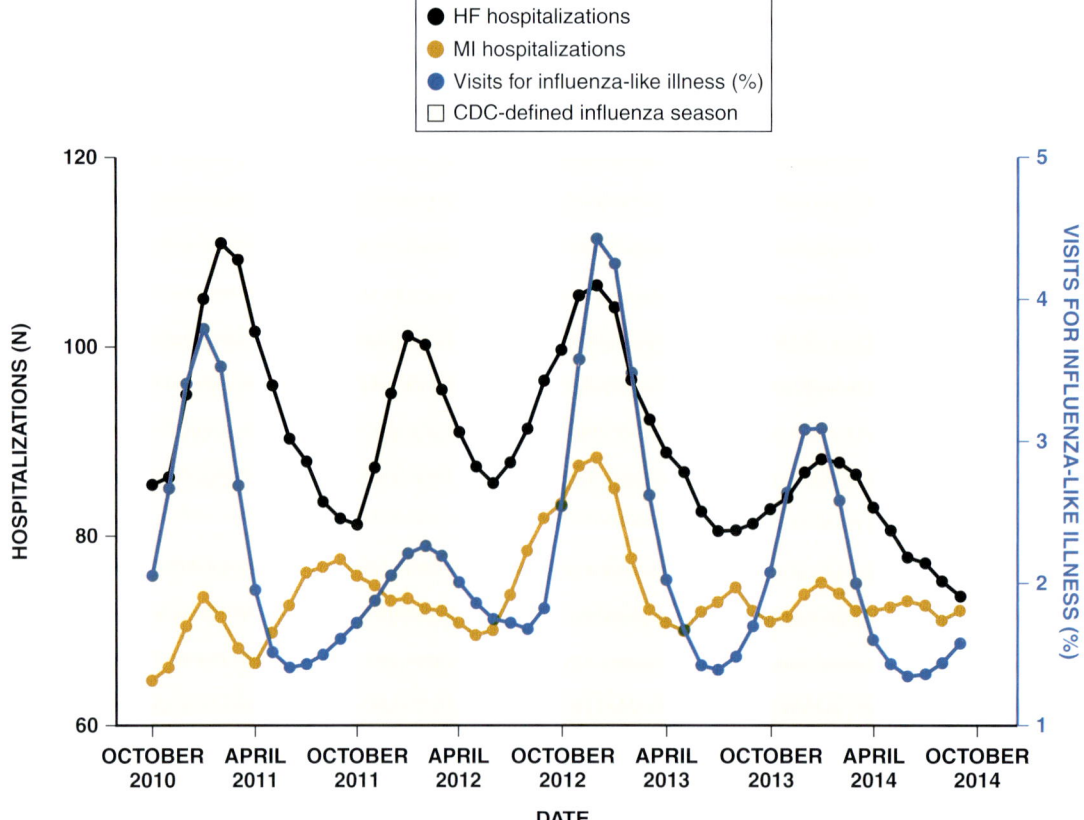

FIGURE 94.1 Association of timing of influenza season with hospitalizations for cardiovascular events. (From Kytömaa S, et al. Association of Influenza-like Illness Activity With Hospitalizations for Heart Failure: The Atherosclerosis Risk in Communities Study. JAMA Cardiol 2019;4(4):363-369.)

Influenza and Arrhythmia Risk

The incidence of cardiac arrest and sudden cardiac death (SCD) show seasonal variation, increasing during the winter in line with peak influenza season, and the likelihood of survival to hospital discharge after cardiac arrest was lowest during the winter.[12,13] A study of 481,516 out-of-hospital cardiac arrests in Japan reported a significant association between cardiac arrests and severe influenza epidemics (relative risk [RR], 1.25; 95% CI, 1.16, 1.34), with a more pronounced effect within 7 days of reported peaks in influenza activity, consistent with previous data on associations of influenza with acute MI. Ventricular tachyarrhythmias detected by implantable cardioverter-defibrillators (ICDs) have exhibited seasonal variation, with positive associations observed during the winter and during increased influenza activity.[14,15]

Because the risk of atrial fibrillation (AF) increases during winter months and colder temperatures,[16] a population case-control study in Taiwan related newly diagnosed AF to influenza infection during the previous year (adjusted OR, 1.18; 95% CI, 1.014 to 1.378; $P = 0.032$). Individuals who received influenza vaccination had a reduced risk for AF compared with unvaccinated people (adjusted OR, 0.881; 95% CI, 0.836 to 0.928; $P < 0.001$).[17]

Influenza and Myocarditis

Sporadic reports have linked myocarditis to influenza infection, varying from asymptomatic to fulminant myocarditis resulting in hemodynamic compromise, HF, or cardiogenic shock, requiring vasopressor or mechanical support. In cases of symptomatic myocarditis, patients typically present within 4 to 7 days of their illness with shortness of breath; pleuritic chest pain; and less frequently with hypotension, syncope, arrhythmia, or fulminant HF. Cases of fulminant myocarditis have been more common during pandemic influenza or during virulent years of seasonal influenza, as was the case during the 2009 H1N1 pandemic and the particularly severe 2017/2018 influenza season. In case series, the majority of influenza-related myocarditis cases involved the A/H1N1 strain, followed by B-type and A/H3N2; HF was the most common complication (84% of cases), and over half of the cases required advanced cardiac support.[18]

Pathophysiology of Influenza and Cardiovascular Disease

Influenza affects the cardiovascular system through multiple mechanisms. Influenza virus has been localized to human coronary endothelial and smooth muscle cells.[19] Infection of mice with influenza A H3N2 virus led to severalfold increased expression of genes for monocyte chemoattractant protein-1 (MCP-1), interleukin-8 (IL-8), tissue factor (TF), plasminogen activator inhibitor 1 (PAI-1), vascular cell adhesion molecule 1 (VCAM-1), intercellular adhesion molecule (ICAM)-1, and E-selectin, whereas endothelial nitric oxide synthase (eNOS) expression decreased in endothelial cells.[19] In *Apo E*-deficient atherosclerotic mice, influenza virus A H3N2 can reside in the atherosclerotic plaques and myocardium, and the virus has been cultured from aorta and myocardium a week after infection in high titers, comparable to pulmonary tissue.[19] Infection also significantly increases plasma levels of proinflammatory cytokines and chemokines and can lead to an exaggerated cellular inflammatory response in atherosclerotic plaque, with a significant increase in plaque macrophage content.[19,20]

Viable virus could be detected in the myocardium of mice infected with influenza A within 12 days of infection, with evidence of oxidative stress-induced mitochondrial damage resulting in a low-energy state.[21] In addition, bacterial superinfection can complicate influenza infection, and likely contribute substantially to the risk in elderly individuals affected by influenza, and provide a rationale for administration of pneumococcal vaccine in this population.[22,23] The ability of influenza infection to directly infect arterial and myocardial tissues and to cause local arterial-level plus systemic proinflammatory effects, prothrombotic effects, and increases in pro-oxidative stress, in conjunction with nonspecific effects induced by demand ischemia, hypoxia, sympathetic stimulation, and myocardial depression, all contribute to an increased risk for multiple cardiovascular adverse outcomes (Fig. 94.2).[24-26]

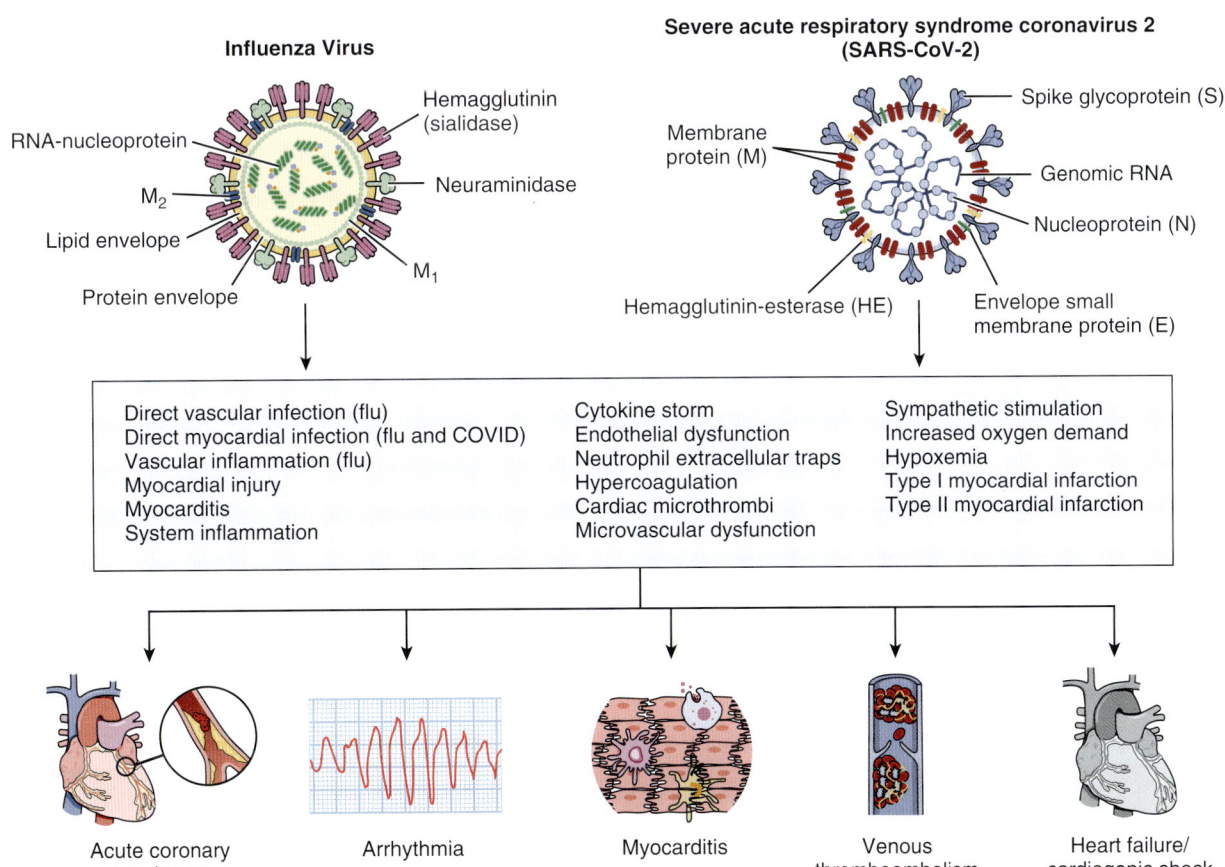

FIGURE 94.2 Mechanisms of acute viral infections on the cardiovascular system.

Influenza Prevention and Therapy

The association between influenza and CVD has stimulated growing interest in the role of influenza vaccination in the prevention of CVD. Several observational and small randomized, clinical trials (RCTs) have suggested that influenza vaccination can protect from adverse cardiovascular outcomes. To prevent influenza illness the CDC recommends annual influenza vaccination for individuals 6 months or older, unless contraindicated. Each year the WHO and the CDC Advisory Committee on Immunization Practices make recommendations for the influenza vaccine composition based on circulating strains in the Southern Hemisphere. Because antigenic mismatch can occur due to antigenic drifts or virus mutations during the period of production of vaccines, vaccine effectiveness (VE) can vary each year, with VE in recent years between 20% and 70%; nevertheless, vaccines confer some protection even during years with a poor antigenic match.

A large meta-analysis of six RCTs (four blinded, two open label) assessed the benefit of influenza vaccination on reducing major adverse cardiovascular events, including cardiovascular death or hospitalization for MI, unstable angina, stroke, HF, or urgent coronary revascularization in 6734 individuals, with numerically fewer deaths in the vaccinated group.[27] During a mean duration of follow-up of 7.9 months, the vaccine recipient group had fewer major adverse cardiovascular events compared with those who received placebo or no vaccination (RR, 0.64; 95% CI, 0.48, 0.86; $P = 0.003$), with an absolute risk difference of 1.74%. The effect was more pronounced in individuals with a recent acute coronary syndrome (ACS) compared with those without recent ACS.

In patients with HF, data on the effects of influenza vaccine on cardiac outcomes rely on observational studies due to the paucity of placebo-controlled trials. In a self-controlled case series from the United Kingdom between 1990 and 2013,[28] vaccinated individuals had a lower risk for hospitalization from cardiovascular (IRR, 0.73; 95% CI, 0.71, 0.76), respiratory infections (IRR 0.83, 95% CI 0.77, 0.90), or any cause (IRR, 0.96; 95% CI, 0.95, 0.98) relative to an adjacent vaccination-free year. Nevertheless, influenza vaccination in patients with HF remains low. In a post hoc analysis of the global PARADIGM-HF trial in over 8000 patients with HF with reduced ejection fraction (HFrEF), only 21% of patients with HF received influenza vaccination in the year of enrollment, with rates varying widely by country from less than 5% to 77%.[29] Vaccination was associated with an adjusted reduced risk for mortality (HR, 0.81; 95% CI, 0.67, 0.97; $P = 0.015$), but not all-cause hospitalizations, cardiovascular death, HF, or cardiopulmonary- or influenza-related hospitalizations. Similar reduction in HF-related outcomes were observed in a nation-wide observational cohort study from Denmark of greater than 130,000 individuals, with reductions in death and hospitalizations.[30] Observational data of influenza vaccination may indicate improved access to care, in addition to reflecting practice variation by region.

Influenza Vaccine Formulations

Influenza vaccine contains two strains from the A-lineage, A/H1N1 and A/H3N2, and either one or two strains from the B-lineage, B/Victoria or B/Yamagata, and are available in several formulations varying in their method of preparation (egg-based, cell culture, recombinant technology), in the amount of and number of vaccine antigens included, and in the presence of adjuvant. The CDC does not recommend preferentially one vaccine formulation over another, but it does emphasize the importance of annual vaccination. Immune responses to influenza vaccine are less robust among older individuals, which is a manifestation of immunosenescence. High-dose influenza vaccine that contains four times the amount of vaccine antigen as standard-dose influenza vaccine has been tested and approved in the United States and other regions for individuals age 65 or older. In a large, RCT of approximately 31,989 medically stable older adults, high-dose influenza vaccine reduced laboratory-confirmed symptomatic influenza by 24% compared with standard-dose vaccine,[31] with a suggestion of reduced risk in serious events caused by cardiac or pulmonary causes (rate ratio, 0.82; 95% CI, 0.73 to 0.93).[32]

The INVESTED trial compared high-dose vaccine with standard-dose vaccine in 5260 high-risk CVD participants; there was no reduction in cardiovascular or pulmonary hospitalizations.[33] Participants were randomized to high-dose trivalent inactivated influenza vaccine or standard-dose quadrivalent inactivated influenza vaccine and treated for up to three influenza seasons. The primary composite endpoint, death or cardiopulmonary hospitalization, did not differ between vaccine groups (HR, 1.06; 95% CI, 0.97, 1.17; $P = 0.21$), and results were consistent across secondary endpoints and within prespecified subgroups, although high-dose vaccine was associated with more mild vaccine-related adverse events such as injection site pain, swelling, and myalgias. The low rates of hospitalizations ascribed to influenza or pneumonia were low overall, suggesting a modest attributable risk of these types of events to the overall risk for hospitalizations in this high-risk patient group.

Antiviral Therapies for Influenza

In addition to vaccination, antiviral agents may reduce the likelihood of influenza-related cardiovascular events, although available data are mostly observational. A large, propensity-matched, retrospective analysis of adults with a prior diagnosis of CVD suggested that treatment with oseltamivir in the first 48 hours after a diagnosis of influenza confers a significant reduction in the incidence of recurrent cardiovascular events (OR, 0.417; 95% CI, 0.349 to 0.498),[34] and at least one other retrospective study suggested potential benefit of oseltamivir in preventing stroke and transient ischemic attack (TIA) (HR, 0.56; 95% CI, 0.42 to 0.74).[35]

SARS-CoV-2 AND COVID-19

Coronavirus Virology and Epidemiology

Coronaviruses (Coronavirinae subfamily) fall into four groups of alpha, beta, gamma, and delta coronaviruses by phylogenetic clustering.[36] Alpha and beta coronaviruses cause infection in humans.[37] Coronaviruses contain four major structural proteins: the spike (S) protein, the nucleocapsid (N) protein, the membrane (M) protein, and the envelope (E) protein.[38] The spike protein, which resembles a crown in cross section and for which the viruses are named, mediates the attachment of the virus to the host cell receptor and subsequent fusion of the virus and cell membrane.

First discovered in the 1960s, the coronavirus family includes seven strains with the ability to infect humans. Four viruses (i.e., HCoV-229E, HCoV-NL63, HCoV-OC43, and HCoV-HKU1) generally cause mild and self-resolving infections. Three other coronaviruses can cause severe and potentially fatal infections (Table 94.1): severe acute respiratory syndrome coronavirus (SARS-CoV), Middle East respiratory syndrome coronavirus (MERS-CoV), and severe acute respiratory syndrome coronavirus 2 (SARS-CoV-2).[39,40]

Severe Acute Respiratory Syndrome Coronavirus and Middle East Respiratory Syndrome. The SARS-CoV virus causing SARS infection

TABLE 94.1 Comparison of Coronaviruses with an Epidemic Potential

VIRUS	RECEPTOR	INCUBATION PERIOD	PREVALENCE OF UNDERLYING CARDIOVASCULAR DISEASE	AVERAGE CASE FATALITY RATE
SARS-CoV	ACE2	2-11 days	10%	10%
MERS-CoV	DPP4	2-13 days	30%	30%
SARS-CoV-2	ACE2	2-14 days	Up to 20% in hospitalized patients	2%-4% (Highly variable, based on multiple factors)

~80% of cases
Usually <50 years old and with few comorbidities

Asymptomatic or mild to moderate disease
Incubation period: ~5 (2–14) days

- Can remain asymptomatic
  Or:
- Fever, fatigue, dry cough
- Bilateral, peripheral, ground glass infiltrates on x-ray
- No or mild dyspnea
- Loss of sense of taste or smell
- Myalgia
- Diarrhea
- Possible cardiac, neurologic, or dermal manifestations

~15% of cases
Often older with risk factors

Severe disease
(usually after day 10)
- Dyspnea
- Oxygen saturation <94%
- Respiratory rate ≥30 per min
- Lung infiltrates area >50%
- Elevated troponin, BNP, and inflammatory markers

~5% of cases
Often older with risk factors

Critical disease
(usually after day 10)
- ARDS
- Acute cardiac injury
- Multi-organ failure
- SIRS/shock

Proinflammatory effects

Prothrombotic effects

FIGURE 94.3 Clinical course and manifestations of COVID-19.

first emerged in November 2002 in the Guangdong Province of China, likely related to a zoonotic transmission from the wild-animal markets. The virus most likely originated from bats with an intermediate host of civet cats.[41] SARS-CoV binds to and uses the angiotensin-converting enzyme 2 (ACE2) to enter host cells. ACE2 is abundantly expressed on the surfaces of endothelial cells of arteries, arterial smooth muscle, pericytes, and the epithelium of the respiratory tract and small intestine.[42] Primarily transmitted from symptomatic patients via respiratory droplets, SARS has an incubation period of 2 to 11 days after exposure,[43] and it affected 8096 people in 29 countries in 2003 with 774 cases of death reported worldwide (and 8 nonfatal cases in the United States). Cardiovascular complications reported with SARS in small case series included tachycardia, hypotension, bradycardia, ACS, MI, and thromboembolic events.[36,44-46]

The MERS-CoV outbreak emerged in Saudi Arabia (SA) in June 2012.[47] This virus also likely originated in bats with dromedary camels acting as the intermediate host for transmission to humans.[47] MERS-CoV enters the host cells through a serine peptidase, dipeptidyl peptidase 4 (DPP4),[42] and is transmitted from patients via respiratory secretions through close contact with an incubation period of 2 to 13 days.[43,48] MERS-CoV has been reported in about 2500 cases in 26 countries with a case fatality rate of 34.4%.[36,49] A systematic review of 637 patients with MERS-CoV showed a high prevalence of comorbidities among these patients including cardiac diseases (30%), hypertension (50%), diabetes (50%), and obesity (16%).[50]

Severe Acute Respiratory Syndrome CORONAVIRUS 2 and COVID-19

On December 31, 2019, a cluster of 27 cases of pneumonia of unknown etiology was reported in Wuhan, China. Patients had symptoms of viral pneumonia including fever, cough, chest discomfort, dyspnea, and bilateral lung infiltrates. The exact source of the initial infection remains unclear, although most of the initial cohort had an epidemiologic link to a wet market in Wuhan. The first genome sequence of the novel causative coronavirus was published on January 10, 2020, and the virus was later named SARS-CoV-2.[36] Human-to-human transmission was confirmed by January 20, 2020, and the disease reached epidemic peak in China by February 2020. On March 11, 2020, the WHO officially declared the global outbreak of COVID-19 as a pandemic.[51] By late March 2021, COVID-19 had affected 127 million and killed over 2.7 million individuals worldwide, and it has caused over 30 million infections and about 550,000 deaths in the United States.

SARS-CoV-2 belongs to the beta-CoVs group and shows about 89% nucleotide identity with bat virus and 79% with human SARS-CoV, and similarly uses ACE2 as the receptor to enter the host cell.[36] Transmission of SARS-CoV-2 occurs mainly by contact with an infected person or contaminated surface, exposure to virus-containing respiratory droplets, and exposure to virus-containing aerosols (<5 μm).[52] Fecal-oral transmission is also a rare route of transmission.[53]

The SARS-CoV-2 infection in adults can be either symptomatic or asymptomatic, and asymptomatic individuals still have the ability to transmit the disease. There are fewer symptomatic cases in children of 15 years old or younger. The primary symptoms of COVID-19 are fever, cough, and shortness of breath, although the full spectrum of symptoms is broad, and can include muscle pain, anorexia, malaise, sore throat, nasal congestion, anosmia, dyspnea, and headache. Symptoms may appear in as few as 2 days or as long as 14 days after exposure (Fig. 94.3).[36] The detected viral load is similar in asymptomatic and symptomatic COVID-19 patients, which explains the high potential for transmission of the virus from asymptomatic or minimally symptomatic patients to other persons.[54] COVID-19 is associated with multiple extrapulmonary manifestations (Fig. 94.4). Gastrointestinal symptoms such as diarrhea, abdominal pain, and vomiting occur in 2% to 10% of COVID-19 patients,[55] and SARS-CoV-2 patients' feces often contain viral RNA.[56]

As an RNA virus, SARS-CoV-2 is susceptible to mutation during replication. Mutations that persist after rounds of replication lead to the emergence of new *variants*[57,57a] and those with different phenotypic characteristics are termed *strains*. Three different nomenclature systems are used for naming and tracking SARS-CoV-2 variants. The World Health Organization (WHO) has introduced a simpler method of using Greek alphabet letters to identify variants of concern and variants of interest. Early in the pandemic, a novel variant, D614G, increased the efficacy of the virus to replicate and its ability to interact with the ACE2 receptor. Another variant, termed *alpha variant,* was initially identified in the United Kingdom and has additional mutations in the spike protein and is more easily transmissible with possibly higher mortality. The beta variant first identified in South Africa, also with mutations in the spike protein, shows high potential for transmissibility and is less likely to be effectively neutralized by convalescent serum, and might be less responsive to early vaccines based on the original circulating virus. The highly contagious delta variant, initially detected in India, has caused significant mortality, and first-generation vaccines may offer less protection against it.

Overall, the emergence of new variants is a cause for concern because they may have higher transmissibility, higher virulence, less susceptibility to treatments using monoclonal antibodies, and the potential ability to evade the body's innate or acquired immune responses, as well as the response to vaccines. Additional booster vaccine doses might become necessary to protect against them. It is yet not clear if new variants will have a different impact on the cardiovascular system.

Epidemiology of COVID-19 and Risk Factors
Comorbidities and COVID-19 Illness

Several comorbidities confer higher risk of requiring critical care from COVID-19, including advanced age, diabetes, hypertension, HF, and atherosclerotic CVD. Advanced age is associated with SARS-CoV-2 infection and worse disease severity, potentially related to immunosenescence, but also due to the presence of other comorbidities that portend a worse prognosis from COVID-19. Hypertension is the most prevalent comorbidity among patients with COVID-19 and affects approximately

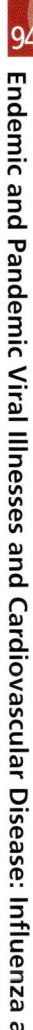

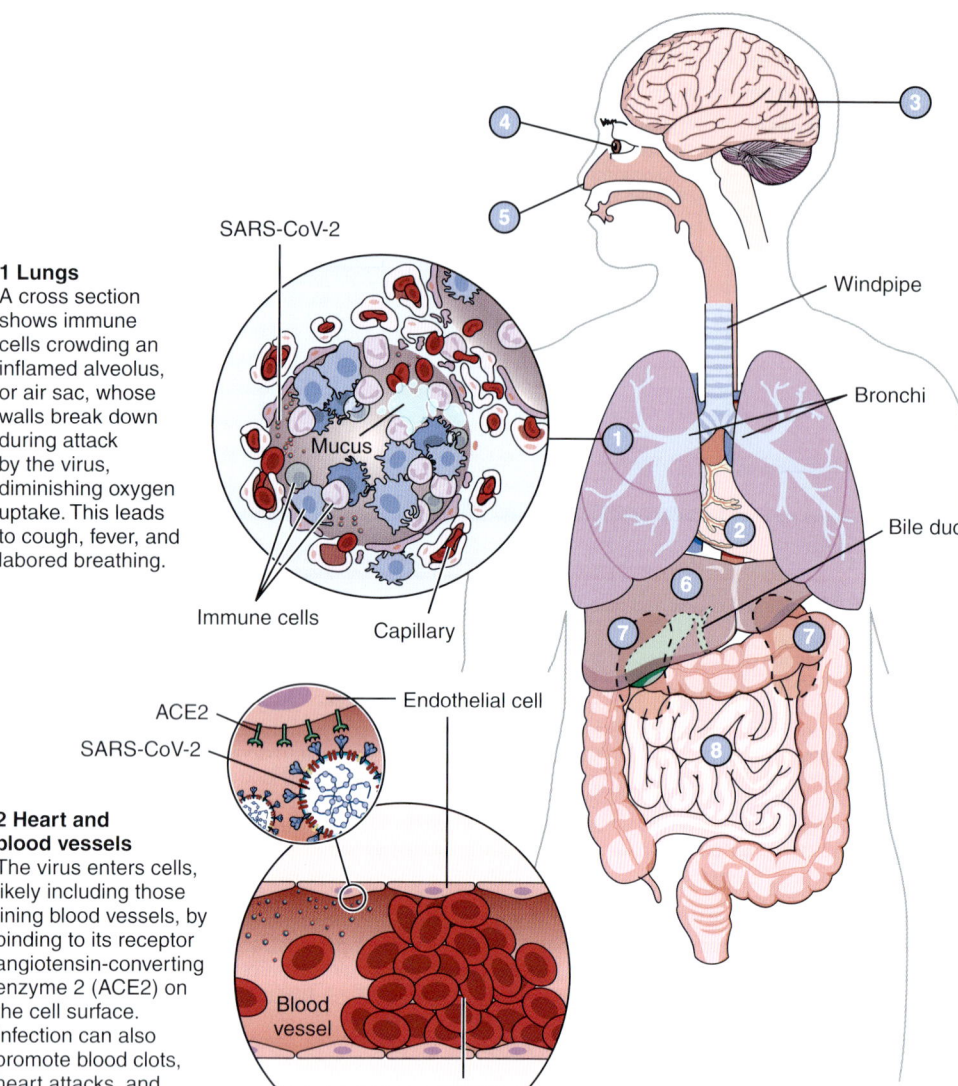

FIGURE 94.4 Extrapulmonary manifestations of COVID-19. (From Wadman M., et al. A rampage through the body. Science 2020;368(6489):356-360.)

30% of patients with severe COVID-19,[58] followed by diabetes mellitus, obesity, CVD, pulmonary disease, and cerebrovascular disease. Hypertension and CVD are associated with increased susceptibility to SARS-CoV-2 infection, and along with diabetes link to more severe COVID-19 and an increased mortality.

Individuals who meet criteria for obesity (body mass index [BMI] ≥30 kg/m^2) also have increased risk for hospitalization for COVID-19, respiratory failure, and higher mortality even after adjustments for age, race, and comorbid conditions.[59] Obese individuals (WHO class I through III) are more likely to require mechanical ventilation or experience in-hospital death compared with nonobese patients (OR, 1.28 [95% CI 1.09 to 1.51], 1.57 [1.29 to 1.91], 1.80 [1.47 to 2.20], respectively). Obesity and age interact significantly, such that the association with obesity and adverse clinical outcomes was stronger for individuals younger than age 50 (p-interaction <0.05).

The mechanism by which increased BMI contributes to an adverse prognosis in COVID-19 is not entirely clear, but it may relate to increased inflammation from adipose tissue, which may stimulate production of inflammatory cytokines and increase the risk for cytokine storm (see later). Moreover, adipose tissue highly expresses ACE2,[60] which may contribute to the increased risk of more severe infection. In patients with more advanced disease, adverse respiratory mechanical factors, such as decreased pulmonary expiratory reserve volume, functional capacity, and respiratory system compliance, may also contribute to severity of disease. Obesity is also often accompanied by other comorbidities known to increase risk for adverse clinical outcomes from COVID-19 illness such as hypertension, diabetes mellitus, and atherosclerotic CVD.

Racial and Ethnic Influences on COVID-19 Illness

Individuals from certain races and ethnic minority groups are at increased risk for COVID-19 and resultant hospitalizations, independent of age or other comorbid conditions.[61] Blacks were 3.6 more likely, Native Americans 3.4 times more likely, and Latinx individuals are 3.2 times more likely to die of COVID-19 when compared with whites, across all age groups, including younger adults who normally exhibit lower mortality rates.[62] Black Americans have a doubled risk of hospitalization from COVID-19 compared with white Americans, after adjustment for age, gender, residence, insurance plan, obesity and Charlson Comorbidity Index score.[63] Once hospitalized, Blacks and whites appear to have similar mortality rates.

Racial and ethnic disparities with COVID-19 infection and prognosis may arise from systemic structural disadvantages. Blacks are disproportionately represented in "essential worker" groups that were exempt from shelter-in-place efforts. Housing disadvantages with larger per household numbers are more common among Blacks and challenge social distancing initiatives, as is the use of public transportation. COVID-19 has exacerbated these disparities in the United States and across the globe.[64]

Clinical Cardiovascular Manifestations of COVID-19

Cardiovascular manifestations of COVID-19 vary, and acute infection links to a wide spectrum of cardiovascular complications, including ACS, stroke, acute-onset HF, arrhythmias, myocarditis, and cardiac arrest. Exactly how the disease leads to these complications remains unclear, although most likely it appears to be linked to the underlying inflammatory response that becomes unbridled in some patients, resulting in an immune-mediated thrombotic state (immunothrombosis).

Atherosclerotic Cardiovascular Syndromes: Acute Coronary Syndromes and Stroke in COVID-19 Patients

Respiratory infections are associated with ACSs, as noted previously for influenza.[26] SARS-CoV-2 can also trigger ACSs and strokes by producing profound proinflammatory and prothrombotic effects (see later). Early limited reports have suggested a higher thrombus burden in COVID-19 patients presenting with ST-elevation MI.[65] A Danish nationwide registry-based study of over 5000 patients with hospitalized COVID-19 revealed that the risk of acute MI and ischemic stroke were 5 and 10 times higher, respectively, during the first 14 days after COVID-19 infection compared with a period preceding known infection.[66]

Myocarditis due to COVID-19

Despite early reports of myocarditis in the setting of COVID-19, its actual incidence in the setting of COVID-19 infection appears quite low, with most evidence limited to case reports or small case series. Symptom presentation of cases thought to be myocarditis related to COVID-19 have varied from fatigue or dyspnea to chest pain or tightness on exertion. There have only been a few reports of fulminant myocarditis, evidenced by ventricular dysfunction and acute HF within a few weeks of confirmed SARS-CoV-2 infection. Although viral particles with the morphology and size of SARS-CoV-2 have been detected in myocardial interstitial macrophages, SARS-CoV-2 genomic material has not been detected in the cardiac myocytes (see later).[67]

COVID-19 and Heart Failure

COVID-19 is associated with increased risk for hospitalization and mortality in patients with prevalent HF and may also increase the risk of developing incident HF, particularly in at-risk individuals. Among 152 patients with a history of HF hospitalized with COVID-19 in a tertiary hospital in Spain, mortality rates were higher compared with those with COVID-19 and without HF ($n = 2928$, 48.7% vs. 19.0%; $P < 0.001$).[68] Of the 77 patients who developed acute HF, only 22.1% had a prior history of it, which supports the potential of the SARS-CoV-2 virus to result in myocardial damage. In a study of 132,312 patients with HF hospitalized between April and June 2020, using data from a large, multicenter, all-payer database inclusive of over 1000 health care entities and health systems in the United States, the in-hospital mortality rate for patients with HF hospitalized for COVID-19 was 24.2% compared with 2.6% in those hospitalized for acute HF and 4.6% in those who were hospitalized for other reasons during the same time frame.[69]

Arrhythmias in COVID-19

COVID-19 is associated with a wide array of arrhythmias. In general, acute infections can cause arrhythmias through multiple possible mechanisms, including direct infection of the myocardium, myocardial injury, myocarditis, hypoxia, ischemia, cytokine storm, and electrolyte disturbances.[70] Interruption of cardiac medications and iatrogenic effects of certain medications (i.e., chloroquine, hydroxychloroquine, azithromycin) used in COVID-19 may also contribute to the arrhythmogenic burden of COVID-19.

Overall, COVID-19-related arrhythmias are heterogeneous and include sinus tachycardia, AF, sinus bradycardia, complete heart block, ventricular tachycardia, ventricular fibrillation arrest, torsade de pointes, and pulseless electrical activity.[70,71] Although patients may develop sinus tachycardia during the infection period, the risk of other types of arrhythmias is lower and varies depending on the severity of the infection and the underlying condition of patients. Tachycardia and palpitation are among common complaints in patients who have postacute sequelae SARS-CoV-2 (PASC, see later) infection. Limited reports from the Lombardy region in Italy and New York City described a temporal increase in out-of-hospital cardiac arrests during COVID-19 early peak activity, which could be ascribed to cardiac arrests or pulmonary embolism (PE).[72,73]

COVID-19 patients who are admitted to an intensive care unit (ICU) more commonly have severe and life-threatening arrhythmias. In a cohort of 700 patients (mean age 50 years, 45% men) with 11% in the ICU, 9 had cardiac arrest, all of which happened in ICU patients, and were due to pulseless electrical activity, asystole, or torsades de pointes, but not ventricular tachycardia or fibrillation.[74] Cardiac arrests, as expected, were associated with increased risk of in-hospital mortality; however, other arrhythmias (25 incident AF events, 9 significant bradyarrhythmias, and 10 nonsustained ventricular tachycardias [NSVTs]) were not.[74] In a large series of patients (3970 patients) admitted early in the pandemic to New York hospitals, new-onset atrial fibrillation/flutter was detected in 4% of COVID-19 patients, which was comparable to the same rate (4%) in a historic comparable cohort of patients hospitalized with influenza.[75] COVID-19 patients who developed atrial fibrillation/flutter were older and had higher levels of inflammatory biomarkers (i.e., C-reactive protein, IL-6), troponin, and D-dimer.[75]

Venous and Arterial Thromboembolism in COVID-19

Patients with COVID-19 exhibit increased rates of deep vein thrombosis (DVT) and PE (Fig. 94.5). A systematic review of 27 radiologic studies with 3342 patients showed high incidence rates of PE on computed tomography (CT) pulmonary angiography and DVT (17% and 15%, respectively).[76] PE was more frequent in patients admitted to the ICU (25%) compared with those not in the ICU (11%). Concomitant DVT was identified in 42% of patients with PE. The established guideline cutoffs for D-dimer used to exclude PE were applicable to patients with COVID-19.[76] Arterial thrombosis is less common in COVID-19 than venous thrombosis. In a retrospective study of 3334 hospitalized COVID-19 patients in New York (March to April 2020), 207 (6%) had venous thromboembolism (VTE) (3% PE and 4% DVT), whereas 11% had arterial thrombosis (2% ischemic stroke, 9% MI, and 1% systemic thromboembolism).[77] Patients with a thrombotic event had higher all-cause mortality than those without (43% vs. 21%; $P < 0.001$).

Multisystem Inflammatory Syndrome in Children

Initial experience with COVID-19 early during the pandemic suggested that children would not encounter the same degree of severity, complications, and sequelae from the SARS-CoV-2 virus. Albeit quite rare, a growing number of cases of an inflammatory shock syndrome in children prompted the CDC to define this manifestation as "multisystem inflammatory syndrome in children" (MIS-C).[78] MIS-C has several features akin to other known syndromes such as Kawasaki disease, Kawasaki shock syndrome, and toxic shock syndrome. It presents with prolonged fever, elevated inflammatory markers, and cardiovascular features such as arrhythmia, myocardial function depression, and valvular dysfunction. A survey that included 55 hospitals in Europe identified 286 cases that met a prespecified definition of persistent fever, inflammation, and cardiac involvement between February and June 2020.[79] Median age was 8.4 years, and 67% were male. Current or prior COVID-19 infection was confirmed in 65% of cases via polymerase chain reaction (PCR) or measurements of IgM or IgG antibodies. Only a minority of patients had preexisting congenital heart disease or autoimmune disorders. Among patients who had cardiac biomarkers checked, the majority had elevated troponin T or natriuretic peptides. Abnormal electrocardiogram (ECG) (primarily abnormal ST or T wave segment) occurred in 35% of cases and ejection fraction was impaired in 34% of cases, with 20% exhibiting sustained left ventricular systolic dysfunction at discharge. Although 30% of the cohort required inotropic support and 15% required mechanical ventilation, most patients had resolution of the acute manifestations and 93% of patients were discharged, suggesting a more benign course in children with MIS-C than adults with COVID-19, despite significant biomarker elevations and cardiovascular features.[80]

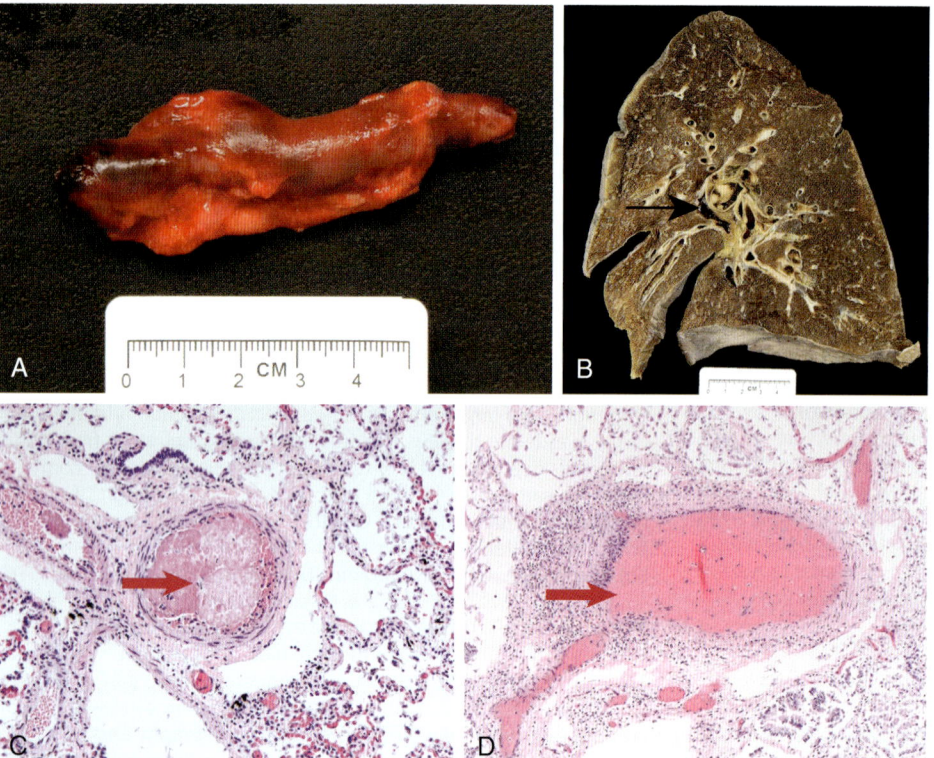

FIGURE 94.5 Gross and microscopic pathology of thromboembolism and vasculitis in COVID-19. **A,** Gross photograph of a deep vein thrombus removed from the femoral vein in a COVID-19 decedent. **B,** Gross photograph of a cross section of the right lung demonstrating extensive fatal thromboemboli (*arrow*) in a COVID-19 decedent. The background lung shows acute diffuse alveolar damage, characteristic of COVID-19 pneumonia. **C,** Photomicrograph of pulmonary thromboemboli (*arrow*) within small pulmonary arteries in the lung of a COVID-19 decedent. Microscopic thrombi/thromboemboli are common postmortem findings in the lungs, even in patients without known premortem clinical thromboembolic signs/symptoms. (Hematoxylin and eosin (H&E)-stained section, 400× original magnification.) **D,** Photomicrograph of vasculitis within a small pulmonary artery within the lung of a COVID-19 decedent. Vasculitis in the lungs is a rare finding in COVID-19 decedents. (H&E-stained section, 400× original magnification.) (Images courtesy Robert Padera, MD, Brigham and Women's Hospital.)

Biomarker Evidence of Myocardial Injury

Increased troponin levels indicate myocardial injury during the acute phase of infection, as defined as serum concentrations above a certain threshold (e.g., >0.03 ng/mL or levels above the 99th percentile upper reference limit), with or without accompanying electrocardiographic or echocardiographic evidence of acute ischemia.[81] Multiple mechanisms can elevate troponin including but not limited to ACSs,[82] type 1 or type 2 MI, myocarditis, cytokine storm, PE, or Takotsubo syndrome (stress-induced cardiomyopathy) with or without cardiogenic shock.[36,82-84] Chronic baseline conditions such as congestive HF or left ventricular hypertrophy can also raise troponin levels.[36,82] Biochemical evidence of myocardial injury portends worse clinical outcomes among hospitalized patients with COVID-19, and more commonly occurs in patients of older age and with comorbidities. Elevated troponin in COVID-19 has been associated with an increased risk for arrhythmias, respiratory failure, and mortality[85]; increased requirements for invasive and noninvasive mechanical ventilation; higher frequency of acute kidney injury, acute respiratory distress syndrome (ARDS), and coagulation disorders; and a greater than fourfold increased risk for death.[86] A multicenter study in 614 patients hospitalized with COVID-19 reported that elevated troponin occurred in 45.3% of patients and was associated with an increased in-hospital mortality (37% vs. 13%; HR, 1.71 [95% CI 1.13 to 2.59]; P = 0.01), independent of concomitant CVD.[87] Similarly, in a larger retrospective study of 2736 hospitalized patients, 36% had biochemical evidence of myocardial injury (any elevation of troponin I above the upper limits of normal), but less than a third had a history of CAD, and was associated with a 75% increased risk for in-hospital mortality.[81] Although evidence of the association of myocardial injury with adverse outcomes is consistent, it is unclear whether cardiac injury is a marker for disease severity or a direct contributor to COVID-19 morbidity and mortality.

Biomarkers Suggestive of Prothrombotic State

Patients with COVID-19 often have elevated levels of D-dimer, the degradation product of cross-linked fibrin monomers and a marker of coagulation and fibrinolysis. High D-dimer levels are associated with PE and VTE (see later). D-Dimer can be elevated in COVID-19 even in the absence of overt evidence of macrovascular thrombus, and elevated D-dimer levels are associated independently with mortality and a higher likelihood for requiring intubation.[88] High D-dimer levels are nonspecific and may indicate a hypercoagulable state, inflammation, pathologic fibrinolysis, microvascular angiopathy, and overall reflect COVID-19 illness severity.

Cardiac Imaging Findings in COVID-19

COVID-19 has been associated with abnormalities of cardiac structure and function in several studies, including echocardiographic evidence of left ventricular dysfunction, regional wall motion abnormalities, and mild reduction in right ventricular function.[89] Several cardiovascular magnetic resonance (CMR) imaging studies have noted myocardial abnormalities that persist after acute infection. In a study of 100 COVID-19 patients (33 of whom had been hospitalized), imaging was performed at a median of 71 days after diagnosis of COVID-19.[90] Pericardial effusion (>10 mm) was observed in 20% (20/100) of patients, and late gadolinium enhancement (LGE), reflecting scarring, was observed in 32% (32/100) (myocardial) and 22% (22/100) (pericardial) of the COVID-19 group. It was significantly more prevalent in COVID-19 patients than in healthy controls or risk factor-matched controls. In addition, other studies have noted high prevalence of myocardial edema post-COVID-19 infection. Whether abnormal CMR imaging findings observed after COVID-19 reflect permanent cardiac injury is unknown at this time due to the lack of long-term studies.

Effects of the COVID-19 Pandemic on Cardiovascular Health More Broadly

In addition to the effects of the disease on individuals infected with COVID-19, the pandemic has influenced cardiovascular health more broadly in the population. Early in the pandemic, a decrease in the incidence of hospitalization for acute MI, including both ST-segment elevation MI (STEMI) and non–ST-segment elevation MI (NSTEMI), by as much as 40% to 50% was noted compared with previous years (Fig. 94.6).[91-94] Northern Italy observed a 20% reduction in hospitalizations for MI during their peak surge of COVID-19 from February to May 2020 when compared with expected hospitalization rates based on historical data.[95] Unfortunately, this was paralleled with an increase in the number of out-of-hospital cardiac deaths.[95] The cause for the decline in acute MI in the overall population during COVID-19 peak surges likely arose for multiple reasons including patient avoidance of medical care due to fear of contracting COVID-19 in the emergency rooms or hospital settings and misdiagnosis or underappreciation of acute MI. Patients with COVID-19 also suffered longer door-to-CT, door-to-needle, and door-to-endovascular therapy times, with higher in-hospital mortality (OR, 4.34; 95% CI, 3.48 to 5.40).[96]

During peak COVID-19 surges, patients may ignore symptoms of myocardial ischemia, exacerbations of HF, or stroke, and delay seeking appropriate medical care. This delay may worsen outcomes and development of serious complications such as ischemic cardiomyopathy, increased risk of SCD, and development of rare but very high risk complications such as postinfarction myocardial rupture, ischemic ventricular septal defects, or ventricular aneurysms. Because of the potential hesitancy of patients to seek cardiovascular care in the setting of a pandemic, it is imperative to optimize safety measures in health care facilities to encourage patients to seek immediate care when facing early signs of heart attack and stroke. During high COVID-19 activity periods, patients should be screened and tested for coinfection and appropriate personal protective equipment should be utilized when performing emergency procedures on patients with unknown COVID-19 status.

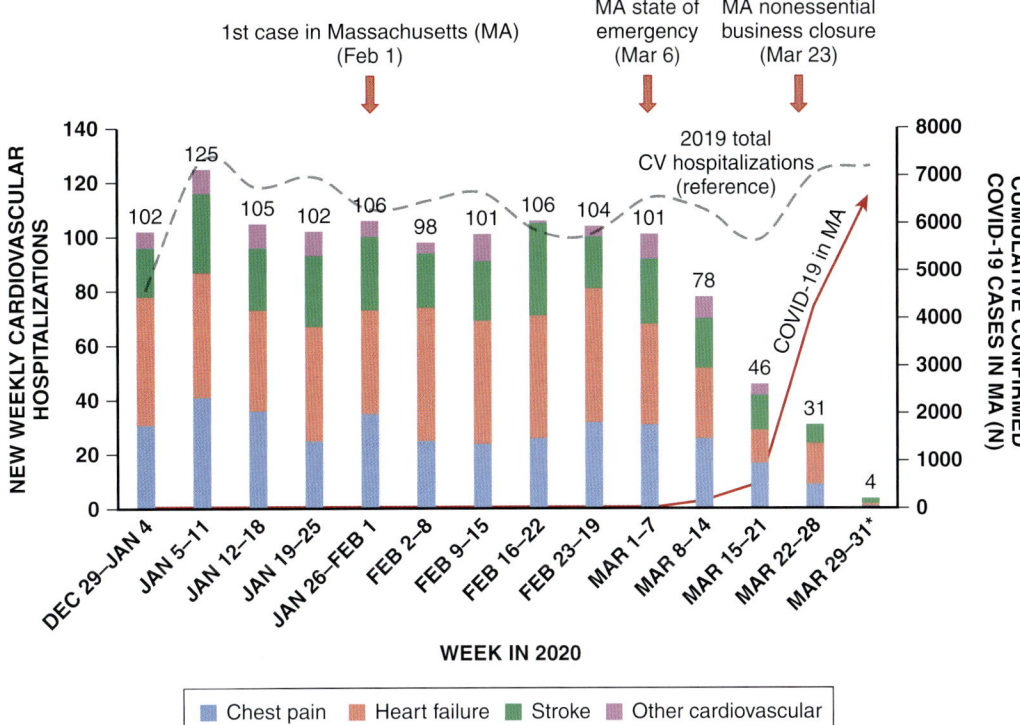

FIGURE 94.6 Decline in non–COVID-19-related cardiovascular hospitalizations during the SARS-CoV-2 pandemic. (From Bhatt AS, et al. Fewer hospitalizations for acute cardiovascular conditions during the COVID-19 pandemic. J Am Coll Cardiol 2020;76(3):280-288.)

MECHANISMS OF COVID-19 CARDIOVASCULAR DISEASE
Direct Effect on Cardiovascular Tissues

SARS-CoV-2 enters cells by binding to the ACE2 receptors in a process that is facilitated by transmembrane serine protease 2 (TMPRSS2). Both ACE2 and TMPRSS2 are present in multiple extrapulmonary tissues and are expressed in high concentrations in vascular tissues.[97] This may explain in part the high affinity of the virus for the circulatory system.[98] The presence of microthrombi in the myocardium parallels the finding of alveolar capillary microthrombi and widespread thrombosis with microangiopathy in pulmonary vessels of COVID-19 patients.[99] Multiple autopsy series have shown the presence of DVT and PE in these patients.[100,101] Major pulmonary and cardiac findings identified on autopsy are listed in Table 94.2. A systemic at review of 41 studies, including 316 autopsy cases, identified a variety of postmortem cardiac manifestations including cardiac dilatation (20%), acute ischemia (8%), intracardiac thrombi (2.5%), pericardial effusion (2.5%), and myocarditis in 1.5% of cases.[102] Direct infection of the myocardial cells with SARS-CoV-2 was extremely rare.

Histopathologic studies of cardiovascular tissues in COVID-19 have been mostly performed in a small series of deceased patients. They are subject to the inherent bias of studying the most severe cases, which likely decreases the findings' generalizability, yet they can provide critical information on the pathogenesis of the disease. SARS-CoV-2 RNA has been identified in a varying fraction of autopsied hearts, and true myocarditis (Fig. 94.7) has been generally rare.[101,103] In a small study of 15 hearts from COVID-19 victims, none revealed true myocarditis, and the virus was detected only in the myocytes of the left atrium of one case (with viral copies much less than lungs).[98] In another study of 104 endomyocardial biopsies performed during peak COID-19 activity in Germany, SARS-CoV-2 RNA was detected only in 5% of cases of clinically suspected myocarditis or new-onset HF.[104] A series of 39 serial autopsies in Germany identified SARS-CoV-2 RNA in 61.5% of cases and no myocarditis.[105] A high viral RNA load was detected in 16 (41%) cases and was associated with a proinflammatory cytokine response but was not associated with increased infiltration of mononuclear cells into the myocardium.[105] Indeed, a series of 40 autopsies in Italy revealed 14 patients with myocyte necrosis (of whom 3 had acute MI and 11 had focal myocyte necrosis).[106] Microthrombi rich in fibrin and terminal complement C5b-9 in myocardial capillaries, arterioles, and small muscular arteries were more common than large epicardial coronary thrombi. This may explain presentations of STEMI in the absence of epicardial coronary obstruction.[107] In contrast with influenza, limited autopsy series have not shown infiltration of atherosclerotic plaques with inflammatory cells and/or plaque rupture after COVID-19.[101]

TABLE 94.2 **Important Pathology Findings in Autopsies of Subjects with COVID-19**

Cardiac Pathology
Cardiomegaly
Cardiac dilation
Lymphocytic epicarditis/pericarditis
Lymphocytic myocarditis
Individual/focal myocyte necrosis
Acute ischemia
Intracardiac thrombi
Intramyocardial microthrombi in capillaries, arterioles, and small arteries
Pericardial effusion
Pulmonary Pathology
Severe endothelial injury
Acute pneumonitis
Interstitial pneumonitis
Interstitial lymphocytic pneumonitis
Incipient interstitial pneumonitis
Diffuse alveolar damage with perivascular T-cell infiltration
Bronchopneumonia with aspiration
Microthrombi in capillaries and small blood vessels
Microangiopathy and intussusceptive angiogenesis
Large pulmonary thromboemboli

Cytokine Storm, Hyperinflammatory Response, and Endothelial Disease in COVID-19

Many patients with COVID-19 are asymptomatic or have mild to moderate disease. However, depending on age and comorbidities, up to 10% to 15% may develop severe disease requiring hospitalization, and up to 5% may need care in an ICU.[108] It is still unknown why some patients remain asymptomatic or have mild symptoms and why others progress to severe disease. Age, comorbidities, viral load, immune response, prior exposure (or lack of exposure) to coronaviruses, and inflammatory response play a role in this process.

Inflammation is an integral part of the innate immune response to infection. The inflammatory response begins after exposure to the pathogens and is expected to react proportionally to the pathogen burden and to return to baseline hemostasis after clearance of infectious burden. The balance between producing sufficient cytokines to clear the infection and avoiding hyperinflammation, which could damage the host cells, is pivotal for this process.[109]

SARS-CoV-2 infection triggers a robust systemic inflammatory response that can initiate a "cytokine storm" with a hyperinflammatory state, as evident by overproduction of a wide array of inflammatory mediators including circulating cytokines and chemokines, such as IL-1α, IL-1β, IL-2, IL-7, IL-6, IL-8, IL-10, tumor necrosis factor (TNF), interferon (IFN)-γ, granulocyte colony-stimulating factor (G-CSF), IFN-inducible protein-10 (IP-10), CCL2 (monocyte chemotactic protein [MCP]-1), CCL3 (macrophage inflammatory protein 1 alpha [MIP1α]), CXC-chemokine ligand 10 (CXCL10), C-reactive protein, ferritin, and D-dimers.[110-117] High serum levels of IL-6, IL-8, and TNF-α levels at the time of hospitalization powerfully predict patient survival ($P < 0.0001$, $P = 0.0205$, and $P = 0.0140$, respectively).[110] The cytokine storm likely contributes to the development of ARDS in COVID-19 patients, which has a mortality rate of up to 40% to 50%.[118] The hyperinflammation state of ARDS is characterized by increased proinflammatory cytokines, increased risk of shock, and poor clinical outcomes including multiorgan failure, and death.[116]

Although the term *cytokine storm* does not have an established definition,[118] it refers broadly to a hyperactive immune response characterized by the release of multiple proinflammatory mediators. However, these mediators are also part of our innate immune response and it is often challenging to distinguish a normal immune response from a dysregulated response leading to damage to host cells.[118] The cytokine response in COVID-19 is not universally exaggerated. In fact, a study of critically ill patients with COVID-19 with ARDS showed lower circulating cytokine levels when compared with patients with bacterial sepsis. The exact role of cytokines in the pathogenesis of COVID-19 remains undetermined and is subject of extensive research. At present, multiple clinical studies are under way to examine the potential benefit of targeting multiple inflammatory pathways in controlling COVID-19 and preventing its complications, noticeably ARDS (Fig. 94.8).[119-121]

Neutrophil extracellular trap (NET) formation may play an important role in the pathology of COVID-19. NETs are multimolecular, DNA-based, netlike structures made up of cytosolic and granule proteins and mitochondrial DNA originating from neutrophils in response to infections.[122] They may trap and limit dissemination of bacteria, fungi, and viruses. The inflammatory response in COVID-19 can activate NET formation.[116] Patients with COVID-19 have higher plasma levels of NET markers than healthy controls, and these markers correlate with

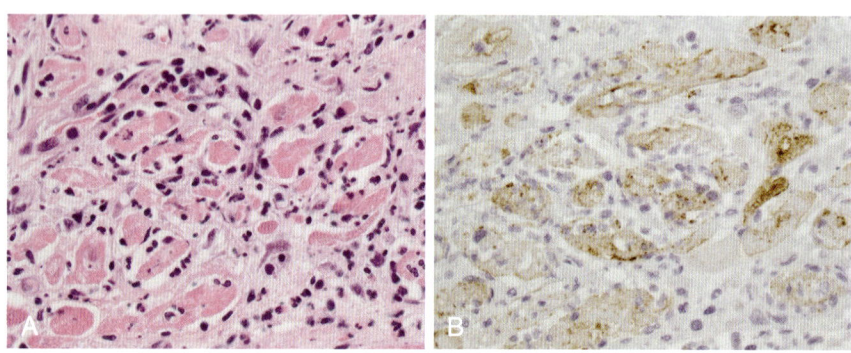

FIGURE 94.7 Lymphocytic myocarditis in COVID-19. **A,** Photomicrograph of lymphocytic myocarditis with myocyte necrosis in the myocardium of a profoundly immunosuppressed COVID-19 decedent. Hematoxylin and eosin–stained section, 400× original magnification. **B,** Photomicrograph of the same field as **(A)** of immunohistochemistry for the nucleocapsid protein of SARS-CoV-2 demonstrating positivity in the dying myocytes, but not in the associated endothelium or inflammatory infiltrate. 400× original magnification. (Images courtesy of Robert Padera, MD, Brigham and Women's Hospital.)

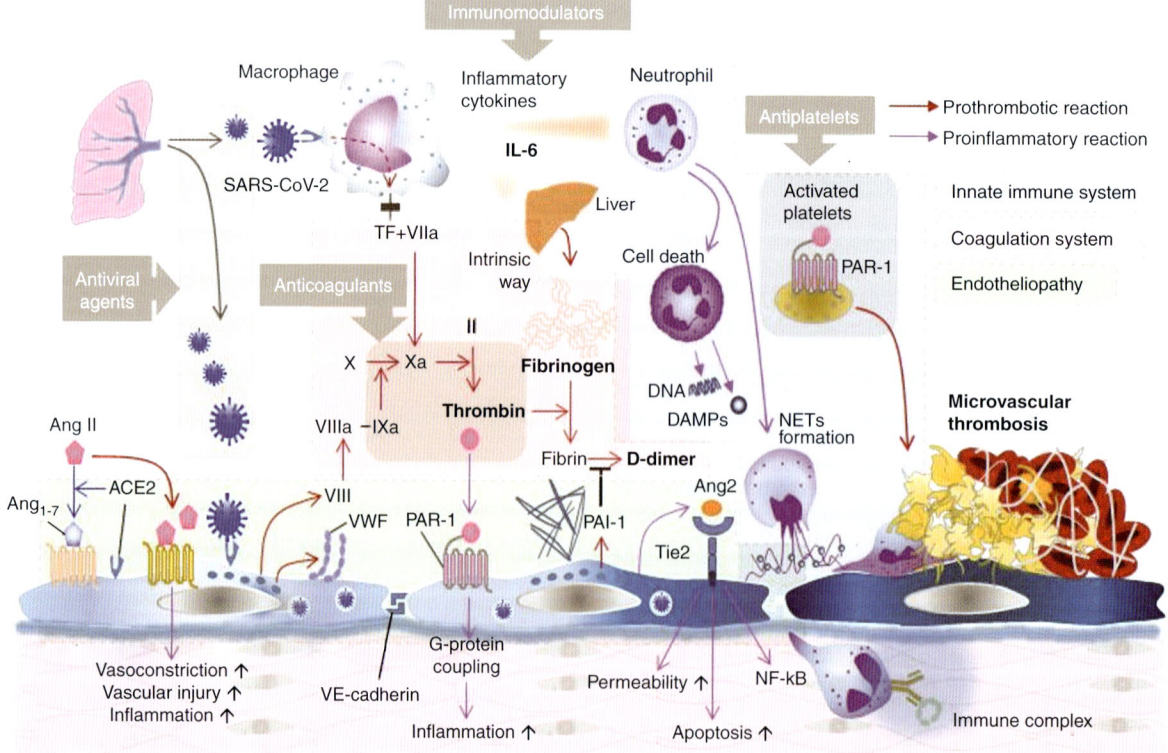

FIGURE 94.8 Pathophysiology of the effect of SARS-CoV-2. (From Connors JM, et al. Thrombosis and COVID-19: controversies and (tentative) conclusions. [published online ahead of print February 4, 2021]. *Clin Infect Dis.* https://doi.org/10.1093/cid/ciab096.)

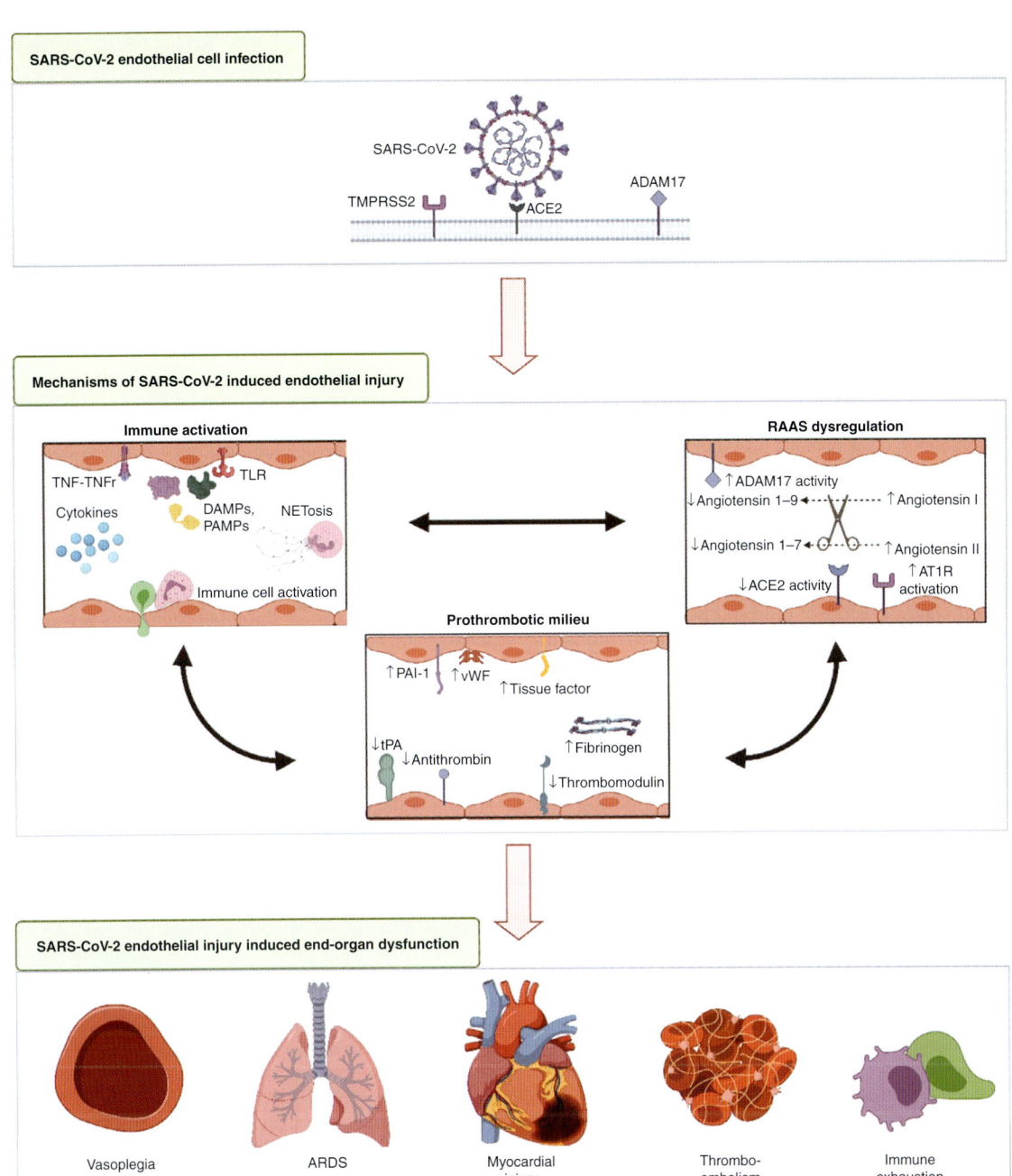

FIGURE 94.9 SARS-CoV-2–induced endothelial injury. Schematic of SARS-CoV-2 infection and proposed resulting endothelial injury, involving immune activation, prothrombotic milieu, and renin-angiotensin-aldosterone system (RAAS) dysregulation. These insults interact with each other to cause end-organ dysfunction that is manifest in many COVID-19 patients. *ADAM17,* A disintegrin and metalloproteinase 17; *ARDS,* acute respiratory distress syndrome; *AT1R,* angiotensin 1 receptor; *DAMPs,* damage-associated molecular patterns; *eNOS,* endothelial nitric oxide; *PAI-1,* plasminogen activator inhibitor-1; *PAMPs,* pathogen-associated molecular patterns; *TLR,* Toll-like receptor; *TMPRSS2,* transmembrane protease serine 2; *TNF,* tumor necrosis factor; *TNFr,* tumor necrosis factor receptor; *tPA,* tissue plasminogen activator; *vWF,* von Willebrand factor. (From Siddiqi HK, et al. COVID-19: a vascular disease. Trends Cardiovasc Med 2021;31:1-5.)

leukocyte numbers, neutrophils, inflammatory cytokines, and in vivo markers of coagulation, fibrinolysis, and endothelial damage. NET formation is associated with an increased risk of requiring respiratory support and worse short-term mortality.[123] A small case series of coronary thrombus samples aspirated during STEMI interventions detected NETs in all 5 patients with COVID-19, whereas it was detected in only 34 of 50 thrombi (68%) retrieved from noninfected controls.[124]

Another small in vitro study showed that neutrophils obtained from COVID-19 patients more readily release NETs compared with neutrophils from healthy individuals. NET production related directly with disease severity and was higher in intubated patients and in those who died later.[125] At autopsy, lungs show neutrophil-platelet accumulation in NET-containing microthrombi. In contrast, NET formation fell during convalescence after COVID-19.[125] SARS-CoV-2 induces a robust immunothrombotic process, which is part of the body's protective response to infections. However, NET formation induces a thrombogenic and cytotoxic environment that can damage epithelial and vascular integrity and likely contributes to rapid pulmonary dysfunction and other complications.[116,126]

COVID-19 can provoke endothelial dysfunction (Fig. 94.9).[116] The normal endothelium has strong and unique anticoagulant, antithrombotic, vasodilatory, antioxidant, and pro-fibrinolytic properties.[116] (see Chapter 24). The release of proinflammatory cytokines during acute infections affect the endothelial cells and switch their homeostatic functions, leading to loss of many of their protective features.[84,116,127] Normally functioning endothelial cells effectively prevent platelet activation by producing nitric oxide, releasing prostacyclin, and expressing CD39 (an ecto-ADPase).[128] Endothelial dysfunction can cause cells to stop generating prostacyclin and produce thromboxane, which is a potent vasoconstrictor prostaglandin with prothrombotic effects. Endothelial injury can also disrupt the endothelial-dependent vasodilatation through impaired NOS expression and lead to production of endothelin-1, a potent vasoconstrictor.[129]

Moreover, the endothelial cells store von Willebrand factor (vWf) and P-selectin in a preformed state in intracellular granules called

Weibel-Palade bodies. Once activated, they can release vWf, which can facilitate platelet aggregates and thrombosis.[130] Additionally, the expression of TF after endothelial injury can activate the coagulation cascade leading to the well-known increased risk of thrombin generation and clot formation in COVID-19.[127]

Treatment of COVID-19 and COVID-19-Related Complications

The treatment of COVID-19 continues to evolve rapidly as more treatments complete testing in randomized trials.

Antiviral Therapy

Early-stage treatments include antivirals and anti-SARS-CoV-2 monoclonal antibodies. Remdesivir is a nucleoside analog that inhibits the RNA-dependent RNA polymerase, and the only U.S. Food and Drug Administration (FDA)-approved antiviral for the treatment of COVID-19. It is currently recommended for patients hospitalized with moderate COVID-19 who require supplemental oxygen, but benefit is not established in patients who require high-flow oxygen, noninvasive ventilation, or mechanical ventilation. Duration of treatment is 5 days, which may be extended to 10 days in the absence of clinical improvement.[131]

Anti-SARS-CoV-2 Monoclonal Antibodies

The FDA has issued emergency use authorizations (EUA) for several monoclonal antibodies. Bamlanivimab plus etesevimab (administered together) were authorized for the treatment of mild to moderate non-hospitalized COVID-19 in adults and pediatric patients (12 years of age or older weighing at least 40 kg).[132] In addition, the FDA has issued an EUA for casirivimab and imdevimab (administered together) for the treatment of mild to moderate non-hospitalized COVID-19 in adults and pediatric patients (12 years of age or older weighing at least 40 kg).[133] Other monoclonal antibodies are currently in development. Potential cardioprotective effects from anti-cytokine treatments are not yet determined due to inconsistency in clinical trial results.

Corticosteroid Therapy

Corticosteroids have shown benefit in the subset of patients with moderate COVID-19 who require supplemental oxygen. In the Randomized Evaluation of COVID-19 Therapy trial, dexamethasone (6 mg once daily for up to 10 days) reduced 28-day mortality, but patients who did not require oxygen did not benefit.[134] In the setting of more severe COVID-19, corticosteroids may negate the adverse inflammatory response that can lead to multiorgan failure. In a meta-analysis of 7 RCTs that enrolled 1703 critically ill patients (including those requiring mechanical ventilation) with COVID-19, use of systemic dexamethasone, hydrocortisone, or methylprednisolone resulted in a 34% reduced risk for all-cause mortality at 28 days.[135]

Other Management Considerations

Role of Anticoagulation in COVID-19

Many observational or smaller studies have investigated which patients with COVID-19 might benefit from anticoagulation or antiplatelet therapy at what dose and what stage of disease with varied results. While awaiting sufficiently powered, properly designed and executed blinded randomized trials, many institutions have adopted escalated-dose prophylaxis in all or specific groups of hospitalized patients with COVID-19. Consensus documents have generally recommended following the available evidence-based medicine recommendations to avoid a widespread usage of higher than prophylactic-dose anticoagulation unless used as part of a research study.[136]

In general, the risk of VTE in hospitalized patients peaked earlier in the pandemic but fell later with the adoption of prophylactic anticoagulation. A large study of nationwide population-based Danish registries suggested that the VTE risk in hospitalized COVID-19 patients is low to moderate and is not significantly higher than the VTE risk in hospitalized SARS-CoV-2-negative and influenza patients.[137] The risk of VTE in the postdischarge period and in outpatient COVID-19 cases may be mildly elevated but much less than the risk in acutely ill and hospitalized patients.

Anticoagulation Strategies in COVID-19

The potential benefit from anticoagulation needs to be balanced against the increased risk of bleeding and thrombocytopenia. There has been a clear paucity of high-quality data and a need for randomized clinical trials to assess the appropriate approach to anticoagulation in various COVID-19 patient populations. A few large studies have addressed these questions.

A large, open-label, adaptive, multiplatform, randomized clinical trial tested therapeutic-dose anticoagulation with heparin vs. usual-care pharmacologic thromboprophylaxis in more than 1000 *critically ill* patients with severe COVID-19. This multiplatform study incorporated data from the Randomized, Embedded, Multifactorial Adaptive Platform Trial for Community-Acquired Pneumonia (REMAP-CAP), the Accelerating COVID-19 Therapeutic Interventions and Vaccines-4 Antithrombotics Inpatient platform trial (ACTIV-4a), and the Antithrombotic Therapy to Ameliorate Complications of COVID-19 (ATTACC) trial.[138] In critically ill COVID-19 patients, an initial strategy of therapeutic dose anticoagulation with heparin did not result in a greater likelihood of survival to hospital discharge or a greater number of days free of intensive care unit (ICU)–level cardiovascular or respiratory organ support when compared to usual-care pharmacologic thromboprophylaxis. The usual-care thromboprophylaxis was determined by the local treating physicians and included either standard low-dose thromboprophylaxis or enhanced intermediate-dose thromboprophylaxis. This trial was stopped early due to meeting futility criteria. Major bleeding happened more often in patients assigned to therapeutic anticoagulation than those assigned to pharmacologic thromboprophylaxis. Major bleeding was infrequent.

Another multiplatform trial by the ATTACC, ACTIV-4a, and REMAP-CAP investigators studied the role of therapeutic anticoagulation in *non-critically ill* hospitalized COVID-19 patients.[139] In this open-label, adaptive, randomized controlled trial, more than 2000 non-critically ill patients hospitalized for COVID-19 were randomized to a pragmatic strategy of therapeutic-dose anticoagulation with heparin vs. usual-care pharmacological thromboprophylaxis (determined by the treating physicians per local protocols). An initial strategy of therapeutic-dose anticoagulation with heparin increased the probability of survival to hospital discharge and reduced the need for organ support. This study was stopped early when therapeutic-dose anticoagulation met the pre-specified criteria of superiority for patients on therapeutic-dose anticoagulation irrespective of baseline D-dimer. Major bleeding occurred infrequently.

The Intermediate vs. Standard-Dose Prophylactic Anticoagulation in Critically-Ill Patients With COVID-19: An Open Label Randomized Controlled Trial (INSPIRATION) was a multicenter randomized trial that compared intermediate-dose (enoxaparin, 1 mg/kg daily) vs. standard-dose prophylactic anticoagulation (enoxaparin, 40 mg daily) in 600 adult patients admitted to the ICU with COVID-19.[140] On 30-day follow up, the primary efficacy outcome (a composite of venous or arterial thrombosis, treatment with extracorporeal membrane oxygenation, or mortality) showed no significant difference between the two groups.

Recommendations and living guidelines for prevention, diagnosis, and treatment of VTE are available (and continuously updated) on the websites of the American College of Cardiology (ACC), International Society on Thrombosis and Haemostasis (ISTH), American Society of Hematology (ASH), and American College of Chest Physicians (ACCP).

Angiotensin-Converting Enzyme Inhibitors and Angiotensin Receptor Blockers in the Setting of COVID-19

On discovery that SARS-CoV-2 uses ACE2 for host cell entry, concerns were raised regarding the potential for ACE inhibitors and ARBs to cause compensatory increases in expression of ACE2 and worsen prognosis among those with COVID-19. Observational studies evaluating outcomes associated with use of ACE inhibitors and ARBs among patients with confirmed COVID-19,[141,142] and RCTs comparing continuation or withdrawal of these agents among those hospitalized with COVID-19, showed no adverse effects on survival and other clinical outcomes.[143,144] Thus continuation of ACE inhibitors and ARBs during COVID-19 illness is recommended for patients treated with these medications.

Prevention of COVID-19: Vaccines

The discovery that neutralizing antibodies to SARS-CoV-2 primarily target the receptor binding domain of the S1 protein, also known as the spike protein, led to development of vaccine candidates within a year of release of the virus genome sequence. Several vaccines have been developed using nucleic acid platforms, non-replicating viral vectored platforms, inactivated virus, or recombinant subunit antigens. In the United States, the FDA has approved BNT162b2-mRNA (Pfizer-BioNTech) mRNA COVID-19 vaccine for people 12 years or older (two injections, 21 days apart) and has issued emergency use authorization for mRNA-1273 (Moderna) vaccine for people 18 years or older (two injections, 28 days apart). The Ad26.COV2.S (Johnson & Johnson's Janssen) vaccine utilizes a viral vector platform with a replication-incompetent recombinant adenovirus type 26 (Ad26) vector and has received an EUA for single-dose administration for people 18 years or older. The AZD1222 (Oxford/AstraZeneca) vaccine is a single injection vaccine that utilizes a viral vector platform with modified adenovirus ChAdOx1 and is used extensively outside of the United States. Gam-COVID-Vac (Sputnik V) is a heterologous recombinant adenovirus (rAd)-based vaccine. It uses vectors rAd26 and rAd5 (both carrying the gene for SARS-CoV-2 glycoprotein S) and is given intramuscularly over a 21-day interval. Other promising and widely used vaccines include CoronaVac (by Sinovac Life Sciences), which contains inactivated SARS-CoV-2 virus, BBV152 (by Bharat Biotech International), which contains whole-virion inactivated SARS-CoV-2, and inactivated adjuvanted BBIBP-CorV (by Sinopharm/BBIBP) vaccines. Multiple other vaccines with various mechanisms of action are under development and investigation.

Vaccines have demonstrated efficacy in reducing COVID-19 morbidity and mortality in randomized clinical trials and in real world studies. Their widespread use has led to significant decrease in incident cases of COVID-19.

As of July 2021, the CDC Vaccine Adverse Event Reporting System (VAERS) received over 1100 reports of myocarditis or pericarditis and confirmed about 70% of these, after receipt of COVID-19 vaccination (primarily mRNA vaccines). The European Economic Area (EEA) has also reported myocarditis cases both with mRNA vaccines and with the AstraZeneca vaccine. Cases have been reported predominantly in young adults, more often in men, and usually after the second dose of the vaccine. Myocarditis, detectable by cardiac magnetic resonance, typically occurs within 3 to 5 days after vaccination and presents with chest discomfort, abnormal ECG, and troponin elevation. Although the exact mechanism is unknown, it is likely immune-mediated and eosinophilic myocarditis has been reported with prior vaccines. The possible incidence of asymptomatic cases, risk factors, management, and long-term effects have yet to be determined. Overall, myocarditis after COVID-19 immunization appears to be rare (~24 per million second doses), often mild, and likely self-resolving in the majority of cases. Treatment is primarily supportive.[145,146]

Rare cases of severe thrombosis with thrombocytopenia have been reported, primarily with the adenovirus-based vaccines, and have been termed *vaccine-induced immune thrombocytopenia and thrombosis* (VITT).[147,148] This syndrome is characterized by arterial or venous thrombosis, and has been reported in the cerebral sinuses (see Fig. 45.2) and splanchnic vessels, among others, in association with mild to severe thrombocytopenia. The mechanism appears to be similar to heparin-induced thrombocytopenia [HIT], and antibodies to platelet factor 4 (PF4)–polyanion have been identified by enzyme-linked immunosorbent assay (ELISA). Most cases have occurred in women under age 50 without recent exposure to heparin, with a peak time of symptom onset of 6 to 14 days after vaccination; and up to one third of initial cases resulted in death. Treatment is similar to that of HIT, including IVIG or non-heparin anticoagulation, although responses to these treatments is uncertain.

Postacute Sequelae SARS-CoV-2 Infection

Certain patients infected with SARS-CoV-2 continue to have symptoms for weeks to months after seeming recovery from the acute phase of the disease. Early reports suggest that up to 10% of COVID-19 patients may experience the "Long COVID syndrome" or PASC. The PASC symptoms are highly variable in variety, severity, and duration.

Preliminary studies suggest that up to 30% of patients may report symptoms as long as 9 months after acute infection.[149] Most common symptoms include but are not limited to fatigue, a decline in functional capacity and exercise tolerance, shortness of breath, sleeping issues, and palpitations. Some patients describe difficulty thinking clearly ("brain fog"), anxiety, and/or depression. The exact predictors, duration, extent of cardiac (or other organs) involvement, and the potential effects of various treatments for PASC require extensive research that has already started.

REFERENCES

Influenza and Cardiovascular Disease

1. Krammer F, Smith GJD, Fouchier RAM, et al. Influenza. *Nat Rev Dis Primers*. 2018;4(1):3.
2. Webster RG, Bean WJ, Gorman OT, et al. Evolution and ecology of influenza a viruses. *Microbiol Rev*. 1992;56(1):152–179.
3. Smith GJ, Vijaykrishna D, Bahl J, et al. Origins and evolutionary genomics of the 2009 swine-origin H1N1 influenza a epidemic. *Nature*. 2009;459(7250):1122–1125.
4. Cohen SA, Chui KK, Naumova EN. Influenza vaccination in young children reduces influenza-associated hospitalizations in older adults, 2002-2006. *J Am Geriatr Soc*. 2011;59(2):327–332.
5. Thompson WW, Shay DK, Weintraub E, et al. Influenza-associated hospitalizations in the United States. *J Am Med Assoc*. 2004;292(11):1333–1340.
6. Smeeth L, Thomas SL, Hall AJ, et al. Risk of myocardial infarction and stroke after acute infection or vaccination. *New Engl J Med*. 2004;351(25):2611–2618.
7. Warren-Gash C, Smeeth L, Hayward AC. Influenza as a trigger for acute myocardial infarction or death from cardiovascular disease: a systematic review. *Lancet Infect Dis*. 2009;9(10):601–610.
8. Kwong JC, Schwartz KL, Campitelli MA, et al. Acute myocardial infarction after laboratory-confirmed influenza infection. *N Engl J Med*. 2018;378(4):345–353.
9. Sandoval C, Walter SD, Krueger P, et al. Risk of hospitalization during influenza season among a cohort of patients with congestive heart failure. *Epidemiol Infect*. 2007;135(4):574–582.
10. Kytomaa S, Hegde S, Claggett B, et al. Association of influenza-like illness activity with hospitalizations for heart failure: the Atherosclerosis risk in communities study. *JAMA Cardiol*. 2019;4(4):363–369.
11. Panhwar MS, Kalra A, Gupta T, et al. Effect of influenza on outcomes in patients with heart failure. *JACC Heart Fail*. 2019;7(2):112–117.
12. Bagai A, McNally BF, Al-Khatib SM, et al. Temporal differences in out-of-hospital cardiac arrest incidence and survival. *Circulation*. 2013;128(24):2595–2602.
13. Herlitz J, Eek M, Holmberg M, Holmberg S. Diurnal, weekly and seasonal rhythm of out of hospital cardiac arrest in Sweden. *Resuscitation*. 2002;54(2):133–138.
14. Madjid M, Connolly AT, Nabutovsky Y, et al. Effect of high influenza activity on risk of ventricular arrhythmias requiring therapy in patients with implantable cardiac defibrillators and cardiac resynchronization therapy defibrillators. *Am J Cardiol*. 2019;124(1):44–50.
15. Muller D, Lampe F, Wegscheider K, et al. Annual distribution of ventricular tachycardias and ventricular fibrillation. *Am Heart J*. 2003;146(6):1061–1065.
16. Loomba RS. Seasonal variation in paroxysmal atrial fibrillation: a systematic review. *J Atr Fibrillation*. 2015;7(5):1201.
17. Chang TY, Chao TF, Liu CJ, et al. The association between influenza infection, vaccination, and atrial fibrillation: a nationwide case-control study. *Heart Rhythm*. 2016;13(6):1189–1194.
18. Sellers SA, Hagan RS, Hayden FG, Fischer 2nd WA. The hidden burden of influenza: a review of the extra-pulmonary complications of influenza infection. *Influenza Other Respir Viruses*. 2017;11(5):372–393.
19. Haidari M, Wyde PR, Litovsky S, et al. Influenza virus directly infects, inflames, and resides in the arteries of atherosclerotic and normal mice. *Atherosclerosis*. 2010;208(1):90–96.
20. Naghavi M, Wyde P, Litovsky S, et al. Influenza infection exerts prominent inflammatory and thrombotic effects on the atherosclerotic plaques of apolipoprotein E-deficient mice. *Circulation*. 2003;107(5):762–768.
21. Lin YH, Platt M, Gilley RP, et al. Influenza causes MLKL-driven cardiac proteome remodeling during convalescence. *Circ Res*. 2021.
22. Metersky ML, Masterton RG, Lode H, et al. Epidemiology, microbiology, and treatment considerations for bacterial pneumonia complicating influenza. *Int J Infect Dis*. 2012;16(5):e321–e331.
23. Musher DM, Rueda AM, Kaka AS, Mapara SM. The association between pneumococcal pneumonia and acute cardiac events. *Clin Infect Dis*. 2007;45(2):158–165.
24. Ng MP, Lee JC, Loke WM, et al. Does influenza a infection increase oxidative damage? *Antioxid Redox Signal*. 2014;21(7):1025–1031.
25. Madjid M, Aboshady I, Awan I, et al. Influenza and cardiovascular disease: is there a causal relationship? *Tex Heart Inst J*. 2004;31(1):4–13.

Influenza Prevention and Therapy

26. Corrales-Medina VF, Madjid M, Musher DM. Role of acute infection in triggering acute coronary syndromes. *Lancet Infect Dis*. 2010;10(2):83–92.
27. Udell JA, Zawi R, Bhatt DL, et al. Association between influenza vaccination and cardiovascular outcomes in high-risk patients: a meta-analysis. *J Am Med Assoc*. 2013;310(16):1711–1720.
28. Mohseni H, Kiran A, Khorshidi R, Rahimi K. Influenza vaccination and risk of hospitalization in patients with heart failure: a self-controlled case series study. *Eur Heart J*. 2017;38(5):326–333.
29. Vardeny O, Claggett B, Udell JA, et al. Influenza vaccination in patients with chronic heart failure: the PARADIGM-HF trial. *JACC Heart Fail*. 2016;4(2):152–158.
30. Modin D, Jorgensen ME, Gislason G, et al. Influenza vaccine in heart failure. *Circulation*. 2019;139(5):575–586.
31. DiazGranados CA, Dunning AJ, Kimmel M, et al. Efficacy of high-dose versus standard-dose influenza vaccine in older adults. *New Engl J Med*. 2014;371(7):635–645.
32. DiazGranados CA, Robertson CA, Talbot HK, et al. Prevention of serious events in adults 65 years of age or older: a comparison between high-dose and standard-dose inactivated influenza vaccines. *Vaccine*. 2015;33(38):4988–4993.
33. Vardeny O, Kim K, Udell JA, et al. Effect of high-dose trivalent vs standard-dose quadrivalent influenza vaccine on mortality or cardiopulmonary hospitalization in patients with high-risk cardiovascular disease: a randomized clinical trial. *J Am Med Assoc*. 2021;325(1):39–49.

34. Casscells SW, Granger E, Kress AM, et al. Use of oseltamivir after influenza infection is associated with reduced incidence of recurrent adverse cardiovascular outcomes among military health system beneficiaries with prior cardiovascular diseases. *Circ Cardiovasc Qual Outcomes*. 2009;2(2):108–115.
35. Madjid M, Curkendall S, Blumentals WA. The influence of oseltamivir treatment on the risk of stroke after influenza infection. *Cardiology*. 2009;113(2):98–107.

Corona viruses

36. Madjid M, Safavi-Naeini P, Solomon SD, Vardeny O. Potential effects of coronaviruses on the cardiovascular system: a review. *JAMA Cardiol*. 2020.
37. Zhang S-F, Tuo J-L, Huang X-B, et al. Epidemiology characteristics of human coronaviruses in patients with respiratory infection symptoms and phylogenetic analysis of HCoV-OC43 during 2010-2015 in Guangzhou. *PloS One*. 2018;13(1):e0191789-e.
38. Fehr AR, Perlman S. Coronaviruses: an overview of their replication and pathogenesis. *Methods Mol Biol*. 2015;1282:1–23.
39. Li W, Hulswit RJG, Kenney SP, et al. Broad receptor engagement of an emerging global coronavirus may potentiate its diverse cross-species transmissibility. *Proc Nat Acad Sci USA*. 2018;115(22):E5135–E5143.
40. Chen N, Zhou M, Dong X, et al. Epidemiological and clinical characteristics of 99 cases of 2019 novel coronavirus pneumonia in Wuhan, China: a descriptive study. *Lancet*. 2020.
41. Berry M, Gamieldien J, Fielding BC. Identification of new respiratory viruses in the new millennium. *Viruses*. 2015;7(3):996–1019.
42. Li F. Structure, function, and evolution of coronavirus spike proteins. *Ann Review Virol*. 2016;3(1):237–261.
43. Su S, Wong G, Shi W, et al. Epidemiology, genetic recombination, and pathogenesis of coronaviruses. *Trends Microbiol*. 2016;24(6):490–502.
44. Peiris JS, Chu CM, Cheng VC, et al. Clinical progression and viral load in a community outbreak of coronavirus-associated SARS pneumonia: a prospective study. *Lancet*. 2003;361(9371):1767–1772.
45. Chong PY, Chui P, Ling AE, et al. Analysis of deaths during the Severe Acute Respiratory Syndrome (SARS) epidemic in Singapore: challenges in determining a SARS diagnosis. *Arch Pathol Lab Med*. 2004;128(2):195–204.
46. Yu CM, Wong RS, Wu EB, et al. Cardiovascular complications of severe acute respiratory syndrome. *Postgrad Med J*. 2006;82(964):140–144.
47. Mohd HA, Al-Tawfiq JA, Memish ZA. Middle East Respiratory Syndrome Coronavirus (MERS-CoV) origin and animal reservoir. *Virol J*. 2016;13(1):87. https://doi.org/10.1186/s12985-016-0544-0.
48. Mackay IM, Arden KE. MERS coronavirus: diagnostics, epidemiology and transmission. *Virol J*. 2015;12(1):222. https://doi.org/10.1186/s12985-015-0439-5.
49. Oh MD, Park WB, Park SW, et al. Middle East respiratory syndrome: what we learned from the 2015 outbreak in the Republic of Korea. *Korean J Intern Med*. 2018;33(2):233–246.
50. Badawi A, Ryoo SG. Prevalence of comorbidities in the Middle East Respiratory Syndrome Coronavirus (MERS-CoV): a systematic review and meta-analysis. *Int J Infect Dis*. 2016;49:129–133.

SARS-CoV-2 and COVID-19

51. Hu B, Guo H, Zhou P, Shi ZL. Characteristics of SARS-CoV-2 and COVID-19. *Nat Rev Microbiol*. 2020.
52. The Lancet Respiratory M. COVID-19 transmission-up in the air. *Lancet Respir Med*. 2020;8(12):1159.
53. Hindson J. COVID-19: faecal-oral transmission? *Nat Rev Gastroenterol Hepatol*. 2020;17(5):259.
54. Zou L, Ruan F, Huang M, et al. SARS-CoV-2 viral load in upper respiratory specimens of infected patients. *N Engl J Med*. 2020.
55. Yeo C, Kaushal S, Yeo D. Enteric involvement of coronaviruses: is faecal–oral transmission of SARS-CoV-2 possible? *Lancet Gastroenterol Hepatol*. 2020;5(4):335–337.
56. Holshue ML, DeBolt C, Lindquist S, et al. First case of 2019 novel coronavirus in the United States. *N Engl J Med*. 2020. https://doi.org/10.1056/NEJMoa2001191.
57. Mascola JR, Graham BS, Fauci AS. SARS-CoV-2 viral variants-tackling a moving target. *J Am Med Assoc*. 2021.
57a. Konings F, Perkins MD, Kuhn JH, et al. SARS-CoV-2 variants of interest and concern naming scheme conducive for global discourse. *Nat Microbiol*. 2021;6:821–823.
58. Schiffrin EL, Flack JM, Ito S, et al. Hypertension and COVID-19. *Am J Hypertens*. 2020;33(5): 373–374.
59. Hendren NS, de Lemos JA, Ayers C, et al. Association of body mass index and age with morbidity and mortality in patients hospitalized with COVID-19: results from the American Heart Association COVID-19 cardiovascular disease registry. *Circulation*. 2021;143(2):135–144.
60. Al-Benna S. Association of high level gene expression of ACE2 in adipose tissue with mortality of COVID-19 infection in obese patients. *Obes Med*. 2020;19:100283.
61. Rentsch CT, Kidwai-Khan F, Tate JP, et al. Patterns of COVID-19 testing and mortality by race and ethnicity among United States veterans: a nationwide cohort study. *PLoS Med*. 2020;17(9):e1003379.
62. Gross CP, Essien UR, Pasha S, et al. Racial and ethnic disparities in population-level Covid-19 mortality. *J Gen Intern Med*. 2020;35(10):3097–3099.
63. Price-Haywood EG, Burton J, Fort D, Seoane L. Hospitalization and mortality among Black patients and white patients with Covid-19. *New Engl J Med*. 2020;382(26):2534–2543.
64. Selden TM, Berdahl TA. COVID-19 and racial/ethnic disparities in health risk, employment, and household composition. *Health Aff*. 2020;39(9):1624–1632.

Cardiovascular Complications of COVID-19

65. Choudry FA, Hamshere SM, Rathod KS, et al. High thrombus burden in patients with COVID-19 presenting with ST-segment elevation myocardial infarction. *J Am Coll Cardiol*. 2020;76(10):1168–1176.
66. Modin D, Claggett B, Sindet-Pedersen C, et al. Acute COVID-19 and the incidence of ischemic stroke and acute myocardial infarction. *Circulation*. 2020;142(21):2080–2082.
67. Sala S, Peretto G, Gramegna M, et al. Acute myocarditis presenting as a reverse Tako-Tsubo syndrome in a patient with SARS-CoV-2 respiratory infection. *Eur Heart J*. 2020;41(19):1861–1862.
68. Rey JR, Caro-Codón J, Rosillo SO, et al. Heart failure in COVID-19 patients: prevalence, incidence and prognostic implications. *Eur J Heart Fail*. 2020;22(12):2205–2215.
69. Bhatt AS, Jering KS, Vaduganathan M, et al. Clinical outcomes in patients with heart failure hospitalized with COVID-19. *JACC Heart Fail*. 2021;9(1):65–73.
70. Dherange P, Lang J, Qian P, et al. Arrhythmias and COVID-19: a review. *JACC Clin Electrophysiol*. 2020;6(9):1193–1204.
71. Gopinathannair R, Merchant FM, Lakkireddy DR, et al. COVID-19 and cardiac arrhythmias: a global perspective on arrhythmia characteristics and management strategies. *J Interv Card Electrophysiol*. 2020;59(2):329–336.
72. Baldi E, Sechi GM, Mare C, et al. Out-of-Hospital cardiac arrest during the Covid-19 outbreak in Italy. *N Engl J Med*. 2020;383(5):496–498.
73. Goyal P, Choi JJ, Pinheiro LC, et al. Clinical characteristics of Covid-19 in New York city. *N Engl J Med*. 2020;382(24):2372–2374.
74. Bhatla A, Mayer MM, Adusumalli S, et al. COVID-19 and cardiac arrhythmias. *Heart Rhythm*. 2020;17(9):1439–1444.
75. Musikantow DR, Turagam MK, Sartori S, et al. Atrial fibrillation in patients hospitalized with COVID-19: incidence, predictors, outcomes and comparison to influenza. *JACC: Clinical Electrophysiology*. 2021.
76. Suh YJ, Hong H, Ohana M, Bompard F, et al. Pulmonary embolism and deep vein thrombosis in COVID-19: a systematic review and meta-analysis. *Radiology*. 2021;298(2):E70–E80.
77. Bilaloglu S, Aphinyanaphongs Y, Jones S, et al. Thrombosis in hospitalized patients with COVID-19 in a New York city health system. *J Am Med Assoc*. 2020;324(8):799–801.
78. Whittaker E, Bamford A, Kenny J, et al. Clinical characteristics of 58 children with a pediatric inflammatory multisystem syndrome temporally associated with SARS-CoV-2. *J Am Med Assoc*. 2020;324(3):259–269.
79. Valverde I, Singh Y, Sanchez-de-Toledo J, et al. Acute cardiovascular manifestations in 286 children with multisystem inflammatory syndrome associated with COVID-19 infection in Europe. *Circulation*. 2021;143(1):21–32.
80. Feldstein LR, Tenforde MW, Friedman KG, et al. Characteristics and outcomes of US children and adolescents with Multisystem Inflammatory Syndrome in Children (MIS-C) compared with severe acute COVID-19. *J Am Med Assoc*. 2021;325(11):1074–1087.
81. Lala A, Johnson KW, Januzzi JL, et al. Prevalence and impact of myocardial injury in patients hospitalized with COVID-19 infection. *J Am Coll Cardiol*. 2020;76(5):533–546.
82. Sandoval Y, Januzzi Jr JL, Jaffe AS. Cardiac troponin for the diagnosis and risk-stratification of myocardial injury in COVID-19: JACC review topic of the week. *J Am Coll Cardiol*. 2020. https://doi.org/10.1016/j.jacc.2020.06.068.
83. Kong N, Singh N, Mazzone S, et al. Takotsubo's syndrome presenting as cardiogenic shock in patients with COVID-19: a case-series and review of current literature. *Cardiovasc Revasc Med*. 2021.
84. Libby P. The heart in COVID-19: primary target or secondary bystander? *JACC Basic Transl Sci*. 2020;5(5):537–542.
85. Guo T, Fan Y, Chen M, et al. Cardiovascular implications of fatal outcomes of patients with Coronavirus Disease 2019 (COVID-19). *JAMA Cardiol*. 2020;5(7):811–818.
86. Shi S, Qin M, Shen B, et al. Association of cardiac injury with mortality in hospitalized patients with COVID-19 in Wuhan, China. *JAMA Cardiol*. 2020.
87. Lombardi CM, Carubelli V, Iorio A, et al. Association of troponin levels with mortality in Italian patients hospitalized with coronavirus disease 2019: results of a multicenter study. *JAMA Cardiol*. 2020;5(11):1274–1280.
88. Short SAP, Gupta S, Brenner SK, et al. D-dimer and death in critically ill patients with coronavirus disease 2019. *Crit Care Med*. 2021.
89. Szekely Y, Lichter Y, Taieb P, et al. Spectrum of cardiac manifestations in COVID-19: a systematic echocardiographic study. *Circulation*. 2020;142(4):342–353.
90. Puntmann VO, Carerj ML, Wieters I, et al. Outcomes of cardiovascular magnetic resonance imaging in patients recently recovered from Coronavirus Disease 2019 (COVID-19). *JAMA Cardiol*. 2020;5(11):1265–1273.
91. Garcia S, Albaghdadi MS, Meraj PM, et al. Reduction in ST-segment elevation cardiac catheterization laboratory activations in the United States during COVID-19 pandemic. *J Am Coll Cardiol*. 2020;75(22):2871–2872.
92. Solomon MD, McNulty EJ, Rana JS, et al. The Covid-19 pandemic and the incidence of acute myocardial infarction. *N Engl J Med*. 2020;383(7):691–693.
93. De Filippo O, D'Ascenzo F, Angelini F, et al. Reduced rate of hospital admissions for ACS during Covid-19 outbreak in northern Italy. *N Engl J Med*. 2020;383(1):88–89.
94. Mafham MM, Spata E, Goldacre R, et al. COVID-19 pandemic and admission rates for and management of acute coronary syndromes in England. *Lancet*. 2020;396(10248):381–389.
95. Campo G, Fortuna D, Berti E, et al. In- and out-of-hospital mortality for myocardial infarction during the first wave of the COVID-19 pandemic in Emilia-Romagna, Italy: a population-based observational study. *The Lancet Regional Health - Europe*. 221;3(100055).
96. Srivastava PK, Zhang S, Xian Y, et al. Acute ischemic stroke in patients with COVID-19: an analysis from get with the guidelines-stroke. *Stroke*. 2021;52(5):1826–1829.
97. Giustino G, Pinney SP, Lala A, et al. Coronavirus and cardiovascular disease, myocardial injury, and arrhythmia: JACC focus seminar. *J Am Coll Cardiol*. 2020;76(17):2011–2023.
98. Sakamoto A, Kawakami R, Kawai K, et al. ACE2 (Angiotensin-Converting Enzyme 2) and TMPRSS2 (Transmembrane Serine Protease 2) expression and localization of SARS-CoV-2 infection in the human heart. *Arterioscler Thromb Vasc Biol*. 2021;41(1):542–544.
99. Ackermann M, Verleden SE, Kuehnel M, et al. Pulmonary vascular endothelialitis, thrombosis, and angiogenesis in Covid-19. *N Engl J Med*. 2020;383(2):120–128.
100. Wichmann D, Sperhake JP, Lutgehetmann M, et al. Autopsy findings and venous thromboembolism in patients with COVID-19: a prospective cohort study. *Ann Intern Med*. 2020;173(4):268–277.
101. Buja LM, Wolf DA, Zhao B, et al. The emerging spectrum of cardiopulmonary pathology of the coronavirus disease 2019 (COVID-19): report of 3 autopsies from Houston, Texas, and review of autopsy findings from other United States cities. *Cardiovasc Pathol*. 2020;48:107233.
102. Roshdy A, Zaher S, Fayed H, Coghlan JG. COVID-19 and the heart: a systematic review of cardiac autopsies. *Front Cardiovasc Med*. 2021;7:626975.
103. Halushka MK, Vander Heide RS. Myocarditis is rare in COVID-19 autopsies: cardiovascular findings across 277 postmortem examinations. *Cardiovasc Pathol*. 2021;50:107300.
104. Escher F, Pietsch H, Aleshcheva G, et al. Detection of viral SARS-CoV-2 genomes and histopathological changes in endomyocardial biopsies. *ESC Heart Fail*. 2020;7(5):2440–2447.
105. Lindner D, Fitzek A, Bräuninger H, et al. Association of cardiac infection with SARS-CoV-2 in confirmed COVID-19 autopsy cases. *JAMA Cardiol*. 2020;5(11):1281–1285.
106. Pellegrini D, Kawakami R, Guagliumi G, et al. Microthrombi as a major cause of cardiac injury in COVID-19: a pathologic study. *Circulation*. 2021.
107. Guagliumi G, Sonzogni A, Pescetelli I, et al. Microthrombi and ST-segment-elevation myocardial infarction in COVID-19. *Circulation*. 2020;142(8):804–809.
108. Guan WJ, Ni ZY, Hu Y, et al. Clinical characteristics of coronavirus disease 2019 in China. *New Eng J Med*. 2020;58(4):711–712.
109. Fajgenbaum DC, June CH. Cytokine storm. *N Engl J Med*. 2020;383(23):2255–2273.
110. Del Valle DM, Kim-Schulze S, Huang HH, et al. An inflammatory cytokine signature predicts COVID-19 severity and survival. *Nat Med*. 2020;26(10):1636–1643.
111. Xu ZS, Shu T, Kang L, et al. Temporal profiling of plasma cytokines, chemokines and growth factors from mild, severe and fatal COVID-19 patients. *Signal Transduct Target Ther*. 2020;5(1):100.
112. Chen Y, Wang J, Liu C, et al. IP-10 and MCP-1 as biomarkers associated with disease severity of COVID-19. *Mol Med*. 2020;26(1):97.
113. Zizzo G, Cohen PL. Imperfect storm: is interleukin-33 the Achilles heel of COVID-19? *Lancet Rheumatol*. 2020;2(12):e779–e790.
114. Ye Q, Wang B, Mao J. The pathogenesis and treatment of the 'Cytokine Storm' in COVID-19. *J Infect*. 2020;80(6):607–613.
115. Hojyo S, Uchida M, Tanaka K, et al. How COVID-19 induces cytokine storm with high mortality. *Inflamm Regen*. 2020;40:37.
116. Libby P, Luscher T. COVID-19 is, in the end, an endothelial disease. *Eur Heart J*. 2020;41(32):3038–3044.
117. Mehta P, Porter JC, Manson JJ, et al. Therapeutic blockade of granulocyte macrophage colony-stimulating factor in COVID-19-associated hyperinflammation: challenges and opportunities. *Lancet Respir Med*. 2020;8(8):822–830.
118. Sinha P, Matthay MA, Calfee CS. Is a "cytokine storm" relevant to COVID-19? *JAMA Intern Med*. 2020;180(9):1152–1154.
119. Tang L, Yin Z, Hu Y, Mei H. Controlling cytokine storm is vital in COVID-19. *Front Immunol*. 2020;11:570993.
120. Quirch M, Lee J, Rehman S. Hazards of the cytokine storm and cytokine-targeted therapy in patients with COVID-19: review. *J Med Internet Res*. 2020;22(8):e20193.

121. Cron RQ, Schulert GS, Tattersall RS. Defining the scourge of COVID-19 hyperinflammatory syndrome. *Lancet Rheumatol*. 2020;2(12):e727–e729.
122. Brinkmann V, Reichard U, Goosmann C, et al. Neutrophil extracellular traps kill bacteria. *Science*. 2004;303(5663):1532–1535.
123. Ng H, Havervall S, Rosell A, et al. Circulating markers of neutrophil extracellular traps are of prognostic value in patients with COVID-19. *Arterioscler Thromb Vasc Biol*. 2020: ATVBAHA120315267.
124. Blasco A, Coronado M-J, Hernández-Terciado F, et al. Assessment of neutrophil extracellular traps in coronary thrombus of a case series of patients with COVID-19 and myocardial infarction. *JAMA Cardiol*. 2020;6(4):1–6.
125. Middleton EA, He X-Y, Denorme F, et al. Neutrophil extracellular traps contribute to immunothrombosis in COVID-19 acute respiratory distress syndrome. *Blood*. 2020;136(10):1169–1179.
126. Hidalgo A. A NET-thrombosis axis in COVID-19. *Blood*. 2020;136(10):1118–1119.
127. Folco EJ, Mawson TL, Vromman A, et al. Neutrophil extracellular traps induce endothelial cell activation and tissue factor production through interleukin-1alpha and cathepsin G. *Arterioscler Thromb Vasc Biol*. 2018;38(8):1901–1912.
128. Marcus AJ, Broekman MJ, Drosopoulos JH, et al. The endothelial cell ecto-ADPase responsible for inhibition of platelet function is CD39. *J Clin Invest*. 1997;99(6):1351–1360.
129. Gupta RM, Libby P, Barton M. Linking regulation of nitric oxide to endothelin-1: the Yin and Yang of vascular tone in the atherosclerotic plaque. *Atherosclerosis*. 2020;292:201–203.
130. Wagner DD. The Weibel-Palade body: the storage granule for von Willebrand factor and P-selectin. *Thromb Haemost*. 1993;70(1):105–110.

Management of COVID-19

131. Goldman JD, Lye DCB, Hui DS, et al. Remdesivir for 5 or 10 Days in patients with severe Covid-19. *New Engl J Med*. 2020;383(19):1827–1837.
132. Gottlieb RL, Nirula A, Chen P, et al. Effect of bamlanivimab as monotherapy or in combination with etesevimab on viral load in patients with mild to moderate COVID-19: a randomized clinical trial. *J Am Med Assoc*. 2021;325(7):632–644.
133. Weinreich DM, Sivapalasingam S, Norton T, et al. REGN-COV2, a neutralizing antibody cocktail, in outpatients with Covid-19. *New Engl J Med*. 2020;384(3):238–251.
134. RECOVERY Collaborative Group, Horby P, Lim WS, et al. Dexamethasone in hospitalized patients with Covid-19. *New Engl J Med*. 2021;384(8):693–704.
135. Sterne JAC, Diaz J, Villar J, et al. Corticosteroid therapy for critically ill patients with COVID-19: a structured summary of a study protocol for a prospective meta-analysis of randomized trials. *Trials*. 2020;21(1):734.
136. Moores LK, Tritschler T, Brosnahan S, et al. Prevention, diagnosis, and treatment of VTE in patients with coronavirus disease 2019: CHEST guideline and expert panel report. *Chest*. 2020;158(3):1143–1163.
137. Dalager-Pedersen M, Lund LC, Mariager T, et al. Venous thromboembolism and major bleeding in patients with COVID-19: a nationwide population-based cohort study. [published online ahead of print January 5, 2021]. *Clin Infect Dis*. https://doi.org/10.1093/cid/ciab003
138. The REMAP-CAP, ACTIV-4a, and ATTACC Investigators. Therapeutic anticoagulation with heparin in critically ill patients with Covid-19. *N Engl J Med*. https://doi.org/10.1056/NEJMoa2103417.
139. The ATTACC, ACTIV-4a, and REMAP-CAP Investigators. Therapeutic anticoagulation with heparin in noncritically ill patients with Covid-19. *N Engl J Med*. https://doi.org/10.1056/NEJMoa2105911.
140. INSPIRATION Investigators, Sadeghipour P, Talasaz AH, Rashidi F, et al. Effect of intermediate-dose vs standard-dose prophylactic anticoagulation on thrombotic events, extracorporeal membrane oxygenation treatment, or mortality among patients with COVID-19 admitted to the intensive care unit: The INSPIRATION randomized clinical trial. *JAMA*. 2021;325(16):1620–1630.
141. Reynolds HR, Adhikari S, Pulgarin C, et al. Renin-angiotensin-aldosterone system inhibitors and risk of Covid-19. *New Engl J Med*. 2020;382(25):2441–2448.
142. Mancia G, Rea F, Ludergnani M, et al. Renin-angiotensin-aldosterone system blockers and the risk of Covid-19. *New Engl J Med*. 2020;382(25):2431–2440.
143. Lopes RD, Macedo AVS, de Barros ESPGM, et al. Effect of discontinuing vs continuing angiotensin-converting enzyme inhibitors and angiotensin II receptor blockers on days alive and out of the hospital in patients admitted with COVID-19: a randomized clinical trial. *J Am Med Assoc*. 2021;325(3):254–264.
144. Cohen JB, Hanff TC, William P, et al. Continuation versus discontinuation of renin-angiotensin system inhibitors in patients admitted to hospital with COVID-19: a prospective, randomised, open-label trial. *Lancet Respir Med*. 2021;9(3):275–284.
145. Diaz GA, Parsons GT, Gering SK, et al. Myocarditis and pericarditis after vaccination for COVID-19. *JAMA*. 2021 Aug 4:e2113443.
146. Montgomery J, Ryan M, Engler R, et al. Myocarditis following immunization with mRNA COVID-19 vaccines in members of the US military. *JAMA Cardiol*. Published online June 29, 2021. https://doi.org/10.1001/jamacardio.2021.2833.
147. Pavord S, Scully M, Hunt BJ, et al. Clinical features of vaccine-induced immune thrombocytopenia and thrombosis. *N Engl J Med*. 2021. https://doi.org/10.1056/NEJMoa2109908. Epub ahead of print. PMID: 34379914.
148. Rizk JG, Gupta A, Sardar P, et al. Clinical characteristics and pharmacological management of COVID-19 vaccine-induced immune thrombotic thrombocytopenia with cerebral venous sinus thrombosis: a review. *JAMA Cardiol*. 2021. https://doi.org/10.1001/jamacardio.2021.3444. Epub ahead of print. PMID: 34374713.
149. Logue JK, Franko NM, McCulloch DJ, et al. Sequelae in adults at 6 months after COVID-19 infection. *JAMA Network Open*. 2021;4(2):e210830-e.

95 Hemostasis, Thrombosis, Fibrinolysis, and Cardiovascular Disease

JEFFREY I. WEITZ

HEMOSTATIC SYSTEM, 1766
Vascular Endothelium, 1766
Platelets, 1767
Coagulation, 1769
Fibrinolytic System, 1770

THROMBOSIS, 1771
Arterial Thrombosis, 1772
Venous Thrombosis, 1772
Inherited Hypercoagulable States, 1772
Acquired Hypercoagulable States, 1773

TREATMENT OF THROMBOSIS, 1775
Antiplatelet Drugs, 1775
Anticoagulants, 1779
Fibrinolytic Drugs, 1787

FUTURE PERSPECTIVES, 1789

REFERENCES, 1789

Hemostasis preserves vascular integrity by balancing the physiologic processes that maintain blood fluidity under normal circumstances and prevent excessive bleeding after vascular injury. Preservation of blood fluidity depends on an intact vascular endothelium and a complex series of regulatory pathways that maintain platelets in a quiescent state and keep the coagulation system in check. In contrast, arrest of bleeding requires rapid formation of hemostatic plugs at sites of vascular injury to prevent exsanguination. Perturbation of hemostasis can lead to thrombosis, which can occur in arteries or veins and causes considerable morbidity and mortality. Arterial thrombosis is the most common cause of acute coronary syndrome, ischemic stroke, and limb gangrene, whereas thrombosis in the deep veins of the leg leads to postthrombotic syndrome and pulmonary embolism (see also Chapter 87).

Most arterial thrombi form on top of disrupted atherosclerotic plaques because plaque rupture exposes thrombogenic material in the core to blood (see also Chapters 24 and 37). This material then triggers platelet aggregation and fibrin formation, which results in the generation of a platelet-rich thrombus that temporarily or permanently occludes blood flow.[1] The consequent reduction in blood flow can cause acute coronary syndrome, transient ischemic attack, ischemic stroke, or acute limb ischemia.

In contrast to arterial thrombi, venous thrombi rarely form at sites of obvious vascular disruption.[2] Although venous thrombi can develop after surgical trauma to veins or arise due to indwelling venous catheters, they usually originate in valve cusps of the deep veins of the calf or in muscular sinuses, where there is stasis. Sluggish blood flow in these veins reduces oxygen supply to the avascular valve cusps. Hypoxemia induces endothelial cells lining the valve cusps to express adhesion molecules, which tether tissue factor–bearing leukocytes and microparticles onto their surface. The tissue factor then induces coagulation.[3] In addition, webs of chromatin released from activated neutrophils, called neutrophil extracellular traps (NETs), also contribute to thrombosis by providing a scaffold that binds platelets and promotes their activation and aggregation and by activating the contact system of coagulation.[4] Impaired blood flow exacerbates local thrombus formation by reducing clearance of activated clotting factors. Thrombi that extend into the proximal veins of the leg can dislodge and travel to the lungs to produce pulmonary embolism.

Arterial and venous thrombi contain platelets and fibrin, but the proportions differ. Arterial thrombi are rich in platelets because of high shear in the injured arteries.[1] In contrast, venous thrombi, which form under low-shear conditions, contain relatively few platelets and consist mostly of fibrin and trapped red cells.[2] Because of the predominance of platelets, arterial thrombi appear white, whereas venous thrombi appear red because of the trapped red cells.

The antithrombotic drugs used for prevention and treatment of thrombosis target components of thrombi and include antiplatelet drugs, which inhibit platelets; anticoagulants, which attenuate coagulation; and fibrinolytic agents, which induce fibrin degradation (Fig. 95.1). With the predominance of platelets in arterial thrombi, strategies to inhibit or treat arterial thrombosis focus mainly on antiplatelet agents, although in the acute setting, anticoagulants and fibrinolytic agents may also be used. For occlusive arterial thrombi that require rapid restoration of blood flow, mechanical and/or pharmacologic methods enable thrombus extraction, compression, or degradation. Although rarely used for this indication, warfarin prevents recurrent ischemic events after acute myocardial infarction. The observations that the addition of low-dose rivaroxaban, an oral factor Xa inhibitor, to dual-antiplatelet therapy reduces recurrent ischemic events and stent thrombosis in patients with acute coronary syndrome, whereas its addition to aspirin reduces the risk of major adverse coronary and limb events in patients with stable coronary or peripheral artery disease, highlight the potential usefulness of anticoagulants on top of antiplatelet agents for secondary prevention (see also Chapters 40 and 43).[5,6]

Anticoagulants are the mainstay for prevention and treatment of venous thromboembolism (VTE), which includes deep vein thrombosis and pulmonary embolism.[2] Antiplatelet drugs are less effective than anticoagulants for prevention of venous thrombosis because of the limited platelet content of venous thrombi. Nonetheless, when given for secondary prevention, aspirin produces about a 30% reduction in risk for recurrent VTE,[7] a finding that highlights the overlap between venous and arterial thrombosis. Selected patients with VTE benefit from fibrinolytic therapy[2]; for example, patients with massive pulmonary embolism achieve more rapid restoration of pulmonary blood flow with systemic or catheter-directed fibrinolytic therapy than with anticoagulant therapy alone (see Chapter 87). Similarly, some patients with extensive iliac and/or femoral vein thrombosis may have a better outcome with catheter-directed fibrinolytic therapy and/or mechanical thrombus extraction in addition to anticoagulants.

This chapter reviews hemostasis and thrombosis and highlights the processes involved in platelet activation and aggregation, blood coagulation, and fibrinolysis. It reviews the major components of the hemostatic system: the vascular endothelium, platelets, and coagulation and fibrinolytic systems. The chapter then focuses on antiplatelet, anticoagulant, and fibrinolytic drugs in common use. It also provides a brief overview of new antithrombotic drugs in advanced stages of development.

HEMOSTATIC SYSTEM

Vascular Endothelium (see also Chapter 24)

A monolayer of endothelial cells lines the intimal surface of the circulatory tree and separates blood from the prothrombotic subendothelial components of the vessel wall. Accordingly, the vascular endothelium encompasses about 10^{13} cells and covers a vast surface area. Rather

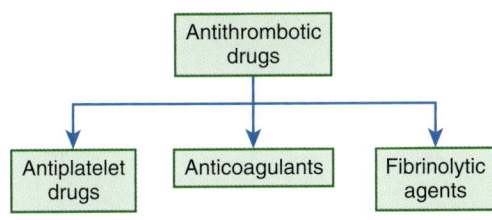

FIGURE 95.1 Classification of antithrombotic drugs.

than serving as a static barrier, healthy vascular endothelium dynamically regulates hemostasis by inhibiting platelets, suppressing coagulation, and promoting fibrinolysis.

Platelet Inhibition

Endothelial cells synthesize prostacyclin and nitric oxide and release them into blood. These mediators not only serve to potently vasodilate but also inhibit platelet activation and subsequent aggregation by stimulating adenylate cyclase and increasing intracellular levels of cyclic adenosine monophosphate (cAMP). In addition, endothelial cells express the ecto-adenosine diphosphatase (ecto-ADPase) CD39 on their surface. This membrane-associated enzyme attenuates platelet activation by degrading ADP.[8]

Anticoagulant Activity

Intact endothelial cells actively regulate thrombin generation. Endothelial cells express heparan sulfate proteoglycans on their surface. Like medicinal heparin, heparan sulfate binds circulating antithrombin and enhances its activity. Heparan sulfate proteoglycans also bind tissue factor pathway inhibitor (TFPI), a naturally occurring inhibitor of coagulation.[9] Additional TFPI becomes tethered to the endothelial cell surface via glycosylphosphatidylinositol anchors. Administration of heparin or low-molecular-weight heparin (LMWH) displaces glycosaminoglycan-bound TFPI from the vascular endothelium, and the released TFPI may contribute to the antithrombotic activity of these drugs by inhibiting tissue factor–bound factor VIIa in a factor Xa–dependent manner.

Endothelial cells are central to the protein C anticoagulant pathway because they express thrombomodulin and endothelial cell protein C receptor (EPCR) on their surfaces.[10] The protein C pathway is initiated when thrombin binds to thrombomodulin. Once bound, the substrate specificity of thrombin is altered such that it no longer acts as a procoagulant but becomes a potent activator of protein C (Fig. 95.2). Activated protein C serves as an anticoagulant by degrading and inactivating activated factor V and factor VIII (factors Va and VIIIa, respectively), key cofactors involved in thrombin generation, in reactions enhanced by protein S. EPCR on the endothelial cell surface promotes this pathway about 20-fold by binding protein C and presenting it to the thrombin-thrombomodulin complex for activation. In addition to its role as an anticoagulant, activated protein C also regulates inflammation and preserves the barrier function of the endothelium.[10]

Fibrinolytic Activity

The vascular endothelium modulates fibrinolysis by synthesizing and releasing tissue and urokinase plasminogen activators (t-PA and u-PA, respectively), which initiate fibrinolysis by converting plasminogen to plasmin.[11] Whereas endothelial cells constitutively express t-PA, they produce u-PA in the settings of inflammation and wound repair. Endothelial cells also produce type 1 plasminogen activator inhibitor (PAI-1), the major regulator of both t-PA and u-PA. Therefore, net fibrinolytic activity depends on the dynamic balance between the release of plasminogen activators and PAI-1. Fibrinolysis localizes to the endothelial cell surface because these cells express annexin II, a coreceptor for plasminogen and t-PA that promotes their interaction. Hence, healthy vessels actively resist thrombosis and help maintain platelets in a quiescent state.[11]

Platelets

Platelets enter the circulation after the fragmentation of bone marrow megakaryocytes. Because they lack nuclei, platelets have a limited

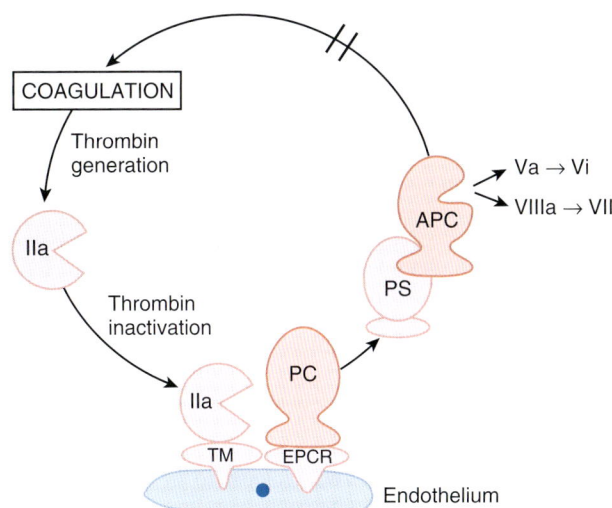

FIGURE 95.2 Protein C pathway. Activation of coagulation triggers thrombin (IIa) generation. Excess thrombin binds to thrombomodulin (TM) on the endothelial cell surface. Once bound, the substrate specificity of thrombin is altered such that it no longer acts as a procoagulant but becomes a potent activator of protein C (PC). The endothelial cell protein C receptor (EPCR) binds protein C and presents it to thrombomodulin-bound thrombin for activation. Activated protein C (APC), together with its cofactor protein S (PS), binds to the activated platelet surface and proteolytically degrades factors Va and VIIIa into inactive fragments (Vi and VIIIi). Degradation of these activated cofactors inhibits thrombin generation (double bar).

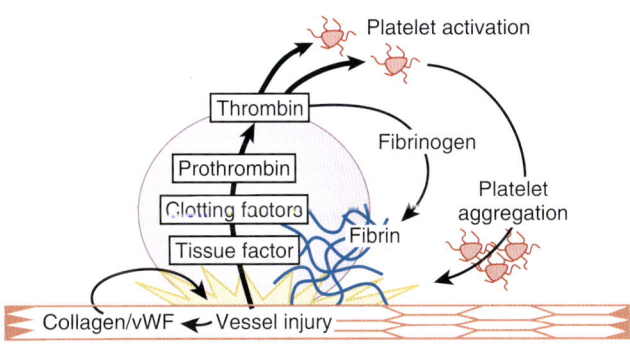

FIGURE 95.3 Central role of thrombin in thrombogenesis. Vascular injury simultaneously triggers platelet adhesion and activation, as well as activation of the coagulation system. Platelet activation is initiated by exposure of subendothelial collagen and von Willebrand factor (vWF), onto which platelets adhere. Adherent platelets become activated and release ADP and thromboxane A_2, platelet agonists that activate ambient platelets and recruit them to the site of injury. Coagulation, which is triggered by tissue factor exposed at the site of injury and enhanced by assembly of clotting factor complexes on the activated platelet surface, results in thrombin generation. Thrombin not only converts fibrinogen to fibrin but also serves as a potent platelet agonist. When platelets are activated, glycoprotein (GP) IIb/IIIa on their surfaces undergoes a conformational change that endows it with the capacity to ligate fibrinogen and mediate platelet aggregation. Fibrin strands then weave the platelet aggregates together to form a platelet/fibrin thrombus.

capacity to synthesize proteins. Thrombopoietin, a glycoprotein synthesized in the liver and kidneys, regulates megakaryocytic proliferation and maturation, as well as platelet production.[12] Once they enter the circulation, platelets have a life span of 7 to 10 days.

Damage to the intimal lining of the vessel exposes the underlying subendothelial matrix. Platelets home to sites of vascular disruption and adhere to the exposed matrix proteins.[13] Adherent platelets undergo activation and not only release substances that recruit additional platelets to the site of injury, but also promote thrombin generation and subsequent fibrin formation (Fig. 95.3). A potent platelet agonist, thrombin amplifies platelet recruitment and activation. Activated platelets then aggregate to form a plug that seals the leak in the vasculature. An understanding of the steps in these highly integrated processes helps pinpoint the sites of action of antiplatelet drugs and rationalizes the usefulness of anticoagulants for the treatment of arterial and venous thrombosis.

Adhesion

Platelets adhere to exposed collagen and von Willebrand factor (vWF) and form a monolayer that supports and promotes thrombin generation and subsequent fibrin formation.[13] These events depend on constitutively expressed receptors on the platelet surface, $\alpha_2\beta_1$ and glycoprotein VI (GP VI), which bind collagen, and GP Ibα and GP IIb/IIIa ($\alpha_{IIb}\beta_3$), which bind vWF. Receptors crowd the platelet surface, but those involved in adhesion are the most abundant. Each platelet has approximately 80,000 copies of GP IIb/IIIa and 25,000 copies of GP Ibα. Receptors cluster in cholesterol-enriched subdomains, which render them more mobile, thereby increasing the efficiency of platelet adhesion and subsequent activation.[1,2]

Under low-shear conditions, collagen can capture and activate platelets on its own. The captured platelets undergo cytoskeletal reorganization, which causes them to flatten out and adhere more closely to the damaged vessel wall. Under high-shear conditions, however, collagen and vWF must act in concert to support optimal platelet adhesion and activation. The vWF synthesized by endothelial cells and megakaryocytes assembles into multimers that range in size from 550 kDa to greater than 10,000 kDa.[1,14] Proteolytic processing of newly secreted vWF by the metalloproteinase ADAMTS13 (A Disintegrin-like And Metalloprotease with ThromboSpondin type 1 motif 13) reduces vWF multimer size, thereby preventing the accumulation of unusually large multimers. Deficiency of ADAMTS13 such as occurs with thrombotic thrombocytopenic purpura (TTP) results in microvascular thrombosis because these exceptionally large vWF multimers tether platelets to the endothelium.

When released from storage in the Weibel-Palade bodies of endothelial cells or the alpha-granules of platelets, most of the vWF enters the circulation, but the vWF released from the abluminal surface of endothelial cells accumulates in the subendothelial matrix, where it binds collagen via its A3 domain.[15] This surface-immobilized vWF can simultaneously bind platelets via its A1 domain. In contrast, circulating vWF does not react with unstimulated platelets. This difference in reactivity reflects the conformation of vWF; circulating vWF is in a coiled conformation, which prevents access of its platelet-binding domain to vWF receptors on the platelet surface, whereas immobilized vWF assumes an elongated shape, which exposes the platelet-binding A1 domain. In their extended conformation, large vWF multimers act as the molecular glue that tethers platelets to the damaged vessel wall with sufficient strength to withstand a higher shear force. Large vWF multimers provide additional binding sites for collagen and heighten platelet adhesion because platelets have more vWF receptors than collagen receptors.

Activation

Adhesion to collagen and vWF initiates signaling pathways that result in platelet activation. These pathways induce cyclooxygenase-1 (COX-1)–dependent synthesis and release of thromboxane A_2 and trigger the release of ADP from storage granules. Thromboxane A_2 is a potent vasoconstrictor and, like ADP, locally activates ambient platelets and recruits them to the site of injury, thereby expanding the platelet plug. To activate platelets, thromboxane A_2 and ADP must bind to their respective receptors on the platelet membrane. The thromboxane receptor (TP) is a G protein–coupled receptor that is found on platelets and the endothelium, which explains why thromboxane A_2 induces vasoconstriction as well as platelet activation.[16] ADP interacts with a family of G protein–coupled receptors on the platelet membrane. The most important of these is $P2Y_{12}$, which is the target of the thienopyridines (clopidogrel and prasugrel) and ticagrelor. $P2Y_1$ also contributes to ADP-induced platelet activation such that maximal ADP-induced platelet activation requires activation of both receptors and cangrelor. A third ADP receptor, $P2X_1$, is an adenosine triphosphate (ATP)-gated calcium channel. Platelet storage granules contain ATP, as well as ADP; the ATP released during the platelet activation process may contribute to the platelet recruitment process in a $P2X_1$-dependent fashion.

Although TP and the various ADP receptors signal through different pathways, they all trigger an increase in the intracellular concentration of calcium in platelets. The increase in calcium induces changes in platelet shape via cytoskeletal rearrangement, granule

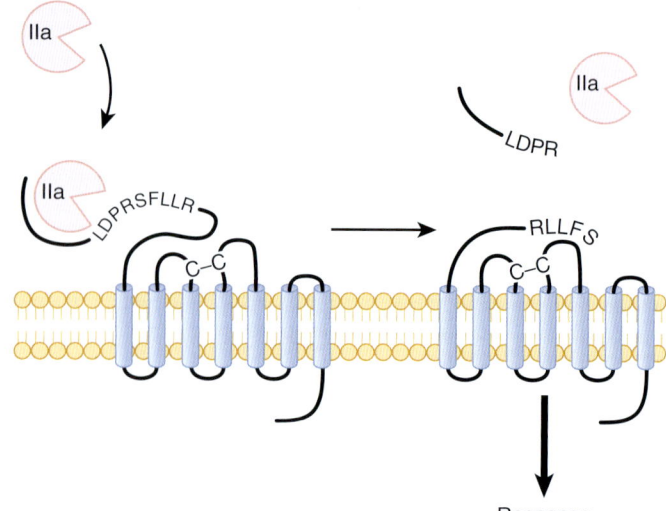

FIGURE 95.4 Activation of PAR-1 by thrombin. Thrombin (IIa) binds to the amino-terminal of the extracellular domain of PAR-1, where it cleaves a specific peptide bond. Cleavage of this bond generates a new amino-terminal sequence that acts as a tethered ligand and binds to the body of the receptor, thereby activating it. Thrombin then dissociates from the receptor. Analogues of the first five or six amino acids of the tethered ligand sequences, known as thrombin receptor agonist peptides, can independently activate PAR-1. *LDPRSFLLR*, Leu-Asp-Pro-Arg-Ser-Phe-Leu-Leu-Arg; *RLLFS*, Arg-Leu-Leu-Phe-Ser.

mobilization and release, and subsequent platelet aggregation. Activated platelets promote coagulation by expressing phosphatidylserine on their surface, an anionic phospholipid that supports the assembly of coagulation factor complexes. Once assembled, these clotting factor complexes trigger a burst of thrombin generation and subsequent fibrin formation. In addition to converting fibrinogen to fibrin, thrombin amplifies platelet recruitment and activation and promotes expansion of the platelet plug. Thrombin binds to protease-activated receptor types 1 and 4 (PAR-1 and PAR-4, respectively) on the platelet surface and cleaves their extended amino-terminal tails (Fig. 95.4), thereby generating new amino-termini that serve as tethered ligands that bind and activate the receptors.[17] Low concentrations of thrombin cleave PAR-1, whereas PAR-4 cleavage requires higher thrombin concentrations. Cleavage of either receptor triggers platelet activation.

In addition to providing a surface on which clotting factors assemble, activated platelets also promote fibrin formation and subsequent stabilization by enhancing the activation of factor V, factor VIII, factor XI, and factor XIII. Thus, a coordinated activation of platelets and coagulation, and formation of the fibrin network that results from the action of thrombin, help anchor the platelet aggregates at the site of injury. Activated platelets also release adhesive proteins, such as vWF, thrombospondin, and fibronectin, which may augment platelet adhesion at sites of injury, as well as growth factors such as platelet-derived growth factor (PDGF) and transforming growth factor-beta (TGF-β), which promote wound healing.

Platelet Aggregation

Aggregation serves as the final step in formation of the platelet plug by linking platelets to each other to form clumps. GP IIb/IIIa mediates these platelet-to-platelet linkages. On nonactivated platelets, GP IIb/IIIa exhibits minimal affinity for its ligands. Upon platelet activation, GP IIb/IIIa undergoes a conformational change that reflects transmission of inside-out signals from its cytoplasmic domain to its extracellular domain.[1,5] This transformation enhances the affinity of GP IIb/IIIa for its ligands, fibrinogen, and, under high-shear conditions, vWF. Arg-Gly-Asp (RGD) sequences located on fibrinogen and vWF, as well as a platelet-binding Lys-Gly-Asp (KGD) sequence on fibrinogen, mediate their interactions with GP IIb/IIIa. When subjected to high shear, circulating vWF elongates and exposes its platelet-binding domain, which enables its interaction with the conformationally activated GP IIb/IIIa.[18] Divalent fibrinogen and multivalent vWF molecules serve as bridges and bind adjacent platelets together. Once bound to GP IIb/IIIa, fibrinogen

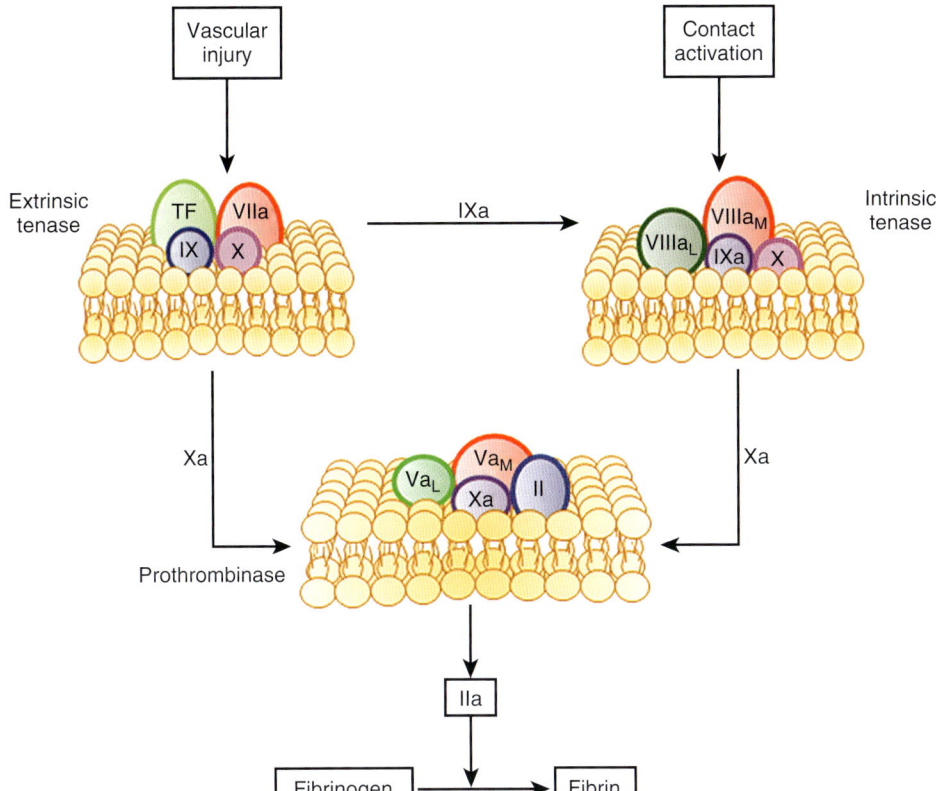

FIGURE 95.5 Coagulation system. Coagulation occurs through the action of discrete enzyme complexes composed of a vitamin K–dependent enzyme and a nonenzyme cofactor. These complexes assemble on anionic phospholipid membranes, such as the surface of activated platelets, in a calcium-dependent manner. Vascular injury exposes tissue factor (TF), which binds factor VIIa to form extrinsic tenase. Extrinsic tenase activates factors IX and X. Factor IXa binds to factor VIIIa to form intrinsic tenase, which activates factor X. Factor Xa binds to factor Va to form prothrombinase, which converts prothrombin (II) to thrombin (IIa). Thrombin then converts soluble fibrinogen to insoluble fibrin.

monocyte-derived microparticles (small membrane vesicles) also provide a source of tissue factor. When tissue factor–bearing monocytes or microparticles bind to platelets or other leukocytes and their plasma membranes fuse, transfer of tissue factor takes place. By binding to the adhesion molecules expressed on activated endothelial cells or to P-selectin on activated platelets, these tissue factor–bearing cells or microparticles can initiate or augment coagulation. This phenomenon probably explains how venous thrombi develop in the absence of obvious vessel wall injury.[2]

An integral membrane protein, tissue factor serves as a receptor for factor VII. Once bound, factor VII undergoes autoactivation, thereby forming the extrinsic tenase complex, which is a potent activator of factors IX and X or is activated by factor Xa. Upon activation, factors IXa and Xa serve as the enzyme components of intrinsic tenase and prothrombinase, respectively.

Intrinsic Tenase
Factor IXa binds to factor VIIIa on anionic cell surfaces to form the intrinsic tenase complex. Factor VIII circulates in blood in complex with vWF. Thrombin cleaves factor VIII and releases it from vWF, thereby converting it to its activated form. Activated platelets express binding sites for factor VIIIa. Once bound, factor VIIIa binds factor IXa in a calcium-dependent manner to form the intrinsic tenase complex, which then activates factor X. The change in catalytic efficiency of factor IXa–mediated activation of factor X that occurs with deletion of individual components of the intrinsic tenase complex highlights their importance. Absence of the membrane surface or factor VIIIa almost completely abolishes enzymatic activity, and the catalytic efficiency of the complete complex is 10^9-fold greater than that of factor IXa alone. Because intrinsic tenase activates factor X at a rate 50- to 100-fold faster than extrinsic tenase does, intrinsic tenase plays a critical role in the amplification of factor Xa and thrombin generation. The bleeding that occurs in patients with hemophilia A or B, which occurs with congenital or acquired deficiency of factor VIII or factor IX, respectively, highlights the importance of intrinsic tenase in hemostasis.

Prothrombinase
Factor Xa binds to factor Va, its activated cofactor, on anionic phospholipid membrane surfaces to form the prothrombinase complex. Activated platelets release factor V from their alpha granules, and this platelet-derived factor V may play a more important role in hemostasis than its plasma counterpart does. Although plasma factor V requires thrombin activation to exert its cofactor activity, the partially activated factor V released from platelets already exhibits substantial cofactor activity. Activated platelets express specific factor Va binding sites on their surface, and bound factor Va serves as a receptor for factor Xa. The catalytic efficiency of activation of prothrombin by factor Xa increases by 10^9-fold when factor Xa is incorporated into the prothrombinase complex. Prothrombin binds to the prothrombinase complex, where it undergoes conversion to thrombin in a reaction that releases prothrombin fragment 1.2 (F1.2). Plasma levels of F1.2 therefore provide a marker of prothrombin activation.

Fibrin Formation
Thrombin, the final effector in coagulation, converts soluble fibrinogen to insoluble fibrin. Fibrinogen is a dimeric molecule, each half

and vWF induce outside-inside signals that augment platelet activation and result in the activation of additional GP IIb/IIIa receptors, thus creating a positive feedback loop. Because GP IIb/IIIa serves as the final effector in platelet aggregation, it is a logical target for potent antiplatelet drugs. Fibrin, the ultimate product of the coagulation system, tethers the platelet aggregates together and anchors them to the site of injury.

Coagulation
Coagulation results in the generation of thrombin, which converts soluble fibrinogen to fibrin.[19] Coagulation occurs through the action of discrete enzyme complexes composed of a vitamin K–dependent enzyme and a nonenzyme cofactor that assemble on anionic phospholipid membranes in a calcium-dependent fashion. Each enzyme complex activates a vitamin K–dependent substrate that becomes the enzyme component of the subsequent complex (Fig. 95.5). Together, these complexes generate a small amount of thrombin that feeds back to amplify its own generation by activating the nonenzyme cofactors and platelets. The phosphatidylserine expressed on the surface of activated platelets provides an anionic surface on which the complexes assemble. The three enzyme complexes involved in thrombin generation are extrinsic tenase, intrinsic tenase, and prothrombinase. Although extrinsic tenase initiates the system under most circumstances, the contact system also plays a role in some situations.

Extrinsic Tenase
This complex forms on exposure of tissue factor–expressing cells to blood.[3] Tissue factor exposure occurs after atherosclerotic plaque rupture because the core of the plaque is rich in cells that express tissue factor. Denuding injury to the vessel wall also exposes the tissue factor constitutively expressed by subendothelial smooth muscle cells. In addition to cells in the vessel wall, cytokine activated monocytes and

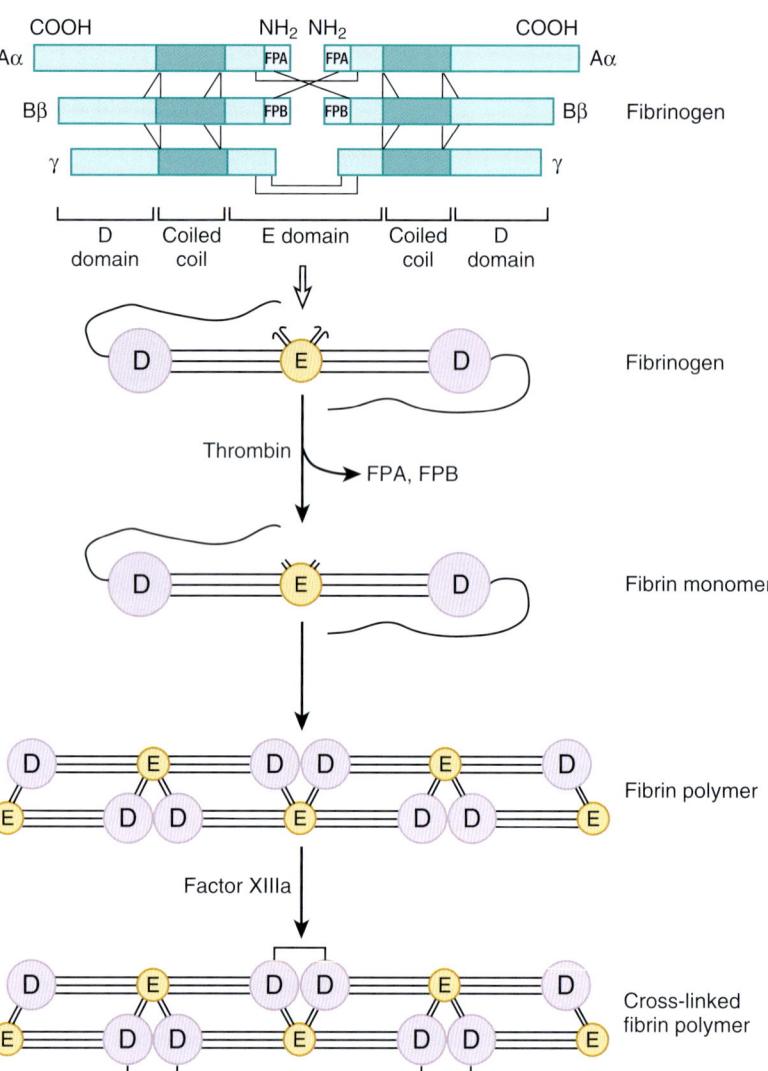

FIGURE 95.6 Fibrinogen structure and conversion of fibrinogen to fibrin. A dimer, each half of the fibrinogen molecule is composed of three polypeptide chains, the Aα, Bβ, and γ chains. Numerous disulfide bonds (lines) covalently link the chains together and join the two halves of the fibrinogen molecule to yield a trinodular structure with a central E domain linked via the coiled-coil regions to two lateral D domains. To convert fibrinogen to fibrin, thrombin cleaves specific peptide bonds at the amino (NH$_2$) terminals of the Aα and Bβ chains of fibrinogen to release fibrinopeptide A (FPA) and fibrinopeptide B (FPB), thereby generating fibrin monomer. Fibrin monomers polymerize to generate protofibrils arranged in a half-staggered overlapping manner. By covalently cross-linking the α and γ chains of adjacent fibrin monomers, factor XIIIa stabilizes the fibrin network and renders it resistant to degradation.

of which is composed of three polypeptide chains, the Aα, Bβ, and γ chains. Numerous disulfide bonds covalently link the chains together and join the two halves of the fibrinogen molecule (Fig. 95.6). Electron micrographic studies of fibrinogen reveal a trinodular structure with a central E domain flanked by two D domains. Crystal structures show symmetry of design with the central E domain, which contains the amino-terminals of the fibrinogen chains joined to the lateral D domains by coiled-coil regions.

Fibrinogen, the most abundant plasma protein involved in coagulation, circulates in an inactive form. Thrombin binds to the amino terminals of the Aα and Bβ chains of fibrinogen, where it cleaves specific peptide bonds to release fibrinopeptide A and fibrinopeptide B and generates fibrin monomers (see Fig. 95.6). Because they are products of the action of thrombin on fibrinogen, plasma levels provide an index of thrombin activity. Release of the fibrinopeptides creates new amino terminals that extend as knobs from the E domain of fibrinopeptides of one fibrin monomer and insert into preformed holes in the D domains of other fibrin monomers. This creates long strands known as protofibrils that consist of fibrin monomers noncovalently linked together in a half-staggered, overlapping manner.

Noncovalently linked fibrin protofibrils are unstable. By covalently cross-linking α- and γ-chains of adjacent fibrin monomers, factor XIIIa stabilizes the fibrin network in a calcium-dependent fashion and renders it relatively resistant to degradation. Factor XIII circulates in blood as a heterodimer consisting of two A and two B subunits. The active site and calcium binding sites of factor XIII are localized to the A subunit. Platelets contain large amounts of factor XIII in their cytoplasm, but platelet-derived factor XIII consists only of A subunits. Both plasma and platelet factor XIII are activated by thrombin.

Contact System

Current thinking views exposure of tissue factor as the sole pathway for activation of coagulation and regards the contact system—which includes factor XII, prekallikrein, and high-molecular-weight kininogen—as unimportant for hemostasis because patients deficient in these factors do not have bleeding problems. However, this concept is changing with emerging evidence that the contact system contributes to thrombosis. There are several mechanisms through which the contact system can be activated. First, blood-contacting medical devices such as stents or mechanical heart valves, and extracorporeal circuits such as those used for cardiopulmonary bypass or extracorporeal membrane oxygenation, trigger clotting by activating factor XII. Factor XIIa converts prekallikrein to kallikrein in a reaction accelerated by high-molecular-weight kininogen, and factor XIIa and kallikrein then feed back to activate additional factor XII. Factor XIIa propagates coagulation by activating factor XI (Fig. 95.7). Second, activated neutrophils extrude web-like structures known as neutrophil extracellular traps (NETs). Composed of nuclear DNA, histones, and proteases, NETs promote coagulation by binding and activating platelets, trapping red blood cells, and activating the contact pathway.[20] Third, polyphosphates released from the dense granules of activated platelets can activate factor XII and promote the inorganic activation of factor XI by thrombin.[21] Thus, surfaces and cells contribute to coagulation at numerous sites in the cascade.

Studies in animals and humans suggest that the contact system contributes to the growth of arterial and venous thrombi. Thus, mice deficient in factor XII or factor XI form small unstable thrombi at sites of arterial or venous damage.[20] Studies in humans undergoing knee arthroplasty have shown that lowering of factor XI levels with an antisense oligonucleotide or inhibiting factor XIa with an antibody reduces the risk of postoperative VTE to a greater extent than enoxaparin.[22,23] These findings identify factor XI and factor XII as potential targets for new anticoagulants.[24]

Fibrinolytic System

Fibrinolysis begins when plasminogen activators convert plasminogen to plasmin, which then degrades fibrin into soluble fragments (Fig. 95.8). Blood contains two immunologically and functionally distinct plasminogen activators, t-PA and u-PA. t-PA mediates intravascular fibrin degradation, whereas u-PA binds to a specific u-PA receptor (u-PAR) on the surface of cells, where it activates cell-bound plasminogen.[11] Consequently, pericellular proteolysis during cell migration and tissue remodeling and repair are the major functions of u-PA.

Regulation of fibrinolysis occurs at two levels. PAI-1 and, to a lesser extent, PAI-2 inhibit the plasminogen activators, whereas alpha$_2$-antiplasmin inhibits plasmin.[11] Endothelial cells synthesize PAI-1, which inhibits both t-PA and u-PA, whereas monocytes and the placenta synthesize PAI-2, which specifically inhibits u-PA. Thrombin-activated fibrinolysis inhibitor (TAFI) also attenuates fibrinolysis and provides a link between fibrinolysis and coagulation.[25] Impaired

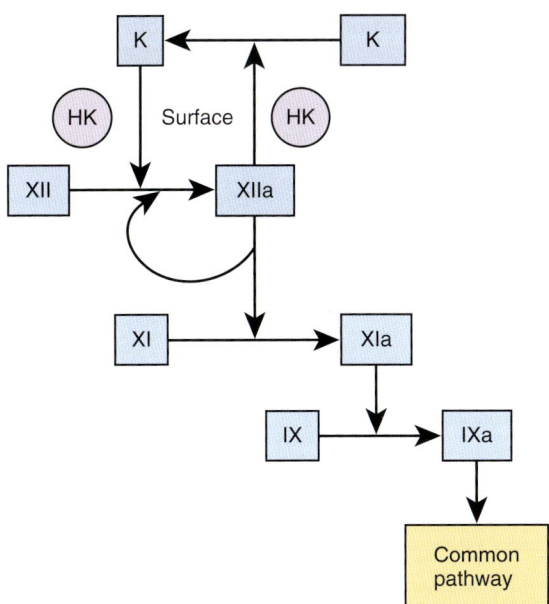

FIGURE 95.7 Contact system. Factor XII is activated by contact with negatively charged surfaces. Factor XIIa converts prekallikrein (PK) to kallikrein (K) and can feed back to activate more factor XII. Similarly, factor XIIa also can feed back to amplify its own generation. Approximately 75% of circulating PK is bound to high-molecular-weight kininogen (HK), which localizes it to anionic surfaces and promotes activation of PK. Factor XIIa propagates clotting by activating factor XI, which then activates factor IX, a process known as autoactivation. The resultant factor IXa assembles into the intrinsic tenase complex, which activates factor X to initiate the common pathway of coagulation.

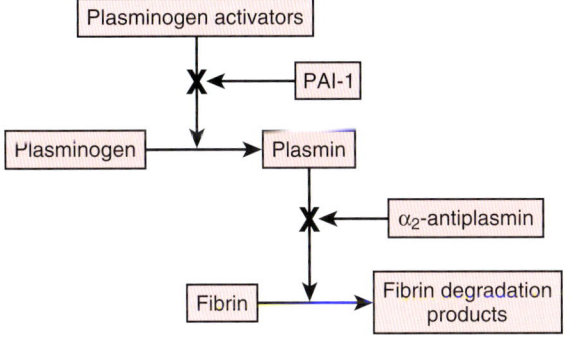

FIGURE 95.8 Fibrinolytic system and its regulation. Plasminogen activators convert plasminogen to plasmin. Plasmin then degrades fibrin into soluble fibrin degradation products. The system is regulated at two levels. Type 1 plasminogen activator inhibitor (PAI-1) inhibits the plasminogen activators, whereas alpha$_2$-antiplasmin serves as the major inhibitor of plasmin.

t-PA has little enzymatic activity in the absence of fibrin, but its activity increases by at least three orders of magnitude when fibrin is present.[11] This increase in activity reflects the capacity of fibrin to serve as a template that binds t-PA and plasminogen and promotes their interaction. t-PA binds fibrin via its finger and second kringle domains, whereas plasminogen binds fibrin via its kringle domains. Kringle domains are loop-like structures that bind Lys residues on fibrin. Degradation of fibrin exposes more Lys residues, which provides additional binding sites for t-PA and plasminogen. Consequently, degrading fibrin stimulates activation of plasminogen by t-PA more than intact fibrin does.

Alpha$_2$-antiplasmin rapidly inhibits circulating plasmin by docking to its first kringle domain and then inhibiting the active site.[11] Because plasmin binds to fibrin via its kringle domains, plasmin generated on the fibrin surface resists inhibition by alpha$_2$-antiplasmin. This phenomenon endows fibrin-bound plasmin with the capacity to degrade fibrin. Factor XIIIa cross-links small amounts of alpha$_2$-antiplasmin onto fibrin, which prevents premature fibrinolysis.

Like fibrin, annexin II on endothelial cells binds t-PA and plasminogen and promotes the interaction of these proteins. Cell surface gangliosides and alpha-enolase may also bind plasminogen and promote its activation by altering its conformation into the more readily activated open form. Plasminogen binds to endothelial cells via its kringle domains. Lipoprotein(a), which also possesses kringle domains, impairs cell-based fibrinolysis by competing with plasminogen for cell surface binding (see also Chapter 27). This phenomenon may explain the association between elevated levels of lipoprotein(a) and atherosclerosis (see also Chapters 25 and 27).[26]

Mechanism of Action of Urokinase Plasminogen Activator

Synthesized as a single-chain polypeptide, single-chain u-PA (scu-PA) has minimal enzymatic activity. Plasmin readily converts scu-PA into an active two-chain form that can bind u-PAR on cell surfaces. Further cleavage at the amino-termini of two-chain u-PA yields a truncated, lower-molecular-weight form that lacks the u-PAR binding domain.[11]

Two-chain forms of u-PA readily convert plasminogen to plasmin in the absence or presence of fibrin. In contrast, scu-PA does not activate plasminogen in the absence of fibrin but can activate fibrin-bound plasminogen because plasminogen adopts a more open and readily activatable conformation when bound to fibrin. Like the higher-molecular-weight form of two-chain u-PA, scu-PA binds cell surface u-PAR, where plasmin can activate it. Many tumor cells elaborate u-PA and express u-PAR on their surface. Plasmin generated on these cells promotes their capacity to metastasize.[11] Inflammatory stimuli such as viruses and cardiovascular risk factors such as smoking and diabetes can trigger cleavage of membrane-bound u-PAR. Soluble u-PAR can cause acute kidney injury by inducing the formation of reactive oxygen species in the kidney tubules. The high levels of soluble u-PAR found in patients with COVID-19 may contribute to their predisposition to acute kidney injury.[27]

Mechanism of Action of Thrombin-Activatable Fibrinolysis Inhibitor

TAFI is synthesized in the liver and circulates in blood in a latent form, where thrombin bound to thrombomodulin can activate it. Unless bound to thrombomodulin, thrombin activates TAFI inefficiently.[25] Activated TAFI (TAFIa) attenuates fibrinolysis by cleaving Lys residues from the carboxy-termini of chains of degrading fibrin, thereby removing binding sites for plasminogen, plasmin, and t-PA. TAFI links fibrinolysis to coagulation in that the thrombin-thrombomodulin complex not only activates TAFI, which attenuates fibrinolysis, but also activates protein C, which mutes thrombin generation (see Fig. 95.2). TAFIa has a short half-life in plasma because the enzyme is unstable.[25] Genetic polymorphisms can result in the synthesis of more stable forms of TAFIa. Persistent attenuation of fibrinolysis by these variant forms of TAFIa may render patients susceptible to thrombosis.[25]

fibrinolysis promotes thrombus accumulation, whereas its excessive activation leads to bleeding.

Mechanism of Action of Tissue Plasminogen Activator

t-PA, a serine protease, contains five discrete domains: a fibronectin-like finger domain, an epidermal growth factor domain, two kringle domains, and a protease domain. Synthesized as a single-chain polypeptide, plasmin converts single-chain t-PA into a two-chain form. Both forms of t-PA convert plasminogen to plasmin. Native Glu-plasminogen is a single-chain polypeptide with a Glu residue at its amino-terminal. Plasmin cleavage near the amino-terminal generates Lys-plasminogen, a truncated form with a Lys residue at its new amino-terminal. t-PA cleaves a single peptide bond to convert single-chain Glu- or Lys-plasminogen into two-chain plasmin, which is composed of a heavy chain containing five kringle domains and a light chain containing the catalytic domain. Because its open conformation exposes the t-PA cleavage site, Lys-plasminogen is a better substrate for t-PA and u-PA than Glu-plasminogen is, which assumes a circular conformation that renders this bond less accessible.

THROMBOSIS

A physiologic host defense mechanism, hemostasis focuses on arrest of bleeding by forming hemostatic plugs composed of platelets and fibrin at sites of vessel injury. In contrast, thrombosis reflects a pathologic process associated with intravascular thrombi that fill and occlude the lumens of arteries or veins.

Arterial Thrombosis (see also Chapter 24)

Most arterial thrombi occur on top of disrupted atherosclerotic plaques. Coronary plaques with a thin fibrous cap and a lipid-rich core are most prone to disruption.[1] Rupture of the fibrous cap exposes thrombogenic material in the lipid-rich core to blood and triggers platelet activation and thrombin generation. The extent of plaque disruption and the content of thrombogenic material in the plaque determine the consequences of the event, but host factors also contribute. Breakdown of the regulatory mechanisms that limit platelet activation and inhibit coagulation can augment thrombosis at sites of plaque disruption. Decreased production of nitric oxide and prostacyclin by diseased endothelial cells can trigger vasoconstriction and platelet activation.[28] Proinflammatory cytokines lower expression of thrombomodulin by endothelial cells, which promotes thrombin generation, and stimulate expression of PAI-1, which inhibits fibrinolysis.[29]

Products of blood coagulation contribute to atherogenesis, as well as to its complications. Microscopic erosions in the vessel wall trigger the formation of tiny platelet-rich thrombi. Activated platelets release PDGF and TGF-β, which promote a fibrotic response.[30] Thrombin generated at the site of injury not only activates platelets and converts fibrinogen to fibrin but also activates the thrombin receptor PAR-1 on smooth muscle cells and induces their proliferation, migration, and elaboration of extracellular matrix. Incorporation of microthrombi into plaque promotes their growth and decreased endothelial cell production of heparan sulfate—which normally limits smooth muscle proliferation—contributes to plaque expansion. The multiple links between atherosclerosis and thrombosis have prompted the term *atherothrombosis*.

Venous Thrombosis (see also Chapter 87)

Venous thrombosis may be caused by genetic or acquired hypercoagulable states or by such factors as advanced age, obesity, or cancer, which are usually acquired and are associated with immobility (Table 95.1). Inherited hypercoagulable states and these acquired risk factors combine to establish the intrinsic risk for thrombosis. Superimposed triggering factors, such as surgery, smoking, pregnancy, or hormonal therapy, modify this risk, and thrombosis occurs when the combination of genetic, acquired, and triggering forces exceeds a critical threshold (Fig. 95.9).

Some acquired or triggering factors entail a higher risk than do others. For example, major orthopedic surgery, neurosurgery, polytrauma, and metastatic cancer entail the highest risk, whereas prolonged bed rest, the presence of antiphospholipid antibodies, and the puerperium are associated with intermediate risk; pregnancy, obesity, long-distance travel, and the use of oral contraceptives or hormonal replacement therapy are mild risk factors. Up to half of patients with VTE before the age of 45 years have inherited hypercoagulable disorders (so-called thrombophilia), particularly those whose event occurred in the absence of risk factors or with minimal provocation, such as after minor trauma or a long-haul flight or with estrogen use. The following sections describe the inherited and acquired hypercoagulable states.

Inherited Hypercoagulable States

Inherited hypercoagulable states fall into two categories. Some are associated with gain-of-function mutations in procoagulant pathways, such as factor V Leiden, the prothrombin gene mutation, and increased levels of procoagulant proteins; others are associated with loss-of-function mutations of endogenous anticoagulant proteins, such as deficiencies of antithrombin, protein C, and protein S.[31] Although all of these inherited hypercoagulable disorders increase the risk for VTE, only increased levels of procoagulant proteins are clearly associated with an increased risk for arterial thrombosis.

TABLE 95.1 Classification of Hypercoagulable States

HEREDITARY	MIXED	ACQUIRED
Loss of Function		
Antithrombin deficiency	Hyperhomocysteinemia	Advanced age
Protein C deficiency		Previous venous thromboembolism
Protein S deficiency		Surgery
Gain of Function		Immobilization
Factor V Leiden		Obesity
Prothrombin gene mutation		Cancer
Elevated factor VIII, IX, or XI levels		Pregnancy, puerperium
		Drug-induced: L-asparaginase, hormonal therapy

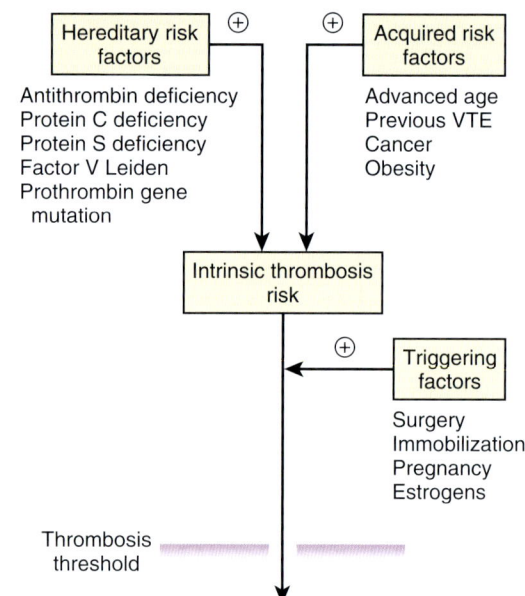

FIGURE 95.9 Thrombosis threshold. Hereditary and acquired risk factors combine to create an intrinsic risk for thrombosis. This risk is increased by extrinsic triggering factors. If the intrinsic and extrinsic forces exceed a critical threshold at which thrombin generation overwhelms protective mechanisms, thrombosis occurs. VTE, venous thromboembolism.

Factor V Leiden

The factor V Leiden mutation, present in about 5% of white individuals, is the most common inherited thrombophilia. Because of a founder effect, the mutation is less common in Hispanics and blacks and rare in Asians. Caused by a point mutation in the factor V gene, the defect results in the synthesis of a factor V molecule with a Gln residue in place of an Arg residue at position 506, one of three sites where activated protein C cleaves factor Va to inactivate it. Consequently, activated factor V Leiden resists rapid proteolysis and persists 10-fold longer in the presence of activated protein C than its wild-type counterpart does. The mutation is inherited in an autosomal dominant fashion. Individuals heterozygous for the factor V Leiden mutation have a fivefold increased risk for VTE; those homozygous for the mutation have a higher risk. However, the absolute risk for venous thrombosis is low with factor V Leiden, and with a yearly risk of 0.1% to 0.3%, patients with this disorder have a lifetime risk for thrombosis of only 5% to 10%.

An activated protein C resistance assay establishes the diagnosis of factor V Leiden in most cases. This assay involves calculation of the ratio of the activated partial thromboplastin time (APTT) measured after the addition of activated protein C divided by that determined before its addition. Use of factor V–deficient plasma increases the specificity of the test. When the clotting assay results are equivocal, genetic testing using a polymerase chain reaction (PCR)–based assay confirms the diagnosis.

Prothrombin Gene Mutation
The second most common thrombophilic disorder, the prothrombin gene mutation, reflects a G-to-A nucleotide transition at position 20210 in the 3′-untranslated region of the prothrombin gene. This mutation causes elevated levels of prothrombin, which enhance thrombin generation. The prevalence of the prothrombin gene mutation is about 3% in white persons and is lower in Asians and blacks. The mutation increases the risk for venous thrombosis to a similar extent as factor V Leiden does. Laboratory diagnosis depends on genetic screening after PCR amplification of the 3′-untranslated region of the prothrombin gene. Although persons heterozygous for this mutation have 30% higher levels of prothrombin than noncarriers do, the wide range of prothrombin levels in healthy individuals precludes the use of this phenotype for carrier identification.

Elevated Levels of Procoagulant Proteins
Elevated levels of factor VIII and other coagulation factors, including fibrinogen and factors IX and XI, appear to be independent risk factors for venous thrombosis. Increased levels of factor VIII are also associated with an up to threefold increase in the risk for myocardial infarction.[31] Although the molecular bases for the high levels of these coagulation factors have yet to be identified, genetic mechanisms probably contribute because these quantitative abnormalities have high heritability.

Antithrombin Deficiency
Synthesized in the liver, antithrombin regulates coagulation by forming a 1:1 covalent complex with thrombin, factor Xa, and other activated clotting factors. Heparan sulfate or heparin accelerates the rate of antithrombin interaction with its target proteases. Inherited antithrombin deficiency is rare; it occurs in approximately 1 in 2000 people and can be due to decreased synthesis of a normal protein or production of a dysfunctional protein. A parallel reduction in the levels of antithrombin antigen and activity identifies deficiencies caused by decreased synthesis, whereas decreased antithrombin activity in the presence of normal antigen levels identifies dysfunctional forms of antithrombin. Comparison of antithrombin activity with or without added heparin identifies variants with impaired heparin-binding capacity.

Acquired antithrombin deficiency results from decreased synthesis, increased consumption, or enhanced clearance. Decreased synthesis can occur in patients with severe hepatic disease, particularly cirrhosis, or in those given L-asparaginase. Increased activation of coagulation can result in antithrombin consumption in disorders such as extensive thrombosis, disseminated intravascular coagulation, severe sepsis, disseminated malignancy, or prolonged extracorporeal circulation. Heparin treatment can also reduce antithrombin levels up to 20% by enhancing the clearance of antithrombin. Severe antithrombin deficiency can develop in some patients with nephrotic syndrome because of loss of protein in urine.

Protein C Deficiency
Thrombin initiates the protein C pathway when it binds thrombomodulin on the endothelial cell surface (see Fig. 95.2). Thrombin bound to thrombomodulin activates protein C approximately 1000-fold more efficiently than free thrombin does.[10] EPCR augments this process 20-fold by binding protein C and presenting it to the thrombin-thrombomodulin complex for activation.[10] Activated protein C then becomes dissociated from the activation complex and decreases thrombin generation by inactivating factors Va and VIIIa on the activated platelet surface. For efficient inactivation of these factors, activated protein C must bind to protein S, its cofactor.

Protein C deficiency can be inherited or acquired. Approximately 1 in 200 adults has heterozygous protein C deficiency inherited in an autosomal dominant fashion, but most have no history of thrombosis. The variable phenotypic expression of hereditary protein C deficiency suggests the existence of other, yet unrecognized, modifying factors. In contrast to antithrombin deficiency, in which the homozygous state is associated with embryonic lethality, homozygous or doubly heterozygous protein C deficiency can occur. Newborns with these disorders often develop purpura fulminans characterized by widespread thrombosis.

Inherited protein C deficiency can result from decreased synthesis of normal protein or from synthesis of dysfunctional forms of protein C. Identification of the type of deficiency requires simultaneous measurement of protein C antigen and activity; reduced synthesis of a normal protein results in a parallel reduction in protein C antigen and activity, whereas synthesis of a dysfunctional protein results in normal antigen with reduced activity.

Acquired protein C deficiency can be due to decreased synthesis or increased consumption. Decreased synthesis can occur in patients with severe liver disease or in those given warfarin. Protein C consumption can occur with severe sepsis, with disseminated intravascular coagulation, and after surgery. Although antithrombin levels can be low in patients with nephrotic syndrome, protein C levels are normal or elevated in such patients.

Protein S Deficiency
Protein S serves as a cofactor for activated protein C (see Fig. 95.2). In addition, protein S may directly inhibit prothrombin activation because of its capacity to bind factors Va and Xa, components of the prothrombinase complex, in the presence of zinc. The importance of the direct anticoagulant activity of protein S is uncertain.

In the circulation, approximately 60% of total protein S is bound to C4b-binding protein, a complement component; only the remaining free 40% is functionally active. Diagnosis of protein S deficiency requires measurement of both the free and bound forms of protein S. Inherited protein S deficiency can result from reduced synthesis of the protein or synthesis of a dysfunctional protein. Acquired protein S deficiency can be due to decreased synthesis, increased consumption, loss, or shift of free protein S to the bound form. Decreased synthesis can occur in patients with severe liver disease or in those given warfarin or L-asparaginase. Increased consumption of protein S occurs in patients with acute thrombosis or disseminated intravascular coagulation. Patients with nephrotic syndrome can excrete free protein S in their urine, which causes decreased protein S activity. Total protein S levels in these patients are often normal because the levels of C4b-binding protein increase, thus shifting more protein S to the bound form. C4b-binding protein levels also increase in pregnancy and with the use of oral contraceptives. This shifts more protein S to the bound form and lowers the levels of free protein S and protein S activity. The consequences of this phenomenon are uncertain.

Other Hereditary Disorders
A polymorphism in the gene that encodes EPCR has been linked to venous thrombosis. Associated with EPCR shedding and high levels of soluble EPCR, this polymorphism reduces endothelial EPCR, and soluble EPCR competes with its endothelial cell counterpart for protein C binding.

A polymorphism in factor XIII that results in more rapid activation by thrombin is associated with a small reduction in the risk for VTE, myocardial infarction, and ischemic stroke in some but not all case-control studies.[32] The frequency of this polymorphism varies among different ethnic populations, and certain environmental factors, such as obesity and estrogen therapy, may augment its protective effect. More work is needed to determine the extent to which this polymorphism modulates the risk for thrombosis.

Acquired Hypercoagulable States (see also Chapter 87)
Acquired hypercoagulable states may develop during surgery and the period of immobilization following it; in persons of advanced age; in

those who are obese, have cancer, are pregnant, or are taking estrogen therapy (oral contraceptive or hormone replacement therapy); or in those with a history of VTE, antiphospholipid syndrome, or hyperhomocysteinemia (see Table 95.1). These conditions can occur in isolation or in conjunction with hereditary hypercoagulable states.

Surgery and Immobilization

Surgery can directly damage veins, and immobilization after surgery leads to stasis in the deep veins of the leg. The risk for VTE in surgical patients depends on the patient's age, the type of surgery, and the presence of active cancer. Patients older than 65 years have a greater risk, and high-risk types of surgery include major orthopedic procedures, neurosurgery, and extensive abdominal or pelvic surgery, especially for cancer. Because the risk for VTE increases up to 20-fold in these patients, they require thromboprophylaxis until they gain full mobility. Hospitalization and nursing home confinement account for approximately 60% of cases of VTE, again reflecting the impact of immobilization. Hospitalization for medical illness accounts for a similar proportion of cases as hospitalization for surgery, thus highlighting the need for thromboprophylaxis in medical patients as well as in surgical patients. Extending thromboprophylaxis after hospital discharge may be beneficial in high-risk medical and surgical patients.[33,34]

Advanced Age

Predominantly a disease of older age, VTE in those younger than 50 years has an incidence of 1 per 10,000 and increases approximately 10-fold per decade thereafter. Men have an overall age-adjusted incidence rate approximately 1.2-fold higher than women. Although incidence rates are higher in women during the reproductive years, after 45 years of age, men have higher incidence rates. Many potential mechanisms may increase the incidence of VTE with advanced age, including decreased mobility, associated diseases, and vascular endothelium that is less resistant to thrombosis. Levels of procoagulant proteins also increase with age.

Obesity

The risk for VTE increases approximately 1.2-fold for every 10-kg/m^2 increase in body mass index, but the basis for the association between obesity and VTE is unclear. Obesity leads to immobility; in addition, adipose tissue, particularly visceral fat, expresses proinflammatory cytokines and adipokines, which may promote coagulation by increasing levels of procoagulant proteins or impair fibrinolysis by elevating levels of PAI-1.

Cancer

Approximately 20% of patients with VTE have cancer.[35] Cancer patients with VTE have reduced survival times compared with those without VTE. Patients with brain tumors, pancreatic cancer, or advanced ovarian or prostate cancer have particularly high rates of VTE. Treatment with chemotherapy, hormonal therapy, and biologic or gastric agents (such as erythropoietin, antiangiogenic drugs) further increases the risk, as do central venous catheters or surgery and immunotherapy for cancer. The pathogenesis of thrombosis in cancer patients is multifactorial and involves a complex interplay between the tumor, patient characteristics, and the hemostatic system. Many types of tumor cells express tissue factor or other procoagulants that can initiate coagulation. In addition to its role in coagulation, tissue factor also acts as a signaling molecule that promotes tumor proliferation and spread.[36] Patient characteristics that contribute to VTE include immobility and venous stasis secondary to extrinsic compression of major veins by tumor. Surgical procedures, central venous catheters, and chemotherapy can injure vessel walls. In addition, tamoxifen and selective estrogen receptor modulators (SERMs) induce an acquired hypercoagulable state by reducing levels of natural anticoagulant proteins.

A proportion of patients with unprovoked VTE have occult cancer. This observation has prompted some experts to recommend extensive screening for cancer in such patients, but the potential harms—including procedure-related morbidity, the psychological impact of false-positive test results, and the cost of screening—offsets any benefits of this approach. Studies comparing extensive cancer screening with little or no screening in patients with unprovoked VTE have not demonstrated a reduction in cancer-related mortality rates with screening.[37] Therefore, unless symptoms suggestive of underlying cancer are present, only age-appropriate screening for breast, cervical, colon, and possibly prostate cancer is indicated because screening for these cancers may reduce mortality rates.

Pregnancy

Pregnant women have a fivefold to sixfold higher risk for VTE than do age-matched nonpregnant women. VTE occurs in approximately 1 in 1000 pregnancies, and in approximately 1 in 1000 women VTE develops in the postpartum period. VTE is the leading cause of maternal morbidity and mortality. Patient-related factors influence the risk for VTE in pregnancy and the puerperium, including age older than 35 years, body mass index higher than 29, cesarean delivery, thrombophilia, or a personal or family history of VTE. Ovarian hyperstimulation and multiparity also increase risk for thrombosis.

More than 90% of deep vein thrombi in pregnancy occur in the left leg, probably because the enlarged uterus compresses the left iliac vein. Hypercoagulability occurs in pregnancy because of the combination of venous stasis and changes in levels of blood proteins. Uterine enlargement reduces venous blood flow from the lower extremities. This is not the only contributor to venous stasis, however, because blood flow from the lower extremities begins to decrease by the end of the first trimester. Systemic factors also contribute to hypercoagulability. Thus, levels of procoagulant proteins, such as factor VIII, fibrinogen, and vWF increase in the third trimester of pregnancy. Coincidentally, suppression of the natural anticoagulant pathways takes place. These changes enhance thrombin generation, as evidenced by elevated levels of F1.2 and thrombin-antithrombin complexes.

About half the episodes of VTE in pregnancy occur in women with thrombophilia. The risk for VTE in women with thrombophilic defects depends on the type of abnormality and the presence of other risk factors. Risk appears highest in women with antithrombin, protein C, or protein S deficiency and lower in those with factor V Leiden or the prothrombin gene mutation. In general, these women have a higher daily risk for VTE in the postpartum period than during pregnancy. The risk during pregnancy is similar in all three trimesters. Therefore, women needing thromboprophylaxis require treatment throughout pregnancy and for at least 6 weeks postpartum.

Estrogen Therapy (see also Chapter 91)

Oral contraceptives, estrogen replacement therapy, and SERMs are all associated with an increased risk for VTE. The relatively high risk for VTE associated with first-generation oral contraceptives prompted the development of low-dose formulations. Currently available low-estrogen combination oral contraceptives contain 20 to 50 μg of ethinyl estradiol and one of several different progestins. Even use of these low-dose combination contraceptives is associated with a threefold to fourfold increased risk for VTE compared with nonusers. In absolute terms this translates to an incidence of 3 to 4 per 10,000 as compared with 5 to 10 per 100,000 in nonusers of reproductive age.

Although smoking increases the risk for myocardial infarction and stroke in women taking oral contraceptives, it is unclear whether smoking affects the risk for VTE. Obesity, however, increases the risk of both arterial and venous thrombosis. The risk for VTE is highest during the first year of oral contraceptive use and persists only for the duration of use. Case-control studies suggest a 20- to 30-fold higher risk for VTE in women with inherited thrombophilia who use oral contraceptives than in nonusers with thrombophilia or users without these defects. Despite the increased risk, routine screening for thrombophilia in young women considering oral contraceptive use is not recommended. Based on the incidence and case fatality rate of thrombotic events, estimates suggest that screening 400,000 women would detect 20,000 factor V Leiden carriers and that prevention of a single death would necessitate withholding oral contraceptives in all these women. Even larger numbers of women with less prevalent thrombophilic defects would require screening.

Hormonal replacement therapy with conjugated equine estrogen, with or without a progestin, is associated with a small increase in the risk for myocardial infarction, ischemic stroke, and VTE. SERMs, such as tamoxifen, are estrogen-like compounds that serve as an estrogen antagonist in the breast but as estrogen agonists in other tissues, such as bone and the uterus. Like estrogens, tamoxifen increases the risk for VTE by threefold to fourfold. The risk is higher in postmenopausal women, particularly those receiving systemic combination chemotherapy. Because of this risk, aromatase inhibitors, which antagonize estrogens by blocking their synthesis from androgens, are sometimes used in place of tamoxifen for the treatment of estrogen receptor–positive breast cancer. Aromatase inhibitors are associated with a lower risk for VTE than tamoxifen. Raloxifene, a SERM used to prevent osteoporosis, increases the risk for VTE threefold when compared with placebo, which contraindicates the use of raloxifene for prevention of osteoporosis in women with a history of VTE.

History of Previous Venous Thromboembolism
A history of previous VTE places patients at risk for recurrence. When anticoagulation treatment stops, patients with unprovoked VTE have a risk for recurrence of approximately 10% at 1 year and 30% at 5 years. This risk appears independent of whether an underlying thrombophilic defect is present, such as factor V Leiden or the prothrombin gene mutation. The risk for recurrent VTE is lower in patients whose incident event occurred in association with a transient major risk factor, such as surgery or trauma. These patients have a risk for recurrence of approximately 1% at 1 year and 5% at 5 years. Patients whose VTE occurred on the background of minor transient or persistent risk factors, such as a long-haul flight or chronic kidney disease, respectively, have an intermediate risk for recurrence. Patients at highest risk for recurrence are those with inherited deficiencies of antithrombin, protein C, or protein S; those with antiphospholipid syndrome; patients with advanced malignancy; or those homozygous for factor V Leiden or the prothrombin gene mutation. Their risk for recurrence likely ranges from 15% at 1 year to up to 50% at 5 years.

Antiphospholipid Syndrome
A heterogeneous group of autoantibodies directed against proteins that bind phospholipid to some antiphospholipid antibodies, known as lupus anticoagulants (LA), prolong phospholipid-dependent coagulation assays. Others, such as anticardiolipin (ACL) antibodies, target cardiolipin, and a subset of ACL antibodies recognizes other phospholipid-bound proteins, particularly beta$_2$-glycoprotein I. Patients with thrombosis in association with a persistent LA and/or ACL antibody have antiphospholipid syndrome. Primary antiphospholipid syndrome occurs in isolation, whereas secondary forms are associated with autoimmune disorders, such as systemic lupus erythematosus or other connective tissue diseases. Patients with antiphospholipid syndrome can have arterial, venous, or placental thrombosis. Arterial thrombosis can cause a transient ischemic attack, stroke, or myocardial infarction. Cerebral vein thrombosis can occur in addition to deep vein thrombosis and pulmonary embolism. Placental thrombosis probably causes pregnancy-related complications that characterize antiphospholipid syndrome. Such complications include fetal loss before 10 weeks of gestation and unexplained fetal death after 10 weeks of gestation, intrauterine growth restriction, preeclampsia, and eclampsia. Treatment with aspirin and/or LMWH during pregnancy may reduce the risk for these complications in women with antiphospholipid syndrome but not in those with other documented thrombophilic defects.

Laboratory diagnosis of antiphospholipid syndrome requires the presence of an LA or ACL antibody on tests taken at least 6 weeks apart. Diagnosis of an LA requires a battery of phospholipid-dependent clotting tests, whereas immunoassays detect ACL antibodies. Only ACL antibodies of medium to high titer and of the IgG or IgM subclass are associated with thrombosis. Approximately 3% to 10% of healthy individuals have ACL antibodies. Such antibodies also occur with certain infections, such as coronavirus disease (COVID-19), mycobacterial pneumonia, malaria, or parasitic disorders, and after exposure to some medications. Frequently, these antibodies are transient and of low titer. Approximately 30% to 50% of patients with systemic lupus erythematosus or other connective tissue disorders have ACL antibodies, and 10% to 20% have LA antibodies.

The mechanism by which antiphospholipid antibodies trigger thrombosis is unclear. These antibodies directly activate endothelial cells in culture and induce the expression of adhesion molecules that can tether tissue factor–bearing leukocytes or microparticles onto their surface. ACL antibodies also interfere with the protein C pathway, inhibit catalysis of antithrombin by endothelial heparan sulfate, and impair fibrinolysis. The relative importance of these mechanisms in humans remains unclear.

HYPERHOMOCYSTEINEMIA
Homocysteine serves as a methyl group donor during the metabolism of methionine, an essential amino acid derived from the diet. The interconversion of methionine and homocysteine depends on the availability of 5-methyltetrahydrofolate, a methyl group donor; vitamin B_{12} and folate, cofactors in the interconversion; and the enzyme methionine synthase. Increased levels of homocysteine can result from increased production or reduced metabolism. Severe hyperhomocysteinemia and cystinuria, which are rare, usually result from deficiency of cystathionine beta-synthetase. The more common mild to moderate hyperhomocysteinemia often results from genetic mutations in methyltetrahydrofolate reductase (MTHFR) in association with nutritional deficiency of folate, vitamin B_{12}, or vitamin B_6. The common C677T and A1298C polymorphisms in MTHFR are associated with reduced enzymatic activity and increased thermolability, respectively, thereby increasing the requirement for nutritional cofactors. Hyperhomocysteinemia can also be associated with certain drugs, such as methotrexate, theophylline, cyclosporine, and most anticonvulsants, as well as with some chronic diseases, such as advanced renal disease, severe hepatic dysfunction, or hypothyroidism.

Although elevated levels of fasting serum homocysteine (>15 mmol/L) were once common, routine fortification of flour in North America with folic acid has lowered homocysteine levels in the general population. Elevated serum homocysteine may be associated with an increased risk for myocardial infarction, stroke, and peripheral artery disease, as well as VTE. Administration of folate along with vitamin B_{12} and vitamin B_6 reduces levels of homocysteine. Nonetheless, randomized trials have shown that such therapy does not lower the risk for recurrent cardiovascular events in patients with coronary artery disease or stroke, nor does it lower the risk for recurrent VTE. Based on these negative trials and the declining incidence of hyperhomocysteinemia, enthusiasm for screening for hyperhomocysteinemia has declined.

TREATMENT OF THROMBOSIS
Antiplatelet Drugs
The commonly used antiplatelet drugs include aspirin, thienopyridines (ticlopidine, clopidogrel, and prasugrel), ticagrelor, cangrelor, dipyridamole, GPIIb/IIIa antagonists, and vorapaxar. Each agent has a distinct site of action (Fig. 95.10).

Aspirin
Aspirin is the most widely used antiplatelet agent worldwide. Because it is an inexpensive and effective drug, aspirin serves as the foundation of most antiplatelet strategies.

Mechanism of Action
Aspirin produces its antithrombotic effect by irreversibly acetylating and inhibiting platelet COX-1 (Fig. 95.10), a critical enzyme in the biosynthesis of thromboxane A_2. At high doses ($\approx$ 1 g/day), aspirin also inhibits COX-2, an inducible COX isoform found in endothelial cells and inflammatory cells.[38] In endothelial cells, COX-2 initiates the synthesis of prostacyclin, a potent vasodilator and inhibitor of platelet activation that antagonizes the effects of thromboxane A_2.

Indications
Aspirin is widely used for secondary prevention in patients with established coronary, cerebrovascular, or peripheral artery disease. In such patients, aspirin produces about a 20% reduction in the risk for cardiovascular death, myocardial infarction, or stroke.[38] Use of aspirin for

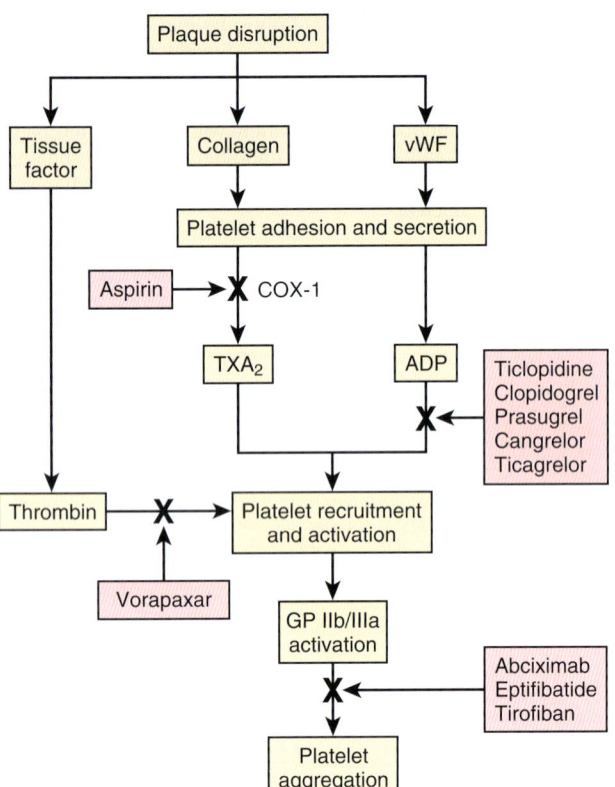

FIGURE 95.10 Sites of action of antiplatelet drugs. Aspirin inhibits the synthesis of thromboxane A_2 (TXA_2) by irreversibly acetylating cyclo-oxygenase 1 (COX-1). The reduced release of TXA_2 attenuates platelet activation and recruitment to the site of vascular injury. Ticlopidine, clopidogrel, and prasugrel irreversibly block $P2Y_{12}$, a key ADP receptor on the platelet surface; cangrelor and ticagrelor are reversible inhibitors of $P2Y_{12}$. Abciximab, eptifibatide, and tirofiban inhibit the final common pathway of platelet aggregation by blocking binding of fibrinogen and vWF to activated GP IIb/IIIa. Vorapaxar inhibits thrombin-mediated platelet activation by targeting protease-activated receptor-1 (PAR-1), the major thrombin receptor on platelets.

primary prevention is more controversial. Metaanalyses suggest that daily aspirin use produces a 20% to 25% reduction in the risk for a first cardiovascular event in patients at moderate to high risk for cardiovascular disease. Recent studies, however, have questioned whether the benefits of daily aspirin for primary cardiac protection outweigh its associated risks for gastrointestinal and intracerebral hemorrhage.[39,40] Consequently, aspirin is no longer recommended for primary cardiac prevention unless the baseline cardiovascular risk is at least 1% per year and 10% at 10 years (see also Chapter 25).[39]

Dosages
Usually administered at dosages of 75 to 325 mg once daily, there is no evidence that higher-dose aspirin is more effective than lower doses, and some meta-analyses suggest reduced efficacy with higher doses.[38] Because the side effects of aspirin, particularly gastrointestinal bleeding, depend on the dosage, daily aspirin dosages of 75 to 150 mg suffice for most indications. Rapid platelet inhibition requires an initial dose of non–enteric-coated aspirin of at least 160 mg.[38]

Side Effects
The most common side effects are gastrointestinal, and they range from dyspepsia to erosive gastritis or peptic ulcers with bleeding and perforation.[38] Use of enteric-coated or buffered aspirin in place of plain aspirin does not eliminate the risk for gastrointestinal side effects. The risk for major bleeding with aspirin is 1% to 3% per year. The concomitant use of aspirin and anticoagulants such as warfarin increases the risk for bleeding. When combined with warfarin or other oral anticoagulants, use of low-dose aspirin (75 to 100 mg daily) is best. Eradication of *Helicobacter pylori* infection and administration of proton pump inhibitors may reduce the risk for aspirin-induced upper gastrointestinal bleeding in patients with peptic ulcer disease.

Patients with a history of aspirin allergy characterized by bronchospasm should not receive aspirin. This problem occurs in approximately 0.3% of the general population but is more common in patients with chronic urticaria or asthma, particularly those with coexisting nasal polyps or chronic rhinitis.[41] Clopidogrel can be used in place of aspirin in such patients. Aspirin overdose is associated with hepatic and renal toxicity.

Aspirin Resistance
The term *aspirin resistance* is used to describe both clinical and laboratory phenomena.[42] A diagnosis of clinical aspirin resistance, defined as failure of aspirin to protect patients from ischemic vascular events, can be made only after such an event occurs. This retrospective diagnosis provides no opportunity to modify therapy. Furthermore, it is unrealistic to expect aspirin, which selectively blocks thromboxane A_2–induced platelet activation, to prevent all vascular events. The biochemical definition of aspirin resistance involves failure of the drug to inhibit thromboxane A_2 synthesis and/or arachidonic acid–induced platelet aggregation. Potential mechanisms for aspirin resistance include poor adherence, reduced or delayed absorption of aspirin due to its enteric coating,[43] thromboxane A_2 generation via pathways distinct from COX-1, increased activity of thromboxane A_2–independent pathways of platelet activation, use of concomitant medications that interfere with the action of aspirin, and pharmacogenetic factors. Tests used for the diagnosis of biochemical aspirin resistance include measurements of thromboxane B_2, the stable metabolite of thromboxane A_2, in serum or in urine, and assessment of arachidonic acid–induced platelet aggregation. These tests have not been standardized, however, and there is no evidence that they identify patients at risk for recurrent vascular events or that resistance can be reversed either by giving higher doses of aspirin or by adding other antiplatelet drugs. Until such information is available, testing for aspirin resistance remains a research tool.

Thienopyridines (see also Chapters 38 to 40)
The thienopyridines include ticlopidine, clopidogrel, and prasugrel, drugs that target $P2Y_{12}$, the key ADP receptor on platelet.

Mechanism of Action
The thienopyridines selectively inhibit ADP-induced platelet aggregation by irreversibly blocking $P2Y_{12}$ (see Fig. 95.10). These prodrugs require metabolic activation by the hepatic cytochrome P-450 (CYP) enzyme system. Therefore, when given in usual doses, ticlopidine and clopidogrel have a delayed onset of action. The metabolic activation of prasugrel is more efficient than that of clopidogrel. Consequently, prasugrel acts more rapidly and produces greater and more predictable inhibition of ADP-induced platelet aggregation than clopidogrel.[44] The active metabolites of the thienopyridines bind irreversibly to $P2Y_{12}$. Consequently, these drugs have prolonged action, which can present problems if patients require urgent surgery. To reduce the risk for bleeding, thienopyridine therapy must be stopped approximately 5 days before surgery.

Indications
When compared with aspirin in patients with recent ischemic stroke, myocardial infarction, or peripheral arterial disease, clopidogrel reduced the risk for cardiovascular death, myocardial infarction, and stroke by 8.7%. Therefore, clopidogrel is marginally more effective than aspirin, but it is more expensive, although the cost of clopidogrel has decreased now that generic forms are available. The combination of clopidogrel and aspirin capitalizes on the capacity of each drug to block complementary pathways of platelet activation. For example, this combination is recommended after stent implantation in coronary arteries. Chapter 41 discusses the use of antiplatelet agents after intervention.

The combination of clopidogrel and aspirin is also effective in patients with unstable angina (see also Chapter 39). In 12,562 such patients, the risk for cardiovascular death, myocardial infarction, or stroke was 9.3% in those randomly assigned to the combination of clopidogrel and aspirin and 11.4% in those given aspirin alone. This 20% relative risk reduction with combination therapy was highly statistically significant. However, combining clopidogrel with aspirin increases the risk for major bleeding to approximately 2% per year, a risk that persists even with a daily aspirin dose of 100 mg or less. Therefore, use of clopidogrel plus aspirin should be restricted to situations in which there is clear evidence of benefit. For example, this combination has not proved to be superior to clopidogrel alone in patients with acute ischemic stroke or to aspirin alone for primary prevention in those at risk for cardiovascular events.

Prasugrel was compared with clopidogrel in 13,608 patients with acute coronary syndromes scheduled to undergo percutaneous coronary intervention (PCI).[44] The incidence of the primary efficacy endpoint—a composite of cardiovascular death, myocardial infarction, and stroke—was significantly lower with prasugrel than with clopidogrel (9.9% and 12.1%, respectively), mainly because of a reduction in the incidence of nonfatal myocardial infarction. The incidence of stent thrombosis was also significantly lower with prasugrel than with clopidogrel (1.1% and 2.4%, respectively). These advantages, however, were at the expense of significantly higher rates of fatal bleeding (0.4% and 0.1%, respectively) and life-threatening bleeding (1.4% and 0.9%, respectively) with prasugrel. Because patients older than 75 years and those with a history of previous stroke or transient ischemic attack have a particularly high risk for bleeding, prasugrel should be avoided in older patients, and the drug is contraindicated in those with a history of cerebrovascular disease. Caution is required if prasugrel is used in patients weighing less than 60 kg or in those with renal impairment.

Dosages

Clopidogrel is given once daily at a dose of 75 mg.[38] Because its onset of action is delayed for several days, 300- to 600-mg loading doses of clopidogrel are given when rapid ADP receptor blockade is desired (see also Chapter 41). After a loading dose of 60 mg, prasugrel is given once daily at a dose of 10 mg.[38] Patients older than 75 years or weighing less than 60 kg should receive a daily prasugrel dose of 5 mg.

Clopidogrel Resistance

The capacity of clopidogrel to inhibit ADP-induced platelet aggregation varies among subjects.[45] This variability reflects, at least in part, genetic polymorphisms in the CYP isoenzymes involved in the metabolic activation of clopidogrel (see also Chapters 8, 38, and 39). The most important of these enzymes is CYP2C19. Clopidogrel-treated patients with the loss-of-function *CYP2C19*2* allele exhibit reduced platelet inhibition in comparison with those with the wild-type *CYP2C19*1* allele and experience a higher rate of cardiovascular events.[46] This is important because estimates suggest that up to 25% of whites, 30% of blacks, and 50% of Asians carry the loss-of-function allele, which may render them resistant to clopidogrel. Even patients with reduced-function *CYP2C19*3*, *CYP2C19*4*, or *CYP2C19*5* alleles may derive less benefit from clopidogrel than do those with the full-function *CYP2C19*1* allele. Patients with polymorphisms in *ABCB1* may exhibit impaired clopidogrel absorption, and polymorphisms in *CYP3A4* can contribute to reduced metabolic activation of clopidogrel. Polymorphisms in both these enzymes have been linked to adverse clinical outcomes. In contrast to their effect on the metabolic activation of clopidogrel, polymorphisms in *CYP2C19* and *CYP3A4* do not appear to influence activation of prasugrel, nor do they affect the response to ticagrelor.

Although concomitant administration of clopidogrel with proton pump inhibitors, which inhibit CYP2C19, reduces the effect of clopidogrel on ADP-induced platelet aggregation, this interaction has questionable clinical significance. Atorvastatin, a competitive inhibitor of CYP3A4, reduced the inhibitory effect of clopidogrel on ADP-induced platelet aggregation in one study, a finding unconfirmed in subsequent investigations.[47]

The influence of genetic polymorphisms on clinical outcomes with clopidogrel has raised the possibility that pharmacogenetic profiling and/or point-of-care platelet function testing could be used to identify clopidogrel-resistant patients so that they could be targeted for more intensive antiplatelet therapy.[48] Although up to 30% of clopidogrel-treated patients have evidence of reduced responsiveness to the drug, randomized clinical trials have failed to show that more intensive antiplatelet therapy improves the outcome in such patients.[49] Consequently, there is no indication for routine clopidogrel resistance testing at this time. Because their antiplatelet effects are more predictable, guidelines recommend prasugrel or ticagrelor instead of clopidogrel for high-risk patients.

Ticagrelor

As an orally active inhibitor of $P2Y_{12}$, ticagrelor differs from the thienopyridines in that it does not require metabolic activation and it produces reversible inhibition of the ADP receptor.

Mechanism of Action

Like the thienopyridines, ticagrelor inhibits $P2Y_{12}$. Because it does not require metabolic activation, ticagrelor has a more rapid onset and offset of action than clopidogrel does and it produces greater and more predictable inhibition of ADP-induced platelet aggregation.

Dosages

Ticagrelor is initiated with an oral loading dose of 180 mg followed by 90 mg twice daily. The dose does not need adjustment in patients with renal impairment, but caution is needed in patients with hepatic impairment or in those receiving potent inhibitors or inducers of CYP3A4 because ticagrelor is metabolized in the liver via CYP3A4. Ticagrelor is usually administered in conjunction with aspirin; the daily aspirin dose should not exceed 100 mg. For secondary prevention at least 1 year after myocardial infarction, the dose of ticagrelor is reduced to 60 mg twice daily.

Side Effects

In addition to bleeding, a side effect of all $P2Y_{12}$ inhibitors, the most common side effects of ticagrelor are dyspnea, which can develop in up to 15% of patients, and bradyarrhythmias. The dyspnea, which tends to occur soon after initiating ticagrelor, is usually self-limited and mild in intensity but can be persistent and may necessitate drug discontinuation in some patients. Although the exact mechanism responsible for these side effects is unknown, they may be adenosine-mediated because ticagrelor inhibits its reuptake.

Although platelet transfusions may be useful to treat serious bleeding complications in patients taking clopidogrel or prasugrel, which bind irreversibly to $P2Y_{12}$, they are not effective for ticagrelor reversal because ticagrelor will bind to the transfused platelets. Bentracimab, an antibody fragment that binds ticagrelor and its metabolite with high affinity and rapidly reverses its inhibitory effects, is under development for ticagrelor reversal prior to urgent surgery or intervention or for patients with serious bleeding.[50]

Indications (see also Chapters 38 and 39)

When compared with clopidogrel in patients with acute coronary syndromes,[46] ticagrelor produced a greater reduction in the primary efficacy endpoint—a composite of cardiovascular death, myocardial infarction, and stroke at 1 year—than did clopidogrel (9.8% and 11.7%, respectively; $P = .001$). This difference reflected a significant reduction in both cardiovascular death (4.0% and 5.1%, respectively; $P = .001$) and myocardial infarction (5.8% and 6.9%, respectively; $P = .005$) with ticagrelor relative to clopidogrel. Rates of stroke were similar with ticagrelor and clopidogrel (1.5% and 1.3%, respectively), and there was no difference in rates of major bleeding. When minor bleeding was added to the major bleeding results, however, ticagrelor showed an increase relative to clopidogrel (16.1% and 14.6%, respectively; $P = .008$). Ticagrelor was also superior to clopidogrel in patients with acute coronary syndrome who underwent PCI or cardiac surgery. Based on these observations, guidelines give preference to ticagrelor over clopidogrel, particularly in higher-risk patients.

Cangrelor (see also Chapter 41)

Cangrelor is a rapidly acting reversible inhibitor of P2Y12 that is administered intravenously. It has an immediate onset of action, a half-life of 3 to 5 minutes, and an offset of action within an hour. Cangrelor is licensed for use in patients undergoing PCI and produces rapid ADP receptor blockade in those who have not received pretreatment with clopidogrel, prasugrel, or ticagrelor.[51]

Dipyridamole

A relatively weak antiplatelet agent on its own,[38] an extended-release formulation of dipyridamole combined with low-dose aspirin, a preparation marketed as Aggrenox, is used for prevention of stroke in patients with transient ischemic attacks.

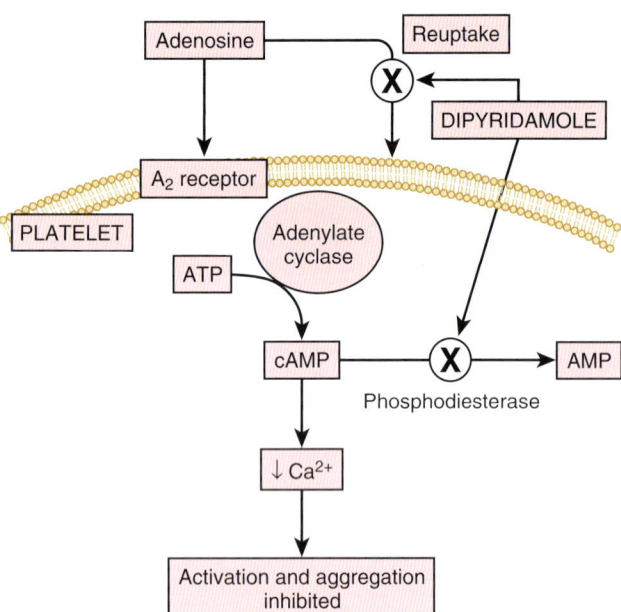

FIGURE 95.11 Mechanism of action of dipyridamole. Dipyridamole increases levels of cAMP in platelets by (1) blocking the reuptake of adenosine, thereby increasing the concentration of adenosine available to bind to the A_2 receptor, and (2) inhibiting phosphodiesterase-mediated cAMP degradation. By promoting calcium uptake, cAMP reduces intracellular levels of calcium. This, in turn, inhibits platelet activation and aggregation.

Mechanism of Action

By inhibiting phosphodiesterase, dipyridamole blocks the breakdown of cAMP. Increased levels of cAMP reduce intracellular calcium and inhibit platelet activation. Dipyridamole also blocks the uptake of adenosine by platelets and other cells. With more extracellular adenosine, there is a further increase in local cAMP levels because the platelet adenosine A_2 receptor and adenylate cyclase are coupled (Fig. 95.11).

Dosages

This fixed combination is given twice daily. Each capsule contains 200 mg of extended-release dipyridamole and 25 mg of aspirin.

Side Effects

Because dipyridamole has vasodilatory effects, caution is necessary in patients with coronary artery disease. Gastrointestinal complaints, headache, facial flushing, dizziness, and hypotension can also occur. These symptoms often subside with continued use of the drug.

Indications

Dipyridamole plus aspirin was compared with aspirin or dipyridamole alone and with placebo in patients with an ischemic stroke or a transient ischemic attack. The combination reduced the risk for stroke by 22.1% in comparison with aspirin and by 24.4% in comparison to dipyridamole.[52] A second trial compared dipyridamole plus aspirin with aspirin alone for secondary prevention in patients with ischemic stroke. Vascular death, stroke, or myocardial infarction occurred in 13% of patients given combination therapy and in 16% of those treated with aspirin alone. Although the combination of dipyridamole plus aspirin compares favorably with aspirin, the combination is not superior to clopidogrel. In a large, randomized trial that compared dipyridamole plus aspirin with clopidogrel for secondary prevention in patients with ischemic stroke, recurrent stroke event rates were similar (9.0% and 8.8%, respectively), as were rates of vascular death, stroke, and myocardial infarction (13.1% in both treatment arms). However, there was a trend toward more hemorrhagic strokes with dipyridamole plus aspirin than with clopidogrel (0.8% and 0.4%, respectively) and more major bleeding (4.1% and 3.8%, respectively).

Although dipyridamole/aspirin can replace aspirin for stroke prevention, because of the vasodilatory effects of dipyridamole and the paucity of data supporting the usefulness of this drug in patients with symptomatic coronary artery disease, dipyridamole/aspirin is contraindicated in such patients; clopidogrel is a better choice in patients with coronary artery disease.

Glycoprotein IIb/IIIa Receptor Antagonists (see also Chapters 38, 39, and 41)

As a class, parenteral GPIIb/IIIa receptor antagonists have a niche in patients with acute coronary syndromes. The three agents in this class are abciximab, eptifibatide, and tirofiban.

Mechanism of Action

A member of the integrin family of adhesion receptors, GPIIb/IIIa is expressed on the surface of platelets and megakaryocytes. With approximately 80,000 copies per platelet, GPIIb/IIIa is the most abundant receptor. GPIIb/IIIa is inactive on resting platelets. With platelet activation, however, inside-outside signal transduction pathways trigger conformational activation of the receptor. Once activated, GPIIb/IIIa binds fibrinogen and, under high-shear conditions, vWF. Once bound, fibrinogen and vWF bridge adjacent platelets together to induce platelet aggregation.

Although abciximab, eptifibatide, and tirofiban all target the GPIIb/IIIa receptor, they are structurally and pharmacologically distinct (Table 95.2).[45] Abciximab is a Fab fragment of a humanized murine monoclonal antibody directed against the activated form of GPIIb/IIIa. Abciximab binds to the activated receptor with high affinity and blocks the binding of adhesive molecules. In contrast to abciximab, eptifibatide and tirofiban are synthetic molecules. Eptifibatide is a cyclical heptapeptide that binds GPIIb/IIIa because it incorporates the KGD motif, whereas tirofiban is a nonpeptidic tyrosine derivative that acts as an RGD mimetic. With its long half-life, abciximab persists on the surface of platelets for up to 2 weeks. Eptifibatide and tirofiban have shorter half-lives.

In addition to targeting the GPIIb/IIIa receptor, abciximab (but not eptifibatide or tirofiban) also inhibits the closely related $\alpha_{v\beta3}$ receptor, which binds vitronectin, and $\alpha_{M\beta2}$, a leukocyte integrin. Inhibition of $\alpha_{v\beta3}$ and $\alpha_{M\beta2}$ may endow abciximab with antiinflammatory and/or antiproliferative properties that extend beyond platelet inhibition.

Dosages

All of the GPIIb/IIIa antagonists are given as an intravenous bolus followed by an infusion. Because of their renal clearance, eptifibatide and tirofiban doses require reduction in patients with renal insufficiency.

Side Effects

In addition to bleeding, thrombocytopenia is the most serious complication. Antibodies directed against neoantigens on GPIIb/IIIa that are exposed on antagonist binding cause thrombocytopenia, which is immune mediated. With abciximab, thrombocytopenia occurs in up to 5% of patients and is severe in approximately 1% of these individuals. Thrombocytopenia is less common with the other two agents and occurs in approximately 1% of patients.

TABLE 95.2 Features of Glycoprotein IIb/IIIa Antagonists

FEATURE	ABCIXIMAB	EPTIFIBATIDE	TIROFIBAN
Description	Fab fragment of humanized mouse monoclonal antibody	Cyclical KGD-containing heptapeptide	Nonpeptidic RGD mimetic
Specific for GP IIb/IIIa	No	Yes	Yes
Plasma half-life	Short (min)	Long (2.5 hr)	Long (2.0 hr)
Platelet-bound half-life	Long (days)	Short (sec)	Short (sec)
Renal clearance	No	Yes	Yes

KGD, Lys-Gly-Asp sequence; *RGD*, Arg-Gly-Asp sequence.

Indications (see also Chapter 41)
Abciximab, eptifibatide, and tirofiban are used occasionally in patients undergoing PCI, particularly those with acute myocardial infarction, whereas tirofiban and eptifibatide are used in high-risk patients with unstable angina.

Vorapaxar
Unlike the other antiplatelet drugs, vorapaxar inhibits PAR-1, the major thrombin receptor on human platelets. Vorapaxar was compared with placebo for secondary prevention in 26,449 patients with previous myocardial infarction, ischemic stroke, or peripheral artery disease.[53] Overall, vorapaxar reduced the risk for cardiovascular death, myocardial infarction, or stroke by 13% but doubled the risk for intracranial bleeding. In the prespecified subgroup of 17,779 patients with previous myocardial infarction, however, vorapaxar reduced the risk for cardiovascular death, myocardial infarction, or stroke by 20% (from 9.7% to 8.1%). The rate of intracranial hemorrhage was higher with vorapaxar than with placebo (0.6% and 0.4%, respectively; $P = .076$), as was the rate of moderate or severe bleeding (3.4% and 2.1%, respectively; $P < .001$). Based on these data, the drug is now licensed for patients younger than 75 years with myocardial infarction who have no history of stroke, transient ischemic attack, or intracranial bleeding and who weigh more than 60 kg.

Anticoagulants
There are parenteral and oral anticoagulants. Currently available parenteral anticoagulants include heparin, LMWH, fondaparinux, a synthetic pentasaccharide, bivalirudin, and argatroban. Currently available oral anticoagulants include warfarin as well as dabigatran etexilate, which is an oral thrombin inhibitor, and rivaroxaban, apixaban, and edoxaban, which are oral factor Xa inhibitors.[54]

Parenteral Anticoagulants
Heparin
A sulfated polysaccharide, heparin is isolated from mammalian tissues rich in mast cells (Table 95.3). Most commercial heparin is derived from porcine intestinal mucosa and is a polymer of alternating D-glucuronic acid and N-acetyl-D-glucosamine residues.[55]

MECHANISM OF ACTION. Heparin acts as an anticoagulant by activating antithrombin (previously known as antithrombin III) and accelerating the rate at which it inhibits clotting enzymes, particularly thrombin and factor Xa. Antithrombin, the obligatory plasma cofactor for heparin, belongs to the serine protease inhibitor (serpin) superfamily. Synthesized in the liver and circulating in plasma at a concentration of 2.6 ± 0.4 μM, antithrombin acts as a suicide substrate for its target enzymes.

To activate antithrombin, heparin binds to the serpin via a unique pentasaccharide sequence found on a third of the chains of commercial heparin (Fig. 95.12). Heparin chains lacking this pentasaccharide sequence have little or no anticoagulant activity.[56] Once bound to antithrombin, heparin induces a conformational change in the reactive center loop of antithrombin that renders it more readily accessible to its target proteases. This conformational change enhances the rate at which antithrombin inhibits factor Xa by at least two orders of magnitude but has little effect on the rate of thrombin inhibition by antithrombin. To promote thrombin inhibition, heparin serves as a template that binds antithrombin and thrombin simultaneously. Formation of this ternary complex brings the enzyme in close apposition to the inhibitor, thereby promoting the formation of a stable covalent thrombin-antithrombin complex.

Only pentasaccharide-containing heparin chains composed of at least 18 saccharide units (which corresponds to a molecular weight of 5400) have sufficient length to bridge thrombin and antithrombin together.[56] With a mean molecular weight of 15,000 and a range of 5,000 to 30,000, almost all the chains of unfractionated heparin are long enough to provide this bridging function. Consequently, by definition, heparin has equal capacity to promote inhibition of thrombin and factor Xa by antithrombin and has an anti–factor Xa–to–anti–factor IIa (thrombin) ratio of 1:1. Heparin causes the release of TFPI from the endothelium. A factor Xa–dependent inhibitor of tissue factor–bound factor VIIa,[9] TFPI may contribute to the antithrombotic activity of heparin. Longer heparin chains induce the release of more TFPI than shorter chains do.

PHARMACOLOGY OF HEPARIN. Heparin requires parenteral administration and is usually administered subcutaneously or by continuous intravenous infusion. If administered subcutaneously for the treatment of thrombosis, the dose must be high enough to overcome the limited bioavailability associated with this method of delivery. In the circulation, heparin binds to the endothelium and to plasma proteins other than antithrombin. Binding of heparin to endothelial cells explains its dose-dependent clearance. At low intravenous doses, the

TABLE 95.3 Comparison of Features of Heparin, Low-Molecular-Weight Heparin, and Fondaparinux

FEATURES	HEPARIN	LMWH	FONDAPARINUX
Source	Biologic	Biologic	Synthetic
Molecular weight	15,000	5000	1500
Target	Xa and IIa	Xa and IIa	Xa
Bioavailability (%)	30	90	100
Half-life (hr)	1	4	17
Renal excretion	No	Yes	Yes
Antidote	Complete	Partial	No
Heparin-induced thrombocytopenia	<5%	<1%	Rare

LMWH, Low-molecular-weight heparin.

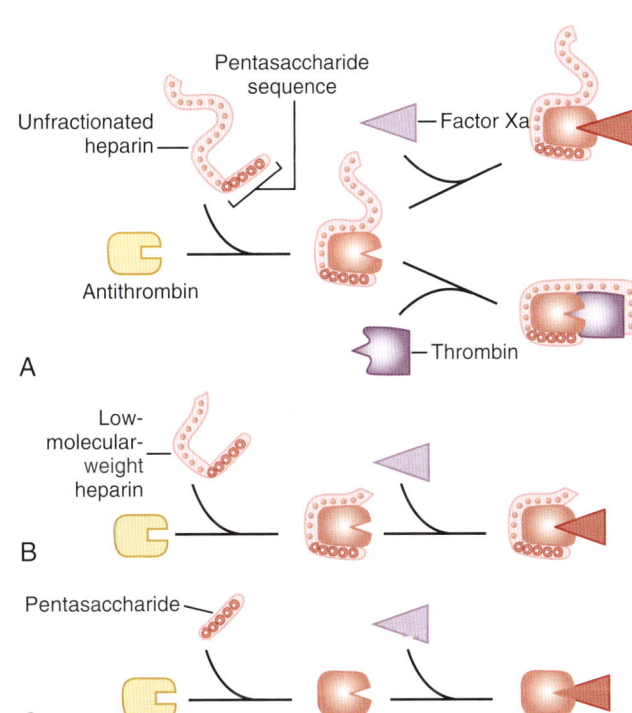

FIGURE 95.12 Mechanism of action of heparin, LMWH, and fondaparinux, a synthetic pentasaccharide. (**A**,) Heparin binds to antithrombin via its pentasaccharide sequence. This induces a conformational change in the reactive center loop of antithrombin that accelerates its interaction with factor Xa. To potentiate thrombin inhibition, heparin must simultaneously bind to antithrombin and thrombin. Only heparin chains composed of at least 18 saccharide units, which corresponds to a molecular weight of 5400, are of sufficient length to perform this bridging function. With a mean molecular weight of 15,000, all the heparin chains are long enough to do this. **B**, LMWH has greater capacity to potentiate factor Xa inhibition by antithrombin than thrombin does because with a mean molecular weight of 4500 to 6000, at least half of the LMWH chains are too short to bridge antithrombin to thrombin. **C**, Fondaparinux, a synthetic pentasaccharide, only accelerates inhibition of factor Xa by antithrombin because it is too short to bridge antithrombin to thrombin.

half-life of heparin is short because it rapidly binds to the endothelium. With higher intravenous doses of heparin, the half-life is longer because heparin clearance is slower once the endothelium is saturated. Clearance is mainly extrarenal; heparin binds to macrophages, which internalize and depolymerize the long heparin chains and secrete shorter chains back into the circulation. Because of its dose-dependent clearance mechanism, the plasma half-life of heparin ranges from 30 to 60 minutes with bolus intravenous doses of 25 and 100 units/kg, respectively.

Once heparin enters the circulation, it binds to plasma proteins other than antithrombin, a phenomenon that reduces the anticoagulant activity of heparin. Some of the heparin-binding proteins found in plasma are acute-phase reactants whose levels are elevated in ill patients. Activated platelets or endothelial cells release other proteins that can bind heparin, such as large multimers of vWF. Activated platelets also release platelet factor 4 (PF4), a highly cationic protein that binds heparin with high affinity. The large amounts of PF4 associated with platelet-rich arterial thrombi can neutralize the anticoagulant activity of heparin. This phenomenon may attenuate heparin's capacity to suppress thrombus growth.

Because levels of heparin binding–proteins in plasma vary from person to person, the anticoagulant response to fixed or weight-adjusted doses of heparin is unpredictable. Consequently, monitoring of coagulation is essential to ensure a therapeutic response, particularly when heparin is administered for the treatment of established thrombosis, because a subtherapeutic anticoagulant response may render patients at risk for recurrent thrombosis, whereas excessive anticoagulation increases the risk for bleeding.

MONITORING THE ANTICOAGULANT EFFECT OF HEPARIN. The APTT or anti-factor Xa level is used to monitor heparin.[57] Although the APTT is the test most often used for this purpose, there are problems with the assay: APTT reagents vary in their sensitivity to heparin, and the type of coagulometer used for testing can influence the results. Consequently, laboratories must establish a therapeutic APTT range with each reagent-coagulometer combination by measuring both the APTT and anti-factor Xa levels in plasma samples collected from heparin-treated patients. With most APTT reagents and coagulometers in current use, heparin levels are therapeutic with a twofold to threefold prolongation of the APTT. Anti-factor Xa levels can also be used to monitor heparin therapy. With this test, therapeutic heparin levels range from 0.3 to 0.7 units/mL. Although this test is gaining in popularity, anti-factor Xa assays have yet to be standardized, and results can vary widely between laboratories.

Up to 25% of patients with VTE are heparin resistant; they require more than 35,000 units/day to achieve a therapeutic APTT. It is useful to measure anti-factor Xa levels in heparin-resistant patients because many will have a therapeutic anti-factor Xa level despite a subtherapeutic APTT. This dissociation in test results occurs because elevated plasma levels of fibrinogen and factor VIII, both acute-phase proteins, shorten the APTT but have no effect on anti-factor Xa levels.[57] Anti-factor Xa levels are better than the APTT for monitoring heparin in patients who exhibit this phenomenon. Patients with congenital or acquired antithrombin deficiency and those with elevated levels of heparin-binding proteins may also need high doses of heparin to achieve a therapeutic APTT or anti–factor Xa level. If there is good correlation between the APTT and the anti–factor Xa level, either test can be used for monitoring heparin therapy.

DOSAGES. For prophylaxis, heparin is usually given in fixed doses of 5000 units subcutaneously two or three times daily. With these low doses, monitoring of coagulation is unnecessary. In contrast, monitoring is essential when the drug is given in higher doses. Fixed-dose or weight-based heparin nomograms are used to standardize heparin regimens and to shorten the time required to achieve a therapeutic anticoagulant response. At least two heparin nomograms have been validated in patients with VTE, and both reduce the time required to achieve a therapeutic APTT. Weight-adjusted heparin nomograms have also been evaluated in patients with acute coronary syndromes. After an intravenous heparin bolus of 5000 units or 70 units/kg, a heparin infusion rate of 12 to 15 units/kg/hr is usually administered. In contrast, weight-adjusted heparin nomograms for patients with VTE use an initial bolus of 5000 units or 80 units/kg, followed by an infusion of 18 units/kg/hr. Thus achievement of a therapeutic APTT requires higher doses of heparin in patients with VTE than in those with acute coronary syndromes. This difference may reflect differences in thrombus burden. Heparin binds to fibrin, and the fibrin content of extensive deep vein thrombi is greater than that of coronary thrombi.

Traditionally, heparin manufacturers in North America measured heparin potency in USP units, with a unit defined as the concentration of heparin that prevents 1 mL of citrated sheep plasma from clotting for 1 hour after the addition of calcium. In contrast, manufacturers in Europe measured heparin potency with anti-Xa assays that use an international heparin standard for comparison. Because of problems with heparin contamination with oversulfated chondroitin sulfate,[55] which the USP assay system does not detect, North American heparin manufacturers now use the anti-Xa assay to measure heparin potency. Use of international units in place of USP units results in a 10% to 15% reduction in the heparin dose. This change is unlikely to affect patient care because dosing of heparin has been done this way in Europe for many years. Furthermore, heparin monitoring ensures a therapeutic anticoagulant response in high-risk situations, such as cardiopulmonary bypass surgery or PCI.

LIMITATIONS OF HEPARIN. Heparin has pharmacokinetic and biophysical limitations (Table 95.4). The pharmacokinetic limitations reflect heparin's propensity to bind in a pentasaccharide-independent fashion to cells and plasma proteins. Binding of heparin to endothelial cells explains its dose-dependent clearance, whereas binding to plasma proteins results in a variable anticoagulant response and can lead to heparin resistance.

The biophysical limitations of heparin reflect the inability of the heparin-antithrombin complex to inhibit factor Xa when it is incorporated into the prothrombinase complex, the complex that converts prothrombin to thrombin, and to inhibit thrombin bound to fibrin. Consequently, factor Xa bound to activated platelets within platelet-rich thrombi can generate thrombin, even in the presence of heparin. Thrombin bound to fibrin protects it from inhibition by the heparin-antithrombin complex. Clot-associated thrombin can then trigger growth of thrombi by locally activating platelets and amplifying its own generation through feedback activation of factors V, VIII, and XI. Neutralization of heparin by the high concentrations of PF4 released from activated platelets within the platelet-rich thrombus further compounds this problem.

SIDE EFFECTS. The most common side effect of heparin is bleeding. Other complications include thrombocytopenia, osteoporosis, and elevated levels of transaminases.

BLEEDING. The risk for heparin-induced bleeding increases with higher heparin doses. Concomitant administration of drugs that affect hemostasis, such as antiplatelet or fibrinolytic agents, increases the risk for bleeding, as does recent surgery or trauma.[58] Protamine sulfate will neutralize heparin in patients with serious bleeding. A mixture of basic polypeptides isolated from salmon sperm, protamine sulfate binds heparin with high affinity to form protamine-heparin complexes that undergo renal clearance. Typically, 1 mg of intravenous protamine

TABLE 95.4 Pharmacokinetic and Biophysical Limitations of Heparin

LIMITATIONS	MECHANISM
Poor bioavailability	Limited absorption of long heparin chains
Dose-dependent clearance	Binds to endothelial cells from subcutaneous injection sites
Variable anticoagulant response	Binds to plasma proteins; levels vary from patient to patient
Reduced activity in the vicinity of platelet-rich thrombi	Neutralized by platelet factor 4 released from activated platelets
Limited activity against factor Xa incorporated into the prothrombinase complex and thrombin bound to fibrin	Reduced capacity of heparin-antithrombin complex to inhibit factor Xa bound to activated platelets and thrombin bound to fibrin

TABLE 95.5 Features of Heparin-Induced Thrombocytopenia

FEATURE	DETAILS
Thrombocytopenia	Platelet count of ≤100,000/μL or a decrease in platelet count of ≥50% from baseline
Timing	Platelet count falls 5 to 14 days after starting heparin
Type of heparin	More common with unfractionated heparin than with low-molecular-weight heparin
Type of patient	More common in surgical patients than in medical patients; more common in women than in men
Thrombosis	Venous thrombosis more common than arterial thrombosis

TABLE 95.6 Management of Heparin-Induced Thrombocytopenia

- Stop all heparin.
- Give an alternative anticoagulant, such as argatroban, bivalirudin, fondaparinux, rivaroxaban, or apixaban.
- Do not give platelet transfusions.
- Do not give warfarin until the platelet count returns to baseline levels; if warfarin was administered, give vitamin K to restore the international normalized ratio to normal.
- Evaluate for thrombosis, particularly deep vein thrombosis.

TABLE 95.7 Advantages of Low-Molecular-Weight Heparin and Fondaparinux over Heparin

ADVANTAGE	CONSEQUENCE
Better bioavailability and longer half-life after subcutaneous injection	Can be given subcutaneously once or twice daily for both prophylaxis and treatment
Dose-independent clearance	Simplified dosing
Predictable anticoagulant response	Monitoring of coagulation is unnecessary in most patients
Lower risk for heparin-induced thrombocytopenia	Safer than heparin for short- or long-term administration
Lower risk for osteoporosis	Safer than heparin for long-term administration

sulfate neutralizes 100 units of heparin. Anaphylactoid reactions to protamine sulfate can occur, but administration by slow intravenous infusion reduces the risk for this problem.[59]

THROMBOCYTOPENIA. Heparin-induced thrombocytopenia (HIT) is an antibody-mediated process triggered by antibodies against neoantigens on PF4 that are exposed when heparin binds to this protein.[60] These antibodies, which are usually of the IgG subtype, bind simultaneously to the heparin-PF4 complex and to platelet Fc receptors. Such binding activates the platelets and generates platelet microparticles. Circulating microparticles are procoagulant because they express anionic phospholipids on their surface and can bind clotting factors, thereby promoting thrombin generation.

Typically, HIT occurs 5 to 14 days after the initiation of heparin therapy, but it may be manifested earlier if the patient has received heparin within the past 3 months (Table 95.5). Even a 50% decrease in the platelet count from the pretreatment value should raise suspicion of HIT in those receiving heparin. HIT is more common in surgical patients than in medical patients and, like many autoimmune disorders, occurs more frequently in females than in males.[60]

HIT is associated with either arterial or venous thrombosis. Venous thrombosis, which is manifested as deep vein thrombosis and/or pulmonary embolism, is more common than arterial thrombosis. Arterial thrombosis manifests as ischemic stroke or acute myocardial infarction. Rarely, platelet-rich thrombi in the distal aorta or iliac arteries can cause critical limb ischemia.

The diagnosis of HIT is established via enzyme-linked assays to detect antibodies against heparin-PF4 complexes or via platelet activation assays. Enzyme-linked assays are sensitive but are not specific and can be positive even in the absence of any clinical evidence of HIT.[61] The most specific diagnostic test is the serotonin release assay. This test involves quantification of serotonin release after exposure of washed platelets loaded with labeled serotonin to patient serum in the absence or presence of various concentrations of heparin. If the patient's serum contains HIT antibody, the addition of heparin induces platelet activation and subsequent serotonin release.

To manage HIT, heparin therapy should be stopped in patients with suspected or documented HIT, and an alternative anticoagulant should be administered to prevent or treat thrombosis (Table 95.6).[61] The agents most often used for this indication are parenteral direct thrombin inhibitors, such as argatroban or bivalirudin, or factor Xa inhibitors, such as fondaparinux, rivaroxaban or apixaban. Patients with HIT, particularly those with associated thrombosis, often have evidence of increased thrombin generation, which can lead to consumption of protein C. If these patients receive warfarin without a concomitant parenteral anticoagulant, the further decrease in protein C levels induced by the vitamin K antagonist can trigger skin necrosis. To avoid this problem, patients with HIT require treatment with a direct thrombin inhibitor, fondaparinux, rivaroxaban, or apixaban until the platelet count returns to normal levels. At this point, low-dose warfarin therapy can be introduced, and the thrombin inhibitor or fondaparinux can be discontinued when the anticoagulant response to warfarin has been therapeutic for at least 2 days.

OSTEOPOROSIS. Treatment with therapeutic doses of heparin for more than a month can cause a reduction in bone density. This occurs in up to 30% of patients treated over the long term with heparin,[62] and symptomatic vertebral fractures occur in 2% to 3% of these individuals. Studies in vitro and in laboratory animals have provided insight into the pathogenesis of heparin-induced osteoporosis. These investigations suggest that heparin causes bone resorption by decreasing bone formation and enhancing bone resorption. Thus, heparin affects the activity of both osteoclasts and osteoblasts.

ELEVATED LEVELS OF TRANSAMINASES. Therapeutic doses of heparin frequently cause a modest elevation in serum levels of hepatic transaminases without a concomitant increase in the level of bilirubin. Levels of transaminases rapidly return to normal when use of the drug is stopped. The mechanism responsible for this phenomenon is unknown.

Low-Molecular-Weight Heparin

Consisting of smaller fragments of heparin, LMWH is prepared from unfractionated heparin by controlled enzymatic or chemical depolymerization. The mean molecular weight of LMWH is around 5000, one third the mean molecular weight of unfractionated heparin.[56] Because of its advantages over heparin (Table 95.7), LMWH has replaced heparin for most indications.

MECHANISM OF ACTION. Like heparin, LMWH exerts its anticoagulant activity by activating antithrombin. With a mean molecular weight of 5000, which corresponds to approximately 17 saccharide units, at least half of the pentasaccharide-containing chains of LMWH are too short to bridge thrombin to antithrombin (see Fig. 95.12). These chains retain the capacity to accelerate inhibition of factor Xa by antithrombin because this activity results largely from the conformational changes in antithrombin evoked by pentasaccharide binding. Consequently, LMWH catalyzes inhibition of factor Xa by antithrombin more than inhibition of thrombin.[63] Depending on their unique molecular weight distributions, LMWH preparations have anti–factor Xa to anti–factor IIa ratios ranging from 2:1 to 4:1 (see Table 95.3).

PHARMACOLOGY OF LOW-MOLECULAR-WEIGHT HEPARIN. Although usually given subcutaneously, LMWH can be administered intravenously if a rapid anticoagulant response is needed. LMWH has pharmacokinetic advantages over heparin. These advantages arise because the shorter heparin chains bind less avidly to endothelial cells, macrophages, and heparin-binding plasma proteins. Reduced binding to endothelial cells and macrophages eliminates the rapid, dose-dependent, and saturable mechanism of clearance that is a characteristic of unfractionated heparin. Instead, clearance of LMWH is not dose dependent and its plasma half-life is longer. Based on measurement of anti–factor Xa levels, LMWH has a plasma half-life of approximately 4 hours. Because of its renal clearance, LMWH can accumulate in patients with renal insufficiency.

LMWH exhibits approximately 90% bioavailability after subcutaneous injection.[63] Because LMWH binds less avidly to heparin-binding proteins in plasma than heparin does, LMWH produces a more predictable dose response, and resistance to LMWH is rare. With a longer half-life and more predictable anticoagulant response, LMWH can be given subcutaneously once or twice daily without monitoring coagulation, even when the drug is administered in treatment doses. These properties render LMWH more convenient than unfractionated heparin. Capitalizing on this feature, studies in patients with VTE have shown that home treatment with LMWH is as effective and safe as in-hospital treatment with continuous intravenous infusions of heparin.[63] Outpatient treatment with LMWH streamlines care, reduces health care costs, and increases patient satisfaction.

MONITORING OF LOW-MOLECULAR-WEIGHT HEPARIN. In most patients, LMWH does not require monitoring of coagulation. If monitoring is necessary, the anti–factor Xa level is measured because most LMWH preparations have little effect on the APTT. Therapeutic anti–factor Xa levels with LMWH range from 0.5 to 1.2 units/mL when measured 3 to 4 hours after drug administration. With prophylactic doses of LMWH, peak anti–factor Xa levels of 0.2 to 0.5 units/mL are desirable.[64]

Situations that may require LMWH monitoring include renal insufficiency and obesity. Monitoring of LMWH in patients with a creatinine clearance of 30 mL/min or less is advisable to ensure that no drug accumulation takes place. Although weight-adjusted LMWH dosages appear to produce therapeutic anti–factor Xa levels in overweight patients, this approach has not been well studied in those with morbid obesity. It may also be advisable to monitor the anticoagulant activity of LMWH during pregnancy because dose requirements can change, particularly in the third trimester. Monitoring should also be considered in high-risk settings, such as when patients with mechanical heart valves are given LMWH for prevention of valve thrombosis.

DOSAGES. The doses of LMWH recommended for prophylaxis or treatment vary depending on the preparation. For prophylaxis, once-daily subcutaneous doses of 4000 to 5000 units are often used, whereas doses of 2500 to 3000 units are given when the drug is administered twice daily. For treatment of VTE, a dose of 150 to 200 units/kg is given if the drug is administered once daily. If a twice-daily regimen is used, a dose of 100 units/kg is given. In patients with unstable angina, LMWH is administered subcutaneously twice daily at a dose of 100 to 120 units/kg. The dose is reduced in patients with renal impairment.

SIDE EFFECTS. The major complication of LMWH is bleeding. Meta-analyses suggest that the risk for major bleeding may be lower with LMWH than with unfractionated heparin. HIT and osteoporosis also are less common with LMWH than with unfractionated heparin.

BLEEDING. The risk for bleeding with LMWH increases when antiplatelet or fibrinolytic drugs are given concomitantly.[58] Recent surgery, trauma, or underlying hemostatic defects also increase the risk for bleeding with LMWH. Although protamine sulfate serves as an antidote for LMWH, it incompletely neutralizes the anticoagulant activity of LMWH because it binds only the longer chains.[56] Because longer chains contribute to thrombin inhibition by antithrombin, protamine sulfate completely reverses the anti–factor IIa activity of LMWH. In contrast, protamine sulfate only partially reverses the anti–factor Xa activity of LMWH because the shorter pentasaccharide-containing chains of LMWH do not bind protamine sulfate. Consequently, continuous intravenous unfractionated heparin may be a better choice than subcutaneous LMWH for patients at high risk for bleeding.

THROMBOCYTOPENIA. The risk for HIT is about fivefold lower with LMWH than with heparin.[55] LMWH binds less avidly to platelets and causes less release of PF4. Furthermore, with lower affinity for PF4 than for heparin, LMWH is less likely to induce the conformational changes in PF4 that trigger the formation of HIT antibodies. LMWH should not be used to treat patients with HIT, because most HIT antibodies exhibit cross-reactivity with LMWH.[55] This in vitro cross-reactivity is not simply a laboratory phenomenon; thrombosis can occur in HIT patients treated with LMWH.

OSTEOPOROSIS. The risk for osteoporosis is lower with long-term LMWH than with heparin.[62] For extended treatment, therefore, LMWH is a better choice than heparin because of the lower risk for osteoporosis and HIT.

Fondaparinux

A synthetic analogue of the antithrombin-binding pentasaccharide sequence, fondaparinux differs from LMWH in several ways (see Table 95.3). Fondaparinux is licensed for thromboprophylaxis in medical, general surgical, and high-risk orthopedic patients and as an alternative to heparin or LMWH for the initial treatment of patients with established VTE. Although fondaparinux is licensed as an alternative to heparin or LMWH in patients with acute coronary syndrome in Europe and Canada, it is not approved for this indication in the United States.

MECHANISM OF ACTION. As a synthetic analogue of the antithrombin-binding pentasaccharide sequence found in heparin and LMWH, fondaparinux has a molecular weight of 1728. Fondaparinux binds only to antithrombin (see Fig. 95.12) and is too short to bridge thrombin to antithrombin. Consequently, fondaparinux catalyzes inhibition of factor Xa by antithrombin and does not enhance the rate of thrombin inhibition.[55]

PHARMACOLOGY OF FONDAPARINUX. (SEE ALSO CHAPTER 41). Fondaparinux exhibits complete bioavailability after subcutaneous injection. With no binding to endothelial cells or plasma proteins, clearance of fondaparinux does not depend on the dosage, and its plasma half-life is 17 hours. The drug is administered subcutaneously once daily. Because of its renal clearance, fondaparinux is contraindicated in patients with creatinine clearance lower than 30 mL/min, and it should be used with caution in those with a creatinine clearance lower than 50 mL/min.[64]

Fondaparinux produces a predictable anticoagulant response after administration in fixed doses because it does not bind to plasma proteins. The drug is given at a dosage of 2.5 mg once daily for prevention of VTE. For initial treatment of established VTE, fondaparinux is given at a dosage of 7.5 mg once daily. The dosage can be reduced to 5 mg once daily for those weighing less than 50 kg and increased to 10 mg for those heavier than 100 kg. When given in these doses, fondaparinux is as effective as heparin or LMWH for the initial treatment of patients with deep vein thrombosis or pulmonary embolism and produces similar rates of bleeding.[55]

Fondaparinux is used at a dosage of 2.5 mg once daily in patients with acute coronary syndromes. When this prophylactic dose of fondaparinux was compared with treatment doses of enoxaparin in patients with non–ST-segment elevation acute coronary syndrome, no difference in the rate of cardiovascular death, myocardial infarction, or stroke was seen at 9 days. The rate of major bleeding, however, was 50% lower with fondaparinux than with enoxaparin, which resulted in a 17% reduction in mortality rates at 1 month with fondaparinux. In patients with acute coronary syndromes who require PCI, there is a risk for catheter thrombosis with fondaparinux unless adjunctive heparin is given.

SIDE EFFECTS. Although fondaparinux can induce the formation of HIT antibodies, HIT rarely occurs.[61] This apparent paradox reflects the fact that induction of HIT requires heparin chains of sufficient length to bind multiple PF4 molecules. Fondaparinux is too short to do so. In contrast to LMWH, there is no cross-reactivity of fondaparinux with HIT antibodies. Consequently, fondaparinux appears to be effective for the treatment of HIT, although large clinical trials supporting its use are lacking.

The major side effect of fondaparinux is bleeding, and it has no antidote. Protamine sulfate has no effect on the anticoagulant activity of fondaparinux because it fails to bind to the drug. Recombinant activated factor VII has reversed the anticoagulant effects of fondaparinux in volunteers, but it is unknown whether this agent controls fondaparinux-induced bleeding.

TABLE 95.8 Comparison of the Properties of Hirudin, Bivalirudin, and Argatroban

PROPERTY	HIRUDIN	BIVALIRUDIN	ARGATROBAN
Molecular mass	7000	1980	527
Site or sites of interaction with thrombin	Active site and exosite 1	Active site and exosite 1	Active site
Renal clearance	Yes	No	No
Hepatic metabolism	No	No	Yes
Plasma half-life (minutes)	60	25	45

Parenteral Direct Thrombin Inhibitors

Heparin and LMWH indirectly inhibit thrombin because they require antithrombin to exert their anticoagulant activity. In contrast, direct thrombin inhibitors do not require a plasma cofactor; instead, they bind directly to thrombin and block its interaction with its substrates. Approved parenteral direct thrombin inhibitors include argatroban and bivalirudin; lepirudin, a recombinant form of hirudin, also falls within this class but is no longer available (Table 95.8). Argatroban is licensed for the treatment of HIT, whereas bivalirudin is approved as an alternative to heparin in patients undergoing PCI, including those with HIT.

Argatroban

Argatroban, a univalent inhibitor that targets the active site of thrombin, is metabolized in the liver.[65] Consequently, it must be used with caution in patients with hepatic insufficiency. Argatroban is administered by continuous intravenous infusion and has a plasma half-life of approximately 45 minutes. The APTT is used to monitor its anticoagulant effect, and the dosage is adjusted to achieve an APTT 1.5 to 3 times the baseline value, but not to exceed 100 seconds. Argatroban also prolongs the international normalized ratio (INR), a feature that can complicate transitioning of patients to warfarin. This problem can be circumvented by using levels of factor X in place of the INR to monitor warfarin. Alternatively, the argatroban infusion can be stopped for 2 to 3 hours before determination of the INR.

Bivalirudin (see also Chapter 41)

A synthetic 20–amino acid analogue of hirudin, bivalirudin is a divalent thrombin inhibitor.[65] Thus, the amino terminal portion of bivalirudin interacts with the active site of thrombin, whereas its carboxy terminal tail binds to exosite 1, the substrate-binding domain on thrombin. Bivalirudin has a plasma half-life of 25 minutes, the shortest half-life of all the parenteral direct thrombin inhibitors. It is degraded by peptidases and is partially excreted via the kidneys. When given in high doses in the cardiac catheterization laboratory, the anticoagulant activity of bivalirudin is monitored with the activated clotting time. With lower doses, its activity can be monitored using the APTT.

Studies comparing bivalirudin with heparin plus a GPIIb/IIIa antagonist suggest that bivalirudin produces less bleeding. This feature, plus its short half-life, renders bivalirudin a potential alternative to heparin in patients undergoing PCI. Bivalirudin has also been used successfully in patients with HIT who require PCI.[65]

Oral Anticoagulants

For over 60 years, the vitamin K antagonists, such as warfarin, were the only available oral anticoagulants. This situation changed with the introduction of the direct oral anticoagulants, which include dabigatran, rivaroxaban, apixaban, and edoxaban.

Warfarin

A water-soluble vitamin K antagonist initially developed as a rodenticide; warfarin is the coumarin derivative most often prescribed in North America. Like other vitamin K antagonists, warfarin interferes with the synthesis of vitamin K–dependent clotting proteins, which include prothrombin (factor II) and factors VII, IX, and X. Warfarin also impairs synthesis of the vitamin K–dependent anticoagulant proteins C and S.[66]

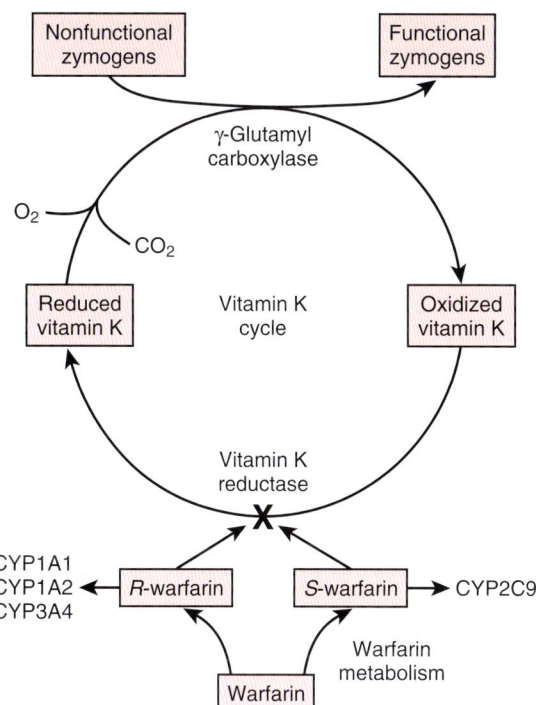

FIGURE 95.13 Mechanism of action of warfarin. A racemic mixture of S- and R-enantiomers, S-warfarin is most active. By blocking vitamin K epoxide reductase, warfarin inhibits the conversion of oxidized vitamin K into its reduced form. This inhibits vitamin K–dependent gamma-carboxylation of factors II, VII, IX, and X because reduced vitamin K serves as a cofactor for a gamma-glutamylcarboxylase, which catalyzes the gamma-carboxylation process, thereby converting prozymogens to zymogens capable of binding calcium and interacting with anionic phospholipid surfaces. S-warfarin is metabolized by CYP2C9. Common genetic polymorphisms in this enzyme can influence the metabolism of warfarin. Polymorphisms in the C1 subunit of vitamin K reductase (*VKORC1*) can also affect susceptibility of the enzyme to warfarin-induced inhibition, thereby influencing warfarin dosage requirements.

MECHANISM OF ACTION. All the vitamin K–dependent clotting factors possess glutamic acid residues at their N-terminals. A posttranslational modification adds a carboxyl group to the gamma carbon of these residues to generate gamma-carboxyglutamic acid. This modification is essential for expression of the activity of these clotting factors because it permits calcium-dependent binding of them to anionic phospholipid surfaces. A vitamin K–dependent carboxylase catalyzes the gamma-carboxylation. Thus, vitamin K from the diet undergoes reduction to vitamin K hydroquinone by vitamin K reductase (Fig. 95.13). Vitamin K hydroquinone serves as a cofactor for the carboxylase enzyme, which in the presence of carbon dioxide, replaces the hydrogen on the gamma carbon of glutamic acid residues with a carboxyl group. During this process, vitamin K hydroquinone is oxidized to vitamin K epoxide, which then undergoes reduction to vitamin K in a reaction catalyzed by vitamin K epoxide reductase.

Warfarin inhibits vitamin K epoxide reductase, thereby blocking the gamma-carboxylation process. This results in the synthesis of partially gamma-carboxylated clotting proteins with little or no biologic activity. Warfarin exerts its anticoagulant activity when the newly synthesized clotting factors with reduced activity gradually replace their fully active counterparts. The antithrombotic effect of warfarin requires a reduction in the functional levels of factor X and prothrombin, clotting factors with half-lives of 24 and 72 hours, respectively.[66] Because the antithrombotic effect of warfarin is delayed, patients with established thrombosis or at high risk for thrombosis require concomitant treatment with a rapidly acting parenteral anticoagulant, such as heparin, LMWH, or fondaparinux.[67]

PHARMACOLOGY. Warfarin is a racemic mixture of R- and S-isomers. It is rapidly and almost completely absorbed from the gastrointestinal tract. Levels of warfarin in blood peak approximately 90 minutes after administration. Racemic warfarin has a plasma half-life of 36 to 42 hours, and more than 97% of circulating warfarin is bound

TABLE 95.9 Frequencies of *CYP2C9* Genotypes and *VKORC1* Haplotypes in Different Populations and Their Effect on Warfarin Dose Requirements

GENOTYPE/HAPLOTYPE	FREQUENCY (%) WHITES	FREQUENCY (%) BLACKS	FREQUENCY (%) ASIANS	DOSE REDUCTION COMPARED WITH WILD-TYPE (%)
CYP2C9				
*1/*1	70	90	95	—
*1/*2	17	2	0	22
*1/*3	9	3	4	34
*2/*2	2	0	0	43
*2/*3	1	0	0	53
*3/*3	0	0	1	76
VKORC1				
Non-A/non-A	37	82	7	—
Non-A/A	45	12	30	26
A/A	18	6	63	50

to albumin. Only the small fraction of unbound warfarin is biologically active.[68]

Warfarin accumulates in the liver, where the two isomers are metabolized via distinct pathways. The more active S-enantiomer of warfarin is primarily metabolized by CYP2C9 (see Fig. 95.12). Two relatively common variants, *CYP2C9*2* and *CYP2C9*3*, encode an enzyme with reduced activity. Approximately 25% of whites have at least one variant allele of *CYP2C9*2* or *CYP2C9*3*; these variant alleles are less common in blacks and Asians (Table 95.9). Patients with one variant allele require 20% to 30% lower maintenance doses of warfarin, whereas those homozygous for these alleles require 50% to 70% lower doses than do those with the wild-type *CYP2C9*1* alleles. Consistent with the decreased warfarin dose requirement, patients with at least one CYP2C9 variant allele are at increased risk for bleeding. Thus, when compared with individuals with no variant alleles, the relative risk for warfarin-associated bleeding in *CYP2C9*2* or *CYP2C9*3* carriers is 1.9 and 1.8, respectively.[68]

Warfarin interferes with the vitamin K cycle by inhibiting the C1 subunit of vitamin K epoxide reductase (VKORCI).[68] Polymorphisms in *VKORC1* can influence the anticoagulant response to warfarin. Several genetic variations of *VKORC1* are in strong linkage disequilibrium and have been designated as non-A haplotypes. *VKORC1* variants are more prevalent than variants of *CYP2C9*. Asians have the highest prevalence of *VKORC1* variants, followed by whites and blacks. Warfarin dose requirements for patients heterozygous or homozygous for the A haplotype are 25% and 50% lower, respectively, than the dose needed for patients with the non-A/non-A haplotype. Polymorphisms in *CYP2C9* and *VKORC1* explain up to 25% of the variability in warfarin dose requirements.[68] These findings prompted the U.S. Food and Drug Administration to amend the prescribing information for warfarin to recommend lower starting doses for patients with the *CYP2C9* and *VKORC1* genetic variants. In addition to genetic factors, fluctuations in the dietary intake of vitamin K, drugs, and various disease states influence the anticoagulant effect of warfarin. Consequently, computerized genotype-based warfarin-dosing algorithms also include pertinent patient characteristics, such as age, body weight, and concomitant medications.[68] Although these algorithms streamline warfarin dosing, randomized trials following time in therapeutic range with genotype-based warfarin dosing have yielded mixed results. It remains unclear whether better dose identification improves patient outcomes in terms of reducing hemorrhagic complications or recurrent thrombotic events.[68]

MONITORING. Warfarin therapy is most often monitored with the prothrombin time, a test sensitive to reductions in the levels of prothrombin, factor VII, and factor X.[69] The test involves the addition of thromboplastin, a reagent that contains tissue factor, phospholipid, and calcium, to citrated plasma and determination of the time until clot formation.

Thromboplastins vary in their sensitivity to reductions in the levels of vitamin K–dependent clotting factors. Consequently, less sensitive thromboplastins will trigger the administration of higher doses of warfarin to achieve a target prothrombin time. This issue can cause problems because higher doses of warfarin increase the risk for bleeding.

The INR was developed to circumvent many of the problems associated with the prothrombin time. To calculate the INR, the patient's prothrombin time is divided by the mean normal prothrombin time, and this ratio is then multiplied by the international sensitivity index (ISI), an index of the sensitivity of the thromboplastin used for determination of the prothrombin time to reductions in levels of the vitamin K–dependent clotting factors. Extremely sensitive thromboplastins have an ISI of 1.0. Most current thromboplastins have ISI values that range from 1.0 to 1.4.[69]

Although the INR has helped standardize anticoagulant practice, problems persist. The precision of INR determination varies depending on reagent-coagulometer combinations, which has led to variability in INR results. Unreliable reporting of the ISI by thromboplastin manufacturers also complicates determination of the INR. Furthermore, every laboratory must establish the mean normal prothrombin time with each new batch of thromboplastin reagent. To accomplish this, the prothrombin time must be measured in fresh plasma samples from at least 20 healthy volunteers via the same coagulometer that is used for patient samples.

For most indications, warfarin is administered at doses that produce a target INR of 2.0 to 3.0. An exception is patients with mechanical heart valves in the mitral position or in patients with a mechanical heart valve in other positions who have additional risk factors for stroke, such as atrial fibrillation, in whom a target INR of 2.5 to 3.5 is recommended. Studies in patients with atrial fibrillation demonstrate an increased risk for ischemic stroke when the INR falls below 1.7 and an increase in bleeding with INR values higher than 4.5. These findings highlight the narrow therapeutic window of vitamin K antagonists. In support of this concept, a study in patients receiving long-term warfarin therapy for unprovoked VTE demonstrated a higher rate of recurrent VTE with a target INR of 1.5 to 1.9 than with a target INR of 2.0 to 3.0.

DOSAGES. Warfarin is usually started at a dose of 5 to 10 mg. Lower doses are used for patients with *CYP2C9* or *VKORC1* polymorphisms that affect the pharmacodynamics or pharmacokinetics of warfarin and render patients more sensitive to the drug. The dose is then titrated to achieve the desired target INR. Because of its delayed onset of action, patients with established thrombosis or those at high risk for thrombosis are given concomitant treatment with a rapidly acting parenteral anticoagulant, such as heparin, LMWH, or fondaparinux. Initial prolongation of the INR reflects a reduction in the functional levels of factor VII. Consequently, concomitant treatment with the parenteral anticoagulant should be continued until the INR has been therapeutic for at least 2 consecutive days. A minimum 5-day course of parenteral anticoagulation is recommended to ensure that the levels of prothrombin have fallen into the therapeutic range with warfarin.

The narrow therapeutic window of warfarin renders frequent monitoring of coagulation necessary to ensure a therapeutic anticoagulant response. Even patients with stable warfarin dose requirements should have their INR determined every 3 to 4 weeks. Although some studies have raised the possibility that testing every 12 weeks may suffice in such patients, these results require confirmation in a larger number of patients.[70] More frequent INR monitoring is necessary with the introduction of new concomitant medications because many drugs enhance or reduce the anticoagulant effects of warfarin.

SIDE EFFECTS. Like all anticoagulants, the major side effect of warfarin is bleeding; a rare complication is skin necrosis. Warfarin crosses the placenta and can cause fetal abnormalities, so it should not be used during pregnancy.

BLEEDING. At least half of the bleeding complications with warfarin occur when the INR exceeds the therapeutic range. Bleeding complications may be mild, such as epistaxis or hematuria, or more severe, such as retroperitoneal or gastrointestinal bleeding. Life-threatening intracranial bleeding can also occur. To minimize the risk for bleeding, the INR should be maintained in the therapeutic range.

In asymptomatic patients whose INR is between 3.5 and 9, warfarin should be withheld until the INR returns to the therapeutic range. If the patient is at high risk for bleeding, sublingual or oral vitamin K can be administered. A vitamin K dose of 1 to 2.5 mg is usually adequate for patients with an INR between 4.9 and 9, whereas 2.5 to 5 mg can be used for those with an INR higher than 9. Higher doses of oral vitamin K (5 to 10 mg) produce more rapid reversal of the INR and may be helpful if the INR is excessively high.

Patients with serious bleeding need additional treatment. These patients require 10 mg of vitamin K by slow intravenous infusion with additional doses of vitamin K until the INR is in the normal range and four factor prothrombin complex concentrate to replace the vitamin K–dependent clotting proteins. Prothrombin complex concentrate is preferred over fresh frozen plasma for warfarin reversal because it normalizes the INR more rapidly and because the volume of administration is much smaller.[71]

Warfarin-treated patients who experience bleeding when their INR is in the therapeutic range require investigation of the cause of the bleeding. Those with gastrointestinal bleeding often have underlying peptic ulcer disease or a tumor. Similarly, investigation of hematuria or uterine bleeding in patients with a therapeutic INR may unmask a tumor of the genitourinary tract.

SKIN NECROSIS. A rare complication of warfarin, skin necrosis usually occurs 2 to 5 days after initiation of therapy. Well-demarcated erythematous lesions form on the thighs, buttocks, breasts, or toes. Typically, the center of the lesion becomes progressively necrotic. Examination of skin biopsy specimens taken from the borders of these lesions reveals thrombi in the microvasculature.

Warfarin-induced skin necrosis occurs in patients with congenital or acquired deficiencies of protein C or protein S or in patients with HIT whose heparin has been stopped but an alternate anticoagulant has not been given.[72,73] Initiation of warfarin therapy in these patients produces a precipitous fall in plasma levels of proteins C or S, thereby eliminating this important anticoagulant pathway before warfarin exerts an antithrombotic effect through lowering the functional levels of factor X and prothrombin. The resultant procoagulant state triggers thrombosis that is localized to the microvasculature of fatty tissues for unknown reasons.

Treatment of warfarin-induced skin necrosis involves discontinuation of warfarin and reversal with vitamin K, if needed. An alternative anticoagulant, such as heparin or LMWH, or fondaparinux or rivaroxaban in patients with HIT, should be given to patients with thrombosis. Protein C concentrates may accelerate healing of the skin lesions in protein C–deficient patients; fresh frozen plasma may be of value for those with protein S deficiency. Occasionally, skin grafting is necessary in those with extensive skin loss. Because of the potential for skin necrosis, patients with known protein C or protein S deficiency require overlapping treatment with a parenteral anticoagulant when initiating warfarin therapy. Warfarin should be started at low doses in these patients, and the parenteral anticoagulant should be continued until the INR is therapeutic for at least 2 to 3 consecutive days. Use of rivaroxaban or apixaban in place of warfarin can simplify management of such patients.

PREGNANCY. Warfarin crosses the placenta and can cause fetal abnormalities or bleeding. The fetal abnormalities include a characteristic embryopathy, which consists of nasal hypoplasia and stippled epiphyses. The risk for embryopathy is highest with warfarin administration in the first trimester of pregnancy. Central nervous system abnormalities can also occur with exposure to warfarin at any time during pregnancy. Finally, maternal administration of warfarin produces an anticoagulant effect in the fetus that can cause bleeding. This is of particular concern at delivery, when trauma to the head during passage through the birth canal can lead to intracranial bleeding. Because of these potential problems, warfarin is contraindicated in pregnancy, particularly in the first and third trimesters. Instead, heparin, LMWH, or fondaparinux can be given during pregnancy for prevention or treatment of thrombosis. Warfarin does not pass into breast milk and thus is safe for nursing mothers.

SPECIAL PROBLEMS. Patients with a lupus anticoagulant (LA) or those who need urgent or elective surgery present special challenges.

Although observational studies suggested that patients with thrombosis complicating antiphospholipid syndrome require higher-intensity warfarin regimens to prevent recurrent thromboembolic events, randomized trials indicated that usual-intensity warfarin treatment (INR of 2.0 to 3.0) is as effective as higher-intensity therapy and produces less bleeding.[74] Monitoring of warfarin can be problematic in patients with antiphospholipid syndrome if the LA prolongs the baseline INR; factor X levels can be used instead of the INR in such patients.

There is no need to stop warfarin treatment before procedures associated with a low risk for bleeding, including dental cleaning, simple dental extraction, cataract surgery, or skin biopsy.[75] In contrast, warfarin must be stopped 5 days before elective invasive procedures associated with a moderate or high risk for bleeding to allow the INR to return to normal levels. Only patients at high risk for thrombosis while not taking warfarin (such as those with mechanical heart valves in the mitral position or atrial fibrillation patients with a prior history of stroke) require bridging with once- or twice-daily subcutaneous injections of LMWH when the INR falls below 2.0. The last dose of LMWH should be given 12 to 24 hours before the procedure, depending on whether LMWH is administered twice or once daily, respectively. Once hemostasis is secure after the procedure, warfarin can be restarted. Thromboprophylaxis with LMWH can be given starting the day after major surgery and should be continued until the INR is therapeutic.

Direct Oral Anticoagulants (see also Chapters 38, 39, 66, and 87)

Direct oral anticoagulants that target thrombin or factor Xa are well established alternatives to warfarin. These drugs have a rapid onset of action and half-lives that permit once- or twice-daily administration. Designed to produce a predictable level of anticoagulation, direct oral anticoagulants are more convenient to administer than warfarin because they are given in fixed doses without the need for routine monitoring of coagulation. As a class, the direct oral anticoagulants are at least as effective as warfarin and produce less serious bleeding, particularly less intracranial hemorrhage.

MECHANISM OF ACTION. Direct oral anticoagulants are small molecules that bind reversibly to the active site of their target enzyme. Table 95.10 summarizes the pharmacologic features of these agents.

DOSAGES. For prevention of stroke in patients with nonvalvular atrial fibrillation, rivaroxaban is given at a dosage of 20 mg once daily, with a reduction to 15 mg once daily in patients with a creatinine clearance of 15 to 49 mL/min; dabigatran is given at a dosage of 150 mg twice daily, with a reduction to 75 mg twice daily in those with a creatinine clearance of 15 to 30 mL/min; apixaban is given at a dosage of 5 mg twice daily, with a reduction to 2.5 mg twice daily for patients with at least two of the "ABC" criteria (i.e., *a*ge over 80 years, *b*ody weight under 60 kg, and *c*reatinine over 1.5 g/dL); and edoxaban is given at a dosage of 60 mg once daily for patients with a creatinine clearance of 50 to 95 mL/min and with a reduction to 30 mg once daily for patients with any one of the following criteria: creatinine clearance 15 to 50 mL/min,

TABLE 95.10 Comparison of the Features of the Direct Oral Anticoagulants

FEATURES	RIVAROX-ABAN	APIXABAN	EDOXABAN	DABIGATRAN
Target	Xa	Xa	Xa	IIa
Molecular weight	436	460	548	628
Prodrug	No	No	No	Yes
Bioavailability (%)	80	60	50	6
Time to peak (hr)	3	3	2	2
Half-life (hr)	7–11	12	9–14	12–17
Renal excretion (%)	33	25	50	80

body weight of 60 kg or less, or use of potent P-glycoprotein inhibitors, such as verapamil or quinidine.

Dabigatran, rivaroxaban, apixaban, and edoxaban are also licensed for treatment of patients with VTE. Dabigatran and edoxaban are started after patients have received at least a 5-day course of treatment with a parenteral anticoagulant such as LMWH; dabigatran is given at a dose of 150 mg twice daily provided the creatinine clearance is over 30 mL/min, and the dosage regimen for edoxaban is identical to that used in patients with atrial fibrillation. In contrast, rivaroxaban and apixaban can be given in all-oral regimens; rivaroxaban is started at a dose of 15 mg twice daily for 21 days and is then reduced to 20 mg once daily thereafter, whereas apixaban is started at a dose of 10 mg twice daily for 7 days and is then reduced to 5 mg twice daily thereafter.[54] For long-term secondary prevention, the dosage of apixaban can be lowered to 2.5 mg twice daily and the dose of rivaroxaban can be lowered to 10 mg once daily, doses that have safety profiles similar to those of placebo and aspirin, respectively.[54]

Dabigatran, rivaroxaban, and apixaban are licensed for thromboprophylaxis after elective hip or knee replacement surgery; edoxaban is not licensed for this indication except in Japan. Thromboprophylaxis is started after surgery and is often continued for 30 days in patients undergoing hip replacement and for 10 to 14 days in patients undergoing knee replacement. In lower-risk patients undergoing hip or knee replacement surgery, a 5-day course of rivaroxaban followed by a 30-day course of aspirin at a dose of 81 mg daily appears to be as effective and safe as extended thromboprophylaxis with rivaroxaban.[76] Dabigatran is given at a dose of 220 mg once daily, whereas rivaroxaban and apixaban are given at doses of 10 mg once daily and 2.5 mg twice daily, respectively. For secondary prevention of adverse cardiac or limb events in patients with coronary or peripheral artery disease, rivaroxaban is given at a dose of 2.5 mg twice daily on top of aspirin (81 or 100 mg once daily).

MONITORING. Although administered without routine monitoring, in some situations determination of the anticoagulant activity of the direct oral anticoagulants can be helpful,[77] including assessment of adherence, detection of accumulation or overdose, identification of bleeding mechanisms, and determination of activity before surgery or intervention. For qualitative assessment of anticoagulant activity, the prothrombin time can be used for factor Xa inhibitors and the APTT for dabigatran. Rivaroxaban and edoxaban prolong the prothrombin time more than apixaban does. In fact, because apixaban has such a limited effect on the prothrombin time, anti–factor Xa assays are needed to assess its activity.[77] The effect of the drugs on tests of coagulation varies depending on the reagents used to perform the tests, and variability increases with conversion of the prothrombin time to an INR. Chromogenic anti–factor Xa assays and the diluted thrombin clotting time or ecarin clotting or chromogenic assays with appropriate calibrators provide quantitative assays to measure plasma levels of the factor Xa inhibitors and dabigatran, respectively.[77]

SIDE EFFECTS. As with any anticoagulant, bleeding is the most common side effect of the direct oral anticoagulants. Although the direct oral anticoagulants are associated with less intracranial bleeding than warfarin is, the risk for gastrointestinal bleeding is higher with dabigatran (at the 150-mg, twice-daily dose), rivaroxaban, and edoxaban (at the 60-mg, once-daily dose) than with warfarin. Dyspepsia occurs in up to 10% of patients treated with dabigatran; this problem improves with time and can be minimized by taking the drug with food.

PERIPROCEDURAL MANAGEMENT. Like warfarin, the direct oral anticoagulants must be stopped before surgical procedures associated with a moderate or high risk for bleeding.[77,78] The drugs should be withheld for 1 to 2 days or longer if renal function is impaired. After surgery, patients should receive thromboprophylaxis with LMWH until hemostasis is restored, at which point the direct oral anticoagulants can be restarted.

Cardiac procedures such as atrial fibrillation ablation or pacemaker implantation can safely be performed without interruption of the direct oral anticoagulants. However, it may be prudent to hold the dose in the morning of the day of the procedure to avoid intervention at peak drug levels.

MANAGEMENT OF BLEEDING. With minor bleeding, withholding one or two doses of drug is usually sufficient.[79,80] With more serious bleeding, the approach is similar to that with warfarin, except that vitamin K administration is of no benefit; the anticoagulant and any antiplatelet drugs should be withheld, the patient should be resuscitated with fluids and blood products as necessary, and the bleeding site should be identified and managed. Coagulation testing will determine the extent of anticoagulation, and renal function should be assessed so that the half-life of the drug can be calculated.[79] Timing of the last dose of anticoagulant is important, and oral activated charcoal may help prevent absorption of drug administered in the past 4 hours particularly in cases of overdose. If bleeding continues or is life-threatening or if it occurs in a critical organ (e.g., the eye) or in a closed space (e.g., the pericardium or retroperitoneum), reversal of the anticoagulant should be considered.

Idarucizumab is licensed for dabigatran reversal in patients with serious bleeding or in those requiring urgent surgery or intervention.[81] A humanized antibody fragment, idarucizumab binds dabigatran with 350-fold higher affinity than that of dabigatran for thrombin to form an essentially irreversible complex that is cleared by the kidneys (Table 95.11). Idarucizumab is given intravenously as a 5-g bolus and is supplied in a box containing two 50-mL vials, each containing 2.5 g of idarucizumab.[81] Idarucizumab rapidly reverses the anticoagulant effects of dabigatran and normalizes the aPTT, diluted thrombin time, or ecarin clot time.[82]

Andexanet alfa is available for reversal of rivaroxaban, apixaban, and edoxaban. A recombinant variant of factor Xa without catalytic activity, andexanet serves as a decoy to sequester oral factor Xa inhibitors until they are cleared from the circulation.[81] Low- or high-dose intravenous andexanet regimens are used. The low-dose regimen starts with a bolus of 400 mg followed by an infusion of 4 mg/min for up to 120 minutes, whereas the high-dose regimen starts with a bolus of 800 mg followed by an infusion of 8 mg/min for up to 120 minutes.

TABLE 95.11 Reversal Agents for Direct Oral Anticoagulants

FEATURE	IDARUCIZUMAB	ANDEXANET ALFA	CIRAPARANTAG
Structure	Humanized antibody fragment	Recombinant human factor Xa variant	Synthetic, small cationic molecule
Mass (Da)	47,776	39,000	573
Mechanism of action	Binds dabigatran with high affinity	Competes with factors Xa for binding	Binds via hydrogen bonds
Target	Dabigatran	Rivaroxaban, apixaban, edoxaban and heparins	Dabigatran, rivaroxaban, apixaban, edoxaban and heparins
Administration	Intravenous bolus	Intravenous bolus followed by a 2-hour infusion	Intravenous bolus
Measurement of reversal	Activated partial thromboplastin time, diluted thrombin time, or ecarin clotting time or chromogenic assay	Calibrated anti-factor Xa assays	Whole-blood clotting time
Elimination	Renal (catabolism)	Not reported	Not reported
Cost	$3,500 per dose in the United States	$25,000 for low dose and double for high dose	Likely to be low

The low-dose regimen is used for reversal of doses of rivaroxaban or apixaban of 10 mg or 5 mg or less, respectively, or for any dose of rivaroxaban or apixaban if the last dose was taken more than 8 hours prior to presentation. The high-dose regimen is used to reverse rivaroxaban or apixaban doses over 10 and 5 mg, respectively, if the last dose was taken less than 8 hours since presentation, or for reversal if the dose of rivaroxaban or apixaban or the timing of the last dose is unknown (see Table 95.11). Andexanet alfa is expensive and is not available in all hospitals. Because of its cost, andexanet alfa is often reserved for reversal in patients with intracranial bleeds or for bleeds into a closed space such as retroperitoneal or pericardial bleeds. If andexanet is unavailable, the results of prospective cohort studies suggest that 4-factor prothrombin complex concentrate (25 to 50 units/kg) also is effective at restoring hemostasis.[81] If there is continued bleeding, activated prothrombin complex concentrate (50 units/kg) or recombinant factor VIIa (90 μg/kg) can be considered.[81]

Neither andexanet alfa nor 4-factor prothrombin complex concentrate has been evaluated for reversal in patients requiring urgent surgery or intervention. Furthermore, andexanet alfa not only reverses oral factor Xa inhibitors but also reverses heparin and LMWH. This could be problematic in patients who require cardiac surgery or vascular surgery, procedures where heparin is used routinely. To circumvent this problem, most surgical procedures and interventions can be done without reversal and 4-factor prothrombin complex concentrate can be given if necessary. For patients requiring surgery to stop bleeding such as those with a ruptured aortic aneurysm or with bleeding secondary to polytrauma, up front 4-factor prothrombin concentrate administration can be considered.

At an earlier stage of development than andexanet, ciraparantag is a synthetic, cationic small molecule that binds rivaroxaban, apixaban, and edoxaban, as well as dabigatran, heparin, LMWH, and fondaparinux. When given as an intravenous bolus to volunteers who took 60 mg of edoxaban, ciraparantag reduced the whole-blood clotting time in a concentration-dependent manner.[81] Because it binds citrate and other calcium chelators, routine tests of coagulation, such as the INR, APTT, or anti–factor Xa activity cannot be used to monitor ciraparantag reversal. Although the whole-blood clotting time may be useful for this purpose, the test is not widely available. Therefore, additional studies are needed before ciraparantag will be approved.

PREGNANCY. As small molecules, the direct oral anticoagulants can all pass through the placenta. Consequently, these agents are contraindicated in pregnancy, and when used by women of childbearing potential, appropriate contraception is important. Small amounts of rivaroxaban pass into breast milk, and it is unknown whether the other direct oral anticoagulants also do so. Therefore, direct oral anticoagulants should not be used in nursing mothers.

Novel Anticoagulants in Development
Although the direct oral anticoagulants represent a major advance over warfarin, the search for more effective and safer anticoagulants continues. Evidence that factor XII and factor XI, components of the contact system, are important for thrombus stabilization and growth has prompted development of anticoagulants that target these factors. Numerous phase 2 studies evaluating antisense oligonucleotides, inhibitory antibodies, and small molecule inhibitors are underway.[24]

Fibrinolytic Drugs (see also Chapter 38)
Used to degrade thrombi, fibrinolytic drugs are administered systemically or are delivered via catheters directly into the substance of the thrombus. Currently approved fibrinolytic agents include streptokinase; acylated plasminogen streptokinase activator complex (anistreplase); urokinase; recombinant t-PA (rt-PA), also known as alteplase or Activase; and two recombinant derivatives of rt-PA, tenecteplase and reteplase. Each of these agents acts by converting the proenzyme, plasminogen, to plasmin, the active enzyme.[11] There are two pools of plasminogen—circulating plasminogen and fibrin-bound plasminogen (Fig. 95.14). Plasminogen activators that preferentially activate fibrin-bound plasminogen are fibrin specific. In contrast, nonspecific plasminogen activators do not discriminate between fibrin-bound

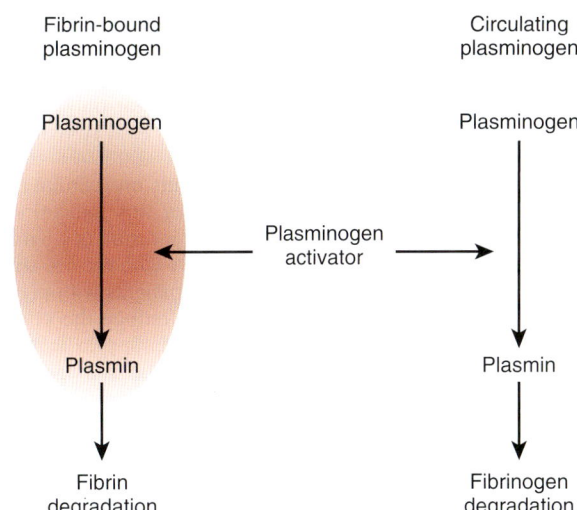

FIGURE 95.14 Consequences of activation of fibrin-bound or circulating plasminogen. The fibrin specificity of plasminogen activators reflects their capacity to distinguish between fibrin-bound and circulating plasminogen, which depends on their affinity for fibrin. Plasminogen activators with high affinity for fibrin preferentially activate fibrin-bound plasminogen. This results in the generation of plasmin on the fibrin surface. Fibrin-bound plasmin, which is protected from inactivation by alpha$_2$-antiplasmin, degrades fibrin to yield soluble fibrin degradation products. In contrast, plasminogen activators with little or no affinity for fibrin do not distinguish between fibrin-bound and circulating plasminogen. Activation of circulating plasminogen results in systemic plasminemia and subsequent degradation of fibrinogen and other clotting factors.

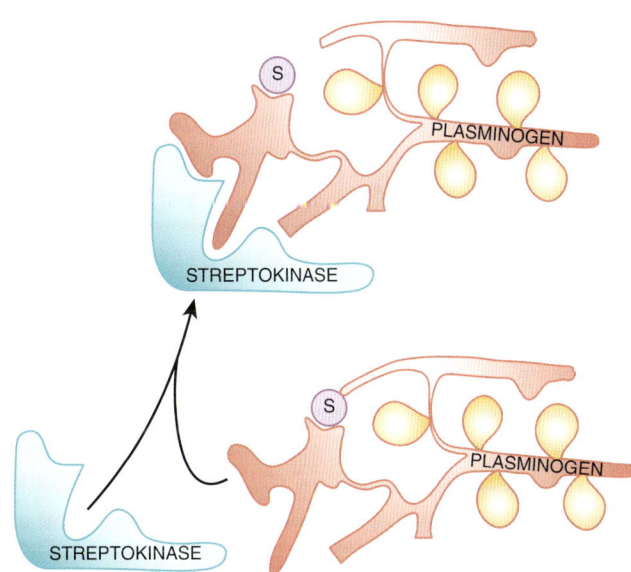

FIGURE 95.15 Mechanism of action of streptokinase. Streptokinase binds to plasminogen and induces a conformational change in plasminogen that exposes its active site. The streptokinase/plasmin(ogen) complex then serves as the activator of additional plasminogen molecules.

and circulating plasminogen.[83] Activation of circulating plasminogen results in the generation of unopposed plasmin, which can trigger the systemic lytic state. Alteplase and its derivatives are fibrin-specific plasminogen activators, whereas streptokinase, anistreplase, and urokinase are nonspecific agents.

Streptokinase
Unlike other plasminogen activators, streptokinase is not an enzyme and does not directly convert plasminogen to plasmin. Instead, it forms a 1:1 stoichiometric complex with plasminogen, thereby inducing a conformational change in plasminogen that exposes its active site (Fig. 95.15). This conformationally altered plasminogen then converts additional plasminogen molecules to plasmin.[84] Streptokinase

has no affinity for fibrin, and the streptokinase-plasminogen complex activates both free and fibrin-bound plasminogen. Activation of circulating plasminogen generates sufficient amounts of plasmin to overwhelm alpha$_2$-antiplasmin. Unopposed plasmin not only degrades fibrin in the occlusive thrombus but also induces a systemic lytic state.[83]

When given systemically to patients with acute myocardial infarction, streptokinase reduces mortality rates. For this indication the drug is usually administered as an intravenous infusion of 1.5 million units over a period of 30 to 60 minutes. Patients who receive streptokinase can form antibodies against it, as can patients with previous streptococcal infection. These antibodies can reduce the effectiveness of streptokinase. Allergic reactions occur in approximately 5% of patients treated with streptokinase. They may be manifested as a rash, fever, chills, and rigors; rarely, anaphylactic reactions can occur. Transient hypotension is common with streptokinase and probably reflects plasmin-mediated release of bradykinin. The hypotension usually responds to leg elevation and administration of intravenous fluids and low doses of vasopressors, such as dopamine or norepinephrine.

Anistreplase

To generate anistreplase, streptokinase is mixed with equimolar amounts of Lys-plasminogen, a plasmin-cleaved form of plasminogen with a Lys residue at its N-terminal. The active site of Lys-plasminogen exposed on combination with streptokinase is then blocked with an anisoyl group. After intravenous infusion, the anisoyl group is removed by deacylation, such that the complex has a half-life of approximately 100 minutes.[85] This allows drug administration via a single bolus infusion. Although it is more convenient to administer, anistreplase offers few mechanistic advantages over streptokinase. Like streptokinase, anistreplase does not distinguish between fibrin-bound and circulating plasminogen. Consequently, anistreplase produces a systemic lytic state. Similarly, allergic reactions and hypotension are just as frequent with anistreplase as they are with streptokinase. When anistreplase was compared with alteplase in patients with acute myocardial infarction, reperfusion was achieved more rapidly with alteplase than with anistreplase. Improved reperfusion was associated with a trend toward better clinical outcomes and reduced mortality rates with alteplase. The modest improvement in outcomes and the high cost of anistreplase have dampened enthusiasm for its use.

Urokinase

Originally isolated from cultured fetal kidney cells and later synthesized using recombinant DNA technology, urokinase is a two-chain serine protease with a molecular weight of 34,000.[11] Urokinase directly converts plasminogen to plasmin. Unlike streptokinase, urokinase is not immunogenic, and allergic reactions are rare. Urokinase produces a systemic lytic state because it does not discriminate between fibrin-bound and circulating plasminogen. Despite many years of use, systemic urokinase has never been evaluated for coronary fibrinolysis; instead, urokinase was mostly used for catheter-directed lysis of thrombi in the deep veins or in peripheral arteries. Because of production problems, urokinase is no longer available.

Alteplase

A recombinant form of single-chain t-PA, alteplase has a molecular weight of 68,000. Plasmin rapidly converts alteplase into its two-chain form. The interaction of alteplase with fibrin is mediated by the finger domain and, to a lesser extent, by the second kringle domain (Fig. 95.16).[11] Alteplase has a considerably higher affinity for fibrin than for fibrinogen. Consequently, the catalytic efficiency of plasminogen activation by alteplase is two to three orders of magnitude higher in the presence of fibrin than in the presence of fibrinogen.[83] Although alteplase preferentially activates plasminogen in the presence of fibrin, it is not as fibrin selective as first thought. Its fibrin specificity is limited because like fibrin, (DD)E, the major soluble degradation product of cross-linked fibrin, binds alteplase and plasminogen with high affinity. As a result, (DD)E is as potent as fibrin as a stimulator of plasminogen activation by alteplase. Plasmin generated on the

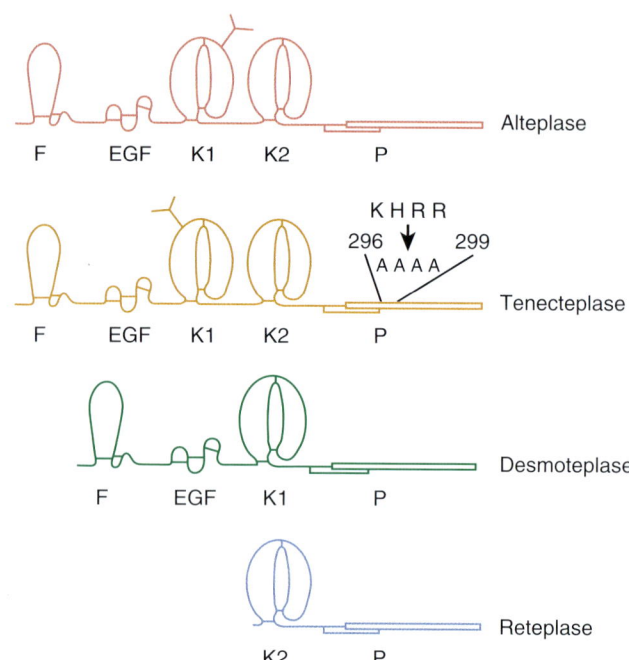

FIGURE 95.16 Domain structures of alteplase, tenecteplase, desmoteplase, and reteplase. The finger (F), epidermal growth factor (EGF), first and second kringles (K1 and K2, respectively), and protease (P) domains are illustrated. The glycosylation site (Y) on K1 has been repositioned in tenecteplase to endow it with a longer half-life. In addition, a tetra-alanine substitution in the protease domain renders tenecteplase resistant to PAI-1 inhibition. Desmoteplase differs from alteplase and tenecteplase in that it lacks a K2 domain. Reteplase is a truncated variant that lacks the F, EGF, and K1 domains.

fibrin surface results in thrombolysis, whereas plasmin generated on the surface of circulating (DD)E degrades fibrinogen. Fibrinogenolysis results in the accumulation of fragment X, a high-molecular-weight clottable fibrinogen degradation product. Incorporation of fragment X into hemostatic plugs formed at sites of vascular injury renders them susceptible to lysis.[86] This phenomenon may contribute to alteplase-induced bleeding.

A trial comparing alteplase with streptokinase for the treatment of patients with acute myocardial infarction demonstrated significantly lower mortality rates with alteplase than with streptokinase, although the absolute difference was small. Patients older than 75 years with anterior myocardial infarction presenting less than 6 hours after the onset of symptoms derived the greatest benefit from alteplase. Acute myocardial infarction or acute ischemic stroke is treated with an intravenous infusion of alteplase over a 60- to 90-minute period. The total dose of alteplase usually ranges from 90 to 100 mg. Allergic reactions and hypotension are rare, and alteplase is not immunogenic.

Tenecteplase

A genetically engineered variant of t-PA, tenecteplase was designed to have a longer half-life than t-PA and to be resistant to inactivation by PAI-1.[85] To prolong its half-life, a new glycosylation site was added to the first kringle domain (see Fig. 95.16). Because addition of this extra carbohydrate side chain reduced fibrin affinity, the existing glycosylation site on the first kringle domain was removed. To render the molecule resistant to inhibition by PAI-1, a tetra-alanine substitution was introduced at residues 296 to 299 in the protease domain, the region responsible for the interaction of t-PA with PAI-1.

Tenecteplase is more fibrin specific than t-PA. Although both agents bind to fibrin with similar affinity, the affinity of tenecteplase for (DD)E is significantly lower than that of t-PA. Consequently, (DD)E does not stimulate systemic plasminogen activation by tenecteplase to the same extent as t-PA does. As a result, tenecteplase produces less fibrinogenolysis than t-PA does.

For coronary fibrinolysis, tenecteplase is administered as a single intravenous bolus. In a large phase III trial that enrolled more than

16,000 patients, the 30-day mortality rate with single-bolus tenecteplase was like that with accelerated-dose t-PA. Although rates of intracranial hemorrhage were also similar with both treatments, patients given tenecteplase had less noncerebral bleeding and a reduced need for blood transfusions in comparison with those treated with t-PA. The improved safety profile of tenecteplase probably reflects its enhanced fibrin specificity.

Reteplase

A recombinant t-PA derivative, reteplase is a single-chain variant that lacks the finger, epidermal growth factor, and first kringle domains (see Fig. 95.16). This truncated derivative has a molecular weight of 39,000.[85] Reteplase binds fibrin with lower affinity than t-PA does because it lacks the finger domain. Because it is produced in *Escherichia coli*, reteplase is not glycosylated; this feature endows it with a plasma half-life longer than that of t-PA. Consequently, reteplase is given as two intravenous boluses separated by 30 minutes. Clinical trials in patients with acute myocardial infarction showed improved 30-day survival rates when reteplase was compared with streptokinase, but its noninferiority compared with alteplase.

Other Fibrinolytic Agents

Other fibrinolytic agents include desmoteplase (see Fig. 95.16), a recombinant form of the full-length plasminogen activator isolated from the saliva of the vampire bat, and alfimeprase, a truncated form of fibrolase, an enzyme isolated from the venom of the southern copperhead snake. Clinical studies with these agents have been disappointing. Desmoteplase, which is more fibrin specific than t-PA, was investigated for the treatment of acute ischemic stroke. Patients initially seen 3 to 9 hours after the onset of symptoms were randomly assigned to one or two doses of desmoteplase or to placebo. Overall response rates were low, and no differences from placebo were noted. Mortality rates were higher with desmoteplase.

Alfimeprase is a metalloproteinase that degrades fibrin and fibrinogen in a plasmin-independent fashion. In the circulation, alpha$_2$-macroglobulin inhibits alfimeprase, so alfimeprase must be delivered via a catheter directly into the thrombus. Despite promising phase II results, studies of alfimeprase for the treatment of peripheral arterial occlusion or for restoration of flow in blocked central venous catheters were stopped because of lack of efficacy. The disappointing results with desmoteplase and alfimeprase highlight the challenges of introducing new fibrinolytic drugs.

FUTURE PERSPECTIVES

Thrombosis in arteries or veins involves interplay among the vessel wall, platelets, the coagulation system, and fibrinolytic pathways. Activation of coagulation also triggers inflammatory pathways that may contribute to thrombosis. A better understanding of the biochemistry of platelet aggregation and blood coagulation and advances in structure-based drug design have identified new targets and prompted the development of novel antithrombotic drugs. Despite these advances, however, arterial and venous thromboembolic disorders remain a major cause of morbidity and death. The search for better targets and more potent, safer, or more convenient antiplatelet, anticoagulant, and fibrinolytic drugs continues.

REFERENCES

Hemostatic and Thrombotic Mechanisms

1. Bäck M, Yurdagul Jr A, Tabas I, et al. Inflammation and its resolution in atherosclerosis: mediators and therapeutic opportunities. *Nat Rev Cardiol*. 2019;16(7):389–406.
2. Chan NC, Weitz JI. Recent advances in understanding, diagnosing and treating venous thrombosis. *F1000Res*. 2020;9:F1000 Faculty Rev-1206.
3. Grover SP, Mackman N. Tissue factor: an essential mediator of hemostasis and trigger of thrombosis. *Arterioscler Thromb Vasc Biol*. 2018;38(4):709–725.
4. Thalin C, Hisada Y, Lundstrom S, et al. Neutrophil extracellular traps: Villains and targets in arterial, venous, and cancer-associated thrombosis. *Arterioscler Thromb Vasc Biol*. 2019;39(9):1724–1738.
5. Eikelboom JW, Connolly SJ, Bosch J, et al. Rivaroxaban with or without aspirin in stable cardiovascular disease. *N Engl J Med*. 2017;377(14):1319–1330.
6. Bonaca MP, Bauersachs RM, Anand SS, et al. Rivaroxaban in peripheral artery disease after revascularization. *N Engl J Med*. 2020;382(21):1994–2004.
7. Simes J, Becattini C, Agnelli G, et al. Aspirin for the prevention of recurrent venous thromboembolism: the inspire collaboration. *Circulation*. 2014;130(13):1062–1071.
8. Fuentes E, Palomo I. Extracellular ATP metabolism on vascular endothelial cells: a pathway with pro-thrombotic and anti-thrombotic molecules. *Vascul Pharmacol*. 2015;751–756.
9. Mast AE. Tissue factor pathway inhibitor: multiple anticoagulant activities for a single protein. *Arterioscl Thromb Vasc Biol*. 2016;36(1):9–14.
10. Griffin JH, Zlokovic BV, Mosnier LO. Activated protein c: Biased for translation. *Blood*. 2015;125(19):2898–2907.
11. Urano T, Castellino FJ, Suzuki Y. Regulation of plasminogen activation on cell surfaces and fibrin. *J Thromb Haemost*. 2018;16(8):1487–1497.
12. Baigger A, Blasczyk R, Figueiredo C. Towards the manufacture of megakaryocytes and platelets for clinical application. *Transfus Med Hemother*. 2017;44(3):165–173.
13. Becker RC, Sexton T, Smyth SS. Translational implications of platelets as vascular first responders. *Circ Res*. 2018;122(3):506–522.
14. Grover SP, Mackman N. Intrinsic pathway of coagulation and thrombosis. *Arterioscler Thromb Vasc Biol*. 2019;39(3):331–338.
15. Lenting PJ, Christophe OD, Denis CV. Von Willebrand factor biosynthesis, secretion, and clearance: connecting the far ends. *Blood*. 2015;125(13):2019–2028.
16. Gurbel PA, Kuliopulos A, Tantry US. G-protein-coupled receptors signaling pathways in new antiplatelet drug development. *Arterioscl Thromb Vasc Biol*. 2015;35(3):500–512.
17. Han X, Nieman MT. The domino effect triggered by the tethered ligand of the protease activated receptors. *Thromb Res*. 2020:19687–19698.
18. Jaffer IH, Weitz JI. The blood compatibility challenge. Part 1: Blood-contacting medical devices: the scope of the problem. *Acta Biomater*. 2019:942–10.
19. Ten Cate H, Hackeng TM, García de Frutos P. Coagulation factor and protease pathways in thrombosis and cardiovascular disease. *Thromb Haemost*. 2017;117(7):1265–1271.
20. Long AT, Kenne E, Jung R, et al. Contact system revisited: an interface between inflammation, coagulation, and innate immunity. *J Thrombosis Haemostasis*. 2016;14(3):427–437.
21. Baker CJ, Smith SA, Morrissey JH. Polyphosphate in thrombosis, hemostasis, and inflammation. *Res Pract Thromb Haemost*. 2019;3(1):18–25.
22. Buller HR, Bethune C, Bhanot S, et al. Factor XI antisense oligonucleotide for prevention of venous thrombosis. *N Engl J Med*. 2015;372(3):232–240.
23. Weitz JI, Bauersachs R, Becker B, et al. Effect of osocimab in preventing venous thromboembolism among patients undergoing knee arthroplasty: the foxtrot randomized clinical trial. *J Am Med Assoc*. 2020;323(2):130–139.
24. Fredenburgh JC, Weitz JI. New anticoagulants: moving beyond the direct oral anticoagulants. *J Thromb Haemost*. 2021;19(1):20–29.
25. Plug T, Meijers JC. Structure-function relationships in thrombin-activatable fibrinolysis inhibitor. *J ThrombHaemost*. 2016;14(4):633–644.
26. Bucci M, Tana C, Giamberardino MA, et al. Lp(a) and cardiovascular risk: investigating the hidden side of the moon. *Nutr Metab CardiovascDis*. 2016;26(11):980–986.
27. Azam TU, Shadid HR, Blakely P, et al. Soluble urokinase receptor (supar) in covid-19-related aki. *J Am Soc Nephrol*. 2020;31(11):2725–2735.
28. Vanhoutte PM, Zhao Y, Xu A, et al. Thirty years of saying no: sources, fate, actions, and misfortunes of the endothelium-derived vasodilator mediator. *Circ Res*. 2016;119(2):375–396.
29. Loghmani H, Conway EM. Exploring traditional and nontraditional roles for thrombomodulin. *Blood*. 2018;132(2):148–158.
30. Leask A. Getting to the heart of the matter: new insights into cardiac fibrosis. *Circ Res*. 2015;116(7):1269–1276.
31. Martinelli I, De Stefano V, Mannucci PM. Inherited risk factors for venous thromboembolism. *Nat Rev Cardiol*. 2014;11(3):140–156.
32. Walton BL, Byrnes JR, Wolberg AS. Fibrinogen, red blood cells, and factor xiii in venous thrombosis. *J Thrombosis Haemostasis*. 2015;13 suppl 1S208-S15.
33. Cohen AT, Harrington RA, Goldhaber SZ, et al. Extended thromboprophylaxis with betrixaban in acutely ill medical patients. *N Engl J Med*. 2016;375(6):534–544.
34. Spyropoulos AC, Ageno W, Albers GW, et al. Rivaroxaban for thromboprophylaxis after hospitalization for medical illness. *N Engl J Med*. 2018;379(12):1118–1127.
35. Mahajan A, Brunson A, White R, et al. The epidemiology of cancer-associated venous thromboembolism: an update. *Semin Thromb Hemost*. 2019;45(4):321–325.
36. Hisada Y, Mackman N. Cancer-associated pathways and biomarkers of venous thrombosis. *Blood*. 2017;130(13):1499–1506.
37. Delluc A, Antic D, Lecumberri R, et al. Occult cancer screening in patients with venous thromboembolism: guidance from the SSC of the ISTH. *J Thromb Haemost*. 2017;15(10):2076–2079.

Treatment of Thrombosis

38. Yeung J, Li W, Holinstat M. Platelet signaling and disease: targeted therapy for thrombosis and other related diseases. *Pharmacol Rev*. 2018;70(3):526–548.
39. Dugani S, Ames JM, Manson JE, et al. Weighing the anti-ischemic benefits and bleeding risks from aspirin therapy: a rational approach. *Curr Atheroscler Rep*. 2018;20(3):15.
40. Raber I, McCarthy CP, Vaduganathan M, et al. The rise and fall of aspirin in the primary prevention of cardiovascular disease. *Lancet*. 2019;393(10186):2155–2167.
41. Wangberg H, White AA. Aspirin-exacerbated respiratory disease. *Curr Opin Immunol*. 2020.669-13.
42. Michelson AD, Bhatt DL. How I use laboratory monitoring of antiplatelet therapy. *Blood*. 2017;130(6):713–721.
43. Bhatt DL, Grosser T, Dong JF, et al. Enteric coating and aspirin nonresponsiveness in patients with type 2 diabetes mellitus. *J Am Coll Cardiol*. 2017;69(6):603–612.
44. Gurbel PA, Myat A, Kubica J, et al. State of the art: oral antiplatelet therapy. *JRSM Cardiovasc Dis*. 2016;52048004016652514.
45. Thomas MR, Storey RF. Clinical significance of residual platelet reactivity in patients treated with platelet p2y12 inhibitors. *Vascul Pharmacol*. 2016:8425–8427.
46. Sabatine MS, Mega JL. Pharmacogenomics of antiplatelet drugs. *Hematology Am Soc Hematol Educ Program*. 2014;(1):343–347.
47. Cuisset T, Quilici J. Cyp-mediated pharmacologic interference with optimal platelet inhibition. *J Cardiovasc Transl Res*. 2013;6(3):404–410.
48. Siller-Matula JM, Trenk D, Schror K, et al. How to improve the concept of individualised antiplatelet therapy with p2y12 receptor inhibitors–is an algorithm the answer? *Thromb Haemost*. 2015;113(1):37–52.
49. Pereira NL, Rihal CS, So DYF, et al. Clopidogrel pharmacogenetics. *Circ Cardiovasc Interv*. 2019;12(4):e007811.
50. Bhatt DL, Pollack CV, Weitz JI, et al. Antibody-based ticagrelor reversal agent in healthy volunteers. *N Engl J Med*. 2019;380(19):1825–1833.
51. Rollini F, Franchi F, Angiolillo DJ. Switching p2y12 receptor inhibiting therapies. *Interv Cardiol Clin*. 2017;6(1):67–89.
52. Kapil N, Datta YH, Alakbarova N, et al. Antiplatelet and anticoagulant therapies for prevention of ischemic stroke. *Clin Appl Thromb Hemost*. 2017;23(4):301–318.
53. Tantry US, Liu F, Chen G, et al. Vorapaxar in the secondary prevention of atherothrombosis. *Expert Rev Cardiovasc Ther*. 2015;13(12):1293–1305.
54. Chan NC, Weitz JI. Antithrombotic agents. *Circ Res*. 2019;124(3):426–436.
55. Mulloy B, Hogwood J, Gray E, et al. Pharmacology of heparin and related drugs. *Pharmacol Rev*. 2016;68(1):76–141.
56. Chandarajoti K, Liu J, Pawlinski R. The design and synthesis of new synthetic low-molecular-weight heparins. *J Thromb Haemost*. 2016;14(6):1135–1145.

57. Baluwala I, Favaloro EJ, Pasalic L. Therapeutic monitoring of unfractionated heparin - trials and tribulations. *Expert Rev Hematol.* 2017;10(7):595–605.
58. Piran S, Schulman S. Management of venous thromboembolism: an update. *Thromb J.* 2016;14(suppl 1):23.
59. Sokolowska E, Kalaska B, Miklosz J, et al. The toxicology of heparin reversal with protamine: past, present and future. *Expert Opin Drug Metab Toxicol.* 2016;12(8):897–909.
60. Greinacher A, Selleng K, Warkentin TE. Autoimmune heparin-induced thrombocytopenia. *J Thromb Haemost.* 2017;15(11):2099–2114.
61. Warkentin TE. Heparin-induced thrombocytopenia. *Curr Opin Crit Care.* 2015;21(6):576–585.
62. Signorelli SS, Scuto S, Marino E, et al. Anticoagulants and osteoporosis. *Int J Mol Sci.* 2019;20(21).
63. Spadarella G, Di Minno A, Donati MB, et al. From unfractionated heparin to pentasaccharide: Paradigm of rigorous science growing in the understanding of the in vivo thrombin generation. *Blood Rev.* 2020;39100613.
64. Babin JL, Traylor KL, Witt DM. Laboratory monitoring of low-molecular-weight heparin and fondaparinux. *Semin Thromb Hemost.* 2017;43(3):261–269.
65. van Es N, Bleker SM, Büller HR, et al. New developments in parenteral anticoagulation for arterial and venous thromboembolism. *Best Pract Res Clin Haematol.* 2013;26(2):203–213.
66. Mega JL, Simon T. Pharmacology of antithrombotic drugs: an assessment of oral antiplatelet and anticoagulant treatments. *Lancet.* 2015;386(9990):281–291.
67. Douketis JD. Navigating the anticoagulant landscape in 2017. *Cleveland Clin J Med.* 2017;84(10):768–778.
68. Fawzy AM, Lip GYH. Pharmacokinetics and pharmacodynamics of oral anticoagulants used in atrial fibrillation. *Expert Opin Drug Metab Toxicol.* 2019;15(5):381–398.
69. Dorgalaleh A, Favaloro EJ, Bahraini M, et al. Standardization of prothrombin time/international normalized ratio (PT/INR). *Int J Lab Hematol.* 2020.
70. Porter AL, Margolis AR, Staresinic CE, et al. Feasibility and safety of a 12-week inr follow-up protocol over 2 years in an anticoagulation clinic: a single-arm prospective cohort study. *J Thromb Thrombolysis.* 2019;47(2):200–208.
71. Milling TJ, Pollack CV. A review of guidelines on anticoagulation reversal across different clinical scenarios - is there a general consensus? *Am J Emerg Med.* 2020;38(9):1890–1903.
72. Dabiri G, Damstetter E, Chang Y, et al. Coagulation disorders and their cutaneous presentations: diagnostic work-up and treatment. *J Am Acad Dermatol.* 2016;74(5):795–804; quiz 805-6.
73. Warkentin TE, Greinacher A. Management of heparin-induced thrombocytopenia. *Curr Opin Hematol.* 2016;23(5):462–470.
74. Arachchillage DRJ, Laffan M. What is the appropriate anticoagulation strategy for thrombotic antiphospholipid syndrome? *Br J Haematol.* 2020;189(2):216–227.
75. Shaw JR, Kaplovitch E, Douketis J. Periprocedural management of oral anticoagulation. *Med Clin North Am.* 2020;104(4):709–726.
76. Anderson DR, Dunbar M, Murnaghan J, et al. Aspirin or rivaroxaban for vte prophylaxis after hip or knee arthroplasty. *N Engl J Med.* 2018;378(8):699–707.
77. Gosselin RC, Adcock DM. Douxfils J an update on laboratory assessment for direct oral anticoagulants (doacs). *Int J Lab Hematol.* 2019;41(S1):33–39.
78. Spyropoulos AC, Al-Badri A, Sherwood MW, et al. Periprocedural management of patients receiving a vitamin k antagonist or a direct oral anticoagulant requiring an elective procedure or surgery. *J Thromb Haemost.* 2016;14(5):875–885.
79. Siegal DM. Managing target-specific oral anticoagulant associated bleeding including an update on pharmacological reversal agents. *J Thromb Thrombolysis.* 2015;39(3):395–402.
80. Tomaselli GF, Mahaffey KW, Cuker A, et al. Acc expert consensus decision pathway on management of bleeding in patients on oral anticoagulants: a report of the American College of Cardiology Task Force on expert consensus decision pathways. *J Am Coll Cardiol.* 2017;70(24):3042–3067. 2017.
81. Shaw JR, Siegal DM. Pharmacological reversal of the direct oral anticoagulants-a comprehensive review of the literature. *Res Pract Thromb Haemost.* 2018;2(2):251–265.
82. Pollack Jr CV, Reilly PA, Eikelboom J, et al. Idarucizumab for dabigatran reversal. *N Engl J Med.* 2015;373(6):511–520.
83. Longstaff C, Kolev K. Basic mechanisms and regulation of fibrinolysis. *J Thrombosis Haemostasis.* 2015;13.suppl 1S98-105.
84. Verhamme IM, Panizzi PR, Bock PE. Pathogen activators of plasminogen. *J Thrombosis Haemostasis.* 2015;13 suppl 1S106-S14.
85. Khasa YP. The evolution of recombinant thrombolytics: current status and future directions. *Bioengineered.* 2017;8(4):331–358.
86. Matosevic B, Knoflach M, Werner P, et al. Fibrinogen degradation coagulopathy and bleeding complications after stroke thrombolysis. *Neurology.* 2013;80(13):1216–1224.

96 Endocrine Disorders and Cardiovascular Disease

BERNADETTE BIONDI

PITUITARY HORMONES AND CARDIOVASCULAR DISEASE, 1791
Growth Hormone, 1791
Cardiovascular Manifestations of Acromegaly, 1791

ADRENAL HORMONES AND CARDIOVASCULAR DISEASE, 1793
Adrenocorticotropic Hormone and Cortisol, 1793
Cushing Disease and Cushing Syndrome, 1793
Primary Hyperaldosteronism, 1794
Addison Disease, 1795
Treatment, 1795

PHEOCHROMOCYTOMA AND PARAGANGLIOMA, 1795
Diagnosis, 1796

PARATHYROID HORMONE AND CARDIOVASCULAR DISEASE, 1796
Hyperparathyroidism, 1796
Hypocalcemia, 1797
Vitamin D, 1797

THYROID HORMONE AND CARDIOVASCULAR DISEASE, 1797
Cellular Mechanisms of Thyroid Hormone Action on the Heart, 1797
Cardiovascular Manifestations of Overt and Subclinical Hyperthyroidism, 1799

Atrial Fibrillation in Overt and Subclinical Hyperthyroidism, 1799
Heart Failure in Overt and Subclinical Hyperthyroidism, 1800
CHD in Hyperthyroidism, 1800
Diagnosis of Overt and Subclinical Hypothyroidism, 1801
Cardiovascular Effects of Overt and Subclinical Hypothyroidism, 1801
Amiodarone and Thyroid Function, 1803
Changes in Thyroid Hormone Metabolism That Accompany Cardiac Disease, 1804

FUTURE PERSPECTIVES, 1804

REFERENCES, 1807

The endocrine system links tightly with many important cardiovascular diseases. As our understanding of the cellular and molecular effects of various hormones has evolved, we understand better the clinical manifestations that arise from excessive secretion of hormone and from glandular failure and subsequent hormone deficiency states.

This chapter reviews the spectrum of cardiac disease states that arise from changes in specific endocrine function. This approach allows us to explore the cellular mechanisms whereby various hormones can alter the cardiovascular system through actions on cardiac myocytes, vascular smooth muscle cells, and other target cells and tissues. In addition, this chapter discusses epidemiological studies and meta-analyses on cardiovascular morbidity and mortality associated with endocrine dysfunction to guide clinicians on the appropriate treatment of these patients.

PITUITARY HORMONES AND CARDIOVASCULAR DISEASE

The pituitary gland consists of two distinct anatomic portions. The anterior pituitary, or adenohypophysis, contains six different cell types; five of them produce polypeptide or glycoprotein hormones, and the sixth consists of nonsecretory chromophobic cells. The posterior pituitary, or neurohypophysis, is the anatomic location of the nerve terminals that secrete vasopressin (antidiuretic hormone) to control water balance or oxytocin, the milk letdown polypeptide.

Growth Hormone

The somatotropic cells secrete human growth hormone (hGH). Excessive secretion of hGH and insulin-like growth factor type 1 (IGF-1) by benign pituitary adenomas leads to the clinical syndrome of gigantism in youth before fusion of the bony epiphysis and to acromegaly in adults after maturation of the long bones.[1] hGH exerts its cellular effects through two major pathways. The first is by binding of the hormone to specific hGH receptors on target cells. Such receptors exist in the heart, skeletal muscle, fat, liver, and kidneys, as well as in many additional cell types throughout fetal development. The second growth-promoting effect of hGH results from stimulation of the synthesis of IGF-1. The liver produces the bulk of IGF-I, but other cell types can produce IGF-1 under the influence of hGH.[2] Shortly after identification of the IGF family, this second messenger was thought to mediate most actions of hGH. The ability to promote glucose uptake and cellular protein synthesis gave rise to the term "insulin-like." IGF-1 binds to its cognate IGF-1 receptor, which localizes on almost all cell types. Genetic experiments have demonstrated that the presence of IGF-1 receptors on cell types links closely to the ability of these cells to divide. Studies in which the IGF-1 receptor was overexpressed in cardiac myocytes reportedly produced an increase in myocyte number and mitotic rate and enhanced the replication of post-differentiated myocytes.

Infusion of hGH or IGF-1 acutely changes cardiac function and hemodynamics. The acute increases in cardiac contractility and cardiac output may result, at least in part, from a decrease in systemic vascular resistance and left ventricular afterload.[3]

Cardiovascular Manifestations of Acromegaly

Acromegaly is a relatively uncommon condition with an annual incidence of 3 to 4 cases/million. Despite its rarity, this disorder is associated with markedly increased morbidity and mortality due to cardiovascular, respiratory, metabolic, and neoplastic complications, especially in undiagnosed and untreated patients.[4,5] The clinical disease activity of patients with an excess of hGH correlates better with serum levels of IGF-1 than with hGH concentrations.

About 60% of acromegalic patients develop cardiovascular disease. Hypertension, insulin resistance, diabetes mellitus, and hyperlipidemia represent the cardiovascular manifestations most frequently associated with acromegaly.[4,5] The Endocrine Society (ES) Clinical Practice Guidelines recommend that acromegalic patients undergo evaluation for associated comorbidities (hypertension, diabetes mellitus, cardiovascular disease, and sleep apnea).[6]

The cardiovascular and hemodynamic effects of acromegaly vary considerably depending on the patient's age and the disease's severity and duration. A specific acromegalic cardiomyopathy develops in patients with persistently increased secretion of hGH and IGF-1; this condition is characterized by a concentric biventricular hypertrophy, diastolic dysfunction, and mitral and aortic valve disease, and can occur even in the absence of cardiovascular risk factors.[3] The natural history of this specific cardiomyopathy has three phases.[3,7] The first phase typically develops in young patients with new onset acromegaly and involves a hyperkinetic syndrome with increased myocardial contractility and enhanced cardiac output. More evident hypertrophy usually develops during the second phase of cardiomyopathy which is associated with impaired diastolic filling and reduced cardiac performance during exercise. Impaired systolic function and low cardiac output progressively develop in the late phase of the disease in patients in whom acromegaly is undiagnosed or under-treated. Heart failure can complicate this late phase of the disease and portend a poor prognosis.[7] Hypertension, type 2 diabetes, and hyperlipidemia may further contribute to the impaired contractile function. Hypertension occurs with a mean prevalence of 33% to 46%, although the mechanism remains poorly understood. Administration of hGH promotes sodium retention and volume expansion while IGF-1 has a potent antinatriuretic effect independent of any effect on aldosterone. Studies of the renin-angiotensin-aldosterone system have shown failure to inhibit release of renin optimally by volume expansion. Impaired glucose tolerance and diabetes mellitus are present in approximately 30% of acromegalic patients. Hyperlipidemia is principally characterized by hypertriglyceridemia and reduced high-density lipoprotein (HDL) cholesterol levels.

Acromegaly increases the prevalence of aortic and mitral valve disease. Patients with active acromegaly have a high prevalence of mitral and aortic abnormalities, which is higher in those with left ventricular hypertrophy. This condition can be considered one of the aspects of acromegalic cardiomyopathy because it is detectable even in young patients and in those with a short duration of the disease and can persist after treatment in cured patients. This persistence is likely to be correlated with the persistence of left ventricular hypertrophy and should be carefully monitored due to the risk of cardiac dysfunction. Progressive mitral regurgitation and increased left ventricular preload and afterload occur in patients with uncontrolled acromegaly. Patients with acromegaly can exhibit dilation of the aortic root, which is greater in men than in women. Left ventricular mass index is positively correlated with the diameter of the aorta, and patients with aortic ectasia usually have a greater left ventricular mass index than patients without this feature.

Although initial reports suggested that accelerated atherosclerosis impairs cardiac function in patients with longstanding acromegaly, a postmortem study revealed significant coronary artery disease in only 11% of patients dying of disease-related causes. Angiography showed normal or dilated coronary arteries in most cases. Fewer than 25% of the patients had positive nuclear stress tests, indicating that atherosclerosis and ischemic heart disease do not likely account for the marked degree of biventricular cardiac hypertrophy, cardiac failure, and cardiovascular mortality.

Abnormalities on the electrocardiogram (ECG), including left-axis deviation, septal Q waves, ST-T wave depression, abnormal QT dispersion, and conduction system defects, develop in up to 50% of patients with acromegaly. A variety of dysrhythmias can occur, including atrial and ventricular ectopic beats, sick sinus syndrome, and supraventricular and ventricular tachycardia.[8] Monitoring shows a fourfold increase in complex ventricular arrhythmias. Signal-averaged ECGs reveal a parallel rise late potential, a finding related to ventricular arrhythmia. Patients with active acromegaly more commonly show these electrophysiologic abnormalities than do treated patients. Patients with newly diagnosed, untreated acromegaly also manifest derangements in cardiac autonomic function, as measured by heart rate recovery and variability.

Acromegalic patients have an increased mortality compared to age- and gender-matched controls.[9] In uncontrolled acromegaly patients, the standardized mortality ratio (SMR) is significantly higher than the general population; however, mortality is strongly related to the disease control, which has normalized with the more frequent use of adjuvant therapy in the last decade.[9] In a 20-year follow-up study, the causes of death shifted from predominantly cardiovascular deaths (about 44%) during the first decade to predominantly cancer-related deaths in the next two decades.[10] Multiple studies have associated an increased risk of cancer of the gastrointestinal tract, colon, or lungs with this increased mortality.

Diagnosis

In 99% of the cases, acromegaly arises from benign adenomas of the anterior pituitary gland. At diagnosis most of these neoplasms are classified as macroadenomas (>10 mm), and patients have historical clinical evidence of having had the disease for longer than 10 years. The biochemical diagnosis of acromegaly depends on demonstrating elevated serum IGF-1 levels and lack of suppression of hGH to less than 1 μg/L following an oral glucose load.[6] Localization of the tumor occurs through magnetic resonance imaging (MRI) of the pituitary gland or computed tomographic (CT) scan when MRI is contraindicated or unavailable.

TREATMENT

Treatment aims to control tumor growth and normalize serum hGH and IGF-1 to reduce the risk of premature mortality and improve the quality of life.[11] Medical therapies include various options ranging from somatostatin analogs (SSAs) and somatostatin receptor ligands (SRLs) to GH, receptor antagonist pegvisomant, and dopamine agonists.[6,11] Pasireotide long-acting release (LAR), a long-acting somatostatin multireceptor ligand, can normalize IGF-1 in acromegalic patients who cannot be controlled with available SRLs; however, hyperglycemia develops in approximately half of the patients.[6,11]

Trans-sphenoidal surgery with resection of the adenoma cures about 50% to 70% of patients. Pre-operative medical therapy with SRLs is recommended to reduce surgical risk in patients with heart failure or severe comorbidities.[6,11]

The cardiovascular complications of acromegaly usually improve with disease modifying treatment and survival increases significantly in patients achieving disease remission, defined as the normalization of serum IGF-1 and serum hGH less than 1 μg/L.[6] hGH and/or IGF-1 levels that remain elevated after surgery mandate medical therapy.[6] Residual tumor mass following surgery may require radiotherapy if medical therapy is unavailable, unsuccessful, or not tolerated.[6] Cardiomyopathy, hypertension, valvular disease, and arrhythmias are the major causes of disease-associated morbidity and mortality. Surgery and medical treatment can all improve left ventricular hypertrophy and arrhythmias in patients who achieve biochemical control during treatment. Hyperglycemia, hypertension, and dyslipidemia should be treated promptly according to standard care. In the presence of a clinically relevant residual tumor that is unsuitable for resection, patients should be switched to pasireotide LAR or pegvisomant, in relation to the glycemia control.[6] Baseline fasting plasma glucose levels could help predict the onset of hyperglycemia during treatment with pegvisomant.

Growth Hormone Deficiency

hGH has an important role in the development of the normal heart and the maintenance of normal structure and function in the adult life. Children with untreated growth hormone deficiency (GHD) have an impaired cardiac structure, body composition, and cardiopulmonary functional capacity which can be restored after GH replacement therapy.[12] Even untreated adults with hGH deficiency have cardiac and endothelial dysfunction, insulin resistance, deranged lipid profile, increased carotid intima-media-thickness, elevated inflammatory markers, increased body fat with abdominal obesity, hypercoagulability, and decreased skeletal muscle mass and strength.[13] Early premature atherosclerosis can develop in hypopituitaric patients not receiving hGH therapy so that GH therapy should be continued after achieving adult height in patients with persistent growth hormone deficiency. Patients with untreated hypopituitarism have a doubled overall mortality, principally due to increased CV mortality.[14] Several reports have documented low IGF-1 levels as well as a blunted response to hypothalamic growth hormone-releasing hormone (GHRH) in patients with congestive heart failure (CHF) and severe LV dysfunction.[3,15] GH deficiency can be detected in about 30% of patients with CHF and is associated with an impaired LV remodeling.[3] A low IGF-1/GH ratio and high NT-proBNP levels were independent predictors of death in HF patients without cachexia, suggesting that low IGF-1 circulating levels in CHF can be linked to a progression of the disease, which GH replacement therapy is able to delay.[15] Treatment with recombinant human replacement therapy can have beneficial effects in patients with CHF (due to either ischemic or idiopathic dilated cardiomyopathy) with a coexisting GH deficiency.[16]

Prolactin Disease

The most common disorder of the anterior pituitary gland is small (<1.0 cm), prolactin-producing pituitary adenomas causing amenorrhea and galactorrhea. Prolactin plays a well-recognized stimulatory role in inflammation; prolactin receptors were localized in human coronary artery plaques, suggesting that prolactin might influence atherogenesis. Because hypothalamic dopamine normally inhibits prolactin secretion, dopamine agonists such as cabergoline and bromocriptine are first-line treatments. Patients with prolactinoma can have an unfavorable cardiovascular and metabolic risk profile. A decreased hypothalamic dopaminergic tone is involved in the pathogenesis of insulin resistance, while an increase in dopaminergic neurotransmission reduces food intake and induces energy expenditure. Moreover, suppression of dopaminergic tone is responsible for weight gain and metabolic abnormalities because the dopamine receptor type 2 is abundantly expressed on human pancreatic beta-cell and adipocytes, suggesting a regulatory role for peripheral dopamine in insulin and adipose functions. Exposure of pancreatic islet to prolactin (PRL) is known to stimulate insulin secretion and beta-cell proliferation. Medical treatment with dopamine-agonists (bromocriptine and cabergoline) can improve insulin resistance and metabolic abnormalities.[17] In a recent prospective study, a 5-mg/dL increment in prolactin was associated with increased odds of incidence of diabetes and hypertension.[18]

Treatment with low-dose cabergoline in hyperprolactinemia has been associated with an increased prevalence of tricuspid regurgitation in a recent meta-analysis.[19] Although the clinical significance of this finding has not been established, a complete echocardiographic evaluation could be indicated in patients treated with elevated doses of cabergoline, particularly for a long period.

ADRENAL HORMONES AND CARDIOVASCULAR DISEASE

Adrenocorticotropic Hormone and Cortisol

The adrenocorticotropic cells in the anterior pituitary synthesize a large protein (pro-opiomelanocortin), which is then processed within the corticotropic cell into a family of smaller proteins that include adrenocorticotrophic hormone (ACTH). The adrenal cortex zona glomerulosa produces aldosterone, and the zona fasciculata produces primarily cortisol and some androgenic steroids. The zona reticularis produces cortisol and androgens as well. ACTH regulates the synthesis of cortisol in both the zona fasciculata and reticularis.

Cushing Disease and Cushing Syndrome

Cushing syndrome results from prolonged and inappropriately high exposure of tissues to glucocorticoids.[20] Excessive cortisol secretion and its attendant clinical disease state can arise from excessive release of ACTH by the pituitary (Cushing disease) or through the adenomatous or rarely malignant neoplastic process arising in the adrenal gland itself (Cushing syndrome).[21] Well-characterized conditions of adrenal glucocorticoid and mineralocorticoid excess appear to result from the excessively high levels of (ectopic) ACTH produced by small cell carcinoma of the lung, carcinoid tumors, pancreatic islet cell tumors, medullary thyroid cancer, and other adenocarcinomas and hematologic malignancies.[20] Clinical signs and symptoms of Cushing syndrome often develop in patients treated with exogenous steroids at doses equivalent to 20 mg of prednisone daily for more than 1 month. Cortisol, a member of the glucocorticoid family of steroid hormones, binds to receptors located within the cytoplasm of many cell types (Fig. 96.1). After binding cortisol these receptors translocate to the nucleus and function as transcription factors. Several cardiac genes contain glucocorticoid response elements in their promoter regions that confer transcriptional-level glucocorticoid responsiveness. Such genes include those that encode voltage-gated potassium channels, as well as protein kinases, which serve to phosphorylate and regulate the voltage-gated sodium channels. In addition, there are more rapidly acting, nontranscriptional pathways by which cortisol may regulate the activity of voltage-gated potassium channels.

Patients with Cushing disease can exhibit a variety of electrocardiographic changes. The duration of the PR interval appears to correlate inversely with adrenal cortisol production rates. The mechanism underlying this correlation may be related to the expression or regulation of the voltage-gated sodium channel (SCN5A). Changes in the ECG, specifically in the PR and QT intervals, may also arise from the direct (nongenomic) effects of glucocorticoids on the voltage-gated potassium channel (Kv1.5) in excitable tissues.

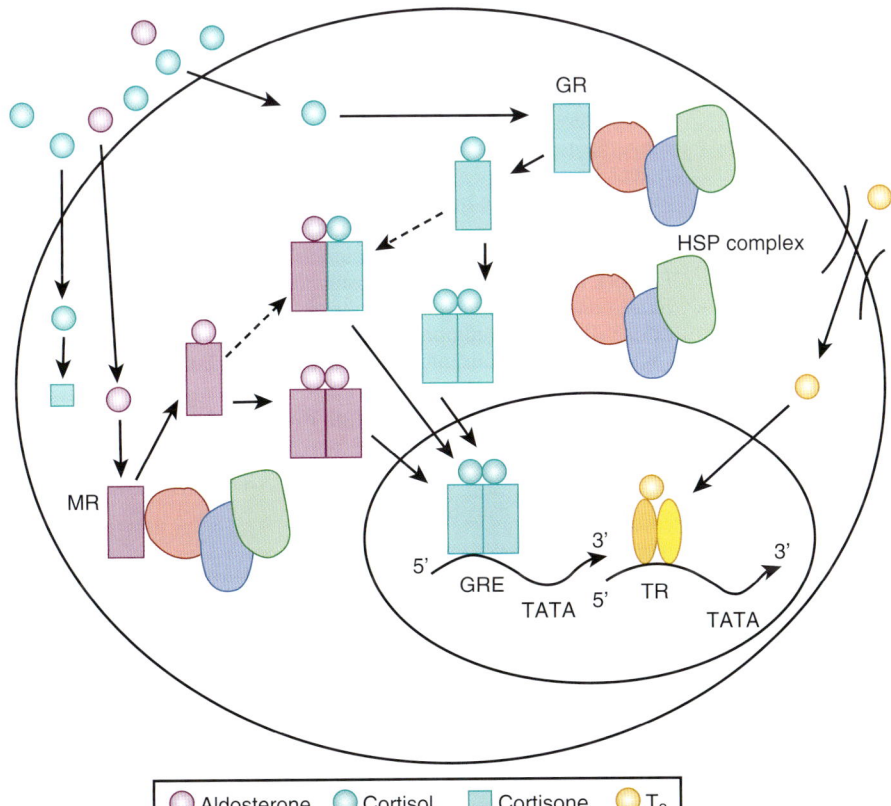

FIGURE 96.1 Generalized mechanism of action of the nuclear hormone receptor. The mineralocorticoid receptor (MR) has similar affinities for aldosterone and cortisol. Circulating levels of cortisol are 100 to 1000 times greater than those of aldosterone. In MR-responsive cells, the enzyme 11-beta-hydroxysteroid dehydrogenase metabolizes cortisol to cortisone, thereby allowing aldosterone to bind to the MR. The MR and glucocorticoid receptor (GR) are cytoplasmic receptors that after binding ligand, translocate to the nucleus and bind to glucocorticoid response elements (GREs) in the promoter regions of responsive genes. Triiodothyronine (T_3) is transported into the cell via specific membrane proteins and binds to thyroid hormone receptors (TRs), which are bound to thyroid hormone response elements in the promoter regions of T_3-responsive genes. HSP, heat shock protein; TATA, TATA box promoter region. (Courtesy Dr. S. Danzi.)

The cardiac effects of Cushing syndrome arise from the effects of glucocorticoids on the heart, liver, skeletal muscle, and fat tissue. The interaction between high cortisol levels and active mineralocorticoid receptor (MR) in cardiomyocytes induces cardiac remodeling and fibrosis, ventricular remodeling, and an impairment of relaxation.[21] It can also stimulate the expression of several pro-inflammatory and adhesion molecules, leading to increased myocardial stiffness and contractile dysfunction. Cortisol-mediated hypertension has multiple mechanisms in patients with Cushing[22]; cardiac structural and functional alterations are more severe in hypertensive patients, suggesting an interaction between the deleterious effects of hypertension and cortisol excess. Chronic cortisol hypersecretion can also cause central obesity, insulin resistance, dyslipidemia, a prothrombotic state, and metabolic syndrome. The prevalence of diabetes mellitus ranges between 18% and 30%.

A two- to fourfold increase in mortality has been reported in Cushing syndrome compared with the general population. This increased cardiovascular morbidity and mortality is largely due to cerebrovascular, peripheral vascular, and coronary artery disease, and CHF.[23–25] The cardiovascular risk may persist even after restoration of eucortisolaemia.[25] Recent evidence suggests an impaired cardiovascular profile even in patients with subclinical Cushing syndrome when compared with the general population; this condition is characterized by an incomplete post-dexamethasone cortisol suppression and adrenal incidentalomas.[26]

Diagnosis
The diagnosis of Cushing disease and Cushing syndrome requires the demonstration of increased cortisol production as reflected by an elevated 24-hour urinary free cortisol or nocturnal salivary cortisol level. ACTH measurement allows assessment of whether the disease is pituitary-, adrenal-, or ectopically based. An abnormal dexamethasone suppression test and a corticotropin-releasing hormone (CRH) test can help establish the cause of Cushing syndrome. Anatomic localization of the suspected lesions using MRI helps confirm laboratory findings.

TREATMENT
Treatment of excessive cortisol production depends on the underlying mechanisms.[27] Initial resection of primary lesion(s) is recommended for underlying Cushing disease (based in the pituitary) and also for Cushing disease related to ectopic and adrenal causes. Trans-sphenoidal selective adenomectomy with or without postoperative radiation therapy can partially or completely reverse the increased ACTH production by the anterior pituitary. Cushing syndrome requires surgical removal of one (adrenal adenoma, adrenal carcinoma) or both (multiple nodular) adrenal glands. Immediately after surgery, cortisol and mineralocorticoid (fludrocortisone [FST]) need to be replaced to prevent adrenal insufficiency.

Drug therapy before or after surgery can help control persistent cortisol production.[27] Pasireotide can decrease ACTH production from a pituitary tumor. The adrenal enzyme inhibitor ketoconazole may be used alone or in combination with metyrapone to enhance control of severe hypercortisolemia. Mitotane is used primarily to treat adrenal carcinoma. Mifepristone is approved in the United States for people with Cushing syndrome who have type 2 diabetes or glucose intolerance. This drug blocks the direct effect of cortisol on tissues and leads to an improvement in hypertension and/or diabetes in 40% to 60% of patients. Etomidate is useful where immediate parenteral action is required and in seriously ill patients who cannot take oral medications. The goal of therapy is the clinical normalization of cortisol levels.[27]

Primary Hyperaldosteronism
Primary hyperaldosteronism (PA) (see also Chapter 26) refers to a group of disorders in which aldosterone production is inappropriately high, relatively autonomous from the major regulators of secretion (angiotensin II and plasma potassium concentration), and non-suppressible by sodium loading.[28,29] It is the most common cause of secondary hypertension, with a prevalence of 20% in patients with resistant hypertension and 10% in those with severe hypertension.[30,31] Hypokalemia in the setting of hypertension should induce a prompt consideration of PA, although most patients with PA are not hypokalemic.[32] Common causes of PA include an adrenal adenoma, unilateral or bilateral adrenal hyperplasia, or, in rare cases, an adrenal carcinoma or an inherited condition: glucocorticoid-remediable aldosteronism (GRA).[28]

Aldosterone's mechanism of action on target tissues resembles that reported for glucocorticoids (see Fig. 96.1). Aldosterone enters cells and binds to the MR, which then translocates to the nucleus and promotes the expression of aldosterone-responsive genes. In addition to kidney cells, in which MRs control sodium transport, in vitro studies on rats have located these receptors in cardiac myocytes. MR is also expressed in vascular smooth muscle cells, endothelial cells, cells within brown adipose tissue, macrophages, and neurons in several brain regions.

In humans, primary aldosteronism causes cardiovascular damage; it can induce development of cardiac hypertrophy, myocardial fibrosis, diastolic dysfunction, and heart failure.[33,34] Stroke, nonfatal myocardial infarction, or atrial fibrillation are more frequent among patients with PA compared with patients with primary hypertension. Patients with PA also have an increased prevalence of metabolic syndrome and diabetes. Death resulting from cardiovascular causes is more common among patients with PA compared with matched control patients with primary hypertension. Fibrosis of the heart, adrenal glands, pancreas, and lungs has been found in autoptic studies in patients with PA.

In light of the cardiorenal and cerebrovascular implications stemming from an unrecognized and untreated PA, early diagnosis and screening are imperative. Primary aldosteronism should be investigated in patients with: (1) severe hypertension, systolic blood pressure ≥180, and diastolic blood pressure ≥110 mm Hg; (2) treatment-resistant hypertension (an office SBP/diastolic blood pressure ≥130/80 mm Hg and prescription of ≥3 antihypertensive medications at optimal doses, including a diuretic or an office SBP/diastolic blood pressure less than 130/80 mm Hg for a patient requiring ≥4 antihypertensive medications); (3) hypertension with spontaneous or diuretic-induced hypokalemia; (4) hypertension with incidentally discovered adrenal tumors; (5) hypertension and sleep apnea; (6) family history of early-onset hypertension or cerebrovascular accident at a young age (<40 years) (Table 96.1).[24,31]

Diagnosis
Plasma aldosterone/renin ratio detects possible PA.[28,31] Patients should have unrestricted dietary salt intake before testing and should be potassium replete. MR antagonists should be withdrawn for at least 4 weeks before testing, especially in patients with mild hypertension; for other drugs (beta-blockers, clonidine, methyldopa, non-steroidal anti-inflammatory drugs, ACE inhibitors, angiotensin receptor blockers, and dihydropyridine calcium blockers) a 2-week withdrawal should be sufficient. Correction of hypokalemia before testing is recommended. An aldosterone-to-renin ratio (ARR) greater than 20 is commonly used as the threshold for positive PA screening, with a sensitivity of 78% and a specificity of 83% in study participants with resistant hypertension.[28] Patients with an abnormal aldosterone/renin ratio undergo one or more confirmatory tests to definitively confirm or exclude the diagnosis.[28] The most commonly used suppression tests use saline loading (either by intravenous infusion or orally), FST, or a captopril challenge.

TABLE 96.1 Patients With a High Risk of Hyperaldosteronism[26,29]

- Severe hypertension: systolic blood pressure ≥180 and diastolic blood pressure ≥110 mm Hg
- Treatment-resistant hypertension
  - Office SBP/diastolic blood pressure ≥130/80 mm Hg and prescription of ≥3 antihypertensive medications at optimal doses, including a diuretic
  - Office SBP/diastolic blood pressure <130/80 mm Hg or prescription of ≥4 antihypertensive medications
- Hypertension with spontaneous or diuretic-induced hypokalemia
- Hypertension with adrenal incidentaloma
- Hypertension and sleep apnea
- Family history of early-onset hypertension or cerebrovascular accident at a young age (<40 years)

Caution should be used when performing confirmatory tests and hypokalemia, if present, should be corrected.

All patients with suspected disease should undergo adrenal CT to search for adrenocortical carcinoma,[28] although the value of CT scanning and MRI are debated because they cannot identify the source of aldosterone excess and micro-APAs (≤10 mm in diameter) are often undetectable by current imaging methods. Therefore, the available guidelines recommend performing adrenal venous sampling (AVS) before surgery to distinguish between unilateral and bilateral adrenal disease. Steroid profiling of adrenal vein and peripheral serum samples can distinguish between adenoma and hyperplasia; peripheral plasma 18-oxocortisol is higher in patients with adenoma than in those with bilateral hyperplasia, whereas cortisol, corticosterone, and dehydroepiandrosterone are lower.[35,36]

TREATMENT (See Also Chapters 26, 50, and 51)

Patients with PA and hypokalemia should receive slow-release potassium chloride supplementation to maintain plasma potassium.[28,31] The aldosterone antagonists, spironolactone or eplerenone (as a second choice) should be used to control hypertension, hypokalemia, and the deleterious CV effects of aldosterone hypersecretion.[28] Gynecomastia and sexual dysfunction can develop in 30% of cases in men; in these cases eplerenone can be used.[28] Close monitoring of electrolytes is essential when MR antagonists are used. Surgical treatment is practicable in young patients (<35 years) with spontaneous hypokalemia, marked aldosterone excess, and unilateral adrenal lesions with evidence of a cortical adenoma on adrenal CT.[28] Unilateral laparoscopic adrenalectomy can cure hypokalemia and improve or cure hypertension in such patients, lowering the risk of incidental CHF and all-cause mortality in a long-term follow-up.[37] Patients with a bilateral disease and those reluctant to undergo surgery should receive medical treatment with MR antagonists. In patients with GRA, low doses of glucocorticoid to lower ACTH and normalize BP and potassium levels represent the first-line treatment. In addition, if BP fails to normalize with glucocorticoid alone, an MR antagonist can be added.

Addison Disease

Primary adrenal insufficiency occurs when the adrenal cortex cannot produce sufficient glucocorticoids and/or mineralocorticoids.[38] Primary adrenal insufficiency arises most commonly from bilateral loss of adrenal function on an autoimmune basis; as a result of infection, hemorrhage, or metastatic malignancy; or in selected cases, from inborn errors of steroid hormone metabolism.[38] Addison disease can manifest itself at any age; it may be associated with other autoimmune disorders (e.g., Hashimoto thyroiditis, type 1 diabetes mellitus, autoimmune gastritis/pernicious anemia, and vitiligo). In contrast, secondary adrenal insufficiency, which results from pituitary-dependent loss of ACTH secretion, leads to a fall in glucocorticoid production, whereas mineralocorticoid production, including aldosterone, remains at relatively normal levels.

The non-cardiac symptoms—including increased pigmentation, abdominal pain with nausea and vomiting, hypoglycemia, and weight loss can be chronic, but tachycardia, hypotension, hyponatremia, hyperkalemia, loss of autonomic tone, cardiovascular collapse, and crisis may develop especially in acutely ill or untreated patients with Addison disease. Delayed treatment of more severe symptoms is likely to increase morbidity and mortality.

Laboratory findings (hyponatremia and hyperkalemia) indicate loss of aldosterone production (high renin levels).[39]

Hyperkalemia can alter findings on the ECG by producing low-amplitude P waves and peaked T waves. Blood pressure measurements uniformly show low diastolic pressure (<60 mm Hg) along with orthostatic changes that reflect loss of volume and acquired autonomic dysfunction. Patients with newly diagnosed, untreated Addison disease have reduced left ventricular end-systolic and end-diastolic dimensions in comparison to controls.

Diagnosis

Acute adrenal insufficiency characteristically occurs in the setting of acute stress, infection, or trauma in patients with chronic autoimmune adrenal insufficiency or in children with congenital abnormalities in cortisol metabolism. It can also develop as a result of bilateral adrenal hemorrhage in patients with severe systemic infection or diffuse intravascular coagulation. Secondary adrenal insufficiency can occur in the setting of hypopituitarism and is usually chronic, but acute changes caused by pituitary hemorrhage (apoplexy) or pituitary inflammation (lymphocytic hypophysitis) can also occur. Acute adrenal insufficiency can develop in patients treated with long-term suppressive doses of corticosteroids (>10 mg of prednisone for more than 1 month) if treatment is stopped precipitously or if an acute severe non–endocrine-related illness arises.

The diagnostic criteria include low cortisol levels (morning cortisol < 140 nmol/L [<5 μg/dL]) or when cortisol levels fail to rise above 500 nmol/L (20 μg /dL) 30 or 60 minutes after an intravenous injection of 250 μg of corticotropin.[39] The simultaneous measurement of plasma renin and aldosterone can help determine mineralocorticoid deficiency.

Treatment

Management of acute Addisonian crisis requires an adequate hydrocortisone replacement therapy (100 mg given as an initial IV bolus, then 100 mg every 8 to 12 hours for the first 24 hours, and tapering of the dose over the next 72 to 96 hours). Large volumes of normal saline with 5% dextrose can help address the intravascular fluid deficit. Potential underlying precipitating causes (including infection, acute cardiac or cerebral ischemia, or intra-abdominal emergency) require identification and treatment. Long-term treatment of adrenal insufficiency consists of oral corticosteroid therapy (hydrocortisone 20 mg) in two divided oral doses per day or prednisone (5 mg/day) administered orally once or twice daily.[39] A dual-release hydrocortisone preparation could be used, when possible, to mimic the cortisol circadian rhythm. Patients with confirmed aldosterone deficiency should receive mineralocorticoid replacement with fluorohydrocortisone (starting dose, 50 to 100 μg in adults). Diuretics and aldosterone antagonists such as spironolactone or eplerenone should be avoided.

PHEOCHROMOCYTOMA AND PARAGANGLIOMA

Pheochromocytomas (PCCs) and paragangliomas (PGLs), also named PPGLs, are tumors arising from neuroectodermal chromaffin cell in adrenal medulla or extra-adrenal paraganglia (see Chapter 26).[40,41] The 2017 WHO classification of adrenal tumors established anatomic criteria for PPGL classification and distinguished between PCCs originating from the adrenal medulla and PGLs originating from extra-adrenal paraganglia.[42] PGLs can be further divided according to clinical and biological behavior into: head and neck PGLs (HNPGLs) that originate from parasympathetic paraganglia and are characterized by a lack of catecholamine secretion, and sympathetic PGLs that originate from sympathetic paraganglia and are biochemically positive.[40–42] Head and neck PGLs are often multifocal, bilateral, sometimes recurrent, and rarely malignant (<5%). Sympathetic PGLs can be found everywhere from the skull base to the pelvic region, even though approximately 85% are located below the diaphragm. Metastatic disease is defined by the presence of PPGLs in nonchromaffin organs and occurs in about 5% to 20% of PCCs and 15% to 35% of sympathetic PGLs.[40]

Different familial autosomal dominant diseases have been identified: neurofibromatosis type 1 (NF1), multiple endocrine neoplasia type 2 (MEN2), von Hippel-Lindau (VHL) syndrome, and Carney triad (PGL, gastric stromal tumors, pulmonary chondromas).[43] When pheochromocytoma coexists with medullary thyroid carcinoma or occasionally with hyperparathyroidism, it is designated as MEN syndrome type 2A. In patients with MEN 2B, pheochromocytoma coexists with medullary thyroid cancer and with mucosal neuromas frequently seen on the lips and tongue. TMEM 127 encoding transmembrane protein 127 has been identified as a new susceptibility gene for PCC.[40,45] These patients have a malignancy rate less than 5% and adrenal catecholamine secreting PCC; bilateral PCCs can develop in a third of patients and rare cases of patients with extra-adrenal abdominal PGL and head and neck PGL have also been reported.[40] Myc-associated factor

X (MAX) adrenal tumors are bilateral in 67% of the cases and have malignant behavior in 25%.[40,45]

PPGLs are expected to have succinate dehydrogenase (SDH*x*) or fumarate hydratase (FH) mutations. About 22% to 70% PPGLs are caused by a single driver germ line mutation in SDHA, SDHB, SDHC, SDHD, and SDHAF2. SDHB-associated tumors can be malignant in more than 30% of the cases.[40] Succinate dehydrogenase gene A (SDHA) mutated paragangliomas PGL may be at high risk of metastases.[44] Next-generation sequencing (NGS) technology could be appropriate for carrying out genetic screening of these individuals.[46]

Clinical manifestations of pheochromocytoma include headache, palpitations, excessive sweating, tremulousness, chest pain, weight loss, and a variety of other constitutional complaints. Hypertension may be sustained or episodic but is usually constant and is paradoxically associated with orthostatic hypotension on arising in the morning. The paroxysmal attacks and classic symptoms result from episodic excessive catecholamine secretion. However, a small, but significant proportion of patients with pheochromocytoma are normotensive. Another rare sign can be the onset of diabetes in younger patients without typical risk factors for diabetes. Hypertensive crises can be induced after accidental tumor manipulation or during anesthesia. As a result of the release of norepinephrine and an increase in systemic vascular resistance, cardiac output is minimally (if at all) increased despite increases in the heart rate. The ECG can show left ventricular hypertrophy (LVH), as well as repolarization abnormalities, findings suggesting left ventricular strain. Although ventricular and atrial ectopy and episodes of supraventricular tachycardia can occur, little distinguishes the LVH from that of essential hypertension.

Patients with sympathetic PPGLs have a higher incidence of cardiovascular events before diagnosis. Impaired left ventricular function and cardiomyopathy can occur in patients with pheochromocytoma. The mechanism underlying this condition is complex and includes increased left ventricular work and LVH from associated hypertension; potential adverse effects of catecholamine excess on myocyte structure and contractility; and changes in coronary arteries, including thickening of the media, which presumably impairs blood flow to the myocardium. Patients with previously diagnosed or undiagnosed disease can show histologic evidence of myocarditis postmortem. The possibility of catecholamine-stimulated tachycardia in turn mediating left ventricular dysfunction should be addressed because treatments designed to slow the heart rate may improve the left ventricular function. Life-threatening cardiovascular manifestations of pheochromocytoma primarily result from hypertensive emergencies, abnormality of cardiac rhythm, and serious ventricular arrhythmias or conduction disturbances. Reversible dilated hypertrophic cardiomyopathy and Takotsubo cardiomyopathy are well established cardiac manifestations of pheochromocytoma. Rarely, pheochromocytoma can arise within the heart, presumably from chromaffin cells, which are part of the adrenergic autonomic paraganglia.

Diagnosis

An increase in norepinephrine, epinephrine, or its metabolites in serum or blood is essential for the diagnosis. Quantitative 24-hour urinary fractionated metanephrine levels are the most reliable screening indicators; they provide a sensitivity of 97% and a specificity of 91%.[43] There are at least four principal secretory profiles in PPGL: adrenergic, noradrenergic, dopaminergic, and silent. PCC and sympathetic PGL usually synthesize and secrete norepinephrine and/or epinephrine, while 23% of parasympathetic paraganglia-derived tumors secrete only dopamine.[40] Chromogranin A can be a useful biomarker in silent PPGLs and for monitoring the disease. Increased plasma levels of methoxytyramine (product of dopamine degradation) could discriminate patients with *SDHx* mutations and predict malignancy.[40] Interfering medications (anti-depressants, some anti-hypertensives, and other medications) and several foods which can cause false-positive elevations of these markers should be ruled out before testing patients with known or suspected PPGL. CT is the first-choice imaging modality because of its excellent spatial resolution for thorax, abdomen, and pelvis. MRI is recommended in patients with metastatic disease and for detection of skull base and neck PGL.[131] I-metaiodobenzylguanidine can localize catecholamine-producing lesions.[123] MIBG SPECT/MRI has the highest sensitivity for adrenal PHEOs. 18F-fluorodeoxyglucose positron emission tomography scanning can visualize metastatic disease. FDOPA is extremely sensitive for patients with head/neck PGLs and particularly useful for patients with SDH mutations and/or biochemically silent PHEO/PGL. Promising results have been found with radiolabeled DOTA peptides (DOTATATE, DOTATOC, and DOTANOC), which target somatostatin receptors on the cell membrane; this tracer is superior to FDOPA PET/CT in the diagnosis of metastatic tumors.[47]

TREATMENT

Definitive treatment of pheochromocytoma requires removal of the lesion.[39] Accurate preoperative localization reduces operative mortality and eliminates the need for exploratory laparotomy. Endoscopic procedures are now standard for small tumors and open resection is indicated for large tumors (e.g., >6 cm) or invasive PCC.[41]

Preoperative pharmacologic treatment should be provided to prevent perioperative cardiovascular complications.[41] It includes 7 to 14 days of alpha-adrenergic blockade (usually with doxazosin, prazosin, or phenoxybenzamine) to normalize blood pressure. Beta-blocking drugs can normalize heart rate but should follow establishment of sufficient alpha blockade. Before surgical treatment, a high-sodium diet and fluid intake should be started to improve blood volume contraction and prevent severe hypotension after tumor removal. Operative intervention requires constant blood pressure monitoring, and intravenous phentolamine or sodium nitroprusside may be required to treat episodic hypertension intraoperatively.[41] Gauges of the success of surgery include effective blood pressure and symptom improvement, as well as measurement of urinary catecholamines 4 weeks after the procedure. Lifelong annual biochemical testing to assess for recurrent or metastatic disease is necessary.

PARATHYROID HORMONE AND CARDIOVASCULAR DISEASE

Diseases of the parathyroid glands can alter the cardiac function through two mechanisms. Parathyroid hormone (PTH), a protein hormone, can itself affect the heart, vascular smooth muscle cells, and endothelial cells. PTH-induced changes in serum calcium levels can also affect the cardiovascular system.[48]

PTH can bind to its receptor and alter the spontaneous beating rate of neonatal cardiac myocytes through an increase in intracellular cyclic adenosine monophosphate (cAMP). PTH can also alter calcium influx and cardiac contractility in adult cardiac myocytes and relaxation of vascular smooth muscle cells. Moreover, a variety of tissues, including cardiac myocytes produce the structurally related PTH-related peptide (PTHrP). PTHrP can bind to the PTH receptor on cardiac cells and stimulate accumulation of cAMP and contractile activity, as well as regulate L-type calcium currents. Long-term treatment with the recombinant human PTH may require monitoring for adverse cardiac effects.

Hyperparathyroidism

In primary hyperparathyroidism (PHPT) hypercalcemia (or high-normal serum calcium levels) occurs in presence of inappropriately normal or elevated PTH concentrations because of an overproduction of PTH. PHPT most often results from adenomatous enlargement of one of the four parathyroid glands.[48] Cardiovascular actions of hypercalcemia include increased cardiac contractility, shortening of the ventricular action potential duration (primarily through changes in phase 2), and blunting of the T wave and changes in the ST segment, occasionally suggesting cardiac ischemia. The QT interval shortens and occasionally the PR interval decreases. Treatment with digitalis glycosides appears to increase sensitivity of the heart to hypercalcemia. Increased PTH levels are associated with an increased risk of incident hypertension.[49] Patients with PHPT generally maintain normal left ventricular systolic function, but severe or chronic disease may impair diastolic function. Changes in left ventricular structure and function can improve after successful parathyroid surgery; higher preoperative PTH levels have been associated with greater improvements.[50] Even patients with normocalcemic PHPT have a higher risk of high blood pressure than subjects with normal PTH.[51]

Excess PTH (as seen in primary and secondary hyperparathyroidism) is associated with a higher incidence of hypertension, left ventricular hypertrophy, heart failure, cardiac arrhythmias, and valvular calcific disease, which may contribute to higher cardiac morbidity and mortality.[52,53] Several observational and population studies have discovered an association between elevated PTH and HF. This relationship may be attributed to the direct effects of PTH on cardiac myocytes, endothelial cells, and vascular smooth muscles. HF is an important predictor of cardiac morbidity and mortality, and there is increasing evidence that elevated PTH levels are an independent risk factor for incident HF.[52]

Hypercalcemia may lead to pathological changes in the heart, including the myocardial interstitium, and conducting systemic as well as calcific deposits in the valve cusps, annuli, and possibly coronary arteries. Although initially observed in fairly longstanding and severe hypercalcemia, so-called metastatic calcifications can also occur in secondary parathyroid disease arising from chronic renal failure, in which the serum calcium-phosphorus product constant is exceeded.

Diagnosis
A simultaneous increase in serum immunoreactive PTH (best represented by the intact PTH assay) with elevation of the serum calcium level establishes the diagnosis of PHPT. Other causes of hypercalcemia include malignancy with an increased level of PTHrP or hypercalcemia arising directly from bony metastases or neoplastic (lymphoma) or non-neoplastic disease (e.g., sarcoidosis) leading to an increase in the synthesis and release of 1,25-dihydroxyvitamin D_3.

TREATMENT
Treatment of hyperparathyroidism is the surgical removal of the parathyroid adenoma.[48] Calcimimetic medications (cinacalcet) can lower PTH concentrations and normalize serum calcium levels. Asymptomatic PHPT, routinely encountered in clinical endocrinology practice, may not require definitive treatment.

Hypocalcemia
Low serum levels of total and ionized calcium directly alter myocyte function. Hypocalcemia prolongs phase 2 of the action potential duration and the QT interval. Severe hypocalcemia can impair cardiac contractility and give rise to a diffuse musculoskeletal syndrome consisting of tetany and rhabdomyolysis. Primary hypoparathyroidism is rare and can develop after surgical removal of the parathyroid glands, as may occur after treatment of thyroid cancer, in the setting of polyglandular dysfunction syndromes, as a result of glandular agenesis (DiGeorge) syndrome, and in the rare heritable pseudohypoparathyroidism disorder. Recombinant human PTH offers a treatment option.[53]

Chronic renal failure is the most common cause of low serum calcium and high PTH levels. In patients suffering from such a condition, the effects of chronically high levels of PTH (secondary hyperparathyroidism) on the heart and cardiovascular system may be both causative and serve as a biomarker in assessing heart failure treatment strategies. In older adult patients with progression of aortic stenosis, a rise in serum PTH and bone remodeling occurs. The ability of PTH to stimulate G protein–coupled receptors may impair myocyte contractility and contribute to LVH. Cinacalcet can treat the secondary hyperparathyroidism associated with chronic renal failure.

Vitamin D
Most body tissues and cells express the vitamin D receptor. 1,25(OH)2D has a wide range of biological actions, including inhibiting cellular proliferation and inducing terminal differentiation, inhibiting angiogenesis, stimulating insulin production, and inhibiting renin production. Observational evidence suggests that lower levels of vitamin D are associated with an increased all-cause and cardiovascular morbidity. Vitamin D deficiency can contribute to coronary risk factors and cardiovascular disease; it predisposes to hypertension, diabetes mellitus and the metabolic syndrome, left ventricular hypertrophy, CHF, stroke, peripheral arterial disease, and chronic vascular inflammation.

THYROID HORMONE AND CARDIOVASCULAR DISEASE

The thyroid gland and the heart share a close relationship that arises in embryology. In ontogeny, the thyroid and heart migrate together. Changes in cardiovascular function across the entire spectrum of thyroid disease illustrate the close physiological relationship between the heart and thyroid.[54,55] Cardiovascular complications commonly occur in both subclinical and overt thyroid dysfunction.

Cellular Mechanisms of Thyroid Hormone Action on the Heart
Diagnosis and management of thyroid hormone–mediated cardiac disease states require understanding of the cellular mechanisms of thyroid hormone on the heart and vascular smooth muscle cells. Thyroid function is regulated by the hypothalamic-pituitary-thyroid (HPT) axis via a feedback mechanism. Secretion of thyroid stimulating hormone (TSH) by the pituitary gland is stimulated by hypothalamic TSH-releasing hormone (TRH), and TSH, in turn, stimulates the thyroid gland to release thyroxine (T_4) and triiodothyronine (T_3). TSH release is regulated directly by the negative feedback of thyroid hormone; this loop maintains the levels of circulating thyroid hormones and TSH in a physiological inverse relationship that defines the HPT axis set-point. This set-point is genetically determined although environmental factors, age, and systemic illness may induce changes in the HPT-axis.[56] The thyroid gland concentrates iodide and, through a series of enzymatic steps, synthesizes predominantly T_4 (about 80%) and a smaller percentage of triiodothyronine [T_3 about 20%]). Although T_4 is the main hormone produced by the thyroid gland, T_3 is the active hormone. Most circulating T_3 derives largely from T_4, thanks to the deiodinases activity in extrathyroidal peripheral tissues; 80% of the extrathyroidal T_3 is produced by deiodination of T_4.[57] Peripheral T_3 availability is regulated by three deiodinase isoforms, namely deiodinase type I (D1), type 2 (D2), and type 3(D3).[57] The most important pathway for T_4 metabolism is its monodeiodination to active T_3 by D2 which catalyzes 5' deiodination and converts T_4 to T_3. The deiodinase activity can change with aging and critical illness and D3 can arise in ischemic tissue.[58]

T_3 accounts for the vast majority of biological effects of TH. It increases myocardial oxygen consumption and tissue thermogenesis, regulates glucose and lipid metabolism, and acts on the heart and vascular smooth muscle cells (Fig. 96.2). Thyroid hormone regulates cardiac inotropy and chronotropy through direct and indirect mechanisms.[58,59] T_3 regulates the expression of genes that encode nuclear receptors and plasma membrane transport proteins within cardiac myocytes. Genomic effects of TH are mediated by TH nuclear receptors that are located in the intracellular compartment. T_3 is transported into the cytoplasm and several families of TH transporters have been identified; variations on binding protein levels can change the peripheral activity of THs.[54,59] The monocarboxylate transporters (MCTs) 8 and 10 are highly specific for iodothyronines and MCT10 has a greater capacity to transport T_3 than MCT8.[60,61] In humans, thyroid hormones bind intracellular DNA-binding proteins that combine as hormone receptor complexes to thyroid hormone response elements (TREs) in the regulatory regions of target genes. There are different subtypes of receptors—TRα1, TRα2, TRβ1, and TRβ2. TRα1 is mostly expressed in the trabecular myocardium. TR α 2 does not bind T_3; however, it is able to bind TRE, thereby exerting a substantial negative effect on gene expression.[54,62] TR β 1 is only weakly expressed in the myocardium. After binding to the promoter regions, T_3 can activate or repress cardiac gene expression to regulate the synthesis of structural and regulatory cardiac proteins, cardiac membrane ion channels, and cell surface receptors, thus providing a molecular mechanism to explain many of the effects of thyroid hormone on the cardiovascular system. Major T_3 targets include myosin heavy chain isoforms because T_3 up-regulates alpha-MHC, the fast myosin, and down-regulates β-MHC, the slow myosin. The human ventricle expresses principally beta-myosin, and limited alterations in isoform expression accompany thyroid disease states; however, changes in

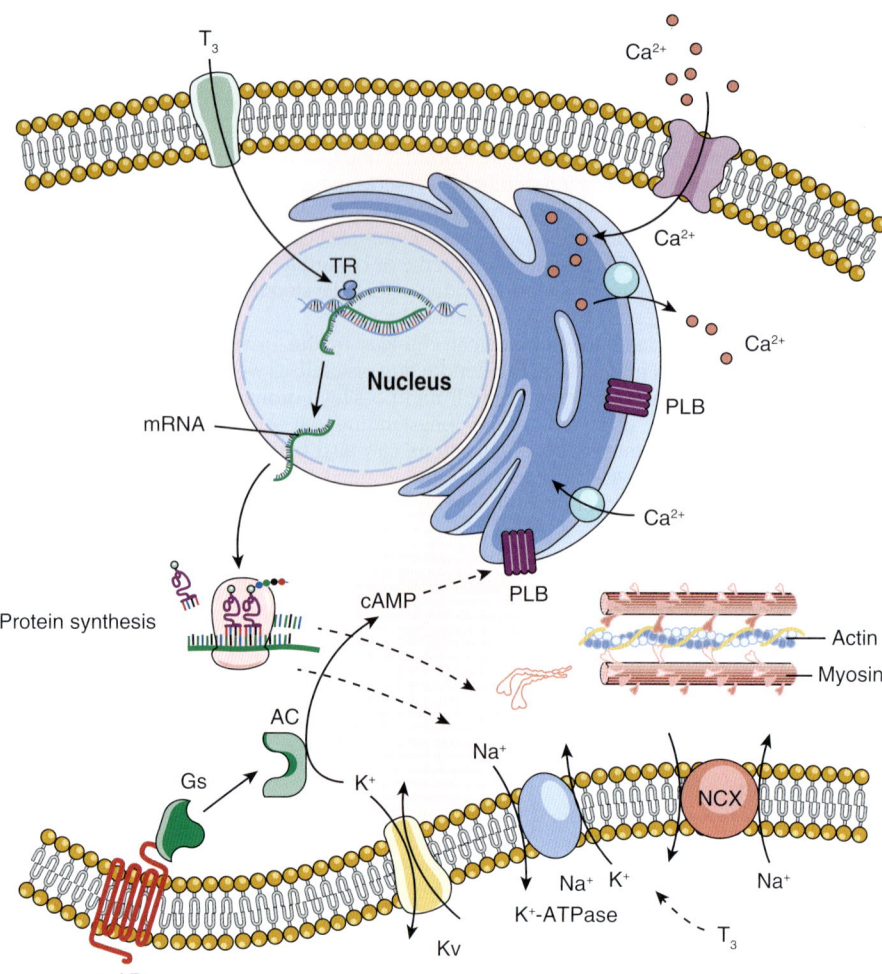

FIGURE 96.2 T_3 enters the cell via specific membrane transporters and binds to nuclear T_3 receptors. The complex binds to thyroid hormone response elements and regulates the transcription of specific genes. Non-nuclear T_3 actions on channels for Na^+, K^+, and Ca^{2+} ions are indicated. *AC*, adenylyl cyclase; *β-AR*, beta-adrenergic receptor; *Gs*, guanine nucleotide–binding protein subunit; *Kv*, voltage-gated potassium channel; *mRNA*, messenger RNA; *NCX*, sodium calcium exchanger; *PLB*, phospholamban; *TR*, T_3 receptor protein.

myosin heavy chain isoform expression can occur in the human atria in various diseases, including CHF and severe hypothyroidism, but are reversible with the appropriate therapy.[63,64] Sarcoplasmic reticulum Ca^{2+}-adenosine triphosphatase (ATPase) (SERCA2) is an important ion pump that determines the magnitude of myocyte calcium cycling (see Chapter 46). Reuptake of calcium into the sarcoendoplasmic reticulum, early in diastole, determines the rate at which the left ventricle relaxes (isovolumic relaxation time). SERCA2 is up-regulated and phospholamban is down-regulated by T_3 (PLB). This molecular mechanism can explain why diastolic function varies inversely across the entire spectrum of thyroid disease states, including even mild subclinical hypothyroidism (Fig. 96.3), contributing to the development of heart failure.[54] Changes in other myocyte genes include Na^+,K^+-ATPase, voltage-gated K^+ channels (Kv1.5 and Kv4.2), Na^+/Ca^{2+} exchanger, beta$_1$-adrenergic receptors, guanosine triphosphate–binding proteins, and the expression of cardiac-specific adenylyl cyclase catalytic subunit isoforms (V,VI).[54,62]

In addition to the well-characterized nuclear effects of thyroid hormone, some cardiac responses to thyroid hormone appear to result from non-transcriptional mechanisms,[65] as suggested by their relatively rapid onset of action, faster than attributable to changes in gene expression and protein synthesis, and non-susceptible to the effects of inhibitors of gene transcription. These indirect effects of TH largely occur at the plasma membrane, regulating ion transporter activity, and include ion channel activation (Na^+,K^+,Ca^{2+}) and regulation of specific signal transduction pathways.

T_3 decreases systemic vascular resistance through vascular smooth-muscle relaxation, which in turn decreases renal perfusion and leads to renin-angiotensin-aldosterone axis activation. T_3 also enhances the release of vasodilatory mediators by increasing metabolic and oxygen consumption. The activation of phosphatidylinositol 3-kinase (PI3K) and serine/threonine protein kinase (AKT) pathways cause the production of endothelial nitric oxide leading to a reduction in systemic vascular resistance through its effects on vascular smooth muscle cells.[66]

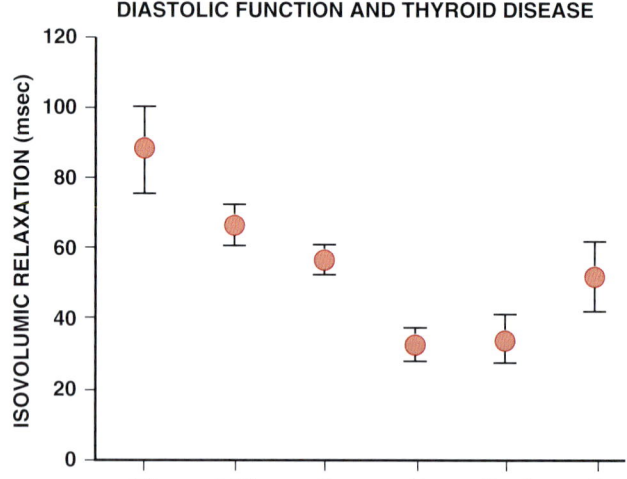

FIGURE 96.3 Diastolic function, as measured by the isovolumic relaxation time, varies over the entire range of thyroid disease, including overt hypothyroidism (OH), subclinical hypothyroidism (SCH), control (C), hyperthyroidism (H), hyperthyroidism after beta-adrenergic blockade (H + P), and hyperthyroidism after treatment to restore normal thyroid function (E).

Diagnosis of Hyperthyroidism

The serum TSH level is the most widely used and sensitive marker for the diagnosis of thyroid dysfunction. Serum TSH levels decrease in hyperthyroidism due to the feedback of excessive T_4 and T_3 serum levels on thyrotropin pituitary synthesis and secretion. Overt hyperthyroidism is a severe clinical disorder induced by TH excess. Serum free thyroxine (FT_4) and or total (TT_3) or free triiodothyronine (FT_3) levels are above their respective reference ranges and serum TSH is suppressed in overt hyperthyroidism. In presence of abnormal TSH levels, measurement of FT_4 and TT_3 or FT_3 can help identify subclinical hyperthyroidism,[67,68] which is defined by subnormal serum TSH and normal serum FT_4 and/or total or FT_3 concentrations, although usually in the mid-to-high normal part of their reference ranges.[67,68] Subclinical hyperthyroidism can be classified into two categories: grade 1 subclinical hyperthyroidism, characterized by low detectable serum TSH levels (e.g., 0.1 to 0.4 mIU/L), and grade 2 subclinical hyperthyroidism in which serum TSH levels are completely undetectable (<0.1 mIU/L)[67,68]; 25% of patients with subclinical hyperthyroidism have grade 2 thyroid dysfunction. Patients with grade 2 subclinical hyperthyroidism are more likely to have an increased risk of progression to overt hyperthyroidism and negative CV adverse events.[67,68]

Overt and subclinical hyperthyroidism result most commonly from increased thyroid hormone synthesis related to Graves disease (GD), toxic adenoma (TA), or toxic multinodular goiter (TMNG). GD, an autoimmune form of hyperthyroidism, is the most common cause of overt and subclinical hyperthyroidism in iodine-replete countries.[67–69] TMNG and TA represent the main causes of thyroid hormone excess in areas with mild to moderate iodine deficiency.[67,68]

Cardiovascular Manifestations of Overt and Subclinical Hyperthyroidism

Changes in myocardial contractility and hemodynamics occur across the entire spectrum of thyroid disease (Table 96.2; see Fig. 96.3). Echocardiographic data indicate that, in humans, newly diagnosed thyrotoxicosis induces an improvement in left ventricular systolic function and an enhancement in left ventricular relaxation, diastolic flow velocities, and isovolumic relaxation time.[70] T_3 excess decreases systemic vascular resistance in arterioles of the peripheral circulation; this drop results in a smaller left ventricular end-systolic volume. A decrease in mean arterial pressure and activation of the renin-angiotensin-aldosterone system increases serum angiotensin-converting enzyme activity and renal sodium reabsorption.[70] The enhanced plasma volume, coupled with increased erythropoietin synthesis expands blood volume; the improvement in diastolic relaxation of the heart contributes to increased left ventricular end-diastolic volume. Despite the marked reduction in systemic vascular resistance, the pulsatile arterial load undergoes a compensatory change and increased aortic input sustains the systolic arterial pressure.[70] Systolic arterial pressure almost invariably increases and diastolic arterial pressure decreases in subjects with overt hyperthyroidism, so that pulse pressure characteristically widens and mean arterial pressure only marginally decreases. Systolic hypertension may develop in up to 30% of hyperthyroid patients and is more pronounced in older patients. The net effect of an increased preload and a decreased afterload yields increased left ventricular stroke volume in hyperthyroidism.[70] In turn, the rise in heart rate and the increased stroke volume combine to cause a two- to threefold increase in cardiac output (see Table 96.2). Therefore, the hyperthyroid heart increases its performance through the modulation of hemodynamic loads; this positive effect on energy metabolism and oxygen consumption improves the left ventricle mechanical efficiency, optimizing its cardiac mechanical-energetic consumption.

Cardiovascular symptoms are an integral and often predominant clinical feature of patients with hyperthyroidism. Most patients experience palpitations resulting from increases in the rate and force of cardiac contractility. The increase in heart rate results from a decrease in parasympathetic stimulation and an increase in sympathetic tone. Heart rates higher than 90 beats/min at rest and during sleep commonly occur, the normal diurnal variation in heart rate is blunted, and the increase during exercise exaggerated.

Subclinical hyperthyroidism may increase heart rate, ventricular mass, arterial stiffness, and left atrial size, especially after long-term exposure to thyroid hormone excess.[67] It may exert unfavorable effects on cardiac morphology, inducing diastolic dysfunction and thereby impairing left ventricle performance (see Table 96.2).[67,68] Sinus tachycardia and atrial premature beats frequently occur in young patients; older patients (>60 years) usually do not have symptoms of adrenergic over-activity, but can develop atrial fibrillation.

Untreated hyperthyroidism is associated with increased CV morbidity and mortality.[67,68] Overt and subclinical hyperthyroidism have been associated with an increased risk of major CV events; this risk is mainly due to higher incidence of HF events.[71] Grade 2 subclinical hyperthyroidism has been associated with an increased risk of AF, HF, and coronary heart disease (CHD) in a meta-analysis assessing individual participant data (IPD) of euthyroid subjects and participants from high-quality prospective studies (see Table 96.2).[72]

Atrial Fibrillation in Overt and Subclinical Hyperthyroidism (see also Chapter 66)

Hyperthyroidism is linked to an increased supraventricular ectopic activity. Atrial fibrillation is a major cause for concern in patients with overt and subclinical hyperthyroidism[70,71] and may be the first symptom of thyroid hormone excess in older adults. T_3 increases systolic depolarization and diastolic repolarization and decreases the action potential duration and the refraction period of the atrial myocardium, as well as the atrial/ventricular nodal refraction period; the reduced inter-atrial action potential duration gives the substrate for atrial arrhythmias.[73]

There is unequivocal evidence that subclinical hyperthyroidism is also associated with an increased risk of atrial fibrillation. In an IPD meta-analysis from five prospective cohort studies, the overall hazard ratio (HR) for incident AF was significantly greater in participants with subclinical hyperthyroidism than in euthyroid controls during a mean follow-up of 8.8 years; grade 2 subclinical hyperthyroidism was associated with a higher risk of AF than grade 1 subclinical hyperthyroidism (see Table 96.2).[67,72] Absolute risks, but not relative risks, increase with aging. Additional analyses have explored whether there is a gradient of risk for developing AF even within the normal reference range of thyroid function tests. Data from the Rotterdam Study have shown that

TABLE 96.2 Effect of Thyroid Disease on Cardiovascular Function and Outcome

	OVERT HYPERTHYROIDISM AND GRADE 2 SUBCLINICAL HYPERTHYROIDISM (<0.1 mIU/L)	OVERT HYPOTHYROIDISM AND GRADE 2 SUBCLINICAL HYPOTHYROIDISM (TSH > 10 mIU/L)
Hypertension	Systolic hypertension Wide pulse pressure	Diastolic hypertension
Cardiac function	CO ↑ Systolic function ↑ Diastolic function ↑ Cardiac workload and LVM in long-term hyperthyroidism ↑ Cardiac preload ↑ Cardiac afterload ↓ Vascular reactivity ↑	CO ↓ Systolic function ↓ Diastolic function ↓ LVM → ↑ Arterial stiffness ↑ Cardiac preload ↓ Cardiac afterload ↑ Vascular reactivity ↓
Thrombogenicity	Coagulability ↑ Fibrinolysis ↑	Unclear
Cardiovascular outcome	Risk of atrial arrhythmias ↑ Risk of AF ↑ Risk of CHD ↑ Risk of HF ↑	Risk of CHD mortality with serum TSH > 7 mIU/L ↑ Risk of HF events with serum TSH > 7 mIU/L ↑

CHD, coronary heart disease; *LVM*, left ventricular mass; *TSH*, Thyroid stimulating hormone.

increasing FT_4 levels within the normal reference range are associated with an increased risk of AF.[74] In a meta-analysis in the Thyroid Studies Collaboration assessing IPD from 11 prospective studies, higher FT_4 levels at baseline in euthyroid individuals were associated with a significant increased risk of AF in age- and gender-adjusted analysis.[75]

Overt and subclinical hyperthyroidism have been associated with increased markers of thrombogenesis (fibrinogen and factor X levels). Hyperthyroid patients have higher von Willebrand antigen levels compared to euthyroid patients, leading to an enhanced platelet plug formation which subsequently decreases with treatment. Stroke is a potential complication of AF in overt hyperthyroidism leading to increased cerebrovascular events; on the contrary insufficient results have been reported in subclinical hyperthyroidism.[72,76]

The first-line treatment of atrial fibrillation and supraventricular tachycardia in patients with thyroid dysfunction should aim primarily to restore a euthyroid state.[68,77–79] Treatment of hyperthyroidism with antithyroid drugs should be the first-line therapy in patients with hyperthyroidism and atrial fibrillation to obtain conversion to sinus rhythm and to improve hemodynamics. A beta1-selective or nonselective agent may help to control the ventricular response. Beta blockers promptly improve the tachycardia-mediated component of ventricular dysfunction. Digitalis may help control the ventricular response in hyperthyroidism-associated atrial fibrillation, but because of the increased rate of digitalis clearance, the decreased sensitivity of drug action resulting from the high cellular levels of Na^+,K^+-ATPase, and the decreased parasympathetic tone, patients usually require higher doses. Anticoagulation, especially with the new non-vitamin K-dependent agents, in patients with hyperthyroidism and AF is controversial. The potential for systemic or cerebral embolization must be weighed against the risk for bleeding and complications. Pharmacological or electrical cardioversion should be considered in patients who do not recover normal rhythm spontaneously within 4 months of normalization of the thyroid function, after evaluation of the patient's age and underlying cardiac status. The ability to restore thyrotoxic patients to a euthyroid state and sinus rhythm justifies TSH testing in most patients with a recent onset of otherwise unexplained atrial fibrillation or other supraventricular arrhythmias.[77–79]

Heart Failure in Overt and Subclinical Hyperthyroidism

The cardiovascular alterations in hyperthyroidism include increased resting cardiac output and enhanced cardiac contractility (see Table 96.2). However, many hyperthyroid patients experience exercise intolerance and exertional dyspnea, caused in part by skeletal and respiratory muscle weakness.[70] The low vascular resistance and increased preload compromise cardiac functional reserve, which cannot rise further to accommodate the demands imposed by submaximal or maximal exercise. Despite the high cardiac output state, hyperthyroid patients have an impaired cardiopulmonary function during effort, which reflects their reduced CV and respiratory reserve during exercise. Nevertheless, a minority of patients have symptoms, including dyspnea on exertion, orthopnea, and paroxysmal nocturnal dyspnea, as well as signs demonstrating peripheral edema, elevated jugular venous pressure, or an S_3. This complex of findings, coupled with failure to increase the left ventricular ejection fraction with exercise, suggests a hyperthyroid cardiomyopathy. The term often used in this setting, *high-output failure*, is not appropriate because although resting cardiac output is as much as two to three times normal, the exercise intolerance does not appear to result from cardiac failure but rather from skeletal muscle weakness and perhaps associated pulmonary hypertension.[70,76] High-output states, however, can increase renal sodium reabsorption and expand plasma volume. Although systemic vascular resistance falls with hyperthyroidism, pulmonary vascular resistance does not, and because of the greater output to the pulmonary circulation, pulmonary arterial pressure increases. This leads to a rise in mean venous pressure, hepatic congestion, and peripheral edema of the type associated with primary pulmonary hypertension or right-sided heart failure. In patients with longstanding hyperthyroidism and marked sinus tachycardia or atrial fibrillation, low cardiac output, impaired cardiac contractility with a low ejection fraction, and pulmonary congestion can develop—all consistent with heart failure.

A review of such cases suggests that the impairment in the left ventricular function results from the prolonged high heart rate and the development of a rate-related heart failure. When the left ventricle becomes dilated, mitral regurgitation may also develop (see Chapter 76). Recognition of this phenomenon is important as treatment aimed at slowing the heart rate or controlling the ventricular response in atrial fibrillation appears to improve left ventricular function, even before initiation of antithyroid therapy. Some patients with hyperthyroidism, similar to the overall CHF population, do not tolerate initiation of beta blockers in full doses. Patients critically ill who develop low cardiac output should be managed in an intensive care unit setting. Subclinical and overt hyperthyroidism are associated with 23% and 25% increased risk of major cardiovascular events (MACEs) respectively.[71] This risk is motivated by heart failure being about 15% to 20% higher respectively in subjects with subclinical hyperthyroidism and overt hyperthyroidism.[71] Pooled IPD data from six prospective cohort studies reported a significant risk of HF events in participants with grade 2 subclinical hyperthyroidism compared to grade 1.[72] Thyroid testing is highly recommended in patients with HF.[68]

CHD in Hyperthyroidism

A subset of thyrotoxic patients can experience angina-like chest pain. In older hyperthyroid patients with known or suspected coronary artery disease, the increase in cardiac work associated with the increase in cardiac output and cardiac contractility can produce myocardial ischemia, which can respond to beta blockers or lead to the restoration of a euthyroid state. Rarely patients, usually younger women, experience a syndrome of chest pain at rest associated with ischemic electrocardiographic changes. Cardiac catheterization has demonstrated that most of these patients have angiographically normal coronary arteries, but coronary vasospasm similar to that found in variant angina can occur (see also Chapters 40 and 91). Myocardial infarction rarely develops and these patients appear to respond to calcium channel–blocking agents or nitroglycerin.

A meta-analysis of IPD data from 10 prospective cohorts reported that grade 2 subclinical hyperthyroidism can increase the risk of CHD mortality (see Table 96.2).[72] The Rotterdam Study showed a higher risk of CVD events even in participants with high-normal FT_4 concentrations.[80]

Pulmonary Hypertension and Autoimmune Cardiovascular Involvement

Hyperthyroidism associates with a substantial degree of pulmonary hypertension (mean pulmonary artery systolic pressure >50 mm Hg).[76] Pulmonary hypertension in turn places a significant degree of stress and afterload on the right ventricle—thus implying that although systemic vascular resistance decreases with thyrotoxicosis, pulmonary vascular resistance does not. Correction of hyperthyroidism usually reduces pulmonary arterial pressure. Severe pulmonary hypertension may also reverse completely after successful treatment of hyperthyroidism. In addition to the reduction in pulmonary blood flow, a specific vasoactive effect of methimazole may explain the improvement in the pulmonary vasculature hemodynamics after treatment of hyperthyroidism.

Autoimmune hyperthyroidism occasionally links to autoimmune cardiovascular involvement. Pulmonary arterial hypertension, myxomatous cardiac valve disease, irreversible dilated cardiomyopathy, and peripartum cardiomyopathy have been reported in patients with GD.[76] Patients with autoimmune thyroid disease may have anticardiolipin antibodies and antiphospholipid syndrome.[76]

TREATMENT OF OVERT AND SUBCLINICAL HYPERTHYROIDISM

Graves disease tends to either resolve spontaneously or worsen with time. Methimazole is appropriate for younger adults with Graves disease, because this autoimmune condition may spontaneously remit

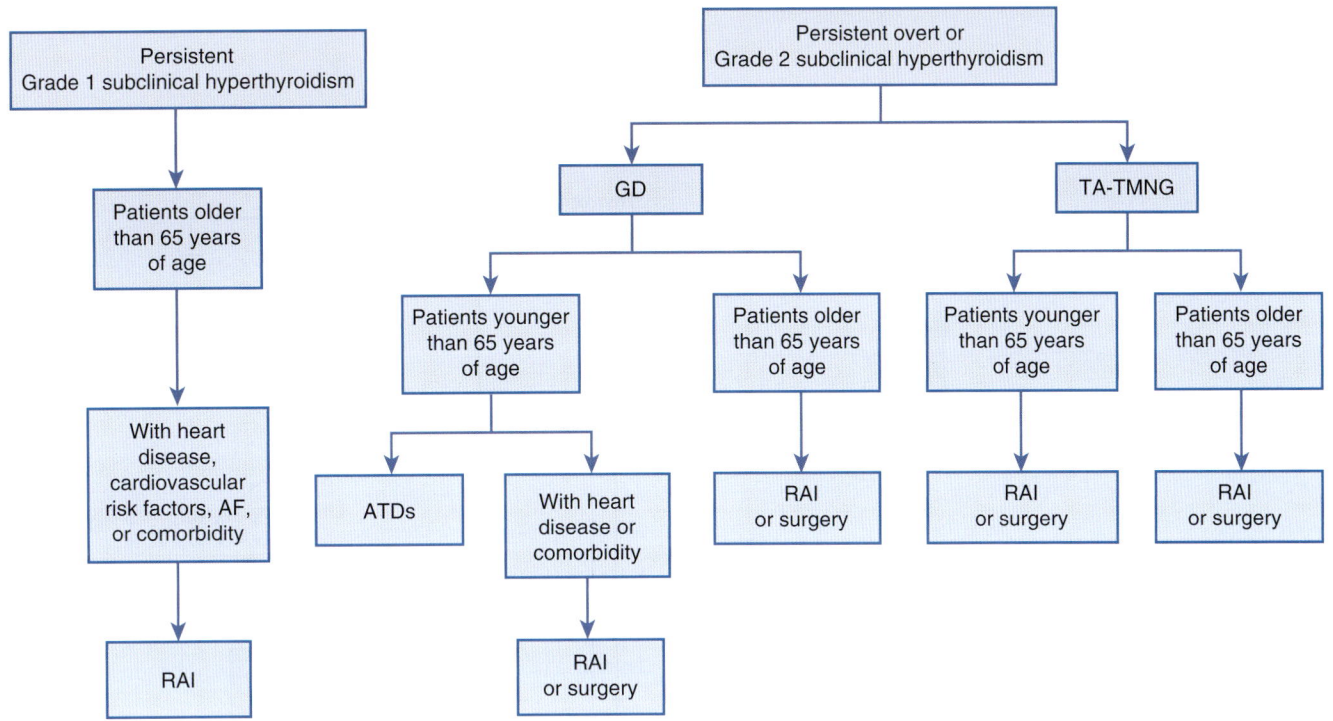

FIGURE 96.4 Treatment of overt and subclinical hyperthyroidism according to the etiology and degree of hyperthyroidism.

after a course of therapy; also patients with milder disease, that is, subclinical hyperthyroidism, are most likely to remit.[69] Radioiodine therapy is appropriate for older individuals with persistent Graves disease who have underlying comorbidities because definitive treatment is necessary to avoid the progression of cardiac disease (Fig. 96.4).[69,81]

Most patients with chronic subclinical hyperthyroidism have multinodular goiters or solitary nodules rather than autoimmune hyperthyroidism. Radioiodine would be the preferred treatment for individuals with overt or subclinical hyperthyroidism with a TMNG or a solitary autonomously functioning nodule.[67,69] Definitive therapy can then be safely performed with iodine-131 alone or in combination with an antithyroid drug (see Fig. 96.4).[67,68] Surgery would typically be reserved for patients with a large goiter and symptoms of compression, coexisting hyperparathyroidism, or suspicion of thyroid malignancy.[67,68] Treatment of subclinical hyperthyroidism is not recommended in asymptomatic younger persons or premenopausal women with milder degrees of lowering serum TSH (i.e., 0.1 to 0.4 mU/L) due to a lack of evidence of harm.[67,68]

Subclinical hyperthyroidism may develop during levothyroxine (L–T_4) therapy with doses that suppress serum TSH. Intentional TSH–suppressive doses of L–T_4 are only indicated in patients with a previous diagnosis of thyroid cancer with high risk of recurrences; the risk–benefit of TSH suppression should be considered in older patients.[82]

THYROID STORM

Patients with thyroid storm, the most severe form of hyperthyroidism, can display altered mental status, fever, gastrointestinal symptoms including pain, nausea, and rarely jaundice, exaggerated tachycardia, new onset supraventricular arrhythmias such as atrial fibrillation or hypotension, and cardiovascular collapse.[83] Takotsubo cardiomyopathy links to severe thyrotoxicosis and may be a manifestation of thyroid storm.

The mortality rate of thyroid storm can be as high as 50% and outcomes vary based on management of the cardiovascular manifestations. These patients require intensive care unit monitoring in addition to the use of antithyroid drugs, potassium iodide, and attention to other coexistent medical problems such as infection, trauma, or drugs such as amiodarone; they may tolerate intravenous administration of beta-adrenergic blocking drugs or calcium channel blockers poorly. The development of hypotensive cardiac arrest or worsening heart failure represents the untoward effects of such agents in patients with thyrotoxic heart disease. As noted above, intensive monitoring, judicious use of esmolol, and standard fluid and volume management with simultaneous treatment to lower T_4 and T_3 can optimize the therapeutic response.[83]

Diagnosis of Overt and Subclinical Hypothyroidism

Overt hypothyroidism is a clinical condition in which TSH is increased and free thyroid hormones (especially FT_4) are low. The term myxedema is reserved for severe and/or complicated thyroid hormone deficiency in adults and is usually used to indicate a nonpitting edema caused by the accumulation of glycosaminoglycans in interstitial tissue. Subclinical hypothyroidism is diagnosed when serum TSH is above the upper limit of the normal reference range and free thyroid hormones are within their respective reference range. Patients may have a mild disease (TSH 4.5 to 9.9 mU/L) or a more severe dysfunction (TSH ≥ 10 mU/L).[84,85] Hashimoto thyroiditis represents the most common cause of acquired subclinical hypothyroidism in the adult. Thyroid surgery, radioiodine therapy, and, in some parts of the world, iodine deficiency are the most common causes of hypothyroidism.

Cardiovascular Effects of Overt and Subclinical Hypothyroidism

Hemodynamic changes occur in hypothyroidism (Fig. 96.5; see Table 96.2). Left ventricular function falls reversibly in hypothyroidism. Cardiac preload decreases due to the impaired diastolic function and decreased blood volume; left ventricular ejection fraction at rest and during exercise and cardiopulmonary exercise testing declines and tends to improve with restoration of euthyroidism.[86] Afterload increases in patients with hypothyroidism as a result of increased systemic vascular resistance, arterial stiffness, and endothelial dysfunction.[87] Systemic vascular resistance may increase as much as 30% and mean arterial pressure rise in up to 20% of patients with diastolic hypertension. Diastolic hypertension in patients with hypothyroidism is associated with a low renin level and a decrease in the hepatic synthesis of renin substrate. Cardiac output may decrease by as much as 30% to 40% in hypothyroidism. Despite the decrease in cardiac output and contractility of the hypothyroid myocardium, studies of myocardial metabolism have shown that the hypothyroid myocardium is energy-inefficient

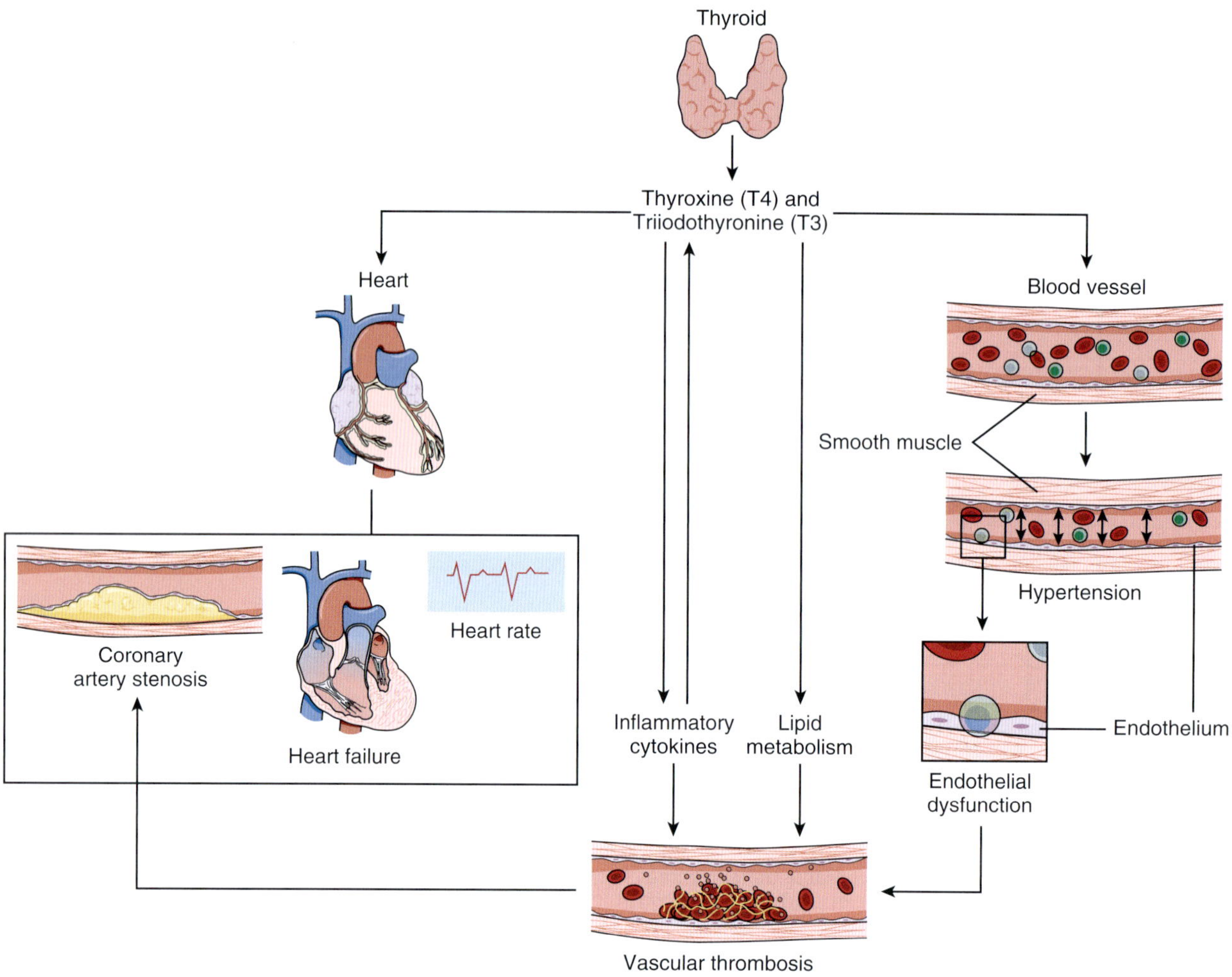

FIGURE 96.5 Effects of thyroid hormones (TH) on the risk of heart failure and coronary heart disease (effects on blood pressure, smooth muscle tone, endothelial function, lipid metabolism, and modulation of inflammatory pathways). (From Razvi S, Jabbar A, Pingitore A, et al. Thyroid hormones and cardiovascular function and diseases. *J Am Coll Cardiol.* 2018;71:1781.)

despite the low level of overall oxygen consumption. Indeed, increased afterload is one of the major factors determining myocardial oxygen consumption.

Pericardial effusions can occur in severe or long-standing hypothyroidism; occasionally, it can be large and cause the appearance of cardiomegaly on chest radiographs. Although rare, tamponade with hemodynamic compromise may occur. Echocardiography demonstrates small to moderate effusions in up to 30% of overtly hypothyroid patients; the effusions tend to resolve within weeks or months after initiation of thyroid hormone replacement therapy.

As a result of the changes in ion channel expression and parasympathetic tone, the ECG in hypothyroidism may show sinus bradycardia, low voltage, and prolongation of the action potential duration and QT interval. The QT prolongation predisposes patients to ventricular arrhythmias, and some patients have acquired torsades de pointes which can improve or completely resolve with thyroid hormone replacement.

Subclinical hypothyroidism can impair left ventricular filling and relaxation (see Fig. 96.3; Table 96.2).[84] It can also impair relaxation of vascular smooth muscle cells, inducing increases in systemic vascular resistance and arterial stiffness, as well as changes in endothelial function by reducing the availability of nitric oxide.[86-89]

Overt and subclinical hypothyroidism can progressively impair cardiac function leading to HF. A pooled analysis on a total of 2068 IPD data from six prospective studies reported an increased risk of HF events in patients with serum TSH greater than 7 to 10 mIU/L.[72,84] Some studies also demonstrate that subclinical hypothyroidism could potentially induce a worsening of the cardiac function in patients with preexisting HF leading to an increase in CV mortality.[90-92] Treatment of hypothyroid patients with restoration of a euthyroid state resolves the CV changes in parallel with return of systemic vascular resistance to lower level (see Table 96.2).[93]

Coronary Heart Disease

Hypothyroidism also increases total and low-density lipoprotein (LDL) cholesterol in proportion to the rise in serum TSH levels.[94] Although thyroid hormone can alter cholesterol metabolism through multiple mechanisms, including a decrease in biliary excretion, the primary mechanism involves changes in the LDL metabolism caused by decreases in the numbers of the hepatic LDL receptor and reduced activity of cholesterol 7α-hydroxylase, an enzyme that lowers cholesterol levels. A recent study reported that the liver-selective thyroid hormone agonist eprotirome can lower cholesterol levels in statin-treated patients, in support of this concept.[95]

Increases in risk factors for atherosclerosis, including hypercholesterolemia, hypertension, endothelial dysfunction, and elevated levels of homocysteine, may elevate the risk for atherosclerosis and coronary and systemic vascular disease in patients with hypothyroidism (see Chapters 25 to 27) (see Fig. 96.5). Myocardial perfusion scans have demonstrated abnormalities suggestive of myocardial ischemia, but these defects appear to resolve with thyroid hormone treatment. A patient-level meta-analysis of several prospective cohort studies providing 542,494 person-years of follow-up has shown that subclinical hypothyroidism is associated with a higher risk of CV events and mortality in people with serum TSH greater than 7 mIU/L levels and even more in those with TSH levels greater than 10 mU/L irrespective of age.[84]

One of the major factors that affects CV risk in SCH populations is age and several observations have concluded that older individuals with grade 1 subclinical hypothyroidism may have a lower risk of CV disease than younger ones.[84] Treatment of mild disease is recommended in young patients with evidence of atherosclerotic cardiovascular disease, heart failure, or associated risk factors. Trials of L–T_4 in mild subclinical hypothyroidism using surrogate markers have shown improvements in the left ventricular function, vascular endothelial function, atherogenic lipid particles, or cardiac mitochondrial function.[84]

TSH screening is advisable in adults, particularly in patients with hypertension, hypercholesterolemia, hypertriglyceridemia, coronary or peripheral vascular disease, and unexplained pericardial or pleural effusions, as well as for various musculoskeletal syndromes or statin-associated myopathy.

TREATMENT OF HYPOTHYROIDISM

Replacement doses of purified preparations of L–T_4 (levothyroxine) are the treatment of choice in hypothyroid patients.[96,97] The optimal replacement dose of L–T_4 should take into account both the age of the patient and the cause of hypothyroidism. Indeed, the L–T_4 dosage should be lower in older adults and higher in patients with a more severe disease, particularly those who have undergone thyroidectomy or prior iodine treatment for GD. In all patients, thyroid hormone replacement should suffice to restore the serum TSH level to normal so that they are clinically and chemically euthyroid. The known effects of thyroid hormone on the heart and cardiovascular system do not support the concept that these patients benefit from maintenance of mild hypothyroidism.

Treatment of hypothyroidism yields predictable responses, especially from a cardiovascular perspective. Stepwise thyroid hormone replacement with L–T_4 incrementally decreases serum TSH, serum cholesterol, and serum creatine-kinase (CK) levels and improves left ventricular performance. Patients less than 50 years with no history of heart disease generally tolerate full replacement doses of L–T_4 (1.5 µg/kg/day) without concern for untoward cardiac effects. Patients greater than 50 years with known or suspected coronary artery disease have more complicated issues. Three major issues arise. Coronary artery bypass graft surgery (CABG) can be performed in patients with unstable angina, left main coronary artery disease, or three-vessel disease with impaired left ventricular function, even in the setting of overt hypothyroidism. Rarely a patient has sufficiently profound hypothyroidism to prolong bleeding times and partial thromboplastin times, which requires preoperative supplementation of clotting factors. Thyroid hormone replacement can be delayed until the postoperative period, when it can be administered in full doses parenterally or orally. Treatment of patients with known stable cardiac disease in whom cardiac revascularization is not clinically indicated should begin with low doses (12.5 µg) of L–T_4 and then stepwise increases (12.5 to 25 µg) every 6 to 8 weeks until the serum TSH level normalizes. Thyroid hormone replacement in this setting and its ability to lower systemic vascular resistance and decrease afterload, as well as improve myocardial efficiency, can actually decrease clinical signs of myocardial ischemia. In patients who, although potentially at risk for coronary artery disease, exhibit no clinical signs or symptoms, thyroid hormone replacement can start at low doses, generally in the range of 25 to 50 µg/day, and then increase by 25 µg every 6 to 8 weeks until the serum TSH level is normal. If signs or symptoms of ischemic heart disease develop, the same recommendations apply as for patients with known underlying heart diseases.

Despite the lack of definitive long-term studies on the outcome of mild-to-moderate hypothyroidism with and without replacement therapy, recommendations for treatment of patients with serum TSH ≥ 7 mIU/L have fallen on the side of replacement treatment with L–T_4.[84] Randomized controlled trials are needed to evaluate the clinical benefits and safety of treatment of SCH in reducing CV risk.

MYXEDEMA COMA

In the rare condition of myxedema coma, characterized by the development of hypothermia, altered mental status, hypotension, bradycardia, and hypoventilation, the need for thyroid hormone replacement is more of an emergency.[98] In patients with severe coma, treatment can be accomplished by intravenous administration of 200 µg of L–T_4 followed by 100 µg of L–T_4 per day to restore vital functions. L–T_3 may also be started simultaneously with L–T_4 in a starting dosage of 10 to 20 µg, followed by 10 µg every 6 hours for 1 or 2 days until the cerebral function of the patient improves. Patients with myxedema coma require intensive care unit monitoring with volume repletion, gentle warming, and ventilatory support in the presence of CO_2 retention. Administration of hydrocortisone (50 to 100 mg three times daily) should be undertaken until the results of serum cortisol testing are obtained. When treated in this manner, hemodynamics, including systemic vascular resistance, cardiac output, and heart rate, improve within 24 to 48 hours. Severe hyponatremia should be corrected with the judicious administration of hypertonic saline solution (50 to 100 mL of 3% sodium chloride) followed by an IV bolus of 40 to 120 mg furosemide. This treatment should be used cautiously to avoid inadvertent correction of hyponatremia with its devastating consequences.

Amiodarone and Thyroid Function

Amiodarone is an iodine-rich antiarrhythmic agent used in the treatment of ventricular and atrial tachyarrhythmias; its 30% iodine content by weight and structural similarity to L–T_4 causes abnormalities in thyroid function test results in as many as 60% of the patients treated for short or long periods. The finding that dronedarone, a noniodinated benzofuran antiarrhythmic, does not alter thyroid function reinforces this concept.

Amiodarone inhibits entry of T_4 into cells and the intracellular conversion of T_4 to T_3 by inhibiting the 5′-monodeiodination of T_4 in the liver and pituitary. Inhibition of T_4 metabolism in the liver decreases serum T_3 and increases serum T_4 levels, whereas serum TSH levels initially remain normal. With more chronic treatment, T_4 synthesis and release from the thyroid gland can be inhibited, thereby producing an increase in TSH levels. Patients with autoimmune thyroid disease or enzymatic defects in thyroid hormone biosynthesis and even some patients without any risk factors can progress to overt chemical and clinical hypothyroidism.[99] The overall prevalence of hypothyroidism in amiodarone-treated patients is between 15% and 30%. Symptoms of hypothyroidism in this setting can be subtle and significant hypothyroidism can occur even in their absence. *Thyroid function should be measured every 3 months in all patients receiving amiodarone.* The effect on thyroid function does not depend on the dose and can occur at any time after initiating treatment; furthermore, because of the high lipid solubility and long half-life of amiodarone, this effect can persist up to 1 year after discontinuing therapy.

Less common but perhaps more challenging is the development of amiodarone-induced thyrotoxicosis (Table 96.3).[99] Although not initially observed in the iodine-replete American population, the experience from more iodine-deficient populations (such as Italy) suggests that it occurs with a prevalence as high as 10%. The onset was often sudden and could occur shortly after initiation of amiodarone therapy, during chronic treatment, or up to 1 year after stopping therapy. Clinical clues to the development of this condition include a new onset or recurrence of ventricular irritability (increased firing of an implantable cardioverter-defibrillator), decreased warfarin dose requirements, or return or worsening of the obstructive physiology of hypertrophic cardiomyopathy (see Chapter 54). Two forms of amiodarone-induced thyrotoxicosis can occur.[99] Type I occurs primarily in patients with preexisting thyroid disease and most commonly in iodine-deficient areas. These patients rarely have an increase in 24-hour radioiodine uptake and frequently some measures of thyroid autoimmunity, including antithyroid antibodies. In contrast, a variety of proinflammatory cytokines, including IL-6, presumably mediate type II thyroiditis. In this case, the toxic effect on the thyroid gland induces a release of preformed thyroid hormone through thyroiditis (type 2 amiodarone-induced thyrotoxicosis). This destructive process can continue for weeks or months and is usually associated with low to absent radioiodine uptake. Further experience has shown that these two types have substantial overlap in many of the distinguishing features. Amiodarone-induced thyrotoxicosis associates with a threefold increased risk for major adverse cardiovascular events, underscoring its clinical importance.[99] Table 96.3 proposes a scheme for thyroid function treatment in patients treated with amiodarone.

Because of the increased thyroidal and total-body iodine content, use of iodine-131 is almost always ineffective. Similarly, treatment with antithyroid drugs has marginal effectiveness. Corticosteroids (prednisone, 20 to 40 mg/day) provide benefit, perhaps with increased usefulness in patients with type II disease who have high serum levels of IL-6. However, corticosteroids can be instituted in all patients because when effective the response usually occurs within 2 to 4 weeks of initiating

TABLE 96.3 Treatment of Amiodarone-Associated Thyroid Dysfunction

Amiodarone-Induced Hypothyroidism (AIH)
- Amiodarone-induced thyrotoxicosis (AIT) can be diagnosed on the basis of classic signs and symptoms of hypothyroidism or hyperthyroidism or by routine (every 3–6 months) thyroid function testing
- Withdrawal of amiodarone is not necessary in patients with hypothyroidism
- L–T_4 treatment can be started at a low dose and progressively increased
- The target serum TSH level during levothyroxine therapy should be balanced with the risk of arrhythmias

Type 1 Amiodarone-Induced Thyrotoxicosis (AIT 1)
- Clinical hypothyroidism with a TSH level higher than 10 mIU/mL should be treated
- The treatment of choice is the use of antithyroid drugs
- Perchlorate at doses not exceeding 1 g/day can be useful in patients with resistant hyperthyroidism
- Total thyroidectomy should be performed in AIT 1 patients with a deterioration of the cardiovascular function or severe underlying cardiac disease and/or in patients with persistent hyperthyroidism unresponsive to medical therapies
- Hyperfunctioning thyroid gland can be definitely treated with thyroidectomy or radioiodine (RAI) treatment
- Euthyroidism should be restored before total thyroidectomy or RAI, when possible

Type 2 Amiodarone-Induced Thyrotoxicosis (AIT 2)
- Amiodarone can be continued only in patients with life-threatening arrhythmias and severe critical illness with poor prognosis
- The first-line treatment is the administration of oral glucocorticoids

Mixed/Indefinite Form of AIT
- Glucocorticoids should be added to thionamides

treatment. In patients unresponsive to glucocorticoids with evidence of hyperthyroidism—including weight loss, tachycardia, palpitations, worsening angina, ventricular tachycardia, or other untoward cardiac effects—treatment with antithyroid therapy (methimazole 10 to 30 mg/day) is variably effective and can cause considerable side effects. Total thyroidectomy can be performed safely and can rapidly reverse hyperthyroidism.[99] Preoperative treatment with beta blockers is indicated, and there have been no reported cases of resulting thyroid storm.

Whether amiodarone-mediated thyroid dysfunction should mandate discontinuation of therapy with the drug is an important issue. There is no evidence that stopping treatment with amiodarone hastens the resolution of chemical hyperthyroidism.

Changes in Thyroid Hormone Metabolism That Accompany Cardiac Disease

In addition to the changes in thyroid function that can result from classic thyroid disease, primary alterations in levels of serum total and free T_3 and occasionally in serum T_4 can accompany a variety of acute and chronic illnesses, including sepsis, starvation, and cardiac disease. In the absence of thyroid gland abnormality, changes in serum T_3 levels result from alterations in thyroid hormone metabolism. Some refer to such cases as nonthyroidal illness.[100] The mechanism for this decrease in serum T_3 levels is multifactorial and in part related to a decrease of 5'-monodeiodination in the liver. Up to 30% of patients with heart failure have a low serum T_3 level, a finding in patients treated with or without amiodarone. In patients with CHF, the fall in serum T_3 levels correlates with the severity of heart failure as assessed by the NYHA classification.[101] In addition, in patients with heart failure and preserved ejection fraction, the serum level of T_3 is inversely proportional to the level of pro-brain natriuretic peptide. The increased levels of inflammatory proteins (interleukins and cytokines such as IL-6, TNF-α, etc.) induce changes in thyroid hormone metabolism, type 2 deiodinase activity, and thyroid hormone receptors expression in patients with heart failure, resulting in the development of tissue hypothyroidism in patients with severe heart failure. Changes occurring in the damaged myocardium and the reactivation of the fetal genotype in HF may suggest that the deleterious effects of hypothyroidism on the myocardium may benefit from T_3 replacement. In addition, TH treatment reduces interstitial fibrosis in animal models of ischemic and non-ischemic heart failure because of the inhibitory effect on metalloproteinases.

An antifibrotic effect of TH is also linked to the T_3-induced inhibition of the profibrotic pathways and supported by the association of low serum T_3 levels with the presence of cardiac fibrosis in patients with idiopathic dilated cardiomyopathy. A population-based study of patients with cardiac disease has shown how a low serum T_3 level strongly predicts all-cause and cardiovascular mortality. These observations led to studies examining the administration of L–T_4, L–T_3, or thyroid hormone analogs in patients with heart failure to potentially improve their prognosis. L–T_3 infusion in patients with chronic and stable dilated cardiomyopathy and low-T_3 syndrome improved cardiac performance and the neurohumoral milieu without a significant increase in myocardial O_2 consumption.[102] Larger multicenter trials for longer periods are needed to provide information on hard clinical outcomes such as mortality, arrhythmias, and hospitalizations before thyroid hormone therapy can be routinely prescribed in patients with heart failure as part of clinical practice.

Children and adults undergoing cardiac surgery with cardiopulmonary bypass demonstrate a predictable fall in serum T_3 levels in the perioperative period, which identifies patients at increased risk for morbidity and mortality. A prospective, randomized study has shown that especially in neonates, administration of T_3 in doses sufficient to restore serum T_3 levels to normal decreases the degree of therapeutic intervention and the need for postoperative inotropic agents.

THYROID HORMONES AND CARDIOPROTECTION

Following uncomplicated acute myocardial infarction (AMI), serum T_3 levels fall by about 20% and reach a nadir after approximately 96 hours. Experimental myocardial infarction in animals produces a similar decrease in serum T_3 levels, and replacement of T_3 levels to normal may increase left ventricular contractile function. Cardioprotection is an emerging target of therapeutic intervention in AMI to minimize irreversible ischemic damage and favor functional recovery of the ischemic-damaged myocardium. Low T_3 induces oxidative stress, increases the apoptotic rate, and is able to depress myocardial function, leading to worsened ventricular dysfunction. There is some evidence in animal studies that thyroid hormones play a critical role in regeneration and repair during adult life. T_3 has a cardioprotective effect, owing to the activation of cytoprotective mechanisms, stimulation of cell growth and neo-angiogenesis, and regulation of mitochondrial dysfunction. Therefore, T_3 increases the post-ischemic recovery of myocardial function. The reduction in myocardial damage and the positive left ventricular remodeling induced by T_3 could delay or improve the evolution toward postischemic irreversible heart failure.

In a recent meta-analysis, patients with ischemic heart disease and concomitant Non-thyroidal illness syndrome (NTIS) or hypothyroidism had a higher risk of all-cause mortality and MACE.[103] However, despite these results, there is a need for future studies to clarify the causal relationship between these events and the association of NTIS or hypothyroidism in patients with ischemic heart disease. In a recent phase 2, randomized, controlled trial of oral T_3 in patients with STEMI and low serum free T_3 levels, the administration of T_3 in replacement doses for 6 months was proved to be safe and effective in reducing regional cardiac dysfunction and significantly increased stroke volume, as compared with no treatment.[104] Future randomized trials are necessary to demonstrate the safety and efficacy of thyroid hormone supplementation in patients with ischemic heart disease and NTIS or hypothyroidism before considering its routine use.

FUTURE PERSPECTIVES

Endocrine dysfunction can be responsible for hypertension, atrial fibrillation, coronary heart disease, and heart failure, increasing cardiovascular mortality. The identification of these disorders is important because appropriate treatment of the specific endocrine deficiency

TABLE 96.4 Clinical Features of Endocrine Dysfunctions: Diagnosis and Cardiovascular Outcome

CLINICAL FEATURES	POSSIBLE DIAGNOSIS	DIAGNOSTIC TESTS
Bradycardia	Hypothyroidism	TSH
Diastolic hypertension		FT_3
Fatigue		FT_4
Increased sensitivity to cold		ABTG
Constipation		ABTPO
Dry skin		Thyroid Doppler ultrasound
Weight gain		
Hoarseness		
Muscle weakness		
Elevated blood cholesterol levels		
Heart failure		
Coronary heart disease		
Systolic hypertension	Hyperthyroidism	TSH
Tachycardia		FT_3
Atrial arrhythmia		FT_4
Weight loss despite increased appetite		TG
Nervousness, anxiety, and irritability		ABTG
Tremor		ABTPO
Sweating		TSHR-Abs
Goiter		Thyroid Doppler ultrasound
Insomnia		Thyroid scan
Heart failure		
Coronary heart disease		
Young onset	Primary aldosteronism	Aldosterone/renin ratio
Sustained blood pressure		Confirmatory tests
Resistant hypertension with or without hypokalemia		Anatomic localization according to etiology
Diuretic-induced hypokalemia		Adrenal venous sampling
Muscle weakness		
Cramping		
Polyuria		
Incidental adrenal mass		
Young stroke		
Sleep apnea		
Family history of early-onset hypertension		
Myocardial fibrosis		
Paroxysmal hypertension	Pheochromocytoma	24-hr urinary fractionated metanephrines
Flushing		Plasma-free metanephrines
Headaches		Chromogranin A methoxytyramine
Sweating		Anatomic localization according to etiology
Palpitations		
Orthostatic hypotension		
Syncope		
Paradoxic blood pressure response to drugs, surgery, or anesthesia		
Incidentally discovered adrenal mass		
Family history of PPGL		
Previous PPGL		
Syndromic feature indicating a pheochromocytoma-related hereditary syndrome		

Continued

TABLE 96.4 Clinical Features of Endocrine Dysfunctions: Diagnosis and Cardiovascular Outcome—cont'd

CLINICAL FEATURES	POSSIBLE DIAGNOSIS	DIAGNOSTIC TESTS
Weight gain with central obesity and rounded face	Cushing syndrome	ACTH and cortisol levels
Pink or purple stretch marks on the skin of the abdomen, thighs, breasts, and arms		24-hr urinary cortisol
Fragile skin that bruises easily		Late-night salivary cortisol
Hypertension		Dexamethasone suppression test
Insulin resistance or type 2 diabetes		CRH test
Dyslipidemia		Anatomic localization according to etiology
Prothrombotic state		
Depression		
Increased pigmentation	Addison disease	ACTH and cortisol levels
Abdominal pain with nausea and vomiting		24-hr urinary cortisol
Hypotension		Intravenous injection of ACTH
Hypoglycemia		Anatomic evaluation according to etiology
Hyponatremia		
Hyperkalemia		
Loss of autonomic tone		
Enlarged hands and feet	Acromegaly	GH
Enlarged facial features		IGF1
Enlarged tongue		GH after oral glucose load
Hypertension		Localization of the tumor according to etiology
Insulin resistance		
Type 2 diabetes mellitus		
Hyperlipidemia		
Incidentally discovered pituitary tumors		
Sleep apnea		
Debilitating arthritis or carpal tunnel syndrome		
Cardiomegaly		
Concentric biventricular hypertrophy		
History of traumatic brain injury, subarachnoid hemorrhage, cranial irradiation, pituitary hemorrhage, or surgery	GH deficiency	GH
		IGF1
Central adiposity		IGF- Binding protein 3
Reduced lean muscle mass		GH-releasing hormone-arginine stimulation test
Impaired neuromuscular function		
Impaired lipid profile		
Depression, anxiety, social isolation		
Fatigue		
Impaired cardiac function		
Accelerated atherogenesis		
Increased risk of hypertension		
Prothrombotic state		
Decreased sweating and thermoregulation		
Changes in memory, processing speed, and attention		
Kidney stones	Primary hyperparathyroidism	Serum calcium level
Excessive urination		Urinary calcium
Abdominal pain		PTH
Bone and joint pain		1,25OH D3
Nausea, vomiting, or loss of appetite		Bone mineral density
Hypercalcemia or high-normal serum calcium levels		Technetium sestamibi scanning
Hypertension		

ACTH, Adrenocorticotrophic hormone; *IGF*, insulin-like growth factor; *PPGL*, pheochromocytoma and paraganglioma; *PTH*, parathyroid hormone *TSH*, thyroid stimulating hormone.

or excess can improve the cardiovascular outcome (Table 96.4). The fact that a variety of naturally occurring hormones have such profound effects on the heart and cardiovascular system also suggests that these actions can be harnessed to treat a variety of cardiovascular diseases. The ability of thyroid hormone to lower cholesterol levels, enhance cardiac contractility (especially diastolic function) via novel transcription-based mechanisms, and at the same time lower systemic vascular resistance provides a platform for developing novel therapies. In addition, the recognition that GH and serum T_3 levels alter in the setting of various forms of cardiac disease and heart failure can provide new biomarkers for assessing novel treatment strategies.

REFERENCES

For references to the older literature, please see the 11th edition of *Braunwald's Heart Disease*..

PITUITARY FUNCTION AND CARDIOVASCULAR DISEASE

Adrenal Function and Cardiovascular Disease

1. Melmed S. Pituitary-tumor endocrinopathies. *N Engl J Med*. 2020;382:937.
2. Higashi Y, Gautam S, Delafontaine P, Sukhanov S. IGF-1 and cardiovascular disease growth. *Horm IGF Res*. 2019;45(6).
3. Isgaard J, Arcopinto M, Karason K, Cittadini A. GH and the cardiovascular system: an update on a topic at heart. *Endocrine*. 2015;48:25.
4. Gadelha MR, Kasuki L, Lim DST, Fleseriu M. Systemic complications of acromegaly and the Impact of the current treatment Landscape: an update. *Endocr Rev*. 2019;40:268.
5. Ramos-Leví AM. Marazuela M Cardiovascular comorbidities in acromegaly: an update on their diagnosis and management. *Endocrine*. 2017;55:346.
6. Katznelson L, Laws Jr ER, Melmed S, et al. Acromegaly: an endocrine society clinical practice guideline. Endocrine Society. *J Clin Endocrinol Metab*. 2014;99:3933.
7. Sharma AN, Tan M, Amsterdam EA, Singh GD. Acromegalic cardiomyopathy: epidemiology, diagnosis, and management. *Clin Cardiol*. 2018;41:419.
8. Dural M, Kabakci G, Cinar N, et al. Assessment of cardiac autonomic functions by heart rate recovery, heart rate variability and QT dynamicity parameters in patients with acromegaly. *Pituitary*. 2014;17:163.
9. Bolfi F, Neves AF, Boguszewski CL. Nogueira N Mortality in acromegaly decreased in the last decade: a systematic review and meta-analysis. *Eur J Endocrinol*. 2018;179:59.
10. Ritvonen E, Loyttyniemi E, Jaatinen P, et al. Mortality in acromegaly: a 20-year follow-up study. *Endocr-Relat Cancer*. 2016;23:469.
11. Melmed S, Bronstein MD. Chanson P Consensus Statement on acromegaly therapeutic outcomes. *Nat Rev Endocrinol*. 2018;14:552.
12. Capalbo D, Barbieri F, Improda N, et al. Growth hormone improves cardiopulmonary capacity and body composition in children with growth hormone deficiency. *J Clin Endocrinol Metab*. 2017;102:4080.
13. Thomas JD, Dattani A, Zemrak F, et al. Characterisation of myocardial structure and function in adult-onset growth hormone deficiency using cardiac magnetic resonance. *Endocrine*. 2016;54(3):778e87.
14. Jasim S, Alahdab F, Ahmed AT, et al. Mortality in adults with hypopituitarism: a systematic review and meta-analysis. *Endocrine*. 2016;56:33.
15. Cittadini A, Marra AM, Arcopinto M, et al. Growth hormone replacement delays the progression of chronic heart failure combined with growth hormone deficiency: an extension of a randomized controlled single-blind study. *JACC Heart Fail1*. 2013;325.
16. Arcopinto M, Salzano A, Giallauria F, et al. Growth hormone deficiency is associated with worse cardiac function, physical performance, and outcome in chronic heart failure: insights from the T.O.S.CA. GHD study. *PloS One*. 2017;12(1):e0170058.
17. Lopez Vicchi F, Luque GM, Brie B, et al. Dopaminergic drugs in type 2 diabetes and glucose homeostasis. *Pharmacol Res*. 2016;109:74.
18. Kate E, Therkelsen BA, Tobin M, et al. Association between prolactin and incidence of cardiovascular risk factors in the framingham heart study. *J Am Heart Assoc*. 2016;5:e002640.
19. Stiles CE, Tetteh-Wayoe ET, Bestwick J, et al. A meta-analysis of the prevalence of cardiac valvulopathy in hyperprolactinemic patients treated with Cabergoline. *J Clin Endocrinol Metab*. 2018.

Adrenal Function and Cardiovascular Disease

20. Lacroix A, Feelders RA, Stratakis CA, Nieman LK. Cushing's syndrome. *Lancet*. 2015;386:913.
21. Kamenický P, Redheuil A, Roux C, et al. Cardiac structure and function in cushing's syndrome: a cardiac magnetic resonance imaging study. *J Clin Endocrinol Metab*. 2014;99:E2144.
22. Isidori AM, Graziadio C, Paragliola RM, et al. ABC Study Group. The hypertension of Cushing's syndrome: controversies in the pathophysiology and focus on cardiovascular complications. *J Hypertens*. 2015;33:44.
23. Javanmard P, Duan D, Geer EB. Mortality in patients with endogenous cushing's syndrome. *Endocrinol Metab Clin North Am*. 2018;47:313.
24. van Haalen FM, Broersen LH, Jorgensen JO, et al. Management of endocrine disease: mortality remains increased in Cushing's disease despite biochemical remission: a systematic review and meta-analysis. *Eur J Endocrinol*. 2015;172:R143.
25. Clayton RN, Jones PW, Reulen RC, et al. Mortality in patients with Cushing's disease more than 10 years after remission: a multicentre, multinational, retrospective cohort study. *Lancet Diabetes Endocrinol*. 2016;4:569.
26. Di Dalmazi G, Pasquali R. Adrenal adenomas, subclinical hypercortisolism, and cardiovascular outcomes. *Curr Opin Endocrinol Diabetes Obes*. 2015;22:163.
27. Nieman LK, Biller BM, Findling JW, et al. Treatment of cushing's syndrome: an endocrine society clinical practice guideline. *J Clin Endocrinol Metab*. 2015;100:2807.
28. Funder JW, Carey RM, Mantero F, et al. The management of primary aldosteronism: case detection, diagnosis, and treatment: an endocrine society clinical practice guideline. *J Clin Endocrinol Metab*. 2016;101:1889.
29. Vaidya A, Mulatero P, Baudrand R, Adler GL. The expanding spectrum of primary aldosteronism: implications for diagnosis, pathogenesis, and treatment. *Endocr Rev*. 2018;39:1057.
30. Monticone S, Burrello J, Tizzani D, et al. Prevalence and clinical manifestations of primary aldosteronism encountered in primary care practice. *J Am Coll Cardiol*. 2017;69:1811.
31. Byrd JB, Turcu AF, Auchus RJ. Primary aldosteronism. Practical approach to diagnosis and management. *Circulation*. 2018;138:823–835.
32. Rehan M, Raizman JE, Cavalier E, et al. Laboratory challenges in primary aldosteronism screening and diagnosis. *Clin Biochem*. 2015;48:377.
33. Monticone S, D'Ascenzo F, Moretti C, et al. Cardiovascular events and target organ damage in primary aldosteronism compared with essential hypertension: a systematic review and meta-analysis. *Lancet Diabetes Endocrinol*. 2018;6:41.
34. Huang WC, Chen YY, Lin YH, et al. TAIPAI study group incidental congestive heart failure in patients with aldosterone-producing adenomas. *J Am Heart Assoc*. 2019;8(24):e012410. 17.
35. Satoh F, Morimoto R, Ono Y, et al. Peripheral plasma 18-oxocortisol can discriminate unilateral adenoma from bilateral diseases in primary aldosteronism patients. *Hypertension*. 2015;65:1096.
36. Williams TA, Peitzsch M, Dietz AS, et al. Genotype-specific steroid profiles associated with aldosterone- producing adenomas. *Hypertension*. 2016;67:139.
37. Hundemer GL, Curhan GC, Yozamp N, et al. Cardiometabolic outcomes and mortality in medically treated primary aldosteronism: a retrospective cohort study. *Lancet Diabetes Endocrinol*. 2018;6:51.
38. Charmandari E, Nicolaides NC, Chrousos GP. Adrenal insufficiency. *Lancet*. 2014;383:2152.
39. Bornstein SR, Allolio B, Arlt W, et al. Diagnosis and treatment of primary adrenal insufficiency: an endocrine society clinical practice guideline. *J Clin Endocrinol Metab*. 2016;101:364.

Pheochromocytoma and Paraganglioma

40. Crona J, Taïeb D, Pacak K. New perspectives on pheochromocytoma and paraganglioma: toward a molecular classification. *Endocr Rev*. 2017;38:489.
41. Lenders JW, Duh QY, Eisenhofer G, et al. Pheochromocytoma and paraganglioma: an endocrine society clinical practice guideline. *J Clin Endocrinol Metab*. 2014;99:1915.
42. Lam AK. Update on adrenal tumours in 2017 World Health Organization (WHO) of endocrine tumours. *Endocr Pathol*. 2017.
43. Martucci VL, Pacak K. Pheochromocytoma and paraganglioma: diagnosis, genetics, management, and treatment. *Curr Probl Cancer*. 2014;38(7).
44. Tufton N, Ghelani R, Srirangalingam U, et al. SDHA mutated paragangliomas may be at high risk of metastasis. *Endocr Relat Cancer*. 2017;24:L43.
45. Bausch B, Schiavi F, Ni Y, et al. European-American-Asian Pheochromocytoma-Paraganglioma Registry Study Group. Clinical characterization of the pheochromocytoma and paraganglioma susceptibility genes SDHA, TMEM127, MAX, and SDHAF2 for gene-informed prevention. *JAMA Oncol*. 2017;3:1204.
46. Toledo RA, Burnichon N, Cascon A, et al. Consensus Statement on next-generation-sequencing-based diagnostic testing of hereditary phaeochromocytomas and paragangliomas. *Nat Rev Endocrinol*. 2017;3:233.
47. Janssen I, Chen CC, Millo CM, et al. PET/CT comparing (68)Ga-DOTATATE and other radiopharmaceuticals and in comparison with CT/MRI for the localization of sporadic metastatic pheochromocytoma and paraganglioma. *Eur J Nucl Med Mol Imaging*. 2016;43:1784.

Parathyroid Function, Calcium Metabolism, and Cardiovascular Disease

48. Bilezikian JP, Brandi ML, Eastell R, et al. Guidelines for the management of asymptomatic primary hyperparathyroidism: summary statement from the Fourth International Workshop. *J Clin Endocrinol Metab*. 2014;99:3561.
49. Yao L, Folsom AR, Pankow JS, et al. Parathyroid hormone and the risk of incident hypertension: the Atherosclerosis Risk in Communities study. *J Hypertens*. 2016;34:196.
50. McMahon D, Carrelli A, Palmeri N, et al. Effect of parathyroidectomy upon left ventricular mass in primary hyperparathyroidism: a meta-analysis. *J Clin Endocrinol Metab*. 2015;100:4399.
51. Chen G, Xue Y, Zhang Q, Wen, et al. Is normocalcemic primary hyperparathyroidism harmful or harmless? *J Clin Endocrinol Metab*. 2015;100:2420.
52. Pepe J, Cipriani C, Sonato C, et al. Cardiovascular manifestations of primary hyperparathyroidism: a narrative review. *Eur J Endocrinol*. 2017;77(6):R297–R308.
53. Bollerslev J, Rejnmark L, Marcocci C. European society of endocrinology clinical guideline: treatment of chronic hypoparathyroidism in adults. *Eur J Endocrinol*. 2015;173:G1–G20.

Thyroid Involvement in Cardiovascular Disease

54. Razvi S, Jabbar A, Pingitore A, et al. Thyroid hormones and cardiovascular function and diseases. *J Am Coll Cardiol*. 2018;71:1781.
55. Cappola AR, Desai AS, Medici M. Thyroid and cardiovascular disease research agenda for enhancing knowledge, prevention, and treatment. *Thyroid*. 2019;29:760.
56. Medici M, Visser WE, Visser TJ, Peeters RP. Genetic determination of the hypothalamic–pituitary–thyroid axis: where do we stand? *Endocr Rev*. 2015;36:214.
57. Bianco AC, Dumitrescu A, Gereben B, et al. Paradigms of dynamic control of thyroid hormone signaling. *Endocr Rev*. 2019;40:1000.
58. de Vries EM, Fliers E. Boelen A. The molecular basis of the non-thyroidal illness syndrome. *J Endocrinol*. 2015;225:R67–R81.
59. Danzi S, Klein I. Thyroid disease and the cardiovascular system. *Endocrinol Metab Clin North Am*. 2014;43:517.
60. Groeneweg S, van Geest FS, Peeters RP, et al. Thyroid hormone transporters. *Endocr Rev*. 2020;41(1).
61. Felmlee MA, Jones RS, Rodriguez-Cruz V, et al. Monocarboxylate transporters (SLC16): function, regulation, and role in health and disease. *Pharmacol Rev*. 2020;72(2):466.
62. Jabbar A, Pingitore A, Pearce SH, et al. Thyroid hormones and cardiovascular disease. *Nat Rev Cardiol*. 2017;14:39.
63. Wan W, Xu X, Zhao W, et al. Exercise training induced myosin heavy chain Isoform alteration in the infarcted heart. *Appl Physiol Nutr Metab*. 2014;39(2):226.
64. Biondi B. The management of thyroid abnormalities in chronic heart failure. *Heart Fail Clin*. 2019;15:393.
65. Davis PJ, Goglia F, Leonard JL. Nongenomic actions of thyroid hormone. *Nat Rev Endocrinol*. 2016;12:111.
66. Gluvic ZM, Obradovic MM, Sudar-Milovanovicc EM, et al. Regulation of nitric oxide production in hypothyroidism. *Biomed Pharmacother*. 2020;124:109881.
67. Biondi B, Cooper DS. Subclinical hyperthyroidism. *N Engl J Med*. 2018;378:2411.
68. Biondi B, Bartalena L, Cooper DS, et al. The 2015 European thyroid association guidelines on diagnosis and treatment of endogenous subclinical hyperthyroidism. *Eur Thyroid J*. 2015;4:149
69. Burch HB, Cooper DS. Management of Graves disease a review. *J Am Med Assoc*. 2015;314:2544.
70. Biondi B, Kahaly G. In: Luster M, Duntas L, Wartofsly L, eds. *Heart in Hyperthyroidism. The Thyroid and its Diseases. A Comprensive Guide for Clinicians*. Springer; 2019:367–375.
71. Selmer C, Olesen JB, Hansen ML, et al. Subclinical and overt thyroid dysfunction and risk of all-cause mortality and cardiovascular events: a large population study. *J Clin Endocrinol Metab*. 2014;99:2372.
72. Floriani C, Gencer B, Collet TH. Rodondi N Subclinical thyroid dysfunction and cardiovascular diseases: 2016 update. *Eur Heart J*. 2018;14:503.
73. Biondi B. Atrial fibrillation and hyperthyroidism. In: Lüscher TF, Camm AJ, Maurer G, Serruys PW, eds. *ESC Textbook of Cardiovascular Medicine*. 3rd ed. European Society of Cardiology.
74. Chaker L, Heeringa J, Dehghan A, et al. Normal thyroid function and the risk of atrial fibrillation: the Rotterdam Study. *J Clin Endocrinol Metab*. 2015;100:3718.
75. Baumgartner C, da Costa BR, Collet TH, et al. Thyroid studies collaboration. Thyroid function within the normal range, subclinical hypothyroidism, and the risk of atrial fibrillation. *Circulation. 8*. 2017;136(22):2100.
76. Biondi B. Impact of hyperthyroidism on the cardiovascular and musculoskeletal systems and management of subclinical Graves' disease. In Graves' disease: a comprehensive guide for clinicians. Editor R. Bahn Springer (New York). Editor R. Bahn Springer (New York) pages 133-146 ISBN 9781493925339.

77. Page RL, Joglar JA, Caldwell MA, et al. Evidence review committee chair 2015 ACC/AHA/HRS guideline for the management of adult patients with supraventricular tachycardia: a report of the American college of cardiology/American heart association task force onclinical practice guidelines and the heart rhythm society. *Circulation*. 2016;13(134):e232.
78. Al-Khatib SM, Arshad A, Balk EM, et al. Risk stratification for arrhythmic events in patients with asymptomatic pre-excitation: a systematic review for the 2015 ACC/AHA/HRS guideline for the management of adult patients with supraventricular tachycardia: a report of the American College of Cardiology/American Heart Association Task Force on clinical practice guidelines and the Heart Rhythm Society. *J Am Coll Cardiol*. 2016;67:1624–1638.
79. January CT, Wann LS, Alpert JS, et al. ACC/AHA task force member 2014. AHA/ACC/HRS guideline for the management of patients with atrial fibrillation: a report of the American college of cardiology/American heart association task force on practice guidelines and the heart rhythm society. *Circulation*. 2014;130. e199–267.
80. Bano A, Chaker L, Mattace-Raso FUS, et al. Thyroid function and the risk of atherosclerotic cardiovascular morbidity and mortality: the Rotterdam Study. *Circ Res*. 2017;121:1392.
81. De Leo S, Lee SY, Braverman LE. Hyperthyroidism. *Lancet*. 2016;388:906.
82. Biondi B, Cooper DS. Thyroid hormone suppression therapy. *Endocrinol Metab Clin North Am*. 2019;48(1):227.
83. Satoh T, Isozaki O, Suzuki A, et al. 2016 guidelines for the management of thyroid storm from the Japan thyroid association and Japan endocrine society (first edition). *Endocr J*. 2016;63:1025.
84. Biondi B, Cappola AR, Cooper DS. Subclinical hypothyroidism: a review. *J Am Med Assoc*. 2019;9(2):153. 322.
85. Peeters RP. Subclinical hypothyroidism. *N Engl J Med*. 2017;376(26):2556.
86. Biondi B , Duntas. Heart in hypothyroidism. The thyroid and its diseases. In: Luster M , Duntas L, Wartofsly L, eds. *A Comprensive Guide for Clinicians*. Springer pp 255-263, 2019.
87. Klein I, Danzi S. Thyroid disease and the heart. *Curr Probl Cardiol*. 2016;41:65.
88. del Busto-Mesa A, Cabrera-Rego JO, Carrero-Fernández L, et al. Changes in arterial stiffness, carotid intima-media thickness, and epicardial fat after L-thyroxine replacement therapy in hypothyroidism. *Endocrinol Nutr*. 2015;62:270.
89. Aziz M, Kandimalla Y, Machavarapu A, et al. Effect of thyroxin treatment on carotid intima-media thickness (CIMT) reduction in patients with subclinical hypothyroidism (sch): a meta-analysis of clinical trials. *J Atheroscler Thromb*. 2017;24:643.
90. Chen S, Shauer A, Zwas DR, et al. The effect of thyroid function on clinical outcome in patients with heart failure. *Eur J Heart Fail*. 2014;16(2):217.
91. Ning N, Gao D, Triggiani V, et al. Prognostic role of hypothyroidism in heart failure a meta-analysis. *Medicine (Baltim)*. 2015;94(30):e1159.
92. Yang G, Wang Y, Ma A, Wang T. Subclinical thyroid dysfunction is associated with adverse prognosis in heart failure patients with reduced ejection fraction. *BMC Cardiovasc Disord*. 2019;19:83.
93. Kong LY, Gao X, Ding XY, et al. Left ventricular end-diastolic strain rate recovered in hypothyroidism following levothyroxine replacement therapy: a strain rate imaging study. *Echocardiography*. 2019;36:707.
94. Sinha RA, Singh BK, Yen PM. Direct effects of thyroid hormones on hepatic lipid metabolism. *Nat Rev Endocrinol*. 2018;14:259.
95. Olsson AG, Chester Ridgway E, Ladenson PW. Reductions in serum levels of LDL cholesterol, apolipoprotein B, triglycerides and lipoprotein(a) in hypercholesterolaemic patients treated with the liver-selective thyroid hormone receptor agonist eprotirome. *J Intern Med*. 2015;277:331.
96. Biondi B, Cooper DS. Thyroid hormone therapy for hypothyroidism. *Endocrine*. 2019;66(1):18.
97. Jonklaas J, Bianco AC, Bauer AJ, et al. American thyroid association task force on thyroid hormone replacement guidelines for the treatment of hypothyroidism: prepared by the American thyroid association task force on thyroid hormone replacement. *Thyroid*. 2014;24:1670.
98. Rizzo LFL, Mana DL, Bruno OD, Wartofsky L. Myxedema coma. *Medicina (B Aires)*. 2017;4(77):321.
99. Bartalena L, Bogazzi F, Chiovato L, et al. 2018 European Thyroid Association (ETA) guidelines for the management of amiodarone-associated thyroid dysfunction. *Eur Thyroid J*. 2018;7(55).
100. Fliers E, Bianco AC, Langouche L, Boelen A. Thyroid function in critically ill patients. *Lancet Diabetes Endocrinol*. 2015;3:816.
101. Rothberger GD, Gadhvi S, Michelakis N, Kumar A, et al. Usefulness of serum triiodothyronine (T3) to predict outcomes in patients hospitalized with acute heart failure. *Am J Cardiol*. 2017;119:599.
102. Vale C, Neves JS, von Hafe M, et al. The role of thyroid hormones in heart failure. *Cardiovasc Drugs Ther*. 2019;33:179–188.
103. Chang CY, Chien YJ, Lin PC, et al. Non-thyroidal illness syndrome and hypothyroidism in ischemic heart disease population: systematic review and meta-analysis. *J Clin Endocrinol Metab*. 2020.
104. Pingitore A, Mastorci F, Piaggi P, et al. Usefulness of triiodothyronine replacement therapy in patients with ST elevation myocardial infarction and borderline/reduced triiodothyronine levels (from the THIRST study). *Am J Cardiol*. 2019;123:905.

97 Rheumatic Diseases and the Cardiovascular System

JUSTIN C. MASON

ATHEROSCLEROSIS AND THE RHEUMATIC DISEASES, 1809
- Endothelial Dysfunction and Vascular Injury, 1809
- Rheumatoid Arthritis, 1810
- Systemic Lupus Erythematosus, 1810

VASCULITIDES, 1812
- Large-Vessel Vasculitis, 1812
- Medium-Vessel Vasculitis, 1816

PERICARDITIS AND MYOCARDITIS, 1818
- Pericarditis, 1818
- Myocarditis, 1819

VALVULAR HEART DISEASE, 1820
- Systemic Lupus Erythematosus, 1820
- Seronegative Spondyloarthropathies, 1821
- Rheumatoid Arthritis, 1821

Takayasu Arteritis, 1821

CARDIAC CONDUCTION DISTURBANCES, 1821
- Systemic Lupus Erythematosus and Sjögren Syndrome, 1821
- Systemic Sclerosis, 1821
- Spondyloarthropathies, 1821
- Rheumatoid Arthritis, 1821

PULMONARY ARTERIAL HYPERTENSION, 1821
- Systemic Sclerosis, 1822
- Systemic Lupus Erythematosus, 1822
- Rheumatoid Arthritis, 1823
- Sjögren Syndrome, 1823
- Takayasu Arteritis, 1823

THROMBOSIS IN THE RHEUMATIC DISEASES, 1823

Antiphospholipid Syndrome, 1824
Behçet Disease, 1824

ANTIRHEUMATIC DRUGS AND CARDIOVASCULAR DISEASE, 1824
- Relationship Between Drug Treatment and Cardiovascular Disease, 1824
- B Cell Depletion, 1825
- Methotrexate, 1826
- Other Disease-Modifying Antirheumatic Drugs, 1826
- Glucocorticoids, 1826
- Statins, 1826
- Nonsteroidal Antiinflammatory Drugs, 1826

FUTURE PERSPECTIVES, 1827

REFERENCES, 1827

The relationship between inflammatory rheumatic diseases and the cardiovascular system has long been recognized. As the treatment of these diseases has improved considerably over the last 30 years and increased survival, the importance and complexity of this interrelationship have achieved prominence. Indeed, we have entered an era in which established anti-rheumatic therapies are being trialed for the treatment of atherosclerosis.[1,2] Patients with multisystem rheumatic diseases may, on occasion, present initially to a cardiovascular physician or surgeon, and early recognition of the immune-mediated basis of the cardiovascular disease reduces morbidity and mortality. The vasculature may represent a primary target organ of the underlying rheumatic disease and can be affected at numerous sites and at micro- and macrovascular levels. Systemic sclerosis (SSc) impacts the microvessels and may be responsible for pulmonary arterial vasculopathy and pulmonary artery hypertension (PAH). Antineutrophil cytoplasmic antibody (ANCA)-associated systemic vasculitides (AASVs) affect arterioles preferentially, while the large-vessel vasculitides affect the aorta and its major branches. Antiphospholipid syndrome (APS) causes both venous and arterial thromboses. Cardiac complications influence morbidity and mortality and in systemic lupus erythematosus (SLE) include coronary arteritis, pericarditis, myocarditis, and valvular heart disease. Renal artery stenosis leading to uncontrolled hypertension is a feature of Takayasu arteritis (TA), and occlusive lesions in the subclavian, axillary, or iliac arteries may lead to limb claudication in patients with TA and giant cell arteritis (GCA). Inflammatory rheumatic diseases have equally important secondary effects on the cardiovascular system. Chronic systemic inflammation predisposes to endothelial dysfunction and increased arterial stiffness, thereby escalating the risk of cardiovascular events. Cardiovascular specialists increasingly recognize the significantly increased prevalence of cardiac dysrhythmias, premature myocardial infarction and stroke in patients suffering from rheumatoid arthritis (RA) and SLE.[3] Many outstanding clinical challenges remain; predominant among them are the development and rigorous evaluation of preventive strategies, early recognition, diagnosis and treatment of patients with rheumatic disease who have the highest risk for cardiovascular complications, alongside improved understanding of the underlying molecular mechanisms.

ATHEROSCLEROSIS AND THE RHEUMATIC DISEASES

Recognition of the role of inflammation in atherosclerosis has highlighted and stimulated study of the potential relationship between systemic inflammatory diseases and premature atherogenesis. This effort has substantially advanced our understanding of the epidemiology and underlying pathogenic mechanisms, revealing novel therapeutic targets. Current priorities include identification of patients most at risk and the development of preventive therapeutic strategies.[4,5] Evidence supporting an association between inflammatory diseases and premature cardiovascular events is best developed for RA and SLE. In addition, ankylosing spondylitis, psoriatic arthritis, AASV, TA, and APS may all associate with premature atherosclerosis. Cardiovascular specialists should consider an underlying inflammatory disease in young patients with otherwise unexplained angina, myocardial infarction, or stroke. Patients with a rheumatic disease who suffer a myocardial infarction have worse outcomes in terms of both heart failure and mortality than the age-matched general population.[3]

Endothelial Dysfunction and Vascular Injury

Homeostatic mechanisms promote a quiescent, antithrombotic, antiadhesive vascular endothelium and control vasodilation and permeability (see Chapters 24 and 36). Prolonged systemic inflammation such as that seen in RA and SLE may promote endothelial injury, increased endothelial apoptosis, and endothelial vasodilator dysfunction.

Traditional risk factors alone do not explain the increased burden of atherosclerosis, but inflammation may exacerbate the effects of classic risk factors.[6] When compared with the general population, patients with systemic inflammatory diseases more commonly exhibit endothelial dysfunction and increased aortic stiffness. Although the results of individual studies vary, effective treatment of the underlying inflammation may not always reverse the endothelial dysfunction or improve the aortic stiffness.[3,6,7] As plaque burden may not increase in rheumatologic diseases, systemic inflammatory environment may promote qualitative changes in plaques that predispose to plaque rupture, a conjecture supported by autopsy studies. Thus, both accelerated atherogenesis and higher-risk plaque may contribute to the observed increased incidence of premature cardiovascular events.[6,8]

Various molecular mechanisms mediate the increased risk for atherosclerotic disease and cardiovascular events. In addition to traditional cardiovascular risk factors, disease-related factors may include effects of the proinflammatory cytokines tumor necrosis factor-alpha (TNF-α), interleukin-1 (IL-1), interferon (IFN)-α, and IL-6 on endothelial activation, leukocyte adhesion, endothelial injury, and permeability. Chronic activation of toll-like receptor signaling, increased endothelial cell apoptosis and diminished capacity for repair may contribute. Autoantibodies (e.g., antiphospholipid antibodies), $CD4^+CD28^-$ cytotoxic T cells, $Th17/T_{REG}$ imbalance, complement deficiency or excessive activation, genetic polymorphisms, and the deleterious effects of drugs, including corticosteroids and cyclosporine, are important.[3,6,8] The potential role for clonal hematopoiesis caused by somatic mutations in bone marrow stem cells also merits further investigation in autoimmune rheumatic disease (see also Chapter 24).[9]

Rheumatoid Arthritis

RA, an autoimmune, symmetric inflammatory polyarthritis with a female-to-male ratio of 3:1, affects up to 1% of the population in the Western world, with the onset of symptoms most commonly occurring between 30 and 50 years of age. Up to 80% of patients have a positive serum rheumatoid factor and/or anti–cyclic citrullinated peptide (CCP) antibodies. A systemic inflammatory response is evident, with low-grade fever, weight loss, raised erythrocyte sedimentation rate (ESR) and C-reactive protein (CRP), hypoalbuminemia, normochromic normocytic anemia, and thrombocytosis.

Atherosclerotic Disease in Rheumatoid Arthritis

A variety of studies have shown subclinical arterial disease with increased carotid intimal-media thickness (IMT) and early plaque development. Although RA independently raises the risk for atherosclerosis, the precise mechanistic relationship between RA and atherogenesis remains unknown. Similarly, the mechanisms and long-term outcomes of abnormalities in myocardial perfusion and coronary flow reserve in patients with RA and nonstenotic epicardial arteries remain to be established.[10] The initial abnormalities in vascular function may occur at or before the onset of RA symptoms.[11] The direct effect of chronic inflammation on vascular endothelium may itself promote atherogenesis, in addition to exacerbating the actions of traditional cardiovascular risk factors.[8,12] Moreover, the systemic inflammatory environment might contribute to the features of plaque and blood that promote cardiovascular events in patients with RA.[13]

Patients with RA have increased classic risk factors for atherosclerosis. Tobacco smoking associates with both cardiovascular risk and the development of RA. Similarly, insulin resistance and the metabolic syndrome are more common in RA. Patients with RA may have a dyslipidemia characterized by high triglyceride levels and low levels of high-density lipoprotein (HDL) and low-density lipoprotein (LDL) cholesterol.[14,15] The risk for myocardial infarction in patients with RA is considered similar to diabetes mellitus, and women with RA are twice as likely as age-matched controls in the general population to suffer myocardial infarction. Although death rates from both heart attack and stroke are comparable to that in the general population, events occur at an earlier age, with 50% of premature deaths in patients with RA being a direct consequence of cardiovascular disease. The excess mortality becomes apparent 7 to 10 years after diagnosis and associates with persistent disease activity and the presence of rheumatoid factor and anti-CCP antibodies. A recent review suggests that patients with RA who suffer a myocardial infarction have worse outcomes.[16] However, this situation is changing, reflecting improved recognition of excess risk.[17]

TREATMENT
Drug therapy for RA has evolved remarkably over the past 25 years, with the focus on biologic therapies and aggressive management of early disease. Clinical trials have demonstrated that this approach reduces symptoms and structural damage to joints. Increasing evidence suggests treatment to target to control synovitis also confers vascular protection.[3,18]

Methotrexate has become the most widely used disease-modifying antirheumatic drug (DMARD), and since its introduction, mortality from myocardial infarction in patients with RA has improved. Sulfasalazine and hydroxychloroquine may confer similar benefit. Patients who do not respond adequately to DMARD therapy should switch to biologic therapies. These include those targeting TNF-α (infliximab, adalimumab, etanercept, certolizumab, and golimumab), the IL-6 receptor (tocilizumab, sarilumab), CTLA4Ig (abatacept), and the B cell–depleting monoclonal antibody rituximab, alongside oral small molecules targeting the Janus kinases (JAK) (baricitinib, tofacitinib, upadacitinib, ruxolitinib).[19,20] An aggressive disease-modifying approach minimizes the use of nonsteroidal antiinflammatory drugs (NSAIDs) and the requirement for corticosteroid therapy. Glucocorticoids may worsen traditional risk factors including insulin resistance, hypertension, and lipid profiles and may hasten carotid plaque formation in RA.[12] Because NSAIDs and cyclooxygenase-2 (COX-2)-selective NSAIDs (coxibs), although effective, may elevate blood pressure and increase the frequency of thrombotic cardiovascular events, their use in patients with cardiovascular complications of inflammatory disease requires caution.[21] However, evidence suggests that NSAID use in patients with RA does not confer an increased risk for cardiovascular events, thus indicating that their anti-inflammatory effects predominate.

Definitive demonstration of the potential cardiovascular benefits of the biologic therapies requires the results of long-term prospective studies (see later). TNF-α promotes vascular endothelial activation and dysfunction and may lead to plaque destabilization, and hence blockade would appear to be an attractive therapeutic option. Infliximab therapy may improve endothelial function as measured by flow-mediated dilation 4 to 12 weeks after infusion, whereas etanercept has been reported to reduce aortic stiffness. Analysis of carotid IMT suggests that TNF-α antagonists reduce systemic inflammation and retard progression of IMT.[12] Tight therapeutic control of RA disease activity per se appears to have a beneficial effect on the risk for myocardial infarction.[18] Treatment of the arthritis must be combined with a careful review of classic risk factors, with appropriate steps taken to modify them. Despite this, too few patients are routinely assessed for cardiovascular risk.[22] Although we lack rigorous trials, most rheumatologists have a low threshold for addition of a statin.[23] Meanwhile, debate continues concerning the pros and cons of disease-specific cardiovascular risk calculators.[22] New guidelines have reviewed such issues.[14]

Systemic Lupus Erythematosus

SLE, a systemic autoimmune disease, predominates in women at a ratio of 9:1 and affects all racial groups but more commonly those of Afro-Caribbean, Asian, and Chinese extraction. Initial constitutional symptoms include night sweats, lethargy, malaise, and weight loss. Mucocutaneous features including the classic butterfly facial rash, oral ulcers, and alopecia are frequent. Serositis, myalgia, arthralgia, and Jaccoud nonerosive arthropathy also occur. Potentially life-threatening complications include glomerulonephritis with renal failure, central nervous system (CNS) involvement with cerebral vasculitis, pneumonitis, shrinking lung syndrome, and PAH. Hematologic involvement includes lymphopenia in most and frequently hemolytic anemia, neutropenia, and thrombocytopenia. Cardiac manifestations of SLE include pericarditis, myocarditis, endocarditis, aortitis, and coronary arteritis. Understanding of the pathogenesis of SLE continues to improve. A defect in apoptotic cell clearance results in the exposure of nuclear antigens to an immune system with hyperreactive B cells. Loss of immune tolerance results in the generation of autoantibodies and immune complexes. Deposition of immune complexes in target organs leads to the activation of complement and tissue injury.[24]

Most patients have high-titer antinuclear antibodies and antibodies against double-stranded DNA (dsDNA). The latter are more specific for the diagnosis of SLE, which is reinforced by the presence of antibodies against one or more nuclear antigens, including Sm, Ro, La, and ribonucleoprotein (RNP). Complement activation and consumption of C3 and C4 leading to reduced plasma levels characterize active disease. The ESR also rises in active disease, while CRP levels typically remain normal except in those with serositis or secondary infection.

Atherosclerotic Disease in Systemic Lupus Erythematosus

The increased risk for myocardial infarction and stroke in patients with SLE is somewhere between 2-fold and 10-fold and up to 50-fold greater than that in the general population. The young age of patients with SLE and cardiovascular disease (67% of female patients with SLE and a first cardiac event are less than 55 years of age) suggests that SLE accelerates arterial disease.[25,26] A study of 1874 cases (9485 person-years follow-up) revealed a 2.66-fold increase in the risk of myocardial infarction, stroke and coronary intervention when compared with the general population. Although the pattern and extent of coronary artery disease in SLE does not appear to differ (Fig. 97.1), the plaques may be more vulnerable to rupture. Patients with SLE have worse outcomes following myocardial infarction than the age-matched general population, with a higher risk for the development of cardiac failure and increased mortality.[8] This difference may result from late diagnosis of ischemic heart disease and a reluctance to treat aggressively.

Hypertension is common in SLE because of renal disease and the widespread use of glucocorticoids. Similarly, patients with SLE commonly have metabolic syndrome, which associates with renal impairment, higher corticosteroid doses, and Korean or Hispanic ethnicity. Patients with SLE also have lipid abnormalities, including high levels of very low-density lipoprotein (VLDL) and triglycerides, elevated or normal LDL cholesterol, reduced HDL cholesterol and impaired cholesterol efflux.[26]

TREATMENT

Mild SLE with rash and arthralgia can be treated with simple analgesics and NSAIDs, with hydroxychloroquine commonly added to minimize flares. Organ involvement, including mild renal impairment, hematologic abnormalities, myositis, arthritis, and cutaneous lesions, requires the addition of prednisone and typically an immunosuppressant such as mycophenolate mofetil (MMF), azathioprine, or methotrexate to aid in controlling the disease and to facilitate steroid sparing. Cyclophosphamide and corticosteroids remain the first-line treatment of life-threatening complications, including myocarditis, cerebritis, severe hematologic involvement, and glomerulonephritis. MMF often replaces cyclophosphamide for lupus nephritis because of its equivalent efficacy and concerns regarding the risk for permanent infertility seen in up to 50% of patients treated with cyclophosphamide.[27] Most rheumatologists and nephrologists consider rituximab an effective treatment of severe SLE, although clinical trials to date have proved disappointing. A variety of regimens have been used, including combinations of rituximab, prednisone, and cyclophosphamide.[28] Belimumab, a monoclonal antibody that binds to the soluble B lymphocyte stimulator and prevents its interaction with B cell surface receptors, has a modest disease-modifying effect in nonrenal SLE. Positive phase III trial data are emerging for belimumab in lupus nephritis, for IFN type 1 receptor antibody anifrolumab and calcineurin inhibitor voclosporin.[29]

Defining effective strategies for prevention of cardiovascular disease in patients with SLE will require long-term prospective trials with adjudicated cardiovascular endpoints. Undertreated and/or persistently active disease associates with accelerated atherogenesis. Therefore, adequate individualized immunosuppressive therapy should minimize cardiovascular complications. Hydroxychloroquine reduces LDL cholesterol and lowers mortality from cardiovascular disease in patients with SLE. Aggressive management of traditional risk factors is also advocated, including regular diligent monitoring and tight blood pressure control. Statins are widely used, particularly in patients with renal impairment. Caution and careful monitoring should be exercised in patients with active myositis, as statin therapy can exacerbate this complication. The clinical data available do not support significant protection against atherosclerosis by statins 2 to 3 years after initiation, although longer-term analysis is awaited.[26]

Atherosclerosis in Association With Other Rheumatic Diseases

The relationship between chronic inflammation and atherogenesis implies that many rheumatic diseases may be associated with premature and increased cardiovascular risk (Table 97.1). Because data in support of this hypothesis derive from relatively small studies, important current clinical challenges include the need to determine (1) which rheumatic diseases pose the greatest cardiovascular threat, (2) a means of identifying subsets of patients most at risk, and (3) evidence-based strategies to minimize cardiovascular events.

Ankylosing spondylitis, psoriatic arthritis, and gout all associate with atherosclerotic disease. Hyperuricemia independently predicts cardiovascular disease, and patients with gout often have hypertension, hyperlipidemia, obesity, and diabetes mellitus. Many drugs used for the treatment of cardiac disease, including diuretics, beta blockers, and low-dose aspirin, can increase serum uric acid levels. In contrast, losartan, angiotensin-converting enzyme (ACE) inhibitors, atorvastatin, and fenofibrate may reduce urate levels. Allopurinol may reduce the risk for congestive cardiac failure and cardiovascular-associated death, whereas an increased risk of cardiovascular death has been reported with febuxostat.[30] In addition to achieving a serum uric acid level lower than 0.36 mmol/L (6 mg/dL), patients with gout should receive dietary advice and aggressive management of cardiovascular risk factors.

Systematic review of articles on cardiovascular disease in psoriatic arthritis has revealed increased traditional risk factors, endothelial dysfunction, aortic stiffness, and subclinical atherosclerosis. The limited data available suggest that adequate suppression of inflammatory disease activity, which leads to improvement in endothelial dysfunction and carotid IMT, should be combined with regular assessment and

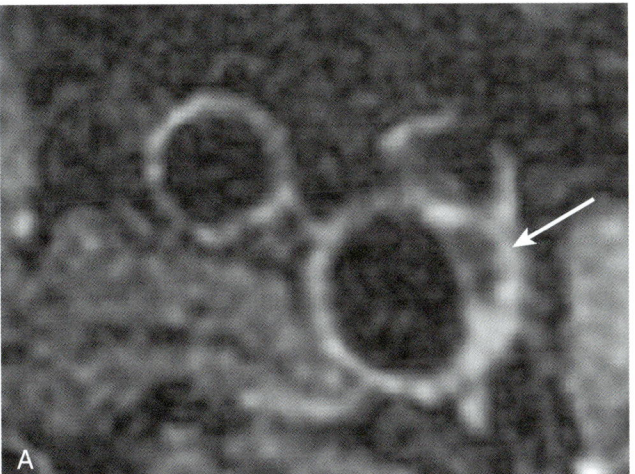 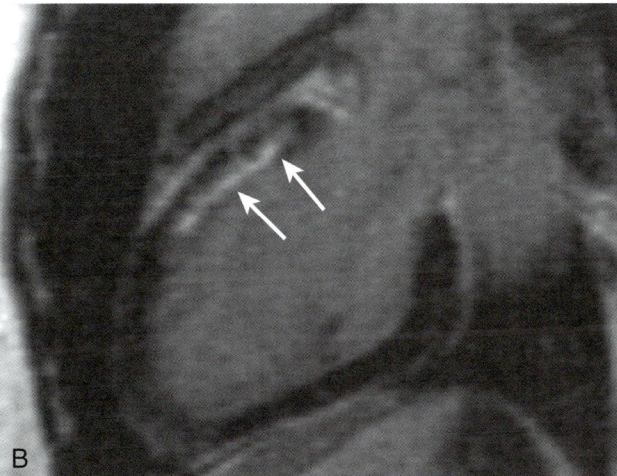

FIGURE 97.1 Atherosclerosis in systemic lupus erythematosus. **A,** Transaxial T2-weighted cardiac magnetic resonance (CMR) of the carotid bifurcation showing atherosclerotic plaque *(arrow)*. The lipid-filled core and fibrous cap can be seen along with evidence of calcification. **B,** CMR showing a two-chamber view in the late phase after gadolinium injection. Subendocardial late gadolinium enhancement is present in the anteroseptal left ventricle *(arrows)* and extends from the base of the heart to the midventricular region, consistent with a previous subendocardial myocardial infarction.

TABLE 97.1 Coronary Artery Involvement and the Rheumatic Diseases

Premature Atherosclerosis
- Systemic lupus erythematosus
- Rheumatoid arthritis
- Ankylosing spondylitis
- Psoriatic arthritis
- Gout
- Takayasu arteritis
- Giant cell arteritis

Coronary Arteritis
- Systemic lupus erythematosus
- Takayasu arteritis
- Kawasaki disease
- Churg-Strauss syndrome
- Polyarteritis nodosa
- Granulomatous polyangiitis
- Rheumatoid arthritis

control of traditional risk factors.[15,31] Patients with ankylosing spondylitis have also demonstrated impaired endothelial function, increased carotid IMT and pulse wave velocity, all of which indicate an increased risk for atherosclerosis.[31] The long-term impact of anti-TNF-α, and the pros and cons associated with increasing use of anti-IL-17 and anti-IL-12/23 therapies on the incidence of cardiovascular events in spondyloarthritides will emerge from international biologic registries.

VASCULITIDES (SEE CHAPTERS 42 AND 43)

The vasculitides, a heterogeneous group of diseases, represent a significant clinical challenge, both diagnostically and therapeutically. The primary systemic vasculitides are classified into large-, medium-, and small-vessel disease. This leaves a small group of unclassified conditions, including Behçet disease, relapsing polychondritis, primary CNS vasculitis, and Cogan syndrome.[32]

The histologic features of vasculitis include perivascular inflammatory infiltrates that may invade the arterial wall, fibrinoid necrosis, thrombosis, fibrosis, and scar formation. Fibrinoid necrosis, a specific feature of the medium- and small-vessel vasculitides, typically affects the tunica media. Complications include stenosis and occlusions resulting in organ ischemia, thrombosis, aneurysm formation, and hemorrhage. Although biopsy is optimal for making the diagnosis, suitable tissue may not always be accessible, or arterial biopsy may present unacceptable hazards, such as in patients with TA. Thus, diagnosis often depends on clinical findings, laboratory indices, and imaging.

The vasculitides have a complex, multifactorial, and poorly understood immunopathogenesis. The endothelium may be subject to complement-mediated injury as a consequence of immune complex deposition in polyarteritis nodosa (PAN) or rheumatoid vasculitis. In the medium- and small-vessel vasculitides, ANCAs may stimulate formation of neutrophil extracellular traps (NETs), which damage the endothelium. The proinflammatory cytokines TNF-α, IL-1, IL-6, and IFN-γ may activate the endothelium and induce the expression of adhesion molecules, including E-selectin, vascular cell adhesion molecule-1 (VCAM-1), and intercellular adhesion molecule-1 (ICAM-1), thereby facilitating leukocyte adhesion and recruitment into the vessel wall and surrounding tissue.

Cardiovascular disease in patients with vasculitis, although relatively rare, can be life-threatening. Aortitis, hypertension, coronary arteritis, valvular heart disease, pericarditis, myocarditis, conduction abnormalities, accelerated atherosclerosis, and cardiac failure can all occur. This section focuses on the vasculitides most likely to be encountered by cardiovascular disease specialists.

Large-Vessel Vasculitis
Giant Cell Arteritis

GCA affects large and medium-sized arteries. The disease affects those older than 50 years, with incidence increasing with age. GCA occurs most commonly in northern Europe, Scandinavia, and the United States in people of northern European ancestry. GCA typically affects extracranial branches of the aorta and, in addition to the temporal arteries, may involve the subclavian and axillary arteries, the thoracic aorta, and, on occasion, the vertebrobasilar circulation, and femoral and iliac arteries. Clinical features include fever, weight loss, malaise, headache, temporal artery thickening with loss of pulsation, scalp tenderness, and jaw claudication. The most feared complication, anterior ischemic optic neuropathy (AION), may be manifested as amaurosis fugax or sudden permanent visual loss. Up to 25% of patients present with systemic features without the classic sign of tenderness and temporal artery involvement. ^{18}F-fluorodeoxyglucose positron emission tomography (FDG-PET) has shown widespread FDG avidity throughout the aorta and subclavian and iliac arteries consistent with inflammation in more than 50% of patients.[33]

Pathogenesis
Histopathologic examination reveals localized fragmentation of the internal elastic lamina closely associated with an inflammatory infiltrate consisting predominantly of IFN-γ-producing CD4+ T lymphocytes, monocytes/macrophages, and occasional characteristic multinucleated giant cells. Activated CD83+ dendritic cells initiate the arterial wall inflammation and colocalize with activated T cells. Local synthesis of mediators such as platelet-derived growth factor leads to proliferation of smooth muscle cells and concentric stenosis of the arterial lumen (Fig. 97.2). Release of matrix metalloproteinases and generation of reactive oxygen species can result in arterial wall injury and aneurysm formation, typically involving the thoracic aorta.

Diagnosis
Biopsy is the definitive means of diagnosis and should be considered for all patients. However, the need for biopsy should not delay treatment. Temporal artery biopsy is positive in up to 80% of patients. Temporal artery ultrasound can reveal a characteristic halo sign with concentric homogeneous thickening of the arterial wall and evidence of flow disturbance and stenosis (see Fig. 97.2).[33]

Cardiovascular Complications
Although relatively rare, severe cardiovascular complications can occur and include aortic dissection and thoracic aortic aneurysms (Table 97.2).[33,34] Imaging and autopsy studies suggest that aortitis and aortic wall thickening are frequent in GCA, although their relationship with the development of aortic aneurysm remains unclear. Those with conventional cardiovascular risk factors including cigarette smoking, poorly controlled disease, and aortic regurgitation have a higher risk. Increased FDG uptake in the thoracic aorta can associate with an increased risk for aortic dilation. In the absence of guidelines, we recommend annual thoracic aortic screening for those with FDG-PET–positive thoracic aortic uptake or magnetic resonance angiography (MRA) or computed tomography angiography (CTA) evidence of aortic wall thickening and every 2 to 3 years in the remainder of patients. CTA and MRA are the optimal imaging techniques.[35] Pericarditis, coronary arteritis, limb ischemia, accelerated atherosclerosis, myocardial infarction, and cerebrovascular accidents all associate with GCA. Yet most outcome studies do not report increased mortality, so the impact of severe cardiovascular disease seems to be small.[36]

Takayasu Arteritis
TA, a granulomatous panarteritis, affects the aorta and its major branches, typically before the age of 40 years. The disease predominates in women, with a female-to-male ratio of up to 10:1. Because the diagnosis is often delayed, substantial arterial injury accrues.

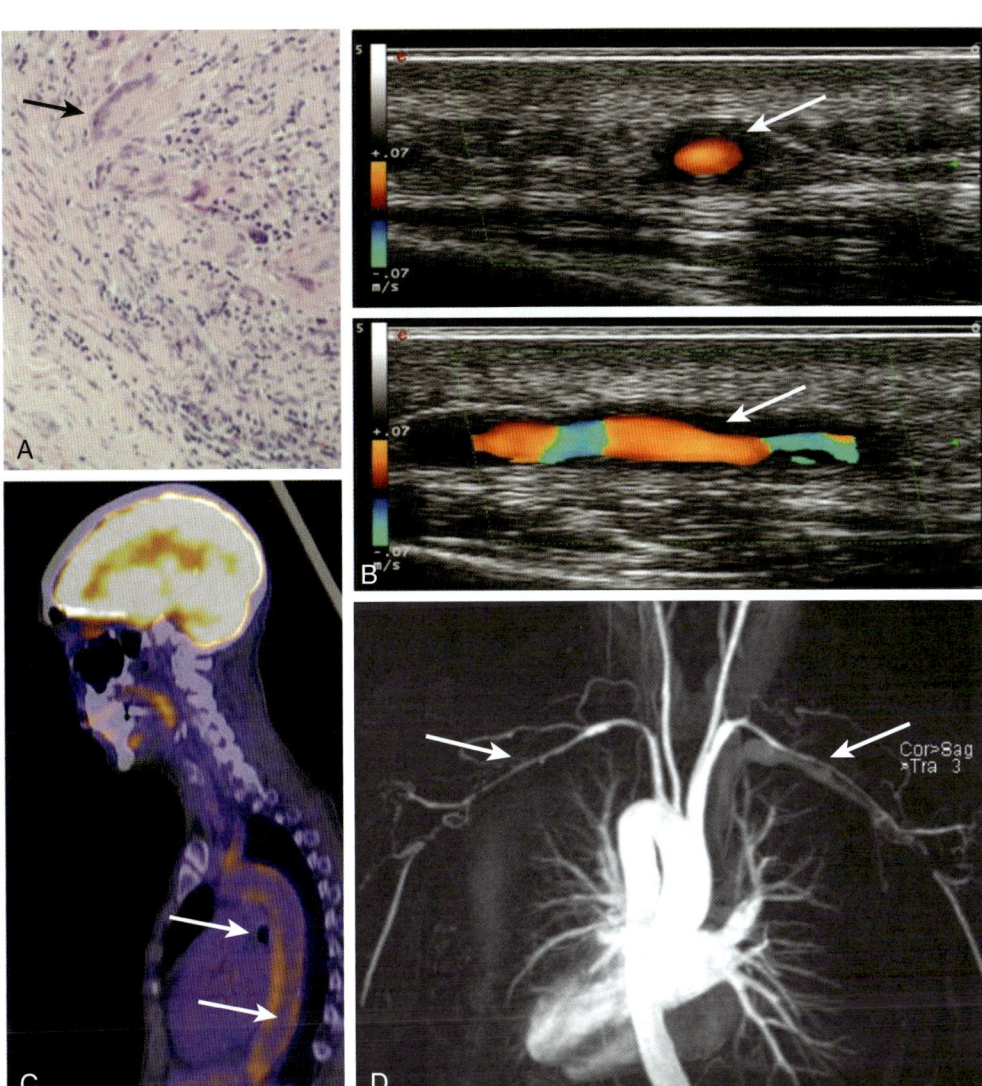

FIGURE 97.2 Giant cell arteritis (GCA). **A,** A temporal artery biopsy specimen stained with hematoxylin-eosin shows evidence of myofibroblast proliferation and vessel occlusion, a focal mononuclear cell inflammatory infiltrate, and the presence of multinucleated giant cells *(arrow)*. **B,** Dark hypoechoic, circumferential wall thickening (halo sign) *(arrows)* is seen around the temporal artery lumen in active GCA in both transverse and longitudinal views. **C,** ^{18}FDG-PET-CT scan demonstrating uptake in the thoracic aorta, consistent with active arteritis. **D,** Magnetic resonance angiogram demonstrating bilateral stenosis of the left subclavian and axillary arteries *(arrows)* in a 60-year-old woman with upper limb ischemic symptoms. (**B** courtesy Dr. Wolfgang Schmidt, Medical Center for Rheumatology Berlin-Buch, Berlin, Germany.)

Presentation is typically nonspecific and associated with fever, night sweats, arthralgia, malaise, profound tiredness, and lethargy. TA may be accompanied by symptoms of upper limb claudication, and carotidynia occurs in up to 25% of patients. The aorta may be involved throughout its length, and even though any branches can be diseased, the most commonly affected are the subclavian and common carotid arteries. More than 90% of patients have stenotic/occlusive arterial lesions, whereas approximately 25% have aneurysms. The pulmonary arteries are involved in up to 50% of patients, and aortic valve regurgitation and coronary arteritis may occur (Fig. 97.3).[37]

TA has severe consequences, with 74% reporting compromised daily activities and 23% unable to work. In our cohort, survival at 15 years is higher than 95%; similarly, in the United States, 94% to 96% survival rates are reported, whereas in Korea the survival rate was 87% at 10 years. In Japan, 15-year survival rates have improved to 96.5%. However, the survival rate fell to 67% in a subset of patients with serious complications and/or a progressive disease course.

Pathogenesis

Arteritic lesions demonstrate adventitial thickening and focal leukocytic accumulation in the media with intimal hyperplasia. The leukocytes include activated dendritic cells, T and B lymphocytes, macrophages, and multinucleated giant cells (see Fig. 97.3). Growth factor–driven mesenchymal cell proliferation leads to intimal hyperplasia and fibrosis and subsequent arterial stenosis or occlusion. Local matrix metalloproteinase synthesis may predispose to aneurysmal dilation.

TABLE 97.2 Cardiovascular Disease in the Systemic Vasculitides

VASCULITIDES	CARDIOVASCULAR COMPLICATIONS
Large-Vessel Vasculitis	
Giant cell arteritis	Thoracic/abdominal artery aneurysm, limb ischemia, pericarditis, coronary arteritis, IHD, MI
Takayasu arteritis	Aortic regurgitation, limb ischemia, aortic stenosis, aortic aneurysm, stroke, hypertension, coronary arteritis and aneurysm, IHD, MI, myocarditis, cardiac failure
Kawasaki disease	Coronary artery aneurysm, MI, myocarditis, pericarditis, valvular dysfunction, cardiac failure
Medium-Vessel Vasculitis	
Eosinophilic granulomatosis with polyangiitis (Churg-Strauss syndrome)	Myocarditis, pericarditis, coronary arteritis, cardiomyopathy, cardiac fibrosis, valvular dysfunction, MI
Polyarteritis nodosa	Myocarditis, pericarditis, coronary arteritis, coronary aneurysm, hypertension, cardiac failure
Wegener granulomatosis (granulomatous polyangiitis)	Myocarditis, pericarditis, coronary arteritis, valvular heart disease, cardiac failure
Microscopic polyangiitis	Pericarditis, coronary microaneurysm, MI

IHD, Ischemic heart disease; *MI,* myocardial infarction.

Diagnosis

Diagnosis of TA depends principally on the physician including the disease in the differential diagnosis. The variable nature of the features of TA and the lack of constitutional symptoms in 30% to 50% of patients initially present a challenge to prompt diagnosis. In addition to improved physician awareness, a list of "red flags" that raise the possibility of TA is helpful (Table 97.3). One's index of suspicion must be high in young patients with an unexplained acute-phase response or hypertension. Similarly, common initial signs, including diminished or absent pulsation or arterial bruits, can suggest the diagnosis.

Laboratory abnormalities during active disease include raised ESR and CRP (in 75% of patients), often accompanied by normochromic normocytic anemia, thrombocytosis, hypergammaglobulinemia, and hypoalbuminemia. No specific autoantibodies or other serologic abnormalities exist. Noninvasive imaging is now the optimal means of diagnosis because tissue biopsy is rarely available. High-resolution ultrasound, cardiac magnetic resonance (CMR), MRA, CTA, and PET have all been studied.[35,38] Although the potential of these techniques is not in doubt, their specificity and sensitivity in the management of TA remain undetermined. ^{18}F-FDG-PET-CT may reveal evidence of active arteritis and lead to early detection of prestenotic disease. Demonstration of arterial wall enhancement, edema, or thickening on MRA and CTA may also facilitate the diagnosis of prestenotic disease, and stenoses and aneurysms can be readily identified and monitored (see Fig. 97.3). Color duplex ultrasound has particular use in assessing the common carotid and proximal subclavian arteries in TA. Homogeneous, bright concentric arterial wall thickening is a typical finding in affected common carotid arteries.

Cardiovascular Complications

In addition to the sequelae associated with cerebral, internal organ, and limb ischemia, aneurysms, PAH, or aortic rupture may develop. Cardiac complications include aortic valve insufficiency, accelerated atherosclerosis, cardiac ischemia, myocarditis, myocardial infarction, and heart failure. Coronary disease is often asymptomatic, as illustrated by the identification of silent myocardial injury in 27% of a cohort that we studied. Thallium stress scintigraphy revealed myocardial perfusion defects in 53%, whereas intra-arterial angiography has shown that up to 30% have coronary artery lesions typically affecting the ostia and proximal segments, with the left main coronary artery being most commonly affected. Ostial vasculitic coronary lesions are typically uncalcified, while more distal calcified lesions reflect secondary accelerated atherosclerosis. Neither MRA nor ^{18}F-FDG-PET-CT reliably identifies coronary arteritis, which is best identified by coronary CTA. Inflammation of the ascending aorta predisposes to coronary artery involvement, as well as to dilation of the aortic root with subsequent aortic valve regurgitation and the need for aortic valve replacement. Left ventricular dysfunction may affect up to 20% and may reflect myocarditis, ischemic heart disease, and hypertension. High blood pressure occurs commonly with renal artery stenosis often in association in TA.

Kawasaki Disease

Kawasaki disease (KD) predominantly affects children younger than 5 years with a peak incidence at 6 to 24 months of age. The vasculitis affects medium and small arteries, notably the coronary arteries. All racial groups may be affected, with the highest incidence is recorded in Asia (20 to 100 per 100,000 children <5 years of age). KD is an

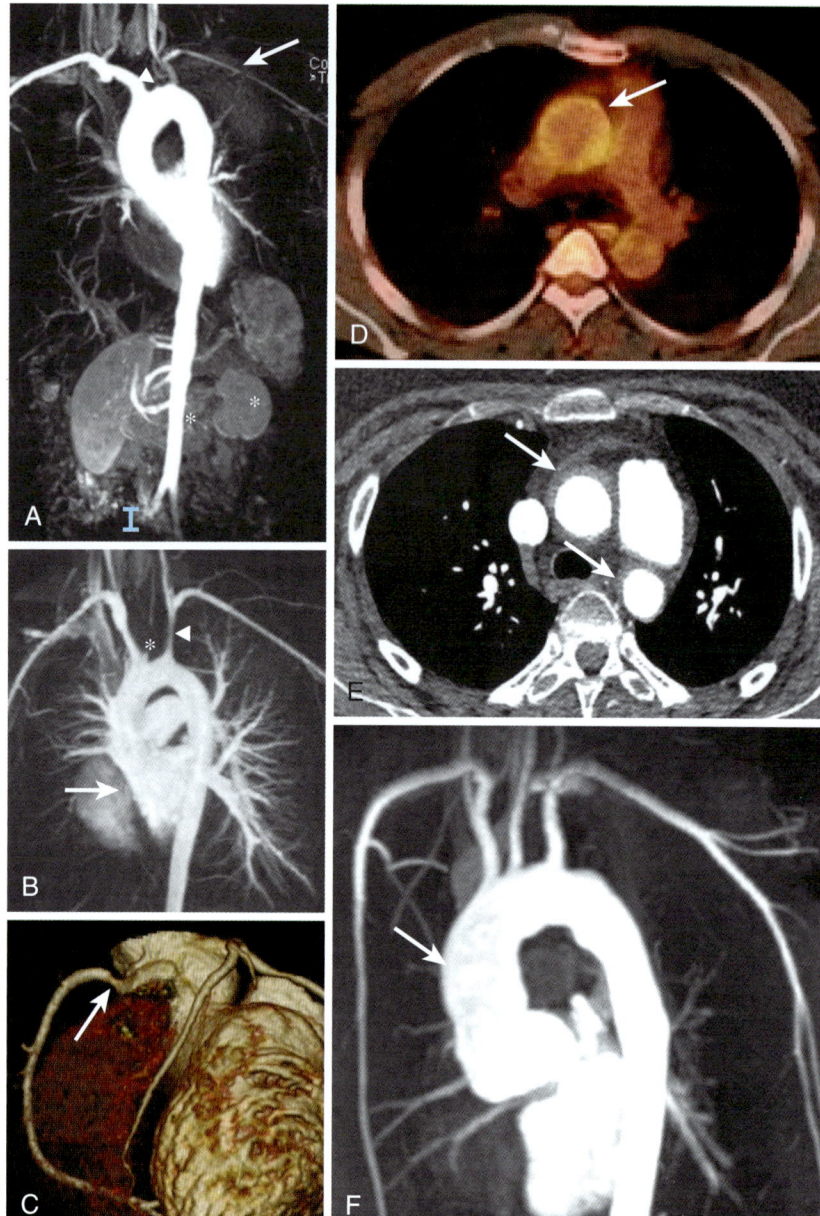

FIGURE 97.3 Takayasu arteritis. **A,** MRA demonstrating occlusion of the left common carotid artery (*arrowhead*), stenosis of the left subclavian artery with collateral formation (*arrow*), occlusion of the left renal artery and an atrophic left kidney (*asterisks*). **B,** MRA demonstrating severe stenosis of the right middle and lower lobe pulmonary arteries (*arrow*). The left common carotid artery is also occluded (*asterisk*) and there is stenosis of the left subclavian artery (*arrowhead*). **C,** Coronary CT angiogram demonstrating proximal ostial stenosis in the right coronary artery (*arrow*). **D,** ^{18}FDG-PET-CT scan demonstrating uptake in the aortic arch (*arrow*), consistent with active arteritis. **E,** CT angiogram demonstrating thickening of the wall of the ascending and descending aorta (*arrows*). **F,** MRA revealing severe dilatation of the ascending aorta (*arrow*) requiring aortic valve replacement.

TABLE 97.3 "Red Flags" for Takayasu Arteritis

In patients younger than 40 years the following may indicative of TA:
Unexplained acute-phase response (raised ESR and/or CRP)
Carotidynia
Hypertension
Discrepant blood pressure between the arms (>10 mm Hg)
Absent/weak peripheral pulse or pulses
Limb claudication
Arterial bruit
Angina

CRP, C-reactive protein; *ESR,* erythrocyte sedimentation rate.

acute self-limited illness that typically resolves within 1 to 2 months, although mortality still remains 1% to 2%. Characteristic initial features include fever of 5 days' duration or longer, bilateral conjunctivitis, and mucocutaneous lesions, including red fissured lips and a strawberry tongue. Cervical lymphadenopathy may be prominent, with erythema affecting the palms and soles and a polymorphous exanthema.

Pathogenesis
The cause of KD is unknown, although occasional seasonal epidemics and increased incidence in siblings suggests infection may trigger the disease and lead to an uncontrolled immunologic response in a genetically susceptiblE host. Tissue specimens show endothelial injury, perhaps caused by proinflammatory cytokines and activated neutrophils. Infiltration of the arterial wall by neutrophils, T cells, and macrophages is associated with the development of arterial stenosis or, more commonly, aneurysms. Coronary artery aneurysms develop in up to 20% of patients during the first month of the illness, and 50% will regress in the following years. A variety of organisms have been implicated, including streptococci, staphylococci, and *Propionibacterium acnes*. Although no definitive evidence supports an infectious cause, the emergence of a Kawasaki-like syndrome in children affected by SARS-Cov-2 has reignited interest.[39]

Diagnosis
Neutrophilia, thrombocytosis, and a raised acute-phase response occur acutely. Echocardiography can detect coronary involvement from the second week of illness and can be used to monitor progress. Coronary angiography is not performed acutely because of the risk of precipitating myocardial infarction, but it can be used after 6 months to establish the degree of coronary artery involvement. The electrocardiogram (ECG) demonstrates abnormalities in up to 50% of patients, including tachycardia, T wave inversion, ST depression, atrioventricular block, and rarely, ventricular arrhythmia.

Cardiovascular Complications
Coronary artery aneurysms develop in up to 25% of untreated patients with KD. Sudden death can occur as a consequence of myocardial infarction following acute coronary thrombosis or rupture of a coronary artery aneurysm. Pericarditis, pericardial effusion, myocarditis, valvular dysfunction, and cardiac failure may all occur, whereas peripheral arterial involvement is less common but may affect the limb, renal, and visceral arteries.

Treatment
Intravenous immunoglobulin (IVIG) 2 g/kg over 10 to 12 hours should be prescribed as soon as diagnosis is made and within 10 days of presentation. Aspirin (30 to 100 mg/kg/day) is given concurrently until the patient is afebrile and then reduced to 3 to 5 mg/kg/day. This treatment combination reduces development of coronary artery aneurysm to 5%, with a significant impact on mortality. Ten to twenty percent of cases are resistant to IVIG. In this event a repeat course is recommended, and this can be combined with prednisone (2 mg/kg/day in divided doses). Alternative therapies for refractory disease, anti-TNF-α monoclonal infliximab (5 mg/kg IV over 2 hours) and the IL-1 receptor antagonist anakinra (100 to 200 mg/day SC), are both the subject of ongoing clinical trials.[40]

Most patients with KD have a good outcome. Yet in up to 20% of those with coronary artery aneurysms, coronary stenoses eventually develop, and these patients require long-term follow-up into adulthood by an experienced cardiologist. Although the risk for long-term complications, including myocardial infarction and sudden death, is greater in those with giant aneurysms, the risk for thrombosis and myocardial infarction still remains increased in those in whom aneurysms have regressed and throughout adult life.

Idiopathic Aortitis
Aortitis can complicate SLE, Cogan syndrome, Behçet disease, human leukocyte antigen (HLA) B27-positive spondyloarthropathy, KD, and GCA. Aortitis may also be idiopathic, although a number of such cases are now recognized to fall within the IgG4-related disease spectrum.[41] The clinical features are nonspecific and include malaise, lethargy, chest pain, fever, and weight loss, and the diagnosis is often missed, or made during incidental imaging or at the time of surgery. The ESR and CRP are typically raised, and the extent of the disease can be demonstrated by ^{18}F-FDG-CT-PET scanning and aortic MRA or CTA (Fig. 97.4). Dilation of the aortic root may require aortic valve and root replacement, whenever possible preceded by immunosuppressive therapy to control aortic wall inflammation. Treatment involves corticosteroids and a steroid-sparing immunosuppressant drug such as azathioprine, methotrexate, or MMF. The B-cell depleting antibody rituximab has proven particularly effective for IgG4-related disease.

Treatment of Large-Vessel Vasculitis
The evidence base for the treatment of large-vessel vasculitis is remarkably small. Although GCA and TA typically respond to steroids, gaining remission requires high doses and a considerable side effect burden. In GCA, the dependence on prednisone and conflicting evidence concerning the efficacy of steroid-sparing drugs, combined with concerns about AION, often result in overtreatment and considerable side effects. Indeed, 86% of patients experience glucocorticoid-related adverse events at 10-year follow-up. Both of these diseases have a high relapse rate when the dose of corticosteroid is tapered, suggesting persistent vasculitis. Potential mechanistic insight comes from the identification of two pathogenic pathways in GCA. Raised plasma IL-17 and Th17 cells in the arterial wall are rapidly reduced by prednisone therapy and remained suppressed as the dose is reduced. In contrast, the Th1-promoting cytokine IL-12 and IFN-γ-producing Th1 cells typically demonstrate corticosteroid resistance, which may account for the reemergence of disease.[33,42] Corticosteroid treatment of GCA should be tapered carefully to maintain remission and minimize side effects. Although the literature is somewhat conflicting, methotrexate may offer corticosteroid-sparing efficacy for those unable to reduce the dose of prednisone sufficiently.[43] Most patients with active TA require steroid-sparing immunosuppressive drugs. Methotrexate, MMF, and azathioprine are the most widely prescribed, and small open-label studies support their use.[37] In patients failing to respond or in those with life-threatening disease such as coronary arteritis or myocarditis, treatment with intravenous pulsed cyclophosphamide is recommended.

GiACTA, a double-blind, placebo-controlled study of the efficacy and safety of anti–IL-6 receptor monoclonal antibody tocilizumab in GCA reported that at 52 weeks, tocilizumab plus either a 26-week or 52-week prednisone taper demonstrated superiority in achieving sustained remission in GCA compared to the prednisone taper control arms alone.[44] While case reports also suggest that anti-TNF-α therapy can treat refractory GCA effectively, two small, randomized, placebo-controlled trials failed to demonstrate a significant clinically useful benefit. In patients with TA who fail to respond adequately to combination therapy with prednisone and steroid-sparing immunosuppressant drugs, including cyclophosphamide, current opinion is that both TNF-α and IL-6 blockade are effective, although clinical trial data is sparse.[45] A review of all published cases of TA treated with TNF-α antagonists found complete remission in 37%, partial remission in 53.5%, and no response in 9.5%. An initial placebo-controlled trial of tocilizumab in TA suggested a beneficial effect.[46] The suppression of both constitutional symptoms and CRP synthesis by tocilizumab complicates disease monitoring and may be falsely reassuring. Follow-up of patients with TA should therefore include angiographic monitoring, preferably with MRI because it avoids radiation exposure.[37]

Critical analysis of the published results suggests that percutaneous angioplasty or bypass surgery requires caution in patients with TA or GCA. Indications for surgical intervention include aneurysmal enlargement with risk for rupture, severe aortic regurgitation or coarctation, stenotic or occlusive lesions resulting in severe symptomatic coronary artery or cerebrovascular disease, uncontrolled hypertension as a consequence of renal artery stenosis, and stenoses leading to critical limb ischemia. Whenever possible, surgery should be delayed until immunosuppression has achieved clinical remission.[47]

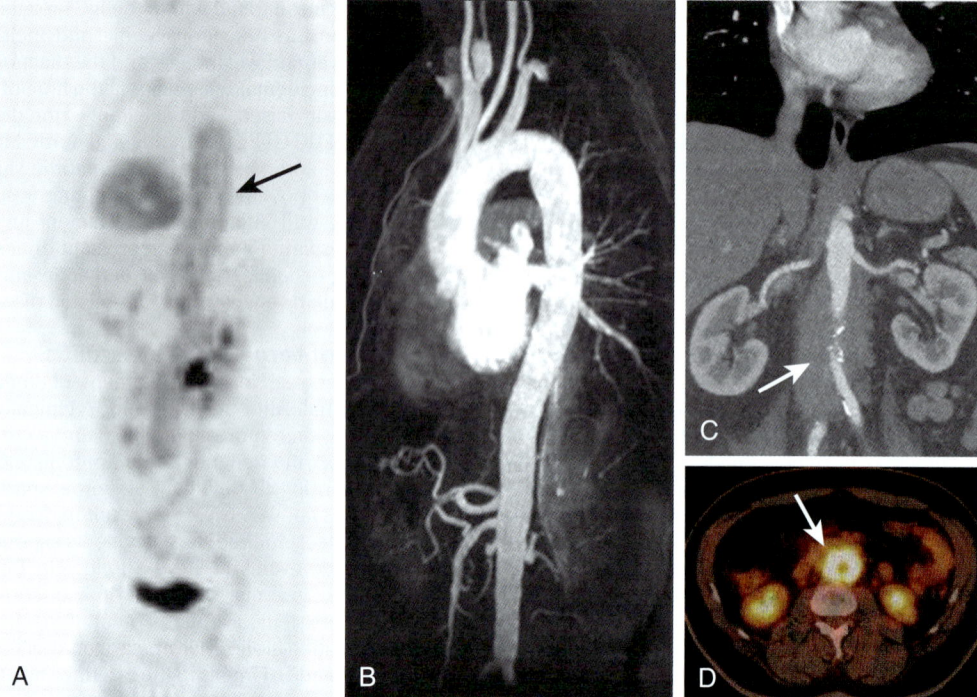

FIGURE 97.4 Idiopathic aortitis. **A,** 18F-FDG-PET scan demonstrating high-grade tracer uptake *(arrow)* in the aorta from below the level of the arch to just above the level of the aortic bifurcation, in keeping with aortitis. The activity is largely concentric around the aortic lumen. **B,** MRA showing aortic ectasia. **C,** IgG4-related disease with inflammatory peri-aortitis encasing the distal aorta below the renal arteries *(arrow)*. Calcification is seen within the aortic wall. **D,** 18F-FDG-PET scan reveals the inflammatory nature of the peri-aortitis with intense tracer uptake *(arrow)*.

Medium-Vessel Vasculitis

The medium-vessel vasculitides include Churg-Strauss syndrome (CSS, eosinophilic granulomatosis with polyangiitis, EGPA), granulomatosis with polyangiitis (GPA; Wegener granulomatosis), and microscopic polyangiitis (MPA). Although these diseases have overlapping features, they represent distinct clinical entities. GPA is most frequently associated with a cytoplasmic ANCA (cANCA) staining pattern that recognizes the antigen proteinase-3, whereas MPA most commonly associates with a perinuclear ANCA (pANCA) directed against myeloperoxidase.[48]

Eosinophilic Granulomatosis With Polyangiitis (Churg-Strauss Syndrome)

EGPA, a systemic small-vessel necrotizing vasculitis with a prevalence of 10 to 14 per million population, encompasses three disease phases. An initial prodrome characterized by allergic rhinitis, sinusitis, and asthma precedes peripheral blood eosinophilia and eosinophilic infiltrative lesions in the lung and myocardium. Some years later, a systemic phase follows with necrotizing vasculitis affecting the skin, peripheral nerves, gastrointestinal tract, and kidney (in 30%). Up to 40% of patients with EGPA are ANCA positive, most typically pANCA. ANCA-negative patients are more likely to suffer cardiopulmonary complications, whereas pANCA-positive patients seem to be more at risk for renal and peripheral nerve involvement. The diagnosis depends on the clinical features, imaging studies, ANCA, and whenever possible, biopsy results. Patients have a markedly raised peripheral eosinophil count and evidence of necrotizing vasculitis, including eosinophilic infiltration (Fig. 97.5).

The diagnosis of EGPA requires consideration of a number of alternatives, including GPA and MPA. A history of asthma, the presence of marked peripheral eosinophilia, and a dense eosinophilic infiltrate highly suggest EGPA. Viral infections, including cytomegalovirus and hepatitis B and C, must be excluded. In light of the eosinophilia, parasitic infestation, particularly by helminths, should be sought and excluded. Eosinophilia in the absence of demonstrable vasculitis may represent idiopathic hypereosinophilic syndrome or an underlying leukoproliferative disorder.

Cardiovascular Complications

Of all the vasculitides, EGPA most likely associates with severe and potentially fatal cardiac disease (see Table 97.2). Cardiac involvement complicates up to 60% of cases, and the disease spectrum includes pericarditis, myocarditis, coronary arteritis, myocardial infarction, cardiac fibrosis, arterial thrombosis, and valvular dysfunction. Cardiac disease is a prominent cause of death. Cardiomyopathy occurs as a result of ischemia secondary to arteritis affecting the intramyocardial arteries or, less frequently, the epicardial coronary arteries. Myocarditis associates with eosinophilic infiltration, fibrosis, and occasionally, granuloma formation. Release of major basic protein and eosinophil-derived neurotoxin by infiltrating eosinophils can lead to direct tissue injury. Myocarditis may result in the development of restrictive, congestive, or dilated cardiomyopathy, or death.

Investigation

Cardiac involvement in EGPA requires urgent investigation, aggressive treatment, and initially, a 12-lead ECG and transthoracic echocardiography (see Fig. 97.5). Common findings include evidence of left ventricular dilation in 30% of patients, reduced shortening fraction, and increased cardiac wall echogenicity. Contrast-enhanced CMR provides the most sensitive means of detecting myocardial involvement.[49] If the diagnosis remains in doubt, endomyocardial biopsy may reveal eosinophilic infiltration with or without fibrosis, although vasculitis is rarely seen and the patchy nature of the disease renders diagnostic yield low.

Treatment

High-dose corticosteroid treatment typically results in a good response and associates with a 90% remission of disease. Relapses occur frequently on tapering steroid therapy, and prednisone-related side effects are common. In the presence of severe disease, including cardiac, gastrointestinal, CNS, and renal involvement, an immunosuppressant drug should be prescribed concomitantly. Although further clinical trials are required, the first choice of drug is pulsed intravenous cyclophosphamide. Once remission is achieved, generally by 3 to 6 months, cyclophosphamide can be replaced by azathioprine or methotrexate. In some patients with milder disease and evidence of steroid side effects, azathioprine or methotrexate should be added to

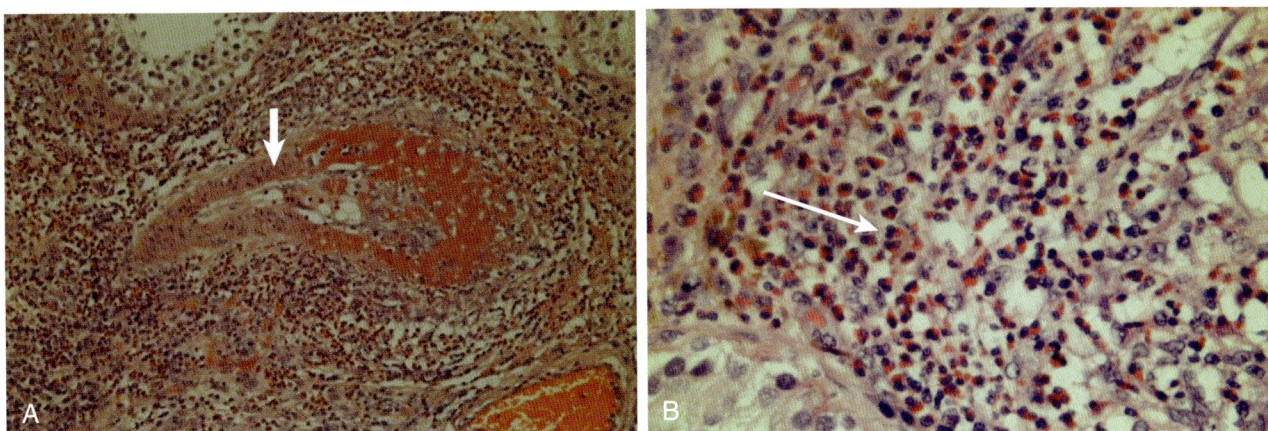

FIGURE 97.5 Churg-Strauss syndrome. **A,** Hematoxylin-eosin staining of a small artery *(arrow)* demonstrates fibrinoid necrosis and a dense perivascular mononuclear cell infiltrate. **B,** At higher magnification the inflammatory cells can be identified as predominantly eosinophils *(arrow)* with scattered macrophages.

aid in steroid tapering. In refractory disease, anecdotal case reports have suggested the effectiveness of IVIG or TNF-α blockade. The anti–IL-5 mAb mepolizumab has demonstrated efficacy in a randomized, placebo-controlled trial[50] and further results from the study of B cell depletion are awaited.[48]

Polyarteritis Nodosa

PAN is an increasingly rare disease characterized by a systemic necrotizing vasculitis of medium-sized arteries complicated by aneurysmal nodules. Viral infections, particularly with cytomegalovirus, human immunodeficiency virus, and hepatitis B and C virus, should be specifically sought and excluded. The classic type of PAN is an ANCA-negative vasculitis with the predominant clinical features including fever, malaise, arthralgia, weight loss, livedo reticularis, cutaneous nodules, and a vasculitic rash. Abdominal, cardiac, and testicular pain may occur, and some patients manifest mononeuritis multiplex. Hematuria, proteinuria, and/or hypertension indicates renal involvement.

The pathogenesis of PAN remains poorly understood. The initial vascular endothelial injury is followed by local release of IL-1 and TNF-α, which predispose to chronic inflammation and augmented leukocyte adhesion molecule expression. Recruitment of neutrophils is followed by monocyte infiltration, local endothelial disruption, thrombosis, and fibrinoid necrosis (Fig. 97.6). The associated arterial wall injury predisposes to aneurysm formation. The diagnosis of PAN is not straightforward. Although a biopsy can be definitive, yield is variable and dependent on an accessible lesion. A deep skin biopsy specimen from an involved nodular site is optimal. Combined sural nerve and muscle biopsy may also be helpful. Occasionally, nodules are detected on a medium-sized peripheral artery that can safely undergo biopsy. Renal biopsy should be approached with caution because of the risk for hemorrhage from microaneurysms. Despite increasing use of noninvasive imaging with CTA or MRA, mesenteric arteriography remains the most accurate way of identifying renal or hepatic microaneurysms.

Cardiovascular Complications

Cardiac involvement in PAN is often subclinical and clinically apparent in only 10% of patients. Congestive cardiac failure is most commonly seen and may reflect myocarditis or coronary arteritis. Alternatively, the underlying cause may be PAN-related renal disease complicated by hypertension. Five percent of patients develop pericarditis, as well as supraventricular tachycardia and valvular disease. Coronary angiography may reveal coronary artery microaneurysms, coronary arteritis, or coronary spasm. Coronary CTA may demonstrate coronary artery aneurysms.

Treatment

Glucocorticoids form the basis of treatment of PAN. In those with cardiac disease, significant proteinuria with or without renal impairment, CNS involvement, gastrointestinal disease, or mononeuritis multiplex, intravenous cyclophosphamide therapy is used initially. Some physicians prefer oral cyclophosphamide, and although side effects are more common, time until relapse may be longer. Six months of cyclophosphamide usually suffices to achieve disease remission, and treatment can be switched to oral azathioprine. In those with refractory disease, infliximab given in combination with methotrexate or azathioprine may provide benefit.

Granulomatosis With Polyangiitis (Wegener Granulomatosis)

GPA is a granulomatous necrotizing vasculitis that commonly affects the sinuses, upper airways, lungs, skin, joints, and kidneys. Diagnosis is based on clinical features, biopsy evidence, and typically a positive cANCA with antibodies against proteinase-3. The disease may be confined to the upper airways or be more generalized and include ocular inflammation, cutaneous vasculitis, arthralgia, cavitating lung lesions (Fig. 97.7), pulmonary hemorrhage, and acute renal failure. Clinical cardiac involvement is rare, although it has been reported in up to 30% of autopsy cases. The most frequently encountered problem is pericarditis, which can lead to hemodynamic compromise and tamponade. The presence of congestive cardiac failure is a poor prognostic sign and associated with 25% mortality in the first year. Underlying causes include coronary arteritis, myocarditis, and occasionally aortitis and valvular heart disease.

Microscopic Polyangiitis

MPA is most commonly associated with glomerulonephritis, renal impairment, and pulmonary hemorrhage. Cardiac disease is rarely clinically significant, but pericarditis occurs in 10% of patients, and congestive cardiac failure develops in up to 18%. Subclinical and occasionally symptomatic acute myocardial infarction can occur. Evidence from case reports and small series shows that this disease also features symptomatic aortitis and coronary artery microaneurysms.

Investigation

Cardiac involvement should initially be investigated noninvasively with modalities that include rest or stress echocardiography. Contrast-enhanced CMR can sensitively detect myocardial pathology, and coronary CTA can demonstrate coronary arteritis and microaneurysms. Echocardiography suggests valvular thickening is a common and typically asymptomatic finding in MPA. Aortic valve regurgitation may occur because of distortion and thickening of valve cusps or from aortic root dilation. On occasion, coronary arteriography may be required, and as for other vasculitides, it should be used cautiously in those suspected of having active coronary arteritis. When possible, steps should be taken to suppress disease activity with immunosuppressive therapy before angiography. Coronary arteritis can cause multiple small areas of myocardial infarction, which often remain clinically silent until the development of congestive cardiac failure. Occasionally, granulomas in conduction tissue precipitate cardiac dysrhythmia.

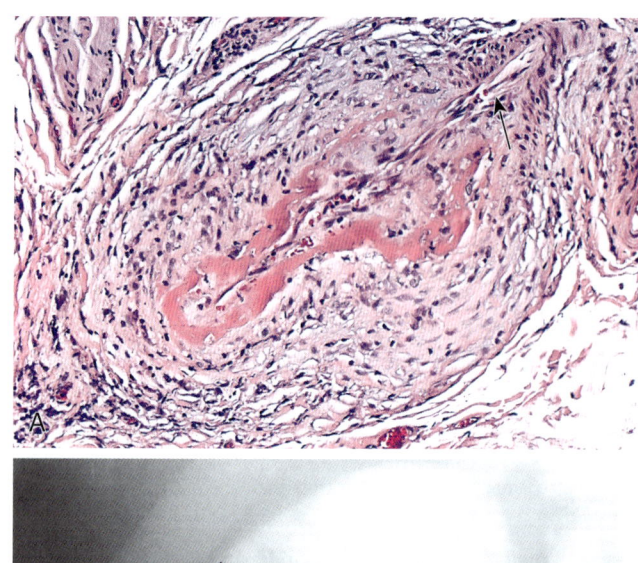
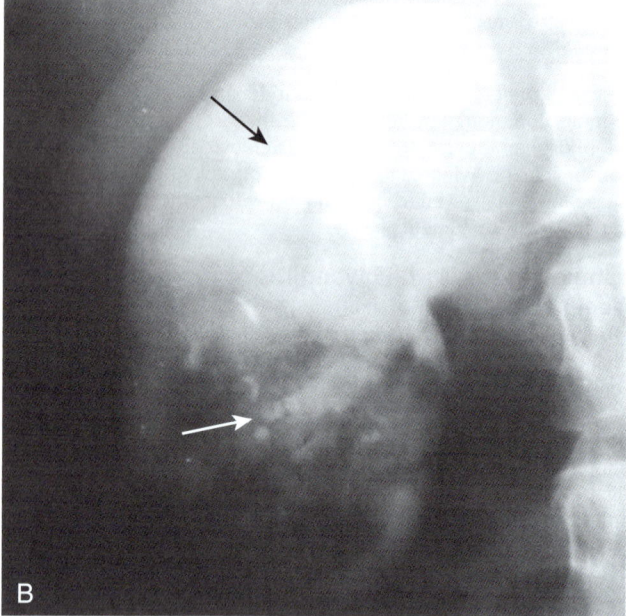

FIGURE 97.6 Polyarteritis nodosa (PAN). **A,** Photomicrograph of a hematoxylin-eosin–stained section of an artery biopsy specimen from a patient with PAN showing segmental fibrinoid necrosis, thrombotic occlusion of the lumen, and a small uninvolved remnant. **B,** Right renal angiogram showing multiple small aneurysms *(white arrow)* and a normal calyceal system *(black arrow)*. (From Mitchell RN. Blood Vessels. In: Kumar V, Abbas A, Aster JC, eds. *Robbins & Cotran Pathologic Basis of Disease.* 9th ed. Philadelphia: Elsevier Saunders; 2014.)

Treatment

For both GPA and MPA, high-dose prednisone (up to 1 mg/kg/day) is recommended at the onset and may be preceded by pulsed intravenous methylprednisolone if indicated. Patients with the most severe disease, including pulmonary hemorrhage, severe cardiac disease, or significant renal impairment, also receive pulsed intravenous cyclophosphamide to induce remission over the first 3 to 6 months, or alternatively B-cell depletion therapy with rituximab. In nonorgan threatening disease, remission can be achieved reliably with prednisolone in combination with methotrexate or MMF. Once remission is achieved, maintenance therapies may include azathioprine, methotrexate or rituximab, with continued prednisone tapering.[51] A range of novel therapies are under investigation including B-cell activating antagonist blisibimod, proteasome inhibitor bortezomib, abatacept targeting T-cell activation, and inhibition of the complement pathway with avacopan a C5a receptor antagonist.[48]

PERICARDITIS AND MYOCARDITIS

Pericarditis

Pericarditis commonly complicates the autoimmune connective tissue diseases, particularly SLE, SSc, and RA. Nonetheless, clinically

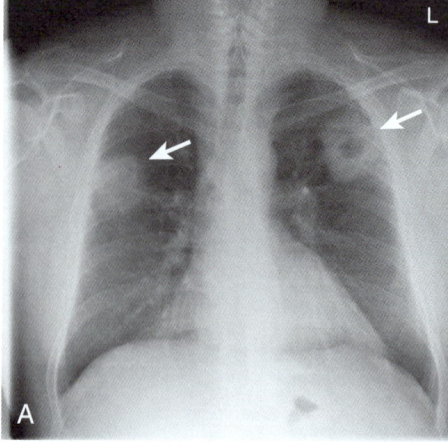
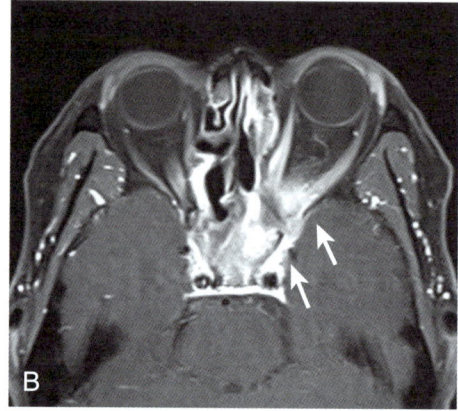
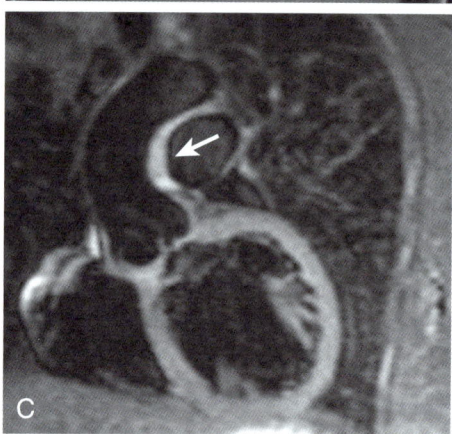

FIGURE 97.7 Granulomatosis with polyangiitis. **A,** Chest radiograph of a 36-year-old man showing pulmonary involvement with evidence of opacification and cavitation in the left upper lobe lesion *(arrows)*. **B,** CT scan of the orbits demonstrating confluent enhancing soft tissue at the left orbital apex as well as enhancing soft tissue opacifying the sinuses bilaterally (left > right) *(arrows)*. **C,** MRA demonstrating aortitis. The wall is thickened and enhancing around the root, extending to the left side of the ascending aorta.

significant pericarditis develops in fewer than 30% of patients. The reported prevalence ranges from 11% to 85%, depending on the type of study used to detect disease. Thus in necropsy studies, prevalence is high with pericardial involvement reported in 40% of individuals with RA, 40% to 80% of those with SLE, and up to 70% of those with SSc. Echocardiography detects pericardial thickening or small effusions in up to 50% of these patients. CMR can also define the extent of pericardial involvement.

Systemic Lupus Erythematosus

In SLE, pericarditis usually associates with disease flare and often with polyserositis. The symptoms are typically mild and consist of chest pain, which is worse on lying flat, and dyspnea, which may have a pleuritic component. Complicated pericarditis is rare, and in only 1% to 2%

is the effusion sufficiently large to cause cardiac tamponade. Constrictive pericarditis or infective pericarditis occur infrequently.

Rheumatoid Arthritis
Clinically significant pericarditis affects only 1% to 2% of patients with RA, more commonly male, seropositive patients. Constrictive pericarditis can develop over a period of months. Hemodynamically significant pericarditis, although reported, is extremely rare in patients being treated with antirheumatic therapy. Indeed, the more aggressive approach to management of RA and the increasing use of biologic therapies appear to have reduced the incidence of symptomatic pericarditis.

Systemic Sclerosis
The two most commonly encountered forms of scleroderma are diffuse cutaneous SSc (dSSc) and limited cutaneous SSc (lSSc). Following an initial vascular inflammatory phase, the predominant lesion is fibrosis, which affects multiple organs. In addition to the severe cutaneous manifestations, common clinical features include arthralgia, telangiectasia, pulmonary fibrosis, PAH, and esophageal dysmotility.[52] Renal crises are common and complicated by hypertension. Aggressive intervention is essential and includes the use of ACE inhibitors and calcium channel antagonists. This approach has transformed the prognosis.[53] Pericardial disease is common and more frequent in those with dSSc and a history of renal crisis. Echocardiography typically demonstrates small pericardial effusions, which are rarely hemodynamically significant. Rapidly accumulating large effusions may occur occasionally.

Pericardial Fluid Analysis
Analysis of pericardial fluid is rarely useful diagnostically unless infective pericarditis is suspected. Immune complexes, antinuclear and anti-dsDNA antibodies, complement consumption, and normal glucose levels have been reported in pericardial exudates from patients with SLE. In RA the pericardial fluid glucose concentration may be lower than that in plasma, and although rheumatoid factor activity is often detected, it is not considered diagnostic.

Treatment
In most cases a small pericardial effusion appears on a routine chest radiograph or echocardiogram and requires no specific treatment. Those with troublesome symptoms of pericarditis can receive a short course of an NSAID unless contraindicated. Colchicine is an important adjunctive therapeutic option in acute and chronic pericarditis. Likewise, low-dose oral prednisone may be required or used as an alternative.[54] Particularly recurrent cases require further optimization of the regular immunosuppressive therapy. Pericardial fluid accumulation may occasionally cause hemodynamic compromise requiring pericardiocentesis or, in recurrent cases, a pericardial window. For immunosuppressed patients, pericardial fluid should be analyzed for an infective cause. Advice should be sought from a microbiologist to ensure that the correct specimens are sent, including those required to exclude tuberculosis.

Myocarditis
Myocarditis is a rare but recognized cause of mortality in patients with autoimmune rheumatic diseases and is most commonly seen in patients with SLE, SSc, EGPA and polymyositis or dermatomyositis. Although most commonly present in those with an established rheumatic disease, myocarditis may be an initial feature requiring consideration of these conditions in the differential diagnosis of those with unexplained heart failure. The most common symptom of myocarditis is recent-onset exertional dyspnea with evidence of hypoxia. A patient rarely presents with severe heart failure at initial evaluation, and echocardiography usually reveals relatively modest changes in ventricular size and function. PAH must be excluded. In addition to standard blood tests, investigations should include: ESR, antinuclear antibody, antibodies against dsDNA and extractable nuclear antigens, rheumatoid factor, a myositis immunoblot screen, and complement factor C3 and C4 levels.

Systemic Lupus Erythematosus
Although the widespread use of more effective immunosuppressive regimens has reduced the prevalence of myocarditis in patients with SLE to fewer than 10%, much of which is subclinical, it remains an important and potentially life-threatening complication. Other potential causes of heart failure include hypertension, ischemic heart disease, valvular heart disease, and complications associated with renal failure.

The initial symptoms of myocarditis vary from low-grade fever, dyspnea, and palpitations to signs of severe heart failure. In addition to complement consumption, a raised ESR, and an increased titer of anti-dsDNA antibodies, the troponin I level may increase markedly. The ECG typically shows nonspecific findings such as sinus tachycardia, ST or T-wave changes. Supraventricular or ventricular tachycardias may also occur. Echocardiography aids in assessment (Fig. 97.8). Functional abnormalities may include segmental, regional, or global wall motion abnormalities; chamber dilation; and a reduced ejection fraction. In contrast, left ventricular hypertrophy in SLE more commonly associates with poorly controlled hypertension, whereas systolic and diastolic abnormalities in left ventricular function can associate with both hypertension and ischemic heart disease. CMR can detect myocarditis and myocardial fibrosis, and gadolinium or adenosine stress first-pass perfusion may demonstrate coronary microvascular dysfunction.[55] Indeed, CMR and PET identify coronary myocardial dysfunction and reduced coronary flow reserve in patients with SLE.

Opinion is divided on the use of endomyocardial biopsy. It will not permit a specific diagnosis of SLE per se. However, biopsy may identify an alternate cause or demonstrate an underlying inflammatory cause and features suggestive of SLE. Histopathologic analysis typically reveals small focal areas of fibrinoid necrosis with infiltration of lymphocytes and plasma cells, along with evidence of the deposition of immune complexes closely associated with myocyte bundles. Immunofluorescent studies may reveal granular staining and deposition of complement in and around myocardial blood vessels. Biopsy may also help exclude other potential causes of cardiomyopathy.

Systemic Sclerosis
Inflammatory myocarditis rarely results in symptomatic cardiomyopathy in patients with SSc; it affects mostly those with prominent skeletal muscle myositis. Echocardiography may demonstrate impaired diastolic and systolic function and a reduced ejection fraction, occasionally severe enough to cause cardiac failure. Endomyocardial biopsy most commonly reveals myocardial fibrosis. The fibrosis occurs focally and affects both ventricles. As with other lesions in SSc, microvascular disease is considered an important pathogenic factor.[52] Reduced coronary flow reserve occurs commonly, and subclinical myocardial ischemia probably contributes importantly to the ventricular dysfunction.

Myositis
Polymyositis and dermatomyositis affect the proximal skeletal muscles and can cause severe weakness. In dermatomyositis, additional characteristic cutaneous manifestations include a violaceous heliotrope rash, Gottron papules, and periungual erythema. In pediatric cases, subcutaneous calcification is common and vasculitis may lead to severe gut ischemia and hemorrhage. In adults, particularly those older than 60 years, dermatomyositis may be paraneoplastic. In severe cases, myositis involves the myocardium and pharyngeal or respiratory muscles and can be life-threatening. Creatine kinase levels rise markedly, and electromyography demonstrates fibrillation and polyphasic action potentials. MRI of the proximal limb muscles helps identify the muscles involved and those most amenable to biopsy. Histopathologic findings include muscle fiber necrosis and regeneration, a predominantly CD8+ T lymphocyte infiltrate, and HLA class I expression. Clinically significant myocarditis affects only 3%. Echocardiography may reveal ventricular dysfunction, whereas endomyocardial biopsy specimens demonstrate interstitial and perivascular lymphocytic infiltrates, contraction band necrosis, variable cardiomyocyte size, and degeneration and patchy fibrosis. Overt cardiac failure is rare; more common are rhythm and

conduction abnormalities, including left anterior hemiblock and right bundle branch block.

Other Causes of Myocarditis
Even though postmortem studies have revealed evidence of myocarditis in patients with RA, it is seldom manifested clinically or causes heart failure. Although heart failure affects patients with RA more than it does age- and sex-matched controls, it predominantly reflects ischemia. Myocarditis also associates rarely with other rheumatic diseases, including ankylosing spondylitis, adult Still disease, GCA, and TA. In the latter it can be life-threatening.[56]

Treatment
Cardiac failure following myocarditis associated with autoimmune disease is treated with standard protocols and supportive interventions (see Chapter 50). Myocarditis in EGPA, TA, and SLE requires urgent corticosteroid treatment and, when severe, intravenous methylprednisolone, up to 1 g/day for 3 days, followed by oral prednisone, up to 1 mg/kg/day. These patients typically receive pulsed intravenous cyclophosphamide. For more modest disease, treatment can include the addition of, or increased dosages of, azathioprine or MMF. Some evidence suggests benefit of IVIG in resistant cases. Management of myocarditis complicating dermatomyositis or polymyositis uses a similar approach. Myocarditis in patients with SSc rarely requires aggressive treatment. Because high-dose corticosteroids increase the risk for renal crisis, early use of intravenous cyclophosphamide is favored.

VALVULAR HEART DISEASE

Clinically significant valvular disease can complicate many rheumatic diseases. Mechanisms may include direct damage to cardiac valve leaflets or aortic valve regurgitation as a consequence of aortitis affecting the ascending aorta.

Systemic Lupus Erythematosus
Valvular abnormalities occur commonly in patients with SLE, and necropsy studies have reported lesions in up to 75%. Verrucous endocarditis (Libman-Sacks endocarditis) and nonspecific valvular thickening occur most commonly. Valvulitis with rapid valvular dysfunction may also happen rarely. Transthoracic echocardiography detects verrucae in 2.5% to 12% and thickening in 4% to 38%, which increases to 30% and 43%, respectively, in those undergoing transesophageal echocardiography. Libman-Sacks lesions typically affect both valve surfaces, most commonly the mitral valve. Active valve lesions contain immunoglobulins, fibrin clumps, areas of focal necrosis, and a leukocytic infiltrate, whereas older healed lesions contain fibrous tissue predisposing to scarring and valve leaflet deformity. These abnormalities may cause valvular regurgitation. Libman-Sacks endocarditis occurs more commonly in SLE complicated by antiphospholipid antibodies and can accompany primary APS.

Libman-Sacks endocarditis is generally asymptomatic and may not cause a murmur. Assessment of SLE patients with a murmur may not be straightforward and requires exclusion of bacterial endocarditis. Echocardiography can help distinguish Libman-Sacks from infectious endocarditis, an important consideration in immunosuppressed patients. In contrast to the typically nonmobile vegetations of Libman-Sacks, bacterial vegetations usually localize at the valve leaflet closure line and demonstrate mobility that is independent of valve leaflet motion.

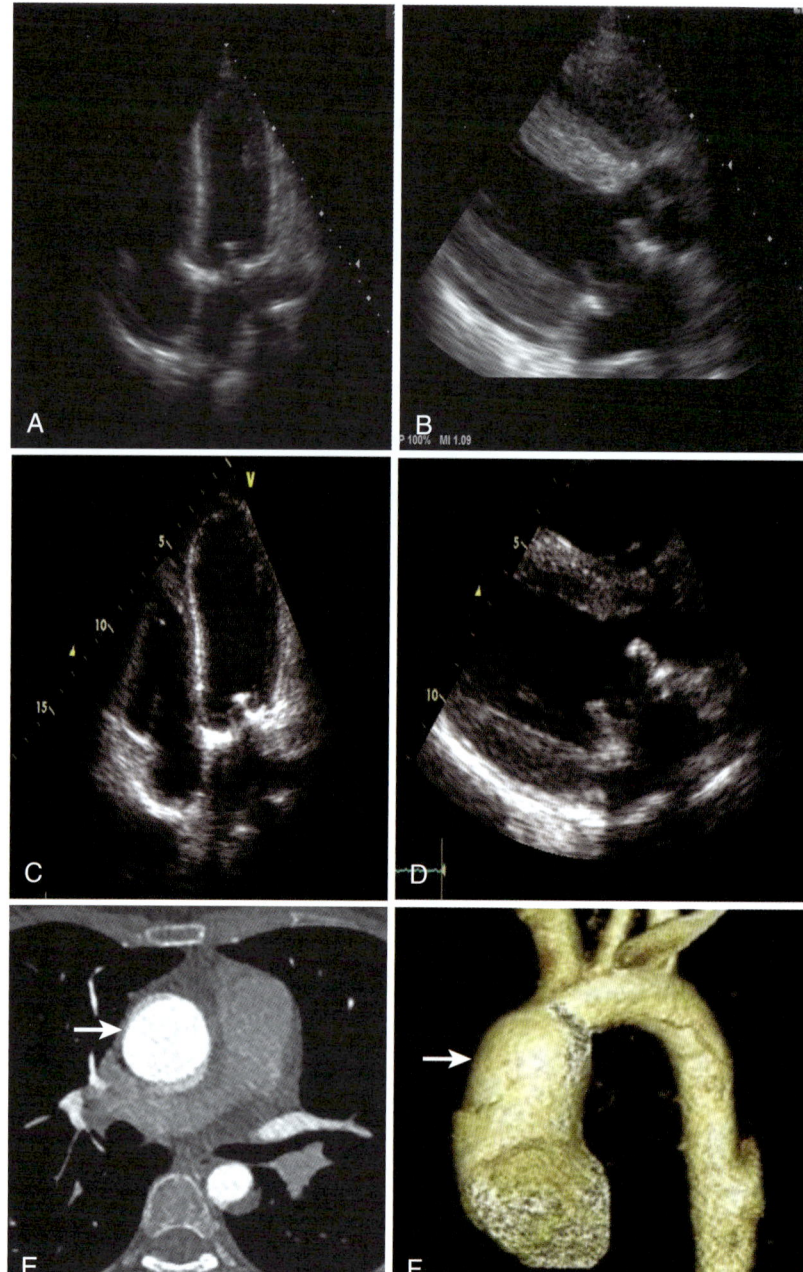

FIGURE 97.8 Myocarditis, aortitis and valvular heart disease. Myocarditis in systemic lupus erythematosus (SLE). **A** and **C,** Four-chamber view, **B** and **D,** Left ventricular view. In a 20-year-old patient with dyspnea and active SLE, the initial echocardiograms (**A** and **C**) showed mild impairment of ventricular function. Following symptomatic deterioration, the echocardiograms were repeated 6 days later (**B** and **D**) and demonstrated markedly increased thickening of the left ventricular wall with a bright signal suggestive of inflammatory infiltration. These findings were associated with substantial deterioration in left ventricular function. **E** and **F**, CTA of aorta in B27-positive ankylosing spondylitis complicated by aortitis and aortic root dilatation *(arrows)*, resulting in aortic regurgitation requiring aortic valve and root replacement.

The presence of Libman-Sacks lesions increases the risk for secondary infective endocarditis, and prophylactic antibiotic prophylaxis should be considered to cover high-risk procedures such as invasive dental treatment (see Chapter 80). Complications of SLE-related valvular disease are rare, with hemodynamic effects seen in fewer than 5%. Valve replacement may be required for symptomatic regurgitation and occasionally for stenosis. The verrucous lesions may also embolize or rupture and lead to a cerebrovascular accident or peripheral embolism. Chordae tendineae rupture may also occur.

Treatment
Most patients require no specific treatment, although annual echocardiography can be used to monitor valve function. The introduction of

corticosteroid therapy may have reduced the prevalence of Libman-Sacks endocarditis, and thus prednisone treatment may be considered in those with early active lesions. Patients with uncomplicated Libman-Sacks endocarditis with valve thickening on the echocardiogram are not routinely anticoagulated. However, in those with associated antiphospholipid syndrome and no previous thrombosis, prophylactic low-dose aspirin is advised. Those with definitive vegetations, previous thrombosis or evidence of embolic phenomena should be considered for lifelong anticoagulation therapy.[57]

Seronegative Spondyloarthropathies

The seronegative spondyloarthropathies include ankylosing spondylitis, postinfectious reactive arthritis, inflammatory bowel disease-related arthritis, and psoriatic arthritis. HLA-B27 is associated with ankylosing spondylitis and reactive arthritis. The spondyloarthropathies share overlapping clinical features, including asymmetric, predominantly large-joint oligoarthritis, ocular inflammation, sacroiliitis, spinal disease, and enthesopathy. Ankylosing spondylitis and reactive arthritis commonly involve the aortic root and valve. Aortic valvulitis leads to aortic cusp thickening and retraction and subsequently to symptomatic aortic regurgitation, which may cause heart failure. Proximal aortitis affecting the ascending aorta leads to aortic root thickening and subsequently to dilation and aortic regurgitation (see Fig. 97.8), the prevalence of which relates to disease duration.

Treatment

Management of the spondyloarthropathies traditionally consisted of NSAIDs and, in more severe cases, the addition of DMARDs such as methotrexate, sulfasalazine, and leflunomide. Although these agents have some efficacy in the treatment of peripheral inflammatory arthritis, they have little effect on spinal inflammation. The use of TNF-α antagonists for ankylosing spondylitis and psoriatic arthropathy, and more recently agents targeting IL-17 and IL-12/23 pathways, is transforming control of these diseases, with beneficial effects on peripheral arthritis, spinal disease, and extra-articular complications, including uveitis.[58] Although evidence is currently limited, the initiation of biologic therapy in those with early signs and symptoms of aortitis may reduce the risk for cardiovascular complications, including aortic regurgitation.

Rheumatoid Arthritis

Valvular thickening commonly associates with RA in echocardiographic studies and at autopsy, but seldom causes clinical problems. Patients with seropositive RA and with prominent extra-articular nodular disease more frequently have valvular lesions. Echocardiography typically reveals mitral valve involvement, with valve thickening, asymptomatic mitral regurgitation, and prolapse being the predominant findings. Histopathologic examination of the valves demonstrates granulomatous nodular lesions. No specific treatment is indicated, although on occasion hemodynamically significant disease develops and requires mitral or aortic valve replacement.

Takayasu Arteritis

Cardiac valve dysfunction commonly complicates TA. In a series of 204 Korean patients, 23% had an abnormality in at least one valve, with regurgitation at the aortic valve found in 18% and at the mitral valve in 7.5%. Inflammation of the ascending aorta predisposes to dilation of the aortic root and aortic valve regurgitation. Approximately 15% of patients require aortic valve replacement with or without aortic root replacement with a graft. If possible, surgery should follow control of disease activity with immunosuppressive therapy.[47]

CARDIAC CONDUCTION DISTURBANCES

A variety of rheumatic diseases cause conduction abnormalities and cardiac rhythm disturbances, in part through a direct effect of systemic inflammation on cardiac electrophysiology.

Systemic Lupus Erythematosus and Sjögren Syndrome

Adult SLE seldom causes primary conduction abnormalities or rhythm disturbance, which may instead result from underlying ischemic heart disease or myocarditis. Female patients with SLE or Sjögren syndrome who test positive for antibodies against the Ro and/or La antigens carry the risk of bearing a child with congenital heart block, which may be complicated by myocarditis. These antibodies can cross the placenta and induce myocardial inflammation and may target the conduction system leading to fibrosis. The precise incidence is not established, but the usual figures quoted are 1 case in 20,000 live births with a range of 11,000 to 25,000. Patients with SLE, the overlap syndromes, and Sjögren syndrome should be screened for anti-Ro and anti-La before pregnancy and be counseled appropriately. The fetus of mothers known to be antibody positive should be screened in utero by echocardiography every 2 weeks from 16 weeks of gestation onward. Incomplete atrioventricular block can reverse, and myocarditis may respond to dexamethasone therapy. Complete atrioventricular block is irreversible and associated with up to 20% mortality, with 65% requiring insertion of a pacemaker.

Systemic Sclerosis

Conduction system disease affects up to 50% of SSc patients. The patchy myocardial fibrosis characteristically associated with SSc may account for the abnormalities seen with disruption of the conduction pathways. Supraventricular arrhythmias are usually benign and amenable to treatment. Ventricular conduction abnormalities also frequently occur in SSc. In these patients, ventricular ectopy is common and closely associated with sudden death.

Spondyloarthropathies

Conduction abnormalities frequently complicate the HLA-B27-related spondyloarthropathies. In ankylosing spondylitis, up to 30% of patients experience conduction system disease, predominantly caused by subaortic fibrosis extending into the septum and affecting the atrioventricular node. Atrioventricular conduction block occurs commonly and may become complete.

Polymyositis and Dermatomyositis

Conduction abnormalities are the most common cardiac manifestation of the myositis syndromes. Left anterior hemiblock and right bundle branch block occur most frequently and occasionally progress to complete heart block. The inflammation and fibrosis associated with polymyositis and dermatomyositis affect the conduction pathways, as demonstrated in 25% of autopsy cases.

Rheumatoid Arthritis

ECG screening studies in patients with RA have revealed arrhythmias or conducting system abnormalities in up to 50%, although they are usually clinically inapparent; RA patients have a twofold increase in sudden cardiac death compared to healthy controls.[59] Rheumatoid myocarditis and cardiac amyloid deposition can cause atrioventricular node conduction block. Similarly, rheumatoid nodules may disrupt the conduction system and cause all types of conduction abnormality.

PULMONARY ARTERIAL HYPERTENSION

PAH (see Chapter 88) is an important complication of the connective tissue diseases and is of concern to rheumatologists as a significant cause of premature mortality (Table 97.4). PAH often manifests late in disease evolution or remains undiagnosed. Furthermore, PAH frequently proves resistant to optimized treatment of the underlying connective tissue diseases. Notwithstanding, increased awareness, recognition of high-risk groups, improved screening and novel therapies point toward a better outlook.

Systemic Sclerosis

SSc is the most resistant of the connective tissue diseases to treatment and has the highest mortality. PAH has very serious prognostic implications and is the most common single cause of SSc-related death. Novel therapeutic options offer renewed hope, and early data suggest improved survival.

Pathogenesis

Arterial remodeling is a central component in the pathogenesis of PAH and follows uncontrolled smooth muscle cell proliferation, deposition of extracellular matrix and subsequent fibrosis, vasoconstriction, and in situ thrombosis that together lead to increased pulmonary vascular resistance. Right ventricular dilation, dysfunction, and failure follow the development of PAH. Because PAH may develop very rapidly, effective screening strategies for patients with SSc are essential to detect PAH and allow early therapeutic intervention.

Screening

The prevalence of PAH in patients with SSc is up to 19%. PAH can occur as an early or late complication, and there is a lack of reliable predictive risk factors. Although more common with lSSc, PAH also frequently occurs in patients with dSSc. Pulmonary fibrosis can also complicate SSc and may exacerbate PAH (Fig. 97.9). Although debate continues regarding the frequency of screening, all patients must undergo an initial assessment, and annual screening is recommended thereafter to facilitate early diagnosis and improve survival. Annual screening should include echocardiography and pulmonary function testing.[60,61] In the latter, a low or falling carbon monoxide diffusing capacity may predict the development of PAH. In those with disease duration of more than 3 years and DLCO less than 60% the DETECT algorithm can be applied.[60,61] Echocardiographically assessed pulmonary artery pressure may miss early asymptomatic disease. The level of NT-pro-brain natriuretic protein (NT-proBNP) should be measured and relates to the degree of right ventricular dysfunction and the severity of PAH. Right-heart catheterization should follow positive screening results.[62]

Treatment and Outcome

The typical initial symptom of PAH is dyspnea. The diverse causes of this symptom often delay diagnosis until clinical evidence of hemodynamic impairment appears. The very poor 3-year survival rate of 47% to 56% also reflects delayed diagnosis, emphasizing the need for early diagnosis and treatment, which may improve outcome.[60] The aims of treatment include improvement in New York Heart Association (NYHA) functional class and quality of life, delay in clinical deterioration, and improved long-term outcome.[62] Although standard PAH outcome measures can assess response to treatment (Chapter 88), not all of them have been validated in patients with SSc and they may be complicated by coexistent conditions, including pulmonary fibrosis and musculoskeletal pain. Supported by clinical trials, treatment targets four main pathways with agents used alone and increasingly in combination.[60,63] Endothelin-1 receptor antagonists include bosentan, ambrisentan and macitentan. Epoprostenol, iloprost, treprostinil and selexipag target the prostacyclin pathway. The phosphodiesterase type 5 (PDE5) antagonists currently used are sildenafil and tadalafil. Riociguat, a soluble guanylate cyclase agonist has also been investigated in SSc PAH. Although efficacious, concerns remain about its safety in SSc.[63] Following clinical trial data, including that from AMBITION which demonstrated enhanced efficacy of ambrisentan and tadalafil in combination versus monotherapy,[63] the majority of specialist centers support the aggressive use of combination therapy in SSc patients considered at high risk of PAH.[60,63]

Systemic Lupus Erythematosus

The prevalence of PAH in patients with SLE varies between studies and was recently estimated to be between 0.5% and 17.5%. These patients are typically females of reproductive age, in whom PAH during pregnancy markedly increases the risk for mortality.

TABLE 97.4 Pulmonary Arterial Hypertension in Rheumatic Diseases

RHEUMATIC DISEASE	FEATURES OF PULMONARY ARTERIAL HYPERTENSION
Systemic sclerosis	Prevalence up to 19%. More common in lSSc. Annual screening recommended (echocardiography and pulmonary function)
	Disease >3 years and DLCO <60%, apply DETECT algorithm
PM/Scl overlap	Annual screening recommended. Survival rate at 3 years of 47%–56%
Systemic lupus erythematosus	Prevalence of 0.5%–17.5%. Survival rate at 3 years of 74%. Thrombotic arteriopathy is the most common underlying cause. 83% of patients have anticardiolipin antibodies. Patients with severe Raynaud phenomenon, anticardiolipin antibodies, and anti-U1RNP require screening
Rheumatoid arthritis	Prevalence data limited; reported to be up to 20%. Clinically significant disease rare, often secondary to COPD, chronic thromboembolic disease, or interstitial lung disease. Improved RA treatment may result in a reduced incidence
Sjögren syndrome	PAH a very rare complication of Sjögren syndrome. Usually occurs late in the course of disease. Prevalence unknown
Takayasu arteritis	Pulmonary arteritis present in up to 50% of patients. PAH prevalence of 12%. CMR or CTA and echocardiography required for screening

CMR, Cardiac magnetic resonance; *COPD*, chronic obstructive pulmonary disease; *CTA*, computed tomography angiography; *lSSc*, limited cutaneous systemic sclerosis; *PAH*, pulmonary artery hypertension; *PM/Scl*, polymyositis/scleroderma; *RNP*, ribonucleoprotein.

Pathogenesis

In situ pulmonary thrombosis or chronic thromboembolic disease leading to thrombotic arteriopathy is the most common cause of PAH in patients with SLE, and 83% of such patients have anticardiolipin antibodies. Additional causes include pulmonary arteritis, underlying interstitial lung disease, and left-sided heart disease secondary to myocarditis, hypertension, or ischemic heart disease.

Clinical Findings and Diagnosis

Dyspnea, which may associate with fatigue, cough, and chest pain, is the typical initial symptom. The development of PAH does not necessarily reflect the duration of SLE or its severity. Limited data concerning predictive features indicate that patients with severe Raynaud phenomenon, anticardiolipin antibodies, and anti-U1RNP antibodies have more susceptibility to develop PAH. These patients should be screened annually with lung function, NT-proBNP levels, and echocardiography to estimate pulmonary artery pressure. Abnormality should be investigated further by right-heart catheterization.[64]

Treatment and Outcome

Management of PAH in patients with SLE uses a dual approach that combines optimized immunosuppression and vasodilator therapy,[65] although protocols vary between centers. Limited evidence supports therapeutic decisions in PAH associated with SLE. In contrast to SSc-related PAH, the response to increased corticosteroids and pulsed intravenous cyclophosphamide can be good, and once response is achieved, switching from cyclophosphamide to azathioprine or MMF can reduce toxicity. Stronger trial evidence is available for the use of the vasodilator therapies mentioned above. In those with anticardiolipin antibodies, life-long anticoagulation with warfarin is indicated. The 3-year survival rate of up to 89% is significantly higher than that in patients with SSc-related PAH.[64]

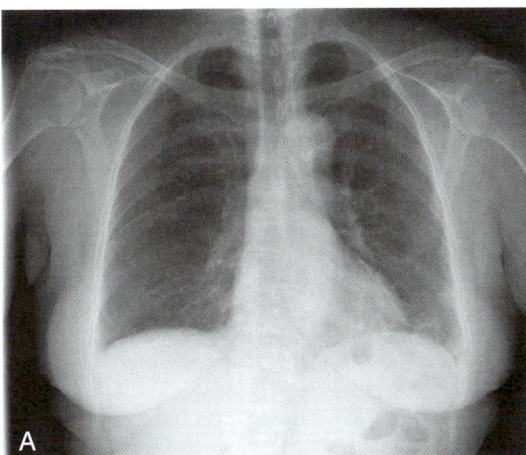
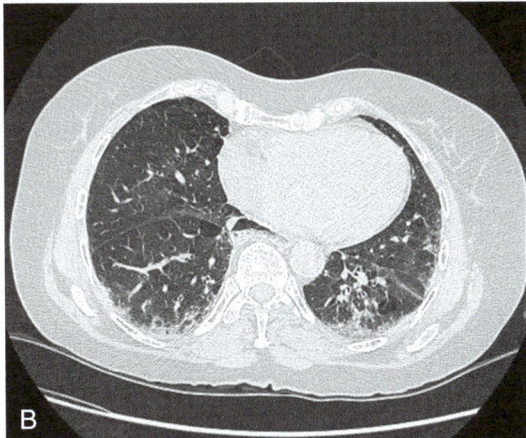
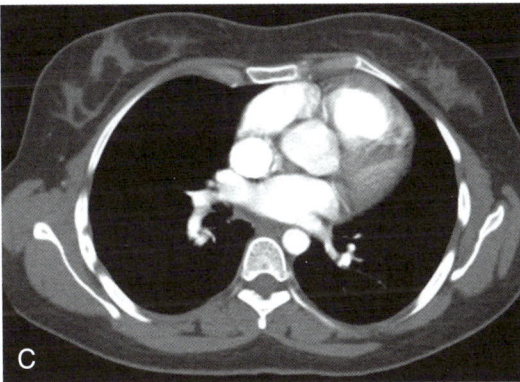

FIGURE 97.9 Systemic sclerosis. **A,** Chest radiograph of a patient with diffuse cutaneous systemic sclerosis showing interstitial shadowing, mainly in the lung bases, along with associated loss of volume, consistent with early pulmonary fibrosis. **B,** CT of the thorax demonstrating ground-glass opacity, subpleural honeycombing with thickening of the interlobular septa, and linear fibrotic bands, in keeping with pulmonary fibrosis. There is also evidence of associated mild traction bronchiectasis. **C,** Pulmonary CTA in a patient with limited cutaneous scleroderma and pulmonary hypertension. The right atrium and right ventricle are enlarged, and there is dilation of the pulmonary trunk.

Rheumatoid Arthritis

Pulmonary complications in RA include pleural effusions, pulmonary nodules, interstitial lung disease, bronchiolitis obliterans, and occasionally PAH. The prevalence of PAH in RA does not differ from that in the general population and does not warrant routine screening.[66] PAH in RA most commonly results from other underlying diseases, including chronic obstructive pulmonary disease, chronic pulmonary thromboembolism, hyperviscosity syndromes, lung surgery, or left-sided heart disease. PAH may also relate to extra-articular manifestations of RA, pulmonary fibrosis, or isolated pulmonary arteritis. Dyspnea is the most common initial symptom, and diagnosis is often delayed, not only because dyspnea is initially attributed to other causes but because of limited exercise capacity in arthritic patients. Diagnosis of PAH by the measures outlined above should be followed by specific investigations such as high-resolution pulmonary CT, CTA, and pulmonary function tests to determine the underlying cause. No specific guidelines inform the treatment of PAH arising as a primary complication of RA. Active RA should be treated aggressively and preferably with biologic agents such as IL-6 receptor antagonists or rituximab. Specific treatment of PAH should also be considered as above.

Sjögren Syndrome

Clinically significant PAH very rarely complicates Sjögren syndrome and usually occurs late, most typically in patients with NYHA functional class III or IV, and the diagnosis is established as described for RA above.[67] Little evidence guides therapeutic decisions, and regimens vary considerably. Therapy with corticosteroids and immunosuppressive drugs, including azathioprine and cyclophosphamide, should be optimized to gain control of the underlying Sjögren syndrome activity. These measures may provide at least transient benefit in PAH, particularly in patients with evidence of active interstitial lung disease. Anecdotal evidence suggests beneficial effects of B cell depletion therapy with rituximab in patients with severe disease and may offer a future approach for those with PAH. In the majority enhanced immunosuppression is combined with standard PAH treatments described above.

Takayasu Arteritis

Pulmonary artery involvement in TA is often overlooked. Yet 50% of patients with TA have evidence of pulmonary arteritis in autopsy studies, and PAH develops in 12%. Even though pulmonary arteritis typically coexists with disease of the aorta, it can be isolated. Systemic hypertension and left ventricular dysfunction may cause secondary PAH. The pulmonary arterial lesions seen include stenoses, occlusions, and aneurysms. PAH may develop acutely early in the disease course or later and more insidiously following progressive pulmonary artery narrowing.[68] When present, symptoms may include dyspnea, chest pain, and peripheral edema. These symptoms are often ascribed to other causes, delaying diagnosis. Unless specifically sought, pulmonary artery involvement can be missed on initial radiologic studies. Dedicated CMR and contrast-enhanced CTA are the most sensitive detection modalities. Abnormalities should be pursued to exclude PAH with echocardiography and other studies as described above.

No available clinical trials guide therapeutic decisions. Aggressive treatment of the underlying arteritis with high-dose corticosteroids and a steroid-sparing drug such as methotrexate is recommended. Pulsed intravenous cyclophosphamide is typically reserved for nonresponders, and biologic therapies including antagonists of TNF-α or IL-6 receptor, should be considered early in refractory disease.[37] Warfarin is often used, particularly in those with evidence of thrombosis or pulmonary infarction. Case reports suggest antagonists of endothelin-1 and PDE5 may help in patients with more severe or resistance PAH. Open reconstructive surgery or percutaneous angioplasty may prove successful.

THROMBOSIS IN THE RHEUMATIC DISEASES (SEE ALSO CHAPTER 95)

Thrombosis is an important pathologic process in many rheumatic diseases and a cause of significant morbidity and mortality. Large-vessel thrombosis, both venous and arterial, can occur in Behçet disease and APS. Thrombosis in situ also occurs in small vessels, principally as the end result of chronic vessel wall hyperplasia or inflammation in diseases such as SSc, the vasculitides, and PAH. Chronic thromboembolic PAH can complicate SLE and SSc.

Activation of the coagulation cascade leading to thrombosis may be caused by abnormalities in the vessel wall, blood constituents, or blood flow (see Chapters 24 and 95). Abnormalities in endothelial function have particular relevance to rheumatic diseases. The prolonged systemic inflammation in patients with SLE, Behçet disease, and the vasculitides can cause endothelial apoptosis, a local inflammatory response, and endothelial activation. Cytokine-mediated endothelial activation disturbs anticoagulant and fibrinolytic mechanisms. Treatment of prothrombotic risk in these diseases requires consideration of approaches that include immunosuppression to control disease activity and minimize endothelial dysfunction, antiplatelet agents, anticoagulation, and the use of statins.

Antiphospholipid Syndrome (see Chapter 95)

APS associates with thrombosis (both arterial and venous) and with first-trimester fetal loss. Laboratory tests demonstrate antiphospholipid antibodies, most commonly anticardiolipin antibodies, anti-beta$_2$-glycoprotein-1 and/or a positive lupus anticoagulant test. Anticardiolipin antibodies, typically of the IgG or IgM isotype and present in medium to high titer, or the lupus anticoagulant should be demonstrated on at least two occasions 12 or more weeks apart. Antiphospholipid antibodies directed against beta$_2$-glycoprotein-1 may activate the endothelium, monocytes, and platelets. This leads to surface expression of cellular adhesion molecules and generation of tissue factor by both monocytes and the vascular endothelium. The increased tissue factor and thromboxane A$_2$ synthesis by platelets results in a procoagulant state. Thrombosis requires a second hit, such as that provided by activation of the complement cascade or intercurrent infection. Laboratory studies have demonstrated that antiphospholipid antibodies enhance leukocyte-endothelial cell interactions and induce thrombosis through inhibition of endothelial nitric oxide (eNOS) activation and nitric oxide biosynthesis. The mechanism involves binding of antibody to domain I of beta$_2$-glycoprotein-1 and impaired eNOS phosphorylation.[69] An important role for aPL-induced NET formation as a driver of thrombosis in APS has also emerged. Moreover, anti-NET antibodies in patients with primary APS may impair NET clearance and activate the complement cascade, novel data that may facilitate patient risk stratification and novel therapeutic approaches.[70]

Cardiovascular Disease

Valvular abnormalities are the most frequently reported cardiac abnormality in patients with APS. The most commonly detected lesions are verrucous (Libman-Sacks) endocarditis and nonspecific valvular thickening (see earlier) (Fig. 97.10). Although lesions are commonly found, clinically significant features are rare. Symptomatic disease is more frequent in those with high antibody titers. Congestive cardiac failure develops in up to 5% of patients, and 13% require cardiac valve replacement. Histologic analysis of the valves reveals deposition of antiphospholipid antibodies with complement activation. Occasionally, amaurosis fugax, transient ischemic attack, or stroke is seen as a consequence of arterial thromboembolism. Coronary thrombosis and myocardial infarction can complicate primary APS in 0.5% to 6% of patients, and intracardiac thrombi can also occur.[69,71] APS in patients with SLE may enhance their risk for myocardial infarction and stroke.

Treatment

Confirmed thrombosis in patients with APS requires anticoagulation. Most centers target an international normalized ratio (INR) of 2.5 to 3.5.[69,71] Some evidence supports the use of low-dose aspirin in patients with SLE complicated by antiphospholipid antibodies. In contrast, low-dose aspirin did not protect against deep venous thrombosis or pulmonary embolic disease in a study of men with primary APS. The role of direct oral anticoagulants (DOACs), including rivaroxaban, compared to vitamin K antagonists for the prevention of APS-related thrombosis remains the subject of on-going research. However, current clinical trial data and guidelines recommend against the use of DOACs in those with a high risk of thrombosis including triple positive patients (anticardiolipin Ab, anti-2-glycoprotein I Ab and lupus anticoagulant positive), while single or double positive patients established on DOACs may continue.[72]

Behçet Disease

Behçet disease occurs throughout the world but most commonly in Turkey, Iran, Japan, and Korea at 80 cases per 100,000 individuals, which falls to 4 to 8 per 100,000 in the United States, France, Germany, and the United Kingdom. This multisystem disorder includes orogenital ulceration, acneiform skin lesions, and arthralgia. It may cause uveitis and blindness in the young. Arthralgia is common, and less frequently, patients suffer from meningoencephalitis, gastrointestinal ulceration, or vascular complications.

The vasculitis associated with Behçet disease predominantly affects the pulmonary arteries and veins, with thrombosis being a prominent clinical feature. Most thrombi are venous and cause superficial thrombophlebitis and deep venous thrombosis, including superior vena cava obstruction, cerebral vein thrombosis, and Budd-Chiari syndrome. In a small number of cases, pulmonary arterial vasculitis leads to in situ pulmonary arterial thrombosis. Although small studies have suggested that thrombosis is linked to the concurrent presence of a prothrombotic condition such as factor V Leiden or prothrombin mutations, this is not thought to be the cause in most. Indirect evidence suggests that the procoagulant state arises from an activated, adhesive, and prothrombotic endothelium due to chronic vascular inflammation. A clinical trial comparing treatment of thrombosis in Behçet disease with anticoagulation, immunosuppression, or a combination of both therapies supports this hypothesis. A higher proportion of patients treated with anticoagulation alone had recurrent thrombosis than did those prescribed immunosuppression.[73] Pulmonary arterial aneurysms are a rare life-threatening complication in Behçet disease (Fig. 97.11), and aneurysms may also occur in other arterial beds. Other cardiovascular complications occur in less than 10% and include pericarditis, myocarditis, intracardiac thrombosis, myocardial infarction, and myocardial aneurysm.

Treatment

The management of Behçet disease has advanced significantly in recent years.[74] The European League Against Rheumatism (EULAR) guidelines recommend immunosuppression for the treatment of thrombosis, an approach typically used in endemic areas. However, first-line treatment of these patients in emergency units in nonendemic areas is usually anticoagulation. This approach is appropriate because the cause of the thrombosis may not be immediately apparent, although patients with aneurysms have a substantial risk for bleeding. Patients should consult a specialist clinic for assessment of the need for long-term anticoagulation, immunosuppressive therapy, and noninvasive angiographic screening for aneurysms. Cardiovascular complications including arterial aneurysms are typically treated aggressively with cyclophosphamide, high-dose prednisone and anticoagulants to reduce inflammatory disease activity before surgical intervention, which may involve stenting via a percutaneous route or open surgical repair.[74] Because the lesions often recur, patients require regular screening. Second line treatments include anti-TNF-α therapy in those with recurrent aneurysms or those who fail to respond to cyclophosphamide (Fig. 97.11). For those with refractory disease, IFN-α has been used successfully, although side-effects are prominent. There is current interest in the use of other biologic agents including those targeting IL-1, IL-17, and IL-12/23.[74]

ANTIRHEUMATIC DRUGS AND CARDIOVASCULAR DISEASE

Drug therapy for the rheumatic diseases has undergone a dramatic transformation over the past 20 years and continues to do so. Contributory factors include advanced biologic insights, more accurate diagnostic tests and imaging data, improved understanding of the mechanistic actions of drugs, and the development of novel targeted therapies. This section emphasizes the beneficial and deleterious effects of antirheumatic drugs on the cardiovascular system.

Relationship Between Drug Treatment and Cardiovascular Disease

Although inflammation contributes to atherogenesis and patients with systemic inflammatory rheumatic diseases have a heightened risk for premature myocardial infarction and stroke, causality remains unproven.[8] The impact of antiinflammatory drugs on atherogenesis and the incidence of cardiovascular events has begun to provide insight in this regard.[4,75] Two recent trials demonstrate that the antiinflammatory effects associated with targeting the inflammasome reduces cardiovascular events.[1,2] Until recently, no clinical trial had convincingly demonstrated a beneficial effect of antiinflammatory drugs on cardiovascular outcomes. Indeed, the traditional NSAIDs or coxibs actually lead to a small but measurable increased risk for thrombosis. However, NSAID use in patients with inflammatory arthritis does not appear to confer increased cardiovascular risk, thus suggesting that their antiinflammatory role predominates.[76] Similarly, statins reduce serum CRP levels, and large clinical trials suggest that in part, statins provide vascular protection independent of their actions on LDL cholesterol, including immunomodulatory and antiinflammatory effects.

INTERLEUKIN-1 INHIBITION AND THE INFLAMMASOME

The CANTOS trial represented a step change in understanding the link between inflammation and atherothrombosis. The interleukin-1β monoclonal antibody canakinumab reduced cardiovascular events in patients with stable coronary artery disease and a baseline high-sensitivity-CRP >2 mg/L, if the hsCRP fell to <2 mg/L or the IL-6 level was reduced to less than the study median after 3 months' treatment (see Chapter 24).[1] Colchicine may act in part by targeting the inflammasome. COLCOT recruited participants to a randomized, double-blind trial of low dose colchicine (0.5 mg daily) within 30 days of myocardial infarction. The significant reduction in the composite primary endpoint of ischemic cardiovascular events in those receiving colchicine versus placebo predominantly reflected a reduction in stroke and in recurrent angina requiring coronary revascularization.[2]

TUMOR NECROSIS FACTOR-ALPHA ANTAGONISTS

TNF-α blockade affords an effective therapy for patients suffering from active RA, psoriatic arthritis, and ankylosing spondylitis. TNF-α can be targeted by monoclonal antibodies given intravenously or subcutaneously, or by subcutaneous injection of etanercept, a soluble TNF receptor fusion protein. The use of these agents is contraindicated in patients with established cardiovascular disease with evidence of NYHA class III and IV cardiac failure, and they should be used with caution in those with mild congestive cardiac failure.[4] In RA the combination of systemic inflammation and traditional risk factors is associated with rapid progression of carotid IMT. Treatment with methotrexate and TNF-α antagonists can reduce this progress,[12] with some evidence for a reduction in cardiovascular events.[77,78] Antiinflammatory treatments can reduce arterial ^{18}F-FDG avidity in patients with RA.[4,8,13,15]

INTERLEUKIN-6 INHIBITION

In light of the role of IL-6 signaling in atherogenesis, tocilizumab and sarilumab—inhibitors of IL-6R signaling—might be expected to have vasculoprotective effects and, at least in the short term, IL-6R inhibition may improve both endothelial function and aortic stiffness. However, these agents may also adversely affect lipid profiles and increase LDL cholesterol, thereby requiring the addition of a statin. Current data suggest that the rate of cardiovascular events in those receiving IL-6R inhibitors is equivalent to that in RA patients prescribed etanercept.[79]

INTERLEUKIN-17 INHIBITION

The role of IL-17A in atherothrombosis remains to be completely defined. Anti-IL-17 immunotherapy is increasingly used for the treatment of psoriasis and psoriatic arthritis. Clinical studies to date have not shown reduced cardiovascular risk.[80,81]

INTERLEUKIN-12 AND INTERLEUKIN-23 INHIBITION

Ustekinumab targets both IL-12 and IL-23 and is licensed for use in psoriasis and psoriatic arthritis. Preliminary clinical data derived from meta-analyses suggest that there might be an increased risk of major adverse cardiovascular events in those with pre-existing cardiovascular disease prescribed anti-IL12/23 antibodies.[4] As IL-23 selective monoclonal antibodies are now also entering clinical practice, cardiovascular risk data must be carefully sought.

B Cell Depletion

Rituximab targets CD20 and depletes B lymphocytes. Initially established as a treatment of B cell lymphoma, rituximab can control RA disease activity and reduce erosions. Similarly, rituximab exhibits efficacy equivalent to that of cyclophosphamide for the treatment of ANCA-associated vasculitis and may exert disease-modulating effects in SLE. Although long-term, adequately powered clinical trials with primary cardiovascular endpoints are required, evidence to date has not identified significant cardiovascular risk associated with rituximab therapy.[75,82] Conflicting results have been reported concerning its effect

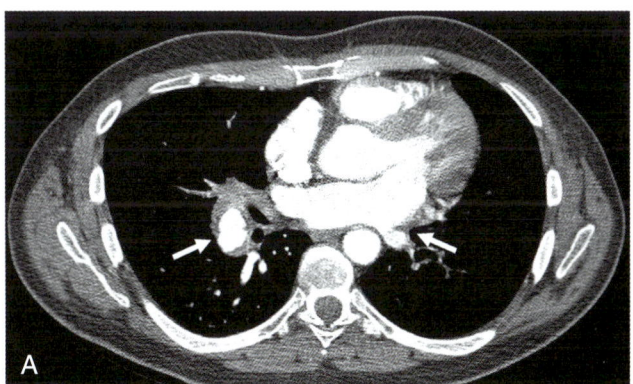

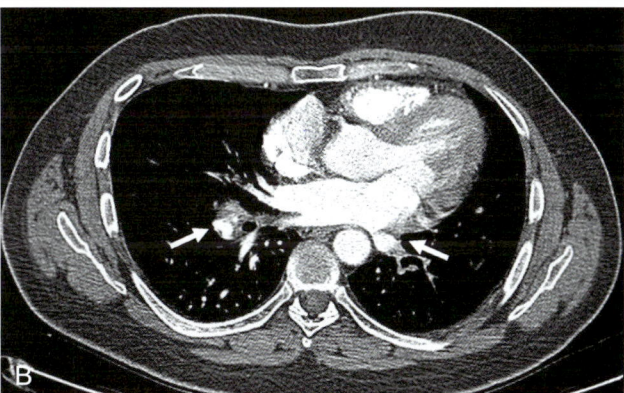

FIGURE 97.11 **A,** CT angiogram of a patient with Behçet disease showing bilateral pulmonary artery aneurysms (*arrows*). **B,** Following 4 months of treatment with tumor necrosis factor-α antagonist infliximab, some reduction in the size of the pulmonary aneurysm on the right is seen. (Courtesy Professor Dorian Haskard, National Heart and Lung Institute, Imperial College London.)

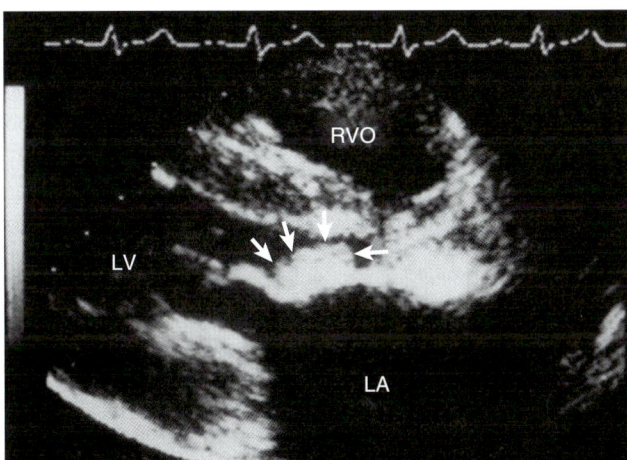

FIGURE 97.10 Parasternal long-axis view of the heart from a patient with SLE and high-titer antiphospholipid antibodies. A massive vegetation is seen on the ventricular surface of the anterior mitral leaflet (*arrows*), but it is not interfering with valve mobility. *LA*, Left atrium; *LV*, left ventricle; *RVO*, right ventricular outflow; *SLE*, systemic lupus erythematosus. (Courtesy Professor Petros Nihoyannopoulos, National Heart and Lung Institute, Imperial College London.)

on lipid profiles and these should be monitored. Following the reports of protective effects of B-cell depletion in mice with experimental atherosclerosis and myocardial infarction, a small phase I/II clinical trial of rituximab in patients suffering acute myocardial infarction showed reduced CRP and BNP (https://clinicaltrials.gov/ Identifier: NCT03072199).[4] Severe cardiovascular complications have occurred following rituximab infusions. Regulatory agency advice is that this treatment should be used with caution and the infusion rate reduced in those with preexisting cardiorespiratory disease and avoided in those with NYHA Class III and IV heart failure.

Methotrexate

Methotrexate in dosages up to 25 mg/wk has proven to be remarkably effective in treatment of RA and other inflammatory arthritides and is frequently used as a steroid-sparing drug in the vasculitides. The majority of clinical evidence suggests that methotrexate has a cardiovascular protective effect in patients with inflammatory arthritis, with those responding to methotrexate therapy demonstrating improvement in endothelial function. A recent consecutive meta-analysis confirmed early reports of a relative risk reduction in cardiovascular mortality in patients with RA and psoriatic arthritis prescribed methotrexate.[77] Novel additional mechanisms potentially underlying vascular protection include activation of an AMP-activated kinase and cyclic AMP response element-binding protein-dependent pathway[83] and beneficial effects on macrophage cholesterol handling.[84] These cardioprotective actions of methotrexate inspired the Cardiovascular Inflammation Reduction Trial (CIRT) in which patients with a previous myocardial infarction or multivessel coronary disease, as well as type 2 diabetes mellitus and/or the metabolic syndrome, were prescribed methotrexate (15 to 20 mg/wk) or placebo. No benefit from methotrexate was detected; this is likely because, and in contrast to CANTOS, CIRT participants had a median CRP of 1.5 mg/L at entry.[1,85] The different findings of CANTOS and CIRT imply that patient stratification and selection are essential for future studies.

Other Disease-Modifying Antirheumatic Drugs

The potential cardiovascular benefits of hydroxychloroquine, an antimalarial drug frequently used for the treatment of RA, SLE, and Sjögren syndrome, have become more widely recognized in recent years. Hydroxychloroquine lowers cholesterol and may improve both endothelial function and aortic stiffness. Clinical studies have demonstrated that hydroxychloroquine reduces the risk for cardiovascular events in patients with both RA and SLE. In contrast, concern regarding a prolonged QT interval, occasional association of high cumulative dosages with restrictive cardiomyopathy and with retinal damage require monitoring.

Cyclosporine continues to be used for the treatment of rheumatic disease on occasion, including polymyositis, Behçet diseases, SLE, and RA, as well as in many patients following organ transplantation. Clinical studies suggest that cyclosporine impairs flow-mediated vasodilation. At least in part, this effect reflects reduced eNOS activity and nitric oxide bioavailability. The adverse cardiovascular effects seen with cyclosporine may also reflect its propensity to induce hypertension and renal impairment. Alternative immunosuppressive drugs, used predominantly in the transplantation scenario, including tacrolimus and rapamycin (sirolimus), appear to have a more favorable vascular profile. JAK inhibitors (tofacitinib, baricitinib) are oral small inhibitors with disease-modifying efficacy in RA and psoriatic arthritis.[20] Data concerning effects of these agents on cardiovascular risk is sparse. A study of tofacitinib in RA reported an increase in cholesterol levels.[86]

Glucocorticoids

Glucocorticoids have undisputed efficacy in the treatment of systemic inflammatory diseases, including RA, SLE, and the vasculitides. Yet the substantial side effect burden concerns patients and physicians alike prompting the increased use of low-dose and rapid taper protocols. The influence of corticosteroid therapy on the progression of atherosclerosis is complex and dependent on the context. Their impact on blood pressure and glucose and lipid metabolism may have a deleterious effect. In contrast, in SLE, evidence suggests that insufficient use of glucocorticoids risks persistently active and/or relapsing disease, thereby leading to an increased risk for accelerated atherogenesis. Thus combination therapy with a steroid-sparing drug such as azathioprine, MMF, methotrexate or biologic agents, which allows prednisone to be tapered to 7.5 mg/day or less, may be optimal.

Statins (see Chapters 25 and 27)

Large primary prevention trials indicate that statins can reduce cardiovascular morbidity and mortality, in part independently of changes in LDL cholesterol.[87] These actions have led to interest in statins as adjunctive therapy for rheumatic diseases, including RA and SLE, for which they have the potential to both reduce disease activity and lower cardiovascular risk.[88] Although meta-analyses indicate some antiinflammatory benefit,[89] clinical trial evidence supporting the routine use of statins in all patients with rheumatic diseases is relatively lacking. The recent Trial of Atorvastatin for the Primary Prevention of Cardiovascular Events in Patients with Rheumatoid Arthritis (TRACE RA) demonstrated the safety of atorvastatin 40 mg daily, a significant fall in the LDL cholesterol and a 34% cardiovascular events (CVE) risk reduction versus placebo, consistent with statin effects in other populations.[23] Although no guidelines exist, most rheumatologists currently consider the cardiovascular risk in patients with RA and SLE as equivalent to that in patients with diabetes mellitus. EULAR has suggested adding a 1.5× multiplier to standard cardiovascular risk calculations, while recent reports have recommended further expansion of the cardiovascular risk prediction score for RA.[75,90] Indications for a statin include an LDL cholesterol level of 190 mg/dL or higher, a long history of RA, a family history of hyperlipidemia, higher age at disease onset, and the presence of any other cardiovascular risk factors.[26]

Nonsteroidal Antiinflammatory Drugs

NSAIDs and coxibs are important and effective drugs for the treatment of pain and inflammation. Concerns regarding atherothrombotic complications have, however, raised reservations regarding their use. As a consequence, patients with rheumatic disease are often denied these medications inappropriately. Although current evidence suggests that both classes have a small, manageable, and dose-dependent risk for cardiovascular complications, establishing the degree of risk and the relative safety profiles between individual drugs is difficult because of clinical trial heterogeneity and a lack of randomized controlled trial data for older NSAIDs. Data overall suggest that no traditional NSAID or COX-2 inhibitor is entirely safe and that naproxen has the best cardiovascular profile as a result of its antiplatelet effects and that diclofenac may have the worst.[14,91] Despite these reservations, the absolute risk for a cardiovascular event is very low, and gastrointestinal bleeding and perforation likely represent the major long-term risk associated with NSAIDs (Table 97.5). Although coxibs are less likely to cause gastrointestinal problems, many guidelines recommend concomitant prescription of a proton pump inhibitor for patients taking either NSAIDs or coxibs for more than 10 to 14 days.

Current data concerning the use of NSAIDs and coxibs in rheumatic diseases are beginning to shift significantly. Data from studies comparing NSAIDs and coxibs in patients with arthritis do not support a class effect based on COX-2 selectivity. Moreover, longitudinal cohort analysis of NSAID use in RA and ankylosing spondylitis reveals only a small increase in cardiovascular events, which was lower than that recorded in the general population and with a low versus high intake of NSAIDs.[76] The difference may reflect the impact of these drugs on inflammation and minimization of an echo effect.[8,13] The study population is important, and few studies have looked in detail at patients with inflammatory arthritis. The Prospective Randomized Evaluation of Celecoxib Integrated Safety versus Ibuprofen or Naproxen (PRECISION) trial enrolled 24,081 RA or osteoarthritis patients with established or significant risk of cardiovascular disease.[21] Following

TABLE 97.5 Cardiovascular Versus Gastrointestinal Risk in Prescribing Nonsteroidal Antiinflammatory Drugs

Patients with CV risk who are taking aspirin should avoid tNSAIDs or coxibs if possible
If essential, consider naproxen plus a PPI if GI risk is low or a coxib in those with significant GI risk
Cardiovascular risk varies between individual tNSAIDs and coxibs
Risk for CV events appears lower in those with inflammatory rheumatic diseases
Patients with cardiac failure or hypertension should avoid tNSAIDs and coxibs
Risk for a CV event with a tNSAID or coxib is <1% in those with <2 classic risk factors
Risk for a CV event may increase in older adults, men, and those with preexisting CV disease
Aspirin use increases the risk for GI events associated with tNSAIDs and coxibs
Coprescription of a PPI reduces the risk for GI events with tNSAIDs and coxibs
PPIs are more effective than H_2 antagonists or misoprostol for gastroprotection
Gastrointestinal risk varies between individual tNSAIDs
Use the lowest effective dose for the shortest period

coxibs, COX-2–selective antiinflammatory drugs; *CV*, cardiovascular; *GI*, gastrointestinal; *PPI*, proton pump inhibitor; *tNSAIDs*, traditional NSAIDs.

prescription of esomeprazole and randomization to moderate dose celecoxib, naproxen or ibuprofen, cardiovascular death, nonfatal stroke, and myocardial infarction were recorded. Although drug discontinuation rates were high, the trial revealed celecoxib to be noninferior to naproxen and ibuprofen with respect to cardiovascular safety and significantly safer than either comparator regarding gastrointestinal risk. These data provide important reassurance concerning the safety of moderate doses of celecoxib.

Wherever possible, NSAIDs and coxibs should be avoided in patients with known ischemic heart disease, previous thrombosis, poorly controlled hypertension, kidney disease, and cardiac failure. In patients in whom antiinflammatory drugs are being considered, an individualized assessment of both gastrointestinal and cardiovascular risk should be made. The patient should be encouraged to use these drugs when required and at the minimally effective dose rather than as a standing dose (see Table 97.5).

FUTURE PERSPECTIVES

The rapid development of novel biologics and small molecules targeting inflammatory pathways offers considerable promise for cardiovascular disease.[92] The current challenge is to design and perform adequately powered randomized clinical trials to investigate the efficacy of individual antiinflammatory drugs in preventing cardiovascular events. These drugs need to be affordable and sufficiently tractable for use in cardiovascular clinical practice. The data from the CANTOS and COLCOT clinical trials provide the impetus for further RCTs. The ultimate aim is to test the hypothesis that a relatively aggressive antiinflammatory approach, alongside conventional therapy, will confer additional benefit in those with known atherosclerotic coronary artery disease in the absence of an underlying rheumatic problem.

REFERENCES
Background
1. Ridker PM, Everett BM, Thuren T, et al. Antiinflammatory therapy with canakinumab for atherosclerotic disease. *N Engl J Med.* 2017;377:1119–1131.
2. Tardif JC, Kouz S, Waters DD, et al. Efficacy and safety of low-dose colchicine after myocardial infarction. *N Engl J Med.* 2019;381:2497–2505.
3. Prasad M, Hermann J, Gabriel SE, et al. Cardiorheumatology: cardiac involvement in systemic rheumatic disease. *Nat Rev Cardiol.* 2015;12:168–176.
4. Ait-Oufella H, Libby P, Tedgui A. Anticytokine immune therapy and atherothrombotic cardiovascular risk. *Arterioscler Thromb Vasc Biol.* 2019;39:1510–1519.
5. Libby P, Pasterkamp G, Crea F, Jang IK. Reassessing the mechanisms of acute coronary syndromes. *Circ Res.* 2019;124:150–160.
6. Skeoch S, Bruce IN. Atherosclerosis in rheumatoid arthritis: is it all about inflammation? *Nat Rev Rheumatol.* 2015;11:390–400.
7. Skeoch S, Williams H, Cristinacce P, et al. Evaluation of carotid plaque inflammation in patients with active rheumatoid arthritis using (18)F-fluorodeoxyglucose PET-CT and MRI: a pilot study. *Lancet.* 2015;385(suppl 1):S91.
8. Mason JC, Libby P. Cardiovascular disease in patients with chronic inflammation: mechanisms underlying premature cardiovascular events in rheumatologic conditions. *Eur Heart J.* 2015;36:482–489.
9. Jaiswal S, Libby P. Clonal haematopoiesis: connecting ageing and inflammation in cardiovascular disease. *Nat Rev Cardiol.* 2020;17:137–144.
10. Erre GL, Buscetta G, Paliogiannis P, et al. Coronary flow reserve in systemic rheumatic diseases: a systematic review and meta-analysis. *Rheumatol Int.* 2018;38:1179–1190.
11. Totoson P, Maguin-Gate K, Nappey M, et al. Microvascular abnormalities in adjuvant-induced arthritis: relationship to macrovascular endothelial function and markers of endothelial activation. *Arthritis Rheumatol.* 2015;67:1203–1213.
12. Del Rincon I, Polak JF, O'Leary DH, et al. Systemic inflammation and cardiovascular risk factors predict rapid progression of atherosclerosis in rheumatoid arthritis. *Ann Rheum Dis.* 2015;74:1118–1123.
13. Libby P, Nahrendorf M, Swirski FK. Leukocytes link local and systemic inflammation in ischemic cardiovascular disease: an expanded "cardiovascular continuum". *J Am Coll Cardiol.* 2016;67:1091–1103.
14. Agca R, Heslinga SC, Rollefstad S, et al. EULAR recommendations for cardiovascular disease risk management in patients with rheumatoid arthritis and other forms of inflammatory joint disorders: 2015/2016 update. *Ann Rheum Dis.* 2017;76:17–28.
15. Ferguson LD, Siebert S, McInnes IB, Sattar N. Cardiometabolic comorbidities in RA and PsA: lessons learned and future directions. *Nat Rev Rheumatol.* 2019;15:461–474.
16. Skielta M, Soderstrom L, Rantapaa-Dahlqvist S, et al. Trends in mortality, co-morbidity and treatment after acute myocardial infarction in patients with rheumatoid arthritis 1998-2013. *Eur Heart J Acute Cardiovasc Care.* 2020;9:931–938.
17. Elbadawi A, Ahmed HH, Elgendy IY, et al. Outcomes of acute myocardial infarction in patients with rheumatoid arthritis. *Am J Med.* 2020.
18. Solomon DH, Reed GW, Kremer JM, et al. Disease activity in rheumatoid arthritis and the risk of cardiovascular events. *Arthritis Rheumatol.* 2015;67:1449–1455.
19. Aletaha D. Precision medicine and management of rheumatoid arthritis. *J Autoimmun.* 2020;110:102405.
20. You H, Xu D, Zhao J, et al. JAK inhibitors: prospects in connective tissue diseases. *Clin Rev Allergy Immunol.* 2020.
21. Nissen SE, Yeomans ND, Solomon DH, et al. Cardiovascular safety of celecoxib, naproxen, or ibuprofen for arthritis. *N Engl J Med.* 2016;375:2519–2529.
22. Semb AG, Ikdahl E, Wibetoe G, Crowson C, Rollefstad S. Atherosclerotic cardiovascular disease prevention in rheumatoid arthritis. *Nat Rev Rheumatol.* 2020;16:361–379.
23. Kitas GD, Nightingale P, Armitage J, et al. A multicenter, randomized, placebo-controlled trial of atorvastatin for the primary prevention of cardiovascular events in patients with rheumatoid arthritis. *Arthritis Rheumatol.* 2019;71:1437–1449.
24. Catalina MD, Owen KA, Labonte AC, et al. The pathogenesis of systemic lupus erythematosus: harnessing big data to understand the molecular basis of lupus. *J Autoimmun.* 2019:102359.
25. Giannelou M, Mavragani CP. Cardiovascular disease in systemic lupus erythematosus: a comprehensive update. *J Autoimmun.* 2017;82:1–12.
26. Liu Y, Kaplan MJ. Cardiovascular disease in systemic lupus erythematosus: an update. *Curr Opin Rheumatol.* 2018;30:441–448.
27. Gatto M, Zen M, Iaccarino L, Doria A. New therapeutic strategies in systemic lupus erythematosus management. *Nat Rev Rheumatol.* 2019;15:30–48.
28. Murphy G, Isenberg DA. New therapies for systemic lupus erythematosus - past imperfect, future tense. *Nat Rev Rheumatol.* 2019;15:403–412.
29. van Vollenhoven R. String of successful trials in SLE: have we cracked the code? *Lupus Sci Med.* 2020;7:e000380.
30. Stamp LK, Dalbeth N. Prevention and treatment of gout. *Nat Rev Rheumatol.* 2019;15:68–70.

Vasculitides
31. Liew JW, Ramiro S, Gensler LS. Cardiovascular morbidity and mortality in ankylosing spondylitis and psoriatic arthritis. *Best Pract Res Clin Rheumatol.* 2018;32:369–389.
32. Watts RA, Robson J. Introduction, epidemiology and classification of vasculitis. *Best Pract Res Clin Rheumatol.* 2018;32:3–20.
33. Dejaco C, Brouwer E, Mason JC, et al. Giant cell arteritis and polymyalgia rheumatica: current challenges and opportunities. *Nat Rev Rheumatol.* 2017;13:578–592.
34. Berti A, Dejaco C. Update on the epidemiology, risk factors, and outcomes of systemic vasculitides. *Best Pract Res Clin Rheumatol.* 2018;32:271–294.
35. Dejaco C, Ramiro S, Duftner C, et al. EULAR recommendations for the use of imaging in large vessel vasculitis in clinical practice. *Ann Rheum Dis.* 2018;77:636–643.
36. Udayakumar PD, Chandran AK, Crowson CS, et al. Cardiovascular risk and acute coronary syndrome in giant cell arteritis: a population-based retrospective cohort study. *Arthritis Care Res (Hoboken).* 2015;67:396–402.
37. Tombetti E, Mason JC. Takayasu arteritis: advanced understanding is leading to new horizons. *Rheumatology (Oxford).* 2019;58:206–219.
38. Tombetti E, Mason JC. Application of imaging techniques for Takayasu arteritis. *Presse Med.* 2017;46:e215–e223.
39. Whittaker E, Bamford A, Kenny J, et al. Clinical characteristics of 58 children with a pediatric inflammatory multisystem syndrome temporally associated with SARS-CoV-2. *J Am Med Assoc.* 2020.
40. Soni PR, Noval Rivas M, Arditi M. A comprehensive update on Kawasaki disease vasculitis and myocarditis. *Curr Rheumatol Rep.* 2020;22:6.
41. Perugino CA, Wallace ZS, Meyersohn N, et al. Large vessel involvement by IgG4-related disease. *Medicine (Baltim).* 2016;95:e3344.
42. Watanabe R, Goronzy JJ, Berry G, et al. Giant cell arteritis: from pathogenesis to therapeutic management. *Curr Treatm Opt Rheumatol.* 2016;2:126–137.
43. Mackie SL, Dejaco C, Appenzeller S, et al. British Society for Rheumatology guideline on diagnosis and treatment of giant cell arteritis. *Rheumatology (Oxford).* 2020;59:e1–e23.
44. Stone JH, Tuckwell K, Dimonaco S, et al. Trial of tocilizumab in giant-cell arteritis. *N Engl J Med.* 2017;377:317–328.
45. Hellmich B, Agueda A, Monti S, et al. 2018 Update of the EULAR recommendations for the management of large vessel vasculitis. *Ann Rheum Dis.* 2020;79:19–30.
46. Nakaoka Y, Isobe M, Takei S, et al. Efficacy and safety of tocilizumab in patients with refractory Takayasu arteritis: results from a randomised, double-blind, placebo-controlled, phase 3 trial in Japan (the TAKT study). *Ann Rheum Dis.* 2018;77:348–354.

47. Mason JC. Surgical intervention and its role in Takayasu arteritis. *Best Pract Res Clin Rheumatol.* 2018;32:112–124.
48. Nakazawa D, Masuda S, Tomaru U, Ishizu A. Pathogenesis and therapeutic interventions for ANCA-associated vasculitis. *Nat Rev Rheumatol.* 2019;15:91–101.
49. Yune S, Choi DC, Lee BJ, et al. Detecting cardiac involvement with magnetic resonance in patients with active eosinophilic granulomatosis with polyangiitis. *Int J Cardiovasc Imaging.* 2016;32(suppl 1):155–162.
50. Wechsler ME, Akuthota P, Jayne D, et al. Mepolizumab or placebo for eosinophilic granulomatosis with polyangiitis. *N Engl J Med.* 2017;376:1921–1932.
51. Yates M, Watts RA, Bajema IM, et al. EULAR/ERA-EDTA recommendations for the management of ANCA-associated vasculitis. *Ann Rheum Dis.* 2016;75:1583–1594.
52. Denton CP, Khanna D. Systemic sclerosis. *Lancet.* 2017;390:1685–1699.
53. Volkmann ER, Varga J. Emerging targets of disease-modifying therapy for systemic sclerosis. *Nat Rev Rheumatol.* 2019;15:208–224.
54. Adler Y, Charron P, Imazio M, et al. 2015 ESC guidelines for the diagnosis and management of pericardial diseases: the task force for the diagnosis and management of pericardial diseases of the European Society of Cardiology (ESC) endorsed by: the European Association for Cardio-Thoracic Surgery (EACTS). *Eur Heart J.* 2015;36:2921–2964.
55. Mavrogeni S, Koutsogeorgopoulou L, Markousis-Mavrogenis G, et al. Cardiovascular magnetic resonance detects silent heart disease missed by echocardiography in systemic lupus erythematosus. *Lupus.* 2018;27:564–571.
56. Bechman K, Gopalan D, Nihoyannopoulos P, Mason JC. A cohort study reveals myocarditis to be a rare and life-threatening presentation of large vessel vasculitis. *Semin Arthritis Rheum.* 2017;47:241–246.
57. Kolitz T, Shiber S, Sharabi I, et al. Cardiac manifestations of antiphospholipid syndrome with focus on its primary form. *Front Immunol.* 2019;10:941.
58. Sieper J, Poddubnyy D, Miossec P. The IL-23-IL-17 pathway as a therapeutic target in axial spondyloarthritis. *Nat Rev Rheumatol.* 2019;15:747–757.
59. Lazzerini PE, Capecchi PL, Laghi-Pasini F. Systemic inflammation and arrhythmic risk: lessons from rheumatoid arthritis. *Eur Heart J.* 2017;38:1717–1727.

Pulmonary Hypertension

60. Denton CP, Wells AU, Coghlan JG. Major lung complications of systemic sclerosis. *Nat Rev Rheumatol.* 2018;14:511–527.
61. Saygin D, Domsic RT. Pulmonary arterial hypertension in systemic sclerosis: challenges in diagnosis, screening and treatment. *Open Access Rheumatol.* 2019;11:323–333.
62. Galie N, Humbert M, Vachiery JL, et al. 2015 ESC/ERS guidelines for the diagnosis and treatment of pulmonary hypertension: the joint task force for the diagnosis and treatment of pulmonary hypertension of the European Society of Cardiology (ESC) and the European Respiratory Society (ERS): endorsed by: association for European Paediatric and Congenital Cardiology (AEPC), International Society for Heart and Lung Transplantation (ISHLT). *Eur Heart J.* 2016;37:67–119.
63. Lee MH, Bull TM. The role of pulmonary arterial hypertension-targeted therapy in systemic sclerosis. *F1000Res.* 2019;8.
64. Hannah JR, D'Cruz DP. Pulmonary complications of systemic lupus erythematosus. *Semin Respir Crit Care Med.* 2019;40:227–234.
65. Kommireddy S, Bhyravavajhala S, Kurimeti K, et al. Pulmonary arterial hypertension in systemic lupus erythematosus may benefit by addition of immunosuppression to vasodilator therapy: an observational study. *Rheumatology (Oxford).* 2015;54:1673–1679.
66. Montani D, Henry J, O'Connell C, et al. Association between rheumatoid arthritis and pulmonary hypertension: data from the French pulmonary hypertension registry. *Respiration.* 2018;95:244–250.
67. Flament T, Bigot A, Chaigne B, et al. Pulmonary manifestations of Sjogren's syndrome. *Eur Respir Rev.* 2016;25:110–123.
68. He Y, Lv N, Dang A, Cheng N. Pulmonary artery involvement in patients with Takayasu arteritis. *J Rheumatol.* 2020;47:264–272.

Management Strategies

69. Petri M. Antiphospholipid syndrome. *Transl Res.* 2020.
70. Zuo Y, Yalavarthi S, Gockman K, et al. Anti-NET antibodies and impaired NET degradation in antiphospholipid syndrome. *Arthritis Rheumatol.* 2020.
71. Oliveira DC, Correia A, Oliveira C. The issue of the antiphospholipid antibody syndrome. *J Clin Med Res.* 2020;12:286–292.
72. Wahl D, Dufrost V. Direct oral anticoagulants in antiphospholipid syndrome: too early or too late? *Ann Intern Med.* 2019;171:765–766.
73. Emmi G, Bettiol A, Silvestri E, et al. Vascular Behcet's syndrome: an update. *Intern Emerg Med.* 2019;14:645–652.
74. Bettiol A, Hatemi G, Vannozzi L, et al. Treating the different phenotypes of behcet's syndrome. *Front Immunol.* 2019;10:2830.
75. Halacoglu J, Shea LA. Cardiovascular risk assessment and therapeutic implications in rheumatoid arthritis. *J Cardiovasc Transl Res.* 2020.
76. Braun J, Baraliakos X, Westhoff T. Nonsteroidal anti-inflammatory drugs and cardiovascular risk - a matter of indication. *Semin Arthritis Rheum.* 2020;50:285–288.
77. Roubille C, Richer V, Starnino T, et al. The effects of tumour necrosis factor inhibitors, methotrexate, non-steroidal anti-inflammatory drugs and corticosteroids on cardiovascular events in rheumatoid arthritis, psoriasis and psoriatic arthritis: a systematic review and meta-analysis. *Ann Rheum Dis.* 2015;74:480–489.
78. Low AS, Symmons DP, Lunt M, et al. Relationship between exposure to tumour necrosis factor inhibitor therapy and incidence and severity of myocardial infarction in patients with rheumatoid arthritis. *Ann Rheum Dis.* 2017;76:654–660.
79. Choy EH, De Benedetti F, Takeuchi T, et al. Translating IL-6 biology into effective treatments. *Nat Rev Rheumatol.* 2020;16:335–345.
80. Baeten D, Sieper J, Braun J, et al. Secukinumab, an interleukin-17A inhibitor, in ankylosing spondylitis. *N Engl J Med.* 2015;373:2534–2548.
81. Mease PJ, McInnes IB, Kirkham B, et al. Secukinumab inhibition of interleukin-17A in patients with psoriatic arthritis. *N Engl J Med.* 2015;373:1329–1339.
82. Cohen MD, Keystone E. Rituximab for rheumatoid arthritis. *Rheumatol Ther.* 2015;2:99–111.
83. Thornton CC, Al-Rashed F, Calay D, et al. Methotrexate-mediated activation of an AMPK-CREB-dependent pathway: a novel mechanism for vascular protection in chronic systemic inflammation. *Ann Rheum Dis.* 2016;75:439–448.
84. Ronda N, Greco D, Adorni MP, et al. Newly identified antiatherosclerotic activity of methotrexate and adalimumab: complementary effects on lipoprotein function and macrophage cholesterol metabolism. *Arthritis Rheumatol.* 2015;67:1155–1164.
85. Ridker PM, Everett BM, Pradhan A, et al. Low-dose methotrexate for the prevention of atherosclerotic events. *N Engl J Med.* 2019;380:752–762.
86. Charles-Schoeman C, Fleischmann R, Davignon J, et al. Potential mechanisms leading to the abnormal lipid profile in patients with rheumatoid arthritis versus healthy volunteers and reversal by tofacitinib. *Arthritis Rheumatol.* 2015;67:616–625.
87. Satoh M, Takahashi Y, Tabuchi T, et al. Cellular and molecular mechanisms of statins: an update on pleiotropic effects. *Clin Sci (Lond).* 2015;129:93–105.
88. Xing B, Yin YF, Zhao LD, et al. Effect of 3-hydroxy-3-methylglutaryl-coenzyme a reductase inhibitor on disease activity in patients with rheumatoid arthritis: a meta-analysis. *Medicine (Baltim).* 2015;94:e572.
89. Li GM, Zhao J, Li B, et al. The anti-inflammatory effects of statins on patients with rheumatoid arthritis: a systemic review and meta-analysis of 15 randomized controlled trials. *Autoimmun Rev.* 2018;17:215–225.
90. Solomon DH, Greenberg J, Curtis JR, et al. Derivation and internal validation of an expanded cardiovascular risk prediction score for rheumatoid arthritis: a Consortium of Rheumatology Researchers of North America Registry Study. *Arthritis Rheumatol.* 2015;67:1995–2003.
91. Schjerning AM, McGettigan P, Gislason G. Cardiovascular effects and safety of (non-aspirin) NSAIDs. *Nat Rev Cardiol.* 2020.
92. Ridker PM. Anticytokine agents: targeting interleukin signaling pathways for the treatment of atherothrombosis. *Circ Res.* 2019;124:437–450.

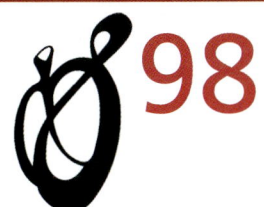

98 Tumors Affecting the Cardiovascular System

DANIEL J. LENIHAN, MICHAEL J. REARDON, AND W. GREGORY HUNDLEY

CLINICAL MANIFESTATION OF CARDIAC TUMORS, 1829
Initial Clinical Decision Making Regarding Cardiac Masses, 1829
Classification of Cardiac Tumors, 1830

BENIGN (NONMALIGNANT) PRIMARY CARDIAC TUMORS, 1830
Simple Benign Tumors, 1830
Complex Benign Tumors, 1834

MALIGNANT PRIMARY CARDIAC TUMORS, 1835
Sarcomas, 1835

SECONDARY CARDIAC TUMORS, 1837
Treatment, 1838

DIRECT AND INDIRECT COMPLICATIONS OF NEOPLASIA, 1838
Pericardial Effusion, 1839

Cardiac Tamponade, 1839
Constrictive Pericarditis, 1839
Superior Vena Cava Syndrome, 1839

FUTURE PERSPECTIVES, 1839

REFERENCES, 1839

Cardiac masses frequently present significant diagnostic and therapeutic clinical challenges. In many cases, a cardiac mass is detected as an incidental finding and the resultant evaluation may culminate in the confirmation of a cardiac tumor; however, this is generally an uncommon event since other cardiac masses, including normal structures (particularly within the right atrium), thrombi, or valvular vegetations are more common.[1,2] This chapter describes the initial symptoms and signs that may indicate a cardiac tumor, followed by an explanation that often includes cardiovascular imaging. Once a cardiac tumor is suspected, the ultimate diagnosis is usually confirmed by a biopsy or surgery as histologic diagnosis has a direct bearing on further treatment planning. The remainder of the chapter focuses on the delineation and potential management of cardiac tumors as well as the overall anticipated outcomes. In many cases, the final pathologic diagnosis is typically confirmed by surgical removal after many difficult decisions regarding investigations and treatment are made in relation to the urgency of the clinical situation and initial presentation.

CLINICAL MANIFESTATION OF CARDIAC TUMORS

Initial Clinical Decision Making Regarding Cardiac Masses

Patients with cardiac tumors may present with no symptoms or physical findings and receive notification of an abnormality on an imaging examination performed for an unrelated indication. Alternatively, patients may experience nonspecific or detailed symptoms or signs that should alert practitioners to the possibility of a cardiac tumor (Table 98.1). The most important consideration in confirming the presence of a cardiac tumor is a high index of suspicion and the integration of symptoms, physical findings, and imaging characteristics in a logical manner to establish a clinically reasonable plan of action. The initial diagnostic test for a patient with concerning symptoms often involves an imaging test (Table 98.2), such as two-dimensional (2D) echocardiography (2D-echo) (see Chapter 16)[3] or cardiac magnetic resonance imaging (cMRI) (see Chapter 19).[4] Depending on the characteristics of this mass and the known comorbidities of the patient, additional imaging may be undertaken.[5] These including three-dimensional (3D) echo with or without contrast (see Chapter 16),[6] cMRI with gadolinium[7] (see Chapter 19), coronary angiography (to define the presence of coronary artery disease) (see Chapter 21),[8] positron emission testing (PET) to provide staging for cancer (see Chapter 18),[8] or computed tomography (CT) (see Chapter 20), including a CT angiogram (CTA) to clarify intrathoracic structures.[9,10] Transesophageal echocardiography (TEE) can also provide very specific anatomical information that is critical to treatment planning (see Chapter 16).[8]

Clinical Scenarios When Evaluating a Cardiac Mass

In assessing a cardiac mass as the initial evaluation for a cardiac tumor, the clinical context in which the image was obtained is critical for making a diagnosis. A differential diagnosis of a cardiac mass is broad and includes tumors, thrombi, infection, and artifacts (Table 98.3). The most important characteristic would be evidence of perfusion into the mass as an indicator of a benign or malignant tumor.[5] When considering typically encountered clinical scenarios, a patient with new-onset heart failure and severe left ventricular (LV) dysfunction, who has a 2D-echo image that shows an apical mass, a cardiac tumor is quite unlikely. This suspicion would be firmly established if there was a severe wall motion abnormality in that region, the mass appeared distinct from the myocardial wall and was lobulated (Fig. 98.1). An LV mass with these characteristics is much more likely to be a thrombus as opposed to a tumor. Additionally, patients treated for cancer with indwelling catheters may experience development of abnormal masses, which may be observed during routine screening for cardiac dysfunction. As shown in Figure 98.2, this right atrial mass seen during transthoracic echocardiogram and then characterized more completely with cardiovascular MRI is consistent with a thrombus.

Another scenario involves a patient with a history of melanoma that is metastatic to other organs, who has routine cardiac imaging and a solid mass is seen in an unusual location. Since there is no wall motion abnormality and no significant valvular disease or clinical signs suggestive of infective endocarditis, a mobile mass on the tricuspid valve is very likely to be a metastatic lesion to the heart (Fig. 98.3). Another imaging characteristic that provides insight indicating a tumor is present is the behavior of the mass during cardiac motion. If a tumor is infiltrating the myocardium, it is unlikely to contract in a normal fashion. An LV myocardial apical mass contracting similarly to the surrounding tissue is likely to be either focal hypertrophy (Fig. 98.4) or LV noncompaction (Fig. 98.5)[11,12] as opposed to a cardiac tumor. Furthermore, progression of an image over time also may indicate the pathologic process. If a cardiac mass changes in size during serial imaging, suspicion of a cardiac tumor is much higher. However, an LV apical mass that is stable for months or years is unlikely to be a malignant cardiac tumor as noted in Figures 98.4 and 98.5.

The exact nature and location of a mass is critical in the determination of the likelihood that it is a tumor. A classic example of this principle is lipomatous hypertrophy of the intraatrial septum (Fig. 98.6). The initial suspicion might be that this is a myxoma or other tumor, but an MRI with specific characteristics that are a hallmark for lipomatous hypertrophy will confirm the diagnosis.[13] Additionally, ridges of tissue including the crista terminalis or the eustachian valve remnant can also mimic cardiac masses.

TABLE 98.1 Range of Clinical Findings That May Indicate a Cardiac Tumor

- Completely asymptomatic but an incidental abnormality on imaging
- Low-grade fevers
- Transient ischemic attack or cerebral vascular event
- Positional dyspnea
- Weight loss
- Peripheral embolic events
- Chest discomfort
- Congestive heart failure
- Upper extremity/neck swelling
- Lower extremity venous thrombosis
- Palpitations
- Arrhythmias
- Pericardial effusion/tamponade

TABLE 98.2 Common Testing That May Indicate the Possibility of a Cardiac Tumor

- Two or three dimensional echocardiography
- Chest x-ray
- Computed tomography (CT)
- CT angiography
- Magnetic resonance imaging
- Transesophageal echocardiography
- Positron emission tomography
- Nuclear scintigraphy

TABLE 98.3 Differential Diagnosis of Cardiac Masses

- Intracardiac thrombus
- Focal myocardial hypertrophy
- Left ventricular noncompaction
- Infectious (abscess)
- Primary cardiac tumor
- Secondary cardiac tumor (metastasis)
- Lipomatous hypertrophy of the septum
- Cyst
- Imaging artifact

Classification of Cardiac Tumors

Cardiac tumors are divided into primary and secondary tumors. Primary cardiac tumors are very rare, with an autopsy incidence of 1:2000.[14] These tumors include benign or malignant neoplasms that may arise from any tissue of the heart. In terms of primary tumors, approximately 80% are benign and these can be grouped as simple or complex, considering the treatment that is typically required. The approximately 20% of primary cardiac tumors remaining are malignant and usually are pathologically described as sarcomas.[15-17] Table 98.4 summarizes some of the pathologic descriptions of cardiac tumors that have been reported, albeit not an exhaustive list, since there have been many very specific pathologic descriptions and it can be difficult to adequately categorize them. Thus, general categories will be discussed in the remainder of this chapter. Figure 98.7 illustrates the types of tumor that may affect different chambers of the heart and pericardium. Secondary or metastatic cardiac tumors are 30 times more common than a primary neoplasm with an autopsy incidence of 1.7% to 14%[18] or 1:100.[14]

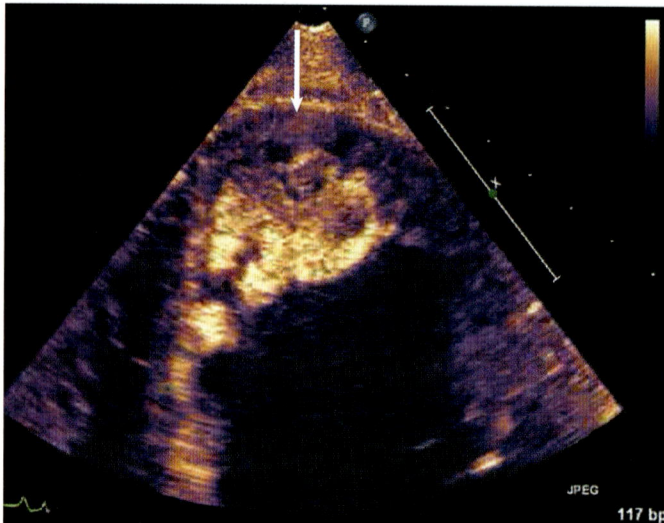

FIGURE 98.1 A large irregular mass noted in the left ventricular apex (*arrow*) in the context of a patient with severe left ventricular dysfunction. The edges are distinct from the myocardium classic for a thrombus.

BENIGN (NONMALIGNANT) PRIMARY CARDIAC TUMORS

The majority (>80%) of the primary cardiac tumors are nonmalignant; however, because of their location these frequently require surgical treatment.[19,20] Myxoma constitutes about 50% of all benign cardiac tumors in adults, but only a small percentage of such tumors in children.[21] Rhabdomyomas are the most common benign tumor in children and account for 40% to 60% of the pediatric cases.[20] Other benign cardiac tumors that have been described include fibromas, lipomas, hemangiomas, papillary fibroelastomas, cystic tumors of the AV node, and paragangliomas.

Simple Benign Tumors
Myxomas
Most myxomas (>80%) are most commonly found in the left atrium and in decreasing frequencies in the right atrium, right ventricle, and left ventricle (Fig. 98.8).[16,22] The incidence of cardiac myxoma peaks at 40 to 60 years of age, with a female to male ratio of approximately 3:1. Most myxomas occur sporadically but may be familial and occasionally these have been described in relation to a particular syndrome called Carney's complex, an autosomal-dominant condition associated with cardiac myxomas, myxomas in other regions (cutaneous or mammary), hyperpigmented skin lesions, hyperactivity of the adrenal or testicular glands, and pituitary tumors. Carney's complex occurs at a younger age and should be considered when cardiac myxomas are discovered in atypical locations in the heart.[15]

Etiology and Pathophysiology
The exact origin of myxoma cells remains uncertain, but they are thought to arise from remnants of subendocardial cells or multipotential mesenchymal cells in the region of the fossa ovalis, which can differentiate along a variety of cell lines. The hypothesis is that cardiac myxoma originates from a pluripotential stem cell, and myxoma cells express a variety of antigens and other endothelial markers. Myxomas typically form a pedunculated mass with a short broad base (85% of myxomas), but sessile forms can also occur.[19] Classically, myxomas appear yellowish, appear white or brownish, and are frequently friable. The tumor size can range from 1 cm to more than 10 cm, and the surface is smooth in the majority of the cases. A villous or papillary form of myxoma has been reported and contains a surface that consists of multiple fine or very fine villous, gelatinous, and fragile extensions that have a tendency to fragment spontaneously and are associated with embolic phenomena.[23] Histologically, myxomas are composed of

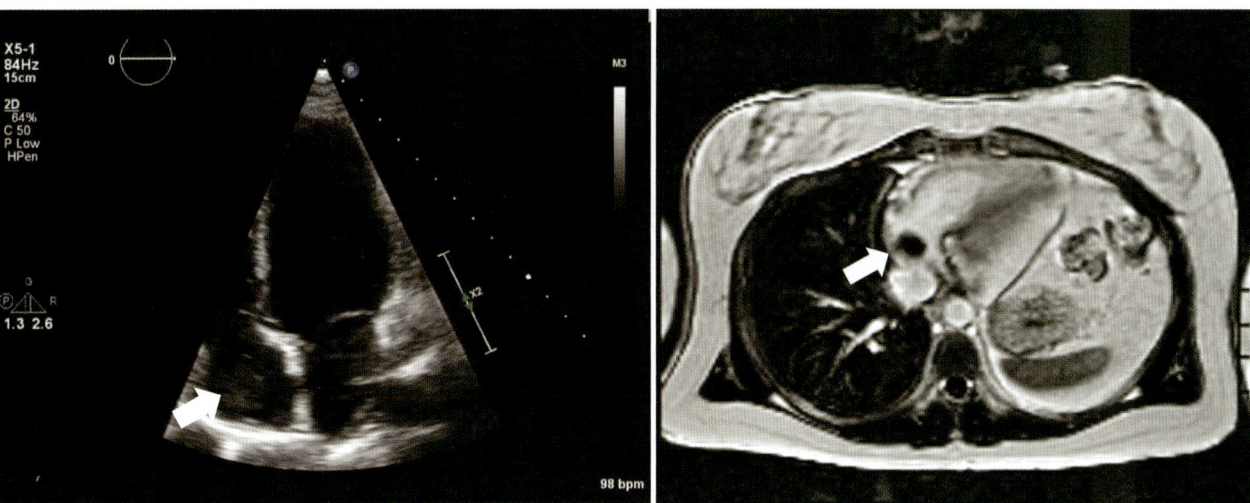

FIGURE 98.2 Differentiation of tumor versus thrombus formation in 48-year-old woman treated for breast cancer. **Left,** Four-chamber echocardiogram with new right atrial mass (*arrow*) that developed after the third round of anthracycline-based chemotherapy administered via an indwelling catheter. **Right,** Late gadolinium enhanced cardiac MRI demonstrating absence of contrast uptake within the mass consistent with a thrombus (*arrow*). The etiology of the thrombus in this case is related to the indwelling catheter (not shown) resting against the wall of the right atrium and serving as a nidus for thrombus formation.

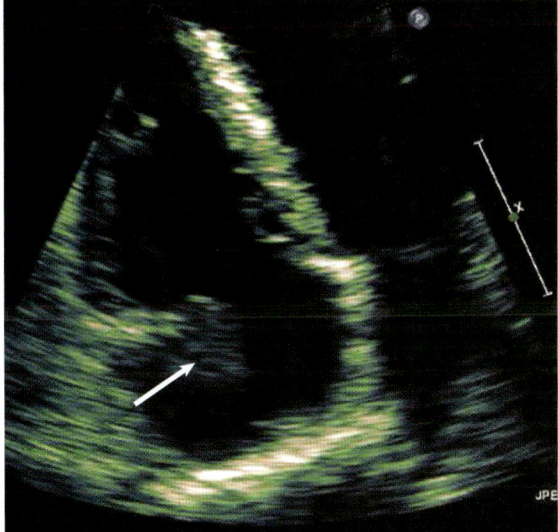

FIGURE 98.3 An irregular mass is noted on the atrial side of the tricuspid valve (*arrow*) in a patient with metastatic melanoma.

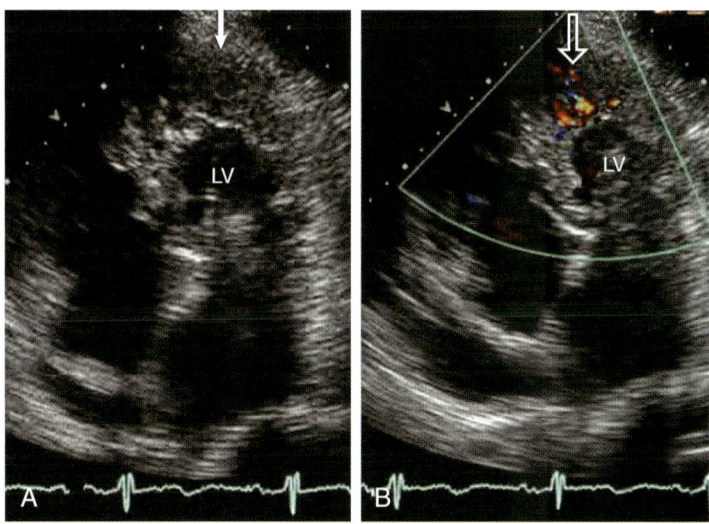

FIGURE 98.5 An apical mass is not solid (*arrow* in **A**) and color flow is detected in "lakes" within the apical mass (*arrow* in **B**). This is typical of noncompaction cardiomyopathy and this area does appear to contract.

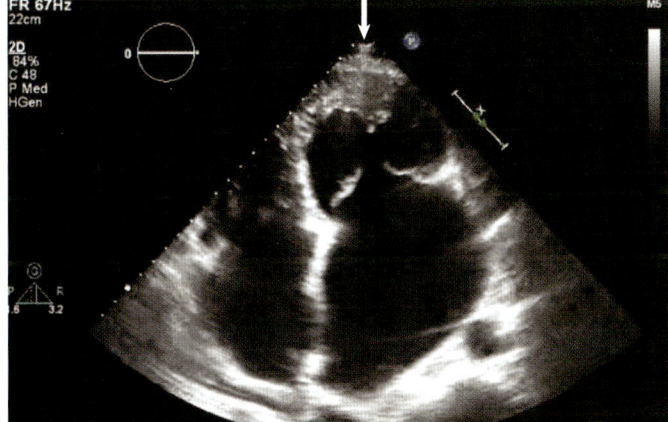

FIGURE 98.4 A four-chamber echo image showing focal apical hypertrophy (*arrow*) that resulted in severe diastolic heart failure. The apical mass contracted and was stable in appearance for years.

spindle and stellate shaped cells with myxoid stroma that may also contain endothelial cells, smooth muscle cells, and other elements surrounded within an acid mucopolysaccharide substance. Calcifications may also be seen in some cases.[19]

Clinical Manifestations

Patients commonly are asymptomatic and the tumor is found as an incidental finding on 2D-echo. When symptoms are present, dyspnea, especially dyspnea that is worse while lying on the left side, should alert the astute clinician to the possibility of a myxoma. Most clinical presentations related to myxoma result from mitral valve obstruction (syncope, dyspnea, and pulmonary edema) followed by embolic manifestations.[16,23] Patients may present with nonspecific symptoms such as fatigue, cough, low-grade fever, arthralgia, myalgia, weight loss, erythematous rash, and laboratory findings of anemia and increased erythrocyte sedimentation rate (ESR), C-reactive protein, and gamma globulin levels. Less commonly they may have thrombocytopenia, clubbing, cyanosis, or Raynaud's phenomenon. Physical exam findings can reveal a systolic murmur or a diastolic murmur suggestive of mitral stenosis. A tumor plop may potentially be heard (a low-pitched diastolic sound heard as the tumor prolapses into the left ventricle).[16,23] In one study, a cardiac auscultation abnormality was detected in 64% of patients,[24] and the most common auscultation

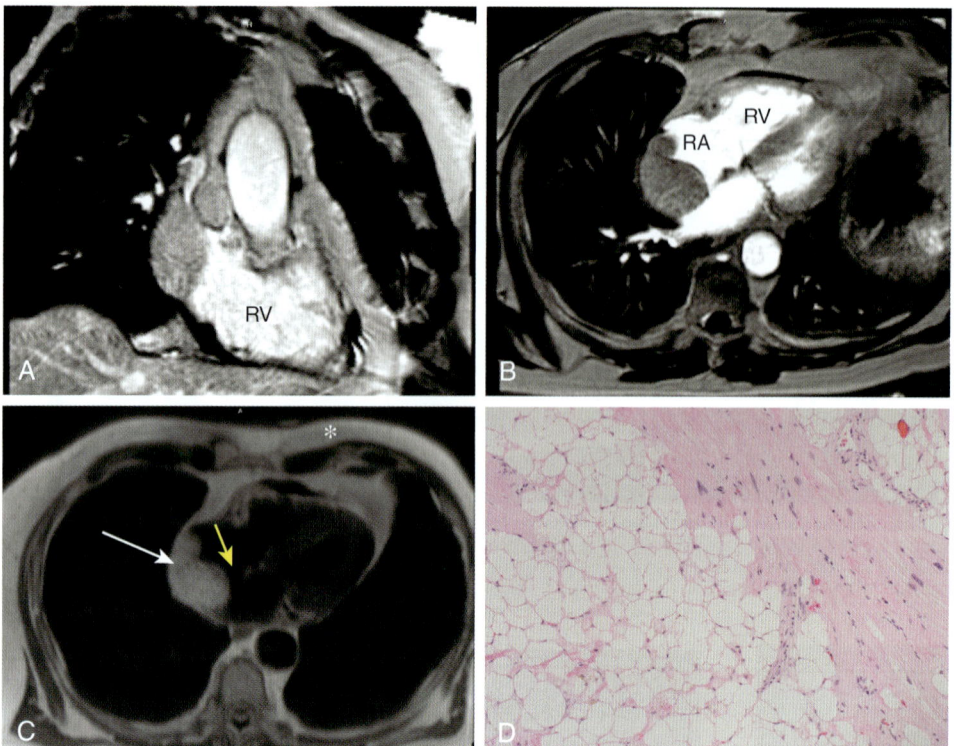

FIGURE 98.6 **A** and **B**, A large intraatrial mass (lipomatous septal hypertrophy) obstructing the inflow into the right atrium. **C**, MRI showing a large intraatrial mass with high intensity signal (*white arrow*) and sparing the region of fossa ovalis (*yellow arrow*). Also noted is the signal intensity is similar to the subcutaneous chest wall fat consistent with lipomatous hypertrophy of the intraatrial septum (*). **D**, There is an admixture of adipocytes, fibrosis, and entrapped hypertrophic cardiomyocytes. The adipocytes have variable size of cytoplasmic vacuolation, demonstrating a "hibernoma" or "brown fat" morphology. *RA*, Right atrium; *RV*, right ventricle.

mitral valve from the tumor. Tumor plop may be confused with a mitral opening snap or a third heart sound and can be detected in up to 15% of cases.[24] Chest examination may reveal fine crepitations consistent with pulmonary edema while there may be peripheral signs of embolic phenomenon. The physical evidence of embolic phenomenon will vary depending on the vascular territory involved. Involvement of cerebral vessels results in neurologic signs; involvement of coronary arteries may result in an acute coronary syndrome; intestinal arterial obstruction may result in ischemic bowel; and peripheral arterial obstruction can result in limb-threatening ischemia.

Laboratory Testing

Laboratory test abnormalities may include anemia, elevated serum gamma globulin, elevated ESR, and elevated serum C-reactive protein, which is present in approximately 75% of the patients.[23] There are no specific electrocardiogram (ECG) findings in myxoma. Chest x-ray findings are also nonspecific and include signs of congestive heart failure, cardiomegaly, and left atrial enlargement. In some cases, the tumor itself may be visible due to calcification.[24] A 2D echo usually should demonstrate a mass in the atrium, with the stalk attached to the interatrial septum but myxomas have been reported in all chambers of the heart.[22] A TEE provides specific delineation of the tumor including the size and origin. CT and MRI scans provide better delineation of the intracardiac mass, the extent of tumor in relation to extracardiac structures, and provide anatomical definition for preoperative planning (Table 98.5).

Treatment

The only definitive treatment of cardiac myxoma is surgical removal. Generally, the myxoma is surgically excised using cardiopulmonary bypass and cardioplegic arrest. The tumor is removed by either right or left atriotomy or combined atriotomy, depending on the site and extent of the tumor. The choice of technique also depends on associated conditions that need surgical intervention, such as valve repair or replacement, and coronary disease if present. Lifelong follow-up is needed, as myxomas have some tendency to recur. The recurrence rate of myxoma has varied but one large experience suggests that is quite low and may be below 1%.[23,25]

Fibroelastoma

Valvular structures may have a papillary fibroelastoma attached, which is often found incidentally. These are small in size, typically less than 2 cm, and most commonly occur on the aortic valve followed by the mitral valve. Rarely these may be found anywhere in the endocardial surface and the majority of fibroelastomas that have been reported are solitary, although multiple ones have been rarely reported.[26] Fibroelastomas may result in embolic phenomena, and when situated on the aortic valve or the left ventricle, can cause coronary ostial occlusion (Fig. 98.9).[27] Grossly, they have a characteristic frond like appearance, resembling a sea anemone, and histologically the tumor has an inner central core of collagen surrounded by a layer of acid mucopolysaccharides and covered by endothelial cells[26]. For the most part, complete surgical resection is recommended for left-sided papillary fibroelastoma primarily because of the high likelihood of systemic embolism, which

TABLE 98.4 Pathologic Description of Cardiac Tumors

Benign
• Myxoma
• Paraganglioma
• Rhabdomyoma
• Fibroma
• Lipoma
• Hemangioma
• Papillary fibroelastoma
• Cystic tumor of the AV node

Malignant
• Sarcoma
• Lymphoma

Metastatic
• Renal cell carcinoma
• Melanoma
• Breast cancer
• Lung cancer
• Sarcoma
• Lymphoma
• Leukemia
• Cervical cancer

findings are a systolic murmur (in 50% of cases) followed by loud first heart sound (32%), an opening snap (26%), and a diastolic murmur (15%).[23] The reason for the systolic murmur may be caused by damage to the valves, failure of the leaflets to coapt, or narrowing of the outflow tract by the tumor. A diastolic murmur is present due to obstruction of the can lead to stroke, myocardial infarction, peripheral embolism, and even sudden death. The decision for surgery in right-sided disease is more difficult as the number of asymptomatic right heart fibroelastomas is unknown and recommendation for surgery depends on the exact location, size, and potential risk to the patient. On imaging, especially echocardiographic imaging, there is a characteristic small, mobile, pedunculated, and very echo dense core that enables it to be differentiated from a vegetation or thrombi. Typically the structure of the valve can be preserved once the tumor is removed. The chance of recurrence appears low and there is no compelling data to continue anticoagulation long term unless there are other indications to do so.[28]

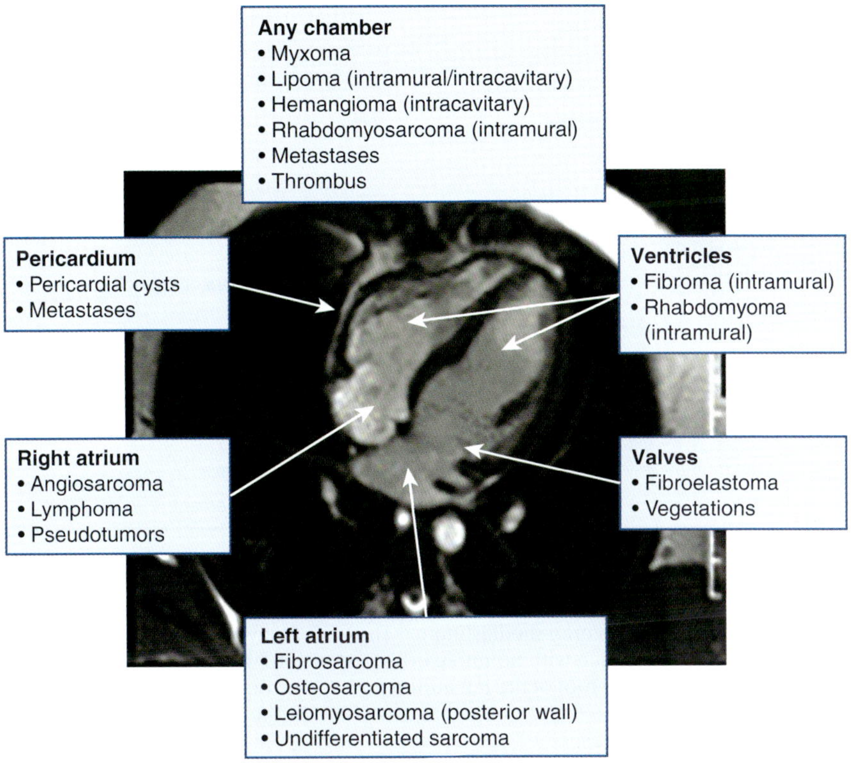

Rhabdomyomas

Rhabdomyomas are usually found in the ventricle and are the most common benign cardiac tumor found in children.[20,21] The majority of these patients have signs of or a family history of tuberous sclerosis.[20] In one study of patients with tuberous sclerosis complex, cardiac tumor was found in 48% of the patients, with an incidence of 66% in patients less than 2 years old.[29] Frequently, these patients are asymptomatic although some patients with rhabdomyoma may present clinically with arrhythmias and heart failure.[20,29] It is possible these tumors may regress with age but can sometimes grow or appear during puberty.[29] As a result of these uncertain outcomes, long-term clinical and echocardiographic follow-up is needed in patients with tuberous sclerosis. Most often, surgery can be avoided, although if arrhythmias become a symptomatic problem, antiarrhythmics and ultimately surgery may have to be considered.[20]

Lipomas

A lipoma is a rare benign cardiac tumor comprising only 3% of all benign tumors.[30] These tend to occur in the left ventricle or the right atrium but may be found anywhere in the heart as well as the pericardium. Although frequently asymptomatic, they may grow large enough to cause obstructive symptoms and require surgical intervention (see Fig. 98.6). Obstruction and compression of the superior vena cava may occur in patients with lipomas involving the right atrium.

Cystic Tumor of the AV Node (Previously Called Mesothelioma)

Because of their location near the atrioventricular node, these cystic tumors can present with varying degree of heart block or even sudden death.[31] Cardiac MRI is particularly useful in the diagnosis of this tumor.[32]

Other Very Rare Benign Cardiac Tumors

There are few very rare reports of hemangioma,[33,34] neurofibroma, teratomas,[35] leiomyoma, and lymphangioma; however, there are not enough data to summarize

FIGURE 98.7 Illustration of tumors or masses in the various chambers and structures of the heart.

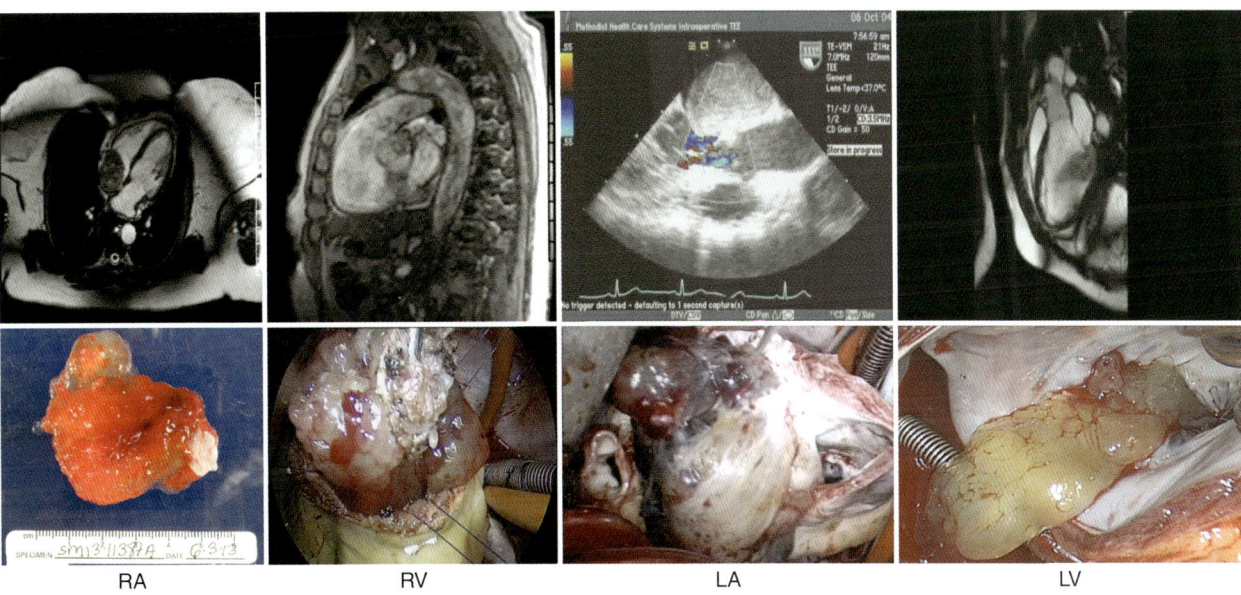

FIGURE 98.8 Myxomas have been reported in every chamber of the heart. Imaging and gross surgical samples are provided from the right atrium (RA), right ventricle (RV), left atrium (LA), and the left ventricle (LV). On all of the gross pictures from each chamber, the outward appearance is generally yellow to gray and can appear soft and villous or perhaps smooth and more solid. Note the lack of thrombus on the surface of each tumor.

TABLE 98.5 Imaging Characteristics of Tumors with Echo, CT, and cMRI

CARDIAC TUMOR	ECHOCARDIOGRAPHY (ECHO)	COMPUTED TOMOGRAPHY (CT)	MAGNETIC RESONANCE IMAGING (cMRI)
Myxoma	Mobile tumor	Narrow base of attachment	Mottled gadolinium contrast enhancement
	Frequently attached fossa ovalis	Heterogeneous with low attenuation	Mobile on cine imaging
	Heterogeneous echogenicity	Possible calcification	Varying (mixture of values on T1 mapping)
Papillary Fibroelastoma	Mobile valve leaflet mass	Mass seen on valve leaflets	Mobile mass on valve leaflets
			Variable gadolinium contrast enhancement
Lipoma	General thickening of interatrial septum	Low attenuation due to fat	High T1 signal
			Fat saturated images with low signal
Rhabdomyoma	Small lobulated hyperechoic intramuscular masses		Multiple masses with homogeneous signal intensity
			Uniform T1 and T2 values
Fibroma	Large intramural mass	Homogeneous with low attenuation	Uniform T1 and T2 values
		Calcification may be present	Isointense on T1-weighted images
		Large intramural mass	Large intramural mass
Hemangioma	Increased echogenicity	Heterogeneous with marked enhancement	Gadolinium enhancement present
Angiosarcoma	Invades across tissue boundaries	Invasive across tissue boundaries; low attenuation	Invasive across tissue boundaries
			Varying or heterogeneous gadolinium enhancement
	Pericardial effusion		Varying or heterogeneous T1 and T2 values
Lymphoma	Low echogenicity masses	Low attenuation masses	Enhancement with gadolinium that may be heterogeneous
	Pericardial effusion		
Metastases	Often multiple masses	Often multiple lesions	Often multiple lesions
	May have pericardial effusion		Gadolinium enhancement

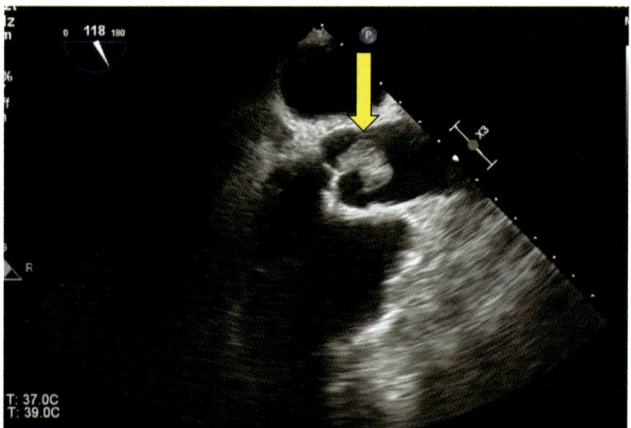

FIGURE 98.9 A large pedunculated mass affixed and above the aortic valve (*arrow*) was a papillary fibroelastoma confirmed at surgery. The valve was repaired successfully without replacement.

expected findings. Typically these tumors will be diagnosed after resection. Complete resection of the tumor is possible in most of the benign primary tumors, compared with malignant tumors, with a perioperative death of 1.4%.[36] Hemangiomas are characteristically vascular and maybe endocardial or epicardial (Fig. 98.10).[37]

Complex Benign Tumors
Paragangliomas
Cardiac paragangliomas are chromaffin-producing tumors arising from the neural crest cells of the sympathetic and parasympathetic chains. Only 1% to 2% occur in the chest and most of these are in the posterior mediastinum.[25] The tumor may be located in the pericardial space with no intracardiac extension[38] but are often located around the roof of the left atrium and aortic root involving the cardiac structures[39] and can occur anywhere in the heart. When paraganglioma is suspected, a coronary CT angiogram or cardiac catheterization is necessary looking for large feeding vessels (Fig. 98.11). If present, this is almost pathognomonic for paraganglioma and diagnostic biopsy should be avoided due to the high risk of bleeding. Paragangliomas are a highly vascular tumor and may present with hypertension and chest pain.[38,40] The tumors originating from the roof of left atrium are often very large and require extensive surgery, including cardiac auto transplantation,[39] and should generally be confined to specialized centers. A coronary angiogram in these patients shows a characteristic "tumor blush" (Fig. 98.11C).[38,40] These tumors are further classified as hormonally active or inactive. Histology cannot reliably determine if the tumor is benign and about 10% will recur with metastatic disease. These tumors were originally referred to as malignant paraganglioma but the term "metastatic paraganglioma" is currently favored. Although large surgical cohorts are lacking, the author's (MR) current experience (Methodist Hospital, Houston, Texas) includes a total of 20 resections in 19 patients with two deaths and one recurrence as metastatic paraganglioma.[41]

Fibromas
These tumors are histologically composed primarily of fibroblasts or collagen. Typically these occur in childhood, although it can also occur in adults.[16,19,42] Most often a fibroma is located in the ventricle and interventricular septum, and patients may present with chest pain, pericardial effusion, heart failure, arrhythmias, and sudden death. Cardiomegaly is frequently seen on chest x-ray, which may also show the calcification within the tumor mass.[42] Frequently these tumors are associated with arrhythmias and might require multimodality treatment with medications, electrophysiologic procedures,

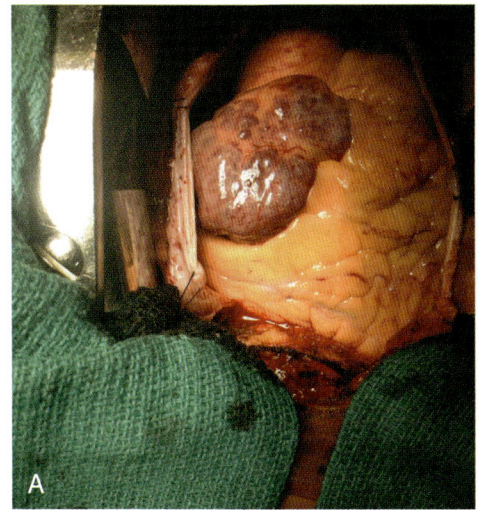
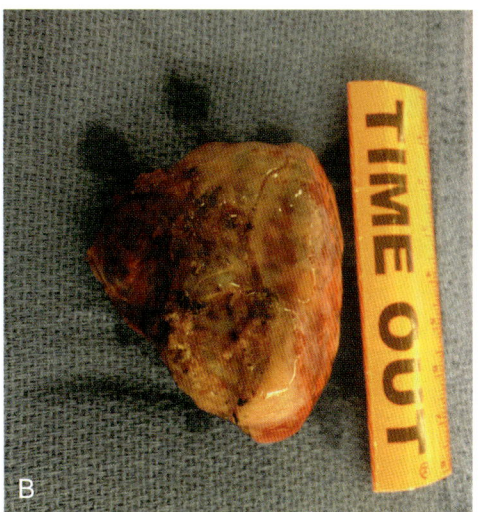
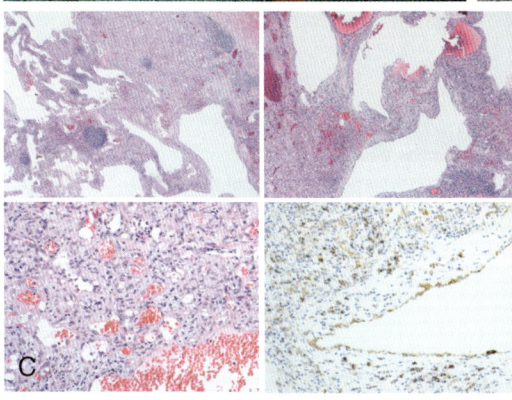
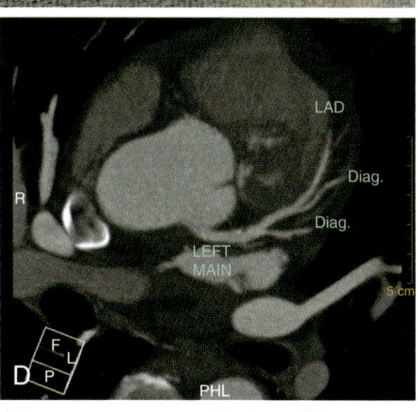

FIGURE 98.10 Primary cardiac hemangioma arising from the right coronary artery at the base of the aorta and right atrium. **A,** Complete resection was possible with uneventful postoperative course. **B,** The resected specimen was easily dissected free from adjacent structures and was supplied by the right coronary artery. **C,** Histologic and immunohistochemical features of the tumor. **Top left,** Low-power view showing large vascular spaces and more solid areas with small capillaries. There is a portion of residual cardiac muscle in the upper right corner (2× magnification). **Top right,** Medium-power view showing that the vascular spaces are lined by an attenuated endothelial lining with cells with small nuclei. Many of the spaces contain blood and fibrin and the intervening areas of capillary proliferation have blood and scattered chronic inflammatory cells (4×magnification). **Bottom left,** High-power view of the capillary rich area showing plump cells lining the vascular spaces (20× magnification). **Bottom right,** CD 31 immunohistochemistry showing strong brown staining of the lining cells of the large spaces and also of the plump cells in the capillary rich areas (20× magnification). **D,** CT angiography showing the mass adjacent to the right coronary artery.

and/or surgery. If surgical resection is performed, fibromas tend not to recur. A distinguishing feature of fibromas, contrasted to rhabdomyoma, is that there is classically calcification within the tumor.[19] Although these tumors can be extremely large when they involve the left ventricle, they tend to push the myocardium away, rather than replace it, allowing for resection of large tumors with preservation of ventricular function.[43]

Treatment

Most tumors, particularly benign masses, are relatively limited in size and do not have extensive adjacent cardiac involvement. The surgical approach, whether via median sternotomy or right thoracotomy, allows complete removal and repair of most resulting defects. However, there is a small group of tumors with complex cardiac involvement. These tumors may invade and obstruct pulmonary veins or the mitral annulus, which renders complete removal impossible with conventional surgical approaches. Pioneered by Reardon and colleagues in Houston, the complete removal of the heart with back table resection and reconstruction of the pulmonary veins and atria offers a potential cure or significant palliation in selected patients. The approach is similar to heart transplant cardiectomy allowing for exposure of the pulmonary veins and complete resection of atrial and even ventricular masses.[44] In their select series there was 100% 1-year survival among patients with benign tumors and 50% survival in patients with malignant tumors (primarily sarcoma).[45]

MALIGNANT PRIMARY CARDIAC TUMORS

Sarcomas

Primary cardiac tumors, both benign and malignant, are rare with a meta-analysis covering 22 studies showing an autopsy incidence of approximately 0.02% while primary cardiac sarcomas make up over 75% of these malignant tumors.[46] Primary cardiac sarcoma constitutes only about 1% of all soft tissue sarcomas.[47] The age of presentation for cardiac sarcomas ranges from 1 to 76 years, with a mean age around 40 years.[17,47] Studies using large U.S. national databases have confirmed the extreme rarity of primary cardiac sarcoma as well is its usual dismal outlook.[48,49] Angiosarcomas and unclassified sarcomas account for approximately 76% of all cardiac sarcomas, of which angiosarcomas are the most common.[50] Rhabdomyosarcoma is the most common form of cardiac sarcoma in children. Leiomyosarcoma, synovial sarcoma, osteosarcoma, fibrosarcoma, myxoid sarcoma, liposarcoma, mesenchymal sarcoma, neurofibrosarcoma, and malignant fibrous histiocytoma are other cardiac sarcomas observed.[15,17,50] Angiosarcomas are predominantly found on the right side while osteosarcomas and unclassified sarcomas are predominantly found on the left side of the heart.[50] Pericardial angiosarcomas are extremely rare.[51] Most published reports are from institutional series and generally have included 30 or fewer surgical cases.[17,52-54] The national French Sarcoma Group found 124 cases of primary cardiac sarcoma over 33 years in France with 81 patients receiving surgical resection.[55] The largest single institution report found 131 primary cardiac sarcoma (PCS) cases over 25 years with 95 patients receiving surgical resection.[56] Three recent large national database studies in the United States have reinforced this rarity. The Surveillance, Epidemiology and End Results (SEER) database had 442 patients with PCS identified over 42 years (1973 to 2015) with only 218 (49.8%) having surgery.[48] The National Cancer Database (NCDB) was queried for 2004 to 2015 finding 617 patients with PSC over this 21-year period and 372 (60.3%) having surgery.[49] An additional study using the NCDB from 2004 to 2016 found 100,317 primary cardiac tumors, of which 826 (0.8%) were malignant and of these, 731 (88.5%) were sarcoma.[57] In this study, surgery was done on 442 (59.2%) of the primary malignant tumors and 225 (50.9%) had multimodality treatment in addition to their surgery.

As a result of this rarity, only a few institutions and even fewer individual physicians have an appreciable experience with treating this disease.[58] It is generally agreed that complete surgical resection is the mainstay of therapy. If surgery cannot be done, the 1-year survival is less than 10%.[59] Knowing when complete resection is possible and who would be an appropriate candidate can be difficult but is important for the clinician to understand. Additionally, the role of neoadjuvant and adjuvant chemotherapy and radiation therapy are poorly defined as most studies have been small, although recent evidence seems to be favoring both.[48,49,60-62] A clinically practical way to consider primary

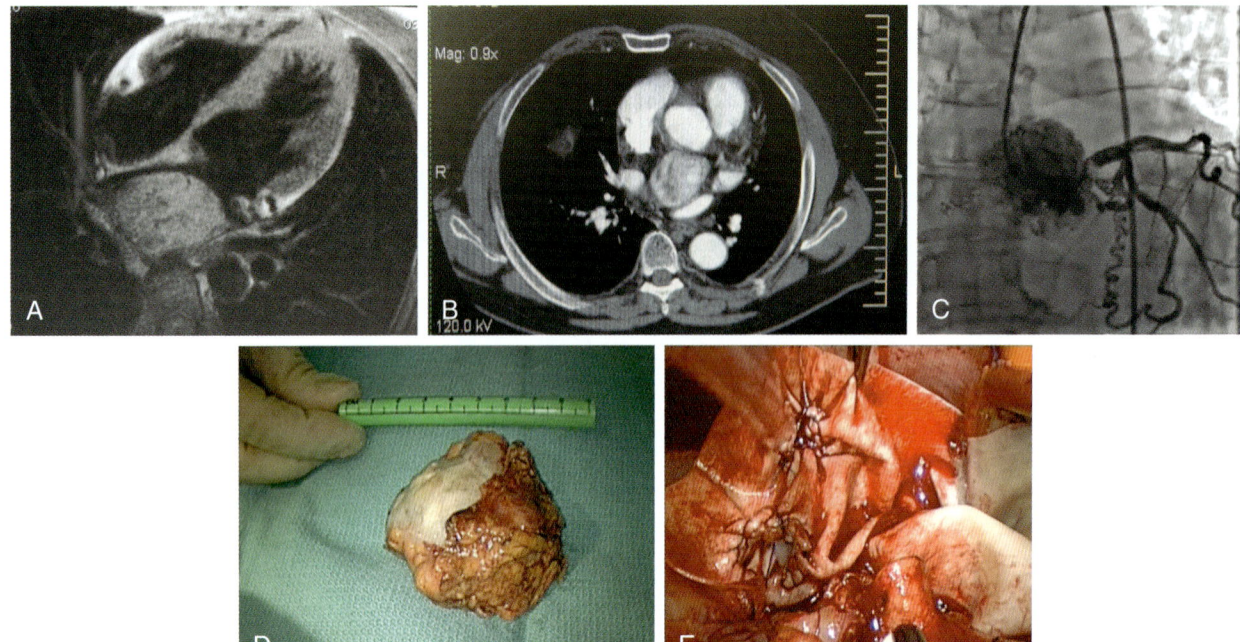

FIGURE 98.11 Imaging and pathology of the presentation for a paraganglioma. **A,** CMR image with a large hypervascular tumor of the left atrium. **B,** CT imaging demonstrates the tumor extends superiorly behind the aorta and pulmonary artery. **C,** Cardiac catheterization image that demonstrates giant vessels feeding the paraganglioma. **D,** Gross specimen, which shows the diffuse nature of the tumor. The smooth portion is part of the left atrial wall that had to be resected. There is no tissue plane between the tumor and the atrial wall. **E,** Posterior left atrial repair with bovine pericardium. (**C** from Chan EY, et al. Management of primary cardiac paraganglioma. J Thorac Cardiovasc Surg 2020;S0022-5223(20):32704-32705.)

cardiac sarcoma is by tumor location since this often determines the clinical presentation, urgency of treatment, and surgical options: (1) right heart, (2) left heart, or (3) pulmonary artery.

Clinical Manifestations

Cardiac tumors commonly cause symptoms by three separate mechanisms: obstruction, embolization, and arrhythmias. Rarely pericardial invasion and tamponade may be the first manifestation of the disease. Both atrial and ventricular tumors, when large enough, may result in obstructive symptoms and cause syncope, chest pain, dyspnea, or heart failure. The most common presenting symptoms include dyspnea, followed by chest pain, cough, syncope, hemoptysis, sudden death, fever, embolic events, and cardiac arrhythmias.[17] Large tumors on the right side, besides causing venous congestion, may also limit cardiac filling with sudden decreases in intravascular volume and potentially precipitating syncope in these patients. Left-sided cardiac tumors, if large enough, can also impair ventricular filling leading to syncope or heart failure (Fig. 98.12). Unfortunately, about 29% of cardiac sarcomas have metastatic disease at the time of presentation, typically in the lung.[17,51] Sarcomas, especially left-sided, are commonly associated with cardiac embolic events[15] and arrhythmia may be an important problem as well. A finding of a cardiac mass with pericardial effusion should raise the suspicion of a malignant cardiac tumor.[51] Commonly, pericardial effusion is due to associated pericardial involvement; however, a malignant effusion is not always proven.

Laboratory Investigations

Regardless of the imaging modalities used, malignant tumors of the heart often involve invasion of the tumor across tissue boundaries or planes including the pericardium, epicardium, endocardium, and valve planes. This feature often distinguishes these tumors from nonmalignant and other normal structures. Due to increasing use of CT scan and better modalities of cardiac imaging, the primary cardiac tumors may be identified at an earlier stage. ECG changes are usually nonspecific; however, heart block, ventricular hypertrophy, bundle branch blocks, atrial flutter, and atrial tachycardia may be present in some cases. Cardiomegaly is a common but nonspecific radiologic finding of cardiac sarcomas.[15] Echo is commonly used in the initial diagnosis of primary

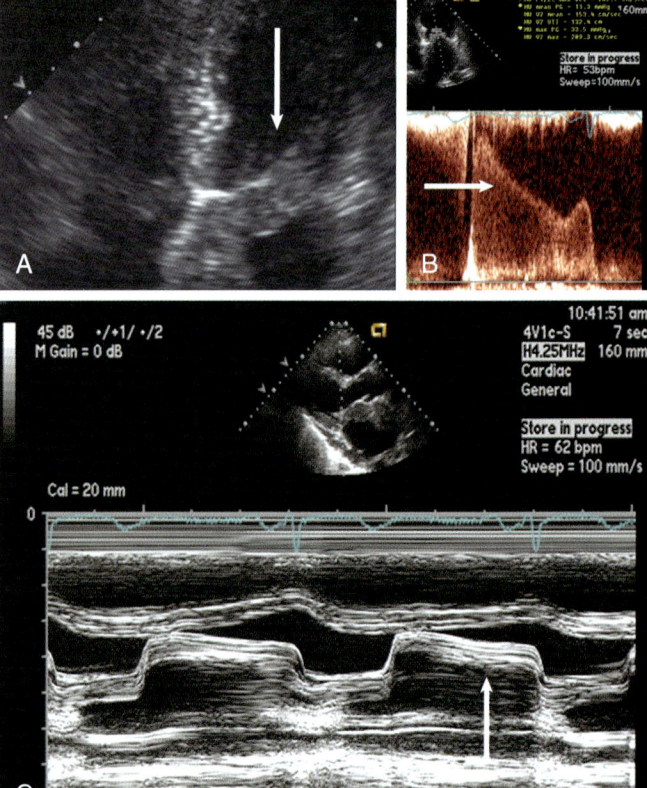

FIGURE 98.12 Echo Doppler images from a patient with sarcoma who presented with heart failure and mitral stenosis. **A,** Four-chamber image with mitral valve thickening (*arrow*). **B,** Increased velocity across the mitral valve showing stenosis (*arrow*). **C,** M-mode showing a classic mitral stenosis pattern.

cardiac tumors with transthoracic 2D, 3D, and contrast imaging being appropriate techniques. However, transthoracic echo has several well-known limitations: operator experience, lung interference due to pulmonary disease, narrow rib spaces, or unfavorable body habitus. TEE can provide more specific and detailed imaging than 2D echo especially structures that are more posterior such as the left atrium. Cross sectional imaging methods, such as CT and MRI, have an important role in the evaluation and further assessment of malignant cardiac tumors, especially in evaluation of myocardial invasion (Fig. 98.13), involvement of mediastinal structures, tissue characterization (Fig. 98.14), and vascularity (Table 98.5).[5,63]

Treatment

A complete resection is the optimal goal for surgical treatment.[15,17,64] Once surgical treatment is completed, adjuvant chemotherapy seems prudent although not widely studied but has shown to improve survival over surgery alone in a SEER database analysis.[48,64] It is possible that neoadjuvant therapy may be useful and has been shown to improve survival with some sarcomas, but this is speculative.[65] The most common chemotherapeutic regimen used for cardiac sarcomas is combined doxorubicin and ifosfamide.[51] A combination of docetaxel and gemcitabine also showed some response in various sarcomas and can be used as an alternative chemotherapeutic regimen.[51] Other treatment options include ifosfamide-epirubicin (doxorubicin) and cyclophosphamide, vincristine, doxorubicin, and dacarbazine (CyVADIC).[47] Unlike other sarcomas, cardiac sarcomas overall have a very poor prognosis with a median survival rate of 6 months to 25 months after diagnosis.[16,19,50] The presence of tumor necrosis and metastases is associated with a poor prognosis[50] as is the presence of a right-sided cardiac sarcoma.[66] Sarcomas other than angiosarcomas, sarcomas on the left side of the heart, and completely resected sarcomas seem to have a better prognosis.[17] At the time of surgical resection, patients with negative surgical margins have a better survival.[66] Low-grade cardiac sarcoma on histologic grading may appear to have a better survival, although in one study there was no significant correlation between the histologic grade and survival.[17,50,67]

Heart Tumor Team

Malignant primary cardiac tumors are rare, are exceedingly complex, and have a dismal survival without treatment. The treatment of primary cardiac tumors requires a multidisciplinary cardiac tumor team including cardio-oncologists, sarcoma oncologists, specialized cardiac surgeons, and imaging experts.[58] The author's (MR) current single institution published experience with primary cardiac sarcoma surgical resection includes 95 patients.[56] The mean survival for the entire group was 20 months. Most deaths are due to metastatic disease suggesting that better biologic treatment is the key to significantly improving survival.

SECONDARY CARDIAC TUMORS

The autopsy incidence of secondary cardiac tumors ranges from 1.7% to 14% (average 7.1%) in cancer patients and 0.7% to 3.5% (average 2.3%) in the general population.[18] In comparison to older series, there is a significant increase in the incidence of cardiac metastases in cancer patients after 1970, predominately due to improvement in imaging modalities (Figs. 98.15 and 98.16). Cardiac metastases can occur either by direct extension, via blood stream, by lymphatics, or by intracavitary diffusion through the inferior vena cava (IVC). Pericardial metastasis (69%) is the most common location followed by epicardial (34%), myocardial (32%), and endocardial metastases (5%).[68] The pericardium is most often involved due to direct invasion by the thoracic cancers, including breast and lung cancer. Abdominal and pelvic tumors may reach the right atrium through the IVC. The most common tumor exhibiting this tendency is renal cell carcinoma.[51] A recent review suggests that lung cancer is the most common cause of cardiac metastasis followed by esophageal cancer and hematologic malignancy.[16] The symptoms of cardiac metastases are extremely variable, depending on

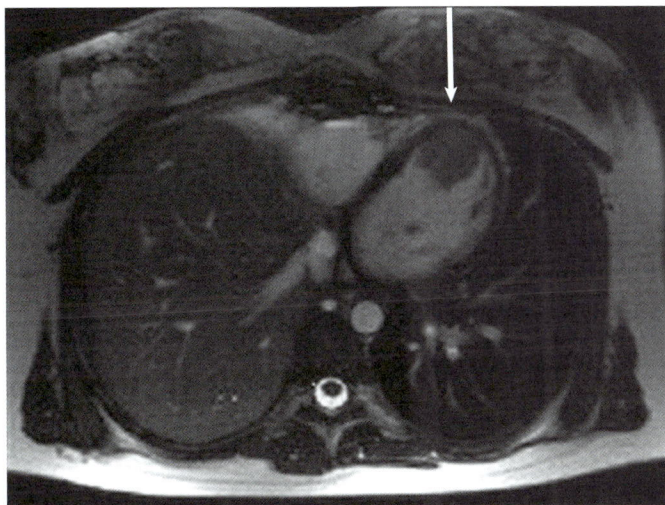

FIGURE 98.13 T_1-weighted cardiac magnetic resonance image of a left ventricular apical tumor of metastatic alveolar cell sarcoma. Note the indistinct nature of the tumor infiltrating the myocardium (*arrow*). This is in contrast to the distinct line that classically separates thrombus from myocardium.

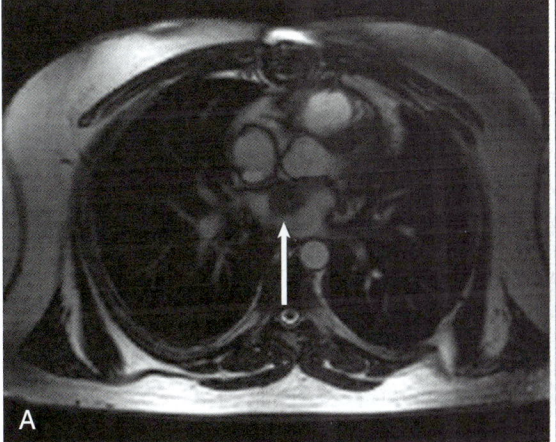 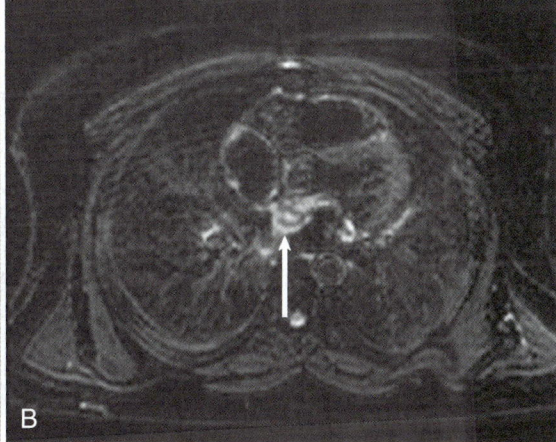

FIGURE 98.14 A, T_2-weighted image of a cardiac magnetic resonance image demonstrating a large left atrial mass near the anterior leaflet of the mitral valve. **B,** Contrast enhancement of the mass confirms a high degree of blood flow strongly suggesting an angiosarcoma.

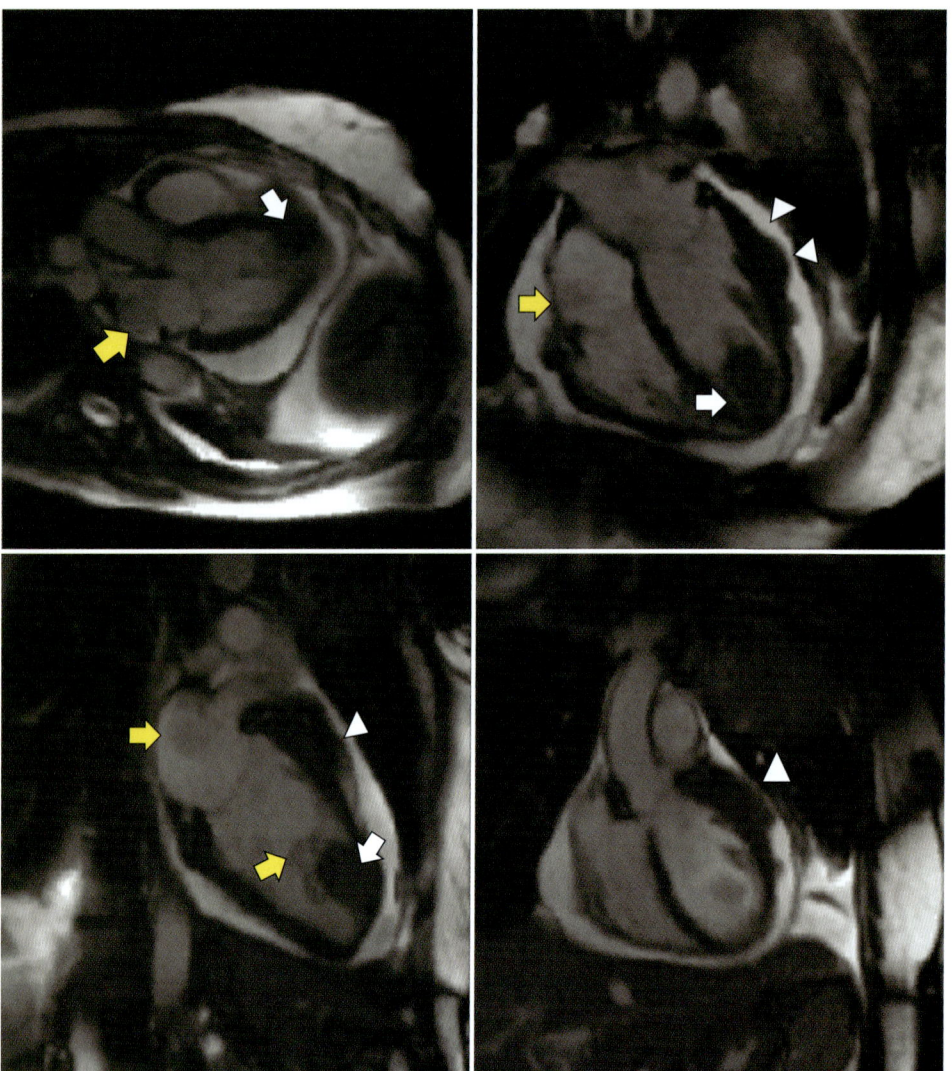

FIGURE 98.15 A 39-nine-year-old with prior history of breast cancer presents with 2-day history of dyspnea and was referred for cardiac MRI after mass seen in LV apex on echocardiography. **Top left,** Three-chamber view. **Top right,** Four-chamber view. **Bottom left,** Two-chamber view. **Bottom right,** Coronal view of the left ventricle. White arrows demonstrate cavitary masses of different texture (*solid white arrows and cystic yellow arrows*). Also, there are pericardial masses (*white triangles*) and a moderate-sized circumferential pericardial effusion. These findings are consistent with metastatic breast cancer.

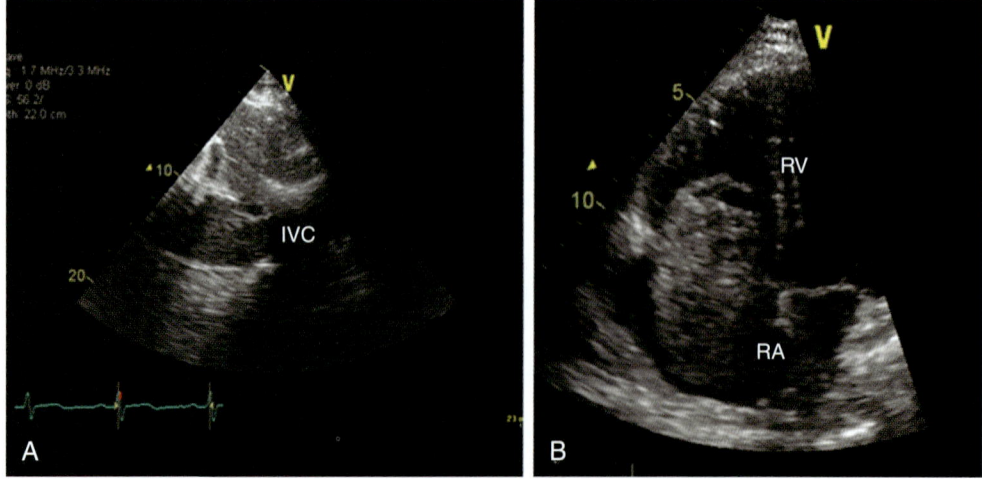

FIGURE 98.16 A, Renal cell carcinoma invading the inferior vena cava (IVC). **B,** Renal cell carcinoma invading the right atrium (RA) and prolapsing into the right ventricle (RV).

the location of the tumor. Dyspnea, palpitations, syncope, chest pain, and peripheral edema are common clinical presentations.[51,68] Heart failure, cardiac arrhythmias, heart blocks, acute myocardial infarction, myocardial rupture, systemic embolization, and superior vena cava syndrome are other manifestations of cardiac metastases. Multiple tumor metastases contributing to both pulmonary and systemic emboli can be observed as shown in Figure 98.15 in a woman with breast cancer. A new heart murmur or any new ECG finding without clear symptoms in a cancer patient should raise the sus-picion of cardiac metastases. Typical ECG findings encountered patients with cardiac metastases are ST-T wave changes (mimicking myocardial ischemia or injury), new atrial fibrillation or flutter, and low voltages with electrical alternans indicating a significant pericardial effusion. The ECG findings of myocardial injury may indicate an invasion of the coronary vessels by tumor.[69]

Treatment

Treatment of metastatic cardiac tumors is usually palliative, as overall prognosis is poor, with >50% of patients dying within one year.[51] Palliative radiotherapy and chemotherapy in chemo-sensitive tumors are recommended.[18] In these patients, end-of-life care should be discussed and all efforts should be made to improve the quality of life (see Chapter 50). In highly selected cases, extraordinary surgical approaches can be attempted, such as auto transplantation, but this is an unusual option. The management of a malignant pericardial effusion is typically individualized to a local center experience and close collaboration between oncology and cardiology is necessary to ensure an optimal treatment plan. Recent data indicate that infusion of selected chemotherapy may be useful in patients who have a malignant effusion,[70] but this is not widely practiced.[71]

DIRECT AND INDIRECT COMPLICATIONS OF NEOPLASIA

Patients with cardiac and noncardiac neoplasia can develop direct and indirect complications that affect the pericardium and the superior vena cava. These topics are discussed briefly in the following section.

Pericardial Effusion

The differential diagnosis of a pericardial effusion in a patient with a known malignancy includes malignant effusion, radiation-induced or drug-induced pericarditis, idiopathic pericarditis, infectious (including tuberculosis, fungal, or bacterial), or iatrogenic, secondary to procedures (see Chapters 56 and 57). It is estimated that approximately 40% of patients with cancer and a pericardial effusion were found to have either radiation-induced or idiopathic and only a minority actually have malignant effusion.[53] Drug-induced pericarditis is typically seen after high-dose anthracycline or cyclophosphamide therapy (see Chapter 57). The management of patients with pericardial effusions secondary to metastatic disease and radiation is discussed in Chapter 86.

Cardiac Tamponade

The diagnosis and management of cardiac tamponade secondary to metastatic disease and radiation is discussed in Chapter 86.

Constrictive Pericarditis

Constrictive or effusive-constrictive pericarditis is a late complication of chest irradiation that may be becoming more common because of the longer survival of patients with breast cancer and Hodgkin disease who typically receive chest irradiation. This topic is covered in detail in Chapter 86.

Superior Vena Cava Syndrome

The superior vena cava (SVC) syndrome refers to clinical signs and symptoms that result from either partial or complete obstruction of blood flow through the SVC. This obstruction most commonly results from tumor infiltration of the vessel wall or from thrombotic occlusion.

FUTURE PERSPECTIVES

The clinical outcomes of patients who have a primary cardiac tumor heavily depend on early detection and prompt, appropriate treatment. It is a frequent phenomenon that cardiac tumors are only discovered after a patient experiences a period of confusing constellation of symptoms that are ultimately connected to an abnormal image that suggests a cardiac tumor. As a result, there is commonly an advanced stage of disease already at the time of diagnosis. Once a primary cardiac tumor is diagnosed, all patients should be managed by a multidisciplinary team including medical oncologists, radiation oncologists, cardiologists, and cardiac surgeons. Over the last few years, increasing use of imaging modalities (e.g., echo, MRI, and CT) has led to an increasing number of incidental findings of primary cardiac tumor. However, current imaging techniques may accurately differentiate tumors from other causes of masses seen on imaging slightly more than 50% of the time. With improvements in echocardiographic and CT/MRI imaging techniques, identification of all cardiac tumors will be done with a higher degree of certainty. No noninvasive technique can identify whether the tumor is benign or malignant and a pathologic sample is needed in all cases. Improvement in surgical technique has led to minimally invasive approaches, but this still entails general anesthesia, a surgical incision, and is a major stress for a patient. Continued refinement in the surgical tools and approaches will lead to less morbidity and mortality. Currently, there are no blood tests available that would point to metastasis, and this gap represents a large unmet clinical need.

REFERENCES

Clinical Manifestations

1. Zaragoza-Macias E, Chen MA, Gill EA. Real time three-dimensional echocardiography evaluation of intracardiac masses. *Echocardiography*. 2012;29:207–219.
2. Mankad R, Herrmann J. Cardiac tumors: echo assessment. *Echo Res Pract*. 2016;3:R65–R77.
3. Auger D, Pressacco J, Marcotte F, et al. Cardiac masses: an integrative approach using echocardiography and other imaging modalities. *Heart*. 2011;97:1101–1109.
4. O'Donnell DH, Abbara S, Chaithiraphan V, et al. Cardiac tumors: optimal cardiac MR sequences and spectrum of imaging appearances. *AJR Am J Roentgenol*. 2009;193:377–387.
5. Kassi M, Polsani V, Schutt RC, et al. Differentiating benign from malignant cardiac tumors with cardiac magnetic resonance imaging. *J Thorac Cardiovasc Surg*. 2019;157:1912–1922.e2.
6. Plana JC. Added value of real-time three-dimensional echocardiography in assessing cardiac masses. *Curr Cardiol Rep*. 2009;11:205–209.
7. Buckley O, Madan R, Kwong R, et al. Cardiac masses, part 1: imaging strategies and technical considerations. *AJR Am J Roentgenol*. 2011;197:W837–W841.
8. Buckley O, Madan R, Kwong R, et al. Cardiac masses, part 2: key imaging features for diagnosis and surgical planning. *AJR Am J Roentgenol*. 2011;197:W842–W851.
9. van Beek EJ, Stolpen AH, Khanna G, Thompson BH. CT and MRI of pericardial and cardiac neoplastic disease. *Canc Imag*. 2007;7:19–26.
10. Yuan SM, Shinfeld A, Lavee J, et al. Imaging morphology of cardiac tumours. *Cardiol J*. 2009;16:26–35.
11. Kohli SK, Pantazis AA, Shah JS, et al. Diagnosis of left-ventricular non-compaction in patients with left-ventricular systolic dysfunction: time for a reappraisal of diagnostic criteria? *Eur Heart J*. 2008;29:89–95.
12. Jacquier A, Thuny F, Jop B, et al. Measurement of trabeculated left ventricular mass using cardiac magnetic resonance imaging in the diagnosis of left ventricular non-compaction. *Eur Heart J*. 2010;31:1098–1104.
13. Xanthos T, Giannakopoulos N, Papadimitriou L. Lipomatous hypertrophy of the interatrial septum: a pathological and clinical approach. *Int J Cardiol*. 2007;121:4–8.
14. Basso C, Rizzo S, Valente M, Thiene G. Cardiac masses and tumours. *Heart*. 2016;102:1230–1245.
15. Neragi-Miandoab S, Kim J, Vlahakes GJ. Malignant tumours of the heart: a review of tumour type, diagnosis and therapy. *Clin Oncol (R Coll Radiol)*. 2007;19:748–756.
16. Ekmektzoglou KA, Samelis GF, Xanthos T. Heart and tumors: location, metastasis, clinical manifestations, diagnostic approaches and therapeutic considerations. *J Cardiovasc Med (Hagerstown)*. 2008;9:769–777.
17. Simpson L, Kumar SK, Okuno SH, et al. Malignant primary cardiac tumors: review of a single institution experience. *Cancer*. 2008;112:2440–2446.
18. Al-Mamgani A, Baartman L, Baaijens M, et al. Cardiac metastases. *Int J Clin Oncol*. 2008;13:369–372.
19. McManus B. Primary tumors of the heart. In: *Braunwald's Heart Disease*. 9th ed. Elsevier; 2011:1638–1650.

Benign Primary Cardiac Tumors

20. Burke A, Virmani R. Pediatric heart tumors. *Cardiovasc Pathol*. 2008;17:193–198.
21. Thomas-de-Montpreville V, Nottin R, Dulmet E, Serraf A. Heart tumors in children and adults: clinicopathological study of 59 patients from a surgical center. *Cardiovasc Pathol*. 2007;16:22–18.
22. Bakaeen FG, Reardon MJ, Coselli JS, et al. Surgical outcome in 85 patients with primary cardiac tumors. *Am J Surg*. 2003;186:641–647; discussion 647.
23. Acebo E, Val-Bernal JF, Gomez-Roman JJ, Revuelta JM. Clinicopathologic study and DNA analysis of 37 cardiac myxomas: a 28-year experience. *Chest*. 2003;123:1379–1385.
24. Pinede L, Duhaut P, Loire R. Clinical presentation of left atrial cardiac myxoma. A series of 112 consecutive cases. *Medicine*. 2001;80:159–172.
25. Yanagawa B, Chan EY, Cusimano RJ, Reardon MJ. Approach to surgery for cardiac tumors: primary simple, primary complex, and primary malignant. *Cardiol Clin*. 2019;37:525–531.
26. Sydow K, Willems S, Reichenspurner H, Meinertz T. Papillary fibroelastomas of the heart. *Thorac Cardiovasc Surgeon*. 2008;56:9–13.
27. Walkes JC, Bavare C, Blackmon S, Reardon MJ. Transaortic resection of an apical left ventricular fibroelastoma facilitated by a thoracoscope. *J Thorac Cardiovasc Surg*. 2007;134:793–794.
28. Abu Saleh WK, Al Jabbari O, Ramlawi B, Reardon MJ. Cardiac papillary fibroelastoma: single-institution experience with 14 surgical patients. *Tex Heart Inst J*. 2016;43:148–151.
29. Jozwiak S, Kotulska K, Kasprzyk-Obara J, et al. Clinical and genotype studies of cardiac tumors in 154 patients with tuberous sclerosis complex. *Pediatrics*. 2006;118:e1146–e1151.
30. Yu K, Liu Y, Wang H, et al. Epidemiological and pathological characteristics of cardiac tumors: a clinical study of 242 cases. *Interact Cardiovasc Thoracic Surg*. 2007;6:636–639.
31. Evans CA, Suvarna SK. Cystic atrioventricular node tumour: not a mesothelioma. *J Clin Pathol*. 2005;58:1232.
32. Tran TT, Starnes V, Wang X, et al. Cardiovascular magnetics resonance diagnosis of cystic tumor of the atrioventricular node. *J Cardiovasc Magn Res*. 2009;11:13.
33. Eftychiou C, Antoniades L. Cardiac hemangioma in the left ventricle and brief review of the literature. *J Cardiovasc Med (Hagerstown)*. 2009;10:565–567.
34. Wu G, Jones J, Sequeira IB, Pepelassis D. Congenital pericardial hemangioma responding to high-dose corticosteroid therapy. *Can J Cardiol*. 2009;25:e139–140.
35. Cohen R, Mirrer B, Loarte P, Navarro V. Intrapericardial mature cystic teratoma in an adult: case presentation. *Clin Cardiol*. 2013;36:6–9.
36. Centofanti P, Di Rosa E, Deorsola L, et al. Primary cardiac tumors: early and late results of surgical treatment in 91 patients. *Ann Thorac Surg*. 1999;68:1236–1241.
37. Abu Saleh WK, Al Jabbari O, Ramlawi B, et al. Case report: cardiac tumor resection and repair with porcine Xenograft. *Methodist Debakey Cardiovasc J*. 2016;12:116–118.
38. Rana O, Gonda P, Addis B, Greaves K. Image in cardiovascular medicine. Intrapericardial paraganglioma presenting as chest pain. *Circulation*. 2009;119:e373–375.
39. Ramlawi B, David EA, Kim MP, et al. Contemporary surgical management of cardiac paragangliomas. *Ann Thorac Surg*. 2012;93:1972–1976.
40. Khalid TJ, Zuberi O, Zuberi L, Khalid I. A rare case of cardiac paraganglioma presenting as anginal pain: a case report. *Cases J*. 2009;2:72.
41. Chan EY, Ali A, Umana JP, et al. Management of primary cardiac paraganglioma. *J Thorac Cardiovasc Surg*. 2020;S0022–S5223(20):32704–5. https://doi.org/10.1016/j.jtcvs.2020.09.100. Epub ahead of print. PMID: 33148444.
42. Burke AP, Rosado-de-Christenson M, Templeton PA, Virmani R. Cardiac fibroma: clinicopathologic correlates and surgical treatment. *J Thorac Cardiovasc Surg*. 1994;108:862–870.
43. Leja MJ, Perryman L, Reardon MJ. Resection of left ventricular fibroma with subacute papillary muscle rupture. *Tex Heart Inst J*. 2011;38:279–281.
44. Reardon MJ, DeFelice CA, Sheinbaum R, Baldwin JC. Cardiac autotransplant for surgical treatment of a malignant neoplasm. *Ann Thorac Surg*. 1999;67:1793–1795.
45. Ramlawi B, Al-Jabbari O, Blau LN, et al. Autotransplantation for the resection of complex left heart tumors. *Ann Thorac Surg*. 2014;98:863–868.

Malignant Primary Tumors

46. Reynen K. Frequency of primary tumors of the heart. *Am J Cardiol*. 1996;77:107.
47. Gupta A. Primary cardiac sarcomas. *Expert Rev Cardiovasc Ther*. 2008;6:1295–1297.
48. Yin K, Luo R, Wei Y, et al. Survival outcomes in patients with primary cardiac sarcoma in the United States. *J Thorac Cardiovasc Surg*. 2021;162(1):107–115.e2.
49. Hendriksen BS, Stahl KA, Hollenbeak CS, et al. Postoperative chemotherapy and radiation improve survival following cardiac sarcoma resection. *J Thorac Cardiovasc Surg*. 2019.
50. Kim CH, Dancer JY, Coffey D, et al. Clinicopathologic study of 24 patients with primary cardiac sarcomas: a 10-year single institution experience. *Human Pathol*. 2008;39:933–938.
51. Yusuf SW, Bathina JD, Qureshi S, et al. Cardiac tumors in a tertiary care cancer hospital: clinical features, echocardiographic findings, treatment and outcomes. *Heart Int*. 2012;7:e4.
52. Randhawa JS, Budd GT, Randhawa M, et al. Primary cardiac sarcoma: 25-year cleveland clinic experience. *Am J Clin Oncol*. 2016;39:593–599.

53. Li H, Xu D, Chen Z, et al. Prognostic analysis for survival after resections of localized primary cardiac sarcomas: a single-institution experience. *Ann Thorac Surg*. 2014;97:1379–1385.
54. Agaimy A, Rosch J, Weyand M, Strecker T. Primary and metastatic cardiac sarcomas: a 12-year experience at a German heart center. *Int J Clin Exp Pathol*. 2012;5:928–938.
55. Isambert N, Ray-Coquard I, Italiano A, et al. Primary cardiac sarcomas: a retrospective study of the French Sarcoma Group. *Eur J Cancer*. 2014;50:128–136.
56. Ramlawi B, Leja MJ, Abu Saleh WK, et al. Surgical treatment of primary cardiac sarcoma: review of a single-institution experience. *Ann Thorac Surg*. 2016;101:698–702.
57. Sultan I, Bianco V, Habertheuer A, et al. Long-term outcomes of primary cardiac malignancies: multi institutional results from the national cancer database. *J Am Coll Cardiol*. 2020;75(18):2338–2347.
58. Lestuzzi C, Reardon MJ. Primary cardiac malignancies: the need for a multidisciplinary approach and the role of the cardio-oncologist. *J Am Coll Cardiol*. 2020;75:2348–2351.
59. Leja MJ, Shah DJ, Reardon MJ. Primary cardiac tumors. *Tex Heart Inst J*. 2011;38:261–262.
60. Abu Saleh WK, Ramlawi B, Shapira OM, et al. Improved outcomes with the evolution of a neoadjuvant chemotherapy approach to right heart sarcoma. *Ann Thorac Surg*. 2017;104:90–96.
61. Wu Y, Million L, Moding EJ, et al. The impact of postoperative therapy on primary cardiac sarcoma. *J Thorac Cardiovasc Surg*. 2018;156:2194–2203.
62. Ravi V, Reardon MJ. Commentary: primary cardiac sarcoma-Systemic disease requires systemic therapy. *J Thorac Cardiovasc Surg*. 2019;S0022-5223(19):32391–32398.
63. Salanitri J, Lisle D, Rigsby C, et al. Benign cardiac tumours: cardiac CT and MRI imaging appearances. *J Med Imaging Radiat Oncol*. 2008;52:550–558.
64. Blackmon SH, Patel AR, Bruckner BA, et al. Cardiac autotransplantation for malignant or complex primary left-heart tumors. *Tex Heart Inst J*. 2008;35:296–300.
65. Pigott C, Welker M, Khosla P, Higgins RS. Improved outcome with multimodality therapy in primary cardiac angiosarcoma. *Nat Clin Pract Oncol*. 2008;5:112–115.
66. Kim MP, Correa AM, Blackmon S, et al. Outcomes after right-side heart sarcoma resection. *Ann Thorac Surg*. 2011;91:770–776.
67. Zhang PJ, Brooks JS, Goldblum JR, et al. Primary cardiac sarcomas: a clinicopathologic analysis of a series with follow-up information in 17 patients and emphasis on long-term survival. *Hum Pathol*. 2008;39:1385–1395.

Secondary Cardiac Tumors and Direct and Indirect Complications of Neoplasia

68. Bussani R, De-Giorgio F, Abbate A, Silvestri F. Cardiac metastases. *J Clin Pathol*. 2007;60:27–34.
69. Yusuf SW, Durand JB, Lenihan DJ. Wrap beats. *Am J Med*. 2007;120:417–419.
70. Maisch B, Ristic A, Pankuweit S. Evaluation and management of pericardial effusion in patients with neoplastic disease. *Prog Cardiovasc Dis*. 2010;53:157–163.
71. El Haddad D, Iliescu C, Yusuf SW, et al. Outcomes of cancer patients undergoing percutaneous pericardiocentesis for pericardial effusion. *J Am Coll Cardiol*. 2015;66:1119–1128.

99 Psychiatric and Psychosocial Aspects of Cardiovascular Disease

KENNETH E. FREEDLAND, ROBERT M. CARNEY, ERIC J. LENZE, AND MICHAEL W. RICH

ACUTE STRESS AND EMOTIONAL AROUSAL, 1841
Stress and Emotional Triggers of Acute Cardiovascular Events, 1841
Cardiovascular Responses to Everyday Stressors and Emotions, 1841
Mechanisms Underlying Acute Stress Effects, 1842

CARDIOVASCULAR CONSEQUENCES OF CHRONIC STRESS, 1842
Childhood Adversity, 1842
Socioeconomic Status, 1842
Occupational Stress and Unemployment, 1842
Social Discrimination and Stigmatization, 1843

Caregiving, 1843
Combinations of Chronic and Acute Stress, 1843

MENTAL HEALTH AND PSYCHIATRIC DISORDERS, 1843
Mechanisms, 1843
Shared Features Across Mental Disorders, 1844
Anxiety, 1844
Posttraumatic Stress Disorder, 1844
Depression, 1844
Cognitive Impairment, 1845

EVALUATION AND MANAGEMENT OF MENTAL HEALTH IN THE CARDIAC PATIENT, 1846
Current Guidelines, 1846

Psychotherapy, 1847
Antidepressant Medications, 1847
Electroconvulsive Therapy, 1850
Transcranial Magnetic Stimulation, 1850
Anxiolytic Medications, 1850
Alternative Medicines and Supplements, 1850
Mindfulness, 1850
Exercise, 1851
Collaborative Care, 1851

SUMMARY AND FUTURE DIRECTIONS, 1851

ACKNOWLEDGMENT, 1851

REFERENCES, 1851

Psychological stress and certain psychiatric disorders can have clinically significant cardiovascular (CV) effects. The CV consequences of acute psychological stress have been examined in naturalistic studies of responses to disasters and personal losses, as well as in controlled laboratory studies. Various forms of chronic stress and adversity, such as unemployment and financial difficulties, have been shown to increase the risk of developing coronary heart disease (CHD) and to exacerbate established CHD. Similarly, multiple psychiatric disorders including anxiety, posttraumatic stress disorder (PTSD), depression, and others have been found to increase the risk of developing CHD and other CV conditions and are associated with increased morbidity and mortality in patients with established CV disease (CVD).

This chapter provides an overview of the CV consequences of stress and psychiatric disorders and discusses the biobehavioral mechanisms that might explain these effects. It also discusses approaches to the evaluation and management of psychiatric comorbidities in cardiac patients, including psychotherapeutic interventions, medications, noninvasive procedures including electroconvulsive therapy (ECT) and transcranial magnetic stimulation (TMS), and other nonpharmacological interventions.

ACUTE STRESS AND EMOTIONAL AROUSAL

Stress and Emotional Triggers of Acute Cardiovascular Events

Cardiac event rates often surge in populations that are exposed *en masse* to extremely stressful events.[1] Acute myocardial infarctions (MIs) increased 35% in Los Angeles after the 1994 Northridge earthquake, and sudden cardiac deaths increased from 4.6 per day during the previous week to 24 on the day of the earthquake. The 1995 Great Hanshin (Kobe) earthquake produced a 3.5-fold increase in acute MIs and a significant increase in fatal MIs. In contrast, the 1989 Loma Prieta earthquake did not affect the rate of acute MIs. Whether a disaster triggers cardiac events may depend on the time of day that it strikes—whereas the Northridge earthquake hit at 4:30 AM, the Loma Prieta earthquake hit at 5:00 PM. Superimposition of an extremely stressful event on the stress of sudden early morning awakening may be especially dangerous for individuals who are at risk for an acute MI.

Cardiac event rates may also increase during wars and terrorist attacks. For example, CV mortality increased 58% on the first day of Iraqi missile attacks on Israel during the 1991 Persian Gulf War, primarily in the targeted cities. In contrast, CV mortality did not increase in New York City on September 11, 2001. Cardiac event rate changes may depend in part on whether the stressful situation is inescapable. Individuals who were in close proximity to the 9/11 attacks were at higher risk for stress-related disorders than were those who were farther away at the time.

Private stressors can also trigger CV events. In a Danish study, the death of a child increased the risk of a first MI by 31% and of a fatal MI by 58%. In the Determinants of MI Onset Study, the risk of MI increased 21-fold after the death of a loved one.[2] A U.K. study of older primary care patients found elevated 30-day rates of MI (rate ratio 2.14) and stroke (rate ratio 2.40) in bereaved compared to matched non-bereaved patients.[3]

Takotsubo cardiomyopathy mostly affects women and is usually associated with transient left ventricular dysfunction (see also Chapters 37, 38, and 50). The onset is preceded by a stressful event in about four out of five cases.[4] The cardiomyopathy frequently resolves within weeks but recurrences are common and patients (especially older ones) who have had this syndrome are at increased risk for mortality.[4]

Emotional triggers have been studied retrospectively in survivors of cardiac events. The trauma of having a cardiac event can affect a patient's recall of antecedent emotions, and recall bias can affect the validity of this type of research. Case-crossover designs, in which patients serve as their own controls, can reduce recall bias. The Determinants of MI Onset Study used this design and found a 2.43-fold increase in the incidence of acute MI within two hours after angry outbursts. A meta-analysis of case-crossover studies found that the risk of MI or acute coronary syndrome (ACS) was 4.74 times higher in the 2 hours after an angry outburst than at other times.[5]

Cardiovascular Responses to Everyday Stressors and Emotions

Ambulatory monitoring studies have documented a variety of CV responses to everyday stressors and negative emotions. For example, in patients with implantable cardioverter-defibrillators (ICDs), anger precedes about 15% of shocks compared to only 3% of control periods. Everyday stressors and negative emotions such as anger, tension, frustration, and sadness can reduce heart rate variability and trigger episodes of myocardial ischemia and ventricular ectopy in patients with CHD.

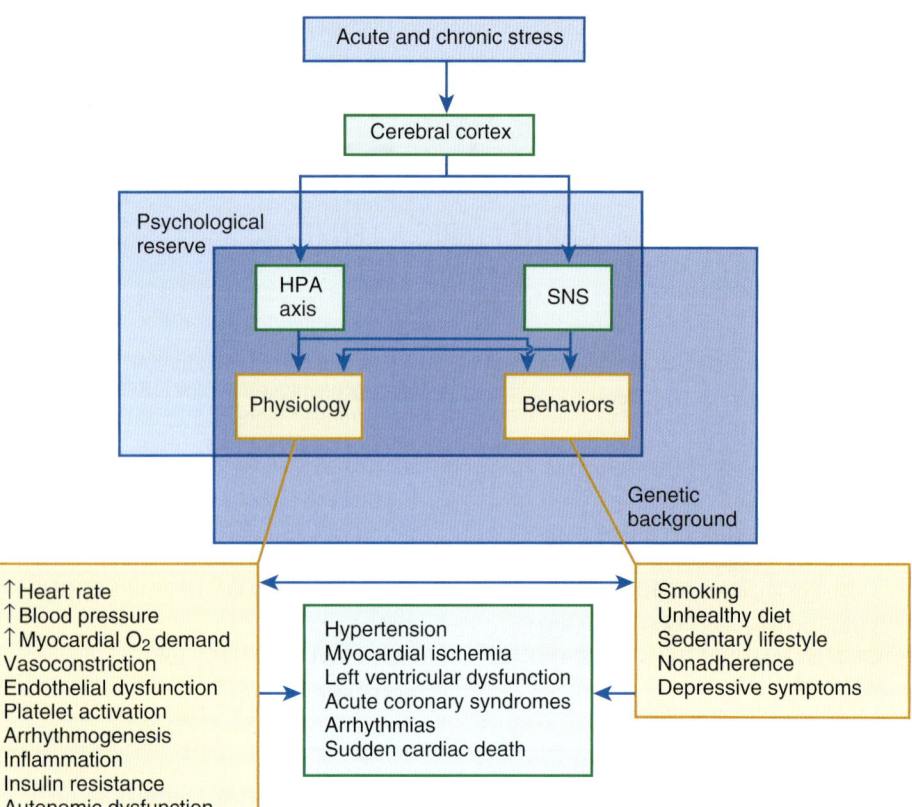

FIGURE 99.1 Potential mechanisms underlying the link between psychological factors and cardiovascular disease. *HPA*, Hypothalamic-pituitary-adrenal axis; *SNS*, sympathetic nervous system. (From Vaccarino V, Bremner JD. *Braunwald's Heart Disease: A Textbook of Cardiovascular Medicine.* 11th ed. Philadelphia, Elsevier, 2019.)

Mechanisms Underlying Acute Stress Effects

Several interrelated biobehavioral mechanisms have been implicated in the CV effects of acute stress. Mental stress-induced myocardial ischemia (MSMI) is accompanied by hemodynamic, neurohormonal, and vascular responses[6] and activation of brain areas involved in stress reactivity and depression (Fig. 99.1).[7] Among 196 patients with coronary disease in the Psychophysiological Investigations of Myocardial Ischemia (PIMI), 58% developed MSMI during mental stress testing. MSMI was accompanied by increases in heart rate, blood pressure, cardiac output, and systemic vascular resistance, a decrease in left ventricular ejection fraction, and wall motion abnormalities. In the more recent Mental Stress Ischemia Prognosis Study (MIPS) of 660 patients with coronary disease, mental stress testing increased the rate-pressure product, arterial stiffness, microvascular constriction, and plasma epinephrine,[8] as well as the inflammatory biomarkers IL-6, MCP-1, and MMP-9.[9] The 106 (16%) patients who developed MSMI had greater hemodynamic and vasoconstrictive responses to mental stress compared to MSMI-negative patients.[8] Normal epicardial coronary arteries and coronary microvessels dilate in response to acute mental stress. Diseased vessels paradoxically constrict in response to mental stress, and resistance vessel dilation is impaired. The coronary microvascular response to mental stress is endothelium-dependent and mediated by nitric oxide.[10]

CARDIOVASCULAR CONSEQUENCES OF CHRONIC STRESS (SEE ALSO CHAPTER 93)

Several sources of chronic stress have been identified as CV risk factors. These include childhood adversity, low socioeconomic status (SES), work stress, discrimination, stigmatization, and caregiving.

Childhood Adversity

Adverse childhood experiences (ACEs) include physical, sexual, and emotional abuse, as well as neglect, economic disadvantage, homelessness, exposure to violent crime, bullying, and other forms of victimization. Over 50% of the U.S. population has had at least one ACE. An American Heart Association scientific statement concluded that there is substantial evidence linking ACEs to cardiometabolic diseases later in life, including heart disease, diabetes, and stroke.[11] A recent analysis of Behavioral Risk Factor Surveillance System (BRFSS) data found dose-response relationships between ACE exposure and the incidence of CVD, as well as asthma, arthritis, chronic obstructive pulmonary disease (COPD), and depression. The associations with CVD and COPD were explained in part by smoking, heavy drinking, and obesity.[12] A separate analysis of BRFSS data also found that high exposure to ACEs was associated with CVD, but only in respondents with a history of depression.[13]

Socioeconomic Status

There has been extensive research on the health effects of low SES, also known as socioeconomic position. Most studies of the long-term effects of SES in childhood are based on parental or household income, education, or occupation. There is growing evidence that low childhood SES increases the risk of CVD in adulthood. For example, a longitudinal population-based cohort study in Finland found that growing up in a family with low SES predicts increased left ventricular mass and impaired diastolic function in middle age.[14]

Most studies associating adult SES with health outcomes use education, income, wealth, occupation, or employment status as indicators.[15] Early studies established that adult SES is related to CVD risk,[16] and more recent studies have strengthened the evidence. For example, a recent report from the Atherosclerosis Risk in Communities Study found that over a 24-year follow-up, the lowest SES group had a 1.92-fold higher risk of developing heart failure compared with the highest SES group after adjusting for income, education, deprivation, CV risk factors, and health care access.[17] A recent Medicare Expenditure Panel Survey report found that the lowest income group had the highest prevalence of cardiac risk factors including obesity, diabetes, hypertension, and physical inactivity. The trend in physical inactivity was particularly concerning, with a 71% increase in the lowest income group over a decade.[18] A study from the Swedish National Diabetes Register reported CV mortality hazard ratios (HRs) of 1.87 for the lowest versus highest income quintiles and 0.84 for individuals with college degrees versus those with less than 10 years of education.[19] SES effects have also been found in recent clinical follow-up studies. For example, low SES was associated with a high risk of all-cause mortality over 4.5 years in a retrospective study of 4503 patients who had been hospitalized with atrial fibrillation.[20]

Occupational Stress and Unemployment

A large body of research has linked various forms of occupational or work-related stress to CVD.[21] The job strain or demand-control model has dominated the research on occupational stress. It hypothesizes that demanding jobs in which the worker has little control are highly stressful, especially in socially unsupportive work environments. There is considerable evidence that job strain is a CV risk factor, at least among men. In an individual-level meta-analysis with 47,045 participants, individuals with job strain were more likely to have elevated Framingham Risk Scores (odds ratio, 1.13). A cumulative meta-analysis of 26 prospective cohort studies reported a HR for incident CHD of 1.34 for the presence versus absence of job strain.

The effort-reward imbalance model identifies another source of occupational stress. The rewards of some highly demanding jobs are insufficient in terms of compensation, job security, prospects for advancement, and/or prestige. The evidence for effort-reward imbalance as a CV risk factor in men is more limited than it is for job strain, and little is known about its effects in women. However, it predicted CV and all-cause mortality in men in the Kuopio Ischemic Heart Disease Risk Factor Study and CV mortality over 25 years in a prospective Finnish cohort study. Job strain predicted and effort-reward imbalance marginally predicted incident CHD in the Whitehall II study of male civil servants in London, but only among employees who were frequently subjected to unfair criticism or other forms of occupational injustice. Occupational injustice itself was an independent predictor of incident CHD, even after adjusting for job strain and effort-reward imbalance.

Job insecurity and unemployment have also been identified as contributors to poor CV health. An individual-level meta-analysis of 13 cohort studies found an adjusted relative risk of high versus low job security of 1.32 for incident CHD, with no differences between men and women or younger and older individuals. The CV risks of job insecurity were partly explained by lower SES and higher prevalence of CHD risk factors among job-insecure individuals.[22] An analysis of nationally representative prospective data on adults aged 51 to 75 years in the Health and Retirement Study showed that the risk of having an acute MI was significantly higher among unemployed than consistently employed workers (HR 1.35), and that there was a dose-response relationship with MI risk and the cumulative number of job losses. The first year of unemployment was an especially high-risk period.

Social Discrimination and Stigmatization
There is inconsistent evidence as to whether various forms of social discrimination and stigmatization, including discrimination based on race, age, sex, or sexual orientation, increase the risk of CVD. Some studies have yielded null or paradoxical results, such as findings from the Jackson Heart Study that racial discrimination among African Americans is associated with a lower risk of all-cause mortality[23] and from the Coronary Artery Risk Development in Young Adults (CARDIA) study that racial discrimination is inversely associated with coronary artery calcification. However, other studies do suggest that chronic exposure to discrimination or stigmatization can have adverse CV consequences.[24] For example, when participants in the National Epidemiological Survey on Alcohol and Related Conditions were grouped by state-level indicators of structural racism, there was a significantly greater past-year prevalence of acute MI among blacks living in states with high levels of structural racism compared to those living in low-structural racism states. Conversely, whites were less likely to have had an acute MI if they lived in a high- rather than a low-structural racism state.[25] Among participants in the Multi-Ethnic Study of Atherosclerosis who were initially free of clinical CVD, those who reported high lifetime levels of racial discrimination had a higher 10-year risk of incident CV events (adjusted HR, 1.36).[26] African American participants in the Jackson Heart Study without hypertension at baseline who experienced medium (HR, 1.49) or high (HR, 1.34) levels of racial discrimination were at increased risk for incident hypertension.[27] Thus, there is growing evidence that racial discrimination increases CVD risks in African Americans.

Caregiving
There has been limited research on the CV effects of chronic stress associated with caregiving for a family member with a debilitating chronic illness such as Alzheimer disease, and much of this work has focused on surrogate outcomes. Nevertheless, there is evidence that stressful caregiving over relatively long periods may promote CVD. In the Reasons for Geographic and Racial Differences in Stroke (REGARDS) study, Framingham Stroke Risk scores averaged 23% higher in participants who reported high caregiver strain compared to those with low or no caregiver strain. The risk was especially high in African American men. Caregiver strain did not affect Framingham CHD Risk scores in this study. Other studies have shown that caregiver stress can contribute to endothelial dysfunction, impairment of the cardiovagal baroreflex,[28] the development or worsening of cardiometabolic syndrome, and the development of carotid plaque.

Combinations of Chronic and Acute Stress
Acute stress is often superimposed on a background of chronic stress and other psychological (e.g., depression) and pathophysiological (e.g., unstable plaque) vulnerabilities. The "perfect storm" model proposes that when mental stress triggers an ACS, it does so in concert with these other factors.[29] Few studies have examined whether the CV effects of acute mental stress differ depending on the background level of chronic stress. However, a recent analysis of MIPS data showed that in patients with stable coronary disease, a high level of chronic psychosocial distress is associated with a blunted hemodynamic response to acute mental stress.[30] In prior studies, blunted CV reactivity to mental stress has been associated with obesity, smoking, and other health risk behaviors.[31]

MENTAL HEALTH AND PSYCHIATRIC DISORDERS
The Diagnostic and Statistical Manual of Mental Disorders (DSM-5)[32] provides a compendium of psychiatric disorders, along with the corresponding ICD-10 codes. Some of these disorders are prevalent in the general adult population, and even more prevalent in populations with chronic medical illness.[33] Conversely, certain medical conditions such as diabetes and CHD are highly prevalent among populations with serious mental illnesses.[34] A small number of psychiatric disorders, including PTSD and several mood and anxiety disorders, are of particular interest in the context of CVD because they have been identified as risk factors for the development of CVD or as predictors of adverse outcomes and poor health-related quality of life in patients with established CVD.

Mechanisms
The search for pathways that link psychiatric disorders to incident cardiac disease and subsequent cardiac events is ongoing, and many candidate mechanisms have been identified. The links between depression and cardiac outcomes have received the most study. Depression is associated with dysregulation of the autonomic nervous system (ANS) and the hypothalamic–pituitary–adrenal (HPA) axis, including higher levels of plasma and urinary catecholamines and cortisol, higher resting and mean 24-hour heart rates, and lower heart rate variability (see Fig. 99.1). Other studies have found elevated proinflammatory cytokines, acute-phase proteins, chemokines, and adhesion molecules, including increased levels of C-reactive protein (CRP), interleukin-6 (IL-6), and tumor necrosis factor (TNF). There is also evidence that depressed patients with CHD have elevated markers of coagulation and platelet activity, especially β-thromboglobulin and platelet factor 4. However, none of these abnormalities is present in every depressed patient,[35] and the proportion of the effect of depression on incident CHD or cardiac events (including mortality) explained by these factors is modest. This suggests that several pathways may be involved and that they differ across individuals.[36]

In addition to the physiological mechanisms, there are behavioral characteristics of depressed patients that likely contribute to the increased risk for CVD and adverse cardiac outcomes. Depressed patients are more likely to be sedentary, to smoke, and to engage in other unhealthy behaviors (e.g., poor diet, higher alcohol consumption) (see Fig. 99.1). Furthermore, depression predicts poor adherence to medication regimens, risk factor modification interventions including dietary regimens and smoking cessation programs, and cardiac rehabilitation.[36]

Shared Features Across Mental Disorders

As discussed below, there is now compelling evidence that a wide range of negative emotional states and psychiatric disorders increase the risk for incident CVD and for cardiac events in patients with established CVD. These observations have led to growing interest in elucidating common elements that might explain the risks. One such effort has been the attempt to identify underlying personality dimensions and temperaments associated with these psychiatric disorders and with the susceptibility to the effects of acute and chronic stress that might explain their CV effects. Type D (distressed) personality, which consists of a combination of neuroticism and social inhibition, is an example. Neuroticism is a personality trait that in itself has been associated with depression and anxiety disorders. The hypothesis that a single underlying personality type explains much of the effect of different negative affective states on CVD is intuitively appealing. It might also be more efficient to study a single unifying disorder than the growing number of negative affective states and disorders (e.g., distress, anger, hostility, depression, general anxiety, panic disorder, phobias, PTSD, vital exhaustion) that have been identified as risk factors for CVD. These disorders are often comorbid, and they share many of the same symptoms and many of the same putative mechanisms that may explain their effect on CVD (e.g., ANS dysfunction, increased inflammatory activity, poor diet, insufficient exercise, smoking). Furthermore, many drugs considered to be primarily antidepressants, and many forms of psychotherapy including cognitive behavior therapy (CBT), are used to treat depression, anxiety disorders, PTSD, and psychosocial distress associated with stressful situations. Thus, there is both mechanistic and therapeutic overlap between these ostensibly distinct psychiatric disorders, suggesting that an integrative approach to their evaluation and management may be warranted. Nonetheless, most research continues to study these affective states and psychiatric disorders individually as separate albeit related entities.

Anxiety

The 12-month prevalence of anxiety disorders in the United States is about 18%, and the lifetime prevalence is about 30% in women and 19% in men. There is evidence that anxiety is a risk factor for incident CHD, as well as atrial and ventricular arrhythmias. However, most studies of anxiety as a risk factor for cardiac morbidity and mortality have used self-report anxiety symptom questionnaires. There have been fewer studies of clinically diagnosed anxiety disorders.

A meta-analysis of 20 studies with nearly 250,000 individuals and a mean follow-up of 11.2 years found that anxious persons had a 26% increased risk for incident CHD (HR = 1.26; CI 1.15–1.38) and a nearly 50% increased risk of cardiac death (HR = 1.48; CI 1.14–1.92), independent of biological and demographic risk factors and health behaviors.[37] A more recent meta-analysis reported a 40% increased risk of developing CHD among anxious persons, but found significant heterogeneity of effect sizes across the studies.[38]

There is also evidence that anxiety is a risk factor for cardiac events in patients with established CHD.[39] However, anxiety is highly comorbid with depression,[40] making it difficult to separate the risks of incident CHD or subsequent cardiac events associated with anxiety from those of depression. Adding to this difficulty, patients with both anxiety and major depressive disorder are likely to be more severely depressed and impaired than depressed patients with little anxiety.[36] Thus, it has been difficult to demonstrate an effect of anxiety independent from depression in many studies.

Some anxiety disorders are associated with a daily experience of mild to moderate anxiety throughout the day. Individuals with specific phobias may be relatively free of anxiety at most times, but they experience anxiety or panic in certain situations such as when exposed to heights or to certain animals. Individuals with agoraphobia have an extreme fear of being away from home or in open spaces, crowds, or places from which it would be difficult to escape in an emergency. Individuals with panic disorder, with or without agoraphobia, experience episodes of extreme anxiety accompanied by highly elevated sympathetic nervous system activity. There is some evidence that these anxiety disorders may differ with respect to their risk for cardiac events and mortality, but not all studies have supported this conclusion. Nearly every review of this literature has concluded that larger, better quality studies are needed to address this question.

A few studies have found that some forms of anxiety may be beneficial in cardiac patients, at least at moderate levels. In one study, patients with a lifetime diagnosis of generalized anxiety disorder tended to have better CV outcomes than those without an anxiety diagnosis. A potential explanation for this finding is that a moderate level of anxiety, while perhaps unpleasant, may motivate patients to follow medical advice and engage in self-care after a diagnosis of heart disease. This may also explain why anxiety symptom questionnaires do not always predict worse outcomes in CHD patients. Much like depression, anxiety has been associated with poor sleep, lower activity level, poor diet, and increased smoking.[36] These factors may help explain poorer prognosis associated with anxiety.

In summary, there is moderate evidence that anxiety is a risk factor for incident CHD and cardiac events in patients with established CHD. However, there are fewer studies of anxiety than of depression as predictors of cardiac outcomes, and not all studies have found anxiety to be a significant independent predictor of incident CHD or cardiac events. Nevertheless, the consensus among most experts is that anxiety is likely to be a risk factor for incident CHD. More research is needed to determine whether this risk differs by type of anxiety disorder and the extent to which the effects of anxiety are independent from those of depression.

Posttraumatic Stress Disorder

PTSD may be triggered by a single traumatic, life-threatening event or by recurrent events. A diagnosis of PTSD requires exposure to a traumatic event, such as a natural disaster, injurious accident, combat, or a life-threatening medical event such as ACS, accompanied by intense fear or panic. This is followed by persistent painful and intrusive memories, nightmares and flashbacks, avoidance behavior, and hyperarousal. The lifetime prevalence of PTSD in the U.S. population is estimated to be as high as 8%, whereas approximately 18% of combat veterans have or will develop this disorder during their lifetime. PTSD is independently associated with an increased risk for incident CHD[41,42] and for recurrent cardiac events following an ACS. There is also evidence that PTSD is associated with increased risk for atrial fibrillation, heart failure, and CV mortality. Along with anxiety and depression, PTSD has been widely reported in patients with an implantable cardioverter defibrillator (ICD). PTSD also increases the long-term risk of mortality in patients with an ICD, independent of cardiac disease severity.

Although there are medications for PTSD, psychotherapeutic interventions may be more effective. The best-established approaches include prolonged exposure therapy and cognitive processing therapy. Prolonged exposure therapy involves repeated exposure to the traumatic event(s), through either guided imagination or stimuli such as photographs or videos. Cognitive processing therapy involves examination of thoughts and beliefs about the trauma and its meaning and consequences. Although these approaches can produce dramatic results in many cases, the response rate is only around 50% and the full remission rate is even lower. Thus, more work is needed to improve PTSD treatment outcomes and to determine whether effective treatment of this disorder reduces the risk for both incident CHD and cardiac events in patients with established CHD.

Depression

Of the psychosocial problems and psychiatric disorders that may be risk factors for incident CHD or for cardiac events in patients with established CHD, depression is by far the best studied. There have been over 100 studies of depression as a risk factor for incident CVD. Many different self-report questionnaires and diagnostic interviews have been used to define depression in these studies. Some studies have focused on older adults, on women or men only, or on patients with cardiac risk factors such as hypertension. Despite the heterogeneity of the methods for assessing and defining depression and of the populations examined, at least six meta-analyses have been performed. Five of them found a 60% to 80% increased risk of incident CHD associated with depression. One reported a more modest level of risk (30%), but all found that depression is a significant risk factor for developing CHD.[36]

Most studies have found that the risks associated with depression remain significant after adjustment for a variety of medical and demographic confounders. For example, Gan and colleagues[43] found that adjustment for established cardiac risk factors including smoking, body mass index (BMI), hypertension, diabetes, physical inactivity, and low SES did not substantially change the risk estimates for depression in their meta-analysis.

A recent cohort study conducted in 21 countries with 145,862 participants found the incidence of MI and CVD mortality to be about 20% higher in those with four or more symptoms of depression (11% of the total sample) compared to non-depressed participants.[44] This represents a lower estimate of risk than those reported in recent meta-analyses. Unlike the meta-analyses, however, these data were collected from many different countries with different standards of living, socioeconomic levels, and medical care. The effect of depression on MI and cardiac mortality was twice as high in urban compared to rural areas, regardless of economic level.

Depression has also been studied as a predictor of cardiac events and mortality in patients with established CHD. The point prevalence of major depression in the adult population is estimated to be about 5%. By contrast, 15% to 20% of patients with medically stable CHD have major depression, and up to 30% have significant depressive symptoms.[36] Over 300 studies have evaluated depression as a risk factor for medical morbidity and mortality in patients with established CHD and at least five meta-analyses have been published.[36]

One of the largest and most recent meta-analyses included 29 studies and found that depression was associated with a 2.7-fold increased risk for cardiac-related mortality, a 2.3-fold increased risk for all-cause mortality, and a 1.6-fold increased risk for CV events.[45] In one of the largest studies of depression and CV mortality in CHD, after extensive adjustment for major cardiac risk factors, including age, sex, smoking, systolic blood pressure, BMI, diabetes, social class, heavy alcohol use, and antidepressant medications, a 2.7-fold increased risk of cardiac death in patients with depression over a median follow-up period of 8 years was reported.

Thus, the preponderance of evidence indicates that depression is an independent risk factor for incident CHD and for cardiac events in persons with known heart disease. However, many established risk factors for CHD have been shown to be associated with depression, such as smoking and sedentary lifestyle.[36] Although residual confounding must be considered as a possible explanation for at least part of the association, after a careful review of the literature, a scientific panel convened by the American Heart Association issued a statement identifying depression as a major risk factor for cardiac morbidity and mortality after an ACS.[46] Correspondingly, the current ACC/AHA Practice Guidelines for the Management of Patients with ST-elevation MI recommend screening for depression, as well as anxiety and sleep disorders, in the post-MI period (Fig. 99.2).[47]

OTHER PSYCHIATRIC DISORDERS

Other psychiatric disorders may also be risk factors for the development of CHD or subsequent cardiac events, as well as early mortality. A study of over 47,000 community-dwelling adults from 17 countries with over 2 million person-years[48] reported the relationships between 16 DSM-IV psychiatric disorders and the risk of onset of 10 physical disorders including heart disease. After adjusting for age, sex, country, education, and smoking, they found significant associations between most of the 16 psychiatric disorders and the subsequent onset of most of the 10 physical conditions, including CVD. They concluded that the "piecemeal" perspective of evaluating a single mental disorder and medical disorder obscures the "broader message" that mental disorders of all types are associated with a wide range of chronic physical conditions, including CVDs. Although the investigators administered a standardized psychiatric diagnostic interview to all participants, they relied on the participants' self-report of the physical conditions, which the investigators acknowledged as a limitation of the study. Nevertheless, the study provides intriguing, suggestive evidence that many psychiatric disorders may be risk factors for a wide range of medical conditions including CVD.

Similarly, Vance and colleagues found that multiple psychiatric illnesses, including psychotic disorders, were associated with an increased risk of adverse cardiac outcomes in over 1.5 million men and 94,000 women military veterans who were receiving care in the Department of Veterans Affairs health system.[49] In addition, they reported that more severe psychiatric disorders had the largest effect sizes, even after controlling for standard CVD risk factors and psychotropic medication use. Weye and colleagues reported on the relationship between specific mental disorders and life expectancy in a population-based cohort study from Denmark that included nearly 7 million participants.[50] They found that the diagnosis of a mental disorder was associated with life expectancies shortened by 11.2 years in males and 7.9 years in females compared to those without mental disorders. The effects were most dramatic for alcohol use, but depression and anxiety disorders also predicted shorter life spans, in many cases in patients with CVD. In a recent study of 108,610 Canadian patients with acute MI, patients with comorbid schizophrenia (N = 1145, 1.1%) had an increased risk for all-cause, 1-year mortality (adjusted HR = 1.55; CI 1.37–1.77).[51] The association of schizophrenia with mortality was attenuated after adjusting for revascularization. Thus, there is ample evidence that many psychiatric disorders are risk markers for CVD, cardiac events, and early mortality.

Cognitive Impairment

The prevalence of cognitive impairment increases with age and with CVD. In addition, many mental disorders, such as depression, are also associated with cognitive impairment. As a result, individuals with comorbid CVD and mental disorders are at substantially increased risk for cognitive impairment. The presence of cognitive impairment complicates management of CV disease, as cognitively impaired individuals have difficulty remembering and following through on treatment plans, adhering to medication regimens, or accurately reporting symptoms. Even mildly cognitively impaired patients can have difficulty with adherence to their medication regimen, and they may need support with medication adherence, getting to appointments, following medical instructions, and making lifestyle changes such as exercising. Thus, it is essential to involve family or other caregivers in medical discussions with cognitively impaired patients. Cognitive impairment also necessitates screening for reversible causes of the impairment, in particular medications. Atropine (for bradyarrhythmias) and tertiary amine tricyclics such as amitriptyline, imipramine, or doxepin (most often for pain or sleep) can cause cognitive impairment and delirium due to their centrally acting antimuscarinic effects. In addition, benzodiazepines can cause cognitive impairment and delirium.

Older patients and patients with mental disorders should be screened for cognitive impairment. Effective approaches to screening include: (i) conducting brief tests of cognitive performance and (ii) asking a corroborative source whether the patient is having difficulties with memory or thinking. A simple screening test for cognitive impairment that takes only 1 to 2 minutes includes questions on orientation ("what is today's date?" "what floor are we on?"), memory (remember three objects, or a name and address; assess recall after 5 minutes), attention and information processing speed ("say the months of the year backwards, starting with December"), and executive function and visuospatial abilities ("please draw a clock face" then "draw the hands to show 10 after 11"). Corroborative sources should be individuals who know the patient well, have frequent contact with them, and can answer questions such as "how much difficulty do they have remembering new information?" and "how much trouble do they have understanding or doing complex things such as finances or shopping?" Family members may either downplay or over-report a patient's cognitive problems and often may note that their remote memory is intact. (This is common in mild to moderate Alzheimer dementia, in which recent but not remote recall is impaired.)

While there is increasing evidence that cognitive impairment can be prevented by CVD risk reduction,[52] once cognitive impairment occurs there are few therapies and they are only modestly effective. Two classes of cognitive enhancing medications, acetylcholinesterase inhibitors and stimulants, are commonly associated with CV effects. Acetylcholinesterase inhibitors include donepezil, rivastigmine, and galantamine. These medications are indicated for patients with dementia. They are also frequently prescribed off-label for patients with mild neurocognitive disorder (a milder level of cognitive impairment that

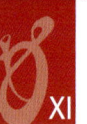

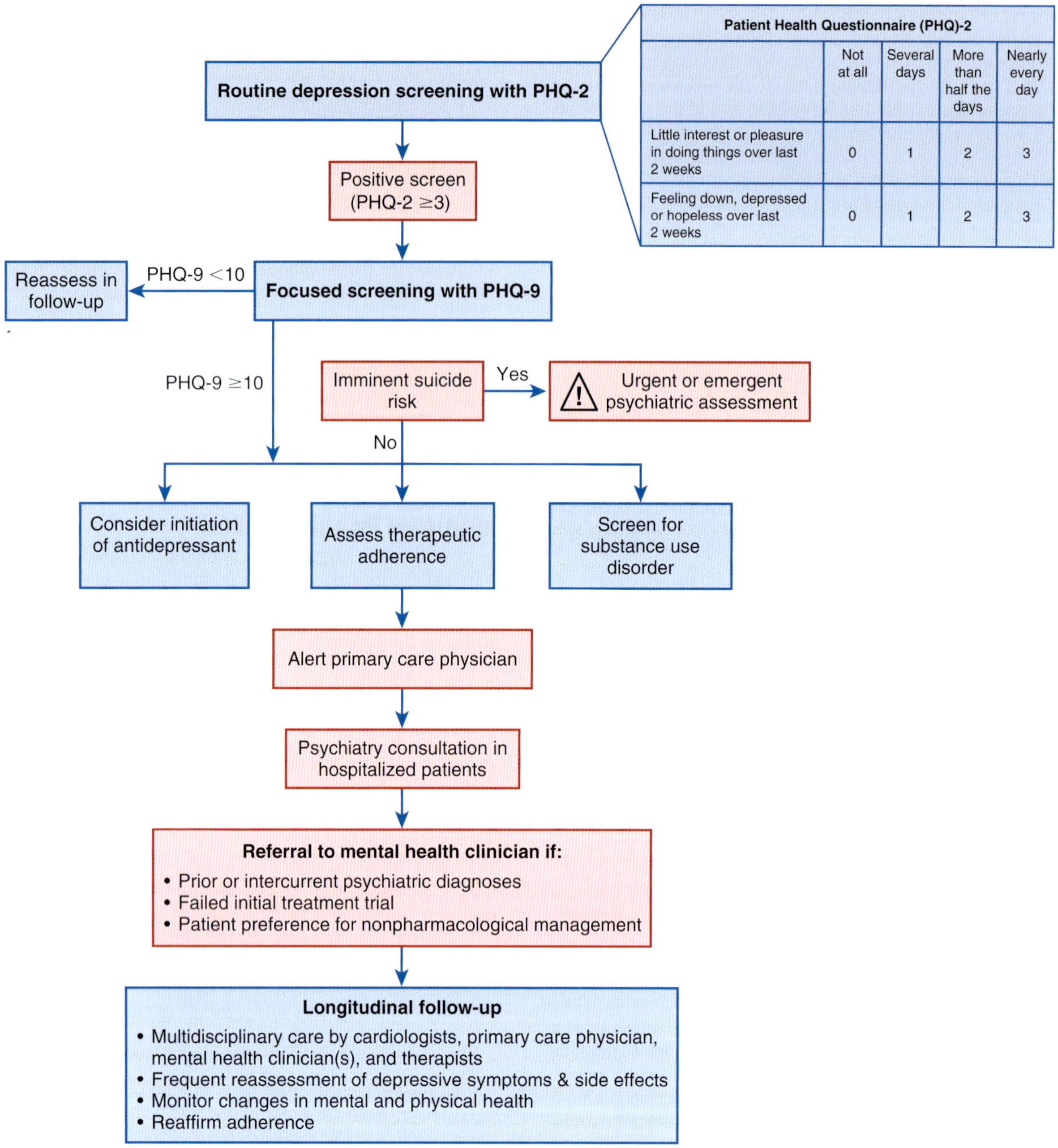

FIGURE 99.2 Guideline-supported routine depression screening pathway in patients with cardiovascular disease. (From Jha MK, Qamar A, Vaduganathan M, et al. Screening and management of depression in patients with cardiovascular disease: JACC state-of-the-art review. *J Am Coll Cardiol.* 2019;73[14]:1827–1845.)

often transitions to dementia) or even for cognitively normal older adults with subjective cognitive complaints. The cholinesterase inhibitors produce modest improvements in memory and other aspects of cognitive function. Their main cardiac effect is bradycardia through increasing cholinergic transmission. They can also increase the PR interval and cause, or be relatively contraindicated in, heart block.[53] As well, these drugs are sometimes poorly tolerated due to side effects of nausea, diarrhea, or depression. Memantine is not a cholinesterase inhibitor but is thought to act via glutamatergic N-methyl-D-aspartate (NMDA) antagonism and is unlikely to produce CV effects.

Stimulants include methylphenidate and amphetamine. They are typically used for attention deficit disorder in children, but many middle-aged and older adult patients take them for longstanding attention deficits or new-onset problems with concentration. They are also used for disorders of excessive somnolence and binge eating, and are sometimes used in stroke (e.g., for apathy) and depression. All of these conditions are more common in patients with CV disorders than in the general adult population; as a result, stimulant use in the CV population is not rare. In children, stimulants are widely regarded as safe, but in adults—particularly older adults—they have been associated with CV complications, including MI, cerebrovascular events, ventricular arrhythmias, and sudden death. Causes of these complications may include increased blood pressure and heart rate and induced vasospasm via increased levels of catecholamines (norepinephrine and dopamine), vasculitis, and prolongation of the QTc interval.[54]

The decision to use cholinesterase inhibitors or stimulants in patients with CVD is often a complex one that requires balancing perceived benefits against the potential safety risks. Ideally, this can be best achieved through a multidisciplinary shared decision-making process involving the cardiologist, psychiatrist and/or geriatrician, and the patient and patient surrogate.

EVALUATION AND MANAGEMENT OF MENTAL HEALTH IN THE CARDIAC PATIENT

Current Guidelines

Although several psychiatric comorbidities are prevalent in patients with CVD and predict adverse outcomes, current cardiology and primary care practice guidelines address only some of them. Several organizations have provided guidance on screening, assessment, and/or treatment of depression and anxiety in patient populations with or at risk for CVD.

> The American Academy of Family Physicians recommends that patients with a recent ACS should be screened for depression, and strongly recommends that patients with clinically significant depression should be treated with antidepressant medications and/or CBT. The screening guidance is based on low-quality evidence, but treatment recommendations are based on moderate-quality evidence.[55] The United States Preventive Services Task Force (USPSTF) found convincing evidence to support depression screening for all adults and older adults in clinical practice settings.[56] The 2016 European Guidelines on Cardiovascular Disease Prevention in Clinical Practice recommend screening and evaluation of patients for depression, anxiety, and other psychiatric conditions (level of evidence B, Class IIa recommendation).[57] The European Society of Cardiology recommends assessment of depression and anxiety in patients after implantation of an ICD (level of evidence C, Class I recommendation).[58] The American College of Cardiology (ACC) and the American Heart Association (AHA) recommend recognition of depression as a risk factor for adverse medical outcomes in patients with an ACS[59] and screening for depression in patients with CHD.[60] In patients with an ST-elevation MI, the ACC and AHA also recommend screening for depression, anxiety, and sleep disorders (level of evidence C, Class I recommendation).[47] When indicated, depressed patients should be treated with CBT or selective serotonin reuptake inhibitors (SSRIs; level of evidence A, Class IIa recommendation), and anxiolytic agents should be used for the short-term treatment of anxiety (level of evidence C, Class IIa recommendation).[47]

Psychotherapy

Psychotherapies such as CBT or interpersonal psychotherapy are as effective as antidepressants for moderate to severe depression in medically well depressed patients. Anxiety disorders also respond well to CBT. CBT for depression is the best studied psychotherapy in patients with heart disease.[61] CBT helps patients identify dysfunctional thoughts, attitudes, and behaviors that may cause or prolong depressed mood and related symptoms. The patient learns to replace their dysfunctional cognitions and behaviors with more adaptive ones. These cognitive and behavioral changes improve the patient's mood. In addition, CBT promotes effective coping and problem-solving strategies, and it encourages patients to use behavioral activation, i.e., increased engagement in pleasant and productive activities, to further improve their mood. Antidepressant medications are often used to augment CBT or other psychotherapeutic interventions for patients who do not have a sufficient response after a month or two of therapy. This stepped-care approach to treating depression has been shown to be more effective than the usual care provided in typical clinical settings.[62]

Patients who are already taking multiple medications for their cardiac and other medical conditions often express a preference for psychotherapy over antidepressants or anxiolytics. In addition, many patients want to discuss problems related to their illness, as well as family, personal, and work-related concerns. Learning more effective ways of coping with their illness may also help improve their quality of life. CBT is an appropriate option for patients who are not only seeking relief from the symptoms of depression or anxiety, but who also want to address the distressing problems, stressors, or losses they are experiencing. If a patient with CVD is motivated to work on his or her problems and is cognitively intact, evidenced-based psychotherapies, such as CBT or interpersonal psychotherapy, are likely to be helpful in improving their depression and anxiety.[61] However, these psychotherapies may not be available in some communities, and psychotherapy is not always covered by medical insurance in the United States. Antidepressant or anxiolytic medications may be the best alternatives for patients who lack access to effective psychotherapeutic services.

Antidepressant Medications

Antidepressant medications are the most common type of treatment for depression and other mental disorders associated with an increased risk for CVD, including PTSD. Antidepressants appear to be more effective (compared to placebo) in patients with moderate or severe depression than in patients with mild depression. This suggests that patients with mild depression are about as likely to improve with watchful waiting as with an antidepressant. Therefore, prior to initiating antidepressant treatment, providers should ensure that patients have sufficiently severe and persistent symptomatology to warrant starting a medication. Such evidence includes: mood is low (or anxious) most of the day, nearly every day; persistent negative thoughts about ones' self (i.e., guilt, worthlessness, hopelessness); symptoms cause persistent distress or functional impairment; and/or symptoms include recurrent thoughts about death (e.g., life is not worth living, it may be better to be dead than alive). Absent such severity markers, antidepressant medications are unlikely to be effective, and psychotherapy or watchful waiting is preferred.

One exception to this precept is for patients already taking an antidepressant, in whom "mild" depression or anxiety may indicate residual symptoms of an inadequately treated illness and should prompt a consideration of whether the antidepressant dose should be increased. As discussed below, antidepressants useful in patients with CVD include SSRIs (paroxetine, fluoxetine, sertraline, and others), mirtazapine, bupropion, venlafaxine, desvenlafaxine, and duloxetine.

Antidepressants act on the brain's monoaminergic neurotransmitter systems: serotonin, norepinephrine, and/or dopamine. Almost all antidepressants bind to and inhibit transporter proteins that are responsible for the reuptake of neurotransmitter into the neuron after it has been released into the synapse, thereby causing an increase in neurotransmitter within the synapse. Most antidepressant drugs block the serotonin transporter (serotonin reuptake inhibitors), the norepinephrine transporter (norepinephrine reuptake inhibitors [NRIs]), or a combination of the two (serotonin-norepinephrine reuptake inhibitors [SNRIs]). The process by which this molecular action reduces depression or other mental disorders remains unknown. Of note, these SNRIs effects are not confined to the brain and the synaptic cleft; for example, serotonin transporters are found in platelets, bone (osteoblasts, osteoclasts), and intestinal absorptive cells. The clinical significance of peripheral SSRI effects is not well understood, although there is substantial evidence for increased bleeding risks due to effects on platelets.

Many antidepressants also have other non-monoaminergic effects on the cholinergic, histaminergic, or alpha-adrenergic systems, which are sometimes called "off-target" effects because they are thought to be unrelated to the drug's therapeutic effects. The original tricyclic antidepressants tended to have widespread effects on these receptors, which were responsible for many of their side effects. For many of the newer antidepressants, the non-monoaminergic effects are minimal or have unknown clinical relevance, and some of these actions, such as sigma-1 receptor agonism, have been the subject of research for possible cardioprotective effects. Table 99.1 summarizes medications commonly used for the treatment of depression in patients with CVD, and general principles for prescribing antidepressant medications are shown in Table 99.2.

Tricyclic Antidepressants

Tricyclics were developed specifically for treating depression and were the first class of medications proven to be effective in patients with depression. They are also used for treating anxiety disorders, including panic disorder, and clomipramine is used for obsessive-compulsive disorder. With the development of newer agents, they are usually reserved for treatment-resistant cases. Tricyclics are frequently used at lower doses for non-psychiatric conditions such as chronic pain, migraine headaches, and insomnia. The mechanism of action is to increase norepinephrine and serotonin levels in the synapse. Representative agents include imipramine, doxepin, desipramine, clomipramine, nortriptyline, and amitriptyline.

The two most salient concerns regarding tricyclics for patients with CVD are their side effects and their potential for inducing QTc prolongation. Tricyclics have anticholinergic effects, which may cause dry mouth, constipation, memory problems, confusion, blurred vision, sexual dysfunction, and decreased urination. They also cause alpha-1 adrenergic blockade, which may lead to orthostatic hypotension, and anti-histaminergic effects, including sedation, increased appetite, and confusion. Generally, the tertiary amine tricyclics—amitriptyline, imipramine, doxepin, and clomipramine—have more significant effects at these receptors and hence more side effects compared to the secondary amine tricyclics nortriptyline and desipramine. For this reason, tertiary amine tricyclics are not recommended for older adults, who are more susceptible to the memory impairment and orthostatic hypotension associated with these medications.

TABLE 99.1 Commonly Used Antidepressant Medications

ANTIDEPRESSANT	TYPICAL DAILY STARTING DOSE	EFFECTIVE DAILY DOSE RANGE	COMMENTS
Selective Serotonin Reuptake Inhibitors (SSRIs)			
Escitalopram	5–10 mg	10–20 mg	Good first-line medications because of safety, tolerability, and ease of use
Sertraline	25–50 mg	50–200 mg	
Citalopram	10–20 mg	20–40 mg	QTc prolongation (avg 13 msec) at doses >20 mg in older adults
			Has mild antihistamine effects at higher doses
Fluoxetine	10–20 mg	20–40 mg	Reduces metabolism of other drugs through CYP2D6 and CYP2B6 (moderate inhibitor)
Paroxetine	10–20 mg	20–40 mg	Reduces metabolism of other drugs through CYP2D6 and CYP2B6 (strong inhibitor)
Fluvoxamine	50 mg	100–300 mg	Reduces metabolism of other drugs through multiple CYP enzymes, particularly CYP2C19 and CYP1A2 (strong interaction)
Serotonin-Norepinephrine Reuptake Inhibitors (SNRIs)			Usually safe but can cause hypertension or orthostatic hypotension
Venlafaxine extended release	37.5–75 mg	150–300 mg	
Desvenlafaxine	50 mg	50–100 mg	
Duloxetine	30–60 mg	60–120 mg	Reduces metabolism of other drugs through CYP2D6 and CYP2B6 (moderate interaction)
Milnacipran	12.5–25 mg	50 mg twice daily	Under patent protection, expensive
Other Antidepressant Medications and Strategies			
Bupropion XL	150 mg	300–450 mg	Reduces metabolism of other drugs through CYP2D6 (strong interaction). Metabolized chiefly by CYP2B6 and can cause ataxia, falls, and rarely seizures at excessively high concentrations
Mirtazapine	7.5–15 mg	30–45 mg	Has strong antihistamine properties so can cause sedation and weight gain, even at low doses (15 mg or less)
Tricyclics	25–50 mg	Based on blood concentration	Pro-arrhythmic effects in ischemic heart disease. Can prolong QTc interval. Nortriptyline and desipramine are better tolerated
Vortioxetine	5 mg	5–20 mg	Well-tolerated alternative to SSRIs but under patent protection, expensive
Vilazodone	10 mg	40 mg	Under patent protection, expensive
Aripiprazole augmentation	2 mg	2–15 mg	Avoid in patients with or at risk for parkinsonism, can cause akathisia or rarely tardive dyskinesia
			Sometimes causes weight gain; recommend following lipids and glucose
Quetiapine augmentation	25 mg	50–300 mg	Can cause sedation and (often) weight gain, recommend monitoring lipids and glucose
Brexpiprazole augmentation	1 mg	2–4 mg	Avoid in patients with or at risk for parkinsonism, can cause akathisia or rarely tardive dyskinesia
			Sometimes causes weight gain; recommend monitoring lipids and glucose

TABLE 99.2 General Principles for Prescribing Antidepressant Medications

1. Start low but use full dose range as needed and as tolerated.
2. Avoid drug-drug interactions when possible but do not stop an antidepressant medication that is helpful.
3. For patients who do not respond, switch to another class of agent. For those who respond partially, consider augmentation treatment.
4. After 1–2 failed trials, refer to psychiatry.
5. Psychotherapy works well in combination with antidepressants.

All tricyclics have quinidine-like properties, leading to an increase in the PR interval, prolongation of the QRS duration and QT interval, and flattening of the T wave on the electrocardiogram (ECG) (see also Chapter 14). These effects are usually only seen at the higher "antidepressant" doses. Tricyclics should be avoided in patients with preexisting cardiac conduction defects, a prolonged QT interval, heart failure, or ischemic heart disease including a recent MI. Additionally, if tricyclics are used for the treatment of depression (as opposed to low doses for migraine, for example), therapeutic drug level monitoring and ECG monitoring are recommended. Importantly, tricyclic medications have been associated with an increased risk of malignant ventricular arrhythmias and sudden cardiac death (see also Chapters 9, 62, and 70). For patients who suffer a cardiac event while being treated with a tricyclic, there is a theoretical concern that abrupt withdrawal from the medication can also be associated with an increased risk of arrhythmias. A practical way to address these competing concerns is to taper the tricyclic medication slowly over two weeks, but more quickly if the patient has ongoing arrhythmias. Similarly, tricyclics should be tapered and stopped if prolongation of the QT interval or significant hypotension becomes problematic; if appropriate, the patient should be treated with an alternative medication such as an SSRI, venlafaxine, or bupropion (see below). These latter medications are preferred in patients who develop new onset depression after an acute MI.

Selective Serotonin Reuptake Inhibitors

The SSRIs include fluoxetine, paroxetine, fluvoxamine, citalopram, escitalopram, and sertraline. As the name implies, SSRIs block reuptake of serotonin into the neuron at the synapse. SSRIs have not been shown to have greater efficacy in the treatment of depression than the older tricyclics, but they have a more favorable side effect profile. Specifically, the SSRIs have no anticholinergic effects (except paroxetine) and no cardiac effects (except citalopram, which increases the QTc interval).

For these reasons, the SSRIs are good first-line antidepressant choices for the cardiac patient population.

Side effects of SSRIs include nausea, diarrhea, headache, insomnia (or sometimes somnolence), agitation, and sexual dysfunction, which may include loss of libido, delayed ejaculation, and erectile dysfunction. Most of these side effects are usually transient, with the exception of sexual dysfunction. Alternative antidepressants that do not cause sexual dysfunction include bupropion or mirtazapine, which are not in the SSRI class. SSRIs, especially fluoxetine, are associated with an increase in risk of bleeding. For cardiac patients taking aspirin or other antiplatelet or anticoagulant medication, this can be a significant concern. Abrupt cessation of an SSRI can result in a discontinuation syndrome, which, while not dangerous, can cause unpleasant symptoms including agitation, nervousness, and physical sensations like electrical shocks. Rarely SSRIs can cause akathisia and other extrapyramidal side effects, as can the antipsychotics. Akathisia includes feelings of restlessness, pacing, and internal stiffness, which are often very uncomfortable. All antidepressant medications carry the warning of an increased risk of suicidal thoughts in children and young adults under the age of 25, although this risk should not preclude their use in such populations.[63]

Based on several short-term trials, SSRIs are generally considered safe and effective in cardiac patients. Although treatment of depression has not been shown to improve cardiac outcomes, in several trials treatment responders appeared to have better cardiac outcomes than nonresponders, suggesting that antidepressant treatment, when effective for depression, improves cardiac outcomes. Conversely, several observational studies have shown an increased risk of cardiac death with longer-term use of SSRIs. A Danish nationwide study, for example, found a significant association between SSRI (as well as tricyclic antidepressant) use and out-of-hospital cardiac arrest, especially for citalopram and nortriptyline, whereas no association was found for other drug classes, such as the NRIs and the serotonin-norepinephrine dual reuptake inhibitors.[64] A prior analysis of the Nurses' Health Study also found that antidepressant use was associated with a threefold increase in the risk of sudden cardiac death, even after adjusting for the severity of depression and risk factors for CHD. In this study, the risk was similar for SSRIs and other antidepressants outside of the SSRI class. These observational data are difficult to interpret given the likelihood of confounding by indication[65]; i.e., the patients for whom antidepressants were prescribed may have had an inherently higher risk for cardiac arrest. Therefore, while it is not possible to make pragmatic recommendations based on these observational studies, it should be recognized that the risk of sudden cardiac death associated with antidepressant use is very low, and that the potential benefits of treating depression outweigh the risks.

Norepinephrine Reuptake Inhibitors

The NRIs block reuptake of norepinephrine into the neuron. Medications in this group include most of the tricyclics, such as nortriptyline and desipramine, as well as reboxetine. These drugs have a relatively favorable side effect profile and may be useful in individuals who do not respond to, or cannot tolerate, SSRIs.

Serotonin and Norepinephrine Dual Reuptake Inhibitors

Several antidepressants have dual reuptake inhibition for SNRIs, including venlafaxine, desvenlafaxine, milnacipran, and duloxetine. There is speculation that by affecting both neurotransmitters, these drugs provide a better treatment response for depression than SSRIs. In an analysis combining multiple studies, the response rate with venlafaxine, defined as at least a 50% reduction in symptoms of depression, was 74%, which was significantly better than SSRIs, with a 61% response rate, and tricyclics, with a 58% response. SNRIs are therefore often used as second-line agents in individuals who do not adequately respond to SSRIs.

Common side effects with SNRIs, including venlafaxine and duloxetine, include dizziness, constipation, dry mouth, headache, and changes in sleep. Rarely a serotonin syndrome may occur, with restlessness, shivering, and sweating. Venlafaxine has also been associated with a dose-dependent increase in blood pressure, which may be problematic for patients with comorbid hypertension or CVD. A recent study found that approximately 10% of previously-normotensive patients developed hypertension with high-dose venlafaxine, and orthostatic hypotension was also common.[66]

Monoamine Oxidase Inhibitors

Drugs that block the monoamine oxidase inhibitor enzyme (MAOI drugs), and therefore boost the monoamines (serotonin, norepinephrine), include selegiline/deprenyl, phenelzine, and tranylcypromine. They have a more favorable CV profile than the tricyclics, with little or no effect on cardiac conduction, although they can be associated with orthostatic hypotension (because of alpha-adrenergic blockade) and anticholinergic and antihistaminergic effects. The older MAOI drugs phenelzine and tranylcypromine in particular can cause potentially life-threatening elevations of blood pressure if taken with foods that are high in tyramine content, including wine, cheese, chocolate, and beer. This risk is much less for selegiline/deprenyl, especially at lower doses where it acts as a more selective MAOI. Drugs that can precipitate hypertensive reactions in a patient taking an MAOI include those with sympathomimetic effects (e.g., amphetamines, ephedrine, cocaine). MAOIs should not be taken with meperidine. Due to the risk of hypertensive crisis, the MAOIs are not recommended for use in cardiac patients, and indeed they are no longer commonly prescribed in general.

Antidepressants with Other Mechanisms of Action

Some drugs act on other neurotransmitter systems or their mechanism of action is poorly understood. Two commonly used drugs are bupropion and mirtazapine. Bupropion primarily acts on dopamine and norepinephrine systems and is used for both depression and smoking cessation. Side effects include weight loss and restlessness, as well as possible increases in blood pressure; in relatively rare cases, high doses can cause seizures or, in older adults, falls. Mirtazapine is a quadracyclic antidepressant that has actions on several different receptor systems. It blocks presynaptic noradrenergic alpha-2 receptors with resultant enhancement of norepinephrine release. Mirtazapine also increases serotonin release. Side effects include sweating and shivering, tiredness, strange dreams, dyslipidemia, weight gain, anxiety, and agitation. It can be associated with antihistaminergic effects and mild orthostatic hypotension. Short-term randomized trials in cardiac patients have not shown an increase in mortality or cardiovascular events associated with these medications.

Other drugs with mixed actions include trazodone and maprotiline. These drugs are rarely used for the treatment of depression, although trazodone is frequently prescribed as a hypnotic because of its sedative effect. The profile of these medications appears safe in terms of anticholinergic side effects and effects on the heart and blood pressure. Trazodone can cause priapism (extended painful erection that requires emergency treatment) in rare cases. It is a safe and often effective medication for induction of sleep that is not habit-forming. It is sometimes preferred to zolpidem and related insomnia medications, for example, when patients have alcohol or substance use disorders or side effects such as sleepwalking or hallucinations from zolpidem or similar drugs.

ANTIDEPRESSANTS AND CARDIAC QTc PROLONGATION. As noted above, tricyclic antidepressants prolong the QTc interval when used at doses sufficient to produce an antidepressant effect. Most of the newer SSRI and SNRI drugs have been studied with respect to QTc prolongation. Citalopram prolongs the QTc interval in a dose-dependent fashion, such that the FDA included a warning in its package insert stating that the drug should not be used at doses greater than 20 mg in older adults because of this risk. There is a similar concern with escitalopram, although at its usual dosing range of 10 to 20 mg it is not considered to produce sufficient QTc prolongation to advise against its use. Other SSRI/SNRI drugs appear to have less or no effect on the QTc interval. For example, a recent study of venlafaxine found no QTc prolongation even at high therapeutic doses.[67] CV clinicians may wish to advise against the use of citalopram when QTc prolongation is a concern (e.g., in older adults), and against escitalopram as an alternative in patients with citalopram-induced QTc prolongation. One exception is if the antidepressant is highly effective for the patient's depression, in which case the medication should be continued with monitoring of the QTc interval.

ANTIDEPRESSANTS AND DRUG-DRUG INTERACTIONS. The above sections described pharmacodynamic (i.e., receptor) effects of antidepressants, but many antidepressants also have relevant pharmacokinetic effects by reducing the metabolism of other drugs through inhibition of hepatic cytochrome P450 (CYP) enzymes (see also Chapter 9).

Thus, cardiac patients may have additional risks related to concomitant drugs whose metabolism is affected by these antidepressants. Drugs prone to cause these interactions include paroxetine and bupropion (strong inhibitors of CYP 2D6, which metabolizes many drugs including beta-blockers and several antiarrhythmic agents), fluoxetine and duloxetine (moderate inhibitors of CYP 2D6), and fluvoxamine (strong inhibitor of CYP 1A2, which metabolizes caffeine and theophylline, and CYP 2C19, which metabolizes clopidogrel). In contrast, escitalopram, sertraline, and venlafaxine have no significant effects on CYP enzymes. The practical implications of these drug-drug interactions remain controversial, in part because many drugs are metabolized by multiple enzymes (e.g., propranolol is metabolized by CYPs 2D6, 2C19, and 1A2) and blocking one enzyme may not have significant effects. However, many pharmacologists believe that these interactions are important, particularly in older adults. They can be avoided by prioritizing drugs without these effects as first-line treatments.

Electroconvulsive Therapy

ECT is used for the treatment of severe depression in patients who have had multiple failed trials of psychotherapy and medication. ECT has an 80% response rate, which is better than for medications, works quickly (within 2 to 3 weeks), and is a safe procedure for most individuals. Cardiologists may be asked to assess patient safety for ECT, as it may cause brief but profound hemodynamic changes, including bradycardia (up to frank asystole, which may last for a few seconds), followed by tachycardia and hypertension. These effects usually resolve within 20 minutes. Rare complications include persistent hypertension, arrhythmias, asystole lasting more than 5 seconds, ischemia, and heart failure. Older age and preexisting CVD, including hypertension, coronary artery disease, heart failure, aortic stenosis, atrial fibrillation, and implanted cardiac devices are associated with increased complication rates. Patients undergoing ECT should be monitored throughout the procedure and until stable after the procedure. With appropriate monitoring and management of medications, almost all patients can safely complete treatment.

While there are no absolute contraindications to ECT, the procedure should be delayed in patients who are hemodynamically unstable or who have new-onset or uncontrolled arrhythmias or hypertension. In patients with stable CHD and controlled hypertension, medications may be continued through the morning of the procedure. For patients with sustained post-ECT hypertension, antihypertensive therapy should be given after ECT and premedication used on the morning of subsequent ECT sessions; medications shown to be effective for this indication include labetalol, nicardipine, and clonidine.

In patients with an implanted pacemaker, the pacemaker should be tested before and after ECT; a magnet should be placed at the patient's bedside in the event that electrical interference leads to pacemaker inhibition and bradycardia. ECT appears safe in patients with an ICD. The detection mode of the ICD should be turned off during ECT, and continuous electrocardiographic monitoring should be maintained, with resuscitative equipment by the patient bedside in the event that external defibrillation is necessary.

Transcranial Magnetic Stimulation

TMS is a noninvasive therapy approved for treatment-resistant depression. It involves exposing the brain to a magnetic field, usually in the prefrontal cortex. It does not require sedation or the induction of a seizure and typically does not have any cardiac effects. It is increasingly being used as it has become more available and as shorter TMS sequences have been shown to be effective.[68]

Anxiolytic Medications

Benzodiazepines

In the 1960s benzodiazepines displaced barbiturates as the most commonly used medications for insomnia, and they were frequently prescribed for patients with anxiety and depression as well. Originally marketed as having less potential for dependence and abuse, this has not subsequently been borne out. Benzodiazepines act on the gamma-aminobutyric acid (GABA)-benzodiazepine receptor complex in the central nervous system, where they have a discrete binding site. This is the same complex that alcohol and the inhibitory transmitter GABA bind to. The most commonly prescribed benzodiazepines today include alprazolam, which is used primarily for anxiety attacks and panic disorder; clonazepam, which is used for epilepsy; and temazepam, which is used for insomnia. Other benzodiazepines include oxazepam, lorazepam, chlordiazepoxide, clorazepate, and diazepam, among others. Benzodiazepines are also used for treating in-patients with alcohol withdrawal, a not uncommon condition in patients hospitalized with CVD. Differences between benzodiazepines are related to the time of onset of action and duration of effect. Benzodiazepines increase sleep time by an average of about 1 hour per night. Side effects from benzodiazepines include daytime drowsiness, dizziness, light-headedness, falls, and memory problems. In addition, use of benzodiazepines is associated with a 60% increase in traffic accidents. This risk is further increased with concurrent alcohol usage and in older adults. In patients with cardiac disease and comorbid chronic pulmonary disease, benzodiazepines should be used with caution due to the potential for respiratory depression. This is of particular concern in obstructive sleep apnea because benzodiazepine-induced reductions in upper airway muscle tone and central nervous system response to hypoxia could result in an increased number and duration of apneic and hypopneic events.[69]

Benzodiazepines are habit-forming. As a result, patients can become resistant to stopping them, and in some cases their use can lead to abuse and addiction. Furthermore, abrupt cessation of benzodiazepines is often associated with a withdrawal syndrome that may include serious adverse events, including seizures and death. Therefore, discontinuation of long-term benzodiazepines should be gradual (e.g., 25% reduction every 2 weeks). The challenges associated with stopping benzodiazepines may lead to their inappropriate chronic use and potential risks from that use, which should be considered when initiating a new prescription.

Non-Benzodiazepine "Z-Drug" Medications

The so-call "Z drugs"—zaleplon, zolpidem, eszopiclone, and zopiclone—act on specific subsets of the GABA receptor and are mainly used for insomnia. Although they are commonly called "nonbenzodiazepine" medications, they have not been shown to be more effective or safe than benzodiazepines. As with benzodiazepines, these medications can cause memory impairment, drowsiness, dizziness, and falls; they can also cause hallucinations and parasomnias such as sleepwalking. Zaleplon has a shorter half-life (1 hour) than zolpidem (2.5 hours) or eszopiclone (6 hours), and is better for promoting sleep onset as opposed to sleep maintenance. As with benzodiazepines, abrupt discontinuation of these medications may be associated with withdrawal symptoms, including serious and even life-threatening adverse events, especially if the drug is taken chronically at high dose.

Medications with Other Mechanisms of Action

Buspirone is effective in treating generalized anxiety disorder and is sometimes used as an augmenting agent in depression. It is an agonist of the serotonin 1A receptor and relatively free of next-day drowsiness and memory impairment, or the potential for dependence or abuse. Buspirone is preferable to the benzodiazepines for the treatment of anxiety in cardiac patients because it lacks respiratory suppressive effects and there are no known adverse cardiac effects. Other side effects are minimal, and include nausea, headache, and lightheadedness.

Alternative Medicines and Supplements

Several natural remedies, including St. John's wort and omega-3 fatty acids, have been used for the treatment of depression and anxiety. However, data from high-quality large controlled studies evaluating the safety and efficacy of these agents are limited.

Mindfulness

Mindfulness is nonjudgmental awareness of one's own present thoughts, emotions, and behaviors. Mindfulness interventions combine elements of traditional meditation and CBT with a goal of learning to moderate emotional responses to day-to-day experiences. Controlled trials have shown reductions in distress and increases in feelings of general well-being in mindfulness groups compared to usual care. There is some evidence that mindfulness may augment the efficacy of antidepressants,[70] and it may help improve lifestyle risk factors, including smoking, diet, weight, and physical activity.[71] However, there is little evidence that mindfulness techniques improve CV outcomes, owing to the paucity of rigorous clinical trials in this area.

Tai chi and yoga are mindfulness techniques with multiple components thought to be helpful for CV health: physical exercise, stress reduction, emotional regulation, improved breathing efficiency, and social support. CV benefits with tai chi include improved blood pressure control, whereas yoga improves multiple CV risk factors including blood pressure, triglycerides, and insulin resistance.[72] Given the widespread availability and popularity of programs that include tai chi or yoga, they can play an important role in enhancing both CV and mental health.

Exercise

Multiple studies over the past 25 years have shown that various types of exercise are associated with salutary effects on depression (see also Chapter 32). Meta-analyses have consistently reported favorable effects of exercise, noting clinically significant benefits in medically well depressed patients. Similarly, a recent meta-analysis revealed that exercise-based cardiac rehabilitation alleviates symptoms of depression and anxiety among patients with recent MI or coronary artery bypass surgery.[73]

Current public health guidelines recommend 30 minutes of moderate intensity aerobic exercise at least 5 days per week, and this also appears to be an effective exercise "dose" to improve the mood of people with mild to moderate depression. Exercise may also be a useful adjunct to antidepressant medication in depressed patients who do not have a complete response to drug therapy.

Collaborative Care

Although depression and anxiety disorders are associated with worse prognosis and quality of life in patients with CVDs, they are infrequently recognized or treated by cardiology providers. Many primary care physicians, cardiologists, and other specialists are now using a collaborative care model to assist in the identification and treatment of psychiatric disorders in their practices. In this model, treatment for depression or anxiety is managed by the primary care physician or specialist, in consultation with a psychiatrist and/or other mental health professional, using a measurement-guided care plan based on evidence-based practice guidelines.[74] Studies in cardiology settings have generally found superior outcomes in patients receiving collaborative versus standard care, although this approach has had less of an impact in settings in which depression screening was already being practiced.[75]

SUMMARY AND FUTURE DIRECTIONS

To date, treatment of depression and anxiety have not been definitively shown to improve CV outcomes. However, recognition and management of these conditions, especially if they are severe or persistent, is essential for promoting patient wellness, enhancing quality of life, and improving patients' ability to adhere to treatments and lifestyle recommendations. In many cases the CV clinician can address the problem without an immediate referral to a mental health professional. Self-reported "anxiety" may reflect concern about their cardiac condition. Educating the patient about their heart disorder, listening to their concerns, and allowing the patient to express their worries often has a therapeutic effect and helps alleviate distress. It is important to determine if the patient is having thoughts of taking his or her own life or is having such severe impairment in functioning that referral to a psychiatrist, psychologist, or social worker is indicated; this depends both on the severity of the condition and the type of treatment that might be appropriate (medications versus psychotherapy or counseling).

Antidepressants useful in patients with CVD include SSRIs (paroxetine, fluoxetine, sertraline, and others), mirtazapine, bupropion, venlafaxine, desvenlafaxine, and duloxetine, with careful monitoring of blood pressure for the latter 3 SNRI drugs. ECT and TMS are alternative nonpharmacological treatment options in selected cases. A healthy lifestyle, including physical activity tailored to patients' functional capabilities, should be recommended to reduce depression, improve well-being, and lower CV risk. Community resources include therapists, counselors, and social workers who can teach stress reduction and mindfulness techniques, either individually or in classes, as well as exercise, tai chi, and yoga classes. There are also many self-help books that patients can purchase to teach themselves these stress reduction techniques.

Numerous stressors, psychosocial factors, and psychiatric disorders have been found to increase the risk of incident CVD and to predict adverse outcomes in established CVD. Although these factors differ in many ways, some of their features overlap and they often co-occur in various combinations. In addition, the clinical presentations of some of these problems are highly heterogeneous. Further research is needed to characterize the highest-risk phenotypes and to identify factors that contribute to their development and persistence. Identification of these phenotypes will facilitate research on the biobehavioral mechanisms that link mental stress, psychosocial distress, and psychiatric disorders to adverse outcomes in CVD. It will also facilitate treatment research and make it possible to identify patients with mental health disorders who are at high risk for adverse cardiac outcomes.

ACKNOWLEDGMENT

The authors gratefully acknowledge Drs. Viola Vaccarino and J. Douglas Bremner, whose chapter on this topic in the prior edition of *Braunwald's Heart Disease: A Textbook of Cardiovascular Medicine* served as the basis for the current chapter.

REFERENCES

Acute Stress, Emotional Arousal, Cardiovascular Consequences of Chronic Stress

1. Zarifeh J, Mulder R. Natural disasters and the risk of cardiovascular disease. In: Alvarenga ME, Byrne D, eds. *Handbook of Psychocardiology*. New York, NY: Springer Berlin Heidelberg; 2016.
2. Mostofsky E, Maclure M, Sherwood JB, et al. Risk of acute myocardial infarction after the death of a significant person in one's life: the determinants of myocardial infarction onset study. *Circulation*. 2012;125(3):491–496.
3. Carey IM, Shah SM, DeWilde S, et al. Increased risk of acute cardiovascular events after partner bereavement: a matched cohort study. *JAMA Intern Med*. 2014;174(4):598–605.
4. Pelliccia F, Pasceri V, Patti G, et al. Long-term prognosis and outcome predictors in takotsubo syndrome: a systematic review and meta-regression study. *JACC Heart Fail*. 2019;7(2):143–154.
5. Mostofsky E, Penner EA, Mittleman MA. Outbursts of anger as a trigger of acute cardiovascular events: a systematic review and meta-analysis. *Eur Heart J*. 2014;35(21):1404–1410.
6. Hammadah M, Alkhoder A, Al Mheid I, et al. Hemodynamic, catecholamine, vasomotor and vascular responses: determinants of myocardial ischemia during mental stress. *Int J Cardiol*. 2017;243:47–53.
7. Bremner JD, Campanella C, Khan Z, et al. Brain mechanisms of stress and depression in coronary artery disease. *J Psychiatr Res*. 2019;109:76–88.
8. Hammadah M, Kim JH, Al Mheid I, et al. Coronary and peripheral vasomotor responses to mental stress. *J Am Heart Assoc*. 2018;7(10):e008532.
9. Hammadah M, Sullivan S, Pearce B, et al. Inflammatory response to mental stress and mental stress induced myocardial ischemia. *Brain Behav Immun*. 2018;68:90–97.
10. Khan SG, Melikian N, Shabeeh H, et al. The human coronary vasodilatory response to acute mental stress is mediated by neuronal nitric oxide synthase. *Am J Physiol Heart Circ Physiol*. 2017;313(3):H578–h583.
11. Suglia SF, Koenen KC, Boynton-Jarrett R, et al. Childhood and adolescent adversity and cardiometabolic outcomes: a scientific statement from the American heart association. *Circulation*. 2018;137(5):e15–e28.
12. Waehrer GM, Miller TR, Silverio Marques SC, et al. Disease burden of adverse childhood experiences across 14 states. *PloS One*. 2020;15(1):e0226134.
13. Salas J, van den Berk-Clark C, Skiöld-Hanlin S, et al. Adverse childhood experiences, depression, and cardiometabolic disease in a nationally representative sample. *J Psychosom Res*. 2019;127:109842.
14. Laitinen TT, Puolakka E, Ruohonen S, et al. Association of socioeconomic status in childhood with left ventricular structure and diastolic function in adulthood: the cardiovascular risk in young finns study. *JAMA Pediatr*. 2017;171(8):781–787.
15. Havranek EP, Mujahid MS, Barr DA, et al. Social determinants of risk and outcomes for cardiovascular disease: a scientific statement from the American Heart Association. *Circulation*. 2015;132(9):873–898.
16. Schultz WM, Kelli HM, Lisko JC, et al. Socioeconomic status and cardiovascular outcomes: challenges and interventions. *Circulation*. 2018;137(20):2166–2178.
17. Vart P, Matsushita K, Rawlings AM, et al. SES, heart failure, and N-terminal pro-b-type natriuretic peptide: the atherosclerosis risk in communities study. *Am J Prev Med*. 2018;54(2):229–236.
18. Valero-Elizondo J, Hong JC, Spatz ES, et al. Persistent socioeconomic disparities in cardiovascular risk factors and health in the United States: medical expenditure Panel Survey 2002-2013. *Atherosclerosis*. 2018;269:301–305.

19. Rawshani A, Svensson AM, Zethelius B, et al. Association between socioeconomic status and mortality, cardiovascular disease, and cancer in patients with type 2 diabetes. *JAMA Intern Med.* 2016;176(8):1146–1154.
20. Kargoli F, Shulman E, Aagaard P, et al. Socioeconomic status as a predictor of mortality in patients admitted with atrial fibrillation. *Am J Cardiol.* 2017;119(9):1378–1381.
21. Sara JD, Prasad M, Eleid MF, et al. Association between work-related stress and coronary heart disease: a review of prospective studies through the job strain, effort-reward balance, and organizational justice models. *J Am Heart Assoc.* 2018;7(9).
22. Virtanen M, Nyberg ST, Batty GD, et al. Perceived job insecurity as a risk factor for incident coronary heart disease: systematic review and meta-analysis. *BMJ (Clinical Research ed).* 2013;347:f4746.
23. Dunlay SM, Lippmann SJ, Greiner MA, et al. Perceived discrimination and cardiovascular outcomes in Older African Americans: insights from the Jackson heart study. *Mayo Clin Proc.* 2017;92(5):699–709.
24. Panza GA, Puhl RM, Taylor BA, et al. Links between discrimination and cardiovascular health among socially stigmatized groups: a systematic review. *PloS One.* 2019;14(6):e0217623.
25. Lukachko A, Hatzenbuehler ML, Keyes KM. Structural racism and myocardial infarction in the United States. *Soc Sci Med.* 2014;103:42–50.
26. Everson-Rose SA, Lutsey PL, Roetker NS, et al. Perceived discrimination and incident cardiovascular events: the multi-ethnic study of atherosclerosis. *Am J Epidemiol.* 2015;182(3):225–234.
27. Forde AT, Sims M, Muntner P, et al. Discrimination and hypertension risk among African Americans in the Jackson heart study. *Hypertension.* 2020. HYPERTENSIONAHA11914492.
28. Wu KK, Bos T, Mausbach BT, et al. Long-term caregiving is associated with impaired cardiovagal baroreflex. *J Psychosom Res.* 2017;103:29–33.
29. Burg MM, Edmondson D, Shimbo D, et al. The "perfect storm" and acute coronary syndrome onset: do psychosocial factors play a role? *Prog Cardiovasc Dis.* 2013;55(6):601–610.
30. Pimple P, Hammadah M, Wilmot K, et al. The relation of psychosocial distress with myocardial perfusion and stress-induced myocardial ischemia. *Psychosom Med.* 2019;81(4):363–371.
31. Phillips AC, Ginty AT, Hughes BM. The other side of the coin: blunted cardiovascular and cortisol reactivity are associated with negative health outcomes. *Int J Psychophysiol.* 2013;90(1):1–7.

Mental Health and Psychiatric Disorders, Evaluation

32. American Psychiatric Association. *DSM-5 Task Force. Diagnostic and Statistical Manual of Mental Disorders: DSM-5.* 5th ed. Washington, DC: American Psychiatric Association; 2013.
33. Thom R, Silbersweig DA, Boland RJ. Major depressive disorder in medical illness: a review of assessment, prevalence, and treatment options. *Psychosom Med.* 2019;81(3):246–255.
34. Janssen EM, McGinty EE, Azrin ST, et al. Review of the evidence: prevalence of medical conditions in the United States population with serious mental illness. *Gen Hosp Psychiatry.* 2015;37(3):199–222.
35. Stewart JC. One effect size does not fit all—is the depression-inflammation link missing in racial/ethnic minority individuals? *JAMA Psychiatry.* 2016;73(3):301–302.
36. Carney RM, Freedland KE. Depression and coronary heart disease. *Nat Rev Cardiol.* 2017;14(3):145–155.
37. Roest AM, Martens EJ, de Jonge P, Denollet J. Anxiety and risk of incident coronary heart disease: a meta-analysis. *J Am Coll Cardiol.* 2010;56(1):38–46.
38. Emdin CA, Odutayo A, Wong CX, et al. Meta-analysis of anxiety as a risk factor for cardiovascular disease. *Am J Cardiol.* 2016;118(4):511–519.
39. Allgulander C. Anxiety as a risk factor in cardiovascular disease. *Curr Opin Psychiatry.* 2016;29(1):13–17.
40. Tully PJ, Cosh SM, Baumeister H. The anxious heart in whose mind? A systematic review and meta-regression of factors associated with anxiety disorder diagnosis, treatment and morbidity risk in coronary heart disease. *J Psychosom Res.* 2014;77(6):439–448.
41. Ahmadi N, Hajsadeghi F, Mirshkarlo HB, et al. Post-traumatic stress disorder, coronary atherosclerosis, and mortality. *Am J Cardiol.* 2011;108(1):29–33.
42. Edmondson D, Kronish IM, Shaffer JA, et al. Posttraumatic stress disorder and risk for coronary heart disease: a meta-analytic review. *Am Heart J.* 2013;166(5):806–814.
43. Gan Y, Gong Y, Tong X, et al. Depression and the risk of coronary heart disease: a meta-analysis of prospective cohort studies. *BMC Psychiatr.* 2014;14:371.
44. Rajan S, McKee M, Rangarajan S, et al. Association of symptoms of depression with cardiovascular disease and mortality in low-, middle-, and high-income countries. *JAMA Psychiatry.* 2020;77(10):1052–1063.
45. Meijer A, Conradi HJ, Bos EH, et al. Adjusted prognostic association of depression following myocardial infarction with mortality and cardiovascular events: individual patient data meta-analysis. *Br J Psychiatry.* 2013;203(2):90–102.
46. Lichtman JH, Froelicher ES, Blumenthal JA, et al. Depression as a risk factor for poor prognosis among patients with acute coronary syndrome: systematic review and recommendations: a scientific statement from the American Heart Association. *Circulation.* 2014;129(12):1350–1369.
47. Antman EM, Anbe DT, Armstrong PW, et al. ACC/AHA guidelines for the management of patients with ST-elevation myocardial infarction—executive summary: a report of the American college of cardiology/American heart association task force on practice guidelines (writing committee to revise the 1999 guidelines for the management of patients with acute myocardial infarction). *Circulation.* 2004;110(5):588–636.
48. Scott KM, Lim C, Al-Hamzawi A, et al. Association of mental disorders with subsequent chronic physical conditions: world mental health surveys from 17 countries. *JAMA Psychiatry.* 2016;73(2):150–158.
49. Vance MC, Wiitala WL, Sussman JB, et al. Increased cardiovascular disease risk in veterans with mental illness. *Circ Cardiovasc Qual Outcomes.* 2019;12(10):e005563.
50. Weye N, Momen NC, Christensen MK, et al. Association of specific mental disorders with premature mortality in the Danish population using alternative measurement methods. *JAMA Netw Open.* 2020;3(6):e206646.
51. Hauck TS, Liu N, Wijeysundera HC, Kurdyak P. Mortality and revascularization among myocardial infarction patients with schizophrenia: a population-based cohort study. *Can J Psychiatry.* 2020;65(7):454–462.
52. Wolters FJ, Chibnik LB, Waziry R, et al. Twenty-seven-year time trends in dementia incidence in Europe and the United States: the alzheimer cohorts consortium. *Neurology.* 2020;95(5):e519–e531.
53. Isik AT, Soysal P, Stubbs B, et al. Cardiovascular outcomes of cholinesterase inhibitors in individuals with dementia: a meta-analysis and systematic review. *J Am Geriatr Soc.* 2018;66(9):1805–1811.
54. Westover AN, Halm EA. Do prescription stimulants increase the risk of adverse cardiovascular events?: a systematic review. *BMC Cardiovasc Disord.* 2012;12:41.

Evaluation and Management of Mental Health in the Cardiac Patient

55. Frost JL, Rich Jr RL, Robbins CW, et al. Depression following acute coronary syndrome events: screening and treatment guidelines from the AAFP. *Am Fam Physician.* 2019;99(12). Online.
56. Siu AL, Bibbins-Domingo K, Grossman DC, et al. Screening for depression in adults: US preventive services task force recommendation statement. *J Am Med Assoc.* 2016;315(4):380–387.
57. Piepoli MF, Hoes AW, Agewall S, et al. European guidelines on cardiovascular disease prevention in clinical practice: the sixth joint task force of the European society of cardiology and other societies on cardiovascular disease prevention in clinical practice (constituted by representatives of 10 societies and by invited experts) developed with the special contribution of the European Association for Cardiovascular Prevention & Rehabilitation (EACPR). *Eur Heart J.* 2016;37(29):2315–2381. 2016.
58. Priori SG, Blomström-Lundqvist C, Mazzanti A, et al. ESC guidelines for the management of patients with ventricular arrhythmias and the prevention of sudden cardiac death: the Task Force for the management of patients with ventricular arrhythmias and the prevention of sudden cardiac death of the European Society of Cardiology (ESC). endorsed by: association for European Paediatric and Congenital Cardiology (AEPC). *Eur Heart J.* 2015;36(41):2793–2867. 2015.
59. Lichtman JH, Froelicher ES, Blumenthal JA, et al. Depression as a risk factor for poor prognosis among patients with acute coronary syndrome: systematic review and recommendations: a scientific statement from the American Heart Association. *Circulation.* 2014;129(12):1350–1369.
60. Lichtman JH, Bigger Jr JT, Blumenthal JA, et al. Depression and coronary heart disease: recommendations for screening, referral, and treatment: a science advisory from the American heart association prevention committee of the council on cardiovascular nursing, council on clinical cardiology, council on epidemiology and prevention, and interdisciplinary council on quality of care and outcomes research: endorsed by the American psychiatric association. *Circulation.* 2008;118(17):1768–1775.
61. Freedland KE, Carney RM, Rich MW, et al. Cognitive behavior therapy for depression and self-care in heart failure patients: a randomized clinical trial. *JAMA Intern Med.* 2015;175(11):1773–1782.
62. Davidson KW, Bigger JT, Burg MM, et al. Centralized, stepped, patient preference-based treatment for patients with post-acute coronary syndrome depression: CODIACS vanguard randomized controlled trial. *JAMA Intern Med.* 2013;173(11):997–1004.
63. Friedman RA. Antidepressants' black-box warning—10 years later. *N Engl J Med.* 2014;371(18):1666–1668.
64. Weeke P, Jensen A, FF, et al. Antidepressant use and risk of out-of-hospital cardiac arrest: a nationwide case-time-control study. *Clin Pharmacol Ther.* 2012;92(1):72–79.
65. Dragioti E, Solmi M, Favaro A, et al. Association of antidepressant use with adverse health outcomes: a systematic umbrella review. *JAMA Psychiatry.* 2019;76(12):1241–1255.
66. Wathra R, Mulsant BH, Thomson L, et al. Hypertension and orthostatic hypotension with venlafaxine treatment in depressed older adults. *J Psychopharmacol.* 2020;34(10):1112–1118.
67. Behlke LM, Lenze EJ, Pham B, et al. The effect of venlafaxine on ECG intervals during treatment for depression in older adults. *J Clin Psychopharmacol.* 2020;40(6):553–559.
68. Janicak PG, Dokucu ME. Transcranial magnetic stimulation for the treatment of major depression. *Neuropsychiatr Dis Treat.* 2015;11:1549–1560.
69. Heck T, Zolezzi M. Obstructive sleep apnea: management considerations in psychiatric patients. *Neuropsychiatr Dis Treat.* 2015;11:2691–2698.
70. Segal ZV, Dimidjian S, Beck A, et al. Outcomes of online mindfulness-based cognitive therapy for patients with residual depressive symptoms: a randomized clinical trial. *JAMA Psychiatry.* 2020;77(6):563–573.
71. Gotink RA, Younge JO, Wery MF, et al. Online mindfulness as a promising method to improve exercise capacity in heart disease: 12-month follow-up of a randomized controlled trial. *PloS One.* 2017;12(5):e0175923.
72. Cramer H, Lauche R, Haller H, et al. Effects of yoga on cardiovascular disease risk factors: a systematic review and meta-analysis. *Int J Cardiol.* 2014;173(2):170–183.
73. Zheng X, Zheng Y, Ma J, et al. Effect of exercise-based cardiac rehabilitation on anxiety and depression in patients with myocardial infarction: a systematic review and meta-analysis. *Heart Lung.* 2019;48(1):1–7.
74. Archer J, Bower P, Gilbody S, et al. Collaborative care for depression and anxiety problems. *Cochrane Database Syst Rev.* 2012;10:Cd006525.
75. Huffman JC, Mastromauro CA, Beach SR, et al. Collaborative care for depression and anxiety disorders in patients with recent cardiac events: the Management of Sadness and Anxiety in Cardiology (MOSAIC) randomized clinical trial. *JAMA Intern Med.* 2014;174(6):927–935.

100 Neuromuscular Disorders and Cardiovascular Disease

WILLIAM J. GROH, ELIZABETH M. MCNALLY, AND GORDON F. TOMASELLI

NEUROMUSCULAR DISEASES, 1853
MUSCULAR DYSTROPHIES, 1853
Duchenne and Becker Muscular Dystrophy, 1853
Myotonic Dystrophies, 1856
Emery-Dreifuss Muscular Dystrophy and Associated Disorders, 1859
Limb-Girdle Muscular Dystrophies, 1861
Facioscapulohumeral Muscular Dystrophy, 1863
Friedreich Ataxia, 1864

LESS COMMON NEUROMUSCULAR DISEASES ASSOCIATED WITH CARDIAC MANIFESTATIONS, 1864
The Periodic Paralyses, 1864
Mitochondrial Disorders, 1866
Spinal Muscular Atrophy, 1868
Myofibrillar Myopathies, 1868
Guillain-Barré Syndrome, 1868
Myasthenia Gravis, 1869

ABCC9-related Intellectual Disability Myopathy Syndrome, 1869
Epilepsy, 1869
Acute Cerebrovascular Disease, 1870

CONCLUSIONS/FUTURE PERSPECTIVES, 1871

REFERENCES, 1871

Neurologic diseases often affect the heart and vascular system, and in many cases, cardiovascular disease limits life expectancy and reduces quality of life in these patients. As such, cardiologists are an integral part of the medical team evaluating and treating patients with primary neurologic disorders. In several disorders, the cardiovascular manifestations are responsible for a greater risk than that attributable to the neurologic manifestations. This chapter reviews those neurologic disorders associated with important cardiovascular manifestations or sequelae.

NEUROMUSCULAR DISEASES

The neuromuscular diseases may be classified based on clinical features, molecular genetics, or pathophysiological consequences. This group includes disorders of muscle proteins dystrophin and sarcoglycans; membrane and filament proteins lamin A/C, emerin, and desmin; nucleotide repeat disorders such as myotonic dystrophy, Friedreich ataxia (FRDA), and spinobulbar muscular atrophy; and mitochondrial and metabolic disorders.

MUSCULAR DYSTROPHIES

Muscular dystrophies are a group of inherited skeletal muscle diseases. Skeletal muscle and the heart are both striated muscles, and many muscular dystrophies have direct effects on cardiac muscle, with manifestations including heart failure, conduction disease and heart block, atrial and ventricular arrhythmias, and sudden death. With improved multidisciplinary care and, more recently, targeted treatment, patients are living longer and an increasing proportion manifest cardiac disease.[1] This section will review the genetics, pathogenesis, clinical presentation, cardiovascular manifestations, evaluation, prognosis, and treatment of muscular dystrophies with major cardiac involvement. These include:
- Duchenne and Becker muscular dystrophies
- Myotonic dystrophies
- Emery-Dreifuss muscular dystrophies and associated disorders
- Limb-girdle muscular dystrophies
- Facioscapulohumeral muscular dystrophy

Duchenne and Becker Muscular Dystrophy
Genetics and Pathogenesis
Duchenne muscular dystrophy (DMD) and Becker muscular dystrophy (BMD) are X-linked recessive disorders caused by mutations in one of the largest genes in the human genome, dystrophin (see also Chapters 7, 52, and 63). *Dystrophin* is located on the short arm of the X chromosome with 79 exons, spanning 2.4 Mb producing a 14 kb mRNA. Variable promoters produce different full-length and shorter versions of dystrophin expressed in muscle and brain, and the short 71 kDa isoform is ubiquitously expressed. Alternative splicing produces other isoforms expressed in the retina, kidney, brain, and peripheral nerves. About 60% of DMD cases are due to deletions of one or more exons; more rarely, duplications, small insertions/deletions, or point mutations produce disease. In DMD, mutations usually disrupt the reading frame or introduce a premature stop codon, leading to the absence of dystrophin. Mutations that maintain the reading frame produce internally truncated, relatively functional proteins, resulting in a milder form of the disease, BMD. Although the skeletal muscle symptoms are less severe, the majority of BMD patients also develop a cardiomyopathy, and it is the leading cause of death in patients with BMD.

The dystrophin protein and its associated glycoproteins provide a structural link between the myocyte cytoskeleton and extracellular matrix linking contractile proteins to the cell membrane (Fig. 100.1B). Absence of dystrophin leads to membrane fragility resulting in myofiber or cardiomyocyte necrosis and eventual loss of cells with fibrotic replacement. Mutations in the genes encoding dystrophin-associated glycoproteins also present with degeneration of cardiac and skeletal muscle. Cardiac myocytes lacking dystrophin are susceptible to mechanical damage.[2] Cardiac involvement is seen in both DMD and BMD and the severity is not correlated with the severity of skeletal muscle involvement. Mutations in specific domains of the dystrophin gene are associated with a higher risk for cardiomyopathy.[3] X-linked dilated cardiomyopathy arises from mutations that primarily affect cardiac dystrophin production which manifests as cardiac involvement without skeletal muscle dysfunction.

Clinical Presentation
DMD is the most common inherited neuromuscular disease, with an incidence of 1 case in 3600 to 6000 live male births.[4] Patients typically present with skeletal muscle weakness before the age of 5 years, which progresses if untreated such that boys become wheelchair-bound by their early teens (Fig. 100.2). Without support, death occurs by age 25 years, primarily from a combination of respiratory dysfunction and heart failure. A multidisciplinary treatment approach, including glucocorticoid steroids, ventilatory support, and cardiac therapy has improved survival rates.[1] BMD is less common than DMD, is associated with a highly variable presentation of skeletal muscle weakness compared to Duchenne (see Fig. 100.2), and carries a better prognosis, with most patients surviving to the age of 40 to 50 years or longer. In both Duchenne and Becker muscular dystrophies,

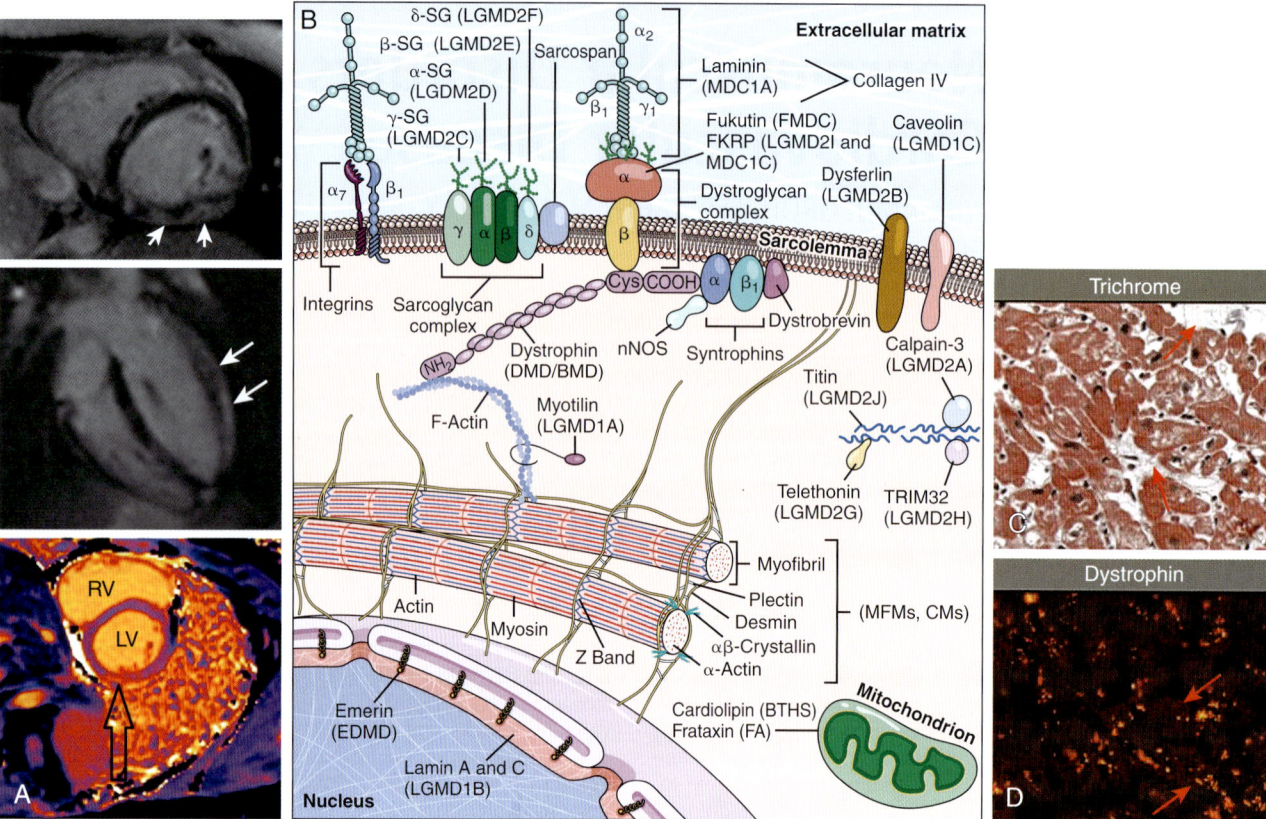

FIGURE 100.1 Cardiac involvement in Duchenne muscular dystrophy. **A** *(top, middle),* Late gadolinium enhancement (LGE) in MR images of a patient with Duchenne muscular dystrophy (*arrows* indicate areas of positive LGE, primarily in the inferior-lateral left ventricle). *Bottom,* T1 mapping shows variation (*orange*) in the LV wall consistent with fibrosis. **B,** Constitution of a cardiomyocyte cell membrane, demonstrating connection between the intramembranous sarcoglycan complex (α, β, γ, δ), dystroglycan complex (α and β), and dystrophin, which is linked to the intracellular actin cytoskeleton. The dystroglycan complex connects to the basal lamina on the extracellular side via laminin and to syntrophins and nitric oxide synthase (nNOS) via dystrobrevin (encoded by the *DTNA* gene). **C,** Trichrome staining of an endomyocardial biopsy sample taken from the patient in **A** showing irregular-sized cardiomyocytes in the presence of diffuse interstitial fibrosis (*red arrows*). **D,** Dystrophin staining: A few cardiomyocytes show discontinuous expression of dystrophin in the cell membrane (*red arrows*), whereas most cardiomyocytes have no dystrophin at all in their membranes. *BMD,* Becker muscular dystrophy; *DMD,* Duchenne muscular dystrophy; *LGMD,* limb-girdle muscular dystrophy. (**A** from Power LC, O'Grady GL, Hornung TS, et al. Imaging the heart to detect cardiomyopathy in Duchenne muscular dystrophy: a review. *Neuromuscul Disord*. 2018;28:717–730; Rochitte CE, Liberato G, Silva MC. Comprehensive assessment of cardiac involvement in muscular dystrophies by cardiac MR imaging. *Magn Reson Imaging Clin N Am*. 2019;27:521–531; **B** modified from Feingold B, Mahle WT, Auerbach S, et al. Management of cardiac involvement associated with neuromuscular diseases: a scientific statement from the American Heart Association. *Circulation*. 2017;136:e200–e231; **C** and **D** from Yilmaz A, Gdynia H-J, Ludolph AC, et al. Images in cardiovascular medicine: cardiomyopathy in a Duchenne muscular dystrophy carrier and her diseased son: similar pattern revealed by cardiovascular MRI. *Circulation*. 2010;121:e237.)

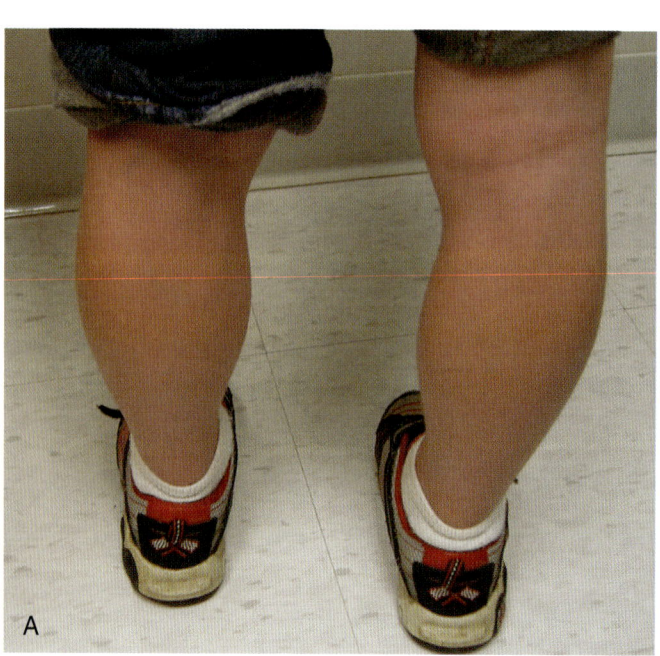
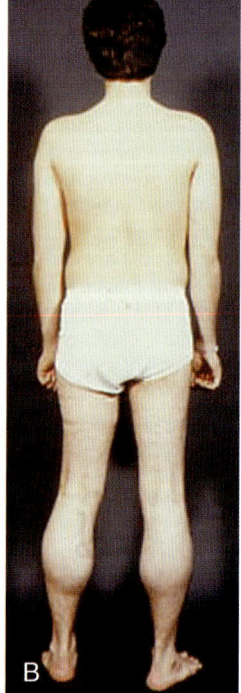

FIGURE 100.2 A, Calf pseudohypertrophy (related to an increase in fat, fibrous tissue, and diseased, poorly functioning muscle) in an 8-year-old boy with Duchenne muscular dystrophy. **B,** Becker muscular dystrophy in a 24-year-old man. Dystrophy of the shoulder girdle and calf pseudohypertrophy are evident. (**A** courtesy Dr. Laurence E. Walsh; **B** courtesy Dr. Robert M. Pascuzzi.)

elevated serum creatine kinase activity is observed, at levels more than 10 and 5 times normal values, respectively. Cardiac troponin T is elevated in up to one-half of patients likely related to immunoreactivity of the assay with diseased skeletal muscle. Cardiac troponin I remains normal in the majority of patients but has been observed to elevate in Duchenne patients with clinical features indicative of cardiomyopathy progression.[5]

Cardiovascular Manifestations

Most patients with DMD develop cardiomyopathy, but symptoms can be masked by activity limits due to skeletal muscle weakness. Sinus tachycardia is the earliest finding in the Duchenne heart, with the onset of clinically apparent cardiomyopathy common after the age of 10. Cardiac involvement can be diagnosed earlier by cardiac magnetic resonance imaging (MRI).[5-7] The majority of patients with DMD 18 years of age or older develop cardiomyopathy with reduced ejection fraction. Early involvement is observed in the inferobasal and lateral left ventricle (LV) (see Fig. 100.1A). As with the skeletal muscle weakness, cardiac involvement in Becker muscular dystrophy is more variable than in DMD, ranging from none or subclinical disease to severe cardiomyopathy requiring transplant. More than one-half of patients with subclinical or benign skeletal muscle disease were noted to have cardiac involvement if carefully evaluated. Progression in the severity of cardiac involvement is common. Cardiomyopathy can initially involve solely the right ventricle. The severity of cardiac involvement in both Duchenne and Becker muscular dystrophy can be independent of skeletal muscle involvement.

Thoracic deformities and a high diaphragm can alter the cardiovascular examination in patients with DMD. A reduction in the anterior-posterior chest dimension is commonly responsible for a systolic impulse displaced to the left sternal border, a grade 1 to 3/6 short midsystolic murmur in the second left interspace, and a loud pulmonary component of the second heart sound. In both Duchenne and Becker types of muscular dystrophy, mitral regurgitation is observed. The presence of mitral regurgitation is related to posterior papillary muscle dysfunction in DMD and to mitral annular dilation in BMD. Female carriers of Duchenne and Becker muscular dystrophy are at increased risk for dilated cardiomyopathy[8,9] and is consistent with increased susceptibility to cardiac injury in DMD carrier mice.[10]

Electrocardiography

In a majority of patients with DMD, the electrocardiogram (ECG) is abnormal (see Chapter 14). The classically described electrocardiographic pattern shows distinctive tall R waves and increased R/S amplitude in V_1 and deep narrow Q waves in the left precordial leads possibly related to the posterolateral left ventricular involvement (Fig. 100.3). Other common findings include a short PR interval and right ventricular hypertrophy. No association between the presence of a dilated cardiomyopathy and electrocardiographic abnormalities has been established. In BMD, electrocardiographic abnormalities are present in up to 75% of the patients. The electrocardiographic abnormalities observed include tall R waves and an increased R/S amplitude in V_1, akin to that seen in DMD. In patients with dilated cardiomyopathy, a left bundle branch block is also common.

Imaging

Clinical care guidelines recommend using screening echocardiography at diagnosis or by the age of 6 years; subsequently every 2 years until the age of 10; and annually thereafter in boys with DMD (this and other cardiac imaging modalities are described more fully in Chapters 16 to 20).[11] Cardiac MRI, especially with gadolinium contrast, is more sensitive in detecting subclinical ventricular involvement and fibrosis. The presence of fibrosis as indicated by late gadolinium enhancement on MRI predicted a subsequent decrement in left ventricular function.[7] Regional abnormalities in the posterobasal and lateral wall typically occur earlier than in other areas (see Fig. 100.1A). A process akin to left ventricular noncompaction can be observed, possibly resulting from compensatory mechanisms in response to the failing dystrophic myocardium. Mitral regurgitation can result from dystrophic changes in the posterior leaflet papillary muscles.

Arrhythmias

In DMD, persistent or labile sinus tachycardia is the most common arrhythmia recognized (see Chapter 65). Atrial arrhythmias, including atrial fibrillation and atrial flutter (see Chapter 66), occur in the setting of respiratory dysfunction and cor pulmonale or are associated with progression of dilated cardiomyopathy. Abnormalities in atrioventricular conduction have been observed, with both short and prolonged PR intervals recognized. Ventricular arrhythmias occur on monitoring in 30% of patients, primarily ventricular premature beats. Complex ventricular arrhythmias have been reported, more commonly in patients with advanced DMD. Sudden death occurs in DMD, typically in patients with end-stage muscular disease, and may occur due to arrhythmias or events like fat emboli.[12] Several follow-up studies have shown a correlation between sudden death and the presence of complex ventricular arrhythmias. The presence of ventricular arrhythmias was not a predictor for all-cause mortality. Arrhythmia manifestations in BMD are typically related to the severity of the associated structural cardiomyopathy. Distal conduction system disease with complete heart block and bundle branch reentry ventricular tachycardia has been observed (see Chapter 67).

Treatment and Prognosis

DMD is a progressive skeletal and cardiac muscle disorder. Glucocorticoid steroids and steroid derivatives are effective in delaying skeletal muscle disease progression and appear to decrease the progression to a dilated cardiomyopathy.[13] They constitute the mainstay of treatment for DMD and are part of the Care Considerations. Deflazacort is an FDA approved glucocorticoid for DMD, although prednisone is still commonly used. A retrospective analysis supports steroid benefit to the heart. The adverse side effects from long-term glucocorticoid treatment include obesity, osteoporosis, and metabolic syndrome. A novel dissociative steroid, vamolorone, is being investigated with initial promising results. Steroid treatment is not routinely recommended in BMD.

A cardiac cause for morbidity and mortality is playing an increasingly significant role in DMD because of improved multidisciplinary support for respiratory issues. There is an equal distribution of cardiac death from heart failure and sudden death. With evidence of reduced left ventricular function, even mildly reduced function, it is reasonable to offer guideline-directed heart failure management. Angiotensin-converting enzyme (ACE) inhibitors and beta blockers can improve left ventricular function in patients treated early. Angiotensin receptor blockers can be used if the patient cannot tolerate ACE inhibitors. The aldosterone antagonist, eplerenone, showed benefit in maintaining cardiac magnetic resonance left ventricular circumferential strain in boys already receiving ACE inhibitors or angiotensin receptor blockers.[14,15] Dosing, age, or clinical status at which pharmacotherapy should be initiated is unclear (see Chapters 49 and 50). Other advanced types of therapy such as implantable cardioverter-defibrillators (ICDs) play an uncertain role but should be considered individually based on clinical presentation using a shared decision-making approach (see Chapter 69). The use of left ventricular mechanical assist devices has been described. Whether heart failure therapies improve long-term outcomes is unclear. However, the age at death has increased, with the majority of patients surviving into their 30s, and recognition and treatment of the associated cardiomyopathy likely plays a role in that success. In patients with Becker muscular dystrophy, an improvement in left ventricular function also is observed after treatment with ACE inhibitors and beta blockers. Screening with left ventricular imaging is recommended as in DMD. Advanced heart failure therapy, including primary prevention ICDs, is appropriate in patients with cardiomyopathy. Patients with Becker muscular dystrophy with advanced heart failure can undergo cardiac transplantation, with expected outcomes similar to those for non–muscular dystrophy cohorts of age-matched patients with dilated cardiomyopathy.[16] Female carriers of Duchenne and BMD do not develop a cardiomyopathy during childhood, and screening can be delayed until later in adolescence. Cardiac transplantation also has been reported in carriers.

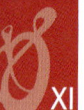

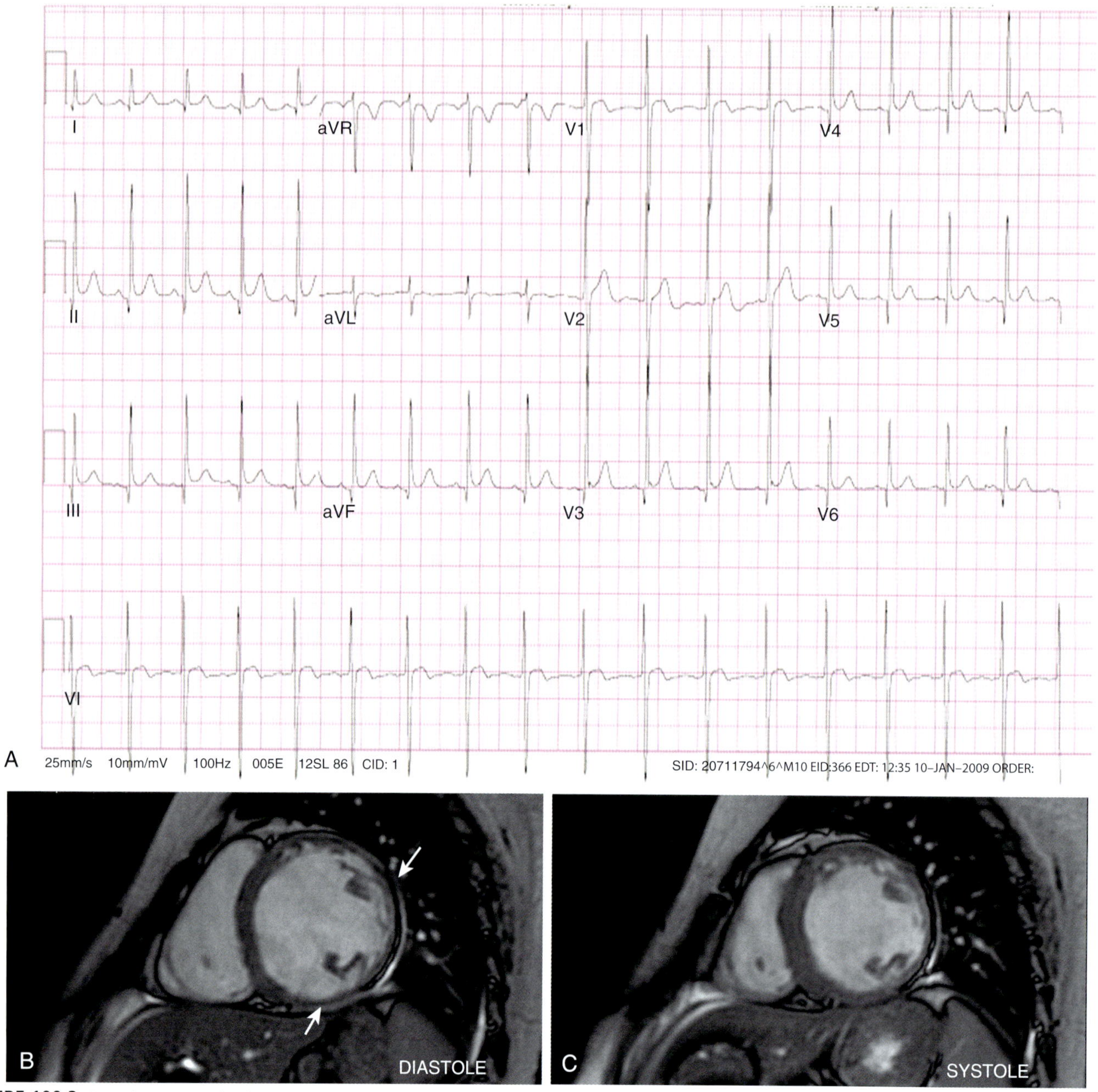

FIGURE 100.3 A, Duchenne muscular dystrophy (DMD) electrocardiogram reveals a short PR interval, an increase in the R/S ratio in the right precordial leads and narrow Q wave in the inferolateral leads. **B** and **C,** Cine sequences in the short axis view in diastole and systole showing dilation and thinning of the left ventricle wall particularly prominent in the inferior and lateral regions. (From Rochitte CE, Liberato G, Silva MC. Comprehensive assessment of cardiac involvement in muscular dystrophies by cardiac MR imaging. *Magn Reson Imaging Clin N Am.* 2019;27:521–531.)

Mutation-targeted treatment for Duchenne includes three forms of antisense mediated exon skipping that have been FDA approved, eteplirsen, golodirsen, and casimersen, and these agents treat different primary gene mutations. Adeno-associated viral gene therapy is in later stages of clinical investigation using microdystrophin, which is designed to convert Duchenne into Becker muscular dystrophy. On the horizon, CRISPR-Cas9-mediated gene editing is being designed to mediate more permanent exon skipping.[17,18]

Myotonic Dystrophies
Genetics and Pathogenesis

The myotonic dystrophies are autosomal dominant disorders characterized by myotonia, which is a delayed muscle relaxation after contraction, weakness, and atrophy of skeletal muscles, and systemic manifestations, including endocrine abnormalities, cataracts, cognitive impairment, and cardiac involvement (Fig. 100.4). Two distinct mutations are responsible for the myotonic dystrophies. In myotonic dystrophy type 1 (Steinert disease), the mutation is an amplified trinucleotide cytosine-thymine-guanine (CTG) repeat on chromosome 19 in the 3′ untranslated region of dystrophia myotonica protein kinase *(DMPK).* Normal individuals have 5 to 37 copies of the repeat, whereas patients with myotonic dystrophy have 50 to several thousand repeats. A direct correlation exists between an increasing number of CTG repeats and earlier age at onset and increasing severity of neuromuscular involvement (Table 100.1). Cardiac involvement including conduction disease, arrhythmias, and age at cardiovascular death also correlate with the length of repeat expansion (Fig. 100.5). It is typical for the CTG repeat to expand as it is passed from parents to offspring, resulting in the characteristic worsening clinical manifestations in subsequent generations, termed *anticipation.* Myotonic dystrophy type 2, also called proximal myotonic myopathy (PROMM), has generally less severe skeletal muscle and cardiac manifestations than type 1. Both congenital presentation and cognitive impairment are lacking in myotonic dystrophy type 2—typically, the most severely involved subsets of the type 1 patients. The genetic

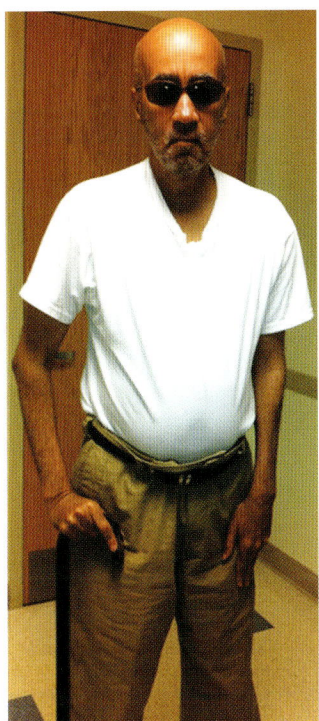

FIGURE 100.4 The patient is a 54-year-old man with myotonic dystrophy type 1. Typical characteristics of balding, thin face, and distal muscle atrophy are evident.

TABLE 100.1 Clinical Manifestation of Myotonic Dystrophy Type I

PHENOTYPE	CLINICAL	CTG LENGTH	ONSET
Congenital	Infantile hypotonia	>1000 (maternal)	Birth
	Respiratory failure		
	Learning disability		
	CV complications		
Childhood onset	Facial weakness	50–1000	1–10 yr
	Myotonia		
	Low IQ		
	Conduction defects		
"Classic DM1"	Myotonia	50–1000	10–30 yr
	Weakness (distal)		
	Conduction defects		
	Insulin resistance		
	Cataracts		
Late onset	Mild myotonia	50–100	20–70 yr
	Cataracts		

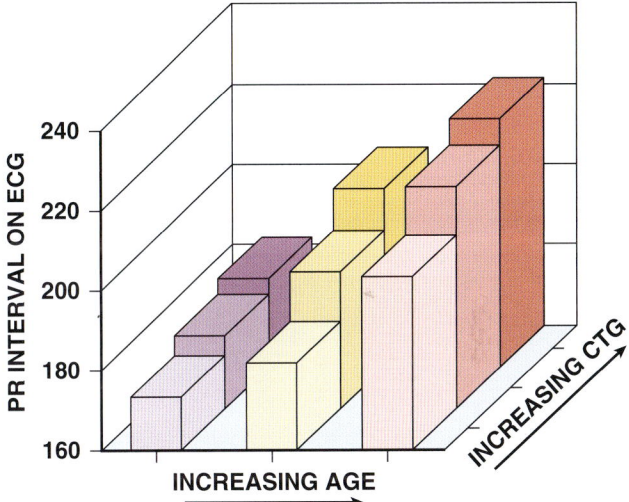

FIGURE 100.5 The relationship between the PR interval on the electrocardiogram and age and cytosine-thymine-guanine (CTG) repeat sequence expansion in 342 patients with myotonic dystrophy type 1. There is a direct relationship between age and CTG repeat sequence expansion and the severity of cardiac conduction disease, as quantified by the PR interval. The relationship suggests that cardiac involvement in myotonic dystrophy type 1 is a time-dependent degenerative process, with the rate of progression modulated by the extent of CTG repeat expansion. (From Groh WJ, Lowe MR, Zipes DP. Severity of cardiac conduction involvement and arrhythmias in myotonic dystrophy type 1 correlates with age and CTG repeat length. *J Cardiovasc Electrophysiol.* 2002;13:444.)

mutation responsible for myotonic dystrophy type 2 is a tetranucleotide repeat expansion, cytosine-cytosine-thymine-guanine (CCTG), found on chromosome 3 in intron 1 of the cellular nucleic acid binding protein (*CNBP* aka *ZNF9*). Intergenerational repeat contraction and expansion has been reported, and there is no apparent relationship between the degree of expansion and clinical severity. The prominent molecular mechanism by which both myotonic dystrophies exert their similar phenotypic presentations is by a toxic RNA gain-of-function effect. Large RNA expansions sequester and alter the function of nuclear RNA–binding proteins, resulting in aberrant mRNA splicing and polyadenylation. Cardiac involvement is related to the resultant dysregulation of multiple cardiac proteins that underlie contraction, calcium handling, excitability, and cell connectivity (Fig. 100.6).[19]

Clinical Presentation

The myotonic dystrophies are the most common inherited neuromuscular disorders in patients presenting as adults. Type 1 is more commonly diagnosed than type 2, except in certain areas of northern Europe. The global incidence of myotonic dystrophy type 1 has been estimated to be 1 in 8000 but higher in certain populations, such as French Canadians. The age at onset of symptoms and diagnosis averages 20 to 25 years. A congenital presentation is seen in severely affected patients with myotonic dystrophy type 1. Common early manifestations are related to weakness in the muscles of the face, neck, and distal extremities. Muscle weakness is progressive. On examination, myotonia can be demonstrated in the grip, thenar muscle group, and tongue (Fig. 100.7). A diagnosis can be made in asymptomatic patients using electromyography and genetic testing. Subcapsular ("Christmas tree") cataracts and early male-pattern baldness are common. Hyperinsulinemia, hyperglycemia, insulin resistance, diabetes, testicular failure, and adrenocortical dysregulation are seen in myotonic dystrophy type 1. Cardiac symptoms typically appear after the onset of skeletal muscle weakness but can be the initial manifestation. Patients with myotonic dystrophy type 2 exhibit muscle weakness, myotonia, cataracts, and endocrine abnormalities, as in type 1; however, age at symptom onset is typically older.

Cardiovascular Manifestations

Histopathology in the myotonic dystrophies shows cardiac myocyte hypertrophy and degeneration with fibrosis and fatty infiltration preferentially targeting the specialized conduction tissue, including the sinus node, atrioventricular node, and His-Purkinje system (Fig. 100.8). Degenerative changes are observed in working atrial and ventricular tissue but only rarely progress to a symptomatic dilated cardiomyopathy. It is not clear if there are differences in the cardiac pathology observed between myotonic dystrophy type 1 and 2. Patients with type 2 myotonic dystrophy typically demonstrate cardiac involvement later in life or not at all. The primary cardiac manifestations of the myotonic dystrophies are arrhythmias.

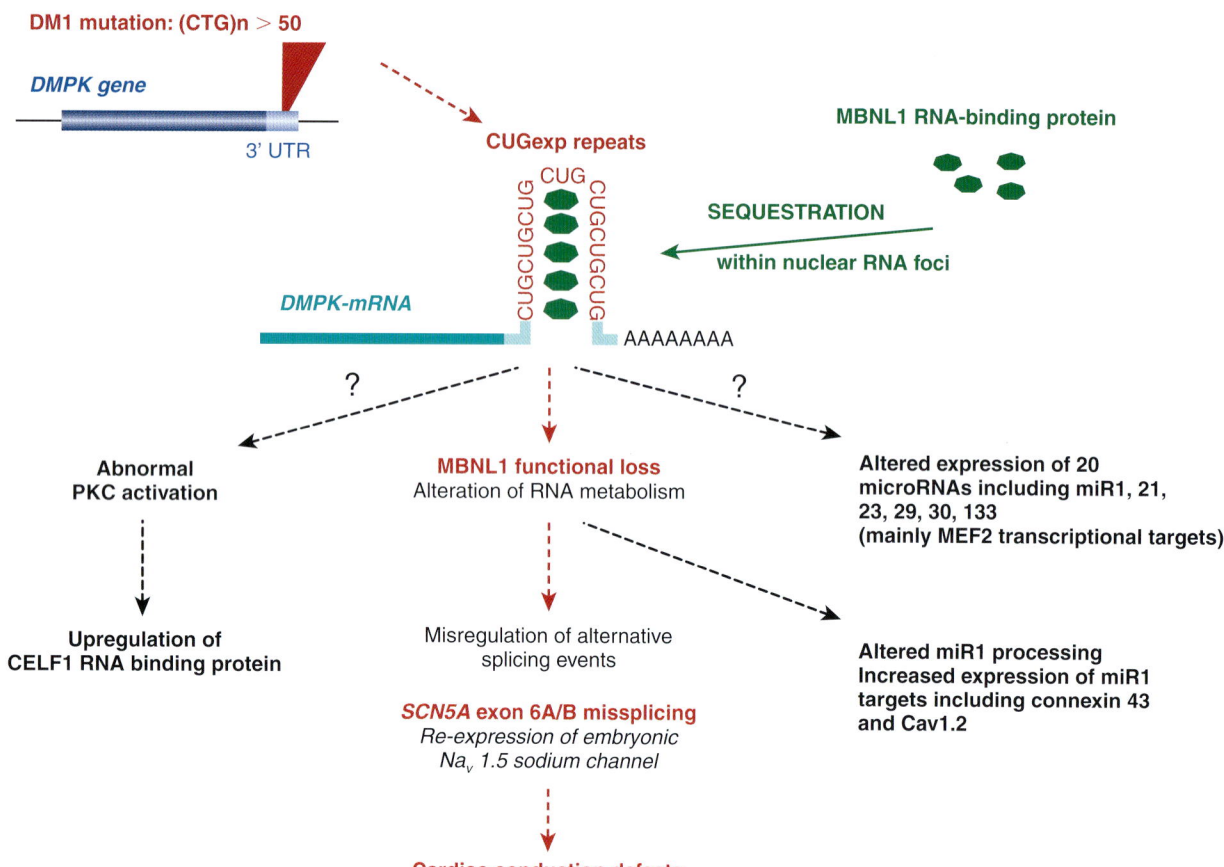

FIGURE 100.6 Multiple molecular mechanisms of cardiac involvement in type 1 myotonic dystrophy. Triplet nucleotide repeats in the 3'UTR of dystrophia myotonica protein kinase (DMPK) disrupt chromatin, can sequester muscle blind 1 (MBNL1), altering mRNA metabolism. Disruption of mRNA splicing and increased expression of microRNAs can cause dysregulation of target genes including sodium, calcium, chloride and gap junction channels, calcium handling proteins, troponins and the insulin receptor. *CELF1,* CUG binding protein Elav-like family member 1; *MEF2,* myocyte enhancer factor; *PKC,* protein kinase C; *UTR,* untranslated region.

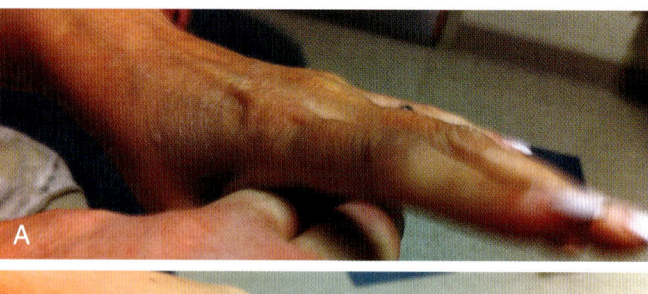
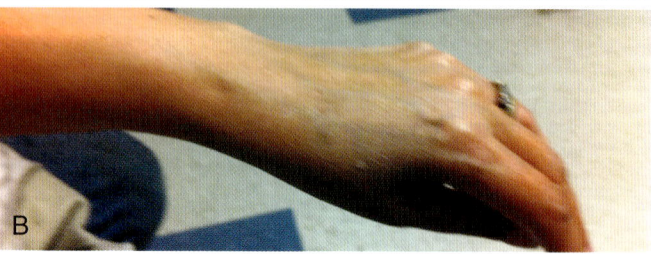

FIGURE 100.7 Grip myotonia in myotonic dystrophy. After exerting a grip **(A)** the patient is unable to fully open the hand **(B)**.

Electrocardiography

A majority of adult patients with myotonic dystrophy type 1 exhibit electrocardiographic abnormalities. In a general middle-aged US myotonic population, abnormal electrocardiographic patterns were seen in 65% of the patients. Abnormalities included first-degree atrioventricular block in 42%, right bundle branch block in 3%, left bundle branch block in 4%, and nonspecific intraventricular conduction delay in 12%. Q-waves not associated with a known myocardial infarction are common. Electrocardiographic abnormalities are less common in younger patients. Conduction disease worsens with advancing age (Fig. 100.9). Electrocardiographic abnormalities are less common in myotonic dystrophy type 2, occurring in approximately 20% of middle-aged patients.

Imaging and Heart Failure

Left ventricular systolic and diastolic dysfunction, left ventricular hypertrophy, mitral valve prolapse, regional wall motion abnormalities, and left atrial dilatation have been reported in patients with myotonic dystrophy type 1 at moderate prevalence rates. Clinical heart failure is observed but is less common than are arrhythmias. Left ventricular hypertrophy and ventricular dilation have been reported in myotonic dystrophy type 2. Cardiac MRI is more sensitive than echocardiography for detection of early cardiac involvement. Myocardial fibrosis is often observed in myotonic dystrophy and is associated with regional abnormalities in LV function. The association of global LV function and conduction abnormalities is more variable.[20-22]

Arrhythmias

A cardiac etiology is second only to respiratory failure as a cause of death in patients with myotonic dystrophy type 1. The major goal of management is evaluation of the risk for serious arrhythmias and sudden death. Patients with myotonic dystrophy type 1 demonstrate a wide range of arrhythmias. At cardiac electrophysiologic study, the most common abnormality found is a prolonged His-ventricular (H-V) interval (Chapter 68). Conduction system disease can progress to symptomatic atrioventricular block and necessitate pacemaker implantation. The prevalence of permanent cardiac pacing in patients with myotonic dystrophy type 1 varies widely between studies based on referral patterns and the indications used for implant. Updated practice guidelines have recognized that asymptomatic conduction abnormalities in neuromuscular diseases such as myotonic dystrophy may warrant special consideration for pacing (Chapter 69).[23] Atrial arrhythmias, primarily atrial fibrillation and atrial flutter (Chapter 66), are the most common arrhythmias observed. Ventricular

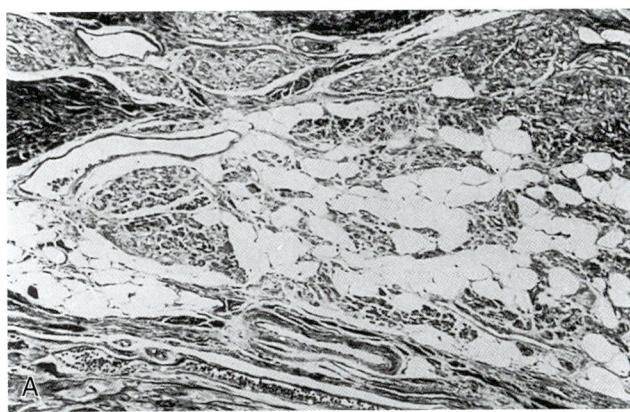
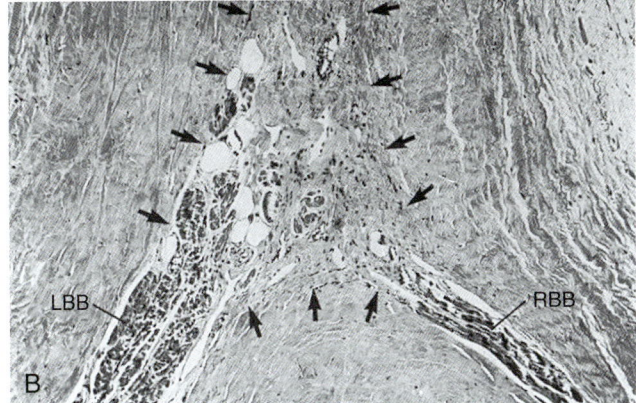

FIGURE 100.8 Histopathologic features of the atrioventricular bundle in myotonic dystrophy. **A,** Fatty infiltration in a specimen from a 57-year-old man (Masson trichrome stain, ×90). **B,** Focal replacement fibrosis and atrophy in a specimen from a 48-year-old woman. *Arrows* demarcate expected size and shape of the branching atrioventricular bundle (hematoxylin-eosin stain, ×90.) *LBB*, left bundle branch; *RBB*, right bundle branch. (From Nguyen HH, Wolfe JT 3rd, Holmes DR Jr, et al. Pathology of the cardiac conduction system in myotonic dystrophy: a study of 12 cases. *J Am Coll Cardiol.* 1988;11:662.)

tachycardia can occur. Patients with myotonic dystrophy type 1 are at risk for ventricular tachycardia occurring as a consequence of reentry in the diseased distal conduction system, as characterized by bundle branch reentry and interfascicular reentry tachycardia (Fig. 100.10). Therapy with right bundle branch or fascicular radiofrequency ablation can be curative (Chapter 67). Sudden death is responsible for 18% to 33% of deaths in myotonic dystrophy type 1; presumably, most are due to arrhythmias. Annual rates of sudden death in population studies vary between 0.25% and 2%. The mechanisms leading to sudden death are not clear. Distal conduction disease producing atrioventricular block can result in the lack of an appropriate escape rhythm and asystole or bradycardia-mediated ventricular fibrillation. Sudden death can occur in myotonic dystrophy type 1 despite pacing, implicating ventricular arrhythmias. Non-arrhythmic causes of sudden death, probably acute respiratory issues, play some role. Arrhythmias and sudden death have been reported in myotonic dystrophy type 2 but seem to be rarer than in type 1.

Treatment and Prognosis

Cardiac manifestations occur in both myotonic dystrophy types 1 and 2, and therefore diagnostic evaluation is essential in both.[24] Cardiac disease is observed at a younger age in myotonic dystrophy type 1 compared with type 2. Annual ECGs are recommended even in patients without symptoms or conduction disease. Echocardiography or other imaging modalities can determine if structural abnormalities are present. Cardiac imaging in adults should be done at diagnosis or with new symptoms. In the absence of significant abnormalities and symptoms, repeat evaluation every 3 to 5 years is appropriate. In the patient with reduced left ventricular function, standard therapy including ACE inhibitors and beta blockers has improved symptoms. There are no data on the role of ACE inhibitors or beta blockers in preventing the development of a cardiomyopathy in myotonic dystrophy. Patients presenting with symptoms indicative of arrhythmias such as syncope and palpitations should undergo an evaluation, often including a cardiac electrophysiologic study, to determine an underlying causative disorder. The role and interval for ambulatory ECG (Holter) monitoring are not clear although periodic surveillance even in the absence of conduction system disease is prudent (Chapter 61). The presence of significant or progressive electrocardiographic abnormalities despite a lack of symptoms is an indication for consideration of prophylactic pacing.[23] The presence of severe electrocardiographic conduction abnormalities and atrial arrhythmias were independent risk factors for sudden death.[25] The strategy of pacing when the H-V interval is 70 milliseconds or more decreased sudden death in a large observational trial using propensity analysis for risk stratification. Patients with significant conduction defects who are candidates for pacemaker implantation should be evaluated for their risk of ventricular arrhythmias. If cardiac MRI reveals fibrosis or if LV dysfunction is present, programmed stimulation of the ventricle may be appropriate. If a ventricular tachyarrhythmia is inducible with a non-aggressive protocol, an ICD may be the preferred cardiac rhythm management device. In patients presenting with wide complex tachycardia, cardiac electrophysiologic study with particular evaluation for bundle branch reentry tachycardia should be done (Chapter 67). The use of cardiac resynchronization therapy may be appropriate in patients requiring ventricular pacing.

Treatment of myotonia, weakness, and muscle pain with sodium channel blocking drugs (mexiletine) in patients with myotonic dystrophy may be required. In the setting of a normal resting ECG and no evidence for cardiac involvement, mexiletine can be used without further evaluation. If the ECG demonstrates any conduction system disease, pacing may be required to safely use sodium channel blocking drugs. In situations in which pacing is not possible or desired, instituting drug therapy with electrocardiographic monitoring may be considered recognizing the risk of progressive conduction system disease. Similarly, the use of Na channel blocking drugs for the treatment of atrial fibrillation is contraindicated in patients with conduction system disease in the absence of a pacemaker.

Anesthesia in patients with myotonic dystrophy increases the risks of decreased gastrointestinal motility, respiratory failure, and arrhythmias. Patients may have unpredictable responses to neuromuscular blocking agents and careful monitoring during the perioperative period is mandatory. Monitored anesthesia during cardiac device implants should be done under an anesthesiologist's care.[24]

The course and prognosis of neuromuscular abnormalities in the myotonic dystrophies is variable.[26] Respiratory failure from progressive muscle dysfunction is the most common cause of death. Some patients, however, are only minimally limited by weakness up to the age of 60 to 70 years. Sudden death can reduce survival rates in patients with myotonic dystrophies, including those minimally symptomatic neuromuscular involvement. Decisions regarding primary prevention cardiac devices need to be made with full consideration of all aspects for the care of the myotonic patient.

Emery-Dreifuss Muscular Dystrophy and Associated Disorders
Genetics and Cardiac Pathology

Emery-Dreifuss muscular dystrophy (EDMD) is a spectrum of rare inherited disorders in which skeletal muscle symptoms are often mild but with cardiac involvement that is both common and serious. The disease (EDMD1) is classically inherited in an X-linked recessive fashion and the gene responsible, *STA*, encodes a nuclear membrane protein termed emerin (Table 100.2). EDMD is also inherited in an autosomal manner, the result of mutations in the *LMNA* gene that encodes the nuclear membrane proteins, lamins A and C. *LMNA* mutations also cause a spectrum of other diseases, including dilated cardiomyopathy and conduction system disease without skeletal muscle involvement and lipodystrophy (Chapter 52).[27] Nuclear membrane proteins such as emerin and lamins A and C provide structural support for the nucleus and interact with the cell's cytoskeletal proteins. The most common pattern of inheritance of LMNA mutations is autosomal dominant with variable expressivity and penetrance. Mutations throughout the *LMNA* gene have been documented in EDMD.

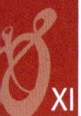

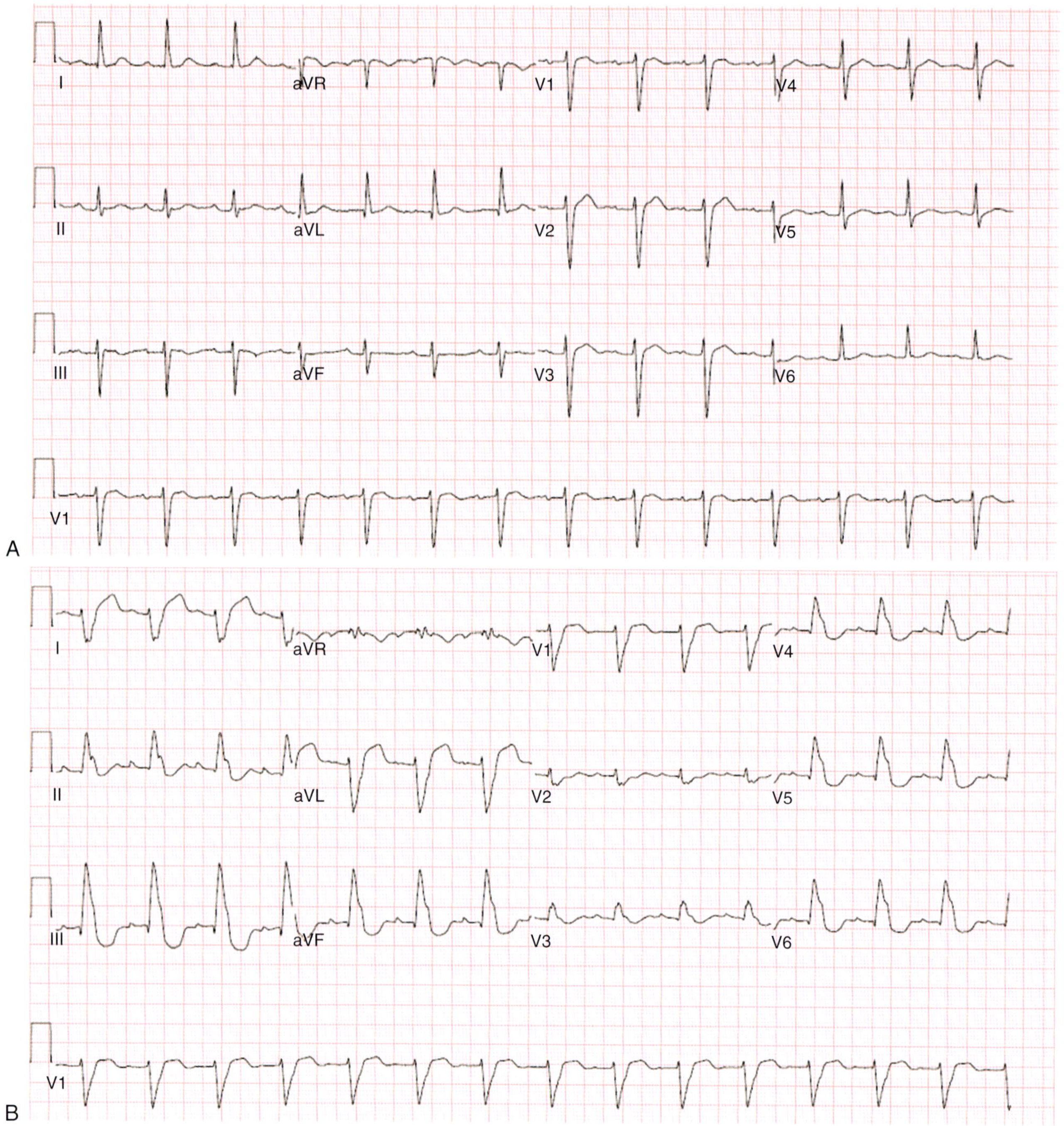

FIGURE 100.9 A and **B,** Electrocardiograms recorded 2 years apart in a 36-year-old woman with myotonic dystrophy (the *top tracings* are older). There is a dramatic increase in the QRS duration, ventricular axis shift, and increase in the PR interval consistent with progressive and severe conduction disease.

Clinical Presentation

EDMD is characterized by a triad of early contractures of the elbow, Achilles tendon, and posterior cervical muscles; slowly progressing muscle weakness and atrophy, primarily in humeroperoneal muscles; and cardiac involvement (Fig. 100.11). The disorder has been labeled "benign X-linked muscular dystrophy" to differentiate the slowly progressive muscular weakness from that of DMD. In the autosomal dominant and recessive inheritance of EDMD, a more variable phenotypic expression and penetrance are typically observed. Mutations in the lamin A/C gene are also responsible for an autosomal dominant familial partial lipodystrophy characterized by marked loss of subcutaneous fat, diabetes, hypertriglyceridemia, and cardiac abnormalities.

Cardiovascular Manifestations

In most patients with EDMD, the cardiac manifestations are the cause of mortality. Arrhythmias and dilated cardiomyopathy are the major manifestations of cardiac disease in EDMD and its associated disorders. In X-linked recessive EDMD, abnormalities in impulse generation and conduction are common. Electrocardiographic abnormalities are usually apparent by age 20 to 30 years, commonly showing first-degree atrioventricular block. The atria appear to be involved earlier than the ventricles, with atrial fibrillation and atrial flutter, or more classically, permanent atrial standstill and junctional bradycardia. Abnormalities in impulse generation or conduction are present in virtually all patients by age 35 to 40 years, and requirement for pacing is typical. Ventricular arrhythmias occur, including sustained ventricular tachycardia and ventricular fibrillation. Sudden death, presumably due to cardiac disorders, before age 50 is observed and has informed the use of primary prevention ICDs.[12,28] Female carriers of X-linked recessive EDMD due to emerin mutations do not exhibit skeletal muscle disease but exhibit late cardiac disease, including conduction abnormalities, and more rarely sudden death. Although arrhythmias are the

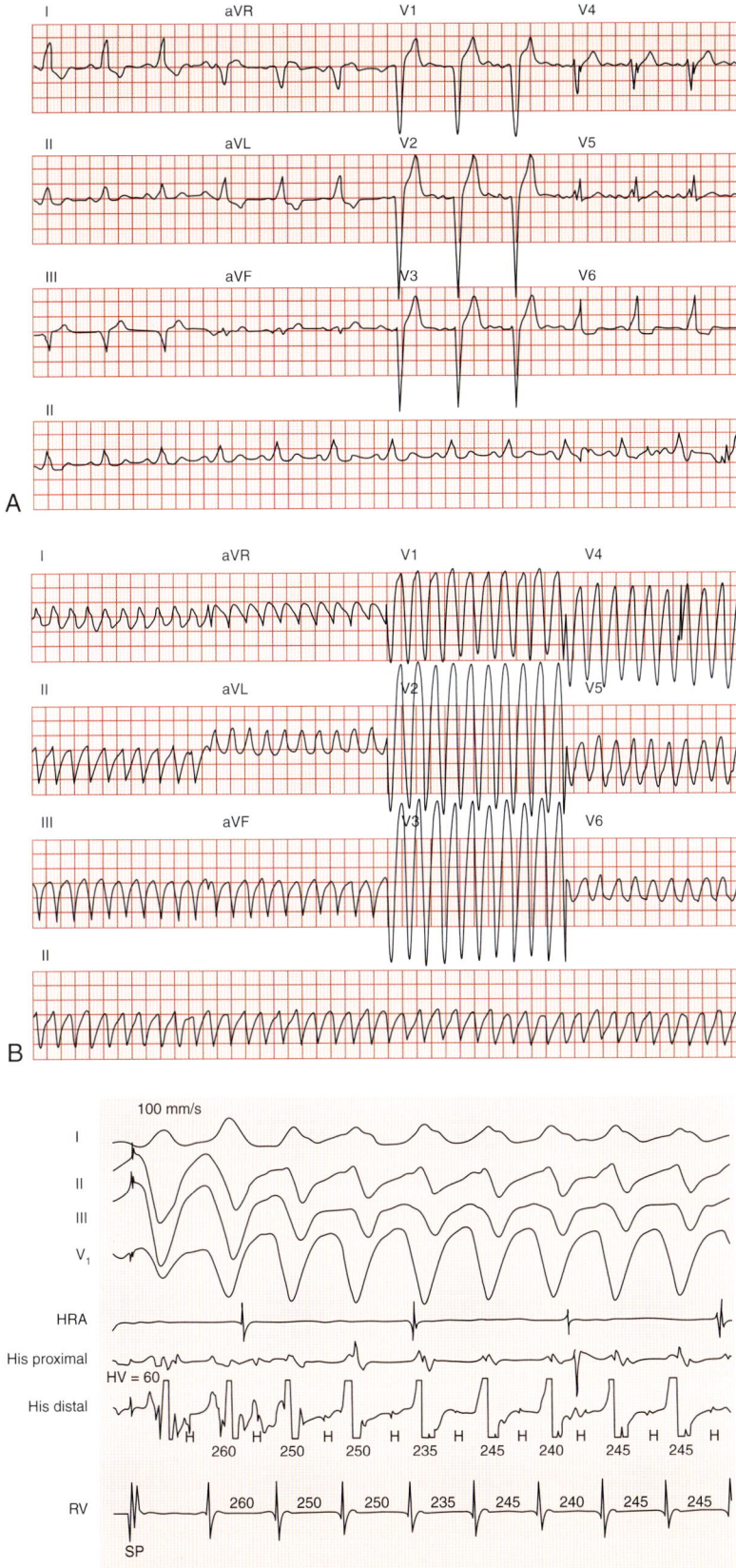

FIGURE 100.10 Bundle branch reentry tachycardia in a 34-year-old woman with myotonic dystrophy type 1 presenting with a symptomatic (recurrent syncope) wide-complex tachycardia. **A,** Electrocardiogram (ECG) showing sinus rhythm and a QRS complex with left bundle branch block. **B,** ECG showing a rapid monomorphic tachycardia easily inducible on electrophysiologic study, with left bundle morphology. **C,** Recordings during electrophysiologic study, including the surface ECG (leads I, II, III, V₁) and intracardiac ECGs (high right atrium, HRA, His proximal, His distal, and right ventricle, RV). A monomorphic ventricular tachycardia is induced with atrial-ventricular (A-V) dissociation and His association, consistent with bundle branch reentry tachycardia. Note, the H-H interval drives the subsequent V-V interval.

most common presentation of cardiac involvement in X-linked recessive EDMD, a dilated cardiomyopathy does occur. The dilated cardiomyopathy is more common in patients in whom the survival time has been improved with cardiac device implantation. Both autopsy and endomyocardial biopsy specimens have shown cardiac fibrosis.

Patients with disorders caused by lamin A and C mutations typically present at 20 to 40 years of age with cardiac conduction disease, atrial fibrillation, and dilated cardiomyopathy. Skeletal muscle disease typically is subclinical or absent. Progressive cardiomyopathy severe enough to require heart transplantation has been reported. Sudden death in those patients with dilated cardiomyopathy occurs. Pacing often is required for symptomatic heart block. ICDs are the appropriate cardiac device for a majority of these patients.

Treatment and Prognosis

Patients should be monitored for development of electrocardiographic conduction abnormalities and arrhythmias. Annual evaluation including an ECG is appropriate. Sinus node dysfunction and atrial standstill are associated with AF often before the development of bradyarrhythmias. AF is associated with a relatively high frequency of embolic stroke, even in the absence of ventricular dysfunction; therefore, anticoagulation should be considered in patients with EDMD with atrial standstill or AF.[29] Sudden death even in patients with pacemakers has been observed. Primary prevention ICD is recommended in patients with EDMD and its associated disorders if significant electrocardiographic conduction disease is present and pacing is being considered.[12,28] The use of biventricular pacing should be considered in patients that require ventricular pacing. Whether ICDs should be considered only in certain subgroups of patients or in all patients with significant conduction disease or cardiomyopathy is not clear. In a large observational European series, risk factors for sudden death and appropriate ICD therapy included non-sustained ventricular tachycardia, left ventricular ejection fraction less than 45% at presentation, male sex, and lamin A or C non–missense mutations.[12] Routine imaging for evaluation of left ventricular function is appropriate in all patients with EDMD and the associated disorders. Although data are limited in this cohort, patients with LV dysfunction should be managed with guideline-recommended medical therapies, including ACEIs or ARBs, neprilysin inhibitors, beta blockers, and diuretics. Advanced HF treatment, including mechanical cardiac support (ventricular assist devices) and heart transplantation should be considered in appropriate patients. Female carriers of X-linked recessive EDMD develop conduction disease, and electrocardiographic monitoring on a routine basis is appropriate. Atrioventricular block can occur with anesthesia.

Limb-Girdle Muscular Dystrophies
Genetics and Pathophysiology

The limb-girdle muscular dystrophies are a group of over 25 muscle disorders with a limb-shoulder and pelvic girdle distribution of weakness, but with otherwise heterogeneous inheritance and genetic causes.[30,31] The naming convention is based on the mode of inheritance, with limb-girdle muscular dystrophy (LGMD)1 being transmitted as an autosomal dominant trait and LGMD2 as autosomal recessive. Within each class, there are subclasses of LGMDs identified by a letter designation. Autosomal recessive (subtypes 2A to 2Z), dominant (subtypes 1A to 1H), and sporadic patterns of inheritance have been observed. Genes involved include those encoding dystrophin-associated glycoproteins,

TABLE 100.2 Inheritance, Gene Locus, Disease Protein, and Cardiac Manifestations of Neuromuscular Disorders

DISEASE	OMIM	HERITANCE	GENE LOCUS	DISEASE PROTEIN	CARDIAC MANIFESTATIONS			
					Cardiomyopathy	Conduction abnormalities	Ventricular arrhythmia	Atrial arrhythmia
Duchenne MD	#310200	X-linked	Xp21	Dystrophin	+++	+	++	+
Becker MD	#300376	X-linked	Xp21	Dystrophin	+++	+	++	+
Limb-girdle MD, types 2C-G, I, J, N,Q	multiple	Autosomal recessive	Various	Sarcoglycans and others	+++	+	++	++
Myotonic dystrophy 1	#160900	Autosomal dominant	19q13	DMPK	+	+++	+	++
Myotonic dystrophy 2	#602668	AD	3q21	ZF9	Rare	+	+	+
Emery-Dreifuss MD, type 1	#310300	XL	Xq28	Emerin	++	+++	+++	++
Limb-girdle MD, type 1B	#150330	AD	1q11-21	Lamin A/C	+	++	+++	++
Fascioscapulohumeral MD	#158900	AD	4q35 D4Z4	DUX4	Rare	Rare	Rare	Rare
Friedreich ataxia	#229300	AR	9q21.11	Frataxin	+++ (HCM)	+++	+++	+
Kearns-Sayre syndrome	#530000	AD	mtDNA	Various	+	+++	+	++

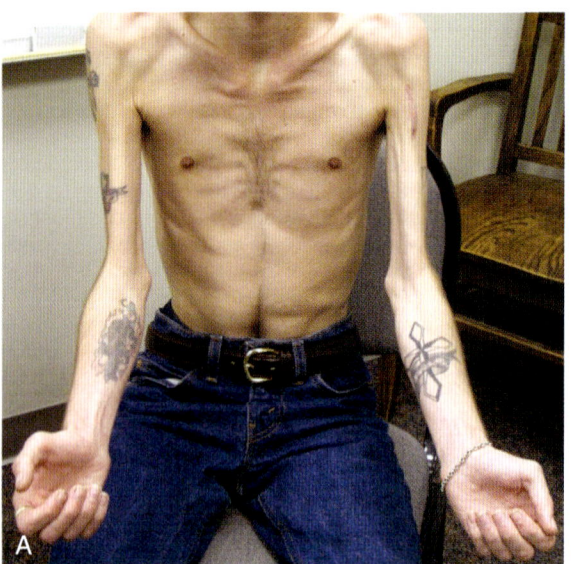
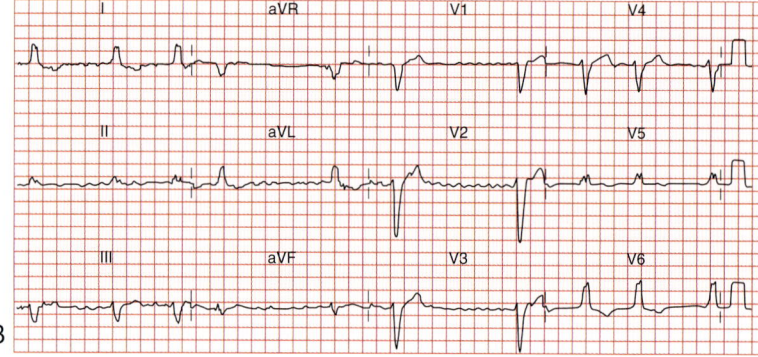

FIGURE 100.11 Emery-Dreifuss muscular dystrophy in a 28-year-old man presenting with syncope. **A,** Contractures of the elbow and atrophy in the humeroperoneal muscles. **B,** Electrocardiogram obtained at initial presentation showed atrial fibrillation with slow ventricular rate and a QRS complex with left bundle branch block. (Courtesy Dr. Robert M. Pascuzzi.)

sarcomeric proteins, sarcolemmal proteins, nuclear membrane proteins, and cellular enzymes. An autosomal dominant LGMD (subtype 1B) with a high prevalence of arrhythmias and a late dilated cardiomyopathy is caused by mutations encoding lamin A/C, as in EDMD. An autosomal recessive or sporadic LGMD associated with a progressive dilated cardiomyopathy is caused by mutations affecting the function of the dystrophin-glycoprotein complex, including sarcoglycan and fukutin-related proteins (subtypes 2C to 2F and 2I, respectively). The sarcoglycans interact with dystrophin-associated glycoproteins to counteract mechanical stress associated with contraction. Fukutin-related proteins affect glycosylation of a dystrophin-associated glycoprotein. An autosomal recessive LGMD associated with a variable onset of a dilated cardiomyopathy is caused by a mutation in a sarcolemmal repair protein termed dysferlin (subtype 2B) (see Fig. 100.1). Other more recently discovered and rarer subtypes of LGMD are variably associated with cardiac abnormalities in limited reports. A new nomenclature has been recommended.[32]

Clinical Presentation

The onset of proximal muscle weakness is variable but usually occurs before age 30. The recessive disorders tend to cause earlier and produce more severe weakness than the dominant disorders. Sarcoglycan-associated LGMDs more prominently affect flexor muscle groups and exhibit a rapidly progressive course, often with wheelchair confinement within a decade. Creatine kinase levels may be moderately to severely elevated. Patients commonly present with complaints of difficulty with walking or running secondary to pelvic girdle involvement. As the disease progresses, involvement of the shoulder muscles and then more distal muscles occurs, with sparing of facial involvement. Independent of the onset of skeletal muscle disease, effects on the heart are usually apparent by the second or third decade of life.

Cardiovascular Manifestations

As with many of the features of the limb-girdle muscular dystrophies, heterogeneity in the presence and degree of cardiac involvement is usual. Importantly, the severity of cardiac involvement may not be correlated with the degree of skeletal muscle impairment. The limb-girdle muscular dystrophies types 2C to 2F, termed *sarcoglycanopathies*, exhibit a dilated cardiomyopathy. Cardiac abnormalities are detected in a majority of patients typically a decade after skeletal muscle symptoms occur. Cardiomyopathy is less common in the subtype 2D than present in the other sarcoglycanopathies. ECGs show similar abnormalities as in Duchenne and Becker muscular dystrophy, including an increased R wave in V_1 and lateral Q waves. Imaging can show a progressive dilated cardiomyopathy. A severe cardiomyopathy, including presentation with heart failure in childhood, can occur. Sudden death associated with the cardiomyopathy has been reported.

LGMD type 2I, caused by mutations in fukutin-related proteins, is associated with a dilated cardiomyopathy. The mutation is also responsible for a form of congenital muscular dystrophy. The age at disease onset and severity of skeletal muscle involvement are variable, with symptoms emerging in some patients during childhood but more typically developing after the age of 20 years. Approximately one-half of patients with LGMD type 2I exhibit cardiac involvement (Fig. 100.12) more commonly reported in males. Cardiac findings include regional wall motion abnormalities or a dilated cardiomyopathy and heart failure. Conduction disease generally does not occur independent of structural cardiac involvement. LGMD type 2A due to calpain 3 mutations and type 2B, due to dysferlin gene mutations, have little cardiac involvement, although abnormalities can be detected on cardiac imaging.

The autosomal dominant LGMD type 1B is caused by mutations in the gene encoding lamins A and C with a clinical phenotype similar to EDMD. Skeletal muscle involvement is mild, with frequent and severe cardiac involvement. Atrioventricular block develops by early middle age, often necessitating pacing. Sudden death is observed even in patients with pacemakers. A progressive dilated cardiomyopathy can occur, typically after the development of conduction disease.

Treatment and Prognosis
Because of the heterogeneous nature of LGMD, specific recommendations for routine cardiac evaluation and therapy are based on the disease type. The frequency and severity of cardiac involvement in LGMD and in particular the laminopathies, mandates an aggressive approach to evaluation and management. This is particularly relevant in view of the often milder skeletal muscle disease in these patients. In addition to a thorough cardiovascular history and physical examination, the recommended evaluation includes resting and ambulatory ECGs, echocardiography, and cardiac MRI with contrast (in cases in which there is any suggestion of cardiac involvement).

Treatment of LV dysfunction even in the absence of clinical HF is appropriate and should include ACEIs or ARBs and beta blockers in the absence of contraindications. Patients with dilated cardiomyopathies respond to standard heart failure therapy. Heart transplantation has been reported. Prophylactic placement of an ICD instead of a pacemaker has been recommended in patients with lamin A and C mutation after conduction disease is observed akin to that in EDMD. In a large observational European series, risk factors for sudden death and appropriate ICD therapy included nonsustained ventricular tachycardia, left ventricular ejection fraction less than 45% at presentation, male sex, and lamin A or C non–missense mutations.[12]

Facioscapulohumeral Muscular Dystrophy
Genetics and Pathophysiology
Facioscapulohumeral muscular dystrophy is the third most common muscular dystrophy after the Duchenne and myotonic types.[33] Underreporting of disease prevalence is likely due to mild subclinical forms. It is an autosomal dominant disorder in which the primary genetic mutation occurs at chromosomal locus 4q35, with a contraction of a D4Z4 repeat sequence that leads to derepression of a retrogene, *DUX4* encoding a transcriptional regulator whose target genes are toxic to skeletal muscle (Table 100.2). *DUX4* derepression may result from repeat contraction induced chromatin hypomethylation (FSHD1, most common form) or as a consequence of a second mutation in SMCHD1, a gene involved in chromatin methylation of the D4Z4 region (FSHD2).

Clinical Presentation
The onset and rates of progression of muscle weakness are highly variable, with a distinct regional pattern starting in the face and periscapular region, then progressing caudally and distally in the upper body, then to the pelvic musculature. Muscle weakness in FSHD tends to be more asymmetric than other muscular dystrophies, except in advanced disease. Respiratory involvement is rare; however, some patients develop restrictive lung disease. In patients with large deletions in the D4Z4 region, high frequency hearing loss and retinal vascular disease with exudative retinopathy (Coats Disease) has been described.[34]

Cardiovascular Manifestations
Cardiac involvement in facioscapulohumeral muscular dystrophy is reported but does not constitute as significant a problem in prevalence or severity as in other muscular dystrophies. Cardiomyopathy, ventricular arrhythmias and symptomatic conduction disease are generally not observed. There are reports of supraventricular tachycardia (SVT) and asymptomatic right bundle branch block.

Treatment and Prognosis
Because significant clinical cardiac involvement is rare in facioscapulohumeral muscular dystrophy, specific monitoring or treatment recommendations are not well defined. Annual ECGs have been recommended.

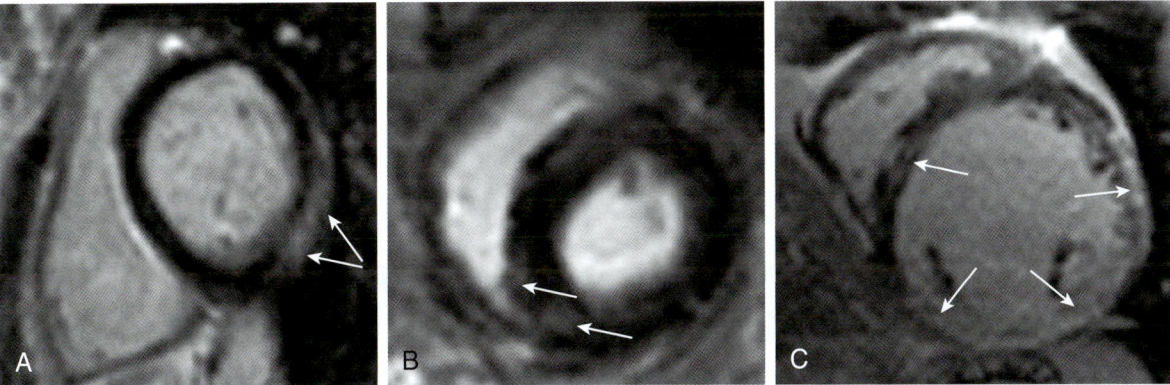

FIGURE 100.12 Cardiac magnetic resonance imaging findings in limb-girdle muscular dystrophy. Late gadolinium enhancement (*arrows*) in limb-girdle muscular dystrophy patients demonstrating focal epicardial (**A**) or midwall (**B**) enhancement. **C,** Patient with limb-girdle muscular dystrophy 2I and advanced dilated cardiomyopathy had extensive myocardial injury/fibrosis. (From Rosales XQ, Moser SJ, Tran T, et al. Cardiovascular magnetic resonance of cardiomyopathy in limb girdle muscular dystrophy 2B and 2I. *J Cardiovasc Magn Reson*. 2011;13:39.)

Friedreich Ataxia

Genetics and Pathophysiology

Friedreich ataxia (FRDA) is an autosomal recessive, multisystem disease characterized by spinocerebellar degeneration. The clinical presentation includes ataxia of the limbs and trunk, dysarthria, loss of deep tendon reflexes, sensory abnormalities, skeletal deformities, diabetes mellitus, and cardiac involvement. The primary genetic abnormality is an unstable trinucleotide repeat expansion (guanine-adenine-adenine, GAA), in the first intron of frataxin gene *(FXN)* that inhibits its transcription. Frataxin is a 210–amino acid mitochondrial protein associated with iron homeostasis. Deficiency of the protein leads to mitochondrial iron aggregation increasing cell susceptibility to oxidative stress. Messenger RNA for frataxin is highly expressed in the heart. Endomyocardial biopsy samples have shown deficient function in mitochondrial respiratory complex subunits and in aconitase, an iron-sulfur protein involved in iron homeostasis. Impaired mitochondrial lipid metabolism also may play a role in the cardiomyopathy in FRDA. Histopathologic examination has revealed myocyte hypertrophy due to proliferation of mitochondria, myocyte degeneration, interstitial fibrosis, active muscle necrosis, bizarre pleomorphic nuclei, and periodic acid–Schiff–(PAS) positive deposition in both large and small coronary arteries. Degeneration and fibrosis in cardiac nerves and ganglia and the conduction system also have been observed. An earlier age at symptom onset, increasing severity of neurologic symptoms, and worsening left ventricular hypertrophy are observed in patients in whom genetic testing shows a larger GAA repeat expansion.

Clinical Presentation

FRDA is one of the most common inherited ataxias. The development of neurologic symptoms before age 25 and typically around puberty is characteristic. Progressive, debilitating ataxia and loss of neuromuscular function, with the patient wheelchair-bound 10 to 20 years after symptom onset, is the usual course. Neurologic symptoms precede cardiac symptoms in most but not all cases.

Cardiovascular Manifestations

FRDA is associated with left ventricular hypertrophy (Fig. 100.13). Asymmetric septal hypertrophy is uncommon and a left ventricular outflow gradient is rare but has been observed. The prevalence of hypertrophy increases, particularly with a younger age at diagnosis and with increasing GAA trinucleotide expansion. ECG abnormalities are present in over 90% of patients with FRDA. Left ventricular hypertrophy is not always present on ECGs despite echocardiographic evidence. Widespread ST deviation and T wave inversions are common as is right axis deviation (Fig. 100.14). Patients with left ventricular hypertrophy without systolic dysfunction typically have no cardiac symptoms. About 10% of patients develop left ventricular systolic dysfunction with an ejection fraction of less than 50%.[35,36] Presentation with a dilated cardiomyopathy has been reported (Fig. 100.15). The dilated cardiomyopathy occurs as a transition from the hypertrophic cardiomyopathy. Atrial arrhythmias including atrial fibrillation and flutter are associated with the progression to a dilated cardiomyopathy. Similarly, ventricular tachycardias are generally coincident with the development of dilated cardiomyopathy. The hypertrophic cardiomyopathy of FRDA is not associated with serious ventricular arrhythmias, as observed in the other types of heritable hypertrophic cardiomyopathies. Myocardial fiber disarray is not commonly observed in the hypertrophic cardiomyopathy of FRDA. Sudden death likely due to ventricular arrhythmias has been reported, but a mechanism has not been well characterized.[12,36]

Treatment and Prognosis

Idebenone, a free radical scavenger, has modest but variable effectiveness for decreasing left ventricular hypertrophy in FRDA. Idebenone does not improve left ventricular systolic function. It is unclear whether the modest improvement in cardiac imaging parameters leads to an alteration in the clinical cardiovascular course. Idebenone and other antioxidants (vitamin E and coenzyme Q10) have been studied and do not improve neurologic outcomes. In a majority of patients with FRDA, neurologic dysfunction is progressive. Heart failure is the most common cause of death.[37] Arrhythmias complicate heart failure deaths in one third of patients. Respiratory dysfunction is the second most common cause of death. Death from heart failure occurs earlier than respiratory death, typically before the age of 30 years. The role of pharmacologic or defibrillator therapy in FRDA and dilated cardiomyopathy has not been evaluated, but such conventional therapy should be considered. Small case series describe cardiac transplantation in FRDA patients with mild neurological disease.[38]

LESS COMMON NEUROMUSCULAR DISEASES ASSOCIATED WITH CARDIAC MANIFESTATIONS

The Periodic Paralyses

Genetics and Clinical Presentation

The primary periodic paralyses are rare, non-dystrophic disorders of autosomal dominant inheritance associated with mutations in ion channel genes.[39] They can be classified into hypokalemic and hyperkalemic periodic paralyses and Andersen-Tawil syndrome (see Chapter 63). In addition, acquired hypokalemic periodic paralysis may complicate thyrotoxicosis, especially in Asian men. All patients present with episodic attacks of flaccid paralysis precipitated by variable environmental stimuli including cold and exercise, or with rest after exercise. The periodic paralyses may be complicated by a late-onset permanent skeletal myopathy. Hypokalemic periodic paralysis is characterized by episodic attacks of weakness exacerbated by carbohydrate load or occurring during rest after exercise and is associated with decreased serum potassium levels at onset. Penetrance is nearly complete in male patients and 50% in female patients. It is caused by point mutations in the dihydropyridine-sensitive calcium channel *(CACNA1S)* or in skeletal muscle sodium channel *(SCN4A)*. Approximately 20% of cases are of uncertain genetic cause. One third of the cases of thyrotoxic hypokalemic periodic paralysis are caused by mutations in an inward rectifier potassium channel, Kir2.6, which is regulated by thyroid hormone. Hyperkalemic periodic paralysis also manifests with episodic weakness but with symptoms worsening with potassium supplementation and decreasing with carbohydrate load. Potassium levels usually are high but may be normal during an attack. Hyperkalemic periodic paralysis is due primarily to mutations in *SCN4A*, but other loci also have been identified. Multiple different mutations

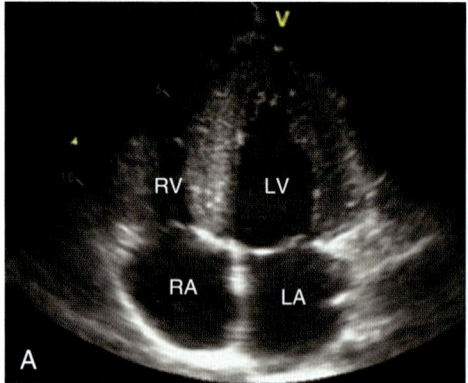
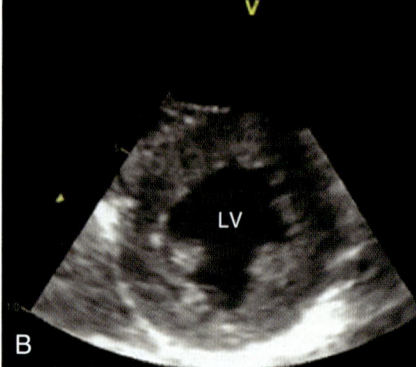

FIGURE 100.13 Hypertrophic cardiomyopathy in Friedreich ataxia. Echocardiographic apical 4-chamber (**A**) and short-axis (**B**) views from a Friedreich ataxia patient with left ventricular hypertrophy (LV wall thickness 15 mm). *LA*, left atrium; *LV*, left ventricle; *RA*, right atrium; *RV*, right ventricle. (From Weidemann F, Störk S, Liu D, et al. Cardiomyopathy of Friedreich ataxia. *J Neurochem.* 2013;126[suppl 1]:88.)

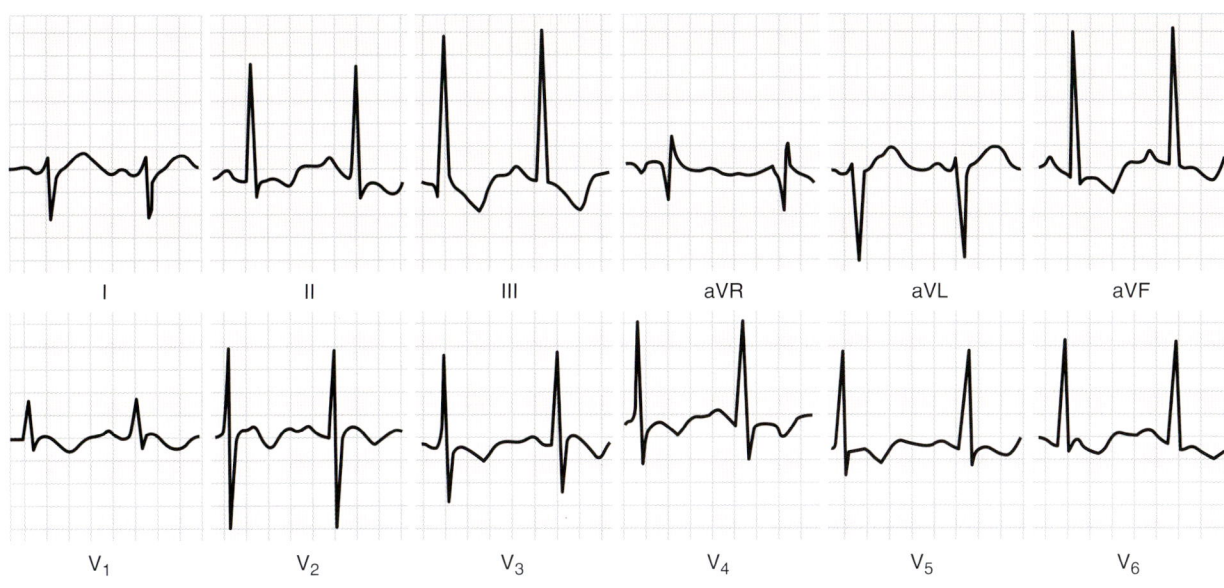

FIGURE 100.14 Electrocardiogram from a 34-year-old man with Friedreich ataxia. Widespread ST and T changes are evident. (Courtesy Dr. Charles Fisch, Indiana University School of Medicine, Indianapolis.)

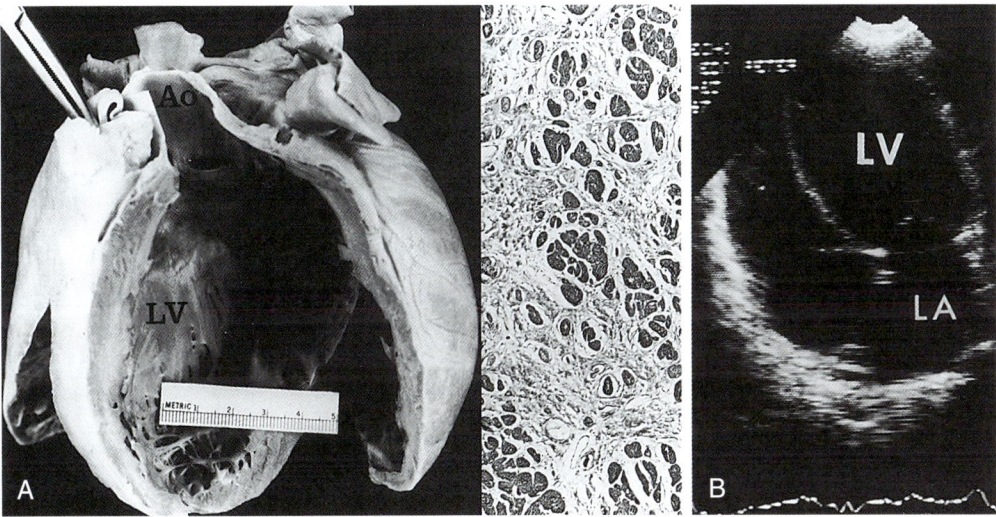

FIGURE 100.15 A, Gross and histologic specimens from a 17-year-old boy with Friedreich ataxia whose electrocardiogram progressed from a normal appearance at age 13 years to a minimally dilated, hypocontractile left ventricle (LV) 3 to 4 years later. The gross specimen *(left)* shows a mildly dilated LV with normal wall thickness. The microscopic section from the left ventricular free wall *(right)* shows marked connective tissue replacement. Although specifically sought, small-vessel coronary artery disease was not identified. **B,** Two-dimensional echocardiogram (apical window) showing the mildly dilated, thin-walled LV. *Ao,* aorta; *LA,* left atrium. (From Child JS, Perloff JK, Bach PM, et al. Cardiac involvement in Friedreich ataxia. *J Am Coll Cardiol.* 1986;7:1370.)

in this gene have been reported that result in a potassium-sensitive failure of inactivation (gain-of-function) in the sodium channel.

Andersen-Tawil syndrome (also designated as long QT syndrome 7) is a distinct periodic paralysis associated with dysmorphic physical features of short stature, low-set ears, micrognathia, hypertelorism, and clinodactyly; abnormalities on the ECG include an abnormal QT-U wave pattern and ventricular arrhythmias (Fig. 100.16).[39] Weakness can be triggered by low, normal, or high potassium levels. It can be inherited in an autosomal dominant fashion or can be sporadic. Phenotypic variability and incomplete penetrance can complicate the diagnosis for a given family. Mutations in the *KCNJ2* gene encoding the inward rectifier potassium channel subunit (Kir2.1), and inward rectifier current (IK1, responsible for maintaining the resting membrane potential) accounts for 60% of cases. The genetic cause(s) in the other 40% of patients is unknown but seemingly involve other proteins contributing to IK1 because the phenotype is indistinguishable from *KCNJ2*-mediated disease. The loss of function of IK1 is responsible for the large and prolonged U-wave.

Cardiovascular Manifestations

The periodic paralyses are associated with ventricular arrhythmias. Most arrhythmias occur in Andersen-Tawil syndrome and less often in hyperkalemic periodic paralysis. Bidirectional ventricular tachycardia (see Fig 100.16) has been observed without digitalis intoxication (Chapters 14 and 63). The episodes of bidirectional ventricular tachycardia are independent of attacks of muscle weakness, do not correlate with serum potassium levels, and can convert to sinus rhythm with exercise. The tachycardia typically is less than 150 beats/min and well tolerated. Andersen-Tawil syndrome is associated with modest prolongation in the QT interval but more specifically a prolonged and prominent U wave. Cardiac conduction abnormalities, atypical of long QT syndromes, have been observed in Andersen-Tawil syndrome. Torsades de pointes is observed in Andersen-Tawil syndrome but is less common than in the other long QT syndromes. Syncope, cardiac arrest, and sudden death have been reported in the periodic paralyses, most prominently in the Andersen-Tawil syndrome. The factors that portend an increased risk of life-threatening arrhythmias are not clear. The frequency of ventricular ectopy or non-sustained ventricular tachycardia on ambulatory monitoring did not differentiate Andersen-Tawil syndrome patients with and without syncope.[40]

Treatment and Prognosis

The episodes of weakness typically respond to measures that normalize potassium levels. Weakness in hyperkalemic periodic paralysis can respond to mexiletine. Weakness in hypokalemic periodic paralysis may respond to acetazolamide. Treatment targeting electrolyte abnormalities usually does not ameliorate arrhythmias or, if it does, affords only transient benefit. Improvement in symptomatic non-sustained ventricular tachycardia associated with a prolonged QT interval has been reported with beta-blocker therapy. Class 1A antiarrhythmic drugs can worsen muscle weakness and exacerbate arrhythmias associated with a prolonged QT interval. Bidirectional ventricular tachycardia, not associated with a prolonged QT interval, may not respond to beta-blocker therapy. Flecainide decreases the frequency of ventricular arrhythmias assessed by ambulatory monitoring and is associated with a good clinical outcome over 2 years in Andersen-Tawil syndrome.[40] Amiodarone and imipramine have also been shown to have efficacy in small series and case reports. The use of ICDs has been reported in Andersen-Tawil syndrome, primarily in those with symptomatic and drug-refractory sustained ventricular arrhythmias. Programming of defibrillators to avoid inappropriate discharges is problematic because ventricular tachycardia is often self-terminating. Prognosis in the Andersen-Tawil syndrome is reasonably good despite frequent episodes of ventricular ectopy.

Mitochondrial Disorders
Genetics and Clinical Presentation

The mitochondrial disorders, also termed mitochondrial myopathies, encephalomyopathies, or respiratory chain disorders, are a heterogeneous group of diseases resulting from abnormalities in mitochondrial function.[41] The list of distinct disorders is extensive and includes deficiencies in electron transport chain proteins, mutations in mitochondrial DNA and tRNA, coenzyme Q10 deficiency, 3-methylglucatonic acidurias and abnormal iron handling. Mitochondrial DNA is inherited maternally, and some of these disorders are thus transmitted from mother to children of both sexes. Many other disorders result from abnormalities in nuclear DNA involved in mitochondrial form and function and are inherited in an autosomal or X-linked fashion. Sporadic cases can occur. Disease severity can vary among family members because both mutant and normal mitochondrial DNA can be present in tissue in variable proportions, a phenomenon termed *heteroplasmy*. Consistent with the energy-generating

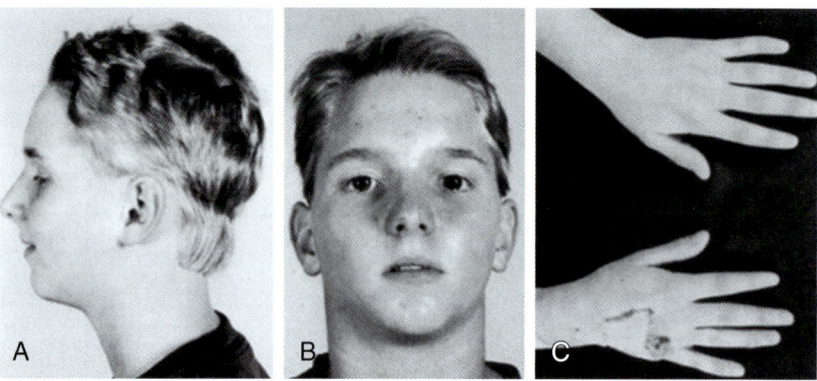

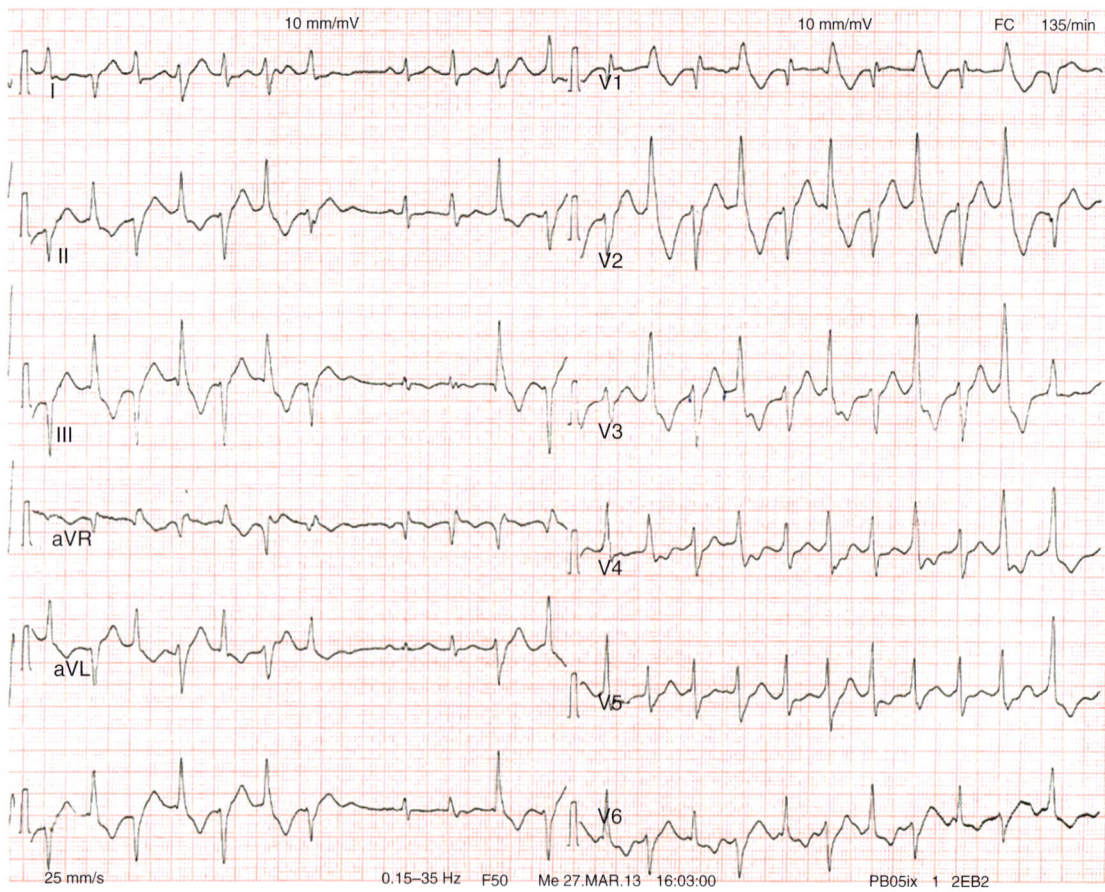

FIGURE 100.16 Andersen-Tawil syndrome. **A** and **B,** An affected patient exhibits characteristic low-set ears, hypertelorism, micrognathia, and clinodactyly of the fifth digits **(C)**. ECG from a patient with Andersen-Tawil syndrome before **(D)** and after flecainide **(E)**. (D and E from Maffe S, Paffoni P, Bergamasco L, et al. Therapeutic management of ventricular arrhythmias in Andersen-Tawil syndrome. *J Electrocardiol*. Jan–Feb 2020;58:37–42.)

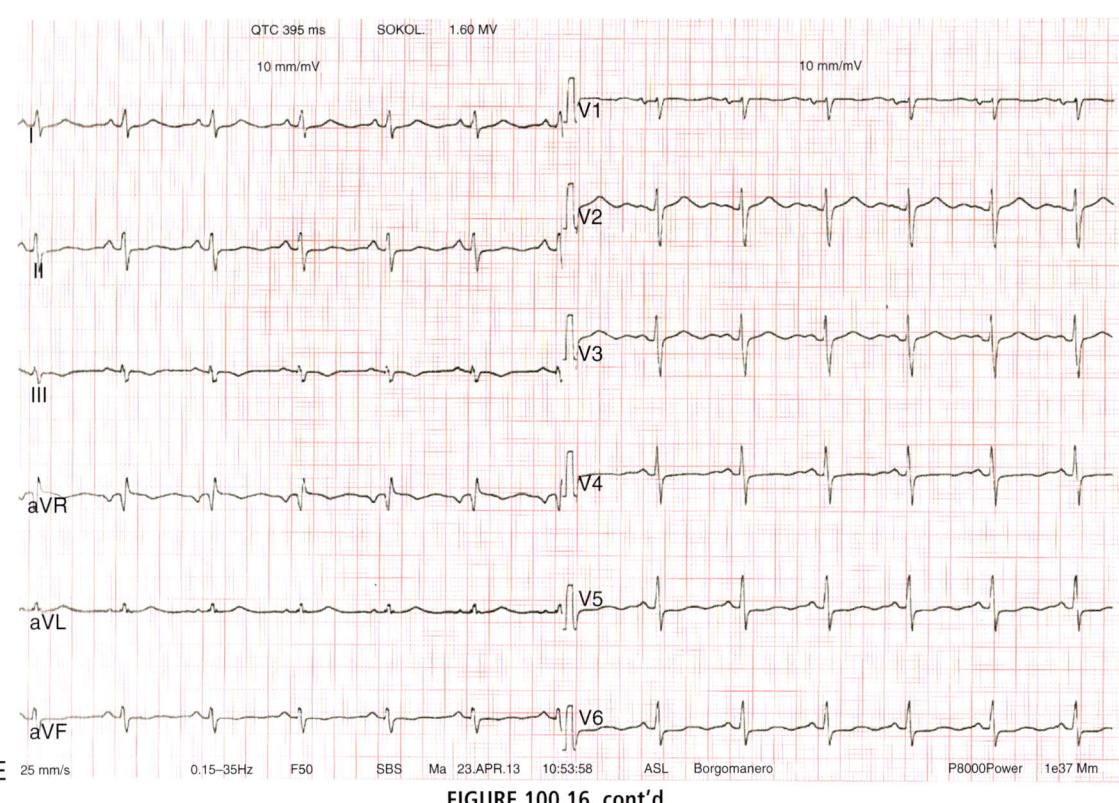

FIGURE 100.16, cont'd

role of mitochondria in all cells, these disorders have systemic manifestations. Tissue with a high respiratory workload such as brain and skeletal muscle, especially extraocular, retinal, and cardiac muscle, are primarily affected. Mitochondrial disorders that have cardiac manifestations may appear as part of several clinical phenotypes. *Chronic progressive external ophthalmoplegia* is characterized by involvement of the extraocular muscles and can also involve oropharyngeal muscles. It is primarily a sporadic disease. *Kearns-Sayre syndrome*, a subtype of chronic progressive external ophthalmoplegia, is characterized by ocular myopathy, pigmentary retinopathy, and age at onset before 20 years. Diabetes, deafness, and ataxia can also be associated. *Myoclonus epilepsy with red ragged fibers* (MERRF) is characterized by myoclonus, seizures, ataxia, dementia, and skeletal muscle weakness. *Mitochondrial myopathy with encephalopathy, lactic acidosis, and strokelike episodes* (MELAS) is the most common of the maternally inherited mitochondrial disorders and is characterized by encephalopathy, subacute stroke-like events, migraine-like headaches, recurrent emesis, extremity weakness, and short stature. *Leber hereditary optic neuropathy* causes subacute blindness, primarily in young men. Other, mitochondrial point mutation disorders, including neuropathy, ataxia, and retinitis pigmentosa *(NARP)* and *Leigh syndrome* (subacute necrotizing encephalomyelopathy) cause neurodegenerative disorders primarily in children. *Barth syndrome* is an X-linked mitochondrial disease manifested by hypotonia, growth retardation, cyclic neutropenia, and 3-methylglutaconic aciduria in children. It is caused by mutations in exons of the nuclear gene encoding tafazzin.

Cardiovascular Manifestations

Patients with mitochondrial myopathy can present with chest pain or, more typically, dyspnea with exertion. In chronic progressive external ophthalmoplegia, most commonly in the Kearns-Sayre syndrome variant, cardiac involvement manifests primarily as conduction abnormalities. In the Kearns-Sayre syndrome, atrioventricular block is observed, usually manifesting after eye involvement. The H-V interval is prolonged, consistent with distal conduction disease. Permanent pacing often is required by early- to mid-adulthood. An increased prevalence of ventricular preexcitation has also been reported. Cardiac MRI demonstrates nonischemic, late gadolinium enhancement in approximately one third of patients and in some cases dilated cardiomyopathy.[41] Mutations in mitochondrial tRNA such as *MERRF* and *MELAS*, are typically associated with hypertrophic (symmetric or asymmetric) cardiomyopathy but dilated cardiomyopathy and rarely arrhythmogenic histiocytoid cardiomyopathy have been observed. Other disorders caused by mitochondrial point mutations can manifest with a similar cardiac phenotype of hypertrophic or dilated cardiomyopathy, often in children. Whether the dilated cardiomyopathy represents a progression from the hypertrophic cardiomyopathy or a separate syndrome is not clear. The dilated cardiomyopathy can result in heart failure and death. More than one half of patients with MELAS had non-ischemic, late gadolinium enhancement on cardiac MRI. Leber hereditary optic neuropathy can be associated with a hypertrophic cardiomyopathy and a short PR interval or preexcitation syndromes (Chapter 65). Barth syndrome is associated with left ventricular non-compaction and endocardial fibroelastosis or a hypertrophic or dilated cardiomyopathy. Heart failure and ventricular arrhythmias occur, often in young children.[42]

Treatment and Prognosis

There are currently no effective treatments for most mitochondrial disorders. There are strategies for managing some of the cardiac manifestations. In Kearns-Sayre syndrome, the implantation of a pacemaker has been advocated when significant or progressive conduction disease is present including in asymptomatic patients. The degree of conduction disease that warrants prophylactic pacing is not clear. ICDs are recommended in patients with both conduction disease and a dilated cardiomyopathy.[42] In the other mitochondrial disorders, an understanding of the potential and specific presentations for cardiac involvement is necessary. Cardiac evaluation, electrocardiography, echocardiography, and other imaging modalities are recommended. Prophylactic or symptomatic heart failure pharmacotherapy, although not studied in these rare diseases, would seem warranted. Improved survival rates in children with Barth syndrome receiving aggressive treatment for cardiomyopathy and neutropenia has been observed.[43]

Spinal Muscular Atrophy
Genetics and Clinical Presentation
Spinal muscular atrophy (SMA) is a lower motor neuron disorder manifesting as progressive, symmetric proximal muscular weakness.[44] It is the leading inherited cause of infant death. SMA is classified clinically by the age at symptom onset and disease severity into type I (Werdnig-Hoffman disease), type II (intermediate form), type III (Kugelberg-Welander disease), and type IV (adult-onset spinal muscular atrophy). SMA is inherited in autosomal recessive fashion or is sporadic. Mutations or deletions in the telomeric survival of motor neuron (SMN) gene are observed in most patients. The loss of functional SMN protein results in premature neuronal cell death.

Cardiovascular Manifestations
The SMN protein has primarily a motor neuron role. However, cardiac abnormalities can be present including sinus tachycardia.[44] Additionally, the profound respiratory muscle weakness that occurs in SMA can impact cardiac function.

Treatment and Prognosis
SMA type 1 is now treated with adeno-associated gene therapy as a one-time intravenous infusion. Onasemnogene abeparvovec is an FDA approved gene therapy for the treatment of SMA type 1 patients under the age of 2. Additionally, nusinersen is an antisense oligonucleotide-based exon skipping therapy also approved for the treatment of SMA, as is the oral small molecule splicing modulator risdiplam. Older symptomatic SMA patients can also receive treatment with nusinersen or risdiplam. Nusinersen is delivered intrathecally and requires repeated dosing, often three times a year. A prolonged lifespan for SMA type 1 patients is now being seen, and whether these treatments will uncover any cardiac defects remains to be seen.[45]

Myofibrillar Myopathies
Genetics and Clinical Presentation
The myofibrillar myopathies arise from mutations in genes encoding proteins of myofibrils. This includes mutations in *DES, CYRAB, MYOT, ZASP, BAG3, DNAJB6, TTN* and *FLNC*. The inheritance patterns can vary and the age of onset is from child to adult, with both familial and sporadic forms. *DES* encodes desmin, an abundant intermediate filament protein, expressed in cardiomyocytes.[46,47] Desmin has multiple functions in the heart and interacts with well over a dozen other proteins involved in contraction, maintenance of cell-cell contacts, apoptosis, and energetics. Acquired disruption of the intermediate filament network is a common pathological consequence in structural heart disease. DES mutation can lead to myopathic process that affects both heart and skeletal muscle.[46] The disorder is inherited primarily in autosomal dominant fashion, but autosomal recessive inheritance, and sporadic mutations have been reported. Typically, symptomatic skeletal muscle abnormalities, manifesting as respiratory dysfunction, will be observed prior to cardiac involvement. For any of the myofibrillar myopathies, muscle biopsy can be diagnostic. Variability in the phenotype is recognized and a cardiomyopathy can develop without obvious skeletal muscle abnormalities. Creatine kinase is mildly elevated in some patients.

FLNC encodes filamin C, a structural protein found at the Z disk and also at the sarcolemma. A distal skeletal myopathy is typically observed. Some variants have little or no skeletal muscle involvement but with serious cardiac issues. FLNC truncations have increased arrhythmia risks.

Cardiovascular Manifestations
The cardiac involvement observed in desmin myopathy typically consists of conduction system disease and, more rarely, ventricular arrhythmias, before the onset of a dilated or restrictive cardiomyopathy. An arrhythmogenic right ventricular cardiomyopathy–like phenotype has been reported.[48] Both sudden death and heart failure–related deaths can occur. Sudden death can occur despite pacemaker implantation.[12]

Similarly, filamin C-associated disease can present with different forms of cardiomyopathy including hypertrophic, restrictive, and dilated. Involvement of the right ventricle can lead to a clinical picture mimicking arrhythmogenic right ventricular cardiomyopathy. The majority of patients have frequent ventricular ectopy on monitoring and are at risk of ventricular arrhythmias and sudden death.

Treatment and Prognosis
The desmin and filamin-C associated myopathies should be considered in the differential diagnosis in individuals or families presenting with a skeletal or cardiac myopathy, including those with an arrhythmogenic right ventricular cardiomyopathy. Monitoring for the development of cardiac conduction and structural heart disease is necessary in affected families. Asymptomatic conduction disease on the ECG predicts future adverse cardiac events in desmin associated myopathies.[12] Primary prevention pacemakers or ICDs should be considered in those patients with significant conduction disease. It is not clear if the presence of conduction disease predicts future adverse cardiac events in filamin-C associated myopathies. Guideline based heart failure pharmacotherapy is recommended in these patients.

Guillain-Barré Syndrome
Clinical Presentation
The Guillain-Barré syndrome is an acute inflammatory demyelinating neuropathy characterized by peripheral, cranial, and autonomic nerve dysfunction (Chapter 102).[49] It is the most common acquired demyelinating neuropathy. Men are more commonly affected than women. In two thirds of affected patients, an acute viral or bacterial illness, or respiratory or gastrointestinal manifestations precede the onset of neurologic symptoms within 6 weeks. The disorder is typically associated with pain, paresthesias, and symmetric limb weakness that progresses proximally and can involve cranial and respiratory muscles. One fourth of affected patients require assisted ventilation.

Cardiovascular Manifestations
Non-ambulant patients are at increased risk for deep vein thrombosis and pulmonary emboli. Cardiac involvement related to accompanying autonomic nervous system dysfunction is seen in one-half of patients. Autonomic dysfunction, characterized by alternating sympathetic and parasympathetic hyperactivity poses a significant risk in Guillain-Barré syndrome patients and increases mortality rates. Moreover, there is no clear association between the severity of motor weakness and the degree and lability of autonomic dysfunction.[50] Cardiovascular manifestations include hypertension, orthostatic hypotension, resting sinus tachycardia, loss of heart rate variability, electrocardiographic ST abnormalities, and both bradycardia and tachycardias. Microneurographic recordings have shown increased sympathetic outflow during the acute illness, which normalizes with recovery. Extreme presentations of autonomic dysfunction have been associated with Takotsubo cardiomyopathy.[51] Life-threatening arrhythmias occur in Guillain-Barré syndrome, primarily in patients requiring assisted ventilation. Arrhythmias observed include asystole, symptomatic bradycardia, rapid atrial fibrillation, and ventricular tachycardia or fibrillation. Asystole commonly was associated with tracheal suctioning. Death may occur as a consequence of an arrhythmia.[52]

Treatment and Prognosis
Supportive care should include deep vein thrombosis prophylaxis in non-ambulant patients. Early plasmapheresis or intravenous immunoglobulin can improve recovery. In severely affected patients, especially those requiring assisted ventilation, cardiac rhythm monitoring is mandatory. It is reasonable to monitor the rhythm via telemetry in all those admitted with Guillain-Barré syndrome. If serious bradycardia or asystole is observed, temporary or permanent pacing can improve survival. Atropine or isoproterenol during tracheal suctioning can be of benefit. Takotsubo cardiomyopathy should be treated with beta blockers and routine treatment for left ventricular dysfunction and cardiac congestion (Chapters 48 and 50). The mortality rate in patients hospitalized with Guillain-Barré syndrome is as high as 15%. In patients who recover from Guillain-Barré syndrome, autonomic function also normalizes, and an increase in the long-term arrhythmia risk has not been observed.

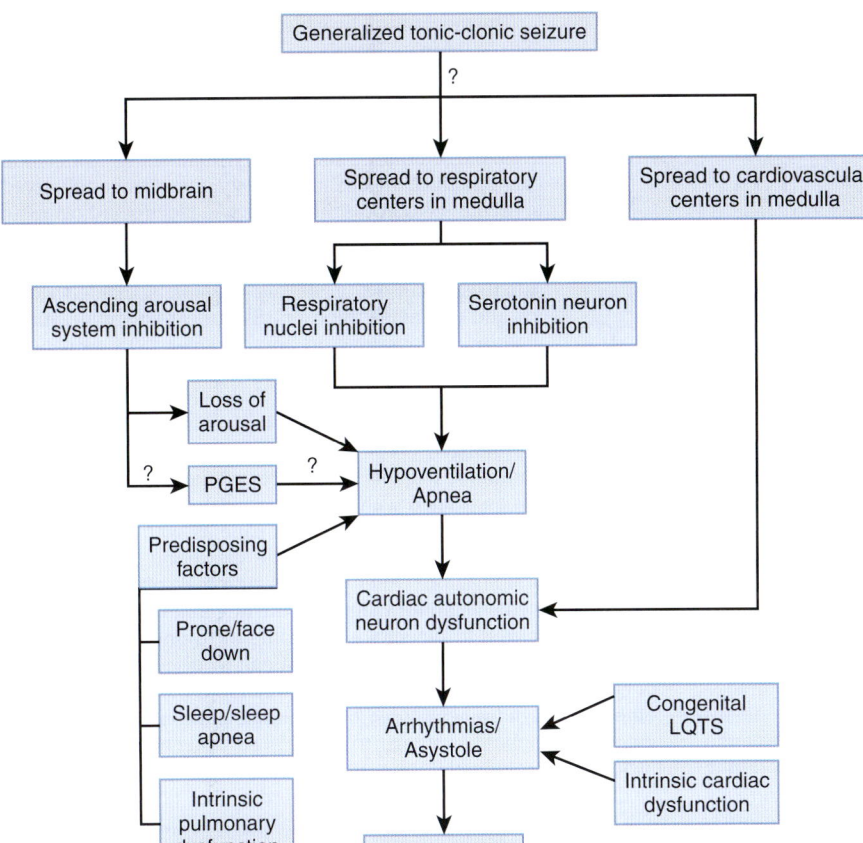

FIGURE 100.17 Pathophysiologic mechanisms underlying sudden unexpected death in epilepsy (SUDEP). SUDEP often results from a generalized tonic-clonic seizure, which leads to inhibition of specific midbrain- and medulla-mediated effects via an unknown pathway. Other factors shown may predispose these patients to SUDEP. *LQTS*, long QT syndrome; *PGES*, postictal generalized EEG suppression. (From Dlouhy BJ, Gehlbach BK, Richerson GB. Sudden unexpected death in epilepsy: basic mechanisms and clinical implications for prevention. *J Neurol Neurosurg Psychiatry.* 2016;87:402.)

Myasthenia Gravis

Clinical Presentation

Myasthenia gravis is a disorder of neuromuscular transmission resulting from production of antibody targeted to the nicotinic acetylcholine receptor or muscle-specific receptor tyrosine kinase.[53] The primary symptom, fluctuating weakness, usually begins with the eye and facial muscles and later can involve the large muscles of the limbs. Patients can present at any age, typically at a younger age in women and at an older age in men. Myasthenia gravis is commonly associated with hyperplasia or a benign or malignant tumor (thymoma) of the thymus gland. Multiple autoimmune diseases can complicate myasthenia gravis. With the development of immune check point inhibitors used in cancer treatment, myasthenia gravis has been associated with immune-related cardiotoxicity with cardiomyopathy and life-threatening ventricular arrhythmias.[54]

Cardiovascular Manifestations

Myocarditis can occur in patients with myasthenia gravis, especially in those with a thymoma (Chapters 55 and 94). The mechanism in myocarditis is a humoral immune response against proteins in striated muscle, including titin, the ryanodine receptor, and a potassium-channel protein (Kv1.4).[53] Up to 16% of patients with myasthenia gravis have cardiac manifestations not explained by another etiologic disorder. Presentation with arrhythmias, which can include atrial fibrillation, atrioventricular block, asystole, ventricular tachycardia, sudden death, or heart failure, is typical. Myasthenic crisis has been associated with stress cardiomyopathy.[55] Autopsy findings are consistent with myocarditis, often giant cell myocarditis. A polymyositis affecting both skeletal and cardiac muscle is seen. In some cases autonomic nervous system dysfunction may be associated with myasthenia gravis.[56]

Treatment and Prognosis

Myasthenia gravis is treated with anticholinesterases and immunosuppressive agents. Thymectomy is often indicated. Anticholinesterase agents may slow the sinus rate and cause heart block and hypotension. Pacing can be necessary. Whether immunosuppressive agents or thymectomy improve associated cardiac disease is unknown. Case reports have described the development of rapidly progressive and fatal heart failure within weeks after thymoma resection in patients in whom histologic examination showed giant cell myocarditis.

Myoglobinopathy

Myoglobinopathy is a recently described adult-onset autosomal dominant progressive centrifugal skeletal myopathy. The skeletal myopathy is variably associated with cardiomyopathy and HF. Myoglobin is highly expressed in the heart, and disease associated mutations have been suggested to accelerate oxygen dissociation from heme and alter the redox state of skeletal and cardiac tissues, increasing superoxide levels.[57] Sarcoplasmic inclusion bodies in both skeletal and cardiac muscle are the hallmark of the disease. The onset of skeletal muscle symptoms is the 5th decade of life with progression with patients becoming non-ambulant over a decade or two. The cause of death in these patients is both respiratory and cardiac failure.

ABCC9-Related Intellectual Disability Myopathy Syndrome

KATP channels (IK-ATP) are heterooctomers of an inwardly rectifying potassium channel, Kir6.x and regulatory sulfonylurea receptor, SURx (Chapter 62). In the pancreas and nerve, K-ATP channels are composed of Kir6.2 (*KCNJ8*) and SUR1 (*ABCC8*). In skeletal and cardiac muscle the channel is formed by the combination of Kir6.2 and SUR2A (*ABCC9*). Mutations in the channel subunits are associated with congenital forms of diabetes and hyperinsulinism as well as Cantu Sydrome.[58] Loss-of-function mutations in *ABCC9* have been described in a syndrome that includes mild intellectual disability, skeletal myopathy characterized by lordosis, facial dysmorphism, reddish-purple skin discoloration (cutis marmorata), abnormal dentition and dilated cardiomyopathy. KATP channel subunits are expressed broadly but the mechanism of production of the manifestations of disease is uncertain. The loss-of-function phenotype suggests that KATP channel activators may be useful in symptom control.

Epilepsy

Cardiovascular Manifestations

Epilepsy is a complex brain disorder characterized by recurrent unprovoked seizures.[59] Patients with epilepsy are at increased risk for sudden death of unknown cause, which has been termed *sudden unexpected death in epilepsy* (SUDEP) (Chapter 70). It is the leading cause of premature death in patients with epilepsy, with an incidence ranging from 0.6 to 9 per 1000 patient-years, depending on the population studied. It accounts for up to 18% of all deaths in people with epilepsy and a lifetime cumulative risk as high as 35% in patients with refractory epilepsy.[60] The mechanisms leading to sudden death in epilepsy are not clear and probably vary. Central or obstructive postictal apnea, mechanical suffocation possibly exacerbated by prone positioning, excessive respiratory secretions, acute pulmonary edema, and arrhythmias all may be involved (Fig. 100.17). A number of drugs affecting the brain prolong the QT interval and may contribute (Chapters 9 and 64).

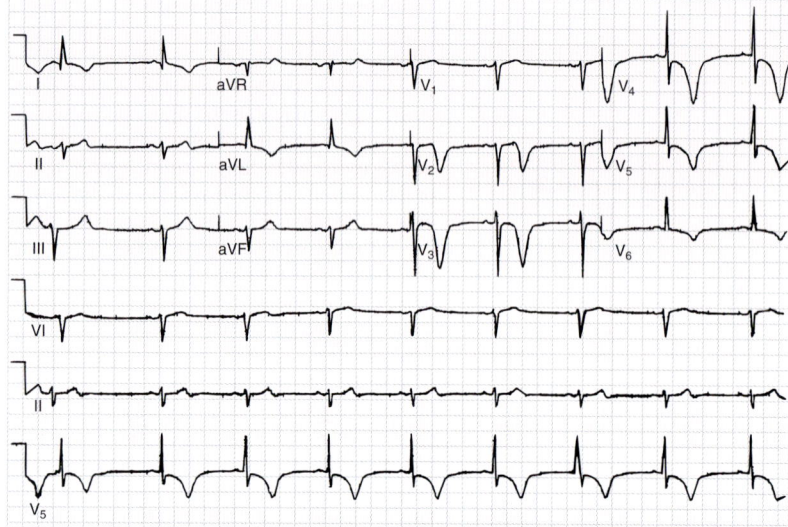

FIGURE 100.18 Electrocardiogram from a patient with cerebral hemorrhage. Deep and symmetric T wave inversions are evident. (Courtesy Dr. Charles Fisch, Indiana University School of Medicine, Indianapolis.)

The role of genetics is an area of active investigation[60] and early repolarization with seizure induced remodeling of cardiac electrophysiology has been suggested.[61–63] A majority of witnessed sudden deaths occur at or in proximity to the time of a seizure. Severe bradycardia with sinus arrest has been documented in monitored patients during seizures, including studies with an implantable loop recorder. Periictal bradycardia is more common in patients with temporal lobe seizures. Whether bradycardia has a role in epileptic patients who experience sudden death is not clear. Ventricular arrhythmia disorders such as long-QT syndrome or right ventricular dysplasia can manifest with symptoms suggestive of epilepsy and could be responsible for a small proportion of sudden deaths. The role of preexisting structural heart disease in SUDEP is uncertain, but the presence of heart disease will increase the arrhythmic risk of seizures. Observational studies have assessed risk factors for SUDEP. These include male sex, onset of epilepsy at a young age, a long duration of epilepsy, high seizure frequency especially of generalized tonic-clonic seizures, and the need for polytherapy to control seizures.

Treatment and Prognosis

A primary rhythm disorder needs to be considered in the differential diagnosis of epilepsy. Patients with poorly controlled epilepsy should be aggressively evaluated and treated at tertiary epilepsy centers. Medications to control seizures may increase the risk of life-threatening cardiac arrhythmias.[61] Particularly in refractory cases, epilepsy surgery should be strongly considered. Patients with ictal bradycardia can require pacemaker implantation. Nighttime supervision of the epileptic patient and supine sleeping positions should be considered although data are limited in support of efficacy of such maneuvers.[64]

Acute Cerebrovascular Disease
Cardiovascular Manifestations

Acute cerebrovascular diseases, including subarachnoid hemorrhage, other stroke syndromes, and head injury, can be associated with severe cardiac manifestations, which represent a major challenge in the management of these patients (Chapter 45). For example, severe adverse cardiac events including acute coronary syndrome, heart failure, and cardiac arrhythmia occur in approximately 20% of patients with ischemic stroke, occurring predominantly within the first 3 days after the event.[65] The patient's age and burden of cardiovascular disease or risk correlate with the individual susceptibility to develop severe cardiovascular complications of stroke. In addition, factors promoting electrical instability such as electrolyte abnormalities and drugs that prolong QT interval, as well as comorbidities that promote autonomic failure (e.g., diabetes) increase the risk of cardiac manifestations of brain injury.

The mechanism by which cardiac abnormalities occur with brain injury is related to autonomic nervous system dysfunction, with both increased sympathetic and parasympathetic output (Chapter 102). Excessive myocardial catecholamine release is primarily responsible for the observed cardiac pathology. Hypothalamic stimulation can reproduce the electrocardiographic changes observed in acute cerebrovascular disease. Electrocardiographic changes associated with hypothalamic stimulation or blood in the subarachnoid space can be diminished with spinal cord transection, stellate ganglion blockade, vagolytics, and adrenergic blockers. Electrocardiographic abnormalities are observed in approximately 70% of patients with subarachnoid hemorrhage. Abnormalities including ST elevation and depression, T-wave inversion, and pathologic Q-waves are observed. Peaked inverted T-waves and a prolonged QT interval can occur in a significant proportion of patients with electrocardiographic abnormalities associated with cerebrovascular disease (Fig. 100.18). Hypokalemia often seen in patients with subarachnoid hemorrhage can increase the likelihood of QT interval prolongation. Other stroke syndromes often are associated with abnormalities on the ECG, but whether these are related to the stroke syndrome or to underlying intrinsic cardiac disease often is difficult to discern. Prolongation of QT interval is more common in subarachnoid hemorrhage than in other stroke syndromes. Closed head trauma can cause electrocardiographic abnormalities similar to those in subarachnoid hemorrhage, including a prolonged QT interval. Myocardial damage with liberation of enzymes and subendocardial hemorrhage or fibrosis at autopsy can occur in the setting of acute cerebral disease. The term *neurogenic stunned myocardium* is used to describe the reversible syndrome. The process can manifest with selective apical involvement, a Takotsubo cardiomyopathy. Cardiac troponin elevation and echocardiographic evidence of left ventricular dysfunction are present in a significant proportion of patients with subarachnoid hemorrhage. Patients with a poorer neurologic status at admission are more likely to have higher peak troponin levels. Women are at higher risk for myocardial necrosis. Pulmonary edema can accompany the acute neurologic insult. The edema can have both a cardiogenic component, related to systemic hypertension and left ventricular dysfunction, and a neurogenic (pulmonary capillary leak) component. Life-threatening arrhythmias can occur in the setting of acute cerebrovascular disease. Ventricular tachycardia or fibrillation has been observed in patients with subarachnoid hemorrhage and head trauma. Torsades de pointes–type ventricular tachycardia can occur (Fig. 100.19) (Chapter 67), often in the setting of a prolonged QT interval and hypokalemia. Stroke syndromes other than subarachnoid hemorrhage appear to be only rarely associated with serious ventricular tachycardias. Atrial arrhythmias, including atrial fibrillation and regular supraventricular tachycardia, have been observed. Atrial fibrillation is most common in patients presenting with acute thromboembolic stroke. Separating an effect from the cause can be difficult. Bradycardias, including sinoatrial block, sinus arrest, and atrioventricular block, occur in up to 10% of patients with subarachnoid hemorrhage.

Treatment and Prognosis

Beta blockers are effective in decreasing myocardial damage and in controlling both supraventricular and ventricular arrhythmias associated with subarachnoid hemorrhage and head trauma. Beta blockers increase the likelihood of bradycardia and cannot be used in patients with hypotension requiring vasopressors. Life-threatening arrhythmias occur primarily in the first day after a neurologic event. Continuous electrocardiographic monitoring during this period is indicated. Careful monitoring of potassium levels, especially in patients with subarachnoid hemorrhage, is warranted. Refractory ventricular arrhythmias have been controlled effectively with stellate ganglion blockade. Electrocardiographic abnormalities reflect unfavorable intracranial factors but do not appear to portend a poor cardiovascular outcome. The magnitude of peak troponin elevation is predictive for adverse

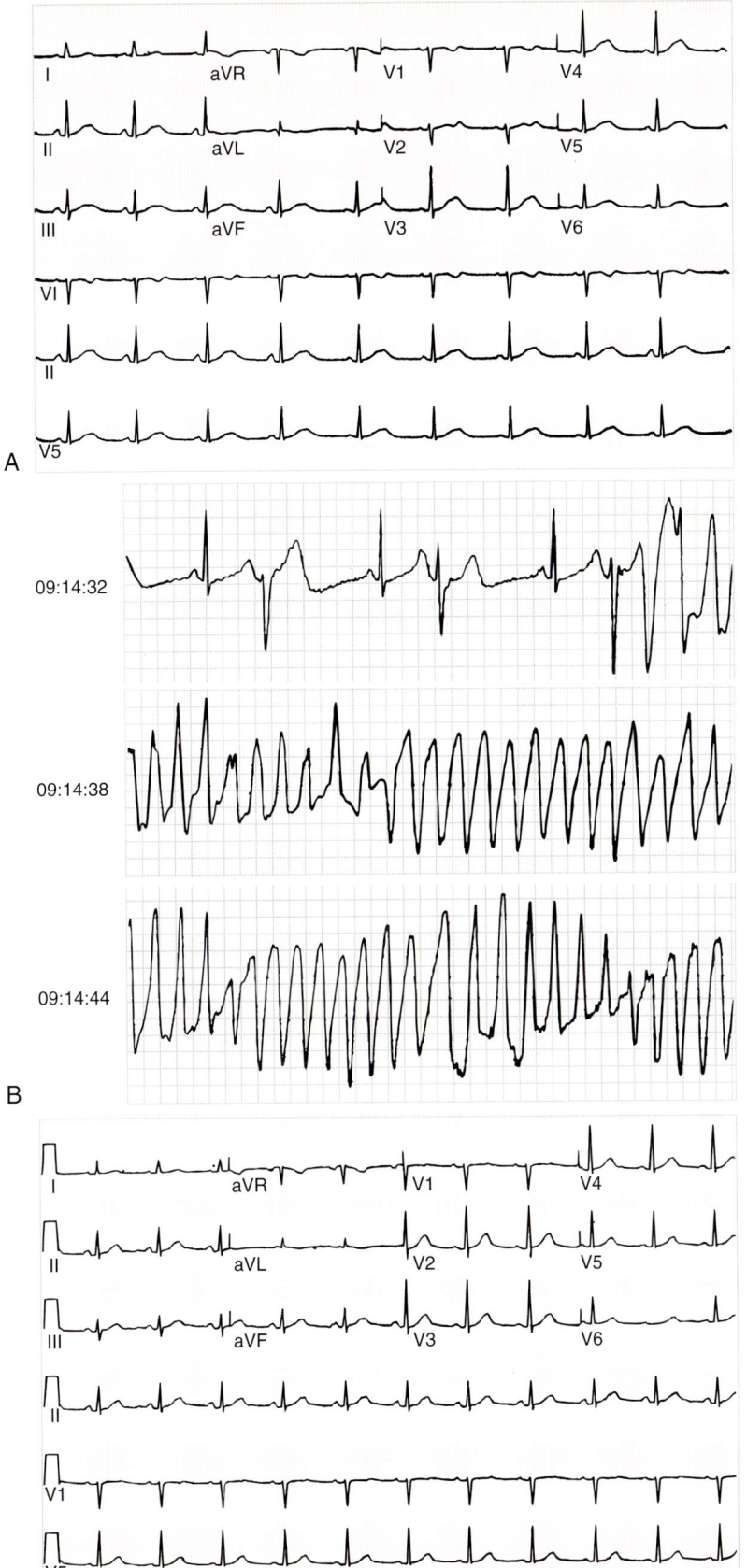

FIGURE 100.19 Cardiac manifestations with cerebral hemorrhage in a 49-year-old patient. **A,** ECG recorded within 3 hours of admission and 4 hours after onset of symptoms. QT interval prolongation is evident. **B,** Electrocardiographic monitoring 6 hours after admission. Ventricular bigeminy precedes the onset of polymorphic ventricular tachycardia. Cardioversion was required. The patient subsequently was treated with a beta-adrenergic blocker without further ventricular tachycardia. **C,** On an ECG obtained 2 weeks after hospital admission, the QT interval has normalized.

patient outcomes, including severe disability at hospital discharge and death.[65] Head injury (blunt trauma or gunshot wound) and cerebrovascular accidents are the leading causes of brain death in patients being considered as heart donors. These donors can manifest electrocardiographic abnormalities, hemodynamic instability, and myocardial dysfunction related primarily to adrenergic storm and not to intrinsic cardiac disease. Experimental studies on whether contractile performance recovers with transplantation are still controversial. Optimization of volume status and inotropic support with careful echocardiographic evaluation and possibly left-heart catheterization can allow the use of some donor hearts that would have otherwise been rejected.

CONCLUSIONS/FUTURE PERSPECTIVES

Neurologic diseases often affect the heart and vascular system, and in many cases, cardiovascular disease limits life expectancy and reduces quality of life in these patients. As such, cardiologists are an integral part in the medical evaluation and treatment of patients with primary neurologic disorders. In several disorders, the cardiovascular manifestations are responsible for a greater risk than that attributable to the neurologic manifestations. An area of ongoing investigation is understanding the mechanisms of cardiac disease produced by neurological and neuromuscular disorders. This work will identify precision diagnostics and therapeutics and has helped to inform biological and gene therapeutic treatment of these disorders.

REFERENCES
Muscular Dystrophies
1. Nikhanj A, Yogasundaram H, Miskew Nichols B, et al. Cardiac intervention improves heart disease and clinical outcomes in patients with muscular dystrophy in a multidisciplinary care setting. *J Am Heart Assoc.* 2020;9:e014004.
2. Kamdar F, Garry DJ. Dystrophin-deficient cardiomyopathy. *J Am Coll Cardiol.* 2016;67:2533–2546.
3. McNally EM, Kaltman JR, Benson DW, et al. Contemporary cardiac issues in Duchenne muscular dystrophy. Working group of the National Heart, Lung, and Blood Institute in collaboration with parent project muscular dystrophy. *Circulation.* 2015;131:1590–1598.
4. Mercuri E, Bonnemann CG, Muntoni F. Muscular dystrophies. *Lancet.* 2019;394:2025–2038.
5. Hor KN, Mah ML, Johnston P, et al. Advances in the diagnosis and management of cardiomyopathy in duchenne muscular dystrophy. *Neuromuscul Disord.* 2018;28:711–716.
6. Power LC, O'Grady GL, Hornung TS, et al. Imaging the heart to detect cardiomyopathy in Duchenne muscular dystrophy: a review. *Neuromuscul Disord.* 2018;28:717–730.
7. Rochitte CE, Liberato G, Silva MC. Comprehensive assessment of cardiac involvement in muscular dystrophies by cardiac MR imaging. *Magn Reson Imaging Clin N Am.* 2019;27:521–531.
8. Adachi K, Hashiguchi S, Saito M, et al. Detection and management of cardiomyopathy in female dystrophinopathy carriers. *J Neurol Sci.* 2018;386:74–80.
9. Ishizaki M, Kobayashi M, Adachi K, et al. Female dystrophinopathy: review of current literature. *Neuromuscul Disord.* 2018;28:572–581.
10. Meyers TA, Heitzman JA, Townsend D. DMD carrier model with mosaic dystrophin expression in the heart reveals complex vulnerability to myocardial injury. *Hum Mol Genet.* 2020;29:944–954.
11. Feingold B, Mahle WT, Auerbach S, et al. Management of cardiac involvement associated with neuromuscular diseases: a scientific statement from the American Heart Association. *Circulation.* 2017;136:e200–e231.
12. Finsterer J, Stollberger C, Maeztu C. Sudden cardiac death in neuromuscular disorders. *Int J Cardiol.* 2016;203:508–515.
13. Birnkrant DJ, Bushby K, Bann CM, et al. Diagnosis and management of Duchenne muscular dystrophy, part 2: respiratory, cardiac, bone health, and orthopaedic management. *Lancet Neurol.* 2018;17:347–361.
14. Bourke JP, Bueser T, Quinlivan R. Interventions for preventing and treating cardiac complications in Duchenne and Becker muscular dystrophy and x-linked dilated cardiomyopathy. *Cochrane Database Syst Rev.* 2018;10:CD009068.
15. Raman SV, Hor KN, Mazur W, et al. Stabilization of early Duchenne cardiomyopathy with aldosterone inhibition: results of the multicenter aidmd trial. *J Am Heart Assoc.* 2019;8:e013501.
16. Wells D, Rizwan R, Jefferies JL, et al. Heart transplantation in muscular dystrophy patients: is it a viable option? *Circ Heart Fail.* 2020;13:e005447.

17. Min YL, Bassel-Duby R, Olson EN. Crispr correction of duchenne muscular dystrophy. *Annu Rev Med.* 2019;70:239–255.
18. Verhaart IEC, Aartsma-Rus A. Therapeutic developments for duchenne muscular dystrophy. *Nat Rev Neurol.* 2019;15:373–386.
19. Wahbi K, Furling D. Cardiovascular manifestations of myotonic dystrophy. *Trends Cardiovasc Med.* 2020;30:232–238.
20. Luetkens JA, von Landenberg C, Isaak A, et al. Comprehensive cardiac magnetic resonance for assessment of cardiac involvement in myotonic muscular dystrophy type 1 and 2 without known cardiovascular disease. *Circ Cardiovasc Imaging.* 2019;12:e009100.
21. Cardona A, Arnold WD, Kissel JT, et al. Myocardial fibrosis by late gadolinium enhancement cardiovascular magnetic resonance in myotonic muscular dystrophy type 1: highly prevalent but not associated with surface conduction abnormality. *J Cardiovasc Magn Reson.* 2019;21:26.
22. Tanawuttiwat T, Wagner KR, Tomaselli G, et al. Left ventricular dysfunction and conduction disturbances in patients with myotonic muscular dystrophy type i and ii. *JAMA Cardiol.* 2017;2:225–228.
23. Kusumoto FM, Schoenfeld MH, Barrett C, et al. 2018 acc/aha/hrs guideline on the evaluation and management of patients with bradycardia and cardiac conduction delay: a report of the American college of cardiology/American heart association task force on clinical practice guidelines and the heart rhythm society. *J Am Coll Cardiol.* 2019;74:e51–e156.
24. McNally EM, Mann DL, Pinto Y, et al. Clinical care recommendations for cardiologists treating adults with myotonic dystrophy. *J Am Heart Assoc.* 2020;9:e014006.
25. Wahbi K, Babuty D, Probst V, et al. Incidence and predictors of sudden death, major conduction defects and sustained ventricular tachyarrhythmias in 1388 patients with myotonic dystrophy type 1. *Eur Heart J.* 2017;38:751–758.
26. Wahbi K, Porcher R, Laforet P, et al. Development and validation of a new scoring system to predict survival in patients with myotonic dystrophy type 1. *JAMA Neurol.* 2018;75:573–581.
27. Muchir A, Worman HJ. Emery-Dreifuss muscular dystrophy: focal point nuclear envelope. *Curr Opin Neurol.* 2019;32:728–734.
28. Wang S, Peng D. Cardiac involvement in Emery-Dreifuss muscular dystrophy and related management strategies. *Int Heart J.* 2019;60:12–18.
29. Limipitikul W, Ong CS, Tomaselli GF. Neuromuscular disease: cardiac manifestations and sudden death risk. *Card Electrophysiol Clin.* 2017;9:731–747.
30. Taghizadeh E, Rezaee M, Barreto GE, et al. Prevalence, pathological mechanisms, and genetic basis of limb-girdle muscular dystrophies: a review. *J Cell Physiol.* 2019;234:7874–7884.
31. Thompson R, Straub V. Limb-girdle muscular dystrophies - international collaborations for translational research. *Nat Rev Neurol.* 2016;12:294–309.
32. Straub V, Murphy A, Udd B, et al. 229th ENMC international workshop: limb girdle muscular dystrophies – Nomenclature and reformed classification Naarden, The Netherlands, 17–19 March 2017. *Neuromuscul Disord.* 2018;28(8):702–710.
33. Hamel J, Tawil R. Facioscapulohumeral muscular dystrophy: update on pathogenesis and future treatments. *Neurotherapeutics.* 2018;15:863–871.
34. Tawil R. Facioscapulohumeral muscular dystrophy. *Handb Clin Neurol.* 2018;148:541–548.
35. Sommerville RB, Vincenti MG, Winborn K, et al. Diagnosis and management of adult hereditary cardio-neuromuscular disorders: a model for the multidisciplinary care of complex genetic disorders. *Trends Cardiovasc Med.* 2017;27:51–58.
36. Arbustini E, Di Toro A, Giuliani L, et al. Cardiac phenotypes in hereditary muscle disorders: JACC state-of-the-art review. *J Am Coll Cardiol.* 2018;72:2485–2506.
37. Kearney M, Orrell RW, Fahey M, et al. Pharmacological treatments for Friedreich ataxia. *Cochrane Database Syst Rev.* 2016;CD007791.
38. McCormick A, Shinnick J, Schadt K, et al. Cardiac transplantation in Friedreich ataxia: extended follow-up. *J Neurol Sci.* 2017;375:471–473.
39. Statland JM, Fontaine B, Hanna MG, et al. Review of the diagnosis and treatment of periodic paralysis. *Muscle Nerve.* 2018;57:522–530.
40. Maffe S, Paffoni P, Bergamasco L, et al. Therapeutic management of ventricular arrhythmias in Andersen-Tawil syndrome. *J Electrocardiol.* 2020;58:37–42.

Other Neuromuscular Diseases

41. El-Hattab AW, Scaglia F. Mitochondrial cardiomyopathies. *Front Cardiovasc Med.* 2016;3:25.
42. Towbin JA, Jefferies JL. Cardiomyopathies due to left ventricular noncompaction, mitochondrial and storage diseases, and inborn errors of metabolism. *Circ Res.* 2017;121:838–854.
43. Kang SL, Forsey J, Dudley D, et al. Clinical characteristics and outcomes of cardiomyopathy in Barth syndrome: the UK experience. *Pediatr Cardiol.* 2016;37:167–176.
44. Nash LA, Burns JK, Chardon JW, et al. Spinal muscular atrophy: more than a disease of motor neurons? *Curr Mol Med.* 2016;16:779–792.
45. Levin AA. Treating disease at the rna level with oligonucleotides. *N Engl J Med.* 2019;380:57–70.
46. Tsikitis M, Galata Z, Mavroidis M, et al. Intermediate filaments in cardiomyopathy. *Biophys Rev.* 2018;10:1007–1031.
47. Brodehl A, Gaertner-Rommel A, Milting H. Molecular insights into cardiomyopathies associated with desmin (des) mutations. *Biophys Rev.* 2018;10:983–1006.
48. Finsterer J, Stollberger C. Arrhythmogenic right ventricular dysplasia in neuromuscular disorders. *Clin Med Insights Cardiol.* 2016;10:173–180.
49. Burakgazi AZ, AlMahameed S. Cardiac involvement in peripheral neuropathies. *J Clin Neuromuscul Dis.* 2016;17:120–128.
50. Hilz MJ, Liu M, Roy S, et al. Autonomic dysfunction in the neurological intensive care unit. *Clin Auton Res.* 2019;29:301–311.
51. Jones T, Umaskanth N, De Boisanger J, et al. Guillain-barre syndrome complicated by Takotsubo cardiomyopathy: an under-recognised association. *BMJ Case Rep.* 2020;13.
52. Gupta S, Verma R, Sethi R, et al. Cardiovascular complications and its relationship with functional outcomes in Guillain-Barre syndrome. *QJM.* 2020;113:93–99.
53. Gilhus NE. Myasthenia gravis. *N Engl J Med.* 2016;375:2570–2581.
54. Hu JR, Florido R, Lipson EJ, et al. Cardiovascular toxicities associated with immune checkpoint inhibitors. *Cardiovasc Res.* 2019;115:854–868.
55. Desai R, Abbas SA, Fong HK, et al. Burden and impact of takotsubo syndrome in myasthenic crisis: a national inpatient perspective on the under-recognized but potentially fatal association. *Int J Cardiol.* 2020;299:63–66.
56. Kocabas ZU, Kizilay F, Basarici I, et al. Evaluation of cardiac autonomic functions in myasthenia gravis. *Neurol Res.* 2018;40:405–412.
57. Olive M, Engvall M, Ravenscroft G, et al. Myoglobinopathy is an adult-onset autosomal dominant myopathy with characteristic sarcoplasmic inclusions. *Nat Commun.* 2019;10:1396.
58. Smeland MF, McClenaghan C, Roessler HI, et al. ABCC9-related intellectual disability myopathy syndrome is a KATP channelopathy with loss-of-function mutations in ABCC9. *Nat Commun.* 2019;10:4457.
59. Krishnamurthy KB. Epilepsy. *Ann Intern Med.* 2016;164. ITC17-32.
60. Chahal CAA, Salloum MN, Alahdab F, et al. Systematic review of the genetics of sudden unexpected death in epilepsy: potential overlap with sudden cardiac death and arrhythmia-related genes. *J Am Heart Assoc.* 2020;9:e012264.
61. Li MCH, O'Brien TJ, Todaro M, et al. Acquired cardiac channelopathies in epilepsy: evidence, mechanisms, and clinical significance. *Epilepsia.* 2019;60:1753–1767.
62. Hayashi K, Kohno R, Akamatsu N, et al. Abnormal repolarization: a common electrocardiographic finding in patients with epilepsy. *J Cardiovasc Electrophysiol.* 2019;30:109–115.
63. Ufongene C, El Atrache R, Loddenkemper T, et al. Electrocardiographic changes associated with epilepsy beyond heart rate and their utilization in future seizure detection and forecasting methods. *Clin Neurophysiol.* 2020;131:866–879.
64. Maguire MJ, Jackson CF, Marson AG, et al. Treatments for the prevention of sudden unexpected death in epilepsy (SUDEP). *Cochrane Database Syst Rev.* 2020;4:CD011792.
65. Scheitz JF, Nolte CH, Doehner W, et al. Stroke-heart syndrome: clinical presentation and underlying mechanisms. *Lancet Neurol.* 2018;17:1109–1120.

101 Interface Between Renal Disease and Cardiovascular Illness

PETER A. MCCULLOUGH

THE CARDIORENAL INTERSECTION, 1873

CHRONIC KIDNEY DISEASE AND CARDIOVASCULAR RISK, 1873

IMPLICATIONS OF ANEMIA DUE TO CHRONIC KIDNEY DISEASE, 1874

CONTRAST-INDUCED ACUTE KIDNEY INJURY, 1875

PREVENTION OF CONTRAST-INDUCED ACUTE KIDNEY INJURY, 1876

CARDIAC SURGERY ASSOCIATED ACUTE KIDNEY INJURY, 1877

ACCELERATION OF VASCULAR CALCIFICATION, 1879

RENAL DISEASE AND HYPERTENSION, 1879

DIAGNOSIS OF ACUTE CORONARY SYNDROMES IN PATIENTS WITH CHRONIC KIDNEY DISEASE, 1880

RENAL DYSFUNCTION AS A PROGNOSTIC FACTOR IN ACUTE CORONARY SYNDROMES, 1880

REASONS FOR POOR OUTCOMES AFTER ACUTE CORONARY SYNDROMES IN PATIENTS WITH RENAL DYSFUNCTION, 1881

TREATMENT OF MYOCARDIAL INFARCTION IN PATIENTS WITH RENAL DYSFUNCTION, 1882

CARDIORENAL SYNDROMES, 1882

CHRONIC KIDNEY DISEASE AND VALVULAR HEART DISEASE, 1887

RENAL FUNCTION AND ARRHYTHMIAS, 1887

CONSULTATIVE APPROACH TO SEVERE KIDNEY DISEASE AND HEMODIALYSIS PATIENTS, 1888

EVALUATION AND MANAGEMENT OF THE RENAL TRANSPLANT RECIPIENT, 1891

SUMMARY, 1891

REFERENCES, 1891

Kidney disease confers increased risks for atherosclerotic cardiovascular disease (CVD), myocardial disease and heart failure (HF), arrhythmias, and valvular disease. Obesity, type 2 diabetes mellitus, hypertension (HTN), and increased longevity contribute to an expanding prevalence pool of patients with chronic kidney disease (CKD). Recognition of the stage of CKD is important in cardiology as it influences the approach to the screening, diagnosis, prognosis, and management of many cardiovascular problems as well as the use of many drugs. Both pharmacologic and interventional management of patients with heart disease can be designed to minimize risk to the kidneys and in some scenarios simultaneously improve the risk of major adverse renal and cardiovascular events.

THE CARDIORENAL INTERSECTION

The heart and kidney are inextricably linked in terms of hemodynamic and regulatory functions. In a normal 70-kg human, each kidney weighs about 130 to 170 g and receives blood flow of 400 mL/min per 100 g, which is approximately 20% to 25% of the cardiac output, allowing the needed flow to maintain glomerular filtration by approximately 1 million nephrons (Fig. 101.1). This flow is several times greater per unit weight than most other organs due to lower vascular resistance. Although the oxygen extraction is low, the kidneys account for about 8% of the total oxygen consumption of the body. The kidney has a central role in electrolyte balance, protein metabolism, and blood pressure regulation. Communication between these two organs occurs at multiple levels, including the sympathetic nervous system (SNS), the renin-angiotensin-aldosterone system (RAAS), vasopressin, endothelin, and the natriuretic peptides.

The obesity pandemic is spawning secondary epidemics of type 2 diabetes mellitus (DM) and HTN often leading to CKD and CVD.[1] Among those with DM for 25 years or more, the prevalence of diabetic nephropathy as a result of microvascular disease in type 1 and type 2 DM is about 50%.[2] Approximately half of all cases of end-stage renal disease (ESRD) result from diabetic nephropathy. All forms of kidney disease have a more rapid progression when there are maladaptive mutations in apoprotein L1 (bound to high-density lipoprotein particles and expressed in the podocytes, proximal tubules, and vascular endothelium). Mutant apoprotein L1 protects against African trypanosomiasis but is associated with both kidney and coronary heart disease (Fig. 101.2).[3] With the aging of the general population and cardiovascular care shifting toward the elderly, age-related decreased renal function comprises a major adverse prognostic factor after CVD events. CKD accelerates the progression of atherosclerosis, myocardial disease, valvular disease, and promotes an array of cardiac arrhythmias leading to sudden death.[4]

CHRONIC KIDNEY DISEASE AND CARDIOVASCULAR RISK

A range of estimated glomerular filtration rate (eGFR) values derived from equations defines CKD.[5] A common definition for CKD stipulates an eGFR of less than 60 mL/min/1.73 m^2 or the presence of kidney damage. With aging (age 20 to 80), the eGFR declines from about 130 to 60 mL/min/1.73 m^2, and a variety of pathobiological processes emerge when the eGFR drops below 60 mL/min/1.73 m^2 or stage 3 CKD (approximately a serum creatinine [Cr] of 1.2 mg/dL in a woman and 1.5 mg/dL in a man). Because Cr is a crude indicator of renal function and often underestimates renal dysfunction in women and the elderly, eGFR or creatinine clearance (CrCl) calculated by the CKD-EPI (Chronic Kidney Disease Epidemiology Collaboration) and Cockcroft-Gault equation, improve the assessment of renal function. CrCl is used most often for drug dosing since it incorporates body weight. For classification of disease, and prognosis, the CKD-EPI equation is preferred because it does not rely on body weight and associates best with adverse outcomes including death. The equation is: eGFR = $141 \times \min(Cr/\kappa, 1)^\alpha \times \max(Cr/\kappa, 1)^{-1.209} \times 0.993^{age (yr)} \times 1.018$ [if female] $\times 1.159$ [if Black]; where: Cr is serum creatinine in mg/dL, κ is 0.7 for females and 0.9 for males, α is -0.329 for females and -0.411 for males, min indicates the minimum of Cr/κ or 1, and max indicates the maximum of Cr/κ or 1.

Another approved blood test reflecting renal filtration function and used in eGFR equations is Cystatin-C.[6] Cystatin C is a 13 kDa protein produced by all nucleated cells. Its low molecular mass and its high isoelectric point allow it to be freely filtered by the glomerulus and 100% reabsorbed by the proximal tubule. The serum concentration of cystatin C correlates with eGFR and, in combination with a stable production rate, provides a sensitive marker of renal filtration function. Serum levels of cystatin C do not depend on weight and height, muscle mass, age or sex, making it less variable than Cr. Furthermore,

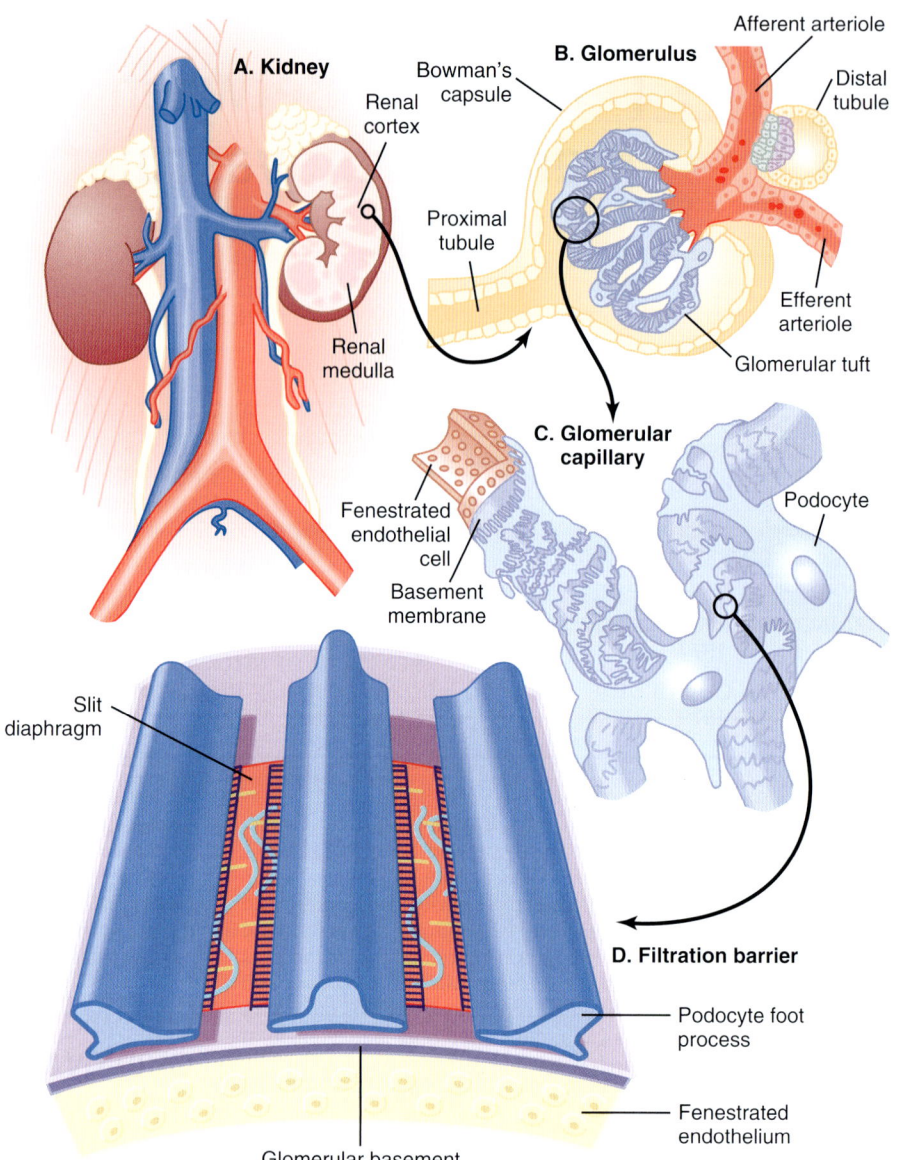

FIGURE 101.1 Normal structure of the glomerular vasculature. Each kidney contains about 1 million glomeruli in the renal cortex (Part A, Kidney). Part B, Glomerulus, shows an afferent arteriole entering Bowman's capsule and branching into several capillaries that form the glomerular tuft; the walls of the capillaries constitute the actual filter. The plasma filtrate (primary urine) is directed to the proximal tubule, whereas the unfiltered blood returns to the circulation through the efferent arteriole. The filtration barrier of the capillary wall contains an innermost fenestrated endothelium, the glomerular basement membrane, and a layer of interdigitating podocyte foot processes (Part C, Glomerular capillary). In Part D, Filtration barrier, a cross section through the glomerular capillary depicts the fenestrated endothelial layer and the glomerular basement membrane with overlying podocyte foot processes. An ultrathin slit diaphragm spans the filtration slit between the foot processes, slightly above the basement membrane. To show the slit diaphragm, the foot processes are drawn smaller than actual scale. (Adapted from Tryggvason K, Patrakka J, Wartiovaara J. Hereditary proteinuria syndromes and mechanisms of proteinuria. *N Engl J Med.* 2006;354[13]:1387–1401.)

measurements can be made and interpreted from a single random sample with reference intervals in women and men being 0.54 to 1.21 mg/L (median 0.85 mg/L, range 0.42 to 1.39 mg/L).

In addition, microalbuminuria at any level of eGFR indicates CKD and occurs as the result of endothelial dysfunction or damage in glomerular capillaries secondary to the metabolic syndrome, DM, and HTN. The most widely accepted definition of microalbuminuria is a random urine albumin/Cr ratio (ACR) of 30 to 300 mg/g. An ACR greater than 300 mg/g is considered gross proteinuria. The random, spot ACR is the office test for microalbuminuria recommended as part of the cardiovascular and renal risk assessment done by cardiologists and other specialists. Microalbuminuria independently predicts CVD risk for those with and without DM. The amount of albumin and protein in the urine is the most important prognostic factor for the rapid progression of CKD to ESRD.[7] In addition both the eGFR and degree of albuminuria contribute independently to the risks of future acute kidney injury (AKI), myocardial infarction (MI), stroke, HF, and death (Fig. 101.3).[8]

IMPLICATIONS OF ANEMIA DUE TO CHRONIC KIDNEY DISEASE

Blood hemoglobin (Hb) concentration is associated with CKD, and CVD. The World Health Organization defines anemia as a Hb level less than 13 g/dL in men and less than 12 g/dL in women: approximately 9% of the general adult population meets this definition. Some 20% of patients with stable coronary disease and 30% to 60% of patients with HF have anemia due to CKD. Hence, anemia is a common and easily identifiable potential cause of constitutional symptoms as well as a potential diagnostic and therapeutic target, particularly in the setting of iron deficiency or reduced availability of vitamin B_{12} or folic acid.

Anemia is associated with multiple adverse outcomes, and decreases tissue oxygen delivery and utilization.[13] The cause of anemia in patients with CKD can be multifactorial due to impairment in iron transport and a relative deficiency of erythropoietin-α (EPO), an erythrocyte stimulating protein (ESP), which is normally produced by renal parenchymal cells in response to blood partial pressure of oxygen under the control of gene regulator hypoxia-inducible factor (HIF). Patients with CKD and HF resist the effects of EPO. In addition, increased circulating levels of hepcidin-25, an inhibitor of the ferroportin receptor, impair iron absorption and utilization throughout the body including the bone marrow. As Hb drops over the course of CKD, HF hospitalizations and death increase. Conversely, those patients who have had a spontaneous rise in Hb whether it be due to improved nutrition, reduced neurohormonal factors, or other unknown reasons, enjoy a significant reduction in endpoints over the next several years. This improvement is associated with a significant reduction in left ventricular mass index, suggesting a favorable change in left ventricular remodeling.

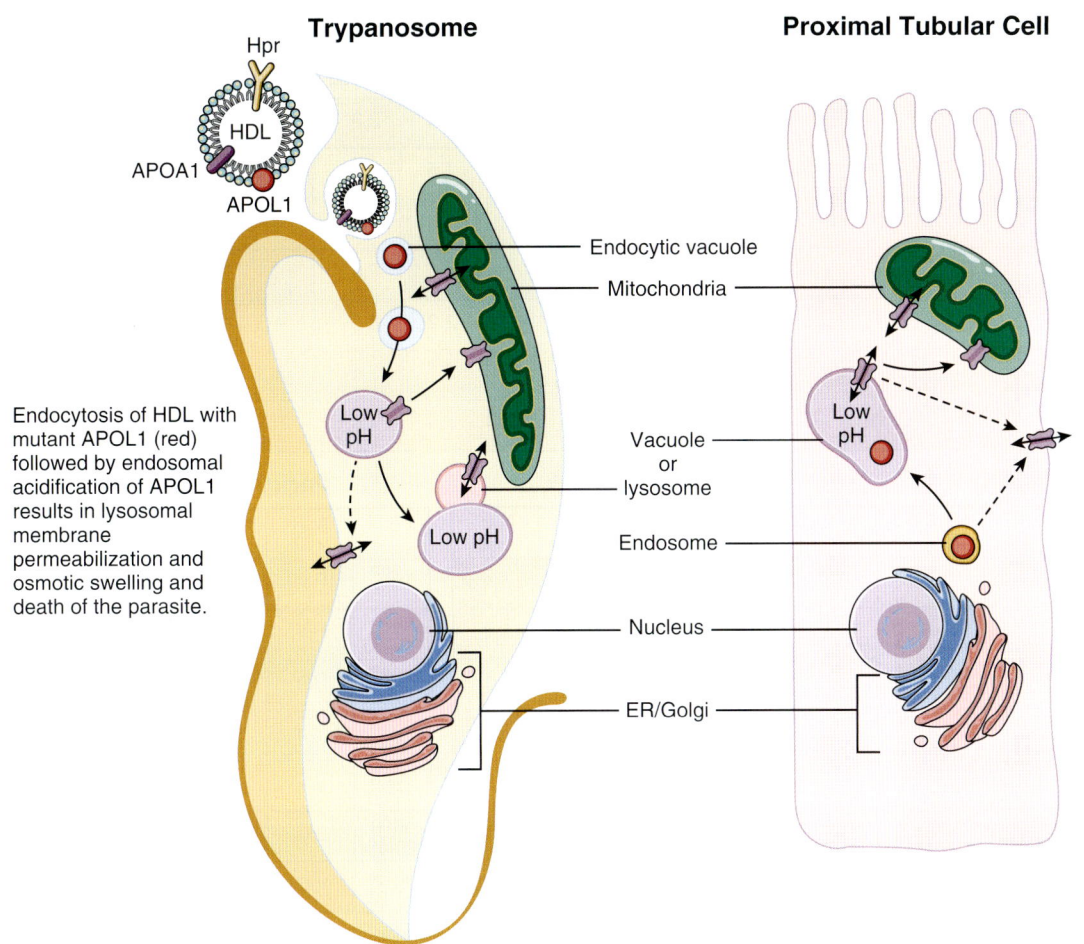

FIGURE 101.2 APOL1 killing mechanisms applied to trypanosomes and normal human kidney cells by intracellular, membrane-associated and intracellular APOL1. (Adapted from Bruggeman LA, O'Toole JF, Sedor JR. Identifying the Intracellular Function of APOL1. *J Am Soc Nephrol.* 2017;28[4]:1008–1011.)

Treatment of anemia with exogenous ESPs (EPO and darbepoetin-α) increasing the Hb level from below 10 g/dL to 12 g/dL has been linked to favorable changes in left ventricular remodeling, improved ejection fraction, improved functional classification, and higher levels of peak oxygen consumption with exercise testing. However, treatment with EPO and supplemental iron which is needed in approximately 70% of cases of ESRD, is associated with three problems: (1) increased platelet activity, thrombin generation, and resultant increased risk of thrombosis; (2) elevated endothelin and asymmetric dimethylarginine which theoretically reduces nitric oxide availability, and can raise blood pressure; and (3) worsened measures of oxidative stress. Randomized trials of ESAs targeting higher levels of Hb in CKD have shown higher rates of CVD events and no improvement in mortality, progression of CKD, or health-related quality of life.[9–11] The Reduction of Events With Darbepoetin Alfa in Heart Failure Trial Failure (RED-HF) randomized, 2278 patients with systolic HF and mild-to-moderate anemia (Hb = 9.0 to 12.0 g/dL) to receive darbepoetin alfa approximately 60 to 600 μg SQ q 2 to 4 weeks (target Hb = 13 g/dL) or placebo and found no reductions in HF hospitalizations or death, but a 35% excess risk of thromboembolic complications with the ESA.[12] When the dose exposure of ESA is taken into account, it appears that cardiovascular drug toxicity and not the Hb accounts for the adverse outcomes reported in ESA trials.[13] As a result of these trials, the current strategy is to use ESA sparingly to maintain a Hb concentration to avoid symptoms and the need for transfusion.

High-dose oral or intravenous iron may overcome the iron-reutilization defect in CKD anemia.[14] In a meta-analysis of 64 trials (including five studies of HF patients) comprising 9004 patients, iron associated with elevations in Hb and reductions in the need for transfusion.[15] Analysis of the five trials of HF patients with iron deficiency (509 patients received iron therapy and 342 controls) showed that intravenous iron is associated with reductions in HF hospitalizations and cardiovascular death (OR 0.39, 95% CI 0.24 to 0.63, $P = 0.0001$) and improvements in multiple measures of functional status.[16] While these results need confirmation in large-scale clinical trials, they support consideration of iron repletion in patients with CKD, anemia, and HF when there is evidence of iron deficiency (iron saturation <20% and ferritin <200 ng/mL).

HIF is short-lived due to a prolylhydroxylase that breaks down this regulator of EPO expression. There are oral HIF prolyl hydroxylase inhibitors that stabilize HIF and allow greater endogenous production of EPO, improved iron transport, and elevated Hb concentrations.[17] Phase III trials have demonstrated efficacy in maintaining Hb along with cardiovascular safety in pre-dialysis CKD and ESRD.[18,19]

CONTRAST-INDUCED ACUTE KIDNEY INJURY (SEE ALSO CHAPTER 21 AND FIG. 21.2)

Iodinated contrast-induced acute kidney injury (CI-AKI) is most commonly defined by the Kidney Disease International Global Outcomes criteria of a ≥0.3 (mg/dL) rise in serum Cr from baseline within 48 hours of intravascular administration or a ≥50% elevation from baseline over the course of hospitalization.[20] The National Cardiovascular Data Registry Cath-PCI ($n = 985,737$ who underwent elective and urgent percutaneous coronary intervention [PCI]) reported 69,658 (7.1%) cases of CI-AKI (Cr rise ≥0.3 mg/dL) and 3005 (0.3%) cases of AKI requiring dialysis.[21] Transient rises in Cr are associated with longer hospital ward and intensive care unit stays, MI, stroke, HF, rehospitalization, and death after coronary angiography, PCI, and angiography followed by cardiac surgery (Fig. 101.4).[22]

Post angiography-AKI has three potential pathophysiologic mechanisms: (1) direct toxicity of iodinated contrast material to nephrons,

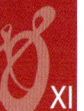

ALL-CAUSE MORTALITY

	ACR <10	ACR 10–29	ACR 30–299	ACR ≥300
eGFR >105	1.1	1.5	2.2	5.0
eGFR 90-105	Ref	1.4	1.5	3.1
eGFR 75-90	1.0	1.3	1.7	2.3
eGFR 60-75	1.0	1.4	1.8	2.7
eGFR 45-60	1.3	1.7	2.2	3.6
eGFR 30-45	1.9	2.3	3.3	4.9
eGFR 15-30	5.3	3.6	4.7	6.6

CARDIOVASCULAR MORTALITY

	ACR <10	ACR 10–29	ACR 30–299	ACR ≥300
eGFR >105	0.9	1.3	2.3	2.1
eGFR 90-105	Ref	1.5	1.7	3.7
eGFR 75-90	1.0	1.3	1.6	3.7
eGFR 60-75	1.0	1.4	2.0	4.1
eGFR 45-60	1.5	2.2	2.8	4.3
eGFR 30-45	2.2	2.7	3.4	5.2
eGFR 15-30	14	7.9	4.8	8.1

KIDNEY FAILURE (ESRD)

	ACR <10	ACR 10–29	ACR 30–299	ACR ≥300
eGFR >105	Ref	Ref	7.8	18
eGFR 90-105	Ref	Ref	11	20
eGFR 75-90	Ref	Ref	3.8	48
eGFR 60-75	Ref	Ref	7.4	67
eGFR 45-60	5.2	22	40	147
eGFR 30-45	56	74	294	763
eGFR 15-30	433	1044	1056	2286

AKI

	ACR <10	ACR 10–29	ACR 30–299	ACR ≥300
eGFR >105	Ref	Ref	2.7	8.4
eGFR 90-105	Ref	Ref	2.4	5.8
eGFR 75-90	Ref	Ref	2.5	4.1
eGFR 60-75	Ref	Ref	3.3	6.4
eGFR 45-60	2.2	4.9	6.4	5.9
eGFR 30-45	7.3	10	12	20
eGFR 15-30	17	17	21	29

PROGRESSIVE CKD

	ACR <10	ACR 10–29	ACR 30–299	ACR ≥300
eGFR >105	Ref	Ref	0.4	3.0
eGFR 90-105	Ref	Ref	0.9	3.3
eGFR 75-90	Ref	Ref	1.9	5.0
eGFR 60-75	Ref	Ref	3.2	8.1
eGFR 45-60	3.1	4.0	9.4	57
eGFR 30-45	3.0	19	15	22
eGFR 15-30	4.0	12	21	7.7

FIGURE 101.3 Relative risks of heart and kidney outcomes in cohorts where eGFR and ACR where measured. *ACR*, Albumin/Cr ratio; *AKI*, Acute kidney injury; *CKD*, chronic kidney disease; *eGFR*, estimated glomerular filtration rate; *ESRD*, end-stage renal disease. (Adapted from Chronic Kidney Disease Prognosis Consortium, Matsushita K, van der Velde M, et al. Association of estimated glomerular filtration rate and albuminuria with all-cause and cardiovascular mortality in general population cohorts: a collaborative meta-analysis. *Lancet.* 2010;375[9731]:2073–2081.)

(2) microshowers of atheroemboli to the kidneys (due to catheter and wire exchanges above the renal arteries), and (3) contrast material- and atheroemboli-induced intrarenal vasoconstriction. Direct toxicity to nephrons with iodinated contrast media appears related to the ionicity and osmolality of the contrast media given in the milieu of CKD.[22] Microshowers of cholesterol emboli may occur in about 50% of percutaneous interventions using an aortic approach; most episodes are clinically silent.[23] However, in approximately 1% of high-risk cases, an acute cholesterol emboli syndrome can develop, manifested by acute renal failure, mesenteric ischemia, decreased microcirculation to the extremities, and, in some cases, embolic stroke. Because there is less trans-aortic movement of wires and catheters, trans-radial coronary intervention is associated with approximately 22% to 50% lower rates of CI-AKI.[24,25] Intrarenal vasoconstriction as a pathological vascular response to contrast media in CKD and perhaps as an organ reaction to superimposed cholesterol microemboli also injure the kidney. Hypoxia triggers activation of the renal SNS and further reduces renal blood flow (Fig. 101.5). The most important predictor of CI-AKI is eGFR less than 60 mL/min/1.73 m^2, a proxy for a reduced number of functioning nephrons that must take on the filtration load with increased oxygen demands in the face of reduced delivery, and hence a greater susceptibility to cytotoxic, ischemic, and oxidative injury.[22]

PREVENTION OF CONTRAST-INDUCED ACUTE KIDNEY INJURY

Patients with preexisting CKD (baseline eGFR <60 mL/min/1.73 m^2), and in particular, those with CKD and DM merit a mitigation strategy for CI-AKI. The presence of CKD, DM, and other risk factors including hemodynamic instability, use of intra-aortic balloon counterpulsation, HF, older age, and anemia in the same patient entail a risk of CI-AKI over 50%.[26] The informed consent process of a high-risk patient before the use of intravascular iodinated contrast should include discussion of CI-AKI. CI-AKI prevention involves consideration of four issues: (1) intravascular volume expansion, (2) choice and quantity of contrast material, (3) trans-radial or femoral approach, and (4) postprocedural monitoring and expectant care.

Because iodinated contrast is water soluble, it is amenable to prevention strategies that expand intravascular volume, increase renal filtration and tubular flow of urine into collecting ducts, and then into the ureters and bladder. CI-AKI responds to intravascular administration of isotonic crystalloid solutions to enhance renal elimination of contrast via the urine. Numerous randomized trials have compared isotonic bicarbonate solutions to intravenous saline. The largest and highest quality trials have shown no differences in the rates of renal outcomes.[27,28] Patient factors should guide the use of either isotonic crystalloid solution. The POSEIDON (Prevention of Contrast Renal Injury with Different Hydration Strategies) trial randomized 396 patients with eGFR less than 60 mL/min/1.73 m^2 and one additional risk factor to a strategy of measurement of left ventricular end-diastolic pressure (LVEDP) and expanding plasma volume versus usual care. Each group had standard of care of normal saline 3 mL/kg for 1 hour before cardiac catheterization. The LVEDP guided approach with more intensive fluid administration during and after the procedure resulted in a 69% relative risk reduction in CI-AKI, p = 0.005. Thus, it is reasonable to consider a 250 mL intravenous administration of normal saline before the procedure and achieve a urine output of approximately 150 mL/hr throughout and after the procedure.

Randomized trials of iodinated contrast agents have demonstrated the lowest rates of CI-AKI with nonionic, iso-osmolar iodixanol. A meta-analysis restricted to 25 head-to-head, prospective, double-blind,

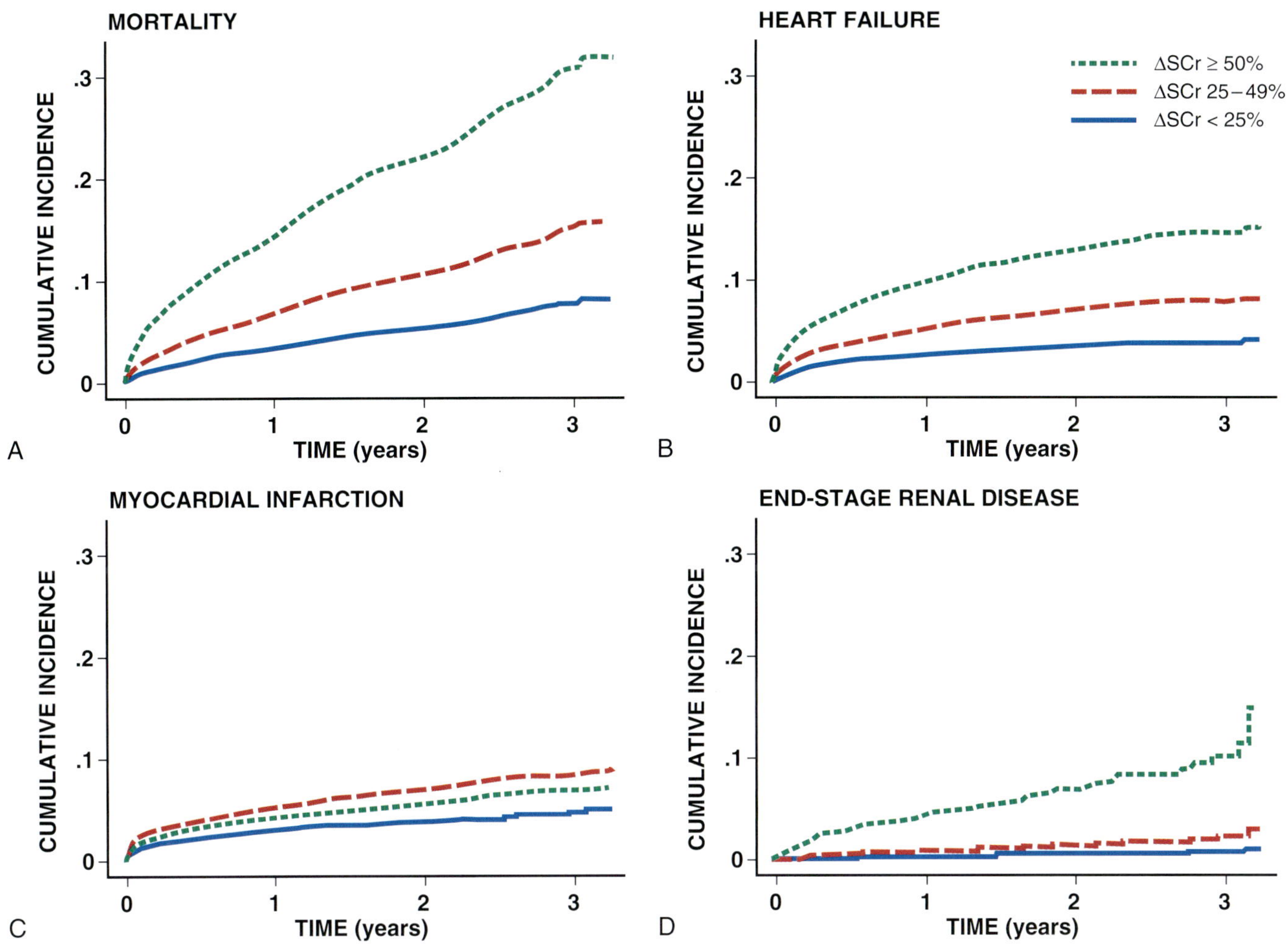

FIGURE 101.4 Cumulative incidence of all-cause mortality (**A**), hospitalization for heart failure (**B**), hospitalization for myocardial infarction (**C**), and end stage renal disease following coronary angiography (**D**), according to severity of acute kidney injury as reflected by magnitude of change in serum creatinine (ΔScr) concentration after coronary angiography. Coronary angiography alone = 4219, with PCI = 8205, with cardiac surgery = 2412. *PCI*, Percutaneous coronary intervention. (Adapted from James MT, Ghali WA, Knudtson ML, et al. Associations between acute kidney injury and cardiovascular and renal outcomes after coronary angiography. *Circulation*. 2011;123[4]:409–416.)

randomized, controlled trials that compared iodixanol with low-osmolar contrast media (LOCM) in adult patients undergoing angiographic examinations with serum Cr values at baseline and following CM administration.[29] The relative risk of CI-AKI (Cr rise ≥0.5 mg/dL) occurring for iodixanol was 0.46, p= 0.004, compared to LOCM as summarized in Figure 101.6. These data indicate that iodixanol (290 mOsm/kg) is less nephrotoxic than LOCM agents with osmolalities ranging from 600 to 800 mOsm/kg when given intra-arterially. However, there appears to be no significant difference in rates of CI-AKI between iodixanol and LOCM when contrast is administered in lower-risk patients or intravenously.[29]

Although it is desirable to limit contrast to the smallest volume possible in any setting, there is disagreement about a "safe" contrast limit. The lower the eGFR, the less contrast material may cause CI-AKI. In general, it is desirable to limit the contrast medium to less than 30 mL for a diagnostic procedure and less than 100 mL for an interventional procedure. If staged procedures are planned, it is advantageous to have more than 10 days between the first and second contrast exposures if CI-AKI has occurred with the first procedure. As mentioned above, the trans-radial approach is associated with significantly lower risk of CI-AKI when controlling for all other factors.[30]

Most trials of preventive strategies for CI-AKI have been small, underpowered, and inconclusive. After many small, suggestive studies, a large (n = 2308) randomized trial of N-acetylcysteine 1200 mg p.o. bid the day before and after the procedure showed no differences in the rates of CI-AKI (12.7% for both groups), ESRD, or other outcomes.[31] This result received support from a larger trial (n = 5177) of diagnostic angiography and PCI demonstrating no impact of N-acetylcysteine or sodium bicarbonate.[32] As a result, neither N-acetylcysteine nor any other drug or intravenous solution is approved for the prevention of CI-AKI.

A suggested algorithm for risk stratification and prevention of CI-AKI is shown in Figure 101.7. An eGFR less than 60 mL/min/1.73 m² mandates preprocedural volume expansion, use of trans-radial access if possible, iodixanol or LOCM as the contrast agent, and minimization of contrast volume. Postprocedural monitoring is critical in the current era of short stays and outpatient procedures. In general, high-risk patients in the hospital should have hydration started 1 to 3 hours before the procedure and continued at least 3 hours afterward. Serum Cr should be measured 24 hours after the procedure. Outpatients, particularly those with eGFR less than 60 mL/min/1.73 m², should have either an overnight stay or discharge to home with 48-hour follow-up and serum Cr measurement. If severe CI-AKI is going to develop, patients usually have a rise of Cr greater than 0.5 mg/dL in the first 24 hours after the procedure. Thus, for those who do not have this degree of serum Cr elevation and are otherwise uncomplicated, discharge to home may be considered. Those patients with eGFR less than 30 mL/min/1.73 m², should have a discussion of the possibility of dialysis and nephrology consultation for possible pre- and post-procedure hemofiltration and dialysis management.

CARDIAC SURGERY ASSOCIATED ACUTE KIDNEY INJURY

AKI occurs in approximately 15% of patients after forms of cardiac surgery with or without use of cardiopulmonary bypass. Rates of AKI are

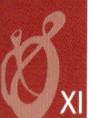

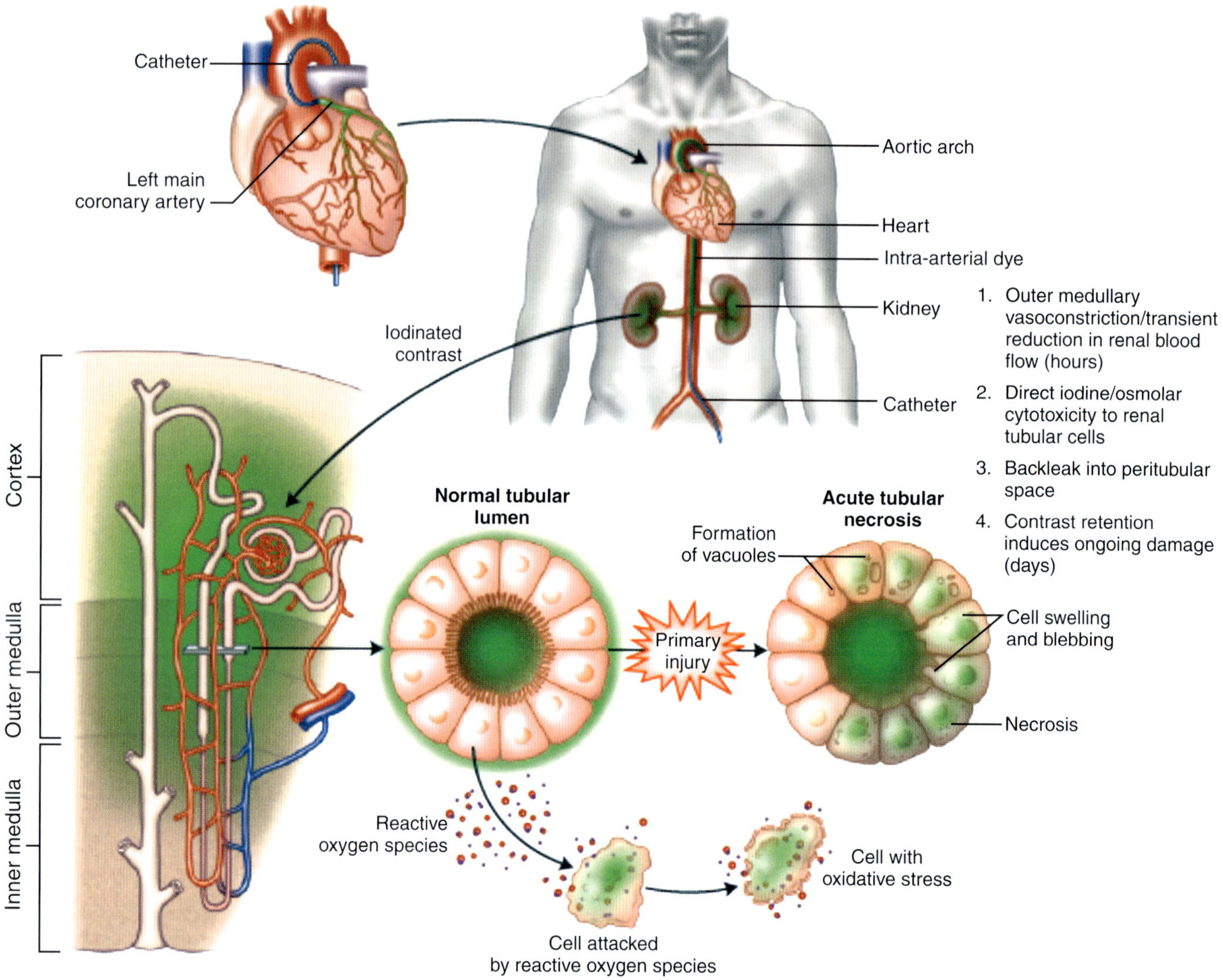

FIGURE 101.5 Pathogenesis of contrast-induced acute kidney injury. (Adapted from Brown JR, McCullough PA. *Contrast Nephropathy and Kidney Injury Textbook of Cardiovascular Intervention.* Springer; 2011.)

Meta-analysis, year	Administration	CI-AKI definition	IOCM	LOCM	RR (95% CI)	P value	RR and 95% CI
McCullough, 2011	IV	≥0.5 mg/dL	158	157	0.968 (0.19–4.97)	0.968	
From, 2010	IV/IA	mixed	3192	3046	0.77 (0.56–1.06)	0.11	
Reed, 2009	IV/IA	mixed	1291	1289	0.79 (0.56–1.12)	0.189	
Heinrich, 2009	IV/IA	≥0.5 mg/dL	1303	1238	0.75 (0.44–1.26)	0.27	
McCullough, 2011	IA	≥0.5 mg/dL	2396	2373	0.46 (0.27–0.79)	0.004	

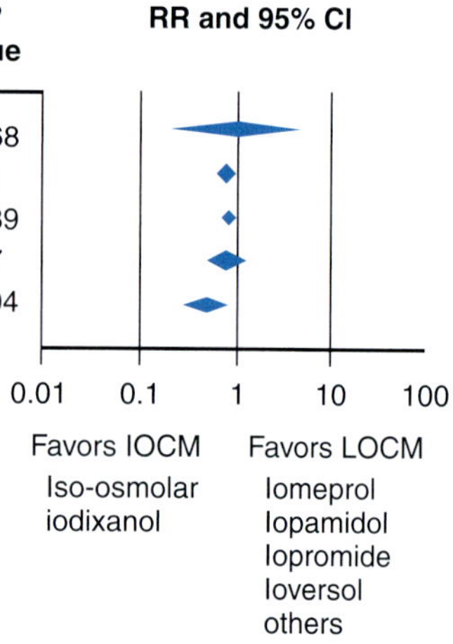

Favors IOCM: Iso-osmolar iodixanol
Favors LOCM: Iomeprol, Iopamidol, Iopromide, Ioversol, others

FIGURE 101.6 Compilation of pooled odds ratios from head-to-head trials for IA, IV, and mixed IA and IV meta-analyses of the incidence of CI-AKI (defined as ≥0.5 mg/dL increase in sCr from baseline) demonstrating a leftward shift in pooled estimates moving from IV, to mixed IV/IA, and IA trials favoring the use of iodixanol. *CI-AKI,* Contrast-induced acute kidney injury. (Adapted from McCullough PA, Brown JR. Effects of intra-arterial and intravenous iso-osmolar contrast medium (iodixanol) on the risk of contrast-induced acute kidney injury: a meta-analysis. *Cardiorenal Med.* 2011;1[4]:220–234.)

higher when coronary angiography is done on the same day or less than 5 days between the angiogram and the surgery.[33] Cardiac surgery exposes patients to many factors including endogenous/exogenous toxins (free heme, catalytic iron), metabolic factors, ischemia and reperfusion, neurohormonal activation, inflammation, and oxidative stress, all of which may contribute to renal tubular injury heralded by reduced urine output and a rise in serum Cr after cardiac surgery.[34] KDIGO (Kidney Disease Global Outcomes) criteria can be used to identify AKI in this patient group (Fig. 101.8).[20] Various blood and urine markers may predict post-operative AKI.[34] Off-pump cardiac surgery

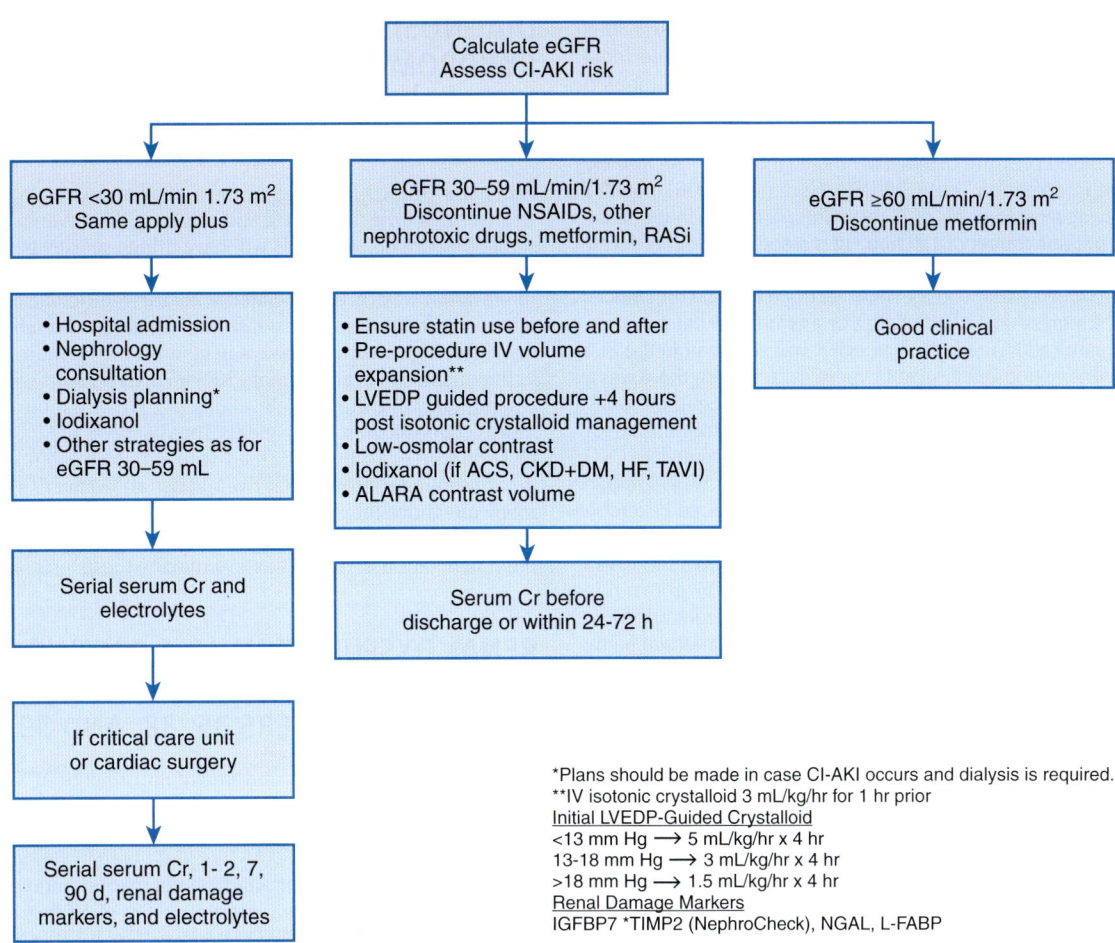

FIGURE 101.7 Algorithm for management of patients receiving iodinated contrast media. *ALARA,* As low as reasonably achievable; *CI-AKI,* contrast-induced acute kidney injury; *CKD,* chronic kidney disease; *Cr,* creatinine; *eGFR,* estimated glomerular filtration rate; *NSAIDs,* nonsteroidal anti-inflammatory agents. (Adapted from McCullough PA, Choi JP, Feghali GA, et al. Contrast-induced acute kidney injury. *J Am Coll Cardiol.* 2016;68[13]:1465–1473.)

Stage	Serum creatinine	Urine output
1	1.5–1.9 × baseline or ≥0.3 mg/dl (≥26.5 mmol/L) increase	<0.5 mL/kg/h for 6–12 h
2	2.0–2.9 × baseline	<0.5 mL/kg/h for >12 h
3	3.0 × baseline, or increase in serum creatinine ≥4.0 mg/dL (≥353.6 mmol/L), or initiation of RRT, or decrease in eGFR <35 mL/min/1.73 m² for patients <18 years	<0.3 mL/kg/h for ≥24 h or anuria for ≥12 h

FIGURE 101.8 Stages of acute kidney injury according to the KDIGO classification. *eGFR,* Estimated glomerular filtration rate; *KDIGO,* kidney disease: Improving global outcomes; *RRT,* renal replacement therapy. (Adapted from KDIGO AKI Work Group. KDIGO clinical practice guideline for acute kidney injury. *Kidney Int Suppl.* 2012;17:1–138.)

does not seem to lower rates of AKI. Trials of natriuretic peptides, corticosteroids, alpha melanocytic stimulating hormone agonists, complement inhibitors, and remote ischemic preconditioning have failed to prevent AKI. Thus, there are no accepted forms of prophylaxis or treatment for cardiac surgery associated with AKI at this time.

ACCELERATION OF VASCULAR CALCIFICATION

When the eGFR falls below 60 mL/min/1.73 m², filtration and elimination of phosphorus falls. In addition, a lower production of 1,25 dihydroxyvitamin D leads to a relative hypocalcemia. Thus, subtle degrees of hyperphosphatemia and hypocalcemia trigger increased release of parathyroid hormone (PTH) causing liberation of calcium and phosphorus from bone. The bone, in turn, produces greater amounts of fibroblast growth factor-23, which directs the kidneys to increase the clearance of phosphorus but also promotes left ventricular hypertrophy (LVH). As a result of this abnormal bone and mineral metabolism, patients with ESRD have markedly increased absolute values and rates of accumulation of arterial calcification as well as LVH. A variety of in vitro stimuli can induce vascular smooth muscle cells to assume osteoblast-like functions, including handling of phosphorus, oxidized low-density lipoprotein cholesterol (LDL-C), vascular calcification factor, PTH, and PTH-related peptide.

No specific strategy to manipulate calcium-phosphorus balance or to treat secondary hyperparathyroidism changes the annual rate of increase in coronary artery calcium score or cardiovascular events.[35-37]

RENAL DISEASE AND HYPERTENSION (SEE ALSO CHAPTER 26)

The kidney is a central regulator of blood pressure and controls intraglomerular pressure through autoregulation. Sodium retention stimulates increases in systemic and renal arteriolar pressure in an attempt to force greater degrees of filtration in the glomerulus. Glomerular injury activates a variety of pathways that further increase systemic blood pressure. This effect sets up a vicious circle of more glomerular and tubulointerstitial injury and worsened HTN. A cornerstone of management of combined CKD and CVD is strict blood pressure control. In most patients with CKD and proteinuria, three or more antihypertensive agents are needed to achieve a goal blood pressure of less than 130/80 mm Hg.[38] The Systolic Blood Pressure Intervention Trial (SPRINT) randomized 9361 patients without DM having a mean eGFR of 71 mL/min/1.72 m^2 and found that a systolic blood pressure target of 120 mm Hg is associated with reduced rates of first occurrence of MI, acute coronary syndrome (ACS), stroke, HF, or death from cardiovascular causes. However, there were no differences in the rates of progression to CKD, ESRD, or any other renal outcome. When a significant (≥20%) reduction in eGFR was seen within the first 6 months of intensive combination antihypertensive therapy, there was a 33% reduction in cardiovascular events and no difference in mortality suggesting the blood pressure reduction should not be compromised for excess concern over Cr.[39] The key lifestyle issues for management of CKD and HTN include dietary changes with sodium restriction, weight reduction of ≥15% to a target body mass index less than 25 kg/m^2, and exercise for 60 min/day most days of the week. Pharmacological therapy aims for strict blood pressure control with an agent that antagonizes the RAAS often in combined action with a thiazide-type diuretic. Dihydropyridine calcium channel blockers alone because of relative afferent arteriolar dilation increase intraglomerular pressure and worsen glomerular injury, and thus should be avoided as singular agents for blood pressure control. Combinations of multiple RAAS-blocking drugs (angiotensin converting enzyme inhibitors [ACEI], angiotensin II receptor blockers [ARB], direct renin inhibitor) provide no additional benefit but cause more complications. Clinical clues such as poorly controlled blood pressure on more than three agents, abdominal bruits, smoking history, peripheral arterial disease, and a marked change in serum Cr with administration of ACEI/ARB should raise the possibility of bilateral renal artery stenosis.[40] Although renal artery stenosis accounts for less than 3% of ESRD cases, it represents a potentially treatable condition (see Chapters 26 and 44). Catheter-based renal sympathetic denervation improves blood pressure in patients with resistant HTN, and additional trials are addressing lesser degrees of HTN and clinical outcomes including major cardiovascular events including HF.[41]

DIAGNOSIS OF ACUTE CORONARY SYNDROMES IN PATIENTS WITH CHRONIC KIDNEY DISEASE (SEE ALSO CHAPTERS 38 AND 39)

Patients with CKD have higher rates of silent ischemia, which cluster with serious arrhythmias, HF, and other cardiac events. About half of stable outpatients with CKD will have a high-sensitivity cardiac troponin I (cTnI) or cTnT above the 99th percentile of normal.[42] The degree of elevation of cTn is associated with left ventricular mass, coronary disease, severity of renal disease, and all-cause mortality.[43] Thus with the use of high-sensitivity assays, in general, cTnI is more advantageous in the diagnostic evaluation of CKD or ESRD patients with acute chest discomfort, while chronic elevations of cTnT are more common and more prognostic in stable patients. The diagnosis of MI in patients with CKD or ESRD can be confirmed with serial troponin measurements demonstrating approximately fivefold rise above the first value since so many are above the 99th percentile of normal at baseline.[44] The skeletal myopathy of CKD can elevate creatine kinase, myoglobin, and some older generation cTnI/cTnT assays, making these tests less desirable.

RENAL DYSFUNCTION AS A PROGNOSTIC FACTOR IN ACUTE CORONARY SYNDROMES (SEE ALSO CHAPTERS 35, 38, AND 39)

Advances in the diagnosis and treatment of acute ACS include early paramedic response and defibrillation, coronary care units, and pharmacotherapy including antiplatelet agents, antithrombotics, beta receptor–blocking agents, RAAS blockade, lipid-lowering therapy, intravenous thrombolytic agents, and percutaneous intervention (Tables 101.1–101.3). CKD patients represent 30.5% of ST segment elevation MI (STEMI) and 42.9% of NSTEMI cases (Fig. 101.9) and have higher rates of in-hospital mortality in a graded fashion with worsened renal function (Fig. 101.10).[45] The degree of CKD is independently associated with 30-day and 1-year mortality after ACS. Reduced baseline

TABLE 101.1 Acute and Chronic Treatments for Coronary Artery Disease in Patients with Chronic Kidney Disease

MEDICATION	USE	CKD POPULATION	PHARMACOLOGY
Antiplatelet Agents			
Aspirin	Acute MI: 160–325 mg by mouth as soon as possible MI prophylaxis: 81–162 mg by mouth once daily PCI: 325 mg by mouth 2 hr pre-surgery, then 160–325 mg by mouth maintenance UA: 75–162 mg by mouth once daily	No specific dosing adjustments in patients with CKD Meta-analysis involving patients on dialysis demonstrated a benefit of aspirin therapy on cardiovascular outcomes	Metabolism: liver, microsomal enzyme system Renal clearance: 80%–100% 24–72 hr Excretion: principally in urine (80%–100%), sweat, saliva, feces
Clopidogrel	UA/NSTEMI: 300–600 mg initial loading dose, followed by 75 mg by mouth once daily with aspirin STEMI: 75 mg by mouth once daily with aspirin 75–162 mg per day Recent MI: 75 mg by mouth once daily	No specific dosing adjustments in patients with CKD	Metabolism: CYP3A4, CYP2C19 (predominantly) and others to generate active metabolite; also by esterase to an inactive metabolite Excretion: urine and feces
Prasugrel	ACS: Loading dose: 60 mg by mouth once Maintenance dose: 10 mg by mouth once daily with aspirin 81–325 mg per day; bleeding risk may increase if weight <60 kg, consider 5 mg by mouth once daily (efficacy/safety not established)	No specific dose adjustments in patients with CKD	Metabolism: liver; CYP450, CYP2B6, CYP2C9/CYP2C19 (minor), CYP3A4 substrate; CYP2B6 (weak) inhibitor Excretion: urine (68%) and feces (27%)
Ticagrelor	ACS with PCI and stent: Starting dose: 180 mg by mouth once Maintenance dose: 90 mg by mouth twice daily To be given for 1 year with aspirin as an alternative option for dual antiplatelet therapy	No specific dose adjustments in patients with CKD	Metabolism: hepatic CYP450 Excretion: bile primarily, urine <1%

Continued

TABLE 101.1 Acute and Chronic Treatments for Coronary Artery Disease in Patients with Chronic Kidney Disease—cont'd

MEDICATION	USE	CKD POPULATION	PHARMACOLOGY
Angiotensin Converting Enzyme Inhibitors			
For example, Captopril, zofenopril, enalapril, ramipril, quinapril, perindopril, lisinopril, benazepril, imidapril, trandolapril, fosinopril	Indicated for the treatment of hypertension, prevention of cardiovascular events including heart failure in those at risk, reduction in the progression of type 1 diabetic nephropathy, and reduction in cardiovascular events in patients post MI with left ventricular dysfunction or heart failure Also indicated for the treatment of heart failure	The dosing schedules may need to be individualized for each dialysis session in order to avoid intradialytic hypotension In general, reduce dose by 50%–75% in ESRD	Elimination: mainly renal with an elimination half-life of 12.6 hr in healthy individuals In patients with impaired renal function (CrCl ≤30 mL/min) a longer half-life and accumulation have been observed without clinical consequences
Angiotensin II Receptor Antagonists			
For example, Losartan, irbesartan, olmesartan, candesartan, valsartan, telmisartan	Indicated for treatment of hypertension, to reduce the progression of type 2 diabetic nephropathy, and reduce cardiovascular events in patients post-MI with left ventricular dysfunction or heart failure Indicated for heart failure in those intolerant to ACE inhibitors	As first-line treatment in the majority of patients with CKD, recommend the use of ACE inhibitors or ARBs; both have been shown to reduce LVH in patients on hemodialysis Levels of ARBs do not change significantly during hemodialysis	Losartan has 88% hepatic and 12% renal clearance
Calcium Channel Blockers			
Dihydropyridines: e.g., Amlodipine, felodipine, nicardipine, nifedipine, nimodipine, nitrendipine Nondihydropyridines: e.g., Diltiazem, verapamil	In UA/NSTEMI, if β-blockers are contraindicated, a non-dihydropyridine CCB should be chosen in the absence of clinically significant left ventricular dysfunction or other contraindications[44]	No specific dose adjustments for patients with CKD The management of chronic CAD in patients on dialysis should follow that of the general population and use of CCBs as indicated The hemodynamic and electrophysiologic effects of CCBs are markedly different from each other and should be evaluated when selecting a suitable therapy	Amlodipine has renal elimination as the major route of excretion with about 60% cleared in the urine Diltiazem undergoes primary liver metabolism
Nitrates			
Nitroglycerin	2% ointment Angina: 0.5–2 inches applied in morning and 6 hr later to truncal skin Heart failure: 1.5 inches, increase by 0.5–1 inch up to 4 inches, every 4 hr Sublingual: 0.4 mg for relief of chest pain in ACS Sublingual: 0.3-0.6 mg every 5 min Maximum: 3 doses within 15 min	No specific dose adjustments for patients with CKD Care must be used to avoid hypotension in low volume states such as dialysis sessions	Metabolism: mainly in liver, extrahepatic sites such as vascular wall, red blood cells Excretion: urine
Antianginal			
Ranolazine	500–1000 mg by mouth twice daily Max: 2000 mg/day	No specific dose adjustments for patients with CKD Prolongs QTc interval Recommend close monitoring	Excretion: urine 73%–75%, feces 25%

ACE, Angiotensin-converting enzyme; *ACS*, acute coronary syndromes; *ARB*, angiotensin-receptor blocker; *CAD*, coronary artery disease; *CCB*, calcium-channel blocker; *CKD*, chronic kidney disease; *CrCl*, creatinine clearance; *ESRD*, end-stage renal disease; *LVH*, left ventricular hypertrophy; *MI*, myocardial infarction; *NSTEMI*, non-ST-elevation myocardial infarction; *PCI*, percutaneous coronary intervention; *STEMI*, ST-elevation myocardial infarction; *UA*, unstable angina.

eGFR also predicts higher rates of AKI, bleeding, the development of HF, recurrent MI, rehospitalization, and stroke in the setting of ACS. Patients with ESRD have the highest mortality after MI of any large, chronic disease population.

REASONS FOR POOR OUTCOMES AFTER ACUTE CORONARY SYNDROMES IN PATIENTS WITH RENAL DYSFUNCTION

Patients with renal dysfunction may have poor cardiovascular outcomes after ACS for four reasons: (1) excess comorbidities associated with CKD and ESRD, in particular DM and left ventricular dysfunction, (2) therapeutic nihilism, (3) toxicity of therapies, and (4) special biological and pathophysiological factors in renal dysfunction that cause worsened outcomes.[46]

The primary defects that promote thrombosis attributable to uremia are cytokine elevation, excess thrombin generation, and decreased platelet aggregation. Hence, patients with CKD and ESRD can have increased rates of coronary thrombotic events and increased bleeding risks at the same time. In patients with renal dysfunction, the risks of bleeding increase with aspirin, unfractionated heparin, low-molecular-weight heparin, direct thrombin inhibitors, anti-factor Xa agents, thrombolytics, glycoprotein IIb/IIIa antagonists, and thienopyridine antiplatelet agents (Tables 101.4 and 101.5). Uremia causes platelet dysfunction by independent mechanisms that add to pharmacologic anti-platelet agents.[47]

Renal dysfunction creates a pro-inflammatory oxidative stress state, and is associated with higher rates of plaque rupture and incident

TABLE 101.2 β-Adrenergic Receptor Blockers in Patients with Chronic Kidney Disease*

MEDICATION	USE	CKD POPULATION	PHARMACOLOGY
Metoprolol	Acute MI Metoprolol tartrate: 2.5–5 mg rapid IV every 2–5 min, up to 15 mg over 10–15 min, then 15 min after last IV and receiving 15 mg IV or 50 mg by mouth every 6 hr for 48 hr, then 50–100 mg by mouth twice daily Angina Metoprolol tartrate: initially 50 mg by mouth twice daily then titrated to 200 mg by mouth twice daily Heart failure Metoprolol succinate: 25–100 mg by mouth once daily, target dose 200 mg/day	No specific dose adjustments for patients with CKD Recommend close monitoring for adverse effects	Dialyzable: Yes. Metabolism: hepatic CYP2D6 Metabolites: inactive Excretion: urine 95%
Esmolol	Immediate control For intraoperative treatment give an 80 mg (approximately 1 mg/kg) bolus dose over 30 s followed by a 150 μg/kg/min infusion, if needed Maximum infusion rate: 300 μg/kg/min Gradual control For postoperative treatment, give loading dosage infusion of 500 μg/kg/min over 1 min followed by a 4 min infusion of 50 μg/kg/min If no effect within 5 min, repeat loading dose and follow with infusion increased to 100 μg/kg/min	No specific dose adjustments for patients with CKD	Metabolism: extensively metabolized by esterase in cytosol of red blood cells Metabolites: major acid metabolite (ASL-8123), methanol (inactive) Excretion: urine <1%–2%
Carvedilol	Hypertension, HF, and post-MI protection: 6.25–25 mg by mouth twice daily Start at 6.25 mg by mouth twice daily, then increase every 3–14 days to 12.5 mg by mouth twice daily, then 25 mg by mouth twice daily, then 50 mg twice daily for weight >85 kg	No specific dose adjustments for patients with CKD In a small study of patients on dialysis with dilated cardiomyopathies, carvedilol improved left ventricular function and decreased hospitalization, cardiovascular deaths and total mortality	Elimination: mainly biliary Excretion: primarily via feces

*Hemodialysis reduces blood levels of atenolol, acebutolol, and nadolol; by contrast, levels of carvedilol and labetalol do not change significantly.
ACS, Acute coronary syndromes; CKD, chronic kidney disease; HF, heart failure; IV, intravenous; MI, myocardial infarction.

thrombotic CVD events. Patients with CKD have more proximal and extensive coronary artery disease (CAD) than the general population; thus, they have larger areas of myocardium at risk for ischemia and dysfunction. Finally, acute on chronic hyperactivation of neurohormonal systems including the RAAS, SNS, endothelin, vasopressin, without adequate counter-regulation by natriuretic peptides, nitric oxide, and other systems may promote worsened ischemia, myocardial dysfunction, and HF.

TREATMENT OF MYOCARDIAL INFARCTION IN PATIENTS WITH RENAL DYSFUNCTION (SEE CHAPTERS 38 AND 39)

Therapies that benefit the general population often yield enhanced benefit in patients with CKD and ESRD include aspirin, beta blockers, ACEI, ARB, aldosterone receptor antagonists.[48] Therapies that require dose adjustment on the basis of CrCl include low-molecular-weight heparins, bivalirudin, and glycoprotein IIb/IIIa antagonists. Given that the major inputs for bleeding risks include older age, low body weight, and renal dysfunction, Tables 101.4 and 101.5 also list agents that are approved in a weight-adjusted dose form and gives the currently recommended dose adjustments for commonly used antiplatelet and antithrombotic agents.[47] Greater utilization of such therapies, despite the heightened risk for complications, might attenuate the excess mortality reported in CKD and ESRD populations. There have been no randomized trials of PCI in patients with CKD or ESRD. However, in the large Swedish Web-system for Enhancement and Development of Evidence-based care in Heart disease Evaluated According to Recommended Therapies (SWEDEHEART) has observed an apparent benefit to revascularization in ACS in CKD groups with eGFR ≥15 mL/min/1.73 m² (Fig. 101.11).[49] Patients with more severe degrees of renal impairment and those on dialysis, although infrequently offered PCI, appeared to have no improvement in survival with interventional management.

CARDIORENAL SYNDROMES (SEE PART VI)

The term cardiorenal syndrome (CRS) refers to disorders of the heart and kidneys whereby acute or chronic dysfunction in one organ may induce acute or chronic dysfunction in the other. Patients with CKD, and in particular ESRD, have three key mechanical contributors to HF: pressure overload (related to HTN), volume overload, and cardiomyopathy (Fig. 101.12). Approximately 20% of patients approaching hemodialysis have a diagnosis of preexisting HF. It is unclear how much of this diagnosis results purely from chronic volume overload from renal failure and how much is due to impaired systolic or diastolic function. CKD influences the blood levels of B-type natriuretic peptide (BNP) and to a greater extent with NT-proBNP.[50] In general, when the eGFR is less than 60 mL/min/1.73 m², higher cut points of 200 pg/mL and 1200 pg/mL should be used in the diagnosis of HF with BNP and NT-proBNP, respectively.

Once acute heart failure is recognized on clinical grounds, approximately 25% of patients will develop a CRS during the hospitalization characterized by a rise in serum Cr ≥0.3 mg/dL and a reduction in urine output (Fig. 101.13). These findings are not associated with markers of acute tubular injury suggesting that they reflect a transient renal hemodynamic problem.[51] Of those, approximately one third return to baseline, one third are left with worsened eGFR, and the final third have progressive cardiorenal disease resulting in either death or the need for renal replacement therapy.[52] Multiple studies have shown

TABLE 101.3 Lipid-Lowering Therapy for Primary and Secondary Prevention in Patients with Chronic Kidney Disease

MEDICATION	USE	CKD POPULATION	PHARMACOLOGY
Rosuvastatin	Cardiovascular event protection 10–40 mg by mouth once daily	Efficacy in LDL-C reduction in CKD demonstrated at doses as low as 2.5 mg daily	Metabolism: liver, CYP450 CYP2C9 Excretion: bile primarily, urine <2%
Simvastatin	Cardiovascular event protection: 20–40 mg by mouth once daily combined with ezetimibe 10 mg by mouth once daily Maximum dose: 40 mg by mouth given at hour of sleep	Consider starting dose at 5 mg in the evening in patients with CKD In SHARP, lipid lowering with statin + ezetimibe was beneficial in patients with CKD In HPS, simvastatin reduced the renal decline in patients with CKD	Metabolism: liver, CYP450 CYP3A4 Excretion: bile primarily, urine <2%
Atorvastatin	Cardiovascular event protection: 10–80 mg by mouth once daily	No specific dose adjustments for patients with CKD Atorvastatin 10 mg in patients with CKD revealed a significantly lower risk of the primary end point (nonfatal MI or cardiac death) when compared with placebo[110] With the TNT and GREACE studies, atorvastatin showed improvement in renal function in patients with CKD	Metabolism: liver, CYP450 CYP3A4 Excretion: bile primarily, urine <2%
Fluvastatin	Cardiovascular event protection: 40 mg by mouth twice daily Extended release: 80 mg by mouth once daily	No specific dose adjustments for patients with CKD Caution for increased risk of rhabdomyolysis A multicenter, randomized, double blind, placebo-controlled trial of fluvastatin was conducted in kidney transplant recipients. Fluvastatin reduced LDL cholesterol levels by 32%. Although the primary end point did not achieve statistical significance, secondary analysis showed that the fluvastatin group experienced fewer cardiac deaths and nonfatal MI than did the placebo group. Coronary intervention procedures were not significantly different between the two groups	Metabolism: liver, CYP450 CYP2C9 isozyme system (75%), and to a lesser extent by CYP3A4 (approximately 20%) and CYP2C8 (approximately 5%) Excretion: bile primarily 90%, urine 5%
Pravastatin	Cardiovascular event protection: Start: 40 mg by mouth once daily, may adjust dose every 4 weeks Maximum dose: 80 mg by mouth once daily	Start at 10 mg by mouth once daily in patients with CKD A randomized trial of pravastatin versus placebo in patients with previous MI and CKD in a secondary analysis showed coronary death or nonfatal MI was lower in patients receiving pravastatin, suggesting that pravastatin is effective for secondary prevention of cardiovascular events in patients with CKD	Metabolism: glucuronidation Excretion: bile primarily 70%, urine 20%
Pitavastatin	Lowering LDL-C and total cholesterol: Start: 1 mg by mouth once daily may adjust every 4 weeks Maximum dose: 4 mg by mouth once daily	Start at 1 mg po qd in patients with CKD	Metabolism: glucuronidation Excretion: bile primarily 79%, urine 15%
Ezetimibe	Lowering LDL-C and total cholesterol: Start 10 mg po qd	Start at 10 mg po qd with no renal dose adjustment, tested in ESRD	Metabolism: glucuronidation Excretion: Bile/feces 78%, urine 11%
Colesevelam hydrochloride	Lowering LDL-C and total cholesterol, improving glycemic control type 2 diabetes: Start 625 mg tabs, 3 tabs po bid	Start at 3 tabs po bid with no renal dose adjustment	Metabolism: no systemic absorption Excretion: feces
Evolocumab Humanized monoclonal IgG2 directed against PCSK9	Cardiovascular event protection: Start 140 mg SQ q 2 weeks or 420 mg SQ q 4 weeks	Start 140 mg SQ q 2 weeks or 420 mg SQ q 4 weeks with no renal dose adjustment	Metabolism: saturable target binding and proteolysis Excretion: none
Alirocumab Humanized monoclonal IgG1 directed against PCSK9	Cardiovascular event protection: Start 75 or 150 mg SQ q 2 weeks or 300 mg SQ q 4 weeks	Start 75 or 150 mg SQ q 2 weeks or 300 mg SQ q 4 weeks with no renal dose adjustment	Metabolism: saturable target binding and proteolysis Excretion: none

ACS, Acute coronary syndromes; *CKD*, chronic kidney disease; *ESRD*, end-stage renal disease; *LDL-C*, low-density lipoprotein cholesterol; *MI*, myocardial infarction.

that the predictors of CRS (type 1) include baseline eGFR, older age, female sex, increased baseline blood pressure, higher initial natriuretic peptide levels, and increased central venous pressure. Because CRS Type 1 in patients with HF rarely occurs in the prehospital phase and more commonly develops after treatment is started in-hospital, initial diuresis followed by inadequate plasma refill from the extravascular tissues has been implicated. Continued administration of loop diuretics, probably by further activating the RAAS and possibly worsening intra-renal hemodynamics, probably contribute to CRS Type 1 when diuresis is not maintained.

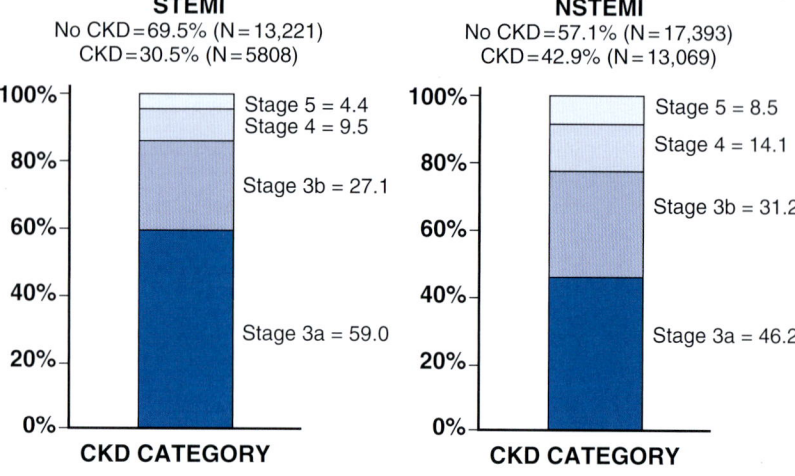

FIGURE 101.9 Prevalence of chronic kidney disease (CKD) and stages 3a, 3b, 4, and 5 (no dialysis) and dialysis presenting with ST segment elevation myocardial infarction (STEMI) and NSTEMI. Stage 3b as estimated glomerular filtration rate (eGFR) 30 to 44 mL/min/1.73 m^2; Stage 4 CKD as eGFR between 15 and 29 mL/min/1.73 m^2, and Stage 5 CKD as an eGFR less than 15 mL/min/1.73 m^2 or dialysis therapy. (Adapted from Fox CS, Muntner P, Chen AY, et al. Acute Coronary Treatment and Intervention Outcomes Network registry. Use of evidence-based therapies in short-term outcomes of ST-segment elevation myocardial infarction and non-ST-segment elevation myocardial infarction in patients with chronic kidney disease: a report from the National Cardiovascular Data Acute Coronary Treatment and Intervention Outcomes Network registry. *Circulation.* 2010;121[3]:357–365.)

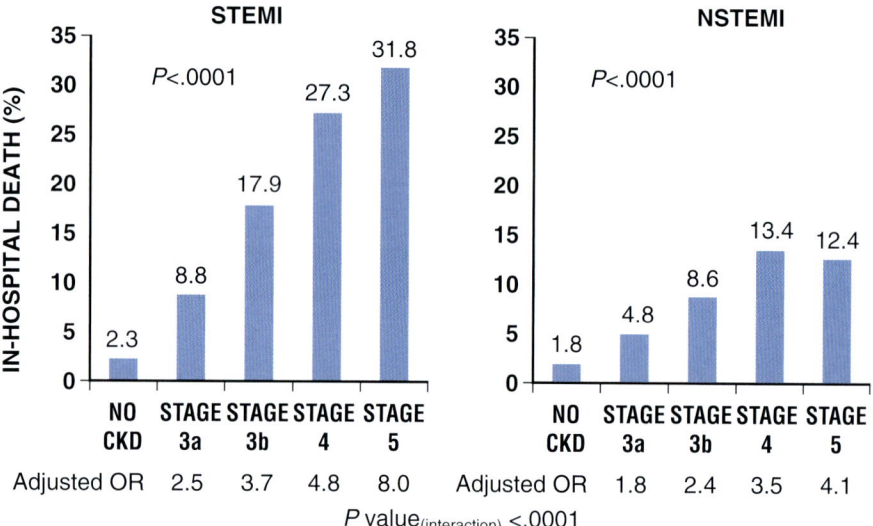

FIGURE 101.10 Crude rates and adjusted odds ratios for death by CKD stages among those presenting with STEMI and NSTEMI, with *P*-trend and *P*-interaction for STEMI versus NSTEMI by CKD stages. Stage 3a CKD was defined as an eGFR between 45 and 59 mL/min/1.73 m^2; Stage 3b as eGFR 30 to 44 mL/min/1.73 m^2; Stage 4 CKD as eGFR between 15 and 29 mL/min/1.73 m^2; and Stage 5 CKD as an eGFR less than 15 mL/min/1.73 m^2 or dialysis therapy. *CKD*, Chronic kidney disease; *eGFR*, estimated glomerular filtration rate; *STEMI*, ST segment elevation myocardial infarction. (Adapted from Fox CS, Muntner P, Chen AY, et al. Use of evidence-based therapies in short-term outcomes of ST-segment elevation myocardial infarction and non-ST-segment elevation myocardial infarction in patients with chronic kidney disease: a report from the National Cardiovascular Data Acute Coronary Treatment and Intervention Outcomes Network registry. *Circulation.* 2010;121[3]:357–365.)

TABLE 101.4 Intravenous Glycoprotein IIb/IIIa Inhibitors for Unstable Angina/NSTEMI, STEMI, PCI

MEDICATION	USE	CKD POPULATION*	PHARMACOLOGY
Abciximab	Adjunct to PCI: 0.25 mg/kg IV bolus over at least 1 min, 10–60 min before start of PCI, then 0.125 µg/kg/min (not to exceed 10 µg/min) continuous IV infusion for 12 hr Unstable angina with PCI planned within 24 hr: 0.25 mg/kg IV bolus over at least 1 min, then 0.125 µg/kg/min (not to exceed 10 µg/min) IV infusion for 18–24 hr concluding 1 hr after PCI	No specific dose adjustments for patients with CKD Abciximab should also be considered as adjunctive therapy in patients with ACS on dialysis In CKD, safety of abciximab has been shown for creatinine levels >152.5 µmol/L Although increased bleeding with abciximab in patients with CKD has been reported, other studies have shown no increase in bleeding for CKD versus no CKD for abciximab in PCI	Metabolism: unknown, but likely by the reticuloendothelial system CYP450: unknown involvement Excretion: urine
Eptifibatide	ACS: 180 µg/kg IV bolus, then 2 µg/kg/min IV for up to 72 hr PCI: 180 µg/kg IV, then a continuous infusion at 2 µg/kg/min with another 180 µg/kg IV bolus 10 min after first bolus Continue infusion for at least 12 hr	Creatinine clearance <50 mL/min and ACS: 180 µg/kg IV, then continuous infusion 1 µg/kg/min Safety and use during hemodialysis is not established	Metabolism: other, minimal CYP450: unknown involvement Excretion: urine 50%
Tirofiban	In patients undergoing PCI, tirofiban is not recommended as an alternative to abciximab[43] ACS: 0.4 µg/kg/min IV for 30 min, then 0.1 µg/kg/min IV for 48–108 hr PCI: Continue 0.1 µg/kg/min IV through procedure and for 12–24 hr after	Creatinine clearance <30 mL/min and ACS: reduce dose to 50% of normal rate Safety and use during hemodialysis not established	Excretion: urine 65% (primarily unchanged), feces 25% (primarily unchanged)

ACS, Acute coronary syndromes; *CKD,* chronic kidney disease; *IV,* intravenous; *NSTEMI,* non-ST-elevation myocardial infarction; *PCI,* percutaneous coronary intervention; *STEMI,* ST-elevation myocardial infarction.
*When a glycoprotein IIb/IIIa antagonist is used, abciximab and tirofiban should be considered preferred agents as no dosing changes are required for abciximab, and dialysis-specific dosing recommendations are available for tirofiban. Increased bleeding but reduced in-hospital mortality in CKD patients with ACS treated with glycoprotein IIb/IIIa antagonists has also been shown.[49]

TABLE 101.5 Antithrombotic Agents for Acute Coronary Syndromes and Other Thrombotic Indications in Patients with Chronic Kidney Disease

MEDICATION	USE	CKD POPULATION	PHARMACOLOGY
Indirect Factor Xa Inhibitors			
Unfractionated heparin	Recommended dosage and desired aPTT values as per institutional protocol PCI: 60–100 units/kg IV given once Target ACT 250–350 sec In patients receiving glycoprotein IIb/IIIa inhibitor, give 50–70 units/kg IV to target ACT 200 sec STEMI, adjunct treatment, streptokinase use: 800 units/hr when <80 kg body weight or 1000 units/hr when >80 kg body weight Start: 5000 units IV, adjust dose to target aPTT 50–75 sec NSTEMI: 12-15 units/kg/hr IV Start: 60–70 units/kg IV; Max 5000 units bolus, max rate 1000 units/hr Adjust dose to target aPTT 50–75 sec	In patients with CKD, suggested starting dose of heparin is 50 IU/kg bolus, then 18 IU/kg/hr Monitor aPTT level and adjust accordingly as per institutional protocol	Metabolism: liver (partial) Metabolites: none Excretion: urine
Low-molecular-weight heparin (e.g., enoxaparin)	Unstable angina, non-Q-wave myocardial infarction: 1 mg/kg subcutaneously twice daily STEMI, aged <75 years: 30 mg IV bolus plus 1 mg/kg subcutaneously, then 1 mg/kg subcutaneously every 12 hr PCI: additional 0.3 mg/kg IV bolus if last subcutaneous administration given >8 hr before balloon inflation STEMI, aged >75 years: 0.75 mg/kg subcutaneously every 12 hr (no IV bolus)	CrCl <30 mL/min STEMI, aged <75 years: 30 mg IV bolus plus 1 mg/kg subcutaneously, then 1 mg/kg subcutaneously once a day STEMI, aged >75 years: 1 mg/kg subcutaneously once a day	Excretion: urine 40%
Direct Factor Xa Inhibitor			
Fondaparinux	Unstable angina/NSTEMI Conservative strategy: 2.5 mg subcutaneously once daily During PCI: add unfractionated heparin 50–60 units/kg IV bolus for prophylaxis of catheter thrombosis[49]	CrCl 30–50 mL/min: use with caution CrCl <30 mL/min: not indicated	Excretion: urine (primarily unchanged)
Direct Thrombin Inhibitors			
Bivalirudin	Intended for use with aspirin 300–325 mg/day 0.75 mg/kg IV bolus initially, followed by continuous infusion at rate of 1.75 mg/kg/hr for duration of procedure Perform ACT 5 min after bolus dose Administer additional 0.3 mg/kg bolus if necessary May continue infusion following PCI beyond 4 hr (optional post-PCI, at discretion of treating healthcare provider) initiated at rate of 0.2 mg/kg/hr for up to 20 hr as needed	CrCl 10–29 mL/min: usual bolus dose, then initial infusion of 1 mg/kg/hr IV up to 4 hr Hemodialysis: usual bolus dose, then initial infusion of 0.25 mg/kg/hr IV up to 4 hr Bivalirudin is a direct thrombin inhibitor with specific dosing adjustments for patients on dialysis and should be preferentially considered	Dialysable: with 25% reduction in levels Excretion: urine
Dabigatran	Indicated for prevention of stroke and thromboembolism associated with nonvalvular atrial fibrillation CrCl >30 mL/min: 150 mg by mouth twice daily	CrCl 15–30 mL/min: 75 mg by mouth twice daily CrCl <15 mL/min or hemodialysis: not indicated For patients currently taking dabigatran, wait 12 hr (CrCl ≥30 mL/min) or 24 hr (CrCl <30 mL/min) after the last dose of dabigatran before initiating treatment with a parenteral anticoagulant If possible, discontinue dabigatran 1–2 days (CrCl ≥50 mL/min) or 3–5 days (CrCl <50 mL/min) before invasive or surgical procedures because of increased risk of bleeding	Metabolism liver esterases and microsomal carboxylesterases Excretion: feces 7%, urine 86%

Continued

TABLE 101.5 Antithrombotic Agents for Acute Coronary Syndromes and Other Thrombotic Indications in Patients with Chronic Kidney Disease—cont'd

MEDICATION	USE	CKD POPULATION	PHARMACOLOGY
Rivaroxaban	Indicated for prevention of stroke and thromboembolism associated with nonvalvular atrial fibrillation, venous thromboembolism (VTE) CrCl >50 mL/min: 15 mg by mouth bid for 3 weeks (acute anticoagulation for VTE) CrCl >50 mL/min: 20 mg by mouth at hour of sleep (chronic anticoagulation)	CrCl 15–50 mL/min: 15 mg by mouth at hour of sleep CrCl <15 mL/min: not indicated	Metabolism: liver CYP450 Excretion: feces 28%, urine 66% Half-life: 5–9 hr or 11–13 hr in elderly
Apixaban	Indicated for prevention of stroke and thromboembolism associated with nonvalvular atrial fibrillation, venous thromboembolism (VTE) 2.5 mg by mouth twice daily (VTE prophylaxis) 5 mg by mouth twice daily (chronic anticoagulation)	age ≥80 years, body weight ≤60 kg, or serum creatinine ≥1.5 mg/dL, the recommended dose is 2.5 mg orally twice daily	Metabolism: liver CYP450 CYP3A4/5 while CYP1A2, 2C8, 2C9, 2C19, and 2J2 are minor Excretion: feces 83%, urine 27%
Edoxaban	Indicated for prevention of stroke and thromboembolism associated with nonvalvular atrial fibrillation, venous thromboembolism (VTE) 60 mg by mouth once daily (VTE prophylaxis) 60 mg by mouth once daily (chronic anticoagulation)	CrCl >95 mL/min: Do not use; increased ischemic stroke compared with warfarin CrCl >50–95 mL/min 60 mg orally once daily CrCl 15–50 mL/min or <60 kg: 30 mg orally once daily	Metabolism: minimal Excretion: urine

ACS, Acute coronary syndromes; *ACT*, activated clotting time; *aPTT*, activated partial thromboplastin time; *CKD*, chronic kidney disease; *CrCl*, creatinine clearance; *IV*, intravenous; *NSTEMI*, non-ST-elevation myocardial infarction; *PCI*, percutaneous coronary intervention; *STEMI*, ST-elevation myocardial infarction.

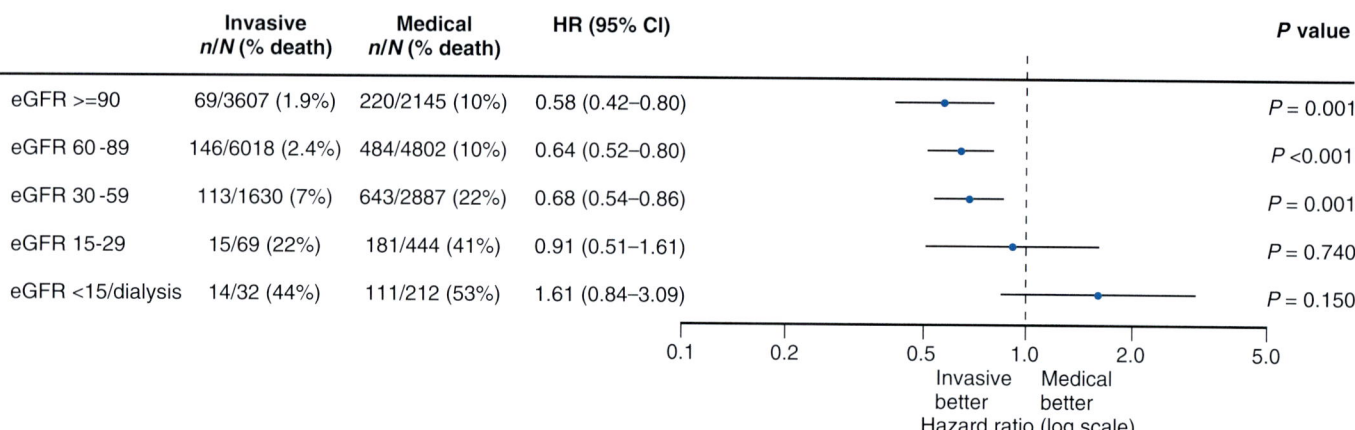

FIGURE 101.11 Estimated hazard ratio for mortality at 1 year for patients treated either medically or with early revascularization. (Adapted from Szummer K, Lundman P, Jacobson SH, et al. Influence of renal function on the effects of early revascularization in non-ST-elevation myocardial infarction: data from the Swedish Web-System for Enhancement and Development of Evidence-Based Care in Heart Disease Evaluated According to Recommended Therapies (SWEDEHEART). *Circulation*. 2009;120[10]:851–858.)

There are no proven strategies for CRS Type 1. Withdrawal of RAAS inhibition with the aim of improving azotemia is associated with increased risk of rehospitalization and mortality.[53] Hence, provided blood pressure is adequate and hyperkalemia is manageable, ACEI/ARB including MRA should be continued despite the development of azotemia.[54] Failed approaches include use of continuous furosemide infusions, low-dose dopamine, nesiritide, and programmatic use of inotropic agents. In the setting of poor arterial perfusion, dobutamine or milrinone are commonly used during hospitalizations to support the patient while ACE/ARB or sacubitril/valsartan, beta-blockers, and diuretics are optimized. Neither agent alone reduces mortality, but they do increase the risk of arrhythmias, and milrinone must be dose adjusted when the eGFR is below 45 mL/min/1.73 m^2 (Table 101.6). Patients with advanced HF have reduced renal blood flow, decreased glomerular filtration rate, enhanced proximal reabsorption of water, increased absorption of sodium along the loop of Henle, and an overall reduced capacity of the nephron to excrete water. Furthermore, reduced effective arterial blood volume stimulates vasopressin release, which plays a dominant role in worsening water retention. Hyponatremia and excess body water can be improved with the use of oral tolvaptan without worsening azotemia.[55]

Treatment efforts should be aimed at reducing congestion within a narrow management window (see Chapters 50 and 51) and improving left ventricular systolic function, often in the hospitalized setting, with the oral and intravenous therapies including diuretics mentioned previously. Observational studies and small trials utilizing continuous veno-venous ultrafiltration have shown mixed results in symptoms, reductions in fluid weight, length of stay, rehospitalization, and death.[56] Until larger trials help define the indicated population, optimal timing and mode of ultrafiltration, and demonstrate longer-term reductions in hospitalization and mortality, ultrafiltration can be considered a last-line approach for the patient with refractory CRS.

The management of the patient who is already receiving dialysis and has HF requires particular care. In general, proven HF therapies, provided they are tolerated, should be employed along with regular and ad hoc dialysis as needed to control volume overload. Clinicians should keep in mind that ACEI are dialyzed but angiotensin receptor blockers are not. Both agents are associated with reductions in mortality in ESRD patients in observational studies. Studies of frequent dialysis performed in the home at lower rates of ultrafiltration have consistently demonstrated lower rates of HF hospitalization and death.[57]

In ambulatory patients with HF with reduced ejection fraction and CKD, administration of sodium glucose cotransporter-2 inhibitors

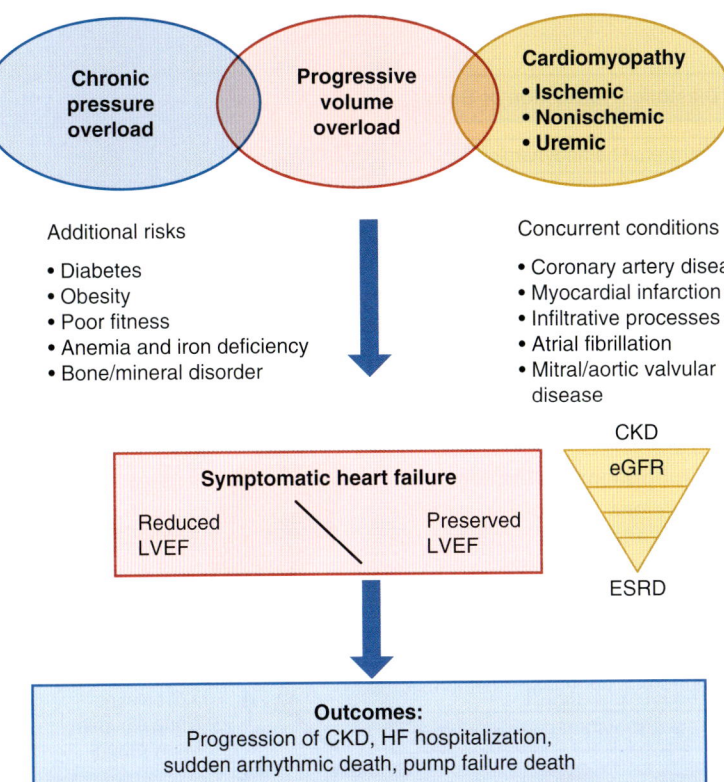

FIGURE 101.12 Pathophysiology of heart failure (HF) in chronic kidney disease (CKD) progressing to end-stage kidney disease (ESRD). Pressure overload implies systemic hypertension. *eGFR*, Estimated glomerular filtration rate; *LVEF*, left ventricular ejection fraction. (Adapted from House AA, Wanner C, Sarnak MJ, et al. Heart failure in chronic kidney disease: conclusions from a Kidney Disease: Improving Global Outcomes (KDIGO) Controversies Conference. Kidney Int. 2019;95[6]:1304–1317.)

(SGLT2i) offers considerable benefit for both HF and renal function.[58] These oral agents approved for use in type 2 diabetes, HF, and diabetic nephropathy induce glycosuria, urinary sodium loss, and a spectrum of secondary metabolic effects in the body. Across multiple trials there are consistent greater than 25% relative risk reductions in HF hospitalization, progression of CKD, ESRD, and cardiovascular death associated with these agents.[59,60]

In summary, CKD and HF present a particularly challenging scenario for clinicians and patients. Among patients with CKD, beta blockers, ACEI/ARB, sacubitril/valsartan, and SGLT2i are associated with both cardiac and renal benefits. Frequent outpatient monitoring and avoidance of overly aggressive diuresis are advised. Dialysis patients, despite having volume reduction with mechanical fluid removal, should have medical therapy with ACEIs or ARBs, beta blockers, and additional agents for blood pressure control if needed. Ideally, ESRD patients with HF would undergo frequent (daily) hemodialysis at home provided self- and partner-care can be delivered without difficulties.

CHRONIC KIDNEY DISEASE AND VALVULAR HEART DISEASE (SEE PART VIII)

CKD mineral and bone disorder (phosphate retention, relative hypocalcemia, increased PTH) are associated with valvular thickening and calcific deposits of the aortic and mitral valves occurs in patients with ESRD.[61] Approximately 80% of patients with ESRD have the murmur of aortic sclerosis and 40% have mitral annular calcification.[62] Patients with CKD and ESRD have rates of valve failure greater than in the general population.[63]

Bacterial endocarditis may develop in patients with ESRD who have temporary dialysis access catheters (see also Chapter 80.)[64] Endocarditis with common pathogens including *Staphylococcus*, *Streptococcus*, and *Enterococcus* in the mitral, aortic, or tricuspid valves, are associated with a risk of cerebral embolism of 40% and a mortality rate of 50% in ESRD.[64] It becomes very difficult to treat given the continued need for dialysis access and the delay in surgical placement of permanent arteriovenous shunts or fistulas. Unfortunately, surgical mortality associated with valve replacement in ESRD related to endocarditis is very high. In the setting of ESRD, when valve surgery is carried out for endocarditis or other causes of valve failure, there has been no difference in survival among those who received tissue or mechanical valve prostheses. Thus, tissue valves are a reasonable choice given the complicating issue of chronic anticoagulation and bleeding with repeated dialysis vascular access.[65]

RENAL FUNCTION AND ARRHYTHMIAS (SEE PART VII)

Uremia, hyperkalemia, acidosis, and disorders of calcium-phosphorous balance all link to higher rates of atrial and ventricular arrhythmias. Given a concurrent substrate of LVH, left ventricular dilation, HF, and valvular disease, it is not surprising that higher rates of virtually all arrhythmias have been reported in CKD, including bradyarrhythmias and heart block. Hypokalemia after hemodialysis can be observed for 6 to 8 hours as the plasma potassium concentration equilibrates from approximately 2.0 mEq/liter to the normal range of 3.5 to 5.5 mEq/liter. During this time, there is an increased risk of sudden cardiac death.[66] There is a general trend to increase the potassium concentration of the dialysis fluid to reduce the large shifts in potassium in ESRD patients. Chronic hyperkalemia between dialysis sessions can be controlled with daily oral potassium binders (patiromer, sodium zirconium cyclosilicate).[67] Caveats for practical management include dose adjustment for many antiarrhythmic medications including dofetilide and sotalol (Table 101.7). One randomized trial failed to find a benefit with prophylactic implantable cardioverter-defibrillator (ICD) insertion in dialysis patients with LVEF ≥35%.[68] Observational studies suggest that ESRD patients who survive a sudden death event have a favorable benefit to risk ratio favoring ICD implantation; however, rates of infection are higher and when they occur are associated with in-hospital mortality of approximately 14%.[69] Of concern, CKD, and ESRD in particular, may cause elevated defibrillation thresholds and failure of ICDs and are associated with high rates of shock and antitachycardia pacing therapy than patients with normal renal function.[70] Until this association

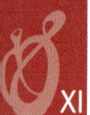

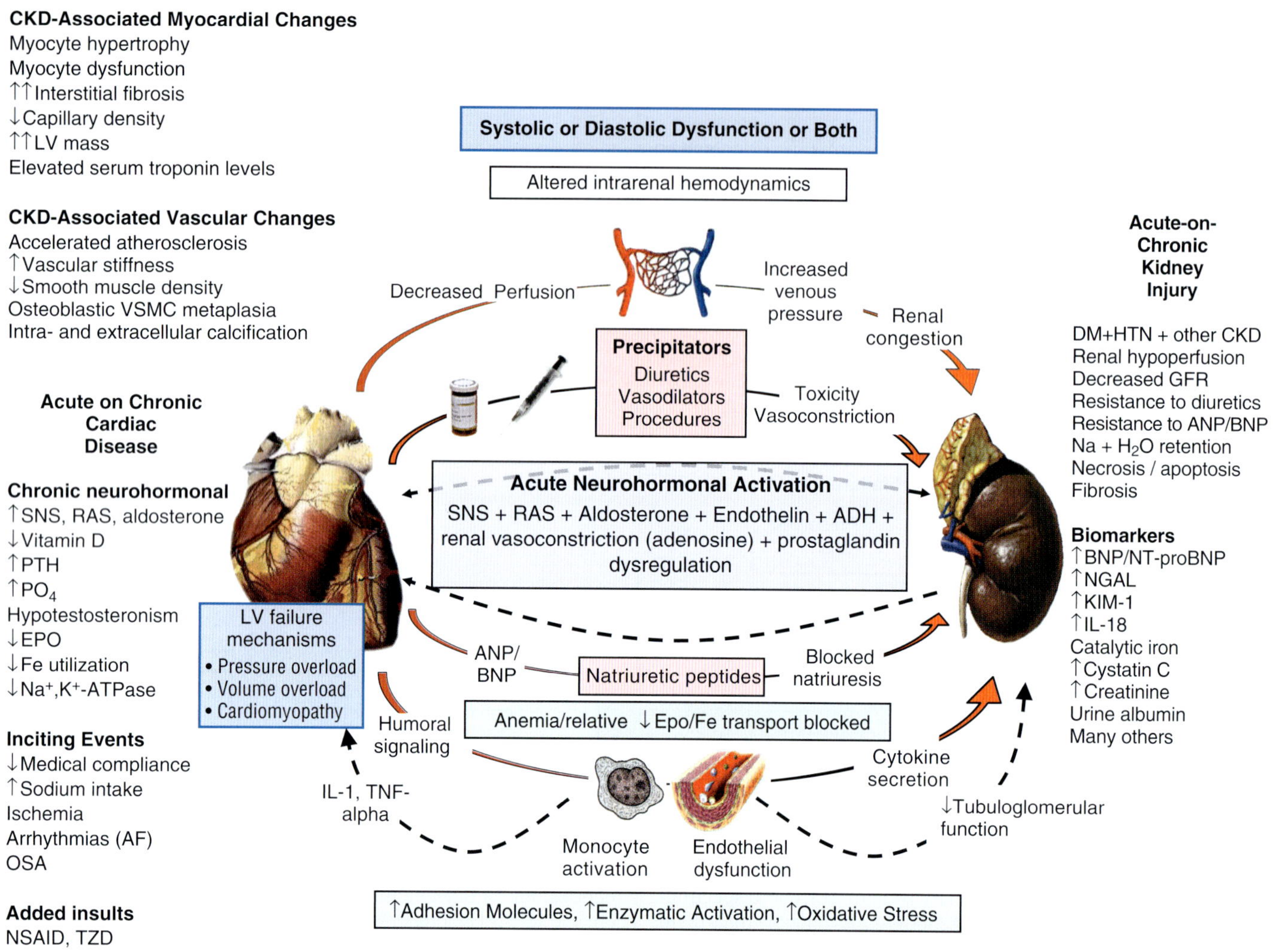

FIGURE 101.13 Pathophysiology of type 1 cardiorenal syndrome or worsening renal function after hospitalization for acutely decompensated heart failure. (Adapted from Herzog CA, Asinger RW, Berger AK, et al. Cardiovascular disease in chronic kidney disease. A clinical update from Kidney Disease: Improving Global Outcomes (KDIGO). *Kidney Int.* 2011;80[6]:572–586.)

is better understood, patients receiving ICDs should have frequent surveillance and consideration for noninvasive programmed stimulation for appropriate antitachycardia and defibrillation therapy.

CONSULTATIVE APPROACH TO SEVERE KIDNEY DISEASE AND HEMODIALYSIS PATIENTS

The prevalence of angiographically significant CAD ranges from 25% in young, non-diabetic hemodialysis patients, to 85% in older ESRD patients with long-standing DM.[71] Of those initiating dialysis, 87% have some structural abnormality on echocardiography including LVH, reduced LVEF, right ventricular hypertrophy or dysfunction, pulmonary HTN, or valvular disease.[72] Thus, many years of CKD must be associated with these progressive changes and we cannot attribute them solely to the dialysis procedure in most patients who are in the first few months of treatment. Cardiac death in dialysis patients younger than age 45 may be 100 times greater than that the general population. Medicare beneficiaries with CKD prior to initiation of dialysis are 60% more likely to have a billing claim submitted for the diagnosis of CVD and 70% more likely to have a claim submitted for "atherosclerotic heart disease." Of those claims incident to dialysis, a substantial proportion, perhaps the majority, have established CAD. In diabetic renal transplant candidates 30% will have one or more lesions with greater than 75% stenosis.[73] When comparing patients who undergo evaluation for CAD, those with ESRD have substantially more numerous, proximal, and severe coronary artery lesions, as well as more severe left ventricular dysfunction. The patient with incipient ESRD on dialysis can be considered the highest cardiovascular risk patient in medicine with expected rates of CHD death that exceed many-fold than that expected for a non-ESRD patient, even those with a burden of several cardiovascular risk factors.

Despite the use of multiple medications, most published series of ESRD patients from either clinical trials or registries indicate the mean systolic blood pressure is approximately 155 mm Hg. Indeed 80% of ESRD patients have HTN, which is adequately controlled in only 30%. Peritoneal dialysis, more frequent in-center, and home hemodialysis are all associated with much better blood pressure control than thrice-weekly hemodialysis.[74] Home hemodialysis for 5 or more days in the week is associated with approximately 45% relative risk reduction in HF but at approximately 25% excess risk of more frequent access site and endovascular infections.[75] Arteriovenous fistulas used for dialysis access cause recirculation of blood in one of the extremities (usually with upper arm), and depending on size and proximity, can account for as much as approximately 25% shunting, resulting in right ventricular volume overload and development of HF.[76] Long-term cardiorenal protection involves two important concepts; blood pressure control, and use of an agent that blocks the RAAS such as an ACEI or ARB as the base of therapy. The RAAS appears to have considerable redundancy and is able to maintain is function, if not increase its overall level of activity, without participation by the kidneys. Hence this hyperactivation of the RAAS is a target for therapy even in anephric patients

TABLE 101.6 Selected Therapies for Heart Failure in Patients with Chronic Kidney Disease

MEDICATION	USE	CKD POPULATION	PHARMACOLOGY
Dobutamine	Acutely decompensated heart failure with low cardiac output. Continuous infusion: 5.0–15 µg/kg/min IV Initial rate 5.0 µg/kg/min IV titrate 5–20 µg/kg/min; no more than 40 µg/kg/min	No specific dose adjustments for patients with CKD Recommend close monitoring for adverse effects including arrhythmias Doses <5.0 µg/kg/min may produce hypotension	Metabolism: methylation of the catechol and hepatic conjugation May increase renal clearance of other drugs in low cardiac output states
Milrinone	Acutely decompensated heart failure with low cardiac output. Loading dose of 50 µg/kg IV over 10 min, then start maintenance: 0.375–0.75 µg/kg/min	Recommended infusion rates (µg/kg/min) CrCl – mL/min/1.73 m^2 [CrCl >50]: No change [50]: 0.43 µg/kg/min [40]: 0.38 µg/kg/min [30]: 0.33 µg/kg/min [20]: 0.28 µg/kg/min [10]: 0.23 µg/kg/min [5]: 0.2 µg/kg/min	Excreted unchanged in the urine
Nesiritide	Acutely decompensated heart failure with pulmonary congestion. 2 µg/kg IV bolus over 1 min, then 0.01 µg/kg/min IV infusion. If hypotension, discontinue until stabilized, then restart at 30% lower dose	No specific dose adjustments for patients with CKD Recommend close monitoring for adverse effects including hypotension	Cleared by: (1) binding to cell surface clearance receptors with subsequent cellular internalization and lysosomal proteolysis; (2) proteolytic cleavage of the peptide by endopeptidases, such as neutral endopeptidase, which are present on the vascular luminal surface; and (3) renal filtration
Nitroprusside	Acutely decompensated heart failure with vasoconstriction 0.25–0.8 mg/kg/min IV	No specific dose adjustments for patients with CKD Recommend close monitoring for adverse effects including hypotension and thiocyanate accumulation	Intraerythrocytic reaction but hepatic and renal function impacts thiocyanate accumulation
Valsartan/Sacubitril	Chronic HF with reduced LVEF sacubitril/valsartan 24/26, 49/51, 97/103 mg orally twice daily	No specific dose adjustments for patients with CKD, monitor Cr, BUN, K$^+$, greater preservation of renal function compared to enalapril over time in HF	Metabolism: Sacubitril converted to LBQ657 by esterases, urine 52%–68%, feces 37%–48% Valsartan urine approximately 13%, feces 86%
Dapagliflozin	Chronic HF with LVEF ≤40% with or without type 2 diabetes	Start 10 mg po qd with eGFR >30 mL/min/1.73 m^2 and continue to ESRD, no dose adjustments based on renal function	Metabolism: glucuronidation in liver, 75% eliminated in urine, 21% in feces
Ivabradine	Chronic HF with LVEF <35% and heart rate >70 start 5 mg orally twice daily and may reduce to 2.5 mg or increase to 7.5 mg twice daily depending on heart rate and tolerability	No specific dose adjustments for patients with CKD	Metabolism: liver CYP450 CYP3A4 Excretion: feces 96%, urine 4%
Hydralazine	Acute and chronic HF, intolerant to RAAS blockers, 25–50 mg by mouth t.i.d. or q.i.d.	Dose q8–16 hr with CrCl <10 mL/min	Hepatic clearance, 25%–40% removed with dialysis
Digoxin	Chronic systolic and diastolic heart failure, atrial fibrillation with rapid ventricular rate 0.25 mg by mouth qd	0.125 mg po qd or q.o.d.	50%–70% excreted unchanged in the urine. The half-life in anuric patients is prolonged to 3.5–5 days. Digoxin is not effectively removed from the body by dialysis
Patiromer	Reduction of potassium and control of hyperkalemia	8.4 g po qd, advance up to 25.2 g po daily, in general take 3 hr away from other medications, can be used in HF, CKD, ESRD	Metabolism: none Elimination: fecal
Sodium Zirconium Cyclosilicate	Reduction of potassium and control of hyperkalemia	5 or 10 g po qd, in general take 2 hr away from other medications, can be used in HF, CKD, ESRD	Metabolism: none Elimination: fecal

CKD, Chronic kidney disease; *CrCl*, creatinine clearance; *eGFR*, estimated glomerular filtration rate; *ESRD*, end-stage renal disease; *HF*, heart failure; *IV*, intravenous; *LVEF*, left ventricular ejection fraction; *RAAS*, renin-angiotensin-aldosterone system.

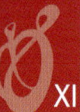

TABLE 101.7 Selected Anti-Arrhythmics in Patients with Chronic Kidney Disease

MEDICATION	USE	CKD POPULATION	PHARMACOLOGY
Amiodarone	Acute ventricular and acute and chronic atrial arrhythmias, First Rapid: 150 mg over 10 min (15 mg/min) Followed by Slow: 360 mg over 6 hr (1 mg/min) Maintenance infusion: 540 mg over the remaining 18 hr (0.5 mg/min) Oral 800–1600 mg/day in divided doses until a total of 10 g has been given; then 200–400 mg/day	No specific dose adjustments for patients with CKD	Eliminated primarily by hepatic metabolism and biliary excretion; negligible renal excretion
Dronedarone	Atrial fibrillation/atrial flutter 400 mg orally twice a day with morning and evening meals	No specific dose adjustments for patients with CKD	Dronedarone is extensively metabolized by the liver
Dofetilide	Atrial fibrillation/atrial flutter 500 µg p.o. bid initially. QTc interval should be measured 2–3 hr after the initial dose. If the QTc >15% of baseline, or if the QTc is >500 msec (550 msec in patients with ventricular conduction abnormalities), dofetilide should be adjusted. Continued monitoring for doses 2–5: QTc interval must be determined 2–3 hr after each subsequent dose of dofetilide for in-hospital doses 2–5. If the measured QTc is >500 msec (550 msec in patients with ventricular conduction abnormalities) dofetilide should be stopped	[CrCl >60 mL/min]: 500 µg bid [40–60 mL/min]: 250 µg twice daily. [20–39 mL/min]: 125 µg twice daily. [<20 mL/min]: Contraindicated	Hepatic metabolism accounts for 20%–30%, 70%–80% renal elimination
Sotalol	Atrial fibrillation/atrial flutter 80–160 mg orally twice a day	CrCl 30–59 mL/min: The dosage interval should be increased to 24 hr. CrCl 10–29 mL/min: The dosage interval should be increased to 36–48 hr. CrCl less than 10 mL/min: Dose should be individualized.	Excreted unchanged in the kidney. Removed with dialysis

CKD, Chronic kidney disease; *CrCl*, creatinine clearance.

since ACEI/ARB can reduce LVH and possibly improve survival. A small trial demonstrated that ramipril can preserve residual urine output in those receiving peritoneal dialysis, which is a consistently favorable finding in ESRD.[77] A case-matched study of ESRD patients found that those who were taking ACEI or ARB had improved survival and this benefit appeared to get larger for longer durations of use.[78] ACEI/ARB therapy may worsen hyperkalemia in patients with ESRD. As tolerated, the clinician should consider adjusting the dialysis regimen to improve potassium removal and/or daily use of oral potassium binders.[79]

With an ACEI/ARB as a base of therapy, the antihypertensive regimen can be further modified according to blood pressure–lowering efficacy and CAD event reduction. Beta-blockers can be used as both an anti-hypertensive and anti-ischemic agents. In those with HF, beta-blockers improve left ventricular ejection fraction, and reduce rates of hospitalization, sudden death, and all-cause mortality. Patients with ESRD who receive beta-blockers after CAD events may have large relative risk reductions in all-cause mortality.

Additional choices of anti-hypertensive or cardioprotective agents should be based on ease of management and compliance, and lack of adverse effects. Guidelines for non-ESRD patients state the optimal office systolic blood pressure should be less than 130 mm Hg. The difficult task in the ESRD patient is to achieve these goals without having hypotension during dialysis sessions. Given the high rates of severe CAD in ESRD, hypotension during dialysis can worsen clinical and subclinical ischemia recognized as chest discomfort, shortness of breath, ST-segment depression on electrocardiography, and elevations of cTn on blood testing.

The goal of LDL-C reduction, in most cases with a statin and ezetimibe, in patients with ESRD is supported by a 17% reduction in major atherosclerotic events shown in the Study of Heart and Renal Protection in patients with predialysis CKD and ESRD.[80] Monoclonal antibodies against proprotein convertase subtilisin kexin 9 (PCSK9) can be used in CKD and ESRD to lower LDL-C in addition to maximally tolerated lipid-lowering therapy.[81] These agents additionally lower lipoprotein (a), which is commonly elevated in ESRD.[82] Colesevelam, a bile-acid sequestrant, also can aid in lowering serum phosphorus. Because of competing risk and reduced survival in CKD and ESRD, there are no trials demonstrating a mortality benefit with lipid-lowering therapy.

In ESRD with DM, blood glucose control to a target glycohemoglobin less than 7% can be expected to reduce rates of microvascular complications (retinopathy) and to a lesser extent, clinically important atherosclerotic disease elsewhere (MI, stroke, CVD death).[89] Patients with ESRD should stop smoking. The use of antiplatelet or antithrombotic agents for the prevention of CVD risk in ESRD requires caution.

In the setting of stable symptomatic CAD, an analysis from the Clinical Outcomes Utilizing Revascularization and Aggressive Drug Evaluation (COURAGE) trial suggested that PCI had no benefit over optimal medical therapy in patients with predialysis CKD.[83] The ISCHEMIA-CKD trial randomized 777 patients with moderate coronary ischemia and CKD (eGFR = 23 mL/min/1.73 m^2) or on dialysis (51%) to an initial invasive strategy consisting of coronary angiography and revascularization (if appropriate) versus medical therapy alone and angiography reserved for those in whom medical therapy had failed.[84] While the rates of MI or cardiovascular death at 2.2 years were high (approximately 36.5%) in both groups, there was no benefit observed with the invasive approach. After symptomatic failure of optimal medical therapy in a patient with ESRD and CAD, the next step is coronary angiography and consideration of revascularization. In the common scenario of multivessel disease, multiple studies have shown that coronary artery bypass graft (CABG) surgery is associated with superior outcomes over PCI with drug-eluting stents probably due to more complete revascularization and protection from recurrent MI.[85] Patients with ESRD undergoing coronary revascularization procedures have increased risk for adverse events including death. Dialysis-dependent patients undergoing CABG face a 4.4-fold increased risk of in-hospital death, a 3.1 times greater risk of mediastinitis, and a 2.6-fold increased risk of stroke compared to those patients undergoing CABG who were not on dialysis.[48]

In summary, patients with ESRD have greater coronary heart disease risk than those with equivalent risk factor status without ESRD. An aggressive approach with medical management for CAD is warranted, even in the case of subclinical CAD. The threshold for diagnostic testing should be low in ESRD patients. When significant multivessel CAD is found, ESRD patients appear to benefit from revascularization with CABG compared to PCI, and if clinically reasonable, should be given that opportunity for improved survival and reduction in future cardiac events.

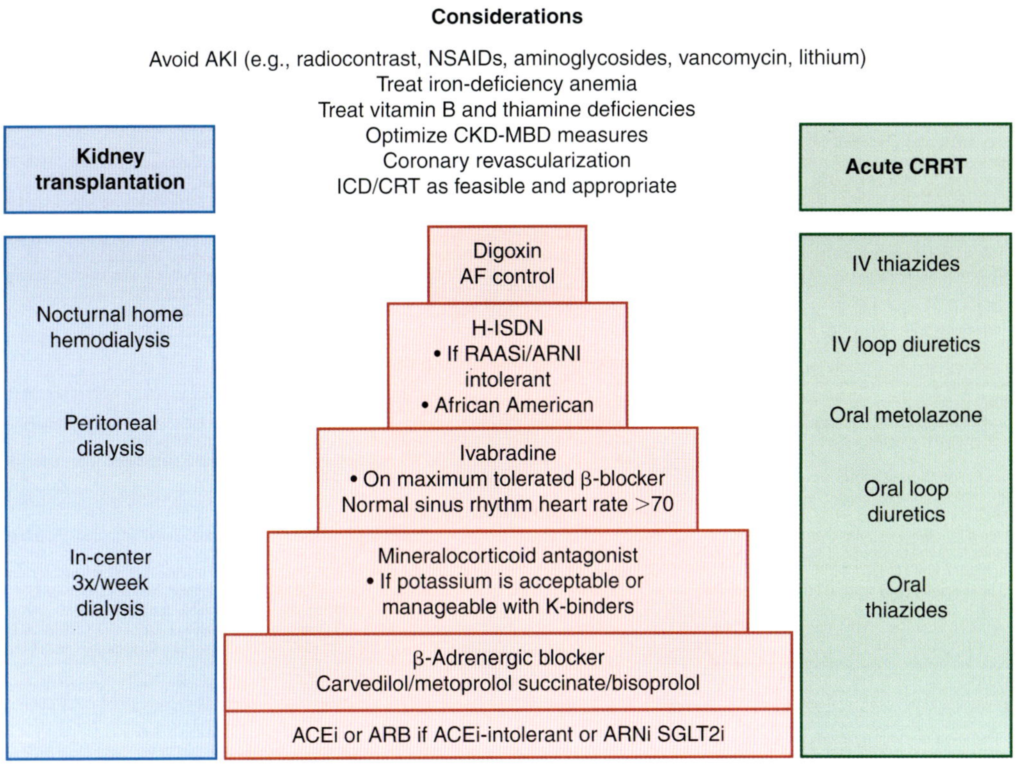
Considerations
Avoid AKI (e.g., radiocontrast, NSAIDs, aminoglycosides, vancomycin, lithium)
Treat iron-deficiency anemia
Treat vitamin B and thiamine deficiencies
Optimize CKD-MBD measures
Coronary revascularization
ICD/CRT as feasible and appropriate
Kidney transplantation
Nocturnal home hemodialysis
Peritoneal dialysis
In-center 3x/week dialysis
Digoxin
AF control
H-ISDN
• If RAASi/ARNI intolerant
• African American
Ivabradine
• On maximum tolerated β-blocker
Normal sinus rhythm heart rate >70
Mineralocorticoid antagonist
• If potassium is acceptable or manageable with K-binders
β-Adrenergic blocker
Carvedilol/metoprolol succinate/bisoprolol
ACEi or ARB if ACEi-intolerant or ARNi SGLT2i
Acute CRRT
IV thiazides
IV loop diuretics
Oral metolazone
Oral loop diuretics
Oral thiazides

FIGURE 101.14 Pharmacotherapy for the prevention and treatment of heart failure with reduced ejection fraction in chronic kidney disease (CKD) progressing to end-stage kidney disease. *ACEi,* Angiotensin-converting enzyme inhibitor; *AF,* atrial fibrillation; *AKI,* acute kidney injury; *ARB,* angiotensin II receptor blocker; *ARNi,* angiotensin receptor neprilysin inhibitor; *CKD-MBD,* chronic kidney disease–mineral bone disorder; *CRT,* cardiac resynchronization therapy; *CRRT,* continuous renal replacement therapy; *H-ISDN,* hydralazine-isosorbide dinitrate; *ICD,* implantable cardioverter-defibrillator; *NSAID,* nonsteroidal anti-inflammatory drug; *RAASi,* renin-angiotensin-aldosterone system inhibitor; *SGLT2i,* sodium glucose cotransporter 2 inhibitor. (Adapted from House AA, Wanner C, Sarnak MJ, et al. Heart failure in chronic kidney disease: conclusions from a Kidney Disease: Improving Global Outcomes (KDIGO) Controversies Conference. *Kidney Int.* 2019;95[6]:1304–1317.)

EVALUATION AND MANAGEMENT OF THE RENAL TRANSPLANT RECIPIENT

Cardiovascular screening is recommended in high-risk CKD patients before renal transplantation.[86] These include persons with DM, men over age 45 years, women over 55 years, previous history of ischemic heart disease, an abnormal electrocardiogram, left ventricular dysfunction, smoking history, and duration of dialysis more than 2 years. Controversies exist regarding the ideal screening test for CAD in ESRD patients. The choice of exercise versus pharmacologic stress and echocardiographic versus nuclear scintigraphic imaging requires individualization. Coronary cardiac computed tomographic angiography may be considered as another screening tool especially in the young with the understanding that it can exclude significant coronary disease and identify very-low-risk patients who may move on to renal transplantation.[87] However, substantial coronary artery calcification can render the interpretation of the computed tomographic angiogram difficult (see Chapter 20.) Coronary angiography and revascularization can be performed with very little loss of renal function in very low eGFR groups if done carefully with staged intervals between the diagnostic procedure and PCI or CABG.[88] After renal transplantation, treatment with lipid-lowering therapy (low potency statins, i.e., fluvastatin, pravastatin), is generally associated with a favorable benefit-to-risk ratio.[89] A meta-analysis of 22 studies (3465 participants) has supported the use of statins in renal transplant recipients for the reduction of cardiovascular events.[90] Finally, renal transplantation confers a relative freedom from the development of HF and associated complications and can be considered as a therapy in the overall schema of managing patients with combined heart and kidney failure (Fig. 101.14).[91]

SUMMARY

Recognition has increased over the last several decades that patients with CKD have a high risk for CVD. Frequent clinical scenarios in which renal function influences care include PCI, cardiac surgery, ACS, HF, valvular disease, and arrhythmias. Further study of the adverse metabolic milieu of CKD is likely to lead to generalizable diagnostic and therapeutic targets for the future management of renal patients with cardiovascular illness.

REFERENCES

Chronic Kidney Disease and Cardiovascular Risk

1. Szczech LA, Stewart RC, Su HL, et al. Primary care detection of chronic kidney disease in adults with type-2 diabetes: the ADD-CKD Study (awareness, detection and drug therapy in type 2 diabetes and chronic kidney disease). *PloS One.* 2014;9(11):e110535.
2. Ritz E, Zeng X-X, Rychlík I. Clinical manifestation and natural history of diabetic nephropathy. *Contrib Nephrol.* 2011;170:19–27.
3. Kruzel-Davila E, Wasser WG, Aviram S, Skorecki K. APOL1 nephropathy: from gene to mechanisms of kidney injury. *Nephrol Dial Transplant.* 2016;31(3):349–358.
4. Herzog CA, Asinger RW, Berger AK, et al. Cardiovascular disease in chronic kidney disease. a clinical update from kidney disease: improving Global Outcomes (KDIGO). *Kidney Int.* 2011;80(6):572–586.
5. Levey AS, Inker LA, Coresh J. GFR estimation: from physiology to public health. *Am J Kidney Dis.* 2014;63(5):820–834.
6. Ferguson TW, Komenda P, Tangri N. Cystatin C as a biomarker for estimating glomerular filtration rate. *Curr Opin Nephrol Hypertens.* 2015;24(3):295–300.
7. Amin AP, Whaley-Connell AT, Li S, et al. The synergistic relationship between estimated GFR and microalbuminuria in predicting long-term progression to ESRD or death in patients with diabetes: results from the Kidney Early Evaluation Program (KEEP). *Am J Kidney Dis.* 2013;61(4 suppl 2):S12–S23.
8. Matsushita K, Coresh J, Sang Y, et al. Estimated glomerular filtration rate and albuminuria for prediction of cardiovascular outcomes: a collaborative meta-analysis of individual participant data. *Lancet Diabetes Endocrinol.* 2015;3(7):514–525.
9. Palmer SC, Navaneethan SD, Craig JC, et al. Meta-analysis: erythropoiesis-stimulating agents in patients with chronic kidney disease. *Ann Intern Med.* 2010;153(1):23–33.
10. Covic A, Nistor I, Donciu MD, et al. Erythropoiesis-stimulating agents (ESA) for preventing the progression of chronic kidney disease: a meta-analysis of 19 studies. *Am J Nephrol.* 2014;40(3):263–279.
11. Collister D, Komenda P, Hiebert B, et al. The effect of erythropoietin-stimulating agents on health-related quality of life in anemia of chronic kidney disease: a systematic review and meta-analysis. *Ann Intern Med.* 2016;164(7):472–478.
12. Swedberg K, Young JB, Anand IS, et al. Treatment of anemia with darbepoetin alfa in systolic heart failure. *N Engl J Med.* 2013;368(13):1210–1219.
13. McCullough PA, Barnhart HX, Inrig JK, et al. Cardiovascular toxicity of epoetin-alfa in patients with chronic kidney disease. *Am J Nephrol.* 2013;37(6):549–558.
14. McCullough PA, Uhlig K, Neylan JF, et al. Usefulness of oral ferric citrate in patients with iron-deficiency anemia and chronic kidney disease with or without heart failure. *Am J Cardiol.* 2018;122(4):683–688.
15. Clevenger B, Gurusamy K, Klein AA, et al. Systematic review and meta-analysis of iron therapy in anaemic adults without chronic kidney disease: updated and abridged Cochrane review. *Eur J Heart Fail.* 2016.
16. Jankowska EA, Tkaczyszyn M, Suchocki T, et al. Effects of intravenous iron therapy in iron-deficient patients with systolic heart failure: a meta-analysis of randomized controlled trials. *Eur J Heart Fail.* 2016.
17. Maxwell PH, Eckardt KU. HIF prolyl hydroxylase inhibitors for the treatment of renal anaemia and beyond. *Nat Rev Nephrol.* 2016;12(3):157–168.
18. Chen N, Hao C, Liu BC, et al. Roxadustat treatment for anemia in patients undergoing long-term dialysis. *N Engl J Med.* 2019;381(11):1011–1022.
19. Liu J, Zhang A, Hayden JC, et al. Roxadustat (FG-4592) treatment for anemia in dialysis-dependent (DD) and not dialysis-dependent (NDD) chronic kidney disease patients: a systematic review and meta-analysis. *Pharmacol Res.* 2020;155:104747.

Contrast-Induced and Intervention-Associated Acute Kidney Injury

20. KDIGO AKI Work Group. KDIGO clinical practice guideline for acute kidney injury. *Kidney Int Suppl.* 2012;17:1–138.

21. Tsai TT, Patel UD, Chang TI, et al. Contemporary incidence, predictors, and outcomes of acute kidney injury in patients undergoing percutaneous coronary interventions: insights from the NCDR cath-PCI registry. *JACC Cardiovasc Interv.* 2014;7(1):1–9.
22. McCullough PA, Choi JP, Feghali GA, et al. Contrast-induced acute kidney injury. *J Am Coll Cardiol.* 2016;68(13):1465–1473.
23. Keeley EC, Grines CL. Scraping of aortic debris by coronary guiding catheters: a prospective evaluation of 1,000 cases. *J Am Coll Cardiol.* 1998;32(7):1861–1865.
24. Kooiman J, Seth M, Dixon S, et al. Risk of acute kidney injury after percutaneous coronary interventions using radial versus femoral vascular access: insights from the Blue Cross Blue Shield of Michigan Cardiovascular Consortium. *Circ Cardiovasc Interv.* 2014;7(2):190–198.
25. Cortese B, Sciahbasi A, Sebik R, et al. Comparison of risk of acute kidney injury after primary percutaneous coronary interventions with the transradial approach versus the transfemoral approach (from the PRIPITENA urban registry). *Am J Cardiol.* 2014;114(6):820–825.
26. Mehran R, Aymong ED, Nikolsky E, et al. A simple risk score for prediction of contrast-induced nephropathy after percutaneous coronary intervention: development and initial validation. *J Am Coll Cardiol.* 2004;44(7):1393–1399.
27. Solomon R, Gordon P, Manoukian SV, et al. Randomized trial of bicarbonate or saline study for the prevention of contrast-induced nephropathy in patients with CKD. *Clin J Am Soc Nephrol.* 2015;10(9):1519–1524.
28. Brar SS, Shen AY, Jorgensen MB, et al. Sodium bicarbonate vs sodium chloride for the prevention of contrast medium-induced nephropathy in patients undergoing coronary angiography: a randomized trial. *J Am Med Assoc.* 2008;300(9):1038–1046.
29. McCullough PA, Brown JR. Effects of intra-arterial and intravenous iso-osmolar contrast medium (iodixanol) on the risk of contrast-induced acute kidney injury: a meta-analysis. *Cardiorenal Med.* 2011;1(4):220–234.
30. Andò G, Gragnano F, Calabrò P, Valgimigli M. Radial vs femoral access for the prevention of acute kidney injury (AKI) after coronary angiography or intervention: a systematic review and meta-analysis. *Catheter Cardiovasc Interv.* 2018;92(7):E518-E526.
31. ACT Investigators. Acetylcysteine for prevention of renal outcomes in patients undergoing coronary and peripheral vascular angiography: main results from the randomized Acetylcysteine for Contrast-induced nephropathy Trial (ACT). *Circulation.* 2011;124(11):1250–1259.
32. Weisbord SD, Gallagher M, Jneid H, et al. Outcomes after angiography with sodium bicarbonate and acetylcysteine. *N Engl J Med.* 2018;378(7):603–614.
33. Tecson KM, Brown D, Choi JW, et al. Major adverse renal and cardiac events after coronary angiography and cardiac surgery. *Ann Thorac Surg.* 2018;105(6):1724–1730.
34. O'Neal JB, Shaw AD, Billings 4th FT. Acute kidney injury following cardiac surgery: current understanding and future directions. *Crit Care.* 2016;20(1):187.

Acceleration of Vascular Calcification

35. Raggi P, Chertow GM, Torres PU, et al. The ADVANCE study: a randomized study to evaluate the effects of cinacalcet plus low-dose vitamin D on vascular calcification in patients on hemodialysis. *Nephrol Dial Transplant.* 2011;26(4):1327–1339.
36. EVOLVE Trial Investigators, Chertow GM, Block GA, et al. Effect of cinacalcet on cardiovascular disease in patients undergoing dialysis. *N Engl J Med.* 2012;367(26):2482–2494.
37. Charytan DM, Fishbane S, Malyszko J, et al. Cardiorenal syndrome and the role of the bone-mineral axis and anemia. *Am J Kidney Dis.* 2015;66(2):196–205.

Renal Disease and Hypertension

38. Khouri Y, Steigerwalt SP, Alsamara M, McCullough PA. What is the ideal blood pressure goal for patients with stage III or higher chronic kidney disease?. *Curr Cardiol Rep.* 2011;13(6):492–501.
39. Beddhu S, Shen J, Cheung AK, et al. Implications of early decline in eGFR due to intensive BP control for cardiovascular outcomes in SPRINT. *J Am Soc Nephrol.* 2019;30(8):1523–1533.
40. Cohen MG, Pascua JA, Garcia-Ben M, et al. A simple prediction rule for significant renal artery stenosis in patients undergoing cardiac catheterization. *Am Heart J.* 2005;150(6):1204–1211.
41. Akinseye OA, Ralston WF, Johnson KC, et al. Renal sympathetic denervation: a comprehensive review [published online ahead of print, 2020 may 3]. *Curr Probl Cardiol.* 2020:100598.

Acute Coronary Syndromes in Patients with Chronic Kidney Disease

42. Twerenbold R, Wildi K, Jaeger C, et al. Optimal cutoff levels of more sensitive cardiac troponin assays for the early diagnosis of myocardial infarction in patients with renal dysfunction. *Circulation.* 2015;131(23):2041–2050.
43. deFilippi C, Seliger SL, Kelley W, et al. Interpreting cardiac troponin results from high-sensitivity assays in chronic kidney disease without acute coronary syndrome. *Clin Chem.* 2012;58(9):1342–1351.
44. Vasudevan A, Singer AJ, DeFilippi C, et al. Renal function and scaled troponin in patients presenting to the emergency department with symptoms of myocardial infarction. *Am J Nephrol.* 2017;45(4):304–309.
45. Fox CS, Muntner P, Chen AY, et al. Acute Coronary Treatment and Intervention Outcomes Network registry. Use of evidence-based therapies in short-term outcomes of ST-segment elevation myocardial infarction and non-ST-segment elevation myocardial infarction in patients with chronic kidney disease: a report from the National Cardiovascular Data Acute Coronary Treatment and Intervention Outcomes Network registry. *Circulation.* 2010;121(3):357–365.
46. McCullough PA. Why is chronic kidney disease the "spoiler" for cardiovascular outcomes?. *J Am Coll Cardiol.* 2003;41(5):725–728.
47. Sica D. The implications of renal impairment among patients undergoing percutaneous coronary intervention. *J Invasive Cardiol.* 2002;14(suppl B):30B-37B.
48. Roberts JK, McCullough PA. The management of acute coronary syndromes in patients with chronic kidney disease. *Adv Chronic Kidney Dis.* 2014;21(6):472–479.
49. Szummer K, Lundman P, Jacobson SH, et al. Influence of renal function on the effects of early revascularization in non-ST-Elevation myocardial infarction: data from the Swedish web-system for enhancement and development of evidence-based care in heart disease evaluated according to recommended therapies (SWEDEHEART). *Circulation.* 2009;120(10):851–858.

Cardiorenal Syndromes

50. McCullough PA, Kluger AY. Interpreting the wide range of NT-proBNP concentrations in clinical decision making. *J Am Coll Cardiol.* 2018;71(11):1201–1203.
51. Rangaswami J, Bhalla V, Blair JEA, et al. American heart association council on the kidney in cardiovascular disease and council on clinical cardiology. Cardiorenal syndrome: classification, Pathophysiology, diagnosis, and treatment strategies: a scientific statement from the American heart association. *Circulation.* 2019;139(16):e840–e878.
52. Haase M, Müller C, Damman K, et al. Pathogenesis of cardiorenal syndrome type 1 in acute decompensated heart failure: workgroup statements from the eleventh consensus conference of the Acute Dialysis Quality Initiative (ADQI). *Contrib Nephrol.* 2013;182:99–116.
53. Oliveros E, Oni ET, Shahzad A, et al. Benefits and risks of continuing angiotensin-converting enzyme inhibitors, angiotensin II receptor antagonists, and mineralocorticoid receptor antagonists during hospitalizations for acute heart failure. *Cardiorenal Med.* 2020;10(2):69–84.
54. Singhania G, Ejaz AA, McCullough PA, et al. Continuation of chronic heart failure therapies during heart failure hospitalization - a review. *Rev Cardiovasc Med.* 2019;20(3):111–120.

55. Gunderson EG, Lillyblad MP, Fine M, et al. Tolvaptan for volume management in heart failure. *Pharmacotherapy.* 2019;39(4):473–485.
56. Costanzo MR, Ronco C, Abraham WT, et al. Extracorporeal ultrafiltration for fluid overload in heart failure: current status and prospects for further research. *J Am Coll Cardiol.* 2017;69(19):2428–2445.
57. Weinhandl ED, Gilbertson DT, Collins AJ. Mortality, hospitalization, and technique failure in daily home hemodialysis and matched peritoneal dialysis patients: a matched cohort study. *Am J Kidney Dis.* 2016;67(1):98–110.
58. Kluger AY, Tecson KM, Barbin CM, et al. Cardiorenal outcomes in the canvas, DECLARE-TIMI 58, and EMPA-REG outcome trials: a systematic review. *Rev Cardiovasc Med.* 2018;19(2):41–49.
59. Kluger AY, Tecson KM, et al. Class effects of SGLT2 inhibitors on cardiorenal outcomes. *Cardiovasc Diabetol.* 2019;18(1):99.
60. Lo KB, Gul F, Ram P, et al. The effects of SGLT2 inhibitors on cardiovascular and renal outcomes in diabetic patients: a systematic review and meta-analysis. *Cardiorenal Med.* 2020;10(1):1–10.
61. Roberts WC, Taylor MA, Shirani J. Cardiac findings at necropsy in patients with chronic kidney disease maintained on chronic hemodialysis. *Medicine (Baltim).* 2012;91(3):165–178.
62. Roberts WC, Taylor MA, Shirani J. Cardiac findings at necropsy in patients with chronic kidney disease maintained on chronic hemodialysis. *Medicine (Baltim).* 2012;91(3):165–178.

Chronic Kidney Disease and Valvular Heart Disease

63. Kim D, Shim CY, Hong GR, et al. Effect of end-stage renal disease on rate of progression of aortic stenosis. *Am J Cardiol.* 2016;117(12):1972–1977.
64. Kamalakannan D, Pai RM, Johnson LB, et al. Epidemiology and clinical outcomes of infective endocarditis in hemodialysis patients. *Ann Thorac Surg.* 2007;83(6):2081–2086.
65. Altarabsheh SE, Deo SV, Dunlay SM, et al. Tissue valves are preferable for patients with end-stage renal disease: an aggregate meta-analysis. *J Card Surg.* 2016.

Renal Function and Arrhythmias

66. Pun PH, Lehrich RW, Honeycutt EF, et al. Modifiable risk factors associated with sudden cardiac arrest within hemodialysis clinics. *Kidney Int.* 2011;79(2):218–227.
67. Palmer BF. Potassium binders for hyperkalemia in chronic kidney disease-diet, renin-angiotensin-aldosterone system inhibitor therapy, and hemodialysis. *Mayo Clin Proc.* 2020;95(2):339–354.
68. Jukema JW, Timal RJ, Rotmans JI, et al. Prophylactic use of implantable cardioverter-defibrillators in the prevention of sudden cardiac death in dialysis patients. *Circulation.* 2019;139(23):2628–2638.
69. Opelami O, Sakhuja A, Liu X, et al. Outcomes of infected cardiovascular implantable devices in dialysis patients. *Am J Nephrol.* 2014;40(3):280–287.
70. Hage FG, Aljaroudi W, Aggarwal H, et al. Outcomes of patients with chronic kidney disease and implantable cardiac defibrillator: primary versus secondary prevention. *Int J Cardiol.* 2013;165(1):113–116.

Consultative Approach to the Hemodialysis Patient

71. De Vriese AS, Vandecasteele SJ, Van den Bergh B, De Geeter FW. Should we screen for coronary artery disease in asymptomatic chronic dialysis patients?. *Kidney Int.* 2012;81(2):143–151.
72. McCullough PA, Roberts WC. Influence of chronic renal failure on cardiac structure. *J Am Coll Cardiol.* 2016;67(10):1183–1185.
73. De Lima JJ, Gowdak LH, de Paula FJ, et al. Coronary artery disease assessment and intervention in renal transplant patients: analysis from the KiHeart cohort. *Transplantation.* 2016;100(7):1580–1587.
74. Kotanko P, Garg AX, Depner T, et al. Effects of frequent hemodialysis on blood pressure: results from the randomized frequent hemodialysis network trials. *Hemodial Int.* 2015;19(3):386–401.
75. McCullough PA, Chan CT, Weinhandl ED, et al. Intensive hemodialysis, left ventricular hypertrophy, and cardiovascular disease. *Am J Kidney Dis.* 2016;68(5S1):S5-S14.
76. Rao NN, Dundon BK, Worthley MI, Faull RJ. The impact of arteriovenous fistulae for hemodialysis on the cardiovascular system. *Semin Dial.* 2016;29(3):214–221.
77. Li PK, Chow KM, Wong TY, et al. Effects of an angiotensin-converting enzyme inhibitor on residual renal function in patients receiving peritoneal dialysis. A randomized, controlled study. *Ann Intern Med.* 2003;139(2):105–112. PubMed PMID: 12859160.
78. Wu CK, Yang YH, Juang JM, et al. Effects of angiotensin converting enzyme inhibition or angiotensin receptor blockade in dialysis patients: a nationwide data survey and propensity analysis. *Medicine (Baltim).* 2015;94(3):e424.
79. McCullough PA, Costanzo MR, Silver M, et al. Novel agents for the prevention and management of hyperkalemia. *Rev Cardiovasc Med.* 2015;16(2):140–155. Review. PubMed PMID: 26198561.
80. Baigent C, Landray MJ, Reith C, et al. The effects of lowering LDL cholesterol with simvastatin plus ezetimibe in patients with chronic kidney disease (Study of Heart and Renal Protection): a randomised placebo-controlled trial. *Lancet.* 2011;377(9784):2181–2192.
81. Charytan DM, Sabatine MS, Pedersen TR, et al. Efficacy and safety of evolocumab in chronic kidney disease in the FOURIER trial. *J Am Coll Cardiol.* 2019;73(23):2961–2970.
82. Watts GF, Chan DC, Pang J, et al. PCSK9 Inhibition with alirocumab increases the catabolism of lipoprotein(a) particles in statin-treated patients with elevated lipoprotein(a). *Metabolism.* 2020;107:154221.
83. Sedlis SP, Jurkovitz CT, Hartigan PM, et al. Optimal medical therapy with or without percutaneous coronary intervention for patients with stable coronary artery disease and chronic kidney disease. *Am J Cardiol.* 2009;104(12):1647–1653.
84. Bangalore S, Maron DJ, O'Brien SM, et al. Management of coronary disease in patients with advanced kidney disease. *N Engl J Med.* 2020;382(17):1608–1618.
85. Ashrith G, Lee VV, Elayda MA, et al. Short- and long-term outcomes of coronary artery bypass grafting or drug-eluting stent implantation for multivessel coronary artery disease in patients with chronic kidney disease. *Am J Cardiol.* 2010;106(3):348–353.
86. Lentine KL, Costa SP, Weir MR, et al. American heart association council on the kidney in cardiovascular disease and council on peripheral vascular disease. cardiac disease evaluation and management among kidney and liver transplantation candidates: a scientific statement from the American heart association and the American college of cardiology foundation. *J Am Coll Cardiol.* 2012;60(5):434–480.
87. Winther S, Svensson M, Jørgensen HS, et al. Diagnostic performance of coronary CT angiography and myocardial perfusion imaging in kidney transplantation candidates. *JACC Cardiovasc Imaging.* 2015;8(5):553–562.
88. Kumar N, Dahri L, Brown W, et al. Effect of elective coronary angiography on glomerular filtration rate in patients with advanced chronic kidney disease. *Clin J Am Soc Nephrol.* 2009;4(12):1907–1913.
89. Riella LV, Gabardi S, Chandraker A. Dyslipidemia and its therapeutic challenges in renal transplantation. *Am J Transplant.* 2012;12(8):1975–1982.
90. Palmer SC, Navaneethan SD, Craig JC, et al. HMG CoA reductase inhibitors (statins) for kidney transplant recipients. *Cochrane Database Syst Rev.* 2014;(1):CD005019.
91. House AA, Wanner C, Sarnak MJ, et al. Heart failure in chronic kidney disease: conclusions from a kidney disease: Improving Global Outcomes (KDIGO) Controversies conference. *Kidney Int.* 2019;95(6):1304–1317.

102 Cardiovascular Manifestations of Autonomic Disorders

JASON S. BRADFIELD AND KALYANAM SHIVKUMAR

OVERVIEW OF ANATOMY AND PHYSIOLOGY OF THE AUTONOMIC NERVOUS SYSTEM, 1893
Sympathetic, Parasympathetic, and Intrinsic Neuronal Control, 1893
Baroreflex, 1894
Chemoreflex, 1895
Diving Reflex, 1896

PATHOPHYSIOLOGY, 1896
Autonomic Dysfunction in the Setting of a Structurally Normal Heart, 1896

Autonomic Dysfunction in the Setting of Intrinsic Cardiac Disease, 1897

PROARRHYTHMIA, 1897
Atrial Fibrillation, 1897
Ventricular Tachycardia/Ventricular Fibrillation, 1897

INVESTIGATIONS AND DIAGNOSIS, 1897
Orthostatic Blood Pressure, 1897
Valsalva Maneuver, 1897
Cold Pressor Test, 1898
Plasma Catecholamines, 1898

NEUROMODULATORY THERAPIES, 1898
Pharmacologic Therapy, 1898
Sympathetic Modulation, 1899
Thoracic Epidural Anesthesia/Percutaneous Stellate Block, 1899
Renal Denervation, 1899
Cardiac Sympathetic Denervation, 1899
Augmentation of Parasympathetic Drive, 1899

FUTURE PERSPECTIVES, 1900

REFERENCES, 1902

The critical role of a balanced autonomic nervous system for appropriate function and responsiveness of the cardiovascular system is often overlooked. The interrelationship of these two systems is often thought of predominantly through the lens of abnormalities in blood pressure and heart rate in response to internal and external stimuli in patients with structurally "normal hearts" or secondary to primary neurologic abnormalities. However, the cardiovascular manifestations of autonomic dysfunction are much more complex. Autonomic dysfunction/dysregulation can be caused by direct cardiac insults, leading to abnormal afferent signaling and local remodeling subsequent progression to cardiac disorders from heart failure to atrial and ventricular arrhythmias and sudden cardiac death.

This chapter reviews cardiovascular autonomic anatomy and physiology in health and disease with further discussion of primary and secondary cardiovascular autonomic dysfunction and how this dysfunction can lead to benign as well as life-threatening disorders.

OVERVIEW OF ANATOMY AND PHYSIOLOGY OF THE AUTONOMIC NERVOUS SYSTEM

The autonomic nervous system regulates heart rate, cardiac contractility, and blood pressure and responds on a beat-to-beat basis to physiologic stress. This real-time response allows individuals to adjust to the external environment as well as to physiologic changes in multiple organ systems. Therefore, the "environment" that the autonomic nervous system is responding to is both internal and external encompassing a broad spectrum of stimuli including cardiovascular afferents, pressure, and volume sensors, as well as postural and visual stimuli.

Sympathetic, Parasympathetic, and Intrinsic Neuronal Control

The anatomy and physiology of the cardiovascular autonomic nervous system is a complex interplay of sympathetic, parasympathetic, and intrinsic neurons in addition to a number of well-established reflexes (Fig. 102.1). In addition to direct afferent and efferent connections between the brain and central nervous system and the heart and vascular system that control all aspects of cardiac physiologic function, visceral integration and reflexes maintain and optimize blood pressure. The sympathetic and parasympathetic systems are often thought of as opposing forces; however the intricate feedback between these systems, the intrinsic cardiac nervous system, and numerous reflex arcs allows for highly refined regulation of cardiac electrical and mechanical function.

Cardiac autonomic nerves can anatomically be broken down into central, intrathoracic, and intrinsic cardiac components.[1,2] The cardiac intrinsic components are located in the epicardial fat pads and cardiac ganglia. These ganglionated plexi include afferent, efferent, and interconnecting neurons. The ganglia (located in the region of the posterior left atrium, aortopulmonary window, anterior/posterior right atrium, and junction of the inferior vena cava and inferior right atrium) give input to the sinus and atrioventricular nodes (Fig. 102.2). The left and right cardiac nerves are a combination of sympathetic and parasympathetic nerves entering and leaving the heart.

From the heart, afferent sensory neurons provide real-time information on cardiac status via parasympathetic (vagal trunk/nodose ganglia) and sympathetic (dorsal root ganglia) tracts to the higher centers. Efferent motor neurons travel from the central system to the epicardial cardiac structures. Sympathetic efferents travel from the intermediolateral spinal cord to the superior, middle, and cervicothoracic (stellate) ganglia. The pre-ganglionic neurons secrete acetylcholine that binds to nicotinic receptors. The post-ganglionic nerves then project from the stellate ganglia (C8-T1) plus T2-T4 to the epicardium of the atria and ventricles where the postganglionic neurons release norepinephrine, which binds to alpha- and beta-adrenergic receptors. Parasympathetic efferents originate in the nucleus ambiguous and medulla oblongata and travel through the vagus nerve to the cardiac ganglia. Approximately 80% of fibers in the vagus nerve are thought to be afferent, however. Parasympathetic pre-ganglionic neurons release acetylcholine to activate nicotinic and muscarinic cholinergic receptors. Post-ganglionic neurons secrete acetylcholine to activate muscarinic receptors in the myocardium and vasculature.

The sympathetic and parasympathetic nervous systems are generally thought of as parallel and separate systems, though there is some crossover between sympathetic and parasympathetic systems as well as afferent and efferent pathways. Identification of neuron types is often only possible by assessment of specific neurotransmitters (which is beyond the scope of this chapter). The antagonization that does occur happens at both pre- and postsynaptic levels. Norepinephrine and acetylcholine impair the release of the other and afferent signals are processed at multiple levels of the system. Further, the cotransmitter neuropeptide Y released from sympathetic nerves can also inhibit acetylcholine.[3] Cardiac electrophysiologic effects of sympathetic and parasympathetic systems are summarized in Table 102.1.[4]

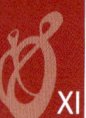

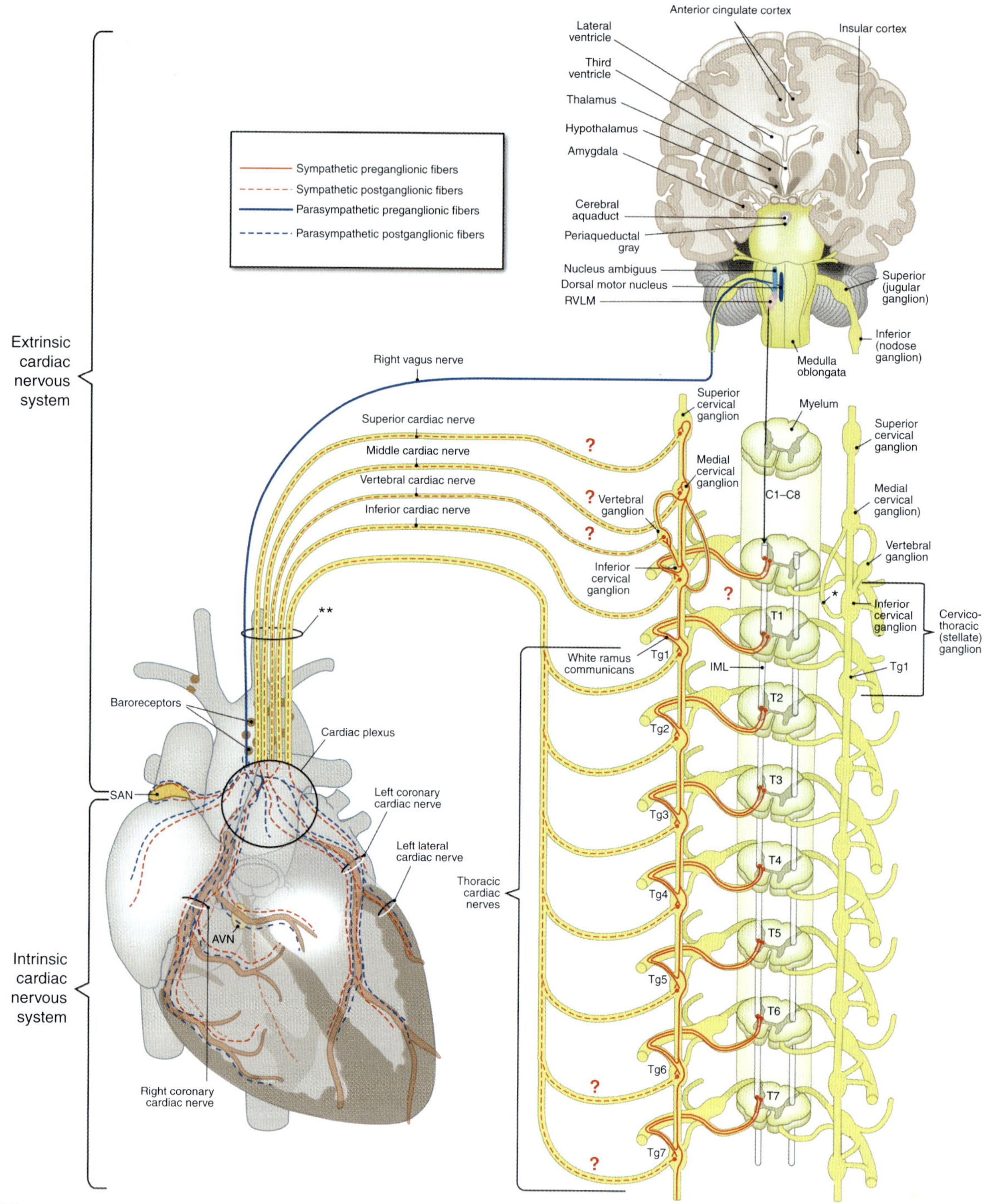

FIGURE 102.1 Overview of cardiac innervation. Schematic drawing of the cardiac autonomic nervous system. Preganglionic cardiac parasympathetic axons arise from neurons in either the nucleus ambiguus or dorsal motor nucleus of the vagus nerve; they run in cardiac branches of the vagus nerve (*solid blue lines*) to synapse in cardiac plexuses and ganglia from where postganglionic fibers (*dashed blue lines*) innervate the sinoatrial node (SAN), atrioventricular node (AVN), coronary arteries, and ventricular myocytes. Preganglionic cardiac sympathetic axons (*solid red lines*) arise from neurons in the intermediolateral cell columns (IMLs) of the upper four or five (possibly six or seven) thoracic spinal segments, that receive modulating input from several forebrain centers (e.g., the insular cortex, anterior cingulate cortex, central nuclei of the amygdala, and several hypothalamic nuclei interneurons); they leave the spinal cord through anterior (ventral) roots, enter the anterior (ventral) rami of spinal nerves and pass to the sympathetic chains through white rami communicantes to synapse in the upper thoracic (Tg) or cervical ganglia; postganglionic fibers (*dashed red lines*) from these ganglia form the sympathetic cardiac nerves. At the heart parasympathetic and sympathetic nerves converge to form the cardiac plexus from which atrial and ventricular autonomic innervation is arranged. The red question marks (?) indicate anatomical structures for which existence and/or involvement in cardiac sympathetic innervation are debated. *Ansa subclavia. **Vagal and sympathetic nerves intermingle before reaching the cardiac plexus and projecting on the heart. *RVLM,* rostral ventrolateral medulla. (From Wink J, et al. Human adult cardiac autonomic innervation: controversies in anatomical knowledge and relevance for cardiac neuromodulation. Auton Neurosci 2020;227:102674.)

Baroreflex

Autonomic innervation of arteries, veins, and capillaries control vascular tone and diameter. Afferent neurons respond to chemical and mechanical stimuli in regions such as the aortic arch and carotid sinus to regulate blood flow, blood pressure, and heart rate via baroreflexes with the ultimate goal of protecting cerebral perfusion.[5] Baroreceptors existing in the walls of major blood vessels (mechanoreceptors in the aortic arch, carotid sinus, origin of the right subclavian artery in addition to low pressure sensors in the atria and pulmonary artery) are activated by stretch related to blood pressure/volume and activate the brain stem predominantly via the vagus nerve. These mechanoreceptors are stretch-dependent, leading to an increased frequency of discharge in the glossopharyngeal nerve and the aortic nerve, which coalesce with the vagus nerve. The low-pressure cardiopulmonary baroreceptors

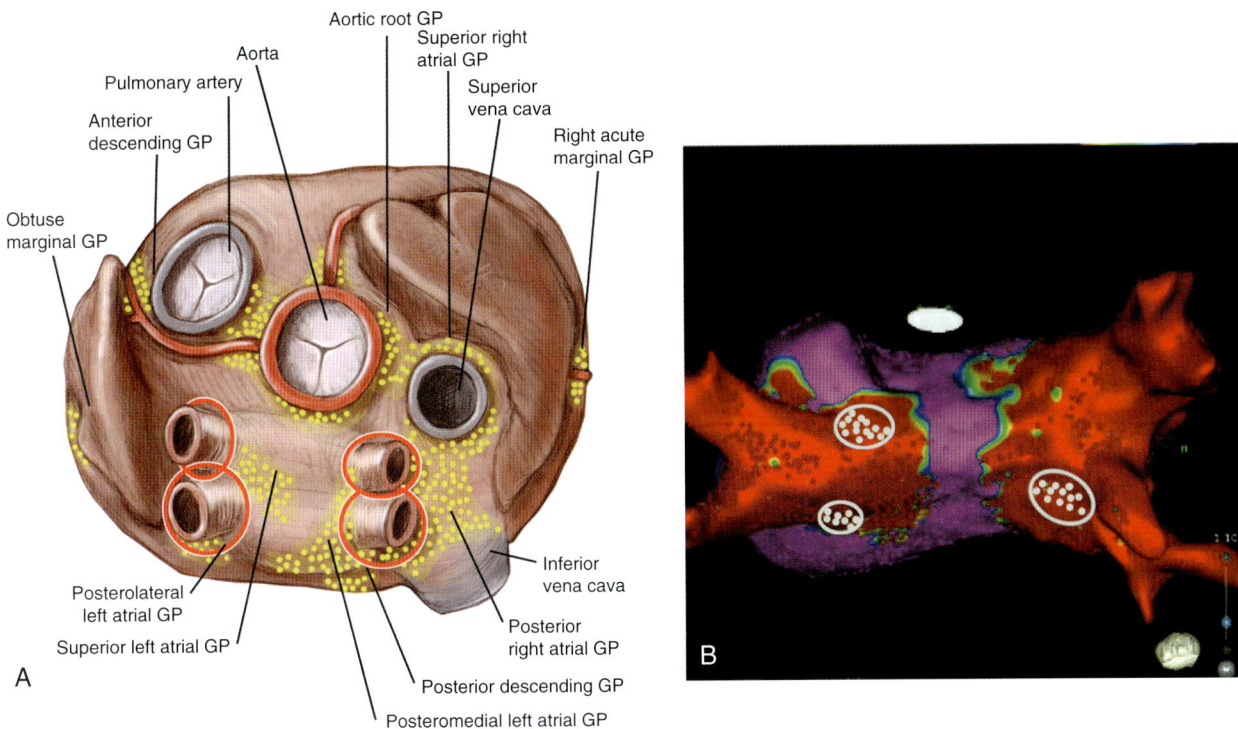

FIGURE 102.2 Intrinsic cardiac nervous system. **A**, Dense network of intrinsic cardiac ganglionated plexi (GP) (*yellow dots*) correlates anatomically with major cardiac vessels. These GP also crudely match ablation sites targeted by most pulmonary vein isolation (PVI) techniques (*red circles*) for atrial fibrillation. **B**, Electroanatomic map of PV after atrial fibrillation ablation, showing correlation of ablation sites with approximated sites of intrinsic cardiac GP (*encircled gray dots*). *Red*, low voltage tissue after pulmonary vein isolation (ablation); *Purple*, normal tissue (not ablated). (From Zhu C, et al. Neuromodulation for ventricular tachycardia and atrial fibrillation: a clinical scenario-based review. JACC Clin Electrophysiol 2019;5:881–896.)

TABLE 102.1 Sympathetic versus Parasympathetic Effects on Heart

CARDIAC PARAMETER	SYMPATHETIC ACTIVATION	PARASYMPATHETIC ACTIVATION	POTENTIAL MECHANISMS
Chronotropy (heart rate)	↑	↓	SNS: Increased SA node phase 4 slope due to increased L-type Ca and I_f currents. PSNS: Less steep phase 4 slope from increased magnitude of ligand-gated K current
Ventricular action potential duration and refractory period	↓	↑	SNS leads to release of NE and beta-adrenergic receptors. Role of cotransmitters unknown. PNS releases ACh, which inhibits NE release and may also increase APD by muscarinic receptor activation
Automaticity	↑	↓	SNS-mediated release of NE and beta-adrenergic receptor activation. Role of cotransmitters unknown. PNS releases ACh, which inhibits NE release and may also increase APD by muscarinic receptor activation
Dispersion of repolarization	↑	↓	SNS: Causes heterogeneity in repolarization in infarcted hearts PNS: Reduces DOR by reducing dispersion in border zone of infarcts
Afterdepolarizations (EADs and DADs)	↑	↓	SNS: Causes calcium overload PNS: Reduces calcium entry

Ach, Acetylcholine; *APD*, action potential duration; *DAD*, delayed after depolarization; *DOR*, dispersion of repolarization; *EAD*, early after depolarization; *NE*, norepinephrine; *PNS*, parasympathetic nervous system activation; *SNS*, sympathetic nervous system activation.
From Wu P, Vaseghi M. The autonomic nervous system and ventricular arrhythmias in myocardial infarction and heart failure. *Pacing Clin Electrophysiol* 2020;43:172–180.

respond to volume, and when volume increases there is a vasodilatory response and drop in blood pressure in addition to a decrease in vasopressin, which leads to an increase in salt and water excretion.

Critical adjustment for postural changes is predominantly controlled through baroreflexes (Fig. 102.3). As vascular pressures change, the relative sympathetic to parasympathetic activity is modified to allow for increased vascular tone, cardiac contractility, and heart rate. Abruptly elevated blood pressure leads to increased stretch of baroreceptors and increased firing, causing decreased sympathetic and increased parasympathetic activity. This change in activity leads to reduced arteriolar resistance and decreased venous tone, as well as decreased heart rate and cardiac contractility.

With standing, less pressure is sensed by the baroreceptors, which leads to vasoconstriction and increased heart rate to prevent drop in blood pressure and associated symptoms. At rest, the baroreflex allows the parasympathetic input to predominate and inhibits sympathetic output. This critical reflex is not consistently present for patients with orthostatic hypotension and vasovagal syncope discussed later. One must recall that the "intrinsic heart rate" of the sinus node is approximately 100 beats per minute (bpm), and what we consider normal resting heart rate (50 to 70 bpm) is the result of elevated parasympathetic input relative to sympathetic. Therefore, heart rate can be raised with decreased parasympathetic stimulation.

Chemoreflex

Chemoreceptors respond to hypoxia and hypercapnia. When activated they lead to vasoconstriction and hyperventilation. There are peripheral (carotid body) and central (brainstem) chemoreceptors. In obstructive sleep apnea, for example, chemoreflexes respond to the recurrent apnea/hypoxia with a sympathetic vasoconstriction and a

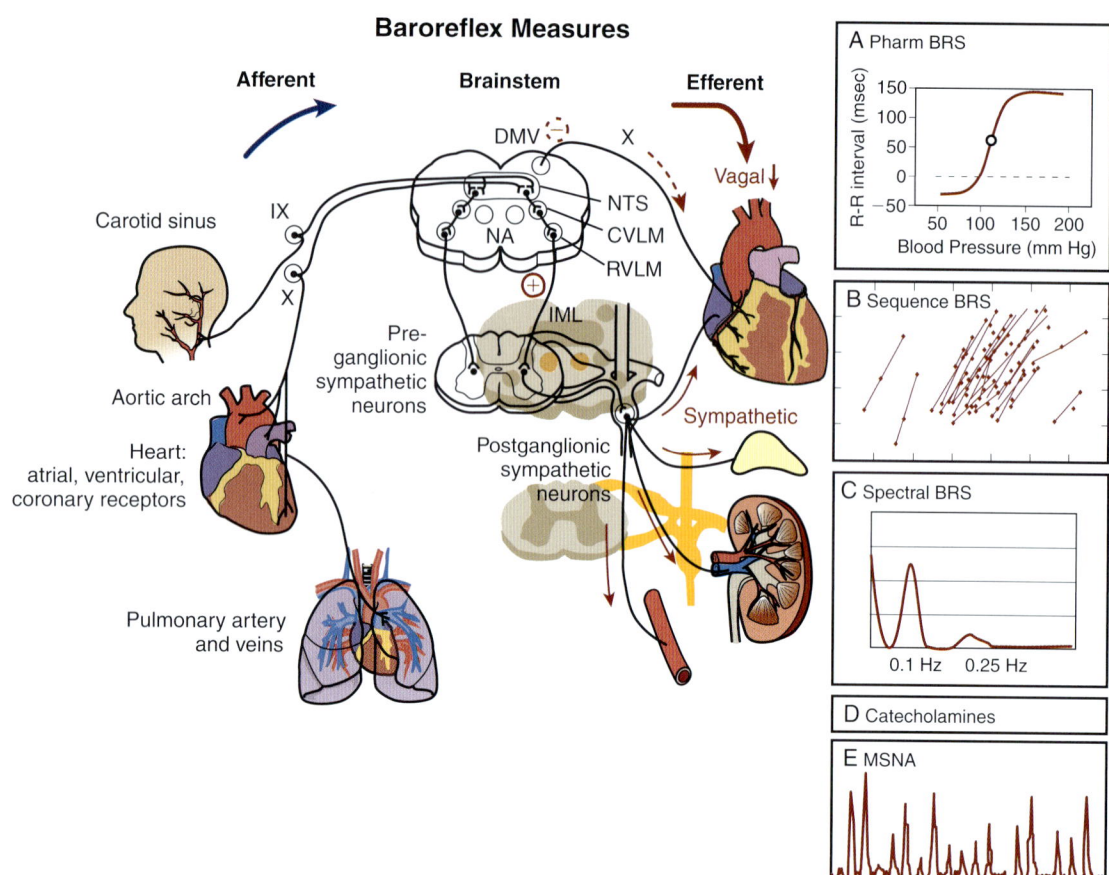

FIGURE 102.3 Diagram of the baroreflex in humans with methods of assessment. **A** to **E**, Five methods of assessing baroreflex sensitivity (BRS). **A**, Baroreflex properties can be assessed by pharmacologic probing with graduated doses of BP-elevating and/or BP-lowering drugs such as phenylephrine and nitroprusside. Changes in slope of the regression line between R-R interval changes and BP changes is referred to as *baroreflex sensitivity*. **B**, The same can be done by using spontaneous fluctuations of BP and R-R intervals, where sequences of heartbeats with increasing or decreasing BP and R-R prolongation are identified and analyzed. **C**, Spectral analysis of HR and BP variability allows assessment of sympathetic and vagal modulation of HR and BP. Cross-spectral transfer function analysis can be used to study the interactions and determine baroreflex sensitivity. **D**, Plasma catecholamine levels are essential markers for sympathetic activity. **E**, Recording of muscle sympathetic nerve activity (MSNA). MSNA is an instantaneous signal of current sympathetic activation, and it allows the estimation of sympathetic baroreflex sensitivity. *CVLM*, Caudal ventrolateral medulla; *DMV*, dorsal motor nucleus of vagus; *IML*, intermediolateral column of spinal cord; *NA*, nucleus ambiguous (vagus); *NTS*, nucleus tractus solitarius; *RVLM*, rostral ventrolateral medulla. (From Robertson D, Robertson RM. Cardiovascular Manifestations of Autonomic Disorders. In Zipes DP, et al., editors. Braunwald's Heart Disease: A Textbook Cardiovascular Medicine. 11th ed. Elsevier; 2019.)

bradycardic response, which is adaptive initially but ultimately can have pathologic consequences.

Diving Reflex

The diving reflex is a powerful reflex in response to diving under water in mammals to allow for prolonged submersion. There is a simultaneous increase in parasympathetic and sympathetic drive. Crucial organ oxygenation is protected including a dramatic bradycardia to decrease myocardial oxygen demand.

PATHOPHYSIOLOGY

Autonomic Dysfunction in the Setting of a Structurally Normal Heart

Autonomic dysregulation can lead to neurally mediated syncope from orthostatic hypotension/vasovagal syncope or carotid sinus syndrome.[6] These are disorders of autonomic reflexes. Other disorders such as postural tachycardia syndrome (POTS) and inappropriate sinus tachycardia (IST) are thought to be in part due to elevated sympathetic activity. These syndromes, which are more common in young women, can have significant overlap. Though not life-threatening, these disorders can significantly impair quality of life.

Vasovagal syncope occurs after upright posture or after painful stimuli or emotional stress. Prodromal symptoms of diaphoresis, a "warm sensation" and nausea, often occur. Vasovagal syncope is reported to occur in over 40% of women and 30% of men by the age of 60 due to lack of effective reflex response to posture and venous pooling or in response to external stimuli. Decreased cardiac output and a potential paradoxical vasodilation with hypotension and possible bradycardia can lead to syncope. Treatment for vasovagal syncope, when episodes are frequent, include lifestyle modification, hydration, lower extremity compression stockings, beta blockers, and fludrocortisone/midodrine. While most vasovagal syncope involves a combination of hypotension and bradycardia (mixed), in some cases patients may have a primary "cardio-inhibitory" response with pronounced bradycardia that responds to pacemaker implantation.

POTS patients have symptoms (lightheadedness, palpitations, etc.) with standing that are associated with a rise in heart rate of ≥30 bpm without an associated drop in systolic blood pressure. POTS is much more prevalent in women (~75%) in the age range of 15 to 25 years, but overall prevalence is low at around 0.2%.[7] A full understanding of mechanism is not clear but has been postulated to involve components of autonomic denervation, hypovolemia, possible autoimmunity, hypervigilance, and deconditioning. In fact, a structured exercise program starting with recumbent exercises can be used as a treatment prior to considering pharmacologic therapies such as beta blockers. IST is a resting heart rate over 100 bpm, or over 90 bpm on average Holter monitor recordings, without reversible cause and associated with symptoms. IST occurs in less than 1.5% of the population. Similar to POTS, the cause is not completely understood. Medical therapy with beta blockers or Ivabradine (an I*f* current blocker) can be utilized to decrease heart rate in some cases.

Neural pathology can secondarily occur in a number of disorders including but not limited to diabetes, Parkinson disease, and multisystem atrophy. Neurologic injury including spinal cord disorders, severe head injury, subarachnoid hemorrhage, and stroke can manifest with distinct cardiac electrophysiologic abnormalities including brady- and tachyarrhythmias.[8,9] In some instances the resulting autonomic dysfunction is transient and can resolve with resolution of the primary pathology, such as in subarachnoid hemorrhage. In more chronic disease states, such as Parkinson or multisystem atrophy, the autonomic manifestations can be chronic and progressive.

Autonomic Dysfunction in the Setting of Intrinsic Cardiac Disease

Autonomic dysfunction can occur due to, and further exacerbate, primary cardiac pathology including myocardial infarction as well as ischemic and nonischemic cardiomyopathy and associated heart failure. These disorders can directly damage cardiac nerves. Subsequent increase in sympathetic (including increased cardiac norepinephrine spillover and increased activation of the renin-angiotensin-aldosterone system in the kidneys) and decrease in parasympathetic output may occur to maintain homeostasis; however, the persistent afferent pathologic signaling can lead to a cycle of worsening cardiac dysfunction and proarrhythmia.[10]

Persistently elevated sympathetic stimulation in heart failure can cause tachycardia, increased afterload, and ventricular remodeling. Subsequent changes can lead to downregulation of beta-1 receptors at the plasma membrane. Cardiac injury can lead to sympathetic nerve death, which is followed by heterogenous nerve sprouting at scar border zones and supersensitivity of denervated regions within the myocardium. The altered myocardium becomes prone to ventricular arrhythmias in the acute and chronic phases of disease. Interestingly, changes are not limited to the heart itself, with evidence that cardiac injury can lead to changes within the stellate ganglia.[11] When parasympathetic dysfunction is present, manifestations include abnormal heart rate response with tachycardia and decreased heart rate variability, which is a marker for increased mortality.[12]

PROARRHYTHMIA

Atrial Fibrillation

Mechanisms of atrial fibrillation (AF) are complex and incompletely understood. Pulmonary vein triggers are well established as the primary target of electrophysiologic intervention and increased ectopy can be triggered by sympathetic stimulation. However, numerous other factors including atrial stretch, fibrosis, altered calcium handling, and autonomic pathology are thought to be involved to varying degrees.

The posterior left atrium is highly innervated by ganglionated plexi with parasympathetic nerves predominating. The data for the relative contribution of vagal stimulation and the ganglionated plexi to the initiation and maintenance of AF is mixed. Vagal nerve stimulation can induce AF, and there are data that injection of botulinum toxin into the fat pads where ganglionated plexi reside can decrease AF episodes. Although relative contributions of the sympathetic and parasympathetic nervous system still need to be fully elucidated, the role of the autonomic nervous system in general is clear, exemplified by the fact that in orthotopic heart transplant patients (complete cardiac denervation), AF is rare, except for patients with active graft rejection.

Ventricular Tachycardia/Ventricular Fibrillation

Parasympathetic dysfunction is associated with sudden death, and reduced heart rate variability and baroreceptor sensitivity are measurable markers of said dysfunction. However, specific data for parasympathetic dysfunction and ventricular tachycardia/ventricular fibrillation (VT/VF) are limited, whereas data for the sympathetic nervous system contributing to ventricular arrhythmias are better defined. Elevated sympathetic afferent and efferent signaling in heart disease leads to elevated norepinephrine and neuropeptide Y release, which is associated with vasoconstriction and cardiac remodeling as well as shortening of action potential and refractory period durations.[13,14] Both right and left stellate stimulation can cause early and late afterdepolarizations, even in normal hearts.[15] Nerve death, nerve sprouting at scar border zones, and supersensitivity, as noted above, can predispose to ventricular ectopy as well as creating a substrate for reentrant arrhythmias.

INVESTIGATIONS AND DIAGNOSIS

Testing to determine autonomic function/dysfunction during health and disease is challenging. While numerous testing measures have been assessed, the sensitivity and specificity of these tests is limited and the tests are not easily incorporated into clinical practice.[16] Heart rate variability, heart rate turbulence, baroreceptor sensitivity, and heart rate recovery have been used with variable success to assess cardiac autonomic dysfunction, but they are beyond the scope of this chapter (see Chapter 61). However, certain clinical assessments can be utilized with limited additional expertise.

Orthostatic Blood Pressure

Change from a supine to standing position can lead to ½ to 1 liter of blood to pool in the lower extremities and splanchnic venous system. This pooling leads to decreased venous return and associated decreased cardiac output. Decreased return and cardiac stroke volume/output leads to decreased afferent baroreceptor activity. The subsequent decrease in parasympathetic and increase in sympathetic tone causes vasoconstriction, increased cardiac contractility, and increased heart rate, which optimizes blood pressure and most importantly protects cerebral profusion. Appropriate orthostatic blood pressure can be easily tested at the bedside. It is important to ensure the patient has been lying flat for 10 minutes before the baseline blood pressure and heart rate are established. On standing, repeat measurements should be obtained at 1, 3, and 5 minutes and correlated with any symptoms (Fig. 102.4).

Tilt table testing can be utilized to assess orthostatic tolerance and the responses are potentially increased given that lower extremity muscle tone is not utilized with tilt table testing (Fig. 102.5). The four phases of vasovagal response seen during a tilt table test are well described by Jardine and colleagues and include early stabilization in response to upright posture, circulatory instability (early presyncope), terminal hypotension, and recovery with resumption of supine posture.[17] Tilt table testing, with prolonged passive postural stress, can be assessed in isolation or with the addition of pharmacologic agents such as isoproterenol or nitrates, though these medications reduce specificity. A "positive" tilt test doesn't define the cause of a patient's syncope but simply shows that the patient has a propensity for this abnormal reflex, which as noted above effects a large percentage of the population over time.

Valsalva Maneuver

The Valsalva maneuver can also be done at the bedside with electrocardiogram, blood pressure, and ideally expiratory pressure monitoring. After baseline measurements are obtained, the patient blows into a closed system to 40 mm Hg for 12 seconds. There is an initial increase in blood pressure due to the expiratory pressure being transmitted to the intrathoracic vessels. Subsequently, there is a fall in systolic blood pressure as the venous return is diminished, as is stroke volume. The fall in blood pressure is sensed and sympathetic simulation and parasympathetic withdrawal brings the blood pressure back up toward baseline and the heart rate elevates. Ultimately, venous return is restored and blood is pumped by a sympathetically activated heart and because the circulation is vasoconstricted, leading to an elevated blood pressure, which then stimulates the baroreceptors and causes sympathetic withdrawal and slowing of the heart rate.[18]

Cold Pressor Test

The cold pressor test involves placing a supine patient's hand in ice water for 3 to 5 minutes after obtaining baseline steady state heart rate and blood pressure. Rise in heart rate and blood pressure due to vasoconstriction in skeletal muscle can be monitored and may be abnormal if autonomic dysfunction is present.

Plasma Catecholamines

Plasma catecholamines including norepinephrine, epinephrine, and dopamine can be easily measured in plasma. However, in currently available assays the utility is limited for the assessment and treatment of most autonomic disorders. Approximately 80% to 90% of norepinephrine undergoes reuptake into neurons with 10% to 20% "spillover" that can be measured. These measurements can however be useful for evaluating for neuroendocrine tumors.

NEUROMODULATORY THERAPIES

Autonomic interventions predominantly target the overactivity of the sympathetic nervous system relative to the parasympathetic.[19] Blockade of the sympathetic nervous system via pharmacologic or interventional/surgical techniques (so-called neuraxial modulation) can reduce the risk of atrial and ventricular arrhythmias and the risk of sudden death. Parasympathetic modulation is also under evaluation to treat the component of dysregulation that contributes to heart failure (see Chapter 47) and atrial (see Chapters 65 and 66) and ventricular arrhythmias (see Chapter 67).

Pharmacologic Therapy

Therapy with beta blockers, angiotensin-converting enzyme inhibitors (ACE-I), angiotensin receptor blockers (ARB), and mineralocorticoid receptor antagonists have significant beneficial autonomic effects. Beta blockers inhibit the effect of norepinephrine on beta receptors and

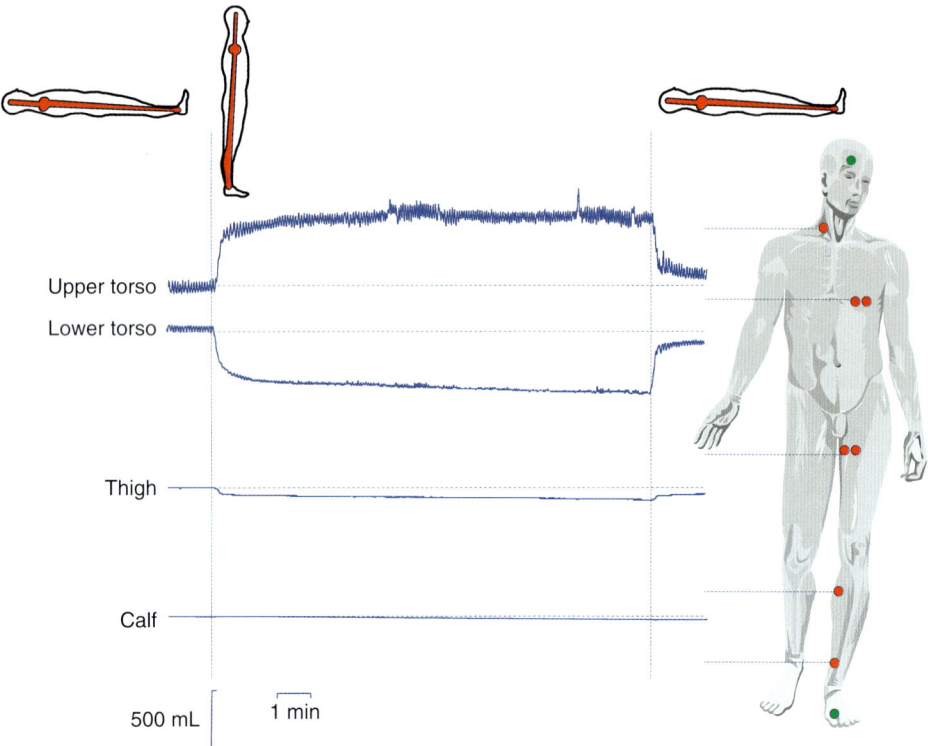

FIGURE 102.4 Orthostatic fluid shifts estimated by impedance. Change in impedance within segments of the human body during upright posture, reflecting shifts in fluid volume from the upper torso to the lower torso and to a lesser degree to the thighs. The increase in fluid in the splanchnic circulation forms the basis for considering studies of an abdominal binder to improve orthostatic tolerance in patients with orthostatic hypotension and orthostatic tachycardia. (From Robertson D, Robertson RM. Cardiovascular Manifestations of Autonomic Disorders. In Zipes DP, et al., editors. Braunwald's Heart Disease: A Textbook Cardiovascular Medicine. 11th ed. Elsevier; 2019.)

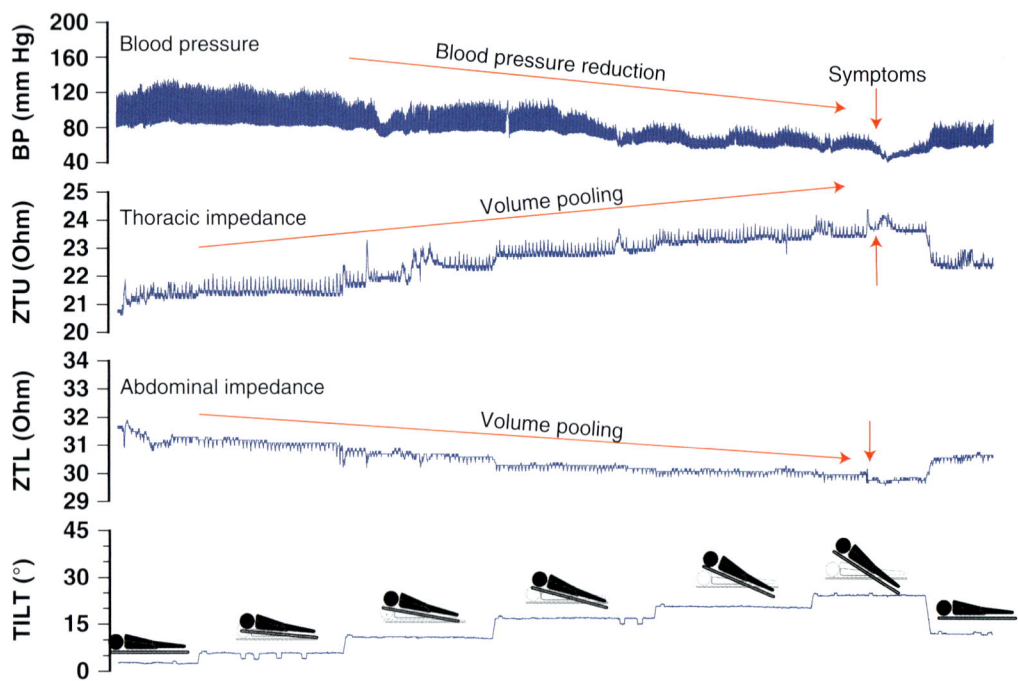

FIGURE 102.5 Impedance assessment of fluid shifts with head-up tilt. Note that with increasing head-up tilt, there is a gradual shift in fluid volume from the chest to the abdomen, reflecting pooling in the splanchnic/mesenteric circulation. Recovery of pooling begins immediately with the assumption of the supine posture. *ZTU, ZTL (ohm),* measure of impedance inversely related to fluid volume in the body segment referred to. (From Robertson D, Robertson RM. Cardiovascular Manifestations of Autonomic Disorders. In Zipes DP, et al., editors. Braunwald's Heart Disease: A Textbook Cardiovascular Medicine. 11th ed. Elsevier; 2019.)

help return the downregulated beta receptors to equilibrium. Additionally, they can inhibit intrinsic pacemaker currents and further reduce heart rate. Blockade of angiotensin II type I receptors inhibit norepinephrine levels, and therefore ACE-I and ARBs have benefit in treating autonomic dysregulation of heart failure when the renin-angiotensin-aldosterone system is upregulated. More extensive discussion of pharmacotherapy for heart failure and arrhythmia management are discussed elsewhere (see Chapters 50 and 64).

Sympathetic Modulation

Data for interventional and surgical autonomic modulation have predominantly been studied for arrhythmia management with limited data for heart failure (Fig. 102.6). Data are strongest for sympathetic denervation with more variable data for parasympathetic modulation to date (Table 102.2).

Thoracic Epidural Anesthesia/Percutaneous Stellate Block

Thoracic epidural anesthesia (TEA) blocks both afferent and efferent communication with the spinal cord. TEA is performed by delivering anesthetic (bupivacaine or ropivacaine) as 1 mL boluses and subsequent continuous infusion via an epidural needle to the T1-T2 or T2-T3 interspaces.

TEA has been shown to prolong myocardial refractory periods and has been utilized for the acute management of refractory ventricular arrhythmias. The largest series was reported by Do and colleagues. This was a multicenter retrospective series of 11 patients that underwent TEA for VT storm. In this series, response rate was modest, with 45% of patients demonstrating complete control of VT/VF and 9% having partial clinical benefit.[20] Clinical markers of success are limited in available data, as patients undergoing TEA did not have significant changes in blood pressure or heart rate that could be monitored for effect. However, patients that had a relative response (decreased arrhythmia burden) to general anesthesia were more likely to have further decrease in arrhythmia burden with TEA. Use of TEA may allow patients to avoid intubation/sedation or be woken from sedation to allow participation in their plan of care.

TEA cannot be utilized in the setting of anticoagulation or use of antiplatelets medications such as clopidogrel. An alternative to TEA that can be considered when anticoagulation or antiplatelets are mandatory is percutaneous stellate ganglion blockade. Stellate block can inhibit both afferent and efferent signaling at the level of the stellate ganglia. A systematic review of 38 cases demonstrated a reduction in ventricular arrhythmias and associated implantable cardioverter-defibrillator (ICD) therapies.[21] Similar to TEA, this procedure can be performed at the bedside. It is performed by injecting lidocaine or bupivacaine, using ultrasound guidance (to avoid the carotid artery or jugular vein) to target the stellate ganglia via a needle inserted in the supraclavicular region at the C6 transverse process.[22]

Renal Denervation

Renal artery denervation (RDN) of afferent and efferent nerves decreases sympathetic output to the heart and has been shown to decrease norepinephrine spillover.[23] Animal data show increased VF threshold and decreased ventricular arrhythmia burden.[24] RDN in its current clinical form (outside of studies of new technology) is performed with a standard open-irrigated cardiac ablation catheter delivering short circumferential ablation lesions within the renal arteries. More RDN-specific catheters and techniques are being evaluated.

RDN has shown promise for the management of atrial and ventricular arrhythmias as well as heart failure. The largest case series utilizing RDN for refractory ventricular arrhythmias was presented by Ukena and colleagues, who showed a significant decrease in ventricular arrhythmia burden at 1 and 3 months in 13 patients from 5 international centers.[25] RDN has also been shown to be adjunctive to cardiac sympathetic denervation (CSD), discussed below.[26] In a series of 10 patients that had failed ablation and CSD, 6 (60%) had clinical benefit from RDN, suggesting that RDN has additional benefits even when other autonomic interventions such as CSD are unsuccessful.

RDN has been utilized to treat AF in greater numbers than for VT and has even been studied in a randomized trial (ERADICATE AF). ERADICATE AF compared ablation alone (n = 148) to ablation and RDN (n = 154) with a significant improvement in freedom from AF in the combined ablation and RDN group (72.1% versus 56.5%) at 12 months' follow-up.[27] Data from a meta-analysis further supports the benefit of RDN for the treatment of AF.[28]

Cardiac Sympathetic Denervation

Cardiac sympathetic denervation (CSD) has been shown to decrease VT/VF in various animal models and clinical series since the 1960s. CSD has been utilized for a variety of disorders including medication-refractory angina, long QT syndrome, and catecholaminergic VT, in addition to more recent data on patients with structural heart disease. CSD is performed by surgical removal of the lower one-third to half of the stellate ganglia and the T2-T4 ganglia and is most commonly performed with video-assisted thoracoscopic techniques.

CSD reduces VT inducibility and increases ventricular ARIs in a porcine model.[29] Further evidence in a canine model demonstrates reduced cardiac norepinephrine levels during ischemia and a significant reduction in VF when the heart is decentralized from the stellate ganglia and spinal cord.[30] CSD has been shown to decrease VT/VF refractory to antiarrhythmic drugs and catheter ablation in patients with structural heart disease. Vaseghi and colleagues followed initial data with intermediate and long-term results of 41 patients that underwent CSD.[31] Of the patients that underwent a bilateral approach, 48% were free of VT/VF at a mean follow-up of 367 days, but 90% had a significant overall reduction in ICD therapies. A subsequent multicenter series assessed 121 patients with a 1-year freedom from sustained ventricular arrhythmias or ICD shocks of 58%. Lower success was seen in patients with more advanced heart failure and slower VT rates.[32]

Augmentation of Parasympathetic Drive

Studies of parasympathetic stimulation for the treatment of heart failure and arrhythmia management have been mixed, and data is stronger for AF than for VT/VF. This may be due to variability in the frequencies, pulse widths, and intensities utilized in available studies that limit interpretation.[33]

Vagal Nerve Stimulation

Vagal nerve stimulation (VNS) has been shown in a porcine infarct model to stabilize electrical heterogeneity and reduce ventricular arrhythmia inducibility.[34] Low level VNS may have benefit for AF as well, with a randomized trial of low level stimulation in 54 patients that underwent cardiac surgery demonstrating a significant reduction in postoperative AF (12% versus 36%) as well as a reduction in inflammatory markers.[35] VNS trials in heart failure have shown mixed results. The ANTHEM Heart Failure trial showed improvements in ejection fraction, symptoms, and quality of life, but other studies have been negative.[36]

Tragal stimulation, via stimulation of the auricular branch of the vagus nerve, is a percutaneous method of increasing vagal tone and has shown benefit for management of AF. Low level stimulation over a 6-month period was associated with a decrease in AF burden compared with a sham control group in 52 patients with paroxysmal AF.[37]

Spinal Cord Stimulation

Spinal cord stimulation (SCS), performed by inserting electrodes in the epidural space, typically at the T2 to T4 level, can increase vagal tone and decrease sympathetic activity. SCS has shown promising

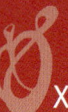

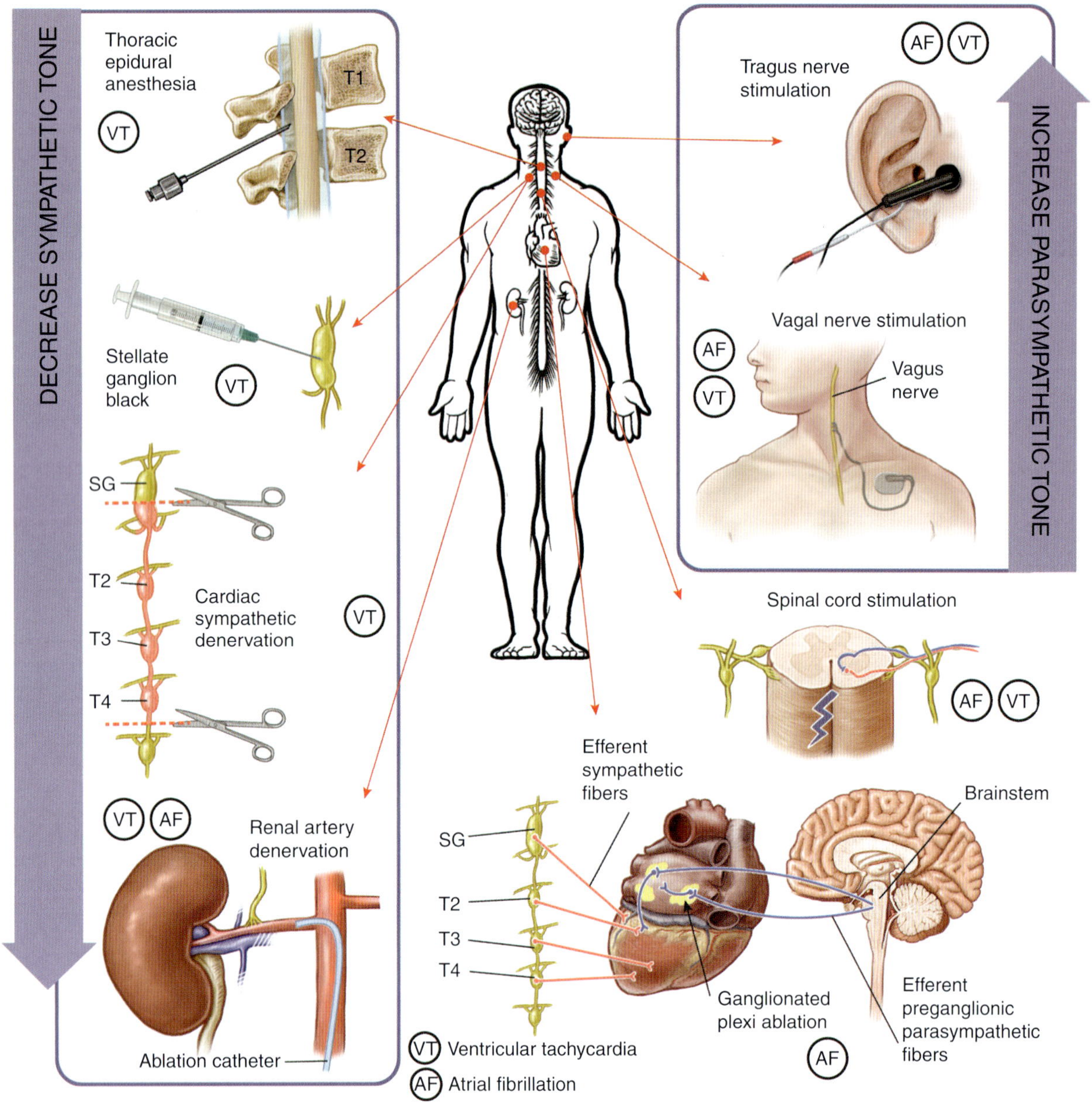

FIGURE 102.6 Schematic demonstrating options for autonomic modulation of arrhythmias. *AF*, Atrial fibrillation; *SG*, stellate ganglia; *T*, thoracic; *VT*, ventricular tachycardia. (From Zhu C, et al. Neuromodulation for ventricular tachycardia and atrial fibrillation: a clinical scenario-based review. JACC Clin Electrophysiol 2019;5:881-896.)

results in animal models with suggestion of improved myocardial function and reduced ventricular arrhythmias with prolonged ventricular refractory periods and decreased left stellate ganglia activity.[38,39] However, clinical studies such as the DEFEAT-HF study did not show significant differences in arrhythmia burden. A canine model of pacing-induced AF suggests SCS may reduce the incidence and burden of AF, but that benefit was only seen early in the disease process.[40]

Baroreceptor Stimulation

Targeting the carotid sinus baroreceptors via the placement of electrodes adjacent to the carotid bodies can increase parasympathetic afferent activity with a goal of augmenting vagal tone.[41] The Baroreflex Activation Therapy for Heart Failure (BEAT-HF) study, which utilized an implanted electrode, led to improvements in functional capacity and quality of life for patients with mild-moderate heart failure without an indication for cardiac resynchronization therapy.[42] No significant data exist to date for this method in the management of atrial or ventricular arrhythmias.

FUTURE PERSPECTIVES

Neurocardiology in general, and specifically assessing the autonomic influences during health and disease, is a growing area of basic, translational, and clinical research with a goal of clinical intervention. However, while our understanding of this complex system is progressing rapidly, there is still a remarkable amount of progress that needs to be made.

A number of autonomic disorders, including vasovagal syncope and IST, have very few efficacious treatments for a symptomatic patient population. Recent data suggest the potential benefit of ganglionated plexi ablation for neutrally mediated syncope.[43,44] Sun and colleagues assessed 57 patients who underwent cardioneural ablation and found that during 36-month follow-up, 91% remained syncope-free.

Novel concepts involving interventions on the autonomic nervous system to treat bradyarrhythmias are also gaining interest. Treatment of bradyarrhythmias (sinus node dysfunction, AV block) has largely been limited to pacemaker implantation, as these disorders were thought

TABLE 102.2 Studies of Autonomic Modulation Targeting the Sympathetic Nervous System

MODALITY	YEAR	CITATION	STUDY TYPE	N	ETIOLOGY OF CMY	TYPE OF VT	FOLLOW-UP	MAIN FINDINGS
Thoracic Epidural Anesthesia								
TEA	2017	Do et al.	Retrospective, multicenter	11	NiCMY (45%), iCMY (27%), other (28%)	VT storm: PMVT (27%), MMVT (73%)	Acute	45% complete response*, 9% partial response*, 45% no response
TEA	2010	Bourke et al.	Retrospective, multicenter	8	iCMY (50%), NiCMY (25%), other (25%)	VT storm: PMVT (37.5%), MMVT (62.5%)	6.2 ± 4.6 mo	≥80% reduction in arrhythmia burden in 6 of 8 patients
Percutaneous Sympathetic Ganglion Block								
SGB (89% Left)	2017	Meng et al.	Retrospective review	38	NiCMY (18%), iCMY (45%), unspecified (29%)	Mixed VT/VF (39%), PMVT (32%), MMVT (11%), VF (18%)	Hospital d/c (6-28 days)	83%-95% relative reduction in VA burden, 80.6% survived to hospital discharge
SGB (50% Bilateral, 50% Left)	2019	Tian et al.	Single-center case series	30	iCMY (57%), NiCMY (33%), idiopathic (7%), LQT (3%)	VT storm (40%), VT+VF storm (50%), VF storm (10%)	72 hr + f/u of 22 ± 16 mo	50% complete response^, 20% partial response^ at 72 hours post TEA. Overall 92% reduction in VA episodes (in patients with ICD)
Surgical Cardiac Sympathetic Denervation in Structural Heart Disease								
LCSD	2010	Bourke et al.	Retrospective, multicenter	9	NiCMY (22%), iCMY (22%), Sarcoid (22%), HCM (22%), ARVC (11%)	VT storm: PMVT (22%), MMVT (78%)	6.2 ± 4.6 mo	33% complete response+, 22% partial response+, 44% no response
BCSD (66%), LCSD (34%)	2014	Vaseghi et al.	Retrospective, single center	41	NiCMY (54%), iCMY (22%), HCM (7%), sarcoid (5%), other (12%)	Refractory VT or VT storm: MMVT (80%), PMVT/VF (20%)	367 ± 251 days	48% had 1-yr survival free of ICD shock after BCSD (30% after LCSD); 90% had reduction in ICD therapies
BCSD	2016	Saenz et al.	Retrospective, multicenter	75	Chagasic cardiomyopathy	MMVT	7 mo (IQR 1-46)	Decrease in ICD shocks from median of 4 (range 2-30) before to 0 (range 0-2) after BCSD
BCSD (81%) LCSD (19%)	2017	Vaseghi et al.	Retrospective, multicenter	121	NiCMY (71%), iCMY (27%), mixed CMY (2%)	Recurrent VT or VT storm	1.5 ± 1.4 years	Reduction in ICD shocks from mean of 18 ± 30 in the year before to 2.0 ± 4.3 after CSD
BCSD	2019	Assis et al.	Retrospective, single center	8	ARVC	Refractory VT	1.9 ± 0.9 years	Reduction in ICD shocks/sustained VT (12.6 ± 18.2 to 0.9 ± 1.4)
BCSD (80%) RCSD (20%)	2019	Okada et al.	Retrospective, single center	5	Cardiac sarcoidosis	Refractory VT	26 mo (IQR 5-29)	Reduction in ICD shocks from median of 5 (in the 6 months preceding CSD) to 0
Renal Sympathetic Denervation								
RDN	2014	Remo et al.	Retrospective, single center	4	iCMY (50%), NiCMY (50%)	Recurrent VT	8.8 mo (IQR 5-11)	Decrease in VT episodes from 11.0 ± 4.2 during the month pre-RDN to 0.3 ± 0.1/month post-RDN
RDN	2015	Armaganijan et al.	Prospective single center	10	Chagas CMY (60%), NiCMY (20%), iCMY (20%)	Refractory VA	6 mo (IQR 18 days, 6 mo)	Reduction in VT/VF episodes from 28.5 to 1, reduction in ICD shocks from 8 to 0
RDN	2016	Ukena et al.	Retrospective, multicenter	13	iCMY (54%), NiCMY (46%)	Refractory VAs: VF (62%), MMVT (54%), PMVT (46%)	12 mo	Reduction in VT/VF episodes from median of 21 in the month pre-RDN to 2 and 0 at 1 and 3 months post-RDN
RDN	2016	Evranos et al.	Propensity score-matched cohort	32	iCMY (62%), NiCMY (38%)	Refractory VA	15 mo (IQR 6-20)	Reduction in VT/VF/ICD therapies in RDN + ablation vs. ablation only group
RDN	2018	Jiang et al.	Prospective case series	8	DCM (63%), iCMY (25%), iCMY (12%)	VT storm or VA episodes on ICD interrogation	15 mo (IQR 6-30)	Reduction in VA episodes from 3.2 to 0.1 per mo
RDN (10% Left-sided only)	2019	Bradfield et al.	Retrospective, single center	10	NiCMY (90%), iCMY (10%)	Recurrent VT/VT storm: MMVT (70%), PMVT (30%)	23 mo	Reduction in ICD therapies (from 29.5 ± 25.2 to 7.1 ± 10.1) 6 mo pre-to 23 mo post-RDN

Continued

TABLE 102.2

Follow-up is given as mean ± standard deviation or median (IQR); months, months of follow-up. *complete response, complete suppression of VT episodes (48 hours after TEA), *partial response (80% to 99% reduction in VT episodes); ^partial response not defined; +complete response = no VA within 1 week of procedure, +partial response = recurrence of VAs that did not fulfill definition of VT storm. *ARVC*, Arrhythmogenic right ventricular cardiomyopathy; *ATP*, anti-tachycardia pacing; *BCSD/LCSD/RCSD*, bilateral/left/right cardiac sympathetic denervation; *CMY*, cardiomyopathy; *CPVT*, catecholaminergic polymorphic ventricular tachycardia; *DCM*, dilated cardiomyopathy; *HCM*, hypertrophic cardiomyopathy; *ICD*, implantable cardioverter defibrillator; *iCMY*, ischemic cardiomyopathy; *LQTS*, long QT syndrome; *MMVT*, monomorphic ventricular tachycardia; *NiCMY*, nonischemic cardiomyopathy; *PMVT*, polymorphic ventricular tachycardia; *RDN*, renal sympathetic denervation; *SGB*, stellate ganglion blockade; *TEA*, thoracic epidural anesthesia; *VF*, ventricular fibrillation; *VT*, ventricular tachycardia.

From Nguyen LH, Vaseghi M. Sympathetic denervation for treatment of ventricular arrhythmias. J Atr Fibrillation 2020;13:2404.

---

to be secondary to irreversible conduction system fibrosis associated with normal aging, previous cardiac surgery (valve replacement, etc.), or other cardiac pathology (myocardial infarction, infiltrative/inflammatory cardiomyopathies). However, recent clinical evidence suggests that in at least a subset of this population cardioneural ablation, targeting specific cardiac ganglia, may increase the sinus rate and/or improve atrioventricular nodal conduction properties.[45]

With regard to primary cardiac disorders that lead to autonomic dysregulation such as myocardial infarction and/or ischemic or nonischemic cardiomyopathy, novel interventions have been developed for the treatment of cardiomyopathy and atrial and ventricular arrhythmias. As these techniques develop and as our understanding of the pathophysiology improves, many of these interventions, which are currently surgical such as CSD, will become catheter-based or even noninvasive. Additionally, while many of these procedures have shown promising results, substantial opportunity exists to optimize the techniques and to further delineate the best targets with comprehensive translational research.

REFERENCES

Overview

1. Hanna P, Rajendran PS, Ajijola OA, et al. Cardiac neuroanatomy - imaging nerves to define functional control. *Auton Neurosci.* 2017;207:48–58.
2. Ardell JL, Armour JA. Neurocardiology: structure-based function. *Compr Physiol.* 2016;6:1635–1653.
3. Dusi V, Zhu C, Ajijola OA. Neuromodulation approaches for cardiac arrhythmias: recent advances. *Curr Cardiol Rep.* 2019;21:32.
4. Wu P, Vaseghi M. The autonomic nervous system and ventricular arrhythmias in myocardial infarction and heart failure. *Pacing Clin Electrophysiol.* 2020;43:172–180.
5. Kaufmann H, Norcliffe-Kaufmann L, Palma JA. Baroreflex dysfunction. *N Engl J Med.* 2020;382:163–178.
6. Feigofsky S, Fedorowski A. Defining cardiac dysautonomia - different types, overlap syndromes; case-based presentations. *J Atr Fibrillation.* 2020;13:2403.

Pathophysiology

7. Sheldon RS, Grubb 2nd BP, Olshansky B, et al. 2015 heart rhythm society expert consensus statement on the diagnosis and treatment of postural tachycardia syndrome, inappropriate sinus tachycardia, and vasovagal syncope. *Heart Rhythm.* 2015;12:e41–e63.
8. Chen Z, Venkat P, Seyfried D, et al. Brain-heart interaction: cardiac complications after stroke. *Circ Res.* 2017;121:451–468.
9. Silvani A, Calandra-Buonaura G, Dampney RA, et al. Brain-heart interactions: physiology and clinical implications. *Philos Trans A Math Phys Eng Sci.* 2016;374.
10. Shivkumar K, Ajijola OA, Anand I, et al. Clinical neurocardiology defining the value of neuroscience-based cardiovascular therapeutics. *J Physiol.* 2016;594:3911–3954.
11. Nakamura K, Ajijola OA, Aliotta E, et al. Pathological effects of chronic myocardial infarction on peripheral neurons mediating cardiac neurotransmission. *Auton Neurosci.* 2016;197:34–40.
12. Sobowale CO, Hori Y, Ajijola OA. Neuromodulation therapy in heart failure: combined use of drugs and devices. *J Innov Card Rhythm Manag.* 2020;11:4151–4159.
13. Ajijola OA, Chatterjee NA, Gonzales MJ, et al. Coronary sinus neuropeptide Y levels and adverse outcomes in patients with stable chronic heart failure. *JAMA Cardiol.* 2020;5:318–325.
14. Herring N, Tapoulal N, Kalla M, et al. Oxford Acute Myocardial Infarction S. Neuropeptide-Y causes coronary microvascular constriction and is associated with reduced ejection fraction following ST-elevation myocardial infarction. *Eur Heart J.* 2019;40:1920–1929.
15. Yagishita D, Chui RW, Yamakawa K, et al. Sympathetic nerve stimulation, not circulating norepinephrine, modulates T-peak to T-end interval by increasing global dispersion of repolarization. *Circ Arrhythm Electrophysiol.* 2015;8:174–185.
16. Goldberger JJ, Arora R, Buckley U, et al. Autonomic nervous system dysfunction: JACC Focus Seminar. *J Am Coll Cardiol.* 2019;73:1189–1206.
17. Jardine DL, Wieling W, Brignole M, et al. The pathophysiology of the vasovagal response. *Heart Rhythm.* 2018;15:921–929.
18. Braunwald's Heart Disease: A Textbook of Cardiovascular Medicine. 11th ed: Elsevier.
19. Hanna P, Shivkumar K, Ardell JL. Calming the nervous heart: autonomic therapies in heart failure. *Card Fail Rev.* 2018;4:92–98.

Arrhythmia

20. Do DH, Bradfield J, Ajijola OA, et al. Thoracic epidural anesthesia can Be effective for the short-term management of ventricular tachycardia storm. *J Am Heart Assoc.* 2017;6.
21. Fudim M, Boortz-Marx R, Ganesh A, et al. Stellate ganglion blockade for the treatment of refractory ventricular arrhythmias: a systematic review and meta-analysis. *J Cardiovasc Electrophysiol.* 2017;28:1460–1467.
22. Fudim M, Boortz-Marx R, Patel CB, et al. Autonomic modulation for the treatment of ventricular arrhythmias: therapeutic use of percutaneous stellate ganglion blocks. *J Cardiovasc Electrophysiol.* 2017;28:446–449.
23. Bradfield JS, Vaseghi M, Shivkumar K. Renal denervation for refractory ventricular arrhythmias. *Trends Cardiovasc Med.* 2014;24:206–213.
24. Zhang WH, Zhou QN, Lu YM, et al. Renal denervation reduced ventricular arrhythmia after myocardial infarction by inhibiting sympathetic activity and remodeling. *J Am Heart Assoc.* 2018;7:e009938.
25. Ukena C, Mahfoud F, Ewen S, et al. Renal denervation for treatment of ventricular arrhythmias: data from an International Multicenter Registry. *Clin Res Cardiol.* 2016;105:873–879.
26. Bradfield JS, Hayase J, Liu K, et al. Renal denervation as adjunctive therapy to cardiac sympathetic denervation for ablation refractory ventricular tachycardia. *Heart Rhythm.* 2020;17:220–227.
27. Steinberg JS, Shabanov V, Ponomarev D, et al. Effect of renal denervation and catheter ablation vs catheter ablation alone on atrial fibrillation recurrence among patients with paroxysmal atrial fibrillation and hypertension: the ERADICATE-AF randomized clinical trial. *J Am Med Assoc.* 2020;323:248–255.
28. Atti V, Turagam MK, Garg J, et al. Renal sympathetic denervation improves clinical outcomes in patients undergoing catheter ablation for atrial fibrillation and history of hypertension: a meta-analysis. *J Cardiovasc Electrophysiol.* 2019;30:702–708.
29. Irie T, Yamakawa K, Hamon D, et al. Cardiac sympathetic innervation via middle cervical and stellate ganglia and antiarrhythmic mechanism of bilateral stellectomy. *Am J Physiol Heart Circ Physiol.* 2017;312:H392–H405.
30. Ardell JL, Foreman RD, Armour JA, et al. Cardiac sympathectomy and spinal cord stimulation attenuate reflex-mediated norepinephrine release during ischemia preventing ventricular fibrillation. *JCI Insight.* 2019;4.
31. Vaseghi M, Gima J, Kanaan C, et al. Cardiac sympathetic denervation in patients with refractory ventricular arrhythmias or electrical storm: intermediate and long-term follow-up. *Heart Rhythm.* 2014;11:360–366.
32. Vaseghi M, Barwad P, Malavassi Corrales FJ, et al. Cardiac sympathetic denervation for refractory ventricular arrhythmias. *J Am Coll Cardiol.* 2017;69:3070–3080.
33. Ardell JL, Nier H, Hammer M, et al. Defining the neural fulcrum for chronic vagus nerve stimulation: implications for integrated cardiac control. *J Physiol.* 2017;595:6887–6903.
34. Vaseghi M, Salavatian S, Rajendran PS, et al. Parasympathetic dysfunction and antiarrhythmic effect of vagal nerve stimulation following myocardial infarction. *JCI Insight.* 2017;2.
35. Stavrakis S, Humphrey MB, Scherlag B, et al. Low-level vagus nerve stimulation suppresses post-operative atrial fibrillation and inflammation: a randomized study. *JACC Clin Electrophysiol.* 2017;3:929–938.
36. Premchand RK, Sharma K, Mittal S, et al. Autonomic regulation therapy via left or right cervical vagus nerve stimulation in patients with chronic heart failure: results of the ANTHEM-HF trial. *J Card Fail.* 2014;20:808–816.
37. Stavrakis S, Humphrey MB, Scherlag BJ, et al. Low-level transcutaneous electrical vagus nerve stimulation suppresses atrial fibrillation. *J Am Coll Cardiol.* 2015;65:867–875.
38. Wang S, Zhou X, Huang B, et al. Spinal cord stimulation protects against ventricular arrhythmias by suppressing left stellate ganglion neural activity in an acute myocardial infarction canine model. *Heart Rhythm.* 2015;12:1628–1635.
39. Howard-Quijano K, Takamiya T, Dale EA, et al. Spinal cord stimulation reduces ventricular arrhythmias during acute ischemia by attenuation of regional myocardial excitability. *Am J Physiol Heart Circ Physiol.* 2017;313:H421–H431.
40. Ardell JL, Cardinal R, Beaumont E, et al. Chronic spinal cord stimulation modifies intrinsic cardiac synaptic efficacy in the suppression of atrial fibrillation. *Auton Neurosci.* 2014;186:38–44.
41. Wang Y, Dai M, Cao Q, et al. Carotid baroreceptor stimulation suppresses ventricular fibrillation in canines with chronic heart failure. *Basic Res Cardiol.* 2019;114:41.

Newer Modulating Therapies

42. Zile MR, Lindenfeld J, Weaver FA, et al. Baroreflex activation therapy in patients with heart failure with reduced ejection fraction. *J Am Coll Cardiol.* 2020;76:1–13.
43. Aksu T, Guler TE, Mutluer FO, et al. Electroanatomic-mapping-guided cardioneuroablation versus combined approach for vasovagal syncope: a cross-sectional observational study. *J Interv Card Electrophysiol.* 2019;54:177–188.
44. Sun W, Zheng L, Qiao Y, et al. Catheter ablation as a treatment for vasovagal syncope: long-term Outcome of Endocardial autonomic modification of the left atrium. *J Am Heart Assoc.* 2016;5:e003471.
45. Rivarola E, Hardy C, Sosa E, et al. Selective atrial vagal denervation guided by spectral mapping to treat advanced atrioventricular block. *Europace.* 2016;18:445–449.

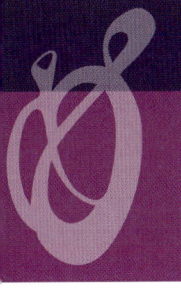

Disclosure Index

The following contributors have indicated that they have a relationship or affiliation that, in the context of their participation in the writing of a chapter for the twelfth edition of *Braunwald's Heart Disease,* could be perceived as a real or apparent conflict of interest, but they do not consider that it has influenced the writing of their chapter.

Codes for the disclosure information (institution[s] and nature of relationship[s]) are provided below.

RELATIONSHIP CODES

A—Stock options or bond holdings in a for-profit corporation or self-directed pension plan
B—Research grants
C—Employment (full or part-time)
D—Ownership or partnership
E—Consulting fees or other remuneration received by the contributor or immediate family
F—Nonremunerative positions, such as board member, trustee, unremunerated consultant, or public spokesperson
G—Receipt of royalties
H—Speakers bureau or CME lectures

INSTITUTION AND COMPANY CODES

001 4D Molecular Therapeutics
002 89Bio
003 ABBIVE
004 Abbott
005 Abbott Laboratories
006 Abbott Lantheus Medical Imaging
007 Abbott Medical
008 Abbott Vascular
009 ABBVIE
010 Abiomed
011 Acasti Pharma
012 ACC & ABIM
013 Acist
014 Acist Medical
015 Actelion Pharmaceuticals
016 Acutus Medical
017 Aetna
018 Afimmune
019 Agepha
020 Agile
021 Alexion Pharmaceuticals
022 AliveCor
023 Alkem Metabolics
024 Allegiant
025 Allergan
026 Alleviant
027 Alnylam
028 Althera
029 AM Pharma
030 Amarin
031 America's Test Kitchen
032 American Board of Internal Medicine
033 American Board of Vascular Medicine
034 American College of Cardiology
035 American College of Cardiology Foundation
036 American Heart Association
037 American Medical Association
038 American Regent
039 American Society of Nuclear Cardiology
040 Amgen
041 Ancora
042 Anthos Therapeutics
043 Anumana
044 Apnimed Inc
045 Apple
046 Applied Therapeutics
047 ARCA Biopharma
048 Arena
049 Arena Pharmaceuticals
050 Aria
051 ARIA CV
052 Arnold and Porter Law Firm
053 AstraZeneca, Inc.
054 AstraZeneca/Bristol Myers Squibb Alliance
055 Atricure
056 Attralus
057 Audentes
058 Avidity
059 AXON Therapies
060 Baim Institute
061 Barnes-Jewish Hospital Foundation
062 Bausch Health
063 Bayer Healthcare
064 Belvoir Publications
065 Beren Therapeutics
066 Beth Israel Deaconess
067 Biosense Webster
068 Biosensors
069 Biosig, Inc
070 Biotronik
071 BMS, Inc
072 Boehringer Ingelheim
073 Boston Biomedical Innovation Center
074 Boston Scientific Corporation
075 Boston Scientific Inc.
076 Boston Pharmaceuticals
077 Bracco
078 Brightseed
079 Bristol Meyers Squibb, Co.
080 BTG EKOS
081 Bunge
082 Calibrate
083 California Institute for Regenerative Medicine (CIRM)
084 Canadian Cardiovascular Society
085 Canadian Institutes of Health Research (CIHR)
086 Cantargia, Inc
087 Cardax
088 Cardiac Booster
089 Cardiac Dimensions
090 Cardiac Dimensions, Inc
091 Cardiac Phoenix
092 CardiaWave
093 Cardiol
094 Cardiology Today
095 Cardior Pharmaceuticals
096 Cardiora
097 Cardurion
098 Cardurion Pharmaceuticals
099 Caristo Diagnostics
100 Cartesian Therapeutics
101 Celladon
102 CellAegis
103 Cellprothera
104 CeloNova
105 Centre for Chronic Disease Control (New Delhi India)
106 Centre intégré universitaire de santé et de services sociaux de la Capitale-Nationale
107 CERC
108 Chiesi
109 Cine-Med Research
110 Civibiopharm

DI-1

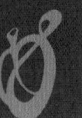

111	Clementia	176	General Electric	244	Milestone Pharmaceuticals
112	Cleveland Clinic	177	Genfit	245	Moderna
113	Cleveland Clinic Foundation	178	Gilead Sciences	246	Motif FoodWorks
114	Colorado Prevention Center	179	GlaxoSmithKline	247	Myocarditis Foundation
115	Columbia University School of Medicine	180	Global Clinical Trial Partners Ltd (GCTP)	248	Myocoskial Solutions Inc.
116	Concept Medical	181	GOED	249	Myokardia
117	Cook Medical	182	GSK	250	National Cancer Institute
118	Corvia	183	Hamni	251	National Heart, Lung and Blood Institute
119	Corvidia Therapeutics	184	Harvard Clinical Research Institute	252	National Human Genome Research Institute
120	CRF	185	Health [at] Scale		
121	Cryolife	186	Heart Rhythm Society	253	Nestle
122	CSL Behring	187	Hikma	254	NeuCures, Inc
123	CVRX	188	HLS Therapeutics	255	Neurotronik
124	CVS Caremark	189	HMP Communications	256	NIH
125	Cytokinetics, Inc.	190	HugoHealth	257	Northwestern University
126	Daiichi Sankyo	191	HumanCo	258	Novartis, Inc.
127	DalCor Pharmaceuticals	192	IBM Watson	259	Novo Nordisk
128	Danone	193	i-Cordis	260	Odonatan health
129	Dartmouth-Hitchcock	194	Idorsia	261	Ohio State University Wexner Medical Center
130	DayTwo	195	Idorsia Pharmaceuticals		
131	Dementi Publishing Co.	196	IFM Therapeutics	262	Olatec Therapeutics
132	Department of Defense	197	Ikaika Therapeutics	263	Omeicos
133	Dewpoint Therapeutics	198	Imbria	264	Opsens
134	Dimagi	199	Impulse Dynamics	265	Optum
135	DINAQOR	200	InCarda	266	OrbusNeich
136	Domicell, LLC	201	Indiana University School of Medicine	267	Ortho-Clinical Diagnostics
137	Dr. Reddy's Laboratories	202	Indigo Agriculture	268	Otsuka Pharmaceuticals
138	Drugs for the Heart	203	Insel Gruppe AG	269	Owkin
139	DSMB	204	Intarcia	270	Path to Improved Risk Stratification
140	Duke University	205	Invitae	271	Patient Centered Outcomes Research Institute (PCORI)
141	Dyrnamix	206	Ionis Pharmaceuticals		
142	East End Medical	207	iRhythm	272	Pava
143	Eastern Virginia Medical School	208	Ironwood	273	PepGen
144	EBR	209	Ischemix	274	Pfizer, Inc.
145	Edwards Lifesciences	210	JanOne	275	PhaseBio
146	Eidos	211	Janssen	276	Philips Medical
147	Eisai	212	Jazz Pharmaceuticals	277	Phillips
148	Eko, Inc	213	Johnson & Johnson	278	Pi-Cardia
149	Element Science	214	Kancera	279	PlaqueTec
150	Eli Lilly and Company	215	Kansas City Heart Rhythm Society	280	PLx Pharma
151	Elsevier	216	KBP Biosciences	281	Population Health Research Institute
152	Elsevier Practice Update Cardiology	217	Kiniksa Pharmaceutical	282	Portola Pharmaceuticals
153	Elysium Health	218	Kowa Pharmaceuticals	283	Private Companies
154	Emory	219	Kowa Research Institute	284	ProAdWise Communications
155	Epirium Bio, Inc	220	Lantheus Medical Imaging	285	Proctor and Gamble
156	Eris Lifesciences	221	Lexicon	286	Prothena
157	Esperion	222	LivaNova	287	Public Health Foundation of India
158	Ethicon	223	London School of Hygiene and Tropical Medicine	288	Pulsecath
159	Facebook			289	Qualcomm
160	Farapulse	224	LQT Therapeutics	290	Quantum Genomics
161	Ferring Pharmaceutical	225	Lupin	291	Quark Pharmaceuticals
162	Filtricine	226	Marfan Foundation	292	Quest Diagnostics
163	Flame	227	Martin and Baughman Law Firm	293	Radcliffe Cardiology
164	Fondation de l'Institut universitaire de cardiologie et de pneumologie de Québec	228	Mayo Clinic	294	Radiometer
		229	McGraw Hill	295	Refactor Health
		230	Medical University of South Carolina	296	Regeneron
165	Fonds de la recherche du Québec – Santé (FRQS)	231	Medicines Company	297	Relationship
		232	MedImmune	298	Renovacor
166	Food and Drug Administration	233	Medscape	299	Research Triangle Institute International
167	Foodome	234	Medscape/Heart.Org	300	Respicardia
168	Forest Labs	235	Medtronic Vascular	301	Roche Diagnostics
169	F-Prime	236	Medtronic, Inc.	302	Roivant Sciences
170	Fractyl	237	Menarini International	303	SAJA Pharmaceuticals
171	France ANR	238	Merck & Co., Inc.	304	Samsung
172	Gaples Institute for Integrative Cardiology	239	Merck-Schering Plough Corp.	305	Sanifit
		240	Mesoblast	306	Sanofi
173	Gates Foundation	241	Metavant Sciences	307	Sanofi Pasteur, Inc.
174	GE Healthcare	242	Microinterventional Devices Inc.	308	Sanofi-Aventis
175	Genentech	243	Microport	309	Sanofi-Regeneron

310 Sarepta	335 Terumo	360 Vanderbilt Univ Med Ctr
311 SCAI	336 the Corpus	361 Variant Bio
312 Sensible Medical	337 The Rockefeller Foundation	362 Venus MedTech
313 Sentara Healthcare	338 The SAFARI-STEMI Trial	363 Vertex
314 Servier	339 Theracos	364 Verve
315 Servier France	340 Thrombolex	365 Verve Therapeutics
316 Shenzhen Center for Health Information in Beijing	341 Tiny Organics	366 Veterans Health Administration
	342 Torrent Pharmaceuticals, India	367 Vifor
317 Shifamed	343 Transverse Medical	368 Vivalink
318 Shockwave	344 TRDRP	369 Vivasure Medical
319 Siegfried and Jensen Law Firm	345 Tremaeu	370 Volumetrix
320 Siemens	346 TripleBlind, Inc	371 vTv Therapeutics
321 SleepImage	347 U.S. Department of Health and Human Services	372 Vwave
322 Sobi Pharmaceuticals		373 Vytronus
323 SOCAR Research	348 United Health	374 Wake Forest Health – Atrium
324 Society for Health Psychology	349 United Therapeutics, Inc.	375 Washington University School of Medicine in St. Louis
325 Spectrum Dynamics	350 Université Laval	
326 Springer	351 University of Arizona	376 WebMD
327 St. Jude Medical	352 University of California	377 WL Gore
328 Stealth BioTherapeutics	353 University of Michigan	378 Wolters-Kluwer
329 Sun Pharmaceuticals	354 University of Washington	379 World Health Organization
330 Synaptic	355 UpToDate (Wolters-Kluwer)	380 World Heart Federation
331 Takeda	356 Uppton	381 Wraser
332 Techsomed, Inc	357 Us2.ai	382 Xbiotech Inc
333 Tenax	358 VA	383 ZOLL
334 Tenaya Therapeutics	359 Valve Medical	384 Zora Biosciences

CONTRIBUTORS

Ackerman, Michael J.: E-005, G-022, G-043, G-075, E-126, E-205, E-224, E-236, G-355
Ades, Philip A.: B-251
Albert, Christine M.: B-005, B-301, E-301, B-327
Albert, Michelle: B-036, C-352
Attia, Zachi: A-022, A-148, A-260, F-186
Bairey Merz, C. Noel: B-299, E-207
Bakris, George L.: E-053, E-063, E-027, E-206, E-238, E-259, E-367, E-216
Balzer, David T.: E-005, E-145, E-236
Beckman, Joshua A.: C-040, C-063, B-079, C-211, C-210, C-258
Bers, Donald M.: E-249
Bhatnagar, Armin: B-256
Bhatt, Deepak L.: B-002, B-008, B-018, B-030, B-040, B-053, B-063, B-072, B-074, B-079, B-087, B-103, B-108, B-122, B-147, B-150, B-158, B-161, B-168, B-170, B-188, B-194, B-195, B-208, B-209, B-211, B-221, B-231, B-236, B-238, B-258, B-249, B-259, B-269, B-275, B-280, B-296, B-306, B-308, B-330, E-034, E-052, E-060, E-064, E-084, E-112, E-140, E-152, E-184, E-189, E-281, E-293, E-311, E-376, F-034, G-151,
Blankstein, Ron: B-040, E-040, G-355
Bohula, Erin A.: B-005, B-040, B-053, B-126, B-147, B-204, B-232, B-238, B-258, B-274, B-296, B-301, B-231, E-040, E-219, E-233, E-259, E-315
Bonaca, Mark P.: B-040, B-053, B-063, B-211, B-221, B-259, B-047, E-040, E-053, E-057, E-063, E-117, E-211, E-221, E-238, E-259, E-274, E-296, E-305, E-381
Bonow, Robert O.: C-257, E-037
Borlaug, Barry A.: E-213, E-050, E-238, E-258, E-150, E-259, B-256, B-234, B-118, B-053, B-240, B-333, B-179
Braunwald, Eugene: B-053, B-126, B-238, B-258, E-040, E-072, E-249, E-259, E-097, E-364
Braverman, Alan C.: F-226, G-355

Brush, John Elliot: C-313, F-143, F-032, F-034, G-131
Calkins, Hugh: E-236, E-067, B-075, E-075, E-055, E-032, E-355, E-007
Canty, John M.: B-256, B-358, E-220, E-289
Carney, Robert M.: E-274, B-251
Chandrashekhar, Y.S.: E-034
Chen, Peng-Shen: E-186
Chung, Mina K.: B-256, B-036, F-186, E-032, G-355, E-171, E-115, E-215, E-036, G-151, C-112
Cooper, Leslie T.: F-093, E-071, E-086, F-247
Creager, Mark A.: B-036, B-078, G-151, C-129, F-380
Cremer, Paul: B-258, B-217, C-322, C-217
Crestanello, Juan A.: C-228, E-236
Curtis, Anne B.: E-008, E-211, E-236, E-244, E-308, E-383
Dangas, George D.: B-008, B-074, B-276
Daubert, James P: B-005, E-005, E-067, E-070, E-074, C-140, E-383, E-373, E-160, E-243, E-277
de Lemos, James A.: B-005, E-035, E-036, E-040, E-296, B-301, E-267, E-320, C-166
Després, Jean-Pierre: C-350, C-106, B-085
Devries, Stephen: C-172
Di Carli, Marcelo F.: B-178, B-325
Dorbala, Sharmila: B-274, B-174, B-056, B-256, B-036, E-274, E-174, E-256, F-040
Duncker, Dirk J.: B-070, B-288, B-369, B-088
Ellenbogen, Kenneth A.: E-012, B-236, E-236, H-236, B-074, E-074, H-074, G-151, H-070, B-067, E-067, F-067
Everett IV, Thomas H.: B-256, C-201
Felker, G. Michael: E-005, B-036, B-048, B-063, E-072, E-079, B-040, E-040, B-125, E-125, B-238, E-236, B-249, B-251, E-258
Fleg, Jerome L.: C-251
Freedland, Kenneth E.: B-251, C-375, E-324
Friedman, Paul: G-228
Gaziano, J. Michael: B-258, E-063

Gaziano, Thomas A.: B-258, C-231, C-040, C-127, C-134, C-379
Genest, Jacques: B-085, B-165, E-238, E-258, E-294, F-084, H-040, H-306
Gillam, Linda: E-276, E-077, E-145, E-036, E-034
Giudicessi, John R.: A-182, A-274
Giugliano, Robert P.: B-040, E-040, B-042, B-126, E-126, E-239, E-030, E-034, E-053, E-072, E-079, E-121, E-124, E-150, E-157, E-178, E-182, E-211, E-221, E-274, E-303, E-304, E-314
Goldberger, Ary L.: B-151, C-066, G-321, B-251
Goldberger, Jeffrey J.: C-270, E-236
Goldhaber, Samuel Z.: E-063, B-072, B-079, B-080, B-126, B-211, B-251, E-072
Gulati, Martha: C-351
Hahn, Rebecca T.: H-008, H-145, H-276, E-008, E-074, H-145, H-276
Hasenfuss, Gerd: F-118, E-315, E-199, E-258, E-053, E-063, E-072
Herrmann, Howard C.: E-005, B-041, B-063, B-074, B-145, B-235, B-318, B-377, E-005, E-145, E-235, D-242
Herrmann, Joerg: G-151, B-250, B-228
Hershberger, Ray E.: G-355, B-251, B-252, C-261
Ho, Carolyn Y.: B-249, E-249, B-079, E-079, E-334
Hsue, Priscilla Y.: D-178, D-238
Hundley, Gregory: B-036, C-374, E-353, D-272, B-250, B-251, E-094
Inzucchi, Silvio E.: E-072, E-053, E-259, E-221, E-157, E-005, E-371, C-151, G-355, G-229
Joynt Maddox, Karen E: B-251, B-256, C-347
Kalman, Jonathan M.: B-067, B-005, B-236, H-067
Kapa, Suraj: A-069, A-346, B-005, B-075, B-211, A-148, A-332
Kern, Morton J.: H-008, H-075, H-276, H-014, H-264
Kinlay, Scott: C-358, R-132, R-256, E-114, F-033
Klein, Allan L.: B-217, E-322, E-274

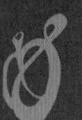

Kloner, Robert A.: B-306, E-306, B-251, B-132, B-344

Krumholz, Harlan M.: B-236, B-213, B-166, B-316, D-190, D-295, E-017, E-149, E-192, E-348, E-227, E-319, E-052, E-159, E-169

Kumbhani, Daram J.: E-034, E-036

Kwong, Raymond Y.: E-236, H-063, B-027, B-249, B-155, G-326

Ky, Bonnie: E-034, E-036, E-125, B-251, B-250, E-301, E-355

Lam, Carolyn S. P.: B-063, B-074, B-053, B-236, B-301, E-005, E-040, E-053, E-063, E-072, E-074, E-118, E-125, E-211, E-236, E-237, E-238, E-249, E-258, E-259, E-301, E-306, E-328, E-233, E-376, A-357

Larose, Eric: B-165, B-164, F-139, F-338

Lasala, John M.: E-005, E-377

Lenihan, Daniel J.: B-248, E-053, E-286, E-146, E-150, E-111, E-125

Leon, Martin B.: B-008, B-074, B-145, B-235, E-362, A-278, D-142, D-359

LeWinter, Martin M.: B-217, E-217

Libby, Peter: A-382, B-036, B-251, B-258, E-382, F-040 F-053, F-060, F-065, F-099, F-100, F-122, F-127, F-133, F-157, F-175, F-218, F-232, F-238, F-258, F-259, F-262, F-274, F-279, F-292

Lindenfeld, JoAnn: B-053, B-312, B-370, E-053, E-004, E-072, E-075, E-123, E-145, E-199, E-372, E-024

Lindman, Brian R.: B-145

Mack, Michael J.: F- 145, F-008, F-236

Madjid, Mohammad: E-307, H-307

Mann, Douglas L.: E-259, E-334, A-334, E-095, E-098, A-098, B-193, D-193, E-199, E-240, E-258, E-298, A-298

Maron, Bradley A.: C-015, G-326, B-256, B-073

Marx, Nikolaus: B-072, E-053, E-063, E-072, E-177, E-219, E-238, E-259, H-040, H-053, H-063, H-072, H-238, H-259, H-274

Mason, Justin C.: E-211, E-258, E-301

Maurer, Mathew S.: E-005, B-027, E-027, E-139, E-182, B-249, B-251, B-206, E-206, B-274

McGuire, Darren K.: E-072, E-306, E-053, E-238, E-274, E-259, E-157, E-004, E-150, E-221, E-268, E-122, E-046, E-241, E-146, E-018

McMurray, John J.V.: H-004, H-023, H-156, H-187, H-225, H-329, H-234, H-284, H-293, H-314, H-336, C-180

McNally, Elizabeth: E-053, E-040, E-125, E-211, E-274, E-205, E-004, E-001, E-273, E-058, D-197

Mehran, Roxana: B-005, B-010, E-034, F-034, E-037, F-037, B-029, B-026, B-049, B-046, A-046, B-053, B-063, B-066, B-068, B-074, E-074, E-083, E-109, B-092, B-102, B-104, B-107, B-108, B-116, F-120, B-122, B-126, B-140, B-195, B-203, E-211, B-235, B-258, B-266, B-276, B-311, F-311, B-343, E-376, B-383

Miller, John M.: E-005, E-067, E-070, E-074, E-236, G-151, C-201

Mirvis, David M.: G-355

Mora, Samia: E-274, E-292

Morady, Fred: A-016

Morris, Alanna A.: A-178, B-251

Morrow, David A.: B-005, B-053, B-126, B-147, B-182, B-238, B-258, B-274, B-296, B-301, B-320, B-331, B-042, B-291, B-384, E-053, E-063, E-238, E-258, E-301, E-200, G-151, G-378

Mozaffarian, Dariush: B-251, B-250, B-173, B-337, B-030, E-081, E-181, E-202, E-246, E-011, E-113, E-031, E-128, E-078, E-082, E-130, E-153, E-162, E-167, E-191, E-341, G-355

Musunuru, Kiran: A-361, A-364, F-364

Myerburg, Robert J.: B-132

Natarajan, Pradeep: B-045, E-045, B-040, B-074, C-363

Nkomo, Vuyisile T.: C-228

Noseworthy, Peter: D-022

O'Gara, Patrick T.: F-145, F-236

Olgin, Jeffrey E.: E-368, B-256, B-271, B-173, B-304

Patton, Kristen K.: C-354

Pellikka, Patricia A.: G-355

Piazza, Gregory: B-080, B-079, B-211, B-282, B-063, E-020, E-040, E-074, E-079, E-340

Pibarot, Philippe: B-145, E-145, B-235, E-235, B-278, B-091

Poirier, Paul: E-005, E-040, E-053, E-063, E-072, E-150, E-201, E-258, E-259, E-308, E-315, F-350, E-062, E-188

Prabhakaran, Dorairaj: F-034, F-379, B-154, B-250, B-251, B-256, B-299, C-287, C-105, C-223, E-342

Rajagopalan, Sanjay: E-259, E-331

Reardon, Michael J.: E-236, E-074, E-008, E-074, E-235, E-377

Redline, Susan: B-212, E-212, E-044, E-147

Rich, Michael W.: B-256, B-061

Ridker, Paul M: B-030, B-036, B-053, B-219, B-251, B-256, B-259, B-274, E-053, E-072, E-122, E-259, E-263, E-019, E-323, E-356, E-163, E-110, E-076, F-256, F-166

Ruberg, Frederick L.: B-027, B-206, B-274, E-021

Sabatine, Marc S.: E-028, B-040, E-042, B-053, E-053, B-063, E-079, E-124, B-126, E-127, E-137, E-141, E-147, E-157, E-196, B-204, E-204, B-211, E-211, B-231, E-231, B-232, E-232, B-238, E-238, B-258, E-258, B-274, B-291

Schermerhorn, Marc: F-235, F-276

Scirica, Benjamin M.: B-054, B-148, B-239, B-259, B-260, B-275, E-025, E-073, E-153, E-158, E-184, E-222, E-237, E-260, E-186, D-186

Seto, Arnold H.: B-013, B-276, H-335, H-176, H-211

Shah, Sanjiv J.: B-015, B-036, B-053, B-118, B-251, B-258, B-274, E-005, E-015, E-040, E-053, E-063, E-072, E-074, E-079, E-123, E-125, E-145, E-147, E-199, E-206, E-208, E-238, E-249, E-258, E-259, E-274, E-296, E-306, E-349, E-283, E-051, E-059, E-096, E-146, E-286, E-317, E-333, E-334, G-326, G-355

Shahanavaz, Shabana: E-008, E-236, E-145

Shivkumar, Kalyanam: C-352, A-254, D-254

Solomon, Scott D.: E-005, B-015, B-027, E-027, B-040, E-040, E-048, B-053, E-053, B-063, E-063, E-072, B-074, B-079, E-079, E-089, E-101, E-118, B-125, E-125, E-126, B-150, E-150, B-182, E-182, B-206, E-208, E-211, E-238, B-249, E-249, E-253, B-258, E-258, B-259, B-300, E-301, B-306, E-306, B-331, E-097, E-095, E-290, B-146, B-255, B-339, E-339, E-334, E-135, E-345, E-103, E-245, E-038, E-310

Sorrentino, Matthew J.: G-355

Starling, Randall C.: B-258, B-005, B-118, B-040, C-166, E-265

Stevenson, William G.: H-005, H-066, H-074, H-070, H-236, E-258, C-036, C-361-, G-152, B-257, B-037

Teerlink, John R.: B-005, E-005, B-040, E-040, B-053, E-053, B-054, E-054, B-063, E-063, B-072, E-072, B-079, E-079, B-125, E-125, B-222, E-222, B-236, E-236, B-238, E-238, B-258, E-258, B-315, E-315, B-327, E-327, C-366

Thompson, Paul D.: A-003, A-005, A-008, A-124, A-176, A-213, A-274, A-285, A-245, B-040, B-157, B-258, E-151

Tomaselli, Gordon F.: F-040, D-136, H-186, H-233

Turakhia, Mintu P.: B-036, B-063, B-079, B-045, E-005, E-063, E-171, E-213, E-236, E-249, E-306, E-274, E-244

Vardeny, Orly: B-053, B-063, B-306, B-166, B-251, E-036, C-358

Weitz, Jeffrey I.: E-063, E-072, E-079, E-126, E-206, E-211, E-238, E-274

Wenger, Nanette Kass: B-053, B-072, B-140, B-251, B-383, B-132

Wu, Justina C.: G-151, E-090

Zeppenfeld, Katja: B-067

Zile, Michael R.: E-005, E-074, E-118, E-123, D-132, E-145, E-150, C-230, E-236, E-258, C-366, E-372, E-144

Index

Note: Page numbers followed by "f" indicate figures, "t" indicate tables, "b" indicate boxes.

A

a wave, 127–128
AAI pacing mode, 1327, 1327f
Abacavir, cardiovascular disease and, in HIV patients, 1605
ABCC9-related intellectual disability myopathy syndrome, 1869
Abciximab
 in myocardial infarction, renal dysfunction and, 1884f
 in percutaneous coronary intervention, 800.e1
 in thrombosis, 1778
Abdomen, examination of, 126
Abdominal pain, in rheumatic fever, 1535
Abdominojugular reflux, 128
Abetalipoproteinemia, 510b
Ablation, cryoballoon catheter, 1281, 1281f–1282f
Absolute benefit, 57–58
Absolute flow reserve, 620, 620f, 620.e1f
Absolute risk reduction, 58
Acarbose, in diabetes mellitus, 562t–563t, 569
Accelerated arteriosclerosis, after transplantation, 438–439, 439f–440f
Accelerated idioventricular rhythm, 1210t, 1292
 electrocardiography in, 1292, 1293f
 electrotherapy in, 1227b
 management of, 1292
Accentuated antagonism, 1178
Accessory pathways
 anatomic considerations, 1264b
 anterograde, 1217b–1218b
 arrhythmias associated with, 1266–1267
 atriofascicular, 1231b–1232b, 1268b–1270b, 1269f
 concealed *vs.* manifest, 1264b
 epidemiology of, 1264, 1264f
 localization, 1266b
 location of, 1231–1232, 1231f
 multiple, 1241f
 radiofrequency catheter ablation of, 1231–1232
 retrograde, 1217b–1218b, 1223b–1224b
 septal, 1231b–1232b
 tachycardias due to, 1264–1270
 unusual forms of, 1268.e1f, 1268b–1270b, 1269f
 WPW ECG, 1264–1266, 1264f–1266f
Accuracy, in biomarkers, 106
ACE inhibitors. *See* Angiotensin-converting enzyme (ACE) inhibitors
Acebutolol, in angina pectoris, 758t
Acetylcholine, of sinoatrial node, 1175.e1b
Acetylsalicylic acid. *See* Aspirin
Acidosis, coronary vascular resistance and, 616b–617b
Acoustic shadowing, in echocardiography, 215b–216b
Acquired atrioventricular block, 1162.e1, 1162.e3t
Acquired immunodeficiency syndrome (AIDS). *See* Human immunodeficiency virus (HIV) infection
Acromegaly, 487
 cardiovascular manifestations of, 1791–1793
 diagnosis of, 1792–1793
 treatment of, 1792b
ACTA2, 812
Actin, 892f, 893, 894f
Action potential. *See* Cardiac action potential
Action potential duration (APD)
 functional reentry and, 1187.e1f, 1185
 in heart failure, 924–925, 925.e1f
Action to Control Cardiovascular Risk in Diabetes (ACCORD) trial, 492
Active fixation leads, 1322b–1323b
Acupuncture, 593b–594b
 in hypertension, 595
Acute Addisonian crisis, 1795b

Acute aortic regurgitation, 1428–1429
 clinical presentation of, 1428–1429, 1428f, 1428b–1429b
 management of, 1428b–1429b
 pathophysiology of, 1428–1429, 1428f, 1428b–1429b
Acute aortic syndromes, 818, 818f
Acute cerebrovascular disease, 1870–1871, 1870f
Acute chest pain. *See* Chest pain
Acute coronary syndrome (ACS). *See also* Myocardial infarction
 acute heart failure and, 956b
 acute stress and, 1841
 in chronic kidney disease, 1880, 1880t–1881t
 in COVID-19 patients, 1757
 in diabetes mellitus, 571–573
 in elderly, 1696–1697
 evaluation of, 124t, 138
 magnetic resonance imaging in, 322b, 323f–324f
 marijuana use and, 1600, 1600b
 myocardial infarction, 636, 638f, 639
 non-ST elevation, 714–738, 715f
  amphetamine use and, 735
  biomarkers in, 717–718, 717f–718f, 718t–720t
  cardiac syndrome X and, 735
  chronic kidney disease and, 733b–734b
  clinical assessment of, 715–718
  cocaine use and, 735
  diabetes mellitus and, 733–734
  early risk stratification in, 735.e1
  electrocardiography in, 716–717
  epidemiology of, 714
  future perspectives in, 735, 735t
  glucose intolerance and, 733–734
  heart failure and, 734
  history of, 715
  invasive imaging of, 719
  management of, 721–732
   anticoagulant therapy in, 726–727, 735.e3
   anti-inflammatory therapies, 728
   anti-ischemic therapy in, 721–723, 723t, 735.e2
   antithrombotic therapy in, 723–726, 723f, 724t, 735.e2, 735.e4t
   bleeding and, 728
   coronary revascularization in, 735.e2
   discharge and posthospital care for, 732
   early hospital care for, 735.e1, 735.e2t
   evidence gaps in, 735.e3
   general measures in, 721
   guidelines on, 735.e1, 735.e1t
   hospital discharge in, 735.e2
   initial evaluation in, 735.e1, 735.e3f
   invasive *vs.* conservative, 728–731, 730f
   ischemia-guided strategy for, 731, 735.e2, 735.e5f
   lipid-lowering therapy in, 731–732, 732f
   performance measures and registries in, 735.e7t
   posthospital care in, 732
   risk factor modification, 735.e3
   timing of invasive approach, 731
  noninvasive testing for, 718–719, 721t
  in older adults, 732–733
  pathophysiology of, 714–715, 716f–717f, 716t
  physical examination in, 716
  Prinzmetal variant angina and, 734
  risk assessment of, 720, 722f
  risk criteria in, 735.e6t
  vasospastic angina, 734–735
  in women, 733
 OCT in, 381–382, 381f–382f
 percutaneous coronary interventions in, 787–793
 reasons for poor outcomes after, 1881–1882, 1884t–1886t

Acute coronary syndrome (ACS) *(Continued)*
 renal dysfunction as prognostic factor in, 1880–1881, 1880t–1883t, 1884f
 suspected, 293–294
 transcatheter aortic valve replacement and, 1436
 in women, 1717
Acute ischemia, electrophysiologic effects of, 1366b
Acute ischemic stroke
 management of, 879–886, 880t
  anticoagulation therapy for, 883–886, 885f
  endovascular therapy for, 881–883, 883f–884f, 884t
  intravenous recombinant tissue plasminogen activator, 880–881, 881f–883f, 881b, 882t
 other modalities for treatment of, 885b–886b
Acute kidney injury
 cardiac surgery associated, 1877–1879, 1879f
 contrast-induced, 1875–1876, 1877f–1878f
Acute limb ischemia (ALI), 854–855, 859
 clinical categories of, 854.e1t
 diagnostic tests in, 854, 854.e2t
 incidence of, 837–838
 pathogenesis of, 854, 854f
 prognosis of, 854, 854.e1f, 854.e1t
 treatment of, 854–855, 855f
Acute myocardial infarction
 cardiovascular disease and, 6–7, 6f
 influenza and, 1752
 pacemakers in
  asystole, 703
  permanent pacing in, 703
  temporary pacing in, 703
 secondary prevention after, 707–710
  anticoagulants as, 709–710, 709.e1f
  antiplatelet agents as, 708
  beta-adrenergic blocking agents as, 709
  calcium channel antagonists as, 710
  cardiac rehabilitation, 707
  depression, 707–708
  hormone therapy as, 710
  lifestyle modification, 707
  modification of lipid profile, 708
  nitrates as, 709
  nonsteroidal antiinflammatory drugs as, 710
  renin-angiotensin-aldosterone system as, 708–709
Acute pericarditis, 1616–1620
 causes of, 1616
 definition of, 1616, 1617t
 diagnosis of, 1618–1619
 differential diagnosis of, 1616
 electrocardiography in, 1616–1617, 1618f
 epidemiology of, 1616
 etiology of, 1617t
 history of, 1616
 laboratory testing in, 1616–1618
 management of, 1618–1619, 1618t–1619t, 1619f
 natural history of, 1618–1619
 physical examination in, 1616
 recurrent, 1619–1620, 1620.e1f
Acute vasospasm, 1100
Adams-Stokes attacks, 1318–1319
Adaptive design, 49–50
Adaptive immunity, in atherosclerosis, 432, 433f
Addison disease, 1795b
Adenoma
 of adrenal gland, 1794b
 of pituitary gland, 1792
Adenosine, 1211.e1t, 1208t–1210t, 1212t, 1214t, 1225, 1225b
 coronary vascular resistance and, 616b–617b
 pregnancy and, 1730f
Adenosine A$_1$ receptor antagonists, for acute heart failure, 971b–972b

Volume 1 pp. 1-888 • **Volume 2** pp. 889-1902

I-1

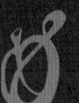

Adenosine A₂ receptor agonists, as coronary vasodilators, 614b
Adenosine diphosphate receptor antagonists, in percutaneous coronary intervention, 799–800, 800.e1t
Adenovirus infection, 1080b–1081b
Adenylyl cyclase, 901–902
ADI pacing mode, reducing right ventricular pacing, 1328b, 1329f
Adipokines, in heart failure, 920.e1f, 920b–921b
Adiponectin, in heart failure, 920b–921b
Adipose tissue
  in heart failure with preserved and mildly reduced ejection, 1011b–1017b
  obesity and, 548
  visceral, as endocrine organ, 549, 550f–551f
Adiposity, causal inference for, 80
Adjunctive pharmacotherapy, in percutaneous coronary intervention, 787.e1, 787.e3t
Ado-trastuzumab Emtansine (T-DM1), 1095
ADRA2C, 1194
ADRB1, 1194
ADRB1 gene, 95t, 98
ADRB2 gene, 95t
Adrenal insufficiency, 1795b
Adrenergic inhibitors. See Beta adrenoceptor-blocking agents (beta blockers)
Adrenergic signaling systems, 899–903, 900t
Adrenocorticotropic hormone, 1793
Adrenomedullin, in heart failure, 920b–921b
Advanced heart failure, statins in, 517
Adventitia, 428, 428f
  in intravascular imaging, 379
AED. See Automated external defibrillator
Aerobic exercise
  capacity, age-associated changes in, 1687b–1690b, 1690f
  in hypertension, 595
African Americans
  heart failure in, 1001
  hypertension in, 1747t
Afterdepolarizations, 1180, 1181f
  delayed, 1180–1181, 1182f
    generation of, role of intracellular Ca²⁺-handling abnormalities in, 1183.e1f, 1181–1183
  early, 1180, 1183
    drugs and, 1183
Afterload, 906
  abrupt increase in, 906–907
Age/aging. See also Older adults
  abdominal aortic aneurysm, 1709.e1
  acute coronary syndromes and, 1696–1697
  acute heart failure and, 946–947
  aortic dissection, 1709.e2
  cardiac rhythm abnormalities and, 1701–1702
  cardiovascular structure and function, associated changes in, 1687–1690, 1688f
    to exercise, 1687b–1690b, 1690f
    left ventricular, 1687b–1690b
    resting cardiac function, 1687b–1690b, 1689f
    vasculature, 1687b–1690b
  central sleep apnea and, 1679–1680
  coronary heart disease and, 1695–1696
  definition of, 1687
  epidemiology of, 25–26
  heart failure and, 933, 1697–1699
  lower extremity peripheral arterial disease and, 1709.e1
  obstructive sleep apnea and, 1679–1680
  STEMI-related mortality and, 636, 636.e1f
  sudden cardiac death and, 1352–1354, 1353f
  syncope and, 1703
  valvular heart disease and, 1699–1701
  venous thromboembolic disease and, 1702–1703, 1774
  visceral obesity and, 550
Air pollution, cardiovascular disease and, 31–37, 32f, 39.e1t
  cardiovascular effects of, 34–36, 35f
    approaches to communicate risk, 37
    arrhythmia, 36
    chronic kidney disease, 36
    diabetes, 36
    heart failure, 36
    hypertension, 35–36
    ischemic heart disease, 35
    mechanistic insights into, 36–37, 36f
    societal and personal strategies, 37
    venous thromboembolism, 36

Air pollution, cardiovascular disease and (Continued)
  cardiovascular mortality and, 34
  composition of, 31–34, 33t
    gaseous pollutants, 33
    household vs. ambient air pollution, 34
    particulate matter, 33–34
Airway, in cardiopulmonary resuscitation, 1372
Ajmaline, 1211.e1t, 1208t–1209t, 1212t, 1216, 1216b
Albiglutide, in diabetes mellitus, 562t–563t, 567
Alcohol, 535, 540t. See also Ethanol
Alcohol consumption, cardiovascular disease and, 459–461, 460f
Alcohol septal ablation, in hypertrophic cardiomyopathy, 1071–1072, 1075f
Alcoholic cardiomyopathy, 1041, 1593–1594
Aldosterone, 1025, 1793f, 1795b
  heart failure and, 983, 993–994
  hypertension and, 475–476
Aldosterone antagonists
  in chronic HFrEF, 1698b
  hyperkalemia due to, 988
  pregnancy and, 1730f
Aldosterone/renin ratio, 1794–1795
Alfimeprase, 1789b
Aliskiren, in heart failure, 996–997
Alkylating agents, cardiotoxic effects of, 1092t, 1094.e1
Alkylating-like agents, cardiotoxic effects of, 1092t, 1094.e1
Alleles, 73
Allen test, 386
Allergic reactions, after coronary angiography, 364b–366b
Allergy, to aspirin, 1776
Alogliptin, in diabetes mellitus, 562t–563t, 566
Alpha adrenoceptor-blocking activity, 759.e1
Alpha-adrenergic receptor subtypes, 901
Alpha-galactosidase A deficiency, 1046
  echocardiography in, 222
Alteplase, 1788, 1788f
Alternans patterns, 171b–172b, 172f
Alternative payment models (APMs), cardiovascular disease and, 65–66
Ambrisentan, in pulmonary arterial hypertension, 1675f
Ambulatory blood pressure monitoring (ABPM), 482–483
Ambulatory electrocardiographic (Holter) recording, 1151–1153, 1154f–1155f, 1162.e2t, 1162.e3t
Ambulatory monitoring, in sudden cardiac death, 1378b–1379b
Amiloride, in heart failure, 983t, 984
Amiodarone, 1211.e1t, 1208t–1209t, 1212t, 1214t, 1220–1222, 1221t
  in atrial fibrillation, 1278
  in heart failure, 1002
  in chronic kidney disease, 1890t
  in pregnancy, 1730f
  thyroid function and, 1803–1804, 1804t
Amiodarone-induced thyrotoxicosis (AIT), 1803, 1804t
AMIOVERT trial, 1336t
Amlodipine, in angina pectoris, 760, 761t
Amniotic fluid embolism, sudden cardiac death and, 1363b–1365b
Amphetamines
  cardiovascular complications of, 1599, 1599b
  in non-ST elevation acute coronary syndromes, 735
Amphotericin B, in infective endocarditis, 1519b–1523b
Ampicillin-sulbactam, in infective endocarditis, 1519b–1523b
Amplatz catheters, 367, 368f
Amplatzer ASD closure device, echocardiography in, 257, 259f
Amplatzer devices, in atrial septal defects, 1589–1590, 1589f, 1590b
Amplatzer duct occluders, in congenital heart disease, 1591, 1591f
Amplatzer vascular plugs, in congenital heart disease, 1591, 1591f
Amylin mimetics, in diabetes mellitus, 562t–563t
Amyloid A, serum, in chest pain evaluation, 603b
Amyloidosis
  advanced circulatory support in, 1058b
  amyloidogenic light chain, 1052, 1058–1059
  amyloidogenic transthyretin, 1052–1053, 1059–1060, 1059t
    TTR silencers, 1060
    TTR stabilizers, 1059–1060

Amyloidosis (Continued)
  arrhythmia, management of, 1058b
  cardiac, 1044, 1052–1061, 1053t
    biomarkers of, 1056b
    biopsy in, 1056b
    clinical features of, 1054
    clinical management of, 1058–1060
    diagnosis of, 1055–1056, 1055f, 1057t
    epidemiology of, 1052–1053
    genotyping in, 1056b
    imaging in, 1056b, 1057f
    magnetic resonance imaging in, 326, 326f–327f
    pathophysiology of, 1053–1054
    prognosis of, 1054
  disease-targeted therapeutics for, 1058–1060
  echocardiography in, 220f, 222
  heart failure, management of, 1058b
  imaging, 284b
  organ transplantation and, 1058b
  radionuclide imaging in, 303–304, 304f–305f
  supportive non-disease-modifying therapies, 1058
Analgesics, for STEMI, 665–666
Analyses, alternative methods of, 46b–47b
Anastrozole, cardiotoxic effects of, 1092t
Andersen-Tawil syndrome (ATS), 1199, 1865, 1866f–1867f
  clinical description and manifestations of, 1199, 1200f
  electrocardiography in, 1199
  genetic basis of, 1192f, 1199b
  KCNJ2-Mediated, phenotypic correlates of, 1199
Andexanet alfa, 1786–1787, 1786t
Androgen deprivation therapy, 1092t, 1096
Anemia
  in chronic kidney disease, 1874–1875
  heart failure and, 977.e1f, 976–977
  prevalence of, 977b–978b
Anesthesia, for noncardiac surgery, 417–418, 417f–418f
  epidural, 418
  monitored anesthesia care in, 418
  regional, 418
  spinal, 418
Aneurysmal disease, atherosclerosis and, 439–440
Aneurysmectomy, left ventricular, 780.e1
Aneurysms
  aortic. See Aortic aneurysm(s)
  coronary artery, 749.e1
  left ventricular, 218b–219b
  sinus of Valsalva, echocardiography in, 244, 248f
Aneurysms-osteoarthritis syndrome, 811, 811t
Angina pectoris. See also Chest pain; Stable ischemic heart disease
  evaluation of, 123–124
  pain, mechanism of, 740.e1
  stable, 739–742
    assessment of, 740
    characteristics of, 739–740, 740.e1f
    classification of, 740
    clinical manifestations of, 739–740
    enhanced external counterpulsation for, 764.e1
    importance of pathophysiologic considerations, 742
    increased myocardial oxygen requirements and, 741–742
    nonpharmacologic treatment approaches to, 764
    pain in, 740–741
    pathophysiology of, 741–742, 741f
    percutaneous coronary intervention in, 786–787
    pharmacologic management of, 757–758, 757t
      beta adrenoceptor-blocking agents for, 757–758, 757f, 757t–758t, 760t
      calcium antagonists for, 758–760
      choice of initial therapy of, 763
      combination therapy in, 764
      integrated approach to, 764
      nitrates for, 760–762, 760.e1f, 762t
      selection of, 763–764
    physical examination in, 741
    relief of, 772
    risk models of, 749
    risk stratification in, 749
    spinal cord stimulation for, 764.e1
    transiently decreased oxygen supply and, 742
    treatment of associated diseases, 749
Angiogenesis, 628
  in plaques, 434–435, 434f
Angiographic stroke volume, 402

Angiography
  in aortic regurgitation, 1423
  in Behçet disease, 1825f
  in constrictive pericarditis, 1627
  coronary, 363–384
    access sites for, 366–367, 366.e1f
    in acute kidney injury, 364b–366b, 365f
    appropriate use criteria for, 364–366
    basic technique for, 367
    catheters for, 367–369, 367f–368f
    complications of, 364b–366b, 365f
    contraindications to, 364b–366b
    contrast media for, 371, 371.e1t
      manual injection of, 371, 371b, 371.e1t
    coronary anatomy and, 372–373
    in coronary artery anomalies, 373–374, 373t
    in dilated cardiomyopathy, 1032
    evaluation of, 375
    high-risk findings from, 748.e1, 748.e1f
    indications for, 363–366, 363.e1t
    patient preparation for, 366
    percutaneous coronary intervention for, 382–383, 382.e1f
    pitfalls of, 374–375, 374.e1f
    projections, 371–372, 372f–373f, 372t
    risks associated with, 363t–364t
    risks related to radiation exposure in, 364b–366b
    selective coronary artery cannulation in, 367b–368b, 368f
    special lesion considerations for, 377–378
      bifurcation lesions, 378
      calcific lesions, 377, 377.e1f, 377.e1t
      chronic total occlusion, 377
      coronary dissections, 378, 378f, 378.e1t
      thrombotic lesions, 377, 378f
    in stable ischemic heart disease, 747–748, 748.e1f
    technique for, 366–371
    ventriculography for, 369–371, 369f–370f, 370t
  limitations of, 748
  in polyarteritis nodosa, 1818f
  in pulmonary embolism, 1644
AngioJet rheolytic thrombectomy catheter, 795.e1, 862–863
Angioplasty. See Percutaneous coronary interventions
Angiopoietin-like protein 3 (ANGPTL3), inhibition of, 520
Angiosarcoma, 1834t
Angiosome-directed revascularization, 865, 865.e1f
Angiotensin II receptor blockers
  in coronary artery disease, chronic kidney disease and, 1880t–1881t
  in hypertension management, 560–561
  pregnancy and, 1730
Angiotensin receptor blockers (ARBs)
  in atrial fibrillation, 1280
  in chronic HFrEF, 1698b
  in COVID-19, 1762–1763
  in heart failure, 991t, 993, 993b
  for heart failure with preserved and mildly reduced ejection, 1024–1025
  in peripheral artery disease, 847–848
  side effects of, 993
  in stable ischemic heart disease, 754b–756b, 756f
Angiotensin receptor neprilysin inhibitors
  in heart failure, 575, 991t, 993–994, 994f
  for heart failure with preserved and mildly reduced ejection, 1025–1026, 1026f–1027f
  side effects of, 994
Angiotensin II, in hypertension, 475, 477
Angiotensin-converting enzyme (ACE) inhibitors
  in atrial fibrillation, 1280
  in chronic HFrEF, 1698b
  in coronary artery disease, chronic kidney disease and, 1880t–1881t
  in COVID-19, 1762–1763
  in heart failure, 989–993, 991f, 991t
  for heart failure with preserved and mildly reduced ejection, 1024
  in hypertension management, 560
  in peripheral artery disease, 847–848
  in pregnancy, 1730
  side effects of, 991–993
  in stable ischemic heart disease, 754b–756b, 757f
Angiotensinogen, 3
Anidulafungin, in infective endocarditis, 1519b–1523b
Anisotropy, 1173
Anistreplase, 1788

Anitschkow cells, 1532b–1533b, 1533f
Ankle-brachial index (ABI), 128, 453
  in peripheral artery disease, 837, 843
Ankylosing spondylitis
  atherosclerosis in, 1811
  conduction disturbances in, 1821
"Ankyrin-B syndrome", 1199–1200
Annuloplasty
  in mitral regurgitation
    direct, 1486b–1488b, 1490f
    indirect, 1486b–1488b, 1490f
  in tricuspid regurgitation, 1490b–1492b, 1492f
Anomalous coronary artery, 352, 353f–354f
  from the pulmonary artery, 1578, 1579f
Anomalous origin of coronary artery, coronary angiography in, 373b–374b, 374f
Anomalous pulmonary venous connection, magnetic resonance imaging in, 330b–332b, 331f
Anomalous termination, coronary angiography in, 373b–374b
Anrep effect, 906–907
Anterograde access, for peripheral artery disease, 864, 864.e1f
Anterolateral papillary muscle, 1456
Anthracyclines, 1091b
  cardiotoxic effects of, 1091–1094, 1092t, 1093f–1094f, 1093b–1094b, 1099, 1102t
  genetics of, 1094.e1, 1094.e2t, 1094.e4t
Antianginal medications, in coronary artery disease, chronic kidney disease and, 1880t–1881t
Antiarrhythmic therapy, 1227
  adenosine as, 1211.e1t, 1208t–1209t, 1212t, 1225, 1225b
  class IA, 1213–1216
    ajmaline as, 1211.e1t, 1208t–1209t, 1212t, 1216, 1216b
    disopyramide as, 1211.e1t, 1208t–1209t, 1212t, 1215–1216, 1215b–1216b
    procainamide as, 1211.e1t, 1208t–1209t, 1212t, 1213–1215, 1213b–1215b
    quinidine as, 1211.e1t, 1208t–1209t, 1212t, 1213, 1213b
  class IB, 1216–1217
    lidocaine as, 1211.e1t, 1208t–1209t, 1212t, 1216–1217, 1216b
    mexiletine as, 1211.e1t, 1208t–1209t, 1212t, 1217, 1217b
    phenytoin as, 1211.e1t, 1208t–1209t, 1212t, 1217
  class IC, 1217–1219
    flecainide as, 1211.e1t, 1208t–1209t, 1212t, 1217–1218, 1217b–1218b
    propafenone as, 1211.e1t, 1208t–1209t, 1212t, 1218–1219, 1218b
  class II, 1219–1220
    beta adrenoceptor-blocking agents as, 1212t, 1219–1220, 1219b
  class III, 1220–1223, 1220b
    amiodarone as, 1211.e1t, 1208t–1209t, 1212t, 1220–1222
    dofetilide as, 1211.e1t, 1208t–1209t, 1212t, 1223, 1223b
    dronedarone as, 1211.e1t, 1208t–1209t, 1212t, 1222, 1222b
    ibutilide as, 1211.e1t, 1208t–1209t, 1212t, 1223, 1223b
    sotalol as, 1211.e1t, 1208t–1209t, 1212t, 1222–1223, 1222b
  class IV, 1223–1225
    diltiazem as, 1211.e1t, 1209t, 1212t, 1223–1225, 1223b–1224b
    verapamil as, 1211.e1t, 1209t, 1212t, 1223–1225, 1223b–1224b
  digoxin as, 1211.e1t, 1209t, 1212t, 1225–1226, 1226b
  drug use during pregnancy, 1212t
  effects of nonantiarrhythmic drugs in, 1227
  efficacy of, 1162.e1
  new, 1227
    vernakalant as, 1227b
    ranolazine as, 1211.e1t, 1209t, 1212t, 1226–1227, 1226b–1227b
  in sudden cardiac death, 1368
Antiarrhythmics Versus Implantable Defibrillators (AVID) trial, 1331–1332
Antibiotic prophylaxis
  in cardiovascular implantable electronic device, 1528
  in rheumatic fever, 1537

Antibody-mediated rejection (AMR), 1137–1138
Anticardiolipin antibodies, 1822
Anticoagulant therapy, 1766. See also Heparin; Warfarin
  for acute ischemic stroke, 883–886, 885f
  in acute limb ischemia, 855
  for acute myocardial infarction, 709–710, 709.e1f
  in heart failure, 1001–1002
  for ischemic stroke, 878–879, 879b
  novel, 1787
  in NSTE-ACS, 723f, 726–728, 735.e3, 735.e4t
  oral, 1783–1787
    dosages of, 1785–1786
    mechanism of action of, 1785
    monitoring of, 1786
    periprocedural management of, 1786
    side effects of, 1786
    in stable ischemic heart disease, 754b–756b
  oral, chronic, 728b
  in peripheral artery disease, 849, 849.e1f
  during pregnancy, 1735–1737, 1785
  for STEMI, 675–679, 675.e1f
    with fibrinolysis, 677
    for patients treated without reperfusion therapy, 677
    for primary percutaneous coronary intervention, 677
  in thrombosis, 1779–1787, 1779f, 1779t–1781t, 1783f, 1784t–1786t
Anticoagulation
  in cancer, 1104
  ongoing trials of
  optimal duration of, 1648
  role of, in COVID-19, 1762
Antidepressant medications, 1847–1850, 1848t
  cardiac QTc prolongation and, 1849
  drug-drug interactions and, 1849–1850
Antidigoxin immunotherapy, 1000.e2
Antigen-presenting cells, 432
Antihyperglycemic medications, in heart failure, 575–576, 576f
Antihypertensive and Lipid-Lowering Treatment to Prevent Heart Attack Trial (ALLHAT), 494
Antihypertensive therapy, 97
  in chronic kidney disease, 1890
  in peripheral artery disease, 847–848
Anti-ischemic therapy, in NSTE-ACS, 721–723, 723t, 735.e2
Antimetabolites, cardiotoxic effects of, 1092t, 1094.e1
Antioxidants
  in ischemic heart disease, 595
  in stable ischemic heart disease, 754b–756b
  vitamins, 539b
Antiphospholipid antibodies, 1824
Antiphospholipid syndrome
  pulmonary embolism and, 1637
  therapy for, 1651
  thrombosis and, 1824
    cardiovascular disease and, 1824, 1825f
    treatment of, 1824
  venous thrombosis and, 1775
Antiplatelet therapy, 1766. See also Aspirin; Dipyridamole; Glycoprotein IIb/IIIa inhibitors; Thienopyridines
  in acute coronary syndromes, 572–573
  for acute myocardial infarction, 708
  in atheroembolism, 856
  in coronary artery disease, chronic kidney disease and, 1880t–1881t
  in coronary heart disease, 561
  in heart failure, 1001–1002
  for ischemic stroke, 878, 878f–879f, 879b
  in NSTE-ACS, 723–726, 723f, 724t
    intravenous, 726
    long-term, 726, 729f–730f
    oral, 723–726, 724b, 735.e3
  in percutaneous coronary intervention, 787.e3t, 799–801
  in peripheral artery disease, 848–849, 848.e2f
  pregnancy and, 1730f
  in stable ischemic heart disease, 771
  for STEMI, 675–679
    combination pharmacologic reperfusion, 679
    with fibrinolysis, 678
    for percutaneous coronary intervention in, 677–678, 678f–679f
    recommendation for, 679, 679.e1f
  for stroke, 877, 877f
  in thrombosis, 1775–1779, 1776f, 1778f, 1778t

Antiproliferative agents, in cardiac transplantation, 1136
Antiretroviral therapy, in HIV patients, cardiovascular disease and, 1608–1609, 1609t
Antirheumatic drugs, cardiovascular disease and, 1824–1827
Antitachycardia pacing (ATP), 1337b–1339b, 1341f
   for monomorphic ventricular tachycardia, 1341f
Antithrombin, deficiency in, 1773
Antithrombotic therapy, 1766, 1767f
   in NSTE-ACS, 723–726, 723f, 724t, 735.e2, 735.e4t
   in percutaneous coronary intervention, 801
   in peripheral artery disease, 848–849
   in prosthetic heart valves, 1498–1499, 1499t
      interruption of, 1498–1499
   for stroke, 877–879
Antithrombotic Trialists' (ATT) Collaboration Meta-analysis, 848
Antithymocyte globulins (ATGs), in cardiac transplantation, 1136
Anti-TNF-α therapy, for giant cell arteritis, 1815
Antiviral therapies
   for COVID-19, 1762
   for influenza, 1754
Anxiety, 1844, 1844b. *See also* Stress
Anxiolytic medications, 1850
AOO pacing mode, 1327, 1327f
Aorta
   abdominal
      examination of, 126
      pulsation of, 130
   abnormalities of, 1582
   anatomy of, 806, 807f
   aneurysm of. *See* Aortic aneurysm(s)
   bacterial infections of, 832–834
   coarctation of. *See* Aortic coarctation
   disease of, 806–836
      echocardiography in, 244–248, 244f–246f, 246t
   dissection of, echocardiography in, 244, 245f–246f, 249f
   evaluation of, 806
   in heart failure with preserved and mildly reduced ejection, 1011b–1017b
   layers of, 806b
   microscopic structure of, 806b, 808f
   palpation of, 807
   physiology of, 806
   primary tumors of, 834, 834.e1f
   transection of, echocardiography in, 245–246
   valve of, echocardiography in, 231–234, 232f
Aortic aneurysm(s), 806–818
   abdominal, 807–810, 807.e1f
      clinical features of, 807
      computed tomographic angiography in, 807–808
      computed tomography in, 807–808, 809f
      diagnostic imaging for, 807–808
      in elderly, 1709.e1
      genetics of, 808
      magnetic resonance angiography in, 807–808
      management of, 809–810
         medical therapy for, 809
         surgery for, 809–810
         surveillance for, 809
      natural history, 809, 809.e1f
      pathogenesis of, 807, 807.e1f
      ruptured, 809
      screening for, 808
      ultrasound in, 807–808, 808.e1f
   echocardiography in, 244, 247f
   thoracic, 810–818
      in aneurysms-osteoarthritis syndrome, 811, 811t
      in aortitis, 814
      in bicuspid aortic valve, 812–813, 814f
      cause of, 810–814
      chest radiography in, 814f–815f, 815
      clinical manifestations of, 813.e1f, 814–815
      computed tomographic angiography in, 815, 816f
      computed tomography in, 813.e1f, 815
      degenerative, 814
      diagnosis of, 815, 815.e1f
      dissection with, 814
      familial, 812, 814f
      genetics of, 810–814, 811t, 812f, 813t
      Kommerell diverticulum, 814
      in Loeys-Dietz syndrome, 811, 811t, 814f
      magnetic resonance angiography in, 815
      management of, 817–818
         aortic arch, 817, 817.e2f
         ascending, 817, 817.e1f, 817.e2f

Aortic aneurysm(s) *(Continued)*
         descending, 817
         endovascular repair for, 817–818
         medical, 818
         surgical treatment for, 817–818
         thoracoabdominal, 817, 817b, 817.e3f
      in Marfan syndrome, 811, 811t, 811.e1f, 813f
      natural history of, 815–816, 815.e1f, 815f–816f
      pathogenesis of, 810–814, 811.e1f
      in syphilis, 814
      transthoracic echocardiography in, 815
      in Turner syndrome, 813, 813.e1f
      in vascular Ehlers-Danlos syndrome, 812
Aortic arch
   anatomy of, 806
   aneurysms of, 817, 817.e2f
Aortic coarctation, 274, 489–490, 1575–1576, 1575f–1577f
   echocardiography in, 244
   magnetic resonance imaging in, 330b–332b, 331f
Aortic dilation
   arterial switch operation and, 1567
   congenital heart disease and, 1551–1552
Aortic dissection, 818–831
   aortic regurgitation in, 822, 822f
   aortography in, 824, 824.e1f
   biomarkers in, 823f, 823b
   cause of, 819–821
   chest pain in, 600, 600t
   chest radiography in, 823, 823.e1f
   classification of, 819, 819f, 819t–820t, 819f–820f
   clinical manifestations of, 821–823
   cocaine and, 1598
   complications of, 821, 822t
   computed tomography in, 815.e1f, 823, 824f
   coronary angiography in, 824
   diagnostic techniques in, 823–824, 823.e1t
   echocardiogram in, 824
   in elderly, 1709.e2
   evaluation of, 824–830, 825f
   imaging modality in, 824
   laboratory findings in, 823
   magnetic resonance imaging in, 823–824, 824.e1f
   management of, 825–827, 826f
      blood pressure reduction in, 827, 827t
      of cardiac tamponade, 827
      definitive therapy for, 827–830, 827f, 827.e1f, 827.e2f, 829t
      follow-up in, 830–831, 830.e3f
      long-term therapy in, 830–831
      surgical, 828b–830b
      type A aortic dissection, 827.e2f, 828b–830b
      type B aortic dissection, 828f–829f, 828b–830b, 829t
   neurologic manifestations of, 822
   pathogenesis of, 819–821
   physical findings in, 821–823, 822f, 822.e1f
   risk factors for, 821t
   symptoms of, 821
   with thoracic aortic aneurysms, 814
   transesophageal echocardiography in, 822f, 824
   transthoracic echocardiography in, 824, 824.e1f
   ultrasound in, 824
   variants of, 831–832. *See also* Aortic intramural hematoma
Aortic impedance, 907b–908b
Aortic intramural hematoma, 831, 831.e2f, 833f
   computed tomography in, 831f–832f, 832, 832.e1f
   echocardiography in, 245–246, 246f
   high-risk features of, 831.e2t
   magnetic resonance imaging in, 831, 831.e2f
   transesophageal echocardiograms in, 831, 831f–832f
Aortic isthmus, anatomy of, 806
Aortic regurgitation, 1419–1429
   acute, 1428–1429
      clinical presentation of, 1428–1429, 1428f, 1428b–1429b
      management of, 1428b–1429b
      pathophysiology of, 1428–1429, 1428f, 1428b–1429b
   in aortic dissection, 822, 822f
   aortic root disease, 1419
   arterial switch operation and, 1567
   ascending aorta, 1419
   assessment of severity of, 1424f
   asymptomatic patients, 1423–1424, 1425f
   bifid pulse in, 129

Aortic regurgitation *(Continued)*
   causes of, 1419, 1420t
   chronic, 1419–1428
      clinical stages of, 1422t
      management of patients with, 1427f
      pathophysiology of, 1419–1420
      treatment of, 1426–1428
   clinical presentation of, 1420–1421
   diagnostic testing of, 1421–1423
   disease course of, 1423–1428
   echocardiography in, 234, 234f, 234.e1f, 234.e2f
   in elderly, 1700b–1701b
   evaluation of, 137–138
   hemodynamics of, 1421f
   indications for aortic valve surgery, 1426t
   in infective endocarditis, 1515–1516
   magnetic resonance imaging in, 328–329, 328f
   mitral regurgitation and, 1482b
   pathology of, 1419
   pathophysiology of, 1420f
   physical examination of, 1420b–1421b
   pregnancy and, 1735
   in rheumatic fever, 1534, 1534t
   symptomatic patients, 1424–1425
   symptoms of, 1420–1421
   transcatheter aortic valve replacement for, 1438
   valvular disease, 1419
Aortic root, anatomy of, 806
Aortic root disease, 1419
Aortic sclerosis, chronic kidney disease and, 1887
Aortic stenosis
   asymptomatic patients with, 1410, 1412f
      clinical outcomes, 1410.e1t
   asymptomatic severe, 1438.e1
   atrial fibrillation and, 1437.e1
   auscultation, 1406
   bicuspid valve and, 1399
   coronary artery disease and, 1437.e1
   diagnosis of, 1430.e1
   echocardiography in, 232–234, 233f–234f, 234b
   in elderly, 1699–1701
   evaluation of, 137
   exercise testing in, 189–190
   magnetic resonance imaging in, 328
   main pathology of, 1430.e1
   management of young, low-risk patient with, 1438
   mild, 1403
   mitral annular calcification and, 1451
   mitral regurgitation and, 1482b
   moderate, 1403, 1438.e1
   multivalve disease and, 1437.e1
   noncardiac surgery and, 411b–412b
   pregnancy and, 1735
   progressive, 1409
   pulsus parvus et tardus in, 130
   rheumatic, 1400–1403
   severe, 1409–1412, 1411t
      assessment of, 1408f
   sudden cardiac death (SCD) and, 1360–1361
   symptomatic patients with, 1410–1412
Aortic valve
   endocarditis of, 1361b
   homografts, 1497
   infective endocarditis of, 1516
Aortic valve disease, 312, 312.e1f
   mitral stenosis and, 1482b
Aortic valve stenosis, 1399–1418
   bicuspid, 1399–1400, 1401f–1402f
   calcific, 1399
      clinical risk factors and, 1400t
      disease mechanisms and time course of, 1403f
      pathogenesis of, 1404f
      pathophysiology of, 1400b–1403b
         hypertrophic myocardial remodeling, 1400b–1403b, 1405f
         left ventricular diastolic function and, 1400b–1403b
         left ventricular systolic function and, 1400b–1403b
         valve obstruction, 1400b–1403b, 1411t
   causes of, 1399–1403
   clinical presentation of, 1403–1408
   diagnostic testing in, 1406–1408
      cardiac catheterization, 1408b
      cardiac computed tomography, 1408b
      cardiac magnetic resonance imaging, 1405f, 1408b

Aortic valve stenosis *(Continued)*
   echocardiography, 1406–1408, 1409f
   exercise stress testing, 1408b
   multimodality imaging for cardiac amyloidosis, 1408b, 1410f
   positron emission tomography, 1408b, 1409f
  disease course of, 1408–1412
  epidemiology of, 1399
  etiology of, 1399–1403
  management of
   balloon valvuloplasty, 1412b–1413b
   medical, 1412b–1413b
   valve replacement in, 1413–1415, 1413t, 1414f
    surgical, 1414, 1415f, 1416f
    transcatheter, 1414–1415, 1415t, 1416f
  physical examination in, 1406
  postprocedural issues of, 1415
  pressure gradient and, 398f–399f, 399–400, 399.e1f, 399.e1t, 399.e2f
  staging, 1408–1412
  symptoms of, 1403–1406
  treatment of, 1412–1415
  types of, 1400f
Aortic valve surgery, with aortic regurgitation, indications for, 1426t
Aortitis
  idiopathic, 1815, 1816f
  thoracic aortic aneurysms in, 814
Aortoarteritis syndromes, 832–834
Aortobifemoral bypass, for peripheral artery disease, 851
Aortography
  in aortic dissection, 824, 824.e1f
  for coronary angiography, 370–371
Aortoiliac disease, endovascular treatment of, 864, 864.e3f
Aortopathies, in congenital heart disease, 1551–1552
APASS (Antiphospholipid Antibody Stroke Study), 879b
Apelin, in heart failure, 920b–921b
Apixaban, 97t
  in atrial fibrillation-associated thromboembolism, 1276
  in chronic kidney disease, 1885t–1886t
  drug interaction with, 97t
  in NSTE-ACS, 727b
Apo CIII, inhibition of, 520
APOB, 72
APOC3 gene, 82b
Apolipoprotein A-I gene defects, 513
Apolipoprotein(s), 503–505, 503t, 506f
Apoptosis, 433
  in heart failure, 920.e1f, 926b–927b
Apparent mineralocorticoid excess states, 485
Argatroban, 1783, 1783t
Arginine vasopressin antagonists, in acute heart failure, 965b
Arginine vasopressin, in heart failure, 917f, 917b
Arm cycle ergometry, 178b–180b
Aromatase inhibitors, cardiotoxic effects of, 1092t, 1096–1097
Arrhythmias
  in adult congenital heart disease, 1545–1549
   bradyarrhythmia, 1547
   demographics and prognosis of, 1545–1546
   diagnostic testing of, 1546
   pacemakers and implantable defibrillators, 1549, 1549t, 1550f
   tachyarrhythmias, 1547–1548
   types of, 1546
   ventricular tachycardia and sudden death, 1548–1549
  air pollution and, 36
  amyloidosis and, 1058b
  in Andersen-Tawil syndrome, 1865
  atrial fibrillation and, 1106.e2, 1737.e3f
  in Becker muscular dystrophy, 1855
  cancer and, 1101–1103
  in cancer survivorship, 1105
  cardiac, 1208–1244
  cardiovascular disease and, 5
  in chronic kidney disease, 1887–1888, 1890t
  cocaine and, 1598–1599
  coronary artery disease and, 780b–781b
  COVID-19 in, 1757
  in Duchenne muscular dystrophy, 1855
  electrotherapy for, 1227–1241
   ablation therapy, for cardiac arrhythmias in, 1229–1241, 1230f, 1230b

Arrhythmias *(Continued)*
   direct-current electrical cardioversion in, 1227–1229
   implantable electrical devices for treatment of cardiac arrhythmias in, 1229
  in Emery-Dreifuss muscular dystrophy, 1860–1861
  in epilepsy, 1869–1870
  ethanol and, 1594
  exercise electrocardiographic testing in, 190b–191b, 191t
  in Friedreich ataxia, 1864
  genetics of, 1191–1207
  in heart failure, 1002
  in HIV patients, 1612–1613
  integrative strategies for, 596–597
  management of, 1104, 1106.e3
  mechanical circulatory support and, 1124.e1
  in myocarditis, 1089
  in myotonic dystrophy, 1858–1859, 1858.e1f, 1861f
  noncardiac surgery and, 411b–412b
  pharmacologic therapy for, 1208–1227
   antiarrhythmic agents in, 1213–1227
   general considerations regarding antiarrhythmic drugs in, 1208–1213, 1209b–1212b, 1209t, 1211f
  in pregnancy, 1731, 1737, 1737.e2f
  single ventricle and, 1581
  stress-induced, 1363
  for sudden cardiac death, 1565–1566
  suppression, 1209b–1212b, 1210t
  surgical therapy for tachyarrhythmias, 1241–1243
   supraventricular tachycardias in, 1241–1242, 1242f
   ventricular tachycardia in, 1242–1243
  ventricular, 699–701
   accelerated idioventricular rhythm in, 700
   fibrillation, 700–701, 701f
   management of, 699–700
   prognosis of, 700–701
   prophylaxis for, 700
   tachycardia, 700–701, 701f
   ventricular premature depolarizations, 699–700
  in women, 1719–1720
Arrhythmogenesis, mechanisms of, 1179–1189, 1180t
  disorders of impulse conduction in, 1183–1186, 1184f
  disorders of impulse formation in, 1179–1183
Arrhythmogenic cardiomyopathy, echocardiography in, 220f, 222
Arrhythmogenic right ventricular cardiomyopathy (ARVC), 1033t, 1036f, 1039–1041, 1039f–1040f, 1189
  approach to genetic evaluation of, 1040
  clinical genetics of, 1040
  diagnosis of, 1039.e2t, 1040
  differential diagnosis of, 1040
  exercise electrocardiographic testing in, 190b–191b
  exercise in, 585
  genomic cause of, 1039–1040, 1039.e3f
  molecular genetics of, 1039b–1040b
  treatment of, 1040–1041, 1041.e1f
Arrhythmogenic right ventricular dysplasia, 1360b
ARRIVE study, 877
Arsenic, cardiovascular effects of, 1601
Artefacts, on echocardiography, 203f, 203b, 256b
Arterial access, for cardiac catheterization, 386–388
  percutaneous femoral artery technique, 386–388, 387f–389f
  percutaneous radial artery technique, 386, 386f–387f, 387.e1f
Arterial conduits, in stable ischemic heart disease, 770–771
Arterial extracellular matrix, 433–434
Arterial grafts, patency of, 771
Arterial stenoses, atherosclerosis and, 435
Arterial stiffness, in hypertension, 478
Arterial switch operation
  long-term complications following, 1567
  pregnancy and, 1739t
  for transposition of great arteries, 1566, 1567f
Arterial thromboembolism, in COVID-19, 1757, 1758f
Arterial tortuosity syndrome, thoracic aortic aneurysm in, 811t
Arteriography, 376b–377b, 628
Arteriography, in thromboangiitis obliterans, 852
Arteriovenous (AV) fistulas, cardiac catheterization and, 386–387
Arteritis
  coronary, sudden cardiac death and, 1357.e1, 1358t
  giant cell. *See* Giant cell arteritis
  Takayasu. *See* Takayasu arteritis

Artery
  layers of, 427–428
  structure of, 425–428
Arthritis, in rheumatic fever, 1533, 1533f
Articulated hypothesis, 57b
Artifacts, on electrocardiography, 173, 173f
Artificial intelligence (AI), 109–111, 311
  cardiovascular disease and, 9–11
  definition of, 109–111, 109.e1f
  fully connected and convolutional neural networks, 110
  implementing into clinical practice, 113–115, 113f–115f
  learning, 109
  optimization and hyperparameters, 110–111
  pitfalls and limitations of, 115, 116f
  reinforcement learning, 110
  supervised learning, 109–110, 109.e1f
  transfer learning, 111
  unsupervised learning, 110
ASCEND study, 877
Ascending aorta, 1419
Ascending thoracic aortic aneurysms, management of, 817, 817.e1f, 817.e2f
Aschoff-Geipel bodies, 1532b–1533b, 1533f
Asian Americans
  hypertension in, 1743
  type 2 diabetes in, 1743
Aspart, in diabetes mellitus, 562t–563t
Aspiration devices, for percutaneous coronary intervention, 795
Aspiration thrombectomy, for peripheral artery disease, 862–863
Aspirin, 463–464, 463f–464f
  allergy to, 1776
  in antiplatelet therapy, 561
  in atrial fibrillation, 1276
  clopidogrel and, combination of, 1777
  in coronary artery disease, chronic kidney disease and, 1880t–1881t
  cost-effectiveness study of, 27
  dosages for, 1776
  drug interactions, 97t
  indications for, 1775–1776
  in Kawasaki disease, 1815
  mechanism of action of, 1775, 1776f
  in NSTE-ACS, 723, 735.e4t
  in percutaneous coronary intervention, 787.e3t, 799
  during pregnancy, 1730f
  resistance to, 1776
  for rheumatic fever, 1537
  side effects of, 1776
  in stable ischemic heart disease, 754b–756b
  for STEMI, 665
  for stroke, 877–878
  in thrombosis, 1775–1776
ASPREE study, 877
Asthma, cardiac, 937
Asthmatic attacks, sudden cardiac death (SCD) and, 1363b–1365b
Atenolol
  in angina pectoris, 758t
  cost-effectiveness study of, 27
Atherectomy
  orbital, 794.e1
  in percutaneous coronary intervention, 794, 794f
  in peripheral artery disease, 863, 863.e1f, 863.e2f
  rotational, 794.e1, 797f
Atheroembolism, 855–856
  clinical features of, 856, 856f
  diagnostic tests for, 856
  pathogenesis of, 855
  treatment of, 856
Atherogenesis
  mechanisms of HIV-related, 1605–1607
  smooth muscle cell death during, 433
Atheroma. *See also* Atherosclerosis
  evolution of, 432–435
Atheromatous plaque, in NSTE-ACS, 714, 716f
Atherosclerosis, 311b–312b, 453, 866
  accelerated, in athletes, 585, 586f
  complication of, 435–438
   arterial stenoses and clinical implications as, 435
   diffuse and systemic nature of plaque susceptibility to rupture and inflammation in, 437–438, 439f
   plaque rupture and thrombosis as, 435–436, 437f

Atherosclerosis *(Continued)*
 thrombosis and atheroma as, 435, 435f–436f
 thrombosis and healing in progression of atheroma, 437
 thrombosis caused by superficial erosion of plaques, 437, 438f
 in endothelial dysfunction, 1809–1810
 in HIV patients, 1606f, 1607, 1611f
 initiation, 428–432
  extracellular lipid accumulation in, 428–430, 429f–430f
  focality of lesion formation in, 431–432, 431f
  intracellular lipid accumulation in, 432
  leukocyte recruitment and retention in, 430–431, 430f
 management of, in heart failure, 996.e1
 NSTE-ACS from, 715
 overview and background of, 425, 426f
 premature, 1809
 in rheumatic diseases, 1809–1812, 1812t
 in rheumatoid arthritis, 1810
 special cases of, 438–440
 stages of, 352f
 systemic lupus erythematosus and, 1810–1812, 1811f
 vascular biology of, 425–441
 in vascular injury, 1809–1810
Atherosclerotic aortic ulcer, penetrating, 831–832, 832. e1f, 834f
Atherosclerotic cardiovascular disease (ASCVD), athletes with, 583–584
Atherosclerotic cardiovascular syndromes, acute coronary syndromes and stroke in COVID-19 patients, 1757
Atherosclerotic plaque, echocardiography in, 244, 247f
Atherothrombosis, 870, 1772
 of carotid artery, 870
 pulmonary embolism and, 1638.e1f, 1637b–1639b
 stable ischemic heart disease and, 753
Athletes
 accelerated atherosclerosis in, 585, 586f
 atherosclerotic cardiovascular disease in, 583–584
 atrial fibrillation in, 584, 585f
 bicuspid aortic valve in, 584
 cardiac troponin in, 584, 584f
 cardiovascular complaints in, 583
 chest pain in, 583
 eccentric left ventricular hypertrophy in, 580, 580f
 eligibility of, 583–585
 myocardial fibrosis in, 585
 noncompaction cardiomyopathy in, 585
 preparticipation screening in, 582
 sudden cardiac death in, 1363–1365, 1383
 valve disease in, 584
 vasovagal syncope in, 583
"Athlete's heart", 579–580, 581f
Athletes, hypertrophic cardiomyopathy in, 1072
Atorvastatin, 97t
 in chronic kidney disease, 1883t
Atria
 electrical remodeling of, 1187
 function of, 911
Atrial arrhythmias
 atrial switch operation and, 1567
 in chronic kidney disease, 1887–1888
 marijuana use and, 1599
Atrial fibrillation, 1101b, 1106.e2, 1187, 1548, 1897
 aortic stenosis and, 1437.e1
 in aortic valve stenosis, 1412b–1413b
 asymptomatic, 1274
 in athletes, 584, 585f
 atrial flutter and, 1252b, 1253f, 1272, 1273f
 catheter ablation of, 1280–1283
  indications for, 1282–1283
  and outcomes of, 1281–1282, 1282f–1283f
  selection of patients, 1282–1283
 causes of, 1274
 classification of, 1272
 clinical features of, 1274
 in congestive heart failure, 1284–1285
 in coronary artery disease, 1283
 device detection of, 1287.e8
 in diabetes mellitus, 556, 576
 diagnosis of, 1275
  electrocardiographic features of, 1272, 1273f–1274f
  exercise electrocardiographic testing, 190b–191b
  laboratory testing in, 1275

Atrial fibrillation *(Continued)*
 in Duchenne muscular dystrophy, 1855
 effects of food and nutrients on, 541t–542t
 in elderly, 1701–1702
 in Emery-Dreifuss muscular dystrophy, 1860–1861
 epidemiology of, 1272–1273
 ethanol-induced, 1594
 in Friedreich ataxia, 1864
 genetic factors of, 1274
 guidelines of, 1287.e1
  cardioversion in, 1287.e4t
  pharmacologic rate control, 1287.e1, 1287.e3t
 heart disease and, 1274
 in heart failure, 1000.e1
 in heart failure with preserved and mildly reduced ejection, 1008, 1024
 in hyperthyroidism, 1287.e6t, 1287.e8
 in hypertrophic cardiomyopathy, 1285, 1287.e6t, 1287.e8
 management of, 1072
 ion channel abnormalities in, 1187b
 lone, 1272
 longstanding, 1272
 management of
  acute, 1277–1279
  angiotensin-converting enzyme (ACE) inhibitors, 1280
  cardioversion in, 1277, 1287.e3
  cryoballoon ablation for, 1281, 1281f–1282f
  long-term, 1279–1280
  pacing in, 1280
  pharmacologic rate control, 1279
  pharmacologic rhythm control, 1279–1280
  radiofrequency catheter ablation in, 1277f
   atrial tachyarrhythmias after, 1280
   atrioventricular node for, 1283–1284
   recurrence after, 1277–1278
  risk factor modification of, 1280
  statins in, 1280
  surgical, 1283
 mechanisms of, 1273–1274
 monogenic (familial), 1187b
 in myocardial infarction, 1287.e6t
 in myotonic dystrophy, 1855
 nonpharmacologic management of, 1280–1284
 obesity and, 1274
 obstructive sleep apnea and, 1274
 in overt hyperthyroidism, 1799–1800
 paroxysmal, 1272
 perioperative, 411b–412b
 permanent, 1272
 persistent, 1272
 physical examination in, 1274
 polygenic factors in, 1187b
 postoperative, 1284, 1287.e5, 1287.e6t
 during pregnancy, 1285, 1287.e6t, 1287.e8
 prevention in, 877
 prevention of thromboembolism of, 1287.e1, 1287.e2t
 in pulmonary disease, 1287.e6t, 1287.e8
 pulmonary veins in, 1277f, 1281
 radiofrequency catheter ablation of, 1237
 with rapid ventricular response, in acute heart failure, 956b
 rheumatic mitral stenosis and, 1446–1447, 1446f
 spatiotemporal organization and focal discharge in, 1187
 stable ischemic heart disease and, 772.e1
 syncope with, 1274
 tachycardia-induced, 1274
 thromboembolic complications of, 1275–1277, 1287.e1t, 1287.e2t
  aspirin, 1276
  direct thrombin inhibitors in, 1276
  factor Xa inhibitors for, 1276
  left atrial appendage, excision or closure of, 1277, 1278f
  low-molecular-weight heparin, 1277
  other antiplatelet agents, 1276
  risk stratification for, 1275–1276, 1275f
  warfarin for, 1276
 ventricular rate during, 1272
 wearable devices and, 118–120
  electrocardiogram, 119–120, 120f
  photoplethysmography detection of irregular rhythm, 118–119, 119f
 in Wolff-Parkinson-White syndrome, 1284, 1287.e6t, 1287.e8

Atrial flutter, 1186–1187, 1235–1236, 1235b–1236b, 1236f, 1252–1257, 1255f
 in aortic valve stenosis, 1412b–1413b
 atrial fibrillation and, 1252b, 1253f, 1272, 1273f
 classification of, 1252–1257
 different types of, 1255f
 in Duchenne muscular dystrophy, 1855
 in Emery-Dreifuss muscular dystrophy, 1860–1861
 epidemiology of, 1252
 in myotonic dystrophy, 1855
 preexcited, acute treatment of, 1268
 variants of, 1256f
Atrial macroreentry, 1252, 1255f
Atrial natriuretic peptide (ANP), in heart failure, 918f, 918b–919b
Atrial paced atrial event, 1327
Atrial pacing, for sinus node dysfunction, 1547
Atrial premature complexes, 1248.e1f, 1246–1247, 1246f–1247f, 1246b–1247b
Atrial pressure, measurements of, 396, 397f
Atrial reentry, 1187
Atrial repolarization, 146
Atrial septal defect (ASD), 1554–1557
 anatomic description and prevalence of, 1554–1555, 1557f–1558f
 clinical features of, 1555–1556
 closure of, techniques for, 1589–1590, 1589f
 coronary sinus, echocardiography in, 258–259
 echocardiography in, 256–259, 256b, 257f
 long-term outcomes and complications of, 1556–1557
 magnetic resonance imaging in, 330b–332b, 331f
 pregnancy and, 1737–1738
 primum, echocardiography in, 258, 259f
 repairs for, 1556, 1558f
 secundum, echocardiography in, 257, 257f–259f
 sinus venosus, echocardiography in, 258, 259f
Atrial switch operation
 Baffle complications in, 1566–1567, 1568f
 long-term outcomes and complications following, 1566–1567, 1568t
 for transposition of great arteries, 1566, 1567f
Atrial tachyarrhythmias, 1236–1237, 1236b–1237b, 1237f
 response to, 1328b, 1329f
Atrial tachycardia, 1234–1235, 1247
 AVNRT/AVRT *vs.*, 1248b–1249b
 inappropriate sinus tachycardia *vs.*, 1248b–1249b, 1249f
Atrioventricular (AV) block, 1156b–1159b, 1315–1319
 advanced, 1317, 1318f
 clinical features of, 1319
 congenital, 1318–1319
 in Emery-Dreifuss muscular dystrophy, 1860–1861
 first-degree, 1315
  electrocardiography for, 1315, 1315f
 management of, 1319
 paroxysmal, 1318
  pause-dependent, 1318
 second-degree, 1315–1317, 1315f, 1315f–1316f, 1316b
  electrocardiography for, 1315f, 1315f–1316f
  type I, 1316f–1317f, 1317b
  type II, 1316f–1317f, 1317b
 tachycardia-dependent, 1318
 third-degree, 1317–1319, 1318f, 1318.e1f
Atrioventricular (AV) bundle
 branching portion of, 1176–1177, 1178f
 penetrating portion of, 1176–1177
Atrioventricular (AV) conduction, anterograde, 1176b
Atrioventricular (AV) dissociation, 1319–1320, 1319b, 1319.e1f
 classification of, 1319, 1319.e1f
 electrocardiographic and clinical features of, 1319–1320
 management of, 1320
 mechanisms of, 1319b
Atrioventricular (AV) nodal ablation, 1237f
Atrioventricular (AV) nodal reentrant tachycardia (AVNRT), 1232–1234, 1232f–1233f
 anatomy, physiology and ECG characteristics, 1259b–1260b, 1262f
 antidromic, 1267, 1267f
 atypical, 1261–1262, 1262f
 chronic therapy in, 1268
 orthodromic, 1266–1267
 treatment of, 1262–1263, 1268–1270
  acute management, 1262
  chronic management, 1263
 typical, 1260–1261, 1260f–1261f, 1261.e1f

Atrioventricular (AV) nodal reentry, 1187
Atrioventricular (AV) node, 1175.e3f, 1175.e3f, 1175–1176, 1175f–1177f
  ablation of, 1283–1284
  arterial supply to, 1175.e4f, 1176, 1176.e1f
  cystic tumors of, 1833
  innervation of, 1177–1178, 1179f
Atrioventricular (AV) reciprocating tachycardia (AVRT), 1187–1188
Atrioventricular septal defects, 1557–1558, 1559f
Atropine, 1209t
  for sinus bradycardia, 1312
Auscultation, 1420b–1421b
Austin Flint murmur, 1420b–1421b, 1445
Autografts, 1497
Autoimmune diseases
  cardiovascular disease in women and, 1710b–1714b
  pericardial involvement in, 1630b–1633b
Autoinflammatory diseases, pericardial involvement in, 1630b–1633b
Automated external defibrillator (AED), 1369, 1373.e1f
Automaticity
  abnormal, 1180
  normal, 1170–1171, 1170f
    passive membrane electrical properties and, 1170b–1171b, 1171f
Autonomic disorders/dysfunction, 1893–1902
  cardiovascular manifestations of, 1893–1902
    pathophysiology of, 1896–1897
    proarrhythmia, 1897
  neuromodulatory therapies, 1898–1900
    pharmacologic therapy, 1898–1899
  in setting of a structurally normal heart, 1896–1897
  testing, 1897
    tilt-table testing, 1897, 1898f
    Valsalva maneuver in, 1897
Autonomic nervous system, 1893
  arrhythmias and, 1183.e1f, 1178–1179, 1179.e1f
  disorders of. See Autonomic disorders/dysfunction
  overview of anatomy and physiology, 1893–1896
    baroreflex, 1894–1895, 1896f
    chemoreflexes, 1895–1896
    diving reflex, 1896
    intrinsic neuronal control, 1893
    parasympathetic, 1893, 1895t
    sympathetic, 1893, 1895t, 1901t
Autonomic remodeling, 1183.e1f, 1178–1179
Autonomic/neurally mediated bradycardia, 1320
Autophagy, in heart failure, 926b–927b, 928f
Autosomal recessive hypercholesterolemia, 510b
Autotaxin, 1400b–1403b
AVID (AVID Investigators) trial, 1332t
AVP antagonists, 983t
Azathioprine
  in cardiac transplantation, 1136
  for systemic lupus erythematosus, 1811b
Azotemia, diuretic-induced, 988

B

B cell, drugs causing depletion of, 1825–1826
Bacterial endocarditis, in chronic kidney disease, 1887
Bacterial infection, myocardial, 1079t, 1081. See also Myocarditis
Bacterial pericarditis, 1630b–1633b
Balanced coronary dominance, in angiographic projection, 372, 372.e1f
Balloon angioplasty, 786
  in percutaneous coronary intervention, 793
  in peripheral artery disease, 860, 861f
Balloon aortic valvuloplasty, 1430
Balloon pulmonary valvuloplasty, for pulmonary stenosis, 1562
Balloon-expandable stents, 793.e1
  in peripheral artery disease, 860
Bandpass filters, 1324b–1326b
Barbeau test, 386
Bare-metal stents (BMS), in peripheral artery disease, 860, 860f–861f
Bariatric surgery, obesity and, 553, 554t, 555f
Baroreceptor(s)
  arterial, 1894–1895
  cardiopulmonary, 1894–1895
  stimulation, 1900
Baroreflex, 1894–1895, 1895t, 1896f
Baroreflex activation therapy, 1114
Baroreflex sensitivity, assessment of, 1896f

Barostim Neo trial, 496–497
Barth syndrome, 1866–1867
BASILICA procedure, 1437
Basiliximab, in cardiac transplantation, 1136
Bayesian reasoning, 54b–55b
Bazett formula, 149
Bcr-Abl targeted therapies, cardiotoxic effects of, 1096
Beals syndrome, thoracic aortic aneurysm in, 811t
Beans, 532, 533f
Becker muscular dystrophy, 1853–1856, 1853f–1854f
Behavior, diet-related, 543
Behçet disease, thrombosis in, 1824, 1825f
  treatment of, 1824
Belimumab, for systemic lupus erythematosus, 1811b
Bempedoic acid, 520
Benzodiazepines, 1850
Benzothiadiazines, in heart failure, 982–983
BEST (Randomized Comparison of Coronary Artery Bypass Surgery and Everolimus-Eluting Stent Implantation in the Treatment of Patients with Multivessel Coronary Artery Disease) trial, 789.e1
Beta adrenoceptor-blocking agents (beta blockers), 1209t, 1219–1220, 1219b
  in abdominal aortic aneurysms, 809
  in acute coronary syndromes, 573
  for acute myocardial infarction, 709
  in angina pectoris, 757–758, 757f, 757t–758t, 760t
    advantages of, 763, 763t
    adverse effects and contraindications of, 758–776
    alpha adrenoceptor-blocking activity of, 759.e1
    characteristics of, 759.e1
    effects on serum lipid levels, 759.e1
    intrinsic sympathomimetic activity of, 759.e1
    lipid solubility of, 759.e1
    potency of, 758
  in aortic dissection, 825–827
  in chronic HFrEF, 1698b
  in chronic kidney disease, 1882t
  drug interactions, 97t
  electrocardiography effects of, 184
  genetic variations in, 996.e1
  in heart failure, 575, 991t, 994–996, 995f
    in arrhythmias, 1002
  for heart failure with preserved and mildly reduced ejection, 1024
  in hypertension management, 561
  in noncardiac surgery, 421, 423t
  in NSTE-ACS, 721–722, 723t
  in pregnancy, 1730
  side effects of, 996
  sinoatrial node and, 1175.e1b
  in stable ischemic heart disease, 754b–756b, 755f
  for STEMI, 666, 680–681, 681f, 681t
  in thoracic aortic aneurysms, 818
Beta-adrenergic receptor, 900–901, 901f
  desensitization of, 903f, 903b
  in heart failure, 926
Beta-adrenergic responses, inhomogeneity in, 634b–635b
Beta-hemolytic streptococci, causing infective endocarditis, antimicrobial therapy for, 1519b–1523b
Betaxolol, for angina pectoris, 758t
Bevacizumab, 1096
  cardiotoxic effects of, 1092t
Beverages, 535
Biased judgments, 60
Bicalutamide, cardiotoxic effects of, 1092t
Bicaval anastomosis technique, 1136
Bicuspid aortic valve (BAV), 1551–1552
  athletes with, 584
  thoracic aortic aneurysms in, 812–813, 814f
Bicuspid aortic valve disease (BAVD), treatment of, 1438
Bicuspid aortic valve stenosis, 1399–1400, 1401f–1402f
Bidis, 21
Bifurcation lesions, percutaneous coronary intervention in, 790–791
Biguanides, for diabetes mellitus, 562t–563t
Bile acid sequestrants, for diabetes mellitus, 562t–563t
Bile acid-binding resins, 519
Biliary colic, 741
Bioabsorbable polymer drug-eluting stents, 794
Biochemical coupling, 1173
BioFreedom stent, 794, 794.e1
Biologic death, 1349, 1350f, 1368. See also Sudden cardiac death
Biologic lipids, 502

Biomarker(s), 102–108
  accuracy in, 106
  in acute heart failure, 954
  in aortic dissection, 823f, 823b
  calibration in, 106
  causality and, 104
  in chest pain evaluation, 602–603
  clinical applications of, 103–105, 103f–104f
  clinical measures of, 105–107
  C-statistics in, 106, 106f
  definition of, 102–105, 103t–104t
  in diagnosis, 103
  discrimination in, 106, 106f
  in drug development, 103
  elevation of, before surgery, 419
  in evaluation, 103
  external validation in, 107
  FDA-NIH BEST Resource, 103t
  future directions in, 91
  in goals for therapy, 103
  in heart failure, 939, 939t, 941f
  of heart failure with preserved and mildly reduced ejection, 1011b–1017b
  high-sensitivity CRP in, 107
  identification of, 105
  impact studies in, 107
  mendelian randomization study of, 79, 79f
  in myocarditis, 1087
  novel technologies in identification of, 87
  in precision medicine, 102–108
  predictive value of, 105–106, 105t
  receiver operating characteristic curve in, 106, 106f
  in registration, 103
  Reynolds Risk Score in, 107
  risk reclassification in, 106–107
  in risk stratification, 103
  sensitivity of, 105–106, 105t
  specificity of, 105–106, 105t
  in targeting of therapy, 103
BIONYX (Bioresorbable Polymer ORSIRO Versus Durable Polymer RESOLUTE ONYX Stents) trial, 794.e1
Biopsy
  in arrhythmogenic right ventricular cardiomyopathy, 1040
  in heart failure, 942
  in sarcoid cardiomyopathy, 1045b
Bioresorbable vascular scaffolds, 794
Bipolar leads, 1322b–1323b
Birth, cardiovascular disease at, 1–2
Bisoprolol
  in angina pectoris, 758t
  in heart failure, 991t–992t, 995f, 995b–996b
Bivalirudin, 1783, 1783t
  in chronic kidney disease, 1885t–1886t
  in NSTE-ACS, 727
  in percutaneous coronary intervention, 787.e3t, 801
  for STEMI, 675, 675f–676f
Biventricular hypertrophy, electrocardiography in, 155, 156f
Biventricular pacing, ameliorative role of, 1326
Black American
  coronary heart disease, 1747
  percutaneous coronary interventions for, 1747
Bleeding
  fondaparinux and, 1781
  heparin and, 1780–1781
    low-molecular-weight, 1782
  management of, 1786–1787
  NSTE-ACS and, 728
  in prosthetic heart valves, 1502b–1503b
  warfarin and, 1784–1785
Blinding, clinical trial, 45
Blood pressure
  in acute heart failure, 954–955, 958, 959f
  ambulatory monitoring, 482–483
  in coronary artery disease, 181b–182b
  excursions, noncardiac surgery and, 411
  heart failure and, 937–938
  management
    for heart failure with preserved and mildly reduced ejection, 1023
    in patients undergoing dialysis, 492–493
  measurement of, 128–129, 129t, 481–483, 481t
  office vs. home, 482
  orthostatic, heart rate and, 1895f, 1897, 1898f
  in peripheral artery disease, 847–848

Blood pressure (Continued)
  reduction of
    in aortic dissection, 827, 827t
    for cardiovascular disease, 448
    in STEMI, 654
Blood pressure levels, updated definitions of, 874t
Blood pressure–lowering medications, for hypertension, 490
Blood supply, factors regulating, 838–839, 839f, 839.e1f
Blood urea nitrogen
  in acute heart failure, 954
  in heart failure, 938b–939b
Blue toe syndrome, atheroembolism and, 856, 856f
Blunt aortic trauma, 821
Blunted systolic pressure peak during, in coronary artery disease, 181b–182b
Body mass index (BMI), epidemiology of, 24, 25f
Boerhaave syndrome, 601
Borrelia burgdorferi infection, myocarditis and, 1081b
Bortezomib, cardiotoxic effects of, 1092t, 1094
Bosentan, in pulmonary arterial hypertension, 1675f
Bowditch effect, 908, 908f
Bowel endoscopy, in ischemia, 867
Brachial artery
  for peripheral artery disease, 864
  for vascular access, 799
Bradyarrhythmias, 701–703, 1183, 1312–1315, 1547, 1702b
  atrioventricular and intraventricular block for, 701–702, 702t
  bifascicular block for, 703
  in cardiac arrhythmias, 1147
  complete (third-degree) atrioventricular block for, 701–702
  first-degree atrioventricular block for, 701
  heart block, 1547
  intraventricular block for, 702–703
  isolated fascicular blocks for, 702–703
  management for, 701
  right bundle branch block for, 703
  second-degree atrioventricular block for, 701
  sinus bradycardia, 701
  sinus node dysfunction, 1547
Bradycardia, pacemakers for, 1321
Bradycardia pacing, NASPE/BPEG generic code for, 1325t
Bradykinin, in heart failure, 920b–921b
Brain (B-type) natriuretic peptide (BNP)
  in acute heart failure, 940, 954
  in cardiovascular disease in women, 1719
  in chest pain evaluation, 603
  in heart failure, 918f, 918b–919b
  in perioperative period, 419–420
  in STEMI, 655
Breast attenuation artifact, 289f
Breast cancer
  radiation therapy for, 1097b
  therapy for, cardiovascular disease in women and, 1710b–1714b
Breathing
  in cardiopulmonary resuscitation, 1372
  Cheyne-Stokes, in heart failure, 999f, 1002–1003
  sleep-disordered, 1002–1003, 1003b, 1678–1686
    cardiac arrhythmias and, 1684–1685
    cardiac function and, 1683–1684
    coronary heart disease and, 1682–1683
    definitions of, 1678, 1679f, 1679t
    future perspectives in, 1685
    heart failure and, 1683–1684, 1684f
    hypertension and, 1681–1682
    pathophysiologic mechanism that link, 1681, 1681f
    pathophysiology of, 1678–1681, 1680f
    recognition for, 1679–1681, 1681.e1f
    risk factors for, 1679–1681
Breathing exercise, for hypertension, 595
Bromocriptine, in diabetes mellitus, 562t–563t
Brugada syndrome, 158, 1171b–1173b, 1188, 1200–1201
  clinical description and manifestations of, 1200–1201
  drug-related, 98
  electrocardiography in, 1307f, 1308, 1362f
  genetic basis of, 1192f, 1201b, 1202f
  SCN5A-mediated, phenotypic correlates of, 1201
  sudden cardiac death and, 1362, 1362f, 1380
Bucindolol, in heart failure, 992t, 995b–996b
Bumetanide, in heart failure, 982, 983t, 985–987

Bundle branch reentrant ventricular tachycardia, 1294–1295, 1297f
Bundle branch reentry tachycardia, in myotonic dystrophy, 1858–1859, 1861f
Bundle branches, 1176–1177, 1178f
Bundle of His, 1176–1177
Bupropion, 1849
Buspirone, 1850

C

c wave, 127–128
C4b-binding protein, 1773
Ca^{2+}/calmodulin-dependent protein kinase II, 899b, 903
CABGPatch trial, 1336t
CACNA1C, 1191b–1193b
CACNA2D1, 1197b
CACNB2b, 1197b, 1204b
CAD. See Coronary artery disease
N-Cadherin, loss of, 1174b–1175b, 1175f
Cadmium, cardiovascular complications of, 1601
Café coronary, 1363b–1365b
Caffeine, 1600–1601
Calcific aortic valve disease (CAVD), 1399, 1400f
  clinical risk factors and, 1400t
  disease mechanisms and time course of, 1403f
  pathogenesis of, 1404f
  pathophysiology of, 1400b–1403b
Calcific pericarditis, chest radiography in, 271
Calcification(s)
  mitral annulus, in chronic kidney disease, 1887
  vascular, kidney injury and, 1879
Calcineurin inhibitors (CNIs), in cardiac transplantation, 1136
Calcium antagonists. See Calcium channel-blocking agents
Calcium (Ca), 539b
  in contraction-relaxation cycle, 895–896, 896f
  in delayed afterdepolarization generation, 1183.e1f, 1181–1183
  release and uptake by sarcoplasmic reticulum, 896–897
Calcium channel, 898–899
  L-type, 898, 1166b–1170b
  molecular structure of, 898
  T-type, 898, 1166b–1170b
  voltage-gated, 1171b–1173b
Calcium channel-blocking agents
  in acute heart failure, 965b
  for acute myocardial infarction, 710
  in angina pectoris, 760, 761t
    advantages of, 763, 763t
    first-generation, 759–760
    second-generation, 760
  in coronary artery disease, chronic kidney disease and, 1880t–1881t
  as coronary vasodilator, 614b
  for heart failure with preserved and mildly reduced ejection, 1024
  for hypertension, 491, 561
  in NSTE-ACS, 722–723, 723t
  for STEMI, 684
Calcium clock model, 1170b–1171b
Calcium leak, in heart failure, 924
Calcium release channel deficiency syndrome, 1203–1204
Calcium sparks, 897b
Calibration, in biomarkers, 106
CALM1, 1191b–1193b
Calmodulin, 897f, 897b
Calmodulinopathic long QT syndrome, 1195
Calsequestrin, 889
Canagliflozin, in diabetes mellitus, 562t–563t, 567
Canakinumab, 9
  cardiovascular disease and, in HIV patients, 1607b
Cancer
  in adult congenital heart disease, 1544
  arrhythmia and, 1101–1103
    atrial fibrillation, 1106.e2
    in cancer survivorship, 1105
    management of, 1104, 1106.e3
  cardiomyopathy/heart failure and, 1099–1100, 1102t
    in cancer survivorship, 1104–1106, 1105.e1f, 1106.e4t
    direct cardiotoxicity concerns, 1106.e1
    indirect cardiotoxicity concerns, 1106.e1
    inflammatory cardiotoxicity concerns, 1106.e1

Cancer (Continued)
    management of, 1103–1104, 1106.e2
    preventive efforts and screening recommendations for, 1106.e1
  cardiovascular care for, 1097
  heart failure in, 1001
  mechanistic overlap between cardiovascular disease and, 1097.e1
  radiation therapy for, 1092t, 1097
  superior vena cava syndrome in, 1837–1838, 1838f
  targeted therapies in, 1095–1096
  therapy for
    cardiotoxicity of, 1091–1094
    managing cardiotoxic effects of, 1091–1098, 1092t
    at risk of or with cardiovascular disease, 1099–1103, 1101f, 1103.e1t
  vascular disease and, 1100, 1102t
    in cancer survivorship, 1105–1106, 1105b
    management of, 1104, 1106.e3
    risk, prevention, and monitoring of, 1106.e1
  venous thrombosis and, 1774
Candesartan, in heart failure, 993.e1f, 991t–992t, 993
Candida spp., causing infective endocarditis, 1506b–1507b
Candidate gene approach, 93b–96b
Cangrelor
  in NSTE-ACS, 726, 735.e6t
  in thrombosis, 1777
Cannabidiol oil, cardiovascular complications, 1600, 1600b
Cannabis, use of, cardiac transplantation and, 1134
Cannon *a* wave, 127–128
Capecitabine, cardiotoxic effects of, 1092t
Capillary perfusion, in peripheral artery disease, 839
CAPRIE (Clopidogrel *versus* Aspirin in Patients at Risk of Ischemic Events) trial, 848
Captopril challenge test, for primary hyperaldosteronism, 485
Captopril, in heart failure, 991t–992t, 993b
Carbohydrates, 535–536, 536f
Carbonic anhydrase inhibitors, 984
Carboplatin, cardiotoxic effects of, 1092t
Carcinoid heart disease, 1048–1049, 1048.e1f
Carcinoid syndrome, tricuspid regurgitation in, 1476
Cardiac action potential, 1163, 1163f–1164f
  fast response and, 1166b–1170b
  membrane voltages during, 1163b–1166b
  phase 0: upstroke (rapid depolarization), 1166b–1170b, 1169f
  phase 1: early rapid repolarization in, 1168.e1f, 1168.e1f, 1166b–1170b
  phase 2: plateau in, 1166b–1170b
  phase 3: final rapid repolarization in, 1166b–1170b
  phase 4: diastolic depolarization in, 1166b–1170b
  phases of, 1164f, 1166–1170, 1167f
  resting membrane potential, 1166b–1170b, 1167f, 1168t
  slow response and, 1166b–1170b
Cardiac allograft vasculopathy
  after cardiac transplantation, 1141–1142, 1142f, 1142t
  patients with, 296b–298b, 297f
Cardiac amyloidosis, 1052–1061, 1053t, 1699
  biomarkers of, 1056b
  biopsy in, 1056b
  clinical features of, 1054
  clinical management of, 1058–1060
  diagnosis of, 1055–1056, 1055f, 1057t
  diagnostic criteria for, 304t
  epidemiology of, 1052–1053
  genotyping in, 1056b
  imaging in, 1056b, 1057f
  multimodality imaging for, 1408b, 1410f
  pathophysiology of, 1053–1054
  prognosis of, 1054
Cardiac arrest, 1367, 1367.e1t
  asystolic, 1366, 1374
  clinical features of patients with, 1367–1369
  definitions of, 1349–1350, 1350f, 1350t
  in-hospital
    noncardiac abnormalities, 1376b
    outcomes, 1367
  management of, 1369–1377
    in bradyarrhythmia and asystolic arrest, 1374
    community-based interventions in, 1369–1371, 1370.e1f
    in-hospital interventions in, 1369, 1370f
    in pulseless electrical activity, 1374

Cardiac arrest (Continued)
  myocardial infarction and, 1375–1376
  onset of, 1367
  out-of-hospital
    advanced cardiac life support in, 1373–1375
    basic life support in, 1371–1372
    chest thump in, 1371
    clinical features of, 1368–1369
    defibrillation-cardioversion in, 1373–1374
    early defibrillation in, 1372–1373, 1373f
    initial assessment in, 1371–1373
    long-term management after, 1376–1377
    outcomes of, 1367
    pharmacotherapy in, 1374
    public safety and, 1383–1384
    survivors of, 1368–1369
  pathophysiology of, 1359f, 1365
    bradyarrhythmias in, 1366, 1370b–1371b
    pulseless electrical activity in, 1366–1367
    tachyarrhythmias in, 1365–1367
  in patients with hemodynamically unstable acute myocardial infarction, 1376
  prevention of, 1377–1383, 1377t, 1378f
  risk identification by QT interval prolongation after, 1376
  sudden, in cardiac arrhythmias, 1148, 1148f
  survivors of, 1162.e5, 1162.e5t, 1368–1369
    blood chemistry in, 1369
    coronary angiography in, 1369
    electrocardiographic changes in, 1368
    exercise testing in, 1365–1366
    hospital course in, 1368
    left ventricular function in, 1368–1369
    long-term prognosis for, 1369
  wearable devices and, 120
Cardiac arrhythmias. *See also* Arrhythmias
  abnormal automaticity and, 1180
  approach to patient with, 1145–1162.e7
    clinical and laboratory testing for, 1148–1155
      cardiac imaging in, 1149, 1152f
      electrophysiologic studies, 1159, 1160f–1161f
      head-up tilt-table testing in, 1155–1162, 1155.e2f
      Holter monitoring and event recording in, 1151–1155, 1151.e1t, 1154f, 1154.e1f, 1154f–1155f, 1162.e2t, 1162.e3t
      in hospital electrocardiographic recording, 1151, 1154f
      insertable loop recorders, 1151–1155
      invasive electrophysiologic testing in, 1156–1159
      resting electrocardiogram in, 1148–1149, 1149f–1152f, 1151t
      resting electrocardiographic recording in, 1148f
      stress electrocardiography in, 1149–1151, 1153f
  guidelines, 1162.e1
    antiarrhythmic therapy efficacy, 1162.e1
    clinical competence, 1162.e1
    diagnosis in, 1162.e1
    electrophysiologic procedures, for diagnosis, 1162.e1
      acquired atrioventricular block, 1162.e1
      cardiac arrest, survivors of, 1162.e5
      chronic intraventricular delay, 1162.e2
      narrow-and wide-QRS complex tachycardia, 1162.e2
      palpitations, 1162.e5
      prolonged QT intervals, 1162.e5
      sinus node function, evaluation of, 1162.e1, 1162.e3t
      unexplained syncope, 1162.e5, 1162.e5t
      Wolff-Parkinson-White syndrome, 1162.e5
    electrophysiologic studies, for therapeutic intervention, 1162.e5, 1162.e6t
    myocardial ischemia, monitoring for, 1162.e1
    pacemaker/ICD function assessment of, 1162.e1
  physical examination in, 1146, 1146f–1148f
  signs and symptoms of, 1146–1148
    aborted sudden cardiac death in, 1148, 1148f
    bradyarrhythmias in, 1147
    consciousness, altered level of, 1147–1148
    general approach in, 1145–1146
    palpitations in, 1146–1147
    presyncope in, 1147–1148
    sudden cardiac arrest in, 1148, 1148f
    syncope in, 1147–1148, 1147.e1
    tachyarrhythmias in, 1156

Cardiac arrhythmias (Continued)
  autonomic nervous system and, 1183.e1f, 1178–1179, 1179.e1f
  cardiac electrical network and, structure and function of, 1175–1179
  deceleration-dependent block and, 1183b–1184b
  decremental conduction and, 1183b–1184b
  delayed afterdepolarizations and, 1180–1181, 1182f
    generation of, role of intracellular Ca^{2+}-handling abnormalities in, 1183.e1f, 1181–1183
  early afterdepolarizations, 1183
  electrical therapy for, 1321
  entrainment and, 1183b–1184b, 1184f
  foundations of cardiac electrophysiology in, 1163–1175
  gap junctions and, 1174b–1175b
  long-QT syndrome and, 1183, 1183.e1f
  mechanisms of, 1163–1170
    disorders of impulse conduction in, 1183–1186, 1184f
    disorders of impulse formation in, 1179–1183
    Na^+/Ca^{2+} exchanger and, 1171b–1173b, 1174f
    reentry and, 1183b–1184b
      anatomic, 1184–1185, 1185f–1186f
      functional, 1187.e1f, 1185–1186, 1188f
    sleep-disordered breathing and, 1684–1685
    tachycardia-dependent block and, 1183b–1184b
    triggered activity and, 1180–1183, 1181f–1182f
Cardiac asthma, 937
Cardiac auscultation, 130–131
  in aortic valve stenosis, 1406
  in pulmonic regurgitation, 1479b–1481b
Cardiac catheterization, 2–3, 3f
  in aortic valve stenosis, 1408b
  arterial access for, 386–388
    percutaneous femoral artery technique, 386–388, 387f–389f
    percutaneous radial artery technique, 386, 386f–387f, 387.e1f
  cardiac output measurements, 393–394
    Fick method for, 393–394, 395f
    thermodilution method for, 393, 394f
  complications of, 386, 386.e1t
    vascular, 386, 386.e1t
  in constrictive pericarditis, 1627
  contraindications for, 385, 385.e1t
  death and, 386
  development, 385
  of heart failure with preserved and mildly reduced ejection, 1011b–1017b, 1014f–1015f, 1014.e1f
  hemodynamic measurements in, 392–393, 394t
  indications for, 385–386, 385.e1t
  left-heart, 390–391, 391f
  pharmacologic challenges for, 407–408
    dobutamine, 407
    isoproterenol, 407–408
    nitric oxide, 408
    nitroprusside, 408
    pulmonary vasodilators, 408
  physiologic and pharmacologic maneuvers with, 405–408
    dynamic exercise in, 406, 406.e1f
    exercise provocation in, 406
    pacing tachycardia in, 406–407
    pharmacologic maneuvers in, 405–408
    static exercise in, 406
  pressure gradients determination in
    in aortic regurgitation, 401–402, 401t, 402f, 402.e1f
    in aortic valve stenosis, 398f–399f, 399–400, 399.e1f, 399.e1t, 399.e2f
    in hypertrophic obstructive cardiomyopathy, 400–401, 400f–401f
    intraventricular, 404, 404.e1f
    in low-flow, low-gradient aortic stenosis, 400, 400.e1f
    in mitral regurgitation, 402, 403f
    in mitral valve stenosis, 401, 401f
    in pulmonary and tricuspid valve stenosis, 401
    in valvular regurgitation, 402–403
  pressure measurements in, 391–392
    aortic and pulmonary artery, 397–398, 398.e1f
    atrial, 396, 397f
    cardiac cycle and generation, 394–395, 395f
    fluid-filled pressure systems, 392, 392.e1t, 394f
    micromanometer catheters for, 392
    normal waveforms in, 395–398, 396f, 396t

Cardiac catheterization (Continued)
  pulmonary capillary wedge pressure in, 396–397, 397f, 397.e1f
  ventricular pressure waveforms, 398
  pressure-volume relationship in, 408, 408f–409f
  in pulmonary arterial hypertension, 1669
  of rheumatic mitral stenosis, 1446
  right-heart, 391, 393f
    Swan-Ganz catheter for, 391, 392f
  septal defects and, 403–405
  shunt and, 403–405
  for syncope, 1392
  for tetralogy of Fallot, 1564
  transseptal, 390, 390f
  vascular closure devices for, 387
  venous access for, 388–390
Cardiac conduction disturbances
  in rheumatic diseases, 1821
  in rheumatoid arthritis, 1821
  in Sjögren syndrome, 1821
  in spondyloarthropathies, 1821
  in systemic lupus erythematosus, 1821
  in systemic sclerosis, 1821
Cardiac contractility modulation, 1114
Cardiac contraction and relaxation, mechanism of, 889–912
  adrenergic signaling systems in, 899–903, 900f, 900t
  afterload in, 906
  atrial function in, 911
  calcium channels in, 898–899
  calcium ion fluxes in, 895–898, 896f
  cholinergic signaling in, 903–904
  contractile cells and proteins in, 889–895, 890f–891f, 891t
  contractile proteins in, 892–894, 892f
  cross-bridge cycle in, 894–895, 894f
  cyclic guanosine monophosphate signaling in, 903b–904b, 904f
  heart volume and, 906
  ion exchangers and pumps in, 899
  left ventricular contraction in, 904, 905f, 906t
  left ventricular filling phases in, 904–906
  left ventricular relaxation in, 904, 905f, 906t
  mitochondrial morphology and function in, 891–892, 891f
  nitric oxide signaling, 903–904
  preload in, 906, 906b
  pressure-volume loops in, 909f, 910, 910b
  right ventricular function in, 911
  sodium channels in, 898–899
  sodium pump in, 899, 899b
  sodium-calcium exchanger in, 899
  venous filling pressure and, 906
  wall stress in, 907–908
Cardiac cycle, 904–906, 905f, 906t
Cardiac death
  magnetic resonance imaging in, 327–328
  sudden, aborted, in cardiac arrhythmias, 1148, 1148f
Cardiac electrical activity, primary prevention in patients with structurally normal hearts or molecular disorders of, 1382–1383
Cardiac electrical network
  arrhythmias and autonomic nervous system and, 1183.e1f, 1178–1179, 1179.e1f
  atrioventricular junctional area and intraventricular conduction system in, 1175–1176
  innervation of atrioventricular node, His bundle, and ventricular myocardium in, 1177–1178, 1179f
  sinoatrial node in, 1175, 1175.e1f, 1175f–1176f
  structure and function of, 1175–1179
Cardiac electrical system, functions of, 1163, 1164f
Cardiac electrophysiology, magnetic resonance imaging in, 330b–332b
Cardiac emboli, 870
Cardiac energetics, in heart failure, 930.e1f, 930b
Cardiac fibroblasts, in heart failure, 928.e1f, 927f, 927b–929b
Cardiac function
  age-associated changes in, resting, 1687b–1690b, 1689t
  sleep-disordered breathing and, 1683–1684
Cardiac imaging
  in cardiac arrhythmias, 1149, 1152f
  cardiovascular disease and, 2
  in myocarditis, 1087, 1087.e1f, 1087.e1t

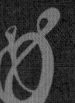

Cardiac implantable electrical devices (CIEDs), 1321
  for atrial fibrillation, 1344
  clinical issues in, 1346–1347
    driving and, 1347
    drug interactions, 1347
    lifestyle issues, 1347
    participation in sports, 1347
    psychosocial issues, 1344f, 1346–1347, 1346.e1t
  device longevity and replacement considerations, 1345b–1346b
  device radiography, 1321, 1321f–1324f
  electromagnetic interference with, 1344–1346, 1345b–1346b, 1345.e1t
  infections of, 1343, 1343.e2f
  types of devices, 1321
Cardiac index, in heart failure, 136
Cardiac innervation, overview of, 1894f
Cardiac magnetic resonance (CMR) imaging
  in aortic regurgitation, 1423, 1425f
  in aortic valve stenosis, 1405f, 1408b
  of heart failure with preserved and mildly reduced ejection, 1011b–1017b, 1013f–1014f
  of primary mitral regurgitation, 1462b
  in pulmonary arterial hypertension, 1668
  in pulmonic regurgitation, 1479b–1481b, 1480f
  of secondary mitral regurgitation, 1466b–1467b
  in sudden cardiac death, 1378b–1379b
  in tricuspid regurgitation, 1476b–1478b
Cardiac masses
  differential diagnosis of, 1830t
  echocardiography in, 253–256, 254t, 255f
  evaluation of, 361
  initial clinical decision making, 1829.e1f, 1829–1830, 1829b, 1830t
  magnetic resonance imaging in, 330b–332b, 332f
Cardiac murmurs, 131–134, 133f
  bedside maneuvers of, 133t, 134
  continuous, 132t, 134
  diastolic, 132–134, 132t
  in infective endocarditis, 1508, 1510t
  in STEMI, 654–655
  systolic, 131–132, 132t, 133f
Cardiac muscle, ion concentrations in, 1163.e1t
Cardiac myocytes
  in heart failure
    apoptosis, 926.e1f, 926b–927b
    hypertrophy, 922–923, 922f–923f
  structure and function of, ethanol on, 1593
Cardiac myosin activators, for acute heart failure, 971b–972b
Cardiac only Timothy syndrome (COTS), 1197, 1198f
Cardiac output
  exercise and, 579
  in heart failure, 937–938
  measurements, in cardiac catheterization, 393–394
    Fick method for, 393–394, 395f
    thermodilution method for, 393, 394f
Cardiac pain, control of, in STEMI, 665–666
Cardiac perforation, implantable cardioverter-defibrillators and, 1343
Cardiac rehabilitation
  additional patient groups in, 591
  comprehensive, 588–592
  cost-effectiveness of, 590–591, 591f
  efforts to reduce participation gap, 591
  in elderly, 1706
  elements of, 588–589, 591t
    facilities, equipment, and technology tools, 588–589
    multidisciplinary team, 588
    patient assessments, 589b
    process, 589b
    structural, 588–589
  evolution of, 588, 589t
  future directions for, 591
  lack of sufficient, 590b–591b
  limitations and potential solutions of, 590b–591b
  longer-term maintenance of, 590b–591b
  low patient referral, enrollment and participation rates of, 590b–591b
  safety of, 590
  value of, 589–591
    physiologic improvements, 589
    recovery from cardiovascular disease event, 589
  wearable devices and, 120
Cardiac Resynchronization in Heart Failure Trial (CARE-HF), 1107b–1110b, 1111f

Cardiac resynchronization therapy (CRT), 1107
  CARE-HF trial of, 1107b–1110b, 1111f
  COMPANION trial of, 1107b–1110b, 1111f
  for congenital heart disease, 1551
  CONTAK CD trial of, 1107b–1110b
  devices for, 1321, 1322f
  guidelines for, 1113
  in heart failure with reduced ejection fraction, 1002
  indications for, 1111
  limitations of, 1111, 1113f
  MADIT-CRT trial of, 1110b–1111b
  MIRACLE ICD trial of, 1107b–1110b
  MIRACLE trial of, 1107b–1110b, 1110f
  MUSTIC trials of, 1107b–1110b, 1108t–1109t
  in patients with narrow QRS complex, 1110b–1111b, 1112t, 1115t
  RAFT trial of, 1110b–1111b
  REVERSE trial of, 1110b–1111b
  target of, 1107–1111
    in NYHA class I and II patients, randomized controlled trials of, 1110–1111, 1110b–1111b
    in NYHA class III and IV patients, randomized controlled trials of, 1107–1110, 1107b–1110b, 1108t–1109t, 1110f–1111f
Cardiac rhythm abnormalities, aging and, 1701–1702
Cardiac sarcoidosis
  criteria to diagnose, 306t
  diagnostic algorithm for, 1045.e1f
  patterns of myocardial perfusion and ^{18}F-FDG images in, 289f
Cardiac structure and function, assessment of, 203–210, 204.e1f, 204.e2f
Cardiac sympathetic denervation (CSD), 1899
Cardiac syndrome X, NSTE-ACS and, 735
Cardiac tamponade, 405, 407f, 1620–1625
  aortic dissection and, 827
  clinical presentation of, 1621
  etiology of, 1617t, 1620
  hemodynamics of, 1620–1621, 1621f–1622f, 1622t
  laboratory testing in, 1622, 1622f–1623f
  management of, 1623–1624, 1624f
  pathophysiology of, 1620–1621, 1620.e1f
  pericardial fluid, analysis of, 1624–1625
  pericardioscopy and percutaneous biopsy, 1625
Cardiac thrombus, magnetic resonance imaging in, 330b–332b, 332f
Cardiac transplantation, 1132
  cardiac donor for, 1134–1135
    donation after circulatory determined death donors, 1135
    evaluation of, 1134–1135
    hepatitis C and drug overdose, 1135, 1135f
  donor allocation system of, 1134, 1134t
  epidemiology of, 1132
  future perspectives for, 1142
  historical aspects of, 1132
  immunosuppression in, 1136–1137
  infection during, 1139–1140
  medical complications and comorbid conditions of, 1140–1142, 1141f, 1141t
    cardiac allograft vasculopathy, 1141–1142, 1142f, 1142t
    diabetes, 1140
    hyperlipidemia, 1141
    hypertension, 1140
    malignancy, 1140, 1142t
    renal insufficiency, 1140–1141
  outcomes after, 1138–1139
    functional, 1139
    rejection and coronary artery vasculopathy, 1138
    survival in, 1138–1139, 1139f–1140f
  potential recipient, evaluation of, 1132–1134
    medical issues, 1132–1134, 1133f
    psychosocial evaluation, 1134
    substance abuse, 1134
  rejection of, 1137–1138, 1137t
    antibody-mediated rejection, 1137–1138
    cellular, 1137
  surgical considerations of, 1136
  in women, 1719
Cardiac troponin I, in chronic kidney disease, 1880
Cardiac-specific troponins I, in NSTE-ACS, 717
Cardioband transcatheter annuloplasty devices, 1490b–1492b

Cardiogenic shock, 938, 938f
  in acute heart failure, 952, 953t, 956b
  in NSTE-ACS, 734
  percutaneous coronary interventions in, 792
  ST-elevation myocardial infarction and, 690–694, 690f
    complications of, 692
    diagnosis of, 691
    intra-aortic balloon counterpulsation for, 691–692, 693f
    mechanical circulatory support for, 691, 692f
    medical management in, 691
    pathologic findings in, 686
    pathophysiology of, 691
    percutaneous left ventricular assist devices for, 691–692
    recommendations for, 693–694
    revascularization in, 692, 694f–695f
    shock teams for, 693
Cardioinhibitory response, 1320
Cardiologist, integrative self-care for, 597
CardioMEMS heart sensor, 1026–1027
Cardiometabolic disease, based discovery to, 90
Cardiomyocytes, 889
Cardiomyopathy, 895b
  alcoholic, 1041, 1593–1594
  approach to clinical genetic evaluation of, 1037–1039, 1038f
  arrhythmogenic
    echocardiography in, 220f, 222
    ventricular tachycardia in, 1299–1302, 1302f
  arrhythmogenic right ventricular, 1033t, 1036f, 1039–1041, 1039f–1040f, 1189
    approach to genetic evaluation of, 1040
    clinical genetics of, 1040
    diagnosis of, 1039.e2t, 1040
    differential diagnosis of, 1040
    exercise testing in, 190b–191b
    genomic cause of, 1039–1040, 1039.e3f
    molecular genetics of, 1039–1040
    treatment of, 1040–1041, 1041.e1f
  cancer and, 1099–1100, 1102t
  in cancer survivorship, 1104–1106, 1105.e1f, 1106.e4t
  classification of, 1031, 1033t
  diabetic, 1041
  dilated, 1032–1043, 1033t, 1034f
    approach to genetic evaluation of, 1040
    in Becker muscular dystrophy, 1853
    cardiac magnetic resonance imaging in, 1032–1035
    clinical genetics of, 1036–1037
    coronary angiography in, 1032
    echocardiography in, 220–221, 220f, 1032, 1034f
    in Emery-Dreifuss muscular dystrophy, 1859
    familial, clinical genetics of, 1035–1037
    genetics of, 1035, 1035f–1036f, 1035.e1t
    in limb-girdle muscular dystrophy, 1861–1862
    in muscular dystrophies, 1853
    pregnancy and, 1732
    therapy for, 1039
  direct cardiotoxicity concerns, 1106.e1
  future perspectives on, 1049
  genetics of, 1031, 1032f, 1034f, 1035.e1t, 1037f, 1038t
  in HIV patients, 1612
  hypertrophic, 1033t, 1062–1076
    atrial fibrillation in, 1285, 1287.e6t, 1287.e8
      management of, 1072
    clinical trials and emerging therapies for, 1073–1075
    definition of, 1062, 1063f–1064f
    diagnosis of, 1062–1063, 1065t
    echocardiography in, 220f–221f, 221–222
    etiology of, 1063, 1065t
    exercise and sports participation and, 1072
    exercise testing in, 190
    in Friedreich ataxia, 1864, 1865f
    genetics of, 1063, 1065t, 1066–1067, 1066f–1067f
    left ventricular hypertrophy in, 1063
    magnetic resonance imaging in, 322–324, 324f
    management of, 1069–1071
      alcohol septal ablation in, 1071–1072, 1075f
      atrial fibrillation and, 1072
      family, 1067–1069, 1070f–1071f
      sudden death and, 1070–1071
      surgical myectomy in, 1071, 1074f
    morphology of, 1062–1063, 1064f
    natural history of, 1066, 1069f

Cardiomyopathy *(Continued)*
　　nonobstructive, 1072
　　obstructive, 1071–1072
　　pathophysiology of, 1063–1066
　　　diastolic dysfunction in, 1063–1065
　　　left ventricular outflow tract obstruction in, 1065, 1068f
　　　phenotype of, 1063
　　　pregnancy and, 1068–1069, 1732
　　　prevalence of, 1063
　　　sudden cardiac death and, 1358t, 1359, 1359b
　　　　prevention of, 1069–1070, 1072f
　　　　risk stratification of, 1069–1070
　　　symptoms in, 1070–1071, 1073f
　　　ventricular tachycardia in, 1302
　hypertrophic obstructive, bifid pulse in, 129
　idiopathic dilated, magnetic resonance imaging in, 326–327, 327f
　indirect cardiotoxicity concerns, 1106.e1
　induced by drugs or toxins, 1593–1602
　　amphetamines, 1599, 1599b
　　arsenic, 1601
　　cadmium, 1601
　　catecholamines, 1599
　　cathinones, 1599
　　cocaine, 1596–1599, 1597f
　　electronic cigarettes, 1595–1596
　　ethanol, 1593–1595, 1594f–1595f
　　future directions for, 1601
　　heavy metals, 1601
　　marijuana, 1599–1600, 1600f
　　mercury, 1601
　　methamphetamines, 1599, 1599b
　　opiates, 1601
　　synthetic cannabinoids, 1600b
　induced, premature ventricular complex, 1291–1292
　infectious, 1033t
　infiltrative, 1033t, 1043–1049. *See also* Amyloidosis; Hemochromatosis
　inflammatory, 1033t
　inflammatory cardiotoxicity concerns, 1106.e1
　ischemic, 779–780, 1033t
　　echocardiography in, 220f, 221
　　patients with, 298–303
　　percutaneous coronary interventions in, 792
　　quantitative myocardial perfusion imaging in, 300f
　　ventricular tachycardia in, 1297–1299
　left ventricular noncompaction, 1041, 1041.e2t
　　diagnosis of, 1829b, 1831f
　　management of, 1041
　magnetic resonance imaging in, 322–326
　management of, 1103–1104, 1106.e2
　mitral regurgitation in, 221f
　noncompaction, in athletes, 585
　nonischemic, ventricular tachycardia in, 1296f, 1299, 1301f
　percutaneous coronary interventions in, 792
　peripartum, 1042, 1086.e1, 1719, 1733f
　　clinical features of, 1042
　　pregnancy and, 1732–1733, 1732.e1f
　　preventive efforts and screening recommendations for, 1106.e1
　pulmonary hypertension and, 1659
　restrictive, 1033t, 1043–1049
　　approach to identifying cause of, 1043–1044
　　clinical genetics of, 1043–1044
　　constrictive pericarditis and, 1044.e1f
　　echocardiography in, 220f, 222, 1044, 1044f
　　idiopathic, 1044
　　molecular genetics of, 1043–1044
　sarcoid, 1044–1046
　　clinical features of, 1044–1045, 1046f
　　diagnosis of, 1045, 1046f–1047f
　　pathology of, 1044, 1045f
　　treatment of, 1045–1046, 1045.e2t
　tachycardia-induced, 1041–1042
　Takotsubo, 1042.e1f, 1042–1043, 1042b, 1043t, 1598
　　electrocardiography in, 168–169
　　magnetic resonance imaging in, 327–328
　　therapy for, 1043
　　in women, 1717
　undiagnosed, 322
Cardio-oncology, 1099–1106.e6, 1091–1098, 1100f–1101f
　care team and clinics of, 1105, 1106f
　future perspectives on, 1097–1098, 1105–1106
　radionuclide imaging in, 310

Cardiopulmonary dynamics, of pulmonary embolism, 1638.e1f, 1637b–1639b, 1640f
Cardiopulmonary exercise testing, 178b–180b
　in heart failure, 942–943, 942b–943b
　of heart failure with preserved and mildly reduced ejection, 1011b–1017b, 1017t
　invasive, in pulmonary arterial hypertension, 1669t–1670t, 1670b
　of pulmonary stenosis, 1562
Cardiopulmonary resuscitation, 1372
　airway in, 1372
　breathing in, 1372
　cardiocerebral resuscitation in, 1372
　circulation in, 1372, 1373.e1f
Cardiorenal syndrome, 1882–1887, 1887f–1888f, 1889t
　in heart failure, 938b–939b, 957
Cardiotoxicity, 1091, 1103
Cardiovascular disease (CVD), 502–524.e1, 1–13, 1751–1765
　access policy and, 62–63
　acute myocardial infarction and, 6–7, 6f
　adrenal hormones and, 1793–1795
　air pollution and, 31–37, 32f, 39.e1t
　　approaches to communicate risk, 37
　　composition of, 31–34, 33t
　　　gaseous pollutants, 33
　　　household *vs.* ambient air pollution, 34
　　　particulate matter, 33–34
　　effects of, 34–36, 35f
　　　arrhythmia, 36
　　　chronic kidney disease, 36
　　　diabetes, 36
　　　heart failure, 36
　　　hypertension, 35–36
　　　ischemic heart disease, 35
　　　societal and personal strategies, 37
　　　venous thromboembolism, 36
　　mechanistic insights into, 36–37, 36f
　　mortality and, 34
　alternative payment models and, 65–66
　arrhythmias and, 5
　artificial intelligence and, 9–11
　assisted circulation, 7–8
　biomarkers of, 453–457
　　homocysteine, 455
　　lipids/lipoproteins, 453–455
　　lipoprotein(a), 455, 455.e1f
　at birth, 1–2
　cardiac imaging and, 2
　care for, 66–68
　climate change and, 37–38, 38f
　clonal hematopoiesis and, 9, 10f
　community interventions for, 467, 467f
　coronary risk factors of, 6–7, 7f
　cost-effective solutions for, 27–29, 28t
　dyslipidemias and, 5–6
　economic burden of, 26–27, 27f
　endocrine disorders and, 1791–1808
　epidemiology of, 1752–1753
　future perspectives in, 1804–1807, 1805t–1806t
　gaps in evidence and future perspectives in, 467–468
　genomics and genetics of, 8
　global burden of, 14–30
　group disparities in, emerging scientific research for, 1748
　health policy in, 62, 63f
　heart failure and, 7
　in heterogeneous populations
　　epidemiology of, 1743–1744
　　management of, 1744–1748
　hypertension and, 3–4
　impact of health care policy in, 62–70
　income and, 67
　inflammation and, 9
　insurance coverage and, 62–63, 63f
　invasive procedures for, 2–3
　lifestyle factors and interventions for, 458–462
　management, 27
　mental health and psychiatric disorders, 1843–1846
　　mechanisms, 1843–1844
　　shared features across, 1844
　metallic pollutants and, 39, 39t
　mobile health, remote monitoring, and wearables for, 467
　mortality from, 15–16, 17f
　　in Central and Eastern Europe and Central Asia, 18f, 19

Cardiovascular disease (CVD) *(Continued)*
　　in East Asia and Pacific, 18f, 19
　　in high-income countries, 18–19, 18f
　　in Latin America and Caribbean, 18f, 19–20
　　in North Africa and Middle East, 18f, 20
　　in South Asia, 18f, 20
　　in sub-Saharan Africa, 18f, 20
　noise pollution and, 38
　nutrition and, 531–546, 532f
　obesity and, 547, 547f–548f
　in older adults, 1687–1709.e2
　in other population groups, 1743–1744
　outcomes of, 66–68
　parathyroid hormone and, 1796–1797
　pathophysiology of, 1753b
　payment and delivery system policy in, 63–66, 64t
　pharmacologic therapies for, 462–465
　　aspirin, 463–464, 463f–464f
　　n-3 fatty acid supplements, 464–465, 466f
　　shared decision-making, 462–463
　physical activity and, 461–462, 461f
　pituitary hormones and, 1791–1793
　precision medicine *vs.* preventive care, 466–467
　prevention of
　　novel approaches to, 465–467
　　primary, 442–470, 443f
　　primordial, 8–9, 442–443, 443f
　　secondary, 442–443, 443f
　　types of, 442–443, 443f
　　in women, 457–458
　psychiatric and psychosocial aspects of, 1841–1852
　public reporting and, 64–65
　in racial and ethnic groups, 1743, 1744f
　in racial and ethnic minorities, 66–68, 66f
　recovery from, 589
　risk assessment, 27–28, 443–445
　　cardiovascular health and life's simple 7, 443–444, 444f, 444b
　　global risk, 444
　　lifetime risk, 445
　　society guidelines for, 445, 446f, 446t
　　vascular imaging in preventive practice, 445, 445.e1f
　risk factors for, 20–26
　　control of, 590
　　enhancing, 451–453
　　traditional, 446–451
　risk of, 66–68
　　nicotine and tobacco products, 525–530
　sex, gender, and genetic differences in, 1710
　stress and emotional arousal, 1841
　　acute, 1841–1842
　　chronic, 1842–1843
　　mechanisms underlying, 1842, 1842f
　　responses to everyday, 1841
　synthetic chemicals and, 38–39
　tests to improve identification and definition of, 416–417
　thyroid hormones and, 1797–1804
　trends in
　　global, 442, 442.e1f
　　in United States, 442
　in urban-rural geography, 67–68, 68f
　value-based payment programs: hospitals, 65
　value-based purchasing: outpatient, 65
　valvular heart disease and, 4–5
　windows of exposure, susceptibility, and vulnerability, 37
　in women, 1710–1722
Cardiovascular events, 590
　fatal and non-fatal, 590, 590f
　hospital readmission of, 590
Cardiovascular examination, 126–134
　blood pressure in, 128–129, 129t
　jugular venous pressure and waveform in, 126–128, 128f, 128t
　pulses in, 129–130, 130f
Cardiovascular health, 443–444, 444f, 444b
　environment on, 31–41, 32f
Cardiovascular implantable electronic device, infections with, 1526–1528, 1527f
Cardiovascular infections
　implantable electronic device, 1526–1528, 1527f
　infective endocarditis, 1505–1525
　left ventricular assist device, 1528
Cardiovascular injury, by smoking, 527

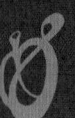

Cardiovascular medicine
  artificial intelligence in, 109–111
    definition of, 109–111, 109.e1f
    fully connected and convolutional neural networks, 110
    implementing into clinical practice, 113–115, 113f–115f
    learning, 109
    optimization and hyperparameters, 110–111
    pitfalls and limitations of, 115, 116f
    reinforcement learning, 110
    supervised learning, 109–110, 109.e1f
    transfer learning, 111
    unsupervised learning, 110
  clinical trials in, 42–52
  clinical uses in, 111–113
    coronary arteriography, 113
    detection, 111
    ECG-based screening, 111
    image interpretation and procedural guidance, 111–113
    natural language processing and structures data analysis, 113
    prevention, 111
    risk scores (deep phenotyping), 113
  human genetics, key principles of, 71–75
  wearable devices in, 117–122
    activity and heart rate tracking for general cardiovascular wellness, 117–118, 118f
    atrial fibrillation, 118–120
      electrocardiogram, 119–120, 120f
      photoplethysmography detection of irregular rhythm, 118–119, 119f
    cardiac arrest and sudden cardiac death, 120
    cardiac rehabilitation and heart failure, 120
    definitions and overview, 117
    evaluation of, 120–121
      activity, exercise, and sleep, 121
      ancillary information, 120, 121f
      heart rate and rhythm notifications, 120–121, 122t
    hypertension, 120
    limitations of, 121
Cardiovascular surgery, 3
Cardiovascular system
  diabetes mellitus and, 556–578
    future perspectives in, 576–577
  mechanisms of acute viral infections on, 1753f
  rheumatic diseases and, 1809–1828
Cardiovascular tissues, direct effect on, 1759b–1762b
Cardioversion, 1227, 1228f
  indication for, 1277, 1287.e4t
  pharmacologic, 1278
Cardioversion shock therapy, defibrillation and, 1337b–1339b, 1339.e1f, 1342f
Carditis, in rheumatic fever, 1534, 1534t
Caregiving, stress from, 1843
Carfilzomib, cardiotoxic effects of, 1092t
Carney's complex, 1830
Carotid artery disease, 774.e1
  surgical treatment of, 774.e1
Carotid artery, pulse of, 128t–129t, 129
Carotid atherosclerosis, in HIV patients, 1604f
Carotid pulse, in STEMI, 654
Carotid sinus hypersensitivity, 1389
Carotid sinus massage, 1391
Carotid ultrasound, in HIV patients, 1607
Carotid-femoral pulse wave velocity (cf-PWV), 478
Carteolol, for angina pectoris, 758t
Carvajal syndrome, 1040
Carvedilol
  for angina pectoris, 758t
  in chronic kidney disease, 1882t
  in heart failure, 991t–992t, 995f, 995b–996b
  for heart failure with preserved and mildly reduced ejection, 1024
CASH trial, 1332t
Caspofungin, for infective endocarditis, 1519b–1523b
CASQ2, 1203b
CAT trial, 1336t
Catecholamine
  cardiovascular complications of, 1599
Catecholaminergic polymorphic ventricular tachycardia (CPVT), 1188–1189, 1201–1203
  clinical description and manifestations of, 1201–1203
  electrocardiography in, 1309
  exercise testing in, 190b–191b

Catecholaminergic polymorphic ventricular tachycardia (CPVT) (Continued)
  genetic basis of, 1203f, 1203b
  sudden cardiac death and, 1362–1363
Catheter ablation
  of atrial fibrillation, 1280–1283
  for interatrial re-entrant tachycardia, 1548
  for sudden cardiac death (SCD), 1380
Catheter aspiration thrombectomy, for peripheral artery disease, 862
Catheter-based mechanical thrombectomy, for acute limb ischemia, 854–855
Catheter-based reperfusion strategies, for STEMI, 671, 671f–673f
Catheter-based therapy, advances in, 1649–1650
Catheter-based thrombolytic therapy, for acute limb ischemia, 854–855
Catheter-directed intra-arterial thrombolysis plus thrombectomy, for acute limb ischemia, 854–855
Catheter-directed thrombolysis, in peripheral artery disease, 862
Catheterization, right heart, in heart failure, 942, 942b
Catheter-related thrombosis, 868
Catheter(s)
  Amplatz, 367, 368f
  for coronary angiography, 367–369, 367f–368f
  Judkins, for coronary angiography, 367, 367f
Cathinones, cardiovascular complications of, 1599
Cathodal stimulation, 1323b–1324b
Causal biomarker, 104
CAV. See Cardiac allograft vasculopathy
Cav1.2, 1171b–1173b
Cav3.1/α_1 G alpha subunits, 1171b–1173b
Caval devices, for tricuspid regurgitation, 1492
Caveolin, 889–891
Cavo-tricuspid isthmus dependent flutter, 1253b–1257b
CCTA. See Coronary computed tomographic angiography
Cefazolin, in infective endocarditis, 1519b–1523b, 1521t
Cefotaxime, for infective endocarditis, from HACEK organisms, 1519b–1523b
Ceftriaxone, for infective endocarditis
  from HACEK organisms, 1519b–1523b
  from streptococcal species, 1519b–1523b
Central aortic stiffness, increased, in heart failure with preserved and mildly reduced ejection, 1011b–1017b
Central dogma, 71
Central sleep apnea (CSA)
  definition of, 1678
  in heart failure with preserved and mildly reduced ejection, 1011b–1017b
  key features of, 1679t
  new implantable therapeutic devices for, 1114
  pathophysiology of, 1679
CentriMag VAD, 1121f, 1125t
Cephalization, 271
Cerebral embolic protection, during transcatheter aortic valve replacement, 1436
Cerebral hemorrhage, 1870f
Cerebral venous/sinus thrombosis (CVST), 870b–873b, 872f
Cerebrovascular disease
  endovascular treatment of, 865–867
  in HIV patients, 1613
Cervical disc disease, chest pain in, 600t
CHADS-VASC score, 877
Chagas disease, 1081
  epidemiology of, 1081–1082, 1081.e1f
  symptoms of, 1082b
  treatment of, 1082
CHARISMA (Clopidogrel for High Atherothrombotic Risk and Ischemic Stabilization, Management, and Avoidance) trial, 848
Chemical ablation, 1239b–1241b
Chemokines, 431
Chemoreceptors, 1895–1896
Chemoreflexes, 1895–1896
Chemotherapy, cardiotoxicity of, 1091b
Chest compressions, in cardiopulmonary resuscitation, 1372
Chest discomfort, recurrent, 703–704
  diagnosis of, 704
  ischemia and reinfarction, 704
  management of, 704
  prognosis of, 704
Chest examination, 126

Chest fluoroscopy, 268b–269b
Chest pain, 599–608
  acute, coronary computed tomography angiography in, 341
  in athletes, 583
  atypical descriptions of, 599
  in biliary colic, 741
  biomarkers in, 602–603
  B-type natriuretic peptides, 603b
  causes of, 599–601, 600t
  clinical evaluation of, 601
  cocaine-induced, 1597
  in costochondritis, 741
  creatine kinase MB isoenzyme in, 603
  D-dimer in, 603b
  decision aids for, 604–605, 604f, 605t
  differential diagnosis of, 740–741
  electrocardiography in, 602, 602t, 605–606, 606t
  in esophageal disorders, 740
  evaluation of, 123–124
  exercise electrocardiographic testing in, 191–192, 192t
  exercise testing in, 605–606
  in gastrointestinal conditions, 601
  history in, 601, 602t
  in hyperthyroidism, 1800
  in infective endocarditis, 1508
  initial assessment in, 601–604
  management of, 603.e3f, 605–607, 606f
    algorithm for diagnostic approach, 604f, 606f
    imaging tests in, 606–607
    treadmill electrocardiography in, 605–606, 606t
  in musculoskeletal disorders, 601
  in myocardial ischemia or infarction, 599
  in neurologic and musculoskeletal disorders, 741
  with normal coronary arteriogram, 777
  in NSTE-ACS, 715
  in pericardial disease, 600
  physical examination in, 601–602
  in pulmonary conditions, 600–601
  radiography in, 602
  stable, coronary computed tomography angiography in, 342–344
  testing strategy for, 603–604, 603.e1f, 603.e2f, 603.e3f
  triage for, 601
  troponins in, 603, 603.e1f
  in vascular disease, 600
Chest radiography, 268–276
  in acquired heart disease, 274–275
  in acute pericarditis, 1617
  advanced imaging, 275–276
  anatomy, 270
  in aortic dissection, 823, 823.e1f
  in calcific pericarditis, 271
  in chest pain, 602
  common anatomic variants, 270–271
  in congenital heart disease, 273–274
  in congestive heart failure, 269t
  in constrictive pericarditis, 1627
  in coronary artery disease, 275
  decubitus views, 268b–269b
  evaluation, 269–273
  frontal, 270, 271f
  in granulomatous polyangiitis, 1818f
  in heart failure, 275, 276f, 938
  inspiration-expiration, 268b–269b
  interpretation of, 270b
  lateral, 268–270
  localization within cardiac silhouette, 271–273, 271f–273f
  normal, 268, 269f
  in pericardial effusion, 271
  portable, 272b–273b, 274f
  in pregnancy, 1725
  in prosthetic heart valves, 1499
  in pulmonary embolism, 1643
  in pulmonary hypertension, 274, 274f–275f
  radiographic densities, 270
  of rheumatic mitral stenosis, 1446
  standard, 268b–269b
  in systemic sclerosis, 1823f
  in thoracic aortic aneurysms, 814f–815f, 815
  in valvular heart disease, 274–275
  variants, 268b–269b
Chest roentgenography
  in pulmonary arterial hypertension, 1667
  in stable ischemic heart disease, 744

Cheyne-Stokes respiration, in heart failure, 935, 999f, 1002–1003
Childhood adversity, 1842
Children
  AV block in, 1318–1319
  multisystem inflammatory syndrome in, 1757
  obesity in, 23
  pericardial disease in, 1630b–1633b
  sudden cardiac death in, 1358t, 1363, 1383
Chimeric antigen receptor T Cells, cardiotoxic effects of, 1092t, 1094–1095
China Antihypertensive Trial in Acute Ischemic Stroke (CATIS), 885b–886b
"CHIP" (Complex High Risk and Indicated Procedures) interventions, 793
Chlorothiazide, in heart failure, 983t
Chlorthalidone, in heart failure, 983t
Cholecystitis, pain in, 601
Cholesterol, 503
  dietary, 538, 539b
  total, 23, 24f
Cholesterol embolism, 855
Cholesteryl ester transfer protein deficiency, 513
Cholesteryl esters, 503
Chorea, Sydenham, 1534
Chronic aortic regurgitation, 1419–1428
  clinical stages of, 1422t
  management of patients with, 1427f
  pathophysiology of, 1419–1420
  treatment of, 1426–1428
    asymptomatic patients, 1426–1427, 1428f
    medical therapy, 1426
    operative procedures, 1427–1428
    surgical treatment, 1426–1428
    symptomatic patients, 1426
Chronic cardiac dilatation, 1615.e1f, 1615b
Chronic hemolytic anemia, in chronic thromboembolic pulmonary hypertension, 1676
Chronic intraventricular delay, 1162.e2, 1162.e3t
Chronic kidney disease
  air pollution and, 36
  in HIV patients, cardiovascular risk factors in, 1605
  management of hypertension in, 492–493
  in NSTE-ACS, 733b–734b
  statins in, 517
Chronic mesenteric ischemia, 867
Chronic obstructive pulmonary disease (COPD), right ventricular hypertrophy in, 155, 155f
Chronic progressive external ophthalmoplegia, 1866–1867
Chronic secondary mitral regurgitation, 4
Chronic thromboembolic pulmonary hypertension, 1640–1641, 1668f, 1672, 1674, 1674f, 1676f
  advanced therapy for, 1648–1651
  pulmonary arterial hypertension and, 1662
Chronic total occlusions, percutaneous coronary intervention in, 789
Chronic venous insufficiency, 1640b–1641b
Chronotropic incompetence, 181b–182b, 1023, 1314, 1314f
Churg-Strauss syndrome (eosinophilic granulomatosis with polyangiitis), 1816–1817, 1817f
  cardiovascular complications of, 1816
  investigation of, 1816
  treatment for, 1816–1817
Chylomicrons, 505b–506b, 507f
CIDS trial, 1332t
Cigarette smoking
  cardiovascular effects, 526–528, 527t, 527b–528b
  cessation, in peripheral artery disease, 847, 849
  in coronary artery disease, 1356
  in HIV patients, cardiovascular risk factors in, 1605b
  in peripheral artery disease, 838, 847
  in stable ischemic heart disease, 751
  by women, cardiovascular disease and, 1710b–1714b
Cilostazol, for peripheral artery disease, 847.e2t, 850–851, 852f, 863
Cinaciguat, for acute heart failure, 971b–972b
Ciraparantag, 1786t, 1787
Circulation, assisted, 7–8
Cisplatin, cardiotoxic effects of, 1092t
Claudication, 838, 840, 840t, 859
Claudication onset time, 843
Cleveland Clinic Prognostic Score, 186b–187b, 189f
Clevidipine, for acute heart failure, 965b

Clinical decision-making
  in cardiology, 53–61.e1
  diagnostic, 53–57, 54f–57f
  framing effects in, 59
  heuristics in, 53–54
  on new findings, clinical practice based, changing, 59
  outcomes and, 57b
  quality of, monitoring, 60
  risk-treatment paradox and, 58
  shared, 59–60
  teaching clinical reasoning, 60–61
  therapeutic, 57–58
Clinical endpoint, definition of, 102, 103t
Clinical research/trials
  in cardiovascular medicine, 42–52
  components of, 43–46
  data safety, 49
  design, 43–44, 44f
    novel approaches to, 49–50
  endpoints, 45–46
  equipoise in, 48
  ethical considerations of, 48–49
  factorial design for, 43
  inclusion and exclusion criteria, 45
  informed consent, 48–49
  interpretation of subgroups, 51–52, 51f
  monitoring of data, 49
  versus other types of studies, 42–43
  phases, 42b–43b, 43f
  post-hoc analyses, 52
  power and sample size, 47–48, 48f
  rationale of, 43
  registration and reporting of, 50
  "response variables", 45–46
  secondary endpoints, 50
  statistical considerations in, 46–48
  study background of, 43
  study execution, 44–45
  types of, 43f
  typical consort diagram in, 50f
  understanding primary results, 50
  use of electronic medical records in, 49
Clonal hematopoiesis, 1097.e1
  cardiovascular disease and, 9, 10f
Clopidogrel, 83
  in arterial thrombosis, 1776
  aspirin and, combination of, 1777
  in coronary artery disease, chronic kidney disease and, 1880t–1881t
  drug interaction with, 97, 97t
  in NSTE-ACS, 724–725, 724b–725b, 725f, 735.e6t
  in percutaneous coronary intervention, 787.e3t, 799–800
  in peripheral artery disease, 847.e2t
  pregnancy and, 1730f
  resistance to, 1777b
  in stable ischemic heart disease, 754b–756b
  for stroke, 878
Clopidogrel in High-Risk Patients with Acute Nondisabling Cerebrovascular Events (CHANCE) trial, 878
Closed mitral valvotomy (CMV), for mitral stenosis, 1449
Closed pericardiocentesis, for cardiac tamponade, 1623
Clozapine, myocarditis and, 1083b
Clubbing, 126
Cluster randomization, 44
Clustering, 110
Coagulation, 1769–1770, 1769f
  mechanical circulatory support and, 1124, 1124b
Cocaethylene, 1598b–1599b
Cocaine, 1596–1599
  aortic dissection and, 1598
  arrhythmias and, 1598–1599
  chest pain and, 1597
  clinical presentation of, 1597–1598
  epidemiology of, 1596
  history of, 1596
  myocardial dysfunction and, 1598
  NSTE-ACS and, 735
  pathophysiology of, 1596–1597
Codeine, drug interaction with, 97t
Coenzyme Q10
  for congestive heart failure, 596
  for dyslipidemia, 596b

Coffee, 534f, 535
Cognitive impairment
  cardiovascular disease and, 1845–1846
  in older adult, 1690b–1693b
Cognitive psychologists, 53
COL3A1, 812
Colchicine, 9
  for acute pericarditis, 1618
Cold pressor test, 1898
Colesevelam, in diabetes mellitus, 562t–563t
Collagen, in heart failure, 927b–929b, 928f
Collateral vessel circulation, coronary angiography in, 376b–377f, 377f
Color Doppler imaging, in infective endocarditis, 1513f–1514f
Color flow Doppler imaging, in aortic regurgitation, 1422–1423
Color M-Mode and flow propagation, 208, 208.e2f
Combined lipoprotein disorders, treatment of, 521–522
Commercial beverages, sugar content in, 467, 467f
Community-based intervention programs, in cardiovascular disease prevention, 28–29
Comorbidity-inflammation-endothelial dysfunction paradigm, 1018b–1020b
Comparison of Medical Therapy, Pacing and Defibrillation in Heart Failure (COMPANION) trial, 1107b–1110b, 1111f, 1336t
Compensatory enlargement, 434
  of atherosclerotic lesion, 425
Competitive atrial pacing, 1331
Competitive sports, for congenital heart disease, 1553–1554
COMPLETE TAVR trial (Staged Complete Revascularization for Coronary Artery Disease vs Medical Management Alone in Patients with AS Undergoing Transcatheter Aortic Valve Replacement), 1437.e1
Comprehensive Cardiac Rehabilitation, 588–592
Comprehensive lifestyle approach, for arrhythmias, 596–597
Computed tomographic angiography (CTA)
  in abdominal aortic aneurysms, 807–808
  in chest pain, 607
  in peripheral artery disease, 845, 845f, 863
  in stable ischemic heart disease, 747f
  in thoracic aortic aneurysms, 813.e1f, 815, 816f
Computed tomography (CT)
  in abdominal aortic aneurysms, 807–808, 809f
  in aortic dissection, 815.e1f, 823, 824f
  in aortic intramural hematoma, 831f–832f, 832, 832.e1f
  in aortic valve stenosis, 1408b
  cardiac, 335–362
    coronary and, basic of, 335–337, 336f
      calcium testing, 337–340
      different types of, 335–337
      radiation principles/patient safety, 335b–337b, 337f
      technical considerations/image acquisition, 335b–337b
    coronary angiography, 340–354
    image acquisition parameters during, 336t
    pre-transcatheter aortic valve replacement, 357–358, 359t
    of primary mitral regurgitation, 1462b
  in cardiac tumors, 1829
  cardiovascular medicine and, 113
  chest, in pulmonary embolism, 1643, 1643f–1644f
  contrast-enhanced, for NSTE-ACS, 721t
  evaluation of cardiac masses, 361
  fractional flow reserve, 347–349, 349f
    clinical effectiveness, 347–349, 350t
    diagnostic accuracy, 347, 347.e1f, 349f
  in heart failure, 943
  in mycotic aneurysms, 833, 835f
  perfusion, 349
  in pericardial effusion and cardiac tamponade, 1622
  in peripheral artery disease, 863
  in pregnancy, 1725
  in stable ischemic heart disease, 746–747, 747f
  in STEMI, 658–659
  for structural heart disease interventions, 357–361
  for transcatheter aortic valve replacement, 1435
Concomitant cardiac diseases, transcatheter aortic valve replacement and, 1437
Conditional probability, 54b–55b
Condoms, 1740–1741

Conduction
  decremental, 1183b–1184b
  safety factor for, 1173
Conduction disturbances, in transcatheter aortic valve replacement, 1437
Conductor fractures, 1341
Confrontational fluid challenge, in pulmonary arterial hypertension, 1670b
Congenital atresia of coronary ostium, coronary angiography in, 373b–374b
Congenital bicuspid aortic stenosis, 1400f
Congenital contractural arachnodactyly, thoracic aortic aneurysm in, 811t
Congenital coronary artery fistulas (CAFs), coronary angiography in, 373b–374b, 375f
Congenital heart disease, 1541–1586, 1737–1740
  in adolescent and adult, 1541–1586
    access and delivery of care for, 1541, 1542t
    arrhythmias in, 1545–1549
    cardiac development of, 1545, 1546f
    cardiac resynchronization for, 1551
    clinical evaluation of, 1542–1543, 1543t–1544t
    competitive sports for, 1553–1554
    exercise and sports participation for, 1553–1554
    exercise testing in, 190–191
    general considerations in, 1541–1544
    genetic considerations of, 1545, 1547t
    great complexity, 1541, 1542t
    heart failure, transplantation, and mechanical circulatory support in, 1549–1550
    individualized exercise programs for, 1553, 1555f, 1556t
    long-term considerations of, 1545–1554
    magnetic resonance imaging in, 330b–332b
    medical therapy for, 1550–1551
    moderate severity, 1541, 1542t
    noncardiac complications in, 1543–1544, 1545t
    noncardiac surgery and, 411b–412b
    palliative care for, 1551
    simple, 1541, 1542t
    transition to care of, 1541–1542
    transplantation for, 1551, 1552f
  anatomy in, 1544–1545
  aortopathies in, 1551–1552
  catheter-based treatment of, 1587–1592
    arterial interventions in, 1588–1589
      pulmonary angioplasty in, 1588–1589, 1588b–1589b
      stenting for coarctation of aorta in, 1589, 1589b
    future perspectives for, 1591–1592, 1591f–1592f
    septal interventions in, 1589–1591
      techniques for closure of atrial septal defects, 1589–1590, 1589f
      techniques for closure of ventricular septal defects, 1590
      treatment of patent ductus arteriosus, 1591, 1591f
    valvular interventions in, 1587–1588
      pulmonary valve replacement in, 1587–1588
      pulmonary valve systems in, 1588, 1588f
      pulmonary valvuloplasty in, 1587, 1587f
  chest radiography in, 273–274
  coronary artery disease and, 296b–298b, 299f
  echocardiography of, 1546
  electrocardiography of, 1543
  nomenclature of, 1544–1545
  pregnancy and, 1552–1553, 1554t
  pulmonary arterial hypertension and, 1658t, 1661–1662
  specific defects of, 1554–1582
    anomalous coronary artery from the pulmonary artery, 1578, 1579f
    atrial septal defects and partial anomalous pulmonary veins, 1554–1557
    atrioventricular septal defects, 1557–1558, 1559f
    coarctation of aorta, 1575–1576, 1575f–1577f
    congenitally corrected transposition of great arteries, 1569–1570, 1569f
    cor triatriatum, 1572–1573, 1572f
    double outlet right ventricle, 1570–1572, 1571f
    Ebstein anomaly of the tricuspid valve, 1560–1562
    interrupted aortic arch, 1576–1577
    left-to-right shunt lesions, 1554, 1556f, 1556t
    patent ductus arteriosus, 1559
    pulmonary stenosis, 1562–1563, 1562f
    single ventricle, 1578–1582
    subvalvular left ventricular outflow tract obstruction, 1573, 1573f–1574f

Congenital heart disease (Continued)
    supravalvar aortic stenosis, 1573–1574
    tetralogy of Fallot, 1563–1566
    transposition of great arteries, 1566–1569
    truncus arteriosus, 1572
    vascular rings, 1577–1578, 1578f
    ventricular septal defects, 1558–1559, 1559t, 1560f
  sudden cardiac death and, 1358t
  supraventricular tachycardia in adults late after surgical repair of, 1268b–1270b, 1270f
  ventricular tachycardia in, 1302
Congenitally corrected transposition of great arteries, 1569–1570, 1569f
  anatomic description and prevalence of, 1569
  clinical features of, 1569, 1569f
  late complications of, 1570
  surgical repairs of, 1569, 1570f
Congestive heart failure
  atrial fibrillation in, 1284
  chest radiography in, 269t
  integrative strategies for, 596
    coenzyme Q10 in, 596
    nutrition and lifestyle, 596
  stroke and, 879b
Conivaptan, in heart failure, 983t
Connective tissue disorders, coronary artery disease and, 780b–781b
Connexins
  of gap junctions, 1174b–1175b
  in sinoatrial node, 1175.e1b
Conotruncal anomalies, magnetic resonance imaging in, 330b–332b
Consciousness, altered level of, in cardiac arrhythmias, 1147–1148
Constrictive pericarditis, 406t, 1625–1630
  cardiac catheterization and angiography in, 1627, 1628f
  clinical presentation of, 1625b–1626b
  computed tomography and cardiac magnetic resonance imaging in, 1627–1628, 1629f
  echocardiography in, 242–244, 242f–243f
  echocardiography-Doppler examination for, 1627, 1627.e1f
  etiology of, 1617t, 1625f, 1625b–1626b
  laboratory testing in, 1627, 1627.e1f
  management of, 1628–1630
  pathophysiology of, 1625b–1626b, 1626f
  physical examination in, 1626–1627
  restrictive cardiomyopathy vs., 1628, 1630t
Contact pathway, 1770, 1771f
Contact system, 1770
Continuous positive airway pressure (CPAP), in acute heart failure, 955–956
Continuous-flow rotary pumps, 1122.e1, 1122.e1f, 1122.e2f
Contraception, 1740–1741, 1740.e1t
Contractile cells, ultrastructure of, 889–891, 890f–891f
Contractile proteins, 892–894, 892f
  abnormalities of, in heart failure, 925, 925t
Contralateral common femoral artery (CFA), 864
Contrast echocardiography, 212–216, 213f–214f, 214f–215f, 215.e1f
Contrast media, in magnetic resonance imaging, 314b–320b
Contrast phlebography, in pulmonary embolism, 1644
Contrast venography, in pulmonary embolism, 1644
Contrast-enhanced angiography, in peripheral artery disease, 845, 846f
Contrast-enhanced computed tomography (CECT), in aortic dissection, 815.e1f, 823, 824f, 827.e1f
Contrast-induced acute kidney injury, 364b–366b, 365f, 1875–1876, 1877f–1878f
  prevention of, 1876–1877, 1878f–1879f
Convolutional neural networks, 110
Cooled-tip radiofrequency ablation, 1230–1231, 1230f, 1230b–1231b
Copeptin, in NSTE-ACS, 718
Copy number variants (CNVs), 73
Cor triatriatum, 1572–1573, 1572f
CoreValve Evolut self-expanding TAVR series, 1435.e1, 1436f
Coronary absence, coronary angiography in, 373b–374b
Coronary angiography, 363–384
  access sites for, 366–367, 366.e1f
  in acute kidney injury, 364b–366b, 365f
  in aortic dissection, 824

Coronary angiography (Continued)
  appropriate use criteria for, 364–366
  basic technique for, 367
  in cardiac arrest, 1369
  catheters for, 367–369, 367f–368f
  complications of, 364b–366b, 365f
  contraindications to, 364b–366b
  contrast media for, 371, 371.e1t
    manual injection of, 371, 371b, 371.e1t
  coronary anatomy and, 372–373
  in coronary artery anomalies, 373–374, 373t
  evaluation of, 375
  indications for, 363–366, 363.e1t
  in NSTE-ACS, 717b, 718
  patient preparation for, 366
  percutaneous coronary intervention for, 382–383, 382.e1f
  pitfalls of, 374–375, 374.e1f
  projections, 371–372, 372f–373f, 372t
  risks associated with, 363t–364t, 364b–366b
  selective coronary artery cannulation in, 367b–368b, 368f
  special lesion considerations for, 377–378
    bifurcation lesions, 378
    calcific lesions, 377, 377.e1f, 377.e1t
    chronic total occlusion, 377
    coronary dissections, 378, 378f, 378.e1t
    thrombotic lesions, 377, 378f
  technique for, 366–371
  ventriculography for, 369–371, 369f–370f, 370t
Coronary arteries
  embolism of, sudden cardiac death (SCD) and, 1357.e1, 1358t
  mechanical abnormalities of, 1357, 1358t
  mechanical obstruction of, 1357.e1
  nonatherosclerotic, abnormalities of, sudden cardiac death (SCD) and, 1357
  spasm of, sudden cardiac death (SCD) and, 1357.e1, 1358t
Coronary arteriography, cardiovascular medicine and, 113
Coronary artery abnormalities, pathology of sudden death caused by, 1363b–1365b, 1364f
Coronary artery bypass grafting (CABG), 353
  in heart failure, 1000
  before noncardiac surgery, 420
  in NSTE-ACS, 731
  in stable ischemic heart disease, 773.e1f, 770–776
    with associated vascular disease, 774
    minimally invasive, 770–772
    percutaneous coronary intervention vs., 775.e1f, 774–775, 775f–776f, 776.e1t
  in women, 1718
Coronary artery calcium, 335, 445, 445.e1f
Coronary artery disease (CAD)
  abnormal pain perception in, 777–778
  aortic stenosis and, 1437.e1
  atrial fibrillation in, 1283
  cardiac arrhythmias and, 780b–781b
  chest radiography in, 275
  clinical features of, 778, 778f
  connective tissue disorders and, 780b–781b
  coronary vasculitis and, 780b–781b
  coronary vasospasm in, 614
  diagnosis of, 745b–746b, 746t
  diagnostic assessment for, 778, 779t
  ethanol and, 1594–1595, 1595f
  evaluation of, 310
  exercise testing in, 180
    assessment of anatomic and functional extent of, 185
    blood pressure in, 181b–182b
    blunted systolic pressure peak during, 181b–182b
    chronotropic incompetence, 181b–182b
    Cleveland Clinic Prognostic Score, 186b–187b, 189f
    diagnostic value in, 184–185
    digitalis glycosides, 184
    for disability assessment, 192b, 193t
    double-product reserve in, 181b–182b
    Duke Treadmill Prognostic Score for, 186b–187b
    exercise prescription, 192
    functional capacity in, 181b–182b
    heart rate recovery in, 181b–182b
    heart rate responses, 181b–182b
    hypotension in, 181b–182b
    induced symptoms in, 180

Coronary artery disease (CAD) *(Continued)*
   lead aVR ST elevation, 182
   peak heart rate, 181b–182b
   pharmacologic influences on interpretation, 184
   post-myocardial infarction evaluation and, 187
   predictive values of, 184–185
   pre-test and post-test disease probability and, 185, 185f
   prognostic value of, 186–187, 188t
   sensitivity and specificity of, 184, 184t
   separate scores for men and women, 186b–187b, 187f–188f
   ST adjustments, 182–183
   ST depression, 182
   ST elevation, 183–184
   ST-segment changes in, 182–184, 183f, 183b–184b
   for therapeutic assessment, 189
   upsloping ST depression, 182
   in women, 185–186, 186f, 186t
  extent of, 748.e1, 748.e2f
  ischemia in, 777–779
  magnetic resonance imaging in, 315t–319t, 320–322
  management of, 779
  manifestations of, 777–781
  mechanical circulatory support for, 1124.e1
  microvascular dysfunction and, 777
  mitral regurgitation secondary to, 780–781
  myocardial bridging in, 780b–781b
  noncardiac surgery and, 410
  obstructive
   integrated invasive assessment in patients without, 748–749
   symptomatic patients without angiographically, 292
  peripheral artery disease and, 774.e1
  physiologic evaluation of, 347–349
  postmediastinal irradiation in, 780b–781b
  pregnancy and, 1734
  prognosis of, 778–779
  spontaneous coronary artery dissection in, 780b–781b
  stable, 294–298
   prior PCI and recurrent symptoms, 294, 295f
   suspected, 290–292
  Takayasu arteritis in, 780b–781b
  vasculopathy in, 780b–781b
Coronary artery ectasia, in stable ischemic heart disease, 749.e1
Coronary artery revascularization, noncardiac surgery and, 420–421
Coronary artery spasm, coronary angiography in, 374–375, 375f
Coronary artery stenosis
  arterial switch operation and, 1567
  fluid mechanics of, 618, 618f
  measurement of, microcirculatory abnormalities and, 623b–627b
  physiologic assessment of, 617–627
   coronary reserve in, 619–622, 619f–620f
   distal coronary pressure in, 618f, 619
   pressure-flow relation in, 617–619, 618f
Coronary artery vasculopathy (CAV), surveillance for, 1138
Coronary blood flow, 609–619
  autoregulation, 609–611, 610f
  collateral circulation and, 627–628, 628.e1f
  endothelin, 612–613
  endothelium-dependent hyperpolarizing factor and, 612
  endothelium-dependent modulation of coronary tone, 612–613, 612.e1t, 614f
  future perspectives for, 635
  myocardial oxygen consumption and, 609, 609.e1f
  nitric oxide, 612
  prostacyclin, 612
  systolic and diastolic variation in, 609, 610f
Coronary care unit (CCU), STEMI and, 679–680
Coronary chronic total occlusions (CTOs), patients with, 296–298, 296f
Coronary collateral circulation, 627–628, 628.e1f
  arteriogenesis and angiogenesis and, 628
  collateral resistance and, 628
  interventions for, 628
Coronary collateral vessels, in stable ischemic heart disease, 749.e1

Coronary computed tomographic angiography (CCTA), 279, 335, 340–354, 445, 445.e1f
  in acute chest pain, 341
  assessment of cardiovascular structure and function, 354–361
  cost-effectiveness data, 343b–344b
  diagnostic accuracy of, 340–341
  guidelines, 350t, 353–354, 355t
  hard clinical outcomes, 342–343, 343f, 343b
  implications of ischemia trial for, 349
  and incident risk, 345–347
  in non-ST elevation myocardial infarction, 341
  patient management considerations, 350–352, 351f
  patient outcomes following, 342
  performance of, 340b
  plaque burden of, 341
  plaque characteristics, 344–345, 344t
   high-risk plaque characteristics, 344–345, 345f
  prognosis of, 341
  prognostic implications of, 341
  prognostic value of, 341
  selecting appropriate candidates for, 342
  special populations, 352–353, 353f
  in stable chest pain, 342–344
  use of invasive angiography following, 343–344
Coronary devices
  balloon angioplasty, 793–796
  coronary stents, 793, 793.e1f
   drug-eluting, 793
   everolimus-eluting, 793, 793–794
   paclitaxel-eluting, 793.e2
   sirolimus-eluting, 793.e2
   zotarolimus-eluting, 793, 793–794
  in percutaneous coronary interventions, 793–796
Coronary disease, in HIV patients, 1607–1610
  clinical presentation of, 1608
  epidemiology of, 1607–1608
  risk factors for, screening for, 1610
   risk assessment models in, 1610
  treatment of, 1608, 1609t
Coronary drug-eluting stents
  bioabsorbable polymers and, 794
  bioresorbable vascular scaffolds and, 794
  everolimus for, 793, 793–794
  paclitaxel for, 793.e2
  sirolimus for, 793.e2
  zotarolimus for, 793, 793–794
Coronary endothelial dysfunction, in heart failure with preserved and mildly reduced ejection, 1017–1018
Coronary flow reserve (CFR), 609–610
  absolute, 620, 620f, 620.e1f
  advantages and limitations of, 620.e1f, 622b
  fractional, 619f, 621–622, 621f, 621.e1f, 621.e2f, 624f, 627f
  instantaneous wave-free ratio, 622, 622f–623f
  pathophysiologic states affecting, 622–627
   coronary microvascular dysfunction, 623b–627b, 625f
   endothelium-dependent vasodilation in, impaired, 623b–627b, 625f–626f
   left ventricular hypertrophy, 623b–627b, 625f
  relative, 620–621, 620f
Coronary heart disease (CHD)
  in diabetes mellitus, 558–574
   mechanistic considerations in, 558, 559t
   prevention of, 558–571, 558.e1t, 558.e2t, 558.e3t
    antiplatelet therapy in, 561
    hypertension management in, 560–561, 560f
    lipid management in, 558–560
   revascularization in, 573–574
  effects of food and nutrients on, 541t–542t
  in elderly, 1695–1696
  for heterogeneous populations, 1747
  management of, in heterogeneous populations, 1747
  sleep-disordered breathing and, 1682–1683
  ventricular tachyarrhythmias in, 1359f
Coronary intravascular imaging, 378–383
Coronary microcirculation, structure and function of, 611f–612f, 614–617, 616f
Coronary microvascular dysfunction, evaluation of, 294f
Coronary obstruction, transcatheter aortic valve replacement and, 1436
Coronary revascularization, in NSTE-ACS, 735.e2
Coronary stenosis, evaluation of, coronary angiography in, 375, 375.e1f, 376t
Coronary vascular resistance
  collateral, 628

Coronary vascular resistance *(Continued)*
  coronary microcirculation and, 611f–612f, 614–617, 616f
  coronary vasospasm in, 614
  determinants of, 611–612, 611f–612f
  diastolic driving pressure, 611b–612b
  extravascular compressive resistance, 611b–612b, 613f
  flow-mediated resistance artery control and, 616–617
  intraluminal physical forces, 615
  metabolic mediators of, 616b–617b
   acidosis, 616b–617b
   adenosine, 616b–617b
   ATP-sensitive potassium channels, 616b–617b
   oxygen sensing, 616b–617b
  minimum, transmural variations in, 611b–612b, 616f
  myogenic regulation and, 615–616, 615.e1f, 617f
  neural control, 613b
   cholinergic innervation, 613b, 615f
   sympathetic innervation, 613b, 615f
  paracrine factors in, 613–614, 614f
  pharmacologic vasodilation and, 614b
   with adenosine A_2 receptor agonists, 614b
   with calcium channel blockers, 614b
   with dipyridamole, 614b
   with nitroglycerin, 614b
   with papaverine, 614b
  right coronary artery flow, 617
Coronary vasculitis, coronary artery disease and, 780b–781b
Coronary vasospasm, 614
Coronavirus; *see also* COVID-19; SARS-CoV-2
  with epidemic potential, 1754t
  and myocarditis, 1080
  timeline of, 1754.e1f
  virology and epidemiology, 1754b–1755b
Corticosteroids
  in acute pericarditis, 1619
  in amiodarone-induced thyrotoxicosis, 1803–1804
  in cardiac transplantation, 1136
  in Churg-Strauss syndrome, 1816–1817
  for COVID-19, 1762
Cortisol, 1793, 1793f
  excess of, 1793, 1793f
  in STEMI, 653
Cortisone, 1793f
Corynebacterium infection, myocarditis and, 1081b
Cost-effectiveness data, coronary computed tomography angiography, 343b–344b
Costochondritis
  angina pectoris *vs.*, 741
  chest pain in, 600t
Cough
  in heart failure, 935
  in STEMI, 654
Covered stents, for peripheral artery disease, 862, 862.e1f
COVID-19, 1751–1765; *see also* Coronavirus; SARS-CoV-2
  arrhythmias in, 1757
  cardiac imaging findings in, 1758
  cardiovascular disease, mechanisms of, 1759b–1762b
  clinical cardiovascular manifestations of, 1757–1762
  clinical course and manifestations of, 1755f
  comorbidities and, 1755–1756
  cytokine storm, hyperinflammatory response, and endothelial disease in, 1759b–1762b
  effects of, on cardiovascular health more broadly, 1758–1762, 1759f, 1759t
  epidemiology of, 1755–1756
  extrapulmonary manifestations of, 1756f
  heart failure and, 1757
  lymphocytic myocarditis in, 1760f
  mechanisms of and development of venous and arterial thrombosis, 1627.e1f
  myocarditis due to, 1757
  other management considerations, 1762–1763
  prevention of, vaccines, 1763
  and pulmonary embolism, 1637
  racial and ethnic influences on, 1756
  related complications, 1762
  as risk factor of stroke, 874b–877b
  risk factors of, 1755–1756
  role of anticoagulation in, 1762
  SARS-CoV-2 and, 1754–1763, 1754b–1755b
  severe acute respiratory syndrome CORONAVIRUS 2 and, 1754b–1755b
  thrombosis, 1638f
  treatment of, 1762
  venous and arterial thromboembolism in, 1757, 1758f

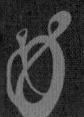

Coxiella burnetii infection, infective endocarditis and, 1510–1511
Coxsackievirus infection, myocarditis and, 1080b–1081b
C-reactive protein (CRP)
　in chest pain evaluation, 603b
　high-sensitivity, 107
　　cardiovascular disease in women and, 1710b–1714b
　in peripheral artery disease, 838
Creatine kinase MB isoenzyme
　in chest pain evaluation, 603
　in STEMI, 655, 657f
Creatine kinase, serum, in hypothyroidism, 1803b
Creatinine, in heart failure, 938b–939b
Critical limb ischemia (CLI), 859
　clinical categories of, 841, 841t
　incidence of, 837–838
Cross-bridge cycling, 894–895, 894f
　calcium effects on, 894–895, 895f
　force transmission, 895
　Frank-Starling effect on, 895
　vs. cardiac contraction-relaxation cycle, 895
Crossover designs, 43
Crosstalk inhibition, 1329.e1f
CRT. See Cardiac resynchronization therapy
Cryoballoon ablation, 1281, 1281f–1282f
Cryoplasty, in peripheral artery disease, 863, 863.e3f
Cryptogenic strokes, 870b–873b, 872f, 872t
C-statistics, in biomarkers, 106, 106f
C-type natriuretic peptide (CNP), in heart failure, 918f, 918b–919b
Culprit Lesion Only PCI *versus* Multivessel PCI in Cardiogenic Shock (CULPRIT-SHOCK) trial, 792
Cushing disease, 1793–1794, 1793f
　diagnosis of, 1794
　treatment of, 1794b
Cushing syndrome, 1793–1794, 1793f
　diagnosis of, 1794
　treatment of, 1794b
Cutis laxa, thoracic aortic aneurysm in, 811t
Cyanosis
　evaluation of, 125
　in pregnancy, 1739–1740
　single ventricle and, 1581–1582
Cyanotic heart disease, pregnancy and, 1739–1740, 1739t
Cyclic adenosine monophosphate (cAMP), 901–903, 964
Cyclophosphamide
　cardiotoxic effects of, 1092t, 1094.e1
　in Churg-Strauss syndrome, 1816–1817
　in polyarteritis nodosa, 1817
　in systemic lupus erythematosus, 1811b
Cyclosporine, 97t
　in cardiac transplantation, 1136
　drug interaction with, 97t
　in rheumatic disease, 1826
CYP2C9, 95t, 97t, 1784
CYP2C19, 83, 95t, 96, 1777b, 1784t
CYP2D6 gene, 95t, 96
CYP3A substrates, 97t
CYP4F2 gene, 95t
Cypher stent, 793.e2
Cyst, hydatid, 1083.e1
Cystatin C, 1873–1874
　in heart failure, 941b
Cystic medial degeneration (CMD), 810
Cytokines, in heart failure, 920b–921b
Cytolytic T cells, 432
Cytoplasm, 889
Cytoskeletal proteins, abnormalities of, in heart failure, 925

D

Dabigatran, 1785–1786
　for atrial fibrillation-associated thromboembolism, 1276
　in chronic kidney disease, 1885t–1886t
　drug interaction with, 97t
Dairy foods, 533f, 535, 540t
DANISH trial, 1336t
Dapagliflozin, in diabetes mellitus, 562t–563t, 567
Daptomycin, in infective endocarditis, 1519b–1523b
Darbepoetin alfa, in anemia, chronic kidney disease and, 1875

Dasatinib, cardiotoxic effects of, 1092t, 1096
DASH diet, for hypertension, 595
Data, missing, 45
Data safety monitoring board (DSMB), 49
Data-monitoring committee (DMC), 49
Daunorubicin, cardiotoxic effects of, 1092t
DDI pacing mode, 1327, 1327f–1328f
　enhancements to, 1328b, 1329f
D-dimer, in chest pain evaluation, 603b
Deafness, diuretic-induced, 988
Death, 1349, 1350f. See also Sudden cardiac death
DEBuT-HT European trial, 496
Deceleration-dependent block, cardiac arrhythmia and, 1183b–1184b
Decompensated heart failure, 952, 953t
Decongestive therapy, with diuretics, for heart failure with preserved and mildly reduced ejection, 1023
Decremental conduction, 1183b–1184b
Dedicated sensing bipoles, integrated *vs.*, 1334b–1335b
Deep venous thrombosis
　classification of, 1640b–1641b
　evolution of oral anticoagulants for, 1647
　extremity, 867–868, 867.e2f
　interventions, 1650–1651
　pulmonary embolism and, 1635–1655, 1636f
Defibrillation
　cardioversion shock therapy, 1337b–1339b, 1339.e1f, 1342f
　mechanism of, 1337b–1339b, 1342f
　waveforms, pacing and, 1323.e1f
DEFINITE trial, 1336t
Definitive therapy, for aortic dissection, 827–830, 827f, 827.e1f, 827.e2f, 829f
Degarelix, cardiotoxic effects of, 1092t
Degenerative aneurysms, 814
Degenerative diseases, 14, 16t
Degenerative mitral stenosis, 1441
Degludec, in diabetes mellitus, 562t–563t
Delirium, in older adult, 1690b–1693b, 1707
Delivery. *See also* Pregnancy
　hemodynamic changes during, 1723–1724
Demand angina, 741–742
Denervation supersensitivity, 1178–1179, 1179.e1f
Deoxyribonucleic acid (DNA), 71
Deprescribing, in elderly, cardiovascular disease in, 1695
Depressed left ventricular function, stable ischemic heart disease and, 772b–773b, 772f–773f
Depression
　cardiovascular disease and, 1844–1845, 1845b, 1846f
　exercise and, 582
　psychotherapy for, 1847
　screening, 1845b
Dermatomyositis, 1819–1820
　cardiac conduction disturbances in, 1821
Descending thoracic aneurysms, management of, 817
Desipramine, drug interaction with, 97t
Desmin, 1174b–1175b
Desmoplakin, mutations in, 1174b–1175b
Desmosome, 1173
Desmoteplase, 1789b
Detemir, in diabetes mellitus, 562t–563t
Detraining, 580, 580f
Device-based heart failure diagnostics, 1114–1116
Diabetes
　after cardiac transplantation, 1140
　air pollution and, 36
　as risk factor of stroke, 874b–877b
Diabetes mellitus, 556
　acute coronary syndromes in, 571–573
　atherosclerotic vascular disease in, 556, 557f–559f
　atrial fibrillation in, 556, 576
　cardiac metabolic alterations in, 574.e1f
　cardiovascular disease and, 448–449
　cardiovascular system and, 556–578
　　future perspectives in, 576–577
　coronary heart disease in, 558–574
　　mechanistic considerations in, 558, 559f
　　prevention of, 558–571, 558.e1t, 558.e2t, 558.e3t
　　　antiplatelet therapy in, 561
　　　hypertension management in, 560–561, 560f
　　　lipid management in, 558–560
　　revascularization in, 573–574
　diagnostic criteria for, 556t
　in elderly, 1705
　epidemiology of, 23, 24f
　estimated number of adults with, 557f

Diabetes mellitus *(Continued)*
　exercise electrocardiographic testing in, 193–194
　glucose management in, 561–571, 562t–563t
　　in acute coronary syndromes, 571–573
　　cardiovascular effects of
　　　more intensive *vs.* less intensive, 569–571
　　　selected medications, 561–569, 564t, 565f
　　dipeptidyl peptidase 4 inhibitors in, 562t–563t, 566–567
　　dopamine D_2 receptor agonists in, 562t–563t
　　glucagon like peptide (GLP)-1 receptor agonists in, 562t–563t, 567, 568f–569f
　　α-glucosidase inhibitors in, 562t–563t, 569
　　in heart failure, 575–576, 576f
　　insulin in, 562t–563t, 566, 572
　　intensive strategies in
　　　in acute coronary syndromes, 571–573
　　　cardiovascular effects on, 569–571
　　metformin in, 561–564
　　meglitinides in, 562t–563t
　　metformin in, 562t–563t, 564b
　　ongoing trials of, 564t, 566b–567b
　　sodium-glucose cotransporter 2 (SGLT2) inhibitors, 562t–563t, 567–569, 570f
　　sulfonylureas in, 562t–563t, 564–566
　　thiazolidinediones in, 562t–563t, 564b–566b
　　treatment guidelines, 571, 572f
　heart failure in, 556, 574–576, 938b–939b
　　mechanistic considerations in, 574–575, 574f
　　prevention and management of, 575–576
　　scope of problem, 574
　in HIV patients, cardiovascular risk factors in, 1605
　hypertension in, 574–575
　ischemic heart disease in, 574–575
　myocardial metabolism and structure in, 574.e1f, 574b–575b
　NSTE-ACS and, 733–734
　percutaneous coronary intervention in, 792
　peripheral artery disease in, 838, 847, 847.e5f
　risk stratification of, 556–558
　stable ischemic heart disease and
　　medical management of, 752
　　percutaneous coronary intervention of, 769b–770b
　　revascularization strategies for, 776f
　　surgical treatment for, 774
　statins in, 516
　type 1, 556
　type 2, 556
　　effects of food and nutrients on, 541t–542t
　　in heterogeneous populations, 1743
Diabetic cardiomyopathy, 1041
"Diagnostic creep", 583
Diagnostic decisions, 53–57, 54f–57f
Diamondback360, 863
Diastole, 905b
Diastolic function/dysfunction, 910
　in acute heart failure, 950
　drug therapeutics and, 99
　echocardiography in, 208–209, 208t–209t, 209.e1f
　hypertrophic cardiomyopathy and, 1063–1065
　magnetic resonance imaging in, 326
　measures of, in heart failure with preserved and mildly reduced ejection, 1011b–1017b, 1013f
　in STEMI, 651
　thyroid disease and, 1797–1798
Diastolic strain, measures of, in heart failure with preserved and mildly reduced ejection, 1011b–1017b, 1013f
Diet
　alcohol in, 535, 540t
　beans in, 532, 533f
　behavior changes due to, 543
　carbohydrates in, 535–536, 536f
　cardiovascular disease and, 458–461
　coffee in, 534f, 535
　dairy foods in, 533f, 535, 540t
　eggs in, 533f, 535
　in elderly, 1706
　epidemiology of, 24–25
　fats in, 536–538, 551–552
　fish in, 533f, 534, 540t
　fruits in, 532, 533f, 540t
　grains in, 532–534, 533f, 540t
　in heart failure, 981
　hypertension and, 476–477
　lipid reduction in, 28–29

Diet (Continued)
  for lipoprotein disorders, 521
  nuts in, 532, 533f, 540t
  patterns in, 539–540, 541t–542t
  in peripheral artery disease, 847
  plant oils in, 535
  poultry in, 535
  red meats in, 533f, 534
  salt reduction in, 28–29
  starches in, 532–534
  sugar-sweetened beverages in, 534f, 535, 540t
  sweets in, 532–534, 540t
  tea in, 534f, 535
  vegetables in, 532, 533f, 540t
Diffuse intimal thickening, 427, 429f
Diffuse ST-segment elevation, in acute pericarditis, 1616–1617, 1618f
Digital subtraction angiography (DSA), in peripheral artery disease, 863, 863.e3f
Digitalis
  electrocardiography effects of, 169, 170f
  in heart failure, 1000.e2
Digitoxin, in heart failure, 999
Digoxin, 1211.e1t, 97t, 1000.e1, 1209t, 1212t, 1214t, 1225–1226, 1226b
  in acute heart failure, 965b
  in cardiorenal syndrome, 1889t
  in chronic HFrEF, 1698b
  complications of, 999–1000
  digitalis toxicity and, 1000.e2
  drug interactions with, 97t, 1000.e1, 1000.e1t
  genetic variations in response to, 996.e2
  in heart failure, 991t, 999
  mechanisms of action of, 1000.e1
  pharmacokinetics and dosing of, 1000.e1
  pregnancy and, 1730f
  therapeutic monitoring of, 1000.e2
Dihydropyridines, in coronary artery disease, chronic kidney disease and, 1880t–1881t
Dilated cardiomyopathy, 1032–1043, 1033t, 1034f
  approach to genetic evaluation of, 1040
  cardiac magnetic resonance imaging in, 1032–1035
  coronary angiography in, 1032
  echocardiography in, 220–221, 220f, 1032, 1034f
  familial, clinical genetics of, 1035–1037
  genetics of, 1035, 1035f–1036f, 1035.e1t
  pregnancy and, 1732
  therapy for, 1039
Diltiazem, 1211.e1t, 1209t, 1212t, 1214t, 1223–1225, 1223b–1224b
  in angina pectoris, 760, 761t
DINAMIT trial, 1336t
Dipeptidyl peptidase 4 inhibitors, in glucose management, 562t–563t, 566–567
Dipyridamole
  as coronary vasodilator, 614b
  dosages for, 1778
  indications for, 1778
  mechanism of action of, 1778, 1778f
  side effects of, 1778
  in thrombosis, 1777–1778
Direct annuloplasty, in mitral regurgitation, 1486b–1488b, 1490f
Direct cardiac mapping, 1159b
Direct renin inhibitors (DRIs), for acute heart failure, 971b–972b
Direct thrombin inhibitors
  in atrial fibrillation-associated thromboembolism prevention, 1276
  in NSTE-ACS, 727
  parenteral, 1783, 1783t
Direct-acting oral anticoagulants (DOACs), in atrial fibrillation-associated thromboembolism prevention, 1276–1277
Directional atherectomy, for peripheral artery disease, 863, 863.e1f, 863.e2f
Disability, in elderly, 1690b–1693b
Discrimination, in biomarkers, 106, 106f
Disease-modifying antirheumatic drug (DMARD), 1810b, 1826
Disopyramide, 1211.e1t, 1209t, 1212t, 1214t, 1215–1216, 1215b–1216b
Distorted probability estimates, decision making and, 60
Diuretics
  in acute heart failure, 961–962, 961t–962t
  carbonic anhydrase inhibitors, 984
  in chronic HFrEF, 1698b

Diuretics (Continued)
  classes of, 982–985, 983t
  decongestive therapy with, for heart failure with preserved and mildly reduced ejection, 1023
  in heart failure, 938b–939b, 985–988, 987f
    complications of, 987–988
    resistance to, 987f, 988–989, 988b–989b
  loop, 982, 982b, 983t, 984f
  mineralocorticoid receptor antagonists, 983–984, 983b
  potassium-sparing, 983t, 984, 985f
  sites of action of, 984f
  thiazide and thiazide-like, 982–983, 983b, 984f
  vasopressin antagonists, 985, 985b
Diving reflex, 1896
D-loop transposition of the great arteries, magnetic resonance imaging in, 330b–332b
DNA sequencing technologies, schematic of, 74f
Dobutamine, 283
  in acute heart failure, 964, 964b
  cardiac catheterization and, 407
  in cardiorenal syndrome, 1886, 1889t
  in myocarditis, 1083b
  for STEMI, 690
Docetaxel, cardiotoxic effects of, 1094.e1
Dofetilide, 1211.e1t, 1209t, 1212t, 1214t, 1223, 1223b
  antiarrhythmics, chronic kidney disease and, 1890t
  for complex congenital heart disease, 1548
  drug interaction with, 97t
  kidney function and, 99
Donation after circulatory determined death (DCD), 1135
Dopamine
  in acute heart failure, 964
  for STEMI, 687–690
Dopamine D₂ receptor agonists, in glucose management, 562t–563t
Doppler echocardiography
  in aortic regurgitation, 1422–1423
  blood flow profile on, 198b–199b, 200f
  color flow, 198b–199b, 199f
  continuous-wave, 198f–199f, 198b–199b
  in heart failure, 943
  in practice, 199–200, 199.e1f
  principles of, 198b–199b, 198.e1f
  in prosthetic heart valves, 1500
  pulsed-wave, 198f–199f, 198b–199b
  stenotic valve on, 200
  stroke volume on, 200, 200f
  tissue, 208, 211f
Doppler ultrasonography, in peripheral artery disease, 844
Double density sign, 270
Double outlet right ventricle, 1570–1572, 1571f
Double-blind study, 45
Double-product reserve, in coronary artery disease, 181b–182b
Down syndrome, 1545
Doxorubicin, cardiotoxic effects of, 1092t, 1093, 1093f
Dressler syndrome, 704–705
Driving, cardiac implantable electrical devices and, 1347
Dronedarone, 1211.e1t, 1209t, 1212t, 1214t, 1222, 1222b
  antiarrhythmics, chronic kidney disease and, 1890t
  in atrial fibrillation, 1280
  in heart failure, 1002b
Drug effects, time course of, 93b–96b, 95f
Drug interactions, cardiac implantable electrical devices and, 1347
Drug overdose, cardiac transplantation and, 1135, 1135f
Drug response, molecular and genetic basis for variable, 96–98
Drug therapy
  adverse reactions to, 92–93
    clinical trials, 92
    minimization of, 98
  cardiomyopathies induced by, 1593–1602
  for cardiovascular disease, 448
  dose adjustments in, 99
  drug elimination in, 93f, 93b–96b, 94t
  drug interactions in, 97t, 99–100
  drug optimization in, 98–100, 99f
  drug targets in, 93b–96b
  elimination half-life in, 95f, 98
  future perspectives for, 100
  in myocarditis, 1083

Drug therapy (Continued)
  pharmacodynamics in, 93–96
  pharmacokinetics in, 93–96, 93f, 93b–96b
  plasma concentration in, 93f
    monitoring of, 98–99, 99f
  risk vs. benefit of, 92–93
  single-nucleotide polymorphism and, 95t
  in visceral obesity, 551, 551t
Drug-coated balloons
  in percutaneous coronary intervention, 795
  for peripheral artery disease, 861–862
Drug-eluting stents, 793
  coronary
    bioabsorbable polymers and, 794
    bioresorbable vascular scaffolds and, 794
    everolimus for, 793, 793–794
    paclitaxel for, 793.e2
    sirolimus for, 793.e2
    zotarolimus for, 793, 793–794
  noncardiac surgery and, 420
  in peripheral artery disease, 860–861
Drug-induced hypertension, 484t, 487–488
  sleep deprivation and sleep-disordered breathing, 487–488
DSC2 gene, 1039b–1040b
DSG2 gene, 1039b–1040b
DSP gene, 1039b–1040b
Dual-antiplatelet therapy
  in percutaneous coronary intervention, 787.e3t
  for vascular disease, 1104
Dual-chamber implantable cardioverter-defibrillators, 1331, 1332b–1333b, 1335
  single-chamber transvenous vs., 1333–1334
Dual-chamber pacemaker, 1321, 1322f, 1327–1328, 1328f
Dual-coil leads, vs. single, 1334b–1335b
Duchenne muscular dystrophy, 1853–1856, 1853f–1854f, 1856f
Duke Activity Scale Index, 413, 415t
Duke criteria, for infective endocarditis, 1510–1511, 1511t
Duke Treadmill Prognostic Score, 186b–187b
Dulaglutide, in diabetes mellitus, 562t–563t, 567
Dunnigan lipodystrophy, 514
Duplex ultrasound, in peripheral artery disease, 844, 844f–845f, 863–864
Dural ectasia, 830
Dynamic "perturbation", during invasive hemodynamic testing, 1011b–1017b
Dyslipidemia, 502
  atherogenic, effects of food and nutrients on, 541t–542t
  cardiovascular disease and, 5–6
  in elderly, 1704–1705, 1704t
  in HIV patients, 1603–1604, 1604t
  integrative strategies for, 595–596
    coenzyme Q10 in, 596b
    dietary fiber in, 596b
    nutrition in, 595–596
    physical activity in, 596
    red yeast rice in, 596b
    stanols in, 596b
    statin intolerance in, 596b
    sterols in, 596b
  management of, 524.e1, 524.e1t
  stable ischemic heart disease and, 751–752
  in women, cardiovascular disease and, 1710b–1714b
Dyslipoproteinemias, 502
  secondary causes of, 514t
Dyspnea
  evaluation of, 124
  in heart failure, 935
  in infective endocarditis, 1508
  mitral stenosis and, 1444–1445
  narcotics for, 1005.e2
  ticagrelor in, 1777

E

Early repolarization syndrome (ERS), 1204, 1308
  clinical description and manifestations of, 1204
  genetic basis of, 1204b
Ebstein anomaly
  pregnancy and, 1738, 1739f
  tricuspid regurgitation in, 1475
  of tricuspid valve, 1560–1562
    anatomic description and prevalence of, 1560, 1560f

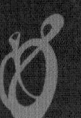

Ebstein anomaly (Continued)
  clinical features and diagnostic testing of, 1560–1561, 1561f
  long-term outcomes and complications of, 1561–1562
    transcatheter atrial septal defect/patent foramen ovale closure, 1561–1562
    tricuspid valve repair and replacement surgery, 1561
    unrepaired, 1561
    ventricular dysfunction, heart failure, and transplantation, 1562
ECG-based screening, in cardiovascular medicine, 111
ECG-gated image interpretation, 287b–288b
Echinocandins, for infective endocarditis, 1519b–1523b
Echinococcosis, myocarditis and, 1083.e1
Echocardiography, 196–267.e1
  acoustic shadowing in, 215b–216b
  for acute aortic regurgitation, 1428f, 1428b–1429b
  in acute cerebrovascular disease, 1870
  in acute heart failure, 954
  in amyloidosis, 220f, 222, 1044f
  in aorta, disease of, 244–248, 244f–246f, 246t
  in aortic aneurysm, 244, 247f
  in aortic coarctation, 244
  in aortic dissection, 244, 245f–246f, 249f, 824
  in aortic intramural hematoma, 245–246, 246f
  in aortic regurgitation, 234, 234f, 234.e1f, 234.e2f, 1421–1423, 1423f
  in aortic stenosis, 232–234, 233f–234f, 234b
  in aortic transection, 245–246
  in aortic valve, 231–234, 232f
  in aortic valve stenosis, 1406–1408, 1409f
  appropriate use criteria for, 266–267, 267.e1
  in arrhythmogenic cardiomyopathy, 220f, 222
  artefacts on, 203f, 203b, 256b
  in atherosclerotic plaque, 244, 247f
  in atrial septal defect, 256–259, 256b, 257f
  in Becker muscular dystrophy, 1855
  in cardiac masses, 253–256, 254t, 255f
  cardiovascular medicine and, 111–113, 112f–113f
  in chest pain, 606–607
  of congenital heart disease, 1546
  in constrictive pericarditis, 242–244, 242f–243f
  contrast, 212–216, 213f–214f, 214f–215f, 215.e1f
    myocardial perfusion contrast-enhanced echocardiography, 214–215, 215f
  in coronary sinus atrial septal defect, 258–259
  of diastolic function, 208.e1t
  in dilated cardiomyopathy, 220–221, 220f, 1032, 1034f
  Doppler
    in acute pericarditis, 1617
    blood flow profile on, 198b–199b, 200f
    color flow, 198b–199b, 199f
    in constrictive pericarditis, 1627, 1627.e1f
    continuous-wave, 198f–199f, 198b–199b
    in heart failure, 943
    in practice, 199–200, 199.e1f
    principles of, 198b–199b, 198.e1f
    pulsed-wave, 198f–199f, 198b–199b
    stenotic valve on, 200
    stroke volume on, 200, 200f
    tissue, 208, 211f
  in Duchenne muscular dystrophy, 1855, 1856f
  in Fabry disease, 222
  in fibromas, 253b, 253.e1f
  future directions of, 265
  handheld, 265–266
  in heart failure, 222–224
  of heart failure with preserved and mildly reduced ejection, 1011b–1017b, 1013f
  in hemochromatosis, 222
  in human immunodeficiency virus (HIV) infection, 252b–253b
  of hypertension, 483
  in hypertrophic cardiomyopathy, 220f–221f, 221–222
  indications for, 131, 133f
  in infective endocarditis, 1530.e2t, 248–253, 251f, 1513, 1516f–1517f, 1517, 1530.e1
  in intracardiac thrombus, 255–256, 256f
  in ischemic cardiomyopathy, 220f, 221
  in left atrium, 204t, 210
  in left ventricle, 204–205, 204t, 205f–206f, 205f
  in left ventricular ejection fraction, 205–206
  in left ventricular noncompaction, 220f, 222, 1829, 1831f

Echocardiography (Continued)
  in lipomas, 253b
  in lipomatous hypertrophy of intraatrial septum, 253b, 1829b, 1832f
  in Loeffler endocarditis, 222
  in mitral inflow patterns, 208, 208.e1f, 208.e2f
  in mitral regurgitation, 229–231, 229b, 230f–231f, 231.e1f
  in mitral stenosis, 227–229, 227f–229f, 229t
  in mitral valve, 226–231, 227f, 227.e1f
  M-mode, 196, 200–203, 203f
  in myocardial infarction, 216–220, 217f–218f, 220f
  in myocardial strain, 206b–208b, 206f–207f, 206.e2f
  in myocarditis, 1087
  in myxoma, 253b, 255f
  noncardiac surgery and, 423
  normal variants on, 256b
  in NSTE-ACS, 716
  in pannus, 256b
  in papillary fibroelastomas, 253b, 255f
  in pericardial cyst, 253b
  in pericardial effusion, 240–242, 240f
  in pericardial hematoma, 241–242, 241f
  in pericardial tumor, 243b, 244f
  in pericardiocentesis, 241b–242b
  in pregnancy, 1725
  of primary mitral regurgitation, 1459–1462
  in primary tumors, 253b
  in primum atrial septal defect, 258, 259f
  in prosthetic regurgitation, 237b–240b, 238f–240f
  in prosthetic valve assessment, 235–240, 236.e1t, 237f–238f
  in pseudoneoplasm, 255
  in pulmonary arterial hypertension, 1668t
  in pulmonary embolism, 247b–248b, 247.e1f, 249f–250f, 1644, 1645f
  in pulmonary hypertension, 248, 250f
  of pulmonary stenosis, 1562
  of pulmonary venous Doppler flow patterns, 208, 208.e2f
  in pulmonic regurgitation, 235, 236f–237f, 1479b–1481b, 1480f
  in pulmonic stenosis, 235
  in pulmonic valve, 235, 235b, 235.e1f
  in regional ventricular function, 213–214
  in restrictive cardiomyopathy, 220f, 222, 1044, 1044f
  in rhabdomyoma, 253b
  of rheumatic mitral stenosis, 1445–1446, 1445f
  in right atrium, 210, 210t–211t
  in right ventricle, 209, 209t–210t, 209f–211f
  in sarcoidosis, 252b–253b, 252.e1f
  in secundum atrial septal defect, 257, 257f–259f
  in sinus of Valsalva aneurysm, 244, 248f
  in sinus venosus atrial septal defect, 258, 259f
  speckle-tracking techniques in, 206b–208b, 206f–207f
  in stable ischemic heart disease
    resting, 744
    stress, 745b–746b
  standard, 200–210, 201f–202f
  stress, 224–226
    in assessment of myocardial viability, 225–226
    coronary flow reserve and perfusion for, 226
    in hypertrophic cardiomyopathy, 221–222
    limitations of, 225–226
    in mitral stenosis, 227–229
    as preoperative test, 417
    protocol for, 225f, 225b
    risk stratification with, 225
    in valvular heart disease, 226, 226f
  in subaortic membrane, 231b–232b, 232f
  in systemic diseases, 252b–253b
  in systemic lupus erythematosus, 1820f
  of systolic function, 205–208, 205f–206f
  in tamponade, 241f, 241b–242b
  in tetralogy of Fallot, 260b, 263f, 1563–1564
  three-dimensional, 212, 214f
  in transcatheter interventions, 260–266, 261f–262f, 264f, 264.e1f
  transesophageal, 210–212, 210t–212t, 213f
  in transposition of the great arteries, 260b, 260.e1f, 262f–263f
  transthoracic, in pregnancy, 1725
  of tricuspid annular plane systolic excursion (TAPSE), 209, 211f
  in tricuspid regurgitation, 235, 236f, 1476b–1478b, 1477f–1478f
  in tricuspid stenosis, 235, 235f, 1473b–1475b

Echocardiography (Continued)
  of tricuspid valve, 202f, 234–235, 234b–235b
  in tumor evaluation, 1829, 1830f–1832f
  in valvular heart disease, 226–240
  in vegetations, 256b
  in ventricular septal defect, 259–260, 260f–262f
  in ventricular twist and torsion, 206b–208b, 206.e3f
E-cigarettes. See Electronic cigarettes
Eclampsia, cardiovascular disease in women and, 1710b–1714b
Ecstasy (3,4-methylenedioxymethamphetamine), cardiovascular complications of, 1599
Ectopic beats, 1248.e1f, 1246–1247, 1246f–1247f, 1246b–1247b
Ectopic fat deposition, 550
Edema
  in heart failure, 135
  lower extremity, in heart failure, 938b
  peripheral, in acute heart failure, 954
Edge-to-edge repair, for primary mitral regurgitation, 1464–1465
Edoxaban, 1785–1786
  in atrial fibrillation-associated thromboembolism prevention, 1276
  in chronic kidney disease, 1885t–1886t
Effect of Ticagrelor on Health Outcomes in Diabetes Mellitus Patients Intervention Study (THEMIS), 848–849
Effective blood flow (EBF), 404
Effusive-constrictive pericarditis, 1630–1633
Eggs, 533f, 535
Ehlers-Danlos syndrome, vascular, thoracic aortic aneurysm in, 811t
Einthoven triangle, 141b–145b
Eisenmenger syndrome, 1582–1585, 1583f–1584f, 1583t–1584t
  sudden cardiac death in, 1361b
Elastin fibers, 433–434
Electrical alternans, 171b–172b, 172b
Electrical cardioversion, 1227
Electrical mechanisms, importance of, 1370b–1371b
Electrical remodeling, of atria, 1187
Electrical storm, 1296
Electrical stunning, 167–168
Electrocardiogram dynamics/analytics, 1155.e1f, 1155.e1f
Electrocardiography (ECG), 141–174.e3
  abnormal, 150–173
    in abnormal atrial activation and conduction, 151b
    in accelerated idioventricular rhythm, 1292, 1293f
    in acromegaly, 1792
    in acute cerebrovascular disease, 1870, 1870f
    in acute heart failure, 954
    in acute pericarditis, 168, 168f, 1616–1617
    in alternans patterns, 171b–172b, 172f
    ambulatory, 1162.e1
    in amyloidosis, 1044, 1044f
    in Andersen-Tawil syndrome, 1199
    artifacts in, 173, 173f
    in atrial abnormalities, 150–152, 151f–152f, 151t
    in atrial fibrillation, 1272, 1273f–1274f
    in Becker muscular dystrophy, 1855, 1856f
    in biventricular hypertrophy, 155, 156f
    in Brugada syndrome, 1307f, 1308
    in cardiac arrest survivors, 1368
    cardiac electrical fields, genesis of, 141b–145b
    in catecholaminergic polymorphic ventricular tachycardia, 1309
    in chest pain evaluation, 602, 602t, 605–606, 606t
    of congenital heart disease, 1543
    in Cushing disease, 1793
    data transformation in, 141b–145b
    digitalis effects on, 169, 170f
    display in, 141b–145b
    drug effects on, 170
    in Duchenne muscular dystrophy, 1855, 1856f
    in early repolarization syndrome, 1308
    in electrical alternans, 171b–172b, 172f
    electrodes and leads systems in, 141b–145b, 142t
      augmented limb, 141b–145b, 143f
      electrical axis and, 141b–145b, 144f
      expanded, 141b–145b
      hexaxial reference frame and, 141b–145b, 144f
      lead vectors and, 141b–145b, 144f
      precordial, 141b–145b
      standard limb, 141b–145b, 143f
    electrolyte and metabolic abnormalities, 170–172

Electrocardiography (ECG) *(Continued)*
    calcium, 170–171
    magnesium, 171b–172b
    potassium, 171–172
  exercise. *See* Exercise testing
  in first-degree atrioventricular block, 1315, 1315f
  future perspectives for, 173–174
  guidelines for, 173–174
    cardioactive drug administration, 174.e2
    patients with known or suspected cardiovascular disease, 174.e1, 174.e2t
    patients without known or suspected cardiovascular disease, 174.e1, 174.e2t
    persons with dangerous or physically demanding occupations, 174.e1
    preoperative evaluation, 174.e1
    screening of athletes, 174.e1
  in heart failure, 938, 938b
  of His bundle pacing, 1326b, 1326.e2f
  in hypercalcemia, 170–171, 170f
  in hyperkalemia, 170–171, 171f
  in hypermagnesemia, 171b–172b
  in hypernatremia, 171b–172b
  in hypertrophic cardiomyopathy, 167, 168f
  in hypocalcemia, 170–171, 170f
  in hypokalemia, 171, 171f
  in hypomagnesemia, 171b–172b
  in hyponatremia, 171b–172b
  in hypothermia, 171f, 171b–172b
  in hypothyroidism, 1802
  indications and clinical value of, 172–173
  in infective endocarditis, 1512–1513
  interatrial block and, 151b
  interpretation of, clinical issues in, 172–173
    computer, 173, 173b
  J wave in, 149
  in J wave syndromes, 1308–1309
  in left anterior fascicular block, 156, 156t, 156b, 157f
  in left atrial abnormality, 151, 151b
  in left bundle branch block, 157–158, 157f, 157f–158b, 158t
  in left posterior fascicular block, 156
  in left ventricular hypertrophy, 152f–153f, 152b–153b, 153t
  in long QT syndrome, 1305f–1306f, 1307–1308
  in multifascicular blocks, 159–160, 159f–160f
  in myocarditis, 1087
  in myotonic dystrophy, 1858, 1860f
  noncardiac surgery and, 423
  in nonspecific intraventricular conduction defect, 160b
  normal, 145–150, 145f–146f, 146t
    variants in, 149–150, 150f
  in NSTE-ACS, 716–717
  P wave in, 145–146
  in pericardial effusion and cardiac tamponade, 1622
  in peri-infarction block, 160b
  persistent juvenile pattern in, 150, 150f
  in premature ventricular complexes, 1288–1289, 1289f–1292f
  of primary mitral regurgitation, 1462b
  principles of, 141b–145b
  in Prinzmetal variant angina, 164f
  processing of, 141b–145b
  pseudoinfarction patterns in, 167, 168f
  in pulmonary arterial hypertension, 1667
  in pulmonary embolism, 1643
  QRS complex in, 147–149, 147b. *See also* QRS complex
  QRST angle in, 149b
  QT interval in, 148–149. *See also* QT interval
  in rate-dependent conduction blocks, 160f, 160b
  reading competency for, 173
  of rheumatic mitral stenosis, 1446
  in right atrial abnormality, 152, 152b
  in right bundle branch block, 157f, 158, 158t
  in right ventricular hypertrophy, 154–155, 154f–155f, 154t, 154b
  in second-degree atrioventricular block, 1315f, 1315f–1316f
  signal acquisition in, 141b–145b
  in stable ischemic heart disease
    exercise, 745b–746b
    resting, 744
  for STEMI, 668b–669b
  stress, in cardiac arrhythmias, 1149–1151, 1153f
  ST-T wave in, 148
  T wave alternans on, 164f

Electrocardiography (ECG) *(Continued)*
  technical errors in, 173
  in torsade de pointes, 1306–1307
  in tricuspid regurgitation, 1476b–1478b
  in tricuspid stenosis, 1473b–1475b
  U wave in, 149
  ventricular activation and, 147–149, 147f, 147b
  in ventricular fibrillation, 1309–1310
  in ventricular flutter, 1309f, 1310
  ventricular gradient in, 149b
  in ventricular tachycardia, 1292, 1292.e1f, 1292.e2f, 1292.e3f, 1294f–1295f
  waveform identification in, 141b–145b
Electroconvulsive therapy, 1850
Electrograms
  implantable cardioverter-defibrillators and, 1338f
  in pacemakers, 1324–1326, 1324b–1326b, 1325f–1326f
Electrolyte disturbances, diuretic-induced, 987–988, 987b
Electromagnetic interference, 1328b, 1344–1346, 1345.e1t
Electronic cigarette or vaping-induced lung injury (EVALI), 529
Electronic cigarettes, 525b, 528–529
  associated lung injury, 1596
  cardiovascular complications of, 1595–1596
  effects of, 1595–1596, 1596b
  cardiovascular disease and, 446–447, 447.e1f
Electronic collimation, 278–279
Electronic decision support, for pulmonary embolism, 1644
Electronic medical records, in clinical trials, 49
Electronic nicotine delivery systems (ENDS), 528–529
Electrophysiologic studies
  complications of, 1159, 1160f–1161f
  for diagnosis, 1162.e1
    acquired atrioventricular block, 1162.e1
    cardiac arrest, survivors of, 1162.e1
    chronic intraventricular delay, 1162.e2
    narrow-and wide-QRS complex tachycardia, 1162.e2
    palpitations, 1162.e5
    prolonged QT intervals, 1162.e5
    sinus node function, evaluation of, 1162.e1, 1162.e3t
    unexplained syncope, 1162.e5, 1162.e5t
    Wolff-Parkinson-White syndrome, 1162.e5
  preoperative, 1243b
  protocol, for syncope, 1393–1394
  for syncope, 1393–1394, 1393t
  for therapeutic intervention, 1162.e5, 1162.e6t
    clinical competence, 1162.e7
Electrophysiology, cardiac, foundations of, 1163–1175
  gap junction channels and intercalated discs in, 1173–1175, 1175f
  ion channels in
    molecular structure of, 1171–1173
    physiology of, 1163–1166, 1164f, 1165f–1166f, 1167f
    normal automaticity in, 1170–1171, 1170f
Electrotherapy, 1227–1241
  ablation therapy, for cardiac arrhythmias, 1229–1241, 1230f, 1230b
  in accelerated idioventricular rhythm, 1227b
  for cardiac arrhythmias, 1321
  direct-current electrical cardioversion in, 1227–1229
Embolectomy, surgical, 1650, 1650f
Embolic protection devices, in percutaneous coronary intervention, 795
Embolism, in infective endocarditis, 1518–1524
Emergency medical service systems, 663, 664f
Emery-Dreifuss muscular dystrophy, 1859–1861, 1861f–1862f, 1862t
Emotional support, in pulmonary embolism, 1651
Empagliflozin, in diabetes mellitus, 562f–563t, 567
Enalapril, in heart failure, 990b–991b, 991t–992t
Encephalomyopathies, 1866–1867
End of life care, 1005.e2
Endemic viral illnesses, 1751–1765
Endocannabinoid system, visceral obesity and, 551
Endocarditis
  in elderly, 1700b–1701b
  infective. *See* Infective endocarditis
  Libman-Sacks, 1820
  Löffler (eosinophilic), 1049
  nonbacterial thrombotic, 1507
  prophylaxis, for patent ductus arteriosus, 1559
  sudden cardiac death (SCD) and, 1358t

Endocrine disorders, cardiovascular disease and, 1791–1808
Endocrine organ, visceral adipose tissue as, 549, 550f–551f
End-of-life decisions, for elderly, cardiovascular disease in, 1694–1695
Endoleaks, 810, 810.e1f
Endomyocardial biopsy
  in heart failure, 942
  of heart failure with preserved and mildly reduced ejection, 1011b–1017b, 1016f
  in myocarditis, 1078t, 1088, 1088f
Endomyocardial disease, 1048
Endomyocardial fibrosis, 1049
  magnetic resonance imaging in, 326
Endotension, 810
Endothelial cell protein C receptor (EPCR), 1767
Endothelial cells
  in artery, 425–426, 426f–427f
  hypertension and, 477
Endothelial dysfunction
  atherosclerosis in, 1809–1810
  in hypertension, 477
Endothelial thrombotic balance, 426f
Endothelin
  coronary blood flow and, 612–613
  in heart failure, 919.e1
Endothelin receptor antagonists
  in acute heart failure, 971b–972b
  in pulmonary arterial hypertension, 1675f
Endothelin-1
  in hypertension, 477
  for pulmonary arterial hypertension, 1664b–1665b
Endothelium
  hypertension and, 477–478
  vascular, in hemostatic system, 1766–1767
Endothelium-dependent hyperpolarizing factor, 612
Endothelium-derived relaxing factor, 612
Endovascular abdominal aortic aneurysm repair, 809–810, 810t
Endovascular therapy, for acute ischemic stroke, 881–883, 883f–884f, 884t
Endpoints, 45–46
  analysis of, 46–47
  clinical decision making and, 59b
  secondary, 50
  surrogate, 45, 102, 103t
ENDS. *See* Electronic nicotine delivery systems
Endurance capacity, 579
Energy balance, 531–532
Energy drinks, 1600–1601
Engineering designs, of ventricular assist devices (VADs), 1122.e1
  continuous-flow rotary pumps, 1122.e1, 1122.e1f, 1122.e2f
  general characteristics of, 1121f, 1122.e1, 1123f–1124f
  pulsatile-flow, volume-displacement pumps, 1122.e1
Enhanced recovery after surgery (ERAS) protocols, regional anesthesia and, 418
Enoxaparin
  in NSTE-ACS, 727
  in percutaneous coronary intervention, 787.e3t, 801
Enoximone, for acute heart failure, 964b–965b
Enrollment, in cardiac rehabilitation, 589f, 589b
Enterococcal species, causing infective endocarditis, 1506b–1507b, 1512t
  antimicrobial therapy for, 1522.e1t–e2t, 1522.e1t–e2t, 1522.e1t–e2t, 1522.e1t–e2t, 1519b–1523b
Enterovirus infection, myocarditis and, 1080b–1081b
Entrainment, cardiac arrhythmia and, 1183b–1184b, 1184f
Environmental exposures, cardiovascular disease and, 26
Eosinophilic granulomatosis with polyangiitis (Churg-Strauss syndrome), 1816–1817, 1817f
  cardiovascular complications of, 1816
  investigation of, 1816
  treatment of, 1816–1817
Epicardial catheter mapping, 1239b–1241b
Epicardial leads, 1322b–1323b
Epidemiologic transitions, in mortality, 14–16, 16t, 17f
Epigenetics, 71, 83–84
Epilepsy, 1869–1870, 1869f
Epinephrine
  in acute heart failure, 964
  for STEMI, 690
Epirubicin, cardiotoxic effects of, 1092t

Eplerenone, 1795b
  in heart failure, 983, 991t–992t
Eptifibatide
  in myocardial infarction, renal dysfunction and, 1884t
  in percutaneous coronary intervention, 800.e1
  in thrombosis, 1778
Equipoise, in clinical trials, 48
ErbB antagonists, 1095, 1095b
Erythema marginatum, 1535, 1535f
Erythropoietin-α, in anemia of chronic kidney disease, 1874
E-selectin, 431
Esmolol
  for angina pectoris, 758t
  in chronic kidney disease, 1882t
Esophageal disorders, angina pectoris *vs.*, 740
Esophageal reflux, chest pain in, 600t
Esophagus
  Mallory-Weiss tears of, 601
  spasm of, 601
Essential myosin light chain (MLC-2), 894
Estrogen replacement therapy
  in stable ischemic heart disease, 752
  in venous thrombosis, 1774
Estrogen-receptor modulators, 1092t, 1096–1097
Eszopiclone, 1850
Ethacrynic acid, in heart failure, 982, 983t
Ethanol, 1593–1595
  arrhythmias and, 1594
  cardiomyopathy, 1593–1594
  coronary artery disease and, 1594–1595, 1595f
  epidemiology of, 1593
  heart failure and, 1593–1594
  history of, 1593
  hypertension and, 1595
  lipid metabolism and, 1594, 1595f
  myocardial injury and, 1593
  pharmacology and pathophysiology of, 1593
  sudden death and, 1594
Ethnic minorities, cardiovascular disease and, 66–68, 66f
EUCLID (Examining Use of Ticagrelor in PAD) trial, 848
EVALI. *See* Electronic cigarette or vaping-induced lung injury
Everolimus, 793
  in cardiac transplantation, 1136–1137
  in drug-eluting stents, 793, 793–794
Evidence-based medicine, definition of, 59
Exaggerated ventricular interaction, 1620–1621
EXCEL trial, 789
Excimer laser angioplasty (ECLA), 794.e1
Excitation-contraction coupling, 895–896, 896f
  alterations of, in heart failure, 923–924, 924f
Exemestane, cardiotoxic effects of, 1092t
Exenatide, in diabetes mellitus, 562t–563t, 567
Exercise, 579–587
  in arrhythmogenic right ventricular cardiomyopathy, 585
  cardiovascular response, age-associated changes in, 1687b–1690b, 1690f
  cardiovascular risks of, 581
  catecholaminergic polymorphic ventricular tachycardia with, 1201–1202
  for congenital heart disease, 1553–1554
  decreased capacity of, 582
  effects of, 580
  guidelines for, 25
  long QT syndrome with, 1193
  in obesity, 552, 552.e1f
  pathology of, 581
  in peripheral artery disease, 850, 850f
  relative and absolute risk of, 581
  as risk factor of stroke, 874b–877b
  screening in, 582–583
  in stable ischemic heart disease, 752–753
  in sudden cardiac death, 1356, 1363–1365
Exercise capacity, cardiovascular disease and, 1710b–1714b
Exercise echocardiography
  of heart failure with preserved and mildly reduced ejection, 1011b–1017b
  of primary mitral regurgitation, 1461–1462
Exercise testing, 175–195, 282–283
  in adult congenital heart disease, 190–191
  arm cycle ergometry, 178b–180b

Exercise testing *(Continued)*
  in arrhythmias, 190b–191b, 191t
  in arrhythmogenic right ventricular cardiomyopathy, 190b–191b
  in atrial fibrillation, 190b–191b
  blood pressure in, 181b–182b
  blunted systolic pressure peak during, 181b–182b
  in cardiac arrest survivors, 1365–1366
  cardiopulmonary, 178b–180b
  in catecholaminergic polymorphic ventricular tachycardia, 190b–191b
  in chest pain, 605–606
  in chest pain units, 191–192, 192t
  chronotropic incompetence, 181b–182b
  Cleveland Clinic Prognostic Score, 186b–187b, 189f
  diagnostic value in, 184–185
  digitalis glycosides, 184
  in disability assessment, 192b, 193t
  double-product reserve in, 181b–182b
  Duke Treadmill Prognostic Score for, 186b–187b
  electrocardiographic lead systems for, 177
  electrocardiography, in stable ischemic heart disease, 745b–746b, 746t
  in exercise prescription, 192
  functional capacity in, 181b, 181b–182b
  in heart failure, 942–943, 942b–943b
  heart rate recovery in, 181b–182b
  heart rate responses, 181b–182b
  in hypertrophic cardiomyopathy, 190
  hypotension during, 181b–182b
  inadequate, 181b–182b
  lead aVR ST elevation, 182
  in long-QT Syndrome, 190b–191b
  myocardial oxygen demand and, 175–177, 176f
  myocardial oxygen supply and, 175–177
  in nonatherosclerotic heart disease, 189–191
  nondiagnostic study, 181b–182b
  pacemaker and, 190b–191b
  patient assessment in, 177, 177t
  patient monitoring during, 179t
  patient preparation for, 177
  peak heart rate, 181b–182b
  in peripheral artery disease, 192–193, 193t
  pharmacologic influences on interpretation, 184
  physiology of, 175–177
  post-myocardial infarction evaluation and, 187
  predictive values of, 184–185
  preoperative, 189
  pre-test and post-test disease probability and, 185, 185t
  prognostic value of, 186–187, 188t
  protocols for, 177–180, 178t
  in pulmonary arterial hypertension, 1669, 1669b
  of rheumatic mitral stenosis, 1446
  risks of, 180
  sensitivity and specificity of, 184, 184t
  separate scores for men and women, 186b–187b, 187f–188f
  six-minute walk, 178b–180b, 180t
  ST adjustments, 182–183
  ST depression, 182
  ST elevation, 183–184
  stationary cycle, 178b–180b, 179t
  stress, in aortic valve stenosis, 1408b
  ST-segment changes in, 182–184, 183f, 183b–184b
  submaximal, 178, 178t
  supervision of, 180
  symptom rating scales for, 177
  technical components of, 177–180
  termination of, 178, 178t
  for therapeutic assessment, 189, 190b–191b
  total-body oxygen uptake and, 175, 176f
  treadmill, 179.e1f, 178b–180b, 179t
  upsloping ST depression, 182
  in valvular heart disease, 189–190
  in ventricular arrhythmias, 190b–191b
  in ventricular preexcitation, 190b–191b
  in women, 185–186, 186f, 186t
Exercise tolerance, noncardiac surgery and, 413
Exercise training, for heart failure with preserved and mildly reduced ejection, 1028
Exercise-induced systolic hypotension, in coronary artery disease, 181b–182b
Exertional compartment syndrome, 840
Exertional leg pain, differential diagnosis of, 840t
Extended-duration anticoagulation, optimal oral anticoagulant for, 1648

External validation, 107
External work rate, 579
Extracardiac phenotyping, of heart failure with preserved and mildly reduced ejection, 1011b–1017b
Extracellular lipid accumulation, in atherosclerosis initiation, 428–430, 429f–430f
Extracellular matrix (ECM), alterations of, in heart failure, 927
Extracorporeal life support (ECLS), 1122f, 1126–1127
Extracorporeal membrane oxygenation (ECMO), 1126–1127
Extracorporeal ultrafiltration (UF), 989
Extracranial carotid disease, endovascular treatment of, 865–866, 865t–866t, 866f, 866.e1f
Extreme frailty, aortic stenosis and, 1431.e1
Extremities
  evaluation of, in STEMI, 655
  examination of, 126
Extremity deep venous thrombosis, treatment of, 867–868, 867.e2f
Ezetimibe, 518
  in coronary heart disease, 559
  in NSTE-ACS, 731–732

F

Fabry disease, 1046–1047, 1046.e1t, 1047.e1f
  echocardiography in, 222
Facioscapulohumeral muscular dystrophy, 1863, 1863.e1f
Factor V, 1769
Factor V Leiden, 1772–1773
  therapy for, 1651
Factor VIII, intrinsic tenase and, 1769
Factor IX, intrinsic tenase and, 1769
Factor Xa inhibitors
  in atrial fibrillation-associated thromboembolism prevention, 1276
  in NSTE-ACS, 727b
  oral, 727b
  in percutaneous coronary intervention, 801
Factor XI, 1768, 1771f
Factor XIII, polymorphism in, venous thrombosis and, 1773
Factorial design, 43
Fallacies, 60
False aneurysms, 806–807
FAME (Fractional Flow Reserve *versus* Angiography for Multivessel Evaluation) trial, 795
Familial atrial fibrillation (FAF), 1204–1205
  clinical description and manifestations of, 1204–1205
  genetic basis of, 1204b–1205b
Familial combined hyperlipidemia, 512
Familial defective apolipoprotein B, 510
Familial glycerolemia, 512
Familial high-density lipoprotein deficiency, 513
Familial hyperchylomicronemia syndrome, 509–510, 512–513
Familial hypertriglyceridemia, 511–512
Familial lipodystrophy, 514
Familial paraganglioma, 486
Familial thoracic aortic aneurysm and dissection syndrome (TAAD), 812, 814f
Family history, cardiovascular disease and, 451, 451f
Famine, 14, 16t
Fas ligand, 433
Fascia adherens, 1173
Fascicular block
  bifascicular, 159, 159f
  left anterior, 156–157, 156t, 157f
  left posterior, 156
  multifascicular, 159–160, 160f
Fast pathway ablation, 1233f, 1233b–1234b
Fatigue, in heart failure, 935
Fats, 536–538
Fatty acids
  monounsaturated, 537f, 538
  polyunsaturated, 537f, 538
  saturated, 536–538, 537f
  trans, 537f, 538
Fatty streak, 432
FBN1 gene, 811
Felodipine, for angina pectoris, 760, 761t

Femoral artery
　access complications of, 799.e1
　　percutaneous technique, for cardiac catheterization, 386–388, 387f–389f
　for vascular access, 798–799
Femoral-popliteal artery disease, endovascular treatment of, 864–865, 864.e3f, 864f–865f
Fetus
　effects of warfarin on, 1785
　undernutrition effects on, 26
Fever, in STEMI, 654
18F-FDG metabolic imaging protocols, 286–288
18F-FDG PET/CT
　versus 99mTc-SPECT MPI, 311.e1f
　imaging in large-vessel vasculitis, 309f
　metabolic imaging protocols, 286–288
　to therapy in aortitis, 310f
Fiber
　dietary, 537f
　in dyslipidemia, 596b
Fibrates, 518
Fibric acid derivatives (fibrates), 518
　for coronary heart disease, 559
Fibrin, formation of, 1769–1770, 1770f
Fibrinogen, 1769–1770, 1770f
　in peripheral artery disease, 838
　serum, in STEMI, 652b
Fibrinolysis, 1766–1790
　anticoagulation with, 677
　antiplatelet therapy with, 678
　prehospital, in STEMI, 663–664
　STEMI and, 668–669
Fibrinolytic activity, vascular endothelium and, 1767
Fibrinolytic drugs, 1787–1789, 1787f
　alteplase as, 1788, 1788f
　anistreplase as, 1788
　reteplase as, 1788–1789
　streptokinase as, 1787–1789, 1787f
　tenecteplase as, 1788–1789
　urokinase as, 1788
Fibrinolytic system, 1770–1771, 1771f
Fibrinolytic therapy, effect of, 669–671, 669f–670f
　comparison of, 670, 670t, 670.e1f
　complications of, 670–671, 671f
　intracoronary fibrinolysis, 671
　late therapy, 671
　on left ventricular function, 670
Fibrinopeptide A, in STEMI, 652b
Fibroblasts, in heart failure, 928.e1f, 927f, 927b–929b
Fibroelastoma, papillary, 1832–1833, 1832.e1f
Fibromas, 1834–1835, 1834f
　echocardiography in, 253b, 253.e1f
Fibromuscular dysplasia (FMD), 488, 853, 853f, 853t
　in renal artery stenosis, 867
Fibrosis, endomyocardial, 1049
Fick method, for cardiac output measurements, 393–394, 395f
Fight-or-flight response, 899–900, 900f, 900t
Filipinos, hypertension in, 1743
Fine particles, 31–32
Finger cuffs, 483
Fingers, examination of, 126
First-degree atrioventricular (AV) block, 1315
　electrocardiography for, 1315, 1315f
Fish, 533f, 534, 540t
Fish eye disease, 513
Fish oils, 519–520
Fixed coupling, in premature ventricular complexes, 1288
Flamm's formula, 404
Flecainide, 1121.e1t, 1209t, 1212t, 1214t, 1217–1218, 1217b–1218b
　in atrial fibrillation, 1280
　in pregnancy, 1730f
Fluconazole, for infective endocarditis, 1519b–1523b
Fludrocortisone suppression test, for primary hyperaldosteronism, 485
Fluid retention, management of, in heart failure, 981–989, 982f
Fluid status, device-based therapies for management of, 989, 989b
Fluid-filled pressure systems, in pressure measurements, 392, 392.e1t
Fluoroquinolones, for infective endocarditis, from HACEK organisms, 1519b–1523b
Fluoroscopy, in pericardial effusion and cardiac tamponade, 1622

5-Fluorouracil, cardiotoxic effects of, 1092t, 1094.e1
Flutamide, cardiotoxic effects of, 1092t
Fluvastatin, in chronic kidney disease, 1883t
Focal atrial tachycardia, 1234f–1235f, 1234b–1235b, 1247–1251, 1248f–1249f
　acute management of, 1251b
　atomic distribution of, 1250–1251, 1251f
　chronic management, 1251b, 1252f
　clinical features of, 1248b
　diagnosis of, 1248–1251
　differential diagnosis of, 1248–1251
　epidemiology of, 1248b
　macroreentrant atrial tachycardia vs., 1248b–1249b
　management of, 1251b
　multifocal atrial tachycardia vs., 1248b–1249b, 1250f
Focal discharge, in atrial fibrillation, 1187
Focal fibromuscular dysplasia, 853
Focal ventricular fibrillation, 1241f
Fondaparinux, 1779t, 1782
　in chronic kidney disease, 1885t–1886t
　mechanism of action of, 1779f, 1782
　in NSTE-ACS, 727b
　in percutaneous coronary intervention, 787.e3t, 801
　pharmacology of, 1782
　in pulmonary embolism, 1646
　side effects of, 1782
Fontaine classification, of peripheral artery disease, 841, 841t
Fontan procedure, pregnancy and, 1738, 1739t
Fontan-associated liver disease, 1582
Food processing, 540–543
Foods, 532–535
Foramen ovale, patent. See Patent foramen ovale
Fosinopril, in heart failure, 991t
FOURIER (Further Cardiovascular Outcomes Research with PCSK9 Inhibition in Subjects with Elevated Risk) trial, 874b–877b
Fractional flow reserve, 619f, 621–622, 621f, 621.e1f, 621.e2f, 624f, 627f
　in percutaneous coronary intervention, 795
　in stable ischemic heart disease, 747, 765, 769f
Frailty, 1431.e1
　in elderly, 1690b–1693b
　extreme, aortic stenosis and, 1431.e1
　in physical examination, 125, 125t
Framing effects, information and, 59
Framingham Risk Score, 28, 1610
Frank-Starling effect, 895, 906
Friction rubs, in STEMI, 655
Friedreich ataxia, 1864, 1864f–1865f, 1864.e1f
Fruits, 532, 533f, 540t
Functional assessment, of pulmonary arterial hypertension, 1669
Functional reentry, 1187.e1f, 1185–1186, 1188f
Funduscopic examination, 126
Fungi, causing infective endocarditis, 1506b–1507b, 1512t
　antimicrobial therapy for, 1519b–1523b
Furosemide
　in heart failure, 982, 983t
　in pregnancy, 1730f
Fusiform aneurysm, 806–807
FXYD proteins, 1171b–1173b

G

G protein, 901, 902f
　inhibitory, 901b
　stimulatory, 901b
　third, 901b
Gadolinium-enhanced magnetic resonance angiography, for pulmonary embolism, 1644
Gallbladder disease, chest pain in, 600t
Ganglionated plexuses, 1179b
Gap junction channels, 1173–1175, 1175f
　alterations in, arrhythmias and, 1174b–1175b
　biochemical coupling and, 1173
　connexins of, 1174b–1175b
Gaseous pollutants, 33
Gastroepiploic artery, cannulation for, 367b–368b, 369f
Gastrointestinal conditions, chest pain in, 601
Gastrointestinal tract, aspirin effects on, 1775–1776
Gated blood pool scans, 284b
Gaucher disease, 1047–1048
Gender
　in acute heart failure, 946–947
　body mass index and, 24, 25f

Gender (Continued)
　hypertension and, 22–23, 22f
　obesity and, 23–24
　tobacco use and, 20–21, 21f
　total cholesterol and, 23, 24f
Gene therapy, for lipoprotein disorders, 522
General appearance, in patient evaluation, 125, 125t
Genetic architecture, 72
Genetic lipoprotein disorders, 509–510, 509t
Genetic susceptibility factors, in rheumatic fever, 1532b–1533b
Genetics
　in abdominal aortic aneurysms, 808
　in Andersen-Tawil syndrome, 1192f, 1199b
　in arrhythmogenic right ventricular cardiomyopathy, 1039b–1040b
　in atrial fibrillation, 1274
　in Brugada syndrome, 1192f, 1201b, 1202f
　in cardiac arrhythmias, 1191–1207
　of cardiovascular disease, 8
　cardiovascular medicine to
　　applications of, 71–86
　　translating, 72t
　in catecholaminergic polymorphic ventricular tachycardia, 1203f, 1203b
　central dogma, 71
　in dilated cardiomyopathy, 1035, 1035f–1036f
　disease risk prediction, 80–81
　DNA in, 71
　in early repolarization syndrome, 1204b
　epidemiologic associations, causal inference of, 77–80
　in familial atrial fibrillation, 1204b–1205b
　in familial hypercholesterolemia, 83
　future perspectives for, 85
　gene discovery, 75–77
　　case-control studies, 75–77
　　family-based studies, 75
　　population-based studies of, 75–77
　genetic architecture, 72
　genetic variation in, 72–73, 72f–73f
　　characterizing, 73–75, 73b–75b
　genome-wide association study for
　　coronary artery disease, 77, 78f
　　lipids, 76–77, 77f
　in heart failure, 921.e1f
　heritability in, 72
　human genetic variation, characterizing, 73–75, 73b–75b
　in hypertrophic cardiomyopathy, 1063, 1065t, 1066–1067, 1066f–1067f
　in idiopathic ventricular fibrillation, 1205.e1f, 1205b
　in long QT syndrome, 1191b–1193b, 1192f
　mendelian randomization principles and applications, 79–80
　next-generation technologies and therapeutics, 83–85
　on-target therapeutic side effect prediction, 82
　pathogenicity assessments and monogenic risk, 80–81, 80t
　population-based discovery of rare protein-coding variants associated
　　with coronary artery disease, 77
　precision medicine, 82–83
　principles of, 71–75
　in progressive cardiac conduction disease, 1205b–1206b
　in restrictive cardiomyopathy, 1043–1044
　in short QT syndrome, 1192f, 1197b
　in sick sinus syndrome, 1206b
　in sudden cardiac death, 1354t, 1355f, 1356, 1377t
　therapeutic response prediction, 81–83
　in Timothy syndrome, 1192f, 1196b–1197b
　visceral obesity and, 550
Genome
　conceptual relationship of, 88f
　therapeutically targeting, 84–85
Genome-wide association study (GWAS), 93b–96b
Genomics, of cardiovascular disease, 8
Genotype, 71
Gentamicin, in infective endocarditis, from streptococcal species, 1519b–1523b, 1520t–1521t
Geriatric domains, pertinent to cardiovascular care, 1690–1693, 1691t
　cognitive impairment in, 1690b–1693b
　delirium in, 1690b–1693b
　disability in, 1690b–1693b

Geriatric domains, pertinent to cardiovascular care *(Continued)*
　　frailty in, 1690b–1693b
　　morbidity, 1690b–1693b, 1692f
　　polypharmacy in, 1690b–1693b
　　sarcopenia in, 1690b–1693b
Geriatric patients. *See* Older adults
Gestational diabetes, cardiovascular disease in women and, 1710b–1714b
Giant cell arteritis, 853, 1812
　　cardiovascular complications of, 1812, 1813t
　　diagnosis of, 1812
　　pathogenesis of, 1812, 1813f
GLA gene, 1046–1047
Glargine, in diabetes mellitus, 562t–563t
Gliclazide, in diabetes mellitus, 562t–563t, 571
Glimepiride, in diabetes mellitus, 562t–563t, 564b–566b
Glipizide, in diabetes mellitus, 562t–563t
Global Group in Chronic Heart Failure (MAGGIC) meta-analysis, 1008
Glomerular filtration rate, in heart failure, 938b–939b
Glomerular vasculature, normal structure of, 1874f
Glossopharyngeal nerve, 1894–1895
Glucagon like peptide (GLP)-1 receptor agonists, in glucose management, 562t–563t, 567, 568f–569f
Glucocorticoids
　　excess of, 1793
　　in polyarteritis nodosa, 1817
　　in rheumatic disease, 1826
Glucose
　　in diabetes mellitus, 561–571, 562t–563t
　　　　in acute coronary syndromes, 571–573
　　　　cardiovascular effects of
　　　　　　more intensive *vs.* less intensive, 569–571
　　　　　　selected medications, 561–569, 564t, 565f
　　　　dipeptidyl peptidase 4 inhibitors in, 562t–563t, 566–567
　　　　dopamine D_2 receptor agonists in, 562t–563t
　　　　glucagon like peptide (GLP)-1 receptor agonists in, 562t–563t, 567, 568f–569f
　　　　α-glucosidase inhibitors, 562t–563t, 569
　　　　in heart failure, 575–576, 576f
　　　　insulin in, 562t–563t, 566, 572
　　　　intensive strategies in
　　　　　　in acute coronary syndromes, 571–573
　　　　　　cardiovascular effects of, 569–571
　　　　meglitinides in, 562t–563t
　　　　metformin in, 561–564, 562t–563t, 564b
　　　　ongoing trials of, 564t, 566b–567b
　　　　sodium-glucose cotransporter 2 (SGLT2) inhibitors, 562t–563t, 567–569, 570f
　　　　sulfonylureas in, 562t–563t, 564–566
　　　　thiazolidinediones in, 562t–563t, 564b–566b
　　　　treatment guidelines, 571, 572f
　　plasma, 23, 24f
Glucose control, during ST-elevation myocardial infarction, 684
Glucose homeostasis, in STEMI, 652b
Glucose intolerance, in NSTE-ACS, 733–734
α-Glucosidase inhibitors, in glucose management, 562t–563t, 569
Glulisine, in diabetes mellitus, 562t–563t
Glyburide (glibenclamide), in diabetes mellitus, 562t–563t, 564b–566b
Glycemic index, 537f
Glycemic load, 537f
Glycerolipids, 503
Glycerophospholipids, 503
Glycogen storage disease, 1047–1048
　　type V, 840
Glycoprotein IIb/IIIa inhibitors
　　in chronic kidney disease, 1881
　　dosages for, 1778
　　indications for, 1779
　　mechanism of action of, 1778
　　in NSTE-ACS, 726b, 735.e4t
　　in percutaneous coronary intervention, 787.e3t, 800–801
　　side effects of, 1778
　　in thrombosis, 1778–1779, 1778t
Glycosides, in heart failure, 999–1000, 999b, 1000.e1
Goldilocks alleles, 76
GORE devices, for atrial septal defects, 1589f, 1590, 1590b
Gorlin formula, 398
Goserelin, cardiotoxic effects of, 1092t
Gout, atherosclerosis in, 1811

Graft stenoses, 851
Grains, 532–534, 533f, 540t
Granulomatosis with polyangiitis (Wegener granulomatosis), 1817, 1818f
　　treatment for, 1818
Great arteries
　　congenitally corrected transposition of, pregnancy and, 1738
　　transposition of, echocardiography in, 260b, 260.e1f, 262f–263f
Grip myotonia, 1858f
GRK5 gene, 95t
Group A streptococcal (GAS) infection, evidence of, 1535–1536, 1535b–1536b
Growth hormone, 1791
Growth hormone deficiency, 1792
Guanadrel, drug interaction with, 97t
Guideline-directed medical therapy (GDMT), for congenital heart disease, 1551
Guillain-Barré syndrome, 1868

H

H_2FPEF score, 1011b–1017b
HACEK organisms, causing infective endocarditis, 1506b–1507b, 1512t
　　antimicrobial therapy for, 1522.e2t, 1519b–1523b
Hakki formula, 399
Handheld echocardiography, 265–266
Haplotype, 73
Harvey, William, 1, 2f
Hasty judgments, 60
HCN4, 1206b
HDL cholesterol, 454
Head and neck, examination of, 125–126
Head injury, 1870–1871
Head-up tilt-table testing, in cardiac arrhythmias, 1155–1162, 1155.e2f
Healing touch, in integrative cardiology, 593b–594b
Health effects, of tobacco products, 525–530
Health policy, 62, 63f
Hearing impairment, diuretic-induced, 988
Heart
　　auscultation of, 130–131
　　contractile performance of, 904–911
　　dynamic auscultation of, 134
　　inspection of, 130
　　muscle of, myocardial infarction and, 639–649, 639.e1t, 642f
　　palpation of, 130
　　total artificial, 1129
　　work of, 909–910
Heart block, 1315–1319, 1547
Heart disease
　　congenital, 1737–1740
　　drug adjustments in, 99
　　integrative approaches to management of patients with, 593–598
　　in racially and ethnically diverse populations, 1743–1750
Heart failure, 1549–1550
　　acute, 946–974, 947f
　　　　acute coronary syndromes in, 956b
　　　　age and, 946–947
　　　　atrial fibrillation in, 956b
　　　　cardiogenic shock in, 952, 953t, 956b
　　　　cardio-renal syndrome in, 957
　　　　comorbidities in, 947
　　　　congestion in, 949
　　　　decompensated, 952, 953t
　　　　definition of, 946
　　　　ejection fraction in, 946, 948f
　　　　epidemiology of, 946–947
　　　　evaluation of, 951–955, 952f
　　　　　　biomarkers in, 954
　　　　　　chest radiography in, 954
　　　　　　classification in, 951–953, 952f, 953t
　　　　　　echocardiogram in, 954
　　　　　　electrocardiogram in, 954
　　　　　　laboratory testing in, 954
　　　　　　natriuretic peptides in, 954
　　　　　　physical examination in, 953–954
　　　　　　risk stratification in, 954–955, 954t
　　　　　　symptoms in, 953, 953t
　　　　gender and, 946–947
　　　　global differences in, 947
　　　　hospitalization in

Heart failure *(Continued)*
　　　　　　mortality and, 954–955
　　　　　　numbers of, 946
　　　　　　post-discharge events and, 954–955
　　　　　　worsening in, 957, 957f
　　　　hypertensive, 952, 953t
　　　　inflammatory mechanisms in, 951
　　　　management of, 955–972
　　　　　　arginine vasopressin antagonists in, 965b
　　　　　　blood pressure in, 958, 959f
　　　　　　calcium channel blockers in, 965b
　　　　　　cardiac myosin activators in, 971b–972b
　　　　　　digoxin in, 965b
　　　　　　direct renin inhibitors in, 971b–972b
　　　　　　diuretics in, 961–962, 961t–962t
　　　　　　dobutamine in, 964, 964b
　　　　　　dopamine in, 964
　　　　　　endothelin receptor antagonists in, 971b–972b
　　　　　　enoximone in, 964b–965b
　　　　　　epinephrine in, 964
　　　　　　hypertonic saline in, 966b
　　　　　　inodilators in, 962t, 963–964
　　　　　　inotropes in, 962t, 963–964
　　　　　　inotropic agents in, 971b–972b
　　　　　　invasive hemodynamic strategy in, 959–960
　　　　　　istaroxime in, 971b–972b
　　　　　　levosimendan in, 965, 965b
　　　　　　milrinone in, 964b–965b
　　　　　　natriuretic peptides in, 971–972
　　　　　　nesiritide in, 963b
　　　　　　neurohormonal antagonists in, 971b–972b
　　　　　　nitrates in, 962–963, 963b
　　　　　　novel therapies in, 966–972, 966t–970t
　　　　　　omecamtiv mecarbil in, 971b–972b
　　　　　　outcomes in, 960–961, 960t
　　　　　　phase I (urgent/emergent care), 955–956, 955f
　　　　　　phase II (hospital care), 956–957
　　　　　　phase III (pre-discharge planning), 957–958, 958t
　　　　　　phase IV (post-discharge management), 958
　　　　　　phosphodiesterase inhibitors in, 964–965
　　　　　　process of care in, 960–961
　　　　　　quality assessment in, 960–961
　　　　　　renal function in, 959
　　　　　　renoprotective agents in, 971b–972b
　　　　　　serelaxin in, 970–971, 971f
　　　　　　sodium nitroprusside in, 963
　　　　　　soluble guanylate cyclase activators and stimulators in, 971b–972b
　　　　　　targeting congestion in, 958–959
　　　　　　ultrafiltration in, 966
　　　　　　vasodilators in, 962–963, 962t
　　　　　　vasopressors in, 965–966
　　　　　　volume status in, 958–959
　　　　myocardial function in, 949–950, 950f
　　　　neurohormonal mechanisms in, 951
　　　　nomenclature of, 946
　　　　pathophysiology of, 947–951, 949f
　　　　with preserved ejection fraction in, 946
　　　　race and, 946–947
　　　　with reduced ejection fraction in, 946
　　　　renal mechanisms in, 950–951, 951f
　　　　right ventricular, 956b
　　　　scope of the problem in, 946, 948t
　　　　vascular mechanisms in, 951
　　advanced, timing of, 944
　　aging and, 933, 1697–1699
　　　　chronic heart failure with reduced ejection fraction
　　　　　　nonmedicinal options for, 1698
　　　　　　pharmacotherapy for, 1698, 1698b
　　　　diagnosis of, 1697
　　　　epidemiology of, 1697
　　　　lifestyle management in, 1697–1698
　　　　pathophysiology of, 1697
　　　　with preserved ejection fraction, 1698–1699
　　　　pulmonary hypertension and, 1699
　　air pollution and, 36
　　amyloidosis and, 1058b
　　approach to patient with, 933–945, 978–981
　　assessment of, 134–137, 934
　　　　biomarkers in, 939, 939t, 941f
　　　　blood chemistry in, 938–940
　　　　blood urea nitrogen in, 938b–939b
　　　　cardiopulmonary exercise testing in, 942–943, 942b–943b
　　　　chest radiography in, 938

Heart failure *(Continued)*
    computed tomography in, 943
    echocardiography in, 943
    electrocardiogram in, 938, 938b
    endomyocardial biopsy in, 942
    imaging in, 943–944
    magnetic resonance imaging in, 943, 944f
    medical history in, 935–938, 935t
    natriuretic peptides in, 940, 940b, 940.e1t
    nuclear imaging in, 943–944
    physical examination in, 935t–936t, 936–938
    right heart catheterization in, 942, 942b
    risk scoring for prognosis, 941–942
    symptoms and signs in, 935–936, 937t
  atrial fibrillation in, 1287.e6t
  blood pressure and, 493–494, 495f, 937–938
  cancer and, 1099–1100, 1102t
  in cancer survivorship, 1104–1106, 1105.e1f, 1106.e4t
  cardiac index in, 136
  cardiac resynchronization therapy for, 223
  cardiogenic shock in, 938
  cardiorenal syndrome in, 938b–939b
  cardiovascular disease and, 7
  catheter ablation in, 1287.e8
  chest radiography in, 275, 275b, 276f
  classification of, 934, 935t, 936f
  clinical features of, 1549
  comorbid condition, detection of, 942
  COVID-19 and, 1757
  definition of, 933–934
  device use in, 1719
  in diabetes mellitus, 556, 574–576
    mechanistic considerations in, 574–575, 574f
    prevention and management of, 575–576
    scope of problem, 574
  in dilated cardiomyopathy, 1032–1043
  direct cardiotoxicity concerns, 1106.e1
  distribution of ejection fraction and, 933
  diuretics in, 938b–939b
  drug adjustments in, 99
  Ebstein anomaly of the tricuspid valve and, 1562
  echocardiography in, 222–224
  edema in, 135
  effects of food and nutrients on, 541t–542t
  epidemiology of, 933–934, 934f, 1549
  ethanol and, 1593–1594
  heart sounds in, 135, 135.e1f
  heart transplantation for, 223–224
  indirect cardiotoxicity concerns, 1106.e1
  in infective endocarditis, 1508
  inflammatory cardiotoxicity concerns, 1106.e1
  influenza and, 1752, 1752f
  in ischemic heart disease, 779–781
  jugular venous pressure in, 135, 135.e1f
  lung ultrasound in, 224, 224.e1f
  management of, 1103–1104, 1106.e2
    in heterogeneous populations, 1746f, 1747–1748
  mechanical causes of, 694–699
    free wall rupture, 694–696
      diagnosis of, 696
      differentiation between ventricular septal rupture and mitral regurgitation, 698
      of interventricular septum, 696–697, 697f, 697f–698f, 697t
      management of, 699, 699f
      of papillary muscle, 697–698, 698f
      pseudoaneurysm, 694–696, 694.e1f
      treatment for, 696
  monitoring and managing, devices for, 1107
    cardiac resynchronization therapy in, 1107
      CARE-HF trial of, 1107b–1110b, 1111f
      COMPANION trial of, 1107b–1110b, 1111f
      CONTAK CD trial of, 1107b–1110b
      indications for, 1111
      limitations of, 1111, 1113f
      MADIT-CRT trial of, 1110b–1111b
      MIRACLE ICD trial of, 1107b–1110b
      MIRACLE trial of, 1107b–1110b, 1110f
      MUSTIC trials of, 1107b–1110b, 1108t–1109t
      in NYHA class I and II patients, randomized controlled trials of, 1110–1111, 1110b–1111b
      in NYHA class III and IV patients, randomized controlled trials of, 1107–1110, 1107b–1110b, 1108t–1109t, 1110f–1111f
      in patients with narrow QRS complex, 1110b–1111b, 1112t, 1115t

Heart failure *(Continued)*
      RAFT trial of, 1110b–1111b
      REVERSE trial of, 1110b–1111b
    implantable devices in, 1113
      implantable hemodynamic monitors, 1116–1117, 1117f
      implantable-cardioverter defibrillators for, randomized controlled trials of, 1111–1113, 1111b–1113b, 1112t
        DANISH trial of, 1111b–1113b
        DEFINITE trial of, 1111b–1113b
        MADIT II trial of, 1111b–1113b
        SCD-HeFT trial of, 1111b–1113b, 1113f
      sudden cardiac death in, 1111–1113
    new implantable therapeutic devices for, 1113–1114
  noncardiac surgery and, 411–412
  NSTE-ACS and, 734
  in older adults, 1001
  outcomes of, 938b–939b
  in overt hyperthyroidism, 1800
  pathophysiology of, 913–924, 1549–1550
    action potential duration in, 924–925, 925.e1f
    adipokines in, 920.e1f, 920b–921b
    adiponectin in, 920b–921b
    adrenomedullin in, 920b–921b
    apelin in, 920b–921b
    apoptosis in, 926.e1f, 926b–927b
    arginine vasopressin in, 917f, 917b
    autophagy in, 926b–927b, 928f
    beta-adrenergic desensitization in, 926
    bradykinin in, 920b–921b
    calcium leak in, 924
    cardiac energetics in, 930.e1f, 930b
    cardiac fibroblasts in, 928.e1f, 927f, 927b–929b
    cardiac myocyte apoptosis in, 926–930, 926b–927b
    cardiac myocyte hypertrophy in, 922–923, 922f–923f
    contractile and regulatory proteins, abnormalities in, 925, 925t
    cytoskeletal proteins, abnormalities in, 925
    endothelin in, 919.e1
    excitation-contraction coupling, alterations in, 923–924, 924f
    inflammatory mediators in, 920b–921b, 921f, 922t
    left ventricular remodeling in, 921–930, 921.e1f, 922t
      reversibility of, 930–931, 930.e2t, 931f, 931b
    left ventricular structure, alterations in, 930, 930.e1t, 931f
    mast cells in, 927f, 927b–929b
    matrix metalloproteinases in, 929.e1, 929.e1t
    metalloproteinases in, tissue inhibitors of, 929.e1, 929.e1t
    mitochondrial biology in, 930.e1f, 930b
    myocardium, alterations in, 926–930, 927f
    natriuretic peptides in, 918f, 918b–919b
    necrosis in, 926b–927b
    neurohormonal mechanisms in, 913–921, 914f
    neuropeptide Y in, 919.e1
    nitric oxide in, 919–921, 919.e2f
    noncoding RNAs in, 929f, 929b–930b
    oxidative stress in, 916f, 916b
    pathogenesis in, 913–930, 914f
    peripheral vasculature, neurohormonal alterations of, 919–921
    renal function, neurohormonal alterations of, 916–919, 917.e1t
    renin-angiotensin system in, 915–916, 915f
    sarcolemmal Ca^{2+} elimination in, 924
    sarcoplasmic reticulum Ca^{2+} reuptake in, 924
    sodium handling in, 924–925, 925.e1f
    sympathetic nervous system in, 913–915, 913f–914f
    T-tubules, alterations in, 924b
    urotensin II in, 919.e1
    vasoconstricting peptides in, 919.e1
  patient history of, 134–135
  patients at high risk for developing, 978–979
  physical examination in, 135
  pleural effusions in, 136–137
  with preserved and mildly reduced ejection fraction, 1007–1030
    atrial fibrillation in, 1008
    biomarkers of, 1011b–1017b
    cardiac catheterization in, 1011b–1017b, 1014–1015f, 1014.e1f
    cardiac magnetic resonance imaging of, 1011b–1017b, 1013f–1014f

Heart failure *(Continued)*
    cardiopulmonary exercise testing of, 1011b–1017b, 1017t
    coronary evaluation of, 1011b–1017b
    device therapy in, 1026–1028
      diagnostic devices, 1026–1027
      therapeutic devices, 1027–1028
    diagnosis of, 1010–1017, 1011t
    diagnostic scores of, 1011b–1017b, 1012f
    echocardiography of, 1011b–1017b, 1013f
    emerging concepts in the treatment of, 1028
    empiric therapy of, 1023–1024
      angiotensin converting enzyme inhibitors, 1024
      angiotensin receptor blockers, 1024–1025, 1025t
      angiotensin receptor neprilysin inhibition, 1025–1026, 1026f–1027f
      atrial fibrillation, 1024
      beta blockers, 1024
      blood pressure management, 1023–1024
      calcium channel blockers, 1024
      decongestive therapy with diuretics, 1023
      mineralocorticoid receptor antagonists, 1025
      renin-angiotensin-aldosterone system inhibitors, 1024
    endomyocardial biopsy of, 1011b–1017b, 1016f
    epidemiology of, 1007–1010
    extracardiac phenotyping in, 1011b–1017b
    general considerations of, 1021–1023
      exclusion of other causes of signs/symptoms, 1021–1023, 1022t–1023t
      mortality reduction in, 1023
      pathophysiologic considerations of therapy, 1023
    hospitalization of, 1009–1010
    incidence of, 1008
    lifestyle modification and exercise training for, 1028
    measures of diastolic function and strain in, 1011b–1017b, 1013f
    molecular mechanisms underlying, 1018b–1020b, 1021f
    mortality of, 1008–1009, 1009f–1010f
    ongoing clinical trials in, 1028
    pathophysiology of, 1017–1020, 1018f–1020f
    prevalence of, 1007, 1007.e1f, 1007.e1t
    prognosis of, 1008–1010
    quality of life in, 1010
    risk factors of, 1008, 1008t, 1009f
    strategies for phenotypic subtyping of, 1018b–1020b, 1022t
    treatment of, 1020–1028
    unsuccessful and potentially harmful treatments in, 1028
  prevalence of, 933, 934f
  preventive efforts and screening recommendations for, 1106.e1
  prognosis for, 941–942
  pulmonary hypertension and, 1659
  pulse pressure in, 136
  quality of life, 942
  radionuclide imaging in patients with, 298–307
    in infiltrative cardiomyopathy: amyloidosis, 303–304, 304f–305f
    in inflammatory cardiomyopathy: sarcoidosis, 304–307, 304f–307f
    left ventricular systolic dysfunction, patients with newly diagnosed, 298
    patients with ischemic cardiomyopathy and, 298–303
  rales in, 135
  rates of, 933
  with reduced ejection fraction (HFrEF), 975–984
    acute decompensation in, 979–981, 981t
    algorithm for, 990f
    atherosclerotic disease management in, 1000
    in cancer patients, 1001
    defining appropriate strategy, 979–981
    diagnostic criteria for, 980t
    end of life care, 1005.e2
    etiology of, 975, 976t
    future perspectives for, 1005
    in geriatric patients, 1001
    integration of palliative care into, 1004–1005, 1005f
    management of
      activity in, 981, 981.e1f
      aliskiren in, 996–997

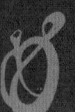

Heart failure *(Continued)*
　　angiotensin receptor blockers in, 991t–992t, 993, 993b
　　angiotensin receptor neprilysin inhibitors in, 991t–992t, 993–994, 994f
　　angiotensin-converting enzyme inhibitors in, 989–993, 991f, 991t–992t
　　anticoagulation and antiplatelet therapy in, 1001–1002
　　arrhythmias in, 1002
　　beta-adrenergic blockers in, 991t–992t, 994–996, 995f
　　cardiac resynchronization therapy in, 1002
　　combination of hydralazine and isosorbide dinitrate in, 997
　　diet in, 981
　　disease management approach in, 1003, 1004f
　　diuretics in, 985–988, 987f
　　extracorporeal ultrafiltration in, 989
　　general measures in, 977t, 979–981
　　in hospitalized patient, 989b
　　implantable cardioverter-defibrillators in, 1002
　　ivabradine in, 991t, 997–998, 997f
　　mineralocorticoid receptor antagonists in, 991t–992t, 996, 996b
　　in patients who remain symptomatic, 998–1000
　　patients with symptomatic and asymptomatic, 979
　　physical activity in, 981.e1f
　　n-3 polyunsaturated fatty acids in, 1000
　　preserved ejection fraction and, 1001
　　to prevent progression, 989–998, 991t
　　in refractory end-stage heart failure, 981t, 1003
　nonmedicinal options for, 1698
　pharmacotherapy for, 1698, 1698b
　prognosis of, 975–978, 976f, 977t
　　anemia and, 977.e1f, 976–977
　　biomarkers and, 977.e1f, 976–978, 977t
　　renal insufficiency and, 978, 978f
　race/ethnicity in, 997f, 1001
　screening for, 978b, 980t
　stages of, 978, 979f, 1004t
　transient left ventricular dysfunction and, 979, 980f
　treatment of symptoms approaching end of life, 1004–1005, 1005.e1t
　in women, 1001
　renal function and, 938b–939b
　in sarcoid cardiomyopathy, 1044–1045
　single ventricle and, 1581
　sleep-disordered breathing and, 1683–1684, 1684f
　sudden cardiac death and, 1358f, 1359–1361, 1360f
　tetralogy of Fallot and, 1565
　thyroid hormone levels in, 1804
　Valsalva maneuver in, 135, 136f
　ventricular assist device in, 223b–224b, 224.e1f
　volume status in, 937
　wearable devices and, 120
　in women, 1718–1719
　　diagnosis of, 1719
　　treatment of, 1719, 1720f
Heart Outcomes Prevention Evaluation (HOPE) study, 494
Heart rate
　in coronary artery disease, 181b–182b
　force-frequency relationship and, 908–909, 908f
　in hyperthyroidism, 1799
　myocardial oxygen consumption and, 609
　orthostatic blood pressure and, 1895f, 1897, 1898f
　peak, 181b–182b
　sodium-calcium exchanger and, 899b
　in STEMI, 653
　variability in, 146
Heart rate variability (HRV), 1114–1116
Heart sounds, 130–131
　in amyloidosis, 1044
　diastolic, 131
　first, 130–131
　　in STEMI, 654
　fourth
　　in heart failure, 135, 135.e1f
　　in STEMI, 654
　in heart failure, 937b
　with prosthetic heart valves, 138
　second, 131
　　in STEMI, 654
　in STEMI, 654

Heart sounds *(Continued)*
　systolic, 131, 131f
　third, 131
　　in heart failure, 135.e1f
　　in STEMI, 654
Heart team
　introduction to, 1431
　modern era, 1438.e1
　role of, 1431
Heart to mediastinum ratio (HMR), assessment of, with ^{123}I-MIBG, 303f
Heart transplantation
　in amyloidosis, 1042
　cardiac allograft vasculopathy after, 223
　echocardiography after, 223–224
　mechanical circulatory support bridge to, 1119
　prior, 353
Heart tumor team, 1837
Heartbeat
　apical, 130
　patient description of, 124
HeartMate II, 1123f, 1127, 1127t–1128t
　clinical trials with, 1127.e2, 1128t
HeartMate 3, 1123f, 1127, 1127t–1128t
HeartWare ventricular assist device, 1127–1129, 1127t–1128t
Heat stroke, myocarditis and, 1083.e1
Heated tobacco products, 529–530
Heavy metals, 1601
Helminths, myocardial infection, 1083
Helper T cells, 432
Hemangioma, primary cardiac, 1834t, 1837f
Hematoma
　aortic. *See* Aortic intramural hematoma
　grading scale, 387.e1f
　retroperitoneal, after cardiac catheterization, 386–387
Hemiarch resection, 817
Hemochromatosis, 222, 1048
Hemodynamic stress, biomarkers of, 742–743
Hemodynamics
　monitoring, noncardiac surgery and, 423
　of pulmonary hypertension, 1658–1659
Hemoglobin
　in heart failure, 938b–939b
　in STEMI, 656
Hemolytic anemia, in prosthetic heart valves, 1503
Hemopericardium, 1630b–1633b
Hemoptysis, in adult congenital heart disease, 1543–1544
Hemorrhagic stroke, effects of food and nutrients on, 541t–542t
Hemostasis, 1766–1790
Hemostatic system, 1766–1771
　anticoagulant activity in, 1767, 1767f
　coagulation in, 1769–1770
　fibrinolytic activity in, 1767
　platelets in, 1767–1769, 1767f
　　inhibition of, 1767
Heparin, 1779–1781, 1779t
　anticoagulant effect of, monitoring of, 1780
　bleeding and, 1780–1781
　dosages for, 1780
　elevated levels of transaminases and, 1781
　limitations of, 1780, 1780t
　low-molecular-weight, 1779t, 1781–1782
　　advantages of, 1781t
　　in atrial fibrillation-associated thromboembolism prevention, 1277
　　bleeding and, 1782
　　dosages of, 1782
　　mechanism of action of, 1779f, 1781
　　monitoring of, 1782
　　osteoporosis and, 1782
　　in percutaneous coronary intervention, 801
　　pharmacology of, 1781–1782
　　side effects of, 1782
　　thrombocytopenia and, 1782
　mechanism of action of, 1779, 1779f
　in NSTE-ACS, 726–727
　　low-molecular-weight, 727
　　unfractionated, 726
　osteoporosis and, 1781
　pharmacology of, 1779–1780
　pregnancy and, 1730f
　side effects of, 1780
　for STEMI

Heparin *(Continued)*
　　disadvantages, 675
　　effects of, 675
　　low-molecular-weight, 675, 677f
　thrombocytopenia and, 1781, 1781t
Heparin reversal, 727
Heparin-induced thrombocytopenia (HIT), 1646
Hepatic function, mechanical circulatory support and, 1123–1124, 1123b–1124b
Hepatitis C virus infection
　in adult congenital heart disease, 1544
　cardiac transplantation and, 1135, 1135f
　myocarditis and, 1080b–1081b
Hereditary pulmonary artery hypertension, 1660–1661, 1660t
hERG/K$_v$11.1 channel blockade, 1197–1199
Herpes zoster
　angina pectoris *vs.*, 741
　chest pain in, 600t
Heteroplasmy, 1866–1867
Heuristics, 53–54
HFA-PEFF score, 1011b–1017b
HFrEF. *See* Heart failure; with reduced ejection fraction
Hibernating myocardium, chronic, 633–635, 633f–634f, 634t
　adaptation *vs.* degeneration in, 634b–635b
　apoptosis in, 634b–635b
　cell survival in, 634b–635b
　contractile response in, 634b–635b
　energetics in, 634b–635b
　metabolism in, 634b–635b
　myofibrillar loss, 634b–635b
Hibernation, short-term, 630, 634t
High triglycerides, stable ischemic heart disease and, 752
High-density lipoproteins, 508–509, 513–514
　biogenesis, disorders of, 513
High-dose dopamine, for acute heart failure, 964b
High-risk populations, cardiovascular disease and, 459, 459f, 459.e1f
High-sensitivity C-reactive protein (hsCRP), 107, 455–457, 457f, 457.e1f
High-sensitivity troponin (hsTnT), in heart failure with preserved and mildly reduced ejection, 1011b–1017b
Hirudin, 1783t
　for STEMI, 675, 676f
His bundle pacing, permanent, 1326b, 1326.e2f
Hispanic Americans
　coronary heart disease, 1747
　hypertension in, 1743
　percutaneous coronary interventions for, 1747
　type 2 diabetes in, 1743
His-Purkinje system, disease of, 1361, 1363b–1365b
History
　in chest pain evaluation, 601, 602t
　in STEMI, 653
Holiday heart syndrome, 1363b–1365b
Holter monitoring and event recording, in cardiac arrhythmias, 1151–1155, 1151.e1t, 1154f, 1154.e1f, 1154f–1155f, 1162.e2t, 1162.e3t
Home Blood Pressure Monitoring (HBPM), 482–483
　clinical practice integration of, 483
Homocysteine, 455
　elevated, as risk factor of stroke, 874b–877b
　stable ischemic heart disease and, 742
Hookah pipes, 21
Hookah/Waterpipe, 527b–528b
HOPE-3 trial, 874b–877b
Hormonal replacement therapy, venous thrombosis and, 1774–1775
Hormone therapy
　cardiotoxicity of, 1096–1097
　in lipoprotein disorders, 513
Hosmer-Lemeshow test, 106
Hospice, in heart failure, 1004
Hospitalization, of heart failure with preserved and mildly reduced ejection, 1009–1010
HPS (Heart Protection Study), 874b–877b
HRV. *See* Heart rate variability
Human immunodeficiency virus (HIV) infection
　arrhythmias in, 1612–1613
　atherosclerosis in, 1606f, 1607, 1611f
　biomarkers of inflammation and coagulation are associated with, 1608t
　cardiomyopathy in, 1612

Human immunodeficiency virus (HIV) infection (Continued)
  cardiovascular abnormalities in, 1603–1614
  cardiovascular disease and, 20
  cardiovascular risk factors for, 1603–1605
    chronic kidney disease, 1605
    diabetes, 1605
    dyslipidemia, 1603–1604
    hypertension, 1605
    lipodystrophy, 1604–1605
    metabolic syndrome, 1604–1605
    obesity, 1604–1605
    smoking, 1605, 1605b
  cerebrovascular disease in, 1613
  coronary disease in, 1607–1610
    clinical presentation of, 1608
    epidemiology of, 1607–1608
    treatment of, 1608, 1609t
  echocardiography in, 252b–253b
  heart failure, 1612
  myocarditis and, 1080b–1081b, 1080.e1
  other cardiovascular conditions associated with, 1610–1613
  pericardial disease, 1630b–1633b
  pulmonary arterial hypertension and, 1661
  pulmonary hypertension in, 1610–1612, 1610b–1612b
  screening for coronary risk factors in, 1610
    risk assessment models in, 1610
  sudden cardiac death in, 1612–1613
  treatment of
    lipids in setting of, 1609–1610, 1609b–1610b
Human NPH, in diabetes mellitus, 562t–563t
Hybrid SPECT/CT scanner, 279
Hydatid cyst, myocarditis and, 1083.e1
Hydralazine
  in cardiorenal syndrome, 1889t
  genetic variations in response to, 996.e1
  in heart failure, 997
  in pregnancy, 1730f
Hydrochlorothiazide, in heart failure, 983t
Hydroxychloroquine
  for rheumatic disease, 1826
  for systemic lupus erythematosus, 1811b
Hydroxymethylglutaryl-coenzyme A reductase inhibitors, 515–517
Hyperaldosteronism, primary, 1794–1795, 1794t
Hypercalcemia
  electrocardiography in, 170–171, 170f
  in hyperparathyroidism, 1796–1797
  in sarcoid cardiomyopathy, 1045
Hypercholesterolemia, 75
  autosomal recessive, 510b
  coronary artery disease and, 75, 76f
  familial, 83, 509–510
  polygenic, 510
Hypercoagulable states
  acquired, 1772f, 1772t, 1773–1775
  classification of, 1772t
  inherited, 1772–1773, 1772f, 1772t
  pulmonary embolism and, 1637
Hypercortisolism (Cushing disease), 486–487
Hypereosinophilic syndromes, 1049
Hyperglycemia, with STEMI, 652b
Hyperhomocysteinemia, venous thrombosis and, 1775
Hypericum perforatum (St. John's wort), 1850.e1
Hyperkalemia
  electrocardiography in, 171, 171f
  mineralocorticoid receptor antagonist-related, 988
  pacing thresholds and, 1323b–1324b
Hyperkalemic periodic paralysis, 1864–1865
Hyperlipidemia
  after cardiac transplantation, 1141
  familial combined, 512
  as risk factor of stroke, 874b–877b
  secondary causes of, 513
    hormonal, 513
    lifestyle as, 514
    liver disease as, 514
    medication as, 514
    metabolic, 514
    renal disorders as, 514
  type I, 512–513
Hyperlipoproteinemia, type IV, 511–512
Hypermagnesemia, electrocardiography in, 171b–172b
Hypernatremia
  electrocardiography in, 171b–172b
  in heart failure, 938b–939b

Hyperparathyroidism, 1796–1797, 1797b
  secondary, 1797
Hypersensitivity vasculitides, atheroembolism and, 856
Hypertensin, 3
Hypertension
  acromegaly and, 1791
  after cardiac transplantation, 1140
  air pollution and, 35–36
  arterial stiffness in, 478
  baroreceptor-activation in, 496–497
  blood pressure-lowering medications for, 490
  cardiovascular (CV) risk and, 471
  cardiovascular disease and, 3–4, 447–448, 447.e1f, 447.e2f
    in women, 1710b–1714b, 1711f–1712f
  chronic kidney disease management of, 492–493
  definition of, 471, 472t
  diagnostic approach to, 480–490
    blood pressure measurement of, 481t
    history and physical examination of, 480–481
  drug-induced, 487–488
  effects of food and nutrients on, 541t–542t
  in elderly
    management of, 1704
    pulmonary, 1699
  endocrine causes of, 484–487
    acromegaly, 487
    apparent mineralocorticoid excess states, 485
    hypercortisolism (Cushing disease), 486–487
    pheochromocytoma, 485–486
    primary hyperaldosteronism, 484–485, 484t
    thyroid dysfunction, 487
  endothelium and, 477–478
  epidemiology of, 22–23, 22f, 471–473, 472f–474f, 473t
  ethanol and, 1595
  factors involved in predisposition to, 478–480
  genetics of, 478, 479t–480t
  in heterogeneous populations, 1743, 1744f–1745f, 1747t
    management of, 1745–1747, 1747t
  in HIV patients, cardiovascular risk factors in, 1605
  immune system in, 478, 479f
  integrative strategies for, 595
    acupuncture in, 595
    aerobic exercise in, 595
    breathing exercise in, 595
    DASH diet in, 595
    meditation in, 595
    potassium in, 595
  laboratory and other complementary tests for, 483–484
    echocardiography, 483
    evaluation of sodium and potassium intake, 483
    renin profiling, 483–484
  lifestyle factors of, 487
  natriuretic peptides and, 477
  noncardiac surgery and, 411
  nonendocrine causes of, 487
  nonlifestyle, nonendocrine causes of, 488–490
    coarctation of aorta, 489–490
    intrinsic kidney disease, 488, 488f–489f
    renovascular hypertension, 488–489
  obesity-related, 478–480
  pathophysiology of, 473–478
  from pheochromocytomas, 1796
  pregnancy and, 1730f
    cardiovascular disease in women and, 1710b–1714b
  pressure natriuresis and salt sensitivity in, 473–474, 475f
  prevalence of, 473
  pulmonary, 1656–1660
    anatomy of, 1656
    approach to diagnosis, 1667–1670, 1667b
    classification of, 1657–1662, 1658f–1659f, 1658t
      chronic thromboembolic pulmonary hypertension, 1668f, 1672, 1674f
      pulmonary arterial hypertension, 1660
      combined pre-and post-capillary, 1662
    definition of, 1656
    future perspectives on, 1676
    hemodynamics of, 1658–1659
    in HIV patients, 1610–1612, 1610b–1612b
    isolated post-capillary clinical classifications, 1659–1660
    normal pulmonary circulation, 1656–1657
    pathobiology of, 1662–1665, 1664f

Hypertension (Continued)
  pathology of, 1661f, 1662
    pre-capillary clinical classifications, 1660–1662
    pulmonary venous system, 1657
  renal disease and, 1879–1880
  renin-angiotensin-aldosterone system and, 474–476, 476f
  as risk factor of stroke, 874t–875t, 874b–877b
  sleep-disordered breathing and, 1681–1682
  sodium intake and, 474
  stable ischemic heart disease and, 749–751
  stage 1, 874b–877b
  sudden cardiac death (SCD) and, 1355
  sympathetic nervous system and, 476–477, 477f
  therapeutic options and approaches for subgroups of, 490–492
    pharmacologic intervention in the older people, 490–492
  wearable devices and, 120
  white-coat, 482
Hypertension in the Very Elderly Trial (HYVET), 494
Hypertensive crisis, 1021
  noncardiac surgery and, 411
Hypertensive emergency, 497–498
Hypertensive heart failure, 952, 953t
Hypertensive systolic pressure, in coronary artery disease, 181b–182b
Hypertensive urgency, 497–498
Hyperthermia, malignant, 1363
Hyperthyroidism, 1798–1799
  atrial fibrillation in, 1287.e6t, 1287.e8, 1799–1800
  CHD in, 1800–1801
  diastolic function in, 1798f
  heart failure in, 1800
  hemodynamic alterations in, 1800
  pulmonary hypertension and, 1800
  subclinical, 1800b–1801b, 1801f
Hypertonic saline solution, for acute heart failure, 966b
Hypertriglyceridemia, familial, 511–512
Hypertrophic cardiomyopathy, 1062–1076
  atrial fibrillation in, management of, 1072
  clinical trials and emerging therapies for, 1073–1075
  definition of, 1062, 1063f–1064f
  diagnosis of, 1062–1063, 1065t
  echocardiography in, 220f–221f, 221–222
  etiology of, 1063, 1065t
  exercise and sports participation and, 1072
  genetics of, 1063, 1065t, 1066–1067, 1066f–1067f
  left ventricular hypertrophy in, 1063
  management of, 1069–1071
    alcohol septal ablation in, 1071–1072, 1075f
    atrial fibrillation and, 1072
    family, 1067–1069, 1070f–1071f
    sudden death and, 1070–1071
    surgical myectomy in, 1071, 1074f
  morphology of, 1062–1063, 1064f
  natural history of, 1066, 1069f
  noncardiac surgery and, 411–412
  nonobstructive, 1072
  obstructive, 1071–1072
  pathophysiology of, 1063–1066
    diastolic dysfunction in, 1063–1065
    left ventricular outflow tract obstruction in, 1065, 1068f
  phenotype of, 1063
  pregnancy and, 1068–1069, 1732
  prevalence of, 1063
  sudden cardiac death and
    prevention of, 1069–1070, 1072f
    risk stratification for, 1069–1070
  symptoms in, 1070–1071, 1073f
Hypertrophic myocardial remodeling, aortic valve stenosis and, 1400b–1403b, 1405f
Hypertrophic obstructive cardiomyopathy, 400–401, 400f–401f
Hyperuricemia, atherosclerosis in, 1811
Hypoalbuminemia, in heart failure, 938b–939b
Hypobetalipoproteinemia, 510b
Hypocalcemia, 1797
  electrocardiography in, 170–171, 170f
Hypocapnia, in central sleep apnea (CSA), 1681
Hypokalemia, electrocardiography in, 171, 171f
Hypomagnesemia
  atrial fibrillation and, 1284
  diuretic-induced, 988
  electrocardiography in, 171b–172b

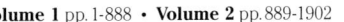

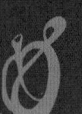

Hyponatremia
 diuretic-induced, 988
 electrocardiography in, 171b–172b
 in heart failure, 938b–939b
Hypoplasia, coronary angiography in, 373b–374b
Hypotension, 1387–1398
 diuretic-induced, 988
 exercise-induced systolic, in coronary artery disease, 181b–182b
 neurally mediated, 1389
 orthostatic, 129, 1387–1388
 orthostatic, definition of, 1896
Hypothalamic-pituitary-adrenal axis, visceral obesity and, 551
Hypothermia
 electrocardiography in, 171f, 171b–172b
 myocarditis and, 1083.e2
Hypothesis
 null, 43–44
 testing, 46
Hypothyroidism, 1801–1803, 1802f
 diastolic function in, 1798f
 in lipoprotein disorders, 513
 subclinical, 1801
 treatment of, 1803b

I

IABP. *See* Intra-aortic balloon pump
IART. *See* Interatrial re-entrant tachycardia
IAST. *See* Inappropriate sinus tachycardia
Ibrutinib, 1104
 cardiotoxic effects of, 1092t
Ibutilide, 1211.e1t, 1209t, 1212t, 1214t, 1223, 1223b
ICDs. *See* Implantable cardioverter-defibrillators
ICU. *See* Intensive care unit
Idarubicin, cardiotoxic effects of, 1092t
Idarucizumab, 1786, 1786t
IDI. *See* Integrated discrimination improvement
Idiopathic acute pericarditis, 1616
Idiopathic pulmonary arterial hypertension, 1658–1659
Idiopathic ventricular fibrillation (IVF), 1205
 clinical description and manifestations of, 1205
 genetic basis of, 1205.e1f, 1205b
Idiopathic VT/PVCs, 1242, 1242b
I$_f$-Channel inhibitor, in heart failure, 997–998
IGF-1. *See* Insulin-like growth factor type 1
IHMs. *See* Implantable hemodynamic monitors
Iliac artery
 aortoiliac disease, 864
 perforated external, with covered stent, 862.e1f
 stenosis in, 861f
Iloprost, in thromboangiitis obliterans, 852–853
ILRs. *See* Implantable loop recorders
Imatinib, 1096
 cardiotoxic effects of, 1092t
Immobilization, venous thrombosis and, 1774
Immune checkpoint inhibitors, cardiotoxic effects of, 1092t, 1094
Immune-modulating agents, cardiotoxic effects of, 1092t
Immune system, in hypertension, 478, 479f
Immunoglobulin (Ig), 430–431
Immunosuppression
 in cardiac transplantation, 1136–1137
 in myocarditis, 1088–1089
Impact studies, in biomarkers, 107
Impaired renal function, in heart failure with preserved and mildly reduced ejection, 1011b–1017b
Impella, 798
Impella device, 1121f, 1125t
Implantable cardioverter-defibrillators (ICDs), 1208, 1331–1333, 1333f
 in cardiovascular disease in women, 1719
 in chronic kidney disease, 1887–1888
 common clinical issues in, 1346–1347
  driving and, 1347
  drug interactions, 1347
  lifestyle issues, 1347
  participation in sports, 1347
  psychosocial issues, 1344f, 1346–1347, 1346.e1t
 complications of, 1343, 1343.e1t
  lead placement, 1343
  leadless pacemaker, 1343
  pocket hematoma and CIED infections, 1343, 1343.e2f

Implantable cardioverter-defibrillators (ICDs) *(Continued)*
  subcutaneous, 1343
  vascular access, 1343
 for congenital heart disease, 1549, 1549t, 1550f
 conventional, 1331
 device longevity and replacement considerations, 1345b–1346b
 device radiography, 1321, 1321f–1324f
 dual-chamber, 1331, 1332b–1333b, 1335
 electrograms and, 1338f
 follow-up and management of, 1343–1347
  device clinic follow-up, 1344
  remote monitoring, 1343–1344, 1343.e3f
 general considerations of, 1336–1339
  antitachycardia pacing, 1337b–1339b, 1341f
  defibrillation and cardioversion shock therapy, 1337b–1339b, 1339.e1f, 1342f
 generators, 1332b–1333b
 in heart failure, 1002, 1111–1113, 1111b–1113b, 1112t
  DANISH trial of, 1111b–1113b
  DEFINITE trial of, 1111b–1113b
  MADIT II trial of, 1111b–1113b
  SCD-HeFT trial of, 1111b–1113b, 1113f
 indications for, 1331–1333
  primary prevention, 1332–1333, 1335f, 1336t, 1337f
  secondary prevention, 1331–1332, 1332t, 1334f–1335f
 lead failure, 1341–1343
  approach to patient, 1343, 1346f
  clinical presentations of, 1341–1343, 1346f
  imaging of, 1343, 1343.e1f
  impedance and impedance trends in diagnosis of, 1342b–1343b, 1342.e1f
 leads of, 1332b–1333b, 1338f
 in myocarditis, 1089
 sensing and detection of, 1334b–1335b, 1334f–1336f, 1336.e1t, 1336.e2f, 1339f–1340f, 1339t
 subcutaneous, 1321, 1331
 in sudden cardiac death, 1377t, 1380f
 system selection of, 1333–1336
  dual- *vs.* single-chamber transvenous, 1333–1334
  transvenous *vs.* subcutaneous, 1334–1336, 1334.e1t
 therapy, 1336–1339
 transvenous, 1331
 transvenous defibrillation leads, 1334b–1335b
  dual *vs.* single coil, 1334b–1335b
  integrated *vs.* dedicated sensing bipoles, 1334b–1335b
 troubleshooting of, 1339–1343
  failure to deliver therapy or delayed therapy, 1340–1341
  shocks, 1339–1340, 1340.e1t, 1344f–1345f
  ventricular oversensing, 1339, 1339b, 1339.e2f
 types of, 1331, 1333f
Implantable hemodynamic monitors (IHMs), 1116–1117, 1117f
Implantable loop recorders (ILRs), 1154.e2f, 1162.e1
Implantable monitors, 1153–1154, 1154.e2f
Implanted devices, atrial fibrillation in, 1287.e6t
IMR. *See* Index of microcirculatory resistance
In hospital electrocardiographic recording, 1151, 1154f
Inactivity, mortality and, 15–16, 16t
Inappropriate sinus tachycardia (IAST), 1234, 1245, 1251–1252, 1252b
 atrial tachycardias *vs.*, 1248b–1249b, 1249f
Inclisiran, in coronary heart disease, 560
Income, cardiovascular disease and, 67
Indapamide, in heart failure, 983t
Index of microcirculatory resistance (IMR), 748
Indirect annuloplasty, in mitral regurgitation, 1486b–1488b, 1490f
Individualized exercise programs, for congenital heart disease, 1553, 1555f, 1556t
Indoor air pollution, 33–34
Inducible NO synthase (iNOS), 1018b–1020b
INE. *See* Inferior nodal extension
Infected aortic aneurysms, 832
Infection
 18F-FDG for, 284b
 atherosclerosis and, 440
Infectious disease, of pericardium, 1630b–1633b
Infectious pulmonary artery hypertension subtypes, 1661

Infective endocarditis, 1505–1525
 aerobic Gram-negative bacilli causing, 1506b–1507b
  antimicrobial therapy for, 1519b–1523b
 anticoagulant therapy for, 884–886
 antimicrobial therapy in, 1519b–1523b
  blood cultures for, 1525
  for dental procedures, 1530.e1t
  for implantable electronic devices, 1526
  for left ventricular assist device infection, 1528
  outpatient management and follow-up evaluation for, 1525, 1526t
 cardiac biomarkers in, 1511b–1512b
 clinical presentation of, 1507–1508
 in congenital heart disease, 1508
 Coxiella burnetii infection and, 1510–1511
 culture-negative, 1506b–1507b, 1512t, 1519b–1523b, 1523t
 diagnosis of, 1510–1523
  complete blood count in, 1511b–1512b
  electrocardiography in, 1512–1513, 1513f
  erythrocyte sedimentation rate (ESR) in, 1511b–1512b, 1512t
  imaging in, 1513–1523, 1513f–1516f, 1516t–1517t
  procalcitonin in, 1511b–1512b
  serum creatinine in, 1511b–1512b
 differential diagnosis of, 1513–1515
 Duke criteria for, 1510–1511, 1511t
 echocardiography in, 248–253, 251f
 embolism in, 1518–1524
 enterococcal species causing, 1506b–1507b
 epidemiology of, 1505–1507
 fungi causing, 1506b–1507b
 guidelines for, 1530.e1
 HACEK organisms causing, 1522.e2t, 1506b–1507b, 1512t, 1519b–1523b
 heart failure and, 1508
 local valvular destruction in, 1515–1516
 microbiology of, 1506b–1507b, 1511b–1512b, 1512t
 mitral regurgitation in, 1508, 1514f
 pathogenesis of, 1507
 perivalvular extension of, 1516–1517
 physical examination in, 1508–1510, 1510t
 predisposing cardiac conditions in, 1507–1508
 in prosthetic heart valves, 1503
  prophylaxis for, 1499
 prosthetic valves and, 1522.e1t–e2t, 1522.e1t–e2t, 1522.e1t–e2t, 1522.e1t–e2t, 1511b–1512b
 radionuclide imaging in, 307–310, 308f–309f
 Staphylococcal species causing, 1506b–1507b, 1512t
 Streptococcal species causing, 1506b–1507b, 1512t
  antimicrobial therapy for, 1519t–1521t, 1519b–1523b
 surgery in, 1530.e1
  ACC/AHA guidelines for, 1530.e2t, 1530.e2t
  European Society of Cardiology guidelines for, 1530.e3t
  indications for and timing of, 1523–1525, 1525t
 symptoms in, 1508, 1509f, 1510t
 thrombotic, 1507
 valvular cardiac conditions and, 1505
 vegetations in, 1513–1515, 1524
Inferior nodal extension (INE), 1175, 1177f
Inferior vena cava (IVC) filters, for massive pulmonary embolism, 1650, 1650f
Infiltrative cardiomyopathy, radionuclide imaging in, 303–304, 304f–305f
Inflammasomes
 inhibition of, 1825b
 in myocarditis, 1085.e1
Inflammation
 18F-FDG for, 284b
 in abdominal aortic aneurysms, 807
 in atherogenesis, 432, 433f
 biomarkers of, 455–457, 457f, 457.e1f
 cardiovascular disease and, 9
 in peripheral artery disease, 838
 in pulmonary embolism, 1637
 in stable ischemic heart disease, 753–756, 753f
Inflammatory cardiomyopathy, radionuclide imaging in, 304–307, 304f–307f
Inflammatory heart disease, ventricular tachycardia in, 1302–1303
Inflammatory mechanisms, in acute heart failure, 951
Inflammatory mediators, in heart failure, 920b–921b, 921f, 922t

Influenza, 1751–1765
　acute myocardial infarction and, 1752
　antiviral therapies for, 1754
　arrhythmia risk and, 1753
　cardiovascular risk and disease, 1751–1754, 1751b–1752b
　epidemiology of, 1752–1753
　heart failure and, 1752, 1752f
　myocarditis and, 1753
　pathophysiology of, 1753b
　prevention and therapy of, 1754
　vaccine formulations, 1754
　virology, 1751b–1752b
Influenza virus infection, myocarditis and, 1080b–1081b
Informed consent, 48–49
Inherited aortopathies, pregnancy and, 1740, 1740.e1f
Innate immunity
　in atherosclerosis, 432, 433f
　in myocarditis, 1085.e1
INOCA. See Ischemia with nonobstructive coronary arteries
Inodilators, for acute heart failure, 962t, 963–964
iNOS. See Inducible NO synthase
Inotropes, in acute heart failure, 962t, 963–964, 971b–972b
Inotropic infusion, 1005.e2
Insertable loop recorders, in cardiac arrhythmias, 1151–1155
Inspiratory crackles, in acute heart failure, 953
InSTIs. See Integrase strand transfer inhibitors
Insulin, in glucose management, 562t–563t, 566, 572
Insulin-like growth factor type 1 (IGF-1), 1791
Insulin resistance, cardiovascular disease and, 448–449
Insulin Resistance Intervention after Stroke (IRIS) trial, 874b–877b
Insurance coverage, 62–63, 63f
Integrase strand transfer inhibitors (InSTIs), 1603, 1604t
Integrated diagnostic approach, for pulmonary embolism, 1644, 1647f
Integrated discrimination improvement (IDI), 106–107
Integrated sensing bipoles, dedicated vs., 1334b–1335b
Integrative cardiology, 593–594
　acupuncture in, 593b–594b
　elements of, 594f
　mind/body therapy in, 593b–594b
　nutrition in, 593b–594b
　supplements in, 593b–594b, 594t
Intensive care, postoperative, noncardiac surgery and, 419b
Intensive care unit (ICU), STEMI and, 679–680
Interatrial block, ECG and, 151b
Interatrial re-entrant tachycardia (IART), 1547–1548, 1548f
Interatrial septum, lipomatous hypertrophy in, echocardiography in, 253b
Intercalated discs, 1173–1175, 1175f
Interference, 1315
Interleukin-1, inhibition of, 1825b
Interleukin-6
　in chest pain evaluation, 603b
　inhibition of, 1825b
Interleukin-12, inhibition of, 1825b
Interleukin-17, inhibition of, 1825b
Interleukin-23, inhibition of, 1825b
Intermediate-density lipoprotein, 505b–506b, 507f
Intermediate-dose dopamine, for acute heart failure, 964b
Intermediate-risk pulmonary embolism, 1639
Intermittent claudication
　pathophysiology of, 839f
　prevalence of, 837–838, 837.e1f
Internal mammary artery grafts, cannulation for, 367b–368b, 369f
Internal work, 909b–910b
Internal work rate, 579
International INTERSTROKE study, 873–874
International Society of Heart and Lung Transplantation (ISHLT), 1132
Interrupted aortic arch, 1576–1577
Intestinal pathway, 505b–506b, 507f
Intima, 427, 428f–429f
　in aorta, 806b, 808f
　intravascular imaging in, 379
Intra-aortic balloon pump (IABP), 7, 1120f, 1125–1126, 1125f, 1126f
Intraatrial septum, lipomatous hypertrophy of, echocardiography in, 1829b, 1832f

Intracardiac shunts, mechanical circulatory support and, 1124.e1
Intracardiac thrombus, echocardiography in, 255–256, 256f
Intramural hematoma, aortic, 831, 831.e2f, 833f
　computed tomography in, 831f–832f, 832, 832.e1f
　echocardiography in, 246f
　high-risk features of, 831.e2t
　magnetic resonance imaging in, 831, 831.e2f
　transesophageal echocardiograms in, 831, 831f–832f
Intraoperative ventricular mapping, 1243b
Intravascular imaging, in percutaneous coronary interventions, 796, 796f–797f, 796t–797t
Intravascular lithotripsy, in peripheral artery disease, 863, 863.e3f
Intravascular Lithotripsy (IVL) System, 794
Intravascular ultrasound, 378–380, 378b–379b, 379f–380f
　in NSTE-ACS, 719
Intravenous beta blockers, 722
Intravenous recombinant tissue plasminogen activator, for acute ischemic stroke, 880–881, 881f–883f, 881b, 882t
Intraventricular conduction delays, 156–160
　acceleration (tachycardia)-dependent block, 160f, 160b
　deceleration (bradycardia)-dependent block, 160f, 160b
Intraventricular conduction disturbance, 1156b–1159b, 1157f
Intrinsic kidney disease, 488, 488f–489f
Intrinsic neuronal control, 1893
Invasive assessment, for STEMI, 668b–669b
Invasive electrophysiologic testing, in cardiac arrhythmias, 1156–1159
Invasive hemodynamic strategy, for acute heart failure, 959–960
Invasive procedures, for cardiovascular disease, 2–3
Investigational leadless devices, 1321
Inwardly rectifying cardiac K+ channels, 1171b–1173b
Iodinated contrast-induced acute kidney injury and, 1875
Iodixanol, contrast-induced acute kidney injury and, 1876–1877
Ion channels, 1171
　abnormalities in, atrial fibrillation and, 1187b
　cardiac pacemaker channel, 1171b–1173b
　electrogenic transporters and, 1171b–1173b
　ionic current modulation and, 1163b–1166b
　membrane voltages of, 1163b–1166b
　molecular structure of, 1171–1173
　Nernst potential of, 1163b–1166b
　permeability ratio of, 1163b–1166b
　physiology of, 1163–1166, 1164f, 1165t–1166t, 1167f
　voltage-gated
　　Ca^{2+}, 1171b–1173b
　　ion flux through, 1163b–1166b, 1167f
　　K^+, 1171b–1173b
　　Na^+, 1171b–1173b, 1172f
Ionic current modulation, 1163b–1166b
IP_3 receptor (IP3R), 1183.e1f, 1181b–1183b
IRIS trial, 1336t
Iron overload (hemochromatosis), magnetic resonance imaging in, 314b–320b, 327–328
Ischemia
　in coronary artery disease, 777–779
　critical limb, 859
　evidence of, 777
Ischemia with nonobstructive coronary arteries (INOCA), 1696–1697
Ischemic cardiomyopathy, 779–780
　echocardiography in, 220f, 221
　patients with, 298–303
　percutaneous coronary interventions in, 792
　quantitative myocardial perfusion imaging in, 300f
Ischemic heart disease, 1242–1243, 1243f
　air pollution and, 35
　integrative strategies for, 594–595
　　antioxidants, 595
　　meditation in, 594
　　mind/heart connection in, 594–595
　　multivitamins, 595
　　nutrition in, 594
　　omega-3 fatty acids, 595
　　tai chi in, 594
　pregnancy-associated, 1733–1734
　radionuclide imaging in patients with, 290–298

Ischemic heart disease (Continued)
　　evaluation before organ transplantation, 292–293
　　patients with known stable coronary artery disease, 294–298
　　perfusion imaging, principles of, 290
　　suspected acute coronary syndrome, 293–294
　　suspected stable coronary artery disease, 290–292
　　symptomatic patients without angiographically obstructive coronary artery disease, 292
　secondary prevention of sudden cardiac death with, 1334f
　stable, 739–762
　　coronary artery bypass grafting for, 770–776
　　diagnosis of
　　　coronary angiography for, 747
　　　coronary computed tomography angiography for, 747f
　　　exercise electrocardiography for, 745b–746b
　　　noninvasive studies for, 744–748
　　　resting electrocardiography for, 744
　　dual-antiplatelet therapy for, 754b–756b
　　evaluation and management of, 742–758
　　　advanced structural coronary imaging in, 748
　　　angiography in, 748, 748.e1f
　　　biochemical tests for, 742–744
　　　biomarkers in, 742–743, 743f
　　　chest roentgenography in, 744
　　　computed tomography in, 746–747, 747f
　　　exercise electrocardiography in, 745b–746b, 746t
　　　functional assessment in, 748
　　　genetic and transcriptomic biomarkers in, 743–744, 744f
　　　inflammatory biomarkers in, 743
　　　invasive assessment in, 748–749
　　　magnetic resonance imaging in, 747–748
　　　noninvasive testing for, 744–748
　　　resting echocardiography in, 744
　　　resting electrocardiography in, 744
　　　stress echocardiography in, 745b–746b
　　　stress myocardial perfusion imaging in, 745b–746b, 746t
　　　stress testing in, 745–746, 745t
　　future perspectives in, 781
　　magnitude of problem with, 739
　　medical management of, 749–757
　　　counseling and changes in lifestyle for, 756–757
　　　risk factors reduction in, 749–756
　　natural history of, 749
　　noninvasive tests for, 746t
　　pathophysiology of, 740f–741f
　　percutaneous coronary intervention for, 766
　　　atrial fibrillation in, 772.e1
　　　cerebrovascular complications in, 772.e1
　　　coronary artery bypass surgery vs., 775.e2f, 774–775, 775f–776f, 776.e1t
　　　early outcome of, 766b
　　　effects on survival, 772–773
　　　fractional flow reserve strategy in, 765, 769f
　　　left ventricular dysfunction, 769b–770b
　　　long-term outcome of, 766b
　　　medical therapy vs., 766–769, 767f–769f
　　　in multivessel disease, 776
　　　myocardial infarction in, 772.e1
　　　operative mortality in, 772
　　　patient selection in, 771f–772f, 772, 772.e2f
　　　perioperative complications, 772
　　　perioperative complications in, 772.e1
　　　previous coronary bypass grafting and, 770–776
　　　renal dysfunction in, 772.e2
　　　reoperation in, 774
　　　revascularization for, 769–770
　　　in single-vessel disease, 776
　　　surgical outcomes and long-term results in, 772–773
　　　in women and older patients, 769b–770b
　　revascularization for, 764–766, 776
　　　fractional flow reserve in, 765
　　　indications for, 780
　　　ischemia and left ventricular dysfunction in, 765, 765.e1t
　　　patient selection for, 765–766
　　　presence and severity of symptoms of, 765
　　　risk associated with, 765–766
　　　significance of coronary lesions in, 765
　　risk factor modification for, 764
　　risk stratification in, 749, 750f

Volume 1 pp. 1-888 • **Volume 2** pp. 889-1902

Ischemic heart disease *(Continued)*
    surgical treatment of, 773–774
        with diabetes, 774
        in older patients, 774
        with renal disease, 774
        in women, 773–774
    stable, percutaneous coronary intervention in, 786–787
    in women, 1714–1716
        diagnosis of, 1715
        interventions and medical therapy for, 1715–1716
        symptoms of, 1714–1715
Ischemic heart failure, myocardial viability imaging to guide revascularization in patients with, 301–303, 301f–302f
Ischemic left ventricular dysfunction, pathophysiology of, 298
Ischemic preconditioning, 666
Ischemic stroke
    classification of, 870–873, 870b–873b, 871t–872t, 872f
    effects of food and nutrients on, 541t–542t
    future directions of, 886b
    prevention and management of, 870–888, 871f, 871t
    secondary prevention of, 878–879
        anticoagulant therapy, 878–879, 879b
        antiplatelet therapy, 878, 878f–879f, 879b
ISHLT. *See* International Society of Heart and Lung Transplantation
Isolated calf deep vein thrombosis, 1640b–1641b
Isolated valvular pulmonary stenosis, 1562
Isoproterenol, cardiac catheterization and, 407–408
Isosorbide 5-mononitrate, for angina pectoris, 762, 762t
Isosorbide dinitrate
    for angina pectoris, 762, 762t
    genetic variations in response to, 996.e1
Isradipine, for angina pectoris, 760, 761t
Istaroxime, for acute heart failure, 971b–972b
Iterative hypothesis testing, 54
Ivabradine, 1211.e1t, 1208t–1209t, 1214t
    in angina pectoris, 763.e1
    in cardiorenal syndrome, 1889t
    in heart failure, 991t, 997–998, 997f
IVF. *See* Idiopathic ventricular fibrillation

J

J wave, 149, 171f, 171b–172b
J wave syndromes, 1308–1309
Jaccoud arthropathy, 1533, 1533f, 1534t
Jarvik 2000, 1130–1131
Jeopardized myocardium, percutaneous coronary interventions in, 787
Jetstream, 862–863
jSR. *See* Junctional sarcoplasmic reticulum
Judkins catheter, for coronary angiography, 367, 367f
Judkins technique, for femoral artery access, 387
Jugular venous pressure (JVP), 126–128
    in acute heart failure, 953
    in heart failure, 135, 136f, 937
    in STEMI, 654
Junctional ectopic tachycardia, 1263f, 1263b
Junctional sarcoplasmic reticulum (jSR), 889
JUP gene, 1039b–1040b
JUPITER (Justification for the Use of Statin in Prevention: An Intervention Trial Evaluating Rosuvastatin), 874b–877b
JVP. *See* Jugular venous pressure

K

Kansas City Cardiomyopathy Questionnaire overall score (KCCQ-OS), 1432.e1
Kaplan-Meier curves, 47f
Karnofsky Index, 1139
Kawasaki disease, 1814–1815
    cardiovascular complications of, 1815
    diagnosis of, 1815
    pathogenesis of, 1815
    treatment of, 1815
KCCQ-OS. *See* Kansas City Cardiomyopathy Questionnaire overall score
KCNE1, 95t, 1198
KCNE2, 1198
KCNE3, 1192f
KCNH2, 1191b–1193b, 1192f, 1194f, 1196f
KCNJ2, 1197b, 1199
KCNQ1, 1191b–1193b, 1192f, 1194f, 1196f

Kearns-Sayre syndrome, 1866–1867
Khat *(Catha edulis)*, cardiovascular complications of, 1599
Kidneys
    in heart failure with preserved and mildly reduced ejection, 1011b–1017b
    hypertension and, 474
"Kissing stents", 864
Kommerell diverticulum, thoracic aortic aneurysms in, 814
Kreteks, 21
Kussmaul sign, 128
    in constrictive pericarditis, 1626–1627
Kv1.5α subunits, 1171b–1173b
KvLQT1 subunit
    α, 1171b–1173b
    mutations in, 1166b–1170b

L

LA conduit strain, 1011b–1017b
LA longitudinal strain, 1011b–1017b
LA reservoir strain, 1011b–1017b
LAA. *See* Left atrial appendage
Labetalol, for angina pectoris, 758t
Labor, hemodynamic changes during, 1723–1724
Lactation
    cardiovascular medications during, 1730f
    pericardial disease during, 1630b–1633b
Lacunar strokes, 870b–873b, 871t–872t
LAE. *See* Left atrial enlargement
Laser atherectomy, for peripheral artery disease, 863, 863.e2f
LBBB. *See* Left bundle branch block
LD. *See* Linkage disequilibrium
LDL cholesterol, 454
LDL-C. *See* Low-density lipoprotein cholesterol
LDLR gene, 75
Leadless pacemakers, 1321
Leaflet clip devices, for tricuspid regurgitation, 1492
Leaflet repair with MitraClip device, in mitral regurgitation, 1485–1488, 1488f–1489f
Learning, 109
Leber hereditary optic neuropathy, 1866–1867
Lecithin-cholesterol acyltransferase deficiency, 513
Left atrial appendage (LAA)
    coronary computed tomography angiography in, 359–361, 360f
    excision or closure of, 1277, 1278f
Left atrial enlargement (LAE), chest radiography in, 269, 269f–270f
Left atrial function, in rheumatic mitral stenosis, 1442–1443
Left atrial pressure, in rheumatic mitral stenosis, 1442, 1444f
Left atrium, 1544–1545
    to aorta assist device, 1121f, 1127
    echocardiography of, 204t, 210
    strain measures of, 1011b–1017b
Left bundle branch area pacing, 1326b, 1326.e2f, 1326.e3f
Left bundle branch block (LBBB)
    clinical significance of, 158
    electrocardiography in, 157–158, 157f, 157b–158b, 158t
    incomplete, 157
    myocardial infarction and, 165, 166f–167f
Left coronary artery, cannulation for, 367–368b, 368f
Left coronary dominance, in angiographic projection, 372, 372.e1f
Left heart structural and functional disorders, 1662
Left main coronary artery disease, percutaneous coronary intervention in, 787–789, 788t–789t, 790f–791f
Left ventricle
    age-associated changes in
        in composition and mass, 1687b–1690b
        in thickness, cavity size, and shape, 1687b–1690b
    aneurysms of, 218b–219b
    to aorta assist device, 1127
    contraction of, 904, 905f, 906t
    echocardiography of, 204–205, 204t, 205f–206f, 205f
    relaxation of, 904, 905f, 906t
    remodeling and function, 1419b–1420b
    thrombus, 218b–219b, 220f
Left ventricular aneurysm, 780, 780.e1f
Left ventricular angiography, of primary mitral regurgitation, 1462b

Left ventricular assist device
    for congenital heart disease, 1551
    patient with, 137.e1f
Left ventricular contractility, myocardial oxygen consumption and, 609
Left ventricular diastolic function, aortic valve stenosis and, 1400b–1403b
Left ventricular ejection fraction (LVEF)
    after myocardial infarction, 218b–219b
    in dilated cardiomyopathy, 221
    on echocardiography, 205–206
    sudden cardiac death (SCD) and, 1356, 1360f
Left ventricular failure, ST-elevation myocardial infarction and, 685–690, 686f
    afterload reduction for, 687
    beta-adrenergic agonists for, 687–690, 688t–689t
    digitalis, 687
    diuretics for, 686–687
    glucose-lowering agents for, 687
    hypoxemia, 686
    nitroglycerin for, 687
    oral vasodilators for, 687
    other positive inotropic agents for, 690
    therapeutic implications for, 686
    vasoactive medications for, 687
    vasopressors for, 690
Left ventricular function/dysfunction, 649–651
    in cardiac arrest survivors, 1368–1369
    percutaneous coronary intervention and, 792, 792.e1f
    in rheumatic mitral stenosis, 1443
    stable ischemic heart disease and, percutaneous coronary intervention in, 769b–770b
Left ventricular hypertrophy (LVH)
    coronary flow reserve and, 623b–627b, 625f
    drug adjustments in, 99
    electrocardiography in, 152–154, 152f–153f, 152b–153b, 153t
    in Friedreich ataxia, 1864, 1864f
    in HIV patients, 1610
    in hypertrophic cardiomyopathy, 1063
Left ventricular noncompaction cardiomyopathy, 1041, 1041.e2t
    echocardiography in, 220f, 1829b, 1831f
Left ventricular outflow tract obstruction, in hypertrophic cardiomyopathy, 1065, 1068f
Left ventricular regional function, echocardiography of, 206b–208b, 207.e1f
Left ventricular remodeling and function
    after myocardial infarction, 218b–219b
    in heart failure, 921–930, 921.e1f, 922t
        reversibility of, 930–931, 930.e2t, 931f, 931b
    in mitral regurgitation, 1486b–1488b, 1490f
Left ventricular response, aortic valve stenosis and, 1400b–1403b
Left ventricular structure, alterations of, in heart failure, 930, 930.e1t, 931f
Left ventricular systolic dysfunction, patients with newly diagnosed, 298
Left ventriculography, for coronary angiography, 369–370, 369f–370f
Left-to-right shunt lesions, 1554, 1556f, 1556t
Leigh syndrome, 1866–1867
Lenègre disease, sudden cardiac death in, 1361, 1363b–1365b
Lepirudin, 1783
Lesion calcification, in percutaneous coronary intervention, 791–792
Lethal arrhythmias
    acute ischemia and initiation of, 1366
    transition from myocardial instability to, 1366
Lethal reperfusion, 668
Letrozole, cardiotoxic effects of, 1092t
Leukocyte, recruitment and retention, in atherosclerosis initiation, 430–431, 430f
Leuprolide, cardiotoxic effects of, 1092t
Lev disease, 1361, 1363b–1365b
Lev-Lenègre disease, 1205
Levosimendan, for acute heart failure, 965, 965b
Levothyroxine, 1803b
LGBT population, cardiovascular disease in, 1744
Libman-Sacks endocarditis, in systemic lupus erythematosus, 1820
Lidocaine, 1211.e1t, 1209t, 1212t, 1214t, 1216–1217, 1216b
    pregnancy and, 1730f
Life expectancy, 25
Lifestyle issues, cardiac implantable electrical devices and, 1347

Lifestyle modification
  in congestive heart failure, 596
  for heart failure with preserved and mildly reduced ejection, 1028
  in lipoprotein disorders, 514
    changes of, 521
  in visceral obesity, 551
Likelihood ratio, 56
Limb-girdle muscular dystrophy, 1861–1863, 1862f–1863f
Limb vascular events, treatment of symptoms and prevention of, 849–851
Linagliptin, in diabetes mellitus, 562t–563t
Linezolid, for infective endocarditis, 1519b–1523b
Linkage disequilibrium (LD), 73, 73t
Lipid-lowering therapy, 515t
  in atheroembolism, 856
  in chronic kidney disease, 1880–1881, 1883t
  in NSTE-ACS, 731–732, 732f
  in peripheral artery disease, 848, 848.e1f, 848.e2f
  in stable ischemic heart disease, 772
Lipid management, guidelines for, 523–524
Lipid metabolism, ethanol and, 1594, 1595f
Lipid risk, pharmacologic management of, 515–521
  bile acid-binding resins in, 519
  ezetimibe in, 518
  fibric acid derivatives in, 518
  fish oils in, 519–520
  hydroxymethylglutaryl-coenzyme A reductase inhibitors in, 515–517
  nicotinic acid in, 518–519
  novel medications in, 520–521
  PCSK9 inhibitors in, 517–518
  phytosterols in, 520
  pure eicosapentaenoic acid in, 519–520
Lipids, 23
  biochemistry of, 502–504, 503t–504t, 505f
  biomarkers and, 107
  dietary reduction of, 28–29
Lipodystrophy
  genetic forms of, 550
  in HIV patients, cardiovascular risk factors in, 1604–1605
Lipomas, 1833, 1834t, 1835f
  echocardiography in, 253b
Lipomatous hypertrophy, echocardiography in, 253b
Lipoprotein(a), 455, 455.e1f, 510
  inhibition of, 520–521
Lipoprotein(s), 504–505, 506f
  causal inference for, 79
  disorders of, 502–524.e1
    definition of, 509
    genetic, 509–510, 509t
    treatment of, 521–522
      in combined lipoprotein disorders, 521–522
      diet as, 521
      gene therapy as, 522
      residual cardiovascular risk, 522
      societal changes in, 522–523
  future perspectives in, 522–523
  high-density, 508–509, 513–514
    disorders of, 513
    in STEMI, 655
    in women, 1710b–1714b
  intermediate-density, 505b–506b, 507f
  low-density, 506–507, 508f, 509–510
    in hypothyroidism, 1802
    receptor gene, 510
    in women, 1710b–1714b
  metabolism of, 505–509
    hepatic pathway in, 505b–506b, 507f
    intestinal pathway in, 505b–506b, 507f
  plasma, composition of, 503t
  processing enzymes in, 504–505, 506f
  receptors of, 504–505, 504t, 506f
  transport of, 502–509, 507f
  triglyceride-rich, 510–513, 511t
  very-low-density, 505b–506b, 507f
Lipoprotein-x, 514
Liraglutide, in diabetes mellitus, 562t–563t, 567
Lisinopril, in heart failure, 991t
Lispro, in diabetes mellitus, 562t–563t
Livedo reticularis, atheroembolism and, 856
Liver disease
  in adult congenital heart disease, 1544
  drug adjustments in, 99
  in lipoprotein disorders, 514
Liver, in heart failure with preserved and mildly reduced ejection, 1011b–1017b

Lixisenatide, in diabetes mellitus, 562t–563t, 567
Lixivaptan, in heart failure, 983t
LMNA gene, 1036
LMWH. See Low-molecular-weight heparin
Local R wave, 1324b–1326b
Loeffler (eosinophilic) endocarditis, echocardiography in, 222
Loeys-Dietz syndrome, 1740
  thoracic aortic aneurysms in, 811, 811t, 814f
Löffler (eosinophilic) endocarditis, 1049
Löffler's cardiomyopathy, 327f
Long QT syndrome (LQTS), 1191–1195, 1305f–1306f, 1307–1308
  auditory triggers of, 1193, 1196f
  calmodulinopathic, 1195
  cardiac arrhythmia and, 1183, 1183.e1f
  clinical description and manifestations of, 1191–1193, 1192f
  exercise electrocardiographic testing in, 190b–191b
  exertion-induced, 1193
  genetic basis of, 1192.e1t-e3t, 1191b–1193b, 1192f
  management of, 1308
  risk stratification for, 1193
  single nucleotide polymorphisms in, 1195
  sleep/rest-related, 1193, 1196f
  sudden cardiac death and, 1191, 1361–1362, 1382–1383
  three canonical, phenotypic correlates for, 1193–1195, 1195f–1196f
Longitudinal magnetization recovery, 314
Long-term care, for elderly, cardiovascular disease in, 1694
Loop diuretics, 982, 982b, 983t, 984f
  genetic variations in response to, 996.e2
Losartan
  drug interaction with, 97t
  in heart failure, 991t–992t, 993
Losmapimod, for STEMI, 684
Lovastatin, drug interaction with, 97t
Low-attenuation plaque, coronary computed tomography angiography in, 344, 344.e1f
Low-density lipoprotein cholesterol (LDL-C)
  effects of food and nutrients on, 541t–542t
  elevated, stroke and, 874b–877b
Low-density lipoproteins, 506–507, 508f, 509–510
  receptor gene, 510
Low-dose dopamine, for acute heart failure, 964b
Low-gradient aortic stenosis
  with preserved LVEF, 1411t, 1412
  with reduced LVEF, 1411–1412, 1411t
  transcatheter aortic valve replacement in, 1437.e1
Low high-density lipoprotein cholesterol, in stable ischemic heart disease, 751–752
Low-molecular-weight heparin (LMWH)
  in NSTE-ACS, 727
  in pregnancy, 1737
  in pulmonary embolism, 1646
  for STEMI, 675, 677f
  for vascular disease, 1100
Low-pressure tamponade, 1621
Low-risk populations, cardiovascular disease and, 458–459
Low-risk pulmonary embolism, 1639
Lower extremities
  deep vein thrombosis, 1640b–1641b, 1641f
  evaluation of, 126
  peripheral arterial disease of, 864–865
    in elderly, 1709.e1
LQTS. See Long QT syndrome
Lung disease, pulmonary arterial hypertension associated with, 1662
Lung function, abnormal, in adult congenital heart disease, 1543–1544
Lung scanning, for pulmonary embolism, 1644
Lung ultrasound, in pulmonary embolism, 1643
Lung, ultrasound of, in heart failure, 224, 224.e1f
LV diastolic dysfunction, 1023
LVEF. See Left ventricular ejection fraction
LVH. See Left ventricular hypertrophy
Lyme disease, myocarditis and, 1081b
Lymphocytic myocarditis, in COVID-19, 1760f
Lymphoma, T cell, 1831f, 1834t

M

MAC. See Mitral annular calcification
Macitentan, for pulmonary arterial hypertension, 1675f
Macronutrients, 535–539

Macrophages, in myocarditis, 1085.e1
Macroreentrant atrial tachycardia, 1252–1257
  focal atrial tachycardia vs., 1248b–1249b
Macula adherens, 1173
MAD. See Mitral annular disjunction
MADIT-CRT. See Multicenter Automatic Defibrillator Implantation Trial with Cardiac Resynchronization Therapy
MADIT II. See Multicenter Automatic Defibrillator Implantation II Trial
MADIT II trial, 1332, 1336t
MADIT trial, 1336t
Magnesium, 539b
  deficiency of, diuretic-induced, 988
  for digitalis toxicity, 1000.e2
Magnetic resonance angiography (MRA)
  in abdominal aortic aneurysms, 807–808
  in large-vessel vasculitis, 1813f–1814f
  in peripheral artery disease, 844, 863.e3f
Magnetic resonance imaging (MRI)
  in acute coronary syndromes, 322b, 323f–324f
  in adult congenital heart disease, 330b–332b
  in anomalous pulmonary venous connection, 330b–332b, 331f
  in aortic dissection, 823–824, 824.e1f
  in aortic intramural hematoma, 831, 831.e2f
  in aortic regurgitation, 328–329, 328f
  in aortic stenosis, 328
  in arrhythmogenic right ventricular cardiomyopathy, 324–325, 325f
  in atrial septal defect, 330b–332b, 331f
  basic physics of, 314–320
  basic principles of, 314–320
  cardiac
    in dilated cardiomyopathy, 1032–1035
    in pulmonary arterial hypertension, 1668
    in sarcoid cardiomyopathy, 1045
  in cardiac amyloidosis, 326, 326f–327f
  in cardiac electrophysiology, 330b–332b
  cardiac implantable electrical devices and, 1345b–1346b
  in cardiac sarcoidosis, 326, 326f
  in cardiac tumors, 1829, 1838f
  cardiovascular, 314–334
  cardiovascular medicine and, 113
  in chest pain, 607
  in coarctation of the aorta, 330b–332b, 331f
  in conotruncal anomalies, 330b–332b
  in constrictive pericarditis, 1627–1628, 1629f
  contrast agents in, 314b–320b
  coronary, 315t–319t
  in coronary artery disease, 320–322
  in coronary revascularization assessment, 320–322
  in diastolic function/dysfunction, 326
  in D-loop transposition of the great arteries, 330b–332b
  in endomyocardial fibrosis, 326
  in heart failure, 943, 944f
  in hypertrophic cardiomyopathy, 322–324, 324f
  in idiopathic dilated cardiomyopathy, 326–327, 327f
  in iron overload, 314b–320b, 327–328
  magnetic field in, 314
  methods of, 314b–320b
  in mitral regurgitation, 329, 329f
  in myocardial infarction, 321f
  in myocardial ischemia, 321f
  in myocardial viability assessment, 320–322
  in myocarditis, 325, 325f
  in NSTE-ACS, 716
  patient safety in, 314b–320b
  in pericardial disease, 329–333, 330f
  in pericardial effusion and cardiac tamponade, 1622
  in peripheral artery disease, 863
  in pulmonary embolism, 1644
  pulse sequences in, 314
  in stable chest pain syndromes, 320, 321f–323f
  in stable ischemic heart disease, 747–748
  in STEMI, 658, 659f
  in sudden death, 330b–332b
  summary of, 315t–319t
  in systemic lupus erythematosus, 1811f
  in T1 mapping, 314b–320b
  in T2 mapping, 314b–320b
  in Takotsubo cardiomyopathy, 327–328
  techniques and future perspectives of, 333, 333f
  in tetralogy of Fallot, 330b–332b
  in tricuspid regurgitation, 329
  in ventricular septal defect, 330b–332b, 331f

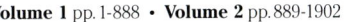
Volume 1 pp. 1-888 • **Volume 2** pp. 889-1902

Malignancy, after cardiac transplantation, 1140, 1142t
Mallory-Weiss tears, 601
Mammalian target of rapamycin (mTOR), in cardiac transplantation, 1136–1137
Marfan syndrome
　pregnancy and, 1740, 1740.e1f
　thoracic aortic aneurysms in, 811, 811t, 811.e1f, 813f
Marijuana, cardiovascular complications, 1599–1600, 1600f
Masked hypertension, phenomenon of, 482
Mass spectrometers, 89
Mass spectrometry, 90f
　applications of, 90
　schematic of tandem, 90f
Massive pulmonary embolism, 1649.e1f
Mast cells, in heart failure, 927f, 927b–929b
Matrix metalloproteinases (MMPs), 434
　in abdominal aortic aneurysms
　in heart failure, 929.e1, 929.e1t
Maximal exercise capacity, 579
Maze procedure, in atrial fibrillation, 1283
McArdle syndrome, 840
MCS. See Mechanical circulatory support
MDMA (3,4-methylenedioxymethamphetamine), cardiovascular complications of, 1599
Mechanical aspiration, percutaneous coronary interventions and, 795.e1
Mechanical circulatory support
　for congenital heart disease, 1551
　in percutaneous coronary interventions, 796–798, 798f
Mechanical circulatory support (MCS), 1119–1131, 1120t
　as bridge to recovery, 1119–1120, 1120f–1122f
　as bridge to transplantation, 1120, 1123f–1124f
　coagulation and, 1124, 1124b
　comorbidity of, 1122–1124
　as destination therapy, 1120–1122
　engineering designs of, 1122.e1
　future perspective of, 1130–1131
　hepatic function and, 1123–1124, 1123b–1124b
　indications and device selection for, 1119–1122
　interagency registry of, 1129–1130, 1130f, 1130t
　long-term, 1127–1129, 1128t
　medical considerations in, 1124
　patient outcomes with, 1124–1129
　patient selection for, 1122–1124
　pulmonary function and, 1123, 1123b
　renal function and, 1122–1123, 1122b–1123b
　right ventricular function and, 1124, 1124b
　temporary, 1124–1127, 1125t
　timing of intervention for, 1122–1124
Mechanical heart valves, maternal and fetal risk in women with, 1736t
Mechanical prostheses, pregnancy and, 1735, 1736t
Mechanical thrombectomy, for peripheral artery disease, 862–863
Mechanically expanded Lotus valve, 1435.e1, 1435.e2f
Media, in intravascular imaging, 379
Medical therapy, plaque progression and, 345b–347b, 347.e1f
Medications, in lipoprotein disorders, 514
Meditation
　in hypertension, 595
　in ischemic heart disease, 594
Mediterranean diet, cardiovascular disease and, 459, 459f, 459.e1f
Meester-Loeys syndrome, thoracic aortic aneurysm in, 811t
Meglitinides, in glucose management, 562t–563t
Melanoma, 1829b, 1831f
MELAS syndrome. See Mitochondrial myopathy with encephalopathy, lactic acidosis, and strokelike episodes (MELAS) syndrome
Melody valve, for congenital heart disease, 1588, 1588f
Membrane clock, 1170
Mendelian randomization
　acyclic graph with assumptions, 79f
　assumption assessments, 80
　principles and applications, 79–80, 79f
Menopause, cardiovascular disease and, 458
Mental status, altered, in STEMI, 655
Mental stress, cardiovascular disease and, 452, 452.e1f
Mercury, cardiovascular effects of, 1601
Mesenteric artery disease, endovascular treatment of, 867, 867.e1f
Mesodermal precardiac cells, 1545
Metabolic agents, in angina pectoris, 763.e1

Metabolic disorders, nutrition and, 531–546, 532f
Metabolic disturbances, diuretic-induced, 987–988, 987b
Metabolic function, in peripheral artery disease, 839
Metabolic syndrome
　cardiovascular disease and, 448–449
　coronary artery disease and, 75
　in HIV patients, cardiovascular risk factors in, 1604–1605
　secondary causes of, 513, 514t
　in women, cardiovascular disease and, 1710b–1714b
Metabolism, in lipoprotein disorders, 514
Metabolome, conceptual relationship of, 88f
Metabolomics
　analytic challenges for, 87–88, 89f
　in cardiovascular medicine, 87–91
　novel technologies in identification of biomarkers, 87
　overview of, 87
　discovery process, 88–90
Metaiodobenzylguanidine (MIBG) scintigraphy, for pheochromocytoma, 486
Metallic pollutants, cardiovascular disease and, 39, 39t
Metalloproteinases, tissue inhibitors, in heart failure, 929.e1, 929.e1t
Metastases, 1834t
Metastatic calcifications, 1797
Metastatic cardiac neoplasms, evaluation of, 310
Metastatic pericardial disease, 1630b–1633b
Metformin
　for diabetes, 1705
　in glucose management, 561–564, 562t–563t, 564b
Methamphetamines, cardiovascular complications of, 1599, 1599b
Methotrexate, 1826
　for rheumatoid arthritis, 1810b
3,4-Methylenedioxymethamphetamine (MDMA), cardiovascular complications of, 1599
Metolazone, in heart failure, 982–983, 983t
Metoprolol
　in angina pectoris, 758t
　in chronic kidney disease, 1882t
　in heart failure, 991t–992t, 995f, 995b–996b
Mexiletine, 1211.e1t, 1209t, 1212t, 1214t, 1217, 1217b
　drug interaction with, 97t
MI. See Myocardial infarction
Micafungin, for infective endocarditis, 1519b–1523b
Microalbuminuria, in chronic kidney disease, 1874
Microbiome, 543
　atherosclerosis and, 440
Micronutrients, 539
MicroRNAs (miRNAs)
　in heart failure, 929f, 929b–930b
　in myocarditis, 1083.e2
Microscopic polyangiitis, 1817
　investigation in, 1817
　treatment for, 1818
Microvascular angina, 777
Microvascular blood flow, evaluation of, coronary angiography in, 376–377, 376t
Microvascular dysfunction, coronary artery disease and, 777
Mifepristone, 1794b
Miglitol, in diabetes mellitus, 562t–563t
Migratory polyarthritis, 1533
Milrinone
　for acute heart failure, 964b–965b
　in cardiorenal syndrome, 1886, 1889t
Mind/body therapy, 593b–594b
Mindfulness, 1850–1851
Mind/heart connection, for ischemic heart disease, 594–595
Mineralocorticoid receptor antagonists (MRAs), 983–984, 983b, 984f
　in heart failure, 991t–992t, 996, 996b
　for heart failure with preserved and mildly reduced ejection, 1023, 1025
　side effects of, 996
Mipomersen, 520
Mirtazapine, 1849
Missing data, 45
Mitochondria, morphology and function of, 891–892, 891f
Mitochondrial disorders, 1866–1867, 1867.e1t
Mitochondrial myopathy with encephalopathy, lactic acidosis, and strokelike episodes (MELAS) syndrome, 1866–1867
Mitophagy, 892
Mitoxantrone, cardiotoxic effects of, 1092t

Mitral annular calcification (MAC)
　degenerative mitral stenosis associated with, 1441, 1450–1452, 1451f, 1451f–1452f
　aortic stenosis associated, 1451
　natural history of, 1451
　treatment of, 1452
　in elderly, 1700b–1701b
Mitral annular disjunction (MAD), 1463
Mitral annulus, in mitral regurgitation, 1455
Mitral balloon valvuloplasty, in mitral stenosis, 1484–1485
　indication for, 1484–1485
　procedure of, 1484b–1485b, 1485f–1486f
Mitral leaflets, in mitral regurgitation, 1455, 1456f
Mitral regurgitation, 1455–1472
　acute, 1470b–1471b
　aortic regurgitation and, 1482b
　aortic stenosis and, 1482b
　aortic valve disease and, 1482b
　echocardiography in, 229–231, 229b, 230f–231f, 231.e1f
　in elderly, 1700b–1701b
　evaluation of, 130, 137
　exercise testing in, 190
　in magnetic resonance imaging, 329, 329f
　mechanisms of, 1456–1458
　mitral annulus in, 1455
　mitral leaflets in, 1455, 1456f
　mitral valve chordae in, 1455–1456
　morphologic classifications of, 1456b–1457b, 1457t, 1458f–1459f
　myocardial infarction and, echocardiography in, 218f, 218b–219b
　papillary muscles in, 1455–1456
　pregnancy and, 1732
　primary, 1458–1465, 1462b
　　auscultation of, 1458b–1459b
　　clinical presentation of, 1458–1462, 1460t
　　dynamic auscultation of, 1458b–1459b
　　echocardiography of, 1459–1462
　　edge-to-edge repair for, 1464–1465
　　exercise echocardiography of, 1461–1462
　　investigational devices for, 1465
　　left ventricular volumes and systolic function in, 1462–1463
　　management of, 1463–1465
　　medical therapy for, 1463
　　mitral annular disjunction, 1463
　　natural history of, 1462–1463
　　physical examination of, 1458–1459
　　quantification of MR severity, 1460–1461, 1461f
　　surgical therapy for, 1463–1464, 1464f–1465f, 1464t
　　symptoms of, 1458, 1463, 1463f
　　transcatheter therapy for, 1464–1465
　　transesophageal echocardiography of, 1461, 1461f
　in rheumatic fever, 1534
　secondary, 1465–1471
　　clinical presentation of, 1466–1467, 1467f
　　to coronary artery disease, 780–781
　　investigational devices for, 1470–1471
　　management of, 1467–1471
　　medical therapy for, 1467
　　pathophysiology of, 1465–1466, 1466f, 1466t
　　surgical therapy for, 1467–1468, 1468f
　　symptoms of, 1466b–1467b
　　transcatheter therapy for, 1468–1470, 1469f–1470f, 1469t
　transcatheter therapies for, 1485–1489
　　devices for, 1485, 1487t
　　direct annuloplasty in, 1486b–1488b, 1490f
　　indirect annuloplasty in, 1486b–1488b, 1490f
　　left ventricular remodeling techniques in, 1486b–1488b, 1490f
　　MitraClip device in, leaflet repair with, 1485–1488, 1488f–1489f
　　rationale for, 1485
　　transcatheter mitral valve replacement in, 1488–1489, 1491f
　type I, 1456b–1457b
　type II, 1456b–1457b
　type III, 1456b–1457b
Mitral stenosis (MS), 1441–1453, 1441.e1f
　aortic valve disease and, 1482b
　definition of disease and severity of, 1441
　echocardiography in, 227–229, 227f–229f, 229t
　in elderly, 1700b–1701b
　epidemiology and secular trends of, 1441
　nonrheumatic, 1441
　rheumatic, 1441

Mitral stenosis (MS) *(Continued)*
  evaluation of, 137
  following interventional and surgical therapies, 1453
  noncardiac surgery and, 411b–412b
  nonrheumatic, 1441, 1450–1453
    degenerative MS related to mitral annular calcification, 1450–1452, 1451f, 1451f–1452f
    radiotherapy-induced mitral stenosis, 1452, 1453f
  pregnancy and, 1734f
  pressure gradient determinations in, 401, 401f
  rheumatic, 1442–1450
    additional diagnostic investigations of, 1446
    associated conditions of, 1446–1447
    atrial fibrillation and, 1446–1447, 1446f
    clinical pathophysiology of, 1442–1443, 1443f
    clinical presentation of, 1444–1445
    diagnosis of, 1444–1446
    echocardiography of, 1445–1446, 1445f
    EKG and chest X-ray of, 1446
    exercise testing of, 1446
    left atrial function, 1442–1443
    left atrial pressure, 1442, 1444f
    left ventricular function, 1443
    medical therapy for, 1448
    natural history of, 1443–1444, 1444t
    pathology of, 1442, 1442f
    physical examination of, 1445
    pregnancy and, 1447
    pulmonary hypertension and, 1447
    right ventricular function, 1443
    transcatheter interventional therapy for, 1448–1449, 1448t, 1449f–1450f
    treatment of, 1448–1450
  stages of, 1444t
  transcatheter therapies in, 1484–1485
    mitral balloon valvuloplasty in, 1484–1485
      indication for, 1484–1485
      procedure of, 1484b–1485b, 1485f–1486f
Mitral valve
  anatomy of, 1455–1456, 1456f
    echocardiography of, 226b–227b, 227f, 227.e1f
  echocardiography of, 226–231, 227f, 227.e1f
  endocarditis of, 1361b
  infective endocarditis involving, 1508, 1514f, 1517
  inflow patterns of, 208, 208.e1f, 208.e2f
  normal physiology of, 1456–1458
Mitral valve area (MVA), 1441
  in stenotic valve orifice calculations, 399
Mitral valve chordae, in mitral regurgitation, 1455–1456
Mitral valve prolapse, sudden cardiac death and, 1358t
Mitral valve replacement (MVR), for mitral stenosis, 1449
MMF. *See* Mycophenolate mofetil
M-mode Doppler echocardiography, in pericardial effusion and cardiac tamponade, 1622
M-mode echocardiography, 196, 200–203, 203f
MMPs. *See* Matrix metalloproteinases
MobiusHD device, for baroreflex amplification, 497
Moderate stenosis, 352
Modern era heart team, 1438.e1
Modified Seldinger technique, for percutaneous femoral artery access, 387, 389f
Molecular genetic allelic heterogeneity, 1036.e1f
Monarthritis, 1533
Monitored anesthesia care, 417–418
Monoamine oxidase inhibitor enzyme, 1849–1850
Monoclonal antibody, 1092t
Monogenic coronary artery disease, 81
Monoleaflet valves, 1495
Monomorphic ventricular tachycardia, antitachycardia pacing for, 1341f
Monophasic pulses, 1323b–1324b
Morbidity, in elderly, 1690b–1693b, 1692f
Morphine, for NSTE-ACS, 722b
Mortality
  cardiovascular disease-related, 15–16, 15f, 17f
    in Central and Eastern Europe and Central Asia, 18f, 19
    in East Asia and Pacific, 18f, 19
    in high-income countries, 18–19, 18f
    in Latin America and Caribbean, 18f, 19–20
    in North Africa and Middle East, 18f, 20
    in South Asia, 18f, 20
    in sub-Saharan Africa, 18f, 20
  cardiovascular disease-related, air pollution and, 34
  epidemiologic transitions of, 14–16, 16f
  obesity and, 15–16, 16t

"Mother rotor" hypothesis, 1189b
Motion artifact, on electrocardiography, 173f
MPI. *See* Myocardial perfusion imaging
MRA. *See* Magnetic resonance angiography
MRAs. *See* Mineralocorticoid receptor antagonists
MRI. *See* Magnetic resonance imaging
MS. *See* Mitral stenosis
Multicenter Automatic Defibrillator Implantation II Trial (MADIT II), 1111b–1113b
Multicenter Automatic Defibrillator Implantation Trial with Cardiac Resynchronization Therapy (MADIT-CRT), 1110b–1111b
Multicenter InSync Randomized Clinical Evaluation (MIRACLE) trial, 1107b–1110b, 1110f
Multicenter InSync-Implantable Cardioverter-Defibrillator Randomized Clinical Evaluation (MIRACLE ICD) trial, 1107b–1110b
Multidisciplinary team, in cardiac rehabilitation, 588
Multielectrode mapping systems, 1239b–1241b
Multifocal ectopic Purkinje-related premature contractions, 1205
Multifocal fibromuscular dysplasia, 853
Multisite Stimulation in Cardiomyopathy Trials (MUSTIC), 1107b–1110b, 1108t–1109t, 1110f
Multisystem atrophy (Shy-Drager syndrome), 1388
Multisystem inflammatory syndrome, in children, 1757
Multivalvular disease, 1481–1483
  aortic stenosis and, 1437.e1
  causes of, 1481t
  surgical treatment of, 1482–1483
Multivessel disease, percutaneous coronary intervention in, 789
Multivitamins, for ischemic heart disease, 595
Murmur, in mitral stenosis, 1445
Muscarinic receptors, sinoatrial node and, 1175.e1b
Muscle
  maximum contractile function in, 910
  in peripheral artery disease, 839
  statin-induced disease of, 1803
Muscular dystrophies, 1853–1864
  Becker muscular dystrophy, 1853–1856, 1853f–1854f
  Duchenne muscular dystrophy, 1853–1856, 1853f–1854f, 1856f
  Emery-Dreifuss muscular dystrophy, 1859–1861, 1861f–1862f, 1862t
  facioscapulohumeral, 1863, 1863.e1f
  limb-girdle, 1861–1863, 1862f–1863f
  myotonic, 1856–1859, 1857f–1861f, 1857t, 1860.e1t
Musculoskeletal disorders, chest pain in, 601
MUSTIC. *See* Multisite Stimulation in Cardiomyopathy Trials
MUSTT trial, 1336t
MVA. *See* Mitral valve area
MVR. *See* Mitral valve replacement
Myasthenia gravis, 1869
MYBPC3 gene, 1063, 1066f
Mycophenolate mofetil (MMF)
  in cardiac transplantation, 1136
  in systemic lupus erythematosus, 1811b
Mycotic aneurysms, 832, 835f
Myectomy, surgical, in hypertrophic cardiomyopathy, 1071, 1074f
Myeloperoxidase, in chest pain evaluation, 603b
MYH7 gene, 1063, 1066f
MYH11, 812
MYLK, 812
Myocardial blush score, for evaluation of microvascular blood flow, 376, 377t
Myocardial bridging
  coronary angiography in, 374, 375f
  in coronary artery disease, 780b–781b
  in stable ischemic heart disease, 749.e1
Myocardial disease, coronary computed tomography angiography in, 354, 356f
Myocardial dysfunction, cocaine-induced, 1598
Myocardial fibrosis, aortic valve disease and, 1400b–1403b, 1405f–1406f
Myocardial flow, risk stratification with, 293f
Myocardial function, in acute heart failure, 949–950, 950f
Myocardial hibernation, 298
  stable ischemic heart disease and, 772b–773b, 773t, 776.e1t
Myocardial infarction (MI)
  acute, 1287.e5, 1287.e6t
  chest pain in, 599
  chronic kidney disease and, 1882, 1884t–1886t, 1886f

Myocardial infarction (MI) *(Continued)*
  classification type of, 637t
  cocaine-related, 1597, 1598f
  collateral circulation in, 647
  complications after, echocardiography in, 218f, 218b–219b, 218.e1f, 220f
  definition of, 636, 637t
  echocardiography in, 216–220, 217f–218f, 218.e1f, 220f
    complications after, 218f, 218b–219b, 218.e1f, 220f
    prognostic indicators after, 219–220
  electrocardiography in, 160–170, 164f, 656–658, 658t
    atrial infarction and, 166, 166f
    differential diagnosis of, 166–170
    localization of, 164–165, 165f
    Q wave on, 162
    QRS changes on, 162, 163f, 164t
    repolarization (ST-T wave) abnormalities on, 161–162, 161f–162f, 161b–162b
    T wave on, 162–163
    U wave on, 164
  exercise testing and, 187
  free wall rupture in, echocardiography in, 218b–219b, 219.e1f
  history in, 653
  left bundle branch block and, 165, 166f–167f
  left ventricular aneurysms after, echocardiography in, 218b–219b
  left ventricular ejection fraction (LVEF) after, 218b–219b
  left ventricular thrombus after, echocardiography in, 218b–219b, 220f
  limitations of, 636–637
  magnetic resonance imaging in, 321f
  mitral regurgitation and, echocardiography in, 218f, 218b–219b
  nausea in, 653
  nonatherosclerotic, 648, 648.e1f
  noncardiac surgery and, 410
  with nonobstructive coronary arteries, 647–649, 648f–649f
  outcome of, 636–637, 639f
  pain in, 653
  pathologic findings of, 638–649, 640t
    apoptosis, 641–643
    cellular, 643–646, 645f
    coagulation necrosis in, 640, 643f 644f
    contraction band necrosis in, 640, 643f–645f
    gross, 639, 639.e1f, 643f
    histologic, 639–640, 640.e1t, 644f–645f
    microscopic, 639–640, 640.e1t, 644f–645f
    myocytolysis, 641
    reperfusion, pathologic changes by, 646, 646.e1f, 648f
    ultrastructural, 639–640, 640.e1t
  pathophysiology of, 649–652
    circulatory regulation, 651, 651f
    diastolic function in, 651
    hemostatic markers, 652b
    infarct expansion, 652
    left ventricular function in, 649–651
    leukocytes in, 646f–647f
    natriuretic peptides in, 655
    platelets in, 652b
    renin-angiotensin-aldosterone system in, 652b
    systolic function in, 649–651, 651f
    thyroid gland in, 652b
    treatment effects on, 646.e1f, 648f, 652
    ventricular dilation in, 652
  with percutaneous coronary intervention, 801–802, 801.e1t
  physical examination in, 653–655
  plaque formation and disruption, 639, 640f
  predisposing factors of, 653
  pregnancy-associated, 1733–1734
  prior, patients with, 295, 296f
  prodromal symptoms in, 653
  prognosis of, echocardiography in, 219–220
  pseudoaneurysm after, echocardiography in, 218b–219b, 218.e1f
  Q wave in, 638, 657
  right bundle branch block and, 165–166, 166f
  right ventricular, 646–647, 657–658
  risk of, ethanol and, 1595
  sinus bradycardia and, 1312
  stable ischemic heart disease and, 772.e1
  ST-elevation (STEMI), management of, 662–712

Myocardial infarction (MI) *(Continued)*
    anticoagulant and antiplatelet therapy as, 675–679, 675.e1f
    arrhythmias in, 699–703, 700t
        bradyarrhythmias, 701–703
        hemodynamic consequences of, 699
        supraventricular tachyarrhythmias, 703
        ventricular, 699–701
    catheter-based reperfusion strategies as, 671, 671f–673f
    complications in, 703–705
        left ventricular aneurysm, 705
        left ventricular thrombus and arterial embolism, 705
        pericardial effusion and pericarditis, 704–705
        recurrent chest discomfort, 703–704
        venous thrombosis and pulmonary embolism, 705
    convalescence, discharge, and post-myocardial infarction care, 705–710
        assessment at hospital discharge, 706–707
        assessment for electrical instability, 707
        assessment of left ventricular function, 706–707
        assessment of myocardial ischemia, 707
        counseling, 706
        hospital course, 706b
        initial findings, 706b
        prophylactic antiarrhythmic therapy, 707, 708f–709f
        risk stratification, 706b
        timing of hospital discharge, 705–707
    in emergency department, 664–667, 665t
        analgesics for, 665–666
        aspirin for, 665
        beta-adrenergic blocking agents for, 666
        control of cardiac pain, 665–666
        nitrates for, 666
        oxygen for, 666
    fibrinolysis, 668–669
    fibrinolytic therapy as, 669–671, 669f–670f
    future perspectives and emerging therapies for, 710
    hemodynamic disturbances, 684–699
        abnormalities, 684–685
        cardiogenic shock in, 690–694, 690f
        hyperdynamic state, 685
        hypotension in prehospital phase, 685
        left ventricular failure in, 685–690, 686f
        mechanical causes of heart failure, 694–699
        pulmonary artery pressure, monitoring of, 684–685, 685t
        right ventricular infarction in, 694, 696f
        subsets, 685, 685t–686t
    hospital, 679–684
        coronary care and intermediate care units, 679–680
        pharmacologic therapy as, 680–684
    infarct
        dynamic nature of, 666–667, 667f
        routine measures for, 667
        size, 666–667
    mortality rates, 663f
    myocardial reperfusion, pathophysiology of, 667–668
        patency of infarct vessel, 668
        reperfusion arrhythmias, 668
        reperfusion injury, 668
    perfusion therapy as, 667–679, 667f
    prehospital, 662–664, 663t
        care, 662
        emergency medical service systems, 663, 664f
        fibrinolysis, 663–664, 665f
    selection of reperfusion strategy, 671–675, 673f
        patients not eligible for, 674–675
        referral for angiography, 673–674, 673f–674f, 674t
    ST-segment elevation (STEMI), 636–638
        anatomy of, 641f–642f, 646–647
        atrial, 647
        atypical features, 653
        auscultation in, 654–655
        blood pressure, 654
        cardiac examination in, 654–655
        cardiac markers in, 659
        carotid pulse in, 654
        chest in, 654
        circadian periodicity in, 653
        clinical features of, 653–659

Myocardial infarction (MI) *(Continued)*
        computed tomography in, 658–659
        differential diagnosis of, 168, 169t, 653
        at a distance, 657
        echocardiography in, 658
        electrocardiography in, 656–659, 658t
        extremity examination in, 655
        fever in, 654
        friction rubs in, 655
        future perspectives of, 659
        general patient appearance in, 653
        heart rate in, 653
        heart sounds in, 654
        hematologic findings in, 655–656
        hemoglobin in, 656
        incidence and care of, 636
        jugular venous pulse in, 654
        laboratory findings in, 655–659
        lipoprotein in, 655
        magnetic resonance imaging in, 658, 659f
        murmurs in, 654–655
        neuropsychiatric findings in, 655
        nuclear imaging in, 658
        outcome of, 636–637, 639f
        palpation in, 654
        radiography in, 658
        rales in, 654
        respiration in, 654
        revascularization for, 1696
        serum markers, 655, 657f
        silent, 653
        size, 659, 659.e1f
        ventricular remodeling in, 651–652
    tamponade after, echocardiography in, 218b–219b
    thrombolytic treatment of, 885b–886b
    thyroid hormone levels after, 1804b
    ventricular remodeling in, 651–652
    ventricular septal defects and, echocardiography in, 218b–219b, 218.e1f
    vomiting in, 653
Myocardial injury
    biomarker evidence of, 1758
    ethanol-induced, 1593
Myocardial ischemia, 609–619, 1392, 1419b–1420b
    aortic valve stenosis and, 1400b–1403b
    chest pain in, 599
    cocaine-related, 1597, 1598f
    collateral circulation and, 627–628
    demand-induced, 629–630
    electrocardiography in, 160–170
        differential diagnosis of, 166–170
        localization of, 164–165
    future perspectives for, 635
    in hyperthyroidism, 1800
    irreversible injury in, 628–629, 629f
    magnetic resonance imaging in, 321f
    metabolic and functional consequences of, 628–635
    monitoring for, 1162.e1
    myocyte death in, 628–629, 629f
    myocyte hypertrophy in, 634.e2f
    myocyte loss in, 634b–635b, 634.e2f
    myofibrillar loss in, 634b–635b
    perioperative, 418–419
    plaque features and, 345b–347b
    radionuclide imaging approaches to assess, 299–301, 300f
    reversible, 629–630, 629.e1f
        cell survival mechanisms in, 634b–635b
        functional consequences of, 630–635, 631f
        myocardial preconditioning and postconditioning in, 629b, 630f
        perfusion-contraction matching in, 630, 631f
        stunned myocardium in, 631f–632f, 631b–633b
        subendocardial, 630
    supply-induced, 629–630
Myocardial metabolic imaging tracers, 280b–281b
Myocardial oxygen consumption
    determinants of, 609, 609.e1f
        coronary autoregulation, 609–611, 610f
        endothelium-dependent modulation of coronary tone, 612–613, 612.e1t, 614f
        endothelin, 612–613
        endothelium-dependent hyperpolarizing factor, 612
        nitric oxide, 612
        prostacyclin, 612
Myocardial oxygen demand, 175–177, 175b–177b, 176f
Myocardial oxygen supply, 175–177, 175b–177b

Myocardial oxygen uptake, 909–910, 909f
Myocardial perfusion, 668b–669b, 669f
Myocardial perfusion contrast-enhanced echocardiography, 214–215, 215f
Myocardial perfusion imaging (MPI), 284–286
    in patient with cardiomyopathy, 299f
    for PET, 286
    with pharmacologic vasodilator stress, for stable ischemic heart disease, 745b–746b, 746t
    stress, in stable ischemic heart disease, 745b–746b, 746t
Myocardial perfusion imaging tracers, 280b–281b, 281f, 287f
    physiologic basis of, 282f
Myocardial postconditioning, 629b, 630f
Myocardial preconditioning, 629b, 630f
Myocardial reperfusion, pathophysiology of, 667–668
    patency of infarct vessel, 668
    reperfusion arrhythmias, 668
    reperfusion injury, 668
Myocardial segmentation model, 287f
Myocardial strain, echocardiography of, 206b–208b, 206f–207f, 206.e2f
Myocardial stunning, 298, 631b–633b, 632f
Myocardial viability
    imaging to guide revascularization in patients with ischemic heart failure, 301–303, 301f
    in magnetic resonance imaging, 320–322
    radionuclide imaging approaches to assess, 299–301, 300f
Myocardial wall stress, myocardial oxygen consumption and, 609
Myocarditis, 1077–1090
    acute, 1086.e1
    bacterial infection in, 1079t, 1081
    chronic active, 1086.e1
    clinical syndromes of, 1086, 1087f
    definition of, 1077
    diagnostic approaches to, 1086–1088
        cardiac imaging, 1087, 1087.e1f, 1087.e1t
        endomyocardial biopsy, 1078t, 1088, 1088f
        laboratory testing, 1087
    drugs and, 1083
    due to COVID-19, 1757
    eosinophilic, 1086.e1
    epidemiology of, 1077–1078, 1078f, 1078t–1079t
    fulminant, 1086.e1
    future perspectives on, 1089–1090
    giant cell, 1086.e1
    heat stroke and, 1083.e1
    helminth infection in, 1083
    hypothermia and, 1083.e2
    influenza and, 1753
    innate immunity in, 1085.e1
    in magnetic resonance imaging, 325, 325f
    microRNAs in, 1083.e2
    pathogenesis of, 1077, 1083–1086, 1084f
    physical agents and, 1083, 1083.e1
    prognosis for, 1088, 1088f
    protozoal infection in, 1081–1082, 1081f–1082f
    radiation and, 1083.e1
    in rheumatic diseases, 1818–1820
    in rheumatic fever, 1534
    sarcoid, 1044–1045
    sudden cardiac death (SCD) and, 1358t, 1360, 1360f
    in systemic lupus erythematosus, 1819, 1820f
    in systemic sclerosis, 1819
    toxins in, 1079t
    treatment of, 1088–1089, 1089f
    viral infection in, 1083.e1f, 1078–1081, 1079f, 1079t, 1083–1085
        acquired immunity and, 1085–1086
        cardiac remodeling and, 1086
        innate immunity and, 1085, 1085f
Myocardium
    oxygen demand of, 175–177, 175b–177b, 176f
    oxygen supply to, 175–177, 175b–177b
    oxygen uptake by, 909–910, 909f
    ventricular, innervation of, 1177–1178, 1179f
Myocardium, contractility of, 906
Myoclonus epilepsy with red ragged fibers (MERRF) syndrome, 1866–1867
Myocyte injury, biomarkers of, 742–743
Myocytes, 889, 891t
    in heart failure
        apoptosis, 926.e1f, 926b–927b
        hypertrophy, 922–926, 922f–923f

Myocytolysis, 169
Myofiber, 889
Myofibril, 889, 890f
Myofibrillar myopathies, 1868
Myoglobinopathy, 1869
Myopericarditis, 1616
Myosin, 892–893, 894f
  light chains of, 892f, 894
  structure and function of, 893–894
Myosin activators, in heart failure, 998
Myosin ATPase activity, 894
Myositis, 1819–1820
Myotonic dystrophies, 1856–1859, 1857f–1861f, 1857t, 1860.e1t
Myxedema coma, 1803b
Myxomas, 1830–1832, 1833f–1834f, 1834t
  echocardiography in, 253b, 255f

N

n-3 fatty acid supplements, 464–465, 466f
n-3 polyunsaturated fatty acids (PUFAs), 538
  in heart failure, 1000
n-6 polyunsaturated fatty acids (PUFAs), 538
$Na^+ K^+$-ATPase, 1171b–1173b, 1174f
Na^+ pump, 1171b–1173b
Na^+/Ca^{2+} exchanger, 1171b–1173b, 1174f
Nadolol, 1209t
  in angina pectoris, 758t
Nafcillin, in infective endocarditis, 1519b–1523b, 1521t–1522t
NAFLD. See Nonalcoholic fatty liver disease
Napkin-ring sign (NRS), coronary computed tomography angiography in, 345, 346f
NARP syndrome, 1866–1867
Narrow- and wide-QRS complex tachycardia, 1162.e2, 1162.e3t
Narrow-complex tachycardia, algorithm for evaluation of, 1260f
Nateglinide, in diabetes mellitus, 562t–563t
Native arteries, progression of disease, 771
Native vessel progression, effects of therapy on, 771
Natriuretic peptides
  in acute heart failure, 971–972
  in heart failure, 918f, 918b–919b, 940, 940b, 940.e1t
    with preserved and mildly reduced ejection, 1011b–1017b
  hypertension and, 477
  in STEMI, 655
Nausea, in STEMI, 653
Naxos disease, 1040
Necrosis
  in heart failure, 926b–927b
  in STEMI, 639.e1f, 640, 644f–645f, 655
Negative predictive value (NPV), 54b–55b
  of biomarkers, 105–106, 105t
Neprilysin, 1025–1026
  for heart failure, 575
Nernst potential, 1163b–1166b
Nesiritide
  in acute heart failure, 963b
  in cardiorenal syndrome, 1889t
Net reclassification index (NRI), 106–107
NETs. See Neutrophil extracellular traps
Network sarcoplasmic reticulum, 889
Neurally mediated hypotension, 1389
Neurally mediated syncope, 1389, 1395–1396, 1396t
  cardioneuroablation for treatment of, 1396–1397
Neurally-mediated bradyarrhythmias, 1320
Neuregulins, 903
Neurogenic pseudoclaudication, 840
Neurogenic stunned myocardium, 1870
Neurohormonal activation, of diuretics, 988
Neurohormonal antagonists, for acute heart failure, 971b–972b
Neurohormonal mechanisms, in acute heart failure, 951
Neurohormonal modulators, for heart failure with preserved and mildly reduced ejection, 1024
Neurologic disorders, 1853–1866, 1853.e1f
  acute cerebrovascular disease, 1870–1871, 1870f–1871f
  epilepsy, 1869–1870, 1869f
  Friedreich ataxia, 1864, 1864f–1865f, 1864.e1f
  Guillain-Barré syndrome, 1868
  mitochondrial disorders, 1866–1867, 1867.e1t
  muscular dystrophies, 1853–1864

Neurologic disorders (Continued)
  Becker muscular dystrophy, 1853–1856, 1853f–1854f
  Duchenne muscular dystrophy, 1853–1856, 1853f–1854f, 1856f
  Emery-Dreifuss muscular dystrophy, 1859–1861, 1861f–1862f, 1862t
  facioscapulohumeral, 1863, 1863.e1f
  limb-girdle, 1861–1863, 1862f–1863f
  myotonic, 1856–1859, 1857f–1861f, 1857t, 1860.e1t
  myasthenia gravis, 1869
  periodic paralyses, 1864–1866, 1866f–1867f
  spinal muscular atrophy, 1868
Neurologic events
  marijuana use and, 1600
  in transcatheter aortic valve replacement, 1436
Neuropathy, ataxia, and retinitis pigmentosa (NARP) syndrome, 1866–1867
Neuropeptide Y, in heart failure, 919.e1
Neurotransmitters, sinoatrial node and, 1175.e1b
Neurotrophic ulcers, 840–841
Neutralizing antibodies, for COVID-19, 1762
Neutrophil extracellular traps (NETs), in pulmonary embolism, 1638.e1f, 1637b–1639b
New-onset chest pain, patients with, 290–291, 290f–291f, 291.e1f
New York Heart Association (NYHA), 1107–1110
Nexus, 1173
Niacin, 518–519
Nicardipine
  in acute heart failure, 965b
  in angina pectoris, 760, 761t
Nicorandil
  in angina pectoris, 763.e1
  in NSTE-ACS, 723t
Nicotiana genus, 525
Nicotine products
  cardiovascular disease risk of, 525–530
  harm reduction and cessation, 529b–530b
  physiologic effects of, 528f
Nicotinic acid, 518–519
Niemann-Pick type C disease, 513
Nifedipine, in angina pectoris, 759, 761t
Nilotinib, cardiotoxic effects of, 1092t, 1096
NIPPV. See Noninvasive intermittent positive-pressure ventilation
Nisoldipine, for angina pectoris, 761t
Nit-Occlud device, for congenital heart disease, 1591, 1591f
Nitrates
  in acute heart failure, 962–963, 963b
  in angina pectoris, 760–762
    adverse reactions to, 762
    cellular mechanism of action, 760.e1
    with cyclic guanosine monophosphate-specific phosphodiesterase type 5 inhibitors, 762
    effects on coronary circulation, 760.e1
    management of, 760.e1
    mechanism of action of, 760, 760.e1f
    preparations and routes of administration of, 762, 762t
    redistribution of blood flow and, 760.e1
    tolerance to, 760.e1
    withdrawal from, 760.e1
  in coronary artery disease, chronic kidney disease and, 1880t–1881t
  in NSTE-ACS, 721, 723t
  for STEMI, 666, 683–684
Nitric oxide (NO), 904, 904f
  cardiac catheterization and, 408
  coronary blood flow and, 612
  in heart failure, 919–921, 919.e2f
  hypertension and, 477
  for pulmonary arterial hypertension, 1664b–1665b
Nitroglycerin
  in angina pectoris, 762, 762t
  in coronary artery disease, chronic kidney disease and, 1880t–1881t
  as coronary vasodilator, 614b
  in noncardiac surgery patients, 422
Nitroprusside
  in acute heart failure, 963
  cardiac catheterization and, 408
  in cardiorenal syndrome, 1889t
NNT. See Number needed to treat
Nodules, subcutaneous, 1534–1535, 1535f
Noise pollution, cardiovascular disease and, 38

Non cavo-tricuspid isthmus-dependent flutter (atypical atrial flutter), 1253b–1257b, 1256f–1257f
Nonalcoholic fatty liver disease (NAFLD), 1011b–1017b
Nonatheromatous coronary artery disease, 780b–781b
Nonbacterial thrombotic endocarditis, 1507
Noncoding RNAs, in heart failure, 929f, 929b–930b
Noncompaction cardiomyopathy, in athletes, 585
Noncoronary obstructive vascular disease, treatment of, 859–869
Noncoronary structures, cardiac CT to, 335
Nondiagnostic electrocardiogram, patients with, 293–294, 295f
Nondihydropyridines, in coronary artery disease, chronic kidney disease and, 1880t–1881t
Noninferiority trials, 59b
  in clinical trials, 44f
  design of, 43–44
Noninvasive imaging, for STEMI, 668b–669b
Noninvasive intermittent positive-pressure ventilation (NIPPV), in acute heart failure, 955–956
Non-invasive radioablation, 1239b–1241b
Nonischemic cardiomyopathy, 1242, 1242b
Nonobstructive plaque, 351–352
Non-Q wave infarctions, 638, 657
Nonreentrant junctional tachycardia, 1263f, 1263b
Non-reentrant ventricular-atrial synchrony, 1331
Nonrheumatic mitral stenosis, 1441, 1450–1453
  degenerative MS related to mitral annular calcification, 1450–1452, 1451f, 1451f–1452f
  radiotherapy-induced mitral stenosis, 1452, 1453f
Nonspecific intraventricular conduction defect, 160b
Non-ST elevation acute coronary syndromes (NSTE-ACS), 714–738, 715f
  amphetamine use and, 735
  biomarkers in, 717–718, 717f–718f, 718t–720t
  cardiac syndrome X and, 735
  chronic kidney disease and, 733b–734b
  clinical assessment of, 715–718
  cocaine use and, 735
  diabetes mellitus and, 733–734
  early risk stratification in, 735.e1
  electrocardiography for, 716–717
  epidemiology of, 714
  future perspectives in, 735, 735t
  glucose intolerance and, 733–734
  heart failure and, 734
  history of, 715
  invasive imaging of, 719
  management of, 721–732
    anticoagulant therapy for, 726–727, 735.e3
    anti-inflammatory therapies, 728
    anti-ischemic therapy for, 721–723, 723t, 735.e2
    antithrombotic therapy for, 723–726, 723f, 724t, 735.e2, 735.e4t, 735.e6t
    bleeding and, 728
    coronary revascularization in, 735.e2
    discharge and posthospital care for, 732
    early hospital care for, 735.e1, 735.e2t
    evidence gaps in, 735.e3
    general measures in, 721
    guidelines on, 735.e1, 735.e1t
    initial evaluation in, 735.e1, 735.e3f
    invasive vs. conservative, 728–731, 730f
    ischemia-guided strategy for, 731, 735.e2, 735.e5f
    lipid-lowering therapy for, 731–732, 732f
    performance measures and registries in, 735.e7t
    risk factor modification, 735.e3
    timing of invasive approach, 731
  noninvasive testing for, 718–719, 721t
  in older adults, 732–733
  pathophysiology of, 714–715, 716f–717f, 716t
  physical examination in, 716
  Prinzmetal variant angina and, 734
  revascularization for, 1696
  risk assessment of, 720, 722f
  risk criteria in, 735.e6t
  vasospastic angina, 734–735
  in women, 733
Non-ST elevation myocardial infarction, coronary computed tomography angiography in, 341
Nonsteroidal antiinflammatory drugs (NSAIDs)
  for acute myocardial infarction, 710
  drug interaction with, 97t
  in heart failure, 935b–936b
  in rheumatic diseases, 1826–1827, 1827t
  in rheumatoid arthritis, 1810b

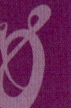

Nonsteroidal mineralocorticoid receptor antagonists (MRAs)
Nonsustained ventricular tachycardia, 1162.e5
Nontachyarrhythmic cardiac arrest, 1371t
Nontargeted liquid chromatography-MS-based metabolite profiling, 90
Nonthrombotic pulmonary embolism, 1639
Norepinephrine
  in acute heart failure, 965
  release of, 900, 900f
  for STEMI, 690
Norepinephrine reuptake inhibitors, 1849
NOS1AP, 1194, 1199
Novacor, 1122
Novel image reconstruction software, 277
Novel PET perfusion tracers, 311.e1f, 311b–312b
Novel SPECT scanners, 277–278, 278.e1f
Novel therapies, for acute heart failure, 966–972, 966t–970t
NPV. See Negative predictive value
NRI. See Net reclassification index
NRS. See Napkin-ring sign
NSAIDs. See Nonsteroidal antiinflammatory drugs
NSTE-ACS. See Non-ST elevation acute coronary syndromes
N-terminal (NT)-pro-brain natriuretic peptide (NT-proBNP)
  in acute heart failure, 954
  in heart failure, 940
  in myocarditis, 1087
  in STEMI, 655
N-terminal pro-BNP, in heart failure with preserved and mildly reduced ejection, 1011b–1017b
Nuclear cardiology, 277–310
  artificial intelligence, 311
  cardiovascular medicine and, 111
  hybrid SPECT/CT, PET/CT, and PET/MR, 279
  machine learning of, 311, 311.e1f
  patient-centered clinical applications, 290–310
  position emission tomography, 278–279
  principles of imaging, 277–288
  radiotracers and protocols, 280–288
  reducing radiation dose, 288–290, 290.e1f, 290.e1t
  single photon emission computed tomography, 277–278
  testing, preparation for, 284b
  translational molecular imaging, 311–312
Nuclear imaging
  in heart failure, 943–944
  in STEMI, 658
Nuclear ventilation/perfusion (V/Q) scintigraphy, for pulmonary arterial hypertension, 1668
Null hypothesis, 43–44
Number needed to treat (NNT), 58
Nutrition
  cardiovascular diseases and, 458–461, 531–546, 532f
  in congestive heart failure, 596
  in dyslipidemia, 595–596
  fetal, 26
  in integrative cardiology, 593b–594b
  in ischemic heart disease, 594
  in metabolic diseases, 531–546, 532f
  in obesity, 551–552, 552t
  personalized, 543
  as risk factor of stroke, 874b–877b
"Nutritionally variant streptococci", causing infective endocarditis, antimicrobial therapy for, 1519b–1523b
Nuts, 532, 533f, 540t
NYHA. See New York Heart Association

O

Obesity, 547–555
  atrial fibrillation in, 1274, 1287.e6t, 1287.e8
  bariatric surgery and, 553, 554t, 555f
  cardiovascular disease and, 449–451, 450f, 547, 547f–548f
  clinical management for, 551–552
    nutritional factors in, 551–552, 552t
    pharmacotherapy in, 552, 553t
    physical activity and exercise in, 552, 552.e1f
    sleep and stress management in, 552
  effects of food and nutrients on, 541t–542t
  in elderly, 1706
  epidemiology of, 23–24, 25f
  in HIV patients, cardiovascular risk factors in, 1604–1605
  hypertension and, 478–480
  mortality and, 15–16, 16t

Obesity *(Continued)*
  in obstructive sleep apnea (OSA), 1678–1679
  risk assessment in, 547–548, 548f–549f, 549t
  as risk factor of stroke, 874b–877b
  severe, 552–554, 553.e1f
  stable ischemic heart disease and, 753
  traditional definition of, 547, 547f–548f
  venous thrombosis and, 1774
  visceral, 549–551
    clinical tools to identify patients with, 551
    key factors associated with, 550–551
    marker of ectopic fat deposition in, 549–550
  in women, cardiovascular disease and, 1710b–1714b
Observational research, 59b
Obstructive atherosclerosis, 864
Obstructive coronary artery disease, pretest probability of, 342, 342f
Obstructive sleep apnea (OSA), 1895–1896
  definition of, 1678
  in heart failure with preserved and mildly reduced ejection, 1011b–1017b
  key features of, 1679t
  pathophysiology of, 1678–1679
  as risk factor of stroke, 874b–877b
  screening questions for, 1681.e1f
OCT. See Optical coherence tomography
Odds, 56
Ohm's law, 1323b–1324b
Older adults, cardiovascular disease in, 1687–1709.e2
  abdominal aortic aneurysm, 1709.e1
  acute coronary syndromes and, 1696–1697
  aortic dissection, 1709.e2
  cardiac rhythm abnormalities, 1701–1702
  heart failure, 1697–1699
  lower extremity peripheral arterial disease, 1709.e1
  noncardiac surgery and perioperative management considerations in, 1706–1709
  precepts of patient-centered care in, 1693–1695
    application of guidelines in, 1693
    diagnosis of, 1693
    management and care coordination in, 1693
    risk assessment of, 1693
    shared decision making in, 1693–1694, 1694f
  syncope, 1703
  valvular heart disease, 1699–1701
  venous thromboembolic disease, 1702–1703
Omecamtiv mecarbil, for acute heart failure, 971b–972b
Omega-3 fatty acids (fish oil)
  in atrial fibrillation, 1280
  in coronary heart disease, 559–560
  in depression, 1850.e1
  in ischemic heart disease, 595
Omeprazole, drug interaction with, 97
OMV. See Open mitral valvotomy
Open mitral valvotomy (OMV), for mitral stenosis, 1449
Open pericardiocentesis, for cardiac tamponade, 1624
Opening snap (OS), in rheumatic mitral stenosis, 1445
Opiates, 1601
Optical coherence tomography (OCT), 380–383, 380b–381b
  in assessment after percutaneous coronary intervention, 382–383, 383f
  in coronary syndrome, 381–382, 381f–382f
  intravascular, for stable ischemic heart disease, 748
  in normal vessel wall, 381, 381f
  in NSTE-ACS, 719
  in plaque morphology, 379.e1t, 381
  in procedure planning and lesion preparation, 382, 382f
  in stable coronary artery disease, 381
Optimal leadless pacemaker candidates, 1328
Optimal medical therapy, revascularization vs., in diabetes, 573
Oral anticoagulants, evolution of, for pulmonary embolism, 1647
Oral anticoagulation, in stable ischemic heart disease, 754b–756b
Oral beta blockers, 722
Oral contraceptives
  cardiovascular disease and, 1710b–1714b
  venous thrombosis and, 1774
Orbital atherectomy, 794.e1
  for peripheral artery disease, 863, 863.e1f, 863.e2f
Organ transplantation
  and amyloidosis, 1058b
  evaluation before, 292–293

Orsiro, 794.e1
Orthostatic hypotension, 1387–1388
  causes of, 1389t
Orthostatic intolerance, 1387–1388
OSA. See Obstructive sleep apnea
Osborn wave, 149, 171f, 171b–172b
Osteoporosis, heparin and, 1781
  low-molecular-weight, 1782
Osteoprotegerin, 435
Ototoxicity, of diuretics, 988
Outcomes, surrogate, 59b
Outdoor air pollution, 33–34
Overdrive acceleration, 1181b–1183b
Overdrive pacing, 1181b–1183b
Overnight oximetry, for pulmonary arterial hypertension, 1667–1668
Overnight polysomnography, of heart failure with preserved and mildly reduced ejection, 1011b–1017b
Overt hyperthyroidism, cardiovascular manifestations of, 1799, 1799t
Overtraining, 582
Overweight, 552–553
Oxacillin, for infective endocarditis, 1519b–1523b, 1521t–1522t
Oxaliplatin, cardiotoxic effects of, 1092t
Oxidative stress, in heart failure, 916f, 916b
Oxygen
  exercise and, 579
  myocardial uptake of, 909–910, 909f
  for STEMI, 666
  total-body uptake of, 175, 176f

P

P value, 59
P waves, 145–146, 145f, 146t
  in atrial abnormalities, 151f–152f, 151b
  atrial activation and, 145–146
  normal, 145–146
  skipped, 1315
$P2Y_{12}$ inhibitors
  for NSTE-ACS, 724, 735.e4t, 735.e6t
  oral, for stable ischemic heart disease, 754b–756b
$P2Y_{12}$ receptor antagonists
  for acute coronary syndromes, 572–573
  in antiplatelet therapy, 561
PAC. See Premature atrial complex
Pace mapping, 1239f
Pacemaker generators, 1321.e1f, 1322b–1323b
Pacemaker/ICD function, assessment of, 1162.e1
Pacemaker-mediated tachycardia (PMT), 1330–1331, 1330.e1f
Pacemaker pulse generators, 1321, 1321f–1322f
Pacemaker syndrome, 1326
Pacemakers, 1321–1348
  in atrial fibrillation, 1275–1276
  for atrioventricular block, 1319
  capture and stimulation of, 1323–1324, 1323b–1324b, 1323.e1f, 1323.e2f, 1324.e1t, 1325f
  for congenital heart disease, 1549, 1549t, 1550f
  conventional, 1321
  device radiography, 1321, 1321f–1324f
  electrograms and sensing function in, 1324–1326, 1324b–1326b, 1325f–1326f
  exercise electrocardiographic testing and, 190b–191b
  for heart block, 1547
  hemodynamic aspects of, 1326, 1326b
  inappropriate discharge rate of, 1179–1180
  indications for, 1322–1323
  lead and generator design, 1322b–1323b, 1325f
  leadless, 1321
  mode and timing cycles of, 1326–1331
    common modes of, 1326–1327, 1326.e3t, 1327f–1328f, 1327f
    definitions of, 1326
    rate responsive pacing, 1327–1328, 1328b, 1329f
    single- or dual-chamber pacing device, 1328
    troubleshooting, 1328–1331, 1329.e1f, 1330t
  for sick sinus syndrome, 1315
  troubleshooting of, 1328–1331, 1329.e1f, 1330t
    failure to capture, 1329, 1330f
    failure to pace, 1330, 1331f
    pacing-induced proarrhythmia, 1331, 1331.e1f
    pseudo-malfunction, 1331
    unexpected drop in pacing rate, 1331, 1332f

Pacemakers (Continued)
  unexpected pacing at or near the upper rate, 1330–1331, 1330.e1f, 1330.e1t
  types of, 1321, 1325f
  types of devices, 1321
Pace-sense malfunctions, 1341
Pacing, 1323
  biventricular, ameliorative role of, 1326
  bradycardia, NASPE/BPEG generic code for, 1325t
  hemodynamic aspects of, 1326, 1326b
  His bundle, 1326b
    permanent, 1326b
  mode and timing cycles of, 1326–1331
    common modes of, 1326–1327, 1326.e3t, 1327f–1328f, 1327f
    definitions of, 1326
    rate responsive pacing, 1327–1328, 1328b, 1329f
    single- or dual-chamber pacing device, 1328
    troubleshooting, 1328–1331, 1329.e1f, 1330t
  rate responsive, 1327–1328, 1328b, 1329f
  right ventricle
    adverse effects of, 1326
    potential deleterious effects of, 1326
  ventricular, 1326
Pacing-induced proarrhythmia, 1331, 1331.e1f
Pacing lead design, 1325f
Pacing rate, unexpected drop in, 1331, 1332f
Pacing stimulus, 1323b–1324b
Pacing thresholds, 1323b–1324b
Paclitaxel
  cardiotoxic effects of, 1092t
  in drug-eluting stents, 793.e2
Paclitaxel-coated balloons and stents, controversy about, 861–862
PAD. See Peripheral artery disease
PAH. See Pulmonary arterial hypertension
Pain
  of aortic dissection, 821
  management of, after noncardiac surgery, 419b
  narcotics for, 1005.e2
Palliative care
  for congenital heart disease, 1551
  in elderly, cardiovascular disease in, 1694–1695
Palpitations, 1156b–1159b, 1162.e5
  in cardiac arrhythmias, 1146–1147
  differential diagnosis of, 1147
  unexplained, 1162.e5t
Panautonomic neuropathy, 1388
Pancreatitis, chest pain in, 600t, 601
Pandemic viral illnesses, 1751–1765
Pandemics, receding, 14, 16t
Panic disorder, chest pain in, 600t, 601
Pannus, echocardiography in, 256b
Papaverine, as coronary vasodilator, 614b
Papillary fibroelastoma, 1832–1833, 1832.e1f, 1834t
  echocardiography in, 253b
Papillary muscles, in mitral regurgitation, 1455–1456
PAPVC. See Partial anomalous pulmonary venous connection
PAR-1. See Protease-activated receptor types 1
Paradoxical embolism, 1639
Paradoxical pulse, 1620–1621
Paraganglioma, 1795–1796, 1796b, 1834, 1834.e1f, 1836f
Parallel group design, 43
Parasympathetic drive, augmentation of, 1899–1900
Parasympathetic nervous systems, 1893, 1895t
Parathyroid hormones, cardiovascular disease and, 1796–1797
Paravalvular aortic regurgitation (PVR), after TAVR, 1431–1432
Paravalvular leak, in prosthetic heart valves, 1501–1503, 1502f
Paravalvular regurgitation, in transcatheter aortic valve replacement, 1437
Parenteral factor Xa antagonists, for STEMI, 675–677
Parietal layer, of pericardium, 1615b
Parkinsonian tremor, electrocardiography of, 173f
Paroxysmal nocturnal dyspnea, in heart failure, 935
Paroxysmal supraventricular tachycardia, 1257–1270
  AVNRT: anatomy, physiology and ECG characteristics, 1259b–1260b
  clinical presentation of, 1258–1263
  ECG characteristics and ECG classification of, 1257–1258, 1258f–1260f
  epidemiology of, 1259b–1260b

Partial anomalous pulmonary veins, 1554–1557
  anatomic description and prevalence of, 1554–1555, 1557f–1558f
  clinical features of, 1555–1556
  long-term outcomes and complications of, 1556–1557
  repairs for, 1556, 1558f
Partial anomalous pulmonary venous connection (PAPVC), 1554–1555
Particulate matter, 33–34
Parvovirus infection, myocardial, 1080b–1081b
Passive fixation leads, 1322b–1323b
Patent ductus arteriosus, 1559
  pregnancy and, 1737–1738
  treatment of, 1591, 1591f
Patent foramen ovale (PFO), management of, 885b–886b, 886t
Patient history, 123–124
  in heart failure, 134–135
Patiromer, 988
PCCD. See Progressive cardiac conduction disease
PCIs. See Percutaneous coronary interventions
PCR. See Polymerase chain reaction
PCSK9. See Proprotein convertase subtilisin-kexin type 9
PCSK9, 82f, 82b
PCWP. See Pulmonary capillary wedge pressure
Peak walking time, 843
Pediatric populations, therapy in, 1651
Penbutolol, for angina pectoris, 758t
Penetrating atherosclerotic aortic ulcer, 831–832, 832.e1f, 834f
Penicillin, in infective endocarditis, 1519t–1521t, 1519b–1523b
Pentoxifylline, for peripheral artery disease, 847.e2t, 850–851
Penumbra Indigo (Penumbra, Almeda, CA) aspiration system, 862
Peptic ulcer disease, chest pain in, 600t, 601
Percutaneous 4TECH TriCinch Coil Tricuspid Valve Repair System early feasibility study, 1490b–1492b
Percutaneous balloon mitral valvuloplasty, 4
  for mitral stenosis, during pregnancy, 1447
  transcatheter interventional therapy vs., 1449–1450
Percutaneous balloon pericardiotomy, in cardiac tamponade, 1624
Percutaneous biopsy, for pericardial effusion and cardiac tamponade, 1625
Percutaneous coronary interventions (PCIs), 3, 786–805
  in acute coronary syndromes, 787–793
  adenosine diphosphate receptor antagonists in, 799–800, 800.e1t
  adjunctive pharmacotherapy in, 787.e1, 787.e3t
  angiographic complications of, 802
  antiplatelet agents in, 799–801
  antithrombin agents in, 801
  aspiration devices for, 795
  aspirin in, 799
  in asymptomatic or minimally symptomatic patients, 787
  atherectomy in, 794, 794f
  balloon angioplasty in, 793
  in bifurcation lesions, 790–791
  bivalirudin in, 801
  in cardiogenic shock, 792
  in cardiomyopathy/left ventricular dysfunction, 792
  in chronic total occlusions, 789
  clinical features of, 787.e1, 787.e2t
  clinical presentations of, 786–787
  contrast-induced acute kidney injury in, 1875
  coronary artery bypass grafting vs., 573–574
  coronary artery bypass surgery vs., 774b–775b
    medical therapy, 775–776
  by coronary artery hemodynamic data, 769
  coronary devices in, 793–796
  coronary physiology in, 795–796, 796f
  coronary stents for, 793, 793.e1f
  excimer laser angioplasty and, 794.e1
  factor Xa inhibitors in, 801
  future perspectives in, 803
  glycoprotein IIb/IIIa inhibitors in, 800–801
  guidelines for, 787.e1
    appropriateness criteria for, 787.e1, 787.e4t, 787.e5t, 787.e6t, 787.e7t, 787.e8t, 787.e9t
    for heterogeneous populations, 1747
  indications for, 786–787

Percutaneous coronary interventions (PCIs) (Continued)
  intravascular imaging in, 796, 796f–797f, 796t–797t
  in ischemic cardiomyopathy, 792
  in jeopardized myocardium, 787
  in left main coronary artery disease, 787–789, 788t–789t, 790f–791f
  lesion calcification in, 791–792
  low-molecular weight heparin in, 801
  mechanical aspiration and, 795.e1
  mechanical circulatory support in, 796–798, 798f
  in moderate to severe angina, 786.e1
  mortality after, 801
  myocardial infarction and, 801–802, 801.e1t
  before noncardiac surgery, 420–421
  no-reflow during, 802
  for NSTE-ACS, 731
  in NSTEMI, 787
  orbital atherectomy and, 794.e1
  outcomes after, 801–803
    benchmarking and procedural volumes, 803, 803.e1t
    early, 801–802
    late, 802
  in patients with diabetes mellitus, 792
  patients with recent myocardial infarction evaluated for potential staged, 294–295
  patient-specific considerations in, 787–793
  preoperative considerations of, 787
  in renal dysfunction, 792–793
  rotational atherectomy and, 794.e1, 797f
  saphenous vein grafts in, 789–790, 791f
  specific lesion subsets in, 787–792
  in stable ischemic heart disease and stable angina, 786–787
  in STEMI, 787
  stents for
    drug-eluting, 793
    everolimus-eluting, 793, 793–794
    paclitaxel-eluting, 793.e2
    sirolimus-eluting, 793.e2
    thrombosis, 802, 802.e1t, 802.e2f
    zotarolimus-eluting, 793, 793–794
  stroke after, 885b–886b
  in three-vessel coronary artery disease, 789
  thrombectomy for, 795
  thrombus and, 792
  urgent revascularization after, 802
  vascular access for, 798–799, 799.e1f, 799.e2f
    complications in, 799
Percutaneous transluminal angioplasty, for peripheral artery disease, 851
Perfusion imaging
  interpretation, 287b–288b, 288t
  principles of, 290
Perfusion therapy, for STEMI, 667–679
Pericardial cyst, echocardiography in, 253b
Pericardial disease, 404, 1615–1629
  acute pericarditis, 1616–1620
    causes of, 1616
    definition of, 1616, 1617t
    diagnosis of, 1618–1619
    differential diagnosis of, 1616
    electrocardiogram (ECG) in, 1616–1617, 1618f
    epidemiology of, 1616
    etiology of, 1617t
    history of, 1616
    laboratory testing in, 1616–1618
    management of, 1618–1619, 1618t–1619t, 1619f
    natural history of, 1618–1619
    physical examination in, 1616
    recurrent, 1619–1620, 1620.e1f
  in children, 1630b–1633b
  constrictive pericarditis, 1625–1630
    cardiac catheterization and angiography for, 1627, 1628f
    clinical presentation of, 1625b–1626b
    computed tomography and cardiac magnetic resonance for, 1627–1628, 1629f
    echocardiography-Doppler examination for, 1627, 1627.e1f
    etiology of, 1617t, 1625f, 1625b–1626b
    laboratory testing in, 1627, 1627.e1f
    management of, 1628–1630
    pathophysiology of, 1625b–1626b, 1626f
    physical examination in, 1626–1627
    from restrictive cardiomyopathy, differentiating, 1628, 1630t

Pericardial disease *(Continued)*
    coronary computed tomography angiography in, 354, 356f
    effusive-constrictive pericarditis, 1630–1633
    during lactation, 1630b–1633b
    metastatic, 1630b–1633b
    pericardial effusion and cardiac tamponade, 1620–1625
        clinical presentation of, 1621
        etiology of, 1617t, 1620
        hemodynamics of, 1620–1621, 1621f–1622f, 1622t
        laboratory testing in, 1622, 1622f–1623f
        management of, 1623–1624, 1624t
        pathophysiology of, 1620–1621, 1620.e1f
        pericardial fluid, analysis of, 1624–1625
        pericardioscopy and percutaneous biopsy, 1625
    pericardium
        anatomy and physiology of, 1615.e1f, 1615b, 1616f
        congenital anomalies of, 1630b–1633b
    in pregnancy, 1630b–1633b
    specific etiologies of, 1630b–1633b
        in autoimmune and autoinflammatory diseases, 1630b–1633b
        hemopericardium, 1630b–1633b
        infectious, 1630b–1633b
        post-cardiac injury syndromes, 1630b–1633b
        primary pericardial tumors, 1630b–1633b
        radiation-induced pericarditis, 1630b–1633b
        with renal disease, 1630b–1633b
        stress cardiomyopathy, 1630b–1633b
    thyroid-associated, 1630b–1633b
Pericardial effusion, 704–705, 1620–1625
    chest radiography in, 271
    clinical presentation of, 1621
    echocardiography in, 240–242, 240f
    etiology of, 1617t, 1620
    hemodynamics of, 1620–1621, 1621f–1622f, 1622t
    in hypothyroidism, 1802
    laboratory testing in, 1622, 1622f–1623f
    management of, 1623–1624, 1624t
    pathophysiology of, 1620–1621, 1620.e1f
    pericardial fluid, analysis of, 1624–1625
    pericardioscopy and percutaneous biopsy in, 1625
Pericardial function, normal, 404–405, 405f, 405.e1f
Pericardial hematoma, echocardiography in, 241–242, 241f
Pericardial knock, in constrictive pericarditis, 1627
Pericardial space or sac, 1615b
Pericardial tamponade, evaluation of, 138
Pericardial tumor, echocardiography in, 243b, 244f
Pericardiectomy, for constrictive pericarditis, 1628–1629
Pericardiocentesis
    in cardiac tamponade, 1623
    echocardiography in, 241b–242b
Pericardioscopy, for cardiac tamponade, 1624–1625
Pericarditis, 600, 704–705
    acute, 1616–1620
        causes of, 1616
        definition of, 1616, 1617t
        diagnosis of, 1618–1619
        differential diagnosis of, 1616
        electrocardiography in, 168, 168f, 1618f
        epidemiology of, 1616
        history of, 1616
        laboratory testing in, 1616–1618
        management of, 1618–1619, 1618t–1619t, 1619f
        natural history of, 1618–1619
        physical examination in, 1616
        recurrent, 1619–1620, 1620.e1f
        STEMI vs., 653
    angina pectoris vs., 741
    chest pain in, 600t
    constrictive, 1625–1630
        cardiac catheterization and angiography in, 1627, 1628f
        clinical presentation of, 1625b–1626b
        computed tomography and cardiac magnetic resonance for, 1627–1628, 1629f
        echocardiography in, 242–244, 242f–243f
        echocardiography-Doppler examination for, 1627, 1627.e1f
        etiology of, 1617t, 1625f, 1625b–1626b
        evaluation of, 139
        laboratory testing in, 1627, 1627.e1f
        magnetic resonance imaging in, 329–330
        management of, 1628–1630

Pericarditis *(Continued)*
    pathophysiology of, 1625b–1626b, 1626f
    physical examination in, 1626–1627
    restrictive cardiomyopathy and, 1044.e1f
    from restrictive cardiomyopathy, differentiating, 1628, 1630t
  effusive-constrictive, 1630–1633
  evaluation of, 138
  radiation-induced, 1630b–1633b
  in rheumatic diseases, 1818–1820
  in rheumatic fever, 1534, 1534t
  in rheumatoid arthritis, 1819
  in systemic lupus erythematosus, 1818–1819
  in systemic sclerosis, 1819
Pericardium
  anatomy and physiology of, 1615.e1f, 1615b, 1616f
  congenital anomalies of, 1630b–1633b
  functions of, 1615b
  lipomas of, 1833, 1835f
Pericytes, 426–427
Peri-infarction block, 160b
Perimyocarditis, 1616
Periodic paralyses, 1864–1866
Peripartum cardiomyopathy, 1042, 1733f
  clinical features of, 1042
  in women, 1719
Peripheral artery disease (PAD), 311b–312b, 837–859
  approach to, 859–860, 860f
    in aortoiliac disease, 864, 864.e3f
    atherectomy for, 863, 863.e1f, 863.e2f
    balloon angioplasty for, 860, 861f
    bare-metal stents for, 860, 860f–861f
    in cervical artery disease, 865–867
    covered stents for, 862, 862.e1f
    cryoplasty for, 863, 863.e3f
    drug-coated balloons for, 861–862
    drug-eluting peripheral stents for, 860–861
    endovascular treatments in, 860
    in extracranial carotid disease, 865–866, 865t–866t, 866f, 866.e1f
    in femoral-popliteal artery disease, 864–865, 864.e3f, 864f–865f
    intravascular lithotripsy for, 863, 863.e3f
    of lower extremities, 864–865
    medical therapy to improve endovascular durability, 863
    in mesenteric artery disease, 867, 867.e1f
    in renal artery disease, 867, 867.e1f
    in subclavian disease, 866–867, 866.e1f
    thrombectomy for, 862–863
    thrombolysis for, 862–863, 862f
    in tibial disease, 865, 865.e1f, 865.e2f
    in vertebral disease, 866–867, 866.e1f
  assessment of, ankle-brachial index in, 128
  asymptomatic, 859
  blood supply in, factors regulating, 838–839, 839f, 839.e1f
  categorization of, 841–842, 841.e1f, 842t
  classification of, 841, 841t
  claudication and, 859
  clinical features of, 840–842
  coronary artery disease and, 774.e1
  critical limb ischemia and, 859
  diagnostic tests in, 847.e1t
  epidemiology of, 837–839, 837.e1f
  evaluation of, 130
  exercise electrocardiographic testing in, 192–193, 193
  guidelines for, 847.e1t, 847.e2t, 847.e3t
  intervention for, 863–864
    vascular access in, 864, 864.e1f, 864.e2f
    vascular imaging in, 863–864, 863.e3f
  longitudinal follow-up in, 847.e1t
  pathophysiology of, 838–839, 838f
  physical examination in, 847.e1t
  physical findings of, 841, 841f
  prognosis of, 845–847, 846f, 846.e1f
  risk factors for, 838, 838t, 838.e1f
  skeletal muscle structure and metabolic function in, 839
  stroke and, 859
  symptoms of, 840–841
  testing for, 842–845
    ankle-brachial index in, 843
    computed tomographic angiography in, 845, 845f
    contrast-enhanced angiography in, 845, 846f
    Doppler ultrasonography in, 844

Peripheral artery disease (PAD) *(Continued)*
    duplex ultrasound imaging in, 844, 844f–845f
    magnetic resonance angiography in, 844
    pulse volume recording in, 843–844
    segmental pressure measurement in, 842–843, 843f
    treadmill exercise, 843
  treatment of, 847–849, 847.e1t, 847.e2t, 847.e3t, 847.e4f
    anticoagulant therapy in, 849, 849.e1f
    antiplatelet monotherapy in, 848
    antiplatelet therapy in, 848–849, 848.e2f
    antithrombotic therapy in, 848–849
    blood pressure control in, 847–848
    in diabetes, 847, 847.e5f
    diet in, 847
    exercise training in, 850, 850f
    lipid-lowering therapy in, 848, 848.e1f, 848.e2f
    percutaneous transluminal angioplasty and stents in, 851
    pharmacotherapy in, 850–851
    risk factor modification in, 847
    smoking cessation in, 847, 849
    surgery for, 851, 852f
    vascular history of, 847.e1t
Peripheral edema, in acute heart failure, 954
Peripheral vascular disease, 837, 859
Peripheral vasculature, neurohormonal alterations of, in heart failure, 919–921
Perivascular fat attenuation, 347, 348f
Permanent His bundle pacing, 1326b, 1326.e2f
Permeability ratio, 1163b–1166b
Personalized medicine, in heart failure, 1000
Pertuzumab, 1095, 1095b
  cardiotoxic effects of, 1092t
Pestilence, 14, 16t
PET. *See* Positron emission tomography
PET/CT scanner, 279
  imaging protocols, 286f
  misregistration artifact on hybrid, 289f
PET MPI tracers, 280b–281b
PET/MR scanner, 279
PET/SPECT dynamic image interpretation, 287b–288b
PGF. *See* Primary graft failure
P-glycoprotein, 97t, 100
PH. *See* Pulmonary hypertension
Pharmacodynamics, 93–96, 94f
  principles, 93b–96b
Pharmacogenetics, 93
  other important effects, 97–98
  in prescribing drugs, 100
Pharmacogenomic principles, 93b–96b
Pharmacogenomics, 93
  in heart failure, 996.e1, 1000
Pharmacokinetics, 93–96, 93f–94f
  high-risk, 96, 96f
Pharmacologic stress, stress testing and, 283, 284f
Pharmacotherapy, obesity and, 552, 553t
Phase I studies, in clinical trial, 42b–43b
Phase II studies, in clinical trial, 42b–43b
Phase III studies, in clinical trial, 42b–43b
Phase IV studies, in clinical trial, 42b–43b
Phenotype, 71
Phenylephrine
  for acute heart failure, 965
  for STEMI, 690
Phenytoin, 1211.e1t, 1209t, 1212t, 1214t, 1217
Pheochromocytoma, 485–486, 1795–1796, 1796b
Phosphodiesterase inhibitors, in acute heart failure, 964–965
Phosphodiesterase type 5 (PDE5) inhibitors, for heart failure with preserved and mildly reduced ejection, 1028
Phospholamban, 897
Phospholemman (PLM), 1171b–1173b
Physical activity, 579
  cardiovascular disease and, 461–462, 461f
  increase, interventions to, 462
  in dyslipidemia, 596
  in heart failure, 981, 981.e1f
  in obesity, 552, 552.e1f
  prescription, in elderly, 1706
  with STEMI, 680
  in women, cardiovascular disease and, 1710b–1714b
Physical agents, myocarditis and, 1083, 1083.e1

Physical appearance, in STEMI, 653
Physical examination, 123–140, 139t, 139b
    abdomen examination in, 126
    in abdominal aortic aneurysms, 807
    in acute heart failure, 953–954
    in amyloidosis, 1044
    in atrial fibrillation, 1274
    in carcinoid heart disease, 1048
    cardiovascular, 126–134
        blood pressure in, 128–129
        cardiac auscultation in, 130–131
        cardiac inspection and palpation in, 130
        jugular venous pressure and waveform in, 126–128, 128f, 128t
        pulses in, 129–130, 129f–130f
    chest examination in, 126, 127f
    in chest pain, 601–602
    extremities examination in, 126
    future directions for, 139
    general, 124–126
    general appearance in, 125, 125t
    head and neck examination in, 125–126
    in heart failure, 135, 935t–936t, 936–938
    skin examination in, 125, 125f
    in STEMI, 653–655
Physical exercise, benefits of, 1553
Physical fitness, in women, cardiovascular disease and, 1710b–1714b
Physical inactivity, 25
    in elderly, 1706
Phytosterols, 520
Pindolol, for angina pectoris, 758t
Pioglitazone, in diabetes mellitus, 562t–563t, 564b–566b
PISA method, 1460
Pitavastatin, in chronic kidney disease, 1883t
Pituitary gland, 1791
    adenoma of, 1792
Pituitary hormones, cardiovascular disease and, 1791–1793
Pivotal studies, in clinical trial, 42b–43b
PKP2 gene, 1039b–1040b
Placebo, randomization to, 48–49
Placement of Aortic Transcatheter Valves (PARTNER) trial, 1430.e1
Plakoglobin, mutations in, 1174b–1175b
Plant oils, 535
Plaque erosion, in NSTE-ACS, 714–715, 716t, 717f
Plaque morphology, OCT in, 379.e1t, 381
Plaque rupture, in NSTE-ACS, 714–715, 716t, 717f
Plaques
    angiogenesis in, 434–435, 434f
    mineralization, 435
Plasma catecholamines, 1898
Plasma D-dimer assay, in pulmonary embolism, 1642
Plasmin, 425–426
Plasminogen activator inhibitor, type 1 (PAI-1), 1767, 1771f
Plastic bronchitis, single ventricle and, 1582
Platelet glycoprotein IIb/IIIa inhibitors, for acute limb ischemia, 854–855
Platelets
    activation of, 1768, 1768f
    adhesion of, 1768
    aggregation of, 1768–1769
    hemostatic system and, 1767–1769, 1767f
    inhibition of, 1767
    in STEMI, 652b
Pleural effusions, in heart failure, 136–137
Pleuritis, chest pain in, 600t
Plexuses, ganglionated, 1179b
PLM. See Phospholemman
PMJ. See Purkinje fiber-myocyte junction
PMT. See Pacemaker-mediated tachycardia
Pneumonia
    in adult congenital heart disease, 1543–1544
    chest pain in, 600t
Pneumothorax, 600–601
    implantable cardioverter-defibrillators and, 1343
POCD. See Postoperative cognitive dysfunction
Pocket hematoma, implantable cardioverter-defibrillators and, 1343, 1343.e2f
POINT study, 878, 878f
Policy interventions, for cardiovascular disease prevention, 28–29
Polyangiitis
    granulomatosis with, 1817, 1818f
    microscopic, 1817

Polyarteritis nodosa, 1817, 1818f
    cardiovascular complications of, 1817
    treatment of, 1817
Polycystic ovary syndrome, cardiovascular disease in women and, 1710b–1714b
Polygenic coronary artery disease, 81, 83, 83f
Polygenic hypercholesterolemia, 510
Polygenic risk scoring, 81, 81f
Polymerase chain reaction (PCR), 76
Polymyositis, 1819–1820
    cardiac conduction disturbances in, 1821
Polypharmacy
    drug interaction in, 99
    in elderly, 1690b–1693b
Polyphenols, 539b
Polypill approach, 465–466
Polysomnography, for obstructive sleep apnea, 485
Polyunsaturated fatty acids, n-3, in heart failure, 1000
Ponatinib, cardiotoxic effects of, 1092t, 1096
Popliteal artery, 865
    occluded, 862f
    stenosis in, 863.e1f
Popliteal artery entrapment syndrome, 853–854
Portal free fatty acid hypothesis, visceral obesity and, 549
Portopulmonary hypertension, pulmonary arterial hypertension associated with, 1662
Position emission tomography (PET), 278–279, 279t
    advantages of, 279t
    imaging of infiltrative and inflammatory processes, 287b–288b, 289f
    photon attenuation and attenuation correction, 287b–288b
    principles, 278f
    protocols, 286–288, 287b–288b
    viability imaging interpretation, 287b–288b, 288f
Positive predictive value (PPV), 54b–55b
    of biomarkers, 105–106, 105t
Positive remodeling, 434
    of atherosclerotic lesion, 425
    coronary computed tomography angiography in, 344, 346f
Positron emission tomography (PET)
    in aortic valve stenosis, 1408b, 1409f
    FDG, in sarcoid cardiomyopathy, 1045, 1047f
    in myocarditis, 1087
    in pulmonary arterial hypertension, 1668–1669
Postacute sequelae SARS-CoV-2 infection, 1763
Post-atrial ventricular blanking, 1327
Post-cardiac injury syndromes, 1630b–1633b
Posteromedial papillary muscle, 1456
Post-hoc analyses, of clinical trial, 52
Postmediastinal irradiation, in coronary artery disease, 780b–781b
Postmenopausal hormone therapy, 458
Postoperative cognitive dysfunction (POCD), 1707
Post-pulmonary embolism syndrome, 1639–1640
Poststreptococcal reactive arthritis, 1533
Postthrombotic syndrome, in pulmonary embolism, 1640b–1641b, 1641f
Post-transcatheter aortic valve replacement, in cardiac computed tomography, 358, 359f
Posttraumatic stress disorder (PTSD), 1844
Postural orthostatic tachycardia syndrome (POTS), 1147–1148, 1388
Postventricular atrial refractory period (PVARP), 1327
Potassium, 538–539
    dietary, 537f, 539
    in digitalis toxicity, 1000.e2
    in hypertension, 595
    supplemental, drug interaction with, 97t
Potassium channels
    ATP-sensitive, coronary vascular resistance and, 616b–617b
    cardiac, inwardly rectifying, 1171b–1173b
    small-conductance, Ca^{2+}-sensitive, 1171b–1173b
    voltage-gated, 1171b–1173b
Potassium-sparing diuretics, 983t, 984, 985f
    for hypertension, 492
Potential energy, in work of the heart, 909f, 909b–910b
POTS. See Postural orthostatic tachycardia syndrome
Poultry, 535
PPM. See Prosthesis-patient mismatch
PPV. See Positive predictive value
PR interval, 145f, 146, 146t
PR segment, 146–147
Pragmatic (large simple) trials, 49

Pramlintide, in diabetes mellitus, 562t–563t
Prasugrel
    in arterial thrombosis, 1777
    in coronary artery disease, chronic kidney disease and, 1880t–1881t
    in NSTE-ACS, 725, 725f, 735.e6t
    in percutaneous coronary intervention, 787.e3t, 800
    ticagrelor vs., 726b
Pravastatin, in chronic kidney disease, 1883t
"Precision Public Health", 467
Predictive value, of biomarkers, 105–106, 105t
Prednisone, for giant cell arteritis, 1815
Preexcitation syndrome, 1187–1188
Pregnancy
    anticoagulation during, 1735–1737
    aortic dissection and, 821
    aortic stenosis and, 1735
    arrhythmias and, 1731, 1737, 1737.e2f
    assisted reproductive technologies, 1727b–1729b
    atrial fibrillation in, 1285, 1287.e6t, 1287.e8
    atrial fibrillation/flutter during, 1737.e3f
    atrial septal defect and, 1737–1738
    cardiac surgery during, 1731
    cardiomyopathy in, 1732–1733, 1732.e1f
    cardiovascular changes in, 1723–1724, 1724t
    cardiovascular disease and, 457–458
    complex congenital lesions in, 1738, 1739t
    congenital heart disease and, 1737–1740
    congenitally corrected transition of the great arteries in, 1738
    coronary artery disease and, 1734
    cyanotic heart disease and, 1739–1740
    dilated cardiomyopathy and, 1732
    Ebstein anomaly and, 1738
    evaluation and testing during, 1724–1729
        chest radiography in, 1725
    Fontan operation and, 1738
    general management principles in, 1729–1731
    heart disease and, 1723–1742
        general management principles in, 1729–1731, 1735t–1736t
        guidelines for, 1735.e1t
    hemodynamic changes of, 1723–1724
    hypertension in, 1730f, 1731–1732, 1731.e1t, 1732f
    hypertrophic cardiomyopathy and, 1068–1069, 1732
    left-sided obstruction in, 1738
    management planning in, 1727–1729
    Marfan syndrome and, 1740, 1740.e1f
    mechanical prostheses and, 1736t
    medical therapy during, 1731, 1735.e1t
    mitral stenosis and, 1734f
    native valvular heart disease and, 1734–1735, 1734f
    normal, cardiac findings during, 1724–1725
    oral anticoagulants and, 1787
    patent ductus arteriosus and, 1737–1738
    pericardial disease in, 1630b–1633b
    peripartum cardiomyopathy and, 1042, 1733f
    preconception counseling for, 1725–1729, 1725t
    prosthetic heart valves in, 1499
    prosthetic valves and, 1735–1737, 1737.e1f
    pulmonary hypertension and, 1676, 1740
    pulmonary stenosis and, 1731
    rheumatic mitral stenosis and, 1447
    risk stratification in, 1725–1727, 1726t, 1727f, 1728t, 1729f
    role of cardiac testing during, 1725
    specific cardiovascular conditions, 1731–1732
    tetralogy of Fallot and, 1738
    timing of complications in women, 1724f
    unoperated complex congenital lesions in, 1738
    valvular heart disease and, 1734–1735, 1734f, 1740.e1t
    venous thrombosis and, 1774
    ventricular septal defect and, 1737–1738
    ventricular tachycardia during, 1737.e4f, 1732
    warfarin and, 1785
    in women with congenital heart disease, 1552–1553, 1554t
Pregnancy-associated hypertension, cardiovascular disease in women and, 1710b–1714b, 1714f
Preload, 906, 906b
    wall stress and, 907b–908b
Premature atrial complex (PAC), 1246b–1247b
Premature menopause, cardiovascular disease and, 457–458

Premature ventricular complexes (PVCs), 1162.e3t, 1239f, 1242f, 1288–1292
 bigeminy, 1288
 clinical features of, 1289
 clinical use of, 1212
 electrocardiography in, 1288–1289, 1289f–1292f
 idiopathic, 1291
 induced cardiomyopathy, 1291–1292
 management of, 1289–1292
 multiform/multifocal, 1288, 1289f
 in structural heart disease, 1291
 trigeminy, 1288
 ventricular arrhythmias and, 1356–1357
Premixed, in diabetes mellitus, 562t–563t
Prescription, 100
Pressure natriuresis
 definition of, 474
 in hypertension, 473–474, 475f
Pressure-volume area, 909
Pressure-volume relation (PVR), of pericardial sac, 1615b
Pressure wave, 392
Pressure-work index, 909
Presyncope, in cardiac arrhythmias, 1147–1148
Pre-transcatheter aortic valve replacement, in cardiac computed tomography, 357–358, 358f, 359t
Pre-transcatheter mitral valve replacement, evaluation, 358–359, 360f
Primary cardiac neoplasms, evaluation of, 310
Primary endpoints, analysis of, 46–47
Primary graft failure (PGF), 1138
Primary hyperaldosteronism, 484–485, 484t
 sleep-disordered breathing associated with, 485
Primary hypertension, 471
 diagnostic approach to, 480–484
  blood pressure measurement of, 481t
  history and physical examination of, 480–481
 therapeutic options and approaches for, 490
  blood pressure guidelines, 490
  dietary approaches, 490, 491t
  effects of lifestyle intervention in older people, 490
  goals of, 490
Primary invasive strategy, for Non-ST-segment elevation ACS, 573
Primary palliative care, in heart failure, 1004
Primary percutaneous coronary intervention
 adjunctive anticoagulation for, 677
 antiplatelet therapy for, 677–678, 678f–679f
Primary pericardial tumors, 1630b–1633b
Primary prevention, for cardiovascular disease, 442–443, 443f
Primary reperfusion therapy, for ST-segment elevation myocardial infarction, 573
Primary stroke center (PSC), key elements of, 880
Primordial prevention, for cardiovascular disease, 442–443, 443f
Primum atrial septal defect, 1554
Prinzmetal variant angina
 electrocardiography in, 164f
 NSTE-ACS and, 734
PRKG1, 812
Proarrhythmia, 1212–1213, 1897
Probability, for clinical decision making, 54b–55b
Probability theory, 54b–55b
Procainamide, 1211.e1t, 1209t, 1212t, 1213–1215, 1213b–1215b, 1214t
 for pregnancy, 1730f
Procoagulant disorders, atheroembolism and, 856
Procoagulant proteins, elevated levels of, 1773
Prodromes, in sudden cardiac death, 1349, 1350f, 1367
Proepicardial organ, 426–427
Prognostic impact studies, 107
PROGRESS (Perindopril Protection Against Recurrent Stroke Study) study, 874b–877b
Progressive aortic stenosis, 1409
Progressive cardiac conduction disease (PCCD), 1205–1206
 clinical description and manifestations of, 1205–1206
 genetic basis of, 1205b–1206b
Progressive fusion, 1183b–1184b
Prolactin disease, 1792–1793
Prolactin-producing pituitary adenomas, 1792–1793
Prolonged QT intervals, 1162.e3t, 1162.e5
Propafenone, 1211.e1t, 1209t, 1212t, 1214t, 1218–1219, 1218b
 in atrial fibrillation, 1280
 drug interaction with, 97t
 for pregnancy, 1730f

Propagation, safety factor for, 1173
Prophylactic Defibrillator Implantation in Patients with Nonischemic Dilated Cardiomyopathy Trial (DEFINITE), 1111b–1113b
Propranolol, 1211.e1t, 1208t–1209t, 1212t, 1214t
 for angina pectoris, 758t
Proprotein convertase subtilisin-kexin type 9 (PCSK9), 510, 1705
 inhibitors of, 517–518
 inhibitors of, in coronary heart disease, 559
Prorenin, in hypertension, 475
Prospective Comparison of ARNI with an ACE-Inhibitor to Determine Impact on Global Mortality and Morbidity in Heart Failure (PARADIGM-HF) trial, 1010
Prospective open-label blinded endpoint (PROBE) design, 45
Prostacyclin
 coronary blood flow and, 612
 in heart failure, 917–918
Prostaglandin E_2 (PGE_2), in heart failure, 917–918
Prostaglandin-I_2, for pulmonary arterial hypertension, 1664b–1665b
Prosthesis-patient mismatch (PPM)
 with prosthetic heart valves, 1500–1501, 1500f–1501f
 in transcatheter aortic valve replacement, 1437
Prosthetic heart valves, 1495–1504
 antithrombotic therapy in, 1498–1499, 1499t
  interruption of, 1498–1499
 assessment of, echocardiography in, 235–240, 236.e1t, 237f–238f
 bioprosthetic
  autografts, 1497
  homografts, 1497
  stented, 1495–1497, 1496f
  stentless, 1496f, 1497
  transcatheter, 1496f, 1497–1498
 bleeding in, 1502b–1503b
 chest radiography in, 1499
 deterioration, structural, 1501, 1502f
 Doppler echocardiography in, 1500
 dysfunction and complication of, evaluation and treatment of, 1500–1503, 1500f–1501f
 evaluation of, 138
 hemolytic anemia in, 1503
 infective endocarditis in, 1503
  prophylaxis for, 1499
 mechanical, 1495, 1496f
  tissue valves vs., 1497b–1498b
 noncardiac surgery and, 411b–412b
 paravalvular leak in, 1501–1503, 1502f
 in pregnancy, 1499, 1735–1737, 1737.e1f
 prosthesis-patient mismatch with, 1500–1501, 1500f–1501f
 replacement procedure
  choice of, 1497b–1498b
  clinical assessment after, 1499
  medical management and surveillance after, 1498–1500
  surgical, transcatheter valves vs., 1500
 thromboembolism in, 1502b–1503b
 thrombosis and, 1496f, 1502f, 1502b–1503b
 tissue, 1495–1498, 1496f
  mechanical valves vs., 1497b–1498b
 types of, 1495–1498
Prosthetic regurgitation, echocardiography in, 237b–240b, 238f–240f
Prosthetic valve endocarditis, 1511b–1512b
 antimicrobial therapy for, 1519t–1521t, 1519b–1523b
Protease-activated receptor types 1 (PAR-1), 1768, 1768f
Proteasome inhibitors, cardiotoxic effects of, 1092t, 1094
Protein C, 1767, 1767f
 deficiency in, 1773
Protein G, 901, 901b
Protein kinase A, 901–903
Protein-losing enteropathy, single ventricle and, 1582
Protein S deficiency, 1773
Protein(s)
 abnormalities of, in heart failure, 925, 925t
 contractile, 892–894, 892f
Proteome, 87
 conceptual relationship of, 88f
Proteomics
 analytic challenges for, 87–88, 89f
 in cardiovascular medicine, 87–91
 novel technologies in identification of biomarkers, 87

Proteomics (Continued)
 overview of, 87
  discovery process, 88–90
  experiment, 90f
Prothrombin gene mutation, 1773
Prothrombinase, 1769
Prothrombotic state, biomarkers suggestive of, 1758
Protozoal infection, myocardial, 1081–1082, 1081f–1082f
Proximal myotonic myopathy, 1856–1857
PSC. See Primary stroke center
Pseudoaneurysms, 806–807
 after myocardial infarction, 218b–219b, 218.e1f
Pseudoinfarction, 656–657
 electrocardiography in, 167, 168f
Pseudo-malfunction, 1331
Pseudoneoplasm, echocardiography in, 255
Psoriatic arthritis, atherosclerosis in, 1811
Psychiatric disorders, 1843–1846
 management of, 1846–1851
  antidepressant medications in, 1847–1850, 1848t
  anxiolytic medications, 1850
  collaborative care, 1851
  current guidelines, 1846–1847, 1847b
  electroconvulsive therapy, 1850
  exercise, 1851
  mindfulness, 1850–1851
  omega-3 fatty acids, 1850.e1
  psychotherapy in, 1847
  St. John's wort, 1850.e1
  transcranial magnetic stimulation, 1850
Psychosocial factors, cardiovascular disease and, 451–453, 452.e1f, 452.e2f
Psychosocial issues, cardiac implantable electrical devices and, 1344f, 1346–1347, 1346.e1t
PTH-related peptide (PTHrP), 1796
PTHrP. See PTH-related peptide
PTSD. See Posttraumatic stress disorder
Public reporting, cardiovascular disease and, 64–65
Pulmonary arterial hypertension (PAH), 1658t, 1660
 chest roentgenogram in, 1667
 in congenital heart disease, 1658t, 1661–1662
 in connective tissue disease, 1661
 echocardiogram for, 1668t
 electrocardiography in, 1667
 genetic counseling, 1673
 hereditary, 1660–1661, 1660t
 in human immunodeficiency virus infection, 1661
 idiopathic, 1658–1659
 initial management of treatment-naïve, 1673
 mechanisms implicated in pathogenesis of, 1663f–1664f
 physical examination in, 1665, 1668t
 in portal hypertension, 1660
 in rheumatic diseases, 1821–1823, 1822t
 in rheumatoid arthritis, 1823
 right heart catheterization for, 1669f
 risk stratification of, 1670, 1670.e1f
 in Sjögren syndrome, 1823
 in systemic lupus erythematosus, 1822
 in systemic sclerosis, 1822, 1822t, 1823f
 systemic sclerosis with, 1661
 in Takayasu arteritis, 1822t, 1823
 therapeutic escalation and end-stage disease, 1673
 treatment for, 1672–1673, 1673t, 1675f
 two-dimensional transthoracic echocardiography, 1667, 1667f
Pulmonary arteries, abnormalities of, 1582
Pulmonary artery (PA) catheterization, noncardiac surgery and, 423
Pulmonary artery pressure
 evaluation of, in cardiac transplantation, 1132–1133
 monitoring of, in STEMI, 684–685, 685t
 in pulmonary embolism, 1638.e1f, 1637b–1639b, 1638f
Pulmonary capillary wedge pressure (PCWP), 396–397, 397f, 397.e1f, 1011b–1017b, 1014.e1f, 1014.e2f
Pulmonary circulation
 effect of aging on, 1657
 normal, 1656–1657
 physiology, 1656–1657, 1657f
 during exercise, 1657
Pulmonary conditions, chest pain in, 600–601
Pulmonary disease, atrial fibrillation in, 1287.e6t, 1287.e8
Pulmonary edema
 high-altitude, 1674–1675
 in STEMI, 653

Pulmonary embolism, 1635–1655, 1636f
  acute, advanced therapy for, 1648–1651
  angina pectoris vs., 741
  anticoagulation therapy in
    dosing and monitoring of warfarin, 1647
    heparin-induced thrombocytopenia in, 1646
    managing bleeding complications from, 1647–1648
    novel oral, 1647, 1649t
    optimal duration of, 1648
    risk stratification, 1647f, 1648t
    selection of, 1648
    warfarin, 1646
    warfarin overlap with heparin, 1647
  cancer and, 1636, 1637t
  cardiopulmonary dynamics of, 1638.e1f, 1637b–1639b, 1638f
  catheter-based therapy, advances in, 1649–1650
  chest computed tomography in, 1643, 1643f–1644f
  chest pain in, 600t
  chest radiography in, 1643
  chronic thromboembolic pulmonary hypertension, 1640–1641
  classification of, 1639–1641, 1640t
  clinical presentation of, 1642, 1642f, 1642t–1643t
  clinical risk factors for, 1636
  contrast phlebography for, 1644
  in COVID-19 infection, 1637, 1637.e1f
  deep vein thrombosis and, 1640b–1641b
  diagnosis of, 1641–1644
  differential diagnosis of, 1642, 1643t
  echocardiography in, 247b–248b, 247.e1f, 249f–250f, 1644, 1645f
  electrocardiogram (ECG) for, 1643
  electronic decision support for, 1644
  emotional support, 1651
  epidemiology of, 1635–1637
  evolution of oral anticoagulants for, 1647
  future perspectives in, 1652–1653
  general considerations in, 1635–1636
  high-risk, 1639, 1648–1649
  hypercoagulable states and, 1637
  integrated diagnostic approach for, 1644, 1647f
  intermediate-risk, 1639
  low-risk, 1639, 1640t
  lung scanning for, 1644
  magnetic resonance imaging for, 1644
  massive, 1640t, 1649.e1f
  nonthrombotic, 1639
  paradoxical, 1639
  pathophysiology of, 1637–1639
  plasma D-dimer assay in, 1642
  prevention of, 1651–1652
    in-hospital prophylaxis, 1651, 1652t
    in-hospital risk factors, 1652, 1652t
    mechanical prophylaxis, 1652
  pulmonary angiography in, 1644
  pulmonary infarction and, 1639, 1641f
  right ventricular hypertrophy in, 155, 155f
  submassive, 1639.e1f, 1640t
  sudden cardiac death (SCD) and, 1363b–1365b
  surgical embolectomy, 1650, 1650f
  therapy for, 1644–1648
    parenteral, 1645–1646
    patients with cancer, 1651
    risk stratification, 1644–1645
  venous thromboembolic and, 1636, 1637t
    long-term complications of, 1637
    other conditions associated with, 1637
    role of coagulation and platelets in, 1638.e1f, 1637b–1639b, 1639f
  venous ultrasonography for, 1644, 1646f
Pulmonary function, mechanical circulatory support and, 1123, 1123b
Pulmonary function tests, in pulmonary arterial hypertension, 1667–1668
Pulmonary hypertension (PH), 1582–1585, 1583t, 1656–1660
  anatomy of, 1656
  angina pectoris vs., 741
  approach to diagnosis, 1667–1670, 1667b
  chest radiography in, 274, 274f–275f
  chronic thromboembolic, 1674, 1676f
  classification of, 1657–1662, 1658f–1659f, 1658t
    chronic thromboembolic pulmonary hypertension, 1668f, 1672, 1674f
    pulmonary arterial hypertension, 1660

Pulmonary hypertension (PH) (Continued)
  combined pre- and post-capillary, 1662
  definition of, 1656
  echocardiography in, 248, 250f
  in elderly, 1699
  future perspectives on, 1676
  hemodynamics of, 1658–1659
  high-altitude pulmonary edema, 1674–1675
  hyperthyroidism and, 1800
  integrated approach to diagnosing, 1671–1672, 1671f–1672f
  isolated post-capillary clinical classifications, 1659–1660
  from left heart disease, 1674
  normal pulmonary circulation, 1656–1657
  pathobiology of, 1662–1665, 1664f
  pathology of, 1661f, 1662
  pathophysiology of, 1665
  patient medical history, 1665
  perioperative management of, 1676
  pre-capillary clinical classifications, 1660–1662
  pregnancy and, 1740
  pulmonary venoocclusive disease, 1671–1672, 1673t
  pulmonary venous system, 1657
  rheumatic mitral stenosis and, 1447
  systemic manifestations of, 1665
Pulmonary infarction, 1639, 1641f
Pulmonary regurgitation, in tetralogy of Fallot, 1564
Pulmonary stenosis, 1562–1563, 1562f
  pregnancy and, 1731
Pulmonary valve
  replacement of, for congenital heart disease, 1587–1588
  stenosis, pressure gradient determination in, 401
Pulmonary valve systems, for congenital heart disease, 1588, 1588f
Pulmonary vascular resistance (PVR), evaluation of, in cardiac transplantation, 1132–1133
Pulmonary vasculature, aortic valve stenosis and, 1400b–1403b
Pulmonary vasodilators, cardiac catheterization and, 408
Pulmonary veins
  in atrial fibrillation, 1277f, 1282
  Doppler flow patterns of, echocardiography of, 208, 208.e2f
  flow patterns of, 208, 208.e1f, 208.e2f
Pulmonary venoocclusive disease, 1671–1672, 1673t
  pulmonary arterial hypertension associated with, 1662
Pulmonary venous system, 1657
Pulmonic flow murmurs, 582
Pulmonic regurgitation, 1479–1481
  auscultation in, 1479b–1481b
  cardiac magnetic resonance imaging in, 1479b–1481b, 1480f
  causes of, 1479
  clinical presentation of, 1479–1481
  echocardiography in, 235, 236f–237f, 1479b–1481b, 1480f
  management of, 1481
  pathology of, 1479
  physical examination in, 1479b–1481b
  radiography in, 1479b–1481b
Pulmonic stenosis, 1479
  causes of, 1479
  chest radiography in, 275f
  clinical presentation of, 1479
  echocardiography in, 235
  management of, 1479
  pathology of, 1479
  physical examination of, 1479
Pulmonic valve disease, evaluation of, 138
Pulsatile-flow pump, 1122.e1
Pulse pressure
  in acute heart failure, 953
  in heart failure, 136
Pulse volume recording, in peripheral artery disease, 843–844
Pulseless electrical activity, 1374
Pulses
  assessment of, 129–130, 129f–130f
  bifid, 129
  bounding, 129
  carotid artery, 128t, 129, 129f
Pulsus alternans, 129–130, 129f
Pulsus paradoxus, 128, 1620–1621
  in pericardial tamponade, 138

Pulsus parvus et tardus, 130
Pure eicosapentaenoic acid, 519–520
Purkinje cells, 891t
Purkinje fiber-myocyte junction (PMJ), 1177
Purkinje fibers, terminal, 1177, 1177.e1f
PVARP. *See* Postventricular atrial refractory period
PVCs. *See* Premature ventricular complexes
PVR. *See* Paravalvular aortic regurgitation; Pressure-volume relation; Pulmonary vascular resistance

Q

Q wave, 147
  infarction, 638, 657
  noninfarction, 166–168, 167t
QRS complex, 147–149, 147b
  changes in, nonspecific, 171b–172b
  duration of, 146t, 147b–148b
  early patterns of, 147f, 147b–148b
  electrical axis and, 147b–148b
  intrinsicoid deflection of, 147b–148b
  mid- and late patterns of, 147b–148b
  normal, 147–148
  ventricular activation and, 147–149, 147f, 147b
  wide, 160t, 160b
QRST angle, 149b
QS complex, 147
QT interval, 145f, 146t, 148–149
  digitalis effect on, 169, 170f
QT-prolonging antiarrhythmics, 97t
Quadruple-valve disease, 1482–1483
Quality of life
  in heart failure with preserved and mildly reduced ejection, 1010
  in pulmonary embolism, 1651
Quality-of-life assessments, in transcatheter aortic valve replacement, 1432, 1432.e3f, 1432.e4f
Quinapril, in heart failure, 991t
Quinidine, 1211.e1t, 97t, 1209t, 1212t, 1213, 1213b, 1214t
  drug interaction with, 97t
  early afterdepolarization and, 1183

R

R wave, 147, 165–166
RAAS. *See* Renin-angiotensin-aldosterone system
RAAS blockers, for hypertension, 491–492
Race/ethnicity
  acute heart failure in, 946–947
  heart failure in, 997f, 1001
  sudden cardiac death in, 1353f, 1354
  visceral obesity in, 550
Racial minorities, cardiovascular disease and, 66–68, 66f
Radial artery
  access, for peripheral artery disease, 864
  percutaneous technique, for cardiac catheterization, 386–388, 386f–387f, 387.e1f
  for vascular access, 799
Radial grafts, cannulation for, 367b–368b, 369f
Radiation dose, reducing, 288–290, 290.e1f, 290.e1t
Radiation-induced heart disease, 1099b–1100b
Radiation-induced pericarditis, 1630b–1633b
Radiation principles/patient safety, cardiac CT, 335b–337b
Radiation therapy
  in cancer, 1092t, 1097
  cardiotoxicity of, 1097
  in myocarditis, 1083.e1
Radiofrequency catheter ablation, 1277f
  atrial tachyarrhythmias after, 1280
  atrioventricular node for, 1283–1284
  recurrence after, 1277–1278
Radiography
  for acute aortic regurgitation, 1428b–1429b
  pacemakers and cardiac implantable electrical devices, 1321, 1321f–1324f
  of primary mitral regurgitation, 1462b
  in pulmonic regurgitation, 1479b–1481b
  in STEMI, 658
  in tricuspid regurgitation, 1476b–1478b
  in tricuspid stenosis, 1473b–1475b
Radionuclide imaging
  in cardio-oncology, 310
  in chest pain, 606–607
  in infective endocarditis, 307–310, 308f–309f
  in patients
    with heart failure, 298–307
    with ischemic heart disease, 290–298

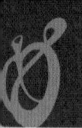

Radionuclide myocardial perfusion imaging, risk stratification with, 291–292, 292f, 292.e1f
Radiotherapy-induced mitral stenosis, 1452, 1453f
Radiotracers, 280–288, 280t, 280b–281b
    imaging protocols of, 283–284
        general principles of, 283–284
    SPECT protocols, 284–286
    stress testing
        physiologic basis for, 281–282, 283f
        protocols, 282–283
RAE. *See* Right atrial enlargement
RAFT. *See* Resynchronization/Defibrillation for Ambulatory Heart Failure Trial
Rales
    in acute heart failure, 953
    in heart failure, 135, 937
    in STEMI, 654
Ramipril, in heart failure, 991t–992t
Randomized clinical trials, 43
Randomized controlled trials, 44
RANKL. *See* Receptor activator of NF-κB ligand
Ranolazine, 1211.e1t, 1208t–1209t, 1212t, 1214t, 1226–1227, 1226b–1227b
    in angina pectoris, 760.e1f, 762–763
    in coronary artery disease, chronic kidney disease and, 1880t–1881t
    in NSTE-ACS, 723t
Rapamycin, in cardiac transplantation, 1136–1137
Rapid ventricular pacing, common causes of, 1330.e1t
Rastelli operation
    long-term complications following, 1568–1569
    for transposition of great arteries, 1566, 1567f
Rate responsive pacing, 1327–1328, 1328b, 1329f
RBBB. *See* Right bundle branch block
RC. *See* Reclassification calibration
RCRI. *See* Revised cardiac risk index
RDN. *See* Renal denervation
Reactive oxygen species (ROS), in heart failure, 916f, 916b
Receiver operating characteristic curve, in biomarkers, 106, 106f
Receptor activator of NF-κB ligand (RANKL), 435
Receptors, toll-like, 1085.e1
Reclassification calibration (RC), 106–107
Recurrent event analysis, 46b–47b
Recurrent pericarditis, 1619–1620, 1620.e1f
Recurrent venous thromboembolism, after discontinuation of anticoagulation, 1648
Red meats, 533f, 534
Red yeast rice, in dyslipidemia, 596b
Reentrant atrial tachycardia, 1234b–1235b, 1235f
Reentry
    anatomic, 1184–1185, 1185f–1186f
        conditions for, 1185b, 1186f
    atrial, 1187
    atrioventricular nodal, 1187
    cardiac arrhythmias and, 1183b–1184b
    functional, 1187.e1f, 1185–1186, 1188f
    sinus, 1187
    tachycardias caused by, ventricular, 1188
Referral, in cardiac rehabilitation, 589f, 589b
Reflex, diving, 1896
Reflex-mediated syncope, 1388–1389, 1396t
Refractory symptoms, general palliation for, 1005.e2
Regional ventricular function, echocardiography of, 213–214
Regulatory myosin light chain (MLC-2), 894
Regulatory proteins, abnormalities of, in heart failure, 925, 925t
Regulatory T cells (Tregs), 432
Regurgitant fraction, 402
Regurgitant stroke volume, 402
Regurgitation
    in elderly
        aortic, 1700b–1701b
        mitral, 1700b–1701b
    valvular
        in cardiac catheterization, 402
        regurgitant fraction in, 402
Rehospitalization problem, in acute heart failure, 960–961
Reiki, 593b–594b
Reinforcement learning, 110
Rejection
    of cardiac transplantation, 1137–1138, 1137t
    surveillance for, 1138
Relative benefit, 57–58

Relative flow reserve, 620–621, 620f
Relative risk reduction, 58
Remodeling
    autonomic, 1183.e1f, 1178–1179, 1179.e1f
    electrical, of atria, 1187
Remote interrogation, 1343–1344
Remote ischemic conditioning (RIC), 668b
Remote monitoring, of implantable cardioverter-defibrillators, 1343–1344, 1343.e3f
Renal artery disease, 488–489
    endovascular treatment of, 867, 867.e1f
Renal cell carcinoma, 1837–1838, 1838f
Renal denervation (RDN), 1899
    in hypertension, 495–496, 496f
Renal disease
    chronic, 1873–1874, 1876f
        acute coronary syndromes, 1880, 1880t–1881t
        anemia and, 1874–1875
        arrhythmias and, 1887–1888, 1890t
        cardiorenal intersection and, 1873, 1874f–1875f
        cardiorenal syndrome, 1882–1887, 1887f–1888f, 1889t
        cardiovascular risk and, 1873–1874, 1876f
        consultative approach to, 1888–1890
        valvular heart disease and, 1887
    coronary artery disease and, 1888
    drug adjustments in, 99
    hypertension and, 1879–1880
    in lipoprotein disorders, 514
    pericardial disease with, 1630b–1633b
Renal failure, chronic, hypocalcemia and, 1797
Renal function/dysfunction
    in acute heart failure, 959
    in adult congenital heart disease, 1544
    in heart failure, 916–919, 917.e1t, 921.e1f, 938b–939b
    mechanical circulatory support and, 1122–1123, 1122b–1123b
    percutaneous coronary interventions in, 792–793
    stable ischemic heart disease and, 769b–770b, 772.e2
Renal insufficiency
    after cardiac transplantation, 1140–1141
    heart failure prognosis and, 978, 978f
Renal mechanisms, in acute heart failure, 950–951, 951f
Renal transplantation, cardiovascular disease and, 1891, 1891f
Renin-angiotensin system, in heart failure, 915–916, 915f
Renin-angiotensin-aldosterone inhibitors
    for heart failure with preserved and mildly reduced ejection, 1024
    in NSTE-ACS, 735.e3
Renin-angiotensin-aldosterone system antagonists
    for acute coronary syndromes, 573
    in coronary heart disease, 560–561
    for heart failure, 575
Renin-angiotensin-aldosterone system (RAAS), 474–476, 476f
    for acute myocardial infarction, 708–709
    genetic variations in, 996.e1
    for STEMI, 681–683, 682f–683f
    in STEMI, 652b
Renin-angiotensin-aldosterone system (RAAS) blockade, for congenital heart disease, 1551
Renin, in hypertension, 475
Renin inhibitors, in heart failure, 996–997
Renin profiling, of hypertension, 483–484
Renoprotective agents, for acute heart failure, 971b–972b
Renovascular hypertension, 488–489
Repaglinide, in diabetes mellitus, 562t–563t
Reperfusion arrhythmias, 668
Reperfusion injury, 668, 668b
Repetitive shocks, 1340
"Repolarization reserve", 1197–1199
Resistant hypertension, 494–497
    nondrug therapy for, 495
Respiratory chain disorders, 1866–1867
Respiratory rate, in STEMI, 654
"Response variables", clinical trials, 45–46
Restenosis, after arterial intervention, 438
Resting echocardiography, in stable ischemic heart disease, 744
Resting electrocardiogram, in cardiac arrhythmias, 1148–1149, 1149.e1t–1152f, 1151t
Resting electrocardiographic recording, in cardiac arrhythmias, 1148f
Resting membrane potential, 1166b–1170b, 1167f, 1168t

Restraining effect, of pericardium, 1615b
Restricted mean survival time, 46b–47b
Restrictive cardiomyopathy, 404, 1033t, 1043–1049
    approach to identifying cause of, 1043–1044
    clinical genetics of, 1043–1044
    constrictive pericarditis *vs.*, 1044.e1f, 1628, 1630t
    echocardiography in, 1044, 1044f
    idiopathic, 1044
    molecular genetics of, 1043–1044
Resynchronization Reverses Remodeling in Systolic Left Ventricular Dysfunction Trial (REVERSE), 1110b–1111b
Resynchronization/Defibrillation for Ambulatory Heart Failure Trial (RAFT), 1110b–1111b
Reteplase, 1789
Retrograde access, for peripheral artery disease, 864, 864.e2f
Retrograde ascending aortic dissection, 821
Revascularization
    in acute limb ischemia, 854–855, 855f
    in stable ischemic heart disease, 764–766, 776
        fractional flow reserve in, 765
        indications for, 780
        patient selection for, 765–766
        percutaneous coronary intervention for, 769b–770b
        presence and severity of symptoms of, 765
        risk associated with, 765–766
        significance of coronary lesions in, 765
Reverse cholesterol transport, 508–509
Revised cardiac risk index (RCRI), 415–416
Reynolds Risk Score, 107
Rhabdomyomas, 1833, 1834t
Rheobase, 1323b–1324b
Rheos Pivotal Trial, 496
Rheumatic arthritis, 1531
Rheumatic diseases
    antirheumatic drugs in, 1824–1827
    atherosclerosis in, 1809–1812, 1812t
    cardiac conduction disturbances in, 1821
    cardiovascular system and, 1809–1828
    future perspectives in, 1827
    pericarditis and myocarditis in, 1818–1820, 1820f
    pulmonary arterial hypertension in, 1821–1823, 1822t
    thrombosis in, 1823–1824
    valvular heart disease in, 1820–1821
    vasculitis in
        large-vessel, 1812–1815, 1813f–1814f, 1814t, 1816f
        medium-vessel, 1816–1818, 1817f–1818f
Rheumatic fever, 1531–1540
    abdominal pain in, 1535
    antibiotic treatment of, 1536
    arthritis for, 1533, 1533f
    carditis in, 1534, 1534t
    clinical features of, 1533–1535, 1534t
    diagnosis of, 1535–1536, 1536t
    epidemiology of, 1531, 1532f
    erythema marginatum in, 1535, 1535f
    general management of, 1536
    genetic susceptibility factor in, 1532b–1533b
    management of, 1536–1537, 1537t
    natural history of, 1536
    pathogenesis of, 1531–1533, 1532b–1533b, 1533f
    prevention of, 1537–1538, 1538t
    socioeconomic status and, 1532b–1533b
    subcutaneous nodules in, 1534–1535, 1535f
    Sydenham chorea in, 1534
    temperature in, 1535
    valvular heart disease and
        aortic valve stenosis and, 1400
        tricuspid regurgitation, 1475
Rheumatic mitral stenosis (RMS), 1441–1450
    additional diagnostic investigations of, 1446
        EKG and chest X-ray, 1446
        exercise testing, 1446
    associated conditions of, 1446–1447
        atrial fibrillation, 1446–1447, 1446f
        pregnancy, 1447
        pulmonary hypertension, 1447
    clinical pathophysiology of, 1442–1443, 1443f
    clinical presentation of, 1444–1445
    diagnosis of, 1444–1446
    echocardiography of, 1445–1446, 1445f
    left atrial function, 1442–1443
    left atrial pressure, 1442, 1444f
    left ventricular function, 1443

Rheumatic mitral stenosis (RMS) (Continued)
  natural history of, 1443–1444, 1444t
  pathology of, 1442, 1442f
  physical examination of, 1445
  right ventricular function, 1443
  treatment of, 1448–1450
    medical therapy, 1448
    transcatheter interventional therapy, 1448–1449, 1448t, 1449f–1450f
Rheumatoid arthritis
  atherosclerosis in, 1810
  cardiac conduction disturbances in, 1821
  pericarditis in, 1819
  pulmonary arterial hypertension in, 1822t, 1823
  sudden cardiac death and, 1363b–1365b
  treatment of, 1810b
  valvular heart disease in, 1821
RIC. See Remote ischemic conditioning
Rifampin, for infective endocarditis, 1519b–1523b
Right atrial enlargement (RAE), chest radiography in, 270
Right atrial inversion, echocardiography of, 241f–242f, 241b–242b
Right atrium, 1544–1545
  echocardiography of, 210, 210t–211t
Right bundle branch block (RBBB)
  clinical significance of, 158–159
  electrocardiography in, 157f, 158–159, 158t, 158b
  incomplete, 158
  myocardial infarction and, 165, 166f
Right coronary artery, cannulation for, 367b–368b
Right coronary dominance, in angiographic projection, 372, 372.e1f
Right heart catheterization
  in heart failure, 942, 942b
  for pulmonary arterial hypertension, 1669f
Right subclavian artery (RSCA), and aortic anomalies, 274
Right ventricle
  echocardiography of, 209, 209t–210t, 209f–211f
  function of, mechanical circulatory support and, 1124, 1124b
  strain measures of, 1011b–1017b
Right ventricle (RV) pacing
  ADI mode to reduce, 1328b, 1329f
  adverse effects of, 1326
  potential deleterious effects of, 1326
Right ventricular cardiomyopathy, 1360b
Right ventricular dysfunction, in pulmonary hypertension, 1665, 1666f
Right ventricular fractional area change, 209, 210f
Right ventricular function, in rheumatic mitral stenosis, 1443
Right ventricular heart failure, 956b
Right ventricular hypertrophy, electrocardiography in, 154–155, 154f–155f, 154t, 154b
Right ventricular infarction, 657–658
  ST-elevation myocardial infarction and, 694, 696f
    diagnosis of, 694
    noninvasive assessment for, 694
    treatment for, 694
Riociguat, for pulmonary arterial hypertension, 1675f
Risk
  prediction of, 57b, 58f
  ratio, 57–58
  stratification, 53
Risk factors, of cardiovascular disease, 20–26
Risk of Paradoxical Embolism (RoPE) Score, 885b–886b, 886t
Risk-treatment paradox, 58
Rituximab, for rheumatoid arthritis, 1825b
Rivaroxaban, 97t, 1785–1786
  in atrial fibrillation-associated thromboembolism prevention, 1276
  in chronic kidney disease, 1885t–1886t
  drug interaction with, 97t
  in NSTE-ACS, 727b
RMS. See Rheumatic mitral stenosis
RNAi, 85
Rofecoxib, withdrawal of, 92–93
Rolofylline, for acute heart failure, 971b–972b
R-on-T ventricular pacing, 1331
ROS. See Reactive oxygen species
Rose Questionnaire, 840
Rosiglitazone, in diabetes mellitus, 562t–563t, 564b–566b
Ross procedure, for thoracic aortic aneurysms, 817

Rosuvastatin, in chronic kidney disease, 1883t
Rotablator, 863
Rotablator Rotational Atherectomy System, 794.e1
Rotational atherectomy, 794.e1, 797f
  for peripheral artery disease, 863, 863.e1f, 863.e2f
Routine screening, for sleep apnea, 1681, 1681.e1f
RSCA. See Right subclavian artery
RSr′ complex, 147
Ruptured abdominal aortic aneurysm, 809
Ryanodine receptors (RyRs), 1183.e1f, 889, 896, 896f, 1181b–1183b
RYR2, 1203, 1203f, 1203b
RyRs. See Ryanodine receptors

S

S wave, 147
S_1 heart sound, in mitral stenosis, 1445
Saccular aneurysm, 806–807
Sacubitril, in cardiorenal syndrome, 1889t
Sacubitril/valsartan
  for chronic HFrEF, 1698b
  for heart failure, 991t–992t
    with preserved and mildly reduced ejection, 1025–1026
Salt, reduction of, 28–29
Salt sensitivity, in hypertension, 473–474, 475f
SAMMPRIS (Stenting and Aggressive Medical Management for Preventing Recurrent Stroke in Intracranial Stenosis) trial, 879b
Saphenous vein grafts
  cannulation for, 367b–368b, 369f
  in percutaneous coronary intervention, 789–790, 791f
Sapien balloon-expandable TAVR series, 1435f, 1435.e1
SAPIEN valve, 1588, 1588f, 1588b
Sarcoglycanopathies, 1862–1863
Sarcoid cardiomyopathy, 1044–1046
  clinical features of, 1044–1045, 1046f
  diagnosis of, 1045, 1046f–1047f
  pathology of, 1044, 1045f
  treatment of, 1045–1046, 1045.e2t
Sarcoidosis
  cardiac, magnetic resonance imaging in, 326, 326f
  echocardiography in, 252b–253b, 252.e1f
  pulmonary hypertension and, 1676
  radionuclide imaging in, 304–307, 304f–307f
  sudden cardiac death and, 1363b–1365b
Sarcolemma, 889
Sarcolemmal Ca^{2+} elimination, in heart failure, 924
Sarcomas, 1835–1837, 1836f
  left heart, 1840.e1, 1840.e1f
  pulmonary artery, 1840.e1
  right heart, 1840.e1
  treatment of, 1840.e1
Sarcomere, 891f, 892–893
  force-length relationship of, 906, 907f
  length of, 895
Sarcopenia, in older adult, 1690b–1693b
Sarcopenic obesity, in heart failure with preserved and mildly reduced ejection, 1011b–1017b
Sarcoplasm, 889
Sarcoplasmic reticulum Ca^{2+} reuptake, in heart failure, 924
Sarcoplasmic reticulum Ca^{2+}-adenosine triphosphatase (ATPase) (SERCA2), 1797–1798
Sarcoplasmic reticulum (SR), 889
  calcium movements and, 896
  calcium release and uptake by, 896–897
  ryanodine receptor and, 896, 896f
  turning off calcium release, 896–897
SARS-CoV-2; see also Coronavirus; COVID-19
  COVID-19 and, 1754–1763, 1754b–1755b
  induced endothelial injury, 1761f
  pathophysiology of effect of, 1760f
Satavaptan, in heart failure, 983t
Saturated fat, 551–552
Saturated fatty acids, 536–538, 537f
SAVR. See Surgical aortic valve replacement
Saxagliptin, in diabetes mellitus, 562t–563t, 566b–567b
SCA. See Sudden cardiac arrest
Scaffolding proteins, 889–891
Scarring, in constrictive pericarditis, 1625b–1626b
Scavenger receptor, 432
SCD. See Sudden cardiac death
SCD-HeFT. See Sudden Cardiac Death-Heart Failure Trial
Scientific Registry of Transplant Recipients, 1132
SCN1B, 1205b–1206b

SCN5A, 1191b–1193b, 1192f, 1196f
SCOUT (Percutaneous Tricuspid Valve Annuloplasty System for Symptomatic Chronic Functional Tricuspid Regurgitation) trial, 1490b–1492b
Screening
  in abdominal aortic aneurysms, 808
  in depression, 1845b
  in heart failure, 978b, 980t
SCS. See Spinal cord stimulation
Second-degree atrioventricular (AV) block, 1315–1317, 1315f, 1315f–1316f, 1316b
  electrocardiography for, 1315f, 1315f–1316f
  type I, 1316f–1317f, 1317b
  type II, 1316f–1317f, 1317b
Second-hand smoke, as risk factor of stroke, 874b–877b
Secondary endpoints, analysis of, 46–47
Secondary hypertension
  diagnostic approach for, 484–490
  endocrine causes of, 484–487
    acromegaly, 487
    apparent mineralocorticoid excess states, 485
    hypercortisolism (Cushing disease), 486–487
    pheochromocytoma, 485–486
    primary hyperaldosteronism, 484–485, 484t
    thyroid dysfunction, 487
  lifestyle factors of, 487
  nonendocrine causes of, 487
  nonlifestyle, nonendocrine causes of, 488–490
    coarctation of aorta, 489–490
    intrinsic kidney disease, 488, 488f–489f
    renovascular hypertension, 488–489
Secondary prevention, for cardiovascular disease, 442–443, 443f
Secondhand smoke, 21
Secundum atrial septal defect, 1554
  echocardiography in, 257, 257f–259f
Sedentary behavior, cardiovascular disease and Seeds, 462, 462.e1f, 533f
Segmental pressure measurement, in peripheral artery disease, 842–843, 843f
Selectins, 431
Selective serotonin reuptake inhibitors, 1848–1849
Selexipag, for pulmonary arterial hypertension, 1675f
Self-expanding first-generation intra-annular Portico TAVR system, 1435.e1, 1435.e2f
Self-expanding stents, for peripheral artery disease, 860
Sensing
  in implantable cardioverter-defibrillators, 1334b–1335b, 1339f–1340f, 1339t
  in pacemakers, 1324–1326, 1324b–1326b, 1325f–1326f
Sensitivity
  of biomarkers, 105–106, 105t
  of test, 54b–55b
SERCA (sarcoendoplasmic reticulum Ca^{2+}-adenosine triphosphatase), 889, 897–898, 898f
Serelaxin, for acute heart failure, 970–971, 971f
Serotonin and norepinephrine dual reuptake inhibitors, 1849
Serotonin, for pulmonary arterial hypertension, 1664b–1665b
Serum biomarkers, in STEMI, 656f
Serum C-reactive protein (CRP), in acute pericarditis, 1617
Serum markers, in STEMI, 655
Severe stenosis, 352
Sex
  in central sleep apnea (CSA), 1681
  in obstructive sleep apnea (OSA), 1679–1680
  sudden cardiac death and, 1353f, 1354
  visceral obesity and, 550
Sex hormone therapy, visceral obesity and, 550
Shared decision making, 59–60, 462–463
SHEP. See Systolic Hypertension in Elderly Program
Shock-component malfunction, 1341–1342
Shock reduction, strategic programming principles for, 1339t
Shock(s), 1339–1340, 1340.e1t, 1344f–1345f
  cardiogenic
    in acute heart failure, 952, 953t
    in heart failure, 938, 938f
    in STEMI, 651, 651f
  unsuccessful, 1340, 1345t
Short QT syndrome, 1197, 1308
  clinical description and manifestations of, 1197
  genetic basis of, 1192f, 1197b
  genotype-phenotype correlates of, 1197
  sudden cardiac death and, 1362b

Shprintzen-Goldberg syndrome, thoracic aortic aneurysm in, 811t
Shunts, coronary computed tomography angiography in, 357, 357f
Shy-Drager syndrome. See Multisystem atrophy
"Sicilian Gambit", 1208
Sick sinus syndrome (SSS), 1206, 1313–1315
  anatomic basis of, 1314
  chronotropic incompetence, 1314, 1314f
  clinical description and manifestations of, 1206
  electrocardiographic recognition of, 1313–1314, 1313f–1314f
  genetic basis of, 1206b
  management of, 1315
Sickle cell disease, pulmonary hypertension and, 1676
Sildenafil
  drug interaction with, 97t
  in pulmonary arterial hypertension, 1675f
Silent ischemia, detection and management of, 779.e1
Silent myocardial ischemia, 779
  mechanism of, 779.e1
Simvastatin
  in chronic kidney disease, 1883t
  drug interaction with, 97t
Single-blind study, 45
Single-cell ribonucleic acid sequencing, 84
Single-chamber implantable cardioverter-defibrillators, dual-chamber transvenous vs., 1333–1334
Single chamber modes, of pacemaker, 1327f
Single-chamber pacing device, 1328
Single-coil leads, dual vs., 1334b–1335b
Single nucleotide polymorphisms (SNPs), 73
  in long QT syndrome, 1195
Single photon emission computed tomography, 277–278
  conventional, 277, 278f
  novel image reconstruction software, 277
  novel SPECT scanners, 277–278, 278.e1f
Single shock, 1340
Single ventricle, 1578–1582
  anatomic description and prevalence of, 1578–1579
  clinical features and diagnostic testing of, 1580–1581, 1581f
  long-term outcomes and complications of, 1581–1582
  surgical palliation of, 1579–1580, 1580f
Sinoatrial conduction time, 1156b–1159b
Sinoatrial exit block, 1312b–1313b, 1313.e1f
Sinoatrial node, 1175, 1175.e1f, 1175f–1176f
  artery supplying, 1175, 1175.e1f, 1175.e2f
  automaticity of, 1170b–1171b
  cellular structure of, 1175.e1b
  connexins in, 1175.e1b
  discharge rate of, 1166b–1170b
  function of, 1175.e1b
  innervation of, 1175.e1b
  neurotransmitters and, 1175.e1b
Sinoatrial node artery, 1175, 1175.e1f, 1175.e2f
Sinoatrial node pacemaking, 1170
Sinus arrest, 1312b–1313b, 1313.e1f
Sinus arrhythmia, 1312–1313, 1312b–1313b, 1313f
  nonrespiratory, 1312b–1313b
  respiratory, 1312b–1313b
Sinus bradycardia, 1312
  clinical features of, 1312
  electrocardiographic recognition of, 1312, 1313f
  management of, 1312
Sinus node dysfunction, 1156b–1159b, 1547
Sinus node function, 1393
  evaluation of, 1162.e1, 1162.e3t
Sinus node recovery time, 1156b–1159b, 1157f
Sinus node reentry, 1251
Sinus of Valsalva aneurysms, echocardiography in, 244, 248f
Sinus pause, 1312b–1313b, 1313.e1f
Sinus reentry, 1187
Sinus rhythm, maintenance of, 1287.e3, 1287.e5t
Sinus venosus atrial septal defect, echocardiography in, 258, 259f
SIPAT. See Stanford Integrated Psychosocial Assessment for Transplantation
SIRIUS (Sirolimus-Eluting Stent in De-Novo Native Coronary Lesions) trial, 793.e2
siRNA-inclisiran, 6
Sirolimus, 793.e2
  in cardiac transplantation, 1136–1137
  in drug-eluting stents, 793.e2

Sitagliptin, in diabetes mellitus, 562t–563t, 566
Sitosterolemia, 510b
Six-minute walk test, 178b–180b, 180t
Sjögren syndrome
  cardiac conduction disturbances in, 1821
  pulmonary arterial hypertension in, 1822t, 1823
Skeletal muscle, in heart failure with preserved and mildly reduced ejection, 1011b–1017b
Skilled nursing facilities, for elderly, cardiovascular disease in, 1694
Skin necrosis, warfarin and, 1785
Skipped P waves, 1315
SLCO1B1 gene, 95t, 98
Sleep apnea
  central, in heart failure, 999f, 1002–1003
  obesity and, 552
  obstructive, 1895–1896
    atrial fibrillation and, 1274
    definition of, 1678
    key features of, 1679t
    pathophysiology of, 1678–1679
    screening questions for, 1681.e1f
    sudden cardiac death and, 1363b–1365b
Sleep deprivation, 487–488
Sleep-disordered breathing, 487–488
  associated with primary hyperaldosteronism, 485
  cardiac disease and, 1678–1686
    cardiac arrhythmias and, 1684–1685
    cardiac function and, 1683–1684
    coronary heart disease and, 1682–1683
    definitions of, 1678, 1679f, 1679t
    future perspectives in, 1685
    heart failure and, 1683–1684, 1684f
    hypertension and, 1681–1682
    pathophysiologic mechanism link, 1681, 1681f
    pathophysiology of, 1678–1681, 1680f
    recognition for, 1679–1681, 1681.e1f
    risk factors for, 1679–1681
  pulmonary arterial hypertension associated with, 1662
Sleep/rest, long QT syndrome and, 1193, 1196f
Slow pathway ablation, 1233f, 1233b–1234b
Slow responses, 1166b–1170b
SMAD3 mutations, 811
Small circuit reentry, 1253b–1257b, 1258f
Smoking
  cardiovascular disease and, 446–447, 447.e1f
  as risk factor of stroke, 874b–877b
Smooth muscle cells
  arterial, 426–427, 427f–428f
  in evolution of atheroma
    death, 433
    migration and proliferation, 432–433, 434f
SNP. See Sodium nitroprusside
SNPs. See Single nucleotide polymorphisms
Social determinants of health, cardiovascular disease and, 451, 451f–452f
Social discrimination, stress and, 1843
Societal changes, for lipoprotein disorders, 522–523
Socioeconomic status
  rheumatic fever and, 1532b–1533b
  stress and, 1842
Sodium channels, 898–899
  molecular structure of, 898
  voltage-gated, 1171b–1173b, 1172f
Sodium, dietary, 537f, 539
Sodium-glucose cotransporter 2 (SGLT2) inhibitors, in glucose management, 562t–563t, 567–569, 570f
Sodium-glucose transporter-2 inhibitors, 984–985, 986f
  in heart failure, 997f, 998, 998b
Sodium handling, in heart failure, 924–925, 925.e1f
Sodium nitroprusside (SNP), in acute heart failure, 963
Soluble guanylate cyclase stimulators
  in acute heart failure, 971b–972b
  in heart failure, 998
Somatic genomics, 83, 84f
Sones, Mason, 363
Sorafenib, cardiotoxic effects of, 1092t, 1096
Sortilin (Sort-1), 435
Sotalol, 1211.e1t, 1209t, 1212t, 1214t, 1222–1223, 1222b
  for angina pectoris, 758t
  antiarrhythmics, chronic kidney disease and, 1890t
  in atrial fibrillation, 1280
  for complex congenital heart disease, 1548
  kidney function and, 99
  for pregnancy, 1730f

SPARCL (Stroke Prevention with Aggressive Reduction in Cholesterol Levels) trial, 874b–877b
Spasm
  coronary artery, sudden cardiac death and, 1357.e1, 1358t
  esophageal, pain in, 601
Spatiotemporal organization, in atrial fibrillation, 1187
Specificity
  of biomarkers, 105–106, 105t
  of test, 54b–55b
Speckle-tracking echocardiography, of heart failure with preserved and mildly reduced ejection, 1011b–1017b, 1013f
SPECT and PET image acquisition, 279
SPECT and PET perfusion tracers, 286
SPECT MPI tracers, 280b–281b
SPECT protocols, 284–286, 285f
Sphingomyelin, 503
Spinal cord stimulation (SCS), 1899–1900
  for angina pectoris, 764.e1
SPIRIT program, 793.e2
Spironolactone, 1795b
  drug interaction with, 97t
  in heart failure, 983, 991t–992t, 996
Spondyloarthropathies
  cardiac conduction disturbances in, 1821
  seronegative
    treatment for, 1821
    valvular heart disease in, 1821
Spontaneous circulation, stabilization of cardiac rhythm after initial return of, 1374–1375
Spontaneous coronary artery dissection, in coronary artery disease, 780b–781b
Spontaneous pneumothorax, chest pain in, 600t
Sports cardiology, 579–587
  atherosclerotic cardiovascular disease and, 583–584
  athletic eligibility and, 583–585
  cardiovascular response to, 579–580, 580f–581f
  clinical problems in, approach to, 581–583
  decreased exercise capacity in, 582
  elevated "cardiac enzymes" in, 584, 584f
  historical perspective of, 579
  myocardial fibrosis in, 585
  screening in, 582–583
  valve disease in, 584
Sports participation, for congenital heart disease, 1553–1554
Sports, participation in, cardiac implantable electrical devices, 1347
Spotty calcifications, coronary computed tomography angiography in, 345
SPRINT. See Systolic Blood Pressure Intervention Trial
SR. See Sarcoplasmic reticulum
SSOC. See Stroke System of Care
SSS. See Sick sinus syndrome
St. John's wort, drug interaction with, 100
St. Jude bileaflet valve, 1495
Stable angina, percutaneous coronary intervention in, 786–787
Stable chest pain, coronary computed tomography angiography in, 342–344
Stable chest pain syndromes, assessment of, 320, 321f–323f
Stable coronary artery disease, optical coherence tomography in, 381
Stable ischemic heart disease, 739–762
  coronary artery bypass grafting in, 770–776
  diagnosis of
    coronary angiography for, 747
    coronary computed tomography angiography for, 747
    exercise electrocardiography for, 745b–746b
    noninvasive studies for, 744–748
    resting electrocardiography for, 744
  dual-antiplatelet therapy in, 754b–756b
  evaluation and management of, 742–758
    advanced structural coronary imaging in, 748
    angiography in, 748, 748.e1f
    biochemical tests in, 742–744
    biomarkers in, 742–743, 743f
    chest roentgenography in, 744
    computed tomography in, 746–747, 747f
    exercise electrocardiography in, 745b–746b, 746t
    functional assessment in, 748
    genetic and transcriptomic biomarkers in, 743–744, 744f
    inflammatory biomarkers in, 743

Stable ischemic heart disease *(Continued)*
    invasive assessment in, 748–749
    magnetic resonance imaging in, 747–748
    noninvasive testing in, 744–748
    resting echocardiography in, 744
    resting electrocardiography in, 744
    stress echocardiography in, 745b–746b
    stress myocardial perfusion imaging in, 745b–746b, 746t
    stress testing, 745–746, 745t
  future perspectives for, 781
  magnitude of problem with, 739
  medical management of, 749–757
    counseling and changes in lifestyle for, 756–757
    risk factors reduction in, 749–756
  natural history of, 749
  noninvasive tests for, 746t
  pathophysiology of, 741f
  percutaneous coronary intervention for, 766
    atrial fibrillation in, 772.e1
    cerebrovascular complications in, 772.e1
    coronary artery bypass surgery *vs.*, 775.e1f-e2f, 775.e1f-e2f, 774–775, 776f, 776.e1t
    early outcome of, 766b
    effects on survival, 772–773
    fractional flow reserve strategy in, 765, 769f
    long-term outcome of, 766b
    medical therapy *vs.*, 766–769, 767f–768f
    in multivessel disease, 776
    myocardial infarction in, 772.e1
    operative mortality in, 772
    patient selection in, 771f–772f, 772, 772.e2f
    perioperative complications in, 772.e1
    previous coronary bypass grafting and, 770–776
    renal dysfunction in, 772.e2
    reoperation in, 774
    revascularization for, 769b–770b
    in single-vessel disease, 776
    surgical outcomes and long-term results in, 772–773
    in women and older patients, 769b–770b
  percutaneous coronary intervention in, 786–787
  revascularization in, 764–766, 776
    fractional flow reserve in, 765
    patient selection for, 765–766
    presence and severity of symptoms of, 765
    risk associated with, 765–766
    significance of coronary lesions in, 765
  risk factor modification for, 764
  risk stratification in, 749, 750f
  surgical treatment of, 773–774
    with diabetes, 774
    in older patients, 774
    with renal disease, 774
    in women, 773–774
Standard coiling, for patent ductus arteriosus treatment, 1591, 1591b
Standard lipid testing, 453–454, 453b–454b
Standard of care, 48–49
Stanford Integrated Psychosocial Assessment for Transplantation (SIPAT), 1134
Stanols, for dyslipidemia, 596b
Staphylococcal species, causing infective endocarditis, 1506b–1507b, 1512t
  antimicrobial therapy for, 1519b–1523b, 1521t–1522t
Starches, 532–534
Starling's law, 906–907
Statin therapy, 445, 446f, 446t
Statins, 462–463, 515–517
  in advanced heart failure, 517
  in atrial fibrillation, 1280
  in chronic kidney disease, 517
  clinical trials with, 516
  in coronary heart disease, 558–560
  in diabetic patients, 516
  in dyslipidemia, 596b
  mechanism of action of, 515
  myopathy induced by, 1803
  in noncardiac surgery patients, 421–422
  in older patients, 517
  in peripheral artery disease, 847.e2t
  pharmacology of, 515, 516t
  for pregnancy, 1730f
  in rheumatic disease, 1826
  risk for diabetes, 516
  in special populations, 516–517
  in women, 517

Stationary cycle testing, 178b–180b, 179t
ST-elevation myocardial infarction (STEMI), management of, 662–712
  anticoagulant and antiplatelet therapy as, 675–679, 675.e1f
  arrhythmias in, 699–703, 700t
    bradyarrhythmias, 701–703
    hemodynamic consequences of, 699
    supraventricular tachyarrhythmias, 703
    ventricular, 699–701
  catheter-based reperfusion strategies as, 671, 671f–673f
  complications in, 703–705
    left ventricular aneurysm, 705
    left ventricular thrombus and arterial embolism, 705
    pericardial effusion and pericarditis, 704–705
    recurrent chest discomfort, 703–704
    venous thrombosis and pulmonary embolism, 705
  convalescence, discharge, and post-myocardial infarction care, 705–710
    assessment at hospital discharge, 706–707
    assessment for electrical instability, 707
    assessment of left ventricular function, 706–707
    assessment of myocardial ischemia, 707
    counseling, 706
    hospital course, 706b
    initial findings, 706b
    prophylactic antiarrhythmic therapy, 707, 708f–709f
    risk stratification, 706b
    timing of hospital discharge, 705–707
  in emergency department, 664–667, 665t
    analgesics for, 665–666
    aspirin for, 665
    beta-adrenergic blocking agents for, 666
    control of cardiac pain, 665–666
    nitrates for, 666
    oxygen for, 666
  fibrinolysis, 668–669
  fibrinolytic therapy as, 669–671, 669f–670f
  future perspectives and emerging therapies for, 710
  hemodynamic disturbances, 684–699
    abnormalities, 684–685
    cardiogenic shock in, 690–694, 690f
    hyperdynamic state, 685
    hypotension in prehospital phase, 685
    left ventricular failure in, 685–690, 686f
    mechanical causes of heart failure, 694–699
    pulmonary artery pressure, monitoring of, 684–685, 685t
    right ventricular infarction in, 694, 696f
    subsets, 685, 685t–686t
  hospital, 679–684
    coronary care and intermediate care units, 679–680
    pharmacologic therapy as, 680–684
  infarct
    dynamic nature of, 666–667, 667f
    routine measures for, 667
    size, 666–667
  mortality rates, 663f
  myocardial reperfusion, pathophysiology of, 667–668
    patency of infarct vessel, 668
    reperfusion arrhythmias, 668
    reperfusion injury, 668
  perfusion therapy as, 667–679, 667f
  prehospital, 662–664, 663t
    care, 662
    emergency medical service systems, 663, 664f
    fibrinolysis, 663–664, 665f
  selection of reperfusion strategy, 671–675, 673f
    patients not eligible for, 674–675
    referral for angiography, 673–674, 673f–674f, 674t
Stem cell transplantation, cardiotoxicity of, 1097
Stent thrombosis, in percutaneous coronary intervention, 802, 802.e1t, 802.e2f
Stented bioprosthetic valves, 1495–1497, 1496f
Stentless bioprosthetic valves, 1496f, 1497
Stent(s)
  in coarctation of aorta, 1589, 1589b
  coronary
    drug-eluting, 793
    everolimus-eluting, 793, 793–794
    noncardiac surgery and, 420–421, 422f
    paclitaxel-eluting, 793.e2

Stent(s) *(Continued)*
    sirolimus-eluting, 793.e2
    zotarolimus-eluting, 793, 793–794
  drug-eluting, noncardiac surgery and, 420
  in peripheral artery disease
    bare-metal, 860, 860f–861f
    covered, 862, 862.e1f
    drug-eluting, 860–861
Sterols, in dyslipidemia, 596b
Stigmatization, stress and, 1843
Stokes-Adams attacks, 1322
Strength-duration curve, 1323b–1324b, 1325f
Streptococcal infection, myocardial, 1081b
Streptococcal species, causing infective endocarditis, 1506b–1507b, 1512t
  antimicrobial therapy for, 1519t–1521t, 1519b–1523b
Streptokinase, 1787–1788, 1787f
Stress
  acute, 1841–1842
  anxiety and, 1844, 1844b
  cardiovascular disease and, 1841
  caregiving, 1843
  chronic, 1842–1843
  obesity and, 552
  occupational, 1842–1843
  posttraumatic, 1844
  sudden cardiac death and, 1356
Stress cardiomyopathy, 649, 649.e1t, 650f, 1630b–1633b
Stress computed tomography perfusion, 349
Stress echocardiography, 224–226
  in assessment of myocardial viability, 225–226
  in cardiac arrhythmias, 1149–1151, 1153f
  coronary flow reserve and perfusion for, 226
  in hypertrophic cardiomyopathy, 221–222
  limitations of, 225–226
  in mitral stenosis, 227–229
  as preoperative test, 417
  protocol for, 225f, 225b
  risk stratification with, 225
  in stable ischemic heart disease, 745b–746b
  in valvular heart disease, 226, 226f
Stress testing
  cardiovascular medicine and, 111
  electrocardiography, in stable ischemic heart disease, 745–746
  nuclear cardiology testing, 284b
  physiologic basis for, 281–282, 283f
  protocols, 282–283
  in stable ischemic heart disease, 745–746, 745t
  for syncope, 1392
Stroke, 870, 1870, 1870.e1f
  in adult congenital heart disease, 1544
  after percutaneous coronary interventions, 885b–886b
  antithrombotic agents for, 877–879
    antiplatelet therapy, 877, 877t
    prevention in atrial fibrillation, 877
  atrial fibrillation-associated, 1274
    aspirin, 1276
    direct thrombin inhibitors in, 1276
    factor Xa inhibitors for, 1276
    left atrial appendage, excision or closure of, 1277, 1278f
    low-molecular-weight heparin, 1277
    other antiplatelet agents, 1276
    risk stratification for, 1275–1276, 1275f
    warfarin for, 1276
  classification of, 870, 871f
  in COVID-19 patients, 1757
  cryptogenic, 870b–873b, 872f, 872t
  hypertension and, 471
  incidence of, 870
  lacunar, 870b–873b, 871t–872t
  management of specific causes of, 885b–886b
  mortality from, 16
  peripheral artery disease and, 859
  prevention of
    aspirin for, 1775–1776
    dipyridamole for, 1777
    thienopyridines for, 1776
  risk factors and prevention of, 873–877, 873t–874t, 874b–877b, 877t
    diabetes, 874b–877b
    exercise, 874b–877b
    hyperlipidemia, 874b–877b
    hypertension, 874t–875t, 874b–877b
    nutrition, 874b–877b

Stroke *(Continued)*
    obesity, 874b–877b
    sleep apnea, 874b–877b
    smoking, 874b–877b
Stroke Belt, 874b–877b
Stroke-heart syndrome, 1870.e1f
Stroke System of Care (SSOC), 879–880
Stroke volume, in work of the heart, 909
Structural valve deterioration (SVD), 1501
"Strut" chordae, 1455–1456
ST-segment elevation myocardial infarction. *See*
    Myocardial infarction (MI); ST-segment elevation
    (STEMI)
ST-T wave
    changes in, nonspecific, 171b–172b
    normal, 148
    ventricular recovery and, 147b–148b
Study execution, in clinical trials, 44–45
Stunned myocardium, 631f–632f, 631b–633b, 668
Subacute bacterial endocarditis, 1552, 1553f
Subaortic membrane, echocardiography in, 231b–232b, 232f
Subarachnoid hemorrhage, 1870
Subcellular microarchitecture, 889–891
Subclavian disease, endovascular treatment of, 866–867, 866.e1f
Subclinical hyperthyroidism, cardiovascular manifestations of, 1799, 1799t
Subclinical leaflet thrombosis, 1438
Subcutaneous implantable cardioverter-defibrillators, 1321, 1331
    complications of, 1343
    transvenous *vs.*, 1334–1336, 1334.e1t
Submassive pulmonary embolism, 1639.e1f, 1640t
Substance abuse, cardiac transplantation and, 1134
Subvalvular left ventricular outflow tract obstruction, 1573, 1573f–1574f
Sudden cardiac arrest (SCA), in cardiac arrhythmias, 1148, 1148f
Sudden cardiac death (SCD), 1349–1386, 1548–1549
    aborted, in cardiac arrhythmias, 1148, 1148f
    with advanced heart disease, 1381–1382
    age and, 1352–1354, 1353f
    anomalous origin of coronary arteries from wrong sinus of Valsalva and, 1357
    arrhythmia and risk stratification for, 1565–1566
    arrhythmias and, 1352, 1354t, 1355f
    asthmatic attacks and, 1363b–1365b
    atherosclerotic coronary artery disease and, 1357, 1359f
    in athletes, 1363–1365
    autonomic remodeling and, 1178–1179, 1179.e1f
    Brugada syndrome and, 1362
    cardiac valve, diseases of, 1358t
    catecholaminergic polymorphic ventricular tachycardia and, 1362–1363
    central nervous system influences in, 1358t, 1363
    in children, 1358t, 1363
    congenital heart disease and, 1358t
    coronary arteritis and, 1357.e1, 1358t
    coronary artery abnormalities and, 1357, 1358t
    coronary artery embolism and, 1357.e1, 1358t
    coronary artery spasm and, 1357.e1, 1358t
    definitions of, 1349–1350, 1350f, 1350t
    early repolarization and, 1362
    electrophysiologic abnormalities and, 1358t, 1361–1363, 1362f
    emerging markers of risk for, 1357
    endocarditis and, 1358t
    epidemiology of, 1350–1357, 1354t
    ethanol and, 1594
    exercise-related, 581
    functional capacity and, 1356
    genetic contributions to, 1352, 1354t
    genetic disorders and, 1354t, 1355f, 1377t
    heart failure and, 1111–1113, 1358t, 1359–1361, 1360f
    heredity and, 1354, 1354t
    in HIV patients, 1612–1613
    hypertension and, 1355
    hypertrophic cardiomyopathy and, 1069–1070, 1358t, 1359, 1359b
    incidence of, 1351f, 1351b
    in infants, 1358t, 1363
    inflammatory, infiltrative, neoplastic, and degenerative diseases of the heart, 1360f, 1360b
    inhomogeneity in, 634b–635b
    left ventricular ejection fraction and, 1356, 1360f

Sudden cardiac death (SCD) *(Continued)*
    lifestyle factors and, 1356
    long-QT syndrome and, 1183, 1361–1362, 1382–1383
    mechanical abnormalities of coronary arteries and, 1357, 1358f
    mechanisms of, 1365
    mitral valve prolapse and, 1358t
    myocarditis and, 1358t, 1360, 1360f
    neuronal imaging to identify patients at risk for, 302.e1f, 302b–303b, 303f
    nonatherosclerotic coronary artery abnormalities and, 1357
    pathology of, 1363b–1365b
    population burden of, 1351b
    postcardiac arrest care, 1375–1376, 1375f
    postcardiac arrest syndrome, 1375–1376, 1375f
    prevention of, 1377–1383, 1377t, 1378f
        in advanced heart disease, 1382f
        after survival from cardiac arrest, 1380–1381, 1380f, 1382f
        antiarrhythmic drugs for, 1379
        in athletes, 1383
        catheter ablation therapy for, 1380
        in children, 1383
        in general population, 1383
        genetic disorders and, 1377t
        implantable cardioverter-defibrillator for, 1377t, 1380f
        individual risk and, 1351f, 1352
        in long-QT syndromes, 1382–1383
        population risk and, 1352
        programmed electrical stimulation for, 1378b–1379b
        secondary, 1377
        subgroup risk and, 1351f, 1352
        surgical intervention for, 1379–1380
        time-dependent risk, 1351f, 1352
    prevention of, in hypertrophic cardiomyopathy, 1069–1070, 1072f
    prodromal symptoms in, 1367
    psychosocial factors and, 1356
    race and, 1353f, 1354
    risk factors for, 1351f–1352f, 1354–1357, 1355f, 1358t
        age and, 1352–1354, 1353f
        ambulatory monitoring for, 1378b–1379b
        family history of, 1354.e1t
        functional capacity and, 1356
        general medical and cardiovascular risk markers, 1377–1379
        heart failure and, 1360–1361, 1360f
        individual, 1351f, 1352
        left ventricular ejection fraction in, 1356
        lifestyle factors and, 1356
        novel proteomic and genomic markers of, 1378b–1379b
        population, 1352
        profile, general, 1354–1356
        programmed electrical stimulation for, 1378b–1379b
        psychosocial factors and, 1356
        race and, 1353f, 1354
        sex and, 1353f, 1354
        subgroup, 1351f, 1352
        time-dependent, 1351f, 1352
        ventricular arrhythmias in, 1356–1357
        ventricular hypertrophy in, 1358t, 1359, 1359b
    risk of, during exercise, 1553
    sex and, 1353f, 1354
    short-QT syndrome and, 1362b
    sleep apnea and, 1363b–1365b
    temperature and, 1352
    time dependence of risk in, 1351–1354
    ventricular arrhythmias and, 1356–1357
    ventricular hypertrophy and, 1359, 1359b
    wearable devices and, 120
    in women, 1719–1720
Sudden Cardiac Death-Heart Failure Trial (SCD-HeFT), 1111b–1113b, 1113f, 1332, 1336b
Sudden death
    implantable cardioverter-defibrillators and, 1331
    magnetic resonance imaging in, 330b–332b
    primary prevention of, 1332–1333, 1335f, 1336t, 1337f
    secondary prevention of, 1331–1332, 1332t, 1334f–1335f
Sudden infant death syndrome, 1358t, 1363
Sudden unexpected death in epilepsy (SUDEP), pathophysiologic mechanisms of, 1869–1870, 1869f
SUDEP. *See* Sudden unexpected death in epilepsy
Sugar-sweetened beverages, 534f, 535, 540t
Sulfonylureas, in glucose management, 562t–563t, 564–566

Sunitinib, 1096, 1096b
    cardiotoxic effects of, 1092t
Superficial thrombophlebitis, treatment of, 1651
Superficial venous thrombosis, 1640b–1641b
Superior vena cava syndrome, 1838.e1f, 1839–1840, 1840.e2f
    treatment of, 868, 868f
Superiority trials, in clinical trials, 43–44, 44f
Supernormal conduction, 1183b–1184b
Supervised exercise training, for peripheral artery disease, 863
Supervised learning, 109–110, 110f
Supplements
    in congestive heart failure, 596
    in dyslipidemia, 596b
    in ischemic heart disease, 595
Supravalvar aortic stenosis, 1573–1574
Supravalvar pulmonic stenosis, arterial switch operation and, 1567
Supraventricular arrhythmia, 1555–1556
    in elderly, 1701–1702
    types, 1246–1270
        atrial flutter, 1252–1257
        atrial premature complexes or ectopic beats, 1248.e1f, 1246–1247, 1246f–1247f, 1246b–1247b
        atrial tachycardias, 1247
        focal atrial tachycardia, 1247–1251, 1248f–1249f
        inappropriate sinus tachycardia, 1251–1252, 1252b
        macroreentrant atrial tachycardia, 1252–1257
        paroxysmal supraventricular tachycardia, 1257–1270
Supraventricular tachyarrhythmias, 703
    atrial flutter and fibrillation, 703
    management for, 703
    sinus tachycardia, 703
Supraventricular tachycardia (SVT), 1241–1242, 1242f, 1245–1251
    assessment of patient with palpitations, 1245–1246
    classification of, 1254t
    definitions of, 1245
    in elderly, 1702b
    paroxysmal, 1218
    supraventricular arrhythmia types, 1246–1270
    ventricular tachycardia *vs.*, 1242–1243, 1293–1294, 1293.e1f, 1295f
Surgery
    atrial fibrillation after, 1283
    bariatric, obesity and, 553, 554t, 555f
    noncardiac, 410–424
        anesthesia for, 417–418, 417b–418b
        arrhythmias and, 411b–412b
        assessment of risk for, 410–412
        beta-adrenergic-blocking agents for, 421, 423t
        complications of, 419–420
        congenital heart disease in adults and, 411b–412b
        coronary artery revascularization and, 420–421
        coronary stenting and, 420–421, 422f
        diagnostic testing for, 412–416, 413f–414f, 415t
            guidelines approach to, 416b
            risk calculators in, 415–416
        electrocardiographic, hemodynamic, and echocardiographic monitoring in, 423
        epidural anesthesia for, 418
        heart failure and, 411–412
        hemodynamics during, 418
        hypertension and, 411
        hypertrophic cardiomyopathy and, 411–412
        ischemic heart disease and, 410–411
        monitored anesthesia care and, 417–418
        myocardial ischemia and, 418
        nitroglycerin in, 422
        nonpharmacologic interventions for, 423
        pharmacologic interventions for, 421–423
        postoperative intensive care for, 419b
        postoperative management in, 418–419
        postoperative pain management in, 419b
        postoperative response to, 418–419
        regional anesthesia for, 418
        spinal anesthesia for, 418
        statin therapy and, 421–422
        temperature and, 423
        transfusion threshold and, 423
        valvular heart disease and, 411b–412b
    in peripheral artery disease, 851
    transcatheter interventional therapy and, 1449
    venous thrombosis after, 1774

Surgical aortic valve replacement (SAVR), 1414, 1415t, 1416f
  patient selection for, 1415, 1417t
Surgical bioprosthetic aortic valve failure, transcatheter aortic valve replacement in, 1437
Surgical reperfusion, for STEMI, 671
Surrogate endpoints, 45, 102, 103t
SVD. *See* Structural valve deterioration
SVT. *See* Supraventricular tachycardia
Swan-Ganz catheter, 391, 392f
Sweets, 532–534, 540t
Sydenham chorea, 1534
Sympathetic innervation, inhomogeneity in, 634b–635b
Sympathetic modulation, 1899, 1900f
Sympathetic nerves, intraventricular route of, 1179f
Sympathetic nervous system, 1893, 1895f, 1901t
  in heart failure, 913–915, 913f–914f
  hypertension and, 476–477, 477f
Sympathetic stimulation
  early afterdepolarization and, 1183
  effects of, 1178, 1179.e1f
SynCardia Total Artificial Heart-Temporary (TAH-t), 1128t, 1129, 1129f
Synchronous cardioversion, 1227
Syncope, 1387–1398
  in atrial fibrillation, 1274
  in cardiac arrhythmias, 1147–1148, 1147.e1t
  cardiac catheterization for, 1392
  cardiac causes of, 1390
  cardiac imaging of, 1392
  cardiac monitoring of, 1392–1393
  carotid sinus massage for, 1391
  causes of, 1388t
    real or apparent transient loss of consciousness, 1388t
  classification of, 1387
  definition of, 1387
  diagnostic tests of, 1390–1394
  differential diagnosis of, 1387
  in elderly, 1703
  electrocardiography for, 1392–1393
  electrophysiologic testing for, 1393–1394, 1393t
  evaluation of, 124, 124t, 1394, 1395f
  history of, 1390–1391, 1391t
  laboratory testing of, 1391
  management of patients with, 1394–1396, 1395f
  neurally mediated, 1389, 1395–1396, 1396t
    in athletes, 583
  neurologic causes of transient loss of consciousness, 1390
  physical examination of, 1390–1391
  reflex-mediated, 1388–1389, 1396t
  stress tests for, 1392
  test to screen for neurologic causes of, 1394
  tilt-table test for, 1391–1392
  unexplained, 1156b–1159b, 1159f, 1162.e5, 1162.e5t
  vascular causes of, 1387–1389
  vasovagal, 1389
Synergy BP-DES, 794.e1
SYNTAX score, classification of coronary segments from, 372.e1t
Synthetic chemicals, cardiovascular disease and, 38–39
Syphilis, thoracic aortic aneurysms in, 814
System 1 thinking, 60
System 2 thinking, 60
Systematic endothelial dysfunction, in heart failure with preserved and mildly reduced ejection, 1017–1018
Systemic hypertension, mechanisms and diagnosis, and treatment of, 471–501
Systemic inflammation
  effects of food and nutrients on, 541t–542t
  in heart failure with preserved and mildly reduced ejection, 1018b–1020b
Systemic lupus erythematosus
  atherosclerosis and, 1810–1812, 1811f
  cardiac conduction disturbances in, 1821
  myocarditis in, 1819, 1820f
  pericarditis in, 1818–1819
  pulmonary arterial hypertension in, 1822
    clinical findings and diagnosis of, 1822
    pathogenesis of, 1822
    treatment and outcome for, 1822
  treatment of, 1811b, 1820–1821
  valvular heart disease in, 1820–1821

Systemic sclerosis
  cardiac conduction disturbances in, 1821
  myocarditis in, 1819
  pericarditis and, 1819
  pulmonary arterial hypertension in, 1822, 1822t, 1823f
    pathogenesis of, 1822
    screening for, 1822, 1823f
    treatment and outcome of, 1822
Systemic vasculature, aortic valve stenosis and, 1400b–1403b, 1407f
Systole, 905b
Systolic Blood Pressure Intervention Trial (SPRINT), 491
Systolic function
  echocardiography of, 205–208, 205f–206f
  in STEMI, 649–651, 651f
Systolic Hypertension in Elderly Program (SHEP), 494

T

T wave, 145f, 148
  inversion of, 164, 164f, 169f
    idiopathic, 169
    primary, 169
    secondary, 166
  in myocardial infarction, 162–163
T wave alternans, 164f
TAAs. *See* Thoracic aortic aneurysms
Tachyarrhythmias, 1236–1237, 1236b–1237b, 1547–1548
  atrial fibrillation, 1548
  in cardiac arrhythmias, 1156
  early afterdepolarization and, 1183
  interatrial re-entrant tachycardia, 1547–1548, 1548f
Tachyarrhythmic cardiac arrest, 1371t
Tachycardia, 1156b–1159b, 1158f
  atrial, 1234–1235
  atrial fibrillation with, 1274
  focal atrial, 1234f–1235f, 1234b–1235b
  interatrial re-entrant, 1547–1548, 1548f
  junctional, 1234
  preexcited, 1267, 1267f
  reciprocating, 1219–1220
  reentrant atrial, 1234b–1235b, 1235f
  ventricular, 1548–1549
    catecholaminergic polymorphic, 1188–1189
    caused by reentry, 1188
  wide QRS, 1293–1294, 1295f
Tachycardia-bradycardia syndrome (TBS), 1314, 1314f
Tachycardia-dependent block, 1183b–1184b
Tachycardia-induced cardiomyopathy, 1041–1042
Tachycardia-mediated cardiomyopathy (TMC), 1248b, 1250f
Tacrolimus, in cardiac transplantation, 1136
TAFI. *See* Thrombin activatable fibrinolysis inhibitor
Tai chi, for ischemic heart disease, 594
Takayasu arteritis, 853, 1812–1814, 1814f
  cardiovascular complications of, 1814
  in coronary artery disease, 780b–781b
  diagnosis of, 1814, 1814t
  pathogenesis of, 1813
  pulmonary arterial hypertension in, 1822t, 1823
  valvular heart disease in, 1821
Takotsubo cardiomyopathy, 1042.e1f, 649, 649.e1t, 650f, 1042–1043, 1042b, 1043f
  electrocardiography in, 168–169
  therapy for, 1043
  in women, 1717
Tamoxifen, cardiotoxic effects of, 1092t, 1096
Tamponade
  after myocardial infarction, 218b–219b
  echocardiography in, 241f, 241b–242b
TandemHeart, 798
TandemHeart pVAD, 1121f, 1125t
Tangier disease, 513
TAO. *See* Thromboangiitis obliterans
TAPSE. *See* Tricuspid annular plane systolic excursion
Targeted therapies, for cancer, 1095–1096
Targeting congestion, in acute heart failure, 958–959
TAVI. *See* Transcatheter aortic valve implantation
TAVR. *See* Transcatheter aortic valve replacement
Taxanes, cardiotoxic effects of, 1092t, 1094.e1
Taxus stent, 793.e2
TB. *See* Tuberculosis
TBS. *See* Tachycardia-bradycardia syndrome
TDI. *See* Tissue Doppler imaging
Tea, 534f, 535
TEE. *See* Transesophageal echocardiography

Temperature, body
  noncardiac surgery and, 423
  in rheumatic fever, 1535
  in STEMI, 654
Tenase
  extrinsic, 1769
  intrinsic, 1769
Tendon of Todaro, 1177f
Tenecteplase, 1788–1789
Terminal cisternae, 889
Terminal Purkinje fibers, 1177, 1177.e1f
Test-ordering strategies, 57b
Tetralogy of Fallot, 1563–1566
  anatomic description and prevalence of, 1563, 1563f
  clinical features and diagnostic testing of, 1563–1564, 1564f–1565f
  echocardiography in, 260b, 263f
  long-term outcomes and complications of, 1564–1566
    anatomic sequalae, 1564–1565, 1565t
    arrhythmia and risk stratification for sudden cardiac death, 1565–1566
    ventricular dilation and dysfunction and heart failure, 1565
  magnetic resonance imaging in, 330b–332b
  pregnancy and, 1738, 1739t
  surgical repair of, 1564
  ventricular tachycardia in, 1302, 1303f
Tetrodotoxin (TTX)-resistant Nav1.5 isoform, 1166b–1170b
TFPI. *See* Tissue factor pathway inhibitor
TGFBR1, mutations in, 811
TGFBR2, mutations in, 811
THALES study, 878, 879f
The Scientific Registry for Transplant Recipients, 1138
Therapeutic decisions, 57–58
Thermodilution method, for cardiac output measurements, 393–394
Thiazide diuretics
  for hypertension, 491
  in hypertension management, 561
Thiazolidinediones, in glucose management, 562t–563t, 564b–566b
Thienopyridines
  in percutaneous coronary intervention, 799–800
  in thrombosis, 1776–1777
    dosages for, 1777
    indications for, 1776–1777
    mechanism of action of, 1776
Third-degree atrioventricular (AV) block, 1317–1319, 1318f, 1318.e1f
Thoracic aortic aneurysms (TAAs), 810–818
  in aneurysms-osteoarthritis syndrome, 811
  in aortitis, 814
  in bicuspid aortic valve, 812–813, 814f
  cause of, 810–814
  chest radiography in, 814f–815f, 815
  clinical manifestations of, 813.e1f, 814–815
  computed tomographic angiography in, 815, 815f–816f
  computed tomography in, 813.e1f, 815
  degenerative, 814
  diagnosis of, 815, 815.e1f
  dissection with, 814
  familial, 812, 814f
  genetics of, 810–814, 811t, 812f, 813t
  in Kommerell diverticulum, 814
  in Loeys-Dietz syndrome, 811, 811t, 814f
  magnetic resonance angiography in, 815
  management of, 817–818
    aortic arch, 817, 817.e2f
    ascending, 817, 817.e1f, 817.e2f
    descending, 817
    endovascular repair for, 817–818
    medical, 818
    surgical treatment for, 817–818
    thoracoabdominal, 817, 817b, 817.e3f
  in Marfan syndrome, 811, 811t, 811.e1f, 813f
  natural history of, 815–816, 815.e1f, 815f–816f
  pathogenesis of, 810–814
  in syphilis, 814
  transthoracic echocardiography in, 815
  in Turner syndrome, 813, 813.e1f
  in vascular Ehlers-Danlos syndrome, 812
Thoracic epidural anesthesia/percutaneous stellate block, 1899
Thoracoabdominal aortic aneurysms, 810
  management of, 817, 817b, 817.e3f

Three-dimensional echocardiography, 212, 214f
Thrombectomy, for percutaneous coronary intervention, 795
Thrombin, 1769–1770, 1770f
Thrombin activatable fibrinolysis inhibitor (TAFI), 1771
  mechanism of action of, 1771
Thromboangiitis obliterans (TAO), 851–853
  clinical features of, 852
  diagnosis of, 852, 852f
  pathology and pathogenesis of, 851–852
  treatment of, 852–853
Thrombocytopenia
  glycoprotein IIb/IIIa receptor antagonists and, 1778
  heparin and, 1781, 1781t
    low-molecular-weight, 1782
Thromboembolic events, in cancer patients, 1100
Thromboembolism
  atrial fibrillation-associated, 1275–1277, 1287.e1, 1287.e1t, 1287.e2t
    aspirin, 1276
    direct thrombin inhibitors in, 1276
    factor Xa inhibitors for, 1276
    left atrial appendage, excision or closure of, 1277, 1278f
    low-molecular-weight heparin, 1277
    other antiplatelet agents, 1276
    risk stratification for, 1275–1276, 1275f
    warfarin, 1276
  in prosthetic heart valves, 1502b–1503b
Thrombolysis
  in massive pulmonary embolism, 1649.e1f
  in peripheral artery disease, 862–863, 862f
Thrombolysis in Myocardial Ischemia (TIMI) risk scores, 720, 722f
Thrombomodulin, 425–426
Thrombosis, 1766–1790
  after myocardial infarction, 218b–219b, 220f
  in antiphospholipid syndrome, 1824, 1825f
  arterial, 1772
  in Behçet disease, 1824, 1825f
  chronic kidney disease and, 1881
  coronary artery, in noncardiac surgery, 418–419
  COVID-19, 1638f
  future perspectives on, 1789
  intracardiac, echocardiography in, 255–256, 256f
  left ventricle, echocardiography in, 218b–219b, 220f
  prosthetic heart, 1496f, 1502f, 1502b–1503b
  in rheumatic diseases, 1823–1824
  stent, coronary, 802, 802.e1t, 802.e2f
  treatment of, 1775–1789
    anticoagulants in, 1779–1787, 1779f, 1779t–1781t, 1783f, 1784t–1786t
    antiplatelet drugs in, 1775–1779, 1776f, 1778f, 1778t
    fibrinolytic drugs in, 1787–1789, 1787f–1788f
  venous, 1772
Thrombotic endocarditis, nonbacterial, 1507
Thromboxane A$_2$, 1768
Thrombus, percutaneous coronary intervention and, 792
Thyroid-associated pericardial disease, 1630b–1633b
Thyroid disease, diastolic function in, 1797–1798, 1798f
Thyroid dysfunction, 487
Thyroid function, amiodarone and, 1803–1804, 1804f
Thyroid gland, in STEMI, 652b
Thyroid hormone
  action of the heart and, cellular mechanisms of, 1797–1799, 1797.e1t, 1798f
  cardiovascular disease and, 1797–1804
  changes in metabolism of, cardiac disease and, 1804, 1804.e1t
Thyroid stimulating hormone (TSH), 1797, 1802
Thyroid storm, 1800b–1801b
TIA. See Transient ischemic attack
Tibial disease, endovascular treatment of, 865, 865.e1f, 865.e2f
Ticagrelor
  in coronary artery disease, chronic kidney disease and, 1880t–1881t
  dosages for, 1777
  indications for, 1777
  mechanism of action of, 1777
  in NSTE-ACS, 725–726, 725f, 735.e6t
  in percutaneous coronary intervention, 787.e3t, 800
  side effects of, 1777
  in stable ischemic heart disease, 754b–756b
  in thrombosis, 1777
Tiered response systems, impact of, 1370–1371, 1370.e1f

Tilting disc valves, 1495
Tilt-table testing (TIT), 1391–1392, 1897, 1898f
  head-up, in cardiac arrhythmias, 1155, 1155.e2f
Timolol, for angina pectoris, 758t
Timothy syndrome (TS), 1196–1197
  clinical description and manifestations of, 1196–1197
  genetic basis of, 1192f, 1196b–1197b
Tirofiban
  in myocardial infarction, renal dysfunction and, 1884t
  in percutaneous coronary intervention, 800.e1
  in thrombosis, 1778
Tissue Doppler imaging (TDI), of heart failure with preserved and mildly reduced ejection, 1011b–1017b, 1013f
Tissue factor pathway inhibitor (TFPI), 1767
Tissue plasminogen activator (t-PA), 1771
  mechanism of action of, 1771
TIT. See Tilt-table testing
Titin, 893, 893f
  in heart failure, 925
TMC. See Tachycardia-mediated cardiomyopathy
TMEM gene, 1039b–1040b
TMVR. See Transcatheter mitral valve replacement
TNNI3 gene, 1063, 1066f
TNNT2 gene, 1063, 1066f
TNR. See True negative rate
Tobacco products
  cardiovascular disease risk of, 525–530
    effects of, 526–530
  epidemiology of, 525b, 526f
  harm reduction and cessation, 529b–530b
  health effects of, 525–530
  heated, 529–530
Tobacco use
  cessation of, 28
  control of, 28
  in elderly, 1705
  epidemiology of, 20–21, 21f
Tocilizumab, 1825b
Toll-like receptors, 1085.e1
Tolvaptan, in heart failure, 983t
Topical nitroglycerin, for angina pectoris, 762
Torsades de pointes
  drug-induced, 98, 1197–1199
    clinical description and manifestations of, 1197
    common ion channel polymorphisms and, 1198–1199
  electrocardiography in, 1306–1307
  variant of, 1363, 1363.e1f
Torsemide, in heart failure, 982, 983t
Total artificial heart, 1129
Total fat, 536, 537f
Total occlusion, 352
Toxin-induced pulmonary arterial hypertension, 1661
Toxins
  cardiomyopathies induced by, 1593–1602
  in myocarditis, 1079t
t-PA. See Tissue plasminogen activator
TPR. See True positive rate
TR. See Tricuspid regurgitation
Tracheobronchitis, 600–601
  chest pain in, 600t
Traditional chemotherapeutic agents, 1091–1094
  anthracyclines, 1091–1094, 1091b, 1093b–1094b
Trandolapril, in heart failure, 991t–992t
Transaminases, elevated levels of, heparin and, 1781
Transcatheter annuloplasty devices, in tricuspid regurgitation, 1490b–1492b
Transcatheter aortic valve implantation (TAVI), 1430
  first case of, 1430.e1, 1430.e1f
Transcatheter aortic valve intervention, in women, 1718
Transcatheter aortic valve replacement (TAVR), 4–5, 1407f, 1414–1415, 1415t, 1416f, 1419, 1430–1440, 1430.e1f
  for aortic regurgitation, 1438
  complications associated, 1436–1437
  concomitant cardiac diseases and, 1437
  coronary obstruction associated, 1436
  early years of, 1430–1431
    introduction to the heart team, 1431
    outcomes in patients not suitable for surgery using, 1430
    patient surgical risk profiles and comorbidity assessments, 1430–1431

Transcatheter aortic valve replacement (TAVR) *(Continued)*
  evidence-based clinical research, 1431–1433
    echocardiographic findings, 1431–1432, 1431.e7f, 1431f–1432f, 1432.e2f
    ecosystem for, 1431, 1431.e2t, 1431.e3t, 1431f–1432f, 1431.e4t, 1431.e6f, 1431.e7f, 1432.e3f, 1432.e4f, 1435f, 1435f–1436f
    key secondary outcomes, 1431
    national registries, 1432–1433, 1432.e4f
    primary clinical endpoints, 1431, 1431.e2t, 1431.e3t, 1432f–1433f
    quality-of-life assessments, 1432, 1432.e3f, 1432.e4f
    randomized clinical trials according to surgical risk strata, 1431
    society-based guidelines and appropriate use criteria, 1433, 1433t, 1434f
  expanded clinical indications of, 1438.e1
    asymptomatic severe aortic stenosis, 1438.e1
    moderate aortic stenosis, 1438.e1
  future directions of, 1438
  gaps and ongoing controversies in, 1437–1438
    durability of, 1437–1438
  history and background of, 1430–1440
    predicate technologies, 1430
    proof-of-concept first-in-human case, 1430
  intraprocedural complications of, 1436
  in low-gradient aortic stenosis, 1437.e1
  modern era heart team, 1438.e1
  next generation valve technology, 1438.e1
  optimal antithrombotic therapies and, 1438
  patient selection for, 1415, 1417t
  postprocedural complications of, 1436–1437
    conduction disturbances, 1437
    neurologic events, 1436
    paravalvular regurgitation, 1437
    prosthesis-patient mismatch, 1437
  procedural maturation of, 1435–1436
    alternative vascular access strategies, 1436
    computed tomography imaging for, 1435
    echocardiography for, 1436
    minimalist approach (including conscious sedation anesthesia), 1436
  in surgical bioprosthetic aortic valve failure, 1437
  technology evolution of, 1433–1435
    accessory devices for, 1435
    anatomy (components) of, 1433–1435
    comparative device *vs.* device studies, 1435
    rapid progression in modern era of, 1435, 1435f–1436f
  vascular complications of, 1436
Transcatheter atrial septal defect, 1561–1562
Transcatheter bioprosthetic valves, 1496f, 1497–1498
Transcatheter interventional therapy
  percutaneous balloon mitral valvuloplasty *vs.*, 1449–1450
  for rheumatic mitral stenosis, 1448–1449, 1448t, 1449f–1450f
Transcatheter mitral valve repair
  secondary (functional) mitral regurgitation, 1114
  in women, 1718
Transcatheter mitral valve replacement (TMVR), in mitral regurgitation, 1488–1489, 1491f
Transcatheter pulmonary valve implantation, for tetralogy of Fallot, 1565
Transcatheter system, development of, 1433–1435
Transcatheter therapy, for secondary mitral regurgitation, 1468–1470, 1469f–1470f, 1469t
Transcatheter tricuspid valve intervention (TTVI), for tricuspid regurgitation, 1490
Transcatheter Valve Therapy (TVT) registry, 1432.e2
Transcaval TAVR procedure, 1436.e1
Transcranial magnetic stimulation, 1850
Transcription, 71
Transcriptome, conceptual relationship of, 88f
Transesophageal echocardiography (TEE), 210–212, 210t–212t, 213f
  in aortic dissection, 822f, 824
  in aortic intramural hematoma, 831, 831f–832f
  in infective endocarditis, 1513, 1514f–1515f
  noncardiac surgery and, 423
  in pericardial effusion and cardiac tamponade, 1622
  of primary mitral regurgitation, 1461, 1461f
Transfemoral access, for TAVR procedures, 1436
Transfer learning, 111
Transfusion threshold, noncardiac surgery and, 423

Transient ischemic attack (TIA), diagnosis and treatment of patients with, 886–887, 886t, 887f
Transient loss of consciousness
 metabolic causes of, 1390
 neurologic causes of, 1390
Translation, 71
Translational molecular imaging, nuclear cardiology and, 311–312
 peripheral arterial disease, 311b–312b
Transmembrane potentials, in heart cells, 1168t, 1176b
Transmural infarction, 638
Transplantation
 cardiovascular disease and, 1891, 1891f
 for congenital heart disease, 1551, 1552f
 Ebstein anomaly of the tricuspid valve and, 1562
Transposition of great arteries, 1566–1569
 anatomic description and prevalence of, 1566, 1567f
 arterial switch operation for, 1566, 1567f
 atrial switch operation for, 1566, 1567f
 clinical features of, 1566
 congenitally corrected, pregnancy and, 1738
 Rastelli operation for, 1566, 1567f
 repaired, pregnancy and, 1738
Transthoracic echocardiography (TTE)
 in aortic dissection, 824
 in cardiac tumors, 1829.e1f
 for congenital heart disease, 1551
 in infective endocarditis, 1513, 1513f
 in pericardial effusion and cardiac tamponade, 1622
 in thoracic aortic aneurysms, 815
Transthyretin amyloid cardiomyopathy (ATTR), 1699
Transthyretin cardiac amyloidosis imaging, 286
Transvenous defibrillation leads, 1334b–1335b
 dual vs. single coil, 1334b–1335b
 integrated vs. dedicated sensing bipoles, 1334b–1335b
Transvenous implantable cardioverter-defibrillators, 1331, 1333f
 subcutaneous vs., 1334–1336, 1334.e1t
Transvenous pacemaker leads, 1321, 1322b–1323b
Transvenous pacemakers, for heart block, 1547
Transvenous pacing, for sinus node dysfunction, 1547
Transvenous system pulse generators, 1321
Transverse magnetization decay, 314
Trastuzumab, 1095, 1095b
 adverse effects of, 98
 cardiotoxic effects of, 1092t
Treadmill testing, 179.e1f, 178b–180b, 179t
 in peripheral artery disease, 843
Treppe effect, 908, 908f
Triadin knockout (TKO) syndrome, 1195–1196
TriAlign system, 1490b–1492b
Triamterene, in heart failure, 983t, 984
Triangle of Koch, 1175.e4f, 1176, 1177f
Trichinosis, myocarditis and, 1083.e1
Tricuspid annular plane systolic excursion (TAPSE), 209, 211f
Tricuspid regurgitation (TR), 1475–1479
 annuloplasty devices for, 1490b–1492b, 1492f
 cardiac magnetic resonance imaging in, 1476b–1478b
 causes of, 1475–1476, 1475t
 caval devices for, 1492
 clinical presentation of, 1476–1478
 diagnosis of, 1476b–1478b
 echocardiography in, 235, 236f, 1476b–1478b, 1477f–1478f
 electrocardiography in, 1476b–1478b
 hemodynamic findings in, 1476b–1478b
 leaflet clip devices for, 1492
 in magnetic resonance imaging, 329
 management of, 1478–1479, 1478t
 pathology of, 1475–1476, 1476f
 pathophysiology of, 1490
 physical examination in, 1476b–1478b
 radiography in, 1476b–1478b
 stages of, 1476, 1477f
 symptoms of, 1476b–1478b
 transcatheter therapies for, 1489–1492, 1493f
 treatment of, 1490–1492, 1491f–1492f
 tricuspid valve replacement devices for, 1492
 valve spacer devices for, 1492
Tricuspid stenosis (TS), 1473–1475
 cardiac catheterization in, 1473b–1475b
 causes of, 1473
 clinical presentation of, 1473–1475
 diagnosis of, 1473
 echocardiography in, 235, 235f, 1473b–1475b
 electrocardiography in, 1473b–1475b

Tricuspid stenosis (TS) (Continued)
 management of, 1475
 pathology of, 1473, 1474f
 pathophysiology of, 1473
 physical examination in, 1473b–1475b
 pressure gradient determination in, 401
 radiography in, 1473b–1475b
 symptoms of, 1473b–1475b, 1474t
Tricuspid valve, 1490
 disease of, evaluation of, 138
 Ebstein anomaly of, 1560–1562
  anatomic description and prevalence of, 1560, 1560f
  clinical features and diagnostic testing of, 1560–1561, 1561f
  long-term outcomes and complications of, 1561–1562
  transcatheter atrial septal defect/patent foramen ovale closure, 1561–1562
  tricuspid valve repair and replacement surgery, 1561
  unrepaired, 1561
  ventricular dysfunction, heart failure, and transplantation, 1562
 echocardiography in, 202f, 234–235, 234b–235b
Tricuspid valve replacement devices, for tricuspid regurgitation, 1492
Tricyclic antidepressants, 1847–1848
Triggered activity, 1180–1183, 1181f–1182f
Triglyceride-rich lipoproteins, 510–513, 511t
Triglycerides, 6, 454–455, 503
Triiodothyronine (T_3), 1797, 1804
 in STEMI, 652b
Trimetazidine, for NSTE-ACS, 723t
Triple-valvular disease, 1482–1483
Triptorelin, cardiotoxic effects of, 1092t
Tropheryma whipplei infection, myocarditis and, 1081b
Troponin
 in acute heart failure, 950, 950f
 in chest pain evaluation, 603, 603.e1f
Troponin complex, 892f, 893
Troponin elevation, patients with, 293–294, 295f
Troponin I
 in athletes, 584, 584f
 in heart failure, 941
 in myocarditis, 1087
 in NSTE-ACS, 719t
 phosphorylation of, 902
 in STEMI, 655
Troponin T, 892f, 893
 in athletes, 584, 584f
 in heart failure, 941
 in myocarditis, 1087
 postoperative myocardial ischemia and, 419
 in STEMI, 655
Troubleshooting
 of implantable cardioverter-defibrillators, 1339–1343
  failure to deliver therapy or delayed therapy, 1340–1341
  shocks, 1339–1340, 1340.e1t, 1344f–1345f
  ventricular oversensing, 1339, 1339b, 1339.e2f
 of pacemakers, 1328–1331, 1329.e1f, 1330t
  failure to capture, 1329, 1330f
  failure to pace, 1330, 1331f
  pacing-induced proarrhythmia, 1331, 1331.e1f
  pseudo-malfunction, 1331
  unexpected drop in pacing rate, 1331, 1332f
  unexpected pacing at or near the upper rate, 1330–1331, 1330.e1f, 1330.e1t
TRPM4, 1205b–1206b
True negative rate (TNR), 54b–55b
True positive rate (TPR), 54b–55b
Truncus arteriosus, 1572
Trypanosoma cruzi, life cycle of, 1081, 1082f
TS. *See* Timothy syndrome; Tricuspid stenosis
TSH. *See* Thyroid stimulating hormone
TTE. *See* Transthoracic echocardiography
TTR gene, 1044
T-tubules, alterations of, in heart failure, 924b
TTVI. *See* Transcatheter tricuspid valve intervention
T-U wave alternans, 171b–172b, 172f
Tuberculosis (TB)
 in acute pericarditis, 1616
 in constrictive pericarditis, 1625b–1626b
 myocardial, 1081b
Tuberculous pericarditis, 1630b–1633b

Tumor necrosis factor-alpha (TNF-α) antagonists, 1825b
 for rheumatoid arthritis, 1810b
Tumor(s)
 of aorta, 834, 834.e1f
 cardiac, 1829–1837
  benign primary, 1830–1835, 1833f–1837f
  cardiac tamponade with, 1839
  classification of, 1830, 1832t
  clinical manifestations of, 1829–1830, 1830t, 1832t
  complications of, 1838–1839
  constrictive pericarditis with, 1839
  diagnosis of, 1830t
  echocardiography in, 1829, 1830f–1831f, 1832–1833, 1833f, 1837f–1838f
  magnetic resonance imaging in, 330b–332b
  malignant, 1835–1837, 1837f–1838f
  metastatic, 1830, 1831f, 1832t, 1836, 1838f
  pericardial effusion with, 1839
  secondary, 1837–1838, 1838f, 1838.e1f
  superior vena cava syndrome with, 1838.e1f, 1839
  valvular disease with, 1829b
 metastatic, cardiac, 1830, 1831f, 1832t, 1836, 1838f
Tunica adventitia, in aorta, 806b, 808f
Tunica intima, 427
Tunica media, 427–428, 428f
 in aorta, 806b, 808f
Turner syndrome, thoracic aortic aneurysms in, 811t, 813, 813.e1f
"Twiddler's syndrome, 1343
Two-dimensional Doppler echocardiography, in pericardial effusion and cardiac tamponade, 1622, 1623f
Two-dimensional transthoracic echocardiography, in pulmonary arterial hypertension, 1667, 1667f
Type A aortic dissection, 827.e2f, 828b–830b
Type B aortic dissection, 828f–829f, 828b–830b, 829t
Type I hyperlipidemia, 512–513
Type III hyperlipoproteinemia, 512
Type IV hyperlipoproteinemia, 511–512
Tyrosine kinase inhibitors, 1095–1096
 cardiotoxic effects of, 1095–1096
 monoclonal antibody, cardiotoxic effects of, 1092t

U

U wave, 145f, 149
 in myocardial infarction, 164
UFH. *See* Unfractionated heparin
UFP. *See* Ultrafine particles
UKPDS. *See* United Kingdom Prospective Diabetes Study
Ularitide, for acute heart failure, 971
Ultrafiltration, for acute heart failure, 966
Ultrafine particles (UFP), 31–32
Ultrasonography
 in abdominal aortic aneurysms, 807–808, 808.e1f
 in aortic dissection, 824
 Doppler
  color flow, 198b–199b, 199f
  continuous-wave, 198f–199f, 198b–199b
  in practice, 199–200, 199.e1f
  principles of, 198b–199b, 198.e1f
  pulsed-wave, 198f–199f, 198b–199b
 of lung, in heart failure, 224, 224.e1f
 principles of, 196–200, 197f–198f
Uncommon diseases, primary prevention in patients with, 1382b
Uncomplicated acute pericarditis, 1616
Uncontrolled primary hypertension, 471
Unemployment, stress and, 1842–1843
Unfractionated heparin (UFH)
 in percutaneous coronary intervention, 787.e3t, 801
 in pregnancy, 1735–1737
 in pulmonary embolism, 1646
Unidirectional block, 1315.e1f
Unipolar leads, 1322b–1323b
United Kingdom Prospective Diabetes Study (UKPDS), 492
United Network of Organ Sharing (UNOS), 1132
UNOS. *See* United Network of Organ Sharing
Unrepaired Ebstein anomaly, 1561
Unsupervised learning, 110
Upper extremity deep vein thrombosis, 1640b–1641b
Urban-rural geography, in cardiovascular disease, 67–68, 68f
Urodilatin
 in acute heart failure, 971
 in heart failure, 918b–919b

Urokinase, 1788
Urokinase plasminogen activator (u-PA)
    mechanism of action of, 1771
    single-chain, 1771
    two-chain, 1771
Urotensin II, in heart failure, 919.e1

V

v wave, 127–128
VAD. *See* Ventricular assist device
Vagal bursting, 1178
Vagal nerve stimulation (VNS), 1899
Vagal nerves, intraventricular route of, 1179f
Vagal stimulation
    effects of, 1178, 1179.e1f
    tonic, 1178
Valsalva maneuver, 1896f, 1897
    in heart failure, 135, 136f
Valsartan
    in cardiorenal syndrome, 1889t
    in heart failure, 991t–992t, 993
Value-based payment programs: hospitals, 65
Value-based purchasing: outpatient, 65
Valve Academic Research Consortium (VARC), 1431.e1
Valve obstruction, aortic valve stenosis and, 1400b–1403b, 1403f, 1411t
Valve replacement, indications for, 1426
Valve spacer devices, for tricuspid regurgitation, 1492
Valvular aortic stenosis
    epidemiology of, 1430
    natural history of, 1430
    treatment alternatives for, 1430
Valvular cardiac conditions, infective endocarditis in, 1505
Valvular disease, 1419
    management of, 1001
Valvular heart disease, 1360–1361
    aging and, 1699–1701
        aortic regurgitation, 1700b–1701b
        aortic stenosis, 1699–1701
        endocarditis, 1700b–1701b
        mitral annular calcification, 1700b–1701b
        mitral regurgitation, 1700b–1701b
        mitral stenosis, 1700b–1701b
    assessment of, 137–138
    in athletes, 584
    cardiovascular disease and, 4–5
    chest radiography in, 274–275
    chronic kidney disease and, 1887
    coronary computed tomography angiography in, 354–361, 356f–357f
    echocardiography in, 226–240
    exercise electrocardiographic testing in, 189–190
    magnetic resonance imaging in, 328–329
    mechanical circulatory support for, 1124.e1
    native, in pregnancy, 1734–1735, 1734f, 1740.e1t
    noncardiac surgery and, 411b–412b
    prevalence of, 1455
    pulmonary hypertension and, 1659–1660
    in rheumatic diseases, 1820–1821
    in rheumatoid arthritis, 1821
    in seronegative spondyloarthropathies, 1821
    in systemic lupus erythematosus, 1820–1821
    in Takayasu arteritis, 1821
    transcatheter therapies for, 1484–1494
        mitral regurgitation, 1485–1489
        mitral stenosis, 1484–1485
        tricuspid regurgitation, 1489–1492
Valvular heart surgery, in women, 1718
Valvular regurgitation
    in cardiac catheterization, 402
    regurgitant fraction in, 402
Valvular stenosis
    calculation of stenotic valve orifice areas in, 398–399, 401
    evaluation of, 398
Valvulitis, 1534
Valvuloplasty, pulmonary, for congenital heart disease, 1587, 1587b
Vancomycin, in infective endocarditis
    from staphylococcal species, 1521t–1522t
    from streptococcal species, 1519b–1523b
Vaping product, associated lung injury, 1596
VARC. *See* Valve Academic Research Consortium
Variable coupling, in premature ventricular complexes, 1288

Vascular access, in peripheral artery disease, 864, 864.e1f, 864.e2f
Vascular closure devices, for percutaneous coronary intervention, 799
Vascular complications, after coronary angiography, 364b–366b
Vascular disease
    cancer and, 1100, 1102t
    in cancer survivorship, 1105–1106, 1105b
    chest pain in, 600
    management of, 1104, 1106.e3
        patients with associated, 774.e1
    risk, prevention, and monitoring of, 1106.e1
Vascular Ehlers-Danlos syndrome, thoracic aortic aneurysm in, 811t, 812
Vascular endothelial growth factor receptor inhibitors, 1096
Vascular imaging, in peripheral artery disease, 863–864, 863.e3f
Vascular injury, atherosclerosis in, 1809–1810
Vascular mechanisms, in acute heart failure, 951
Vascular reperfusion, 668
Vascular rings, 1577–1578, 1578f
Vasculature, age-associated changes in, 1687b–1690b, 1690f
Vasculitis, 851–853
    large-vessel, 1812–1815, 1813f–1814f, 1814t, 1816f
        treatment of, 1815
    medium-vessel, 1816–1818, 1817f–1818f
    radionuclide imaging in, 309b–310b, 310f
Vasculopathy, in coronary artery disease, 780b–781b
Vasoconstricting peptides, in heart failure, 919.e1
Vasodepressor response, 1320
Vasodilators
    in acute heart failure, 962–963, 962t
    in peripheral artery disease, 851
Vasopressin antagonists, 985, 985b
Vasopressors, in acute heart failure, 965–966
Vasoreactivity testing, in pulmonary arterial hypertension, 1670b
Vasospasm, 426
Vasospastic angina, NSTE-ACS and, 734–735
Vasovagal syncope, 1389
    in athletes, 583
    carotid sinus hypersensitivity, 1389
Vaughan Williams classification, 1208
VCG. *See* Vectorcardiogram
VDD pacing mode, 1327, 1327.e1f
Vectorcardiogram (VCG), 141b–145b
Vegetables, 532, 533f, 540t
Vegetations, echocardiography in, 256b
Vein graft occlusion, effects of therapy on, 771
Venous access, for cardiac catheterization
    percutaneous brachial vein access, 389
    percutaneous femoral vein access, 388–389
    percutaneous internal jugular vein access, 389–390
Venous claudication, 840
Venous conduits, in stable ischemic heart disease, 770–771
Venous disease, endovascular treatment of, 867–868
Venous filling pressure, 906
Venous grafts, patency of, 771
Venous insufficiency, differentiating lymphedema from, 1640b–1641b
Venous thoracic outlet syndrome, 868
Venous thromboembolism
    air pollution and, 36
    in COVID-19, 1757, 1758f
Venous thrombosis/thromboembolism, 1772
    advanced age and, 1774
    antiphospholipid syndrome and, 1775
    antithrombin deficiency and, 1773
    cancer and, 1774
    in elderly, 1702–1703
    elevated levels of procoagulant proteins and, 1773
    factor V Leiden in, 1772–1773
    factor XIII polymorphism and, 1773
    high-risk patients with active cancer, 1652
    history of previous, 1775
    hypercoagulable states and
        acquired, 1772f, 1772t, 1773–1775
        inherited, 1772–1773, 1772f, 1772t
    hyperhomocysteinemia and, 1775b
    in-hospital prophylaxis, 1651–1652
    obesity and, 1774
    in pediatric population, 1636–1637
    pregnancy and, 1774

Venous thrombosis/thromboembolism *(Continued)*
    prophylaxis
        at hospital discharge, 1651–1652
        in major orthopedic surgery, 1652
    protein C deficiency, 1773
    protein S deficiency and, 1773
    prothrombin gene mutation and, 1773
    risk of, in cancer patients, 1100
    surgery and immobilization and, 1774
Venous ultrasonography, for pulmonary embolism, 1644, 1646f
Venous waveform, 127–128, 128f, 128t
Veno-venous ultrafiltration, in cardiorenal syndrome, 1886
Ventricular arrhythmias, 699–701, 1237–1241, 1237b–1239b, 1238f, 1240f–1241f, 1288–1295
    accelerated idioventricular rhythm in, 700
    in Andersen-Tawil syndrome, 1865
    in chronic kidney disease, 1887–1888
    diagnosis of, exercise electrocardiographic testing, 190b–191b
    in Duchenne muscular dystrophy, 1855
    in elderly, 1702b
        implantable cardioverter-defibrillators, 1702b
    fibrillation, 700–701, 701f
    management of, 699–700
    marijuana use and, 1599–1600
    prior, patients with, 295, 296f
    prognosis of, 700–701
    prophylaxis for, 700
    tachycardia, 700–701, 701f
    ventricular premature depolarizations, 699–700
Ventricular assist device (VAD)
    design of, 1122
        CentriMag VAD, 1121f, 1125t
        extracorporeal, 1119, 1122f, 1125t
        HeartMate 3, 1123f, 1127, 1127t–1128t
        HeartMate II, 1127, 1127t–1128t
        HeartWare HVAD, 1127–1129, 1127t–1128t
        Impella, 1121f, 1125t
        Jarvik 2000, 1130–1131
        Novacor, 1122
        paracorporeal, 1119
    echocardiography for, 223b–224b, 224.e1f
    infection of, 1528
Ventricular dilation
    single ventricle and, 1581
    tetralogy of Fallot and, 1565
Ventricular dysfunction
    atrial switch operation and, 1566
    Ebstein anomaly of the tricuspid valve and, 1562
    single ventricle and, 1581
    tetralogy of Fallot and, 1565
Ventricular escape pacing, 1331
Ventricular fibrillation, 1189, 1897
    clinical features of, 1310
    electrocardiography in, 1309
    management of, 1310
Ventricular filling pressures, as a target for monitoring, 1116, 1116f
Ventricular flutter, 1310
    electrocardiography in, 1309f, 1310
Ventricular function, assessment of, 310
Ventricular gradient, 149b
Ventricular hypertrophy, sudden cardiac death (SCD) and, 1358t, 1359, 1359b
Ventricular oversensing, 1339, 1339b, 1339.e2f
Ventricular pacing, 1326
Ventricular preexcitation, diagnosis of, exercise electrocardiographic testing, 190b–191b
Ventricular remodeling, 651–652
Ventricular sensed or paced event, 1327
Ventricular septal defect (VSD), 1558–1559, 1559t, 1560f
    closure of, techniques for, 1590–1591, 1590b–1591b
    echocardiography in, 259–260, 260f–262f
    magnetic resonance imaging in, 330b–332b, 331f
    myocardial infarction and, 218b–219b, 218.e1f
    pregnancy and, 1737–1738
Ventricular tachycardia (VT), 1242–1243, 1242f, 1288–1309, 1548–1549, 1897
    in acute myocardial infarction, 1304
    in acute myocardial ischemia, 1304
    in arrhythmogenic right ventricular cardiomyopathy, 1299–1302, 1302f
    bidirectional, 1309
    bundle branch reentrant, 1294–1295, 1297f
    in cardiac sarcoidosis, 1302–1303

Index

Ventricular tachycardia (VT) (Continued)
  in Chagas disease, 1303
  clinical features of, 1295–1296
  in congenital heart disease, 1302
  electrocardiography in, 1292, 1292.e1f, 1292.e2f, 1292.e3f, 1294f–1295f
  focal origin, 1295
  in hypertrophic cardiomyopathy, 1302
  idiopathic, 1293t, 1303–1304
    annular, 1304
    crux, 1304
    fascicular (left septal), 1298f, 1304
    outflow tract, 1303–1304
    papillary muscle, 1304
  in inflammatory heart disease, 1302–1303
  in ischemic cardiomyopathy, 1297–1299
  management of, 1296–1297, 1296.e1t, 1300t
    acute, 1295–1296, 1298f
    long-term therapy, 1297, 1299f
  monomorphic, 1292–1294
  in myocarditis, 1303
  in nonischemic dilated cardiomyopathy, 1296f, 1299, 1301f
  polymorphic, 1304
  postinfarction, 1242f–1243f
  pregnancy and, 1732
  scar-related, 1294
  supraventricular tachycardia vs., 1241–1242, 1242f, 1293–1294, 1293.e1f, 1295f
  in tetralogy of Fallot, 1302, 1303f
Ventricular undersensing, 1327.e1f
Ventriculophasic sinus arrhythmia, 1312b–1313b
Verapamil, 1211.e1t, 1208t–1209t, 1212t, 1214t, 1223–1225, 1223b–1224b
  in angina pectoris, 760, 761t
  drug interaction with, 97t
  in hypertrophic cardiomyopathy, 1071
Vericiguat
  for acute heart failure, 971b–972b
  for heart failure with preserved and mildly reduced ejection, 1028
Vertebral disease, endovascular treatment of, 866–867, 866.e1f
Very-low-density lipoprotein, 505b–506b, 507f
VF zone, 1336
VGS. See Viridans group streptococci
Viability testing, 18F-FDG for, 284b
Vildagliptin, in diabetes mellitus, 562t–563t, 566
Viral infection, myocardial, 1083.e1f, 1078–1081, 1079f, 1079t, 1083–1085
  acquired immunity and, 1085–1086
  cardiac remodeling and, 1086
  innate immunity and, 1085, 1085f
Viral pericarditis, 1630b–1633b
Virchow, Rudolf, 425
Viridans group streptococci (VGS), causing infective endocarditis, 1506b–1507b
  antimicrobial therapy for, 1519t–1521t, 1519b–1523b
Visceral adiposity, increased, in heart failure with preserved and mildly reduced ejection, 1011b–1017b
Visceral obesity, 549–551
  clinical tools to identify patients with, 551
  key factors associated with, 550–551
    age and sex, 550
    drugs, 551, 551t
    ethnicity, 550
    genetics, 550
    hypothalamic-pituitary-adrenal axis and endocannabinoid system, 551
    lifestyle, 551
    sex hormones, 550
  marker of ectopic fat deposition in, 549–550
    portal free fatty acid hypothesis, 549
    visceral adipose tissue as endocrine organ, 549, 550f–551f
Visceral pericardium, 1615b
Vitamin D, 539b
  deficiency of, 1797
Vitamin K antagonists, 1783
Vitamin(s)
  antioxidant, 539b
  for stable ischemic heart disease, 754b–756b

VKORC1, 95t, 1784t, 1784b
VNS. See Vagal nerve stimulation
Voglibose, in diabetes mellitus, 562t–563t
Voltage-gated channels
  Ca^{2+}, 1171b–1173b
  ion flux through, 1163b–1166b, 1167f
  K^+, 1171b–1173b
  Na^+, 1171b–1173b, 1172f
Volume status
  in acute heart failure, 958–959
  in heart failure, 937
Volume-displacement pumps, 1122.e1
Vomiting, in STEMI, 653
von Willebrand factor (vWF), 1768
VOO pacing mode, 1326, 1327f
Voodoo death, 1363
Vorapaxar
  in peripheral artery disease, 847.e2t
  in stable ischemic heart disease, 754b–756b
  in thrombosis, 1779
Voriconazole, in infective endocarditis, 1519b–1523b
VSD. See Ventricular septal defect
VT. See Ventricular tachycardia
VVI pacing mode, 1326, 1327f
vWF. See von Willebrand factor

W

Waistline, as indicator of obesity, 547–548, 548f–549f, 549t
Wall stress, 907–908, 907f
  peak systolic, 907b–908b
  preload and, 907b–908b
"Wandering wavelet" hypothesis, 1189
WARCEF trial, 879b
Warfarin, 1783–1785
  in acute limb ischemia, 855
  in atheroembolism, 856
  in atrial fibrillation-associated thromboembolism prevention, 1276
  bleeding and, 1784–1785
  dosages for, 1784, 1784t
  drug interaction with, 97, 97t
  mechanism of action of, 1783, 1783f
  monitoring of, 1784
  pharmacology of, 1783–1784
  during pregnancy, 1730f, 1735–1737, 1785
  side effects of, 1784
  skin necrosis and, 1785
Warfarin "bridging", in pulmonary embolism, 1647
Warfarin embryopathy, 1735–1737
Warfarin fetopathy, 1735–1737
WASID (Warfarin-Aspirin Symptomatic Intracranial Disease) trial, 879b
WATCH (Warfarin and Antiplatelet Therapy in Chronic Heart Failure) trial, 879b
Wave break, cardiac fibrillation and, 1189b
WAVE (Warfarin Antiplatelet Vascular Evaluation) trial, 849
WCH. See White-coat hypertension
Wearable devices, in cardiovascular medicine, 117–122
  activity and heart rate tracking for general cardiovascular wellness, 117–118, 118f
  atrial fibrillation, 118–120
    electrocardiogram, 119–120, 120f
    photoplethysmography detection of irregular rhythm, 118–119, 119f
  cardiac arrest and sudden cardiac death, 120
  cardiac rehabilitation and heart failure, 120
  definitions and overview, 117
  evaluation of, 120–121
    activity, exercise, and sleep, 121
    ancillary information, 120, 121f
    heart rate and rhythm notifications, 120–121, 122f
  hypertension, 120
  limitations of, 121
Wegener granulomatosis (granulomatosis with polyangiitis), 1817, 1818f
  treatment for, 1818
Weight loss, atrial fibrillation in, 1287.e6t, 1287.e8
Wheezing, in STEMI, 654

Whipple disease
  myocarditis and, 1081b
  sudden cardiac death and, 1363b–1365b
White blood cell (WBC) count
  in acute pericarditis, 1617
  in STEMI, 655–656
White-coat hypertension (WCH), 482
Whole-body PET imaging, 311.e2f, 311b–312b
Wide-complex tachycardia
  differential diagnosis of, 1270
  regular, 1270t
Wilkins score, 1446
Williams, Vaughan, 1208
Win ratio, 46b–47b
Wolff-Parkinson-White (WPW) syndrome, 1162.e3t, 1162.e5, 1231f
  asymptomatic, 1268–1270
  atrial fibrillation in, 1284, 1287.e6t, 1287.e8
  ECG, 1264–1266, 1264f–1266f
  sudden cardiac death in, 1361
Women
  acute coronary syndrome in, 1717
  arrhythmias in, 1719–1720
  cardiac transplantation in, 1719
  cardiovascular disease in, 1710b–1722
    age and, 1710b–1714b
    assessment of risks for, 1714
    dyslipidemia and, 1710b–1714b
    eclampsia, preeclampsia, and pregnancy-associated hypertension in, 1710b–1714b
    family history and, 1710b–1714b
    functional hypothalamic amenorrhea and, 1710b–1714b
    gestational diabetes and, 1710b–1714b
    high-sensitivity C-reactive protein and, 1710b–1714b
    obesity and, 1710b–1714b
    polycystic ovary syndrome and, 1710b–1714b
    premature menopause and premature ovarian insufficiency, 1710b–1714b
    prevention of, 1720
    reproductive hormones, 1710b–1714b
    sleep apnea, 1710b–1714b
  cardiovascular risk factors in, 1710–1714
    age of menarche, 1710b–1714b
  coronary artery bypass grafting in, 1718
  delays in care of, 1715
  heart failure in, 1001, 1718–1719
  diagnosis of, 1719
  ischemia with no obstructive coronary artery disease, 1716–1717, 1716f
  ischemic heart disease in, 1714–1716
    interventions and medical therapy for, 1715–1716
    nonobstructive, 1717, 1717t
    obstructive coronary artery disease, 1716–1717
  mechanical circulatory support, 1719
  peripheral arterial disease in, 1718
  statins in, 517
  sudden cardiac death in, 1719–1720
  Takotsubo cardiomyopathy in, 1717
  transcatheter aortic valve intervention in, 1718
  transcatheter mitral valve repair in, 1718
  valvular heart surgery in, 1718
Women's Health Study, 877
WPW. See Wolff-Parkinson-White

Y

Yoga, 597

Z

Z drug medications, 1850
Z-lines, 891f
Zaleplon, 1850
Zolpidem, 1850
Zopiclone, 1850
Zotarolimus, 793
Zotarolimus-eluting stent, 793, 793–794